DEDICATION

To Our Families

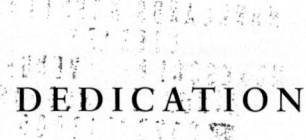

Diane, Rachel, Sara, Catherine, Rebecca, John, Andrew K. Andrew M. and Adam;
Stephanie, Hart, Jaelin, Devon, and Jamie

CONTRIBUTORS

Cynthia K. Aaron, MD, FACMT, FACEP
Professor of Emergency Medicine and Pediatrics
Program Director, Medical Toxicology
Department of Emergency Medicine
Wayne State University School of Medicine
Detroit Medical Center
Regional Poison Center at Children's Hospital of Michigan
Detroit, MI

Wissam Abouzgheib, MD, FCCP
Attending Physician
Department of Pulmonary and Critical Care
Sparks Health System
Fort Smith, AR

Gregory A. Abrahamian, MD
Associate Professor of Surgery
Department of Surgery
University of Texas Health Science Center at San Antonio
San Antonio, TX

Konstantin Abramov, MD
Assistant Professor of Medicine
Division of Renal Medicine
UMass Memorial Medical Center
Worcester, MA

Christopher D. Adams, PharmD, BCPS
Clinical Pharmacist
Department of Pharmacy Services
Brigham and Women's Hospital
Boston, MA

Suresh Agarwal, MD, FACS, FCCM
Chief, Surgical Critical Care
Associate Professor of Surgery
Boston Medical Center
Boston, MA

Lauren Alberta-Wszolek, MD
Assistant Professor of Medicine
Division of Dermatology
University of Massachusetts Medical School
Worcester, MA

Alfred Aleguas Jr, PharmD, DABAT
Managing Director
Northern Ohio Poison Center
Rainbow Babies & Children's Hospital
Cleveland, OH

Satya Allaparthi, MD
Fellow in Robotic and Laparoscopic Urology
Department of Urology/Surgery
UMass Memorial Medical Center
Worcester, MA

Gilman B. Allen, MD
Assistant Professor
Director, Medical Intensive Care Unit
Department of Medicine
Division of Pulmonary and Critical Care Medicine
University of Vermont
Fletcher Allen Health Care
Burlington, VT

Luis F. Angel, MD
Associate Professor of Medicine
Department of Medicine
University of Texas Health Sciences Center at San Antonio
San Antonio, TX

Kevin E. Anger, PharmD, BCPS
Clinical Pharmacy Specialist in Critical Care
Department of Pharmacy Services
Brigham and Women's Hospital
Boston, MA

Derek C. Angus, MD, MPH
Professor and Vice Chair for Research
Department of Critical Care Medicine
University of Pittsburgh Medical Center
Pittsburgh, PA

Neil Aronin, MD
Professor of Medicine and Cell Biology
Chief of Endocrinology and Metabolism
Department of Medicine
University of Massachusetts Medical School
Worcester, MA

Samuel J. Asirvatham, MD, FACC, FHRS
Professor of Medicine and Pediatrics
Division of Cardiovascular Diseases
Mayo Clinic College of Medicine
Rochester, MN

Seth M. Arum, MD, FACE
Assistant Professor of Medicine
Department of Endocrinology
UMass Memorial Medical Center
Worcester, MA

Philip J. Ayvazian, MD
Assistant Professor
Department of Urology
UMass Memorial Medical Center
Worcester, MA

Riad Azar, MD
Associate Professor of Medicine
Department of Internal Medicine
Division of Gastroenterology
Washington University School of Medicine
Barnes Jewish Hospital
St. Louis, MO

Ruben J. Azocar, MD
Associate Professor and Residency Program Director
Department of Anesthesiology
Boston University Medical Center
Boston, MA

Ednan K. Bajwa, MD, MPH
Associate Director, Medical ICU
Department of Pulmonary and Critical Care
Massachusetts General Hospital
Boston, MA

K.C. Balaji, MD
Professor, Department of Surgery
Division of Urology
UMass Memorial Medical Center
Worcester, MA

Jerry P. Balikian, MD, FACR
Professor and Vice Chair of Radiology
Department of Radiology
University of Massachusetts Medical School
Worcester, MA

Ian M. Ball, MD, DABEM, FRCPC
Assistant Professor
Program in Critical Care Medicine and
Departments of Clinical Pharmacology/Toxicology
and Emergency Medicine
Queen's University Kingston
Ontario, Canada

Meyer S. Balter, MD, FRCPC
Professor
Department of Medicine
University of Toronto
Director, Asthma Education Clinic
Mount Sinai Hospital
Toronto, Ontario, Canada

Gisela I. Banauch, MD, MS
Assistant Professor of Medicine Division of Pulmonary,
Allergy, Critical Care and Sleep Medicine
University of Massachusetts Medical School
UMass Memorial Medical Center
Worcester, MA

Daniel T. Baran, MD
Region Medical Director
Merck
Adjunct Professor of Medicine, Cell Biology, and Orthopedics
UMass Memorial Medical Center
Worcester, MA

Stephen L. Barnes, MD, FACS
Associate Professor and Chief, Division of Acute
Care Surgery
Department of Surgery
University of Missouri
Columbia, MO

Suzanne J. Baron, MD
Cardiology Fellow
Department of Cardiology
Massachusetts General Hospital
Boston, MA

Thaddeus C. Bartter, MD, FCCP
Professor of Medicine
Department of Medicine
Division of Pulmonary and Critical Care
University of Arkansas for the Medical Sciences
Little Rock, AR

Amit Basu, MD
Assistant Professor of Surgery and Attending Physician
Department of Surgery
University of Pittsburgh Medical Center
Thomas E Starzl Transplantation Institute
Pittsburgh, PA

Kenneth L. Baughman, MD (DECEASED)

Richard C. Becker, MD
Professor of Medicine
Department of Medicine
Duke University School of Medicine
Durham, NC

Robert W. Belknap, MD
Assistant Professor of Medicine
Division of Infectious Diseases
Denver Health and Hospital Authority
University of Colorado
Denver, CO

Isabelita R. Bella, MD
Associate Professor of Clinical Neurology
Department of Neurology
University of Massachusetts Medical School
UMass Memorial Medical Center
Worcester, MA

Andrew C. Bernard, MD
Associate Professor of Surgery
Department of Surgery
University of Kentucky Healthcare
Lexington, KY

Megan Bernstein, MD
Resident
Department of Dermatology
University of Massachusetts Medical School
Worcester, MA

Mary T. Bessesen, MD
Associate Professor of Medicine
Department of Medicine
University of Colorado at Denver
Department of Veterans Affairs Medical Center—Denver
Denver, CO

Michael C. Beuhler, MD
Medical Director
Department of Emergency Medicine
Carolinas Poison Center
Charlotte, NC

Bonnie J. Bidinger, MD
Assistant Professor of Medicine
Department of Internal Medicine
Division of Rheumatology
University of Massachusetts Medical School
UMass Memorial Medical Center
Worcester, MA

Steven B. Bird, MD
Associate Professor
Department of Emergency Medicine
Division of Medical Toxicology
University of Massachusetts Medical School
Worcester, MA

Bruce R. Bistrian, MD, PhD
Professor of Medicine
Harvard Medical School
Department of Medicine
Beth Israel Deaconess Medical Center
Boston, MA

Robert M. Black, MD
Professor of Clinical Medicine
UMass Medical School
Chief, Nephrology
Division of Renal Medicine
St. Vincent Hospital
Worcester, MA

Ernest F.J. Block, MD, MBA, FACS, FCCM
Professor of Surgery, University of Central Florida
Department of Acute Care Surgery
Holmes Regional Medical Center
Melbourne, FL

Jeremiah Boles, MD
Hematology/Oncology Fellow
Department of Medicine
Division of Hematology/Oncology
University of North Carolina at Chapel Hill
Chapel Hill, NC

Naomi F. Botkin, MD
Assistant Professor of Medicine
Division of Cardiovascular Medicine
UMass Memorial Medical Center
Worcester, MA

Suzanne F. Bradley, MD
Professor
Department of Internal Medicine
Division of Infectious Diseases and Geriatric Medicine
Veterans Affairs Ann Arbor
University of Michigan Healthcare Systems
Ann Arbor, MI

William F. Bria, MD
Chief Medical Information Officer
Department of Medical Affairs
Shriners Hospital for Children
Tampa, FL

Veronica Brito, MD
Pulmonary and Critical Care Medicine Fellow
Department of Medicine
Winthrop-University Hospital
Mineola, NY

Traci L. Buescher, RN
Department of Heart Rhythm Services
Mayo Clinic
Rochester, MN

Keith K. Burkhart, MD, FACMT, FAACT, FACEP
Senior Advisor for Medical Toxicology
FDA Center for Drug Evaluation and Research
Office of New Drugs
Silver Spring, MD

Michael J. Burns, MD, FACEP, FACMT
Chief of Emergency Medicine
Saint Vincent Hospital
Worcester, MA
Division of Medical Toxicology
Department of Emergency Medicine
Beth Israel Deaconess Medical Center
Boston, MA

Tuesday E. Burns, MD
Assistant Professor of Psychiatry
Department of Psychiatry
Eastern Virginia Medical School
Norfolk, VA

Scott W. Byram, MD
Assistant Professor of Anesthesiology
Department of Anesthesiology
Loyola University Medical Center
Maywood, IL

Brian T. Callahan, MD
Interventional Radiology Fellow
Department of Radiology
Harvard Medical School
Beth Israel Deaconess Medical Center
Boston, MA

Christine Campbell-Reardon, MD
Associate Professor of Medicine
Department of Pulmonary and Critical Care Medicine
Boston University School of Medicine
Boston Medical Center
Boston, MA

Christopher P. Cannon, MD
TIMI Study Group
Cardiovascular Division
Brigham and Women's Hospital
Associate Professor of Medicine, Harvard Medical School
Boston, MA

Jason P. Caplan, MD
Chief of Psychiatry
Department of Psychiatry
Creighton University School of Medicine at St. Joseph's
Hospital and Medical Center
Phoenix, AZ

Raphael A. Carandang, MD
Assistant Professor
University of Massachusetts Medical School
Department of Neurology and Surgical Intensive Care
UMass Memorial Medical Center
Worcester, MA

Paul A. Carpenter, MD
Associate Professor
Clinical Research Division
Fred Hutchinson Cancer Research Center
Seattle, WA

Karen C. Carroll, MD
Professor Pathology and Medicine
Department of Pathology
Division of Medical Microbiology
Johns Hopkins Hospital
Baltimore, MD

David A. Chad, MD
Associate Professor of Neurology
Harvard Medical School
Department of Neurology
Massachusetts General Hospital
Neuromuscular Diagnostic Center
Boston, MA

Eugene Chang, MD
Martin Boyer Professor of Medicine
Department of Medicine, Section of Gastroenterology
University of Chicago
Chicago, IL

Steven Y. Chang, MD, PhD
Assistant Professor of Medicine
Division of Pulmonary & Critical Care Medicine
Director of the Medical Intensive Care Unit
University of Medicine & Dentistry of New Jersey—New Jersey Medical School
Newark, NJ

Michael L. Cheatham, MD, FACS, FCCM
Director, Surgical Intensive Care Units
Department of Surgical Education
Orlando Regional Medical Center
Orlando, FL

Sarah H. Cheeseman, MD
Professor of Medicine, Pediatrics, Microbiology and Molecular Genetics
University of Massachusetts Medical School
Division of Infectious Diseases
UMass Memorial Medical Center
Worcester, MA

Annabel A. Chen-Tournoux, MD
Cardiology Fellow
Department of Medicine
Division of Cardiology
Massachusetts General Hospital
Boston, MA

William K. Chiang, MD
Chief of Service and Associate Professor of Emergency Medicine
Department of Emergency
Bellevue Hospital Center
New York, NY

Victor G. Cimino, MD, FACS
Associate Professor
Department of Surgery
Loyola University Medical Center
Maywood, IL

Mary Dawn T. Co, MD
Assistant Professor of Medicine
University of Massachusetts Medical School
UMass Memorial Medical Center
Worcester, MA

Shawn Cody, MSN, MBA, RN
Associate Chief Nursing Officer for Critical Care
UMass Memorial Medical Center
Worcester, MA

Felipe B. Collares, MD, MSc
Interventional Radiologist
Department of Radiology
Beth Israel Deaconess Medical Center
Instructor in Radiology
Harvard Medical School
Boston, MA

Bryan R. Collier, MD
Assistant Professor of Surgery
Division of Trauma & Surgical Critical Care
Vanderbilt University Medical Center
Nashville, TN

Nancy A. Collop, MD
Professor of Medicine
Department of Medicine
Emory University
Atlanta, GA

John B. Cone, MD, FACS, FCCM
Professor of Surgery
Norma & Nolie Mumey Chair in General Surgery
Department of Surgery
University of Hospital of Arkansas
Little Rock, AR

Sara E. Cosgrove, MD
Associate Professor of Medicine
Division of Infectious Disease
Johns Hopkins Medical Institutions
Baltimore, MD

Filippo Cremonini, MD, PhD
Attending Physician
Department of Gastroenterology
Beth Israel Deaconess Medical Center
Harvard Medical School
Boston, MA

Jonathan F. Critchlow, MD
Assistant Professor of Surgery
Harvard University
Beth Israel Deaconess Medical Center
Boston, MA

Ruy J. Cruz Jr, MD, PhD
Assistant Professor of Surgery
Department of Surgery
University of Pittsburgh Medical Center
Pittsburgh, PA

Frederick J. Curley, MD
Associate Professor of Medicine
University of Massachusetts Medical School
Lung, Allergy & Sleep Specialists
Hopedale, MA

Armagan Dagal, MD, FRCA
Assistant Professor
Department of Anesthesiology and Pain Medicine
University of Washington, Harborview Medical Center
Seattle, WA

Seth T. Dahlberg, MD
Associate Professor of Medicine and Radiology
Department of Medicine and Radiology
University of Massachusetts Medical School
Division of Cardiology
UMass Memorial Medical Center
Worcester, MA

Frank F. Daly, MBBS
Clinical Toxicologist and Emergency Physician
Department of Emergency Medicine
Royal Perth Hospital
Western Australia, Australia

Jennifer S. Daly, MD
Professor of Medicine
Clinical Chief, Infectious Diseases and Immunology
Department of Medicine
University of Massachusetts Medical School
Worcester, MA

Lloyd E. Damon, MD
Professor of Clinical Medicine
Department of Medicine
University of California, San Francisco
San Francisco, CA

Raul E. Davaro, MD
Associate Professor, Clinical Medicine
Department of Medicine
University of Massachusetts Medical School
Worcester, MA

Wellington J. Davis III, MD
Assistant Professor of Surgery and Pediatrics
Section of Plastic and Reconstructive Surgery
St. Christopher's Hospital for Children
Philadelphia, PA

Ronald J. DeBellis, PharmD, FCCP
Professor and Chair
Department of Pharmacy Practice
Albany College of Pharmacy and Health Sciences—Vermont
Colchester, VT

G. William Dec, MD
Chief, Cardiology Division
Massachusetts General Hospital
Department of Cardiology
Boston, MA

Paul F. Dellaripa, MD
Assistant Professor of Medicine
Harvard Medical School
Division of Rheumatology
Brigham and Women's Hospital
Boston, MA

Gregory J. Della Rocca, MD, PhD, FACS
Assistant Professor
Co-Director, Orthopaedic Trauma Service
Department of Orthopaedic Surgery
University of Missouri
Columbia, MO

Thomas G. DeLoughery, MD, FACP
Professor of Medicine, Pathology and Pediatrics
Department of Hematology
Oregon Health and Science University
Portland, OR

Mario De Pinto, MD
Assistant Professor
Department of Anesthesiology
University of Washington
Harborview Medical Center
Seattle, WA

Mark Dershwitz, MD, PhD
Professor and Vice Chair of Anesthesiology
Professor of Biochemistry & Molecular Pharmacology
UMass Memorial Medical Center
Worcester, MA

Akshay S. Desai, MD
Instructor in Medicine
Harvard Medical School
Associate Physician
Cardiovascular Division
Department of Medicine
Brigham and Women's Hospital
Boston, MA

Asha Devereaux, MD, MPH
Pulmonary Physician
Sharp Coronado Hospital
Coronado, CA

Christopher R. DeWitt, MD
Medical Toxicologist and Emergency Physician
Department of Emergency and British Columbia Poison Center
Saint Paul's Hospital
University of British Columbia
Vancouver, BC

Peter Doelken, MD
Associate Professor
Department of Medicine
Division of Pulmonary, Critical Care, Allergy & Sleep Medicine
Medical University of South Carolina
Charleston, SC

Robert P. Dowsett, FACEM
Senior Staff Specialist
Department of Emergency Medicine
Westmead Hospital
Wentworthville, NSW, Australia

David A. Drachman, MD
Professor of Neurology
Chairman Emeritus
Department of Neurology
University of Massachusetts Medical School
Worcester, MA

David F. Driscoll, PhD
Vice President
Stable Solutions LLC
Easton Industrial Park
Easton, MA

Cathy Dudick, MD, FACS
Medical Director, Surgical Intensive Care Unit
Department of Surgery
Jersey Shore University Medical Center
Neptune, NJ

David L. Dunn, MD, PhD
Vice President for Health Sciences
Professor of Surgery, Microbiology and Immunology
University at Buffalo, School of Medicine Biomedical Sciences
Buffalo, NY

Cheryl H. Dunnington, RN, MS, CCRN
Operations Director, eICU Support Center Program
Critical Care Operations
UMass Memorial Medical Center
Worcester, MA

Kevin Dwyer, MD, FACS
Director of Trauma
Vice-Chair of Surgery
Stamford Hospital
Stamford, CT

Steven B. Edelstein, MD
Professor of Anesthesiology
Vice-Chairman Education & Compliance
Department of Anesthesiology
Loyola University Medical Center
Loyola University Stritch School of Medicine
Maywood, IL

W. Thomas Edwards, PhD, MD
Director, Fellowship in Pain Medicine
Associate Professor of Anesthesiology
Department of Anesthesiology
University of Washington
Harborview Medical Center
Seattle, WA

Richard T. Ellison III, MD
Professor of Medicine, Molecular Genetics and Microbiology
University of Massachusetts Medical School
Department of Medicine
Division of Infectious Diseases and Immunology
UMass Memorial Medical Center
Worcester, MA

Ashkan Emadi, MD, PhD
Adjunct Faculty
Division of Adult Hematology
Department of Internal Medicine
Johns Hopkins Hospital
Johns Hopkins University
Baltimore, MD

Charles H. Emerson, MD
Professor Emeritus of Medicine
Department of Medicine
UMass Memorial Medical Center
Worcester, MA

Timothy A. Emhoff, MD
Chief, Trauma, Surgical Critical Care
Department of Surgery
UMass Memorial Medical Center
Worcester, MA

Jennifer L. Englund, MD
Medical Toxicology Fellow
Department of Emergency Medicine
Division of Medical Toxicology
University of Massachusetts Medical School
Worcester, MA

Robert M. Esterl Jr, MD
Professor of Surgery
Department of Surgery
University of Texas Health Science Center at San Antonio
San Antonio, TX

Salomao Faintuch, MD, MSc
Instructor in Radiology
Harvard Medical School
Department of Interventional Radiology
Beth Israel Deaconess Medical Center
Boston, MA

Pang-Yen Fan, MD
Associate Professor of Medicine
Division of Renal Medicine
University of Massachusetts Medical School
Medical Director, Renal Transplant Program
UMass Memorial Medical Center
Worcester, MA

James C. Fang, MD
Professor of Medicine
Cardiovascular Division
Case Western Reserve University
Cleveland, OH

John Fanikos, RPh, MBA
Assistant Director of Pharmacy
Department of Pharmacy
Brigham and Women's Hospital
Boston, MA

Harrison W. Farber, MD
Professor of Medicine
Department of Pulmonary Center
Boston University School of Medicine
Boston, MA

Khaldoun Faris, MD
Associate Director of Surgical Intensive Care Unit
Department of Anesthesiology
University of Massachusetts Medical School
UMass Memorial Medical Center
Worcester, MA

Alan P. Farwell, MD
Associate Professor of Medicine
Director, Endocrine Clinics
Department of Endocrinology, Diabetes and Nutrition
Boston University School of Medicine
Boston Medical Center
Boston, MA

Alan M. Fein, MD, FACP, FCCP, FCCM
Clinical Professor of Medicine
Chief of Pulmonary, Sleep and Critical Care Medicine
Hofstra North Shore—LIJ School of Medicine
ProHEALTH Care Associates, LLP
Lake Success, NY

Philip Fidler, MD, FACS
Associate Director, Burn Center
Department of Surgery
Washington Hospital Center
Washington, DC

Michael A. Fifer, MD
Director, Cardiac Catheterization Laboratory
Division of Cardiology
Department of Medicine
Massachusetts General Hospital
Boston, MA

Robert W. Finberg, MD
Professor and Chair, Department of Medicine
University of Massachusetts Medical School
Department of Medicine
UMass Memorial Medical Center
Worcester, MA

Kimberly A. Fisher, MD
Assistant Professor of Medicine
University of Massachusetts Medical School
UMass Memorial Medical Center
Worcester, MA

Marc Fisher, MD
Professor of Neurology
University of Massachusetts Medical School
UMass Memorial Medical Center
Worcester, MA

Patrick F. Fogarty, MD
Director, Penn Comprehensive Hemophilia and Thrombosis Program
Department of Medicine
University of Pennsylvania
Philadelphia, PA

Dorrie K. Fontaine, PhD, RN, FAAN
Dean and Professor
School of Nursing
University of Virginia
Charlottesville, VA

Nancy M. Fontneau, MD
Associate Professor of Clinical Neurology
University of Massachusetts Medical School
UMass Memorial Medical Center
Worcester, MA

Marsha D. Ford, MD
Director, Carolinas Poison Center
Department of Emergency Medicine
Carolinas Medical Center
Charlotte, NC

Keith J. Foster, PharmD, BCPS
Clinical Pharmacist Surgical Intensive Care Unit
Department of Pharmacy
UMass Memorial Medical Center
Worcester, MA

Joseph J. Frassica, MD
VP and Chief Medical Information Officer
Philips Healthcare
Senior Consultant Massachusetts General Hospital
Research Affiliate Massachusetts Institute of Technology
Cambridge, MA

R. Brent Furbee, MD
Medical Director
Indiana Poison Center
Indiana University Health Methodist Hospital
Indianapolis, IN

Shrawan G. Gaitonde, MD
Surgery Resident
Department of Surgery
University Hospital/University of Cincinnati
Cincinnati, OH

Richard L. Gamelli, MD, FACS
Dean, Stritch School of Medicine
Loyola University Chicago
Senior Vice President
Loyola University Medical Center
Maywood, IL

Michael Ganetsky, MD
Clinical Instructor, Harvard Medical School
Clinical Director, Division of Medical Toxicology
Department of Emergency Medicine
Beth Israel Deaconess Medical Center
Boston, MA

Joseph J. Gard, MD
Cardiology Fellow
Department of Internal Medicine
Division of Cardiovascular Diseases
Mayo Clinic
Rochester, MN

James Geiling, MD, FACP, FCCP, FCCM
Professor of Medicine
Dartmouth Medical School
Hanover, NH;
Chief, Medical Service
VA Medical Center
White River Junction, VT

Debra Gerardi, RN, MPH, JD
CEO
EHCCO, LLC
Principal, Debra Gerardi and Associates
Half Moon Bay, CA

Edith S. Geringer, MD
Psychiatrist
Department of Psychiatry
Massachusetts General Hospital
Boston, MA

Terry Gernsheimer, MD
Medical Director of Transfusion
Seattle Cancer Care Alliance and University of Washington Medical Center
Professor of Medicine
Division of Hematology
Puget Sound Blood Center
Department of Medical Education
Seattle, WA

John G. Gianopoulos, MD
System Chair of Maternal/Fetal Medicine
Department of OB/GYN
Cook County Health and Hospital System
Chicago, IL

Michael M. Givertz, MD
Associate Professor of Medicine
Harvard Medical School
Medical Director, Heart Transplant and Circulatory Assist Program
Cardiovascular Division
Brigham and Women's Hospital
Boston, MA

Richard H. Glew, MD
Professor of Medicine, Molecular Genetics and Microbiology
Vice Chair, Medicine—Undergraduate Medical Education and Faculty Affairs
Department of Medicine
UMass Memorial Medical Center
Worcester, MA

Dori Goldberg, MD
Assistant Professor of Medicine
Division of Dermatology
Department of Medicine
University of Massachusetts Medical School
UMass Memorial Medical Center
Worcester, MA

Andrew J. Goodwin, MD
Clinical and Research Fellow
Department of Pulmonary and Critical Care
Brigham and Women's Hospital
Boston, MA

Kim L. Goring, MMBS
Assistant Professor of Medicine
Department of Internal Medicine
Division of Pulmonary, Critical Care and Sleep Medicine
Howard University Hospital
Washington, DC

Robert M. Gougelet, MD
Assistant Professor of Medicine (Emergency Medicine)
Director, New England Center of Emergency Preparedness
Department of Emergency Medicine
Dartmouth Hitchcock Medical Center
Lebanon, NH

Andis Graudins, MBBS, PhD, FACEM, FACMT
Professor of Emergency Medicine Research and Clinical Toxicology
Faculty of Medicine Nursing and Health Sciences
Monash University
Department of Emergency Medicine
Monash Medical Centre
Clayton, Victoria, Australia

Barth A. Green, MD
Professor and Chairman
Department of Neurological Surgery
Jackson Memorial/University of Miami
Miami, FL

Damian J. Green, MD
Research Associate
Clinical Research Division
Fred Hutchinson Cancer Research Center
Seattle, WA

Bruce Greenberg, MD
Assistant Professor
Department of Medicine
University of Massachusetts Medical School
Worcester, MA

Bonnie C. Greenwood, PharmD, BCPS
Staff Development and Perioperative Services Manager
Department of Pharmacy
Brigham and Women's Hospital
Boston, MA

Ronald F. Grossman, MD
Professor of Medicine
University of Toronto
Credit Valley Hospital
Mississauga, Ontario, Canada

Rainer W.G. Gruessner, MD
Professor of Surgery
Department of Surgery
University of Arizona
Tucson, AZ

Chandra Prakash Gyawali, MD, MRCP
Associate Professor of Medicine
Division of Gastroenterology
Department of Medicine
Washington University School of Medicine
Barnes-Jewish Hospital
St. Louis, MO

Ammar Habib, MD
Internal Medicine Resident
Department of Internal Medicine
Mayo Clinic
Rochester, MN

Shirin Haddady, MD
Assistant Professor of Medicine and Neurology
Department of Medicine
University of Massachusetts Medical School
UMass Memorial Medical Center
Worcester, MA

Pegge M. Halandras, MD
Assistant Professor
Department of Surgery
Division of Vascular Surgery and Endovascular Therapy
Loyola University Chicago Stritch School of Medicine
Maywood, IL

Wiley R. Hall, MD
Assistant Professor in Neurology and Surgery
Director of Neuroscience Critical Care
University of Massachusetts Medical School
Medical Director of the Neuro/Trauma ICU
Neurology Department
UMass Memorial Medical Center
Worcester, MA

Stephen B. Hanauer, MD
Professor of Medicine and Clinical Pharmacology
Department of Gastroenterology
University of Chicago
Chicago, IL

Charles William Hargett, III, MD
Associate in Medicine
Division of Pulmonary & Critical Care
Duke University Medical Center
Durham, NC

David M. Harlan, MD
Chief, Diabetes Division
Co-Director, Diabetes Center of Excellence
Department of Medicine
UMass Memorial Medical Center
University of Massachusetts School of Medicine
Worcester, MA

Laura Harrell, MD, MS
Assistant Professor of Medicine
Department of Gastroenterology
University of Chicago Medical Center
Chicago, IL

Lawrence J. Hayward, MD, PhD
Professor of Neurology
Department of Neurology
University of Massachusetts Medical School
Worcester, MA

Kennon Heard, MD
Associate Professor
Rocky Mountain Poison and Drug Center, Denver Health
Department of Emergency Medicine
University of Colorado School of Medicine
Denver, CO

Stephen O. Heard, MD
Professor and Chair
University of Massachusetts Medical School
Department of Anesthesiology
UMass Memorial Medical Center
Worcester, MA

John E. Heffner, MD
Garnjobst Chair and Professor of Medicine
Department of Medicine
Providence Portland Medical Center
Portland, OR

Jeremy S. Helphenstine, DO
Clinical Instructor
Toxicology Fellow
Department of Emergency Medicine
Emory School of Medicine
Atlanta, GA

Robert J. Heyka, MD
Director, Outpatient Hemodialysis
Department of Nephrology & Hypertension
Cleveland Clinic Foundation
Cleveland, OH

Thomas L. Higgins, MD, MBA, FACP, FCCM
Professor of Medicine
Department of Anesthesia and Surgery
Interim Chair
Department of Medicine
Baystate Medical Center
Springfield, MA

Nicholas Hill, MD
Chief
Department of Pulmonary, Critical Care and Sleep Division
Tufts Medical Center
Boston, MA

John B. Holcomb, MD, FACS
Vice Chair and Professor
Department of Surgery
Memorial Hermann Hospital
Houston, TX

Judd E. Hollander, MD
Professor, Clinical Research Director
Department of Emergency Medicine
Hospital of the University of Pennsylvania
Philadelphia, PA

Helen M. Hollingsworth, MD
Associate Professor of Medicine
Department of Pulmonary Allergy and Critical Care Medicine
Boston Medical Center
Boston, MA

Shelley A. Holmer, MD
Clinical Associate
Department of Psychiatry
Duke University Medical Center
Durham, NC

Donough Howard, MD
Consultant Rheumatologist
Hermitage Medical Clinic
Dublin, Ireland

Michael D. Howell, MD, MPH
Director, Critical Care Quality
Beth Israel Deaconess Medical Center
Boston, MA

Rolf D. Hubmayr, MD
Professor
Department of Medicine and Physiology
Mayo Clinic
Rochester, MN

Abhinav Humar, MD
Professor of Surgery
Division Chief, Transplant Surgery
Department of Surgery
University of Pittsburgh
Pittsburgh, PA

Thomas L. Husted, MD
Assistant Professor of Surgery
Department of Surgery
University of Cincinnati
Cincinnati, OH

Richard S. Irwin, MD, Master FCCP
Professor of Medicine and Nursing
University of Massachusetts
Chair, Critical Care
UMass Memorial Medical Center
Worcester, MA

John M. Iskander
Fellow in Gastroenterology
Division of Gastroenterology
St. Louis, MO

Eric M. Isselbacher, MD
Professor of Medicine
Harvard Medical School
Co-Director, Thoracic Aortic Center
Massachusetts General Hospital
Boston, MA

Rao R. Ivatury, MD
Chair
Department of Surgery
Division of Trauma, Critical Care, Emergency Surgery
Virginia Commonwealth University
Richmond, VA

William L. Jackson Jr, MD, MBA
Medical Director, Adult Critical Care
Inova Health System
Falls Church, VA

Eric W. Jacobson, MD
Associate Professor of Medicine
University of Massachusetts Medical School
Senior Vice President, Clinical Research and Regulatory Affairs
Chief Medical Officer
Synta Pharmaceuticals Corp.
Lexington, MA

Donald H. Jenkins, MD, FACS
Trauma Director
Associate Professor of Surgery
Division of Trauma, Critical Care and Emergency General Surgery
Mayo Clinic
Rochester, MN

Jing Ji, MD
Neurology Resident
Department of Neurology
University of Massachusetts Medical School
Worcester, MA

Tun Jie, MD, MS
Assistant Professor of Surgery
Department of Surgery
University of Arizona, College of Medicine
Tucson, AZ

Thanjira Jiranantakan, MD
Preventive and Social Medicine Department
Siriraj Hospital Faculty of Medicine
Mahidol University, Thailand
Medical Toxicology Fellow
Department of Clinical Pharmacology and Medical Toxicology
San Francisco General Hospital, University of California
The California Poison Control System—San Francisco Division
San Francisco, CA

Paul G. Jodka, MD
Assistant Professor of Medicine and Anesthesiology
Tufts University School of Medicine
Adult Critical Care Division
Baystate Medical Center
Springfield, MA

Scott B. Johnson, MD, FACS, FCCP
Associate Professor
Chief of General Thoracic Surgery
Department of Cardiothoracic Surgery
University of Texas Health Science Center, San Antonio
San Antonio, TX

Sreenivasa S. Jonnalagadda, MD, FASGE
Professor of Medicine
Director of Pancreatic and Biliary Endoscopy
Washington University School of Medicine
Division of Gastroenterology
St. Louis, MO

Bryan S. Judge, MD
Associate Program Director
Assistant Professor
Spectrum Health
Grand Rapids MERC/Michigan State University Program in Emergency Medicine
Grand Rapids, MI

Eias E. Jweied, MD, PhD
Cardiovascular/Thoracic Surgeon
Department of Cardiothoracic and Vascular Surgical Associates, S.C.
Advocate Christ Medical Center
Oak Lawn, IL

Marc J. Kahn, MD
Professor of Medicine
SR. Associate Dean
Department of Medicine
Tulane University School of Medicine
New Orleans, LA

Raja Kandaswamy, MD
Axline Professor of Surgery
Director of the University of Florida Institute of Transplantation
Department of Surgery
Shands Hospital—University of Florida Gainesville
Gainesville, FL

Abhishek Katiyar, MD
Medical and Toxicology and Emergency Medicine
Department of Emergency Medicine
UIC/Advocate Christ Hospital
Oak Lawn, IL

Carol A. Kauffman, MD
Professor Internal Medicine
University of Michigan Medical School
Chief, Infectious Diseases
Veterans Affairs Ann Arbor Healthcare System
Ann Arbor, MI

Christoph R. Kaufmann, MD, MPH
Professor of Surgery, East Tennessee State University
Department of Trauma and Emergency Surgery
Johnson City Medical Center
Johnson City, TN

Shubjeet Kaur, MD
Clinical Professor and Vice Chair
Department of Anesthesiology
University of Massachusetts Medical School
UMass Memorial Medical Center
Worcester, MA

Glenn Kershaw, MD
Associate Professor of Clinical Medicine
Division of Renal Medicine
University of Massachusetts Medical School
UMass Memorial Medical Center
Worcester, MA

Mark A. Kirk, MD
Medical Toxicology Fellowship Director
Department of Emergency Medicine
University of Virginia
Charlottesville, VA

Meghan S. Kolodziej, MD
Instructor in Psychiatry
Department of Psychiatry
Brigham and Women's Hospital
Boston, MA

Scott E. Kopec, MD
Assistant Professor of Medicine
Division of Pulmonary, Allergy and Critical Care Medicine
UMass Memorial Medical Center
University of Massachusetts Medical School
Worcester, MA

Bruce A. Koplan, MD
Assistant Professor of Medicine
Harvard Medical School
Cardiac Arrhythmia Service
Department of Cardiac Arrhythmia
Brigham and Women's Hospital
Boston, MA

Richard Kremsdorf, MD
Clinical Professor of Medicine, Voluntary
University of California, San Diego School of Medicine
President
Five Rights Consulting, Inc.
San Diego, CA

Stephen J. Krinzman, MD
Assistant Professor of Medicine
Division of Pulmonary, Allergy, and Critical Care Medicine
University of Massachusetts Medical School
UMass Memorial Medical Center
Worcester, MA

Gowri Kularatna, MD
Fellow in Gastroenterology
Washington University School of Medicine/Barnes Jewish Hospital
Division of Gastroenterology
St. Louis, MO

Sonal Kumar, MD
Internal Medicine Resident
Department of Internal Medicine
Barnes Jewish Hospital
St. Louis, MO

Margaret Laccetti, PhD, RN, AOCN, ACHPN
Director, Nursing Professional Development
UMass Memorial Medical Center
Worcester MA

Hoa Thi Lam, BS
Research Assistant
Department of Child Psychiatry
Massachusetts General Hospital
Boston, MA

Robert A. Lancy, MD, MBA
Chief of Cardiac Surgery
Department of Cardiac Surgery
Bassett Medical Center
Cooperstown, NY

Angeline A. Lazarus, MD
Professor of Medicine
Department of Pulmonary Medicine
Division of Pulmonary
National Naval Medical Center
Bethesda, MD

Jason Lee-Llacer, MD
Fellow
Department of Critical Care Medicine and Anesthesia
George Washington University
Washington, DC

Anthony J. Lembo, MD
Associate Professor of Medicine
Department of Medicine
Beth Israel Deaconess Med Center
Boston, MA

James A. de Lemos, MD
CCU and Cardiology Fellowship Director
Department of Cardiology/Medicine
The University of Texas Southwestern Medical Center
Dallas, TX

Adam B. Lerner, MD
Director, Cardiac Anesthesia
Department of Anesthesia and Critical Care
Beth Israel Deaconess Medical Center
Boston, MA

Phillip A. Letourneau, MD
Research Fellow/General Surgery Resident
Department of Surgery
University of Texas Medical School at Houston
Houston, TX

Howard B. Levene, MD, PhD
Assistant Professor of Neurological Surgery
Department of Neurosurgery
University of Miami Hospital
Miami, FL

Nikki A. Levin, MD, PhD
Associate Professor of Medicine
Division of Dermatology
University of Massachusetts Medical School
Worcester, MA

Stephanie M. Levine, MD
Professor of Medicine
Department of Medicine
University of Texas Health Science Center at San Antonio
San Antonio, TX

William J. Lewander, MD
Professor and Associate Vice Chair of Pediatric Emergency Medicine
The Warren Alpert Medical School of Brown University
Department of Emergency Medicine
Rhode Island Hospital
Providence, RI

Daniel H. Libraty, MD
Associate Professor
Department of Medicine/Infectious Diseases
University of Massachusetts Medical School
Worcester, MA

Craig M. Lilly, MD
Professor of Medicine, Anesthesiology and Surgery
Department of Medicine
University of Massachusetts Medical School
UMass Memorial Medical Center
Worcester, MA

Sonia Lin, PharmD, BCPS
Clinical Pharmacy Specialist
Department of Pharmacy
University of Colorado Hospital
Aurora, CO

Christopher H. Linden, MD
Professor, Department of Emergency Medicine
Division of Medical Toxicology
University of Massachusetts Medical School
UMass Memorial Medical Center
Worcester, MA

Michael Linenberger, MD, FACP
Professor, Division of Hematology
Department of Medicine
University of Washington
Associate Member, Clinical Research Division
Fred Hutchinson Cancer Research Center
Seattle Cancer Care Alliance
Seattle, WA

Mark S. Link, MD
Professor of Medicine
Department of Cardiac Electrophysiology
Tufts Medical Center
Boston, MA

Carol F. Lippa, MD
Professor of Neurology
Department of Neurology
Drexel University College of Medicine
Philadelphia, PA

Alan Lisbon, MD
Associate Professor, Anaesthesia, Harvard Medical School
Department of Anaesthesia, Critical Care and Pain Medicine
Beth Israel Deaconess Medical Center
Boston, MA

Mauricio Lisker-Melman, MD
Professor of Medicine
Director, Hepatology Program
Department of Internal Medicine
Division of Gastroenterology
Washington University School of Medicine
Barnes-Jewish Hospital
St. Louis, MO

N. Scott Litofsky, MD, FACS
Professor and Chief
Director of Neuro-Oncology and Radiosurgery
Division of Neurological Surgery
University of Missouri School of Medicine
Columbia, MO

Afroza Liton, MD
Fellow
Department of Infectious Disease
University of Massachusetts
UMass Memorial Medical Center
Worcester, MA

Frederic F. Little, MD
Assistant Professor of Medicine
Pulmonary Center and Department of Pulmonary, Allergy, and Critical Care Medicine
Boston University School of Medicine
Attending Physician
Boston Medical Center
Boston, MA

Nancy Y.N. Liu, MD
Associate Professor of Clinical Medicine
Department of Medicine
Division of Rheumatology
University of Massachusetts Medical School
Worcester, MA

Randall R. Long, MD, PhD
Cheshire Medical Center/Dartmouth Hitchcock Keene
Keene, NH

Robert B. Love, MD, FACS
Professor and Vice Chairman
Department of Thoracic and Cardiothoracic
Loyola University Medical Center
Maywood, IL

Matthew W. Lube, MD
Assistant Professor of Surgery and Surgical Clerkship Director
University of Central Florida College of Medicine
Associate Director of Medical Education
Department of Surgical Education
Orlando Regional Medical Center
Orlando, FL

Fred A. Luchette, MD, MSc
The Ambrose and Gladys Bowyer Professor of Surgery
Stritch School of Medicine
Medical Director, General Surgery III Service
Department of Surgery
Maywood, IL

Alice D. Ma, MD
Associate Professor of Medicine
Department of Medicine
Division Hematology/Oncology
University of North Carolina
Chapel Hill, NC

Theresa R. (Roxie) Macfarlan, RN, MSN, CCRN, ACNP-BC
Advanced Practice Nurse 2
Department of Thoracic-Cardiovascular Postoperative Intensive Care Unit
University of Virginia Health System
Charlottesville, VA

J. Mark Madison, MD
Professor of Medicine and Physiology
Chief, Division of Pulmonary, Allergy and Critical Care Medicine
UMass Memorial Medical Center
University of Massachusetts Medical School
Worcester, MA

Ajai K. Malhotra, MBBS, MD, MS, DNB, FRCS
Associate Professor and Vice Chair
Associate Medical Director, Level 1 Trauma Center
Department of Surgery
Division of Trauma, Critical Care and Emergency General Surgery
Virginia Commonwealth University Medical Center
Richmond, VA

Atul Malhotra, MD
Associate Professor of Medicine
Department of Medicine
Brigham and Women's Hospital
Boston, MA

Samir Malkani, MD
Clinical Associate Professor of Medicine
Division of Diabetes
Department of Medicine
UMass Memorial Medical Center
Worcester, MA

Avinash V. Mantravadi, MD
Resident Physician
Department of Otolaryngology—Head and Neck Surgery
Loyola University Medical Center
Maywood, IL

Paul E. Marik, MD, FCCM, FCCP
Professor of Medicine
Department of Pulmonary and Critical Care Medicine
Eastern Virginia Medical School and Norfolk General Hospital
Eastern Virginia Medical School Internal Medicine
Norfolk, VA

William L. Marshall, MD
Associate Professor of Medicine
Department of Medicine
UMass Memorial Medical Center
Worcester, MA

Arthur J. Matas, MD
Professor of Surgery
Department of Surgery
University of Minnesota
Minneapolis, MN

Paul H. Mayo, MD
Professor of Clinical Medicine
Hofstra Northshore—LIJ School of Medicine
Long Island Jewish Medical Center
New Hyde Park, NY

Guy Maytal, MD
Director of Urgent Care and Primary Care Psychiatry
Department of Psychiatry
Massachusetts General Hospital
Boston, MA

Melanie Maytin, MD
Instructor in Medicine
Department of Cardiovascular Medicine
Brigham and Women's Hospital
Boston, MA

Kathleen M. McCauley, PhD, RN, ACNS-BC, FAAN, FAHA
Associate Dean for Academic Programs
Class of 1965 25th Reunion Term Professor of Cardiovascular Nursing
Cardiovascular Clinical Specialist
University of Pennsylvania School of Nursing
Hospital of the University of Pennsylvania
Philadelphia, PA

Sara L. Merwin, MPH
Assistant Professor of Medicine
Department of Medicine
Hofstra North Shore—LIJ School of Medicine
North Shore University Hospital
Manhasset, NY

Marco Mielcarek, MD
Assistant Professor
University of Washington
Assistant Member
Department of Medical Oncology
Fred Hutchinson Cancer Research Center
Seattle, WA

Ross Milner, MD
Associate Professor of Surgery
Chief, Division of Vascular Surgery and Endovascular Therapy
Department of Vascular Surgery
Loyola University Medical Center
Maywood, IL

Ann L. Mitchell, MD
Associate Professor of Clinical Neurology
Department of Neurology
University of Massachusetts Medical School
UMass Memorial Medical Center
Worcester, MA

Lawrence C. Mohr Jr, MD, ScD, FACP, FCCP
Professor of Medicine, Biometry and Epidemiology
Director, Environmental Biosciences Program
Medical University of South Carolina
Charleston, SC

Takki Momin, MD
Vascular Surgery Fellow
Department of Vascular Surgery
Georgetown University/Washington Hospital Center
Washington, DC

Jahan Montague, MD
Assistant Professor of Medicine
Department of Nephrology
UMass Memorial Medical Center
Worcester, MA

Bruce Montgomery, MD
Associate Professor
Department of Medicine, Oncology
University of Washington
VA Puget Sound HCS
Seattle, WA

Majaz Moonis, MD, MRCP(1), DM, FRCP (Edin)
Professor of Neurology
Director, Stroke Services
Director, Vascular Fellowship Program
UMass Memorial Medical Center
Worcester, MA

John P. Mordes, MD
Professor of Medicine
Department of Medicine/Endocrinology
UMass Memorial Medical Center
University of Massachusetts Medical School
Worcester, MA

David A. Morrow, MD, MPH
Director, Samuel A. Levine Cardiac Unit
Department of Cardiovascular Medicine
Brigham and Women's Hospital
Harvard Medical School
Boston, MA

James B. Mowry, PharmD, DABAT, FAACT
Director, Indiana Poison Center
Department of Emergency Medicine and Trauma Center
Methodist Hospital, Indiana University Health
Indianapolis, IN

Saori A. Murakami, MD
Psychiatrist
Massachusetts General Hospital, McLean Hospital
Boston, MA

Michael C. Muzinich, MD
Neurosurgical Resident
Department of Neurological Surgery
University Hospital and Clinics
Columbia, MO

John G. Myers, MD
Associate Professor
Department of Surgery
University of Texas Health Science Center, San Antonio
San Antonio, TX

Shashidhara Nanjundaswamy, MD, MBBS, MRCP, DM
Assistant Professor
Department of Neurology
University of Massachusetts Medical School
Worcester, MA

Lena M. Napolitano, MD, FACS, FCCP, FCCM
Professor of Surgery
Department of Surgery
University of Michigan
Ann Arbor, MI

Jaishree Narayanan, MD, PhD
Associate Professor Clinical Neurology
Department of Neurology
UMass Memorial Medical Center
Worcester, MA

Theresa A. Nester, MD
Associate Medical Director
Puget Sound Blood Center
Department of Laboratory Medicine
University of Washington Medical Center
Puget Sound Blood Center
Seattle, WA

Michael S. Niederman, MD
Professor of Medicine
SUNY at Stony Brook
Chairman, Department of Medicine
Winthrop-University Hospital
Mineola, NY

Dominic J. Nompleggi, MD, PhD
Associate Professor of Medicine and Surgery
University of Massachusetts Medical School
Chief, Division of Gastroenterology
Director, Adult Nutrition Support Service
UMass Memorial Medical Center
Worcester, MA

Sean E. Nork, MD
Associate Professor
Department of Orthopaedics & Sports Medicine
Harborview Medical Center, University of Washington
Seattle, WA

Robert L. Norris, MD, FACEP
Associate Professor
Department of Surgery
Chief, Division of Emergency Medicine
Stanford University Medical Center
Palo Alto, CA

Richard A. Oeckler, MD, PhD
Assistant Professor of Medicine and Physiology
Department of Pulmonary and Critical Care Medicine
Mayo Clinic
Rochester, MN

Patrick T. O'Gara, MD
Executive Medical Director of the Carl J. and Ruth Shapiro Cardiovascular Center
Associate Professor
Harvard Medical School
Director, Clinical Cardiology
Brigham and Women's Hospital
Boston, MA

Paulo J. Oliveira, MD, FCCP
Director, Advanced Bronchoscopic and Pleural Procedures
Assistant Professor of Medicine
Division of Pulmonary, Allergy and Critical Care Medicine
UMass Memorial Medical Center
Worcester, MA

Kent R. Olson, MD, FACEP, FAACT, FACMT
Medical Director, San Francisco Division
California Poison Control System
Clinical Professor of Medicine and Pharmacy
University of California, San Francisco
San Francisco, CA

Steven M. Opal, MD
Professor of Medicine
Warren Alpert Medical School of Brown University
Memorial Hospital of Rhode Island
Division of Infectious Disease
Pawtucket, RI

Achikam Oren-Grinberg, MD, MS
Director of Critical Care Echocardiography
Department of Anesthesia, Critical Care & Pain Medicine
Beth Israel Deaconess Medical Center
Boston, MA

David Ost, MD, MPH
Associate Professor
Department of Pulmonary Medicine
The University of Texas M.D. Anderson Cancer Center
Houston, TX

Mickey M. Ott, MD
Assistant Professor in Surgery
Division of Trauma & Surgical Critical Care
Vanderbilt University Medical Center
Nashville, TN

John A. Paraskos, MD
Professor of Medicine
Department of Medicine
University of Massachusetts Medical School
UMass Memorial Medical Center
Worcester, MA

Polly E. Parsons, MD
Professor and Chair of Medicine
Department of Medicine
University of Vermont College of Medicine
Fletcher Allen Health Care
Burlington, VT

Laura Santos Pavia, MD
Resident in Anesthesiology
Boston Medical Center
Boston University School of Medicine
Boston, MA

Marie T. Pavini, MD, FCCP
Intensivist
Department of Intensive Care Unit
Rutland Regional Medical Center
Rutland, VT

David Paydarfar, MD
Professor of Neurology and Physiology
Department of Neurology
University of Massachusetts Medical School
Worcester, MA

William D. Payne, MD
Professor of Surgery
Director, Liver Transplant
Department of Surgery
University of Minnesota
Minneapolis, MN

Randall S. Pellish, MD
Assistant Professor of Medicine
Division of Gastroenterology
University of Massachusetts Medical School
Worcester, MA

Alexis C. Perkins, MD
Chief Resident
Department of Dermatology
University of Massachusetts Medical School
Worcester, MA

Catherine A. Phillips, MD
Associate Professor of Clinical Neurology
University of Massachusetts Medical School
Department of Neurology
UMass Memorial Medical Center
Worcester, MA

Ryan F. Porter, MD
Resident Physician
Department of Internal Medicine
Washington University School of Medicine
Barnes-Jewish Hospital
St. Louis, MO

Louis G. Portugal, MD, FACS
Associate Professor of Surgery
Department of Surgery
The University of Chicago
Chicago, IL

Joseph A. Posluszny Jr, MD
Research Fellow
Department of Burn and Shock Trauma Institute
Loyola University Medical Center
Maywood, IL

Melvin R. Pratter, MD
Head, Division of Pulmonary and Critical Care Medicine
Department of Medicine
Cooper University Hospital
Camden, NJ

David J. Prezant, MD
Chief Medical Officer
Special Advisor to the Fire Commissioner for Health Policy
Co-Director WTC Medical Monitoring & Treatment Programs
New York City Fire Department
Professor of Medicine
Albert Einstein College of Medicine
Pulmonary Division
Brooklyn, NY

Timothy A. Pritts, MD, PhD
Associate Professor of Surgery
Department of Surgery
Division of Trauma and Critical Care
University of Cincinnati
Cincinnati, OH

John T. Promes, MD
Director, Trauma Services
Department of Medical Center
Orlando Regional Medical Center
Orlando, FL

Donald S. Prough, MD
Professor and Chair
Anesthesiology
UTMB Anesthesiology
Galveston, TX

Leon M. Ptaszek, MD, PhD
Clinical Fellow
Department of Medicine
Cardiology Division
Massachusetts General Hospital
Boston, MA

Juan Carlos Puyana, MD
Associate Professor of Surgery
Department of Surgery
University of Pittsburgh Medical Center
Pittsburgh, PA

John Querques, MD
Assistant Professor of Psychiatry
Harvard Medical School
Associate Director, Psychosomatic Medicine—Consultation Psychiatry Fellowship Program
Department of Psychiatry
Massachusetts General Hospital
Boston, MA

Sunil Rajan, MD, FCCP
Department of Medicine
Pulmonary Medicine and Critical Care
Pulmonary Associates of Richmond, Inc.
Midlothian, VA

Paula D. Ravin, MD
Associate Professor of Clinical Neurology
Department of Neurology
UMass Memorial Medical Center
Worcester, MA

Justin L. Regner, MD
Assistant Professor of Surgery
Division of Trauma and Critical Care
University of Arkansas Medical School
Little Rock, AR

Harvey S. Reich, MD, FACP, FCCP
Director, Critical Care Medicine
Department of Critical Care Medicine
Rutland Regional Medical Center
Rutland, VT

Randall R. Reves, MD, MSc
Medical Director of the Denver Metro Tuberculosis Control Program
Department of Medicine and Public Health
Denver Public Health Department
Denver, CO

John Ricotta, MD, FACS
Professor of Surgery, Georgetown University
Harold H. Hawfield Chair of Surgery
Department of Surgery
Washington Hospital Center
Washington, DC

Teresa A. Rincon, BSN, RN, CCRN-E
Nurse Director
Sutter Health System
Sacramento-Sierra Region eICU
Sacramento, CA

Ray Ritz, BA, RRT, FAARC
Director of Respiratory Care
Department of Respiratory Care
Beth Israel Deaconess Medical Center
Boston, MA

Kimberly A. Robinson, MD, MPH
Assistant Professor of Medicine
Division of Pulmonary, Critical Care
Marlborough Hospital
Marlborough, MA

Mark J. Rosen, MD
Division of Pulmonary, Critical Care and Sleep Medicine
North Shore University and Long Island Jewish Health System
Professor of Medicine
Hofstra North Shore—Long Island Jewish School of Medicine
New Hyde Park, NY

Aldo A. Rossini, MD
Professor of Medicine
Emeritus
Department of Medicine
University of Massachusetts Medical School
Worcester, MA

Alan L. Rothman, MD
Professor
Department of Medicine
UMass Memorial Medical Center
Worcester, MA

Marc S. Sabatine, MD, MPH
Vice Chair TIMI Study Group
Associate Professor of Medicine
Harvard Medical School
Associate Cardiologist
Division of Cardiovascular Medicine
Brigham and Women's Hospital
Boston, MA

Marjorie S. Safran, MD
Professor of Clinical Medicine
Department of Endocrinology
University of Massachusetts Medical School
UMass Memorial Medical Center
Worcester MA

Steven A. Sahn, MD
Professor of Medicine and Division Director
Division of Pulmonary, Critical Care, Allergy and Sleep Medicine
The Medical University of South Carolina
Charleston, SC

Todd W. Sarge, MD
Instructor in Anaesthesia
Harvard Medical School
Department of Anesthesia, Critical Care and Pain Medicine
Beth Israel Deaconess Medical Center
Boston, MA

Benjamin M. Scirica, MD, MPH
Associate Physician and Investigator
Department of Medicine
Cardiovascular Division
TIMI Study Group
Brigham and Women's Hospital
Boston, MA

Douglas Seidner, MD
Associate Professor of Medicine
Division of Gastroenterology, Hepatology and Nutrition
Director, Vanderbilt Center for Human Nutrition
Vanderbilt University Medical Center
Nashville, TN

Michael G. Seneff, MD
Associate Professor
Department of Anesthesiology and Critical Care Medicine
The George Washington University Hospital
Washington, DC

M. Michael Shabot, MD
System Chief Medical Officer
Department of Executive Officers
Memorial Hermann Healthcare System
Houston, TX

Violet L. Shaffer, MA, BA
Research Vice President and Global Industry Service Director
Department of Research
Gartner, Inc.
Stamford, CT

Samir R. Shah, MD
Plastic Surgery Fellow
Department of Plastic Surgery
Loyola University Medical Center
Maywood, IL

Sajid Shahul, MD
Assistant Program Director
Associate Director Cardiac Surgical Intensive Care Unit
Beth Israel Deaconess Medical Center
Harvard Medical School
Boston, MA

Michael W. Shannon, MD, MPH, FAAP, FACEP (DECEASED)
Chief and Chair, Division of Emergency Medicine
Director, Center for Biopreparedness
Co-Director, Pediatric Environmental Health Center
Professor of Pediatrics, Harvard Medical School
Children's Hospital Boston
Division of Emergency Medicine
Boston, MA

Richard D. Shih, MD
Emergency Medicine Program Director
Department of Emergency Medicine
Morristown Memorial Hospital
Morristown, NJ

Andrew F. Shorr, MD, MPH
Associate Director, Pulmonary and Critical Care
Department of Medicine
Washington Hospital Center
Washington, DC

Sara J. Shumway, MD
Professor of Cardiothoracic Surgery
Vice-Chief
Division of Cardiothoracic Surgery
Surgical Director, Lung Transplantation
Department of Surgery
University of Minnesota Medical Center, Fairview
Minneapolis, MN

Samy S. Sidhom, MD, MPH
Clinical Associate
Tufts University School of Medicine
Clinical Fellow
Division of Pulmonary, Critical Care and Sleep Medicine
Tufts Medical Center
Boston, MA

Anupam Singh, MD
Assistant Professor of Medicine, GI Hospitalist
Department of Medicine
Division of Gastroenterology
UMass Memorial Medical Center
Worcester, MA

Inder M. Singh, MD
Fellow
Division of Digestive Diseases
University of California, Los Angeles
Los Angeles, CA

Jagmeet P. Singh, MD, PhD
Associate Professor of Medicine
Department of Cardiac Arrhythmia Service
Massachusetts General Hospital
Boston, MA

Marco L.A. Sivilotti, MD, MSc, FRCPC, FACEP, FACMT
Associate Professor, Department of Emergency Medicine and of Pharmacology & Toxicology
Queen's University
Kingston, Ontario, Canada

Brian S. Smith, PharmD, BCPS
Director, Education and Clinical Services
Department of Pharmacy
UMass Memorial Medical Center
Worcester, MA

Craig S. Smith, MD
Assistant Professor of Medicine
University of Massachusetts Medical School
Director of Cardiac Critical Care Unit
UMass Memorial Medical Center
Worcester, MA

Dorsett D. Smith, MD, FCCP, FACP, FACOEM
Clinical Professor of Medicine
Department of Respiratory Diseases and Critical Care Medicine
University of Washington
Seattle, WA

Heidi L. Smith, MD
Instructor of Medicine
University of Massachusetts Medical School
Worcester, MA
Director, Clinical Affairs
Mass Biologics
Boston, MA

Howard G. Smith, MD, FACS
Director of Burn Services
Orlando Regional Medical Center
Associate Professor of Surgery
University of Central Florida College of Medicine
Orlando, FL

Jason W. Smith, MD
Fellow, Cardiothoracic Surgery
Department of Cardiovascular and Thoracic Surgery
Loyola University Medical Center
Maywood, IL

Jennifer Smith, MD
Banner Good Samaritan Medical Center
Phoenix, AZ

Dustin L. Smoot, MD
Associate Consultant
Department of Trauma, Critical Care and General Surgery
Mayo Clinic
Rochester, MN

Nicholas A. Smyrnios, MD
Professor of Medicine
Director, Medical Intensive Care Units
Division of Pulmonary, Allergy, and Critical Care Medicine
University of Massachusetts Medical School
Worcester, MA

Patrick D. Solan, MD
Surgery Resident
Department of Surgery
University Hospital/University of Cincinnati
Cincinnati, OH

Dennis I. Sonnier, MD
Surgery Resident
Department of Surgery
University Hospital/University of Cincinnati
Cincinnati, OH

Brennan M.R. Spiegel, MD, MSHS
Assistant Professor of Medicine
VA Greater Los Angeles Healthcare System
David Geffen School of Medicine at UCLA
Co-Director, Center for the Study of Digestive Healthcare Quality and Outcomes
Los Angeles, CA

Amy E. Spooner, MD
Instructor in Medicine
Harvard Medical School
Department of Medicine
Division of Cardiology
Massachusetts General Hospital
Boston, MA

Judith A. Stebulis, MD
Assistant Professor of Medicine
Department of Medicine
Division of Rheumatology
University of Massachusetts Medical School
Worcester, MA

Michael L. Steer, MD
Professor, Department of Surgery
Tufts University School of Medicine
Boston, MA

M. Kathryn Steiner, MD
Assistant Professor
Department of Medicine
University of Massachusetts Medical School
UMass Memorial Medical Center
Worcester, MA

Jay S. Steingrub, MD, FACP, FCCP
Professor of Medicine
Tufts University School of Medicine
Boston, MA
Director of Medical Intensive Care Unit
Baystate Medical Center
Department of Medicine
Springfield, MA

Theodore A. Stern, MD
Professor of Psychiatry in the field of Psychosomatic Medicine
Consultation
Harvard Medical School
Chief, Psychiatric Consultation Service
Director, Office for Clinical Careers
Department of Psychiatry
Massachusetts General Hospital
Boston, MA

Garrick C. Stewart, MD
Cardiovascular Medicine Fellow
Department of Cardiovascular Medicine
Brigham and Women's Hospital
Boston, MA

Michael B. Streiff, MD, FACP
Associate Professor of Medicine
Division of Hematology
Medical Director, Johns Hopkins Anticoagulation Management Service and Outpatient Clinics
Johns Hopkins Medical Institutions
Baltimore, MD

Mark L. Sturdevant, MD
Assistant Professor of Surgery
Recanati/Miller Transplant Institute
Mount Sinai Medical Center
Mount Sinai College of Medicine
New York, NY

David E.R. Sutherland, MD, PhD
Professor and Head, Division of Transplantation
Director, Diabetes Institute for Immunology and Transplantation
Golf Classic "fore" Diabetes Research Chair
Department of Surgery
University of Minnesota
Minneapolis, MN

Colin T. Swales, MD
Associate Medical Director
Transplant Division
Hartford Hospital
Hartford, CT

Joan M. Swearer, PhD, ABPP
Clinical Professor of Neurology and Psychiatry
Department of Neurology
University of Massachusetts Medical School
Worcester, MA

Daniel Talmor, MD, MPH
Associate Professor of Anaesthesia
Department of Anesthesia, Critical Care and Pain Medicine
Beth Israel Deaconess Medical Center
Boston, MA

Victor F. Tapson, MD
Professor of Pulmonary and Critical Care Medicine
Director, Pulmonary Vascular Disease Center
Department of Medicine
Duke University Medical Center
Durham, NC

Usha B. Tedrow, MD, MSc
Director, Clinical Cardiac Electrophysiology Program
Cardiovascular Division
Brigham and Women's Hospital
Boston, MA

Milton Tenenbein, MD, FRCPC, FAAP, FAACT, FACMT
Professor of Pediatrics and Pharmacology
Director of Emergency Services
University of Manitoba
Children's Hospital
Winnipeg, Manitoba, Canada

Jeffrey J. Teuteberg, MD
Associate Director, Cardiac Transplantation
Department of Cardiovascular Institute
University of Pittsburgh
Pittsburgh, PA

John A. Thompson, MD
Professor of Medicine
University of Washington
Seattle Cancer Care Alliance
Seattle, WA

Michael J. Thompson, MD
Associate Professor of Medicine
Division of Endocrinology
Department of Medicine
The George Washington University
Washington, DC

Mark Tidswell, MD
Assistant Professor of Medicine and Surgery
Tufts University School of Medicine
Department of Adult Critical Care
Baystate Medical Center
Springfield, MA

Robert M. Tighe, MD
Medical Instructor
Department of Medicine
Duke University
Durham, NC

Mira Sofia Torres, MD
Assistant Professor
Fellowship Program Director
Division of Endocrinology
University of Massachusetts Medical School
UMass Memorial Medical Center
Worcester, MA

Ulises Torres, MD
Assistant Professor of Surgery
Director of Trauma Education and Outreach
Division of Trauma and Surgical Critical Care
Department of Surgery
University of Massachusetts Medical School
UMass Memorial Medical Center
Worcester, MA

Matthew J. Trainor, MD
Assistant Professor of Medicine
Department of Medicine
University of Massachusetts Medical School
UMass Memorial Medical Center
Worcester, MA

Arthur L. Trask, MD, FACS
Adjunct Professor of Surgery
Department of Surgery
Uniformed Services University for Health Sciences
Springfield, MO

Todd W. Trask, MD
Director, Neurosurgery Intensive Care Unit
Department of Neurosurgery
Methodist Neurological Institute
Houston, TX

Christoph Troppmann, MD, FACS
Professor of Surgery
Department of Surgery
University of California
Davis Medical Center
Sacramento, CA

Patrick Troy, MD
Fellow
Department of Pulmonary, Critical Care and Sleep Medicine
Beth Israel Deaconess Medical Center
Boston, MA

Cynthia B. Umali, MD (DECEASED)
Department of Radiology
UMass Memorial Medical Center
Worcester, MA

Gaurav A. Upadhyay, MD
Cardiac Fellow
Division of Cardiology
Massachusetts General Hospital
Boston, MA

Craigan T. Usher, MD
Clinical Fellow in Psychiatry
Harvard Medical School
Massachusetts General Hospital/McLean Hospital Child & Adolescent
Psychiatry Fellow
Boston, MA

Javier C. Waksman, MD
Associate Professor of Medicine
Department of Medicine
University of Colorado—Denver
Aurora, CO

J. Matthias Walz, MD, FCCP
Assistant Professor of Anesthesiology and Surgery
Department of Anesthesiology
Division of Critical Care Medicine
University of Massachusetts Medical School
UMass Memorial Medical Center
Worcester, MA

Michael Y. Wang, MD
Associate Professor
Department of Neurosurgery
University of Miami Hospital
Jackson Memorial Hospital
Miami, FL

Richard Y. Wang, DO
Senior Medical Officer
Division Laboratory Sciences
National Center for Environmental Health
Centers for Disease Control and Prevention
Atlanta, GA

Wahid Y. Wassef, MD, MPH
Director of Endoscopy
UMass Memorial Medical Center
Associate Professor of Clinical Medicine
University of Massachusetts Medical School
Department of Medicine
Division of Gastroenterology
UMass Memorial Medical Center
Worcester, MA

Paul M. Wax, MD, FACMT
Clinical Professor of Surgery (Emergency Medicine)
University of Texas, Southwestern
Paradise Valley, AZ
Toxicology
University of Texas
Dallas, TX

John P. Weaver, MD
Associate Professor
University of Massachusetts Medical School
Department of Surgery
Division of Neurosurgery
UMass Memorial Medical Center
Worcester, MA

Mireya Wessolossky, MD
Assistant Professor
Department of Medicine/Infectious Diseases
UMass Memorial Medical Center
Worcester, MA

Matthew J. Wieduwilt, MD, PhD
Clinical Fellow
Division of Hematology and Oncology
University of California, San Francisco Medical Center
San Francisco, CA

Christopher H. Wigfield, MD, FRCS
Assistant Professor, Cardiothoracic Surgery
Department of Thoracic and Cardiovascular Surgery
Loyola University Medical Center
Maywood, IL

Mark M. Wilson, MD
Associate Director of Medical ICU
Associate Professor
Department of Medicine
Division of Pulmonary, Allergy and Critical Care Medicine
University of Massachusetts Medical School
UMass Memorial Medical Center
Worcester, MA

Ann E. Woolfrey, MD
Associate Professor
Department of Clinical Research
Fred Hutchinson Cancer Research Center
Seattle, WA

Shan Yin, MD, MPH
Fellow, Medical Toxicology
Rocky Mountain Poison and Drug Center
Denver Health
Denver, CO

Luke Yip, MD
US Food and Drug Administration, CDER
Division of Anesthesia, Analgesia, and Addiction Products
Silver Spring, MD
Denver Health and Hospital Authority
Department of Medicine, Medical Toxicology
Rocky Mountain Poison & Drug Center
Denver, CO

Firas E. Zahr, MD
Cardiovascular Fellow
Department of Cardiovascular Medicine
University of Pittsburgh Medical Center
Pittsburgh, PA

Rebecca J. Zapatochny Rufo, DNSc, RN, CCRN
Resurrection eICU® Program Operations Director
Department of eICU
Resurrection Healthcare
Holy Family Medical
Des Plaines, IL

John K. Zawacki, MD
Professor of Medicine
Department of Medicine
Division of Gastroenterology
University of Massachusetts Medical School
UMass Memorial Medical Center
Worcester, MA

Chad A. Zender, MD, FACS
Assistant Professor
Department of Otolaryngology
University Hospitals Case Western Reserve
Cleveland, OH

Iva Zivna, MD
Assistant Professor
Department of Infectious Disease
University of Massachusetts Medical School
UMass Memorial Medical Center
Worcester, MA

Gary R. Zuckerman, DO
Associate Professor of Medicine
Division of Gastroenterology
Department of Internal Medicine
Barnes-Jewish Hospital
Washington University School of Medicine
St. Louis, MO

Marc S. Zumberg, MD, FACS
Associate Professor of Medicine
Department of Medicine
Division of Hematology/Oncology
Slands Hospital/University of Florida
Gainesville, FL

PREFACE

It is with great pleasure that we present the seventh edition of *Irwin and Rippe's Intensive Care Medicine*. As with previous editions, the editorial challenge that we faced with the seventh edition was to continue to ensure that the textbook evolved as the field has evolved and improved to meet the varied and rigorous demands placed on it by the diverse group of specialty physicians and nonphysicians practicing in the adult intensive care environment without losing strengths that have made previous editions so useful and popular. We hope and believe that the seventh edition of *Irwin and Rippe's Intensive Care Medicine* has risen to meet these challenges.

Over the past 27 years since the publication of the first edition of our textbook, dramatic changes have occurred in virtually every area of critical care, and these are reflected in the evolution of our textbook. While our textbook initially focused primarily on medical intensive care, it now provides an interdisciplinary emphasis on anesthesia, surgery, trauma, and neurointensive care as well as medical intensive care with strong collaboration across all these disciplines. With this edition, a critical care nursing-centric section has been added. This reflects the reality that intensive care medicine has inevitably become more interdisciplinary and collaborative.

The seventh edition is approximately the same length as the previous edition. To make this happen, we challenged every section editor and author to carefully balance edited materials emphasizing new evidence-based as well as state-of-the-art information by discarding outdated information. All of our section editors and chapter authors have done a superb job meeting this challenge. All chapters in every section have been updated with recent references and other materials that reflect current information, techniques, and principles. New chapters have been added to reflect emerging areas of interest. As stated earlier, an entirely new section has been added on "Nursing Issues in the ICU" that was ably coedited by Dorrie Fontaine and Shawn Cody. This section was meant to focus on issues related to collaboration, healthy work environments, and the expanding roles of nurses not the specifics of nursing care that have been brilliantly covered in textbooks of ICU nursing; and Dorrie and Shawn have admirably succeeded in this regard. Another new section on "Critical Care Consequences of Weapons (or Agents) of Mass Destruction" reflects the changing realities of our world and has been ably edited by Larry Mohr.

Evidenced-based medicine continues to play an ever more prominent role in all branches of medicine including critical care. With this in mind, we have asked every chapter author to make recommendations that specifically reflect recent trials with a particular emphasis on randomized prospective controlled trials. Authors have summarized such evidence, when the data have allowed, with helpful tables.

In medical intensive care, important changes and advances have occurred since the publication of the sixth edition. These include managing our ICUs according to the following guiding principles: (i) making our ICUs safer for our patients; (ii) decreasing variability by following clinical practice guidelines based upon the best available evidence to ensure better outcomes for our patients; and (iii) doing more with less to decrease the cost of caring for our patients. While these principles have always been espoused, it has become clear that we must more consistently follow them. With respect to specific issues, the day-to-day use of ultrasonography by critical care specialists is a very recent change and this is reflected in the liberal use of ultrasonographic images throughout the book and a new chapter entitled Interventional Ultrasound; these are prominently featured in the procedure and monitoring chapters. Moreover, there is an imperative to increasingly utilize information technology in the everyday practice of intensive care medicine. This not only includes using electronic medical records, computer physician order entry, and clinical decision support tools but also tele-ICU. All of these issues are covered in the section entitled "Contemporary Challenges in the Intensive Care Unit" edited by Craig Lilly.

In coronary care, rapid advances in techniques and interventions continue to occur. These changes are reflected in the "Cardiovascular Problems and Coronary Care" section of the seventh edition. It is interesting to see how cardiovascular intensive care has dramatically changed since the publication of our first few editions, as the advances in cardiology and cardiac surgery became known from the large, multicenter, randomized controlled clinical trials. We welcome Akshay Desai who has joined Patrick O'Gara as co-section editor for this section.

Equally important advances have occurred in surgical critical care, including new therapies and techniques in a variety of conditions treated in this environment. Our "Surgical Problems in the Intensive Care Unit" section remains a great strength of this book. Fred Luchette did his usual magnificent job on this edition. We recognize Arthur Trask and Stephen Barnes who have done an admirable job of updating the "Shock and Trauma" section of the textbook as well.

While our textbook has been updated and broadened to include new understandings, information and techniques, our goal has been to maintain the practical, clinically oriented approach that readers have come to expect from previous editions. Our editorial focus remains on clinically relevant studies and information that readers have found so useful in the previous six editions.

As in the past, our textbook opens with a detailed section on commonly performed "Procedures and Techniques in the Intensive Care Unit." This section, along with the "Minimally Invasive Monitoring" section, has also been simultaneously published as a smaller book entitled "Procedures, Techniques, and Minimally Invasive Monitoring in Intensive Care Medicine. All chapters in these sections have been updated with new figures and descriptions of techniques which have been added to reflect changes since the sixth edition of the textbook. We are indebted that section editors Stephen Heard and Alan Lisbon who have done a superb job on these sections.

The "Pharmacology, Overdoses, and Poisoning" section, consisting of 29 chapters, remains a great strength of this book and essentially represents a textbook on these topics embedded into our larger book. In this edition, we welcome new section editors Luke Yip and Kennon Heard who have joined Steven Bird as section editors for this outstanding and comprehensive section.

Because intensive care cannot be divorced from public policy, we continue to emphasize this with a major section of our textbook entitled "Contemporary Challenges in the Intensive Care Unit." This section includes not only more ethical and legal issues but also issues related to ICU organization and management, economics, safety, and information technology. With this edition, we welcome Craig Lilly, who has done an outstanding job on this section.

Our team of section editors continue to do a wonderful job coordinating large bodies of information that comprise the core of modern intensive care. Many of our section editors have been with us for one or more editions. Richard Ellison III (Infectious Disease), Neil Aronin (Endocrinology), Stephanie Levine (Transplantation), Dominic Nompleggi (Metabolism/ Nutrition), Mark Madison (Pulmonary), John Querques (Psychiatry), and Joseph Frassica (Appendix, Calculations Commonly used in Critical Care) all fall into this category and have done their usual, excellent job. A new table on Antidotes has been added to the Appendix based on the efforts of Luke Yip, Jeremy Helphenstine, Jerry Thomas, and Ian Ball.

Some new section editors have joined us for the seventh edition and done great work. In addition to the individuals that we have already mentioned, we would like to specifically acknowledge the excellent efforts by the following new section editors or co-section editors: Pang-Yen Fan (Renal), Dominic Nompleggi (Gastrointestinal Problems), Patrick Fogarty (Hematologic Problems), David Paydarfar (Neurologic Problems), David Harlan (Endocrine Problems), and Nancy Liu (Rheumatologic, Immunologic and Dermatologic Problems).

As with previous editions, our emphasis remains on clinical management. Discussions of basic pathophysiology are also included and guided and supplemented by extensive references to help clinicians and researchers who wish to pursue more in-depth knowledge of these important areas. When therapies reflect institutional or individual bias or are considered controversial, we have attempted to indicate this.

We hope and believe that the outstanding efforts of many people over the past 4 years have continued to result in an evidence-based and state-of-the-art and comprehensive textbook that will elucidate the important principles in intensive care and will continue to guide and support the best efforts of practitioners in this challenging environment in their ongoing efforts to diagnosis and treat complicated diseases and relieve human suffering.

Richard S. Irwin, MD, Master FCCP
James M. Rippe, MD

ACKNOWLEDGMENTS

Numerous outstanding individuals have made significant contributions to all phases of writing and production of this textbook and deserve special recognition and thanks. First and foremost is our managing editor, Elizabeth Grady. Beth literally lives and breathes this textbook as it works its way through the production cycle every 4 years. She is the guiding and organizing force behind this textbook. It would simply not be possible without Beth's incredible organizational skills, good humor, and enormous energy. She has guided this book through six editions—this book is as much hers as it is ours.

Our administrative assistants, office assistant, and clinical coordinators, Carol Moreau, Debra Adamonis, Karen Barrell, Mary Garabedian, and Cynthia French have helped us continue to coordinate and manage our complex professional and personal lives and create room for the substantial amount of time required to write and edit. Our section editors have devoted enormous skill, time, and resources to every edition of this textbook. We have very much appreciated their deep commitment to this book and to advancing the field of intensive care medicine.

Our editors at Lippincott Williams & Wilkins including Brian Brown, executive editor, have been a source of great help and encouragement. As with the last edition, Nicole Dernoski continues to be extremely helpful and accommodating in supervising and coordinating all phases of production in an outstanding way.

Lastly, we are grateful to Indu Jawwad and her staff for the outstanding job they have done copyediting the manuscript for this edition.

Our families support our efforts with unfailing encouragement and love. To them, and the many others who have helped in ways too numerous to count, we are deeply grateful.

Richard S. Irwin, MD, Master FCCP
James M. Rippe, MD

CONTENTS

SECTION IV ■ PULMONARY PROBLEMS IN THE INTENSIVE CARE UNIT

SECTION V ■ RENAL PROBLEMS IN THE INTENSIVE CARE UNIT

SECTION VI ■ INFECTIOUS DISEASE PROBLEMS IN THE INTENSIVE CARE UNIT

SECTION IX ■ HEMATOLOGIC AND ONCOLOGIC PROBLEMS IN THE INTENSIVE CARE UNIT

SECTION X ■ PHARMACOLOGY, OVERDOSES, AND POISONINGS

SECTION XI ■ SURGICAL PROBLEMS IN THE INTENSIVE CARE UNIT

SECTION XII ■ SHOCK AND TRAUMA

SECTION XIV ■ TRANSPLANTATION

SECTION XV ■ METABOLISM/NUTRITION

SECTION XVI ■ RHEUMATOLOGIC, IMMUNOLOGIC, AND DERMATOLOGIC PROBLEMS IN THE INTENSIVE CARE UNIT

SECTION XVII ■ PSYCHIATRIC ISSUES IN INTENSIVE CARE

SECTION XVIII ■ NURSING

SECTION I ■ PROCEDURES, TECHNIQUES, AND MINIMALLY INVASIVE MONITORING

STEPHEN O. HEARD

CHAPTER 1 ■ AIRWAY MANAGEMENT AND ENDOTRACHEAL INTUBATION

J. MATTHIAS WALZ, SHUBJEET KAUR AND STEPHEN O. HEARD

In the emergency room and critical care environment, management of the airway to ensure optimal ventilation and oxygenation is of prime importance. Although initial efforts should be directed toward improving oxygenation and ventilation without intubating the patient (see Chapter 59) [1], these interventions may fail and the placement of an endotracheal tube may be required. Although endotracheal intubation is best left to the trained specialist, emergencies often require that the procedure be performed before a specialist arrives. Because intubated patients are commonly seen in the intensive care unit (ICU) and coronary care unit, all physicians who work in these environments should be skilled in the techniques of airway management, endotracheal intubation, and management of intubated patients.

ANATOMY

An understanding of the techniques of endotracheal intubation and potential complications is based on knowledge of the anatomy of the respiratory passages [2]. Although a detailed anatomic description is beyond the scope of this book, an understanding of some features and relationships is essential to performing intubation.

Nose

The roof of the nose is partially formed by the cribriform plate. The anatomic proximity of the roof to intracranial structures dictates that special caution be exercised during nasotracheal intubations. This is particularly true in patients with significant maxillofacial injuries.

The mucosa of the nose is provided with a rich blood supply from branches of the ophthalmic and maxillary arteries, which allow air to be warmed and humidified. Because the conchae provide an irregular, highly vascularized surface, they are particularly susceptible to trauma and subsequent hemorrhage. The orifices from the paranasal sinuses and nasolacrimal duct open onto the lateral wall. Blockage of these orifices by prolonged nasotracheal intubation may result in sinusitis.

Mouth and Jaw

The mouth is formed inferiorly by the tongue, alveolar ridge, and mandible. The hard and soft palates compose the superior surface, and the oropharynx forms the posterior surface. Assessment of the anatomic features of the mouth and jaw is essential before orotracheal intubation. A clear understanding of the anatomy is also essential when dealing with a patient who has a difficult airway and when learning how to insert airway devices such as the laryngeal mask airway (LMA; discussed in Management of the Difficult Airway section).

Nasopharynx

The base of the skull forms the roof of the nasopharynx, and the soft palate forms the floor. The roof and the posterior walls of the nasopharynx contain lymphoid tissue (adenoids), which may become enlarged and compromise nasal airflow or become injured during nasal intubation, particularly in children. The Eustachian tubes enter the nasopharynx on the lateral walls and may become blocked secondary to swelling during prolonged nasotracheal intubation.

Oropharynx

The soft palate defines the beginning of the oropharynx, which extends inferiorly to the epiglottis. The palatine tonsils protrude from the lateral walls and in children occasionally become so enlarged that exposure of the larynx for intubation becomes difficult. A large tongue can also cause oropharyngeal obstruction. Contraction of the genioglossus muscle normally moves the tongue forward to open the oropharyngeal passage during inspiration. Decreased tone of this muscle (e.g., in the anesthetized state) can cause obstruction. The oropharynx connects the posterior portion of the oral cavity to the hypopharynx.

Hypopharynx

The epiglottis defines the superior border of the hypopharynx, and the beginning of the esophagus forms the inferior boundary. The larynx is anterior to the hypopharynx. The pyriform sinuses that extend around both sides of the larynx are part of the hypopharynx.

Larynx

The larynx (Fig. 1.1) is bounded by the hypopharynx superiorly and is continuous with the trachea inferiorly. The thyroid, cricoid, epiglottic, cuneiform, corniculate, and arytenoid cartilages compose the laryngeal skeleton. The thyroid and cricoid cartilages are readily palpated in the anterior neck. The cricoid cartilage articulates with the thyroid cartilage and is joined to it by the cricothyroid ligament. When the patient's head is extended, the cricothyroid ligament can be pierced with a scalpel or large needle to provide an emergency airway (see

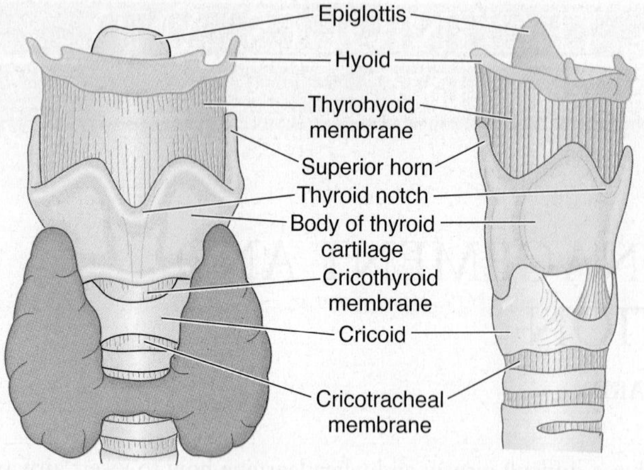

FIGURE 1.1. Anatomy of the larynx, anterior, and lateral aspects. [From Ellis H: *Anatomy for Anaesthetists*. Oxford, Blackwell Scientific, 1963, with permission.]

Chapter 12). The cricoid cartilage completely encircles the airway. It is attached to the first cartilage ring of the trachea by the cricotracheal ligament. The anterior wall of the larynx is formed by the epiglottic cartilage, to which the arytenoid cartilages are attached. Fine muscles span the arytenoid and thyroid cartilages, as do the vocal cords. The true vocal cords and space between them are collectively termed the *glottis* (Fig. 1.2). The glottis is the narrowest space in the adult upper airway. In children, the cricoid cartilage defines the narrowest portion of the airway. Because normal phonation relies on the precise apposition of the true vocal cords, even a small lesion can cause hoarseness. Lymphatic drainage to the true vocal cords is sparse. Inflammation or swelling caused by tube irritation or trauma may take considerable time to resolve. The superior and recurrent laryngeal nerve branches of the vagus nerve innervate the structures of the larynx. The superior laryngeal nerve supplies sensory innervation from the inferior surface of the epiglottis to the superior surface of the vocal cords. From its takeoff from the vagus nerve, it passes deep to both branches of the carotid artery. A large internal branch pierces the thyrohyoid membrane just inferior to the greater cornu of the hyoid. This branch can be blocked with local anesthetics for oral or nasal intubations in awake patients. The recurrent laryngeal branch of the vagus nerve provides sensory innervation below the cords. It also supplies all the muscles of the larynx except the cricothyroid, which is innervated by the external branch of the superior laryngeal nerve.

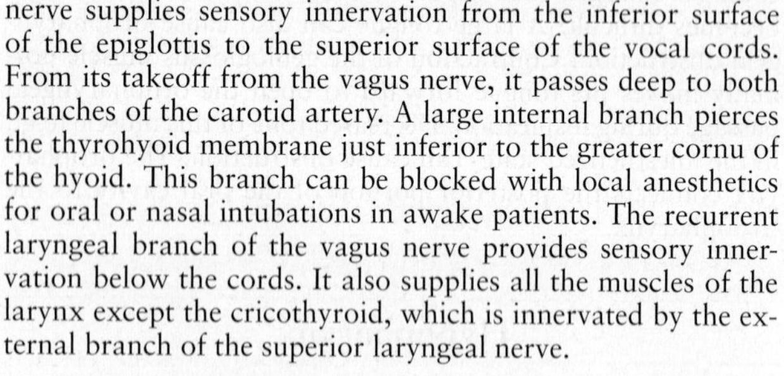

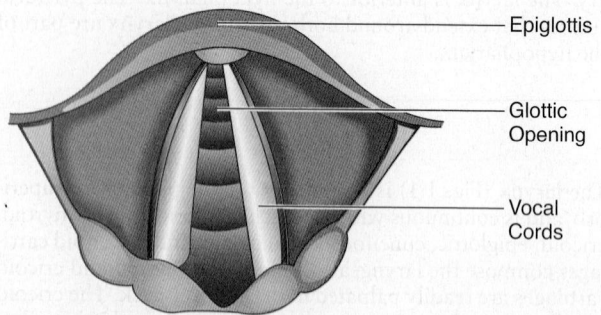

FIGURE 1.2. Superior view of the larynx (inspiration). [From Stoelting RH, Miller RD: *Basics of Anesthesia*. 2nd ed. New York, Churchill Livingstone, 1989, with permission.]

Trachea

The adult trachea averages 15 cm long. Its external skeleton is composed of a series of C-shaped cartilages. It is bounded posteriorly by the esophagus and anteriorly for the first few cartilage rings by the thyroid gland. The trachea is lined with ciliated cells that secrete mucus; through the beating action of the cilia, foreign substances are propelled toward the larynx. The carina is located at the fourth thoracic vertebral level (of relevance when judging proper endotracheal tube positioning on chest radiograph). The right main bronchus takes off at a less acute angle than the left, making right main bronchial intubation more common if the endotracheal tube is in too far.

EMERGENCY AIRWAY MANAGEMENT

In an emergency situation, establishing adequate ventilation and oxygenation assumes primary importance [3]. Too frequently, inexperienced personnel believe that this requires immediate intubation; however, attempts at intubation may delay establishment of an adequate airway. Such efforts are time consuming, can produce hypoxemia and arrhythmias, and may induce bleeding and regurgitation, making subsequent attempts to intubate significantly more difficult and contributing to significant patient morbidity and even mortality [4,5]. Some simple techniques and principles of emergency airway management can play an important role until the arrival of an individual who is skilled at intubation.

Airway Obstruction

Compromised ventilation often results from upper airway obstruction by the tongue, by substances retained in the mouth, or by laryngospasm. Relaxation of the tongue and jaw leading to a reduction in the space between the base of the tongue and the posterior pharyngeal wall is the most common cause of upper airway obstruction. Obstruction may be partial or complete. The latter is characterized by total lack of air exchange. The former is recognized by inspiratory stridor and retraction of neck and intercostal muscles. If respiration is inadequate, the head-tilt–chin-lift or jaw-thrust maneuver should be performed. In patients with suspected cervical spine injuries, the jaw-thrust maneuver (without the head tilt) may result in the least movement of the cervical spine. To perform the head-tilt maneuver, place a palm on the patient's forehead and apply pressure to extend the head about the atlanto-occipital joint. To perform the chin lift, place several fingers of the other hand in the submental area and lift the mandible. Care must be taken to avoid airway obstruction by pressing too firmly on the soft tissues in the submental area. To perform the jaw thrust, lift up on the angles of the mandible [3] (Fig. 1.3). Both of these maneuvers open the oropharyngeal passage. Laryngospasm can be treated by maintaining positive airway pressure using a face mask and bag valve device (see the following section). If the patient resumes spontaneous breathing, establishing this head position may constitute sufficient treatment. If obstruction persists, a check for foreign bodies, emesis, or secretions should be performed [6].

Use of Face Mask and Bag Valve Device

If an adequate airway has been established and the patient is not breathing spontaneously, oxygen can be delivered via face mask and a bag valve device. It is important to establish a

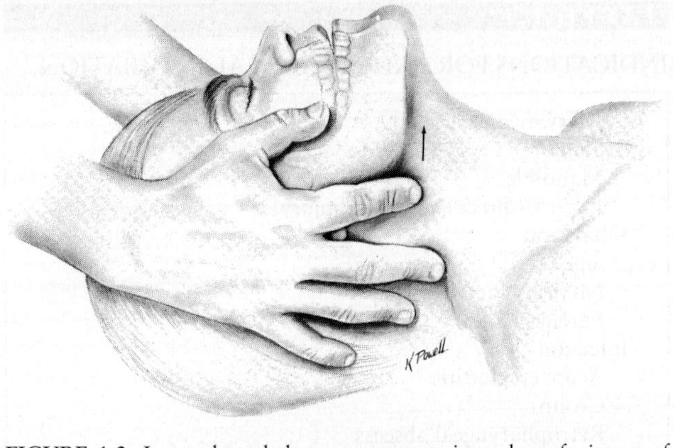

FIGURE 1.3. In an obtunded or comatose patient, the soft tissues of the oropharynx become relaxed and may obstruct the upper airway. Obstruction can be alleviated by placing the thumbs on the maxilla with the index fingers under the ramus of the mandible and rotating the mandible forward with pressure from the index fingers *(arrow)*. This maneuver brings the soft tissues forward and therefore frequently reduces the airway obstruction.

tight fit with the face mask, covering the patient's mouth and nose. To perform this procedure apply the mask initially to the bridge of the nose and draw it downward toward the mouth, using both hands. The operator stands at the patient's head and presses the mask onto the patient's face with the left hand. The thumb should be on the nasal portion of the mask, the index finger near the oral portion, and the rest of the fingers spread on the left side of the patient's mandible so as to pull it slightly forward. The bag is then alternately compressed and released with the right hand. A good airway is indicated by the rise and fall of the chest; moreover, lung–chest wall compliance can be estimated from the amount of pressure required to compress the bag. The minimum effective insufflation pressure should be used to decrease the risk of insufflating the stomach with gas and subsequently increase the risk of aspiration.

Airway Adjuncts

If proper positioning of the head and neck or clearance of foreign bodies and secretions fails to establish an adequate airway, several airway adjuncts may be helpful if an individual who is skilled in intubation is not immediately available. An oropharyngeal or nasopharyngeal airway occasionally helps

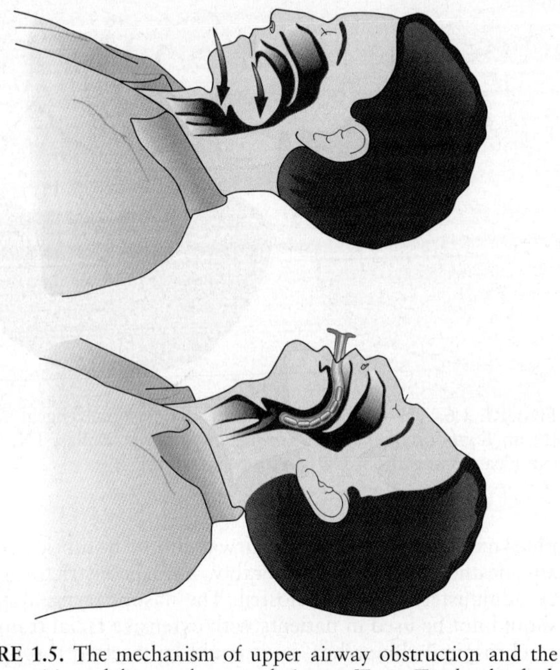

FIGURE 1.5. The mechanism of upper airway obstruction and the proper position of the oropharyngeal airway. [From *Textbook of advanced cardiac life support*. Dallas, TX, American Heart Association, 1997, with permission.]

to establish an adequate airway when proper head positioning alone is insufficient (Figs. 1.4 and 1.5). The oropharyngeal airway is semicircular and made of plastic or hard rubber. The two types are the Guedel airway, with a hollow tubular design, and the Berman airway, with airway channels along the sides. Both types are most easily inserted by turning the curved portion toward the palate as it enters the mouth. It is then advanced beyond the posterior portion of the tongue and rotated downward into the proper position (Fig. 1.5). Often, depressing the tongue or moving it laterally with a tongue blade helps to position the oropharyngeal airway. Care must be exercised not to push the tongue into the posterior pharynx, causing or exacerbating obstruction. Because insertion of the oropharyngeal airway can cause gagging or vomiting, or both, it should be used only in unconscious patients.

The nasopharyngeal airway is a soft tube approximately 15 cm long, which is made of rubber or plastic (Figs. 1.4 and 1.6). It is inserted through the nostril into the posterior

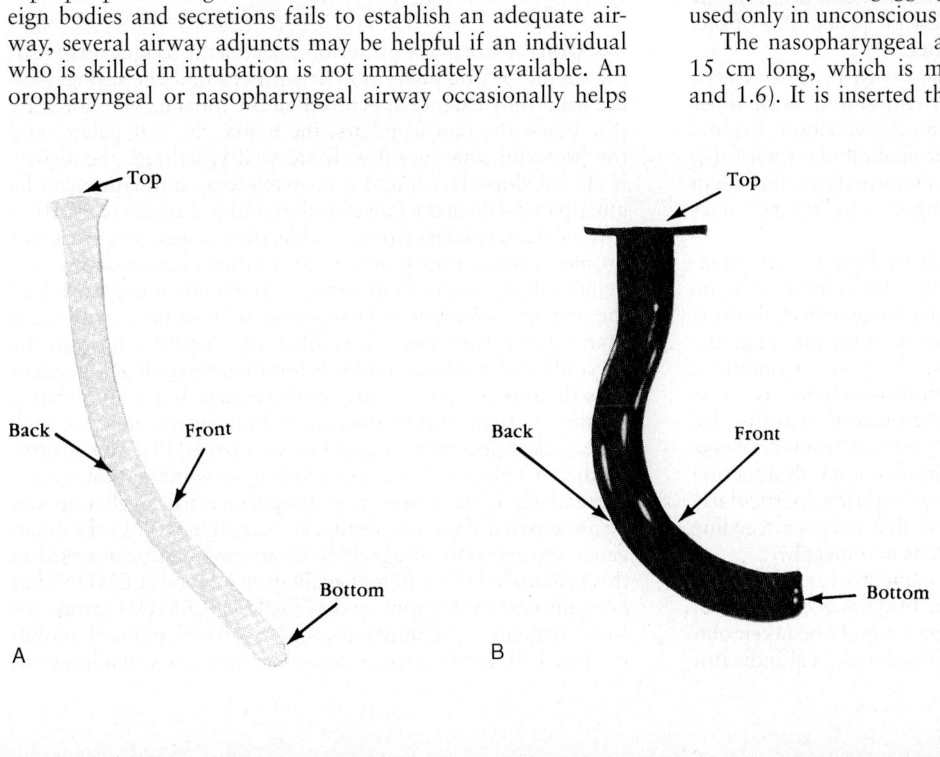

FIGURE 1.4. Nasopharyngeal (**A**) or oropharyngeal (**B**) airways can be used to relieve soft tissue obstruction if elevating the mandible proves ineffective.

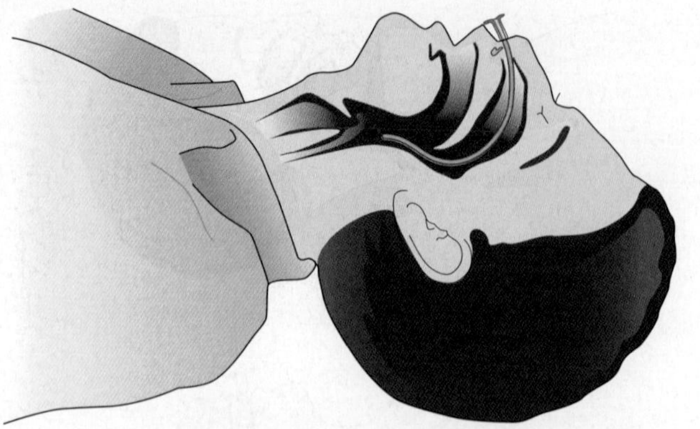

FIGURE 1.6. The proper position of the nasopharyngeal airway. [From *Textbook of advanced cardiac life support*. Dallas, TX, American Heart Association, 1997, with permission.]

pharynx. Before insertion, the airway should be lubricated with an anesthetic gel, and, preferably, a vasoconstrictor should be administered into the nostril. The nasopharyngeal airway should not be used in patients with extensive facial trauma or cerebrospinal rhinorrhea, as it could be inserted through the cribriform plate into the brain.

INDICATIONS FOR INTUBATION

The indications for endotracheal intubation can be divided into four broad categories: (a) acute airway obstruction, (b) excessive pulmonary secretions or inability to clear secretions adequately, (c) loss of protective reflexes, and (d) respiratory failure (Table 1.1).

TABLE 1.1

INDICATIONS FOR ENDOTRACHEAL INTUBATION

Acute airway obstruction
Trauma
Mandible
Larynx (direct or indirect injury)
Inhalation
Smoke
Noxious chemicals
Foreign bodies
Infection
Acute epiglottitis
Croup
Retropharyngeal abscess
Hematoma
Tumor
Congenital anomalies
Laryngeal web
Supraglottic fusion
Laryngeal edema
Laryngeal spasm (anaphylactic response)
Access for suctioning
Debilitated patients
Copious Secretions
Loss of protective reflexes
Head injury
Drug overdose
Cerebrovascular accident
Respiratory failure
Hypoxemia
Acute respiratory distress syndrome
Hypoventilation
Atelectasis
Secretions
Pulmonary edema
Hypercapnia
Hypoventilation
Neuromuscular failure
Drug overdose

Preintubation Evaluation

Even in the most urgent situation, a rapid assessment of the patient's airway anatomy can expedite the choice of the proper route for intubation, the appropriate equipment, and the most useful precautions to be taken. In the less emergent situation, several minutes of preintubation evaluation can decrease the likelihood of complications and increase the probability of successful intubation with minimal trauma.

Anatomic structures of the upper airway, head, and neck must be examined, with particular attention to abnormalities that might preclude a particular route of intubation. Evaluation of cervical spine mobility, temporomandibular joint function, and dentition is important. Any abnormalities that might prohibit alignment of the oral, pharyngeal, and laryngeal axes should be noted.

Cervical spine mobility is assessed by flexion and extension of the neck (performed only after ascertaining that no cervical spine injury exists). The normal range of neck flexion–extension varies from 165 to 90 degrees, with the range decreasing approximately 20% by age 75 years. Conditions associated with decreased range of motion include any cause of degenerative disk disease (e.g., rheumatoid arthritis, osteoarthritis, ankylosing spondylitis), previous trauma, or age older than 70 years. Temporomandibular joint dysfunction can occur in any form of degenerative arthritis (particularly rheumatoid arthritis), in any condition that causes a receding mandible, and in rare conditions such as acromegaly.

Examination of the oral cavity is mandatory. Loose, missing, or chipped teeth and permanent bridgework are noted, and removable bridgework and dentures should be taken out. Mallampati et al. [7] (Fig. 1.7) developed a clinical indicator based on the size of the posterior aspect of the tongue relative to the size of the oral pharynx. The patient should be sitting, with the head fully extended, protruding the tongue and phonating [8]. When the faucial pillars, the uvula, the soft palate, and the posterior pharyngeal wall are well visualized, the airway is classified as class I, and a relatively easy intubation can be anticipated. When the faucial pillars and soft palate (class II) or soft palate only (class III) are visible, there is a greater chance of problems visualizing the glottis during direct laryngoscopy. Difficulties in orotracheal intubation may also be anticipated if (a) the patient is an adult and cannot open his or her mouth more than 40 mm (two-finger breadths), (b) the distance from the thyroid notch to the mandible is less than three-finger breadths (less than or equal to 7 cm), (c) the patient has a high arched palate, or (d) the normal range of flexion–extension of the neck is decreased (less than or equal to 80 degrees) [9]. The positive predictive values of these tests alone or in combination are not particularly high; however, a straightforward intubation can be anticipated if the test results are negative [10]. In the emergency setting, only about 30% of airways can be assessed in this fashion [11]. A different evaluation method (LEMON) has been devised by Murphy and Walls [12]. LEMON stands for *l*ook, *e*valuate, *M*allampati class, *o*bstruction, and *n*eck mobility (Fig. 1.7). In the emergency setting, there are still limitations

L Look externally
Look at the patient externally for characteristics that are known to cause difficult laryngoscopy, intubation or ventilation.

E Evaluate the 3-3-2 rule
In order to allow alignment of the pharyngeal, laryngeal, and oral axes and therefore simple intubation, the following relationships should be observed. The distance between the patient's incisor teeth should be at least 3 finger breadths (3), the distance between the hyoid bone and the chin should be at least 3 finger breadths (3), and the distance between the thyroid notch and the floor of the mouth should be at least 2 finger breadths (2).

1 – Inter-incisor distance in fingers
2 – Hyoid mental distance in fingers
3 – Thyroid to floor of mouth in fingers

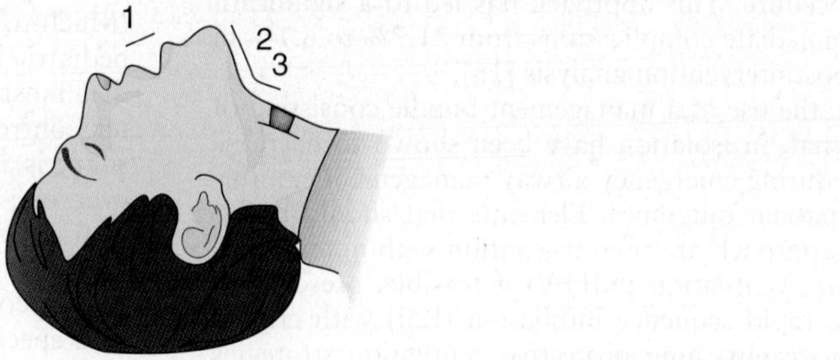

M Mallampati
The hypopharynx should be visualized adequately. This has been done traditionally by assessing the Mallampati classification. The patient is sat upright, told to open the mouth fully and protrude the tongue as far as possible. The examiner then looks into the mouth with a light torch to assess the degree of hypopharynx visible. In the case of a supine patient, Mallampati score can be estimated by getting the patient to open the mouth fully and protrude the tongue and a laryngoscopy light can be shone into the hypopharynx from above.

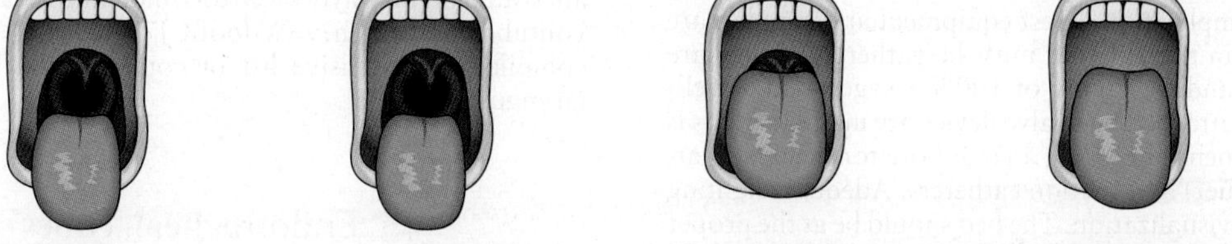

Class I: soft palate, uvula, fauces, pillars visible | Class II: soft palate, uvula, fauces visible | Class III: soft palate, base of uvula visible | Class IV: hard palate only visible

O Obstruction?
Any condition that can cause obstruction of the airway will make laryngoscopy and ventilation difficult. Such conditions are epiglottis, peritonsillar abscesses, and trauma.

N Neck mobility
This is a vital requirement for successful intubation. It can be assessed easily by getting the patient to place his or her chin down onto the chest and then to extend the neck so the patient is looking towards the ceiling. Patients in hard collar neck immobilization obviously have no neck movement and are therefore harder to intubate.

FIGURE 1.7. The LEMON airway assessment method. [From Reed MJ, Dunn MJ, McKeown DW: Can an airway assessment score predict difficulty at intubation in the emergency department? *Emerg Med J* 22(2):99–102, 2005, with permission.]

with the use of LEMON since it is difficult to ascertain the Mallampati class. Nonetheless, using elements of LEMON that could be incorporated into the emergency evaluation of patients, Reed et al. [13] found that large incisors, a reduced interincisor distance, and a reduced distance between the thyroid and floor of the mouth were associated with a limited laryngoscopic view in emergency department patients. Whenever possible, patients in need of elective and emergent airway management should be assessed for indicators of difficult mask ventilation as this may significantly influence the decision on the primary approach to airway management. In the largest analysis published to date, five independent predictors of impossible mask ventilation were identified by the authors; these include neck radiation changes, male sex, a diagnosis of sleep apnea, Mallampati class III or IV airway, and the presence of a beard [14]. Among these factors, neck radiation changes were the most significant predictor of impossible mask ventilation.

Education and Intubation Management

Emergent intubation in the acute care setting is associated with a high complication rate. It is therefore important to provide adequate training to practitioners working in this environment, and have an adequate number of trained personnel be available to assist the operator. Furthermore, a standardized approach to emergency airway management can improve patient outcomes. Although training on a mannequin is an important first step in acquiring competency in performing endotracheal intubation, an investigation including nonanesthesia trainees has shown that approximately 50 supervised endotracheal intubations in the clinical setting are needed to achieve a 90% probability of competent performance [15]. Whenever possible, residents and licensed independent practitioners should be supervised by an attending physician trained in emergency airway management during the procedure. This approach has led to a significant reduction in immediate complications from 21.7% to 6.1% in one pre- and postintervention analysis [16].

In addition, the use of a management bundle consisting of interventions that, in isolation have been shown to decrease complications during emergency airway management can further improve patient outcomes. Elements that should be included in this approach are preoxygenation with noninvasive positive pressure ventilation (NIPPV) if feasible, presence of two operators, rapid sequence intubation (RSI) with cricoid pressure, capnography, lung protective ventilation strategies (LPVS), fluid loading prior to intubation unless contraindicated, and preparation and early administration of sedation and vasopressor use if needed [17].

EQUIPMENT FOR INTUBATION

Assembly of all appropriate equipment before attempted intubation can prevent potentially serious delays in the event of an unforeseen complication. Most equipment and supplies are readily available in the ICU but must be gathered so they are immediately at hand. A supply of 100% oxygen and a well-fitting mask with attached bag valve device are mandatory, as is suctioning equipment, including a large-bore tonsil suction attachment (Yankauer) and suction catheters. Adequate lighting facilitates airway visualization. The bed should be at the proper height, with the headboard removed and the wheels locked. Other necessary supplies include gloves, Magill forceps, oral and nasal airways, laryngoscope handle and blades (straight and curved), endotracheal tubes of various sizes, stylet, tongue depressors, a syringe for cuff inflation, and tape for securing the endotracheal tube in position. Table 1.2 is a checklist of supplies needed.

TABLE 1.2

EQUIPMENT NEEDED FOR INTUBATION

Supply of 100% oxygen
Face mask
Bag valve device
Suction equipment
Suction catheters
Large-bore tonsil suction apparatus (Yankauer)
Stylet
Magill forceps
Oral airways
Nasal airways
Laryngoscope handle and blades (curved, straight; various sizes)
Endotracheal tubes (various sizes)
Tongue depressors
Syringe for cuff inflation
Headrest
Supplies for vasoconstriction and local anesthesia
Tape
Tincture of benzoin

Laryngoscopes

The two-piece laryngoscope has a handle containing batteries that power the bulb in the blade. The blade snaps securely into the top of the handle, making the electrical connection. Failure of the bulb to illuminate suggests improper blade positioning, bulb failure, a loose bulb, or dead batteries. Modern laryngoscope blades with fiberoptic lights obviate the problem of bulb failure. Many blade shapes and sizes are available. The two most commonly used blades are the curved (MacIntosh) and straight (Miller) blades (Fig. 1.8). Although pediatric blades are available for use with the adult-sized handle, most anesthesiologists prefer a smaller handle for better control in the pediatric population. The choice of blade shape is a matter of personal preference and experience; however, one study has suggested that less force and head extension are required when performing direct laryngoscopy with a straight blade [18]. Recently, video assisted laryngoscopes have become widely available in many perioperative and acute care specialties. These have been shown to improve the success rate for difficult endotracheal intubation performed by experienced physicians [19], as well as the rate of successful intubation by untrained individuals when performing normal intubations [20]. Several online tutorials are available demonstrating the use of video laryngoscopes. Two of them can be found here: Turk M, Gravenstein D (2007): Storz DCI Video Laryngoscope. Retrieved March 15, 2010, from University of Florida Department of Anesthesiology, Center for Simulation, Advanced Learning and Technology Web site: http://vam.anest.ufl.edu/airwaydevice/storz/index.html and http://www.youtube.com/watch?v=WdooBCJ79Xc&NR=1. Hagberg has compiled an extensive list of commercially available video-laryngoscopes [21].

Endotracheal Tubes

The internal diameter of the endotracheal tube is measured using both millimeters and French units. This number is stamped on the tube. Tubes are available in 0.5-mm increments, starting at 2.5 mm. Lengthwise dimensions are also marked on the tube in centimeters, beginning at the distal tracheal end.

Selection of the proper tube diameter is of utmost importance and is a frequently underemphasized consideration. The resistance to airflow varies with the fourth power of the radius of the endotracheal tube. Thus, selection of an inappropriately small tube can significantly increase the work of breathing. Moreover, certain diagnostic procedures (e.g., bronchoscopy) done through endotracheal tubes require appropriately large tubes (see Chapter 9). In general, the larger the patient, the larger the endotracheal tube that should be used. Approximate guidelines for tube sizes and lengths by age are summarized in Table 1.3. Most adults should be intubated with an endotracheal tube that has an inner diameter of at least 8.0 mm, although occasionally nasal intubation in a small adult requires a 7.0-mm tube.

Endotracheal Tube Cuff

Endotracheal tubes have low-pressure, high-volume cuffs to reduce the incidence of ischemia-related complications. Tracheal ischemia can occur any time cuff pressure exceeds capillary pressure (approximately 32 mm Hg), thereby causing inflammation, ulceration, infection, and dissolution of cartilaginous rings. Failure to recognize this progressive degeneration sometimes results in erosion through the tracheal wall (into the

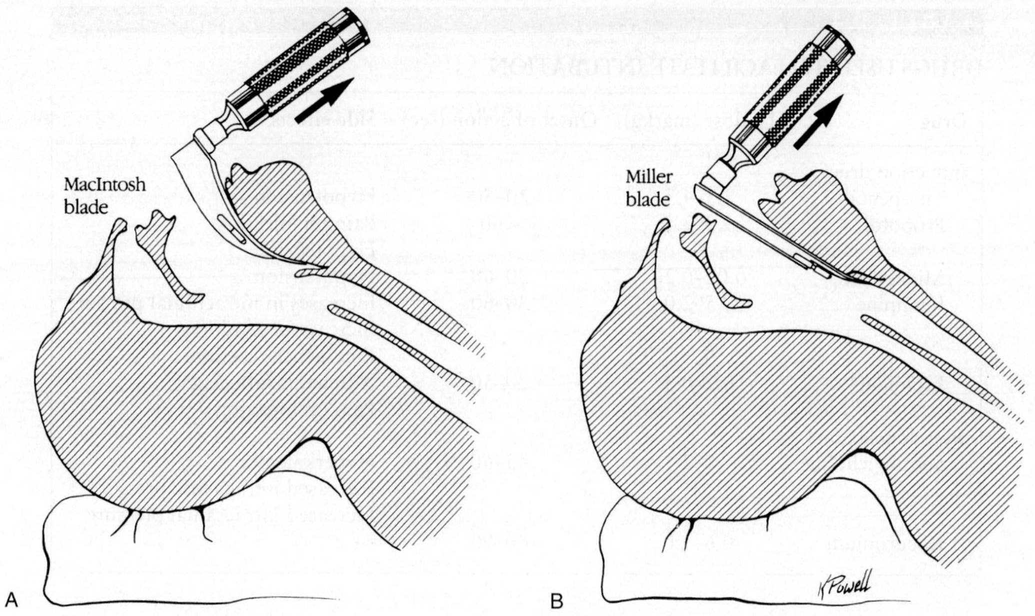

FIGURE 1.8. The two basic types of laryngoscope blades, MacIntosh (A) and Miller (B). The MacIntosh blade is curved. The blade tip is placed in the vallecula and the handle of the laryngoscope pulled forward at a 45-degree angle. This allows visualization of the epiglottis. The Miller blade is straight. The tip is placed posterior to the epiglottis, pinning the epiglottis between the base of the tongue and the straight laryngoscope blade. The motion on the laryngoscope handle is the same as that used with the MacIntosh blade.

innominate artery if the erosion was anterior or the esophagus if the erosion was posterior) or long-term sequelae of tracheomalacia or tracheal stenosis. With cuff pressures of 15 to 30 mm Hg, the low-pressure, high-volume cuffs conform well to the tracheal wall and provide an adequate seal during positive-pressure ventilation. Although low cuff pressures can cause some damage (primarily ciliary denudation), major complications are rare. Nevertheless, it is important to realize that a low-pressure, high-volume cuff can be converted to a high-pressure cuff if sufficient quantities of air are injected into the cuff.

ANESTHESIA BEFORE INTUBATION

Because patients who require intubation often have a depressed level of consciousness, anesthesia is usually not required. If intubation must be performed on the alert, responsive patient, sedation or general anesthesia exposes the individual to potential pulmonary aspiration of gastric contents because protective reflexes are lost. This risk is a particularly important consideration if the patient has recently eaten and must be

TABLE 1.3

DIMENSIONS OF ENDOTRACHEAL TUBES BASED ON PATIENT AGE

Age	Internal diameter (mm)	French unit	Distance between lips and location in midtrachea of distal end (cm)[a]
Premature	2.5	10–12	10
Full term	3.0	12–14	11
1–6 mo	3.5	16	11
6–12 mo	4.0	18	12
2 y	4.5	20	13
4 y	5.0	22	14
6 y	5.5	24	15–16
8 y	6.5	26	16–17
10 y	7.0	28	17–18
12 y	7.5	30	18–20
≥14 y	8.0–9.0	32–36	20–24

[a] Add 2 to 3 cm for nasal tubes.
From Stoelting RK: Endotracheal intubation, in Miller RD (ed): *Anesthesia*. 2nd ed. New York, Churchill Livingstone, 1986, p. 531, with permission.

TABLE 1.4

DRUGS USED TO FACILITATE INTUBATION

Drug	IV dose (mg/kg)	Onset of action (sec)	Side effects
Induction drugs			
Thiopental	2.5–4.5	20–50	Hypotension
Propofol	1.0–2.5	<60	Pain on injection Hypotension
Midazolam	0.02–0.20	30–60	Hypotension
Ketamine	0.5–2.0	30–60	Increases in intracranial pressure Increase in secretions Emergence reactions
Etomidate	0.2–0.3	20–50	Adrenal insufficiency Pain on injection
Muscle relaxants			
Succinylcholine	1–2	45–60	Hyperkalemia Increased intragastric pressure Increased intracranial pressure
Rocuronium	0.6–1.0	60–90	—

weighed against the risk of various hemodynamic derangements that might occur secondary to tracheal intubation and initiation of positive-pressure ventilation. Laryngoscopy in an inadequately anesthetized patient can result in tachycardia and an increase in blood pressure. This may be well tolerated in younger patients but may be detrimental in a patient with coronary artery disease or raised intracranial pressure. Sometimes laryngoscopy and intubation may result in a vasovagal response, leading to bradycardia and hypotension. Initiation of positive-pressure ventilation in a hypovolemic patient can lead to hypotension from diminished venous return.

Some of these responses can be attenuated by providing local anesthesia to the nares, mouth, and/or posterior pharynx before intubation. Topical lidocaine (1% to 4%) with phenylephrine (0.25%) or cocaine (4%, 200 mg total dose) can be used to anesthetize the nasal passages and provide local vasoconstriction. This allows the passage of a larger endotracheal tube with less likelihood of bleeding. Aqueous lidocaine–phenylephrine or cocaine can be administered via atomizer, nose dropper, or long cotton-tipped swabs inserted into the nares. Alternatively, viscous 2% lidocaine can be applied via a 3.5-mm endotracheal tube or small nasopharyngeal airway inserted into the nose. Anesthesia of the tongue and posterior pharynx can be accomplished with lidocaine spray (4% to 10%) administered via an atomizer or an eutectic mixture of local anesthetics cream applied on a tongue blade and oral airway [22]. Alternatively, the glossopharyngeal nerve can be blocked bilaterally with an injection of a local anesthetic, but this should be performed by experienced personnel.

Anesthetizing the larynx below the vocal cords before intubation is controversial. The cough reflex can be compromised, increasing the risk of aspiration. However, tracheal anesthesia may decrease the incidence of arrhythmias or untoward circulatory responses to intubation and improve patient tolerance of the endotracheal tube. Clinical judgment in this situation is necessary. Several methods can be used to anesthetize these structures. Transtracheal lidocaine (4%, 160 mg) is administered by cricothyroid membrane puncture with a small needle to anesthetize the trachea and larynx below the vocal cords. Alternatively, after exposure of the vocal cords with the laryngoscope, the cords can be sprayed with lidocaine via an atomizer. Aerosolized lidocaine (4%, 6 mL) provides excellent anesthesia to the mouth, pharynx, larynx, and trachea [23]. The superior laryngeal nerve can be blocked with 2 mL of 1.0% to 1.5% lidocaine injected just inferior to the greater cornu of the hyoid bone. The rate of absorption of lidocaine differs by method, being greater with the aerosol and transtracheal techniques. The patient should be observed for signs of lidocaine toxicity (circumoral paresthesia, agitation, and seizures).

If adequate topical anesthesia cannot be achieved or if the patient is not cooperative, general anesthesia may be required for intubation. Table 1.4 lists common drugs and doses that are used to facilitate intubation. Ketamine and etomidate are two drugs that are used commonly because cardiovascular stability is maintained. Caution should be exercised when using etomidate in patients with signs and symptoms consistent with severe sepsis or septic shock. In an analysis of risk factors of relative adrenocortical deficiency in intensive care patients needing mechanical ventilation, single bolus etomidate administration was independently associated with relative adrenocortical deficiency [24]. Similarly, when studied for rapid sequence intubation in acutely ill patients both ketamine and etomidate provided adequate intubating conditions but the percentage of patients with adrenal insufficiency was significantly higher in the etomidate group [25]. Lastly, post hoc analysis of the corticosteroid therapy of septic shock study revealed an increased rate of death at 28 days among patients who received etomidate before randomization in both groups (hydrocortisone group and in the placebo group), as compared with patients who did not receive etomidate [26]. Taken together these findings warrant a careful analysis of risks and benefits before etomidate is used to facilitate endotracheal intubation in acutely ill patients with, or at risk for, severe sepsis.

Use of opioids such as morphine, fentanyl, sufentanil, alfentanil, or remifentanil allow the dose of the induction drugs to be reduced and may attenuate the hemodynamic response to laryngoscopy and intubation. Muscle relaxants can be used to facilitate intubation, but unless the practitioner has extensive experience with these drugs and airway management, alternative means of airway control and oxygenation should be used until an anesthesiologist arrives to administer the anesthetic and perform the intubation. Although the use of muscle relaxants is associated with improved laryngoscopy grade during intubation, their use may not be associated with a decrease in overall airway related complications, hypotension or hypoxemia.

Recent reviews have extolled the virtue of rapid sequence intubation (RSI) [27,28]: The process by which a drug such as etomidate, thiopental, ketamine, or propofol (Table 1.4) is administered to the patient to induce anesthesia and is followed immediately by a muscle relaxant to facilitate intubation. Although numerous studies exist in the emergency medicine literature attesting to the safety and efficacy of this approach, the practitioner who embarks on this route to intubation in the ICU must be knowledgeable about the pharmacology and side effects of the agents used *and* the use of rescue methods should attempt(s) at intubation fail. Again, experience and an approached based on a validated algorithm will increase patient safety. In a recent analysis of 6,088 trauma patients undergoing emergency airway management in a single center over 10 years, intubation by anesthesiologists experienced in the management of trauma patients utilizing a modification of the American Society of Anesthesiologists difficult airway algorithm was very effective, resulting in a rate of surgical airway management in only 0.3% of patients included in the analysis [29].

TECHNIQUES OF INTUBATION

In a true emergency, some of the preintubation evaluation is necessarily neglected in favor of rapid control of the airway. Attempts at tracheal intubation should not cause or exacerbate hypoxia. Whenever possible, an oxygen saturation monitor should be used. Preoxygenation (denitrogenation), which replaces the nitrogen in the patient's functional residual capacity with oxygen, can maximize the time available for intubation. During laryngoscopy, apneic oxygenation can occur from this reservoir. Preoxygenation is achieved by providing 100% oxygen at a high flow rate via a tight-fitting face mask for 3.5 to 4.0 minutes. Extending the time of preoxygenation from 4 to 8 minutes does not seem to increase the PaO_2 to a clinically relevant extent and may actually reduce the PaO_2 in the interval from 6 to 8 minutes in some patients [30]. In patients who are being intubated for airway control, preoxygenation is usually efficacious; whereas, the value of preoxygenation in patients with acute lung injury is less certain [31]. Whenever possible, NIPPV should be utilized as the mode of preoxygenation prior to intubation of hypoxemic patients. This approach has been shown to be more effective than the standard approach in maintaining SpO_2 values before, during and even after the intubation procedure resulting [32]. In obese patients, use of the 25-degree head-up position improves the effectiveness of preoxygenation [33].

Just before intubation, the physician should assess the likelihood of success for each route of intubation, the urgency of the clinical situation, the likelihood that intubation will be prolonged, and the prospect of whether diagnostic or therapeutic procedures such as bronchoscopy will eventually be required. Factors that can affect patient comfort should also be weighed. In the unconscious patient in whom a secure airway must be established immediately, orotracheal intubation with direct visualization of the vocal cords is generally the preferred technique. In the conscious patient, direct laryngoscopy or awake fiberoptic intubation may be performed after adequate topicalization of the airway. Alternatively, blind nasotracheal intubation is an option but requires significant skill by the clinician. Nasotracheal intubation should be avoided in patients with coagulopathies or those who are anticoagulated for medical indications. In trauma victims with extensive maxillary and mandibular fractures and inadequate ventilation or oxygenation, cricothyrotomy may be mandatory (see Chapter 12). In patients with cervical spine injury or decreased neck mobility, intubation using the flexible bronchoscope or specialized laryngoscope (Bullard) may be necessary. Many of these techniques require considerable skill and should be performed only by those who are experienced in airway management [34].

Specific Techniques and Routes of Endotracheal Intubation

Orotracheal Intubation

Orotracheal intubation is the technique most easily learned and most often used for emergency intubations in the ICU. Traditional teaching dictates that successful orotracheal intubation requires alignment of the oral, pharyngeal, and laryngeal axes by putting the patient in the "sniffing position" in which the neck is flexed and the head is slightly extended about the atlanto-occipital joint. However, a magnetic resonance imaging (MRI) study has called this concept into question, as the alignment of these three axes could not be achieved in any of the three positions tested: neutral, simple extension, and the "sniffing position" [35]. In addition, a randomized study in elective surgery patients examining the utility of the sniffing position as a means to facilitate orotracheal intubation failed to demonstrate that such positioning was superior to simple head extension [36].

In a patient with a full stomach, compressing the cricoid cartilage posteriorly against the vertebral body can reduce the diameter of the postcricoid hypopharynx. This technique, known as *Sellick's maneuver*, may prevent passive regurgitation of stomach contents into the trachea during intubation [37]. However, an MRI study of awake volunteers demonstrated that the esophagus was lateral to the larynx in more than 50% of the subjects. Moreover, cricoid pressure *increased* the incidence of an unopposed esophagus by 50% and caused airway compression of greater than 1 mm in 81% of the volunteers [38]. These findings are in contrast to a more recent MRI study demonstrating that the location and movement of the esophagus is irrelevant to the efficacy of Sellick's maneuver to prevent gastric regurgitation into the pharynx. Of note, compression of the alimentary tract was demonstrated with midline and lateral displacement of the cricoid cartilage relative to the underlying vertebral body [39]. In addition, cadaver studies have demonstrated the efficacy of cricoid pressure [40] and clinical studies have shown that gastric insufflation with gas during mask ventilation is reduced when cricoid pressure is applied [41]. In aggregate, these data suggest that it is prudent to continue to use cricoid pressure in patients suspected of having full stomachs. In addition, placing the patient in the partial recumbent or reverse Trendelenburg position may reduce the risk of regurgitation and aspiration.

The laryngoscope handle is grasped in the left hand while the patient's mouth is opened with the gloved right hand. Often, when the head is extended in the unconscious patient, the mouth opens; if not, the thumb and index finger of the right hand are placed on the lower and upper incisors, respectively, and moved past each other in a scissor-like motion. The laryngoscope blade is inserted on the right side of the mouth and advanced to the base of the tongue, pushing it toward the left. If the straight blade is used, it should be extended below the epiglottis. If the curved blade is used, it is inserted in the vallecula.

With the blade in place, the operator should lift forward in a plane 45 degrees from the horizontal to expose the vocal cords (Figs. 1.2 and 1.8). This motion decreases the risk of the blade striking the upper incisors and either chipping or dislodging teeth. Both lips should be swept away from between the teeth and blade to avoid soft tissue damage. The endotracheal tube is then held in the right hand and inserted at the right corner of the patient's mouth in a plane that intersects with the laryngoscope blade at the level of the glottis. This prevents the endotracheal tube from obscuring the view of the vocal cords. The endotracheal tube is advanced through the vocal cords until the cuff just disappears from sight. The cuff is inflated with enough air

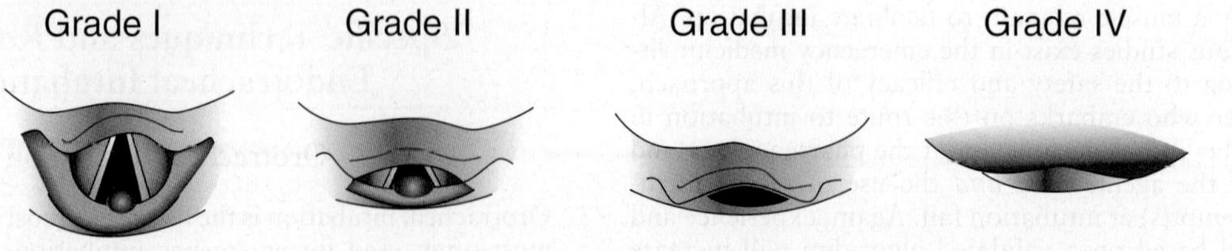

FIGURE 1.9. The four grades of laryngeal view during direct laryngoscopy. Grade I: the entire glottis is seen. Grade II: only the posterior aspect of the glottis is seen. Grade III: only the epiglottis is seen. Grade IV: the epiglottis is not visualized. [From Cormack RS, Lehane J: Difficult tracheal intubation in obstetrics. *Anaesthesia* 39:1105–1111, 1984, with permission.]

to prevent a leak during positive-pressure ventilation with a bag valve device.

A classification grading the view of the laryngeal aperture during direct laryngoscopy has been described [42] and is depicted in Figure 1.9. Occasionally, the vocal cords cannot be seen entirely; only the corniculate and cuneiform tubercles, interarytenoid incisure, and posterior portion of the vocal cords or only the epiglottis is visualized (grades II to IV view; Fig. 1.9). In this situation, it is helpful to insert the soft metal stylet into the endotracheal tube and bend it into a hockey-stick configuration. The stylet should be bent or coiled at the proximal end to prevent the distal end from extending beyond the endotracheal tube and causing tissue damage. The stylet should be lubricated to ensure easy removal. The BURP maneuver (*b*ackward–*u*pward–*r*ightward *p*ressure on the larynx) improves the view of the laryngeal aperture [43]. Alternatively, a control-tip endotracheal tube can be used. This tube has a nylon cord running the length of the tube attached to a ring at the proximal end, which allows the operator to direct the tip of the tube anteriorly. Another aid is a stylet with a light (light wand). With the room lights dimmed, the endotracheal tube containing the lighted stylet is inserted into the oropharynx and advanced in the midline. When it is just superior to the larynx, a glow is seen over the anterior neck. The stylet is advanced into the trachea, and the tube is threaded over it. The light intensity is diminished if the wand enters the esophagus [44]. The gum elastic bougie (flexible stylet) is another alternative device that can be passed into the larynx; once in place, the endotracheal tube is advance over it and the stylet is removed. Endotracheal tubes and stylets are now available that have a fiberoptic bundle intrinsic to the tube or the stylet that can be attached to a video monitor. If the attempt to intubate is still unsuccessful, the algorithm that is described in the Management of the Difficult Airway section should be followed.

Proper depth of tube placement is clinically ascertained by observing symmetric expansion of both sides of the chest and auscultating equal breath sounds in both lungs. The stomach should also be auscultated to ensure that the esophagus has not been entered. If the tube has been advanced too far, it will lodge in one of the main bronchi (particularly the right bronchus), and only one lung will be ventilated. If this error goes unnoticed, the nonventilated lung may collapse. A useful rule of thumb for tube placement in adults of average size is that the incisors should be at the 23-cm mark in men and the 21-cm mark in women [45]. Alternatively, proper depth (5 cm above the carina) can be estimated using the following formula: (height in cm/5) minus 13 [46]. Palpation of the anterior trachea in the neck may detect cuff inflation as air is injected into the pilot tube and can serve as a means to ascertain correct tube position. Measurement of end-tidal carbon dioxide by standard capnography if available or by means of a calorimetric chemical detector of end-tidal carbon dioxide (e.g., Easy Cap II, Nellcor, Inc., Pleasanton, CA) can be used to verify correct endotracheal tube placement or detect esophageal intubation. The latter device is attached to the proximal end of the endotracheal tube and changes color on exposure to carbon dioxide. An additional method to detect esophageal intubation uses a bulb that attaches to the proximal end of the endotracheal tube [47]. The bulb is squeezed. If the tube is in the trachea, the bulb reexpands, and if the tube is in the esophagus, the bulb remains collapsed. It must be remembered that none of these techniques is foolproof. Bronchoscopy is the only method to be absolutely sure the tube is in the trachea. After estimating proper tube placement clinically, it should be confirmed by chest radiograph or bronchoscopy because the tube may be malpositioned. The tip of the endotracheal tube should be several centimeters above the carina (T-4 level). It must be remembered that flexion or extension of the head can advance or withdraw the tube 2 to 5 cm, respectively.

Nasotracheal Intubation

Many of the considerations concerning patient preparation and positioning outlined for orotracheal intubation apply to nasal intubation as well. Blind nasal intubation is more difficult to perform than oral intubation, because the tube cannot be observed directly as it passes between the vocal cords. However, nasal intubation is usually more comfortable for the patient and is generally preferable in the awake, conscious patient. Nasal intubation should not be attempted in patients with abnormal bleeding parameters, nasal polyps, extensive facial trauma, cerebrospinal rhinorrhea, sinusitis, or any anatomic abnormality that would inhibit atraumatic passage of the tube.

As previously discussed in Airway Adjuncts section, after the operator has alternately occluded each nostril to ascertain that both are patent, a topical vasoconstrictor and anesthetic are applied to the nostril that will be intubated. The nostril may be dilated with lubricated nasal airways of increasing size to facilitate atraumatic passage of the endotracheal tube. The patient should be monitored with a pulse oximeter, and supplemental oxygen should be given as necessary. The patient may be either supine or sitting with the head extended in the sniffing position. The tube is guided slowly but firmly through the nostril to the posterior pharynx. Here the tube operator must continually monitor for the presence of air movement through the tube by listening for breath sounds with the ear near the open end of the tube. The tube must never be forced or pushed forward if breath sounds are lost, because damage to the retropharyngeal mucosa can result. If resistance is met, the tube should be withdrawn 1 to 2 cm and the patient's head repositioned (extended further or turned to either side). If the turn still cannot be negotiated, the other nostril or a smaller tube should be tried. Attempts at nasal intubation should be abandoned and oral intubation performed if these methods fail.

Once positioned in the oropharynx, the tube should be advanced to the glottis while listening for breath sounds through the tube. If breath sounds cease, the tube is withdrawn several centimeters until breath sounds resume, and the plane of entry is adjusted slightly. Passage through the vocal cords should be timed to coincide with inspiration. Entry of the tube into

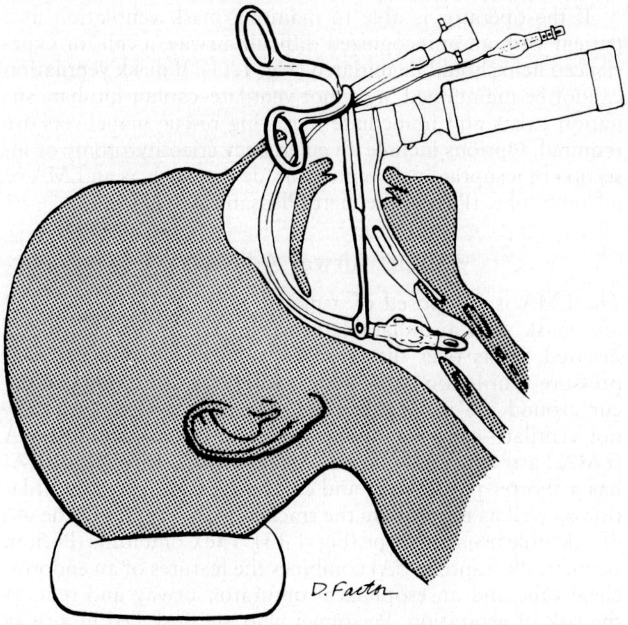

FIGURE 1.10. Magill forceps may be required to guide the endotracheal tube into the larynx during nasotracheal intubation. [From Barash PG, Cullen BF, Stoelting RK: *Clinical Anesthesia*. 2nd ed. Philadelphia, PA, JB Lippincott Co, 1992, with permission.]

the larynx is signaled by an inability to speak. The cuff should be inflated and proper positioning of the tube ascertained as previously outlined.

Occasionally, blind nasal intubation cannot be accomplished. In this case, after adequate topical anesthesia, laryngoscopy can be used to visualize the vocal cords directly and Magill forceps used to grasp the distal end of the tube and guide it through the vocal cords (Fig. 1.10). Assistance in pushing the tube forward is essential during this maneuver, so that the operator merely guides the tube. The balloon on the tube should not be grasped with the Magill forceps.

Occasionally, one may not be able to successfully place the endotracheal tube in the trachea. The technique of managing a difficult airway is detailed later.

Management of the Difficult Airway

A difficult airway may be recognized (anticipated) or unrecognized at the time of the initial preintubation airway evaluation. Difficulty managing the airway may be the result of abnormalities such as congenital hypoplasia, hyperplasia of the mandible or maxilla, or prominent incisors; injuries to the face or neck; acromegaly; tumors; and previous head and neck surgery. Difficulties ventilating the patient with a mask can be anticipated if two of the following factors are present: age older than 55 years, body mass index greater than 26 kg per m^2, beard, lack of teeth, and a history of snoring [48]. When a difficult airway is encountered, the algorithm as detailed in Figure 1.11

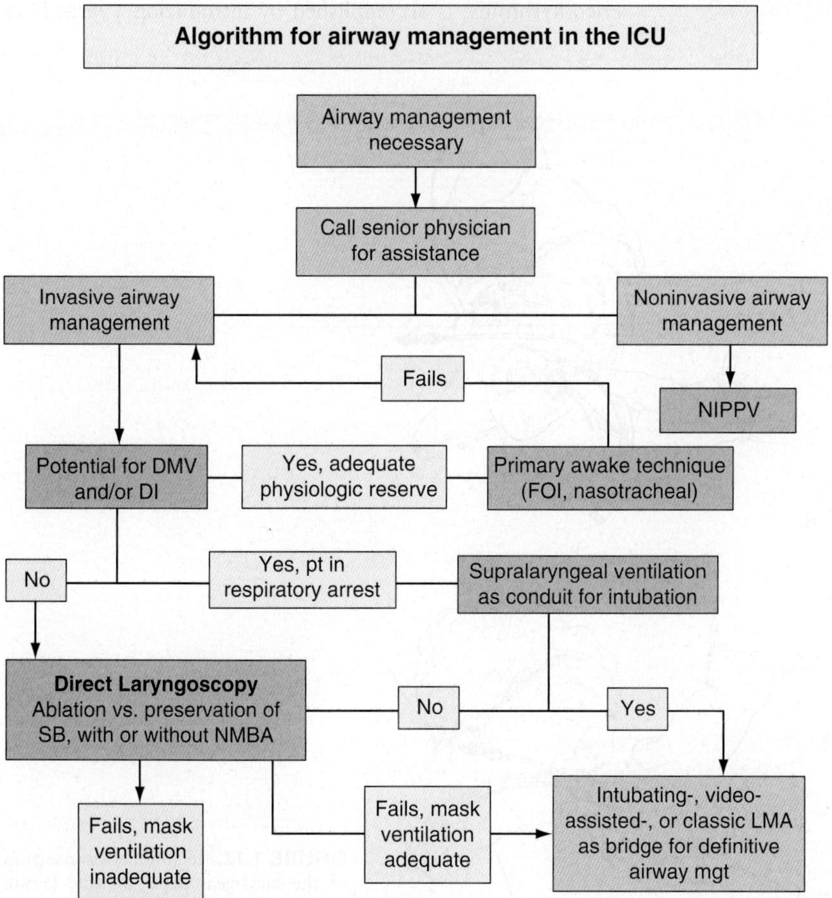

FIGURE 1.11. Modification of the difficult airway algorithm. ASA DAA, American Society of Anesthesiologists difficult airway algorithm; DMV, difficult mask ventilation; FOI, fiberoptic intubation; LMA, laryngeal mask airway; NIPPV, noninvasive positive pressure ventilation; NMBA, neuromuscular blocking agents; SB, spontaneous breathing. [From Walz JM, Zayaruzny M, Heard SO, et al. *Chest* 131(2):608–620, 2007, with permission.]

should be followed [49]. When a difficult airway is recognized before the patient is anesthetized, an awake tracheal intubation is usually the best option. Multiple techniques can be used and include (after adequate topical or local anesthesia) direct laryngoscopy, LMA (or variants), blind or bronchoscopic oral or nasal intubation, retrograde technique, rigid bronchoscopy, lighted stylet, or a surgical airway.

Flexible Bronchoscopic Intubation

Flexible bronchoscopy is an efficacious method of intubating the trachea in difficult cases. It may be particularly useful when the upper airway anatomy has been distorted by tumors, trauma, endocrinopathies, or congenital anomalies. This technique is sometimes valuable in accident victims in whom a question of cervical spine injury exists and the patient's neck cannot be manipulated. An analogous situation exists in patients with severe degenerative disk disease of the neck or rheumatoid arthritis with markedly impaired neck mobility. After adequate topical anesthesia is obtained as described in the section Anesthesia before Intubation, the bronchoscope can be used to intubate the trachea via either the nasal or oral route. An appropriately sized warmed and lubricated endotracheal tube that has been preloaded onto the bronchoscope is advanced through the vocal cords into the trachea and positioned above the carina under direct vision. The flexible bronchoscope has also been used as a stent over which endotracheal tubes are exchanged and as a means to assess tracheal damage periodically during prolonged intubations. (A detailed discussion of bronchoscopy is found in Chapter 9.) Intubation by this technique requires skill and experience and is best performed by a fully trained operator.

If the operator is able to maintain mask ventilation in a patient with an unrecognized difficult airway, a call for experienced help should be initiated (Fig. 1.11). If mask ventilation cannot be maintained, a cannot ventilate–cannot intubate situation exists and immediate lifesaving rescue maneuvers are required. Options include an emergency cricothyrotomy or insertion of a supraglottic ventilatory device, such as an LMA or a Combitube. (Puritan Bennett, Pleasanton, CA.)

Other Airway Adjuncts

The LMA is composed of a plastic tube attached to a shallow mask with an inflatable rim (Fig. 1.12). When properly inserted, it fits over the laryngeal inlet and allows positive-pressure ventilation of the lungs. Although aspiration can occur around the mask, the LMA can be lifesaving in a cannot ventilate–cannot intubate situation. An intubating LMA (LMA-Fastrach, LMA North America, Inc., San Diego, CA) has a shorter plastic tube and can be used to provide ventilation as well as to intubate the trachea with or without the aid of a flexible bronchoscope (Fig. 1.13). The Combitube (Puritan Bennett, Pleasanton, CA) combines the features of an endotracheal tube and an esophageal obturator airway and reduces the risk of aspiration. Personnel who are unskilled in airway management can easily learn how to use the LMA and the Combitube together [50].

Cricothyrotomy

In a truly emergent situation, when intubation is unsuccessful, a cricothyrotomy may be required. The technique is described in detail in Chapter 12. The quickest method, needle cricothyrotomy, is accomplished by introducing a large-bore

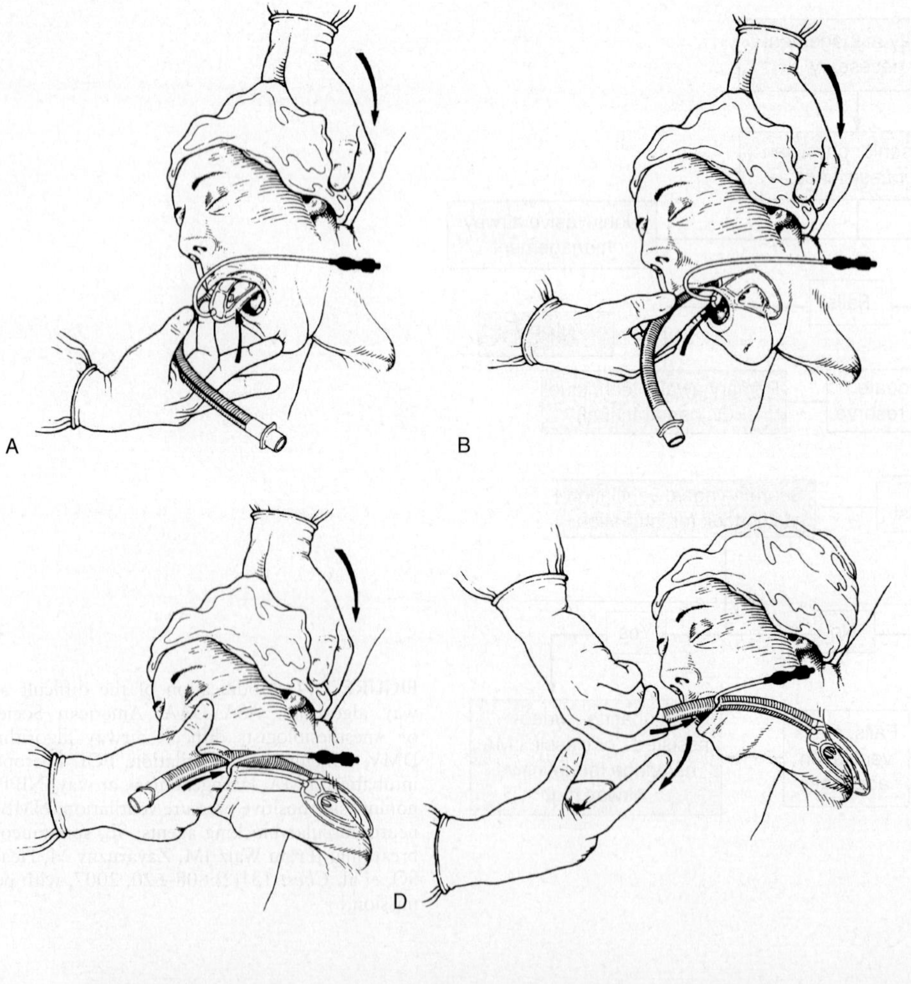

FIGURE 1.12. Technique for insertion of the laryngeal mask airway. [From Civetta JM, Taylor RW, Kirby RR: *Critical Care*. 3rd ed. Philadelphia, PA, Lippincott–Raven Publishers, 1997, with permission.]

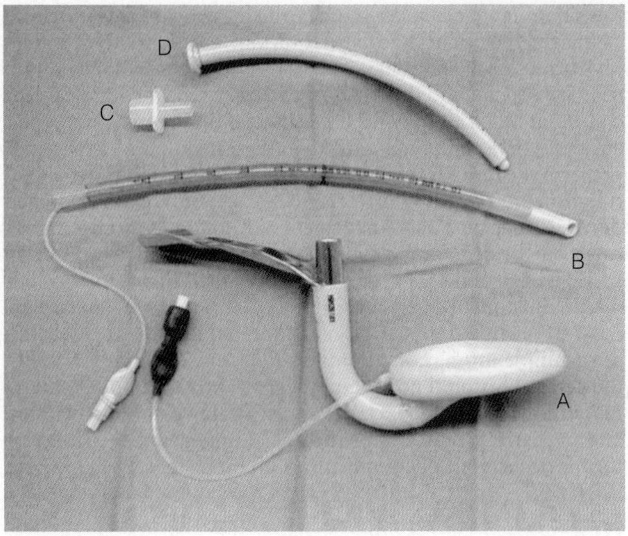

FIGURE 1.13. The laryngeal mask airway (LMA)-Fastrach (A) has a shorter tube than a conventional LMA. A special endotracheal tube (B) [without the adapter (C)] is advanced through the LMA-Fastrach into the trachea. The extender (D) is attached to the endotracheal tube, and the LMA-Fastrach is removed. After the extender is removed, the adapter is placed back on the tube.

(i.e., 14-gauge) catheter into the airway through the cricothyroid membrane while aspirating with a syringe attached to the needle of the catheter. When air is aspirated, the needle is in the airway and the catheter is passed over the needle into the trachea. The needle is attached to a high-frequency jet ventilation apparatus. Alternatively, a 3-mL syringe barrel can be connected to the catheter. Following this, a 7-mm inside diameter endotracheal tube adapter is fitted into the syringe and is connected to a high-pressure gas source or a high-frequency jet ventilator. An algorithm with suggestions for the management of the difficult airway is provided in Figure 1.11.

Management of the Airway in Patients with Suspected Cervical Spine Injury

Any patient with multiple trauma who requires intubation should be treated as if cervical spine injury were present. In the absence of severe maxillofacial trauma or cerebrospinal rhinorrhea, nasal intubation can be considered. However, in the profoundly hypoxemic or apneic patient, the orotracheal approach should be used. If oral intubation is required, an assistant should maintain the neck in the neutral position by ensuring axial stabilization of the head and neck as the patient is intubated [51]. A cervical collar also assists in immobilizing the cervical spine. In a patient with maxillofacial trauma and suspected cervical spine injury, retrograde intubation can be performed by puncturing the cricothyroid membrane with an 18-gauge catheter and threading a 125-cm Teflon-coated (0.025-cm diameter) guidewire through the catheter. The wire is advanced into the oral cavity, and the endotracheal tube is then advanced over the wire into the trachea. Alternatively, the wire can be threaded through the suction port of a 3.9-mm bronchoscope.

Airway Management in the Intubated Patient

Securing the Tube

Properly securing the endotracheal tube in the desired position is important for three reasons: (a) to prevent accidental extubation, (b) to prevent advancement into one of the main bronchi, and (c) to minimize damage to the upper airway, larynx, and trachea caused by patient motion. The endotracheal tube is usually secured in place with adhesive tape wrapped around the tube and applied to the patient's cheeks. Tincture of benzoin sprayed on the skin provides greater fixation. Alternatively, tape, intravenous (IV) tubing, or umbilical tape can be tied to the endotracheal tube and brought around the patient's neck to secure the tube. Care must be taken to prevent occlusion of neck veins. Other products (e.g., Velcro straps) to secure the tube are available. A bite block can be positioned in patients who are orally intubated to prevent them from biting down on the tube and occluding it. Once the tube has been secured and its proper position verified, it should be plainly marked on the portion protruding from the patient's mouth or nose so that advancement can be noted.

Cuff Management

Although low-pressure cuffs have markedly reduced the incidence of complications related to tracheal ischemia, monitoring cuff pressures remains important. The cuff should be inflated just beyond the point where an audible air leak occurs. Maintenance of intracuff pressures between 17 and 23 mm Hg should allow an adequate seal to permit mechanical ventilation under most circumstances while not compromising blood flow to the tracheal mucosa. The intracuff pressure should be checked periodically by attaching a pressure gauge and syringe to the cuff port via a three-way stopcock. The need to add air continually to the cuff to maintain its seal with the tracheal wall indicates that (a) the cuff or pilot tube has a hole in it, (b) the pilot tube valve is broken or cracked, or (c) the tube is positioned incorrectly, and the cuff is between the vocal cords. The tube position should be reevaluated to exclude the latter possibility. If the valve is broken, attaching a three-way stopcock to it will solve the problem. If the valve housing is cracked, cutting the pilot tube and inserting a blunt needle with a stopcock into the lumen of the pilot tube can maintain a competent system. A hole in the cuff necessitates a change of tube.

Tube Suctioning

A complete discussion of tube suctioning can be found in Chapter 62. Routine suctioning should not be performed in patients in whom secretions are not a problem. Suctioning can produce a variety of complications, including hypoxemia, elevations in intracranial pressure, and serious ventricular arrhythmias. Preoxygenation should reduce the likelihood of arrhythmias. Closed ventilation suction systems (Stericath) may reduce the risk of hypoxemia but have not been shown to reduce the rate of ventilator-associated pneumonia (VAP) compared to open suction systems [52].

Humidification

Intubation of the trachea bypasses the normal upper airway structures responsible for heating and humidifying inspired air. It is thus essential that inspired air be heated and humidified (see Chapter 62).

Tube Replacement

At times, endotracheal tubes may need to be replaced because of an air leak, obstruction, or other problems. Before attempting to change an endotracheal tube, one should assess how difficult it will be. After obtaining appropriate topical anesthesia or IV sedation and achieving muscle relaxation, direct laryngoscopy can be performed to ascertain whether there will be difficulties in visualizing the vocal cords. If the cords can be seen, the defective tube is removed under direct visualization and reintubation performed using the new tube. If the cords cannot be seen on direct laryngoscopy, the tube can be changed over an airway exchange catheter (e.g., Cook Critical Care, Bloomington, IN) which allows insufflation of oxygen via either standard oxygen tubing or a bag valve device [53].

COMPLICATIONS OF ENDOTRACHEAL INTUBATION

Table 1.5 is a partial listing of the complications associated with endotracheal intubation. Factors implicated in the etiology of complications include tube size, characteristics of the tube and cuff, trauma during intubation, duration and route of intubation, metabolic or nutritional status of the patient, tube motion, and laryngeal motor activity.

During endotracheal intubation, traumatic injury can occur to any anatomic structure from the lips to the trachea. Possible complications include aspiration; damage to teeth and dental work; corneal abrasions; perforation or laceration of the pharynx, larynx, or trachea; dislocation of an arytenoid cartilage; retropharyngeal perforation; epistaxis; hypoxemia; myocardial ischemia; laryngospasm with noncardiogenic pulmonary edema; and death [5,54]. Many of these complications can be avoided by paying careful attention to technique and ensuring that personnel with the greatest skill and experience perform the intubation. Complications during endotracheal intubation vary according to the location of the patient in need of emergency airway management. Although the complication rates on the regular hospital floor and in the ICU appear to be high at around 28% for both locations, they can be modified with standardized algorithms as outlined previously. The most frequent complications encountered in these two settings are multiple intubation attempts and esophageal intubation in the general hospital units, and severe hypoxemia and hemodynamic collapse in the ICU. Presence of acute respiratory failure and presence of shock appear to be an independent risk factor for the occurrence of complications in the latter setting [55,56].

TABLE 1.5

COMPLICATIONS OF ENDOTRACHEAL INTUBATION

Complications during intubation
Spinal cord injury
Excessive delay of cardiopulmonary resuscitation
Aspiration
Damage to teeth and dental work
Corneal abrasions
Perforation or laceration of
Pharynx
Larynx
Trachea
Dislocation of an arytenoid cartilage
Passage of endotracheal tube into cranial vault
Epistaxis
Cardiovascular problems
Ventricular premature contractions
Ventricular tachycardia
Bradyarrhythmias
Hypotension
Hypertension
Hypoxemia
Complications while tube is in place
Blockage or kinking of tube
Dislodgment of tube
Advancement of tube into a bronchus
Mechanical damage to any upper airway structure
Problems related to mechanical ventilation (see Chapter 58)
Complications following extubation
Immediate complications
Laryngospasm
Aspiration
Intermediate and long-term complications
Sore throat
Ulcerations of lips, mouth, pharynx, or vocal cords
Tongue numbness (hypoglossal nerve compression)
Laryngitis
Vocal cord paralysis (unilateral or bilateral)
Laryngeal edema
Laryngeal ulcerations
Laryngeal granuloma
Vocal cord synechiae
Tracheal stenosis

Complications During Intubation

A variety of cardiovascular complications can accompany intubation. Ventricular arrhythmias have been reported in 5% to 10% of intubations. Ventricular tachycardia and ventricular fibrillation are uncommon but have been reported. Patients with myocardial ischemia are susceptible to ventricular arrhythmias, and lidocaine prophylaxis (100 mg IV bolus) before intubation may be warranted in such individuals. Bradyarrhythmias can also be observed and are probably caused by stimulation of the laryngeal branches of the vagus nerve. They may not require therapy but usually respond to IV atropine (1 mg IV bolus). Hypotension or hypertension can occur during intubation. In the patient with myocardial ischemia, short-acting agents to control blood pressure (nitroprusside, nicardipine) and heart rate (esmolol) during intubation may be needed.

Complications While the Tube is in Place

Despite adherence to guidelines designed to minimize damage from endotracheal intubation, the tube can damage local structures. Microscopic alterations to the surface of the vocal cords can occur within 2 hours after intubation. Evidence of macroscopic damage can occur within 6 hours. As might be expected, clinically significant damage typically occurs when intubation is prolonged. The sudden appearance of blood in tracheal secretions suggests anterior erosion into overlying vascular structures, and the appearance of gastric contents suggests posterior erosion into the esophagus. Both situations require urgent bronchoscopy, and it is imperative that the mucosa underlying the cuff be examined. Other complications include tracheomalacia and stenosis and damage to the larynx. Failure to secure the endotracheal tube properly or patient agitation can contribute to mechanical damage.

Another complication is blockage or kinking of the tube, resulting in compromised ventilation. Placing a bite block in the patient's mouth can minimize occlusion of the tube caused by the patient biting down on it. Suctioning can usually solve blockage from secretions, although changing the tube may be necessary.

Unplanned extubation and endobronchial intubation are potentially life threatening. Judicious use of sedatives and analgesics and appropriately securing and marking the tube should minimize these problems. Daily chest radiographs with the head always in the same position can be used to assess the position of the tube. Other complications that occur while the tube is in position relate to mechanical ventilation (e.g., pneumothorax) and are discussed in detail in Chapter 58.

Complications After Extubation

Sore throat occurs after 40% to 100% of intubations. Using a smaller endotracheal tube may decrease the incidence of postextubation sore throat and hoarseness. Ulcerations of the lips, mouth, or pharynx can occur and are more common if the initial intubation was traumatic. Pressure from the endotracheal tube can traumatize the hypoglossal nerve, resulting in numbness of the tongue that can persist for 1 to 2 weeks. Irritation of the larynx appears to be due to local mucosal damage and occurs in as many as 45% of individuals after extubation. Unilateral or bilateral vocal cord paralysis is an uncommon but serious complication following extubation.

Some degree of laryngeal edema accompanies almost all endotracheal intubations. In adults, this is usually clinically insignificant. In children, however, even a small amount of edema can compromise the already small subglottic opening. In a newborn, 1 mm of laryngeal edema results in a 65% narrowing of the airway. Laryngeal ulcerations are commonly observed after extubation. They are more commonly located at the posterior portion of the vocal cords, where the endotracheal tube tends to rub. Ulcerations become increasingly common the longer the tube is left in place. The incidence of ulceration is decreased by the use of endotracheal tubes that conform to the anatomic shape of the larynx. Laryngeal granulomas and synechiae of the vocal cords are extremely rare, but these complications can seriously compromise airway patency. Surgical treatment is often required to treat these problems.

A feared late complication of endotracheal intubation is tracheal stenosis. This occurs much less frequently now that high-volume, low-pressure cuffs are routinely used. Symptoms can occur weeks to months after extubation. In mild cases, the patient may experience dyspnea or ineffective cough. If the airway is narrowed to less than 5 mm, the patient presents with stridor. Dilation may provide effective treatment, but in some instances surgical intervention is necessary.

EXTUBATION

The decision to extubate a patient is based on (a) a favorable clinical response to a carefully planned regimen of weaning from mechanical ventilation (see Chapter 60), (b) recovery of consciousness following anesthesia, or (c) sufficient resolution of the initial indications for intubation.

Technique of Extubation

The patient should be alert, lying with the head of the bed elevated to at least a 45-degree angle. The posterior pharynx must be thoroughly suctioned. The procedure is explained to the patient. The cuff is deflated, and positive pressure is applied to expel any foreign material that has collected above the cuff as the tube is withdrawn. Supplemental oxygen is then provided.

In situations in which postextubation difficulties are anticipated, equipment for emergency reintubation should be assembled at the bedside. Some clinicians have advocated the "leak test" as a means to predict the risk of stridor after extubation. The utility of this procedure is limited in routine practice, but for patients with certain risk factors (e.g., traumatic intubation, prolonged intubation, and previous accidental extubation), a leak volume of greater than 130 mL or 12% of the tidal volume has a sensitivity and specificity of 85% and 95%, respectively, for the development of postextubation stridor [57]. Probably the safest means to extubate the patient if there are concerns about airway edema or the potential need to reintubate a patient with a difficult airway is to use an airway exchange catheter. This device is inserted through the endotracheal tube, and then the tube is removed over the catheter. Supplemental oxygen can be provided via the catheter to the patient, and the catheter can be used as a stent for reintubation if necessary.

One of the most serious complications of extubation is laryngospasm, and it is more likely to occur if the patient is not fully conscious. The application of positive pressure can sometimes relieve laryngospasm. If this maneuver is not successful, a small dose of succinylcholine (by the IV or intramuscular route) can be administered. Succinylcholine can cause severe hyperkalemia in a variety of clinical settings; therefore, only clinicians who are experienced with its use should administer it. Ventilation with a mask and bag unit is needed until the patient has recovered from the succinylcholine.

Tracheostomy

The optimal time of conversion from an endotracheal tube to a tracheostomy remains controversial. The reader is referred to Chapter 12 for details on tracheostomy.

References

1. Caples SM, Gay PC: Noninvasive positive pressure ventilation in the intensive care unit: a concise review. *Crit Care Med* 33:2651–2658, 2005.
2. Snell RS, Katz J: *Clinical Anatomy for Anesthesiologists*. Norwalk, CT, Appleton and Lange, 1988.
3. Fowler RA, Pearl RG: The airway: emergent management for nonanesthesiologists. *West J Med* 176:45–50, 2002.
4. Mort TC: The incidence and risk factors for cardiac arrest during emergency tracheal intubation: a justification for incorporating the ASA Guidelines in the remote location. *J Clin Anesth* 16:508–516, 2004.
5. Mort TC: Emergency tracheal intubation: complications associated with repeated laryngoscopic attempts. *Anesth Analg* 99:607–613, 2004, table of contents.
6. 2005 American Heart Association Guidelines for cardiopulmonary resuscitation and emergency cardiovascular care. *Circulation* 112:IV-1–IV-5, 2005.
7. Mallampati SR, Gatt SP, Gugino LD, et al: A clinical sign to predict difficult tracheal intubation: a prospective study. *Can Anaesth Soc J* 32:429–434, 1985.
8. Lewis M, Keramati S, Benumof JL, et al: What is the best way to determine oropharyngeal classification and mandibular space length to predict difficult laryngoscopy? *Anesthesiology* 81:69–75, 1994.
9. Gal TJ: Airway management, in Miller RD (ed): *Anesthesia*. 6th ed. Philadelphia, PA, Churchill Livingstone, 2005, pp 1617–1652.
10. Tse JC, Rimm EB, Hussain A: Predicting difficult endotracheal intubation in surgical patients scheduled for general anesthesia: a prospective blind study. *Anesth Analg* 81:254–258, 1995.
11. Levitan RM, Everett WW, Ochroch EA: Limitations of difficult airway prediction in patients intubated in the emergency department. *Ann Emerg Med* 44:307–313, 2004.
12. Murphy MF, Walls RM: *Manual of emergency airway management*. Chicago, IL, Lippincott, Williams and Wilkins, 2000.
13. Reed MJ, Dunn MJ, McKeown DW: Can an airway assessment score predict difficulty at intubation in the emergency department? *Emerg Med J* 22:99–102, 2005.
14. Kheterpal S, Martin L, Shanks AM, et al: Prediction and outcomes of impossible mask ventilation: a review of 50,000 anesthetics. *Anesthesiology* 110:891–897, 2009.
15. Mulcaster JT, Mills J, Hung OR, et al: Laryngoscopic intubation: learning and performance. *Anesthesiology* 98:23–27, 2003.
16. Schmidt UH, Kumwilaisak K, Bittner E, et al: Effects of supervision by attending anesthesiologists on complications of emergency tracheal intubation. *Anesthesiology* 109:973–977, 2008.
17. Jaber S, Jung B, Corne P, et al: An intervention to decrease complications related to endotracheal intubation in the intensive care unit: a prospective, multiple-center study. *Intensive Care Med* 36:248–255, 2010.

18. Hastings RH, Hon ED, Nghiem C, et al: Force, torque, and stress relaxation with direct laryngoscopy. *Anesth Analg* 82:456–461, 1996.
19. Lim TJ, Lim Y, Liu EH: Evaluation of ease of intubation with the GlideScope or Macintosh laryngoscope by anaesthetists in simulated easy and difficult laryngoscopy. *Anaesthesia* 60:180–183, 2005.
20. Nouruzi-Sedeh P, Schumann M, Groeben H: Laryngoscopy via Macintosh blade versus GlideScope: success rate and time for endotracheal intubation in untrained medical personnel. *Anesthesiology* 110:32–37, 2009.
21. Hagberg CA: Current concepts in the management of the difficult airway. in *Anesthesiology news*. New York, McMahon Publishing, 2010.
22. Larijani GE, Cypel D, Gratz I, et al: The efficacy and safety of EMLA cream for awake fiberoptic endotracheal intubation. *Anesth Analg* 91:1024–1026, 2000.
23. Venus B, Polassani V, Pham CG: Effects of aerosolized lidocaine on circulatory responses to laryngoscopy and tracheal intubation. *Crit Care Med* 12:391–394, 1984.
24. Malerba G, Romano-Girard F, Cravoisy A, et al: Risk factors of relative adrenocortical deficiency in intensive care patients needing mechanical ventilation. *Intensive Care Med* 31:388–392, 2005.
25. Jabre P, Combes X, Lapostolle F, et al: Etomidate versus ketamine for rapid sequence intubation in acutely ill patients: a multicentre randomised controlled trial. *Lancet* 374:293–300, 2009.
26. Sprung CL, Annane D, Keh D, et al: Hydrocortisone therapy for patients with septic shock. *N Engl J Med* 358:111–124, 2008.
27. Reynolds SF, Heffner J: Airway management of the critically ill patient: rapid-sequence intubation. *Chest* 127:1397–1412, 2005.
28. Mace SE: Challenges and advances in intubation: rapid sequence intubation. *Emerg Med Clin North Am* 26:1043–1068, x, 2008.
29. Stephens CT, Kahntroff S, Dutton RP: The success of emergency endotracheal intubation in trauma patients: a 10-year experience at a major adult trauma referral center. *Anesth Analg* 109:866–872, 2009.
30. Mort TC, Waberski BH, Clive J: Extending the preoxygenation period from 4 to 8 mins in critically ill patients undergoing emergency intubation. *Crit Care Med* 37:68–71, 2009.
31. Mort TC: Preoxygenation in critically ill patients requiring emergency tracheal intubation. *Crit Care Med* 33:2672–2675, 2005.
32. Baillard C, Fosse JP, Sebbane M, et al: Noninvasive ventilation improves preoxygenation before intubation of hypoxic patients. *Am J Respir Crit Care Med* 174:171–177, 2006.
33. Dixon BJ, Dixon JB, Carden JR, et al: Preoxygenation is more effective in the 25 degrees head-up position than in the supine position in severely obese patients: a randomized controlled study. *Anesthesiology* 102:1110–1115, 2005; discussion 5A.
34. Hastings RH, Marks JD: Airway management for trauma patients with potential cervical spine injuries. *Anesth Analg* 73:471–482, 1991.
35. Adnet F, Borron SW, Dumas JL, et al: Study of the "sniffing position" by magnetic resonance imaging. *Anesthesiology* 94:83–86, 2001.
36. Adnet F, Baillard C, Borron SW, et al: Randomized study comparing the "sniffing position" with simple head extension for laryngoscopic view in elective surgery patients. *Anesthesiology* 95:836–841, 2001.
37. Sellick BA: Cricoid pressure to control regurgitation of stomach contents during induction of anesthesia. *Lancet* 2:404, 1961.
38. Smith KJ, Dobranowski J, Yip G, et al: Cricoid pressure displaces the esophagus: an observational study using magnetic resonance imaging. *Anesthesiology* 99:60–64, 2003.
39. Rice MJ, Mancuso AA, Gibbs C, et al: Cricoid pressure results in compression of the postcricoid hypopharynx: the esophageal position is irrelevant. *Anesth Analg* 109:1546–1552, 2009.
40. Salem MR, Joseph NJ, Heyman HJ, et al: Cricoid compression is effective in obliterating the esophageal lumen in the presence of a nasogastric tube. *Anesthesiology* 63:443–446, 1985.
41. Lawes EG, Campbell I, Mercer D: Inflation pressure, gastric insufflation and rapid sequence induction. *Br J Anaesth* 59:315–318, 1987.
42. Cormack RS, Lehane J: Difficult tracheal intubation in obstetrics. *Anaesthesia* 39:1105–1111, 1984.
43. Ulrich B, Listyo R, Gerig HJ, et al: The difficult intubation. The value of BURP and 3 predictive tests of difficult intubation. *Anaesthesist* 47:45–50, 1998.
44. Agro F, Hung OR, Cataldo R, et al: Lightwand intubation using the Trachlight: a brief review of current knowledge. *Can J Anaesth* 48:592–599, 2001.
45. Owen RL, Cheney FW: Endobronchial intubation: a preventable complication. *Anesthesiology* 67:255–257, 1987.
46. Cherng CH, Wong CS, Hsu CH, et al: Airway length in adults: estimation of the optimal endotracheal tube length for orotracheal intubation. *J Clin Anesth* 14:271–274, 2002.
47. Kasper CL, Deem S: The self-inflating bulb to detect esophageal intubation during emergency airway management. *Anesthesiology* 88:898–902, 1998.
48. Langeron O, Masso E, Huraux C, et al: Prediction of difficult mask ventilation. *Anesthesiology* 92:1229–1236, 2000.
49. Benumof JL: Laryngeal mask airway and the ASA difficult airway algorithm. *Anesthesiology* 84:686–699, 1996.
50. Yardy N, Hancox D, Strang T: A comparison of two airway aids for emergency use by unskilled personnel. The Combitube and laryngeal mask. *Anaesthesia* 54:181–183, 1999.
51. Criswell JC, Parr MJ, Nolan JP: Emergency airway management in patients with cervical spine injuries. *Anaesthesia* 49:900–903, 1994.
52. Subirana M, Sola I, Benito S: Closed tracheal suction systems versus open tracheal suction systems for mechanically ventilated adult patients. *Cochrane Database Syst Rev* (4):CD004581, 2007.
53. Loudermilk EP, Hartmannsgruber M, Stoltzfus DP, et al: A prospective study of the safety of tracheal extubation using a pediatric airway exchange catheter for patients with a known difficult airway. *Chest* 111:1660–1665, 1997.
54. Schwartz DE, Matthay MA, Cohen NH: Death and other complications of emergency airway management in critically ill adults. A prospective investigation of 297 tracheal intubations. *Anesthesiology* 82:367–376, 1995.
55. Benedetto WJ, Hess DR, Gettings E, et al: Urgent tracheal intubation in general hospital units: an observational study. *J Clin Anesth* 19:20–24, 2007.
56. Jaber S, Amraoui J, Lefrant JY, et al: Clinical practice and risk factors for immediate complications of endotracheal intubation in the intensive care unit: a prospective, multiple-center study. *Crit Care Med* 34:2355–2361, 2006.
57. Jaber S, Chanques G, Matecki S, et al: Post-extubation stridor in intensive care unit patients. Risk factors evaluation and importance of the cuff-leak test. *Intensive Care Med* 29:69–74, 2003.

CHAPTER 2 ■ CENTRAL VENOUS CATHETERS

JASON LEE-LLACER AND MICHAEL G. SENEFF

The art and science of central venous catheter (CVC) insertion, maintenance, and management continues to evolve. Increased emphasis on patient safety and prevention of nosocomial complications has focused attention on the impact of CVCs on patient health. Catheter-related infection (CRI), often with a resistant organism such as methicillin-resistant *Staphylococcal aureus* or vancomycin-resistant *enterococci* (VRE) remains an important cause of increased patient morbidity and mortality, and it is simply inexcusable for institutions not to fully adapt proven protocols and procedures that have been shown to significantly reduce CRI and other catheter complications [1]. Patient safety is also the main impetus for increased availability of simulation laboratories [2,3] for operator training in the use of portable ultrasound [4,5] to facilitate catheter insertion. Insertion of CVCs is a procedure at the crossroads of the controversy of the need for training versus patient safety.

Training of physicians in the United States has been guided for years by the mantra "see one, do one, teach one," but this approach can no longer be defended as the best practice. Different institutions have developed different solutions, ranging from specially designated "catheter teams" responsible for all hospital-wide catheter insertions, to well equipped simulation laboratories that provide certification of competence and which have been shown to reduce subsequent clinical complications [2].

Because of the availability and relatively low cost of portable ultrasound units, many nonradiologists have been performing bedside image-guided central venous cannulation. Ultrasound guidance allows visualization of the vessel showing its precise location and patency in real time. It is especially useful for patients with suboptimal body habitus, volume depletion, shock, anatomic deformity, previous cannulation, underlying coagulopathy, and intravenous drug use. The use of ultrasound guidance has significantly decreased the failure rate, complication rate, and the number of attempts in obtaining central venous access and, as a result, has become routine in many centers [4,6]. Experts all over the world argue that ultrasound guidance should be viewed as standard of care for all CVC insertions, a recommendation met with resistance by many clinicians [6,7].

In 2001, the Agency for Healthcare Research and Quality Report listed bedside ultrasonography during central venous access as one of the "Top 11 Highly Proven" patient safety practices that are not routinely used in patient care, and it recommended all CVC insertions be guided by real-time, dynamic ultrasound [8]. The Third Sonography Outcomes Assessment Program (SOAP-3) trial, a concealed, randomized, controlled multicenter study, had an odds ratio 53.5 times higher for success with ultrasound guidance compared with the landmark technique. It also demonstrated a significantly lower average number of attempts and average time of catheter placement [9].

Given the existing data and recommendations, it appears no longer defensible to lack an active ultrasound training and utilization program in the intensive care unit (ICU). Ultrasound can be used in obtaining central venous access from multiple sites, especially the internal jugular and femoral veins (FV) [6,10]. Ultrasound has been less useful in cannulating the subclavian vein [11]. The subclavian vein is more difficult to access using ultrasound due to its deeper and posterior location to the clavicle which prevents the transmission of ultrasound waves. The subclavian vein may be accessed at the midpoint of the clavicle using a long-axis view or by a supraclavicular approach. Similarly, the infraclavicular axillary vein, which lies a few centimeters lateral to the subclavian vein, can be accessed with the short-axis ultrasound view [12].

Because of the success of ultrasound, some experts have argued for the complete elimination of all nonultrasound-guided CVC insertions. Although we recognize that even very experienced operators will benefit from ultrasound (if nothing else, by detection of anatomic variations and thrombosed vessels), it is not yet feasible to insist on 100% ultrasound availability. We also feel that there are still circumstances where standard subclavian catheterization is warranted and that this access site should not be abandoned. Therefore, it is important that one learns to obtain CVC via landmark techniques.

In this chapter, we review the techniques and complications of the various routes available for central venous catheterization, and present a strategy for catheter management that incorporates all of the recent advances.

INDICATIONS AND SITE SELECTION

Like any medical procedure, CVC has specific indications and should be reserved for the patient who has potential to benefit from it. After determining that CVC is necessary, physicians often proceed with catheterization at the site they are most experienced with, which might not be the most appropriate route in that particular patient. Table 2.1 lists general priorities in site selection for different indications of CVC; the final choice of site in a particular patient should vary based on individual institutional and operator experiences. In general, we recommend that all internal jugular and femoral vein cannulations

TABLE 2.1

INDICATIONS FOR CENTRAL VENOUS CATHETERIZATION (CVC)

Indication	Site selection: First	Second	Third
1. Pulmonary artery catheterization	RIJV	LSCV	LIJV
With coagulopathy	IJV	FV	
With pulmonary compromise or high-level positive end-expiratory pressure (PEEP)	RIJV	LIJV	EJV
2. Total parenteral nutrition (TPN)	SCV	IJV (tunneled)	
Long term (surgically implanted)	SCV	PICC	
3. Acute hemodialysis/plasmapheresis	IJV	FV	
4. Cardiopulmonary arrest	FV	SCV	IJV
5. Emergency transvenous pacemaker	RIJV	SCV	
6. Hypovolemia, inability to perform peripheral IV	IJV	SCV	FV
7. Preoperative preparation	IJV	SCV	AV/PICC
8. General purpose venous access, vasoactive agents, caustic medications, radiologic procedures	IJV	SCV	FV
With coagulopathy	IJV	EJV	FV
9. Emergency airway management	FV	SCV	IJV
10. Inability to lie supine	FV	EJV	AV/PICC
11. Central venous oxygen saturation monitoring	IJV	SCV	
12. Fluid management of ARDS (CVP monitoring)	IJV	EJV	SCV

AV, antecubital vein; EJV, external jugular vein; FV, femoral vein; IJV, internal jugular vein; L, left; PICC, peripherally inserted central venous catheter; R, right; SCV, subclavian vein. IJV and FV assume ultrasound guidance. see text for details.

be performed under ultrasound guidance. As noted earlier, we feel the traditional subclavian route offers many advantages for central access and should not be abandoned. However, only experienced operators should use the traditional infraclavicular approach; others should use ultrasound guidance with a modified approach that is described later.

Volume resuscitation alone is not an indication for CVC. A 2.5-inch, 16-gauge catheter used to cannulate a peripheral vein can infuse twice the amount of fluid as an 8-inch, 16-gauge CVC [13]. However, peripheral vein cannulation can be impossible in the hypovolemic, shocked individual. Previously, we recommended the subclavian vein (SCV) as the most reliable central site because it remains patent due to its fibrous attachments to the clavicle. But recently, use of real-time ultrasound-guided CVC placement by direct visualization of the internal jugular vein (IJV) has increased success rate and decreased complications in the shocked or hypovolemic patient [5,6].

Long-term total parenteral nutrition is best administered through SCV catheters, which should be inserted by interventional radiology or surgically implanted if appropriate. The IJV is the preferred site for acute hemodialysis, and the SCV should be avoided because of the relatively high incidence of subclavian stenosis following temporary dialysis, which then limits options for an AV fistula should long-term dialysis become necessary [14,15]. The FV is also suitable for acute short-term hemodialysis or plasmapheresis in nonambulatory patients [16].

Emergency trans-venous pacemakers and flow-directed pulmonary artery catheters are best inserted through the right IJV because of the direct path to the right ventricle. This route is associated with the fewest catheter tip malpositions. The SCV is an alternative second choice for pulmonary artery catheterization even in many patients with coagulopathy [17]. The left SCV is preferred to the right SV due to a less torturous route to the heart. The reader is referred to Chapter 4 for additional information on the insertion and care of pulmonary artery catheters.

Preoperative CVC is desirable in a wide variety of clinical situations. One specific indication for preoperative right ventricular catheterization is the patient undergoing a posterior craniotomy or cervical laminectomy in the sitting position. These patients are at risk for air embolism, and the catheter can be used to aspirate air from the right ventricle [18]. Neurosurgery is the only common indication for (but used only rarely) antecubital approach, as IJV catheters are in the operative field and theoretically can obstruct blood return from the cranial vault and increase intracranial pressure. Subclavian catheters are an excellent alternative for preoperative neurosurgical patients if pneumothorax is ruled out prior to induction of general anesthesia.

Venous access during cardiopulmonary resuscitation warrants special comment. Peripheral vein cannulation in circulatory arrest may prove impossible, and circulation times of drugs administered peripherally are prolonged when compared with central injection [19]. Drugs injected through femoral catheters also have a prolonged circulation time unless the catheter tip is advanced beyond the diaphragm, although the clinical significance of this is debated. Effective drug administration is an extremely important element of successful cardiopulmonary resuscitation, and all physicians should understand the appropriate techniques for establishing venous access. It is logical to establish venous access as quickly as possible, either peripherally or centrally if qualified personnel are present. Prolonged attempts at arm vein cannulation are not warranted, and under these circumstances, the FV is a good alternative. Despite the potential of longer drug circulation times, the FV is recommended for access in a code situation as cardiopulmonary resuscitation (CPR) is interrupted the least with its placement. If circulation is not restored after administration of appropriate drugs and defibrillation, central access should be obtained by the most experienced operator available with a minimum interruption of CPR. Emergency ultrasound-guided femoral CVC placement has been shown to be slightly faster with fewer complications than the landmark technique [20].

The placement of CVC is now common in patients with severe sepsis, septic shock, or acute respiratory distress syndrome (ARDS), to monitor central venous pressure (CVP) and central venous oxygen saturation ($ScvO_2$). Rivers showed a 16% absolute reduction of in-hospital mortality with early goal-directed therapy for patients with severe sepsis, which included keeping the $ScvO_2$ greater than 70% [21]. Early goal-directed therapy was subsequently shown to be achievable in "real-world" settings [22]. For these patients, the relationship between superior vena caval and inferior vena caval oxygen saturations has not been definitively elucidated [23]. Likewise, the ARDS network reported that CVP monitoring using a CVC is as effective as a pulmonary artery catheter in managing patients with acute lung injury and ARDS [24]. Because many of these patients are on high levels of positive end expiratory pressure (PEEP) and at high risk for complications from pneumothorax, IJV catheterization under ultrasound guidance represents the safest approach.

GENERAL CONSIDERATIONS AND COMPLICATIONS

General considerations for CVC independent of the site of insertion are the need for signed informed consent, insuring patient comfort and safety, ultrasound preparation, catheter tip location, vascular erosions, catheter-associated thrombosis, air and catheter embolism, and the presence of coagulopathy. Catheter-associated infection is reviewed separately.

Informed Consent

It seems intuitively obvious that a signed informed consent is mandatory before CVC insertion, but in clinical practice, it is not that straightforward. CVC insertions in the ICU are extremely common, occur at all hours of the day, and may be crucial for early and appropriate resuscitation and commencement of care. Many critically ill patients, especially in urban settings, have no available family members or legal net of kin. Obtaining informed consent for these patients may inappropriately delay completion of the procedure and impact quality of care. Because of these considerations, there is no uniform clinical or legal opinion regarding the necessity of individual informed consent prior to all CVC insertions or other ICU procedures [25]. Some institutions have dealt with this matter by developing a single general "consent form for critical care" that is signed one time for each individual ICU admission and covers all commonly performed bedside procedures. A recent review reported that 14% of all surveyed ICUs used such a consent form, and overall consent practice varied widely. In general, providers in medical ICUs sought consent for CVC insertion more often than providers in surgical ICUs [25]. Given the lack of agreement on this topic, it seems prudent to make a few recommendations: (1) Written informed consent should be obtained prior to all truly elective CVC insertion or other procedures (2). Whenever possible, competent patients or legal next of kin of incompetent/incapacitated patients should be thoroughly informed of the indications, risks, and benefits of emergency CVC insertion prior to the performance of the procedure. If informed consent is not possible prior to CVC insertion, then consent should be obtained as soon as possible after completion of the procedure. A signed consent form is always preferable, but sometimes not feasible. Oral consent should be documented in the procedure note by the person obtaining assent. (3) Emergent CVC placement should not be delayed inappropriately by efforts to obtain consent—oral or written. Patients and family should be told as soon as possible after insertion why the CVC was required. (4) A general consent form that is signed one time as close as possible to ICU admission is a reasonable way to try and inform patients of the benefits/risks of procedures without incurring unnecessary delays or consumption of clinical time. This form can also serve as a useful reference for patients and families of all the various common procedures that are performed in the ICU. (5) Finally, it is good practice to document the practice that is used in the ICU "Policies and Procedures" book and the rationale for it.

Patient Comfort and Safety

Many patients requiring CVC have an unstable airway or are hemodynamically unstable. These considerations should impact preparation and choice of site. For example, many patients are claustrophobic and will not tolerate their face being covered; others who are dyspneic will not tolerate lying flat. In our experience, significant physiologic decompensation or even "code blues" may occur during CVC placement because the operator is focused on establishing access and/or interprets the silent patient as one who is having no problems. Every patient should be specifically assessed prior to CVC regarding their positioning, airway, and hemodynamic stability. On more than one occasion, we have placed a femoral catheter because a patient could not lie flat or needed emergency venous access for endotracheal intubation. Once the patient is stabilized, the appropriate site/catheter can then be inserted under less unstable/rigorous conditions.

Ultrasound Preparation

Ultrasound enables immediate identification of anatomic variation, confirmation of vessel patency, and direct visualization of the needle entering the vessel. The difference between vein and artery can be determined by compressibility, shape, Doppler flow, and increasing size with the Valsalva or other maneuvers. Veins are usually ovoid in shape, completely compressible, and have thin walls; in contrast, arteries are circular, difficult to compress, and have thick walls.

When performing ultrasound, the same general technique is followed regardless of the site of puncture [6]. A quick, nonsterile survey should be made with the vascular probe to quickly identify the presence of a suitable vein for catheterization. After sterile preparation of the patient and site, the vascular probe should be used with a sterile probe cover kit. This kit contains a sterile sleeve, sterile jelly, and rubber bands. To apply the sterile sleeve, have an assistant place nonsterile jelly inside the sleeve and then place probe in the sleeve. Extend the sleeve over the cord and fasten the sleeve with rubber bands. One band should be fastened toward the head of the probe to ensure the jelly remains in place for optimal imaging. Sterile jelly is then applied to the tip of probe on the outside of sleeve.

The target vessels may be visualized using a transverse or longitudinal view. The transverse approach is technically easier than the longitudinal approach and is the best approach for beginners. The transverse view allows identification of the target vein in relation to the artery, which helps decrease risk of unintentional puncture of the artery. Once identified, the vein should be centered underneath the probe. An 18-gauge needle should slowly be advanced with the skin puncture site proximal to the probe, so that vessel puncture is directly visualized. With this approach, the needle traverses diagonally across the ultrasound plane and appears as single bright echogenic foci on ultrasound image. Needle position may be better ascertained by slightly moving the needle back and forth displacing the surrounding soft tissue and possible tenting of vessel wall. It is important to note the depth of the vessel on the ultrasound image to be mindful of how far to penetrate safely with the needle. The return of blood flow confirms intravascular placement of the needle tip, and CVC placement may proceed in the usual fashion. It is good practice to confirm guidewire placement within the vein as well. The longitudinal approach gives more information but is more difficult. When using the longitudinal approach, the plane of the ultrasound and of the needle must be perfectly aligned and is best for one operator to be holding both probe and needle. First, the vein artery must be visualized using the transverse view. The probe should then be turned 90 degrees to image just the vein in the long-axis view. Enter the skin just adjacent to the probe at a 45-degree angle. The needle and needle tip can be directly viewed as it is advanced through the vessel. Once in place, advance the guidewire under direct visualization.

Mobile Catheter Cart

Availability of a mobile catheter cart that contains all necessary supplies and that can be wheeled to the patient's bedside is good practice and likely reduces overall catheter infection rate by decreasing breaks in sterile technique [26]. In our experience, the mobile cart is also an excellent way to standardize all catheter insertions, facilitate communication of procedural tasks (such as use of a time-out), and allow for staff to timely complete mandatory forms.

Catheter Tip Location

Catheter tip location is a very important consideration in CVC placement. The ideal location for the catheter tip is the distal innominate or proximal superior vena cava (SVC), 3 to 5 cm proximal to the caval–atrial junction. Positioning of the catheter tip within the right atrium or right ventricle should be avoided. Cardiac tamponade secondary to catheter tip perforation of the cardiac wall is uncommon, but two thirds of patients suffering this complication die [27]. Perforation likely results from vessel wall damage from infused solutions combined with catheter tip migration that occurs from the motion of the beating heart as well as patient arm and neck movements. Migration of catheter tips can be impressive: 5 to 10 cm with antecubital catheters and 1 to 5 cm with IJV or SCV catheters [28,29]. Other complications from intracardiac catheter tip position include provocation of arrhythmias from mechanical irritation and infusion of caustic medications or unwarmed blood [30].

Correct placement of the catheter tip is relatively simple, beginning with an appreciation of anatomy. The caval–atrial junction is approximately 16 to 18 cm from right-sided skin punctures and 19 to 21 cm from left-sided insertions and is relatively independent of patient gender and body habitus [31,32]. Insertion of a standard 20-cm triple-lumen catheter to its full length frequently places the tip within the heart, especially following right-sided insertions. A chest radiograph should be obtained following every initial CVC insertion to ascertain catheter tip location and to detect complications. The right tracheobronchial angle is the most reliable landmark on plain film chest X-ray for the upper margin of the SVC, and is always at least 2.9 cm above the caval–atrial junction. The catheter tip should lie about 1 cm below this landmark, and above the right upper cardiac silhouette to ensure placement outside of the pericardium [33].

Vascular Erosions

Large-vessel perforations secondary to CVCs are uncommon and often not immediately recognized. Vessel perforation typically occurs 1 to 7 days after catheter insertion. Patients usually present with sudden onset of dyspnea and often with new pleural effusions on chest radiograph [34]. Catheter stiffness, position of the tip within the vessel, and the site of insertion are important factors causing vessel perforation. The relative importance of these variables is unknown. Repeated irritation of the vessel wall by a stiff catheter tip or infusion of hyperosmolar solutions may be the initiating event. Vascular erosions are more common with left IJV and EJV catheters, because for anatomical reasons the catheter tip is more likely to be positioned laterally under tension against the SVC wall [35]. Positioning of the catheter tip within the vein parallel to the vessel wall must be confirmed on chest radiograph. Free aspiration of blood from one of the catheter ports is not always sufficient to rule out a vascular perforation.

Air and Catheter Embolism

Significant air and catheter embolism are rare and preventable complications of CVC. Catheter embolism can occur at the time of insertion when a catheter-through- or over-needle technique is used and the operator withdraws the catheter without simultaneously retracting the needle. It more commonly occurs with antecubital or femoral catheters after insertion, because they are prone to breakage when the agitated patient vigorously bends an arm or leg. Prevention, recognition, and management of catheter embolism are covered in detail elsewhere [36].

Air embolism is of greater clinical importance, often goes undiagnosed, and may prove fatal. This complication is totally preventable with compulsive attention to proper catheter insertion and maintenance. Factors resulting in air embolism during insertion are well known, and methods to increase venous pressure, such as use of the Trendelenburg position, should not be forgotten. Catheter disconnection and passage of air through a patent tract after catheter removal are more common causes of catheter-associated air embolism. An air embolus should be suspected in any patient with an indwelling or recently discontinued CVC who develops sudden unexplained hypoxemia or cardiovascular collapse, often after being moved or transferred out of bed. A characteristic mill wheel sound may be auscultated over the precordium. Treatment involves placing the patient in the left lateral decubitus position and using the catheter to aspirate air from the right ventricle. Hyperbaric oxygen therapy to reduce bubble size has a controversial role in treatment [37]. The best treatment is prevention which can be effectively achieved through comprehensive nursing and physician-in-training educational modules and proper supervision of inexperienced operators [38].

Coagulopathy

Central venous access in the patient with a bleeding diathesis can be problematic. The SCV and IJV routes have increased risks in the presence of coagulopathy, but the true risk is frequently overestimated and it is not known at what degree of abnormality it becomes unacceptable. A coagulopathy is generally defined as an international normalized ratio (INR) greater than 1.5 or platelet count less than 50,000. Although it is clear that safe venipuncture is possible (even with the subclavian approach) with greater degrees of coagulopathy [39], the literature is also fraught with case reports of serious hemorrhagic complications. In patients with severe coagulopathy, IJV cannulation under ultrasound guidance has proven to be very safe, while the FV offers a viable alternative for general-purpose venous access. In nonemergent patients, peripherally inserted central venous catheters (PICC) can be used.

Thrombosis

Catheter-related thrombosis is very common but usually of little clinical significance. The spectrum of thrombotic complications includes a fibrin sleeve surrounding the catheter from its point of entry into the vein distal to the tip, mural thrombus, a clot that forms on the wall of the vein secondary to mechanical or chemical irritation, or occlusive thrombus, which blocks flow and may result in collateral formation. All of these lesions are usually clinically silent; therefore, studies that do not use venography or color flow Doppler imaging to confirm the diagnosis underestimate its incidence. Using venography, fibrin sleeve formation can be documented in a majority of catheters, mural thrombi in 10% to 30%, and occlusive thrombi in 0% to 10% [40–45]. In contrast, clinical symptoms of thrombosis occur in only 0% to 3% of patients. The incidence of thrombosis probably increases with duration of catheterization but does not appear reliably related to the site of insertion. However, the clinical importance of femoral vein catheter-associated thrombosis compared to upper extremity thrombosis caused by IJ and SCV catheters is unknown [46]. The presence of catheter-associated thrombosis is also associated with a higher incidence of infection [47].

ROUTES OF CENTRAL VENOUS CANNULATION

Antecubital Approach

The antecubital veins are used in the ICU for CVC with PICC and midline catheters. Use of PICCs in critically ill adults is becoming increasingly important. Specialized nursing teams are now able to insert PICCs at beside with use of real-time ultrasonography and sterile technique thereby increasing safety and reducing the potential for infection. There are now triple lumen catheters that may be inserted with this approach. PICCs may be useful in ICU patients undergoing neurosurgery, with coagulopathy, or in the rehabilitative phase of critical illness for which general purpose central venous access is required for parenteral nutrition or long-term medication access (Table 2.1) [48,49]. Although many hospitals have a designated "PICC" insertion team, they may have significant work hour limitations that delay insertion of catheters and result in significant delays in delivery of care or throughput. For that reason, we believe intensivists should be familiar with the antecubital route, and as a result, the technique of percutaneous insertion of catheters using the basilic vein is described later.

Anatomy

The basilic vein is preferred for CVC because it is almost always of substantial size and the anatomy is predictable. The basilic vein provides an unimpeded path to the central venous circulation via the axillary vein [50,51]. The basilic vein is formed at the ulnar aspect of the dorsal venous network of the hand. It may be found in the medial part of the antecubital fossa, where it is usually joined by the median basilic vein. It then ascends in the groove between the biceps brachii and pronator teres on the medial aspect of the arm to perforate the deep fascia distal to the midportion of the arm, where it joins the brachial vein to become the axillary vein.

Technique of Cannulation

Several kits are available for antecubital CVC. The PICC and midline catheters are made of silicone or polyurethane and, depending on catheter stiffness and size, are usually placed through an introducer. The method described below is for a PICC inserted through a tear-away introducer.

The success rates from either arm are comparable, though the catheter must traverse a greater distance from the left. With the patient's arm at his or her side, the antecubital fossa is prepared with chlorhexidine and draped using maximum barrier precautions (mask, cap and sterile gown, gloves and large drape covering the patient). A tourniquet is placed proximally by an assistant and a portable ultrasound device used to identify the basilic or its main branches. A vein can be distinguished from an artery by visualizing compressibility, color flow, and Doppler flow (Fig. 2.1). After a time-out and administration of local anesthesia subcutaneously, venipuncture is performed with the thin wall entry needle a few centimeters proximal to the antecubital crease to avoid catheter breakage and embolism. When free backflow of venous blood is confirmed, the tourniquet is released and the guidewire carefully threaded into the vein for a distance of 15 to 20 cm. Leaving the guidewire in place, the thin-wall needle is withdrawn and the puncture site enlarged with a scalpel blade. The sheath-introducer assembly is threaded over the guidewire with a twisting motion, and the guidewire removed. Next, leaving the sheath in place, the dilator is removed, and the introducer is now ready for PICC insertion. The length of insertion is estimated by measuring the distance along the predicted vein path from the venipuncture site to the manubriosternal junction, using the measuring tape provided in the kit. The PICC is typically supplied with an inner obturator that provides stiffness for insertion. The PICC is trimmed to the desired length and flushed with saline and the obturator is inserted into the PICC up to the tip. The PICC/obturator assembly is inserted through the introducer to the appropriate distance, the introducer peeled away, and the obturator removed. The PICC is secured in place and a chest X-ray obtained to determine tip position.

If resistance to advancing the PICC is met, options are limited. Techniques such as abducting the arm are of limited value. If a catheter-through- or over-needle device has been used, the catheter must never be withdrawn without simultaneously retracting the needle to avoid catheter shearing and embolism. If the catheter cannot be advanced easily, another site should be chosen.

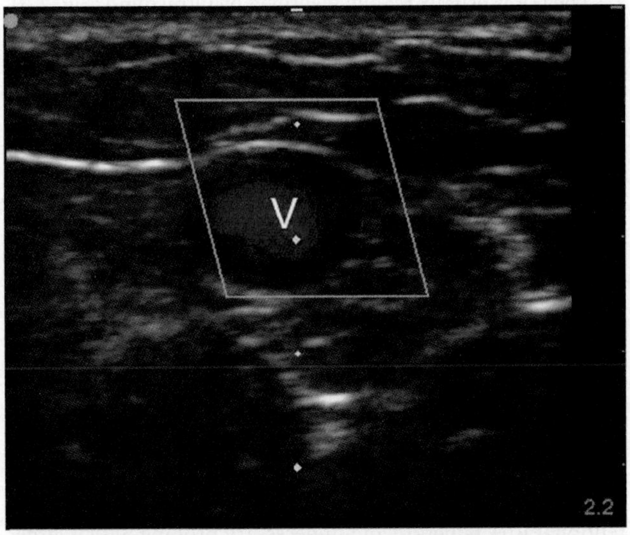

FIGURE 2.1. Ultrasound view of the basilica vein at the antecubital fossa.

Success Rate and Complications

Using the above-mentioned technique, PICC catheters have a 75% to 95% successful placement rate. Overall, PICCs appear to be at least as safe as CVCs, but important complications include sterile phlebitis, thrombosis (especially of the SCV and IJV), infection, limb edema, and pericardial tamponade. Phlebitis may be more common with antecubital CVCs, probably due to less blood flow in these veins as well as the proximity of the venipuncture site to the skin [52,53]. The risk of pericardial tamponade may also be increased if the catheter tip is inserted too deep because of greater catheter tip migration occurring with arm movements [54]. Complications are minimized by strict adherence to recommended techniques for catheter placement and care.

Internal Jugular Approach

The IJV has been used for venous access in pediatric and adult patients for many years but its use in some circumstances has been limited by a relatively lower rate of success due to its compressibility and propensity to collapse in hypovolemic conditions. In our opinion, ultrasound has had its greatest impact by improving the efficiency of IJV cannulation, since real-time direct visualization of the vein is easily obtained. This minimizes the impact of hypovolemia or anatomical variations on overall success, and has rendered the need for EJV catheterization almost extinct. Furthermore, under ultrasound guidance, the central approach is almost always used, and as a result, we will no longer review the anterior or posterior approaches. In general, these techniques will differ only in the point of skin puncture (Fig. 2.2), and readers are referred to previous editions of this text for a thorough description of these approaches.

Anatomy

The IJV emerges from the base of the skull through the jugular foramen and enters the carotid sheath dorsally with the internal carotid artery (ICA). It then courses posterolaterally to the artery and runs beneath the sternocleidomastoid (SCM) muscle. The vein lies medial to the anterior portion of the SCM muscle superiorly and then runs beneath the triangle formed by the two heads of the muscle in its medial portion before entering the SCV near the medial border of the anterior scalene muscle at the sternal border of the clavicle. The junction of the right IJV (which averages 2 to 3 cm in diameter) with the right SCV forming the innominate vein follows a straight path to the SVC. As a result, catheter malposition and looping of the catheter inserted through the right IJV are unusual. In contrast, a catheter passed through the left IJV must negotiate a sharp turn at the left jugulosubclavian junction, which results in a greater percentage of catheter malpositions [55]. This sharp turn may also produce tension and torque at the catheter tip, resulting in a higher incidence of vessel erosion.

Knowledge of the structures neighboring the IJV is essential as they may be compromised by a misdirected needle. The ICA runs medial to the IJV but, rarely, may lie directly posterior or, rarely, anterior. Behind the ICA, just outside the sheath, lie the stellate ganglion and the cervical sympathetic trunk. The dome of the pleura, which is higher on the left, lies caudal to the junction of the IJV and SCV. Posteriorly, at the root of the neck, course the phrenic and vagus nerves. The thoracic duct lies posterior to the left IJV and enters the superior margin of the SCV near the jugulosubclavian junction. The right lymphatic duct has the same anatomical relationship but is much smaller,

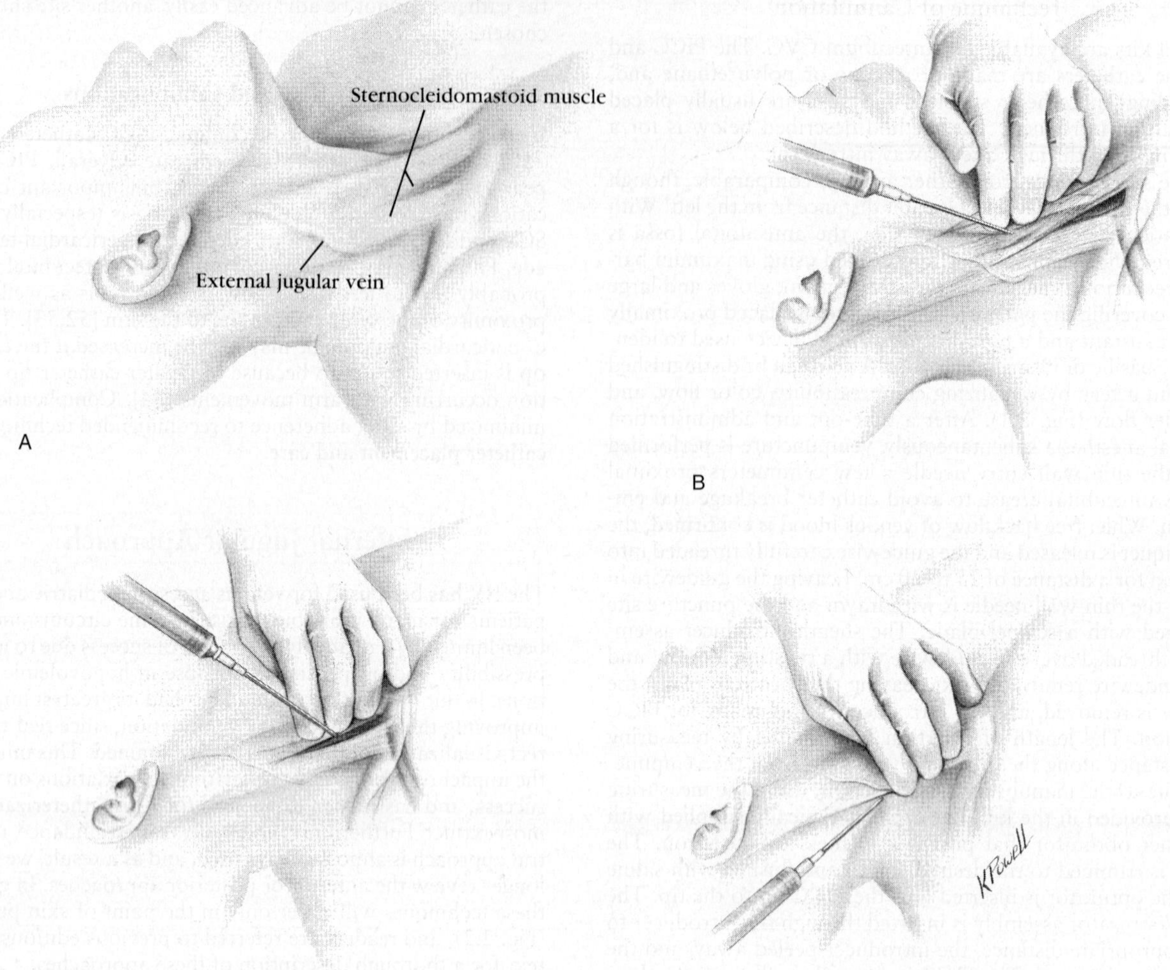

FIGURE 2.2. Surface anatomy and various approaches to cannulation of the internal jugular vein. A: Surface anatomy. B: Anterior approach. C: Central approach. D: Posterior approach. The external jugular vein is also shown.

and chylous effusions typically occur only with left-sided IJV cannulations.

Technique of Cannulation

With careful preparation of equipment and attention to patient comfort and safety as described earlier, the patient is placed in a 15-degree Trendelenburg position to distend the vein and minimize the risk of air embolism. The head is turned gently to the contralateral side. The surface anatomy is identified, especially the angle of the mandible, the two heads of the SCM, the clavicle, the EJV, and the trachea (Fig. 2.2). We recommend preliminary ultrasound examination of the IJV before skin preparation to quickly identify anatomical variations and suitability for catheterization. The probe should initially be placed in the center of the triangle formed by the clavicle and two heads of the SCM. If on the ultrasound the IJV is very small, thrombosed, or there is a significant anatomical variant, it is best to choose another site since successful cannulation is directly dependent on cross-sectional luminal size of the vessel. The neck is then prepared with chlorhexidine and fully draped, using maximum barrier precautions. Before the procedure is begun, a time-out is performed.

The IJV is usually readily identified by ultrasound (Fig. 2.3), and if the anatomy is normal and the IJV of substantial size, use of a finder needle is not required. The operator can directly visualize the needle entering the vein, and then proceed with insertion of the guidewire and catheter as described later. It is important not to be "mesmerized" or to have a false sense of confidence because ultrasound is being used. Always follow standard catheterization technique and always confirm (using multiple techniques) venous puncture. For example, it is good practice to document that the needle or short cannula is in the IJV through the use of manometry or to visualize the guidewire within the vein by using ultrasound before proceeding with catheter insertion.

If ultrasound is unavailable, skin puncture is at the apex of the triangle formed by the two muscle bellies of the SCM and the clavicle. The ICA pulsation is usually felt 1 to 2 cm medial to this point, beneath or just medial to the sternal head of the SCM. The skin at the apex of the triangle is infiltrated with 1% lidocaine using the smallest needle available. Use of a small-bore finder needle to locate the IJV should prevent unintentional ICA puncture and unnecessary probing with a larger bore needle. To avoid collapsing the IJV, the operator should maintain minimal to no pressure on the ICA with the left hand

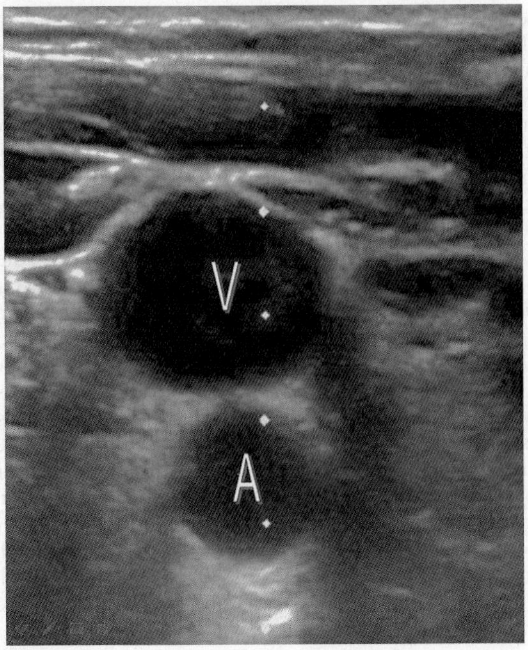

FIGURE 2.3. Ultrasound appearance of the right internal jugular vein and normal relationship with the internal carotid artery.

and insert the finder needle with the right hand at the apex of the triangle at a 45-degree angle with the frontal plane, directed at the ipsilateral nipple. The needle is advanced steadily with constant negative pressure in the syringe, and venipuncture occurs within 1 to 5 cm. If venipuncture does not occur on the initial attempt, negative pressure should be maintained and the needle slowly withdrawn, as often, the needle will compress the vein on advancement and penetrate the back wall without blood return. Once the needle is pulled back past the posterior wall of the vessel, it achieves free flow of blood from the vessel. If the first attempt is unsuccessful, the operator should reassess patient position, landmarks, and techniques to ensure that he or she is not doing anything to decrease IJV lumen size (see later). Subsequent attempts may be directed slightly laterally or medially to the initial direction, as long as the ICA is not entered. If venipuncture does not occur after three to five attempts, further attempts are unlikely to be successful and only increase complications [56–58].

When venipuncture has occurred with the finder needle, the operator can either withdraw the finder needle and introduce the large-bore needle in the identical plane or leave the finder needle in place and introduce the larger needle directly superior to it. Leaving the finder needle in place has been shown to facilitate successful puncture with the introducer needle [59]. Many kits provide both an 18-gauge thin-wall needle through which a guidewire can be directly introduced and a 16-gauge catheter-over-needle device. With the latter apparatus, the catheter is threaded over the needle into the vein, the needle withdrawn, and the guidewire inserted through the catheter. Both techniques are effective; the choice is strictly a matter of operator preference. Regardless of which large-bore needle is used, once venipuncture has occurred the syringe is removed after ensuring that the backflow of blood is not pulsatile and the hub is then occluded with a finger to prevent air embolism or excessive bleeding. The guidewire, with the J-tip oriented appropriately, is then inserted and should pass freely up to 20 cm, at which point the thin-wall needle or catheter is withdrawn. The tendency to insert the guidewire deeper than 15 to 20 cm should be avoided, as it is the most common cause of ventricular arrhythmias during insertion and also poses a risk for cardiac perforation. Furthermore, if the patient has an IVC filter in place, the guidewire can become entangled in the filter. Occasionally, the guidewire does not pass easily beyond the tip of the thin-wall needle. The guidewire should then be withdrawn, the syringe attached, and free backflow of blood reestablished and maintained while the syringe and needle are brought to a more parallel plane with the vein. The guidewire should then pass easily. If resistance is still encountered, rotation of the guidewire during insertion often allows passage, but extensive manipulation and force lead only to complications.

With the guidewire in place, a scalpel is used to make two 90-degree stab incisions at the skin entry site to facilitate passage of the 7-Fr vessel dilator. The dilator is inserted down the wire to the hub, ensuring that control and sterility of the guidewire is not compromised. The dilator is then withdrawn and pressure used at the puncture site to control oozing and prevent air embolism down the needle tract. The proximal and middle lumens of a triple-lumen catheter are flushed with saline and capped. The catheter is then inserted over the guidewire, ensuring that the operator has control of the guidewire, either proximal or distal to the catheter, at all times to avoid intravascular loss of the wire. The catheter is then advanced 15 to 17 cm (17 to 19 cm for left IJV) into the vein, the guidewire withdrawn, and the distal lumen capped. The catheter is sutured securely to limit tip migration and bandaged in a standard manner. A chest radiograph should be obtained to detect complications and tip location.

Success Rates and Complications

Non–ultrasound-guided IJV catheterization is associated with a high rate of successful catheter placement. Elective procedures are successful more than 90% of the time, generally within the first three attempts, and catheter malposition is rare. Use of ultrasound clearly improves the success rate, decreases the number of attempts and complications, avoids unnecessary procedures by identifying unsuitable anatomy, and minimally impacts insertion time. Emergent IJV catheterization is less successful and is not the preferred technique during airway emergencies or other situations that may make it difficult to identify landmarks in the neck.

The incidence and types of complications are similar regardless of the approach. Operator inexperience appears to increase the number of complications, but to an undefined extent, and probably does not have as great an impact as it does on the incidence of pneumothorax in subclavian venipuncture [60].

The overall incidence of complications in IJV catheterization (without ultrasound guidance) is 0.1% to 4.2%. Important complications include ICA puncture, pneumothorax, vessel erosion, thrombosis, and infection. Although the impact of ultrasound use on other complications has not been conclusively demonstrated, it has been shown to significantly reduce the number of attempts and the incidence of arterial puncture, which is by far the most common complication [6]. In the absence of a bleeding diathesis, arterial punctures are usually benign and are managed conservatively by applying local pressure for 10 minutes. Even in the absence of clotting abnormalities, a sizable hematoma may form, frequently preventing further catheterization attempts or, rarely, exerting pressure on vital neck structures [61,62]. Unrecognized arterial puncture can lead to catheterization of the ICA with a large-bore catheter or introducer and can have disastrous consequences, especially if heparin is subsequently administered [63]. Management of carotid cannulation with a large-bore catheter, such as a 7-Fr introducer, is controversial. Options include pulling the catheter and applying pressure, percutaneous closure devices, internal stent grafting, or surgical repair [64,65]. Some experts advise administration of anticoagulants to prevent thromboembolic complications, whereas others advise the opposite. Our approach is to remove small bore catheters and avoid heparinization if possible, as hemorrhage appears to be a greater risk than thromboembolism. For larger bore catheters and complicated cases, we involve interventional radiology and vascular surgery before removal, and individualize the management based on the circumstances.

Pneumothorax, which may be complicated by blood, infusion of intravenous fluid, or tension, is considered an unusual adverse consequence of IJV cannulation; however, it has an incidence of 1.3% in a large meta-analysis, statistically the same as 1.5% found for subclavian puncture [66]. It usually results from a skin puncture too close to the clavicle or, rarely, from other causes. Logically, ultrasound should decrease or even eliminate pneumothorax as a complication during IJV catheterization.

An extraordinary number of case reports indicate that any complication from IJV catheterization is possible, even the intrathecal insertion of a pulmonary artery catheter [67]. In reality, the IJ route is reliable, with a low incidence of major complications. Operator experience is not as important a factor as in SCV catheterization; the incidence of catheter tip malposition is low, and patient acceptance is high. It is best suited for acute, short-term hemodialysis and for elective or urgent catheterizations in volume-replete patients, especially pulmonary artery catheterizations and insertion of temporary transvenous pacemakers. It is not the preferred site during airway emergencies, for parenteral nutrition, or for long-term catheterization because infectious complications are higher with IJV compared with SCV catheterizations.

External Jugular Vein Approach

The EJV is now rarely used for CVC, but in selected cases, it remains an excellent alternative. The main advantages to the EJV route for CVC are that it is part of the surface anatomy, the risk of hemorrhage is low even in the presence of coagulopathy, and the risk of pneumothorax is all but eliminated. The main disadvantage is the unpredictability of passage of the catheter to the central compartment.

Anatomy

The EJV is formed anterior and caudal to the ear at the angle of the mandible by the union of the posterior auricular and retromandibular veins (Fig. 2.2). It courses obliquely across the anterior surface of the SCM, then pierces the deep fascia just posterior to the SCM and joins the SCV behind the medial third of the clavicle. In 5% to 15% of patients, the EJV is not a distinct structure but a venous plexus, in which case it may receive the ipsilateral cephalic vein. The EJV varies in size and contains valves throughout its course. Its junction with the SCV may be at a severe, narrow angle that can be difficult for a catheter to traverse [50,51].

Technique

The EJV should be cannulated using the 16-gauge catheter-over-needle, since guidewire manipulations are often necessary, and secure venous access with a catheter is preferable. The patient is placed in a comfortable supine position with arms to the side and head turned slightly to the contralateral side. The right EJV should be chosen for the initial attempt and can be identified where it courses over the anterior portion of the clavicular belly of the SCM. After skin preparation with chlorhexidine, use of maximum barrier precautions, administration of local anesthesia subcutaneously and a time-out, venipuncture is performed with the 16-gauge catheter-over-needle using the left index finger and thumb to distend and anchor the vein. Skin puncture should be well above the clavicle and the needle advanced in the axis of the vein at 20 degrees to the frontal plane. The EJV may be more difficult to cannulate than expected because of its propensity to roll and displace rather than puncture in response to the advancing needle. A firm, quick thrust is often required to effect venipuncture. When free backflow of blood is established, the needle tip is advanced a few millimeters further into the vein and the catheter is threaded over the needle. The catheter may not thread its entire length because of valves, tortuosity, or the SCV junction, but should be advanced at least 3 to 5 cm to secure venous access. The syringe and needle can then be removed and the guidewire, J-tip first, threaded up to 20 cm and the catheter removed. Manipulation and rotation of the guidewire, especially when it reaches the SCV junction, may be necessary but should not be excessive. Various arm and head movements are advocated to facilitate guidewire passage; abduction of the ipsilateral arm and anterior–posterior pressure exerted on the clavicle may be helpful. Once the guidewire has advanced 20 cm, two 90-degree skin stabs are made with a scalpel, and the vein dilator inserted to its hub, maintaining control of the guidewire. The triple-lumen catheter is then inserted an appropriate length (16 to 17 cm on the right, 18 to 20 cm on the left). The guidewire is withdrawn, the catheter bandaged, and a chest radiograph obtained to screen for complications and tip placement.

Success Rates and Complications

Central venous catheterization via the EJV is successful in 80% of patients (range 75% to 95%) [68,69]. Inability to perform venipuncture accounts for up to 10% of failures [70,71] and the remainders are a result of catheter tip malpositioning. Failure to position the catheter tip is usually due to inability to negotiate the EJV–SCV junction, loop formation, or retrograde passage down the ipsilateral arm. Serious complications arising from the EJV approach are rare and almost always associated with catheter maintenance rather than venipuncture. A local hematoma forms in 1% to 5% of patients at the time of venipuncture [72] but has little consequence unless it distorts the anatomy leading to catheterization failure. External jugular venipuncture is safe in the presence of coagulopathy. Infectious, thrombotic, and other mechanical complications are no more frequent than with other central routes.

Femoral Vein Approach

The FV has many practical advantages for CVC; it is directly compressible, it is remote from the airway and pleura, the technique is relatively simple, and the Trendelenburg position is not required during insertion. During the mid-1950s, percutaneous catheterization of the IVC via a femoral vein approach became popular until 1959 when Moncrief [73] and Bansmer et al. [74] reported a high incidence of complications, especially infection and thrombosis, after which, it was largely abandoned. In the subsequent two decades, FV cannulation was restricted to specialized clinical situations. Interest in short-term (<48 hour) FV catheterization was renewed by positive experiences during the Vietnam conflict and with patients in the emergency department [75]. Some reports on long-term FV catheterization [76] suggest an overall complication rate no higher than that with other routes, although deep vein thrombosis remains a legitimate concern. Furthermore, Centers for Disease Control and Prevention (CDC) guidelines for the prevention of catheter-related bloodstream infection recommend against the use of the femoral site for catheterization if possible [77].

Anatomy

The FV (Fig. 2.4A) is a direct continuation of the popliteal vein and becomes the external iliac vein at the inguinal ligament. At

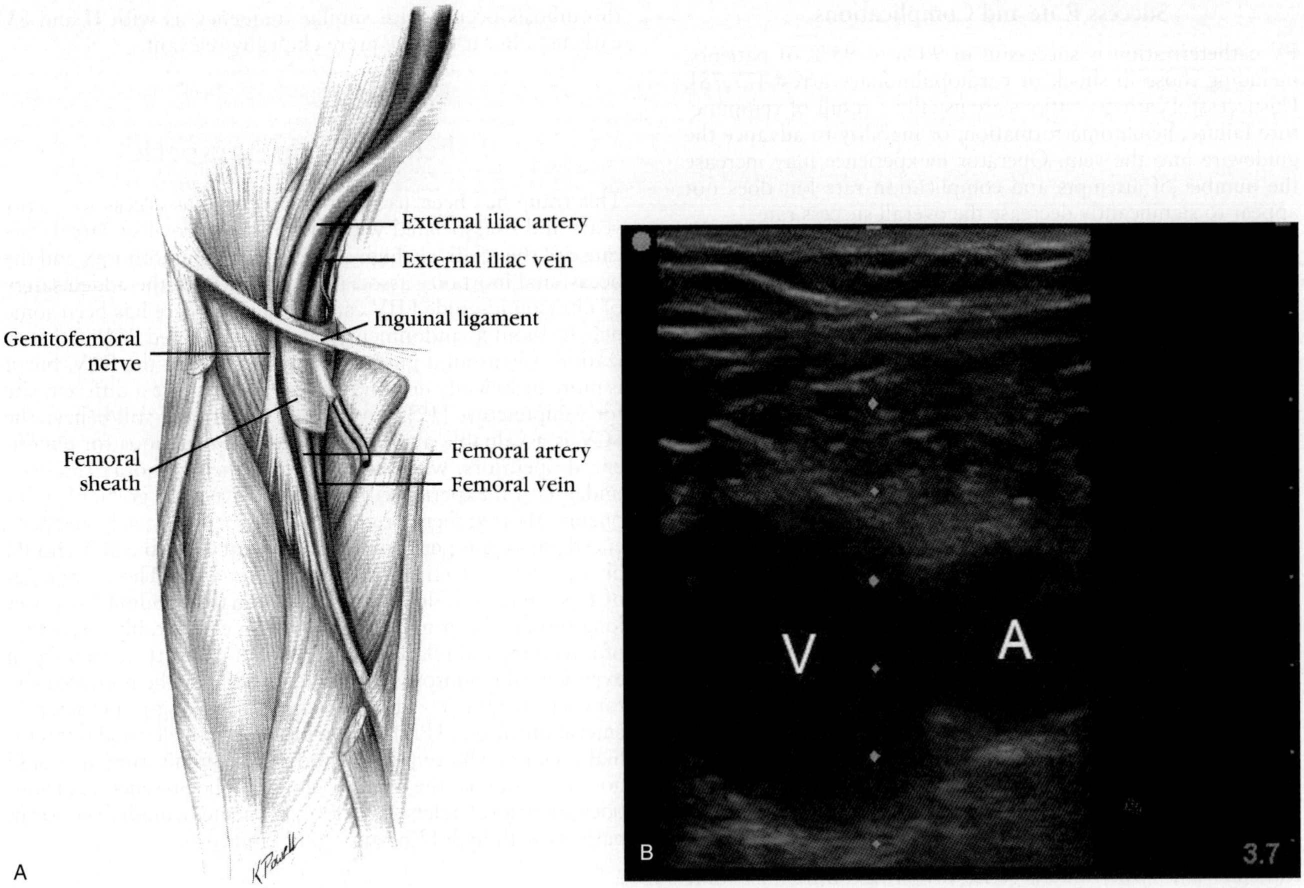

FIGURE 2.4. A: Anatomy of the femoral vein. B: Ultrasound appearance of femoral vein and artery.

the inguinal ligament, the FV lies within the femoral sheath a few centimeters from the skin surface. The FV lies medial to the femoral artery, which in turn lies medial to the femoral branch of the genitofemoral nerve. The medial compartment contains lymphatic channels and Cloquet's node. The external iliac vein courses cephalad from the inguinal ligament along the anterior surface of the iliopsoas muscle to join its counterpart from the other leg and form the (IVC) anterior to and to the right of the fifth lumbar vertebra. Using ultrasound, the femoral vein can be readily identified by placing the probe a few centimeters caudal to the inguinal ligament, just medial to the arterial pulsation (Fig. 2.4B).

Technique

Femoral vein cannulation is the easiest of all central venous procedures to learn and perform. Either side is suitable, and the side chosen is based on operator convenience. Ultrasound guidance is not usually required but for elective situations, we believe it is optimal practice. Ultrasound confirms the anatomy, identifies the depth needed for venipuncture, rules out preexisting thrombosis, and should not unduly delay time to catheterization. It may be particularly useful in the obese [21]. The patient is placed in the supine position (if tolerated) with the leg extended and slightly abducted at the hip. Excessive hair should be clipped with scissors and the skin prepped with chlorhexidine. Maximum barrier precautions should be used. The FV lies 1 to 1.5 cm medial to the arterial pulsation, and the overlying skin is infiltrated with 1% lidocaine. In a patient without femoral artery pulsations, the FV can be located by dividing the distance between the anterior superior iliac spine and the pubic tubercle is divided into three equal segments. The femoral artery is usually found where the medial segment meets the two lateral ones, and the FV lies 1 to 1.5 cm medial. Following a time-out, an 18-gauge thin-wall needle is inserted at this point, 2 to 3 cm inferior to the inguinal ligament, ensuring that venipuncture occurs caudal to the inguinal ligament, which minimizes the risk of retroperitoneal hematoma in the event of arterial puncture. While maintaining constant back pressure on the syringe, the needle, tip pointed cephalad, is advanced at a 45-degree angle to the frontal plane. Insertion of the needle to its hub is sometimes required in obese patients. Blood return may not occur until slow withdrawal. If the initial attempt is unsuccessful, landmarks should be reevaluated and subsequent attempts oriented slightly more medial or lateral. A common error is to direct the needle tip too medially, toward the umbilicus. The femoral vessels lie in the sagittal plane at the inguinal ligament (Fig. 2.4), and the needle should be directed accordingly. If unintentional arterial puncture occurs, pressure is applied for 5 to 10 minutes.

When venous blood return is established, the syringe angle is depressed slightly and free aspiration of blood reconfirmed. The syringe is removed, ensuring that blood return is not pulsatile. The guidewire should pass easily and never forced, although rotation and minor manipulation are sometimes required. The needle is then withdrawn, two scalpel blade stab incisions made at 90 degrees at the guidewire insertion site, and the vein dilator inserted over the wire to the hub. The dilator is then withdrawn and a catheter appropriate to clinical requirements inserted, taking care never to lose control of the guidewire. The catheter is secured with a suture and bandage applied.

Success Rate and Complications

FV catheterization is successful in 90% to 95% of patients, including those in shock or cardiopulmonary arrest [77,78]. Unsuccessful catheterizations are usually a result of venipuncture failure, hematoma formation, or inability to advance the guidewire into the vein. Operator inexperience may increase the number of attempts and complication rate but does not appear to significantly decrease the overall success rate.

Three complications occur regularly with FV catheterization: arterial puncture with or without local bleeding, infection, and thromboembolic events. Other reported complications are rare and include scrotal hemorrhage, right lower quadrant bowel perforation, retroperitoneal hemorrhage, puncture of the kidney, and perforation of IVC tributaries. These complications occur when skin puncture sites are cephalad to the inguinal ligament or when long catheters are threaded into the FV.

Femoral artery puncture occurs in 5% to 10% of adults. Most arterial punctures are uncomplicated, but major hematomas may form in 1% of patients, especially in the presence of anticoagulants, fibrinolytics, or antithrombotic agents. As is the case with other routes, ultrasound should essentially eliminate this complication. Even in the presence of coagulopathy, arterial puncture with the 18-gauge thin-wall needle is usually of minor consequence, but there is a potential for life-threatening thigh or retroperitoneal hemorrhage [79]. Arteriovenous fistula and pseudoaneurysm are rare chronic complications of arterial puncture; the former is more likely to occur when both femoral vessels on the same side are cannulated concurrently [80].

Infectious complications with FV catheters are probably more frequent than SCV catheters but comparable to IJV catheters [81–83]. Modern series involving both short- and long-term FV catheterization in adults and children have reported significant CRI rates of about 5% or less [77,84]. Further evidence that the inguinal site is not inherently "dirty" is provided by experience with femoral artery catheters, which have an infection rate comparable to that with radial artery catheters [85]. Although more recent reports suggest that a catheter properly placed and cared for has a similar rate of infection regardless of venipuncture site, CDC guidelines recommend avoidance of the femoral site unless absolutely necessary [77,86].

Two reports in 1958 highlighted the high incidence of FV catheter-associated deep venous thrombosis, but these studies were primarily autopsy based and prior to modern technological advances. Catheter-associated thrombosis is a risk of all CVCs, regardless of the site of insertion, and comparative studies using contrast venography, impedance plethysmography, or Doppler ultrasound suggest that FV catheters are no more prone to thrombosis than upper extremity catheters. Pulmonary emboli have been reported following CVC-associated upper extremity thrombosis [46] and the relative risk of femoral catheter-related thrombosis is unknown. Clearly, the potential thromboembolic complications of FV catheters cannot be discounted [87], but they do not warrant total abandonment of this approach.

In summary, available evidence supports the view that the FV may be cannulated safely in critically ill adults. It is particularly useful for inexperienced operators because of the high rate of success and lower incidence of major complications. FV catheterizations may be performed during airway emergencies and cardiopulmonary arrest, in patients with coagulopathy, in patients who are unable to lie flat, and for access during renal replacement therapy. The most common major complication during FV catheterization is arterial puncture, which can be lessened or eliminated by ultrasound guidance. Infection is no more common than with IJV catheters. Catheter-associated thrombosis occurs with similar frequency as with IJ and SV catheters, but it may be more clinically relevant.

Subclavian Vein Approach

This route has been used for central venous access for many years and is associated with the most controversy, largely because of the relatively high incidence of pneumothorax and the occasional mortality associated with it. With the added safety of ultrasound-guided IJV catheterization, there has been some debate about abandonment of landmark guided SCV catheterization. Ultrasound guidance is possible with the SCV, but it is more technically demanding and may require a different site for venipuncture [12]. Given these factors, we still believe the SCV is a valuable alternative in certain situations for experienced operators, who should have a pneumothorax rate well under 1%. Inexperienced operators have a far greater rate of pneumothorax; therefore, in settings where relatively inexperienced physicians perform the majority of CVC, the SCV should be used more selectively or perhaps, not at all. The advantages of this route include consistent identifiable landmarks, easier long-term catheter maintenance with a comparably lower rate of infection, and relatively high patient comfort. Assuming an experienced operator is available, the SCV is the preferred site for CVC in patients with hypovolemia, for long-term total parenteral nutrition (TPN), and in patients with elevated intracranial pressure who require hemodynamic monitoring. It should not be considered the primary choice in the presence of thrombocytopenia (platelets <50,000), for acute hemodialysis, or in patients with high PEEP (i.e., >12 cm H_2O).

Anatomy

The SCV is a direct continuation of the axillary vein, beginning at the lateral border of the first rib, extending 3 to 4 cm along the undersurface of the clavicle and becoming the brachiocephalic vein where it joins the ipsilateral IJV at Pirogoff's confluence behind the sternoclavicular articulation (Fig. 2.5). The vein is 1 to 2 cm in diameter, contains a single set of valves just distal to the EJV junction, and is fixed in position directly beneath the clavicle by its fibrous attachments. These attachments prevent collapse of the vein, even with severe volume depletion. Anterior to the vein throughout its course lie the subclavius muscle, clavicle, costoclavicular ligament, pectoralis muscles, and epidermis. Posteriorly, the SCV is separated from the subclavian artery and brachial plexus by the anterior scalenus muscle, which is 10 to 15 mm thick in the adult. Posterior to the medial portion of the SCV are the phrenic nerve and internal mammary artery as they pass into the thorax. Superiorly, the relationships are the skin, platysma, and superficial aponeurosis. Inferiorly, the vein rests on the first rib, Sibson's fascia, the cupola of the pleura (0.5 cm behind the vein), and pulmonary apex [88]. The thoracic duct on the left and right lymphatic duct cross the anterior scalene muscle to join the superior aspect of the SV near its union with the IJV.

The clavicle presents a significant barrier for ultrasound visualization of the SCV, which mandates using a different approach [12]. Typically, we identify the axillary/subclavian vein junction by placing the probe inferior to the clavicle in the deltopectoral groove. We usually initially produce an axial view of the vein by placing the probe in the cranial–caudal direction. The probe is then rotated 90 degrees to produce a longitudinal view of the vein, which is maintained during venipuncture and guidewire insertion (Fig. 2.6). Although this method is usually successful it tends to be more time consuming and in our experience, not as useful.

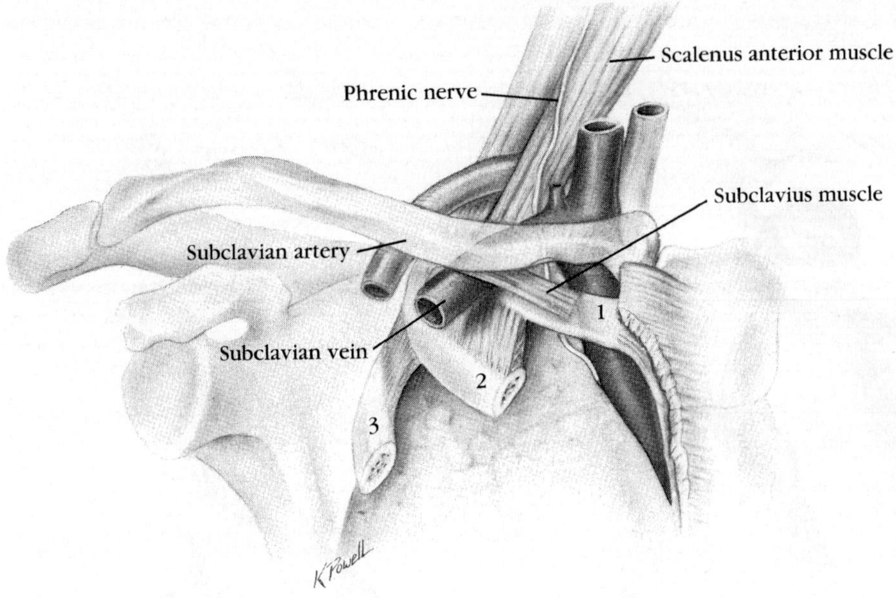

FIGURE 2.5. Anatomy of the subclavian vein and adjacent structures.

Technique

Although there are many variations, the SCV may be cannulated using surface landmarks by two basic techniques: the infraclavicular [89] or supraclavicular [90,91] approach (Fig. 2.7). The differences in success rate, catheter tip malposition, and complications between the two approaches are negligible, although catheter tip malposition and pneumothorax may be less likely with supraclavicular cannulation [92,93]. In general, when discussing the success rate and incidence of complications of SV catheterization, there is no need to specify the approach used.

The 18-gauge thin-wall needle is preferable for SCV cannulation. The patient is placed in a 15- to 30-degree Trendelenburg position, and in our experience, use of a small bedroll between the scapulae tends move the humeral head out of the plane of needle insertion. The head is turned slightly to the contralateral side and the arms are kept to the side. The pertinent landmarks are the clavicle, the two muscle bellies of the SCM, the suprasternal notch, the deltopectoral groove, and the manubriosternal junction. For the infraclavicular approach (Fig. 2.7), the operator is positioned next to the patient's shoulder on the side to be cannulated. For reasons cited earlier, the left SCV should be chosen for pulmonary artery catheterization; otherwise, the success rate appears to be equivalent regardless of the side chosen. Skin puncture is 2 to 3 cm caudal to the clavicle at the deltopectoral groove, corresponding to the area where the clavicle turns from the shoulder to the manubrium. Skin puncture should be distant enough from the clavicle to avoid a downward angle of the needle in clearing the inferior surface of the clavicle, which also obviates any need to bend the needle. The path of the needle is toward the suprasternal notch. Using maximum barrier precautions, the skin is prepped with chlorhexidine. After skin infiltration and liberal injection of the clavicular periosteum with 1% lidocaine and a time-out, the 18-gauge thin-wall needle is mounted on a 10-mL syringe. Skin puncture is accomplished with the needle bevel up, and the needle is advanced in the plane already described until the tip abuts the clavicle. The needle is then

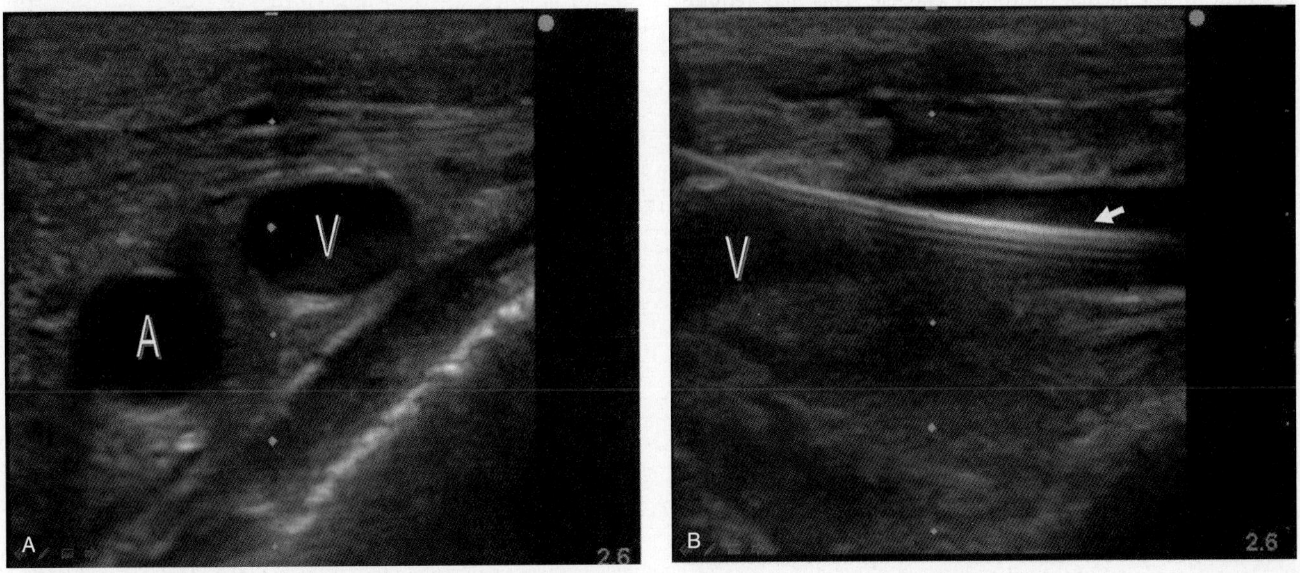

FIGURE 2.6. Ultrasound view of the subclavian vein. **A:** Axial view; **B:** longitudinal view. See text for details.

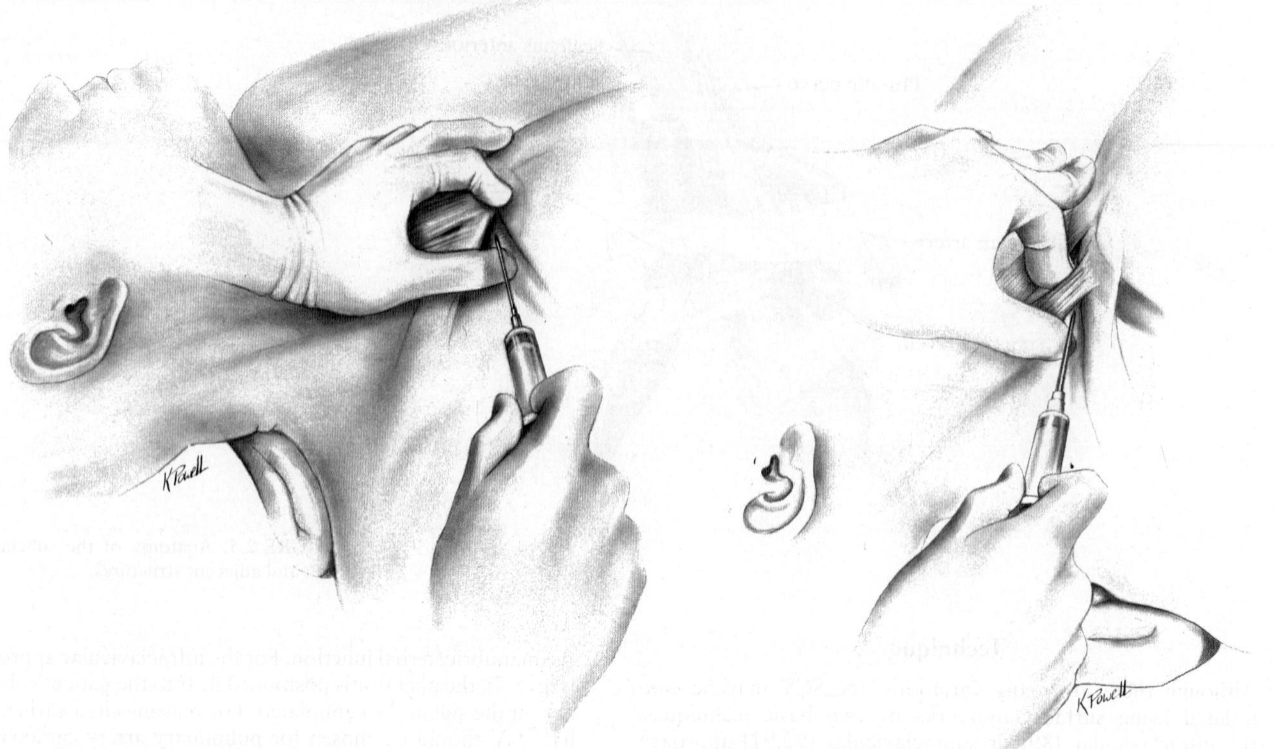

A B

FIGURE 2.7. A: Patient positioning for subclavian cannulation. B: Cannulation technique for supraclavicular approach.

"walked" down the clavicle until the inferior edge is cleared. To avoid pneumothorax, it is imperative the needle stay parallel to the floor and not angle down toward the chest. This is accomplished by using the operator's left thumb to provide downward displacement in the vertical plane after each attempt, until the needle advances under the clavicle.

As the needle is advanced further, the inferior surface of the clavicle should be felt hugging the needle. This ensures that the needle tip is as superior as possible to the pleura. The needle is advanced toward the suprasternal notch during breath holding or expiration, and venipuncture occurs when the needle tip lies beneath the medial end of the clavicle. This may require insertion of the needle to its hub. Blood return may not occur until slow withdrawal of the needle. If venipuncture is not accomplished on the initial thrust, the next attempt should be directed slightly more cephalad. If venipuncture does not occur by the third or fourth attempt, another site should be chosen, as additional attempts are unlikely to be successful and may result in complications.

When blood return is established, the bevel of the needle is rotated 90 degrees toward the heart. The needle is anchored firmly with the left hand while the syringe is detached with the right. Blood return should not be pulsatile, and air embolism prophylaxis is necessary at all times. The guidewire is then advanced through the needle to 15 cm and the needle withdrawn. To increase the success rate of proper placement of the catheter, the J-wire tip should point inferiorly [94]. The remainder of the procedure is as previously described. Triple-lumen catheters should be sutured at 15 to 16 cm on the right and 17 to 18 cm on the left to avoid intracardiac tip placement [31,32,95].

For the supraclavicular approach (Fig. 2.7), the important landmarks are the clavicular insertion of the SCM muscle and the sternoclavicular joint. The operator is positioned at the head of the patient on the side to be cannulated. The site of skin puncture is the claviculosternocleidomastoid angle, just above the clavicle and lateral to the insertion of the clavicular head of the SCM. The needle is advanced toward or just caudal to the contralateral nipple just under the clavicle. This corresponds to a 45-degree angle to the sagittal plane, bisecting a line between the sternoclavicular joint and clavicular insertion of the SCM. The depth of insertion is from just beneath the SCM clavicular head at a 10- to 15-degree angle below the coronal plane. The needle should enter the jugulosubclavian venous bulb after 1 to 4 cm, and the operator may then proceed with catheterization.

Success and Complication Rates

Subclavian vein catheterization is successful in 90% to 95% of cases, generally on the first attempt [96]. The presence of shock does not alter the success rate as significantly as it does during IJV catheterization [97]. Unsuccessful catheterizations are a result of venipuncture failure or inability to advance the guidewire or catheter. Catheter tip malposition occurs in 5% to 20% of cases and tends to be more frequent with the infraclavicular approach. Malposition occurs most commonly to the ipsilateral IJV and contralateral SCV and is usually correctable without repeat venipuncture.

The overall incidence of noninfectious complications varies depending on the operator's experience and the circumstances under which the catheter is inserted. Large series involving several thousand SCV catheters have reported an incidence of major complications of 1% to 3%, with an overall rate of 5%. In smaller, probably more clinically relevant studies, the major complication rate has ranged from 1% to 10% [98–100]. Factors resulting in a higher complication rate are operator inexperience, multiple attempts at venipuncture, emergency conditions, variance from standardized technique, and body mass index. Major noninfectious complications include pneumothorax, arterial puncture, and thromboembolism. There are many case reports of isolated major complications involving neck structures or the brachial plexus; the reader is referred elsewhere for a complete listing of reported complications [11].

Pneumothorax accounts for one fourth to one half of reported complications, with an incidence of about 1.5%. The incidence varies inversely with the operator's experience and the number of "breaks" in technique. There is no magic figure whereby an operator matures from inexperienced to experienced. Fifty catheterizations are cited frequently as a cutoff number [101], but it is reasonable to expect an operator to be satisfactorily experienced after having performed fewer. For the experienced operator, a pneumothorax incidence of less than 1% is expected. Most pneumothoraces are a result of lung puncture at the time of the procedure, but late-appearing pneumothoraces have been reported.

Most pneumothoraces will require thoracostomy tube drainage with a small chest tube and a Heimlich valve but some can be managed conservatively with 100% oxygen and serial radiographs or needle aspiration only [1]. Rarely, a pneumothorax is complicated by tension, blood, infusion of intravenous fluid (immediately or days to weeks after catheter placement), chyle, or massive subcutaneous emphysema. Bilateral pneumothoraces can occur from unilateral attempts at venipuncture. Pneumothorax can result in death, especially when it goes unrecognized [102].

Subclavian artery puncture occurs in 0.5% to 1.0% of cases, constituting one fourth to one third of all complications. Arterial puncture is usually managed easily by applying pressure above and below the clavicle. Bleeding can be catastrophic in patients with coagulopathy, especially thrombocytopenia. As with other routes, arterial puncture may result in arteriovenous fistula or pseudoaneurysm.

Clinical evidence of central venous thrombosis, including SVC syndrome, development of collaterals around the shoulder girdle, and pulmonary embolism, occurs in 0% to 3% of SCV catheterizations, but routine phlebography performed at catheter removal reveals a much higher incidence of thrombotic phenomena. The importance of the discrepancy between clinical symptoms and radiologic findings is unknown, but upper extremity thrombosis, even if asymptomatic, is not a totally benign condition [46]. Duration of catheterization, catheter material, and patient condition probably impact the frequency of thrombosis, but to an uncertain degree.

In summary, the SCV is an extremely reliable and useful route for CVC, but because of the relatively high rate of pneumothorax and the increased success rate of ultrasound-guided IJV catheterization, its use should be limited to those operators skilled in the technique. Inexperienced operators should use an alternative site. Experienced operators should continue to use this route for certain indications (Table 2.1) but should scrupulously avoid it in patients who cannot tolerate a pneumothorax (severe lung disease, one lung), or in patients with severe coagulopathy, especially platelets <50,000. Ultrasound guidance may be helpful, but requires a higher skill level and a different approach to catheterization.

INFECTIOUS COMPLICATIONS

Tremendous advances in the understanding of the pathophysiology, causes, and prevention of CRI have occurred in recent years and have led to corresponding dramatic improvements in catheter technology, insertion, and management. Table 2.2 summarizes current recommendations or interventions that have been shown to reduce the risk of CRI. This section reviews these recommendations, focusing on the epidemiology, pathogenesis, diagnosis, management, and prevention of central CRI.

Definitions and Epidemiology

Consensus regarding the definition and diagnosis of CRI is a necessary initial step in discussing catheter-related infectious complications. The semiquantitative culture method described by Maki et al. [103] for culturing catheter segments is the most accepted technique for diagnosing CRI. Which catheter segment to culture (the tip or intradermal segment) is still controversial; out of convenience, most centers routinely culture the catheter tip. If semiquantitative methods are used, catheter contamination (probably occurring at time of withdrawal) is defined as less than 15 colony-forming units (CFUs) per culture plate. CRI is a spectrum: growth of greater than or equal to 15 CFUs is identified as significant colonization (all other cultures negative and no clinical symptoms); local or exit-site infection (skin site with erythema, cellulitis, or purulence); catheter-related bacteremia (systemic blood cultures positive for identical organism on catheter segment and no other source); and catheter-related sepsis or septic shock. Alternative methods to diagnose CRI include differential time to positivity [104] and direct Gram [105] or acridine-orange staining [106] of catheters. Using the differential time to positivity, blood

TABLE 2.2

STEPS TO MINIMIZE CENTRAL VENOUS CATHETERIZATION (CVC)-RELATED INFECTION

1. Institution-supported standardized education, with knowledge assessment, of all physicians involved in CVC insertion and care
2. Site preparation with approved chlorhexidine-based preparation
3. Maximal barrier precautions during catheter insertion
4. Use of mobile procedure carts, safety checklist, empowerment of staff
5. Strict protocols for catheter maintenance (including bandage and tubing changes), preferably by dedicated IV catheter team
6. Appropriate site selection, avoiding heavily colonized or anatomically abnormal areas; use of SCV for anticipated CVC of >4 d
7. For anticipated duration of catheterization exceeding 96 hr, use of silver-impregnated cuff, sustained release chlorhexidine gluconate patch, and/or antibiotic/antiseptic-impregnated catheters
8. Prompt removal of any catheter which is no longer required
9. Remove pulmonary artery catheters and introducers after 5 d
10. Replace any catheter not placed with sterile precautions within 48 hr (i.e., catheter placed in emergency)
11. Use multilumen catheters only when indicated; remove when no longer needed
12. Avoid "routine" guidewire exchanges
13. Use surgically implanted catheters or PICCs for long term (i.e., >3 wk) or permanent CVC

CVC, central venous catheterization; PICC, peripherally inserted central catheter; SCV, subclavian vein.

TABLE 2.3

INFECTION RATES FOR VARIOUS INTRAVASCULAR CATHETERS

Device	IVD-related BSIs per 1,000 days (95% CI)
Peripheral IV catheters	0.6 (0.2–0.9)
Midline catheters	0.2 (0.0–0.5)
Arterial catheters	1.4 (0.8–2.0)
PICCs	0.8 (0.4–1.2)
Nontunneled CVCs	
Nonmedicated	2.9 (2.6–3.2)
Medicated; Chlorhexadine–silver sulfadiazine	1.3 (1.0–1.7)
Medicated; minocycline–rifampin	1.2 (0.3–2.1)
Tunneled CVCs	2.1 (1.0–3.2)
Pulmonary artery catheters	3.3 (1.9–4.6)
Nontunneled hemodialysis catheters	6.1 (4.9–7.4)

Adapted from Maki DG, Kluger DM, Crnich CJ: The risk of bloodstream infection in adults with different intravascular devices: a systematic review of 200 published prospective studies. *Mayo Clin Proc* 81:1159–1171, 2006.

BSI, bloodstream infection; CI, confidence interval; CVC, central venous catheter; IVD, intravascular device; PICC, peripherally inserted central venous catheter.

cultures are drawn from the catheter and a peripheral vein. If the time to positive culture is greater than 120 minutes longer for the peripheral cultures, a diagnosis of CRI is made. This method has good sensitivity, specificity, and the advantage of faster diagnosis.

The morbidity and economic costs associated with CRI are truly impressive. Estimates vary because the overall incidence of CRI is impacted by so many independent variables, including type of ICU, catheter type and composition, duration of catheterization, and site of insertion. Furthermore, critical care practice is extremely dynamic, and the frequency and type of intravascular catheters used changes over time, rendering much of the data, somewhat out of date. Intravascular devices are now the single most important cause of health-care associated bloodstream infection in the United States and Europe, with an estimated incidence of 250,000 to 500,000 cases annually in the United States alone [107]. More than 5 million CVCs are inserted annually in the United States, accounting for 15 million CVC-days. Approximately 3% to 9% of all CVCs will become infected during clinical use, and the National Healthcare Safety Network reports rates of CVC-associated bloodstream infections varying from 1.2 to 5.5 per 1,000 catheter-days depending on the location of the patient [108]. A recently completed systematic review of the literature reported BSI rates for all intravascular devices [108] (Table 2.3); noncuffed, nontunneled CVCs had an average BSI rate of 2.9 per 1,000 catheter-days. When BSI does occur, often with a resistant organism such as methicillin-resistant *Staphylococcus aureus* (MRSA) and VRE, it increases healthcare costs by as much as $20,000 to 40,000, prolongs ICU and hospital stay by several days, and may increase attributable mortality [109–111]. Importantly, it has been estimated that as many as 50% of CRIs are preventable [112], which should serve as a powerful impetus and render it indefensible for critical care physicians not to implement everything possible to minimize CRI.

Pathophysiology of Catheter Infection

Assuming that they are not contaminated during insertion, catheters can become infected from four potential sources: the skin insertion site, the catheter hub(s), hematogenous seeding, and infusate contamination. Animal and human studies have shown that catheters are most commonly infected by bacteria colonizing the skin site, followed by invasion of the intradermal catheter tract. Once the external surface of the intradermal catheter is infected, bacteria can quickly traverse the entire length and infect the catheter tip, sometimes encasing the catheter in a slime layer known as a biofilm (coagulase-negative staph). From the catheter tip, bacteria may shed into the bloodstream, potentially creating metastatic foci of infection [113]. The pathophysiology of most catheter infections explains why guidewire exchanges are not effective in preventing or treating CRI: the colonized tract and, in many cases, biofilm, remain intact and quickly reinfect the new catheter [114].

The catheter hub(s) also becomes colonized but contributes to catheter-related infectious complications less frequently than the insertion site [115,116]. Hub contamination may be relatively more important as a source of infection for certain types of catheters (hemodialysis) and the longer the catheter remains in place [117]. Hematogenous seeding of catheters from bacteremia is an infrequent cause of CRI.

Site Preparation and Catheter Maintenance

That the majority of CRIs are caused by skin flora highlights the importance of site sterility during insertion and catheter maintenance. Organisms that colonize the insertion site originate from the patient's own skin flora or the hands of operators. Thorough hand washing and scrupulous attention to aseptic technique is mandatory during catheter insertion. A prospective study proved that a nonsterile cap and mask, sterile gown, and a large drape covering the patient's head and body (maximal (triple) sterile barriers, compared to sterile gloves and small drape) reduced the catheter-related bloodstream infection rate sixfold and were highly cost-effective [118]. If a break in sterile technique occurs during insertion, termination of the procedure and replacement of contaminated equipment is mandatory. Use of a mobile catheter cart that can be wheeled to the patient bedside facilitates maintenance of the sterile environment.

Chlorhexidine is a superior disinfectant and should be used instead of iodine-based solutions [119,120]. Proper application includes liberally scrubbing the site using expanding concentric circles. Excessive hair should be clipped with scissors prior to application of the antiseptic, as shaving can cause minor skin lacerations and disruption of the epidermal barrier to infection.

Care of the catheter after insertion is extremely important in minimizing infection, and all medical personnel should follow standardized protocols [121]. The number of piggyback infusions and medical personnel handling tubing changes and manipulation of the catheter site should be minimized. Replacement of administration sets every 72 to 96 hours is safe and cost-efficient [122], unless there are specific recommendations for the infusate (e.g., propofol). Transparent polyurethane dressings have become more popular than gauze and tape, but have not been found to be superior. It is recommended that the transparent dressing be changed every 7 days or sooner if damp or soiled. Addition of a silver-impregnated cuff or chlorhexidine sponge has been shown to reduce the rate of CRI and is cost-effective [123,124]. Application of iodophor or polymicrobial ointments to the skin site at the time of insertion or during dressing changes does not convincingly reduce the overall incidence of catheter infection, and certain polymicrobial ointments may increase the proportion of *Candida* infections [125].

Frequency of Catheter-Related Infection

Observing the above-mentioned recommendations for catheter insertion and maintenance will minimize catheter-associated infection. Colonization of the insertion site can begin within 24 hours and increases with duration of catheterization; 10% to 40% of catheters may eventually become colonized [126]. Catheter-associated bacteremia occurs in 3% to 8% of catheters [101,127–129], although some studies incorporating newer catheter technologies and procedures have demonstrated rates of catheter-associated bacteremia of 2% or less [130–132]. Overall, catheter-infection rates are best expressed as number of episodes per 1,000 days, and although each ICU should strive for perfection (it is possible to attain and maintain the "holy grail" of zero CRIs over an extended period of time [1]), each ICU should definitely reach or exceed an appropriate benchmark. The NHSN publishes average rates of CRIs for different types of ICUs [109]. Table 2.3 provides national references from published literature that has the added advantage of unique data for each specific catheter type [108].

Type of Catheter

The data presented earlier are derived from large studies and are not necessarily applicable to any given catheter in any specific ICU because of variations in definitions, types of catheters, site of insertion, duration of catheterization, types of fluid infused, and policies regarding routine guidewire changes, all of which have been implicated at some point as important factors in the incidence of CRI. The duration of catheterization in combination with the type of catheter are major factors; the site of insertion is less important. Guidewire changes have an important role in evaluation of the febrile catheterized patient, but routine guidewire changes do not prevent infection. Under ideal conditions, all of these factors are less important. Long-term TPN catheters can be maintained for months with low rates of infection, and there is no cutoff time at which colonization and clinical infection accelerate. Today, when the need for long-term catheterization is anticipated, surgically implanted catheters should be used. These catheters have low infection rates and are never changed routinely [133]. PICCs are also an acceptable option for patients requiring long-term CVC.

Catheters inserted percutaneously in the critical care unit, however, are not subject to ideal conditions and have a finite lifespan. For practical purposes, multilumen catheters have replaced single-lumen catheters for many indications for central venous access. Because catheter hubs are a potential source of infection and triple-lumen catheters can require three times the number of tubing changes, it was widely believed that they would have a higher infection rate. Studies have presented conflicting results, but overall the data support the view that triple-lumen catheters have a modestly higher rate of infection [134–136]. If used efficiently, however, they provide greater intravascular access per device and can decrease the total number of catheter days and exposure to central venipuncture. A slight increase in infection rate per catheter is therefore justifiable from an overall risk–benefit analysis, if multilumen catheters are used only when multiple infusion ports are truly indicated.

Finally, it was hoped that routine subcutaneous tunneling of short-term CVCs, similar to long-term catheters, might be an effective way to minimize CRI. This approach is rational since the long subcutaneous tract acts to stabilize the catheter and perhaps act as a barrier to bacterial invasion, and great technical skill is not required. A meta-analysis did not support the routine practice of tunneling all percutaneously inserted CVCs [137], and it is not a common practice. However, further studies of the tunneling of short-term IJV and FV catheters are warranted, especially hemodialysis catheters, since these sites have a higher infection rate and past studies have generally favored this approach [108,138].

Duration of Catheterization

The length of catheterization should be based solely on the need for continued catheterization of the patient. No catheter should be left in longer than absolutely necessary. Most data suggest that the daily risk of infection remains relatively constant and routine replacement of CVCs without a clinical indication does not reduce the rate of CRI [137,139]. Multiple clinical and experimental studies have also demonstrated that guidewire exchanges neither decrease nor increase infectious risk [140].

The above-mentioned recommendations do not necessarily apply to other special-use catheters, which can be exposed to different clinical situations and risk. Pulmonary artery catheters (PACs) and the introducer should be removed after 96 to 120 hours because of the increased risk of infection after this time [141]. These catheters are at greater risk for infection because patients are sicker, the introducer used for insertion is shorter, and catheter manipulations are frequent.

Catheters inserted for acute temporary hemodialysis historically have had a higher rate of infection than other percutaneously placed catheters. Factors contributing to the increased rate have not been completely elucidated, but logically patient factors probably influence the incidence of infection more than the type of catheter or site of insertion [84]. For acutely ill, hospitalized patients, temporary dialysis catheters should be managed similarly to other multilumen catheters, recognizing that the underlying propensity for infection is distinctly higher [108]. As mentioned earlier, perhaps this is the area that tunneling of catheters should be more thoroughly investigated. For ambulatory outpatients, long-term experience with double-lumen, Dacron-cuffed, silicone CVCs inserted in the IJV has been positive [142].

Site of Insertion

The condition of the site is more important than the location. Whenever possible, sites involved by infection, burns, or other dermatologic processes, or in close proximity to a heavily colonized area (e.g., tracheostomy) should not be used as primary access. Data tends to support that PICC and SCV catheters are associated with the lowest rate of CRI, and IJV and FV catheters the highest [101].

Guidewire Exchanges

Guidewire exchanges have always been theoretically flawed as a form of infection control, because although a new catheter is placed, the site, specifically the intradermal tract, remains the same. Studies have shown that when the tract and old catheter are colonized, the new catheter invariably also becomes infected. Alternatively, if the initial catheter is not colonized, there is no reason the new catheter will be more resistant to subsequent infection than the original one. In neither situation will a guidewire change prevent infection. However, guidewire changes continue to have a valuable role for replacing defective catheters, exchanging one type of catheter for another, and in the evaluation of a febrile patient with an existing central catheter. In the latter situation, the physician can assess the sterility of the catheter tract without subjecting the patient to a new venipuncture. However one decides to use guidewire exchanges, they must be performed properly. Using maximal barriers, the catheter should be withdrawn until an intravascular segment is exposed, transected sterilely, and the guidewire inserted through the distal lumen. The catheter fragment can then be removed (always culture the tip) and a new catheter threaded over the guidewire. To ensure sterility, most operators should re-prep the site and change gloves before inserting the new catheter or introducer over the guidewire. Insertion of the guidewire through the distal hub of the existing catheter is not appropriate.

NEW CATHETER TECHNOLOGIES

Improvements in catheter technology continue to play an important role in minimizing catheter complications. Catheter material is an important factor in promoting thrombogenesis and adherence of organisms. Most catheters used for CVC are composed of flexible silicone (for surgical implantation) and polyurethane (for percutaneous insertion), because research has shown these materials are less thrombogenic. Knowledge of the pathogenesis of most CRI has stimulated improvements designed to interrupt bacterial colonization of the skin site, catheter, and intradermal tract, and migration to the catheter tip. Antibiotic and antiseptic impregnated catheters represent a major advance in catheter management. Catheters differ from one another by the type of antibiotic or antiseptic with which they are impregnated. Clinical results with these commercially available catheters have been variable [143,144], likely due to varying practices and the baseline infection rate. Good randomized controlled trials comparing the various types of antiseptic catheters with each other are lacking, but we believe that current evidence supports using one of the above catheters if the baseline CRI rate remains high after instituting infection control practices [101,132,133]. The preponderance of data indicates that in real-life practice, these catheters decrease the rate of CRI and improve patient safety, likely at a neutral or favorable cost [129,145]. The emergence of resistant organisms and allergic reactions has not yet been a problem, but ongoing surveillance is needed.

SYSTEMS-BASED MEASURES

Not surprisingly, evidence is pointing to systems-based factors as being more important in reducing the incidence of CRI than any new technology. At Johns Hopkins, the addition of five systems-based changes reduced the CRI rate from 11.3 to 0 per 1,000 catheter days. These simple interventions were: education of physicians and nurses of evidence-based infection control practices, creation of a central catheter insertion cart which contained every item needed for insertion of a catheter, daily questioning of whether catheters could be removed, a bedside checklist for insertion of catheters, and empowering nurses to stop procedures where the infection control guidelines were not being followed [146]. Similar interventions in Pennsylvania reduced their CRI rate from 4.31 to 1.36 per 1,000 catheter days [147]. A statewide initiative in Michigan, the Keystone Project, implemented these strategies on a large scale over the entire state with equally impressive results [1]. Despite the fact that these and other simple systems interventions and implementation require very little capital outlay, many ICUs have yet to adopt them [148,149].

MANAGEMENT OF THE FEBRILE PATIENT

Patients with a CVC frequently develop fever. Removal of the catheter in every febrile patient is neither feasible nor clinically indicated, as the fever is often unrelated to the catheter. Management must be individualized (Fig. 2.7) and depends on type of catheter, duration of catheterization, anticipated need for continued central venous access, risk of establishing new central venous access, and underlying medical condition and prognosis. All critical care units must have protocols for managing the febrile, catheterized patient [150]. Decisions to remove, change over a guidewire, or leave catheters in place must be based on a fundamental knowledge of risks and benefits for catheters inserted at each site.

Catheter sites in the febrile patient should always be examined. Clinical infection of the site mandates removal of the catheter and institution of antibiotics. Surgically implanted catheters are not easily removed or replaced and can often be left in place while the infection is cleared with antibiotics, unless tunnel infection is present. Percutaneously inserted CVCs are relatively easily removed, and the risks of leaving a catheter in place through an infected site outweigh the risk of replacement at a new site, except in very unusual circumstances.

In patients with severe sepsis or septic shock, CVCs should be considered a possible source. If all catheter sites appear normal and a noncatheter source of infection is implicated, appropriate antibiotics are initiated and the catheters left in place. The usual guidelines for subsequent catheter management should be followed, and this rarely results in treatment failure. In contrast, if a noncatheter source cannot be identified, then central catheters in place more than 3 days should be managed individually, with attention to duration of catheterization (Table 2.3). Only for patients with excessive risks for new catheter placement (i.e., severe coagulopathy), guidewire exchange of the catheter is justifiable after obtaining blood cultures through the catheter and a peripheral site and semiquantitative culture of a catheter segment. If within the next 24 hours an alternative source for sepsis is found, or if the catheter segment culture is negative and the patient improves and stabilizes, the guidewire catheter can be left in place and the risk of catheter insertion avoided. Alternatively, if the catheter culture becomes positive, especially if the same organism is identified on peripheral blood cultures, the cutaneous tract is also infected and the guidewire catheter should be removed and alternative access achieved.

The most common situation is the stable febrile patient with a CVC in place (Table 2.4). As mentioned earlier, if a noncatheter source for fever is identified, appropriate antibiotics are given and the catheter is left in place, assuming it is still needed and the site is clinically uninvolved. In the patient

TABLE 2.4

APPROACH TO THE FEBRILE PATIENT WITH A CENTRAL VENOUS CATHETER

1. Catheter no longer needed—remove and culture tip
2. Patient with severe sepsis or septic shock (catheter >72 hr)—promptly remove catheter and culture tip
3. Patient with severe sepsis or septic shock (catheter <72 h)—initiate antibiotics, remove catheter if no improvement in 12–24 h
4. Stable patient (catheter >72 h)—guidewire exchange with tip culture if culture with ≥15 CFU—remove catheter

with no obvious source of fever [1], indications for the CVCs should be reviewed and the catheter withdrawn if it is no longer required. Otherwise, the physician must decide between observation, potential premature withdrawal, and a guidewire change of the catheter. If the catheter is less than 72 hours old, observation is reasonable, as it is very unlikely that the catheter is already infected unless breaks in sterile technique occurred during insertion. For catheters that are at least 72 hours old, guidewire exchanges are rational but, in our opinion, not mandatory. An appropriately performed guidewire change allows comparison of catheter segment cultures to other clinical cultures without subjecting the patient to repeat venipuncture. If within the next 24 hours an alternative source for fever is identified, and/or the initial catheter segment culture is negative, then the guidewire catheter can be left in place.

When catheter-related bacteremia does develop, antibiotic therapy is necessary for a period of 7 to 14 days. Even in patients treated for 14 days, metastatic infection can develop. Catheter-related fever, infection, and septicemia is a complicated disease, and the expertise of an infectious disease consultant may be required to assist with the decision on how long to continue antibiotic therapy.

References

1. Pronovost P, Needham D, Berenholtz S, et al: An intervention to decrease catheter-related bloodstream infections in the ICU. *N Engl J Med* 356:2725–2731, 2007.
2. Barsuk JH, McGaghie WC, Cohen ER, et al: Simulation-based mastery learning reduces complications during central venous catheter insertion in a medical intensive care unit. *Crit Care Med* 37:2697–2701, 2009.
3. Blitt RC, Reed SF, Britt LD: Central line simulation: a new training algorithm. *Am Surg* 73:680–682, 2007.
4. Abboud PA, Kendall JL: Ultrasound guidance for vascular access. *Emerg Med Clin North Am* 22(3):749–773, 2004.
5. Denys BG, Uretsky BF, Reddy PS: Ultrasound-assisted cannulation of the internal jugular vein. A prospective comparison to the external landmark-guided technique. *Circulation* 87(5):1557–1562, 1993.
6. Feller-Kopman D: Ultrasound-guided internal jugular access: a proposed standardized approach and implications for training and practice. *Chest* 132(1):302–309, 2007.
7. Calvert N, Hind D, McWilliams RG, et al: The effectiveness and cost-effectiveness of ultrasound locating devices for central venous access: a systematic review and economic evaluation. *Health Technol Assess* 7:1–84, 2003.
8. Rothschild JM: Ultrasound guidance of central vein catheterization. In: Making health care safer: A critical analysis of patient safety practices. Agency for Healthcare Research and Quality. Available at http://www.ahrq.gov/clinic/ptsafety/chap21.htm .
9. Milling TJ Jr., Rose J, Briggs WM, et al: Randomized, controlled clinical trial of point-of-care limited ultrasonography assistance of central venous cannulation: the Third Sonography Outcomes Assessment Program (SOAP-3) Trial. *Crit Care Med* 33(8):1764–1769, 2005.
10. Maecken T, Grau T: Ultrasound imaging in vascular access. *Crit Care Med* 35[5, Suppl]:S178–S185, 2007.
11. Mansfield PF, Hohn DC, Fornage BD, et al: Complications and failures of subclavian-vein catheterization. *New Engl J Med* 331:1735–1738, 1994.
12. Sandhu NS: Transpectoral ultrasound-guided catheterization of the axillary vein: an alternative to standard catheterization of the subclavian vein. *Anesth Analg* 99:183–187, 2004.
13. Graber D, Dailey RH: Catheter flow rates updated. *J Am Coll Emerg Physicians* 6:518, 1977.
14. Schwab SJ, Quarles D, Middleton JP, et al: Hemodialysis-associated subclavian vein stenosis. *Kidney Int* 38:1156, 1988.
15. Cimochowski G, Sartain J, Worley E, et al: Clear superiority of internal jugular access over subclavian vein for temporary dialysis. *Kidney Int* 33:230, 1987.
16. Firek AF, Cutler RE, St John Hammond PG: Reappraisal of femoral vein cannulation for temporary hemodialysis vascular access. *Nephron* 47:227, 1987.
17. Doerfler ME, Kaufman B, Goldenberg AS: Central venous catheter placement in patients with disorders of hemostasis. *Chest* 110:185, 1996.
18. Dripps RD, Eckenhoff JE, Vandam LD: *Introduction to Anesthesia: The Principles of Safe Practice*. 6th ed. Philadelphia, PA, WB Saunders, 1982.
19. Emerman CL, Pinchak AC, Hancock D, et al: Effect of injection site on circulation times during cardiac arrest. *Crit Care Med* 16:1138, 1988.
20. Hilty WM, Hudson PA, Levitt MA, et al: Real-time ultrasound-guided femoral vein catheterization during cardiopulmonary resuscitation. *Ann Emerg Med* 3:331–336, 1997.
21. Rivers E, Nguyen B, Havstad S, et al: Early goal-directed therapy in the treatment of severe sepsis and septic shock. *N Engl J Med* 345:1368, 2001.
22. Trzeciak S, Dellinger RP, Abate NL, et al: Translating research to clinical practice: a 1-year experience with implementing early goal-directed therapy for septic shock in the emergency department. *Chest* 129:225, 2006.
23. Davison D, Chawla L, Selassie L, et al: Femoral based central Venous oxygen saturation is not a reliable substitute for subclavian/internal jugular based central venous oxygen saturation in critically ill patients. *Chest* 138:76–83, 2010.
24. The National Heart, Lung, and Blood Institute Acute Respiratory Distress Syndrome (ARDS) Clinical Trials Network: Comparison of two fluid management strategies in acute lung injury. *N Engl J Med* 354:1–12, 2006.
25. Stuke L, Jennings A, Gunst M, et al: Universal consent practices in academic intensive care units (ICUs). *J Intensive Care Med* 25:46–52, 2010.
26. Harting BP, Talbot TR, Dellit TH, et al: University health system consortium quality performance study of the insertion and care of central venous catheters. *Infect Control Hosp Epidemiol* 29:440–442, 2008.
27. Long R, Kassum D, Donen N, et al: Cardiac tamponade complicating central venous catheterization for total parenteral nutrition: a review. *J Crit Care* 2:39, 1987.
28. Curelaru I, Linder LE, Gustavsson B: Displacement of catheters inserted through internal jugular veins with neck flexion and extension. A preliminary study. *Intensive Care Med* 6:179, 1980.
29. Wojciechowski J, Curelaru I, Gustavsson B, et al: "Half-way" venous catheters. III. Tip displacements with movements of the upper extremity. *Acta Anaesthesiol Scand* 81:36–39, 1985.
30. Marx GF: Hazards associated with central venous pressure monitoring. *N Y State J Med* 69:955, 1969.
31. Andrews RT, Bova DA, Venbrux AC: How much guidewire is too much? Direct measurement of the distance from subclavian and internal jugular vein access sites to the superior vena cava-atrial junction during central venous catheter placement. *Crit Care Med* 28:138, 2000.
32. Czepizak CA, O'Callaghan JM, Venus B: Evaluation of formulas for optimal positioning of central venous catheters. *Chest* 107:1662, 1995.
33. Aslamy Z, Dewald CL, Heffner JE: MRI of central venous anatomy: implications for central venous catheter insertion. *Chest* 114:820, 1998.
34. Robinson JF, Robinson WA, Cohn A, et al: Perforation of the great vessels during central venous line placement. *Arch Intern Med* 155:1225, 1995.
35. Duntley P, Siever J, Korwes ML, et al: Vascular erosion by central venous catheters. Clinical features and outcome. [Review] [44 refs]. *Chest* 101:1633, 1992.
36. Doering RB, Stemmer EA, Connolly JE: Complications of indwelling venous catheters, with particular reference to catheter embolus. *Am J Surg* 114:259, 1967.
37. Orebaugh SL: Venous air embolism: clinical and experimental considerations. [Review] [94 refs]. *Crit Care Med* 20:1169, 1992.
38. Ely EW, Hite RD, Baker AM, et al: Venous air embolism from central venous catheterization: a need for increased physician awareness. *Crit Care Med* 27:2113, 1999.
39. Mumtaz H, Williams V, Hauer-Jensen M, et al: Central venous catheter placement in patients with disorders of hemostasis. *Am J Surg* 180:503, 2000.
40. Brismar B, Hardstedt C, Jacobson S: Diagnosis of thrombosis by catheter phlebography after prolonged central venous catheterization. *Ann Surg* 194:779, 1981.

41. Efsing HO, Lindblad B, Mark J, et al: Thromboembolic complications from central venous catheters: a comparison of three catheter materials. *World J Surg* 7:419, 1983.
42. Axelsson CK, Efsen F: Phlebography in long-term catheterization of the subclavian vein. A retrospective study in patients with severe gastrointestinal disorders. *Scand J Gastroenterol* 13:933, 1978.
43. Bonnet F, Loriferne JF, Texier JP, et al: Evaluation of Doppler examination for diagnosis of catheter-related deep vein thrombosis. *Intensive Care Med* 15:238, 1989.
44. Prandoni P, Polistena P, Bernardi E, et al: Upper-extremity deep vein thrombosis. Risk factors, diagnosis, and complications. *Arch Intern Med* 157:57, 1997.
45. Raad II, Luna M, Khalil SA, et al: The relationship between the thrombotic and infectious complications of central venous catheters. *JAMA* 271:1014, 1994.
46. Munoz FJ, Mismeti P, Poggio R, et al: Clinical outcome of patients with upper-extremity deep vein thrombosis. Results from the RIETE registry. *Chest* 133:143–148, 2008.
47. Timsit JF, Farkas JC, Boyer JM, et al: Central vein catheter-related thrombosis in intensive care patients: incidence, risks factors, and relationship with catheter-related sepsis. *Chest* 114:207, 1998.
48. Ng PK, Ault MJ, Maldonado LS: Peripherally inserted central catheters in the intensive care unit. *J Intensive Care Med* 11:49, 1996.
49. Merrell SW, Peatross BG, Grossman MD, et al: Peripherally inserted central venous catheters. Low-risk alternatives for ongoing venous access. *West J Med* 160:25, 1994.
50. Netter FH: *Atlas of Human Anatomy.* New Jersey, Summit, 1989.
51. Williams PL, Warwick R: *Gray's Anatomy*. 8th ed. Philadelphia, PA WB Saunders, 1980.
52. Raad I, Davis S, Becker M, et al: Low infection rate and long durability of nontunneled silastic catheters. A safe and cost-effective alternative for long-term venous access. *Arch Intern Med* 153:1791, 1993.
53. Duerksen DR, Papineau N, Siemens J, et al: Peripherally inserted central catheters for parenteral nutrition: a comparison with centrally inserted catheters. *J Parenter Enteral Nutr* 23:85, 1999.
54. Gustavsson B, Curelaru I, Hultman E, et al: Displacements of the soft, polyurethane central venous catheters inserted by basilic and cephalic veins. *Acta Anaesthesiol Scand* 27:102, 1983.
55. Malatinsky J, Faybik M, Griffith M, et al: Venipuncture, catheterization and failure to position correctly during central venous cannulation. *Resuscitation* 10:259, 1983.
56. Goldfarb G, Lebrec D: Percutaneous cannulation of the internal jugular vein in patients with coagulopathies: an experience based on 1,000 attempts. *Anesthesiology* 56:321, 1982.
57. Johnson FE: Internal jugular vein catheterization. *N Y State J Med* 78:2168, 1978.
58. Sznajder JI, Zveibil FR, Bitterman H, et al: Central vein catheterization. Failure and complication rates by three percutaneous approaches. *Arch Intern Med* 146:259, 1986.
59. Tripathi M, Pandey M: Anchoring of the internal jugular vein with a pilot needle to facilitate its puncture with a wide bore needle: a randomised, prospective, clinical study. *Anaesthesia* 61:15, 2006.
60. Eisenhauer ED, Derveloy RJ, Hastings PR: Prospective evaluation of central venous pressure (CVP) catheters in a large city-county hospital. *Ann Surg* 196:560, 1982.
61. Klineberg PL, Greenhow DE, Ellison N: Hematoma following internal jugular vein cannulation. *Anesth Intensive Care* 8:94, 1980.
62. Briscoe CE, Bushman JA, McDonald WI: Extensive neurological damage after cannulation of internal jugular vein. *Br Med J* 1:314, 1974.
63. Schwartz AJ, Jobes CR, Greenhow DE, et al: Carotid artery puncture with internal jugular cannulation. *Anesthesiology* 51:S160, 1980.
64. Nicholson T, Ettles D, Robinson G: Managing inadvertent arterial catheterization during central venous access procedures. *Cardiovasc Interven Radiol* 27:21, 2004.
65. Shah PM, Babu SC, Goyal A, et al: Arterial misplacement of large-caliber cannulas during jugular vein catheterization: case for surgical management. *J Am Coll Surg* 198:939, 2004.
66. Ruesch S, Walder B, Tramer MR: Complications of central venous catheters: internal jugular versus subclavian access—a systematic review. [Review] [53 refs]. *Crit Care Med* 30:454, 2002.
67. Nagai K, Kemmotsu O: An inadvertent insertion of a Swan-Ganz catheter into the intrathecal space. *Anesthesiology* 62:848, 1985.
68. Schwartz AJ, Jobes DR, Levy WJ, et al: Intrathoracic vascular catheterization via the external jugular vein. *Anesthesiology* 56:400, 1982.
69. Blitt CD, Carlson GL, Wright WA, et al: J-wire versus straight wire for central venous system cannulation via the external jugular vein. *Anesth Analg* 61:536, 1982.
70. Giesy J: External jugular vein access to central venous system. *JAMA* 219:1216, 1972.
71. Riddell GS, Latto IP, Ng WS: External jugular vein access to the central venous system – a trial of two types of catheter. *Br J Anaesth* 54:535, 1982.
72. Jobes DR, Schwartz AJ, Greenhow DE, et al: Safer jugular vein cannulation: recognition of arterial puncture and preferential use of the external jugular route. *Anesthesiology* 59:353, 1983.
73. Moncrief JA: Femoral catheters. *Ann Surg* 147:166, 1958.
74. Bansmer G, Keith D, Tesluk H: Complications following use of indwelling catheters of inferior vena cava. *JAMA* 167:1606, 1958.
75. Dailey RH: "Code Red" protocol for resuscitation of the exsanguinated patient. *J Emerg Med* 2:373, 1985.
76. Kruse JA, Carlson RW: Infectious complications of femoral vs internal jugular and subclavian vein central venous catheterization. *Crit Care Med* 19:843, 1991.
77. O'Grady NP, Alexander M, Burns LA, et al: Guidelines for the prevention of catheter-related infections. *Morb Mortal Weekly Rep*, in press.
78. Deshpande KS, Hatem C, Ulirch HL, et al: The incidence of infectious complication of central venous catheters at the subclavian, internal jugular, and femoral sites in an intensive care unit population. *Crit Care Med* 33:13, 2005.
79. Dailey RH: Femoral vein cannulation: a review. [Review] [26 refs]. *J Emerg Med* 2:367, 1985.
80. Sharp KW, Spees EK, Selby LR, et al: Diagnosis and management of retroperitoneal hematomas after femoral vein cannulation for hemodialysis. *Surgery* 95:90, 1984.
81. Fuller TJ, Mahoney JJ, Juncos LI, et al: Arteriovenous fistula after femoral vein catheterization. *JAMA* 236:2943, 1976.
82. Norwood S, Wilkins HE 3rd, Vallina VL, et al: The safety of prolonging the use of central venous catheters: a prospective analysis of the effects of using antiseptic-bonded catheters with daily site care. *Crit Care Med* 28:1376, 2000.
83. Goetz AM, Wagener MM, Miller JM, et al: Risk of infection due to central venous catheters: effect of site of placement and catheter type. *Infect Control Hosp Epidemiol* 19:842, 1998.
84. Parienti JJ, Thirion M, Megarbane B, et al: Femoral vs jugular venous catheterization and risk of nosocomial events in adults requiring acute renal replacement therapy. A randomized controlled trial. *JAMA* 299:2413–2422, 2008.
85. Stenzel JP, Green TP, Fuhrman BP, et al: Percutaneous femoral venous catheterizations: a prospective study of complications. *J Pediatr* 114:411, 1989.
86. Russell JA, Joel M, Hudson RJ, et al: Prospective evaluation of radial and femoral artery catheterization sites in critically ill adults. *Crit Care Med* 11:936, 1983.
87. Lorente L, Jimenez A, Santana M, et al: Microorganisms responsible for intravascular catheter-related bloodstream infection according to the catheter site. *Crit Care Med* 35:2424–2427, 2007.
88. Lynn KL, Maling TM: A major pulmonary embolus as a complication of femoral vein catheterization. *Br J Radiol* 50:667, 1977.
89. Moosman DA: The anatomy of infraclavicular subclavian vein catheterization and its complications. *Surg Gynecol Obstet* 136:71, 1973.
90. Eerola R, Kaukinen L, Kaukinen S: Analysis of 13 800 subclavian vein catheterizations. *Acta Anaesthesiol Scand* 29:193, 1985.
91. James PM Jr, Myers RT: Central venous pressure monitoring: misinterpretation, abuses, indications and a new technique. *Ann Surg* 175:693, 1972.
92. MacDonnell JE, Perez H, Pitts SR, et al: Supraclavicular subclavian vein catheterization: modified landmarks for needle insertion. *Ann Emerg Med* 21:421, 1992.
93. Dronen S, Thompson B, Nowak R, et al: Subclavian vein catheterization during cardiopulmonary resuscitation. A prospective comparison of the supraclavicular and infraclavicular percutaneous approaches. *JAMA* 247:3227, 1982.
94. Sterner S, Plummer DW, Clinton J, et al: A comparison of the supraclavicular approach and the infraclavicular approach for subclavian vein catheterization. *Ann Emerg Med* 15:421, 1986.
95. Park HP, Jeon Y, Hwang JW, et al: Influence of orientations of guidewire tip on the placement of subclavian venous catheters. *Acta Anaesthesiol Scand* 49:1460, 2005.
96. McGee WT, Ackerman BL, Rouben LR, et al: Accurate placement of central venous catheters: a prospective, randomized, multicenter trial. *Crit Care Med* 21:1118, 1993.
97. Seneff MG: Central venous catheterization: a comprehensive review. *J Intensive Care Med* 2:218, 1987.
98. Simpson ET, Aitchison JM: Percutaneous infraclavicular subclavian vein catheterization in shocked patients: a prospective study in 172 patients. *J Trauma-Injury Inf Crit Care* 22:781, 1982.
99. Herbst CA Jr: Indications, management, and complications of percutaneous subclavian catheters. An audit. *Arch Sur* 113:1421, 1978.
100. Bernard RW, Stahl WM: Subclavian vein catheterizations: a prospective study. I. Non-infectious complications. *Ann Surg* 173:184, 1971.
101. Taylor RW, Palagiri AV: Central venous catheterization. *Crit Care Med* 35:1390–1396, 2007.
102. Despars JA, Sassoon CS, Light RW: Significance of iatrogenic pneumothoraces. *Chest* 105:1147, 1994.
103. Matz R: Complications of determining the central venous pressure. *N Engl J Med* 273:703, 1965.
104. Maki DG, Weise CE, Sarafin HW: A semiquantitative culture method for identifying intravenous-catheter-related infection. *N Engl J Med* 296:1305, 1977.
105. Raad I, Hanna HA, Alakech B, et al: Differential time to positivity: a useful method for diagnosing catheter-related bloodstream infections [see comment] [summary for patients in *Ann Intern Med* 2004;140(1):I39; PMID: 14706995]. *Ann Intern Med* 140:18, 2004.

106. Cooper GL, Hopkins CC: Rapid diagnosis of intravascular catheter-associated infection by direct Gram staining of catheter segments. *N Engl J Med* 312:1142, 1985.
107. Zufferey J, Rime B, Francioli P, et al: Simple method for rapid diagnosis of catheter-associated infection by direct acridine orange staining of catheter tips. *J Clin Microbiol* 26:175, 1988.
108. Maki DG, Kluger DM, Crnich CJ: The risk of bloodstream infection in adults with different intravascular devices: a systematic review of 200 published prospective studies. *Mayo Clin Proc* 81:1159–1171, 2006.
109. Edwards JR, Peterson KD, Banerjee S, et al: National Healthcare Safety Network (NHSN) report: data summary fro 2006 through 2008, issued December 2009. *Am J Infect Control* 37:783–805, 2009.
110. Warren DK, Quadir WW, Hollenbeak CS, et al: Attributable cost of catheter-associated bloodstream infections among intensive care patients in a nonteaching hospital. *Crit Care Med* 34:2084–2089, 2006.
111. Blot SI, Depuydt P, Amnemans L, et al: Clinical and economic outcomes in critically ill patients with nosocomial catheter-related bloodstream infections. *Clin Infect Dis* 41:1591–1598, 2005.
112. Wenzel RP, Edmond MB: The impact of hospital-acquired bloodstream infections. *Emerg Infect Dis* 7:172–177, 2001.
113. Harbarth S, Sax H, Gastmeier P: The preventable proportion of nosocomial infections: an overview of published reports. *J Hosp Infect* 54:258–266, 2003.
114. Passerini L, Lam K, Costerton JW, et al: Biofilms on indwelling vascular catheters. *Crit Care Med* 20:665, 1992.
115. Olson ME, Lam K, Bodey GP, et al: Evaluation of strategies for central venous catheter replacement. *Crit Care Med* 20:797, 1992.
116. Maki DG, Cobb L, Garman JK, et al: An attachable silver-impregnated cuff for prevention of infection with central venous catheters: a prospective randomized multicenter trial. *Am J Med* 85:307, 1988.
117. Moro ML, Vigano EF, Cozzi Lepri A: Risk factors for central venous catheter-related infections in surgical and intensive care units. The Central Venous Catheter-Related Infections Study Group [erratum appears in *Infect Control Hosp Epidemiol* 1994;15(8):508–509]. *Infect Control Hosp Epidemiol* 15:253, 1994.
118. Raad I, Costerton W, Sabharwal U, et al: Ultrastructural analysis of indwelling vascular catheters: a quantitative relationship between luminal colonization and duration of placement. *J Infect Dis* 168:400, 1993.
119. Raad II, Hohn DC, Gilbreath BJ, et al: Prevention of central venous catheter-related infections by using maximal sterile barrier precautions during insertion. *Infect Control Hosp Epidemiol* 15:231, 1994.
120. Mimoz O, Pieroni L, Lawrence C, et al: Prospective, randomized trial of two antiseptic solutions for prevention of central venous or arterial catheter colonization and infection in intensive care unit patients. *Crit Care Med* 24:1818, 1996.
121. Maki DG, Ringer M, Alvarado CJ: Prospective randomised trial of povidone-iodine, alcohol, and chlorhexidine for prevention of infection associated with central venous and arterial catheters. *Lancet* 338:339, 1991.
122. Parras F, Ena J, Bouza E, et al: Impact of an educational program for the prevention of colonization of intravascular catheters. *Infect Control Hosp Epidemiol* 15:239, 1994.
123. Maki DG, Botticelli JT, LeRoy ML, et al: Prospective study of replacing administration sets for intravenous therapy at 48- vs 72-hour intervals. 72 hours is safe and cost-effective. *JAMA* 258:1777, 1987.
124. Maki DG, Cobb L, Garman JK, et al: An attachable silver-impregnated cuff for prevention of infection with central venous catheters: a prospective randomized multicenter trial. *Am J Med* 85:307, 1988.
125. Timsit JF, Schwebel C, Bouadma L, et al: Chlorhexadine-impregnated sponges and less frequent dressing changes for prevention of catheter-related infections in critically ill adults. *JAMA* 301:1231–1241, 2009.
126. Hill RL, Fisher AP, Ware RJ, et al: Mupirocin for the reduction of colonization of internal jugular cannulae—a randomized controlled trial. *J Hosp Infect* 15:311, 1990.
127. Miller JJ, Venus B, Mathru M: Comparison of the sterility of long-term central venous catheterization using single lumen, triple lumen, and pulmonary artery catheters. *Crit Care Med* 12:634, 1984.
128. Arnow PM, Quimosing EM, Beach M: Consequences of intravascular catheter sepsis. *Clin Infect Dis* 16:778, 1993.
129. Veenstra DL, Saint S, Sullivan SD: Cost-effectiveness of antiseptic-impregnated central venous catheters for the prevention of catheter-related bloodstream infection. *JAMA* 282:554, 1999.
130. Hanley EM, Veeder A, Smith T, et al: Evaluation of an antiseptic triple-lumen catheter in an intensive care unit. *Crit Care Med* 28:366, 2000.
131. Flowers RH 3rd, Schwenzer KJ, Kopel RF, et al: Efficacy of an attachable subcutaneous cuff for the prevention of intravascular catheter-related infection. A randomized, controlled trial. *JAMA* 261:878, 1989.
132. Kamal GD, Pfaller MA, Rempe LE, et al: Reduced intravascular catheter infection by antibiotic bonding. A prospective, randomized, controlled trial. *JAMA* 265:2364, 1991.
133. Collin GR: Decreasing catheter colonization through the use of an antiseptic-impregnated catheter: a continuous quality improvement project. *Chest* 115:1632, 1999.
134. Clarke DE, Raffin TA: Infectious complications of indwelling long-term central venous catheters. [Review] [48 refs]. *Chest* 97:966, 1990.
135. McCarthy MC, Shives JK, Robison RJ, et al: Prospective evaluation of single and triple lumen catheters in total parenteral nutrition. *JPEN: J Parenter Enteral Nutr* 11:259, 1987.
136. Clark-Christoff N, Watters VA, Sparks W, et al: Use of triple-lumen subclavian catheters for administration of total parenteral nutrition. *JPEN: J Parenter Enteral Nutr* 16:403, 1992.
137. Randolph AG, Cook DJ, Gonzales CA, et al: Tunneling short-term central venous catheters to prevent catheter-related infection: a meta-analysis of randomized, controlled trials. *Crit Care Med* 26:1452, 1998.
138. Farkas JC, Liu N, Bleriot JP, et al: Single- versus triple-lumen central catheter-related sepsis: a prospective randomized study in a critically ill population. *Am J Med* 93:277, 1992.
139. Eyer S, Brummitt C, Crossley K, et al: Catheter-related sepsis: prospective, randomized study of three methods of long-term catheter maintenance. *Crit Care Med* 18:1073, 1990.
140. Cobb DK, High KP, Sawyer RG, et al: A controlled trial of scheduled replacement of central venous and pulmonary-artery catheters. *N Engl J Med* 327:1062, 1992.
141. Badley AD, Steckelberg JM, Wollan PC, et al: Infectious rates of central venous pressure catheters: comparison between newly placed catheters and those that have been changed. *Mayo Clin Proc* 71:838, 1996.
142. Rello J, Coll P, Net A, et al: Infection of pulmonary artery catheters. Epidemiologic characteristics and multivariate analysis of risk factors. [Review] [37 refs]. *Chest* 103:132, 1993.
143. Moss AH, Vasilakis C, Holley JL, et al: Use of a silicone dual-lumen catheter with a Dacron cuff as a long-term vascular access for hemodialysis patients. *Am J Kidney Dis* 16:211, 1990.
144. Kalfon P, de Vaumas C, Samba D, et al: Comparison of silver-impregnated with standard multi-lumen central venous catheters in critically ill patients. *Crit Care Med* 35:1032–1039, 2007.
145. Brun-Boisson C, Doyon F, Sollet JP, et al: Prevention of intravascular catheter-related infection with newer chlorhexidine-silver sulfadiazine-coated catheters: a randomized controlled trial. *Intensive Care Med* 30: 837–843, 2004.
146. Darouiche RO, Raad II, Heard SO, et al: A comparison of two antimicrobial-impregnated central venous catheters. Catheter Study Group. *N Engl J Med* 340:1, 1999.
147. Berenholtz SM, Pronovost PJ, Lipsett PA, et al: Eliminating catheter-related bloodstream infections in the intensive care unit. *Crit Care Med* 32:2014–2020, 2004.
148. Centers for Disease Control and Prevention (CDC): Reduction in central line-associated bloodstream infections among patients in intensive care units–Pennsylvania, April 2001-March 2005. *MMWR Morb Mortal Wkly Rep* 54:1013, 2005.
149. Krein SL, Hofer TP, Kowalski CP, et al: Use of central venous catheter-related bloodstream infection prevention practices by US hospitals. *Mayo Clin Proc* 82:672–676, 2007.
150. O'Grady NP, Barie PS, Bartlett JG, et al: Guidelines for evaluation of new fever in critically ill adult patients: 2008 update from the American College of Critical Care Medicine and the Infectious Diseases Society of America. *Crit Care Med* 36:1330–1349, 2008.

CHAPTER 3 ■ ARTERIAL LINE PLACEMENT AND CARE

JASON LEE-LLACER AND MICHAEL G. SENEFF

Arterial catheterization remains an extremely important skill for critical care physicians. The most common indications for inserting an arterial catheter remain the need for close blood pressure monitoring and frequent blood gas sampling in unstable and ventilated patients. Newer technologies that necessitate arterial access continue to mature. For example, arterial pulse contour analysis can now be used to predict fluid responsiveness and compute cardiac output more reliably and less invasively in appropriately selected patients [1]. Although it is likely that advancements in current noninvasive technology, such as transcutaneous PCO_2 monitoring and pulse oximetry, will decrease the need for arterial catheter placement, intensivists will always need to be knowledgeable in the setup and interpretation of arterial catheter systems. In this chapter, we review the principles of hemodynamic monitoring and discuss the indications, routes, and management of arterial cannulation.

INDICATIONS FOR ARTERIAL CANNULATION

Arterial catheters should be inserted only when they are specifically required and removed immediately when no longer needed. Too often they are left in place for convenience to allow easy access to blood sampling, which leads to increased laboratory testing and excessive diagnostic blood loss [2,3]. Protocols incorporating guidelines for arterial catheterization and alternative noninvasive monitoring, such as pulse oximetry and end tidal CO_2, have realized significant improvements in resource utilization and cost savings, without impacting the quality of care [4].

The indications for arterial cannulation can be grouped into four broad categories (Table 3.1): (1) hemodynamic monitoring (blood pressure and/or cardiac output/pulse contour analysis); (2) frequent arterial blood gas sampling; (3) diagnostic or therapeutic/interventional radiology procedures, including intra-aortic balloon pump (IABP) use, arterial administration of drugs, vascular stenting and embolization, and (4) continuous cardiac output monitoring.

Noninvasive, indirect blood pressure measurements determined by auscultation of Korotkoff sounds distal to an occluding cuff (Riva–Rocci method) are generally accurate, although systolic readings are consistently lower compared to a simultaneous direct measurement. In hemodynamically unstable patients, however, indirect techniques may significantly underestimate blood pressure. Automated noninvasive blood pressure measurement devices can also be inaccurate, particularly in rapidly changing situations, at the extremes of blood pressure, and in patients with dysrhythmias [5]. For these reasons, direct blood pressure monitoring is usually required for unstable patients. Rapid beat-to-beat changes can easily be monitored and appropriate therapeutic modalities initiated, and variations in individual pressure waveforms may prove diagnostic. Waveform inspection can rapidly diagnose electrocardiogram lead disconnect, indicate the presence of aortic valve disease, help determine the effect of dysrhythmias on perfusion, and reveal the impact of the respiratory cycle on blood pressure (pulsus paradoxus). In addition, in mechanically ventilated patients, responsiveness to fluid boluses may be predicted by calculating the systolic pressure variation (SPV) or pulse pressure variation (PPV) from the arterial waveform, and stroke volume variation (SVV) from the pulse contour analysis. In patients on volume-controlled mechanical ventilation, all of these techniques have been shown to predict, with a high degree of accuracy, patients likely to respond (with an increase in stroke volume) to fluid volume challenge [1].

Recent advances allow continuous CO monitoring using arterial pulse contour analysis. This method relies on the assumption that the contour of the arterial pressure waveform is proportional to the stroke volume [6]. This, however, does not take into consideration the differing impedances among the arteries of individuals and different disease states and therefore requires calibration with another method of determining cardiac output [7]. This is usually done with lithium dilution or transpulmonary thermodilution methods. A different pulse contour analysis device has been introduced which does not require an additional method of determining CO for calibration, but instead estimates impedance based upon a proprietary formula that uses waveform and patient demographic data [7]. This method has significant limitations (i.e., atrial fibrillation) and there is concern that the device may not be accurate in clinical situations with dynamic changes in vascular tone (i.e., sepsis) [8]. Further data and comparison among the methods in authentic and diverse clinical situations are required before definitive recommendations can be made.

Management of complicated patients in critical care units typically requires multiple laboratory and arterial blood gas determinations. In these situations, arterial cannulation permits routine laboratory tests without multiple needle sticks and vessel trauma. In our opinion, an arterial catheter for blood gas determination should be placed when a patient requires two or more measurements daily.

EQUIPMENT, MONITORING, TECHNIQUES, AND SOURCES OF ERROR

The equipment necessary to display and measure an arterial waveform has not changed and includes (a) an appropriate intravascular catheter; (b) fluid-filled noncompliant tubing with stopcocks; (c) transducer; (d) a constant flush device; and (e) electronic monitoring equipment. Using this equipment, intravascular pressure changes are transmitted through the hydraulic (fluid-filled) elements to the transducer, which converts mechanical displacement into a proportional electrical signal.

TABLE 3.1

INDICATIONS FOR ARTERIAL CANNULATION

Hemodynamic monitoring
Acutely hypertensive or hypotensive patients
Use of vasoactive drugs
Multiple blood sampling
Ventilated patients
Limited venous access
Diagnostic or interventional radiology procedures
Intra-arterial drugs
Vascular stenting
Intra-aortic balloon pump use
Arterial embolization
Continuous cardiac output monitoring

The signal is amplified, processed, and displayed as a waveform by the monitor. Undistorted presentation of the arterial waveform is dependent on the performance of each component, and an understanding of potential problems that can interfere with overall fidelity of the system.

The major problems inherent to pressure monitoring with a catheter system are inadequate dynamic response, improper zeroing and zero drift, and improper transducer/monitor calibration. Most physicians are aware of zeroing techniques but do not appreciate the importance of dynamic response in ensuring system fidelity. Catheter-tubing-transducer systems used for pressure monitoring can best be characterized as underdamped second-order dynamic systems with mechanical parameters of elasticity, mass, and friction [9]. Overall, the dynamic response of such a system is determined by its resonant frequency and damping coefficient (zeta). The resonant or natural frequency of a system is the frequency at which it oscillates when stimulated. When the frequency content of an input signal (i.e., pressure waveform) approaches the resonant frequency of a system, progressive amplification of the output signal occurs—a phenomenon known as ringing [10]. To ensure a flat frequency response (accurate recording across a spectrum of frequencies), the resonant frequency of a monitoring system should be at least five times higher than the highest frequency in the input signal [9]. Physiologic peripheral arterial waveforms have a fundamental frequency of 3 to 5 Hz and therefore the resonant frequency of a system used to monitor arterial pressure should ideally be greater than 20 Hz to avoid ringing and systolic overshoot.

The system component most likely to cause amplification of a pressure waveform is the hydraulic element. A good hydraulic system will have a resonant frequency between 10 and 20 Hz, which may overlap with arterial pressure frequencies. Thus amplification can occur, which may require damping to accurately reproduce the waveform [11].

The damping coefficient is a measure of how quickly an oscillating system comes to rest. A system with a high damping coefficient absorbs mechanical energy well (i.e., compliant tubing), causing a diminution in the transmitted waveform. Conversely, a system with a low damping coefficient results in underdamping and systolic overshoot. Damping coefficient and resonant frequency together determine the dynamic response of a recording system. If the resonant frequency of a system is less than 7.5 Hz, the pressure waveform will be distorted no matter what the damping coefficient. On the other hand, a resonant frequency of 24 Hz allows a range in the damping coefficient of 0.15 to 1.1 without resultant distortion of the pressure waveform [9].

Although there are other techniques [12], the easiest method to test the damping coefficient and resonant frequency of a monitoring system is the fast-flush test (also known as the square wave test). This is performed at the bedside by briefly opening and closing the continuous flush device, which produces a square wave displacement on the monitor followed by a return to baseline, usually after a few smaller oscillations (Fig. 3.1). Values for the damping coefficient and resonant frequency can be computed by printing the wave on graph paper [9], but visual inspection is usually adequate to ensure a proper frequency response. An optimum fast-flush test results in one undershoot followed by small overshoot, then settles to the patient's waveform.

For peripheral pulse pressure monitoring, an adequate fast-flush test usually corresponds to a resonant frequency of 10 to 20 Hz coupled with a damping coefficient of 0.5 to 0.7. To ensure the continuing fidelity of a monitoring system, dynamic response validation by fast-flush test should be performed frequently: at least every 8 hours, with every significant change in patient hemodynamic status, after each opening of the system (zeroing, blood sampling, tubing change), and whenever the waveform appears damped [9].

With consideration of the above concepts, components of the monitoring system are designed to optimize the frequency response of the entire system. The 18- and 20-gauge catheters used to gain vascular access are not a major source of distortion but can become kinked or occluded by thrombus, resulting in overdamping of the system. Standard, noncompliant tubing is provided with most disposable transducer kits and should be as short as possible to minimize signal amplification [10]. Air bubbles in the tubing and connecting stopcocks are a notorious source of overdamping of the tracing and can be cleared by flushing through a stopcock. Currently available disposable transducers incorporate microchip technology, are very reliable, and have relatively high resonant frequencies [13]. The transducer is attached to the electronic monitoring equipment by a cable. Modern monitors have internal calibration, filter artifacts, and print the display on request. The digital readout display is usually an average of values over time and therefore does not accurately represent beat-to-beat variability. Monitors provide the capability to freeze a display with on-screen calibration to measure beat-to-beat differences in amplitude

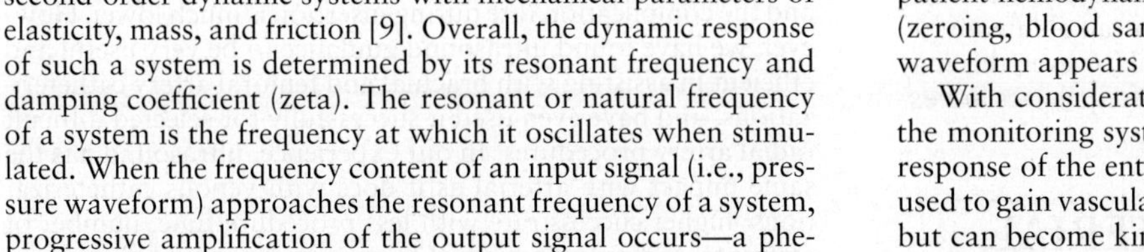

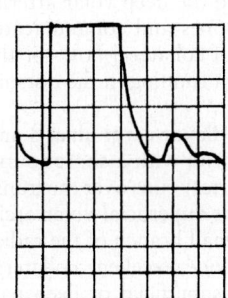

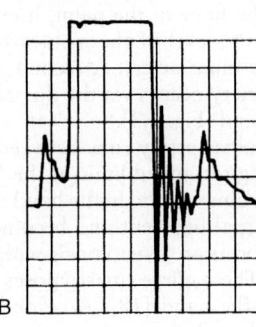

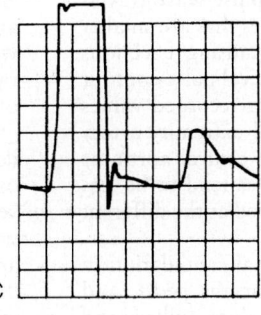

FIGURE 3.1. Fast-flush test. **A:** Overdamped system. **B:** Underdamped system. **C:** Optimal damping.

precisely. This allows measurement of the effect of ectopic beats on blood pressure, PPV, SPV, or assessment of the severity of pulsus paradoxus.

When presented with pressure data or readings believed to be inaccurate, or which are significantly different from indirect readings, a few quick checks can ensure system accuracy. Improper zeroing of the system, because of either change in patient position or zero drift, is the single most important source of error. Zeroing can be checked by opening the transducer stopcock to air and aligning with the midaxillary line, confirming that the monitor displays zero. Zeroing should be repeated with patient position changes, (a transducer that is below the zero reference line will result in falsely high readings and vice versa), when significant changes in blood pressure occur, and routinely every 6 to 8 hours because of zero drift. Disposable pressure transducers incorporate semiconductor technology and are very small, yet rugged and reliable, and due to standardization, calibration of the system is not necessary [13]. Transducers are faulty on occasion, however, and calibration may be checked by attaching a mercury manometer to the stopcock and applying 100, 150, and/or 200 mm Hg pressure. A variation of ±5 mm Hg is acceptable. If calibration is questioned and the variation is out of range, or a manometer is not available for testing, the transducer should be replaced.

If zero referencing and calibration are correct, a fast-flush test will assess the system's dynamic response. Overdamped tracings are usually caused by problems that are correctable, such as air bubbles, kinks, clot formation, overly compliant tubing, loose connections, a deflated pressure bag, or anatomical factors affecting the catheter. An underdamped tracing results in systolic overshoot and can be secondary to excessive tubing length or patient factors such as increased inotropic or chronotropic state. Many monitors can be adjusted to filter out frequencies above a certain limit, which can eliminate frequencies in the input signal causing ringing. However, this may also cause inaccurate readings if important frequencies are excluded.

TECHNIQUE OF ARTERIAL CANNULATION

Site Selection

Several factors are important in selecting the site for arterial cannulation. The ideal artery has extensive collateral circulation that will maintain the viability of distal tissues if thrombosis occurs. The site should be comfortable for the patient, accessible for nursing care and insertion, and close to the monitoring equipment. Sites involved by infection or disruption in the epidermal barrier should be avoided. Certain procedures, such as coronary artery bypass grafting, may dictate preference for one site over another. Larger arteries and catheters provide more accurate (central aortic) pressure measurements. Physicians should also be cognizant of differences in pulse contour recorded at different sites. As the pressure pulse wave travels outward from the aorta, it encounters arteries that are smaller and less elastic, with multiple branch points, causing reflections of the pressure wave. This results in a peripheral pulse contour with increased slope and amplitude, causing recorded values to be artificially elevated. As a result, distal extremity artery recordings yield higher systolic values than central aortic or femoral artery recordings. Diastolic pressures tend to be less affected, and mean arterial pressures measured at the different sites are similar [14].

The most commonly used sites for arterial cannulation in adults are the radial, femoral, axillary, dorsalis pedis, and brachial arteries. Additional sites include the ulnar, axillary and superficial temporal arteries. Peripheral sites are cannulated percutaneously with a 2-inch, 20-gauge, nontapered Teflon catheter-overneedle and larger arteries using the Seldinger technique with a prepackaged kit, typically containing a 6-inch, 18-gauge Teflon catheter, appropriate introducer needles, and guidewire.

Arterial catheterization is performed by physicians from many different specialties and usually the procedure to be performed dictates the site chosen. For example, insertion of an IABP is almost always performed through the femoral artery regardless of the specialty of the physician performing the procedure. Critical care physicians need to be facile with arterial cannulation at all sites, but the radial and femoral arteries are used successfully for more than 90% of all arterial catheterizations performed in the ICU. Although each site has unique complications, available data do not indicate a preference for any one site [15–17]. Radial artery cannulation is usually attempted initially unless the patient is in shock, on high dose vasopressors, and/or pulses are not palpable. If this fails, femoral artery cannulation should be performed. If catheterization at these two sites proves unsuccessful or not appropriate, then the dorsalis pedis, brachial, and axillary artery are the recommended alternative sites. Which of these is chosen depends on the exact clinical situation and the experience and expertise of the operator.

Use of Portable Ultrasound

Bedside ultrasound has not had as great an impact on arterial as it has on venous catheterization because vessel puncture is based on a palpable "landmark" that guides needle placement, and the complication rate during insertion is much lower. However, we have found ultrasound guidance to be very useful and efficient in assisting with brachial and femoral artery catheterizations, and have even used it successfully for selected difficult radial artery procedures. In our experience, ultrasound has the same impact with arterial as it does with venous catheterizations; higher success rate with less procedure time, number of attempts, and complications. Operator technique of ultrasound for arterial is the same as for venous catheterization and the reader is referred to Chapter 2 for a description of ultrasound equipment and technique. Ultrasound images for each of the major arterial routes are shown in Figure 3.2.

Radial Artery Cannulation

A thorough understanding of normal arterial anatomy and common anatomical variants greatly facilitates insertion of catheters and management of unexpected findings at all sites. The radial artery is one of two final branches of the brachial artery. It courses over the flexor digitorum sublimis, flexor pollicis longus, and pronator quadratus muscles and lies just lateral to the flexor carpi radialis in the forearm. As the artery enters the floor of the palm, it ends in the deep volar arterial arch at the level of the metacarpal bones and communicates with the ulnar artery. A second site of collateral flow for the radial artery occurs via the dorsal arch running in the dorsum of the hand (Fig. 3.3).

The ulnar artery runs between the flexor carpi ulnaris and flexor digitorum sublimis in the forearm, with a short course over the ulnar nerve. In the hand the artery runs over the transverse carpal ligament and becomes the superficial volar arch, which forms an anastomosis with a small branch of the radial artery. These three anastomoses provide excellent collateral flow to the hand [18]. A competent superficial or deep palmar arch must be present to ensure adequate collateral flow.

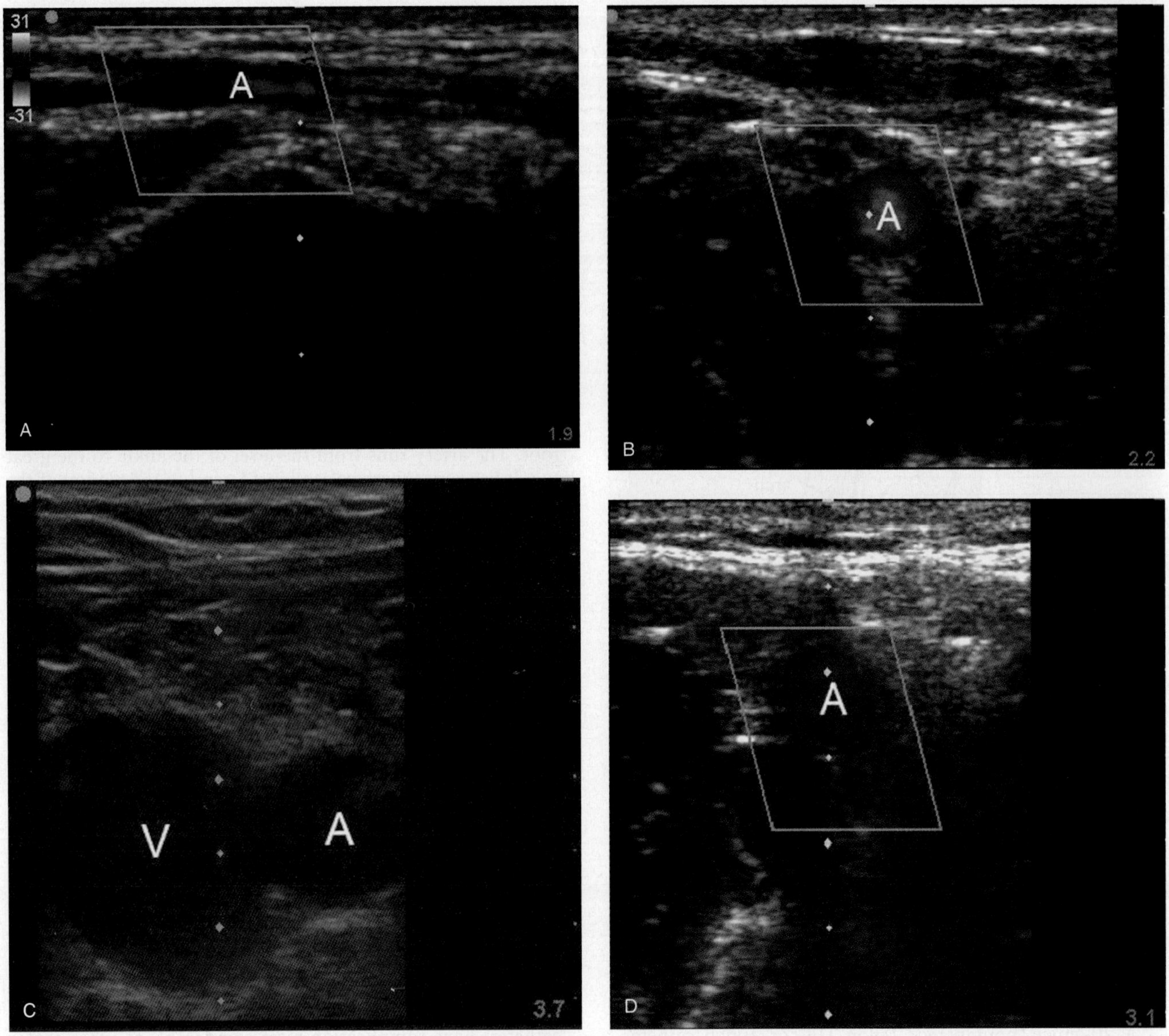

FIGURE 3.2. Portable ultrasound images. A. Radial artery longitudinal view. B. Brachial artery axial view. C. Femoral artery axial view. D. Axillary artery axial view. See text for details.

At least one of these arches may be absent in up to 20% of individuals.

Modified Allen's Test

Hand ischemia is a rare but potential devastating complication of radial artery catheterization that may require amputation [19]. Hand ischemia is rare because of the rich collateral circulation described earlier that insures perfusion even if one of the main arteries thrombose. Historically, the modified Allen's test [20], described in previous editions of this text, was used prior to radial catheterization to detect patients' in whom the collateral circulation may not be intact and presumably at increased risk for hand ischemia. However, as a screening tool the Allen's test has never had very good predictive value [21] and our institution, as well as many others, has abandoned its routine use. The best way to prevent hand ischemia is to avoid radial catheterization in patients at increased risk (i.e., high dose vasopressor therapy, scleroderma, vasculopathy) and to perform clinical evaluation of hand perfusion at each nursing shift change. *Any* change in the hand distal to a radial artery catheter that suggests decreased perfusion (color or temperature change, paresthesias, loss of capillary refill) should prompt *immediate* removal of the catheter and further investigation if the changes do not reverse.

Percutaneous Insertion

The hand is positioned in 30 to 60 degrees of dorsiflexion with the aid of a roll of gauze and armband, avoiding hyperabduction of the thumb. The volar aspect of the wrist is prepared (alcoholic chlorhexidine) and draped using sterile technique, and approximately 0.5 mL of lidocaine is infiltrated on both sides of the artery through a 25-gauge or smaller needle. Lidocaine serves to decrease patient discomfort and may decrease the likelihood of arterial vasospasm [22]. The catheter over the needle approach (e.g., radial or brachial site) necessitates cap, mask, sterile gloves and a small fenestrated drape; whereas, the Seldinger technique (i.e., femoral approach) requires maximum barrier precautions. A time out confirming correct patient,

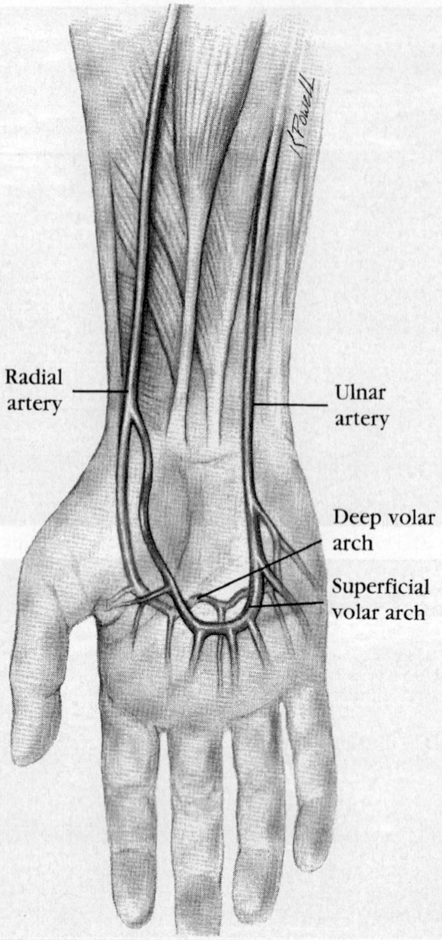

FIGURE 3.3. Anatomy of the radial artery. Note the collateral circulation to the ulnar artery through the deep volar arterial arch and dorsal arch.

correct site, correct equipment and informed consent is necessary before the procedure begins.

A 20-gauge, nontapered, Teflon 1½- or 2-inch catheter-overneedle apparatus is used for puncture. Entry is made at a 30- to 60-degree angle to the skin approximately 3 to 5 cm proximal to the distal wrist crease. Ultrasound image of the radial artery at this position is shown in Figure 3.2A. The needle and cannula are advanced until blood return is noted in the hub, signifying intra-arterial placement of the tip of the needle. A small amount of further advancement is necessary for the cannula to enter the artery as well. With this accomplished, needle and cannula are brought flat to the skin and the cannula advanced to its hub with a firm, steady rotary action. Correct positioning is confirmed by pulsatile blood return on removal of the needle. If the initial attempt is unsuccessful, subsequent attempts should be more proximal, rather than closer to the wrist crease, as the artery is of greater diameter [18], although this may increase the incidence of catheters becoming kinked or occluded [23].

If difficulty is encountered when attempting to pass the catheter, carefully replacing the needle and slightly advancing the whole apparatus may remedy the problem. Alternately, a fixation technique can be attempted (Fig. 3.3). Advancing the needle and catheter through the far wall of the vessel purposely transfixes the artery. The cannula is then pulled back with the needle partially retracted within the catheter until vigorous arterial blood return is noted. The catheter can then be advanced into the arterial lumen, using the needle as a reinforcing stent.

Catheters with self-contained guidewires to facilitate passage of the cannula into the artery are available (Fig. 3.4). Percutaneous puncture is made in the same manner, but when blood return is noted in the catheter hub the guidewire is passed through the needle into the artery, serving as a stent for subsequent catheter advancement. The guidewire and needle are then removed and placement confirmed by pulsatile blood return. The cannula is then secured firmly, attached to transducer tubing, and the site bandaged. Video instruction for the insertion of a radial arterial line is available at www.nejm.org [24].

Dorsalis Pedis Artery Cannulation

Dorsalis pedis artery catheterization is uncommon in most critical care units; compared with the radial artery, the anatomy is less predictable and the success rate is lower [25]. The dorsalis pedis artery is the main blood supply of the dorsum of the foot. The artery runs from the level of the ankle to the great toe. It lies very superficial and just lateral to the tendon of the extensor hallucis longus. The dorsalis pedis anastomoses with branches from the posterior tibial (lateral plantar artery) and, to a lesser extent, peroneal arteries, creating an arterial arch network analogous to that in the hand.

Use of a catheter with self-contained guidewire is recommended for dorsalis pedis catheterization. The foot is placed in plantar flexion and prepared in the usual fashion. Vessel entry is obtained approximately halfway up the dorsum of the foot where the palpable pulse is strongest; advancement is the same as with cannulation of the radial artery. Patients usually find insertion here more painful but less physically limiting. Systolic pressure readings are usually 5 to 20 mm Hg higher with dorsalis pedis catheters than radial artery catheters, but mean pressure values are generally unchanged.

Brachial Artery Cannulation

The brachial artery is cannulated in the bicipital groove proximal to the antecubital fossa at a point where there is no collateral circulation (Fig. 3.2B). In theory, clinical ischemia should be a greater risk, but in most series brachial artery catheters have complication rates comparable to other routes [17,18,26,27]. Even when diminution of distal pulses occurs, because of either proximal obstruction or distal embolization, clinical ischemia is unlikely [26]. An additional anatomic consideration is that the median nerve lies in close proximity to the brachial artery and may be punctured in 1% to 2% of cases [27]. This usually causes only transient paresthesias, but median nerve palsy has been reported. Median nerve palsy is a particular risk in patients with coagulopathy because even minor bleeding into the fascial planes can produce compression of the median nerve [28]. Coagulopathy should be considered a relative contraindication to brachial artery cannulation. Given all these considerations, brachial artery cannulation should only be considered if the radial, femoral, and dorsalis pedis sites are not available or appropriate.

Cannulation of the brachial artery is best performed using a prepackaged kit designed for larger arteries (see femoral artery cannulation). The brachial artery is punctured by extending the arm at the elbow and locating the pulsation a few centimeters proximal to the antecubital fossa, just medial to the bicipital tendon. Once the catheter is established, the elbow must be kept in full extension to avoid kinking or breaking the catheter. Clinical examination of the hand, and Doppler studies if indicated, should be repeated daily while the brachial catheter is in place. The catheter should be promptly removed if diminution of any pulse occurs or there is evidence of embolism. An

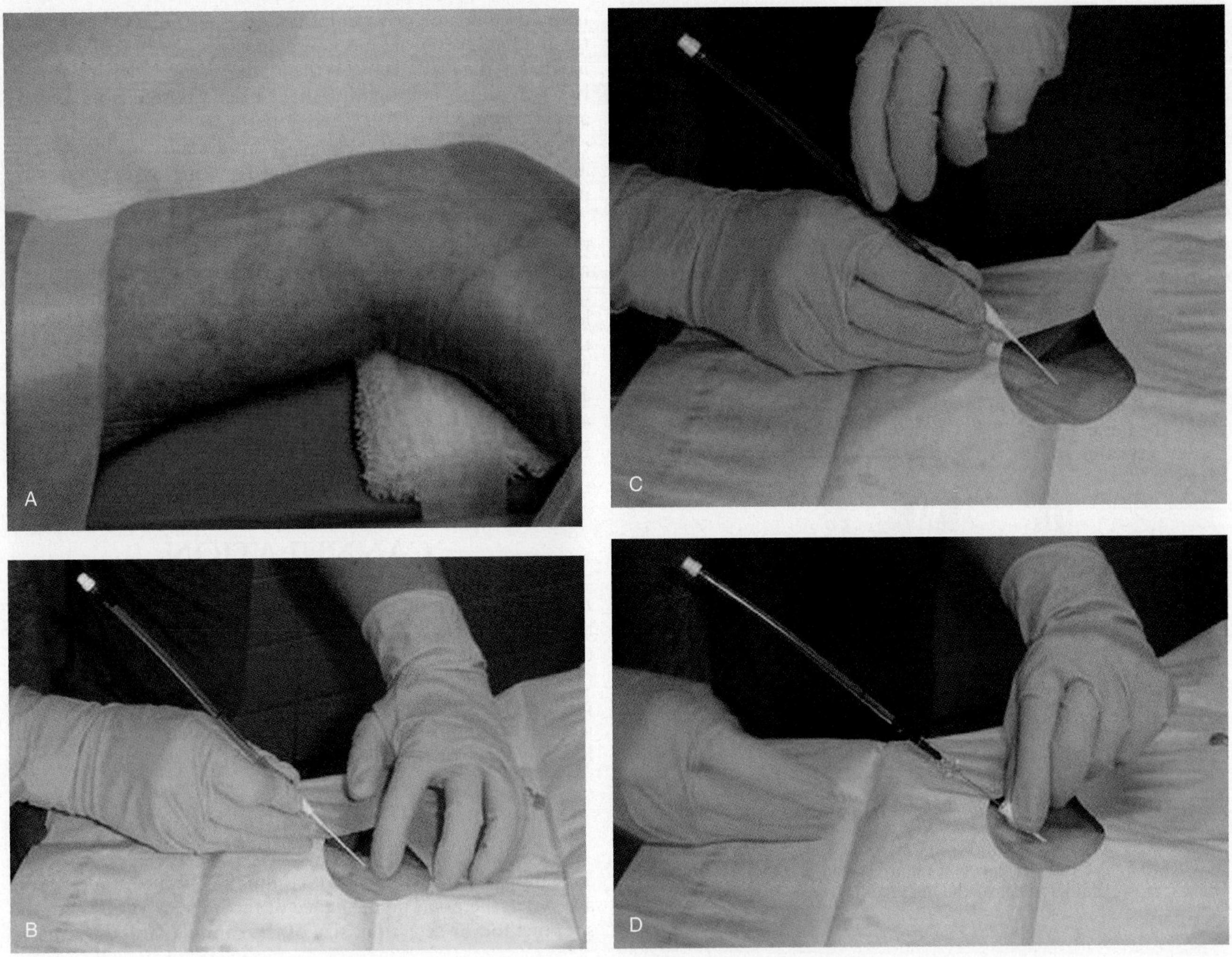

FIGURE 3.4. Cannulation of the radial artery. **A:** A towel is placed behind the wrist, and the hand is immobilized with tape. **B:** The catheter-needle-guidewire apparatus is inserted into the skin at a 30- to 60-degree angle. **C:** The guidewire is advanced into the artery after pulsatile blood flow is obtained. **D:** The catheter is advanced over the guidewire into the artery. [From Irwin RS, Rippe JM: *Manual of Intensive Care Medicine.* 4th ed. Philadelphia, PA: Lippincott Williams & Wilkins, 2006:17, with permission.]

additional concern is air embolism (see later) since placement of a 6-inch catheter puts the tip in the axillary artery.

Femoral Artery Cannulation

The femoral artery is usually the next alternative when radial artery cannulation fails or is inappropriate [15–17]. The femoral artery is large and often palpable when other sites are not, and the technique of cannulation is easy to learn. The most common reason for failure to cannulate is severe atherosclerosis or prior vascular procedures involving both femoral arteries, in which case axillary or brachial artery cannulation is appropriate. Complications unique to this site are rare but include retroperitoneal hemorrhage and intra-abdominal viscus perforation. These complications occur because of poor technique (puncture above the inguinal ligament) or in the presence of anatomical variations (i.e., large inguinal hernia). Ischemic complications from femoral artery catheters are very rare.

The external iliac artery becomes the common femoral artery at the inguinal ligament (Fig. 3.5). The artery courses under the inguinal ligament near the junction of the medial and the middle third of a straight line drawn between the pubis and the anterior superior iliac spine (Fig. 3.2C). The artery is cannulated using the Seldinger technique and any one of several available prepackaged kits. Kits contain the equivalent of a 19-gauge thin-wall needle, appropriate guidewire, and a 6-inch, 18-gauge Teflon catheter. The patient lies supine with the leg extended and slightly abducted. Skin puncture should be 3 to 5 cm caudal to the inguinal ligament to minimize the risk of retroperitoneal hematoma or bowel perforation, which can occur when needle puncture of the vessel is cephalad to the inguinal ligament. The thin-wall needle is directed, bevel up, cephalad at a 45-degree angle. When arterial blood return is confirmed, the needle and syringe may need to be brought down against the skin to facilitate guidewire passage. The guidewire should advance smoothly, but minor manipulation and rotation is sometimes required if the wire meets resistance at the needle tip or after it has advanced into the vessel. Inability to pass the guidewire may be due to an intimal flap over the needle bevel or atherosclerotic plaques in the vessel. In the latter instance, cannulation of that femoral artery may prove impossible. When the guidewire will not pass beyond the needle tip it should be withdrawn and blood return

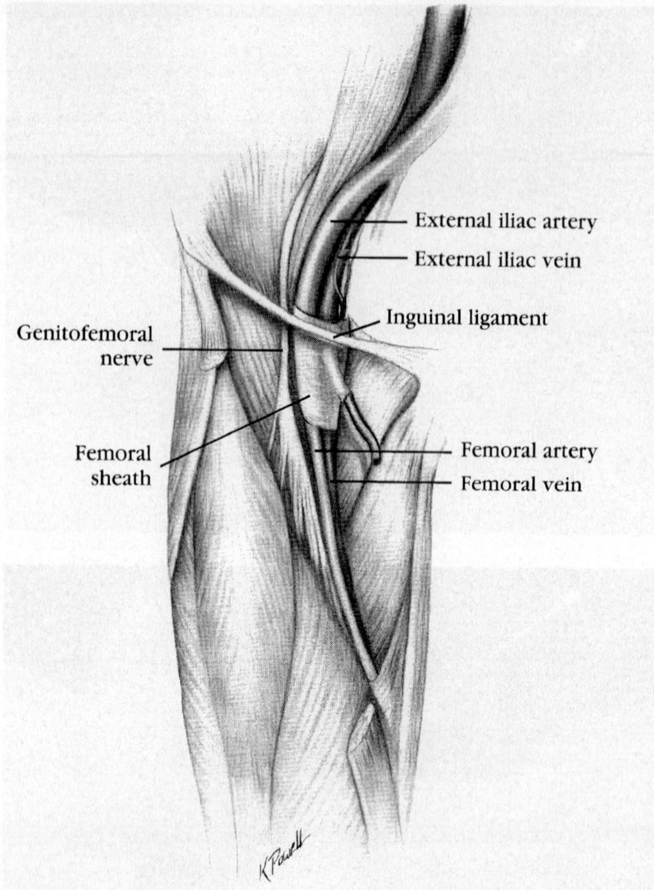

FIGURE 3.5. Anatomy of the femoral artery and adjacent structures. The artery is cannulated below the inguinal ligament.

reestablished by advancing the needle or repeat vascular puncture. The guidewire is then inserted, the needle withdrawn and the catheter threaded over the guidewire to its hub. The guidewire is withdrawn, the catheter sutured securely and connected to the transducer tubing.

Axillary Artery Cannulation

Axillary artery catheterization in the ICU occurs infrequently, but centers experienced with it report a low rate of complications [15,17,29]. The axillary artery is large and frequently palpable when all other sites are not and has a rich collateral circulation. The tip of a 6-inch catheter inserted through an axillary approach lies in the subclavian artery, and thus accurate central pressures are obtained. The central location of the tip makes cerebral air embolism a greater risk, therefore left axillary catheters are preferred for the initial attempt, since air bubbles passing into the right subclavian artery are more likely to traverse the aortic arch. Caution should be exercised in flushing axillary catheters, which is best accomplished manually using low pressures and small volumes.

The axillary artery begins at the lateral border of the first rib as a continuation of the subclavian artery and ends at the inferior margin of the teres major muscle, where it becomes the brachial artery. The optimal site for catheterization is the junction of the middle and lower third of the vessel, which usually corresponds to its highest palpable point in the axilla. At this point, the artery is superficial and is located at the inferior border of the pectoralis major muscle (Fig. 3.2D). The artery is enclosed in a neurovascular bundle, the axillary sheath, with the medial, posterior, and lateral cords of the brachial plexus. Medial to the medial cord is the axillary vein. Not surprisingly, brachial plexus neuropathies have been reported from axillary artery cannulation [30]. Coagulopathy is a relative contraindication, as the axillary sheath can rapidly fill with blood from an uncontrolled arterial puncture, resulting in a compressive neuropathy.

The axillary artery is cannulated using the Seldinger technique and a prepackaged kit. The arm is abducted, externally rotated, and flexed at the elbow by having the patient place the hand under his or her head. The artery is palpated at the lower border of the pectoralis major muscle and fixed against the shaft of the humerus. After site preparation and local infiltration with lidocaine, the thin-wall needle is introduced at a 30- to 45-degree angle to the vertical plane until return of arterial blood. The remainder of the catheterization proceeds as described for femoral artery cannulation.

COMPLICATIONS OF ARTERIAL CANNULATION

Arterial cannulation is a relatively safe invasive procedure. Although estimates of the total complication rate range from 15% to 40%, clinically relevant complications occur in 5% or less (Table 3.2). Risk factors for infectious and noninfectious complications have been identified [31,32] (Table 3.3), but the clinical impact of most of these factors is minimal, given the overall low incidence of complications.

Thrombosis

Thrombosis is the single most common complication of intra-arterial catheters. The incidence of thrombosis varies with the site, method of detection, size of the cannula, and duration of

TABLE 3.2

COMPLICATIONS ASSOCIATED WITH ARTERIAL CANNULATION

Site	Complication
All sites	Pain and swelling
	Thrombosis
	Asymptomatic
	Symptomatic
	Embolization
	Hematoma
	Hemorrhage
	Limb ischemia
	Catheter-related infection including bacteremia
	Diagnostic blood loss
	Pseudoaneurysm
	Heparin-associated thrombocytopenia
Radial artery	Cerebral embolization
	Peripheral neuropathy
Femoral artery	Retroperitoneal hemorrhage
	Bowel perforation
	Arteriovenous fistula
Axillary artery	Cerebral embolization
	Brachial plexopathy
Brachial artery	Median nerve damage
	Cerebral embolization

TABLE 3.3

FACTORS PREDISPOSING TO COMPLICATIONS WITH ARTERIAL CANNULATION

Large tapered cannulas (>20 gauge except at the large artery sites)
Hypotension
Coagulopathy
Low cardiac output
Multiple puncture attempts
Use of vasopressors
Atherosclerosis
Hypercoagulable state
Placement by surgical cutdown
Site inflammation
Intermittent flushing system
Bacteremia

cannulation. Thrombosis is common with radial and dorsalis pedis catheters, but clinical sequelae are rare because of the collateral circulation [31,32]. When a 20-gauge nontapered Teflon catheter with a continuous 3 mL per hour heparinized-saline flush is used to cannulate the radial artery for 3 to 4 days, thrombosis of the vessel can be detected by Doppler study in 5% to 25% of cases [32]. Use of a flush solution containing heparin is no longer standard at our institution because of concern for heparin-induced thrombocytopenia; the incidence of thrombosis does not appear to be significantly higher using saline flush [33,34].

Thrombosis often occurs after catheter removal. Women represent a preponderance of patients who experience flow abnormalities following radial artery cannulation, probably because of smaller arteries and a greater tendency to exhibit vasospasm [23]. Most patients eventually recanalize, generally by 3 weeks after removal of the catheter. Despite the high incidence of Doppler-detected thrombosis, clinical ischemia of the hand is rare and usually resolves following catheter removal. Symptomatic occlusion requiring surgical intervention occurs in fewer than 1% of cases, but can be catastrophic with tissue loss or amputation of the hand [19]. Most patients who develop clinical ischemia have an associated contributory cause, such as prolonged circulatory failure with high-dose vasopressor therapy [31]. We consider the femoral artery the most appropriate first choice in these patients.

Regular inspection of the extremity for unexplained pain or signs of ischemia and immediate removal of the catheter minimize significant ischemic complications. If evidence of ischemia persists after catheter removal, anticoagulation, thrombolytic therapy, embolectomy, surgical bypass, or cervical sympathetic blockade are treatment options and should be pursued aggressively [19,31].

Cerebral Embolization

Continuous flush devices used with arterial catheters are designed to deliver 3 mL per hour of fluid from an infusion bag pressurized to 300 mm Hg. Lowenstein [35] demonstrated that with rapid flushing of radial artery lines with relatively small volumes of radiolabeled solution, traces of the solution could be detected in the central arterial circulation in a time frame representative of retrograde flow. Chang [4,36] demonstrated that injection of greater than 2 mL of air into the radial artery of small primates resulted in retrograde passage of air into the vertebral circulation. Factors that increase the risk for retrograde passage of air are patient size and position (air travels up in a sitting patient), injection site, and flush rate. Air embolism has been cited as a risk mainly for radial arterial catheters but logically could occur with all arterial catheters, especially axillary and brachial artery catheters. The risk is minimized by clearing all air from tubing before flushing, opening the flush valve for no more than 2 to 3 seconds, and avoiding overaggressive manual flushing of the line.

Diagnostic Blood Loss

Diagnostic blood loss (DBL) is patient blood loss that occurs due to frequent blood sampling obtained for laboratory testing. The significance of DBL is underappreciated. It is a particular problem in patients with standard arterial catheter setups that are used as the site for sampling, because 3 to 5 mL of blood is typically wasted (to avoid heparin/saline contamination) every time a sample is obtained. In patients with frequent arterial blood gas determinations, DBL can be substantial and result in a transfusion requirement [37]. There are several ways to minimize DBL, including tubing systems employing a reservoir for blood sampling, continuous intra-arterial blood gas monitoring, point of care microchemistry analysis and the use of pediatric collection tubes. Given the expense and risks of blood component therapy, every ICU should have a blood conservation policy in place that includes minimizing DBL. Protocols that are designed to optimize laboratory utilization have resulted in significant cost savings and reduced transfusion requirements [38].

Other Mechanical and Technical Complications

Other noninfectious complications reported with arterial catheters are pseudoaneurysm formation, hematoma, local tenderness, hemorrhage, neuropathies, and catheter embolization [17]. Heparin-associated thrombocytopenia (HAT) is a risk of any arterial catheter in institutions where heparin is still used as a standard continuous flush solution [39]. Although heparin containing flush solutions may have a slightly reduced rate of vessel thrombosis and catheter occlusions [40] (especially radial), in our opinion the risk of HAT outweighs any benefit. Our institution has used saline-only flush solutions for many years and we have not noticed an increase in thrombotic or other complications.

Infection

Infectious sequelae are the most important clinical complications occurring because of arterial cannulation, and many of the concepts and definitions applied to central venous catheter–related infection (Chapter 2) are also relevant to arterial catheters.

Catheter-associated infection is usually initiated by skin flora that invades the intracutaneous tract, causing colonization of the catheter, and ultimately, bacteremia. An additional source of infection from pressure-monitoring systems is contaminated infusate, which is at greater risk for infection than central venous catheters because (a) the transducer can become colonized because of stagnant flow, (b) the flush solution is infused at a slow rate (3 mL per hour) and may hang for several days, and (c) multiple blood samples are obtained by several different personnel from stopcocks in the system, which can serve as entry sites for bacteria.

Appreciation of the mechanisms responsible for initiating arterial catheter–related infection is important in understanding how to minimize infection. Thorough operator and site preparation is paramount and triple barrier protection is appropriate for all larger artery insertions. Chlorhexadine should be used for skin preparation [41] and use of a chlorhexidine soaked dressing at the insertion site is excellent practice. Breaks in sterile technique during insertion mandate termination of the procedure and replacement of compromised equipment. Nursing personnel should follow strict guidelines when drawing blood samples or manipulating tubing. Blood withdrawn to clear the tubing prior to drawing samples should not be reinjected unless a specially designed system is in use [42]. Inspection of the site at the start of every nursing shift is mandatory, and the catheter should be removed promptly if abnormalities are noted. Routine change of the pressure monitoring system does not reduce infectious complications and may simply be another opportunity to introduce colonization.

Historically, it was always felt that arterial catheters had a lower risk for infection than central venous catheters, but that is probably no longer true. Impressive reductions in overall Catheter Related Infections (CRI) have occurred as a result of increased research, better technology, and an emphasis on patient safety, leading to a convergence of infectious risks for arterial and central venous catheters [43,44]. Using modern techniques, arterial catheter–related colonization may occurs in up to 5% to 10% of catheters but the incidence of catheter-related bacteremia should be in the range of 0.5 to 2.0 per 1,000 catheter-days [15,16,43–45]. The site of insertion does not appear to be an important factor impacting on the incidence of infection [15–17,25] but duration is likely important [44]. We believe 7 days is an appropriate time to reassess the need for and the location of arterial catheterization [44] but each institution should determine its own catheter-associated infection rate so that rational policies can be formulated based on existing local infection rates.

When arterial catheter infection does occur, *Staphylococcus* species are commonly isolated. Gram-negative organisms are less frequent, but predominate in contaminated infusate or equipment-related infection. Infection with *Candida* species is a greater risk in prolonged catheterization of the glucose-intolerant patient on multiple systemic broad-spectrum antibiotics. Catheter-associated bacteremia should be treated with a 7- to 14-day course of appropriate antibiotics. In complicated cases, longer courses are sometimes necessary.

The optimal evaluation of febrile catheterized patients can be a challenging problem (see Chapter 2). If the site appears abnormal or the patient is in septic shock with no other etiology, the catheter should be removed. More specific guidelines are difficult to recommend, and individual factors should always be considered. In general, arterial catheters in place less than 5 days will not be the source of fever unless insertion was contaminated. Catheters in place 7 days or longer should be changed to a different site given the safety of arterial cannulation and the small but measurable chance of infection. Guidewire exchanges should only be used to change a malfunctioning or damaged catheter.

RECOMMENDATIONS

Either the radial or femoral artery is an appropriate initial site for percutaneous arterial cannulation. Most centers have more experience with radial artery cannulation, but femoral artery catheters are reliable and have a comparable incidence of complication. In our opinion, the femoral artery should be used first in shocked patients, especially when vasopressors are infusing, because of the risk of tissue loss with radial or dorsalis pedis catheters. In more than 90% of patients, the radial or femoral site is adequate to achieve arterial pressure monitoring. When these sites are not appropriate, the dorsalis pedis artery is a good alternative, but cannulation is frequently not possible, especially if radial artery cannulation failed because of poor perfusion. Under these circumstances, the brachial followed by the axillary artery can be safely cannulated; when a coagulopathy is present, ultrasound guidance should be used to avoid complications. Arterial catheters can be left in place until there is clinical indication to remove them, but infection rate increases proportionally. Iatrogenic anemia and overutilization of blood tests are a real phenomenon associated with arterial catheters, which should be discontinued promptly when no longer required for patient management.

References

1. Marik PE, Cavallazzi R, Vasu T, et al: Dynamic changes in arterial waveform derived variables and fluid responsiveness in mechanically ventilated patients: A systematic review of the literature. *Crit Care Med* 37:2642–2647, 2009.
2. Low LL, Harrington GR, Stoltzfus DP. The effect of arterial lines on blood-drawing practices and costs in intensive care units. *Chest* 108:216, 1995.
3. Zimmerman JE, Seneff MG, Sun X, et al: Evaluating laboratory usage in the intensive care unit: patient and institutional characteristics that influence frequency of blood sampling. *Crit Care Med* 25:737, 1997.
4. Clark JS, Votteri B, Ariagno RL, et al: Noninvasive assessment of blood gases. *Am Rev Respir Dis* 145:220, 1992.
5. Bur A, Hirschl MM, Herkner H, et al: Accuracy of oscillometric blood pressure measurement according to the relation between cuff size and upper-arm circumference in critically ill patients. *Crit Care Med* 28:371, 2000.
6. Hirschl MM, Kittler H, Woisetschlager C, et al: Simultaneous comparison of thoracic bioimpedance and arterial pulse waveform-derived cardiac output with thermodilution measurement. *Crit Care Med* 28:1798, 2000.
7. Chaney JC, Derdak S: Minimally invasive hemodynamic monitoring for the intensivist: current and emerging technology. *Crit Care Med* 30:2338, 2002.
8. Mayer J, Boldt J, Poland R, et al: Continuous arterial pressure waveform-based cardiac output using the FloTrac/Vigileo: a review and meta-analysis. *J Cardiothorac Vasc Anesth* 23:401–406, 2009.
9. Gardner RM: Direct arterial pressure monitoring. *Curr Anaesth Crit Care* 1:239, 1990.
10. Boutros A, Albert S: Effect of the dynamic response of transducer-tubing system on accuracy of direct blood pressure measurement in patients. *Crit Care Med* 11:124, 1983.
11. Rothe CF, Kim KC: Measuring systolic arterial blood pressure. Possible errors from extension tubes or disposable transducer domes. *Crit Care Med* 8:683, 1980.
12. Billiet E, Colardyn F: Pressure measurement evaluation and accuracy validation: the Gabarith test. *Intensive Care Med* 24:1323, 1998.
13. Gardner RM: Accuracy and reliability of disposable pressure transducers coupled with modern pressure monitors. *Crit Care Med* 24:879, 1996.
14. Pauca AL, Wallenhaupt SL, Kon ND, et al: Does radial artery pressure accurately reflect aortic pressure? *Chest* 102:1193, 1992.
15. Gurman GM, Kriemerman S: Cannulation of big arteries in critically ill patients. *Crit Care Med* 13:217, 1985.
16. Russell JA, Joel M, Hudson RJ, et al: Prospective evaluation of radial and femoral artery catheterization sites in critically ill adults. *Crit Care Med* 11:936, 1983.
17. Scheer BV, Perel A, Pfeiffer UJ: Clinical review: complications and risk factors of peripheral arterial catheters used for haemodynamic monitoring in anaesthesia and intensive care medicine. *Critical Care* 6;199–204, 2002.
18. Mathers LH: Anatomical considerations in obtaining arterial access. *J Intensive Care Med* 5:110, 1990.
19. Valentine RJ, Modrall JG, Clagett GP: Hand ischemia after radial artery cannulation. *J Am Coll Surg* 201:18, 2005.
20. Allen EV: *Thromboangiitis obliterans*: Method of diagnosis of chronic occlusive arterial lesions distal to the wrist with illustrative cases. *Am J Med Sci* 178:237, 1929.
21. Glavin RJ, Jones HM: Assessing collateral circulation in the hand—four methods compared. *Anaesthesia* 44:594, 1989.
22. Giner J, Casan P, Belda J, et al: Pain during arterial puncture. *Chest* 110:1443, 1996.
23. Kaye J, Heald GR, Morton J, et al: Patency of radial arterial catheters. *Am J Crit Care* 10:104, 2001.
24. Tegtmeyer K, Brady G, Lai S, et al: Videos in clinical medicine. Placement of an arterial line. *N Engl J Med* 354:e13, 2006.
25. Martin C, Saux P, Papazian L, et al: Long-term arterial cannulation in ICU patients using the radial artery or dorsalis pedis artery. *Chest* 119:901, 2001.

26. Barnes RW, Foster EJ, Janssen GA, et al: Safety of brachial arterial catheters as monitors in the intensive care unit–prospective evaluation with the Doppler ultrasonic velocity detector. *Anesthesiology* 44:260, 1976.
27. Mann S, Jones RI, Millar-Craig MW, et al: The safety of ambulatory intra-arterial pressure monitoring: a clinical audit of 1000 studies. *Int J Cardiol* 5:585, 1984.
28. Macon WL IV, Futrell JW: Median-nerve neuropathy after percutaneous puncture of the brachial artery in patients receiving anticoagulants. *N Engl J Med* 288:1396, 1973.
29. Brown M, Gordon LH, Brown OW, et al: Intravascular monitoring via the axillary artery. *Anesth Intensive Care* 13:38, 1984.
30. Sabik JF, Lytle BW, McCarthy PM, et al: Axillary artery: an alternative site of arterial cannulation for patients with extensive aortic and peripheral vascular disease. *J Thorac Cardiovasc Surg* 109:885–891, 1995.
31. Wilkins RG: Radial artery cannulation and ischaemic damage: a review. *Anaesthesia* 40:896, 1985.
32. Weiss BM, Gattiker RI: Complications during and following radial artery cannulation: a prospective study. *Intensive Care Med* 12:424, 1986.
33. Clifton GD, Branson P, Kelly HJ, et al: Comparison of normal saline and heparin solutions for maintenance of arterial catheter patency. *Heart Lung* 20:115, 1990.
34. Hook ML, Reuling J, Luettgen ML, et al: Comparison of the patency of arterial lines maintained with heparinized and nonheparinized infusions. The Cardiovascular Intensive Care Unit Nursing Research Committee of St. Luke's Hospital. *Heart Lung* 16:693, 1987.
35. Lowenstein E, Little JW 3rd, Lo HH: Prevention of cerebral embolization from flushing radial-artery cannulas. *N Engl J Med* 285:1414, 1971.
36. Chang C, Dughi J, Shitabata P, et al: Air embolism and the radial arterial line. *Crit Care Med* 16:141, 1988.
37. Smoller BR, Kruskall MS: Phlebotomy for diagnostic laboratory tests in adults. Pattern of use and effect on transfusion requirements. *N Engl J Med* 314:1233, 1986.
38. Roberts DE, Bell DD, Ostryzniuk T, et al: Eliminating needless testing in intensive care–an information-based team management approach. *Crit Care Med* 21:1452, 1993.
39. Warkentin TE, Greinacher A: Heparin-induced thrombocytopenia: recognition, treatment, and prevention: the Seventh ACCP Conference on Antithrombotic and Thrombolytic Therapy. *Chest* 126:311S, 2004.
40. Randolph AG, Cook DJ, Gonzales CA, et al: Benefit of heparin in peripheral venous and arterial catheters: systematic review and meta-analysis of randomised controlled trials. *BMJ* 316:969, 1998.
41. Mimoz O, Pieroni L, Lawrence C, et al: Prospective, randomized trial of two antiseptic solutions for prevention of central venous or arterial catheter colonization and infection in intensive care unit patients. *Crit Care Med* 24:1818, 1996.
42. Peruzzi WT, Noskin GA, Moen SG, et al: Microbial contamination of blood conservation devices during routine use in the critical care setting: results of a prospective, randomized trial. *Crit Care Med* 24:1157, 1996.
43. Maki DG, Kluger DM, Crnich CJ. The risk of bloodstream infection in adults with different intravascular devices: a systematic review of 200 published prospective studies. *Mayo Clin Proc* 81:1159–1171, 2006.
44. Lucet JC, Bouadma L, Zahar JR, et al: Infectious risk associated with arterial catheters compared with central venous catheters. *Crit Care Med* 38:1030–1035, 2010.
45. Traore O, Liotier J, Souweine B: Prospective study of arterial and central venous catheter colonization and of arterial-and central venous catheter-related bacteremia in intensive care units. *Crit Care Med* 33:1276, 2005.

CHAPTER 4 ■ PULMONARY ARTERY CATHETERS

HARVEY S. REICH

Since their introduction into clinical practice in 1970 by Swan et al. [1], balloon-tipped, flow-directed pulmonary artery (PA) catheters have found widespread use in the clinical management of critically ill patients. However, in recent years, both the safety and efficacy of these catheters have been brought into question. In this chapter, I review the physiologic basis for their use, some history regarding their development and use, the concerns raised about their use, and suggestions for appropriate use of the catheters and the information obtained from them.

PHYSIOLOGIC RATIONALE FOR USE OF THE PULMONARY ARTERY CATHETER

In unstable situations, during which hemodynamic changes often occur rapidly, clinical evaluation may be misleading [2]. PA catheters allow for direct and indirect measurement of several major determinants and consequences of cardiac performance—preload, afterload, cardiac output (CO)—thereby supplying additional data to aid in clinical decision making [3].

Cardiac function depends on the relationship between muscle length (preload), the load on the muscle (afterload), and the intrinsic property of contractility. Until the development of the flow-directed PA catheter, there was no way to assess all of these by using one instrument in a clinically useful way at bedside. The catheter allows the reflection of right ventricular (RV) preload (right atrial pressure), RV afterload (PA pressure), left ventricular preload—PA occlusion pressure (PAOP) or pulmonary capillary wedge pressure (PCWP)—and contractility (stroke volume or CO). Left ventricular afterload is reflected by the systemic arterial pressure. This information allows the calculation of numerous parameters, including vascular resistances. No other tool allows the gathering of such a large amount of information.

CONTROVERSIES REGARDING USE OF THE PULMONARY ARTERY CATHETER

Despite all of the advantages of the PA catheter, a number of clinical studies have been published in the past decade that have shown either no benefit or an increased risk of morbidity or mortality associated with its use. (See Table 4.1 for a summary of the evidence for its utility.) Consequently, a number of clinicians have elected to minimize the use of this monitoring device.

Furthermore, the relationship of central venous (CV) pressure and PA pressure to predict ventricular filling was studied

TABLE 4.1

EVIDENCE BASIS FOR THE PA CATHETER

Authors	Year	N	Design	Outcomes
Lower morbidity/mortality				
Rao et al. [4]	1983	733/364	Historical controls/cohort	Lower mortality
Hesdorffer et al. [5]	1987	61/87	Historical controls/cohort	Lower mortality
Shoemaker et al. [6]	1988	146	RCT	Lower mortality
Berlauk et al. [7]	1991	89	RCT	Lower morbidity
Fleming et al. [8]	1992	33/34	RCT	Lower morbidity
Tuchschmidt et al. [9]	1992	26/25	RCT	Decreased LOS; trend toward lower mortality
Boyd et al. [10]	1993	53/54	RCT	Lower mortality
Bishop et al. [11]	1995	50/65	RCT	Lower mortality
Schiller et al. [12]	1997	53/33/30	Retrospective cohort	Lower mortality
Wilson et al. [13]	1999	92/46	RCT	Lower mortality
Chang et al. [14]	2000	20/39	Prospective retrospective cohort	Lower morbidity
Polonen et al. [15]	2000	196/197	RCT	Decreased morbidity
Friese et al. [16]	2006	51379 (no PAC)/ 1933 (PAC)	Retrospective analysis of National Trauma Data Bank	Improved survival in patients older than 60 or with ISS 25—75 and severe shock
No difference				
Pearson et al. [17]	1989	226	RCT	No difference
Isaacson et al. [18]	1990	102	RCT	No difference
Joyce et al. [19]	1990	40	RCT	No difference
Yu et al. [20]	1993	35/32	RCT	No difference
Gattinoni et al. [21]	1995	252/253/257	RCT	No difference
Yu et al. [22]	1995	89	RCT	No difference
Durham et al. [23]	1996	27/31	Prospective cohort	No difference
Afessa et al. [24]	2001	751	Prospective observational	No difference
Rhodes et al. [25]	2002	201	RCT	No difference
Richard [26]	2003	676	RCT	No difference
Yu et al. [27]	2003	1,010	Prospective cohort	No difference
Sandham et al. [28]	2003	997/997	RCT	No difference in mortality; increased risk of pulmonary embolism in PA group
Sakr et al. [29]	2005	3,147	Observational cohort	No difference
Harvey et al. [30]	2005	519/522	RCT	No difference in mortality
Binanay et al. [31]	2005	433	RCT	No difference in mortality
The National Heart, Lung and Blood Institute ARDS Clinical Trials Network [32]	2006	513/487	RCT	No difference in mortality or organ function
Higher or worse morbidity/mortality				
Tuman et al. [33]	1989	1094	Controlled prospective cohort	Increased ICU stay with PAC
Guyatt [34]	1991	33/148	RCT	Higher morbidity
Hayes et al. [35]	1994	50	RCT	Higher mortality
Connors et al. [36]	1996	5,735	Prospective cohort	Higher mortality
Valentine et al. [37]	1998	60	RCT	Increased morbidity
Stewart et al. [38]	1998	133/61	Retrospective cohort	Increased morbidity
Ramsey et al. [39]	2000	8,064/5,843	Retrospective cohort	Higher mortality
Polanczyk et al. [40]	2001	215/215	Prospective cohort	Increased morbidity
Chittock et al. [41]	2004	7,310	Observational cohort	Increased mortality in low severity; decreased mortality in high severity
Peters et al. [42]	2003	360/690	Retrospective case control	Increased risk of death
Cohen et al. [43]	2005	26,437/735	Retrospective cohort	Increased mortality

ICU, intensive care unit; ISS, injury security score; LOS, length of stay; PA, pulmonary artery; PAC, pulmonary artery catheter; RCT, randomized control trial.

TABLE 4.2

GENERAL INDICATIONS FOR PULMONARY ARTERY CATHETERIZATION

Management of complicated myocardial infarction
Hypovolemia versus cardiogenic shock
Ventricular septal rupture versus acute mitral regurgitation
Severe left ventricular failure
Right ventricular infarction
Unstable angina
Refractory ventricular tachycardia
Assessment of respiratory distress
Cardiogenic versus noncardiogenic (e.g., acute respiratory distress syndrome) pulmonary edema
Primary versus secondary pulmonary hypertension
Assessment of shock
Cardiogenic
Hypovolemic
Septic
Pulmonary embolism
Assessment of therapy in selected individuals
Afterload reduction in patients with severe left ventricular function
Inotropic agent
Vasopressors
Beta-blockers
Temporary pacing (ventricular vs. atrioventricular)
Intra-aortic balloon counterpulsation
Mechanical ventilation (e.g., with positive end-expiratory pressure)
Management of postoperative open-heart surgical patients
Assessment of cardiac tamponade/constriction
Assessment of valvular heart disease
Perioperative monitoring of patients with unstable cardiac status during noncardiac surgery
Assessment of fluid requirements in critically ill patients
Gastrointestinal hemorrhage
Sepsis
Acute renal failure
Burns
Decompensated cirrhosis
Advanced peritonitis
Management of severe preeclampsia

Adapted from JM Gore, JS Alpert, JR Benotti, et al: *Handbook of Hemodynamic Monitoring*. Boston, MA, Little, Brown, 1984.

in normal volunteers by Kumar et al. [44] who found there was a poor correlation between initial CV pressure and PAOP, with both respective end diastolic ventricular volume and stroke volume indices. Their data call into question the basic tenet of the theoretical benefit of the PA catheter.

INDICATIONS FOR PULMONARY ARTERY CATHETER USE

Clinicians who use a PA catheter for monitoring should understand the fundamentals of the insertion technique, the equipment used, and the data that can be generated. The Pulmonary Artery Catheter Education Program (PACEP) has been developed by seven specialty organizations, along with the NHLBI and the FDA and is available at http://www.pacep.org.

The use of the PA catheter for monitoring has four central objectives: (a) to assess left or right ventricular function, or both, (b) to monitor changes in hemodynamic status, (c) to guide treatment with pharmacologic and nonpharmacologic agents, and (d) to provide prognostic information. The conditions in which PA catheterization may be useful are characterized by a clinically unclear or rapidly changing hemodynamic status. Table 4.2 is a partial listing of the indications. Use of PA catheters in specific disease entities is discussed in other chapters.

CATHETER FEATURES AND CONSTRUCTION

The catheter is constructed from polyvinylchloride and has a pliable shaft that softens further at body temperature. Because polyvinylchloride has a high thrombogenicity, the catheters are generally coated with heparin. Heparin bonding of catheters, introduced in 1981, has been shown to be effective in reducing catheter thrombogenicity [45,46] but can cause heparin-induced thrombocytopenia. The standard catheter length is 110 cm, and the most commonly used external diameter is 5 or 7 French (Fr) (1 Fr = 0.0335 mm). A balloon is fastened 1 to 2 mm from the tip (Fig. 4.1); when inflated, it guides the catheter (by virtue of fluid dynamic drag) from the greater

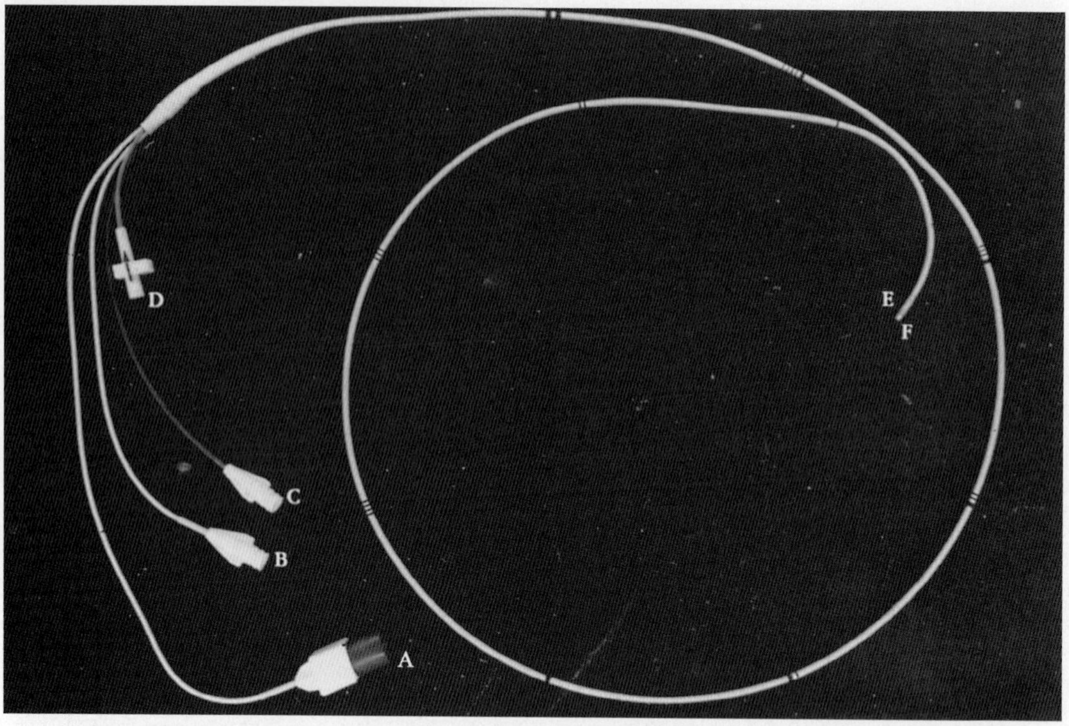

FIGURE 4.1. Quadruple-lumen pulmonary artery catheter. **A:** Connection to thermodilution cardiac output computer. **B:** Connection to distal lumen. **C:** Connection to proximal lumen. **D:** Stopcock connected to balloon at the catheter tip for balloon inflation. **E:** Thermistor. **F:** Balloon. Note that the catheter is marked in 10-cm increments.

intrathoracic veins through the right heart chambers into the PA. When fully inflated in a vessel of sufficiently large caliber, the balloon protrudes above the catheter tip, thus distributing tip forces over a large area and minimizing the chances for endocardial damage or arrhythmia induction during catheter insertion (Fig. 4.2). Progression of the catheter is stopped when it impacts in a PA slightly smaller in diameter than the fully inflated balloon. From this position, the PAOP is obtained. Balloon capacity varies according to catheter size, and the operator must be aware of the individual balloon's maximal inflation volume as recommended by the manufacturer. The balloon is usually inflated with air, but filtered carbon dioxide should be used in any situation in which balloon rupture might result in access of the inflation medium to the arterial system (e.g., if a right-to-left intracardiac shunt or a pulmonary arteriovenous fistula is suspected). If carbon dioxide is used, periodic deflation and reinflation may be necessary, since carbon dioxide diffuses through the latex balloon at a rate of approximately 0.5 cm^3 per minute. Liquids should never be used as the inflation medium.

A variety of catheter constructions is available, each designed for particular clinical applications. Double-lumen catheters allow balloon inflation through one lumen, and a distal opening at the tip of the catheter is used to measure intravascular pressures and sample blood. Triple-lumen catheters have a proximal port terminating 30 cm from the tip of the catheter, allowing simultaneous measurement of right atrial and PA or occlusion pressures. The most commonly used PA catheter in the ICU setting is a quadruple-lumen catheter, which has a lumen containing electrical leads for a thermistor positioned at the catheter surface 4 cm proximal to its tip (Fig. 4.1) [47]. The thermistor measures PA blood temperature and allows thermodilution CO measurements. A five-lumen catheter is also available, with the fifth lumen opening 40 cm from the tip of the catheter. The fifth lumen provides additional central venous access for fluid or medication infusions when peripheral access is limited or when drugs requiring infusion into a large vein (e.g., dopamine, epinephrine) are used. Figure 4.2 shows the balloon on the tip inflated.

Several special-purpose PA catheter designs are available. Pacing PA catheters incorporate two groups of electrodes on the catheter surface, enabling intracardiac electrocardiographic (ECG) recording or temporary cardiac pacing [48]. These catheters are used for emergency cardiac pacing, although it is often difficult to position the catheter for reliable simultaneous cardiac pacing and PA pressure measurements. A five-lumen catheter allows passage of a specially designed 2.4-Fr bipolar pacing electrode (probe) through the additional lumen (located 19 cm from the catheter tip) and allows emergency temporary intracardiac pacing without the need for a separate central venous puncture. The pacing probe is Teflon coated to allow easy introduction through the pacemaker port lumen; the intracavitary part of the probe is heparin impregnated to reduce the risk of thrombus formation. One report demonstrated satisfactory ventricular pacing in 19 of 23 patients using this catheter design (83% success rate) [49]. When a pacing probe is not in use, the fifth lumen may be used for additional central venous access or continuous RV pressure monitoring.

Continuous mixed venous oxygen saturation measurement is clinically available using a fiberoptic five-lumen PA catheter [50]. Segal et al. [51] described a catheter that incorporates Doppler technology for continuous CO determinations. Catheters equipped with a fast-response (95 milliseconds) thermistor and intracardiac ECG-monitoring electrodes are also available. These catheters allow determination of the RV ejection fraction and RV systolic time intervals in critically ill patients [52–55]. The calculated RV ejection fraction has correlated well with simultaneous radionuclide first-pass studies [54].

Aside from the intermittent determination of CO by bolus administration of cold injectate, PA catheters have been adapted to determine near continuous CO by thermal pulses generated by a heating filament on the catheter to produce

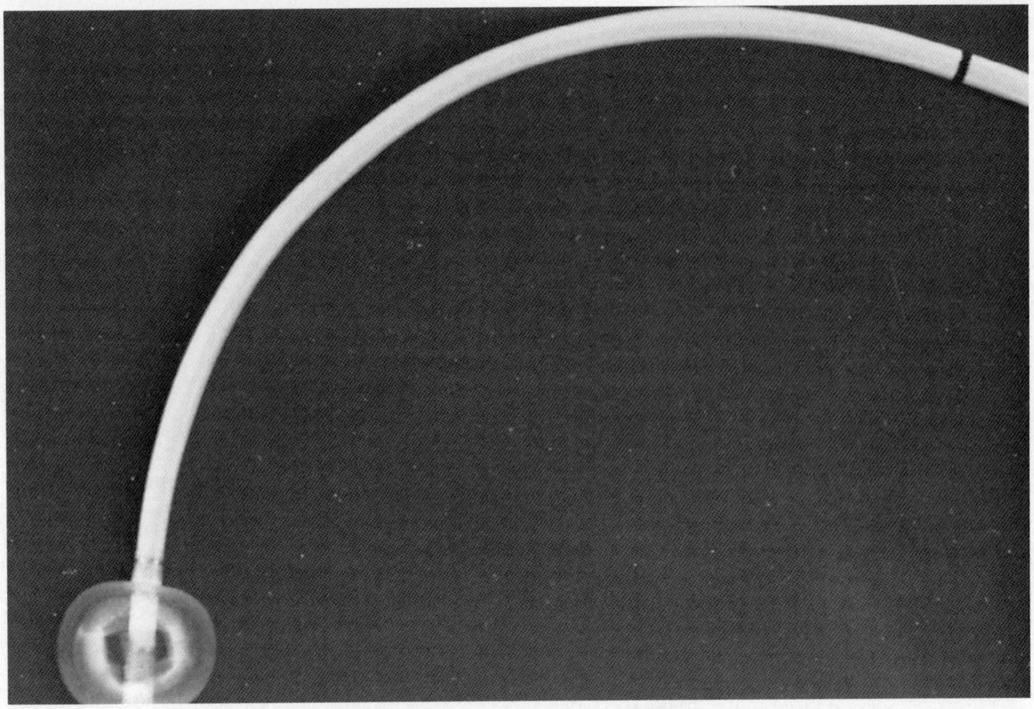

FIGURE 4.2. Balloon properly inflated at the tip of a pulmonary artery catheter. Note that the balloon shields the catheter tip and prevents it from irritating cardiac chambers on its passage to the pulmonary artery.

temperature changes [56]. The accuracy and reliability of CO determination by this heating–cooling cycle have been confirmed by several studies [57–60].

Pressure Transducers

Hemodynamic monitoring requires a system able to convert changes in intravascular pressure into electrical signals suitable for interpretation. The most commonly used hemodynamic monitoring system is a catheter-tubing–transducer system. A fluid-filled intravascular catheter is connected to a transducer by a fluid-filled tubing system. (For more details, see the discussion in Chapters 3 and 26.)

INSERTION TECHNIQUES

General Considerations

Manufacturers' recommendations should be carefully followed. All catheter manufacturers have detailed insertion and training materials.

PA catheterization can be performed in any hospital location where continuous ECG and hemodynamic monitoring are possible and where equipment and supplies needed for cardiopulmonary resuscitation are readily available. Fluoroscopy is not essential, but it can facilitate difficult placements. Properly constructed beds and protective aprons are mandatory for safe use of fluoroscopic equipment. Meticulous attention to sterile technique is of obvious importance; all involved personnel must wear sterile caps, gowns, masks, and gloves, and the patient must be fully covered by sterile drapes.

The catheter should be inserted percutaneously (not by cutdown) into the basilic, brachial, femoral, subclavian, or internal jugular veins by using techniques described in Chapter 2. Threading the catheter into the PA is more difficult from the basilica, brachial, or femoral vein.

Typical Catheter Insertion Procedure

The procedures for typical catheter insertion are as follows:

1. Prepare and connect pressure tubing, manifolds, stopcocks, and transducers. Remove the sterile balloon-tipped catheter from its container. Balloon integrity may be tested by submerging the balloon in a small amount of fluid and checking for air leaks as the balloon is inflated (using the amount of air recommended by the manufacturer). Deflate the balloon.
2. After a time out, insert a central venous cannula or needle into the vein as described in Chapter 2. Using the Seldinger technique, thread the guidewire contained in the catheter kit into the vein and remove the catheter or needle (Figs. 4.3 and 4.4).
3. Make a small incision with a scalpel to enlarge the puncture site (Fig. 4.5). While holding the guidewire stationary, thread a vessel dilator-sheath apparatus (the size should be 8 Fr if a 7-Fr catheter is to be used) over the guidewire and advance it into the vessel, using a twisting motion to get through the puncture site (Fig. 4.6). The dilator and sheath should only be advanced until the tip of the sheath is in the vessel—estimated by the original depth of the cannula or needle required to access the vein. At that point, the dilator and guidewire are held stationary and the sheath is advance off the dilator into the vessel. Advancing the dilator further may cause great vessel or cardiac damage.
4. Remove the guidewire and vessel dilator, leaving the introducer sheath in the vessel (Fig. 4.7). Suture the sheath in place.
5. Pass the proximal portion of the catheter to an assistant and have that person attach the stopcock-pressure tubing-transducer system to the right atrial and PA ports of the

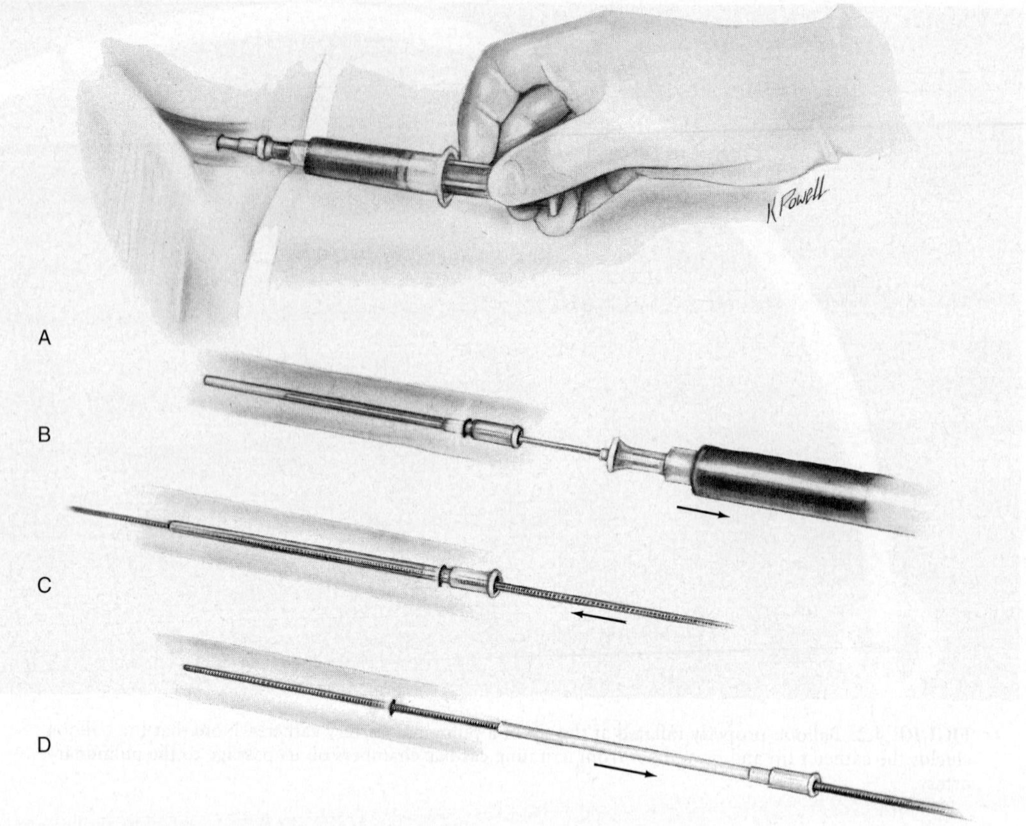

FIGURE 4.3. **A:** Easy blood aspiration has been demonstrated using the guidewire introducer needle. **B:** The inner needle is removed. **C:** The spring guidewire is advanced, soft end first, through the cannula into the vessel. **D:** With the guidewire held in place, the cannula is withdrawn from the vessel by being pulled over and off the length of the guidewire.

PA catheter. Flush the proximal and distal catheter lumens with normal saline.

6. If a sterile sleeve adapter is to be used, insert the catheter through it and pull the adapter proximally over the catheter to keep it out of the way. Once the catheter is advanced to its desired intravascular location, attach the distal end of the sleeve adapter to the introducer sheath hub.
7. Pass the catheter through the introducer sheath into the vein (Fig. 4.8). Advance it, using the marks on the catheter shaft indicating 10-cm distances from the tip, until the tip is in the right atrium. This requires advancement of

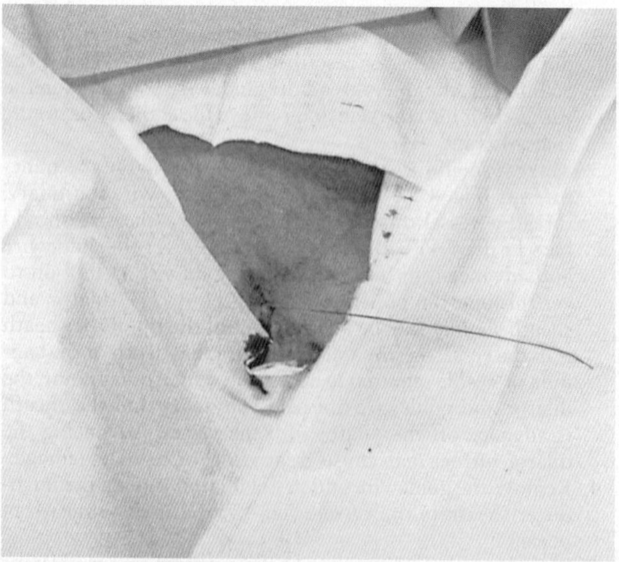

FIGURE 4.4. The spring guidewire, stiff end protruding, is now located in the subclavian vein.

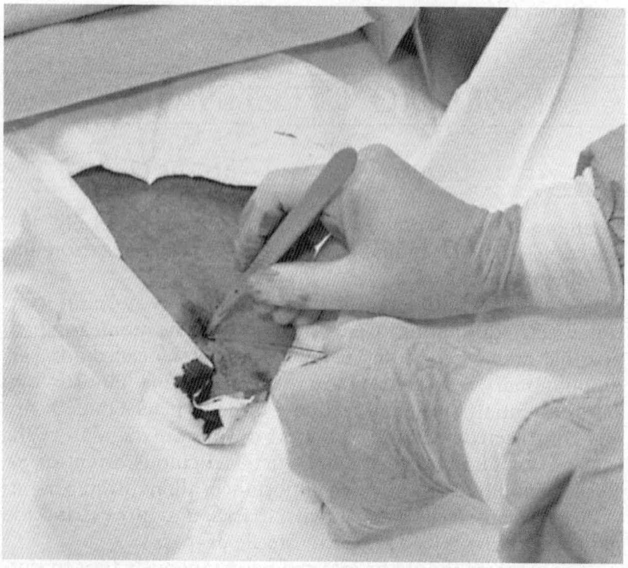

FIGURE 4.5. A small incision is made with a scalpel to enlarge the puncture site.

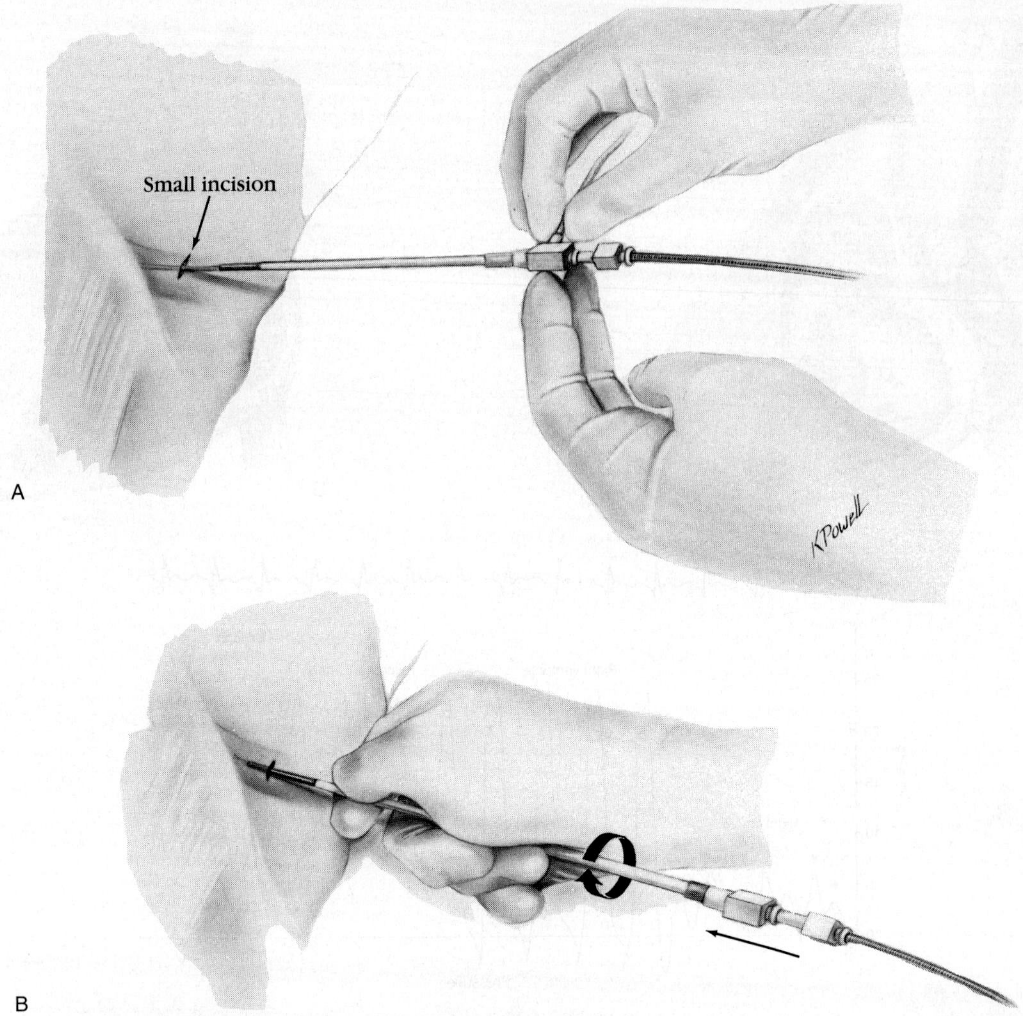

FIGURE 4.6. **A:** The vessel dilator-sheath apparatus is threaded over the guidewire and advanced into the vessel. **B:** A twisting motion is used to thread the apparatus into the vessel.

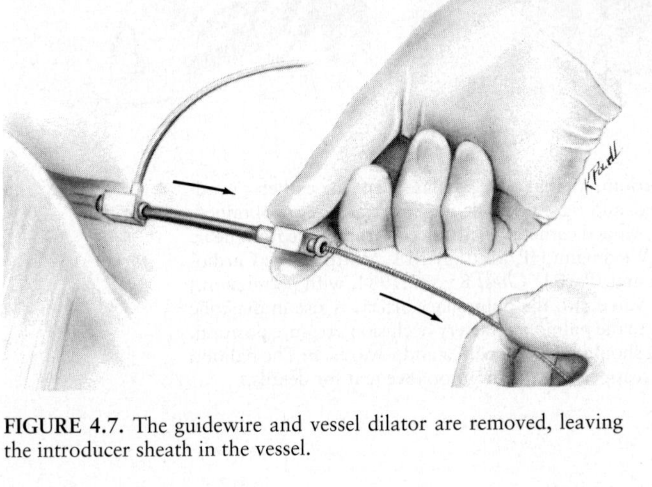

FIGURE 4.7. The guidewire and vessel dilator are removed, leaving the introducer sheath in the vessel.

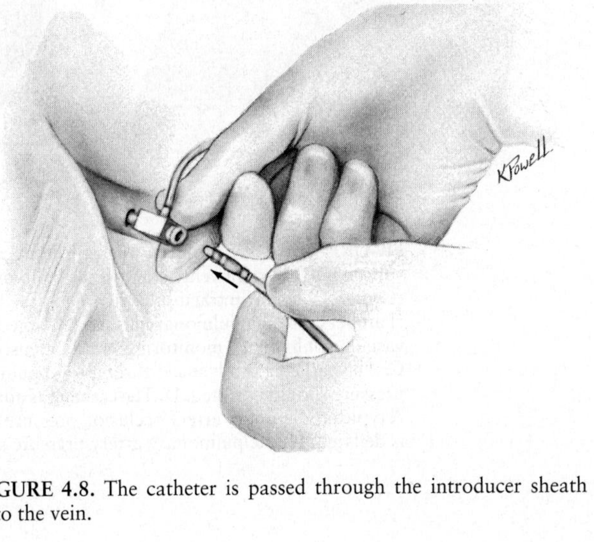

FIGURE 4.8. The catheter is passed through the introducer sheath into the vein.

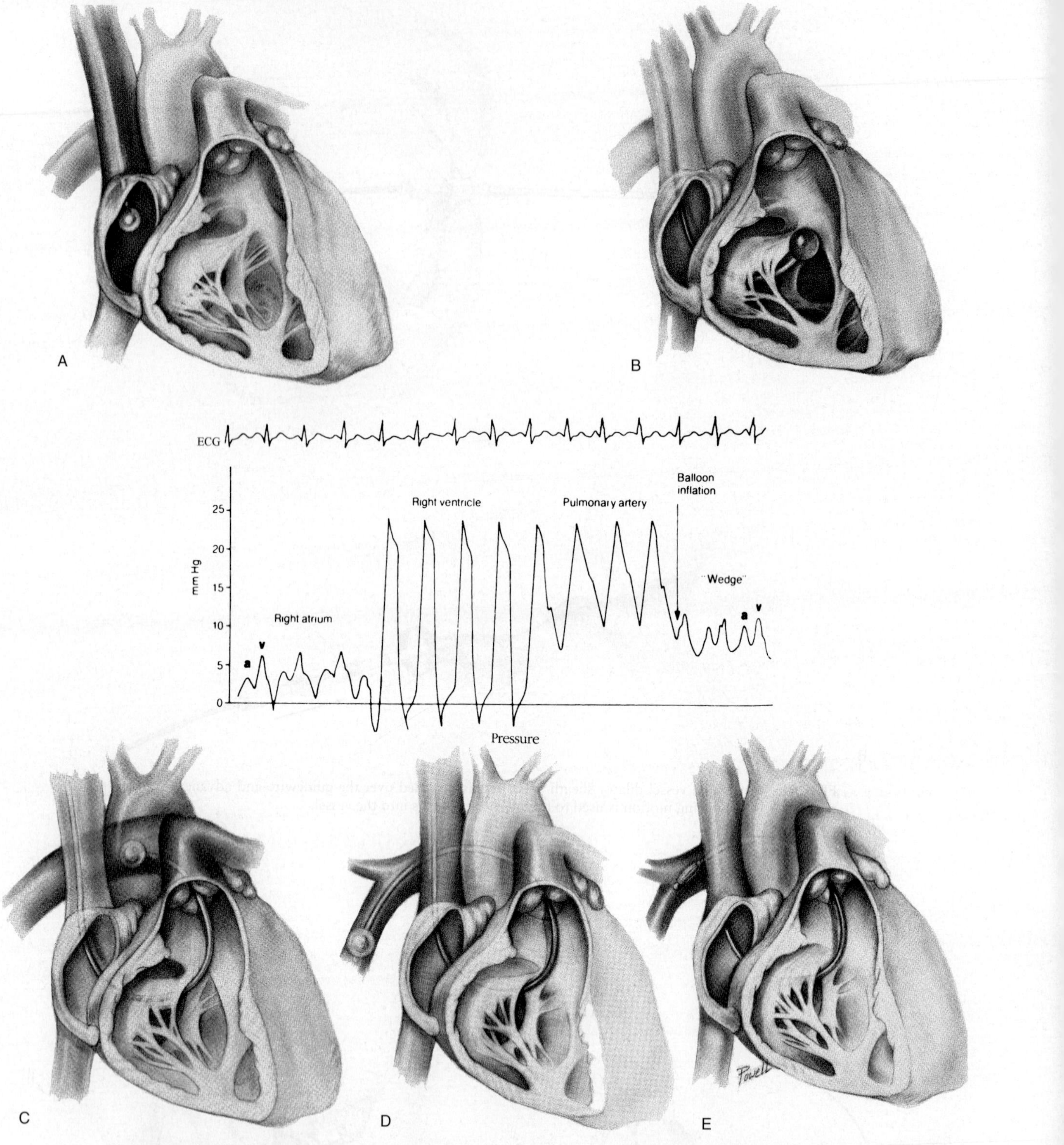

FIGURE 4.9. **A:** With the catheter tip in the right atrium, the balloon is inflated. **B:** The catheter is advanced into the right ventricle with the balloon inflated, and right ventricle pressure tracings are obtained. (*Center*): Waveform tracings generated as the balloon-tipped catheter is advanced through the right heart chambers into the pulmonary artery. [Adapted from Wiedmann HP, Matthay MA, Matthey RA: Cardiovascular pulmonary monitoring in the intensive care unit (Part 1) *Chest* 85:537;1984, with permission.] **C:** The catheter is advanced through the pulmonary valve into the pulmonary artery. A rise in diastolic pressure should be noted. **D:** The catheter is advanced to the pulmonary artery occlusion pressure position. A typical pulmonary artery occlusion pressure tracing should be noted with a and v waves. **E:** The balloon is deflated. Phasic pulmonary artery pressure should reappear on the monitor. (See text for details.)

approximately 35 to 40 cm from the left antecubital fossa, 10 to 15 cm from the internal jugular vein, 10 cm from the subclavian vein, and 35 to 40 cm from the femoral vein. A right atrial waveform on the monitor, with appropriate fluctuations accompanying respiratory changes or cough, confirms proper intrathoracic location (Fig. 4.9, center). If desired, obtain right atrial blood for oxygen saturation from the distal port. Flush the distal lumen with saline and record the right atrial pressures. (Occasionally, it is necessary to inflate the balloon to keep the tip from adhering to the atrial wall during blood aspiration.)

8. With the catheter tip in the right atrium, inflate the balloon with the recommended amount of air or carbon dioxide (Fig. 4.9A). Inflation of the balloon should be associated with a slight feeling of resistance—if it is not, suspect balloon rupture and do not attempt further inflation or advancement of the catheter before properly reevaluating balloon integrity. If significant resistance to balloon inflation is encountered, suspect malposition of the catheter in a small vessel; withdraw the catheter and readvance it to a new position. Do not use liquids to inflate the balloon, as they might be irretrievable and could prevent balloon deflation.
9. With the balloon inflated, advance the catheter until a RV pressure tracing is seen on the monitor (Fig. 4.9, center). Obtain and record RV pressures. Catheter passage into and through the RV is an especially risky time in terms of arrhythmias. Maintaining the balloon inflated in the RV minimizes ventricular irritation (Fig. 4.9B), but it is important to monitor vital signs and ECG throughout the entire insertion procedure. Elevating the head of the bed to 5 degrees and a right tilt position will facilitate the passage of the catheter through the right ventricle and minimize the generation of arrhythmias [61].
10. Continue advancing the catheter until the diastolic pressure tracing rises above that in the RV (Fig. 4.9, center), indicating PA placement (Fig. 4.9C). If a RV trace still appears after the catheter has been advanced 15 cm beyond the original distance needed to reach the right atrium, suspect curling in the ventricle; deflate the balloon, withdraw it to the right atrium, then reinflate it and try again. Advancement beyond the PA position results in a fall on the pressure tracing from the levels of systolic pressure noted in the RV and PA. When this is noted, record the PAOP (Fig. 4.9, center, D) and deflate the balloon. Phasic PA pressure should reappear on the pressure tracing when the balloon is deflated. If it does not, pull back the catheter with the deflated balloon until the PA tracing appears. With the balloon deflated, blood may be aspirated for oxygen saturation measurement. Watch for intermittent RV tracings indicating slippage of the catheter backward into the ventricle.
11. Carefully record the balloon inflation volume needed to change the PA pressure tracing to the PAOP tracing. If PAOP is recorded with an inflation volume significantly lower than the manufacturer's recommended volume, or if subsequent PAOP determinations require decreasing amounts of balloon inflation volume as compared with an initial appropriate amount, the catheter tip has migrated too far peripherally and should be pulled back immediately.
12. Secure the catheter in the correct PA position by suturing or taping it to the skin to prevent inadvertent advancement. Apply a transparent dressing with a chlorhexidine sponge if indicated.
13. Order a chest radiograph to confirm catheter position; the catheter tip should appear no more than 3 to 5 cm from the midline. To assess whether peripheral catheter migration has occurred, daily chest radiographs are recommended to supplement pressure monitoring and checks on balloon inflation volumes. An initial cross-table lateral radiograph may be obtained in patients on positive end-expiratory pressure (PEEP) to rule out superior placements.

Special Considerations

In certain disease states (right atrial or RV dilatation, severe pulmonary hypertension, severe tricuspid insufficiency, low CO syndromes), it may be difficult to position a flow-directed catheter properly. These settings may require fluoroscopic guidance to aid in catheter positioning. Infusion of 5 to 10 mL of cold saline through the distal lumen may stiffen the catheter and aid in positioning. Alternatively, a 0.025-cm guidewire 145 cm long may be used to stiffen the catheter when placed through the distal lumen of a 7-Fr PA catheter. This manipulation should be performed only under fluoroscopic guidance by an experienced operator. Rarely, nonflow-directed PA catheters (e.g., Cournand catheters) may be required. Because of their rigidity, these catheters have the potential to perforate the right heart and must be placed only under fluoroscopy by a physician experienced in cardiac catheterization techniques.

PHYSIOLOGIC DATA

Measurement of a variety of hemodynamic parameters and oxygen saturations is possible using the PA catheter. A summary of normal values for these parameters is found in Tables 4.3 and 4.4.

Pressures

Right Atrium

With the tip of the PA catheter in the right atrium (Fig. 4.9A), the balloon is deflated and a right atrial waveform recorded (Fig. 4.10). Normal resting right atrial pressure is 0 to 6 mm Hg. Two major positive atrial pressure waves, the a wave and v wave, can usually be recorded. On occasion, a third positive wave, the c wave, can also be seen. The a wave is due to atrial contraction and follows the simultaneously recorded ECG P wave [62,63]. The a wave peak generally follows the peak of

TABLE 4.3

NORMAL RESTING PRESSURES OBTAINED DURING RIGHT HEART CATHETERIZATION

Cardiac chamber	Pressure (mm Hg)
Right atrium	
Range	0–6
Mean	3
Right ventricle	
Systolic	17–30
Diastolic	0–6
Pulmonary artery	
Systolic	15–30
Diastolic	5–13
Mean	10–18
Pulmonary artery occlusion (mean)	2–12

Adapted from JM Gore, JS Alpert, JR Benotti, et al: *Handbook of Hemodynamic Monitoring*. Boston, MA, Little, Brown, 1984.

TABLE 4.4

APPROXIMATE NORMAL OXYGEN SATURATION AND CONTENT VALUES

Chamber sampled	Oxygen content (vol%)	Oxygen saturation (%)
Superior vena cava	14.0	70
Inferior vena cava	16.0	80
Right atrium	15.0	75
Right ventricle	15.0	75
Pulmonary artery	15.0	75
Pulmonary vein	20.0	98
Femoral artery	19.0	96
Atrioventricular oxygen content difference	3.5–5.5	—

Adapted from JM Gore, JS Alpert, JR Benotti, et al: *Handbook of Hemodynamic Monitoring*. Boston, MA, Little, Brown, 1984.

the electrical P wave by approximately 80 milliseconds [64]. The v wave represents the pressure generated by venous filling of the right atrium while the tricuspid valve is closed. The peak of the v wave occurs at the end of ventricular systole when the atrium is maximally filled, corresponding to the point near the end of the T wave on the ECG. The c wave is due to the sudden motion of the atrioventricular valve ring toward the right atrium at the onset of ventricular systole. The c wave follows the a wave by a time equal to the ECG P–R interval. The c wave is more readily visible in cases of P–R prolongation [64]. The x descent follows the c wave and reflects atrial relaxation. The y descent is due to rapid emptying of the atrium after opening of the tricuspid valve. The mean right atrial pressure decreases during inspiration with spontaneous respiration (secondary to a decrease in intrathoracic pressure), whereas the a and v waves and the *x* and *y* descents become more prominent. Once a multilumen PA catheter is in position, right atrial blood can be sampled and pressure monitored using the proximal lumen. It should be noted that the pressures obtained via the proximal lumen may not accurately reflect right atrial pressure due to positioning of the lumen against the atrial wall or within the introducer sheath. The latter problem is more frequently encountered in shorter patients [65].

Right Ventricle

The normal resting RV pressure is 17 to 30/0 to 6 mm Hg, recorded when the PA catheter crosses the tricuspid valve (Fig. 4.9B). The RV systolic pressure should equal the PA systolic pressure (except in cases of pulmonic stenosis or RV outflow tract obstruction). The RV diastolic pressure should equal the mean right atrial pressure during diastole when the tricuspid valve is open. Introduction of the catheter with a pacing lumen allows continuous monitoring of RV hemodynamics when the pacing wire is not in place. Using special catheters, RV end-diastolic volume index and RV ejection fraction can be accurately measured [66–69].

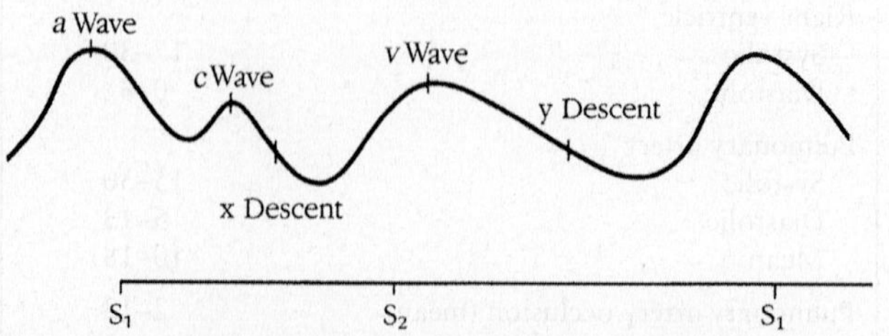

FIGURE 4.10. Stylized representation of a right atrial waveform in relation to heart sounds. (See text for discussion of a, c, and v waves and *x* and *y* descents.) S_1, first heart sound; S_2, second heart sound.

Pulmonary Artery

With the catheter in proper position and the balloon deflated, the distal lumen transmits PA pressure (Fig. 4.9E). Normal resting PA pressure is 15 to 30/5 to 13 mm Hg, with a mean pressure of 10 to 18 mm Hg. The PA waveform is characterized by a systolic peak and diastolic trough with a dicrotic notch due to closure of the pulmonic valve. The peak PA systolic pressure occurs in the T wave of a simultaneously recorded ECG.

Since the pulmonary vasculature is normally a low-resistance circuit, PA diastolic pressure (PADP) is closely related to mean PAOP (PADP is usually 1 to 3 mm Hg higher than mean PAOP) and thus can be used as an index of left ventricle filling pressure in patients in whom an occlusion pressure is unobtainable or in whom PADP and PAOP have been shown to correlate closely. However, if pulmonary vascular resistance is increased, as in pulmonary embolic disease, pulmonary fibrosis, or reactive pulmonary hypertension (see Chapter 56), PADP may markedly exceed mean PAOP and thus become an unreliable index of left heart function [64]. Similar provisos apply when using PA mean pressure as an index of left ventricular function.

Pulmonary Artery Occlusion Pressure

An important application of the balloon flotation catheter is the recording of PAOP. This measurement is obtained when the inflated balloon impacts a slightly smaller branch of the PA (Fig. 4.9D). In this position, the balloon stops the flow, and the catheter tip senses pressure transmitted backward through the static column of blood from the next active circulatory bed—the pulmonary veins. Pulmonary venous pressure is a prime determinant of pulmonary congestion and thus of the tendency for fluid to shift from the pulmonary capillaries into the interstitial tissue and alveoli. Also, pulmonary venous pressure and PAOP closely reflect left atrial pressure (except in rare instances, such as pulmonary veno-occlusive disease, in which there is obstruction in the small pulmonary veins), and serve as indices of left ventricular filling pressure [70,71]. The PAOP is required to assess left ventricular filling pressure, since multiple studies have demonstrated that right atrial (e.g., central venous) pressure correlates poorly with PAOP [72].

The PAOP is a phase-delayed, amplitude-dampened version of the left atrial pressure. The normal resting PAOP is 2 to 12 mm Hg and averages 2 to 7 mm Hg below the mean PA pressure. The PAOP waveform is similar to that of the right atrium, with a, c, and v waves and *x* and *y* descents (Fig. 4.10). However, in contradistinction to the right atrial waveform, the PAOP waveform demonstrates a v wave that is slightly larger than the a wave [14]. Because of the time required for left atrial mechanical events to be transmitted through the pulmonary vasculature, PAOP waveforms are further delayed when recorded with a simultaneous ECG. The peak of the a wave follows the peak of the ECG P wave by approximately 240 milliseconds, and the peak of the v wave occurs after the ECG T wave has been inscribed. Occlusion position is confirmed by withdrawing a blood specimen from the distal lumen and measuring oxygen saturation. Measured oxygen saturation of 95% or more is satisfactory [71]. The lung segment from which the sample is obtained will be well ventilated if the patient breathes slowly and deeply.

A valid PAOP measurement requires a patent vascular channel between the left atrium and catheter tip. Thus, the PAOP approximates pulmonary venous pressure (and therefore left atrial pressure) only if the catheter tip lies in zone 3 of the lungs [62,73]. (The lung is divided into three physiologic zones, dependent on the relationship of PA, pulmonary venous, and alveolar pressures. In zone 3, the PA and pulmonary venous pressure exceed the alveolar pressure, ensuring an uninterrupted column of blood between the catheter tip and the pulmonary veins.) If, on portable lateral chest radiograph, the catheter tip is below the level of the left atrium (posterior position in supine patients), it can be assumed to be in zone 3. This assumption holds if applied PEEP is less than 15 cm H_2O and the patient is not markedly volume depleted. Whether the catheter is positioned in zone 3 may also be determined by certain physiologic characteristics (Table 4.5). A catheter occlusion outside zone 3 shows marked respiratory variation, an unnaturally smooth vascular waveform, and misleading high pressures.

With a few exceptions [74], estimates of capillary hydrostatic filtration pressure from PAOP are acceptable [75]. It should be noted that measurement of PAOP does not take into account capillary permeability, serum colloid osmotic pressure, interstitial pressure, or actual pulmonary capillary resistance [75,76]. These factors all play roles in the formation of pulmonary edema, and the PAOP should be interpreted in the context of the specific clinical situation.

Mean PAOP correlates well with left ventricular end-diastolic pressure (LVEDP), provided the patient has a normal mitral valve and normal left ventricular function. In myocardial infarction, conditions with decreased left ventricular compliance (e.g., ischemia, left ventricular hypertrophy), and conditions with markedly increased left ventricular filling pressure (e.g., dilated cardiomyopathy), the contribution of atrial contraction to left ventricular filling is increased. Thus, the LVEDP may be significantly higher than the mean left atrial pressure or PAOP [62].

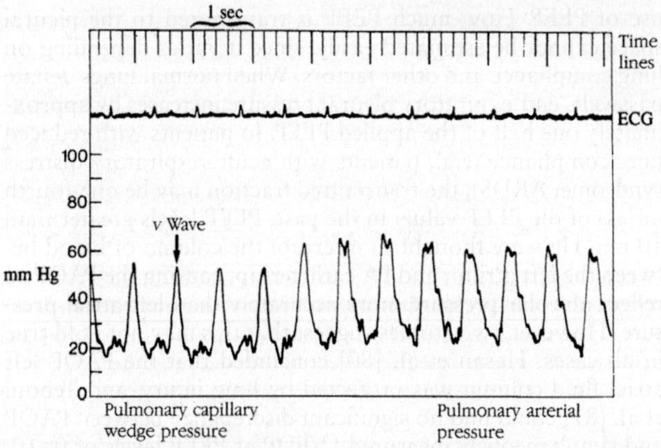

FIGURE 4.11. Pulmonary artery and pulmonary artery occlusion tracings with giant v waves distorting with pulmonary artery recording. ECG, electrocardiogram.

The position of the catheter can be misinterpreted in patients with the presence of giant v waves. The most common cause of these v waves is mitral regurgitation. During this condition, left ventricular blood floods a normal-sized, noncompliant left atrium during ventricular systole, causing giant v waves in the occlusion pressure tracing (Fig. 4.11). The giant v wave of mitral regurgitation may be transmitted to the PA tracing, yielding a bifid PA waveform composed of the PA systolic wave and the v wave. As the catheter is occluded, the PA systolic wave is lost, but the v wave remains. It is important to note that the PA systolic wave occurs earlier in relation to the QRS complex of a simultaneously recorded ECG (between the QRS and T waves) than does the v wave (after the T wave).

Although a large v wave is not diagnostic of mitral regurgitation and is not always present in this circumstance, acute mitral regurgitation remains the most common cause of giant v waves in the PAOP tracing. Prominent v waves may occur whenever the left atrium is distended and noncompliant due to left ventricular failure from any cause (e.g., ischemic heart disease, dilated cardiomyopathy) [77,78] or secondary to the increased pulmonary blood flow in acute ventricular septal defect [79]. Acute mitral regurgitation is the rare instance when the PA end-diastolic pressure may be lower than the computer-measured mean occlusion pressure [64].

End expiration provides a readily identifiable reference point for PAOP interpretation because pleural pressure returns to baseline at the end of passive deflation (approximately equal to atmospheric pressure). Pleural pressure can exceed the normal resting value with active expiratory muscle contraction or

TABLE 4.5

CHECKLIST FOR VERIFYING POSITION OF PULMONARY ARTERY CATHETER

	Zone 3	Zone 1 or 2
PAOP contour	Cardiac ripple (A + V waves)	Unnaturally smooth
PAD versus PAOP	PAD > PAOP	PAD < PAOP
PEEP trial	ΔPAOP < ½ΔPEEP	ΔPAOP > ½ΔPEEP
Respiratory variation of PAOP	< ½ P_{ALV}	≥ ½Δ P_{ALV}
Catheter-tip location	LA level or below	Above LA level

LA, left atrium; PAD, pulmonary artery diastolic pressure; P_{ALV}, alveolar pressure; PAOP, pulmonary artery occlusion pressure; PEEP, positive end-expiratory pressure.
Adapted from RJ Schultz, GF Whitfield, JJ LaMura, et al: The role of physiologic monitoring in patients with fractures of the hip. *J Trauma* 25:309, 1985.

use of PEEP. How much PEEP is transmitted to the pleural space cannot be estimated easily, since it varies depending on lung compliance and other factors. When normal lungs deflate passively, end-expiratory pleural pressure increases by approximately one half of the applied PEEP. In patients with reduced lung compliance (e.g., patients with acute respiratory distress syndrome; ARDS), the transmitted fraction may be one-fourth or less of the PEEP value. In the past, PEEP levels greater than 10 mm Hg were thought to interrupt the column of blood between the left atrium and PA catheter tip, causing the PAOP to reflect alveolar pressure more accurately than left atrial pressure. However, two studies suggest that this may not hold true in all cases. Hasan et al. [80] concluded that the PAOP left atrial fluid column was protected by lung injury, and Teboul et al. [81] could find no significant discrepancy between PAOP and simultaneously measured LVEDP at PEEP levels of 0, 10, and 16 to 20 cm H_2O in patients with ARDS. They hypothesize that (a) a large intrapulmonary right-to-left shunt may provide a number of microvessels shielded from alveolar pressure, allowing free communication from PA to pulmonary veins, or (b) in ARDS, both vascular and lung compliance may decrease, reducing transmission of alveolar pressure to the pulmonary microvasculature and maintaining an uninterrupted blood column from the catheter tip to the left atrium.

Although it is difficult to estimate precisely the true transmural vascular pressure in a patient on PEEP, temporarily disconnecting PEEP to measure PAOP is not recommended. Because the hemodynamics have been destabilized, these measurements will be of questionable value. Venous return increases acutely after discontinuation of PEEP [81], and abrupt removal of PEEP will cause hypoxia, which may not reverse quickly on reinstitution of PEEP [82]. Additional discussion of measurement and interpretation of pulmonary vascular pressures on PEEP is found in Chapter 58.

Cardiac Output

Thermodilution Technique

A catheter equipped with a thermistor 4 cm from its tip allows calculation of CO by using the thermodilution principle [47,83]. The thermodilution principle holds that if a known quantity of cold solution is introduced into the circulation and adequately mixed (passage through two valves and a ventricle is adequate), the resultant cooling curve recorded at a downstream site allows calculation of net blood flow. CO is inversely proportional to the integral of the time-versus-temperature curve.

In practice, a known amount of cold or room temperature solution (typically 10 mL of 0.9% saline in adults and 5 mL of 0.9% saline in children) is injected into the right atrium via the catheter's proximal port. The thermistor allows recording of the baseline PA blood temperature and subsequent temperature change. The resulting curve is usually analyzed by computer, although it can be analyzed manually by simple planimetric methods. Correction factors are added by catheter manufacturers to account for the mixture of cold indicator with warm residual fluid in the catheter injection lumen and the heat transfer from the catheter walls to the cold indicator.

Reported coefficients of variation using triplicate determinations, using 10 mL of cold injectate and a bedside computer, are approximately 4% or less. Variations in the rate of injection can also introduce error into CO determinations, and it is thus important that the solution be injected as rapidly as possible. Careful attention must be paid to the details of this procedure; even then, changes of less than 10% to 15% above or below an initial value may not truly establish directional validity. Thermodilution CO is inaccurate in low-output states, tricuspid regurgitation, and in cases of atrial or ventricular septal defects [84].

Normal values for arterial–venous oxygen content difference, mixed venous oxygen saturation, and CO can be found in Table 4.6.

Analysis of Mixed Venous Blood

CO can be approximated merely by examining mixed venous (PA) oxygen saturation. Theoretically, if CO rises, then the mixed venous oxygen partial pressure will rise, since peripheral tissues need to exact less oxygen per unit of blood. Conversely, if CO falls, peripheral extraction from each unit will increase to meet the needs of metabolizing tissues. Serial determinations of mixed venous oxygen saturation may display trends in CO. Normal mixed venous oxygen saturation is 70% to 75%; values of less than 60% are associated with heart failure and values of less than 40% with shock [85]. Potential sources of error in this determination include extreme low-flow states where poor mixing may occur, contamination of desaturated mixed venous blood by saturated pulmonary capillary blood when the sample is aspirated too quickly through the nonwedged catheter

TABLE 4.6

SELECTED HEMODYNAMIC VARIABLES DERIVED FROM RIGHT HEART CATHETERIZATION

Hemodynamic variable	Normal range
Arterial–venous content difference	3.5–5.5 mL/100 mL
Cardiac index	2.5–4.5 L/min/m^2
Cardiac output	3.0–7.0 L/min
Left ventricular stroke work index	45–60 g/beat/m^2
Mixed venous oxygen content	18.0 mL/100 mL
Mixed venous saturation	75% (approximately)
Oxygen consumption	200–250 mL/min
Pulmonary vascular resistance	120–250 dynes/sec/cm^{-5}
Stroke volume	70–130 mL/contraction
Stroke volume index	40–50 mL/contraction/m^2
Systemic vascular resistance	1,100–1,500 dynes/sec/cm^2

Adapted from JM Gore, JS Alpert, JR Benotti, et al: *Handbook of Hemodynamic Monitoring*. Boston, MA, Little, Brown, 1984.

TABLE 4.7

HEMODYNAMIC PARAMETERS IN COMMONLY ENCOUNTERED CLINICAL SITUATIONS (IDEALIZED)

	RA	RV	PA	PAOP	AO	CI	SVR	PVR
Normal	0–6	25/0–6	25/6–12	6–12	130/80	≥2.5	1,500	≤250
Hypovolemic shock	0–2	15–20/0–2	15–20/2–6	2–6	≤90/60	<2.0	>1,500	≤250
Cardiogenic shock	8	50/8	50/35	35	≤90/60	<2.0	>1,500	≤250
Septic shock								
Early	0–2	20–25/0–2	20–25/0–6	0–6	≤90/60	≥2.5	<1,500	<250
Late[a]	0–4	25/4–10	25/4–10	4–10	≤90/60	<2.0	>1,500	>250
Acute massive pulmonary embolism	8–12	50/12	50/12–15	≤12	≤90/60	<2.0	>1,500	>450
Cardiac tamponade	12–18	25/12–18	25/12–18	12–18	≤90/60	<2.0	>1,500	≤250
AMI without LVF	0–6	25/0–6	25/12–18	≤18	140/90	≤2.5	1,500	≤250
AMI with LVF	0–6	30–40/0–6	30–40/18–25	>18	140/90	>2.0	>1,500	>250
Biventricular failure secondary to LVF	>6	50–60/ >6	50–60/25	18–25	120/80	~2.0	>1,500	>250
RVF secondary to RVI	12–20	30/12–20	30/12	<12	≤90/60	<2.0	>1,500	>250
Cor pulmonale	>6	80/ >6	80/35	<12	120/80	~2.0	>1,500	>400
Idiopathic pulmonary hypertension	0–6	80–100/0–6	80–100/40	<12	100/60	<2.0	>1,500	>500
Acute ventricular septal rupture[b]	6	60/6–8	60/35	30	≤90/60	<2.0	>1,500	>250

[a]Hemodynamic profile seen in approximately one third of patients in late septic shock.
[b]Confirmed by appropriate RA–PA oxygen saturation step-up. See text for discussion.
AMI, acute myocardial infarction; AO, aortic; CI, cardiac index; LVF, left ventricular failure; PA, pulmonary artery; PAOP, pulmonary artery occlusion pressure; PVR, pulmonary vascular resistance; RA, right atrium; RV, right ventricle; RVF, right ventricular failure; RVI, right ventricular infarction; SVR, systemic vascular resistance.
Adapted from Gore JM, Alpert JS, Benotti JR, et al: *Handbook of Hemodynamic Monitoring*. Boston, MA, Little, Brown, 1984.

[86] or in certain disease states (e.g., sepsis) where microcirculatory shunting may occur. Fiberoptic reflectance oximetry PA catheters can continuously measure and record mixed venous oxygen saturations in appropriate clinical situations [50,87].

Derived Parameters

Useful hemodynamic parameters that can be derived using data with PA catheters include the following:

1. Cardiac index = CO (L/minute)/BSA (m^2)
2. Stroke volume = CO (L/minute)/heart rate (beats/minute)
3. Stroke index = CO (L/minute)/[heart rate (beats/minute) × BSA (m^2)]
4. Mean arterial pressure (mmHg) = [(2 × diastolic) + systolic]/3
5. Systemic vascular resistance (dyne/second/cm^{-5}) = ([mean arterial pressure − mean right atrial pressure (mm Hg)] × 80)/CO (L/minute)
6. Pulmonary arteriolar resistance (dyne/second/cm^{-5}) = ([mean PA pressure − PAOP (mm Hg)] × 80)/CO (L/minute)
7. Total pulmonary resistance (dyne/second/cm^{-5}) = ([mean PA pressure (mm Hg)] × 80)/CO (L/minute)
8. Left ventricular stroke work index = 1.36 (mean arterial pressure − PAOP) × stroke index/100
9. Do_2 (mL/minute/m^2) = cardiac index × arterial O_2 content × 10

Normal values are listed in Table 4.6.

CLINICAL APPLICATIONS OF THE PULMONARY ARTERY CATHETER

Normal Resting Hemodynamic Profile

The finding of normal CO associated with normal left and right heart filling pressures is useful in establishing a noncardiovascular basis to explain abnormal symptoms or signs and as a baseline to gauge a patient's disease progression or response to therapy. Right atrial pressures of 0 to 6 mm Hg, PA systolic pressures of 15 to 30 mm Hg, PADPs of 5 to 12 mm Hg, PA mean pressures of 9 to 18 mm Hg, PAOP of 5 to 12 mm Hg, and a cardiac index exceeding 2.5 L per minute per m^2 characterize a normal cardiovascular state at rest.

Table 4.7 summarizes specific hemodynamic patterns for a variety of disease entities in which PA catheters have been indicated and provide clinical information that can impact patient care.

COMPLICATIONS

Minor and major complications associated with bedside balloon flotation PA catheterization have been reported (Table 4.8). During the 1970s, in the first 10 years of clinical catheter use, a number of studies reported a relatively high incidence of certain complications. Consequent revision of guidelines for PA catheter use and improved insertion and maintenance techniques resulted in a decreased incidence of these complications

TABLE 4.8

COMPLICATIONS OF PULMONARY ARTERY CATHETERIZATION

Associated with central venous access
Balloon rupture
Knotting
Pulmonary infarction
Pulmonary artery perforation
Thrombosis, embolism
Arrhythmias
Intracardiac damage
Infections
Miscellaneous complications

in the 1980s [88]. The majority of complications are avoidable by scrupulous attention to detail in catheter placement and maintenance.

Complications Associated with Central Venous Access

The insertion techniques and complications of central venous cannulation are discussed in Chapter 2. Reported local vascular complications include local arterial or venous hematomas, unintentional entry of the catheter into the carotid system, atrioventricular fistulas, and pseudoaneurysm formation [89–91]. Adjacent structures, such as the thoracic duct, can be damaged, with resultant chylothorax formation. Pneumothorax can be a serious complication of insertion, although the incidence is relatively low (1% to 2%) [64,89,92]. The incidence of pneumothorax is higher with the subclavian approach than with the internal jugular approach in some reports [93], but other studies demonstrate no difference between the two sites [94,95]. The incidence of complications associated with catheter insertion is generally considered to be inversely proportional to the operator's experience.

Balloon Rupture

Balloon rupture occurred more frequently in the early 1970s than it does now and was generally related to exceeding recommended inflation volumes. The main problems posed by balloon rupture are air emboli gaining access to the arterial circulation and balloon fragments embolizing to the distal pulmonary circulation. If rupture occurs during catheter insertion, the loss of the balloon's protective cushioning function can predispose to endocardial damage and attendant thrombotic and arrhythmic complications.

Knotting

Knotting of a catheter around itself is most likely to occur when loops form in the cardiac chambers and the catheter is repeatedly withdrawn and readvanced [96]. Knotting is avoided if care is taken not to advance the catheter significantly beyond the distances at which entrance to the ventricle or PA would ordinarily be anticipated. Knotted catheters usually can be extricated transvenously; guidewire placement [97], venotomy, or more extensive surgical procedures are occasionally necessary.

Knotting of PA catheters around intracardiac structures [98] or other intravascular catheters [99] has been reported. Rarely, entrapment of a PA catheter in cardiac sutures after open-heart surgery has been reported, requiring varying approaches for removal [100].

Pulmonary Infarction

Peripheral migration of the catheter tip (caused by catheter softening and loop tightening over time) with persistent, undetected wedging in small branches of the PA is the most common mechanism underlying pulmonary ischemic lesions attributable to PA catheters [101]. These lesions are usually small and asymptomatic, often diagnosed solely on the basis of changes in the chest radiograph demonstrating an occlusion-shaped pleural-based density with a convex proximal contour [102].

Severe infarctions are usually produced if the balloon is left inflated in the occlusion position for an extended period, thus obstructing more central branches of the PA, or if solutions are injected at relatively high pressure through the catheter lumen in an attempt to restore an apparently damped pressure trace. Pulmonary embolic phenomena resulting from thrombus formation around the catheter or over areas of endothelial damage can also result in pulmonary infarction.

The reported incidence of pulmonary infarction secondary to PA catheters in 1974 was 7.2% [101], but recently reported rates of pulmonary infarction are much lower. Boyd et al. [103] found a 1.3% incidence of pulmonary infarction in a prospective study of 528 PA catheterizations. Sise et al. [104] reported no pulmonary infarctions in a prospective study of 319 PA catheter insertions. Use of continuous saline flush solutions and careful monitoring of PA waveforms are important reasons for the decreased incidence of this complication.

Pulmonary Artery Perforation

A serious and feared complication of PA catheterization is rupture of the PA leading to hemorrhage, which can be massive and sometimes fatal [105–107]. Rupture may occur during insertion or may be delayed a number of days [107]. PA rupture or perforation has been reported in approximately 0.1% to 0.2% of patients [93,108,109], although recent pathologic data suggest the true incidence of PA perforation is somewhat higher [110]. Proposed mechanisms by which PA rupture can occur include (a) an increased pressure gradient between PAOP and PA pressure brought about by balloon inflation and favoring distal catheter migration, where perforation is more likely to occur; (b) an occluded catheter tip position favoring eccentric or distended balloon inflation with a spearing of the tip laterally and through the vessel; (c) cardiac pulsation causing shearing forces and damage as the catheter tip repeatedly contacts the vessel wall; (d) presence of the catheter tip near a distal arterial bifurcation where the integrity of the vessel wall against which the balloon is inflated may be compromised; and (e) simple lateral pressure on vessel walls caused by balloon inflation (this tends to be greater if the catheter tip was occluded before inflation began). Patient risk factors for PA perforation include pulmonary hypertension, mitral valve disease, advanced age, hypothermia, and anticoagulant therapy. In patients with these risk factors and in whom PADP reflects PAOP reasonably well, avoidance of subsequent balloon inflation altogether constitutes prudent prophylaxis.

Another infrequent but life-threatening complication is false aneurysm formation associated with rupture or dissection of the PA [111]. Technique factors related to PA hemorrhage are distal placement or migration of the catheter; failure to remove large catheter loops placed in the cardiac chambers during insertion; excessive catheter manipulation; use of stiffer catheter designs; and multiple overzealous or prolonged balloon inflations. Adherence to strict technique may decrease the incidence of this complication. In a prospective study reported in 1986, no cases of PA rupture occurred in 1,400 patients undergoing PA catheterization for cardiac surgery [94].

PA perforation typically presents with massive hemoptysis. Emergency management includes immediate occlusion arteriogram and bronchoscopy, intubation of the unaffected lung, and consideration of emergency lobectomy or pneumonectomy. PA catheter balloon tamponade resulted in rapid control of bleeding in one case report [112]. Application of PEEP to intubated patients may also tamponade hemorrhage caused by a PA catheter [113,114].

Thromboembolic Complications

Because PA catheters constitute foreign bodies in the cardiovascular system and can potentially damage the endocardium, they are associated with an increased incidence of thrombosis. Thrombi encasing the catheter tip and aseptic thrombotic vegetations forming at endocardial sites in contact with the catheter have been reported [103,115]. Extensive clotting around the catheter tip can occlude the pulmonary vasculature distal to the catheter, and thrombi anywhere in the venous system or right heart can serve as a source of pulmonary emboli. Subclavian venous thrombosis, presenting with unilateral neck vein distention and upper extremity edema, may occur in up to 2% of subclavian placements [116,117]. Venous thrombosis complicating percutaneous internal jugular vein catheterization is fairly commonly reported, although its clinical importance remains uncertain [118]. Consistently damped pressure tracings without evidence of peripheral catheter migration or pulmonary vascular occlusion should arouse suspicion of thrombi at the catheter tip. A changing relationship of PADP to PAOP over time should raise concern about possible pulmonary emboli.

If an underlying hypercoagulable state is known to exist, if catheter insertion was particularly traumatic, or if prolonged monitoring becomes necessary, one should consider cautiously anticoagulating the patient.

Heparin-bonded catheters reduce thrombogenicity [45] and are commonly used. However, an important complication of heparin-bonded catheters is heparin-induced thrombocytopenia (HIT) [119,120]. Routine platelet counts are recommended for patients with heparin-bonded catheters in place. Because of the risk of HIT, some hospitals have abandoned the use of heparin-bonded catheters.

Rhythm Disturbances

Atrial and ventricular arrhythmias occur commonly during insertion of PA catheters [121]. Premature ventricular contractions occurred during 11% of the catheter insertions originally reported by Swan et al. [1].

Studies have reported advanced ventricular arrhythmias (three or more consecutive ventricular premature beats) in approximately 30% to 60% of patients undergoing right heart catheterization [93,117,122–124]. Most arrhythmias are self-limited and do not require treatment, but sustained ventricular arrhythmias requiring treatment occur in 0% to 3% of patients [103,123,124]. Risk factors associated with increased incidence of advanced ventricular arrhythmias are acute myocardial ischemia or infarction, hypoxia, acidosis, hypocalcemia, and hypokalemia [92,123]. A right lateral tilt position (5-degree angle) during PA catheter insertion is associated with a lower incidence of malignant ventricular arrhythmias than is the Trendelenburg position [61].

Although the majority of arrhythmias occur during catheter insertion, arrhythmias may develop at any time after the catheter has been correctly positioned. These arrhythmias are due to mechanical irritation of the conducting system and may be persistent. Ventricular ectopy may also occur if the catheter tip falls back into the RV outflow tract. Evaluation of catheter-induced ectopy should include a portable chest radiograph to evaluate catheter position and assessment of the distal lumen pressure tracing to ensure that the catheter has not slipped into the RV. Lidocaine may be used but is unlikely to ablate the ectopy because the irritant is not removed [125]. If the arrhythmia persists after lidocaine therapy or is associated with hemodynamic compromise, the catheter should be removed. Catheter removal should be performed by physicians under continuous ECG monitoring, since the ectopy occurs almost as frequently during catheter removal as during insertion [126,127].

Right bundle branch block (usually transient) can also complicate catheter insertion [128]. Patients undergoing anesthesia induction, those in the early stages of acute anteroseptal myocardial infarction, and those with acute pericarditis appear particularly susceptible to this complication. Patients with preexisting left bundle branch block are at risk for developing complete heart block during catheter insertion, and some have advocated the insertion of a temporary transvenous pacing wire, a PA catheter with a pacing lumen, or pacing PA catheter with the pacing leads on the external surface of the catheter [129]. However, use of an external transthoracic pacing device should be sufficient to treat this complication.

Intracardiac Damage

Damage to the right heart chambers, tricuspid valve, pulmonic valve, and their supporting structures as a consequence of PA catheterization has been reported [130–133]. The reported incidence of catheter-induced endocardial disruption detected by pathologic examination varies from 3.4% [115] to 75% [134], but most studies suggest a range of 20% to 30% [117,131,132]. These lesions consist of hemorrhage, sterile thrombus, intimal fibrin deposition, and nonbacterial thrombotic endocarditis. Their clinical significance is not clear, but there is concern that they may serve as a nidus for infectious endocarditis.

Direct damage to the cardiac valves and supporting chordae occurs primarily by withdrawal of the catheters while the balloon is inflated [1]. However, chordal rupture has been reported despite balloon deflation [113]. The incidence of intracardiac and valvular damage discovered on postmortem examination is considerably higher than that of clinically significant valvular dysfunction.

Infections

Catheter-related septicemia (the same pathogen growing from blood and the catheter tip) was reported in up to 2% of patients undergoing bedside catheterization in the 1970s [135]. However, the incidence of septicemia related to the catheter appears to have declined in recent years, with a number of studies suggesting a septicemia rate of 0% to 1% [93,136,137]. In situ time of more than 72 to 96 hours significantly increases the risk of catheter-related sepsis. Right-sided septic endocarditis has been reported [133,138], but the true incidence of this complication is unknown. Becker et al. [130] noted two cases of left ventricular abscess formation in patients with PA catheters and *Staphylococcus aureus* septicemia. Incidence of catheter colonization or contamination varies from 5% to 20%, depending on the duration of catheter placement and the criteria used to define colonization [137–139]. In situ catheter-related bloodstream infection may be diagnosed by either differential time to positivity or quantitative blood cultures [140]. With the former method, paired blood cultures are drawn from a peripheral vein and the catheter. If the catheter blood culture turns positive two or more hours sooner than the peripheral blood culture, the catheter is the likely cause of the bacteremia. With the other method, positive quantitative blood cultures drawn from the catheter are sensitive, specific, and predictive of catheter-related bacteremia [141].

Pressure transducers have also been identified as an occasional source of infection [142]. The chance of introducing infection into a previously sterile system is increased during injections for CO determinations and during blood withdrawal. Approaches to reduce the risk of catheter-related infection include use of a sterile protective sleeve and antibiotic bonding to the catheter [94,143,144]. Scheduled changes of catheters do not reduce the rate of infection [145].

Other Complications

Rare miscellaneous complications that have been reported include (a) hemodynamically significant decreases in pulmonary blood flow caused by balloon inflation in the central PA in postpneumonectomy patients with pulmonary hypertension in the remaining lung [146], (b) disruption of the catheter's intraluminal septum as a result of injecting contrast medium under pressure [147], (c) artifactual production of a midsystolic click caused by a slapping motion of the catheter against the interventricular septum in a patient with RV strain and paradoxic septal motion [148], (d) thrombocytopenia secondary to heparin-bonded catheters [119,120], and (e) dislodgment of pacing electrodes [149]. Multiple unusual placements of PA catheters have also been reported, including in the left pericardiophrenic vein, via the left superior intercostal vein into the abdominal vasculature, and from the superior vena cava through the left atrium and left ventricle into the aorta after open-heart surgery [150–152].

GUIDELINES FOR SAFE USE OF PULMONARY ARTERY CATHETERS

Multiple revisions and changes in emphasis to the original recommended techniques and guidelines have been published [88,153,154]. These precautions are summarized as follows:

1. Avoiding complications associated with catheter insertion.
   a. Inexperienced personnel performing insertions must be supervised. Many hospitals require that PA catheters be inserted by a fully trained intensivist, cardiologist, or anesthesiologist. Use of ultrasound guidance is recommended.
   b. Keep the patient as still as possible. Restraints or sedation may be required but the patient should be fully monitored with ECG and pulse oximetry.
   c. Strict sterile technique is mandatory. A chlorhexidine skin prep solution and maximum barrier precautions are recommended.
   d. Examine the postprocedure chest radiograph for pneumothorax (especially after subclavian or internal jugular venipuncture) and for catheter tip position.
2. Avoiding balloon rupture.
   a. Always inflate the balloon gradually. Stop inflation if no resistance is felt.
   b. Do not exceed recommended inflation volume. At the recommended volume, excess air will automatically be expelled from a syringe with holes bored in it that is constantly attached to the balloon port. Maintaining recommended volume also helps prevent the accidental injection of liquids.
   c. Keep the number of inflation–deflation cycles to a minimum.
   d. Do not reuse catheters designed for single usage, and do not leave catheters in place for prolonged periods.
   e. Use carbon dioxide as the inflation medium if communication between the right and left sides of the circulation is suspected.
3. Avoiding knotting. Discontinue advancement of the catheter if entrance to right atrium, RV, or PA has not been achieved at distances normally anticipated from a given insertion site. If these distances have already been significantly exceeded, or if the catheter does not withdraw easily, use fluoroscopy before attempting catheter withdrawal. Never pull forcefully on a catheter that does not withdraw easily.
4. Avoiding damage to pulmonary vasculature and parenchyma.
   a. Keep recording time of PAOP to a minimum, particularly in patients with pulmonary hypertension and other risk factors for PA rupture. Be sure the balloon is deflated after each PAOP recording. There is never an indication for continuous PAOP monitoring.
   b. Constant pressure monitoring is required each time the balloon is inflated. It should be inflated slowly, in small increments, and must be stopped as soon as the pressure tracing changes to PAOP or damped.
   c. If an occlusion is recorded with balloon volumes significantly less than the inflation volume recommended on the catheter shaft, withdraw the catheter to a position where full (or nearly full) inflation volume produces the desired trace.
   d. Anticipate catheter tip migration. Softening of the catheter material with time, repeated manipulations, and cardiac motion make distal catheter migration almost inevitable.
      i. Continuous PA pressure monitoring is mandatory, and the trace must be closely watched for changes from characteristic PA pressures to those indicating a PAOP or damped tip position.
      ii. Decreases over time in the balloon inflation volumes necessary to attain occlusion tracings should raise suspicion regarding catheter migration.
      iii. Confirm satisfactory tip position with chest radiographs immediately after insertion and at least daily.
   e. Do not use liquids to inflate the balloon. They may prevent deflation, and their relative incompressibility may increase lateral forces and stress on the walls of pulmonary vessels.
   f. Hemoptysis is an ominous sign and should prompt an urgent diagnostic evaluation and rapid institution of appropriate therapy.
   g. Avoid injecting solutions at high pressure through the catheter lumen on the assumption that clotting is the cause of the damped pressure trace. First, aspirate from the catheter. Then consider problems related to catheter position, stopcock position, transducer dome, transducers, pressure bag, flush system, or trapped air bubbles. Never flush the catheter in the occlusion position.
5. Avoiding thromboembolic complications.
   a. Minimize trauma induced during insertion.
   b. Consider the judicious use of anticoagulants in patients with hypercoagulable states or other risk factors.
   c. Avoid flushing the catheter under high pressure.
   d. Watch for a changing PADP–PAOP relationship, as well as for other clinical indicators of pulmonary embolism.
6. Avoiding arrhythmias.
   a. Constant ECG monitoring during insertion and maintenance, as well as ready accessibility of all supplies for performing cardiopulmonary resuscitation, defibrillation, and temporary pacing, are mandatory.
   b. Use caution when catheterizing patients with an acutely ischemic myocardium or preexisting left bundle branch block.
   c. When the balloon is deflated, do not advance the catheter beyond the right atrium.
   d. Avoid over manipulation of the catheter.
   e. Secure the introducer in place at the insertion site.
   f. Watch for intermittent RV pressure tracings when the catheter is thought to be in the PA position. An unexplained ventricular arrhythmia in a patient with a PA catheter in place indicates the possibility of catheter-provoked ectopy.
7. Avoiding valvular damage.
   a. Avoid prolonged catheterization and excessive manipulation.
   b. Do not withdraw the catheter when the balloon is inflated.
8. Avoiding infections.
   a. Use meticulously sterile technique on insertion.

b. Avoid excessive number of CO determinations and blood withdrawals.
c. Avoid prolonged catheterization.
d. Remove the catheter if signs of phlebitis develop. Culture the tip and use antibiotics as indicated.

SUMMARY

Hemodynamic monitoring enhances the understanding of cardiopulmonary pathophysiology in critically ill patients. Nonetheless, the risk-to-benefit profile of PA catheterization in various clinical circumstances remains uncertain. Recent large trials have concluded that there may be no outcome benefit to patients with PA catheters used as part of clinical decision making. There is increasing concern that PA catheterization may be overused and that the data obtained may not be optimally used, or perhaps in specific groups may increase morbidity and mortality. A recent meta-analysis of 13 randomized clinical trials concludes that the use of the PA catheter neither increased overall mortality or hospital days nor conferred benefit. The authors conclude that despite nearly 20 years of randomized clinical trials involving the PA catheter, there has not been a clear strategy in its use which has lead to improved survival [155].

Although there are open trials involving the PA catheter listed in the clinical trials registry, these are focused on elements of catheter data interpretation or comparisons of hemodynamics obtained from the PA catheter to other methods of obtaining these measurements [156]. There are no further randomized clinical trials looking at the PA catheter and patient outcomes recruiting patients at this time.

Until the results of future studies are available, clinicians using hemodynamic monitoring should carefully assess the risk-to-benefit ratio on an individual patient basis. The operator should understand the indications, insertion techniques, equipment, and data that can be generated before undertaking PA catheter insertion. PA catheterization must not delay or replace bedside clinical evaluation and treatment.

References

1. Swan HJC, Ganz W, Forrester J, et al: Catheterization of the heart in man with use of a flow-directed balloon-tipped catheter. *N Engl J Med* 283:447, 1970.
2. Connors AF, McCaffree DR, Gray BA: Evaluation of right heart catheterization in the critically ill patient without acute myocardial infarction. *N Engl J Med* 308:263, 1983.
3. Gorlin R: Current concepts in cardiology: practical cardiac hemodynamics. *N Engl J Med* 296:203, 1977.
4. Rao TK, Jacobs KH, El-Etr AA: Reinfarction following anesthesia in patients with myocardial infarction. *Anesthesiology* 59:499, 1983.
5. Hesdorffer CS, Milne JF, Meyers AM, et al: The value of Swan-Ganz catheterization and volume loading in preventing renal failure in patients undergoing abdominal aneurysmectomy. *Clin Nephrol* 28:272, 1987.
6. Shoemaker WC, Appel PL, Kram HB, et al: Prospective trial of supranormal values of survivors as therapeutic goals in high-risk surgical patients. *Chest* 94:1176, 1988.
7. Berlauk JF, Abrams JH, Gilmour IL, et al: Preoperative optimization of cardiovascular hemodynamics improves outcome in peripheral vascular surgery: a prospective, randomized clinical trial. *Ann Surg* 214:289, 1991.
8. Fleming A, Bishop M, Shoemaker W, et al: Prospective trial of supernormal values as goals of resuscitation in severe trauma. *Arch Surg* 127:1175, 1992.
9. Tuchschmidt J, Fried J, Astiz M, et al: Elevation of cardiac output and oxygen delivery improves outcome in septic shock. *Chest* 102:216, 1992.
10. Boyd O, Grounds RM, Bennett ED: A randomized clinical trial or the effect of deliberate perioperative increase of oxygen delivery on mortality in high-risk surgical patients. *JAMA* 270:2699, 1993.
11. Bishop MH, Shoemaker WC, Appel PL, et al: Prospective randomized trial of survivor values of cardiac index, oxygen delivery, and oxygen consumption as resuscitation endpoints in severe trauma. *J Trauma* 38:780, 1995.
12. Schiller WR, Bay RC, Garren RL, et al: Hyperdynamic resuscitation improves in patients with life-threatening burns. *J Burn Care Rehabil* 18:10, 1997.
13. Wilson J, Woods I, Fawcett J, et al: Reducing the risk of major elective surgery: randomized controlled trial of preoperative optimization of oxygen delivery. *BMJ* 318:1099, 1999.
14. Chang MC, Meredith JW, Kincaid EH, et al: Maintaining survivors' of left ventricular power output during shock resuscitation: a prospective pilot study. *J Trauma* 49:26, 2000.
15. Polonen P, Ruokonen E, Hippelainen M, et al: A prospective, randomized study of goal-oriented hemodynamic therapy in cardiac surgical patients. *Anesth Analg* 90:1052, 2000.
16. Friese RS, Shafi S, Gentilello LM: Pulmonary artery catheter use is associated with reduced mortality in severely injured patients: a National Trauma Data Bank analysis of 53,312 patients. *Crit Care Med* 34:1597, 2006.
17. Pearson KS, Gomez MN, Moyers, JR, et al: A cost/benefit analysis of randomized invasive monitoring for patients undergoing cardiac surgery. *Anesth Analg* 69:336, 1989.
18. Isaacson IJ, Lowdon JD, Berry AJ, et al: The value of pulmonary artery and central venous monitoring in patients undergoing abdominal aortic reconstructive surgery: a comparative study of two selected, randomized groups. *J Vasc Surg* 12:754, 1990.
19. Joyce WP, Provan JL, Ameli FM, et al: The role of central hemodynamic monitoring in abdominal aortic surgery: a prospective randomized study. *Eur J Vasc Surg* 4:633, 1990.
20. Yu M, Levy M, Smith P: Effect of maximizing oxygen delivery on morbidity and mortality rates in critically ill patients. *Crit Care Med* 21:830, 1993.
21. Gattinoni L, Brazzi L, Pelosi P, et al: A trial of goal-oriented hemodynamic therapy in critically ill patients. *N Engl J Med* 333:1025, 1995.
22. Yu M, Takanishi D, Myers SA, et al: Frequency of mortality and myocardial infarction during maximizing oxygen delivery: a prospective, randomized trial. *Crit Care Med* 23:1025, 1995.
23. Durham RM, Neunaber K, Mazuski JE, et al: The use of oxygen consumption and delivery as endpoints for resuscitation in critically ill patients. *J Trauma* 41:32, 1996.
24. Afessa B, Spenser S, Khan W, et al: Association of pulmonary artery catheter use with in-hospital mortality. *Crit Care Med* 29:1145, 2001.
25. Rhodes A, Cusack RJ, Newman PJ, et al: A randomized, controlled trial of the pulmonary artery catheter in critically ill patients. *Intensive Care Med* 28:256, 2002.
26. Richard C: Early use of the pulmonary artery catheter and outcomes in patients with shock and acute respiratory distress syndrome: a randomized controlled trial. *JAMA* 290:2713, 2003.
27. Yu DT, Platt R, Lanken PN, et al: Relationship of pulmonary artery catheter use to mortality and resource utilization in patients with severe sepsis. *Crit Care Med* 31:2734, 2003.
28. Sandham JD, Hull RD, Brant RF, et al: A randomized, controlled trial of the use of pulmonary-artery catheters in high-risk surgical patients. *N Engl J Med* 348:5, 2003.
29. Sakr Y, Vincent JL, Reinhart K, et al: Use of the pulmonary artery catheter is not associated with worse outcome in the ICU. *Chest* 128:2722, 2005.
30. Harvey S, Harrison DA, Singer M, et al: Assessment of the clinical effectiveness of pulmonary-artery catheters in management of patients in intensive care (PAC-Man): a randomized controlled trial. *Lancet* 366:472, 2005.
31. Binanay C, Califf RM, Hasselblad V, et al: Evaluation study of congestive heart failure and pulmonary artery catheterization effectiveness: the ESCAPE trial. *JAMA* 294:1625, 2005.
32. The National Heart, Lung and Blood Institute ARDS Clinical Trials Network: Pulmonary artery versus central venous catheter to guide treatment of acute lung injury. *New Engl J Med* 354:2213, 2006.
33. Tuman KJ, McCarthy RJ, Spiess BD, et al: Effect of pulmonary artery catheterization on outcome in patients undergoing coronary artery surgery. *Anesthesiology* 70:199, 1989.
34. Guyatt G: A randomized control trial of right heart catheterization in critically ill patients. Ontario Intensive Care Study Group. *J Intensive Care Med* 6:91, 1991.
35. Hayes MA, Timmins AC, Yau H, et al: Elevation of systemic oxygen delivery in the treatment of critically ill patients. *N Eng J Med* 330:1717, 1994.
36. Connors AF, Speroff T, Dawson NV, et al: The effectiveness of right heart catheterization in the initial care of critically ill patients. *JAMA* 276:889, 1996.
37. Valentine RJ, Duke ML, Inman MH, et al: Effectiveness of pulmonary artery catheters in aortic surgery: a randomized trial. *J Vasc Surg* 27:203, 1998.
38. Stewart RD, Psyhojos T, Lahey SJ, et al: Central venous catheter use in low risk coronary artery bypass grafting. *Ann Thorac Surg* 66:1306, 1998.
39. Ramsey SD, Saint S, Sullivan SD, et al: Clinical and economic effects of pulmonary artery catheterization in nonemergent coronary artery bypass graft surgery. *J Cardiothorac Vasc Anesth* 14:113, 2000.
40. Polanczyk CA, Rohde LE, Goldman L, et al: Right heart catheterization and cardiac complications in patients undergoing noncardiac surgery: an observational study. *JAMA* 286:348, 2001.

41. Chittock DR, Dhingra VK, Ronco JJ, et al: Severity of illness and risk of death associated with pulmonary artery catheter use. *Crit Care Med* 32:911, 2004.
42. Peters SG, Afessa B, Decker PA, et al: Increased risk associated with pulmonary artery catheterization in the medical intensive care unit. *J Crit Care* 18:166, 2003.
43. Cohen MG, Kelley RV, Kong DF, et al: Pulmonary artery catheterization in acute coronary syndromes: insights from the GUSTO IIb and GUSTO III trials. *Am J Med* 118:482, 2005.
44. Kumar A, Anel R, Bunnell E: Pulmonary artery occlusion pressure and central venous pressure fail to predict ventricular filling volume, cardiac performance, or the response to volume infusion in normal subjects. *Crit Care Med* 32:691, 2004.
45. Hoar PF, Wilson RM, Mangano DT, et al: Heparin bonding reduces thrombogenicity of pulmonary-artery catheters. *N Engl J Med* 305:993, 1981.
46. Mangano DT: Heparin bonding long-term protection against thrombogenesis. *N Engl J Med* 307:894, 1982.
47. Forrester JS, Ganz W, Diamond G, et al: Thermodilution cardiac output determination with a single flow-directed catheter. *Am Heart J* 83:306, 1972.
48. Chatterjee K, Swan JHC, Ganz W, et al: Use of a balloon-tipped flotation electrode catheter for cardiac monitoring. *Am J Cardiol* 36:56, 1975.
49. Simoons ML, Demey HE, Bossaert LL, et al: The Paceport catheter: a new pacemaker system introduced through a Swan–Ganz catheter. *Cathet Cardiovasc Diagn* 15:66, 1988.
50. Baele PL, McMechan JC, Marsh HM, et al: Continuous monitoring of mixed venous oxygen saturation in critically ill patients. *Anesth Analg* 61:513, 1982.
51. Segal J, Pearl RG, Ford AJ, et al: Instantaneous and continuous cardiac output obtained with a Doppler pulmonary artery catheter. *J Am Coll Cardiol* 13:1382, 1989.
52. Vincent JL, Thirion M, Bumioulle S, et al: Thermodilution measurement of right ventricular ejection fraction with a modified pulmonary artery catheter. *Intensive Care Med* 12:33, 1986.
53. Guerrero JE, Munoz J, De Lacalle B, et al: Right ventricular systolic time intervals determined by means of a pulmonary artery catheter. *Crit Care Med* 20:1529, 1992.
54. Dhainaut JF, Brunet F, Monsallier JF, et al: Bedside evaluation of right ventricular performance using a rapid computerized thermodilution mode. *Crit Care Med* 15:148, 1987.
55. Vincent JL: Measurement of right ventricular ejection fraction. *Intensive Care World* 7:133, 1990.
56. Nelson, LD: The new pulmonary arterial catheters: Right ventricular ejection fraction and continuous cardiac output. *Critical Care Clin* 12:795, 1996.
57. Boldt J, Mendes T, Wollbruck M, et al: Is continuous cardiac output measurement using thermodilution reliable in the critically ill patient? *Crit Care Med* 22:1913, 1994.
58. Haller M, Zollner C, Briegel J, et al: Evaluation of a new continuous thermodilution cardiac output monitor in critically ill patients: a prospective criterion standard study. *Crit Care Med* 23:860, 1995.
59. Mihaljevic T, von Segesser L, Tonz M, et al: Continuous verses bolus thermodilution cardiac output measurements: a comparative study. *Crit Care Med* 23:944, 1995.
60. Munro H, Woods C, Taylor B, et al: Continuous invasive cardiac output monitoring: The Baxter/Edwards Critical-Care Swan Ganz IntelliCath and Vigilance system. *Clin Intensive Care* 5:52, 1994.
61. Keusch DJ, Winters S, Thys DM: The patient's position influences the incidence of dysrhythmias during pulmonary artery catheterization. *Anesthesiology* 70:582, 1989.
62. Marini JJ: Hemodynamic monitoring with the pulmonary artery catheter. *Crit Care Clin* 2:551, 1986.
63. Barry WA, Grossman W: Cardiac catheterization, in Braunwald E (ed): *Heart Disease: A Textbook of Cardiovascular Medicine*. Vol 1. Philadelphia, PA, WB Saunders, 1988; p 287.
64. Sharkey SW: Beyond the occlusion: clinical physiology and the Swan-Ganz catheter. *Am J Med* 83:111, 1987.
65. Bohrer H, Fleischer F: Errors in biochemical and haemodynamic data obtained using introducer lumen and proximal port of Swan-Ganz catheter. *Intensive Care Med* 15:330, 1989.
66. Huford WE, Zapol WM: The right ventricle and critical illness: a review of anatomy, physiology, and clinical evaluation of its function. *Intensive Care Med* 14:448, 1988.
67. Diebel LN, Wilson RF, Tagett MG, et al: End diastolic volume: a better indicator of preload in the critically ill. *Arch Surg* 127:817, 1992.
68. Martyn JA, Snider MT, Farago LF, et al: Thermodilution right ventricular volume: a novel and better predictor of volume replacement in acute thermal injury. *J Trauma* 21:619, 1981.
69. Reuse C, Vincent JL, Pinsky MR, et al: Measurements of right ventricular volumes during fluid challenge. *Chest* 98:1450, 1990.
70. Lange RA, Moore DM, Cigarroa RG, et al: Use of pulmonary capillary occlusion pressure to assess severity of mitral stenosis: is true left atrial pressure needed in this condition? *J Am Coll Cardiol* 13:825, 1989.
71. Alpert JS: The lessons of history as reflected in the pulmonary capillary occlusion pressure. *J Am Coll Cardiol* 13:830, 1989.
72. Forrester JS, Diamond G, McHugh TJ, et al: Filling pressures in the right and left sides of the heart in acute myocardial infarction. *N Engl J Med* 285:190, 1971.
73. O'Quin R, Marini JJ: Pulmonary artery occlusion pressure: clinical physiology, measurement, and interpretation. *Am Rev Respir Dis* 128:319, 1983.
74. Timmis AD, Fowler MB, Burwood RJ, et al: Pulmonary edema without critical increase in left atrial pressure in acute myocardial infarction. *BMJ* 283:636, 1981.
75. Holloway H, Perry M, Downey J, et al: Estimation of effective pulmonary capillary pressure in intact lungs. *J Appl Physiol* 54:846, 1983.
76. Dawson CA, Linehan JH, Rickaby DA: Pulmonary microcirculatory hemodynamics. *Ann NY Acad Sci* 384:90, 1982.
77. Pichard AD, Kay R, Smith H, et al: Large V waves in the pulmonary occlusion pressure tracing in the absence of mitral regurgitation. *Am J Cardiol* 50:1044, 1982.
78. Ruchs RM, Heuser RR, Yin FU, et al: Limitations of pulmonary occlusion V waves in diagnosing mitral regurgitation. *Am J Cardiol* 49:849, 1982.
79. Bethen CF, Peter RH, Behar VS, et al: The hemodynamic simulation of mitral regurgitation in ventricular septal defect after myocardial infarction. *Cathet Cardiovasc Diagn* 2:97, 1976.
80. Hasan FM, Weiss WB, Braman SS, et al: Influence of lung injury on pulmonary occlusion-left atrial pressure correlation during positive end-expiratory pressure ventilation. *Annu Rev Respir Dis* 131:246, 1985.
81. Teboul JL, Zapol WM, Brun-Buisson C, et al: A comparison of pulmonary artery occlusion pressure and left ventricular end diastolic pressure during mechanical ventilation with PEEP in patients with severe ARDS. *Anesthesiology* 70:261, 1989.
82. DeCampo T, Civetta JM: The effect of short-term discontinuation of high-level PEEP in patients with acute respiratory failure. *Crit Care Med* 7:47, 1979.
83. Ganz W, Swan HJC: Measurement of blood flow by thermodilution. *Am J Cardiol* 29:241, 1972.
84. Grossman W: Blood flow measurement: the cardiac output, in Grossman W (ed): *Cardiac Catheterization and Angiography*. Philadelphia, Lea & Febiger, 1985; p 116.
85. Goldman RH, Klughaupt M, Metcalf T, et al: Measurement of central venous oxygen saturation in patients with myocardial infarction. *Circulation* 38:941, 1968.
86. Pace NL: A critique of flow-directed pulmonary artery catheterization. *Anesthesiology* 47:455, 1977.
87. Rayput MA, Rickey HM, Bush BA, et al: A comparison between a conventional and a fiberoptic flow-directed thermal dilution pulmonary artery catheter in critically ill patients. *Arch Intern Med* 149:83, 1989.
88. Matthay MA, Chatterjee K: Bedside catheterization of the pulmonary artery: risks compared with benefits. *Ann Intern Med* 109:826, 1988.
89. McNabb TG, Green CH, Parket FL: A potentially serious complication with Swan-Ganz catheter placement by the percutaneous internal jugular route. *Br J Anaesth* 47:895, 1975.
90. Hansbroyh JF, Narrod JA, Rutherford R: Arteriovenous fistulas following central venous catheterization. *Intensive Care Med* 9:287, 1983.
91. Shield CF, Richardson JD, Buckley CJ, et al: Pseudoaneurysm of the brachiocephalic arteries: a complication of percutaneous internal jugular vein catheterization. *Surgery* 78:190, 1975.
92. Patel C, LaBoy V, Venus B, et al: Acute complications of pulmonary artery catheter insertion in critically ill patients. *Crit Care Med* 14:195, 1986.
93. Damen J, Bolton D: A prospective analysis of 1,400 pulmonary artery catheterizations in patients undergoing cardiac surgery. *Acta Anaesthesiol Scand* 14:1957, 1986.
94. Senagere A, Waller JD, Bonnell BW, et al: Pulmonary artery catheterization: a prospective study of internal jugular and subclavian approaches. *Crit Care Med* 15:35, 1987.
95. Nembre AE: Swan-Ganz catheter. *Arch Surg* 115:1194, 1980.
96. Lipp H, O'Donoghue K, Resnekov L: Intracardiac knotting of a flow-directed balloon catheter. *N Engl J Med* 284:220, 1971.
97. Mond HG, Clark DW, Nesbitt SJ, et al: A technique for unknotting an intracardiac flow-directed balloon catheter. *Chest* 67:731, 1975.
98. Meister SG, Furr CM, Engel TR, et al: Knotting of a flow-directed catheter about a cardiac structure. *Cathet Cardiovasc Diagn* 3:171, 1977.
99. Swaroop S: Knotting of two central venous monitoring catheters. *Am J Med* 53:386, 1972.
100. Loggam C, Sanborn TA, Christian F: Ventricular entrapment of a Swan-Ganz catheter: a technique for nonsurgical removal. *J Am Coll Cardiol* 13:1422, 1989.
101. Foote GA, Schabel SI, Hodges M: Pulmonary complications of the flow-directed balloon-tipped catheter. *N Engl J Med* 290:927, 1974.
102. Wechsler RJ, Steiner RM, Kinori F: Monitoring the monitors: the radiology of thoracic catheters, wires and tubes. *Semin Roentgenol* 23:61, 1988.
103. Boyd KD, Thomas SJ, Gold J, et al: A prospective study of complications of pulmonary artery catheterizations in 500 consecutive patients. *Chest* 84:245, 1983.
104. Sise MJ, Hollingsworth P, Bumm JE, et al: Complications of the flow directed pulmonary artery catheter: a prospective analysis of 219 patients. *Crit Care Med* 9:315, 1981.
105. Barash PG, Nardi D, Hammond G, et al: Catheter-induced pulmonary artery perforation: mechanisms, management and modifications. *J Thorac Cardiovasc Surg* 82:5, 1981.

106. Pape LA, Haffajee CI, Markis JE, et al: Fatal pulmonary hemorrhage after use of the flow-directed balloon-tipped catheter. *Ann Intern Med* 90:344, 1979.
107. Lapin ES, Murray JA: Hemoptysis with flow-directed cardiac catheterization. *JAMA* 220:1246, 1972.
108. McDaniel DD, Stone JG, Faltas AN, et al: Catheter induced pulmonary artery hemorrhage: diagnosis and management in cardiac operations. *J Thorac Cardiovasc Surg* 82:1, 1981.
109. Shah KB, Rao TL, Laughlin S, et al: A review of pulmonary artery catheterization in 6245 patients. *Anesthesiology* 61:271, 1984.
110. Fraser RS: Catheter-induced pulmonary artery perforation: pathologic and pathogenic features. *Hum Pathol* 18:1246, 1987.
111. Declen JD, Friloux LA, Renner JW: Pulmonary artery false-aneurysms secondary to Swan-Ganz pulmonary artery catheters. *AJR Am J Roentgenol* 149:901, 1987.
112. Thoms R, Siproudhis L, Laurent JF, et al: Massive hemoptysis from iatrogenic balloon catheter rupture of pulmonary artery: successful early management by balloon tamponade. *Crit Care Med* 15:272, 1987.
113. Slacken A: Complications of invasive hemodynamic monitoring in the intensive care unit. *Curr Probl Surg* 25:69, 1988.
114. Scuderi PE, Prough DS, Price JD, et al: Cessation of pulmonary artery catheter-induced endobronchial hemorrhage associated with the use of PEEP. *Anesth Analg* 62:236, 1983.
115. Pace NL, Horton W: Indwelling pulmonary artery catheters: their relationship to aseptic thrombotic endocardial vegetations. *JAMA* 233:893, 1975.
116. Dye LE, Segall PH, Russell RO, et al: Deep venous thrombosis of the upper extremity associated with use of the Swan-Ganz catheter. *Chest* 73:673, 1978.
117. Elliot CG, Zimmerman GA, Clemmer TP: Complications of pulmonary artery catheterization in the care of critically ill patients: a prospective study. *Chest* 76:647, 1979.
118. Chastre J, Cornud F, Bouchama A, et al: Thrombosis as a complication of pulmonary artery catheterization via the internal jugular vein. *N Engl J Med* 306:278, 1982.
119. Laster JL, Nichols WK, Silver D: Thrombocytopenia associated with heparin-coated catheters in patients with heparin-associated antiplatelet antibodies. *Arch Intern Med* 149:2285, 1989.
120. Laster JL, Silver D: Heparin coated catheters and heparin-induced thrombocytopenia. *J Vasc Surg* 7:667, 1988.
121. Geha DG, Davis NJ, Lappas DG: Persistent atrial arrhythmias associated with placement of a Swan-Ganz catheter. *Anesthesiology* 39:651, 1973.
122. Sprung CL, Jacobs JL, Caralis PV, et al: Ventricular arrhythmias during Swan-Ganz catheterization of the critically ill. *Chest* 79:413, 1981.
123. Sprung CL, Pozen PG, Rozanski JJ, et al: Advanced ventricular arrhythmias during bedside pulmonary artery catheterization. *Am J Med* 72:203, 1982.
124. Iberti TJ, Benjamin E, Grupzi L, et al: Ventricular arrhythmias during pulmonary artery catheterization in the intensive care unit. *Am J Med* 78:451, 1985.
125. Sprung CL, Marical EH, Garcia AA, et al: Prophylactic use of lidocaine to prevent advanced ventricular arrhythmias during pulmonary artery catheterization: prospective, double blind study. *Am J Med* 75:906, 1983.
126. Johnston W, Royster R, Beamer W, et al: Arrhythmias during removal of pulmonary artery catheters. *Chest* 85:296, 1984.
127. Damen J: Ventricular arrhythmia during insertion and removal of pulmonary artery catheters. *Chest* 88:190, 1985.
128. Morris D, Mulvihill D, Lew WY: Risk of developing complete heart block during bedside pulmonary artery catheterization in patients with left bundle branch block. *Arch Intern Med* 147:2005, 1987.
129. Lavie CJ, Gersh BJ: Pacing in left bundle branch block during Swan-Ganz catheterization [letter]. *Arch Intern Med* 148:981, 1988.
130. Becker RC, Martin RG, Underwood DA: Right-sided endocardial lesions and flow-directed pulmonary artery catheters. *Cleve Clin J Med* 54:384, 1987.
131. Lange HW, Galliani CA, Edwards JE: Local complications associated with indwelling Swan-Ganz catheters. *Am J Cardiol* 52:1108, 1983.
132. Sage MD, Koelmeyer TD, Smeeton WMI: Evolution of Swan-Ganz catheter related pulmonary valve nonbacterial endocarditis. *Am J Forensic Med Pathol* 9:112, 1988.
133. Rowley KM, Clubb KS, Smith GJW, et al: Right sided infective endocarditis as a consequence of flow directed pulmonary artery catheterization. *N Engl J Med* 311:1152, 1984.
134. Ford SE, Manley PN: Indwelling cardiac catheters: an autopsy study of associated endocardial lesions. *Arch Pathol Lab Med* 106:314, 1982.
135. Prochan H, Dittel M, Jobst C, et al: Bacterial contamination of pulmonary artery catheters. *Intensive Care Med* 4:79, 1978.
136. Pinella JC, Ross DF, Martin T, et al: Study of the incidence of intravascular catheter infection and associated septicemia in critically ill patients. *Crit Care Med* 11:21, 1983.
137. Michel L, Marsh HM, McMichan JC, et al: Infection of pulmonary artery catheters in critically ill patients. *JAMA* 245:1032, 1981.
138. Greene JF, Fitzwater JE, Clemmer TP: Septic endocarditis and indwelling pulmonary artery catheters. *JAMA* 233:891, 1975.
139. Myers ML, Austin TW, Sibbald WJ: Pulmonary artery catheter infections: a prospective study. *Ann Surg* 201:237, 1985.
140. Hanna R, Raad II: Diagnosis of catheter-related bloodstream infection. *Curr Infect Dis Rep* 7:413, 2005.
141. Chatzinikolaou I, Hanna R, Darouiche R, et al: Prospective study of the value of quantitative culture of organisms from blood collected through central venous catheters in differentiating between contamination and bloodstream infection. *J Clin Microbiol* 44:1834, 2006.
142. Weinstein RA, Stamm WE, Kramer L: Pressure monitoring devices: overlooked source of nosocomial infection. *JAMA* 236:936, 1976.
143. Singh SJ, Puri VK: Prevention of bacterial colonization of pulmonary artery catheters. *Infect Surg* 1984;853.
144. Heard SO, Davis RF, Sherertz RJ, et al: Influence of sterile protective sleeves on the sterility of pulmonary artery catheters. *Crit Care Med* 15:499, 1987.
145. Cobb DK, High KP, Sawyer RG, et al: A controlled trial of scheduled replacement of central venous and pulmonary artery catheters. *N Engl J Med* 327:1062, 1992.
146. Berry AJ, Geer RT, Marshall BE: Alteration of pulmonary blood flow by pulmonary artery occluded pressure measurement. *Anesthesiology* 51:164, 1979.
147. Schluger J, Green J, Giustra FX, et al: Complication with use of flow-directed catheter. *Am J Cardiol* 32:125, 1973.
148. Isner JM, Horton J, Ronan JAS: Systolic click from a Swan-Ganz catheter: phonoechocardiographic depiction of the underlying mechanism. *Am J Cardiol* 42:1046, 1979.
149. Lawson D, Kushkins LG: A complication of multipurpose pacing pulmonary artery catheterization via the external jugular vein approach [letter]. *Anesthesiology* 62:377, 1985.
150. McLellan BA, Jerman MR, French WJ, et al: Inadvertent Swan-Ganz catheter placement in the left pericardiophrenic vein. *Cathet Cardiovasc Diagn* 16:173, 1989.
151. Allyn J, Lichtenstein A, Koski EG, et al: Inadvertent passage of a pulmonary artery catheter from the superior vena cava through the left atrium and left ventricle into the aorta. *Anesthesiology* 70:1019, 1989.
152. Lazzam C, Sanborn TA, Christian F: Ventricular entrapment of a Swan-Ganz catheter: a technique for nonsurgical removal. *J Am Coll Cardiol* 13:1422, 1989.
153. Ginosar Y, Sprung CL: The Swan–Ganz catheter: twenty-five years of monitoring. *Crit Care Clin* 12:771, 1996.
154. Wiedermann HP, Matthay MA, Matthay RA: Cardiovascular-pulmonary monitoring in the intensive care unit, 2. *Chest* 85:656, 1984.
155. Shah MR, Hasselblad V, Stevenson LW, et al: Impact of the pulmonary artery catheter in critically ill patients. *JAMA* 294:1664, 2005.
156. http://www.clinicaltrials.gov. Accessed January 23, 2011.

CHAPTER 5 ■ TEMPORARY CARDIAC PACING

SETH T. DAHLBERG

Temporary cardiac pacing may be urgently required for the treatment of cardiac conduction and rhythm disturbances commonly seen in patients treated in the intensive care unit (ICU). Therefore, ICU personnel should be familiar with the indications and techniques for initiating and maintaining temporary cardiac pacing as well as the possible complications of this procedure. Recommendations for training in the performance of transvenous pacing have been published by a Task Force of the American College of Physicians, American Heart Association and American College of Cardiology [1]. Competence in the performance of transvenous pacing also requires the operator to have training in central venous access (Chapter 2) and hemodynamic monitoring (Chapters 4 and 26) [2–5].

INDICATIONS FOR TEMPORARY CARDIAC PACING

As outlined in Table 5.1, temporary pacing is indicated in the diagnosis and management of a number of serious rhythm and conduction disturbances.

Bradyarrhythmias

The most common indication for temporary pacing in the ICU setting is a hemodynamically significant or symptomatic bradyarrhythmia such as sinus bradycardia or high-grade atrioventricular (AV) block.

Sinus bradycardia and AV block are commonly seen in patients with acute coronary syndromes, hyperkalemia, myxedema, or increased intracranial pressure. Infectious processes such as endocarditis or Lyme disease [6] may impair AV conduction. Bradyarrhythmias also result from treatment or intoxication with digitalis, antiarrhythmic, beta-blocker, or calcium channel blocker medications and may also result from exaggerated vasovagal reactions to ICU procedures such as suctioning of the tracheobronchial tree in the intubated patient. Bradycardia-dependent ventricular tachycardia may occur in association with ischemic heart disease.

Tachyarrhythmias

Temporary cardiac pacing is used less often for the prevention and termination of supraventricular and ventricular tachyarrhythmias.

Atrial pacing may be effective in terminating atrial flutter and paroxysmal nodal supraventricular tachycardia [7,8]. Atrial pacing in the ICU setting is most frequently performed when temporary epicardial electrodes have been placed during cardiac surgery. A critical pacing rate (usually 125% to 135% of the flutter rate) and pacing duration (usually about 10 seconds) are important in the successful conversion of atrial flutter to sinus rhythm.

In some clinical situations, pacing termination of atrial flutter may be preferable to synchronized cardioversion, which requires sedation with its attendant risks. Pacing termination is the treatment of choice for atrial flutter in patients with epicardial atrial wires in place after cardiac surgery. It may be preferred as the means to convert atrial flutter in patients on digoxin and those with sick sinus syndrome, as these groups often demonstrate prolonged sinus pauses after DC cardioversion.

Temporary pacing may be required for the prevention of paroxysmal polymorphic ventricular tachycardia in patients with prolonged QT intervals (torsades de pointes), particularly when secondary to drugs [9,10]. Temporary cardiac pacing is the treatment of choice to stabilize the patient while a type I antiarrhythmic agent exacerbating ventricular irritability is metabolized. In this situation, the pacing rate is set to provide a mild tachycardia. The effectiveness of cardiac pacing probably relates to decreasing the dispersion of refractoriness of the ventricular myocardium (shortening the QT interval).

Temporary ventricular pacing may be successful in terminating ventricular tachycardia. If ventricular tachycardia must be terminated urgently, cardioversion is mandated (Chapter 6). However, in less urgent situations, conversion of ventricular tachycardia via rapid ventricular pacing may be useful. The success of this technique depends on the setting in which ventricular tachycardia occurs. "Overdrive" ventricular pacing is often effective in terminating monomorphic ventricular tachycardia in a patient with remote myocardial infarction or in the absence of heart disease. This technique is less effective when ventricular tachycardia complicates acute myocardial infarction or cardiomyopathy. Rapid ventricular pacing is most successful in terminating ventricular tachycardia when the ventricle can be "captured" (asynchronous pacing for 5 to 10 beats at a rate of 50 beats per minute greater than that of the underlying tachycardia). Extreme caution is advised, as pacing may result in acceleration of ventricular tachycardia or degeneration to ventricular fibrillation; a cardiac defibrillator should be immediately available at the bedside.

DIAGNOSIS OF RAPID RHYTHMS

Temporary atrial pacing electrodes may be helpful for the diagnosis of tachyarrhythmias when the morphology of the P wave and its relation to the QRS complexes cannot be determined from the surface electrocardiogram (ECG) [11–13]. A recording of the atrial electrogram is particularly helpful in a rapid, regular, narrow-complex tachycardia in which the differential diagnosis includes atrial flutter with rapid ventricular response, and AV nodal reentrant or other supraventricular

TABLE 5.1

INDICATIONS FOR ACUTE (TEMPORARY) CARDIAC PACING

A.	**Conduction disturbances**
1.	Symptomatic persistent third-degree AV block with inferior myocardial infarction
2.	Third-degree AV block, new bifascicular block (e.g., right bundle branch block and left anterior hemiblock, left bundle branch block, first-degree AV block), or alternating left and right bundle branch block complicating acute anterior myocardial infarction
3.	Symptomatic idiopathic third-degree AV block, or high-degree AV block
B.	**Rate disturbances**
1.	Hemodynamically significant or symptomatic sinus bradycardia
2.	Bradycardia-dependent ventricular tachycardia
3.	AV dissociation with inadequate cardiac output
4.	Polymorphic ventricular tachycardia with long QT interval (torsades de pointes)
5.	Recurrent ventricular tachycardia unresponsive to medical therapy

AV, atrioventricular.

tachycardia. This technique may also assist in the diagnosis of wide-complex tachycardias in which the differential diagnosis includes supraventricular tachycardia with aberrant conduction, sinus tachycardia with bundle branch block, and ventricular tachycardia.

To record an atrial ECG, the ECG limb leads are connected in the standard fashion and a precordial lead (usually V_1) is connected to the proximal electrode of the atrial pacing catheter or to an epicardial atrial electrode. A multichannel ECG rhythm strip is run at a rapid paper speed, simultaneously demonstrating surface ECG limb leads as well as the atrial electrogram obtained via lead V_1. This rhythm strip should reveal the conduction pattern between atria and ventricles as antegrade, simultaneous, retrograde, or dissociated.

ACUTE MYOCARDIAL INFARCTION

Temporary pacing may be used therapeutically or prophylactically in acute myocardial infarction [14]. Recommendations for temporary cardiac pacing have been provided by a Task Force of the American College of Cardiology and the American Heart Association (Table 5.2) [15]. Bradyarrhythmias unresponsive to medical treatment that result in hemodynamic compromise require urgent treatment. Patients with anterior infarction and bifascicular block or Mobitz type II second-degree AV block, while hemodynamically stable, may require a temporary pacemaker, as they are at risk for sudden development of complete heart block with an unstable escape rhythm.

Prophylactic temporary cardiac pacing has aroused debate for the role it may play in complicated anterior wall myocardial infarction [16]. Thrombolytic therapy or percutaneous coronary intervention, when indicated, should take precedence over placement of prophylactic cardiac pacing, as prophylactic pacing has not been shown to improve mortality. Transthoracic (transcutaneous) cardiac pacing is safe and usually effective [17–20] and would be a reasonable alternative to prophylactic transvenous cardiac pacing, particularly soon after the administration of thrombolytic therapy.

When right ventricular involvement complicates inferior myocardial infarction, cardiac output may be very sensitive to ventricular preload and AV synchrony. Therefore, AV sequential pacing is frequently the pacing modality of choice in patients with right ventricular infarction [21,22].

EQUIPMENT AVAILABLE FOR TEMPORARY PACING

Several methods of temporary pacing are currently available for use in the ICU. Transvenous pacing of the right ventricle or right atrium with a pacing catheter or modified pulmonary artery catheter is the most widely used technique; intraesophageal, transcutaneous, and epicardial pacing are also available.

Transvenous Pacing Catheters

Some of the many transvenous pacing catheters available for use in the critical care setting are illustrated in Figure 5.1. Pacing catheters range in size from 4 Fr (1.2 mm) to 7 Fr (2.1 mm). In urgent situations, or where fluoroscopy is unavailable, a flow-directed flexible balloon-tipped catheter (Fig. 5.1, top) may be placed in the right ventricle using ECG guidance. After gaining access to the central venous circulation, the catheter is passed into the vein and the balloon inflated. After advancing the catheter into the right ventricle, the balloon can be deflated and the catheter tip advanced to the right ventricular apex. Although the balloon-tipped catheter may avoid the need for fluoroscopy, placement may be ineffective in the setting of low blood flow during cardiac arrest or in the presence of severe tricuspid regurgitation. Stiff catheters (Fig. 5.1, middle) are easier to manipulate but require insertion under fluoroscopic guidance.

A flexible J-shaped catheter (Fig. 5.1, bottom), designed for temporary atrial pacing, is also available [23]. This lead is positioned by "hooking" it in the right atrial appendage under fluoroscopic guidance, providing stable contact with the atrial endocardium. Either the subclavian or internal jugular venous approach may be used.

A multilumen pulmonary artery catheter is available with a right ventricular lumen. Placement of a small (2.4 Fr) bipolar pacing lead through the right ventricular lumen allows intracardiac pressure monitoring and pacing through a single catheter [24]. Details on its use and insertion are described in Chapter 4.

Esophageal Electrode

An esophageal "pill" electrode allows atrial pacing and recording of atrial depolarizations without requiring central venous

TABLE 5.2

ACC/AHA RECOMMENDATIONS FOR TREATMENT OF ATRIOVENTRICULAR AND INTRAVENTRICULAR CONDUCTION DISTURBANCES DURING STEMI

Intraventricular conduction	AV conduction													
	Normal		First-degree AV block				Mobitz I second-degree AV block				Mobitz II second-degree AV block			
			AMI		Non-AMI		AMI		Non-AMI		AMI		Non-AMI	
	Action	Class	Action	Class	Action	Class	Action	Class	Action	Class	Action	Class	Action	Class
Normal	OB	1	OB	1	OB	1	OB	2B	OB	2A	OB	3	OB	3
	A	3	A	3	A	3	A*	3	A	3	A	3	A	3
	TC	3	TC	2B	TC	2B	TC	1	TC	1	TC	1	TC	1
	TV	3	TV	3	TV	3	TV	3	TV	3	TV	2A	TV	2A
Old or new fascicular block (LAFB or LPFB)	OB	1	OB	2B	OB	2B	OB	2B	OB	2B	OB	3	OB	3
	A	3	A	3	A	3	A*	3	A	3	A	3	A	3
	TC	2B	TC	1	TC	2A	TC	1	TC	1	TC	1	TC	1
	TV	3	TV	3	TV	3	TV	3	TV	3	TV	2A	TV	2B
Old BBB	OB	1	OB	3	OB	3	OB	3	OB	3	OB	3	OB	3
	A	3	A	3	A	3	A*	3	A	3	A	3	A	3
	TC	2B	TC	1	TC	1	TC	1	TC	1	TC	1	TC	1
	TV	3	TV	2B	TV	2B	TV	2B	TV	2B	TV	2A	TV	2A
New BBB	OB	3	OB	3	OB	3	OB	3	OB	3	OB	3	OB	3
	A	3	A	3	A	3	A*	3	A	3	A	3	A	3
	TC	1	TC	1	TC	1	TC	1	TC	1	TC	2B	TC	2B
	TV	2B	TV	2A	TV	2A	TV	2A	TV	2A	TV	1	TV	1

Fascicular block + RBBB	OB	3	OB	3	OB	3	OB	3	OB	3	OB	3	OB	3
	A	3	A	3	A	3	A*	3	A	3	A	3	A	3
	TC	1	TC	1	TC	1	TC	1	TC	1	TC	2B	TC	2B
	TV	2B	TV	2A	TV	2A	TV	2A	TV	2A	TV	1	TV	1
Alternating left and right BBB	OB	3	OB	3	OB	3	OB	3	OB	3	OB	3	OB	3
	A	3	A	3	A	3	A*	3	A	3	A	3	A	3
	TC	2B	TC	2B	TC	2B	TC	2B	TC	2B	TC	2B	TC	2B
	TV	1	TV	1	TV	1	TV	1	TV	1	TV	1	TV	1

Notes: This table is designed to summarize the atrioventricular (column headings) and intraventricular (row headings) conduction disturbances that may occur during acute anterior or nonanterior STEMI, the possible treatment options, and the indications for each possible therapeutic option.

LAFB, left anterior fascicular block; LPFB, left posterior fascicular block; RBBB, right bundle-branch block; BBB, bundle-branch block; OB, observe; A, atropine; TC, transcutaneous pacing; TV, temporary transvenous pacing; STEMI, ST elevation myocardial infarction; AV, atrioventricular; and MI, myocardial infarction; AMI, anterior myocardial infarction; non-AMI, nonanterior myocardial infarction.

Action: There are four possible actions, or therapeutic options, listed and classified for each bradyarrhythmia or conduction problem:

1. Observe: continued ECG monitoring, no further action planned.
2. A and A*: Atropine administered at 0.6 to 1.0 mg IV every 5 minutes to up to 0.04 mg/kg. In general, because the increase in sinus rate with atropine is unpredictable, this is to be avoided unless there is symptomatic bradycardia that will likely respond to a vagolytic agent, such as sinus bradycardia or Mobitz I, as denoted by the asterisk in the table.
3. TC: Application of transcutaneous pads and standby transcutaneous pacing with no further progression to transvenous pacing imminently planned.
4. TV: Temporary transvenous pacing. It is assumed, but not specified in the table, that at the discretion of the clinician, transcutaneous pads will be applied and standby transcutaneous pacing will be in effect as the patient is transferred to the fluoroscopy unit for temporary transvenous pacing.

Class: Each possible therapeutic option is further classified according to ACC/AHA criteria as Class 1: indicated, Class 2A: probably indicated, 2B: possibly indicated, and Class 3: not indicated.

Level of Evidence: This table was developed from (1) published observational case reports and case series; (2) published summaries, not meta-analyses, of these data; and (3) expert opinion, largely from the prereperfusion era. There are no published randomized trials comparing different strategies of managing conduction disturbances after STEMI. Thus, the level of evidence for the recommendations in this table is C.

How to Use the Table:

Example: 54-year-old man is admitted with an anterior STEMI and a narrow QRS on admission. On day 1, he develops a right bundle-branch block (RBBB), with a PR interval of 0.28 seconds.

1. RBBB is an intraventricular conduction disturbance, so look at row "New bundle-branch block."
2. Find the column for "First-Degree AV Block."
3. Find the "Action" and "Class" cells at the convergence.
4. Note that "Observe" and "Atropine" are class 3, not indicated; transcutaneous pacing (TC) is class 1. Temporary transvenous pacing (TV) is class 2B.

From Antman EM, Anbe DT, Armstrong PW, et al: ACC/AHA guidelines for the management of patients with ST-elevation myocardial infarction—executive summary. A report of the American College of Cardiology/American Heart Association Task Force on Practice Guidelines (Writing Committee to revise the 1999 guidelines for the management of patients with acute myocardial infarction). *J Am Coll Cardiol* 44:671–719, 2004, with permission.

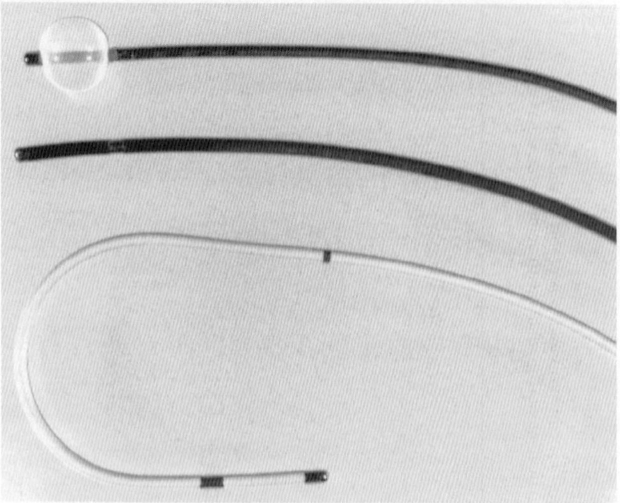

FIGURE 5.1. Cardiac pacing catheters. Several designs are available for temporary pacing in the critical care unit. **Top:** Balloon-tipped, flow-directed pacing wire. **Middle:** Standard 5 Fr pacing wire. **Bottom:** Atrial J-shaped wire.

cannulation. As mentioned earlier, detecting atrial depolarization aids in the diagnosis of tachyarrhythmias. Esophageal pacing has also been used to terminate supraventricular tachycardia and atrial flutter [25]. Because the electrode can be uncomfortable and may not give consistent, stable capture, the esophageal electrode is typically limited to short-term use for diagnosis of arrhythmias in pediatric patients.

Transcutaneous External Pacemakers

Transcutaneous external pacemakers have external patch electrodes that deliver a higher current (up to 200 mA) and longer pulse duration (20 to 40 milliseconds) than transvenous pacemakers. External pacing can be implemented immediately and the risks of central venous access avoided. Some patients may require sedation for the discomfort of skeletal muscle stimulation from the high cutaneous current. Transcutaneous external pacemakers have been used to treat brady-asystolic cardiac arrest, symptomatic bradyarrhythmias, and overdrive pacing of tachyarrhythmias and prophylactically for conduction abnormalities during myocardial infarction. They may be particularly useful when transvenous pacing is unavailable, as in the prehospital setting, or relatively contraindicated, as during thrombolytic therapy for acute myocardial infarction [17–19,26–28]. When continued pacing is needed, transvenous pacing is preferable.

Epicardial Pacing

The placement of epicardial electrodes requires open thoracotomy. These electrodes are routinely placed electively during cardiac surgical procedures for use during the postoperative period [12,13]. Typically, both atrial and ventricular electrodes are placed for use in diagnosis of postoperative atrial arrhythmias and for AV pacing. Because ventricular capture is not always reliable, in patients with underlying asystole or an unstable escape rhythm additional prophylactic transvenous pacing should be considered.

Pulse Generators for Temporary Pacing

Newer temporary pulse generators are now capable of ventricular, atrial, and dual chamber sequential pacing with adjustable ventricular and atrial parameters that include pacing modes (synchronous or asynchronous), rates, current outputs (mA), sensing thresholds (mV), and AV pacing interval/delay (milliseconds). Since these generators have atrial sensing/inhibiting capability, they are also set with an upper rate limit (to avoid rapid ventricular pacing while "tracking" an atrial tachycardia); in addition, an atrial pacing refractory period may be programmed (to avoid pacemaker-mediated/endless-loop tachyarrhythmias).

Earlier dual chamber pulse generators may be limited to sensing only ventricular depolarization (DVI mode). Without atrial sensing, if the intrinsic atrial rate exceeds the atrial pacing rate, the atrial pacing stimulus will fail to capture and AV sequential pacing will be lost with AV dissociation. Consequently, with these models, the pacing rate must be set continuously to exceed the intrinsic atrial rate to maintain AV sequential pacing.

CHOICE OF PACING MODE

A pacing mode must be selected when temporary cardiac pacing is initiated. Common modes for cardiac pacing are outlined in Table 5.3. The mode most likely to provide the greatest hemodynamic benefit should be selected. In patients with hemodynamic instability, establishing ventricular pacing is of paramount importance prior to attempts at AV sequential pacing.

TABLE 5.3

COMMON PACEMAKER MODES FOR TEMPORARY CARDIAC PACING

AOO	Atrial pacing: pacing is asynchronous
AAI	Atrial pacing, atrial sensing: pacing is on demand to provide a minimum programmed atrial rate
VOO	Ventricular pacing: pacing is asynchronous
VVI	Ventricular pacing, ventricular sensing: pacing is on demand to provide a minimum programmed ventricular rate
DVI	Dual-chamber pacing, ventricular sensing: atrial pacing is asynchronous, ventricular pacing is on demand following a programmed AV delay
DDD	Dual-chamber pacing and sensing: atrial and ventricular pacing is on demand to provide a minimum rate, ventricular pacing follows a programmed AV delay, and upper-rate pacing limit should be programmed

Ventricular pacing effectively counteracts bradycardia and is most frequently used in ICU patients; however, it cannot restore normal cardiac hemodynamics because it disrupts AV synchrony [29–31]. In patients with noncompliant ventricles (ischemic heart disease, left ventricular hypertrophy, aortic stenosis, and right ventricular infarction), loss of the atrial contribution to ventricular stroke volume (the atrial "kick") during ventricular pacing may result in increased atrial pressure, intermittent mitral and tricuspid regurgitation with reduced cardiac output and blood pressure.

In addition to the hemodynamic benefit of atrial or AV sequential pacing, the risk of atrial fibrillation or flutter may be reduced because of decreased atrial size and/or atrial pressure [32,33]. This suggests that patients with intermittent atrial fibrillation may be better maintained in normal sinus rhythm with atrial or AV sequential pacing, rather than ventricular demand pacing.

PROCEDURE TO ESTABLISH TEMPORARY PACING

After achieving venous access, most often via the internal jugular or subclavian approach (Chapter 2), the pacing catheter is advanced to the central venous circulation and then positioned in the right heart using fluoroscopic or ECG guidance [34]. To position the electrode using ECG guidance, the patient is connected to the limb leads of the ECG machine, and the distal (negative) electrode of the balloon-tipped pacing catheter is connected to lead V_1 with an alligator clip or a special adaptor supplied with the lead. Lead V_1 is then used to continuously monitor a unipolar intracardiac electrogram. The morphology of the recorded electrogram indicates the position of the catheter tip (Fig. 5.2). The balloon is inflated in the superior vena cava, and the catheter is advanced while observing

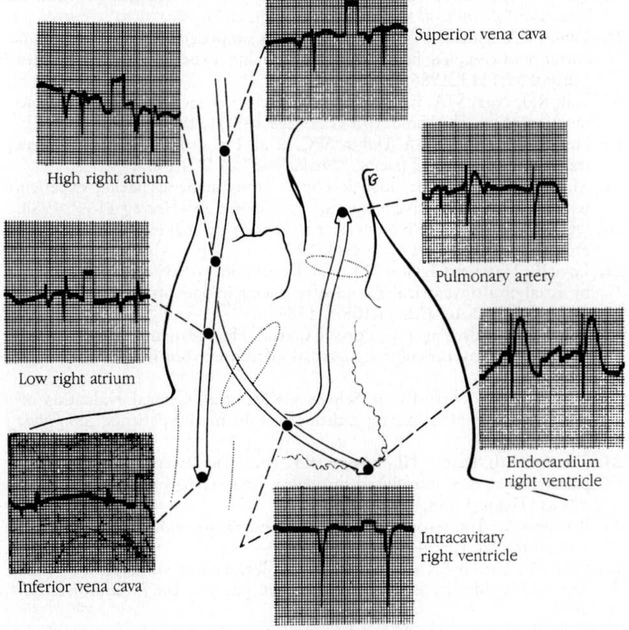

FIGURE 5.2. Pattern of recorded electrogram at various locations in the venous circulation. (From Harthorne JW, McDermott J, Poulin FK: Cardiac pacing, in Johnson RA, Haber E, Austen WG (eds): *The Practice of Cardiology: The Medical and Surgical Cardiac Units at the Massachusetts General Hospital.* Boston, Little, Brown, 1980, with permission.)

the recorded intracardiac electrogram. When the tip of the catheter reaches the right ventricle, the balloon is deflated and the catheter advanced to the right ventricular apex. ST segment elevation of the intracardiac electrogram due to a current of injury indicates contact of the catheter tip with the ventricular endocardium.

After the tip of the pacing catheter is satisfactorily inserted in the right ventricular apex, the leads are connected to the ventricular output connectors of the pulse generator, with the pacemaker box in the off position. The pacemaker is then set to asynchronous mode (VOO) and the ventricular rate set to exceed the patient's intrinsic ventricular rate by 10 to 20 beats per minute. The threshold current for ventricular pacing is set at 5 to 10 mA. Then the pacemaker is switched on. Satisfactory ventricular pacing is evidenced by a wide QRS complex, with ST segment depression and T wave inversion immediately preceded by a pacemaker depolarization (spike). With pacing from the apex of the right ventricle, the paced rhythm usually demonstrates a pattern of left bundle branch block on the surface ECG [35].

Ventricular pacing is maintained as the output current for ventricular pacing is slowly reduced. The pacing threshold is defined as the lowest current at which consistent ventricular capture occurs. With the ventricular electrode appropriately positioned at or near the apex of the right ventricle, a pacing threshold of less than 0.5 to 1.0 mA should be achieved. If the output current for continuous ventricular pacing is consistently greater than 1 to 1.5 mA, the pacing threshold is too high. Possible causes of a high pacing threshold include relatively refractory endomyocardial tissue (fibrosis) or, most commonly, unsatisfactory positioning of the pacing electrode. The tip of the pacing electrode should be repositioned in the region of the ventricular apex until satisfactory ventricular capture at a current of less than 1.0 mA is consistently maintained. After the threshold current for ventricular pacing has been established at a satisfactory level, the ventricular output is set to exceed the threshold current at least threefold. This guarantees uninterrupted ventricular capture despite any modest increase in the pacing threshold.

The pacemaker is now in VOO mode. However, the pacing generator generally should be set in the VVI ("demand") mode, as this prevents pacemaker discharge soon after an intrinsic or spontaneous premature depolarization, while the heart lies in the electrically vulnerable period for induction of sustained ventricular arrhythmias [36]. To set the pacemaker in VVI mode, the pacing rate is set at 10 beats per minute less than the intrinsic rate and the sensitivity control is moved from asynchronous to the minimum sensitivity level. The sensitivity is gradually increased until pacing spikes appear. This level is the sensing threshold. The sensitivity is then set at a level slightly below the determined threshold and the pacing rate reset to the minimum desired ventricular rate.

If AV sequential pacing is desired, the atrial J-shaped pacing catheter should be advanced into the right atrium and rotated anteromedially to achieve a stable position in the right atrial appendage; however, positioning the atrial catheter usually requires fluoroscopy [34,37]. The leads are then connected to the atrial output of the pulse generator. The atrial current is set to 20 mA and the atrial pacing rate adjusted to at least 10 beats per minute greater than the intrinsic atrial rate. The AV interval is adjusted at 100 to 200 milliseconds (shorter intervals usually provide better hemodynamics), and the surface ECG is inspected for evidence of atrial pacing (electrode depolarization and capture of the atrium at the pacing rate).

Atrial capture on ECG is indicated by atrial depolarization (P waves) immediately following the atrial pacing spikes. In patients with intact AV conduction, satisfactory atrial capture can be verified by shutting off the ventricular portion of the pacemaker and demonstrating AV synchrony during atrial pacing.

As long as the atrial pacing rate continually exceeds the intrinsic sinus rate, the atrial P wave activity should track with the atrial pacing spike.

The dual-chamber temporary pacemaker may not have atrial sensing capability. If not, the pacemaker will function in a DVI mode (Table 5.3). Should the intrinsic atrial rate equal or exceed the atrial pacing rate, the atrial stimulus will fail to capture and AV sequential pacing will be lost. If the pacemaker has atrial sensing capability, the atrial sensing threshold should be determined and an appropriate level set. The pacer will then function in the DDD mode. The DDD mode is usually preferred, as it provides optimum cardiac hemodynamics through a range of intrinsic atrial rates. In this mode, an upper-rate limit must be set to prevent rapid ventricular pacing in response to a paroxysmal supraventricular tachycardia.

COMPLICATIONS OF TEMPORARY PACING

Transvenous pacing in the ICU setting is most often performed via the internal jugular or subclavian approach. Appropriate selection of the optimal route requires an understanding of the results and complications of each technique [38,39].

Complications of temporary pacing from any venous access route include pericardial friction rub, arrhythmia, right ventricular perforation, cardiac tamponade, infection, unintentional arterial injury, diaphragmatic stimulation, phlebitis, and pneumothorax. Using predominantly the subclavian or internal jugular approaches, Donovan and Lee reported a 7% rate of serious complications related to temporary cardiac pacing [40]. The Mayo Clinic experience revealed that percutaneous cannulation of the right internal jugular vein provided the simplest, most direct route to the right-sided cardiac chambers [41].

Complications of internal jugular venous cannulation may include pneumothorax, carotid arterial injury, venous thrombosis, and pulmonary embolism (Chapter 2) [42]. These risks are minimized by knowledge of anatomic landmarks, adherence to proved techniques, use of a small-caliber needle to localize the vein before insertion of the large-caliber needle and use of ultrasound assistance (for full discussion see Chapter 2). Full-dose systemic anticoagulation, thrombolytic therapy, and prior neck surgical procedures are relative contraindications to routine internal jugular vein cannulation [43].

Percutaneous subclavian venipuncture is also frequently used for insertion of temporary pacemakers [36,44]. This approach should be avoided in patients with severe obstructive lung disease or a bleeding diathesis (including thrombolytic therapy), in whom the risk of pneumothorax or bleeding is increased.

Although insertion of a pacing lead via the brachial vein may reduce the risk of central arterial injury or hematoma formation in the patient receiving thrombolytic therapy or full-dose anticoagulation, motion of the patient's arm relative to the torso may result in an unstable position of the pacing electrode [41]. The risk of infection may also be increased with this approach. The femoral venous approach is used for electrophysiologic studies or during cardiac catheterization when the catheter is left in place for only a few hours. This approach is less desirable when long-term cardiac pacing is required, since there is a risk of deep venous thrombosis or infection around the catheter approach [45]. Central venous access by the subclavian or internal jugular route provides more stable long-term positioning of the pacing lead.

References

1. Francis GS, Williams SV, Achord JL, et al: Clinical competence in insertion of a temporary transvenous ventricular pacemaker: a statement for physicians from the ACP/ACC/AHA Task Force on Clinical Privileges in Cardiology. *Circulation* 89:1913–1916, 1994.
2. Sankaranarayanan R, Msairi A, Davis G: Ten years on: has competence and training in temporary transvenous cardiac pacing improved? *Brit J Hosp Med* 68:384–387, 2007.
3. Birkhahn RH, Gaeta TJ, Tloczkowski J, et al: Emergency medicine-trained physicians are proficient in the insertion of transvenous pacemakers. *Ann Emerg Med* 43:469–474, 2004.
4. Rajappan K, Fox KF: Temporary cardiac pacing in district general hospitals–sustainable resource or training liability? *QJM: Int J Med* 96:783–785, 2003.
5. Murphy JJ, Frain JP, Stephenson CJ: Training and supervision of temporary transvenous pacemaker insertion. *Br J Clin Pract* 49:126–128, 1995.
6. McAlister HF, Klementowicz PT, Andrews C, et al: Lyme carditis: an important cause of reversible heart block. *Ann Intern Med* 110:339–345, 1989.
7. Deo R, Berger R: The clinical utility of entrainment pacing. *J Cardiovasc Electrophysiol* 20:466–470, 2009.
8. Aronow WS: Treatment of atrial fibrillation and atrial flutter: Part II. *Cardiol Rev* 16:230–239, 2008.
9. Khan IA: Long QT syndrome: diagnosis and management. *Am Heart J* 143:7–14, 2002.
10. Passman R, Kadish A: Polymorphic ventricular tachycardia, long Q-T syndrome, and torsades de pointes. *Med Clin North Am* 85:321–341, 2001.
11. Waldo AL: *Cardiac arrhythmias: their mechanisms, diagnosis, and management*. Philadelphia, PA, J.B. Lippincott, 1987.
12. Reade MC: Temporary epicardial pacing after cardiac surgery: a practical review: part 1: general considerations in the management of epicardial pacing [erratum appears in *Anaesthesia* 62(6):644, 2007]. [Review] [26 refs]. *Anaesthesia* 62:264–271, 2007.
13. Reade MC: Temporary epicardial pacing after cardiac surgery: a practical review. Part 2: Selection of epicardial pacing modes and troubleshooting. *Anaesthesia* 62:364–373, 2007.
14. Brady WJ Jr, Harrigan RA: Diagnosis and management of bradycardia and atrioventricular block associated with acute coronary ischemia. *Emerg Med Clin North Am* 19:371–384, xi–xii, 2001.
15. Antman EM, Anbe DT, Armstrong PW, et al: ACC/AHA guidelines for the management of patients with ST-elevation myocardial infarction—executive summary. A report of the American College of Cardiology/American Heart Association Task Force on Practice Guidelines (Writing Committee to revise the 1999 guidelines for the management of patients with acute myocardial infarction). *J Am Coll Cardiol* 44:671–719, 2004.
16. Lamas GA, Muller JE, Zoltan GT, et al: A simplified method to predict occurrence of complete heart block during acute myocardial infarction. *Am J Cardiol* 57:1213, 1986.
17. Falk RH, Ngai STA: External cardiac pacing: Influence of electrode placement on pacing threshold. *Crit Care Med* 14:931, 1986.
18. Hedges JR, Syverud SA, Dalsey WC, et al: Prehospital trial of emergency transcutaneous cardiac pacing. *Circulation* 76:1337, 1987.
19. Madsen JK, Meibom J, Videbak R, et al: Transcutaneous pacing: experience with the zoll noninvasive temporary pacemaker. *Am Heart J* 116:7, 1988.
20. Dunn DL, Gregory JJ: Noninvasive temporary pacing: experience in a community hospital. *Heart Lung* 1:23, 1989.
21. Love JC, Haffajee CI, Gore JM, et al: Reversibility of hypotension and shock by atrial or atrioventricular sequential pacing in patients with right ventricular infarction. *Am Heart J* 108:5, 1984.
22. Topol EJ, Goldschlager N, Ports TA, et al: Hemodynamic benefit of atrial pacing in right ventricular myocardial infarction. *Ann Intern Med* 96:594, 1982.
23. Littleford PO, Curry RC Jr, Schwartz KM, et al: Clinical evaluation of a new temporary atrial pacing catheter: Results in 100 patients. *Am Heart J* 107:237, 1984.
24. Simoons ML, Demey HE, Bossaert LL, et al: The Paceport catheter: a new pacemaker system introduced through a Swan-Ganz catheter. *Cathet Cardiovasc Diagn* 15:66, 1988.
25. Benson DW. Transesophageal electrocardiography and cardiac pacing: the state of the art. *Circulation* 75:86, 1987.
26. Luck JC, Grubb BP, Artman SE, et al: Termination of sustained ventricular tachycardia by external noninvasive pacing. *Am J Cardiol* 61:574, 1988.
27. Kelly JS, Royster RL, Angert KC, et al: Efficacy of noninvasive transcutaneous cardiac pacing in patients undergoing cardiac surgery. *Anesthesiology* 70:747, 1989.
28. Blocka JJ: External transcutaneous pacemakers. *Ann Emerg Med* 18:1280, 1989.
29. Romero LR, Haffajee CI, Doherty P, et al: Comparison of ventricular function and volume with A-V sequential and ventricular pacing. *Chest* 80:346, 1981.

30. Knuse I, Arnman K, Conradson TB, et al: A comparison of the acute and long-term hemodynamic effects of ventricular inhibited and atrial synchronous ventricular inhibited pacing. *Circulation* 65:846, 1982.
31. Murphy P, Morton P, Murtaugh G, et al: Hemodynamic effects of different temporary pacing modes for the management of bradycardias complicating acute myocardial infarction. *Pacing Clin Electrophysiol* 15:1–396, 1992.
32. Neto VA, Costa R, Da Silva KR, et al: Temporary atrial pacing in the prevention of postoperative atrial fibrillation. *Pacing Clin Electrophysiol* 30[Suppl 1]:S79–S83, 2007.
33. Levy T, Fotopoulos G, Walker S, et al: Randomized controlled study investigating the effect of biatrial pacing in prevention of atrial fibrillation after coronary artery bypass grafting. *Circulation* 102:1382–1387, 2000.
34. Harthorne JW, McDermott J, Poulin FK: Cardiac pacing, in Johnson RA, Haber E, Austen WG (eds): *The Practice of Cardiology: The Medical and Surgical Cardiac Units at the Massachusetts General Hospital*. Boston, Little, Brown, 1980.
35. Morelli RL, Goldschlager N: Temporary transvenous pacing: resolving postinsertion problems. *J Crit Illness* 2:73, 1987.
36. Donovan KD: Cardiac pacing in intensive care. *Anaesth Intensive Care* 13:41, 1984.
37. Holmes DR Jr: Temporary cardiac pacing, in Furman S, Hayes DL, Holmes DR, Jr (eds): *A Practice of Cardiac Pacing*. Mount Kisco, NY, Futura, 1989.
38. Murphy JJ: Current practice and complications of temporary transvenous cardiac pacing. *BMJ* 312:1134, 1996.
39. Cooper JP, Swanton RH: Complications of transvenous temporary pacemaker insertion. *Br J Hosp Med* 53:155–161, 1995.
40. Donovan KD, Lee KY: Indications for and complications of temporary transvenous cardiac pacing. *Anaesth Intensive Care* 13:63, 1984.
41. Hynes JK, Holmes DR, Harrison CE: Five year experience with temporary pacemaker therapy in the coronary care unit. *Mayo Clin Proc* 58:122, 1983.
42. Chastre J, Cornud F, Bouchama A, et al: Thrombosis as a complication of pulmonary-artery catheterization via the internal jugular vein: Prospective evaluation by phlebography. *N Engl J Med* 306:278, 1982.
43. Austin JL, Preis LK, Crampton RS, et al: Analysis of pacemaker malfunction and complications of temporary pacing in the coronary care unit. *Am J Cardiol* 49:301, 1982.
44. Linos DA, Mucha P Jr, van Heerden JA: Subclavian vein: a golden route. *Mayo Clin Proc* 55:315, 1980.
45. Nolewajka AJ, Goddard MD, Brown TC: Temporary transvenous pacing and femoral vein thrombosis. *Circulation* 62:646, 1980.

CHAPTER 6 ■ CARDIOVERSION AND DEFIBRILLATION

MARK S. LINK AND NAOMI F. BOTKIN

The use of electric shock to terminate arrhythmia is one of the critical findings of the last century and underlies much of the modern treatment of arrhythmias. Thanks to the pioneering work of Zoll et al. [1] and Lown et al. [2] in the second half of the twentieth century, the use of electric shock gained widespread acceptance. Although incorporating the same mechanism and physics, *Cardioversion* refers to the use of direct-current electric shock to terminate arrhythmias other than ventricular fibrillation, while *Defibrillation* refers to the termination of ventricular fibrillation. Cardioversion shocks are synchronized to the QRS to avoid the initiation of ventricular fibrillation which may result from shocks on the T-wave while defibrillation occurs with unsynchronized shocks.

PHYSIOLOGY OF ARRHYTHMIA AND SHOCK

Arrhythmias may be due to reentry, increased automaticity, or triggered activity. Reentry refers to the phenomenon in which a wave of excitation travels repeatedly over a closed pathway or circuit of conduction tissue. Reentry requires slow conduction in a portion of myocardium so that by the time the impulse exits the slowly conducting portion the remaining myocardium has repolarized and is hence able to be depolarized again.

Many of the commonly encountered arrhythmias are due to a fixed reentrant mechanism, including atrial flutter, atrioventricular (AV) nodal reentrant tachycardia (AVNRT), AV reentrant tachycardia (AVRT), and most ventricular tachycardias. Atrial fibrillation, once thought exclusively reentrant, has been shown to be caused by foci in the pulmonary veins in many individuals [3]. Atrial fibrillation may also be secondary to functional reentry. Ventricular fibrillation is also due to functional reentry. Cardioversion and defibrillation terminate these arrhythmias by simultaneously depolarizing all excitable tissue, disrupting the process of reentry.

Arrhythmias may also be due to disorders of impulse formation (increased automaticity or triggered activity). These include sinus tachycardia, focal atrial tachycardia, and idiopathic ventricular tachycardias. Sinus tachycardia is a physiologic response and not a pathologic tachycardia; thus, sinus tachycardia will not respond to cardioversion, but atrial tachycardias and ventricular tachycardias generally will terminate.

Insight into the effect of shock on fibrillating myocardial cells has grown in the past few decades. Although it was initially thought that all activation fronts had to be terminated simultaneously to stop atrial and ventricular fibrillation [4], it is now believed that if the vast majority of myocardium is silenced, the remaining mass is insufficient to perpetuate the arrhythmia [5]. The effect of shock on fibrillating myocardium is complex and is dependent on multiple factors including energy, waveform, and myocardial refractory state [6]. Electric shocks at low energy levels may fail to terminate atrial and ventricular fibrillation [7]. Atrial and ventricular arrhythmias may also be terminated by the shock and then reinitiated shortly thereafter. And finally, ventricular fibrillation can be triggered in patients not already in this rhythm if shock occurs on the vulnerable portion of the T wave. Thus, synchronization of shocks with the R wave will minimize the risk.

INDICATIONS AND CONTRAINDICATIONS

Cardioversion and defibrillation are performed for a variety of reasons in the intensive care setting. In the case of hemodynamic instability due to tachyarrhythmia of nearly any type, the urgent use of shock is strongly indicated. One must be careful, however, not to shock sinus tachycardia, which is commonly present in patients who are hypotensive for noncardiac reasons. Acute congestive heart failure and angina that are secondary to an acute tachyarrhythmia are also indications for urgent cardioversion; however, there is usually sufficient time to provide some sedation. Care must be taken not to shock tachycardias that are secondary to the heart failure or chest pain. In the absence of hemodynamic instability or significant symptoms, cardioversion is usually considered elective and the risks and benefits of the procedure must be carefully weighed.

Extreme caution should be exercised in patients with digitalis toxicity or electrolyte imbalance because of the increased risk of ventricular tachycardia or fibrillation after being shocked. Patients with severe sinus node disease may exhibit significant bradyarrhythmia after cardioversion from atrial fibrillation. In addition, patients who have been in atrial fibrillation for greater than 48 hours are at risk for thromboembolism after cardioversion; appropriate measures should be taken to minimize this risk (see later).

CLINICAL COMPETENCE

A clinical competence statement by the American College of Cardiology and American Heart Association outlines the cognitive and technical skills required for the successful and safe performance of elective external cardioversion (Table 6.1). A minimum of eight cardioversions should be supervised before a physician is considered competent to perform the procedure independently. In addition, a minimum of four procedures should be performed annually to maintain competence [8].

Methods

Patient Preparation

In the case of unconsciousness due to tachyarrhythmia, the shock must be performed urgently. In more elective settings, patient safety and comfort become paramount. As with any procedure, informed consent should be obtained. Patients should refrain from eating and drinking for several hours to decrease the risk of regurgitation and aspiration. Constant heart rhythm monitoring should be used throughout the procedure and a 12-lead electrocardiogram should be obtained before and after the shock.

Medications with rapid onset and short half-life are favored for achieving analgesia, sedation, and amnesia. The combination of a benzodiazepine, such as midazolam, and a narcotic, such as fentanyl, is a common choice in the absence of anesthesiology assistance. Propofol is often used when an anesthesiologist is present to assist with airway management and sedation. Existing hospital policies for monitoring during moderate sedation should be followed, including frequent assessment of blood pressure and pulse oximetry. Supplemental oxygen is delivered via nasal cannula or face mask.

Shock Waveforms

Defibrillators that employ biphasic waveforms have largely replaced those using monophasic waveforms. Advantages of biphasic waveforms are lower defibrillation thresholds, meaning shocks using biphasic waveforms require less energy to achieve defibrillation [6], and they are less likely to cause skin burns and myocardial damage. Both biphasic truncated exponential waveform and biphasic rectilinear waveform are commercially available, with the former being more common. Randomized trials comparing the two types of biphasic waveforms in the cardioversion of atrial fibrillation have failed to show any significant difference in efficacy [9–11].

The efficacy of biphasic shocks in the termination of ventricular fibrillation has been well established [12,13]. Furthermore, clinical studies of atrial fibrillation cardioversion have established the superiority of biphasic over monophasic waveform shocks [14,15]. For instance, one study demonstrated the equivalent efficacy of a 120 to 200 J biphasic sequence with a 200 to 360 J monophasic sequence [15]. Biphasic waveforms allow fewer shocks to be given and a lower total energy delivery

TABLE 6.1

COGNITIVE AND TECHNICAL SKILLS NECESSARY FOR PERFORMING EXTERNAL CARDIOVERSION

Physicians should have knowledge of the following:
- Electrophysiologic principles of cardioversion
- Indications for the procedure
- Anticoagulation management
- Proper use of antiarrhythmic therapy
- Use of sedation and the management of overdose
- Direct current cardioversion equipment, including the selection of appropriate energy and synchronization.
- Treatment of possible complications, including advanced cardiac life support (ACLS), defibrillation, and pacing
- Proper placement of paddles or pads
- Appropriate monitor display and recognition of arrhythmias
- Ability to differentiate failure to convert atrial fibrillation from an immediate recurrence of atrial fibrillation
- Baseline 12-lead electrocardiogram reading, recognition of acute changes, drug toxicity, and contraindications

Physicians should have the following technical skills:
- Proper preparation of skin and electrode placement, including application of saline jelly or saline soaked gauze
- Achievement of artifact-free monitored strips and synchronization signal/marker
- Technically acceptable 12-lead electrocardiograms before and after cardioversion
- Temporary pacing and defibrillation capabilities
- Ability to perform advanced cardiac life support, including proper airway management

From Tracy CM, Akhtar M, DiMarco JP, et al: American College of Cardiology/American Heart Association 2006 Update of the Clinical Competence Statement on invasive electrophysiology studies, catheter ablation, and cardioversion: A report of the American College of Cardiology/American Heart Association/American College of Physicians-American Society of Internal Medicine Task Force on Clinical Competence. *Circulation* 114:1654–1668, 2006.

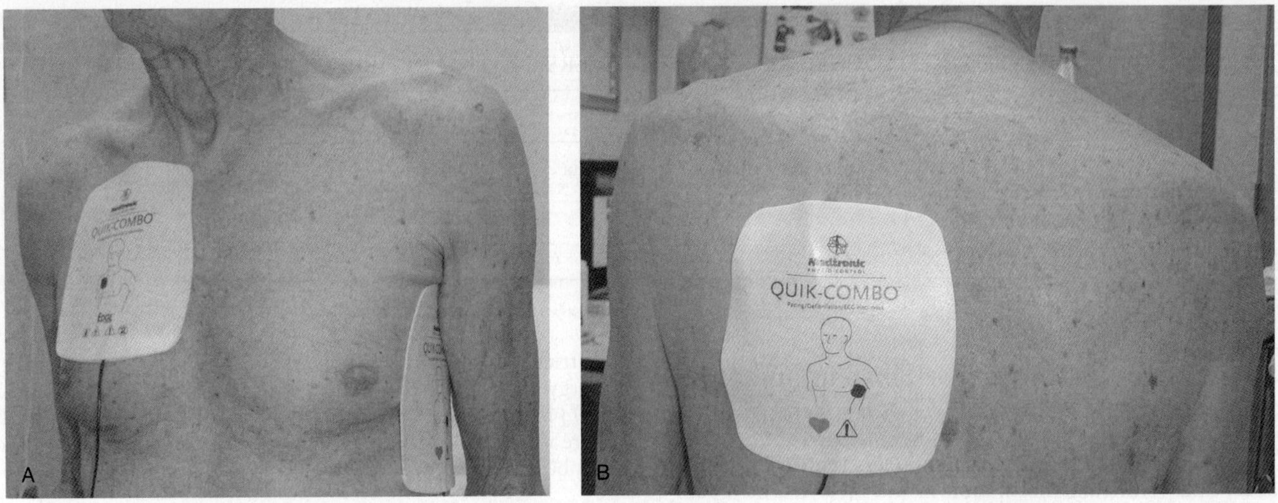

FIGURE 6.1. A: Self-adhesive defibrillator pads in the anterior and lateral positions. **B:** Self-adhesive defibrillator pad in the posterior position. When posterior positioning is used, the second pad is placed anteriorly.

[14]. Whether or not this translates into a significant clinical advantage remains to be demonstrated. However, there is evidence that biphasic shocks result in less dermal injury [14]. Although an animal model suggested better maintenance of cardiac function after biphasic shocks [16], human data on myocardial function are unavailable.

Electrodes

Until recently, hand-held paddles were the only available means of cardioversion or defibrillation. Self-adhesive pads have become more common in the past few years, although paddles may still be used. Limited data are available comparing the two modalities, but one study suggested the superiority of paddles over pads in cardioverting atrial fibrillation [17]). This phenomenon might be explained by the lower transthoracic impedance achieved with paddles [18]. Whichever modality is used, impedance can be minimized by avoiding positioning over breast tissue, by clipping body hair when it is excessive [19], by delivering the shock during expiration, and by firm pressure on the pads or paddles.

The optimal anatomic placement of pads and paddles is controversial; however, the general principal holds that the heart must lie between the two electrodes [6]. Both anterior–lateral and anterior–posterior placements are acceptable (Fig. 6.1). The anterior paddle is placed on the right infraclavicular chest. In anterior–lateral placement, the lateral paddle should be located lateral to the left breast and should have a longitudinal orientation, since this results in a lower transthoracic impedance than horizontal orientation [20]. When anterior–posterior positioning is used, the posterior pad is commonly located to the left of the spine at the level of the lower scapula, although some physicians favor placement to the right of, or directly over, the spine. There are data to suggest that anterior–posterior placement is more successful in the cardioversion of atrial fibrillation than anterior–lateral positioning when monophasic waveforms are used [21]. It is thought that anterior–posterior positioning directs more of the delivered energy to the atria than anterior–lateral placement. However, a study employing biphasic waveforms failed to show any difference of success with anterior–lateral compared with anterior–posterior pad positions [22].

Using the Defibrillator

External defibrillators are designed for easy operation. After the patient is adequately prepared and the electrodes are applied, attention may be turned to the device itself. If the QRS amplitude on the rhythm tracing is small and difficult to see, a different lead should be selected. If cardioversion—rather than defibrillation—is to be performed, the synchronization function should be selected. Many defibrillators require that external leads be applied for synchronization. The appropriate initial energy is selected. Finally, the capacitor is charged, the area is cleared, and the shock is delivered. One should be aware that the synchronization function is automatically deselected after each shock in most devices, meaning that it must be manually reselected prior to any further shock delivery if another synchronized shock is desired.

Table 6.2 provides a checklist for physicians involved in cardioversion. Table 6.3 gives recommendations for the initial energy selection for defibrillation and cardioversion of various arrhythmias. Recommendations specific to each device are available in the manufacturers' manuals and should be consulted by physicians unfamiliar with their particular device.

TABLE 6.2

CHECKLIST FOR PERFORMING CARDIOVERSION

Preparing the patient:
1. Ensure NPO status
2. Obtain informed consent
3. Apply self-adhesive pads (clip hair if needed)
4. Apply external lead
5. Achieve adequate sedation and analgesia
6. Monitor vital signs and cardiac rhythm throughout

Performing the cardioversion:
1. Select initial energy appropriate for specific device
2. Select the synchronization function
3. Confirm that arrhythmia is still present
4. Charge, clear, and deliver shock
5. If no change in rhythm, escalate energy as appropriate

NPO, nil per os.

TABLE 6.3

SUGGESTED INITIAL ENERGY FOR CARDIOVERSION AND DEFIBRILLATION

Rhythm	Monophasic (J)	Biphasic (J)
Ventricular fibrillation, pulseless ventricular tachycardia	360	120–200
Ventricular tachycardia with pulse	100	100
Atrial fibrillation	200	100–200
Atrial flutter	50–100	50

Treatment of Ventricular Fibrillation and Pulseless Ventricular Tachycardia

The algorithm for the treatment of pulseless ventricular tachycardia and ventricular fibrillation in the most recently published American Heart Association guidelines contains some important changes from the previous guidelines [23]. Rather than beginning with three sequential shocks, the guidelines recommend only one shock followed by five cycles of cardiopulmonary resuscitation (CPR) before the rhythm is reassessed [6]. This change was prompted by new data demonstrating that a single biphasic shock was more efficacious than three monophasic shocks in termination of ventricular fibrillation. In addition, three sequential shocks involve a substantial interruption in CPR, which has been shown to be associated with a decreased odds of survival [24]. In the 2010 algorithm, vasopressors (epinephrine or vasopressin) may be given before or after the second shock, and antiarrhythmics such as amiodarone and lidocaine may be considered before or after the second shock (Table 6.4). Both ventricular fibrillation and pulseless

TABLE 6.4

TREATMENT OF VENTRICULAR FIBRILLATION AND PULSELESS VENTRICULAR TACHYCARDIA

Assess airway, breathing, and circulation
Assess rhythm
Deliver 1 shock
- Monophasic: 360 J
- Biphasic: use device specific energy; if unknown, maximum energy

Resume compressions immediately and perform five cycles of CPR
Check rhythm—if still VT/VF, shock again
- Monophasic: 360 J
- Biphasic: same as first shock or higher dose

Resume compressions immediately and perform five cycles of CPR
Give a vasopressor during CPR, either before or after the second shock
- Epinephrine 1 mg IV/IO, repeat every 3–5 min, OR
- Vasopressin 40 U IV/IO may replace First or second dose of epinephrine

Check rhythm—if still VT/VF, shock again
Consider an antiarrhythmic before or after second shock:
- Amiodarone 300 mg IV/IO once, then consider additional 150 mg once OR
- Lidocaine 1 to 1.5 mg/kg first dose, then 0.5 to 0.75 mg/kg IV/IO, maximum three doses.

IO, intraosseous; IV, intravenous; VF, ventricular fibrillation; VT, ventricular tachycardia.

ventricular tachycardia are treated with unsynchronized, high-energy shocks of 120 to 200 J with biphasic defibrillators (or 360 J in the case of devices that use monophasic waveforms). If there is any confusion regarding which energy should be used it is best to shock with the highest available energy.

Treatment of Wide Complex Tachycardia with a Pulse

When a pulse is present, a regular, wide complex tachycardia may be ventricular tachycardia, supraventricular tachycardia with aberrant conduction, or a supraventricular tachycardia with preexcitation. If signs of instability are present (such as chest pressure, altered mental status, hypotension, or heart failure) and are thought to be secondary to the tachycardia, urgent cardioversion is indicated. A starting energy of 100 J is recommended when a monophasic shock waveform is being used. The optimal initial energy with biphasic devices is unknown but it would seem reasonable to begin at 100 J. The energy should be escalated with each successive shock, such as 200, 300, and 360 J [25].

If the patient is stable, however, one might consider enlisting the assistance of an expert in distinguishing between ventricular and supraventricular arrhythmia. If this is not possible, it is generally safest to assume a ventricular etiology. Stable ventricular tachycardia may be treated initially with antiarrhythmic agents such as amiodarone, lidocaine, or procainamide. Elective cardioversion can be performed if necessary, once sedation and analgesia are assured.

Wide complex tachycardia that appears irregular is usually atrial fibrillation with aberrant conduction but may also be polymorphic ventricular tachycardia or torsades de pointes. If the arrhythmia is atrial fibrillation, treatment should follow the recommendations for atrial fibrillation (see later). However, if the Wolff–Parkinson–White Syndrome is suspected, AV nodal blocking agents are contraindicated and procainamide or ibutilide should be used. If the patient is hypotensive or in shock or if the rhythm is thought to be polymorphic ventricular tachycardia then an unsynchronized shock is advised.

Treatment of Supraventricular Tachycardia

The most common narrow complex tachycardia is sinus tachycardia, which is an appropriate cardiac response to some other physiologic condition. Atrial fibrillation and atrial flutter are the next most common, followed by AVNRT, AV-reciprocating tachycardia (AVRT) and atrial tachycardia. Supraventricular tachycardia—defined as a nonventricular tachycardia other than sinus tachycardia—should be suspected when the arrhythmia starts suddenly, when it is more rapid than maximal sinus rates (220-age), and when P waves are absent or closely follow the QRS. Initial therapy involves vagal maneuvers and adenosine. If these fail, nondihydropyridine calcium channel antagonists or beta-blockers may terminate the arrhythmia. Cardioversion is indicated only rarely for clinical instability, usually in patients with underlying heart disease in whom the initial therapies fail.

Treatment of Atrial Fibrillation and Flutter

Rate Control

Although the majority of patients with atrial fibrillation and flutter remain hemodynamically stable, many develop bothersome symptoms such as palpitations, chest pressure, and, occasionally, pulmonary edema. However, a rapid ventricular response is usually secondary to—rather than the cause of heart failure and ischemia. Beta-blockers and nondihydropyridine calcium channel antagonists are used to slow the ventricular response rate by slowing AV nodal conduction. Many patients become asymptomatic or minimally symptomatic with adequate rate control, allowing the decision about cardioversion to be made electively.

Electrical Cardioversion

Cardioversion for atrial fibrillation or flutter is usually performed electively. The risk of thromboembolism dictates a thoughtful decision about treatment options. When cardioversion is performed, an appropriate initial starting dose is 100 to 200 J for monophasic waveform shock and 120 to 200 J for biphasic shock. Atrial flutter responds to lower energy, so a starting dose of 50 to 100 J is recommended with a monophasic waveform. The ideal starting energy for biphasic devices is unknown, so 50 to 100 J is reasonable. If atrial fibrillation or flutter fails to terminate, shock energy should be escalated. For most defibrillators, the synchronization function must be selected after each shock.

Anticoagulation

Patients with atrial fibrillation or flutter may develop thrombus in the left atrial appendage or left atrial cavity, leading to thromboembolism during or after cardioversion. One study demonstrated a risk of pericardioversion thromboembolism of 5.3% in patients who were not anticoagulated and 0.8% in those who were [26].

There is general agreement that cardioversion of patients who have been in atrial fibrillation for less than 24 to 48 hours is very unlikely to cause thromboembolism. Current guidelines indicate that pericardioversion anticoagulation with heparin or low molecular weight heparin is optional in these patients [27]. Individuals in atrial fibrillation or flutter for greater than 48 hours are at risk for thromboembolism. In these individuals, a transesophageal echocardiogram is necessary to exclude left atrial thrombus in all but the most emergent cases [28,29]. Alternatively, one can therapeutically anticoagulate for at least 3 weeks prior to cardioversion. Most physicians will anticoagulate for a few weeks after cardioversion, as the risk of thromboembolism still exists during this period.

Pharmacologic Cardioversion

Cardioversion can be achieved not only electrically but also pharmacologically. Pharmacologic cardioversion is used mainly for atrial fibrillation and flutter of relatively short duration. Although electrical cardioversion is quicker and has a higher probability of success, pharmacologic cardioversion does not require sedation. The risk of thromboembolism with pharmacologic cardioversion has not been well established but is thought to be similar to that of electric shock because it is the return of sinus rhythm rather than the shock itself that is believed to precipitate thromboembolism [30,31].

Dofetilide, flecainide, ibutilide, propafenone, amiodarone, and quinidine have been demonstrated to have some degree of efficacy in restoring sinus rhythm [27]. Each of these medications has potential toxicities including malignant arrhythmias and hypotension. The risks and benefits should be carefully weighed when selecting a pharmacologic agent. Although beta-blockers and calcium channel antagonists are often believed to facilitate cardioversion, their efficacy has not been established in controlled trials.

Management of Resistant Atrial Fibrillation

Electrical cardioversion is unsuccessful in up to 10% of atrial fibrillation and atrial flutter, most often because of early recurrences of arrhythmia. The duration of atrial fibrillation is inversely related to the probability of successful cardioversion.

When cardioversion fails to even temporarily terminate the arrhythmia, the operator's technique should be reviewed and modified. Electrode position may be altered, from anterior–posterior to anterior–lateral or vice versa. Firmer pressure may be employed via the paddles or pads. If a device that delivers monophasic waveform shocks is being employed, it may be exchanged for one that delivers biphasic waveform shocks. Ibutilide may be initiated prior to another attempt at cardioversion [32]. Other antiarrhythmic agents may reduce the recurrence of arrhythmia.

Complications of Defibrillation and Cardioversion

Burns

Shock can cause first-degree burns and pain at the paddle or pad site. One study documented moderate to severe pain in nearly one quarter of patients undergoing cardioversion. Pain was directly related to total energy delivered and number of shocks [33]. Another study showed a lower rate of dermal injury with biphasic rather than monophasic shocks, probably due to the lower energy necessary with biphasic shocks [14]. The lowest effective energy should be used to minimize skin injury. In addition, saline-soaked gauzes between the skin and the paddles, rather than conductive gel, will minimize burns.

Thromboembolism

Cardioversion of atrial fibrillation and atrial flutter carries a risk of thromboembolism. Up to 7% of patients in atrial fibrillation who undergo cardioversion without receiving anticoagulation may experience this complication [26], and anticoagulation is standard of care for those in atrial fibrillation or flutter for those in arrhythmias more than 48 hours [27].

Arrhythmia

Bradyarrhythmias such as sinus arrest and sinus bradycardia are common immediately after shock and are almost always short lived. Patients who have atrial fibrillation may have concomitant sinus node dysfunction that is masked by the atrial fibrillation and unmasked by cardioversion.

Ventricular tachycardia and ventricular fibrillation can occasionally be precipitated by shock, particularly in patients with digitalis toxicity or hypokalemia [34,35]. Elective cardioversion should therefore be avoided in patients with these conditions. If cardioversion or defibrillation must be performed urgently, one should anticipate the ventricular arrhythmias to be more refractory to shock than usual.

Myocardial Damage

Occasionally, one may see transient ST segment elevations on postshock electrocardiograms [36]. This is unlikely to signify myocardial injury. Although a study of cardioversion using higher-than-usual energy levels demonstrated an increase in creatine-kinase–MB levels above that expected from skeletal muscle damage in 10% of patients, there was no elevation in troponin-T or -I seen [37]. This observation suggests that clinically significant myocardial damage from cardioversion or defibrillation is unlikely. Nonetheless, it has been suggested that any two consecutive shocks be delivered no less than 1 minute apart to minimize the chance of myocardial damage [38]. Of course, this recommendation applies only to nonemergent situations.

Miscellaneous Topics

Patients with Implanted Pacemakers and Defibrillators

Patients with implanted pacemakers and defibrillators may undergo external cardioversion and defibrillation safely. However, one must be aware of the possibility that external energy delivery may alter the programming of the internal device. Furthermore, energy may be conducted down an internal lead, causing local myocardial injury and a resultant change in the pacing or defibrillation threshold. The paddles or pads used for external electric shock should never be placed over the device. In addition, interrogation of the device immediately after any external shock delivery is recommended.

Chest Thump

The use of a manual "thump" on the chest to successfully terminate ventricular tachycardia was described in several patients in 1970 [39]. Unfortunately, this technique may inadvertently trigger ventricular fibrillation if the blow happens to fall during the vulnerable period of the ventricle [40]. A chest thump is extremely unlikely to terminate ventricular fibrillation [41,42]. For these reasons, chest thump is considered a therapy of last resort, administered only to a pulseless patient when a defibrillator is unavailable and unlikely to become available soon. It should not be administered when a pulse is present unless a defibrillator is immediately available.

Cardioversion and Defibrillation in Pregnancy

Cardioversion and defibrillation have been performed in all trimesters of pregnancy without obvious adverse fetal effects or premature labor [43]. It has been suggested that the fetal heart rhythm be monitored during cardioversion [44].

References

1. Zoll PM, Linenthal AJ, Gibson W, et al: Termination of ventricular fibrillation in man by externally applied electric countershock. *N Engl J Med* 254:727–732, 1956.
2. Lown B, Amarasingham R, Neuman J: New method for terminating cardiac arrhythmias. Use of synchronized capacitor discharge. *JAMA* 182:548–555, 1962.
3. Haissaguerre M, Jais P, Shah DC, et al: Spontaneous initiation of atrial fibrillation by ectopic beats originating in the pulmonary veins. *N Engl J Med* 339:659–666, 1998.
4. Wiggers CJ: The mechanism and nature of ventricular fibrillation. *Am Heart J* 20:399–412, 1940.
5. Zipes DP, Fischer J, King RM, et al: Termination of ventricular fibrillation in dogs by depolarizing a critical amount of myocardium. *Am J Cardiol* 36:37–44, 1975.
6. Link MS Chair, Atkins DL, Passman RS, et al: Part 6: Electrical therapies: automated external defibrillators, defibrillation, cardioversion, and pacing. 2010 American Heart Association Guidelines for Cardiopulmonary Resuscitation and Emergency Cardiovascular Care. *Circulation* 122:S706–S719, 2010.
7. Chen PS, Shibata N, Dixon EG, et al: Comparison of the defibrillation threshold and the upper limit of ventricular vulnerability. *Circulation* 73:1022–1028, 1986.
8. Tracy CM, Akhtar M, DiMarco JP, et al: American College of Cardiology/American Heart Association Clinical Competence Statement on invasive electrophysiology studies, catheter ablation, and cardioversion: A report of the American College of Cardiology/American Heart Association/American College of Physicians-American Society of Internal Medicine Task Force on Clinical Competence. *Circulation* 102:2309–2320, 2000.
9. Neal S, Ngarmukos T, Lessard D, et al: Comparison of the efficacy and safety of two biphasic defibrillator waveforms for the conversion of atrial fibrillation to sinus rhythm. *Am J Cardiol* 92:810–814, 2003.
10. Kim ML, Kim SG, Park DS, et al: Comparison of rectilinear biphasic waveform energy versus truncated exponential biphasic waveform energy for transthoracic cardioversion of atrial fibrillation. *Am J Cardiol* 94:1438–1440, 2004.
11. Alatawi F, Gurevitz O, White RD, et al: Prospective, randomized comparison of two biphasic waveforms for the efficacy and safety of transthoracic biphasic cardioversion of atrial fibrillation. *Heart Rhythm* 2:382–387, 2005.
12. van Alem AP, Chapman FW, Lank P, et al: A prospective, randomised and blinded comparison of first shock success of monophasic and biphasic waveforms in out-of-hospital cardiac arrest. *Resuscitation* 58:17–24, 2003.
13. Schneider T, Martens PR, Paschen H, et al: Multicenter, randomized, controlled trial of 150-J biphasic shocks compared with 200- to 360-J monophasic shocks in the resuscitation of out-of-hospital cardiac arrest victims. Optimized Response to Cardiac Arrest (ORCA) Investigators. *Circulation* 102:1780–1787, 2000.
14. Page RL, Kerber RE, Russell JK, et al: Biphasic versus monophasic shock waveform for conversion of atrial fibrillation: the results of an international randomized, double-blind multicenter trial. *J Am Coll Cardiol* 39:1956–1963, 2002.
15. Scholten M, Szili-Torok T, Klootwijk P, et al: Comparison of monophasic and biphasic shocks for transthoracic cardioversion of atrial fibrillation. *Heart* 89:1032–1034, 2003.
16. Tang W, Weil MH, Sun S, et al: The effects of biphasic and conventional monophasic defibrillation on postresuscitation myocardial function. *J Am Coll Cardiol* 34:815–822, 1999.
17. Kirchhof P, Monnig G, Wasmer K, et al: A trial of self-adhesive patch electrodes and hand-held paddle electrodes for external cardioversion of atrial fibrillation (MOBIPAPA). *Eur Heart J* 26:1292–1297, 2005.
18. Dodd TE, Deakin CD, Petley GW, et al: External defibrillation in the left lateral position–a comparison of manual paddles with self-adhesive pads. *Resuscitation* 63:283–286, 2004.
19. Sado DM, Deakin CD, Petley GW, et al: Comparison of the effects of removal of chest hair with not doing so before external defibrillation on transthoracic impedance. *Am J Cardiol* 93:98–100, 2004.
20. Deakin CD, Sado DM, Petley GW, et al: Is the orientation of the apical defibrillation paddle of importance during manual external defibrillation? *Resuscitation* 56:15–18, 2003.
21. Kirchhof P, Eckardt L, Loh P, et al: Anterior-posterior versus anterior-lateral electrode positions for external cardioversion of atrial fibrillation: a randomised trial. *Lancet* 360:1275–1279, 2002.
22. Walsh SJ, McCarty D, McClelland AJ, et al: Impedance compensated biphasic waveforms for transthoracic cardioversion of atrial fibrillation: a multi-centre comparison of antero-apical and antero-posterior pad positions. *Eur Heart J* 26:1298–1302, 2005.
23. Field JM Co-Chair, Hazinski MF, Co-Chair, Sayre MR, et al: Part 1: Executive summary: 2010 American Heart Association Guidelines for Cardiopulmonary Resuscitation and Emergency Cardiovascular Care. *Circulation* 122:S640–S656, 2010.
24. Eftestol T, Sunde K, Steen PA: Effects of interrupting precordial compressions on the calculated probability of defibrillation success during out-of-hospital cardiac arrest. *Circulation* 105:2270–2273, 2002.
25. Neumar RW Chair, Otto CW, Link MS, et al: Part 8: Adult advanced cardiovascular life support. 2010 American Heart Association Guidelines for Cardiopulmonary Resuscitation and Emergency Cardiovascular Care. *Circulation* 122:S729–S767, 2010.
26. Bjerkelund CJ, Orning OM: The efficacy of anticoagulant therapy in preventing embolism related to D.C. electrical conversion of atrial fibrillation. *Am J Cardiol* 23:208–216, 1969.
27. Fuster V, Ryden LE, Cannom DS, et al: ACC/AHA/ESC 2006 Guidelines for the Management of Patients with Atrial Fibrillation: a report of the American College of Cardiology/American Heart Association Task Force on Practice Guidelines and the European Society of Cardiology Committee for Practice Guidelines (Writing Committee to Revise the 2001 Guidelines for the Management of Patients With Atrial Fibrillation): developed in collaboration with the European Heart Rhythm Association and the Heart Rhythm Society. *Circulation* 114:e257–e354, 2006.

28. Klein AL, Grimm RA, Murray RD, et al: Use of transesophageal echocardiography to guide cardioversion in patients with atrial fibrillation. *N Engl J Med* 344:1411–1420, 2001.
29. Klein AL, Grimm RA, Jasper SE, et al: Efficacy of transesophageal echocardiography-guided cardioversion of patients with atrial fibrillation at 6 months: a randomized controlled trial. *Am Heart J* 151:380–389, 2006.
30. Manning WJ, Leeman DE, Gotch PJ, et al: Pulsed Doppler evaluation of atrial mechanical function after electrical cardioversion of atrial fibrillation. *J Am Coll Cardiol* 13:617–623, 1989.
31. O'Neill PG, Puleo PR, Bolli R, et al: Return of atrial mechanical function following electrical conversion of atrial dysrhythmias. *Am Heart J* 120:353–359, 1990.
32. Oral H, Souza JJ, Michaud GF, et al: Facilitating transthoracic cardioversion of atrial fibrillation with ibutilide pretreatment. *N Engl J Med* 340:1849–1854, 1999.
33. Ambler JJ, Sado DM, Zideman DA, et al: The incidence and severity of cutaneous burns following external DC cardioversion. *Resuscitation* 61:281–288, 2004.
34. Lown B, Kleiger R, Williams J: Cardioversion and digitalis drugs: changed threshold to electric shock in digitalized animals. *Circ Res* 17:519–531, 1965.
35. Aberg H, Cullhed I: Direct current countershock complications. *Acta Med Scand* 183:415–421, 1968.
36. Van Gelder IC, Crijns HJ, Van der Laarse A, et al: Incidence and clinical significance of ST segment elevation after electrical cardioversion of atrial fibrillation and atrial flutter. *Am Heart J* 121:51–56, 1991.
37. Lund M, French JK, Johnson RN, et al: Serum troponins T and I after elective cardioversion. *Eur Heart J* 21:245–253, 2000.
38. Dahl CF, Ewy GA, Warner ED, et al: Myocardial necrosis from direct current countershock. Effect of paddle electrode size and time interval between discharges. *Circulation* 50:956–961, 1974.
39. Pennington JE, Taylor J, Lown B: Chest thump for reverting ventricular tachycardia. *N Engl J Med* 283:1192–1195, 1970.
40. Yakaitis RW, Redding JS: Precordial thumping during cardiac resuscitation. *Crit Care Med* 1:22–26, 1973.
41. Pellis T, Kette F, Lovisa D, et al: Utility of pre-cordial thump for treatment of out of hospital cardiac arrest: a prospective study. *Resuscitation* 80:17–23, 2009.
42. Madias C, Maron BJ, Alsheikh-Ali AA, et al: Precordial thump for cardiac arrest is effective for asystole but not for ventricular fibrillation. *Heart Rhythm* 6:1495–1500, 2009.
43. Schroeder JS, Harrison DC: Repeated cardioversion during pregnancy. Treatment of refractory paroxysmal atrial tachycardia during 3 successive pregnancies. *Am J Cardiol* 27:445–446, 1971.
44. Meitus ML: Fetal electrocardiography and cardioversion with direct current countershock. Report of a case. *Dis Chest* 48:324–325, 1965.

CHAPTER 7 ■ PERICARDIOCENTESIS

CRAIG S. SMITH AND RICHARD C. BECKER

Pericardiocentesis is a potentially life-saving procedure performed in the critical care setting. In contrast to other cardiac conditions, however, there is a paucity of randomized clinical data to help guide physicians in the diagnosis and management of pericardial diseases. This chapter reviews the indications for emergent and urgent pericardiocentesis, summarizes the pathobiology of pericardial effusions, and provides a step-by-step approach to pericardiocentesis, including management of patients following the procedure.

INDICATIONS FOR PERICARDIOCENTESIS

The initial management of patients with a known or suspected pericardial effusion is largely determined by clinical status. In the absence of hemodynamic instability or suspected purulent bacterial pericarditis, there is no need for emergent or urgent pericardiocentesis. Diagnostic pericardiocentesis may be performed to establish the etiology of an effusion, although only after thorough noninvasive workup is completed before consideration of an invasive procedure [1]. While the etiology of effusions varies widely in the literature depending upon patient population, a diagnosis based on initial examination alone was highly predictive of effusion etiology in one study [2]. In another large series of patients, between 50% and 60% of moderate to large effusions were due to a previously established medical condition [3]. In addition, the clinical context in which diagnostic pericardiocentesis is performed affects its predictive value, with greater diagnostic yield for large effusions than for acute pericarditis [4–6]. Primarily due to the routine use of echocardiographic guidance, the major (1.2%) and minor (3.5%) complications of pericardiocentesis have significantly decreased over the past several decades, with successful single needle passage rates approaching 90% and relief of tamponade in over 97% [7]. As a result, the 2004 European Society of Cardiology (ESC) recommends pericardiocentesis as the method of choice for pericardial fluid removal/sampling [8]. Surgical intervention is recommended for recurring large effusions for which repeated pericardiocentesis has not been effective, loculated or posterior effusions of hemodynamic consequence, purulent pericarditis, traumatic hemopericardium, constrictive pericarditis, and effusions due to aortic dissection [8]. Whenever possible, elective pericardiocentesis should be performed by an experienced operator using echocardiographic guidance. While generally safe, it should be performed in a location with adequate physiologic monitoring to assess any hemodynamic sequelae from complications and to aid in the diagnosis of effusive-constrictive pericarditis.

In contrast to diagnostic pericardiocentesis, the management of hemodynamically compromised patients requires emergent removal of pericardial fluid to restore adequate ventricular filling (preload) and hasten clinical stabilization. Aggressive fluid resuscitation and inotropic agents have been the mainstay of medical management for cardiac tamponade. These measures are largely ineffective and should be used only as a bridge to pericardial drainage [9,10]. The exact method and timing of pericardiocentesis is ultimately dictated by the patient's overall degree of instability. While echocardiographic and fluoroscopic guidance is preferred, unguided (or blind) pericardiocentesis may be required in patients with severe hypotension not responsive to temporizing measures. In this setting, there are no absolute contraindications to the procedure, and it should be performed without delay at the patient's bedside.

Urgent pericardiocentesis is indicated for patients with an established effusion who are initially hypotensive but respond quickly to hemodynamic support. Unlike acute tamponade, subacute tamponade is more likely to present with protean symptoms such as dyspnea and fatigue. Patients with preexisting hypertension may not demonstrate severe hypotension due to a persistent sympathetic response. Echocardiographic assessment of effusion size, hemodynamic impact, and optimal percutaneous approach are of paramount importance [11]. The procedure should be performed within several hours of presentation while careful monitoring and support continue. As in elective circumstances, pericardiocentesis in these patients should be undertaken with appropriate visual guidance, the method of which depends on the physician's expertise and resources.

Three additional points must be stressed regarding patients undergoing expedited pericardiocentesis. First, coagulation parameters—prothrombin time, partial thromboplastin time, and platelet count (>50,000 per μL)—should be checked and, when possible, quickly normalized prior to the procedure. If clinically feasible, the procedure should be postponed until the international normalized ratio is less than 1.4. An anti-Xa level is recommended for patients receiving low-molecular-weight heparin. For emergent pericardiocentesis performed on anticoagulant therapy, prolonged and continuous drainage is recommended. Second, many critical care specialists and cardiologists advocate performance of all pericardiocentesis procedures in the catheterization laboratory with concomitant right heart pressure monitoring to document efficacy of the procedure and to exclude a constrictive element of pericardial disease, although excessive delays must be avoided (see Chapter 34). Finally, efforts to ensure a cooperative and stationary patient during the procedure greatly facilitate the performance, safety, and success of pericardiocentesis.

The clinical presentation of hemodynamically significant pericardial effusions varies widely among patients. A comprehensive understanding requires knowledge of normal pericardial anatomy and physiology.

ANATOMY

The pericardium is a membranous structure with two layers: the visceral and parietal pericardium. The visceral pericardium is a monolayer of mesothelial cells adherent to the epicardial surface by a loose collection of small blood vessels, lymphatics, and connective tissue. The parietal pericardium is a relatively inelastic 2 mm dense outer network of collagen and elastin with an inner surface of mesothelial cells. It is invested around the great vessels and defines the shape of the pericardium, with attachments to the sternum, diaphragm, and anterior mediastinum while anchoring the heart in the thorax [12]. Posteriorly, the visceral epicardium is absent, with the parietal epicardium attached directly to the heart at the level of the vena cavae [13]. The potential space between the visceral and parietal mesothelial cell layers normally contains 15 to 50 mL of serous fluid, which is chemically similar to plasma ultrafiltrate, in the atrioventricular (AV) and interventricular grooves [14]. The pericardium is relatively avascular, but is well innervated and may produce significant pain with vagal responses during procedural manipulation or inflammation [15].

Because of the inelastic physical properties of the pericardium, the major determinant of when and how pericardial effusions come to clinical attention is directly related to the speed of accumulation. Effusions that collect rapidly (over minutes to hours) may cause hemodynamic compromise with volumes of 250 mL or less. These effusions are usually located posteriorly and are often difficult to detect without echocardiography or other imaging modalities such as multislice computed tomography or cardiac magnetic resonance imaging . In contrast, effusions developing slowly (over days to weeks) allow for dilation of the fibrous parietal membrane. Volumes of 2,000 mL or greater may accumulate without significant hemodynamic compromise. As a result, chronic effusions may present with symptoms such as cough, dyspnea, dysphagia, or early satiety owing to compression of adjacent thoracic structures. Conversely, intravascular hypovolemia, impaired ventricular systolic function, and ventricular hypertrophy with decreased elasticity of the myocardium (diastolic dysfunction) may exacerbate hemodynamic compromise without significant effusions present.

PROCEDURE

Since the first blind (or closed) pericardiocentesis performed in 1840 [16], numerous approaches to the pericardial space have been described. Marfan [17] performed the subcostal approach in 1911, which then became the standard approach for unguided pericardiocentesis as it is extrapleural and avoids the coronary and internal mammary arteries.

The advent of clinically applicable ultrasonography has opened a new chapter in diagnostic and therapeutic approaches to pericardial disease, allowing clinicians to quantitate and localize pericardial effusions quickly and noninvasively [18,19]. Callahan et al. [20,21] at the Mayo Clinic established the efficacy and safety of two-dimensional echocardiography to guide pericardiocentesis. While direct quantification of total fluid accumulation with echo is not yet possible, circumferential effusions of more than 10 mm are considered large (500 mL), and the ESC recommends pericardiocentesis of effusions of more than 20 mm, regardless of the presence of hemodynamic compromise (class IIa indication) [8]. Typically, at least 250 mL of fluid is required for safe pericardiocentesis. The routine use of echocardiography has resulted in two major trends in clinical practice: First, two-dimensional echocardiography is commonly used to guide pericardiocentesis, with success rates comparable to those of traditionally fluoroscopic-guided procedures [22–24]. Second, approaches other than the traditional subxiphoid method have been investigated owing to the ability to clearly define the anatomy (location and volume) of each patient's effusion [20,21]. In one series of postsurgical patients, the subxiphoid approach was the most direct route in only 12% of effusions [25]. With the use of echo guidance, apical pericardiocentesis and parasternal pericardiocentesis are increasingly performed with success rates comparable to those of the subxiphoid approach. In the apical approach, the needle is directed parallel to the long axis of the heart toward the aortic valve. Parasternal pericardiocentesis is performed with needle insertion 1 cm lateral to the sternal edge to avoid internal mammary laceration. All approaches employ a Seldinger technique of over-the-wire catheter insertion. As the subxiphoid approach remains the standard of practice and is the preferred approach for unguided emergent pericardiocentesis, it will be described later.

Regardless of the approach used, confirmation of appropriate positioning is mandatory and preferably performed before a dilation catheter is advanced over the wire. Direct visualization of the needle with either echocardiography or fluoroscopy and injection of agitated saline (echo guided) or a small amount of contrast (fluoroscopy guided) should be performed to confirm the correct position. Contrast layering inferiorly and not entering circulation or causing a myocardial stain confirms correct positioning.

In addition to two large-bore peripheral intravenous lines for aggressive resuscitative efforts, standard electrocardiographic monitoring is mandatory. Historically, an electrocardiographic (ECG) lead directly attached to the puncture needle has been used to detect contact with the myocardium via the appearance of a large "injury current" (ST elevation).

TABLE 7.1

MATERIALS FOR PERCUTANEOUS PERICARDIOCENTESIS

Site preparation
Antiseptic
Gauze
Sterile drapes and towels
Sterile gloves, masks, gowns, caps
5-mL or 10-mL syringe with 25-gauge needle
1% lidocaine (without epinephrine)
Code cart
Atropine (1-mg dose vial)
Procedure
No. 11 blade
20-mL syringe with 10 mL of 1% lidocaine (without epinephrine)
18-gauge, 8-cm, thin-walled needle with blunt tip
Multiple 20- and 40-mL syringes
Hemostat
Electrocardiogram machine
Three red-top tubes
Two purple-top (heparinized) tubes
Culture bottles
Postprocedure
Suture material
Scissors
Sterile gauze and bandage

Because a suboptimally grounded needle could fibrillate the heart (and the widespread availability of echocardiography), many cardiologists have abandoned this practice and the 2004 ESC guidelines consider it an inadequate safeguard [8,26].

The materials required for bedside pericardiocentesis are listed in Table 7.1 (Fig. 7.1). Table 7.2 (Fig. 7.2) lists the materials required for simultaneous placement of an intrapericardial drainage catheter. The materials are available in prepackaged kits or individually.

The subxiphoid approach for pericardiocentesis is as follows:

1. *Patient preparation.* Assist the patient in assuming a comfortable supine position with the head of the bed elevated to approximately 45 degree from the horizontal plane. Extremely dyspneic patients may need to be positioned fully upright, with a wedge if necessary. Elevation of the thorax allows free-flowing effusions to collect inferiorly and anteriorly, sites that are safest and easiest to access using the subxiphoid approach.
2. *Needle entry site selection.* Locate the patient's xiphoid process and the border of the left costal margin using inspection and careful palpation. The needle entry site should be 0.5 cm to the (patient's) left of the xiphoid process and 0.5 to 1.0 cm inferior to the costal margin (Fig. 7.3). It is helpful to estimate (by palpation) the distance between the skin surface and the posterior margin of the bony thorax: This helps guide subsequent needle insertion. The usual distance is 1.0 to 2.5 cm, increasing with obesity or protuberance of the abdomen.
3. *Site preparation.* Strict sterile techniques must be maintained at all times in preparation of the needle entry site. Prepare a wide area in the subxiphoid region and lower thorax with a chlorhexidine solution. Use maximum barrier precautions and use a large fenestrated drape to cover the field. After performing a time out, raise a 1- to 2-cm subcutaneous wheal by infiltrating the needle entry site with 1% lidocaine solution (without epinephrine). To facilitate needle entry, incise the skin with a no. 11 blade at the selected site after achieving adequate local anesthesia.
4. *Insertion of the needle apparatus.* The angle of entry with respect to the skin should be approximately 45 degree in the subxiphoid area. Direct the needle tip superiorly, aiming for the patient's left shoulder. Continue to advance the needle posteriorly while alternating between aspiration and

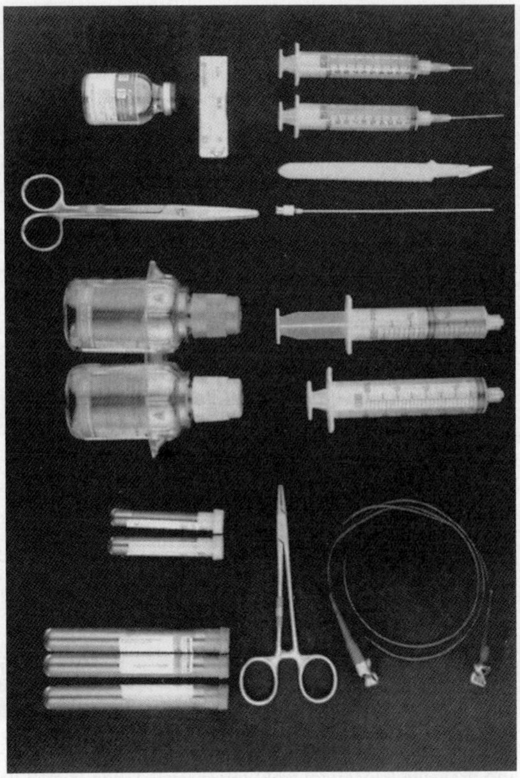

FIGURE 7.1. Materials required for pericardiocentesis (*clockwise from upper left*): 1% lidocaine solution, suture material, 10-mL syringe with 25-gauge needle, 10-mL syringe with 22-gauge needle, no. 11 blade, 18-gauge 8-cm thin-walled needle, 20-mL syringe, 30-mL syringe, alligator clip, hemostat, three red-top tubes, two purple-top tubes, culture bottles, scissors.

TABLE 7.2

MATERIALS FOR INTRAPERICARDIAL CATHETER

Catheter placement
Teflon-coated flexible J-curved guidewire
6 Fr dilator
8 Fr dilator
8 Fr, 35-cm flexible pigtail catheter with multiple fenestrations (end and side holes)
Drainage system[a]
Three-way stopcock
Sterile intravenous tubing
500-mL sterile collecting bag (or bottle)
Sterile gauze and adhesive bag (or bottle)
Suture material

[a] System described allows continuous drainage.

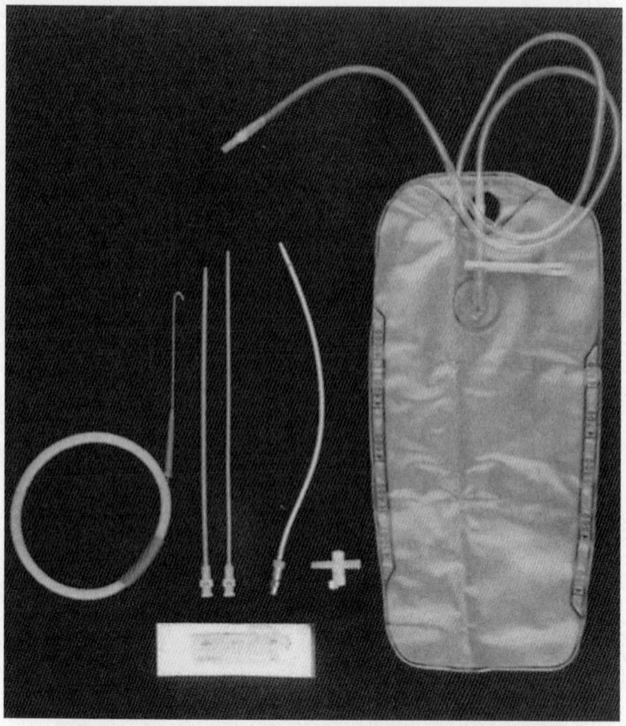

FIGURE 7.2. Materials required for intrapericardial catheter placement and drainage (*clockwise from lower left*): Teflon-coated flexible 0.035-in J-curved guidewire, 8 Fr dilator, 6.3 Fr dilator, 8 Fr catheter with end and side holes (35-cm flexible pigtail catheter not shown), three-way stopcock, 500-mL sterile collecting bag and tubing, suture material.

injection of lidocaine (with a half-filled 20-mL syringe of 1% lidocaine), until the tip has passed just beyond the posterior border of the bony thorax (Fig. 7.3). The posterior border usually lies within 2.5 cm of the skin surface. If the needle tip contacts the bony thorax, inject lidocaine after aspirating to clear the needle tip and anesthetize the periosteum. Then, walk the needle behind the posterior (costal) margin.

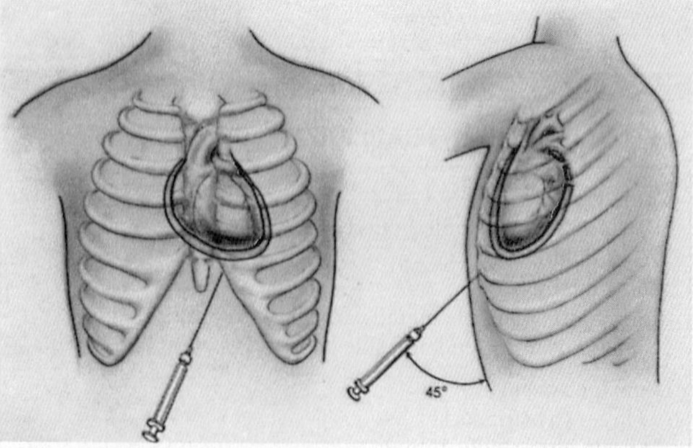

FIGURE 7.3. Insertion of the needle apparatus. After the subxiphoid region and lower thorax are prepared and adequate local anesthesia is given, the pericardiocentesis needle is inserted in the subxiphoid incision. The angle of entry (with the skin) should be approximately 45 degree. The needle tip should be directed superiorly, toward the patient's left shoulder.

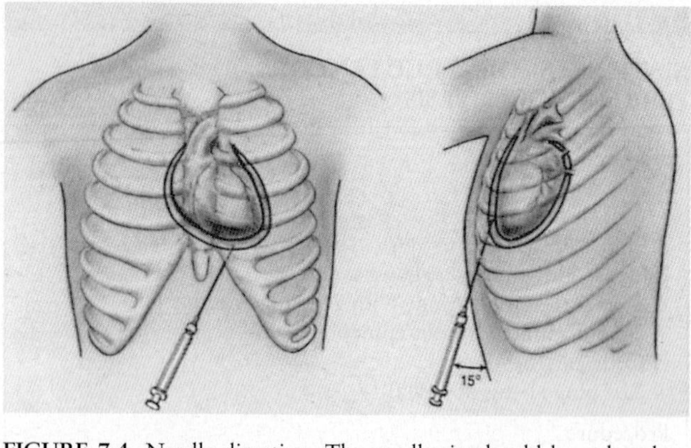

FIGURE 7.4. Needle direction. The needle tip should be reduced to 15 degree once the posterior margin of the bony thorax has been passed. Needle advancement: The needle is advanced toward the left shoulder slowly while alternating between aspiration and injection. A "give" is felt, and fluid is aspirated when the pericardial space is entered.

5. *Needle direction.* Once under the costal margin, reduce the angle of contact between the needle and skin to 15 degree: This will be the angle of approach to the pericardium; the needle tip, however, should still be directed toward the patient's left shoulder. A 15-degree angle is used regardless of the height of the patient's thorax (whether at 45 degree or sitting upright) (Fig. 7.4).
6. *Needle advancement.* Advance the needle slowly while alternating between aspiration of the syringe and injection of 1% lidocaine solution. Obtain a baseline lead V tracing and monitor a continuous ECG tracing for the presence of ST-segment elevation or premature ventricular contractions (evidence of epicardial contact) as the needle is advanced. Advance the needle along this extrapleural path until either
   a. a "give" is felt, and fluid is aspirated from the pericardial space (usually 6.0 to 7.5 cm from the skin) (Fig. 7.4). Some patients may experience a vasovagal response at this point and require atropine intravenously to increase their blood pressure and heart rate or
   b. ST-segment elevation or premature ventricular contractions are observed on the electrocardiographic lead V tracing when the needle tip contacts the epicardium. If ST-segment elevation or premature ventricular complexes occur, immediately (and carefully) withdraw the needle toward the skin surface while aspirating. Avoid any lateral motion, which could damage the epicardial vessels. Completely withdraw the needle if no fluid is obtained during the initial repositioning.

   If sanguineous fluid is aspirated, the differentiation between blood and effusion must be made immediately. In addition to confirming catheter position by saline or contrast as described above (or pressure transduction), several milliliters of fluid can be placed on a gauze and observed for clotting. Intrinsic fibrinolytic activity in the pericardium prevents subacute/chronic effusions from clotting, where frank hemorrhage or intraventricular blood will overwhelm fibrinolysis.

The patient's hemodynamic status should improve promptly with removal of sufficient fluid. Successful relief of tamponade is supported by (a) a fall in intrapericardial pressure to levels between −3 and +3 mm Hg, (b) a fall in right atrial pressure and a separation between right and left ventricular diastolic pressures, (c) augmentation of cardiac output, (d) increased systemic blood pressure, and (e) reduced

TABLE 7.3

DIAGNOSTIC STUDIES PERFORMED ON PERICARDIAL FLUID

Hematocrit
White blood cell count with differential
Glucose
Protein
Gram's stain
Routine aerobic and anaerobic cultures
Smear and culture for acid-fast bacilli
Cytology
Cholesterol, triglyceride
Amylase
Lactate dehydrogenase
Special cultures (viral, parasite, fungal)
Antinuclear antibody
Rheumatoid factor
Total complement, C3

pulsus paradoxus to physiologic levels (10 mm Hg or less). An improvement may be observed after removal of the first 50 to 100 mL of fluid. If the right atrial pressure remains elevated after fluid removal, an effusive-constrictive process should be considered. The diagnostic studies performed on pericardial fluid are outlined in Table 7.3. Several options exist for continued drainage of the pericardial space. The simplest approach is to use large-volume syringes and aspirate the fluid by hand. This approach is not always practical (i.e., in large-volume effusions), however, and manipulation of the needle apparatus may cause myocardial trauma. Alternatively, most pericardiocentesis kits include materials and instructions for a catheter-over-needle technique for inserting an indwelling pericardial drain via the Seldinger technique.

7. *Pericardial drain Placement (Fig. 7.5).* Create a track for the catheter by passing a 6 French (Fr) dilator over a firmly held guidewire. After removing the dilator, use the same technique to pass an 8 Fr dilator. Then advance an 8 Fr flexible pigtail (or side hole) catheter over the guidewire into the pericardial space. Remove the guidewire. Passage of the dilators is facilitated by use of a torquing (clockwise/counterclockwise) motion. Proper positioning of the catheter using radiography, fluoroscopy, or bedside echocardiography can be used to facilitate fluid drainage.
8. *Drainage system* [27,28]. Attach a three-way stopcock to the intrapericardial catheter and close the system by attaching the stopcock to the sterile collecting bag with the connecting tubing. The catheter may also be connected to a transducer, allowing intrapericardial pressure monitoring. The system may be secured as follows:
   a. Suture the pigtail catheter to the skin, making sure the lumen is not compressed. Cover the entry site with a sterile gauze and dressing.
   b. Secure the drainage bag (or bottle) using tape at a level approximately 35 to 50 cm below the level of the heart. Echocardiography or fluoroscopic guidance may be used to reposition the pigtail catheter, facilitating complete drainage of existing pericardial fluid.

It is recommended to drain fluid in sequential steps of less than 1,000 mL to avoid acute right-ventricular dilation—a rare but serious complication [8,29]. Drainage is recommended until pericardial pressure is subatmospheric with inspiration. The catheter should be flushed manually every 4 to 6 hours using 10 to 15 cc of normal saline solution until volume of aspiration falls to less than 25 mL per day [30].

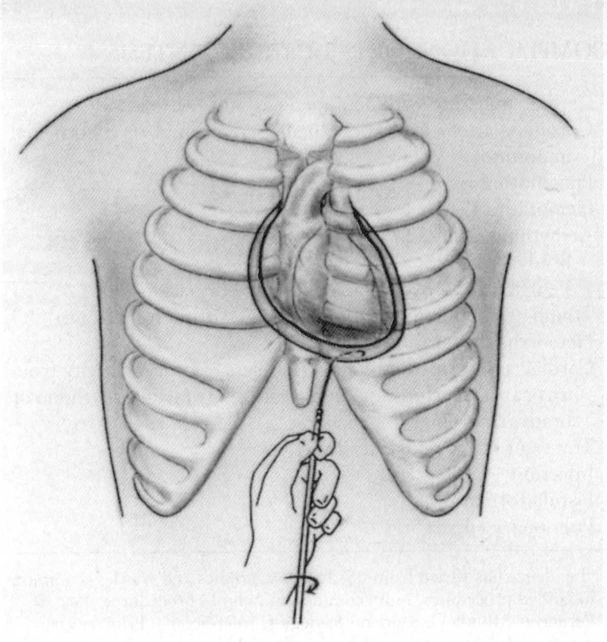

FIGURE 7.5. Placement technique. Holding the needle in place, a Teflon-coated, 0.035-in guidewire is advanced into the pericardial space. The needle is then removed. After a series of skin dilations, an 8Fr, 35-cm flexible pigtail catheter is placed over the guidewire into the pericardial space. Passage of dilators and the pigtail catheter is facilitated by a gentle clockwise/counterclockwise motion.

SHORT-TERM AND LONG-TERM MANAGEMENT

After pericardiocentesis, close monitoring is required to detect evidence of recurrent tamponade and procedure-related complications. Table 7.4 lists the most common serious complications associated with pericardiocentesis [1,8,31,32]. Factors associated with an increased risk of complications include (a) small effusion (less than 250 mL), (b) posterior effusion, (c) loculated effusion, (d) maximum anterior clear space (by echocardiography) less than 10 mm, and (e) unguided percutaneous approach. All patients undergoing pericardiocentesis should have a portable chest radiograph performed immediately after the procedure to exclude the presence of pneumothorax. A transthoracic two-dimensional echocardiogram should be obtained within several hours to evaluate the adequacy of pericardial drainage and confirm catheter placement. As pericardiocentesis typically does not remove all of the effusion (and active bleeding or secretion may occur), the pericardial catheter is typically left in for 24 to 72 hours or until drainage subsides. Extended catheter drainage is safe and is associated with a trend toward lower recurrence rates over a 4-year follow-up [30]. Catheter drainage of more than 100 mL per day after 3 days may need to be considered for surgical intervention, sclerosing agents, or percutaneous balloon pericardotomy.

The long-term management of patients with significant pericardial fluid collections is beyond the scope of this chapter

TABLE 7.4

COMPLICATIONS OF PERICARDIOCENTESIS

Cardiac puncture with hemopericardium
Coronary artery laceration (hemopericardium or myocardial infarction)
Pneumothorax
Hemothorax
Arrhythmias
Bradycardia
Ventricular tachycardia/ventricular fibrillation
Trauma to abdominal organs (liver, gastrointestinal tract)
Hemorrhagic peritonitis
Cardiac arrest (predominantly pulseless electrical activity from myocardial perforation, but occasionally tachyarrhythmia or bradyarrhythmia)[a]
Transient biventricular dysfunction
Infection
Fistula formation
Pulmonary edema

[a]Incidence has varied from 0% to 5% in studies and was less common in guided procedures, more common in "blind" procedures.

Permayer-Miulda G, Sagrista- Savleda J, Soler-Soler J: Primary acute pericardial disease: a prospective study of 231 consecutive patients. *Am J Cardiol* 56:623, 1985.

Wong B, Murphy J, Chang CJ, et al: The risk of pericardiocentesis. *Am J Cardiol* 44:1110, 1979.

Krikorian JG, Hancock EW: Pericardiocentesis. *Am J Med* 65:808, 1978.

TABLE 7.5

COMMON CAUSES OF PERICARDIAL EFFUSION

Idiopathic
Malignancy (primary, metastatic; solid tumors, hematologic)
Uremia
Graft versus host disease
Extramedullary hematopoiesis
Postpericardiotomy syndrome
Connective tissue disease
Trauma
Blunt
Penetrating
Infection
Viral (including HIV)
Bacterial
Fungal
Tuberculosis
Aortic dissection
Complication of cardiac catheterization, percutaneous coronary intervention, or pacemaker insertion
Myxedema
Postirradiation

(see Chapter 34); however, the indications for surgical intervention have been reviewed briefly earlier in the chapter. The etiology of the pericardial effusion (Table 7.5) and the patient's functional status are of central importance for determining the preferred treatment. Aggressive attempts at nonsurgical management of chronically debilitated patients or those with metastatic disease involving the pericardium may be appropriate [33,34]. Percutaneous balloon pericardotomy or pericardial sclerosis with tetracycline, cisplatin, and other agents has benefited carefully selected patients with malignant pericardial disease [35–37]. Patients with a guarded prognosis who fail aggressive medical therapy should be offered the least invasive procedure.

References

1. Permayer-Miulda G, Sagrista-Sauleda J, Soler-Soler J: Primary acute pericardial disease: a prospective study of 231 consecutive patients. *Am J Cardiol* 56:623, 1985.
2. Levy PY, Corey R, Berger P, et al: Etiologic diagnosis of 204 pericardial effusions. *Medicine (Baltimore)* 82:385, 2003.
3. Sagrista-Sauleda J, Merce J, Permanyer-Miralda G, et al: Clinical clues to the causes of large pericardial effusions. *Am J Med* 109:95, 2000.
4. Corey GR, Campbell PT, van Trigt P, et al: Etiology of large pericardial effusions. *Am J Med* 95:209, 1993.
5. Permanyer-Miralda G, Sagrista-Sauleda J, Soler-Soler J. Primary acute pericardial disease: a prospective series of 231 consecutive patients. *Am J Cardiol* 56:623, 1985.
6. Zayas R, Anguita M, Torres F, et al: Incidence of specific etiology and role of methods for specific etiologic diagnosis of primary acute pericarditis. *Am J Cardiol* 75:378, 1995.
7. Quinones M, Douglas P, Foster E, et al: ACC/AHA clinical competence statement on echocardiography: a report of the American College of Cardiology/American Heart Association/American College of Physicians-American Society of Internal Medicine Task Force on Clinical Competence. *J Am Coll Cardiol* 41(4):687–708, 2003.
8. Maisch B, Seferović PM, Ristić AD, et al: Guidelines on the diagnosis and management of pericardial diseases. The task force on the diagnosis and management of pericardial diseases of the European Society of Cardiology. *Eur Heart J* 25(7):587–610, 2004.
9. Callahan M: Pericardiocentesis in traumatic and non-traumatic cardiac tamponade. *Ann Emerg Med* 13:924, 1984.
10. Spodick DH: Medical treatment of cardiac tamponade, in Caturelli G (ed): *Cura Intensive Cardiologica.* Rome, TIPAR Poligrafica, 1991, pp 265–268.
11. Cheitlin MD, Armstrong WF, Aurigemma GP, et al: ACC/AHA/ASE 2003 guideline for the clinical application of echocardiography. *J Am Coll Cardiol* 42(5):954–970, 2003.
12. Spodick DH: Macrophysiology, microphysiology, and anatomy of the pericardium: a synopsis. *Am Heart J* 124:1046–1051, 1992.
13. Roberts WC, Spray TL: Pericardial heart disease: a study of its causes, consequences, and morphologic features, in Spodick D (ed): *Pericardial Diseases.* Philadelphia, FA Davis, 1976, p 17.
14. Shabatai R: Function of the pericardium, in Fowler NO (ed): *The Pericardium in Health and Disease.* Mount Kisco, NY, Futura, 1985, p 19.
15. Little W, Freeman G: Pericardial disease. *Circulation* 113:1622–1632, 2006.
16. Schuh R: Erfahrungen uber de Paracentese der Brust und des Herz Beutels. *Med Jahrb Osterr Staates Wien* 33:388, 1841.
17. Marfan AB: Poncitian du pericarde par l espigahe. *Ann Med Chir Infarct* 15:529, 1911.
18. Tibbles CD, Porcaro W: Procedural applications of ultrasound. *Emerg Med Clin North Am* 22:797, 2004.
19. Rifkin RD, Mernoff DB: Noninvasive evaluation of pericardial effusion composition by computed tomography. *Am Heart J* 149:1120, 2005.
20. Callahan JA, Seward JB, Nishimura RA: 2-dimensional echocardiography-guided pericardiocentesis: experience in 117 consecutive patients. *Am J Cardiol* 55:476, 1985.
21. Callahan JA, Seward JB, Tajik AJ: Pericardiocentesis assisted by 2-dimensional echocardiography. *J Thorac Cardiovasc Surg* 85:877, 1983.
22. Tsang TSM, Freeman WK, Sinak LJ, et al: Echocardiographically guided pericardiocentesis: evolution and state-of-the-art technique. *Mayo Clin Proc* 73:647, 1998.
23. Callahan JA, Seward JB, Tajik AJ: Cardiac tamponade: pericardiocentesis directed by two-dimensional echocardiography. *Mayo Clin Proc* 60:344, 1985.
24. Tsang TS, Enriquez-Sarano M, Freeman WK, et al: Consecutive 1127 therapeutic echocardiographically guided pericardiocentesis: clinical profile, practice patterns, and outcomes spanning 21 years. *Mayo Clin Proc* 77:429, 2002.
25. Fagan S, Chan KL: Pericardiocentesis. *Chest* 116:275–276, 1999.
26. Tweddell JS, Zimmerman AN, Stone CM, et al: Pericardiocentesis guided by a pulse generator. *J Am Coll Cardiol* 14(4):1074–1083, 1989.

27. Kapoor AS: Technique of pericardiocentesis and intrapericardial drainage, in Kapoor AS (ed): *International Cardiology*. New York, Springer-Verlag, 1989, p 146.
28. Patel AK, Kogolcharoen PK, Nallasivan M, et al: Catheter drainage of the pericardium: practical method to maintain long-term patency. *Chest* 92:1018, 1987.
29. Armstrong WF, Feigenbaum H, Dillon JC: Acute right ventricular dilation and echocardiographic volume overload following pericardiocentesis for relief of cardiac tamponade. *Am Heart J* 107:1266–1270, 1984.
30. Tsang TS, Barnes ME, Gersh BJ, et al: Outcomes of clinically significant idiopathic pericardial effusion requiring intervention. *Am J Cardiol* 91(6):704–707, 2002.
31. Wong B, Murphy J, Chang CJ, et al: The risk of pericardiocentesis. *Am J Cardiol* 44:1110, 1979.
32. Krikorian JG, Hancock EW: Pericardiocentesis. *Am J Med* 65: 808, 1978.
33. Shepherd FA, Morgan C, Evans WK, et al: Medical management of malignant pericardial effusion by tetracycline sclerosis. *Am J Cardiol* 60:1161, 1987.
34. Morm JE, Hallonby D, Gonda A, et al: Management of uremia pericarditis: a report of 11 patients with cardiac tamponade and a review of the literature. *Ann Thorac Surg* 22:588, 1976.
35. Reitknecht F, Regal AM, Antkowiak JG, et al: Management of cardiac tamponade in patients with malignancy. *J Surg Oncol* 30:19, 1985.
36. Maisch B, Ristic AD, Pankuweit S, et al: Neoplastic pericardial effusion. Efficacy and safety of intrapericardial treatment with cisplatin. *Eur Heart J* 23:1625, 2002.
37. Ziskind AA, Pearce AC, Lemon CC, et al: Percutaneous balloon pericardiotomy for the treatment of cardiac tamponade and large pericardial effusions: description of technique and report of the first 50 cases. *J Am Coll Cardiol* 21:1–5, 1993.

CHAPTER 8 ■ CHEST TUBE INSERTION AND CARE

ULISES TORRES AND ROBERT A. LANCY

Chest tube insertion involves placement of a sterile tube into the pleural space to evacuate air or fluid into a closed collection system to restore negative intrathoracic pressure, promote lung expansion, and prevent potentially lethal levels of pressure from developing in the thorax. In order to avoid all the potential life-threatening complications that can result from the insertion of a chest tube, a clear concept of physiopathology and anatomy has to be established, followed by a visualization of the different steps in order to proceed with a safe practice [1].

PLEURAL ANATOMY AND PHYSIOLOGY

The pleural space is a potential space that separates the visceral and parietal pleura with a thin layer of lubricating fluid. Although up to 500 mL per day may enter the pleural space, 0.1 to 0.2 mL per kg surrounds each lung in the pleural space at any given time. These two layers are lined by an extensive lymphatic network that ultimately drains into the thoracic duct via the mediastinal and intercostal lymph nodes. These lymphatics prevent the accumulation of this pleural fluid. It is estimated that this mechanism allows clearance of up to 20 mL per hour per hemithorax of pleural fluid in a 70-kg human. The elastic recoil of the chest wall and lung creates a subatmospheric pressure in the space, between −5 and −10 cm H_2O, which binds the lung to the chest wall [2,3].

Drainage of the pleural space is necessary when the normal physiologic processes are disrupted by increased fluid entry into the space due to alterations in hydrostatic pressures (e.g., congestive heart failure) or oncotic pressures or by changes in the parietal pleura itself (e.g., inflammatory diseases). A derangement in lymphatic drainage, as with lymphatic obstruction by malignancy, may also result in excess fluid accumulation and disruption of the pleural and lung parenchymal anatomy, creating accumulation of air and/or blood.

CHEST TUBE PLACEMENT

Indications

The indications for closed intercostal drainage include a variety of disease processes in the hospital setting (Table 8.1). The procedure may be performed to palliate a chronic disease process or to relieve an acute, life-threatening process. Chest tubes also may provide a vehicle for pharmacologic interventions, as when used with antibiotic therapy for treatment of an empyema or instillation of sclerosing agents to prevent recurrence of malignant effusions.

Pneumothorax

Accumulation of air in the pleural space is the most common indication for chest tube placement. Symptoms include tachypnea, dyspnea, and pleuritic pain, although some patients (in particular, those with a small spontaneous pneumothorax) may be asymptomatic. Physical findings include diminished breath sounds and hyperresonance to percussion on the affected side.

Diagnosis is often confirmed by chest radiography. The size of a pneumothorax may be estimated, but this is at best a rough approximation of a three-dimensional space using a two-dimensional view. Although the gold standard for the identification of a pneumothorax (independent of location within the thorax) is a computed tomography (CT) scan of the chest, ultrasound (US) identification has been shown to have the same sensitivity as that of a CT scan. Furthermore, US estimates of the extension of the pneumothorax correlate well with CT scan [4]. The sensitivity of detecting a pneumothorax with US ranges from 86% to 89%, compared to a range of 28% to 75% with a supine chest X-ray [4–6].

The decision to insert a chest tube for a pneumothorax is based on the patient's overall clinical status and may be aided by serial chest radiographs. Tube decompression is indicated in those who are symptomatic, who have a large or expanding

TABLE 8.1

INDICATIONS FOR CHEST TUBE INSERTION

Pneumothorax
Primary or spontaneous
Secondary
Chronic obstructive pulmonary disease
Pneumonia
Abscess/empyema
Malignancy
Traumatic
Iatrogenic
Central line placement
Positive-pressure ventilation
Thoracentesis
Lung biopsy
Hemothorax
Traumatic
Blunt
Penetrating (trauma or biopsy)
Iatrogenic
Malignancy
Pulmonary arteriovenous malformation
Blood dyscrasias
Ruptured thoracic aortic aneurysm
Empyema
Parapneumonic
Posttraumatic
Postoperative
Septic emboli
Intra-abdominal infection
Chylothorax
Traumatic
Surgical
Congenital
Malignancy
Pleural effusion
Transudate
Exudate (malignancy, inflammatory)

pneumothorax, who are being mechanically ventilated (the latter of whom may present acutely with deteriorating oxygenation and an increase in airway pressures, necessitating immediate decompression), or in patients where there is no capability for serial chest radiographs or the absence of trained personnel (off-hour shifts and geographic location) for the emergency placement of a chest tube [3].

A small, stable, asymptomatic pneumothorax can be followed with serial chest radiographs. Reexpansion occurs at the rate of approximately 1.25% of lung volume per day [7].

Persistent leaking of air into the pleural space with no route of escape will ultimately collapse the affected lung, flatten the diaphragm, and eventually produce contralateral shift of the mediastinum. Compression of the contralateral lung and compromise of venous return result in progressive hypoxemia and hypotension. Emergency decompression with a 14- or 16-gauge catheter in the midclavicular line of the second intercostal space may be lifesaving while preparations for chest tube insertion are being made.

Hemothorax

Accumulation of blood in the pleural space can be classified as spontaneous, iatrogenic, or traumatic. Attempted thoracentesis or tube placement may result in injury to the intercostal or internal mammary arteries or to the pulmonary parenchyma. Up to a third of patients with traumatic rib fractures may have an accompanying pneumothorax or hemothorax [8]. Pulmonary parenchymal bleeding from chest trauma is often self-limited due to the low pressure of the pulmonary vascular system. However, systemic sources (intercostal, internal mammary or subclavian arteries, aorta, or heart) may persist and become life threatening.

Indications for open thoracotomy in the setting of traumatic hemothorax include initial blood loss greater than 1,500 mL or continued blood loss exceeding 500 mL over the first hour, 200 mL per hour after 2 to 4 hours, or 100 mL per hour after 6 to 8 hours, or in an unstable patient who does not respond to volume resuscitation [9–11]. Placement of large-bore [36 to 40 French (Fr)] drainage tubes encourages evacuation of blood and helps determine the need for immediate thoracotomy.

Spontaneous pneumothoraces may result from necrotizing pulmonary infections, pulmonary arteriovenous malformations, pulmonary infarctions, primary and metastatic malignancies of the lung and pleura, and tearing of adhesions between the visceral and parietal pleurae.

Empyema

Empyemas are pyogenic infections of the pleural space that may result from numerous clinical conditions, including necrotizing pneumonia, septic pulmonary emboli, spread of intra-abdominal infections, or inadequate drainage of a traumatic hemothorax. Pyothorax as a complication of pneumonia is less common now than in the preantibiotic era, with the common organisms now being *Staphylococcus aureus* and anaerobic and gram-negative microbes.

Definitive management includes evacuation of the collection and antibiotic therapy. Large-bore drainage tubes (36 to 40 Fr) are used, and success is evidenced by resolving fever and leukocytosis, improving clinical status, and eventual resolving drainage. The tube can then be removed slowly over several days, allowing a fibrous tract to form. If no improvement is seen, rib resection and open drainage may be indicated. Chronic empyema may require decortication or, in more debilitated patients, open-flap drainage (Eloesser procedure). Fibrinolytic enzymes (urokinase or streptokinase) can also be instilled through the tube to facilitate drainage of persistent purulent collections or for hemothorax or malignant effusions [12–14].

Chylothorax

A collection of lymphatic fluid in the pleural space is termed *chylothorax*. Because of the immunologic properties of lymph, the collection is almost always sterile. As much as 1,500 mL per day may accumulate and may result in hemodynamic compromise or adverse metabolic sequelae as a result of loss of protein, fat, and fat-soluble vitamins. The diagnosis is confirmed by a fluid triglyceride level greater than 110 mg per dL or a cholesterol–triglyceride ratio of less than 1 [15,16]. Primary causes of chylothorax include trauma, surgery, malignancy, and congenital abnormalities [17].

Treatment involves tube drainage along with aggressive maintenance of volume and nutrition. With central parenteral nutrition and intestinal rest (to limit flow through the thoracic duct), approximately 50% will resolve without surgery [18]. Open thoracotomy may be necessary to ligate the duct and close the fistula; in the cases when the abdominal lymphatics are patent, percutaneous catheterization and embolization of the thoracic duct can be perform with good results [19].

Pleural Effusion

Management of a pleural effusion often begins with thoracentesis to identify the collection as either a transudative or exudative process. Treatment of *transudative* pleural effusions is aimed at controlling the underlying cause (e.g., congestive heart failure, nephrotic syndrome, and cirrhosis). Tube thoracostomy may be helpful in controlling a temporary ventilatory or compliance-related issue, but it is not usually the solution. *Exudative* pleural effusions, however, often require tube drainage.

Sometimes it is necessary to perform chemical pleurodesis in order to develop apposition of pleural surfaces. Agents that can be used include bleomycin, doxycycline, and talc [20–22].

CONTRAINDICATIONS

Large bullous disease of the lung may be mistaken for a pneumothorax, a circumstance in which attempted pleural tube placement may result in significant morbidity. CT scanning is indicated in these instances to clearly analyze the anatomy. Likewise, an apparent pleural effusion may be a lung abscess or consolidated pulmonary parenchyma (e.g., pneumonia and atelectasis). Again, CT scanning or ultrasonography may prove to be helpful in delineating the pathology before tube placement.

History of a process that will promote pleural symphysis (such as a sclerosing procedure, pleurodesis, pleurectomy, or previous thoracotomy on the affected side) should raise caution and prompt evaluation with CT scanning to help identify the exact area of pathology and to direct tube placement away from areas where the lung is adherent to the chest wall. In a postpneumonectomy patient, the pleural tube should be placed above the original incision, as the diaphragm frequently rises to this height.

The possibility of herniation of abdominal contents through the diaphragm in patients with severe blunt abdominal trauma or stab wounds in the vicinity of the diaphragm requires more extensive evaluation before tube placement. In addition, coagulopathies should be corrected before tube insertion in a nonemergent setting. A clinical study showed that placement of chest tubes under emergency conditions (e.g., trauma) using the lateral approach results in more tube misplacements than using the anterior approach. Although no clinical or functional consequences were observed after the misplaced tubes were repositioned, the risk of malpositioning should be considered if the patient is obese, has large breasts, or has a clear history of cardiomegaly [23].

TECHNIQUE

Chest tube insertion requires knowledge not only of the anatomy of the chest wall and intrathoracic and intra-abdominal structures, but also of general aseptic technique. The procedure should be performed or supervised only by experienced personnel, because the complications of an improperly placed tube may have immediate life-threatening results. Before tube placement, the patient must be evaluated thoroughly by physical examination and chest films to avoid insertion of the tube into a bulla or lung abscess, into the abdomen, or even into the wrong side. Particular care must be taken before and during the procedure to avoid intubation of the pulmonary parenchyma.

The necessary equipment is provided in Table 8.2. Sterile technique is mandatory whether the procedure is performed in the operating room, in the intensive care unit, in the emergency room, or on the ward. Detailed informed consent is obtained, and a time-out is performed to make sure all the equipment is ready and available and that the procedure is being done on the correct side and correct patient.

TABLE 8.2

CHEST TUBE INSERTION EQUIPMENT

Chlorhexidine or povidone–iodine solution
Sterile towels and drapes with full body cover
Sterile sponges
1% lidocaine without epinephrine (40 mL)
10-mL syringe
18-, 21-, and 25-gauge needles
2 Kelly clamps, one large and one medium
Mayo scissors
Standard tissue forceps
Towel forceps
Needle holder
0-Silk suture with cutting needle
Scalpel handle and no. 10 blade
Chest tubes (24, 28, 32, and 36 Fr)
Chest tube drainage system (filled appropriately)
Petrolatum gauze
2-in. nonelastic adhesive tape
Sterile gowns and gloves, masks, caps

Careful titration of parenteral narcotics or benzodiazepines and careful, generous administration of local anesthetic agents provide for a relatively painless procedure. Standard, large-bore drainage tubes are made from either Silastic or rubber. Silastic tubes are either right angled or straight, have multiple drainage holes, and contain a radiopaque stripe with a gap to mark the most proximal drainage hole. They are available in sizes ranging from 6 to 40 Fr, with size selection dependent on the patient population (6 to 24 Fr for infants and children) and the collection being drained (24 to 28 Fr for air, 32 to 36 Fr for pleural effusions, and 36 to 40 Fr for blood or pus). Small-caliber Silastic tubes have been increasingly employed for chest drainage, particularly after open-heart surgery, to decrease pain and encourage earlier ambulation [24].

Before performing the procedure, it is important to review the steps to be taken and to ensure that all necessary equipment is available. Patient comfort and safety are paramount. There are three techniques for insertion of a thoracostomy tube. The first two direct techniques require a surgical incision and are (i) blunt dissection and (ii) trocar puncture. Only the former technique has been discussed as the latter is not commonly employed. The third technique is the percutaneous method, which can also be done at the bedside with US guidance.

1. With the patient supine and the head of the bed adjusted for comfort, the involved side is elevated slightly with the ipsilateral arm brought up over the head (Fig. 8.1). Supplemental oxygen is administered as needed. Localize the borders of the triangle of safety whenever possible (A: below level of axillary vessels; B: above fifth intercostal space at the anterior border of the latissimus dorsi; C: lateral border of pectoralis major) [25].
2. The tube is usually inserted through the fourth or fifth intercostal space in the anterior axillary line. An alternative entry site (for decompression of a pneumothorax) is the second intercostal space in the midclavicular line, but for cosmetic reasons and to avoid the thick pectoral muscles, the former site is preferable in adults.
3. Under sterile conditions, the area is prepared with 2% chlorhexidine in 70% isopropyl alcohol, and after allowing it to dry, it is draped to include the nipple, which serves as a landmark, as well as the axilla. A 2- to 3-cm area is infiltrated with 1% lidocaine to raise a wheal two fingerbreadths below the intercostal space to be penetrated. (This

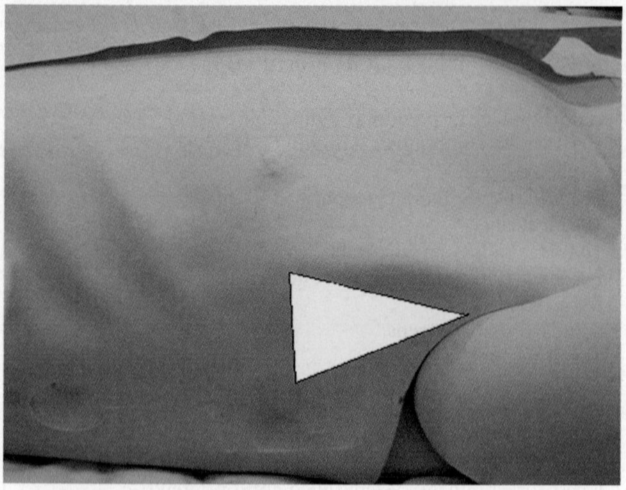

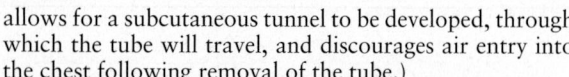

FIGURE 8.1. Positioning of the patient with the arm flexed over the head. Identification of the triangle of safety.

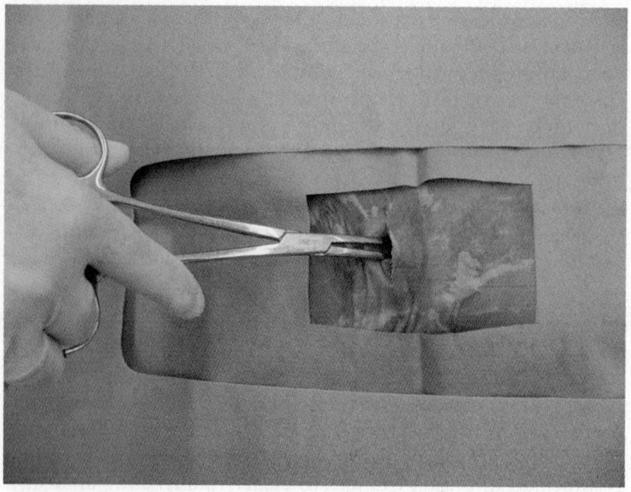

FIGURE 8.2. Dissection with Kelly clamp.

allows for a subcutaneous tunnel to be developed, through which the tube will travel, and discourages air entry into the chest following removal of the tube.)

4. A 2-cm transverse incision is made at the wheal, and additional lidocaine is administered to infiltrate the tissues through which the tube will pass, including a generous area in the intercostal space (especially the periosteum of the ribs above and below the targeted interspace). Care should be taken to anesthetize the parietal pleura fully, as it (unlike the visceral pleura) contains pain fibers. Each injection of lidocaine should be preceded by aspiration of the syringe to prevent injection into the intercostal vessels. Up to 30 to 40 mL of 1% lidocaine may be needed to achieve adequate local anesthesia.
5. To confirm the location of air or fluid, a thoracentesis is then performed at the proposed site of tube insertion. If air or fluid is not aspirated, the anatomy should be reassessed and chest radiographs and CT scans reexamined before proceeding.
6. A short tunnel is created to the chosen intercostal space using Kelly clamps and the intercostal muscles are bluntly divided (Fig. 8.2).
7. The closed clamp is carefully inserted through the parietal pleura, hugging the superior portion of the lower rib to prevent injury to the intercostal bundle of the rib above. The clamp is placed to a depth of less than 1 cm to prevent injury to the intrathoracic structures and is spread open approximately 2 cm.
8. A finger is inserted into the pleural space to explore the anatomy and confirm proper location and lack of pleural symphysis. Only easily disrupted adhesions should be broken. Bluntly dissecting strong adhesions may tear the lung and initiate bleeding.
9. The end of the chest tube is grasped with the clamp and guided with the finger through the tunnel into the pleural space. Once the tip of the tube is in the pleural space, the clamp is removed and the chest tube is advanced and positioned apically for a pneumothorax and dependently for fluid removal (Fig. 8.3A, B). All holes must be confirmed to be within the pleural space. The use of undue pressure or force to insert the tube should be avoided (Fig. 8.4A, B).
10. The location of the tube should be confirmed by observing the flow of air (seen as condensation within the tube) or

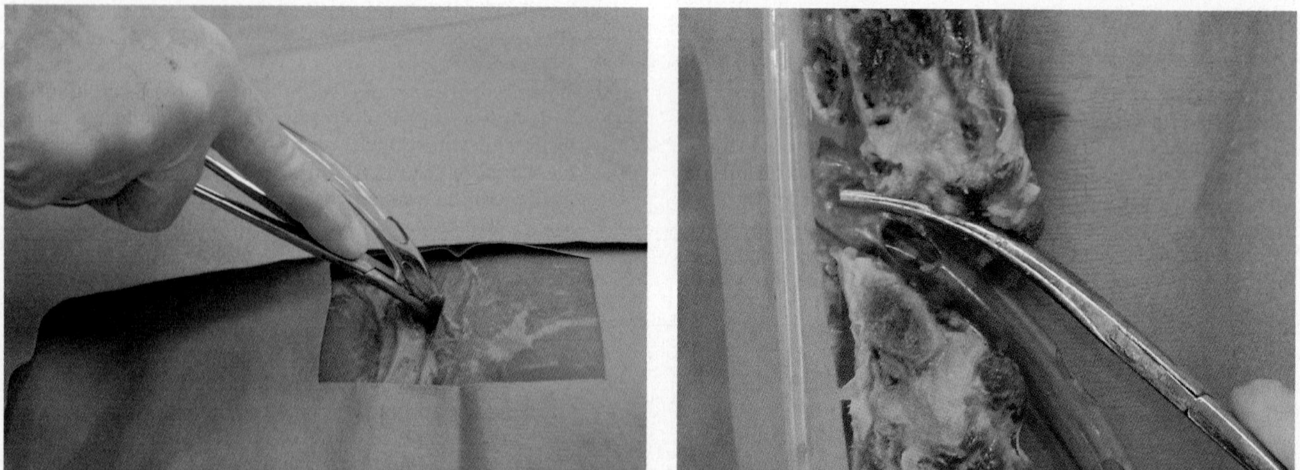

FIGURE 8.3. A, B: The clamp penetrates the intercostal muscle. The end of the chest tube is grasped with a Kelly clamp and guided with a finger through the chest incision. The clamp can be placed above or bellow the tube.

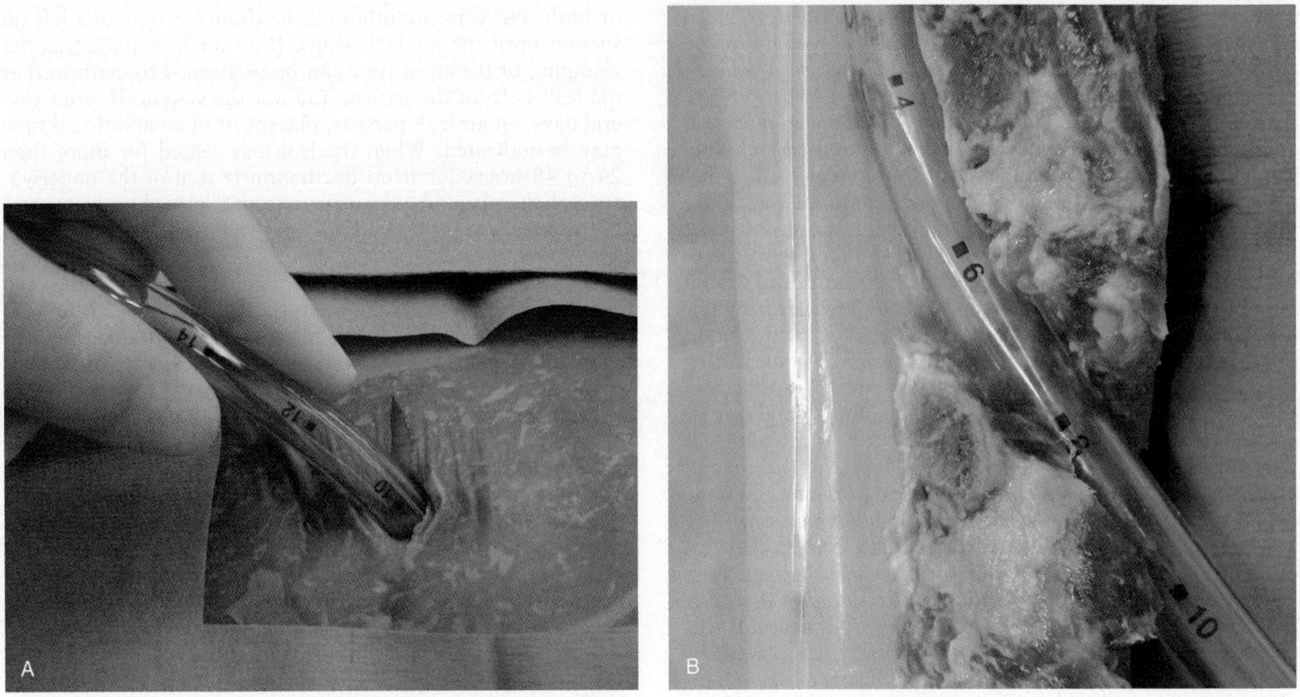

FIGURE 8.4. A, B: Advance the tube once the clamp has been removed.

fluid from the tube. It is then sutured to the skin securely to prevent slippage (Fig. 8.5). A simple suture to anchor the tube can be used or a horizontal mattress suture can be used to allow the hole to be tied closed when the tube is removed. An occlusive petrolatum gauze dressing is applied, and the tube is connected to a drainage apparatus and securely taped to the dressing and to the patient. All connections between the patient and the drainage apparatus must also be tight and securely taped.

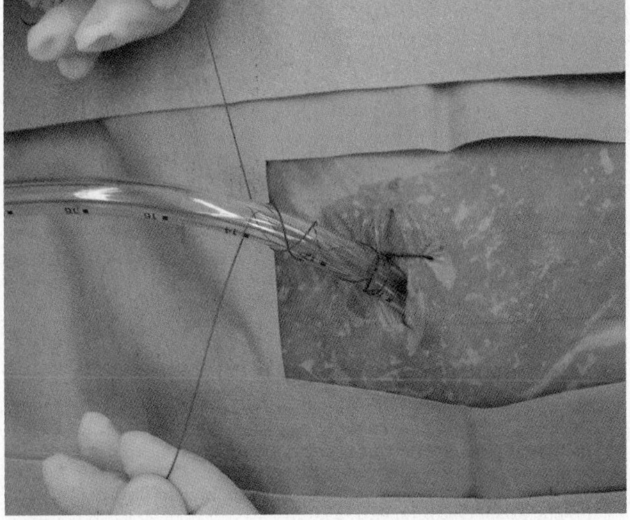

FIGURE 8.5. The tube is securely sutured to the skin with a 1–0 or 2–0 silk suture. This suture is left long, wrapped around the tube, and secured with tape. To seal the tunnel, the suture is tied when the tube is pulled out.

COMPLICATIONS

Chest tube insertion may be accompanied by significant complications. In one series, insertion and management of pleural tubes in patients with blunt chest trauma carried a 9% incidence of complications. Insertion alone is usually accompanied by a 1% to 2% incidence of complications even when performed by experienced personnel [26] (Table 8.3). The use of small-caliber, less rigid, Silastic drains has been found to be safe and efficacious as the more rigid, conventional chest tubes [27], and they allow both more mobility and earlier discharge when used in open-heart surgery patients [28].

CHEST TUBE MANAGEMENT AND CARE

While a chest tube is in place, the tube and drainage system must be checked daily for adequate functioning. Most institutions use a three-chambered system that contains a calibrated collection trap for fluid, an underwater seal unit to allow escape of air while maintaining negative pleural pressure, and

TABLE 8.3

COMPLICATIONS OF CHEST TUBE INSERTION

Unintentional tube placement into vital structures (lung, liver, spleen, etc.)
Bleeding
Reexpansion pulmonary edema
Residual pneumothorax
Residual hemothorax
Empyema

a suction regulator. Suction is routinely established at 15 to 20 cm water, controlled by the height of the column in the suction regulator unit, and maintained as long as an air leak is present. The drainage system is examined daily to ensure that appropriate levels are maintained in the underwater seal and suction regulator chambers. If suction is desired, bubbling should be noted in the suction regulator unit. Connections between the chest tube and the drainage system should be tightly fitted and securely taped. For continuous drainage, the chest tube and the tubing to the drainage system should remain free of kinks, should not be left in a dependent position, and should never be clamped. If problems are encountered with repetitive kinking, a corrugated tubing splint can be used around the chest tube to improve the resistance [29]. The tube can be milked and gently stripped, although with caution, as this may generate negative pressures of up to 1,500 mm Hg and can injure adjacent tissues [30]. Irrigation of the tube is discouraged. Dressing changes should be performed every 2 or 3 days and as needed. Adequate pain control is mandatory to encourage coughing and ambulation to facilitate lung reexpansion.

Chest films can be obtained to evaluate the progress of drainage and to ensure that the most proximal drainage hole has not migrated from the pleural space (a situation that may result in pneumothorax or subcutaneous emphysema). If this occurs and the pathologic process is not corrected, replacement of the tube is usually indicated, especially if subcutaneous emphysema is developing. Mandatory routine daily chest X-rays are not indicated to monitor chest tubes in the intensive care unit unless there is a clinical necessity [31]. A tube should never be readvanced into the pleural space, and if a tube is to be replaced, it should always be at a different site rather than the same hole. If a pneumothorax persists, increasing the suction level may be beneficial, but an additional tube may be required if no improvement results; other etiologies should be considered after this point and further evaluation with a CT scan of the chest. Proper positioning may also be confirmed by chest CT scanning [32].

CHEST TUBE REMOVAL

Indications for removal of chest tubes include resolution of the pneumothorax or fluid accumulation in the pleural space, or both. For a pneumothorax, the drainage system is left on suction until the air leak stops. If an air leak persists, brief clamping of the chest tube can be performed to confirm that the leak is from the patient and not the system. If, after several days, an air leak persists, placement of an additional tube may be indicated. When the leak has ceased for more than 24 to 48 hours (or if no fluctuation is seen in the underwater seal chamber), the drainage system is placed on water seal by disconnecting the wall suction, followed by a chest film several hours later. If no pneumothorax is present and no air leak appears in the system with coughing, deep breathing, and reestablishment of suction, the tube can be removed. For fluid collections, the tube can be removed when drainage is less than 200 cc per 24 hours or lesser [33], unless sclerotherapy is planned.

Tube removal is often preceded by oral or parenteral analgesia at an appropriate time interval [34]. The suture holding the tube to the skin is cut. At end-inspiration, the tube is pulled out and the hole simultaneously covered with occlusive petrolatum gauze dressing at peak inspiration or end expiration the chest tube is pulled [35]. A chest radiograph is performed immediately to check for a pneumothorax if there are clinical signs and symptoms or if the patient is at high risk for reaccumulation; otherwise, a nonurgent chest radiograph can be ordered and repeated 24 hours later to rule out reaccumulation of air or fluid [36].

RELATED SYSTEMS

Percutaneous aspiration of the pleural space to relieve a pneumothorax without an active air leak has been reported. Although successful in up to 75% cases of needle-induced or traumatic pneumothoraces, the success rate is less for those with a spontaneous pneumothorax [37,38]. Small-bore catheters placed via Seldinger technique or using a trocar have been successful for treatment of spontaneous and iatrogenic pneumothoraces [39–41].

Heimlich valves (one-way flutter valves that allow egress of air from pleural tubes or catheters) have also gained popularity because ambulation is facilitated and outpatient care can be provided to those with persistent air leaks [42,43].

References

1. *Advanced Trauma life Support for Doctors, Manual for Coordinators & Faculty* [CD-ROM, thoracic trauma]. Chicago, American College of Surgeons, 2009, p 421.
2. Quigley RL: Thoracentesis and chest tube drainage. *Crit Care Clin* 11(1): 111–126, 1995.
3. Iberti TJ, Stern PM: Chest tube thoracostomy. *Crit Care Clin* 8(4):879–895, 1992.
4. Soldati G, Testa A, Sher S, et al: Occult traumatic pneumothorax: diagnostic accuracy of lung ultrasonography in the emergency department. *Chest* 133(1):204–211, 2008.
5. Wilkerson RG, Stone MB: Sensitivity of bedside ultrasound and supine anteroposterior chest radiographs for the identification of pneumothorax after blunt trauma. *Acad Emerg Med* 17(1):11–17, 2010.
6. Blasivas M, Lyon M, Duggal S: A prospective comparison of supine chest radiography and bedside ultrasound for the diagnosis of traumatic pneumothorax. *Acad Emerg Med* 12(9):844–849, 2005.
7. Kircher LT Jr, Swartzel RL: Spontaneous pneumothorax and its treatment. *JAMA* 155:24, 1954.
8. Ziegler DW, Agarwal NN: The morbidity and mortality of rib fractures. *J Trauma* 37:975, 1994.
9. Sandrasagra FA: Management of penetrating stab wounds of the chest: assessment of the indications for early operation. *Thorax* 33:474, 1978.
10. McNamara JJ, Messersmith JK, Dunn RA, et al: Thoracic injuries in combat casualties in Vietnam. *Ann Thorac Surg* 10:389, 1970.
11. Boyd AD: Pneumothorax and hemothorax, in Hood RM, Boyd AD, Culliford AT (eds): *Thoracic Trauma*. Philadelphia, PA, WB Saunders, 1989, p 133.
12. Bouros D, Schiza S, Patsourakis G, et al: Intrapleural streptokinase versus urokinase in the treatment of complicated parapneumonic effusions: a prospective double-blind study. *Am J Respir Crit Care Med* 155:291, 1997.
13. Roupie E, Bouabdallah K, Delclaux C, et al: Intrapleural administration of streptokinase in complicated purulent pleural effusion: a CT-guided strategy. *Intensive Care Med* 22:1351, 1996.
14. Robinson LA, Moulton AL, Fleming WH, et al: Intrapleural fibrinolytic treatment of multiloculated thoracic empyemas. *Ann Thorac Surg* 57:803, 1994.
15. Staats RA, Ellefson RD, Budahn LL, et al: The lipoprotein profile of chylous and unchylous pleural effusions. *Mayo Clin Proc* 55:700, 1980.
16. Miller JI Jr: Chylothorax and anatomy of the thoracic duct, in Shields TW (ed): *General Thoracic Surgery*. Philadelphia, PA, Lea & Febiger, 1989, p 625.
17. Bessone LN, Ferguson TB, Burford TH: Chylothorax. *Ann Thorac Surg* 12:527, 1971.
18. Ross JK: A review of the surgery of the thoracic duct. *Thorax* 16:12, 1961.
19. Cope C, Salem R, Kaiser LR: Management of chylothorax by percutaneous catheterization and embolization of the thoracic duct: prospective trial. *J Vasnc Interv Radiol* 10(9):1248–1254, 1999.
20. Hausheer FH, Yarbro JW: Diagnosis and treatment of malignant pleural effusions. *Semin Oncol* 12:54, 1985.
21. Milanez RC, Vargas FS, Filomeno LB, et al: Intrapleural talc for the treatment of malignant pleural effusions secondary to breast cancer. *Cancer* 75:2688, 1995.
22. Heffner JE, Standerfer RJ, Torstveit J, et al: Clinical efficacy of doxycycline for pleurodesis. *Chest* 105:1743, 1994.

23. Kang SN: Rib fractures, pneumothorax, haemothorax and chest drain insertion. *Br J Hosp Med (Lond)* 68(9):M158–M928, 2007.
24. Huber-Wagner S, Körner M, Ehrt A, et al: Emergency chest tube placement in trauma care—which approach is preferable? *Resuscitation* 72(2):226–233, 2007.
25. Daly RC, Mucha P, Pairolero PC, et al: The risk of percutaneous chest tube thoracostomy for blunt thoracic trauma. *Ann Emerg Med* 14:865, 1985.
26. Millikan JS, Moore EE, Steiner E, et al: Complications of tube thoracostomy for acute trauma. *Am J Surg* 140:738, 1980.
27. Ishikura H, Kimura F: The use of flexible silastic drains after chest surgery: novel thoracic drainage. *Ann Thorac Surg* 81:231, 2006.
28. Frankel TL, Hill PC, Stamou SB, et al: Silastic drains versus conventional chest tubes after coronary artery bypass. *Chest* 124:108, 2003.
29. Konstantakos AK: A simple and effective method of preventing inadvertent occlusion of chest tube drains: the corrugated tubing splint. *Ann Thorac Surg* 79:1070–1071, 2005.
30. Landolfo K, Smith P: Postoperative care in cardiac surgery, in Sabiston DC, Spencer FC (eds): *Surgery of the Chest.* 6th ed. Philadelphia, PA, WB Saunders, 1996, p 230.
31. Silverstein DS, Livingston DH, Elcavage J, et al: The utility of routine daily chest radiography in the surgical Intensive care unit. *J Trauma* 35:643–646, 1993.
32. Cameron EW, Mirvis SE, Shanmuganathan K, et al: Computed tomography of malpositioned thoracostomy drains: a pictorial essay. *Clin Radiol* 52:187, 1997.
33. Younes RN, Gross JL, Aguiar S, et al: When to remove a chest tube? A randomized study with subsequent prospective consecutive validation. *J Am Coll Surg* 195:658–662, 2002.
34. Puntillo KA: Effects of intrapleural bupivacaine on pleural chest tube removal pain: a randomized controlled trial. *Am J Crit Care* 5:102, 1996.
35. Bell R, Ovadia P, Abdullah F, et al: Chest tube removal: end-inspiration or end expiration? *J Trauma* 50:674–676, 2001.
36. Pizano LR, Houghton D, Cohn S, et al: When should chest radiograph be obtained after CT removal in mechanically ventilated patients? A prospective study. *J Trauma* 1073–1077, 2002.
37. Delius RE, Obeid FN, Horst HM, et al: Catheter aspiration for simple pneumothorax. *Arch Surg* 124:883, 1989.
38. Andrevit P, Djedaini K, Teboul JL, et al: Spontaneous pneumothorax: comparison of thoracic drainage vs. immediate or delayed needle aspiration. *Chest* 108:335, 1995.
39. Conces DJ, Tarver RD, Gray WC, et al: Treatment of pneumothoraces utilizing small caliber chest tubes. *Chest* 94:55, 1988.
40. Peters J, Kubitschek KR: Clinical evaluation of a percutaneous pneumothorax catheter. *Chest* 86:714, 1984.
41. Minami H, Saka H, Senda K, et al: Small caliber catheter drainage for spontaneous pneumothorax. *Am J Med Sci* 304:345, 1992.
42. McKenna RJ Jr, Fischel RJ, Brenner M, et al: Use of the Heimlich valve to shorten hospital stay after lung reduction surgery for emphysema. *Ann Thorac Surg* 61:1115, 1996.
43. Ponn RB, Silverman HJ, Federico JA: Outpatient chest tube management. *Ann Thorac Surg* 64:1437, 1997.

CHAPTER 9 ■ BRONCHOSCOPY

STEPHEN J. KRINZMAN, PAULO J. OLIVEIRA AND RICHARD S. IRWIN

Since its commercial introduction for clinical use in 1968, flexible bronchoscopy has had a dramatic impact on the approach and management of patients with a wide variety of respiratory problems [1]. Because of its safety, low complication rate [2], and comfort [3], flexible bronchoscopy has largely replaced rigid bronchoscopy as the procedure of choice for most endoscopic evaluations of the airway. However, rigid bronchoscopy is indicated for (a) brisk hemoptysis (200 mL per 24 hours); (b) extraction of foreign bodies; (c) endobronchial resection of granulation tissue that might occur after traumatic and/or prolonged intubation; (d) biopsy of vascular tumors (e.g., bronchial carcinoid), in which brisk and excessive bleeding can be controlled by packing; (e) endoscopic laser surgery; and (f) dilation of tracheobronchial strictures and placement of airway stents [1,4]. In the last two decades, there has been renewed interest in the use of rigid bronchoscopy by pulmonologists, driven by the advent of dedicated endobronchial prostheses (airway stents) in the early 1990s and the application of advanced bronchoscopic modalities (laser photoresection, electrocautery, and cryotherapy) for the management of both malignant and benign central airway obstructions [5,6]. These advances in bronchoscopy have fused older techniques and instruments, such as rigid bronchoscopy, with novel applications of flexible bronchoscopy, spurring the development of the field of interventional pulmonology. In an attempt to establish uniformity in the training and performance of bronchoscopy and advanced interventions, the American College of Chest Physicians recently published comprehensive guidelines for interventional pulmonary procedures [7].

DIAGNOSTIC INDICATIONS

General Considerations

Because flexible bronchoscopy can be performed easily even in intubated patients, the same general indications apply to critically ill patients on ventilators and noncritically ill patients; however, only the indications most commonly encountered in critically ill patients are discussed here. Where relevant, the potential application of advanced bronchoscopic diagnostic and therapeutic interventions in the intensive care unit (ICU) setting are also discussed.

Common Indications

Hemoptysis

Hemoptysis is one of the most common clinical problems for which bronchoscopy is indicated [8,9] (see Chapter 53 for a detailed discussion). Whether the patient complains of blood streaking or massive hemoptysis (expectoration of greater than 600 mL in 48 hours), bronchoscopy should be considered to localize the site of bleeding and diagnose the cause. Localization of the site of bleeding is crucial if definitive therapy, such as surgery, becomes necessary, and it is also useful to guide angiographic procedures. Bronchoscopy performed within 48 hours of the time when bleeding stops is more likely to localize the site of bleeding (34% to 91%) compared with delayed bronchoscopy (11% to 52%) [10]. Bronchoscopy is more likely to identify a bleeding source in patients with moderate or severe hemoptysis [11]. Whenever patients have an endotracheal or tracheostomy tube in place, hemoptysis should always be evaluated, because it may indicate potentially life-threatening tracheal damage. Unless the bleeding is massive, a flexible bronchoscope, rather than a rigid bronchoscope, is the instrument of choice for evaluating hemoptysis. In the setting of massive hemoptysis, the patient is at risk for imminent decompensation and death due to asphyxiation. Stabilization of the patient, focusing on establishment of a secure airway, and timely communication with pulmonology, thoracic surgery, anesthesiology, and interventional radiology is of utmost importance. This coordinated, multidisciplinary effort should focus on rapid transfer to the operation room (OR) suite for rigid bronchoscopy. The rigid bronchoscope is ideal in this situation because it provides a secure route for ventilation, serves as a larger conduit for adequate suctioning, and can quickly isolate the lung in the case of a lateralized bleeding source. In most situations, once an adequate airway has been established and initial suctioning of excessive blood has been performed, the flexible bronchoscope can be inserted through the rigid bronchoscope to more accurately assess and localize the source of bleeding beyond the main bronchi [12].

Diffuse Parenchymal Disease

The clinical setting influences the choice of procedure. When diffuse pulmonary infiltrates suggest sarcoidosis, carcinomatosis, or eosinophilic pneumonia, transbronchoscopic lung forceps biopsy should be considered initially because it has an extremely high yield in these situations (see Chapter 69). Transbronchial lung biopsy has a low yield for the definitive diagnosis of inorganic pneumoconiosis and pulmonary vasculitides [13]; when these disorders are suspected, surgical lung biopsy is the procedure of choice. In the case of pulmonary fibrosis and acute interstitial pneumonitis, transbronchial biopsy usually does not provide adequate tissue for a specific histologic diagnosis, although by excluding infection the procedure may provide sufficient information to guide therapy.

Ventilator-Associated Pneumonia

The ability to determine the probability of ventilator-associated pneumonia (VAP) is very limited, with a sensitivity of only 50% and a specificity of 58% [14]. Quantitative cultures obtained via bronchoscopy may thus play an important role in the diagnostic strategy. Quantitative cultures of bronchoalveolar lavage (BAL) fluid and protected specimen brush (PSB), with thresholds of 10^4 colony-forming units (CFU) per mL and 10^3 CFU per mL, respectively, are most commonly employed prior to initiation of antimicrobial therapy. Cultures of bronchial washings do not add to the diagnostic yield of quantitative BAL culture alone [15]. For a brief description of how to perform BAL and obtain PSB cultures, see the "Procedure" section, given later in the chapter.

For BAL, an evidence-based analysis of 23 prior investigations yields a sensitivity of 73% and a specificity of 82%, indicating that BAL cultures fail to diagnose VAP in almost one-fourth of all cases [16]. A similar analysis of PSB cultures indicates a very wide range of results, with a sensitivity of 33% to greater than 95% and a median of 67%, and a specificity of 50% to 100% with a median of 95% [17,18]. PSB is thus more specific than it is sensitive, and negative results may not be sufficient to exclude the presence of VAP [19]. Blind protected telescoping catheter specimens yield similar results to bronchoscopically directed PSB cultures [20,21]. It is critical to note that colony counts change very quickly with antibiotic therapy. Within 12 hours of starting antibiotic therapy, 50% of all significant bacterial species initially identified in significant numbers had colony counts reduced to below the "pathogenic" threshold level. After 48 hours of therapy, only 14% of isolates are still present above threshold values [22]. It is therefore essential to obtain quantitative cultures before starting or changing antibiotics.

Despite the greater accuracy of quantitative bronchoscopic cultures, prospective randomized trials of early invasive diagnostic strategies employing bronchoscopy and quantitative lower respiratory tract cultures for VAP have not demonstrated significant advantages in mortality or other major clinical end points [23,24] over simpler methods. The largest such trial [24] found that compared to therapy based on nonquantitative endotracheal aspirates, patients randomized to bronchoscopy with quantitative cultures had no improvement in mortality, duration of mechanical ventilation, or length of ICU or hospital stay. On the basis of these findings, routine use of bronchoscopy in immunocompetent adults with suspected VAP cannot be recommended.

Pulmonary Infiltrates in Immunocompromised Patients

When an infectious process is suspected, the diagnostic yield depends on the organism and the immune status of the patient. In immunocompetent patients, BAL has a sensitivity of 87% for detecting respiratory pathogens [19], and a negative BAL quantitative culture has a specificity of 96% in predicting sterile lung parenchyma. Numerous recent investigations have examined the utility of bronchoscopy in immunocompromised patients. Most of these investigations have found that the diagnostic yield of BAL in such patients is approximately 50% and that the results of BAL lead to a change in treatment in 17% to 38% of patients. In one prospective multicenter trial [25], BAL was the only conclusive diagnostic study in 33% of patients. Although it is difficult to distinguish respiratory decompensation caused by bronchoscopy from the natural history of the patients' underlying disease, the same study found that 48% of patients developed deterioration in respiratory status after bronchoscopy and 27% of patients were intubated. Transbronchial biopsy may add little to the diagnostic yield of BAL in immunocompromised patients, with an incremental yield of 7% to 12% [26–29]. In some series, the major complication rate of transbronchial biopsy was greater than the diagnostic utility, including a 14% incidence of major bleeding requiring intubation [29]. BAL has a relatively poor sensitivity for detecting fungal infections in this population (40%) [26]. In AIDS patients, the sensitivity of lavage or transbronchial lung biopsy for identifying all opportunistic organisms can be as high as 87% [30,31]. Transbronchial biopsy adds significantly to the diagnostic yield in AIDS patients and may be the sole means of making a diagnosis in up to 24% of patients, including diagnoses of *Pneumocystis jirovecii, Cryptococcus neoformans, Mycobacterium tuberculosis,* and nonspecific interstitial pneumonitis [32]. Lavage alone may have a sensitivity of up to 97% for the diagnosis of *P. jirovecii* pneumonia [33]. However, because induced sputum samples can also be positive for *P. jirovecii* in up to 79% of cases [33], induced expectorated sputum, when available, should be evaluated first for this organism before resorting to bronchoscopy.

Acute Inhalation Injury

In patients exposed to smoke inhalation, flexible nasopharyngoscopy, laryngoscopy, and bronchoscopy are indicated to identify the anatomic level and severity of injury. Prophylactic intubation should be considered if considerable upper airway mucosal injury is noted early; acute respiratory failure is more likely in patients with mucosal changes seen at segmental or lower levels [34]. Upper airway obstruction is a life-threatening problem that usually develops during the initial 24 hours after inhalation injury. It correlates significantly with increased size of cutaneous burns, burns of the face and neck, and rapid intravenous fluid administration, and also portends a greater mortality [35].

Blunt Chest Trauma

Patients may present with atelectasis, pulmonary contusion, hemothorax, pneumothorax, pneumomediastinum, or hemoptysis. Prompt bronchoscopic evaluation of such patients has a diagnostic yield of 53%; findings may include tracheal or bronchial laceration or transection (14%), aspirated material (6%), supraglottic tear with glottic obstruction (2%), mucus plugging (15%), and distal hemorrhage (13%) [36]. Many of these diagnoses may not be clinically evident and require surgical intervention.

Postresectional Surgery

Flexible bronchoscopy can identify a disrupted suture line causing bleeding and pneumothorax following surgery and an exposed endobronchial suture causing cough. In these postpneumonectomy situations, the location of dehiscence and the subsequent bronchopleural fistula (BPF) is easily identified visually via flexible bronchoscopy at the stump site. However, when the BPF occurs in the setting of acute respiratory distress syndrome (ARDS) or necrotizing pneumonia, localization at the segmental and subsegmental level can be more challenging. Readers are referred to Chapter 57, which comprehensively covers this topic.

Assessment of Intubation Damage

When a nasotracheal or orotracheal tube of the proper size is in place, the balloon can be routinely deflated and the tube withdrawn over the bronchoscope to look for subglottic damage. The tube is withdrawn up through the vocal cords and over the flexible bronchoscope and glottic and supraglottic damage sought. This technique may by useful after reintubation for stridor, or when deflation of the endotracheal tube cuff does not produce a significant air leak, suggesting the potential for life-threatening upper airway obstruction when extubation takes place. The flexible bronchoscope may readily identify mechanical problems such as increased airway granulation tissue leading to airway obstruction, tracheal stenosis at pressure points along the artificial airway–tracheal interface, and tracheobronchomalacia.

THERAPEUTIC INDICATIONS

Atelectasis

When atelectasis occurs in critically ill patients who had a normal chest film on admission, mucus plugging is the most likely cause [37]. Bronchoscopy has a success rate of up to 89% in cases of lobar atelectasis, but only produced clinical improvement in 44% of patients when performed for retained secretions [38]. One randomized trial found no advantage of bronchoscopy over a very aggressive regimen of frequent chest physiotherapy, recruitment maneuvers, saline nebulization, and postural drainage [39]. This study also found that the presence of air bronchograms on the initial chest X-ray predicted relative failure of either intervention to resolve the atelectasis. Occasionally, the direct instillation of acetylcysteine (Mucomyst) through the bronchoscope may be necessary to liquefy the thick, tenacious inspissated mucus [40]. Because acetylcysteine may induce bronchospasm in patients with asthma, these patients must be pretreated with a bronchodilator.

Foreign Bodies

Although the rigid bronchoscope is considered by many to be the instrument of choice for removing foreign bodies, devices with which to grasp objects are available for use with the flexible bronchoscope [41]. A review of flexible bronchoscopy in the management of tracheobronchial foreign bodies in adults from the Mayo Clinic demonstrated a success rate of 89% [42]. The success of flexible bronchoscopy in foreign body removal can be enhanced by rigorous preprocedure preparation, assuring the availability of appropriate ancillary grasping equipment, practicing a "dry run," and ensuring that a bronchoscopist with experience in foreign body removal is involved. It is also important to have an appreciation for situations in which rigid bronchoscopy with added ancillary interventions, such as laser therapy or cryotherapy, might be useful (e.g., an embedded foreign body with significant granulation tissue reaction at risk for bleeding) [43].

Endotracheal Intubation

In patients with ankylosing spondylitis and other mechanical problems of the neck, the flexible bronchoscope may be used as an obturator for endotracheal intubation. The bronchoscope with an endotracheal tube passed over it can be passed transnasally (after proper local anesthesia) or transorally. The tube can then be advanced over the scope.

Hemoptysis

On rare occasions where brisk bleeding threatens asphyxiation, endobronchial tamponade may stabilize the patient before definitive therapy is performed (see Chapter 53). With the use of the flexible bronchoscope, usually passed through a rigid bronchoscope or endotracheal tube, a Fogarty catheter with balloon is passed into the bleeding lobar orifice. When the balloon is inflated and wedged tightly, the patient may be transferred to surgery or angiography for bronchial arteriography and bronchial artery embolization [44]. Other bronchial blocking and lung separation techniques have been described and reviewed in the literature [45]. The wire-guided endobronchial blocker (Arndt blocker) is a dedicated bronchial blocker that has a wire loop at its distal end, which—when looped around the distal end of the flexible bronchoscope—can be guided to the bleeding airway, inflated, and its position adjusted under direct visualization. More simple techniques that take advantage of the flexible bronchoscope's ability to act as a stylet for a single-lumen endotracheal tube can be used to separate the lung. One can use the bronchoscope to preferentially intubate the right main or left main bronchus in an acute, emergent situation. Hemostasis may also be achieved by using flexible bronchoscopy to apply oxidized regenerated cellulose mesh to the bleeding site, instill thrombin/thrombin–fibrinogen preparations, and more traditionally, perform iced saline lavage or apply topical epinephrine (1:20,000) to temporize the bleeding [10,46]. There have also been reports of treating hemoptysis by instilling cyanoacrylate through a catheter in the working channel of the flexible bronchoscope [47]. In the case of a visibly bleeding endobronchial tumor, hemostasis can be attained with laser photocoagulation (Nd-YAG laser), electrocautery, or argon plasma coagulation.

Central Obstructing Airway Lesions

Some patients with cancer and others with benign lesions that obstruct the larynx, trachea, and major bronchi can be treated by electrocautery, laser photoresection, argon plasma coagulation, cryotherapy, or photodynamic therapy applied through the bronchoscope (rigid or flexible) [48–55]. Flexible bronchoscopy can also be used to place catheters that facilitate endobronchial delivery of radiation (brachytherapy). Metal or silicone endobronchial stents can be placed bronchoscopically to relieve stenosis of large central airways. Adequate insertion of stents and relief of stenosis (especially due to extrinsic compression) is typically accompanied by dilation of the airway via rigid bronchoscopy or with balloon dilation applied with the aid of flexible bronchoscopy. Several issues regarding airway stents should be noted: silicone stents can only be placed via rigid bronchoscopy and metal stents should generally not be used in the setting of a nonmalignant central airway obstruction because they are associated with excessive growth of granulation tissue with subsequent worsening of airway obstruction and can be very challenging to remove once this complication occurs [51]. The primary goal of the interventions described earlier for the management of malignant central airway obstruction is palliative. Multiple case reports have confirmed that these interventions improve quality of life by relieving symptoms of dyspnea almost immediately [52–55]. In many instances, these procedures also facilitate liberation from mechanical ventilation and downgrading of the level of care from the ICU. It appears that in intubated ICU patients, flexible bronchoscopy performed at the bedside with stent deployment and resective interventions, when necessary, is just as effective as rigid bronchoscopic interventions in the appropriately selected patient [54].

Closure of Bronchopleural Fistula

After placement of a chest tube, drainage of the pleural space, and stabilization of the patient (e.g., infection and cardiovascular and respiratory systems), bronchoscopy can be used to visualize a proximal BPF or localize a distal BPF; it can also be used in attempts to close the BPF [56]. Please see Chapter 57, which comprehensively covers this topic.

Percutaneous Dilatational Tracheostomy

Flexible bronchoscopic guidance is extremely helpful during bedside percutaneous tracheostomy [57,58]. Please see Chapter 12, which comprehensively covers this topic.

COMPLICATIONS

When performed by a trained specialist, *routine* flexible bronchoscopy is extremely safe. Mortality should not exceed 0.1%, and overall complications should not exceed 8.1% [2]. The rare deaths have been due to excessive premedication or topical anesthesia, respiratory arrest from hemorrhage, laryngospasm or bronchospasm, and cardiac arrest from acute myocardial infarction [59,60]. Nonfatal complications occurring within 24 hours of the procedure include fever (1.2% to 24%) [2,61], pneumonia (0.6% to 6%) [2], vasovagal reactions (2.4%) [2], laryngospasm or bronchospasm (0.1% to 0.4%) [2], cardiac arrhythmias (0.9% to 4%) [2,62], pneumothorax, anesthesia-related problems (0.1%) [2], and aphonia (0.1%) [2]. Fever may occur in up to 24% of patients after bronchoscopy and appears to be cytokine mediated and uncommonly indicative of a true infection or bacteremia [61]. Transient bacteremias often occur (15.4% to 33%) after rigid bronchoscopy [63], probably due to trauma to the teeth and airways. Most investigations have found that the incidence of bacteremia after transoral flexible bronchoscopy is much lower (0.7%) [64]. Current guidelines by the American Heart Association for respiratory tract procedures recommend prophylactic antibiotics only when incision or biopsy of the respiratory tract mucosa is anticipated. Prophylaxis is further restricted to patients with high-risk cardiac conditions (prosthetic valves, prior history of infective endocarditis, congenital heart disease, and cardiac transplantation with valvulopathy) only and no distinction is made between rigid and flexible bronchoscopy [65].

Although routine bronchoscopy is extremely safe, critically ill patients appear to be at higher risk of complications. Patients with asthma are prone to develop laryngospasm and bronchospasm. Bone marrow and stem cell transplant recipients are more likely to develop major bleeding during bronchoscopy (0% to 14%) [28,66], particularly if PSB or transbronchial lung biopsy is performed (7% to 14% vs. 1.5% for BAL alone) [29,66]. Patients with uremia are at increased risk of bleeding [67]. One investigation found that aspirin use did not increase bleeding risk after transbronchial biopsy [68]. In critically ill, mechanically ventilated patents, bronchoscopy causes a transient decrease in PaO_2 (partial arterial oxygen pressure) of approximately 25% [69], and transbronchial lung biopsy is more likely to result in pneumothorax (7% to 23%) [70], particularly in patients with ARDS (up to 36%) [71]. Patients with ARDS also have more pronounced declines in oxygenation, with a mean decrease of more than 50% in the PaO_2 [69].

CONTRAINDICATIONS

Bronchoscopy should not be performed (a) unless an experienced bronchoscopist is available; (b) when the patient will not or cannot cooperate; (c) when adequate oxygenation cannot be maintained during the procedure; (d) in unstable cardiac patients [72–74]; and (e) in untreated symptomatic patients with asthma [75]. The impact of coagulation parameters and antiplatelet agents on bleeding risk during transbronchial biopsy remains controversial [68,76]. In patients with recent cardiac ischemia, the major complication rate is low (3% to 5%) and is similar to that of other critically ill populations [77,78]. Although patients with stable carbon dioxide retention can safely undergo bronchoscopy with a flexible instrument [79], premedication, sedation during the procedure, and supplemental oxygen must be used with caution. The major contraindications to rigid bronchoscopy include inability to tolerate general anesthesia, an unstable cervical spine, limited range of motion at the spine, any condition that inhibits opening of the jaw, and an inexperienced operator and staff [5].

Consideration of bronchoscopy in neurologic and neurosurgical patients requires attention to the effects of bronchoscopy on intracranial pressure (ICP) and cerebral perfusion pressure (CPP). In patients with head trauma, bronchoscopy causes the ICP to increase by at least 50% in 88% of patients and by at least 100% in 69% of patients despite the use of deep sedation and paralysis [80]. Because mean arterial pressure tends to rise in parallel with ICP, there is often no change in CPP. No significant neurologic complications have been noted in patients with severe head trauma [80,81] or with space-occupying intracranial lesions with computed tomographic evidence of elevated ICP [82]. Bronchoscopy in such patients should be accompanied by deep sedation, paralysis, and medications for cerebral protection (thiopental and lidocaine). Cerebral hemodynamics should be continuously monitored to ensure that ICP and CPP are within acceptable levels. Caution is warranted in patients with markedly elevated baseline ICP or with borderline CPP.

PROCEDURE

Airway and Intubation

In nonintubated patients, flexible bronchoscopy can be performed by the transnasal or transoral route with a bite block [1]. There has also been a relatively recent interest in performing noninvasive ventilation-assisted flexible bronchoscopy via face mask, first described in eight immunocompromised patients with infiltrates and severe hypoxemia (PaO_2/FIO_2 <100) [83]. The procedure was well tolerated with either maintenance of or an improvement in oxygenation noted throughout, and none of the patients required intubation. Since then, multiple case reports and small randomized controlled trials using similar applications of noninvasive ventilation during bronchoscopy in expanded patient populations with severe hypoxemia (PaO_2/FIO_2 <200) have been described with similar outcomes [84,85]. Thus, it appears that this technique, augmented by BAL, appears to be a safe, effective, and viable option of obtaining an early and accurate diagnosis of pneumonia in nonintubated, otherwise marginal, patients with severe hypoxemia. In intubated and mechanically ventilated patients, the flexible bronchoscope can be passed into the tube through a swivel adapter with a rubber diaphragm that will prevent loss of the delivered respiratory gases [86]. To prevent dramatic increases in airway resistance and an unacceptable loss of tidal volumes, the lumen of the endotracheal tube should be at least 2 mm larger than the outer diameter of the bronchoscope [87,88]. Thus, flexible bronchoscopy with an average adult-sized instrument (outside diameter of scope 4.8 to 5.9 mm) can be performed in a ventilated patient if there is an endotracheal tube in place that is 8 mm or larger in internal diameter. If the endotracheal tube is smaller, a pediatric bronchoscope (outside diameter 3.5 mm) or intubation endoscope (outside diameter 3.8 mm) must be used. Both diagnostic and therapeutic interventions via flexible bronchoscopy have also been performed more frequently in the last decade through laryngeal mask airways used to secure the airway in spontaneously breathing and generally anesthetized individuals [89].

Premedication

Topical anesthesia may be achieved by hand-nebulized lidocaine and lidocaine jelly as a lubricant [1] and by instilling approximately 3 mL of 1% or 2% lidocaine at the main carina and, if needed, into the lower airways. Lidocaine is absorbed through the mucus membranes, producing peak serum concentrations that are nearly as high as that when the equivalent dose is administered intravenously, although toxicity is rare if the total dose does not exceed 6 to 7 mg per kg. In 2000, a study performed in otherwise healthy patients with asthma demonstrated the safety of topical lidocaine doses up to 8.2 mg per kg in this population [90] and subsequently led to this upper limit being recommended by the British Thoracic Society in their guidelines for diagnostic flexible bronchoscopy [91]. In patients with hepatic or cardiac insufficiency, lidocaine clearance is reduced, and the dose should be decreased to a maximum of 4 to 5 mg per kg [92,93]. Administering nebulized lidocaine prior to the procedure substantially increases the total lidocaine dose without improving cough or patient comfort [94]. Moderate sedation with incremental doses of midazolam, titrated to produce light sleep, produces amnesia in more than 95% of patients, but adequate sedation may require a total of greater than 20 mg in some subjects [95]. Cough suppression is more effective when narcotics are added to benzodiazepine premedication regimens [95]. Premedication with intravenous atropine has not been found to reduce secretions, decrease coughing, or prevent bradycardia [96,97] and has been associated with greater hemodynamic fluctuations when compared to placebo [98]. Propofol [99] and fospropofol [100] have also been used with success during moderate sedation for bronchoscopy, and may have the advantage of more rapid onset and shorter recovery time.

Mechanical Ventilation

Maintaining adequate oxygenation and ventilation while preventing breath stacking and positive end expiratory pressure (auto-PEEP) may be challenging when insertion of the bronchoscope reduces the effective lumen of the endotracheal tube by more than 50%. PEEP caused by standard scopes and tubes will approach 20 cm H_2O with the potential for barotrauma [87]. The inspired oxygen concentration must be temporarily increased to 100% prior to starting the procedure [87]. Expired volumes should be constantly monitored to ensure that they are adequate [88]. Meeting these ventilatory goals may require increasing the high-pressure limit in volume-cycled ventilation to near its maximal value, allowing the ventilator to overcome the added resistance caused by the bronchoscope. Although this increases the measured peak airway pressure, the alveolar pressure is not likely to change significantly because the lung is protected by the resistance of the bronchoscope [88]. Alternatively, decreasing the inspiratory flow rate in an attempt to decrease measured peak pressures may paradoxically increase alveolar pressures by decreasing expiratory time and thus increasing auto-PEEP. Suctioning should be kept to a minimum and for short periods of time because it will decrease the tidal volumes being delivered [87].

Quantitative Cultures

BAL is performed by advancing the bronchoscope until the tip wedges tightly in a distal bronchus from the area of greatest clinical interest. If the disease process is diffuse, perform the procedure in the right middle lobe because this is the area from which the best returns are most consistently obtained. Three aliquots of saline, typically 35 to 50 mL, are then instilled and withdrawn; in some protocols, the first aliquot is discarded to prevent contamination with more proximal secretions. A total instilled volume of 100 mL with at least 5% to 10% retrieved constitutes an adequate specimen [101]. PSB may be performed through a bronchoscope by advancing the plugged catheter assembly until it projects from the bronchoscope. When the area of interest is reached (e.g., purulent secretions can be seen), the distal plug is ejected and the brush is then fully advanced beyond the protective sheath. After the specimen is obtained, the brush is pulled back into the sheath and only then is the catheter assembly removed from the bronchoscope.

References

1. Sackner MA: Bronchofiberscopy. *Am Rev Respir Dis* 111:62, 1975.
2. Pereira W Jr, Kovnat DM, Snider GL: A prospective cooperative study of complications following flexible fiberoptic bronchoscopy. *Chest* 73:813, 1978.
3. Rath GS, Schaff JT, Snider GL: Flexible fiberoptic bronchoscopy: techniques and review of 100 bronchoscopies. *Chest* 63:689, 1973.
4. Prakash UBS, Stuffs SE: The bronchoscopy survey: some reflections. *Chest* 100:1660, 1991.
5. Bolliger CT, Mathur PN. *Interventional Bronchoscopy. Progress in Respiratory Research*, Vol 30. Basel, Switzerland, Karger, 2000.
6. Wahidi MM, Ernst A: Role of the interventional pulmonologist in the intensive care unit. *J Intensive Care Med* 20(3):141–146, 2005.

7. Ernst A, Silvestri GA, Johnstone D: Interventional pulmonary procedures, guidelines from the American College of Chest Physicians. *Chest* 123:1693–1717, 2003.
8. Khan MA, Whitcomb ME, Snider GL: Flexible fiberoptic bronchoscopy. *Am J Med* 61:151, 1976.
9. Selecky PA: Evaluation of hemoptysis through the bronchoscope. *Chest* 73[Suppl]:741, 1978.
10. Dweik RA, Stoller JK: Role of bronchoscopy in massive hemoptysis. *Clin Chest Med* 20(1):89–105, 1999.
11. Hirshberg B, Biran I, Glazer M, et al: Hemoptysis: etiology, evaluation, and outcome in a tertiary referral hospital. *Chest* 112:440–444, 1997.
12. Susanto I: Managing a patient with hemoptysis. *J Bronchol* 9:40–45, 2002.
13. Schnabel A, Holl-Ulrich K, Dahloff K, et al: Efficacy of transbronchial biopsy in pulmonary vasculitides. *Eur Respir J* 10:2738–2743, 1997.
14. Fartoukh M, Maitre B, Honore S, et al: Diagnosing pneumonia during mechanical ventilation: the clinical infection score revisited. *Am J Respir Crit Care Med* 168:173, 2003.
15. Pinckard JK, Kollef M, Dunne WM: Culturing bronchial washings obtained during bronchoscopy fails to add diagnostic utility to culturing the bronchoalveolar lavage fluid alone. *Diagn Microbiol Infect Dis* 43:99, 2002.
16. Torres A, El-Ebiary M: Bronchoscopic BAL in the diagnosis of ventilator-associated pneumonia. *Chest* 117:198, 2000.
17. Baughman RP: Protected-specimen brush technique in the diagnosis of ventilator associated pneumonia. *Chest* 117:203S, 2000.
18. Grossman RF, Fein A: Evidence-based assessment of diagnostic tests for ventilator associated pneumonia. *Chest* 117:177S, 2000.
19. Kirtland SH, Corley DE, Winterbauer RH, et al: The diagnosis of ventilator associated pneumonia: a comparison of histologic, microbiologic, and clinical criteria. *Chest* 112:445, 1997.
20. Brun-Bruisson C, Fartoukh M, Lechapt E, et al: Contribution of blinded protected quantitative specimens to the diagnostic and therapeutic management of ventilator-associated pneumonia. *Chest* 128:533, 2005.
21. Wood AY, Davit AJ, Ciraulo DL, et al: A prospective assessment of diagnostic efficacy of blind protected bronchial brushings compared to bronchoscope assisted lavage, bronchoscope-directed brushings, and blind endotracheal aspirates in ventilator assisted pneumonia. *J Trauma* 55:825, 2003.
22. Prats E, Dorca J, Pujol M, et al: Effects of antibiotics on protected specimen brush sampling in ventilator associated pneumonia. *Eur Respir J* 19:944, 2002.
23. Shorr AF, Sherner JH, Jackson WL, et al: Invasive approaches to the diagnosis of ventilator-associated pneumonia: a meta-analysis. *Crit Care Med* 33:46, 2005.
24. Canadian Critical Care Trials Group: A randomized trial of diagnostic techniques for ventilator-associated pneumonia. *N Engl J Med* 355:2619, 2006.
25. Azoulay, E, Mokart, D, Rabbat A, et al: Diagnostic bronchoscopy in hematology and oncology patients with acute respiratory failure: prospective multicenter data. *Crit Care Med* 36:100, 2008.
26. Jain O, Sunder S, Mile Y, et al: Role of flexible bronchoscopy in immunocompromised patients with lung infiltrates. *Chest* 125:712, 2004.
27. Patel N, Lee P, Kim J, et al: The influence of diagnostic bronchoscopy on clinical outcomes comparing adult autologous and allogeneic bone marrow transplant recipients. *Chest* 127:1388, 2005.
28. White P, Bonacum JT, Miller CB: Utility of fiberoptic bronchoscopy in bone marrow transplant patients. *Bone Marrow Transplant* 20:681, 1997.
29. Hofmeister CC, Czerlanis C, Forsythe S, et al: Retrospective utility of bronchoscopy after hematopoietic stem cell transplant. *Bone Marrow Transplant* 38:693, 2006.
30. Emanuel D, Peppard J, Stover D, et al: Rapid immunodiagnosis of cytomegalovirus pneumonia by bronchoalveolar lavage using human and murine monoclonal antibodies. *Ann Intern Med* 104:476, 1986.
31. Broaddus C, Dake MD, Stulbarg MS, et al: Bronchoalveolar lavage and transbronchial biopsy for the diagnosis of pulmonary infections in the acquired immunodeficiency syndrome. *Ann Intern Med* 102:747, 1985.
32. Raoof S, Rosen MJ, Khan FA: Role of bronchoscopy in AIDS. *Clin Chest Med* 20:63, 1999.
33. Hopewell PC: Pneumocystis carinii pneumonia: diagnosis. *J Infect Dis* 157:1115, 1988.
34. Brandstetter RD: Flexible fiberoptic bronchoscopy in the intensive care unit. *Intensive Care Med* 4:248, 1989.
35. Haponik EF, Meyers DA, Munster AM, et al: Acute upper airway injury in burn patients: serial changes of flow-volume curves and nasopharyngoscopy. *Am Rev Respir Dis* 135:360, 1987.
36. Hara KS, Prakash UBS: Fiberoptic bronchoscopy in the evaluation of acute chest and upper airway trauma. *Chest* 96:627, 1989.
37. Mahajan VK, Catron PW, Huber GL: The value of fiberoptic bronchoscopy in the management of pulmonary collapse. *Chest* 73:817, 1978.
38. Kreider ME, Lipson DA: Bronchoscopy for atelectasis in the ICU: a case report and review of the literature. *Chest* 124:344, 2003.
39. Marini JJ, Pierson DJ, Hudson LD: Acute lobar atelectasis: a prospective comparison of fiberoptic bronchoscopy and respiratory therapy. *Am Rev Respir Dis* 119:971, 1979.
40. Lieberman J: The appropriate use of mucolytic agents. *Am J Med* 49:1, 1970.
41. Cunanan OS: The flexible fiberoptic bronchoscope in foreign body removal: experience in 300 cases. *Chest* 73:725, 1978.
42. Swanson KL, Prakash UB, McDougall JC, et al: Airway foreign bodies in adults. *J Bronchol* 10:107–111, 2003.
43. Mehta AC, Rafanan AL: Extraction of airway foreign body in adults. *J Bronchol* 8:123–131, 2001.
44. Schramm R, Abugameh A, Tscholl D, et al: Managing pulmonary artery catheter-induced pulmonary hemorrhage by bronchial occlusion. *Ann Thorac Surg* 88:284–287, 2009.
45. Campos JH: An update on bronchial blockers during lung separation techniques in adults. *Anesth Analg* 97:1266–1274, 2003.
46. Valipour A, Kreuzer A, Koller H, et al: Bronchoscopy-guided topical hemostatic tamponade therapy for the management of life threatening hemoptysis. *Chest* 127:2113, 2005.
47. Battacharyya P, Dutta A, Samanta AN, et al: New procedure: bronchoscopic endobronchial sealing, a new mode for managing hemoptysis. *Chest* 121:2066–2069, 2002.
48. Seijo LM, Sterman DH: Interventional pulmonology. *N Engl J Med* 344:740, 2001.
49. Beamis J: Interventional pulmonology techniques for treating malignant large airway obstruction: an update. *Curr Opin Pulm Med* 11:292, 2005.
50. Ernst A, Feller-Kopman D, Becker HD, et al: Central airway obstruction. *Am J Respir Crit Care Med* 169:1278–1297, 2004.
51. Swanson KL, Edell ES, Prakash UB, et al: Complications of metal stent therapy in benign airway obstruction. *J Bronchol* 14:90–94, 2007.
52. Colt HG, Harrell JH: Therapeutic rigid bronchoscopy allows level of care changes in patients with acute respiratory failure from central airways obstruction. *Chest* 112:202–206, 1997.
53. Shaffer JP, Allen JN: The use of expandable metal stents to facilitate extubation in patients with large airway obstruction. *Chest* 114:1378–1382, 1998.
54. Saad CP, Murthy S, Krizmanich G, et al: Self-expandable metallic airway stents and flexible bronchoscopy. *Chest* 124:1993–1999, 2003.
55. Lippmann M, Rome L, Eiger G, et al: Utility of tracheobronchial stents in mechanically ventilated patients with central airway obstruction. *J Bronchol* 9:301–305, 2002.
56. Lois M, Noppen M: Bronchopleural fistulas, an overview of the problem with special focus on endoscopic management. *Chest* 128:3955–3965, 2005.
57. Madi JM, Trottier SJ: Percutaneous dilatational tracheostomy technique. *J Bronchol* 10:146–149, 2003.
58. Bardell T, Drover JW: Recent developments in percutaneous tracheostomy: improving techniques and expanding roles. *Curr Opin Crit Care* 11:326–332, 2005.
59. Credle WF, Smiddy JF, Elliott RC: Complications of fiberoptic bronchoscopy. *Am Rev Respir Dis* 109:67, 1974.
60. Suratt PM, Smiddy JF, Gruber B: Deaths and complications associated with fiberoptic bronchoscopy. *Chest* 69:747, 1976.
61. Krause A, Hohberg B, Heine F, et al: Cytokines derived from alveolar macrophages induce fever after bronchoscopy and bronchoalveolar lavage. *Am J Respir Crit Care Med* 155:1793, 1997.
62. Stubbs SE, Brutinel WM: Complications of bronchoscopy, in Prakash USB (ed): *Bronchoscopy*. New York, Lippincott Williams & Wilkins, 1994, p 357.
63. Burman SO: Bronchoscopy and bacteremia. *J Thorac Cardiovasc Surg* 40:635, 1960.
64. Yigla M, Oren I, Solomonov A, et al: Incidence of bacteraemia following fiberoptic bronchoscopy. *Eur Respir J* 14:789, 1999.
65. Wilson M, Taubert KA, Gewitz M, et al: Prevention of endocarditis, guidelines from the American Heart Association. *Circulation* 116:1736–1754, 2007.
66. Dunagan DP, Baker AM, Hurd DD: Bronchoscopic evaluation of pulmonary infiltrates following bone marrow transplantation. *Chest* 111:135, 1997.
67. Zavala DC: Pulmonary hemorrhage in fiberoptic transbronchial biopsy. *Chest* 70:584, 1976.
68. Herth FJ, Becker HD, Ernst A: Aspirin does not increase bleeding complications after transbronchial biopsy. *Chest* 122:1461, 2002.
69. Trouillet JL, Guiguet M, Gibert C, et al: Fiberoptic bronchoscopy in ventilated patients: evaluation of cardiopulmonary risk under midazolam sedation. *Chest* 97:927, 1990.
70. O'Brien JD, Ettinger NA, Shevlin D: Safety and yield of transbronchial biopsy in mechanically ventilated patients. *Crit Care Med* 25:440, 1997.
71. Bulpa PA, Dive AM, Mertens L, et al: Combined bronchoalveolar lavage and transbronchial lung biopsy: safety and yield in ventilated patients. *Eur Respir J* 21:489, 2003.
72. Shrader DL, Lakshminarayan S: The effect of fiberoptic bronchoscopy on cardiac rhythm. *Chest* 73:821, 1978.
73. Lundgren R, Haggmark S, Reiz S: Hemodynamic effects of flexible fiberoptic bronchoscopy performed under topical anesthesia. *Chest* 82:295, 1982.
74. Luck JC, Messeder OH, Rubenstein MJ, et al: Arrhythmias from fiberoptic bronchoscopy. *Chest* 74:139, 1978.
75. Sahn SA, Scoggin C: Fiberoptic bronchoscopy in bronchial asthma: a word of caution. *Chest* 69:39, 1976.
76. Chinsky K: Bleeding risk and bronchoscopy: in search of the evidence in evidence-based medicine. *Chest* 127:1875, 2005.
77. Dweik RA, Mehta AC, Meeker DP, et al: Analysis of the safety of bronchoscopy after recent acute myocardial infarction. *Chest* 110:825, 1996.

78. Dunagan DP, Burke HL, Aquino SL, et al: Fiberoptic bronchoscopy in coronary care unit patients: indications, safety and clinical implications. *Chest* 114:1660, 1998.
79. Salisbury BG, Metzger LF, Altose MD, et al: Effect of fiberoptic bronchoscopy on respiratory performance in patients with chronic airways obstruction. *Thorax* 30:441, 1975.
80. Kerwin AJ, Croce MA, Timmons SD, et al: Effects of fiberoptic bronchoscopy on intracranial pressure in patients with brain injury; a prospective clinical study. *J Trauma* 48:878, 2000.
81. Peerless JR, Snow N, Likavec MJ, et al: The effect of fiberoptic bronchoscopy on cerebral hemodynamics in patients with severe head injury. *Chest* 108:962, 1995.
82. Bajwa MK, Henein S, Kamholz SL: Fiberoptic bronchoscopy in the presence of space-occupying intracranial lesions. *Chest* 104:101, 1993.
83. Antonelli M, Conti G, Riccioni L, et al: Noninvasive positive-pressure ventilation via face mask during bronchoscopy with BAL in high-risk hypoxemic patients. *Chest* 110:724–728, 1996.
84. Antonelli M, Conti G, Rocco M, et al: Noninvasive positive-pressure ventilation vs conventional oxygen supplementation in hypoxemic patients undergoing diagnostic bronchoscopy. *Chest* 121:1149–1154, 2002.
85. Antonelli M, Pennisi MA, Conti G: New advances in the use of noninvasive ventilation for acute hypoxaemic respiratory failure. *Eur Respir J* 22[Suppl 42]:65s–71s, 2003.
86. Reichert WW, Hall WJ, Hyde RW: A simple disposable device for performing fiberoptic bronchoscopy on patients requiring continuous artificial ventilation. *Am Rev Respir Dis* 109:394, 1974.
87. Lindholm C-E, Ollman B, Snyder JV, et al: Cardiorespiratory effects of flexible fiberoptic bronchoscopy in critically ill patients. *Chest* 74:362, 1978.
88. Lawson RW, Peters JI, Shelledy DC: Effects of fiberoptic bronchoscopy during mechanical ventilation in a lung model. *Chest* 118:824, 2000.
89. Sung A, Kalstein A, Radhakrishnan P, et al: Laryngeal mask airway: use and clinical applications. *J Bronchol* 14:181–188, 2007.
90. Langmack EL, Martin RJ, Pak J, et al: Serum lidocaine concentration in asthmatics undergoing research bronchoscopy. *Chest* 117:1055–1060, 2000.
91. Honeybourne D, Jabb J, Bowie P, et al: British Thoracic Society guidelines on diagnostic flexible bronchoscopy. *Thorax* 56[Suppl I]:i1–i21, 2001.
92. Milman N, Laub M, Munch EP, et al: Serum concentrations of lignocaine and its metabolite monoethylglycinexylidide during fiberoptic bronchoscopy in local anesthesia. *Respir Med* 92:40, 1998.
93. Bose AA, Colt HG: Lidocaine in bronchoscopy: practical use and allergic reactions. *J Bronchology* 15:163–166, 2008.
94. Stolz D, Chhajed PN, Leuppi J, et al: Nebulized lidocaine for flexible bronchoscopy: a randomized, double-blind, placebo-controlled trial. *Chest* 128:1756, 2005.
95. Williams TJ, Bowie PE: Midazolam sedation to produce complete amnesia for bronchoscopy: 2 years' experience at a district hospital. *Respir Med* 93:361, 1999.
96. Cowl CT, Prakash UBS, Kruger BR: The role of anticholinergics in bronchoscopy: a randomized clinical trial. *Chest* 118:188, 2000.
97. Williams T, Brooks T, Ward C: The role of atropine premedication in fiberoptic bronchoscopy using intravenous midazolam sedation. *Chest* 113:113, 1998.
98. Malik JA, Gupta D, Agarwal AN, et al: Anticholinergic premedication for flexible bronchoscopy—a randomized, double-blind, placebo-controlled study of atropine and glycopyrrolate. *Chest* 136:347–354, 2009.
99. Crawford M, Pollock J, Anderson K, et al: Comparison of midazolam with propofol for sedation in outpatient bronchoscopy. *Br J Anaesth* 70:419–422, 1993.
100. Silvestri GA, Vincent BD, Wahidi MM, et al: A phase-3, randomized, double blind study to assess the efficacy and safety of fospropofol disodium injection for moderate sedation in patients undergoing flexible bronchoscopy. *Chest* 135:41–47, 2009.
101. Meyer KC: The role of bronchoalveolar lavage in interstitial lung disease. *Clin Chest Med* 25:637, 2004.

CHAPTER 10 ■ THORACENTESIS

MARK M. WILSON AND RICHARD S. IRWIN

Thoracentesis is an invasive procedure that involves the introduction of a needle, cannula, or trocar into the pleural space to remove accumulated fluid or air. Although a few prospective studies have critically evaluated the clinical value and complications associated with it [1–3], most studies concerning thoracentesis have dealt with the interpretation of the pleural fluid analyses [4,5].

INDICATIONS

Although history (cough, dyspnea, or pleuritic chest pain) and physical findings (dullness to percussion, decreased breath sounds, and decreased vocal fremitus) suggest that an effusion is present, chest radiography or ultrasonic examination is essential to confirm the clinical suspicion. Thoracentesis can be performed for diagnostic or therapeutic reasons. When done for diagnostic reasons, the procedure should be performed whenever possible before any treatment has been given to avoid confusion in interpretation [5]. Analysis of pleural fluid has been shown to yield clinically useful information in more than 90% of cases [2]. The four most common diagnoses for symptomatic and asymptomatic pleural effusions are malignancy, congestive heart failure, parapneumonia, and postoperative sympathetic effusions. A diagnostic algorithm for evaluation of a pleural effusion of unknown etiology is presented in Figure 10.1. In patients whose pleural effusion remains undiagnosed after thoracentesis and closed pleural biopsy, thoracoscopy should be considered for visualization of the pleura and directed biopsy. Thoracoscopy has provided a positive diagnosis in more than 80% of patients with recurrent pleural effusions that are not diagnosed by repeated thoracentesis, pleural biopsy, or bronchoscopy.

Therapeutic thoracentesis is indicated to remove fluid or air that is causing cardiopulmonary embarrassment or to relieve severe symptoms. Definitive drainage of the pleural space with a thoracostomy tube must be done for a tension pneumothorax (PTX) and should be considered for a PTX that is slowly enlarging, any size PTX in the mechanically ventilated patient, hemothorax, or the instillation of a sclerosing agent after drainage of a recurrent malignant pleural effusion.

CONTRAINDICATIONS

Absolute contraindications to performing a thoracentesis are an uncooperative patient, the inability to identify the top of the rib clearly under the percutaneous puncture site, a lack of expertise in performing the procedure, and the presence of a coagulation abnormality that cannot be corrected. Relative

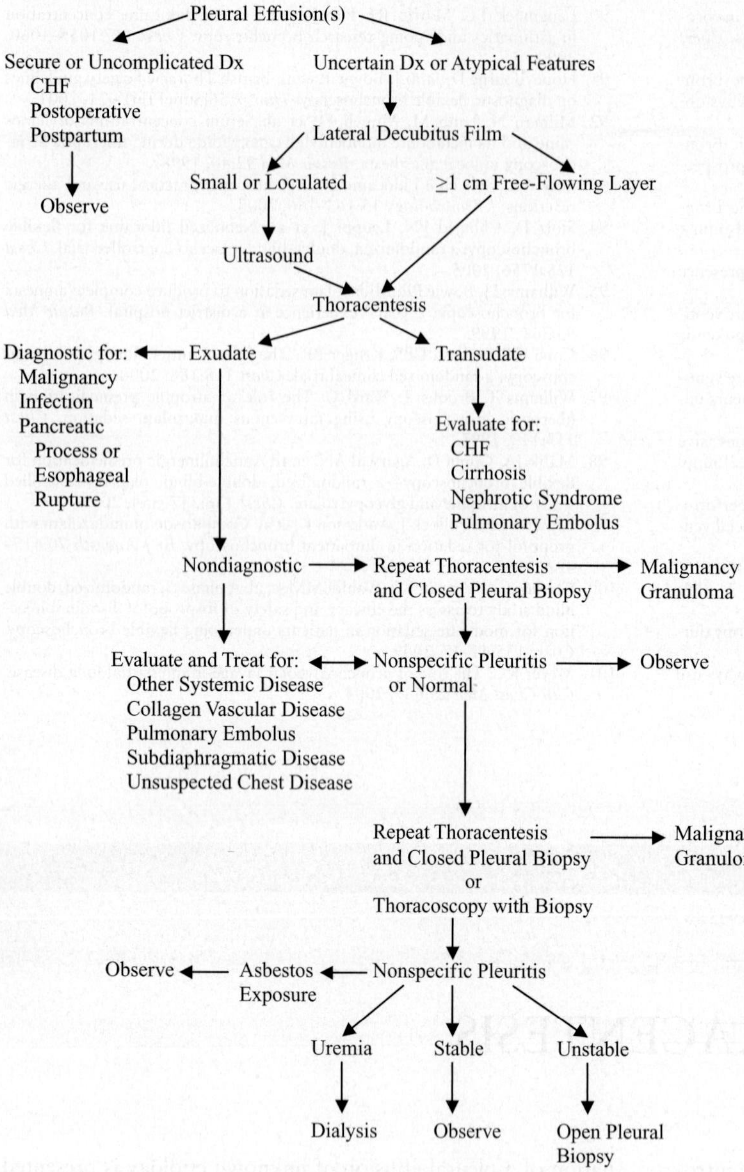

FIGURE 10.1. Diagnostic algorithm for evaluation of pleural effusion. CHF, congestive heart failure; Dx, diagnosis. [Adapted from Smyrnios NA, Jederlinic PJ, Irwin RS: Pleural effusion in an asymptomatic patient. Spectrum and frequency of causes and management considerations. *Chest* 97:192, 1990.]

contraindications to a thoracentesis include entry into an area where known bullous lung disease exists, a patient who is on positive end-expiratory pressure, and a patient who has only one "functioning" lung (the other having been surgically removed or that has severe disease limiting its gas exchange function). In these settings, it may be safest to perform the thoracentesis under ultrasonic guidance.

COMPLICATIONS

A number of prospective studies have documented that complications associated with the procedure are not infrequent [1,2]. The overall complication rate has been reported to be as high as 50% to 78%, and can be further categorized as major (15% to 19%) or minor (31% to 63%) [2,3]. Complication rates appear to be inversely related to experience level of the operator; the more experienced, the fewer the complications [6]. Although death due to the procedure is infrequently reported, complications may be life threatening [1].

Major complications include PTX, hemopneumothorax, hemorrhage, hypotension, and reexpansion pulmonary edema. The reported incidence of PTX varies between 3% and 30% [1–3,6,7], with up to one-third to one-half of those with demonstrated PTX requiring subsequent intervention. Various investigators have reported associations between PTX and underlying lung disease (chronic obstructive pulmonary disease, prior thoracic radiation, prior thoracic surgery, or lung cancer) [8,9], needle size and technique [3,8], number of passes required to obtain a sample [8], aspiration of air during the procedure, experience level of the operator [1,3,6], use of a vacuum bottle [9], size of the effusion [2,8], and mechanical ventilation versus spontaneously breathing patients. Some of the above-mentioned studies report directly contradictory findings compared to other similar studies. This is most apparent in the reported association between PTX and therapeutic thoracentesis [3,8], which was not supported by subsequent large prospective trials [8,9]. The most likely explanation for this discrepancy in the literature concerning the presumed increased risk for PTX for therapeutic over diagnostic procedures is the generally lower experience level of the operator in the first group. Small sample sizes also limit the generalization of reported findings to allow for the delineation of a clear risk profile for the development of a PTX due to thoracentesis. The presence of baseline lung disease, low experience level of the operator with the procedure, and the use of positive-pressure mechanical ventilation appear for now to be the best-established risk factors in the literature. Further research involving more patients is needed.

Although PTX is most commonly due to laceration of lung parenchyma, room air may enter the pleural space if the thoracentesis needle is open to room air when a spontaneously breathing patient takes a deep breath. (Intrapleural pressure is subatmospheric.) The PTX may be small and asymptomatic, resolving spontaneously, or large and associated with respiratory compromise, requiring chest tube drainage. Hemorrhage can occur from laceration of an intercostal artery or inadvertent puncture of the liver or spleen even if coagulation studies are normal. The risk of intercostal artery laceration is greatest in the elderly because of increased tortuosity of their vessels. This last complication is potentially lethal, and open thoracotomy may be required to control the bleeding.

Hypotension may occur during the procedure (as part of a vasovagal reaction or tension PTX) or hours after the procedure (most likely due to reaccumulation of fluid into the pleural space or the pulmonary parenchyma from the intravascular space). Hypotension in the latter settings responds to volume expansion; it can usually be prevented by limiting pleural fluid drainage to 1.5 L or less. Other major complications are rare, and include implantation of tumor along the needle tract of a previously performed thoracentesis, venous and cerebral air embolism (so-called pleural shock) [10,11], and inadvertent placement of a sheared-off catheter into the pleural space [1].

Minor complications include dry tap or insufficient fluid, pain, subcutaneous hematoma or seroma, anxiety, dyspnea, and cough [2]. Reported rates for these minor complications range from 16% to 63% and depend on the method used to perform the procedure, with higher rates associated with the catheter-through-needle technique [2,3]. Dry tap and insufficient fluid are technical problems, and they expose the patient to increased risk of morbidity because of the need to perform a repeat thoracentesis. Under these circumstances, it is recommended that the procedure be repeated under direct sonographic guidance. Pain may originate from parietal pleural nerve endings from inadequate local anesthesia, inadvertent scraping of rib periosteum, or piercing an intercostal nerve during a misdirected needle thrust.

PROCEDURES

General Considerations

The most common techniques for performing thoracentesis are catheter-over-needle, needle-only, and needle under direct sonographic guidance. The catheter-through-needle technique has been used much less frequently over the past decade.

Technique for Diagnostic (Needle-Only or Catheter-Over-Needle) Removal of Freely Flowing Fluid

The technique for diagnostic removal of freely flowing fluid is as follows:

1. Obtain a lateral decubitus chest radiograph to confirm a free-flowing pleural effusion.
2. Describe the procedure to the patient and obtain written informed consent. Operators should be thoroughly familiar with the procedure they will be performing and should receive appropriate supervision from an experienced operator before performing thoracentesis on their own.
3. With the patient sitting, arms at sides, mark the inferior tip of the scapula on the side to be tapped. This approximates the eighth intercostal space and should be the lowest interspace punctured, unless it has been previously determined by sonography that a lower interspace can be safely entered or chest radiographs and sonography show the diaphragm to be higher than the eighth intercostal space.
4. Position the patient sitting at the edge of the bed, comfortably leaning forward over a pillow-draped, height-adjusted, bedside table (Fig. 10.2). The patient's arms should be crossed in front to elevate and spread the scapulae. An assistant should stand in front of the patient to prevent any unexpected movements.
5. Percuss the patient's posterior chest to determine the highest point of the effusion. The interspace below this point should be entered in the posterior axillary line, unless it is below the eighth intercostal space. Gently mark the superior aspect of the rib in the chosen interspace with your fingernail. (The inferior portion of each rib contains an intercostal artery and should be avoided.)
6. Cleanse the area with 2% chlorhexidine in 70% isopropyl alcohol and allow it to dry. Using sterile technique, drape the area surrounding the puncture site.
7. Anesthetize the superficial skin with 2% lidocaine using a 25-gauge needle. Change to an 18- to 22-gauge, 2-in.-long needle and generously anesthetize the deeper soft tissues, aiming for the top of the rib. Always aspirate through the syringe as the needle is advanced and before instilling lidocaine to ensure that the needle is not in a vessel or the pleural space. Carefully aspirate through the syringe as the pleura is approached. (The rib is 1 to 2 cm thick.) Fluid enters the syringe on reaching the pleural space. The patient may experience discomfort as the needle penetrates the well-innervated parietal pleura. Be careful not to instill anesthetic into the pleural space; it is bactericidal for most organisms, including *Mycobacterium tuberculosis.* Place a gloved finger at the point on the needle where it exits the skin (to estimate the required depth of insertion) and remove the needle.
8. Attach a three-way stopcock to a 20-gauge, 1.5-in.-long needle and to a 50-mL syringe. The valve on the stopcock should be open to the needle to allow aspiration of fluid during needle insertion.
9. Insert the 20-gauge needle (or the catheter-over-needle apparatus) into the anesthetized tract with the bevel of the needle down and always aspirate through the syringe as the needle/catheter-over-needle apparatus is slowly advanced. When pleural fluid is obtained using the needle-only technique, stabilize the needle by attaching a clamp to the needle where it exits the skin to prevent further advancement of the needle into the pleural space. Once pleural fluid is obtained with the catheter-over-needle technique, direct the needle-catheter apparatus downward to ensure that the catheter descends to the most dependent area of the pleural space. Advance the catheter forward in a single smooth motion as the inner needle is simultaneously pulled back out of the chest.
10. Once pleural fluid can easily be obtained, fill a heparinized blood gas syringe from the side port of the three-way stopcock for measurement of fluid pH [12]. Express all air bubbles from the sample, cap it, and place it in a bag containing iced slush for immediate transport to the laboratory.
11. Fill the 50-mL syringe and transfer its contents into the appropriate collection tubes and containers [12]. Always maintain a closed system during the procedure to prevent room air from entering the pleural space. For most diagnostic studies, 50 to 100 mL should be ample fluid [13–15].

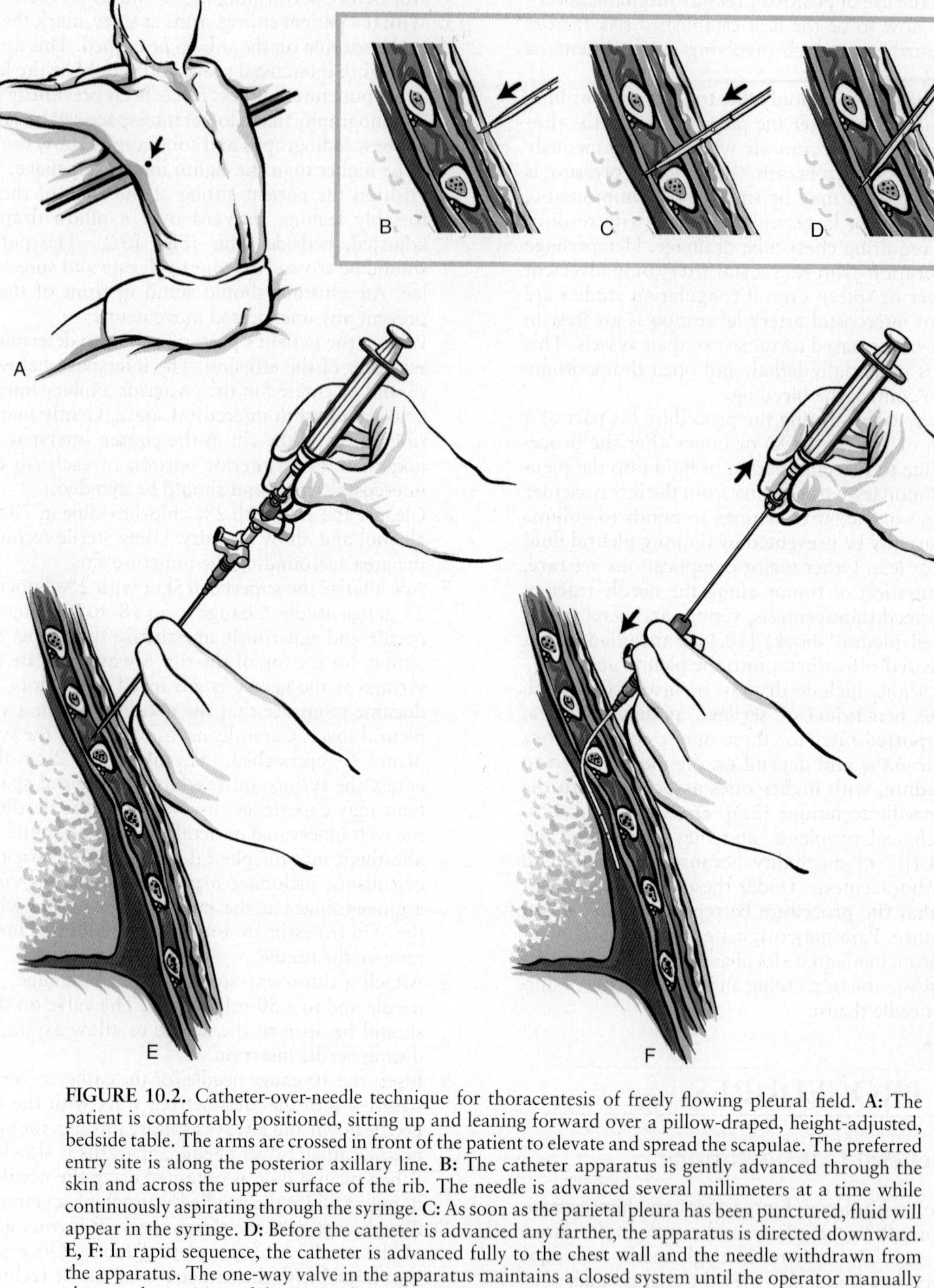

FIGURE 10.2. Catheter-over-needle technique for thoracentesis of freely flowing pleural field. A: The patient is comfortably positioned, sitting up and leaning forward over a pillow-draped, height-adjusted, bedside table. The arms are crossed in front of the patient to elevate and spread the scapulae. The preferred entry site is along the posterior axillary line. B: The catheter apparatus is gently advanced through the skin and across the upper surface of the rib. The needle is advanced several millimeters at a time while continuously aspirating through the syringe. C: As soon as the parietal pleura has been punctured, fluid will appear in the syringe. D: Before the catheter is advanced any farther, the apparatus is directed downward. E, F: In rapid sequence, the catheter is advanced fully to the chest wall and the needle withdrawn from the apparatus. The one-way valve in the apparatus maintains a closed system until the operator manually changes the position of the stopcock to allow drainage of the pleural fluid.

Always ensure that the three-way stopcock has the valve closed toward the patient when changing syringes.

12. When the thoracentesis is completed, remove the needle (or catheter) from the patient's chest as he or she hums or performs a Valsalva maneuver. Apply pressure to the wound for several minutes and then apply a sterile bandage.
13. A routine chest radiograph after thoracentesis is generally not indicated for most asymptomatic, nonventilated patients. Obtain a postprocedure upright end-expiratory chest radiograph if air was aspirated during the procedure, PTX is suspected by developing signs or symptoms, or multiple needle passes were required [16–19].

Technique for Therapeutic Removal of Freely Flowing Fluid

To perform the technique for therapeutic removal of freely flowing fluid, steps 1 to 7 should be followed as described previously. Removal of more than 100 mL pleural fluid generally involves placement of a catheter into the pleural space to minimize the risk of PTX from a needle during this longer procedure. Commercially available kits generally use a catheter-over-needle system, although catheter-through-needle systems are still available in some locations. Each kit should have a specific set of instructions for performing this procedure. Operators should be thoroughly familiar with the recommended procedure for the catheter system that they will be using and should receive appropriate supervision from an experienced operator before performing thoracentesis on their own.

Technique for Thoracentesis by Directed Guidance

Ultrasound guidance has long been used to assist thoracentesis for loculated or small-volume pleural effusions. In recent years, dynamic (real-time) sonographic scanners have become more readily available, and coupled with brief physician training time, ultrasound-assisted thoracentesis is rapidly becoming standard of practice for free-flowing effusions as well [20–23]. The protocol is similar to that described for the needle-only technique, but the needle can be inserted under direct guidance after localization of the effusion. The use of a catheter is optional in this setting. Of important note is that mandatory use of ultrasound for choosing the thoracentesis site and/or for guiding the procedure, the rate of PTX in one study decreased from 8.6% to 1.1% [21].

Technique for Removal of Freely Moving Pneumothorax

The technique for removal of freely moving PTX is as follows:

1. Follow the same catheter-over-needle protocol described for removing freely moving fluid, but position the patient supine with the head of the bed elevated to 30 to 45 degrees.
2. Prepare the second or third intercostal space in the anterior midclavicular line (which avoids hitting the more medial internal mammary artery) for the needle and catheter insertion.
3. Have the bevel of the needle facing up and direct the needle upward so that the catheter can be guided toward the superior aspect of the hemithorax.
4. Air can be actively withdrawn by syringe or pushed out when intrapleural pressure is supra-atmospheric (e.g., during a cough) as long as the catheter is intermittently open to the atmosphere. In the latter setting, air can leave but not reenter if the catheter is attached to a one-way check-valve apparatus (Heimlich valve) or if it is put to underwater seal.
5. When local anesthesia and skin cleansing are not possible because a tension PTX is life threatening, perform the procedure without them. If a tension PTX is known or suspected to be present and a chest tube is not readily available, quickly insert a 14-gauge needle and 16-gauge catheter according to the above technique to avoid puncturing the lung. If a tension PTX is present, air escapes under pressure. When the situation has stabilized and the tension PTX has been diagnosed, leave the catheter in place until a sterile chest tube can be inserted.

INTERPRETATION OF PLEURAL FLUID ANALYSIS

To determine the etiology of a pleural effusion, a number of tests on pleural fluid are helpful. The initial determination should be to classify the effusion as a transudate or an exudate, using the criteria discussed later. Additional studies can then be ordered to help establish a final diagnosis for the etiology of the pleural effusion, especially in the setting of an exudate.

Transudates Versus Exudates

A transudate is biochemically defined by meeting all of the following classic (Light's) criteria [24]: pleural fluid–serum total protein ratio of less than 0.5, pleural fluid–serum lactate dehydrogenase (LDH) ratio of less than 0.6, and pleural fluid LDH of less than two-thirds the normal serum level. Transudates are generally caused by hydrostatic or oncotic pressure imbalances or from migration of fluid from peritoneal or retroperitoneal spaces to the pleural space. An exudate is present when any of the foregoing criteria for transudates is not met. Exudates arise through a variety of mechanisms that result primarily from inflammation of the lung or pleura, impaired lymphatic drainage, or migration of fluid from the peritoneal space.

A wide variety of alternative diagnostic criteria have been studied since Light's original work was published. Abbreviated criteria with similar diagnostic accuracy, but without the need for concurrent serum measurements, have been proposed [4,25]. Meta-analysis indicates that a classic transudate can be identified with equal accuracy by the combination of both pleural fluid cholesterol of less than 45 mg per dL and a pleural fluid LDH less than 0.45 times the upper limit of normal for serum LDH.

If a transudate is present, generally no further tests on pleural fluid are indicated (Table 10.1). One exception to this is the transudative pleural effusion due to urinothorax [26]. An acidotic transudate is characteristic of a urinothorax, and elevated pleural fluid creatinine confirms the diagnosis. If an exudate is identified, further laboratory evaluation is generally warranted (Fig. 10.1). If subsequent testing does not narrow the differential diagnosis and tuberculous pleuritis is a diagnostic consideration, a percutaneous pleural biopsy should be considered [27]. Thoracoscopy-guided pleural biopsy should be considered in patients with pleural effusion of unknown etiology despite the above-listed evaluation.

Selected Tests That Are Potentially Helpful to Establish Etiology for a Pleural Effusion

pH

Pleural fluid pH determinations may have diagnostic and therapeutic implications [28–30]. For instance, the differential diagnosis associated with a pleural fluid pH of less than 7.2 is consistent with systemic acidemia, bacterially infected effusion (empyema), malignant effusion, rheumatoid or lupus effusion, tuberculous effusion, ruptured esophagus, noninfected parapneumonic effusion that needs drainage, and urinothorax. Pleural effusions with a pH of less than 7.2 are potentially sclerotic and require consideration for chest tube drainage to aid resolution [31,32].

Amylase

A pleural fluid amylase level that is twice the normal serum level or with an absolute value of greater than 160 Somogyi units may be seen in patients with acute and chronic pancreatitis, pancreatic pseudocyst that has dissected or ruptured into the pleural space, primary and metastatic cancer, and esophageal rupture. Salivary isoenzymes predominate with malignancy and esophageal rupture, whereas intrinsic pancreatic disease is characterized by the presence of pancreatic isoenzymes.

TABLE 10.1

CAUSES OF PLEURAL EFFUSIONS

ETIOLOGIES OF EFFUSIONS THAT ARE VIRTUALLY ALWAYS TRANSUDATES	*Malignancies*[b]
Congestive heart failure	Carcinoma
Nephrotic syndrome	Lymphoma
Hypoalbuminemia	Mesothelioma
Urinothorax	Leukemia
Trapped lung	Chylothorax
Cirrhosis	*Chronically Increased Negative Intrapleural Pressure*
Atelectasis	Atelectasis
Peritoneal dialysis	Trapped lung
Constrictive pericarditis	Cholesterol effusion
Superior vena caval obstruction	*Iatrogenic*
ETIOLOGIES OF EFFUSIONS THAT ARE TYPICALLY EXUDATES	Drug-induced (nitrofurantoin and methotrexate)
Infections	Esophageal perforation
Parapneumonic	Esophageal sclerotherapy
Tuberculous pleurisy	Central venous catheter misplacement or migration
Parasites (amebiasis, paragonimiasis, and echinococcosis)	Enteral feeding tube in space
Fungal disease	*Connective Tissue Disease*
Atypical pneumonias (virus, *Mycoplasma*, Q fever, and *Legionella*)	Lupus pleuritis
Nocardia and *Actinomyces*	Rheumatoid pleurisy
Subphrenic abscess	Mixed connective tissue disease
Hepatic abscess	Churg–Strauss syndrome
Splenic abscess	Wegener's granulomatosis
Hepatitis	Familial Mediterranean fever
Spontaneous esophageal rupture	*Endocrine Disorders*
Noninfectious Inflammations	Hypothyroidism[c]
Pancreatitis	Ovarian hyperstimulation syndrome
Benign asbestos pleural effusion	*Lymphatic Disorders*
Pulmonary embolism[a]	Malignancy
Radiation therapy	Yellow nail syndrome
Uremic pleurisy	Lymphangioleiomyomatosis
Sarcoidosis	*Movement of Fluid from Abdomen to Pleural Space*
Postcardiac injury syndrome	Pancreatitis
Hemothorax	Pancreatic pseudocyst
Acute respiratory distress syndrome	Meigs' syndrome
	Carcinoma
	Chylous ascites

[a] 10% to 20% may be transudates.
[b] More than 20% are transudates.
[c] Occasional transudates.
Adapted from Sahn SA: The pleura. *Am Rev Respir Dis* 138:184, 1988.

Glucose

A low pleural fluid glucose value is defined as less than 50% of the normal serum value. In this situation, the differential diagnosis includes rheumatoid and lupus effusion, bacterial empyema, malignancy, tuberculosis, and esophageal rupture [32].

Triglyceride and Cholesterol

Chylous pleural effusions are biochemically defined by a triglyceride level greater than 110 mg per dL and the presence of chylomicrons on a pleural fluid lipoprotein electrophoresis [32]. The usual appearance of a chylous effusion is milky, but an effusion with elevated triglycerides may also appear serous. The measurement of a triglyceride level is therefore important. Chylous effusions occur when the thoracic duct has been disrupted somewhere along its course. The most common causes are trauma and malignancy (e.g., lymphoma). A pseudochylous effusion appears grossly milky because of an elevated cholesterol level, but the triglyceride level is normal. Chronic effusions, especially those associated with rheumatoid and tuberculous pleuritis, are characteristically pseudochylous.

Cell Counts and Differential

Although pleural fluid white blood cell count and differential are never diagnostic of any disease, it would be distinctly unusual for an effusion other than one associated with bacterial pneumonia to have a white blood cell count exceeding 50,000 per μL. In an exudative pleural effusion of acute origin, polymorphonuclear leukocytes predominate early, whereas mononuclear cells predominate in chronic exudative effusions. Although pleural fluid lymphocytosis is nonspecific, severe lymphocytosis (>80% of cells) is suggestive of tuberculosis or malignancy. Finally, pleural fluid eosinophilia is nonspecific and most commonly associated with either blood or air in the pleural space.

A red blood cell count of 5,000 to 10,000 cells per μL must be present for fluid to appear pinkish. Grossly bloody effusions containing more than 100,000 red blood cells per mm^3 are most consistent with trauma, malignancy, or pulmonary infarction. To distinguish a traumatic thoracentesis from a preexisting hemothorax, several observations are helpful. First, because a preexisting hemothorax has been defibrinated, it does not form a clot on standing. Second, a hemothorax is suggested when a pleural fluid hematocrit value is 30% or more of the serum hematocrit value.

Cultures and Stains

To maximize the yield from pleural fluid cultures, anaerobic and aerobic cultures should be obtained. Because acid-fast stains may be positive in up to 20% of tuberculous effusions, they should always be performed in addition to Gram-stained smears. By submitting pleural biopsy pieces to pathology and microbiology laboratories, it is possible to diagnose up to 90% of tuberculous effusions percutaneously [24].

Cytology

Malignancies can produce pleural effusions by implantation of malignant cells on the pleura or impairment of lymphatic drainage secondary to tumor obstruction. The tumors that most commonly cause pleural effusions are lung, breast, and lymphoma. Pleural fluid cytology should be performed for an exudative effusion of unknown etiology, using at least 60 to 150 mL fluid [13,14,33]. If initial cytology results are negative and strong clinical suspicion exists, additional samples of fluid can increase the chance of a positive result to approximately 60% to 70%. The addition of a pleural biopsy increases the yield to approximately 80%. In addition to malignancy, cytologic examination can definitively diagnose rheumatoid pleuritis, whose pathognomonic picture consists of slender, elongated macrophages and giant, round, multinucleated macrophages, accompanied by amorphous granular background material.

References

1. Seneff MG, Corwin RW, Gold LH, et al: Complications associated with thoracentesis. *Chest* 89:97–100, 1986.
2. Collins TR, Sahn SA: Thoracocentesis: clinical value, complications, technical problems, and patient experience. *Chest* 91:817–822, 1987.
3. Grogan DR, Irwin RS, Channick R, et al: Complications associated with thoracentesis: a prospective randomized study comparing three different methods. *Arch Intern Med* 150:873–877, 1990.
4. Heffner JE, Brown LK, Barbieri CA: Diagnostic value of tests that discriminate between exudative and transudative pleural effusions. *Chest* 111:970–980, 1997.
5. Romero-Candeira S, Fernandez C, Martin C, et al: Influence of diuretics on the concentration of proteins and other components of pleural transudates in patients with heart failure. *Am J Med* 110:681–686, 2001.
6. Bartter T, Mayo PD, Pratter MR, et al: Lower risk and higher yield for thoracentesis when performed by experimental operators. *Chest* 103:1873–1876, 1993.
7. Colt HG, Brewer N, Barbur E: Evaluation of patient-related and procedure-related factors contributing to pneumothorax following thoracentesis. *Chest* 116:134–138, 1999.
8. Raptopoulos V, Davis LM, Lee G, et al: Factors affecting the development of pneumothorax associated with thoracentesis. *AJR Am J Roentgenol* 156:917–920, 1991.
9. Petersen WG, Zimmerman R: Limited utility of chest radiograph after thoracentesis. *Chest* 117:1038–1042, 2000.
10. Wilson MM, Curley FJ: Gas embolism (Pt I). Venous gas emboli. *J Intensive Care Med* 11:182–204, 1996.
11. Wilson MM, Curley FJ: Gas embolism (Pt II). Arterial gas embolism and decompression sickness. *J Intensive Care Med* 11:261–283, 1996.
12. Rahman NM, Mishra EK, Davies HE, et al: Clinically important factors influencing the diagnostic measurement of pleural fluid pH and glucose. *Am J Respir Crit Care Med* 178:483–490, 2008.
13. Sallach SM, Sallach JA, Vasquez E, et al: Volume of pleural fluid required for diagnosis of pleural malignancy. *Chest* 122:1913–1917, 2002.
14. Abouzgheib W, Bartter T, Dagher H, et al: A prospective study of the volume of pleural fluid required fro accurate diagnosis of malignant pleural effusion. *Chest* 135:999–1001, 2009.
15. Swiderek J, Morcos S, Donthireddy V, et al: Prospective study to determine the volume of pleural fluid required to diagnose malignancy. *Chest* 137:68–73, 2010.
16. Aleman C, Alegre J, Armadans L, et al: The value of chest roentgenography in the diagnosis of pneumothorax after thoracentesis. *Am J Med* 107:340–343, 1999.
17. Capizzi SA, Prakash UB: Chest roentgenography after outpatient thoracentesis. *Mayo Clin Proc* 73:948–950, 1998.
18. Doyle JJ, Hnatiuk OW, Torrington KG, et al: Necessity of routine chest roentgenography after thoracentesis. *Ann Intern Med* 124:816–820, 1996.
19. Terres RT: Thoracentesis. *N Engl J Med* 356:641, 2007.
20. Feller-Kopman D: Therapeutic thoracentesis: the role of ultrasound and pleural manometry. *Curr Opin Pulm Med* 13:312–318, 2007.
21. Duncan DR, Morganthaler TI, Ryu JH, et al: Reducing iatrogenic risk in thoracentesis: establishing best practice via experimental training in a zero-risk environment. *Chest* 135:1315–1320, 2009.
22. Mayo PH, Goltz HR, Tafreshi M, et al: Safety of ultrasound-guided thoracentesis in patients receiving mechanical ventilation. *Chest* 125:1059–1062, 2004.
23. Barnes TW, Morgenthaler TI, Olson EJ, et al: Sonographically guided thoracentesis and rate of pneumothorax. *J Clin Ultrasound* 33:442–446, 2005.
24. Light RW, MacGregor MI, Luchsinger PC, et al: Pleural effusions: the diagnostic separation of transudates and exudates. *Ann Intern Med* 77:507–513, 1972.
25. Gonlugur U, Gonlugur TE: The distinction between transudates and exudates. *J Biomed Sci* 12:985–990, 2005.
26. Garcia-Pachon E, Padilla-Navas I: Urinothorax: a case report and review of the literature with emphasis on biochemical analysis. *Respiration* 71:533–536, 2004.
27. Maskell NV, Gleeson FJO, Davies R: Standard pleural biopsy versus CT-guided cutting-needle biopsy for diagnosis of malignant disease in pleural effusions: a randomized controlled trial. *Lancet* 361:1326–1330, 2003.
28. Burrows CM, Mathews WC, Colt HG: Predicting survival in patients with recurrent symptomatic malignant pleural effusions: an assessment of the prognostic values of physiologic, morphologic, and quality of life measures of extent of disease. *Chest* 117:73–78, 2000.
29. Heffner JE, Nietert PJ, Barbieri C: Pleural fluid pH as a predictor of survival for patients with malignant pleural effusions. *Chest* 117:79–86, 2000.
30. Heffner JE, Nietert PJ, Barbieri C: Pleural fluid pH as a predictor of pleurodesis failure: analysis of primary data. *Chest* 117:87–95, 2000.
31. Heffner JE, Heffner JN, Brown LK: Multilevel and continuous pleural fluid pH likelihood ratios for draining parapneumonic effusions. *Respiration* 72:351–356, 2005.
32. Jimenez Castro D, Diaz Nuevo G, Sueiro A, et al: Pleural fluid parameters identifying complicated parapneumonic effusions. *Respiration* 72:357–364, 2005.
33. Heffner JE, Klein JS: Recent advances in the diagnosis and management of malignant pleural effusions. *Mayo Clin Proc* 83:235–250, 2008.

CHAPTER 11 ■ ARTERIAL PUNCTURE FOR BLOOD GAS ANALYSIS

KIMBERLY A. ROBINSON AND RICHARD S. IRWIN

Analysis of a sample of arterial blood for pH_a, partial arterial carbon dioxide pressure ($PaCO_2$), partial arterial oxygen pressure (PaO_2), bicarbonate, and percentage oxyhemoglobin saturation is performed with an arterial blood gas (ABG) analysis. Because an ABG can be safely and easily obtained and furnishes rapid and accurate information on how well the lungs and kidneys are working, it is the single most useful laboratory test in managing patients with respiratory and metabolic disorders. One should not rely on oximetry alone to evaluate arterial oxygen saturation (SaO_2) fully. Given the shape of the oxyhemoglobin saturation curve, there must be a substantial fall in PaO_2 before SaO_2 is altered to any appreciable degree, and it is not possible to predict the level of PaO_2 and $PaCO_2$ reliably using physical signs such as cyanosis [1] and depth of breathing [2]. In addition, a discrepancy between SaO_2 measured by pulse oximetry and that calculated by the ABG can aid in the diagnosis of carboxyhemoglobinemia and methemoglobinemia.

Unsuspected hypoxemia or hypercapnia (acidemia) can cause a constellation of central nervous system and cardiovascular signs and symptoms. The clinician should have a high index of suspicion that a respiratory or metabolic disorder, or both, is present in patients with these findings and is most appropriately evaluated by obtaining an ABG. Although acute hypercapnia to 70 mm Hg (pH 7.16) and hypoxemia to less than 30 mm Hg may lead to coma and circulatory collapse, chronic exposures permit adaptation with more subtle effects [3]. Thus, the ABG provides the most important way of making a diagnostic assessment regarding the nature and severity of a respiratory or metabolic disturbance and of following its course over time.

Normal range of values for pH_a is 7.35 to 7.45 and for $PaCO_2$, 35 to 45 mm Hg [4]. For PaO_2, the accepted predictive regression equation in nonsmoking, upright, normal individuals aged 40 to 74 years is as follows [5]: $PaO_2 = 108.75 - (0.39 \times \text{age in years})$.

DRAWING THE ARTERIAL BLOOD GAS SPECIMEN

Percutaneous Arterial Puncture

The conventional technique of sampling arterial blood using a glass syringe is described in detail, because it is the standard to which all other methods are compared. The pulsatile arterial vessel is easily palpated in most cases. If a large enough needle is used, entry is apparent as the syringe fills spontaneously by the pressurized arterial flow of blood, without the need for applying a vacuum or using a vacuum-sealed collecting tube. It is logical to preferentially enter arteries that have the best collateral circulation so that if spasm or clotting occurs, the distal tissue is not deprived of perfusion. Logic also dictates that puncture of a site where the artery is superficial is preferable, because entry is easiest and pain is minimized. The radial artery best fulfills the criteria discussed earlier in the chapter; it is very superficial at the wrist, and the collateral circulation to the hand by the ulnar artery provides sufficient collateral blood flow in approximately 92% of normal adults in the event of total occlusion of the radial artery [6].

The absence of a report of total occlusion of the radial artery after puncture for ABG in an adult with normal hemostasis and the absence of significant peripheral vascular disease attest to the safety of the percutaneous arterial puncture. It also suggests that determining the adequacy of collateral flow to the superficial palmar arch by Allen's test [7], a modification of Allen's test [8] (see Chapter 3), or Doppler ultrasound [6] before puncture is not routinely necessary in patients with normal hemostasis and the absence of significant peripheral vascular disease. If radial artery sites are not accessible, dorsalis pedis, posterior tibial, superficial temporal (in infants), brachial, and femoral arteries are alternatives (see Chapter 3).

Contraindications

Brachial and especially femoral artery punctures are not advised in patients with abnormal hemostatic mechanisms because adequate vessel tamponade may not be possible in that these vessels are not located superficially, risking greater chance of complications [9]. If frequent sampling of superficial arteries in the same situation becomes necessary, arterial cannulation is recommended (see Chapter 3). Moreover, any vessel that has been reconstructed surgically should not be punctured for fear of forming a pseudoaneurysm, compromising the integrity of an artificial graft site or seeding the foreign body that could become a nidus for infection. This should also include avoidance of a femoral arterial puncture on the same side as a transplanted kidney.

The conventional recommended radial artery technique is as follows:

1. Put on protective gloves and sit in a comfortable position facing the patient.
2. With the patient's hand supinated and the wrist slightly hyperextended, palpate the radial artery. Severe hyperextension may obliterate the pulse.
3. Cleanse the skin with an alcohol swab.
4. With a 25-gauge needle, inject enough 1% lidocaine intradermally to raise a small wheal at the point where the skin puncture is to be made. The local anesthetic makes subsequent needle puncture with a 22-gauge needle less painful and often painless [10]. If local anesthesia is not given, however, the potential pain and anxiety, if associated with breath holding, may cause substantial blood gas changes. Thirty-five seconds of breath holding in normal subjects has been associated with a fall in PaO_2 of 50 mm Hg and a pH of 0.07 and a rise in $PaCO_2$ of 10 mm Hg [11].

5. Attach a needle no smaller than 22 gauge to a glass syringe that can accept 5 mL blood.
6. Wet the needle and syringe with a sodium heparin solution (1,000 units per mL). Express all excess solution.
7. With the needle, enter the artery at an angle of approximately 30 degrees to the long axis of the vessel. This insertion angle minimizes the pain associated with unintentional contact with the periosteum below the artery.
8. As soon as the artery is entered, blood appears in the syringe. Allow the arterial pressure to fill the syringe with at least 3 mL of blood. Do not apply suction by pulling on the syringe plunger.
9. Immediately after obtaining the specimen, expel any tiny air bubbles to ensure that the specimen will be anaerobic and then cap the syringe.
10. Roll the blood sample between both palms for 5 to 15 seconds to mix the heparin and blood. Apply pressure to the puncture site for 5 minutes or longer, depending on the presence of a coagulopathy. If the arterial sample was obtained from the brachial artery, compress this vessel so that the radial pulse cannot be palpated.
11. Immerse the capped sample in a bag of ice and water (slush) and immediately transport it to the blood gas laboratory.
12. Write on the ABG slip the time of drawing and the conditions under which it was drawn (e.g., fraction of inspired oxygen, ventilator settings, and the patient's position and temperature).

Deviations from these recommended techniques may introduce the following errors:

1. The syringe material may influence the results of PaO_2 [12–14]. The most accurate results have been consistently obtained using a glass syringe. If plastic is used, the following errors may occur: (a) falsely low PaO_2 values may be obtained because plastic allows oxygen to diffuse to the atmosphere from the sample whenever the PO_2 exceeds 221 mm Hg; (b) plastic syringes with high surface area to volume ratios (e.g., 1-mL tuberculin syringes) worsen gas permeability errors as compared to standard 3-mL syringes. For this reason, butterfly infusion kits with their long, thin tubing should not be used [15]; (c) plastic syringes tenaciously retain air bubbles, and extra effort is necessary to remove them [13]; (d) plastic impedes smooth movement of the plunger that can have an impact on the clinician's confidence that arterial rather than venous blood has been sampled.
2. If suction is applied for plunger assistance, gas bubbles may be pulled out of the solution. If they are expelled, measured PaO_2 and $PaCO_2$ tensions may be falsely lowered [16].
3. Although liquid heparin is a weak acid, plasma pH is not altered because it is well buffered by hemoglobin. Mixing liquid heparin with blood dilutes dissolved gasses, shifting their concentration to that of heparin (PO_2 approximately 150 mm Hg and PCO_2 less than 0.3 mm Hg at sea level and room temperature). The degree of alteration depends on the amount of heparin relative to blood and the hemoglobin concentration [16–19]. The dilutional error is no greater than 4% if a glass syringe and 22-gauge needle are only wetted with approximately 0.2 mL heparin and 3 to 5 mL blood collected. Any less heparin risks a clotted and unusable sample. Dilutional errors are avoided with the use of crystalline heparin, but this preparation is difficult to mix and increases the risk of clotting the specimen.
4. If an ABG specimen is not analyzed within 1 minute of being drawn or not immediately cooled to 2°C, the PO_2 and pH fall and PCO_2 rises because of cellular respiration and consumption of oxygen by leukocytes, platelets, and reticulocytes [20]. This is of particular concern in patients with leukemia (leukocytes greater than 40×10^9 per L) or thrombocytosis ($1,000 \times 10^9$ per L) [21].
5. Unintentional sampling of a vein normally causes a falsely low PaO_2. A venous PO_2 greater than 50 mm Hg can be obtained if the sampling area is warmed. The PO_2 of "arterialized" venous blood can approximate PaO_2 when blood flow is greatly increased by warming, compromising the time for peripheral oxygen extraction.

Complications

Using the conventional radial artery technique described earlier in the chapter, complications are unusual. They include a rare vasovagal episode, local pain, and limited hematomas. An expanding aneurysm of the radial artery and reflex sympathetic dystrophy [22] have been reported even more rarely after frequent punctures [23].

MEASUREMENTS FROM THE ARTERIAL BLOOD GAS SPECIMEN

Although pH, PCO_2, PO_2, bicarbonate, and SaO_2 are all usually reported, it is important to understand that the bicarbonate and SaO_2 are calculated, not directly measured. Although the calculated bicarbonate value is as reliable as the measured pH and PCO_2 values, given their immutable relationship through the Henderson–Hasselbalch equation, the calculated SaO_2 is often inaccurate because of the many variables that cannot be corrected (e.g., 2,3-diphosphoglycerate and binding characteristics of hemoglobin).

The patient in the intensive care unit often requires serial ABG measurements to follow the progression of critical illness and guide therapy. Although it is understandable to interpret fluctuations in the ABG data as a sign of the patient's condition worsening or improving, depending on the trend, it is also important to appreciate that modest fluctuations may be due to deviations in the collection of the ABG specimen. Therefore, routine monitoring of ABGs without an associated change in patient status may not be warranted and may lead to an unproductive, lengthy, and expensive search for the cause.

When electrolytes and other blood values are measured from the unused portion of an ABG sample, clinicians should be aware of the following: Traditional liquid and crystalline heparins for ABG sampling are sodium-heparin salts that artificially increase plasma sodium concentrations. Calcium and potassium bind to the negatively charged heparins, spuriously lowering their values. Lithium or electrolyte-balanced heparin is now available that contains physiologic concentrations of sodium and potassium that should be used whenever sodium, potassium, ionized magnesium, ionized calcium, chloride, glucose, and lactate are measured in an ABG specimen [24–26]. Although lithium or electrolyte-balanced heparin minimizes the errors in electrolyte concentrations, dilutional error may still exist if excessive amounts are used for anticoagulation.

By convention, ABG specimens are analyzed at 37°C. Although no studies have demonstrated that correction for the patient's temperature is clinically necessary, blood gases drawn at temperatures greater than 39°C should probably be corrected for temperature [27]. Because the solubility of oxygen and carbon dioxide increases as blood is cooled to 37°C, the hyperthermic patient is more acidotic and less hypoxemic than uncorrected values indicate. Therefore, for each 1°C that the patient's temperature is greater than 37°C, PaO_2 should be increased 7.2%, $PaCO_2$ increased 4.4%, and pH decreased 0.015. Temperature correction for pH and $PaCO_2$ in the hypothermic patient is controversial. Although correction back to the patient's temperature may result in better preservation of cerebral blood flow, intracranial pressure can be adversely affected in selected populations. The reader is referred elsewhere for more information [28]. However, PaO_2 values must be corrected for temperature lest significant hypoxemia be overlooked. The PaO_2 at 37°C is decreased by 7.2% for each degree that the patient's temperature is less than 37°C.

It should also be noted that transport of an ABG specimen to the laboratory via a pneumatic tube system can result in alterations in PaO_2 secondary to contamination with room air. This effect is presumed to be due to pressure changes within the pneumatic tube system because the use of pressure-tight transport containers obliterates the effect [29]. If a pneumatic tube system is to be used, one must be sure that all air bubbles are carefully expelled from the ABG specimen and that a pressure-tight transport container is used. Otherwise, it may be best to hand-carry samples to the laboratory [29–31].

PHYSICIAN RESPONSIBILITY

Even when the ABG values of pH, PCO_2, PO_2, and bicarbonate appear consistently reliable, the clinician should periodically check the accuracy of the blood gas samples because the bicarbonate is calculated, not directly measured. Aliquots of arterial blood can be sent simultaneously for ABG analysis and to the chemistry laboratory for a total (T) CO_2 content. Accuracy of the blood gas laboratory's values can be checked using Henderson's simple mathematical equation that is a rearrangement of the Henderson–Hasselbalch equation: $[H^+] = 25 \times PaCO_2/HCO_3^-$. $[H^+]$ is solved by using the pH measured in the blood gas laboratory (Table 11.1). Measured arterial TCO_2 should be close to the calculated bicarbonate value. Venous TCO_2 should not be used in this exercise because it is often and normally up to 5 mEq per L greater than arterial TCO_2.

TABLE 11.1

RELATION BETWEEN [H+] AND PH OVER A NORMAL RANGE OF PH VALUES[a]

pH	$[H^+]$ (nM/L)
7.36	44
7.37	43
7.38	42
7.39	41
7.40	40
—	
7.41	39
7.42	38
7.43	37
7.44	36

[a]Note that pH 7.40 corresponds to hydrogen ion concentration of 40 nM/L and that, over the small range shown, each deviation in pH of 0.01 units corresponds to opposite deviation in $[H^+]$ of 1 nM/L. For pH values between 7.28 and 7.45, $[H^+]$ calculated empirically in this fashion agrees with the actual value obtained by means of logarithms to the nearest nM/L (nearest 0.01 pH unit). However, in the extremes of pH values, less than pH 7.28 and greater than pH 7.45, the estimated $[H^+]$ is always lower than the actual value, with the discrepancy reaching 11% at pH 7.10 and 5% at pH 7.50. Modified from Kassirer J, Bleich H: Rapid estimation of plasma carbon dioxide tension from pH and total carbon dioxide content. *N Engl J Med* 171:1067, 1965.

ALTERNATIVES

Many situations may arise whereby arterial blood samples are not available. For example, severe peripheral vascular disease makes radial arterial puncture difficult, or the patient refuses arterial blood sampling or cannulation. In general, in the absence of circulatory failure or limb ischemia, central and peripheral venous blood may substitute for arterial when monitoring acid–base and ventilatory status. In hemodynamically stable patients, pH_a is, on average, 0.03 units higher than central venous pH (pH_{cv}) and $PaCO_2$ is lower than central venous carbon dioxide ($P_{cv}CO_2$) by 5 mm Hg [32], and changes in each are tightly correlated [33]. Regression analysis reveals $pH_a = (1.027 \times pH_{cv}) - 0.156$ and $PaCO_2 = (0.754 \times P_{cv}CO_2) + 2.75$. In shock, the accentuated discrepancy may be due to increased carbon dioxide generated by the buffering of acids in conditions characterized by increased lactic acid production.

It must be made clear that in the absence of warming a sampling area to collect "arterialized" venous blood, an arterial sample is still necessary for evaluation of accurate oxygenation status for precise measurements of PO_2 and alveolar–arterial oxygen gradient determination. Once the oxygenation and acid–base status have been identified, pulse oximetry can be used to follow trends in SaO_2 in stable or improving patients because serial ABGs are costly and risk vessel injury with repeated arterial punctures.

Some progress has been made in the area of noninvasive measurement of gas exchange. This includes oximetry, transcutaneous PO_2 and PCO_2 ($P_{tc}CO_2$) measurement, end-tidal CO_2, and indwelling intravascular electrode systems. Measurement of end-tidal CO_2 requires a closed system of gas collection (i.e., ventilator circuit or noninvasive mask ventilation) that is not always possible. Thus, there has been increased focus on transcutaneous measurement of carbon dioxide tension. These systems require localized heating of the skin by a heating element to increase local perfusion. Studies have suggested improvement in the ability of transcutaneous systems to accurately assess SpO_2 and $P_{tc}CO_2$ in critically ill patients as long as the $PaCO_2$ is less than 56 mm Hg [34,35].

POINT-OF-CARE TESTING

Blood gas analysis is now routinely performed at the bedside with point-of-care testing (POCT) devices. Advantages of POCT include convenience and rapid turnaround time, theoretically improving the quality of patient care. With regard to pH, PO_2, and PCO_2, several studies have verified a high correlation between POCT results and conventional analysis methods [36,37].

References

1. Comoroe J, Botelho S: The unreliability of cyanosis in the recognition of arterial anoxemia. *Am J Med Sci* 214:1, 1947.
2. Mithoefer J, Bossman O, Thibeault D, et al: The clinical estimation of alveolar ventilation. *Am Rev Respir Dis* 98:868, 1968.
3. Weiss E, Faling L, Mintz S, et al: Acute respiratory failure in chronic obstructive pulmonary disease I. Pathophysiology. *Disease-a-Month* 1, October 1969.
4. Raffin T: Indications for arterial blood gas analysis. *Ann Intern Med* 105:390, 1986.
5. Cerveri I, Zoia M, Fanfulla F, et al: Reference values of arterial oxygen tension in the middle-aged and elderly. *Am J Respir Crit Care Med* 152:934, 1995.
6. Felix WJ, Sigel B, Popky G: Doppler ultrasound in the diagnosis of peripheral vascular disease. *Semin Roentgenol* 4:315, 1975.

7. Allen E: Thromboangiitis obliterans: methods of diagnosis of chronic occlusive arterial lesions distal to the wrist, with illustrative cases. *Am J Med Sci* 178:237, 1929.
8. Bedford R: Radial arterial function following percutaneous cannulation with 18- and 20-gauge catheters. *Anesthesiology* 47:37, 1977.
9. Macon WI, Futrell J: Median-nerve neuropathy after percutaneous puncture of the brachial artery in patients receiving anticoagulants. *N Engl J Med* 288:1396, 1973.
10. Giner J, Casan P, Belda J, et al: Pain during arterial puncture. *Chest* 110:1143, 1996.
11. Sasse S, Berry R, Nguyen T: Arterial blood gas changes during breath-holding from functional residual capacity. *Chest* 110:958, 1996.
12. Janis K, Gletcher G: Oxygen tension measurements in small samples: sampling errors. *Am Rev Respir Dis* 106:914, 1972.
13. Winkler J, Huntington C, Wells D, et al: Influence of syringe material on arterial blood gas determinations. *Chest* 66:518, 1974.
14. Ansel G, Douce F: Effects of syringe material and needle size on the minimum plunger-displacement pressure of arterial blood gas syringes. *Respir Care* 27:147, 1982.
15. Thelin O, Karanth S, Pourcyrous M, et al: Overestimation of neonatal Po_2 by collection of arterial blood gas values with the butterfly infusion set. *J Perinatol* 13:65, 1993.
16. Adams A, Morgan-Hughes J, Sykes M: pH and blood gas analysis: methods of measurement and sources of error using electrode systems. *Anaesthesia* 22:575, 1967.
17. Bloom S, Canzanello V, Strom J, et al: Spurious assessment of acid-base status due to dilutional effect of heparin. *Am J Med* 79:528, 1985.
18. Hansen J, Simmons D: A systematic error in the determination of blood Pco_2. *Am Rev Respir Dis* 115:1061, 1977.
19. Bloom S, Canzanello V, Strom J, et al: Spurious assessment of acid-base status due to dilutional effect of heparin. *Am J Med* 79:528, 1985.
20. Eldridge F, Fretwell L: Change in oxygen tension of shed blood at various temperatures. *J Appl Physiol* 20:790, 1965.
21. Schmidt C, Mullert-Plathe O: Stability of Po_2, Pco_2 and pH in heparinized whole blood samples: influence of storage temperature with regard to leukocyte count and syringe material. *Eur J Clin Chem Clin Biochem* 30:767, 1992.
22. Criscuolo C, Nepper G, Buchalter S: Reflex sympathetic dystrophy following arterial blood gas sampling in the intensive care unit. *Chest* 108:578, 1995.
23. Mathieu A, Dalton B, Fischer J, et al: Expanding aneurysm of the radial artery after frequent puncture. *Anesthesiology* 38:401, 1973.
24. Burnett R, Covington A, Fogh-Anderson N: Approved IFCC recommendations on whole blood sampling, transport and storage for simultaneous determination of pH, blood gases and electrolytes. *Eur J Clin Chem Clin Biochem* 33:247, 1995.
25. Lyon M, Bremner D, Laha T, et al: Specific heparin preparations interfere with the simultaneous measurement of ionized magnesium and ionized calcium. *Clin Biochem* 28:79, 1995.
26. Toffaletti J, Thompson T: Effects of blended lithium-zinc heparin on ionized calcium and general clinical chemistry tests. *Clin Chem* 41:328, 1995.
27. Curley F, Irwin R: Disorders of temperature control, I. hyperthermia. *J Intensive Care Med* 1:5, 1986.
28. Kollmar R, Georgiadis D, Schwab S: Alpha-stat versus pH-stat guided ventilation in patients with large ischemic stroke treated by hypothermia. *Neurocrit Care* 10:173, 2009.
29. Collinson PO, John CM, Gaze DC, et al: Changes in blood gas samples produced by a pneumatic tube system. *J Clin Pathol* 55(2):105, 2002.
30. Astles JR, Lubarsky D, Loun B, et al: Pneumatic transport exacerbates interference of room air contamination in blood gas samples. *Arch Pathol Lab Med* 120(7):642, 1996.
31. Lu JY, Kao JT, Chien TI, et al: Effects of air bubbles and tube transportation on blood oxygen tension in arterial blood gas analysis. *J Formos Med Assoc* 102(4):246, 2003.
32. Adrogue H, Rashad M, Gorin A, et al: Assessing acid-base status in circulatory failure; differences between arterial and central venous blood. *N Engl J Med* 320:1312, 1989.
33. Philips B, Peretz D: A comparison of central venous and arterial blood gas values in the critically ill. *Ann Intern Med* 70:745, 1969.
34. Senn O, Clarenbach CF, Kaplan V, et al: Monitoring carbon dioxide tension and arterial oxygen saturation by a single earlobe sensor in patients with critical illness or sleep apnea. *Chest* 128:1291, 2005.
35. Cuvelier A, Grigoriu B, Molano LC, et al: Limitations of transcutaneous carbon dioxide measurements for assessing long-term mechanical ventilation. *Chest* 127:1744, 2005.
36. Sediame S, Zerah-Lancner F, d'Ortho MP, et al: Accuracy of the i-STAT bedside blood gas analyser. *Eur Respir J* 14(1):214, 1999.
37. Kampelmacher MJ, van Kesteren RG, Winckers EK: Instrumental variability of respiratory blood gases among different blood analysers in different laboratories. *Eur Respir J* 10(6):1341, 1997.

CHAPTER 12 ■ TRACHEOSTOMY

SCOTT E. KOPEC AND TIMOTHY A. EMHOFF

Although reports of performing tracheostomy date back to the first century BC [1], it was not performed regularly until the 1800s when used by Trousseau and Bretonneau in the management of diphtheria. In the early 1900s, this procedure was used to treat difficult cases of respiratory paralysis from poliomyelitis. Largely because of improvements in tubes and advances in clinical care, endotracheal intubation has become the treatment of choice for short-term airway management.

Although tracheostomy is occasionally required in critically ill and injured patients who cannot be intubated for various reasons (e.g., cervical spine injury, upper airway obstruction, laryngeal injury, and anatomic considerations), the most common use of this procedure today is to provide long-term access to the airway in patients who are dependent on mechanical ventilation. With improvements in critical care medicine over the past 30 years, more patients are surviving the initial episodes of acute respiratory failure, trauma, and extensive surgeries and are requiring prolonged periods of mechanical ventilation. It is now common practice to expeditiously convert these patients from translaryngeal intubation to tracheostomy. Tracheostomy is becoming a very common procedure in the intensive care unit (ICU). The prevalence of tracheostomies in ICU patients ranges from 8% to more than 30% [2,3].

In this chapter we review the indications, contraindications, complications, and techniques associated with tracheostomy. We also discuss the timing of converting an orally intubated patient to tracheostomy.

INDICATIONS

The indications for tracheostomy can be divided into three general categories: (i) to bypass obstruction of the upper airway, (ii) to provide an avenue for tracheal toilet and removal of retained secretions, and (iii) to provide a means for ventilatory support. These indications are summarized in Table 12.1 [4–10].

Anticipated prolonged ventilatory support, especially patients receiving mechanical ventilation via translaryngeal intubation, is the most common indication for placing a tracheostomy in the ICU. There are several advantages and disadvantages of both translaryngeal intubation and tracheostomy in patients requiring prolonged ventilator support,

TABLE 12.1

INDICATIONS FOR TRACHEOSTOMY [4–10]

Upper airway obstruction
- Laryngeal dysfunction: Vocal cord paralysis
- Trauma: Upper airway obstruction due to hemorrhage, edema, or crush injury; unstable mandibular fractures; injury to the larynx; cervical spine injuries
- Burns and corrosives: Hot smoke, caustic gases, corrosives
- Foreign bodies
- Congenital anomalies: Stenosis of the glottic or subglottic area
- Infections: Croup, epiglottitis, Ludwig's angina, deep neck space infections
- Neoplasms: Laryngeal cancer
- Postoperative: Surgeries of the base of the tongue and hypopharynx; rigid fixation of the mandibular
- Obstructive sleep apnea

Tracheal toilet
- Inability to clear secretions: Generalized weakness, altered mental status, excess secretions
- Neuromuscular disease
- Ventilatory support: Prolonged or chronic

Kremer B, Botos-Kremer A, Eckel H, et al: Indications, complications, and surgical technique for pediatric tracheostomies. *J Pediatr Surg* 37:1556, 2002.
Bjure J: Tracheotomy: A satisfactory method in the treatment of acute epiglottis. A clinical and functional follow-up study. *Int J Pediatr Otorhinolaryngol* 3:37, 1981.
Hanline MH Jr: Tracheotomy in upper airway obstruction. *South Med J* 74:899, 1981.
Taicher S, Givol M, Peleg M, et al: Changing indications for tracheostomy in maxillofacial trauma. *J Oral Maxillofac Surg* 54:292, 1996.
Guilleminault C, Simmons FB, Motta J, et al: Obstructive sleep apnea syndrome and tracheostomy. *Arch Intern Med* 141:985, 1981.
Burwell C, Robin E, Whaley R, et al: Extreme obesity associated with alveolar hypoventilation. *Am J Med* 141:985, 1981.
Yung MW, Snowdon SL: Respiratory resistance of tracheostomy tubes. *Arch Otolaryngol* 110:591, 1984.

and these are summarized in Table 12.2 [11–13]. Most authors feel that when the procedure is performed by a skilled surgical group, the potential benefits of tracheostomy over translaryngeal intubation for most patients justify the application despite its potential risks. However, there are no detailed clinical trials consistently confirming the advantages of tracheostomy in patients requiring prolonged mechanical ventilation. In a retrospective and a nonrandomized study, there were conflicting data regarding mortality in patients with respiratory failure of more than 1 week with regard to receiving a tracheostomy or continuing with an endotracheal tube [2,3].

CONTRAINDICATIONS

There are no absolute contraindications to tracheostomy. Relative complications include uncorrected coagulopathy, high levels of ventilator support (i.e., high levels of positive

TABLE 12.2

ADVANTAGES AND DISADVANTAGES OF INTUBATION AND TRACHEOSTOMY [11–13]

Advantages	Disadvantages
Translaryngeal intubation	
Reliable airway during urgent intubation	Bacterial airway colonization
Avoidance of surgical complications	Inadvertent extubation
Lower initial cost	Laryngeal injury
	Tracheal stenosis
	Purulent sinusitis (nasotracheal intubations)
	Patient discomfort
Tracheostomies	
Avoids direct injury to the larynx	Complications (see Table 12.3)
Facilitates nursing care	Bacterial airway colonization
Enhances patient mobility	Cost
More secure airway	Surgical scar
Improved patient comfort	Tracheal and stomal stenosis
Permits speech	
Provides psychologic benefit	
More rapid weaning from mechanical ventilation	
Better oral hygiene	
Decreased risk of nosocomial pneumonia	

end-expiratory pressure [PEEP]), and abnormal anatomy of the upper airway. However, a prospective cohort study has demonstrated that percutaneous tracheostomy can be safely preformed in patients with refractory coagulopathy from liver disease [14]. Morbidly obese patients with body mass index greater than 30 kg per m^2 also appear to be at higher risk for complications with both open tracheostomy [15] and percutaneous tracheostomy [16]. In patients with severe brain injury, percutaneous tracheostomy can be safely performed without significantly further increasing intracranial pressure [17].

Certain conditions warrant special attention before anesthesia and surgery. In patients undergoing conversion from translaryngeal intubation to a tracheostomy for prolonged ventilatory support, the procedure should be viewed as an elective or semielective procedure. Therefore, the patient should be as medically stable as possible, and all attempts should be made to correct the existing coagulopathies, including uremia. Ventilator settings should be reduced to where tube exchange during the tracheostomy is safe because during the exchange positive pressure is temporarily lost for some period of time. If not already on 5 cm H_2O of PEEP, placing the patient supine and using 5 or 7.5 cm H_2O of PEEP temporarily is a good test to decide if the patient will tolerate the exchange. For obvious reasons, emergent tracheostomies for upper airway obstruction may need to be preformed when the patient is unstable or has a coagulopathy.

TIMING OF TRACHEOSTOMY

When to perform a tracheostomy on an intubated, critically ill patient has continued to remain very controversial. Older recommendations range from performing a tracheostomy after just 3 days of translaryngeal intubation due to the risk of mucosal damage to the larynx and vocal cords [18] to more than 21 days on the basis of reported high complication rates of open tracheostomies [19]. In 2003, Heffner recommended a more up-to-date approach regarding the timing of converting an intubated patient to a tracheostomy [11]. This recommendation takes into account the very low mortality and morbidity associated with placing a tracheostomy, plus the advantages and disadvantages of both translaryngeal intubation and tracheostomy. In summary, if a patient remains ventilator dependent after a week of translaryngeal intubation, a tracheostomy can be considered. Whether to perform the procedure or not should depend on the anticipated duration of ventilatory support and the benefits of a tracheostomy in that specific patient. If the patient appears to have minimal barriers to weaning and appears likely to be successfully weaned and extubated within 7 days, tracheostomy should be avoided. In those patients whom it appears unlikely that they will successfully be weaned and extubated in 7 days, tracheostomy should be strongly considered. For those patients whose ability to wean and be extubated is unclear, the patient's status should be readdressed daily [11].

Over the past several years there has been momentum to perform a tracheostomy early, that is, after 1 week of mechanical ventilation. Fueling this was a meta-analysis [20], which suggested advantages to "early tracheostomy," performed within 7 days of translaryngeal intubation over a "late tracheostomy" (>7 days) in critically ill patients requiring mechanical ventilation. The meta-analysis combined five prospective studies and included 406 patients and suggested that early tracheostomy resulted in a decrease in length of ICU stay by an average of 15.3 days and a decrease in duration of mechanical ventilation by an average of 8.5 days [20]. Potential reasons for the decrease in duration of mechanical ventilation include easier weaning due to less dead space, less resistance, and less obstruction due to mucus plugging in patients with tracheostomies. There was no significant increase in hospital mortality or risk of hospital-acquired pneumonia. However, there are obvious limitations to the meta-analysis. Since this meta-analysis, several other studies have revealed conflicting data. Table 12.3 summarizes several studies comparing early versus late tracheostomy [20–28]. In summary, it remains unclear if early tracheostomy has any impact on mortality, length of ICU stay, days on mechanical ventilation, or ventilatory-associated pneumonia. Until more definitive data are available, Heffner's 2003 recommendations [11] appear to make the most sense for most medical and surgical patients on prolonged mechanical ventilation.

TABLE 12.3

STUDIES EVALUATING EARLY (≤7 DAYS) VERSUS LATE (>7 DAYS) TRACHEOSTOMY

Study	No. of patients	Study type	Patient type	Results
Rodriquez et al., 1990	106	Prospective Randomized	Surg	Decreased ICU LOS and MV days with early tracheostomy
Sugarman et al., 1997	127	Prospective Randomized	Surg, Trauma	No difference in mortality, VAP rate, or ICU LOS
Brook et al., 2000	90	Prospective Observational	Med, Surg	Decreased MV days and hospital costs
Rumbak et al., 2004	120	Prospective	Med	Decreased mortality, VAP 2004 rate, ICU LOS, and MV days with early trach
Griffiths et al., 2005		Meta-analysis	Med, Surg	Decreased MV days and ICU LOS with early trach, no difference in mortality or VAP rate
Scales et al., 2008	10,927	Retrospective Cohort	Med, Surg	Decreased mortality, MV days, ICU LOS with early trach
Blot et al., 2008	123	Prospective Randomized	Med, Surg	No difference in mortality, VAP rate, or ICU LOS
Durbin et al., 2010	641	Meta-analysis	Med, Surg	No difference in mortality, VAP rate, or MV days
Terragni et al., 2010	419	Prospective Randomized	Med, Surg	No difference in VAP rate ICU LOS or mortality, but decreased MV days

LOS, length of stay; Med, medicine patients; MV, mechanical ventilation; Surg, surgery patients; VAP, ventilator-associated pneumonia.

Early tracheostomy may be beneficial in some specific instances. Patients with blunt, multiple-organ trauma have a shorter duration of mechanical ventilation, fewer episodes of nosocomial pneumonia [29], and a significant reduction in hospital costs [30] when the tracheostomy is performed within 1 week of their injuries. Similar benefits have been reported in patients with head trauma and poor Glasgow Coma Score [31–33], acute spine trauma [34,35], and thermal injury [36] if a tracheostomy is performed within a week after the injury. Also, patients with facial injuries may require early tracheostomy to allow or facilitate facial fracture surgery, fixation, and immobilization.

PROCEDURES

Emergency Tracheostomy

Emergency tracheostomy is a moderately difficult procedure requiring training and skill, experience, adequate assistance, time, lighting, and proper equipment and instrumentation. When time is short, the patient is uncooperative, anatomy is distorted, and the aforementioned requirements are not met, tracheostomy can be very hazardous. Emergency tracheostomy comprises significant risks to nearby neurovascular structures, particularly in small children in whom the trachea is small and not well defined. The risk of complications from emergency tracheostomy is two to five times higher than for elective tracheostomy [37,38]. Nonetheless, there are occasional indications for emergency tracheostomy [39], including transected trachea, anterior neck trauma with crushed larynx [40], severe facial trauma, acute laryngeal obstruction or near-impending obstruction, and pediatric (younger than 12 years) patients requiring an emergency surgical airway in whom an cricothyrotomy is generally not advised. In emergency situations when there is inadequate time or personnel to perform an emergency tracheostomy, a cricothyrotomy may be a more efficient and expedient manner to provide an airway.

Cricothyrotomy

Cricothyrotomy (cricothyroidotomy) was condemned in Jackson's [41] 1921 article on high tracheostomies because of excessive complications, particularly subglottic stenoses [42]. He emphasized the importance of the cricoid cartilage as an encircling support for the larynx and trachea. However, a favorable report of 655 cricothyrotomies, with complication rates of only 6.1% and no cases of subglottic stenoses [43], prompted reevaluation of cricothyrotomy for elective and emergency airway access. Further reports emphasized the advantages of cricothyrotomy over tracheostomy. These include technical simplicity, speed of performance, low complication rate [43–47], suitability as a bedside procedure, usefulness for isolation of the airway for median sternotomy [46,48], radical neck dissection [49], lack of need to hyperextend the neck, and formation of a smaller scar. Also, because cricothyrotomy results in less encroachment on the mediastinum, there is less chance of esophageal injury and virtually no chance of pneumothorax or tracheal arterial fistula [47]. Despite these considerations, many authorities currently recommend that cricothyrotomy should be used as an elective long-term method of airway access only in highly selective patients [41,43,49–51]. Use of cricothyrotomy in the emergency setting, particularly for managing trauma, is not controversial [52–54]. Emergency cricothyrotomy is useful because it requires a small number of instruments and less training than tracheostomy and can be performed quickly as indicated as a means of controlling the airway in an emergency when oral or nasotracheal intubation is nonsuccessful or contraindicated. The cricothyroid membrane is higher in the neck than the tracheal rings and therefore closer to the surface and more accessible. In emergency situations, translaryngeal intubations fail because of massive oral or nasal hemorrhage or regurgitation, structural deformities of the upper airway, muscle spasm and clenched teeth, and obstruction by foreign body through the upper airway [52]. Cricothyrotomy finds its greatest use in trauma management, axial or suspected cervical spine injury, alone or in combination with severe facial trauma, where nasotracheal and orotracheal intubation is both difficult and hazardous. Thus cricothyrotomy has an important role in emergency airway management [53].

Use and Contraindications

Cricothyrotomy should not be used to manage airway obstruction that occurred immediately after endotracheal extubation because the obstruction may be found below the larynx [41,43,53]; likewise, with primary laryngeal trauma or diseases such as tumor or an infection, cricothyrotomy may prove to be useless. It is contraindicated in infants and children younger than 10 to 12 years under all circumstances because stenosis and even transection are possible [53]. In this age group, percutaneous transtracheal ventilation may be a temporizing procedure until the tracheostomy can be performed.

Anatomy

The cricothyroid space is no larger than 7 to 9 mm in its vertical dimension, smaller than the outside diameter of most tracheostomy tubes (outside diameter 10 mm). The cricothyroid artery runs across the midline in the upper portion, and the membrane is vertically in the midline. The anterior superior edge of the thyroid cartilage is the laryngeal prominence. The cricothyroid membrane is approximately 2 to 3 cm below the laryngeal prominence and can be identified as an indentation immediately below the thyroid cartilage. The lower border of the cricothyroid membrane is the cricoid cartilage [47,48,52,55]. A description of the cricothyrotomy procedure is contained in standard surgical texts.

Complications

The report of incidents of short- and long-term complications of cricothyrotomy ranges from 6.1% [43] for procedures performed in elective, well-controlled, carefully selected cases to greater than 50% [53,56] for procedures performed under emergency or other suboptimal conditions. The incidence of subglottic stenosis after cricothyrotomy is 2% to 3% [42,44]. This major complication occurs at the tracheostomy or cricothyrotomy site, but not at the cuff site [57]. Necrosis of cartilage due to iatrogenic injury to the cricoid cartilage or pressure from the tube on the cartilage may play a role [54]. Possible reasons that subglottic stenoses may occur more commonly with cricothyrotomy than with tracheostomy are as follows: the larynx is the narrowest part of the laryngotracheal airway; subglottic tissues, especially in children, are intolerant of contact; and division of the cricothyroid membrane and cricoid cartilage destroy the only complete rings supporting the airway [42]. Furthermore, the range of tube sizes is limited due to the rigidity of the surrounding structures (cricoid and thyroid cartilage), and the curvature of the tracheostomy tube at this level may obstruct the airway due to potential posterior membrane impingement [58]. Prior laryngotracheal injury, as with prolonged translaryngeal intubation, is a major risk factor for the development of subglottic stenosis after cricothyrotomy [42,44].

The association of cricothyrotomy with these possible complications leads most authorities to consider replacing a cricothyrotomy within 48 to 72 hours with a standardized tracheostomy procedure. This is commonly done by an open surgical tracheostomy (OST), which occurs between the second and third tracheal rings, as compared to a percutaneous dilational tracheostomy (PDT), which usually occurs between the cricoid cartilage and the first ring or the first and second rings [58].

TRACHEOSTOMY PROCEDURES IN THE INTENSIVE CARE UNIT

Tracheostomy is one of the most common surgical ICU procedures and is commonly performed for weaning purposes and for airway protection for patients requiring prolonged ventilation. There are two major techniques for tracheostomy, open and percutaneous, with various modifications of each. The different surgical tracheostomy techniques are well described in the references for this chapter [59–62].

Open Surgical Tracheostomy

In OST the patient's neck is extended and the surgical field is exposed from the chin to several inches below the clavicle. This area is prepped and draped, and prophylactic antibiotics are administered at the discretion of the surgeon. A vertical or horizontal incision may be used; however, a horizontal incision will provide a better cosmetic result. The platysma muscle is divided in line with the incision and the strap muscles are separated in the midline. The thyroid isthmus is then mobilized superiorly or divided as needed to access the trachea. In the event of a low-lying cricoid cartilage, dissection on the anterior wall of the trachea helps to mobilize the trachea out of the mediastinum, and also the use of a cricoid hook will elevate the trachea to expose the second or third tracheal ring. Following identification of the second or third tracheal ring, a vertical tracheostomy is created or a tracheal flap (Bjork flap) is fashioned to create a fistulous tract by suturing the tracheal mucosal flap to the skin in the incision.

Variations on this technique include the use of retention sutures through the lateral aspect of the tracheal walls for retraction purposes during tracheostomy tube insertion and for expeditious reinsertion of a tracheostomy tube in the event of accidental tube decannulation [61,63].

Percutaneous Dilational Techniques

The PDT are divided into several techniques; however, all are alike in that they depend on the basic technique of guidewire placement through the anterior tracheal wall, followed by dilation over this guidewire to create a tracheal stoma. This is all accomplished with provision of adequate monitoring of O_2 saturations as well as adequate monitoring of cardiac rhythm and blood pressure. To be assured of early successful tracheal cannulation within the operating room, use end-tidal CO_2 monitoring via the fresh tracheostomy tube and in the ICU by capnography [64]. There are several different modifications from the original technique that was described by Ciaglia et al. [65] in 1988. There modifications are described in details elsewhere [62].

Both techniques, PDT and OST, can be performed in either the ICU or the operating room. There have been several meta-analyses comparing OST with PDT, most showing no significant difference in mortality or major complications between the two methods of performing the tracheostomy. Freeman et al. [66] reviewed multiple prospective controlled studies published between 1991 and 1999 totaling 236 patients and concluded that there is no difference in mortality between PDT and OST, and PDT was associated with less bleeding and stomal infections and was performed quicker. Delancy et al. [67] also concluded that there was no significant difference in mortality and major complications between PDT and OST in a meta-analysis consisting of 17 randomized trials and a total of 1,212 patients. They also showed a decrease in stomal infections in the PDT group, but no difference in bleeding complications. Similar findings were demonstrated by meta-analysis studies by Higgins and Punthakee [68] and Oliver et al. [69]. However, Dulguerov et al. [70] reviewed 3,512 patients from 48 studies performed between 1960 and 1996 and concluded that OST was more favorable than PDT. Subsequent critiques of these papers indicate the inherent weakness of heterogeneous patient populations and the use of case series and nonrandomized studies in meta-analyses [71–73]. It is likely that experience and technical modifications allow both the techniques to be performed in appropriate patients with the same degree of safety and efficiency (<1% procedure-related mortality) [74].

Other factors have been used to justify the use of one procedure over the other such as cost efficiency [75,76], bleeding, infection, procedural time, and estimated time from the decision to proceed to successful completion of the procedure [74]. Each factor can be used to justify one procedure over another, but it is likely that institutional practice variations and operator experience are more important in the selection of one procedure over another. This is particularly relevant with respect to the target population where ICU daily expenses far outweigh the procedural costs of either technique [77], and the expected patient mortality can reach as high as 35% [78].

It is probably more important to judiciously use the institutional resources and the operator experience in providing the "best" tracheal technique for these compromised patients. It is possible that the target population may vary from one institution to another (cardiac vs. trauma vs. neurosurgical vs. medical ICU patients), which may influence the decision to perform one technique over another. Patient body habitus also plays a large role in selection: difficulty palpating tracheal rings in a short, thick-necked patient makes percutaneous tracheostomy not only difficult but dangerous. This patient is better served in an operating room setting where optimum sedation/paralysis (if needed) and positioning can be accomplished while directly exposing the anterior trachea, mobilizing it if necessary to access the airway with an appropriately sized, sometimes custom-made, tube.

Nonetheless, there are certain distinct advantages of PDT that can be outlined as follows: (a) easier access for timing of the procedure; (b) reduced operating room and manpower utilization; (c) less expensive than OST (even if both the procedures are performed in the ICU); (d) no requirement for transportation of critically ill patients to an operating room; (e) improved cosmetic result; and (f) possibly reduced stomal infection, bleeding, and reduced tracheal secretions in the parastomal area due to the tight fitting of the stoma around the tracheostomy tube.

We do recommend considering performing OST instead of PST in the following patients: (a) patients with more severe respiratory distress (FIO_2 >0.60, positive end-expiratory pressure >10, and complicated translaryngeal intubation or a nonpalpable cricoid cartilage or a cricoid cartilage <3 cm above the sternal notch [75]); (b) obese patients with abundant pretracheal subcutaneous fat; (c) patients with large goiters; (d) abnormal airways secondary to congenital-acquired conditions; (e) the need for the constant attendance of a second physician to monitor ventilation or circulatory abnormalities; (f) abnormal bleeding diathesis that cannot be adequately corrected by coagulation factors [79].

TUBES AND CANNULAS

Characteristics of a good tracheostomy tube are flexibility to accommodate varying patient anatomies, inert material, wide internal diameter, the smallest external diameter possible, a smooth surface to allow easy insertion and removal, and sufficient length to be secured once placed, but not so long as to impinge the carina or other tracheal parts [80]. Until the late 1960s, when surgeons began to experiment with silicone and other synthetic materials, tracheostomy tubes and cannulas were made of metal. At present, almost all tracheostomy tubes are made of synthetic material. One disadvantage of a silicone tube over a metal one is the increased thickness of the tube wall, resulting in a larger outer diameter. Silicone tubes are available with or without a cuff. The cuff allows occlusion of the airway around the tube, which is necessary for positive-pressure ventilation. It may also minimize aspiration. In the past, cuffs were associated with a fairly high incidence of tracheal stenosis caused by ischemia and necrosis of the mucus membrane and subsequent cicatricial contracture at the cuff site [81,82]. High-volume, low-pressure cuffs diminish pressure on the wall of the trachea, thereby minimizing (but not eliminating) problems due to focal areas of pressure necrosis [83]. Cuff pressures should always be maintained at less than 30 cm H_2O, as higher pressures impair mucosal capillary blood flow leading to ischemic injury to the trachea [84]. Cuff pressures should be checked with a manometer daily in critically ill patients. Once the patient is weaned from mechanical ventilation, the cuff should be deflated or consideration should be given to placing an uncuffed tracheostomy tube until the patient can be decannulated. If the only purpose of the tube is to secure the airway (sleep apnea) or provide access for suctioning secretions, a tube without a cuff can be placed. A comprehensive review of tracheostomy tubes can be found elsewhere [85].

POSTOPERATIVE CARE

The care of a tracheostomy tube after surgery is important. Highlighted below are some specific issues that all intensivists need to know when caring for patients with tracheostomies.

Wound and Dressing Care

Daily examinations of the stoma are important in identifying infections or excoriations of the skin at the tracheostomy site [86]. In addition, keeping the wound clean and free of blood and secretions is very important, especially in the immediate posttracheostomy period. Dressing changes should be preformed at least twice a day and when the dressings are soiled. Some authors recommend cleaning the stoma with 1:1 mixture of hydrogen peroxide and sterile saline [86]. When changing dressings and tapes, special care is needed to avoid accidental dislodging of the tracheostomy tube. Sutures, placed either for fixation and/or through the rings themselves for exposure, should be removed as soon as practical, usually after 1 week when an adequate stoma has formed, to facilitate cleaning the stomal area. Malodorous tracheal "stomatitis" that can lead to an enlarging stoma around the tube should be treated with topical antimicrobial dressings such as 0.25% Dakin's solution to facilitate resolution.

Inner Cannulas

The inner cannulas should be used at all times in most tracheostomy tubes in the ICU. Bivona now makes a tracheostomy tube that is lined with silicone and does not require an inner cannula. In other tracheotomy tubes, inner cannulas serve to extend the life of the tracheostomy tubes by preventing the buildup secretions within the tracheostomy. The inner cannulas can be easily removed and either cleaned or replaced with a sterile, disposable one. Disposable inner cannulas have the advantage of quick and efficient changing, a decrease in nursing time, decreased risk of cross-contamination, and guaranteed sterility [87]. The obturator should be kept at the bedside at all times in the event that reinsertion of the tracheostomy is necessary.

Humidification

One of the functions of the upper airway is to moisten and humidify inspired air. Because tracheostomies bypass the upper airway, it is vital to provide patients who have tracheostomies with warm, humidified air. Humidification of inspired gases prevents complications in patients with tracheostomies. Failure to humidify the inspired gases can obstruct the tube by inspissated secretions, impair mucociliary clearance, and decrease cough [88].

Suctioning

Patients with tracheostomies frequently have increased amounts of airway secretions coupled with decreased ability to clear them effectively. Keeping the airways clear of excess secretions is important in decreasing the risk of lung infection and airway plugging [86]. Suctioning is frequently required in patients with poor or ineffective cough. Suction techniques should remove the maximal amount of secretions while causing the least amount of airway trauma [89]. Routine suctioning, however, is not recommended [90]. In the patient who requires frequent suctioning because of secretions, who otherwise appears well, without infection and without tracheitis, the tube itself may be the culprit. Downsizing the tube or even a short trial (while being monitored) with the tube removed may result in significantly less secretions, obviating the need for the tube.

Tracheostomy Tube Changes

Tracheostomy tubes do not require routine changing. In fact, there may be significant risks associated with routine tracheostomy tube changes, especially if this is performed within a week of the initial procedure and by inexperienced caregivers. A survey of accredited otolaryngology training programs suggested a significant incidence of loss of airway and deaths associated with routine changing of tracheostomy tubes within 7 days of initial placement, especially if they are changed by inexperienced physicians [91]. In general, the tube needs to be changed only under the following conditions: (a) there is a functional problem with it, such as an air leak in the balloon; (b) when the lumen is narrowed due to the buildup of dried secretions; (c) when switching to a new type of tube; or (d) when downsizing the tube prior to decannulation. Ideally, a tracheostomy tube should not be changed until 7 to 10 days after its initial placement. The reason for this is to allow the tracheal stoma and the tract to mature. Patients who have their tracheostomy tube changed before the tract is fully mature risk having the tube misplaced into the soft tissue of the neck. If the tracheostomy tube needs to be replaced before the tract has had time to mature, the tube should be changed over a guide, such as a suction catheter or tube changer [92].

Oral Feeding and Swallowing Dysfunction Associated with Tracheostomies

Great caution should be exercised before initiating oral feedings in patients with tracheostomy. Numerous studies have demonstrated that patients are at a significantly increased risk for aspiration when a tracheostomy is in place.

Physiologically, patients with tracheostomies are more likely to aspirate because the tracheostomy tube tethers the larynx, preventing its normal upward movement needed to assist in glottic closure and cricopharyngeal relaxation [93]. Tracheostomy tubes also disrupt normal swallowing by compressing the esophagus and interfering with deglutition [94], decreasing duration of vocal cord closure [95], and resulting in uncoordinated laryngeal closure [96]. In addition, prolonged orotracheal intubation can result in prolonged swallowing disorders even after the endotracheal tube is converted to a tracheostomy [97]. It is therefore not surprising that more than 65% of patients with tracheostomies aspirate when swallowing [98,99]. It is felt that 77% of the episodes are clinically silent [100,101].

Before attempting oral feedings in a patient with a tracheostomy, several objective criteria must be met. Obviously, the patient must be consistently alert, appropriate, and able to follow complex commands. The patient should also have adequate cough and swallowing reflexes, adequate oral motor strength, and a significant respiratory reserve [102]. These criteria are probably best assessed by a certified speech therapist. However, bedside clinical assessment may only identify 34% of the patients at high risk for aspiration [103]. Augmenting the bedside swallowing evaluation by coloring feedings or measuring the glucose in tracheal secretions does not appear to increase the sensitivity in detecting the risk of aspiration [104,105]. A video barium swallow may identify between 50% and 80% of patients with tracheostomies, who are at a high risk, to aspirate oral feeding [101,103]. A laryngoscopy to observe directly a patient's swallowing mechanics, coupled with a video barium swallow, may be more sensitive in predicting which patients are at risk for aspiration [103]. Scintigraphic studies may be the most sensitive test to determining which patients are aspirating [106], and it is much easier to perform than endoscopy. Plugging of the tracheostomy [106] or using a Passy–Muir valve [107] may reduce aspiration in patients with tracheostomies who are taking oral feedings, but this is not a universal finding [108].

Because of the high risk for aspiration and the difficulty assessing which patients are at high risk to aspirate, we do not institute oral feedings in our patients with tracheostomy in the ICU. We believe that the potential risks of a percutaneous endoscopically placed gastrostomy feeding tube or maintaining a nasogastric feeding tube are much less than the risk of aspiration of oral feedings and its complications (i.e., recurrent pneumonia, acute respiratory distress syndrome, and prolonged weaning).

Discharging Patients with Tracheotomies from the ICU to the General Ward

Two relatively recent studies have raised concern about the safety of patients, who have been weaned from mechanical ventilation, who are transferred from the ICU to the general hospital ward with the tracheostomy in place [109,110]. Fernandez et al. retrospectively showed an increased mortality in patients with tracheostomy tubes versus those decannulated prior to transfer out of the ICU, especially among patients with a poorer overall prognosis [109]. Martinez et al. prospectively studied 73 patients who received tracheostomies, who were without neurologic injury, and who were transferred from the ICU to the general ward [110]. Thirty-five of these patients were decannulated prior to transfer to the wards. The decannulated group had a significantly lower mortality. Factors found to be associated with increased mortality in patients not decannulated prior to transfer include body mass index greater than 30 kg per m^2 and tenacious secretions.

Patients with tracheostomies who are transferred to the general medical wards do need special attention. We suggest that these patients be safely cared for on the general ward, provided there is a multidisciplinary team approach between physicians, nurses, and respiratory therapist.

COMPLICATIONS

Tracheostomies, whether inserted by percutaneous dilatation or open surgical procedure, are associated with a variety of complications. These complications are best grouped by the time of occurrence after the placement and are divided into immediate, intermediate, and late complications (Table 12.4). The reported incidence of complications varies from as low

TABLE 12.4

COMPLICATIONS OF TRACHEOSTOMIES [13]

Immediate complications (0–24 h)
Tube displacement
Arrhythmia
Hypotension
Hypoxia/hypercapnia
Loss of airway control
Pneumothorax
Pneumomediastinum
Acute surgical emphysema
Major hemorrhage
Bacteremia
Esophageal injury (*uncommon*)
Cardiorespiratory arrest (*uncommon*)
Tracheolaryngeal injury (*uncommon*)
Crushed airway from dilational tracheostomy (*uncommon*)
Intermediate complications (from day 1 to day 7)
Persistent bleeding
Tube displacement
Tube obstruction (mucus, blood)
Major atelectasis
Wound infection/cellulitis
Late complications (>day 7)
Tracheoinnominate artery fistula
Tracheomalacia
Tracheal stenosis
Necrosis and loss of anterior tracheal cartilage
Tracheoesophageal fistula
Major aspiration
Chronic speech and swallowing deficits
Tracheocutaneous fistula

Conlan AA, Kopec SE: Tracheostomy in the ICU. *J Intensive Care Med* 15:1, 2000.
Angel LF, Simpson CB: Comparison of surgical and percutaneous dilational tracheostomy. *Clin Chest Med* 24:423, 2003.
Epstein SK: Late complications of tracheostomy. *Respir Care* 50:542, 2005.
Durbin CG: Early complications of tracheostomy. *Respir Care* 50:511, 2005.

as 4% [111] to as high as 39% [28], with reported mortality rates from 0.03% to 0.6% [70,112]. Complication rates appear to decrease with increasing experience of the physician performing the procedure [113]. Posttracheostomy mortality and morbidity is usually due to iatrogenic tracheal laceration [114], hemorrhage, tube dislodgment, infection, or obstruction. Neurosurgical patients have a higher posttracheostomy complication rate than other patients [115,116]. Tracheostomy is more hazardous in children than in adults, and carries special risks in the very young, often related to the experience of the surgeon [117]. A comprehensive understanding of immediate, intermediate, and late complications of tracheostomy and their management is essential for the intensivist.

Obstruction

Obstruction of the tracheostomy tube is a potentially life-threatening complication. The tube may become plugged with clotted blood or inspissated secretions. In this case, the inner cannula should be removed immediately and the patient suctioned. Should that fail, it may be necessary to remove the outer cannula also, a decision that must take into consideration the reason the tube was placed and the length of time it has been in place. Obstruction may also be due to angulation of the distal end of the tube against the anterior or posterior tracheal wall. An undivided thyroid isthmus pressing against the angled tracheostomy tube can force the tip against the anterior tracheal wall, whereas a low superior transverse skin edge can force the tip of the tracheostomy tube against the posterior tracheal wall. An indication of this type of obstruction is an expiratory wheeze. Division of the thyroid isthmus and proper placement of transverse skin incisions prevent anterior or posterior tube angulation and obstruction [118].

Tube Displacement/Dislodgment

Dislodgment of a tracheostomy tube that has been in place for 2 weeks or longer is managed simply by replacing the tube. If it cannot be immediately replaced or if it is replaced and the patient cannot be ventilated (indicating that the tube is not in the trachea), orotracheal intubation should be performed. Immediate postoperative displacement can be fatal if the tube cannot be promptly replaced and the patient cannot be reintubated.

Dislodgment in the early postoperative period is usually caused by one of several technical problems. Failure to divide the thyroid isthmus may permit the intact isthmus to ride up against the tracheostomy tube and thus displace it [118]. Excessively low placement of the stoma (i.e., below the second and third rings) can occur when the thoracic trachea is brought into the neck by overextending the neck or by excessive traction on the trachea. When the normal anatomic relationships are restored, the trachea recedes below the suprasternal notch, causing the tube to be dislodged from the trachea [118,119]. The risk of dislodgment of the tracheostomy tube, a potentially lethal complication, can be minimized by (a) transection of the thyroid isthmus at surgery, if indicated; (b) proper placement of the stoma; (c) avoidance of excessive neck hyperextension and/or tracheal traction; (d) application of sufficiently tight tracheostomy tube retention tapes; and (e) suture of the tracheostomy tube flange to the skin in patients with short necks. Some surgeons apply retaining sutures to the trachea for use in the early postoperative period in case the tube becomes dislodged, allowing the trachea to be pulled into the wound for reintubation. Making a Bjork flap involves suturing the inferior edge of the trachea stoma to the skin, thus allowing a sure pathway for tube placement. Bjork flaps, however, tend to interfere with swallowing and promote aspiration [120]. Reintubation of a tracheostomy can be accomplished by using a smaller, beveled endotracheal tube and then applying a tracheostomy tube over the smaller tube, using the Seldinger technique [121]. Using a nasogastric tube as a guidewire has also been described [92].

If a tracheostomy becomes dislodged within 7 to 10 days of surgery, we recommend translaryngeal endotracheal intubation to establish a safe airway. The tracheostomy tube can then be replaced under less urgent conditions, with fiberoptic guidance if needed.

Subcutaneous Emphysema

Approximately 5% of patients develop subcutaneous emphysema after tracheostomy [121]. It is most likely to occur when dissection is extensive and/or the wound is closed tightly. Partial closure of the skin wound is appropriate, but the underlying tissues should be allowed to approximate naturally. Subcutaneous emphysema generally resolves over the 48 hours after tracheostomy, but when the wound is closed tightly and the patient is coughing or on positive-pressure ventilation, pneumomediastinum, pneumopericardium, and/or tension pneumothorax may occur [118].

Pneumothorax and Pneumomediastinum

The cupola of the pleura extends well into the neck, especially in patients with emphysema; thus, the pleura can be damaged during tracheostomy. This complication is more common in the pediatric age group because the pleural dome extends more cephalad in children [1]. The incidence of pneumothorax after tracheostomy ranges from 0% to 5% [1,111,121]. Many surgeons routinely obtain a postoperative chest radiograph.

Hemorrhage

Minor postoperative fresh tracheostomy bleeding occurs in up to 37% of cases [1] and is probably the most common complication of this procedure. Postoperative coughing and straining can cause venous bleeding by dislodging a clot or ligature. Elevating the head of the bed, packing the wound, and/or using homeostatic materials usually controls minor bleeding. Major bleeding can occur in up to 5% of tracheotomies and is due to hemorrhage from the isthmus of the thyroid gland, loss of a ligature from one of the anterior jugular veins, or injury to the transverse jugular vein that crosses the midline just above the jugular notch [122]. Persistent bleeding may require a return to the operating room for management. Techniques to decrease the likelihood of early posttracheostomy hemorrhage include (a) use of a vertical incision; (b) careful dissection in the midline, with care to pick up each layer of tissue with instruments rather than simply spread tissues apart; (c) liberal use of ligatures rather than electrocautery; and (d) careful division and suture ligation of the thyroid isthmus. Late hemorrhage after tracheostomy is usually due to bleeding granulation tissue or another relatively minor cause. However, in these late cases, a tracheoinnominate artery fistula needs to be ruled out.

Tracheoinnominate Artery Fistula

At one point, it had been reported that 50% of all tracheostomy bleeding occurring more than 48 hours after the procedure was due to an often fatal complication of rupture of the innominate artery caused by erosion of the tracheostomy tube at its tip or cuff into the vessel [121]. However, because the advent of the low-pressure cuff, the incidence of this complication has decreased considerably and occurs less than 1% of the time [123].

Eighty-five percent of tracheoinnominate fistulas occur within the first month after tracheostomy [124], although they have been reported as late as 7 months after operation. Other sites of delayed exsanguinating posttracheostomy hemorrhage include the common carotid artery, superior and inferior thyroid arteries, aortic arch, and innominate vein [124]. Rupture and fistula formation are caused by erosion through the trachea into the artery due to excessive cuff pressure or by angulation of the tube tip against the anterior trachea. Infection and other factors that weaken local tissues, such as malnourishment and steroids, also seem to play a role [125]. The innominate artery rises to about the level of the sixth ring anterior to the trachea, and low placement of the stoma can also create close proximity of the tube tip or cuff to the innominate artery. Rarely, an anomaly of the innominate, occurring with an incidence of 1% to 2% [124], is responsible for this disastrous complication. Pulsation of the tracheostomy tube is an indication of potentially fatal positioning [124]. Initially, hemorrhage from a tracheoinnominate fistula is usually not exsanguinating. Herald bleeds must be investigated promptly using fiberoptic tracheoscopy. If a tracheoinnominate fistula seems probable (minimal tracheitis, anterior pulsating erosions), the patient should be taken to the operating room for evaluation. Definitive management involves resection of the artery [126]. The mortality rate approaches 100%, even with emergent surgical intervention [127]. Sudden exsanguinating hemorrhage may be managed by hyperinflation of the tracheostomy cuff tube or reintubation with an endotracheal tube through the stoma, attempting to place the cuff at the level of the fistula. A lower neck incision with blind digital compression on the artery may be part of a critical resuscitative effort [128]. If a tracheoinnominate artery fistula is suspected, the patient should be evaluated in the operating room and preparations should be made for a possible sternotomy.

Misplacement of Tube

Misplacement of the tube error occurs at the time of surgery or when the tube is changed or replaced through a fresh stoma. If not recognized, associated mediastinal emphysema and tension pneumothorax can occur, along with alveolar hypoventilation. Injury to neurovascular structures, including the recurrent laryngeal nerve, is possible [119]. The patient must be orally intubated or the tracheostoma recannulated. Some advise placing retaining sutures in the trachea at the time of surgery. The availability of a tracheostomy set at the bedside after tracheostomy facilitates emergency reintubation.

Stomal Infections

An 8% to 12% incidence of cellulitis or purulent exudate is reported with tracheostomy [1,121]. The risk of serious infection is less than 0.5% [111]. Attention to the details of good stoma care and early use of antibiotics are advised. However, prophylactic antibiotics are not recommended [129].

Tracheoesophageal Fistula

Tracheoesophageal fistula caused by injury to the posterior tracheal wall and cervical esophagus occurs in less than 1% of patients, more commonly in the pediatric age group. Early postoperative fistula is a result of iatrogenic injury during the procedure [121,128]. The chances of creating a fistula can be minimized by entering the trachea initially with a horizontal incision between two tracheal rings (the second and third), thereby eliminating the initial cut into a hard cartilaginous ring [118]. A late tracheoesophageal fistula may be due to tracheal necrosis caused by tube movement or angulation, as in neck hyperflexion, or excessive cuff pressure [119,121,128]. A tracheoesophageal fistula should be suspected in patients with cuff leaks, abdominal distention, recurrent aspiration pneumonia, and reflux of gastric fluids through the tracheostomy site. It may be demonstrated on endoscopy and contrast studies. Tracheoesophageal fistulas require surgical repair. For patients who could not tolerate a major surgical procedure, placement of an esophageal and a tracheal stent may be used [130–132].

Tracheal Stenosis

Some degree of tracheal stenosis is seen in 40% to 60% of patients with tracheostomies [112,133]. However, 3% to 12% of these stenoses are clinically significant enough to require intervention [134]. Stenosis most commonly occurs at the level of the stoma or just above the stoma, but distal to the vocal cords [127]. The stenosis typically results from bacterial infection or chondritis of the anterior and lateral tracheal walls. Granulation tissue usually develops first. Ultimately the granulation tissue matures, becoming fibrous and covered with a layer of epithelium. The granulation tissue itself can also result in other complications, such as obstructing the airway at the level of the stoma, making changing the tracheostomy tube difficult, and occluding tube fenestrations. Identified risk factors for developing tracheal stenosis include sepsis, stomal infections, hypotension, advanced age, male gender, corticosteroid use, excess motion of the tracheostomy tube, oversized tube, prolonged placement, elevated cuff pressures, and excessive excision of the anterior trachea cartilage [127,135]. Using properly sized tracheostomy tubes, inflating cuffs only when indicated, and maintaining intracuff pressures to less than 15 to 20 mm Hg may decrease the incidence of tracheal stenosis [136]. Tracheal stenosis, as well as other long-term complications, appears to be less with the percutaneous procedure [137–139].

Treatment options for granulation tissue include topical strategies (such as topical antibiotic or steroids, silver nitrate, and polyurethane form dressings) or surgical strategies (laser excision, electrocautery, and surgical removal) [127]. Treatment options for symptomatic tracheal stenosis include dilatation with a rigid bronchoscopy with coring, intralumen laser excision, or surgical resection with end-to-end tracheal anastomosis [140].

Tracheomalacia

Tracheomalacia is a weakening of the tracheal wall resulting from ischemic injury to the trachea, followed by chondritis, then destruction, and necrosis of the tracheal cartilage [127]. Consequently, there is collapse of the affected portion of the trachea with expiration, resulting in airflow limitation, air trapping, and retention of airway secretions. Tracheomalacia may ultimately result in the patient failing to wean from mechanical ventilation. A short-term therapeutic approach to tracheomalacia is to place a longer tracheostomy tube to bypass the area of malacia. Long-term treatment options include stenting, tracheal resection, or tracheoplasty [127].

Dysphagia and Aspiration

The major swallowing disorder associated with tracheostomy is aspiration (see the section Oral Feeding and Swallowing Dysfunction). Because of the high risk for aspiration, we do not recommend oral feeding in ICU patients with tracheostomies.

Tracheocutaneous Fistula

Although the tracheostoma generally closes rapidly after decannulation, a persistent fistula may occasionally remain, particularly when the tracheostomy tube is present for a prolonged period. If this complication occurs, the fistula tract can be excised and the wound closed primarily under local anesthesia [141].

CONCLUSION

Tracheostomy is one of the most common surgical procedures preformed in the ICU and appears to be the airway of choice for patients requiring mechanical ventilation for more than 1 to 2 weeks. The exact timing for converting patients to tracheostomy is not entirely clear, so the physician must weight the risks and benefits of tracheostomy versus translaryngeal intubation and estimate the expected duration of mechanical ventilation for each individual patient. The physician performing the tracheostomy procedure needs to assess each patient to determine the best technique (whether it be performed bedside percutaneously or open in the operating room) for that specific patient. The patient's medical condition, the physician's experience with the various techniques, and the hospital's resources all need to be considered in determining the type of procedure performed.

References

1. Goldstein SI, Breda SD, Schneider KL: Surgical complications of bedside tracheotomy in an otolaryngology residency program. *Laryngoscope* 97:1407, 1987.
2. Clec'h C, Alberti C, Vincent F, et al: Tracheostomy does not improve the outcome of patients requiring mechanical ventilation: a propensity analysis. *Crit Care Med* 35:132, 2007.
3. Combes A, Luyt CE, Nieszkowska A, et al: Is tracheostomy associated with better outcomes for patients requiring long-term mechanical ventilation? *Crit Care Med* 25:802, 2007.
4. Kremer B, Botos-Kremer A, Eckel H, et al: Indications, complications, and surgical technique for pediatric tracheostomies. *J Pediatr Surg* 37:1556, 2002.
5. Bjure J: Tracheotomy: A satisfactory method in the treatment of acute epiglottis. A clinical and functional follow-up study. *Int J Pediatr Otorhinolaryngol* 3:37, 1981.
6. Hanline MH Jr: Tracheotomy in upper airway obstruction. *South Med J* 74:899, 1981.
7. Taicher S, Givol M, Peleg M, et al: Changing indications for tracheostomy in maxillofacial trauma. *J Oral Maxillofac Surg* 54:292, 1996.
8. Guilleminault C, Simmons FB, Motta J, et al: Obstructive sleep apnea syndrome and tracheostomy. *Arch Intern Med* 141:985, 1981.
9. Burwell C, Robin E, Whaley R, et al: Extreme obesity associated with alveolar hypoventilation. *Am J Med* 141:985, 1981.
10. Yung MW, Snowdon SL: Respiratory resistance of tracheostomy tubes. *Arch Otolaryngol* 110:591, 1984.
11. Heffner JE: Tracheostomy application and timing. *Clin Chest Med* 24:389, 2003.
12. Durbin CG: Indications for and timing of tracheostomy. *Respir Care* 50:483, 2005.
13. Conlan AA, Kopec SE: Tracheostomy in the ICU. *J Intensive Care Med* 15:1, 2000.
14. Auzinger G, O'Callaghan GP, Bernal W, et al: Percutaneous tracheostomy in patients with severe liver disease and a high incidence of refractory coagulopathy: a prospective trial. *Crit Care* 11:R110, 2007.
15. El Solh AA, Jaafar W: A comparative study of the complications of surgical tracheostomy in morbidly obese critically ill patients. *Crit Care* 11:R3, 2007.
16. Aldawood AS, Arabi YM, Haddad S: Safety of percutaneous tracheostomy in obese critically ill patients: a prospective cohort study. *Anaesth Intensive Care* 36:69, 2008.
17. Milanchi S, Magner D, Wilson MT, et al: Percutaneous tracheostomy in neurosurgical patients with intracranial pressure monitoring is safe. *J Trauma Injury Infect Crit Care* 65:73, 2008.
18. Colice GL: Resolution of laryngeal injury following translaryngeal intubation. *Am Rev Respir Dis* 142(2, Pt 1):361, 1992.
19. Marsh HM, Gillespie DJ, Baumgartner AE: Timing of tracheostomy in the critically ill patient. *Chest* 96:190, 1989.
20. Griffiths J, Barber VS, Morgan L, et al: Systematic review and meta-analysis of studies of the timing of tracheostomy in adult patients undergoing artificial ventilation. *BMJ* 330:1243, 2005.
21. Rodriguez JL, Steinberg SM, Luchetti FA, et al: Early tracheostomy for primary airway management in the surgical critical care setting. *Surgery* 108:655, 1990.
22. Sugerman HJ, Wolfe L, Pasquele MD, et al: Multicenter, randomized, prospective trial on early tracheostomy. *J Trauma* 43:741, 1997.
23. Brook AD, Sherman G, Malen J, et al: Early versus late tracheostomy in patients who require prolonged mechanical ventilation. *Am J Crit Care* 9:352, 2000.
24. Rumbak MJ, Newton M, Truncale T, et al: A prospective, randomized study comparing early percutaneous dilatational tracheostomy to prolonged translaryngeal intubation in critically ill medical patients. *Crit Care Med* 32:1689, 2004.
25. Scales DC, Thiruchelvam D, Kiss A, et al: The effect of tracheostomy timing during critical illness on long-term survival. *Crit Care Med* 36:2547, 2008.
26. Blot F, Similowski T, Trouillet JL, et al: Early tracheostomy versus prolonged endotracheal intubation in unselected severely ill ICU patients. *Intens Care Med* 34:1779, 2008.
27. Durbin CG, Perkins MP, Moores LK: Should tracheostomy be performed as early as 72 hours in patients requiring prolonged mechanical ventilation? *Respir Care* 55:76, 2010.
28. Terragni PP, Antonelli M, Fumagalli R, et al: Early vs late tracheostomy for prevention of pneumonia in mechanically ventilated adult ICU patients. *JAMA* 303:1483, 2010.
29. Lesnik I, Rappaport W, Fulginiti J, et al: The role of early tracheostomy in blunt, multiple organ trauma. *Am Surg* 58:346, 1992.
30. Armstrong PA, McCarthy MC, Peoples JB: Reduced use of resources by early tracheostomy in ventilator-dependent patients with blunt trauma. *Surgery* 124:763, 1998.
31. Teoh WH, Goh KY, Chan C: The role of early tracheostomy in critically ill neurosurgical patients. *Ann Acad Med Singapore* 30:234, 2001.
32. Koh WY, Lew TWK, Chin NM, et al: Tracheostomy in a neuro-intensive care setting: indications and timing. *Anaesth Intensive Care* 25:365, 1997.
33. D'Amelio LF, Hammond JS, Spain DA, et al: Tracheostomy and percutaneous endoscopic gastrostomy in the management of the head-injured patient. *Am Surg* 60:180, 1994.
34. Berney S, Opdam H, Bellomo R, et al: As assessment of early tracheostomy after anterior cervical stabilization in patients with acute cervical spine trauma. *J Trauma* 64:749, 2008.
35. Romero J, Vari A, Gambarrutta C, et al: Tracheostomy timing in traumatic spinal cord injury. *Eur Spine J* 18:1452, 2009.
36. Sellers BJ, Davis BL, Larkin PW, et al: Early predictors of prolonged ventilator dependence in thermally injured patients. *J Trauma* 43:899, 1997.
37. Stock CM, Woodward CG, Shapiro BA, et al: Perioperative complications of elective tracheostomy in critically ill patients. *Crit Care Med* 14:861, 1986.
38. Skaggs JA, Cogbill CL: Tracheostomy: management, mortality, complications. *Am Surg* 35:393, 1969.
39. *American College of Surgeons Committee on Trauma: Advanced Trauma Life Support Course for Physicians, Instructor Manual.* Chicago, American College of Surgeons, 1985, p 159.
40. Kline SN: Maxillofacial trauma, in Kreis DJ, Gomez GA (eds): *Trauma Management.* Boston, Little, Brown, 1989.
41. Jackson C: High tracheotomy and other errors: the chief causes of chronic laryngeal stenosis. *Surg Gynecol Obstet* 32:392, 1921.
42. Esses BA, Jafek BW: Cricothyroidotomy: a decade of experience in Denver. *Ann Otol Rhinol Laryngol* 96:519, 1987.
43. Brantigan CO, Grow JB: Cricothyroidotomy: elective use in respiratory problems requiring tracheotomy. *J Thorac Cardiovasc Surg* 71:72, 1976.
44. Cole RR, Aguilar EA: Cricothyroidotomy versus tracheotomy: an otolaryngologist's perspective. *Laryngoscope* 98:131, 1988.
45. Boyd AD, Romita MC, Conlan AA, et al: A clinical evaluation of cricothyroidotomy. *Surg Gynecol Obstet* 149:365, 1979.
46. Sise MJ, Shacksord SR, Cruickshank JC, et al: Cricothyroidotomy for long term tracheal access. *Ann Surg* 200:13, 1984.
47. O'Connor JV, Reddy K, Ergin MA, et al: Cricothyroidotomy for prolonged ventilatory support after cardiac operations. *Ann Thorac Surg* 39:353, 1985.

48. Lewis GA, Hopkinson RB, Matthews HR: Minitracheotomy: a report of its use in intensive therapy. *Anesthesia* 41:931, 1986.
49. Pierce WS, Tyers FO, Waldhausen JA: Effective isolation of a tracheostomy from a median sternotomy wound. *J Thorac Cardiovasc Surg* 66:841, 1973.
50. Morain WD: Cricothyroidotomy in head and neck surgery. *Plast Reconstr Surg* 65:424, 1980.
51. Kuriloff DB, Setzen M, Portnoy W, et al: Laryngotracheal injury following cricothyroidotomy. *Laryngoscope* 99:125, 1989.
52. Hawkins ML, Shapiro MB, Cue JI, et al: Emergency cricothyrotomy: a reassessment. *Am Surg* 61:52, 1995.
53. Mace SE: Cricothyrotomy. *J Emerg Med* 6:309, 1988.
54. Robinson RJS, Mulder DS: Airway control, in Mattox KL, Feliciano DV, Moore EE (eds): *Trauma*. New York, McGraw-Hill, 2000, p 171.
55. Cutler BS: Cricothyroidotomy for emergency airway, in Vander Salm TJ, Cutler BS, Wheeler HB (eds): *Atlas of Bedside Procedures*. Boston, Little, Brown, 1988, p 231.
56. Erlandson MJ, Clinton JE, Ruiz E, et al: Cricothyrotomy in the emergency department revisited. *J Emerg Med* 7:115, 1989.
57. Brantigan CO, Grow JB: Subglottic stenosis after cricothyroidotomy. *Surgery* 91:217, 1982.
58. Epstein SK: Anatomy and physiology of tracheostomy. *Respir Care* 50:476, 2005.
59. DeBoisblanc BP: Percutaneous dilational tracheostomy techniques. *Clin Chest Med* 24:399, 2003.
60. Lams E, Ravalia A: Percutaneous and surgical tracheostomy. *Hosp Med* 64:36, 2003.
61. Walts PA, Murthy SC, DeCamp MM: Techniques of surgical tracheostomy. *Clin Chest Med* 24:413, 2003.
62. Kopec SE, McNamee CJ: Tracheostomy, in Irwin RS, Rippe JM (eds): *Intensive Care Medicine*. 6th ed. Lippincott, Williams, and Wilkins, Philadelphia, 2005, p 112.
63. Durbin CG: Technique for performing tracheostomy. *Respir Care* 50:488, 2005.
64. Mallick A, Venkatanath D, Elliot SC, et al: A prospective randomized controlled trial of capnography vs. bronchoscopy for Blue Rhino percutaneous tracheostomy. *Anaesthesia* 58:864, 2003.
65. Ciaglia P, Firsching R, Syniec C: Elective percutaneous dilatational tracheostomy: a new simple beside procedure. Preliminary report. *Chest* 87:715, 1985.
66. Freeman BD, Isabella K, Lin N, et al: A meta-analysis of prospective trials comparing percutaneous and surgical tracheostomy in critically ill patients. *Chest* 118:412, 2000.
67. Delancy A, Bagshaw SM, Nalos M: Percutaneous dilatational tracheostomy versus surgical tracheostomy in critically ill patients: a systemic review and meta-analysis. *Crit Care* 10:R55, 2006.
68. Higgins KM, Punthakee X: Meta-analysis comparison of open versus percutaneous tracheostomy. *Laryngoscope* 117:447, 2007.
69. Oliver ER, Gist A, Gillespie MB: Percutaneous versus surgical tracheostomy: an updated meta-analysis. *Laryngoscope* 117:1570, 2007.
70. Dulguerov P, Gysin C, Perneger TV, et al: Percutaneous or surgical tracheostomy: a meta-analysis. *Crit Care Med* 27:1617, 1999.
71. Anderson JD, Rabinovici R, Frankel HL: Percutaneous dilational tracheostomy vs open tracheostomy. *Chest* 120:1423, 2001.
72. Heffner JE: Percutaneous dilational vs standard tracheostomy: a meta-analysis but not the final analysis. *Chest* 118:1236, 2000.
73. Susanto I: Comparing percutaneous tracheostomy with open surgical tracheostomy. *BMJ* 324:3, 2002.
74. Angel LF, Simpson CB: Comparison of surgical and percutaneous dilational tracheostomy. *Clin Chest Med* 24:423, 2003.
75. Massick DD, Yao S, Powell DM, et al: Bedside tracheostomy in the intensive care unit: a perspective randomized trial comparing surgical tracheostomy with endoscopically guided percutaneous dilational tracheotomy. *Laryngoscope* 111:494, 2001.
76. McHenry CR, Raeburn CD, Lange RL, et al: Percutaneous tracheostomy: a cost-effective alternative to standard open tracheostomy. *Am Surg* 63:646, 1997.
77. Garland A: Improving the ICU: part 1. *Chest* 127:2151, 2005.
78. Combes A, Luyt CE, Trouillet JL, et al: Adverse effects on a referral intensive care unit's performance of accepting patients transferred from another intensive care unit. *Crit Care Med* 33:705, 2005.
79. Stocchetti N, Parma A, Lamperti M, et al: Neurophysiologic consequences of three tracheostomy techniques: a randomized study in neurosurgical patients. *J Neurosurg Anesthesiol* 12:307, 2000.
80. Lewis RJ: Tracheostomies: indications, timing, and complications. *Clin Chest Med* 13:137, 1992.
81. Cooper JD, Grillo HC: The evolution of tracheal injury due to ventilatory assistance through cuffed tubes: a pathologic study. *Ann Surg* 169:334, 1969.
82. Stool SE, Campbell JR, Johnson DG: Tracheostomy in children: the use of plastic tubes. *J Pediatr Surg* 3:402, 1968.
83. Grillo HZ, Cooper JD, Geffin B, et al: A low pressured cuff for tracheostomy tubes to minimize tracheal inner injury. *J Thorac Cardiovasc Surg* 62:898, 1971.
84. Seegobin RD, van Hasselt GL: Endotracheal cuff pressure and tracheal mucosal blood flow, endoscopic study of effects of four large volume cuffs. *BMJ* 288:965, 1984.
85. Hess DR: Tracheostomy tubes and related appliances. *Respir Care* 50:497, 2005.
86. Wright SE, van Dahn K: Long-term care of the tracheostomy patient. *Clin Chest Med* 24:473, 2003.
87. Crow S: Disposable tracheostomy inner cannula. *Infect Control* 7:285, 1986.
88. Forbes AR: Temperature, humidity and mucous flow in the intubated trachea. *Br J Anaesth* 46:29, 1974.
89. Shekelton M, Nield DM: Ineffective airway clearance related to artificial airway. *Nurs Clin North Am* 22:167, 1987.
90. Lewis RM: Airway clearance techniques for patients with artificial airways. *Respir Care* 47:808, 2002.
91. Tabaee A, Lando T, Rickert S, et al: Practice patterns, safety, and rationale for tracheostomy tube changes: a survey of otolaryngology training programs. *Laryngoscope* 117:573, 2007.
92. Young JS, Brady WJ, Kesser B, et al: A novel method for replacement of the dislodged tracheostomy tube: the nasogastric tube guidewire technique. *J Emerg Med* 14:205, 1996.
93. Bonanno PC: Swallowing dysfunction after tracheostomy. *Ann Surg* 174:29, 1971.
94. Betts RH: Posttracheostomy aspiration. *N Engl J Med* 273:155, 1965.
95. Shaker R, Dodds WJ, Dantas EO: Coordination of deglutitive glottic closure with oropharyngeal swallowing. *Gastroenterol* 98:1478, 1990.
96. Buckwater JA, Sasaki CT: Effect of tracheostomy on laryngeal function. *Otolaryngol Clin North Am* 21:701, 1988.
97. Devita MA, Spierer-Rundback MS: Swallowing disorders in patients with prolonged intubation or tracheostomy tubes. *Crit Care Med* 18:1328, 1990.
98. Cameron JL, Reynolds J, Zuidema GD: Aspiration in patients with tracheostomies. *Surg Gynecol Obstet* 136:68, 1973.
99. Bone DK, Davis JL, Zuidema GD, et al: Aspiration pneumonia. *Ann Thorac Surg* 18:30, 1974.
100. Panmunzio TG: Aspiration of oral feedings in patients with tracheostomies. AACN Clin Issues. *Adv Pract Acute Crit Care* 7:560, 1996.
101. Elpern EH, Scott MG, Petro L, et al: Pulmonary aspiration in mechanically ventilated patients with tracheostomies. *Chest* 105:563, 1994.
102. Godwin JE, Heffner JE: Special critical care considerations in tracheostomy management. *Clin Chest Med* 12:573, 1991.
103. Tolep K, Getch CL, Criner GJ: Swallowing dysfunction in patients receiving prolonged mechanical ventilation. *Chest* 109:167, 1996.
104. Metheny NA, Clouse RE: Bedside methods for detecting aspiration in tube-fed patients. *Chest* 111:724, 1997.
105. Thompson-Henry S, Braddock B: The modified Evan's blue dye procedure fails to detect aspiration in the tracheostomized patient: five case reports. *Dysphagia* 10:172, 1995.
106. Muz J, Hamlet S, Mathog R, et al: Scintigraphic assessment of aspiration in head and neck cancer patients with tracheostomy. *Head Neck* 16:17, 1994.
107. Dettelbach MA, Gross RD, Mahlmann J, et al: Effect of the Passy-Muir valve on aspiration in patients with tracheostomy. *Head Neck* 17:297, 1995.
108. Leder SB, Tarro JM, Burell MI: Effect of occlusion of a tracheostomy tube on aspiration. *Dysphagia* 11:254, 1996.
109. Fernandez R, Bacelar N, Hernandez G, et al: Ward mortality in patients discharged from the ICU with tracheostomy may depend on patient's vulnerability. *Intens Care Med* 34:1878, 2008.
110. Martinez GH, Fernandez R, Casado MS, et al: Tracheostomy tube in place at intensive care unit discharge is associated with increased ward mortality. *Respir Care* 54:1644, 2009.
111. Goldenberg D, Ari EG, Golz A, et al: Tracheostomy complications: a retrospective study of 1130 cases. *Otolaryngol Head Neck Surg* 123:495, 2000.
112. Walz MK, Peitgen K, Thurauf N, et al: Percutaneous dilatational tracheostomy—early results and long-term outcome of 326 critically ill patients. *Intensive Care Med* 24:685, 1998.
113. Petros S, Engelmann L: Percutaneous dilatational tracheostomy in a medical ICU. *Intensive Care Med* 23:630, 1997.
114. Massard G, Rouge C, Dabbagh A, et al: Tracheobronchial lacerations after intubation and tracheostomy. *Ann Thorac Surg* 61:1483, 1996.
115. Dunham CM, LaMonica C: Prolonged tracheal intubation in the trauma patient. *J Trauma* 24:120, 1984.
116. Miller JD, Kapp JP: Complications of tracheostomies in neurosurgical patients. *Surg Neurol* 22:186, 1984.
117. Shinkwin CA, Gibbin KP: Tracheostomy in children. *J R Soc Med* 89:188, 1996.
118. Kirchner JA: Avoiding problems in tracheotomy. *Laryngoscope* 96:55, 1986.
119. Kenan PD: Complications associated with tracheotomy: prevention and treatment. *Otolaryngol Clin North Am* 12:807, 1979.
120. Malata CM, Foo IT, Simpson KH, et al: An audit of Bjork flap tracheostomies in head and neck plastic surgery. *Br J Oral Maxillofac Surg* 34:42, 1996.
121. Heffner JE, Miller KS, Sahn SA: Tracheostomy in the intensive care unit, 2: complications. *Chest* 90:430, 1986.
122. Muhammad JK, Major E, Wood A, et al: Percutaneous dilatational tracheostomy: hemorrhagic complications and the vascular anatomy of the anterior neck. *Int J Oral Maxillofac Surg* 29:217, 2000.
123. Schaefer OP, Irwin RS: Tracheoarterial fistula: an unusual complication of tracheostomy. *J Intensive Care Med* 10:64, 1995.

124. Mamikunian C: Prevention of delayed hemorrhage after tracheotomy. *Ear Nose Throat J* 67:881, 1988.
125. Oshinsky AE, Rubin JS, Gwozdz CS: The anatomical basis for post-tracheotomy innominate artery rupture. *Laryngoscope* 98:1061, 1988.
126. Keceligil HT, Erk MK, Kolbakir F, et al: Tracheoinnominate artery fistula following tracheostomy. *Cardiovasc Surg* 3:509, 1995.
127. Epstein SK: Late complications of tracheostomy. *Respir Care* 50:542, 2005.
128. Thomas AN: The diagnosis and treatment of tracheoesophageal fistula caused by cuffed tracheal tubes. *J Thorac Cardiovasc Surg* 65:612, 1973.
129. Myers EN, Carrau RL: Early complications of tracheostomy. Incidence and management. *Clin Chest Med* 12:589, 1991.
130. Dartevelle P, Macchiarini P: Management of acquired tracheoesophageal fistula. *Chest Surg Clin North Am* 6:819, 1996.
131. Albes JM, Prokop M, Gebel M, et al: Bifurcate tracheal stent with foam cuff for tracheo-esophageal fistula: utilization of reconstruction modes on spiral computer tomography. *Thorac Cardiovasc Surg* 42:367, 1994.
132. Wolf M, Yellin A, Talmi YP, et al: Acquired tracheoesophageal fistula in critically ill patients. *Ann Otol Rhinol Laryngol* 109(8, Pt 1):731, 2000.
133. Dollner R, Verch M, Schweiger P, et al: Laryngotracheoscopic findings in long-term follow-up after Griggs tracheostomy. *Chest* 122:206, 2002.
134. Streitz JM, Shapshay SM: Airway injury after tracheostomy and endotracheal intubation. *Surg Clin North Am* 71:1211, 1991.
135. Stauffer JL, Olsen DE, Petty TL: Complications and consequences of endotracheal intubation and tracheostomy: a prospective study of 150 critically ill adult patients. *Am J Med* 70:65, 1981.
136. Arola MK, Puhakka H, Makela P: Healing of lesions caused by cuffed tracheotomy tubes and their late sequelae: a follow-up study. *Acta Anaesthesiol Scand* 24:169, 1980.
137. Friedman Y, Franklin C: The technique of percutaneous tracheostomy: using serial dilation to secure an airway with minimal risk. *J Crit Illn* 8:289, 1993.
138. Crofts SL, Alzeer A, McGuire GP, et al: A comparison of percutaneous and operative tracheostomies in intensive care patients. *Can J Anaesth* 42:775, 1995.
139. Hill BB, Zweng TN, Manley RH, et al: Percutaneous dilational tracheostomy: report of 356 cases. *J Trauma* 41:38, 1996.
140. Zietek E, Matyja G, Kawczynski M: Stenosis of the larynx and trachea: diagnosis and treatment. *Otolaryngol Pol* 55:515, 2001.
141. Hughes M, Kirchner JA, Branson RJ: A skin-lined tube as a complication of tracheostomy. *Arch Otolaryngol* 94:568, 1971.

CHAPTER 13 ■ GASTROINTESTINAL ENDOSCOPY

ANUPAM SINGH, RANDALL S. PELLISH AND WAHID Y. WASSEF

Gastrointestinal (GI) endoscopy has evolved into an essential diagnostic and therapeutic tool for the treatment of critically ill patients in the new millennium. Innovations in the field continue to emerge. This chapter reviews general aspects of current indications and contraindications, provides an update of emerging technologies, and concludes by discussing potential future directions in the field.

INDICATIONS

The indications for GI endoscopy in the intensive care unit (ICU) are summarized in Table 13.1 and are divided into those for (a) evaluation of the upper GI tract (esophagus, stomach, and duodenum); (b) evaluation of the pancreaticobiliary tract; (c) evaluation of the mid-GI tract (jejunum and ileum); and (d) evaluation of the lower GI tract (colon and rectum).

Evaluation of the Upper Gastrointestinal Tract

Common indications for evaluation of the upper GI tract in the ICU include, but are not limited to, upper GI bleeding (UGIB), caustic or foreign body ingestion, and placement of feeding tubes. Evaluation of the GI tract in ICU patients with clinically insignificant bleeding or chronic GI complaints should generally be postponed until their medical/surgical illnesses improve. One exception in this group of patients is if anticoagulation or thrombolytic therapy is being contemplated.

Upper Gastrointestinal Bleeding

With an estimated 300,000 admissions annually, acute UGIB is one of the most common medical emergencies [1]. It is defined as the presence of melena, hematemesis, or blood in the nasogastric (NG) aspirate. Studies have shown improved outcomes with urgent endoscopic management in critically ill patients with hemodynamic instability or continuing transfusion requirements [2,3]. Urgent evaluation allows differentiation between nonvariceal (peptic ulcer, esophagitis, Mallory–Weiss tear, and angiodysplasia) and variceal lesions (esophageal or gastric varices), therefore promoting targeted therapy [4,5]. Furthermore, urgent evaluation allows the identification and stratification of stigmata of bleeding, promoting appropriate triage and risk stratification. Finally, urgent evaluation allows the early identification of patients who may require surgical or radiologic intervention [6,7].

Foreign Body Ingestions

Foreign body ingestions (FBI) can be divided into two groups: (i) food impactions and (ii) caustic ingestion. Food impactions constitute the majority of FBI. Although most will pass spontaneously, endoscopic removal will be needed for 10% to 20% of cases, and 1% of patients will ultimately require surgery [8]. Evaluation is crucial to determine the underlying cause of the obstruction (strictures, rings, and carcinoma). Although caustic ingestions constitute only a small number of FBI, they are frequently life threatening, especially when they occur intentionally in adults, and warrant endoscopic evaluation to prognosticate and triage this group of patients [9].

Feeding Tubes

Enteral nutrition improves outcomes in critically ill patients and is preferred over parenteral nutrition in patients with a functional GI tract [10]. Although nasoenteric and oroenteric feeding tubes may be used for short-term enteral nutrition, these tubes are felt to carry a higher risk of aspiration, displacement, and sinus infections than endoscopically placed percutaneous tubes. Percutaneous endoscopic gastrostomy (PEG) [11] is appropriate for most patients in the ICU when there is a reversible disease process likely to require more than 4 weeks of enteral nutrition (e.g., neurologic injury,

TABLE 13.1

INDICATIONS FOR GASTROINTESTINAL (GI) ENDOSCOPY

Upper GI endoscopy
Upper GI bleeding (variceal or nonvariceal)
Caustic or foreign body ingestion
Placement of feeding or drainage tubes
Endoscopic retrograde cholangiopancreatography
Severe gallstone pancreatitis
Severe cholangitis
Bile leak
Lower GI endoscopy
Lower GI bleeding
Decompression of nontoxic megacolon or sigmoid volvulus
Unexplained diarrhea in the immunocompromised (graft vs. host disease and cytomegalovirus infection)

tracheostomy, and neoplasms of the upper aerodigestive tract) [12]. PEG with jejunostomy tube and direct percutaneous endoscopic jejunostomy (PEJ) tubes are appropriate for select patients in the ICU with high risk of aspiration. This includes patients with severe gastroesophageal reflux disease and those with gastroparesis. Enteral feeding beyond the ligament of Treitz with a nasojejunal tube or a jejunostomy tube has been demonstrated to be beneficial in patients with necrotizing pancreatitis. Occasionally, endoscopic gastrostomies or jejunostomies may be indicated for decompression in patients with GI obstruction [13]. Although these procedures are technically simple and can be performed at the bedside under moderate sedation, the risks and benefits should always be weighed carefully in this critically ill group of patients [14].

Evaluation of the Pancreaticobiliary Tract

The indications for evaluation of the pancreaticobiliary tract by endoscopic retrograde cholangiopancreatography (ERCP) in critically ill patients are described in detail in Chapter 97 and only briefly discussed here. Indications include biliary tract obstruction by gallstones [15–17], pancreatic duct leaks, and bile duct leaks (generally a postoperative or traumatic complication) [18–20]. ERCP with sphincterotomy and/or stenting is the treatment of choice. When conventional ERCP is unsuccessful, the recent introduction of miniature endoscopes (cholangioscopes or pancreatic scopes) with direct endoscopic visualization into these ductal systems has proved to be beneficial through the use of advanced techniques such as electrohydraulic lithotripsy (EHL), laser lithotripsy, and glue [21]. Unfortunately, this technique is limited by its lack of availability at all centers and the great deal of experience that is needed for its proper use.

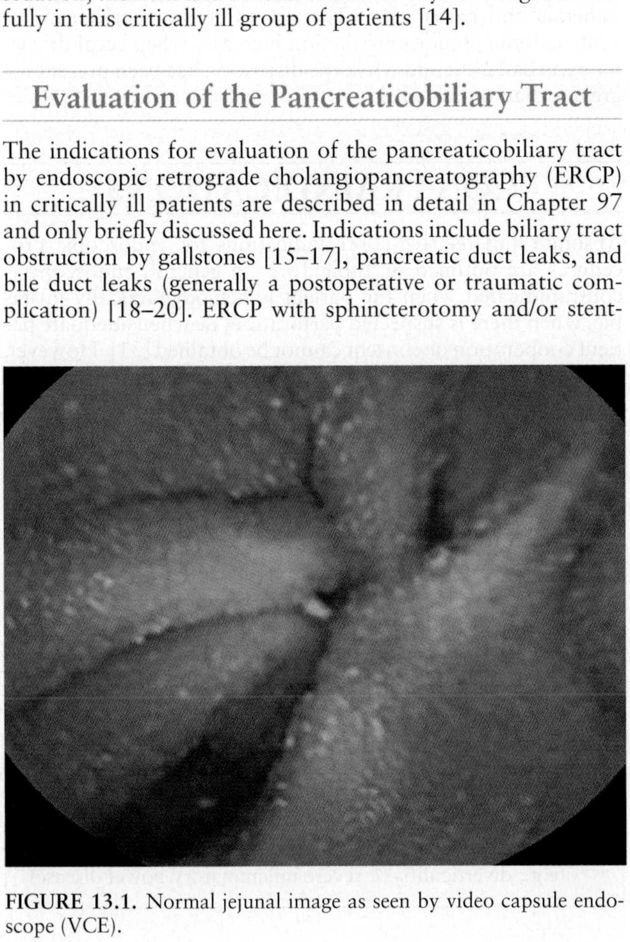

FIGURE 13.1. Normal jejunal image as seen by video capsule endoscope (VCE).

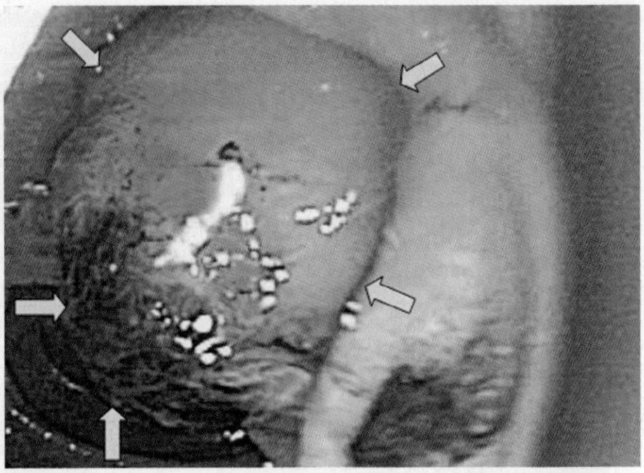

FIGURE 13.2. Tumor seen in proximal jejunum during double-balloon enteroscopy (DBE). (Courtesy: David Cave, MD: Professor of Medicine, University of Massachusetts Medical School.)

Evaluation of the Mid-Gastrointestinal Tract (Jejunum and Ileum)

Persistent, obscure GI bleeding is the most common indication for evaluation of this portion of the GI tract. Although this area of the GI tract had been difficult to evaluate in the past, this is no longer the case. The advent of the wireless video capsule endoscope (VCE), the double-balloon endoscope (DBE), and the spiral endoscope has made this area of the GI tract easily accessible. VCE is usually the first test performed to look for possible sites of bleeding in the jejunum and ileum (Fig. 13.1). If bleeding or lesions are identified, the DBE (Fig. 13.2) or the spiral endoscope (Fig. 13.3) would be used to implement therapy.

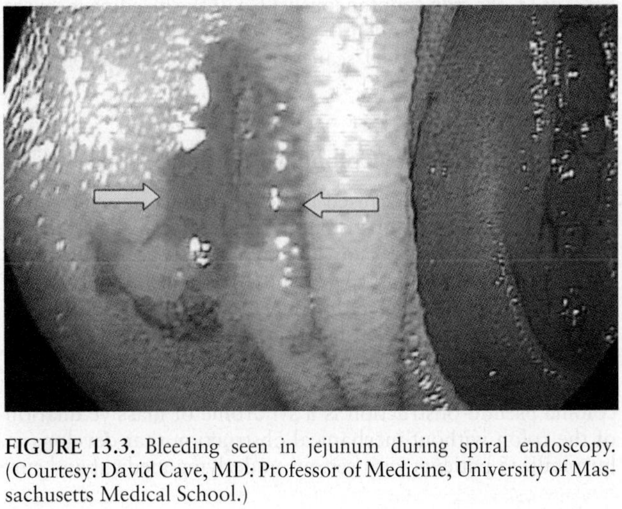

FIGURE 13.3. Bleeding seen in jejunum during spiral endoscopy. (Courtesy: David Cave, MD: Professor of Medicine, University of Massachusetts Medical School.)

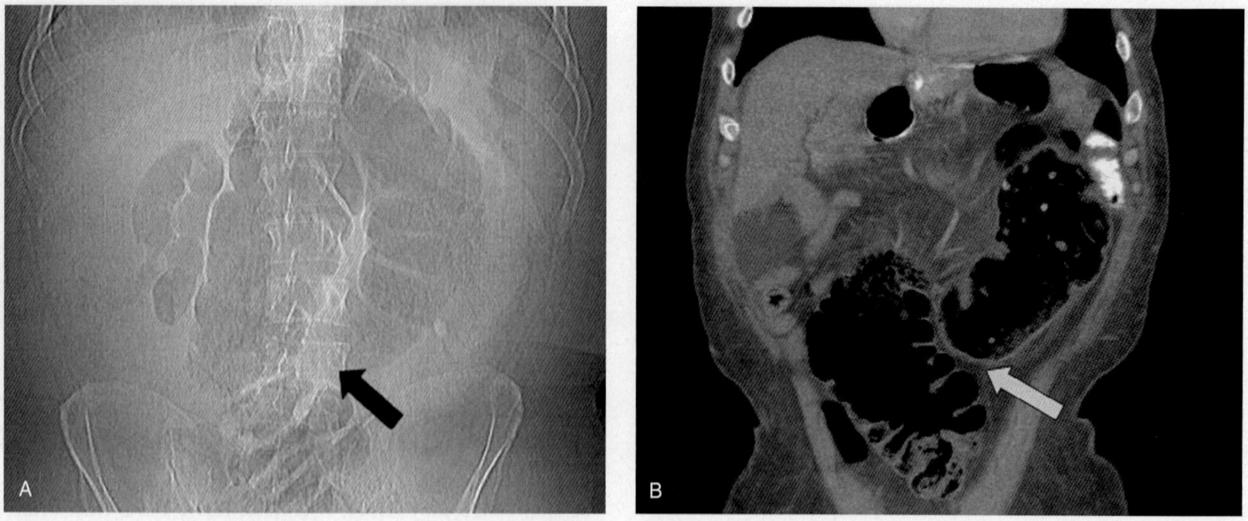

FIGURE 13.4. **A:** X-ray showing cecal volvulus. (Courtesy: Milliam Kataoka, MD, Radiology Fellow, UMass Memorial Medical Center.) **B:** CT scan showing cecal volvulus. (Courtesy: Milliam, MD, Radiology Fellow, UMass Memorial Medical Center.)

Evaluation of the Lower Gastrointestinal Tract

Colonoscopic evaluation is urgently needed in ICU patients in cases of severe lower GI bleeding (LGIB), acute colonic distention, and at times for the evaluation of infection (*Cytomegalovirus* [CMV] and *Clostridium difficile*) in the immunocompromised patients [22,23].

Severe LGIB is predominantly a disease of the elderly. It is defined as bleeding from a source distal to the ligament of Treitz for less than 3 days [24]. Common causes include, but are not limited to, diverticular bleeding, ischemic colitis, and vascular abnormalities (arteriovenous malformations, AVMs). However, as many as 11% of patients initially suspected to have an LGIB are ultimately found to have a UGIB [25]. Therefore, UGIB sources should always be considered first in patients with LGIB, particularly in patients with unstable hemodynamics. Once an upper GI source has been excluded, colonoscopy should be performed to evaluate the lower GI tract and administer appropriate therapy. Although urgent colonoscopy within 24 to 48 hours has shown to decrease the length of hospital stay [26] and endoscopic intervention is often successful, 80% to 85% of LGIBs stop spontaneously [27]. If the bleeding is severe or a source cannot be identified at colonoscopy, a technetium (TC)-99m red blood cell scan with or without angiography should be considered [28].

Acute Colonic Distention

This condition can be caused by acute colonic obstruction or acute colonic pseudo-obstruction. Acute colonic obstruction can be caused by neoplasms, diverticular disease, and volvulus [29]. Volvulus (Fig. 13.4A and B) is a "closed-loop obstruction" and is considered an emergency because unlike the other causes of colonic obstruction, it can rapidly deteriorate from obstruction to ischemia, perforation, and death. However, if identified and treated early, it can be reversed. Acute colonic pseudo-obstruction is a syndrome of massive dilation of the colon without mechanical obstruction that develops in hospitalized patients with serious underlying medical and surgical conditions due to impaired colonic motility. Increasing age, cecal diameter, delay in decompression, and status of the bowel significantly influence mortality, which is approximately 40% when ischemia or perforation is present. Evaluation of the markedly distended colon in the ICU setting involves excluding mechanical obstruction and other causes of toxic megacolon, such as *C. difficile* infection, and assessing for signs of ischemia and perforation. The risk of colonic perforation in acute colonic pseudo-obstruction increases when cecal diameter exceeds 12 cm and when the distention has been present for greater than 6 days [30].

CONTRAINDICATIONS

Absolute and relative contraindications for endoscopic procedures are outlined in Table 13.2. In general, endoscopy is contraindicated when the patient is hemodynamically unstable, when there is suspected perforation, or when adequate patient cooperation or consent cannot be obtained [31]. However, there are exceptions to these rules. In these cases, resuscitation and endoscopic intervention would need to go on simultaneously.

TABLE 13.2

CONTRAINDICATIONS TO ENDOSCOPY

Absolute contraindications
Suspected or impending perforated viscus
Risks to the patient outweigh benefits of the procedure
Relative contraindications
Adequate patient cooperation or consent cannot be obtained
Hemodynamic instability or myocardial infarction
Inadequate airway protection or hypoxemia
Severe coagulopathy or thrombocytopenia
Inflammatory changes with increased risk of perforation (e.g., diverticulitis or severe inflammatory bowel disease)

PERIPROCEDURAL CARE

Key elements of planning interventional endoscopic procedures include appropriate resuscitation and reversal of coagulopathies [32]. Proper sedation may simply involve light sedation in some patients [33]. However, in uncooperative, confused, or hypoxemic patients, it may require endotracheal intubation with deep sedation or general anesthesia. Although endotracheal intubation does not significantly alter the risk of acquired pneumonia or cardiovascular events [33,34], it does generate controlled conditions during the procedure and may help prevent massive aspiration (especially in patients with variceal bleeding). Antibiotics need to be considered in patients with ascites and those with a history of endocarditis [35].

Upper Gastrointestinal Endoscopy

Upper Gastrointestinal Bleeding

In all patients with upper GI bleeding, an empty stomach is crucial for thorough evaluation and identification of the bleeding lesion. Through proper identification and treatment, studies have shown a reduction in the risk of rebleeding and in the need for surgical intervention [36]. Gastric lavage with an NG tube or through use of the endoscope can clear the stomach of blood and clot partially. At times, the use of the prokinetic agents such as erythromycin (250 mg in 50 mL of normal saline IV, 20 minutes prior to the procedure) may also be helpful. Studies have in fact shown that this approach may improve the endoscopic visualization, improve the outcome, and decrease the need for "second-look" endoscopy [37]. Although metoclopramide may theoretically have a similar effect, the use of this agent has not been studied extensively. If a variceal hemorrhage is suspected, on the basis of a clinical history or physical examination suggesting portal hypertension, adjunctive therapy should be initiated immediately in the absence of contraindications. Both somatostatin analogues (octreotide) or vasopressin and its analogues have been used intravenously (IV) to reduce portal pressures and prevent recurrent bleeding. A recent meta-analysis slightly favored octreotide over terlipressin/vasopressin in the control of esophageal variceal bleeding [38]. Octreotide is usually given as a onetime bolus of 50 to 100 μg IV, followed by 25 to 50 μg IV per hour for 3 to 5 days. In addition, prophylactic antibiotics should be given to patients with active esophageal variceal bleeding for the prevention of bacterial infections [39]. In contrast to nonvariceal hemorrhage, volume resuscitation should be performed judiciously in variceal bleeding as volume repletion can theoretically increase portal pressures.

If the bleeding source is found to be a peptic ulcer, the intervention will depend on the specific endoscopic findings [7]. If an actively bleeding or a nonbleeding visible vessel is identified in the crater of the ulcer, endoscopic hemostatic techniques are recommended. If the ulcer has a clean base with no signs of active bleeding, endoscopic intervention is not indicated. A number of endoscopic methods have been developed for hemostasis, including injection therapy, thermal cautery therapy, and mechanical hemostasis with clips (Table 13.3). The combination of injection therapy with thermal coaptive therapy is superior to either alone [1,40]. Although no single solution for endoscopic injection therapy appears superior to another, an epinephrine–saline solution is usually injected in four quadrants surrounding the lesion. Heater probe and multipolar electrocoagulation instruments are subsequently applied with firm pressure to achieve optimal coaptation. Mechanical hemostasis, with hemoclips, has been a more recent addition for hemostasis therapy (Fig. 13.5A and B). Controlled trials comparing clipping alone with other endoscopic hemostatic techniques for nonvariceal UGIB are limited. Current evidence suggests that the hemoclip is not superior to other endoscopic modalities in terms of initial hemostasis, rebleeding rate, emergency surgery, and the mortality rate for treatment of peptic ulcer bleed [41]. However, they may be especially useful in the treatment of critically ill patients [42] and patients with coagulopathy. Argon plasma coagulation (APC) is a noncoaptive technique that provides cautery to tissues by means of ionized argon gas. This method is most commonly used in the treatment of AVMs. The YAG laser has fallen out of favor in the acute management of high-risk patients because of its poor portability and associated high cost.

TABLE 13.3

ENDOSCOPIC METHODS FOR HEMOSTATIS

Thermal methods of hemostasis
Heater probe
Multipolar electrocoagulation (bicap)
Neodymium yttrium-aluminium-garnet (YAG) laser
Argon plasma coagulation
Injection therapy for hemostasis
Distilled water or saline
Epinephrine (adrenaline)
Sclerosants (Cyanoacrylate, polidocanol, ethanol, ethanolamine oleare, sodium tetradecyl sulfate, sodium morrhuate)
Thrombin Fibrin-glue
Mechanical methods
Clips
Band ligation
Detachable loops

Whatever method of hemostasis is used, patients with nonvariceal UGIB need to be placed on antisecretory therapy with a proton pump inhibitor (PPI) following endoscopic hemostasis [2,40]. IV administration of a PPI is a faster way to achieve gastric acid suppression than is oral administration of the same agent. Peak suppression after IV administration occurs within hours, compared with several days later after oral administration. This is crucial because it can reduce the risk of rebleeding and the need for surgery [43,44]. The PPIs currently approved for IV use in the United States include pantoprazole, lansoprazole, and esomeprazole [45].

If the bleeding is found to be caused by esophageal varices, endoscopic variceal ligation (EVL) has become the procedure of choice [46]. With this technique, the varix is suctioned into a banding device attached to the tip of the endoscope and a rubber band is then deployed at its base to obliterate the varix. In contrast, endoscopic sclerotherapy (EST) causes obliteration by injection of a sclerosing agent (e.g., sodium morrhuate) in or around the bleeding varix. A meta-analysis by Laine and Cook [47] suggested that EVL was superior to EST in all major outcomes (recurrent bleeding, local complications such as ulcers or strictures, time to variceal obliteration, and survival). However, EST is effective in controlling active bleeding in more than 90% of cases and can be injected even with poor visualization during an active bleed.

Endoscopic methods (EST, EVL, and injection of fibrin glue) have also been used for the treatment of bleeding gastric varices in small and mostly uncontrolled studies. However, these methods carry a considerable risk of rebleeding and mortality. Patients with bleeding gastric varices generally require urgent

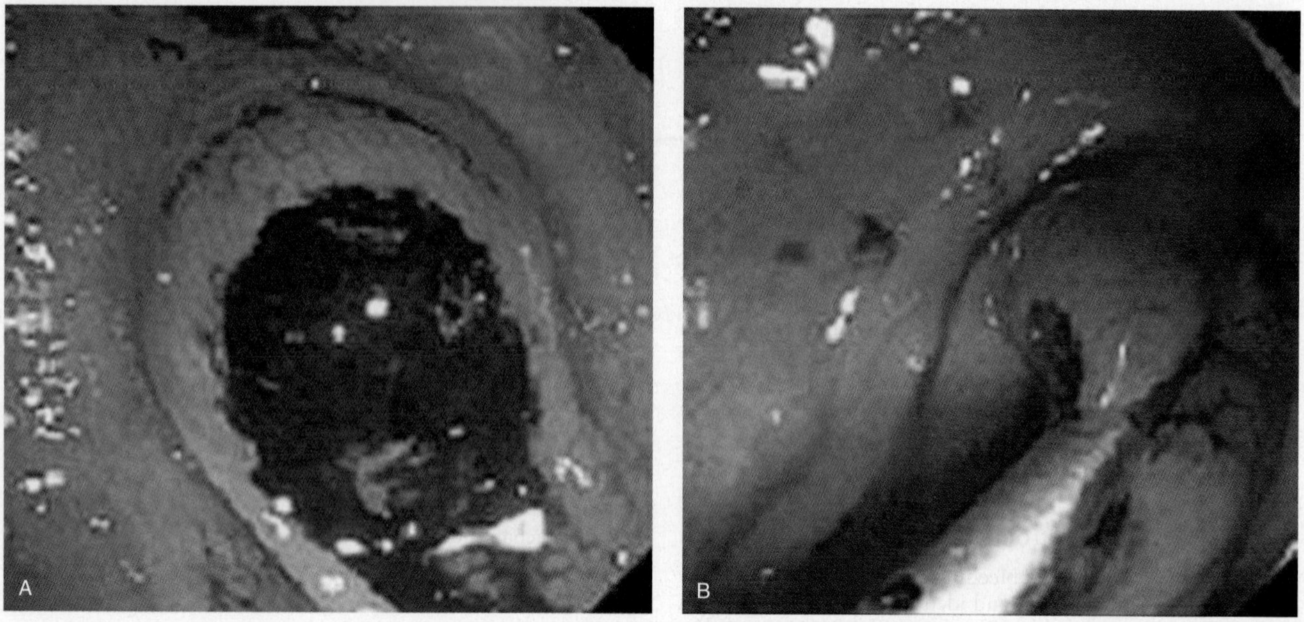

FIGURE 13.5. A: Postpolypectomy bleeding. B: Hemostasis by hemoclip for postpolypectomy bleeding.

placement of a transjugular intrahepatic portosystemic shunt (TIPS) [48].

Enteric Feeding Tubes

Please see Chapter 16 for more detail on the placement of enteric feeding tubes.

Pancreaticobiliary Endoscopy (Refer to Chapter 97)

Small Bowel Endoscopy

The techniques are essentially the same as those for upper GI endoscopy. Please refer to that section for details.

Lower Gastrointestinal Endoscopy

Unlike any of the other types of endoscopies previously discussed, this is the only one requiring a preprocedure bowel preparation. In urgent situations, this can be done through a technique known as a rapid purge. This technique is usually achieved by drinking 4 L or more polyethylene glycol–based solutions over a 2- to 3-hour period. Approximately one-third of hospitalized patients require an NGT for this type of preparation [49]. Metoclopramide (10 mg IV × 1), administered prior to starting the preparation, may help to control nausea and promote gastric emptying [25].

Lower Gastrointestinal Bleeding

The endoscopic treatment options for LGIB are similar to those for UGIB (see earlier in the chapter) and should be based on the stigmata of bleeding that are identified. Hemostasis is usually approached through a combination approach of injection therapy with clipping or coagulation therapy.

Decompressive Endoscopy

A water-soluble contrast enema or computed tomography (CT) should be the initial procedure to perform in patients with acute colon distention. This will establish the presence or absence of mechanical obstruction. Subsequently, the patient should undergo resuscitation with IV fluids (IVF), frequent repositioning, NG and rectal tube placement, correction of metabolic imbalances, and discontinuation of medications known to slow intestinal transit [50]. If conservative measures are unsuccessful, decompressive endoscopy with minimal inflation of air resolves acute obstruction of the colon in the majority of cases (81%) [51]. Despite a high recurrence rate (23% to 57%), colonoscopy is often considered the initial procedure of choice in the absence of intestinal ischemia [52,53]. This may be reduced with the placement of a decompression tube beyond the splenic flexure [54]. In patients with mechanical obstruction, self-expanding metallic stents (SEMS) can be placed with good outcome [55]. In patients with nonmechanical obstruction, medical therapy with the parasympathomimetic agent neostigmine should be considered. On the basis of a double-blind, placebo-controlled, randomized trial, the parasympathomimetic agent neostigmine has been shown to reduce colonic distention significantly, reduce recurrence, and cause minimal risk [56]. This agent should only be given in the absence of contraindications and under close cardiorespiratory monitoring with atropine at the bedside. Percutaneous, endoscopic, or surgical cecostomy presents another alternative if the aforementioned interventions are unsuccessful.

COMPLICATIONS

Although major complications of endoscopic procedures are infrequent, critically ill patients may be particularly sensitive to adverse outcomes due to multiple comorbidities. Complications can be divided into two groups: (i) general complications and (ii) specific complications (Table 13.4).

FUTURE DIRECTIONS

With the start of the new millennium, rapid advances have been made in the development of new techniques [57]. Natural orifice transluminal endoscopic surgery (NOTES) is such

TABLE 13.4

COMPLICATIONS OF ENDOSCOPY

General complications
- Complications of conscious sedation (cardiopulmonary, allergic, paradoxical reactions)
- Bleeding (e.g., treatment of lesions, sphincterotomy)
- Perforation (caused by endoscope, accessories, or air insufflation)
- Aspiration
- Myocardial ischemia

Specific complications (examples)
- Endoscopic retrograde cholangiopancreatography: Pancreatitis, cholangitis, perforation
- Sclerotherapy: Ulceration, mediastinitis
- Stenting procedures: Stent migration

a technique. It involves the use of a natural orifice (such as stomach, rectum, vagina, or urethra) for intraperitoneal access to perform a variety of procedures in the retroperitoneum, such as liver biopsy, cystogastrostomy, appendectomy, cholecystectomy, nephrectomy, and tubal ligation. In the ICU setting, this type of a procedure is being evaluated for a number of potential scenarios: (i) the evaluation of suspected abdominal sepsis and ischemia at the bedside [58]; (ii) the feasibility of transgastric mapping of the diaphragm and implantation of a percutaneous electrode for therapeutic diaphragmatic stimulation in difficult-to-wean ICU patients [59]; and (iii) direct J-tube placement in selected patients without the need for surgery. Whatever role NOTES will have in the future of the critical care population, it is already changing how we approach a number of GI problems and will be a part of the ever-evolving management of the critically ill population in the future to expedite and improve their care.

References

1. Wassef W: Upper gastrointestinal bleeding. *Curr Opin Gastroenterol* 20:538–545, 2004.
2. Adler DG, Leighton JA, Davila RE, et al: ASGE guideline: the role of endoscopy in acute non-variceal upper-GI hemorrhage. *Gastrointest Endosc* 60:497–504, 2004.
3. Chak A, Cooper GS, Lloyd LE, et al: Effectiveness of endoscopy in patients admitted to the intensive care unit with upper GI hemorrhage. *Gastrointest Endosc* 53:6–13, 2001.
4. Kupfer Y, Cappell MS, Tessler S: Acute gastrointestinal bleeding in the intensive care unit. The intensivist's perspective. *Gastroenterol Clin North Am* 29:275–307, 2000.
5. Beejay U, Wolfe MM: Acute gastrointestinal bleeding in the intensive care unit. The gastroenterologist's perspective. *Gastroenterol Clin North Am* 29:309–336, 2000.
6. Laine L, Peterson WL: Bleeding peptic ulcer. *N Engl J Med* 331:717–727, 1994.
7. Cheung FK, Lau JY: Management of massive peptic ulcer bleeding. *Gastroenterol Clin North Am* 38(2):231–243, 2009.
8. Eisen GM, Baron TH, Dominitz JA, et al: Guideline for the management of ingested foreign bodies. *Gastrointest Endosc* 55:802–806, 2002.
9. Poley JW, Steyerberg EW, Kuipers EJ, et al: Ingestion of acid and alkaline agents: outcome and prognostic value of early upper endoscopy. *Gastrointest Endosc* 60:372–377, 2004.
10. Eisen GM, Baron TH, Dominitz JA, et al: Role of endoscopy in enteral feeding. *Gastrointest Endosc* 55:699–701, 2002.
11. Fan AC, Baron TH, Rumalla A: Comparison of direct percutaneous endoscopic jejunostomy and PEG with jejunal extension. *Gastrointest Endosc* 56:890–894, 2002.
12. DeLegge MH, McClave SA, DiSario JA, et al: Ethical and medicolegal aspects of PEG-tube placement and provision of artificial nutritional therapy. *Gastrointest Endosc* 62:952–959, 2005.
13. Herman LL, Hoskins WJ, Shike M: Percutaneous endoscopic gastrostomy for decompression of the stomach and small bowel. *Gastrointest Endosc* 38:314–318, 1992.
14. Hallenbeck J: Reevaluating PEG tube placement in advanced illnesses. *Gastrointest Endosc* 62:960–961, 2005.
15. Sharma VK, Howden CW: Metaanalysis of randomized controlled trials of endoscopic retrograde cholangiography and endoscopic sphincterotomy for the treatment of acute biliary pancreatitis. *Am J Gastroenterol* 94:3211–3214, 1999.
16. Adler DG, Baron TH, Davila RE, et al: ASGE guideline: the role of ERCP in diseases of the biliary tract and the pancreas. *Gastrointest Endosc* 62:1–8, 2005.
17. Lai EC, Mok FP, Tan ES, et al: Endoscopic biliary drainage for severe acute cholangitis. *N Engl J Med* 326:1582–1586, 1992.
18. Kaffes AJ, Hourigan L, De Luca N, et al: Impact of endoscopic intervention in 100 patients with suspected postcholecystectomy bile leak. *Gastrointest Endosc* 61:269–275, 2005.
19. Sandha GS, Bourke MJ, Haber GB, et al: Endoscopic therapy of bile leak based on a new classification: results in 207 patients. *Gastrointest Endosc* 60:567–574, 2004.
20. Lubezky N, Konikoff FM, Rosin D, et al: Endoscopic sphincterotomy and temporary internal stenting for bile leaks following complex hepatic trauma. *Br J Surg* 93:78–81, 2006.
21. Judah JR, Draganov PV: Intraductal biliary and pancreatic endoscopy: an expanding scope of possibility. *World J Gastroenterol* 14(20):3129–3136, 2008.
22. Southworth M, Taffet SL, Levien DH, et al: Colonoscopy in critically ill patients. What conditions call for it? *Postgrad Med* 88:159–163, 1990.
23. Oomori S, Takagi S, Kikuchi T, et al: Significance of colonoscopy in patients with intestinal graft-versus-host disease after hematopoietic stem cell transplantation. *Endoscopy* 37:346–350, 2005.
24. Davila RE, Rajan E, Adler DG, et al: ASGE guideline: the role of endoscopy in the patient with lower GI-bleeding. *Gastrointest Endosc* 62:656–660, 2005.
25. Jensen DM, Machicado GA: Diagnosis and treatment of severe hematochezia. The role of urgent colonoscopy after purge. *Gastroenterology* 95:1569–1574, 1988.
26. Strate LL, Syngal S: Timing of colonoscopy: impact on length of hospital stay in patients with acute lower GI bleeding. *Am J Gastroenterol* 98:317–322, 2003.
27. Farrell JJ, Friedman LS: Review article: the management of lower gastrointestinal bleeding. *Aliment Pharmacol Ther* 21:1281–1298, 2005.
28. Strate LL, Syngal S: Predictors of utilization of early colonoscopy vs. radiography for severe lower intestinal bleeding. *Gastrointest Endosc* 61:46–52, 2005.
29. Frizelle FA, Wolff BG: Colonic volvulus. *Adv Surg* 29:131–139, 1996.
30. Saunders MD, Kimmey MB: Colonic pseudo-obstruction: the dilated colon in the ICU. *Semin Gastrointest Dis* 14(1):20–27, 2003.
31. American Society for Gastrointestinal Endoscopy: Appropriate use of gastrointestinal endoscopy. *Gastrointest Endosc* 52:831–837, 2000.
32. ASGE Standards of Practice Committee: Levy MJ, Anderson MA, Baron TH, et al: Position statement on routine laboratory testing before endoscopic procedures. *Gastrointest Endosc* 68:827–832, 2008.
33. ASGE Standards of Practice Committee: Lichenstein DR, Jagannath S, Baron TH, et al: Sedation and anesthesia in GI endoscopy. *Gastrointest Endosc* 68(5):815–826, 2008.
34. Wassef W, Rullan R: Interventional endoscopy. *Curr Opin Gastroenterol* 21:644–652, 2005.
35. ASGE Standards of Practice Committee: Bannerjee S, Shen B, Baron TH, et al: Antibiotic prophylaxis for GI endoscopy. *Gastrointest Endosc* 67:791–798, 2008.
36. Kahi CJ, Jensen DM, Sung JJY, et al: Endoscopic therapy versus medical therapy for bleeding peptic ulcer with adherent clot: a metaanalysis. *Gastroenterology* 129:855–862, 2005.
37. Frossard JL, Spahr L, Queneau PE, et al: Erythromycin intravenous bolus infusion in acute upper gastrointestinal bleeding: a randomized, controlled, double-blind trial. *Gastroenterology* 123:17–23, 2002.
38. Corley DA, Cello JP, Akisson W, et al: Octreotide for acute esophageal variceal bleeding: a metaanalysis. *Gastroenterology* 120:946–954, 2001.
39. Soares-Weiser K, Brezis M, Tur-Kaspa R, et al: Antibiotic prophylaxis for cirrhotic patients with gastrointestinal bleed. *Cochrane Database Syst Rev* CD002907, 2002.
40. Barkun A, Bardou M, Marshall JK, et al: Consensus recommendations for managing patients with nonvariceal upper gastrointestinal bleeding. *Ann Intern Med* 139:843–857, 2003.
41. Yuan Y, Wang C, Hunt RH: Endoscopic clipping for acute nonvariceal upper-GI bleeding: a meta-analysis and critical appraisal of randomized controlled trials. *Gastrointest Endosc* 68(2):339–351, 2008.
42. Goto H, Ohta S, Yamaguchi Y, et al: Prospective evaluation of hemoclip application with injection of epinephrine in hypertonic saline solution for hemostasis in unstable patients with shock caused by upper GI bleeding. *Gastrointest Endosc* 56:78–82, 2002.
43. Bardou M, Toubouti Y, Benhaberou-Brun D, et al: Meta analysis: proton-pump inhibition in high-risk patients with acute peptic ulcer bleeding. *Aliment Pharmacol Ther* 21:677–686, 2005.

44. Leontiadis GI, Sharma VK, Howden CW: Systematic review and metaanalysis of proton pump inhibitor therapy in peptic ulcer bleeding. *BMJ* 330:568–570, 2005.
45. Baker DE: Intravenous proton pump inhibitors. *Rev Gastroenterol Disord* 6(1):22–34, 2006.
46. Qureshi W, Adler DG, Davila R, et al: ASGE guideline: the role of endoscopy in the management of variceal hemorrhage, updated July 2005. *Gastrointest Endosc* 62:651–655, 2005.
47. Laine L, Cook D: Endoscopic ligation compared with sclerotherapy for treatment of esophageal variceal bleeding: a metaanalysis. *Ann Intern Med* 123:280–287, 1995.
48. Sharara AI, Rockey DC: Gastroesophageal variceal bleed. *N Engl J Med* 345:669–681, 2001.
49. Elta GH: Technological review. Urgent colonoscopy for acute lower-GI bleeding. *Gastrointest Endosc* 59:402–408, 2004.
50. Eisen GM, Baron TH, Dominitz JA, et al: Acute colonic pseudo-obstruction. *Gastrointest Endosc* 56:789–792, 2002.
51. Grossmann EM, Longo WE, Stratton MD, et al: Sigmoid volvulus in Department of Veterans Affairs Medical Centers. *Dis Colon Rectum* 43:414–418, 2000.
52. Martinez Ares D, Yanez Lopez J, Souto Ruzo J, et al: Indication and results of endoscopic management of sigmoid volvulus. *Rev Esp Enferm Dig* 95:544–548, 2003.
53. Saunders MD, Kimmey MB: Systematic review: acute colonic pseudo-obstruction. *Aliment Pharmacol Ther* 22:917–925, 2005.
54. Geller A, Petersen BT, Gostout CJ: Endoscopic decompression for acute colonic pseudo-obstruction. *Gastrointest Endosc* 44:144–150, 1996.
55. Dronamraju SS, Ramamurthy S, Kelly SB, et al: Role of self-expanding metallic stents in the management of malignant obstruction of the proximal colon. *Dis Colon Rectum* 52(9):1657–1661, 2009.
56. Ponec RJ, Saunders MD, Kimmey MB: Neostigmine for the treatment of acute colonic pseudo-obstruction. *N Engl J Med* 341:137–141, 1999.
57. Mallery S, Van Dam J: Endoscopic practice at the start of the new millennium. *Gastroenterology* 118:S129–S147, 2000.
58. Onders RP, McGee MF, Marks J, et al: Natural orifice transluminal endoscopic surgery (NOTES) as a diagnostic tool in the intensive care unit. *Surg Endosc* 21(4):681–683, 2007.
59. Onders R, McGee MF, Marks J, et al: Diaphragm pacing with natural orifice transluminal endoscopic surgery: potential for difficult-to-wean intensive care unit patients. *Surg Endosc* 21(3):475–479, 2007.

CHAPTER 14 ■ PARACENTESIS AND DIAGNOSTIC PERITONEAL LAVAGE

LENA M. NAPOLITANO

ABDOMINAL PARACENTESIS

Indications

Abdominal paracentesis is a simple procedure that can be easily performed at the bedside in the intensive care unit and may provide important diagnostic information or therapy in critically ill patients with ascites. As a *diagnostic* intervention, abdominal paracentesis with removal of 20 mL of peritoneal fluid is performed to determine the etiology of the ascites or to ascertain whether infection is present, as in spontaneous bacterial peritonitis [1]. It can also be used in any clinical situation in which the analysis of a sample of peritoneal fluid might be useful in ascertaining a diagnosis and guiding therapy. The evaluation of ascites should therefore include a diagnostic paracentesis with ascitic fluid analysis.

As a *therapeutic* intervention, abdominal paracentesis is usually performed to drain large volumes of abdominal ascites, termed large-volume paracentesis (LVP), with removal of more than 5 L of ascitic fluid [2]. Ascites is the most common presentation of decompensated cirrhosis, and its development heralds a poor prognosis, with a 50% 2-year survival rate. Effective first-line therapy for ascites includes sodium restriction (2 g per day), use of diuretics, and LVP. When tense or refractory ascites is present, LVP is safe and effective, and has the advantage of producing immediate relief from ascites and its associated symptoms [3]. LVP can be palliative by diminishing abdominal pain from distention or improving pulmonary function by allowing better diaphragmatic excursion in patients who have ascites refractory to aggressive medical management. LVP is also used for percutaneous decompression of resuscitation-induced abdominal compartment syndrome related to the development of acute tense ascites [4].

Refractory ascites occurs in 10% of patients with cirrhosis and is associated with substantial morbidity and a 1-year survival of less than 50% [5,6]. For patients with refractory ascites, transjugular intrahepatic portosystemic shunt (TIPS) is superior to LVP for long-term control of ascites, but it is associated with greater encephalopathy risk and does not affect mortality [7,8].

Techniques

Before abdominal paracentesis is initiated, a catheter must be inserted to drain the urinary bladder, and correction of any underlying coagulopathy or thrombocytopenia should be considered. A consensus statement from the International Ascites Club states that "there are no data to support the correction of mild coagulopathy with blood products prior to therapeutic paracentesis, but caution is needed when severe thrombocytopenia is present" [3]. The practice guideline from the American Association for the Study of Liver Diseases states that routine correction of prolonged prothrombin time or thrombocytopenia is not required when experienced personnel perform paracentesis [9]. This has been confirmed in a study of 1,100 LVPs in 628 patients [10]. But in critically ill patients, there is still uncertainty as to the optimal platelet count and prothrombin time for the safe conduct of paracentesis.

The patient must next be positioned correctly. In critically ill patients, the procedure is performed in the supine position with the head of the bed elevated at 30 to 45 degrees. If the patient is clinically stable and therapeutic LVP is being performed, the patient can be placed in the sitting position, leaning slightly forward, to increase the total volume of ascites removed.

The site for paracentesis on the anterior abdominal wall is then chosen (Fig. 14.1). The preferred site is in the lower

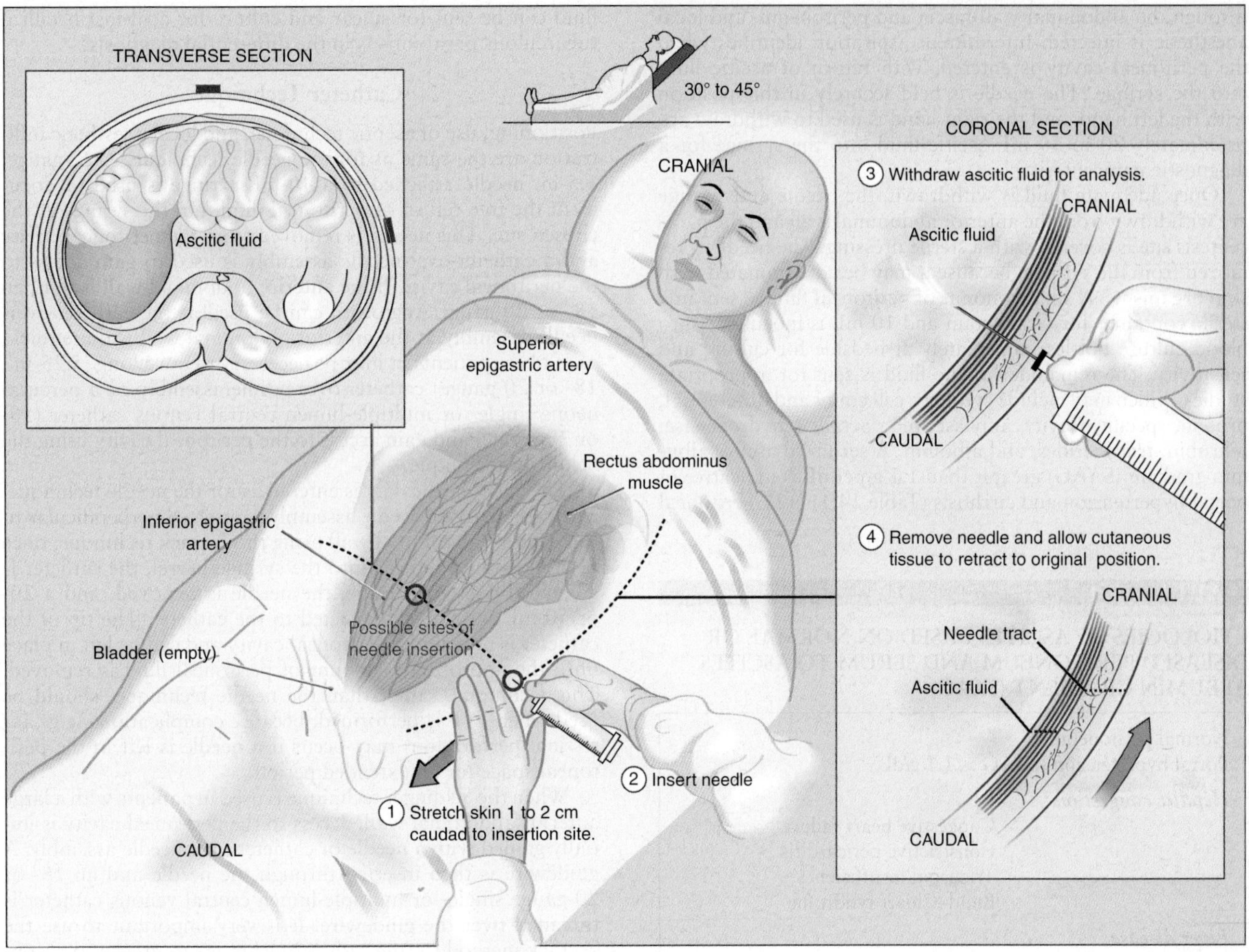

FIGURE 14.1. Suggested sites for paracentesis.

abdomen, just lateral to the rectus abdominis muscle and inferior to the umbilicus. It is important to stay lateral to the rectus abdominis muscle to avoid injury to the inferior epigastric artery and vein. In patients with chronic cirrhosis and caput medusae (engorged anterior abdominal wall veins), these visible vascular structures must be avoided. Injury to these veins can cause significant bleeding because of the underlying portal hypertension and may result in hemoperitoneum. The left lower quadrant of the abdominal wall is preferred over the right lower quadrant for abdominal paracentesis because critically ill patients often have cecal distention. The ideal site is therefore in the left lower quadrant of the abdomen, lateral to the rectus abdominis muscle in the midclavicular line and inferior to the umbilicus. It has also been determined that the left lower quadrant is significantly thinner and the depth of ascites greater compared with the infraumbilical midline position, confirming the left lower quadrant as the preferred location for paracentesis [11].

If the patient had previous abdominal surgery limited to the lower abdomen, it may be difficult to perform a paracentesis in the lower abdomen and the upper abdomen may be chosen. The point of entry, however, remains lateral to the rectus abdominis muscle in the midclavicular line. If there is concern that the ascites is loculated because of a previous abdominal surgery or peritonitis, abdominal paracentesis should be performed under ultrasound guidance to prevent iatrogenic complications.

Abdominal paracentesis can be performed by the needle technique, by the catheter technique, or with ultrasound guidance. Diagnostic paracentesis usually requires 20 to 50 mL peritoneal fluid and is commonly performed using the needle technique. However, if large volumes of peritoneal fluid are required, the catheter technique is used because it is associated with a lower incidence of complications. LVP should always be performed with the catheter technique. Ultrasound guidance can be helpful in diagnostic paracentesis using the needle technique or in LVP using the catheter technique.

Needle Technique

With the patient in the appropriate position and the access site for paracentesis determined, the patient's abdomen is prepared with 2% chlorhexidine and sterile aseptic technique is used. If necessary, intravenous sedation is administered to prevent the patient from moving excessively during the procedure (see Chapter 20). Local anesthesia, using 1% or 2% lidocaine with 1:200,000 epinephrine, is infiltrated into the site. A skin wheal is created with the local anesthetic, using a short 25- or 27-gauge needle. Then, using a 22-gauge, 1.5-in. needle, the local anesthetic is infiltrated into the subcutaneous tissues and anterior abdominal wall, with the needle perpendicular to the skin. Before the anterior abdominal wall and peritoneum are infiltrated, the skin is pulled taut inferiorly, allowing the peritoneal cavity to be entered at a different location than the skin entrance site, thereby decreasing the chance of ascitic leak. This is known as the *Z-track technique*. While tension is maintained inferiorly on the abdominal skin, the needle is advanced through the abdominal wall fascia and peritoneum, and local anesthetic is injected. Intermittent aspiration identifies when the peritoneal cavity is entered, with return of ascitic fluid into the syringe. The needle is held securely in this position with the left hand, and the right hand is used to withdraw approximately 20 to 50 mL ascitic fluid into the syringe for a diagnostic paracentesis.

Once adequate fluid is withdrawn, the needle and syringe are withdrawn from the anterior abdominal wall and the paracentesis site is covered with a sterile dressing. The needle is removed from the syringe, because it may be contaminated with skin organisms. A small amount of peritoneal fluid is sent in a sterile container for Gram stain and 10 mL is inoculated into blood culture bottles immediately at bedside for culture and sensitivity. The remainder of the fluid is sent for appropriate studies, which may include cytology, cell count and differential, protein, specific gravity, amylase, pH, lactate dehydrogenase, bilirubin, triglycerides, and albumin. A serum to ascites albumin gradient (SAAG) greater than 1.1 g per dL is indicative of portal hypertension and cirrhosis (Table 14.1) [12]. Peritoneal fluid can be sent for smear and culture for acid-fast bacilli if tuberculous peritonitis is in the differential diagnosis.

TABLE 14.1

ETIOLOGIES OF ASCITES BASED ON NORMAL OR DISEASED PERITONEUM AND SERUM TO ASCITES ALBUMIN GRADIENT (SAAG)

Normal peritoneum	
Portal hypertension (SAAG > 1.1 g/dL)	
Hepatic congestion	
	Congestive heart failure
	Constrictive pericarditis
	Tricuspid insufficiency
	Budd–Chiari syndrome
Liver disease	
	Cirrhosis
	Alcoholic hepatitis
	Fulminant hepatic failure
	Massive hepatic metastases
Hypoalbuminemia (SAAG < 1.1 g/dL)	
	Nephrotic syndrome
	Protein-losing enteropathy
	Severe malnutrition with anasarca
Miscellaneous conditions (SAAG < 1.1 g/dL)	
	Chylous ascites
	Pancreatic ascites
	Bile ascites
	Nephrogenic ascites
	Urine ascites
	Ovarian disease
Diseased peritoneum infections (SAAG < 1.1 g/dL)	
	Bacterial peritonitis
	Tuberculous peritonitis
	Fungal peritonitis
	HIV-associated peritonitis
Malignant conditions	
	Peritoneal carcinomatosis
	Primary mesothelioma
	Pseudomyxoma peritonei
	Hepatocellular carcinoma
Other rare conditions	
	Familial Mediterranean fever
	Vasculitis
	Granulomatous peritonitis
	Eosinophilic peritonitis

Catheter Technique

Positioning, use of aseptic technique, and local anesthetic infiltration are the same as for the needle technique. A 22-gauge, 1.5-in. needle attached to a 10-mL syringe is used to document the free return of peritoneal fluid into the syringe at the chosen site. This needle is removed from the peritoneal cavity and a catheter-over-needle assembly is used to gain access to the peritoneal cavity. If the anterior abdominal wall is thin, an 18- or 20-gauge Angiocath can be used as the catheter-over-needle assembly. If the anterior abdominal wall is quite thick, as in obese patients, it may be necessary to use a long (5.25-in., 18- or 20-gauge) catheter-over-needle assembly or a percutaneous single- or multiple-lumen central venous catheter (18- or 20-gauge) and gain access to the peritoneal cavity using the Seldinger technique.

The peritoneal cavity is entered as for the needle technique. The catheter-over-needle assembly is inserted perpendicular to the anterior abdominal wall using the Z-track technique; once peritoneal fluid returns into the syringe barrel, the catheter is advanced over the needle, the needle is removed, and a 20- or 50-mL syringe is connected to the catheter. The tip of the catheter is now in the peritoneal cavity and can be left in place until the appropriate amount of peritoneal fluid is removed. This technique, rather than the needle technique, should be used when LVP is performed, because complications (e.g., intestinal perforation) may occur if a needle is left in the peritoneal space for an extended period.

When the Seldinger technique is used in patients with a large anterior abdominal wall, access to the peritoneal cavity is initially gained with a needle or catheter-over-needle assembly. A guidewire is then inserted through the needle and an 18- or 20-gauge single- or multiple-lumen central venous catheter is threaded over the guidewire. It is very important to use the Z-track method for the catheter technique to prevent development of an ascitic leak, which may be difficult to control and may predispose the patient to peritoneal infection.

Ultrasound Guidance Technique

Patients who have had previous abdominal surgery or peritonitis are predisposed to abdominal adhesions, and it may be quite difficult to gain free access into the peritoneal cavity for diagnostic or therapeutic paracentesis. Ultrasound-guided paracentesis can be very helpful in this population, and in patients where the traditional technique fails, by providing accurate localization of the peritoneal fluid collection and determining the best abdominal access site. This procedure can be performed using the needle or catheter technique as described earlier in the chapter, depending on the volume of peritoneal fluid to be drained. Once the fluid collection is localized by the ultrasound probe, the abdomen is prepared and draped in the usual sterile fashion. A sterile sleeve can be placed over the ultrasound probe so that there is direct real-time ultrasound visualization of the needle or catheter as it enters the peritoneal cavity. The needle or catheter is thus directed to the area to be drained, and the appropriate amount of peritoneal or ascitic fluid is removed. If continued drainage of a loculated peritoneal fluid collection is desired, the radiologist can place a chronic indwelling peritoneal catheter using a percutaneous guidewire technique (see Chapter 22).

The use of ultrasound guidance for drainage of loculated peritoneal fluid collections has markedly decreased the incidence of iatrogenic complications related to abdominal paracentesis. If the radiologist does not identify loculated ascites on the initial ultrasound evaluation and documents a large amount of peritoneal fluid that is free in the abdominal cavity, he or she can then indicate the best access site by marking the anterior abdominal wall with an indelible marker. The paracentesis can then be performed by the clinician and repeated whenever necessary. This study can be performed at the bedside in the intensive care unit with a portable ultrasound unit. A video for the correct procedural technique for paracentesis is available for review [13].

Complications

The most common complications related to abdominal paracentesis are bleeding and persistent ascitic leak. Because most patients in whom ascites have developed also have some component of chronic liver disease with associated coagulopathy and thrombocytopenia, it is very important to consider correction of any underlying coagulopathy before proceeding with abdominal paracentesis. In addition, it is very important to select an avascular access site on the anterior abdominal wall. The Z-track technique is very helpful in minimizing persistent ascitic leak and should always be used. Another complication associated with abdominal paracentesis is intestinal or urinary bladder perforation, with associated peritonitis and infection. Intestinal injury is more common when the needle technique is used. Because the needle is free in the peritoneal cavity, iatrogenic intestinal perforation may occur if the patient moves or if intra-abdominal pressure increases with Valsalva maneuver or coughing. Urinary bladder injury is less common and underscores the importance of draining the urinary bladder with a catheter before the procedure. This injury is more common when the abdominal access site is in the suprapubic location; therefore, this access site is not recommended. Careful adherence to proper technique of paracentesis minimizes associated complications.

In patients who have large-volume chronic abdominal ascites, such as that secondary to hepatic cirrhosis or ovarian carcinoma, transient hypotension and paracentesis-induced circulatory dysfunction (PICD) may develop during LVP. PICD is characterized by worsening hypotension and arterial vasodilation, hyponatremia, azotemia, and an increase in plasma renin activity. Evidence is accumulating that PICD is secondary to an accentuation of an already established arteriolar vasodilation with multiple etiologies, including the dynamics of paracentesis (the rate of ascitic fluid extraction), release of nitric oxide from the vascular endothelium, and mechanical modifications due to abdominal decompression [14].

PICD is associated with increased mortality and may be prevented with the administration of plasma expanders. It is very important to obtain reliable peripheral or central venous access in these patients so that fluid resuscitation can be performed if PICD develops during the procedure. A study randomized 72 patients to receive albumin or saline after total paracentesis [15]. The incidence of PICD was significantly higher in the saline group compared with the albumin group (33.3% vs. 11.4%, $p = 0.03$). However, no significant differences were found when less than 6 L of ascitic fluid was evacuated (6.7% vs. 5.6%, $p = 0.9$). Significant increases in plasma renin activity were found 24 hours and 6 days after paracentesis when saline was used, whereas no changes were observed with albumin. Albumin was more effective than saline in the prevention of PICD, but it is not required when less than 6 L of ascitic fluid is evacuated. Therefore, the administration of albumin intravenously (6 to 8 g per L of ascites removed) is recommended with LVP (>6 L).

There have been nine prospective randomized controlled trials ($n = 806$) on the use of plasma expanders for therapeutic paracentesis [1]. In a recent systematic review, there was no significant difference between therapeutic paracentesis with or without volume expansion with albumin, nor with nonalbumin plasma expanders compared with albumin for hyponatremia, renal impairment, encephalopathy, or death. However, these studies did not specifically examine prevention of PICD (defined by an increase in plasma renin activity or aldosterone concentration), and some studies have determined that albumin prevented PCID more effectively than synthetic plasma expanders [15,16].

Randomized trials comparing terlipressin (a vasoconstrictor) with albumin in PICD in cirrhosis documented that both terlipressin and albumin prevented paracentesis-induced renal impairment in these patients [17,18]. Terlipressin may be as effective as intravenous albumin in preventing PICD in patients with cirrhosis. Midodrine and octreotide in combination or alone have shown conflicting results for improving systemic and renal hemodynamics and renal function in patients with cirrhosis-related complications, including the prevention of PICD, and additional studies are warranted [19].

LVP is only transiently therapeutic; the underlying chronic disease induces reaccumulation of the ascites. Percutaneous placement of a tunneled catheter is a viable and safe technique to consider in patients who have symptomatic malignant ascites that require frequent therapeutic paracentesis for relief of symptoms [20].

DIAGNOSTIC PERITONEAL LAVAGE

Before the introduction of diagnostic peritoneal lavage (DPL) by Root et al. [21] in 1965, nonoperative evaluation of the injured abdomen was limited to standard four-quadrant abdominal paracentesis. Abdominal paracentesis for the evaluation of hemoperitoneum was associated with a high false-negative rate. This clinical suspicion was confirmed by Giacobine and Siler [22] in an experimental animal model of hemoperitoneum documenting that a 500-mL blood volume in the peritoneal cavity yielded a positive paracentesis rate of only 78%. The initial study by Root et al. [21] reported 100% accuracy in the identification of hemoperitoneum using 1-L peritoneal lavage fluid. Many subsequent clinical studies confirmed these findings, with the largest series reported by Fischer et al. [23] in 1978. They reviewed 2,586 cases of DPL and reported a false-positive rate of 0.2%, false-negative rate of 1.2%, and overall accuracy of 98.5%. Since its introduction in 1965, DPL has been a cornerstone in the evaluation of hemoperitoneum due to blunt and penetrating abdominal injuries. However, it is nonspecific for determination of the type or extent of organ injury.

Recent advances have led to the use of ultrasound (focused assessment with sonography in trauma [FAST]; Fig. 14.2) and rapid helical computed tomography (CT) in the emergent evaluation of abdominal trauma and have significantly decreased the use of DPL in the evaluation of abdominal trauma to less than 1% [24–26]. FAST has replaced DPL as the initial screening modality of choice for severe abdominal trauma in more than 80% of North American centers surveyed [27] and FAST is now taught in the Advanced Trauma Life Support course [28]. Practice management guidelines from the Eastern Association for the Surgery of Trauma recommend FAST be considered the initial diagnostic modality to exclude hemoperitoneum [29]. DPL remains a valuable adjunct to modern imaging techniques in early trauma assessment, particularly in hemodynamically unstable patients with initial FAST examination that is negative or equivocal and in the assessment of potential hollow visceral injury in blunt abdominal trauma [30]. Diagnostic peritoneal aspiration, without a full lavage, has also been utilized successfully in these circumstances [31].

Indications

The primary indication for DPL is evaluation of blunt abdominal trauma in patients with associated hypotension. If the initial

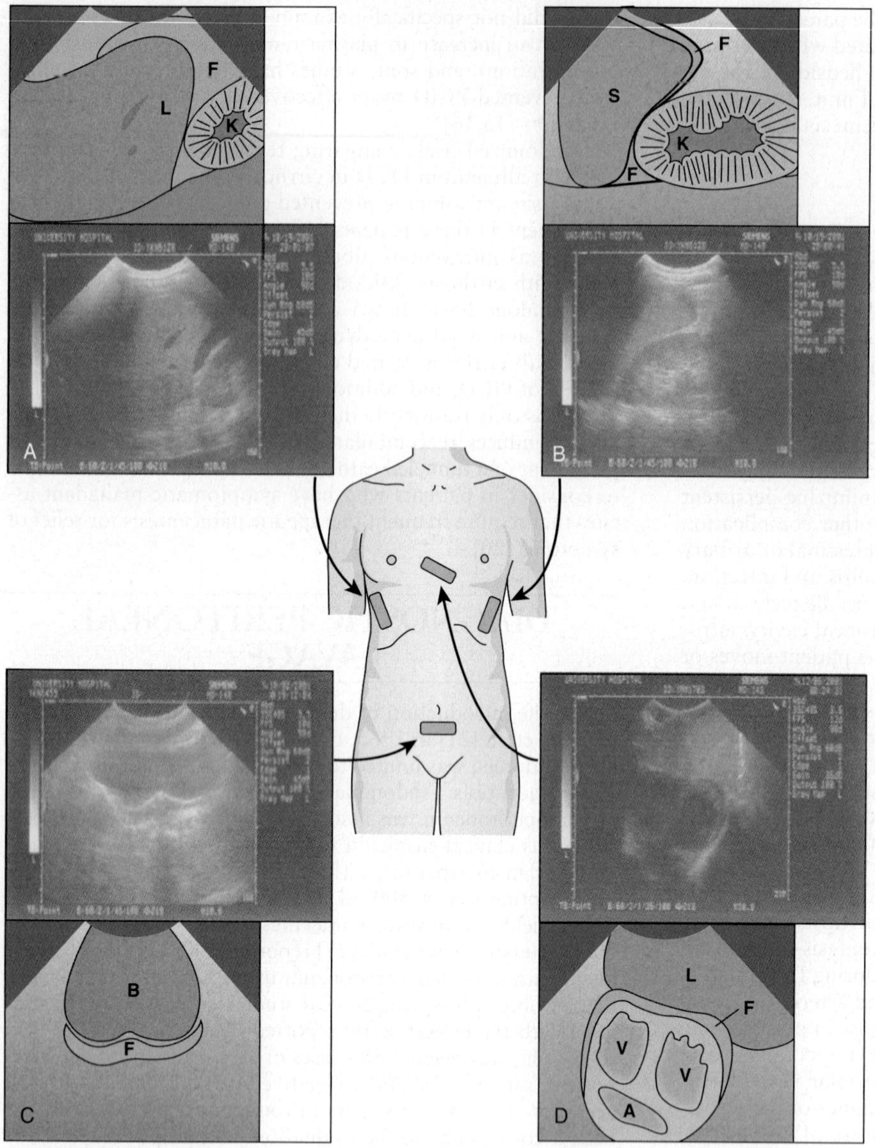

FIGURE 14.2. The FAST examination.

FAST examination is positive for hemoperitoneum, surgical intervention (laparotomy) is required. If the FAST examination is negative or equivocal, DPL should be considered. If the patient is hemodynamically stable and can be transported safely, CT scan of the abdomen and pelvis is the diagnostic method of choice. If the patient is hemodynamically unstable or requires emergent surgical intervention for a craniotomy, thoracotomy, or vascular procedure, it is imperative to determine whether there is a coexisting intraperitoneal source of hemorrhage to prioritize treatment of life-threatening injuries. FAST or DPL can be used to diagnose hemoperitoneum in patients with multisystem injury, who require general anesthesia for the treatment of associated traumatic injuries. Patients with associated thoracic or pelvic injuries should also have definitive evaluation for abdominal trauma, and DPL can be used in these individuals. DPL can also be used to evaluate for traumatic hollow viscus injury, and a cell count ratio (defined as the ratio between white blood cell (WBC) and red blood cell (RBC) count in the lavage fluid divided by the ratio of the same parameters in the peripheral blood) less than or equal to 1 has a specificity of 97% and sensitivity of 100% [32].

DPL can also be used to evaluate penetrating abdominal trauma; however, its role differs from that in blunt abdominal trauma [33]. A hemodynamically unstable patient with abdominal penetrating injury requires no further investigation and immediate laparotomy should be undertaken. Instead, the role of DPL in the *hemodynamically stable* patient with penetrating abdominal injury is to identify hemoperitoneum and hollow viscus or diaphragmatic injury. DPL has also been recommended as the initial diagnostic study in stable patients with penetrating trauma to the back and flank, defining an RBC count greater than 1,000 per μL as a positive test [34]. Implementation of this protocol decreased the total celiotomy rate from 100% to 24%, and the therapeutic celiotomy rate increased from 15% to 80%.

DPL may prove to be useful in evaluation for possible peritonitis or ruptured viscus in patients with an altered level of consciousness but no evidence of traumatic injury. DPL can be considered in critically ill patients with sepsis to determine if intra-abdominal infection is the underlying source. When DPL is used to evaluate intra-abdominal infection, a WBC count greater than 500 per μL of lavage fluid is considered positive. DPL can also serve a therapeutic role. It is very effective in rewarming patients with significant hypothermia. It may potentially be used therapeutically in pancreatitis, fecal peritonitis, and bile pancreatitis, but multiple clinical studies have not documented its efficacy in these cases.

DPL should not be performed in patients with clear signs of significant abdominal trauma and hemoperitoneum associated with hemodynamic instability. These patients should undergo emergent celiotomy. Pregnancy is a relative contraindication to DPL; it may be technically difficult to perform because of the gravid uterus and is associated with a higher risk of complications. Bedside ultrasound evaluation of the abdomen in the pregnant trauma patient is associated with least risk to the woman and to the fetus. An additional relative contraindication to DPL is multiple previous abdominal surgeries. These patients commonly have multiple abdominal adhesions, and it may be very difficult to gain access to the free peritoneal cavity. If DPL is indicated, it must be performed by the open technique to prevent iatrogenic complications such as intestinal injury.

Techniques

Three techniques can be used to perform DPL: (i) the closed percutaneous technique, (ii) the semiclosed technique, and (iii) the open technique. The closed percutaneous technique, introduced by Lazarus and Nelson [35] in 1979, is easy to perform, can be done rapidly, is associated with a low complication rate, and is as accurate as the open technique. It should not be used in patients who have had previous abdominal surgery or a history of abdominal adhesions. The open technique entails the placement of the peritoneal lavage catheter into the peritoneal cavity under direct visualization. It is more time consuming than the closed percutaneous technique. The semiclosed technique requires a smaller incision than does the open technique and uses a peritoneal lavage catheter with a metal stylet to gain entrance into the peritoneal cavity. It has become less popular as clinicians have become more familiar and skilled with the Lazarus–Nelson closed technique.

The patient is placed in the supine position for all three techniques. A catheter is placed into the urinary bladder and a nasogastric tube is inserted into the stomach to prevent iatrogenic bladder or gastric injury. The nasogastric tube is placed on continuous suction for gastric decompression. The skin of the anterior abdominal wall is prepared with 2% chlorhexidine solution and sterilely draped, leaving the periumbilical area exposed. Standard aseptic technique is used throughout the procedure. Local anesthesia with 1% or 2% lidocaine with 1:200,000 epinephrine is used as necessary throughout the procedure. The infraumbilical site is used unless there is clinical concern of possible pelvic fracture and retroperitoneal or pelvic hematoma, in which case the supraumbilical site is optimal.

Closed Percutaneous Technique

With the closed percutaneous technique, local anesthesia is infiltrated inferior to the umbilicus and a 5-mm skin incision is made just at the inferior umbilical edge. An 18-gauge needle is inserted through this incision and into the peritoneal cavity, angled toward the pelvis at approximately a 45-degree angle with the skin. The penetration through the linea alba and then through the peritoneum is felt as two separate "pops." A J-tipped guidewire is passed through the needle and into the peritoneal cavity, again directing the wire toward the pelvis by maintaining the needle at a 45-degree angle to the skin. The 18-gauge needle is then removed and the DPL catheter inserted over the guidewire into the peritoneal cavity, using a twisting motion and guided inferiorly toward the pelvis. The guidewire is then removed, and a 10-mL syringe is attached to the catheter for aspiration. If free blood returns from the DPL catheter before the syringe is attached or if gross blood returns in the syringe barrel, hemoperitoneum has been documented, the catheter is removed, and the patient is quickly transported to the operating room for emergent celiotomy. If no gross blood returns on aspiration through the catheter, peritoneal lavage is performed using 1 L Ringer's lactate solution or normal saline that has been previously warmed to prevent hypothermia. The fluid is instilled into the peritoneal cavity through the DPL catheter; afterward, the peritoneal fluid is allowed to drain out of the peritoneal cavity by gravity until the fluid return slows. A minimum of 250 mL lavage fluid is considered a representative sample of the peritoneal fluid [36]. A sample is sent to the laboratory for determination of RBC count, WBC count, amylase concentration, and presence of bile, bacteria, or particulate matter. When the lavage is completed, the catheter is removed and a sterile dressing applied over the site. Suture approximation of the skin edges is not necessary when the closed technique is used for DPL.

Semiclosed Technique

Local anesthetic is infiltrated in the area of the planned incision and a 2- to 3-cm vertical incision made in the infraumbilical or supraumbilical area. The incision is continued sharply down through the subcutaneous tissue and linea alba, and the peritoneum is then visualized. Forceps, hemostats, or Allis clamps are used to grasp the edges of the linea alba and elevate the fascial edges to prevent injury to the underlying abdominal structures. The DPL lavage catheter with a metal inner stylet is inserted through the closed peritoneum into the peritoneal cavity at a 45-degree angle to the anterior abdominal wall, directed toward the pelvis. When the catheter–metal stylet assembly is in the peritoneal cavity, the DPL catheter is advanced into the pelvis and the metal stylet removed. A 10-mL syringe is attached to the catheter, and aspiration is conducted as previously described. When the lavage is completed, the fascia must be reapproximated with sutures, the skin closed, and a sterile dressing applied.

Open Technique

After the administration of appropriate local anesthetic, a vertical midline incision approximately 3 to 5 cm long is made. This incision is commonly made in the infraumbilical location, but in patients with presumed pelvic fractures or retroperitoneal hematomas or in pregnant patients, a supraumbilical location is preferred. The vertical midline incision is carried down through the skin, subcutaneous tissue, and linea alba under direct vision. The linea alba is grasped on either side using forceps, hemostats, or Allis clamps, and the fascia is elevated to prevent injury to the underlying abdominal structures. The peritoneum is identified, and a small vertical peritoneal incision is made to gain entrance into the peritoneal cavity. The DPL catheter is then inserted into the peritoneal cavity under direct visualization and advanced inferiorly toward the pelvis. It is inserted without the stylet or metal trocar. When in position, a 10-mL syringe is attached for aspiration. If aspiration of the peritoneal cavity is negative (i.e., no gross blood returns), peritoneal lavage is performed, as described earlier in the chapter. As in the semiclosed technique, the fascia and skin must be reapproximated to prevent dehiscence or evisceration, or both.

A prospective randomized study documented that the Lazarus–Nelson technique of closed percutaneous DPL can be performed faster than the open procedure [37]. The procedure times with the closed technique varied from 1 to 3 minutes, compared with 5 to 24 minutes for the open technique. It was documented that the closed percutaneous technique was as accurate as the open procedure and was associated with a lower incidence of wound infections and complications. The closed percutaneous technique, using the Seldinger technique, should therefore be used initially in all patients except those who have had previous abdominal surgery or in pregnant patients. This has been confirmed in a study of 2,501 DPLs performed over a 75-month period for blunt or penetrating abdominal trauma [38]. The majority (2,409, or 96%) were performed using the closed percutaneous technique, and 92 (4%) were done open because of pelvic fractures, previous scars, or pregnancy. Open DPL was less sensitive than closed DPL in patients who sustained blunt trauma (90% vs. 95%), but slightly more sensitive in determining penetration (100% vs. 96%). Overall, there were few (21, or 0.8%) complications, and the overall sensitivity, specificity, and accuracy were 95%, 99%, and 98%, respectively, using an RBC count of 100,000 per μL in blunt trauma and 10,000 per μL in penetrating trauma as the positive threshold. A meta-analysis concluded that the closed DPL technique is comparable to the standard open DPL technique in terms of accuracy and major complications, with the advantage of reduced performance time with closed DPL, which is offset by increased technical difficulties and failures [39].

A DPL modification [40] that resulted in more rapid infusion and drainage of lavage fluid used cystoscopy irrigation tubing for instillation and drainage of the lavage fluid, saving an average of 19 minutes per patient for the DPL completion. This modification can be applied to the closed percutaneous or open DPL technique to decrease the procedure time in critically ill patients.

Interpretation of Results

The current guidelines for interpretation of positive and negative results of DPL are provided in Table 14.2. A positive result can be estimated by the inability to read newsprint or typewritten print through the lavage fluid as it returns through clear plastic tubing. This test is not reliable, however, and a quantitative RBC count in a sample of the peritoneal lavage fluid must be performed [41]. For patients with nonpenetrating abdominal trauma, an RBC count greater than 100,000 per μL of lavage fluid is considered positive and requires emergent celiotomy. Fewer than 50,000 RBCs per μL is considered negative and RBC counts of 50,000 to 100,000 per μL are considered indeterminate. The guidelines for patients with penetrating abdominal trauma are much less clear with clinical studies using an RBC count of greater than 1,000 or 10,000 per μL to greater than 100,000 per μL as the criterion for a positive DPL in patients with penetrating thoracic or abdominal trauma. The lower the threshold the more sensitive the test, but the higher the nontherapeutic laparotomy rate.

Determination of hollow viscus injury by DPL is much more difficult. A WBC count greater than 500 per μL of lavage fluid or an amylase concentration greater than 175 units per dL of lavage fluid is usually considered positive. These studies, however, are not as accurate as the use of RBC count in the lavage fluid to determine the presence of hemoperitoneum. One study in patients with blunt abdominal trauma determined that the WBC count in lavage fluid has a positive predictive value of only 23% and probably should not be used as an indicator of a positive DPL [42]. Other studies analyzed alkaline phosphatase levels in DPL fluid to determine if this assay is helpful in the diagnosis of hollow viscus injuries [43,44], but the results have been variable. A prospective study used a diagnostic algorithm of initial abdominal ultrasound, followed by helical CT and subsequent DPL (if CT was suggestive of blunt bowel or mesenteric injury) using a cell count ratio (defined as the ratio between WBC and RBC count in the lavage fluid divided by the ratio of the same parameters in the peripheral blood) greater than or equal to 1 to determine the need for laparotomy in patients with blunt abdominal injuries [45]. This proposed algorithm had a high accuracy (100%) while requiring the performance of DPL in only a few (2%) patients.

It must be stressed that DPL is not accurate for determination of retroperitoneal visceral injuries or diaphragmatic injuries [46]. The incidence of false-negative DPL results is

TABLE 14.2

INTERPRETATION OF DIAGNOSTIC PERITONEAL LAVAGE RESULTS

POSITIVE
Nonpenetrating abdominal trauma
Immediate gross blood return via catheter
Immediate return of intestinal contents or food particles
Aspiration of 10 mL blood via catheter
Return of lavage fluid via chest tube or urinary catheter
Red blood cell (RBC) count >100,000/μL
White blood cell (WBC) count >500/μL
Cell count ratio (defined as the ratio between WBC and RBC count in the lavage fluid divided by the ratio of the same parameters in the peripheral blood) ≥1
Amylase >175 U/100 mL
Penetrating abdominal trauma
Immediate gross blood return via catheter
Immediate return of intestinal contents or food particles
Aspiration of 10 mL blood via catheter
Return of lavage fluid via chest tube or Foley catheter
RBC count used is variable, from >1,000/μL to >100,000/μL
WBC count >500/μL
Amylase >175 U/100 mL
NEGATIVE
Nonpenetrating abdominal trauma
RBC count <50,000/μL
WBC count <100/μL
Cell count ratio (defined as the ratio between WBC and RBC count in the lavage fluid divided by the ratio of the same parameters in the peripheral blood) <1
Amylase <75 U/100 mL
Penetrating abdominal trauma
RBC count used is variable, from <1,000/μL to <50,000/μL
WBC count <100/μL
Amylase <75 U/100 mL

approximately 30% in patients who sustained traumatic diaphragmatic rupture. In addition, DPL is insensitive in detecting subcapsular hematomas of the spleen or liver that are contained, with no evidence of hemoperitoneum. Although DPL is now used in the evaluation of nontraumatic intra-abdominal pathology, the criteria for positive lavage in these patients have not yet been established. Additional clinical studies are needed.

Complications

Complications of DPL by the techniques described here include malposition of the lavage catheter, injury to the intra-abdominal organs or vessels, iatrogenic hemoperitoneum, wound infection or dehiscence, evisceration, and possible unnecessary laparotomy. DPL is a very valuable technique, however, and if it is performed carefully, with attention to detail, these complications are minimized. In the largest series published to date, with more than 2,500 DPLs performed, the complications rate was 0.8% [38]. Wound infection, dehiscence, and evisceration are more common with the open technique; therefore, the closed percutaneous technique is recommended in all patients who do not have a contraindication to this technique. Knowledge of all techniques is necessary, however, because the choice of technique should be based on the individual patient's presentation.

References

1. Wong CL, Holroyd-Leduc J, Thorpe KE, et al: Does this patient have bacterial peritonitis or portal hypertension? How do I perform a paracentesis and analyze the results? *JAMA* 299(10):1166–1178, 2008.
2. Hou W, Sanyal AJ: Ascites: diagnosis and management. *Med Clin North Am* 93(4):801–817, 2009.
3. Moore KP, Wong F, Gines P, et al: The management of ascites in cirrhosis: report on the consensus conference of the International Ascites Club. *Hepatology* 38(1):258, 2003.
4. Parra MW, Al-Khayat H, Smith HG, et al: Paracentesis for resuscitation-induced abdominal compartment syndrome: an alternative to decompressive laparotomy in the burn patient. *J Trauma* 60(5):1119, 2006.
5. Velamati PG, Herlong HF: Treatment of refractory ascites. *Curr Treat Options Gastroenterol* 9(6):530–537, 2006.
6. Garcia-Tsao G, Lim JK, Members of Veterans Affairs Hepatitis C Resource Center Program. Management and treatment of patients with cirrhosis and portal hypertension: recommendations from the Department of Veterans Affairs Hepatitis C Resource Center Program and the National Hepatitis C Program. *Am J Gastroenterol* 104(7):1802–1829, 2009.
7. Saab S, Nieto JM, Lewis SK, et al: TIPS versus paracentesis for cirrhotic patients with refractory ascites. *Cochrane Database Syst Rev* (4):CD004889, 2006.
8. Salerno F, Camma C, Enea M, et al: Transjugular intrahepatic portosystemic shunt for refractory ascites: a meta-analysis of individual patient data. *Gastroenterology* 133(3):825–834, 2007.
9. Runyon BA: Management of adult patients with ascites caused by cirrhosis. *Hepatology* 39:841, 2004.
10. Grabau CM, Crago SF, Hoff LK, et al: Performance standards for therapeutic abdominal paracentesis. *Hepatology* 40:484, 2004.
11. Sakai H, Sheer TA, Mendler MH, et al: Choosing the location for non-image guided abdominal paracentesis. *Liver Int* 25(5):984, 2005.
12. McGibbon A, Chen GI, Peltekian KM, et al: An evidence-based manual for abdominal paracentesis. *Dig Dis Sci* 52(12):3307–3315, 2007.
13. Thomsen TW, Shaffer RW, White B, et al: Paracentesis. Videos in Clinical Medicine. *N Engl J Med* 355:e21, 2006. Available at: http://content.nejm.org/cgi/video/355/19/e21/
14. Sola-Vera J, Such J: Understanding the mechanisms of paracentesis-induced circulatory dysfunction. *Eur J Gastroenterol Hepatol* 16(3):295, 2004.
15. Sola-Vera J, Minana J, Ricart E, et al: Randomized trial comparing albumin and saline in the prevention of paracentesis-induced circulatory dysfunction in cirrhotic patients with ascites. *Hepatology* 37(5):1147, 2003.
16. Umgelter A, Reindl W, Wagner KS, et al: Effects of plasma expansion with albumin and paracentesis on haemodynamics and kidney function in critically ill cirrhotic patients with tense ascites and hepatorenal syndrome: a prospective uncontrolled trial. *Crit Care* 12(1):R4, 2008.
17. Singh V, Kumar R, Nain CK, et al: Terlipressin versus albumin in paracentesis-induced circulatory dysfunction in cirrhosis: a randomized study. *J Gastroenterol Hepatol* 21(1 Pt 2):303, 2006.
18. Lata J, Marecek Z, Fejfar T, et al: The efficacy of terlipressin in comparison with albumin in the prevention of circulatory changes after the paracentesis of tense ascites. A randomized multicentric study. *Hepatogastroenterology* 54(79):1930–1933, 2007.
19. Karwa R, Woodis CB: Midodrine and octreotide in treatment of cirrhosis-related hemodynamic complications. *Ann Pharmacother* 43(4):692–699, 2009.
20. Rosenberg SM: Palliation of malignant ascites. *Gastroenterol Clin North Am* 35(1):189, xi, 2006.
21. Root H, Hauser C, McKinley C, et al: Diagnostic peritoneal lavage. *Surgery* 57:633, 1965.
22. Giacobine JW, Siler VE: Evaluation of diagnostic abdominal paracentesis with experimental and clinical studies. *Surg Gynecol Obstet* 110:676, 1960.
23. Fischer R, Beverlin B, Engrav L, et al: Diagnostic peritoneal lavage 14 years and 2586 patients later. *Am J Surg* 136:701, 1978.
24. Ollerton JE, Sugrue M, Balogh Z, et al: Prospective study to evaluate the influence of FAST on trauma patient management. *J Trauma* 60(4):785, 2006.
25. Kirkpatrick AW, Sirois M, Laupland KB, et al: Prospective evaluation of hand-held focused abdominal sonography for trauma (FAST) in blunt abdominal trauma. *Can J Surg* 48(6):453, 2005.
26. Fang JF, Wong YC, Lin BC, et al: Usefulness of multidetector computed tomography for the initial assessment of blunt abdominal trauma patients. *World J Surg* 30(2):176, 2006.
27. Boulanger BR, Kearney PA, Brenneman FD, et al: FAST utilization in 1999: results of a survey of North American trauma centers. *Am Surg* 66:1049–1055, 2000.
28. American College of Surgeons Committee on Trauma: *Advanced Trauma Life Support for Doctors*. 8th ed. Chicago, American College of Surgeons, 2008.
29. Hoff WS, Holevar M, Nagy KK, et al: Practice management guidelines for the evaluation of blunt abdominal trauma: the EAST practice management guidelines work group. *J Trauma* 53:602–615, 2002.
30. Cha JY, Kashuk JL, Sarin EL, et al: Diagnostic peritoneal lavage remains a valuable adjunct to modern imaging techniques. *J Trauma* 67(2):330–334, 2009; discussion 334–336.
31. Kuncir EJ, Velmahos GC: Diagnostic peritoneal aspiration—the foster child of DPL: a prospective observational study. *Int J Surg* 5(3):167–171, 2007.
32. Fang JF, Chen RJ, Lin BC: Cell count ratio: new criterion of diagnostic peritoneal lavage for detection of hollow organ perforation. *J Trauma* 45(3):540, 1998.
33. Sriussadaporn S, Pak-art R, Pattaratiwanon M, et al: Clinical uses of diagnostic peritoneal lavage in stab wounds of the anterior abdomen: a prospective study. *Eur J Surg* 168(8–9): 490, 2002.
34. Pham TN, Heinberg E, Cuschieri J, et al: The evaluation of the diagnostic work-up for stab wounds to the back and flank. *Injury* 40(1):48–53, 2009.
35. Lazarus HM, Nelson JA: A technique for peritoneal lavage without risk or complication. *Surg Gynecol Obstet* 149:889, 1979.
36. Sweeney JF, Albrink MH, Bischof E, et al: Diagnostic peritoneal lavage: volume of lavage effluent needed for accurate determination of a negative lavage. *Injury* 25:659, 1994.
37. Howdieshell TR, Osler RM, Demarest GB: Open versus closed peritoneal lavage with particular attention to time, accuracy and cost. *Am J Emerg Med* 7:367, 1989.
38. Nagy KK, Roberts RR, Joseph KT, et al: Experience with over 2500 diagnostic peritoneal lavages. *Injury* 31:479, 2000.
39. Hodgson NF, Stewart TC, Girotti MJ: Open or closed diagnostic peritoneal lavage for abdominal trauma? A metaanalysis. *J Trauma* 48(6):1091, 2000.
40. Cotter CP, Hawkins ML, Kent RB, et al: Ultrarapid diagnostic peritoneal lavage. *J Trauma* 29:615, 1989.
41. Gow KW, Haley LP, Phang PT: Validity of visual inspection of diagnostic peritoneal lavage fluid. *Can J Surg* 39:114, 1996.
42. Soyka J, Martin M, Sloan E, et al: Diagnostic peritoneal lavage: is an isolated WBC count greater than or equal to 500/mm^3 predictive of intra-abdominal trauma requiring celiotomy in blunt trauma patients? *J Trauma* 30:874, 1990.
43. Megison SM, Weigelt JA: The value of alkaline phosphatase in peritoneal lavage. *Ann Emerg Med* 19:5, 1990.
44. Jaffin JH, Ochsner G, Cole FJ, et al: Alkaline phosphatase levels in diagnostic peritoneal lavage as a predictor of hollow visceral injury. *J Trauma* 34:829, 1993.
45. Menegaux F, Tresallet C, Gosgnach M, et al: Diagnosis of bowel and mesenteric injuries in blunt abdominal trauma: a prospective study. *Am J Emerg Med* 24(1):19, 2006.
46. Fischer RP, Freeman T: The inadequacy of peritoneal lavage in diagnosing acute diaphragmatic rupture. *J Trauma* 16:538, 1976.

CHAPTER 15 ■ GASTROESOPHAGEAL BALLOON TAMPONADE FOR ACUTE VARICEAL HEMORRHAGE

MARIE T. PAVINI AND JUAN CARLOS PUYANA

Gastroesophageal variceal hemorrhage is an acute and catastrophic complication that occurs in one-third to one-half of patients with portal pressures greater than 12 mm Hg [1]. Because proximal gastric varices and varices in the distal 5 cm of the esophagus lie in the superficial lamina propria, they are more likely to bleed and respond to endoscopic treatment [2]. Variceal rupture is likely a factor of size, wall thickness, and portal pressure, and may be predicted by Child-Pugh class, red wale markings indicating epithelial thickness, and variceal size [1]. Although urgent endoscopy, sclerotherapy, and band ligations are considered first-line treatments, balloon tamponade remains a valuable intervention in the treatment of bleeding esophageal varices. Balloon tamponade is accomplished using a multilumen tube, approximately 1 m in length, with esophageal and gastric cuffs that can be inflated to compress esophageal varices and gastric submucosal veins, thereby providing hemostasis through tamponade, while incorporating aspiration ports for diagnostic and therapeutic usage.

HISTORICAL DEVELOPMENT

In 1930, Westphal described the use of an esophageal sound as a means of controlling variceal hemorrhage. In 1947, successful control of hemorrhage by balloon tamponade was achieved by attaching an inflatable latex bag to the end of a Miller–Abbot tube. In 1949, a two-balloon tube was described by Patton and Johnson. A triple-lumen tube with gastric and esophageal balloons, as well as a port for gastric aspiration, was described by Sengstaken and Blakemore in 1950. In 1955, Linton and Nachlas engineered a tube with a larger gastric balloon capable of compressing the submucosal veins in the cardia, thereby minimizing flow to the esophageal veins, with suction ports above and below the balloon. The Minnesota tube was described in 1968 as a modification of the Sengstaken–Blakemore tube, incorporating the esophageal suction port, which will be described later. Several studies have published combined experience with tubes such as the Linton–Nachlas tube; however, the techniques described here are limited to the use of the Minnesota and Sengstaken–Blakemore tubes.

ROLE OF BALLOON TAMPONADE IN THE MANAGEMENT OF BLEEDING ESOPHAGEAL VARICES

Treatment of portal hypertension to prevent variceal rupture includes primary and secondary prophylaxis. Primary prophylaxis consists of beta-blockers, band ligation, and endoscopic surveillance, whereas secondary prophylaxis includes nitrates, transjugular intrahepatic portosystemic shunt (TIPS), and surgical shunt [3]. Management of acute variceal bleeding involves multiple simultaneous and sequential modalities. Balloon tamponade is considered a temporary bridge within these modalities. Self-expanding metal stents as an alternative to balloon tamponade are currently under investigation [4].

Splanchnic vasoconstrictors such as somatostatin, octreotide, terlipressin (the only agent shown to decrease mortality), or vasopressin (with nitrates to reduce cardiac side effects) decrease portal blood flow and pressure, and should be administered as soon as possible [5–7]. In fact, Pourriat et al. [8] advocate administration of octreotide by emergency medical personnel before patient transfer to the hospital. Recombinant activated factor VII has been reported to achieve hemostasis in bleeding esophageal varices unresponsive to standard treatment, and may also be considered [9]. Emergent therapeutic endoscopy in conjunction with pharmacotherapy is more effective than pharmacotherapy alone and is also performed as soon as possible. Band ligation has a lower rate of rebleeding and complications when compared with sclerotherapy, and should be performed preferentially, provided visualization is adequate to ligate varices successfully [3,10]. Tissue adhesives such as polidocanol and cyanoacrylate delivered through an endoscope are being used and studied outside the United States.

Balloon tamponade is performed to control massive variceal hemorrhage, with the hope that band ligation or sclerotherapy and secondary prophylaxis will then be possible (Fig. 15.1). If bleeding continues beyond these measures, TIPS [11] is considered. Shunt surgery [12] may be considered if TIPS is contraindicated. Other alternatives include percutaneous transhepatic embolization, emergent esophageal transection with stapling [13], esophagogastric devascularization with esophageal transection and splenectomy, and hepatic transplantation. If gastric varices are noted, therapeutic options include endoscopic administration of the tissue adhesive cyanoacrylate, TIPS, balloon-occluded retrograde transvenous obliteration [14], balloon-occluded endoscopic injection therapy [15], and devascularization with splenectomy, shunt surgery, and liver transplantation.

INDICATIONS AND CONTRAINDICATIONS

A Minnesota or Sengstaken–Blakemore tube is indicated in patients with a diagnosis of esophageal variceal hemorrhage, in which neither band ligation nor sclerotherapy is technically possible, readily available, or has failed [16]. If at all possible, making an adequate anatomic diagnosis is critical before

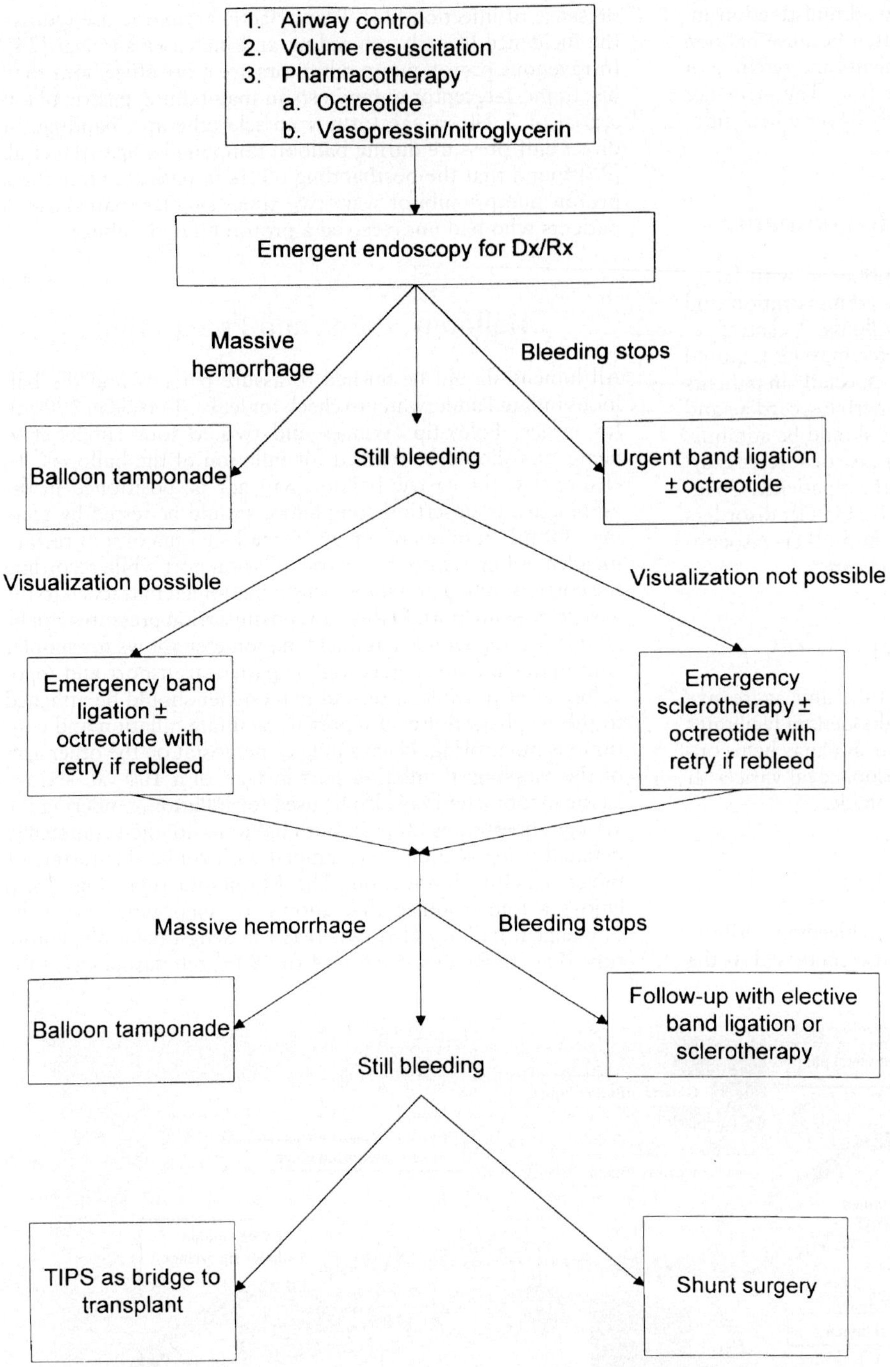

FIGURE 15.1. Management of esophageal variceal hemorrhage. Dx, diagnosis; Rx, therapy; TIPS, transjugular intrahepatic portosystemic shunt.

any of these balloon tubes are inserted. Severe upper gastrointestinal bleeding attributed to esophageal varices in patients with clinical evidence of chronic liver disease results from other causes in up to 40% of cases. The observation of a white nipple sign (platelet plug) is indicative of a recent variceal bleed. A balloon tube is contraindicated in patients with recent esophageal surgery or esophageal stricture [17]. Some authors do not recommend balloon tamponade when a hiatal hernia is present, but there are reports of successful hemorrhage control in some of these patients [18]. If there is no other option, it may be practical to titrate to the lowest effective balloon pressures especially if repeated endoscopic sclerotherapy has been performed as there is increased risk of esophageal perforation [19].

TECHNICAL AND PRACTICAL CONSIDERATIONS

Airway Control

Endotracheal intubation (see Chapter 1) is imperative in patients with upper gastrointestinal bleeding and hemodynamic compromise, encephalopathy, or both. The incidence of aspiration pneumonia is directly related to the presence of encephalopathy or impaired mental status [20]. Suctioning of pulmonary secretions and blood that accumulates in the hypopharynx is facilitated in patients who have been intubated.

Sedatives and analgesics are more readily administered in intubated patients, and may be required often because balloon tamponade is poorly tolerated in most patients and retching or vomiting may lead to esophageal rupture [21]. The incidence of pulmonary complications is significantly lower when endotracheal intubation is routinely used [22].

Hypovolemia, Shock, and Coagulopathy

Adequate intravenous access should be obtained with large-bore venous catheters for blood product administration and fluid resuscitation with crystalloids and colloids. A central venous catheter or pulmonary artery catheter may be required to monitor intravascular filling pressures, especially in patients with severe cirrhosis, advanced age, or underlying cardiac and pulmonary disease. Packed red blood cells should be administered keeping four to six units available in case of severe recurrent bleeding, which commonly occurs in these patients. Coagulopathies, thrombocytopenia, or qualitative platelet disorders should be treated emergently. Octreotide and other vasoconstrictive therapies should be initiated as indicated.

Clots and Gastric Decompression

If time permits, placement of an Ewald tube and aggressive lavage and suctioning of the stomach and duodenum facilitates endoscopy, diminishes the risk of aspiration, and may help control hemorrhage from causes other than esophageal varices. It should be removed prior to balloon tamponade.

Infection and Ulceration

Mortality is increased if infection is present in bleeding cirrhotic patients. The rate of early rebleeding is also increased in the presence of infection [23]. Prophylactic antibiotic use reduces the incidence of early rebleeding and increases survival [24]. Intravenous proton pump inhibitors are more efficacious than histamine-2-receptor antagonists in maintaining gastric pH at a goal of 7. Ulcers can form from sclerotherapy, banding, or direct cuff pressure during balloon tamponade. Shaheen et al. [25] found that the postbanding ulcers in patients receiving a proton pump inhibitor were two times smaller than those in patients who had not received a proton pump inhibitor.

Balloons, Ports, and Preparation

All lumens should be flushed to assure patency and the balloons inflated underwater to check for leaks. Two clean 100-mL (or larger) Foley-tip syringes and two to four rubber-shod hemostats should be readied for inflation of the balloons. To ensure that the gastric balloon will not be positioned in the esophagus, preinsertion compliance should be tested by placing 100-mL aliquots of air up to the listed maximum recommended volumes into the gastric inflation port while recording the corresponding pressures using a manometer attached to the gastric pressure port. In this way, postinsertion pressures can be compared. A portable handheld manometer allows for simpler continuous monitoring as well as patient transport and repositioning. If possible, a second manometer should be attached to the esophageal pressure port to facilitate inflation and continuous monitoring. Place a plug or hemostat on the other arm of the esophageal inflation port instead of a 100-mL syringe as the manometer may also be used for inflation, rendering the syringe superfluous [26,27]. Both balloons are then completely deflated using suction and clamped with rubber hemostats or plugged before lubrication. The Minnesota tube (Fig. 15.2) enjoys a fourth lumen that allows for suctioning above the esophageal balloon [18], whereas the Sengstaken–Blakemore tube (Fig. 15.3) must have a 14 to 18 French nasogastric tube

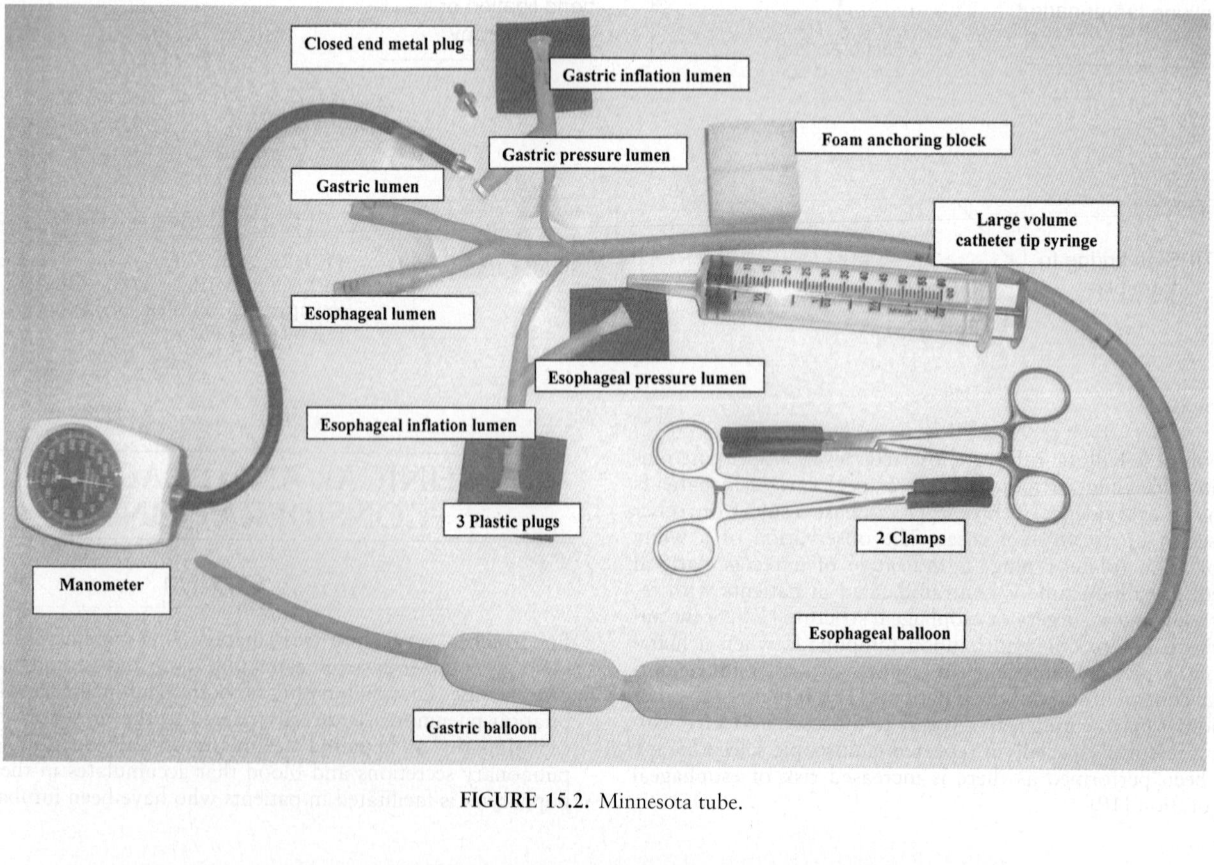

FIGURE 15.2. Minnesota tube.

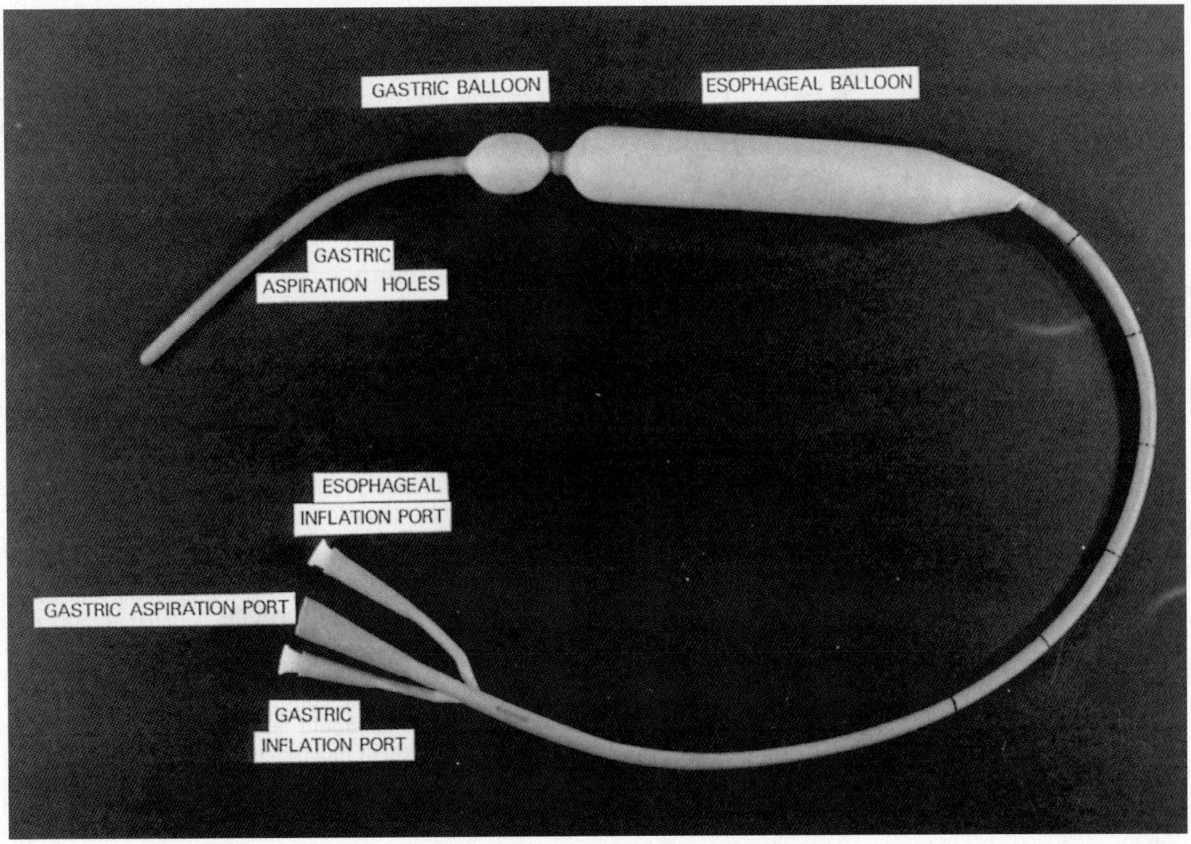

FIGURE 15.3. Sengstaken–Blakemore tube.

secured a few centimeters proximal to the esophageal balloon to be used for esophageal decompression. The nasogastric tube should be used even if the esophageal balloon is not inflated because inflation of the gastric balloon precludes proper drainage of esophageal secretions [28]. If the patient is to be placed in an aircraft (i.e., for evacuation), water should be instilled into balloon(s) instead of air [29].

Insertion and Placement of the Tube

The head of the bed should be elevated to reduce the risk of aspiration. Oral suction should be readied and the correct length of the tube to reach the patient's stomach should be selected (usually 45 to 60 cm orally). If the patient is not intubated, head down with left lateral positioning should be attained to minimize the risk of aspiration [17]. If using a Minnesota tube, the esophageal aspiration port should be set to continuous suction and the tube generously lubricated with lidocaine jelly prior to inserting it through the nose or mouth into the stomach. However, the nasal route is not recommended in patients with coagulopathy or thrombocytopenia. In the difficult insertion, the tube may be placed endoscopically [30] or with a guidewire [31]. Duarte described a technique of placing the tube in a longitudinally split Ewald tube [32]. Auscultation in the epigastrium while air is injected through the gastric lumen verifies the position of the tube, but the position of the gastric balloon must be confirmed at this time radiologically or by ultrasound if it is more expedient [33] as high placement can lead to esophageal rupture and low placement to duodenal rupture [34]. The manometer is then connected to the gastric pressure port and the gastric balloon is inflated with no more than 80 mL of air. A pressure of greater than 15 mm Hg at this stage suggests esophageal placement [27,35]. A (portable) radiograph must be obtained that includes the upper abdomen and lower chest (Figs. 15.4 and 15.5). When it is documented that the gastric balloon is below the diaphragm, it should be further inflated with air in 100 mL aliquots to a volume of 250 to 300 mL. The gastric balloon of the Minnesota tube can be inflated to 450 to 500 mL. If the change in manometric pressure for an aliquot is more than 15 mm Hg of the preinsertion pressure or if the gastric balloon is underinflated causing upward migration, erroneous esophageal placement should be considered. Record tube insertion depth (i.e., at the teeth). Tube balloon inlets should be clamped with rubber-shod hemostats after insufflation. Hemorrhage is frequently controlled with insufflation of the gastric balloon alone without applying traction, but in patients with torrential hemorrhage, it is necessary to apply traction (vide infra). If the bleeding continues, the manometer attached to the esophageal pressure port is used to inflate the esophageal balloon to a pressure of approximately 45 mm Hg. Some authors inflate the esophageal balloon in all patients immediately after insertion. If there is still bleeding, deflate the esophageal balloon, apply more traction, and reinflate in the event that it is a gastric variceal bleed. Pressures should be monitored and maintained.

Fixation and Traction Techniques

Fixation and traction on the tube depend on the route of insertion. When the nasal route is used, attachment of a sponge rubber cuff around the tube at the nostril prevents skin and cartilage necrosis. When traction is required, the tube should be attached to a cord that is passed over a catcher's mask for

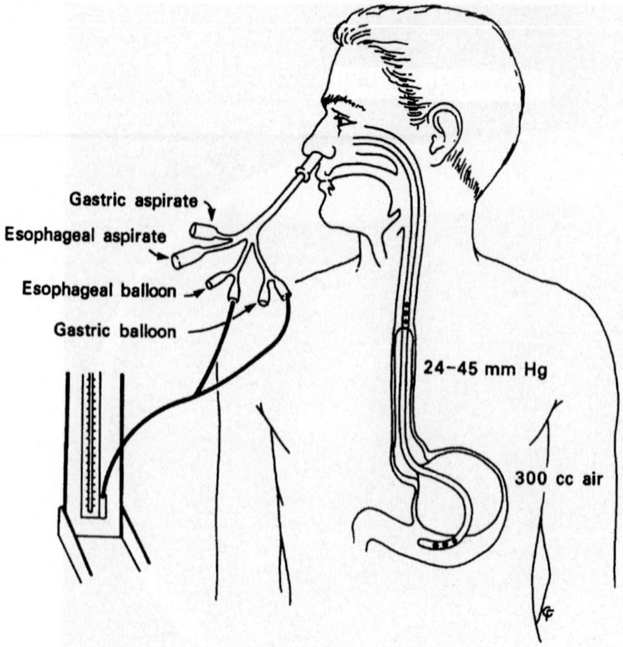

FIGURE 15.4. Proper positioning of the Minnesota tube.

maximum transportability [36] or a pulley in a bed with an overhead orthopedic frame and aligned directly as it comes out of the nose to avoid contact with the nostril. This type of system allows maintenance of traction with a known weight of 500 to 1,500 g either temporarily with IV fluid bags [17] or more permanently with block weights. When the tube is inserted through the mouth, traction is better applied by placing a football helmet on the patient and attaching the tube to the face mask of the helmet after a similar weight is applied for tension. Pressure sores can occur on the head and forehead if the helmet does not fit properly or if it is used for a prolonged period. Several authors recommend overhead traction for either oral or nasal insertion [37].

Maintenance, Monitoring, and Care

Periodically flush ports to ensure patency. To reduce encephalopathy, the gastric aspiration port should be used to thoroughly lavage the stomach before being set to low intermittent suction. It may be used later for medication administration. The esophageal port may be set to intermittent or continuous suction, depending on the extent of bleeding and drainage [35]. Tautness and inflation should be checked often and at least 1 hour after insertion, allowing for only transient fluctuations of as much as 30 mm Hg with respirations and esophageal spasm. Sedation or a pressure decrease may be necessary if large pressure fluctuations persist. If repositioning of the tube is required, assure that the esophageal balloon is deflated. Soft restraints should also be in use and the head of the bed elevated. The tube is left in place a minimum of 24 hours with gastric balloon tamponade maintained continuously for up to 48 hours. The esophageal balloon should be deflated for 5 minutes every 6 hours to help prevent mucosal ischemia and esophageal necrosis. Radiographic assurance of correct placement should be obtained every 24 hours and when dislodgement is suspected (Fig. 15.5). Watch for localized cervical edema, which may signal obstruction or malpositioning [38]. A pair of scissors should be kept with the apparatus in case rapid decompression becomes necessary as balloon migration can acutely obstruct the airway or rupture the esophagus. It is advisable to take care not to utilize bare hemostats and to clamp at the thicker portion of the ports as it is possible for the lumen to become obliterated and the tube thus impacted [39].

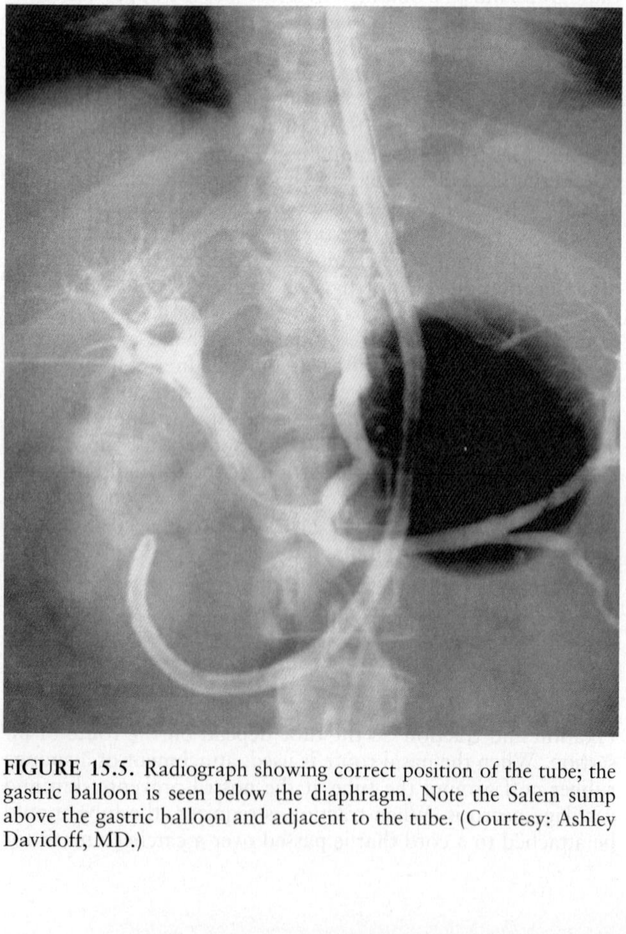

FIGURE 15.5. Radiograph showing correct position of the tube; the gastric balloon is seen below the diaphragm. Note the Salem sump above the gastric balloon and adjacent to the tube. (Courtesy: Ashley Davidoff, MD.)

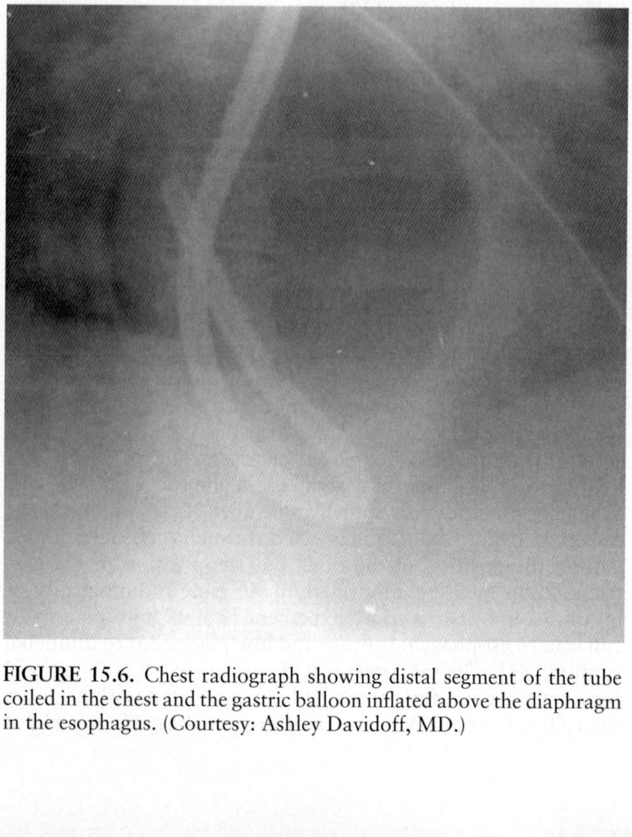

FIGURE 15.6. Chest radiograph showing distal segment of the tube coiled in the chest and the gastric balloon inflated above the diaphragm in the esophagus. (Courtesy: Ashley Davidoff, MD.)

Removal of the Tube

Once hemorrhage is controlled, the esophageal balloon is deflated first. This may be done incrementally over time if desired. The gastric balloon is left inflated for an additional 24 to 48 hours and may be deflated if there is no evidence of bleeding. The tube is left in place 24 hours longer. If bleeding recurs, the balloon is reinflated. The tube is removed if no further bleeding occurs. Primary therapy and secondary prophylaxis, as described previously, should be considered because balloon tamponade is a bridge intervention and rebleeding can occur in up to two thirds of patients within 3 months without therapy [3].

COMPLICATIONS

Rebleeding when the cuff(s) is deflated should be anticipated. The highest risk of rebleeding is in the first few days after balloon deflation. By 6 weeks, the risk of rebleeding returns to premorbid risk level. Independent predictors of mortality in patients undergoing balloon tamponade, described by Lee et al. [40], include blood transfusion greater than 10 units, coagulopathy, presence of shock, Glasgow Coma Score, and total volume of sclerosing agent (ethanolamine).

Aspiration pneumonia is the most common complication of balloon tamponade. The severity and fatality rate is related to the presence of impaired mental status and encephalopathy in patients with poor control of the airway. The incidence ranges from 0% to 12%. Acute laryngeal obstruction and tracheal rupture are the most severe of all complications and the worst examples of tube migration or malpositioning. Migration of the tube occurs when the gastric balloon is not inflated properly after adequate positioning in the stomach or when excessive traction (>1.5 kg) is used, causing migration cephalad to the esophagus or hypopharynx. Mucosal ulceration of the gastroesophageal junction is common and is directly related to prolonged traction time (>36 hours). Perforation of the esophagus is reported as a result of misplacing the gastric balloon above the diaphragm (Fig. 15.6). The incidence of complications that are a direct cause of death ranges from 0% to 20%.

ACKNOWLEDGMENTS

The authors thank Claire LaForce (Rutland Regional Medical Center, Rutland, VT) for her help in collecting references.

References

1. Rikkers LF: Surgical complications of cirrhosis and portal hypertension, in Townsend CM, Beauchamp RD, Evers BM, et al: (eds): *Sabiston's Textbook of Surgery*. 17th ed. Philadelphia, WB Saunders, 2004, p 1175.
2. Tsokos M, Turk EE: Esophageal variceal hemorrhage presenting as sudden death in outpatients. *Arch Pathol Lab Med* 126:1197, 2002.
3. Zaman A, Chalasani N: Bleeding caused by portal hypertension. *Gastroenterol Clin North Am* 34:623, 2005.
4. Zehetner J, Shamiyeh A, Wayand W, et al: Results of a new method to stop acute bleeding from esophageal varices; implantation of a self-expanding stent. *Surg Endosc* 22:2149–2152, 2008.
5. Sandford NL, Kerlin P: Current management of oesophageal varices. *Aust N Z J Med* 25:528, 1995.
6. Stein C, Korula J: Variceal bleeding: what are the options? *Postgrad Med* 98:143, 1995.
7. Erstad B: Octreotide for acute variceal bleeding. *Ann Pharmacother* 35:618, 2001.
8. Pourriat JL, Leyacher S, Letoumelin P, et al: Early administration of terlipressin plus glyceryl trinitrate to control active upper gastrointestinal bleeding in cirrhotic patients. *Lancet* 346:865, 1995.
9. Romero-Castro R, Jimenez-Saenz M, Pellicer-Bautista F, et al: Recombinant-activated factor VII as hemostatic therapy in eight cases of severe hemorrhage from esophageal varices. *Clin Gastroenterol Hepatol* 2:78, 2004.
10. Avgerinos A, Armonis A, Manolakpoulos S, et al: Endoscopic sclerotherapy versus variceal ligation in the long-term management of patients with cirrhosis after variceal bleeding: a prospective randomized study. *J Hepatol* 26:1034, 1997.
11. Banares R, Casado M, Rodriquez-Laiz JM, et al: Urgent transjugular intrahepatic portosystemic shunt for control of acute variceal bleeding. *Am J Gastroenterol* 93:75, 1998.
12. Lewis JJ, Basson MD, Modlin IM: Surgical therapy of acute esophageal variceal hemorrhage. *Dig Dis Sci* 10[Suppl 1]:46, 1992.
13. Mathur SK, Shah SR, Soonawala ZF, et al: Transabdominal extensive oesophagogastric devascularization with gastro-oesophageal stapling in the management of acute variceal bleeding. *Br J Surg* 84:413, 1997.
14. Kitamoto M, Imamura M, Kamada K, et al: Balloon-occluded retrograde transvenous obliteration of gastric fundal varices with hemorrhage. *AJR Am J Roentgenol* 178:1167, 2002.
15. Shiba M, Higuchi K, Nakamura K, et al: Efficacy and safety of balloon-occluded endoscopic injection sclerotherapy as a prophylactic treatment for high-risk gastric fundal varices: a prospective, randomized, comparative clinical trial. *Gastrointest Endosc* 56:522, 2002.
16. Burnett DA, Rikkers LF: Nonoperative emergency treatment of variceal hemorrhage. *Surg Clin North Am* 70:291, 1990.
17. McCormick PA, Burroughs AK, McIntyre N: How to insert a Sengstaken-Blakemore tube. *Br J Hosp Med* 43:274, 1990.
18. Minocha A, Richards RJ: Sengstaken-Blakemore tube for control of massive bleeding from gastric varices in hiatal hernia. *J Clin Gastroenterol* 14:36, 1992.
19. Chong CF: Esophageal rupture due to Sengstaken-Blakemore tube misplacement. *World J Gastroenterol* 11(41):6563–6565, 2005.
20. Pasquale MD, Cerra FB: Sengstaken-Blakemore tube placement. *Crit Care Clin* 8:743, 1992.
21. Zeid SS, Young PC, Reeves JT: Rupture of the esophagus after introduction of the Sengstaken-Blakemore tube. *Gastroenterology* 36:128–131, 1959.
22. Cello JP, Crass RA, Grendell JH, et al: Management of the patient with hemorrhaging esophageal varices. *JAMA* 256:1480, 1986.
23. Papatheodoridis GV, Patch D, Webster JM, et al: Infection and hemostasis in decompensated cirrhosis: a prospective study using thromboelastography. *Hepatology* 29:1085, 1999.
24. Pohl J, Pollmann K, Sauer P, et al: Antibiotic prophylaxis after variceal hemorrhage reduces incidence of early rebleeding. *Hepatogastroenterology* 51(56):541, 2004.
25. Shaheen NJ, Stuart E, Schmitz S, et al: Pantoprazole reduces the size of postbanding ulcers after variceal band ligation: a randomized control trial. *Hepatology* 41:588, 2005.
26. Greenwald B: Two devices that facilitate the use of the Minnesota tube. *Gastroenterol Nurs* 27:268–270, 2004.
27. Bard, Inc: Bard Minnesota four lumen esophagogastric tamponade tube for the control of bleeding from esophageal varices [package insert], 1997.
28. Boyce HW: Modification of the Sengstaken-Blackmore balloon tube. *Nord Hyg Tidskr* 267:195, 1962.
29. Pinto-Marques P, Romaozinho J, Ferreira M, et al: Esophageal perforation-associated risk with balloon tamponade after endoscopic therapy. Myth or reality? *Hepatogastroenterology* 53:536–539, 2006.
30. Lin TC, Bilir BM, Powis ME: Endoscopic placement of Sengstaken-Blakemore tube. *J Clin Gastroenterol* 31(1):29–32, 2000.
31. Wilcox G, Marlow J: A special maneuver for passage of the Sengstaken-Blakemore tube. *Gastrointest Endosc* 30(6):377, 1984.
32. Duarte B: Technique for the placement of the Sengstaken-Blakemore tube. *Surg Gynecol Obstet* 168(5):449–450, 1989.
33. Lock G, Reng M, Messman H, et al: Inflation and positioning of the gastric balloon of a Sengstaken-Blakemore tube under ultrasonographic control. *Gastrointest Endosc* 45(6):538, 1997.
34. Kandel G, Gray R, Mackenzie RL, et al: Duodenal perforation by a Linton-Nachlas balloon tube. *Am J Gastroenterol* 83(4):442–444, 1988.
35. Isaacs K, Levinson S: Insertion of the Minnesota tube, in Drossman D (ed): *Manual of Gastroenterologic Procedures*. 3rd ed. New York, Raven Press, 1993, pp 27–35.
36. Kashiwagi H, Shikano S, Yamamoto O, et al: Technique for positioning the Sengstaken-Blakemore tube as comfortably as possible. *Surg Gynecol Obstet* 172(1):63, 1991.
37. Hunt PS, Korman MG, Hansky J, et al: An 8-year prospective experience with balloon tamponade in emergency control of bleeding esophageal varices. *Dig Dis Sci* 27:413, 1982.
38. Juffe A, Tellez G, Eguaras M, et al: Unusual complication of the Sengstaken-Blakemore tube. *Gastroenterology* 72(4, Pt 1):724–725, 1977.
39. Bhasin DK, Zargar SA, Mandal M, et al: Endoscopic removal of impacted Sengstaken-Blakemore tube. *Surg Endosc* 3(1):54–55, 1989.
40. Lee H, Hawker FH, Selby W, et al: Intensive care treatment of patients with bleeding esophageal varices: results, predictors of mortality, and predictors of the adult respiratory distress syndrome. *Crit Care Med* 20:1555, 1992.

CHAPTER 16 ■ ENDOSCOPIC PLACEMENT OF FEEDING TUBES

LENA M. NAPOLITANO

INDICATIONS FOR ENTERAL FEEDING

Nutritional support is an essential component of intensive care medicine (see Chapters 190–192). It has become increasingly evident that nutritional support administered via the enteral route is far superior to total parenteral nutrition [1–11]. The Society of Critical Care Medicine/American Society for Parenteral and Enteral Nutrition Guidelines for the Provision and Assessment of Nutrition Support Therapy in the Adult Critically Ill Patient [1], the Canadian Clinical Practice Guidelines for Nutrition Support in Critically Ill Adults [2], the European Society for Clinical Nutrition and Metabolism (ESPEN) Guidelines on Enteral Nutrition for Intensive Care [3], and the Practice Management Guidelines for Nutritional Support of the Trauma Patient [4] all strongly recommend that enteral nutrition be used in preference to parenteral nutrition.

Provision of nutrition through the enteral route aids in prevention of gastrointestinal mucosal atrophy, thereby maintaining the integrity of the gastrointestinal mucosal barrier. Other advantages of enteral nutrition are preservation of immunologic gut function and normal gut flora, improved use of nutrients, and reduced cost. Some studies suggest that clinical outcome is improved and infectious complications are decreased in patients who receive enteral nutrition compared with parenteral nutrition.

An evidence-based consensus statement on the management of critically ill patients with severe acute pancreatitis also recommended that enteral nutrition be used in preference to parenteral nutrition [12]. A systematic review also concluded that patients with severe acute pancreatitis should begin enteral nutrition early because such therapy modulates the stress response, promotes more rapid resolution of the disease process, and improves outcome [13].

Although there are absolute or relative contraindications to enteral feeding in selected cases, most critically ill patients can receive some or all of their nutritional requirements via the gastrointestinal tract. Even when some component of nutritional support must be provided intravenously (IV), feeding via the gut is desirable.

Several developments—including new techniques for placement of feeding tubes, availability of smaller caliber, minimally reactive tubes, and an increasing range of enteral formulas—have expanded the ability to provide enteral nutritional support to critically ill patients. Enteral feeding at a site proximal to the pylorus may be absolutely or relatively contraindicated in patients with increased risk of pulmonary aspiration, but feeding more distally (particularly distal to the ligament of Treitz) decreases the likelihood of aspiration. Other relative or absolute contraindications to enteral feeding include fistulas, intestinal obstruction, upper gastrointestinal hemorrhage, and severe inflammatory bowel disease or intestinal ischemia. Enteral feeding is not recommended in patients with severe malabsorption or early in the course of severe short-gut syndrome.

ACCESS TO THE GASTROINTESTINAL TRACT

After deciding to provide enteral nutrition, the clinician must decide whether to deliver the formula into the stomach, duodenum, or jejunum, and determine the optimal method for accessing the site, which is based on the function of the patient's gastrointestinal tract, duration of enteral nutritional support required, and risk of pulmonary aspiration. Gastric feeding provides the most normal route for enteral nutrition, but it is commonly poorly tolerated in the critically ill patient because of gastric dysmotility with delayed emptying [14]. Enteral nutrition infusion into the duodenum or jejunum may decrease the incidence of aspiration because of the protection afforded by a competent pyloric sphincter; however, the risk of aspiration is not completely eliminated by feeding distal to the pylorus [15–17]. Infusion into the jejunum is associated with the lowest risk of pulmonary aspiration. An advantage of this site of administration is that enteral feeding can be initiated early in the postoperative period, because postoperative ileus primarily affects the colon and stomach and only rarely involves the small intestine. However, the early use of postpyloric feeding instead of gastric feeding in critically ill adult patients with no evidence of impaired gastric emptying was not associated with significant clinical benefits [18,19].

TECHNIQUES

Enteral feeding tubes can be placed via the transnasal, transoral, or percutaneous transgastric or transjejunal routes. If these procedures are contraindicated or unsuccessful, the tube may be placed by endoscopy, using endoscopic and laparoscopic technique, or surgically via a laparotomy [20].

Nasoenteric Route

Nasoenteric tubes are the most commonly used means of providing enteral nutritional support in critically ill patients. This route is preferred for short- to intermediate-term enteral support when eventual resumption of oral feeding is anticipated. It is possible to infuse enteral formulas into the stomach using a conventional 16- or 18-French (Fr) polyvinyl chloride nasogastric tube, but patients are usually much more comfortable if a small-diameter silicone or polyurethane feeding tube is used. Nasoenteric tubes vary in luminal diameter (6 to 14 Fr) and length, depending on the desired location of the distal orifice: stomach, 30 to 36 in.; duodenum, 43 in.; jejunum, at least 48 in. Some tubes have tungsten-weighted tips designed to facilitate passage into the duodenum via normal peristalsis; others have a stylet. Most are radiopaque. Some tubes permit gastric decompression while delivering formula into the jejunum.

Nasoenteric feeding tubes should be placed with the patient in a semi-Fowler's or sitting position. The tip of the tube should be lubricated, placed in the patient's nose, and advanced to the posterior pharynx. If the patient is alert and can follow instructions, the patient should be permitted to sip water as the tube is slowly advanced into the stomach. To avoid unintentional airway placement and serious complications, position of the tube should be ascertained after it has been inserted to 30 cm. Acceptable means of documenting intraesophageal location of the tube include a chest radiograph or lack of CO_2 detection through the lumen of the tube by capnography or colorimetry. If the tube is in the airway, CO_2 will be detected and the tube must be removed. Alternatively, commercial systems are now available to track tube progression from the esophagus through the stomach to the duodenum by electromagnetic means. Proper final placement of the tube in the stomach must be confirmed by chest or upper abdominal radiograph before tube feeding is begun. The following methods to assess final tube placement are unreliable and do not assess tube misdirection into the lower respiratory tract: auscultation over the left upper quadrant with air insufflation through the tube, assessment of pH with gastric content aspiration, and easy passage of the tube to its full length with the absence of gagging and coughing [21,22]. The tube should be securely taped to the nose, forehead, or cheek without tension.

Delayed gastric emptying has been confirmed in critically ill patients and may contribute to gastric feeding intolerance. One study randomized 80 critically ill patients to gastric feeding with erythromycin (200 mg IV every 8 hours as a prokinetic agent) or through a transpyloric feeding tube and identified that the two were equivalent in achieving goal caloric requirements [23]. Spontaneous transpyloric passage of enteral feeding tubes in critically ill patients is commonly unsuccessful secondary to the preponderance of gastric atony. The addition of a tungsten weight to the end of enteral feeding tubes and the development of wire or metal stylets in enteral feeding tubes are aimed at improving the success rate for spontaneous transpyloric passage. Once the tube is documented to be in the stomach, various bedside techniques including air insufflation, pH-assisted, magnet-guided [24], and spontaneous passage with [25] or without motility agents may help to facilitate transpyloric feeding tube passage.

IV metoclopramide and erythromycin have been recommended as prokinetic agents. But a Cochrane Database Systematic Review concluded that doses of 10 or 20 mg of IV metoclopramide were equally ineffective in facilitating transpyloric feeding tube placement [26]. No matter which techniques are used to facilitate transpyloric passage of enteral feeding tubes, these tubes must be inserted by skilled practitioners using defined techniques [27,28].

If the tube does not pass into the duodenum on the first attempt, placement can be attempted under endoscopic assistance or fluoroscopic or electromagnetic guidance. The latter method requires specialized equipment. Endoscopic placement of nasoenteral feeding tubes is easily accomplished in the critically ill patient and can be performed at the bedside using portable equipment [29–33]. Transnasal or transoral endoscopy can be used for placement of nasoenteral feeding tubes in critically ill patients [33]. The patient is sedated appropriately (see Chapter 20), and topical anesthetic is applied to the posterior pharynx with lidocaine or benzocaine spray. A 43- to 48-in.-long nasoenteric feeding tube with an inner wire stylet is passed transnasally into the stomach. The endoscope is inserted and advanced through the esophagus into the gastric lumen. An endoscopy forceps is passed through the biopsy channel of the endoscope and used to grasp the tip of the enteral feeding tube. The endoscope, along with the enteral feeding tube, is advanced distally into the duodenum as far as possible (Fig. 16.1).

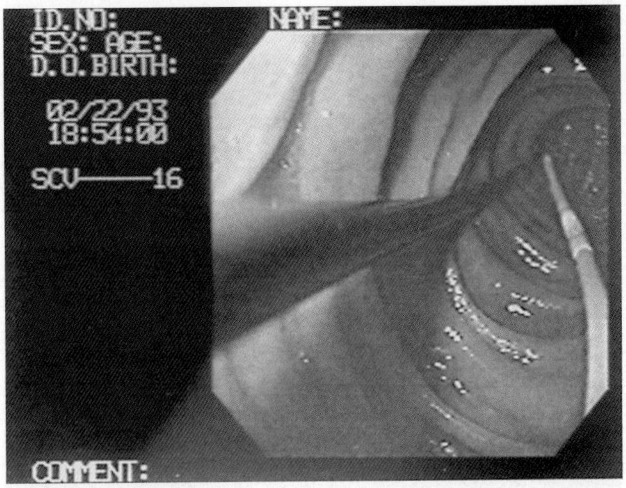

FIGURE 16.1. Endoscopic placement of nasoenteral feeding tube. Endoscopy forceps and gastroscope advance the feeding tube in the duodenum.

The endoscopy forceps and feeding tube remain in position in the distal duodenum as the endoscope is withdrawn back into the gastric lumen. The endoscopy forceps are opened, the feeding tube released, and the endoscopy forceps withdrawn carefully back into the stomach. On first pass, the feeding tube is usually lodged in the second portion of the duodenum. The portion of the feeding tube that is redundant in the stomach is advanced slowly into the duodenum using the endoscopy forceps to achieve a final position distal to the ligament of Treitz (Fig. 16.2). An abdominal radiograph is obtained at the completion of the procedure to document the final position of the nasoenteral feeding tube. Endoscopic placement of postpyloric enteral feeding tubes is highly successful, eliminates the risk of transporting the patient to the radiology department for fluoroscopic placement, and allows prompt achievement of nutritional goals because enteral feeding can be initiated immediately after the procedure.

The recent development of ultrathin endoscopes (outer diameter 5.1 to 5.9 mm vs. 9.8 mm in standard gastroscope) has enabled nasoenteric feeding tube placement via transnasal endoscopy using an over-the-wire technique. A 90% success rate was documented with endoscopic procedure duration of approximately 13 minutes, shorter than fluoroscopic procedure duration and without the need for additional sedation [34]. Unsedated transnasal ultrathin endoscopy can also be used for feeding tube or percutaneous endoscopic gastrostomy (PEG) placement in patients who are unable to undergo transoral endoscopy, that is, those who have partial or complete occlusion of the mouth [35].

Electromagnetic guidance employs a feeding tube with a guidewire that emits electromagnetic waves. A box with three receivers that is placed on the patient's xiphoid process triangulates the position of the tube. The clinician is able to "view" the tip on a monitor as it passes down the esophagus through the stomach and into the duodenum. Although the manufacturer asserts an x-ray after the procedure is not necessary, the practice at many institutions is to obtain an x-ray to confirm placement of the tube.

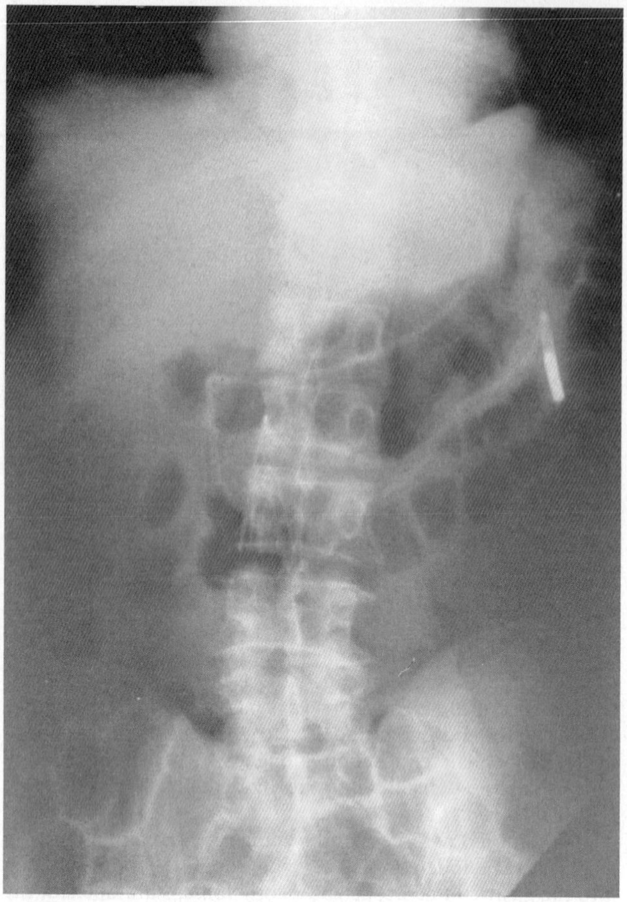

FIGURE 16.2. Abdominal radiograph documenting the optimal position of an endoscopically placed nasoenteral feeding tube, past the ligament of Treitz.

Percutaneous Route

PEG tube placement, introduced by Ponsky et al. [36] in 1990, has become the procedure of choice for patients requiring prolonged enteral nutritional support. PEG tubes range in size from 20 to 28 Fr. PEG rapidly replaced open gastrostomy as the method of choice for enteral nutrition. Unlike surgical gastrostomy, PEG does not require general anesthesia and laparotomy and eliminates the discomfort associated with chronic nasoenteric tubes. This procedure can be considered for patients who have normal gastric emptying and low risk for pulmonary aspiration, and can be performed in the operating room, in an endoscopy unit, or at the bedside in the intensive care unit with portable endoscopy equipment.

PEG should not be performed in patients with near or total obstruction of the pharynx or esophagus, in the presence of coagulopathy, or when transillumination is inadequate. Relative contraindications are ascites, gastric cancer, and gastric ulcer. Previous abdominal surgery is not a contraindication. The original method for PEG was the pull technique; more recent modifications are the push and introducer techniques.

Pull Technique

The pull technique is performed with the patient in the supine position. The abdomen is prepared and draped. The posterior pharynx is anesthetized with a topical spray or solution (e.g., benzocaine spray or viscous lidocaine), and IV sedation (e.g., 1 to 2 mg of midazolam; see Chapter 20) is administered. A prophylactic antibiotic, usually a first-generation cephalosporin, is administered before the procedure. The fiberoptic gastroscope is inserted into the stomach, which is then insufflated with air. The lights are dimmed, and the assistant applies digital pressure to the anterior abdominal wall in the left subcostal area approximately 2 cm below the costal margin, looking for the brightest transillumination (light reflex). The endoscopist should be able to clearly identify the indentation in the stomach created by the assistant's digital pressure on the anterior abdominal wall (digital reflex); otherwise, another site should be chosen.

When the correct spot has been identified, the assistant anesthetizes the anterior abdominal wall. The endoscopist then introduces a polypectomy snare through the endoscope. A small incision is made in the skin, and the assistant introduces a large-bore catheter–needle stylet assembly into the stomach and through the snare. The snare is then tightened securely around the catheter. The inner stylet is removed, and a looped insertion wire is introduced through the catheter and into the stomach. The cannula is slowly withdrawn so that the snare grasps the wire. The gastroscope is then pulled out of the patient's mouth with the wire firmly grasped by the snare. The end of the transgastric wire exiting the patient's mouth is then tied to a prepared gastrostomy tube. The assistant pulls on the end of the wire exiting from the abdominal wall while the endoscopist guides the lubricated gastrostomy tube into the posterior pharynx and the esophagus. With continued traction, the gastrostomy tube is pulled into the stomach so that it exits on the anterior abdominal wall. The gastroscope is reinserted into the stomach to confirm adequate placement of the gastrostomy tube against the gastric mucosa and to document that no bleeding has occurred. The intraluminal portion of the tube should contact the mucosa, but excessive tension on the tube should be avoided because this can lead to ischemic necrosis of the gastric wall. The tube is secured to the abdominal wall using sutures. Feedings may be initiated immediately after the procedure or 24 hours later.

Push Technique

The push technique is similar to the pull technique. The gastroscope is inserted and a point on the anterior abdominal wall localized, as for the pull technique. Rather than introducing a looped insertion wire, however, a straight guidewire is snared and brought out through the patient's mouth by withdrawing the endoscope and snare together. A commercially developed gastrostomy tube (Sachs–Vine) with a tapered end is then passed in an aboral direction over the wire, which is held taut. The tube is grasped and pulled out the rest of the way. The gastroscope is reinserted to check the position and tension on the tube.

Introducer Technique

The introducer technique uses a peel-away introducer technique originally developed for the placement of cardiac pacemakers and central venous catheters. The gastroscope is inserted into the stomach and an appropriate position for placement of the tube is identified. After infiltration of the skin with local anesthetic, a 16- or 18-gauge needle is introduced into the stomach. A J-tipped guidewire is inserted through the needle into the stomach and the needle is withdrawn. Using a twisting motion, a 16-Fr introducer with a peel-away sheath is passed over the guidewire into the gastric lumen [37,38]. The guidewire and introducer are removed, leaving in place the sheath that allows placement of a 14-Fr Foley catheter. The sheath is peeled away after the balloon is inflated with 10 mL of normal saline. Some advocate this as the optimal method for PEG in patients with head and neck cancer, related to an overall lower rate of complications in this patient population [39].

Percutaneous Endoscopic Gastrostomy/Jejunostomy

If postpyloric feeding is desired (especially in patients at high risk for pulmonary aspiration), a PEG/jejunostomy may be performed. The tube allows simultaneous gastric decompression and duodenal/jejunal enteral feeding [40]. A second, smaller feeding tube can be attached and passed through the gastrostomy tube and advanced endoscopically into the duodenum or jejunum. When the PEG is in position, a guidewire is passed through it and grasped using endoscopy forceps. The guidewire and endoscope are passed into the duodenum as distally as possible. The jejunal tube is then passed over the guidewire through the PEG into the distal duodenum, advanced into the jejunum, and the endoscope is withdrawn. An alternative method is to grasp a suture at the tip of the feeding tube or the distal tip of the tube itself and pass the tube into the duodenum, using forceps advanced through the biopsy channel of the endoscope. This obviates the need to pass the gastroscope into the duodenum, which may result in dislodgment of the tube when the endoscope is withdrawn.

Direct Percutaneous Endoscopic Jejunostomy

Jejunostomy tubes can be placed endoscopically by means of a PEG with jejunal extension (PEG-J) or by direct percutaneous jejunostomy (PEJ) [41,42]. Because the size of the jejunal extension of the PEG-J tube is significantly smaller than that of the direct PEJ, some have suggested that the PEJ provides more stable jejunal access for those who require long-term jejunal feeding. Unfortunately, a low success rate (68%) and a high adverse event rate (22.5%) have been documented in the largest series to date [43].

Fluoroscopic Technique

Percutaneous gastrostomy and gastrojejunostomy can also be performed using fluoroscopy [44–46]. The stomach is insufflated with air using a nasogastric tube or a skinny needle if the patient is obstructed proximally. Once the stomach is distended and position is checked again with fluoroscopy, the stomach is punctured with an 18-gauge needle. A heavy-duty wire is passed and the tract is dilated to 7 Fr. A gastrostomy tube may then be inserted into the stomach. An angiographic catheter is introduced and manipulated through the pylorus. The percutaneous tract is then further dilated and the gastrojejunostomy tube is advanced as far as possible.

Complications

The most common complication after percutaneous placement of enteral feeding tubes is infection, usually involving the cutaneous exit site and surrounding tissue [47]. Gastrointestinal hemorrhage has been reported, but it is usually due to excessive tension on the tube, leading to necrosis of the stomach wall. Gastrocolic fistulas, which develop if the colon is interposed between the anterior abdominal wall and the stomach when the needle is introduced, have been reported. Adequate transillumination aids in avoiding this complication. Separation of the stomach from the anterior abdominal wall can occur, resulting in peritonitis when enteral feeding is initiated. In most instances, this complication is caused by excessive tension on the gastrostomy tube. Another potential complication is pneumoperitoneum, secondary to air escaping after puncture of the stomach during the procedure, and is usually clinically insignificant. If the patient develops fever and abdominal tenderness, a Gastrografin study should be obtained to exclude the presence of a leak.

All percutaneous gastrostomy and jejunostomy procedures described here have been established as safe and effective. The method is selected on the basis of the endoscopist's experience and training and the patient's nutritional needs.

SURGICAL PROCEDURES

Since the advent of PEG, surgical placement of enteral feeding tubes is usually performed as a concomitant procedure as the last phase of a laparotomy performed for another indication. Occasionally, an operation solely for tube placement is performed in patients requiring permanent tube feedings when a percutaneous approach is contraindicated or unsuccessful. In these cases, the laparoscopic approach to enteral access should be considered [48]. Laparoscopic gastrostomy was introduced in 2000, 10 years after the PEG. Patients who are not candidates for PEG, due to head and neck cancer, esophageal obstruction, large hiatal hernia, gastric volvulus, or overlying intestine or liver, should be considered for laparoscopic gastrostomy or jejunostomy.

Gastrostomy

Gastrostomy is a simple procedure when performed as part of another intra-abdominal operation. It should be considered when prolonged enteral nutritional support is anticipated after surgery.

Complications are quite common after surgical gastrostomy. This may reflect the poor nutritional status and associated medical problems in many patients who undergo this procedure. Potential complications include wound infection, dehiscence, gastrostomy disruption, internal or external leakage, gastric hemorrhage, and tube migration.

Needle–Catheter Jejunostomy

The needle–catheter jejunostomy procedure consists of the insertion of a small (5-Fr) polyethylene catheter into the small intestine at the time of laparotomy for another indication. Kits containing the necessary equipment for the procedure are available from commercial suppliers. A needle is used to create a submucosal tunnel from the serosa to the mucosa on the antimesenteric border of the jejunum. A catheter is inserted through the needle and then the needle is removed. The catheter is brought out through the anterior abdominal wall and the limb of the jejunum is secured to the anterior abdominal wall with sutures. The tube can be used for feeding immediately after the operation. The potential complications are similar to those associated with gastrostomy, but patients may have a higher incidence of diarrhea. Occlusion of the needle–catheter jejunostomy is common because of its small luminal diameter, and elemental nutritional formulas are preferentially used.

Transgastric Jejunostomy

Critically ill patients who undergo laparotomy commonly require gastric decompression and a surgically placed tube for enteral nutritional support. Routine placement of separate gastrostomy and jejunostomy tubes is common in this patient population and achieves the objective of chronic gastric decompression and early initiation of enteral nutritional support through the jejunostomy. Technical advances in surgically placed enteral feeding tubes led to the development of transgastric jejunostomy [49] and duodenostomy tubes, which allow simultaneous decompression of the stomach and distal feeding into the

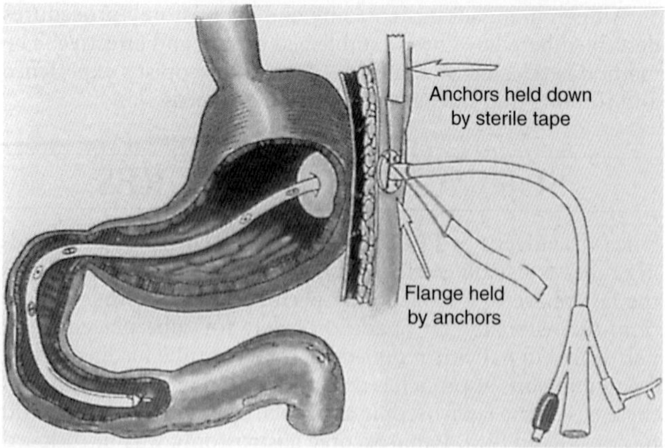

FIGURE 16.3. Transgastric duodenal feeding tube, which allows simultaneous gastric decompression and duodenal feeding, can be placed percutaneously (with endoscopic or fluoroscopic assistance) or surgically.

duodenum or jejunum. The advantage of these tubes is that only one enterotomy into the stomach is needed, eliminating the possible complications associated with open jejunostomy tube placement. In addition, only one tube is necessary for gastric decompression and jejunal feeding, eliminating the potential complications of two separate tubes for this purpose.

The transgastric jejunostomy tube is placed surgically in the same manner as a gastrostomy tube, and the distal portion of the tube is advanced manually through the pylorus into the duodenum, with its final tip resting as far distally as possible in the duodenum or jejunum (Fig. 16.3). The transgastric jejunostomy tube is preferred to transgastric duodenostomy tube because it is associated with less reflux of feedings into the stomach and a decreased risk of aspiration pneumonia. Surgical placement of transgastric jejunostomy tubes at the time of laparotomy is recommended for patients who likely require prolonged gastric decompression and enteral feeding.

DELIVERING THE TUBE-FEEDING FORMULA

The enteral formula can be delivered by intermittent bolus feeding, gravity infusion, or continuous pump infusion. In the intermittent bolus method, the patient receives 300 to 400 mL of formula every 4 to 6 hours. The bolus is usually delivered with the aid of a catheter-tipped, large-volume (60-mL) syringe. The main advantage of bolus feeding is simplicity. This approach is often used for patients requiring prolonged supplemental enteral nutritional support after discharge from the hospital. Bolus feeding can be associated with serious side effects, however. Bolus enteral feeding into the stomach can cause gastric distention, nausea, cramping, and aspiration. The intermittent bolus method should not be used when feeding into the duodenum or jejunum because boluses of formula can cause distention, cramping, and diarrhea.

Gravity-infusion systems allow the formula to drip continuously during 16 to 24 hours or intermittently during 20 to 30 minutes, four to six times per day. This method requires constant monitoring because the flow rate can be extremely irregular. The main advantages of this approach are simplicity, low cost, and close simulation of a normal feeding pattern.

Continuous pump infusion is the preferred method for the delivery of enteral nutrition in the critically ill patient. A peristaltic pump can be used to provide a continuous infusion of formula at a precisely controlled flow rate, which decreases problems with distention and diarrhea. Gastric residuals tend to be smaller with continuous pump-fed infusions, and the risk of aspiration may be decreased. In adult burn and trauma patients, continuous feedings are associated with less stool frequency and shorter time to achieve nutritional goals [50,51].

MEDICATIONS

When medications are administered via an enteric feeding tube, it is important to be certain that the drugs are compatible with each other and with the enteral formula. In general, medications should be delivered separately rather than as a combined bolus. For medications that are better absorbed in an empty stomach, tube feedings should be suspended for 30 to 60 minutes before administration.

Medications should be administered in an elixir formulation via enteral feeding tubes whenever possible to prevent occlusion of the tube. Enteral tubes should always be flushed with 20 mL of saline after medications are administered. To use an enteral feeding tube to administer medications dispensed in tablet form, often the pills must be crushed and delivered as slurry mixed with water. This is inappropriate for some medications, however, such as those absorbed sublingually or formulated as a sustained-released tablet or capsule.

COMPLICATIONS

Enteral tube placement is associated with few complications if practitioners adhere to appropriate protocols and pay close attention to the details of the procedures [52].

Nasopulmonary Intubation

Passage of an enteral feeding tube into the tracheobronchial tree most commonly occurs in patients with diminished cough or gag reflexes due to obtundation, altered mental status, or other causes such as the presence of endotracheal intubation. The presence of a tracheostomy or endotracheal tube does not guarantee proper placement. A chest (or upper abdominal) radiograph should always be obtained before initiating tube feedings with a new tube to ensure that the tube is properly positioned. Endotracheal or transpulmonary placement of a feeding tube can be associated with pneumothorax, hydrothorax, pneumonia, pulmonary hemorrhage, abscess formation, or death. A chest radiograph or a means of detecting CO_2 through the tube after it has been inserted 30 cm should be obtained to prevent inadvertent placement of small-bore feeding tubes into the lungs.

Aspiration

Pulmonary aspiration is a serious and potentially fatal complication of enteral nutritional support [53]. The incidence of this complication is variable and depends on the patient population studied. The two most common bedside tests for detecting aspiration in tube-fed patients include adding dye to the formula and observing for its appearance in tracheobronchial secretions, and using glucose oxidase reagent strips to test tracheobronchial secretions for glucose-containing enteral formula [54]. No large prospective clinical trials have validated the use and safety of bedside monitors for aspiration, and their use should be abandoned. Nonrecumbent positioning is an evidence-based method for aspiration prevention that needs to be initiated in all patients receiving enteral nutrition.

Major risk factors for aspiration include obtundation or altered mental status, absence of cough or gag reflexes, delayed gastric emptying, gastroesophageal reflux, and feeding in the supine position. The risk of pulmonary aspiration is minimized when the enteral feeding tube is positioned in the jejunum past the ligament of Treitz.

Gastrointestinal Intolerance

Delayed gastric emptying is sometimes improved by administering the prokinetic agents metoclopramide (10 to 20 mg IV) or erythromycin (200 mg IV). Dumping syndrome (i.e., diarrhea, distention, and abdominal cramping) can limit the use of enteral feeding. Dumping may be caused by delivering a hyperosmotic load into the small intestine.

Diarrhea in critically ill patients should not be attributed to intolerance of enteral feeding until other causes are excluded. Other possible etiologies for diarrhea include medications (e.g., magnesium-containing antacids and quinidine), alterations in gut microflora due to prolonged antibiotic therapy, antibiotic-associated colitis, ischemic colitis, viral or bacterial enteric infection, electrolyte abnormalities, and excessive delivery of bile salts into the colon. Diarrhea can also be a manifestation of intestinal malabsorption because of enzyme deficiencies or villous atrophy [55].

Even if diarrhea is caused by enteral feeding, it can be controlled in nearly 50% of cases by instituting a continuous infusion of formula (if bolus feedings are used), slowing the rate of infusion, changing the formula, adding fiber to the enteral formula, or adding antidiarrheal agents (e.g., tincture of opium).

Metabolic Complications

Prerenal azotemia and hypernatremia can develop in patients fed with hyperosmolar solutions. The administration of free water, either added to the formula or as separate boluses to replace obligatory losses, can avert this situation. Deficiencies of essential fatty acids and fat-soluble vitamins can develop after prolonged support with enteral solutions that contain minimal amounts of fat. Periodic enteral supplementation with linoleic acid or IV supplementation with emulsified fat can prevent this [56]. The amount of linoleic acid necessary to prevent chemical and clinical fatty acid deficiency has been estimated to be 2.5 to 20.0 g per day.

Bacterial Contamination

Bacterial contamination of enteral solutions [57–59] occurs when commercial packages are opened and mixed with other substances, and more commonly, it occurs with hospital-formulated and powdered feeds that require preparation compared to commercially prepared, ready-to-feed enteral formulas supplied in cans. The risk of contamination also depends on the duration of feeding. Contaminated formula may also play a significant role in the etiology of diarrhea in patients receiving enteral nutrition.

Occluded Feeding Tubes

Precipitation of certain proteins when exposed to an acid pH may be an important factor leading to the solidifying of formulas. Most premixed intact protein formulas solidify when acidified to a pH less than 5. To prevent occlusion of feeding tubes, the tube should be flushed with saline before and after checking residuals. Small-caliber nasoenteric feeding tubes should be flushed with 20 mL of saline every 4 to 6 hours to prevent tube occlusion, even when enteral feedings are administered by continuous infusion.

Medications are a frequent cause of clogging. When administering medications enterally, liquid elixirs should be used, if available, because even tiny particles of crushed tablets can occlude the distal orifice of small-caliber feeding tubes. If tablets are used, it is important to crush them to a fine powder and solubilize them in liquid before administration. In addition, tubes should be flushed with saline before and after the administration of any medications.

Several maneuvers are useful for clearing a clogged feeding tube. The tube can be irrigated with warm saline, a carbonated liquid, cranberry juice, or a pancreatic enzyme solution (e.g., Viokase). Commonly, a mixture of lipase, amylase, and protease (Pancrease) dissolved in sodium bicarbonate solution (for enzyme activation) is instilled into the tube with a syringe and the tube clamped for approximately 30 minutes to allow enzymatic degradation of precipitated enteral feedings. The tube is then vigorously flushed with saline. The pancreatic enzyme solution was successful in restoring tube patency in 96% of cases where formula clotting was the likely cause of occlusion and use of cola or water had failed [60,61]. Prevention of tube clogging with flushes and pancreatic enzyme are therefore the methods of choice in maintenance of chronic enteral feeding tubes.

References

1. Martindale RG, McClave SA, Vanek VW, et al: American College of Critical Care Medicine; ASPEN Board of Directors. Guidelines for the provision and assessment of nutrition support therapy in the adult critically ill patient: Society of Critical Care Medicine and American Society for Parenteral and Enteral Nutrition. *Crit Care Med* 37(5):1757–1761, 2009.
2. Heyland DK, Dhaliwal R, Drover JW, et al: Canadian clinical practice guidelines for nutrition support in mechanically ventilated, critically ill adult patients. *JPEN J Parenter Enteral Nutr* 27(5):355, 2003.
3. Kreymann KG, Berger MM, Duetz NEP, et al: ESPEN guidelines on enteral nutrition: intensive care. *Clin Nutr* 25(2):210, 2006.
4. Jacobs DG, Jacobs DO, Kudsk KA, et al: Practice management guidelines for nutritional support of the trauma patient. *J Trauma* 57:660, 2004.
5. Gramlich L, Kichian K, Pinlla J, et al: Does enteral nutrition compared to parenteral nutrition result in better outcomes in critically ill adult patients? A systematic review of the literature. *Nutrition* 20(10):843, 2004.
6. Heyland DK, Dhaliwal R, Day A, et al: Validation of the Canadian clinical practice guidelines for nutrition support in mechanically ventilated, critically ill adult patients: results of a prospective observational study. *Crit Care Med* 32(11):2260, 2004.
7. Dhaliwal R, Jurewitch B, Harrietha D, et al: Combination enteral and parenteral nutrition in critically ill patients: harmful or beneficial? A systematic review of the evidence. *Intensive Care Med* 30(8):1666, 2004.
8. Mackenzie SL, Zygun DA, Whitmore BL, et al: Implementation of a nutrition support protocol increases the proportion of mechanically ventilated patients reaching enteral nutrition targets in the adult intensive care unit. *JPEN J Parenter Enteral Nutr* 29(2):74, 2005.
9. Napolitano LM, Bochicchio G: Enteral feeding in the critically ill. *Curr Opin Crit Care* 6:1, 2000.
10. Marik PE, Zaloga GP: Early enteral nutrition in acutely ill patients: a systematic review. *Crit Care Med* 29(12):2264, 2001.
11. Zaloga GP: Parenteral and enteral nutrition in adult inpatients with functioning gastrointestinal tracts: assessment of outcomes. *Lancet* 367(9516):1101, 2006.
12. Nathens AB, Curtis JR, Beale RJ, et al: Management of the critically ill patient with severe acute pancreatitis. *Crit Care Med* 32:2524, 2004.
13. McClave SA, Chang WK, Dhaliwal R, et al: Nutrition support in acute pancreatitis: a systematic review of the literature. *JPEN J Parenter Enteral Nutr* 30(2):143, 2006.
14. Ritz MA, Fraser R, Edwards N, et al: Delayed gastric emptying in ventilated critically ill patients: measurement by 13 C-octanoic acid breath test. *Crit Care Med* 29:1744, 2001.
15. McClave SA, DeMeo MT, DeLegge MH, et al: North American Summit on aspiration in the critically ill patient: consensus statement. *JPEN J Parenter Enteral Nutr* 26[6 Suppl]:S80, 2002.

16. Esparza J, Boivin MA, Hartshorne MF, et al: Equal aspiration rates in gastrically and transpylorically fed critically ill patients. *Intensive Care Med* 27:660, 2001.
17. Marik PE, Zaloga GP: Gastric versus post-pyloric feeding: a systematic review. *Crit Care* 7(3):R46, 2003.
18. Ho KM, Dobb GJ, Webb SA: A comparison of early gastric and post-pyloric feeding in critically ill patients: a meta-analysis. *Intensive Care Med* 32(5):639–649, 2006.
19. White H, Sosnowski K, Tran K, et al: A randomized controlled comparison of early post-pyloric versus early gastric feeding to meet nutritional targets in ventilated intensive care patients. *Crit Care* 13(6):R187, 2009.
20. Haslam D, Fang J: Enteral access for nutrition in the intensive care unit. *Curr Opin Clin Nutr Metab Care* 9(2):155, 2006.
21. Burns SM, Carpenter R, Blevins C, et al: Detection of inadvertent airway intubation during gastric tube insertion: capnography versus a colorimetric carbon dioxide detector. *Am J Crit Care* 15:1, 2006.
22. Araujo-Preza CE, Melhado ME, Gutierrez PJ, et al: Use of capnography to verify feeding tube placement. *Crit Care Med* 30:2255, 2002.
23. Boivin MA, Levy H: Gastric feeding with erythromycin is equivalent to transpyloric feeding in the critically ill. *Crit Care Med* 29:1916, 2001.
24. Boivin M, Levy H, Hayes J: A multicenter, prospective study of the placement of transpyloric feeding tubes with assistance of a magnetic device. The Magnet-Guided Enteral Feeding Tube Study Group. *JPEN J Parenter Enteral Nutr* 24:304, 2000.
25. Levy H, Hayes J, Boivin M, et al: Transpyloric feeding tube placement in critically ill patients using electromyogram and erythromycin infusion. *Chest* 125(2):587–591, 2004.
26. Silva CC, Saconato H, Atallah AN: Metoclopramide for migration of nasoenteral rube. *Cochrane Database Syst Rev* 4:CD003353, 2002.
27. Phipps LM, Weber MD, Ginder BR, et al: A randomized controlled trial comparing three different techniques of nasojejunal feeding tube placement in critically ill children. *JPEN J Parenter Enteral Nutr* 29(6):420, 2005.
28. Lee AJ, Eve R, Bennett MJ: Evaluation of a technique for blind placement of post-pyloric feeding tubes in intensive care: application in patients with gastric ileus. *Intensive Care Med* 32(4):553, 2006.
29. Foote JA, Kemmeter PR, Prichard PA, et al: A randomized trial of endoscopic and fluoroscopic placement of postpyloric feeding tubes in critically ill patients. *JPEN J Parenter Enteral Nutr* 28(3):154, 2004.
30. Freeman C, Delegge MH: Small bowel endoscopic enteral access. *Curr Opin Gastroenterol* 25(2):155–159, 2009.
31. Dranoff JA, Angood PJ, Topazian M: Transnasal endoscopy for enteral feeding tube placement in critically ill patients. *Am J Gastroenterol* 94(10):2902, 1999.
32. Napolitano LM, Wagel M, Heard SO: Endoscopic placement of nasoenteric feeding tubes in critically ill patients: a reliable alternative. *J Laparoendosc Adv Surg Tech A* 8:395, 1998.
33. Kulling D, Bauerfeind P, Fried M: Transnasal versus transoral endoscopy for the placement of nasoenteral feeding tubes in critically ill patients. *Gastrointest Endosc* 52:506, 2000.
34. Fang JC, Hilden K, Holubkov R, et al: Transnasal endoscopy vs. fluoroscopy for the placement of nasoenteric feeding tubes in critically ill patients. *Gastrointest Endosc* 62(5):661, 2005.
35. Vitale MA, Villotti G, D'Alba L, et al: Unsedated transnasal percutaneous endoscopic gastrostomy placement in selected patients. *Endoscopy* 37(1):48, 2005.
36. Ponsky JL, Gauderer MWL, Stellato TA, et al: Percutaneous approaches to enteral alimentation. *Am J Surg* 149:102, 1985.
37. Dormann AJ, Glosemeyer R, Leistner U, et al: Modified percutaneous endoscopic gastrostomy (PEG) with gastropexy—early experience with a new introducer technique. *Z Gastroenterol* 38:933, 2000.
38. Maetani I, Tada T, Ukita T, et al: PEG with introducer or pull method: A prospective randomized comparison. *Gastrointest Endosc* 57(7):837, 2003.
39. Foster J, Filocarno P, Nava H, et al: The introducer technique is the optimal method for placing percutaneous endoscopic gastrostomy tubes in head and neck cancer patients. *Surg Endosc* 21(6):897–901, 2007.
40. Melvin W, Fernandez JD: Percutaneous endoscopic transgastric jejunostomy: a new approach. *Am Surg* 71(3):216, 2005.
41. Fan AC, Baron TH, Rumalla A, et al: Comparison of direct percutaneous endoscopic jejunostomy and PEG with jejunal extension. *Gastrointest Endosc* 56(6):890, 2002.
42. Shetzline MA, Suhocki PV, Workman MJ: Direct percutaneous endoscopic jejunostomy with small bowel enteroscopy and fluoroscopy. *Gastrointest Endosc* 53(6):633, 2001.
43. Maple JT, Petersen BT, Baron TH, et al: Direct percutaneous endoscopic jejunostomy: outcomes in 307 consecutive attempts. *Am J Gastroenterol* 100(12):2681, 2005.
44. Ho SG, Marchinkow LO, Legiehn GM, et al: Radiological percutaneous gastrostomy. *Clin Radiol* 56:902, 2001.
45. Giuliano AW, Yoon HC, Lomis NN, et al: Fluoroscopically guided percutaneous placement of large-bore gastrostomy and gastrojejunostomy tubes: review of 109 cases. *J Vasc Interv Radiol* 11:239, 2001.
46. Galaski A, Peng WW, Ellis M, et al: Gastrostomy tube placement by radiological versus endoscopic methods in an acute care setting: a retrospective review of frequency, indications, complications and outcomes. *Can J Gastroenterol* 23(2):109–114, 2009.
47. Schrag SP, Sharma R, Jaik NP, et al: Complications related to percutaneous endoscopic gastrostomy (PEG) tubes. A comprehensive clinical review. *J Gastrointestin Liver Dis* 16(4):407–418, 2007.
48. Edelman DS: Laparoendoscopic approaches to enteral access. *Semin Laparosc Surg* 8:195, 2001.
49. Shapiro T, Minard G, Kudsk KA: Transgastric jejunal feeding tubes in critically ill patients. *Nutr Clin Pract* 12:164, 1997.
50. Hiebert J, Brown A, Anderson R, et al: Comparison of continuous vs intermittent tube feedings in adult burn patients. *JPEN J Parenter Enteral Nutr* 5:73, 1981.
51. Steevens EC, Lipscomb AF, Poole GV, et al: Comparison of continuous vs. intermittent nasogastric enteral feeding in trauma patients: perceptions and practice. *Nutr Clin Pract* 17(2):118, 2002.
52. Baskin WN: Acute complications associated with bedside placement of feeding tubes. *Nutr Clin Pract* 21(1):40–55, 2006.
53. Rassias AJ, Ball PA, Corwin HL: A prospective study of tracheopulmonary complications associated with the placement of narrow-bore enteral feeding tubes. *Crit Care* 2:25, 1998.
54. Maloney JP, Ryan TA: Detection of aspiration in enterally fed patients: A requiem for bedside monitors of aspiration. *JPEN J Parenter Enteral Nutr* 26[6, Suppl]:S34, 2002.
55. Trabal J, Leyes P, Hervas S, et al: Factors associated with nosocomial diarrhea in patients with enteral tube feeding. *Nutr Hosp* 23(5):500–504, 2008.
56. Dodge JA, Yassa JG: Essential fatty acid deficiency after prolonged treatment with elemental diet. *Lancet* 2(8206):1256–1257, 1980.
57. McKinlay J, Wildgoose A, Wood W, et al: The effect of system design on bacterial contamination of enteral tube feeds. *J Hosp Infect* 47:138, 2001.
58. Okuma T, Nakamura M, Totake H, et al: Microbial contamination of enteral feeding formulas and diarrhea. *Nutrition* 16:719, 2000.
59. Lucia Rocha Carvalho M, Beninga Morais T, Ferraz Amaral D, et al: Hazard analysis and critical control point system approach in the evaluation of environmental and procedural sources of contamination of enteral feedings in three hospitals. *JPEN J Parenter Enteral Nutr* 24(50):296, 2000.
60. Williams TA, Leslie GD: A review of the nursing care of enteral feeding tubes in critically ill adults. *Intensive Crit Care Nurs* 21(1):5, 2005.
61. Bourgalt AM, Heyland DK, Drover JW, et al: Prophylactic pancreatic enzymes to reduce feeding tube occlusions. *Nutr Clin Pract* 18(5):398–401, 2003.

CHAPTER 17 ■ CEREBROSPINAL FLUID ASPIRATION

JOHN P. WEAVER

This chapter presents guidelines for safe cerebrospinal fluid (CSF) aspiration for the emergency department or the intensive care physician, and provides a basic understanding of the indications, techniques, and potential complications of these procedures.

Physicians and supervised physician extenders routinely and safely perform CSF aspiration procedures with necessary equipment and sterile supplies readily accessible in most acute hospital patient care units. Most CSF aspirations are performed using local anesthesia alone, without sedation. Because it may be a painful and anxiety-provoking procedure, sedation may be required for an uncooperative patient or for the pediatric population [1,2]. Radiographic imaging (fluoroscopy or ultrasound) is needed in situations in which external anatomic landmarks provide inadequate guidance for safe needle placement or when needle placement using external landmarks alone has proved to be unsuccessful due to anatomic variations caused by trauma, operative scar, congenital defects, or degenerative changes. Fluoroscopy may be used for complicated lumbar puncture, C1–2 puncture, and myelography. Computed tomography (CT) or magnetic resonance imaging (MRI) may be used for stereotactic placement of ventricular catheters. Clinicians should recognize the need for specialized equipment and training in certain cases.

CEREBROSPINAL FLUID ACCESS

Diagnostic Objectives

CSF analysis continues to be a major diagnostic tool in many diseases. The most common indication for CSF sampling is the suspicion of a cerebral nervous system (CNS) infection. CSF is also analyzed for the diagnosis of subarachnoid hemorrhage (SAH), demyelinating diseases, CNS spread of neoplasm, and CNS degenerative conditions. CSF access is necessary for neurodiagnostic procedures, such as myelography and cisternography, and studies for device patencies (tube studies) that require injection of contrast agents. CSF access for pressure recording is also important in the diagnosis of normal-pressure hydrocephalus, benign intracranial hypertension, and head injury.

CSF is an ultrafiltrate of plasma and is normally clear and colorless. Its analysis is a sample of the fluid surrounding the brain and spinal cord. Abnormalities of color and clarity can reflect the presence of cells, protein, hemosiderin, or bilirubin that indicates pathologic processes. The diagnostic tests performed on the aspirated CSF depend on the patient's age, history, and differential diagnosis. A basic profile includes glucose and protein values, a blood cell count, Gram stain, and aerobic and anaerobic cultures. CSF glucose depends on blood glucose levels and is usually equivalent to two-thirds of the serum glucose. It is slightly higher in neonates. Glucose is transported into the CSF via carrier-facilitated diffusion, and changes in spinal fluid glucose concentration lag blood levels by about 2 hours. Increased CSF glucose is nonspecific and usually reflects hyperglycemia. Hypoglycorrhachia can be the result of any inflammatory or neoplastic meningeal disorder, and it reflects increased glucose use by nervous tissue or leukocytes and inhibited transport mechanisms. Elevated lactate levels caused by anaerobic glycolysis in bacterial and fungal meningitis usually accompany lower glucose concentrations.

CSF protein content is usually less than 0.5% of that in plasma with an intact blood–brain barrier. Albumin constitutes up to 75% of CSF protein, and immunoglobulin G (IgG) is the major component of the γ-globulin fraction. IgG freely traverses a damaged blood–brain barrier. Although often nonspecific, elevated CSF protein is an indicator of CNS pathology. There is a gradient of total protein content in the spinal CSF column, with the highest level normally found in the lumbar subarachnoid space at 20 to 50 mg per dL. This is followed by the cisterna magna at 15 to 25 mg per dL and the ventricles at 6 to 12 mg per dL. A value exceeding 500 mg per dL is compatible with an intraspinal tumor or spinal compression causing a complete subarachnoid block, meningitis, or bloody CSF [3]. Low protein levels are seen in healthy children younger than 2 years, pseudotumor cerebri, acute water intoxication, and leukemic patients.

A normal CSF cell count includes no erythrocytes and a maximum of five leukocytes per milliliter. A greater number of white blood cells (WBCs) are normally found in children (up to 10 per milliliter, mostly lymphocytes). Pathologically, increased WBCs are present in infection, leukemia, Guillian–Barré syndrome, hemorrhage, encephalitis, and multiple sclerosis (MS).

Hemorrhage

A *nontraumatic* SAH in the adult population may be due to a ruptured aneurysm. A paroxysmal severe headache is the classic symptom of aneurysm rupture, but atypical headaches reminiscent of migraine are not uncommon. Warning leaks or a sentinel headache occurring at least 4 weeks prior to the diagnosis of SAH was reported by Beck et al. [4] in 17.3% of patients with subsequent diagnosis of SAH.

Leblanc [5] reported that up to 50% of patients with a warning "leak" headache are undiagnosed after evaluation by their physician and 55% of patients with premonitory warning headaches had normal CT findings, but all had a positive finding of SAH on lumbar puncture. Lumbar puncture is indicated with such presenting headache if the head CT is normal and if the clinical history and presentation are typical for aneurysm rupture.

A lumbar puncture should not be performed without prior CT if the patient has any focal neurologic deficit. The neurologic abnormality might indicate the presence of an intracranial mass lesion, and lumbar puncture can increase the likelihood of downward transtentorial herniation. SAH can also cause acute obstructive hydrocephalus by intraventricular extension or obstruction to CSF resorptive mechanisms at the arachnoid granulations. The CT scan would demonstrate ventriculomegaly, which is best treated by CSF access and diversion using a ventricular catheter.

A traumatic lumbar puncture presents a diagnostic dilemma, especially in the context of diagnosing suspected SAH. Differentiating characteristics include a decreasing red blood cell count in tubes collected serially during the procedure, the presence of a fibrinous clot in the sample, and a typical ratio of about 1 leukocyte per 700 red blood cells. Xanthochromia is more indicative of SAH and is quickly evaluated by spinning a fresh CSF sample and comparing the color of the supernatant to that of water. In performing this test, the use of a spectrophotometer is much more sensitive than by visual inspection. Spinal fluid accelerates red blood cell hemolysis, and hemoglobin products are released within 2 hours of the initial hemorrhage, creating the xanthochromia. Associated findings, such as a slightly depressed glucose level, increased protein, and an elevated opening pressure, are also more suggestive of the presence of an SAH.

Infection

CSF evaluation is the single most important aspect of the laboratory diagnosis of meningitis. The analysis usually includes a Gram stain, blood cell count with white cell differential, protein and glucose levels, and aerobic and anaerobic cultures with antibiotic sensitivities. With suspicion of tuberculosis or fungal meningitis, the fluid is analyzed by acid-fast stain, India ink preparation, cryptococcal antigen, and culture in appropriate media. More extensive cultures may be performed in the immunocompromised patient.

Immunoprecipitation tests to identify bacterial antigens for *Streptococcus pneumoniae*, streptococcus group B, *Haemophilus influenzae*, and *Neisseria meningitidis* (meningococcus) allow rapid diagnosis and early specific treatment. Polymerase chain reaction testing can be performed on CSF for rapid identification of several viruses, particularly those commonly responsible for CNS infections in patients with acquired immunodeficiency syndrome. Polymerase chain reaction testing exists for herpes, varicella zoster, cytomegalovirus, and Epstein–Barr virus, as well as toxoplasmosis and *Mycobacterium tuberculosis* [6]. If the clinical suspicion is high for meningitis, administration of broad-spectrum antibiotic therapy should be initiated without delay following CSF collection [7].

Shunt Malfunction

A ventriculoperitoneal shunt is the most commonly encountered implanted system for CSF diversion. The system consists of a ventricular catheter connected to a reservoir and valve mechanism at the skull and a catheter that passes in the subcutaneous soft tissue in the neck and anterior chest wall to the peritoneum. The distal tubing can be alternatively inserted in the jugular vein, the pleura, or even the urinary bladder. Proximal shunt failure of the ventricular catheter may occur due to choroid plexus obstruction or cellular debris from CSF infection. Valve or distal tubing obstruction occurs also from cellular debris, from disconnection, poor CSF absorption, or formation of an intra-abdominal pseudocyst.

The clinical presentation of an obstructed shunt is variable. It may be slowly progressive and intermittent, or there may be a rapid decline in mentation progressing into a coma. A CT scan should be performed immediately to determine ventricular size. Ventriculomegaly is a reliable indicator of a malfunctioning shunt; however, the CT scan should be compared with previous studies because the ventricular system in a shunted patient is often congenitally or chronically abnormal.

Aspiration from the reservoir or valve system of a shunt can be performed to determine patency and collect CSF to diagnose an infectious process. The necessity of and procedure for a shunt tap is best left to a neurosurgeon. Shunt aspiration is an invasive procedure that carries a risk of contaminating the system with skin flora, and the resultant shunt infection requires a lengthy hospitalization for shunt externalization, antibiotic treatment, and replacement of all hardware. Therefore, CSF collection by shunt tap should be performed very selectively and after other potential sources of infection have been evaluated. When shunt failure is due to distal obstruction, aspiration of CSF may temper neurologic impairment and even be lifesaving until surgical revision can be performed.

Normal-Pressure Hydrocephalus

Serial lumbar punctures or continuous CSF drainage via a lumbar subarachnoid catheter can be used as provocative diagnostic tests to select patients who would benefit from a shunt for CSF diversion. The results have a positive predictive value if the patient's gait improves. Lumbar CSF access may also be used for infusion tests, measurement of CSF production rate, pressure–volume index, and outflow resistance or absorption. Some studies suggest that these values are also predictive of therapeutic CSF diversion [8–10].

Benign Intracranial Hypertension (Pseudotumor Cerebri)

Benign intracranial hypertension occurs in young persons, often obese young women. Intracranial pressure (ICP) is elevated without focal deficits and in the absence of ventriculomegaly or intracranial mass lesions [11]. The condition causes blindness, and most patients demonstrate some visual loss. Etiologic factors for childhood presentation include chronic middle ear infection, dural sinus thrombosis, head injury, vitamin A overdosage, tetracycline exposure, internal jugular venous thrombosis, and idiopathic causes. Some authors have proposed a broader definition of the "pseudotumor cerebri syndrome" on the basis of the underlying pathophysiologic mechanism of the presumed CSF circulation disorder [12].

Lumbar puncture demonstrates an elevated ICP (up to 40 cm H_2O), and CSF dynamics demonstrates an increase in outflow resistance. Serial daily punctures can be therapeutic, with CSF aspirated until closing pressure is within normal limits (<20 cm H_2O). In some cases, this can restore the balance between CSF formation and absorption; other cases require medical therapy, such as weight loss, steroids, acetazolamide, diuretics, and glycerol. If all these therapeutic interventions fail, placement of a permanent shunting system may be necessary.

Neoplasms

The subarachnoid space can be infiltrated by various primary or secondary tumors, giving rise to symptoms of meningeal irritation. CSF cytology can determine the presence of neoplastic cells, although their complete identification is not always possible. Systemic neoplasms, such as melanoma or breast cancer, have a greater propensity to metastasize into the CSF spaces than do primary CNS tumors and may even present primarily as meningeal carcinomatosis. Ependymoma, medulloblastoma or primitive neuroectodermal tumor, germinoma, and high-grade glioma are the most commonly disseminated primary tumors. Hematopoietic cancers such as leukemia and lymphoma also frequently infiltrate the subarachnoid spaces with little or no parenchymal involvement. CSF sampling is useful for an initial diagnostic and screening tool in the neurologically intact patient who harbors a tumor type with high risk of CNS relapse. Lymphoma cells in primary CNS lymphoma are present in increased number and pleocytosis correlates with positive cytology [13]. A generous amount of CSF or multiple samples may be required for diagnosis and cisternal puncture may enhance the diagnosis if the lumbar CSF is nondiagnostic. Acute leukemias that tend to invade the CNS include acute lymphocytic leukemia, acute nonlymphocytic leukemia, acute myelogenous leukemia, acute myelomonocytic leukemia, and acute undifferentiated leukemia [14].

Myelography

Lumbar puncture is the most common means of access for lumbar and cervical myelography because the density of contrast material is higher than CSF and may be directed by gravity to the area of interest. Cervical C1–2 puncture had been a usual access route for cervical myelography, but now, it is often reserved for patients in whom a successful lumbar puncture is not possible due to extensive arachnoiditis, epidural tumor, severe spinal stenosis, or CSF block.

Other Neurologic Disorders

There is extensive literature on CSF changes in demyelinating diseases, including MS. Typical lumbar puncture findings are normal ICP, normal glucose levels, mononuclear pleocytosis, and elevated protein levels due to increased endothelial permeability. Immunoelectrophoresis reveals elevated IgG and oligoclonal bands that suggest inflammation in the CNS and may be a sign of MS [15,16].

CSF findings described in other disease states include elevated tau protein and decreased β-amyloid precursor protein in Alzheimer's disease and the presence of anti-GM1 antibodies and cytoalbumin dissociation in Guillain–Barré syndrome [17].

Therapeutic Intervention

Fistulas

CSF leaks occur due to a variety of nontraumatic and traumatic etiologies. Orthostatic headaches are a characteristic symptom of CSF leak, and rhinorrhea may be evident. Iatrogenic postoperative CSF leaks may occur following surgery at the skull base as a result of dural or bony defects. CSF fistulas following middle cranial fossa or cerebellopontine angle surgery occur infrequently, and CSF usually leaks through the auditory tube to the nasopharynx. Dural closure in the posterior fossa following suboccipital craniectomy is often difficult and not watertight. A fistula in that area usually results in a pseudomeningocele, which is clinically apparent as subcutaneous swelling at the incision site. Leaks following lumbar surgery are unusual, but they may occur as a result of recent myelography, dural tear, or inadequate dural closure [18]. In pediatric patients, repair of meningoceles or other spina bifida defects are more likely to present with a CSF leak because of dural or fascial defects.

The most common presentation of a CSF fistula follows trauma. Basilar skull fractures that traverse the ethmoid or frontal sinuses can cause CSF rhinorrhea. Fractures along the long axis of the petrous bone usually involve the middle ear, causing the hemotympanum noted on examination and CSF otorrhea if the tympanic membrane is ruptured. Most CSF leaks present within 48 hours, but delayed leaks are not uncommon because the fistula can be occluded with adhesions, hematoma, or herniated brain tissue, which temporarily tamponades the defect.

The diagnosis of a leak may be easily made on clinical examination; however, at times, the nature of a "drainage fluid" is uncertain and laboratory characterization is necessary. Dipping the fluid for glucose is misleading because nasal secretions are positive for glucose. A chloride level often shows a higher value than in peripheral blood, but identification of β_2-transferrin is the most accurate diagnostic for CSF. This protein is produced by neuraminidase in the brain and is uniquely found in the spinal and perilymph fluids [19].

Elevation of the patient's head is the primary treatment of CSF leak. Placement of a lumbar drainage catheter or daily lumbar punctures should be used if conservative therapy fails. The use of a continuous lumbar drainage by a catheter is somewhat controversial because of the potential for intracranial contamination from the sinuses if the ICP is lowered. To help prevent such complications, the lumbar drain collection bag can be maintained no lower than the patient's shoulder level and the duration of drainage should not exceed 5 days.

Intracranial Hypertension

Intracranial hypertension can cause significant neurologic morbidity or even death. Access to the intracranial CSF space is useful for diagnosis and treatment [20]. A ventriculostomy is commonly used both as an ICP monitor and as a means to treat intracranial hypertension by CSF drainage. An ICP-measuring device should be placed following traumatic brain injury for patients who exhibit a Glasgow Coma Scale score less than 8, a motor score less than 6 (not aphasic), and with initial CT findings of diffuse brain edema, intercranial hematoma, cortical contusions, or absent or compressed basal cisterns [21]. ICP monitoring can also be indicated in cerebrovascular diseases, including aneurysmal SAH, spontaneous cerebral hematoma, ischemic and hypoxic cerebral insults, and intraventricular hemorrhage. Obstructive hydrocephalus is another major indication for placement of a ventricular catheter for drainage and monitoring. ICP may be elevated due to cerebral edema that surrounds tumors, intracranial hematomas, stroke, and traumatic contusions, or that occurs postoperatively or following cranial radiation therapy. Diffuse brain swelling also occurs in the setting of inflammatory and infectious disorders such as Reye's syndrome or meningitis, or as a result of hyperthermia, carbon dioxide retention, or intravascular congestion.

Drug Therapy

The CSF can be a route of administration for medications such as chemotherapeutic agents and antibiotics. Treatment of lymphoma and leukemia often involves intrathecal injections of various agents, which may be infused through a lumbar route or an intraventricular injection via an implanted reservoir. Meningeal carcinomatosis is treated by intrathecal chemotherapy (e.g., methotrexate). Serial injections of small amounts are performed in an attempt to minimize neurotoxicity, and the use of a ventricular reservoir may be less traumatic for the patient than that of multiple lumbar punctures. Treatment of meningitis and ventriculitis may include intrathecal antibiotics in addition to systemic therapy. Careful dosage and administration are recommended, especially if the ventricular route is used, as many antibiotics can cause seizures or an inflammatory ventriculitis when given intrathecally.

TECHNIQUES OF CEREBROSPINAL FLUID ACCESS

There are several techniques for CSF aspiration. All procedures should be performed using sterile technique (including sterile gloves and a mask), and the skin is prepared with antiseptic solution and draped with sterile towels.

Lumbar Puncture

Lumbar puncture is a common procedure that is readily performed by the general practitioner at the bedside and can be performed in any hospital or outpatient setting where commercially prepared lumbar puncture trays are available. In patients with advanced spinal degeneration, extensive previous lumbar surgery for congenital defects and the assistance of a radiologist for needle placement using fluoroscopy or ultrasonography may be required. Contraindications to lumbar puncture include skin infection at the entry site, anticoagulation or blood dyscrasias, papilledema in the presence of supratentorial masses, posterior fossa lesions, and known spinal subarachnoid block or spinal cord arteriovenous malformations.

In adults, CSF aspirations are adequately performed under local anesthesia using 1% lidocaine without premedication. In the pediatric population, however, sedation is often required and allows for a smoother procedure. This is also true in the case of anxious, confused, or combative adult patients.

Oral or rectal chloral hydrate may be used in small children, and moderate sedation using intravenous midazolam and fentanyl or dexmedetomidine can be highly successful in appropriately monitored adults and children when performed in a monitored setting by an experienced individual. The application of a topical anesthetic, such as EMLA cream (2.5% lidocaine and 2.5% prilocaine), preceding injection can also be useful. Conversely, it has been demonstrated in a controlled clinical trial that in the neonatal population, injection of a local anesthetic for lumbar puncture is probably not required and does not reduce perceived stress or discomfort [22].

Figures 17.1 and 17.2 depict some of the steps for lumbar puncture. The patient is placed in the lateral knee-chest position or with the patient sitting leaning forward over a bedside table. The sitting position may be preferred for obese patients in whom adipose tissue can obscure the midline or in elderly patients with significant lumbar degenerative disease. Following a time-out (correct patient, procedure, site, and equipment), the local anesthetic is injected subcutaneously using a 25- or 27-gauge needle. A 1.5-in. needle is then inserted through the skin wheal and additional local anesthetic is injected along the midline, thus anesthetizing the interspinous ligaments and muscles. This small anesthetic volume is usually adequate; however, a more extensive field block is accomplished by additional injections on each side of the interspinous space near the lamina [23].

The point of skin entry is midline at the level of the superior iliac crests, which is usually between the spinous processes of L3 to L4. Lower needle placement at L4 to L5 or L5 to S1 is required in children and neonates to avoid injury to the conus medullaris, which lies more caudal than in adults. The needle is advanced with the stylet or obturator in place to maintain needle patency and prevent iatrogenic intraspinal epidermoid tumors. The bevel of the needle should be parallel to the longitudinal fibers of the dura and spinal column. The needle should be oriented rostrally at an angle of about 30 degrees to the skin and virtually aimed toward the umbilicus. When properly oriented, the needle passes through the following structures before entering the subarachnoid space: skin, superficial fascia, supraspinous ligament, interspinous ligament, ligamentum flavum, epidural space with its fatty areolar tissue and internal vertebral plexus, dura, and arachnoid membrane (Fig. 17.3). The total depth varies from less than 1 in. in the very young patient to as deep as 4 in. in the obese adult. The kinesthetic sensations of passing through the ligaments into the epidural

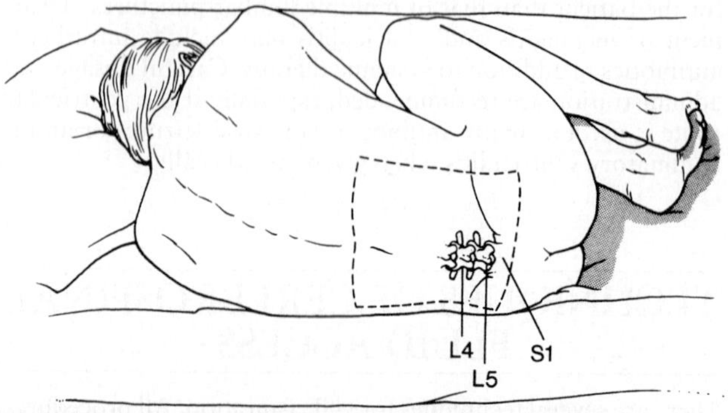

FIGURE 17.1. Patient in the lateral decubitus position with back on the edge of the bed and knees, hips, back, and neck flexed. [From Davidson RI: Lumbar puncture, in VanderSalm TJ (ed): *Atlas of Bedside Procedures.* 2nd ed. Boston, Little, Brown, 1988, with permission.]

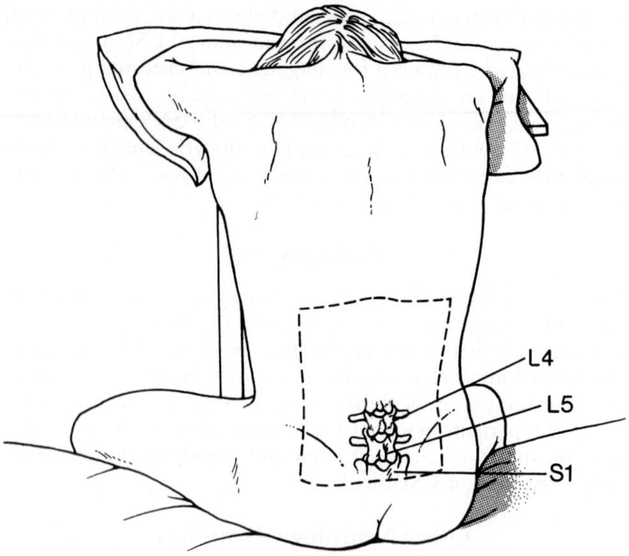

FIGURE 17.2. Patient sitting on the edge of the bed leaning on bedside stand. [From Davidson RI: Lumbar puncture, in VanderSalm TJ (ed): *Atlas of Bedside Procedures.* 2nd ed. Boston, Little, Brown, 1988, with permission.]

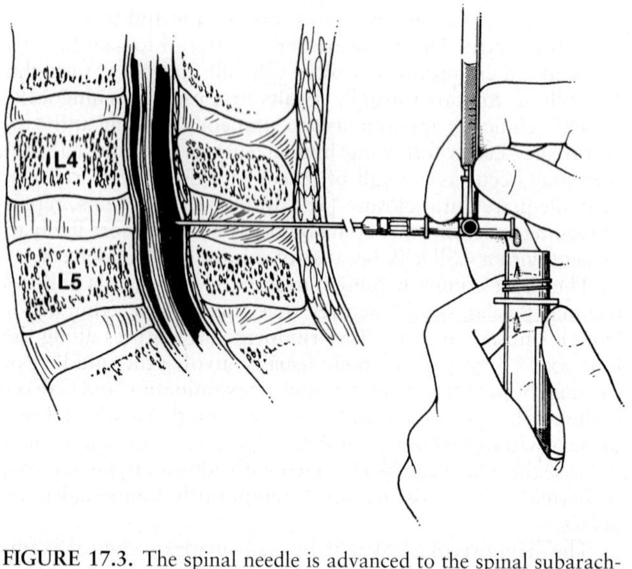

FIGURE 17.3. The spinal needle is advanced to the spinal subarachnoid space and cerebrospinal fluid samples collected after opening pressure is measured. [From Davidson RI: Lumbar puncture, in VanderSalm TJ (ed): *Atlas of Bedside Procedures.* 2nd ed. Boston, Little, Brown, 1988, with permission.]

space followed by dural puncture are quite consistent and recognized with practice. Once intradural, the bevel of the needle is redirected in a cephalad direction in order to improve CSF flow. A spinal needle no smaller than 22 gauge should be used for pressure measurement. The opening pressure is best measured with the patient's legs relaxed and extended partly from the knee-chest position. Pressure measurements may be difficult in children and may be estimated using CSF flow rate [24].

Once CSF is collected, the closing pressure is measured prior to needle withdrawal. It is best to replace the stylet in the needle prior to exiting the subarachnoid space. CSF pressure measurements are not accurate if performed in the sitting position due to the hydrostatic pressure of the CSF column above the entry point or if a significant amount of CSF was lost when the stylet is first withdrawn. If necessary, the pressure could be measured by reclining the patient to the lateral position once entry in the CSF space has been secured.

Although a lumbar puncture is typically safe, there are a number of potential complications and risks involved. Hemorrhage is uncommon but can be seen in association with bleeding disorders and anticoagulation therapy. Spinal SAH has been reported in such conditions, resulting in blockage of CSF outflow with subsequent back and radicular pain, sphincter disturbances, and even paraparesis [25]. Spinal subdural hematoma is likewise very infrequent, but it is associated with significant morbidity that may require prompt surgical intervention. Infection by introduction of the patient's skin flora or the operator's mouth or nose flora into the subarachnoid spaces, causing meningitis, is uncommon and preventable if aseptic techniques (including mask) are used. Risks of infection are increased in serial taps or placement of lumbar catheters for the treatment of CSF fistulas.

Postural headache is the most common complication following lumbar puncture. Its reported frequency varies from 1% to 70% [26]. It is thought to be due to excessive leakage of CSF into the paraspinous spaces, resulting in intracranial hypotension with stretching and expansion of the pain-sensitive intracerebral veins. MRI has demonstrated a reduced CSF volume following lumbar puncture, but with no significant brain displacement and no correlation with headache [27]. Psychologic factors and previous history of headaches seem to strongly influence the patient's risk of and tolerance to headache [28]. A smaller needle size, parallel orientation to the dural fibers, a paramedian approach, and stylet reinsertion prior to withdrawal of the spinal needle have also been reported to decrease the risk of headache after lumbar puncture [29].

The choice of needle type has been the subject of literature debate. Several needle tip designs are available, including the traditional Quincke needle with a beveled cutting tip, the Sprotte needle with a pencil point and side hole, and the Whitacre needle, which is similar to the Sprotte needle but with a smaller side hole. The use of an atraumatic needle seems to be adequate for the performance of a diagnostic lumbar puncture and is probably associated with a lower risk of a postpuncture headache [30,31].

Postdural puncture headache typically develops within 72 hours and lasts 3 to 5 days. Conservative treatment consists of bed rest, hydration, and analgesics. Non-phenothiazine antiemetics are administered if the headache is associated with nausea. If the symptoms are more severe, methylxanthines (caffeine or theophylline) are prescribed orally or parenterally. These agents are successful in up to 85% of patients [32]. Several other pharmacologic agents are discussed in the literature, but none seems to be as effective as caffeine. If the headache persists or is unaffected, an epidural blood patch is then recommended because it is one of the most effective treatments for this condition [33]. Epidural injection of other agents, such as saline, dextran, or adenocorticotropic hormone, has also been described and may be valuable under certain conditions (e.g., sepsis or acquired immunodeficiency syndrome) [34].

An uncommon sequela of lumbar puncture or continuous CSF drainage is hearing loss. Drainage decreases ICP, which is transmitted to the perilymph via the cochlear aqueduct and can cause hearing impairment [35]. The rate of occurrence of this complication is reported to be 0.4%, but is probably higher because it goes unrecognized and seems reversible. There are a few documented cases of irreversible hearing loss [36].

Transient sixth-nerve palsy has also been reported, probably due to nerve traction following significant CSF removal. Neurovascular injury can occur uncommonly in the setting of a subarachnoid block due to spinal tumors. In this situation, CSF drainage leads to significant traction and spinal coning with subsequent neurologic impairment [37,38].

Lateral Cervical (C1–2) Puncture

The C1–2 or lateral cervical puncture was originally developed for percutaneous cordotomy. It may be used for myelography or aspiration of CSF if the lumbar route is inaccessible. It is most safely performed with fluoroscopic guidance with the patient supine, the head and neck flexed, and the lateral neck draped. The skin entry point is 1 cm caudal and 1 cm dorsal to the tip of the mastoid process. The site is infiltrated with a local anesthetic, and the spinal needle is introduced and directed toward the junction of the middle and posterior thirds of the bony canal to avoid an anomalous vertebral or posterior inferior cerebellar artery that may lie in the anterior half of the canal. The stylet should be removed frequently to check for CSF egress. When the procedure is performed under fluoroscopy, the needle is seen to be perpendicular to the neck and just under the posterior ring of C1. The same sensation is recognized when piercing the dura as in a lumbar puncture and the bevel is then directed cephalad in a similar fashion. Complications of the lateral cervical puncture include injury to the spinal cord or the vertebral artery and irritation of a nerve root, causing local pain and headache.

Cisternal Puncture

A cisternal puncture provides CSF access via the cisterna magna when other routes are not possible. A preoperative lateral skull radiograph is performed to ensure normal anatomy. The patient is positioned sitting with the head slightly flexed. The hair is removed in the occipital region and the area prepared, draped, and infiltrated with lidocaine. The entry point is in the midline between the external occipital protuberance in the upper margin of the spinous process of C2 or via an imaginary line through both external auditory meati. The spinal needle is directed through a slightly cephalad course and usually strikes the occipital bone. It is then redirected more caudally in a stepwise fashion until it passes through the atlanto-occipital membrane and dura, producing a "popping" sensation. The cisterna magna usually lies 4 to 6 cm deep to the skin; the needle should not be introduced beyond 7.0 to 7.5 cm from the skin to prevent injury to the medulla or the vertebral arteries. The procedure can be performed relatively safely in a cooperative patient as the cisterna magna is a large CSF space; however, it is rarely practiced due to the greater potential morbidity.

Aspiration of Reservoirs and Shunts

An implanted reservoir or shunt system should not be accessed without prior consultation with a neurosurgeon, despite the apparent simplicity of the procedure itself. Violating implanted systems carries several risks, including infection, which can result in a lengthy hospitalization, prolonged antibiotic course,

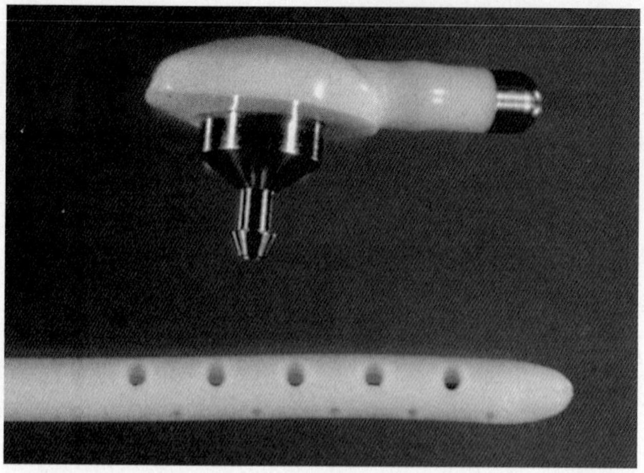

FIGURE 17.4. Close-up view of ventricular reservoir in the calvarial burr hole, the funneled base connected directly to the proximal end of the ventricular catheter. The distal perforated end is shown.

and several operative procedures for shunt externalization, hardware removal, and insertion of a new shunt system.

Subcutaneous reservoirs in ventriculoatrial or ventriculoperitoneal shunting systems are located proximal to the unidirectional valve and can be accessed percutaneously. The reservoirs are usually button-sized, measuring approximately 7 to 10 mm in diameter and 2 mm in height. They can be located in the burr hole directly connected to the ventricular catheter (Fig. 17.4) or as an integral part of the valve system (Fig. 17.5). Indications for reservoir taps have been previously discussed.

The procedure can be performed in any hospital or outpatient setting. Gloves, mask, antiseptic solution, razor, sterile drapes, 23- or 25-gauge needle (short hub or butterfly), tuberculin syringe, and sterile collection tubes are readied. The patient can be in any comfortable position that allows access to the reservoir. Sedation may be required for toddlers, but is otherwise unnecessary. Reference to a skull radiograph may be helpful in localization. The reservoir is palpated, overlying hair is removed preferably with a clipper rather than a razor and the skin cleansed. Local anesthesia is usually not required and the use of topical anesthetic creams is occasionally considered. The needle is inserted perpendicular to the skin and into the reservoir, to a total depth of 3 to 5 mm. A manometer is then connected to the needle or butterfly tubing for pressure measurement. CSF collection is performed and drug injection is performed only if CSF flow is demonstrated. A "dry tap" usually indicates faulty placement or catheter obstruction. Occasionally, an old reservoir may have retracted into the burr hole and not be palpable or may be too calcified for needle penetration and some older shunting systems may not even have a reservoir. Risks and complications of shunt aspiration include improper insertion, contamination with skin flora, introduction of blood in the shunt system, and choroid plexus hemorrhage due to vigorous aspiration.

Lumboperitoneal Shunt

Lumboperitoneal shunts are placed via percutaneous insertion of a lumbar subarachnoid catheter or through a small skin incision. They are tunneled subcutaneously around the patient's flank to the abdomen, where the distal catheter enters the peritoneal cavity through a separate abdominal incision. A reservoir or valve or both may be used and are located on the lateral aspect of the flank. Careful palpation between the two incisions usually reveals the tubing path and reservoir placement in the nonobese patient. The patient is placed in lateral decubitus position and a pillow under the dependent flank may be of assistance. The same technique as described for a ventricular shunt is then performed. Fluid aspiration should be particularly gentle as an additional risk of this procedure is nerve root irritation.

Ventricular Reservoirs

Ventricular reservoirs are inserted as part of a blind system consisting of a catheter located in a CSF space, usually the lateral ventricle, and without distal runoff. Such systems are placed for CSF access purposes only, such as for instillation of antibiotics or chemotherapeutic agents, or CSF aspiration for treatment and monitoring. Ommaya reservoirs are dome-shaped structures (Fig. 17.6) with a diameter of 1 to 2 cm and have a connecting port placed at their base or side. They are placed subcutaneously and attached to a ventricular

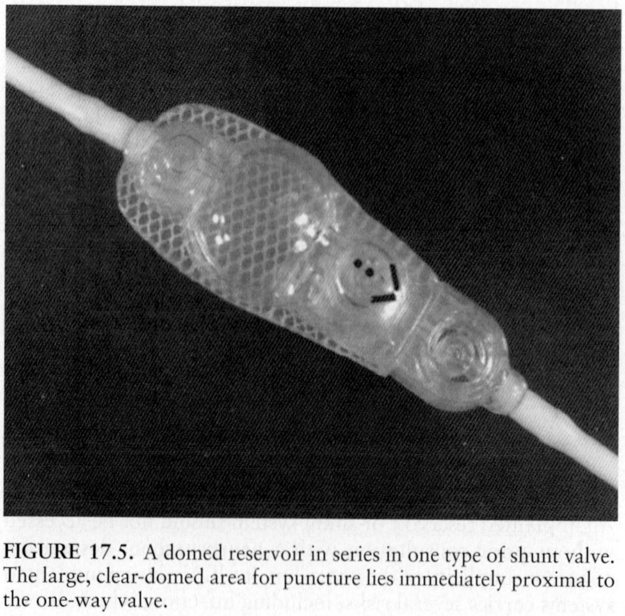

FIGURE 17.5. A domed reservoir in series in one type of shunt valve. The large, clear-domed area for puncture lies immediately proximal to the one-way valve.

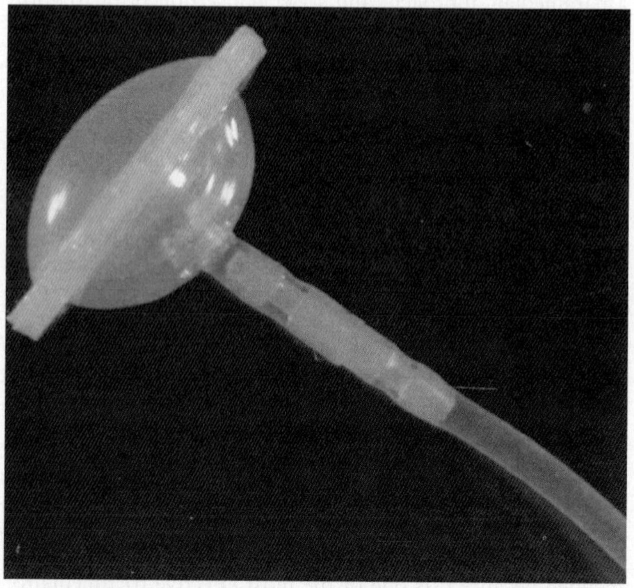

FIGURE 17.6. Close-up view of a ventricular (Ommaya) double-domed reservoir, the caudal half of which is designed to lie within the burr hole.

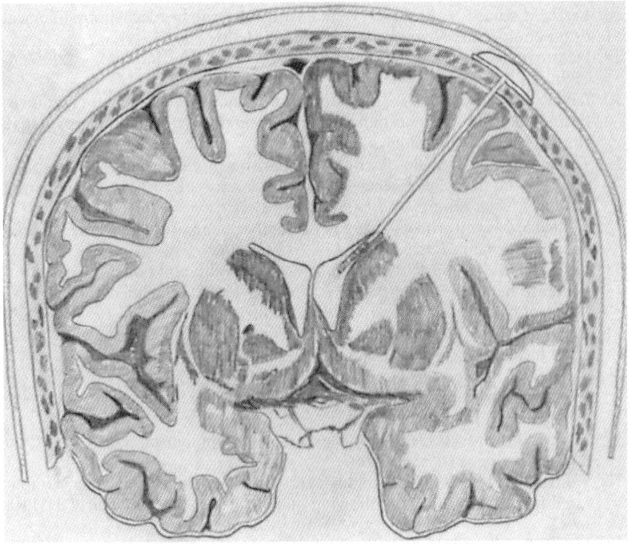

FIGURE 17.7. Coronal section through the brain at the level of the frontal horns, illustrating the subgaleal/epicalvarial location at the reservoir, with the distal perforated part of the catheter lying within the ventricle.

subarachnoid catheter (Fig. 17.7). Aspiration technique is essentially the same as from a shunt reservoir; however, the Ommaya reservoir is often larger and differs in shape from many shunt reservoirs. It is accessed, preferably, with a 25-gauge needle or butterfly. CSF is allowed to flow by gravity if possible; a volume equal to that to be instilled is removed and held for analysis or reinjection. The antibiotic or chemotherapeutic agent is injected; 1 mL of CSF or sterile saline can be used to flush the dose into the ventricle, or gentle barbotage of the reservoir may be performed to achieve the same goal. Risks and complications are essentially the same as in shunt aspirations (i.e., infection, bleeding, and improper insertion), with the addition of chemical ventriculitis or arachnoiditis.

Ventriculostomy

A ventriculostomy is a catheter placed in the lateral ventricle for CSF drainage or ICP monitoring and treatment. It is performed by a neurosurgeon in the operating room or at the bedside in the intensive care unit or emergency department. It is usually performed through the nondominant hemisphere and into the frontal horn of the lateral ventricle. An alternate approach is to cannulate the occipital horn or trigone through an occipital entry point located 6 cm superior to the inion and 4 cm from the midline. Premedication is not necessary unless the patient is very anxious or combative. Radiographic guidance is typically not required unless the procedure is being performed stereotactically. CT or MRI stereotaxy is needed if the ventricles are very small, as in diffuse brain swelling or slit ventricle syndrome. Complications of ventriculostomy placement include meningitis or ventriculitis, scalp wound infection, intracranial hematoma or cortical injury, and failure to cannulate the ventricle.

Lumbar Drainage

Continuous CSF drainage via a lumbar catheter is useful in the treatment of CSF fistulas and as a provocative test to demonstrate the potential effects of shunting in normal-pressure hydrocephalus or ventriculomegaly of various etiologies. Commercially available lumbar drainage kits are closed sterile systems that drain into a replaceable collection bag. Catheter placement is performed just as in lumbar puncture; however, a large-bore Tuohy needle is used, through which the catheter is threaded once CSF return has been confirmed. Needle orientation follows the same guidelines as discussed for a lumbar puncture and is even more important in the case of this large-gauge needle. Epidural catheter kits could also be used, although the catheters tend to be slightly stiffer and have a narrower diameter. Complications include hemorrhage in the epidural or subarachnoid space, infection, inability to aspirate CSF, CSF leak, nerve root irritation, and, most ominously, a supratentorial subdural hematoma secondary to overdrainage. This complication tends to be more common in elderly individuals. The potential for overdrainage is significant because of the large diameter of the catheter and because the amount of drainage depends on the cooperation of the patient and the nursing staff.

SUMMARY

Of the various techniques available for CSF access, lumbar puncture is the procedure most commonly and safely performed by the general practitioner. Other techniques are described that may require the assistance of a radiologist, neurologist, anesthesiologist, or neurosurgeon.

References

1. Hollman GA, Schultz MM, Eickhoff JC, et al: Propofol-fentanyl versus propofol alone for lumbar puncture sedation in children with acute hematologic malignancies: propofol dosing and adverse events. *Pediatr Crit Care Med* 9:616, 2007.
2. Dilli D, Dallar Y, Sorguç N: Comparison of ketamine plus midazolam versus ketamine for sedation in children during lumbar puncture. *Clin J Pain* 25:349, 2009.
3. Wood J: Cerebrospinal fluid: techniques of access and analytical interpretation, in Wilkins R, Rengachary S (eds): *Neurosurgery*. 2nd ed. New York, McGraw-Hill, 1996, p 165.
4. Beck J, Raabe A, Szelenyi, et al: Sentinel headache and the risk of rebleeding after aneurysmal subarachnoid hemorrhage. *Stroke* 27:2733, 2006.
5. Leblanc R: The minor leak preceding subarachnoid hemorrhage. *J Neurosurg* 66:35, 1981.
6. D'Arminio-Monteforte A, Cinque P, Vago L, et al: A comparison of brain biopsy and CSF PCR in the diagnosis of CNS lesions in AIDS patients. *J Neurol* 244:35, 1997.
7. Fitch M, van de Beek D: Emergency diagnosis and treatment of adult meningitis. *Lancet Infect Dis* 7:191, 2007.
8. Albeck MJ, Borgesen SE, Gjerris F, et al: Intracranial pressure and cerebrospinal fluid outflow conductance I healthy subjects. *J Neurosurg* 74:597, 1991.
9. Lundar T, Nornes H: Determination of ventricular fluid outflow resistance in patients with ventriculomegaly. *J Neurol Neurosurg Psychiatry* 53:896, 1990.
10. Walchenback R, Geiger E, Thomeer R, et al: The value of temporary external lumbar CSF drainage in predicting the outcome of shunting on normal pressure hydrocephalus. *J Neurol Neurosurg Psychiatry* 72:503, 2002.
11. Ball AK, Clarke CE: Idiopathic intracranial hypertension. *Lancet Neurol* 5:433, 2006.
12. Johnston I, Hawke S, Halmagyi J, et al: The pseudotumor syndrome: disorders of cerebrospinal fluid circulation causing intracranial hypertension without ventriculomegaly. *Arch Neurol* 48:740, 1991.
13. Fischer L, Jahnke K, Martus P, et al: The diagnostic value of cerebrospinal fluid pleocytosis and protein in the detection of lymphomatous meningitis in primary central nervous system lymphomas. *Haematologica* 91:429, 2006.
14. Bigner SH, Johnston WWW: The cytopathology of cerebrospinal fluid, I. Non-neoplastic condition, lymphoma and leukemia. *Acta Cytol* 25:335, 1981.
15. Fishman RA: *Cerebrospinal Fluid in Diseases of the Nervous System*. 2nd ed. Philadelphia, WB Saunders, 1992.
16. Link H, Huang Y: Oligoclonal bands in multiple sclerosis cerebrospinal fluid: an update on methodology and clinical usefulness. *J Neuroimmunol* 180:17, 2006.

17. Fagan AM, Roe CM, Xiong C, et al: Cerebrospinal fluid tau/β-amyloid 42 ratio as a prediction of cognitive decline in nondemented older adults. *Arch Neurol* 64:343, 2007.
18. Agrillo U, Simonetti G, Martino V: Postoperative CSF problems after spinal and lumbar surgery: general review. *J Neurosurg Sci* 35:93, 1991.
19. Nandapalan V, Watson ID, Swift AC: β_2-Transferrin and CSF rhinorrhea. *Clin Otolaryngol* 21:259, 1996.
20. Lyons MK, Meyer FB: Cerebrospinal fluid physiology and the management of increased intracranial pressure. *Mayo Clin Proc* 65:684, 1990.
21. American Association of Neurological Surgeons, Congress of Neurological Surgeons, Joint Section on Neurotrauma and Critical Care: guidelines for the management of severe traumatic brain injury. 3rd edition. *J Neurotrauma* 24:S1, 2007.
22. Porter FL, Miller JP, Cole FS, et al: A controlled clinical trial of local anesthesia for lumbar punctures in newborns [see comments]. *Pediatrics* 88:663, 1991.
23. Wilkinson HA: Technical note: anesthesia for lumbar puncture. *JAMA* 249:2177, 1983.
24. Ellis RW III, Strauss LC, Wiley JM, et al: A simple method of estimating cerebrospinal fluid pressure during lumbar puncture. *Pediatrics* 89:895, 1992.
25. Scott EW, Cazenave CR, Virapongse C: Spinal subarachnoid hematoma complicating lumbar puncture: diagnosis and management. *Neurosurgery* 25:287, 1989.
26. Strupp M, Brandt T: Should one reinsert the stylet during lumbar puncture? *N Engl J Med* 336:1190, 1997.
27. Grant F, Condon B, Hart I, et al: Changes in intracranial CSF volume after lumbar puncture and their relationship to post-LP headache. *J Neurol Neurosurg Psychiatry* 54:440, 1991.
28. Lee T, Maynard N, Anslow P, et al: Post-myelogram headache: physiological or psychological? *Neuroradiology* 33:155, 1991.
29. Peterman S: Post myelography headache: a review. *Radiology* 200:765, 1996.
30. Lavi R, Rowe JM, Avivi I: Traumatic vs. atraumatic 22 G needle for therapeutic and diagnostic lumbar puncture in the hematologic patient: a prospective clinical trial. *Haematologica* 92:1007, 2007.
31. Torbati S, Katz D, Silka P, et al: Comparison of blunt versus sharp spinal needles used in the emergency department in rates of post-lumbar puncture headache. *Ann Emerg Med* 54:S73, 2009.
32. Ahmed SV, Jayawarna C, Jude E: Post lumbar puncture headache: diagnosis and management. *Postgrad Med J* 82:713, 2006.
33. van Kooten F, Oedit R, Bakker S, et al: Epidural blood patch in post dural puncture headache: a randomized, observer-blind, controlled clinical trial. *J Neurol Neurosurg Psychiatry* 79:553, 2007.
34. Choi A, Laurito CE, Cunningham FE: Pharmacologic management of post-dural headache. *Ann Pharmacother* 30:831, 1996.
35. Walsted A, Salomon G, Thomsen J: Hearing decrease after loss of cerebrospinal fluid: a new hydrops model? *Acta Otolaryngol* 111:468, 1991.
36. Michel O, Brusis T: Hearing loss as a sequel of lumbar puncture. *Ann Otol Rhinol Laryngol* 101:390, 1992.
37. Wong MC, Krol G, Rosenblum MK: Occult epidural chloroma complicated by acute paraplegia following lumbar puncture. *Ann Neurol* 31:110, 1992.
38. Mutoh S, Aikou I, Ueda S: Spinal coning after lumbar puncture in prostate cancer with asymptomatic vertebral metastasis: a case report. *J Urol* 145:834, 1991.

CHAPTER 18 ■ PERCUTANEOUS SUPRAPUBIC CYSTOSTOMY

SATYA ALLAPARTHI, K.C. BALAJI AND PHILIP J. AYVAZIAN

Percutaneous suprapubic cystostomy was described four centuries ago; safety of the procedure was first demonstrated by Garson and Peterson in 1888. The first modern method was the Campbell trocar set, described in 1951 [1]. It is used to divert urine from the bladder when standard urethral catheterization is impossible or undesirable [2]. In emergency situations, the majority of these patients are men with urethral stricture or complex prostatic disease or patients with trauma with urethral disruption. Complete urethral transection associated with a pelvic fracture is an absolute indication for emergent suprapubic cystostomy. The procedure for placement of a small-diameter catheter is rapid, safe, and easily accomplished at the bedside under local anesthesia. This chapter first addresses methods for urethral catheterization before discussing the percutaneous approach.

URETHRAL CATHETERIZATION

Urethral catheterization remains the principal method for bladder drainage. The indications for the catheter should be clarified because they influence the type and size of catheter to be used [3]. A history and physical examination with particular attention to the patient's genitourinary system are important.

Catheterization may be difficult with male patients in several instances. Patients with lower urinary tract symptoms (e.g., urinary urgency, frequency, nocturia, decreased stream, and hesitancy) may have benign prostatic hypertrophy. These patients may require a larger bore catheter, such as 20 or 22 French (Fr). When dealing with urethral strictures, a smaller bore catheter should be used, such as 12 or 14 Fr. Patients with a history of prior prostatic surgery such as transurethral resection of the prostate, open prostatectomy, or radical prostatectomy may have an irregular bladder neck as a result of contracture after surgery. The use of a coudé-tip catheter, which has an upper deflected tip, may help in negotiating the altered anatomy after prostate surgery. The presence of a high-riding prostate or blood at the urethral meatus suggests urethral trauma. In this situation, urethral integrity must be demonstrated by retrograde urethrogram before urethral catheterization is attempted.

Urethral catheterization for gross hematuria requires large catheters, such as 22 or 24 Fr, which have larger holes for irrigation and removal of clots. Alternatively, a three-way urethral catheter may be used to provide continuous bladder irrigation to prevent clotting. Large catheters impede excretion of urethral secretions, however, and can lead to urethritis or epididymitis if used for prolonged periods.

Technique

In male patients, after the patient is prepared and draped, 10 mL of a 2% lidocaine hydrochloride jelly is injected retrograde into the urethra. Anesthesia of the urethral mucosa requires 5 to 10 minutes after occluding the urethral meatus either with a penile clamp or manually to prevent loss of the jelly [4]. The balloon of the catheter is tested, and the catheter tip is covered with a water-soluble lubricant. After stretching the penis upward and perpendicular to the body, the catheter is inserted into the urethral meatus. The catheter is advanced up to the hub to ensure its entrance into the bladder. To prevent urethral trauma, the balloon is not inflated until urine is observed draining from the catheter. Irrigation of the catheter with normal saline helps verify the position. A common site of resistance to catheter passage is the external urinary sphincter within the membranous urethra, which may contract voluntarily. Any other resistance may represent a stricture, necessitating urologic consultation. In patients with prior prostate surgery, an assistant's finger placed in the rectum may elevate the urethra and allow the catheter to pass into the bladder.

In female patients, short, straight catheters are preferred. Typically, a smaller amount of local anesthesia is used. Difficulties in catheter placement occur after urethral surgery or vulvectomy, or with vaginal atrophy or morbid obesity. In these cases, the meatus is not visible and may be retracted under the symphysis pubis. Blind catheter placement over a finger located in the vagina at the palpated site of the urethral meatus may be successful.

When urologic consultation is obtained, other techniques for urethral catheterization can be used. Flexible cystoscopy may be performed to ascertain the reason for difficult catheter placement and for insertion of a guidewire. A urethral catheter can then be placed over the guidewire by the Seldinger technique. Filiforms and followers are useful for urethral strictures.

Indications

On occasion, despite proper technique (as outlined previously), urethral catheterization is unsuccessful. These are the instances when percutaneous suprapubic cystotomy is necessary. Undoubtedly, the most common indication for percutaneous suprapubic cystotomy is for the management of acute urinary retention in men. Other indications for a percutaneous suprapubic cystotomy in the intensive care unit are provided in Table 18.1.

Contraindications

The contraindications to percutaneous suprapubic cystotomy are provided in Table 18.2. An inability to palpate the bladder or distortion of the pelvic anatomy from previous surgery or trauma makes percutaneous entry of the bladder difficult. In these situations, the risks of penetrating the peritoneal cavity become substantial. The bladder may not be palpable if the patient is in acute renal failure with oliguria or anuria, has a small contracted neurogenic bladder, or is incontinent. When the bladder is not palpable, it can be filled in a retrograde manner with saline to distend it. In men, a 14-Fr catheter is placed in the fossa navicularis just inside the urethral meatus and the balloon is filled with 2 to 3 mL of sterile water to occlude the urethra. Saline is injected slowly into the catheter until the bladder is palpable and then the suprapubic tube may be placed. In patients with a contracted neurogenic bladder, it is impossible to adequately distend the bladder by this approach. For these patients, ultrasonography is used to locate the bladder and allow the insertion of a 22-gauge spinal needle. Saline is instilled into the bladder via the needle to distend the bladder enough for suprapubic tube placement (Fig. 18.1).

In patients with previous lower abdominal surgery, ultrasonographic guidance is often necessary before a percutaneous cystotomy can be performed safely. Previous surgery can lead to adhesions that can hold a loop of intestine in the area of insertion. Other relative contraindications include patients with coagulopathy, a known history of bladder tumors, or active hematuria and retained clots. In patients with bladder tumors, percutaneous bladder access should be avoided because tumor cell seeding can occur along the percutaneous tract. Suprapubic cystotomy tubes are small in caliber and therefore do not function effectively with severe hematuria and retained clots. Instead, open surgical placement of a large-caliber tube is necessary if urethral catheterization is impossible.

TABLE 18.1

COMMON INDICATIONS FOR PERCUTANEOUS CYSTOTOMY

Unsuccessful urethral catheterization in the setting of acute urinary retention
History of prostate surgery
Presence or suspected urethral trauma
Urethral stricture
Severe hypospadias
Periurethral abscess
Presence of severe urethral, epididymal, or prostate infection

TABLE 18.2

RELATIVE CONTRAINDICATIONS TO PERCUTANEOUS SUPRAPUBIC CYSTOTOMY

Nonpalpable bladder
Previous lower abdominal surgery
Coagulopathy
Known bladder tumor
Clot retention

Technique

There are two general types of percutaneous cystotomy tubes that range in size from 8 to 14 Fr [5,6]. The first type uses an obturator with a preloaded catheter. Examples include the Stamey catheter (Cook Urological, Spencer, IN) and the Bonanno catheter (Beckton Dickinson and Co, Franklin Lakes, NJ) [7]. The Stamey device is a polyethylene Malecot catheter with a luer lock hub that fits over a hollow needle obturator (Fig. 18.2A). When the obturator is locked to the hub of the catheter, the Malecot flanges are pulled inward (closed) and the system is ready for use. The Bonanno catheter uses a flexible 14-Fr Teflon tube, which is inserted over a hollow 18-gauge obturator (Fig. 18.2B). The obturator locks into the catheter hub and extends beyond the catheter tip. When the obturator is withdrawn, the tube pigtails in the bladder. One advantage to the Stamey catheter is that the flanges provide a secure retaining system. The Bonanno catheter generally induces fewer bladder spasms, however, and is better tolerated.

The second type of percutaneous cystotomy tube consists of a trocar and sheath, which are used to penetrate the abdominal wall and bladder [8,9]. One of the most popular systems is the Lawrence suprapubic catheter (Rusch, Duluth, GA). This system allows a standard Foley catheter to be placed after removal of the trocar (Fig. 18.2C).

The patient is placed in the supine position; a towel roll may be placed under the hips to extend the pelvis. Trendelenburg position may help to move the abdominal contents away from the bladder. The bladder is palpated to ensure that it is distended. The suprapubic region is prepared with 2%

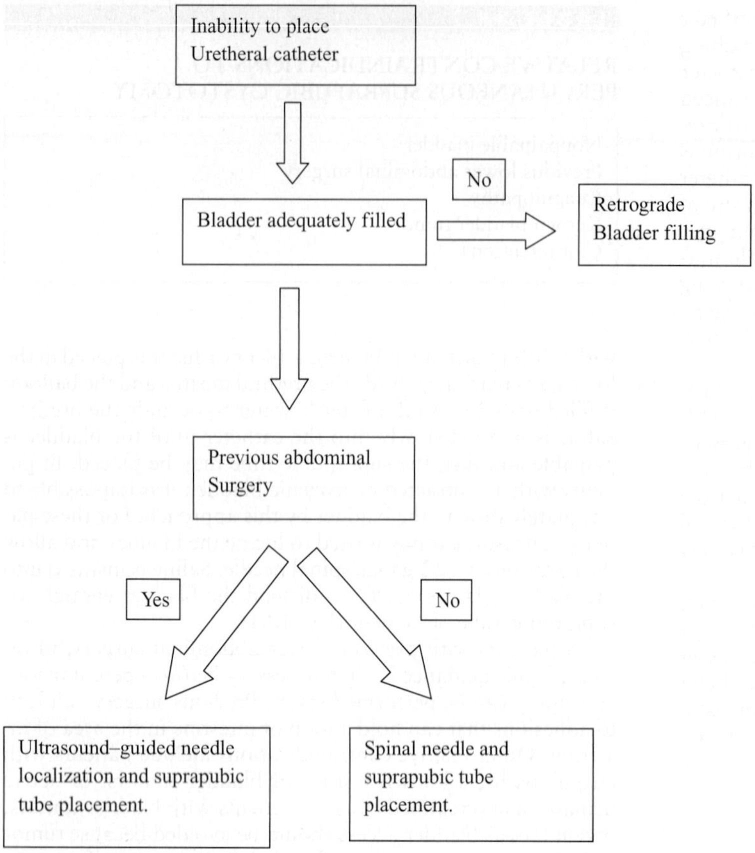

FIGURE 18.1. Algorithm for percutaneous suprapubic tube placement.

chlorhexidine/10% povidone–iodine solution and draped with sterile towels. The insertion site is several centimeters above the symphysis pubis in the midline: this approach avoids the epigastric vessels. In obese patients with a large abdominal fat pad, the fold is elevated. The needle should be introduced into the suprapubic crease, where the fat thickness is minimal. One percent lidocaine is used to anesthetize the skin, subcutaneous tissues, rectus fascia, and retropubic space. A 22-gauge spinal needle with a 5-mL syringe is directed vertically and advanced until urine is aspirated. If the bladder is smaller or the patient had previous pelvic surgery, the needle is directed at a 60-degree caudal angle. Insertion of the cystotomy tube is predicated on the feasibility of bladder puncture and after the angle and depth of insertion are established with the spinal needle (Fig. 18.3).

At the site of bladder puncture, a small 2-mm incision is made with a no. 11 blade. The catheter mounted on the obturator is advanced into the bladder. Two hands are used to grasp the system to provide a forceful, but controlled, thrust through the abdominal wall. One hand can be positioned on the obturator at a site marking the depth of the bladder. A syringe attached to the end of the obturator is used to aspirate urine and confirm obturator placement. Once the bladder is penetrated, the entire system is advanced 2 to 3 cm. This prevents the catheter tip from withdrawing into the retropubic space when the bladder decompresses. After unlocking the obturator from the catheter, the obturator acts as a guide while the catheter is advanced into the bladder. When using a Stamey catheter, the catheter can be gently withdrawn until the Malecot flanges meet resistance against the anterior bladder wall. The Stamey catheter is then advanced 2 cm back into the bladder to allow for movement. This maneuver pulls the catheter away from the bladder trigone and helps reduce bladder spasms.

The same general technique applies to placement of the Lawrence suprapubic catheter system. After the bladder is penetrated, urine appears at the hub of the suprapubic catheter introducer (trocar plus sheath). The trocar is then removed and a Foley catheter is inserted. The Foley catheter balloon is inflated to secure it in the bladder. Pulling the tab at the top of the peel-away sheath allows the remaining portion of the sheath to be removed away from the catheter.

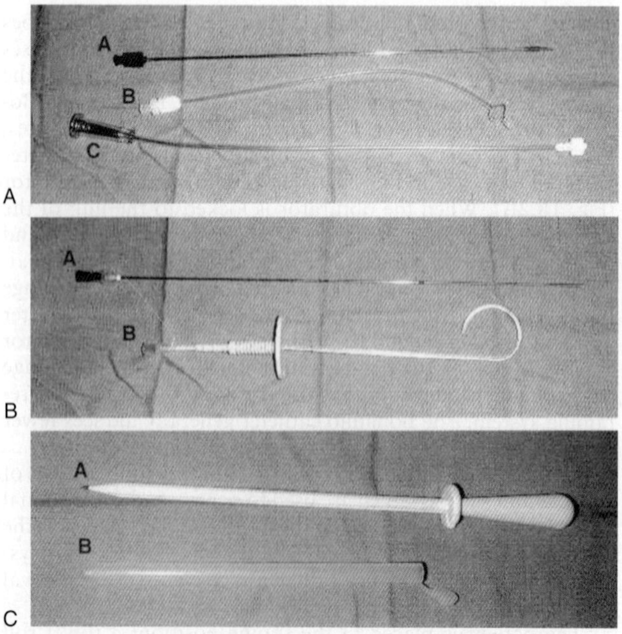

FIGURE 18.2. A: Stamey suprapubic cystostomy trocar set (A is the obturator, B is the Malecot catheter, and C is the drainage tube). **B:** Bonanno catheter set (A is the obturator and B is the catheter). **C:** Lawrence suprapubic catheter (A is the trocar and B is the sheath).

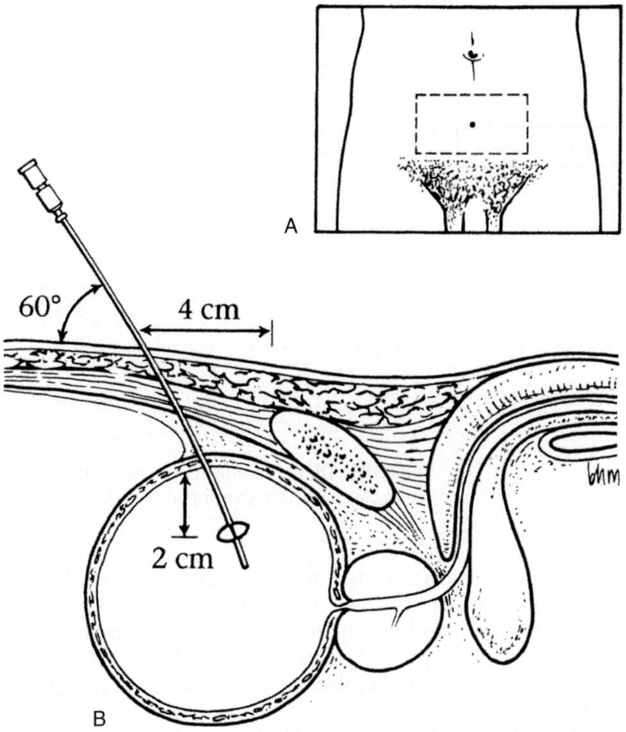

FIGURE 18.3. Technique of suprapubic trocar placement. **A:** Area to be shaved, prepared, and draped before trocar placement. **B:** Position of the Stamey trocar in the bladder. The angle, distance from the pubis, and position of the catheter in relation to the bladder wall are demonstrated.

The patency of the catheter is assessed by irrigating the bladder after decompression. The catheter can be fixed with a simple nylon suture and sterile dressing. The Bonanno catheter contains a suture disk. The Lawrence suprapubic catheter does not require extra fixation because the balloon on the Foley catheter secures it in place.

IMAGE-GUIDED PERCUTANEOUS SUPRAPUBIC CYSTOSTOMY

Ultrasound provides physicians with a twofold increase in success rates for suprapubic bladder needle aspiration and was sensitive in evaluating and confirming bladder distention [10]. It is readily available, can be performed at the bedside, is easy to perform, and poses no additional risk to the patient [11,12]. Ultrasound visualization of a full bladder is easy to learn and provides a well-defined image of the bladder (Fig. 18.4). The bladder is located beneath the abdominal muscles in the lower midline position, anterior to the uterus in females. A full bladder is easy to visualize as a midline symmetrical hypoechoic image under the abdominal rectus muscles in the suprapubic abdominal region. The bladder is best visualized when it is distended, using 3.5-, 5.0-, or 7.5-MHz transducer probes on transabdominal transverse and longitudinal axial planes. Ultrasound can establish the presence of fluid in and surrounding the bladder, as well as provide dimensions of depth and size of the bladder itself. Tenting of the bladder wall can be seen by ultrasound as the needle pushes against the bladder before penetration occurs and the catheter can be seen within the bladder once the cystostomy tube placement has been performed.

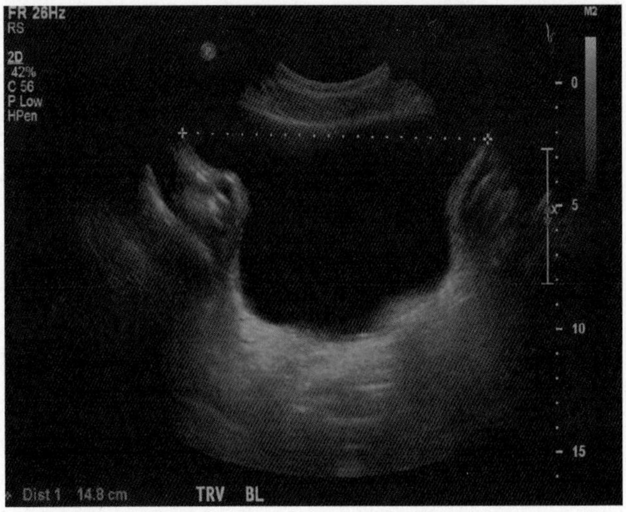

FIGURE 18.4. Ultrasound image of full bladder.

SUPRAPUBIC CATHETER CARE

Bladder spasms occur commonly after suprapubic catheter placement. When using a Stamey catheter or a Foley catheter, bladder spasms can be prevented by withdrawing the tube until it meets the anterior bladder wall and then advancing 2 cm back into the bladder. Persistent bladder spasms can be treated with anticholinergic therapy (e.g., oxybutynin and hyoscyamine). This medication should be discontinued before removing the suprapubic tube to prevent urinary retention.

A suprapubic tube that ceases to drain is usually caused by kinking of the catheter or displacement of the catheter tip into the retropubic space. If necessary, suprapubic catheters may be replaced either by using an exchange set (available for Stamey catheters) or by dilating the cystotomy tract. Closure of the percutaneous cystotomy tract is generally prompt after the tube is removed. Prolonged suprapubic tube use can lead to a mature tract, which may take several days to close. If the tract remains open, bladder decompression via a urethral catheter may be required.

COMPLICATIONS

Placement of suprapubic cystotomy tubes is generally safe with infrequent complications. Possible complications are provided in Table 18.3 [13]. Bowel complications are severe, but rare, with this procedure [14]. Penetration of the peritoneal cavity or bowel perforation produces peritoneal or intestinal symptoms and signs. This complication may be avoided by attempting the procedure on well-distended bladders, using a midline

TABLE 18.3

COMPLICATIONS OF PERCUTANEOUS CYSTOTOMY

Peritoneal and bowel perforation
Hematuria
Retained or calcified catheter
Bladder stones
Postobstructive diuresis
Hypotension
Bladder perforation and infection of space of Retzius

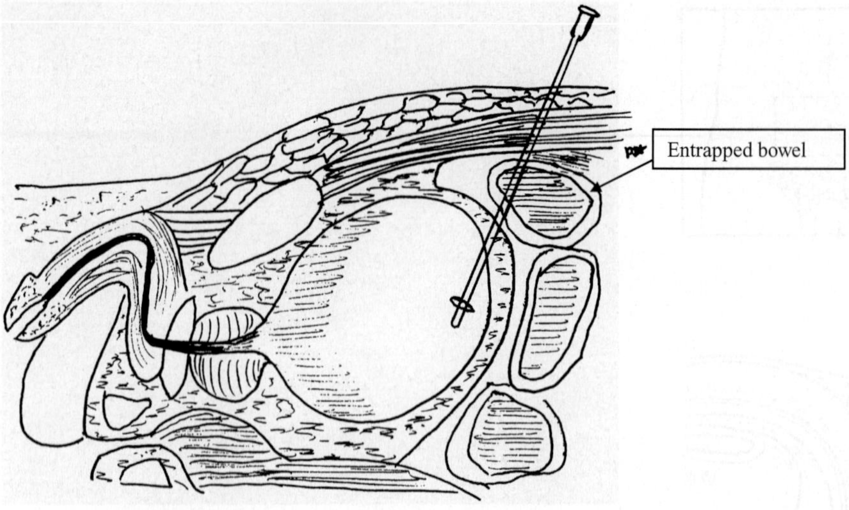

FIGURE 18.5. Placement of the suprapubic tube can perforate entrapped bowel.

approach no more than 4 cm above the pubis or under image guidance.

In patients who have had previous lower abdominal or pelvic surgery, an ultrasound may be used to properly place the suprapubic tube and rule out entrapped bowel (Fig. 18.5). Patients who develop peritoneal symptoms and signs require a full evaluation of the location of not only the suprapubic tube (by a cystogram) but also the cystotomy tract. A kidney–ureter–bladder radiograph and computed tomography scans may be helpful.

Hematuria is the most common complication after suprapubic tube placement. Rarely, this requires open cystotomy for placement of a large-caliber tube for irrigation. Hematuria can result secondary to laceration of blood vessels or rapid decompression of a chronically distended bladder, and the risk of hematuria may be reduced by gradual bladder decompression. Another risk with decompression of chronically distend bladder is postobstructive diuresis.

Complications associated with the catheter include loss of a portion of the catheter in the bladder, calcification of the catheter, or bladder stone formation. These complications may be avoided by preventing prolonged catheter use. Beyond 4 weeks, evaluation and replacement or removal of catheter is advisable.

When chronically distended bladders are decompressed, patients are at risk for postobstructive diuresis [15]. Patients who are at greatest risk include those with azotemia, peripheral edema, congestive heart failure, and mental status changes. Patients with postobstructive diuresis (i.e., urine outputs >200 mL per hour) require frequent monitoring of vital signs and intravenous fluid replacement.

Hypotension rarely occurs after suprapubic tube placement. It may be caused by a vasovagal response or bleeding, alleviated by fluid administration. Another rare, but possible, complication is a through-and-through bladder perforation that is treated conservatively with bladder decompression.

References

1. Hodgkinson CP, Hodari AA: Trocar suprapubic cystostomy for postoperative bladder drainage in the female. *Am J Obstet Gynecol* 96(6):773–783, 1966.
2. Wein AJ, Kavoussi LR, Novick AC, et al: *Campbell-Walsh Urology Ninth Edition Review*. Philadelphia, PA, Saunders/Elsevier, 2007.
3. Brosnahan J, Jull A, Tracy C: Types of urethral catheters for management of short-term voiding problems in hospitalised adults. *Cochrane Database Syst Rev* (1):Cd004013, 2004.
4. Siderias J, Guadio F, Singer AJ: Comparison of topical anesthetics and lubricants prior to urethral catheterization in males: a randomized controlled trial. *Acad Emerg Med* 11(6):703–706, 2004.
5. Irby Iii P, Stoller M: Percutaneous suprapubic cystostomy. *J Endourol* 7(2):125–130, 1993.
6. Lawrentschuk N, Lee D, Marriott P, et al: Suprapubic stab cystostomy: a safer technique. *Urology* 62(5):932–934, 2003.
7. Bonanno PJ, Landers DE, Rock DE: Bladder drainage with the suprapubic catheter needle. *Obstet Gynecol* 35(5):807–812, 1970.
8. O'brien WM, Pahira JJ: Percutaneous placement of suprapubic tube using peel-away sheath introducer. *Urology* 31(6):524–525, 1988.
9. Chiou RK, Morton JJ, Engelsgjerd JS, et al: Placement of large suprapubic tube using peel-away introducer. *J Urol* 153(4):1179–1181, 1995.
10. Munir V, Barnett P, South M: Does the use of volumetric bladder ultrasound improve the success rate of suprapubic aspiration of urine? *Pediatr Emerg Care* 18(5):346, 2002.
11. Aguilera PA, Choi T, Durham BA: Ultrasound-guided suprapubic cystostomy catheter placement in the emergency department. *J Emerg Med* 26(3):319–321, 2004.
12. Lee MJ, Papanicolaou N, Nocks BN, et al: Fluoroscopically guided percutaneous suprapubic cystostomy for long-term bladder drainage: an alternative to surgical cystostomy. *Radiology* 188(3):787–789, 1993.
13. Dogra P, Goel R: Complication of percutaneous suprapubic cystostomy. *Int Urol Nephrol* 36(3):343–344, 2004.
14. Liau S, Shabeer U: Laparoscopic management of cecal injury from a misplaced percutaneous suprapubic cystostomy. *Surg Laparosc Endosc Percutan Tech* 15(6):378, 2005.
15. Nyman MA, Schwenk NM, Silverstein MD: Management of urinary retention: rapid versus gradual decompression and risk of complications. *Mayo Clin Proc* 72(10):951–956, 1997.

CHAPTER 19 ■ ASPIRATION OF THE KNEE AND SYNOVIAL FLUID ANALYSIS

BONNIE J. BIDINGER AND ERIC W. JACOBSON

Arthrocentesis is a safe and relatively simple procedure that involves the introduction of a needle into a joint space to remove synovial fluid. It constitutes an essential part of the evaluation of arthritis of unknown cause, frequently with the intent to rule out a septic process [1–3].

Ropes and Bauer [4] first categorized synovial fluid as *inflammatory* or *noninflammatory* in 1953. In 1961, Hollander et al. [5] and Gatter and McCarty [6] coined the term *synovianalysis* to describe the process of joint fluid analysis and were instrumental in establishing its critical role in the diagnosis of certain forms of arthritis. Septic arthritis and crystalline arthritis can be diagnosed by synovial fluid analysis alone. They may present similarly but require markedly different treatments, thus necessitating early arthrocentesis and prompt synovial fluid analysis.

INDICATIONS

Arthrocentesis is performed for diagnostic and therapeutic purposes. The main indication for arthrocentesis is to assist in the evaluation of arthritis of unknown cause. In the intensive care unit, it is most commonly performed to rule out septic arthritis. As many types of inflammatory arthritis mimic septic arthritis, synovial fluid analysis is essential in differentiating the various causes of inflammatory arthritis [4,7] (Table 19.1). Therefore, patients presenting with acute monoarthritis or oligoarthritis require prompt arthrocentesis with subsequent synovial fluid analysis, preferably before initiation of treatment.

Arthrocentesis is also used for therapeutic purposes. In a septic joint, serial joint aspirations are required to remove accumulated inflammatory or purulent fluid. This accomplishes complete drainage of a closed space and allows serial monitoring of the total white blood cell count, Gram stain, and culture to assess treatment response. Inflammatory fluid contains many destructive enzymes that contribute to cartilage and bony degradation; removal of the fluid may slow this destructive process [8,9]. Additionally, arthrocentesis allows for injection of long-acting corticosteroid preparations into the joint space, which may be a useful treatment for various inflammatory and noninflammatory forms of arthritis [10].

Before performing arthrocentesis, it must be ascertained that the true joint is inflamed and an effusion is present. This requires a meticulous physical examination to differentiate arthritis from periarticular inflammation. Bursitis, tendinitis, and cellulitis all may mimic arthritis. In the knee, the examination begins with assessment of swelling. A true effusion may cause bulging of the parapatellar gutters and the suprapatellar pouch [11]. The swelling should be confined to the joint space. To check for small effusions, the bulge test is performed [12]. Fluid is stroked from the medial joint line into the suprapatellar pouch and then from the suprapatellar pouch down along the lateral joint line. If a bulge of fluid is noted at the medial joint line, a small effusion is present (Fig. 19.1). If a large effusion is present, one can detect a ballotable patella by pushing it against the femur with the right index finger while applying pressure to the suprapatellar pouch with the left hand [13]. Comparison with the opposite joint is helpful. Many texts describe joint examination and assessment for fluid in the knee and other joints [11–13].

CONTRAINDICATIONS

Absolute contraindications to arthrocentesis include local infection of the overlying skin or other periarticular structures and severe coagulopathy [1–3,10]. If coagulopathy is present and septic arthritis is suspected, every effort should be made to correct the coagulopathy (with fresh-frozen plasma or alternate factors) before joint aspiration. Therapeutic anticoagulation is not an absolute contraindication, but every effort should be made to avoid excessive trauma during aspiration in this circumstance. Known bacteremia is a contraindication because inserting a needle into the joint space disrupts capillary integrity, allowing joint space seeding [14]. However, if septic arthritis is strongly suspected, joint aspiration is indicated. The presence of articular instability (e.g., that seen with badly damaged joints) is a relative contraindication, although the presence of a large presumed inflammatory fluid may still warrant joint aspiration.

COMPLICATIONS

The major complications of arthrocentesis are iatrogenically induced infection and bleeding, both of which are extremely rare [1]. The risk of infection after arthrocentesis has been estimated to be less than 1 in 10,000 [15]. Hollander [16] reported an incidence of less than 0.005% in 400,000 injections. Strict adherence to aseptic technique reduces the risk of postarthrocentesis infection. Significant hemorrhage is also extremely rare. Correction of prominent coagulopathy before arthrocentesis reduces this risk.

Another potential complication of arthrocentesis is direct injury to the articular cartilage by the needle. This is not quantifiable, but any injury to the cartilage could be associated with degenerative change over time. To avoid cartilaginous damage, the needle should be pushed in only as far as necessary to obtain fluid and excessive movement of the needle during the procedure should be avoided.

Other complications include discomfort from the procedure itself, allergic reactions to the skin preparation or local anesthetic, and in the case of steroid injection, postinjection flare and local soft-tissue atrophy from the glucocorticoid [17].

TABLE 19.1

COMMON CAUSES OF NONINFLAMMATORY AND INFLAMMATORY ARTHRITIDES

Noninflammatory	Inflammatory

Osteoarthritis
Trauma/internal derangement
Avascular necrosis
Hemarthrosis
Malignancy
Benign tumors
  Osteochondroma
  Pigmented villonodular synovitis
	Rheumatoid arthritis
	Spondyloarthropathies
	  Psoriatic arthritis
	  Reiter's syndrome/reactive arthritis
	  Ankylosing spondylitis
	  Ulcerative colitis/regional enteritis
	Crystal-induced arthritis
	  Monosodium urate (gout)
	  Calcium pyrophosphate dihydrate (pseudogout)
	  Hydroxyapatite
	Infectious arthritis
	  Bacterial
	  Mycobacterial
	  Fungal
	Connective tissue diseases
	  Systemic lupus erythematosus
	  Vasculitis
	  Scleroderma
	  Polymyositis
	Hypersensitivity
	  Serum sickness

TABLE 19.2

ARTHROCENTESIS EQUIPMENT

Procedure	Equipment
Skin preparation and local anesthesia	2% chlorhexidine in 70% isopropyl alcohol Ethyl chloride spray For local anesthesia—1% lidocaine; 25-gauge, 1.5-in needle; 22-gauge, 1.5-in. needle; 5-mL syringe Sterile sponge/cloth
Arthrocentesis	Gloves 20- to 60-mL syringe (depending on size of effusion) 18- to 22-gauge, 1.5-in. needle Sterile sponge/cloth Sterile clamp Sterile bandage
Collection	15-mL anticoagulated tube (with sodium heparin or ethylene-diaminetetraacetic acid) Sterile tubes for routine cultures Slide, cover slip

TECHNIQUE

Joint aspiration is easily learned. A sound knowledge of the joint anatomy, including the bony and soft-tissue landmarks used for joint entry, is needed. Strict aseptic technique must be followed to minimize risk of infection, and relaxation of the muscles surrounding the joint should be encouraged because muscular contraction can impede the needle's entry into the joint.

Most physicians in the intensive care unit can aspirate the knee because it is one of the most accessible joints. Other joints should probably be aspirated by an appropriate specialist, such as a rheumatologist or an orthopedic surgeon. Certain joints are quite difficult to enter blindly and are more appropriately entered using radiologic guidance, such as with fluoroscopy or computed tomography; these include the hip, sacroiliac, and temporomandibular joints. Many texts describe in detail the aspiration technique of other joints [3,16–18]. The technique for knee aspiration is as follows:

1. Describe the procedure to the patient, including the possible complications, and obtain written informed consent.
2. Collect all items needed for the procedure (Table 19.2).
3. With the patient supine and the knee fully extended, examine the knee to confirm the presence of an effusion, as described previously.
4. Identify landmarks for needle entry. The knee may be aspirated from a medial or lateral approach. The medial approach is more commonly used and is preferred when small effusions are present. Identify the superior and inferior borders of the patella. Entry should be halfway between the borders, just inferior to the undersurface of the patella (Fig. 19.2). The entry site may be marked with pressure from

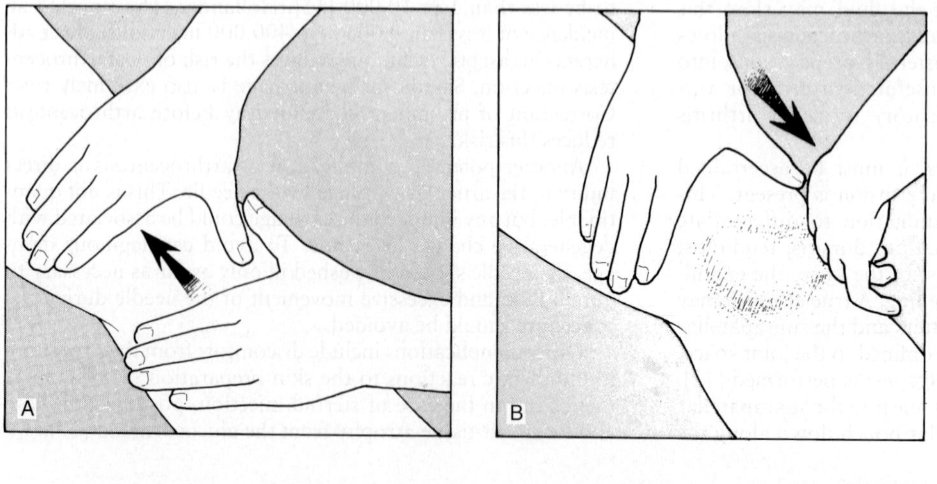

FIGURE 19.1. The bulge test. **A:** Milk fluid from the suprapatellar pouch into the joint. **B:** Slide the hand down the lateral aspect of the joint line and watch for a bulge medial to the joint.

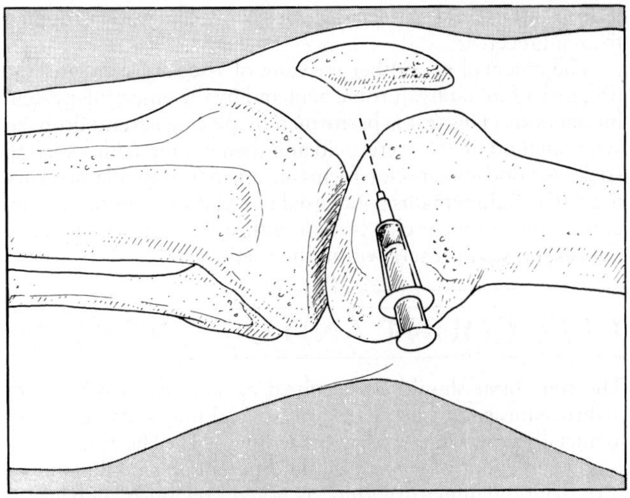

FIGURE 19.2. Technique of aspirating the knee joint. The needle enters halfway between the superior and inferior borders of the patella and is directed just inferior to the patella.

the end of a ballpoint pen with the writing tip retracted. An indentation mark should be visible.

5. Cleanse the area with 2% chlorhexidine in 70% isopropyl alcohol and allow the area to dry. Practice universal precautions: wear gloves at all times while handling any body fluid, although they need not be sterile for routine knee aspiration. Do not touch the targeted area once it has been cleaned.
6. Apply local anesthesia. A local anesthetic (1% lidocaine) may be instilled subcutaneously with a 25-gauge, 1.5-in. needle. Once numbing has occurred, deeper instillation of the local anesthetic to the joint capsule can be performed. Some physicians may use ethyl chloride as an alternative anesthetic. However, this agent provides only superficial anesthesia of the skin. To use, spray ethyl chloride directly onto the designated area and stop when the first signs of freezing are evident in order to limit potential for skin damage.
7. To enter the knee joint, use an 18- to 22-gauge, 1.5-in. needle with a 20- to 60-mL syringe. Use a larger gauge needle particularly if septic arthritis is suspected as the aspirated fluid may be purulent and more difficult to aspirate. Use a quick thrust through the skin and on through the capsule to minimize pain. Avoid hitting periosteal bone, which causes significant pain, or cartilage, which causes cartilaginous damage. Aspirate fluid to fill the syringe. If the fluid appears purulent or hemorrhagic, try to tap the joint dry, which will remove mediators of inflammation that may perpetuate an inflammatory or destructive process. If the syringe is full and more fluid remains, a sterile hemostat may be used to clamp the needle, thus stabilizing it, while switching syringes. When the syringes have been switched, more fluid can be withdrawn. The syringes must be sterile.
8. On occasion, effusions can be difficult to aspirate. Reasons for this include increased fluid viscosity, fibrin and other debris impeding flow through the needle, loculated fluid, and use of a needle with an inappropriately small gauge. Additionally, the fluid may not be accessible by the approach being used [19]. At times, one can obtain a small drop of joint fluid by using continuous suction as the needle is withdrawn from the joint space [17]. This small specimen can then be sent for Gram stain, culture, and if possible, crystal analysis.
9. When the fluid has been obtained, quickly remove the needle and apply pressure to the needle site with a piece of sterile gauze. When bleeding has stopped, remove the gauze, clean the area with alcohol, and apply an adhesive bandage. If the patient is receiving anticoagulation therapy or has a bleeding diathesis, apply prolonged pressure.
10. Document the amount of fluid obtained and perform gross examination, noting the color and clarity. A string sign may be performed at the bedside to assess fluid viscosity (see the following section). Send fluid for cell count with differential count, Gram stain, routine culture, specialized cultures for *Gonococcus*, *Mycobacterium*, and fungus, if indicated, and polarized microscopic examination for crystal analysis. Other tests, such as glucose and complement determinations, are generally not helpful. Use an anticoagulated tube to send fluid for cell count and crystal analysis. Sodium heparin and ethylenediaminetetraacetic acid are appropriate anticoagulants. Lithium heparin and calcium oxalate should be avoided because they can precipitate out of solution to form crystals, thus potentially giving a false-positive assessment for crystals [6,20]. Fluid may be sent for Gram stain and culture in the syringe capped with a blunt tip or in a sterile redtop tube.

SYNOVIAL FLUID ANALYSIS

Synovial fluid analysis is identical for all joints and begins with bedside observation of the fluid. The color, clarity, and viscosity of the fluid are characterized. Synovial fluid is divided into noninflammatory and inflammatory types on the basis of the total nucleated cell count. A white blood cell count less than or equal to 2,000 per μL indicates a *noninflammatory fluid* and a count greater than 2,000 per μL indicates an *inflammatory fluid*. Table 19.3 shows how fluid is divided into major categories on the basis of appearance and cell count.

TABLE 19.3

JOINT FLUID CHARACTERISTICS

Characteristic	Normal	Noninflammatory	Inflammatory	Septic
Color	Clear	Yellow	Yellow or opalescent	Variable—may be purulent
Clarity	Transparent	Transparent	Translucent	Opaque
Viscosity	Very high	High	Low	Typically low
Mucin clot	Firm	Firm	Friable	Friable
White blood cell count per μL	200	200–2,000	2,000–100,000	>50,000, usually >100,000
Polymorphonuclear cells (%)	<25	<25	>50	>75
Culture	Negative	Negative	Negative	Usually positive

GROSS EXAMINATION

Color

Color and clarity should be tested using a clear glass tube. Translucent plastic, as used in most disposable syringes, interferes with proper assessment [1]. Normal synovial fluid is colorless. Noninflammatory and inflammatory synovial fluid appears yellow or straw colored. Septic effusions frequently appear purulent and whitish. Depending on the number of white blood cells present, pure pus may be extracted from a septic joint. Hemorrhagic effusions appear red or brown. If the fluid looks like pure blood, the tap may have aspirated venous blood. The needle is removed, pressure is applied, and the joint is reentered from an alternate site. If the same bloody appearance is noted, the fluid is a hemorrhagic effusion and probably not related to the trauma of the aspiration. If any question remains, the hematocrit of the effusion is compared with that of peripheral blood. The hematocrit in a hemorrhagic effusion is typically lower than that of peripheral blood. In the case of a traumatic tap, the hematocrit of the fluid should be equal to that of peripheral blood. For causes of a hemorrhagic effusion, refer to Table 19.4.

Clarity

The clarity of synovial fluid depends on the number and types of cells or particles present. Clarity is tested by reading black print on a white background through a glass tube filled with the synovial fluid. If the print is easily read, the fluid is transparent. This is typical of normal and noninflammatory synovial fluid. If the black print can be distinguished from the white background, but is not clear, the fluid is translucent. This is typical of inflammatory effusions. If nothing can be seen through the fluid, it is opaque. This occurs with grossly inflammatory, septic, and hemorrhagic fluids.

Viscosity

The viscosity of synovial fluid is a measure of the hyaluronic acid content. Degradative enzymes such as hyaluronidase are released in inflammatory conditions, thus destroying hyaluronic acid and other proteinaceous material, resulting in a thinner, less viscous fluid. Highly viscous fluid, on the other hand, can be seen in myxedematous or hypothyroid effusions.

Viscosity can be assessed at the bedside using the string sign [1]. A drop of fluid is allowed to fall from the end of the needle or syringe and the length of the continuous string that forms is estimated. Normal fluid typically forms at least a 6-cm continuous string. Inflammatory fluid does not form a string; instead, it drops off the end of the needle or syringe like water dropping from a faucet.

The mucin clot, another measure of viscosity, estimates the presence of intact hyaluronic acid and hyaluronic acid–protein interactions. This test is performed by placing several drops of synovial fluid in 5% acetic acid and then mixing with a stirring stick. A good mucin clot forms in normal, noninflammatory fluid. The fluid remains condensed in a clot resembling chewed gum. A poor mucin clot is seen with inflammatory fluid; the fluid disperses diffusely within the acetic acid.

TABLE 19.4

CAUSES OF A HEMORRHAGIC EFFUSION

Trauma (with or without fracture)
Hemophilia and other bleeding disorders
Anticoagulant therapy
Tumor (metastatic and local)
Hemangioma
Pigmented villonodular synovitis
Ehlers-Danlos syndrome
Scurvy

CELL COUNT AND DIFFERENTIAL

The cell count should be obtained as soon as possible after arthrocentesis, as a delay of even several hours may cause an artificially low white blood cell count [21]. The total white blood cell count of synovial fluid differentiates noninflammatory from inflammatory fluid, as noted previously. In general, the higher the total white blood cell count, the more likely the joint is to be infected. This is not absolute, however, and there is considerable overlap. For instance, a total white cell count greater than 100,000 per μL may be seen in conditions other than infection, whereas a total white blood cell count of 50,000 per μL may be due to infection, crystalline disease, or systemic inflammatory arthropathy [28]. The technique for the cell count is identical to that used with peripheral blood. The fluid may be diluted with normal saline for a manual count, or an automated counter may be used. Viscous fluid with excessive debris may clog a counter or give falsely elevated results, thus making the manual procedure somewhat more accurate.

The differential white blood cell count is also performed using the technique used for peripheral blood, typically using Wright's stain. The differential is calculated on the basis of direct visualization. The differential count includes cells typically seen in peripheral blood, such as polymorphonuclear cells, monocytes, and lymphocytes, as well as cells localized to the synovial space. In general, the total white blood cell count and the polymorphonuclear cell count increase with inflammation and infection. Septic fluid typically has a differential of greater than 75% polymorphonuclear cells (see Table 19.3).

In addition to distinguishing polymorphonuclear cells from monocytes and lymphocytes, Wright's stain can detect other cells in synovial fluid that can be useful in establishing a diagnosis. For instance, iron-laden chondrocytes, which are seen in hemochromatosis, may be picked up by Wright's stain, as may be fat droplets and bone marrow spicules, which are suggestive of trauma or a fracture into the joint [19].

CRYSTALS

All fluid should be assessed for the presence of crystals. As with cell count, crystal analysis should be performed as soon as possible after arthrocentesis. A delay is associated with a decreased yield [21]. One drop of fluid is placed on a slide and covered with a coverslip; this is examined for crystals using a compensated polarized light microscope. The presence of intracellular monosodium urate (MSU) or calcium pyrophosphate dihydrate (CPPD) crystals confirms a diagnosis of gout or pseudogout, respectively. MSU crystals are typically long and needle shaped: they may appear to pierce through a white blood cell. The crystals are strongly negatively birefringent, appearing yellow when parallel to the plane of reference. Typically, CPPD crystals are small and rhomboid. The crystals are weakly positively birefringent, appearing blue when oriented parallel to the plane of reference. Rotating the stage of the microscope by 90 degrees and thereby the orientation of the crystals (now perpendicular to the plane of reference) changes their color:

TABLE 19.5

CLASSIFICATION OF HYPERURICEMIA

Primary hyperuricemia
Idiopathic
Enzymatic defects (e.g., hypoxanthine guanine phosphoribosyl- transferase deficiency)
Secondary hyperuricemia
Increased production of uric acid
Increased de novo purine synthesis
Excessive dietary purine intake
Increased nucleic acid turnover (myeloproliferative/lymphoproliferative disorders, psoriasis, hemolytic anemia, ethyl alcohol abuse)
Decreased renal excretion of uric acid
Medications
Diuretics
Low-dose salicylates
Pyrazinamide
Ethambutol
Cyclosporine
Chronic renal failure
Hyperacidemia (lactic acidosis, ketoacidosis, starvation, ethyl alchohol abuse)
Lead nephropathy

MSU crystals turn blue and CPPD crystals turn yellow. Refer to Tables 19.5 and 19.6 for a classification of hyperuricemia and conditions associated with CPPD deposition disease.

In addition to MSU and CPPD crystals, other less common crystals may induce an inflammatory arthropathy. Basic calcium crystals (e.g., hydroxyapatite) and oxalate crystals are two such types. Much like MSU crystals in gout, hydroxyapatite crystals can incite acute articular and periarticular inflammation, which can be difficult to distinguish clinically from septic arthritis and cellulitis, respectively [22]. On light microscopy, however, crystals appear as clumps of shiny nonbirefringent globules, and with alizarin red S stain, the clumps appear red-orange [22,23]. If hydroxyapatite is suspected, alizarin red S stain must be requested specifically from the laboratory as it is not a routine component of the crystal analysis. Calcium oxalate crystals can also induce an inflammatory arthritis. This is generally seen in patients on long-term hemodialysis [24–26], but may also be seen in young patients with primary oxalosis [22]. Synovial fluid typically reveals characteristic bipyramidal crystals as well as polymorphic forms [22].

TABLE 19.6

CONDITIONS ASSOCIATED WITH CALCIUM PYROPHOSPHATE DIHYDRATE DEPOSITION DISEASE

Hereditary
Sporadic (idiopathic)
Aging
Metabolic diseases
Hyperparathyroidism
Hypothyroidism
Hypophosphatemia
Hypomagnesemia
Hemochromatosis
Amyloidosis
Trauma

The yield for all crystals can be increased by spinning the specimen and examining the sediment. If the fluid cannot be examined immediately, it should be refrigerated to preserve the crystals. It is important to note that even in the presence of crystals, infection must be considered because crystals can be seen concomitantly with a septic joint.

Other crystals include cryoimmunoglobulins in patients with multiple myeloma and essential cryoglobulinemia [27], and cholesterol crystals in patients with chronic inflammatory arthropathies, such as rheumatoid arthritis. Cholesterol crystals are a nonspecific finding and appear as platelike structures with a notched corner.

GRAM STAIN AND CULTURE

The Gram stain is performed as with other body fluids. It should be performed as soon as possible to screen for the presence of bacteria. It has been reported that the sensitivity of synovial fluid Gram stain in septic arthritis ranges between 50% and 75% for nongonococcal infection and less than 10% for gonococcal infection [28]. Specificity is much higher; this suggests that a positive Gram stain, despite a negative culture, should be considered evidence of infection. In fact, it is not uncommon for only the Gram stain to be positive in the setting of infection [28]. However, the absence of bacteria by the Gram stain does not rule out a septic process.

Synovial fluid in general should be cultured routinely for aerobic and anaerobic bacterial organisms. A positive culture confirms septic arthritis. In certain circumstances (e.g., in chronic monoarticular arthritis), fluid may be cultured for the presence of mycobacteria, fungus, and spirochetes. If disseminated gonorrhea is suspected, the laboratory must be notified because the fluid should be plated directly onto chocolate agar or Thayer–Martin medium. Just as Gram stain of synovial fluid in gonococcal infection is often negative, so too is synovial fluid culture. Synovial fluid culture is positive approximately 10% to 50% of the time, versus 75% to 95% of the time for nongonococcal infection [28]. However, cultures of genitourinary sites and mucosal sites in gonococcal infection are positive approximately 80% of the time [29]. Therefore, when suspicion of gonococcal arthritis is high (e.g., in a young, healthy, sexually active individual with a dermatitis-arthritis syndrome), the diagnosis must often be confirmed by a positive culture from the urethra, cervix, rectum, or pharynx.

In addition to documenting infection and identifying a specific organism, synovial fluid culture can be useful in determining antibiotic sensitivities and subsequent treatment. Furthermore, serial synovial fluid cultures can help in assessing response to therapy. For example, a negative follow-up culture associated with a decrease in synovial fluid polymorphonuclear cell count is highly suggestive of improvement.

Other studies on synovial fluid (e.g., glucose, protein, lactate dehydrogenase, complement, and immune complexes) are generally not helpful. Specifically, in a study by Shmerling et al. [30], the investigators observed that synovial fluid glucose and protein were "highly inaccurate." The synovial fluid glucose and protein misclassified effusions as inflammatory versus noninflammatory 50% of the time. By contrast, synovial fluid cell count and differential were found to be reliable and complementary; sensitivity and specificity of cell count was 84% for both and for the differential was 75% and 92%, respectively [30]. Although synovial fluid lactate dehydrogenase was also found to be accurate, it did not offer any additional information above and beyond the cell count and differential. A more recent critical appraisal of synovial fluid analysis was conducted by Swan et al. [31] in 2002. Through a detailed survey of the literature, the authors confirmed the diagnostic value of synovial fluid analysis in cases of acute arthritis when an infectious or crystalline etiology is suspected, as well as in cases of intercritical gout. The usefulness of other synovial fluid assays was not supported by the literature.

Of note, there are special stains for synovial fluid that can be helpful as the clinical picture warrants; these include Congo red staining for amyloid arthropathy. Amyloid deposits display an apple-green birefringence with polarized light [32]. Prussian blue stain for iron deposition may reveal iron in synovial lining cells in hemochromatosis [19]. However, neither of these studies should be considered a routine component of synovial fluid analysis.

References

1. Gatter RA: *A Practical Handbook of Joint Fluid Analysis*. Philadelphia, Lea & Febiger, 1984.
2. Stein R: *Manual of Rheumatology and Outpatient Orthopedic Disorders*. Boston, Little, Brown, 1981.
3. Krey PR, Lazaro DM: *Analysis of Synovial Fluid*. Summit, NJ, CIBA-GEIGY, 1992.
4. Ropes MW, Bauer W: *Synovial Fluid Changes in Joint Disease*. Cambridge, MA, Harvard University Press, 1953.
5. Hollander JL, Jessar RA, McCarty DJ: Synovianalysis: an aid in arthritis diagnosis. *Bull Rheum Dis* 12:263, 1961.
6. Gatter RA, McCarty DJ: Synovianalysis: a rapid clinical diagnostic procedure. *Rheumatism* 20:2, 1964.
7. Schumacher HR: Synovial fluid analysis. *Orthop Rev* 13:85, 1984.
8. Greenwald RA: Oxygen radicals, inflammation, and arthritis: pathophysiological considerations and implications for treatment. *Semin Arthritis Rheum* 20:219, 1991.
9. Robinson DR, Tashjian AH, Levine L: Prostaglandin E2 induced bone resorption by rheumatoid synovia: a model for bone destruction in RA. *J Clin Invest* 56:1181, 1975.
10. Gray RG, Tenenbaum J, Gottlieb NL: Local corticosteroid injection treatment in rheumatic disorders. *Semin Arthritis Rheum* 10:231, 1981.
11. Polley HF, Hunder GG: *Rheumatologic Interviewing and Physical Examination of the Joints*. 2nd ed. Philadelphia, WB Saunders, 1978.
12. Doherty M, Hazelman BL, Hutton CW, et al: *Rheumatology Examination and Injection Techniques*. London, WB Saunders, 1992.
13. Moder KG, Hunder GG: History and physical examination of the musculoskeletal system, in Harris ED Jr, Budd RC, Firestein GS, et al: (eds): *Kelley's Textbook of Rheumatology*. 7th ed. Philadelphia, Elsevier Saunders, 2005, p 483.
14. McCarty DJ Jr: A basic guide to arthrocentesis. *Hosp Med* 4:77, 1968.
15. Gottlieb NL, Riskin WG: Complications of local corticosteroid injections. *JAMA* 243:1547, 1980.
16. Hollander JL: Intrasynovial steroid injections, in Hollander JL, McCarty DL Jr (eds): *Arthritis and Allied Conditions*. 8th ed. Philadelphia, Lea & Febiger, 1972, p 517.
17. Wise C: Arthrocentesis and injection of joints and soft tissues, in Harris ED Jr, Budd RC, Firestein GS, et al: (eds): *Kelley's Textbook of Rheumatology*. 7th ed. Philadelphia, Elsevier Saunders, 2005, p 692.
18. Canoso JJ: Aspiration and injection of joints and periarticular tissues, in Hochberg MC, Silman AJ, Smolen JS, et al: (eds): *Rheumatology*. 3rd ed. London, Philadelphia, Elsevier, 2003, p 233.
19. Schumacher HR Jr: Synovial fluid analysis, in Katz WA (ed): *Diagnosis and Management of Rheumatic Diseases*. 2nd ed. Philadelphia, JB Lippincott, 1988, pp 248–255.
20. Tanphaichitr K, Spilberg I, Hahn B: Lithium heparin crystals simulating calcium pyrophosphate dihydrate crystals in synovial fluid [letter]. *Arthritis Rheum* 9:966, 1976.
21. Kerolus G, Clayburne G, Schumacher HR Jr: Is it mandatory to examine synovial fluids promptly after arthrocentesis? *Arthritis Rheum* 32:271, 1989.
22. Reginato AJ, Schumacher HR Jr: Crystal-associated arthropathies. *Clin Geriatr Med* 4(2):295, 1988.
23. Paul H, Reginato AJ, Schumacher HR: Alizarin red S staining as a screening test to detect calcium compounds in synovial fluid. *Arthritis Rheum* 26:191, 1983.
24. Hoffman G, Schumacher HR, Paul H, et al: Calcium oxalate microcrystalline associated arthritis in end stage renal disease. *Ann Intern Med* 97:36, 1982.
25. Reginato AJ, Feweiro JL, Barbazan AC, et al: Arthropathy and cutaneous calcinosis in hemodialysis oxalosis. *Arthritis Rheum* 29:1387, 1986.
26. Schumacher HR, Reginato AJ, Pullman S: Synovial fluid oxalate deposition complicating rheumatoid arthritis with amyloidosis and renal failure. Demonstration of intracellular oxalate crystals. *J Rheumatol* 14:361, 1987.
27. Dornan TL, Blundell JW, Morgan AG: Widespread crystallization of paraprotein in myelomatosis. *QJM* 57:659, 1985.
28. Shmerling RH: Synovial fluid analysis. A critical reappraisal. *Rheum Dis Clin North Am* 20(2):503, 1994.
29. Mahowald ML: Gonococcal arthritis, in Hochberg MC, Silman AJ, Smolen JS, et al: (eds): *Rheumatology*. 3rd ed. London, Mosby, 2003, p 1067.
30. Shmerling RH, Delbanco TL, Tosteson ANA, et al: Synovial fluid tests. What should be ordered? *JAMA* 264:1009, 1990.
31. Swan A, Amer H, Dieppe P: The value of synovial fluid assays in the diagnosis of joint disease: a literature survey. *Ann Rheum Dis* 61(6):493, 2002.
32. Lakhanpal S, Li CY, Gertz MA, et al: Synovial fluid analysis for diagnosis of amyloid arthropathy. *Arthritis Rheum* 30(4):419, 1987.

CHAPTER 20 ■ ANESTHESIA FOR BEDSIDE PROCEDURES

MARK DERSHWITZ

When a patient in an intensive care unit (ICU) requires a bedside procedure, it is usually the attending intensivist, as opposed to a consultant anesthesiologist, who directs the administration of the necessary hypnotic, analgesic, and/or paralytic drugs. Furthermore, unlike in the operating room, the ICU usually has no equipment for the administration of gaseous (e.g., nitrous oxide) or volatile (e.g., isoflurane) anesthetics. Anesthesia for bedside procedures in the ICU is thus accomplished via a technique involving total intravenous anesthesia (TIVA).

COMMON PAIN MANAGEMENT PROBLEMS IN ICU PATIENTS

Dosing of Agent

Selecting the proper dose of an analgesic to administer is problematic for several reasons, including difficulty in assessing the effectiveness of pain relief, pharmacokinetic (PK) differences between the critically ill and other patients, and normal physiologic changes associated with aging.

Assessing the Effectiveness of Pain Relief

Critically ill patients are often incapable of communicating their feelings because of delirium, obtundation, or endotracheal intubation. This makes psychologic evaluation quite difficult because surrogate markers of pain intensity (e.g., tachycardia, hypertension, and diaphoresis) are inherent in the host response to critical illness.

Pharmacokinetic Considerations

Most of the pressors and vasodilators administered in the ICU by continuous intravenous (IV) infusion have a relatively straightforward PK behavior: they are water-soluble molecules that are bound very little to plasma proteins. In contrast, the hypnotics and opioids used in TIVA have high lipid solubility and most are extensively bound to plasma proteins, causing their PK behavior to be far more complex. Figure 20.1 shows the disappearance curves of fentanyl and nitroprusside after bolus injection. The fentanyl curve has three phases: (i) a very rapid phase (with a half-life of 0.82 minutes) lasting about 10 minutes, during which the plasma concentration decreases more than 90% from its peak value; (ii) an intermediate phase (with a half-life of 17 minutes) lasting from about 10 minutes to an hour; and (iii) finally a terminal, very slow phase (with a half-life of 465 minutes) beginning about an hour after bolus injection. After a single bolus injection of fentanyl, the terminal phase occurs at plasma concentrations below which there is a pharmacologic effect. However, after multiple bolus injections or a continuous infusion, this latter phase occurs at therapeutic plasma concentrations. Thus, fentanyl behaves as a short-acting drug after a single bolus injection, but as a very long-lasting drug after a continuous infusion of more than an hour in duration (i.e., fentanyl accumulates). Thus, it is inappropriate to speak of the half-life of fentanyl.

The disappearance curve of nitroprusside has two phases: (i) a very rapid phase (with a half-life of 0.89 minute) lasting about 10 minutes, during which the plasma concentration decreases more than 85% from its peak value, and (ii) a terminal phase (with a half-life of 14 minutes). It may be slightly slower in offset as compared with fentanyl during the initial 10 minutes after a bolus injection, but it does not accumulate at all even after a prolonged infusion.

The PK behavior of the lipid-soluble hypnotics and analgesics given by infusion may be described by their context-

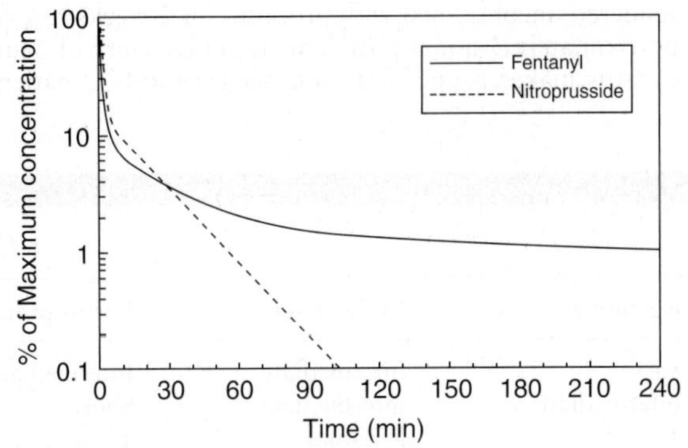

FIGURE 20.1. The time courses, on a semilogarithmic scale, of the plasma concentrations of fentanyl [1] and nitroprusside [2] following a bolus injection. Each concentration is expressed as the percentage of the peak plasma concentration. The fentanyl curve has three phases with half-lives of 0.82, 17, and 465 minutes. The nitroprusside curve has two phases with half-lives of 0.89 and 14 minutes.

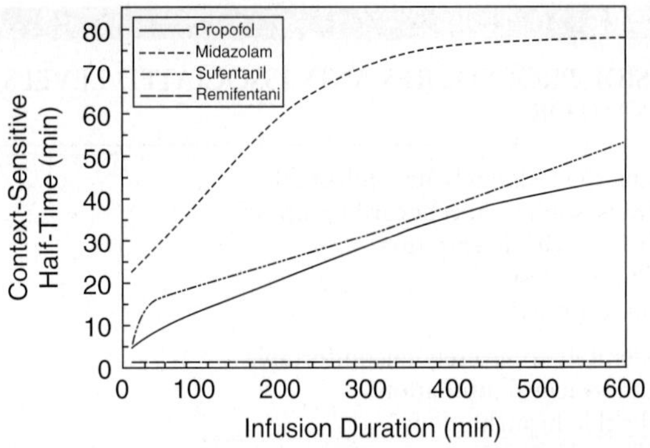

FIGURE 20.2. The context-sensitive half-times for propofol [4], midazolam [5], sufentanil [6], and remifentanil [7] as a function of infusion duration.

sensitive half-times (CSHTs). This concept may be defined as follows: when a drug is given as an IV bolus followed by an IV infusion designed to maintain a constant plasma drug concentration, the time required for the plasma concentration to fall by 50% after termination of the infusion is the CSHT [3]. Figure 20.2 depicts the CSHT curves for the medications most likely to be used for TIVA in ICU patients.

PK behavior in critically ill patients is unlike that in normal subjects for several reasons. Because ICU patients frequently have renal and/or hepatic dysfunction, drug excretion is significantly impaired. Hypoalbuminemia, common in critical illness, decreases protein binding and increases free drug concentration [8]. Because free drug is the only moiety available to tissue receptors, decreased protein binding increases the pharmacologic effect for a given plasma concentration. It is therefore more important in ICU patients that the doses of medications used for TIVA are individualized for a particular patient.

Physiologic Changes Associated with Aging

People 65 years of age and older comprise the fastest growing segment of the population and constitute the majority of patients in many ICUs. Aging leads to (a) a decrease in total body water and lean body mass; (b) an increase in body fat and, hence, an increase in the volume of distribution of lipid-soluble drugs; and (c) a decrease in drug clearance rates, due to reductions in liver mass, hepatic enzyme activity, liver blood flow, and renal excretory function. There is a progressive, age-dependent increase in pain relief and electroencephalographic suppression among elderly patients receiving the same dose of opioid as younger patients. There is also an increase in central nervous system (CNS) depression in elderly patients following administration of identical doses of benzodiazepines.

Selection of Agent

Procedures performed in ICUs today (Table 20.1) span a spectrum that extends from those associated with mild discomfort (e.g., esophagogastroscopy) to those that are quite painful (e.g., orthopedic manipulations, wound debridement, and tracheostomy). Depending on their technical difficulty, these procedures can last from minutes to hours. To provide a proper anesthetic, medications should be selected according to the nature of the procedure and titrated according to the patient's response to surgical stimulus. In addition, specific disease states should be considered in order to maximize safety and effectiveness.

TABLE 20.1

BEDSIDE PROCEDURES AND ASSOCIATED LEVELS OF DISCOMFORT

Mildly to moderately uncomfortable
Transesophageal echocardiography[a]
Transtracheal aspiration
Thoracentesis[a]
Paracentesis[a]
Moderately to severely uncomfortable
Endotracheal intubation[a]
Flexible bronchoscopy[a]
Thoracostomy[a]
Bone marrow biopsy
Colonoscopy
Peritoneal dialysis catheter insertion[a]
Peritoneal lavage[a]
Percutaneous gastrostomy[a]
Percutaneous intra-aortic balloon insertion[a]
Extremely painful
Rigid bronchoscopy
Debridement of open wounds
Dressing changes
Orthopedic manipulations
Tracheostomy[a]
Pericardiocentesis/pericardial window[a]
Open lung biopsy
Ventriculostomy[a]

[a]Procedures in which the level of discomfort may be significantly mitigated by the use of local anesthesia.

Head Trauma

Head-injured patients require a technique that provides effective, yet brief, anesthesia so that the capacity to assess neurologic status is not lost for extended periods of time. In addition, the technique must not adversely affect cerebral perfusion pressure. If the effects of the anesthetics dissipate too rapidly, episodes of agitation and increased intracranial pressure (ICP) may occur that jeopardize cerebral perfusion. In contrast, if the medications last too long, there may be difficulty in making an adequate neurologic assessment following the procedure.

Coronary Artery Disease

Postoperative myocardial ischemia following cardiac and noncardiac surgery strongly predicts adverse outcome [9]. Accordingly, sufficient analgesia should be provided during and after invasive procedures to reduce plasma catecholamine and stress hormone levels.

Renal and/or Hepatic Failure

Risk of an adverse drug reaction is at least three times higher in patients with azotemia than in those with normal renal function. This risk is magnified by excessive unbound drug or drug metabolite(s) in the circulation and changes in the target tissue(s) induced by the uremic state.

Liver failure alters many drug volumes of distribution by impairing synthesis of the two major plasma-binding proteins: albumin and α_1-acid glycoprotein. In addition, reductions in hepatic blood flow and hepatic enzymatic activity decrease drug clearance rates.

CHARACTERISTICS OF SPECIFIC AGENTS USED FOR BEDSIDE PROCEDURES

Hypnotics

The characteristics of the hypnotics are provided in Table 20.2, whereas their recommended doses are provided in Table 20.3. When rapid awakening is desired, propofol and etomidate are the hypnotic agents of choice. Ketamine may be useful when a longer duration of anesthesia is needed. Midazolam is rarely used alone as a hypnotic; however, its profound anxiolytic and amnestic effects render it useful in combination with other agents.

Propofol

Description. Propofol is a hypnotic agent associated with pleasant emergence and little hangover. It has essentially replaced thiopental for induction of anesthesia, especially in outpatients. It is extremely popular because it is readily titratable and has more rapid onset and offset kinetics than midazolam. Thus, patients emerge from anesthesia more rapidly after propofol than after midazolam, a factor that may make propofol the preferred agent for sedation and hypnosis in general and for patients with altered level of consciousness in particular.

The CSHT for propofol is about 10 minutes following a 1-hour infusion, and the CSHT increases about 5 minutes for each additional hour of infusion for the first several hours, as shown in Figure 20.2. Thus, the CSHT is about 20 minutes after a 3-hour infusion. The CSHT rises much more slowly for infusions longer than a day; a patient who is sedated (but not rendered unconscious) with propofol for 2 weeks recovers in approximately 3 hours [10]. This rapid recovery of neurologic status makes propofol a good sedative in ICU patients,

TABLE 20.2

CHARACTERISTICS OF INTRAVENOUS HYPNOTIC AGENTS[a]

	Propofol	Etomidate	Ketamine	Midazolam	Fospropofol
Onset	Fast	Fast	Fast	**Intermediate**	**Intermediate**
Duration	Short	Short	Intermediate	Intermediate	Short
Cardiovascular effects	↓	**None**	↑	Minimal	↓
Respiratory effects	↓	↓	**Minimal**	↓	↓
Analgesia	None	None	**Profound**	None	None
Amnesia	Mild	Mild	**Profound**	**Profound**	Mild

[a]The listed doses should be reduced 50% in elderly patients. Entries in bold type indicate noteworthy differences among the drugs.

TABLE 20.3

USUAL DOSES OF INTRAVENOUS ANESTHETIC AGENTS GIVEN BY CONTINUOUS INFUSION[a]

	Propofol	Etomidate	Ketamine	Midazolam	Sufentanil	Remifentanil
Bolus dose (mg/kg)	1–2	0.2–0.3	1–2	0.05–0.15	0.5–1.5	0.5–1.5
Infusion rate (μg/kg/min)	100–200	NR[b]	25–100	0.25–1.5	0.01–0.03	0.05–0.5

[a]The "usual doses" are for patients without preexisting tolerance and significant cardiovascular disease. The required doses will be higher in patients with tolerance, and should be reduced in elderly patients and in patients with decreased cardiovascular function. In all cases, the medications should be titrated to specific endpoints as described in the text.
[b]Not recommended due to the possibility of prolonged adrenal suppression.

especially those with head trauma, who may not tolerate mechanical ventilation without pharmacologic sedation.

Even though recovery following termination of a continuous infusion is faster with propofol than with midazolam, a comparative trial showed that the two drugs were roughly equivalent in effectiveness for overnight sedation of ICU patients [11]. For long-term sedation (e.g., more than 1 day), however, recovery is significantly faster in patients given propofol.

In spontaneously breathing patients sedated with propofol, respiratory rate appears to be a more predictable sign of adequate sedation than hemodynamic changes. The ventilatory response to rebreathing carbon dioxide during a maintenance propofol infusion is similar to that induced by other sedative drugs (i.e., propofol significantly decreases the slope of the carbon dioxide response curve). Nevertheless, spontaneously breathing patients anesthetized with propofol are able to maintain normal end-tidal carbon dioxide values during minor surgical procedures.

Bolus doses of propofol in the range of 1 to 2 mg per kg induce loss of consciousness within 30 seconds. Maintenance infusion rates of 100 to 200 μg per kg per minute are adequate in younger subjects to maintain general anesthesia, whereas doses should be reduced by 20% to 50% in elderly individuals.

Adverse Effects

Cardiovascular. Propofol depresses ventricular systolic function and lowers afterload, but has no effect on diastolic function [12,13]. Vasodilation results from calcium channel blockade. In patients undergoing coronary artery bypass surgery, propofol (2 mg per kg IV bolus) produced a 23% fall in mean arterial blood pressure, a 20% increase in heart rate, and a 26% decrease in stroke volume. In pigs, propofol caused a dose-related depression of sinus node and His-Purkinje system functions, but had no effect on atrioventricular node function or on the conduction properties of atrial and ventricular tissues. In patients with coronary artery disease, propofol administration may be associated with a reduction in coronary perfusion pressure and increased myocardial lactate production [14].

Neurologic. Propofol may improve neurologic outcome and reduce neuronal damage by depressing cerebral metabolism. Propofol decreases cerebral oxygen consumption, cerebral blood flow, and cerebral glucose utilization in humans and animals to the same degree as that reported for thiopental and etomidate [15]. Propofol frequently causes pain when injected into a peripheral vein. Injection pain is less likely if the injection site is located proximally on the arm or if the injection is made via a central venous catheter.

Metabolic. The emulsion used as the vehicle for propofol contains soybean oil and lecithin and supports bacterial growth; iatrogenic contamination leading to septic shock is possible. Currently available propofol preparations contain ethylenediaminetetraacetic acid (EDTA), metabisulfite, or benzyl alcohol as a bacteriostatic agent. Because EDTA chelates trace metals, particularly zinc, serum zinc levels should be measured daily during continuous propofol infusions. Hyperlipidemia may occur, particularly in infants and small children. Accordingly, triglyceride levels should be monitored daily in this population whenever propofol is administered continuously for more than 24 hours.

Fospropofol

Fospropofol is a water-soluble prodrug of propofol. Fospropofol is metabolized to propofol by the action of alkaline phosphatase. The peak hypnotic effect occurs in about 10 minutes following a bolus injection. The kinetic disposition of liberated propofol differs from that of injected propofol emulsion, with the former being slower for reasons that are as yet unexplained [16,17]. Apparent advantages of an aqueous solution of fospropofol are the reduced risk of bacterial contamination as compared to propofol emulsion and the absence of a lipid load that has been associated with organ toxicity during long-term infusions of propofol emulsion. Although fospropofol does not usually cause pain at the site of injection, it commonly causes a burning sensation distant to the site of injection, typically in the perineum or buttocks. Although it is currently approved for procedural sedation only, it may find utility for sedation or anesthesia in the ICU.

Because the molecular weight of fospropofol is higher than that of propofol, its administered dose is necessarily higher. The package label is unfortunately written in terms of dosing in volume units; because virtually every other medication used in the ICU is dosed in terms of an infusion rate that is a function of the body mass, such doses will be used here. The marketed preparation contains 3.5% fospropofol (35 mg per mL). The manufacturer recommends a bolus dose of 6.5 mg per kg followed by repeat injections of 1.6 mg per kg no more often than every 4 minutes; an infusion rate of 400 μg per kg per minute following the bolus dose would be equivalent. Furthermore, the manufacturer recommends that the doses be decreased by 25% in persons older than 65 years or with severe systemic disease. These dose recommendations are designed to achieve procedural sedation and not general anesthesia. As with propofol, the dose will likely need to be increased two- to threefold to induce and maintain general anesthesia; however, no such study in human beings has yet been published.

Etomidate

Description. Etomidate has onset and offset PK characteristics similar to propofol and an unrivaled cardiovascular profile, even in the setting of cardiomyopathy [18]. Not only does etomidate lack significant effects on myocardial contractility, but baseline sympathetic output and baroreflex regulation of sympathetic activity are well preserved. Etomidate depresses in a dose-related manner cerebral oxygen metabolism and blood flow without changing the intracranial volume–pressure relationship.

Etomidate is particularly useful (rather than thiopental or propofol) in certain patient subsets: patients with hypovolemia, those with multiple trauma with closed-head injury, and those with low ejection fraction, severe aortic stenosis, left main coronary artery disease, or severe cerebral vascular disease. Etomidate may be contraindicated in patients with established or evolving septic shock because of its inhibition of cortisol synthesis (see later).

Adverse Effects

Metabolic. Etomidate, when given by prolonged infusion, may increase mortality associated with low plasma cortisol levels [19]. Even single doses of etomidate can produce adrenal cortical suppression lasting 24 hours or more in normal patients undergoing elective surgery [20]. These effects are more pronounced as the dose is increased or if continuous infusions are used for sedation. Etomidate-induced adrenocortical suppression occurs because the drug blocks the 11β-hydroxylase that catalyzes the final step in the synthesis of cortisol. It is also noteworthy that etomidate causes the highest incidence of postoperative nausea and vomiting of any of the IV anesthetic agents.

In 2005, Jackson warned against the use of etomidate in patients with septic shock [21]. Since then, there have been several studies that have attempted to confirm or refute the safety of etomidate in critically ill patients, including those with sepsis. Unfortunately, some of these studies purportedly confirmed the danger of etomidate [22–25], whereas others support its continued use in patients with sepsis [26–30].

Ketamine

Description. Ketamine induces a state of sedation, amnesia, and marked analgesia in which the patient experiences a strong feeling of dissociation from the environment. It is unique among the hypnotics in that it reliably induces unconsciousness by the intramuscular route. Ketamine is rapidly metabolized by the liver to norketamine, which is pharmacologically active. Ketamine is both slower in onset and offset as compared with propofol or etomidate following IV infusion.

Many clinicians consider ketamine to be the analgesic of choice in patients with a history of bronchospasm. In the usual dosage, it decreases airway resistance, probably by blocking norepinephrine uptake, which in turn stimulates β-adrenergic receptors in the lungs. In contrast to many β-agonist bronchodilators, ketamine is not arrhythmogenic when given to patients with asthma receiving aminophylline.

Ketamine may be safer than other hypnotics or opioids in unintubated patients because it depresses airway reflexes and respiratory drive to a lesser degree. It may be particularly useful for procedures near the airway, where physical access and ability to secure an airway are limited (e.g., gunshot wounds to the face). Because ketamine increases salivary and tracheobronchial secretions, an anticholinergic (e.g., 0.2 mg glycopyrrolate) should be given prior to its administration. In patients with borderline hypoxemia despite maximal therapy, ketamine may be the drug of choice because it does not inhibit hypoxic pulmonary vasoconstriction.

Another major feature that distinguishes ketamine from most other IV anesthetics is that it stimulates the cardiovascular system (i.e., raises heart rate and blood pressure). This action appears to result from both direct stimulation of the CNS with increased sympathetic nervous system outflow and blockade of norepinephrine reuptake in adrenergic nerves.

Because pulmonary hypertension is a characteristic feature of acute respiratory distress syndrome (ARDS), drugs that increase right ventricular afterload should be avoided. In infants with either normal or elevated pulmonary vascular resistance, ketamine does not affect pulmonary vascular resistance as long as constant ventilation is maintained, a finding also confirmed in adults.

Cerebral blood flow does not change when ketamine is injected into cerebral vessels. In mechanically ventilated pigs with artificially produced intracranial hypertension in which ICP is on the shoulder of the compliance curve, 0.5 to 2.0 mg per kg IV ketamine does not raise ICP; likewise, in mechanically ventilated preterm infants, 2 mg per kg IV ketamine does not increase anterior fontanelle pressure, an indirect monitor of ICP [31,32]. Unlike propofol and etomidate however, ketamine does not lower cerebral metabolic rate. It is relatively contraindicated in patients with an intracranial mass, with increased ICP, or who have suffered recent head trauma.

Adverse Effects

Psychologic. Emergence phenomena following ketamine anesthesia have been described as floating sensations, vivid dreams (pleasant or unpleasant), hallucinations, and delirium. These effects are more common in patients older than 16 years, in females, after short operative procedures, after large doses (>2 mg per kg IV), and after rapid administration (>40 mg per minute). Pre- or concurrent treatment with benzodiazepines or propofol usually minimizes or prevents these phenomena [33].

Cardiovascular. Because ketamine increases myocardial oxygen consumption, there is risk of precipitating myocardial ischemia in patients with coronary artery disease if ketamine is used alone. On the other hand, combinations of ketamine plus diazepam, ketamine plus midazolam, or ketamine plus sufentanil are well tolerated for induction in patients undergoing coronary artery bypass surgery. Repeated bolus doses are often associated with tachycardia. This can be reduced by administering ketamine as a constant infusion.

Ketamine produces myocardial depression in the isolated animal heart. Hypotension has been reported following ketamine administration in hemodynamically compromised patients with chronic catecholamine depletion.

Neurologic. Ketamine does not lower the minimal electroshock seizure threshold in mice. When administered with aminophylline, however, a clinically apparent reduction in seizure threshold is observed.

Midazolam

Description. Although capable of inducing unconsciousness in high doses, midazolam is more commonly used as a sedative. Along with its sedating effects, midazolam produces anxiolysis, amnesia, and relaxation of skeletal muscle.

Anterograde amnesia following midazolam (5 mg IV) peaks 2 to 5 minutes after IV injection and lasts 20 to 40 minutes. Because midazolam is highly (95%) protein bound (to albumin), drug effect is likely to be exaggerated in ICU patients. Recovery from midazolam is prolonged in obese and elderly patients and following continuous infusion because it accumulates to a significant degree. In patients with renal failure, active conjugated metabolites of midazolam may accumulate and delay recovery. Although flumazenil may be used to reverse excessive sedation or respiratory depression from midazolam, its duration of action is only 15 to 20 minutes. In addition, flumazenil may precipitate acute anxiety reactions or seizures, particularly in patients receiving chronic benzodiazepine therapy.

Midazolam causes dose-dependent reductions in cerebral metabolic rate and cerebral blood flow, suggesting that it may be beneficial in patients with cerebral ischemia.

Because of its combined sedative, anxiolytic, and amnestic properties, midazolam is ideally suited for both brief, relatively painless procedures (e.g., endoscopy) and prolonged sedation (e.g., during mechanical ventilation).

Adverse Effects

Respiratory. Midazolam (0.15 mg per kg IV) depresses the slope of the carbon dioxide response curve and increases the dead space–tidal volume ratio and arterial P_{CO_2}. Respiratory depression is even more marked and prolonged in patients with chronic obstructive pulmonary disease (COPD). Midazolam also blunts the ventilatory response to hypoxia.

Cardiovascular. Small (<10%) increases in heart rate and small decreases in systemic vascular resistance are frequently observed after administration of midazolam. It has no significant effects on coronary vascular resistance or autoregulation.

Neurologic. Because recovery of cognitive and psychomotor function may be delayed for up to 24 hours, midazolam as the sole hypnotic may not be appropriate in situations where rapid return of consciousness and psychomotor function are a high priority.

Opioids

Morphine

Description. Pain relief by morphine and its surrogates is relatively selective in that other sensory modalities (touch, vibration, vision, and hearing) are not obtunded. Opioids blunt pain by (i) inhibiting pain processing by the dorsal horn of the spinal cord, (ii) decreasing transmission of pain by activating descending inhibitory pathways in the brain stem, and (iii) altering the emotional response to pain by actions on the limbic cortex.

Various types of opioid receptors (denoted by Greek letters) have been discovered in the CNS. The classical pharmacologic effects of morphine such as analgesia and ventilatory depression are mediated by μ-receptors. Other μ-effects include sedation, euphoria, tolerance and physical dependence, decreased gastrointestinal motility, biliary spasm, and miosis. The κ-receptor shares a number of effects with the μ-receptor, including analgesia, sedation, and ventilatory depression. The δ-receptor is responsible for mediating some of the analgesic effects of the endogenous opioid peptides, especially in the spinal cord. Few of the clinically used opioids have significant activity at δ-receptors at the usual analgesic doses.

Morphine is a substrate for the P-glycoprotein, a protein responsible for the transport of many molecules out of cells. The combination of slow CNS penetration due to lower lipid solubility and rapid efflux accounts for the slow onset of morphine's CNS effects. Peak analgesic effects may not occur for more than an hour after IV injection; hence, the plasma profile of morphine does not parallel its clinical effects [34].

Morphine is unique among the opioids in causing significant histamine release after IV injection that occurs almost immediately. The beneficial effect of giving morphine to a patient with acute pulmonary edema is far more related to this hemodynamic effect rather than to its analgesic and sedating effects.

Adverse Effects

Gastrointestinal. Constipation, nausea, and/or vomiting are well-described side effects of morphine administration. Reduced gastric emptying and bowel motility (both small and large intestines), often leading to adynamic ileus, appear to be mediated both peripherally (by opioid receptors located in the gut) and centrally (by the vagus nerve).

Cardiovascular. Hypotension is not unusual following morphine administration, especially if it is given rapidly (i.e., 5 to 10 mg per minute). In patients pretreated with both H_1- and H_2-antagonists, the hypotensive response following morphine administration is significantly attenuated, despite comparable increases in plasma histamine concentrations. These data strongly implicate histamine as the mediator of these changes.

Respiratory. Morphine administration is followed by a dose-dependent reduction in responsiveness of brain stem respiratory centers to carbon dioxide. Key features of this phenomenon include a reduction in the slope of the ventilatory and occlusion pressure responses to carbon dioxide, a rightward shift of the minute ventilatory response to hypercarbia, and an increase in resting end-tidal carbon dioxide and the apneic threshold (i.e., the P_{CO_2} value below which spontaneous ventilation is not initiated without hypoxemia). The duration of these effects often exceeds the time course of analgesia. In addition to blunting the carbon dioxide response, morphine decreases hypoxic ventilatory drive. Morphine administration in patients with renal failure has been associated with prolonged respiratory depression secondary to persistence of its active metabolite, morphine-6-glucuronide [35].

The administration of small doses of IV naloxone (40 μg) to patients in order to reverse the ventilatory depressant effect of morphine may produce some adverse effects. Anecdotal reports describe the precipitation of vomiting, delirium, arrhythmias, pulmonary edema, cardiac arrest, and sudden death subsequent to naloxone administration in otherwise healthy patients after surgery. Furthermore, the duration of action of naloxone is shorter than any of the opioids it may be used to antagonize (except remifentanil). Recurring ventilatory depression therefore remains a distinct possibility, and in the spontaneously breathing patient, it is a source of potential morbidity.

Reversal with a mixed opioid agonist–antagonist agent such as nalbuphine or butorphanol appears to be safer than with naloxone. Mixed opioid agonist–antagonist agents may either increase or decrease the opioid effect, depending on the dose administered, the particular agonist already present, and the amount of agonist remaining.

For bedside procedures in the ICU, many of these problems can be obviated by using a shorter acting opioid.

Neurologic. Morphine has little effect on cerebral metabolic rate or cerebral blood flow when ventilation is controlled. Morphine may affect cerebral perfusion pressure adversely by lowering mean arterial pressure.

Fentanyl and Its Congeners

Description. Fentanyl, sufentanil, and remifentanil enter and leave the CNS much more rapidly than does morphine, thereby causing a much faster onset of effect after IV administration. The only significant difference among these agents is their PK behavior.

Fentanyl may be useful when given by intermittent bolus injection (50 to 100 μg), but when given by infusion, its duration becomes prolonged [36]. For TIVA in ICU patients in whom rapid emergence is desirable, sufentanil or remifentanil is the preferred choice for continuous infusion. When the procedure is expected to be followed by postoperative pain, sufentanil is preferred. Figure 20.2 shows that its CSHT is similar to that of propofol for infusions of up to 10 hours. When the procedure is expected to be followed by minimal postoperative pain (e.g., bronchoscopy), remifentanil is preferred. Its CSHT is about 4 minutes regardless of the duration of the infusion.

Remifentanil owes its extremely short duration to rapid metabolism by tissue esterases, primarily in skeletal muscle [37]. Its PK behavior is unchanged in the presence of severe hepatic [38] or renal [39] failure.

Sufentanil infusion for TIVA may be initiated with a 0.5 to 1.5 μg per kg bolus followed by an infusion at 0.01 to 0.03 μg per kg per minute. If given with a propofol infusion, the two infusions may be stopped simultaneously as governed by the curves in Figure 20.2. Remifentanil infusion for TIVA may be initiated with a 0.5 to 1.5 μg per kg bolus followed by an infusion at 0.05 to 0.5 μg per kg per minute. The remifentanil infusion should be continued until after the procedure is completed; if the patient is expected to have postoperative pain, another opioid should be given because the remifentanil effect will dissipate within a few minutes.

Adverse Effects

Cardiovascular. Although fentanyl, sufentanil, and remifentanil do not affect plasma histamine concentrations, bolus doses can be associated with hypotension, especially when infused rapidly (i.e., <1 minute). This action is related to medullary vasomotor center depression and vagal nucleus stimulation.

Neurologic. Fentanyl and sufentanil have been reported to increase ICP in ventilated patients following head trauma. They may adversely affect cerebral perfusion pressure by lowering mean arterial pressure. All of the fentanyl derivatives may cause chest wall rigidity when a large bolus is given rapidly. This effect may be mitigated by neuromuscular blocking (NMB) agents as well as by coadministration of a hypnotic agent.

NEUROMUSCULAR BLOCKING AGENTS

There are two pharmacologic classes of NMB agents (see Chapter 25): depolarizing agents (e.g., succinylcholine) and nondepolarizing agents (e.g., vecuronium and cisatracurium). Succinylcholine is an agonist at the nicotinic acetylcholine receptor of the neuromuscular junction. Administration of succinylcholine causes an initial intense stimulation of skeletal muscle, manifested as fasciculations, followed by paralysis due to continuing depolarization. Nondepolarizing agents are competitive antagonists of acetylcholine at the neuromuscular junction; they prevent acetylcholine, released in response to motor nerve impulses, from binding to its receptor and initiating muscle contraction. Distinctions among the nondepolarizing agents are made on the basis of PK differences as well as by their cardiovascular effects.

NMB agents are used to facilitate endotracheal intubation and improve surgical conditions by decreasing skeletal muscle tone. Prior to intubation, the administration of an NMB agent results in paralysis of the vocal cords, increasing the ease with which the endotracheal tube may be inserted and decreasing the risk of vocal cord trauma. During surgery, the decrease in skeletal muscle tone may aid in surgical exposure (as during abdominal surgery), decrease the insufflation pressure needed during laparoscopic procedures, and make joint manipulation easier during orthopedic surgery. NMB agents should *not* be used to prevent patient movement, which is indicative of inadequate anesthesia. Dosing of NMB agents should be based on monitoring evoked twitch response; ablation of two to three twitches of the train-of-four is sufficient for the majority of surgical procedures and permits easy reversal.

PRACTICAL CONSIDERATIONS FOR TIVA

Electing to perform common procedures (e.g., tracheostomy and percutaneous gastrostomy) in the ICU instead of the operating room represents a potential cost saving of tremendous scope. Not only does this strategy eradicate costly operating room time and support resources, it eliminates misadventures that sometimes occur in hallways and on elevators. Cost analyses estimate an average overall cost reduction of 50% or more compared with traditional operative procedures [40]. TIVA represents the most cost-effective method of facilitating this.

In most patients, safe and effective TIVA may be achieved via the infusions of propofol plus sufentanil or propofol plus remifentanil. Premedication with midazolam decreases the required propofol doses and decreases the likelihood of recall for intraoperative events. Bolus doses should not be used in hemodynamically unstable patients, and lower bolus doses should be used in elderly individuals. NMB agents are also given if needed.

The opioid infusion rate is titrated to minimize signs of inadequate analgesia (e.g., tachycardia, tachypnea, hypertension, sweating, and mydriasis), although differentiation of pain from the sympathetic responses to critical illness is difficult. The propofol infusion rate is titrated to the endpoint of loss of consciousness; the depth of anesthesia monitors that are based on analysis of the electroencephalogram waveform (bispectral index (BIS), patient state index (PSI), or spectral entropy) facilitate locating this endpoint more accurately. Loss of consciousness should be achieved prior to the initiation of muscle paralysis. It is possible for patients to be completely aware of intraoperative events at times when there is no change in hemodynamics or any manifestation of increased sympathetic activity [41,42]. Hence, administering an opioid to blunt incisional pain without inducing loss of consciousness with a hypnotic is inappropriate.

The following additional points deserve consideration in this context:

1. In subhypnotic doses, propofol is less effective than midazolam in producing amnesia. In the absence of coadministration of a benzodiazepine, propofol must cause unconsciousness in order to reliably prevent recall. Prompt treatment of patient responses (movement, tachycardia, and hypertension) is important.
2. Medications infused for TIVA should be given via a carrier IV fluid running continuously at a rate of at least 50 mL per hour. This method not only helps deliver medication into the circulation, but also serves as another monitor of occlusion of the drug delivery system. Occlusion of the infusion line for more than a few minutes may lead to patient awareness.
3. To take advantage of the known CSHT values for the TIVA agents, communication with the surgeon during the procedure is important in order to anticipate the optimum time for stopping the infusions. The sufentanil and propofol infusions are stopped in advance of the end of the procedure, whereas remifentanil is infused until the procedure is complete.
4. To maintain reasonably constant propofol and sufentanil blood concentrations, the maintenance infusion rates should be decreased during the procedure because the plasma concentrations increase over time at constant infusion rates. An approximate guideline is a 10% reduction in infusion rate every 30 minutes.
5. Strict aseptic technique is important especially during the handling of propofol.

References

1. Shafer SL, Varvel JR, Aziz N, et al: Pharmacokinetics of fentanyl administered by computer-controlled infusion pump. *Anesthesiology* 73:1091, 1990.
2. Vesey CJ, Sweeney B, Cole PV: Decay of nitroprusside. II: in vivo. *Br J Anaesth* 64:704, 1990.
3. Hughes MA, Glass PS, Jacobs JR: Context-sensitive half-time in multicompartment pharmacokinetic models for intravenous anesthetic drugs. *Anesthesiology* 76:334, 1992.
4. Shafer A, Doze VA, Shafer SL: Pharmacokinetics and pharmacodynamics of propofol infusions during general anesthesia. *Anesthesiology* 69:348, 1988.
5. Persson P, Nilsson A, Hartvig P, et al: Pharmacokinetics of midazolam in total i.v. anaesthesia. *Br J Anaesth* 59:548, 1987.
6. Hudson RJ, Bergstrom RG, Thomson IR, et al: Pharmacokinetics of sufentanil in patients undergoing abdominal aortic surgery. *Anesthesiology* 70:426, 1989.
7. Egan TD, Lemmens HJ, Fiset P, et al: The pharmacokinetics of the new short acting opioid remifentanil (GI87084B) in healthy adult male volunteers. *Anesthesiology* 79:881, 1993.
8. Koch-Weser J, Sellers EM: Binding of drugs to serum albumin. *N Engl J Med* 294:311, 1976.
9. Mangano DT, Browner WS, Hollenberg M: Association of perioperative myocardial ischemia with cardiac morbidity and mortality in men undergoing noncardiac surgery. *N Engl J Med* 323:1781, 1990.
10. Barr J, Egan TD, Sandoval NF, et al: Propofol dosing regimens for ICU sedation based upon an integrated pharmacokinetic-pharmacodynamic model. *Anesthesiology* 95:324, 2001.
11. Ronan KP, Gallagher TH, Hamby BG: Comparison of propofol and midazolam for sedation in intensive care unit patients. *Crit Care Med* 23:286, 1995.
12. Pagel PS, Warltier DC: Negative inotropic effects of propofol as evaluated by the regional preload recruitable stroke work relationship in chronically instrumented dogs. *Anesthesiology* 78:100, 1993.
13. Pagel PS, Schmeling WT, Kampine JP, et al: Alteration of canine left ventricular diastolic function by intravenous anesthetics in vivo: ketamine and propofol. *Anesthesiology* 76:419, 1992.
14. Mayer N, Legat K, Weinstabl C, et al: Effects of propofol on the function of normal, collateral-dependent, and ischemic myocardium. *Anesth Analg* 76:33, 1993.
15. Van Hemelrijck J, Fitch W, Mattheussen M, et al: Effect of propofol on cerebral circulation and autoregulation in baboons. *Anesth Analg* 71:49, 1990.
16. Gibiansky E, Struys MM, Gibiansky L, et al: Aquavan® injection, a water-soluble prodrug of propofol, as a bolus injection: a phase I dose-escalation comparison with Diprivan® (Part 1). *Anesthesiology* 103:718, 2005.
17. Struys MM, Vanluchene AL, Gibiansky E, et al: Aquavan® injection, a water-soluble prodrug of propofol, as a bolus injection: a phase I dose-escalation comparison with Diprivan® (Part 2). *Anesthesiology* 103:730, 2005.
18. Goading JM, Wang JT, Smith RA, et al: Cardiovascular and pulmonary responses following etomidate induction of anesthesia in patients with demonstrated cardiac disease. *Anesth Analg* 58:40, 1979.
19. Ledingham IM, Finlay WEI, Watt I, et al: Etomidate and adrenocortical function. *Lancet* 1:1434, 1983.
20. Fragen RJ, Shanks CA, Molteni A, et al: Effects of etomidate on hormonal responses to surgical stress. *Anesthesiology* 61:652, 1984.
21. Jackson WJ: Should we use etomidate as an induction agent for endotracheal intubation in patients with septic shock? A critical appraisal. *Chest* 127:1031, 2005.
22. Mohammad Z, Afessa B, Finkielman JD: The incidence of relative adrenal insufficiency in patients with septic shock after the administration of etomidate. *Crit Care* 10:R105, 2006.
23. Cotton BA, Guillamondegui OD, Fleming SB, et al: Increased risk of adrenal insufficiency following etomidate exposure in critically injured patients. *Arch Surg* 143:62, 2008.
24. Tekwani KL, Watts HF, Chan CW, et al: The effect of single-bolus etomidate on septic patient mortality: a retrospective review. *West J Emerg Med* 9:195, 2008.
25. Cuthbertson BH, Sprung CL, Annane D, et al: The effects of etomidate on adrenal responsiveness and mortality in patients with septic shock. *Intensive Care Med* 35:1868, 2009.
26. Ray DC, McKeown DW: Effect of induction agent on vasopressor and steroid use, and outcome in patients with septic shock. *Crit Care* 11:R56, 2007.
27. de Jong MF, Beishuizen A, Spijkstra JJ, et al: Predicting a low cortisol response to adrenocorticotrophic hormone in the critically ill: a retrospective cohort study. *Crit Care* 11:R61, 2007.
28. Riché FC, Boutron CM, Valleur P, et al: Adrenal response in patients with septic shock of abdominal origin: relationship to survival. *Intensive Care Med* 33:1761, 2007.
29. Tekwani KL, Watts HF, Rzechula KH, et al: A prospective observational study of the effect of etomidate on septic patient mortality and length of stay. *Acad Emerg Med* 16:11, 2009.
30. Jabre P, Combes X, Lapostolle F, et al: Etomidate versus ketamine for rapid sequence intubation in acutely ill patients: a multicentre randomised controlled trial. *Lancet* 374:293, 2009.
31. Pfenninger E, Dick W, Ahnefeld FW: The influence of ketamine on both normal and raised intracranial pressure of artificially ventilated animals. *Eur J Anaesthesiol* 2:297, 1985.
32. Friesen RH, Thieme RE, Honda AT, et al: Changes in anterior fontanel pressure in preterm neonates receiving isoflurane, halothane, fentanyl, or ketamine. *Anesth Analg* 66:431, 1987.
33. White PF: Pharmacologic interactions of midazolam and ketamine in surgical patients. *Clin Pharmacol Ther* 31:280, 1982.
34. Dershwitz M, Walsh JL, Morishige RJ, et al: Pharmacokinetics and pharmacodynamics of inhaled versus intravenous morphine in healthy volunteers. *Anesthesiology* 93:619, 2000.
35. Aitkenhead AR, Vater M, Achola K, et al: Pharmacokinetics of single-dose intravenous morphine in normal volunteers and patients with end-stage renal failure. *Br J Anaesth* 56:813, 1984.
36. Shafer SL, Varvel JR: Pharmacokinetics, pharmacodynamics, and rational opioid selection. *Anesthesiology* 74:53, 1991.
37. Dershwitz M, Rosow CE: Remifentanil: an opioid metabolized by esterases. *Exp Opin Invest Drugs* 5:1361, 1996.
38. Dershwitz M, Hoke JF, Rosow CE, et al: Pharmacokinetics and pharmacodynamics of remifentanil in volunteer subjects with severe liver disease. *Anesthesiology* 84:812, 1996.
39. Hoke JF, Shlugman D, Dershwitz M, et al: Pharmacokinetics and pharmacodynamics of remifentanil in subjects with renal failure compared to healthy volunteers. *Anesthesiology* 87:533, 1997.
40. Barba CA, Angood PB, Kauder DR, et al: Bronchoscopic guidance makes percutaneous tracheostomy a safe, cost effective, and easy to teach procedure. *Surgery* 118:879, 1995.
41. Ausems ME, Hug CC Jr, Stanski DR, et al: Plasma concentrations of alfentanil required to supplement nitrous oxide anesthesia for general surgery. *Anesthesiology* 65:362, 1986.
42. Philbin DM, Rosow CE, Schneider RC, et al: Fentanyl and sufentanil anesthesia revisited: How much is enough? *Anesthesiology* 73:5, 1990.

CHAPTER 21 ■ INTERVENTIONAL ULTRASOUND

GISELA I. BANAUCH AND PAUL H. MAYO

INTRODUCTION

Ultrasonography has major applications in critical care medicine. When used at the bedside by the intensivist who is in charge of the clinical management of the case, it allows for immediate diagnosis and management decisions to be made at the point of care. Bedside, intensivist-performed ultrasound differs substantially from standard radiology or cardiology performed ultrasonography in that the intensivist acquires the image, interprets the image, and promptly applies the results to the clinical situation. This avoids the time delay and clinical disassociation implicit to ultrasonography that is performed on a consultative basis by radiology or cardiology services.

The scope of practice of critical care ultrasonography encompasses those aspects of the discipline that have utility to diagnosis and management of the critically ill patient. A summary of the important elements that are required for competence in the field have been presented in a recent consensus statement [1]. Ultrasonography may be divided into two general categories of application in critical care management: (i) to guide diagnosis and management and (ii) for purposes of procedural guidance. The two are often related. For example, ultrasonography may be used to diagnose a pleural effusion. Ultrasonography is then used to guide thoracentesis, which in turn is useful in identifying the cause of the pleural effusion and therefore its management. This chapter reviews the use of ultrasonography for procedural guidance in the intensive care unit (ICU). For detailed review of critical care ultrasonography, the reader is referred to comprehensive texts on the subject [2,3].

A major responsibility of the intensivist is to safely perform a wide variety of invasive procedures that may be associated with significant complications. The proceduralist has a specific target, such as a vascular structure or body compartment (e.g., pleural, peritoneal, or pericardial), and seeks to avoid injury to adjacent structures while assuring accurate placement of the needle. Inaccurate placement of the needle may injure adjacent structures with potential major morbidity or even life-threatening complication, as well as lead to failure of either diagnostic effort or essential vascular or body cavity access.

This discussion assumes that the reader is fully trained in physical tasks of the procedure (proper sterile technique, needle manipulation, wire insertion, dilation etc.). These are reviewed in other chapters of this text specific to each procedure. Ultrasonography is used to augment the safety and success rate of the operator who is fully competent in the mechanical aspects of the procedure.

The use of ultrasonography for procedural guidance is based on a simple principle. The safety and success of needle insertion is augmented by the ability to image the target; to identify and therefore avoid adjacent structures; and if required, to guide real-time needle insertion. The alternative is to rely on off-line analysis of standard radiography images and/or on landmark technique. Intuitively, ultrasound guidance is an attractive alternative to traditional technique. It is now in widespread use in the critical care community. This chapter reviews the use of ultrasonography for the guidance of a variety of procedures that are commonly performed by the intensivist.

GENERAL PRINCIPLES

1. To maximize the utility of ultrasonography, the operator should have basic knowledge of ultrasound physics, machine control, transducer manipulation, image acquisition, ultrasound anatomy, image orientation, and image interpretation. In addition, the intensivist must have full capability in all the mechanical aspects of the procedure.
2. The machine should be carefully positioned such that the operator may view the screen and the procedure site without untoward head movement; this often requires rearrangement of cluttered equipment that typically surrounds the patient bed in the critical care unit. Machine position for ergonomic efficiency is particularly important when using ultrasonography for real-time image-guided needle insertion. Room lighting and angle of the ultrasound machine's screen should be adjusted to minimize screen glare. Before starting the procedure, machine settings should be set for optimal image quality with attention to gain, depth, and image orientation. Many modern machines are designed such that the structure of interest is best visualized if it is placed in the center of the screen. Some machines have automated image optimization software so that the operator does not need to adjust controls beyond pushing a single control button. The resulting image may not, in fact, be optimal, and it may need further readjustment.
3. In situations where real-time guidance is required (e.g., vascular access) or when there is need for scanning while maintaining a sterile field, ultrasound procedure guidance requires that the operator use a purpose-designed sterile probe cover. The use of covers made from sterile gloves or sterile intravenous skin covers is strongly discouraged. They frequently fail during the procedure, while the operator's attention is focused on the sonographic image or on needle direction and insertion on the sterile field. Well-designed sterile transducer covers are low cost and come with sterile ultrasound coupling medium.
4. By standard convention, guidance of thoracic, abdominal, and vascular procedures requires that the screen orientation marker be placed on the left of the screen. Guidance of procedures related to the heart, such as pericardiocentesis or transvenous pacemaker insertion, is performed with the screen orientation marker placed on the right of the screen. This convention relates purely to common usage patterns. When scanning from the head of the patient, as with internal jugular venous (IJV) access, the operator needs to decide on how to orient the screen marker in reference to the transducer. We suggest that the orientation marker be

on the left of the screen and that the corresponding marker on the transducer always be held such that it is pointed toward the left side of the examiner (unless scanning the vessel in longitudinal axis when the transducer marker is directed cephalad). It is important to understand and standardize orientation and transducer marker position so that the operator can direct the needle in predictable fashion during real-time guidance of needle insertion.

5. Whenever planning an ultrasound-guided procedure, the operator should explore the structure of interest before prepping and draping the patient. This allows for optimal site selection before site preparation. If the procedure aims to cannulate a vessel (e.g., central venous or arterial catheterization), the potential target should be evaluated on both sides of the body unless absolute contraindications exist on one side (e.g., arteriovenous fistula in the upper extremity would preclude radial arterial catheterization on that side). Multiple studies have documented significant anatomic variability in vascular lumina, positioning, and location with respect to adjacent structures for both venous and arterial targets [4–9].
6. Initially, vascular structures should be imaged in their transverse axis, as this approach is best to differentiate the artery and the vein [10]. Features such as compressibility, pulsation, luminal variation with respiratory effort, and/or respiratory maneuvers can all be used to help distinguish arterial from venous vessels. The cross-sectional ultrasonographic view usually displays the vein in close proximity to its accompanying artery, thus facilitating comparison of vessel changes with dynamic maneuvers, such as compression and Valsalva. Detection of vessel pulsatility requires a steady imaging plane for at least a few seconds. Pulsatility is sometimes diminished with hypotension. Differentiation of arterial from venous structures is challenging especially when the patient's perfusion is maintained with a nonpulsatile ventricular assist device (impeller device). The much less compressible, thicker arterial walls, as well as the lack of vessel lumen variability with respiratory effort and/or respiratory maneuvers, provide the most reliable features that differentiate arterial from venous structures in this situation. Color and spectral Doppler analysis may occasionally be required to distinguish the vein from the artery in situations of difficult anatomy or in the subclavian position.
7. For pleural or abdominal access, initial orientation should always be achieved in the longitudinal image plane. The variable position of the diaphragm in the critically ill patient makes is easiest to differentiate intrathoracic from intra-abdominal fluid collections using longitudinal image planes.
8. Whenever possible, the operator should document relevant ultrasound images during the procedure. This may be as simple as capturing a frozen video image that can be placed in the chart. Depending on system capability, video clips may be captured and stored off line. Image documentation is important for quality review and billing purposes. However, it may not be practical in all situations, particularly during hectic resuscitation efforts.
9. Ultrasound guidance of procedures requires specific training. The cognitive aspects of the field are straightforward, and can be easily learned from books, audiovisual sources, courses, or via e-learning program. Image interpretation and acquisition require a component of hands on scanning under the supervision of a skilled bedside instructor. Real-time guidance of needle insertion is a complex psychomotor skill that requires practice. Unfortunately, this is often achieved with the experiential approach; that is, the inexperienced operator is expected to perform the procedure the first time on an actual patient. To avoid this, we strongly recommend that training in real-time needle insertion take place on an ultrasound manikin. Ultrasound-capable vascular access manikins of excellent design are now commercially available [11]. Trainees may practice ultrasound control of the needle and targeted vascular access multiple times before their first effort at the patient bedside. This is imperative for patient safety and comfort as well as for operator confidence.

Ultrasound Guidance of Vascular Access

Vascular access is a major responsibility of the intensivist. Insertion of catheters of varying size and function requires central venous cannulation, accurate ongoing measurement of arterial pressure and waveform requires arterial line insertion, whereas peripheral venous (PV) access is a routine requirement of patient care. Considerations such as obesity or unusual body habitus (e.g., kyphoscoliosis or genetic disease) and coagulopathy may present special challenges. PV access may be difficult in patients due to obesity, intravenous drug use, or chemotherapy. Ultrasound is uniquely useful for guidance of all forms of vascular access.

A benefit of ultrasound guidance of vascular access is that it allows the operator to identify contraindications to vascular access that are not apparent by simple physical examination. For example, marked respiratory effort may completely obliterate internal jugular and subclavian vein lumina during inspiration in the volume-depleted patient. Such intermittent luminal collapse precludes successful vascular access and cannot be identified, except with ultrasonography. The presence of a thrombus in the femoral vein (FV) frequently cannot be detected by physical examination, but it is readily identified ultrasonographically and contraindicates cannulation at that site. Ultrasonography thus warns the operator to redirect attention to less complication-prone sites.

SPECIFIC PROCEDURES

Internal Jugular Venous Access

Several studies report that ultrasound guidance of IJV access is superior to landmark technique, with lower complication and higher success rate [12]. The reasons for this are obvious. Landmark technique may be straightforward in a slender subject, but much less so in an obese subject. Asymmetric IJV size and variation in IJV position relative to the carotid occur in up to 30% of the normal population and cannot be appreciated by surface physical examination [13,14]. A national quality organization has stated that ultrasound guidance of IJV access is required for patient safety purposes [15]. The Residency Review Committee has stated that training in this technique is highly recommended during critical care fellowship training; this will likely be followed by it becoming a mandatory requirement.

In guiding IJV access, ultrasonography should be used in a methodical fashion in order to maximize its utility as follows:

1. Vascular access requires the use of a linear ultrasound transducer typically of 7.5 MHz frequency. This allows for adequate resolution of structures that are relatively near the surface of the body. Lower frequency transducers, which penetrate more deeply at the cost of reduced resolution, are not suitable for guidance of vascular access. The patient should be placed in Trendelenburg in order to distend the vein as much as possible.
2. The operator should perform a preliminary scan of both sides of the neck before the sterile preparation. This allows for identification of aberrant anatomy and/or thrombus, and determination of the best site, angle, and depth of needle penetration. The IJV is usually lateral to the carotid

artery when scanning the anterior neck, and is differentiated from the carotid artery by its larger size, thin wall, and lack of characteristic pulsation, easy compressibility, size fluctuation with respiration or respiratory maneuvers, and the presence of thin mobile venous valves. Color Doppler may be used to confirm, but it is not generally required. The examination of the vein starts with a two-dimensional (2-D) study to examine the anatomy and observe for visible echogenic thrombus. The 2-D examination is followed by compression of the vessel to exclude isoechoic thrombus not visible on 2-D imaging. A fully compressible IJV indicates that there is no thrombus at the site of the examination. In order to ensure patency of the vessel along the length that will be traversed by the central venous catheter, several sites along the course of the vessel must be examined and then compressed. The presence of an ipsilateral thrombus contraindicates line insertion, whereas the presence of a contralateral thrombus is of concern, as the proposed IJV insertion may itself predispose to thrombus. This may yield bilateral IJV thrombus, which is undesirable.

3. The preprocedure scan should include examination of the anterior lung (with the patient in supine position) in order to rule out pneumothorax *before* the procedure. The transducer is held perpendicular to the chest wall in order to examine the rib interspaces of the upper anterior chest. The pleural interface is identified between the rib shadows. Presence of lung sliding, lung pulse, or B-lines rules out pneumothorax with a high level of certainty [16]. The examination may be accomplished with similar result, using a low-frequency abdominal or cardiac transducer, or using a high-frequency vascular transducer that is used to guide vascular access. Following the procedure, the operator again examines the anterior chest for pneumothorax. The finding of pneumothorax following the procedure, when none existed before, is strong evidence for procedural mishap. The preprocedure chest examination should include both lungs to cover the very rare eventuality that the patient has a contralateral pneumothorax before the procedure.
4. Before the sterile field is established, the ultrasound machine must be positioned to allow optimal hand–eye coordination for the operator. Because the operator normally stands on the side of the IJV to be cannulated, next to the patient's head and facing the patient's feet, the optimal position for the ultrasound machine is on the operator's side of the patient, immediately adjacent to the patient's lower chest or upper abdomen. Inadequate placement of the ultrasound screen makes efficient hand–eye coordination very difficult. With an inappropriately placed ultrasound screen, the operator needs to rotate his or her head in order to compare changes in the ultrasound image with changes in needle insertion depth and angle. With a well-placed ultrasound screen, the operator needs to only move his or her head up or down in order to compare ultrasonographic image changes with changes in needle angle and insertion depth on the sterile field. The chance of accidentally changing the ultrasonographic imaging plane (thus losing the ultrasound image essential for real-time guidance) during head rotation is much greater than the chance of an inadvertent change in scanning plane during a simple up-and-down movement of the head.
5. Following preliminary scanning and appropriate placement of the ultrasound unit, the patient is prepared with standard sterile technique. The transducer is covered with a purpose-designed sterile transducer cover. The operator has a choice at this point. A helper may hold the transducer while the operator introduces the needle, or the operator may hold the transducer in one hand while guiding the needle with the other. The latter is the preferred technique. The ability to manipulate the transducer and needle in tandem is advantageous. A variation of ultrasound guidance of vascular access is the "mark-and-stick" technique wherein the operator identifies the vessel and marks an appropriate site for line insertion. The needle is introduced without the benefit of real-time guidance. Although this yields higher success rate than traditional landmark method, it is inferior to real-time guidance [12] and so is not discussed further.
6. The operator needs to decide whether to use transverse or longitudinal scanning plane for real-time needle guidance. This is based on personal preference and training background. Some skilled operators prefer longitudinal approach, as they maintain that it is easier to identify the needle in long axis and therefore to guide it into the vessel. Many operators prefer the transverse plane. In either case, maximal safety is achieved by maintaining clear identification of the needle tip throughout the procedure [17].
7. There are two general approaches to real-time guidance in the transverse scanning plane. The first, which is conceptually easier, is to insert the needle very close to the transducer and angle down toward the vessel, with the goal of identifying the needle tip as it enters the scanning plane and the vessel. This technique results in a very acute angle at which the vessel is accessed, which sometimes makes it difficult to thread the guidewire. Alternatively, the needle may be introduced at some distance from the target vessel. The transducer is then moved toward the needle until the needle tip is identified. The transducer and needle tip are then moved forward in tandem, with the needle tip adjusted at the appropriate angle. In this manner, visual control of the needle tip is maintained throughout its forward movement. In addition, the angle at which the vessel is accessed tends to be less acute, making it easier to thread the guidewire. With the longitudinal scanning method, the transducer is used to obtain a longitudinal image of the target vessel. The needle is introduced along the longitudinal midline of the transducer and kept in full view while it is moved toward the vessel wall. The longitudinal approach tends to result in the least acute angle at which the vessel is accessed, making it easiest to thread the guidewire into the vessel successfully even when the vessel is located relatively far from the skin surface, for example, in the obese patient.
8. A vexing problem with IJV access is vessel compression. Under ultrasound guidance, the advancing needle may compress the anterior wall of the IJV, often to the extent that the vascular lumen is effaced. With further forward movement of the needle, it passes through the posterior wall of the vessel. Frequently, as the needle is slowly withdrawn, the vessel lumen opens up, blood enters the needle and syringe, and the wire is passed without problem. Whether minor needle insertion through the posterior wall has any clinical implication or not has not been determined. It may be avoided by downward orientation of the bevel and careful attention to angulation of the needle, as well as positioning the patient in Trendelenburg. Extensive head rotation or head extension and the presence of a laryngeal mask airway all reduce IJV diameter and move the vein into a position anterior to the carotid artery, thus increasing the risk of inadvertent arterial puncture [18–20].
9. Following wire insertion and before dilation of the vessel, the location of the wire in a venous vessel should be documented. This is best achieved in a longitudinal view of the vessel. If the wire is found to be in the artery (an occasional event, particularly with a less experienced operator), it may be removed without great consequence to the patient. However, inadvertent dilation of the carotid artery may have catastrophic effect. Positive identification of the wire within the vein adds only a short additional time to the procedure and avoids a rare, but dangerous, complication.

10. Generally, a postprocedure chest radiograph is used to document proper position of the venous catheter. Ultrasonography may be used as an alternative method [21]. Identification of suboptimal line position with ultrasonography allows repositioning while the sterile field is still in place, unlike a delayed chest radiograph. However, identification of line position with ultrasonography adds several minutes to the procedure and requires a high level of ultrasound training.
11. Following the procedure, the operator should examine the anterior chest in order to rule out procedure-related pneumothorax. The presence of sliding lung, lung pulse, and/or B-lines excludes pneumothorax. This underlines the importance of performing ultrasonography both *before* and *after* the procedure. The loss of lung sliding, lung pulse, and/or B-lines *following* IJV central venous access, when they were present immediately before the procedure, is strong evidence for a procedure-related pneumothorax. Ultrasonography is more accurate than standard supine chest radiography for the detection of pneumothorax, and has similar accuracy as chest computerized tomography [22].

Subclavian Venous Access

Ultrasonography may be used to guide SCV access [23,24]. The authors' opinion is that ultrasound guidance of SCV access may not augment safety or success in patients with normal anatomy. However, it does have utility in patients with challenging anatomy or coagulopathy. It also requires a higher skill level than IJV or FV access. It should only be used by the operator who has a high level of competence in real-time needle guidance. The pleural surface is in close proximity to the SCV and so accurate identification and precise control of the needle tip are required in order to avoid a pneumothorax. Many of the principles described for IJV insertion apply to the SCV. What follows are concerns that are specific to this site:

1. The SCV is more difficult to locate than the IJV. One strategy is to scan the upper chest with the transducer in longitudinal scanning plane in order to locate the clavicle. Once this is done, the transducer is moved laterally along the clavicle until the vessel is seen to appear from under the clavicle. Further lateral movement of the transducer will image the SCV independent of the clavicle. At this point, the transducer is rotated 90 degrees to obtain a long axis view of the vein. This is the appropriate orientation for real-time guidance of needle insertion. The subclavian artery is located immediately adjacent to the vein, and most often deep to it. Unfortunately, the vein may not be compressible due to anatomic constraint, so it may be challenging to differentiate the artery from the vein. Observation of respirophasic changes, venous valves, and the use of color and pulse wave Doppler all have utility in making the critical distinction between the two structures. It is difficult to visualize SCV thrombus, as compression study is often not possible. Lack of respirophasic changes and/or lack of color Doppler flow augmentation on compression of the ipsilateral arm suggest the possibility of thrombus.
2. In order to minimize operator head movement during the insertion, the ultrasound machine should be positioned immediately adjacent to the patient's axilla on the side that is contralateral to the side at which access will be attempted (e.g., adjacent to the patient's right axilla if the left SCV has been chosen for venous access).
3. Ultrasound guidance of SCV access should be performed with the vein imaged in its long axis so that the entire needle and its tip can be visualized real time throughout the insertion. Any loss of needle tip control runs the risk of pleural or arterial puncture. For the experienced landmark operator, ultrasound guidance of SCV access presents a psychologic challenge. The operator is so used to relying on the clavicle as a definitive structural guide during insertion that it is difficult to perform the access at a lateral site that ignores the clavicle landmark completely. More lateral puncture sites, however, are anatomically less risky for both arterial and pleural puncture, whereas vessel lumen is reduced only by 25% [25].
4. Because the puncture site of the subclavian vein is considerably more lateral for ultrasound-guided punctures compared to landmark-guided punctures, the tip of the central venous catheter may not reach to the superior vena cava when a short catheter is used. This is especially true when the left subclavian vein is used for access.
5. For safety purposes, the operator should use the same precautions as with the IJV insertion by checking for pneumothorax before and after the procedure and by documenting that the wire is within the vein before dilation. Unlike the IJV and FV, where wire identification is straightforward, identification of the wire in the subclavian vein may be difficult, as the clavicle may block easy identification. A useful technique is to image the ipsilateral IJV and follow it down to the medial supraclavicular area. Downward rotation of the probe reveals the confluence of the IJV and the SCV with wire identification.

Femoral Venous Access

Ultrasonography may be used to guide FV access [26], and has the same rationale as for the IJV. It reduces complication rate and improves success rate. It has particular utility in emergency situations that mandate immediate venous access. A trained operator can safely establish venous access very rapidly using ultrasound guidance. Many of the principles described for IJV insertion apply to the FV site. What follows are concerns that are specific to this site:

1. The safe site for FV access should be at the common femoral vein (CVF) level. Immediately below the inguinal crease, the FV rotates so that it is posterior to the artery (then becoming the superficial FV). Attempts at access at this level risk arterial injury. In the worst-case scenario, the needle passes through the artery into the vein. Following dilation, the catheter is passed through the artery and rests, as a fully functional venous line, in the vein. Subsequently, it is removed with no special precaution as the operator believes that it was a well-placed venous line. Major arterial bleeding ensues. Ultrasonography allows identification of the CFV in a position that is medial to the vein at a site close to the inguinal ligament. This is the appropriate site for needle puncture. The position of the vein remains side by side with the artery for a longer distance caudally if the leg is rotated externally (similar to optimal positioning for insertion using the landmark technique [27]).
2. Identification of the vein and artery is straightforward and is based on methods outlined in the discussion on IJV access. The vessel should be imaged in transverse plane and the needle guided into it under real-time ultrasound control. The wire should be documented within the vein before dilation.

Peripheral Venous Access

Ultrasound guidance for PV access improves success rates and reduces complications [28]. Site-specific considerations for ultrasound-guided PV insertion follow:

1. The operator must have knowledge of the complex venous anatomy of the upper extremity. Accessing PVs may be

performed using both cross-sectional and longitudinal scanning techniques. The advantage of the latter is that the needle is visualized along its entire length so that it may be guided accurately into a small venous structure.

Arterial Access

Principles for ultrasound guidance of arterial access are similar to those for ultrasound guidance of venous access. Particular points of importance for each arterial access site follow.

Radial Artery

Ultrasound-guided radial arterial cannulation has been shown to significantly increase success on the first attempt [29], and is especially valuable in hypotensive and grossly edematous patients. In the patient without edema, the artery is located quite superficially at the wrist. Color Doppler imaging can help in its identification. The artery is accompanied by two easily collapsible venous structures, the venae comitantes. Wrist extension beyond 60 degrees reduces vessel diameter, thus making cannulation more difficult [8].

Femoral Artery

Ultrasound guidance for femoral arterial access has been proved valuable in obese and hypotensive patients [30]. The technique is also of benefit in coagulopathic patients. In addition, ultrasound allows selection of a vessel site that is less affected by atherosclerotic changes, as well as permits prompt detection of complications due to catheterization, such as pseudoaneurysm, hematoma, or arteriovenous fistula [31,32].

Ultrasound Guidance of Pleural Access

Pleural fluid collections are frequently encountered in critically ill patients. Ultrasound guidance of thoracentesis reduces the risk of pneumothorax [33]. Ultrasound-guided thoracentesis is safe for patients on mechanical ventilatory support [34,35]. Ultrasound guidance for pleural access and device insertion should incorporate the following points:

1. Prior to establishing the sterile field, a comprehensive scan of the hemithorax should be undertaken with the aim of identifying a safe site, angle, and depth for needle insertion. It is of paramount importance that the operator's first action be a differentiation between peritoneal and retroperitoneal structures and pleural structures. This requires unequivocal identification of the diaphragm. In the intubated, sedated patient, the diaphragm is often located more cranially than in the awake, upright patient. The prudent operator first proceeds with identification of the kidney and the adjacent liver or spleen in the longitudinal axis. The operator then scans more cranially, identifying the curvilinear diaphragm with its characteristic respiratory movement. Positive identification of the diaphragm avoids inadvertent subdiaphragmatic needle insertion with its potentially lethal effect. Pleural fluid, unless loculated, assumes a dependent position in the hemithorax. In the supine patient, the fluid is posterior in location. Ultrasonographically, pleural fluid appears as a hypoechoic space that is subtended by typical anatomic boundaries (inside of chest wall and diaphragm) and associated with typical dynamic findings (lung flapping, diaphragmatic movement, plankton sign, and mobile elements within the fluid, such as septations). Complex effusions, such as empyema or hemothorax, may be difficult to identify by the inexperienced ultrasonographer. Before proceeding with thoracentesis, operators must be completely confident in their identification of fluid within the thorax.
2. It is important that the patient maintain the same position between ultrasonographic site localization and actual device insertion. If the patient changes position between ultrasonographic site localization and actual device insertion, free-flowing fluid may redistribute to a different area in the hemithorax. A large pleural effusion is easy to locate by scanning in the midaxillary line. It may be more difficult to identify a safe access site in patients with smaller effusions, as the mattress blocks appropriate transducer position in the supine patient. In this situation, the operator may need to reposition the patient for better access.
3. When localizing a safe access site and angle, the operator should explore its extent in all three dimensions. This requires imaging the collection in two orthogonal planes (typically, a longitudinal and a coronal plane). A moderate-sized collection that tracks into an interlobar fissure may appear to have a considerable extent, with a wide separation between parietal and visceral pleural surface, if its long axis is imaged; however, an orthogonal scan in a coronal plane will quickly reveal the small lateral extent of such a collection. When determining where to insert the device, the operator must take into consideration not only the optimal point on the thoracic skin, but also the angle with the thorax in which the ultrasound transducer provides the image of the collection's largest extent. This optimal transducer angle for imaging of the collection must then be reproduced without continuous ultrasonographic guidance during insertion of the device. Reproduction of the optimal imaging angle assures that the largest extent of the fluid collection is accessed during device insertion. In this manner, fluid collections with a separation between visceral and parietal pleural surfaces of 15 mm or more can be accessed safely [34].
4. The hypoechoic space between parietal and visceral pleura is usually presumed to contain fluid; however, gelatinous contents can occasionally present with a similar ultrasonographic image [36]. If sterile transducer sheaths are available during the procedure, the operator can image the intrathoracic device position if no fluid return is achieved, thus assuring access to the intended space. If color Doppler signals are imaged in the hypoechoic space on preinsertion scanning, this also assures liquid rather than gelatinous intrathoracic contents [37].

If a pleural device is inserted in order to perform medical pleurodesis, the extent of pleurodesis can be assessed in follow-up pleural ultrasound 1 to 2 days later and repeat ultrasound-guided local pleurodesis can then be performed in locules with persistent fluid content [38].

Ultrasound Guidance of Pericardiocentesis

Pericardiocentesis may be performed safely with ultrasound guidance [39]. The intensivist performs pericardiocentesis for diagnostic purposes. Alternatively, pericardiocentesis may be a lifesaving procedure if the patient has pericardial tamponade. The skills required for performance of ultrasound-guided pericardiocentesis are similar to those required for thoracentesis and paracentesis. The operator must identify a safe site, angle, and depth for needle insertion that avoids injury to structures adjacent to the pericardial fluid. This requires that the operator examine the heart from multiple windows: parasternal, apical, and subcostal. Using ultrasonography, the operator identifies the largest area of fluid collection. This is often at the apical four-chamber view, or in large effusions, from a parasternal view. The subcostal approach is frequently prohibited by the presence of the liver in a blocking position, a feature that is easily recognized with ultrasonography. The use of fluoroscopy to guide pericardiocentesis is typically limited to the subcostal approach. The liver is not easily identified using fluoroscopy, so hepatic laceration is a hazard that is not readily apparent when using fluoroscopy. In addition, the apical or parasternal windows frequently reveal a larger fluid collection target than does the subcostal approach. Some concerns specific to pericardiocentesis are as follows:

1. Lacerations of the myocardium or a coronary artery are specific potentially lethal complications of pericardiocentesis. Site selection requires that there be sufficient fluid to allow safe needle insertion. In making this determination, the operator must observe for cardiac movement that occurs during contractile cycle, which is respirophasic or results from cardiac swinging within the effusion. A minimum of 10 mm of space within the effusion is required for safe needle insertion. Large effusions may allow the operator to select an angle of approach that is free of any cardiac structure. The presence of interposed liver may preclude a subcostal approach. Aerated lung does not permit transmission of ultrasound so that the ultrasonographic visualization of the heart precludes injury to interposed aerated lung. Consolidated lung has a specific ultrasonographic appearance, and must not be interposed in the planned needle track. A coexisting pleural effusion may be interposed between the pericardial effusion and the needle insertion site. The pleural effusion should be removed before the pericardial fluid is accessed.
2. Once the site is selected, it should be marked without placing traction on the skin that may cause inadvertent site movement on release of the traction. The depth of needle penetration is a critical measurement. Compression artifact caused by firm pressure of the transducer in the obese or edematous patient may cause an underestimation of the depth of needle penetration. This needs to be factored into the depth estimate; otherwise the operator will not be able to access the pericardial fluid, out of mistaken concern that the needle has been inserted too far. Angle selection is determined by the location of the fluid. Whenever possible, it should be perpendicular to the skin surface, as this is the easiest angle to duplicate with the needle and syringe assembly.
3. Unlike thoracentesis and paracentesis, it is important to include the transducer with full sterile cover into the set up of the sterile field. The intensivist should be prepared to rescan the target site just before needle insertion in order to document the correct angle for needle insertion, recheck depth in case of initial failure due to compression artifact, and check for proper device position immediately following catheter insertion.
4. Real-time guidance of needle insertion is not necessary for safe performance of pericardiocentesis, similar to thoracentesis and paracentesis. A final confirmatory scan is performed immediately before needle insertion and the needle is placed with free-hand technique duplicating the angle defined by the transducer. Aspiration of fluid is followed by wire insertion and device insertion via Seldinger technique. Correct catheter position may be verified by injection of agitated saline solution.

Ultrasound Guidance of Paracentesis

Peritoneal fluid collections commonly occur in the critically ill. Ultrasound guidance improves the safety of peritoneal access, especially in patients with peritoneal adhesions or difficult anatomy (e.g., morbid obesity and massive subcutaneous edema [40]). Many of the principles described for ultrasound-guided pleural access also apply to ultrasound-guided peritoneal access. Specifically, a comprehensive scan of the abdomen should first ascertain the area of maximal intraperitoneal fluid, and the patient should maintain the same position between the ultrasonographic site localization and the actual procedure so as to avoid fluid redistribution. The operator should explore the extent of the peritoneal fluid collection using two orthogonal planes. In addition, the operator who accesses the peritoneal space under ultrasound guidance should bear in mind the following:

1. The best site, angle, and depth for needle penetration are determined at the bedside. The needle–syringe assembly must duplicate the angle at which the transducer was held when determining the best angle of attack. Normally, an area superior to and medial to the left anterosuperior iliac spine contains some of the free intra-abdominal fluid in the left paracolic gutter (similar to the area identified with the landmark technique). Because the sigmoid colon courses retroperitoneally at this location, the risk of large bowel injury is less than that on the contralateral side, which contains the intraperitoneal cecum. Perihepatic and perisplenic fluid collections also occur in patients with ascites, but the risk of solid organ injury is higher in these locations, and the operator should have experience prior to attempting puncture at these subdiaphragmatic sites.
2. In the edematous patient, compression of the subcutaneous tissue leads to an underestimation of the soft-tissue distance that needs to be traversed prior to entering the peritoneal space (so-called compression artifact). Any ultrasonographic measurement of the distance between the skin and the peritoneal cavity should thus be performed from an image acquired while the transducer is applied to the skin with minimal pressure.

Other Ultrasound-Guided Procedures

Beyond vascular access, thoracentesis, paracentesis, and pericardiocentesis, ultrasonography may be used to guide other procedures of interest to the intensivist as follows:

1. Aspiration and biopsy of solid and fluid-filled structures. Ultrasonography allows the intensivist to identify a fluid-filled structure such as an abscess [41]. With knowledge of surrounding anatomy, a safe site, angle, and depth of needle penetration may be identified for access. Similarly, solid lesions may be accessed for aspiration and biopsy [42].
2. Airway management. Ultrasonography may be used to document endotracheal tube placement and diagnose inadvertent main stem bronchial intubation [43]. Ultrasonography is useful in performing percutaneous tracheostomy to screen for dangerous vascular aberrancy and guide tracheal access.
3. Transvenous pacemaker insertion. Ultrasonography may be used to guide transvenous pacemaker insertion. The subcostal window permits visualization of the IVC, right atrium, and right ventricle. The pacemaker wire may be manipulated into position under real-time guidance.
4. Lumbar puncture. Ultrasonography may be used to guide lumbar puncture [44]. This has application in the patients with difficult anatomy.

CONCLUSION

Ultrasonography is a useful technique in guiding a variety of procedures that are routine to critical care medicine. These include vascular access, thoracentesis, paracentesis, and pericardiocentesis. Competence in ultrasonographic guidance is a useful skill for the intensivist as it improves the safety, comfort, and efficiency of these common procedures.

References

1. Mayo PH, Beaulieu Y, Doelken P, et al: American College of Chest Physicians/La Societe de Reanimation de Langue Francaise statement on competence in critical care ultrasonography. *Chest* 135:1050–1060, 2009.
2. Levitov A, Mayo PH, Slonim AD (eds): *Critical Care Ultrasonography*. 1st ed. New York, McGraw-Hill, 2009.
3. Lichtenstein DA: *General Ultrasound in the Critically Ill*. 1st ed. Berlin, Springer, 2002.
4. Sibai AN, Loutfi E, Itani M, et al: Ultrasound evaluation of the anatomical characteristics of the internal jugular vein and carotid artery—facilitation of internal jugular vein cannulation. *Middle East J Anesthesiol* 19:1305–1320, 2008.
5. Turba UC, Uflacker R, Hannegan C, et al: Anatomic relationship of the internal jugular vein and the common carotid artery applied to percutaneous transjugular procedures. *Cardiovasc Intervent Radiol* 28:303–306, 2005.
6. Fortune JB, Feustel P: Effect of patient position on size and location of the subclavian vein for percutaneous puncture. *Arch Surg* 138:996–1000, 2003.
7. Kitagawa N, Oda M, Totoki T, et al: Proper shoulder position for subclavian venipuncture: a prospective randomized clinical trial and anatomical perspectives using multislice computed tomography. *Anaesthesiology* 101:1306–1312, 2004.
8. Mizukoshi K, Shibasaki M, Amaya F, et al: Ultrasound evidence of the optimal wrist position for radial artery cannulation. *Can J Anaesth* 56:427–431, 2009.
9. Rodriguez-Niedenfuhr M, Vazquez T, Nearn L, et al: Variations of the arterial pattern in the upper limb revisited: a morphological and statistical study, with a review of the literature. *J Anat* 199:547–566, 2001.
10. Kumar A, Chuan A: Ultrasound guided vascular access: efficacy and safety. *Best Pract Res Clin Anaesthesiol* 23:299–311, 2009.
11. Barsuk JH, McGaghie WC, Cohen ER, et al: Use of simulation-based mastery learning to improve the quality of central venous catheter placement in a medical intensive care unit. *J Hosp Med* 4:397–403, 2009.
12. Milling TJ Jr, Rose J, Briggs WM, et al: Randomized, controlled clinical trial of point-of-care limited ultrasonography assistance of central venous cannulation: the Third Sonography Outcomes Assessment Program (SOAP-3) Trial. *Crit Care Med* 33:1764–1769, 2005.
13. Gordon AC, Saliken JC, Johns D, et al: US-guided puncture of the internal jugular vein: complications and anatomic considerations. *J Vasc Interv Radiol* 9:333–338, 1998.
14. Karakitsos D, Labropoulos N, De Groot E, et al: Real-time ultrasound-guided catheterisation of the internal jugular vein: a prospective comparison with the landmark technique in critical care patients. *Crit Care* 10(6):R162, 2006.
15. Rothschild JM. Ultrasound guidance of central vein catheterization. In: On making health care safer: a critical analysis of patient safety practices. Rockville, MD: *AHRQ Publications*, Chapter 21:245–55, 2001.
16. Lichtenstein DA, Mezière GA: Relevance of lung ultrasound in the diagnosis of acute respiratory failure: the BLUE protocol. *Chest* 134:117–125, 2008.
17. Chapman GA, Johnson D, Bodenham AR: Visualisation of needle position using ultrasonography. *Anesthesia* 61:148–158, 2006.
18. Maecken T, Grau T: Ultrasound imaging in vascular access. *Crit Care Med* 35:S178–S185, 2007.
19. Feller-Kopman D: Ultrasound-guided internal jugular access: a proposed standardized approach and implications for training and practice. *Chest* 132:302–309, 2007.
20. Troianos CA, Kuwik RJ, Pasqual JR, et al: Internal jugular vein and carotid artery anatomic relation as determined by ultrasonography. *Anesthesiology* 85:43–48, 1996.
21. Vezzani A, Brusasco C, Palermo S, et al: Ultrasound localization of central vein catheter and detection of postprocedural pneumothorax: an alternative to chest radiography. *Crit Care Med* 38:533–538, 2010.
22. Lichtenstein DA, Mezière G, Lascols N, et al: Ultrasound diagnosis of occult pneumothorax. *Crit Care Med* 33:1231–1238, 2005.
23. Orihashi K, Imai K, Sato K, et al: Extrathoracic subclavian venipuncture under ultrasound guidance. *Circ J* 69:1111–1115, 2005.
24. Brooks AJ, Alfredson M, Pettigrew B, et al: Ultrasound-guided insertion of subclavian venous access ports. *Ann R Coll Surg Engl* 87:25–27, 2005.
25. Galloway S, Bodenham A: Ultrasound imaging of the axillary vein—anatomical basis for central venous access. *Br J Anaesth* 90:589–595, 2003.
26. Prabhu MV, Juneja D, Gopal PB, et al: Ultrasound-guided femoral dialysis access placement: a single-center randomized trial. *Clin J Am Soc Nephrol* 5:235–239, 2010.
27. Werner SL, Jones RA, Emerman CL: Effect of hip abduction and external rotation on femoral vein exposure for possible cannulation. *J Emerg Med* 35:73–75, 2008.
28. Gregg SC, Murthi SB, Sisley AC, et al: Ultrasound-guided peripheral intravenous access in the intensive care unit. *J Crit Care* 2009. Available at: 10.1016/j.jcrc.2009.09.003.
29. Shiloh AL, Eisen LA: Ultrasound-guided arterial catheterization: a narrative review. *Intensive Care Med* 36:214–221, 2010.
30. Dudeck O, Teichgraeber U, Podrabsky P, et al: A randomized trial assessing the value of ultrasound-guided puncture of the femoral artery for interventional investigations. *Int J Cardiovasc Imaging* 20:363–368, 2004.
31. Gabriel M, Pawlaczyk K, Waliszewski K, et al: Location of femoral artery puncture site and the risk of postcatheterization pseudoaneurysm formation. *Int J Cardiol* 120:167–171, 2007.
32. Kreuger K, Zaehringer M, Strohe D, et al: Postcatheterization pseudoaneurysm: results of US-guided percutaneous thrombin injection in 240 patients. *Radiology* 236:1104–1110, 2005.
33. Gordon CE, Feller-Kopman D, Balk EM, et al: Pneumothorax following thoracentesis: a systematic review and meta-analysis. *Arch Intern Med* 170(4):332–339, 2010.
34. Lichtenstein D, Hulot J, Rabiller A, et al: Feasibility and safety of ultrasound-aided thoracentesis in mechanically ventilated patients. *Intensive Care Med* 25:955–958, 1999.
35. Mayo PH, Goltz HR, Tafreshi M, et al: Safety of ultrasound-guided thoracentesis in patients receiving mechanical ventilation. *Chest* 125:1059–1062, 2004.
36. Tu CY, Hsu WH, Hsia TC, et al: Pleural effusions in febrile medical ICU patients: chest ultrasound study. *Chest* 126:1274–1280, 2004.
37. Wu R, Yang P, Kuo S, Luh K: "Fluid color" sign: a useful indicator for discrimination between pleural thickening and pleural effusion. *J Ultrasound Med* 14:767–769, 1995.
38. Sartori S, Tombesi P, Tassinari D, et al: Sonographically guided small-bore chest tubes and sonographic monitoring for rapid sclerotherapy of recurrent malignant pleural effusions. *J Ultrasound Med* 23:1171–1176, 2004.
39. Silvestry FE, Kerber RE, Brook MM, et al: Echocardiography-guided interventions. *J Am Soc Echocardiogr* 22:213–231, 2009.
40. Nazeer SR, Dewbre H, Miller AH: Ultrasound-assisted paracentesis performed by emergency physicians vs the traditional technique: a prospective, randomized study. *Am J Emerg Med* 23:363–367, 2005.
41. Chen HJ, Yu YH, Tu CY, et al: Ultrasound in peripheral pulmonary air-fluid lesions. Color Doppler imaging as an aid in differentiating empyema and abscess. *Chest* 135:1426–1432, 2009.
42. Pang JA, Tsang V, Hom BL, et al: Ultrasound-guided tissue-core biopsy of thoracic lesions with Trucut and Surecut needles. *Chest* 91:823–828, 1987.
43. Lichtenstein DA, Lascols N, Prin S, et al: The "lung pulse": an early sign of complete atelectasis. *Intensive Care Med* 29:2187–2192, 2003.
44. Nomura JT, Leech SJ, Shenbagamurthi S, et al: A randomized controlled trial of ultrasound-assisted lumbar puncture. *J Ultrasound Med* 26:1341–1348, 2007.

CHAPTER 22 ■ INTERVENTIONAL RADIOLOGY: PERCUTANEOUS DRAINAGE TECHNIQUES

BRIAN T. CALLAHAN, SALOMAO FAINTUCH AND FELIPE B. COLLARES

Over the past decade, image-guided percutaneous drainage procedures have become accepted as safe and effective alternatives to surgery for the first-line treatment of symptomatic fluid collections in the body. Image guidance typically provided by sonography or computed tomography (CT) allows for precise localization of fluid collections, improved drainage techniques, and faster patient recovery. Rapid imaging localization and percutaneous treatment has played a major role in decreasing the morbidity and mortality associated with surgical exploration [1–4].

GENERAL AIMS

The aim of the interventional radiologist is to detect and localize symptomatic fluid collections, ascertain if additional imaging or laboratory tests are needed, and determine what, if any, intervention is required. Close communication between interventional and critical care staff is essential to accomplish these goals. Image-guided aspiration or drainage procedures can alleviate symptoms due to mass effect or inflammation, provide fluid samples for laboratory characterization, and cause reduction in sepsis [5]. A list of fluid collections amenable to image-guided procedures is provided in Table 22.1.

DIAGNOSTIC IMAGING

CT and ultrasound are the two main imaging modalities used for percutaneous image guidance. Magnetic resonance imaging (MRI)-guided drainage is available at some academic institutions, but limited by availability, cost, and paucity of MRI-compatible devices. The choice between CT and ultrasound is ultimately determined by operator experience, availability of equipment, and nature of the collection such as size, location, and presence of septations. Advantages of ultrasound include portability, lack of radiation, low cost, and real-time visualization of needle placement into a collection. Ultrasound can also be readily combined with fluoroscopic guidance techniques. Limitations of ultrasound include poor visualization of deep collections secondary to large body habitus, bone, overlying bowel gas, or surgical dressings. CT provides excellent visualization of the fluid collection and its relation to vital structures, allowing for the safest percutaneous access route to be chosen. For deep collections such as those located in the pelvis or retroperitoneal space, CT is particularly well suited [6]. There is typically a shorter learning curve to master CT-guided procedures, especially given the availability of commercially produced skin grids to help aid needle placement. The main limitations of CT include radiation exposure, cost, and lack of real-time visualization of needle placement. The recent advent of CT fluoroscopy allowing the operator to obtain rapid sequential images of needle position without having to leave the patient is a major step forward for helping to resolve some of these technical issues [5]. Table 22.2 is a summary of the advantages and limitations of CT versus sonography [7].

TABLE 22.1

FLUID COLLECTIONS SUCCESSFULLY TREATED WITH PERCUTANEOUS DRAINAGE

Sterile	Nonsterile
Ascites	
Hematoma	Enteric abscess
Lymphocele	Lung abscess and empyema
Pancreatic pseudocyst	Ruptured appendicitis
Postsurgical seroma	Pancreatic abscess
Urinoma	Tubo-ovarian abscess
Multilocular fluid collections	Cholecystitis

INDICATIONS

The indications for image-guided drainage and aspiration include, but are not limited to, fluid sampling to assess infected versus sterile collections, reduction of microorganism burden due to extraction of contaminated material, and relief of pressure symptoms secondary to excess fluid accumulation. In the critically ill patient, catheter drainage may stabilize the patient's condition so that a more definitive surgical procedure can be performed at a later time [8,9]. Abscess size is an important determinant of the need for percutaneous drainage. Many patients with abscesses smaller than 4 cm in diameter can be treated conservatively with broad-spectrum antibiotics, hydration, and bowel rest [10]. If a small collection is unresponsive to initial antibiotic therapy, a drainage procedure should be considered. In patients with abscesses larger than 4 cm, studies have shown that percutaneous catheter placement is beneficial and less invasive than surgical intervention [10].

CONTRAINDICATIONS

Contraindications are divided into absolute and relative. Absolute contraindications for percutaneous drainage include absence of a safe access route or uncorrectable coagulopathy. An uncooperative or unwilling patient may also cause termination of a procedure. Often, the study may be rescheduled

TABLE 22.2

ADVANTAGES AND LIMITATIONS OF COMPUTED TOMOGRAPHY (CT) AND ULTRASOUND

	Advantages	Limitations
CT	Excellent 2-D and 3-D (with reformatting) spatial resolution Images not obscured by overlying structures	Radiation exposure Lack of real-time image guidance Procedures take longer Higher cost
US	No radiation required, real time visualization of anatomy and needle placement Portability allows bedside procedures Low cost	Overlying structures (i.e., bowel gas, real-time visualization of bone) may obscure target More difficult to master Need cooperative patient

to allow for general anesthesia or deep sedation to be provided for patient safety. The utmost care should be taken to avoid transgression of major blood vessels, pleura, pancreas, and spleen. One should also avoid prolonged drainage of sterile collections due to the risk of secondary infection [11]. In patients with relative contraindications, procedures may require more planning or additional time, but are usually amenable to treatment. For example, a transenteric (small bowel) route may allow for needle aspiration of a collection previously thought to be inaccessible [12]. If no direct route is available, the liver, kidney, and stomach may be safely transgressed during needle aspiration or catheter placement. Recent advances in technique such as transgluteal, transvaginal, or transrectal sampling provide more options for draining difficult-to-reach collections [13–15].

RISKS, BENEFITS, AND ALTERNATIVES

Overall complications associated with percutaneous drainage are reported to be less than 15% [16]. These include damage to vital structures, bleeding, and infection among others. Mortality (ranging from 1% to 6%) is frequently secondary to sepsis or multiorgan failure rather than the drainage procedure itself. Depending on the location and physical properties of an infected or sterile collection, percutaneous drainage is curative in 75% to 90% of cases [6,16,17]. In approximately 10% of cases, percutaneous drainage can serve as a temporizing measure allowing surgery to be postponed or performed in a single step [10]. Patients whose drainage collections contain feculent material or a fistulous communication tend to respond poorly, and further surgical intervention may be required. Indications for surgery also include visceral perforation, peritonitis, uncontrolled sepsis, and lack of improvement or deterioration of clinical status following several days of medical treatment [18].

PREPROCEDURE PREPARATION

Regardless of the study to be performed, certain basic principals apply to all patients about to undergo a drainage procedure. After review of the risks, benefits, and alternatives to the procedure, informed consent should be obtained from the patient or health care proxy. The radiologist should review the case with the referring physician to determine if the procedure is medically indicated or if other treatment alternatives exist. A comprehensive history and physical examination is taken, including review of previous and current imaging studies to evaluate fluid collection size, location, and complexity. Determination of the imaging modality used to characterize the fluid collection depends on location and operator preference. Once the collection has been localized, the access route is planned. The basic tenets of surgical drainage are followed using established surgical routes to find the shortest and least invasive path while avoiding lung, pleura, bowel, and other vital structures. Prior to the procedure, the patient should stop all anticoagulant medications, given the benefits of the drainage procedure outweigh the risk to the patient from thrombosis. For example, clopidogrel (Plavix), an antiplatelet agent, should be held for 7 to 10 days before the procedure [19]. For patients receiving vitamin K antagonists such as Coumadin, guidelines recommend bridging anticoagulation with therapeutic dose low-molecular-weight heparin (given subcutaneously) or intravenous unfractionated heparin (given intravenously) [19,20]. The goal is to maintain the international normalized ratio (INR) less than 1.5. It is believed that anticoagulants can be safely restarted 6 to 8 hours following the procedure. Coagulation parameters should also be obtained within a few days before the procedure and corrected if necessary. In a nonemergent situation, the prothrombin time (PT) should be less than 15 seconds, the partial thromboplastin time less than 35 seconds, platelet count greater than 75,000 per mL and INR less than 1.5. In emergent situations where the PT is elevated, fresh-frozen plasma should be given. Platelet transfusions can be administered just prior to the procedure to raise levels to an acceptable value.

The patient should have nothing to eat for 4 to 6 hours prior to the study to reduce the risk of aspiration during moderate sedation. Transient bacteremia associated with percutaneous drainage of an infected collection may require prophylactic treatment with antibiotics. Initial coverage should utilize a broad-spectrum antibiotic before more selective therapy can be deduced from fluid Gram stain and culture. If intravenous contrast is required to visualize a collection, the patient's renal function (blood urea nitrogen [BUN] and creatinine) should be evaluated. If elevated (serum creatinine >1.5 mg per dL), the patient may require hydration and pretreatment with sodium bicarbonate and oral or intravenous *N*-acetylcysteine (Mucomyst) [21]. Low osmolality contrast agents may also be used to help reduce the risk of contrast-induced nephrotoxicity. In patients with a history of prior "contrast reaction," the incident should be discussed to determine if symptoms were truly an anaphylactic reaction. In the setting of a validated contrast reaction, the risks and benefits of the study should be weighed and discussed with both the patient and the referring physician. If a decision is made to precede with intravenous contrast administration, these patients are usually pretreated with a combination of a steroid and an antihistamine. Oral contrast may be given to patients prior to CT to better delineate bowel loops. Reports of unopacified bowel mistaken for an abscess collection are not uncommon.

EQUIPMENT

With the advent of portable, high-resolution ultrasound machines, diagnostic or therapeutic procedures may now be performed at the bedside. Drainage of ascites, pleural effusions, and placement of cholecystostomy tubes are just some of procedures performed at our institution when the patient is too unstable to transport. All procedures must be performed under sterile conditions, with patient monitoring and sedation performed by a qualified nurse. For most procedures, convenient premade sterile kits are available, containing drapes, skin preparation, lidocaine, blades, sharps containers, and additional instruments tailored to the intervention to be performed. A variety of different-size and -configuration needles, guidewires, and catheters should be available to the radiologist during the procedure.

PATIENT CONSENT AND PREPROCEDURE REVIEW

After a thorough explanation of the risks, benefits, and alternatives of the procedure, informed consent should be obtained from the patient or a health care proxy [22].

A careful review of the procedure "time-out" should be held just prior to gaining access to confirm patient identity, site, review allergies and to verify the procedure to be performed.

ANESTHESIA AND MONITORING

Most image-guided drainage procedures can be performed with local anesthesia alone or in combination with moderate sedation. Typically, local anesthesia is achieved using subcutaneous infiltration with 1% to 2% lidocaine using a thin 25-gauge needle. At our institution, we have found that addition of sodium bicarbonate (75 mg per mL mixed in a 1:10 ratio) to lidocaine reduces the pain perception of an intradermal injection [23]. Longer acting agents such as tetracaine gel or bupivacaine (lasting 4 to 8 hours) are available for procedures lasting more than a couple hours. For moderate sedation, the procedure is typically performed using a combination of intravenous fentanyl and midazolam (Versed). The interventional radiologist should be familiar with these drug protocols and their reactions, and conscious sedation certification is recommended. In procedures where balloon dilation is performed or if patients are unable to hold still for long periods of time, general anesthesia may be required. The patient should be well hydrated, and vital signs must be continuously monitored during the procedure as well as during the patient's recovery. It is imperative that the interventional suite is equipped with basic monitoring equipment, including pulse oximetry, blood pressure monitoring devices, and electrocardiography. For the infrequent event of cardiopulmonary resuscitation, a defibrillator, backboard, and code cart supplied with the necessary medications for advanced life support should always be available.

STERILE TECHNIQUE

Regardless of known risk factors, universal precautions against contact exposure should be applied to all patients, including wearing of sterile gloves, impermeable gowns, and a face mask with shield. Hands should be washed with an antibacterial surgical scrub before starting the procedure. All equipment should be placed on a sterile field within easy reach, such as a bedside table. Proper preparation of the patient's skin using an antimicrobial product is essential in reducing the number of microorganisms present. Preferred antiseptics include 70% alcohol, 10% povidone–iodine, or a chlorhexidine-containing product [24]. Skin preparation should be performed in a way that preserves skin integrity and prevents injury to the skin. Shaving is no longer recommended because it may create breaks in the skin where bacteria can multiply and grow. The skin prep should be large enough to allow for extension of the incision or placement of adjacent drainage sites. Creating and maintaining a sterile field by placing sterile surgical drapes around the patient's incision large enough to prevent inadvertent contamination is essential.

PROCEDURES

General Considerations

In principle, a unilocular collection with a well-developed cavity wall is best suited for percutaneous drainage. After localization of the collection with either CT or ultrasound, the patient is placed on the imaging table in the optimal position that affords the shortest and safest approach to the collection being entered. For multiloculated or semisolid collections, multiple drain placements may be required. If possible, drains should be inserted into the most dependent portion of the collection.

Diagnostic or Therapeutic Aspiration

CT and ultrasound used alone or with fluoroscopic guidance can be used to localize the collection. After appropriate patient positioning and selection of the skin insertion site, local anesthesia with 1% lidocaine is administered and a small incision made with a no. 11 scalpel. After the skin entrance site is widened with a surgical forceps, a 22- or 20-gauge needle can be advanced into the collection under image guidance. For a hematoma or viscous collection, 16- or 18-gauge large-bore needles can be used [2,25]. Aspiration of fluid confirms position, and can be sent for culture, Gram stain, and cytology if needed. Additional laboratory tests can be added such as in the case of evaluating fluid for amylase in a peripancreatic collection or creatinine in suspected urinomas. The aspiration needle may be left in place to serve as a guide for parallel catheter placement or a conduit for introduction of a guidewire.

Catheter Selection

Multiple types of drainage catheters are available on the market. These come in different sizes, configurations, and materials. Selection of the appropriate catheter is largely governed by the size, location, and physical properties of the collection to be drained. The two major catheter designs include sump and nonsump varieties. A sump catheter is well suited for abscess drainage and ranges in size from 8 to 14 French (Fr). The catheter contains a small lumen that allows ingress of irrigant or air for drainage and a larger outer lumen designed to prevent side-hole blockage when the catheter is apposed against an abscess cavity wall [26]. Smaller bore nonsump catheters are usually more flexible than sump catheters allowing for guidewire placement into difficult-to-reach fluid collections. Limitations of nonsump catheters include smaller side holes and internal bores, limiting their effectiveness in draining viscous collections, such as pus or hematoma. The largest caliber catheter that can be safely and comfortably inserted should be used to help drain viscous fluid and prevent blockage from debris.

Therapeutic Catheter Drainage

Broadly, catheter drainage systems can be introduced using the trocar or Seldinger technique. The trocar system consists of an 8- to 16-Fr pigtail catheter coaxially loaded over a hollow metal stiffener with a sharp inner stylet. Under image guidance, the trocar system is advanced together into the fluid collection. Once the catheter has reached the desired location, the inner stylet is removed and aspiration performed confirming position within the collection. Next, the catheter is advanced off the cannula into the cavity, assuming its pigtail configuration. Most CT drainages are performed using this system. Advantages of the trocar technique include a single pass and less chance of access loss. The trocar technique is well suited to large, easily accessible collections, and can be performed quickly and safely at the bedside under ultrasound guidance. Given the rigidity of the system, the trocar system is not recommended for drainage procedures where the collection is small or difficult to access.

An alternative to the trocar system for drain placement is the use of the Seldinger technique (Fig. 22.1). The Seldinger system involves two steps starting with insertion of an 18- to 20-gauge sheathed needle into a collection under image guidance. Following aspiration of fluid to confirm position, the needle is removed and a 0.035-in. guidewire is advanced through the sheath into the cavity [27]. The guidewire is subsequently used for tract dilatation and placement of 8- to 12-Fr drainage catheters. This technique is best performed under continuous image guidance such a fluoroscopy as guidewire access can easily be lost in inexperienced hands. If this occurs, cavity decompression may make guidewire reentry nearly impossible. It is recommended not to evacuate the cavity before the catheter has been secured in position.

Fixing the Catheter

A wide variety of catheters containing various types of self-locking detention devices are available on the market. The most frequently used self-locking mechanism consists of a string that when pulled, forms a pigtail at the catheter's internal end. The string can then be locked in position fixing the pigtail in place to prevent accidental dislodgement. A second type of locking device, a Malecot or "mushroom" catheter can be deployed when the abscess cavity does not contain enough room for pigtail formation. For drainage, the catheter should be connected to a bag with intervening stopcock to allow for irrigation. Further security can be achieved by fixing the catheter to the skin with tape and sutures or a commercially available external fixation device. We have found adhesive external devices to be particularly well suited to catheter fixation without the need for additional skin suturing.

Management of the Catheter

The patient with a percutaneous drainage catheter requires regular monitoring. A team approach requiring communication

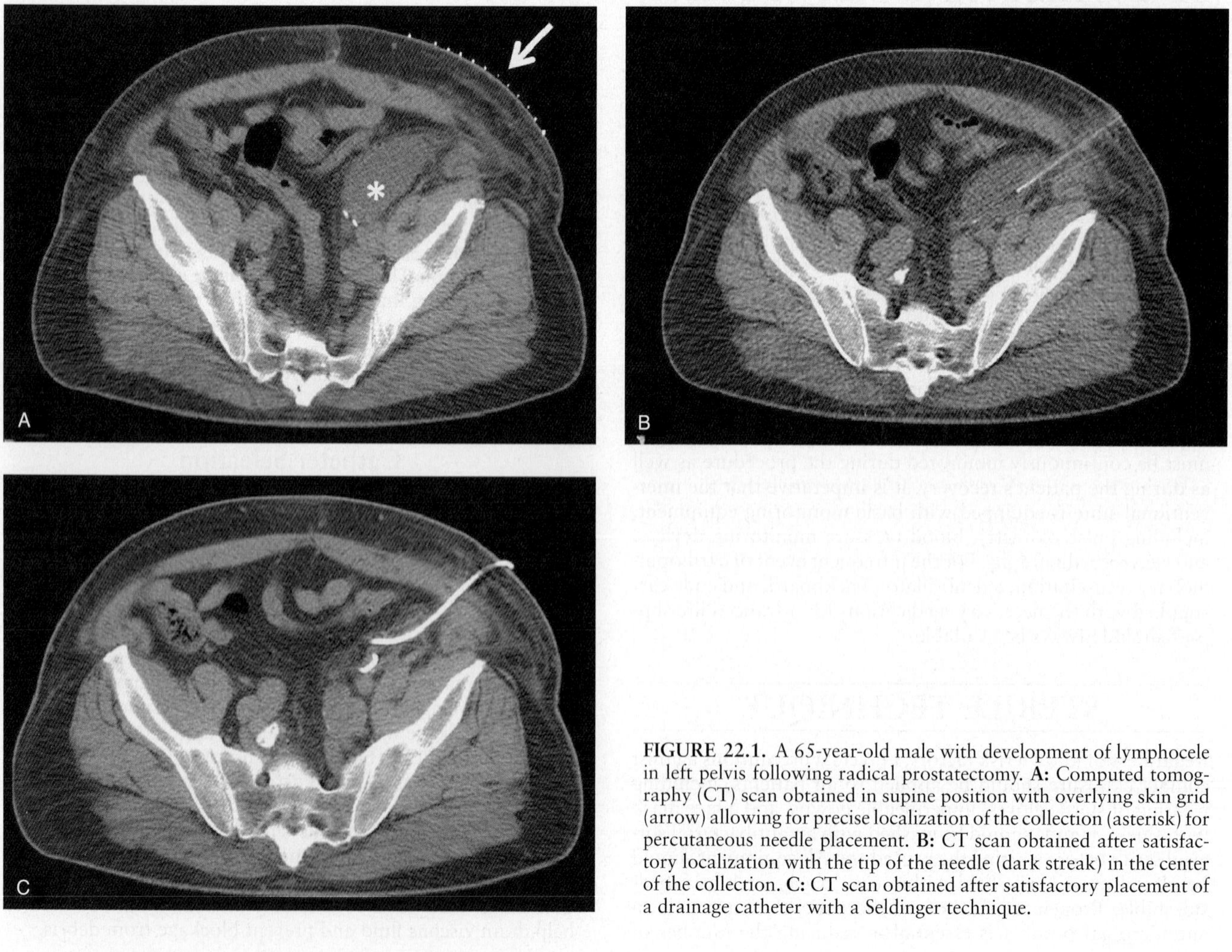

FIGURE 22.1. A 65-year-old male with development of lymphocele in left pelvis following radical prostatectomy. A: Computed tomography (CT) scan obtained in supine position with overlying skin grid (arrow) allowing for precise localization of the collection (asterisk) for percutaneous needle placement. B: CT scan obtained after satisfactory localization with the tip of the needle (dark streak) in the center of the collection. C: CT scan obtained after satisfactory placement of a drainage catheter with a Seldinger technique.

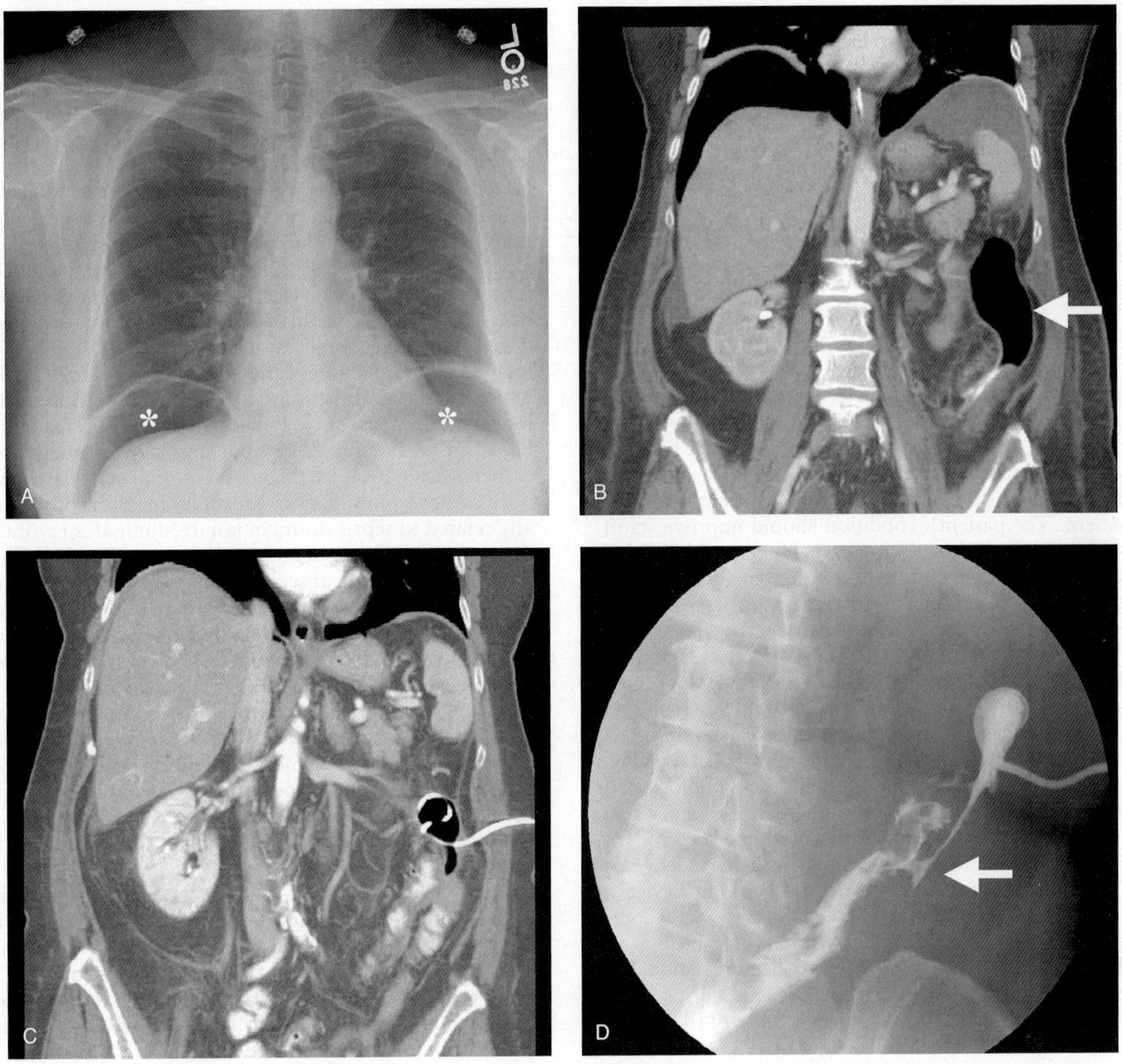

FIGURE 22.2. A 63-year-old female status post–recent sigmoid resection presenting with abdominal pain. A: Chest x-ray showing large amount of free intraperitoneal air (asterisks) concerning for bowel perforation. B: Computed tomography (CT) scan obtained with oral contrast shows large gas and fluid containing collection (arrow) from leak at the surgical anastomosis. C: CT scan performed after satisfactory position of drainage catheter into the collection. D: Due to high drainage output (>50 cc per day), abscessogram was performed demonstrating a fistulous communication (arrow) with the descending colon.

between interventional and critical care staff is critical to prevent catheter malfunction. Daily rounds should be conducted to ensure the catheter is draining and not kinked or dislodged. During rounds, the skin insertion site, catheter tubing, amount of drainage, and body temperature should be evaluated. It is useful to mark the level of the skin insertion on the catheter during initial placement to allow for easy assessment of catheter dislodgement. Most catheters are connected to a bag for external drainage, allowing for evaluation of fluid volume and consistency. Gentle irrigation of the abscess cavity with 10 to 20 mL of sterile saline is recommended three to four times daily to ensure patency. Vigorous irrigation is not recommended as expansion of the abscess cavity may lead to transient bacteremia [28]. Dressing changes should also be performed daily. In anticipation of the patient's discharge from the hospital, family members are instructed in catheter care or a visiting nursing service is arranged. The patient and his or her family should be instructed in catheter care and to how to recognize any potential or existing malfunction. The patient is advised to return to the department in the event of abdominal pain, leakage from the catheter entry site, fever, or chills. When long-term drainage is anticipated, catheters should be exchanged approximately every 3 months to avoid blockage from encrustation or debris.

Patient Response

Following complete evacuation of purulent material from an infected cavity, improved clinical response should be seen in a matter of hours to several days [8,12]. Parameters of improving clinical status include defervescence, reduction in pain, and resolution of leukocytosis. If there is no improvement after 2 to 3 days, suspicion should be raised for an undrained collection, catheter malfunction, or fistula formation. In such cases, follow-up imaging using CT, ultrasound, or fluoroscopy with contrast injection into the collection is recommended. Abscesses containing loculations are more difficult to drain than are unilocular collections. Several techniques have been employed to treat multiloculated collections including placement of additional drains or use of guidewires or fibrinolytic agents (such as urokinase) to break up septations [29]. Semisolid collections such as necrotic tumors, infected hematomas, or pancreatic abscesses are also more resistant to drainage and may require surgical debridement.

Removal of the Catheter

Early removal of the drainage catheter is one of the more common causes of postprocedural morbidity and mortality. Therefore, it is essential for the interventional radiologist to be familiar with guidelines for catheter removal. The most important factor to consider prior to drain removal is the clinical status of the patient. The patient's condition should improve significantly within 24 to 48 hours after catheter removal [3,6,10]. The percutaneous drainage catheter should remain in place until the cavity is undetectable on imaging and the volume of drainage is less than 10 cc on two consecutive days. Daily rounds by the interventional staff should carefully assess the patient for resolution of fever, absence of elevated white blood cell count, or other signs of clinical improvement. If the patient fails to respond to treatment, the catheter should be examined to rule out displacement or kinking. Continuous high drainage (>50 mL per day) should alert the radiologist for a possible fistulous tract to bowel, pancreas, or biliary tree, and the appropriate imaging modality should be used for further evaluation [8,30]. Catheter removal is achieved by cutting or untying the string that fixates the locking device in place.

Follow-up imaging on simple collections is typically not required; however, enteric or complex collections should be evaluated with CT or an abscessogram (Fig. 22.2) prior to discharge to document resolution or decreased size of the abscess cavity.

Clinical Outcome and Complications

Depending on the location and makeup of an infected or sterile collection, image-guided percutaneous drainage is successful in 70% to 90% of cases. Overall complications are reported to be less than 15% [1–4], but most are minor. Major complications (5% to 7% complication rate) include infection, bleeding, septicemia, injury to adjacent structures such as bowel and death. Inadvertent contamination of a previously sterile collection is also a possibility with prolonged catheter drainage [11]. Enteric transgression can usually be treated conservatively with delayed catheter removal to allow for a mature fistulous tract to develop. Minor complications (3% to 5% complication rate) include pain, infection of the skin insertion site, transient bacteremia, and malfunction of the catheter secondary to kinking, dislodgement, or clogging with debris, such as blood clots. Pain can be minimized by judicious use of analgesics. Daily catheter evaluation by the interventional staff can serve to reduce catheter malfunction. Mortality from the procedure, usually related to sepsis or organ failure, compares favorably with the surgical literature rates of 10% to 20% [31]. The recurrence rate following abscess drainage has been estimated to be between 5% and 10%. Recurrence may be due to early catheter removal, failure to completely drain a loculated collection or fistulous communication with the bowel, pancreatic duct, or biliary system. Fistulas should be suspected if there is high output from the catheter (>50 mL per day) or the drainage fluid contains feculent material. When the patient fails to respond to treatment or sepsis is not resolving, repeat imaging with CT or ultrasound should be performed to determine the cause. Repeat drainage of these cavities has been shown to be successful in 50% of patients with the need for surgical drainage reduced by half [3,32].

In conclusion, image-guided percutaneous drainage has been established as the first-line treatment for sterile or infected fluid collections in the abdomen and pelvis. Awareness of the advantages and limitations of the procedure together with an integrated management approach between interventional and critical care staff will serve to benefit the patient and improve clinical outcomes.

References

1. Bufalari A, Giustozzi G, Moggi L: Postoperative intraabdominal abscesses: percutaneous versus surgical treatment. *Acta Chir Belg* 96:197, 1996.
2. vanSonnenberg E, Ferrucci JT, Mueller PR, et al: Percutaneous drainage of abscesses and fluid collections: technique, results and applications. *Radiology* 142:1, 1982.
3. Nakamoto DA, Haaga JR: Percutaneous drainage of postoperative intraabdominal abscesses and collections, in Cope C (ed): *Current Techniques in Interventional Radiology*. Philadelphia, PA, Current Medicine, 1995.
4. vanWaes P, Feldberg M, Mali W, et al: Management of loculated abscesses that are difficult to drain: a new approach. *Radiology* 147:57, 1983.
5. Krebs TL, Daly B, Wong JJ, et al: Abdominal and pelvis therapeutic procedures using CT-fluoroscopic guidance. *Semin Intervent Radiol* 16:191, 1999.
6. Harisinghani MG, Gervais DA, Hahn PF, et al: CT-guided transgluteal drainage of deep pelvic abscesses: indications, technique, procedure-related complications, and clinical outcome. *RadioGraphics* 22:1353, 2002.
7. Yeung E: Percutaneous abdominal biopsy, in Allison DJ, Adam A (eds): *Balliere's Clinical Gastroenterology*. London, Balliere Tindall, 1992, p 219.
8. vanSonnenberg E, Wing VW, Casola G, et al: Temporizing effect of percutaneous drainage of complicated abscesses in critically ill patients. *AJR Am J Roentgenol* 142:821, 1984.
9. Bernini A, Spencer MP, Wong WD, et al: Computed tomography-guided percutaneous abscess drainage in intestinal disease. *Dis Colon Rectum* 40:1009, 1997.
10. Siewert B, Tye G, Kruskal J, et al: Impact of CT-guided drainage in the treatment of diverticular abscesses: size matters. *Am J Roentgenol* 186:680, 2006.
11. Walser EM, Nealon WH, Marroquin S, et al: Sterile fluid collections in pancreatitis: catheter drainage versus simple aspiration. *Cardiovasc Intervent Radiol* 29:102, 2006.
12. vanSonnenberg E, Gerhard R, Wittich MD, et al: Percutaneous abscess drainage: update. *World J Surg* 25:362, 2001.
13. Walser E, Raza S, Hernandez A, et al: Sonographically guided transgluteal drainage of pelvic abscesses. *Am J Roentgenol* 181:498, 2003.
14. Kuligowska E, Keller E, Ferrucci JT: Treatment of pelvic abscesses: value of one-step sonographically guided transrectal needle aspiration and lavage. *Am J Roentgenol* 164:201, 1995.
15. Sudakoff GS, Lundeen SJ, Otterson MF: Transrectal and transvaginal sonographic intervention of infected pelvic fluid collections: a complete approach. *Ultrasound Q* 21:175, 2005.
16. vanSonnenberg E, Mueller PR, Ferrucci JT Jr: Percutaneous drainage of 250 abdominal abscesses and fluid collections. Part I. Results, failures, and complications. *Radiology* 151:337, 1984.
17. Lambiase RE, Deyoe L, Cronan JJ, et al: Percutaneous drainage of 335 consecutive abscesses: results of primary drainage with 1-year follow-up. *Radiology* 184:167, 1992.
18. Jacobs D: Diverticulitis. *N Engl J Med* 357:2057, 2007.
19. Kearon C, Hirsh MD: Management of Anticoagulation before and elective surgery. *N Engl J Med* 336(21):1506, 1997.
20. Douketis JD, Berger PB, Dunn AS, et al: The perioperative management of antithrombic therapy. *Chest* 133:299S, 2008.
21. Pannu N, Wiebe N, Tonelli M, et al: Prophylaxis strategies for contrast-induced neuropathy. *JAMA* 295(23):2765, 2006.
22. Appelbaum PS, Grisso T: Assessing patients' capacities to consent to treatment. *N Engl J Med* 319(25):1635, 1988.
23. Palmon SC, Lloyd AT, Kirsch JR: The effect of needle gauge and lidocaine pH on pain during intradermal injection. *Anesth Analg* 86:379, 1998.
24. Peterson AF, Rosenberg A, Alatary SD: Comparative evaluation of surgical scrub preparations. *Surg Gynecol Obstet* 146(1):163, 1978.

25. vanSonnenberg E, Mueller PR, Ferrucci JT, Jr: Percutaneous drainage of 250 abdominal abscesses and fluid collections. Part II Current procedural concepts. *Radiology* 151:343, 1984.
26. vanSonnenberg E, Mueller P, Ferrucci JT, et al. Sump pump catheter for percutaneous abscess and fluid drainage by trocar or seldinger technique. *Am J Roentgenol* 139:613, 1982.
27. Harisinghani MG, Gervais DA, Maher MM, et al: Transgluteal approach for percutaneous drainage of deep pelvic abscesses: 154 cases. *Radiology* 228:701, 2003.
28. Hassinger SM, Harding G, Wongworawat D: High pressure pulsatile lavage propagates bacteria into soft tissue. *Clin Orthop Relat Res* 439:27, 2005.
29. Lahorra JM, Haaga JR, Stellato T, et al: Safety of intracavity urokinase with percutaneous abscess drainage. *Am J Roentgenol* 160:171, 1993.
30. Hui GC, Amaral J, Stephens D, et al: Gas distribution in intraabdominal and pelvic abscesses on CT is associated with drainability. *Am J Roentgenol* 184:915, 2005.
31. Deveney CW, Lurie K, Deveney KE: Improved treatment of intra-abdominal abscess: a result of improved localization, drainage, and patient care, not technique. *Arch Surg* 123:1126, 1988.
32. Gervais DA, Ho CH, O'Neill MJ, et al: Recurrent abdominal and pelvic abscesses: incidence, results of repeated percutaneous drainage, and underlying causes in 956 drainages. *Am J Roentgenol* 182:463, 2004.

CHAPTER 23 ■ CARDIOPULMONARY RESUSCITATION

BRUCE GREENBERG AND JOHN A. PARASKOS

HISTORY

Since the introduction of cardiopulmonary resuscitation (CPR), we have been forced to rethink our definitions of life and death. Although sporadic accounts of attempted resuscitations are recorded from antiquity, until recently no rational quarrel could be found with the sixth-century BC poetic fragment of Ibycus, "You cannot find a medicine for life once a man is dead" [1]. Until 1960, successful resuscitation was largely limited to artificial ventilation for persons who had undergone respiratory arrest due to causes such as near-drowning, smoke inhalation, and aspiration. Such attempts were likely to succeed if performed before cardiac arrest had resulted from hypoxia and acidosis. Emergency thoracotomy with "open heart massage" was rarely resorted to and was occasionally successful if definitive therapy was readily available [2]. Electric reversal of ventricular fibrillation (VF) by externally applied electrodes was described in 1956 by Zoll et al. [3]. This ability to reverse a fatal arrhythmia without opening the chest challenged the medical community to develop a method of sustaining adequate ventilation and circulation long enough to bring the electric defibrillator to the patient's aid. By 1958, adequate rescue ventilation became possible with the development of the mouth-to-mouth technique described by Safar et al. [4] and Elam et al. [5]. In 1960, Kouwenhoven et al. [6] described "closed chest cardiac massage," thus introducing the modern era of CPR. The simplicity of this technique—"all that is needed are two hands"—has led to its widespread dissemination. The interaction of this technique of sternal compression with mouth-to-mouth ventilation was developed as basic CPR. The first national conference on CPR was sponsored by the National Academy of Sciences in 1966 [7]. Instruction in CPR for both professionals and the public soon followed through community programs in basic life support (BLS) and advanced cardiac life support (ACLS). Standards for both BLS and ACLS were set in 1973 [8] and have been updated periodically.

For individuals with adequately preserved cardiopulmonary and neurologic systems, the cessation of breathing and cardiac contraction may be reversed if CPR and definitive care are quickly available. The short period during which the loss of vital signs may be reversed is often referred to as *clinical death*. If ventilation and circulation are not restored before irreversible damage to vital structures occurs, then irreversible death occurs. This is referred to as *biologic death*. In difficult circumstances, the best single criterion (medical and legal) for the ultimate death of the functioning integrated human individual (i.e., the person) is brain death [9,10]. By this criterion, we can make decisions as to the appropriateness of continuing "life-sustaining" techniques.

EFFICACY

The value of standardized CPR continues to undergo considerable scrutiny. Unfortunately, it appears that its efficacy is limited (Table 23.1). CPR does not seem to go beyond short-term sustenance of viability until definitive therapy can be administered. This was the stated goal of Kouwenhoven et al. [6]. The benefit of rapid initiation of CPR has been demonstrated in numerous studies [11–14]. Data from prehospital care systems in Seattle showed that 43% of patients found in VF were discharged from the hospital if CPR (i.e., BLS) was applied within 4 minutes and defibrillation (i.e., ACLS) within 8 minutes. If the onset of CPR is delayed, or if the time to defibrillation is longer than 10 minutes, the probability is greater that the patient will be in asystole or in *fine* VF and will convert to asystole. Survival decreases as each minute passes without return of spontaneous circulation (ROSC).

Even though patients experiencing cardiac arrest in the hospital can be expected to receive CPR and definitive therapy well within the 4- and 8-minute time frames, the outcomes of in-hospital cardiac arrests are poor (Table 23.1).

Recognizing the importance of early defibrillation, it is imperative that all first-response systems provide defibrillation, by either using emergency medical technicians capable of performing defibrillation or equipping and training emergency personnel with automatic or semiautomatic defibrillators [26]. The development of inexpensive, small, lightweight, easy-to-use, voice-prompted defibrillators allows early access to defibrillation, before the arrival of emergency medical services (EMS). Where these have been made available, and where first

TABLE 23.1

EXPERIMENTAL AND ALTERNATE TECHNIQUES OF CARDIOPULMONARY RESUSCITATION (CPR)

Researcher [Reference]	Technique	Notes
Taylor et al. [15]	Longer compression	Proposed use of longer duration to 40%–50% of the duration compression–relaxation cycle
Chandra et al. [14,16]	Simultaneous chest compression and lung inflation	High airway pressures of 60–110 mm Hg are used to augment carotid flow, requiring intubation and a mechanical ventilator. Its use has not met with universal success
Harris et al. [17]	Abdominal binding	Abdominal binding increases intrathoracic pressure by redistributing blood into the thorax during CPR. Studies have demonstrated adverse effects on coronary perfusion, cerebral oxygenation, and canine resuscitation
Redding [18]		
Koehler et al. [19]		
Chandra et al. [20]		
Ralston et al. [21]	Interposed abdominal	Abdominal compression is released when the sternum is compressed. Higher oxygen delivery and cerebral and myocardial blood flows are reported. One study suggests an improved survival and neurologic outcome
Barranco et al. [22]	Simultaneous chest	Simultaneous chest and abdominal compression provided higher intrathoracic pressures in compression in humans
Maier et al. [23]	High-impulse CPR	At compression rates of 150/min (with moderate force and brief duration), cardiac output in dogs increased as the coronary flow remained as high as 75% of prearrest values. High impulse and high compression rates can result in rescuer fatigue and increased injury
Cohen et al. [24]	Active compression	Forceful rebound using a plunger-like device resulted in improved hemodynamics. Clinical results are equivocal
Halperin et al. [25]	Vest inflation	Circumferential chest pressure with an inflatable vest showed improved hemodynamics and survival in dogs

responders have been trained in their use, survival rates have been dramatically improved [27].

Although the current approach is modestly successful for VF, CPR techniques have most likely not yet been optimized, and further improvement is greatly needed. Cardiac output has been measured at no better than 25% of normal during conventional CPR in humans [28]. In animal models, myocardial perfusion and coronary flow have been measured at 1% to 5% of normal [29]. Cerebral blood flow has been estimated to be 3% to 15% of normal when CPR is begun immediately [30], but it decreases progressively as CPR continues [31] and intracranial pressures rise. Despite these pessimistic findings, complete neurologic recovery has been reported in humans even after prolonged administration of CPR [32].

Researchers continue to evaluate new approaches and techniques, and further refinements in the delivery of CPR can be expected. Although research in improved CPR techniques and devices should be encouraged, research in this field is difficult. Animal models vary, and animal data may not be valid in humans. Before new CPR techniques can be adopted, they must have been demonstrated, ideally in humans, to improve either survival or neurologic outcome.

MECHANISMS OF BLOOD FLOW DURING RESUSCITATION

Any significant improvement in CPR technique would seem to require an understanding of the mechanism by which blood flows during CPR. However, there is no unanimity among researchers in this area. It is of interest that significant advances seem to have been made by research groups holding very different ideas concerning the basic mechanism of blood flow during CPR. Indeed, it is possible that several mechanisms are operative, which of these is most important may vary according to a patient's size and chest configuration.

Cardiac Compression Theory

In 1960, when Kouwenhoven et al. [6] reported on the efficacy of closed chest cardiac massage, most researchers accepted the theory that blood is propelled by compressing the heart trapped between the sternum and the vertebral columns. According to this theory, during sternal compression, the intraventricular pressures would be expected to rise higher than the pressures elsewhere in the chest. With each sternal compression, the semilunar valves would be expected to open and the atrioventricular (AV) valves to close. With sternal release, the pressure in the ventricles would be expected to fall and the AV valves to open, allowing the heart to fill from the lungs and systemic veins. Indeed, a transesophageal echocardiographic study in humans also supports this theory [33]. If the cardiac compression mechanism were operative, ventilation would best be interposed between sternal compressions so as not to interfere with cardiac compression. Also, the faster the sternal compression, the higher the volume of blood flow, assuming that the ventricles could fill adequately. The theory of cardiac compression was first brought into question in 1962, when Weale and Rothwell-Jackson [34] demonstrated that during chest compression, there is a rise in venous pressure almost equal to that of the arterial pressure. The following year, Wilder et al. [35] showed that ventilating synchronously with chest compression produced higher arterial pressures than alternating ventilation and compression. It was more than a decade, however, before more data confirmed these initial findings.

Thoracic Pump Theory

In 1976, Criley et al. [36] reported that during cardiac arrest, repeated forceful coughing is capable of generating systolic pressures comparable with those of normal cardiac activity. This finding strongly suggested that high intrathoracic pressures are capable of sustaining blood flow, independent of sternal compression. Subsequently, Niemann et al. [37,39] proposed that the propulsion of blood during sternal compression is due to the same mechanism of increased intrathoracic pressure. Studies using pressure measurements [13] and angiography [39] support this hypothesis, as do most echocardiographic studies [40]. According to this theory, the heart serves as a conduit only during CPR. Forward flow is generated by a pressure gradient between intrathoracic and extrathoracic vascular structures. Flow to the arterial side is favored by functional venous valves and greater compressibility of veins, compared to arteries, at their exit points from the thorax. The thoracic pump theory provides the rationale for experimental attempts at augmenting forward flow by increasing intrathoracic pressure.

EXPERIMENTAL AND ALTERNATIVE TECHNIQUES OF CPR

Several experimental and alternate techniques of CPR are presented in Table 23.2 [14,19–25].

Interposed Abdominal Compression CPR

Interposed abdominal compression CPR was developed by Ralston et al. [21] and Babbs et al. [41]. This technique includes manual compression of the abdomen by an extra rescuer during the relaxation phase of chest compression (Fig. 23.1). The mid-abdomen is compressed at a point halfway between the xiphoid process and the umbilicus with a force of approximately 100 mm Hg of external pressure. This pressure is estimated to be equivalent to that required to palpate the aortic pulse in a subject with a normal pulse. Two randomized clinical trials

TABLE 23.2

SUMMARY OF BASIC LIFE SUPPORT ABCD MANEUVERS FOR INFANTS, CHILDREN, AND ADULTS (NEWBORN INFORMATION NOT INCLUDED)

Maneuver	Adult Lay rescuer: 8 y HCP: adolescent and older	Child Lay rescuers: 1–8 y HCP: 1 y–adolescent	Infant Younger than 1 y of age
Airway	Head tilt–chin lift (HCP: suspected trauma, use jaw thrust)		
Breathing: initial	2 breaths at 1 s/breath	2 effective breaths at 1 s/breath	
HCP: rescue breathing without chest compressions	10–12 breaths/min (approximate)	12–20 breaths/min (approximate)	
HCP: rescue breaths for CPR with advanced airway		8–10 breaths/min (approximate)	
Foreign body airway obstruction	Conscious: abdominal thrusts Unconscious: CPR		Infant conscious: back slaps and chest thrusts Infant unconscious: CPR
Circulation HCP: pulse check (≤10 s)	Carotid		Brachial or femoral
Compression landmarks	Lower half of the sternum, between nipples		Just below the nipple line (lower half of the sternum)
Compression method: Push hard and fast Allow complete recoil	Heel of one hand, other hand on top	Heel of one hand or as for adults	Two or three fingers HCP (two rescuers): two thumb–encircling hands
Compression depth	$1^1/_2$–2 in	Approximately one-third to one-half the depth of the chest	
Compression rate	Approximately 100/min		
Compression-to-ventilation ratio	30:2 (one or two rescuers)	30:2 (single rescuer) HCP: 15:2 (two rescuers)	
Defibrillation: AED	Use adult pads Do not use child pads	Use AED after 5 cycles of CPR (out of hospital) Use pediatric system for children 1–8 y if available HCP: for sudden collapse (out of hospital) or in-hospital arrest use AED as soon as available	No recommendation for infants <1 y of age

Note: Maneuvers used by only health care providers are indicated by "HCP." AED, automatic external defibrillator.
Adapted from ECC Committee, Subcommittees and Task Forces of the American Heart Association: 2005 American Heart Association Guidelines for Cardiopulmonary Resuscitation and Emergency Cardiovascular Care. *Circulation* 112[24, Suppl]:IV1–203, 2005.

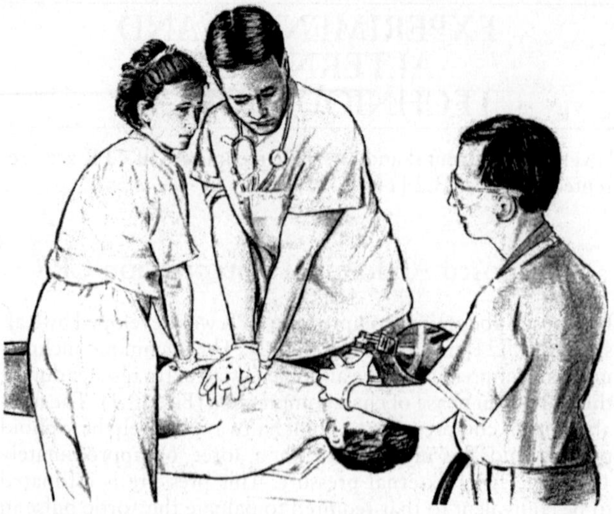

FIGURE 23.1. Interposed abdominal compression cardiopulmonary resuscitation. It is more convenient when the interposed chest and abdominal compressions are performed from opposite sides of the patient. [From Guidelines 2000 for cardiopulmonary resuscitation and emergency cardiovascular care. *Circulation* 102[Suppl 8]:I-1, 2000, with permission. Copyright 2000, American Heart Association.]

have demonstrated a statistically significant improvement in outcome measures for in-hospital cardiac arrest [42,43], but no improvement has been shown for out-of-hospital arrest [44]. On the basis of these findings, interposed abdominal compression CPR is recommended as an option for in-hospital cardiac arrest when sufficient personnel trained in the technique are available. However, it should be emphasized that the safety and efficacy of interposed abdominal compression CPR in patients with recent abdominal surgery, pregnancy, or aortic aneurysm has not been studied.

Open-Chest CPR

One of the first forms of successful CPR was open-chest CPR. It was shown to be effective when definitive care was rapidly available and is associated with survival rates, largely in operating room arrests, ranging from 16% to 37% [2]. Mechanistically, open-chest CPR clearly involves cardiac compression without use of a thoracic gradient. Weale and Rothwell-Jackson [34] demonstrated lower venous pressures and higher arterial pressures than with closed-chest compression. There is considerable evidence that open-chest CPR may be more efficacious than closed-chest CPR in terms of cardiac output and cerebral and myocardial preservation. One study has suggested increased ROSC with open-chest CPR [45]. Clearly, some patients with penetrating chest trauma are not likely to respond to chest compression and are candidates for open-chest CPR. Several studies suggest a benefit from thoracotomy in these patients [46]. If open-chest CPR is to be used, it should be used early in the sequence. Patients with blunt chest and abdominal trauma may also be candidates for open-chest CPR. Obviously, this technique should not be attempted unless adequate facilities and trained personnel are available.

Cardiopulmonary Bypass for Unresponsive Arrest

Cardiopulmonary bypass is certainly not a form of routine life support; however, it has been considered as a possible adjunct to artificial circulation. It is an indispensable adjunct to cardiac surgery and is being used more frequently for invasive procedures as a standby in case of sudden cardiac collapse. In dog models, bypass has been shown capable of providing near-normal end-organ blood flow with improved ability to resuscitate and neurologic status [47]. Emergency bypass can be instituted with femoral artery and vein access, without thoracotomy [48]. Lack of study in humans, timely access, and cost are issues to consider before bypass can be recommended for wider use in cardiac arrest.

INFECTIOUS DISEASES AND CPR

The fear provoked by the spread of human immunodeficiency virus (HIV) may lead to excessive caution when dealing with strangers. The effect of this fear on CPR is serious and must be addressed at some length [49].

The public's fear can be counteracted only by continued education and by stressing the facts. Health care workers have more opportunities for exposure to patients with HIV and their concerns must be adequately addressed [50].

Saliva has not been implicated in the transmission of HIV even after bites, percutaneous inoculation, or contamination of open wounds with saliva from HIV-infected patients [51,52]. Hepatitis B–positive saliva has also not been demonstrated to be infectious when applied to oral mucus membranes or through contamination of shared musical instruments or CPR training manikins used by hepatitis B carriers. However, it is not impossible that the mouth-to-mouth technique may result in the exchange of blood between the patient and the rescuer if there are open lesions or trauma to the buccal mucosa or lips. Diseases such as tuberculosis, herpes, and respiratory viral infections are potentially spread during mouth-to-mouth ventilation. Infections thought to have been transmitted by CPR include *Helicobacter pylori*, *Mycobacterium tuberculosis*, meningococcus, herpes simplex, *Shigella*, *Streptococcus*, *Salmonella*, and *Neisseria gonorrhoeae*. There have been no cases reported of transmission of HIV, hepatitis B virus, hepatitis C virus, or cytomegalovirus. The impact of these facts is different for lay people and health care professionals, and different for those carrying infection and for those at risk of infection [53].

Implications for Rescuers With Known or Potential Infection

Potential rescuers who know or highly suspect that they are infected with a serious pathogenic organism should not perform mouth-to-mouth ventilation if another rescuer is available who is less likely to be infectious or if the circumstances allow for any other immediate and effective method of ventilation, such as using mechanical ventilation devices.

Implications for Health Care Professionals

Although the probability of a rescuer becoming infected with HIV during CPR seems minimal, all those called on to provide CPR in the course of their employment should have ready access to mechanical ventilation devices. Bag–valve–mask devices should be available as initial ventilation equipment, and early endotracheal intubation should be encouraged when possible. Masks with one-way valves and plastic mouth and nose covers with filtered openings are available and provide some protection from transfer of oral fluids and aerosols. S-shaped mouthpieces, masks without one-way valves, and handkerchiefs provide little, if any, barrier protection and should not be considered for routine use. With these guidelines in mind, health care professionals are reminded that they have a special moral and ethical, and in some instances legal, obligation to provide CPR, especially in the setting of their occupational duties.

Implications for Manikin Training in Cardiopulmonary Resuscitation

The guidelines of the American Heart Association (AHA) specify that students or instructors should not actively participate in CPR training sessions with manikins if they have dermatologic lesions on their hands or in oral or circumoral areas, if they are known to be infected with hepatitis or HIV, or if they have reasons to believe that they are in the active stage of any infectious process. In routine ventilation training, instructors should not allow participants to exchange saliva by performing mouth-to-mouth ventilation in sequence without barrier mouthpieces. Special plastic mouthpieces and specialized manikins protect against such interchange of mucus.

Training in CPR for People With Chronic Infections

If a potentially infectious person is to be trained in CPR, commonsense precautions should be taken to protect other participants from any risk of infection. The chronically infected individual should be given a separate manikin for practice that is adequately disinfected before anyone else uses it. The chronically infected trainee should be made aware of the preceding guidelines for potential rescuers with infections. In addition, the potential risk of infection for the immunocompromised rescuer should not be ignored.

An agency that requires successful completion of a CPR course as a prerequisite for employment must decide whether to waive its requirement for an employee who is unable to complete a CPR course for whatever reason. That agency must also determine whether a chronically infected person should continue to work in a situation in which CPR administration is a duty of employment.

STANDARD PROCEDURES AND TEAM EFFORT

The distinctive function of the intensive care unit (ICU) is to serve as a locus of concentrated expertise in medical and nursing care, life-sustaining technologies, and treatment of complex multiorgan system derangement. Historically, it was the development of effective treatment for otherwise rapidly fatal arrhythmias during acute myocardial infarction that impelled the medical community to establish ICUs [54]. Rapid response by medical personnel has been facilitated by constant professional attendance and the development of widely accepted guidelines for resuscitation. Each member of the professional team is expected to respond in accordance with these guidelines.

Avoiding the need for CPR and ACLS by early intervention is a goal of rapid response teams (RRT). RRT, also called medical evaluation teams (MET), have been consistently shown to decrease hospital code rates [55]. Some studies have found a decrease in hospital mortality with the use of RRT, though this has not been found in all studies. How RRT can best be organized and implemented, as well as which hospitals benefit most, is yet to be determined [56].

The skills necessary to perform adequately during a cardiac or respiratory arrest and to interface smoothly with ACLS techniques cannot be learned from reading texts and manuals. CPR courses taught according to AHA guidelines allow hands-on experience that approximates the real situation and tests the psychomotor skills needed in an emergency. All those who engage in patient care should be trained in BLS. Those whose duties require a higher level of performance should be trained in ACLS as well. As these skills deteriorate with disuse, they need to be updated. It is worth noting that there is no "certification" in BLS or ACLS. Issuance of a "card" is neither a license to perform these techniques nor a guarantee of skill, but simply an acknowledgment that an individual attended a specific course and passed the required tests. If employers or government agencies require such a card of their health workers, it is by their own mandate.

The ensuing discussion of BLS and ACLS techniques follows the recommendations and guidelines established by the AHA and presented in a supplement to volume 112 of *Circulation* [57].

BASIC LIFE SUPPORT FOR ADULTS WITH AN UNOBSTRUCTED AIRWAY

BLS is meant to support the circulation and respiration of those who have experienced cardiac or respiratory arrest. After recognizing and ascertaining its need, definitive help is summoned without delay and CPR is initiated.

Respiratory Arrest

Respiratory arrest may result from airway obstruction, near-drowning, stroke, smoke inhalation, drug overdose, electrocution, or physical trauma. In the ICU, pulmonary congestion, respiratory distress syndrome, and mucus plugs are frequent causes of primary respiratory arrests. The heart usually continues to circulate blood for several minutes, and the residual oxygen in the lungs and blood may keep the brain viable. Early intervention by opening the airway and providing ventilation may prevent cardiac arrest and may be all that is required to restore spontaneous respiration. In the intubated patient, careful suctioning of the airway and attention to the ventilator settings are required.

Cardiac Arrest

Cardiac arrest results in rapid depletion of oxygen in vital organs. After 6 minutes, brain damage is expected to occur, except in cases of hypothermia (e.g., near-drowning in cold water). Therefore, early bystander CPR (within 4 minutes) and rapid ACLS with attempted defibrillation (within 8 minutes) are essential in improving survival and neurologic recovery rates [58].

The sequence of steps in CPR may be summarized as the ABCs of CPR: *a*irway, *b*reathing, and *c*irculation. This mnemonic is useful in teaching the public, but it should be remembered that each step is preceded by *assessment* of the need for intervention: before opening the airway, the rescuer determines unresponsiveness; before breathing, the rescuer determines breathlessness; before circulation, the rescuer determines pulselessness (Table 23.2).

Assessment and Determination of Unresponsiveness and Alerting of Emergency Medical Services

A person who has undergone cardiac arrest may be found in an apparently unconscious state (i.e., an unwitnessed arrest) or may be observed to suddenly lapse into apparent unconsciousness (i.e., a witnessed arrest). In either case, the rescuer must react promptly to assess the person's responsiveness by attempting to wake and communicate with the person by tapping or gently shaking and shouting. The rescuer should summon the nearby staff for help. If no other person is immediately available, the rescuer should call the hospital emergency line for the resuscitation team to respond (e.g., "code blue").

In the ICU, nearly all arrests should be witnessed. Early recognition of cardiac and respiratory arrests is facilitated by electronic and video monitoring. Unfortunately, it is quite possible for a patient to become lost behind this profusion of electronic signals, the dependability of which varies widely. For several precious minutes, a heart with pulseless electric activity (PEA) continues to provide a comforting electronic signal, while the brain suffers hypoxic damage. A high frequency of false alarms due to loose electrodes or other artifacts may dangerously raise the threshold of awareness and prolong the response time of the ICU team. The overall efficacy of the monitoring devices, therefore, depends highly on meticulous skin preparation and care of electrodes, transducers, pressure cables, and the like.

Sudden apparent loss of consciousness, occasionally with seizures, may be the first signal of arrest and requires prompt reaction. After determining unresponsiveness, the pulse is assessed. If the carotid pulse cannot be palpated in 5 to 10 seconds and a defibrillator is not immediately available, a precordial thump can be considered and is performed by striking the lower third of the sternum with the fist, from a height of approximately 8 in (or the span of the stretched fingers of one hand). However, there is a lack of evidence supporting its use. The thump should not be performed by BLS providers and the AHA has not recommended for or against its use [57]. If the pulse does not return and a defibrillator is not immediately available, the rescuer should proceed with establishing the airway (see the next section).

Opening the Airway and Determining Breathlessness

After establishing unresponsiveness and positioning the individual on his or her back (Fig. 23.2), the next step is to open the airway and check for spontaneous breathing (see Chapter 1). In a monitored arrest with VF or tachycardia, this step is taken after initial attempts to defibrillate. Meticulous attention to establishing an airway and supplying adequate ventilation is essential to any further resuscitative effort. The team leader must carefully monitor the adequacy of ventilation, as well as direct the resuscitative effort. The leadership role is best accomplished if the leader does not directly perform procedures.

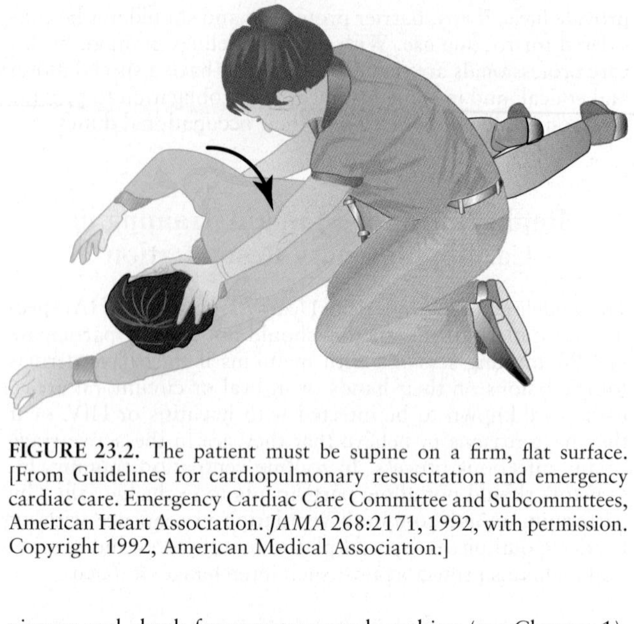

FIGURE 23.2. The patient must be supine on a firm, flat surface. [From Guidelines for cardiopulmonary resuscitation and emergency cardiac care. Emergency Cardiac Care Committee and Subcommittees, American Heart Association. *JAMA* 268:2171, 1992, with permission. Copyright 1992, American Medical Association.]

The head tilt–chin lift maneuver (Figs. 23.3 and 23.4) is usually successful in opening the airway. The head is tilted backward by a hand placed on the forehead. The fingers of the other hand are positioned under the mandible and the chin is lifted upward. The teeth are almost approximated, but the mouth is not allowed to close. Because considerable cervical hyperextension occurs, this method should be avoided in patients with cervical injuries or suspected cervical injuries. The jaw-thrust maneuver (Fig. 23.5) provides the safest initial approach to opening the airway of a patient with a cervical spine injury; it usually allows excellent airway opening with a minimum of cervical extension. The angles of the mandible are grasped using both hands and lifting upward, thus tilting the head gently backward.

After opening the airway, the rescuer should take 3 to 5 seconds to determine if there is spontaneous air exchange. This is accomplished by placing an ear over the patient's mouth and nose while watching to see if the patient's chest and abdomen rise and fall ("look, listen, and feel"; see Fig. 23.4). If

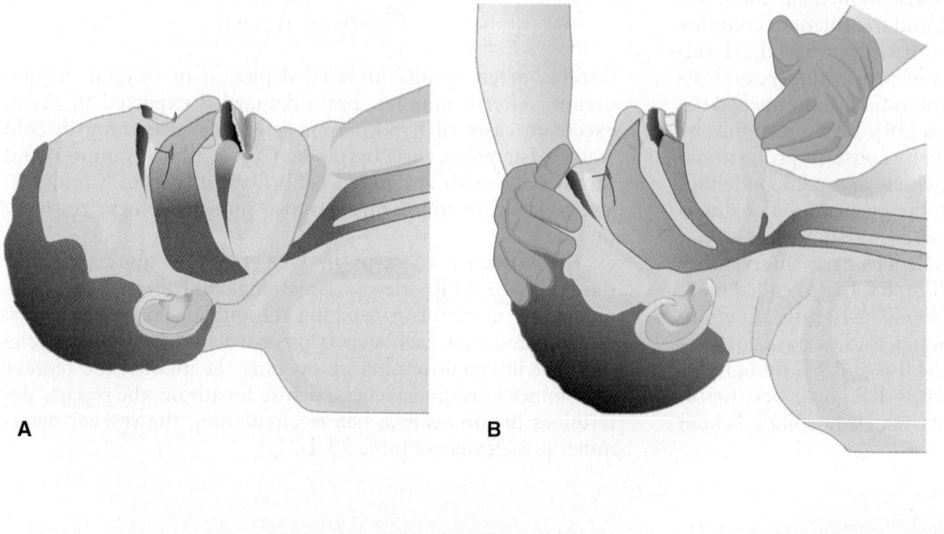

FIGURE 23.3. Opening the airway. **A:** Airway obstruction caused by tongue and epiglottis. **B:** Opening the airway with the head tilt–chin lift maneuver. [From *BLS for Healthcare Providers*, American Heart Association, 2006, with permission. Copyright 2006, American Heart Association.]

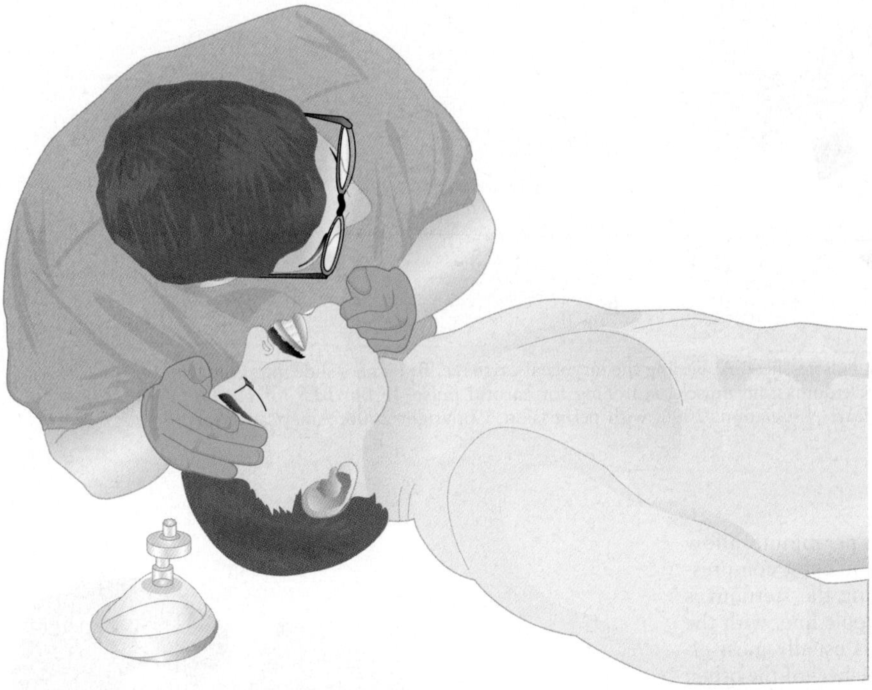

FIGURE 23.4. Determining breathlessness. Open the airway and "look, listen, and feel." [From *BLS for Healthcare Providers*, American Heart Association, 2006, with permission. Copyright 2006, American Heart Association.]

the rescuer fails to see movement, hear respiration, or feel the rush of air against the ear and cheek, rescue breathing should be initiated.

Rescue Breathing

If spontaneous breathing is absent, rescue breathing with an airway–mask–bag unit must be initiated (see Chapter 1). If equipment is immediately available and the rescuer is trained, intubation and ventilatory adjuncts should be used initially. Each breath should be delivered during 1 second, allowing the patient's lungs to deflate between breaths. Thereafter, the rate of 10 to 12 breaths per minute is maintained for as long as necessary, with tidal volumes of approximately 700 mL. Delivering the breath during 1 second helps to prevent gastric insufflation compared with faster delivery. Melker et al. [59] demonstrated airway pressures well in excess of those required to open the lower esophageal sphincter when quick breaths are used to ventilate patients. If the patient wears dentures, they are usually best left in place to assist in forming an adequate seal.

If air cannot be passed into the patient's lungs, another attempt at opening the airway should be made. The jaw-thrust maneuver may be necessary. If subsequent attempts at ventilation are still unsuccessful, the patient should be considered to have an obstructed airway and attempts should be made to dislodge a potential foreign body obstruction.

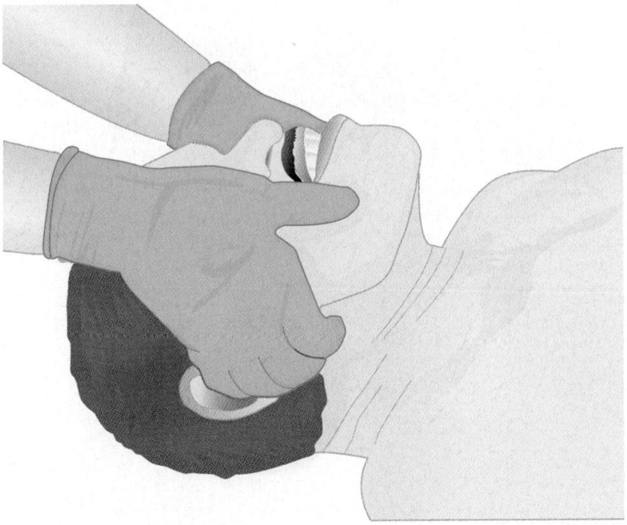

FIGURE 23.5. Jaw-thrust maneuver: opening the airway with minimal extension of the neck. [From *BLS for Healthcare Providers*, American Heart Association, 2006, with permission. Copyright 2006, American Heart Association.]

Determining Pulselessness

In the adult, the absence of a central pulse is best determined by palpating the carotid artery (Fig. 23.6), although rarely the carotid pulse may be absent because of localized obstruction. If a pulse is not felt after 10 seconds of careful searching, chest compression is initiated, unless electric countershock for ventricular arrhythmia or artificial pacing for asystole is immediately available. Although lay rescuers are no longer expected to perform a pulse check because it has been shown that checking the carotid pulse by a lay person is an inaccurate method of confirming the presence or absence of circulation, it is the position of the AHA that *health care providers* should continue to be taught and to perform a pulse check. Therefore, rescuers should start CPR if the victim is unconscious (unresponsive), not moving and not breathing [60].

Chest Compression

Artificial circulation depends on adequate chest compression through sternal depression. Recent recommendations of CPR

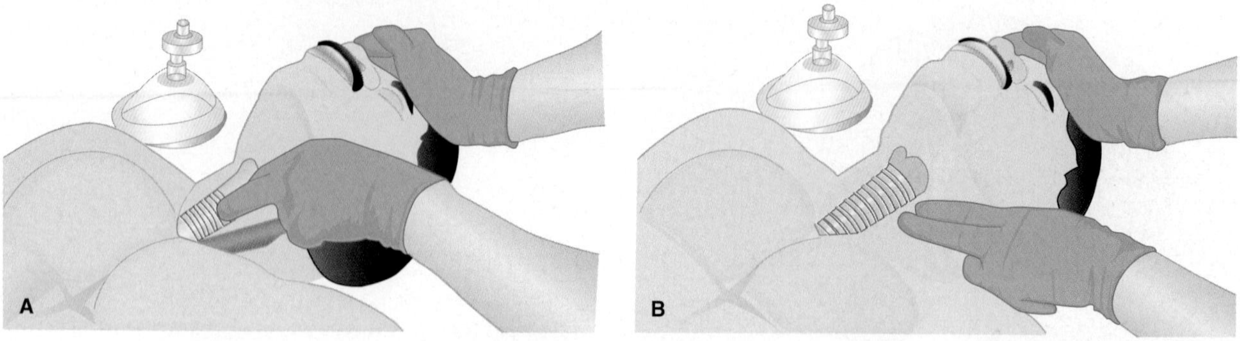

FIGURE 23.6. Determining pulselessness. A: Feeling the laryngeal cartilage. B: Fingers slide into groove between trachea and sternocleidomastoid muscle, searching for carotid pulse. [From *BLS for Healthcare Providers*, American Heart Association, 2006, with permission. Copyright 2006, American Heart Association.]

are "push hard at a rate of 100 compressions per minute, allow full chest recoil, and minimize interruptions in chest compressions" [60]. The safest manner of depressing the sternum is with the heel of the rescuer's hand at the nipple line, with the fingers kept off the rib cage (Fig. 23.7). It is usually most effective to cover the heel of one hand with the heel of the other, the heels being parallel to the long axis of the sternum. If the rescuer's hands are placed either too high or too low on the sternum, or if the fingers are allowed to lie flat against the rib cage, broken ribs and organ laceration can result. Although it is important to allow the chest to recoil to its normal position after each compression, it is not advisable to lift the hands from the chest or change their position.

The rescuer's elbows should be kept locked and the arms straight, with the shoulders directly over the patient's sternum (Fig. 23.7). This position allows the rescuer's upper body to provide a perpendicularly directed force for sternal depression. The sternum is depressed 1.5 to 2.0 in (4 to 5 cm) at a rate of approximately 100 compressions per minute. In large patients, a slightly greater depth of sternal compression may be needed to generate a palpable carotid or femoral pulse. At the end of each compression, pressure is released and the sternum is allowed to return to its normal position. Equal time should be allotted to compression and relaxation with smooth movements, avoiding jerking or bouncing the sternum. Manual and automatic chest compressors are available for fatigue-free sternal compression and are used by some EMS crews and emergency room and ICU personnel. Whether using hinged manually operated devices or compressed air-powered plungers, the rescuer must be constantly vigilant about proper placement and adequacy of sternal compression. An experimental device using a plunger-like suction device may improve flow by facilitating sternal rebound and thoracic vascular filling; this has been referred to as *active compression–decompression CPR*.

Ventilation and sternal compression should not be interrupted except under special circumstances. Warranted interruptions include execution of ACLS procedures (e.g., endotracheal intubation and placement of central venous lines) or an absolute need to move the patient. Even in these limited circumstances, interruption of CPR should be minimized. In a retrospective analysis of the VF waveform, interruption of CPR was associated with a decreased probability of conversion of VF to another rhythm [61].

New data suggest that chest compression-only CPR is as effective as standard CPR (chest compression plus rescue breathing) for out-of-hospital arrest [62,63]. Subgroup analysis in one study suggested a trend for increased survival to hospital discharge for chest compression-only CPR if the cause of the arrest was cardiac in origin or the rhythm was shockable [62].

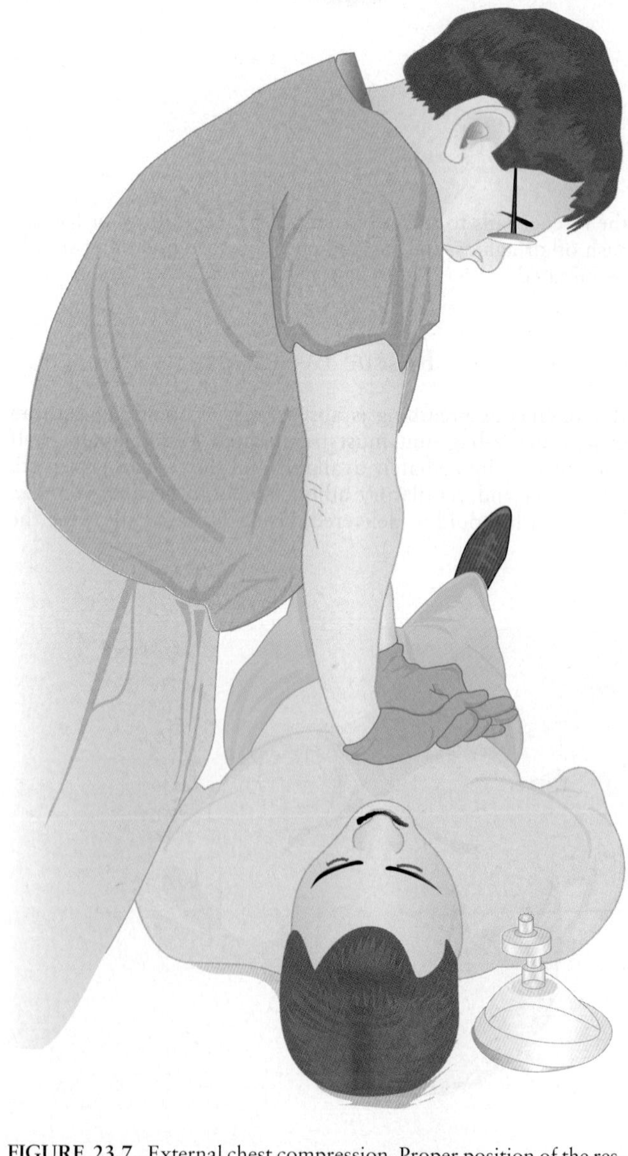

FIGURE 23.7. External chest compression. Proper position of the rescuer: place heel of the hand on the breast bone at the nipple line with shoulders directly over the patient's sternum and elbows locked. [From *BLS for Healthcare Providers*, American Heart Association, 2006, with permission. Copyright 2006, American Heart Association.]

Whether chest compression-only therapy supplants standard therapy will require further research.

Two-Rescuer CPR

The combination of artificial ventilation and circulation can be delivered more efficiently and with less fatigue by two rescuers. One rescuer, positioned at the patient's side, performs sternal compressions, while the other, positioned at the patient's head, maintains an open airway and performs ventilation. This technique should be mastered by all health care workers called on to perform CPR. Lay people have not been routinely taught this method in the interest of improving retention of basic skills. The compression rate for two-rescuer CPR, as for one-rescuer CPR, is approximately 100 compressions per minute. The new recommendation of the compression-to-ventilation ratio is 30 to 2. In an animal model of cardiac arrest, a compression-to-ventilation ratio of 30 to 2 was associated with significantly shorter time to ROSC [64]. The only exception to this recommendation is when two health care workers are providing CPR to a child or infant (except newborns); in this instance, a 15 to 2 compression-to-ventilation ratio should be used [60]. When the rescuer performing compressions is tired, the two rescuers should switch responsibilities with the minimum possible delay.

Complications of BLS Procedures

Proper application of CPR should minimize serious complications, but serious risks are inherent in BLS procedures and should be accepted in the context of cardiac arrest. Awareness of these potential complications is important to the postresuscitative care of the arrest patient.

Gastric distention and regurgitation are common complications of artificial ventilation without endotracheal intubation. These complications are more likely to occur when ventilation pressures exceed the opening pressure of the lower esophageal sphincter. In mask ventilation, 1 second should be allowed for air delivery. Although an esophageal obturator airway may decrease the threat of distention and regurgitation during its use, the risk is increased at the time of its removal. To obviate this risk, the trachea should be intubated and protected with an inflated cuff before the esophageal cuff is deflated and the esophageal obturator removed.

Complications of sternal compression and manual thrusts include rib and sternal fractures, costochondral separation, flail chest, pneumothorax, hemothorax, hemopericardium, subcutaneous emphysema, mediastinal emphysema, pulmonary contusions, bone marrow and fat embolism, and lacerations of the esophagus, stomach, inferior vena cava, liver, or spleen [65]. Although rib fractures are common during CPR, especially in the elderly, no serious sequelae are likely unless tension pneumothorax occurs and is not recognized. The more serious complications are unlikely to occur in CPR if proper hand position is maintained and exaggerated depth of sternal compression is avoided. Overzealous or repeated abdominal or chest thrusts for relief of airway obstruction are more likely to cause fractures or lacerations. For this reason, abdominal thrust is not recommended for the infant younger than 1 year.

Monitoring the Effectiveness of Basic Life Support

The effectiveness of rescue effort is assessed regularly by the ventilating rescuer, who notes the chest motion and the escape of expired air. Unintentional hyperventilation is frequent during CPR, with studies in clinical situations showing that patients are commonly ventilated at a rate of 18 to 30, far faster than recommended. The adequacy of circulation is assessed by noting an adequate carotid pulse with sternal compressions.

Animal and clinical studies suggest that the best guides to the efficacy of ongoing CPR efforts are aortic diastolic pressure and myocardial perfusion pressure (aortic diastolic minus right atrial diastolic) [66–68]. In instrumented patients for whom systemic arterial pressure (with or without central venous pressure) is available, attempts should be made to optimize myocardial perfusion pressure during CPR.

Pupillary response, if present, is a good indicator of cerebral circulation. However, fixed and dilated pupils should not be accepted as evidence of irreversible or biologic death. Ocular diseases, such as cataracts, and a variety of drugs (e.g., atropine and ganglion-blocking agents) interfere with the pupillary light reflex. The decision to cease BLS should be made only by the physician in charge of the resuscitation effort; this decision should not be made until it is obvious that the patient's cardiovascular system will not respond with ROSC to adequate administration of ACLS, including electric and pharmacologic interventions. Remediable problems such as airway obstruction, severe hypovolemia, and pericardial tamponade should also have been reasonably excluded by careful attention to ACLS protocols. Published guidelines in the literature suggest that BLS can be stopped if all of the following are present: the event was not witnessed by EMS personnel, no AED has been used, and there is no ROSC in the prehospital setting [57].

PEDIATRIC RESUSCITATION

Most infants and children who require resuscitation have had a primary respiratory arrest. Cardiac arrest results from the ensuing hypoxia and acidosis; therefore, the focus of pediatric resuscitation is airway maintenance and ventilation. The outcomes for CPR in children with cardiac arrest are poor because the cessation of cardiac activity is usually the manifestation of prolonged hypoxia. Brain damage is, therefore, all too common. Respiratory arrest, if treated before cessation of cardiac activity has supervened, carries a much better prognosis [69]. It is for this reason that it is recommended to provide the initial steps of CPR for infants and children before taking the time to telephone for emergency assistance. The first minute of CPR will allow opening of the airway and the beginning of artificial ventilation. If an obstructed airway is found, attempts at dislodging a foreign body should not be delayed. In children with a history of cardiac disease or arrhythmias, or in previously healthy children who are witnessed to have a sudden collapse, a primary arrhythmic event is more likely and immediate activation of the EMS system may be beneficial.

Effective techniques for ventilation and chest compression vary with the child's size. Infant procedures are applicable to patients who are smaller than an average child of 1 year. Child techniques are applicable to patients who are of a size similar to the average child of 1 to 8 years. Adult techniques are appropriate for patients who appear larger than the typical child of 8 years of age.

If the child is found to be apneic, he or she is placed in the supine position and the head tilt–chin lift maneuver is used to open the airway (Fig. 23.8). Overextension of the neck is unnecessary and is best avoided. Some believe that overextension of the child's flexible neck may obstruct the trachea; however, there are no data to support this. The jaw-thrust maneuver should be used if an adequate airway is not obtained with the head tilt–chin lift maneuver or if neck injury is suspected.

Artificial ventilation of the infant requires the rescuer's mouth to cover both the mouth and the nose to make an effective seal. If the child's face is too large to allow a tight seal to

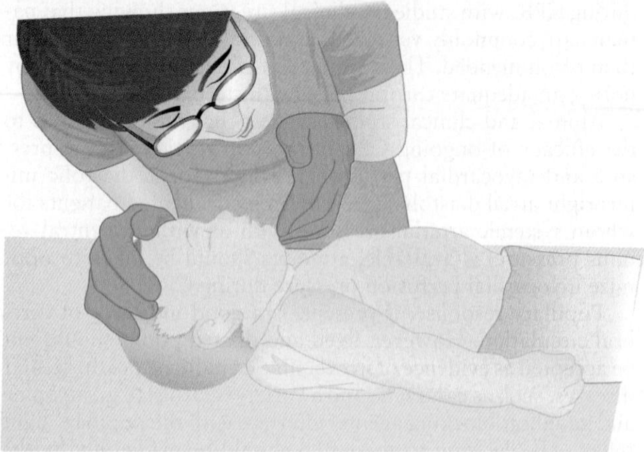

FIGURE 23.8. Head tilt–chin lift in the infant: opening the airway. [From *BLS for Healthcare Providers*, American Heart Association, 2006, with permission. Copyright 2006, American Heart Association.]

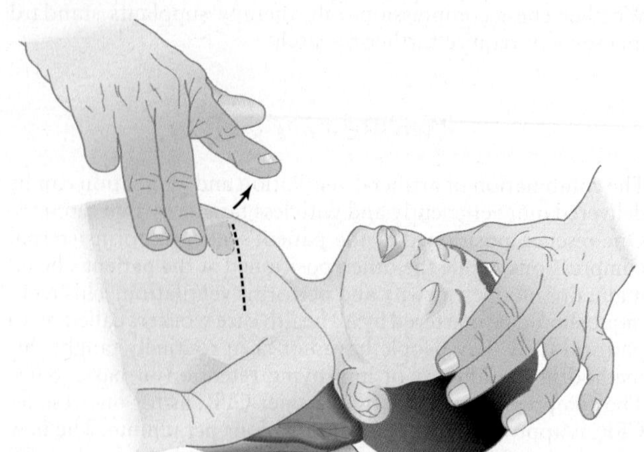

FIGURE 23.9. Locating finger position for sternal compression in the infant, using an imaginary line between the nipples. [From Standards and guidelines for cardiopulmonary resuscitation (CPR) and emergency cardiac care (ECC). *JAMA* 255:2843, 1986, with permission. Copyright 1986, American Medical Association.]

be made over both the mouth and the nose, the mouth alone is covered, as for the adult.

The lung volume of the pediatric patient is small enough that a "puff" of air from the airway–mask–bag unit apparatus might be adequate to inflate the lungs. However, the smaller diameter of the tracheobronchial tree and any pulmonary disease that may be contributing to the arrest usually provide considerable resistance to airflow. Therefore, a surprising amount of inspiratory pressure may be needed to move adequate air into the lungs. This is especially true for the child who may have edematous respiratory passages. Accordingly, adequacy of ventilation must be monitored by observing the rising and falling of the chest and feeling and listening for the exhaled air from the child's mouth and nose. Excessive ventilatory volumes may exceed esophageal opening pressure and cause gastric distention.

Gastric decompression is dangerous and should be avoided until the patient has been intubated and the cuff inflated to protect the respiratory tract from aspiration. If the gastric distention is so severe that ventilation is greatly compromised, the child's body should be turned to one side before pressure on the abdomen is applied. It is preferable to use a gastric tube with suction whenever possible.

The ventilation rate for infants is approximately 20 breaths per minute (one every 3 seconds), whereas the rate for children can be 12 to 20 breaths per minute (one every 3 to 5 seconds). Adolescents are ventilated at the adult rate of 10 to 12 breaths per minute (one every 5 seconds). If artificial circulation is not necessary, more rapid ventilatory rates are acceptable.

Artificial circulation is instituted in the absence of a palpable pulse. The pulse of the larger child can easily be detected at the carotid artery, as in the adult. The neck of the infant, however, is too short and fat for reliable palpation of the carotid artery. Palpation of the precordium is also unreliable; some infants have no precordial impulse in spite of adequate cardiac output. It is recommended, therefore, that the presence of an infant's pulse be determined by palpating the brachial artery between the elbow and the shoulder.

To apply chest compression in an infant, the rescuer's index finger is placed on the sternum, just below the intermammary line. The proper area for compression is one fingerbreadth below the intermammary line on the lower sternum, at the location of the middle and ring fingers (Fig. 23.9). Using two or three fingers, the sternum is compressed approximately one-third to one-half the depth of the thorax. Alternatively, for chest compressions in the infant, the *two thumb–encircling hands* technique may be used when two rescuers are available (Fig. 23.10). The frequency of sternal compressions for infants and children is 100 per minute. During one-rescuer support, the ratio of compression to ventilation is 30 to 2 for infants and children [60].

OBSTRUCTED AIRWAY

An unconscious patient can experience airway obstruction when the tongue falls backward into the pharynx. Alternatively, the epiglottis may block the airway when the pharyngeal muscles are lax. In the sedated or ill patient, regurgitation of stomach contents into the pharynx is a frequent cause of respiratory arrest. Blood clots from head and facial injuries are another source of pharyngeal and upper airway obstruction. Even otherwise healthy people may have foreign body obstruction from poorly chewed food, large wads of gum, and so forth. The combination of attempting to swallow inadequately chewed food, drinking alcohol, and laughing is particularly conducive to pharyngeal obstruction. Children's smaller airways are likely to obstruct with small nuts or candies.

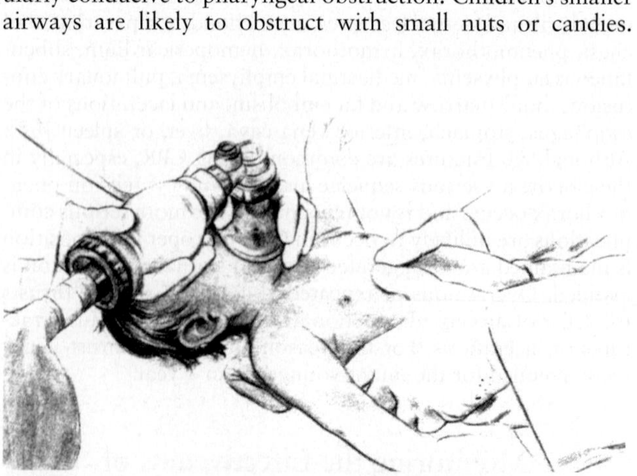

FIGURE 23.10. Chest compression in the infant using the two thumb–encircling hands technique. (Two rescuers are required.) [From Guidelines 2000 for cardiopulmonary resuscitation and emergency cardiovascular care. *Circulation* 102[Suppl 8]:I-1, 2000, with permission. Copyright 2000, American Heart Association.]

Children are also prone to airway obstruction by placing toys or objects such as marbles or beads in their mouths.

Patients who experience partial obstruction with reasonable gas exchange should be encouraged to continue breathing efforts with attempts at coughing. A patient whose obstruction is so severe that air exchange is obviously markedly impaired (cyanosis with lapsing consciousness) should be treated as having complete obstruction.

Patients who experience complete obstruction may still be conscious. They are unable to cough or vocalize. A subdiaphragmatic abdominal thrust may force air from the lungs in sufficient quantity to expel a foreign body from the airway [70].

If the person is still standing, the rescuer stands behind the person and wraps his or her arms around the person's waist. The fist of one hand is placed with the thumb side against the person's abdomen in the midline, slightly above the umbilicus and well below the xiphoid process (Fig. 23.11). The fist is grasped with the other hand and quickly thrust inward and upward. It may be necessary to repeat the thrust six to ten times to clear the airway. Each thrust should be a separate and distinct movement.

If the patient is responsive and lying down, he or she should be positioned face up in the supine position. The rescuer kneels beside or astride the person's thighs and places the heel of one hand against the person's abdomen, slightly above the navel and well below the xiphoid process. The other hand is placed directly on top of the first and pressed inward and upward with a quick forceful thrust. If the patient is unresponsive, CPR should be initiated.

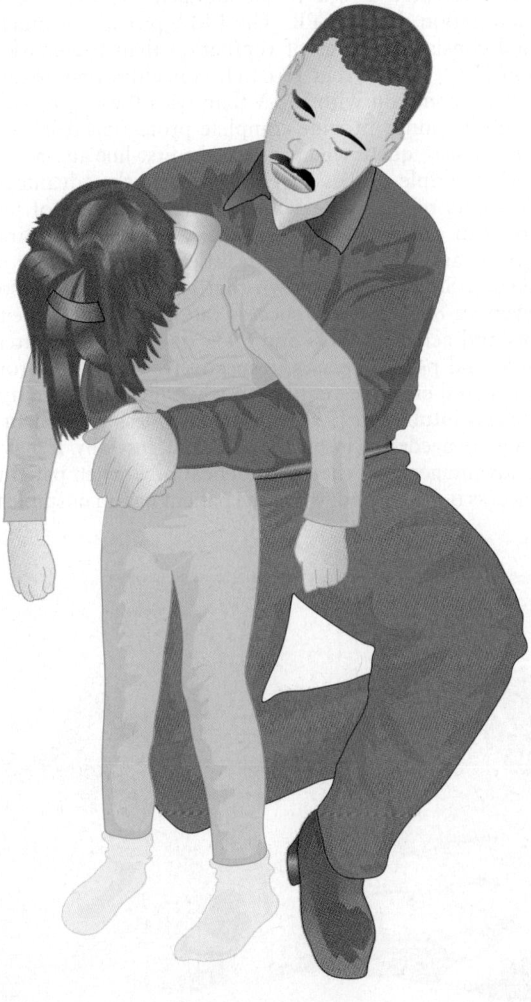

FIGURE 23.11. Abdominal thrust with conscious patient standing: rescuer standing behind individual with foreign body airway obstruction. [From *BLS for Healthcare Providers*, American Heart Association, 2006, with permission. Copyright 2006, American Heart Association.]

If attempted rescue breathing in an arrested patient fails to move air into the lungs, an obstructed airway must be presumed to be present. It may simply be due to the tongue or epiglottis, rather than a foreign body. If the airway remains closed after repositioning the head, other maneuvers to open the airway, including the jaw-thrust and tongue-jaw lift, must be used. Chest thrusts may be substituted for abdominal thrusts in patients in advanced stages of pregnancy, in patients with severe ascites, or in the markedly obese. The fist is placed in midsternum for the erect and conscious patient. For the supine patient, the hand is positioned on the lower sternum, as for external cardiac compression. Each thrust is delivered slowly and distinctly.

If attempts at dislodging a foreign body or relieving airway obstruction fail, special advanced procedures are necessary to provide oxygenation until direct visualization, intubation, or tracheostomy is accomplished.

ADVANCED CARDIAC LIFE SUPPORT IN ADULTS

The use of adjunctive equipment, more specialized techniques, and pharmacologic and electric therapy in the treatment of a person who has experienced cardiac or respiratory arrest is generally referred to as *ACLS*. These techniques and their interface with BLS and the EMS are considered in the AHA's ACLS teaching program. An improvement in survival after in-hospital cardiac arrest has been demonstrated after medical house officers were trained in ACLS [71]. An in-depth discussion is available in the ACLS text published by the AHA.

The focus of the following sections is on the techniques and medications used in the initial resuscitative efforts. The demarcation from therapies more commonly reserved for the ICU is often indistinct; indeed, it is expected to vary with the experience of the prehospital team and the degree of physician supervision. In general, most ACLS measures should be applied by trained personnel operating within an EMS system in the community, in transport, or in the hospital setting.

Airway and Ventilatory Support

Oxygenation and optimal ventilation are prerequisites for successful resuscitation (see Chapter 1). Supplemental oxygen should be administered as soon as it becomes available, beginning with 100%. In the postresuscitation period, the amount of administered oxygen may be decreased as guided by the arterial blood partial pressure of oxygen.

Emergency ventilation commonly begins with the combined use of a mask and oral airway. Mouth-to-mask ventilation is very effective as long as an adequate seal is maintained between the mask and the face. Most masks are best fitted by flaring the top and molding it over the bridge of the nose. The inflated rim is then carefully molded to the cheeks as the mask is allowed to recoil. Relatively firm pressure is required to maintain the seal. Masks with one-way valves also provide a measure of isolation from the patient's saliva and breath aerosol. Bag–valve–mask ventilation requires strong hands and a self-inflating bag. The bag should be connected to a gas reservoir and to oxygen so that 100% oxygen delivery can be approximated. It cannot be overemphasized that the success of this method depends on airway patency and an adequate seal between the mask and the face. Equally important is adequate compression of the bag to deliver the required tidal volume. It is advisable that everyone who uses this technique practice on a recording ventilating manikin to assess the adequacy of the method in his or her hands. Many people will discover that their hands are not large enough or strong enough to deliver 700 mL air. Some may have to squeeze the bag between their elbow and chest wall to supply adequate ventilation. If two people are available to ventilate, one should secure the mask while the other uses both hands to attend to the bag.

The mask design should include the following features:

- The use of transparent material, which allows the rescuer to assess lip color and to observe vomitus, mucus, or other obstructing material in the patient's airway.
- A cushioned rim around the mask's perimeter to conform to the patient's face and to facilitate a tight seal.
- A standard 15- to 22-mm connector, which allows the use of additional airway equipment.
- A comfortable fit to the rescuer's hand.
- An oxygen insufflation inlet, which allows oxygen supplementation during mouth-to-mask ventilation.
- A one-way valve, which allows some protection during mouth-to-mask ventilation.
- Availability in appropriate sizes and shapes, for various-sized faces. Most adults will be accommodated by a standard medium-sized (no. 4) oval-shaped mask.

Ventilating bags must be designed to include the following features:

- A self-refilling bag, which allows operation independent of a fresh gas source.
- A fresh gas inlet, which allows ambient air or supplemental oxygen to flow into the reservoir bag through a valve inlet.
- A nipple for oxygen connection, located near the gas inlet valve.
- An oxygen reservoir bag.
- Availability in pediatric and adult sizes.
- A nonrebreathing valve directing flow to the patient during inhalation and to the atmosphere during exhalation. The valve casing should be transparent to allow visual inspection of its function. A pop-off feature is often present to prevent high airway pressures; however, such valves should have provision to override the pop-off feature because higher airway pressures are sometimes required to ventilate lungs with unusually high resistances, especially in children.
- Reservoir tubing that can be attached to the fresh gas inlet valve, which allows an accumulation of oxygen to refill the reservoir bag during the refill cycle. Such a reservoir allows delivered oxygen to approach 100%; without it, the self-refilling bag can deliver only 40% to 50% oxygen.

Oxygen-powered resuscitators allow the pressure of compressed oxygen tanks at 50 psi to drive lung inflation. They are usually triggered by a manual control button, and the oxygen can be delivered through a mask or tube for ease of ventilation. These devices deliver oxygen at a flow rate of 100 L per minute and allow airway pressures of 60 cm H_2O. However, when used with masks and unprotected airways (not separated from the esophagus by an inflated cuff), these devices are likely to cause gastric distention and poor ventilation. They are not as reliable as mouth-to-mask or valve–bag–mask ventilation. When used in adults, they should be recalibrated to deliver flows of no more than 40 L per minute to avoid opening the lower esophageal sphincter. A relief valve that opens at approximately 60 cm H_2O and vents any excess volume into the atmosphere should be present. In addition, an alarm that sounds whenever the relief valve pressure is exceeded should be present. This alarm warns the rescuer that the patient requires higher inspiratory pressures and may not be adequately ventilated. Barotrauma is likely to occur in infants and children. Children often have high airway resistances and are difficult to ventilate with these resuscitators. These devices should be avoided in general and should not be used with infants or children.

Endotracheal intubation is required if the patient cannot be rapidly resuscitated or when adequate spontaneous ventilation does not resume quickly. Experienced personnel should attempt intubation. Resuscitative efforts should not be interrupted for more than 30 seconds with each attempt. Cricoid pressure should be applied, when possible, by a second person during endotracheal intubation to protect against regurgitation of gastric contents. The prominence inferior to that of the thyroid cartilage is the cricoid cartilage. Downward pressure should be applied with the thumb and index finger (Fig. 23.12) until the cuff of the endotracheal tube is inflated.

Once the patient is intubated and the trachea is protected from regurgitation, faster inspiratory flow rates are possible. However, hyperventilation should be avoided. Checking arterial blood gases will assist in the determination of an adequate minute ventilation. Increasing the respiratory rate may be detrimental [72].

The laryngeal mask airway (LMA) has been effective for maintaining airway patency during anesthesia since 1988 and has been accepted as one of the adjuncts for airway control and ventilation during CPR. The LMA provides a more stable and consistent means of ventilation than bag–mask ventilation [73]. The current research concludes that regurgitation is less common with LMA than with the bag-mask, and although it cannot provide complete protection from aspiration, it is less frequent when used as the first-line airway device [73,74]. Multiple studies have documented the advantages of LMA for its relative ease with insertion and ease of use by a variety of personnel: nurses, medical students, respiratory therapists, and EMS, many with little prior experience using the device. Studies have shown that inexperienced personnel achieved an 80% to 94% success rate on first placement attempts and achieved 98% and 94% on subsequent attempts of adult and pediatric cases, respectively. The LMA provides adequate and effective ventilation when measured against endotracheal intubation [75]. Additionally, less equipment and training are needed to insert the device successfully. It may also have advantages over the endotracheal tube when patient airway access is obstructed, when the patient has an unstable neck

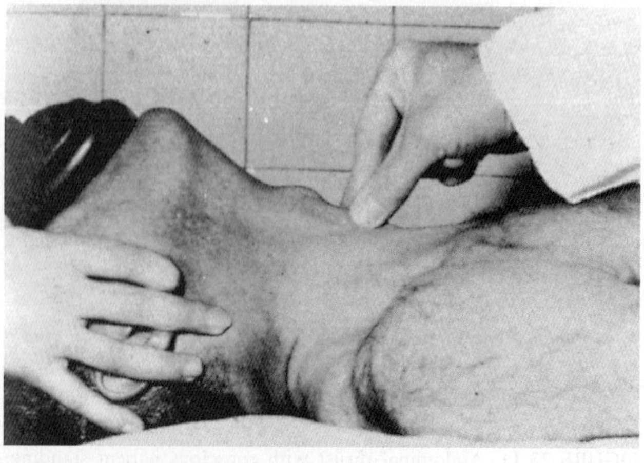

FIGURE 23.12. Cricoid pressure: application of downward pressure over the cricoid with neck extended. [From Sellick BA: Cricoid pressure to control regurgitation of stomach contents during induction of anaesthesia. *Lancet* 2:404, 1961, with permission.]

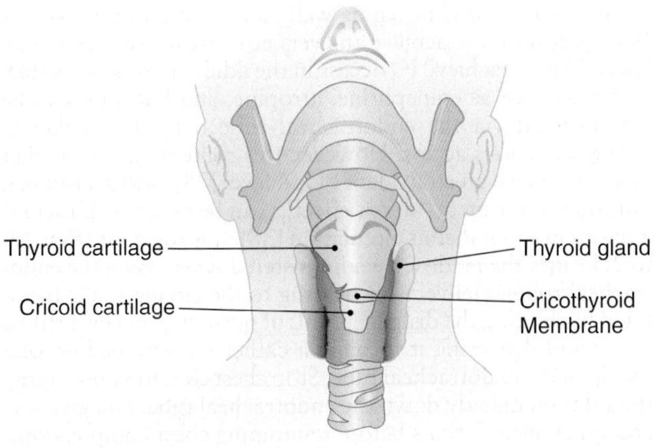

FIGURE 23.13. Landmarks for locating the cricothyroid membrane for use of transtracheal catheter ventilation or cricothyrotomy. [From *Textbook of Advanced Cardiac Life Support*. Chicago, American Heart Association, 1987, with permission. Copyright American Heart Association.]

injury, or when suitable positioning of the patient for endotracheal intubation is unattainable. LMA insertion has been successful when attempts at endotracheal intubation by experts were unsuccessful [75]. Endotracheal tubes can be fiberoptically inserted through an established LMA.

Relative contraindications for LMA use include the patient with an increased risk of aspiration pneumonitis. Examples of such situations include morbid obesity, pregnancy, recent food ingestion, gastrointestinal obstruction, and hiatal hernia. Despite these considerations, oxygenation and ventilation during cardiac arrest receive top priority and the LMA should be used if it is the fastest and efficient means of providing airway patency.

If attempts at relieving an obstructed airway have failed, several advanced techniques may be used to secure the airway until intubation or tracheostomy is successfully performed. In transtracheal catheter ventilation, a catheter is inserted over a needle through the cricothyroid membrane (Fig. 23.13). The needle is removed and intermittent jet ventilation initiated (see Chapter 1). In cricothyrotomy, an opening is made in the cricothyroid membrane with a knife (see Chapter 12). Tracheostomy, if still necessary, is best performed in the operating room by a skilled surgeon after the airway has already been secured by one of the aforementioned techniques.

Circulatory Support

Chest compression should not be unduly interrupted while adjunctive procedures are instituted. The rescuer coordinating the resuscitation effort must ensure that adequate pulses are generated by the compressor. The carotid or femoral pulse should be evaluated every few minutes.

Mechanical chest compressors seem useful in the hands of experienced resuscitators. It is important that such devices be correctly calibrated to provide a stroke of 1.5 to 2.0 in. The position of the press on the sternum must be checked frequently to ensure adequate compression with a minimum of damage. The press may be a manually operated hinged device or may be powered by compressed gas (usually 100% oxygen). The plunger is mounted on a backboard and is associated with a time–pressure-cycled ventilator. This device is programmed to deliver CPR using a compression duration that is 50% of the cycle length. Such units allow the patient to be harnessed to the backboard, fixing the location of the plunger. When used properly, with careful monitoring of patient position, this device facilitates CPR during transport. An acceptable electrocardiogram (ECG) can often be recorded with the compressor in operation, and defibrillation can be delivered during the downstroke of chest compression, without delays in CPR.

ECG monitoring is necessary during resuscitation to guide appropriate electric and pharmacologic therapy. Until ECG monitoring allows diagnosis of the rhythm, the patient should be assumed to be in VF (see the section "Ventricular Fibrillation and Pulseless Ventricular Tachycardia").

Most defibrillators currently marketed have built-in monitoring circuitry in the paddles or pads (quick look). On application of the defibrillator paddles, the patient's ECG is displayed on the monitor screen. This facilitates appropriate initial therapy. For continuous monitoring beyond the first few minutes, a standard ECG monitoring unit should be used.

ECG monitoring must never be relied on without frequent reference to the patient's pulse and clinical condition. What appears on the monitor screen to be VF or asystole must not be treated as such unless the patient is found to be without a pulse. An apparently satisfactory rhythm on the monitor must be accompanied by an adequate pulse and blood pressure.

Defibrillation

Electric defibrillation is the definitive treatment for most cardiac arrests. It should be delivered as early as possible and repeated frequently until VF or pulseless VT has been terminated.

Electric defibrillation involves passing an electric current through the heart and causing synchronous depolarization of the myofibrils. As the myofibrils repolarize, the opportunity arises for the emergence of organized pacemaker activity.

Proper use of the defibrillator requires special attention to the following:

1. *Selection of proper energy levels* (see the section "Clinical Settings"). This lessens myocardial damage and arrhythmias occasioned by unnecessarily high energies. For biphasic defibrillators, the energy should be 120 to 200 J. For the monophasic defibrillators, the energy should be 360 J [57].
2. *Proper asynchronous mode*. The proper mode must be selected if the rhythm is VF. The synchronizing switch must be deactivated or the defibrillator will dutifully await the R wave that will never come. For rapid pulseless VT (approximately 150 to 200 beats per minute), it is best not to attempt synchronization with the R wave because this increases the likelihood of delivering the shock on the T wave. If the countershock should fall on the T wave and induce VF, another unsynchronized countershock must be delivered promptly after confirming pulselessness.
3. *Proper position of the paddles or pads*. This allows the major energy of the electric arc to traverse the myocardium. The anterolateral position requires that one paddle or pad be placed to the right of the upper sternum, just below the clavicle. The other paddle or pad is positioned to the left of the nipple in the left midaxillary line. In the anteroposterior position, one paddle or pad is positioned under the left scapula with the patient lying on it. The anterior paddle or pad is positioned just to the left of the lower sternal border.
4. *Adequate contact between paddles or pads and skin*. This should be ensured, using just enough electrode paste to cover the paddle face without spilling over the surrounding skin. The rescuer should hold the paddles with firm pressure (approximately 25 lb). The pressure should be delivered using the forearms; leaning into the paddles should be avoided for fear that the rescuer may slip. If defibrillator electrode paddles are used, the skin must be carefully prepared according to the manufacturer's directions.

5. *No contact with anyone other than the patient.* The rescuer must be sturdily balanced on both feet and not standing on a wet floor. CPR must be discontinued with no one remaining in contact with the patient. It is the responsibility of the person defibrillating to check the patient's surroundings, ensure the safety of all participants, loudly announce the intention to countershock, and depress both buttons. The use of an automatic or semiautomatic defibrillator does not decrease the operator's need for diligence.
6. If no skeletal muscle twitch or spasm has occurred, the equipment, contacts, and synchronizer switch used for elective cardioversions should be rechecked.

Electric energy delivered in a biphasic waveform is clearly superior to monophasic waveforms for implantable defibrillators (see Chapter 6), but there is a paucity of evidence to show that one waveform is superior over another with regard to ROSC or survival to hospital discharge. External defibrillators are now available with biphasic waveforms.

Electronic Pacemaker

Pacemaker therapy requiring positioning of transvenous or transthoracic electrodes is time consuming, technically demanding, and usually interferes with adequate performance of CPR. External pacing equipment often allows myocardial capture with some discomfort and skeletal muscle contraction [76]. Obviously, this is unimportant during asystole or bradycardic cardiac arrest. Unfortunately, pacing does not produce a perfusing rhythm in most cases of cardiac arrest. Patients who respond to emergency pacing are those with severe bradycardias or conduction block who have reasonably well-preserved myocardial function [77].

Venous Access

Venous access with a reliable intravenous (IV) route must be established early in the course of the resuscitative effort to allow for the administration of necessary drugs and fluids. However, initial defibrillation attempts and CPR should not be delayed for the placement of an IV line. Peripheral venous access through antecubital veins is often more convenient because it is less likely to interfere with other rescue procedures. Cannulation of such veins may be difficult, however, because of venous collapse or constriction. A large-bore catheter system should be used because needles in the vein are apt to become dislodged during CPR. A long catheter may be threaded into the central circulation. Alternatively, the extremity may be elevated for 10 to 20 seconds and 20 mL of flush solution used to help entry of the drug into the central circulation [78]. Lower extremity peripheral veins should be avoided because it is questionable whether drugs enter into the central circulation from such veins during CPR [79].

Central venous access offers a more secure route for drug administration and should be attempted if initial resuscitative efforts are not successful. Femoral vein cannulation is apparently difficult to achieve during CPR, and flow into the thorax is slower than with upper torso access. If the femoral vein is successfully cannulated, a long line should be placed into the vena cava above the level of the diaphragm. Internal jugular or subclavian routes are preferable, but central venous catheterization at these sites should not be allowed to delay defibrillation attempts or interfere with CPR. They should be placed by experienced operators.

Although central lines may be associated with an increased incidence of complications for patients receiving fibrinolytic therapy, they are not an absolute contraindication to its use.

In infants and children as well as adults, the intraosseous (IO) route is easy to achieve and very effective for venous access. Special kits to achieve IO access in the adult are now available.

Drugs such as epinephrine, atropine, and lidocaine can be administered via the endotracheal tube if there is delay in achieving venous access. However, this route requires a higher dose to achieve an equivalent blood level [38], and a sustained duration of action (a "depot effect") can be expected if there is a return in spontaneous circulation [38]. It is suggested that 2.0 to 2.5 times the IV dose be administered when using the endotracheal route. Delivery of the drug to the circulation is facilitated by diluting the drug in 10 mL of normal saline or distilled water and delivering it through a catheter positioned beyond the tip of the endotracheal tube. Stop chest compressions, spray the solution quickly down the endotracheal tube, and give several quick insufflations before reinitiating chest compressions. Intracardiac injection of epinephrine is to be avoided.

Correction of Hypoxia

Hypoxia should be corrected early during CPR with administration of the highest possible oxygen concentration. Inadequate perfusion, decreased pulmonary blood flow, pulmonary edema, atelectasis, and ventilation–perfusion mismatch all contribute to the difficulty in maintaining adequate tissue oxygenation. Inadequate tissue oxygenation results in anaerobic metabolism, the generation of lactic acid, and the development of metabolic acidosis.

Correction of Acidosis

Correction of acidosis must be considered when the arrest has lasted for more than several minutes. *Metabolic acidosis* develops because of tissue hypoxia and conversion to anaerobic metabolism. *Respiratory acidosis* occurs because of apnea or hypoventilation with intrapulmonary ventilation–perfusion abnormalities; the marked decrease in pulmonary blood flow that exists even with well-performed CPR also contributes.

Sodium bicarbonate reacts with hydrogen ions to buffer metabolic acidosis by forming carbonic acid and then carbon dioxide and water. Each 50 mEq sodium bicarbonate generates 260 to 280 mm Hg carbon dioxide, which can be eliminated only through the expired air. Because carbon dioxide of exhaled gas during CPR is decreased, the carbonic acid generated by sodium bicarbonate cannot be effectively eliminated. Paradoxic intracellular acidosis is likely to result, and arterial blood gases may not correctly reflect the state of tissue acidosis. The sodium and osmolar load of bicarbonate is high; excessive administration results in hyperosmolarity, hypernatremia, and worsened cellular acidosis. With these concerns in mind, the AHA guidelines suggest that sodium bicarbonate be avoided until successful resuscitation has reestablished a perfusing rhythm [80]. In the postresuscitative state, the degree of acidosis can be better estimated from blood gases and the acidemia corrected with hyperventilation and possibly bicarbonate administration. Sodium bicarbonate is of questionable value in treating the metabolic acidosis during cardiac arrest; it has not been shown to facilitate ventricular defibrillation or survival in cardiac arrest [81,82]. In any case, bicarbonate should not be used during cardiac arrest until at least 10 minutes have passed, the patient is intubated, and the patient has not responded to initial defibrillation and drug intervention. An exception is the patient with known preexisting hyperkalemia in whom administration of bicarbonate is recommended. The use of bicarbonate may also be of value in patients who have a known preexisting bicarbonate-responsive acidosis or a tricyclic antidepressant overdosage, or to alkalinize the urine in drug overdosage. When bicarbonate is used, 1 mEq per kg may be given as the initial dose. When possible, further therapy should be guided by the calculated base deficit. To avoid iatrogenically induced alkalosis, complete correction of the calculated base deficit should be avoided.

Volume Replacement

Increased central volume is often required during CPR, especially if the initial attempts at defibrillation have failed. PEA is particularly likely to be caused either by acute severe hypovolemia (e.g., exsanguination) or by a cardiovascular process for which volume expansion may be a lifesaving temporizing measure (e.g., pericardial tamponade, pulmonary embolism, and septic shock). The usual clues for hypovolemia, such as collapsed jugular and peripheral veins and evidence of peripheral vasoconstriction, are unavailable during cardiac arrest; furthermore, dry mucus membranes and absence of normal secretions (tears and saliva) are unreliable in acute hypovolemia. Most physical findings of tamponade, pulmonary embolism, or septic shock are absent during arrest. Therefore, one must be guided by an appropriate clinical history and have a low threshold to administer volume during CPR.

Simple crystalloids, such as 5% dextrose in water (D_5W), are inappropriate for rapid expansion of the circulatory blood volume. Isotonic crystalloids (0.9% saline and Ringer's lactate), colloids, or blood are necessary for satisfactory volume expansion. Crystalloids are more readily available, easier to administer, and less expensive than colloids. They are also free of the potential to cause allergic reactions or infections. Colloids are more likely to sustain intravascular volume and oncotic pressure.

If the patient has a weak pulse, simple elevation of the legs may help by promoting venous return to the central circulation. Volume challenges should be given as needed until pulse and blood pressure have been restored or until there is evidence of volume overload.

DRUG THERAPY

Sympathomimetic Drugs and Vasopressors

Sympathomimetic drugs act either directly on adrenergic receptors or indirectly by releasing catecholamines from nerve endings. Most useful during cardiac emergencies are the adrenergic agents, which include the endogenous biogenic amines epinephrine, norepinephrine, and dopamine, and the synthetic agent isoproterenol and its derivative dobutamine [57]. Of note, none of the sympathomimetics can be administered in a line with an alkaline infusion. Extravasation of any agent with α-adrenergic activity can result in tissue necrosis, so they should be infused via a central venous catheter if possible. If extravasation does occur, 5 to 10 mg phentolamine in 10 to 15 mL saline should be infiltrated as soon as possible into the area of extravasation.

Epinephrine

Epinephrine is a naturally occurring catecholamine that has both α- and β-activities. Although epinephrine is the pressor agent used most frequently during CPR, the evidence that it improves the outcome in humans is scant.

Indications for the use of epinephrine include all forms of cardiac arrest because its α-vasoconstrictive activity is important in raising the perfusion pressure of the myocardium and brain. The importance of α-adrenergic activity during resuscitation has been noted in several studies [83], whereas administration of pure β-agonists (e.g., isoproterenol or dobutamine) has been shown to be ineffective [84]. The β-action of epinephrine is theoretically useful in asystole and bradycardic arrests by increasing heart rate. The β-effect has also been touted to convert asystole to VF or to convert "fine" VF to "coarse." Coarse or wide-amplitude VF is easier to convert to a perfusing rhythm than fine or small-amplitude VF. However, this may be primarily due to the shorter time course of the arrest in patients still manifesting wide-amplitude rather than small-amplitude VF.

Epinephrine is best administered IV. As soon as possible after failed ventricular defibrillation attempts (or if defibrillation is not an option), an adult in cardiac arrest should be given a 1-mg dose at a 1 to 10,000 dilution (10 mL). It should be given in the upper extremity or centrally (see the earlier discussion in the section "Venous Access"), and may be repeated every 5 minutes. If a peripheral line is used, the drug should be administered rapidly and followed by a 20-mL bolus of IV fluid and elevation of the extremity. It should not be administered in the same IV line as an alkaline solution. If an IV line has not been established, the endotracheal route may be used, but the intracardiac route should be avoided because it is prone to serious complications such as intramyocardial injection, coronary laceration, and pneumothorax. An IV infusion of 1 to 10 μg per minute can also be given for inotropic and pressor support. Two multicenter trials evaluating the effectiveness of high-dose epinephrine in cardiac arrest failed to demonstrate an improvement in survival or neurologic outcome [85,86].

Risks in the use of epinephrine and other α-agonists include tissue necrosis from extravasation and inactivation from admixture with bicarbonate.

Norepinephrine

Norepinephrine is a potent α-agonist with β-activity. Its salutary α-effects during CPR are similar to those of epinephrine [87]. However, there are no data to support the belief that it is superior to epinephrine during an arrest.

The major effect of norepinephrine is on the blood vessels. Initial coronary vasoconstriction usually gives way to coronary vasodilatation, probably as a result of increased myocardial metabolic activity. In a heart with compromised coronary reserve, this may cause further ischemia. During cardiac arrest, its usefulness, like that of epinephrine, is most likely due to peripheral vasoconstriction with an increase in perfusion pressure. In patients with spontaneous circulation who are in cardiogenic shock (when peripheral vasoconstriction is often already extreme), its effect is more difficult to predict. Norepinephrine also causes considerable renal and mesenteric vasoconstriction, whereas dopamine at low infusion rates causes vasodilatation in these vascular beds.

Indications for the use of norepinephrine during cardiac arrest are similar to those for epinephrine, although there does not appear to be any reason to prefer it to epinephrine. Norepinephrine appears to be most useful in the treatment of shock caused by inappropriate decline in peripheral vascular resistance, such as septic shock and neurogenic shock. It is administered by IV infusion and titrated to an adequate perfusion pressure. Bitartrate, 4 to 8 mg (2 to 4 mg of the base), should be diluted in 500 mL D_5W or 5% dextrose in normal saline. A typical starting infusion rate is 0.5 μg per minute and most adults respond to 2 to 12 μg per minute, but some require rates up to 30 μg per minute. Abrupt termination of the infusion (as may occur in transport) may lead to sudden severe hypotension.

Precautions to the use of norepinephrine include its inappropriate use in hypovolemic shock and in patients with already severe vasoconstriction. Intra-arterial pressure monitoring is strongly recommended when using norepinephrine because indirect blood pressure measurement is often incorrect in patients with severe vasoconstriction. In patients with myocardial ischemia or infarction, the myocardial oxygen requirements are increased by all catecholamines, but especially by norepinephrine because of its marked afterload-increasing properties. Unless the increased oxygen delivery occasioned by the rise in perfusion pressure outweighs the increase in myocardial oxygen requirement caused by the afterload increase, norepinephrine is likely to have deleterious effects. Heart rate, rhythm, ECG evidence for ischemia, direct systemic and pulmonary pressures, urine output, and cardiac output should be closely monitored when using this drug in patients with myocardial ischemia or infarction.

Isoproterenol

This synthetic catecholamine has almost pure β-adrenergic activity. Its cardiac activity includes potent inotropic and chronotropic effects, both of which will increase the myocardium's oxygen demand. In addition to bronchodilatation, the arterial beds of the skeletal muscles, kidneys, and gut dilate, resulting in a marked drop in systemic vascular resistance. Cardiac output can be expected to increase markedly unless the increased myocardial oxygen demand results in substantial myocardial ischemia. Systolic blood pressure is usually maintained because of the rise in cardiac output, but the diastolic and mean pressures usually decrease. As a result, coronary perfusion pressure drops at the same time that the myocardial oxygen requirement is increased. This combination can be expected to have deleterious effects in patients with ischemic heart disease, especially during cardiac arrest. The main clinical usefulness of isoproterenol is in its ability to stimulate pacemakers within the heart.

Indications for isoproterenol are primarily in the setting of atropine-resistant, hemodynamically significant bradyarrhythmias, including profound sinus and junctional bradycardia, as well as various forms of high-degree AV block. It should be used only as an interim measure, until effective transcutaneous or IV pacing can be instituted. If the aortic diastolic pressure is already low, epinephrine is likely to be better tolerated as a stimulus to pacemakers. *Under no circumstances should isoproterenol be used during cardiac arrest.*

Isoproterenol is administered by titration of an IV solution. One mg isoproterenol (Isuprel) is diluted with either 250 mL D_5W (4 mg per mL) or 500 mL D_5W (2 mg per mL). The infusion rate should be only rapid enough to effect an adequate perfusing heart rate (2 to 20 μg per minute, or 0.05 to 0.5 μg per kg per minute). Depending on the adequacy of cardiac reserve, a target heart rate as low as 50 to 55 beats per minute may be satisfactory. Occasionally, more rapid rates are necessary.

Precautions in the use of isoproterenol are largely due to the increase in myocardial oxygen requirement, with its potential for provoking ischemia; *this effect, coupled with the possibility of dropping the coronary perfusion pressure, makes isoproterenol a dangerous selection in the coronary patient.* The marked chronotropic effects may cause tachycardia and provoke serious ventricular arrhythmias, including VF. Isoproterenol is usually contraindicated if tachycardia is already present, especially if the arrhythmia may be secondary to digitalis toxicity. If significant hypotension develops with its use, it may be combined with another β-agonist with α-activity. However, switching to dopamine or epinephrine is usually preferable; better yet is the use of pacing for rate control.

Dopamine

This naturally occurring precursor of norepinephrine has α-, β-, and dopamine-receptor–stimulating activities. The dopamine-receptor activity dilates renal and mesenteric arterial beds at low doses (1 to 2 μg per kg per minute). β-adrenergic activity is more prominent with doses from 2 to 10 μg per kg per minute, whereas α-adrenergic activity is predominant at doses greater than 10 μg per kg per minuteα It has not been shown that these dose ranges have relevance in the clinical setting. Indications for the use of dopamine are primarily significant hypotension and cardiogenic shock.

Dopamine is administered by IV titration in the range of 2 to 20 μg per kg per minute. Rarely, a patient may need in excess of 20 μg per kg per minute. A 200-mg ampule is diluted to 250 or 500 mL in D_5W or 5% dextrose in normal saline for a concentration of 800 or 400 mg per mL. As with all catecholamine infusions, the lowest infusion rate that results in satisfactory perfusion should be the goal of therapy.

Precautions for dopamine are similar to those for other catecholamines. Tachycardia or ventricular arrhythmias may require reduction in dosage or discontinuation of the drug. If significant hypotension occurs from the dilating activity of dopaminergic or β-active doses, small amounts of an α-active drug may be added. Dopamine may increase myocardial ischemia.

Dobutamine

Dobutamine is a potent synthetic β-adrenergic agent that differs from isoproterenol in that tachycardia is less problematic. Unless ischemia supervenes, cardiac output will increase, as will renal and mesenteric blood flow.

Dobutamine is indicated primarily for the short-term enhancement of ventricular contractility in the patient with heart failure. It may be used for stabilization of the patient after resuscitation or for the patient with heart failure refractory to other drugs. It may also be used in combination with IV nitroprusside, which lowers peripheral vascular resistance and thereby left ventricular afterload. Although nitroprusside lowers peripheral resistance, dobutamine maintains the perfusion pressure by augmenting the cardiac output.

Dobutamine is administered by slow-titrated IV infusion. A dose as low as 0.5 μg per kg per minute may prove to be effective, but the usual dose range is 2.5 to 10.0 μg per kg per minute. A 250-mg vial is dissolved in 10 mL of sterile water and then to 250 or 500 mL D_5W for a concentration of 1.0 or 0.5 μg per mL.

Precautions for dobutamine are similar to those for other β-agonists. Dobutamine may cause tachycardia, ventricular arrhythmias, myocardial ischemia, and extension of infarction. It must be used with caution in patients with coronary artery disease.

Vasopressin

Vasopressin is not a catecholamine, but a naturally occurring antidiuretic hormone. In high doses, it is a powerful constrictor of smooth muscles and as such has been studied as an adjunctive therapy for cardiac arrest in an attempt to improve perfusion pressures and organ flows. Vasopressin may be especially useful in prolonged cardiac arrest as it remains effective as a vasopressor even in severe acidosis [88]. It may be used as a first agent in arrest in lieu of epinephrine or as the second agent if the first dose of epinephrine failed to cause a return in pulse. The dose of vasopressin is 40 units IV or IO.

Antiarrhythmic Agents

Antiarrhythmic agents have been thought to play an important role in stabilizing the rhythm in many resuscitation situations; however, the data in support of their value are scanty. Although lidocaine, bretylium, and procainamide had been considered useful in counteracting the tendency to ventricular arrhythmias, convincing evidence of benefit to their use for pulseless VT and VF is wanting. On the basis of recent studies, amiodarone has gained considerable acceptance for the emergency treatment of refractory VT and VF.

Amiodarone

Amiodarone is a benzofuran derivative that is structurally similar to thyroxine and contains a considerable level of iodine. Gastrointestinal absorption is slow; therefore, when given orally, the onset of action is delayed while the drug slowly accumulates in adipose tissue. The mean elimination half-life is 64 days (range, 24 to 160 days). IV administration allows rapid onset of action, with therapeutic blood levels achieved with 600 mg given over 24 hours.

Amiodarone decreases myocardial contractility, and it also causes vasodilatation, which counterbalances the decrease in contractility. In general, it is therefore well tolerated even by those with myocardial dysfunction.

Amiodarone given IV has been successful in terminating a variety of reentrant and other types of supraventricular and ventricular rhythms. In a major study of out-of-hospital cardiac arrest due to ventricular arrhythmias refractory to shock, patients were initially treated with either amiodarone (246 patients) or placebo (258 patients). Patients given amiodarone had a higher incidence of bradycardia (41% vs. 25%) and hypotension (59% vs. 48%), but also a higher rate of survival to hospital admission (44% vs. 34%) [89]. This study did not demonstrate an increase in survival to hospital discharge or in neurologic status. On the basis of this study, amiodarone has been given status as an option for use after defibrillation attempts and epinephrine in refractory ventricular arrhythmias during cardiac arrest. It is also an option for ventricular rate control in rapid atrial arrhythmias in patients with impaired left ventricular function when digitalis has proved ineffective. Other optional uses are for control of hemodynamically stable VT, polymorphic VT, preexcited atrial arrhythmias, and wide-complex tachycardia of uncertain origin. It may also be useful for chemical cardioversion of atrial fibrillation or as an adjunct to electric cardioversion of refractory paroxysmal supraventricular tachycardia (PSVT) and atrial fibrillation or flutter.

Administration in cardiac arrest (pulseless VT or VF) is by rapid IV infusion of 300 mg diluted in 20 to 30 mL of saline or D_5W. Supplementary infusions of 150 mg may be used for recurrent or refractory VT or VF.

Administration for rhythms with a pulse is by IV infusion of 150 mg given during 10 minutes, followed by infusion of 1 mg per minute for 6 hours and then 0.5 mg per minute. Supplemental infusions of 150 mg may be given for recurrent or resistant arrhythmias to a total maximum dose of 2 g during 24 hours.

Lidocaine

This antiarrhythmic agent has been used for ventricular arrhythmias, such as premature ventricular complexes and VT. Premature ventricular complexes are not unusual in apparently healthy people and most often are benign. Even in the patient with chronic heart disease, premature ventricular complexes and nonsustained VT are usually asymptomatic, and controversy exists concerning the need to treat under these circumstances. The situation is different for patients with myocardial ischemia or recent myocardial infarction, who are much more likely to progress from premature ventricular complexes to sustained VT or VF. There is some evidence for the efficacy of prophylactic lidocaine in reducing primary VF in patients with acute myocardial infarction. However, the toxic-to-therapeutic ratio is not favorable enough to warrant its routine use in patients with suspected acute myocardial infarction [90].

Administration of lidocaine begins with an IV bolus. The onset of action is rapid. Its duration of action is brief, but may be prolonged by continuous infusion. A solution of lidocaine, typically 20 mg per mL (2%), should be prepared for IV administration. Prefilled syringes are available for bolus injection (see the section "Ventricular Fibrillation and Pulseless Ventricular Tachycardia" for current dosing recommendations). If the patient has suffered an acute myocardial infarction and has had ventricular arrhythmias, the infusion is continued for hours to days and tapered slowly. If the cause of the arrhythmia has been corrected, the infusion may be tapered more rapidly.

Precautions should be taken against excessive accumulation of lidocaine. The dosage should be reduced in patients with low cardiac output, congestive failure, hepatic failure, and age older than 70 years because of the decreased liver metabolism of the drug. Toxic manifestations are usually neurologic, and can vary from slurred speech, tinnitus, sleepiness, and dysphoria to localizing neurologic symptoms. Frank seizures may occur with or without preceding neurologic symptoms and may be controlled with short-acting barbiturates or benzodiazepines. Conscious patients should be warned about possible symptoms of neurologic toxicity and asked to report them immediately if they occur. Enlisting the patient's aid may also allay the fear that could otherwise develop from unexpected neurologic symptoms. Excessive blood levels can significantly depress myocardial contractility.

Procainamide

Procainamide hydrochloride is an antiarrhythmic agent with quinidine-like activity. Like quinidine, it is useful in suppressing a wide variety of ventricular and supraventricular arrhythmias. It is effective against reentrant as well as ectopic arrhythmogenic mechanisms. It has somewhat less vagolytic effect than quinidine and does not cause the rise in digoxin level seen with quinidine. Procainamide is sometimes of use in the critical care setting for the suppression of ventricular arrhythmias not effectively treated by amiodarone or lidocaine or in patients who cannot be treated with either of these two agents. It may also be used in patients with supraventricular arrhythmias causing hemodynamic compromise or worsening ischemia.

Procainamide is administered either orally or by IV injection. For serious arrhythmias in the critical care setting, IV injection is preferable. An infusion of 20 mg per minute (0.3 mg per kg per minute) is given up to a loading dose of 17 mg per kg (1.2 g for a 70-kg patient) or until the arrhythmia is suppressed, hypotension develops, or the QRS widens by 50% of its original width. A maintenance infusion may then be started at 1 to 4 mg per minute. The dosage should be lowered in the presence of renal failure. Blood levels of procainamide and its metabolite *N*-acetylprocainamide should be monitored in patients with renal failure or patients who are receiving more than 3 mg per minute for more than 24 hours. Infusions as low as 1.4 mg per kg per hour may be needed in patients with renal insufficiency.

Precautions in the use of procainamide include its production of systemic hypotension, disturbance in AV conduction, and decreased ventricular contractility. IV infusion must be carefully monitored, with frequent blood pressure determinations and measurement of ECG intervals PR, QRS, and QT. Hypotension usually responds to slowing the infusion rate. If the QRS interval increases by more than 50% of its initial width, procainamide infusion should be discontinued. Widened QRS signifies toxic blood levels and may herald serious AV conduction abnormalities and asystole. This is particularly true of patients with digitalis intoxication and those with antecedent AV conduction abnormalities. A marked increase in QT interval may predispose a patient to torsades de pointes. Patients who have ventricular arrhythmias of the torsades variety or ventricular arrhythmias associated with bradycardias should not be treated with procainamide.

Adenosine

Adenosine is an endogenous purine nucleoside that depresses AV nodal conduction and sinoatrial nodal activity. Because of the delay in AV nodal conduction, adenosine is effective in terminating arrhythmias that use the AV node in a reentrant circuit (e.g., PSVT) [91]. In supraventricular tachycardias, such as atrial flutter or atrial fibrillation, or atrial tachycardias that do not use the AV node in a reentrant circuit, blocking transmission through the AV node may prove helpful in clarifying the diagnosis [92,93]. However, the use of adenosine in wide-complex tachycardia of uncertain origin to discriminate between VT and supraventricular tachycardia with aberrancy is discouraged. The half-life of adenosine is less than 5 seconds because it is rapidly metabolized.

Administration is by IV bolus of 6 mg given during 1 to 3 seconds, followed by a 20-mL saline flush. An additional dose of 12 mg may be given if no effect is seen within 1 to 2 minutes. Patients taking theophylline may need higher doses.

Side effects caused by adenosine are transient and may include flushing, dyspnea, and angina-like chest pain (even in the absence of coronary disease). Sinus bradycardia and ventricular ectopy are common after terminating PSVT with adenosine, but the arrhythmias are typically short lived so as to be clinically unimportant. The reentrant tachycardia may recur after the effect of adenosine has dissipated and may require additional doses of adenosine or a longer acting drug, such as verapamil or diltiazem.

Theophylline and other methylxanthines, such as theobromine and caffeine, block the receptor responsible for adenosine's electrophysiologic effect; therefore, higher doses may be required in their presence. Dipyridamole and carbamazepine, on the other hand, potentiate and may prolong the effect of adenosine; therefore, other forms of therapy may be advisable.

Verapamil and Diltiazem

Unlike other calcium channel–blocking agents, verapamil and diltiazem increase refractoriness in the AV node and significantly slow conduction. This action may terminate reentrant tachycardias that use the AV node in the reentrant circuit (e.g., PSVT). These drugs may also slow the ventricular response in patients with atrial flutter or fibrillation and even in patients with multifocal atrial tachycardia. They should be used only in patients in whom the tachycardia is known to be supraventricular in origin.

Administration of verapamil is by IV bolus of 2.5 to 5.0 mg during 2 minutes. In the absence of a response, additional doses of 5 to 10 mg may be given at 15- to 30-minute intervals to a maximum of 20 mg. The maximum cumulative dose is 20 mg. Diltiazem may be given as an initial dose of 0.25 mg per kg with a follow-up dose of 0.35 mg per kg, if needed. A maintenance infusion of 5 to 15 mg per hour may be used to control the rate of ventricular response in atrial fibrillation.

Verapamil and diltiazem should be used for arrhythmias known to be supraventricular in origin and in the absence of preexcitation. Both verapamil and diltiazem may decrease myocardial contractility and worsen congestive heart failure or even provoke cardiogenic shock in patients with significant left ventricular dysfunction. They should, therefore, be used with caution in patients with known cardiac failure or suspected diminished cardiac reserve and in the elderly. If worsened failure or hypotension develops after the use of these agents, calcium should be administered, as described in the section "Other Agents."

Magnesium

Cardiac arrhythmias and even sudden cardiac death have been associated with magnesium deficiency [91]. Hypomagnesemia decreases the uptake of intracellular potassium and may precipitate VT or fibrillation. Routine use of magnesium in cardiac arrest or after myocardial infarction is not recommended. Magnesium may be of value for patients with torsades de pointes, even in the absence of hypomagnesemia.

Magnesium is administered IV. For rapid administration during VT or VF with suspected or documented hypomagnesemia, 1 to 2 g may be diluted in 100 mL of D_5W and given during 1 to 2 minutes. A 24-hour infusion of magnesium may be used for peri-infarction patients with documented hypomagnesemia. A loading dose of 1 to 2 g is diluted in 100 mL D_5W and slowly given during 5 minutes to 1 hour, followed by an infusion of 0.5 to 1 g per hour during the ensuing 24 hours. Clinical circumstances and the serum magnesium level dictate the rate and duration of the infusion. Hypotension or asystole may occur with rapid administration.

Other Agents

Additional drugs occasionally found useful or necessary during resuscitation or in the immediate postresuscitation period include atropine, calcium, nitroprusside, and nitroglycerine; these agents are discussed in the following sections. Many other drugs may be required in particular circumstances and are discussed in other parts of this text. An incomplete list of these drugs includes beta-blockers, ibutilide, propafenone, flecainide, sotalol, digoxin, antibiotics, thiamine, thyroxine, morphine, naloxone, adrenocorticoids, fibrinolytic agents, anticoagulants, antiplatelet agents, and dextrose.

Atropine Sulfate

Atropine is an anticholinergic drug that increases heart rate by stimulating pacers and facilitating AV conduction that is suppressed by excessive vagal tone.

Atropine is indicated primarily in bradycardias causing hemodynamic difficulty or associated with ventricular arrhythmias (see Fig. 23.17). Atropine may be useful in AV block at the nodal level. It is also used in asystole and bradycardic arrests in the hope that decreased vagal tone will allow the emergence of an effective pacemaker [57].

Atropine is administered by IV bolus. If a rapid, full vagolytic response is desired, as in asystole or bradycardic arrest, 1 mg should be administered IV at once. If a satisfactory response has not occurred within several (3 to 5) minutes, additional 1-mg doses should be given in a bolus, to a maximum dose of 3 mg (0.04 mg per kg). For bradycardia with a pulse, the initial dose should be 0.5 mg repeated every 5 minutes until the desired effect is obtained, to a maximum dose of 3 mg (0.04 mg per kg). Atropine may be given by the endotracheal route at doses 2.5 times the IV dose.

Precautions for atropine include the requirement that an inordinately rapid heart rate not be produced. Patients with ischemic heart disease are likely to have worsened ischemia or ventricular arrhythmias if the rate is too rapid. Uncommonly, a patient will have a paradoxic slowing of rate with atropine; this is more likely to occur with smaller first doses and is caused by a central vagal effect. This effect is rapidly counteracted by additional atropine. In this situation, the next dose of atropine should be given immediately. If additional atropine does not correct the problem, the patient may require judicious use of isoproterenol or pacemaker therapy.

Calcium

Calcium's positive inotropic effect has led to its use in cardiac arrest. The contractile state of the myocardium depends in part on the intracellular concentration of the calcium ion. Transmembrane calcium flux serves an important regulatory function in both active contraction and active relaxation. The use of calcium in cardiac arrest is based on an early report by Kay and Blalock [94] in which several pediatric cardiac surgical patients were successfully resuscitated, apparently with the aid of calcium. However, several field studies have failed to demonstrate an improvement in survival or neurologic outcome with the use of calcium versus a control [95]. In addition, after standard doses of calcium administered during cardiac arrest, many patients are found to have very high calcium blood levels [96]. This is apparently due to the markedly contracted volume of distribution of the ion in the arrested organism. In addition, calcium has the theoretic disadvantage of facilitating postanoxic tissue damage, especially in the brain and heart. Digitalis toxicity may be exacerbated by the administration of calcium.

Calcium is indicated only in those circumstances in which calcium has been shown to be of benefit [57]: calcium channel blocker toxicity, severe hyperkalemia, severe hypocalcemia, arrest after multiple transfusions with citrated blood, fluoride toxicity, and while coming off heart–lung bypass after cardioplegic arrest.

Calcium is available as calcium chloride, calcium gluceptate, and calcium gluconate. The gluconate salt is unstable and less frequently available. The chloride salt provides the most direct source of calcium ion and produces the most rapid effect. The gluceptate and gluconate salts require hepatic degradation to release the free calcium ion. Calcium chloride is, therefore, the best choice. It is highly irritating to tissues and must be injected into a large vein with precautions to avoid extravasation. Calcium chloride is available in a 10% solution. An initial dose of 250 to 500 mg may be administered slowly during several minutes. It may be repeated as necessary at 10-minute intervals if strong indications exist.

Precautions for calcium use include the need for slow injection without extravasation. If bicarbonate has been administered through the same line, it must be cleared before introducing the calcium. If the patient has a rhythm, rapid injection may result in bradycardia. Calcium salts must be used with caution in patients receiving digitalis.

Sodium Nitroprusside

This is a rapidly acting dilator of both arteries and veins. Systemic arterial dilatation decreases impedance to left ventricular outflow (afterload reduction), thereby diminishing resistance to left ventricular ejection and improving cardiac output. Venous dilatation simultaneously provides preload reduction by withholding blood from the central circulation and reducing left ventricular filling pressure and volume. Myocardial oxygen consumption drops and subendocardial blood flow may rise as the ventricular wall stress is lowered. In addition, the lowered left ventricular filling pressures cause a decrease in pulmonary capillary pressure and pulmonary congestion. Although vasodilators are most commonly used in the critical care unit, they are occasionally needed in the emergency room to aid in the stabilization of the resuscitated patient with severe left ventricular dysfunction.

Nitroprusside is indicated in any situation in which cardiac output is severely reduced, causing either cardiogenic shock with elevated systemic vascular resistance or pulmonary congestion from elevated left ventricular filling pressure. Patients with aortic or mitral regurgitation or a left-to-right shunt from a ventricular septal rupture are apt to respond well especially to nitroprusside infusion. Nitroprusside has also become a preferred treatment for patients in hypertensive crisis.

Nitroprusside is administered by IV infusion. The onset of action is rapid so that the effects of dose change become apparent within several minutes. For patients with severe left ventricular failure, infusion should begin at 10 μg per minute, with increments of 5 to 10 μg per minute at 5-minute intervals. Most patients respond to a total dose of 50 to 100 μg per minute, although an occasional patient requires a significantly higher dose. Patients in hypertensive crisis may be started at 50 μg per minute and may require as much as 400 to 1,000 μg per minute. Nitroprusside is available in 50-mg vials of dihydrate. The drug should be dissolved in 5 mL of D_5W and diluted to a volume of 250 to 1,000 mL in D_5W. Because of the instability of the reconstituted solution, it is recommended that it be used within 4 hours. The solution should be wrapped in opaque material because nitroprusside will deteriorate more rapidly with exposure to light.

Precautions for nitroprusside include hypotension, usually secondary to excessive dosage. Although most patients with hypotension cannot tolerate nitroprusside, some can be given nitroprusside with volume repletion. Nitroprusside is converted to cyanide in the blood, which is metabolized to thiocyanate by the liver. Thiocyanate is cleared by the kidney and can accumulate in renal failure. Signs and symptoms of thiocyanate toxicity (more likely in liver failure) include nausea, tinnitus, blurred vision, and delirium; signs of cyanide toxicity include elevated superior vena cava, or mixed venous oxygen saturation and a lactic acidosis. Nitroprusside should be discontinued if the latter two signs are observed.

Nitroglycerin

Like nitroprusside, nitroglycerin is a vasodilator that may prove to be useful in the emergency treatment of the postresuscitation patient. It may be given sublingually, transdermally, or IV, depending on the situation and desired dose. Unlike nitroprusside, nitroglycerin is a more potent dilator of venous capacitance vessels than of arterioles; therefore, it is more a preload reducer than an afterload reducer. Coronary dilatation does occur and may be particularly beneficial in patients with coronary spasm and acute ischemia. Myocardial ischemia is reversed through the lowering of preload and myocardial oxygen consumption as well as by coronary dilatation.

Sublingual or transdermal nitroglycerin is indicated for angina. The sublingual route is preferable. For persistent or frequently recurring ischemia unrelieved by other routes of administration, an infusion of nitroglycerin is often effective. It is useful for suspected coronary spasm. An infusion of nitroglycerin may also be used for preload reduction in patients with left ventricular failure. It may be given together with an infusion of nitroprusside, especially if ischemia has not been reversed by the hemodynamic effects of nitroprusside alone.

Nitroglycerin is administered by a sublingual tablet or spray (0.3 to 0.4 mg) or by a transdermal patch or ointment. For rapid effect, the sublingual route should be used. It may be repeated every 3 to 5 minutes, if pain relief or ST-segment deviation has not occurred. If ischemia persists, an infusion should be started and titrated to achieve the desired result. A 50-mg bolus of nitroglycerin may be given before the initiation of an IV drip. Two 20-mg vials may be diluted in 250 mL D_5W for a concentration of 160 μg per mL. The infusion is started at 10 to 20 mg per minute and increased by 5 to 10 μg every 5 to 10 minutes until the desired effect is achieved (e.g., fall in left ventricular pressure to 15 to 18 mm Hg, relief of chest pain, or return of ST segments to baseline). Although most patients respond to 50 to 200 μg per minute, an occasional patient will require 500 μg per minute or more; however, the maintenance of high plasma levels of nitroglycerin may induce tolerance. *Whenever possible, intermittent dosing with nitrate-free periods is recommended, and the use of the lowest effective dose is advised.*

Precautions for nitroglycerin use include hypotension and syncope, especially if the patient has had an acute myocardial infarction, is volume depleted, has either restriction to left ventricular filling (e.g., pericardial constriction or tamponade, hypertrophic disease, mitral stenosis, pulmonic stenosis, or pulmonary hypertension) or obstruction to left ventricular outflow (e.g., aortic stenosis, pulmonic stenosis, or hypertrophic obstructive cardiomyopathy). Rapid titration of IV nitroglycerin in patients with left ventricular failure requires careful hemodynamic monitoring to ensure efficacy and safety. The hypotensive patient may be placed in the Trendelenburg position and given volume replacement. Rarely, a patient with severe obstructive coronary disease develops worsened ischemia with nitroglycerin through a coronary steal mechanism. If ischemia is persistent in spite of maximal tolerated nitroglycerin dose, attempts should be made to decrease the dose, and other modalities of therapy, including heparin or cardiac catheterization, should be considered with a view to early revascularization.

CLINICAL SETTINGS

The procedures involved in the resuscitation of a person who has experienced cardiovascular or respiratory collapse are all part of a continuum progressing from the initial recognition of the problem and the institution of CPR to intervention with defibrillators, drugs, pacemakers, transport, and postresuscitative evaluation and care (Figs. 23.14 to 23.17). The following sections focus on the pharmacologic and electric interventions appropriate to various clinical settings common in cardiac arrest.

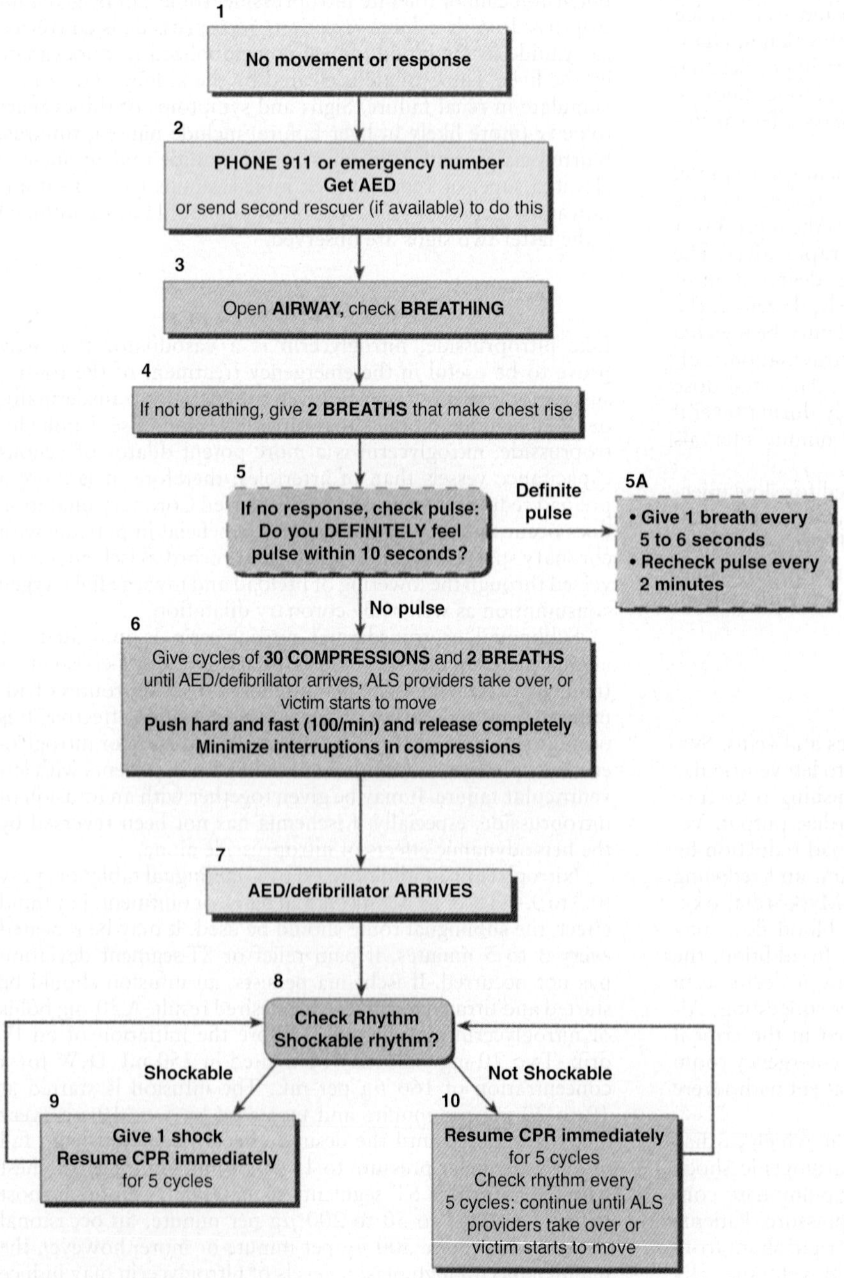

FIGURE 23.14. Adult basic life support health care provider algorithm. [From *Circulation* 112[Suppl 24]:IV-19–34, 2005, with permission. Copyright 2005, American Heart Association guidelines for cardiopulmonary resuscitation and emergency cardiovascular care.]

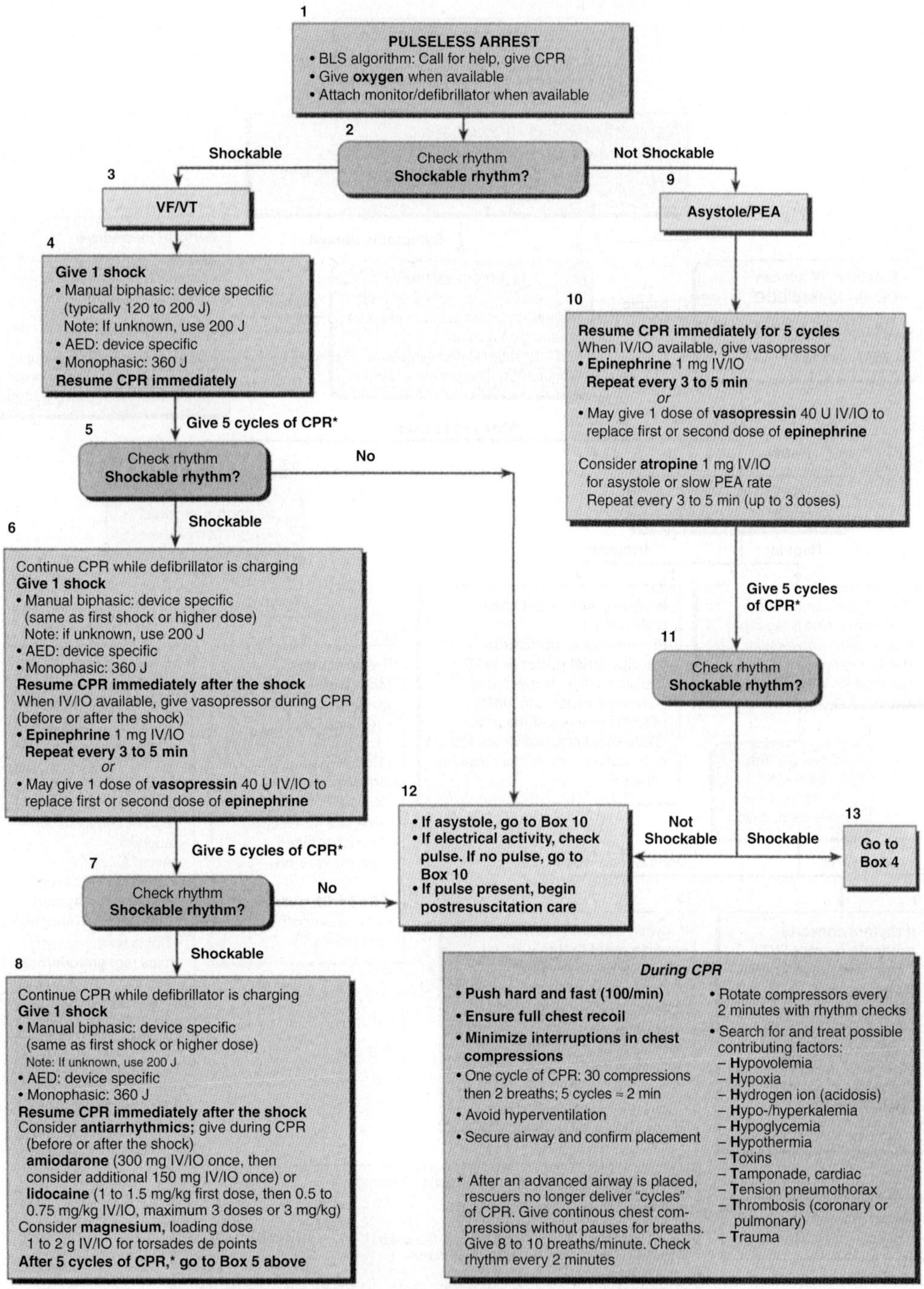

FIGURE 23.15. Advanced cardiac life support pulseless arrest algorithm. [From *Circulation* 112[Suppl 24]:IV-58–66, 2005, with permission. Copyright 2005, American Heart Association guidelines for cardiopulmonary resuscitation and emergency cardiovascular care.]

Ventricular Fibrillation and Pulseless Ventricular Tachycardia

Electric defibrillation is the most important intervention in treating these arrhythmias (see Chapter 6). The sooner it is administered, the more likely it is to succeed. If a defibrillator is not immediately available and an adult cardiac arrest is witnessed, a precordial thump is recommended by some authors [97]; however, no recommendation for or against its use is made in the recent AHA guidelines [57]. Many witnessed arrests in the emergency room will be in monitored patients; the rescuer, however, must never rely solely on the monitored signal but must always confirm the need for CPR by determining the absence of a pulse. Quick-look paddles or pads should confirm the diagnosis of VF or VT and a countershock should be attempted (120 to 200 J for biphasic defibrillators and 360 J for monophasic defibrillators). CPR should be resumed without rechecking the rhythm or a pulse. After 2 minutes or about 5 cycles of CPR, the rhythm should be rechecked. If VF or VT is still present, another shock is applied at the same energy level. CPR is again resumed immediately, and if an IV line is

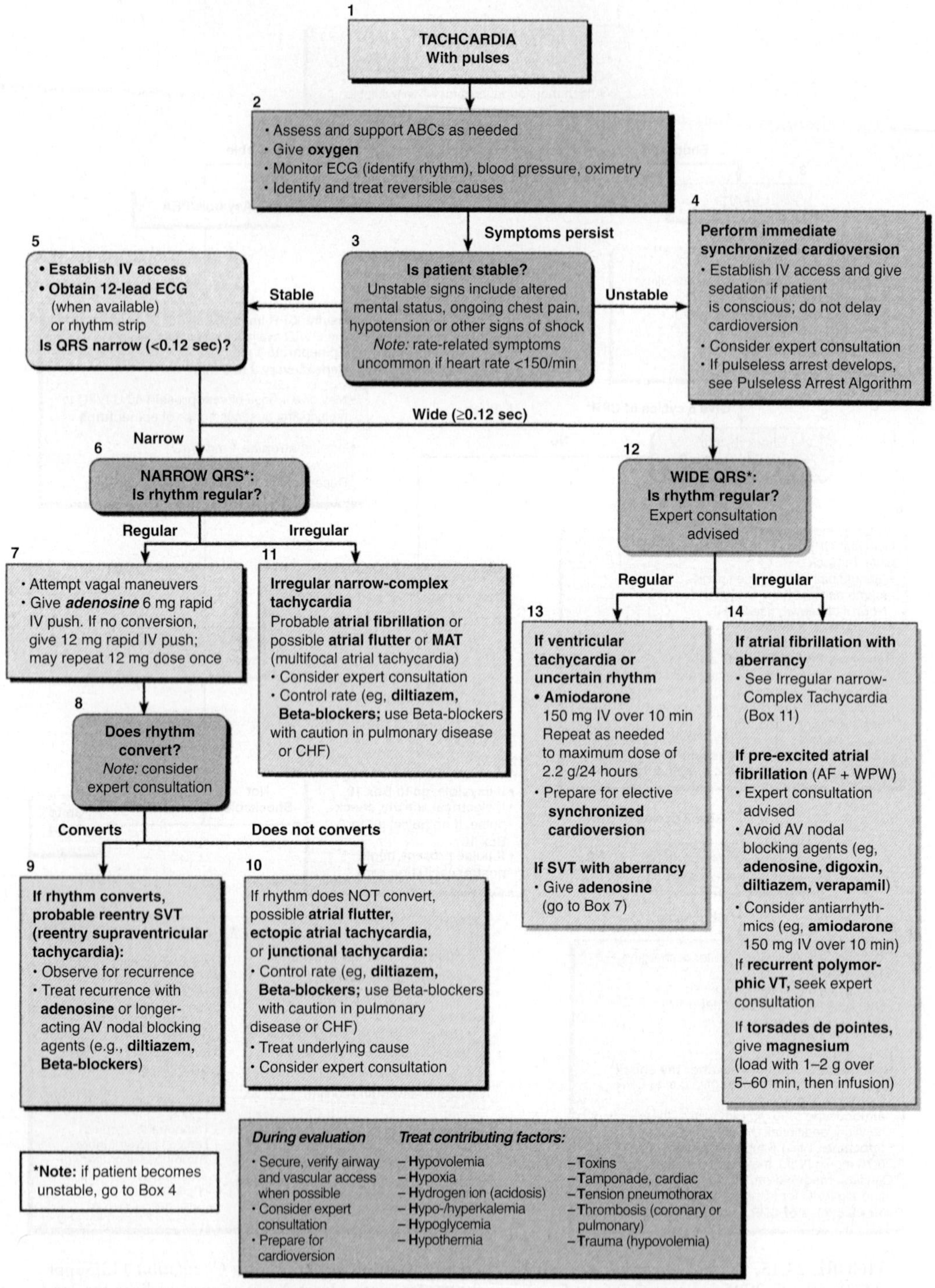

FIGURE 23.16. Advanced cardiac life support tachycardia algorithm. [From *Circulation* 112[Suppl 24]:IV-67–77, 2005, with permission. Copyright 2005, American Heart Association guidelines for cardiopulmonary resuscitation and emergency cardiovascular care.]

available, vasopressors (epinephrine, 1 mg IV, or IO every 3 to 5 minutes, or vasopressin 40 units, IV/IO) are administered. After another 5 cycles of CPR, the rhythm is checked again. If VF or VT is still present, another shock is applied.

After the second shock, if the patient remains in VF or VT, consideration should be given to the administration of an antiarrhythmic agent: amiodarone (300 mg IV/IO once with an additional dose of 150 mg IV/IO if necessary) or lidocaine (1.0 to 1.5 mg per kg IV/IO followed by additional doses of 0.5 to 0.75 mg per kg, if necessary, up to a total dose of 3 mg per kg).

Adequacy of ventilation should be assessed with an arterial blood gas determination, if possible. Sodium bicarbonate is of questionable value during cardiac arrest but should be administered if the patient is known to have preexisting hyperkalemia.

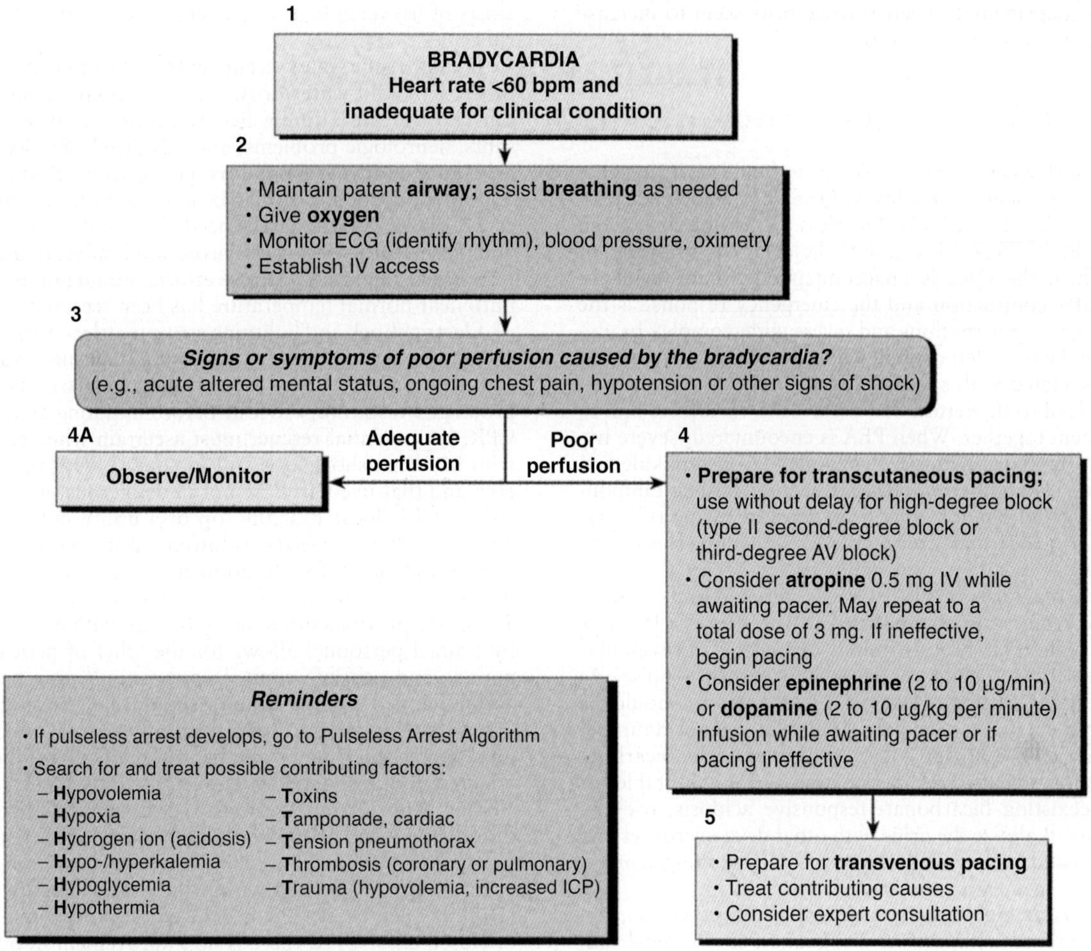
1
BRADYCARDIA
Heart rate <60 bpm and
inadequate for clinical condition
2
• Maintain patent airway; assist breathing as needed
• Give oxygen
• Monitor ECG (identify rhythm), blood pressure, oximetry
• Establish IV access
3
Signs or symptoms of poor perfusion caused by the bradycardia?
(e.g., acute altered mental status, ongoing chest pain, hypotension or other signs of shock)
4A
Adequate perfusion
Observe/Monitor
Poor perfusion
4
• Prepare for transcutaneous pacing; use without delay for high-degree block (type II second-degree block or third-degree AV block)
• Consider atropine 0.5 mg IV while awaiting pacer. May repeat to a total dose of 3 mg. If ineffective, begin pacing
• Consider epinephrine (2 to 10 μg/min) or dopamine (2 to 10 μg/kg per minute) infusion while awaiting pacer or if pacing ineffective
5
• Prepare for transvenous pacing
• Treat contributing causes
• Consider expert consultation
Reminders
• If pulseless arrest develops, go to Pulseless Arrest Algorithm
• Search for and treat possible contributing factors:
– Hypovolemia
– Hypoxia
– Hydrogen ion (acidosis)
– Hypo-/hyperkalemia
– Hypoglycemia
– Hypothermia
– Toxins
– Tamponade, cardiac
– Tension pneumothorax
– Thrombosis (coronary or pulmonary)
– Trauma (hypovolemia, increased ICP)

FIGURE 23.17. Bradycardia algorithm. [From *Circulation* 112[Suppl 24]:I-V-67–77, 2005, with permission. Copyright 2005, American Heart Association guidelines for cardiopulmonary resuscitation and emergency cardiovascular care.]

Asystole

Asystole is obviously the end result of any pulseless rhythm. When asystole is the presenting rhythm, it is often the termination of untreated VF. In the prehospital setting, many cases of asystole are related to delayed initiation of BLS or ACLS. Primary asystole associated with increased parasympathetic tone is less common, but does occur. Whether this rhythm occurs as the initial rhythm or follows on VT or fibrillation, it carries a very poor prognosis. Less than 1% to 2% of patients can be expected to revert successfully to a perfusing rhythm. Even more rarely will such patients leave the hospital with reasonable neurologic integrity or significant long-term survival; their best hope lies in the early discovery and treatment of a reversible cause for cardiovascular collapse, such as hypovolemia. Occasionally, asystole develops due to excessive vagal tone, such as is seen with induction of anesthesia, during surgical procedures, or with stimulation of the carotid body, bladder, biliary, or gastrointestinal tract. Unfortunately, most patients with asystole have severe coronary artery disease and are unlikely to be saved.

In patients with apparent asystole, CPR is initiated and an IV line is established as soon as possible (Fig. 23.15). Either epinephrine (1 mg IV/IO and repeated every 3 to 5 minutes) or vasopressin (1 dose of 40 U IV/IO to replace the first or second dose of epinephrine) is administered. Atropine at a dose of 1 mg IV/IO may also be considered. After 5 cycles of CPR, the rhythm is rechecked. If asystole persists, the aforementioned sequence is repeated.

It has been demonstrated that VF may masquerade as asystole in several leads and for minutes at a time [98]. It is therefore important to check at least two different lead configurations at 90-degree orientation to confirm the diagnosis of asystole. Routine shocking of asystole, however, is discouraged because of the possibility of increasing parasympathetic tone and thus decreasing further any chance of return of spontaneous rhythm. No improvement in survival has been demonstrated with the use of shocks for presumed asystole [99].

As in other forms of arrest, neither sodium bicarbonate nor calcium has been shown to be of benefit; these agents should be considered only under specific circumstances (see previous discussion).

Temporary artificial pacing is of no likely benefit in asystole—either primary or that following countershock. Pacing with endocardial, percutaneous transthoracic, or external transcutaneous electrodes has led to pitifully few long-term survivals in these cases.

The use of isoproterenol in an attempt to stimulate pacemakers through its β-adrenergic agonist effects has not proved to be beneficial. Indeed, its peripheral β-stimulation produces a decrease in arterial resistance and perfusion pressure that is likely to be detrimental, whereas α-agonists seem to increase myocardial and cerebral perfusion.

Pulseless Electric Activity

PEA is present when an arrest patient is found to have organized ECG ventricular complexes (QRS) not associated with a palpable pulse (Fig. 23.15). Pulseless VT is not considered a form of PEA. Electromechanical dissociation is a form of PEA in which the QRS is unaccompanied by any evidence of ventricular contraction and the emergency response is the same. Bradyasystolic rhythms and severe wide-complex bradycardias may be considered along with PEA. These arrhythmias may be associated with specific clinical states that if reversed early, may lead to the return of a pulse. It is, therefore, best to consider them together. When PEA is encountered, severe hypovolemia, hypoxia, acidosis, hyperkalemia or hypokalemia, hypoglycemia, hypothermia, drug overdose, cardiac tamponade, massive pulmonary embolism, tension pneumothorax, and severe myocardial contractile dysfunction should be considered.

With the diagnosis of PEA, CPR is initiated and, as soon as possible, volume is administered in the form of IV crystalloid or colloid. If PEA is indeed caused by intravascular volume depletion, a fluid challenge may return a pulse. As described in the section "Asystole," vasopressors should be administered every 3 to 5 minutes if a pulse has not returned. In bradycardic PEA, atropine is given as in asystole. Bicarbonate is used for preexisting hyperkalemia and is acceptable for known preexisting bicarbonate-responsive acidosis, tricyclic overdose, to alkalinize the urine with other drug overdoses and in intubated and well-ventilated patients with prolonged arrest intervals.

In patients at high risk for pericardial effusions (i.e., patients hospitalized with known malignancy, severe renal failure, recent myocardial infarction, or recent cardiac catheterization), pericardiocentesis should be attempted early in the course of CPR if the patient is not responding to volume administration and α-agonists. In prehospital arrests, pericardial tamponade is rare, but an attempt at pericardiocentesis is warranted if there is no favorable response to volume or α-agonists. Echocardiography, when available, almost always confirms or excludes the possibility of tamponade and may be useful in delineating the volume status as well as the function of the ventricles.

Special Situations

Patients who have nearly drowned in cold water may recover after prolonged periods of submersion. Apparently, the hypothermia and bradycardia of the diving reflex may serve to protect against organ damage [100]. Successful resuscitation has been described after considerable periods of submersion [100]. Because it is often difficult for bystanders and rescuers to estimate the duration of submersion, in most cases it is warranted to initiate CPR at the scene, unless physical evidence exists of irreversible death, such as putrefaction or dependent rubor.

Hypothermia may occur with environmental exposures other than cold-water drowning. The body's ability to maintain temperature is diminished by alcohol, sedation, antidepressants, neurologic problems, and advanced age. Because of the associated bradycardia and oxygen-sparing effects, prolonged hypothermia and arrest may be tolerated with complete recovery. A longer period may be needed to establish breathlessness and pulselessness because of profound bradycardia and slowed respiratory rate. Resuscitative efforts should not be abandoned until near-normal temperature has been reestablished.

Electric shock and lightning strike may lead to tetanic spasm of respiratory muscles or convulsion, causing respiratory arrest. VF or asystole may occur from the electric shock or after prolonged respiratory arrest. Before initiating assessment and CPR, the potential rescuer must ascertain whether the person who has been shocked is still in contact with the electric energy and that live wires are not in dangerous proximity. If the individual is located at the top of a utility pole, CPR is best instituted after the person is lowered to the ground [101].

Open-chest CPR with thoracotomy should be applied early in cases of penetrating chest trauma associated with cardiac arrest (see previous discussion). In such patients, thoracotomy by trained personnel allows for the relief of pericardial tamponade and possible control of exsanguinating hemorrhage. Well-equipped trauma centers should have multidisciplinary teams that can provide early, definitive surgical treatment. The unanswered question is whether another subgroup of patients who have not responded to conventional ACLS techniques (including defibrillation attempts and drugs) would benefit from thoracotomy and open-chest CPR. Animal studies suggest that survival may be improved over closed-chest compression if open-chest CPR is used within the first 15 minutes of arrest [102]. If open-chest CPR is delayed until 20 minutes or more of closed-chest CPR, there is no improvement in outcome despite improved hemodynamics. In patients with out-of-hospital arrest in whom open-chest CPR was attempted after 30 minutes of conventional CPR, survival did not improve [103].

Open-chest CPR may also be indicated in blunt trauma with cardiac arrest and cardiac arrest due to hypothermia, pulmonary embolism, pericardial tamponade, or abdominal hemorrhage in which initiation of conventional therapy and closed-chest CPR is not proving effective. In the aforementioned cases, the decision to use open-chest CPR presupposes quick availability of definitive surgical intervention. Early surgical exploration is indicated in penetrating abdominal trauma with deterioration and cardiac arrest in which aortic cross-clamping may provide temporary control of abdominal hemorrhage.

Induced therapeutic hypothermia (32°C to 34°C) for 12 to 24 hours improves survival and neurologic outcome in comatose patients who have survived an out-of-hospital VF arrest [104,105]. Hypothermia may also be beneficial for in-hospital arrests. Lower cardiac index and hyperglycemia tend to occur more frequently in hypothermic patients. Shivering must be prevented to reduce metabolic rate. Please see Chapter 64 on hypothermia for an in-depth discussion of induced therapeutic hypothermia.

References

1. Ibycus: "Chrysippus," quoted, in Strauss MB (ed): *Familiar Medical Quotations*. Boston, Little, Brown and Company, 1968.
2. Stephenson HE Jr: *Cardiac Arrest and Resuscitation*. St. Louis, Mosby, 1958.
3. Zoll PM, Linenthal AJ, Gibson W, et al: Termination of ventricular fibrillation in man by externally applied electrical countershock. *N Engl J Med* 254:727, 1956.
4. Safar P, Escarraga L, Elam JO: A comparison of the mouth to mouth and mouth to airway methods of artificial respiration with the chest pressure arm-lift method. *N Engl J Med* 258:671, 1958.
5. Elam JO, Green DG, Brown ES, et al: Oxygen and carbon dioxide exchange and energy cost of expired air resuscitation. *JAMA* 167:328, 1958.
6. Kouwenhoven WB, Jude JR, Knickerbocker GG: Closed chest cardiac massage. *JAMA* 173:1064, 1960.

7. Cardiopulmonary resuscitation: statement by the Ad Hoc Committee on Cardiopulmonary Resuscitation of the Division of Medical Sciences, National Academy of Sciences—National Research Council. *JAMA* 198:372, 1966.
8. Standards for cardiopulmonary resuscitation (CPR) and emergency cardiac care (ECC). *JAMA* 227[Suppl]:833, 1974.
9. Guidelines for the determination of death: report of the medical consultants on the diagnosis of death to the President's Commission for the Study of Ethical Problems in Medicine and Biomedical and Behavioral Research. *JAMA* 246:2184, 1981.
10. Wijdicks EFM: The diagnosis of brain death. *N Engl J Med* 344:1215, 2001.
11. Copley DP, Mantle JA, Roger WJ, et al: Improved outcome for prehospital cardiopulmonary collapse with resuscitation by bystanders. *Circulation* 56:902, 1977.
12. Holmberg M, Holmberg S, Herlitz J: Effect of bystander cardiopulmonary resuscitation in out-of-hospital cardiac arrest patients in Sweden. *Resuscitation* 47:59, 2000.
13. Rudikoff MT, Maughan WL, Effron M, et al: Mechanisms of blood flow during cardiopulmonary resuscitation. *Circulation* 61:345, 1980.
14. Chandra N, Weisfeldt ML, Tsitlik J, et al: Augmentation of carotid flow during cardiopulmonary resuscitation by ventilation at high airway pressure simultaneous with chest compression. *Am J Cardiol* 48:1053, 1981.
15. Taylor GJ, Tucker WM, Greene HL, et al: Importance of prolonged compression during cardiopulmonary resuscitation in man. *N Engl J Med* 296:1515, 1977.
16. Chandra N, Rudikoff M, Weisfeldt ML: Simultaneous chest compression and ventilation at high airway pressure during cardiopulmonary resuscitation. *Lancet* 1:175, 1980.
17. Harris LC Jr, Kirimli B, Safar P: Augmentation of artificial circulation during cardiopulmonary resuscitation. *Anesthesiology* 28:730, 1967.
18. Redding JS: Abdominal compression in cardiopulmonary resuscitation. *Anesth Analg* 50:668, 1971.
19. Koehler RC, Chandra N, Guerci AD, et al: Augmentation of cerebral perfusion by simultaneous chest compression and lung inflation with abdominal binding after cardiac arrest in dogs. *Circulation* 67:266, 1983.
20. Chandra N, Snyder LD, Weisfeldt ML: Abdominal binding during cardiopulmonary resuscitation in man. *JAMA* 246:351, 1981.
21. Ralston SH, Babbs CF, Niebauer MJ: Cardiopulmonary resuscitation with interposed abdominal compression in dogs. *Anesth Analg* 61:645, 1982.
22. Barranco F, Lesmes A, Irles JA, et al: Cardiopulmonary resuscitation with simultaneous chest and abdominal compression: comparative study in humans. *Resuscitation* 20:67, 1990.
23. Maier GW, Tyson GS Jr, Olsen CO, et al: The physiology of external cardiac massage: high-impulse cardiopulmonary resuscitation. *Circulation* 70:86, 1984.
24. Cohen TV, Goldner BG, Maccaro PC, et al: A comparison of active compression–decompression cardiopulmonary resuscitation for cardiac arrest occurring in the hospital. *N Engl J Med* 329:1918, 1993.
25. Halperin HR, Guerci AD, Chandra N, et al: Vest inflation without simultaneous ventilation during cardiac arrest in dogs: improved survival from prolonged cardiopulmonary resuscitation. *Circulation* 74:1407, 1986.
26. Emergency Cardiac Care Committee: Automatic external defibrillators and advanced cardiac life support: a new initiative from the American Heart Association. *Am J Emerg Med* 9:91, 1991.
27. Valenzuela TD, Roe DJ, Nichol G, et al: Outcomes of rapid defibrillation by security officers after cardiac arrest in casinos. *N Engl J Med* 343:1206, 2000.
28. Del Guercio LR, Feins NR, Cohn JD, et al: Comparison of blood flow during external and internal cardiac massage in man. *Circulation* 31[Suppl 1]:171, 1965.
29. Luce JM, Ross BK, O'Quin RJ, et al: Regional blood flow during cardiopulmonary resuscitation in dogs using simultaneous and non-simultaneous compression and ventilation. *Circulation* 67:258, 1983.
30. Jackson RE, Joyce K, Danosi SF, et al: Blood flow in the cerebral cortex during cardiac resuscitation in dogs. *Ann Emerg Med* 13:657, 1984.
31. Sharff JA, Pantley G, Noel E: Effect of time on regional organ perfusion during two methods of cardiopulmonary resuscitation. *Ann Emerg Med* 13:649, 1984.
32. Krug JJ: Cardiac arrest secondary to Addison's disease. *Ann Emerg Med* 15:735, 1986.
33. Pell AC, Guly UM, Sutherland GR, et al: Mechanism of closed chest cardiopulmonary resuscitation investigated by transesophageal echocardiography. *J Accid Emerg Med* 11:139, 1994.
34. Weale FE, Rothwell-Jackson RL: The efficiency of cardiac massage. *Lancet* 1:990, 1962.
35. Wilder RJ, Weir D, Rush BF, et al: Methods of coordinating ventilation and closed chest cardiac massage in the dog. *Surgery* 53:186, 1963.
36. Criley JM, Blaufuss AJ, Kissel GL: Cough-induced cardiac compression. *JAMA* 236:1246, 1976.
37. Niemann JT, Rosborough JP, Brown D, et al: Cough-CPR: documentation of systemic perfusion in man and in an experimental model—a "window" to the mechanism of blood flow in external CPR. *Crit Care Med* 8:141, 1980.
38. Haehnel J, Lindner KH, Ahnefeld FW: Endobronchial administration of emergency drugs. *Resuscitation* 17:261, 1989.
39. Niemann JT, Rosborough JP, Hausknecht M, et al: Pressure-synchronized cineangiography during experimental cardiopulmonary resuscitation. *Circulation* 64:985, 1981.
40. Werner JA, Greene HL, Janko CL, et al: Visualization of cardiac valve motion in man during external chest compression using two-dimensional echocardiography: implications regarding the mechanism of blood flow. *Circulation* 63:1417, 1981.
41. Babbs CF, Ralston SH, Geddes LA: Theoretical advantages of abdominal counterpulsation in CPR as demonstrated in a simple electrical model of the circulation. *Ann Emerg Med* 13:660, 1984.
42. Sack JB, Kesselbrenner MB, Bregman D: Survival from in-hospital cardiac arrest with interposed abdominal counterpulsation during cardiopulmonary resuscitation. *JAMA* 267:379, 1992.
43. Ward KR, Sullivan RJ, Zelenak RR, et al: A comparison of interposed abdominal compression CPR and standard CPR by monitoring end-tidal PCO_2. *Ann Emerg Med* 18:831, 1989.
44. Mateer JR, Steuven HA, Thompson BM, et al: Pre-hospital IAC-CPR versus standard CPR: paramedic resuscitation of cardiac arrests. *Am J Emerg Med* 3:143, 1985.
45. Takino M, Okada Y: The optimum timing of resuscitative thoracotomy for non-traumatic out-of-hospital cardiac arrest. *Resuscitation* 26:69, 1993.
46. Bodai BI, Smith JP, Ward RE, et al: Emergency thoracotomy in the management of trauma—a review. *JAMA* 249:1891, 1983.
47. Levine R, Gorayeb M, Safar P, et al: Emergency cardiopulmonary bypass after cardiac arrest and prolonged closed-chest CPR in dogs. *Ann Emerg Med* 16:620, 1987.
48. Hartz R, LoCicero J III, Sanders JH Jr, et al: Clinical experience with portable cardiopulmonary bypass in cardiac arrest patients. *Ann Thorac Surg* 50:437, 1990.
49. Ornato JP, Hallagan LF, McMahon SB, et al: Attitudes of BCLS instructors about mouth-to-mouth resuscitation during the AIDS epidemic. *Ann Emerg Med* 19:151, 1990.
50. Block AJ: The physician's responsibility for the care of AIDS patients: an opinion. *Chest* 94:1283, 1988.
51. Fox PC, Wolff A, Yeh CK, et al: Saliva inhibits HIV-1 infectivity. *J Am Dent Assoc* 116:635, 1988.
52. Sande MH: Transmission of AIDS: the case against casual contagion. *N Engl J Med* 314:380, 1986.
53. Risk of infection during CPR training and rescue: supplemental guidelines. *JAMA* 262:2714, 1989.
54. Adgey AAJ, Geddes JS, Webb SW, et al: Acute phase of myocardial infarction. *Lancet* 2:501, 1971.
55. Konrad D, Jaderling G, Bell M, et al: Reducing in-hospital cardiac arrests and hospital mortality by introducing a medical emergency team. *Intensive Care Med* 36:100–106, 2010.
56. Winters BD, Pham JC, Hunt EA, et al: Rapid responses systems: a systematic review. *Crit Care Med* 35:1238–1243, 2007.
57. ECC Committee, Subcommittees and Task Forces of the American Heart Association: 2005 American Heart Association Guidelines for Cardiopulmonary Resuscitation and Emergency Cardiovascular Care. *Circulation* 112[24 Suppl]:IV1–203, 2005.
58. Thompson RG, Hallstrom AP, Cobb LA: Bystander-initiated cardiopulmonary resuscitation in the management of ventricular fibrillation. *Ann Intern Med* 90:737, 1979.
59. Melker R, Cavallaro D, Krischer J: One-rescuer CPR—a reappraisal of present recommendations for ventilation. *Crit Care Med* 9:423, 1981.
60. 2005 American Heart Association guidelines for cardiopulmonary resuscitation and emergency cardiovascular care. *Circulation* 112:III-5–III-16, 2005.
61. Eftestol T, Sunde K, Steen PA: Effects of interrupting precordial compressions on the calculated probability of defibrillation success during out-of-hospital cardiac arrest. *Circulation* 105:2270, 2002.
62. Rea TD, Fahrenbruch C, Culley L, et al: CPR with chest compression alone or with rescue breathing. *N Engl J Med* 363:423–433, 2010.
63. Svensson L, Bohm K, Castren M, et al: Compression-only CPR or standard CPR in out-of-hospital arrest. *N Engl J Med* 363:434–442, 2010.
64. Dorph E, Wik L, Stromme TA, et al: Oxygen delivery and return of spontaneous circulation with ventilation: compression ratio 2:30 versus chest compressions only CPR in pigs. *Resuscitation* 60:309, 2004.
65. Powner DJ, Holcombe PA, Mello LA: Cardiopulmonary resuscitation-related injuries. *Crit Care Med* 12:54, 1984.
66. Sanders AB, Ewy GA, Taft TV: Prognosis and therapeutic importance of the aortic diastolic pressure in resuscitation from cardiac arrest. *Crit Care Med* 12:871, 1984.
67. Michael JR, Guerci AD, Koehler RC, et al: Mechanisms by which epinephrine augments cerebral and myocardial perfusion during cardiopulmonary resuscitation in dogs. *Circulation* 69:822, 1984.
68. Paradis NA, Martin GB, Rivers EP, et al: Coronary perfusion pressure and the return of spontaneous circulation in cardiopulmonary resuscitation in humans. *JAMA* 263:1106, 1990.
69. Ludwig S, Kettrick RG, Parker M: Pediatric cardiopulmonary resuscitation. *Clin Pediatr* 23:71, 1984.
70. Heimlich HJ, Uhtley MH: The Heimlich maneuver. *Clin Symp* 31:22, 1979.
71. Lowenstein SR, Sabyan EM, Lassen CF, et al: Benefits of training physicians in advanced cardiac life support. *Chest* 89:512, 1986.

72. Aufderheide TP, Lurie KG: Death by hyperventilation: a common and life-threatening problem during cardiopulmonary resuscitation. *Crit Care Med* 32[Suppl]:S345, 2004.
73. Stone BJ, Chantler PJ, Baskett PJ: The Incidence of regurgitation during: cardiopulmonary resuscitation: a comparison between the bag valve mask and laryngeal mask airway. *Resuscitation* 38:3–6, 1998.
74. Kokkinis K: The use of the Laryngeal Mask Airway in CPR. *Resuscitation* 27:9, 1994.
75. Samarkandi AH, Seraj MA, Dawlatly A, et al: The role of laryngeal mask airway in cardiopulmonary resuscitation. *Resuscitation* 28:103, 1994.
76. Zoll PM, Zoll RH, Falk RH, et al: External noninvasive temporary cardiac pacing: clinical trials. *Circulation* 71:937, 1985.
77. Clinton JE, Zoll PM, Zoll R, et al: Emergency noninvasive external pacing. *J Emerg Med* 2:155, 1985.
78. Emerman CL, Pinchak AC, Hancock D, et al: Effect of injection site on circulation times during cardiac arrest. *Crit Care Med* 16:1138, 1988.
79. Kuhn GJ, White BC, Swetnam RE, et al: Peripheral vs central circulation times during CPR: a pilot study. *Ann Emerg Med* 10:417, 1981.
80. Jaffe A: Cardiovascular pharmacology I. *Circulation* 74[Suppl]:IV–70, 1986.
81. Guerci AD, Chandra N, Johnson E, et al: Failure of sodium bicarbonate to improve resuscitation from ventricular fibrillation in dogs. *Circulation* 74[Suppl]:IV–75, 1986.
82. Dybrik T, Strand T, Steen PA: Buffer therapy during out-of-hospital cardiopulmonary resuscitation. *Resuscitation* 29:89, 1995.
83. Otto CW, Yakaitis RW, Redding JS, et al: Comparison of dopamine, dobutamine, and epinephrine in CPR. *Crit Care Med* 9:640, 1981.
84. Niemann JT, Haynes KS, Garner D, et al: Postcountershock pulseless rhythms: response to CPR, artificial cardiac pacing, and adrenergic agonists. *Ann Emerg Med* 15:112, 1986.
85. Stiell IG, Hebert PC, Weitzman BN, et al: High-dose epinephrine in adult cardiac arrest. *N Engl J Med* 327:1045, 1992.
86. Brown CG, Martin DR, Pepe PE, et al: A comparison of standard-dose and high-dose epinephrine in cardiac arrest outside the hospital. *N Engl J Med* 327:1051, 1992.
87. Robinson LA, Brown CG, Jenkins J, et al: The effect of norepinephrine versus epinephrine on myocardial hemodynamics during CPR. *Ann Emerg Med* 18:336, 1989.
88. Lindner KH, Prengel AW, Brinkmann A, et al: Vasopressin administration in refractory cardiac arrest. *Ann Intern Med* 124:1061, 1996.
89. Kudenchuk PJ, Cobb LA, Copass M, et al: Amiodarone for resuscitation after out-of-hospital cardiac arrest due to ventricular fibrillation. *N Engl J Med* 341:871, 1999.
90. MacMahon S, Collins R, Peto R, et al: Effects of prophylactic lidocaine in suspected acute myocardial infarction: an overview of results from the randomized controlled trials. *JAMA* 260:1910, 1988.
91. Teo KK, Yusuf S, Collins R, et al: Effects of intravenous magnesium in suspected acute myocardial infarction: overview of randomised trials. *BMJ* 303:1499, 1991.
92. DiMarco JP, Sellers TD, Berne RM, et al: Adenosine: electrophysiologic effects and therapeutic use for terminating paroxysmal supraventricular tachycardia. *Circulation* 68:1254, 1983.
93. DiMarco JP, Sellers TD, Lerman BB, et al: Diagnostic and therapeutic use of adenosine in patients with supraventricular tachyarrhythmias. *J Am Coll Cardiol* 6:417, 1985.
94. Kay JH, Blalock A: The use of calcium chloride in the treatment of cardiac arrest in patients. *Surg Gynecol Obstet* 93:97, 1951.
95. Stueven HA, Thompson BM, Aprahamian C, et al: Use of calcium in prehospital cardiac arrest. *Ann Emerg Med* 12:136, 1983.
96. Dembo DH: Calcium in advanced life support. *Crit Care Med* 9:358, 1981.
97. Caldwell G, Millar G, Quinn E, et al: Simple mechanical methods of cardioversion: a defense of the precordial thump and cough version. *BMJ* 291:627, 1985.
98. Ewy GA, Dahl CF, Zimmerman M, et al: Ventricular fibrillation masquerading as ventricular standstill. *Crit Care Med* 9:841, 1981.
99. Thompson BM, Brooks RC, Pionkowski RS, et al: Immediate countershock treatment of asystole. *Ann Emerg Med* 13:827, 1984.
100. Southwick FS, Dalgish PH: Recovery after prolonged asystolic cardiac arrest in profound hypothermia. A case report and literature review. *JAMA* 243:1250, 1980.
101. Gordon AS, Ridolpho PF, Cole JE: *Definitive Studies on Pole-Top Resuscitation*. Camarillo, CA, Research Resuscitation Laboratories, Electric Power Research Institute, 1983.
102. Safar P, Abramson NS, Angelos M, et al: Emergency cardiopulmonary bypass for resuscitation from prolonged cardiac arrest. *Am J Emerg Med* 8:55, 1990.
103. Geehr EC, Lewis FR, Auerbach PS: Failure of open-heart massage to improve survival after prehospital non-traumatic cardiac arrest [letter]. *N Engl J Med* 314:1189, 1986.
104. The Hypothermia After Cardiac Arrest Study Group: Mild therapeutic hypothermia to improve the neurologic outcome after cardiac arrest. *N Engl J Med* 346:549, 2000.
105. Benard SA, Gray TW, Buist MD, et al: Treatment of comatose survivors of out-of-hospital cardiac arrest with induced hypothermia. *N Engl J Med* 346:557, 2000.

CHAPTER 24 ■ MANAGEMENT OF PAIN IN THE CRITICALLY ILL PATIENT

ARMAGAN DAGAL, MARIO DE PINTO AND W. THOMAS EDWARDS

Pain in critically ill patients should be systematically observed and regularly assessed. All means of analgesic interventions should be evaluated in a coordinated, individualized, and goal-oriented interdisciplinary manner.

Pain may stem from acute medical or surgical illness as well as preexisting medical conditions. Mechanical ventilation, placement of indwelling tubes and catheters, procedures performed such as placement of chest tubes, intracranial pressure (ICP) monitors, and turning and suctioning are also causes of pain [1,2]. Exposure to high levels of pain has negative psychologic and physiologic consequences, and its effective management is important in the maintenance of patient's dignity [3–5].

Despite numerous improvement initiatives over the past two decades, pain is very common and often not treated appropriately in critically ill patients. It is estimated that as many as 70% of patients experience moderate-intensity procedure-related or postoperative pain during their stay in the hospital intensive care unit (ICU) [6–9]. Pain is frequently treated inappropriately because of fears of depressing spontaneous ventilation, inducing opioid dependence, and precipitating cardiovascular instability. Moreover, many clinicians often poorly understand the methods for assessing pain, the techniques for optimally treating it, and the benefits of its effective management. State-of-the-art pain management means not only decreasing pain intensity, but also reducing analgesics' side effects, which may indeed facilitate patient recovery and is likely to shorten ICU and hospital stay [10–12]. Recent studies also suggest that effective acute pain management may help in reducing the development of chronic pain [13].

In 2005, the American Pain Society (APS) published the following guidelines for quality improvement in acute and cancer pain management [14]:

- Recognize, identify, and treat pain promptly.
- Involve patients and families in the pain management plan.
- Improve treatment patterns.
- Reassess and adjust the pain management plan as needed.
- Monitor processes and outcomes of pain management.

The primary goal of this structured approach to pain management was to prevent pain through the administration of analgesics at regular intervals and before performing potentially painful procedures.

Implementation of the APS guidelines in 120 postcardiac surgery patients over a 3-month period revealed that 95% of them had effective pain relief during every ICU staff shift for the first 6 days after surgery [15]. Data also revealed dramatically improved side-effect profile and reduced length of hospital stay. Implementation of a similar pain management protocol in a medical ICU resulted in a decrease in ventilator days (from 10.3 to 8.9) and significant reductions of average hospital costs.

ICU pain management strategies may also incorporate the application of regional analgesia techniques (neuraxial and peripheral nerve blocks) when possible. Regional analgesia, when used appropriately, helps reduce the total amount of opioid analgesics necessary to achieve adequate pain control and the development of potentially dangerous side effects.

EVALUATION OF PAIN

It is difficult to perform assessment of pain in the ICU. Structured approaches to pain assessment are mandatory for favorable patient outcome.

Pain assessment tools are useful to monitor for deterioration or improvements over time, and evaluate and titrate analgesic therapy appropriately [5,16].

There are several newly proposed methods available for pain assessment in the ICU. The chosen strategy should be adapted to the patient's capacity to interact with the practitioner in order to provide assessment of static (rest) and dynamic pain (while moving the affected part or while taking deep breaths or coughing).

Assessment of pain should include determining cause, type, intensity, duration, site, and prior response to therapy. Categorization of pain into somatic, visceral, neuropathic in nature, or identification of specific sites, such as focal bone pain as opposed to allodynia or diffuse bowel distention, is important because it helps in determining the most effective type of intervention.

In general, appropriate assessment of pain improves the overall quality of pain management.

Subjective Pain Assessment

The Visual Analog Scale (VAS) is a 10-cm horizontal line, anchored by textual descriptors and/or pictures at each end. An end-point descriptor such as "no pain" (a score of 0) is marked at the left end and "worst pain imaginable" (a score of 10) is marked at the right end.

The Numerical Rating Scale (NRS) is a horizontal line with a scale from 0 to 10. Patients are asked to choose a number that relates to their pain intensity, where 0 represents no pain and 10 the worst imaginable pain. The NRS can be administered verbally or visually.

The Faces Pain Scale (FPS) was first developed by Wong and Baker and is recommended for those aged 3 and older. An explanation is given to the patient that each face is a person who feels happy because he or she has no pain or sad because he or she has some or a lot of pain. The patient is then asked to choose the face that best describes how they feel from six possible options.

It has been shown that the NRSs have the least variance and may be the preferred tool overall. Mechanically ventilated and sedated patients will be unable to use the VAS ruler or other self-report pain assessment tools. Once sedation has ceased, some patients may be alert enough to use a VAS ruler. This should be attempted as an option for these patients. If psychomotor abilities are impaired at this point, an NRS or FPS may prove to be more helpful.

Objective Pain Assessment

When the patient is critically ill, sedated, and/or ventilated, pain severity can be estimated only by observing the behavioral and physiologic responses to pain:

- The Behavioral Pain Scale (BPS) is the earliest and most widely tested pain assessment tool for sedated patients. The BPS was developed by Payen et al. There are three component domains: "facial expression," "upper limb movement," and "compliance with ventilation." Patients are scored from 1 to 4 on each section, giving a total score between 3 (no pain) and 12 (maximum pain) [17].
- The Critical Care Pain Observation Tool (CPOT) was designed by Gelinas et al. The CPOT has four domains: "facial expression," "body movement," "muscle tension," and "compliance with ventilation." Patients are scored in each section between 0 and 2, giving an overall score of 0 (no pain) to 8 (maximum pain).
- The Non-Verbal Pain Scale (NVPS) was developed by Odhner et al. The NVPS incorporates three behavioral domains and two physiologic domains. The behavioral domains are "face," "activity (movement)," and "guarding." The first physiologic domain considers vital signs and the second incorporates other physiologic indicators including skin color and temperature, perspiration, and pupillary changes. Again, specific descriptors are given to enable the assessors to rate a patient's pain from 0 to 2 within each domain, giving a total pain score between 0 (no pain) and 10 (maximum pain).

None of these tools can be regarded as gold standard and they require further evaluation and research to investigate the impact of their use on pain management in clinical practice. Nonetheless, they offer a consistent and systematic approach that might improve pain management in ICUs.

Analgesic trials can be another assessment tool if pain is suspected in ICU patients. They involve administration of a low dose of an analgesic followed by observation of the patient's pain-related behavior [5,18].

FORMULATION OF A TREATMENT PLAN

It is important to understand the characteristics of the pathologic process responsible for pain in order to establish the most effective therapy.

Character and Site

Pain can be categorized as follows:

- *Nociceptive pain:* It occurs in response to a noxious stimulus and continues only in the presence of a persistent noxious stimulus. It is transmitted through nonmyelinated C-sensory fibers and small myelinated A-fibers via the dorsal root ganglion and spinothalamic pathways in the spinal cord to the thalamus, periaqueductal gray, and other centers in the brain [19]. Nociceptive pain is often dull, aching, sharp, or tender.

- *Somatic pain:* It is due to nociceptive signals arising from the musculoskeletal system.
- *Visceral pain:* It is due to a disease process or abnormal function of an internal organ or its covering (parietal pleura, pericardium, and peritoneum). It can be frequently associated with nausea, vomiting, sweating, and changes in heart rate and blood pressure.

  Inflammatory pain occurs in response to tissue injury and the subsequent inflammatory reaction. In order to help healing of the injured body part, the sensory nervous system undergoes a profound change as a result; normally innocuous stimuli now produce pain, and responses to noxious stimuli are both exaggerated and prolonged [20]. This is secondary to plasticity in nociceptors and central nociceptive pathways [21,22]. Ablation of a specific set of nociceptor neurons, such as the one expressing the tetrodotoxin-resistant sodium channel Nav1.8, eliminates inflammatory pain, but leaves neuropathic pain intact, indicating a fundamental difference in the neuronal pathways responsible for these pain states [23,24].
- *Neuropathic pain:* It can be burning, tingling, or electric in character. Patients with neuropathic pain may describe positive or negative neurologic phenomena. Positive phenomena include spontaneous pain (arising without stimulus) and evoked pains (abnormal response to stimulus). Negative phenomena include impaired sensation to touch or thermal stimuli. Neuropathic pain is initiated or caused by a primary lesion or dysfunction in the central or peripheral nervous system (CNS or PNS).

Central neuropathic pain most commonly results from spinal cord injury, stroke, or multiple sclerosis [25].

Peripheral neuropathic pain can be caused by [26] the following:

- Trauma (e.g., complex regional pain syndrome (CRPS) and chronic postsurgical pain)
- Infection (e.g., postherpetic neuralgia and HIV-induced neuropathy)
- Ischemia (e.g., diabetic neuropathy and central "poststroke" pain)
- Cancer (e.g., invasion and compression of peripheral nerve structures)
- Chemically induced (e.g., chemotherapy-induced neuropathy)

Neural damage to either the PNS or the CNS provokes maladaptive responses in nociceptive pathways that drive spontaneous pain and sensory amplification. This maladaptive plasticity leads to persistent changes and, therefore, needs to be considered a disease state of the nervous system in its own right, independent of the etiologic factor(s) that triggered it. Studies suggest that peripheral and central sensitization mechanisms are also involved. In the PNS, they include altered gene expression and changes in ion channels that lead to ectopic activity. In the CNS, the regulation of many genes also changes. In addition, synaptic facilitation and loss of inhibition at multiple levels of the neuraxis produce central amplification. Neuronal cell death and aberrant synaptic connectivity provide the structural basis for persistently altered processing of both nociceptive and innocuous afferent input. Highly organized neuroimmunologic interactions as a result of neural damage play an important part in the development of persistent neuropathic pain. Genetically determined susceptibility is also likely to unveil the risk of developing neuropathic pain [24].

Hyperalgesia (the lowering of pain threshold and an increased response to noxious stimuli), allodynia (the evocation of pain by non-noxious stimuli), hyperpathia (explosive pains evoked in areas with an increased sensory threshold when the stimulus exceeds the threshold), dysesthesia (spontaneous or evoked unpleasant abnormal sensation), and paresthesia (spontaneous or evoked abnormal sensation) are typical elements of neuropathic pain.

MEDICAL MANAGEMENT

Consequences of inadequate sedation and analgesia in the ICU may result in excessive pain and anxiety, agitation, self-removal of tubes and catheters, violence toward caregivers, myocardial ischemia, patient-ventilator asynchrony, hypoxemia, and pain-related immunosuppression. In contrast, excessive and/or prolonged sedation can lead to skin breakdown, nerve compression, delirium, unnecessary testing for altered mental status, prolonged mechanical ventilation and associated problems such as ventilator-associated pneumonia (VAP), and perhaps post-traumatic stress disorder (PTSD). Balanced treatment using both nonpharmacologic and pharmacologic methods are imperative for pain management in the ICU [27,28]. Improvement in quality of care results in a reduction of the time spent on mechanical ventilation and length of stay in the ICU.

Nonpharmacologic Treatments

Nonpharmacologic interventions are easy to provide, safe, and economical. They may include attention to proper positioning of patients to avoid pressure points, stabilization of fractures, and elimination of irritating physical stimulation (e.g., avoiding traction on the endotracheal tube).

Several mechanisms have been proposed to explain how to inhibit or modulate the ascending transmission of a noxious stimulus from the periphery or, conversely, to stimulate descending inhibitory control from the brain [29].

They include the following:

1. Gate control theory
2. "Busy-line" effect
3. Production of endogenous opioids at the periaqueductal gray, reticular activating system, and spinal gate
4. Activation of monoaminergic neurons in the thalamus, hypothalamus, and brain stem
5. Activation of second-order neurons in the dorsal horn, selective inhibition of abnormally hypersensitive neurons in the dorsal horn, and increased release of γ-aminobutyric acid (GABA) in spinal neurons
6. Descending inhibition from supraspinal centers via the pretectal zone and posterior columns

Stimulation-produced analgesia (SPA) is a term that describes noninvasive or minimally invasive techniques such as acupuncture, electroacupuncture (EA), transcutaneous electric nerve stimulation (TENS), acupressure and spinal cord stimulation (SCS), peripheral nerve stimulation (PNS), deep-brain stimulation, and motor cortex stimulation. Evidence suggests that these modalities are useful as a sole or supplementary analgesic technique for both acute and chronic painful conditions [29].

Peripherally applied heat causes local vasodilation that promotes circulatory removal of biomediators of pain from the site of injury, whereas cold application decreases the release of pain-inducing chemicals [30].

Modifications of the ICU environment, such as creating units with single rooms, decreasing noise, and providing music and appropriate lighting that better reflect a day–night orientation [31], may help patients achieve normal sleep patterns and also improve pain control. For the cognitively intact ICU patients, provision of sensory and procedural information may improve their ability to cope with the discomfort.

Pharmacologic Treatments

The pharmacologic characteristics of the ideal analgesic medication include easy titration, rapid onset and offset of action without accumulation, and no side effects.

Nonsteroidal Anti-Inflammatory Drugs

Cyclooxygenase (COX) is located in all cells. It metabolizes arachidonic acid to generate prostaglandin H_2. A number of enzymes further modify this product to generate bioactive lipids (prostanoids) such as prostacyclin, thromboxane A_2, and prostaglandins D_2, E_2, and F_2. Three isoforms COX-1, COX-2, and COX-3 have been described. COX-1 is ubiquitous and constitutive. COX-2 is present in areas of inflammation and located in inflammatory cells. COX-3 is a splice variant, found centrally, and its inhibition is thought to be responsible for the action of acetaminophen [32].

It is now recognized that COX-2 is expressed in normal endothelial cells in response to shear stress and its inhibition is associated with suppression of prostacyclin synthesis. Inhibition of COX-2 results in prothrombotic inclination on endothelial surfaces and an increase in sodium and water retention, leading to edema, as well as exacerbations of heart failure and hypertension. Loss of the protective effects of COX-2 upregulation in the setting of myocardial ischemia and infarction leads to a larger infarct size, greater thinning of the left ventricular wall in the infarct zone, and an increased tendency to myocardial rupture [33,34].

Blockade of the proinflammatory mediators by nonsteroidal anti-inflammatory drugs (NSAIDs) reduces the inflammatory response (and subsequent pain). Classically, their effect is anti-inflammatory, analgesic, and antipyretic because of the direct inhibition of prostaglandin production. Adding NSAIDs to intravenous (IV) opioid-based patient-controlled analgesia (PCA) reduces opioid consumption by 30% to 50% and results in a significant reduction in the incidence of nausea, vomiting, and sedation [35].

On the other hand, the nonspecific blockade of COX inhibits the physiologic role of COX-1 and results in clinically significant deterioration of renal function and risk of development of peptic ulceration and upper gastrointestinal (GI) hemorrhage, bronchospasm, and platelet dysfunction. A meta-analysis published in 2002 showed that the risk of GI hemorrhage is related to the patient and drug-related factors, and is irrespective of the type of NSAID used. Patients who smoke, those with history of GI hemorrhage, and those taking anticoagulants are at increased risk [36].

Current evidence indicates that selective COX-2 inhibitors have important adverse cardiovascular effects that include increased risk for myocardial infarction, stroke, heart failure, and hypertension. The risk for these adverse effects is likely to be greatest in patients with a history of or at high risk for cardiovascular disease. In these patients, COX-2 inhibitors for pain relief should be used only if there are no alternatives and then only in the lowest dose and shortest duration necessary [37]. Currently, celecoxib is available for clinical use worldwide, whereas parecoxib is available only outside the United States.

Opioid-sparing properties of NSAIDs have not been studied in critically ill patients, so it is unclear if potential benefits outweigh potential risks such as GI bleeding or renal failure. Therefore, until more evidence for such agents becomes available, the clinician must carefully judge the risks and benefits on an individual basis.

Acetaminophen

Acetaminophen is an analgesic and antipyretic. It may also have anti-inflammatory properties. The mechanism of action of acetaminophen remains unknown. The greater sensitivity of cells containing COX-3 to acetaminophen is frequently cited as indicating that the target of action of acetaminophen is COX-3. Recent research indicates that acetaminophen inhibits prostaglandin synthesis in cells that have a low rate of synthesis and low levels of peroxide. When the levels of arachidonic acid are low, acetaminophen appears to be a selective COX-2 inhibitor. Acetaminophen has predominant effects on the CNS because the peroxide and arachidonic acid levels in the brain are lower than at peripheral sites of inflammation [38]. It is available in oral, rectal, and parenteral formulations. The parenteral formulation is not yet available in the United Sates although approval of the Food and Drug Administration (FDA) is pending. Acetaminophen is an effective adjuvant to opioid analgesia, and a reduction in opioid requirement by 20% to 30% can be achieved when combined with a regular regimen of oral or rectal acetaminophen.

It has been shown that 1 g of acetaminophen significantly reduces postoperative morphine consumption over a 6-hour period. Doses greater than 1,000 mg have been reported to have a superior effect when compared to lower doses. IV acetaminophen has been shown to reduce PCA morphine requirements after spinal surgery [39] and hip arthroplasty.

Its side-effect profile is comparable to placebo [40]; hypersensitivity reactions are rare. Major concerns with acetaminophen administration relate to the potential for hepatotoxicity, which, however, is extremely rare following therapeutic dosing [41]. In patients with severe liver disease, the elimination half-life can be prolonged. A reduced dose of 1 g three times a day with short duration of therapy is recommended. Prospective studies administering acetaminophen to patients consuming alcohol have found no increased evidence of liver injury [42]. In a recent study, nonallergic hypotension has been reported in a cohort of ICU patients on therapeutic doses of acetaminophen. The authors indicated brain injury and sepsis as the potential risk factors for this type of hypotensive reaction [43].

Opioids

For the critically ill patient, opioids remain the main pharmacologic method for the treatment of pain. Despite their extensive side-effect profile, there are no therapeutic alternatives available currently (Table 24.1).

Opiates refer to the nonpeptide synthetic morphine-like drugs while the term opioid is more generic, encompassing all substances that produce morphine-like actions. Opioids can be loosely divided into four groups:

- Naturally occurring, endogenously produced opioid peptides (e.g., dynorphin and Met-enkephalin)
- Opium alkaloids, such as morphine, purified from the poppy (*Papaver somniferum*)
- Semisynthetic opioids (modifications to the natural morphine structure) such as diacetylmorphine (heroin), hydromorphone, oxycodone, and oxymorphone
- Synthetic derivatives with structure unrelated to morphine, which include the phenylpiperidine series (e.g., pethidine and fentanyl), methadone series (e.g., methadone and dextropropoxyphene), benzomorphan series (e.g., pentazocine), and semisynthetic thebaine derivatives (e.g., etorphine and buprenorphine)

TABLE 24.1

GUIDELINES FOR FRONT-LOADING INTRAVENOUS ANALGESIA

Drug	Total front-load dose	Increments	Cautions
Morphine	0.08–0.12 mg/kg	0.03 mg/kg q 10 min	Bradycardia/hypotension (histamine) Nausea/vomiting Biliary colic Acute/chronic renal failure Elderly Bronchospasm
Methadone	0.08–0.12 mg/kg	0.03 mg/kg q 15 min	Accumulation/sedation Elderly
Hydromorphone	0.02 mg/kg	25–50 μg/kg q 10 min	Same as morphine Dosing errors
Fentanyl	1–3 μg/kg	0.5–2.00 μg/kg/h	Accumulation/sedation Elderly skeletal muscle rigidity
Remifentanil	0.25–1.00 μg/kg	0.05–2.00 μg/kg/min	Bradycardia/hypotension Pain on discontinuation Skeletal muscle rigidity
Ketamine	0.2–0.5 mg/kg	0.5–2.0 mg/kg/h	Delirium Increased ICP High myocardial O_2 requirement Hypotension Decreased CO

CO, cardiac output; ICP, intracranial pressure; q, every.

Snyder et al. in 1973 reported on the presence of specific binding sites for opioids, providing the first evidence of distinct receptors for opioids. There are several types of opioid receptors. They differ in their potency, selective antagonism, and stereospecificity of opiate action. With a recent addition, the opioid receptor subtypes are listed as μ (MOP), κ (KOP) and δ (DOP) and nociception/orphanin FQ (N/OFQ) peptide receptor (NOP).

Opioids bind to the CNS and peripheral tissue receptors. μ1-Receptors mediate analgesia, whereas μ2-receptor binding produces respiratory depression, nausea, vomiting, constipation, and euphoria. κ-Receptor activation causes sedation, miosis, and spinal analgesia. In addition to analgesia, opioid receptors may provide mild-to-moderate anxiolysis. Opioids have no reliable amnestic effect on patients. Opioid administration is associated with a dose-dependent, centrally mediated respiratory depression. The respiratory rate is reduced, whereas the tidal volume is initially preserved. The ventilatory response to hypoxia is eradicated and the CO_2–response curve is shifted to the right. Opioids facilitate patients' compliance to the ventilator due to their cough-suppressant effects. Despite minimal cardiovascular effects in normovolemic patients, they may generate hypotension via decreased sympathetic tone, and thus may decrease heart rate and systemic vascular resistance in critically ill patients. Additionally, opioids increase venous capacitance, thereby decreasing venous return. Hypotension clearly is more pronounced in hypovolemic patients.

Opioid-induced ileus is a common problem in critically ill patients.

Morphine

Morphine has poor lipid solubility and thus has a relatively slow onset of action (5 to 10 minutes). The standard IV dose is 5 to 10 mg and the approximate half-life is 3 hours. However, with repeated dosing or continuous infusions, half-life kinetics become unreliable. Morphine is conjugated by the liver to metabolites that include morphine-6-glucuronide, a potent metabolite with 20 times the activity of morphine. Both morphine and morphine-6-glucuronide are eliminated by the kidney; therefore, renal dysfunction results in a prolonged drug effect.

Morphine may also cause hypotension due to vasodilatation (secondary to the release of histamine).

Fentanyl

Fentanyl is highly lipid soluble with rapid onset of action (1 minute) and rapid redistribution into peripheral tissues, resulting in a short half-life (0.5 to 1.0 hour) after a single dose. The duration of action with small doses (50 to 100 μg) is short as a result of redistribution from the brain to other tissues. Larger or repeated doses, including the doses delivered via a continuous infusion, alter the context-sensitive half-time and result in drug accumulation and prolonged effects of the drug. The hepatic metabolism of fentanyl creates inactive metabolites that are renally excreted, making this drug a more attractive choice in patients with renal insufficiency. Fentanyl causes minor hemodynamic changes and does not affect inotropy.

Hydromorphone

Hydromorphone is a semisynthetic opioid that is five- to tenfold more potent than morphine, but with a similar duration of action. It has minimal hemodynamic effects, lacks a clinically significant active metabolite, and causes minor to no histamine release [44]. Recently published data (Chang et al.) suggest that patients who received IV hydromorphone have a greater decrease in pain than those given an equianalgesic dose of IV morphine [45].

Methadone

Methadone is a synthetic opioid agent with properties similar to morphine. It can be given enterally and parenterally. Methadone is an attractive choice for opioid analgesia due to its long half-life and low cost. It produces *N*-methyl-D-aspartate (NMDA) antagonism, which makes it ideal for neuropathic pain. Although methadone is not the drug of choice for an acutely ill patient whose hospital course is rapidly changing, it is a good alternative for the patient who has preexisting opioid tolerance or prolonged ventilatory wean. It may help facilitate the tapering of opioid infusions [46,47]. Metabolized in the liver, 40% of the drug is eliminated from kidney and free from active metabolites. It does not accumulate in renal failure.

Oxycodone

Oxycodone is effective for postoperative pain management. It has a higher bioavailability and a slightly longer half-life than oral morphine. When transferring patients from parenteral morphine to oral oxycodone, the dose should be based on a 1:1.5 ratio (i.e., 1 mg IV morphine = 0.5 to 0.7 mg oral oxycodone). Individual patient variability and incomplete cross-tolerance requires careful titration [48].

The use of controlled-release oxycodone (OxyContin) is indicated for the treatment of moderate-to-severe pain when continuous analgesia is required for prolonged periods. The release of oxycodone from the OxyContin capsule is biphasic; there is a rapid initial absorption phase within 37 minutes followed by a slow absorption phase over 6.2 hours. Peak pain relief for OxyContin capsules occurs at approximately 1 hour and lasts for 12 hours, with peak plasma concentrations at 2 to 3 hours after administration.

Remifentanil

Remifentanil (a derivative of fentanyl) is a powerful analgesic with ultrashort duration of action. It is metabolized by nonspecific esterases to remifentanil acid, which has negligible activity in comparison. Its metabolism is independent from hepatorenal function. The context-sensitive half-time of remifentanil is consistently short (3.2 minutes), even after an infusion of long duration up to 72 hours [49].

In terms of safety, efficacy, and speed of onset and offset, remifentanil has been reported to have a better profile when compared to fentanyl [50]. When a morphine-based pain and sedation regimen was compared to another based on remifentanil, the mean duration of mechanical ventilation and extubation time were significantly shorter in the remifentanil group [51]. Breen et al. [52] compared a remifentanil-based analgesia–sedation regimen with a midazolam-based one, to which fentanyl or morphine could be added for analgesia, in a group of critically ill patients requiring prolonged mechanical ventilation for up to 10 days. The remifentanil-based sedation regimen was associated with significantly reduced duration of mechanical ventilation by more than 2 days.

Rozendaal et al. reported that in patients with anticipated short-term mechanical ventilation, a remifentanil–propofol analgesia–sedation regimen provides better control of sedation and agitation and reduces weaning time compared to conventional regimens. In addition, patients on a remifentanil–propofol-based regimen are almost twice as likely to be extubated and discharged from the ICU within the first 3 days of treatment than patients on conventional regimens [53].

In addition, remifentanil does not exert significantly prolonged clinical effects when it is administered to ICU patients with renal failure or chronic liver disease [49]. On the basis of these studies, it can be concluded that remifentanil is effective for providing both analgesia and sedation in critically ill patients, even those suffering from multiple organ failure. However, further data are needed to better guide clinicians on the use of this drug in ICU patients.

OPIOID SIDE EFFECTS

Opioid-related adverse effects occur commonly in the ICU [54].

Opioid-induced respiratory depression is generally dose related and is most deleterious for the spontaneously breathing ICU patients. Incidence of opioid-induced nausea and vomiting is low in the ICU. High-dose fentanyl may cause muscle rigidity. Opioid-induced hypotension occurs most commonly in patients who are hemodynamically unstable, are volume depleted, or have a high sympathetic tone. The use of morphine is associated with histamine release; therefore, hypotension, urticaria, pruritus, flushing, and bronchospasm are possible. Fentanyl can safely be used in patients with a suspected allergy to morphine. Excessive sedation from opioids is most often seen with the use of continuous infusions, particularly in patients with end-stage renal disease who are receiving fentanyl or morphine. Methadone may cause excessive sedation if the dose is not titrated downward after the first 5 days of therapy or if a human cytochrome P450 inhibitor is concomitantly administered. QTc-interval prolongation and the risk of development of torsades de pointes can occur with high doses of methadone because of its effects on the hERG channel, particularly if the chlorbutanol-containing IV formulation is used. Opioids may cause hallucinations, agitation, euphoria, sleep disturbances, and delirium [55]. Methadone may be the least likely drug to cause delirium because of its antagonistic activity at the NMDA receptor [56]. The effects of opioids on ICP in patients with traumatic brain injury remain unclear. Gastric retention and ileus are common in patients who are critically ill and receiving opioids, with prokinetic therapy and/or postpyloric access required in patients prescribed enteral nutrition. Prophylactic use of a stimulant laxative reduces the incidence of constipation. Methylnaltrexone, an opioid antagonist specific to peripheral receptors, may have a role in treating opioid-induced constipation that fails to respond to laxative therapy [57]. The possibility of developing an addiction problem in adult patients receiving long-term opioids is extremely low.

OPIOIDS ADMINISTRATION METHODS

Opioid analgesics administered by either continuous infusion or titration to effect provide better pain control and less drug-related adverse effects. "As needed" protocols make it difficult to achieve adequate analgesic plasma concentrations with resultant poor pain control.

When a continuous infusion is used, a sedation vacation protocol allows more effective analgesic titration with a lower total dose of opioid used. Daily awakening may also be associated with a shorter duration of ventilation and ICU stay. For patients in whom a long recovery and a prolonged ventilatory wean are anticipated, it is appropriate to use a long-acting medication (e.g., methadone) to achieve adequate background pain control in combination with bolus doses of a short-acting opioid for management of breakthrough pain.

Conventional Routes of Administration (Oral, Intramuscular, and Subcutaneous)

Because of first-pass metabolism in the liver, larger doses of medications are required when oral preparations are used. Immediate-release oral opioids (e.g., morphine, oxycodone, and hydromorphone) are preferred because onset analgesia is obtained in 45 to 60 minutes. Fixed-interval dosing (e.g., every 4 hour) is preferable to a "when required" regimen to ensure adequate relief of moderate-to-severe pain.

The rectal route is rarely used in the ICU. Drugs absorbed from the lower half of the rectum bypass the portal vein and first-pass metabolism in the liver. Suppository formulations containing morphine, oxycodone, hydromorphone, and oxymorphone are available.

Intramuscular injections of opioids are useful if there is a lack of personnel trained to administer IV injections or if venous access is difficult. The intramuscular injection of morphine takes 30 to 60 minutes to be effective. Absorption of intramuscular opioids is variable and depends on the injection site, especially in the critically ill patients.

Subcutaneous injection via an indwelling cannula in the subcutaneous tissue of the upper outer aspect of the arm or thigh is a useful alternative route of administration. The rate of absorption of morphine after subcutaneous injection is similar to that of an intramuscular injection; therefore, the guidelines for titration are the same (Fig. 24.1).

Advanced Methods of Administration

The *IV route* is the preferred route of administration. There is less variability in blood levels when the IV route is used, making it easier to titrate the drug to effective analgesia concentration.

IV infusions are a commonly used method. An opioid infusion at a fixed rate takes five half-lives of the drug to reach 98% of a steady-state concentration. Therefore, a front-loading dose is needed to achieve adequate pain relief more rapidly before starting the infusion. If breakthrough pain occurs, more IV bolus doses may be needed to reestablish pain relief before the infusion rate is increased.

Five-Point Global Scale	None A little = 1 Some = 2 A lot = 3 The worst = 4
Verbal Quantitative Scale	0.......5.......10 None Worst imaginable
Visual Pain Analog Scale	No Worst .... Pain Pain Place a mark on the line

FIGURE 24.1. Several scales that can be useful for the evaluation of patient "self-reports" of pain before and after treatment. [From Stevens DS, Edwards WT: Management of pain in the critically ill. *J Intensive Care Med* 5:258, 1990, with permission.]

IV PCA allows the patient to self-administer a predetermined dose of opioid within the limits of a lockout period. This results in less variability in the blood levels of the drug, thereby enabling titration of the drug to effect [58].

The *epidural* and *intrathecal* routes of administration provide a more rapid analgesia due to the application of the drug directly within the CNS.

Patient-controlled epidural analgesia (PCEA) regimens allow better titration of the medication. In general, the analgesic efficacy of neuraxial opioids is greater than that achieved with parenteral opioid administration, resulting in superior pain relief despite the smaller doses used in the subarachnoid or epidural space (e.g., subarachnoid morphine 0.1 mg = epidural morphine 1 mg = IV morphine 10 mg). Opioid solutions with preservative-free formulations should be used for neuraxial administration to avoid potential neurotoxicity.

Highly lipid-soluble opioids (e.g., fentanyl and buprenorphine) have been formulated as a skin patch for transdermal delivery, especially in the management of severe pain in chronic and palliative care. Fentanyl patches are usually not a recommended modality for acute analgesia because of their 12- to 24-hour delay to peak effect and similar lag time to complete offset once the patch is removed. However, it is appropriate to continue its use in the ICU if the patient has a known history of using this formulation of the medication prior to admission.

Technological advances have led to the development of a transdermal delivery system that uses ionophoresis for the management of acute postoperative and post-trauma pain. This is a compact, self-contained, and self-adhesive system, which is applied to the patient's upper arm or chest. The system is preprogrammed and uses an imperceptible electric field to deliver 40 μg of fentanyl over 10 minutes and is unresponsive to additional dose requests during this time; patients can initiate up to 6 doses per hour for a 24-hour period or a maximum of 80 doses per system, whichever occurs first. Numerous trials have already demonstrated fentanyl iontophoretic transdermal system (ITS) to be better than placebo and therapeutically comparable with a standard morphine IV PCA. The pharmacokinetics is similar to those of IV fentanyl [59,60]. Its release waits completion of further clinical trials.

Other Drugs

Adjuvants are compounds which by themselves have undesirable side effects or low potency, but in combination with opioids, allow a reduction of opioid dosing for pain control.

Ketamine

Ketamine is a dissociative anesthetic also used for sedation. It possesses strong analgesic properties. It acts both centrally and peripherally by inhibition of glutamate activation via noncompetitive antagonism at the phencyclidine receptor of the NMDA channel. Nitric oxide (NO) synthase inhibition also contributes to its effects.

Water- and lipid-soluble characteristics of ketamine hydrochloride enable the IV, intramuscular, subcutaneous, epidural, oral, rectal, and transnasal routes of administration. It has a rapid onset and short duration of action [61]. Following metabolism in the liver, norketamine is produced, which is significantly less potent (20% to 30%) when compared to ketamine.

In subanesthetic or low doses (0.1 to 0.5 mg per kg IV), ketamine demonstrates significant analgesic efficacy without significant adverse pharmacologic effects. There is evidence that low-dose ketamine may play an important role in postoperative pain management when used as an adjunct to opioids, local anesthetics, and other analgesic agents [62–64]. Administration of regular benzodiazepines should be considered to minimize the psychomimetic side effects associated with its use.

Subhypnotic doses of ketamine administered as infusions have been used for critically ill ICU patients who are very difficult to sedate with opioid and benzodiazepine infusions. Because of its potential adverse effects, ketamine is not recommended for routine sedation and analgesia of the critically ill patient, but it can be useful for more difficult situations and/or when short surgical procedures with intense pain, such as placement of chest tubes, dressing changes, and/or wound debridement in burn patients, are necessary.

α_2-Adrenergic Agonists

α_2-Adrenergic activation represents an intrinsic mechanism of pain control at the level of the CNS. α_2-Adrenergic receptors exist in large numbers in the substantia gelatinosa of the spinal cord dorsal horn in humans. Agonists produce their pain control effect on those receptors.

Clonidine

Clonidine produces analgesia after systemic, epidural, or intrathecal administration. It has a short duration of action after a single dose and may produce sedation, bradycardia, and hypotension. Clonidine improves opioid analgesia and potentiates the effect of local anesthetic [65,66].

Dexmedetomidine

Dexmedetomidine is a centrally acting α_2-agonist with sedative and analgesic properties. It has a much greater affinity for α_2-receptors than clonidine. The sedative properties are facilitated through the locus coeruleus in the CNS. Analgesic effects occur via activation of the α_2-receptors and through potentiation of the action of opioids [67]. The drug causes no significant effect on the respiratory drive even when used with opioids. Dexmedetomidine has a biphasic effect on the cardiovascular system. The initial bolus injection is associated with vasoconstrictive effects, causing bradycardia and hypertension. Continuous infusion is associated with hypotension secondary to vasodilation caused by central sympatholysis. Studies conducted in postoperative ICU patients demonstrated successful short-term sedation and analgesic sparing [68]. There are a few studies examining long-term administration to critically ill, mechanically ventilated patients with encouraging results [69]. Suggested dosing recommendation would be a loading dose of 1 μg per kg over 10 minutes followed by an infusion at a rate of 0.2 to 0.7 μg per kg per hour.

Anticonvulsants

Gabapentin and *pregabalin* are licensed for the management of neuropathic pain.

Despite its structural similarity to GABA, gabapentin does not bind to GABA receptors. It has a high affinity for α_2/δ-subunits of voltage-dependent calcium channels, resulting in postsynaptic inhibition of the calcium influx and thereby reducing the presynaptic excitatory neurotransmitter release [70]. It markedly decreases postoperative opioid consumption when given at the time of anesthetic induction [71]. Several randomized controlled trials (RCTs) using different pain models have shown a positive effect of the gabapentinoids on postoperative pain in humans. Single doses of gabapentin up to 1,200 mg have been shown to reduce pain scores and/or morphine consumption after abdominal and vaginal hysterectomy, lower limb arthroplasty, and laparoscopic cholecystectomy. Different meta-analyses have confirmed these effects, which persist for up to 24 hours after surgery [72]. Common side effects of these medications include dizziness and drowsiness, which should not limit its use in ICU. Gabapentin has minimal drug interactions.

Pregabalin has the same mechanism of action as that of gabapentin. It has higher efficacy due to its linear pharmacokinetics. In addition, pregabalin appears to have a faster onset of action, which is due in part to its smaller volume of distribution.

Perioperative gabapentinoids (gabapentin/pregabalin) reduce postoperative pain, opioid requirements, and the incidence of opioid-related adverse effects, but increase the risk of sedation.

REGIONAL ANALGESIA TECHNIQUES

Recent studies suggest that advances in perioperative anesthesia and analgesia improve pain relief, patient satisfaction, and outcome in surgical and trauma patients. Neuraxial anesthesia and peripheral nerve blockade have the potential to reduce or eliminate the physiologic stress response to surgery and trauma, decreasing the possibility of surgical complications and improving outcomes.

When used alone or in combination with other treatment modalities, regional analgesia techniques are an invaluable tool to address pain-related problems in critically ill patients, but the indications for their use must be established correctly. ICU patients are at risk for numerous complications and the use of an inappropriate regional analgesia technique can cause a deterioration of the patient's clinical status, affecting a potentially favorable outcome.

The purpose of this section is to discuss risk and benefits of neuraxial and peripheral nerve blockade for the management of pain in the critically ill patient.

General Considerations

The use of ultrasound (US) technology in regional anesthesia allows a easier and more reliable identification of neural structures, the safe administration of lower doses of local anesthetic, and the insertion of nerve catheters even in the heavily sedated ICU patients. Ultrasound-guided (USG) techniques have reduced misplacement and failure rates in clinical practice. Effective identification of the needle allows for the reduction of the amount of administered drug volumes, which may be of importance in the critically ill, children, and patients who need more than one block, especially for those who have undergone multisite surgery or sustained multitrauma [73].

Regional analgesia techniques also effectively block sympathetic outflow. Many studies show that surgically related stress is reduced when regional anesthesia and analgesia techniques are used, neuraxial techniques in particular. The use of neuraxial analgesia has also been reported to decrease the rate of postoperative myocardial infarctions, shorten postoperative and post-traumatic ileus, improve the outcome, and shorten the length of ICU stay [74].

The use of such techniques may also reduce the incidence of chronic pain in patients undergoing surgical procedures, such as limb amputations and thoracotomies, two procedures in particular associated with the development of chronic persistent postsurgical pain [75].

Nerve Blocks for Thoracic and Abdominal Wall

Intercostal Nerve Blocks

Single and continuous intercostal nerve blocks are used to provide analgesia in patients with thoracic injuries and rib fractures and for the treatment of postoperative pain. Excellent pain relief and improvement in pulmonary mechanics have been reported [76].

Intercostal nerve blocks are associated with risk of pneumothorax and systemic local anesthetic toxicity. The patient's coagulation status must be checked to prevent the risk of bleeding and hematoma formation subsequent to the laceration of an intercostal vessel.

Continuous intercostal nerve blockade after thoracotomy using an extrapleural catheter consistently results in better pain relief and preservation of pulmonary function than the use of systemic opioids and appears to be at least as effective as the relief provided by the epidural approach. The ease of the extrapleural approach and the low incidence of complications suggest that this technique should be used more frequently. Other methods of intercostal nerve blockade appear to be less effective. The use of a multifaceted approach to post-thoracotomy analgesia that includes intercostal nerve blockade has been shown to be beneficial in the immediate postoperative period, as well as reduce the incidence of chronic pain.

Major pulmonary resections, which have been managed with a minithoracotomy and intrapleural intercostal nerve blocks, have been shown to be associated with reduced postoperative pain and improved outcome. However, a recently published study in thoracotomy patients did not find a measurable difference in pain relief between intercostal catheters and epidural analgesia [77].

Although not frequently used, intercostal nerve blocks can be extremely useful in the ICU patient, especially when used as a single injection for painful procedures (e.g., placement of chest tubes), or as an infusion when the patient's hemodynamic conditions do not allow the use of thoracic epidural analgesia (TEA).

Paravertebral Block

Paravertebral nerve blocks (PVBs) provide analgesia for thoracic and upper abdominal pain. Paravertebral nerve blockade can be performed with a single injection or a continuous catheter technique [78]. Injection of contrast material into a paravertebral catheter shows flow of the dye laterally into the intercostal space, as well as up and down the ipsilateral paravertebral space, leading to the spreading of local anesthetics over several dermatomal levels.

The advantages of PVBs are similar to those of the intercostal nerve block technique. Analgesia can be obtained without widespread cardiovascular effects because only unilateral sympathetic blockade is produced.

Because the site of injection is medial to the scapula, this block is easier to perform at high thoracic levels than the intercostal nerve blocks. In contrast to routine intercostal blocks, the posterior primary ramus of the intercostal nerve is also covered with the paravertebral approach, providing analgesia of the posterior spinal muscles and the costovertebral ligaments.

Failure rate after PVB in adults varies from 6.1% to 10.7% and compares favorably with other regional procedures. In a prospective study of 319 adult patients, the incidence of complications after thoracic or lumbar PVB was reported to be as follows: hypotension 5%, vascular puncture 3.8%, pleural puncture 0.9%, and pneumothorax 0.3% [79,80].

Interpleural Analgesia

Interpleural blockade is a technique by which an amount of local anesthetic is injected into the thoracic cage between the parietal and visceral pleura to produce ipsilateral somatic block of multiple thoracic dermatomes. Local anesthetic solutions can be administered as single or intermittent boluses, or as continuous infusions via an indwelling interpleural catheter. It has been shown to provide safe, high-quality analgesia after cholecystectomy, thoracotomy, renal surgery, breast surgery, and some invasive radiologic procedures of the renal and hepatobiliary system. It has also been used successfully in the treatment of pain from multiple rib fractures, herpes zoster, CRPS, thoracic and abdominal cancer, and pancreatitis [80].

There are several methods proposed for the detection of the entry of the needle into the pleural space. All of them involve the detection of the "negative pressure" of the intrapleural space [81]. If a posterior approach is not possible, an anterior approach could be used. The catheter may also be positioned in the interpleural space under direct vision during surgery.

The risk of pneumothorax is 2%. The risk of systemic local anesthetic toxicity is 1.3%. Pleural inflammation increases the risk of toxicity. Interpleural blocks have no clinically significant adverse effect on respiratory muscle function; on the contrary, they are more likely to be beneficial in the presence of painful conditions compromising pulmonary function.

It has been suggested that local anesthetic solution diffuses outward with the interpleural technique blocking multiple intercostal nerves, the sympathetic chain of the head, neck and upper extremity, the brachial plexus, splanchnic nerves, the phrenic nerve, the celiac plexus, and ganglia. As the injected local anesthetic diffuses out through both layers of the pleura, direct local effects on the diaphragm, lung, pericardium, and peritoneum may also contribute to some of its analgesic activity [81].

Transversus Abdominis Plexus Block

Incisional pain represents a considerable portion of postoperative pain following abdominal operations. The abdominal wall consists of three muscle layers: external oblique, internal oblique, transversus abdominis, and their corresponding fascial sheaths. The skin, muscles, and parietal peritoneum of the anterior abdominal wall are innervated by the lower six thoracic nerves and the first lumbar nerve. The anterior primary rami of these nerves exit their respective intervertebral foramina and extend over the vertebral transverse process. They then pierce the musculature of the lateral abdominal wall to travel through a neurofascial plane between the internal oblique and transversus abdominis muscles.

Deposition of local anesthetic dorsal to the midaxillary line blocks both the lateral cutaneous branch and the lateral cutaneous afferents, thus facilitating blockade of the entire anterior abdominal wall. The transversus abdominis plane (TAP) thus provides a space into which local anesthetic can be deposited to achieve myocutaneous sensory blockade.

This regional technique has been shown to provide good postoperative analgesia for a variety of procedures involving the abdominal wall [82]. The use of a fine-gauge, blunt-tipped, short-bevel needle, and USG has been proposed to reduce the incidence of possible complications (intraperitoneal injection with bowel injury/hematoma, liver laceration, transient femoral nerve palsy, accidental intravascular injection, infection, and catheter breakage). In addition, with USG techniques, upper and lower portions of the abdominal wall can be preferentially blocked [83].

Peripheral Nerve Blocks for the Upper Extremities

Severe trauma to the shoulders and arms is frequently present in acutely injured ICU patients. These injuries may be associated with blunt chest trauma requiring mechanical ventilation; they usually augment pain overall, especially during positioning [84]. If the orthopedic injury is part of a complex trauma with closed-head injury causing alterations of the mental status so that opioid-based analgesia regimens may mask the underlined neurologic condition, adequate analgesia can be provided with blocks of the brachial plexus.

Continuous brachial plexus blocks consistently provide superior analgesia with minimal side effects, promoting earlier hospital discharge and possibly improving rehabilitation after major surgery [85].

Peripheral nerve injury is a rare complication of regional anesthesia for the upper extremities. A large study from France reported 0.04% overall risk of a serious adverse event after peripheral nerve block [86]. Several retrospective studies reported the incidence to be between 0.5% and 1.0%, whereas prospective studies published higher incidence rates between 10% and 15% [87].

Current evidence suggests that peripheral nerve blocks should not be routinely performed in most adults during general anesthesia (GA) or heavy sedation especially when using the interscalene approach. However, the risk-to-benefit ratio of performing a peripheral nerve block under these conditions versus using high doses of opioids to maintain adequate analgesia should be carefully considered in select ICU patients [88].

Furthermore, the advent of USG techniques, in combination with injection pressure monitoring and electric nerve stimulation, may help to significantly minimize possible serious complications in heavily sedated patients with increased success rate and potential benefits overall.

Peripheral Nerve Blocks for the Lower Extremities

Lower extremity injuries are also commonly present in critically ill ICU patients.

Reid et al. recently conducted a study to compare the accuracy, success rates, and complications of USG femoral nerve blocks (FNBs) with the fascial pop (FP) technique in an emergency department. The result of this study favors the use of USG FNB. A similar study, conducted by Marhofer et al. has demonstrated a clear benefit in the use of US over a peripheral nerve stimulator when performing a three-in-one nerve block.

FNB is the preferred analgesic technique following injuries of the knee. Compared to epidural analgesia, it has a favorable morbidity profile, it allows early mobilization, and there is no need for urinary catheterization. In addition, with USG, the technique is simple and easy to perform compared to the epidural blocks [89]. FNB and catheters are helpful in the management of acute pain following femoral fractures as well as after surgical stabilization [90].

Easy visualization of the sciatic nerve proximal to the popliteal fossa, before it divides into common peroneal nerve medially and tibial nerve laterally with USG, makes the lateral approach to the sciatic nerve an ideal approach for management of pain secondary to distal tibia, ankle, and foot fractures [91]. This block can be conveniently performed in the supine position and enables more secure placement of a peripheral nerve catheter with high success rate.

Epidural Analgesia

Epidural analgesia is the most frequently used regional anesthesia technique in the ICU [92] and has been reported to provide better pain relief than parenteral opioid administration [93]. However, literature data report conflicting evidence regarding reduction of mortality with the use of epidural analgesia. The largest meta-analysis (CORTRA) [74] to date and analysis of the Medicare claims database [94] indicate a reduction in perioperative mortality with perioperative neuraxial anesthesia. Procedure-specific meta-analyses and specific RCTs, however, have not demonstrated benefit from epidural anesthesia and analgesia regarding reduction in mortality. It is important to note that these specific meta-analyses and individual RCTs lack sufficient sample size due to the relatively low incidence of mortality (0.2% to 5%) overall [95].

A meta-analysis of more than 5,000 surgical patients [96] has shown that postoperative epidural analgesia reduces the time to extubation, length of ICU stay, incidence of renal failure, morphine consumption during the first 24 hours, and maximal glucose and cortisol blood concentrations, and improves forced vital capacity. Many of these benefits may be relevant to ICU patients; they have been demonstrated to be actually beneficial in cardiac surgery [97] and thoracic trauma patients [98], as well as patients with severe acute pancreatitis [99].

Whether sepsis, with or without positive blood cultures, should be an absolute contraindication for the use of epidural analgesia is still a matter of debate [100]. In patients with ischemic heart disease, high thoracic epidural analgesia (HTEA) has been shown to improve systolic and diastolic myocardial function [101]. Furthermore, Ferguson et al. have concluded, in a recently published prospective randomized trial, that PCEA offers superior postoperative pain control after laparotomy for gynecologic surgery compared to traditional IV PCA [102].

TEA exerts a remarkable influence on the cardiovascular system. It reduces the risk of perioperative dysrhythmias except postoperative atrial fibrillation. In cardiac surgical patients, with improved left ventricular function, the left ventricular global and regional wall motions are better preserved. TEA has been associated with a reduction of cardiac oxygen consumption without jeopardizing coronary perfusion pressure with an increase of the diameter of stenotic coronary segments. As a result, TEA reduces the overall incidence of myocardial infarction. It produces functional hypovolemia by inhibiting the vasoconstrictor sympathetic outflow; moreover, it interferes with the integrity of renin–angiotensin system, but increments vasopressin plasma concentration. Despite causing hypotension, TEA has a beneficial outcome during hemorrhagic shock [103].

Issues of consent, coagulopathy, and infection can be addressed easily in elective conditions; they become a major problem in patients with multiple trauma or extremely painful conditions (e.g., acute pancreatitis).

A study published in Sweden reports the risk of hematoma to be 1.3 to 2.7 per 100,000 [104]. The current recommendations of the American Society of Regional Anesthesia should be followed [105].

Placing epidural catheters safely and confirming the presence of an adequate sensory block can be difficult in critically ill, sedated, and anesthetized patients. Awake and cooperative patients usually facilitate the placement of an epidural catheter, minimizing the possibility of undesirable complications. Current recommendations suggest that the possibility to miss systemic local anesthetic toxicity under GA or heavy sedation is not a valid reason not to perform a neuraxial block in this group of patients. However, neuraxial regional anesthesia should be performed rarely in patients whose sensorium is compromised by GA or heavy sedation [88]. The overall risk of neuraxial anesthesia should be weighed against its expected benefit.

Positioning the patient for the procedure may also represent a challenge depending on the underlying injury and the number and position of tubes, catheters, or external fixation devices present. Strict asepsis should always be maintained for neuroaxial procedures.

Bolus injections of long-acting local anesthetics, such as bupivacaine and ropivacaine, or the discontinuation of continuous infusions every morning can help neurologic and sensory assessment.

The most common side effects of thoracic epidural blocks are bradycardia and hypotension related to sympathetic block; this can be more pronounced with intermittent bolus dosing in patients with hypovolemia or shock. Continuous low-rate local anesthetic and/or opioid (morphine) infusions can be safely used in this particular clinical setting.

Currently, sepsis and bacteremia are considered contraindications to neuraxial blockade. Fever and increased white blood cell count alone in the absence of positive blood cultures do not provide a reliable diagnosis of bacteremia. High levels of the serum markers C-reactive protein, procalcitonin, and interleukin-6/8 have been shown to indicate bacterial sepsis with a high degree of sensitivity and specificity and can guide the decision as to whether or not to place an epidural catheter [106].

Because high-risk patients seem to profit most from epidural analgesia and the current literature does not address the specific problem of the critically ill patient with multiple comorbidities and organ failure, logic suggests that in carefully selected and closely monitored patients epidural analgesia may have significant benefits. Further research is needed before clear recommendations can be made.

INFLUENCE OF PAIN MANAGEMENT ON COMPLICATIONS, OUTCOME, LENGTH OF HOSPITAL STAY, AND CHRONIC PAIN

Pain leads to development of increased catabolism, immunosuppression, and prolonged sympathetic response as a result of the combination of tissue injury and pain that leads to increased morbidity and mortality. These effects can be subclassified as follows.

Cardiovascular Effects

- Increased heart rate
- Increased blood pressure
- Increased stroke volume
- Increased myocardial O_2 demands and reduced supply leading to myocardial ischemia

Respiratory Effects

- Stimulation of respiration causing initial hypocapnia and respiratory alkalosis
- Diaphragmatic splinting and hypoventilation, atelectasis, hypoxia, and hypercapnia
- Development of chest infection

Endocrine Effects

- Catabolic and anabolic changes
- Decrease in insulin production
- Reduction in testosterone level
- Fluid retention

Metabolic Effects

- Raised blood sugar level

Gastrointestinal effects

- Delayed gastric emptying
- Nausea
- Reduced GI motility and ileus

Coagulation

- Immobility
- Increased blood viscosity
- Hypercoagulability and deep vein thrombosis (DVT)

A meta-analysis published in the year 2000 has concluded that epidural analgesia prevents postoperative major complications and may decrease postoperative mortality [74]. Other studies have reported that epidural anesthesia may selectively prevent the occurrence of respiratory and cardiovascular complications [107–109].

Recent prospective trials, including a significant number of patients, have failed to confirm the beneficial effect of epidural anesthesia on postoperative morbidity and mortality after major abdominal or orthopedic surgery. Such a discrepancy is thought to be the result of improved postoperative medical care. As an example, previously reported 50% reduction in DVT with epidural analgesia is no longer a valid criterion due to the recent introduction of low-molecular-weight heparin (LMWH) for management of DVT prophylaxis, which decreases the risk by more than 80%. Similarly, the use of prophylactic antibiotics and aggressive physiotherapy significantly reduces the postoperative pulmonary complications, and the preventive effect of epidural analgesia on chest infections has become less important.

Consequently, there is no significant evidence to consider epidural analgesia beneficial for the prevention of morbidity, but as part of a multimodal pain management process, it may facilitate recovery from surgery. The superior quality of pain relief provided by epidural analgesia combined with parenteral analgesia does indeed have a positive impact on mobilization, bowel function, and early food intake that results in a significant improvement in postoperative quality of life [110]. In orthopedic surgery, regional analgesia may provide a functional benefit, allowing better patient involvement with physical therapy and shorter recovery.

Hebl et al. [111] have published their findings on the improvements in perioperative outcomes following peripheral nerve block after major orthopedic surgery. These include significantly shorter hospital stay, earlier ambulation, improved joint range of motion, lower perioperative pain scores, and a reduction in postoperative nausea and vomiting when compared with patients treated with traditional postoperative IV opioids (PCA). These patients also had significantly lower opioid requirements when compared with controls, as well as significant reduction in urinary retention and postoperative ileus [111].

Although the risk factors are difficult to identify, patients who experience severe pain and, above all, persistence of postoperative pain several days after the expected duration are prone to develop chronic pain.

Postoperative chronic pain is defined as persisting pain, without relapse or pain-free interval, 2 months after the surgical insult. Chronic pain syndromes have been described commonly after breast surgery, inguinal hernia repair, cholecystectomy, thoracic surgery, cardiac surgery, and limb or organ amputation. Its incidence has been recorded to be up to 60% [112]. With such a high incidence, it is very important to provide good postoperative and post-trauma pain control to prevent the occurrence of chronic pain syndromes.

CONCLUSIONS

Pain control in critically ill patients is of paramount importance. Achieving adequate levels of analgesia in trauma and surgery patients decreases the stress response and improves morbidity and mortality.

Individual units and acute pain teams should employ pain assessment techniques for patients with cognition impairment.

Lack of education, fear of possible side effects, and inappropriate use of medications contribute to the ineffective treatment of pain in critically ill ICU patients. The expertise of pain management specialists and anesthesiologists is often necessary for the management of these complex situations.

Choosing the treatment plan that best fits the patient's clinical conditions is mandatory. A potentially favorable outcome can be altered if inappropriate pain modalities are chosen and used.

A rational multimodal approach including the use of nonpharmacologic, pharmacologic, and regional analgesia techniques is desirable and often needed. The continued use of these techniques extended into the postoperative period may shorten recovery time and speed discharge.

Always assess and monitor the effects of a treatment modality on the patient's pain and clinical conditions as well. Be prepared to make changes in therapy as needed.

Regional analgesia techniques (epidural and peripheral nerve blockade), although proved to be safe and effective, are underused in the management of pain in critically ill patients. They allow a decrease in the overall use of opioid analgesics and sedatives and reduce the possibility of developing potentially dangerous side effects. A correct indication, as well as an appropriate timing for their use, is required in order to increase their beneficial effects.

The availability of new technologies (e.g., ultrasonography) improves the quality and safety of upper and lower extremity peripheral nerve blocks even in heavily sedated ICU patients.

References

1. Sessler CN, Wilhelm W: Analgesia and sedation in the intensive care unit: an overview of the issues. *Crit Care* 12[Suppl 3]:S1, 2008.
2. Sessler CN, Grap MJ, Brophy GM: Multidisciplinary management of sedation and analgesia in critical care. *Semin Respir Crit Care Med* 22(2):211–226, 2001.
3. Blakely WP, Page GG: Pathophysiology of pain in critically ill patients. *Crit Care Nurs Clin North Am* 13(2):167–179, 2001.
4. Summer GJ, Puntillo KA: Management of surgical and procedural pain in a critical care setting. *Crit Care Nurs Clin North Am* 13(2):233–242, 2001.
5. Herr K, Coyne PJ, Key T, et al: Pain assessment in the nonverbal patient: position statement with clinical practice recommendations. *Pain Manag Nurs* 7(2):44–52, 2006.
6. Dolin SJ, Cashman JN, Bland JM: Effectiveness of acute postoperative pain management: I. Evidence from published data. *Br J Anaesth* 89(3):409–423, 2002.
7. Apfelbaum JL, Chen C, Mehta SS, et al: Postoperative pain experience: results from a national survey suggest postoperative pain continues to be undermanaged. *Anesth Analg* 97(2):534–540, table of contents, 2003.
8. Puntillo KA, White C, Morris AB, et al: Patients' perceptions and responses to procedural pain: results from Thunder Project II. *Am J Crit Care* 10(4):238–251, 2001.
9. Gelinas C, Johnston C: Pain assessment in the critically ill ventilated adult: validation of the Critical-Care Pain Observation Tool and physiologic indicators. *Clin J Pain* 23(6):497–505, 2007.
10. Bonnet F, Marret E: Postoperative pain management and outcome after surgery. *Best Pract Res Clin Anaesthesiol* 21(1):99–107, 2007.
11. Basse L, Hjort Jakobsen D, Billesbolle P, et al: A clinical pathway to accelerate recovery after colonic resection. *Ann Surg* 232(1):51–57, 2000.
12. Kehlet H, Jensen TS, Woolf CJ: Persistent postsurgical pain: risk factors and prevention. *Lancet* 367(9522):1618–1625, 2006.
13. Kehlet H, Wilmore DW: Multimodal strategies to improve surgical outcome. *Am J Surg* 183(6):630–641, 2002.
14. Gordon DB, Dahl JL, Miaskowski C, et al: American Pain Society recommendations for improving the quality of acute and cancer pain management: American Pain Society Quality of Care Task Force. *Arch Intern Med* 165(14):1574–1580, 2005.
15. Reimer-Kent J: From theory to practice: preventing pain after cardiac surgery. *Am J Crit Care* 12(2):136–143, 2003.
16. Gelinas C, Fortier M, Viens C, et al: Pain assessment and management in critically ill intubated patients: a retrospective study. *Am J Crit Care* 13(2):126–135, 2004.
17. Payen JF, Bru O, Bosson JL, et al: Assessing pain in critically ill sedated patients by using a behavioral pain scale. *Crit Care Med* 29(12):2258–2263, 2001.
18. Herr K: Pain assessment in cognitively impaired older adults. *Am J Nurs* 102(12):65–67, 2002.
19. De Pinto M, Dunbar PJ, Edwards WT: Pain management. *Anesthesiol Clin* 24(1):19–37, vii, 2006.
20. Juhl GI, Jensen TS, Norholt SE, et al: Central sensitization phenomena after third molar surgery: a quantitative sensory testing study. *Eur J Pain* 12(1):116–127, 2008.
21. Huang J, Zhang X, McNaughton PA: Inflammatory pain: the cellular basis of heat hyperalgesia. *Curr Neuropharmacol* 4(3):197–206, 2006.
22. Hucho T, Levine JD: Signaling pathways in sensitization: toward a nociceptor cell biology. *Neuron* 55(3):365–376, 2007.
23. Abrahamsen B, Zhao J, Asante CO, et al: The cell and molecular basis of mechanical, cold, and inflammatory pain. *Science* 321(5889):702–705, 2008.
24. Costigan M, Scholz J, Woolf CJ: Neuropathic pain: a maladaptive response of the nervous system to damage. *Annu Rev Neurosci* 32:1–32, 2009.
25. Ducreux D, Attal N, Parker F, et al: Mechanisms of central neuropathic pain: a combined psychophysical and fMRI study in syringomyelia. *Brain* 129[Pt 4]:963–976, 2006.
26. Dworkin RH, Backonja M, Rowbotham MC, et al: Advances in neuropathic pain: diagnosis, mechanisms, and treatment recommendations. *Arch Neurol* 60(11):1524–1534, 2003.
27. Brush DR, Kress JP: Sedation and analgesia for the mechanically ventilated patient. *Clin Chest Med* 30(1):131–141, ix, 2009.
28. Sessler CN, Pedram S: Protocolized and target-based sedation and analgesia in the ICU. *Crit Care Clin* 25(3):489–513, viii, 2009.
29. Kotzé A, Simpson KH: Stimulation-produced analgesia: acupuncture, TENS and related techniques. *Anaesth Intensive Care Med* 9(1):29–32, 2008.
30. French SD, Cameron M, Walker BF, et al: Superficial heat or cold for low back pain. *Cochrane Database Syst Rev* (1):CD004750, 2006.
31. Cepeda MS, Carr DB, Lau J, et al: Music for pain relief. *Cochrane Database Syst Rev* (2):CD004843, 2006.
32. Hebbes C, Lambert D: Non-opioid analgesic drugs. *Anaesth Intensive Care Med* 9(2):79–83, 2008.
33. Timmers L, Sluijter JP, Verlaan CW, et al: Cyclooxygenase-2 inhibition increases mortality, enhances left ventricular remodeling, and impairs systolic function after myocardial infarction in the pig. *Circulation* 115(3):326–332, 2007.
34. Jugdutt BI: Cyclooxygenase inhibition and adverse remodeling during healing after myocardial infarction. *Circulation* 115(3):288–291, 2007.
35. Marret E, Kurdi O, Zufferey P, et al: Effects of nonsteroidal antiinflammatory drugs on patient-controlled analgesia morphine side effects: meta-analysis of randomized controlled trials. *Anesthesiology* 102(6):1249–1260, 2005.
36. Lewis SC, Langman MJ, Laporte JR, et al: Dose-response relationships between individual nonaspirin nonsteroidal anti-inflammatory drugs (NANSAIDs) and serious upper gastrointestinal bleeding: a meta-analysis based on individual patient data. *Br J Clin Pharmacol* 54(3):320–326, 2002.
37. Antman EM, Bennett JS, Daugherty A, et al: Use of nonsteroidal antiinflammatory drugs: an update for clinicians: a scientific statement from the American Heart Association. *Circulation* 115(12):1634–1642, 2007.

38. Kam P, So A: COX-3: Uncertainties and controversies. *Curr Anaesth Crit Care* 20(1):50–53, 2009.
39. Hernandez-Palazon J, Tortosa JA, Martinez-Lage JF, et al: Intravenous administration of propacetamol reduces morphine consumption after spinal fusion surgery. *Anesth Analg* 92(6):1473–1476, 2001.
40. Barden J, Edwards J, Moore A, et al: Single dose oral paracetamol (acetaminophen) for postoperative pain. *Cochrane Database Syst Rev* (1):CD004602, 2004.
41. Benson GD, Koff RS, Tolman KG: The therapeutic use of acetaminophen in patients with liver disease. *Am J Ther* 12(2):133–141, 2005.
42. Kuffner EK, Green JL, Bogdan GM, et al: The effect of acetaminophen (four grams a day for three consecutive days) on hepatic tests in alcoholic patients—a multicenter randomized study. *BMC Med* 5:13, 2007.
43. Mrozek S, Constantin JM, Futier E, et al: Acetaminophene-induced hypotension in intensive care unit: a prospective study. *Ann Fr Anesth Reanim* 28(5):448–453, 2009.
44. Jacobi J, Fraser GL, Coursin DB, et al: Clinical practice guidelines for the sustained use of sedatives and analgesics in the critically ill adult. *Crit Care Med* 30(1):119–141, 2002.
45. Chang AK, Bijur PE, Meyer RH, et al: Safety and efficacy of hydromorphone as an analgesic alternative to morphine in acute pain: a randomized clinical trial. *Ann Emerg Med* 48(2):164–172, 2006.
46. Fredheim OM, Moksnes K, Borchgrevink PC, et al: Clinical pharmacology of methadone for pain. *Acta Anaesthesiol Scand* 52(7):879–889, 2008.
47. Lugo RA, MacLaren R, Cash J, et al: Enteral methadone to expedite fentanyl discontinuation and prevent opioid abstinence syndrome in the PICU. *Pharmacotherapy* 21(12):1566–1573, 2001.
48. Blumenthal S, Min K, Marquardt M, et al: Postoperative intravenous morphine consumption, pain scores, and side effects with perioperative oral controlled-release oxycodone after lumbar discectomy. *Anesth Analg* 105(1):233–237, 2007.
49. Breen D, Wilmer A, Bodenham A, et al: Offset of pharmacodynamic effects and safety of remifentanil in intensive care unit patients with various degrees of renal impairment. *Crit Care* 8(1):R21–R30, 2004.
50. Muellejans B, Lopez A, Cross MH, et al: Remifentanil versus fentanyl for analgesia based sedation to provide patient comfort in the intensive care unit: a randomized, double-blind controlled trial [ISRCTN43755713]. *Crit Care* 8(1):R1-R11, 2004.
51. Dahaba AA, Grabner T, Rehak PH, et al: Remifentanil versus morphine analgesia and sedation for mechanically ventilated critically ill patients: a randomized double blind study. *Anesthesiology* 101(3):640–646, 2004.
52. Breen D, Karabinis A, Malbrain M, et al: Decreased duration of mechanical ventilation when comparing analgesia-based sedation using remifentanil with standard hypnotic-based sedation for up to 10 days in intensive care unit patients: a randomised trial [ISRCTN47583497]. *Crit Care* 9(3):R200–R210, 2005.
53. Rozendaal FW, Spronk PE, Snellen FF, et al: Remifentanil-propofol analgo-sedation shortens duration of ventilation and length of ICU stay compared to a conventional regimen: a centre randomised, cross-over, open-label study in the Netherlands. *Intensive Care Med* 35(2):291–298, 2009.
54. Riker RR, Fraser GL: Adverse events associated with sedatives, analgesics, and other drugs that provide patient comfort in the intensive care unit. *Pharmacotherapy* 25[5 Pt 2]:8S–18S, 2005.
55. Gaudreau JD, Gagnon P, Roy MA, et al: Opioid medications and longitudinal risk of delirium in hospitalized cancer patients. *Cancer* 109(11):2365–2373, 2007.
56. Benitez-Rosario MA, Feria M, Salinas-Martin A, et al: Opioid switching from transdermal fentanyl to oral methadone in patients with cancer pain. *Cancer* 101(12):2866–2873, 2004.
57. Thomas J, Karver S, Cooney GA, et al: Methylnaltrexone for opioid-induced constipation in advanced illness. *N Engl J Med* 358(22):2332–2343, 2008.
58. Hudcova J, McNicol E, Quah C, et al: Patient controlled opioid analgesia versus conventional opioid analgesia for postoperative pain. *Cochrane Database Syst Rev* (4):CD003348, 2006.
59. Power I: Fentanyl HCl iontophoretic transdermal system (ITS): clinical application of iontophoretic technology in the management of acute postoperative pain. *Br J Anaesth* 98(1):4–11, 2007.
60. Grond S, Hall J, Spacek A, et al: Iontophoretic transdermal system using fentanyl compared with patient-controlled intravenous analgesia using morphine for postoperative pain management. *Br J Anaesth* 98(6):806–815, 2007.
61. Liu LL, Gropper MA: Postoperative analgesia and sedation in the adult intensive care unit: a guide to drug selection. *Drugs* 63(8):755–767, 2003.
62. Subramaniam K, Subramaniam B, Steinbrook RA: Ketamine as adjuvant analgesic to opioids: a quantitative and qualitative systematic review. *Anesth Analg* 99(2):482–495, table of contents, 2004.
63. Zakine J, Samarcq D, Lorne E, et al: Postoperative ketamine administration decreases morphine consumption in major abdominal surgery: a prospective, randomized, double-blind, controlled study. *Anesth Analg* 106(6):1856–1861, 2008.
64. Elia N, Tramer MR: Ketamine and postoperative pain—a quantitative systematic review of randomised trials. *Pain* 113(1–2):61–70, 2005.
65. Farmery AD, Wilson-MacDonald J: The analgesic effect of epidural clonidine after spinal surgery: a randomized placebo-controlled trial. *Anesth Analg* 108(2):631–634, 2009.
66. Andrieu G, Roth B, Ousmane L, et al: The efficacy of intrathecal morphine with or without clonidine for postoperative analgesia after radical prostatectomy. *Anesth Analg* 108(6):1954–1957, 2009.
67. Szumita PM, Baroletti SA, Anger KE, et al: Sedation and analgesia in the intensive care unit: evaluating the role of dexmedetomidine. *Am J Health Syst Pharm* 64(1):37–44, 2007.
68. Martin E, Ramsay G, Mantz J, et al: The role of the alpha2-adrenoceptor agonist dexmedetomidine in postsurgical sedation in the intensive care unit. *J Intensive Care Med* 18(1):29–41, 2003.
69. Venn M, Newman J, Grounds M: A phase II study to evaluate the efficacy of dexmedetomidine for sedation in the medical intensive care unit. *Intensive Care Med* 29(2):201–207, 2003.
70. Bian F, Li Z, Offord J, et al: Calcium channel alpha2-delta type 1 subunit is the major binding protein for pregabalin in neocortex, hippocampus, amygdala, and spinal cord: an ex vivo autoradiographic study in alpha2-delta type 1 genetically modified mice. *Brain Res* 1075(1):68–80, 2006.
71. Hurley RW, Cohen SP, Williams KA, et al: The analgesic effects of perioperative gabapentin on postoperative pain: a meta-analysis. *Reg Anesth Pain Med* 31(3):237–247, 2006.
72. Seib RK, Paul JE: Preoperative gabapentin for postoperative analgesia: a meta-analysis. *Can J Anaesth* 53(5):461–469, 2006.
73. Wiebalck A, Grau T: Ultrasound imaging techniques for regional blocks in intensive care patients. *Crit Care Med* 35[5 Suppl]:S268–S274, 2007.
74. Rodgers A, Walker N, Schug S, et al: Reduction of postoperative mortality and morbidity with epidural or spinal anaesthesia: results from overview of randomised trials. *BMJ* 321(7275):1493, 2000.
75. Jenewein J, Moergeli H, Wittmann L, et al: Development of chronic pain following severe accidental injury. Results of a 3-year follow-up study. *J Psychosom Res* 66(2):119–126, 2009.
76. Osinowo OA, Zahrani M, Softah A: Effect of intercostal nerve block with 0.5% bupivacaine on peak expiratory flow rate and arterial oxygen saturation in rib fractures. *J Trauma* 56(2):345–347, 2004.
77. Allen MS, Halgren L, Nichols FC, III, et al: A randomized controlled trial of bupivacaine through intracostal catheters for pain management after thoracotomy. *Ann Thorac Surg* 88(3):903–910, 2009.
78. Eid HE: Paravertebral block: an overview. *Curr Anaesth Crit Care* 20(2): 65–70, 2009.
79. Lonnqvist PA, MacKenzie J, Soni AK, et al: Paravertebral blockade. Failure rate and complications. *Anaesthesia* 50(9):813–815, 1995.
80. Dravid RM, Paul RE: Interpleural block—part 2. *Anaesthesia* 62(11):1143–1153, 2007.
81. Dravid RM, Paul RE: Interpleural block—part 1. *Anaesthesia* 62(10):1039–1049, 2007.
82. Belavy D, Cowlishaw PJ, Howes M, et al: Ultrasound-guided transversus abdominis plane block for analgesia after Caesarean delivery. *Br J Anaesth* 103(5):726–730, 2009.
83. Hebbard P: Subcostal transversus abdominis plane block under ultrasound guidance. *Anesth Analg* 106(2):674–675, 2008; author reply 5.
84. Schulz-Stübner S, Boezaart A, Hata JS: Regional analgesia in the critically ill. *Crit Care Med* 33(6):1400–1407, 2005.
85. Capdevila X, Ponrouch M, Choquet O: Continuous peripheral nerve blocks in clinical practice. *Curr Opin Anaesthesiol* 21(5):619–623, 2008.
86. Auroy Y, Benhamou D, Bargues L, et al: Major complications of regional anesthesia in France: The SOS Regional Anesthesia Hotline Service. *Anesthesiology* 97(5):1274–1280, 2002.
87. Sorenson EJ: Neurological injuries associated with regional anesthesia. *Reg Anesth Pain Med* 33(5):442–448, 2008.
88. Neal JM, Bernards CM, Hadzic A, et al: ASRA Practice Advisory on Neurologic Complications in Regional Anesthesia and Pain Medicine. *Reg Anesth Pain Med* 33(5):404–415, 2008.
89. Davies AF, Segar EP, Murdoch J, et al: Epidural infusion or combined femoral and sciatic nerve blocks as perioperative analgesia for knee arthroplasty. *Br J Anaesth* 93(3):368–374, 2004.
90. Chalmouki G, Lekka N, Lappas T, et al: Perioperative pain management in femoral shaft fractures. Continuous femoral nerve block vs systemic pain therapy. *Reg Anesth Pain Med* 33(5):e77, 2008.
91. Gray AT, Huczko EL, Schafhalter-Zoppoth I: Lateral popliteal nerve block with ultrasound guidance. *Reg Anesth Pain Med* 29(5):507–509, 2004.
92. Schulz-Stübner S: The critically ill patient and regional anesthesia. *Curr Opin Anaesthesiol* 19(5):538–544, 2006.
93. Werawatganon T, Charuluxanun S: Patient controlled intravenous opioid analgesia versus continuous epidural analgesia for pain after intra-abdominal surgery. *Cochrane Database Syst Rev* (1):CD004088, 2005.
94. Wu CL, Hurley RW, Anderson GF, et al: Effect of postoperative epidural analgesia on morbidity and mortality following surgery in medicare patients. *Reg Anesth Pain Med* 29(6):525–533, 2004; discussion 15–19.
95. Liu SS, Wu CL: Effect of postoperative analgesia on major postoperative complications: a systematic update of the evidence. *Anesth Analg* 104(3):689–702, 2007.
96. Guay J: The benefits of adding epidural analgesia to general anesthesia: a metaanalysis. *J Anesth* 20(4):335–340, 2006.
97. Liu SS, Block BM, Wu CL: Effects of perioperative central neuraxial analgesia on outcome after coronary artery bypass surgery: a meta-analysis. *Anesthesiology* 101(1):153–161, 2004.
98. Bulger EM, Edwards T, Klotz P, et al: Epidural analgesia improves outcome after multiple rib fractures. *Surgery* 136(2):426–430, 2004.

99. Bernhardt A, Kortgen A, Niesel H, et al: Using epidural anesthesia in patients with acute pancreatitis—prospective study of 121 patients. *Anaesthesiol Reanim* 27(1):16–22, 2002.
100. Low JH: Survey of epidural analgesia management in general intensive care units in England. *Acta Anaesthesiol Scand* 46(7):799–805, 2002.
101. Jakobsen CJ, Nygaard E, Norrild K, et al: High thoracic epidural analgesia improves left ventricular function in patients with ischemic heart. *Acta Anaesthesiol Scand* 53(5):559–564, 2009.
102. Ferguson SE, Malhotra T, Seshan VE, et al: A prospective randomized trial comparing patient-controlled epidural analgesia to patient-controlled intravenous analgesia on postoperative pain control and recovery after major open gynecologic cancer surgery. *Gynecol Oncol* 114(1):111–116, 2009.
103. Clemente A, Carli F: The physiological effects of thoracic epidural anesthesia and analgesia on the cardiovascular, respiratory and gastrointestinal systems. *Minerva Anestesiol* 74(10):549–563, 2008.
104. Moen V, Dahlgren N, Irestedt L: Severe neurological complications after central neuraxial blockades in Sweden 1990–1999. *Anesthesiology* 101(4):950–959, 2004.
105. Horlocker TT, Wedel DJ, Rowlingson JC, et al: Regional anesthesia in the patient receiving antithrombotic or thrombolytic therapy: American Society of Regional Anesthesia and Pain Medicine Evidence-Based Guidelines (Third Edition). *Reg Anesth Pain Med* 35(1):64–101, 2010.
106. Luzzani A, Polati E, Dorizzi R, et al: Comparison of procalcitonin and C-reactive protein as markers of sepsis. *Crit Care Med* 31(6):1737–1741, 2003.
107. Ballantyne JC, Carr DB, deFerranti S, et al: The comparative effects of postoperative analgesic therapies on pulmonary outcome: cumulative meta-analyses of randomized, controlled trials. *Anesth Analg* 86(3):598–612, 1998.
108. Beattie WS, Badner NH, Choi P: Epidural analgesia reduces postoperative myocardial infarction: a meta-analysis. *Anesth Analg* 93(4):853–858, 2001.
109. Meissner A, Rolf N, Van Aken H: Thoracic epidural anesthesia and the patient with heart disease: benefits, risks, and controversies. *Anesth Analg* 85(3):517–528, 1997.
110. Carli F, Mayo N, Klubien K, et al: Epidural analgesia enhances functional exercise capacity and health-related quality of life after colonic surgery: results of a randomized trial. *Anesthesiology* 97(3):540–549, 2002.
111. Hebl JR, Dilger JA, Byer DE, et al: A pre-emptive multimodal pathway featuring peripheral nerve block improves perioperative outcomes after major orthopedic surgery. *Reg Anesth Pain Med* 33(6):510–517, 2008.
112. Perttunen K, Tasmuth T, Kalso E: Chronic pain after thoracic surgery: a follow-up study. *Acta Anaesthesiol Scand* 43(5):563–567, 1999.

CHAPTER 25 ■ THERAPEUTIC PARALYSIS

KHALDOUN FARIS

The most common indications for the use of neuromuscular blocking agents (NMBAs) in the intensive care unit (ICU) include emergency or elective intubations, optimization of patient–ventilator synchrony, management of increased intracranial pressure, reduction of oxygen consumption, and treatment of muscle spasms associated with tetanus. According to the American College of Critical Care Medicine and the Society of Critical Care Medicine clinical practice guidelines for sustained neuromuscular blockade in the adult critically ill patient, these medications should be used only when all other means of optimizing a patient's condition have been used. This recommendation is based on the concern that the administration of NMBAs may worsen patient outcome when administered during a course of critical illness, particularly if the patient is receiving systemic steroids at the same time [1]. In a recent international multicenter trial, 13% of patients on mechanical ventilation received NMBAs for at least 1 day, which was associated with a longer duration of mechanical ventilation, longer weaning time and stay in the ICU, and higher mortality [2].

In addition to the pharmacology of the most commonly administered agents, we briefly review the biology of the neuromuscular junction (NMJ), its alterations during the course of critical illness, and the resulting implications for the use of depolarizing and nondepolarizing NMBAs. Recommendations for administration of NMBAs to ICU patients on based on available evidence are provided.

PHARMACOLOGY OF NMBAS

The NMJ consists of the motor nerve terminus, acetylcholine (ACh), and muscle end plate. In response to neuronal action potentials, ACh is released from presynaptic axonal storage vesicles into the synapse of the NMJ. Both the presynaptic membrane and the postsynaptic end plate contain specialized nicotinic ACh receptors (nAChRs). The chemical signal is converted into an electric signal by binding of two ACh molecules to the receptor ($\alpha\delta$- and $\alpha\varepsilon$-subunits), causing a transient influx of sodium and calcium, and efflux of potassium from muscle cells. This depolarization propagates an action potential that results in a muscle contraction. Unbound ACh is quickly hydrolyzed in the synapse by the enzyme acetylcholinesterase to acetic acid and choline, thus effectively controlling the duration of receptor activation. A repolarization of the motor end plate and muscle fiber then occurs.

THE NICOTINIC ACETYLCHOLINE RECEPTOR

The nAChR is built of five subunit proteins, forming an ion channel. This ionic channel mediates neurotransmission at the NMJ, autonomic ganglia, spinal cord, and brain. During early development, differentiation and maturation of the NMJ and transformation of the nAChR take place: fetal nAChRs gradually disappear with a rise of new, functionally distinct, mature nAChRs.

These mature nAChRs (also termed *adult, innervated, ε-containing*) have a subunit composition of two α, β, ε, *and* δ in the synaptic muscle membrane. The only structural difference from the fetal nAChR is in substitution of the γ for the ε-subunit, although functional, pharmacologic, and metabolic characteristics are quite distinct. Mature nAChRs have a shorter burst duration and a higher conductance to Na^+, K^+, and Ca^{2+} and are metabolically stable with a half-life averaging about 2 weeks. The two α-, β-, δ-, and ε/γ-subunits interact to form a channel and an extracellular binding site for ACh and other mediators as well. As mentioned previously, simultaneous binding of two ACh molecules to $\alpha\delta$- and $\alpha\varepsilon$-subunits of an nAChR initiates opening of the channel and a flow of cations down their electrochemical gradient. In the absence of ACh or other mediators, the stable closed state (a major function of ε/γ-subunits) normally precludes channel opening [3].

Adult skeletal muscle retains the ability to synthesize not only adult, but also fetal (often called *immature* or *extrajunctional*)-type nAChRs. The synthesis of fetal nAChRs may be triggered in response to altered neuronal input, such as loss of nerve function or prolonged immobility, or in the presence of certain disease states. The major difference between fetal- and adult-type nAChRs is that fetal receptors migrate across the entire membrane surface and adult ones are mostly confined to the muscle end plate. In addition, these fetal nAChRs have a much shorter half-life, are more ionically active with prolonged open channel time that exaggerates the K^+ efflux, and are much more sensitive to depolarizing agents such as succinylcholine and resistant to nondepolarizing neuromuscular blockers.

The functional difference between depolarizing and nondepolarizing neuromuscular blockers lies in their interaction with AChRs. Depolarizing neuromuscular blockers are structurally similar to ACh and bind to and activate AChRs. Nondepolarizing neuromuscular blockers are competitive antagonists.

DEPOLARIZING NEUROMUSCULAR BLOCKERS

Succinylcholine is the only depolarizing neuromuscular blocker in clinical use. Its use is limited to facilitating rapid-sequence intubation in the emergency setting. Succinylcholine mimics the effects of ACh by binding to the ACh receptor and inducing a persistent depolarization of the muscle fiber. Muscle contraction remains inhibited until succinylcholine diffuses away from the motor end plate and is metabolized by serum (pseudo-) cholinesterase [4]. The clinical effect of succinylcholine is a brief excitatory period, with muscular fasciculations followed by neuromuscular blockade and flaccid paralysis. The intravenous dose of succinylcholine is 1 to 1.5 mg per kg and offers the most rapid onset of action (60 to 90 seconds) of the NMBAs. Recovery to 90% muscle strength after an intravenous dose of 1 mg per kg takes from 9 to 13 minutes. Succinylcholine is also suitable for intramuscular administration, most frequently for the treatment of laryngospasm in pediatric patients without intravenous access; however, there are several limitations. First, the required dose is higher (4 mg per kg) and time to maximum twitch depression is significantly longer (approximately 4 minutes). Second, the duration of action of succinylcholine after intramuscular injection is prolonged.

Potential adverse drug events associated with succinylcholine include hypertension, arrhythmias, increased intracranial and intraocular pressure, hyperkalemia, malignant hyperthermia, myalgias, and prolonged paralysis. Neuromuscular blockade can persist for hours in patients with genetic variants of pseudocholinesterase isoenzymes [5]. Contraindications to succinylcholine use include major thermal burns, significant crush injuries, spinal cord transection, malignant hyperthermia, and upper or lower motor neuron lesions. Caution is also advised in patients with open-globe injuries, renal failure, serious infections, and near-drowning victims [6].

NONDEPOLARIZING NMBAS

Nondepolarizing NMBAs function as competitive antagonists and inhibit ACh binding to postsynaptic nAChRs on the motor end plate. They are categorized into two classes on the basis of chemical structure: benzylisoquinoliniums and aminosteroids. Within each of these classes, the therapeutic agents may further be categorized as short-acting, intermediate-acting, or long-acting agents. The benzylisoquinolinium agents commonly used in the critical care setting include atracurium, cisatracurium, and doxacurium, whereas the aminosteroid agents include vecuronium, rocuronium, pancuronium, and pipecuronium.

The nondepolarizing NMBAs are administered by the intravenous route and have volumes of distribution (V_ds) ranging from 0.2 to 0.3 L per kg in adults.

A clinical relationship exists between the time to onset of paralysis and neuromuscular blocker dosing, drug distribution, and ACh-receptor sensitivity. An important factor to consider is V_d, which may change as a result of disease processes. Cirrhotic liver disease and chronic renal failure often result in an increased V_d and decreased plasma concentration for a given dose of water-soluble drugs. However, drugs dependent on renal or hepatic excretion may have a prolonged clinical effect. Therefore, a larger initial dose but smaller maintenance dose may be appropriate.

Alterations in V_d affect both peak neuromuscular blocker serum concentrations and time to paralysis. The pharmacokinetic and pharmacodynamic principles of commonly used NMBAs are summarized in Table 25.1.

Atracurium

Atracurium is an intermediate-acting nondepolarizing agent. Neuromuscular paralysis typically occurs between 3 and 5 minutes and lasts for 25 to 35 minutes after an initial bolus dose. Atracurium undergoes ester hydrolysis as well as Hofmann degradation, a nonenzymatic breakdown process that occurs at physiologic pH and body temperature, independent of renal or hepatic function. Renal and hepatic dysfunction should not affect the duration of neuromuscular paralysis. The neuroexcitatory metabolite laudanosine is renally excreted. Laudanosine is epileptogenic in animals and may induce central nervous system (CNS) excitation in patients with renal failure who are receiving prolonged atracurium infusions. Atracurium may induce histamine release after rapid administration.

Cisatracurium

Cisatracurium and atracurium are similar intermediate-acting nondepolarizing agents. A bolus dose of 0.2 mg per kg of cisatracurium usually results in neuromuscular paralysis within 1.5 to 2.5 minutes and lasts 45 to 60 minutes. When compared with atracurium, cisatracurium is three times as potent and has a more desirable adverse drug event profile, including lack of histamine release, minimal cardiovascular effects, and less interaction with autonomic ganglia. It also undergoes ester hydrolysis as well as Hofmann degradation. However, plasma laudanosine concentrations after cisatracurium administration are five to ten times lower than those detected after atracurium administration [7,8].

Rocuronium

Rocuronium is the fastest onset, shortest acting aminosteroidal NMBA. A bolus dose of 0.6 mg per kg usually results in neuromuscular paralysis within 60 to 90 seconds. It may be considered an alternative to succinylcholine for rapid-sequence intubation (0.8 to 1.2 mg per kg), although, even with large doses, the onset of action is slower as compared to succinylcholine [9]. Rocuronium is primarily eliminated in the liver and

TABLE 25.1

PHARMACOKINETIC AND PHARMACODYNAMIC PRINCIPLES OF NONDEPOLARIZING NEUROMUSCULAR BLOCKERS[a]

	Benzylisoquinolinium agents		
	Cisatracurium (Nimbex)	**Atracurium (Tracrium)**	**Doxacurium (Nuromax)**
Introduced	1996	1983	1991
95% Effective dose (mg/kg)	0.05	0.25	0.025–0.030
Initial dose (mg/kg)	0.1–0.2	0.4–0.5	Up to 0.1
Onset (min)	2–3	3–5	5–10
Duration (min)	45–60	25–35	120–150
Half-life (min)	22–31	20	70–100
Infusion dose (μg/kg/min)	2.5–3.0	4–12	0.3–0.5
Recovery (min)	90	40–60	120–180
% Renal excretion	Hofmann elimination	5–10 (Hofmann elimination)	70
Renal failure	No change	No change	↑Effect
% Biliary excretion	Hofmann elimination	Minimal	Unclear
Hepatic failure	Minimal to no change	Minimal to no change	?
Active metabolites	None, but laudanosine	None, but laudanosine	?
Histamine hypotension	No	Dose-dependent	No
Vagal block tachycardia	No	No	No
Ganglionic block hypotension	No	Minimal to none	No
Prolonged block reported	Rare	Rare	Yes

	Aminosteroidal agents			
	Pancuronium (Pavulon)	**Vecuronium (Norcuron)**	**Pipecuronium (Arduan)**	**Rocuronium (Zemuron)**
Introduced	1972	1984	1991	1994
95% Effective dose (mg/kg)	0.07	0.05	0.05	0.30
Initial dose (mg/kg)	0.1	0.1	0.085–0.100	0.6–1.0
Onset (min)	2–3	3–4	5	1–2
Duration (min)	90–100	35–45	90–100	30
Half-life (min)	120	30–80	100	—
Infusion dose (μg/kg/min)	1–2	1–2	0.5–2.0	10–12
Recovery (min)	120–180	45–60	55–160	20–30
% Renal excretion	45–70	50	50+	33
Renal failure	↑ Effect	↑ Effect	↑ Duration	Minimal
% Biliary excretion	10–15	35–50	Minimal	<75
Hepatic failure	Mild ↑ effect	Mild ↑ effect	Minimal	Moderate
Active metabolites	3-OH and 17-OH pancuronium	3-desacetyl vecuronium	None	None
Histamine hypotension	No	No	No	No
Vagal block tachycardia	Modest to marked	No	No	At high doses
Ganglionic block hypotension	No	No	No	No
Prolonged ICU block	Yes	Yes	No	No

↑, increased; ICU, intensive care unit.
[a]Modified from Grenvik A, Ayres SM, Holbrook PR, et al: *Textbook of Critical Care*. 4th ed. Philadelphia, WB Saunders, 2000; Watling SM, Dasta JF: Prolonged paralysis in intensive care unit patients after the use of neuromuscular blocking agents: a review of the literature. *Crit Care Med* 22(5):884, 1994.

bile. Hepatic or renal dysfunction may reduce drug clearance and prolong recovery time.

Vecuronium

An initial intravenous bolus dose of 0.1 mg per kg of vecuronium typically results in neuromuscular paralysis within 3 to 4 minutes and lasts for 35 to 45 minutes. Vecuronium lacks vagolytic effects, such as tachycardia and hypertension, and produces negligible histamine release. Hepatic metabolism produces three active metabolites, the most significant being 3-desacetyl vecuronium, with 50% to 70% activity of the parent drug. Both vecuronium and its active metabolites are renally excreted. There is potential for prolonged neuromuscular paralysis in patients with renal dysfunction receiving vecuronium by continuous infusion [10].

Pancuronium

Pancuronium is a long-acting nondepolarizing agent that is structurally similar to vecuronium. Unique features of pancuronium are its vagolytic and sympathomimetic activities and potential to induce tachycardia, hypertension, and increased cardiac output. Pancuronium is primarily excreted unchanged (60% to 70%) in the urine and bile, whereas the remaining 30% to 40% is hydroxylated by the liver to 3-hydroxy pancuronium. It has 50% activity of the parent drug and is renally eliminated. Renal dysfunction may result in the accumulation of pancuronium and its metabolites [11].

Doxacurium

Doxacurium is the most potent nondepolarizing agent available, but it has the slowest onset (as long as 10 minutes). It is practically devoid of histaminergic, vagolytic, or sympathomimetic effects. Doxacurium undergoes minimal hepatic metabolism, and excretion occurs unchanged in both the urine and the bile, with significantly prolonged effects seen in patients with renal dysfunction and, to a lesser extent, hepatic disease [12,13].

Pipecuronium

Pipecuronium is structurally related to pancuronium and its duration of action is 90 to 100 minutes, making it the longest acting NMBA. It is metabolized to 3-desacetyl pipecuronium by the liver, and both the parent compound and the metabolite are renally excreted. When compared with pancuronium, pipecuronium has a longer duration of action, less histamine release, and minimal cardiovascular effects [14].

REVERSAL AGENTS

The clinical effects of nondepolarizing neuromuscular blockers can be reversed by acetylcholinesterase inhibitors (anticholinesterases). These agents increase the synaptic concentration of ACh by preventing its synaptic degradation and allow it to competitively displace nondepolarizing NMBAs from postsynaptic nAChRs on the motor end plate. Because anticholinesterase drugs (e.g., neostigmine, edrophonium, and pyridostigmine) also inhibit acetylcholinesterase at muscarinic receptor sites, they are used in combination with the antimuscarinic agents (e.g., atropine or glycopyrrolate) to minimize adverse muscarinic effects (e.g., bradycardia, excessive secretions, and bronchospasm) while maximizing nicotinic effects. Typical combinations include neostigmine and glycopyrrolate (slower acting agents) and edrophonium and atropine (faster acting agents). The depth of neuromuscular blockade determines how rapidly neuromuscular activity returns [15,16].

Sugammadex is a new and novel agent (modified γ-cyclodextrin) that reverses rocuronium and other aminosteroid NMBAs by selectively binding and encapsulating the NMBA [16]. One of the advantages of sugammadex is the rapid reversal of the profound neuromuscular block, induced by the high dose of rocuronium needed for the rapid-sequence induction [17,18]—an effect that is equivalent to, if not better than, the spontaneous recovery from succinylcholine. Hence, rocuronium/sugammadex may prove to be an effective and safer alternative to succinylcholine in cases of the difficult airway and contraindications to the use of succinylcholine. Sugammadex is also useful as a reversal agent whenever the blockade is profound and there is an advantage for a timely reversal [18]. It is approved for use in Europe, but not in the United States. The nonapproval of the Food and Drug Administration (FDA) was based on concerns related to hypersensitivity and allergic reactions. However, a recently published *Cochrane* systemic review concluded that sugammadex was not only effective but also equally safe when compared with placebo and neostigmine [19].

DRUG INTERACTIONS

A substantial number of medications commonly used in clinical practice have the potential for interaction with NMBAs. These interactions typically influence the degree and duration of clinical effects through either potentiation of or resistance to neuromuscular blockade. The most clinically relevant drug interactions with NMBA are discussed here and summarized in Table 25.2.

Aminoglycosides and other antibiotics (e.g., tetracyclines, clindamycin, and vancomycin) have the ability to potentiate neuromuscular blockade and prolong the action of nondepolarizing agents through mechanisms including the inhibition of presynaptic ACh release, reduction of postsynaptic receptor sensitivity to ACh, blockade of cholinergic receptors, and impairment of ion channels. Penicillin and cephalosporin antibiotics do not interact with NMBAs and thus do not influence the degree of neuromuscular blockade.

Local, inhalational, and intravenous anesthetic and sedative agents may potentiate neuromuscular blockade. Local anesthetics reduce ACh release and decrease muscle contractions through direct membrane effects, whereas inhalational anesthetics desensitize the postsynaptic membrane and also depress muscle contractility.

Cardiovascular drugs such as furosemide, procainamide, quinidine, beta-blockers, and calcium channel blockers have the ability to potentiate neuromuscular blocking effects. The role of the calcium ion in the release of ACh from vesicles into the synapse has been well established, although the exact interaction between calcium channel blockers and NMBAs remains to be determined. Verapamil, a calcium channel blocker, has local analgesic effects and direct skeletal muscle effects, but its significance in drug interaction with NMBAs remains to be defined.

Chronic antiepileptic therapy, specifically phenytoin and carbamazepine, can increase the resistance to neuromuscular blocking effects, whereas the acute administration of phenytoin potentiates neuromuscular blockade. Chronic phenytoin therapy appears to induce an upregulation of ACh receptors, resulting in decreased postsynaptic sensitivity. Carbamazepine has been shown to induce resistance and shorten recovery times in combination with both pancuronium and vecuronium, possibly resulting from competition at the NMJ [4,20].

MONITORING OF NMBAS

Current guidelines recommend the routine monitoring of depth of neuromuscular blockade in critically ill patients [1]. It is important to remember that NMBAs have no analgesic and sedative effect. Careful clinical monitoring of the patient for signs consistent with inadequate sedation or analgesia—such as tachycardia, hypertension, salivation, and lacrimation—while receiving NMBAs is important. A recommendation to use monitors such as the Bispectral Index or the Patient State Index to ensure adequate depth of sedation while receiving NMBAs seems plausible; however, more studies are needed to determine whether these monitors are reliable and cost-effective in the critical care setting and whether they contribute to improved outcomes [21–23]. The modality of choice to monitor the depth of nondepolarizing neuromuscular blockade at present is train-of-four (TOF) monitoring. To determine the depth of blockade, four supramaximal stimuli are applied to a peripheral nerve (ideally, the ulnar nerve to assess an evoked response of the adductor pollicis muscle) every 0.5 seconds (2 Hz). Each

TABLE 25.2

DRUG INTERACTIONS WITH NEUROMUSCULAR BLOCKING AGENTS[a]

Therapeutic agent	Potential interaction
Antibiotics	
Aminoglycosides	Potentiate blockade; decreased acetylcholine release
Tetracyclines	Potentiate blockade
Clindamycin and lincomycin	Potentiate blockade
Vancomycin	Potentiate blockade
Sedative/anesthetics	Potentiate blockade
Cardiovascular agents	
Furosemide	Low doses: potentiate blockade; high doses: antagonize blockade
Beta-blockers	Potentiate blockade
Procainamide	Potentiate blockade
Quinidine	Potentiate blockade
Calcium channel blockers	Potentiate blockade
Methylxanthines	Antagonize blockade
Antiepileptic drugs	Acute: potentiate blockade; chronic: resistance to blockade
Phenytoin	
Carbamazepine	Resistance to blockade
Ranitidine	Antagonize blockade
Lithium	Potentiate blockade
Immunosuppressive agents	
Azathioprine	Mild antagonism; phosphodiesterase inhibition
Cyclosporin	Potentiate blockade
Corticosteroids	Potentiate steroid myopathy
Local anesthetics	Potentiate blockade

[a]Adapted from Buck ML, Reed MD: Use of nondepolarizing neuromuscular blocking agents in mechanically ventilated patients. *Clin Pharm* 10(1):32, 1991.

stimulus in the train causes the muscle to contract, and "fade" in the response provides the basis for evaluation. To obtain the TOF ratio, the amplitude of the fourth response is divided by the amplitude of the first response. Before administration of a nondepolarizing muscle relaxant, all four responses are ideally the same: the TOF ratio is 1 to 1. During a partial nondepolarizing block, the ratio decreases (fades) and is inversely proportional to the degree of blockade [24].

Three prospective clinical trials have examined the question whether the routine use of TOF monitoring in the ICU will increase the cost-effectiveness and decrease the incidence of prolonged neuromuscular weakness. TOF monitoring for vecuronium appears to improve the outcome and decrease the cost of therapy. However, these outcomes could not be demonstrated for the benzylisoquinolinium agents, atracurium, and cisatracurium [25–27].

ADVERSE EFFECTS OF DEPOLARIZING AND NONDEPOLARIZING NMBAS IN CRITICALLY ILL PATIENTS

Significant progress has been made in the recent past in our understanding of the changes in regulation and distribution of ACh receptors during a course of critical illness. The majority of patients hospitalized in an ICU will undergo postsynaptic upregulation of nAChRs due to immobility, upper and/or lower motor neuron lesions, and/or pharmacologic denervation (such as NMBAs and aminoglycoside antibiotics). As previously outlined, immature receptors are not confined to the NMJ proper, but can be found over the entire surface of skeletal muscle (Fig. 25.1). This will lead to increased sensitivity to depolarizing NMBAs and decreased sensitivity to nondepolarizing NMBAs. Furthermore, these changes in receptor distribution and physiology put the patient at a heightened risk for succinylcholine-induced hyperkalemia. This is based on the fact that immature (fetal) and α7nAChRs are low conductance channels with prolonged opening times and significantly higher potassium efflux into the systemic circulation as compared to mature (adult) nAChRs. Furthermore, succinylcholine is metabolized more slowly as compared to ACh, thus prolonging the "open" state of the immature receptors. Upregulation of receptors during periods of immobilization has been described as early as 6 to 12 hours into the disease process. Therefore, it seems advisable to avoid succinylcholine in critically ill patients beyond 48 to 72 hours of immobilization and/or denervation. In contrast, a reduction in the number of postsynaptic nAChRs will result in resistance to depolarizing and increased sensitivity to nondepolarizing NMBAs. For conditions associated with the potential for ACh receptor upregulation, see Table 25.3.

INTENSIVE CARE UNIT–ACQUIRED WEAKNESS

ICU-acquired weakness (ICUAW) is a relatively new term used to describe all weaknesses developed in critically ill patients after the onset of illness and in the absence of any identifiable causes. ICUAW is further classified into three entities:

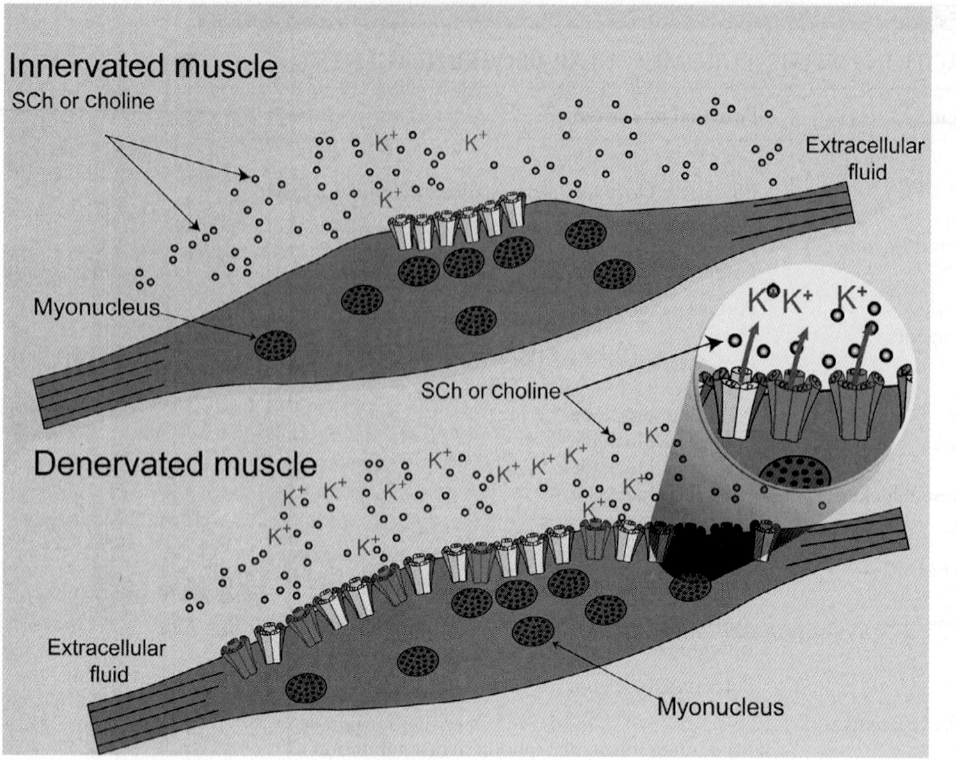

FIGURE 25.1. Schematic of the succinylcholine (SCh)-induced potassium release in an innervated (*top*) and denervated (*bottom*) muscle. In the innervated muscle, the systemically administered SCh reaches all of the muscle membrane, but depolarizes only the junctional ($\alpha 1$, $\beta 1$, δ, ε) receptors because acetylcholine receptors (AChRs) are located only in this area. With denervation, the muscle (nuclei) expresses not only extrajunctional ($\alpha 1$, $\beta 1$, δ, γ) AChRs, but also α7AChRs throughout the muscle membrane. Systemic succinylcholine, in contrast to acetylcholine released locally, can depolarize all of the upregulated AChRs, leading to massive efflux of intracellular potassium into the circulation, resulting in hyperkalemia. The metabolite of SCh, choline, and possibly succinylmonocholine can maintain this depolarization via α7AChRs, enhancing the potassium release and maintaining the hyperkalemia. [From Martyn JA, Richtsfeld M. Succinylcholine-induced hyperkalemia in acquired pathologic states: etiologic factors and molecular mechanisms. *Anesthesiology* 104:158, 2006, with permission.]

critical illness polyneuropathy (CIP), critical illness myopathy (CIM), and critical illness neuromyopathy (CINM) [28,29] (See Chapter 180). These conditions occur in up to 50% to 70% of patients meeting diagnostic criteria for the systemic inflammatory response syndrome as well as in patients immobilized and on mechanical ventilation for more than a week [30]. They manifest as limb weakness and difficulty in weaning from the mechanical ventilator. Nondepolarizing muscle relaxants of both classes, aminosteroids and benzylisoquinoliniums, have been associated with the development of these neuromuscular disorders [31]; however, the etiology appears to be multifactorial and includes alterations in microvascular blood flow in conditions of sepsis/systemic inflammatory response syndrome and the concomitant administration of corticosteroids [30]. There is evidence suggesting that high-dose corticosteroids have direct physiologic effects on muscle fibers, resulting in a typical myopathy with loss of thick-filament proteins. Atrophy and weakness are observed primarily in muscles of trunk and extremities, and functional denervation of muscle with NMBAs in conjunction with corticosteroid therapy seems to heighten the risk of myopathy [31]. Furthermore, both methylprednisolone and hydrocortisone antagonize nAChRs, possibly potentiating the effects of NMBAs [32]. A differential diagnosis of weakness in ICU patients is presented in Table 25.4.

TABLE 25.3

CONDITIONS ASSOCIATED WITH THE POTENTIAL FOR NICOTINIC ACETYLCHOLINE RECEPTOR UPREGULATION

Severe infection/SIRS
Muscle atrophy associated with prolonged immobility
Thermal injury
Upper and/or lower motor neuron defect
Prolonged pharmacologic or chemical denervation (e.g., NMBAs, magnesium, aminoglycoside antibiotics, and clostridial toxins)

NMBAs, neuromuscular blocking agents; SIRS, systemic inflammatory response syndrome.

Critical Illness Polyneuropathy

Electrophysiologic findings of CIP are consistent with a primary, axonal degeneration, resulting in reduction in amplitudes of the compound muscle action potential and sensory

TABLE 25.4

WEAKNESS IN INTENSIVE CARE UNIT PATIENTS: ETIOLOGIES AND SYNDROMES[a]

Prolonged recovery from neuromuscular blocking agents (secondary to parent drug, drug metabolite, or drug–drug interaction)
Myasthenia gravis
Eaton–Lambert syndrome
Muscular dystrophy
Guillain–Barré syndrome
Central nervous system injury or lesion
Spinal cord injury
Steroid myopathy
Mitochondrial myopathy
Human immunodeficiency virus–related myopathy
Critical illness myopathy
Disuse atrophy
Critical illness polyneuropathy
Severe electrolyte toxicity (e.g., hypermagnesemia)
Severe electrolyte deficiency (e.g., hypophosphatemia)

[a]Adapted from Murray MJ, Cowen J, DeBlock H, et al: Clinical practice guidelines for sustained neuromuscular blockade in the adult critically ill patient. *Crit Care Med* 30(1):142, 2002, with permission.

TABLE 25.5

RECOMMENDATIONS FOR ADMINISTRATION OF NEUROMUSCULAR BLOCKING AGENTS (NMBAS) TO ICU PATIENTS[a]

1. Develop, use, and document a standardized approach for administering and monitoring NMBA
2. Use NMBA only after optimizing ventilator settings and sedative and analgesic medication administration
3. Establish the indications and clinical goals of neuromuscular blockade, and evaluate at least daily
4. Select the best NMBA on the basis of patient characteristics:
   A. Use intermittent NMBA therapy with pancuronium, doxacurium, or other suitable agent if clinical goals can be met
   B. If continuous infusion is required and renal or hepatic dysfunction is present, select atracurium or cisatracurium, and avoid vecuronium
5. Use the lowest effective dose for the shortest possible time (<48 h if possible), particularly if corticosteroids are concomitantly administered
6. Administer adequate analgesic and/or sedative medication during neuromuscular blockade, and monitor clinically and by bispectral array EEG if available
7. Systematically anticipate and prevent complications, including provision of eye care, careful positioning, physical therapy, and DVT prophylaxis
8. Avoid the use of medications that affect NMBA actions. Promptly recognize and manage conditions that affect NMBA actions
9. Adjust NMBA dosage to achieve clinical goals (i.e., patient–ventilator synchrony, apnea, or complete paralysis)
10. Periodically (i.e., at least once or twice daily) perform NMBA dosage reduction, and preferably cessation (drug holiday) if clinically tolerated, to determine whether neuromuscular blockade is still needed and to perform physical and neurologic examination
11. Periodically perform and document a clinical assessment in which spontaneous respiration, as well as limb movement, and/or the presence of DTRs are observed during steady-state infusion and/or during dosage reduction/cessation. With deep blockade, muscle activity may be present only during dosage reduction/cessation
12. Perform and document scheduled (i.e., every 4–8 h) TOF testing for patients receiving vecuronium NMBA and/or undergoing deep neuromuscular blockade (i.e., apnea or complete paralysis), and adjust dosage to achieve one-fourth or more twitches. If clinical goals cannot be met when one-fourth or more twitches are present during steady-state infusion, demonstrate one-fourth or more twitches during dosage reduction/cessation. Consider TOF testing in all patients

DTR, deep tendon reflexes; DVT, deep venous thrombosis; EEG, electroencephalogram; TOF, train of four.
[a]Modified from Gehr LC, Sessler CN: Neuromuscular blockade in the intensive care unit. *Semin Respir Crit Care Med* 22:175, 2001, with permission.

nerve action potential. Although several case reports have suggested that NMBAs are causative agents in the etiology of this disorder, prospective studies of CIP have not confirmed a correlation between the use of NMBAs, steroids, and CIP [33]. It seems plausible, however, that NMBAs contribute to nerve and muscle damage during a course of critical illness. Their use should be avoided whenever possible until more prospective data demonstrating their safety in critically ill patients are available [34] (See Chapter 180).

Critical Illness Myopathy

CIM can occur in association with, or independently from, CIP. A group of several myopathies of critical illness are now thought to be part of the same syndrome; these include acute quadriplegic myopathy, critical care myopathy, acute corticosteroid myopathy, acute hydrocortisone myopathy, acute myopathy in severe asthma, and acute corticosteroid and pancuronium-associated myopathy [35]. The major feature of this syndrome is flaccid, diffuse weakness, involving all limb muscles and neck flexors, and often the facial muscles and diaphragm. As with CIP, this can result in difficulty to wean from the mechanical ventilator. The syndrome is more difficult to diagnose than CIP, and diagnostic evaluations include electrophysiologic studies, muscle biopsy, and laboratory evaluations (plasma creatine kinase levels). Again, there is no definitive evidence suggesting that NMBAs are causative agents for this syndrome, but rather a component in a multifactorial etiology. However, the incidence of CIP and CIM appears to be higher in ICUs where these agents are more frequently used [36].

The question whether CIP and CIM increase hospital mortality was recently addressed by Latronico et al. [37]. Although only limited data are available suggesting that CIP increases ICU and hospital mortality in critically ill patients, CIP and CIM appear to be important causes of increased morbidity during and after acute care hospital stay [37] (See Chapter 180).

SUMMARY AND RECOMMENDATIONS

Although there is currently insufficient evidence to demonstrate an unequivocal link between the use of NMBAs and an increase in morbidity and mortality in critically ill patients, it seems prudent to perform a careful risk–benefit analysis prior to the administration of this class of drugs in the ICU setting. Indeed, a recent prospective, randomized study of patients in the early stage of the acute respiratory distress syndrome demonstrated that use of cisatracurium was associated with improved survival without an increase in ICUAW [38]. Nonetheless, more prospective data are needed to identify proper indications, selection of agents, and doses in the ICU setting. Concomitant use of drugs predisposing patients for the development of CIM-like steroids and aminoglycoside antibiotics should alert the clinician for the increased risk of CIP/CIM in this setting. Succinylcholine can subject patients who are immobilized with upper and lower motor neuron lesions or with burns to a markedly increased risk for succinylcholine-induced hyperkalemia, and should be avoided in the ICU whenever possible. For recommendations for the administration of NMBAs to ICU patients, please see Table 25.5.

ACKNOWLEDGMENTS

We thank Dr. Jerry D. Thomas and Dr. Greg A. Bauer for the significant contributions to previous revisions of this chapter.

References

1. Murray MJ, Cowen J, DeBlock H, et al: Clinical practice guidelines for sustained neuromuscular blockade in the adult critically ill patient. *Crit Care Med* 30(1):142–156, 2002.
2. Arroliga A, Frutos-Vivar F, Hall J, et al: Use of sedatives and neuromuscular blockers in a cohort of patients receiving mechanical ventilation. *Chest* 128(2):496–506, 2005.
3. Naguib M, Flood P, McArdle JJ, et al: Advances in neurobiology of the neuromuscular junction: implications for the anesthesiologist. *Anesthesiology* 96:202, 2002.
4. Taylor P: *Agents Acting at the Neuromuscular Junction and Autonomic Ganglia.* 10th ed. New York, McGraw-Hill, 2001.
5. Pantuck EJ: Plasma cholinesterase: gene and variations. *Anesth Analg* 77(2):380–386, 1993.
6. Wadbrook PS: Advances in airway pharmacology. Emerging trends and evolving controversy. *Emerg Med Clin North Am* 18(4):767–788, 2000.
7. Eastwood NB, Boyd AH, Parker CJ, et al: Pharmacokinetics of 1R-cis 1'R-*cis* atracurium besylate (51W89) and plasma laudanosine concentrations in health and chronic renal failure. *Br J Anaesth* 75(4):431–435, 1995.
8. Newman PJ, Quinn AC, Grounds RM, et al: A comparison of cisatracurium (51W89) and atracurium by infusion in critically ill patients. *Crit Care Med* 25(7):1139–1142, 1997.
9. Wright PM, Caldwell JE, Miller RD: Onset and duration of rocuronium and succinylcholine at the adductor pollicis and laryngeal adductor muscles in anesthetized humans. *Anesthesiology* 81(5):1110–1115, 1994.
10. Conway EE, Jr: Persistent paralysis after vecuronium administration. *N Engl J Med* 327(26):1882, 1992.
11. Reeves ST, Turcasso NM: Nondepolarizing neuromuscular blocking drugs in the intensive care unit: a clinical review. *South Med J* 90(8):769–774, 1997.
12. Basta SJ, Savarese JJ, Ali HH, et al: Clinical pharmacology of doxacurium chloride. A new long-acting nondepolarizing muscle relaxant. *Anesthesiology* 69(4):478–486, 1988.
13. Fisher DM, Reynolds KS, Schmith VD, et al: The influence of renal function on the pharmacokinetics and pharmacodynamics and simulated time course of doxacurium. *Anesth Analg* 89(3):786–795, 1999.
14. Atherton DP, Hunter JM: Clinical pharmacokinetics of the newer neuromuscular blocking drugs. *Clin Pharmacokinet* 36(3):169–189, 1999.
15. McManus MC: Neuromuscular blockers in surgery and intensive care, Part 2. *Am J Health Syst Pharm* 58(24):2381–2395, 2001.
16. Naguib M: Sugammadex: another milestone in clinical neuromuscular pharmacology. *Anesth Analg* 104(3):575–581, 2007.
17. Lee C, Jahr JS, Candiotti KA, et al: Reversal of profound neuromuscular block by sugammadex administered three minutes after rocuronium: a comparison with spontaneous recovery from succinylcholine. *Anesthesiology* 110(5):1020–1025, 2009.
18. Rex C, Wagner S, Spies C, et al: Reversal of neuromuscular blockade by sugammadex after continuous infusion of rocuronium in patients randomized to sevoflurane or propofol maintenance anesthesia. *Anesthesiology* 111(1):30–35, 2009.
19. Abrishami A, Ho J, Wong J, et al: Sugammadex, a selective reversal medication for preventing postoperative residual neuromuscular blockade. *Cochrane Database Syst Rev* (4):CD007362, 2009.
20. Booij LH: Neuromuscular transmission and its pharmacological blockade. Part 2: Pharmacology of neuromuscular blocking agents. *Pharm World Sci* 19(1):13–34, 1997.
21. Nasraway SS Jr, Wu EC, Kelleher RM, et al: How reliable is the Bispectral Index in critically ill patients? A prospective, comparative, single-blinded observer study. *Crit Care Med* 30(7):1483–1487, 2002.
22. Schneider G, Heglmeier S, Schneider J, et al: Patient State Index (PSI) measures depth of sedation in intensive care patients. *Intensive Care Med* 30(2):213–216, 2004.
23. Vivien B, Di Maria S, Ouattara A, et al: Overestimation of Bispectral Index in sedated intensive care unit patients revealed by administration of muscle relaxant. *Anesthesiology* 99(1):9–17, 2003.
24. Naguib M, Lien CA: Pharmacology of muscle relaxants and their antagonists, in Miller RD (ed): *Miller's Anesthesia.* 6th ed. New York, Churchill Livingstone, 2005.
25. Baumann MH, McAlpin BW, Brown K, et al: A prospective randomized comparison of train-of-four monitoring and clinical assessment during continuous ICU cisatracurium paralysis. *Chest* 126(4):1267–1273, 2004.
26. Rudis MI, Sikora CA, Angus E, et al: A prospective, randomized, controlled evaluation of peripheral nerve stimulation versus standard clinical dosing of neuromuscular blocking agents in critically ill patients. *Crit Care Med* 25(4):575–583, 1997.
27. Strange C, Vaughan L, Franklin C, et al: Comparison of train-of-four and best clinical assessment during continuous paralysis. *Am J Respir Crit Care Med* 156(5):1556–1561, 1997.
28. Stevens RD, Marshall SA, Cornblath DR, et al: A framework for diagnosing and classifying intensive care unit–acquired weakness. *Crit Care Med* 37[10 Suppl]:S299–S308, 2009.
29. Vincent JL, Norrenberg M: Intensive care unit–acquired weakness: framing the topic. *Crit Care Med* 37[10 Suppl]:S296–S298, 2009.
30. Bolton CF: Neuromuscular manifestations of critical illness. *Muscle Nerve* 32(2):140–163, 2005.
31. Larsson L, Li X, Edstrom L, et al: Acute quadriplegia and loss of muscle myosin in patients treated with nondepolarizing neuromuscular blocking agents and corticosteroids: mechanisms at the cellular and molecular levels. *Crit Care Med* 28(1):34–45, 2000.
32. Kindler CH, Verotta D, Gray AT, et al: Additive inhibition of nicotinic acetylcholine receptors by corticosteroids and the neuromuscular blocking drug vecuronium. *Anesthesiology* 92(3):821–832, 2000.
33. Berek K, Margreiter J, Willeit J, et al: Polyneuropathies in critically ill patients: a prospective evaluation. *Intensive Care Med* 22(9):849–855, 1996.
34. Latronico N, Fenzi F, Recupero D, et al: Critical illness myopathy and neuropathy. *Lancet* 347(9015):1579–1582, 1996.
35. Lacomis D, Zochodne DW, Bird SJ: Critical illness myopathy. *Muscle Nerve* 23(12):1785–1788, 2000.
36. Lacomis D, Petrella JT, Giuliani MJ: Causes of neuromuscular weakness in the intensive care unit: a study of ninety-two patients. *Muscle Nerve* 21(5):610–617, 1998.
37. Latronico N, Shehu I, Seghelini E: Neuromuscular sequelae of critical illness. *Curr Opin Crit Care* 11(4):381–390, 2005.
38. Papazian L, Forel J-M, Gacouin A, et al: Neuromuscular blockers in early acute respiratory distress syndrome. *N Engl J Med* 363(12):1107–1116, 2010.

SECTION II ■ MINIMALLY INVASIVE MONITORING

ALAN LISBON

CHAPTER 26 ■ ROUTINE MONITORING OF CRITICALLY ILL PATIENTS

PATRICK TROY, NICHOLAS A. SMYRNIOS AND MICHAEL D. HOWELL

A key difference between intensive care units (ICUs) and other hospital units is the level of detail with which patients are routinely monitored. This careful monitoring alerts the health care team to changes in the patient's severity of illness—helping to both diagnose disease and assess prognosis. Careful monitoring also helps the health care team safely apply therapies such as volume resuscitation, vasoactive infusions, and mechanical ventilation.

This chapter deals with the routine, predominantly noninvasive monitoring that is often done for many patients in ICUs. It examines the indications for, the technology of, and problems encountered in the routine monitoring of temperature, blood pressure, ECG rhythm, ST segments, respiratory rate, and oxygen and carbon dioxide levels. In addition, it reviews noninvasive monitoring of tissue perfusion, with particular attention to gastric tonometry, sublingual capnometry, and transcutaneous oxygen and carbon dioxide monitoring.

MONITORING SYSTEMS

When ICUs came into being in the late 1950s, nurses monitored patients' vital signs intermittently. Continuous measurement was either unavailable or necessitated invasive procedures. Now, however, nearly all routine vital signs can now be monitored accurately, noninvasively, and continuously. As a result, patients now are monitored more intensively and continuously in the ICU than in any other part of the hospital, with the possible exception of the operating room.

Over the past decades, the trend in monitoring systems has been toward multipurpose systems that integrate monitoring of a variety of parameters. Multipurpose systems eliminate the need for multiple, freestanding devices—reducing clutter and improving workflow ergonomics at the bedside. These systems also interface critical care information systems to provide more efficient data management, quality improvement reports, and in some cases prospective data-driven alerts.

TEMPERATURE MONITORING

Temperature changes in the critically ill are associated with significant morbidity and mortality [1] (see Chapters 65 and 66)—making it clinically important to recognize an abnormal temperature. In one surgical ICU study, rectal temperatures on admission were normal in only 30% of patients, were above 37.6°C in 38%, and were below 36.8°C in 32% [2]. An abnormal temperature is frequently the earliest clinical sign of infection, inflammation, central nervous system dysfunction, or drug toxicity. Unfortunately, the type of thermometer and the site where the temperature is taken can affect the accuracy of this vital measurement. Clinicians should understand the impact of the thermometer type and the measurement site on how to interpret the patient's reported temperature.

Indications for Temperature Monitoring

The Society of Critical Care Medicine's Task Force on Guidelines' recommendations for care in a critical care setting grades temperature monitoring as an essential service for all critical care units [3]. Critically ill patients are at high risk for temperature disorders because of debility, impaired control of temperature, frequent use of sedative drugs, and a high predisposition to infection. All critically ill patients should have core temperature measured at least intermittently. Patients with marked temperature abnormalities should be considered for continuous monitoring; patients undergoing active interventions to alter temperature, such as breathing heated air or using a cooling–warming blanket, should have continuous monitoring to prevent overtreatment or undertreatment of temperature disorders.

Measurement Sites

The goal of temperature measurements is generally to estimate *core temperature*—the deep body temperature that is carefully regulated by the hypothalamus so as to be independent of transient small changes in ambient temperature. Core temperature exists more as a physiologic concept than as the temperature of an anatomic location. An ideal measurement site would be protected from heat loss, painless and convenient to use, and would not interfere with the patient's ability to move and communicate. No one location provides an accurate measurement of core temperature in all clinical circumstances.

Sublingual Temperature Measurements

Sublingual temperature measurements are convenient, but suffer numerous limitations. Although open-mouth versus closed-mouth breathing and use of nasogastric tubes do not alter temperature measurement [4], oral temperature is obviously altered if measured immediately after the patient has consumed hot or cold drinks. Falsely low oral temperatures may occur because of cooling from tachypnea. Sixty percent of sublingual temperatures are more than 1°F lower than simultaneously measured rectal temperatures; 53% differ by 1° to 2°F, and 6% differ by more than 2°F. Continuous sublingual measurement is not generally practical. Sublingual measurement is best suited for intermittent monitoring when some inaccuracy can be tolerated.

Axillary Temperature Measurements

Axillary temperatures are commonly used as an index of core temperature. Although some studies indicate close approximation of the axillary site with pulmonary artery temperatures [5], temperatures average 1.5° to 1.9°C lower than tympanic temperatures [6]. Positioning the sensor over the axillary artery may improve accuracy. The accuracy and precision of axillary temperature measurements are less than at other sites [6], perhaps due in part to the difficulty of maintaining a good probe position.

Rectal Temperature Measurements

Rectal temperature is the most widely accepted standard of measuring core temperature in clinical use. Before a rectal thermometer is inserted, a digital rectal examination should be performed because feces can blunt temperature measurement. Readings are more accurate when the sensor is passed more than 10 cm (4 in) into the rectum. Rectal temperature correlates well in most patients with distal esophageal, bladder, and tympanic temperatures [7]. Rectal temperatures typically respond to induced changes in temperature more slowly than other central measurement sites [8]. Reusable, electronic, sheath-covered rectal thermometers have been associated with the transmission of *Clostridium difficile* and vancomycin-resistant *Enterococcus,* so disposable probes are generally preferred.

Esophageal Temperature Measurements

Esophageal temperature is usually measured with an electric, flexible temperature sensor. On average, esophageal temperatures are 0.6°C lower than rectal temperatures [9]. However, the measured temperature can vary greatly depending on the position of the sensor in the esophagus. In the proximal esophagus, temperature is influenced by ambient air [10]. During hypothermia, temperatures in different portions of the esophagus may differ by up to 6°C [10]. Because of the proximity of the distal esophagus to the great vessels and heart, the distal esophageal temperature responds rapidly to changes in core temperature [11]. Changes in esophageal temperature may inaccurately reflect changes in core temperature when induced temperature change occurs because of the inspiration of heated air, gastric lavage, or cardiac bypass or assist [11].

Tympanic Temperature Measurements

Health care providers can measure tympanic temperature with specifically designed thermometers that are commonly used in the ICU. However, several studies have demonstrated poor correlation with ICU patients' core temperatures [12,13]. Accuracy depends in part on operator experience—but even when trained, experienced ICU nurses use tympanic thermometers, the variability in repeated measurements was more than 0.5°F in 20% of patients [14]. Unlike temporal artery measurements, which are not known to have complications, tympanic temperature measurements come with some risk. Perforation of the tympanic membrane and bleeding from the external canal due to trauma from the probe have been reported.

Temporal Artery Measurements

Temporal artery measurements are not known to have complications. Their accuracy is reviewed later.

Urinary Bladder Temperature Measurements

Providers can easily measure the urinary bladder temperature with a specially designed temperature probe embedded in a Foley catheter [6–8]. In patients undergoing induced hypothermia and rewarming, bladder temperatures correlate well with great vessel and rectal temperatures [7,8]. Bladder temperature under steady-state conditions is more reproducible than that taken at most other sites [7].

Central Circulation Temperature Measurements

ICU practitioners can measure the temperature of blood in the pulmonary artery using a thermistor-equipped pulmonary artery catheter. The temperature sensor is located at the distal tip and can record accurate great vessel temperatures once the catheter is in place in the pulmonary artery. Pulmonary artery temperatures have generally been accepted as the gold standard for accurate measures of core temperature, although readings might be expected to differ from core temperature when heated air was breathed or warm or cold intravenous fluids were infused. However, this understanding may not be true in neurosurgical patients. A study in patients undergoing neurosurgical procedures with induced hypothermic circulatory arrest found that pulmonary arterial temperature measurement was not effective in assessing core brain temperature with a correlation coefficient of 0.63. A greater degree of correlation was found in bladder temperature [15]. Inserting a central venous thermistor specifically to monitor temperature is probably warranted only when other sites are felt to be unreliable and accurate, rapid, continuous temperature measurements are critical to the patient's management.

Types of Thermometers

Mercury Thermometers

Although mercury thermometers were historically been the most common type in clinical use, environmental and health concerns related to mercury have resulted in several state and local legislative efforts to phase out this type of thermometer. Mercury and other liquid–expansion-based thermometers can give a falsely low measurement when the thermometer is left in place for too short a period; falsely high temperatures result from failure to shake the mercury down.

Liquid Crystal Display Thermometers

Liquid crystal display (LCD) thermometers contain liquid crystals embedded in thin adhesive strips that are directly attached to the patient's skin. LCD thermometers are most commonly applied to the forehead for ease of use and steady perfusion, but can be applied to any area of the skin. Like all skin temperature measurements, they may poorly reflect core temperature when the skin is hypoperfused or patients have vasomotor instability. Forehead skin temperature is typically lower than core temperatures by 2.2°C [16], and changes in LCD forehead temperature lag behind changes in core temperature by more than 12 minutes [17]. LCD skin thermometry is probably best used in patients with stable, normal hemodynamics who are not expected to experience major temperature shifts and in whom the trend of temperature change is more important than the accuracy of the measurement.

Standard Digital Thermometers: Thermocouples and Thermistors

Electric thermometers convert an electrical temperature signal into digital displays, frequently by use of thermocouples and thermistors as probes. Thermocouples and thermistors can be fashioned into thin wires and embedded in flexible probes that are suitable for placing in body cavities to measure deep temperature.

Thermocouples consist of a junction of two dissimilar metals. The voltage change across the junction can be precisely related to temperature. The measuring thermocouple must be calibrated against a second constant-temperature junction for absolute temperature measurements. In the range of 20° to 50°C, thermocouples may have a linearity error of less than 0.1 [18].

Thermistors consist of semiconductor metal oxides in which the electrical resistance changes inversely with temperature. A linearity error of up to 4°C may occur over the temperature range of 20° to 50°C, but this can be substantially reduced by mathematical adjustments and electrical engineering techniques [18]. Semiconductors measure temperature by taking advantage of the fact that the base-to-emitter voltage change is temperature dependent, whereas the collector current of the silicon resistor is constant. Thermistors are more sensitive, faster responding, and less linear than thermocouples or semiconductors [18].

Infrared Emission Detection Thermometers

Tympanic Thermometers. Commonly used in a hospital setting, infrared emission detection tympanic thermometers use a sensor that detects infrared energy emitted by the core-temperature tissues behind the tympanic membrane. Infrared emissions through the tympanic membrane vary linearly with temperature. Operator technique is important: errors due to improper calibration, setup, or poor probe positioning can significantly alter temperatures [19]. Measurements are most accurate when the measuring probe blocks the entrance of ambient air into the ear canal and when the midposterior external ear is tugged posterosuperiorly so as to direct the probe to the anterior, inferior third of the tympanic membrane. Studies are mixed on whether tympanic thermometers provide accurate core temperature measurements, ranging from a 4% clinically meaningful error rate [14] to a finding that 21% of tympanic readings might result in delays in therapy for or evaluation of fever [20].

Temporal Artery Thermometers. Infrared technology can also measure temperature over the temporal artery. A probe is passed over the forehead and searches for the highest temperature; some systems also scan the area behind the ear. An algorithm estimates ambient heat loss and blood cooling to calculate core temperature. The device is convenient, painless, and provides a rapid reading. Although one small study of normothermic patients found good correlation with pulmonary artery temperatures [5], another study in patients with a broader temperature range found that 89% of measurements differed from pulmonary artery temperatures by more than 0.5°C, the amount the author's had specified a priori as clinically significant [21].

Selecting the Measurement Site

The site used to monitor temperature must be an individualized choice, but certain generalizations can be made. When intermittent temperature measurement is all that is clinically needed (e.g., in routine monitoring), or the consequences of inaccurate measurement are low, rectal or sublingual measurement may be preferred. If less accuracy is required, tympanic, temporal, or axillary sites may be chosen. When more accurate measurement is needed, bladder, esophageal, and rectal temperatures in general appear to be most accurate and reproducible—although rectal temperatures may lag behind other temperatures when the patient's status is changing quickly [7,13]. However, routine measurement of esophageal temperatures would necessitate inserting an esophageal probe in all patients. In addition, small changes in probe position can affect the accuracy of esophageal measurements, so this mode is probably best used in patients undergoing active, aggressive temperature management in centers with substantial experience with the modality. Meanwhile, rectal probes may be extruded or may be refused by patients. The third option, bladder temperature monitoring, is simplified by the fact that most critically ill patients have an indwelling Foley catheter. Monitoring the bladder temperature in these patients requires only a thermistor-equipped catheter. Patients with a thermistor-tipped pulmonary artery catheter already in place require no additional temperature monitoring.

Patient Safety and Temperature Monitoring

Therapeutic hypothermia is increasingly prevalent in ICU settings (Chapter 65]). Some devices used to induce hypothermia are closed-looped systems. Since core temperature probes can fail (for example, dislodgement of a rectal probe to a position outside the patient), practitioners should consider monitoring core temperature from two sites when temperature is being actively manipulated.

ARTERIAL BLOOD PRESSURE MONITORING

The first recorded blood pressure measurement occurred in 1733 and—somewhat surprisingly—was intra-arterial pressure monitoring. The Reverend Stephen Hales placed a 9-foot brass tube in a horse's crural artery and found a blood pressure of about 8 feet 3 inches. This was obviously not clinically applicable. In the mid-1800s, Carl Ludwig recorded the first arterial pressure waveforms, but it was not until 1881 that the first noninvasive blood pressure recordings were made. In 1896, Riva-Rocci developed and popularized the mercury sphygmomanometer, which was then adopted and disseminated at least in part by Harvey Cushing. In 1905, Korotkoff developed techniques for detecting diastolic pressure by listening for what are now called Korotkoff sounds. More clinical techniques of direct blood pressure measurement by intra-arterial cannula were initially developed in the 1930s and popularized in the 1950s [22]. These measurements were soon accepted as representing true systolic and diastolic pressures.

Since that time, a variety of invasive and alternative indirect methods have been developed that equal and even surpass auscultation in reproducibility and ease of measurement. This section examines the advantages and disadvantages of various methods of arterial pressure monitoring and provides recommendations for their use in the ICU.

Noninvasive (Indirect) Blood Pressure Measurement

Providers can indirectly monitor blood pressure using a number of techniques, most of which describe the external pressure applied to block flow to an artery distal to the occlusion. These methods therefore actually detect blood *flow*, not intra-arterial pressure, although one method describes the pressure required to maintain a distal artery with a transmural pressure gradient of zero. These differences in what is actually measured are the major points of discrepancy between direct and indirect measurements.

Indirectly measured pressures vary depending on the size of the cuff used. Cuffs of inadequate width and length can provide falsely elevated readings. Bladder width should equal 40% and bladder length at least 60% of the circumference of the extremity measured [23]. Anyone who makes indirect pressure measurements must be aware of these factors and carefully select the cuff to be used.

Manual Methods

Auscultatory (Riva-Rocci) Pressures

The traditional way to measure blood pressure involves inflating a sphygmomanometer cuff around an extremity and auscultating over an artery distal to the occlusion. Sounds from the vibrations of the artery under pressure (Korotkoff sounds) indicate systolic and diastolic pressures. The level at which the sound first becomes audible is taken as the systolic pressure. The point at which there is an abrupt diminution in or disappearance of sounds is used as diastolic pressure. This method, still commonly used in the ICU, yields an acceptable value in most situations. Its advantages include low cost, time-honored reliability, and simplicity. Disadvantages include operator variability, susceptibility to environmental noise, and the absence of Korotkoff sounds when pressures are very low. Auscultatory pressures also correlate poorly with directly measured pressures at the extremes of pressure [24].

Manual Oscillation Method

When a cuff is slowly deflated and blood first begins to flow through the occluded artery, the artery's walls begin to vibrate. This vibration can be detected as an oscillation in pressure and has served as the basis for the development of several automated blood pressure monitoring devices. However, it also continues to be used in manual blood pressure measurement. The first discontinuity in the needle movement of an aneroid manometer indicates the presence of blood flow in the distal artery and is taken as systolic pressure [25]. The advantages of the oscillation method are its low cost and simplicity. The disadvantages include the inability to measure diastolic pressure, poor correlation with directly measured pressures [25], and lack of utility in situations in which Riva-Rocci measurements are also unobtainable. Aneroid manometers may also be inaccurate: in one study, 34% of all aneroid manometers in use in one large medical system gave inaccurate measurements, even when more lenient standards were used than those advocated by the National Bureau of Standards and the Association for the Advancement of Medical Instrumentation [26]. In the same survey, 36% of the devices were found to be mechanically defective—pointing out the need for regular maintenance. Although the manometers themselves can also be used for auscultatory measurements, oscillometric readings probably provide no advantage over auscultation in the ICU.

Palpation, Doppler, and Pulse-Oximetric Methods

Systolic pressures can be measured any method that detects flow in a distal artery as the blood pressure cuff is slowly deflated. Palpation of the radial artery is the most commonly used technique; it is most useful in emergency situations in which Korotkoff sounds cannot be heard and an arterial line is not in place. The inability to measure diastolic pressure makes the palpation method less valuable for ongoing monitoring. In addition, palpation obtains no better correlation with direct measurements than the previously described techniques. In one study, variation from simultaneously obtained direct pressure measurements was as high as 60 mm Hg [24]. Like other indirect methods, palpation tends to underestimate actual values to greater degrees at higher levels of arterial pressure. Any method which detects blood flow distal to a sphygmomanometer cuff may be used in this fashion. Doppler machines are commonly used and may be particularly useful in situations where the pulse is not palpable or environmental noise precludes auscultation. Pulse oximeters have been similarly used and correlate well with other methods; the point at which a plethysmographic trace appears is taken as the systolic pressure [27].

Automated Methods

Automated indirect blood pressure devices operate on one of several principles: Doppler flow, infrasound, oscillometry, volume clamp, arterial tonometry, and pulse wave arrival time.

Doppler Flow

Systems that operate on the Doppler principle take advantage of the change in frequency of an echo signal when there is movement between two objects. Doppler devices emit brief pulses of sound at a high frequency that are reflected back to the transducer [28]. The compressed artery exhibits a large amount of wall motion when flow first appears in the vessel distal to the inflated cuff. This causes a change in frequency of the echo signal, known as a *Doppler shift*. The first appearance of flow in the distal artery represents systolic pressure. In an uncompressed artery, the small amount of motion does not cause a change in frequency of the reflected signal. Therefore, the disappearance of the Doppler shift in the echo signal represents diastolic pressure [29].

Infrasound

Infrasound devices use a microphone to detect low-frequency (20 to 30 Hz) sound waves associated with the oscillation of the arterial wall. These sounds are processed by a minicomputer, and the processed signals are usually displayed in digital form [30].

Oscillometry

Oscillometric devices operate on the same principle as manual oscillometric measurements. The cuff senses pressure fluctuations caused by vessel wall oscillations in the presence of pulsatile blood flow [31]. Maximum oscillation is seen at mean pressure, whereas wall movement greatly decreases below diastolic pressure [32]. As with the other automated methods described, the signals produced by the system are processed electronically and displayed in numeric form.

Volume Clamp Technique

The volume clamp method avoids the use of an arm cuff. A finger cuff is applied to the proximal or middle phalanx to keep the artery at a constant size [33]. The pressure in the cuff is changed as necessary by a servocontrol unit strapped to the wrist. The feedback in this system is provided by a photoplethysmograph that estimates arterial size. The pressure needed to keep the artery at its *unloaded volume* can be used to estimate the intra-arterial pressure [34].

Arterial Tonometry

Arterial tonometry provides continuous noninvasive measurement of arterial pressure, including pressure waveforms. It slightly compresses the superficial wall of an artery (usually the radial). Pressure tracings obtained in this manner are similar to intra-arterial tracings. A generalized transfer function can convert these tracings to an estimate of aortic pressure [35]. This method has not yet achieved widespread clinical use. One available system studied in ICU patients had approximately one third of MAP readings which differed by $\geq$10 mm Hg compared with intra-arterial pressure measurements and was associated with significant drift during the course of the study [36]. However, more studies of a different system reported more accurate readings in patients undergoing anesthesia [37], including those with induced hypotension [38].

Utility of Noninvasive Blood Pressure Measurements

Only four of the methods described previously (infrasound, oscillometry, Doppler flow, volume clamp) are associated with significant clinical experience. Of these, methods that use infrasound technology correlate least well with direct measures of arterial blood pressure [31,39]. Therefore, infrasound is rarely used in systems designed for critical care.

Although they have not been consistently accurate, automated methods have the potential to yield pressures as accurate as values derived by auscultation. Commonly used oscillometric methods can correlate to within 1 mm Hg of the directly measured group average values [31] but may vary substantially from intra-arterial pressures in individual subjects, particularly at the extremes of pressure. One study revealed as good a correlation with directly measured pressures as Riva-Rocci pressures have traditionally obtained [31]. Another study demonstrated that mean arterial pressures determined by auscultation were extremely close to those measured by automated devices [40].

When volume clamp methods using a finger cuff have been compared with standard methods [41,42], these devices have been found to respond rapidly to changes in blood pressure and give excellent correlation in group averages. In one study looking at a large number of measurements, 95% of all measurements using this method were within 10 mm Hg of the directly measured values [43]. Studies by Aitken et al. [42] and Hirschl et al. [41] demonstrated acceptable correlation of volume clamp technique with systolic pressures measured directly. However, other studies have shown clinically significant differences between the volume clamp technique and invasively measured pressures in patients undergoing anesthesia [44].

One of the proposed advantages of automated noninvasive monitoring is patient safety. Avoiding arterial lines eliminates the risk of vessel occlusion, hemorrhage, and infection. Automated methods, however, have complications of their own. Ulnar nerve palsies have been reported with frequent inflation and deflation of a cuff [45]. Decreased venous return from the limb and eventually reduced perfusion to that extremity can also be seen when the cuff is set to inflate and deflate every minute [45,46].

In summary, automated noninvasive blood pressure forms a major component of modern critical care monitoring. Oscillometric and Doppler-based devices are adequate for frequent blood pressure checks in patients without hemodynamic instability, in patient transport situations in which arterial lines cannot be easily used, and in the severely burned patient, in whom direct arterial pressure measurement may lead to an unacceptably high risk of infection [47]. Automated noninvasive blood pressure monitors have a role in following trends of pressure change [48] and when group averages, not individual measurements, are most important. In general, they have significant limitations in patients with rapidly fluctuating blood pressures and may diverge substantially from directly measured intra-arterial pressures. Given these limitations, critical care practitioners should be wary of relying solely on these measurements in patients with rapidly changing hemodynamics or in whom very exact measurements of blood pressure are important.

Direct Invasive Blood Pressure Measurement

Direct blood pressure measurement is performed with an intra-arterial catheter. Chapter 3 reviews insertion and maintenance of arterial catheters. Here, we discuss the advantages and disadvantages of invasive monitoring compared with noninvasive means.

Arterial catheters contain a fluid column that transmits the pressure back through the tubing to a transducer. A low-compliance diaphragm in the transducer creates a reproducible volume change in response to the applied pressure change. The volume change alters the resistance of a Wheatstone bridge and is thus converted into an electrical signal. Most systems display the pressure in both wave and numeric forms.

Problems in Direct Pressure Monitoring

System-Related Problems. Several technical problems can affect the measurement of arterial pressure with the arterial line. Transducers must be calibrated to zero at the level of the heart. Improper zeroing can lead to erroneous interpretation. Thrombus formation at the catheter tip can occlude the catheter, making accurate measurement impossible. This problem can be largely eliminated by using a 20-gauge polyurethane catheter, rather than a smaller one, with a slow, continuous heparin flush [49], although this may be associated with heparin-induced thrombocytopenia [50]. Because movement may interrupt the column of fluid and prevent accurate measurement, the patient's limb should be immobile during readings.

The frequency response of the system is a phenomenon not only of transducer design but also of the tubing and the fluid in it. The length, width, and compliance of the tubing all affect the system's response to change. Small-bore catheters are preferable because they minimize the mass of fluid that can oscillate and amplify the pressure [51]. The compliance of the system (the change in volume of the tubing and the transducer for a given change in pressure) should be low [51]. In addition, bubbles in the tubing can affect measurements in two ways. Large amounts of air in the measurement system damp the system response and cause the system to underestimate the pressure [52]. This is usually easily detectable. Small air bubbles cause an increase in the compliance of the system and can significantly amplify the reported pressure [51,52].

Arterial Catheter Infections. Recent data challenge the classical perception that that arterial catheters are less likely to become infected [53] than central venous catheters. A prospective cohort study examined 321 arterial and 618 central venous catheters and found that arterial catheter colonization occurred with similar incidence to central venous catheter colonization [54]. Another recent study found similar results [55]. There is good evidence to support a link between the incidence of catheter colonization and catheter related blood stream infections [56]. Although one study suggested that full barrier precautions did not reduce the incidence of arterial line infection, interpretation of this trial is complex [57]. Taken together, the weight of evidence suggests that arterial catheters are an important potential source for infection in the critically ill patient and should be treated similar to central venous catheters in this setting.

Finally, the location within the hospital where the procedure is performed is important as catheters placed in non-ICU locations may be associated with an increased risk of colonization versus those placed in the ICU [54].

Site Selection. The radial artery is the most common site of arterial cannulation for pressure measurement. This site is accessible and can be easily immobilized to protect both the catheter and the patient. The major alternative site is the femoral artery. Both sites are relatively safe for insertion [58,59]. The ulnar, brachial, dorsalis pedis, and axillary arteries are also used with some frequency [60]. Mechanical complications such as bleeding and nerve injury are discussed in Chapter 11. How should a provider choose a site? Although there are a number of theoretical considerations about comparing blood pressures from one site to another, there is little data in critically ill patients. A systematic review of 19,617 radial, 3,899 femoral, and 1,989 axillary cannulations found that serious complications occurred infrequently (<1% of cannulations) and were similar between the sites [60]. In 14 septic surgical patients on vasopressors, radial pressures were significantly lower than femoral arterial pressures. In 11 of the 14 patients, vasopressor dose was reduced based on the femoral pressure without untoward consequences; after vasopressors were discontinued, radial and femoral pressures equalized. The authors concluded that clinical management based on radial artery pressures may lead to excessive vasopressor administration [61]. Similar significant differences in systolic pressures between the radial and femoral sites were found in the reperfusion phase of liver transplantation, although MAPs did not differ [62]. However, another somewhat larger observational study in critically ill patients [63] found no clinically meaningful differences in blood pressures between the sites. Although data are sparse, mean arterial pressure readings between the radial and femoral sites are probably interchangeable in many or most patients. There may be a preference toward using femoral arterial pressure readings in patients with vasopressor resistant shock, but this decision should be balanced by the risks of the femoral approach.

Should the risk of infection drive site selection? The data are mixed. Earlier work suggested that there was no difference in infection rates between the femoral and radial sites [60]. More recently, a prospective observational study of 2,949 catheters in the intensive care unit found the incidence of catheter related blood stream infection was significantly higher for femoral access (1.92/1,000 catheter-days) than for radial access (0.25/1,000 catheter-days) (odds ratio, 1.9; $p = 0.009$]. Localized skin infections were also significantly increased in femoral versus radial arterial catheters. In addition, femoral arterial catheter blood stream infections may have an increased association with gram negative bacteria when compared to the radial site, similar to previous data from central venous catheters [64].

Advantages

Despite technical problems, direct arterial pressure measurement offers several advantages. Arterial lines actually measure the end-on pressure propagated by the arterial pulse. In contrast, indirect methods report the external pressure necessary either to obstruct flow or to maintain a constant transmural vessel pressure. Arterial lines can also detect pressures at which Korotkoff sounds are either absent or inaccurate. Arterial lines provide a continuous measurement, with heartbeat-to-heartbeat blood pressures. In situations in which frequent blood drawing is necessary, indwelling arterial lines eliminate the need for multiple percutaneous punctures. Finally, analysis of the respiratory change in systolic or pulse pressure may provide important information on cardiac preload and fluid responsiveness.

Conclusions

Indirect methods of measuring the blood pressure estimate the arterial pressure by reporting the external pressure necessary to either obstruct flow or maintain a constant transmural vessel size. Arterial lines measure the end-on pressure propagated by the arterial pulse. Direct arterial pressure measurement offers several advantages in many but not all patients. Although an invasive line is required, the reported risk of complications is low [60]. Arterial lines provide a heartbeat-to-heartbeat measurement, can detect pressures at which Korotkoff sounds are either absent or inaccurate, and do not require repeated inflation and deflation of a cuff. In addition, they provide easy access for phlebotomy and blood gas sampling, and they may provide additional information about cardiac status. However, particular care should be taken with aseptic technique and line site maintenance, since the reported incidence of arterial line infection approaches that of central venous catheterization. Regardless of the method used, the mean arterial pressure should generally be the value used for decision making in most critically ill patients.

ELECTROCARDIOGRAPHIC MONITORING

Almost all ICUs in the United States routinely perform continuous electrocardiographic (ECG) monitoring. Continuous ECG monitoring combines the principles of ECG, which have been known since 1903, with the principles of biotelemetry, which were first put into practical application in 1921 [65]. Here we review the principles of arrhythmia monitoring, automated arrhythmia detection, and the role of automated ST segment analysis.

ECG monitoring in most ICUs is done over hard-wired apparatus. Skin electrodes detect cardiac impulses and transform them into an electrical signal, which is transmitted over wires directly to the signal converter and display unit. This removes the problems of interference and frequency restrictions seen in telemetry systems. Although this comes at the cost of reduced patient mobility, mobility is often not an immediate concern for this group of patients.

Arrhythmia Monitoring in the ICU

The American Heart Association's Practice Standards guideline considers continuous ECG monitoring a Class I intervention for all patients with indications for intensive care, regardless of whether the patient's primary admitting diagnosis related to a cardiac problem [66]. Approximately 20% of ICU patients in a general ICU have significant arrhythmias, mostly atrial fibrillation or ventricular tachycardia [67]. There is also a substantial incidence of arrhythmia following major surgery [68]. Although no studies address whether monitoring for arrhythmias in a general ICU population alters outcomes, this monitoring is generally accepted and considered standard care [66]. In postmyocardial infarction patients, on the other hand, the data is compelling. Arrhythmia monitoring was shown to improve the prognosis of patients admitted to the ICU for acute myocardial infarction (AMI) many years ago [69]. It has been a standard of care in the United States since that time. Although ventricular tachycardia and fibrillation after myocardial infarction have declined in frequency over the years, they still occur in about 7.5% of patients [70]. Monitoring enables the rapid detection of these potentially lethal rhythms.

Evolution of Arrhythmia Monitoring Systems for Clinical Use

After ICUs implemented continuous ECG monitoring, practitioners recognized some deficiencies with the systems. Initially, the responsibility for arrhythmia detection was assigned to specially trained coronary care nurses. Despite this, several studies documented that manual methods failed to identify arrhythmias, including salvos of VT, in up to 80% of cases [71]. This failure was probably due to an inadequate number of staff nurses to watch the monitors, inadequate staff education, and faulty monitors [72]. Subsequently, monitors equipped with built-in rate alarms that sounded when a preset maximum or minimum rate was detected proved inadequate because some runs of VT are too brief to exceed the rate limit for a given time interval [71,73]. Ultimately, computerized arrhythmia detection systems were incorporated into the monitors. The software in these systems is capable of diagnosing arrhythmias based on recognition of heart rate, variability, rhythm, intervals, segment lengths, complex width, and morphology [74]. These systems have been validated in coronary care and general medical ICUs [71,75]. Computerized arrhythmia detection systems are well accepted by nursing personnel, who must work most closely with them [76].

Ischemia Monitoring

Just as simple monitoring systems can miss episodes of VT and ventricular fibrillation, they can fail to detect significant episodes of myocardial ischemia. This is either because the episode is asymptomatic or because the patient's ability to communicate is impaired by intubation or altered mental status. ECG monitoring systems with automated ST segment analysis have been devised to attempt to deal with this problem.

In most ST segment monitoring systems, the computer initially creates a template of the patient's normal QRS complexes. It then recognizes the QRS complexes and the J points of subsequent beats and compares an isoelectric point just before the QRS with a portion of the ST segment 60 to 80 milliseconds after the J point [77]. It compares this relationship to that of the same points in the QRS complex template. The system must decide whether the QRS complex in question was generated and conducted in standard fashion or whether the beats are aberrant, which negates the validity of comparison. Therefore, an arrhythmia detection system must be included in all ischemia monitoring systems. Standard systems can monitor three leads simultaneously. These leads are usually chosen to represent the three major axes (anteroposterior, left-right, and craniocaudal]. The machine can either display these axes individually or sum up the ST segment deviations and display them in a graph over time [77].

Automated ST segment analysis has gained widespread popularity among cardiologists. Since 1989, the American Heart Association has recommended that ischemia monitoring be included in new monitoring systems developed for use in the coronary care unit [78]. In patients admitted for suspected acute coronary syndromes, ischemia is both frequently silent and strongly associated with adverse events after discharge [66]. Although noting that no randomized clinical trials document improved patient outcomes when automated ST segment monitoring is used to detect ischemia, the American Heart Association recommends ST segment monitoring for patients with a number of primary cardiac issues (for example, acute coronary syndromes), based on expert opinion. The guidelines make no statement regarding ST segment monitoring for ICU patients [66].

Newer Techniques

Because conventional three-lead monitoring detects only about one third of transient ischemic events in patients with unstable coronary syndromes [79], some authors have advocated the use of continuous 12-lead ECG systems in the care of acute coronary syndromes. However, continuous 12-lead ECG monitoring can be impractical given the large number of leads required, patient discomfort, interference with medical procedures and proclivity to motion artifact. Some systems based on the dipole hypothesis of vectorcardiography allow the derivation of a 12-lead ECG from four recording electrodes and a reference electrode. Good correlation has been demonstrated between the EASI system and traditional 12-lead ECG in detection of ST segment deviation in acute myocardial ischemia and also in analyzing cardiac rhythm [80]. Other proposed enhancements to continuous ECG monitoring include signal-averaged ECG, QT dispersion, QT interval beat-to-beat variability, and heart rate variability [81]. Although associated with subsequent arrhythmic events, these have not yet reached common clinical use.

Technical Considerations

As with any other biomedical measurement, technical problems can arise when monitoring cardiac rhythms. Standards have been devised to guide manufacturers and purchasers of ECG-monitoring systems [82].

The possibility of electrical shock exists whenever a patient is directly connected to an electrically operated piece of equipment by a low-resistance path. Electrical shocks would most commonly occur with improper grounding of equipment when a device such as a pacemaker is in place. Necessary precautions to avoid this potential catastrophe include (a) periodic checks to ensure that all equipment in contact with the patient is at the same ground potential as the power ground line; (b) insulating exposed lead connections; and (c) using appropriately grounded plugs [83]. Each hospital's biomedical engineering department should have a documented preventive maintenance plan for all equipment in the unit.

The size of the ECG signal is important for accurate recognition of cardiac rate and rhythm. Several factors may affect signal size. The amplitude can be affected by mismatching between skin-electrode and preamplifier impedance. The combination of high skin-electrode impedance, usually the result of poor contact between the skin and electrode, with low-input impedance of the preamplifier can decrease the size of the ECG signal. Good skin preparation, site selection, and conducting gels can promote low skin-electrode impedance. A high preamplifier input impedance or the use of buffer amplifiers can also improve impedance matching and thereby improve the signal obtained. Another factor that affects complex size is critical damping, the system's ability to respond to changes in the input signal. An underdamped system responds to changes in input with displays that exaggerate the signal, called *overshoot*. An overdamped system responds slowly to a given change and may underestimate actual amplitude. The ECG signal can also be affected by the presence of inherent, unwanted voltages at the point of input. These include the common mode signal, a response to surrounding electromagnetic forces; the direct current skin potential produced by contact between the skin and the electrode; and a potential caused by internal body resistance. Finally, the ECG system must have a frequency response that is accurate for the signals being monitored. Modern, commercially available systems have incorporated features to deal with each of these problems.

Personnel

The staff's ability to interpret the information received is crucial to effective ECG monitoring [78]. Primary interpretation may be by nurses or technicians under the supervision of a physician. All personnel responsible for interpreting ECG monitoring should have formal training developed cooperatively by the hospital's medical and nursing staffs. At a minimum, this training should include basic ECG interpretation skills and arrhythmia recognition. Hospitals should also establish and adhere to formal protocols for responding to and verifying alarms. Finally, a physician should be available in the hospital to assist with interpretation and make decisions regarding therapy.

Principles of Telemetry

Intensive care patients frequently continue to require ECG monitoring after they are released from the ICU, and many postoperative critical care patients begin mobilization while in the ICU. At this point, increased mobility is important to allow physical and occupational therapy as well as other rehabilitation services. Telemetry systems can facilitate this.

Telemetry means measurement at a distance biomedical telemetry consists of measuring various vital signs, including heart rhythm, and transmitting them to a distant terminal [84]. Telemetry systems in the hospital consist of four major components [84]: (a) A signal transducer detects heart activity through skin electrodes and converts it into electrical signals; (b) a radio transmitter broadcasts the electrical signal; (c) a radio receiver detects the transmission and converts it back into an electrical signal; and (d) the signal converter and display unit present the signal in its most familiar format. Continuous telemetry requires an exclusive frequency so the signal can be transmitted without interruption from other signals, which means the hospital system must have multiple frequencies available to allow simultaneous monitoring of several patients. The telemetry signal may be received in one location or simultaneously in multiple locations, depending on staffing practices. The signal transducer and display unit should also be equipped with an automatic arrhythmia detection and alarm system to allow rapid detection and treatment of arrhythmias. Notably, telemetry systems may be subject to interference by cellular phones [85] or other radio equipment.

Summary

The American Heart Association recommends continuous ECG monitoring for the detection of arrhythmias as a Class I intervention for all ICU patients [66]. Because ICU staff can miss a large percentage of arrhythmias when they use monitors without computerized arrhythmia detection systems, these computerized systems should be standard equipment in ICUs, especially those which care for patients with AMI. It appears that computerized monitoring devices can also detect a significant number of arrhythmias not noted manually in noncardiac patients. A large percentage of these lead to an alteration in patient care. Automated ST segment analysis facilitates the early detection of ischemic episodes. Telemetry provides close monitoring of recuperating patients while allowing them increased mobility.

RESPIRATORY MONITORING

Critical care personnel should monitor several primary respiratory parameters, including respiratory rate, tidal volume or minute ventilation, and oxygenation in critically ill patients. Routine monitoring of carbon dioxide levels would be desirable, but the technology for monitoring these parameters is not yet developed enough to consider mandatory continuous monitoring. In mechanically ventilated patients, many physiologic functions can be monitored routinely and continuously by the ventilator. This section does not discuss monitoring by the mechanical ventilator (see Chapter 31) but examines devices that might be routinely used to monitor the aforementioned parameters continuously and noninvasively.

Respiratory Rate, Tidal Volume, and Minute Ventilation

Clinical examination of the patient often fails to detect clinically important changes in respiratory rate and tidal volume [86]. Physicians, nurses, and hospital staff frequently report inaccurate respiratory rates, possibly because they underestimate the measurement's importance [87]. In another study, ICU staff had a greater than 20% error more than one-third of the time when the recorded respiratory rate was compared with objective tracings [88]. This is particularly surprising since the respiratory rate is an especially important predictor of outcome in many severity of illness scores such as the APACHE series [89]. In fact, respiratory rate has been called "the neglected vital sign [90]." Providers' clinical assessment of tidal volume and minute ventilation is similarly inaccurate [91]. Therefore, objective monitoring must be used because clinical evaluation is inaccurate.

Impedance Monitors

ICUs commonly use impedance monitors to measure respiratory rates and approximate tidal volume. These devices typically use ECG leads and measure changes in impedance generated by the change in distance between leads as a result of the thoracoabdominal motions of breathing. Obtaining a quality signal requires placing the leads at points of maximal change in thoracoabdominal contour or using sophisticated computerized algorithms. Alarms can then be set for a high and low rates or for a percentage drop in the signal that is thought to correlate with a decrease in tidal volume.

In clinical use, impedance monitors suffer confounding problems. They have failed to detect obstructive apnea when it has occurred and falsely detected apnea when it has not [92,93]. About one third of all apnea alarms from this technology are false-positives [94]. In situations with moving patients, they are even less accurate for the quantification of respiratory rate [95]. Impedance monitors are poor detectors of obstructive apnea because they may count persistent chest wall motion as breaths when the apneic patient struggles to overcome airway obstruction [92,93]. In general, respiratory rate monitoring in the ICU therefore results in a very high fraction of clinically irrelevant alarms: in one study, only 4% of respiratory alarms were deemed clinically relevant [96]. Although impedance monitors offer the advantage of being very inexpensive when ECG is already in use, they lack accuracy when precise measurements of apnea, respiratory rate, or tidal volume are required.

Respiratory Inductive Plethysmography

Respiratory inductive plethysmography (RIP) measures changes in the cross-sectional area of the chest and abdomen that occur with respiration and processes these signals into respiratory rate and tidal volume. This technology may be familiar to providers and patients because it is often used in polysomnograms. Typically, two elastic bands with embedded wire are placed above the xiphoid and around the abdomen. As the cross-sectional area of the bands changes with respiration, the self-inductance of the coils changes the frequency of attached oscillators. These signals are generally calibrated to a known gas volume, or may be internally calibrated so that further measurements reflect a percentage change from baseline rather than an absolute volume. RIP can accurately measure respiratory rate and the percentage change in tidal volume, as well as detect obstructive apnea [97–99]. RIP has been used to follow lung volumes in patients undergoing high-frequency oscillatory ventilation [100]. These measurements are more accurate than impedance measurements [93]. However, some studies have found problems with RIP's estimation of lung volumes. Notably, RIP must be calibrated against a known gas volume in order to provide tidal volume estimates. This calibration is not always accurate and may result in errors of >10% in 5% to 10% of patients even in highly controlled circumstances [97,101]. In mechanically ventilated patients, RIP had significant measurement drift (25 cm^3/min) and imprecise volume estimates. Only about two thirds of tidal volume estimates were accurate to within 10% of the reference value [102].

In addition to displaying respiratory rate and percentage change in tidal volume, RIP can provide asynchronous and paradoxical breathing measurements and alarms, which are common during early weaning and may be helpful in predicting respiratory failure [103]. The noninvasive nature of the tidal volume measurement may be helpful in patients in whom technical problems or leaks make it difficult to directly measure expired volume (e.g., patients with bronchopleural fistulas]. In addition, RIP can display changes in functional residual capacity, which permits health care providers to assess the effect of changing positive end-expiratory pressure (PEEP). Providers can determine the presence and estimation of the amount of auto (intrinsic) PEEP by observing the effect of applied (extrinsic) PEEP on functional residual capacity [104], with the caveats noted earlier regarding possible inaccuracy of volume measurements.

RIP systems are available with central station configurations, which have been used in noninvasively monitored respiratory care units; these units have allowed ICU-level patients to be safely moved to a less-expensive level of care [105]. Compared with impedance methods, RIP is more accurate and offers a variety of other useful measurements but is less convenient and more expensive.

Other Methods

Although health care providers can also use pneumotachometers, capnographs, and electromyography to accurately measure respiratory rate, these methods are not commonly used in the ICU. A pneumotachometer requires complete collection of exhaled gas and, therefore, either intubation or use of a tight-fitting face mask is not practical simply for monitoring. A second alternative, capnography, works exceedingly well as a respiratory rate monitor. Because it does not require intubation or a face mask, it can be a useful tool in many circumstances. Capnography is discussed in more detail later. A third option, surface electromyography of respiratory muscles can be used to calculate respiratory rate accurately [106] but cannot detect obstructive apnea or provide a measure of tidal volume. Electromyography works well in infants but presents difficulties in adults, especially in obese adults and those with edema.

Recently, substantial research has focused on better ways to noninvasively monitor respiratory rate. All of these need clinical validation in a critical care setting, but examples of potentially emerging technologies include mechanical contact sensors placed in either patient beds or pillows, acoustical respiratory monitoring, and photoplethysmography.

Measurements of Gas Exchange

Pulse Oximetry

Clinical estimation of hypoxemia is exceptionally unreliable [107,108]. Pulse oximeters measure the saturation of hemoglobin in the tissue during the arterial and venous phases of pulsation and mathematically derive arterial saturation. Meta-analysis of 74 oximeter studies suggests that these estimates are usually accurate within 5% of simultaneous gold standard measurements [109]. However, up to 97% of physicians and nurses who use pulse oximeters do not understand their underlying fundamental principles [110]. This section reviews the essential technology involved in pulse oximetry and practical problems that limit its use.

Theory. Oximeters distinguish between oxyhemoglobin and reduced hemoglobin on the basis of their different absorption of light. Oxyhemoglobin absorbs much less red (±660 nm) and slightly more infrared (±910 to 940 nm) light than nonoxygenated hemoglobin. Oxygen saturation thereby determines the ratio of red to infrared absorption. When red and infrared light are directed from light-emitting diodes (LEDs) to a photodetector across a pulsatile tissue bed, the absorption of each wavelength by the tissue bed varies cyclically with pulse. During diastole, absorption is due to the nonvascular tissue components (e.g., bone, muscle, and interstitium) and venous blood. During systole, absorption is determined by all of these components and arterialized blood. The pulse amplitude accounts for only 1% to 5% of the total signal [111]. Thus, the difference between absorption in systole and diastole is in theory due to the presence of arterialized blood. The change in ratio of absorption between systole and diastole can then be used to calculate an estimate of arterial oxygen saturation. Absorption is typically measured hundreds of times per second. Signals usually are averaged over several seconds and then displayed numerically. The algorithm used for each oximeter is determined by calibration on human volunteers. Most oximeters under ideal circumstances measure the saturation indicated by the pulse oximeter (SpO_2) to within 2% of arterial oxygen saturation [112].

Cooximeters perform measurements on whole blood obtained from an artery or a vein. They frequently measure absorbance at multiple wavelengths and compute the percentage of oxyhemoglobin, deoxyhemoglobin, methemoglobin, and carboxyhemoglobin (COHb) in total hemoglobin based on different absorption spectra. They are mostly free of the artifacts that limit the accuracy of tissue oximeters and are regarded as the gold standard by which other methods of assessing saturation are measured.

Technology. Many manufacturers market pulse oximeters. Because of the variety of manufacturers, the numerous algorithms used, and the diverse patient populations studied, it is difficult to generalize the studies performed with one particular instrument, with its specific version of software, in one defined group of patients, to critically ill patients in general. The reader should always check with an oximeter's manufacturer before generalizing the following discussion to his or her oximeter and patient population.

Problems Encountered in Use. Because pulse oximeters are ubiquitous, all ICU providers must understand their limitations. A meta-analysis of problems encountered in pulse oximetry trials found that severe hypoxemia, dyshemoglobinemia, low perfusion states, skin pigmentation, and hyperbilirubinemia may affect the accuracy of pulse oximeter readings [109]. Any process that affects or interferes with the absorption of light between the LEDs and photodetector, alters the quality of pulsatile flow, or changes the hemoglobin may distort the oximeter's calculations. Pulse oximeters should be able to obtain valid readings in 98% of patients in an operating room or postanesthesia care unit [113]. Table 26.1 lists the problems that must be considered in clinical use.

Calibration. Manufacturers use normal volunteers to derive pulse oximeter calibration algorithms. This creates three problems. First, manufacturers use different calibration algorithms, which results in a difference in SpO_2 of up to 2.7% between different manufacturers' oximeters used to measure the same

TABLE 26.1

CONDITIONS ADVERSELY AFFECTING ACCURACY OF OXIMETRY

May result in poor signal detection	
Probe malposition	No pulse
Motion	Vasoconstriction
Hypothermia	Hypotension
Falsely lowers SpO_2	**Falsely raises SpO_2**
Nail polish	Elevated carboxyhemoglobin
Dark skin	Elevated methemoglobin
Ambient light	Ambient light
Elevated serum lipids	Hypothermia
Methylene blue	
Indigo carmine	
Indocyanine green	

SpO_2, saturation indicated by the pulse oximeter.

patient [114]. Second, manufacturers define SpO_2 differently for calibration purposes. Calibration may or may not account for the interference of small amounts of dyshemoglobinemia (e.g., methemoglobin or COHb). For example, if an oximeter is calibrated on the basis of a study of nonsmokers with a 2% COHb level, the measured SpO_2 percentage would differ depending on whether the value used to calibrate SpO_2 included or excluded the 2% COHb [114]. Third, it is difficult, for ethical reasons, for manufacturers to obtain an adequate number of validated readings in people with an SpO_2 of less than 70% to develop accurate calibration algorithms in this saturation range. Most oximeters give less precise readings in this saturation range [115]. Unless better calibration algorithms become available, oximeters should be considered unreliable when SpO_2 is less than 70%, although this may have little clinical impact since emergent intervention is usually required for all SpO_2 readings <70%.

Measurement sites. Careful sensor positioning is crucial to obtaining accurate results from a pulse oximeter [116]. Practitioners can obtain accurate measurements from fingers, forehead, and earlobes. The response time from a change in the partial pressure of arterial oxygen (PaO_2) to a change in displayed SpO_2 is delayed in finger and toe probes compared with ear, cheek, or glossal probes [117,118]. Forehead edema, wetness, and head motion may result in inaccurate forehead SpO_2 values [119]. Motion and perfusion artifacts are the greatest problems with finger or toe measurements. The earlobe is believed to be the site least affected by vasoconstriction artifact [120], but paradoxically the finger may give a better signal in times of hypoperfusion [109].

Fingernails. Long fingernails may prevent correct positioning of the finger pulp over the LEDs used in inflexible probes and therefore produce inaccurate SpO_2 readings without affecting the pulse rate [121]. Synthetic nails have produced erroneous results [112]. Adhesive tape, even when placed over both sides of a finger, did not affect measured SpO_2 [122]. Since pulse oximetry depends fundamentally on color, nail polish may falsely lower SpO_2. In a 1988 study, blue, green, and black polish showed greater decreases than red or purple [123]. However, a 2002 study with a newer-generation oximeter did not find this effect [124]. In addition, placing the probe sideways across the fingernail bed appeared to ameliorate any effect of fingernail polish in one study [125].

Skin color. The effect of skin color on SpO_2 was assessed in a study of 655 patients [126]. Although patients with the darkest skin had significantly less accurate SpO_2 readings, the mean inaccuracy in SpO_2 (compared with cooximetry) between subjects with light skin and those with the darkest skin was only 0.5%, a clinically insignificant difference. Pulse oximeters, however, encountered difficulties in obtaining readings in darker-skinned patients; 18% of patients with darker skin triggered warning lights or messages versus 1% of lighter skinned patients. A study of 284 patients with a newer generation oximeter also found that skin color did not affect measurement accuracy. Poor-quality readings were found more often in darker skinned patients, although this was a rare event (<1% of all patients) [127]. Thus, dark skin may prevent a measurement from being obtained, but when the oximeter reports an error-free value, the value is generally accurate enough for clinical use [128].

Ambient light. Ambient light that affects absorption in the 660- or 910-nm wavelengths, or both, may affect calculations of saturation and pulse. Xenon arc surgical lights [129], fluorescent lights [130], and fiberoptic light sources [131] have caused falsely elevated saturation but typically obvious dramatic elevations in reported pulse. An infrared heating lamp [132] has produced falsely low saturations and a falsely low pulse, and a standard 15-W fluorescent bulb resulted in falsely low saturation without a change in heart rate [133]. Interference from surrounding lights should be suspected by the presence of pulse values discordant from the palpable pulse or ECG, or changes in the pulse-saturation display when the probe is transiently shielded from ambient light with an opaque object. Most manufacturers have now modified their probes to minimize this problem. Studies report that ambient lighting has little or no effect on newer generation oximeters [134], although this varies among manufacturers [135].

Hyperbilirubinemia. Bilirubin's absorbance peak is maximal in the 450-nm range but has tails extending in either direction [136]. Bilirubin, therefore, does not typically affect pulse oximeters that use the standard two-diode system [136,137]. However, it may greatly interfere with the measurement of saturation by cooximeters. Cooximeters typically use four to six wavelengths of light and measure absolute absorbance to quantify the percentage of all major hemoglobin variants. Serum bilirubin values as high as 44 mg per dL had no effect on the accuracy of pulse oximeters but led to falsely low levels of oxyhemoglobin measured by cooximetry [136].

Dyshemoglobinemias. Conventional (two-diode) pulse oximeters cannot detect the presence of methemoglobin, COHb, or fetal hemoglobin. Fetal hemoglobin may confound readings in neonates but is rarely a problem in adults. On the other hand, acquired methemoglobinemia—although uncommon—is seen in routine practice, largely due to the use of methemoglobinemia-inducing drugs such as topical anesthetics [138]. Because methemoglobin absorbs more light at 660 nm than at 990 nm, it affects pulse oximetry readings [139]. Moreover, higher levels of methemoglobin tend to bias the reading toward 85% to 90% [140]. COHb is typically read by a two-diode oximeter as 90% oxyhemoglobin and 10% reduced hemoglobin [141], resulting in false elevations of SpO_2. A gap between pulse oximetry and pO_2 or cooximetrically measured oxygen saturation may suggest elevated COHb levels, particularly in patients with smoke inhalation or potential carbon monoxide poisoning [142]. Because COHb may routinely be 10% in smokers, pulse oximetry may fail to detect significant desaturation in this group of patients. Oxygen saturation in smokers, when measured by cooximetry, was on average 5%

lower than pulse oximetric values [143]. Hemolytic anemia may also elevate COHb up to 2.6% [144]. Because other etiologies of COHb are rare in the hospital and the half-life of COHb is short, this problem is unusual in the critical care setting except in newly admitted patients, patients with active hemolysis, or those on COHb-inducing drugs such as sodium nitroprusside [145]. More recently, some pulse oximeters that use multi-wavelength technology have been able to successfully report methemoglobin and COHb levels [146].

Anemia. Few clear data are available on the effect of anemia on pulse oximetry. In dogs, there was no significant degradation in accuracy until the hematocrit was less than 10% [147]. In one study of humans who had hemorrhagic anemia, there appeared to be little effect on pulse oximetry accuracy [148].

Lipids. Patients with elevated chylomicrons and those receiving lipid infusions may have falsely low SpO_2 because of interference in absorption by the lipid [149]. This also affects cooximetry and may lead to spurious methemoglobin readings [150].

Hypothermia. Good-quality signals may be unobtainable in 10% of hypothermic patients [151]. The decrease in signal quality probably results from hypothermia-induced vasoconstriction. When good-quality signals could be obtained, SpO_2 differed from cooximetry-measured saturation by only 0.6% [151] in one series.

Intravascular dyes. Methylene blue, used to treat methemoglobinemia, has a maximal absorption at 670 nm and therefore falsely lowers measured SpO_2 [152]. Indocyanine green and indigo carmine also lower SpO_2, but the changes are minor and brief [153]. Fluorescein has no effect on SpO_2 [153]. Because of the rapid vascular redistribution of injected dyes, the effect on oximetry readings typically lasts only 5 to 10 minutes [154]. Patent V dye, which is used to visualize lymphatics in sentinel node mapping, confounds pulse oximetry, an effect which may persist for more than 90 minutes [155].

Motion artifact. Shivering and other motions that change the distance from diode to receiver may result in artifact. Oximeters account for motion by different algorithms. Some oximeters display a warning sign, others stop reporting data, and others display erroneous values. The display of a plethysmographic waveform rather than a signal strength bar helps to indicate to providers that artifact has distorted the pulse signal and lowered the quality of the SpO_2 reading. Newer generation oximeters appear to have significantly less susceptibility to motion artifact than earlier models [156].

Hypoperfusion. During a blood pressure cuff inflation model of hypoperfusion, most oximeters remained within 2% of control readings [157]. Increasing systemic vascular resistance and decreasing cardiac output can also make it harder to obtain a good-quality signal. In one series, the lowest cardiac index and highest systemic vascular resistance at which a signal could be detected were 2.4 L per minute per m^2 and 2,930 dynes second per cm^5 per m^2, respectively [158]. Warming the finger [159] or applying a vasodilating cream [158] tended to extend the range of signal detection in individual patients. The oximeter's ability to display a waveform and detect perfusion degradation of the signal was crucial in determining when the readings obtained were valid [157].

Pulsatile venous flow. In physiologic states in which venous and capillary flows become pulsatile, the systolic pulse detected by the oximeter may no longer reflect the presence of just arterial blood. In patients with severe tricuspid regurgitation, the measured saturation may be falsely low, especially with ear probes [160].

Indications. The Society of Critical Care Medicine considers pulse oximetry (or transcutaneous oxygen measurement) essential monitoring for all ICU patients receiving supplemental oxygen [161]. Unsuspected hypoxemia is common in critically ill patients. Sixteen percent of patients not receiving supplemental oxygen in the recovery room have saturations of less than 90% [162]. In 35% of patients, saturations of less than 90% develop during transfer out of the operating room [163]. Because of the high frequency of hypoxemia in critically ill patients, the frequent need to adjust oxygen flow, and the unreliability of visual inspection to detect mild desaturation, oximeters should be used in most critically ill patients for routine, continuous monitoring. In one study that randomized more than 20,000 operative and perioperative patients to continuous or no oximetric monitoring, the authors concluded that oximetry permitted detection of more hypoxemic events, prompted increases in the fraction of oxygen in inspired air, and significantly decreased the incidence of myocardial ischemia but did not significantly decrease mortality or complication rates [164].

Oximeters have been used in the ICU for reasons other than continuous monitoring. For example, oximeters may be helpful during difficult intubations. Once desaturation occurs, attempts to intubate should be postponed until manual ventilation restores saturation. Note, however, that oximetry is not helpful in promptly detecting inadvertent esophageal intubation because desaturation may lag significantly behind apnea in preoxygenated patients [165]. Oximeters can be useful in detecting systolic blood pressure (see arterial pressure monitoring earlier), and have been used in other clinical applications with varying degrees of success. Notably, a normal SpO_2 reading should *not* be used to exclude pulmonary embolism [166].

Capnography

Capnography involves the measurement and display of expired PCO_2 concentrations. This section reviews the technology, the sources of difference between end-tidal PCO_2 ($EtCO_2$) and $PaCO_2$, and the indications for capnography in the ICU.

Technology. Expired PCO_2 concentration is usually determined by infrared absorbance or mass spectrometry. The infrared technique relies on the fact that carbon dioxide has a characteristic absorbance of infrared light, with maximal absorbance near a wavelength of 4.28 mm. A heated wire with optical filters is used to generate an infrared light of appropriate wavelength. When carbon dioxide passes between a focused beam of light and a semiconductor photodetector, an electronic signal can be generated that, when calibrated, accurately reflects the PCO_2 of the tested gas.

A mass spectrometer bombards gas with an electron stream. The ion fragments that are generated can be deflected by a magnetic field to detector plates located in precise positions to detect ions that are characteristic of the molecule being evaluated. The current generated at the detector can be calibrated to be proportional to the partial pressure of the molecule being evaluated.

The two techniques have different strengths. Mass spectrometers can detect the partial pressures of several gases simultaneously and can monitor several patients at once. Infrared techniques measure only PCO_2 and are usually used on only one patient at a time. The calibration and analysis time required for mass spectrometry is significantly longer than with infrared techniques. Infrared systems respond to changes in approximately 100 milliseconds, whereas mass spectrometers take 45 seconds to 5 minutes to respond [167]. Although costs vary widely, mass spectrometers are in general far more expensive and are most frequently purchased to be the central component of a carbon dioxide monitoring system. In the operating room, mass spectrometry has the advantage of being able to measure the partial pressure of anesthetic gases, and the need for a technical specialist to oversee its operation can be more easily justified. For these reasons, mass spectrometry has achieved much more popularity in the operating room than in the ICU.

Gases can be sampled by mainstream or sidestream techniques. Mainstream sampling involves placing the capnometer directly in line in the patient's respiratory circuit. All air leaving the patient passes through the capnometer. The sidestream sampling techniques pump 100 to 300 mL expired air per minute through thin tubing to an adjacent analyzing chamber.

The mainstream method can be used only on patients who are intubated or wearing a tight-fitting face or nose mask. Mainstream sampling offers the advantage of almost instantaneous analysis of sampled air, but it increases the patient's dead space and adds weight to the endotracheal tube. Sidestream sampling removes air from the expiratory circuit, altering measurement of tidal volume. Slower aspirating flow rates and longer tubing lengths significantly worsen the ability to detect a rapid rise in carbon dioxide and cause delay between physiologic changes in the patient and the display of changes on the monitor [168]. When the delay exceeds the respiratory cycle time, the generated data are inaccurate [168]. Located near the mouth or nose, sidestream sampling lines are also prone to clogging with secretions, saliva, or water condensation. Sidestream sampling can be used in nonintubated patients to detect cyclic changes in carbon dioxide concentrations. Because of these issues, accurate sidestream sampling requires short sampling tubes and attention to the possibility of clogged sample lines.

Differences Between End-Tidal and Arterial Carbon Dioxide. The PCO_2 in exhaled air measured at the mouth changes in a characteristic pattern in normal people that reflects the underlying physiologic changes in the lung (Fig. 26.1). During inspiration, the PCO_2 is negligible, but it rises abruptly with expiration. The rapid rise reflects mixing and the washout of dead-space air with air from perfused alveoli, which contain higher levels of CO_2. A plateau concentration is reached after dead-space air has been exhaled. The plateau level is determined by the mean alveolar PCO_2, which is in equilibration with pulmonary artery PCO_2. The end-alveolar plateau level of PCO_2 measured during the last 20% of exhalation is the $EtCO_2$. In normal people at rest, the difference between $EtCO_2$ and $PaCO_2$ is ± 1.5 mm Hg. A difference exists because of the presence of dead space and a normal physiologic shunt. Changes in dead space or pulmonary perfusion alters ventilation–perfusion ratio and changes the relationship between end-tidal and arterial PCO_2 values. As dead space increases, the $EtCO_2$ represents more the (lower) PCO_2 of nonperfused alveoli, thereby diverging from the $PaCO_2$ value. As perfusion decreases, fewer alveoli are perfused, creating a similar effect.

In most equipment, the $EtCO_2$ level is determined by a computerized algorithm. Because algorithms are imperfect, a waveform display is considered essential for accurate interpretation of derived values [168]. In slowly breathing patients, cardiac pulsations may cause the intermittent exhalation of small amounts of air at the end of the lungs' expiratory effort. This results in oscillations that may obscure the plateau phase. An irregular respiratory pattern or large increases in dead space can also distort the plateau phase. Visual inspection of traces can detect situations in which algorithms are prone to produce errors [167].

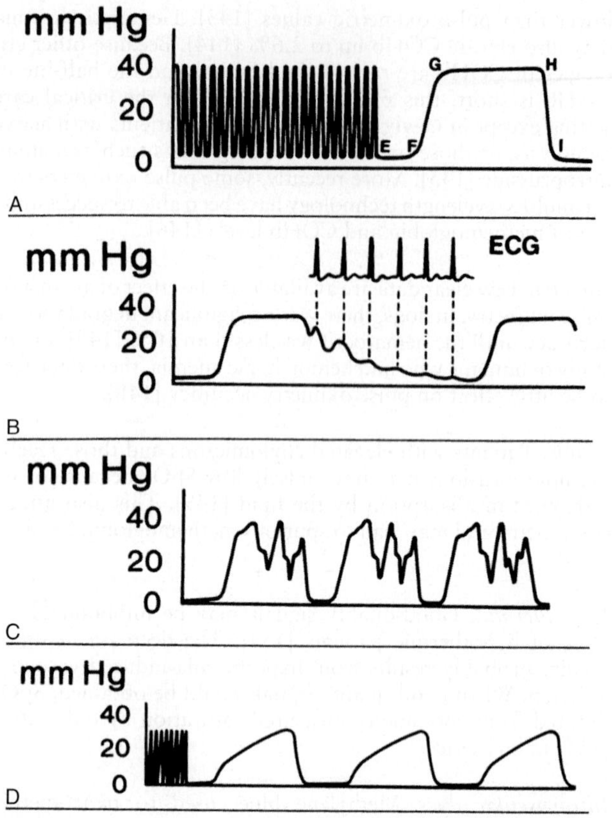

FIGURE 26.1. Normal and abnormal capnograms. In the normal capnogram (**A**), on the right of the trace, the paper speed has been increased. The *EF* segment is inspiration. The *FG* segment reflects the start of expiration with exhalation of dead space gas. The *GH* segment is the alveolar plateau. End-tidal values are taken at point *H*. *HI* is the beginning of inspiration. In the abnormal capnograms, the alveolar plateau is distorted and the end-tidal point cannot be clearly determined because of cardiac oscillations (**B**), erratic breathing (**C**), and obstructive airway disease (**D**). ECG, electrocardiogram. (Modified from Stock MC: Noninvasive carbon dioxide monitoring. *Crit Care Clin* 4:511, 1988.)

Indications. In the ICU, capnography is most useful for (1) detection of extubation, (2) determining the presence or absence of respiration, and (3) detecting return of spontaneous circulation after cardiac arrest. Such determinations do not require that $EtCO_2$ be measured accurately, only that changes be detected reliably. Alarms for apnea and tachypnea can be set and relied on, although capnography cannot discriminate between obstructive and central apnea. Capnography is a useful adjunct for detecting unintentional extubation, malposition of the endotracheal tube, or absence of perfusion. Cyclic variation of $EtCO_2$ is absent in esophageal intubation or disconnection from the ventilator [169]. Although pharyngeal intubation with adequate ventilation may produce a normal capnogram. Capnography can demonstrate the return of circulation after cardiopulmonary arrest or bypass. In full cardiac arrest, $EtCO_2$ is low because of lack of perfusion; a rapid rise in $EtCO_2$ indicates return of circulation and successful delivery of CO_2 to the alveoli [170]. Capnography or capnometry is also frequently used to help detect esophageal intubation [171].

$EtCO_2$ measurements are unreliable indicators of $PaCO_2$ in critically ill patients. Since these patients undergo rapid changes in dead space fraction and pulmonary perfusion, the relationship of $EtCO_2$ to arterial $PaCO_2$ may change rapidly and unpredictably. In one study of anesthetized, stable, generally healthy adults, $PaCO_2$ could not be reliably determined from end-tidal values [172]. In patients undergoing weaning from mechanical ventilation, $EtCO_2$ was also shown to have no predictable relationship to $PaCO_2$[173]. Although end-tidal and arterial values correlated well ($r = 0.78$) and rarely differed by more than 4 mm Hg, changes in $EtCO_2$ correlated poorly with changes in arterial PCO_2 ($r^2 = 0.58$]. Because of changes in dead space and perfusion, arterial and end-tidal measurements at times moved unpredictably in opposite directions. Although theoretically attractive, the use of end-tidal carbon dioxide measurements to evaluate changes in ventilation-perfusion mismatch in response to ventilator changes has failed to yield consistent clinical benefits [174].

Capnography has been helpful in the operating room in detecting air and pulmonary embolism as well as malignant hyperthermia [167]. In these situations, the capnograph does not provide a diagnosis; it records a change that, if limits are exceeded, signals an alarm. The responsibility for accurately interpreting the subtleties of changes in the capnogram remains the task of an experienced physician.

Conclusions. Capnography is of limited use in the critically ill patient. In any patient with changing cardiac output, fluctuating respiratory function, or chronic lung disease, it should not be used to replace $PaCO_2$ monitoring. It has been used to assess correct endotracheal tube placement (or inadvertent extubation) and offers rapid information about the return of spontaneous circulation after cardiac arrest. It does, however, monitor respiratory rate accurately and may be useful in some circumstances for that function. Capnography may be better suited to the operating room, where its value is increased because of its ability to help detect endotracheal tube malposition, air embolism, pulmonary embolism, and malignant hyperthermia, and where there is a highly skilled anesthesiologist immediately available to interpret subtle changes in the capnogram.

NONINVASIVE TISSUE PERFUSION MONITORING

Bedside providers usually monitor tissue perfusion based on clinical signs such as skin temperature and capillary refill time. However, several noninvasive technologies provide quantitative data about overall or regional tissue perfusion. Unlike most of the other monitoring technologies described in this chapter, clinical adoption of these techniques has been relatively limited and heterogeneous [175]. This section reviews three such technologies that measure local pCO_2 or pO_2: gastric tonometry, sublingual capnometry, and transcutaneous oxygen and carbon dioxide monitoring. Measurements from each of these techniques correlate meaningful clinical outcomes such as patient survival.

Physiology: Why Regional pO_2 and pCO_2 Reflects Tissue Perfusion and Not Just Global Gas Exchange

At first glance, it would appear that measurement of pO_2 or pCO_2 in the skin, stomach, or tongue would reflect global gas exchange and might be used for noninvasive blood gas estimation. In some cases, this is true. In healthy adults, for example, transcutaneously measured pO_2 and CO_2 ($PtcO_2$ and $PtcCO_2$) accurately reflect PaO_2 and $PaCO_2$ [176]. The measured transcutaneous values of oxygen and carbon dioxide are typically 10 mm Hg lower [177] and 5 to 23 mm Hg higher [178] than arterial values, respectively.

However, local pO_2 and pCO_2 therefore depend not only on global gas exchange, cardiac output, and oxygen content, but also on regional blood flow and oxygen delivery to the site of measurement. Under normal circumstances, oxygen delivery far exceeds consumption. In critical illness, however, regional hypoperfusion or inadequate regional delivery of oxygen may occur for any number of reasons: hypotension, regional vasoconstriction, low cardiac output states, anemia, vascular occlusion, etc. If there is no flow to the region, there can be no delivery of oxygen and no elimination of carbon dioxide by the vasculature—thus creating lower local pO_2 and higher local pCO_2 than in the arterial circulation. When tissue is hypoperfused, local metabolism then further alters local pO_2 and pCO_2. As cellular processes use available oxygen for the production of adenosine triphosphate (ATP), local pO_2 falls. When these cells use ATP faster than they replenish it, they liberate hydrogen ions (H^+) and reduce local pH. (Alternatively, cells may produce lactic acid through the anaerobic metabolic pathway.) These addition hydrogen ions are then buffered by tissue bicarbonate, generating CO_2: $H^+ + HCO_3^- \rightarrow H_2O_3 \rightarrow H_2O + CO_2$. This increases local pCO_2 above corresponding global/arterial values [179]. For these reasons, local pO_2 and pCO_2 therefore vary not only with global gas exchange, but also with local tissue perfusion.

Gastric Tonometry

Gastric tonometry, probably the most commonly used of the three perfusion monitoring techniques discussed in this section, assesses regional splanchnic perfusion based on the stomach's mucosal pCO_2. The splanchnic circulation has several properties which make this region particularly useful to assess in critically ill patients. Early in the development of shock states, the splanchnic circulation vasoconstricts, shunting cardiac output toward other core organs. Although this helps to prevent circulatory collapse, it may also result in intestinal mucosal ischemia—increasing the risk of gastric stress ulceration, mesenteric ischemia, and translocation of gut bacteria into the systemic circulation [180]. The gut is particularly sensitive to hypoperfusion and so may provide earlier warning of occult hypoperfusion than other vascular beds—leading some to liken it to a coal miner's canary [181]. Gastric tonometry measures gastric luminal pCO_2 and estimates gastric intramucosal pCO_2 and pH (pHi).

Technical Considerations

Development. Early measurements of visceral mucosal pH required operative implantation of monitors and focused on the gallbladder, urinary bladder, and small bowel [182,183]. Development of silastic tubing [184]—which is exceptionally permeable to O_2 and CO_2—and confirmation that gases in tissue equilibrate rapidly with fluid in the lumen of a hollow viscus [185] allowed development of the modern gastrointestinal tonometer.

Technique. The upper gastrointestinal catheter is inserted with standard technique for nasogastric tube placement, and placement is confirmed radiographically. The stopcock is flushed with fluid to eliminate any trapped air, the balloon is filled to the manufacturer's specifications with fluid, and the tonometer lumen is closed to the outside environment. The fluid is allowed to equilibrate with the fluid in the lumen of the organ being monitored, a process believed to require approximately

90 minutes, although formulas are available to correct the values obtained with 30 to 90 minutes of equilibration [186]. After adequate time for equilibration, the dead space (usually 1.0 mL) is aspirated and discarded, and the fluid in the balloon is completely aspirated under anaerobic conditions. An ABG sample is taken simultaneously, and both samples are sent for analysis. The pCO_2 of the tonometer sample is measured directly. Providers can then calculate an arterial/mucosal pCO_2 gap or, using the HCO_3^- of arterial blood and the modified Henderson–Hasselbalch equation, pHi [187,188].

An air-based tonometer has also gained popularity. This device operates on the same principles as the saline-based tonometer, but automatically aspirates small amounts of air from a semipermeable balloon. This is substantially more convenient than the saline-based device, and allows semicontinuous measurement of gastric mucosal pCO_2. Results are generally similar to saline-based tonometry [189].

Technical Limitations. Several issues may confound the clinical use of gastric tonometry. Two of these apply only to saline-based tonometry. The fluid in the tonometer balloon requires 90 minutes for full equilibration with the fluid in the stomach. In a rapidly changing patient, this time window may not be appropriately timely. In addition, manufacturers calibrate blood gas analyzers to measure pCO_2 in blood, not saline. pCO_2 measurements in tonometer saline, therefore, may vary based on the blood gas analyzer used [190]. Other limitations apply to the general principle of measure gastric luminal pCO_2 to estimate mucosal perfusion. Tonometrically derived gastric pHi can be affected by the acid-secretory status of the stomach. In one study, mean gastric pHi was 7.30 in untreated normal volunteers but 7.39 in a similar group treated with ranitidine [191]. This was because the pCO_2 in the gastric fluid of the treated patients was 42 ± 4 mm Hg, compared with 52 ± 14 mm Hg in the untreated group. The difference in carbon dioxide content of the fluid is thought to be due to production of carbon dioxide by the conversion of secreted H^+ and HCO_3^- into water and carbon dioxide. Enteral feeding may also affect pHi reading. Tube feedings may lead to increased production of carbon dioxide through the interaction of secreted hydrogen ions and HCO_3^-. Some suggest temporarily discontinuing tube feeds before doing pHi measurements [192], although the pCO_2 affect appears to diminish after 24 hours of continuous feeding [193]. Finally, pHi is a calculated variable which uses the systemic arterial bicarbonate value; this probably does not reflect regional perfusion [188]. The present consensus favors the use of arterial-gastric pCO_2 gap rather than pHi [189,194].

Clinical Usefulness and Limitations. pHi correlates well with a number of clinically important endpoints. Changes in pHi during weaning from mechanical ventilation predict weaning failure [195]. Intraoperative and postoperative cardiac surgery patients have been particularly well studied, and in that group gastric pHi appears to predict complications well [196,197]. Most importantly, pHi predicts mortality in septic [198], acutely injured [199], and general ICU patients [200].

For a diagnostic tool to be *therapeutically* useful, however, we must be able to act on its results in a way that improves patient outcome [201]. Therapeutic protocols based on gastric tonometry have produced conflicting results. A randomized, controlled trial of 260 ICU patients, reported in 1992, found that gastric pHi-based therapy had no effect on mortality of patients with a low admission pHi but was associated with reduced mortality in patients with a normal admission pHi [202]. However, interpretation of this finding is severely limited because the authors did not analyze the results in an intention-to-treat fashion, thus abandoning many of the benefits of randomization [203], and 21 patients were withdrawn from the study due to protocol noncompliance by treating physicians. A subsequent randomized, controlled trial of 210 general ICU patients, reported in 2000, found no difference between intervention and control arms [204]. In patients with a normal initial pHi, there was a nonsignificant trend toward increased 30-day mortality in the group treated based on pHi. One patient in the intervention group was excluded from analysis due to a conversion to comfort-measures-only status 5 hours after enrollment. A 2005 study randomized 151 trauma patients to pHi-driven therapy, splanchnic ischemia/reperfusion-based protocol, or usual care. The authors found no significant differences in mortality, organ dysfunction, ventilator days, or length of stay. Analysis was intention-to-treat [205]. Other, smaller randomized trials have generally found no effect [206].

Alternative Regional pCO_2 Measurement: Sublingual Capnometry. Sublingual capnometry operates on the same fundamental principles as gastric tonometry. A sensor is placed under the tongue and CO_2 diffuses across a semipermeable membrane into a dye, which fluoresces differently based on CO_2 concentration. A fiberoptic cable transmits light of the appropriate wavelength and detects the resulting fluorescence, which is proportional to CO_2 concentration in the sensor [175]. Results from this technique correlate with gastric tonometry [207] and patient outcome [208]. No randomized intervention trials based on sublingual capnometry have yet been published. Although sublingual capnometry was entering non-research clinical use, the manufacturer recalled the commercially available sublingual capnometry device in 2004 after an outbreak of *Burkholderia cepacia* related to contaminated sublingual probes [209].

Summary. Although gastric tonometry predicts many important clinical outcomes, high-quality data does not support gastric-tonometry–based resuscitation. The Surviving Sepsis Campaign's 2004 guidelines for hemodynamic management of septic shock—representing eleven international professional societies—concludes that these results make gastric tonometry "of interest largely as a research tool rather than as a useful clinical monitor for routine use [194]." Researchers are actively investigating the use of sublingual capnometry, a similar technology, as a potential resuscitation endpoint.

Transcutaneous Oxygen and Carbon Dioxide Measurement in Adults

Transcutaneous measurements of the partial pressures of oxygen ($PtcO_2$) and carbon dioxide ($PtcCO_2$) are frequently used for neonatal blood gas monitoring but have not gained widespread clinical acceptance in adult ICUs [175]. In adults, similar to gastric tonometry, $PtcO_2$ and $PtcCO_2$ reflect *local* tissue oxygen and carbon dioxide levels and therefore blur the boundary between assessment of global gas exchange and regional tissue perfusion monitoring. More recently, measurements of transcutaneous hemoglobin oxygen saturation (StO_2) have entered the research and clinical realms.

This section refers only to transcutaneous monitoring in adults.

Technique

Oxygen and carbon dioxide diffuse out of the capillaries, into the interstitium, and through the skin. The skin usually resists O_2 and CO_2 diffusion, but heating the skin promotes diffusion by changing the structure of the stratum corneum, shifting the oxygen dissociation curve, and promoting arterialization of dermal capillaries [175]. Transcutaneous systems take advantage of these properties to measure partial pressures of oxygen ($PtcO_2$) and carbon dioxide ($PtcCO_2$). Typically, a unit less than 1 inch in diameter is attached with an airtight seal to the skin with an adhesive. An electrode heats the skin to improve gas exchange; a temperature sensor measures skin temperature at the skin surface and adjusts the heater to provide a constant temperature—typically about 44°C. Oxygen and carbon dioxide diffuse out of the capillaries into the interstitium and through the skin to measuring electrodes.

Technical Limitations

Because units use electrodes for partial pressure measurement, problems with calibration and electrode drift during prolonged monitoring can clearly alter measurements. Drift may alter readings by up to 12% over a 2-hour period [210]. Because of the heating requirement, probe sites must be changed at least every 4 hours to prevent burns [211]. Units must be recalibrated whenever the probe temperature is changed and every 4 to 6 hours to prevent artifact from electrode drift. Many units take 15 to 60 minutes to warm the skin and establish stable readings. Probes must be firmly attached to the skin, or leaks from the surrounding atmosphere lower $PtcCO_2$ and alter $PtcO_2$ values. Adhesion is a problem in diaphoretic patients.

Thick or edematous skin provides a diffusion barrier that amplifies differences between arterial and transcutaneous pO_2 and pCO_2. The longer the distance the gases must diffuse to be measured, the more important are the effects of temperature, perfusion, and local metabolism. This appears to be the fundamental reason why transcutaneous measurements are usually more closely related to arterial values in neonates than in adults. Edema, burns, abrasions, or scleroderma would all be expected to alter transcutaneous values.

Clinical Usefulness and Limitations

Because $PtcO_2$ and $PtcCO_2$ reflect local pO_2 and pCO_2, they change in response both to regional perfusion/oxygen delivery and to global derangements. In stable, healthy adults without hemodynamic or respiratory instability, $PtcO_2$ and $PtcCO_2$ accurately reflect PaO_2 and $PaCO_2$ [176,210]. The measured transcutaneous values of oxygen and carbon dioxide are typically 10 mm Hg lower [177] and 5 to 23 mm Hg higher [212] than arterial values, respectively. In stable patients, it may be reasonable to use transcutaneously measured values as surrogates for arterial pO_2 and pCO_2. However, systemic hypoperfusion due to low cardiac output, regional hypoperfusion due to sepsis or shock, and local hypoperfusion due to cutaneous vasoconstriction caused by medication or cold produces discrepancies. In these cases, transcutaneous measurements cease to reflect arterial values and better track oxygen delivery and tissue metabolism [213]. For these reasons, many authors have argued against relying on $PtcO_2$ and $PtcCO_2$ to estimate arterial pO_2 and pCO_2 in critically ill adults [213,214].

Several studies have demonstrated the value of transcutaneous oxygen measurements as indices of perfusion or oxygen delivery. When PaO_2 remains constant, a decrease in $PtcO_2$ is probably due to changes in perfusion. Changes in local perfusion and metabolism may cause $PtcO_2$ values to fall to zero and $PtcCO_2$ values to climb to more than 30 mm Hg above arterial values [212]. During cardiac decompensation and arrest, $PtcO_2$ correlates best with cardiac output [215]. In hemorrhagic shock, the ratio of $PtCO_2$ to PaO_2 decreases, even though PaO_2 may remain normal [216]. Because the measurements are very sensitive to changes in flow, they can be useful in predicting or warning of imminent change before a blood pressure response is seen. In a small series of high-risk perioperative patients, declines in the $PtCO_2/PaO_2$ ratio predicted subsequent hemodynamic collapse [217]. Transcutaneous $PtcO_2$ also correlates with mortality. In emergency department patients with severe sepsis or septic shock, $PtcO_2$ was lower in nonsurvivors than survivors [218]. In trauma patients, $PtcO_2$ values were significantly higher in survivors than nonsurvivors ($p < 0.001$) with an area under the receiver operating characteristics curve of 0.74 for predicting in-hospital mortality [219].

Ongoing Development

More recent work has focused on the use of near-infrared spectroscopy to measure tissue hemoglobin oxygen saturation. This technique, rather than quantifying partial pressures of oxygen, instead measures the percent of microvascular hemoglobin saturated with oxygen. It has shown clinical correlations with invasive hemodynamic measures in sepsis [220] and severity of shock in trauma [221]. Further research is required to define the role of StO_2 as a potential resuscitation endpoint.

Summary

Transcutaneous monitors have little role in the ICU as simple tools to replace other means of measuring arterial gas. They predictably reflect arterial pO_2 and pCO_2 values only in hemodynamically stable patients, who are least likely to demand intensive care or to benefit from ICU monitoring. As monitors of trends in PCO_2 and PO_2, they can be regarded as effective only in the sense that they typically do not produce false-negative alarms—that is, if the arterial values change, the transcutaneous values reflect the change. So many other factors, such as changes in tissue edema and perfusion, may result in alterations in transcutaneous trends that the supervising staff can initially determine only that *something* has changed. An accurate interpretation of the clinical event usually requires reassessment of either cardiac status or arterial gases.

Therefore, transcutaneous monitors are inadequate cardiac monitors and inadequate pulmonary monitors but are good cardiopulmonary monitors. When perfusion is stable, values reflect gas exchange. When gas exchange is stable, values reflect perfusion. When both are unstable, the results cannot be interpreted without additional information. The use of near infrared spectroscopy to measure tissue hemoglobin oxygenation—StO_2—is a promising development, but one that requires further clinical study.

References

1. Peres Bota D, Lopes Ferreira F, Melot C, et al: Body temperature alterations in the critically ill. *Intensive Care Med* 30:811–816, 2004.
2. Kholoussy AM, Sufian S, Pavlides C: Central peripheral temperature gradient: its value and limitations in the management of critically ill surgical patients. *Am J Surg* 140(5):609–612, 1980.
3. Haupt MT, Bekes CE, Brilli RJ, et al: Guidelines on critical care services and personnel: recommendations based on a system of categorization of three levels of care. *Crit Care Med* 31:2677–2683, 2003.
4. Heinz J: Validation of sublingual temperatures in patients with nasogastric tubes. *Heart Lung* 14(2):128–130, 1985.
5. Myny D, De Waele J, Defloor T, et al: Temporal scanner thermometry: a new method of core temperature estimation in ICU patients. *Scott Med J* 50:15–18, 2005.
6. Cork RC, Vaughan RW, Humphrey LS: Precision and accuracy of intraoperative temperature monitoring. *Anesth Analg* 62(2):211–214, 1983.
7. Bone ME, Feneck RO: Bladder temperature as an estimate of body temperature during cardiopulmonary bypass. *Anaesthesia* 43(3):181–185, 1988.
8. Ramsay JG, Ralley FE, Whalley DG: Site of temperature monitoring and prediction of afterdrop after open heart surgery. *Can Anaesth Soc J* 32(6):607–612, 1985.

9. Crocker BD, Okumura F, McCuaig DI: Temperature monitoring during general anaesthesia. *Br J Anaesth* 52(12):1223–1229, 1980.
10. Severinghaus JW: Temperature gradients during hypothermia. *Ann N Y Acad Sci* 80:515–521, 1962.
11. Vale RJ: Monitoring of temperature during anesthesia. *Int Anesthesiol Clin* 19(1):61–84, 1981.
12. Giuliano KK, Scott SS, Elliot S, et al: Temperature measurement in critically ill orally intubated adults: a comparison of pulmonary artery core, tympanic, and oral methods. *Crit Care Med* 27:2188–2193, 1999.
13. Moran JL, Peter JV, Solomon PJ, et al: Tympanic temperature measurements: are they reliable in the critically ill? A clinical study of measures of agreement. *Crit Care Med* 35:155–164, 2007.
14. Amoateng-Adjepong Y, Del Mundo J, Manthous CA: Accuracy of infrared tympanic thermometer. *Chest* 115(4):1002–1005, 1999.
15. Camboni D, Philipp A, Schebesch KM, et al: Accuracy of core temperature measurement in deep hypothermic circulatory arrest. *Interact Cardiovasc Thorac Surg* 7:922–924, 2008.
16. Burgess GE III, Cooper JR, Marino RJ, et al: Continuous monitoring of skin temperature using a liquid-crystal thermometer during anesthesia. *South Med J* 71:516, 1978.
17. Roberts NH: The comparison of surface and core temperature devices. *J Am Assoc Nurse Anesth* 48:53, 1980.
18. Silverman RW, Lomax P: The measurement of temperature for thermoregulatory studies. *Pharmacol Ther* 27:233, 1985.
19. Terndrup TE, Rajk J: Impact of operator technique and device on infrared emission detection tympanic thermometry. *J Emerg Med* 10:683, 1992.
20. Farnell S, Maxwell L, Tan S, et al: Temperature measurement: comparison of non-invasive methods used in adult critical care. *J Clin Nurs* 14:632–639, 2005.
21. Suleman MI, Doufas AG, Akca O, et al: Insufficiency in a new temporal-artery thermometer for adult and pediatric patients. *Anesth Analg* 95:67–71, 2002, table of contents.
22. Pierce EC: Percutaneous arterial catheterization in man with special reference to aortography. *Surg Gynecol Obstet* 93:56, 1951.
23. Carrol GC: Blood pressure monitoring. *Crit Care Clin* 4:411, 1988.
24. Van Bergen FH, Weatherhead S, Treloar AE, et al: Comparison of direct and indirect methods of measuring arterial blood pressure. *Circulation* 10:481, 1954.
25. Bruner JM, Krenis LJ, Kunsman JM, et al: Comparison of direct and indirect methods of measuring arterial blood pressure: Pt III. *Med Instrum* 15:182, 1981.
26. Bailey RH, Knaus VL, Bauer JH: Aneroid sphygmomanometers: an assessment of accuracy at a university hospital and clinics. *Arch Intern Med* 151:1409, 1991.
27. Talke P, Nichols RJ Jr, Traber DL: Does measurement of systolic blood pressure with a pulse oximeter correlate with conventional methods? *J Clin Monit* 6:5–9, 1990.
28. Zagzebski JA, ed: *Physics and Instrumentation in Doppler and B-Mode Ultrasonography*. Orlando, FL: Grune & Stratton, 1986.
29. Hochberg HM, Salomon H: Accuracy of automated ultrasound blood pressure monitor. *Curr Ther Res Clin Exp* 13:129, 1971.
30. Puritan BC: *Infrasonde Model D4000 Electronic Blood Pressure Monitor Operating Manual*. Los Angeles: Puritan Bennett Corporation.
31. Nystrom E, Reid KH, Bennett R, et al: A comparison of two automated indirect arterial blood pressure meters: with recordings from a radial arterial catheter in anesthetized surgical patients. *Anesthesiology* 62:526, 1985.
32. Borow KM, Newberger JW: Non-invasive estimation of central aortic pressure using the oscillometric method for analyzing systemic artery pulsatile blood flow: comparative study of indirect systolic, diastolic, and mean brachial artery pressure with simultaneous direct ascending aortic pressure measurements. *Am Heart J* 103:879, 1982.
33. Van Egmond J, Hasenbros M, Crul JF: Invasive v. non-invasive measurement of arterial pressure. *Br J Anaesth* 57:434, 1985.
34. Bogert LW, van Lieshout JJ: Non-invasive pulsatile arterial pressure and stroke volume changes from the human finger. *Exp Physiol* 90:437–446, 2005.
35. O'Rourke MF, Adji A: An updated clinical primer on large artery mechanics: implications of pulse waveform analysis and arterial tonometry. *Curr Opin Cardiol* 20:275–281, 2005.
36. Steiner LA, Johnston AJ, Salvador R, et al: Validation of a tonometric noninvasive arterial blood pressure monitor in the intensive care setting. *Anaesthesia* 58:448–454, 2003.
37. Janelle GM, Gravenstein N: An accuracy evaluation of the T-Line Tensymeter (continuous noninvasive blood pressure management device) versus conventional invasive radial artery monitoring in surgical patients. *Anesth Analg* 102:484–490.2006.
38. Szmuk P, Pivalizza E, Warters RD, et al: An evaluation of the T-Line Tensymeter continuous noninvasive blood pressure device during induced hypotension. *Anaesthesia* 63:307–312, 2008.
39. Reder RF, Dimich I, Cohen ML: Evaluating indirect blood pressure measurement techniques: a comparison of three systems in infants and children. *Pediatrics* 62:326, 1978.
40. Yelderman M, Ream AK: Indirect measurement of mean blood pressure in the anesthetized patient. *Anesthesiology* 50:253, 1979.
41. Hirschl MM, Binder M, Herkner H, et al: Accuracy and reliability of noninvasive continuous finger blood pressure measurement in critically ill patients. *Crit Care Med* 24:1684, 1996.
42. Aitken HA, Todd JG, Kenny GN: Comparison of the Finapres and direct arterial pressure monitoring during profound hypotensive anesthesia. *Br J Anaesth* 67:36, 1991.
43. Rutten AJ, Isley AH, Skowronski GA, et al: A comparative study of the measurement of mean arterial blood pressure using automatic oscillometers, arterial cannulation and auscultation. *Anaesth Intensive Care* 14:58, 1986.
44. Stokes DN, Clutton-Brock T, Patil C, et al: Comparison of invasive and non-invasive measurements of continuous arterial pressure using the Finapres. *Br J Anaesth* 67:26–35, 1991.
45. Sy WP: Ulnar nerve palsy possibly related to use of automatically cycled blood pressure cuff. *Anesth Analg* :687, 1981.
46. Betts EK: Hazard of automated noninvasive blood pressure monitoring. *Anesthesiology* :717, 1981.
47. Bainbridge LC, Simmons HM, Elliot D: The use of automatic blood pressure monitors in the burned patient. *Br J Plast Surg* :322, 1990.
48. Hutton P, Prys-Roberts C: An assessment of the Dinamap 845. *Anaesthesia* :261, 1984.
49. Gardner RM, Schwarz R, Wong HC: Percutaneous indwelling radial-artery catheters for monitoring cardiovascular function. *N Engl J Med* :1227, 1974.
50. McNulty I, Katz E, Kim KY: Thrombocytopenia following heparin flush. *Prog Cardiovasc Nurs* 20:143–147, 2005.
51. Rothe CF, Kim KC: Measuring systolic arterial blood pressure: possible errors from extension tubes or disposable transducer domes. *Crit Care Med* :683, 1980.
52. Shinozaki T, Deane RS, Mazuzan JE: The dynamic responses of liquid filled catheter systems for direct measurements of blood pressure. *Anesthesiology*: 498, 1980.
53. Mermel LA, Farr BM, Sherertz RJ, et al: Guidelines for the management of intravascular catheter-related infections. *Clin Infect Dis* 32:1249–1272, 2001.
54. Koh DB, Gowardman JR, Rickard CM, et al: Prospective study of peripheral arterial catheter infection and comparison with concurrently sited central venous catheters. *Crit Care Med* 36:397–402, 2008.
55. Traore O, Liotier J, Souweine B: Prospective study of arterial and central venous catheter colonization and of arterial- and central venous catheter-related bacteremia in intensive care units. *Crit Care Med* 33:1276–1280, 2005.
56. Fraenkel DJ, Rickard C, Lipman J: Can we achieve consensus on central venous catheter-related infections? *Anaesth Intensive Care* 28:475–490, 2000.
57. Rijnders BJ, Van Wijngaerden E, Wilmer A, et al: Use of full sterile barrier precautions during insertion of arterial catheters: a randomized trial. *Clin Infect Dis* 36:743–748, 2003.
58. Davis FM, Stewart JM: Radial artery cannulation. *Br J Anaesth* :41, 1980.
59. Russell JA, Joel M, Hudson RJ: Prospective evaluation of radial and femoral artery catheterization sites in critically ill adults. *Crit Care Med* :936, 1983.
60. Scheer B, Perel A, Pfeiffer UJ: Clinical review: complications and risk factors of peripheral arterial catheters used for haemodynamic monitoring in anaesthesia and intensive care medicine. *Crit Care* 6:199–204, 2002.
61. Dorman T, Breslow MJ, Lipsett PA, et al: Radial artery pressure monitoring underestimates central arterial pressure during vasopressor therapy in critically ill surgical patients. *Crit Care Med* 26:1646–1649, 1998.
62. Arnal D, Garutti I, Perez-Pena J, et al: Radial to femoral arterial blood pressure differences during liver transplantation. *Anaesthesia* 60:766–771, 2005.
63. Mignini MA, Piacentini E, Dubin A: Peripheral arterial blood pressure monitoring adequately tracks central arterial blood pressure in critically ill patients: an observational study. *Crit Care* 10:R43, 2006.
64. Lorente L, Santacreu R, Martin MM, et al: Arterial catheter-related infection of 2,949 catheters. *Crit Care* 10:R83, 2006.
65. Winters SR: Diagnosis by wireless. *Sci Am* :465, 1921.
66. Drew BJ, Califf RM, Funk M, et al: Practice standards for electrocardiographic monitoring in hospital settings: an American Heart Association scientific statement from the Councils on Cardiovascular Nursing, Clinical Cardiology, and Cardiovascular Disease in the Young: endorsed by the International Society of Computerized Electrocardiology and the American Association of Critical-Care Nurses. *Circulation* 110:2721–2746, 2004.
67. Reinelt P, Karth GD, Geppert A, et al: Incidence and type of cardiac arrhythmias in critically ill patients: a single center experience in a medical-cardiological ICU. *Intensive Care Med* 27:1466–1473, 2001.
68. Brathwaite D, Weissman C: The new onset of atrial arrhythmias following major noncardiothoracic surgery is associated with increased mortality. *Chest* 114:462–468, 1998.
69. Kimball JT, Killip T: Aggressive treatment of arrhythmias in acute myocardial infarction: procedures and results. *Prog Cardiovasc Dis* :483, 1968.
70. Henkel DM, Witt BJ, Gersh BJ, et al: Ventricular arrhythmias after acute myocardial infarction: a 20-year community study. *Am Heart J* 151:806–812, 2006.
71. Vetter NJ, Julian DG: Comparison of arrhythmia computer and conventional monitoring in coronary-care unit. *Lancet* :1151, 1975.

72. Holmberg S, Ryden L, Waldenstrom A: Efficiency of arrhythmia detection by nurses in a coronary care unit using a decentralized monitoring system. *Br Heart J* :1019, 1977.
73. Romhilt DW, Bloomfield SS, Chou T: Unreliability of conventional electrocardiographic monitoring for arrhythmia detection in coronary care units. *Am J Cardiol* :457, 1973.
74. Watkinson WP, Brice MA, Robinson KS: A computer-assisted electrocardiographic analysis system: methodology and potential application to cardiovascular toxicology. *J Toxicol Environ Health* :713, 1985.
75. Alcover IA, Henning RJ, Jackson DL: A computer-assisted monitoring system for arrhythmia detection in a medical intensive care unit. *Crit Care Med* :888, 1984.
76. Badura FK: Nurse acceptance of a computerized arrhythmia monitoring system. *Heart Lung* :1044, 1980.
77. Clements FM, Bruijn NP: Noninvasive cardiac monitoring. *Crit Care Clin* : 435, 1988.
78. Mirvis DM, Berson AS, Goldberger AL: Instrumentation and practice standards for electrocardiographic monitoring in special care units. *Circulation* : 464, 1989.
79. Drew BJ, Pelter MM, Adams MG, et al: 12-lead ST-segment monitoring vs single-lead maximum ST-segment monitoring for detecting ongoing ischemia in patients with unstable coronary syndromes. *Am J Crit Care* 7:355–363, 1998.
80. Wehr G, Peters RJ, Khalife K, et al: A vector-based, 5-electrode, 12-lead monitoring ECG (EASI) is equivalent to conventional 12-lead ECG for diagnosis of acute coronary syndromes. *J Electrocardiol* 39:22–28, 2006.
81. Balaji S, Ellenby M, McNames J, et al: Update on intensive care ECG and cardiac event monitoring. *Card Electrophysiol Rev* 6:190–195, 2002.
82. Association for the Advancement of Medical I: *American National Standard for Cardiac Monitors, Heart Rate Meters, and Alarms (EC 13–1983)*. Arlington, VA: ANSI/AAMI, 1984.
83. Starmer CF, Whalen RE, McIntosh HD: Hazards of electric shock in cardiology. *Am J Cardiol* :537, 1964.
84. Pittman JV, Blum MS, Leonard MS: *Telemetry Utilization for Emergency Medical Services Systems*. Atlanta, Georgia Institute of Technology, 1974.
85. Tri JL, Severson RP, Firl AR, et al: Cellular telephone interference with medical equipment. *Mayo Clin Proc* 80:1286–1290, 2005.
86. Mithoefer JC, Bossman OG, Thibeault DW, et al: The clinical estimation of alveolar ventilation. *Am Rev Respir Dis* 98:868–871, 1968.
87. McFadden JP, Price RC, Eastwood HD: Raised respiratory rate in elderly patients: a valuable physical sign. *Br J Med* :626, 1982.
88. Krieger B, Feinerman D, Zaron A: Continuous noninvasive monitoring of respiratory rate in critically ill patients. *Chest* :632, 1986.
89. Knaus WA, Wagner DP, Draper EA, et al: The APACHE III prognostic system. Risk prediction of hospital mortality for critically ill hospitalized adults. *Chest* 100:1619–1636, 1991.
90. Cretikos MA, Bellomo R, Hillman K, et al: Respiratory rate: the neglected vital sign. *Med J Aust* 188:657–659, 2008.
91. Semmes BJ, Tobin MJ, Snyder JV, et al: Subjective and objective measurement of tidal volume in critically ill patients. *Chest* 87:577–579, 1985.
92. Shelly MP, Park GR: Failure of a respiratory monitor to detect obstructive apnea. *Crit Care Med* :836, 1986.
93. Sackner MA, Bizousky F, Krieger BP: Performance of impedance pneumograph and respiratory inductive plethysmograph as monitors of respiratory frequency and apnea. *Am Rev Respir Dis* :A41, 1987.
94. Wiklund L, Hok B, Stahl K, et al: Postanesthesia monitoring revisited: frequency of true and false alarms from different monitoring devices. *J Clin Anesth* 6:182–188, 1994.
95. Lovett PB, Buchwald JM, Sturmann K, et al: The vexatious vital: neither clinical measurements by nurses nor an electronic monitor provides accurate measurements of respiratory rate in triage. *Ann Emerg Med* 45:68–76, 2005.
96. Tsien CL, Fackler JC: Poor prognosis for existing monitors in the intensive care unit. *Crit Care Med* 25:614–619, 1997.
97. Chadha TS, Watson H, Birch S, et al: Validation of respiratory inductive plethysmography using different calibration procedures. *Am Rev Respir Dis* 125:644–649, 1982.
98. Sackner MA, Watson H, Belsito AS: Calibration of respiratory inductive plethysmograph during natural breathing. *J Appl Physiol* :410, 1989.
99. Tobin MJ, Jenouri G, Lind B: Validation of respiratory inductive plethysmography in patients with pulmonary disease. *Chest* :615, 1983.
100. Wolf GK, Arnold JH: Noninvasive assessment of lung volume: respiratory inductance plethysmography and electrical impedance tomography. *Crit Care Med* 33:S163–S169, 2005.
101. Stradling JR, Chadwick GA, Quirk C, et al: Respiratory inductance plethysmography: calibration techniques, their validation and the effects of posture. *Bull Eur Physiopathol Respir* 21:317–324, 1985.
102. Neumann P, Zinserling J, Haase C, et al: Evaluation of respiratory inductive plethysmography in controlled ventilation: measurement of tidal volume and PEEP-induced changes of end-expiratory lung volume. *Chest* 113:443–451, 1998.
103. Tobin MJ, Guenther SM, Perez W: Konno-Mead analysis of ribcage-abdominal motion during successful and unsuccessful trials of weaning from mechanical ventilation. *Am Rev Respir Dis* :1320, 1987.
104. Hoffman RA, Ershowsky P, Krieger BP: Determination of auto-PEEP during spontaneous and controlled ventilation by monitoring changes in end-expiratory thoracic gas volume. *Chest* :613, 1989.
105. Krieger BP, Ershowsky P, Spivack D: One year's experience with a noninvasively monitored intermediate care unit for pulmonary patients. *JAMA* 264:1143–1146, 1990.
106. O'Brien MJ, Van Eykern LA, Oetomo SB, et al: Transcutaneous respiratory electromyographic monitoring. *Crit Care Med* 15:294–299, 1987.
107. Mower WR, Sachs C, Nicklin EL: A comparison of pulse oximetry and respiratory rate in patient screening. *Respir Med* :593, 1996.
108. Brown LH, Manring EA, Korengay HB: Can prehospital personnel detect hypoxemia without the aid of pulse oximetry. *Am J Emerg Med* :43, 1996.
109. Jensen LA, Onyskiw JE, Prasad NG: Meta-analysis of arterial oxygen saturation monitoring by pulse oximetry in adults. *Heart Lung* 27:387–408, 1998.
110. Stoneham MD, Saville GM, Wilson IH: Knowledge about pulse oximetry among medical and nursing staff. *Lancet* :1339, 1994.
111. Huch A, Huch R, Konig V: Limitations of pulse oximetry. *Lancet* :357, 1988.
112. New W: Pulse oximetry. *J Clin Monit* :126, 1985.
113. Moller JT, Pederen T, Rasmussen LS: Randomized evaluation of pulse oximetry in 20,802 patients: I. Design, demography, pulse oximeter failure rate, and overall complications rate. *Anesthesiology* :436, 1993.
114. Choe H, Tashiro C, Fukumitsu K: Comparison of recorded values from six pulse oximeters. *Crit Care Med* :678, 1989.
115. Severinghaus JW, Naifeh KH, Koh SO: Errors in 14 pulse oximeters during profound hypoxia. *J Clin Monit* :72, 1989.
116. Barker SJ, Hyatt J, Shah NK: The effect of sensor malpositioning on pulse oximetry accuracy during hypoxemia. *Anesthesiology* :248, 1993.
117. Severinghaus JW, Naifeh KH. Accuracy of responses of six pulse oximeters to profound hypoxia. *Anesthesiology* :551, 1987.
118. Reynolds LM, Nicolson SC, Steven JM: Influence of sensor site location on pulse oximetry kinetics in children. *Anesth Analg* :751, 1993.
119. Cheng EY, Hopwood MB, Kay J: Forehead pulse oximetry compared with finger pulse oximetry and arterial blood gas measurement. *J Clin Monit* : 223, 1988.
120. Evans ML, Geddes LA: An assessment of blood vessel vasoactivity using photoplethysmography. *Med Instrum* :29, 1988.
121. Tweedie IE: Pulse oximeters and finger nails. *Anaesthesia* :268, 1989.
122. Read MS: Effect of transparent adhesive tape on pulse oximetry. *Anesth Analg* :701, 1989.
123. Cote CJ, Goldstein EA, Fuchsman WH: The effect of nail polish on pulse oximetry. *Anesth Analg* :683, 1988.
124. Brand TM, Brand ME, Jay GD: Enamel nail polish does not interfere with pulse oximetry among normoxic volunteers. *J Clin Monit Comput* 17:93–96, 2002.
125. Chan MM, Chan MM, Chan ED: What is the effect of fingernail polish on pulse oximetry? *Chest* 123:2163–2164, 2003.
126. Ries AL, Prewitt LM, Johnson JJ: Skin color and ear oximetry. *Chest* :287, 1989.
127. Adler JN, Hughes LA, Vivilecchia R, et al: Effect of skin pigmentation on pulse oximetry accuracy in the emergency department. *Acad Emerg Med* 5:965–970, 1998.
128. Bothma PA, Joynt GM, Lipman J: Accuracy of pulse oximetry in pigmented patients. *S Afr Med J* :594, 1996.
129. Costarino AT, Davis DA, Keon TP: Falsely normal saturation reading with the pulse oximeter. *Anesthesiology* :830, 1987.
130. Hanowell L, Eisele JH Jr, Downs D: Ambient light affects pulse oximeters. *Anesthesiology* :864, 1987.
131. Block FE Jr: Interference in a pulse oximeter from a fiberoptic light source. *J Clin Monit* :210, 1987.
132. Brooks TD, Paulus DA, Winkle WE: Infrared heat lamps interfere with pulse oximeters. *Anesthesiology* :630, 1984.
133. Amar D, Neidzwski J, Wald A: Fluorescent light interferes with pulse oximetry. *J Clin Monit* :135, 1989.
134. Fluck RR Jr, Schroeder C, Frani G, et al: Does ambient light affect the accuracy of pulse oximetry? *Respir Care* 48:677–680, 2003.
135. Gehring H, Hornberger C, Matz H, et al: The effects of motion artifact and low perfusion on the performance of a new generation of pulse oximeters in volunteers undergoing hypoxemia. *Respir Care* 47:48–60, 2002.
136. Beall SN, Moorthy SS: Jaundice, oximetry, and spurious hemoglobin desaturation. *Anesth Analg* :806, 1989.
137. Veyckemans F, Baele P, Guillaume JE: Hyperbilirubinemia does not interfere with hemoglobin saturation measured by pulse oximetry. *Anesthesiology* : 118, 1989.
138. Moore TJ, Walsh CS, Cohen MR: Reported adverse event cases of methemoglobinemia associated with benzocaine products. *Arch Intern Med* 164:1192–1196, 2004.
139. Watcha MF, Connor MT, Hing AV: Pulse oximetry in methemoglobinemia. *Am J Dis Child* :845, 1989.
140. Reynolds KJ, Palayiwa E, Moyle JTB: The effect of dyshemoglobins on pulse oximetry: I. Theoretical approach. II. Experimental results using an in vitro system. *J Clin Monit* :81, 1993.
141. Barker SJ, Tremper KK: The effect of carbon monoxide inhalation on pulse oximetry and transcutaneous PO_2. *Anesthesiology* :677, 1987.

142. Buckley RG, Aks SE, Eshom JL: The pulse oximetry gap in carbon monoxide intoxication. *Ann Emerg Med* :252, 1994.
143. Glass KL, Dillard TA, Phillips YY: Pulse oximetry correction for smoking exposure. *Mil Med* :273, 1996.
144. Coburn RF, Williams WJ, Kahn SB: Endogenous carbon monoxide production in patients with hemolytic anemia. *J Clin Invest* :460, 1966.
145. Lopez-Herce J, Borrego R, Bustinza A, et al: Elevated carboxyhemoglobin associated with sodium nitroprusside treatment. *Intensive Care Med* 31:1235–1238, 2005.
146. Barker SJ, Badal JJ: The measurement of dyshemoglobins and total hemoglobin by pulse oximetry. *Curr Opin Anaesthesiol* 21:805–810, 2008.
147. Lee SE, Tremper KK, Barker SJ: Effects of anemia on pulse oximetry and continuous mixed venous oxygen saturation monitoring in dogs. *Anesth Analg* :S130, 1988.
148. Jay GD, Hughes L, Renzi FP: Pulse oximetry is accurate in acute anemia from hemorrhage. *Ann Emerg Med* :32, 1994.
149. Cane RD, Harrison RA, Shapiro BA: The spectrophotometric absorbance of intralipid. *Anesthesiology* :53, 1980.
150. Sehgal LR, Sehgal HL, Rosen AL, et al: Effect of Intralipid on measurements of total hemoglobin and oxyhemoglobin in whole blood. *Crit Care Med* 12:907–909, 1984.
151. Gabrielczyk MR, Buist RJ: Pulse oximetry and postoperative hypothermia: an evaluation of the Nellcor N-100 in a cardiac surgical intensive care unit. *Anaesthesia* :402, 1988.
152. Rieder HU, Frei FJ, Zbinden AM: Pulse oximetry in methemoglobinemia: failure to detect low oxygen saturation. *Anaesthesia* :326, 1989.
153. Scheller MS, Unger RJ, Kelner MJ: Effects of intravenously administered dyes on pulse oximetry readings. *Anesthesiology* :550, 1986.
154. Unger R, Scheller MS: More on dyes and pulse oximeters. *Anesthesiology* : 148, 1987.
155. Koivusalo AM, Von Smitten K, Lindgren L: Sentinel node mapping affects intraoperative pulse oximetric recordings during breast cancer surgery. *Acta Anaesthesiol Scand* 46:411–414, 2002.
156. Barker SJ: "Motion-resistant" pulse oximetry: a comparison of new and old models. *Anesth Analg* 95:967–972, 2002. [Table of contents.]
157. Morris RW, Nairn M, Torda TA: A comparison of fifteen pulse oximeters: I: a clinical comparison. II: a test of performance under conditions of poor perfusion. *Anaesth Intensive Care* :62, 1989.
158. Palve H, Vuori A: Pulse oximetry during low cardiac output and hypothermia states immediately after open heart surgery. *Crit Care Med* :66, 1989.
159. Paulus DA: Cool fingers and pulse oximetry. *Anesthesiology* :168, 1989.
160. Stewart KG, Rowbottom SJ: Inaccuracy of pulse oximetry in patients with severe tricuspid regurgitation. *Anaesthesia* :668, 1991.
161. Critical Care Services and Personnel: Recommendations based on a system of categorization into two levels of care. American College of Critical Care Medicine of the Society of Critical Care Medicine. *Crit Care Med* 27:422–426, 1999.
162. Smith DC, Canning JJ, Crul JF: Pulse oximetry in the recovery room. *Anaesthesia* :345, 1989.
163. Tyler IL, Tantisera B, Winter PM: Continuous monitoring of arterial oxygen saturation with pulse oximetry during transfer to the recovery room. *Anesth Analg* :1108, 1985.
164. Moller JT, Johannenssen NW, Espersen K: Randomized evaluation of pulse oximetry in 20,802 patients: II. Perioperative events and postoperative complications. *Anesthesiology* :423, 1993.
165. Guggenberger H, Lenz G, Federle R: Early detection of inadvertent esophageal intubation: pulse oximetry vs. capnography. *Acta Anaesthesiol Scand* :112, 1989.
166. Stein PD, Goldhaber SZ, Henry JW, et al: Arterial blood gas analysis in the assessment of suspected acute pulmonary embolism. *Chest* 109:78–81, 1996.
167. Stock MC: Noninvasive carbon dioxide monitoring. *Crit Care Clin* :511, 1988.
168. Schena J, Thompson J, Crone R: Mechanical influences on the capnogram. *Crit Care Med* :672, 1984.
169. Murray IP, Modell JM: Early detection of endotracheal tube accidents by monitoring of carbon dioxide concentration in respiratory gas. *Anesthesiology* :344, 1983.
170. Garnett AR, Ornato JP, Gonzalez ER, et al: End-tidal carbon dioxide monitoring during cardiopulmonary resuscitation. *Jama* 257:512–515, 1987.
171. Grmec S: Comparison of three different methods to confirm tracheal tube placement in emergency intubation. *Intensive Care Med* 28:701–704, 2002.
172. Raemer DB, Francis D, Philip JH: Variation in PCO_2 between arterial blood and peak expired gas during anesthesia. *Anesth Analg* :1065, 1983.
173. Morley TF, Giaimo J, Maroszan E: Use of capnography for assessment of the adequacy of alveolar ventilation during weaning from mechanical ventilation. *Am Rev Respir Dis* :339, 1993.
174. Jardin F, Genevray B, Pazin M: Inability to titrate PEEP in patients with acute respiratory failure using end tidal carbon dioxide measurements. *Anesthesiology* :530, 1985.
175. Lima A, Bakker J: Noninvasive monitoring of peripheral perfusion. *Intensive Care Med* 31:1316–1326, 2005.
176. Rooth G, Hedstrand U, Tyden H: The validity of the transcutaneous oxygen tension method in adults. *Crit Care Med* :162, 1976.
177. Gothgen I, Jacobsen E: Transcutaneous oxygen tension measurement: I. Age variation and reproducibility. *Acta Anaesthesiol Scand* :66, 1978.
178. Tremper KK, Waxman K, Shoemaker WC: Use of transcutaneous oxygen sensors to titrate PEEP. *Ann Surg* :206, 1981.
179. Cerny V, Cvachovec K: Gastric tonometry and intramucosal pH–theoretical principles and clinical application. *Physiol Res* 49:289–297, 2000.
180. Reilly PM, Wilkins KB, Fuh KC, et al: The mesenteric hemodynamic response to circulatory shock: an overview. *Shock* 15:329–343, 2001.
181. Dantzker DR: The gastrointestinal tract. The canary of the body? *Jama* 270:1247–1248, 1993.
182. Bergofsky EM: Determination of tissue O_2 tensions by hollow visceral tonometers: effects of breathing enriched O_2 mixtures. *J Clin Invest* :193, 1964.
183. Dawson AM, Trenchard D, Guz A: Small bowel tonometry: assessment of small gut mucosal oxygen tension in dog and man. *Nature* :943, 1965.
184. Kivisaari J, Niinikoski J: Use of Silastic tube and capillary sampling technic in the measurement of tissue pO_2 and pCO_2. *Am J Surg* :623, 1973.
185. Fiddian-Green RG, Pittenger G, Whitehouse WM: Back-diffusion of CO_2 and its influence on the intramural pH in gastric mucosa. *J Surg Res* :39, 1982.
186. Fiddian-Green RG: Tonometry: theory and applications. *Intensive Care World* :1, 1992.
187. Fiddian-Green RG: Gastric intramucosal pH, tissue oxygenation and acid-base balance. *Br J Anaesth* 74:591–606, 1995.
188. Schlichtig R, Mehta N, Gayowski TJ: Tissue-arterial PCO_2 difference is a better marker of ischemia than intramural pH (pHi) or arterial pH-pHi difference. *J Crit Care* 11:51–56, 1996.
189. Marshall AP, West SH: Gastric tonometry and monitoring gastrointestinal perfusion: using research to support nursing practice. *Nurs Crit Care* 9:123–133, 2004.
190. Riddington D, Venkatesh B, Clutton-Brock T, et al: Measuring carbon dioxide tension in saline and alternative solutions: quantification of bias and precision in two blood gas analyzers. *Crit Care Med* 22:96–100, 1994.
191. Heard SO, Helsmoortel CM, Kent JC: Gastric tonometry in healthy volunteers: effect of ranitidine on calculated intramural pH. *Crit Care Med* :271, 1991.
192. Marik PE, Lorenzana A: Effect of tube feedings on the measurement of gastric intramucosal pH. *Crit Care Med* :1498, 1996.
193. Marshall AP, West SH: Gastric tonometry and enteral nutrition: a possible conflict in critical care nursing practice. *Am J Crit Care* 12:349–356, 2003.
194. Beale RJ, Hollenberg SM, Vincent JL, et al: Vasopressor and inotropic support in septic shock: an evidence-based review. *Crit Care Med* 32:S455–S465, 2004.
195. Mohsenifar Z, Hay A, Hay J, et al: Gastric intramural pH as a predictor of success or failure in weaning patients from mechanical ventilation. *Ann Intern Med* 119:794–798, 1993.
196. Fiddian-Green RG, Baker S: Predictive value of the stomach wall pH for complications after cardiac operations: comparison with other monitoring. *Crit Care Med* :153, 1987.
197. Landow L, Phillips DA, Heard SO: Gastric tonometry and venous oximetry in cardiac surgery patients. *Crit Care Med* :1226, 1991.
198. Friedman G, Berlot G, Kahn RJ, et al: Combined measurements of blood lactate concentrations and gastric intramucosal pH in patients with severe sepsis. *Crit Care Med* 23:1184–1193, 1995.
199. Kirton OC, Windsor J, Wedderburn R, et al: Failure of splanchnic resuscitation in the acutely injured trauma patient correlates with multiple organ system failure and length of stay in the ICU. *Chest* 113:1064–1069, 1998.
200. Maynard N, Bihari D, Beale R, et al: Assessment of splanchnic oxygenation by gastric tonometry in patients with acute circulatory failure. *Jama* 270:1203–1210, 1993.
201. Keenan SP, Guyatt GH, Sibbald WJ, et al: How to use articles about diagnostic technology: gastric tonometry. *Crit Care Med* 27:1726–1731, 1999.
202. Gutierrez G, Palizas F, Doglio G, et al: Gastric intramucosal pH as a therapeutic index of tissue oxygenation in critically ill patients. *Lancet* 339:195–199, 1992.
203. Heritier SR, Gebski VJ, Keech AC: Inclusion of patients in clinical trial analysis: the intention-to-treat principle. *Med J Aust* 179:438–440, 2003.
204. Gomersall CD, Joynt GM, Freebairn RC, et al: Resuscitation of critically ill patients based on the results of gastric tonometry: a prospective, randomized, controlled trial. *Crit Care Med* 28:607–614, 2000.
205. Splanchnic hypoperfusion-directed therapies in trauma: a prospective, randomized trial. *Am Surg* 71:252–260, 2005.
206. Ivatury RR, Simon RJ, Islam S, et al: A prospective randomized study of end points of resuscitation after major trauma: global oxygen transport indices versus organ-specific gastric mucosal pH. *J Am Coll Surg* 183:145–154, 1996.
207. Marik PE: Sublingual capnography: a clinical validation study. *Chest* 120:923–927, 2001.

208. Marik PE, Bankov A: Sublingual capnometry versus traditional markers of tissue oxygenation in critically ill patients. *Crit Care Med* 31:818–822, 2003.
209. Press Release: Nellcor announces nationwide voluntary recall of all Capno-Probe sublingual sensors. Nellcor, Inc., 2004. Accessed April 21, 2006, at http://www.fda.gov/cdrh/recalls/recall-082404-pressrelease.html.
210. Wimberley PD, Pedersen KG, Thode J: Transcutaneous and capillary pCO_2 and pO_2 measurements in healthy adults. *Clin Chem*:1471, 1983.
211. Wimberley PD, Burnett RW, Covington AK, et al: Guidelines for transcutaneous pO_2 and pCO_2 measurement. *J Int Fed Clin Chem* 2:128–135, 1990.
212. Eletr S, Jimison H, Ream AK: Cutaneous monitoring of systemic PCO_2 on patients in the respiratory intensive care unit being weaned from the ventilator. *Acta Anaesthesiol Scand* :123, 1978.
213. Tremper KK, Shoemaker WC: Transcutaneous oxygen monitoring of critically ill adults, with and without low flow shock. *Crit Care Med* 9:706–709, 1981.
214. Hasibeder W, Haisjackl M, Sparr H, et al: Factors influencing transcutaneous oxygen and carbon dioxide measurements in adult intensive care patients. *Intensive Care Med* 17:272–275, 1991.
215. Tremper KK, Waxman K, Bowman R, et al: Continuous transcutaneous oxygen monitoring during respiratory failure, cardiac decompensation, cardiac arrest, and CPR. Transcutaneous oxygen monitoring during arrest and CPR. *Crit Care Med* 8:377–381, 1980.
216. Shoemaker WC, Fink S, Ray CW: Effect of hemorrhagic shock on conjunctival and transcutaneous oxygen tensions in relation to hemodynamic and oxygen transport changes. *Crit Care Med* :949, 1984.
217. Nolan LS, Shoemaker WC: Transcutaneous O_2 and CO_2 monitoring of high risk surgical patients during the perioperative period. *Crit Care Med*: 762, 1982.
218. Shoemaker WC, Wo CC, Yu S, et al: Invasive and noninvasive haemodynamic monitoring of acutely ill sepsis and septic shock patients in the emergency department. *Eur J Emerg Med* 7:169–175, 2000.
219. Shoemaker WC, Wo CC, Lu K, et al: Outcome prediction by a mathematical model based on noninvasive hemodynamic monitoring. *J Trauma* 60:82–90, 2006.
220. Mesquida J, Masip J, Gili G, et al: Thenar oxygen saturation measured by near infrared spectroscopy as a noninvasive predictor of low central venous oxygen saturation in septic patients. *Intensive Care Med* 35:1106–1109, 2009.
221. Crookes BA, Cohn SM, Bloch S, et al: Can near-infrared spectroscopy identify the severity of shock in trauma patients? *J Trauma* 58:806–813; discussion 813–816, 2005.

CHAPTER 27 ■ MINIMALLY INVASIVE HEMODYNAMIC MONITORING

ANDREW J. GOODWIN, EDNAN K. BAJWA AND ATUL MALHOTRA

INTRODUCTION

The assessment of cardiac output (CO) has historically been vital to the management of critically ill patients. The underlying nature of shock in a hypotensive patient may not be obvious clinically and is often multifactorial. In these circumstances, it is crucial to characterize what type of shock (i.e., distributive, cardiogenic, hypovolemic) is playing a role in a patient's presentation as well as how they will respond to interventions, such as volume loading. Determination of CO is thought to be a critical component of this process and thus has long been a matter of interest to clinicians.

The physical exam can be unreliable in assessing hemodynamics in systolic heart failure [1] and in critically ill patients without recent myocardial infarction [2]. As such, more dependable measurements may be required to treat such patients optimally. Since its introduction [3], the flow-directed pulmonary artery catheter (PAC) has been useful in obtaining measurements of CO and has been used both diagnostically as well as to gauge response to treatment. For many years, the PAC thermodilution technique was considered to be the "gold standard" of ICU hemodynamic measurement. This philosophy has been called into question over the last several years in light of mounting evidence that clinicians may be using the PAC ineffectively [4] and that morbidity and mortality in a variety of clinical situations are not improved with its use [5–7], but instead may be worsened [8,9].

In light of these studies, many clinicians have begun to question the importance and the credibility of the PAC. Some postulate that the lack of improvement in morbidity and mortality stems from the deleterious complications that are inherent to an invasive procedure. Others have shown that even when oxygen delivery in critically ill patients is known and is optimized or even increased to supranormal levels, there is no corresponding improvement in outcomes [10]. This gives rise to the notion that once tissue hypoperfusion results in organ dysfunction, a cycle of inflammation ensues which leads to irreversible organ damage if not corrected early. This concept has been described as "cytopathic hypoxia" where hypoperfusion leads to the disruption of the intracellular utilization of oxygen such that delivery of normal or supranormal amounts of oxygen to a cell will not restore its function [11,12]. More recently, some intensivists have questioned the notion of "cytopathic hypoxia" although the concept of mitochondrial failure in some ICU patients is relatively well accepted. Some data have emerged that suggest that correction of hypoperfusion and inadequate oxygen delivery early in the course of sepsis improves outcomes [13,14]. Interestingly, these studies did not use PACs, but instead used central venous oxygen saturation as a surrogate for CO and oxygen utilization. Two other possibilities may explain the failure of RCTs to show benefit to the PAC. Considerable data suggest inadequate knowledge among practitioners regarding the optimal use of PAC, making any hope of improving outcome unlikely under such circumstances. Alternatively, the failure of PAC trials may reflect failure of the protocols used to guide PAC treatment rather than failure of the PAC per se [15].

Many are focusing on alternative and less invasive methods of determining cardiac function. These methods can be divided into two broad categories: measurements of cardiac function and measurements of indices of oxygen delivery and/or tissue perfusion as surrogates for CO. The goal of this research has been to develop feasible minimally invasive techniques that provide accurate measurements in the ICU patient. In some cases, these studies have focused on adapting monitoring technology that is already routinely used in this patient population.

In this chapter, we focus on several emerging technologies being used to determine CO and tissue perfusion in the ICU. The methods of Doppler echocardiography, pulse contour analysis, partial carbon dioxide rebreathing, and gastric tonometry represent the modalities best studied to date. Consideration will also be given to new and developing methods such as sublingual capnometry and biomarkers. Given its known limitations in critically ill patients, thoracic bioimpedance will not be discussed in detail in this chapter. We will conclude with a summary of practice recommendations and future directions.

CARDIAC OUTPUT

CO is the amount of blood flow through the cardiovascular system over a period of time. Traditionally, it is reported in liters per minute and can be normalized for body surface area to provide the cardiac index. In the normal subject, CO is directly related to a subject's metabolic rate and oxygen consumption ($\dot{V}O_2$). The fundamental principles of CO will be described in more detail elsewhere in this text. The therapy for a hypotensive patient with diminished CO (cardiogenic shock) is fundamentally different from the therapy for a patient with diminished vascular tone (distributive shock). Therefore, an accurate knowledge of these variables is vital to the effective treatment of hypotension. The systemic vascular resistance is calculated from the ratio of pressure gradient (mean arterial pressure minus central venous pressure) to flow rate (CO). This formula assumes an Ohmic resistor (i.e., one with a linear pressure flow relationship). Because a fall in systemic vascular resistance could represent a decrease in blood pressure or a rise in CO, we favor the use of the primary measured variables in hemodynamic assessments. We would also suggest caution in the interpretation of changes in systemic vascular resistance in isolation, without consideration for underlying mechanism (e.g., changes in CO).

Traditionally, a number of techniques have been used for the assessment of cardiac function. Jugular venous pulsations, S3 gallop, and skin temperature have all been used to estimate CO with mixed results [16–18]. The pulmonary artery occlusion pressure (PAOP) and central venous pressure (CVP) have also been used as surrogates for left and right ventricular function, respectively. The PAOP is commonly used to establish the diagnosis of left heart failure in the hypotensive patient and is often used to guide resuscitation. Magder et al. demonstrated that the CVP could provide useful information about the volume status of critically ill patients [19,20]. Because the majority of the blood volume is in the systemic veins, and the right ventricle is the major determinant of CO, some would argue that the CVP should receive more attention as the focus of hemodynamic resuscitation protocols [21]. Unfortunately, PAOP and CVP only represent the end-diastolic pressures of their respective chambers. These variables do not always accurately translate into systolic function and CO. In addition, invasive assessment of PAOP [22,23] and clinical assessment of CVP [24] have been notoriously difficult to assess accurately and reliably.

Over the last few decades, considerable research has been devoted to the accurate measurement of CO by minimally invasive means. At present, there exist several modalities that are able to provide estimates of CO on a continuous or near-continuous basis. As described later, some have been established enough to warrant increasing use in clinical settings (esophageal Doppler, pulse contour analysis) while the clinical usefulness of others is still unclear (partial carbon dioxide rebreathing).

Esophageal Doppler

Background

To date, the esophageal Doppler (ED) has been one of the most rigorously studied noninvasive CO measurement modalities. Side et al. described ED in 1971 and it was later refined by Singer et al. [25,26]. This technique uses a Doppler probe placed in the esophagus to measure blood flow in the descending thoracic aorta. The ED uses the Doppler Shift principle, which implies that when a transmitted sound wave is impeded by a structure, the reflected sound wave will vary in a frequency dependent manner with the structure's characteristics. In the case of a fluid filled tube, such as the aorta, the magnitude of Doppler shift will vary in direct proportion to the velocity of flow in the tube (Fig. 27.1). Thus, the reflected sound wave can be used to determine flow velocity in the descending aorta. Multiplying this flow velocity by the ejection time and the cross-sectional area of the aorta provides an estimate of the stroke volume (SV). As this measurement does not account for the component of total stroke volume that travels to the coronary, carotid, and subclavian arteries, a correction factor must be applied to estimate the total SV. CO is then calculated by multiplying corrected stroke volume by the heart rate. The original versions of the ED system provided only Doppler shift data; therefore, the cross-sectional area of the aorta was estimated from a nomogram based on a patient's height, weight, and age. Subsequently, a combined Doppler and ultrasound probe has been introduced to provide estimates of both aortic flow velocity and cross-sectional area [27]. The descending aortic cross-sectional area measured by this model correlated very well with that measured by transesophageal echocardiography. In addition, aortic blood flow measured with this model was well correlated with CO as measured by thermodilution [27].

Beyond providing an estimate of CO, ED systems can provide information about the preload and the contractility of the heart. Singer et al. analyzed the flow-velocity waveform derived from an ED system and discovered that the corrected flow time (FT_c) correlated with preload [26,28] (Fig. 27.2). These studies further demonstrated that as preload was increased or

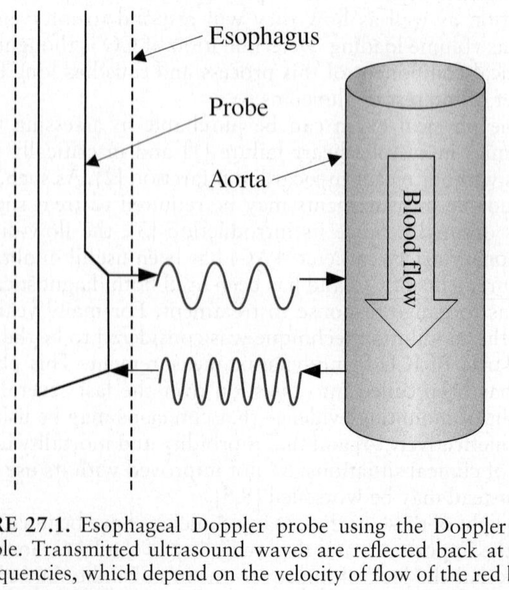

FIGURE 27.1. Esophageal Doppler probe using the Doppler Shift principle. Transmitted ultrasound waves are reflected back at varying frequencies, which depend on the velocity of flow of the red blood cells they encounter.

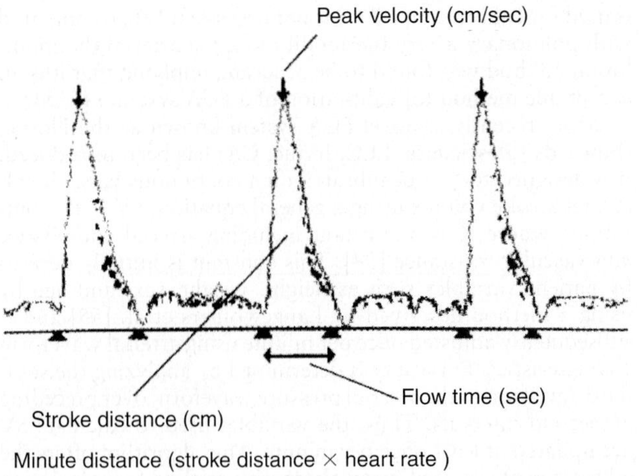

FIGURE 27.2. Esophageal Doppler flow-velocity waveform. (Adapted from Marik PE: Pulmonary artery catheterization and esophageal doppler monitoring in the ICU. *Chest* 116:1085–1091, 1999, with permission.)

decreased, the corrected flow time increased or decreased, respectively [26,28]. It is not clear, however, if following trends in FT_c in response to volume loading is superior to following trends to SV [29]. Wallmeyer et al. described a correlation between the peak velocity measured by Doppler and contractility measured by electromagnetic catheter measured flow [30]. Singer et al. further substantiated this finding by demonstrating that dobutamine infusions increased peak flow velocities measured by an ED system in a dose-dependent fashion [31]. These observations suggest that an experienced operator may be able to extrapolate useful hemodynamic parameters beyond the CO, through careful data synthesis.

Clinical Utility

The clinical usefulness of the ED system is still being determined. The majority of recent studies that have compared this system to the "gold standard" of thermodilution have been performed in either intraoperative or postoperative settings and have revealed mixed results. One single-center study of 35 patients that compared ED measurements of CO to simultaneous measurements of CO by thermodilution during off-pump coronary artery bypass graft showed very poor correlation between the two techniques [32]. Other studies, including a meta-analysis of 11 trials, have shown that ED systems are better at following changes in CO in response to fluid challenges than they are at measuring the absolute CO [33–35]. The authors of the meta-analysis also made an important point when discussing the reliability of comparing ED systems to thermodilution. They argued that the poor reproducibility inherent in the thermodilution technique will likely affect the limits of agreement between ED systems and thermodilution even if ED systems were reliable [33]. This concept was described by Bland and Altman [36] and has important implications when comparing the accuracy of absolute CO measured by any system when compared to thermodilution.

Advantages and Disadvantages

While comparing ED systems to thermodilution, technical advantages and disadvantages deserve consideration (Table 27.1). One advantage of the ED system is that it is continuous. Unlike the traditional bolus thermodilution techniques, an ED system can continuously display CO, which allows earlier recognition of hemodynamic deterioration or improvement in system responsiveness to a therapeutic intervention. In addition, an ED

TABLE 27.1

ADVANTAGES AND DISADVANTAGES OF THE ESOPHAGEAL DOPPLER SYSTEM FOR CARDIAC OUTPUT MONITORING

Concept: Doppler probe in the esophagus measures stroke volume in the descending aorta to estimate cardiac output.
Advantages
Continuous
Short set-up time
Low incidence of iatrogenic complications
Ability to leave in place for extended periods
Minimal training period required
Minimal infection risk
Disadvantages
High up-front cost
Can only be used in the intubated patient
May require frequent repositioning if patient is moved
High interobserver variability

probe can be placed in minutes and has been associated with a low incidence of major iatrogenic complications [37–39]. Some data suggest that once inserted, an esophageal probe can be left in situ safely for more than 2 weeks [40]. One study determined that the training required to become proficient in the use of ED consisted of no more than 12 patients [41]. Furthermore, as the esophagus is a nonsterile environment, it is logical to assume that the infectious risk of ED probe use is less than that of a PAC placed percutaneously.

There are also technical disadvantages to the ED system. One is the high up-front cost of the system itself as compared to the PAC apparatus. This cost may represent a very real limitation in the number of systems that a facility can purchase and maintain. This financial obstacle must be balanced with the likelihood that multiple patients would have need of this system simultaneously, which would necessitate multiple systems. Another disadvantage of this system is that it can only be used in the intubated patient. Although a large percentage of critically ill and/or surgical patients who would benefit from this system fit this criterion, the nonintubated patient would be more problematic. Additional concerns would include the likely need for repositioning or recalibration in the ICU patient. Though surgical patients are often immobile, ICU patients are often repositioned frequently to prevent skin breakdown or to facilitate improved oxygenation. Such movements will increase the chance of probe position changes that will require frequent calibration and repositioning. Finally, Roeck et al. suggested that there is significant interobserver variability when measuring changes in stroke volume in response to fluid challenges with ED [35]. Poor reproducibility may limit the utility of this system.

Future Research

As the ED is used more widely, outcome data will be crucial. To date, the majority of research has focused on the technique's validity and feasibility. One notable study which compared intraoperative ED use with conventional monitoring during femoral neck fracture repair found a faster recovery time and significantly shorter hospital stay in the ED group [42]. Similarly, Gan et al. demonstrated in a prospective randomized trial of patients undergoing major elective surgery that stroke volume optimization using ED shortened hospital length of stay and resumption of PO intake as compared to conventional intraoperative care [43]. This latter finding may be due to less gut hypoperfusion which has also been demonstrated with the use of ED [44]. A recent meta-analysis of nine trials of perioperative ED use also found improvements in length of stay as well as time to resuming an oral diet [45].

Although the above-mentioned data suggest that perioperative outcomes are improved with the use of ED, there are no robust parallel data for nonoperative ICU patients. The ultimate use of ED will depend on further outcome data, availability of equipment and local experience and expertise.

Pulse Contour Analysis

Background

Pulse Contour Analysis (PCA) is another modality for measuring CO noninvasively that has been extensively studied. This method relies on the theory, first described by Frank in the early part of the twentieth century, that SV and CO can be derived from the characteristics of an aortic pressure waveform [46]. Wesseling et al. eventually published in 1983 an algorithm to link mathematically SV and the pressure waveform [47]. This original version calculated SV continuously by dividing the area under the curve of the aortic pressure waveform by the aortic impedance. As aortic impedance varies between patients, it had to be measured using another modality to initially calibrate the PCA system. The calibration method usually employed was arterial thermodilution. Aortic impedance, however, is not a static property. It is based on the complex interaction of the resistive and compliant elements of each vascular bed, which are often dynamic, especially in hemodynamically unstable patients. Since the first PCA algorithm was introduced, several unique algorithms have been created to model accurately the properties of the human vascular system for use in PCA systems.

PCA involves the use of an arterial placed catheter with a pressure transducer, which can measure pressure tracings on a beat-to-beat basis. Such catheters are now routinely used in operating rooms and ICUs as they provide a continuous measurement of blood pressure that is superior to intermittent noninvasive measurements in hemodynamically unstable patients. These catheters are interfaced with a PCA system, which uses its unique algorithm as well as the initial aortic impedance calibration data from a thermodilution measurement of CO to provide a continuously displayed measurement of CO. Obviously, the reliability of a PCA system depends upon the accuracy of the algorithm that it employs. Because each algorithm is unique in the weight that it ascribes to each element of vascular conductivity, it is impossible to ensure that a system will be able to reproduce the results of another system under similar conditions [48]. Keeping this in mind, one cannot conclude that all systems are equally reliable.

PiCCO (Pulsion SG, Munich, Germany) is a PCA system that has received considerable attention in the literature. Numerous studies have demonstrated good correlation between this system and pulmonary thermodilution in both critically ill and surgical patients [49–53]. Notably, this system did not require recalibration during these study periods, which were performed under static ventricular loading conditions. The system involves the placement of a femoral arterial catheter that is passed into the abdominal aorta. In addition to a pressure transducer, the catheter also contains a thermistor for arterial thermodilution. The system is calibrated by injecting cold saline via a central venous catheter at the right atrium in a manner similar to pulmonary arterial thermodilution. Instead of using a thermistor in the pulmonary artery, however, the thermistor on the femoral arterial catheter allows calculation of CO. This initial value of CO is then used to calibrate the PCA system that is attached to the arterial catheter. Because the arterial catheter is used for calibration, a PAC is not necessary. When compared with pulmonary artery thermodilution, the arterial thermodilution method was found to be accurate, implying that it is an acceptable method for calibration of a PCA system [49–51].

More recently, a novel PCA system known as the Flotrac (Edwards Lifesciences, LLC, Irvine, CA) has been introduced. It is designed to "autocalibrate" on a continuous basis. It calculates stroke volume using a general equation: $SV = K \times$ pulsatility, where K is a constant including arterial compliance and vascular resistance [54]. This constant is initially derived by patient variables such as height, weight, sex, and age by using a method described by Langewouters et al. [55] and is subsequently adjusted once per minute using arterial waveform characteristics. Pulsatility is determined by analyzing the standard deviation of the arterial pressure waveform over preceding 20-second intervals. Thus, the variables used to calculate SV are updated at least once per minute. This algorithm offers the advantage of not needing an alternative method for calculating CO for calibration purposes. When compared to pulmonary artery catheter thermodilution in a postcardiac surgery setting, this system showed good correlation over a wide range of COs. In addition, it appears that a radial artery catheter is just as accurate as a femoral artery catheter in this setting, which is another advantage of this system [54].

Clinical Utility

As mentioned earlier, the initial trials studying PCA systems used data from static ventricular loading conditions. Both the critically ill and the intraoperative patient, however, often experience rapid changes in ventricular preload. The accuracy of the PiCCO system with dynamic changes in preload was addressed in a subsequent study, which used a modified algorithm. Felbinger et al. showed that changes in CO in response to preload could be accurately measured in a cardiac surgical ICU population when compared to pulmonary thermodilution [56].

Although being able to monitor changes in CO during volume loading is important, being able to predict *a priori* when a patient would benefit from volume loading is perhaps more useful. Pulse pressures commonly vary throughout the respiratory cycle. Pulse pressure variation (PPV) is defined as the result of the minimum pulse pressure subtracted from the maximum pulse pressure divided by the mean of these two pressures.

$$PPV = \frac{\text{Pulse Pressure}_{\max} - \text{Pulse Pressure}_{\min}}{\text{Pulse Pressure}_{\text{mean}}} \qquad (1)$$

The magnitude of the PPV in a patient can predict preload responsiveness [57–59]. Analogous to PPV, an additional piece of data that PCA systems can provide is the stroke volume variation (SVV). The SVV represents the change in percentage of SV over a preceding time period as a result of changes in SV due to ventilation. So far, the ability to use SVV to determine preload responsiveness has yielded mixed results. Reuter et al. found that SVV reliably decreased as cardiac index increased in response to preloading with colloids in ventilated postoperative cardiac surgical patients [60]. This finding supports the argument that the magnitude of SVV may be used to predict preload responsiveness. It is important to note that the tidal volumes used in this study were supraphysiologic (15 mL per kg), which results in a larger SVV and a resultant increase in the accuracy of this approach. Subsequently, another study used a smaller tidal volume (10 mL per kg) in a similar patient population and could not demonstrate a reliable relationship between SVV and an increase in cardiac index in response to preloading [61]. This finding suggests that when using lower tidal volume ventilation strategies, which are optimal for acute respiratory

TABLE 27.2

ADVANTAGES AND DISADVANTAGES OF THE PULSE CONTOUR ANALYSIS METHOD FOR CARDIAC OUTPUT MONITORING

Concept: Arterial catheter used to determine stroke volume from aortic pressure waveforms.
Advantages
Continuous
Uses catheters that are already commonly used in ICU patients
Does not require calibration with pulmonary artery catheter
Disadvantages
Likely unable to determine preload responsiveness during low tidal volume ventilation
Questionable accuracy during large changes in blood pressure
Questionable accuracy during vasoconstrictor use

distress syndrome (ARDS), PCA-derived SVV should not be used to estimate preload responsiveness.

Advantages and Disadvantages

Overall, the pulse contour analysis system offers several advantages over the traditional "gold standard" of pulmonary artery thermodilution (Table 27.2). Depending on the system, only an arterial catheter (Flotrac) or an arterial catheter and a central venous catheter (PiCCO) are required, both of which are commonly in place in critically ill and surgical patients. Thus, PACs and their possible risks can be avoided when using these systems. The PCA systems also provide a continuous measurement of CO as opposed to the intermittent nature of traditional thermodilution systems.

As with any system, there are disadvantages to the PCA system as well. The ability to use this system to determine preload responsiveness is questionable in patients who are being managed with recommended ventilatory strategies. In addition, some data suggest that in patients who have marked changes in blood pressure, the algorithm is not able to model adequately the changes in vascular resistance and compliance and, therefore, the accuracy of the measured CO declines [62]. Furthermore, a similar breakdown in the accuracy of measured CO has been suggested during the administration of vasoconstrictors [63], which are common in the critically ill patient.

Future Research

The clinical utility of the pulse contour analysis system is still being determined. Future studies that may help in defining the system's clinical role could focus on several points. First, a better understanding of how changes in blood pressure and vasoconstrictor use affect the accuracy of a particular system's algorithm will help to determine when a system needs to be recalibrated to maintain its accuracy. In addition, an analysis of how SVV predicts preload responsiveness at lower tidal volumes will provide more applicable information. Finally, a paucity of data regarding how PCA systems affect patient outcomes exists at present. Comparisons between the outcomes seen with this system and pulmonary artery thermodilution may provide convincing evidence about the real usefulness of PCA. In particular, the common question "will the patient respond to fluids?" may be replaced by the question "should the patient be given fluids?" once adequate outcome data are available.

Partial Carbon Dioxide Rebreathing Method

Background

The Fick equation for calculating CO has been known for over a 100 years. Its underlying principle states that for a gas (X) whose uptake in the lung is transferred completely to the blood, the ratio of that gas's consumption (VX) to the difference between the arterial (C_aX) and venous (C_vX) contents of the gas will equal the CO. In its original form, Fick used the example of oxygen (O_2) and described the following equation:

$$\text{Cardiac Output} = \frac{\dot{V}O_2}{C_aO_2 - C_vO_2} \quad (2)$$

For this equation to be accurate, several conditions must exist. The first is that blood flow through the pulmonary capillaries must be constant. In order for this to occur, the right and left ventricular outputs must be equal (i.e., steady state) and there must be no respiratory variation of pulmonary capillary flow. Another condition critical to this method's accuracy is an absence of shunts. As this method is dependent upon using gas exchange to calculate CO, any blood that does not participate in gas exchange will result in underestimation of CO. Furthermore, oxygen uptake by the lung itself must be minimal to maintain the integrity of this equation.

Although possible, the accurate measurement of $\dot{V}O_2$ is clinically challenging, especially in patients who require high FiO_2 [64]. This prompted investigators to focus on using carbon dioxide production ($\dot{V}CO_2$) in place of $\dot{V}O_2$ [65–67]. As $\dot{V}O_2$ is equal to $\dot{V}CO_2$ divided by the respiratory quotient, they determined that CO could be calculated by $\dot{V}CO_2$ divided by the arteriovenous difference between O_2 concentrations as well as the respiratory quotient (R). To measure O_2 concentrations continuously, arterial and venous oximeters were used to measure oxygen saturation (SO_2) and concentration was determined based on measured hemoglobin (Hgb) levels. This technique, therefore, relied upon the assumption that both R and hemoglobin levels remained constant during the measurement period.

$$\dot{V}O_2 = \frac{\dot{V}CO_2}{R} \quad (3)$$

$$C_aO_2 = 13.4 \times \text{Hgb} \times S_aO_2 \quad (4)$$

$$CO = \frac{\dot{V}CO_2}{13.4 \times \text{Hgb} \times R \times [S_aO_2 - S_vO_2]} \quad (5)$$

Using this method, one study found good correlation with CO determined by thermodilution [67]. The drawback to this approach, however, is the need for an invasive central venous catheter to measure accurately venous oxygen saturations as well as initially to calibrate the system and determine R. Subsequently, the partial carbon dioxide rebreathing method was introduced in an attempt to avoid the need for such catheters.

The partial CO_2 rebreathing method is based upon the Fick equation for CO_2 [68]:

$$CO = \frac{\dot{V}CO_2}{C_vCO_2 - C_aCO_2} \quad (6)$$

When using this method, a disposable rebreathing loop is placed between the endotracheal tube and the ventilator resulting in the rebreathing of carbon dioxide. A carbon dioxide sensor, an airflow sensor, and an arterial noninvasive pulse oximeter are then used to gather data before and after a period of CO_2 rebreathing. The CO_2 sensor and airflow monitor allow for the calculation of produced carbon dioxide ($\dot{V}CO_2$) both before and during the rebreathing period. Because CO does not change from baseline during rebreathing conditions [69], one can generate the following equation [68]:

$$CO = \frac{\dot{V}CO_{2_{baseline}}}{C_vCO_{2_{baseline}} - C_aCO_{2_{baseline}}} = \frac{\dot{V}CO_{2_{rebreathing}}}{C_vCO_{2_{rebreathing}} - C_aCO_{2_{rebreathing}}} \quad (7)$$

Gedeon et al. [70] determined that subtracting the rebreathing ratio from the baseline ratio yields the following equation [68]:

$$CO = \frac{\dot{V}CO_{2_{baseline}} - \dot{V}CO_{2_{rebreathing}}}{\left[C_vCO_{2_{baseline}} - C_aCO_{2_{baseline}}\right] - \left[C_vCO_{2_{rebreathing}} - C_aCO_{2_{rebreathing}}\right]} \quad (8)$$

As CO_2 diffuses rapidly into the blood, one can further assume that the mixed venous CO_2 concentration (C_vCO_2) remains unchanged between baseline and rebreathing conditions, that is, $C_vCO_{2_{baseline}} = C_vCO_{2_{rebreathing}}$. This allows for further simplification of the equation to the following [68]:

$$CO = \frac{\Delta\dot{V}CO_2}{\Delta C_aCO_2} \quad (9)$$

C_aCO_2 can be estimated from end-tidal carbon dioxide ($etCO_2$) and the carbon dioxide dissociation curve. Therefore, ΔC_aCO_2 can be substituted for by $\Delta etCO_2$ multiplied by the slope (S) of the dissociation curve [68]:

$$CO = \frac{\Delta\dot{V}CO_2}{\Delta etCO_2 \times S} \quad (10)$$

An estimate of CO can now be calculated using data that can be measured before and after a period of rebreathing, in addition to S, which can be determined from a carbon dioxide dissociation curve. It is important to note that the estimate of CO calculated using equation 10 only accounts for the blood that is able to participate in gas exchange. Any blood involved in a right to left intrapulmonary shunt is not considered by this equation; therefore, a correction factor must be incorporated to account for this shunted blood. This is determined by a partial rebreathing system by using the data collected from the noninvasive arterial oximeter, the FiO_2, and the PaO_2 as determined by arterial blood gases. These data allow one to determine an estimate of shunted blood using Nunn's iso-shunt tables [71].

Clinical Utility

So far, the results of comparisons between partial CO_2 rebreathing techniques and alternative methods of measuring CO have been mixed at best. Although some studies have demonstrated reasonable agreement with the "gold standard" of thermodilution [72–74], others have shown poor agreement [52,75,76]. One of these studies [76] did demonstrate good reproducibility of the results obtained from the partial rebreathing method despite the fact that they did not correlate with results obtained by thermodilution. One could infer from this that the method may have been appropriately precise but that something in its algorithm, that is, estimation of shunt or estimation of C_aCO_2 from $etCO_2$, prevented it from obtaining accurate results. This may be encouraging evidence that the partial rebreathing method can be an acceptable technique in certain clinical situations as the accuracy of currently marketed systems is improved.

Determining which clinical situations are appropriate for the partial rebreathing method is critical when considering its use. Because the method's accuracy depends upon an estimate of C_aCO_2 from $etCO_2$ as well as an estimate of shunt, clinical situations that affect these estimates may not be appropriate for using this method. For instance, post-operative cardiac surgical patients tend to have increased pulmonary dead space and shunt [77] and may not be an appropriate population for partial CO_2 rebreathing monitor use [76]. In addition, some data suggest that the correlation between this method and thermodilution declines as the amount of venous admixture from shunting increases in animal models [78]. In order for C_aCO_2 to be estimated accurately by $etCO_2$, gas exchange needs to be somewhat homogenous throughout the lung. One of the hallmarks of acute lung injury (ALI) and ARDS is a heterogeneous pattern of injury and fibrosis. This heterogeneity results in a large variation of gas exchange throughout the lung. Consequently, the $etCO_2$ may be a poor estimate of C_aCO_2 leading to an important source of error. Indeed, one study, which compared the partial CO_2 rebreathing method to thermodilution in patients with varying degrees of ALI, found poor agreement between the two methods [79]. The disagreement intensified with worsening severity of ALI. Finally, significant variations in tidal volume during a period of measurement will often markedly affect the accuracy of $\dot{V}CO_2$ on a breath-to-breath basis. Consequently, the accuracy of measured CO is limited in situations of varying tidal volume such as pressure support ventilation [80].

Advantages and Disadvantages

The most notable advantage of the partial CO_2 rebreathing method is its true noninvasive nature. With the exception of the arterial blood gases used to estimate shunt, this method does not require any additional invasive procedures. In addition, CO can be measured on a near-continuous basis. However, the disadvantages of the system are substantial (Table 27.3). It is challenging to use in patients who are not intubated or in intubated patients with spontaneous ventilation. Its accuracy is questionable in patients with intrapulmonary shunt and lung injury, which are both common findings in the ICU. Because the technique raises arterial PCO_2, its safety in patients with hypercapnia or increased intracranial pressure is unknown. Each system also represents an important fixed cost but can only be used by one patient at any given time. The limited clinical utility of these systems may not justify this expenditure.

TABLE 27.3

ADVANTAGES AND DISADVANTAGES OF THE PARTIAL CARBON DIOXIDE REBREATHING METHOD FOR CARDIAC OUTPUT MONITORING

Concept: Using exhaled carbon dioxide to determine cardiac output using a modified Fick equation
Advantages
Truly noninvasive
Nearly continuous
Disadvantages
High up-front cost
Can only be used in the intubated patient
Questionable accuracy in patients with lung injury
Unclear risk in patients with hypercapnia or increased intracranial pressure

Future Research

At present, the clinical applicability of partial CO_2 rebreathing systems is not completely known. Future research should focus on further examining the accuracy of these systems in patients with lung injury as the current data are limited. Improvements of existing algorithms for shunt and C_aCO_2 estimation could also aid in increasing this method's generalizability. Finally, determining if this method's noninvasive nature truly makes a difference in clinical outcomes should be an important focus of upcoming investigation. In critically ill patients, there may be no major advantage to using monitoring techniques that avoid central lines and arterial lines since these are nearly ubiquitous in the ICU.

OXYGEN DELIVERY AND TISSUE PERFUSION

Although directly measuring CO can provide information vital to the management of critically ill patients, one can also argue that accurate knowledge of oxygen delivery and/or adequacy of tissue perfusion can be similarly useful. Proponents of this concept are less interested in the absolute CO as long as adequate oxygen is delivered to tissues. One of the traditional techniques used to assess oxygen delivery is the mixed venous oxygen saturation ($S_{mv}O_2$). The $S_{mv}O_2$ is measured by sampling blood from the pulmonary artery, which is representative of the venous return from both the superior and inferior vena cava after sufficient mixing. $S_{mv}O_2$ is dependent on both systemic oxygen delivery (DO_2) as well as systemic oxygen consumption ($\dot{V}O_2$). Because $\dot{V}O_2$ does not dramatically change in the absence of major metabolic derangements, decreases in $S_{mv}O_2$ can be considered to be due to decreases in DO_2 (and, thereby, CO) in many patients. As a result, investigators have focused on the clinical utility of measuring $S_{mv}O_2$ as a surrogate means of monitoring CO [81,82]. Pearson et al. found that $S_{mv}O_2$ monitoring did not improve length of ICU stay or length of vasopressor requirement when compared to traditional pulmonary artery catheter use and CVP monitoring. In addition, $S_{mv}O_2$ monitoring cost more [83].

Another potential drawback of $S_{mv}O_2$ monitoring is the need for PAC and the possible associated risks. Because many critically ill patients receive central venous catheters, some research has focused on using central venous oxygen saturations ($S_{cv}O_2$) rather than $S_{mv}O_2$. One early study found that $S_{cv}O_2$ tended to be approximately 5% to 10% lower than $S_{mv}O_2$ in humans [84]. While studying dogs, Reinhart et al. found good correlation ($r = 0.96$) between the two [85]. So far, clinical data using this variable are limited, however, the previously mentioned landmark trial by Rivers et al. used $S_{cv}O_2$ among other variables with success [13,14].

In addition to estimating oxygen delivery, recent research has focused on estimating tissue perfusion as a guide for resuscitative therapy. With this approach, the adequacy of blood and oxygen delivery is assessed by measuring markers of hypoperfusion of accessible organs. We will focus on three modalities that have demonstrated considerable promise in this field to date: gastric tonometry, sublingual capnometry, and cardiac biomarkers.

Gastric Tonometry

Background

Mounting evidence that early correction of hypoperfusion in shock improves mortality [13,14,86] has led investigators to focus on the development of methods for its early detection. Tissue levels of CO_2 rise early in the setting of hypoperfusion [87–89]. The level of CO_2 in a tissue is determined by the balance between the concentration of arterial CO_2(C_aCO_2), blood flow to the tissue, and CO_2 production by the tissue. In a state of hypoperfusion, CO_2 increase is thought to be multifactorial. Carbon dioxide production increases in hypoperfused tissue to buffer the increase in hydrogen ions generated by the hydrolysis of ATP during glycolysis [90]. In addition, the low flow state seen in hypoperfusion results in an impaired clearance of CO_2 causing a further increase in tissue CO_2 concentrations [91]. This impaired clearance is likely the largest contributor to tissue hypercapnia in states of hypoperfusion [92]. The complex mucosal circulation of the gut results in the recirculation of CO_2 as well as arteriovenous O_2 shunting, which is exacerbated by the low-flow state of hypoperfusion. As a result, the gut mucosa is one of the earliest regions in the body affected by hypoperfusion. This characteristic combined with the relatively easy accessibility of the gut makes gastric tonometry an appealing choice for the early detection of shock [93].

Tonometry is based on the principle that gases will equilibrate between semipermeable compartments over time. Gastric tonometry involves placing a nasogastric tube tipped with a fluid or air filled balloon into the lumen of the stomach and allowing its contents to equilibrate with the fluid in the stomach. This gastric fluid, in turn, is in equilibrium with the mucosal lining the stomach. Therefore, by sampling the steady state contents of the balloon, one can estimate the partial pressure of CO_2 in the gastric mucosa ($P_{gm}CO_2$). The original set-ups used saline in the balloon, which required approximately 90 minutes for equilibration. Once equilibrated, the saline was aspirated and its PCO_2 was determined. Newer automated models use air in place of saline, which results in shorter equilibration times (less than 20 minutes) and improved precision [94–96]. Many of the early studies performed with gastric tonometry used the $P_{gm}CO_2$ to determine the intramucosal pH (pH_i) by estimating the tissue bicarbonate levels from serum bicarbonate and solving the Henderson–Hasselbach equation. Recent focus has shifted away from this approach due to the introduction of error by estimating intramucosal bicarbonate from serum bicarbonate. Instead, the PCO_2 gap ($P_{gm}CO_2$–P_aCO_2) has been proposed as an alternative measure of tissue perfusion that is less influenced by the systemic acid–base status [97].

Clinical Utility

Given its relatively noninvasive nature, gastric tonometry would be an ideal candidate for a safe modality for the guidance of resuscitation in shock. Indeed, many studies have attempted to explore this technique's ability to guide therapy in situations of hypoperfusion. Silva et al. measured changes in PCO_2 gap in addition to changes in systemic hemodynamic variables in response to fluid challenges in septic patients. They found that while cardiac index increased in response to fluid loading, indices of global oxygen delivery such as $S_{mv}O_2$ did not. The PCO_2 gap, however, was noted to significantly fall in response to fluid challenges [98]. This implies that gastric tonometry may provide a more reliable and less invasive means of monitoring response to resuscitation than monitoring traditional global variables of oxygenation such as $S_{mv}O_2$. Jeng et al. monitored $P_{gm}CO_2$ in a small series of burn patients and found that changes in $P_{gm}CO_2$ often preceded more traditional signs of hypoperfusion such as changes in mean arterial pressure and urine output [99].

In perhaps the best-known trial using this modality, Gutierrez et al. randomized 260 critically ill patients in the ICU to a standard therapy arm and a protocol arm in which patients received additional therapy aimed at improving oxygen delivery whenever pH_i fell below 7.35 [100]. These authors found a significant increase in 28-day survival in a subset of the protocol group whose pH_i was greater than 7.35 on admission. Although this study suggested that gastric tonometry could be used to improve survival in a select group of patients, perhaps its most relevant point is that early correction of hypoperfusion is crucial to improving survival. Barquist et al. compared the effects of a pH_i guided splanchnic therapy with that of a non-pH_i–guided therapy in trauma patients. They found that patients in the splanchnic therapy group had fewer organ failures, which was associated with shorter length of both ICU and hospital stays [101]. Unfortunately, a similar "splanchnic-oriented therapy" failed to show significant clinical benefit when compared to conventional therapy in trauma patients in a more recent study [102].

Not all studies, however, have demonstrated the usefulness of gastric tonometry as a resuscitative guide. In one notable article comparing pH_i-guided therapy with therapy guided by global oxygen delivery indices in trauma patients, Ivatury et al. did not find any significant difference in overall mortality [103]. In their analysis, however, they pointed out that the time to optimization of pH_i was significantly longer in nonsurvivors. This implies that the resuscitative therapy used or the clinical condition of the nonsurvivors likely resulted in a delay of pH_i optimization and that this delay was most responsible for their outcome. Gomersall et al. also compared pH_i-guided therapy with conventional treatment in 210 ICU patients [104]. They, too, found no significant change in mortality although this study may have been underpowered [105].

Although the ideal use of gastric tonometry is guidance of resuscitation in shock, many studies using this modality have demonstrated its prognostic utility. Levy et al. analyzed how pH_i and PCO_2 gap on admission to the ICU and at 24 hours correlated with outcome in 95 critically ill patients [86]. They found that the nonsurvivor group had significantly lower pH_i values on admission and at 24 hours as compared to the survivor group. In addition, the PCO_2 gap at 24 hours independently predicted 28-day survival. These findings supported those of Maynard et al. who compared pH_i with other global measures of perfusion in 83 patients with acute circulatory failure. In their study, pH_i was found to be a better predictor of outcome than lactate and other global measures of perfusion [106]. Interestingly, mortality may not be the only outcome that can be predicted through the use of gastric tonometry. Lebuffe et al. demonstrated that the intraoperative gap between gastric and end-tidal CO_2 can predict postoperative morbidity in high-risk patients undergoing major surgery [107]. The relationship between pH_i and outcome of ventilator weaning has also been studied [108–111]. In these studies, a low baseline pH_i and a significant drop in pH_i during weaning were associated with failure to wean and failed extubations. It is not entirely clear if the witnessed drop in pH_i is due to splanchnic ischemia from diverted blood flow to facilitate increased work of breathing or if it is related to increased P_aCO_2.

Thus far, studies have suggested that gastric tonometry may be a promising modality for the treatment and prognosis of shock with numerous advantages over traditional methods (Table 27.4). It is relatively noninvasive and can provide early information regarding the development of hypoperfusion that may be more reliable than global indices of oxygen delivery. Insufficient sample sizes and the inability of some treatment protocols to raise pH_i may explain some of the negative results derived from the studies performed to date. Critics of this modality question the validity of using gastric intramucosal pH as a surrogate for the entire splanchnic circulation [112]. Others wonder if the information obtained from gastric tonometry could be determined less invasively by the base deficit/excess [113]. This particular question was partially addressed by Totapally who showed that base excess responded very slowly to changes in intravascular changes in hemorrhagic shock in rats. Alternatively, esophageal PCO_2 gap was seen to reflect changes in intravascular volume more closely [114]. One major concern for this modality is its inability to accurately measure $P_{gm}CO_2$ during enteral feeding. This may limit gastric tonometry's use in patients with protracted critical illness.

TABLE 27.4

ADVANTAGES AND DISADVANTAGES OF GASTRIC TONOMETRY

Concept: Using a semipermeable balloon in the lumen of the stomach to estimate gastric mucosal perfusion
Advantages
Low risk of infection
May provide signs of early shock before traditional methods
Provides evidence of response to therapy before traditional markers
Disadvantages
Not continuous, takes up to 20 min per measurement
Does not reveal the cause of hypoperfusion (i.e., cardiogenic vs. distributive)

Future Research

The future study of gastric tonometry should focus in several directions. First, it should be used to help determine effective protocols for increasing gut mucosal perfusion. Poorly outlined and/or ineffective protocols were potential flaws in both the Guitierrez and the Ivatury studies [100,103]. A clearly delineated and effective protocol for optimizing pH_i or PCO_2 gap would allow for a more meaningful comparison between conventional and gastric-tonometry–guided treatment. Furthermore, once a reliable protocol has been determined, gastric tonometry may be used to validate further the increasing evidence that early restoration of perfusion and oxygen delivery in shock is crucial to outcomes. Finally, the ability of gastric tonometry to predict not only mortality but also ability to wean from mechanical ventilation should be further explored as this may help to guide determining goals of care and family decision making.

Sublingual Capnometry

Background

In attempts to further explore the clinical utility of guiding resuscitative therapy by tissue CO_2 levels, investigators have begun to focus on using alternative sites for measurement. One site that appears to be particularly promising due to its easy accessibility and, thus far, its accuracy, is the sublingual mucosa. After Sato et al. demonstrated that esophageal pH_i correlated well with gastric pH_i in a rodent model [115], Jin revealed that the more proximal sublingual mucosa developed hypercapnia to a similar degree as gastric mucosa in a model of hemorrhagic shock [116]. These authors went on to show not only a close correlation between increases in sublingual PCO_2 ($P_{sl}CO_2$) and decreases in arterial pressure and cardiac index [117] but also demonstrated that reversal of shock led to a correction of $P_{sl}CO_2$ comparable to that of $P_{gm}CO_2$ and more rapidly than the traditional marker of hypoperfusion, lactate [118].

The most widely clinically studied sublingual capnometry system is the Capnoprobe SL Monitoring System (Nellcor; Pleasanton, CA) which is a CO_2-sensing optode. This device is a CO_2-permeable capsule filled with a buffered solution of fluorescent dye. The capsule is attached to an optic fiber and is placed under the tongue. As CO_2 diffuses into the capsule, the pH of the buffered solution is altered by production of carbonic acid (H_2CO_3). This change in pH results in an alteration of the fluorescent emissions from the solution, which is ultimately sensed as a change in projected light by the attached optic fiber. Hence, by calibrating wavelengths of light with known partial pressures of CO_2, one can measure PCO_2 with this system. To ensure the highest possible accuracy of the device, it must be placed securely under the tongue with the mouth closed. An open mouth allows the entrance of light and ambient air to the optode, which can significantly alter accuracy. The reliable range of a well-seated and calibrated probe is 30 to 150 mm Hg [119].

Clinical Utility

Using this probe, researchers began to further investigate the comparability of sublingual capnometry and gastric tonometry as well as the clinical utility of capnometry. In one validation study, Marik demonstrated close correlation between $P_{gm}CO_2$ and $P_{sl}CO_2$ ($r = 0.78$; $p < 0.001$) in a heterogeneous population of 76 ICU patients [120]. Furthermore, Marik and Bankov went on to show that in another ICU population of 54 patients, $P_{sl}CO_2$ and $P_{sl}CO_2$–P_aCO_2 gap were better predictors of outcome than lactate or $S_{mv}O_2$. These authors specifically found that a $P_{sl}CO_2$–P_aCO_2 gap greater than 25 mm Hg was the best discriminator of outcome. In addition, they found that $P_{sl}CO_2$ and $P_{sl}CO_2$–P_aCO_2 gap were more responsive to treatment measures than were lactate and $S_{mv}O_2$ [121]. Weil et al. also demonstrated the prognostic abilities of sublingual capnometry when they found that a $P_{sl}CO_2$ <70 mm Hg had a positive predictive value of 93% for survival [122].

Unfortunately, in 2004 Nellcor initiated a voluntary recall of the Capnoprobe device after reports of Burkholderia cepacia being cultured from patients using this device as well as from unused devices themselves. As such, there is currently no system commercially available for sublingual capnography. Further insight into its clinical utility will have to wait until this technology is again available for clinical use.

Conclusion

In summary, the existing research regarding the clinical utility of sublingual capnometry appears promising. This technique may provide similar accuracy to gastric tonometry while being less invasive and providing results on a more instantaneous basis. In addition, it does not require discontinuation of enteral feeding during measurement periods, as some have advocated for gastric tonometry. If sublingual capnography is safely made available again, it may replace the use of lactate and $S_{mv}O_2$ as markers of hypoperfusion and as resuscitative guides. Further research into this technique's effect on patient outcome would also be warranted in the future.

Cardiac Biomarkers

Background

Cardiac biomarkers are molecules, usually proteins, which are specifically released from the heart into the blood and can be used to judge both cardiac function and dysfunction. Myocardial dysfunction is commonly seen early in the course of sepsis [123] and may be related to elevated levels of proinflammatory cytokines such as interleukin-1 and tumor necrosis factor-α, which have been shown to be cardiodepressant [124]. However, due to a concomitant increase in left ventricular ejection fraction (LVEF) caused by afterload reduction from systemic vasodilation, diagnosis of myocardial dysfunction early in sepsis can be difficult by traditional echocardiography. The study of cardiac biomarkers in the ICU setting is becoming an increasingly popular method of determining early cardiac dysfunction. As they can be obtained from a peripheral venous blood sample, they represent completely noninvasive and potentially valuable data that may assist in prognostication as well as in guiding management. To date, research has focused primarily on two proteins: troponin and B-type natriuretic peptide (BNP).

Troponin

Troponin T (TnT) and Troponin I (TnI) are cardiac-specific contractile proteins that have been studied extensively in the context of myocardial ischemia. Both have been shown to be superior to the traditional creatinine kinase MB (CK-MB) in diagnosing myocardial injury in certain clinical contexts [125–127]. As such, they have become part of the mainstay for diagnosing acute myocardial infarction today. Less is known about their role in the ICU in patients who are not undergoing myocardial infarction due to coronary plaque rupture. Several authors have observed an elevated level of troponin in ICU patients who are not undergoing an acute coronary syndrome [128,129]. One recent prospective case control study showed that 17 out of 20 patients (85%) with systemic inflammatory response syndrome (SIRS), sepsis, or septic shock had elevations in TnI. Furthermore, of the six patients who died in the study, five had elevated TnI levels. Ten of the seventeen patients with elevated TnI levels had no evidence of important coronary artery disease by coronary angiography, stress echocardiography, or autopsy [130]. Interestingly, in this study there were patients with a normal LVEF by echocardiography who had increased TnI levels. This suggests that TnI may be able to detect myocardial dysfunction even when echocardiography cannot. Troponin has also been studied as a prognostic marker in sepsis. Spies et al. measured serum TnT levels in 26 septic patients in a surgical ICU. They found that elevated TnT levels within the first 24 hours of sepsis were associated with a significantly higher mortality rate when compared to normal TnT levels [131]. Thus, troponin may be useful for detection of occult myocardial dysfunction as well as for prognostication in ICU patients in the absence of an acute coronary syndrome. These promising early findings as well as the development of more sensitive troponin assays [132] should lead to further research into the utility of troponin in the ICU.

BNP

The natriuretic peptides are a family of hormones that exert a wide range of biologic functions including diuresis and vasodilation. Two members of this family, atrial natriuretic peptide (ANP) and B-type (or brain) natriuretic peptide (BNP), are secreted by the atria and the ventricles, respectively. Their secretion is stimulated by myocardial stretch induced by increased filling volumes. Each hormone is derived from a prohormone that is cleaved into the biologically active C-terminal component and the biologically quiescent but longer lasting N-terminal component. In recent years, research has suggested that BNP can be a valuable surrogate for left ventricular end-diastolic pressure and left ventricular ejection fraction and can correlate with New York Heart Association heart failure class in patients with congestive heart failure (CHF) [133–137]. Until recently, however, little was known about the role of BNP as a marker of myocardial dysfunction in the critically ill population. Prompted by data that suggest that BNP can correlate with pulmonary artery occlusion pressure (PAOP) in patients with severe CHF [138,139], Tung et al. investigated the utility of using BNP as a surrogate for pulmonary artery catheter placement in a heterogeneous population in shock. Although BNP levels did not correlate with cardiac index or PAOP in this study, they did find that a BNP level of

<350 pg per mL had a 95% negative predictive value for the diagnosis of cardiogenic shock [140]. This suggests that although BNP should not be used in place of PAOP, a low BNP level may obviate the need for PAC placement.

This study also demonstrated that BNP levels have prognostic significance among the critically ill. The median BNP level at the time of PAC placement was significantly higher in the nonsurvivor population as compared with survivors. In addition, a multivariate analysis showed that a BNP concentration in the highest log-quartile was the strongest predictor of mortality with an odds ratio of 4.5. This was an even stronger predictor of mortality than the APACHE II scores [140]. The prognostic utility of BNP was further validated by Brueckmann et al. when these authors found that elevated N-terminal proBNP (NT-proBNP) levels on day 2 were significantly correlated with an increased mortality rate in patients with severe sepsis. These authors did not, however, find prognostic significance with N-terminal proANP (NT-proANP). Interestingly, the levels of NT-proBNP, NT-proANP, and troponin I were all found to be significantly lower in patients being treated with drotrecogin alfa (activated) than in those not receiving it [141]. This suggests that drotrecogin alfa (activated) may provide some cardioprotective effect in severe sepsis, perhaps through its proposed anti-inflammatory properties [142]. However, the sample size did not allow assessment of mortality benefit from APC.

Conclusion

In summary, the study of cardiac biomarkers in the ICU is still in the early stages. Till date, the majority of data suggests that troponin and BNP may have some prognostic significance in critically ill patients without CHF. Neither has been shown to be able to guide management, so far, although some data suggest that low BNP levels may exclude cardiogenic shock thereby preventing the need for a diagnostic PA line. Larger trials may further prove this concept in the future allowing for less invasive management of a select population of patients. Furthermore, a better understanding of the effect of drotrecogin alfa (activated) on cardiac biomarkers may provide some insight into the nature of the myocardial dysfunction seen in sepsis.

PRACTICE RECOMMENDATIONS

Independent of which cardiac monitoring technique is employed, a strategy that should be utilized in all patients with shock is early intervention. Mounting evidence suggests that mitochondrial failure may play a role in late shock [11,12] and efforts to correct hemodynamic derangements and augment oxygen delivery early in shock have shown promising results, thus far [13]. The optimal method for cardiac monitoring, however, is yet to be determined. At present, pulmonary artery thermodilution remains the "gold standard"; however, increasing interest has been given to less invasive monitoring modalities. Till date, the most substantial research has focused on ED, pulse contour analysis (Table 27.5), and gastric tonometry systems. Although there remains some question whether the absolute CO determined by ED is accurate, most studies have proven its reliability in monitoring trends in CO in response to therapeutic interventions. This ability to monitor trends may be sufficient for the management of patients in shock. Pulse contour analysis systems have also proven to be useful in monitoring trends in response to interventions. In addition, PCA systems do not require additional invasive procedures other than an arterial catheter, which is commonly used in patients with shock.

Despite these positive attributes, both ED and PCA systems do not provide a direct measure of tissue perfusion, which is, arguably, the most important variable to follow. Alternatively, gastric tonometry, and by extension sublingual capnometry, do not focus on the absolute CO but instead measure indices of tissue perfusion. This quality combined with noninvasiveness, makes these techniques appealing as replacements of thermodilution. The partial carbon dioxide rebreathing method has not yet sufficiently demonstrated its applicability to the critically ill patient. Confounding clinical features such as ALI are commonly found in this population and would likely impair the validity of existing systems. Finally, although BNP has not shown the ability to replace the PAC to date, there is some evidence that suggests that patients with a low BNP may not need one for diagnostic purposes. At present, use of any of these modalities must be performed cautiously. The majority of data available regarding these techniques has focused on comparing their accuracy with that of thermodilution. Few studies have addressed patient outcomes. Ultimately, before definite recommendations can be made, further research focusing on clinical outcomes will be necessary.

TABLE 27.5

SUMMARY OF RECOMMENDATIONS BASED ON RANDOMIZED CONTROLLED CLINICAL TRIALS

Early intervention in shock is beneficial
Esophageal Doppler can be used to follow trends in cardiac output
Pulse contour analysis can reliably estimate cardiac output in perioperative patients
Stroke volume variation cannot reliably be used to estimate preload responsiveness during low tidal volume ventilation

FUTURE DIRECTIONS

As medical technology continues to advance at an explosive rate, it is easy to imagine that ICU practice will completely change in the not too distant future. The next generation of intensivists and likely younger members of this generation may find themselves looking back with awe at the "archaic" methods of current practice. At present, there are many technologies that are still in their early stages but may one day provide useful clinical information. A few of these deserve mention.

Magnetic resonance imaging (MRI) has become a common fixture in many large hospitals and is routinely used in a variety of clinical settings due to its improved accuracy over computed tomography (CT) in defining soft tissue structure. The role of MRI continues to expand as clinicians and researchers develop new ways to use its capabilities. One area in which MRI has shown particular promise is that of cardiac MRI. Although this technique is still being primarily used experimentally, early results have demonstrated its ability to assess both cardiac function as well as viability [143–145]. As more data become available, one can envision the possibility of more routine use of MRI to assess cardiac function in the ICU. In addition, advances in nuclear magnetic resonance (NMR) spectroscopy have made it possible to estimate arterial oxygen supply (DO_2) as well as skeletal muscle reoxygenation, mitochondrial ATP production, and oxygen consumption($\dot{V}O_2$) [146]. Although cost and the technical difficulties of using MRI in the ICU may be prohibitive, there clearly exists potential in this arena.

Although traditional two-dimensional transthoracic echocardiography is certainly not a new technology, recently there has been new interest in this technique among intensivists. Echocardiography has historically fallen under the domain of cardiologists who are formally trained to perform and interpret these useful studies. This technique can provide a wealth of information about systolic function, valvular dysfunction and pericardial disease in critically ill patients [147]. More and more, noncardiology intensivists are now learning how to perform, at least, basic exams to help quickly guide initial management decisions. For example, some bedside ultrasound devices used for central line placement, also have probes, which allow at least cursory examination of cardiac function (e.g., to exclude pericardial tamponade). However, the authors are aware of instances of erroneous information being gathered from such devices when used in untrained hands. Therefore, a more formal education in echocardiography would likely be beneficial for intensivists who do not have access to immediate echocardiography by an expert.

Finally, as in other areas of medicine, in the coming years emerging technology may substantially impact critical care through insights gained in the fields of proteomics, genomics, and metabolomics. These techniques use next-generation technologies of mass spectroscopy and microarray analysis to isolate and compare which proteins, genes, and other molecular markers are preferentially expressed during different disease states. Through analysis of these patterns, it may be possible to better understand the mechanisms behind diseases such as sepsis and ARDS. Ultimately such technologies could theoretically be used in the field of hemodynamic monitoring if such patterns could be associated with specific hemodynamic states. Ideally, for example, a simple blood or urine test could reveal a biomarker pattern consistent with cardiogenic shock that would take the place of invasive measuring of CO. Determining these expression patterns as well as refining the technique such that the information could be obtained in a timely manner will be important and challenging obstacles to overcome.

References

1. Thomas JT, Kelly RF, Thomas SJ, et al: Utility of history, physical examination, electrocardiogram, and chest radiograph for differentiating normal from decreased systolic function in patients with heart failure [see comment]. *Am J Med* 112(6):437–445, 2002.
2. Connors AF Jr, McCaffree DR, Gray BA: Evaluation of right-heart catheterization in the critically ill patient without acute myocardial infarction. *N Engl J Med* 308(5):263–267, 1983.
3. Swan HJ, Ganz W, Forrester J, et al: Catheterization of the heart in man with use of a flow-directed balloon-tipped catheter. *N Engl J Med* 283(9):447–451, 1970.
4. Iberti TJ, Fischer EP, Leibowitz AB, et al: A multicenter study of physicians' knowledge of the pulmonary artery catheter. pulmonary artery catheter study group [see comment]. *JAMA* 264(22):2928–2932, 1990.
5. Richard C, Warszawski J, Anguel N, et al: Early use of the pulmonary artery catheter and outcomes in patients with shock and acute respiratory distress syndrome: a randomized controlled trial [see comment]. *JAMA* 290(20):2713–2720, 2003.
6. Gore JM, Goldberg RJ, Spodick DH, et al: A community-wide assessment of the use of pulmonary artery catheters in patients with acute myocardial infarction. *Chest* 92(4):721–727, 1987.
7. Anonymous: Pulmonary-artery versus central venous catheter to guide treatment of acute lung injury. *N Engl J Med* 354(21):2213–2224, 2006.
8. Connors AF Jr, Speroff T, Dawson NV, et al: The effectiveness of right heart catheterization in the initial care of critically ill patients. SUPPORT investigators [see comment]. *JAMA* 276(11):889–897, 1996.
9. Binanay C, Califf RM, Hasselblad V, et al: Evaluation study of congestive heart failure and pulmonary artery catheterization effectiveness: the ESCAPE trial [see comment]. *JAMA* 294(13):1625–1633, 2005.
10. Gattinoni L, Brazzi L, Pelosi P, et al: A trial of goal-oriented hemodynamic therapy in critically ill patients. SvO2 collaborative group [see comment]. *N Engl J Med* 333(16):1025–1032, 1995.
11. Schwartz DR, Malhotra A, Fink M: Cytopathic hypoxia in sepsis: an overview. *Sepsis* 2:279–289, 1998.
12. Fink M: Cytopathic hypoxia in sepsis [review] [100 refs]. *Acta Anaesthesiol Scand Suppl* 110(Suppl 110):87–95, 1997.
13. Rivers E, Nguyen B, Havstad S, et al: Early goal-directed therapy in the treatment of severe sepsis and septic shock [see comment]. *N Engl J Med* 345(19):1368–1377, 2001.
14. Trzeciak S, Dellinger RP, Abate NL, et al: Translating research to clinical practice: a 1-year experience with implementing early goal-directed therapy for septic shock in the emergency department [article]. *Chest* 129(2):225–232, 2006.
15. Sandham JD, Hull RD, Brant RF, et al: A randomized, controlled trial of the use of pulmonary-artery catheters in high-risk surgical patients. *N Engl J Med* 348(1):5–14, 2003.
16. Rame JE, Dries DL, Drazner MH: The prognostic value of the physical examination in patients with chronic heart failure [review] [36 refs]. *Congest Heart Fail* 9(3):170–175, 2003.
17. Kaplan LJ, McPartland K, Santora TA, et al: start with a subjective assessment of skin temperature to identify hypoperfusion in intensive care unit patients. *J Trauma* 50(4):620–627, 2001.
18. Joly HR, Weil MH: Temperature of the great toe as an indication of the severity of shock. *Circulation* 39(1):131–138, 1969.
19. Magder S, Georgiadis G, Tuck C: Respiratory variations in right atrial pressure predict response to fluid challenge. *J Crit Care* 7:76–85, 1992.
20. Magder S, Lagonidis D, Erice F: The use of respiratory variations in right atrial pressure to predict the cardiac output response to PEEP. *J Crit Care* 16(3):108–114, 2001.
21. Magder S: More respect for the CVP. *Intensive Care Med* 24(7):651–653, 1998.
22. Morris AH, Chapman RH, Gardner RM: Frequency of technical problems encountered in the measurement of pulmonary artery wedge pressure. *Crit Care Med* 12(3):164–170, 1984.
23. Marik P, Heard SO, Varon J: Interpretation of the pulmonary artery occlusion (wedge) pressure: physician's knowledge versus the experts' knowledge [comment]. *Crit Care Med* 26(10):1761–1764, 1998.
24. Eisenberg PR, Jaffe AS, Schuster DP: Clinical evaluation compared to pulmonary artery catheterization in the hemodynamic assessment of critically ill patients. *Crit Care Med* 12(7):549–553, 1984.
25. Side CD, Gosling RG: Non-surgical assessment of cardiac function. *Nature* 232(5309):335–336, 1971.
26. Singer M, Clarke J, Bennett ED: Continuous hemodynamic monitoring by esophageal doppler. *Crit Care Med* 17(5):447–452, 1989.
27. Cariou A, Monchi M, Joly LM, et al: Noninvasive cardiac output monitoring by aortic blood flow determination: evaluation of the sometec dynemo-3000 system [see comment]. *Crit Care Med* 26(12):2066–2072, 1998.
28. Singer M, Bennett ED: Noninvasive optimization of left ventricular filling using esophageal doppler. *Crit Care Med* 19(9):1132–1137, 1991.
29. Bundgaard-Nielsen M, Ruhnau B, Secher NH, et al: flow-related techniques for preoperative goal-directed fluid optimization. *Br J Anaesth* 98(1):38–44, 2007.
30. Wallmeyer K, Wann LS, Sagar KB, et al: The influence of preload and heart rate on doppler echocardiographic indexes of left ventricular performance: comparison with invasive indexes in an experimental preparation. *Circulation* 74(1):181–186, 1986.
31. Singer M, Allen MJ, Webb AR, et al: effects of alterations in left ventricular filling, contractility, and systemic vascular resistance on the ascending aortic blood velocity waveform of normal subjects. *Crit Care Med* 19(9):1138–1145, 1991.
32. Sharma J, Bhise M, Singh A, et al: Hemodynamic measurements after cardiac surgery: transesophageal doppler versus pulmonary artery catheter. *J Cardiothorac Vasc Anesth* 19(6):746–750, 2005.
33. Dark PM, Singer M: The validity of trans-esophageal doppler ultrasonography as a measure of cardiac output in critically ill adults [review] [23 refs]. *Intensive Care Med* 30(11):2060–2066, 2004.
34. Kim K, Kwok I, Chang H, et al: comparison of cardiac outputs of major burn patients undergoing extensive early escharectomy: esophageal doppler monitor versus thermodilution pulmonary artery catheter. *J Trauma* 57(5):1013–1017, 2004.
35. Roeck M, Jakob SM, Boehlen T, et al: Change in stroke volume in response to fluid challenge: assessment using esophageal doppler [see comment]. *Intensive Care Med* 29(10):1729–1735, 2003.
36. Bland JM, Altman DG: Statistical methods for assessing agreement between two methods of clinical measurement [see comment]. *Lancet* 1(8476):307–310, 1986.
37. Daniel WG, Erbel R, Kasper W, et al: Safety of transesophageal echocardiography. A multicenter survey of 10,419 examinations. *Circulation* 83(3):817–821, 1991.
38. Singer M: Esophageal doppler monitoring of aortic blood flow: beat-by-beat cardiac output monitoring [review] [73 refs]. *Int Anesthesiol Clin* 31(3):99–125, 1993.
39. Valtier B, Cholley BP, Belot JP, et al: Noninvasive monitoring of cardiac output in critically ill patients using transesophageal doppler. *Am J Respir Crit Care Med* 158(1):77–83, 1998.
40. Gan TJ, Arrowsmith JE: The oesophageal doppler monitor [comment]. *BMJ* 315(7113):893–894, 1997.
41. Lefrant JY, Bruelle P, Aya AG, et al: Training is required to improve the reliability of esophageal doppler to measure cardiac output in critically ill patients. *Intensive Care Med* 24(4):347–352, 1998.

42. Sinclair S, James S, Singer M: Intraoperative intravascular volume optimisation and length of hospital stay after repair of proximal femoral fracture: randomised controlled trial [see comment]. *BMJ* 315(7113):909–912, 1997.
43. Gan TJ, Soppitt A, Maroof M, et al: Goal-directed intraoperative fluid administration reduces length of hospital stay after major surgery. *Anesthesiology* 97(4):820–826, 2002.
44. Mythen MG, Webb AR: Perioperative plasma volume expansion reduces the incidence of gut mucosal hypoperfusion during cardiac surgery. *Arch Surg* 130(4):423–429, 1995.
45. Phan TD, Ismail H, Heriot AG, et al: improving perioperative outcomes: fluid optimization with the esophageal doppler monitor, a metaanalysis and review. *J Am Coll Surg* 207(6):935–941, 2008.
46. Frank O: Wellen- und windkesselthrorie [estimation of the strok volume of the human heart using the "windkessel" theory]. *Zaitech Biol* 90:405–409, 1930.
47. Wesseling KH, de Wit B, Weber JAP, et al: a simple device for the continuous measurement of cardiac output. *Adv Cardiovasc Phys* 5:16–52, 1983.
48. Pinsky MR: Probing the limits of arterial pulse contour analysis to predict preload responsiveness [comment]. *Anesth Analg* 96(5):1245–1247, 2003.
49. Della Rocca G, Costa MG, Pompei L, et al: Continuous and intermittent cardiac output measurement: pulmonary artery catheter versus aortic transpulmonary technique [see comment]. *Br J Anaesth* 88(3):350–356, 2002.
50. Della Rocca G, Costa MG, Coccia C, et al: Cardiac output monitoring: aortic transpulmonary thermodilution and pulse contour analysis agree with standard thermodilution methods in patients undergoing lung transplantation. *Can J Anaesth* 50(7):707–711, 2003.
51. Godje O, Hoke K, Goetz AE, et al: Reliability of a new algorithm for continuous cardiac output determination by pulse-contour analysis during hemodynamic instability. *Crit Care Med* 30(1):52–58, 2002.
52. Mielck F, Buhre W, Hanekop G, et al: Comparison of continuous cardiac output measurements in patients after cardiac surgery. *J Cardiothorac Vasc Anesth* 17(2):211–216, 2003.
53. Rauch H, Muller M, Fleischer F, et al: Pulse contour analysis versus thermodilution in cardiac surgery patients [miscellaneous article]. *Acta Anaesthesiol Scand* 46(4):424–429, 2002.
54. Manecke J, Gerard R, Auger WR: Cardiac output determination from the arterial pressure wave: clinical testing of a novel algorithm that does not require calibration. *J Cardiothorac Vasc Anesth* 21(1):3–7, 2007.
55. Langewouters GJ, Wesseling KH, Goedhard WJA: The pressure dependent dynamic elasticity of 35 thoracic and 16 abdominal human aortas in vitro described by a five component model. *J Biomech* 18(8):613–620, 1985.
56. Felbinger TW, Reuter DA, Eltzschig HK, et al: Cardiac index measurements during rapid preload changes: a comparison of pulmonary artery thermodilution with arterial pulse contour analysis. *J Clin Anesth* 17(4):241–248, 2005.
57. Gunn SR, Pinsky MR: Implications of arterial pressure variation in patients in the intensive care unit [review] [26 refs]. *Curr Opin Crit Care* 7(3):212–217, 2001.
58. Michard F, Teboul JL: Using heart-lung interactions to assess fluid responsiveness during mechanical ventilation [review] [47 refs]. *Crit Care* 4(5):282–289, 2000.
59. Michard F, Teboul JL: Predicting fluid responsiveness in ICU patients: a critical analysis of the evidence [review] [36 refs]. *Chest* 121(6):2000–2008, 2002.
60. Reuter DA, Felbinger TW, Schmidt C, et al: Stroke volume variations for assessment of cardiac responsiveness to volume loading in mechanically ventilated patients after cardiac surgery [see comment]. *Intensive Care Med* 28(4):392–398, 2002.
61. Wiesenack C, Prasser C, Rodig G, et al: stroke volume variation as an indicator of fluid responsiveness using pulse contour analysis in mechanically ventilated patients [see comment]. *Anesth Analg* 96(5):1254–1257, 2003.
62. Goedje O, Hoeke K, Lichtwarck-Aschoff M, et al: Continuous cardiac output by femoral arterial thermodilution calibrated pulse contour analysis: comparison with pulmonary arterial thermodilution [see comment]. *Crit Care Med* 27(11):2407–2412, 1999.
63. Rodig G, Prasser C, Keyl C, et al: Continuous cardiac output measurement: pulse contour analysis vs thermodilution technique in cardiac surgical patients. *Br J Anaesth* 82(4):525–530, 1999.
64. Ultman JS, Bursztein S: Analysis of error in the determination of respiratory gas exchange at varying FIO_2. *J Appl Physiol* 50(1):210–216, 1981.
65. Mahutte CK, Jaffe MB, Sassoon CS, et al: cardiac output from carbon dioxide production and arterial and venous oximetry. *Crit Care Med* 19(10):1270–1277, 1991.
66. Mahutte CK, Jaffe MB, Chen PA, et al: Oxygen Fick and modified carbon dioxide Fick cardiac outputs. *Crit Care Med* 22(1):86–95, 1994.
67. Lynch J, Kaemmerer H: Comparison of a modified Fick method with thermodilution for determining cardiac output in critically ill patients on mechanical ventilation. *Intensive Care Med* 16(4):248–251, 1990.
68. Berton C, Cholley B: Equipment review: new techniques for cardiac output measurement—oesophageal doppler, Fick principle using carbon dioxide, and pulse contour analysis [review] [30 refs]. *Crit Care* 6(3):216–221, 2002.
69. Murias GE, Villagra A, Vatua S, et al: Evaluation of a noninvasive method for cardiac output measurement in critical care patients. *Intensive Care Med* 28(10):1470–1474, 2002.
70. Gedeon A, Forslund L, Hedenstierna G, et al: a new method for noninvasive bedside determination of pulmonary blood flow. *Med Biol Eng Comput* 18(4):411–418, 1980.
71. Benatar SR, Hewlett AM, Nunn JF: The use of iso-shunt lines for control of oxygen therapy. *Br J Anaesth* 45(7):711–718, 1973.
72. Neviere R, Mathieu D, Riou Y, et al: Carbon dioxide rebreathing method of cardiac output measurement during acute respiratory failure in patients with chronic obstructive pulmonary disease. *Crit Care Med* 22(1):81–85, 1994.
73. Odenstedt H, Stenqvist O, Lundin S: Clinical evaluation of a partial CO2 rebreathing technique for cardiac output monitoring in critically ill patients [see comment]. *Acta Anaesthesiol Scand* 46(2):152–159, 2002.
74. Binder JC, Parkin WG: Non-invasive cardiac output determination: comparison of a new partial-rebreathing technique with thermodilution. *Anaesth Intensive Care* 29(1):19–23, 2001.
75. Botero M, Kirby D, Lobato EB, et al: Measurement of cardiac output before and after cardiopulmonary bypass: comparison among aortic transit-time ultrasound, thermodilution, and noninvasive partial CO_2 rebreathing. *J Cardiothorac Vasc Anesth* 18(5):563–572, 2004.
76. Nilsson LB, Eldrup N, Berthelsen PG: Lack of agreement between thermodilution and carbon dioxide-rebreathing cardiac output. *Acta Anaesthesiol Scand* 45(6):680–685, 2001.
77. Hachenberg T, Tenling A, Nystrom SO, et al: Ventilation-perfusion inequality in patients undergoing cardiac surgery. *Anesthesiology* 80(3):509–519, 1994.
78. de Abreu MG, Quintel M, Ragaller M, et al: partial carbon dioxide rebreathing: a reliable technique for noninvasive measurement of nonshunted pulmonary capillary blood flow. *Crit Care Med* 25(4):675–683, 1997.
79. Valiatti JL, Amaral JL: Comparison between cardiac output values measured by thermodilution and partial carbon dioxide rebreathing in patients with acute lung injury. *Sao Paulo Med J* 122(6):233–238, 2004.
80. Tachibana K, Imanaka H, Takeuchi M, et al: Noninvasive cardiac output measurement using partial carbon dioxide rebreathing is less accurate at settings of reduced minute ventilation and when spontaneous breathing is present [see comment]. *Anesthesiology* 98(4):830–837, 2003.
81. Cason CL, DeSalvo SK, Ray WT: Changes in oxygen saturation during weaning from short-term ventilator support after coronary artery bypass graft surgery. *Heart Lung* 23(5):368–375, 1994.
82. Magilligan DJ Jr, Teasdall R, Eisinminger R, et al: mixed venous oxygen saturation as a predictor of cardiac output in the postoperative cardiac surgical patient. *Ann Thorac Surg* 44(3):260–262, 1987.
83. Pearson KS, Gomez MN, Moyers JR, et al: A cost/benefit analysis of randomized invasive monitoring for patients undergoing cardiac surgery [see comment]. *Anesth Analg* 69(3):336–341, 1989.
84. Lee J, Wright F, Barber R, et al: central venous oxygen saturation in shock: a study in man. *Anesthesiology* 36(5):472–478, 1972.
85. Reinhart K, Rudolph T, Bredle DL, et al: Comparison of central-venous to mixed-venous oxygen saturation during changes in oxygen supply/demand. *Chest* 95(6):1216–1221, 1989.
86. Levy B, Gawalkiewicz P, Vallet B, et al: Gastric capnometry with air-automated tonometry predicts outcome in critically ill patients. *Crit Care Med* 31(2):474–480, 2003.
87. Fink MP: Tissue capnometry as a monitoring strategy for critically ill patients: just about ready for prime time [see comment]. *Chest* 114(3):667–670, 1998.
88. Sato Y, Weil MH, Tang W: Tissue hypercarbic acidosis as a marker of acute circulatory failure (shock) [review] [76 refs]. *Chest* 114(1):263–274, 1998.
89. Marik P: Gastric tonometry: the canary sings once again [see comment]. *Crit Care Med* 26(5):809–810, 1998.
90. Krebs HA, Woods HF, Alberti KGMM: Hyperlactataemia and lactic acidosis. *Essays Biochem* 1:81–103, 1970.
91. Neviere R, Chagnon JL, Teboul JL, et al: Small intestine intramucosal PCO(2) and microvascular blood flow during hypoxic and ischemic hypoxia [see comment]. *Crit Care Med* 30(2):379–384, 2002.
92. Creteur J: Gastric and sublingual capnometry. *Curr Opin Crit Care* 12(3): 272–277, 2006.
93. Fiddian-Green RG, Baker S: Predictive value of the stomach wall pH for complications after cardiac operations: comparison with other monitoring. *Crit Care Med* 15(2):153–156, 1987.
94. Graf J, Konigs B, Mottaghy K, et al: in vitro validation of gastric air tonometry using perfluorocarbon FC 43 and 0.9% sodium chloride. *Br J Anaesth* 84(4):497–499, 2000.
95. Barry B, Mallick A, Hartley G, et al: Comparison of air tonometry with gastric tonometry using saline and other equilibrating fluids: an in vivo and in vitro study. *Intensive Care Med* 24(8):777–784, 1998.
96. Tzelepis G, Kadas V, Michalopoulos A, et al: comparison of gastric air tonometry with standard saline tonometry. *Intensive Care Med* 22(11):1239–1243, 1996.
97. Schlichtig R, Mehta N, Gayowski TJ: Tissue-arterial PCO_2 difference is a better marker of ischemia than intramural pH (pHi) or arterial pH–pHi difference. *J Crit Care* 11(2):51–56, 1996.
98. Silva E, De Backer D, Creteur J, et al: effects of fluid challenge on gastric mucosal PCO_2 in septic patients. *Intensive Care Med* 30(3):423–429, 2004.
99. Jeng JC, Jaskille AD, Lunsford PM, et al: improved markers for burn wound perfusion in the severely burned patient: the role for tissue and gastric PCO_2. *J Burn Care Res* 29(1):49–55, 2008.

100. Gutierrez G, Palizas F, Doglio G, et al: Gastric intramucosal pH as a therapeutic index of tissue oxygenation in critically ill patients. *Lancet* 339(8787):195–199, 1992.
101. Barquist E, Kirton O, Windsor J, et al: The impact of antioxidant and splanchnic-directed therapy on persistent uncorrected gastric mucosal pH in the critically injured trauma patient. *J Trauma* 44(2):355–360, 1998.
102. Miami Trauma Clinical Trials G: Splanchnic hypoperfusion-directed therapies in trauma: a prospective, randomized trial. *Am Surg* 71(3):252–260, 2005.
103. Ivatury RR, Simon RJ, Islam S, et al: A prospective randomized study of end points of resuscitation after major trauma: global oxygen transport indices versus organ-specific gastric mucosal pH. *J Am Coll Surg* 183(2):145–154, 1996.
104. Gomersall CD, Joynt GM, Freebairn RC, et al: Resuscitation of critically ill patients based on the results of gastric tonometry: a prospective, randomized, controlled trial [see comment]. *Crit Care Med* 28(3):607–614, 2000.
105. Heard SO: Gastric tonometry: the hemodynamic monitor of choice (pro). *Chest* 123(5 Suppl):469S–474S, 2003.
106. Maynard N, Bihari D, Beale R, et al: Assessment of splanchnic oxygenation by gastric tonometry in patients with acute circulatory failure [see comment]. *JAMA* 270(10):1203–1210, 1993.
107. Lebuffe G, Vallet B, Takala J, et al: A European, multicenter, observational study to assess the value of gastric-to-end tidal PCO_2 difference in predicting postoperative complications. *Anesth Analg* 99(1):166–172, 2004.
108. Mohsenifar Z, Hay A, Hay J, et al: Gastric intramural pH as a predictor of success or failure in weaning patients from mechanical ventilation [see comment]. *Ann Intern Med* 119(8):794–798, 1993.
109. Bouachour G, Guiraud MP, Gouello JP, et al: Gastric intramucosal pH: an indicator of weaning outcome from mechanical ventilation in COPD patients. *Eur Respir J* 9(9):1868–1873, 1996.
110. Bocquillon N, Mathieu D, Neviere R, et al: Gastric mucosal pH and blood flow during weaning from mechanical ventilation in patients with chronic obstructive pulmonary disease. *Am J Respir Crit Care Med* 160(5, Pt 1): 1555–1561, 1999.
111. Hurtado FJ, Beron M, Olivera W, et al: Gastric intramucosal pH and intraluminal PCO2 during weaning from mechanical ventilation. *Crit Care Med* 29(1):70–76, 2001.
112. Uusaro A, Lahtinen P, Parviainen I, et al: gastric mucosal end-tidal PCO2 difference as a continuous indicator of splanchnic perfusion. *Br J Anaesth* 85(4):563–569, 2000.
113. Boyd O, Mackay CJ, Lamb G, et al: Comparison of clinical information gained from routine blood-gas analysis and from gastric tonometry for intramural pH. *Lancet* 341(8838):142–146, 1993.
114. Totapally BR, Fakioglu H, Torbati D, et al: esophageal capnometry during hemorrhagic shock and after resuscitation in rats [see comment]. *Crit Care* 7(1):79–84, 2003.
115. Sato Y, Weil MH, Tang W, et al: Esophageal PCO_2 as a monitor of perfusion failure during hemorrhagic shock. *J Appl Physiol* 82(2):558–562, 1997.
116. Jin X, Weil MH, Sun S, et al: Decreases in organ blood flows associated with increases in sublingual PCO_2 during hemorrhagic shock. *J Appl Physiol* 85(6):2360–2364, 1998.
117. Nakagawa Y, Weil MH, Tang W, et al: Sublingual capnometry for diagnosis and quantitation of circulatory shock. *Am J Respir Crit Care Med* 157(6 Pt 1):1838–1843, 1998.
118. Povoas HP, Weil MH, Tang W, et al: Comparisons between sublingual and gastric tonometry during hemorrhagic shock [see comment]. *Chest* 118(4):1127–1132, 2000.
119. Maciel AT, Creteur J, Vincent JL: Tissue capnometry: does the answer lie under the tongue? [review] [81 refs]. *Intensive Care Med* 30(12):2157–2165, 2004.
120. Marik PE: Sublingual capnography: a clinical validation study [see comment]. *Chest* 120(3):923–927, 2001.
121. Marik PE, Bankov A: Sublingual capnometry versus traditional markers of tissue oxygenation in critically ill patients [see comment]. *Crit Care Med* 31(3):818–822, 2003.
122. Weil MH, Nakagawa Y, Tang W, et al: Sublingual capnometry: a new noninvasive measurement for diagnosis and quantitation of severity of circulatory shock [see comment]. *Crit Care Med* 27(7):1225–1229, 1999.
123. Price S, Anning PB, Mitchell JA, et al: myocardial dysfunction in sepsis: mechanisms and therapeutic implications [review] [93 refs]. *Eur Heart J* 20(10):715–724, 1999.
124. Scire CA, Caporali R, Perotti C, et al: Plasma procalcitonin in rheumatic diseases [review] [30 refs]. *Reumatismo* 55(2):113–118, 2003.
125. Gerhardt W, Katus H, Ravkilde J, et al: S-troponin T in suspected ischemic myocardial injury compared with mass and catalytic concentrations of S-creatine kinase isoenzyme MB [see comment]. *Clin Chem* 37(8):1405–1411, 1991.
126. Katus HA, Remppis A, Neumann FJ, et al: Diagnostic efficiency of troponin T measurements in acute myocardial infarction [see comment]. *Circulation* 83(3):902–912, 1991.
127. Parrillo JE: Myocardial depression during septic shock in humans. *Crit Care Med* 18(10):1183–1184, 1990.
128. Fernandes Junior CJ, Iervolino M, Neves RA, et al: Interstitial myocarditis in sepsis. *Am J Cardiol* 74(9):958, 1994.
129. Piper RD: Myocardial dysfunction in sepsis [review] [36 refs]. *Clin Exp Pharmacol Physiol* 25(11):951–954, 1998.
130. Ammann P, Fehr T, Minder EI, et al: Elevation of troponin I in sepsis and septic shock [see comment]. *Intensive Care Med* 27(6):965–969, 2001.
131. Spies C, Haude V, Fitzner R, et al: Serum cardiac troponin T as a prognostic marker in early sepsis. *Chest* 113(4):1055–1063, 1998.
132. Reichlin TMD, Hochholzer WMD, Bassetti SMD, et al: Early diagnosis of myocardial infarction with sensitive cardiac troponin assays. *N Engl J Med* 361(9):858–867, 2009.
133. Omland T, Aakvaag A, Bonarjee VV, et al: Plasma brain natriuretic peptide as an indicator of left ventricular systolic function and long-term survival after acute myocardial infarction. Comparison with plasma atrial natriuretic peptide and N-terminal proatrial natriuretic peptide [see comment]. *Circulation* 93(11):1963–1969, 1996.
134. Krishnaswamy P, Lubien E, Clopton P, et al: Utility of B-natriuretic peptide levels in identifying patients with left ventricular systolic or diastolic dysfunction [see comment]. *Am J Med* 111(4):274–279, 2001.
135. Maisel AS, Koon J, Krishnaswamy P, et al: Utility of B-natriuretic peptide as a rapid, point-of-care test for screening patients undergoing echocardiography to determine left ventricular dysfunction. *Am Heart J* 141(3):367–374, 2001.
136. Maisel AS, Krishnaswamy P, Nowak RM, et al: Rapid measurement of B-type natriuretic peptide in the emergency diagnosis of heart failure [see comment, summary for patients in *J Fam Pract.* 2002 51(10):816; PMID: 12401145]. *N Engl J Med* 347(3):161–167, 2002.
137. Vasan RS, Benjamin EJ, Larson MG, et al: Plasma natriuretic peptides for community screening for left ventricular hypertrophy and systolic dysfunction: the Framingham heart study. *JAMA* 288(10):1252–1259, 2002.
138. Kazanegra R, Cheng V, Garcia A, et al: A rapid test for B-type natriuretic peptide correlates with falling wedge pressures in patients treated for decompensated heart failure: a pilot study. *J Card Fail* 7(1):21–29, 2001.
139. Park MH, Scott RL, Uber PA, et al: Usefulness of B-type natriuretic peptide levels in predicting hemodynamic perturbations after heart transplantation despite preserved left ventricular systolic function. *Am J Cardiol* 90(12):1326–1329, 2002.
140. Tung RH, Garcia C, Morss AM, et al: Utility of B-type natriuretic peptide for the evaluation of intensive care unit shock [see comment]. *Crit Care Med* 32(8):1643–1647, 2004.
141. Brueckmann M, Huhle G, Lang S, et al: Prognostic value of plasma N-terminal pro-brain natriuretic peptide in patients with severe sepsis [see comment]. *Circulation* 112(4):527–534, 2005.
142. Nacira S, Meziani F, Dessebe O, et al: Activated protein C improves lipopolysaccharide-induced cardiovascular dysfunction by decreasing tissular inflammation and oxidative stress. *Crit Care Med* 37(1):246–255, 2009.
143. Lee VS, Resnick D, Tiu SS, et al: MR imaging evaluation of myocardial viability in the setting of equivocal SPECT results with (99 m) tc sestamibi. *Radiology* 230(1):191–197, 2004.
144. Chiu CW, So NM, Lam WW, et al: Combined first-pass perfusion and viability study at MR imaging in patients with non-ST segment-elevation acute coronary syndromes: feasibility study. *Radiology* 226(3):717–722, 2003.
145. Kitagawa K, Sakuma H, Hirano T, et al: Acute myocardial infarction: myocardial viability assessment in patients early thereafter comparison of contrast-enhanced MR imaging with resting (201)tl SPECT. Single photon emission computed tomography. *Radiology* 226(1):138–144, 2003.
146. Carlier PG, Brillault-Salvat C, Giacomini E, et al: How to investigate oxygen supply, uptake, and utilization simultaneously by interleaved NMR imaging and spectroscopy of the skeletal muscle. *Magn Reson Med* 54(4):1010–1013, 2005.
147. Price S, Nicol E, Gibson DG, et al: echocardiography in the critically ill: Current and potential roles. *Int Care Med* 32:48–59, 2006.

CHAPTER 28 ■ NEUROLOGIC MULTIMODAL MONITORING

RAPHAEL A. CARANDANG, WILEY R. HALL AND DONALD S. PROUGH

Neurologic function is a major determinant of quality of life. Injury or dysfunction can have a profound effect on a patient's ability to be alert, communicate, and interact with his or her environment meaningfully, and function as an independent human being. The brain is a highly complex organ with specialized areas of function and is exquisitely sensitive to metabolic and physical insults such as hypoxemia, acidosis, trauma, and hypoperfusion. The goal of neurocritical care is to protect the brain and preserve neurologic functions in the critically ill patient. The impetus for multimodal monitoring of brain function arises from both its importance and vulnerability and also the difficulty in obtaining a satisfactory assessment of function in the setting of numerous insults and processes including toxic and metabolic encephalopathy, sedation and chemical restraints, and primary central nervous system (CNS) processes like stroke and traumatic brain injury.

There has been rapid growth and there continues to be much interest in the field as numerous devices and modalities are developed to monitor brain function and processes including intracranial pressure (ICP) monitoring, electroencephalography, and corticography, global and regional brain tissue oxygen monitoring, cerebral blood flow measurements, and neurochemical and cellular metabolism assessment with microdialysis.

As with any diagnostic or therapeutic tool, an understanding of the indications, limitations, risks and benefits of an intervention are essential in the effective utilization, interpretation, and application of the obtained information to the management of the individual patient. Important characteristics of monitoring devices include the ability to detect important abnormalities (sensitivity), to differentiate between dissimilar disease states (specificity), and to prompt changes in care that alter long-term prognosis (Table 28.1). Limitations of techniques include risks to patients (during placement, use, and removal), variability errors in generation of data (e.g., calibration and drift), and inherent trade-offs between specificity and sensitivity. Monitors with high specificity—values fall outside of threshold levels only when a disease state is unequivocally present—are unlikely to detect less profound levels of disease, while monitors with high sensitivity (will detect any value outside of the normal range) are likely to demonstrate small deviations from normal, which may be trivial in individual patients. The advantage of multimodal monitoring is it increases the sensitivity and accuracy of our detection of physiologic and cellular changes that signal further impending clinical deterioration by using different monitoring modalities in a complementary fashion. A legitimate concern raised by some is that the vastly larger amounts of data generated by these devices requires computer-supported data analyses which is costly and time-consuming and may overwhelm the ill-prepared clinician and detract whatever benefits may be gained from the new technology [1]. Most agree that careful consideration should go into selecting the appropriate patient to monitor, the modalities to use, and that determining the most beneficial application of these technologies requires further prospective study.

The compelling theoretical importance of brain monitoring is based on the high vulnerability of the brain to hypoxic and ischemic injuries. The brain uses more oxygen and glucose per weight of tissue than any large organ, yet has no appreciable reserves of oxygen or glucose. The brain is thus completely dependent on uninterrupted cerebral blood flow (CBF) to supply metabolic substrates that are required for continued function and survival and to remove toxic byproducts. Even transient interruptions in CBF, whether local or global, can injure or kill neural cells. These perturbations may not result in immediate cell death, but can initiate metabolic or cellular processes (e.g., gene transcription, secondary injury) that may lead to cell death days, months, or years after the insult. Therefore, clinical monitoring of neuronal well-being should emphasize early detection and reversal of potentially harmful conditions. Although there is limited conclusive data to demonstrate that morbidity and mortality are reduced by the information gathered from current neurologic monitoring techniques, most clinicians caring for patients with critical neurologic illness have confidence that their use improves management. In this chapter, we review currently available techniques with emphasis on the current scientific literature and indications for utilization.

GOALS OF BRAIN MONITORING

Monitoring devices cannot independently improve outcome. Instead, they contribute physiologic data that can be integrated into a care plan that, while frequently adding risks (associated with placement, use, and removal), may lead to an overall decrease in morbidity and mortality.

Neurologic monitoring can be categorized into three main groups: (i) Monitors of neurologic function (e.g., neurologic examination, EEG, evoked potentials, functional MRI), (ii) Monitors of physiologic parameters (e.g., ICP, cerebral blood flow, transcranial Doppler), and (iii) Monitors of cellular metabolism (e.g., $SjvO_2$, NIRS, Brain tissue oxygen tension, Microdialysis, PET, MRSPECT). Most categorizations are arbitrary and obviously overlaps and inter-relationships between modalities (e.g., blood flow and electrical activity, oxygenation, and perfusion) blur the lines of distinction. All categories provide information that may be useful in assessing the current status of the brain and nervous system and in directing therapies as well as monitoring responses to interventions, but it cannot be overemphasized that the data obtained from these monitoring devices should always be interpreted in relation to the overall clinical picture of the individual patient.

TABLE 28.1

GLOSSARY OF NEUROLOGIC MONITOR CHARACTERISTICS

Term	Definition
Bias	Average difference (positive or negative) between monitored values and "gold standard" values
Precision	Standard deviation of the differences (bias) between measurements
Sensitivity	Probability that the monitor will demonstrate cerebral ischemia when cerebral ischemia is present
Positive predictive value	Probability that cerebral ischemia is present when the monitor suggests cerebral ischemia
Specificity	Probability that the monitor will not demonstrate cerebral ischemia when cerebral ischemia is not present
Negative predictive value	Probability that cerebral ischemia is not present when the monitor reflects no cerebral ischemia
Threshold value	The value used to separate acceptable (i.e., no ischemia present) from unacceptable (i.e., ischemia present)
Speed	The time elapsed from the onset of actual ischemia or the risk of ischemia until the monitor provides evidence

CEREBRAL ISCHEMIA

Given the brain's dependence and sensitivity to perturbations in oxygenation many if not all monitors are concerned with the detection of cerebral ischemia defined as cerebral delivery of oxygen (CDO_2) insufficient to meet metabolic needs. Cerebral ischemia is traditionally characterized as global or focal, and complete or incomplete (Table 28.2). Systemic monitors readily detect most global cerebral insults, such as hypotension, hypoxemia, or cardiac arrest. Brain-specific monitors can provide additional information primarily in situations, such as stroke, SAH with vasospasm, and TBI, in which systemic oxygenation and perfusion appear to be adequate but focal cerebral oxygenation may be impaired.

The severity of ischemic brain damage has traditionally been thought to be proportional to the magnitude and duration of reduced CDO_2. For monitoring to influence long-term patient morbidity and mortality, prompt recognition of reversible cerebral hypoxia/ischemia is essential. Numerous animal studies and human studies using different imaging techniques such as PET, MRI, and SPECT have concluded that the ischemic threshold for reversible injury or penumbra is a cerebral blood flow of 20 mL per 100 g per minute below which tissue is at risk for irreversible damage [2,3]. The tolerable duration of more profound ischemia is inversely proportional to the severity of CBF reduction (Fig. 28.1). Ischemia and hypoxemia initiate a cascade of cellular reactions that involve multiple pathways including energy failure from anaerobic glycolysis with accumulation of lactic acid and increase in lactate/pyruvate ratios, loss of ion homeostasis and failure of ATP-dependent ion pumps to maintain ion gradients. This leads to sodium and calcium influx into the cell and activation of enzymes such as phospholipases that result in further membrane and cytoskeletal damage, glutamate release and excitotoxicity, lipoperoxidases and free fatty acid breakdown, and free-radical formation and inflammation with microvascular changes. Endonucleases which alter gene regulation and protein synthesis and activate the caspase pathways that trigger apoptosis are also released [4,5]. Other proteins synthesized in response to altered oxygen delivery, such as hypoxia inducible factors (HIF), have been identified as adaptive mechanisms that respond to variations in oxygen partial pressure [6] and may be protective. These multiple pathways and cellular mediators and their interactions are potential areas for therapeutic intervention. Byproducts of these reactions provide potential biomarkers for secondary injury that can be used for monitoring. Our current understanding of the utility of this data is still evolving and currently when a cerebral monitor detects ischemia, the results must be carefully interpreted. Often, all that is known is that cerebral oxygenation in the region of the brain that is assessed by that monitor has fallen below a critical threshold. Such information neither definitively implies

TABLE 28.2

CHARACTERISTICS OF TYPES OF CEREBRAL ISCHEMIC INSULTS

Characteristics	Examples
Global, incomplete	Hypotension, hypoxemia, cardiopulmonary resuscitation
Global, complete	Cardiac arrest
Focal, incomplete	Stroke, subarachnoid hemorrhage with vasospasm

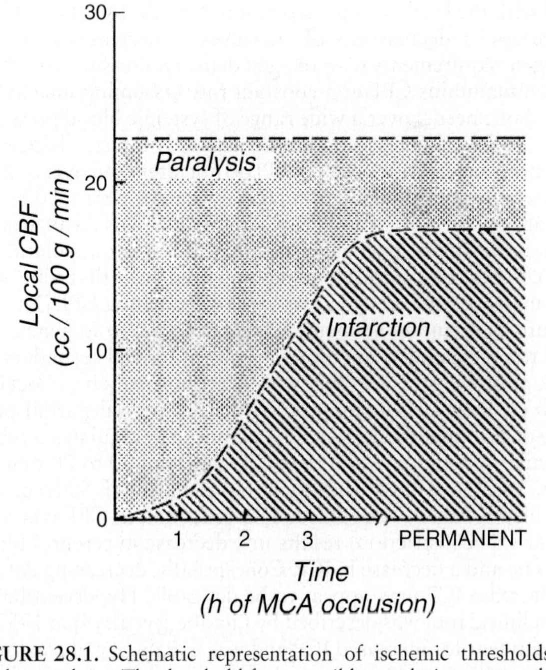

FIGURE 28.1. Schematic representation of ischemic thresholds in awake monkeys. The threshold for reversible paralysis occurs at local cerebral blood flow (local CBF) of approximately 23 mL/100 m/min. Irreversible injury (infarction) is a function of the magnitude of blood flow reduction and the duration of that reduction. Relatively severe ischemia is potentially reversible if the duration is sufficiently short. (From Jones TH, Morawetz RB, Crowell RM, et al: Thresholds of focal cerebral ischemia in awake monkeys. *J Neurosurg* 54:773–782, 1981, with permission.)

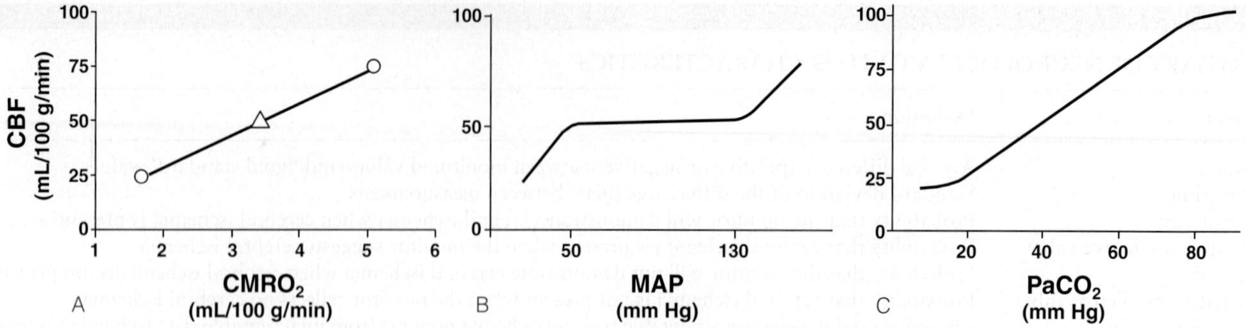

FIGURE 28.2. A: The normal relationship between the cerebral metabolic rate of oxygen consumption ($CMRO_2$) and cerebral blood flow (CBF) is characterized by closely couple changes in both variables. Normally, CBF is 50 mL per 100 g per minute in adults (*open triangle*). As $CMRO_2$ increases of decreases, CBF changes in a parallel fashion (*solid line*). **B:** Effect of mean arterial pressure (MAP) on CBF. Note that changes in MAP produce little change in CBF over a broad range of pressures. If intracranial pressure (ICP) exceeds normal limits, substitute cerebral perfusion pressure on the horizontal axis. **C:** Effect of $PaCO_2$ on CBF. Changes in $PaCO_2$ exert powerful effects on cerebral vascular resistance across the entire clinically applicable range of values.

that ischemia will necessarily progress to infarction nor does it clearly define what biochemical or genetic transcriptional changes may subsequently occur. Also, because more severe ischemia produces neurologic injury more quickly than less severe ischemia, time and dose effects must be considered. More important, if regional ischemia involves structures that are not components of the monitored variable, then infarction could develop without warning.

In healthy persons, CBF is tightly regulated through multiple pathways such that CDO_2 is adjusted to meet the metabolic requirements of the brain. In the normal, "coupled" relationship, CBF is dependent on the cerebral metabolic rate for oxygen ($CMRO_2$), which varies directly with body temperature and with the level of brain activation (Fig. 28.2A). As $CMRO_2$ increases or decreases, CBF increases or decreases to match oxygen requirements with oxygen delivery. Pressure autoregulation maintains CBF at a constant rate (assuming unchanged metabolic needs) over a wide range of systemic blood pressures (Fig. 28.2B). If pressure autoregulation is intact, changes of cerebral perfusion pressure (CPP) do not alter CBF over a range of pressures of 50 to 130 mm Hg. CPP can be described by the equation $CPP = MAP - ICP$, where MAP equals mean arterial pressure. After neurologic insults (e.g., TBI), autoregulation of the cerebral vasculature may be impaired such that CBF may not increase sufficiently in response to decreasing CPP [7]. This failure to maintain adequate CDO_2 can lead to ischemia and add to preexisting brain injury, a process termed secondary injury, at blood pressures that would not normally be associated with cerebral ischemia/injury. Normally, arterial partial pressure of carbon dioxide, ($PaCO_2$) significantly regulates cerebral vascular resistance over a range of $PaCO_2$ of 20 to 80 mm Hg (Fig. 28.2C). CBF is acutely halved if $PaCO_2$ is halved, and doubled if $PaCO_2$ is doubled. This reduction in CBF (via arteriolar vasoconstriction) results in a decrease in cerebral blood volume and a decrease in ICP. Conceptually, decreasing $PaCO_2$ to decrease ICP may appear to be desirable. Hyperventilation as a clinical tool was described by Lundberg et al. [8] in 1959 as a treatment for increased ICP and was a mainstay of treatment for over 40 years. However, in healthy brain, there are limits to maximal cerebral vasoconstriction with falling $PaCO_2$ (as well as vasodilation with increasing $PaCO_2$), such that, as CBF decreases to the point of producing inadequate CDO_2, local vasodilatory mechanisms tend to restore CBF and CDO_2. As a consequence, in healthy brain, hyperventilation does not produce severe cerebral ischemia; however, after TBI, hypocapnia can generate cerebral ischemia as reflected in decreased $PbtO_2$ and $SjvO_2$ [9,10]. For this reason, hyperventilation has fallen out of favor as a treatment modality for intracranial hypertension. If hyperventilation is required to acutely reduce ICP to bridge a patient to emergent surgery for example, administration of an increased inspired oxygen concentration can markedly increase $SjvO_2$ (Fig. 28.3). In response to decreasing arterial oxygen content (CaO_2), whether the reduction is secondary to a decrease of hemoglobin (Hgb) concentration or of arterial oxygen saturation (SaO_2), CBF normally increases, although injured brain tissue has impaired ability to increase CBF [11].

TECHNIQUES OF NEUROLOGIC MONITORING

Neurologic Examination

Frequent and accurately recorded neurologic examinations are an essential aspect of medical care, but are often limited in patients with moderate-to-severe neurologic compromise. Neurologic examination quantifies three key characteristics: level of consciousness, focal brain dysfunction, and trends in neurologic function. Recognition of changing consciousness or new focal deficits may warn of a variety of treatable conditions, such as progression of intracranial hypertension, new mass lesions such as expansion of intraparenchymal contusions or subdural hematoma and systemic complications of intracranial pathology, such as hyponatremia.

The GCS score, originally developed as a tool for the assessment of impaired consciousness [12], has also been used as a prognostic tool for patients with TBI [13]. The GCS score at the time of initial hospitalization is used to characterize the severity of TBI, with severe TBI defined as a GCS score less than or equal to 8, moderate TBI as a GCS score of 9 to 12, and mild TBI as that associated with a GCS score greater than 12. Lower GCS scores are generally associated with poorer long-term outcomes, although correlation to individual patients with TBI is difficult because of the significant variations in mortality rates and functional outcome [14]. Significant concern has arisen regarding the validity of the initial GCS score on presentation given the aggressive prehospital management of these patients over the last decade or so, that includes sedation and intubation in the field or the administration of paralytics and sedatives in

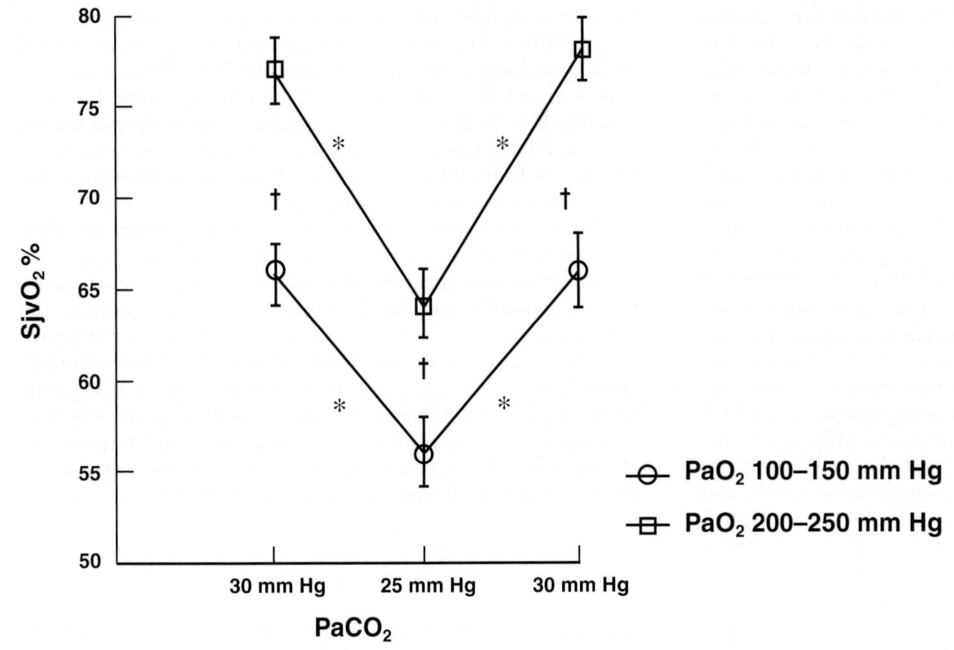

FIGURE 28.3. The effect of hyperoxia on percentage of oxygen saturation of jugular venous blood ($SjvO_2$) at two levels of $PaCO_2$. *$p < 0.001$ for $SjvO_2$ at $PaCO_2$ 25–30 mm Hg at each PaO_2. †$p < 0.001$ for $SjvO_2$ between PaO_2 at each $PaCO_2$ level. (From Thiagarajan A, Goverdhan PD, Chari P, et al: The effect of hyperventilation and hyperoxia on cerebral venous oxygen saturation in patients with traumatic brain injury. *Anesth Analg* 87:850–853, 1998, with permission.)

the emergency room. Some authors have reported a loss of predictive value of the GCS score from 1997 onwards and call for a critical reconsideration of its use [15]. Other studies done have looked at GCS in the field versus GCS upon arrival and have found good correlation and prognostic value in predicting outcome and have even found the changes in scores from field GCS to arrival GCS to be highly predictive of outcome in patients with moderate to severe TBI [16]. Many centers use the best GCS or postresuscitation GCS in the first 24 hours or just the motor component of the GCS instead of initial GCS given these issues. Nevertheless, the GCS score is popular as a quick, reproducible estimate of level of consciousness (Table 28.3), has become a common tool for the serial monitoring of consciousness, and has been incorporated into various outcome models, such as the Trauma score, APACHE II, and the Trauma-Injury Severity score. The GCS score, which includes eye opening, motor responses in the best functioning limb, and verbal responses is limited and by no means replaces a thoughtful and focused neurologic examination. It should be supplemented by recording pupillary size and reactivity, cranial nerve examination and more detailed neurologic testing depending on the relevant neuroanatomy involved in the disease process. Even so, the use of serial GCS determinations remains a common tool in the management of patients with neurologic dysfunction.

Systemic Monitoring

Although not specific to neurologic monitoring, systemic parameters, including blood pressure, arterial oxygen saturation (SaO_2), $PaCO_2$, serum glucose concentration, and temperature, have clinical relevance in the management of patients with neurologic dysfunction or injury. The relationships between these systemic variables and long-term outcome after neurologic insults are closely linked and are subject to continuing research.

Perhaps the most important systemic monitor is blood pressure, as CBF is dependent on the relationship between CPP and cerebral vascular resistance (CVR), and can be modeled generally by the equation: CBF = CPP/CVR. As previously discussed, CBF is maintained relatively constant over a wide range of blood pressures (pressure autoregulation) through arteriolar changes in resistance (assuming no change in brain metabolism) in healthy individuals. After brain injury, autoregulation may become impaired, especially in traumatically brain-injured patients. Chesnut et al. [17,18] reported that even brief periods of hypotension (systolic blood pressure less than 90 mm Hg) worsened outcome after TBI, and recommended that systolic blood pressure be maintained greater than 90 mm Hg (with possible benefit from higher pressures). These recommendations have also been promoted by the Brain Trauma Foundation for patients with severe TBI [19]. To achieve this goal, the use of vasoactive substances, such as norepinephrine, may be required [20]. Nevertheless, optimal blood pressure management

TABLE 28.3

GLASGOW COMA SCALE

Component	Response	Score
Eye opening	Spontaneously	4
	To verbal command	3
	To pain	2
	None	1
		Subtotal: 1–4
Motor response (best extremity)	Obeys verbal command	6
	Localizes pain	5
	Flexion-withdrawal	4
	Flexor (decorticate posturing)	3
	Extensor (decerebrate posturing)	2
	No response (flaccid)	1
		Subtotal: 1–6
Best verbal response	Oriented and converses	5
	Disoriented and converses	4
	Inappropriate words	3
	Incomprehensive sounds	2
	No verbal response	1
		Subtotal: 1–5
		Total: 3–15

for patients with TBI has yet to be defined. Some clinical data suggest that the influence of hypotension on outcome after TBI is equivalent to the influence of hypotension on outcome after non-neurologic trauma [21]. Proposed treatment protocols include CPP greater than 70 mm Hg [22], greater than 60 mm Hg [23], or greater than 50 mm Hg [24]. The augmentation of CPP above 70 mm Hg with fluids and vasopressors has, however, been associated with increased risk of acute respiratory distress syndrome and is not universally recommended [23].

Another essential step in insuring adequate CDO_2 is the maintenance of adequate CaO_2, which in turn is dependent on Hgb and SaO_2; therefore, anemia and hypoxemia can reduce CDO_2, which would normally result in compensatory increases in CBF. However, these compensatory mechanisms are limited. As SaO_2 (or PaO_2) decreases below the compensatory threshold, $SjvO_2$ and jugular venous oxygen content ($CjvO_2$), which reflect the ability of CDO_2 to supply $CMRO_2$, also decrease. The correlation is most evident below a PaO_2 of approximately 60 mm Hg, the PaO_2 at which SaO_2 is 90% and below which SaO_2 rapidly decreases. In contrast, as Hgb is reduced by normovolemic hemodilution, $SjvO_2$ remains relatively constant unless severe anemia is produced [25].

The management of arterial CO_2 in patients with neurologic injury has changed dramatically in the past 10 years. Although hyperventilation as a management strategy for increased ICP was routine in the 1990s, it is now reserved for acute or life-threatening increases in the intensive care unit (ICU) and is no longer recommended for routine use. Having been associated with cerebral ischemia in children and adults [9,10] with severe TBI, hyperventilation is least likely to be harmful when combined with monitoring, such as $SjvO_2$ or $PbtO_2$, that can identify cerebral ischemia.

Hyperglycemia increased injury in experimental TBI [26] and was associated with worse outcome in clinical TBI [27,28], although it is difficult to distinguish between elevated glucose causing worsened outcome versus increased severity of TBI inducing more elevated glucose levels [29]. In critically ill patients requiring mechanical ventilation, elevated glucose levels were associated with worsened outcomes [30], and current recommendations are to tightly control serum glucose in critically ill patients in the medical and surgical ICU [31]. Caution must be exercised in the brain injured patient as there is also evidence to suggest that hypoglycemia can be more detrimental than hyperglycemia and microdialysis studies in traumatic brain injury patients found that extracellular glucose concentration is low after TBI and is associated with markers for tissue distress and poor outcome [32].

The monitoring and management of body temperature remains an important aspect of care for critically ill patients. Hypothermia and hyperthermia should be considered separately in this context. The use of hypothermia as a treatment for brain injury, while demonstrating benefit in animals [33] and in some phase II human studies, has not shown consistent benefit in larger studies [34] and is not recommended for general use in TBI [35,36]. Although the largest clinical trials (NABISH-1 and Hypothermia Pediatric Head Injury Trial Investigators and the Canadian Critical Care Trials Group) were negative [37,38], there were numerous smaller human trials and meta-analyses that suggested improved neurologic outcomes with hypothermia in TBI. Some authors suggest that the failure of these trials was because of poor protocol design and lack of proper management of the side effects of hypothermia [39,40]. In contrast, induced hypothermia after resuscitation from cardiac arrest (secondary to ventricular tachycardia or fibrillation) has improved outcome in some trials [41,42]. Research into this complex area is ongoing, and clinical practice is likely to undergo further refinement.

Hyperthermia is common in critically ill patients, occurring in up to 90% of patients with neurologic disease, related to both diagnosis and length of stay [43,44]. Hyperthermia is generally associated with poorer outcome when associated with neurologic injury in adults and children [45], but a causal link with adverse outcome (as with serum glucose levels) is lacking. It is unclear whether increased temperatures result in worsened long-term neurologic outcome, or whether a greater severity of brain injury is associated with more frequent or severe increases in systemic temperature.

The method of temperature monitoring is important. Thermal gradients exist throughout the body, and the site of measurement influences the diagnosis of hypothermia, normothermia, or hyperthermia. Measurements of systemic temperature may underestimate brain temperature. In studies of temperature monitoring by site, variations of up to 3°C have been identified between the brain and other routinely used monitoring sites, emphasizing the importance of monitoring site selection in patients with neurologic injury and the need to appreciate the difference between brain temperature and the active site of measurement used clinically for a given patient.

EEG/Electrocorticography

Electroencephalographic (EEG) monitoring has long been used in neurology for diagnosis and intraoperative monitoring, but has less frequently been used as a neurologic monitoring technique in critically ill patients. EEG is indicated in response to suspicion of a new or progressive abnormality such as cerebral ischemia or new onset of seizures. The cortical EEG or electrocorticography, which is altered by mild cerebral ischemia and abolished by profound cerebral ischemia, can be used to indicate potentially damaging cerebral hypoperfusion. More recent research has documented its utility in the detection of cortical spreading depression and peri-infarct depolarizations (proposed to be early indicators of delayed ischemic injury) in the acutely injured human cortex in traumatic brain injury and subarachnoid hemorrhage [46,47]. The EEG can document seizures, either convulsive or nonconvulsive, and provide information as to the efficacy of antiseizure therapy. Other functions include defining the depth or type of coma, documenting focal or lateralizing intracranial abnormalities, and the diagnosis of brain death.

If the EEG is to be used for monitoring, care must be taken and weaknesses of the technique appreciated [48]. In the ICU, electrical noise from other equipment may produce artifacts and interfere with technically adequate tracings. Continuous EEG recording was cumbersome in the past owing to the sheer volume of data (300 pages per hour of hard copy on as many as 16 channels), but techniques for digital recording and networking direct computer recording of EEG data are now available given adequate computer power and storage. Scalp fixation has also been a significant limiting factor, although newer fixation techniques are easier to apply and more stable. Techniques of mathematical data analysis, such as rapid Fourier analysis, can be used to determine the relative amplitude in each frequency band (delta—less than 4 Hz, theta—4 to 8 Hz, alpha—8 to 13 Hz, beta—greater than 13 Hz), which can then be displayed graphically in formats such as the compressed spectral array or density spectral array. Alpha variability has been found to predict vasospasm/delayed cerebral ischemia in subarachnoid hemorrhage patients [49] and the percentage of alpha variability was found to have prognostic value in traumatic brain injury [50]. Analytic software has been developed that processes the raw EEG signal to provide single number interpretation of the "depth of sedation." These devices have been recommended for use during general anesthesia as a means to reduce the risk of awareness [51], although the scientific justification for this claim is not conclusive. The American Society of Anesthesiologists has developed a practice advisory on this issue [52]. Use of this type of monitoring has also been implemented by some for use in the ICU for monitoring sedation levels in the critically ill, the utility of which has yet to be proven [53,54]. All devices use proprietary analysis of an EEG signal (either spontaneous or evoked, with or without electromyogram monitoring), which is converted to a single number that is intended to correspond to an awareness level based on an arbitrary scale. The future role and evidence of improved patient outcomes with this monitoring modality remain unclear. A more detailed discussion of the clinical indications, technical aspects, and limitations can be found in a recent review [55].

EVOKED POTENTIALS

Sensory-evoked potentials (EPs), which include somatosensory-evoked potentials (SSEPs), brainstem auditory EPs, and visual EPs, can be used as qualitative threshold monitors to detect severe neural ischemia. Unlike EEG that records the continuous, spontaneous activity of the brain, EPs evaluate the responses of the brain to specific stimuli. To record SSEPs, stimuli are applied to a peripheral nerve, usually the median nerve at the wrist or posterior tibial nerve at the ankle, by a low-amplitude current of approximately 20 milliseconds in duration. The resultant sensory (afferent) nerve stimulation and resultant cortical response to the stimulus are recorded at the scalp. Repeated identical stimuli are applied and signal averaging is used to remove the highly variable background EEG and other environmental electrical noise and thereby visualize reproducible evoked responses (Fig. 28.4).

EPs are described in terms of the amplitude of cortical response peaks and the conduction delay (latency) between the stimulus and the appearance of response waveform. Because peripheral nerve stimulation can be uncomfortable, SSEPs are usually obtained from sedated or anesthetized patients. SSEPs are unaffected by neuromuscular blocking agents but may be significantly influenced by sedative, analgesic, and anesthetic agents, often in a dose-dependent manner. In general, however, the doses of drugs required to influence EPs are sufficient to produce general anesthesia and are not usually clinically important in the ICU. If a patient is undergoing EP monitoring and requires large doses of analgesic or sedative agents, potential impairment of monitoring should be considered. Motor EPs represent a method of selectively evaluating descending motor tracts. Stimulation of proximal motor tracts (cortical or spinal) and evaluation of subsequent responses yield information that can be used for intraoperative and early postoperative neurosurgical management. Induction of motor EP and its interpretation is exquisitely sensitive to sedative, analgesic, and anesthetic drugs, making clinical use difficult when drugs are given concurrently. Despite these limitations, motor EP evaluation has been successfully used for the management of neuro-ICU patients and may become more common as techniques and equipment improve [56,57].

The sensitivity of EP monitoring is similar to that of EEG monitoring. EPs, especially brainstem auditory EPs, are relatively robust, although they can be modified by trauma, hypoxia, or ischemia. Because obliteration of EPs occurs only under conditions of profound cerebral ischemia or mechanical trauma, EP monitoring is one of the most specific ways in which to assess neurologic integrity in specific monitored pathways. However, as with the discussion of cerebral ischemia, there is a dose–time interaction that ultimately determines the magnitude of cerebral injury. As a result, neurologic deficits occur that have not been predicted by changes in EPs, and severe changes in EPs may not be followed by neurologic deficits. The most definitive indication for SSEPs is in the prognostication of anoxic brain injury from cardiac arrest. The absence of the N20 response on bilateral SSEPs of the median nerve within 3 days postarrest has been found to be a reliable predictor of negative outcome or recovery of consciousness in anoxic postarrest coma and is part of the AAN practice parameter in the prognostication of postanoxic coma [58].

INTRACRANIAL PRESSURE MONITORING

The symptoms and signs of intracranial hypertension are neither sensitive nor specific. Usually, the physical findings associated with increasing ICP (e.g., Cushing's response–hypertension and Cushing's triad–hypertension, reflex bradycardia, and alterations in respiratory function) become apparent only when intracranial hypertension has become sufficiently severe to injure the brain. Likewise, papilledema is a late development and is often difficult to identify clinically. Because ICP cannot otherwise be adequately assessed, direct

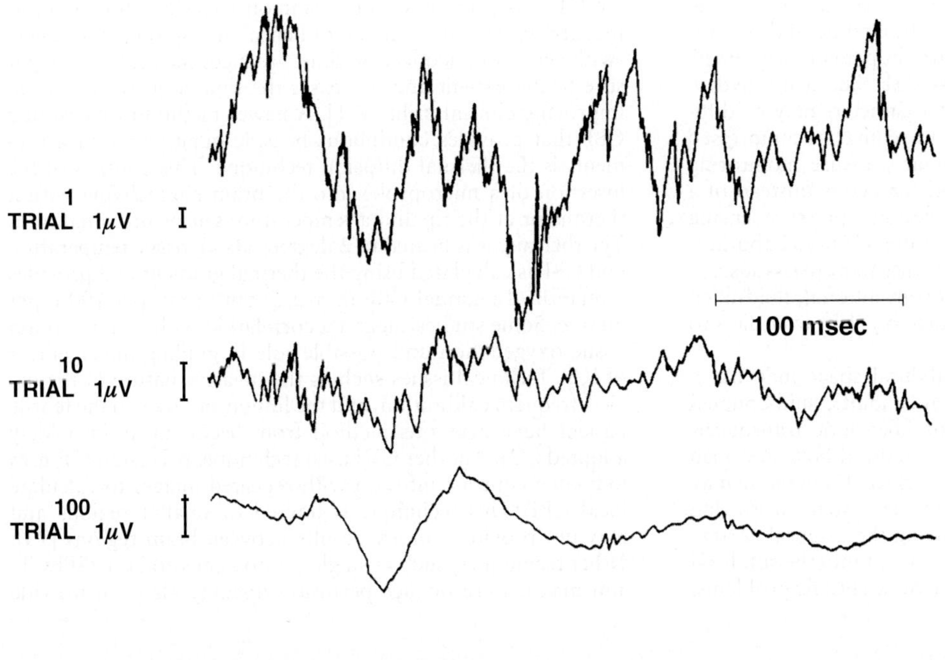

FIGURE 28.4. Averaging reduces background noise. After 100 trials, this visual evoked potential (EP) is relatively noise-free. The same EP is hard to distinguish after only 10 trials and would be impossible to find in the original unaveraged data. (From Nuwer MR: *Evoked Potential Monitoring in the Operating Room*. New York, Raven Press, 1986, p 29, with permission.)

measurement and monitoring of ICP has become a common intervention, especially in the management of TBI [59], and less commonly after critical illnesses such as SAH or stroke. Although there is no class 1 evidence that the use of this technique improves outcomes, there is a large body of clinical evidence supporting its use to guide therapeutic interventions in traumatic brain injury that have potential risks (such as aggressive osmotherapy, induced hypothermia and barbiturate coma), to aid in the detection intracranial mass lesions and to provide prognostic data [60]. ICP monitoring has been found to improve outcome prediction in TBI and next to clinical parameters such as age, GCS motor score and abnormal pupillary responses, the proportion of hourly ICP recordings greater than 20 mm Hg was the next most significant predictor of outcome in an analysis done of the National Traumatic Coma Data Bank [61]. Despite this, the debate continues on how to use ICP data to change patient care and reduce morbidity and mortality. It is unlikely that a large randomized clinical trial will ever be done given the lack of clinical equipoise. The Brain Trauma Foundation/American Association of Neurosurgeons Guidelines recommend ICP monitoring in all patients with severe TBI (GCS <8) and an abnormal CT scan or a normal scan with patients who are greater than 40 years old, have motor posturing, or a systolic BP <90 mm Hg [62,63]. Because pressure gradients may exist among various sites within the calvarium, it may be advantageous to monitor in or adjacent to the most severely damaged hemisphere [64], some even recommend bilateral ICP monitoring to circumvent this problem [65].

ICP functions as the outflow pressure apposing MAP (CPP = MAP − ICP) when ICP exceeds jugular venous pressure. Because the skull is not distensible, the brain, cerebrospinal fluid (CSF), and cerebral blood volume have little room to expand without increasing ICP. It is important to appreciate that some increase in intracranial volume is possible without much change in ICP, but when the compensatory mechanisms are exhausted, even small changes in volume can lead to significant increases in pressure. Although CBF cannot be directly inferred from knowledge of MAP and ICP, severe increases in ICP reduce CPP and CBF. ICP monitoring provides temporally relevant, quantitative information. The problems associated with ICP monitoring fall generally into three categories: direct morbidity due to monitor placement (e.g., intracranial hemorrhage, cortical damage, and infection), inaccurate measurement, and misinterpretation or inappropriate use of the data. Clinically, one of three sites is used to measure ICP: a lateral ventricle, the brain parenchyma, and much less commonly the subdural space. Ventricular catheterization, when performed using strict asepsis, is the method of choice for ICP monitoring and CSF drainage [66] in patients with acute intracranial hypertension and excess CSF (i.e., acute hydrocephalus). In practice, intraventricular catheters may be difficult to place if cerebral edema or brain swelling has compressed the ventricular system. Intraventricular pressure monitoring can also be performed with fiber-optic catheters (instead of a hollow catheter) that use a variable reflectance pressure sensing system (transducer tip) to measure pressure (Camino Laboratories, San Diego, CA). These fiber-optic catheters are less susceptible to short-term malfunction than conventional, fluid-filled catheters but may slowly and unpredictably drift over days to weeks [67].

Pressure monitoring from the subdural space may use a fluid-coupled bolt (simple transcranial conduit), fluid-coupled subdural catheters (or reservoirs), or fiber-optic transducer-tipped catheters (see earlier). Because subdural bolts are open tubes facing end-on against the brain surface, brain tissue may herniate into the system, obstructing the system, distorting measurements, and potentially damaging the cerebral cortex. Reservoir systems require surgical placement into the subdural space. Fiber-optic systems do not have these specific problems, but fixation and equipment reliability are practical issues. This technique is used uncommonly for these reasons.

Intraparenchymal placement of a fiber-optic catheter is also possible and is associated with complications similar to ventricular fiber-optic catheters. Complications are generally noted to be highest with ventriculostomies (when compared with fiber-optic catheter usage), and complications of ICP monitoring are associated with a worse GCS score.

Management decisions based on ICP data are the focus of ongoing debate and study. Clinical studies after TBI have demonstrated that increased ICP is associated with worsened outcome [68]. Therefore, control of ICP has been considered by some clinicians to be the primary focus of treatment [24], while other clinicians have considered restoration of CPP (by increasing MAP) to be the primary goal of medical management [21]. To date, the ideal approach has not been established by outcome trials; therefore, practice patterns remain variable [69]. Clinical experience with ICP monitoring of head-injured patients has resulted in publication of clinical guidelines using an evidence-based approach (Fig. 28.5) [70].

CEREBRAL BLOOD FLOW MONITORING

The first quantitative clinical method of measurement of CBF, the Kety–Schmidt technique, calculated global CBF from the difference between the arterial and jugular bulb concentration curves of an inhaled, inert gas as it equilibrated with blood and brain tissue. Later techniques used extracranial gamma detectors to measure regional cortical CBF from washout curves after intracarotid injection of a radioisotope such as 133-xenon (Xe 133). Carotid puncture was avoided by techniques that measured cortical CBF after inhaled or intravenous administration of Xe 133, using gamma counting of exhaled gas to correct clearance curves for recirculation of Xe 133. Because Xe is radiodense, saturation of brain tissue increases radiographic density in proportion to CBF. Imaging of the brain after equilibration with stable (nonradioactive) Xe provides a regional estimate of CBF that includes deep brain structures. Clinical studies of CBF after TBI performed using stable xenon computed tomography (CT) have prompted a radical revision of conventional understanding by demonstrating that one third of patients had evidence of cerebral ischemia within 8 hours of trauma. Although slow in becoming a routine clinical tool, Xe CT is becoming a more common technique for monitoring CBF in patients. The use of helical and spiral CT scanners (with very short acquisition times) reduces the radiation exposure to the patient and decreases the time needed for a scan, improving clinical utility [71]. A newer method of measuring CBF that provides continuous bedside quantitative measurements is the thermal diffusion technique. This consists of the insertion of a microprobe into the brain parenchyma with a thermistor at the tip and a temperature sensor proximal to it. The thermistor is heated to 2 degrees above tissue temperature and CBF is calculated using the thermal gradient and provides a quantified regional CBF measurement in mL per 100 g per minute. Some studies suggest a correlation with regional brain tissue oxygenation and possible role in guiding management of ICP. Technical issues such as the invasive nature of the device, frequent calibration, and the limitations seen in the febrile patient have kept this method from becoming more widely adopted [72]. Another CT-based technique, perfusion CT, uses iodinated contrast infusion with repeated images to calculate local CBF. This technique is limited to smaller regions and may not provide uniform results between brain regions [73]. Other techniques, such as single-photon emission CT (SPECT) and magnetic resonance perfusion imaging also can provide

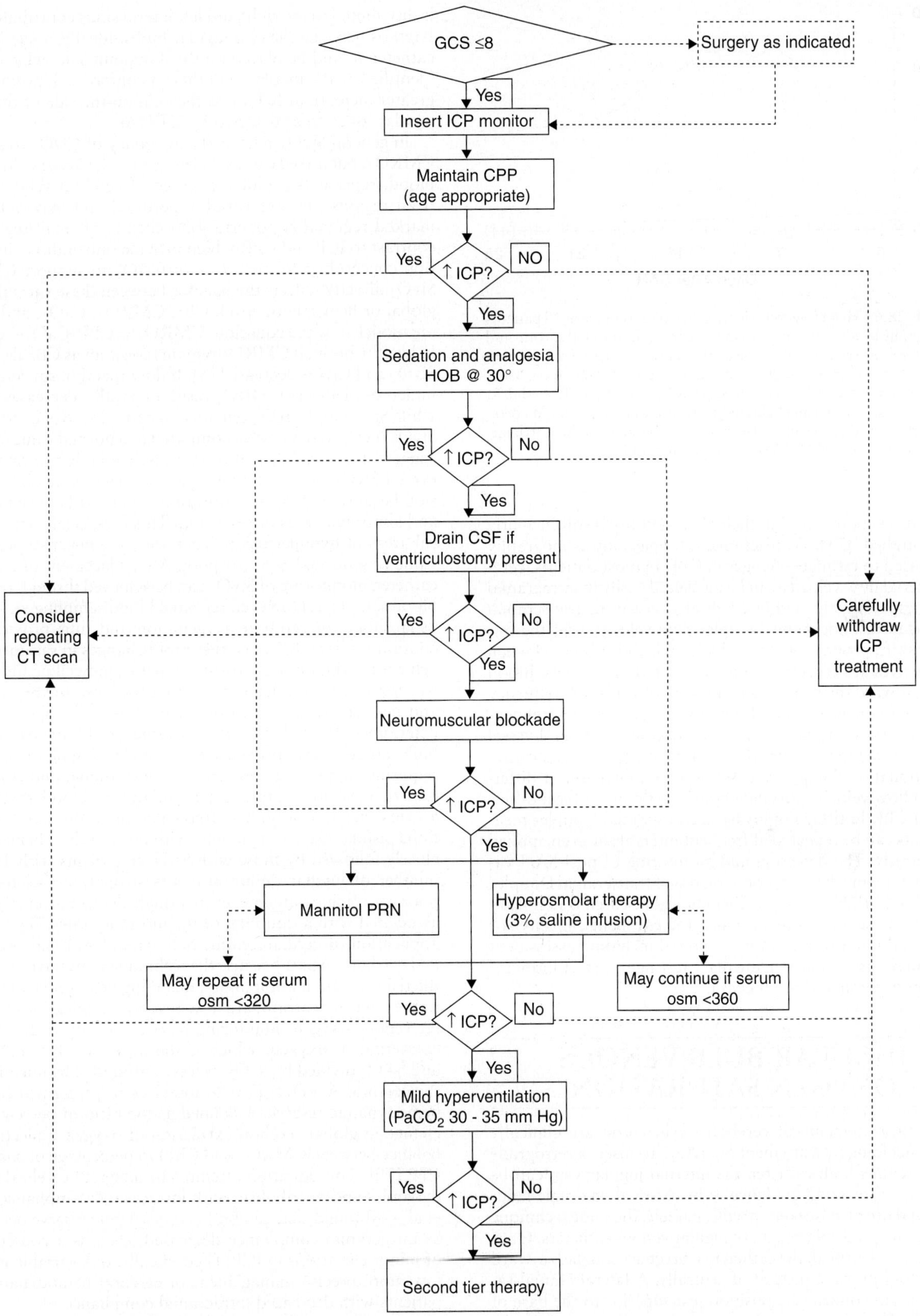

FIGURE 28.5. Critical pathway for treatment of intracranial hypertension in the pediatric patient with severe head injury. ICP, intracranial pressure. (From Adelson PD, Bratton SL, Carney NA, et al: Critical pathway for the treatment of established intracranial hypertension in pediatric traumatic brain injury. *Ped Crit Care Med* 4(3)[Suppl]:S65–S67, 2003, with permission.)

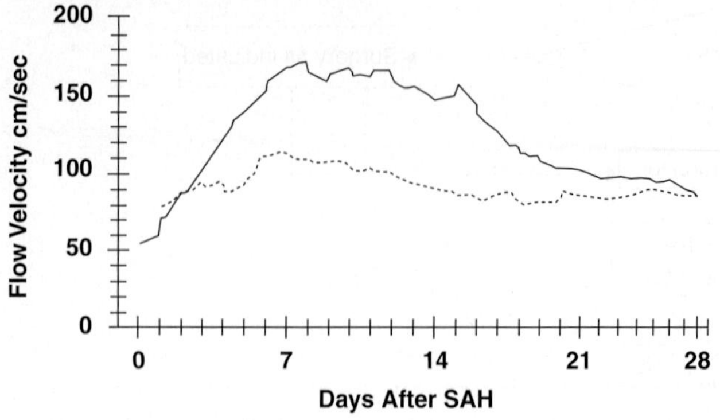

FIGURE 28.6. Mean flow velocity (FV, in cm/sec) curves of 18 patients with laterally localized aneurysms (arising from the internal carotid and middle cerebral arteries). The side of the ruptured aneurysm (*continuous line*) shows a higher FV than the unaffected side (*dotted line*). SAH, subarachnoid hemorrhage. (From Seiler RW, Grolimund P, Aaslid R, et al: Cerebral vasospasm evaluated by transcranial ultrasound correlated with clinical grade and CT-visualized subarachnoid hemorrhage. *J Neurosurg* 64:594–600, 1986, with permission.)

information about CBF, but their clinical utility is still currently being studied [71]. Transcranial Doppler ultrasonography can be used to estimate changes in CBF. In most patients, cerebral arterial flow velocity can be measured easily in intracranial vessels, especially the middle cerebral artery, using transcranial Doppler ultrasonography. Doppler flow velocity uses the frequency shift, proportional to velocity, which is observed when sound waves are reflected from moving red blood cells. Blood moving toward the transducer shifts the transmitted frequency to higher frequencies; blood moving away, to lower frequencies. Velocity is a function of both blood flow rate and vessel diameter. If diameter remains constant, changes in velocity are proportional to changes in CBF; however, intersubject differences in flow velocity correlate poorly with intersubject differences in CBF. Entirely noninvasive, transcranial Doppler measurements can be repeated at frequent intervals or even applied continuously. The detection and monitoring of post-SAH vasospasm remains the most common use of transcranial Doppler (Fig. 28.6) [74]. However, further clinical research is necessary to define those situations in which the excellent capacity for rapid trend monitoring can be exploited including assessment of vascular autoregulation, ancillary testing to detect intracranial hypertension and brain death.

JUGULAR BULB VENOUS OXYGEN SATURATION

Several measurements of cerebral oxygenation are clinically useful, including measurement of $SjvO_2$. To insert a retrograde jugular venous bulb catheter, the internal jugular vein can be located by ultrasound guidance or by external anatomic landmarks and use of a "seeker" needle, namely, the same technique used for antegrade placement of jugular venous catheters. Once the vessel is identified, the catheter is directed cephalad, toward the mastoid process, instead of centrally. A lateral cranial radiograph can confirm the position just superior to the base of the skull. The decision to place a jugular bulb catheter in the left or right jugular bulb is important. Simultaneous measurements of $SjvO_2$ in the right and left jugular bulb demonstrate differences in saturation [75], suggesting that one jugular bulb frequently is dominant, carrying the greater portion of cerebral venous blood. Differences in the cross-sectional areas of the vessels that form the torcula and the manner in which blood is distributed to the right and left lateral sinus contribute to differences between the two jugular bulbs. Ideally, a jugular bulb catheter should be placed on the dominant side, which can be identified as the jugular vein that, if compressed, produces the greater increase in ICP or as the vein on the side of the larger jugular foramen as detected by CT [76].

In general $SjvO_2$ reflects the adequacy of CDO_2 to support $CMRO_2$, but mixed cerebral venous blood, like mixed systemic blood, represents a global average of cerebral venous blood from regions that are variably perfused and may not reflect marked regional hypoperfusion/ischemia of small regions. In contrast to ICP and CPP, which provide only indirect information concerning the adequacy of CDO_2 to support $CMRO_2$, $SjvO_2$ directly reflects the balance between these variables on a global or hemispheric level. CBF, $CMRO_2$, CaO_2, and $CjvO_2$ are modeled by the equation: $CMRO_2 = CBF\,(CaO_2 - CjvO_2)$. In healthy brain, if $CMRO_2$ remains constant as CBF decreases, $SjvO_2$ and $CjvO_2$ decrease [25]. If flow-metabolism coupling is intact, decreases in $CMRO_2$ result in parallel decreases in CBF while $SjvO_2$ and $CjvO_2$ remain constant [25]. Abnormally low $SjvO_2$ (i.e., less than 50%, compared to a normal value of 65%) suggests the possibility of cerebral ischemia; but normal or elevated $SjvO_2$ does not prove the adequacy of cerebral perfusion because of possible saturation averaging between normal and abnormal areas of perfusion. This is especially true for focal areas of hypoperfusion. Therefore, the negative predictive value of a normal $SjvO_2$ is poor. After placement of a jugular catheter, monitoring of $SjvO_2$ can be achieved through repeated blood sampling. However, repeated blood sampling yields only "snapshots" of cerebral oxygenation and thus provides discontinuous data that may miss rapid changes in saturation. To achieve continuous monitoring of $SjvO_2$, indwelling fiber-optic oximetric catheters have been used. Because oxyhemoglobin and deoxyhemoglobin absorb light differently, $SjvO_2$ can be determined from differential absorbance. Oximetric jugular bulb catheters have proven somewhat challenging to maintain, requiring frequent recalibration, repositioning, and confirmation of measured saturation by analyzing blood samples in a cooximeter. The highest frequency of confirmed desaturation episodes occurs in patients with intracerebral hematomas, closely followed by those with SAH. In patients with TBI, the number of jugular desaturations is strongly associated with poor neurologic outcome; even a single desaturation episode is associated with a doubling of the mortality rate [77]. Clinical application of jugular venous bulb cannulation has been limited, perhaps in part because the technique is invasive, although the risks of cannulation injury, including hematoma and injury to the adjacent carotid, are low. Several modifications of jugular venous oxygen monitoring have been proposed. Cerebral extraction of oxygen, which is the difference between SaO_2 and $SjvO_2$ divided by SaO_2, is less confounded by anemia than the cerebral A-VDO_2 [78]. Another concept, termed cerebral hemodynamic reserve, is defined as the ratio of percentage of change in global cerebral extraction of oxygen (reflecting the balance between $CMRO_2$ and CBF) to percentage of change in CPP [79]. This equation attempts to integrate cerebral hemodynamics and metabolism with intracranial compliance. Cruz et al. [78] found that cerebral hemodynamic reserve decreased as intracranial compliance decreased, even as a consequence of minor elevations in ICP. Theoretically, this variable may allow more precise management of cerebral hemodynamics in patients with decreased intracranial compliance.

BRAIN TISSUE OXYGEN TENSION

Another promising technique for monitoring the adequacy of CDO_2 is direct assessment of $PbtO_2$. Monitoring of $PbtO_2$ overcomes one important limitation of $SjvO_2$ monitoring, which is that the global saturation measurements provide no information about regional or focal tissue oxygenation. Only relatively profound focal global ischemia causes $SjvO_2$ to decrease to less than the accepted critical threshold of 50%. Even severe regional ischemia may not result in desaturation if venous effluent from other regions is normally saturated, in part because the absolute flow of poorly saturated blood returning from ischemic regions is by definition less per volume of tissue than flow from well-perfused regions, resulting in a smaller percentage of poorly oxygenated to well-oxygenated blood. Intracranial, intraparenchymal probes have been developed that monitor only $PbtO_2$ or that also monitor brain tissue PCO_2 and pH [79]. Modified from probes designed for continuous monitoring of arterial blood gases, intraparenchymal probes can be inserted through multiple-lumen ICP monitoring bolts. Although these probes provide no information about remote regions, they nevertheless provide continuous information about the region that is contiguous to the probe. They also carry the theoretical risk of hematoma formation, infection, and direct parenchymal injury. Evaluation of $PbtO_2$ after severe TBI has shown that low partial pressures ($PbtO_2$ less than 10 mm Hg for greater than 15 minutes) powerfully predict poor outcomes and that $PbtO_2$ probes are safe [80,81]. Both $PbtO_2$ and $SjvO_2$ may reflect changes in cerebral oxygenation secondary to alterations in CBF (Fig. 28.7) [82]. However, comparisons of simultaneous $PbtO_2$ and $SjvO_2$ monitoring suggest that each monitor detects cerebral ischemia that the other fails to detect. In 58 patients with severe TBI, the two monitors detected 52 episodes in which $SjvO_2$ decreased to less than 50% or $PbtO_2$ decreased to less than 8 mm Hg; of those 52 episodes, both monitored variables fell below the ischemic threshold in 17, only $SjvO_2$ reflected ischemia in 19, and only $PbtO_2$ reflected ischemia in 16 (Fig. 28.8) [83]. Ongoing research will determine the role of $PbtO_2$ monitoring and the relationship between $PbtO_2$ monitoring and $SjvO_2$ monitoring in critical neurologic illness. Recent single-center prospective studies comparing brain tissue oxygen directed protocols in traumatic brain injury with historical controls report reduced mortality as well as improved 6-month clinical outcomes [84,85]. A randomized multicenter clinical trial is in the planning stages but has not started recruiting patients yet (BOOST-2).

NEUROCHEMICAL MONITORING

Neuronal injury is associated with the release or production of chemical markers such as free radicals, inflammatory mediators, metabolic products, and excitatory amino acids [4]. Neurochemical monitoring via microdialysis allows assessment of the chemical milieu of cerebral extracellular fluid, provides valuable information about neurochemical processes in various neuropathologic states, and is used clinically in the management of severe TBI [86] and SAH [87,88]. There is data to suggest that chemical changes detected by microdialysis precede secondary neurologic injury and clinical worsening in intracranial hypertension, subarachnoid hemorrhage, and ischemic stroke. Substances monitored via microdialysis include energy-related metabolites such as glucose, lactate, pyruvate, adenosine, and xanthine; neurotransmitters such as glutamate, aspartate, gamma-amino butyric acid; markers of tissue damage such as glycerol and potassium [89], and alterations in membrane phospholipids by oxygen radicals [90]. Lactate levels and lactate/pyruvate ratios are reliable markers of ischemia and have been found to correlate well with PET, cerebral perfusion pressure and jugular venous bulb oxygen saturation values and associated with outcome in traumatic brain injury and subarachnoid hemorrhage. Elevations of the excitatory neurotransmitter glutamate have been found in hypoxic-ischemic injury seen in low CBF, jugular venous bulb desaturation, seizures and low CPP, and correlated with poor outcome in TBI. The magnitude of release of these substances correlates with the extent of ischemic damage. The time-dependent changes of these substances and the clinical implications are being evaluated, and their incorporation into standard practice is being studied. Certain issues related to quantification, bedside presentation of data, implantation strategies, and standardization of protocols need to be addressed. An excellent review of the current status, issues surrounding potential future developments and

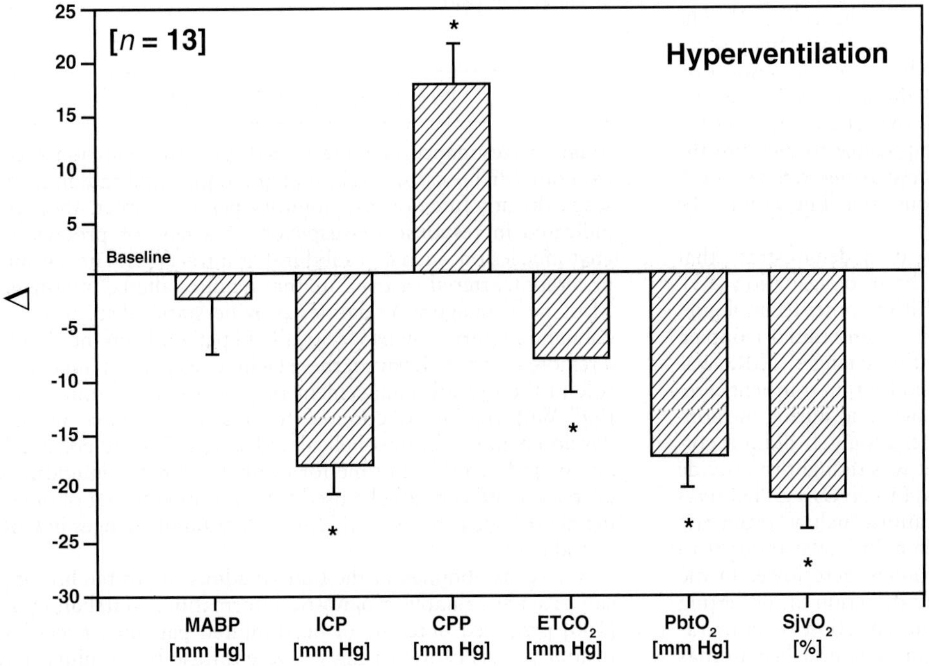

FIGURE 28.7. The effect of hyperventilation-induced hypocapnia on changes in mean arterial blood pressure (MABP), intracranial pressure (ICP), cerebral perfusion pressure (CPP), end-tidal CO_2 ($ETCO_2$), $PtiO_2$, and jugular bulb oximetry ($SjvO_2$). $*p < 0.05$; before hyperventilation versus 10 minutes later. (From Unterberg AW, Kiening KL, Härtl R, et al: Multimodal monitoring in patients with head injury: evaluation of the effects of treatment on cerebral oxygenation. *J Trauma* 42:S32–S37, 1997, with permission.)

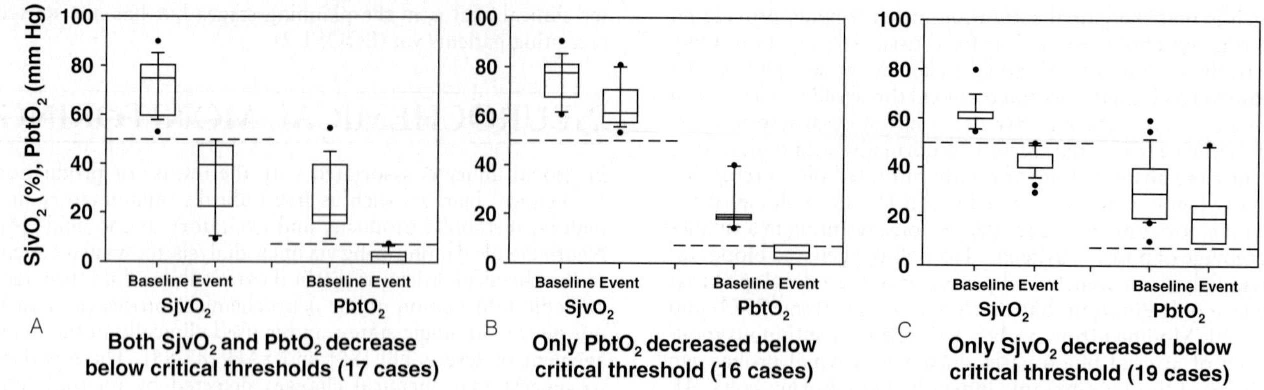

FIGURE 28.8. Changes in jugular venous oxygen saturation ($SjvO_2$) and brain tissue PO_2 ($PbtO_2$) during 52 episodes of cerebral hypoxia/ischemia. The horizontal line across the box plot represents the median, and the lower and upper ends of the box plot are the 25th percentile and 75th percentile, respectively. The error bars mark the 10th and 90th percentiles. The closed circles indicate any outlying points. **A:** Summary of the 17 cases in which both $SjvO_2$ and $PbtO_2$ decreased to less than their respective thresholds, as defined in the text. **B:** Summary of the 16 cases in which $PbtO_2$ decreased to less than the defined threshold; but $SjvO_2$; although decreased, did not decrease to less than 50%. **C:** Summary of the 19 cases in which $SjvO_2$ decreased to less than the threshold, but $PbtO_2$ remained at greater than 10 torr. (From Gopinath SP, Valadka AB, Uzura M, et al: Comparison of jugular venous oxygen saturation and brain tissue PO_2 as monitors of cerebral ischemia after head injury. *Crit Care Med* 27:2337–2345, 1999, with permission.)

methodological aspects of microdialysis are discussed in detail in a recent article [91].

NEAR-INFRARED SPECTROSCOPY

Theoretically, the best monitor of brain oxygenation would be a noninvasive device that characterizes brain oxygenation in real time: near-infrared spectroscopy (NIRS) might eventually offer the opportunity to assess the adequacy of brain oxygenation continuously and noninvasively, although to date the use of the technique in adults has been limited.

Near-infrared light penetrates the skull and, during transmission through or reflection from brain tissue, undergoes changes in intensity that are proportional to the relative concentrations of oxygenated and deoxygenated hemoglobin in the arteries, capillaries, and veins within the field [92]. The absorption (A) of light by a chromophore (i.e., hemoglobin) is defined by Beer's Law: $A = abc$, where a is the absorption constant, b is the path length of the light, and c is the concentration of the chromophore, namely, oxygenated and deoxygenated hemoglobin. Because it is impossible to measure the path length of NIRS light in tissue, approximations as to relative lengths and arterial versus venous contribution must be made.

Extensive preclinical and clinical data demonstrate that NIRS detects qualitative changes in brain oxygenation [93]. Studies have been done comparing NIRS to other technologies and assessing its correlation with EEG, transcranial Doppler, $PbtO_2$ and jugular venous O_2 saturation changes. NIRS was found to correlate with EEG, TCD, and PtO_2 in transient cerebral hypoxia, subarachnoid hemorrhage, and during intraoperative monitoring for carotid endarterectomy. It did not correlate well with $SjvO_2$ [94] values but was thought to provide complementary focal oxygenation data to $SjvO_2$'s global oxygenation assessment. Clinical applications include traumatic brain injury where an rSO_2 of less than 55% was thought to suggest inadequate CPP and NIRS values were lower in the high ICP group of patients vasospasm detection in the setting of subarachnoid hemorrhage, and the detection of intracranial hemorrhages such as subdural and epidural hematomas but studies are not definitive [95]. Despite the promise and enthusiasm generated by NIRS, many problems remain with the technology including tissue penetration, spatial and temporal resolution, artifacts from subcutaneous blood flow and methods of quantitative analysis which need to be resolved [96]. Therefore, validation studies suggest that NIRS may be more useful for qualitatively monitoring trends of brain tissue oxygenation than for actual quantification and its current clinical use is limited to a few centers and is adjunctive at best [93,97]. Some of the liabilities of near-infrared spectroscopy may be overcome by optoacoustic monitoring of cerebral venous saturation. Optoacoustic monitoring of cerebral venous saturation depends on the generation by near-infrared light of ultrasonic signals in blood. The acoustic signals are then transmitted linearly through tissue and bone and provide a focused, depth-resolved signal that reflects venous oxygenation [98].

NEUROIMAGING

Magnetic resonance imaging (MRI), positron emission spectroscopy (PET) scans, cerebral angiography, and radionuclide scans do not function as monitors per se. Rather, they are indicated in response to suspicion of a new or progressive anatomic lesion, such as a subdural or intracerebral hematoma or cerebral arterial vasospasm, that requires altered treatment. Most neuroimaging modalities provide static, discontinuous data and require moving a critically ill patient from the ICU to a remote location. Even so, these techniques play an important role in the overall management of patients with brain injury [99]. With the introduction of portable CT scanners and the development of ultrafast helical and spiral CT scanners, availability and acquisition time for evaluations have significantly decreased and can now be used for serial monitoring of ongoing neurologic processes and for evaluation of changes in CBF (see above).

CT scans obtained at the time of admission to the hospital can provide valuable prognostic information. Marshall et al. [100] predicted outcome of head-injured patients in relation to four grades of increasingly severe diffuse brain injury and

TABLE 28.4

OUTCOME AT DISCHARGE IN RELATION TO INTRACRANIAL DIAGNOSIS (% OF PATIENTS)

Outcome	DI I	DI II	DI III	DI IV	Evacuated mass	Nonevacuated mass
GR	27.0	8.5	3.3	3.1	5.1	2.8
MD	34.6	26.0	13.1	3.1	17.7	8.3
SD	19.2	40.7	26.8	18.8	26.0	19.4
PVS	9.6	11.2	22.9	18.8	12.3	16.7
Death	9.6	13.5	34.0	56.2	38.8	52.8
Total	100	100	100	100	100	100

GR, good recovery; MD, moderate disability; SD, severe disability; PVS, persistent vegetative state; DI, diffuse injury; DI categories I to IV represent increasingly severe classes of diffuse brain injury.
From Marshall LF, Marshall SB, Klauber MR, et al: A new classification of head injury based on computerized tomography. *J Neurosurg* 75:S14–S20, 1991, with permission.

the presence of evacuated or nonevacuated intracranial mass lesions (Table 28.4). Normal CT scans at admission in patients with GCS scores less than 8 are associated with a 10% to 15% incidence of ICP elevation [101,102]; however, the risk of ICP elevation increases in patients older than age 40 years, those with unilateral or bilateral motor posturing, or those with systolic blood pressure less than 90 mm Hg [101].

Although MRI often provides better resolution than CT scans, the powerful magnetic fields make the use of ferrous metals impractical (and dangerous), a ubiquitous component of life-support equipment. To address this issue, MRI-compatible ventilators, monitors, and infusion pumps have been developed, although the logistics of transport and the time required for scans continues to make this technique difficult for repeated monitoring. Recent advances in MRI technology, such as diffusion-weighted imaging, magnetic resonance spectroscopy (carbon labeled, phosphorus labeled, and nitrogen labeled), phase-contrast angiography, and functional MRI provide information about oxidative metabolic pathways, cerebral blood volume, functional CBF, and neuronal activation [99,103,104]. These techniques, while undergoing further evaluation and validation, may one day prove useful in evaluating brain injury and its management. Recent clinical evidence of brain mitochondrial dysfunction after TBI, despite apparently adequate CDO_2, suggests that functional cellular evaluation and associated therapy may someday be as important as maintaining CDO_2 [105]. In addition to providing information regarding ischemia and defining tissue at risk, MRI-based Diffusion Tensor Imaging has been found to be helpful in further defining the anatomy of fiber tracts that have been damaged and has also been found to have prognostic value in severe TBI [106]. Functional MRI provides information regarding neural activity, localization and the physiology of brain function but is currently in use only for neurosurgical planning, brain mapping and in the investigation of neurobehavioral aspects and neuropsychologic sequelae of disorders such as Alzheimer's disease, stroke, multiple sclerosis, brain tumors, and traumatic brain injury.

MULTIMODAL MONITORING STRATEGIES

With technological advances and active ongoing research the field of neurologic monitoring is developing rapidly. Multimodal monitoring takes into account the limitations of each monitoring modality and compensates by combining different techniques into a generalized strategy that help to further elucidate the pathophysiology and underlying cellular mechanisms of disease and focuses care on the physiologic aspects of disease. This concept is not new (consider the operating room and the role of the anesthesiologist) and is becoming more common in the management of brain injury [107] as well as other neurologic diseases. It is hoped that the use of these regimented techniques will lead to improvements in patient outcome [108].

References

1. Wright WL: Multimodal monitoring in the ICU: When could it be useful? *Journal of Neurological Sciences* 261:10–15, 2007.
2. Baron JC: Perfusion thresholds in human cerebral ischemia: Historical perspective and therapeutic implications. *Cerebrovascular Diseases* 11:2–8, 2001.
3. Cunningham AS, Salvador R, Coles JP, et al: Physiological thresholds for irreversible tissue damage in contusional regions following traumatic brain injury. *Brain* 128:1931–1942, 2005.
4. Carmichael ST: Gene expression changes after focal stroke, traumatic brain and spinal cord injuries. *Curr Opin Neurol* 16:699–704, 2003.
5. Enriquez P, Bullock R: Molecular and cellular mechanisms in the pathophysiology of severe head injury. *Curr Pharm Des* 10:2131–2143, 2004.
6. Acker T, Acker H: Cellular oxygen sensing need in CNS function: physiological and pathological implications. *J Exp Biol* 207:3171–3188, 2004.
7. Hlatky R, Furuya Y, Valadka AB, et al: Dynamic autoregulatory response after severe head injury. *J Neurosurg* 97:1054–1061, 2002.
8. Lundberg N, Kjällquist Å, Bien C: Reduction of increased intracranial pressure by hyperventilation. *Acta Psychiatr Neurol (Scand)* 34[Suppl]: 5–57, 1959.
9. Marion DW, Puccio A, Wisniewski SR, et al: Effect of hyperventilation on extracellular concentrations of glutamate, lactate, pyruvate, and local cerebral blood flow in patients with severe traumatic brain injury. *Crit Care Med* 30:2619–2625, 2002.
10. Coles JP, Minhas PS, Fryer TD, et al: Effect of hyperventilation on cerebral blood flow in traumatic head injury: clinical relevance and monitoring correlates. *Crit Care Med* 30:1950–1959, 2002.
11. Tommasino C, Moore S, Todd MM: Cerebral effects of isovolemic hemodilution with crystalloid or colloid solutions. *Crit Care Med* 16:862–868, 1988.
12. Teasdale G, Jennett B: Assessment of coma and impaired consciousness: a practical scale. *Lancet* 2:81–84, 1974.
13. Langfitt TW: Measuring the outcome from head injuries. *J Neurosurg* 48:673–678, 1978.
14. Udekwu P, Kromhout-Schiro S, Vaslef S, et al: Glasgow Coma Scale score, mortality, and functional outcome in head-injured patients. *J Trauma* 56:1084–1089, 2004.
15. Balestreri M, Czosnyka M, Chatfield DA, et al: Predictive value of Glasgow Coma Scale after brain trauma: change in trend over the past ten years. *J Neurol Neurosurg Psychiatry* 75:161–162, 2004.
16. Davis DP, Serrano JA, Vilke GM, et al: The predictive value of field versus arrival GCS and TRISS calculations in moderate to severe TBI. *J Trauma Injury Infection Crit Care* 60:985–990, 2006.

17. Chesnut RM, Marshall SB, Piek J, et al: Early and late systemic hypotension as a frequent and fundamental source of cerebral ischemia following severe brain injury in the traumatic coma data bank. *Acta Neurochir* 59:121–125, 1993.
18. Chesnut RM, Ghajar J, Mass AIR, et al: Management and prognosis of severe traumatic brain injury. Part II. Early indications of prognosis in severe traumatic brain injury. *J Neurotrauma* 17:555–627, 2000.
19. Bullock RM, Chesnut RM, Clifton GL, et al: Resuscitation of blood pressure and oxygenation. *J Neurotrauma* 17:471–478, 2000.
20. Johnston AJ, Steiner LA, Chatfield DA, et al: Effect of cerebral perfusion pressure augmentation with dopamine and norepinephrine on global and focal brain oxygenation after traumatic brain injury. *Intensive Care Med* 30:791–797, 2004.
21. Shafi S, Gentilello L: Hypotension does not increase mortality in brain-injured patients more than it does in non-brain-injured patients. *J Trauma* 59:830–834, 2005.
22. Bullock RM, Chesnut RM, Clifton GL, et al: Guidelines for cerebral perfusion pressure. *J Neurotrauma* 17:507–511, 2000.
23. Brain Trauma Foundation, American Association of Neurological Surgeons Congress of Neurological Surgeons Joint Section on Neurotrauma and Critical Care. Guidelines for the management of severe traumatic brain injury: cerebral perfusion pressure. 3–14-2003. Brain Trauma Foundation, Inc. Available from the Agency for Healthcare Research and Quality (AHRQ), http://www.guideline.gov/summary/summary.aspx?doc_id=3794 Retrieved December 5, 2006.
24. Grande PO, Asgeirsson B, Nordstrom CH: Physiologic principles for volume regulation of a tissue enclosed in a rigid shell with application to the injured brain. *J Trauma* 42:S23–S31, 1997.
25. Feldman Z, Robertson CS: Monitoring of cerebral hemodynamics with jugular bulb catheters. *Crit Care Clin* 13:51–77, 1997.
26. Kinoshita K, Kraydieh S, Alonso O, et al: Effect of posttraumatic hyperglycemia on contusion volume and neutrophil accumulation after moderate fluid-percussion brain injury in rats. *J Neurotrauma* 19:681–692, 2002.
27. Jeremitsky E, Omert LA, Dunham CM, et al: The impact of hyperglycemia on patients with severe brain injury. *J Trauma* 58:47–50, 2005.
28. Cochran A, Scaife ER, Hansen KW, et al: Hyperglycemia and outcomes from pediatric traumatic brain injury. *J Trauma* 55:1035–1038, 2003.
29. Rovlias A, Kotsou S: The influence of hyperglycemia on neurological outcome in patients with severe head injury. *Neurosurgery* 46:335–343, 2000.
30. Van den Berghe G, Wouters P, Weekers F, et al: Intensive insulin therapy in critically ill patients. *N Engl J Med* 345:1359–1367, 2001.
31. Van Den Berghe G, Wouters PJ, Bouillon R, et al: Outcome benefit of intensive insulin therapy in the critically ill: insulin dose versus glycemic control. *Crit Care Med* 31:359–366, 2003.
32. Vespa PM, McArthur D, O'Phelan K, et al: Persistently low ECF glucose correlates with poor outcome 6 months after human traumatic brain injury. *J Cereb Blood Flow Metab* 23:865–877, 2003.
33. Clifton GL, Jiang JY, Lyeth BG, et al: Marked protection by moderate hypothermia after experimental traumatic brain injury. *J Cereb Blood Flow Metab* 11:114–121, 1991.
34. Clifton G: Hypothermia and severe brain injury. *J Neurosurg* 93:718–719, 2000.
35. McIntyre LA, Fergusson DA, Hebert PC, et al: Prolonged therapeutic hypothermia after traumatic brain injury in adults: a systematic review. *JAMA* 289:2992–2999, 2003.
36. Henderson WR, Dhingra VK, Chittock DR, et al: Hypothermia in the management of traumatic brain injury. A systematic review and meta-analysis. *Intensive Care Med* 29:1637–1644, 2003.
37. Clifton Gl, Miller ER, Choi SC, et al: Lack of effect of induction of hypothermia after acute brain injury. *N Engl J Med* 344:556–563, 2001.
38. Hutchison JS, Ward RE, Lacroix J, et al: Hypothermia therapy after traumatic brain injury in children. *N Engl J Med* 358:2447–2456, 2008.
39. Polderman K, Ely EW, Badr AE, et al: Induced hypothermia for TBI: considering conflicting results of meta analysis and moving forward. *Intensive Care Med* 30:1860–1864, 2004.
40. Peterson K, Carson S, Carney N: Hypothermia treatment for traumatic brain injury: a systematic review and meta analysis. *J Trauma* 25:62–71, 2008.
41. Hypothermia After Cardiac Arrest Study Group: Mild therapeutic hypothermia to improve the neurologic outcome after cardiac arrest. *N Engl J Med* 346:549–556, 2002.
42. Bernard SA, Gray TW, Buist MD, et al: Treatment of comatose survivors of out-of-hospital cardiac arrest with induced hypothermia. *N Engl J Med* 346:557–563, 2002.
43. Kilpatrick MM, Lowry DW, Firlik AD, et al: Hyperthermia in the neurosurgical intensive care unit. *Neurosurgery* 47:850–856, 2000.
44. Schwarz S, Hafner K, Aschoff A, et al: Incidence and prognostic significance of fever following intracerebral hemorrhage. *Neurology* 54:354–361, 2000.
45. Natale JE, Joseph JG, Helfaer MA, et al: Early hyperthermia after traumatic brain injury in children: risk factors, influence on length of stay, and effect on short-term neurologic status. *Crit Care Med* 28:2608–2615, 2000.
46. Fabricius M, Fuhr S, Bhatia R, et al: Cortical spreading depression and peri infarct depolarization in acutely injured human cerebral cortex. *Brain* 129:778–790, 2006.
47. Drier JP, Woitzik J, Fabricius M, et al: Delayed ischemic neurological deficits after subarachnoid hemorrhage are associated with clusters of spreading depolarizations. *Brain* 129:3224–3237, 2006.
48. Nuwer M: Assessment of digital EEG, quantitative EEG, and EEG brain mapping: report of the American Academy of Neurology and the American Clinical Neurophysiology Society. *Neurology* 49:277–292, 1997.
49. Vespa PM, et al: *Electroencephalogr Clin Neurophysiol* 103:607–615, 1997.
50. Vespa PM, Boscardin WJ, Becker DP, et al: Early persistent impaired percent alpha variability on continuous EEG monitoring as predictive of poor outcome in TBI. *J Neurosurgery* 97:84–92, 2002.
51. Preventing and managing the impact of anesthesia awareness. *JCAHO Sentinel Event Alert* 2004. Available from the Joint Commission on Accreditation of Healthcare Organizations, http://www.jointcommission.org/SentinelEvents/SentinelEventAlert/seq_32.htm Retrieved December 5, 2006.
52. American Society of Anesthesiologists practice advisory for intraoperative awareness and brain function monitoring. *House of Delegates*. 10-25-2005. Available from the American Society of Anesthesiologists, http://www.asahg.org/publicationsandServices/AwareAdvisoryFinalOct5.pdf Retrieved December 5, 2006.
53. Nasraway SA Jr, Wu EC, Kelleher RM, et al: How reliable is the bispectral index in critically ill patients? A prospective, comparative, single-blinded observer study. *Crit Care Med* 30:1483–1487, 2002.
54. Bruhn J, Bouillon TW, Shafer SL: Electromyographic activity falsely elevates the bispectral index. *Anesthesiology* 92:1485–1487, 2000.
55. Friedman D, Claasen J, Hirsch LJ: Continuous EEG monitoring in the ICU. *Anesth Analg* 109:506–523, 2009.
56. Lotto ML, Banoub M, Schubert A: Effects of anesthetic agents and physiologic changes on intraoperative motor evoked potentials. *J Neurosurg Anesthesiol* 16:32–42, 2004.
57. Schwarz S, Hacke W, Schwab S: Magnetic evoked potentials in neurocritical care patients with acute brainstem lesions. *J Neurol Sci* 172:30–37, 2000.
58. Wijdicks EF, Hijdra A, Young GB, et al: Practice parameter: prediction of outcome in comatose survivors after cardiopulmonary resuscitation (an evidence-based review): report of the quality standards subcommittee of the American Academy of Neurology. *Neurology* 67:203–210, 2006.
59. Marion DW, Spiegel TP: Changes in the management of severe traumatic brain injury: 1991–1997. *Crit Care Med* 28:16–18, 2000.
60. Smith M: Monitoring Intracranial pressure in traumatic brain injury. *Anesth Analg* 106:240–248, 2008.
61. Marmarou A, Anderson RL, Ward JD, et al: Impact of ICP instability and hypotension on outcome in patients with severe head trauma. *J Neurosurg* 75:S59–S66, 1991.
62. Bullock RM, Chesnut RM, Clifton GL, et al: Management and prognosis of severe traumatic brain injury. Part I. Guidelines for the management of severe traumatic brain injury. *J Neurotrauma* 17:449–553, 2000.
63. Bullock RM, Chesnut RM, Clifton GL, et al: Indications for intracranial pressure monitoring. *J Neurotrauma* 17:479–491, 2000.
64. Sahuquillo J, Poca MA, Arribas M, et al: Interhemispheric supratentorial intracranial pressure gradients in head-injured patients: are they clinically important? *J Neurosurg* 90:16–26, 1999.
65. Chambers IR, Kane PJ, Signorini DF, et al: Bilateral ICP monitoring: its importance in detecting the severity of secondary insults. *Acta Neurochir Suppl* 71:42–43, 1998.
66. Bullock RM, Chesnut RM, Clifton GL, et al: Recommendations for intracranial pressure monitoring technology. *J Neurotrauma* 17:497–506, 2000.
67. Martinez-Manas RM, Santamarta D, de Campos JM, et al: Camino intracranial pressure monitor: prospective study of accuracy and complications. *J Neurol Neurosurg Psychiatry* 69:82–86, 2000.
68. Juul N, Morris GF, Marshall SB, et al: Intracranial hypertension and cerebral perfusion pressure: influence on neurological deterioration and outcome in severe head injury. *J Neurosurg* 92:1–6, 2000.
69. Robertson CS: Management of cerebral perfusion pressure after traumatic brain injury. *Anesthesiology* 95:1513–1517, 2001.
70. Adelson PD, Bratton SL, Carney NA, et al: Guidelines for the acute medical management of severe traumatic brain injury in infants, children, and adolescents. Chapter 17. Critical pathway for the treatment of established intracranial hypertension in pediatric traumatic brain injury. *Pediatr Crit Care Med* 4:S65–S67, 2003.
71. Latchaw RE: Cerebral perfusion imaging in acute stroke. *J Vasc Interv Radiol* 15:S29–S46, 2004.
72. Jaeger M, Siehke M, Meixenberger J, et al: Correlation of continuously monitored regional cerebral blood flow and brain tissue oxygen. *Acta Neurochir* 147:51–56, 2005.
73. Sase S, Honda M, Machida K, et al: Comparison of cerebral blood flow between perfusion computed tomography and xenon-enhanced computed tomography for normal subjects: territorial analysis. *J Comput Assist Tomogr* 29:270–277, 2005.
74. Qureshi AI, Sung GY, Razumovsky AY, et al: Early identification of patients at risk for symptomatic vasospasm after aneurysmal subarachnoid hemorrhage. *Crit Care Med* 28:984–990, 2000.
75. Lam JMK, Chan MSY, Poon WS: Cerebral venous oxygen saturation monitoring: is dominant jugular bulb cannulation good enough? *Br J Neurosurg* 10:357–364, 1996.

76. Metz C, Holzschuh M, Bein T, et al: Monitoring of cerebral oxygen metabolism in the jugular bulb: reliability of unilateral measurements in severe head injury. *J Cereb Blood Flow Metab* 18:332–343, 1998.
77. Gopinath SP, Robertson CS, Contant CF, et al: Jugular venous desaturation and outcome after head injury. *J Neurol Neurosurg Psychiatry* 57:717–723, 1994.
78. Cruz J, Jaggi JL, Hoffstad OJ: Cerebral blood flow and oxygen consumption in acute brain injury with acute anemia: an alternative for the cerebral metabolic rate of oxygen consumption? *Crit Care Med* 21:1218–1224, 1993.
79. Zauner A, Doppenberg EMR, Woodward JJ, et al: Continuous monitoring of cerebral substrate delivery and clearance: initial experience in 24 patients with severe acute brain injuries. *Neurosurgery* 41:1082–1093, 1997.
80. Maloney-Wilensky E, Gracias V, Itkin A, et al: Brain tissue oxygen and outcome after severe TBI: a systematic review. *Crit Care Med* 37:2057–2063, 2009.
81. van den Brink WA, van Santbrink H, Steyerberg EW, et al: Brain oxygen tension in severe head injury. *Neurosurgery* 46:868–878, 2000.
82. Unterberg AW, Kiening KL, Härtl R, et al: Multimodal monitoring in patients with head injury: evaluation of the effects of treatment on cerebral oxygenation. *J Trauma* 42:S32–S37, 1997.
83. Gopinath SP, Valadka AB, Uzura M, et al: Comparison of jugular venous oxygen saturation and brain tissue PO_2 as monitors of cerebral ischemia after head injury. *Crit Care Med* 27:2337–2345, 1999.
84. Stiefel MF, Spiotta A, Gracias VH, et al: Reduced mortality in patients with severe TBI treated with brain tissue oxygen monitoring. *J Neurosurg* 103:805–811, 2005.
85. Narotam PK, Morrison JF, Nathoo N, et al: Brain tissue oxygen monitoring in traumatic brain injury and major trauma: outcome analysis of a brain tissue oxygen directed therapy. *J Neurosurg* 111:672–682, 2009.
86. Mazzeo AT, Bullock R: Effect of bacterial meningitis complicating severe head trauma upon brain microdialysis and cerebral perfusion. *Neurocrit Care* 2:282–287, 2005.
87. Sarrafzadeh AS, Sakowitz OW, Kiening KL, et al: Bedside microdialysis: a tool to monitor cerebral metabolism in subarachnoid hemorrhage patients? *Crit Care Med* 30:1062–1070, 2002.
88. Bellander BM, Cantais E, Enblad P, et al: Consensus meeting on microdialysis in neurointensive care. *Intensive Care Med* 30:2166–2169, 2004.
89. Johnston AJ, Gupta AK: Advanced monitoring in the neurology intensive care unit: microdialysis. *Cur Opin Crit Care* 8:121–127, 2002.
90. Peerdeman SM, Girbes AR, Vandertop WP: Cerebral microdialysis as a new tool for neurometabolic monitoring. *Intensive Care Med* 26:662–669, 2000.
91. Hillered L, Vespa PM, Hovda DA: Translational neurochemical research in acute human brain injury: The current status and potential future of cerebral Microdialysis. *J Neurotrauma* 22:3–41, 2005.
92. Ferrari M, Mottola L, Quaresima V: Principles, techniques, and limitations of near infrared spectroscopy. *Can J Appl Physiol* 29:463–487, 2004.
93. Pollard V, Prough DS, DeMelo AE, et al: Validation in volunteers of a near-infrared spectroscope for monitoring brain oxygenation in vivo. *Anesth Analg* 82:269–277, 1996.
94. Unterberg A, Rosenthal A, Schneider GH, et al. Validation of monitoring of cerebral oxygenation by near-infrared spectroscopy in comatose patients, in Tasubokawa T, Marmarou A, Robertson C, et al (eds): *Neurochemical Monitoring in the Intensive Care Unit*. New York, Springer-Verlag, 1995 pp 204–210.
95. Arnulphi M, Calaraj A, Slavin KV: Near Infrared technology in neuroscience: past, present and future. *Neurological Research* 31:605–614, 2009.
96. Nicklin SE, Hassan IA-A, Wickramasinghe YA, et al: The light still shines, but not that brightly? the current status of perinatal near infrared spectroscopy. *Arch Dis Child* 88:F263–F268, 2003.
97. Henson LC, Calalang C, Temp JA, et al: Accuracy of a cerebral oximeter in healthy volunteers under conditions of isocapnic hypoxia. *Anesthesiology* 88:58–65, 1998.
98. Petrov YY, Prough DS, Deyo DJ, et al: Optoacoustic, noninvasive, real-time, continuous monitoring of cerebral blood oxygenation: an in vivo study in sheep. *Anesthesiology* 102:69–75, 2005.
99. Newberg AB, Alavi A: Neuroimaging in patients with head injury. *Semin Nucl Med* 33:136–147, 2003.
100. Marshall LF, Marshall SB, Klauber MR, et al: A new classification of head injury based on computerized tomography. *J Neurosurg* 75:S14–S20, 1991.
101. Narayan RK, Kishore PRS, Becker DP, et al: Intracranial pressure: to monitor or not to monitor? A review of our experience with severe head injury. *J Neurosurg* 56:650–659, 1982.
102. Eisenberg HM, Gary HE Jr, Aldrich EF, et al: Initial CT findings in 753 patients with severe head injury. A report from the NIH traumatic coma data bank. *J Neurosurg* 73:688–698, 1990.
103. Kemp GJ: Non-invasive methods for studying brain energy metabolism: what they show and what it means. *Dev Neurosci* 22:418–428, 2000.
104. Watson NA, Beards SC, Altaf N, et al: The effect of hyperoxia on cerebral blood flow: a study in healthy volunteers using magnetic resonance phase-contrast angiography. *Eur J Anaesthesiol* 17:152–159, 2000.
105. Verweij BH, Muizelaar P, Vinas FC, et al: Impaired cerebral mitochondrial function after traumatic brain injury in humans. *J Neurosurg* 93:815–820, 2000.
106. Tollard E, Galanaud D, Perlbarg V, et al: Experience of diffusion tensor imaging and H-spectroscopy for outcome prediction in severe TBI. *Crit Care Med* 37:1448–1455, 2009.
107. De Georgia MA, Deogaonkar A: Multimodal monitoring in the neurological intensive care unit. *Neurologist* 11:45–54, 2005.
108. Elf K, Nilsson P, Enblad P: Outcome after traumatic brain injury improved by an organized secondary insult program and standardized neurointensive care. *Crit Care Med* 30:2129–2134, 2003.

CHAPTER 29 ■ ECHOCARDIOGRAPHY IN THE INTENSIVE CARE UNIT

ACHIKAM OREN-GRINBERG, SAJID SHAHUL AND ADAM B. LERNER

INTRODUCTION

Echocardiography was introduced to the operating suite in the 1970s, with epicardial echocardiography as its initial application. Transesophageal echocardiography (TEE) during surgery was first described in 1980 but did not become commonplace until the mid-1980s. Since then, TEE has evolved to become a widely used and versatile modality for diagnosis and monitoring of critically ill patients. As such, its use has expanded into the perioperative period and the intensive care unit (ICU). Echocardiography provides both anatomic and functional information about the heart; systolic and diastolic function, cavity size, and valvular function [1].

Ease of use, availability of diagnostic information within 10 to 15 minutes from the start of examination, high-quality imaging in most patients, and low complication rates have all led to the pervasive use of echocardiography in the perioperative environment and increasing use in the ICU [2–8]. However, patient safety and optimal outcome depend heavily on a thorough understanding of both the strengths and limitations of the available technologies and their applications.

BASIC TERMINOLOGY OF ECHOCARDIOGRAPHY TECHNIQUES

A sonographer must use different echocardiographic imaging techniques and hemodynamic modalities to achieve a diagnosis or management plan. The following is a list of the basic techniques used during an echocardiographic study.

Two-Dimensional Echocardiography

Two-dimensional (2D) echocardiography is the backbone of the echocardiographic examination [9]. Using 2D, a complete visualization of the beating heart is achieved by displaying anatomic structures in real-time tomographic images. By aiming the ultrasound probe at the heart, exactly oriented anatomic "slices" are obtained. Information acquired includes cardiac chamber sizes, global and regional systolic function, and valvular anatomy.

M-Mode Echocardiography

M-mode or motion-mode images are a continuous 1D graphic display that can be derived by selecting any of the individual sector lines from which a 2D image is constructed [9]. It is useful for quantification of myocardial wall and chambers sizes, which in turn can be used to estimate left ventricle (LV) mass and chamber volumes, respectively. Though very limited, M-mode can also be used to determine fractional shortening, a rough estimate of left ventricular systolic function. In addition, since it has high temporal resolution, M-mode is helpful in assessing the motion of rapidly moving cardiac structures such as cardiac valves.

Doppler Echocardiography

Doppler echocardiography is used to supplement 2D and M-mode echocardiography. It can provide functional information regarding intracardiac hemodynamics; systolic and diastolic flows, blood velocities and volumes, severity of valvular lesions, location and severity of intracardiac shunts, and assessment of diastolic function. The four types of Doppler modalities used include continuous-wave, pulsed-wave, color flow mapping, and tissue Doppler [9]. Continuous-wave Doppler is used for measuring high-pressure gradient/high-velocity flows such as seen in aortic stenosis. When using continuous wave Doppler, the ultrasound probe continuously transmits and receives sound waves. This increases the maximum limit of blood velocity that can be evaluated before exceeding the Nyquist limit. The Nyquist limit represents the maximum flow velocity that can be evaluated by Doppler and is dependent on both equipment and imaging variables. Continuous wave Doppler can evaluate higher flows but does so at the expense of spatial specificity. This is referred to as "range ambiguity." Pulsed-wave Doppler is used for measuring lower-pressure gradient/lower-velocity flows such as in mitral stenosis. In this mode, the ultrasound probe sends out a pulse of sound and then waits to receive reflected waves. This lowers the Nyquist limit and the maximum velocities that can be interrogated but allows for precise spatial resolution. Color flow mapping is useful for screening valves for stenosis or regurgitation, quantifying the degree of valvular regurgitation, imaging systolic and diastolic flow, and detection of intracardiac shunts. Doppler tissue imaging has been introduced as a new method of quantifying segmental and global left ventricular function. It records systolic and diastolic velocities within the myocardium and at the corners of the mitral annulus and is useful for studying diastolic function and contractile asynchrony of the LV [10].

Contrast Echocardiography

Contrast echocardiography is used to enhance the diagnostic quality of the echocardiogram [11]. It may be used to improve assessment of global function and regional wall motion abnormalities by 2D echocardiography. Although approved only for LV opacification, recent clinical studies suggest a potential use in assessing myocardial perfusion [12,13].

Transesophageal Versus Transthoracic Echocardiography

Although transthoracic echocardiography (TTE) is a less invasive way to image cardiac structures, suboptimal acoustic windows lead to low-quality images in many critically ill patients. These suboptimal acoustic windows are due to obesity, pulmonary disease, the presence of chest tubes, drains and wound dressings, and limitations on patient positioning. Using TTE in the ICU can be challenging; one study found the echocardiographic examination to be inadequate in approximately 50% of patients on mechanical ventilation and 60% of all ICU patients [8]. The relatively low percentage of adequate imaging improves when TTE is used as a **monitoring tool**, which does not require the same quality of images, and not as a diagnostic tool. In a report of more than 200 ICU patients, TTE used as a monitoring tool provided 2D images of acceptable quality in 97% of patients [14].

In contrast to TTE, TEE is more invasive but consistently provides images of better quality. In up to 40% of patients, TEE may provide additional unexpected diagnoses that are missed by TTE [4,15]. Recent advances in ultrasound imaging, which include harmonic imaging, digital acquisition, and contrast endocardial enhancement, have improved the diagnostic yield of TEE [16,17].

CONTRAINDICATIONS TO PERFORMING TEE

Although TEE is safe [18,19], there are several contraindications to probe insertion. These include significant esophageal or gastric pathology; mass or tumors, strictures, diverticulum, Mallory-Weiss tears, recent esophageal or gastric surgery, upper gastrointestinal bleeding, and dysphagia or odynophagia not previously evaluated. Esophageal varices are not an absolute contraindication, and a risk–benefit analysis of each case must be carried out before performing TEE in any individual patient [20]. Practitioners must be aware of the potential for severe bleeding, in particular when a coagulation abnormality exists. Cervical spinal injury is another relative contraindication requiring careful risk–benefit analysis.

COMPLICATIONS AND SAFETY OF TEE

TEE is considered a moderately invasive procedure and complications are rare. In one study of ICU patients, complication rates reached 1.6% and included hypotension following sedation for probe insertion, oropharyngeal bleeding in a coagulopathic patient, and aspiration during tracheal intubation performed prior to TEE [19]. Another study in 2,508 ICU patients reported a complication rate of 2.6%. In this study, there was no examination-related mortality. Complications included transient hypotension or hypertension, circulatory deterioration, hypoxemia, arrhythmias, vomiting, coughing, superficial mucous membrane lesions, displacement of a tracheostomy tube and accidental removal of a duodenal feeding tube [18]. A large European multicenter study of 10,419 examinations reported a complication rate of 2.5% with one (0.01%) case of fatal hematemesis due to a malignant tumor [2]. In addition, in 0.88% of the reported cases, the TEE exam had to be prematurely terminated due to either patient intolerance or because of cardiac, pulmonary, or bleeding events [2].

Common Indications for TEE in the ICU

In 1996, a task force created by the American Society of Anesthesiologists and the Society of Cardiovascular Anesthesiologists published guidelines regarding the indications for TEE [21]. Three categories of evidence-based clinical indications were identified. For indications grouped into category I, TEE was judged to be *frequently* useful in improving clinical outcomes. To date, there is only a single category I indication for TEE in the ICU. That indication is for "unstable patients with unexplained hemodynamic disturbance, suspected valve disease, or thromboembolic problems (if other tests or monitoring techniques have not confirmed the diagnosis or patients are too unstable to undergo other tests)" [21]. This indication, however, encompasses a significant proportion of ICU patients and in practice, clinicians use echocardiography in the ICU for many other indications. These are summarized in Table 29.1.

ECHOCARDIOGRAPHIC EVALUATION OF HEMODYNAMIC INSTABILITY

Hemodynamic instability is an extremely common event in every ICU. Determining the cause of such can sometimes be more challenging than one would expect. Echocardiography can be used successfully in the diagnosis, monitoring, and management of the unstable patient in the ICU. Using echocardiography to determine the etiology of hemodynamic instability requires assessment of cardiac function, volume status, valvular function, and extracardiac processes.

ASSESSMENT OF CARDIAC FUNCTION

Systolic dysfunction of either ventricular chamber must be considered in every unstable patient. The etiology of dysfunction may often times be discerned from the echocardiographic evaluation allowing for appropriate therapy to be initiated.

TABLE 29.1

COMMON INDICATIONS FOR PERFORMING TEE IN THE ICU

Assessment of LV systolic function	Evaluation of valvular pathology
Hemodynamic management	Determination of source of emboli
Evaluation of pericardial tamponade	Evaluation of endocarditis
Evaluation of pulmonary embolism	Evaluation of chest trauma
Evaluation of aortic dissection	Evaluation of hypoxemia

Assessment of Left Ventricular Systolic Function

Use of several echocardiographic assessment modalities is necessary for evaluation of left ventricular systolic function. These modalities include quantitative as well as qualitative assessments.

Quantitative Assessment of Left Ventricular Systolic Function

Volumetric Method Using Geometric Models. Quantitative assessment of left ventricular systolic function relies on volume assessment using 2D tomographic images. To determine the volume at end diastole (LVEDV) and end systole (LVESV), the endocardial borders in two orthogonal tomographic planes are traced at end diastole and end systole. Several geometric assumptions and formulas have been developed (e.g., truncated ellipse, "bullet" formula, cylinder, and cone) to determine the LVEDV and LVESV based on these 2D images. Once LVEDV and LVESV have been determined, the stoke volume, and thus cardiac output (CO) can be calculated:

$$SV = LVEDV - LVESV$$
$$CO = SV \times HR$$

In addition, ejection fraction (EF) can be calculated from these volumes using the formula:

$$EF = SV/LVEDV \times 100\%$$

These formulas work optimally in a symmetrically contracting ventricle; the presence of regional wall motion abnormalities decreases accuracy. In addition, foreshortening of the LV cavity is a common source of underestimation of LV end-diastolic and end-systolic volumes and can similarly impact the accuracy of systolic function assessment with these formulas [1,22]. Lastly, since the models depend on accurate endocardial border definition, their use requires adequate visualization. Incomplete endocardial definition is described in 10% to 20% of routine echocardiographic studies [23] and may reach 25% in ICU patients [24]. This challenge is even greater in patients requiring mechanical ventilation in which imaging can be particularly challenging. These challenges have limited the use of the geometric models and formulas for assessment of LV systolic function.

Discs Method (Simpson's Rule). Another method for volumetric assessment of LV systolic function is the discs method, which may be more accurate than the other volumetric methods described above, particularly in the presence of distorted LV geometry [9]. In this method the ventricle is divided into a series of discs of equal height and each disc volume is calculated as follows:

$$\text{Disc volume} = \text{disc height} \times \text{disc area}$$

The ventricular volume can be calculated from the sum of the volumes. This technique requires true apical images, which in clinical practice may be difficult to achieve. Foreshortening of the ventricular apex will result in inaccurate assessment of the left ventricular EF and CO (Fig. 29.1).

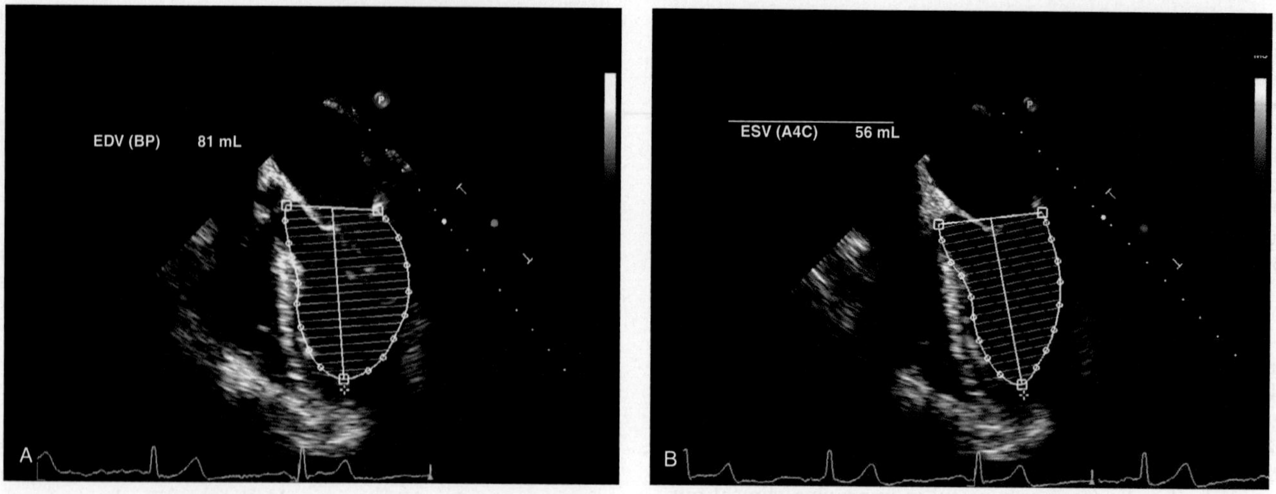

FIGURE 29.1. Calculation of cardiac output using the disc method (Simpson's rule). TEE Mid-esophageal 4-chamber view in diastole (**A**) and systole (**B**) is shown. Using the Simpson's rule, LVEDV (81 mL) and LVESV (56 mL) were calculated by the echocardiographic computer. From these volumes, the cardiac output was calculated to be 1.7 L/min (81–56 mL) × 69 beats per minute.

Qualitative Assessment of Left Ventricular Systolic Function

2D Evaluation of Ventricular Systolic Function. Using 2D imaging, two of the most important questions regarding hemodynamic stability can be rapidly answered; are the ventricles contracting well and are they adequately filled. Using 2D, an experienced observer can qualitatively evaluate systolic function. This should be assessed from multiple tomographic planes and attention must be given to obtaining adequate endocardial definition. Normal ventricular contraction consists of simultaneous myocardial thickening and endocardial excursion toward the center of the ventricle. It is important to look for this myocardial thickening; infarcted myocardium may be pulled inward by surrounding, normal myocardium. There is some regional heterogeneity of normal wall motion with the proximal lateral and inferolateral (or posterior) walls contracting somewhat later than the septum and inferior wall [25]. For qualitative assessment of overall systolic function, the echocardiographer integrates the degree of wall thickening and endocardial motion in all tomographic views and reaches a conclusion about overall LV systolic function and EF. Although different institutions use different standards, severe LV systolic dysfunction is usually defined as an EF <30%, moderate dysfunction 30% to 45%, mild depression 45% to 55%, and normal >55%. This method of EF estimation is of great clinical utility and can be performed with good correlation to quantitative measurements. There are however, a few potential pitfalls to 2D assessment of EF that must be considered:

1. Accurate assessment requires satisfactory endocardial border definition. Qualitative EF estimation becomes inaccurate when the endocardium is inadequately defined.
2. Accurate estimation of EF depends on the experience of the echocardiographer.
3. In asynchronous contraction (paced-rhythm, conduction defects, etc.), assessment of EF is more difficult.

Despite its limitations, 2D qualitative assessment is the most widely used technique for assessment of LV systolic function due to its ease of application in the clinical setting. In the operating room, after completing the TEE exam, most physicians monitor LV systolic function continuously with 2D imaging using the transgastric (TG) midpapillary short-axis view. This allows for quick assessment of regional wall motion abnormalities in all coronary arterial circulatory beds as well as rudimentary evaluation of volume status [26]. However, it is important to remember that this view alone is never satisfactory for assessing overall systolic function.

Regional Left Ventricular Function

Most commonly, abnormal regional wall motion is the result of coronary artery disease and resultant ischemia/infarction. Abnormal wall motion is a continuum of conditions consisting of hypokinesis, akinesis, and dyskinesis. With dyskinesis, the affected wall segment moves away from the center of the ventricle during systole. To standardize echocardiographic evaluations of wall motion, a 17-segment model of the LV has been defined [25]. These 17 segments are evaluated separately for the presence and degree of regional wall motion abnormality. When the etiology of the wall motion abnormality is CAD, the location of the coronary lesion can be usually predicted from the location of the regional wall motion abnormality.

Contrast Echocardiography

Recent innovations have been made to overcome some of the technical obstacles related to endocardial border detection and image quality. Intravenous echocardiographic contrast agents that opacify the left side of the heart can markedly improve visualization of the LV cavity and enhance endocardial definition. These agents can aid assessment of regional and global LV functions [27–30]. They also have the potential to "salvage" nondiagnostic TTEs in ICU patients. One study demonstrated a "salvage" rate of 51% [31] and another 77% of nondiagnostic TTEs [32]. In addition to improving visualization and assessment of LV function, assessment of myocardial perfusion defects with intravenous contrast has been reported with various imaging techniques and modalities [33–35].

Doppler Assessment of Left Ventricular Systolic Function

Doppler spectral profiles can be used to evaluate left ventricular function quantitatively. This evaluation of left ventricular systolic function is based on calculation of stroke volume (SV) and CO.

Stroke Volume—the volume of blood ejected during each cardiac cycle is a key indicator of cardiac performance. SV can be calculated by using pulse wave Doppler (PWD) to measure the instantaneous blood velocity recorded during systole from an area in the heart where a cross-sectional area (CSA) can be easily determined. The left ventricular outflow tract (LVOT) is most commonly used because its cross section is essentially a circle. By measuring the diameter of the LVOT and assuming a circular geometry, the CSA is calculated as $\pi(D/2)^2$. Any cardiac chamber or structure that has a measurable CSA may be used; mitral valve annulus, right ventricular outflow tract outflow, and tricuspid annulus are some examples. By tracing the outline of the PWD profile, the echocardiographic computer can calculate the integral of velocity by time or the velocity–time integral (VTI). The VTI is the distance (commonly referred as the *stroke distance*) that the average red cell has traveled during the systolic ejection phase. SV (cm^3) is then calculated by multiplying the VTI (stroke distance in cm) by the CSA in cm^2 of the conduit (i.e., LVOT, aorta, mitral valve annulus, pulmonary artery) through which the blood has traveled [36–42]; SV = CSA × VTI. CO is then easily derived by multiplying the calculated SV by the heart rate: CO (cm^3/min) = SV × HR (Fig. 29.2).

This approach to SV and CO calculations has shown very good correlation with thermodilution-derived CO measurements [43]. There are however, several potential sources of error:

1. CSA determination often leads to the greatest source of error. When using any diameter for CSA determination, any error in measurement will be squared (CSA = $\pi(D/2)^2$). This translates to a 20% error in calculation of CO for each 2-mm error when measuring a 2.0-cm diameter LV outflow tract [25]. Studies have shown that while the Doppler velocity curves can be recorded consistently with little interobserver measurement variability (2% to 5%), the variability in 2D LVOT diameter measurements for CSA is significantly greater (8% to 12%) [44].
2. The Doppler signal is assumed to have been recorded at a parallel or near parallel intercept angle, called θ, to blood flow. The Doppler equation has a cos θ term in its denominator. With an intercept angle of 0 degree, the cos θ term equals 1. Deviations up to 20 degrees in intercept angle are acceptable since only a 6% error in measurement is introduced.
3. Velocity and diameter measurements should be made at the same anatomic site. When the two are measured at different places, the accuracy of SV and CO calculations is decreased.
4. Although the pattern of flow is assumed to be laminar, in reality the flow profile is parabolic. This does have some impact on velocity-based calculations [25]. However, in routine clinical practice this factor is of little significance and can be essentially ignored.

Determination of Left Ventricular *d*P/*dt*

The changing rate of left ventricular pressure (dP/dt) is an important parameter in the assessment of myocardial systolic function. Traditionally, dP/dt was derived from the left ventricular pressure curve acquired at cardiac catheterization using a micromanometer catheter recording. It has been shown that echocardiography can be used accurately and reliably to assess dP/dt by performing Doppler assessment of mitral regurgitant jet [45,46]. Using continuous wave Doppler, a spectral display of the mitral regurgitation (MR) jet is obtained. From the spectral display, information about the rate of pressure development within the LV can be derived using measurements undertaken in the early phase of systole (the upstroke of the velocity curve is used for calculations). Determination of dP/dt using the MR spectral jet is done by calculation of the time required for the MR jet velocity to go from 1 m per second to 3 m per second. The time between these two points represents the time that it takes for a 32 mm Hg pressure change to occur in the left ventricular cavity. This is based on the modified Bernoulli equation ($P = 4v^2$), which relates pressure to velocity. Thus, in going from 1 m per second to 3 m per second:

$$\mathrm{P} = 4v_{\mathrm{B}}^2 - 4v_{\mathrm{A}}^2(4(3^2) - 4(1^2) = 32)$$

where v_{B} is velocity of 3 m/s.

dP/dt is then is calculated using the formula:

$$dP/dt = 32\,\mathrm{mm\,Hg} \div \mathrm{time\,(seconds)}.$$

A depressed ventricle will take a longer time to develop this pressure gradient—a lower dP/dt. Normal dP/dt value is >1,200 mm Hg per second (or time ≤27 milliseconds),

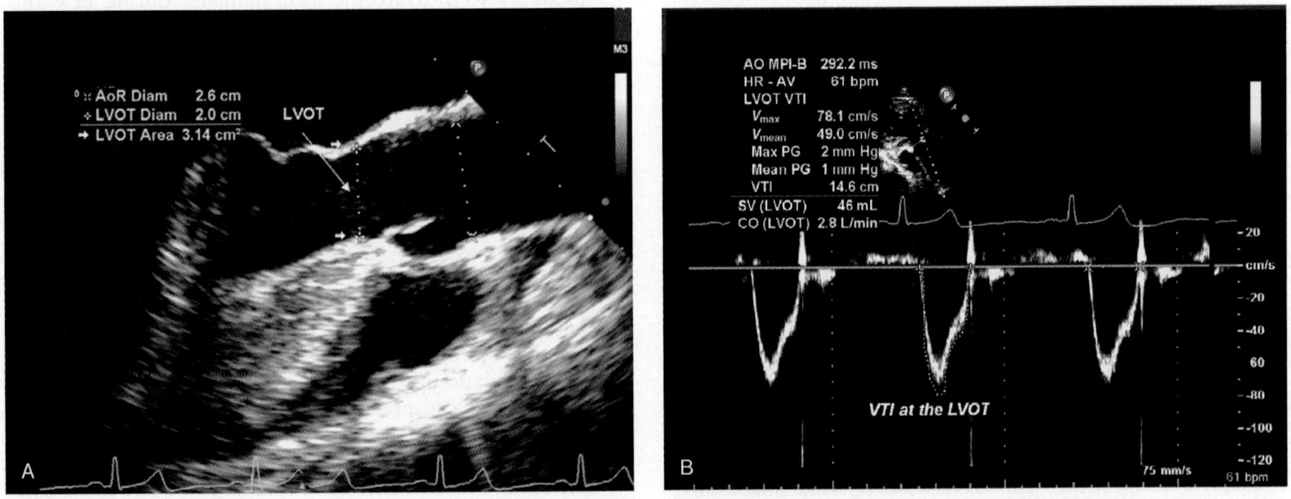

FIGURE 29.2. Calculation of CO using spectral Doppler approach. **A:** Mid-esophageal long-axis view of LVOT. LVOT measurement is 2.0 cm. The CSA is calculated as $\pi(D/2)^2$ to be 3.14 cm^2. **B:** Transgastric long-axis view using a PWD directed through the aortic valve opening. VTI is calculated by the computer through tracing the outer envelope of the spectral signal and is determined to be 14.6 cm. **SV** is the product of CSA and VTI: 3.14 × 14.6 = 46 mL. CO = SV × HR: 46 × 61 = 2.8 L/min.

moderately depressed systolic function value range between 1,000 and 1,200 mm Hg per second, and when dP/dt is decreased bellow 1,000 mm Hg per second, left ventricular systolic function is severely depressed [47,48].

ASSESSMENT OF PATIENT VOLUME STATUS

One of the most challenging and crucial tasks in the management of a hemodynamically unstable patient is to predict accurately whether the patient would benefit from fluid therapy. Overhydration may lead to pulmonary edema, hypoxia, and worsening outcome and therefore should be avoided. A novel and effective method for determining this "fluid responsiveness" is through the assessment of "dynamic parameters." Examples of such dynamic parameters are stroke volume variation (SVV) and pulse pressure variation (PPV). These parameters can be readily assessed with echocardiography.

SVV and PPV are caused by the interaction of the cardiac and respiratory systems; that is, the changes in intrathoracic pressure during controlled ventilation have an impact on SV and therefore, arterial pressure. The increase in intrathoracic pressure during the inspiratory phase of positive pressure ventilation leads to simultaneous but different physiologic effects on the left and right sides of the heart. In the left side, SV increases as blood is pushed forward out of the pulmonary veins into the LV. In addition, the increased intrathoracic pressure leads to improved "afterload matching" for the LV, which increases SV by functionally decreasing afterload. The interventricular septum is shifted toward the right ventricle (RV) also increasing LV SV. On the right side, right ventricular inflow decreases secondary to compression of the inferior vena cava (IVC). The rightward shift of the septum also decreases RV SV. At the beginning of the exhalation phase, SV decreases since both the pulmonary veins and the RV are relatively "empty." In hypovolemic patients, the magnitude of these cyclical or dynamic changes is increased and this serves as the basis for the accurate assessment of fluid responsiveness using these parameters [49–54].

In addition to preload, other factors affecting SVV and PPV include chest wall compliance and ventilation parameters, including tidal volumes and airway pressures. In situations wherein chest wall compliance and respiratory parameters are held relatively constant, SVV can be used as a guide to establishing whether a given patient will respond to fluid loading by increasing CO.

Limitations to this technique include the following:

1. Need for positive pressure ventilation with either total paralysis or heavy sedation preventing from the patient to initiate the ventilator.
2. Effect of cardiac rhythm. In patients with cardiac arrhythmia, the beat-to-beat variation in SV and hence in BP may no longer reflect the effects of mechanical ventilation. This is particularly true in patients with atrial fibrillation or frequent extrasystoles. In patients with few-and-far-between extrasystoles, the arterial pressure curve can still be analyzed if the cardiac rhythm is regular during at least one respiratory cycle.
3. Effect of tidal volume. Increasing tidal volume will result in increasing the mean airway pressure and, hence, in decreasing the mean cardiac preload (leftward shift on the Frank–Starling curve). Therefore, a patient operating on the flat portion of the Frank–Starling curve (i.e., insensitive to changes in preload) may operate on the steep portion and hence become sensitive to changes in preload (in essence leading to false-positive reading of this index) if the tidal volume is increased. Conversely, using lung-protective ventilation with low tidal volume may lead to minimal pleural pressure changes over a single respiratory cycle. In this case, inspiration will not induce any significant change in LV SV, even in fluid-responsive patients (leading to a false-negative reading). This may explain why the SVV has been found to be a reliable predictor of fluid responsiveness in patients with tidal volume ranging between 8 and 15 mL per kg [49,55,56].

Three echocardiographic indices have been shown to reliably assess fluid responsiveness based on the dynamic parameter approach:

1. ***Aortic Flow Index***: The increase in SV during positive pressure ventilation as described earlier leads to increased peak flow across the LVOT, the aortic valve and descending aorta. Similarly, the decrease in SV during exhalation leads to decrease in peak flow across these structures. The aortic flow index can efficiently predict fluid responsiveness in patients ventilated with positive pressure. To calculate the aortic flow index, one has to use the pulse wave Doppler to sample flow at the ascending aorta. This will generate a series of peak flow spectral displays that are increased during inspiration and decreased during exhalation (Fig. 29.3). The formula to calculate the aortic flow index is

   $$\text{Aortic flow index} = (\text{PEAK max}_{ins} - \text{PEAK min}_{exp})/\text{mean} \times 100$$

   An index of >12% has been shown to discriminate between fluid responders and nonresponders with high sensitivity and specificity (100% and 89%, respectively) [57]. This index can be calculated rapidly by either TTE or TEE.
2. ***Superior Vena Cava Collapsibility Index***: This concept is similar to other dynamic parameters. During the inspiratory phase of positive pressure ventilation, the superior vena cava (SVC) collapses due to increase in the intrathoracic pressure. The SVC re-expands back to its baseline during exhalation. The degree of collapsibility depends on the degree of hypovolemia; as less volume circulates in the intravascular compartment the SVC will be susceptible to the increase in intrathoracic pressure, and thus this phenomenon is exacerbated in a state of hypovolemia. The SVC index can be calculated with TEE only by using either 2D or M-mode modality to measure the SVC diameter during PPV (Fig. 29.4). The formula to calculate this index is

   $$\text{SVC collapsibility index} = (D\text{max}_{exp} - D\text{min}_{ins})/D\text{max}_{exp} \times 100$$

   An index of >36% has been shown to predict fluid responsiveness with high sensitivity and specificity (90% and 100%, respectively) [58] and can be very useful in predicting the need for fluid therapy in hemodynamically unstable patients.
3. ***Inferior Vena Cava Collapsibility Index***: The rationale behind the IVC collapsibility index is similar to other dynamic parameters. The physiology, however, is slightly different. The increased intrathoracic pressure during positive pressure ventilation as compared to the extrathoracic pressure leads to reduced pressure gradient to venous return. This, in turn, leads to decrease in systemic venous return and as a consequence to increase in the volume of the extrathoracic venous blood. The end result is an increase in extrathoracic IVC diameter during positive pressure breath, followed by a decrease in its diameter during exhalation [59,60]. Recently, IVC collapsibility during positive pressure ventilation has been used to predict fluid responsiveness similar to the

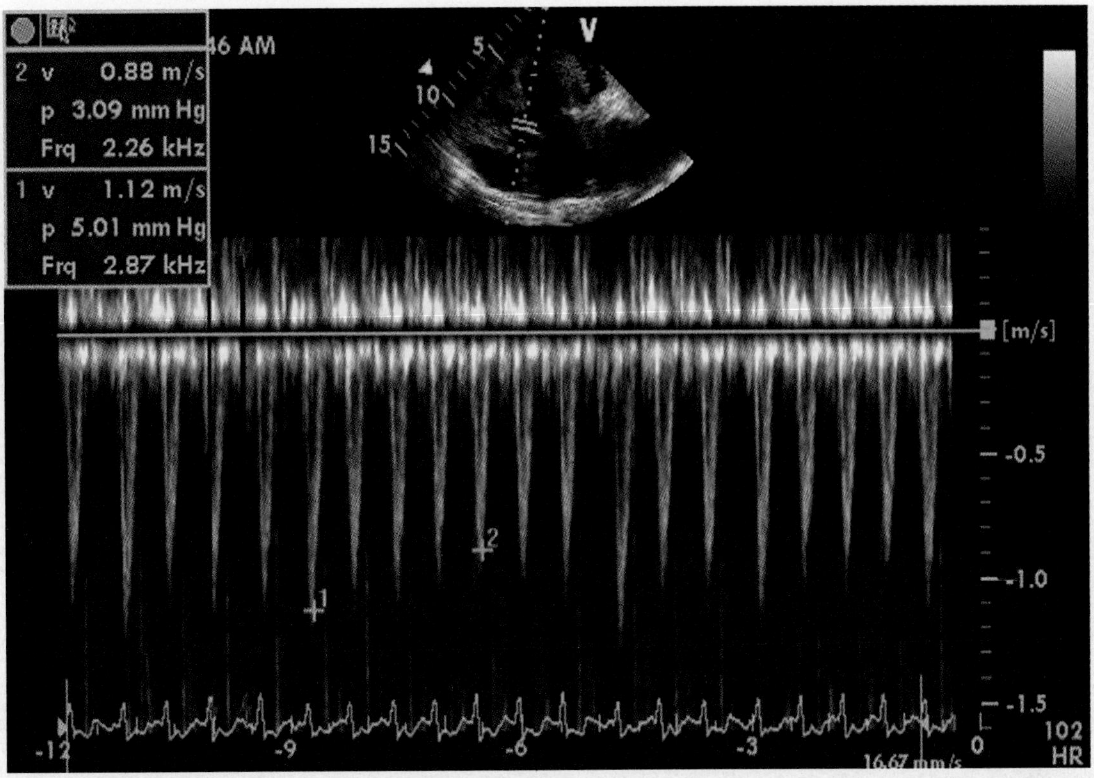

FIGURE 29.3. TEE deep transgastric view assessment of aortic flow index. The pulse-wave Doppler sample volume is positioned at the LVOT level, demonstrating spectral displays of peak flows during PPV. The peak flows vary with respiration; increased during positive pressure breath (1) and decreased during exhalation (2). The aortic flow index is calculated as the difference between the peaks flows divided by their mean. In this example, the aortic flow index = (PEAK max_{ins} − PEAK min_{exp})/mean × 100 = (1.12 − 0.88/1) × 100 = 24%. This indicated severe hypovolemia and fluid resuscitation initiated.

aortic flow index and other dynamic parameters [61]. In this study, the change in IVC diameter during positive pressure ventilation (ΔD_{IVC}) was defined as the difference between the maximum and the minimum IVC diameter over the mean and expressed as percentage: $\Delta D_{IVC} = (D_{IVCmax} - D_{IVCmin})/\text{mean} \times 100\%$. In this study, a threshold ΔD_{IVC} value of 12% allowed identification of fluid responders with positive and negative predictive values of 93% and 92%, respectively. To assess for IVC collapsibility, the IVC is visualized in the subcostal view, and the IVC diameter is measured 3 cm from the right atrium by either 2D or M-mode technique.

ASSESSMENT OF LEFT VENTRICULAR PRELOAD

Preload is defined as the myocardial fiber length at end diastole [43]. LV end-diastolic volume (LVEDV) is one of several clinical variables used to assess preload. Accurate preload estimation is one of the main challenges faced when caring for critically ill patients, even to the most experienced physician. Traditionally, preload has been assessed using physical examination, clinical assessment of end-organ perfusion, and direct measurement of intravascular pressures. Echocardiography can be used efficiently to supplement clinical assessment.

A. *2D Echo Method*: LV diameter measured with 2D echo can be used to extrapolate LV volume at end-diastole, and thus estimate preload. These measurements can be compared with reported estimates of normal ventricular dimensions to define degrees of ventricular enlargement. A single measurement, however, is of limited value in defining the preload state of any given patient. A patient with a history of cardiomyopathy, as an example, will have an increased LV end-diastolic diameter compared to a normal patient. To define such a patient as having adequate or excess preload is not justifiable. Serial measurements of LV diameter are more useful clinically in assessing changes over time and in response to therapies such as intravenous fluid challenge or diuresis. A number of studies that have compared echocardiographic estimates of preload with PAOP have shown the potential superiority of the echocardiographic method [62–64]. This method seems to perform well in detecting decreased end-diastolic volumes and hypovolemia. However, when used to diagnose high preload or fluid overload, they may not be as reliable [43]. In the operating room, both end-diastolic areas and volumes correlated well with thermodilution cardiac index in patients undergoing coronary artery bypass grafting [65] and liver transplantation [66], while PAWP showed no correlation.

B. ***Pulsed Wave Doppler Method***: Preload estimation can be assessed by Doppler echocardiography. The velocity profile of blood flow through the mitral valve during diastole is normally biphasic. In a young individual with normal LV compliance and relaxation, the early, passive filling phase, represented by the *E*-wave, exceeds the component of filling due to atrial contraction, represented by the A-wave. The

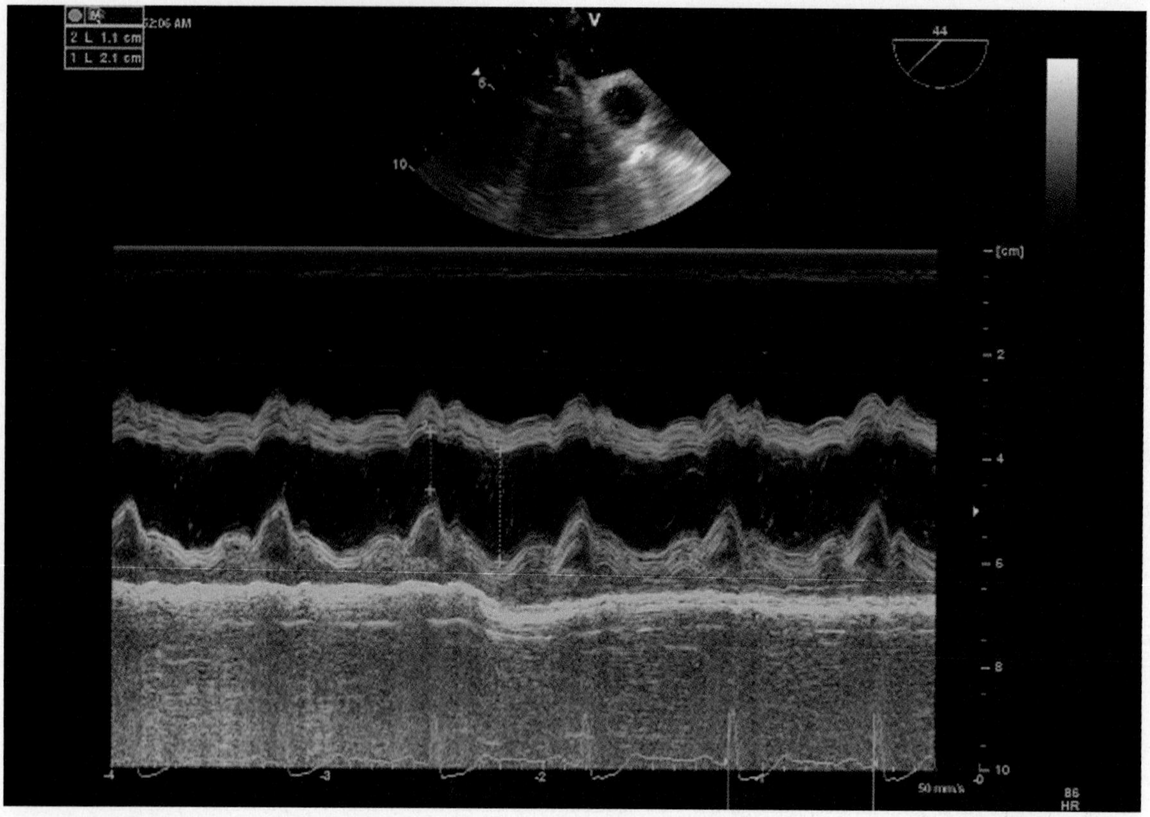

FIGURE 29.4. TEE upper esophageal view of the superior vena cava M-mode. SVC collapsibility index = $(Dmax_{exp} - Dmin_{ins})/Dmax_{exp} \times 100 = (2.1 - 1.1)/2.1 \times 100 = 47\%$, indicating hypovolemia and fluid responsiveness.

magnitude of theses flows and their ratio varies with age in normal individuals [25] (Fig. 29.5).

Using the peak *E/A velocity* ratio, LV end-diastolic pressure (LVEDP) can be roughly estimated. With this technique, a ratio >2 is associated with LVEDP >20 mm Hg [67]. It is possible to estimate PAWP more accurately by using the equation [68]:

$$\text{PAWP} = 18.4 + [17.1 \cdot \ln(E\,\text{peak}/A\,\text{peak})]$$

One study demonstrated that measurement of transmitral and pulmonary venous flows by Doppler can be used to estimate LV-filling pressure in critically ill patients under mechanical ventilation [69]. In this study, an E/A ratio >2 had a positive predictive value of 100% for a PAWP value >18 mm Hg. However, a large E/A ratio may also be seen in young healthy subjects. In this population, LV elastic myocardial relaxation is rapid, which allows for almost complete LV filling during early diastole. This can lead to high E/A ratio without elevation of left atrial (LA) pressure [70]. Therefore, any interpretation of transmitral flow must take into account the patient's age. In addition, heart rate also modifies the transmitral flow pattern. Since tachycardia shortens diastolic filling time, atrial contraction may occur before early filling is completed. This will potentially result in a higher peak A-wave velocity than when the heart rate is slower. Furthermore, the transmitral E- and A-waves can overlap, making interpretation of the transmitral indices impossible [71]. Thus, in tachycardic patients a low E/Aratio does not necessarily relate to a low PAOP.

EVALUATION OF RIGHT VENTRICULAR FUNCTION AND PRELOAD

Right ventricular systolic dysfunction is another potential cause of hypotension. In practice, estimates of RV function are made from qualitative assessments of 2D imaging. Using either TEE (mid-esophageal four-chamber view) or TTE (apical and subcostal views), the right ventricular free wall can be visualized and its thickening and displacement can be noted. In situations where right ventricular dysfunction is the sole cause of hypotension, whether directly from states causing myocardial dysfunction or as a result of a secondary issue such as a pulmonary embolus, the LV is typically underfilled. Preload of the RV is also estimated from either qualitative or quantitative assessment of ventricular size while again understanding that single measurements of such dimensions are of limited usefulness.

ASSESSMENT OF VALVULAR ETIOLOGIES OF HEMODYNAMIC INSTABILITY

Abnormalities of valvular function can, on occasion, be the primary cause of hypotension. Although valvular stenoses can certainly have impact on hemodynamics in the ICU patient, they are rarely the direct cause of hypotension. For this

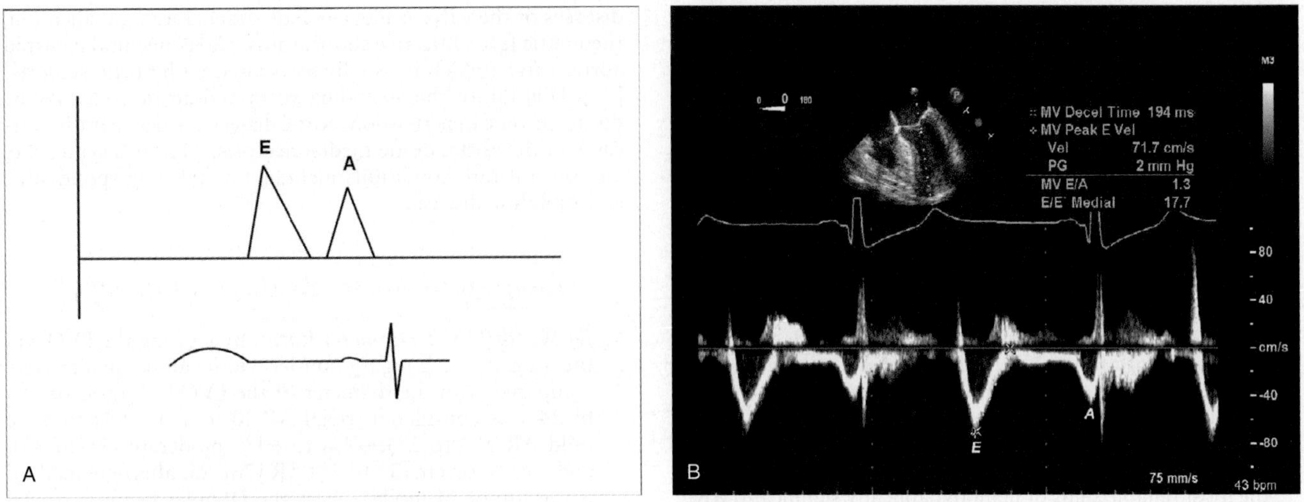

FIGURE 29.5. **A**: Schematic representation of transmitral inflow profile showing *E*- and *A* waves during diastole. **B**: TEE mid-esophageal four-chamber view of transmitral inflow showing *E*- and *A* waves.

reason, this section will concentrate on evaluation of regurgitant valvular lesions.

Echocardiographic Evaluation of Mitral Regurgitation

Echocardiographic evaluation of MR includes assessment of valve anatomy, severity of regurgitation, LA enlargement due to volume overload, ventricular function, and the severity of pulmonary arterial hypertension. The mitral apparatus includes the anterior and posterior leaflets, the annulus, chordae tendineae, and the papillary muscles with their supporting LV walls. The etiology of MR could be a result of anatomical or functional changes in the mitral valve and its supporting structures. Anatomical changes in mitral valve leaflet pathology can be caused by rheumatic disease, endocarditis, myxomatous disease, infiltrative diseases, such as amyloid, sarcoid, mucopolysaccharidosis, and collagen-vascular disorders, such as systemic lupus erythematosus and rheumatoid arthritis. Functional changes in the mitral annulus leading to dilation, secondary to LA as well as LV dilation, may result in MR due to incomplete leaflet coaptation. MR can also occur as a result of chordal tear or elongation, which leads to inadequate tensile support of the closed leaflet(s) in systole with prolapse of the leaflet(s) into the left atrium [44]. Papillary muscle rupture can occur in the setting of acute myocardial infarction and frequently leads to cardiogenic shock from acute, severe MR. Partial rupture is more common and better tolerated.

The Carpentier classification is commonly used to define the pathophysiologic mechanism leading to the regurgitation: normal, restrictive, or excessive leaflet motion [72].

- *Class I—Normal leaflet motion*: the most common cause of MR wherein leaflet motion is normal and there is mitral annular dilation and papillary muscle dysfunction due to myocardial ischemia. In most cases, the MR jet is centrally directed into the left atrium.
- *Class II—Excessive leaflet motion*: Characterized by excessive leaflet motion ranging from leaflet *billowing* wherein a portion of a leaflet projects above the annulus in systole while the coaptation point remains below the mitral annulus, to *prolapse* wherein the excursion of a leaflet tip is above the level of the mitral annulus during systole, to *flail*, where a leaflet flows freely into the left atrium, frequently as a consequence of ruptured chordae tendineae. Typically, the MR jet is eccentrically directed away from the affected leaflet.
- *Class III—Restrictive leaflet motion*: Characterized by restriction of the leaflet, most commonly as a result of left ventricular dilation that displaces the papillary muscle away from the mitral valve annulus and in this way prevents leaflet coaptation. The direction of the MR jet may be central or eccentrically directed toward the side of the more affected leaflet. Mitral valvular systolic anterior motion (SAM), which is discussed later, is also considered as an example of restricted leaflet motion

Mitral Regurgitation Assessment

1. ***2D Examination***: Basic 2D assessment may provide clues for the presence of MR. Structural leaflet abnormality or coaptation defects may be obvious in some cases. Indirect signs of MR should also be sought. These include LV and LA enlargement and signs of pulmonary arterial hypertension; elevated PA pressures estimated from Doppler interrogation of Tricuspid regurgitation (TR) jets as an example.
2. ***Doppler Flow Examination***: Doppler flow examination is the most common method used to screen and evaluate MR. MR is graded as trivial, mild, moderate, or severe, which corresponds to the angiography scores of 1+, 2+, 3+, and 4+. A visual assessment of the area of the MR color map provides a rough estimate of the severity of regurgitation. However, this simple visual assessment has limitations. As an example, eccentric MR jets that run along an LA wall may appear less severe (the Coanda effect). In addition, color gain settings—a technical issue—can have significant impact on the size of the MR color map. Low color gains will increase the size where as high gains will reduce it. This is sometimes referred to as the "dial-a-jet" phenomenon. Typically, color flow velocity limits should be set in the 50 to 60 cm per second range when evaluating MR. As mentioned in the prior section, MR jet direction has important clinical implications. Centrally directed jets usually result from annular dilation or ischemic and dysfunctional

papillary muscle. Eccentric jets are caused almost exclusively by structural abnormalities of the mitral apparatus. As a consequence, eccentric jets are unlikely to improve after improving myocardial ischemia.

Quantification of Mitral Regurgitation

A. ***Vena Contracta Width***: The vena contracta is the narrow contracted portion of the MR jet seen just below the mitral leaflets. The width of this jet has been shown to correlate well with the severity of MR [73]. Widths of <3 mm correspond to mild MR, 3 to 5 mm with moderate MR, and more than 7 mm with severe MR [74]. Limitation includes the situation where there are multiple MR jets or the presence of eccentric jets.
B. ***Pulmonary Vein Flow Reversal***: Blunting or reversal of the systolic component of pulmonary venous inflow is one of the most reliable signs of hemodynamically significant MR. Systolic flow reversal is associated with severe MR whereas blunting is usually associated with moderate or moderate-to-severe MR. Limitations includes the inability to use this in the presence of atrial fibrillation where there is systolic blunting of flow due to loss of atrial relaxation, independent of the degree of MR.
C. ***Proximal Isovelocity Surface Area Method (PISA)***: The PISA method is based on the principle that a regurgitant jet accelerates in layers of concentric shells proximal to the regurgitant orifice. Immediately adjacent to the orifice, these shells have small area with high-velocity flow and at increasing distance from the orifice they have larger area and lower velocities [44]. By interrogating this area with color Doppler, the regurgitant volume can be calculated. The regurgitant volume of blood is the product of the shell area (PISA) and the aliasing velocity. Since this regurgitant volume is passing through a defect in the mitral valve, the regurgitant orifice area (ROA) can be calculated as follows: ROA = regurgitant volume ÷ VTI_{MRjet}.

Systolic Anterior Motion: SAM of the mitral valve represents an important diagnosis that must be considered in the unstable patient. MV SAM is caused when a venturi effect of blood flow at high velocity through a narrowed space between the anterior mitral valve leaflet and LV septum causes the MV leaflet(s) to be displaced toward the LVOT, causing obstruction to systolic flow. Patients at risk for developing SAM include those with hypertrophied LV septums, whether asymmetric or symmetric, patients with small LV diameters, patients with redundant mitral apparatus tissue and patients with hypercontractile left ventricles. 2D imaging of the mitral leaflet and LVOT will show movement of the leaflet into the path of blood flow. Color Doppler imaging will reveal "color aliasing" of blood flow, the Doppler equivalence of turbulence, in the LVOT. In addition, SAM frequently prevents normal coaptation of the mitral leaflets resulting in significant, usually anteriorly directed, eccentric MR. Continuous wave Doppler interrogation of the outflow tract from deep gastric windows will reveal a high-velocity flow profile, often "dagger" shaped, which can be used to quantify a pressure gradient across the obstruction. The response of this process to therapeutic interventions can be followed using these echocardiographic assessments.

Assessing Aortic Regurgitation

Causes of aortic regurgitation (AR) can be divided into abnormalities of the aortic valve leaflets and the aorta. Primary diseases of the valve leaflets include degenerative calcification, rheumatic fever, infective endocarditis, and congenital bicuspid aortic valve (which is usually associated with aortic stenosis) [75]. Dilation of the ascending aorta and aortic root may be due to chronic hypertension, aortic dissection, degenerative diseases of the aorta, cystic medial necrosis, Marfan's syndrome, and several rare conditions including ankylosing spondylitis, and syphilitic disease.

Evaluation of Aortic Regurgitation Severity

A. ***Jet Width/LVOT Diameter Ratio***: By viewing the LVOT in the long axis, the regurgitant jet width can be qualitatively compared with the diameter of the LVOT. A ratio of 1% to 24% is considered trivial AR (0 to 1^+), 25% to 46% mild AR (1^+ to 2^+), 47% to 64% moderate (2^+ to 3^+), and >65% severe (3^+ to 4^+) AR [76]. An alternate method is the use of M-mode, where the Doppler beam is placed perpendicular to the outflow tract. The regurgitant jet can be seen within the LVOT boundaries during diastole. Dividing the regurgitant jet width by the LVOT width can then be used as outlined to grade the AR.
B. ***Jet Area/LVOT Area Ratio***: Using a short-axis view of the aortic valve, the area of the regurgitant jet can be compared with the area of the LVOT. A ratio of <4% is considered trivial AR (0 to 1^+), 4% to 24% mild (1^+ to 2^+), 25% to 59% moderate (2^+ to 3^+), and >60% severe (3^+ to 4^+) AR [77].
C. ***Vena Contracta***: The vena contracta width of an aortic insufficiency (AI) jet can be measured in the long-axis view of the jet. A vena contracta width of more than 6 mm has been associated with severe AR [78].
D. ***Slope of Aortic Regurgitant Jet Velocity Profile***: The velocity of the regurgitant jet is directly correlated to the pressure gradient between the aorta and the LV in diastole. The more severe the AR, the faster the velocity profile will approach zero as the gradient between the aorta and the LV decreases rapidly. Using this principle, the slope of the rate of decay of the velocity jet can be used as a measure of regurgitation severity. A measurement of the pressure half time of this decay (the time interval between maximal AR gradient and the time it takes to half the maximal gradient). A pressure half-time of less than 200 ms corresponds to severe, 200 to 500 ms moderate, and >500 ms mild AR [79,80]. A potential pitfall of this grading technique is that it may be influenced by other pathologies that influence the gradient between the aorta and LV, such as diastolic dysfunction.

Assessing Tricuspid Regurgitation

Tricuspid regurgitation may be the result of leaflet abnormalities due to myxomatous disease or destruction from endocarditis. More frequently, increases in TR may be secondary to processes that impact right ventricular and tricuspid annular dimensions. Such examples include both acute and chronic volume overload and acute and chronic increases to RV afterload. Examples of the latter include pulmonary embolus and primary or secondary pulmonary artery hypertension. TR is typically quantified by assessing color map area and with vena contracta width as described in the assessment of MR. Evaluation for RV enlargement and systolic function is important. Continuous wave Doppler interrogation of the TR jet allows for quantification of systolic pulmonary arterial pressures and partial assessment of RV afterload. This is performed by adding an actual or estimate of CVP to the maximum pressure of the TR jet.

EXTRACARDIAC CAUSES OF HEMODYNAMIC INSTABILITY

Pericardial Tamponade

Cardiac tamponade is a clinical and hemodynamic diagnosis; echocardiography may however, be assistance in equivocal cases. Chronic, or slowly accumulating effusions can become very large (>1,000 mL) without significant increase in pericardial pressures. In the acute setting, however, even a small volume of fluid (50 to 100 mL) may lead to significant increase in pericardial pressure and tamponade physiology. The echocardiographic diagnosis of tamponade first requires demonstration of an effusion. From there, the examination should focus on identifying cardiac chamber collapse. As the pericardial pressure increases, the cardiac chambers will show collapse in sequence from lowest pressure to highest; the atria will collapse first, followed by the RV and then LV. Furthermore, the collapse of each chamber will be most pronounced during the portion of the cardiac cycle during which the pressure is the lowest in that chamber; ventricular systole for the atria and ventricular diastole for the ventricles. This collapse can be evaluated with M-mode interrogation of the chamber walls. Pulsed-wave Doppler echocardiographic interrogation of ventricular inflow, across both the mitral and tricuspid valves, can also be used to assess for the effects of respiratory variation on ventricular filling—the echocardiographic equivalent of pulsus paradoxus. In the setting of tamponade, the peak LV inflow velocities will decrease by more than 25% with spontaneous inspiration while peak RV velocities will decrease by more than 25% during expiration [44] (Fig. 29.6).

Pulmonary Embolus

Diagnosis of pulmonary embolism (PE) in ICU patients can be extremely challenging. TTE has been described as a routine screening test in patients with suspected PE. When TTE

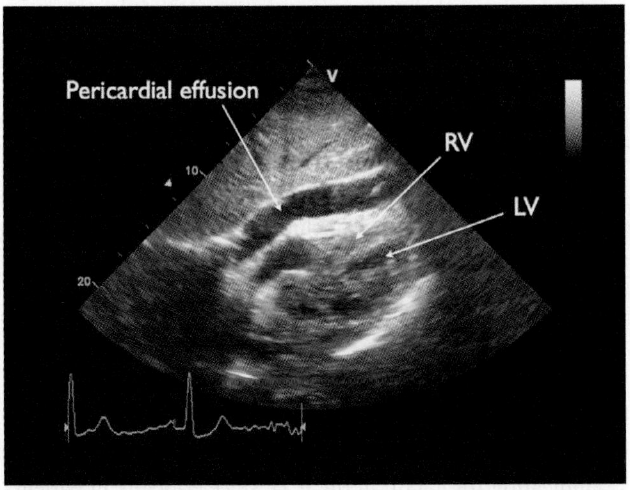

FIGURE 29.6. Transthoracic subcostal view demonstrating large pericardial effusion with end-diastolic right-ventricular chamber collapse making the echocardiographic diagnosis of tamponade. RV, right ventricle; LV, left ventricle.

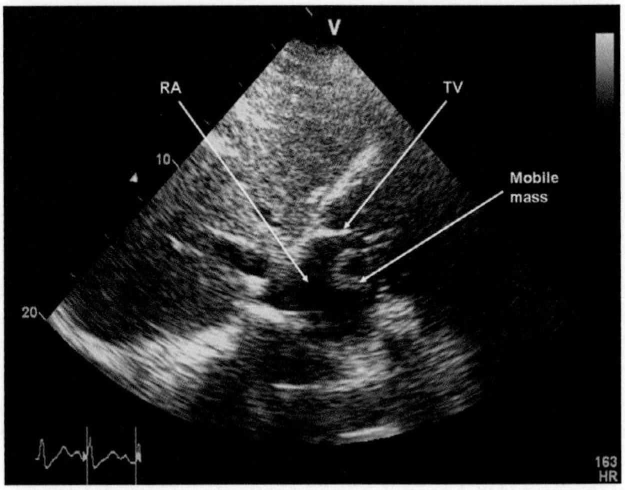

FIGURE 29.7. Transthoracic echocardiography subcostal view focusing on the right atrium demonstrating a mobile mass in the atrium making the diagnosis of emboli in transit in a patient with acute cardiovascular collapse. RA, right atrium; TV, tricuspid valve.

is nondiagnostic and the clinician has high level of suspicion, or there is evidence of RV overload or hemodynamic instability, TEE examination is indicated [81]. In these circumstances, TEE has a sensitivity of 80% and a specificity of 100%. 2D echo visualization of the main and proximal right and left pulmonary arteries may allow visualization of an embolus lodged in those locations. The left pulmonary artery may be difficult to visualize as the left bronchus is frequently interposed between the TEE probe and the artery. When the PE is not extensive and easily diagnosed by echocardiography, several indirect echocardiographic signs may suggest the presence of one. These include evidence of acute right ventricular pressure overload with elevated PA pressures, right ventricular dilation, right ventricular systolic dysfunction, and increased tricuspid regurgitation. In situations where the echocardiogram can not definitively make the diagnosis of PE, the exam findings can aid the clinician in guiding therapy (Fig. 29.7).

Aortic Dissection

Aortic dissection is a life-threatening condition where an intimal tear in the aortic wall allows passage of blood into a "false" lumen between the intima and the media. The mortality rate for acute aortic dissection is as high as a 1% per hour among untreated patients in the first 48 hours [82]. A rapid and correct diagnosis is paramount for improving survival rate. TEE has become a standard modality for the evaluation of suspected aortic dissection due to its availability, low cost, and noninvasiveness [83]. In addition, TEE can be used to diagnose other dissection-related cardiac and noncardiac complications such as AI, coronary occlusion, pericardial effusion with or without tamponade, and hemothorax.

Diagnosis of an ascending aortic dissection can prove to be very challenging due to imaging-related issues. The ascending aorta and aortic arch are areas where imaging artifacts due to reverberation and refraction are common. These artifacts can mimic the appearance of dissection flaps. Furthermore, at the level of the distal ascending aorta and proximal arch, the left mainstem bronchus crosses between the esophagus and aorta, causing image degradation. As an end result, imaging from different tomographic planes and angles is mandatory to insure accurate reporting. To distinguish artifact from dissection

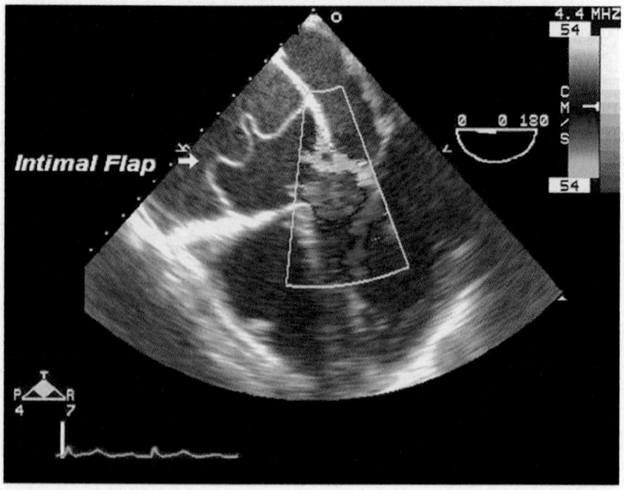

FIGURE 29.8. TEE mid-esophageal four chamber view (zooming on the aortic valve) showing acute aortic dissection with an intimal flap (arrow). The color Doppler showing severe aortic regurgitation.

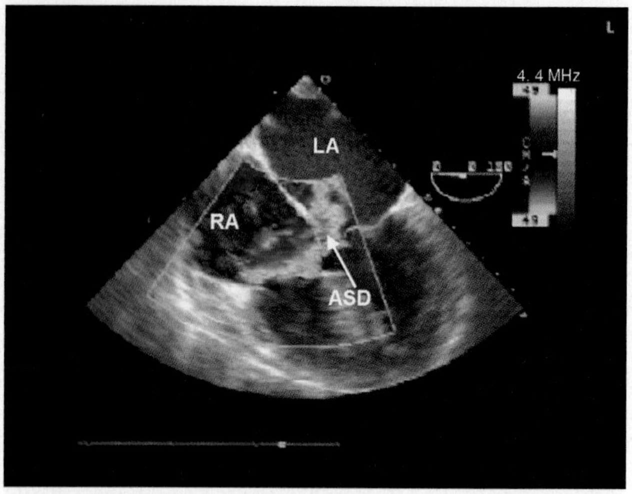

FIGURE 29.9. TEE mid-esophageal four chamber view showing a left to right shunt through an atrial septal defect (*arrow*). LA, left atrium; RA, right atrium; ASD, atrial septal defect.

flap, the echocardiographer should establish whether or not the linear echodensity conforms to the limits of the aorta or if it seems to disregard such anatomic boundaries as would an artifact. Color Doppler imaging can be used to establish whether or not blood flow respects or ignores the echodensity.

Usually, an intimal flap creates a true and false lumen. Identification of these lumina is frequently an important goal of TEE evaluation but can create a diagnostic challenge for the sonographer. There are several indirect findings that can help differentiate the lamina. First, the true lumen usually expands during systole and is slightly compressed during diastole [84]. Second, spontaneous echo contrast or thrombus may be seen in the false lumen as a result of stagnant flow; however, this may occasionally be misleading as in some instances it may be the true lumen where flow is stagnant. In addition, the true lumen is usually smaller than the false lumen, especially in chronic dissection [85,86]. Several communications between the true and false lamina can often be identified by color Doppler. Although some of these communications represent entry sites allowing blood to flow from the true to the false lumen, others are exit sites with bidirectional flow. Identification of the starting point of a dissection can have ramifications for deciding therapy (Fig. 29.8).

ECHOCARDIOGRAPHIC EVALUATION OF HYPOXEMIA

Assessment of unexplained hypoxemia and the inability to wean from ventilatory support is another potential use of echocardiography in the ICU. Etiologies of hypoxemia that can be diagnosed by echocardiography include intracardiac right to left shunting, pulmonary embolus, and LV pathologies such as LV systolic and/or diastolic dysfunction and mitral valvular abnormalities which can lead to pulmonary edema. The echocardiographic evaluation of pulmonary embolus and of LV and mitral valvular pathologies has been discussed earlier.

Intracardiac shunt is defined as an abnormal communication between two cardiac chambers and is characterized by blood flow across the defect [44]. The direction and volume of flow is determined by the pressure gradient across the defect and the size of the defect. A chronic left-to-right shunt may lead to right-sided volume overload and, over time, right-sided pressure overload from irreversible pulmonary arterial hypertension. This right-sided pressure increase may then lead to right-to-left shunting through the same defect. In clinical practice, right-to-left shunt is more commonly seen in settings where right-sided pressure acutely increases over left-sided pressures and typically involves defects in the interatrial septum. The diagnosis of an intracardiac shunt can be made with color flow Doppler. Typically, the flow across an atrial septal defect (ASD) is of low velocity because of the small pressure difference between the chambers. A significant right-to-left shunt will occur when right atrial pressure exceeds LA as with severe pulmonary arterial hypertension. Other echocardiographic signs consistent with an ASD are biatrial and RV enlargement. The ratio of pulmonary to systemic blood flow, Q_p/Q_s, can be determined by Doppler flow measurements. To calculate Q_p/Q_s, it is necessary to measure SV form the left and right sides of the heart. Transpulmonary flow, Q_p, can be calculated by measurement of the pulmonary artery CSA and VTI at the same site. Systemic flow, Q_s, is calculated from the measurement of LVOT CSA and VTI as outlined earlier (Fig. 29.9).

$$Q_p/Q_s = \frac{CSA_{PA} \times VTI_{PA}}{CSA_{LVOT} \times VTI_{LVOT}}$$

ECHOCARDIOGRAPHIC ASSESSMENT FOR SOURCES OF EMBOLI

Several disease processes, including intracardiac mass and shunt, are potential sources of systemic emboli leading to acute vascular occlusive events. Echocardiography can be very useful in the diagnosis or exclusion of the heart as a source of systemic emboli.

Cardiac masses: the three basic types of cardiac masses include vegetation, thrombus, and tumor, all of which are known causes of emboli.

A. *Vegetation*: suspected infective endocarditis is a common indication for a TEE in the ICU, since critically ill patients are at a high risk for bacteremia. Endocarditis is a diagnosis based on a combination of findings from physical examination, laboratory findings (most importantly bacteremia), and echocardiographic examination. The purpose of the echocardiographic exam is to identify valvular lesions that may be consistent with endocarditis, to evaluate any functional abnormality associated with the affected valve, to assess the impact of the valvular disease on chamber function and dimensions, and to discover other complications of endocarditis such as paravalvular abscess and pericardial effusion. All valves have to be carefully inspected as more than one valve can be involved. Echocardiographic evaluation of valvular endocarditis involves multiple acoustic windows and 2D views, since the vegetation may be seen only in a certain tomographic planes. Most commonly, the vegetation is attached to the upstream, lower pressure side of the valve leaflet. It appears as an abnormal, echogenic, irregular mass attached to a leaflet [44]. Although vegetations can be attached to any part of the leaflet, attachment to the coaptation point is most common.

B. ***Thrombus***: Intracardiac thrombi form in areas of blood stasis or low flow. Examples of this within the ventricles include ventricular aneurysm, pseudoaneurysm, and areas adjacent to severely hypokinetic or akinetic wall segments. LA thrombi are usually associated with atrial enlargement, mitral stenosis, and atrial fibrillation. Most LA thrombi are found in the LA appendage, which is best visualized by TEE. Thrombi are usually more echogenic than the underlying myocardium and have a shape distinct from the endocardial border. Imaging from several tomographic planes is frequently necessary to rule out artifact that may mimic thrombus. Again, color Doppler can be used to establish whether or not blood flow respects the apparent boundaries of the suspected thrombus to attempt to distinguish it from an echo artifact.
C. *Cardiac Tumors*: Nonprimary tumors, which are about twenty times more common than primary cardiac tumors, can involve the heart by either metastatic or lymphatic spread, or invasion from neighboring malignancies. They can invade all structures of the heart; the pericardium, epicardium, myocardium and endocardium. About 75% of metastatic cardiac tumors involve the pericardium and epicardium and most commonly present as pericardial effusion. A definite diagnosis usually cannot be made from the echocardiographic images alone. A probable diagnosis can sometimes be made by incorporating the clinical information along with the echocardiographic images. Renal cell carcinoma has a propensity to develop "finger-like" projections that may extend up the IVC into the right atrium. Occasionally, uterine tumors may present in a similar manner
D. ***Shunts***: As described earlier, right-to-left shunting can play a role in hypoxemia. In addition, any right to left communications can allow for paradoxical emboli to travel from the systemic venous to arterial circulation. This can lead to stroke or vascular occlusive disease of one or several organs.

IMPACT OF ICU ECHOCARDIOGRAPHY ON PATIENT MANAGEMENT

Indications for performing a TEE study vary significantly depending on patient type: for patients in the medical and neurosurgical ICUs, most TEE studies are performed to rule out or confirm bacterial endocarditis (medical ICU) and/or a cardiac source of emboli (neurosurgical ICU). In contrast, in medical-surgical and coronary ICU patients the most common indications are for diagnosing aortic dissection, valvular dysfunction, or hemodynamic instability [18].

A recent review of 21 studies evaluating the impact of TEE on patient management demonstrated that out of 2,508 critically ill patients, TEE findings had therapeutic implications, either surgical interventions or changes in medical therapy, in 68.5% of patients. [18] 5.6% of patients underwent a surgical intervention without additional investigations following their TEE. In 62.9% of patients, the TEE study had a therapeutic, nonsurgical impact. Included within this group was the institution or dose adjustment of inotropic or vasopressor drugs, antibiotics, anticoagulation, thrombolysis, fluid administration, and the initiation of advanced hemodynamic monitoring. This represents the largest reported series evaluating the use of TEE in a noncardiac surgical ICU setting.

The current body of literature that focuses on the use of echocardiography in the ICU lacks prospective, randomized controlled studies demonstrating efficacy in decreasing morbidity and mortality and cost-effectiveness. However, this literature does point to the potential benefits that may be gained by the availability of echocardiography in ICUs. It also demonstrates the potential benefit of more widespread and advanced training in echocardiography for intensive care physicians.

FUTURE POTENTIAL USE OF ECHOCARDIOGRAPHY IN TRAUMA PATIENTS IN THE ICU

Recently, hand-carried ultrasound (HCU) devices have been introduced into clinical use [87–89]. These devices are attractive because of their size, portability, and cost. They may be easily stored in the ICU, which makes them immediately available for bedside use. Portable echocardiograms performed at the bedside can help the physician to diagnose and manage critically ill patients. Although overall image and color flow qualities of hand-carried echocardiographic devices are not equivalent to the standard full-featured machines, they have been found to compare well with standard platforms for the identification of cardiac pathology [90]. Reports in the literature regarding the use of these devices are mixed. Early reports showed favorable results in the outpatient setting [88], when used on hospital rounds [89], and in a small cohort of ICU patients [87]. Some of these reports have shown a good correlation between these devices and standard echocardiographic equipment for the evaluation of wall motion abnormalities and valvular regurgitation. [91,92] In addition, data from a few studies have shown a high level of agreement between hand-carried device examination and standard echocardiographic examination [87,89,93–95]. In one study, examination with a HCU device was able to evaluate and answer 85% of clinical questions presented by the referring physician. Of those questions, 86% were later confirmed as correctly answered [96]. Although one study has demonstrated the relative equivalence of the HCU device with regards to 2D imaging, even in mechanically ventilated patients [97], other studies have shown it to be inferior to standard echocardiography when comparing spectral Doppler capabilities [98]. Other reports have shown that HCU imaging may lead to inadequate evaluation of pulmonary hypertension, valvular disease, and LV outflow tract obstruction in severely ill patients [96,97]. In ICU cohorts, several reports have demonstrated similar shortcomings. [96,98]

In addition to cardiac evaluation, the HCU can be used in the ICU to aid in placing central venous catheters and arterial lines as well as for ultrasound guidance of pleurocentesis and paracentesis. The day when the HCU becomes an extension of the traditional physical exam may not be far off. It is also not unreasonable to imagine the HCU used by the hospital code team for better diagnosis and patient management during resuscitative efforts.

CONCLUSION

Echocardiography is an important tool for diagnosis and monitoring of the critically ill. With time, utilization of echocardiography is likely to become even more widespread. It is quickly establishing itself as a highly efficient and reliable clinical tool. The echo examination can be performed in numerous clinical settings and in a diverse patient population, including the most complex. Technical advancements in this field will potentially improve the imaging quality and clinical capabilities and allow for implementation of this tool in new situations and settings. With this in mind, proper education and implementation of utilization guidelines becomes increasingly important. To achieve optimal clinical results, clinicians must be well aware of the limitation as well as the benefits of each modality and when and how they should be used. An important step toward achieving this will be inclusion of echocardiographic training within critical care fellowships.

References

1. Cahalan MK, Litt L, Botvinick EH: Advances in noninvasive cardiovascular imaging: implications for the anesthesiologist. *Anesthesiology* 66:356–372, 1987.
2. Daniel WE, Erbel R, Kasper W, et al: Safety of transesophageal echocardiography. A multicenter survey of 10,419 examinations. *Circulation* 83:817–821, 1991.
3. Sohn DW, Shin GJ, Oh JK, et al: Role of transesophageal echocardiography in hemodynamically unstable patients. *Mayo Clin Proc* 70:925–931, 1995.
4. Hwang JJ, Shyu KG, Chen JJ, et al: Usefulness of transesophageal echocardiography in the treatment of critically ill patients. *Chest* 104:861–866, 1993.
5. Khoury AF, Afridi I, Quinones MA, et al: Transesophageal echocardiography in critically ill patients: feasibility, safety and impact on management. *Am Heart J* 127:1363–1371, 1994.
6. Heidenreich PA, Stainback RF, Redberg RF, et al: Transesophageal echocardiography predicts mortality in critically ill patients with unexplained hypotension. *J Am Coll Cardiol* 26:152–158, 1995.
7. Poelaert JI, Trouerbach J, De Buyzere M, et al: Evaluation of transesophageal echocardiography as a diagnostic and therapeutic aid in a critical care setting. *Chest* 107:774–779, 1995.
8. Vignon P, Mentec H, Terre S, et al: Diagnostic accuracy and therapeutic impact of transthoracic and transesophageal echocardiography in mechanically ventilated patients in the ICU. *Chest* 106:1829–1834, 1994.
9. Gottdiener JS, Bednarz J, Devereux R, et al: American society of echocardiography recommendations for use of echocardiography in clinical trials. *J Am Soc Echocardiogr* 17:1086–1119, 2004.
10. Nagueh SF, Appleton CP, Gillebert TC, et al: Recommendations for the evaluation of left ventricular diastolic function by echocardiography. *J Am Soc Echocardiogr* 22:107–133, 2009.
11. Mulvagh SL, De Maria AN, Feinstein SB, et al: Contrast echocardiography: current and future applications. *J Am Soc Echocardiogr* 13:331–342, 2000.
12. Mor-Avi V, Caiani EG, Collins KA, et al: Combined assessment of myocardial perfusion and regional left ventricular function by analysis of contrast-enhanced power modulation images. *Circulation* 104:352–357, 2001.
13. Porter TR, Xie F, Silver M, et al: Real-time perfusion imaging with low mechanical index pulse inversion Doppler imaging. *J Am Coll Cardiol* 10:748–753, 2001.
14. Jensen MB, Sloth E, Larsen KM, et al: Transthoracic echocardiography for cardiopulmonary monitoring in intensive care. *Eur J Anaesthesiol* 21:700–707, 2004.
15. Pearson AC, Castello R, Labovitz AJ: Safety and utility of transesophageal echocardiography in the critically ill patient. *Am Heart J* 119:1083–1089, 1990.
16. Beaulieu Y, Marik PE: Bedside ultrasonography in the ICU part 1. *Chest* 128(2):881–895, 2005.
17. Joseph MX, Disney PJS, Da Costa R, et al: Transthoracic echocardiography to identify or exclude cardiac cause of shock. *Chest* 126(5):1592–1597, 2004.
18. Huttemann E, Schelenz C, Kara F, et al: The use and safety of transoesophageal echocardiography in the general ICU—a mini review. *Acta Anaesthesiol Scand* 48:827–836, 2004.
19. Colreavy FB, Donovan K, Lee KY, et al: Transesophageal echocardiography in critically ill patients. *Crit Care Med* 30:989–996, 2002.
20. Lobato EB, Urdaneta F: Transesophageal echocardiography in the intensive care unit, in Perrino RSA Jr (ed): *A Practical Approach to Transesophageal Echocardiography*. Philadelphia, Lippincott Williams & Wilkins, 2003, pp 272–285.
21. Thys DM, Abel M, Bollen BA, et al: Practice guidelines for perioperative transesophageal echocardiography: a report by the American Society of Anesthesiologists and the Society of Cardiovascular Anesthesiologists task force on transesophageal echocardiography. *Anesthesiology* 84(4):986–1006, 1996.
22. Chuang ML, Hibberd MG, Salton CJ, et al: Importance of imaging method over imaging modality in noninvasive determination of left ventricular volumes and ejection fraction: assessment by two-and-three-dimensional echocardiography and magnetic resonance imaging. *J Am Coll Cardiol* 35:477–484, 2000.
23. Crouse IJ, Cheirif J, Hanly DE, et al: Opacification and border delineation improvement in patients with suboptimal endocardial border definition in routine echocardiography: results of the phase III Albunex multicenter trial. *J Am Coll Cardiol* 22:1494–1500, 1993.
24. Reilly JP, Tunick PA, Timmermans RJ, et al: Contrast echocardiography clarifies uninterpretable wall motion in intensive care unit patients. *J Am Coll Cardiol* 35:485–490, 2000.
25. Feigenbaum H, Armstrong WF, Ryan T: Evaluation of systolic and diastolic function of the left ventricle, in *Feigenbaum's Echocardiography*. Philadelphia, Lippincott Williams & Wilkins, 2005, pp 138–180.
26. Walton SJ, Reeves ST, Dorman BH Jr: Ventricular systolic performance and pathology, in Perrino AJ, Reeves ST (eds): *Transesophageal Echocardiography*. Philadelphia, Lippincott Williams & Wilkins, 2003, pp 37–55.
27. Cohen JL, Cheirif J, Segar DS, et al: Improved left ventricular endocardial border delineation and opacification with OPTISON (FS069), a new echocardiographic contrast agent. Results of phase III multicenter trial. *J Am Coll Cardiol* 32:746–752, 1998.
28. Kitzman DW, Goldman ME, Gillam LD, et al: Efficacy and safety of the novel ultrasound contrast agent perflutren (Definity) in patients with suboptimal baseline left ventricular echocardiographic images. *Am J Cardiol* 86:669–674, 2000.
29. Malhotra V, Nwogu J, Bondmass MD, et al: Is the technically limited echocardiographic study an endangered species? Endocardial border definition with native tissue harmonic imaging and Optison contrast: a review of 200 cases. *J Am Soc Echocardiogr* 13:771–773, 2000.
30. Spencer KT, Bednarz J, Mor-Avi V, et al: The role of echocardiographic harmonic imaging and contrast enhancement for improvement of endocardial border delineation. *J Am Soc Echocardiogr* 13:131–138, 2000.
31. Nash PJ, Kassimatis KC, Borowski AG, et al: Salvage of nondiagnostic transthoracic echocardiograms on patients in intensive care units with intravenous ultrasound contrast. *Am J Cardiol* 94:409–411, 2004.
32. Costa JM, Tsutsui JM, Nozawa E, et al: Contrast echocardiography can save nondiagnostic exams in mechanically ventilated patients. *Echocardiography: J CV Ultrasound Allied Tech* 22(5):389–394, 2005.
33. Heinle SK, Noblin J, Goree-Best P, et al: Assessment of myocardial perfusion by harmonic power Doppler imaging at rest and during adenosine stress. *Circulation* 102:55–60, 2000.
34. Porter TR, Li S, Kricsfeld D, et al: Detection of myocardial perfusion in multiple echocardiographic windows with one intravenous injection of microbubbles using transient response second harmonic imaging. *J Am Coll Cardiol* 29:791–799, 1997.
35. Porter TR, Li S, Jiang L, et al: Real-time visualization of myocardial perfusion and wall thickening in human beings with intravenous ultrasonographic contrast and accelerated intermittent harmonic imaging. *J Am Soc Echocardiogr* 12:266–271, 1999.
36. Darmon PL, Hillel Z, Mograder A, et al: Cardiac output by transesophageal echocardiography using continuous-wave Doppler across the aortic valve. *Anesthesiology* 80:796–805, 1994.
37. Gorcsan J III, Dianna P, Ball BS, et al: Intraoperative determination of cardiac output by transesophageal continuous wave Doppler. *Am Heart J* 123:171–176, 1992.
38. Maslow AD, Haering J, Comunale M, et al: Measurement of cardiac output by pulsed wave Doppler of the right ventricular outflow tract. *Anesth Analg* 83:466–471, 1996.
39. Muhiuden IA, Kuecherer HF, Lee E, et al: Intraoperative estimation of cardiac output by transesophageal pulsed Doppler echocardiography. *Anesthesiology* 74:9–14, 1991.
40. Perrino AC, Harris SN, Luther MA: Intraoperative determination of cardiac output using multiplane transesophageal echocardiography: a comparison to thermodilution. *Anesthesiology* 89(2):350–357, 1998.
41. Savino JS, Troianos CA, Aukbur S, et al: Measurements of pulmonary blood flow with transesophageal two-dimensional and Doppler echocardiography. *Anesthesiology* 75:445–451, 1991.
42. Steward WJ, Jiang L, Mich R, et al: Variable effects of changes in flow rate through the aortic, pulmonary, and mitral valves on valve area and flow velocity: impact on quantitative Doppler flow calculations. *J Am Coll Cardiol* 6:653–662, 1985.

43. Brown JM: Use of echocardiography for hemodynamic monitoring. *Crit Care Med* 30(6):1361–1364, 2002.
44. Otto CM: *Textbook of Clinical Echocardiography*. 2nd ed. Philadelphia, W.B. Saunders Company, 2000.
45. Bargiggia GS, Bertucci C, Recusani F, et al: A new method for estimating left ventricular dP/dt by continuous wave Doppler-echocardiography. Validation studies at cardiac catheterization. *Circulation* 80:1287–1292, 1989.
46. Pai RG, Bansal RC, Shah PM: Doppler-derived rate of left ventricular pressure rise. Its correlation with the postoperative left ventricular function in mitral regurgitation. *Circulation* 82:514–520, 1990.
47. Chen C, Rodriguez L, Guerrero L, et al: Noninvasive estimation of the instantaneous first derivative of left ventricular pressure using continuous-wave Doppler echocardiography. *Circulation* 83:2101–2110, 1991.
48. Reynolds T: Left ventricular systolic function, in *The Echocardiographer's Pocket Reference*. Arizona, Arizona Heart Institute, 2000, pp 383–384.
49. Reuter DA, Felbinger TW, Schmidt C, et al: Stroke volume variations for assessment of cardiac responsiveness to volume loading in mechanically ventilated patients after cardiac surgery. *Intensive Care Med* 28:392–398, 2002.
50. Kramer A, Zygun D, Hawes H, et al: Pulse pressure variation predicts fluid responsiveness following coronary artery bypass surgery. *Chest* 126:1563–1568, 2004.
51. Bendjelid K, Romand JA: Fluid responsiveness in mechanically ventilated patients: a review of indices used in intensive care. *Intensive Care Med* 29:352–360, 2003.
52. Lopes MR, Oliveira MA, Pereira VO, et al: Goal-directed fluid management based on pulse pressure variation monitoring during high-risk surgery: a pilot randomized controlled trial. Crit Care 11:R100, 2007.
53. Berkenstadt H, Margalit N, Hadani M, et al: Stroke volume variation as a predictor of fluid responsiveness in patients undergoing brain surgery. *Anesth Analg* 92:984–989, 2001.
54. Michard F: Volume management using dynamic parameters. *Chest* 128:1902–1903, 2005.
55. Tavernier B, Makhotine O, Lebuffe G: Systolic pressure variation as a guide to fluid therapy in patients with sepsis-induced hypotension. *Anesthesiology* 89:1313–1321, 1998.
56. Michard F, Boussat S, Chemla D: Relation between respiratory changes in arterial pulse pressure and fluid responsiveness in septic patients with acute circulatory failure. *Am J Respir Crit Care Med* 162:134–138, 2000.
57. Feissel M, Michard F, Mangin I, et al: Respiratory changes in aortic blood velocity as an indicator of fluid responsiveness in ventilated patients with septic shock. *Chest* 119:867–873, 2001.
58. Vieillard-Baron A, Chergui K, Rabiller A, et al: Superior vena caval collapsibility as a gauge of volume status in ventilated septic patients. *Intensive Care Med* 30:1734–1739, 2004.
59. Natori H, Tamaki S, Kira S: Ultrasonographic evaluation of ventilatory effect on inferior vena caval configuration. *Am Rev Respir Dis* 120:421–427, 1979.
60. Mitaka C, Nagura T, Sakanishi N, et al: Two-dimensional echocardiographic evaluation of inferior vena cava, right ventricle, and left ventricle during positive pressure ventilation with varying levels of positive end-expiratory pressure. *Crit Care Med* 17:205–210, 1989.
61. Feissel M, Michard F, Faller JP, et al: The respiratory variation in inferior vena cava diameter as a guide to fluid therapy. *Intensive Care Med* 30:1834–1837, 2004.
62. Dalibon N, Schlumberger S, Saada M, et al: Haemodynamic assessment of hypovolaemia under general anaesthesia in pigs submitted to graded haemorrhage and retransfusion. *Br J Anaesth* 82(1):97–103, 1999.
63. Clements FM, Harpole DH, Quill T, et al: Estimation of left ventricular volume and ejection fraction by two-dimensional transoesophageal echocardiography: comparison of short axis imaging and simultaneous radionuclide angiography. *Br J Anaesth* 64:331–336, 1990.
64. Jardin F, Valtier B, Beauchet A, et al: Invasive monitoring combined with two-dimensional echocardiographic study in septic shock. *Int Care Med* 20:550–554, 1994.
65. Thys DM, Hillel Z, Goldman ME, et al: A comparison of hemodynamic indices derived by invasive monitoring and two-dimensional echocardiography. *Anesthesiology* 67:630–634, 1987.
66. Tuchy GL, Gabriel A, Muller C, et al: Titrating the preload by using the rapid infusion system: use of echocardiography during orthotopic liver transplantation. *Transplant Proc* 25:1858–1860, 1993.
67. Channer KS, Culling W, Wilde P, et al: Estimation of left ventricular end-diastolic pressure by pulsed Doppler ultrasound. *Lancet* 1:1005–1007, 1986.
68. Vanoverschelde JL, Robert AR, Gerbaus A, et al: Noninvasive estimation of pulmonary arterial wedge pressure with Doppler transmitral flow velocity pattern in patients with known heart disease. *Am J Cardiol* 75:383–389, 1995.
69. Boussuges A, Blanc P, Molenat F, et al: Evaluation of left ventricular filling pressure by transthoracic Doppler echocardiography in the intensive care unit. *Crit Care Med* 30(2):362–367, 2002.
70. Appleton CP, Hatle LK: The natural history of left ventricular filling abnormalities: assessment by two-dimensional and Doppler echocardiography. *Echocardiography* 9:437–457, 1992.
71. Sohn DW, Choi YJ, Oh BH, et al: Estimation of left ventricular end-diastolic pressure with the difference in pulmonary venous and mitral A durations is limited when mitral E and A waves are overlapped. *J Am Soc Echocardiogr* 12:106–112, 1999.
72. Carpentier A: Cardiac valve surgery—the "French correction". *J Thorac Cardiovasc Surg* 86(3):323–337, 1983.
73. Lambert AS: Mitral regurgitation, in Perrino AC Jr (ed): *A Practical Approach to Transesophageal Echocardiography*. Philadelphia, PA, Lippincott Williams & Wilkins, 2003.
74. Zoghbi WA, Enriquez-Sarano M, Foster E, et al: Recommendations for evaluation of the severity of native valvular regurgitation with two-dimensional and Doppler echocardiography. *J Am Soc Echocardiogr* 16:777–802, 2003.
75. Nyuan D, Johns RA: Anesthesia for cardiac surgery procedures, in Miller RD (ed): *Miller's Anesthesia*. 6th ed. Philadelphia, Elsevier, Churchill Livingston, 2005.
76. Perry J, Helmcke F, Nanda N, et al: Evaluation of aortic insufficiency by Doppler color flow mapping. *J Am Coll Cardiol* 9:952–959, 1987.
77. Cohen IS: *A Practical Approach to Transesophageal Echocardiography*, Perrino AC Jr (ed): Philadelphia, PA, Lippincott Williams & Wilkins, 2003.
78. Willett DL, Hall SA, Jessen ME, et al: Assessment of aortic regurgitation by transesophageal color Doppler imaging of the vena contracta: validation against an intraoperative aortic flow probe. *J Am Coll Cardiol* 37:1450–1455, 2001.
79. Labovitz AJ, Ferrara RP, Kern MJ, et al: Quantitative evaluation of aortic insufficiency by continuous wave Doppler echocardiography. *J Am Coll Cardiol* 8:1341–1347, 1986.
80. Cohen IS: Aortic regurgitation, in Perrino AC Jr (ed): *A Practical Approach to Transesophageal Echocardiography*. Philadelphia, PA, Lippincott Williams & Wilkins, 2003, pp 177–187.
81. Bobato EB, Urdanet F: Transesophageal echocardiography in the intensive care unit, in Perrino A Jr (ed): *A Practical Approach to Transesophageal Echocardiography*. Philadelphia, PA, Lippincott Williams & Wilkins, 2003, pp 272–285.
82. Hirst AE Jr, Johns VJ Jr, Kime SW Jr: Dissecting aneurysm of the aorta: a review of 585 cases. *Medicine* 37:217–279, 1985.
83. Payne KJ, Yarbrough WM, Ikonomidis JS, et al: Transesophageal echocardiography of the thoracic aorta, in Perrino AC Jr (ed): *A Practical Approach to Transesophageal Echocardiography*. Philadelphia, PA, Lippincott Williams & Wilkins, 2003, pp 251–271.
84. Iliceto S, Nanda NC, Rizzon P, et al: Color Doppler evaluation of aortic dissection. *Circulation* 75:748–755, 1987.
85. Erbel R, Mohr-Kahaly S, Oelert H, et al: Diagnostic strategies in suspected aortic dissection: comparison of computed tomography, aortography, and transesophageal echocardiography. *Am J Card Imaging* 4:157–172, 1990.
86. Mohr-Kahaly S, Erbel R, Rennollet H, et al: Ambulatory follow-up of aortic dissection by transesophageal two-dimensional and color-coded Doppler echocardiography. *Circulation* 80:24–33, 1989.
87. Firstenberg MS, Cardon L, Jones P, et al: Initial clinical experience with an ultra-portable echocardiograph for the rapid diagnosis and evaluation of critically ill patients [Abstract]. *J Am Soc Echocardiogr* 13:489, 2000.
88. Bruce CJ, Zummach PL, Prince DP, et al: Personal ultrasound imager: utility in the cardiology outpatient setting [Abstract]. *Circulation* 102:II364, 2000.
89. Pandian NG, Ramasamy S, Martin P, et al: Ultrasound stethoscope as an extension of clinical examination during hospital patient rounds: preliminary experience with a hand-held miniaturized echocardiography instrument [Abstract]. *J Am Soc Echocardiogr* 13:486, 2000.
90. DeCara JM, Lang RM, Spencer KT: The hand-carried echocardiographic device as an aid to the physical examination. *Echocardiography: J CV Ultrasound Allied Tech* 20(5):477–485, 2003.
91. Masuyama T, Yamamoto K, Nishikawa N, et al: Accuracy of ultraportable hand-carried echocardiography system in assessing ventricular function and valvular regurgitation [Abstract]. *Circulation* 102:II364, 2000.
92. Rugolotto M, Hu BS, Liang DH, et al: Validation of new small portable ultrasound device (SPUD): a comparison study with standard echocardiography [Abstract]. *Circulation* 102:II364, 2000.
93. Rugolotto M, Hu BS, Liang DH, et al: Rapid assessment of cardiac anatomy and function with a new hand-carried ultrasound device (OptiGo): a comparison with standard echocardiography. *Eur J Echocardiogr* 2:262–269, 2001.
94. Pritchett AM, Bruce CJ, Bailey KR, et al: Personal ultrasound imager: extension of the cardiovascular physical examination [Abstract]. *J Am Soc Echocardiogr* 13:485, 2000.
95. Alexander JH, Peterson ED, Chen Ay, et al: Feasibility of point-of-care echo by non-cardiologist physicians to assess left ventricular function, pericardial effusion, mitral regurgitation, and aortic valvular thickening [Abstract]. *Circulation* 104:II-334, 2001.
96. Goodkin GM, Spevack DM, Tunick PA, et al: How useful is hand-carried bedside echocardiography in critically ill patients? *J Am Coll Cardiol* 37:2019–2022, 2001.
97. Vignon P, Chastagner C, Francois B, et al: Diagnostic ability of hand-held echocardiography in ventilated critically-ill patients. *Crit Care* 7:R84–R91, 2003.
98. Vignon P, Frank MB, Lesage J, et al: Hand-held echocardiography with Doppler capability for the assessment of critically-ill patients: is it reliable? *Intensive Care Med* 30(4):718–723, 2004.

CHAPTER 30 ■ MONITORING GASTROINTESTINAL TRACT FUNCTION

RUBEN J. AZOCAR, LAURA SANTOS PAVIA AND SURESH AGARWAL

Gastrointestinal system function is of paramount importance for the maintenance of the body's homeostasis, which is not only limited to the important functions of digestion and absorption but also closely related to immune function. Monitoring the gastrointestinal tract function remains largely based on clinical exam and a few diagnostic tests. The majority of the tests that are available have been primarily used for research purposes and are not available at the bedside of the critically ill patient (Table 30.1).

This chapter examines the diagnostic modalities available, on an organ system basis, for assessing abnormalities in the critically ill patient.

ESOPHAGUS

Tests of Esophageal Motility and Lower Esophageal Sphincter Function

Impaired tubular esophageal motility is involved in the pathogenesis of gastroesophageal reflux disease (GERD) which might cause nosocomial pneumonias in the critically ill.

Esophageal manometry has been used extensively to study GERD in critically ill patients. One study, of 15 critically ill patients, demonstrated that low esophageal sphincter (LES) pressure (mean 2.2 ± 0.4 mm Hg) and poor motor response to reflux correlated with the presence of GERD. Furthermore, low LES pressures were associated with frequent reflux episodes (60% of untreated patients) and decreased esophageal motility [1].

In a more recent 24-hour manometric study, the authors demonstrated that propulsive esophageal motility is impaired in critically ill patients receiving sedation and postulated that 24-hour motility studies appear to be a valuable and feasible method to analyze and quantify esophageal motor disorders in critically ill patients [2].

Twenty-four–hour pH and impedance monitoring further elucidates the function of the LES and the amount of gastric reflux a patient is experiencing. Over a 24-hour period, the pH should not drop below 4 frequently or for a prolonged duration (6% of total time in the supine patient, 10% of total time in the upright patient).

Both barium swallow and real-time fluoroscopy yield functional and anatomic data about the esophagus and the swallowing mechanisms. Similarly, an isotope swallow, using a technetium-99 colloid and a gamma camera, may provide data regarding esophageal physiology.

STOMACH

Tests of Gastric and Duodenal Motility

Delayed gastric emptying (GE) is common during critical illness. Patients receiving enteral nutrition are frequently assessed to evaluate feeding tolerance and prevent nosocomial pneumonias.

Traditionally this is done by quantification of gastric residual volumes (GRV), which despite being easy to perform, are a poor predictor of the patient's ability to tolerate enteral nutrition. In addition, a recent article suggests that the use of residual volumes as a marker of risk for aspiration in critically ill patients has poor validity [3].

Reflectometry (RFT) of gastric contents seems to provide complementary information on the adequacy of gastric emptying [4] by differentiating gastric contents from feeding formula when measuring GRVs. This model implies the measurement of the Brix value (BV) of the gastric aspirate at several time points. The BV is the refractive index of a substance, which is the degree of deviation or refraction of a beam of light when passing obliquely through a solution [5]. Chang et al. [6] studied 36 patients receiving continuous enteral nutrition. Based on the data collected, the authors created and algorithm using BVs and GRV, which suggest values at which enteral feedings can be safety continued. RFT uses an inexpensive handheld instrument (refractometer) similar to a small telescope. A drop of the solution is placed in the viewing window and the BV is read thought the eyepiece. The use of RFT is simple, inexpensive, and quick, but it has not been compared with what is consider the gold standard, gamma scintigraphy.

Gamma scintigraphy is a quantitative method to measuring gastric motility by administering radiolabeled solid food (usually greater than 200 kcal) and measuring transit after 2 to 4 hours. The administration of liquids may not be relevant as liquids may empty from the stomach even as solid food remains behind. The feasibility of scintigraphy testing for the critically ill patient makes is difficult as it is often impractical to transport these individuals to the nuclear radiology suite for this study.

Breath tests are a novel and useful bedside technique to assess gastric emptying of both solids and liquids by using ^{13}C- or ^{14}C-labeled octanoic acid. The absorption of the labeled octanoic acid in the small intestine and subsequent metabolism in the liver produce $^{13}CO_2$, which can be measured in the exhaled air. The delivery of the 13-octanoic acid into the duodenum is the rate-limiting step for these processes. As such, measurement of $^{13}CO_2$ levels correlates with the rate of gastric emptying. Ritz et al. [7] founded that gastric emptying of a caloric-dense liquid meal is slow in 40 to 45 of unselected mechanically ventilated patients by using the 13-octanoic acid breath test. They concluded that this test is a useful bedside adjunct to measure gastric emptying in ventilated, critically ill patients.

Gastroduodenal manometry has also been used to study the effects of critical illness in gastric motor activity. Nguyen demonstrated that in critical illness in addition to impaired proximal and distal gastric motor activity, the association between the two regions was also abnormal which interferes with meal distribution and affects GE [8]. Similar data was observed by Chapman et al. who noted that in critical illness there is slower GE probably associated by fewer anterograde waves

TABLE 30.1

TESTS FOR MONITORING GASTROINTESTINAL FUNCTION

Organ	Function	Test
Esophagus	Motility/LES function	Barium swallow Isotope swallow Esophageal manometry Esophageal pH and impedance
Stomach	Motility	Gastric residuals Refractometry Gastroduodenal manometry Breath tests Acetaminophen absorption test
	Mucosal permeability and ischemia	Gastric tonometry Laser Doppler flowmetry Near-infrared spectrometry Positron emission tomography Microdialysis Orthogonal polarization spectrometry Sidestream Dark Field
Small intestine	Absorption	Stool analysis: fecal pH, fecal osmotic gap, steatorrhea Carbohydrates absorption tests (D-xylose, L-rhamnose) Acetaminophen absorption test Breath tests
Pancreas	Exocrine functions	Fecal fat concentration Amylase/lipase Secretin tests
Liver	Liver function test	**Static tests** Transaminases Bilirubin Albumin Lactate Coagulation tests **Dynamic test** MEGX ICG Breath tests
	Hepatic blood flow tests	ICG MEGX
	Cholestasis	Transaminases Bilirubin Alkaline phosphatase Gamma glutamyl transpeptidase Ultrasound HIDA

HIDA, hepatic iminodiacetic acid; ICG, indocyanine green; LES, low esophageal sphincter; MEGX, monoethylglycinexylidide.

and more retrograde waves as recorded when measuring the antroduodenal motility [9].

The acetaminophen absorption test may also be used to assess gastric emptying, by administering 1,000 mg of acetaminophen and measuring serum concentrations of acetaminophen over a 1-hour period to construct an area under the curve (AUC) absorption model. This AUC is then compared to a known AUC model constructed from healthy volunteers. The utility of this test may be quite variable in the critically ill patient given differences in volume of distribution, hepatic metabolism, and renal clearance [5].

Other novel methods to assess GE include the use of ultrasound and gastric impedance monitoring (GIM). Ultrasound has used different equipment and different methods to assess GE, which has not allowed standardization or validation despite its obvious benefits of availability, lack of radiation and good interobserver agreement. GIM, which measures increases in impedance as the stomach fills, and declines as it empties, seems to be a promising tool. However, the time needed to complete and the requirement of a fasting state for baseline may interfere with its use in the clinical setting.

Tests of Mucosal Permeability and Ischemia

Microcirculatory dysfunction plays an important role in the pathogenesis of the systemic inflammatory response, sepsis, and shock. Global hemodynamic measurements do not assess oxygen delivery at the microcirculatory level. Gut ischemia at this level causes changes in permeability leading to bacterial translocation that may initiate, perpetuate, and aggravate sepsis and multisystem organ failure (MOF). Many methods have been used to study the gut microcirculation. Unfortunately, most of them have failed to be applicable in the clinical setting or have flaws in the data collected.

Tonometry

Although the diagnosis of bowel ischemia may be done by a variety of different methods, gastric tonometry is the simplest, most practical, and least invasive [10]. It attempts to determine the perfusion status of the gastric mucosa by measuring the local PCO_2 [11]. As perfusion to the stomach decreases, the PCO_2 in the tonometer will increase. Once cellular anaerobic respiration starts, the hydrogen ions titrate with bicarbonate, with the end result of more CO_2 production by mass action. By estimating the PCO_2 gap (the difference between gastric mucosa and arterial CO_2) the gastric perfusion can be assessed [12]. Unfortunately, the use of the technique has not gained widespread popularity despite many clinical studies that have validated gastric tonometry as a valuable and easily accessible prognostic tool [13,14]. This may be explained by the possibility of error in the determination of the PCO_2 and interoperator variability [15,16]. Other pitfalls include multiple local effects, including increased gastric secretions and refluxed duodenal contents; both of which can increase CO_2 measurement and lead to false PCO_2 measurement, and that this technique may only represent one region of perfusion [11].

Recently, the measurement of carbon dioxide in the sublingual mucosa by sublingual capnometry has been advocated as a monitor for tissue oxygenation and as an end-point for resuscitation [17]. Studies have demonstrated a good correlation between gastric mucosal and sublingual mucosa PCO_2. In addition, sublingual mucosa PCO_2 seems to respond faster to therapeutic interventions [18].

Laser Doppler Flowmetry

Laser Doppler flowmetry (LDP), which estimates gastric and jejunal blood perfusion by integrating red blood cell content and velocity, correlates well with absolute blood flow. The flowmeter consists of a laser source, a fiberoptic probe, and a photodetector with a signal-processing unit. The laser conducts through the tissue by a flexible fiberoptic guide. The probe contains an optic fiber for transmission of laser light to the tissue and two fibers for collecting the reflected scattered light. The signal-processing unit consists of a photodetector and an analog circuit to analyze the frequency spectrum of the scattered light. By determining the instantaneous mean Doppler frequency and the fraction of backscattered light that is Doppler shifted, the signal-processing unit provides a continuous output proportional to the number of red blood cells moving in the measuring volume and the mean velocity of these cells. Measurements are considered satisfactory if (a) the measurement is stable for 15 seconds; (b) the measurement is free of motion artifacts; (c) pulse waves can be clearly identified; and (d) the reading is reproducible. Although LDP is relatively easy to use and it is noninvasive, it does not account for blood flow heterogeneity, a major parameter of microcirculation [19].

Near-Infrared Spectometry

Near-infrared spectrometry (NIRS) has been used to measure local tissue blood flow and oxygenation at the cellular level [20]. Local oxygen delivery and oxygen saturation can be determined by comparing the differences in the absorption spectrum of oxyhemoglobin with its deoxygenated counterpart, deoxyhemoglobin [21]. Puyana et al. [22] reported using NIRS to measure tissue pH in a model of experimental shock and showed that NIRS gut pH correlated with the pH obtained by microelectrodes. This technology has progressed to the measurement of muscle tissue oxygenation and microcirculation by measuring thenar muscle oxygenation saturation with promising results [23].

POSITRON EMISSION TOMOGRAPHY

Positron emission tomography may also be used to evaluate regional blood flow. Fluoromisonidazole accumulation has been used to demonstrate abdominal splanchnic perfusion and regional oxygenation of the liver in pigs; however, the lack of portability of this technique makes it difficult to use for monitoring in the intensive care unit (ICU) [14].

MICRODIALYSIS

Microdialysis measurement of mucosal lactate is a novel way to assess gut mucosal ischemia. Tenhunen et al. [24] inserted microdialysis catheters into the lumen of the jejunum, the jejunal wall, and the mesenteric artery and vein of pigs. Subsequently, the animals were subjected to nonischemic hyperlactataemia or an episode of mesenteric ischemia and reperfusion. The lactate levels from the jejunal wall and the jejunal lumen were compared. The gut wall lactate was increased in both the nonischemic and the ischemic lactataemia whereas the lactate measured from the jejunal lumen only was altered significantly during true ischemia.

Microdialysates of other substances have also been measured, including glucose and glycerol, showing that, while lactate levels increase with ischemia, intestinal wall glucose levels drop with the same stressor. Glycerol was increased, but the changes were seen later than the changes in lactate [25]. Similarly, increases in the lactate/pyruvate ratio in both intraperitoneal or intraluminal placed microdialysis catheters have correlated with hypoperfusion [26]. As glucose from the splanchnic circulation is inhibited, pyruvate accumulates in the tissue and, in the setting of inadequate oxygen delivery, is broken down to lactate. Using glycerol as a marker, Sollingard et al. [27] suggested that gut luminal microdialysis could serve as a valuable tool for surveillance not only during ischemia, but also after the ischemic insult. This group has also suggested that gut luminal lactate measured by this technique correlates well with changes in the permeability of the intestinal mucosa after ischemia [28].

The assessment of the barrier function using colon submucosal microdialysis with a radioactive tracer substance has also been reported. No data comparing these results with local tissue chemistry have been reported [29].

These data support the idea that microdialysis could be a potentially useful method to monitor gut ischemia. However, even under investigational conditions, technical difficulties were reported in up to 15% of cases by either damage to the microdialysate membrane, dislocation of the probe, or incorrect placement [30].

ORTHOGONAL POLARIZATION SPECTROMETRY AND SIDESTREAM DARK FIELD

Recently devices able to allow the microcirculation to be visualized directly have been used clinically [31]. Orthogonal polarization spectrometry (OPS) and the sidestream dark field provide high-contrast images of the microvasculature. Both devices are based on the principle that green light penetrates a tissue and that then green light is absorbed by red blood cells (RBCs) hemoglobin contained in superficial vessels. Therefore, capillaries and venules can be visualized if they contain RBCs. The easiest assessment method is the microvascular flow index. The image is divided into four quadrants and the flow is characterized and scored as absent (0), intermittent (1), sluggish (2), or normal (3). The values of the quadrants are then averaged. Clinical studies suggest that this is a good method to assess microcirculation in critically ill patients. Those patients with more severe alterations have a higher mortality and that if these alterations persist they may lead to MOF [32–34]. In most studies, the sublingual circulation has been the site chosen. An attempt to use this method for gut ischemia by assessment of the villi microvasculature per se was not successful. Likely causes include blood flow redistribution, heterogenicity of the intestine microcirculation, and suboptimal OPS imaging, which resulted in large interobserver differences in the quantification of vessel density [35].

SMALL INTESTINE

Tests of Intestinal Absorption

Clinically, the recognition of malabsorption in the ICU is associated with a variety of signs and symptoms. On physical exam, abdominal distention, abdominal pain, and increased flatulence may be present. Isolated carbohydrate malabsorption may result in increased gas production, which can lead to flatulence, bloating, and abdominal distention. Likewise, diarrhea may indicate a problem with absorption of nutrients, but again it is nonspecific and other potential causes should be examined. Steatorrhea may indicate pancreatic insufficiency. It is also important to elicit the past medical history since it can provide useful information in regards to primary (i.e., lactose intolerance) or secondary (i.e., chronic pancreatitis) malabsorptive problems.

Malabsorption can be detected by a variety of tests. Stool analysis may provide information regarding carbohydrate and fat malabsorption. Bacterial fermentation of malabsorbed carbohydrates may result in an acidic fecal pH. Eherer and Fordtran [36] found that when diarrhea was caused by carbohydrate malabsorption (lactulose or sorbitol), the fecal fluid pH was always less than 5.6 and usually less than 5.3. Other causes of diarrhea rarely caused fecal pH to be as low as 5.6 and never caused a pH less than 5.3.

Another measurement is of fecal osmolarity. Assuming the fecal osmolality is similar to that of the serum, the fecal osmotic gap can be calculated. A sample is taken from the stool supernatant and if the value is greater than 50 to 100 mOsm, it would suggest the presence of an unmeasured solute. Although this solute may be a malabsorbed carbohydrate, other compounds, such as sorbitol, or ions, such as sulfates, may yield similar results.

Steatorrhea is defined as the presence of at least 7 g of fat in a 24-hour stool collection [37]. Sudan II stain is a simple screen testing and it is helpful to detect those patients with mild degrees of steatorrhea (7 to 20 g per 24 hours). The gold standard is represented by quantitative fecal fat analysis [38]. Stool is collected over 2 to 3 days while the patient ingests 75 to 100 g of fat within 24 hours. Normal values are less than 7 g per day. However, this test is laborious and may not help with differentiating diagnoses.

D-Xylose Uptake

The D-xylose test has been used in the diagnosis of malabsorption. This pentose sugar of vegetable origin is incompletely absorbed in the small intestine by a passive mechanism. The test consists in the ingestion of a 25 g dose of D-xylose and the subsequent measurement of the levels in the serum or urine. In normal individuals, a serum sample taken 1 to 2 hours after ingestion will reveal a level of 25 mg per dL and a 5-hour urine collection will result in at least 4 g of this substance. Many entities such celiac disease, alterations in gastrointestinal motility, and impaired function of the pylorus will result in abnormal results. In the critically ill, renal function may be altered and may alter the results of the urine test. Chiolero et al. [39] studied the intestinal absorption of D-xylose in critically ill patients that were tolerating enteral feeding. They introduced D-xylose to the stomach or the jejunum and found that although the levels in plasma in all patients in the study increased indicating proper gastric emptying, in those receiving the compound in the stomach, the levels of D-xylose were lower than normal, indicating delays or depression in absorption. These results were similar to a prior study in trauma and septic patients. In that study, in both groups the D-xylose test showed abnormal results at the onset of the illness with resolution by 1 to 3 weeks after trauma or resolution of sepsis. Interestingly, enteral feedings were tolerated by these patients before the test results returned to normal [40]. As the patients in both studies were tolerating tube feeds even with abnormal D-xylose test results, Chiolero et al. [39] suggested that this test may not be a good indicator to determine the capacity of patients to tolerate enteral feeds. This does confirm that absorption of D-xylose stays depressed for a prolonged period of time in the critically ill.

Johnson et al. [41] also found decreased absorption in the septic population when compared with healthy individuals. They used an oral test solution that contained 5 g of lactulose, 1 g of L-rhamnose, 0.5 g of D-xylose, and 0.2 g of 3-*O*-methyl-D-glucose. L-rhamnose is absorbed by passive diffusion and therefore particularly sensitive to changes of the absorptive capacity of the gut when compared with D-xylose and 3-*O*-methyl-D-glucose, which depend on specific carrier mechanisms. The authors found that septic patients had decreased L-rhamnose/3-*O*-methyl-D-glucose ratios when compared with normal individuals, a result consistent with decrease absorptive capacity during sepsis. They also used the lactulose/L-rhamnose ratio to assess permeability of the gut. This group concluded that the changes in the absorptive capacities of the gut may contribute to the pathophysiology of sepsis.

Other Tests

The rapid absorption of acetaminophen at the jejunal level can also aid the assessment of the absorptive capacity of the gut. It has, however, been used more to assess gastric emptying [5] and tube feeding location for enteral feeding [42]. From these data, it appears that either carbohydrate absorption tests or the acetaminophen test could be used to a monitor absorption in the critically ill. No correlation has been established between tolerating tube feeds and the degree of absorption. The role of this test may be to monitor improvement of absorptive function of the gastrointestinal tract after critical illness.

Breath tests are a simple and safe alternative to diagnose many gastrointestinal conditions including malabsorption. Most of the data are from the gastroenterology literature and are used to diagnose specific gastrointestinal pathologies. However, it seems feasible to apply this test to the critically ill population. These tests are based on the appearance of a metabolite of a specific test substance in the breath [43]. Both hydrogen gas excretion and carbon dioxide appearance on breath tests are available.

If carbohydrates are not absorbed in the small intestine, they are fermented in the colon by colonic bacteria. This process results in the production of hydrogen. For example, in cases of lactose intolerance, this disaccharide will reach the colon and a peak on the end-expiratory hydrogen of more of

20 ppm over baseline by either gas chromatography or portable hydrogen analyzers at 2 to 3 hours indicates malabsorption for this carbohydrate [44]. A similar test using a nonabsorbable carbohydrate, such as lactulose, has been used for the diagnosis of bacterial overgrowth in which the peak of hydrogen occurs earlier but is less pronounced. The use of carbon dioxide that results from the fermentation of labeled substances has also been reported. The use of both radioactive ^{14}C and stable ^{13}C compounds has been described. However, since the nonradioactive substances can be detected by mass spectrometry and do not involve radiation exposure, they seem to be preferred over the radioactive ones [45].

In critically ill patients ^{13}C-acetate has been studied to evaluate intestinal absorption [12]. Acetate possesses interesting properties that allow its use for absorption purposes since it is readily absorbed by the intestinal mucosa and it is metabolized through oxidative metabolism by nearly all body tissues. Acetate is converted into acetyl–CoA and then oxidized to CO_2. When marked acetate is provided, the $^{13}CO_2$ is then measured in the breath by mass spectometry. ^{13}C-acetate was provided by intravenous infusion and enterally at both gastric and jejunal levels. Surprisingly, the kinetics of all three routes was similar (the gastric group was delayed but probably secondary to the time for gastric emptying), indicating a rapid absorption and metabolism. The authors concluded that further studies are needed in this area before this particular breath test can be used to assess tolerance of enteral feeding [15]. C-octanoic acid has been used to assess gastric emptying in the critically ill and was discussed in the motility section [3]. Other breath tests have been use to assess absorption anomalies [44]. In the case of bile acid malabsorption and bacterial overgrowth, cholylglycine (glycocholic acid) is not absorbed at the ileum and the glycine is cleaved from the labeled cholylglycine by colonic bacteria. Glycine is then absorbed and metabolized into CO_2. The CO_2 can be detected in the breath and 4.5% of the radioactivity is seen in the breath over the subsequent 6 hours. To differentiate between bacterial overgrowth and bile acid malabsorption a stool collection is needed to detect bile acid losses.

In pancreatic insufficiency mixed triglycerides that are hydrolyzed to glycerol and fatty acid are then absorbed and finally metabolized in the liver where they release labeled CO_2. This test indirectly measures intraluminal fat digestion by pancreatic enzymes. Other substances such as triolein, hiolein, tripalmitin, and labeled starch have been use for this purpose but are not sensitive enough for patients with mild disease [44].

PANCREAS

Although the pancreas performs both endocrine and exocrine functions, only the functions affecting the digestive tract are discussed here. Although diabetes mellitus may decrease gastric motility, the diagnosis and management of endocrine disorders will be dealt with elsewhere (see Section VIII).

Fecal Fat Concentration

As discussed in the digestion and absorption section, in the presence of pancreatic steatorrhea, fecal fat concentration is elevated [37,38]. Diarrhea resolves and fecal fat concentration abates once the individual is challenged with enzyme replacement therapy.

Amylase/Lipase

These simple blood tests are elevated in the presence of acute pancreatic inflammation. Although not indicative of the severity of injury, they do indicate that injury is present. Pancreatitis will be covered in other portions of this text (see Chapter 99).

Secretin Test

The secretin test is a direct measurement of pancreatic exocrine function that measures the intraduodenal secretion of bicarbonate, amylase, and trypsin after exogenous administration of secretin. Generally, bicarbonate and amylase secretion will increase in adults, whereas the increase of bicarbonate, amylase, and trypsin will increase in children. In the presence of chronic pancreatitis, concentrations and quantity will be diminished; in contrast to pancreatic cancer, which presents with diminished volume but normal concentration. The maintenance of normal concentrations in pancreatic cancer is attributed to normal pancreatic function in the nonmalignant portions of the pancreas.

LIVER

Liver function includes vital functions of metabolism, synthesis, detoxification, and excretion. It is then, not surprising that patients with deteriorating liver function will have a more complex course during critical illness. Traditionally, tests related to measuring the products of liver synthesis have been use to assess liver function and damage in a static fashion, but as it will be discussed, tests that evaluate the liver function in a more dynamic fashion are also available.

Tests of Liver Injury and Static Function

In the critically ill, different levels of dysfunction can be manifest ranging from mild elevation of the transaminases to profound hepatic failure. It is difficult to separate completely those tests that assess liver injury from those that are related to its function as some will suggest the insult to the organ as well as the alteration on its function, particularly in the acute setting. The tests described in this section are considered "static" and will reflect an injury that has occurred and changes on the liver's function, but they do not assess current functionality, particularly in the patient with chronic liver failure. However, in a critically ill patient with no prior liver problems these tests are helpful in detecting an ongoing morbid process in the liver.

Transaminases

Serum glutamic-oxaloacetic transaminase (SGOT), or aspartate aminotransferase (AST), and serum glutamate-pyruvate transaminase (SGPT), or alanine aminotransferase (ALT), are enzymes that are present in all organism cells; however, they are found in highest concentration in the hepatocyte: SGPT in the cytoplasm and SGOT in the cytoplasm as well as the mitochondria. Therefore, as injury and necrosis of the hepatocyte occurs the enzymes levels in the plasma will increase reflecting the damage to this organ. The rate and the level of the elevation are usually related to the onset of the dysfunction and its severity. Severe ischemic hepatitis is characterized by an acute elevation of the aminotransferases to at least 20 times the upper limit of normal [45].

Bilirubin

One of the main functions of the liver is to conjugate and excrete bilirubin, a product of erythrocyte breakdown. Therefore, either elevations of the bilirubin clinically (jaundice, icterus, dark urine) or by laboratory testing should raise the clinical suspicion of liver dysfunction or injury. It is possible to determine if the bilirubin has already been conjugated, and this helps in searching for the causes of the hyperbilirubinemia. Unconjugated (or indirect) hyperbilirubinemia is the result of excess production of bilirubin (e.g., hemolysis) or decreased hepatic uptake. Conjugated hyperbilirubinemia results when intrinsic parenchymal injury or biliary obstruction exists. Acute changes of the conjugated bilirubin levels are related to acute hepatocyte injury in situations such as viral hepatitis or ischemic hepatitis and will be related to the increase in the transaminases. This should alert the clinician of injury and dysfunction of the liver. Tests to study cholestasis are described in a separate section of this chapter. However, it should be remembered that biliary obstruction may also lead to hepatic dysfunction.

Lactate

The ability of the liver to clear lactate is profound. Greater than 99% of lactate is cleared by first pass metabolism by a healthy liver. Inability to clear lactate may be an indicator of poor organ perfusion and anaerobic metabolism, and this metabolite can be used as a resuscitation parameter. If other indicators of resuscitation are optimized and the arterial lactate levels remain elevated, this may indicate severe liver dysfunction and injury, particularly in patients in shock.

Albumin

Liver function may also be evaluated by measuring its ability to synthesize a variety of proteins. Albumin is the most common protein measured when evaluating liver synthetic ability. Although hepatocellular dysfunction may be the cause of hypoalbuminemia, the protein concentration also varies in a variety of diseases/acute injury phases (e.g., burns, nephrotic syndrome, etc.) and can be nonspecific. It is a better marker to assess the degree of chronic hepatic failure than acute dysfunction and it does not reflect injury.

Coagulation Studies

More sensitive and specific measurements of hepatic function include evaluation of the coagulation cascade and the production of specific coagulation factors. If the prothrombin time (PT) is elevated, one of two conditions exists: vitamin K deficiency or deficiency in vitamin K dependent factors (II, VII, IX, and X). If vitamin K has been replaced and the PT remains elevated, this is very specific for liver dysfunction. This is not a sensitive test, as the PT remains normal as long as 20% of the liver remains intact. Far more sensitive, although more time consuming and costly, is the measurement of factor V levels. Factor V, produced in the liver, is not vitamin K dependent, and its deficiency is both sensitive and specific for hepatocellular synthetic dysfunction.

Dynamic or Qualitative Tests of Liver Function

Although the tests discussed in the earlier section are very important in detecting and helping the clinician assess liver dysfunction, they are not perfect as some are nonspecific (lactate, coagulation disorders, albumin levels) or reflect past damage (transaminases) in assessing the current state of liver functionality. Figg et al. [46] compared the Pugh's classification, which is based in clinical and laboratory data, with dynamic or qualitative methods of hepatic function and found that the Pugh's classification seemed to be a reliable indicator of the degree of chronic liver disease but could not replace qualitative metabolic markers particularly isozyme-specific markers. Although the quantitative tests may be more complicated to perform and more expensive than conventional tests, they may prove superior in monitoring the degree of liver dysfunction by monitoring the liver's metabolic or clearance functions [47]. Different tests have been used in an attempt to have a dynamic or "real-time" assessment of the liver's metabolic or clearance functions and complement the information provided by the static tests.

Monoethylglycinexylidide

The hepatic metabolism of lidocaine by sequential oxidative *N*-dealkylation by the cytochrome P450 system into its major metabolite; monoethylglycinexylidide (MEGX) is a dynamic liver function test [48]. Because of the high extraction ratio of lidocaine by the liver, this test not only evaluates liver metabolic capacity but also hepatic blood flow [49]. Detection of this metabolite can be accomplished by different techniques such as immunoassay based on the fluorescence polarization immunoassay technique, high performance liquid chromatography, and gas liquid chromatography [49]. Fluorescence polarization immunoassay technique may cross react with another metabolite (3-OH-MEGX). The other two tests are specific for MEGX.

This test has been useful in patients with end-stage liver disease in which a MEGX level at 15 or 30 minutes of less than 10 mg per L indicates poor 1-year survival. In liver transplant recipients, a change in the levels may indicate a deterioration of the graft function. In critically ill patients, a rapid decrease in MEGX test values have been associated not only with liver dysfunction but with the development of multisystem organ failure and an enhanced systemic inflammatory response [49]. McKindley et al. [50] reported on the pharmacokinetics of lidocaine and MEGX in a rat model of endotoxic shock. They found that the metabolism of both compounds was altered and attributed the results to both the reduced hepatic blood flow and altered function of the cytochrome P450 system, particularly cytochrome P450–3A4. Chandel et al. [51] also report the use of this test in an animal model of hypovolemic shock. They found that the MEGX levels were significantly lower in shocked animals. Once the animals were resuscitated with Ringer's lactate, the MEGX levels were higher but still lower than the control group. They concluded that shock produced significant depression of hepatocyte function and that MEGX seemed a suitable tool for clinical evaluation and therapeutic intervention after shock.

Dyes

Another dynamic test of liver function is related to the rate of elimination of dyes such as indocyanine green (ICG) and/or bromsulphthalein [52]. Most of the data in the critically ill come from the use of ICG. This dye is a water-soluble inert compound that is injected intravenously. In the plasma, it binds to albumin and is then selectively taken up by hepatocytes. The ICG is then excreted into the bile via an adenosine triphosphate (ATP)-dependent transport process. This compound is not metabolized and does not undergo enterohepatic recirculation. The excretion rate of ICG into the bile reflects the hepatic excretory function and the hepatic energy status and justifies its use as a tool for assessment of liver function [53]. In a study comparing cirrhotic and noncirrhotic patients, Hashimoto and Watanabe [54] found that ICG clearance was proportional to liver parenchymal cell volume and is related to the hepatic dysfunction in cirrhotic patients. Traditionally, the ICG clearance has been measured by a series of blood samples and subsequent laboratory analysis. NIRS has also been used to measure hepatic ICG clearance with promising results in the assessment of hepatic parenchymal dysfunction [55].

Fortunately, bedside techniques have become available to measure the plasma disappearance rate (PDR) of ICG.

Von Spiegel et al. [56] compared the clearance method of a transpulmonary indicator dilution technique with an arterial fiberoptic thermistor catheter that assessed the ICG-circulating curve in patients undergoing liver transplantation. They found that both methods were effective in detecting onset and maintenance of graft function in these patients. Newer technology allows the use of assessment of ICG PDR transcutaneously. In two separate publications, Sakka et al. [57,58] suggested that this technology, when compared with invasive methods, reflected ICG blood clearance with sufficient accuracy in critically ill patients to be used as a surrogate. In contrast, in a model of hyperdynamic porcine endotoxemia the PDR of ICG failed to accurately substitute for direct short-term measurements of ICG excretion [59]. The authors suggested that normal values of PDR of ICG should be interpreted with caution in early, acute inflammatory conditions. As mentioned before, ICG clearance also aids with the evaluation of the hepatic energy status since the excretion into bile is energy dependent. Chijiiwa et al. [60] correlated the biliary excretion of ICG with the ATP levels in liver samples obtained from patients with biliary obstruction, and in a second study, they were able to correlate those variables with the biliary acid output [61]. They concluded that biliary bile acid output and ICG excretion are valuable parameters of hepatic energy status, which is essential for organ viability. ICG can be considered a valuable tool to assess liver function in patients after liver transplantation, at risk to develop, or with ongoing liver injury to assess damage and recovery and to assess the energy status of the liver.

Radiological Studies

Another method to assess functional liver reserve is with the use of technetium-99 diethylenetriamine penta-acetic acid galactosyl human serum albumin (99mTc-DTPA-GSA) clearance. Studies using hepatic scintigraphy and more recently single-proton emission computer tomography (SPECT) scan have been described [62,63]. Hwang et al. [63] demonstrated the use of this test as a reflection of hepatic function and also suggested that predicting residual hepatic values was a good indicator of postoperative hepatic function and early prognosis after liver resection. Kira et al. [62] showed that using this test before and after transjugular intrahepatic portosystemic shunt was useful to evaluate changes in hepatic functional reserve and evaluate the degree of portosystemic shunt. At this time, the test is mostly used as a predictor of liver function after liver resection and not used in the critically ill [64].

Breath Tests

The use of breath tests as qualitative measurement of liver function has also been described. The principle behind these tests is similar to the description of breaths tests used for monitoring of gut absorption described earlier. As the carbon marked compound is metabolized, the resulting marked carbon dioxide can be measured in the breath. As liver function declines, less of the marked CO_2 will be detected in the breath. In an animal model of hepatectomy, Ishii et al. [65] injected L-[1-(13)C] methionine and L-[1-(13)C] phenylalanine intravascularly and measured the exhaled $^{13}CO_2$ over 15 minutes. They concluded that this test could qualitatively evaluate liver dysfunction. In a human study, Kobayashi et al. [66] demonstrated that the use of the ^{13}C phenylalanine test correlated well with ICG clearance test, Child Pugh's classification, and standard liver blood tests, suggesting that this test is a useful noninvasive method to determine liver functional reserve. Koeda et al. [67] studied the validity of the ^{13}C phenylalanine breath test in both chronic cirrhosis and acute hepatitis patients and concluded that in both groups this test allows the noninvasive evaluation of hepatic function. Hepatic dysfunction associated with obstructive jaundice in a rat model was also evaluated using this test. As similar results were achieved, the authors concluded that this test could be used to measure hepatic dysfunction associated with obstructive jaundice [68]. Reports of the use of other marked compounds to assess liver function using the breath test principles, such as ^{13}C-methacetin [69], L-[1,2–13C] Ornithine [70], and L-[1–130 C] alanine [71] have been described with promising results.

Other dynamic tests that are available include the antipyrine clearance test [46,47], the caffeine clearance test [47], and the pharmacokinetics of acetaminophen. Zapater et al. [72] reported a higher AUC concentration and lower clearance and higher elimination half-life in cirrhotics when compared with healthy volunteers.

Blood Flow Tests

Tests to determine hepatic blood flow are also useful. Xylocaine metabolism also evaluates hepatic blood flow [35]. The use of ICG has also been described for this purpose. The use of intravenous infusions of ICG seemed more reliable and accurate in evaluation of hepatic blood flow than with the use of boluses or intravenous injections of galactose [59]. Apparently with the use of boluses, extrahepatic accumulation of the dye occurs and alters the results [60]. More recently, pulse dye-densitometry (PDD) has been used in the critically ill patient instead of blood tests. Mizushima et al. [61] measured effective hepatic blood volume (EHBV) and cardiac output (CO) using ICG-PDD [61]. They found that in septic patients, the EHBF/CO ratio was lower than that of nonseptic patients, suggesting that inadequate splanchnic perfusion or metabolic changes occur in septic patients. In addition, the lower EHBF/CO ratio was related to a fatal outcome in septic patients. The authors concluded that PDD could be a clinically useful method of assessing splanchnic conditions in critically ill patients. Dysfunction in one of the components of the gastrointestinal system, in this case the liver, manifested by decreased metabolic [35–37] capacities or hepatic blood flow [36,61] are related to shock states and are probably an integral part of the multiorgan system failure (MOSF) cascade, highlighting the relationship of the gastrointestinal system with immunity.

Tests of Cholestasis

In patients with conjugated hyperbilirubinemia but without other indicators of liver dysfunction or injury, biliary obstruction should be suspected. Alkaline phosphatase (AP), like SGOT and SGPT, is found in a variety of different organs, but has its highest concentration in the liver. As such, it is most often elevated in situations where cholestasis is present. AP is more specific than gamma glutamyl transpeptidase (GTT) for biliary tree inflammation, as GGT is sensitive to even mild liver inflammation and/or activation of the cytochrome P-450 enzymes.

Further workup may include radiological evaluation. Hepatic iminodiacetic acid (HIDA) scan may also prove valuable in differentiating the cause of cholestasis. The test reveals many facets of hepatic function with respect to its ability to conjugate bile: If the liver does not actively uptake tracer, than its ability to conjugate bile must be questioned. In addition, when conjugation is not an issue, definitive anatomic localization of biliary obstruction is possible. In addition, in the presence of a functional sphincter of Oddi, it is possible to diagnose acute cholecystitis. Further assessment of biliary architecture can be made with ultrasonography. Not only can one determine the architecture of the liver and gallbladder, but one can also determine the amount of intra- and extrahepatic biliary dilatation, further delineating the source of biliary obstruction.

CONCLUSIONS

Gastrointestinal function is of vital importance in the critically ill patient. These functions are not limited to the mere absorption of nutrients but are closely related with the immune system, particularly in the critically ill patient. Despite its importance, monitoring of intestinal function is limited, providing anatomic and physiologic information rather than an assessment of pathophysiologic change. Assessment of absorption by sugar absorption tests and breath tests, of motility by manometry, and of ischemia by tonometry and microdialysis are promising modalities that may help monitor the functions of the gastrointestinal tract.

References

1. Heyland DK, Cook DJ, Guyatt GH: Enteral nutrition in the critically ill patient: a critical review of the evidence. *Intensive Care Med* 19:435–442, 1993.
2. Kölbel CB, Rippel K, Klar H, et al: Esophageal motility disorders in critically ill patients: a 24-hour manometric study. *Intensive Care Med* 26(10):1421–1427, 2000.
3. McClave SA, Lukan JK, Stafer JA, et al: Poor validity of residual volumes as a marker for risk of aspiration in critically ill patients. *Crit Care Med* 33:449–450, 2005.
4. Chang WK, McClave SA, Lee MS: Monitoring bolus nasogastric tube feeding by the Brix value determination and residual volume measurement of gastric contents. *J Parenter Enteral Nutr* 28:105–112, 2004.
5. Moreira TV, McQuiggan M: Methods for the assessment of gastric emptying in critically ill, enterally fed adults. *Nut Clin Pract* 24:261–273, 2009.
6. Chang WK, McCLave SA, Caho YC: Continuous nasogastric tube feeding: monitoring by combined use of refractometry and traditional gastric residual volumes. *Clin Nutr* 23:105–112, 2004.
7. Ritz MA, Frazer R, Edwards N, et al: Delayed gastric emptying in ventilated critically ill patients: measurement by 13C-octanoic acid breath test. *Crit Care Med* 29:1744–1749, 2001.
8. Nguyen NQ, Fraser RJ, Bryant LK, et al: Diminished functional association between proximal and distal gastric motility in critically ill patients. *Intensive Care Med* 34:1246–1255, 2008.
9. Chapman MJ, Fraser RJ, Bryant LK, et al: Gastric emptying and the organization of antro-duodenal pressures in the critically ill. *Neurogastroenterol Motil* 20:27–35, 2008.
10. Pastores SM, Katz DP, Kvetan V: Splanchnic ischemia and gut mucosal injury in sepsis and multisystem organ dysfunction syndrome. *Am J Gastroenterol* 91:1697–1710, 1996.
11. Heard SO: Gastric tonometry: the hemodynamic monitor of choice (Pro). *Chest* 123(469S):469–474, 2003.
12. Schlichtig R, Mehta N, Gayowski TJ: Tissue arterial PCO_2 difference is a better marker of ischemia than intramural pH (Phi) or arterial pH-Phi difference. *J Crit Care* 11:51–56, 1996.
13. Kirton OC, Windsor J, Wedderburn R, et al: Failure of splanchnic resuscitation in the acutely injured trauma patient correlates with multiple organ system failure and length of stay in the ICU. *Chest* 113:1064–1069, 1998.
14. Maynard N, Bihari D, Bealae R, et al: Assessment of splanchnic oxygenation by gastric tonometry in patients with acute circulatory failure. *JAMA* 270:1203–1210, 1993.
15. Takala J, Parviainen I, Siloaho M, et al: Saline PCO_2 is an important source of error in the assessment of gastric intramucosal pH. *Crit Care Med* 22:1877–1879, 1994.
16. Knichwitz G, Kuhmann M, Brodner G, et al: Gastric tonometry: precision and reliability are improved by a phosphate buffered solution. *Crit Care Med* 24:512–516, 1996.
17. Marik PE: Sublingual capnometry: a non-invasive measure of microcirculation dysfunction and tissue hypoxia. *Physiol Meas* 27:R37–R47, 2006.
18. Marik PE: Regional carbon dioxide monitoring to assess the adequacy of tissue perfusion. *Curr Opin Crit Care* 11:245–251, 2005.
19. De Backer D, Dubois MJ: Assessment of the microcirculatory flow in patients in the intensive care unit. *Curr Opin Crit Care* 7:200–203, 2001.
20. Yuh-Chin TW: Monitoring oxygen delivery in the critically ill. *Chest* 128(S554):554–560, 2005.
21. Cohn SM, Crookes BA, Proctor KG: Near-infrared spectrometry in resuscitation. *J Trauma* 54:S199–S202, 2003.
22. Puyana JC, Soller BR, Zhang S, et al: Continuous measurement of gut pH with near-infrared spectroscopy during hemorrhagic shock. *J Trauma* 46:9–15, 1999.
23. Nanas S, Gerovasili V, Renieris P, et al: Non-invasive assessment of the microcirculation in critically ill patients. *Anaesth Intensive Care* 37:733–739, 2009.
24. Tenhunen JJ, Kosunen H, Alhava E, et al: Intestinal luminal microdialysis: a new approach to assess gut mucosal ischemia. *Anesthesiology* 91:1807–1815, 1999.
25. Sommer T, Larsen JF: Detection of intestinal ischemia using a microdialysis technique in an animal model. *World J Surg* 27:416–420, 2003.
26. Sommer T, Larsen JF: Intraperitoneal and intraluminal microdialysis in the detection of experimental regional intestinal ischaemia. *BJS* 91:855–861, 2004.
27. Sollingard E, Ingebjorg SJ, Bakkelund K, et al: Gut luminal microdialysis of glycerol as a marker of intestinal ischemic injury and recovery. *Crit Care Med* 33:2278–2285, 2005.
28. Solligard E, Juel IS, Spigset O, et al: Gut luminal lactate measured by microdialysis mirrors permeability of the intestinal mucosa after ischemia. *Shock* 29:245–251, 2008.
29. Cibicek N, Zivna H, Zadak Z: Colon submucosal microdialysis: a novel in vivo approach in barrier function assessment—a pilot study in rats. *Physiol Res* 56(5):611–617, 2007.
30. Sommer T, Larsen JF: Validation of intramural intestinal microdialysis as a detector of intestinal ischemia. *Scand J Gastroenterol* 39:493–499, 2004.
31. De Backer D, Hollenberg S, Boerma C, et al: How to evaluate the microcirculation: report of a round table conference. *Crit Care* 11:R101, 2007. Available at http://ccform.com/content//11/5/R101
32. De Backer D, Creteur J, Preiser JC, et al: Microvascular blood flow is altered in patients with sepsis. *Am J Resp Crit Care Med* 166:98–104, 2002.
33. Trzeciak S, Dellinger RP, Parrillo JE, et al: Early microcirculatory perfusion derangements in patients with severe sepsis and septic shock: relationship to hemodynamics, oxygen transport, and survival. *Ann Emerg Med* 49:88–98, 2007.
34. Sakr Y, Dubois MJ, De Backer D, et al: Persistent microcirculatory alterations are associated with organ failure and death in patients with septic shock. *Crit Care Med* 32:1825–1833, 2004.
35. Brancht H, Krejci V, Hiltebrant: Orthogonal polarization spectroscopy to detect mesenteric hypoperfusion. *Intensive Care Med* 34:1883–1890, 2008.
36. Eherer AJ, Fordtran JS: Fecal osmotic gap and pH in experimental diarrhea of various causes. *Gastroenterology* 103:545–551, 1992.
37. Weinstein WM, Hawkey CJ, Bosch JM (eds): *Clinical Gastroenterology and Hepatology*. Philadelphia, PA, Elsevier, 2005.
38. Farrell JJ: Overview and diagnosis of malabsorption syndrome. *Semin Gastrointest Dis* 13:182–190, 2002.
39. Chiolero RL, Revelly JP, Berger MM: Labeled acetate to assess intestinal absorption in critically ill patients. *Crit Care Med* 31:853–857, 2003.
40. Singh G, Harkema JM Mayberry AJ: Severe depression of gut absorptive capacity in patients following trauma or sepsis. *J Trauma* 36:803–809, 1994.
41. Johnson JD, Harvey CJ, Menzies IS, et al: Gastrointestinal permeability and absorptive capacity in sepsis. *Crit Care Med* 24:1144–1149, 1996.
42. Berger MM, Werner D, Revelly JP: Serum paracetamol concentration: an alternative to x-rays to determine feeding tube location in the critically ill. *J Parenter Entreal Nutr* 27:151–155, 2003.
43. Swart GR, van den Berg JW: 13C breath test in gastroenterological practice. *Scand J Gastroenterol Suppl* 225:13–18, 1998.
44. Romagnuolo J, Schiller D, Bailey RJ: Using breath tests wisely in a gastroenterology practice: an evidence-based review if indications and pitfalls in interpretation. *Am J Gastroenterology* 97:1113–1116, 2002.
45. Seeto RK, Fenn B, Rockey DC: Ischemic hepatitis: clinical presentation and pathogenesis. *Am J Med* 109:109–113, 2000.
46. Figg WD, Dukes GE, Lesene HR, et al: Comparison of quantitative methods to assess hepatic function: Pugh's classification, indocyanine green, antipyrine and dextromorphan. *Pharmacotherapy* 15:693–700, 1995.
47. Burra P, Masier A: Dynamic tests to study liver function. *Eur Rev Med Pharmacol Sci* 8:19–21, 2004.
48. Tanaka E, Inomata S, Yasuhara H: The clinical importance of conventional and qualitative liver function test in liver transplantation. *J Clin Pharm Ther* 25:411–419, 2000.
49. Oellerich M, Amstrong VW: The MEGX test: a toll for real-time assessment of hepatic function. *Drug Monit* 23:81–92, 2001.
50. McKindley DS, Boulet J, Sachdeva K, et al: Endotoxic shock alters the pharmacokinetics of lidocaine and monoethylglycinexylidide. *Shock* 17:199–204, 2002.
51. Chandel B, Shapiro MJ, Kurtz M, et al: MEX (monoethylglycinexylidide): a novel in vivo test to measure early hepatic dysfunction after hypovolemic shock. *Shock* 3:51–53, 1995.
52. Tichy JA, Loucka M, Trefny ZM: The new clearance methods for hepatic diagnosis. *Prague Med Rep* 106:229–242, 2005.
53. Faybik P, Hetz H: Plasma disappearance rate of indocyanine green in liver dysfunction. *Transpl Proc* 38:801–802, 2006.
54. Hashimoto M, Watanabe G: Hepatic parenchymal cell volume and the indocyanine green tolerance test. *J Surg Res* 92:222–227, 2000.
55. El-Desoky A, Seifalian AM, Cope M, et al: Experimental study of liver dysfunction evaluated by direct indocyanine green clearance using near infrared spectroscopy. *Br J Surg* 86:1005–1011, 1999.

56. Von Spiegel T, Scholz M, Wietasch G, et al: Perioperative monitoring of indocyanine green clearance and plasma disappearance rate in patients undergoing liver transplantation. *Anaesthesist* 51:359–366, 2002.
57. Sakka SG, Reinhart K, Meir-Hellman A: Comparison of invasive and noninvasive measurements of indocyanine green plasma disappearance rate in critically ill patients with mechanical ventilation and stable hemodynamics. *Intensive Care Med* 26:1553–1556, 2000.
58. Sakka SG, van Hout N: Relation between indocyanine green (ICG) plasma disappearance rate and ICG blood clearance in critically ill patients. *Intensive Care Med* 32:766–769, 2006.
59. Stehr A, Ploner F, Traeger K: Plasma disappearance of indocyanine green: a marker for excretory liver function? *Intensive Care Med* 31:1719–1722, 2005.
60. Chijiiwa K, Watanabe M, Nakno K, et al: Biliary indocyanine green excretion as predictor of hepatic adenosine triphosphate levels in patients with obstructive jaundice. *Am J Surg* 179:161–169, 2000.
61. Chijiiwa K, Mizuta A, Ueda J, et al: Relation of biliary acid output to hepatic adenosine triphosphate level and biliary indocyanine green excretion in humans. *World J Surg* 26:457–461, 2002.
62. Kira T, Tomiguchi S, Kira M, et al: Quantitative evaluation of hepatic functional reserve using technetium 99 DTPA-galactosyl human serum albumin before and after transjugular intrahepatic portosystemic shunt. *Eur J Nucl Med* 24:1268–1272, 1997.
63. Hwang EH, Taki J, Shuke N, et al: Preoperative assessment of residual hepatic functional reserve using 99mTc-DTPA-galactosyl-human serum albumin dynamic SPECT. *J Nucl Med* 40:1644–1651, 1999.
64. Scheneider PD: Preoperative assessment of live function. *Surg Clin North Am* 84:355–373, 2004.
65. Ishii Y, Asai S, Kohno T, et al: (13) CO_2 peak value of L-[1-(13)C] phenylalanine breath test reflects hepatopathy. *J Surg Res* 86:130–135, 1999.
66. Kobayashi T, Kubota K, Imamura H, et al: Hepatic phenylalanine metabolism measured by the [13C] phenylalanine breath test. *Eur J Clin Invest* 31:356–361, 2001.
67. Koeda N, Iwai M, Kato A, et al: Validity of 13C-phenylalanine breath test to evaluate functional capacity of hepatocyte in patient with liver cirrhosis and acute hepatitis. *Aliment Parmacol Ther* 21:851–859, 2005.
68. Aoki M, Ishii Y, Ito A, et al: Phenylalanine breath test as a method to evaluate hepatic dysfunction in obstructive jaundice. *J Surg Res* 130:119–123, 2006.
69. Klatt S, Taut C, Mayer D, et al: Evaluation of the 13C-methacetin breath test for quantitative liver function testing. *Z Gastroenterol* 35:609–614, 1997.
70. Aoki M, Ishii Y, Asai S, et al: Ornithine breath test as a method to evaluate functional liver volume. *J Surg Res* 124:9–13, 2005.
71. Suzuki S, Ishii Y, Asai S, et al: 1-[1-(13)C] alanine is a useful substance for the evaluation of liver function. *J Surg Res* 103:13–18, 2002.
72. Zapater P, Lasso de la Vega MC, Horga JF: Pharmacokinetic variations of acetaminophen according to liver dysfunction and portal hypertension status. *Aliment Pharmacol Theory* 1:29–36, 2004.

CHAPTER 31 ■ RESPIRATORY MONITORING DURING MECHANICAL VENTILATION

TODD W. SARGE, RAY RITZ AND DANIEL TALMOR

Respiratory function may be simply classified into ventilation and oxygenation, where ventilation and oxygenation are quantified by the ability of the respiratory system to eliminate carbon dioxide and form oxyhemoglobin, respectively. The goal of respiratory monitoring in any setting is to allow the clinician to ascertain the status of the patient's ventilation and oxygenation. The clinician must then use the data appropriately to correct the patient's abnormal respiratory physiology. As with all data, it is imperative to remember that interpretation and appropriate intervention are still the onus of the clinician, who must integrate these data with other pieces of information (i.e., history and physical examination) to make a final intervention. In the acutely ill patient, the principal intervention with regard to respiratory function and monitoring usually involves the initiation, modification, or withdrawal of mechanical ventilatory support. This chapter focuses on respiratory monitoring for the mechanically ventilated patient.

Mechanical ventilation entails the unloading of the respiratory system by the application of positive pressure to achieve the goal of lung insufflation (i.e., inspiration) followed by the release of pressure to allow deflation (i.e., expiration). These simplified goals of mechanical ventilation are achieved in spite of complex and dynamic interactions of mechanical pressure with the physical properties of the respiratory system, namely elastance (E_{rs}) and resistance (R_{rs}). Furthermore, the patient's neurologic and muscular conditions can also affect the goals of respiration, and they need to be monitored and evaluated as well. This chapter focuses on three specific areas in monitoring the mechanically ventilated patient: (a) the evaluation of gas exchange, (b) respiratory mechanics, and (c) respiratory neuromuscular function.

GAS EXCHANGE

Basic Physics of Gas Exchange

As mentioned earlier, the primary function of the respiratory system is gas exchange (i.e., elimination of carbon dioxide while instilling oxygen to form oxyhemoglobin). Inadequate ventilation and oxygenation within the intensive care setting are typically caused by hypoventilation, diffusion impairment, or shunt and ventilation–perfusion (V–Q) mismatch.

Hypoventilation is defined as inadequate alveolar ventilation, and it is commonly caused by drugs, neurologic impairment, or muscle weakness/fatigue, which results in hypercarbia, according to the following equation:

$$P_aCO_2 = (\dot{V}_{CO_2}/V_A)k$$

where P_aCO_2 is the arterial partial pressure of carbon dioxide, $\dot{V}_{CO_2}$ the production of carbon dioxide in the tissues, $\dot{V}_A$ the alveolar ventilation, and k the constant. Fortunately, the institution of mechanical ventilatory support readily corrects hypoventilation while the underlying cause is determined and corrected.

Diffusion impairment is a result of inadequate time for the exchange of oxygen across the capillary–alveolar membrane. This may occur due to pathologic thickening of the membrane or high-output cardiac states such as sepsis. However, the relative clinical significance of diffusion impairment in the intensive care unit (ICU) is debatable. This is because the hypoxemia that results from the acute exacerbation of diffusion impairment is usually corrected by supplemental oxygen therapy. Furthermore, P_aCO_2 is rarely affected by diffusion impairments because it is highly soluble and is eliminated in multiple forms, such as bicarbonate.

The most common cause of hypoxemia in the ICU is ventilation–perfusion ($\dot{V}$–$\dot{Q}$) mismatch. One manifestation of $\dot{V}$–$\dot{Q}$ mismatch is shunting. The true shunt fraction is the amount of cardiac output that results in venous blood mixing with end-arterial blood without participating in gas exchange. This has little effect on carbon dioxide tension; however, increases in shunt can lead to hypoxemia. The true shunt is expressed by the shunt equation as follows:

$$Q_s/Q_t = (C_c - C_a)/(C_c - C_v)$$

where Q_s and Q_t are the shunt and total blood flows, and C_c, C_a, and C_v represent the oxygen contents of pulmonary end-capillary, arterial, and mixed venous blood, respectively. The absolute oxygen content of arterial and mixed venous blood is calculated according to the oxygen content equation:

$$C_x = (1.34 \times \mathrm{Hb} \times S_xO_2) + (P_xO_2 \times 0.003)$$

where C_x, S_xO_2, and P_xO_2 are the oxygen content, saturation, and partial pressure of oxygen within arterial and mixed venous blood, respectively. The oxygen content of end-capillary blood is estimated by the alveolar gas equation as follows:

$$C_c = (P_{atm} - P_{H_2O}) \times F_iO_2 + P_aCO_2/\mathrm{RQ}$$

where P_{atm} and P_{H_2O} are the partial pressures of the atmosphere and water (typically 760 and 47 at sea level), respectively; while F_iO_2 is the concentration of inspired oxygen; P_aCO_2 the arterial partial pressure of carbon dioxide; and RQ the respiratory quotient. The significance of true shunt is the fact that it is not amenable to supplemental oxygen therapy. Shunted blood reenters the circulation and dilutes oxygenated blood, resulting in a lower partial pressure of oxygen (P_aO_2) in the arterial system. Increasing the F_iO_2 will not improve oxygenation since the shunted fraction of blood does not meet alveolar gas.

V–Q mismatch is the result of inequality of the normal ventilation/perfusion ratio within the lung. V–Q mismatch is a spectrum of abnormal ratios signifying inadequate gas exchange at the alveolar level. It is possible with supplemental oxygen to overcome hypoxemia that is caused by an abnormal ratio of ventilation and perfusion, which differentiates this form of hypoxemia from true shunt. However, in the extreme, as the V–Q ratio in any alveolus approaches zero (i.e., ventilation approaches zero), it approaches true shunt as described above. At the other end of the spectrum, as the ratio in any alveolus approaches infinity (i.e., as perfusion approaches zero), it becomes physiologic "dead space," which denotes alveoli that are ventilated but not perfused. Dead space is described in greater detail later in this chapter.

Direct Blood Gas Analysis

Monitors of gas exchange in the mechanically ventilated patient are typically directed at measurements of gas content and their gradients from the ventilator circuit to the alveolus and from the alveolus to the end-artery. As with most monitors, sources of error abound at many points as gases flow down their concentration gradients. The most accurate assessment of gas exchange is direct measurement from an arterial blood sample. This provides the partial pressures of carbon dioxide (P_aCO_2) and oxygen (P_aO_2) in the blood as well as the pH, base deficit, and co-oximetry of other substances such as carboxyhemoglobin and methemoglobin. Advantages of arterial blood gas (ABG) analysis include the fact that it is a fairly exact representation of the current state of the patient with regard to acid–base status, oxygenation, and ventilation. However, the limitations of blood gas analysis as a tool for monitoring gas exchange are numerous, including the fact that it is invasive, wasteful (blood), and noncontinuous (i.e., it is only a snapshot of the patient's condition at the time the ABG is drawn).

Central and peripheral venous blood gas sampling has been proposed as an acceptable surrogate to arterial blood for monitoring pH, P_aCO_2, and base deficit [1]. The obvious advantage is mitigation of the invasiveness (i.e., patients are not required to have arterial access or punctures), while the disadvantages are the need for correlation and inability to assess oxygenation. With the exception of patient's undergoing cardiopulmonary resuscitation [2], good correlation has been observed between arterial and venous pH and P_aCO_2 in patients with acute respiratory disease, with one study noting an average difference of 0.03 for pH and 5.8 for P_aCO_2 [1]. Another study in mechanically ventilated trauma patients also demonstrated good correlation between arterial and central venous pH, P_aCO_2, and base deficit; however, the authors concluded that the limits of agreement (−0.09 to 0.03 for pH and −2.2 to 10.9 for P_aCO_2) represented clinically significant ranges that could affect management and therefore should not be used in initial resuscitation efforts of trauma patients [3].

Pulse Oximetry

Without question, pulse oximetry has been the most significant advance in respiratory monitoring in the past three decades. On the basis of established oxyhemoglobin dissociation curve (Fig. 31.1), pulse oximetry allows for the continuous, noninvasive estimate of a patient's oxyhemoglobin and is expressed as a percentage of total hemoglobin. A detailed explanation of pulse oximetry including the physics and limitations is provided in Chapter 26.

Expired Carbon Dioxide Measurements

Capnometry is the quantification of the carbon dioxide concentration in a sample of gas. Capnography is the continuous

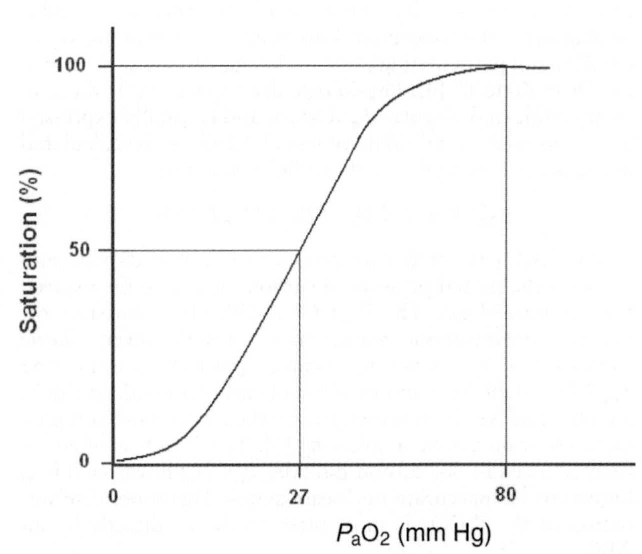

FIGURE 31.1. This is a schematic demonstrating a normal hemoglobin dissociation curve with 50% saturation at P_aO_2 of 27 mm Hg and approaching 100% saturation at a P_aO_2 of 80 mm Hg.

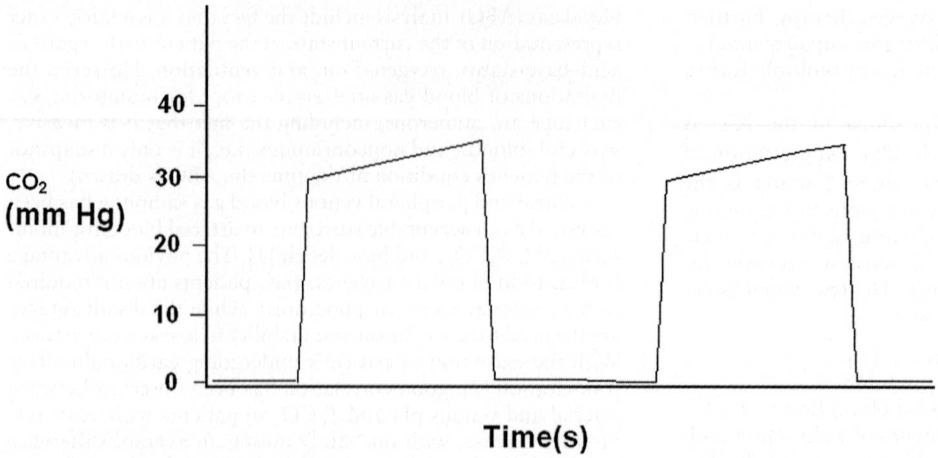

FIGURE 31.2. This is a schematic representation of a capnograph waveform with the expiratory plateau delineating the end-tidal CO_2 between 30 and 40 mm Hg.

plotting of carbon dioxide over time to create a waveform (Fig. 31.2). When capnography is performed on continuous samples of gas from the airway circuit, a waveform is created whereby the plateau is reported as the maximum pressure in millimeters Hg and termed end-tidal carbon dioxide, or $P_{et}CO_2$. Although continuous capnography has limited usefulness in the ICU, capnometry has many clinical uses such as early detection of esophageal intubation. For a detailed explanation of capnography and its uses, please refer to Chapter 26.

Dead Space Measurements

Dead space is defined as any space in the respiratory system that is ventilated but not perfused, such that no gas exchange can occur. Measurement of dead space is a marker of respiratory efficiency with regard to carbon dioxide elimination. Dead space can be subdivided into several categories including alveolar and anatomic. Anatomic dead space is the sum of the inspiratory volume that does not reach the alveoli and, therefore, participate in gas exchange. For mechanically ventilated patients, the anatomic dead space includes the proximal airways, trachea, endotracheal tube, and breathing circuit up to the Y-adapter. In normal human subjects, anatomic dead space in cubic centimeters is approximately two to three times the ideal body weight in kilograms, or 150 to 200 cm^3. Alveolar dead space is the conceptual sum of all alveoli that are ventilated but not participating in gas exchange, otherwise described as "West Zone 1" [4]. Physiologic dead space (V_d) is the sum of anatomic and alveolar dead space and is usually expressed as a ratio of the total tidal volume (V_t) and can be calculated at the bedside using the modified Bohr equation:

$$V_d/V_t = P_aCO_2 - P_{exp}CO_2/P_aCO_2$$

where P_aCO_2 is the partial pressure of carbon dioxide and $P_{exp}CO_2$ the partial pressure of carbon dioxide in the expired tidal volume of gas. The $P_{exp}CO_2$ is difficult to measure, often requiring metabolic monitoring systems. However, *volume capnography* is a novel and simple approach to estimating $P_{exp}CO_2$, involving measurements of carbon dioxide at the Y-adapter, and has been shown to correlate with more complex methods of metabolic monitoring [5]. The P_aCO_2 is often estimated as end-tidal carbon dioxide, $P_{et}CO_2$, however this is known to be inaccurate in disease states. Therefore, determination of the P_aCO_2 is most often measured directly by an ABG.

Physiologic dead space, V_d/V_t, is often increased in critical illnesses that cause respiratory failure, such as acute respiratory distress syndrome (ARDS) and chronic obstructive pulmonary disease (COPD). V_d/V_t can also increase with dynamic hyperinflation or auto-PEEP, as well as with overaggressive application of extrinsic positive end-expiratory pressure (PEEP) due to overinflation of alveoli impeding pulmonary artery blood flow—effectively increasing the West Zone 1 volume. Serial measurements of V_d/V_t have been shown to correlate with outcome in ARDS [6] and have been used to monitor the degree of respiratory compromise in critically ill patients [7]. However, these data have not translated into changes in treatment. Furthermore, Mohr et al. [8] found no appreciable difference in V_d/V_t while studying a series of posttracheostomy patients successfully weaned from mechanical ventilation compared with those who had failed weaning.

PULMONARY MECHANICS

Basic Pulmonary Variables

Modern ventilators allow manipulation and measurement of the airway pressures (P_{aw}), including peak, plateau, mean and end-expiratory; volumes (V); and flows ($\dot{V}$). Integration of these measurements allows assessment of the mechanical components of the respiratory system. The mechanical components are influenced by various disease states, and understanding these relationships may allow delivery of more appropriate ventilator support. The airway pressure (P_{aw}) is described by the equation of motion and must be equal to all opposing forces. For the relaxed respiratory system ventilating at normal frequencies, the major forces that oppose P_{aw} are the elastive and resistive properties of the respiratory system as they relate to the tidal volume (V_t) and flow ($\dot{V}$), respectively:

$$P_{aw} = E_{rs}V_t + R_{rs}(\dot{V})$$

where E_{rs} and R_{rs} are the elastance and resistance of the respiratory system, respectively.

Constant flow inflation in a relaxed, ventilator-dependent patient produces a typical picture as depicted in Figure 31.3 [9]. The rapid airway occlusion method at end inflation results in zero flow and a drop in P_{aw} from the peak value (peak inspiratory pressure, PIP) to a lower initial value and then a gradual decrease over the rest of the inspiratory period until a plateau pressure (P_{plat}) is observed. The P_{plat} measured at the airway represents the static end-inspiratory recoil of the entire respiratory system [10].

Measurement of the pleural pressures would allow further partitioning of these pressures into the lung (i.e., transpulmonary pressure, P_L) and chest wall (i.e., pleural pressure, P_{pl})

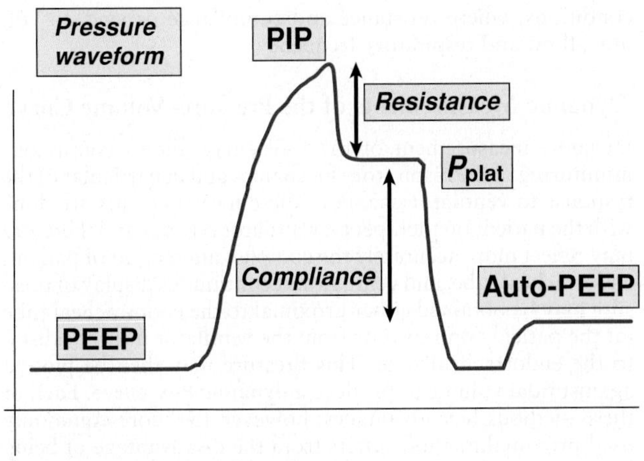

FIGURE 31.3. Schematic drawing of an airway pressure waveform delineating PEEP, auto-PEEP, peak inspiratory pressure (PIP), plateau pressure (P_{plat}), resistance, and compliance.

components using the equation:

$$P_{\text{aw}} = P_{\text{L}} + P_{\text{pl}}$$

Unfortunately, direct measurements of pleural pressure are not practical in the intensive care setting. Therefore, pleural pressures have often been estimated by esophageal balloon catheters measuring the pressure in the esophagus (P_{es}), which lies in the proximity of the pleura at mid-lung height. This alters the earlier equation as follows:

$$P_{\text{aw}} = P_{\text{L}} + P_{\text{es}}$$

where P_{es} is esophageal pressure.

These partitioned pressures are presented graphically in Figure 31.4.

Compliance and Elastance

The static compliance ($C_{\text{st,rs}}$) of the respiratory system and its reciprocal, elastance ($E_{\text{st,rs}}$), are easily measured at the bedside using the aforementioned end-inspiratory airway occlusion method to produce zero flow and thus negate the resistive forces within the system. The elastance of the respiratory system ($E_{\text{st,rs}}$) is simply the pressure gradient between the total PEEP (PEEP_{t}) and the plateau pressure (P_{plat}) divided by the tidal volume (V_{t}) to yield the following equation:

$$E_{\text{st,rs}} = (P_{\text{plat}} - \text{PEEP}_{\text{t}})/V_{\text{t}}$$

$E_{\text{st,rs}}$ may also be separated into its lung (E_{L}) and chest wall (E_{cw}) components by applying this equation to the P_{L} and P_{es} tracings obtained using P_{es} tracings (see Fig. 31.4) and by the equation:

$$E_{\text{st,rs}} = E_{\text{L}} + E_{\text{cw}}$$

The relative contributions of the lung and chest wall to the total elastance may be dependent on the etiology of respiratory failure. By way of example, pulmonary edema, either cardiogenic or as a result of ARDS, will lead to an elevated lung E_{st} and reduced compliance. ARDS of a nonpulmonary origin, for example, sepsis, may also lead to edema of the chest wall and abdominal distension. Both of these will lead to an additional increase in the $E_{\text{st,rs}}$ as a result of an increase in the elastance of the chest wall.

Resistance

According to Ohm's law, resistance is a function of the airway pressure gradient (ΔP_{aw}) divided by flow ($\dot{V}$). Airway resistance can be measured in ventilator-dependent patients by using the technique of rapid airway occlusion during constant flow

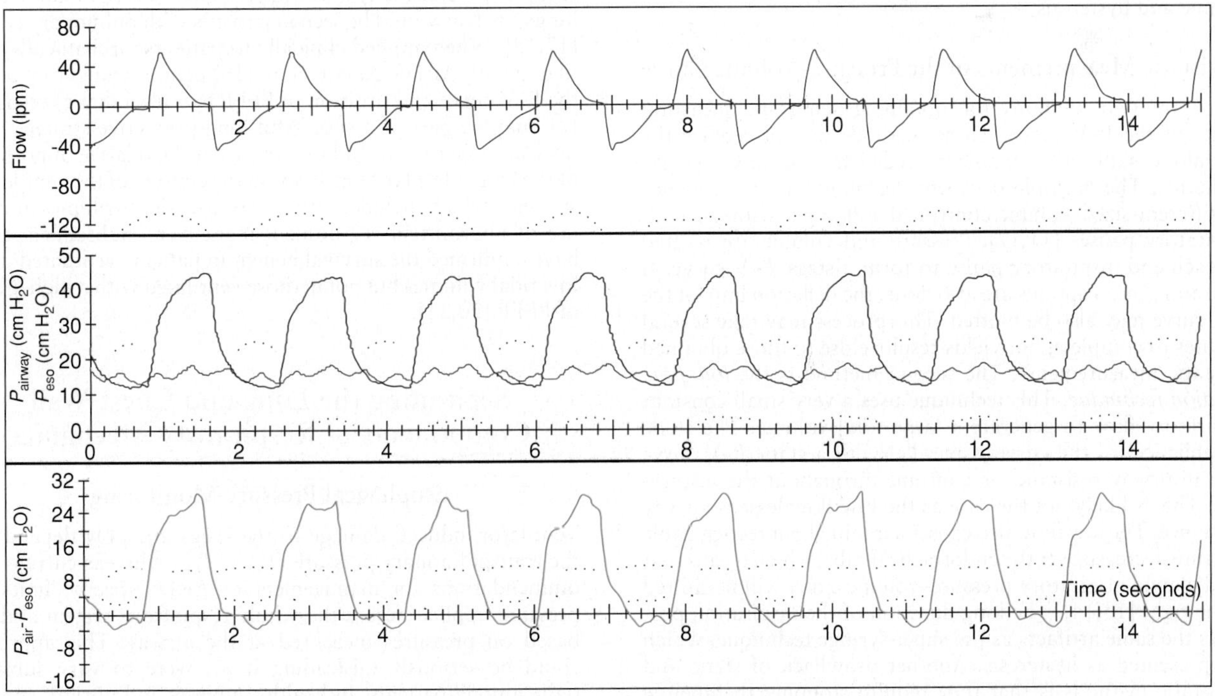

FIGURE 31.4. Esophageal pressure tracing (P_{eso}) can be seen superimposed on the airway pressure tracing (P_{air}) during pressure control ventilation (PCV). Transpulmonary pressure has been estimated as the difference between these pressures with specific assumptions.

inflation. The maximum resistance (R_{max}) of the respiratory system is calculated by

$$R_{max} = [P_{peak} - P_{plat}]/\dot{V}$$

And the minimum resistance (R_{min}) of the respiratory system can be computed by dividing

$$R_{min} = [P_{peak} - PEEP_t]/\dot{V}$$

R_{min} reflects ohmic airway resistance, while the difference between R_{max} and R_{min} (ΔR) reflects both the viscoelastic properties (stress relaxation) and the time–constant variability within the respiratory tissues (*pendelluft effect*).

Pressure–Volume Curves

Static Measurements of the Pressure–Volume Curve

The gold standard of pressure–volume (P–V) curve measurement is the super-syringe method. Using a large calibrated syringe, increments of volume of 50 ± 100 mL gas are used to inflate the lung up to a total volume of 1,000 ± 2,000 mL. After each increment, the static airway pressure is measured during a pause lasting a few seconds during which there is no flow, and the pressure is the same in the entire system from the super-syringe to the alveoli. The lung is then deflated in the same manner and the pressure at each decrement of gas is recorded and the inspiratory and expiratory P–V curves are plotted. Continued oxygen uptake from the blood during this slow inflation–deflation cycle, coupled with equalization of the partial pressure of CO_2 in the blood and alveoli, will lead to a decrease in the deflation volume as compared with the inflation volume of gas. This artifact may appear to contribute to the phenomena of hysteresis. The more important mechanical cause of hysteresis is based on the slow inflation of the lung during the P–V curve maneuver. This slow inflation recruits or opens up areas of the lung with slow time constants and collapsed alveoli. This again will lead to a decreased expiratory volume and hysteresis.

Semistatic Measurements of the Pressure–Volume Curve

There are two methods for obtaining semistatic measurements of the P–V curve. These methods do not require the specialized skill and equipment needed for the super-syringe technique. The *multiple occlusion technique* uses a sequence of different-sized volume-controlled inflations with an end-inspiratory pauses [11,12]. Pressure and volume are plotted for each end-inspiratory pause to form a static P–V curve. If expiratory interruptions are also done, the deflation limb of the P–V curve may also be plotted. This process may take several minutes to complete, but yields results close to those obtained by static measurements. The second method is the *low-flow inflation technique*. This technique uses a very small constant inspiratory flow to generate a large total volume. The slope (compliance) of the curve is parallel with a static P–V curve only if airway resistance is constant throughout the inspiration. This is likely not the case as the low flow lessens airway resistance. The low flow also causes a minimal but recognizable pressure decrease over the endotracheal tube, which means that the dynamic inspiratory pressure–volume curve will be shifted to the right [13,14]. The long duration of the inspiration produces the same artifacts as the super-syringe technique, which is represented as hysteresis. Another drawback of static and semistatic methods is that they require stopping therapeutic ventilation while the maneuver is performed. The question has been raised, therefore, if these maneuvers are relevant in predicting the mechanical behavior of the lung under dynamic conditions, where resistance and compliance depend on volume, flow, and respiratory frequency.

Dynamic Measurements of the Pressure–Volume Curve

Dynamic measurement of the P–V curve allows continuous monitoring of the respiratory mechanics and in particular of the response to ventilator changes. These measurements are done with the patient on therapeutic ventilator settings and therefore may reflect more accurately the complex interaction of patient, endotracheal tube, and ventilator. A continuous display of pressure may be obtained either proximal to the endotracheal tube (at the patient connector or from the ventilator itself) or distal to the endotracheal tube. This pressure may then be plotted against tidal volume to produce a dynamic P–V curve. Each of these methods has advantages; however, the more commonly used proximal method suffers from the disadvantage of being heavily influenced by the resistance of the endotracheal tube. Neither the peak pressure nor the end-expiratory pressures are accurately recorded, and this will lead to an underestimation of compliance [12].

Clinical Use of the Pressure–Volume Curve

There is a characteristic shape to the static respiratory system P–V curve of patients with injured lungs. This shape includes an S-shaped inflation curve with an upper and lower inflection point (UIP and LIP, respectively; Fig. 31.5), an increased recoil pressure at all lung volumes, and reduced compliance (Fig. 31.6), which is seen in the slope of the inflation curve between LIP and UIP. The LIP has often been considered the critical opening pressure of collapsed lung units and has been used as a method of setting the optimal PEEP in patients with acute lung injury (ALI). The pressure at UIP, in turn, was considered to indicate alveolar overdistension that should not be exceeded during mechanical ventilation [15]. These ideas have been challenged for multiple reasons. Accurate identification of the LIP and UIP is challenging even for experienced clinicians [16]. In addition, changes in the P–V curve are not specific for alveolar collapse and have been observed in saline-filled lungs, such as would be seen in patients with pulmonary edema [17,18]. When applied clinically to patients mechanically ventilated with ARDS, Amato et al. [19] demonstrated that use of the P–V curve and titration of PEEP to a level that exceeds the LIP may be part of a successful lung-protective strategy. It is unclear from this study, however, what the relative importance of the higher levels of PEEP was in the context of the ventilatory strategy, which included delivery of low tidal volumes and the use of intermittent recruitment maneuvers. Subsequent trials have confirmed the survival benefit in patients ventilated using low tidal volumes but not in those ventilated with a higher level of PEEP [20,21].

Separating the Lung and Chest Wall Components of Respiratory Mechanics

Esophageal Pressure Monitoring

Ventilator-induced damage to the lungs arguably depends on the transpulmonary pressure ($P_{aw} - P_{pl}$), whereas current recommendations for management of ARDS specify limits for pressure applied across the whole respiratory system and are based on pressures measured at the airway. This approach could be seriously misleading if P_{pl} were to vary substantially among patients. In healthy subjects and upright spontaneously breathing patients, P_{pl} is often estimated by measuring esophageal pressure (P_{es}); however, this is rarely done in patients with acute injury, possibly because of a widespread, but

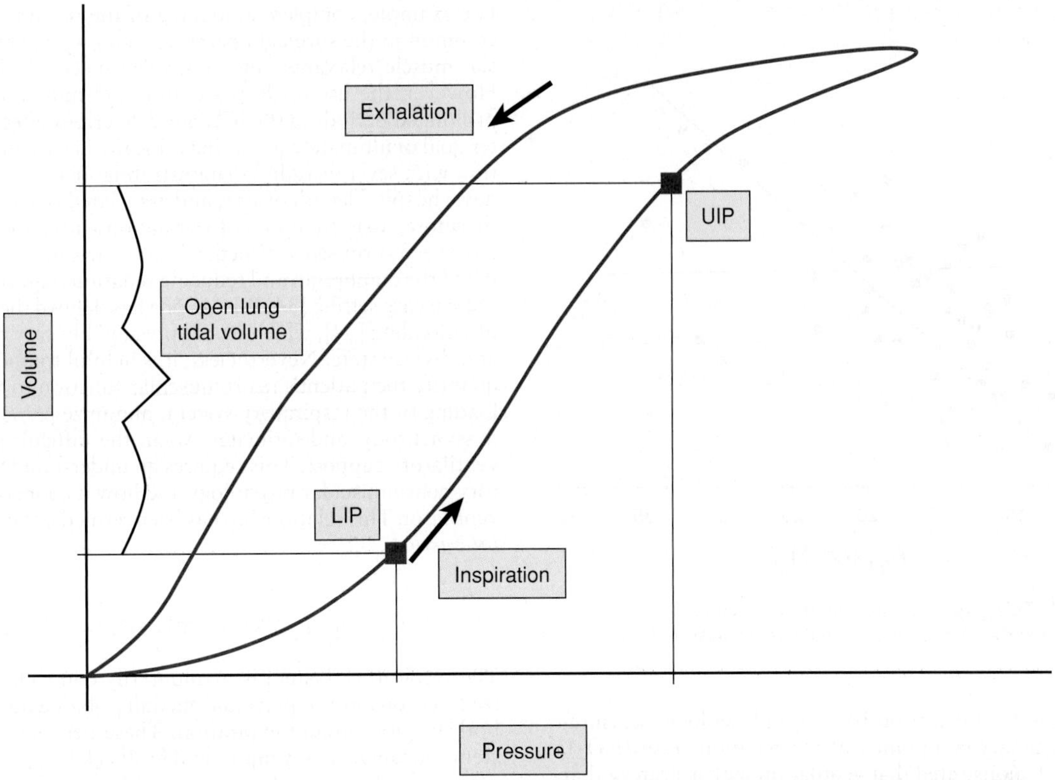

FIGURE 31.5. Schematic representation of normal pressure–volume curve (PV curve) with upper and lower inflection points (UIP and LIP, respectively) delineating the more compliant portion of the inspiratory limb and corresponding tidal volume that has been proposed as an "open lung" approach to ventilation in ARDS.

untested, belief that artifacts make P_{es} unreliable as an estimate of P_{pl} [22]. However, in a lung-injured canine model, Pelosi et al. [23] demonstrated good correlation at mid-lung height between an esophageal balloon catheter measuring the pressures in the esophagus (P_{es}) and the pleural pressures measured by pressure-transducing wafers inserted directly in the thorax. Although the absolute values of the esophageal pressures were not identical with the pleural pressures, Pelosi noted the excursions of esophageal pressure were the same as those observed in the directly measured pleural pressures. The authors therefore concluded that the changes in esophageal pressures were

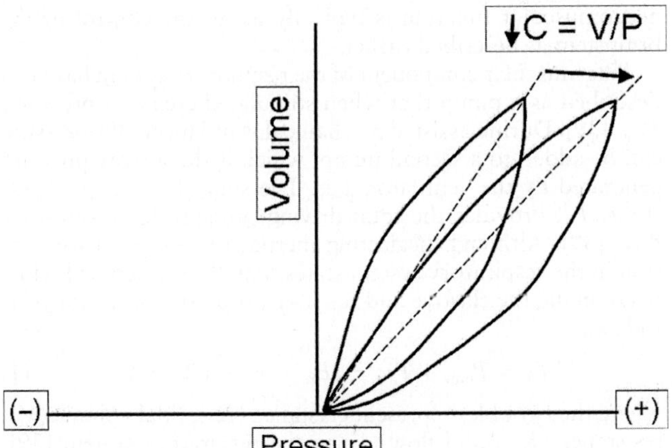

FIGURE 31.6. Schematic representation of altered compliance (C) and the effect on the volume–pressure (V/P) curve as occurs with pulmonary edema.

accurate, but the absolute values were not [23]. Others have postulated the explicit assumption that absolute values of P_{es}, corrected for a positional artifact, may reliably reflect an effective P_{pl} in critically ill patients [24].

Variations in P_{pl} may have contributed to inconsistent outcomes among clinical trials of ventilation strategies in ARDS. Although one large-scale randomized trial demonstrated a survival benefit from use of low tidal volume ventilation, results from other studies have been equivocal [20,25,26]. It is possible that in some patients with high P_{pl}, low tidal volume ventilation coupled with inadequate levels of PEEP results in cyclic alveolar collapse at end-expiration. In such cases, resulting atelectrauma might negate the benefit of limiting tidal volume. Similarly, higher levels of PEEP have been shown to be lung protective in numerous animal models of ARDS but have demonstrated inconsistent benefit in clinical investigations [19,21]. This too may reflect failure to account for P_{pl}, leading to under- or overapplication of PEEP in some patients as well as misinterpretation of high-plateau airway pressures as evidence of lung overdistension [27,28]. Measuring P_{es} to estimate transpulmonary pressure may allow mechanical ventilator settings to be individualized to accommodate variations in lung and chest wall mechanical characteristics. Such an individual approach may reduce the risk of further lung injury in ARDS [22,27,29]. This was the hypothesis of a recent single-center, randomized control trial (EPVENT Trial) of 61 patients by Talmor et al. in which ARDS and ALI patients with low tidal lung-protective ventilation were randomized to a high or low PEEP. Unique when compared with prior trials, the intervention group received PEEP based on the contribution of the chest wall as measured by esophageal pressure manometry. The control group received PEEP based on the PEEP/F_iO_2 tables from earlier trials that were created from expert opinion

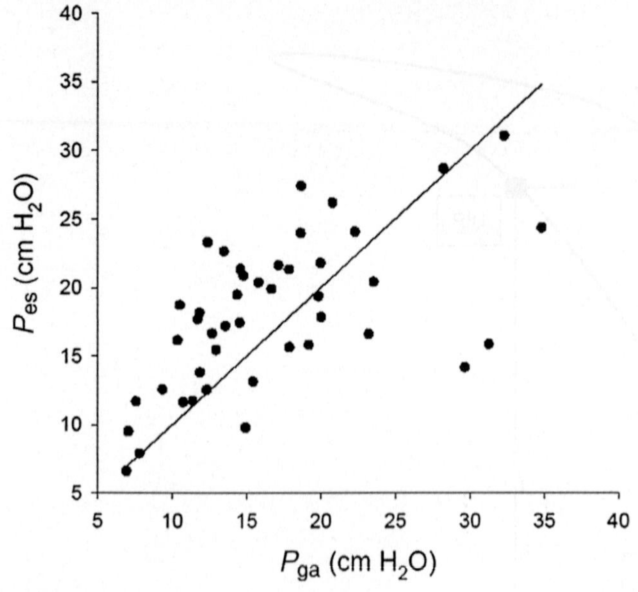

FIGURE 31.7. This graph demonstrates the correlation between pressures measured in the esophagus (P_{es}) and gastric pressure (P_{ga}).

and without individualization based on physiologic measurements. The primary end point was oxygenation (P_aO_2/F_iO_2). The authors demonstrated that ventilation with a strategy that used esophageal pressures measurements to determine PEEP settings was superior as evidenced by improved oxygenation, compliance, and a trend toward improved mortality [30].

Gastric Pressure

Esophageal pressure monitoring is not a trivial task, requiring specialized equipment and experienced operators. Gastric pressure may provide a reasonable surrogate measure for P_{pl}. In an earlier study, Talmor et al. [24] have demonstrated that there is a correlation between pressure measured in the esophagus and gastric pressures (Fig. 31.7). This relationship may be particularly important in patients having ARDS with extrapulmonary causes, where abdominal distension may contribute significantly to alveolar collapse.

Bladder Pressure

An alternative measurement of intra-abdominal pressure may be obtained by measuring pressure in the urinary bladder [31]. Instilling 50 to 100 mL of sterile water through the Foley catheter, clamping the catheter, and measuring the resulting bladder pressure has been shown to correlate well with intra-abdominal pressure measured through a gastric tube [32]. These pressures have also been shown to correlate well with esophageal pressures [33]. Studies are still required to validate use of any of these measurements in the clinical care of patients with respiratory failure.

Respiratory Neuromuscular Function

During mechanical ventilation, the goal of the clinician is to unload the patient's failing respiratory system and thereby reduce the work of breathing in the setting of respiratory failure [34]. Obviously, this goal is temporary with the later goal of weaning mechanical ventilation once the patient begins to recover from his or her disease process. To accomplish these goals, the clinician needs to have an understanding of the patient's respiratory function, which impacts each of these goals differently. For example, complete unloading of the respiratory system is common in the surgical operating room with general anesthesia, muscle relaxants, and controlled mechanical ventilation. However, the use of deep sedation and muscle relaxants for prolonged periods in the ICU has deleterious effects on the latter goal of ultimately preparing critically ill patients for extubation with several studies demonstrating increases in ventilator days, hospital length of stay, and associated costs [35–37]. Furthermore, assisted modes of ventilation with partial unloading have been surmised as beneficial for maintaining the conditioning of the diaphragm and reducing sedation requirements in the critical care setting [34,38]. No one has defined the ideal degree of unloading [34], which would presumably vary by individual and disease state. Nevertheless, it is helpful to understand and quantify the patient's neuromuscular function to facilitate unloading of the respiratory system, minimize patient–ventilator dyssynchrony, and ultimately wean the difficult patient from ventilatory support. This requires an understanding of respiratory neuromuscular physiology and how it cooperates with the ventilator. This relationship has been termed *patient–ventilator interaction*.

Respiratory Neuromuscular Anatomy

The respiratory system is involuntarily controlled by specialized neurons in the pons and medulla oblongata that control both inspiration and expiration. These neurons in the brainstem coordinate many inputs and feedback loops to control respiration and ensure adequate gas exchange. The specific types of feedback can be mechanical, chemical, reflex, and behavioral, all of which directly affect the neurons rate and intensity of neural firing [39]. Together these neurons and their feedback loops constitute the respiratory control center. Under normal resting conditions, neurons in the inspiratory center stimulate contraction of the diaphragm and intercostal muscles through the phrenic and spinal nerves, which creates a negative force in the chest cavity relative to the airway (i.e., a pressure gradient), thus allowing air to flow into the lungs (Fig. 31.8). Subsequent exhalation is typically passive, and air is exhaled as a consequence of lung and chest wall elastance. However, when the respiratory center is stimulated in the presence of carbon dioxide, acidosis, or hypoxemia, exhalation can be made more active by contraction of abdominal and chest wall muscles. The cerebral cortex has the ability to take control of the respiratory system by overriding the brainstem to change the frequency, depth, and rhythm of respirations. This is of minimal concern in the mechanically ventilated patient, whose cerebral cortex is sedated, by either medications or illness, such that respiratory neuromuscular function is typically under the control of the brainstem as described earlier.

The muscular component of the respiratory system has been described as a pump that when stimulated creates a pressure, P_{mus} [39]. During assisted mechanical ventilation, this pressure can be added to a second pump, which is the airway pressure generated by the ventilator, P_{aw}. The sum of these two pressures, P_T, provides the total driving pressure for inspiratory flow [39]. Although neglecting inertia, the equation for motion in the respiratory system states that P_T is dissipated while overcoming the elastive and resistive properties of the lungs as follows:

$$P_T = P_{mus} + P_{aw} = (E_{rs} \times V_t) + (R_{rs} \times \dot{V}) \quad (1)$$

where the variables represent elastance (E_{rs}), tidal volume (V_t), resistance (R_{rs}), and flow ($\dot{V}$) in the respiratory system [39]. Since the ventilator-generated pressure, P_{aw}, is intended to unload the patient's respiratory muscles, it should be synchronous with the neural impulses generated by the respiratory center and thus P_{mus}. To be synchronous with the patient's neural

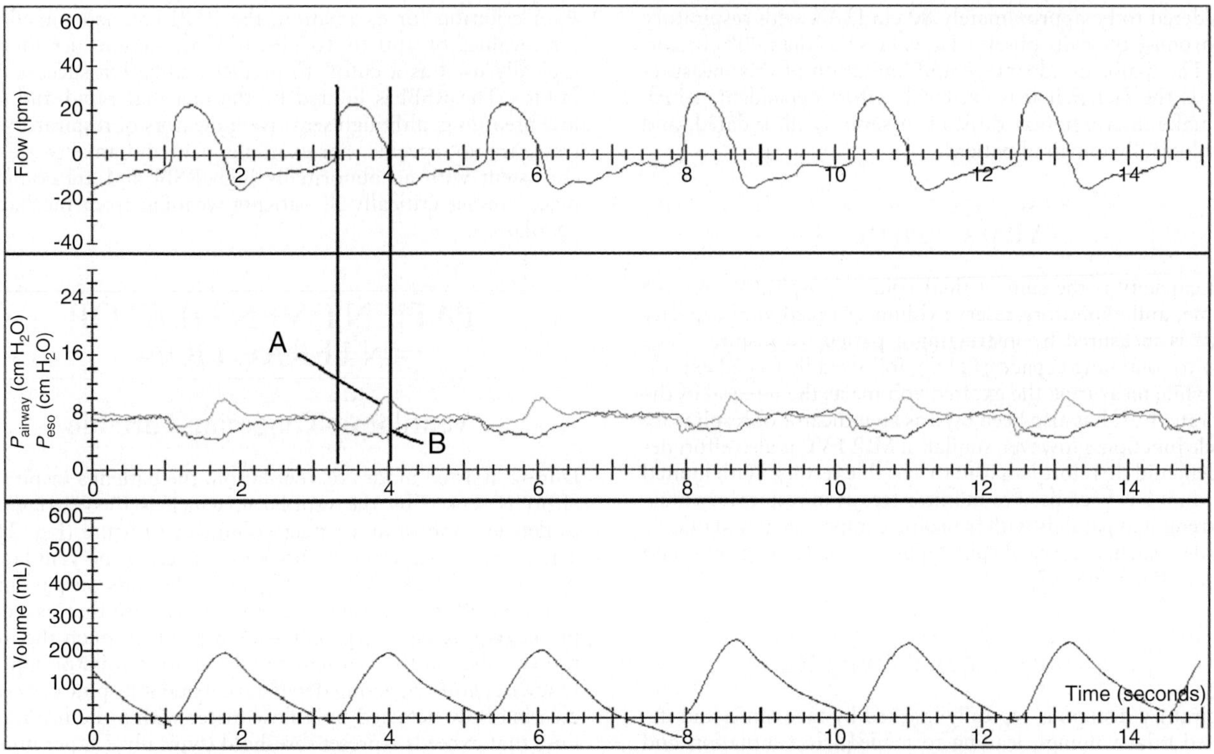

FIGURE 31.8. Spontaneous ventilation with continuous positive airway pressure (CPAP) at 7.5 mm Hg. Airway and esophageal pressure tracings are superimposed and marked as A and B, respectively. Note the onset of inspiration and flow, marked by the first vertical line, as esophageal (P_{eso}) and airway (P_{air}) pressures separate, creating a pressure gradient. Flow then ceases, as marked by the second vertical line, when the expiratory valve is opened on the ventilator and airway pressure quickly decreases.

inspiration, the ventilator would need to initiate support simultaneously with the patient's neural firing at the onset of inspiration, continue this support throughout the neural firing, and stop support at the end of neural firing. In reality, this goal is virtually impossible, as currently there is no practical monitor for efferent motor neurons of the respiratory system. Rather than monitoring neural impulses, modern ventilators sense changes in pressure and flow within the circuit in an effort to match the patient's respiratory cycle. The variables that we discuss regarding the patient–ventilator interaction include ventilator triggering, cycling-off, and delivery of gas between these two events (i.e., the posttrigger phase). However, it is essential to first define some of the measures of respiratory drive and effort that are commonly used to assess patient–ventilator interaction and weaning such as work of breathing, pressure–time product (PTP), airway occlusion pressure, maximal inspiratory force, vital capacity (VC), and rapid shallow breathing index (RSBI).

Work of Breathing

Patient respiratory effort is typically discussed and quantified via some measure of the patient's "work of breathing." *Work* is defined as the force acting on an object to cause displacement of that object. Therefore, mechanical work of breathing includes the measurement of a force required to create a change in volume of gas and is expressed in Joules per liter. However, measurements that are based on volume frequently fail to account for the work done by the diaphragm and respiratory muscles during isometric contraction against a closed valve [40], as occurs before triggering in some assisted modes of ventilation. The PTP, which measures swings in intrathoracic pressure by an esophageal pressure monitor and correlates with oxygen requirements of breathing, is considered superior for quantifying a patient's effort and degree of unloading [34]. This is a calculation of the difference in the time integrals between esophageal pressure, P_{es}, during assisted breathing and the recoil pressure of the chest wall during passive breathing at a similar tidal volume and flow [40].

Airway Occlusion Pressure

Airway occlusion pressure at 0.1 seconds ($P_{0.1}$) is an indicator of respiratory drive and is determined by measuring the pressure in the airway a tenth of a second after the onset of inspiration beginning at functional residual capacity (FRC). This has been shown to correlate well with work of breathing during pressure support ventilation [40]. Therefore, several authors have advocated its use as a potential predictor for discontinuation of mechanical ventilation [41–44]. The threshold value for $P_{0.1}$ of 6 cm H_2O appeared to delineate success versus failure in one such study, although this value was variable among authors. Although the utility of this measurement is still debated, it has been incorporated into several commercially available ventilators.

Maximal Inspiratory Force

Maximal inspiratory pressure (MIP), also known as negative inspiratory force, is another marker of respiratory muscle function and strength and is determined by measuring the maximum pressure that can be generated by the inspiratory muscles against an occluded airway beginning FRC. A normal value is considered to be approximately 80 cm H_2O, with respiratory compromise typically observed at values less than 40% of normal. The major disadvantage and limitation of this measurement is the fact that it is extremely effort dependent, which can make interpretation difficult in severely ill, sedated, and neurologically impaired patients.

Vital Capacity

Vital capacity is the sum of tidal volume, inspiratory reserve volume, and expiratory reserve volume. Forced vital capacity (FVC) is measured by instructing a patient to inspire maximally to total lung capacity (TLC), followed by forced expiration while measuring the expired volume as the integral of the flow rate. FVC has also been used as an indicator of respiratory muscle function. However, similar to MIP, FVC is also effort dependent and therefore can lead to variable results. With limited success, it has been used to monitor trends in respiratory muscle strength in patients with neurologic impairment and muscle disorders such as cervical spine injury, myasthenia gravis, and Guillain-Barre [45–47].

Frequency/Tidal Volume Ratio

Respiratory distress is typically marked by tachypnea and decreased tidal volumes, leading to inadequate ventilation and increases in P_aCO_2 secondary to disproportionate ventilation of anatomic dead space and inadequate alveolar ventilation. Therefore, the ratio of frequency to tidal volume, also known as the RSBI, has been used to gauge respiratory distress and facilitate weaning and readiness for extubation [43,48–50]. As a criterion for extubation, the RSBI has had mixed success. Values of 100 to 105 breaths per minute per liter are typically used as a cutoff to predict extubation success from failure. The RSBI is limited by the fact that rapid and shallow breathing, although sensitive indicators of respiratory distress, are not specific. For example, pain and anxiety are also consistent with an abnormally high RSBI and are commonplace among critically ill patients weaning from mechanical ventilation.

PATIENT VENTILATOR INTERACTION

Ventilator–Triggering Variable

During assisted modes of ventilation, the patient's inspiratory effort is sensed by the ventilator, which is then "triggered" to deliver support at a preset volume or pressure (Fig. 31.9). There are two distinct methods of triggering the ventilator—pressure and flow. *Pressure triggering* depends on patient inspiratory effort, creating a change in pressure that exceeds a preset requirement (typically—2 cm H_2O) to open the inspiratory valve on the ventilator and initiate ventilator support. Likewise, *flow triggering* depends on patient inspiratory effort, creating flow detected by a flow meter within the inspiratory limb that exceeds a preset threshold (typically 2 L per minute) for triggering the ventilator support. The significant difference between these two triggering criteria is the presence of a closed demand valve in the inspiratory limb in pressure-triggered ventilators. In general, flow triggering has been considered superior to pressure-triggered algorithms in that it is believed that the

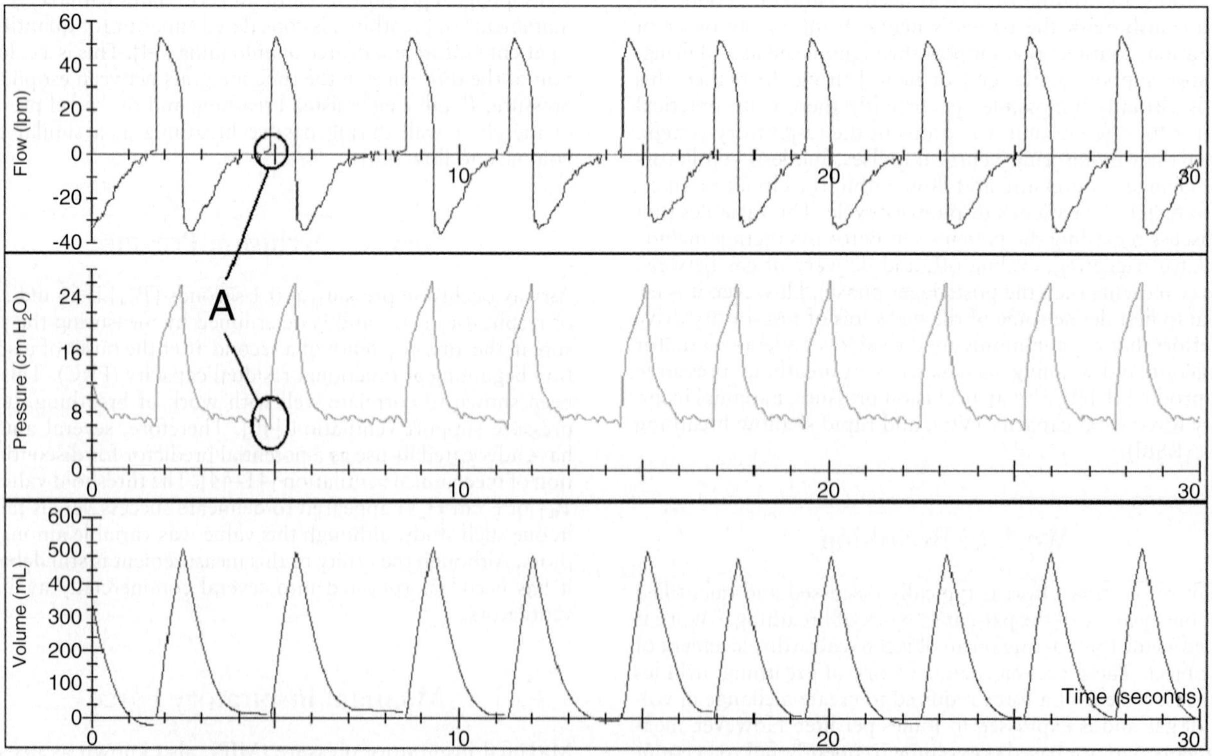

FIGURE 31.9. Normal triggering in assisted-control ventilation. The circles marked A denote the pressure and flow that correspond to patient neural inspiration that is detected by the ventilator and leads to delivery of a mechanical breath.

work of breathing is less in a system that does not require an initial inspiratory effort against this closed valve. Many studies have compared flow triggering and pressure triggering with respect to work of breathing with most showing significant advantages in favor of flow-triggered systems [51–53]. This is partially explained by the fact that flow-triggering results in improved responsiveness with shorter delay between onset of diaphragm contraction and ventilator triggering [53].

The main variable that can be controlled on the ventilator with regard to triggering is termed *sensitivity*. Typical values for pressure triggering are 1 to 2 cm H_2O, while those for flow triggering are 2 to 3 L per minute. The sensitivity threshold is important because it is required to strike a balance between two main problems associated with triggering. First, if the sensitivity is set too low, patients may experience autotriggering, in which pressure and flow changes that occur from sources of artifact such as cardiac oscillations, water in the circuit, patient movement, or resonance within the system lead to irregular breathing patterns and dyssynchrony. Second, sensitivity settings that are too high will lead to ineffective triggering, which has the consequences of increased and wasted work and energy (Fig. 31.10). Ineffective triggering is also common in the setting of dynamic hyperinflation, as seen in obstructive disorders such as asthma and COPD. In the setting of obstructive diseases, dynamic hyperinflation leads to elevations in the intrinsic PEEP ($PEEP_i$) above a critical threshold such that the patient's respiratory drive is insufficient to overcome the elastic recoil of the lung and chest wall and trigger the ventilator [34]. Clearly, this is also disadvantageous to the patient in terms of work of breathing and may contribute to ventilator dyssynchrony. Leung et al. [54] demonstrated that ineffective trigger attempts required 38% increases in patient effort as compared to successfully triggered breaths. Obviously, autotriggering and ineffective triggering can create a challenge to the clinician when attempting to optimize the ventilator settings. In general, it is helpful to reduce the trigger threshold to a point where the delay between neural firing and ventilator support is minimized without allowing autotriggering to occur.

Cycle-Off Variable

Neurons in the respiratory center continue firing beyond ventilator triggering and throughout inspiration. The cessation of firing is an important time point in the respiratory cycle and marks the beginning of expiration. The neural inspiratory time is often variable from breath to breath [34]. This can lead to considerable dyssynchrony in controlled modes of ventilation such as assisted-control, pressure-control, and intermittent mandatory ventilation, where "cycling-off" of the ventilator into expiration is a function of the inspiratory time (T_i) and is generally constant from one breath to the next. This can lead to increased sedation requirements that are inconsistent with the goal of ventilator weaning, as mentioned earlier. Ideally, the ventilator should be able to detect the end of neural firing and react accordingly to halt the inspiratory pressure supplied. This is one of the goals and advantages of the "supportive" modes of ventilation such as "pressure support ventilation." That is, supportive modes of ventilation have the ability to detect patient expiration and stop ventilator inspiration such that the T_i is variable. This can be accomplished by measuring flow or pressure changes within the circuit. As neural firing ceases and P_{mus} decreases to baseline with muscle relaxation, total pressure and thus flow should decrease according to the elastive and resistive properties of the lung according to the equation of motion previously described. Typically, support modes have

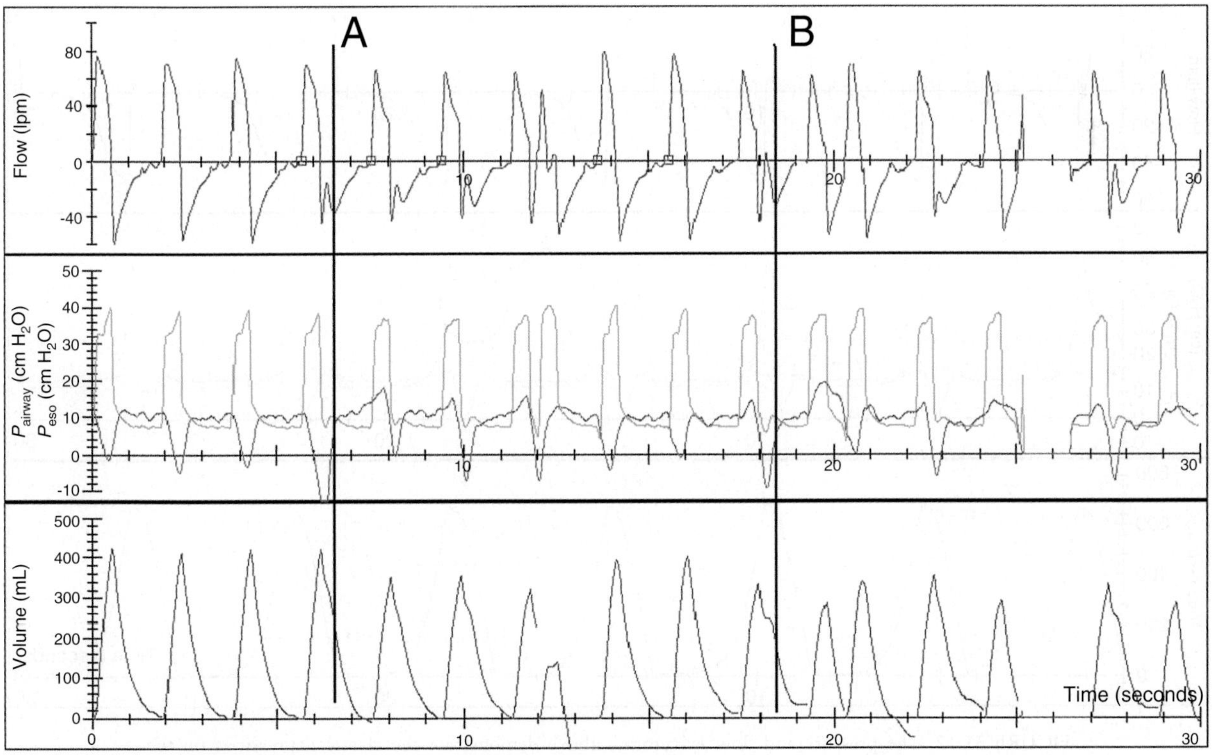

FIGURE 31.10. This pressure and flow tracing demonstrated failed trigger attempts that can be appreciated by the negative deflections in the expiratory limbs in the flow waveform and delineated by lines A and B.

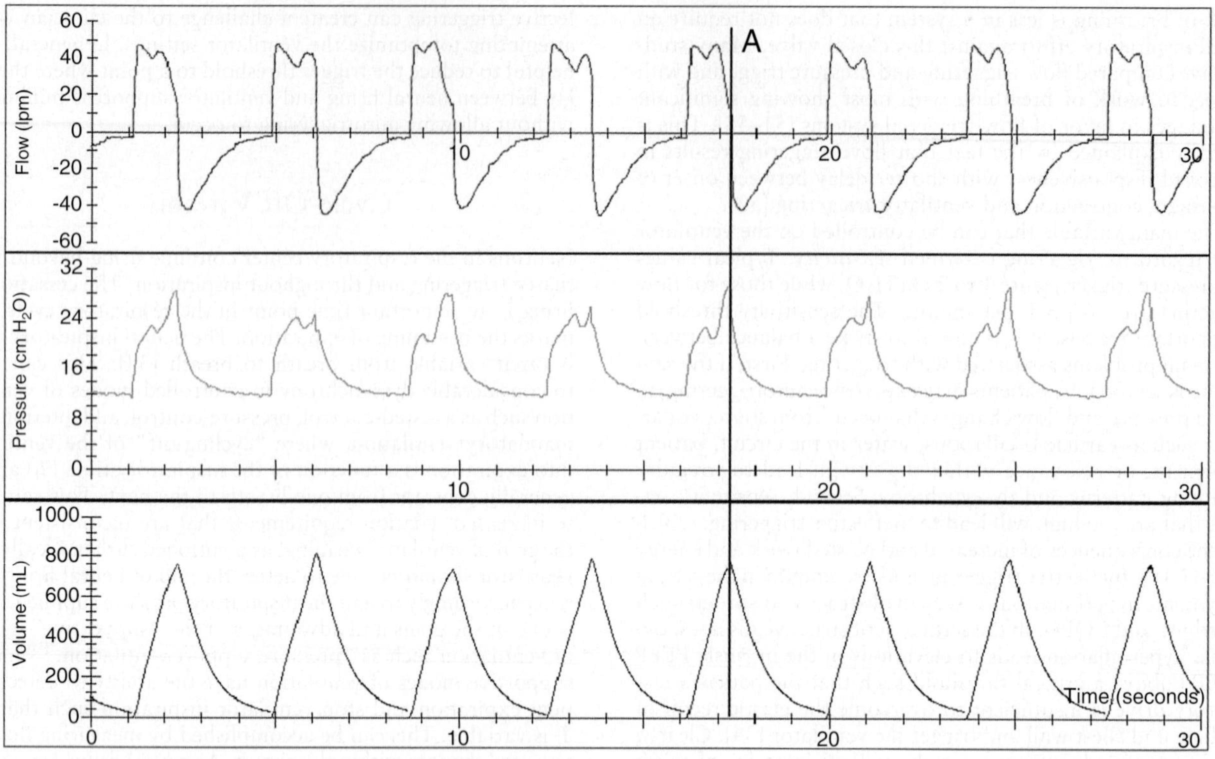

FIGURE 31.11. The pressure and flow waveforms demonstrate active recruitment of expiratory muscles to terminate ventilator inspiration. Note the time point marked by line A in which flow decreases rapidly corresponding to a sharp increase in the airway pressure due to active exhalation.

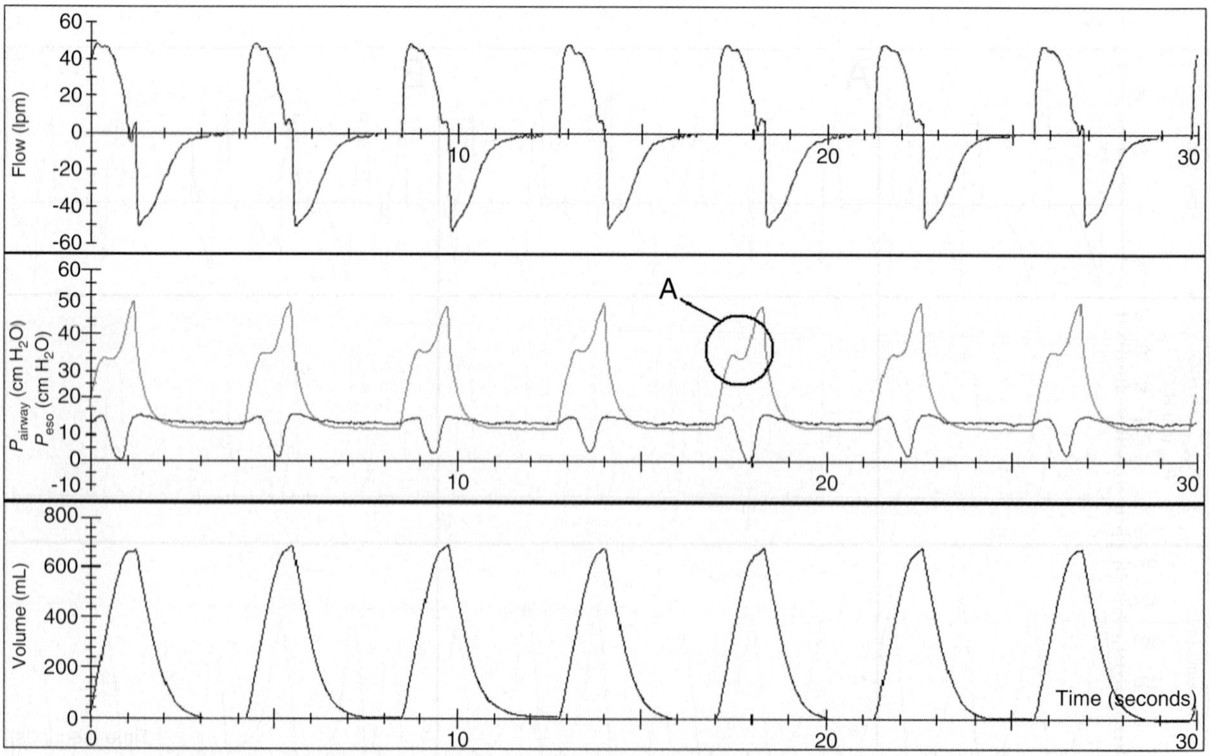

FIGURE 31.12. The pressure and flow waveforms above demonstrate the classic depressions on the inspiratory airway (P_{air}) pressure tracing in a patient with an elevated respiratory drive as highlighted by circle A. P_{eso}, esophageal pressure.

software that detects a preset decrement in flow, which in turn leads to cycling off the inspiratory support. This preset threshold can be an absolute value of flow or a percentage of maximum flow in the circuit, or both. Often, an increase in pressure that exceeds the programmed support level will also signal the ventilator to stop inspiration and open the expiratory valve as well.

Just as with triggering, the cycle-off variable can be a source of serious tribulations with the patient–ventilator interaction. For example, in the setting of decreased lung elastance, such as emphysematous lung disease, flow may not diminish enough to be detected properly despite a drop in P_{mus} at the end of neural inspiratory time. This can lead to patient discomfort and was studied by Jubran et al. [55], who noticed that 5 out of 12 patients with COPD required active exhalation to cycle off the ventilator during pressure support ventilation at 20 cm H_2O. Active exhalation is counterproductive to both the primary goal of respiratory muscle unloading and ventilator synchrony (Fig. 31.11). Furthermore, active exhalation will increase transpulmonary pressure, which can lead to premature airway closure and increased intrinsic $PEEP_i$ as closing capacity increases.

Inspiratory Flow Variable

Inspiratory flow is now being recognized as an important parameter in assisted modes of ventilation. Critically ill patients in acute respiratory failure often have elevated respiratory drives that appear to demand greater flow to overcome the resistance of the failing respiratory system and ventilator breathing circuit [34]. Classically, this appears as a depression on the inspiratory limb of the airway pressure tracing and has been described by some practitioners as "flow hunger" (Fig. 31.12). Clinically, the response has been to increase flow, which typically ranges between 30 and 80 L per minute during assisted modes of mechanical ventilation in an effort to decrease the work of breathing and intrinsic PEEP in these situations. However, a recent series of studies has shown that this may in fact be counterproductive due to a phenomenon now recognized as "flow-associated tachypnea" [34]. Puddy and Younes [56] demonstrated this phenomenon by adjusting inspiratory flow in awake volunteers breathing on a volume-cycled ventilator in assisted-control mode in which inspiratory T_i was variable. Laghi et al. [57] later delineated the contributions of flow, tidal volume, and inspiratory time in their study in which flow was increased from 60 to 90 L per minute and balanced with tidal volume settings of 1.0 and 1.5 L to maintain a constant inspiratory time, where frequency did not change. Furthermore, they were able to show that imposed ventilator inspiratory time during mechanical ventilation can determine frequency independently of delivered inspiratory flow and tidal volume. Therefore, the clinician must consider the counteracting variables of flow, tidal volume, and inspiratory time when attempting to ventilate patients with elevated respiratory drive in acute respiratory failure and how one may negatively influence the other.

SUMMARY

Respiratory monitoring is a complicated task in the critically ill patient who requires mechanical ventilation. The clinician must carefully balance a plethora of data acquired from studying variables of gas exchange, pulmonary mechanics, neuromuscular function, and patient ventilator interactions. Skilled intensive-care–trained personnel must then process these data so that a plan of respiratory support, often with mechanical ventilation, can be instituted. This plan must proceed in such a way that the patient is safely ventilated and oxygenated without imposing the undue harm that is associated with injurious and careless methods of ventilation.

References

1. Kelly AM, Kyle E, McAlpine R: Venous pCO(2) and pH can be used to screen for significant hypercarbia in emergency patients with acute respiratory disease. *J Emerg Med* 22(1):15–19, 2002.
2. Weil MH, Rackow EC, Trevino R, et al: Difference in acid-base state between venous and arterial blood during cardiopulmonary resuscitation. *N Engl J Med* 315(3):153–156, 1986.
3. Malinoski DJ, Todd SR, Slone S, et al: Correlation of central venous and arterial blood gas measurements in mechanically ventilated trauma patients. *Arch Surg* 140(11):1122–1125, 2005.
4. West JB, Dollery CT, Naimark A: Distribution of blood flow in isolated lung; relation to vascular and alveolar pressures. *J Appl Physiol* 19:713–724, 1964.
5. Kallet RH, Daniel BM, Garcia O, et al: Accuracy of physiologic dead space measurements in patients with acute respiratory distress syndrome using volumetric capnography: comparison with the metabolic monitor method. *Respir Care* 50(4):462–467, 2005.
6. Kallet RH, Alonso JA, Pittet JF, et al: Prognostic value of the pulmonary dead-space fraction during the first 6 days of acute respiratory distress syndrome. *Respir Care* 49(9):1008–1014, 2004.
7. Wathanasormsiri A, Preutthipan A, Chantarojanasiri T, et al: Dead space ventilation in volume controlled versus pressure controlled mode of mechanical ventilation. *J Med Assoc Thai* 85[Suppl 4]:S1207–S1212, 2002.
8. Mohr AM, Rutherford EJ, Cairns BA, et al: The role of dead space ventilation in predicting outcome of successful weaning from mechanical ventilation. *J Trauma* 51(5):843–848, 2001.
9. Bates JH, Rossi A, Milic-Emili J: Analysis of the behavior of the respiratory system with constant inspiratory flow. *J Appl Physiol* 58(6):1840–1848, 1985.
10. Polese G, Rossi A, Appendini L, et al: Partitioning of respiratory mechanics in mechanically ventilated patients. *J Appl Physiol* 71(6):2425–2433, 1991.
11. Iotti GA, Braschi A, Brunner JX, et al: Respiratory mechanics by least squares fitting in mechanically ventilated patients: applications during paralysis and during pressure support ventilation. *Intensive Care Med* 21(5):406–413, 1995.
12. Stenqvist O: Practical assessment of respiratory mechanics. *Br J Anaesth* 91(1):92–105, 2003.
13. Lu Q, Vieira SR, Richecoeur J, et al: A simple automated method for measuring pressure–volume curves during mechanical ventilation. *Am J Respir Crit Care Med* 159(1):275–282, 1999.
14. Servillo G, Coppola M, Blasi F, et al: The measurement of the pressure–volume curves with computerized methods. *Minerva Anestesiol* 66(5):381–385, 2000.
15. Roupie E, Dambrosio M, Servillo G, et al: Titration of tidal volume and induced hypercapnia in acute respiratory distress syndrome. *Am J Respir Crit Care Med* 152(1):121–128, 1995.
16. Harris RS, Hess DR, Venegas JG: An objective analysis of the pressure–volume curve in the acute respiratory distress syndrome. *Am J Respir Crit Care Med* 161(2, Pt 1):432–439, 2000.
17. Hubmayr RD: Perspective on lung injury and recruitment: a skeptical look at the opening and collapse story. *Am J Respir Crit Care Med* 165(12):1647–1653, 2002.
18. Martin-Lefevre L, Ricard JD, Roupie E, et al: Significance of the changes in the respiratory system pressure–volume curve during acute lung injury in rats. *Am J Respir Crit Care Med* 164(4):627–632, 2001.
19. Amato MB, Barbas CS, Medeiros DM, et al: Effect of a protective-ventilation strategy on mortality in the acute respiratory distress syndrome. *N Engl J Med* 338(6):347–354, 1998.
20. Ventilation with lower tidal volumes as compared with traditional tidal volumes for acute lung injury and the acute respiratory distress syndrome. The Acute Respiratory Distress Syndrome Network. *N Engl J Med* 342(18): 1301–1308, 2000.
21. Brower RG, Lanken PN, MacIntyre N, et al: Higher versus lower positive end-expiratory pressures in patients with the acute respiratory distress syndrome. *N Engl J Med* 351(4):327–336, 2004.
22. de Chazal I, Hubmayr RD: Novel aspects of pulmonary mechanics in intensive care. *Br J Anaesth* 91(1):81–91, 2003.
23. Pelosi P, Goldner M, McKibben A, et al: Recruitment and derecruitment during acute respiratory failure: an experimental study. *Am J Respir Crit Care Med* 164(1):122–130, 2001.
24. Talmor D, Sarge T, O'Donnell CR, et al: Esophageal and transpulmonary pressures in acute respiratory failure. *Crit Care Med* 34(5):1389–1394.

25. Brochard L, Roudot-Thoraval F, Roupie E, et al: Tidal volume reduction for prevention of ventilator-induced lung injury in acute respiratory distress syndrome. The Multicenter Trail Group on Tidal Volume reduction in ARDS. *Am J Respir Crit Care Med* 158(6):1831–1838, 1998.
26. Stewart TE, Meade MO, Cook DJ, et al: Evaluation of a ventilation strategy to prevent barotrauma in patients at high risk for acute respiratory distress syndrome. Pressure- and Volume-Limited Ventilation Strategy Group. *N Engl J Med* 338(6):355–361, 1998.
27. Matthay MA, Bhattacharya S, Gaver D, et al: Ventilator-induced lung injury: in vivo and in vitro mechanisms. *Am J Physiol Lung Cell Mol Physiol* 283(4):L678–L682, 2002.
28. Terragni PP, Rosboch GL, Lisi A, et al: How respiratory system mechanics may help in minimising ventilator-induced lung injury in ARDS patients. *Eur Respir J Suppl* 42:15s–21s, 2003.
29. Milic-Emili J, Mead J, Turner JM, et al: Improved technique for estimating pleural pressure from esophageal balloons. *J Appl Physiol* 19(2):207–211, 1964.
30. Talmor D, Sarge T, Malhotra A, et al: Mechanical ventilation guided by esophageal pressure in acute lung injury. *N Engl J Med* 359(20):2095–2104, 2008.
31. Malbrain ML: Abdominal pressure in the critically ill: measurement and clinical relevance. *Intensive Care Med* 25(12):1453–1458, 1999.
32. Collee GG, Lomax DM, Ferguson C, et al: Bedside measurement of intra-abdominal pressure (IAP) via an indwelling naso-gastric tube: clinical validation of the technique. *Intensive Care Med* 19(8):478–480, 1993.
33. Chieveley-Williams S, Dinner L, Puddicombe A, et al: Central venous and bladder pressure reflect transdiaphragmatic pressure during pressure support ventilation. *Chest* 121(2):533–538, 2002.
34. Tobin MJ, Jubran A, Laghi F: Patient–ventilator interaction. *Am J Respir Crit Care Med* 163(5):1059–1063, 2001.
35. Carson SS, Kress JP, Rodgers JE, et al: A randomized trial of intermittent lorazepam versus propofol with daily interruption in mechanically ventilated patients. *Crit Care Med* 34(5):1326–1332, 2006.
36. Kress JP, Pohlman AS, O'Connor MF, et al: Daily interruption of sedative infusions in critically ill patients undergoing mechanical ventilation. *N Engl J Med* 342(20):1471–1477, 2000.
37. Prielipp RC, Coursin DB, Wood KE, et al: Complications associated with sedative and neuromuscular blocking drugs in critically ill patients. *Crit Care Clin* 11(4):983–1003, 1995.
38. Le Bourdelles G, Viires N, Boczkowski J, et al: Effects of mechanical ventilation on diaphragmatic contractile properties in rats. *Am J Respir Crit Care Med* 149(6):1539–1544, 1994.
39. Kondili E, Prinianakis G, Georgopoulos D: Patient–ventilator interaction. *Br J Anaesth* 91(1):106–119, 2003.
40. Jubran A: Advances in respiratory monitoring during mechanical ventilation. *Chest* 116(5):1416–1425, 1999.
41. Capdevila X, Perrigault PF, Ramonatxo M, et al: Changes in breathing pattern and respiratory muscle performance parameters during difficult weaning. *Crit Care Med* 26(1):79–87, 1998.
42. Murciano D, Boczkowski J, Lecocguic Y, et al: Tracheal occlusion pressure: a simple index to monitor respiratory muscle fatigue during acute respiratory failure in patients with chronic obstructive pulmonary disease. *Ann Intern Med* 108(6):800–805, 1988.
43. Sassoon CS, Mahutte CK: Airway occlusion pressure and breathing pattern as predictors of weaning outcome. *Am Rev Respir Dis* 148(4, Pt 1):860–866, 1993.
44. Sassoon CS, Te TT, Mahutte CK, et al: Airway occlusion pressure. An important indicator for successful weaning in patients with chronic obstructive pulmonary disease. *Am Rev Respir Dis* 135(1):107–113, 1987.
45. Chevrolet JC, Deleamont P: Repeated vital capacity measurements as predictive parameters for mechanical ventilation need and weaning success in the Guillain-Barre syndrome. *Am Rev Respir Dis* 144(4):814–818, 1991.
46. Loveridge BM, Dubo HI: Breathing pattern in chronic quadriplegia. *Arch Phys Med Rehabil* 71(7):495–499, 1990.
47. Rieder P, Louis M, Jolliet P, et al: The repeated measurement of vital capacity is a poor predictor of the need for mechanical ventilation in myasthenia gravis. *Intensive Care Med* 21(8):663–668, 1995.
48. Krieger BP, Isber J, Breitenbucher A, et al: Serial measurements of the rapid-shallow-breathing index as a predictor of weaning outcome in elderly medical patients. *Chest* 112(4):1029–1034, 1997.
49. Vallverdu I, Calaf N, Subirana M, et al: Clinical characteristics, respiratory functional parameters, and outcome of a two-hour T-piece trial in patients weaning from mechanical ventilation. *Am J Respir Crit Care Med* 158(6):1855–1862, 1998.
50. Yang KL, Tobin MJ: A prospective study of indexes predicting the outcome of trials of weaning from mechanical ventilation. *N Engl J Med* 324(21):1445–1450, 1991.
51. Aslanian P, El Atrous S, Isabey D, et al: Effects of flow triggering on breathing effort during partial ventilatory support. *Am J Respir Crit Care Med* 157(1):135–143, 1998.
52. Barrera R, Melendez J, Ahdoot M, et al: Flow triggering added to pressure support ventilation improves comfort and reduces work of breathing in mechanically ventilated patients. *J Crit Care* 14(4):172–176, 1999.
53. Branson RD, Campbell RS, Davis K Jr, et al: Comparison of pressure and flow triggering systems during continuous positive airway pressure. *Chest* 106(2):540–544, 1994.
54. Leung P, Jubran A, Tobin MJ: Comparison of assisted ventilator modes on triggering, patient effort, and dyspnea. *Am J Respir Crit Care Med* 155(6):1940–1948, 1997.
55. Jubran A, Van de Graaff WB, Tobin MJ: Variability of patient–ventilator interaction with pressure support ventilation in patients with chronic obstructive pulmonary disease. *Am J Respir Crit Care Med* 152(1):129–136, 1995.
56. Puddy A, Younes M: Effect of inspiratory flow rate on respiratory output in normal subjects. *Am Rev Respir Dis* 146(3):787–789, 1992.
57. Laghi F, Karamchandani K, Tobin MJ: Influence of ventilator settings in determining respiratory frequency during mechanical ventilation. *Am J Respir Crit Care Med* 160(5, Pt 1):1766–1770, 1999.

SECTION III ■ CARDIOVASCULAR PROBLEMS AND CORONARY CARE

AKSHAY S. DESAI • PATRICK T. O'GARA

CHAPTER 32 ■ APPROACH TO THE PATIENT WITH HYPOTENSION AND HEMODYNAMIC INSTABILITY

MICHAEL M. GIVERTZ AND JAMES C. FANG

Hypotension and hemodynamic instability are frequently encountered clinical problems in the intensive care setting. When the mean arterial blood pressure falls below approximately 60 mm Hg, end-organ perfusion becomes compromised and is manifested clinically as cool skin, decreased urine output, and altered mental status. Cornerstones of management include volume resuscitation and therapy directed toward the underlying cause of hypotension (e.g., cardiac pacing for bradycardia, cardioversion or defibrillation for tachyarrhythmias, blood transfusion for gastrointestinal bleeding, corticosteroids for adrenal insufficiency). When these measures fail to restore blood pressure and vital organ perfusion or while awaiting their availability, administration of intravenous vasoactive agents may be necessary. This chapter reviews the general management of the hypotensive patient with an emphasis on coronary care and the pharmacologic properties of commonly used vasopressor and positive inotropic agents. An overview of shock (see Chapter 157), volume resuscitation (see Chapter 158), sepsis (see Chapter 159), the use of intra-aortic balloon counterpulsation and mechanical circulatory support devices (see Chapter 45) are discussed elsewhere.

GENERAL APPROACH TO THE HYPOTENSIVE PATIENT IN THE CORONARY CARE UNIT

The assessment of the hypotensive patient begins with accurate measurement of the blood pressure and rapid correlation with clinical signs of hypoperfusion. Blood pressure should be measured in both arms and confirmed by another examiner. This practice is especially important when automated devices are used to make these measurements in the setting of tachyarrhythmias or respiratory distress. In patients with peripheral arterial disease, upper extremity blood pressure should also be compared to measurements in the legs in the supine position. In rare circumstances, true central aortic pressure may differ significantly from peripherally obtained blood pressures and can only be confirmed by invasive measurement during diagnostic catheterization. This situation should be suspected when clinical features of hypoperfusion do not accompany low blood pressure.

Hypotension is generally defined as a mean arterial pressure of less than 60 mm Hg and/or a systolic blood pressure less than 100 mm Hg. However, higher values may be consistent with clinically relevant hypotension if there are concomitant clinical signs of hypoperfusion such as mental confusion, oliguria, pallor, and cool extremities. If clinically relevant hypotension cannot be rapidly corrected, invasive monitoring with an arterial line should be considered, especially if vasoactive medications are employed. Central venous catheterization should also be considered to monitor intravascular volume, since volume status is often dynamic in the hypotensive patient and multiple mechanisms of hypotension may be simultaneously present. Foley catheterization should also be employed to assess hourly urine output as a surrogate for end-organ perfusion.

The history and physical examination should be directed toward establishing the primary mechanism and etiology of hypotension. Primary mechanisms include hypovolemia, low cardiac output, and vasodilation. Assessing volume status is critical; if not discernible from the bedside evaluation (jugular venous pressure, skin turgor, urine output, orthostasis), invasive measurement of the central venous pressure should be obtained with placement of a central venous catheter. If there are clinical reasons to suggest a dissociation of right and left ventricular hemodynamics (i.e., right ventricular infarction), pulmonary artery catheterization may be required to measure the left ventricular filling pressure. Warm well-perfused skin and extremities despite hypotension may suggest low systemic vascular resistance and a vasodilatory state, whereas cool clammy skin and extremities suggest vasoconstriction as a compensatory response to a low output syndrome. A narrow pulse pressure may also suggest reduced cardiac output. If a putative mechanism of hypotension cannot be ascertained from bedside assessment, pulmonary artery catheterization can be used to characterize the hemodynamic profile. This strategy is especially useful when more than one mechanism is present (for example, a large myocardial infarction complicated by pneumonia, leading to cardiogenic and vasodilatory shock).

Initial management strategies are directed at the primary etiology of hypotension and addressed later in this chapter. In general, therapy is guided by the primary pathophysiologic mechanism underlying the hypotension (e.g., volume resuscitation for hypovolemia, positive inotropes for low cardiac output, vasopressors for vasoplegia). The pace and aggressiveness of therapeutic intervention are guided by the presence or absence of clinical signs of hypoperfusion. For example, holding vasodilators may be sufficient in the hypotensive patient without changes in mental status or urine output. In contrast, the acutely hypotensive patient with clinical shock needs rapid resuscitation with intravascular volume expansion and usually vasoactive therapy.

ADRENERGIC RECEPTOR PHYSIOLOGY

Most vasopressor and positive inotropic agents currently available for use are sympathomimetic amines that exert their action by binding to and stimulating adrenergic receptors. To better understand the similarities and differences among these agents, a basic knowledge of adrenergic receptor distribution and function is required [1].

The adrenergic receptors that are most relevant to the management of hypotension are the α_1, β_1, and β_2 receptors. α_1-Adrenergic receptors are present in smooth muscle cells of many vascular beds, including the arterioles supplying the skin, mucosa, skeletal muscle, and kidneys, as well as the peripheral veins. α_1-Adrenergic stimulation causes vasoconstriction and is the most common mechanism of vasopressor action. The presence of α_1 receptors has also been demonstrated in the myocardium, where stimulation appears to result in a positive inotropic effect with little change in heart rate. β_1-Adrenergic receptors are the predominant adrenergic receptor type in the heart and they mediate positive inotropic, chronotropic and lusitropic responses. Stimulation of β_2-adrenergic receptors causes relaxation of smooth muscle cells in bronchial, gastrointestinal, and uterine muscle, as well as vasodilation in skeletal muscle. β_3-adrenergic receptors, which are located mainly in adipose tissue, are involved in the regulation of lipolysis and thermogenesis and do not play a role in hemodynamic stability. Other relevant receptors are the dopaminergic receptors (DA_1 and DA_2), which mediate renal, coronary, cerebral, and mesenteric vasodilation, and cause a natriuretic response.

The receptor selectivity of sympathomimetic amines can be drug and dose dependent. For example, β_2 receptors are more sensitive to epinephrine than are α_1 receptors. Thus, at low doses of epinephrine, the vasodilatory effect of β_2 receptors predominates, whereas at high doses, α_1-mediated vasoconstriction overcomes the β_2 effect and increases systemic vascular resistance. The dose-dependent actions of dopamine have also been well established.

The overall clinical effects of vasoactive agents depend not only on the outcome of direct adrenergic receptor stimulation, but also on the reflex response of homeostatic forces. For example, stimulation of β_1-adrenergic receptors by norepinephrine would be expected to cause an increase in heart rate; however, norepinephrine-mediated α_1-adrenergic stimulation induces a reflex increase in vagal tone that cancels out its positive chronotropic effects. The action of some drugs (e.g., dopamine and ephedrine) is further complicated by their ability to stimulate release of stored endogenous catecholamines.

COMMONLY USED VASOPRESSORS AND POSITIVE INOTROPES

The armamentarium of vasoactive agents has changed little since the 1980s. Commonly used drugs with vasopressor activity are dopamine, epinephrine, norepinephrine, phenylephrine, and ephedrine. Vasopressin is a newer alternative to adrenergic vasopressors. Agents with positive inotropic activity that are useful for the treatment of hypotension include dobutamine, dopamine, epinephrine, and isoproterenol. Table 32.1 summarizes the receptor activity and hemodynamic effects of these drugs.

Dopamine

Dopamine is an endogenous catecholamine that functions as a central neurotransmitter and a synthetic precursor of norepinephrine and epinephrine. When administered intravenously, the effects of dopamine are mediated by dose-dependent stimulation of dopaminergic and adrenergic receptors, and by stimulation of norepinephrine release from nerve terminals.

At low doses (less than 5 μg per kg per minute), dopamine predominantly stimulates dopaminergic receptors in renal, mesenteric, and coronary vessels with minimal adrenergic effects. In normal subjects, so-called renal-dose dopamine augments renal blood flow, glomerular filtration rate, and natriuresis, with little effect on blood pressure. Low-dose dopamine has frequently been used by itself or in combination with other drugs as a renoprotective agent. However, the efficacy and safety of this strategy remain controversial [2]. Although a recent study demonstrated renal vasodilatory effects of dopamine in patients with heart failure [3], a randomized placebo-controlled trial in 328 critically ill patients with evidence of early renal dysfunction demonstrated no protective effect of low-dose dopamine on renal function and no difference in ICU or hospital length of stay [4]. Moderate doses of dopamine (5 to 10 μg per kg per minute) stimulate β_1-adrenergic receptors in the myocardium, augmenting cardiac output by increasing contractility and, to a lesser extent, heart rate (Fig. 32.1). In addition, venoconstriction mediated by serotonin and dopaminergic receptors may occur [5]. At higher doses (greater than 10 μg per kg per minute), α_1-adrenergic

TABLE 32.1

DOSE RANGE, RECEPTOR ACTIVITY, AND PREDOMINANT HEMODYNAMIC EFFECTS OF VASOACTIVE DRUGS COMMONLY USED TO TREAT HYPOTENSION

Drug	Dose range	Dopaminergic	α_1	β_1	β_2	Heart rate	Cardiac output	Systemic vascular resistance
Dobutamine	2.5–20 μg/kg/min	–	+	+++	++	↔↑	↑↑	↓
Dopamine	1–5 μg/kg/min	+++	–	–	–	↔	↔	↔
	5–10 μg/kg/min	++	+	++	–	↑	↑↑	↔↑
	10–20 μg/kg/min	++	+++	++	–	↑↑	↔↑	↑↑
Epinephrine	1–10 μg/min	–	+++	++	++	↑↑	↑	↑↑
Isoproterenol	2–10 μg/min	–	–	+++	+++	↑↑	↑↑	↓
Norepinephrine	0.5–30 μg/min	–	+++	++	–	↔	↔	↑↑
Phenylephrine	40–180 μg/min	–	+++	–	–	↔	↔	↑↑
Ephedrine	10–25 mg IV q5–10 min	–	++	++	++	↑	↔	↑↑
Vasopressin	0.01–0.05 U min	–	–	–	–	↔	↔↓	↑↑

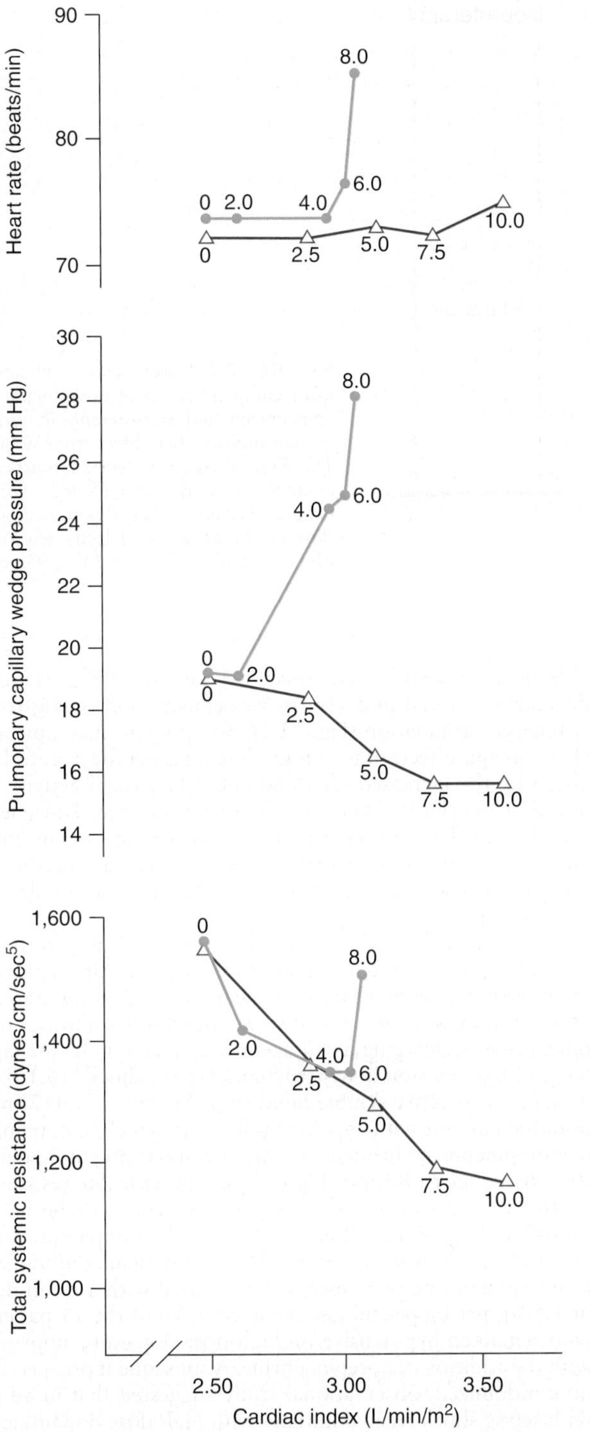

FIGURE 32.1. Comparative effects of dopamine (*closed circles*) and dobutamine (*open triangles*) on heart rate, pulmonary capillary wedge pressure, and total systemic resistance in patients with advanced heart failure. The numbers shown on the figures are infusion rates in μg per kg per minute. These data demonstrate that dopamine at doses greater than 2 to 4 μg/kg/min exerts a vasoconstrictor effect and increases heart rate and left ventricular filling pressure. [Adapted from Leier CV, Heban PT, Huss P, et al: Comparative systemic and regional hemodynamic effects of dopamine and dobutamine in patients with cardiomyopathic heart failure. *Circulation* 58:466–475, 1978, with permission.]

receptor stimulation predominates, resulting in systemic arteriolar vasoconstriction. The overall effects of dopamine at the highest doses resemble those of norepinephrine (see later). However, it should be remembered that there is a great deal of overlap in the dose-dependent effects of dopamine in critically ill patients [1,2].

Moderate- to high-dose dopamine is a mainstay in the treatment of hypotension. In studies of fluid-resuscitated patients with septic shock, dopamine produced a mean increase in mean arterial pressure of approximately 25%, primarily owing to an increase in cardiac index and, to a lesser extent, systemic vascular resistance [2]. In the setting of hyperdynamic septic shock when excessive vasodilation is the primary source of hypotension, addition or substitution of a more potent α-adrenergic agonist such as norepinephrine may be more effective. Moreover, evidence of worsening splanchnic oxygen utilization with the use of high-dose dopamine has made it a less attractive agent.

By itself or in combination with other agents, dopamine may be used at moderate doses in the management of patients with acute decompensated heart failure and hypotension. Venodilating agents (e.g., nitroprusside and nitroglycerin) may be added to moderate the tendency of dopamine to increase cardiac-filling pressures [6]. Dopamine may also be combined with dobutamine for added inotropic effects or used at low doses to augment diuresis [7], although the benefits of "renal-dose" dopamine remain controversial and other agents may be more effective for preserving renal function in critically ill patients [8].

The use of dopamine is associated with several adverse effects, including tachycardia, tachyarrhythmias, and excessive vasoconstriction. Although these effects are generally dose dependent, in individual patients there may be substantial overlap of receptor affinity such that even at low doses dopamine may result in toxicity. In patients with ischemic heart disease, increased myocardial oxygen consumption coupled with some degree of coronary vasoconstriction with high-dose dopamine can result in myocardial ischemia. As with other positive inotropes, dopamine can increase flow to poorly oxygenated regions of the lung and cause shunting and hypoxemia. In addition, dopamine has been shown to depress minute ventilation in normoxic heart failure patients [9]. When dopamine is used in patients with acute decompensated heart failure, increased venous tone and pulmonary arterial pressure may exacerbate pulmonary edema in the setting of already high cardiac filling pressures. Despite these caveats, oxygen saturation generally remains constant due to improved hemodynamics.

There is mounting evidence that dopamine adversely effects splanchnic perfusion at doses usually required to treat septic shock. A small, randomized study of patients with sepsis using selective splanchnic and hepatic cannulation showed that infusion of dopamine was associated with a disproportionate increase in splanchnic oxygen delivery compared with oxygen extraction (65% vs. 16%). In contrast, norepinephrine produced better-matched increases in oxygen delivery and extraction (33% vs. 28%) [10]. Another study showed that in patients with septic shock randomly assigned to treatment with norepinephrine or dopamine, gastric intramucosal pH worsened significantly in patients treated with dopamine despite similar improvements in mean arterial pressure [11]. Thus, the use of dopamine in septic shock may be associated with splanchnic shunting, impairment of gastric mucosal oxygenation, and increased risk of gastrointestinal bleeding [2].

Epinephrine

Epinephrine is an endogenous catecholamine that is a potent nonselective agonist of α- and β-adrenergic receptors.

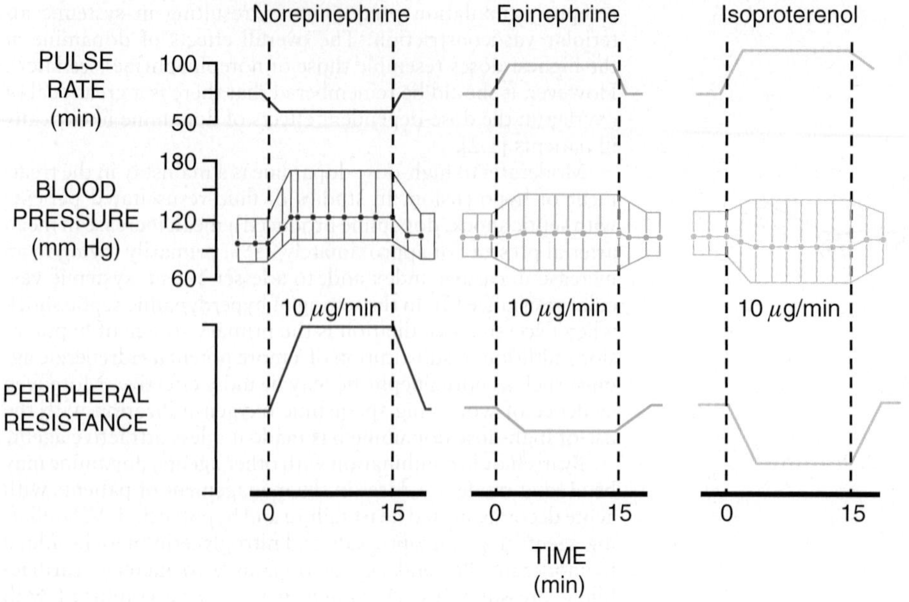

FIGURE 32.2. Cardiovascular effects of intravenous infusions of norepinephrine, epinephrine, and isoproterenol in normal human subjects. [Modified from Westfall TC, Westfall DP: Adrenergic agonists and antagonists, in Brunton LL (ed): *Goodman & Gilman's The Pharmacological Basis of Therapeutics*. 11th ed. New York, McGraw-Hill, 2005, pp 237–295, with permission.]

Stimulation of myocardial β_1 and β_2 receptors increases contractility and heart rate, resulting in a rise in cardiac output (Fig. 32.2). Cardiac output is further augmented by an increase in venous return as a result of α_1-mediated venoconstriction. Blood flow to skeletal muscles is increased owing to β_2-mediated vasodilation. With very low-dose infusions of epinephrine (0.01 to 0.05 μg per kg per minute), β-adrenergic–mediated positive chronotropic and inotropic effects predominate. Diastolic blood pressure and overall peripheral vascular resistance may actually decrease owing to vasodilation in skeletal muscle. With higher doses of epinephrine, stimulation of α-adrenergic receptors in precapillary resistance vessels of the skin, mucosa, and kidneys outweighs β_2-mediated vasodilation in skeletal muscle, causing increased mean and systolic blood pressure [1].

Epinephrine plays a central role in cardiovascular resuscitation (see Chapter 23) and the management of anaphylaxis (see Chapter 194). Epinephrine is also used to reverse hypotension with or without bradycardia after cardiopulmonary bypass or cardiac transplantation [12]. Because of its adverse effects on splanchnic and renal blood flow and potential for inducing myocardial ischemia and tachyarrhythmias, epinephrine has generally been regarded as a second-line agent in the management of septic shock [2,13]. However, a recent randomized trial showed no difference in efficacy or safety between epinephrine alone versus norepinephrine plus dobutamine in patients with septic shock [14]. For patients with symptomatic bradycardia and hypotension who have failed atropine or external pacing, epinephrine may be used to stabilize the patient while awaiting more definitive therapy (e.g., transvenous placement of a temporary or permanent pacemaker) [15]. When used to treat hypotension, epinephrine is given as a continuous infusion starting at a low dose (0.5 to 1.0 μg per minute) and titrating up to 10 μg per minute as needed. Continuous infusions of epinephrine may cause restlessness, tremor, headache, and palpitations. Epinephrine should be avoided in patients taking β-adrenergic antagonists, as unopposed α-adrenergic vasoconstriction may cause severe hypertension and cerebral hemorrhage.

Norepinephrine

Norepinephrine is an endogenous catecholamine that is a potent β_1- and α_1-adrenergic agonist, with little β_2 activity. The main cardiovascular effect of norepinephrine is dose-dependent arterial and venous vasoconstriction owing to α-adrenergic stimulation (Fig. 32.2). The positive inotropic and chronotropic effects of β_1 stimulation are generally counterbalanced by the increased afterload and reflex vagal activity induced by the elevated systemic vascular resistance. Thus, heart rate and cardiac output usually do not change significantly, although cardiac output may increase or decrease depending on vascular resistance, left ventricular function, and reflex responses [5].

Norepinephrine, when infused at doses ranging from 0.5 to 30.0 μg per minute, is a potent vasopressor. Although generally reserved as a second-line agent or used in addition to other vasopressors in cases of severe distributive shock, norepinephrine is emerging as an agent of choice for the management of hypotension in hyperdynamic septic shock [14,16]. In a small, prospective double-blind trial, Martin et al. [17] randomized patients with hyperdynamic septic shock to dopamine or norepinephrine titrated to a mean arterial pressure greater than or equal to 80 mm Hg or systemic vascular resistance greater than 1,100 dynes per second per cm^{-5}, or both. Although only 5 of 16 patients randomized to dopamine were able to achieve these endpoints, 15 of 16 patients randomized to norepinephrine were successfully treated with a mean dose of 1.5 μg per kg per minute. Moreover, 10 of the 11 patients who remained hypotensive on high-dose dopamine improved with the addition of norepinephrine. A subsequent prospective, nonrandomized, observational study suggested that in adults with septic shock treated initially with high-dose dopamine or norepinephrine, the use of norepinephrine was associated with improved survival [18]. In the setting of sepsis, norepinephrine improves renal blood flow and urine output [19], although large doses may be required to achieve these effects due to α-receptor downregulation [2].

Adverse effects of norepinephrine include increased myocardial oxygen consumption causing ischemia and renal and mesenteric vasoconstriction. Renal ischemia, may be of particular concern in patients with hemorrhagic shock. Norepinephrine can also cause necrosis and sloughing at the site of intravenous injection owing to drug extravasation. Norepinephrine is relatively contraindicated in patients with hypovolemia. As previously discussed, the overall effect of norepinephrine on gut mucosal oxygenation in septic patients compares favorably with that of high-dose dopamine.

Phenylephrine

Phenylephrine is a synthetic sympathomimetic amine that selectively stimulates α_1-adrenergic receptors. When administered intravenously, phenylephrine causes dose-dependent arterial vasoconstriction and increases peripheral vascular resistance. As blood pressure rises, activation of vagal reflexes causes slowing of the heart rate.

Phenylephrine, infused at 40 to 180 μg per minute, is commonly used in the management of anesthesia-induced hypotension [20,21] and hyperdynamic septic shock. Its rapid onset of action, short duration, and primary vascular effects make it an ideal agent for treating hemodynamically unstable patients in the intensive care setting. However, there are few data regarding its relative efficacy compared with older vasopressors such as norepinephrine and dopamine. In one small study of fluid-resuscitated patients with septic shock, the addition of phenylephrine to dobutamine or dopamine increased mean arterial pressure and systemic vascular resistance without a change in heart rate [22]. In addition, urine output improved while serum creatinine remained stable. The absence of β-adrenergic agonist activity at usual doses (phenylephrine activates β receptors only at much higher doses) makes phenylephrine an attractive agent for the management of hypotension in clinical situations where tachycardia or tachyarrhythmias, or both, limit the use of other agents [2]. As with other vasopressors, high-dose phenylephrine may cause excessive vasoconstriction. In addition, patients with poor ventricular function may not tolerate the increased afterload induced by α_1-stimulation [22]. Compared to epinephrine and norepinephrine, phenylephrine is less likely to decrease microcirculatory blood flow in the gastrointestinal tract [23].

Ephedrine

Ephedrine is a naturally occurring sympathomimetic amine derived from plants. Its pharmacologic action results from direct nonselective activation of adrenergic receptors, as well as stimulation of norepinephrine release from storage sites. Although ephedrine is less potent and longer acting (half-life, 3 to 6 hours) than epinephrine, its hemodynamic profile is similar and includes cardiac stimulation and peripheral vasoconstriction.

Ephedrine is rarely used in the critical care setting except in the temporary treatment of hypotension induced by spinal anesthesia [20]. Ephedrine does not appear to compromise uterine blood flow and is considered by some to be the vasopressor of choice in the treatment of anesthesia-induced hypotension in the obstetric patient [24]. However, prophylactic use in pregnant woman undergoing Caesarian section is not recommended as it may cause hypertension and tachycardia [25]. Ephedrine can be administered in doses of 10 to 25 mg, given as an intravenous bolus every 5 to 10 minutes, with the total dose not to exceed 150 mg in 24 hours. In healthy women undergoing elective cesarean delivery that develop hypotension, pharmacogenomic data suggests that β_2-adrenoceptor genotype may affect dose requirements [26]. Adverse effects of ephedrine include myocardial ischemia and excessive vasoconstriction.

Isoproterenol

Isoproterenol is a synthetic sympathomimetic amine with potent nonselective β-adrenergic activity and little effect on α-adrenergic receptors. Its major cardiovascular effect is increased cardiac output owing to direct positive inotropic and chronotropic effects (Fig. 32.2). Isoproterenol also increases heart rate by increasing atrioventricular nodal conduction. Systemic and pulmonary vascular resistances decrease owing to β_2-mediated vasodilation in skeletal muscle and pulmonary vasculature, respectively. Reduced peripheral resistance typically causes a fall in mean arterial and diastolic blood pressure, whereas systolic blood pressure is unchanged or rises modestly owing to increased cardiac output. Coronary blood flow remains unchanged, which in the face of increased myocardial oxygen demand can produce ischemia in patients with ischemic heart disease. In addition, stimulation of myocardial β_2-receptors can cause arrhythmias via increased dispersion of repolarization [27].

Stimulation of β-adrenergic receptors in the heart by isoproterenol increases the risk of excessive tachycardia, tachyarrhythmias, and myocardial ischemia. Given the likelihood of toxicity and the availability of alternative drugs, isoproterenol is no longer used as an inotropic agent; rather, its use is limited to the temporary treatment of hemodynamically significant bradycardia unresponsive to atropine while awaiting more definitive treatment with an external or transvenous pacemaker. The starting infusion rate for isoproterenol is 1 μg per minute, and this can be titrated up to 10 μg per minute to achieve the desired response (e.g., for bradycardia, titrated to a heart rate of 60 beats per minute or higher, depending on the blood pressure response). Other uses for isoproterenol include "chemical" overdrive pacing for torsades de pointes refractory to magnesium [28], and temporary inotropic and chronotropic support after cardiac transplantation [29]. Side effects of isoproterenol include palpitations, headache, flushing, and rarely paradoxical bradycardia [30].

Dobutamine

Dobutamine is a synthetic sympathomimetic amine that was derived from isoproterenol in an attempt to create a less arrhythmogenic positive inotrope with minimal vascular effects. Although initially thought to be a selective β_1-adrenergic agonist, its mechanism of action appears to be more complex. Dobutamine is available for clinical use as a mixture of two enantiomeric forms with different pharmacologic properties. Ruffolo et al. [31] showed that although both stereoisomers are nonselective β-agonists, the positive isomer is several times more potent. In addition, the two isomers have opposing effects on α-adrenergic receptors: the positive isomer is an α-antagonist and the negative isomer is a potent α_1-agonist. The overall effect of the racemic mixture is potent nonselective β- and mild α-adrenergic stimulation [31].

Cardiac contractile force is enhanced by β_1- and α-adrenergic stimulation. Heart rate may also increase, but to a lesser extent than occurs with isoproterenol or dopamine (Fig. 32.1). In contrast to dopamine, dobutamine decreases cardiac filling pressures, making it a preferred agent in the treatment of patients with acute decompensated heart failure [32]. Systemic vascular resistance is modestly reduced or may remain unchanged, as α_1-mediated vasoconstriction is counterbalanced by β_2-mediated vasodilation and reflex withdrawal of sympathetic tone that typically occurs in response to increased cardiac output. Dobutamine has no effect on dopaminergic receptors; however, renal blood flow often increases in proportion to the increase in cardiac output [33].

Dobutamine, by itself or in combination with other vasoactive drugs, is useful in the temporary support of myocardial function in patients with hypotension and poor end-organ perfusion, including those with acute decompensated heart failure as well as patients with concomitant septic shock and depressed cardiac function. In patients with cardiogenic shock, the effect of dobutamine on systemic vascular resistance and blood pressure is difficult to predict. Therefore, when used in this setting, it is often administered in combination with dopamine [7].

Dobutamine is generally initiated at an infusion rate of 2 μg per kg per minute and can be titrated up to 15 μg per kg per minute or higher to achieve the desired hemodynamic or clinical effects, or both. Side effects that may limit dose titration include increased heart rate and exacerbation of supraventricular and ventricular arrhythmias. As with other positive inotropic agents, increased myocardial oxygen consumption can worsen cardiac ischemia, and short-term dobutamine therapy has been associated with excess mortality [34]. Although systolic and mean arterial blood pressures typically increase, hypotension may occur if dobutamine is administered to a volume-depleted patient. Some patients with advanced heart failure may be resistant to dobutamine owing to β-receptor hyporesponsiveness or may develop tolerance after several days of a continuous infusion [35]. Chronic dobutamine therapy may also cause an eosinophilic or hypersensitivity myocarditis [36], leading to further hemodynamic deterioration.

Vasopressin

Arginine vasopressin, an antidiuretic hormone, has emerged as a potential alternative to adrenergic vasopressors for the treatment of refractory vasodilatory shock. The mechanism of action of vasopressin has not been fully elucidated, but likely involves binding to V_1 receptors on vascular smooth muscle cells. Although it has minimal pressor activity in normal subjects, vasopressin has been shown to improve blood pressure in patients with sepsis [37] and in patients with vasodilatory shock after cardiopulmonary bypass [38] (Table 32.2). In these initial studies, vasopressin was initiated at a dose of 0.1 U per minute; for subjects maintaining a mean arterial pressure greater than 70 mm Hg, vasopressin was tapered to 0.01 U per minute and then discontinued. Notably, many patients in these studies were poorly responsive to intravenous catecholamine support and had inappropriately low vasopressin levels before treatment consistent with a defect in baroreflex-mediated vasopressin secretion. It remains unclear, however, whether the benefits of vasopressin are confined to patients with relative vasopressin deficiency, hypersensitivity, or both.

Russell et al. [39] randomized 778 patients with septic shock who were receiving a minimum of 5 μg per minute of norepinephrine to receive either low-dose vasopressin (0.01 to 0.03 U per minute) or norepinephrine (5 to 15 μg per minute) in addition to open-label vasopressors. After 28 days, there was no significant difference in mortality rates between the vasopressin and norepinephrine groups (35.4% and 39.3%, respectively; $p = 0.26$) (Fig. 32.3). However, in patients with less severe septic shock (prospectively defined as those receiving treatment with less than 15 μg per minute of norepinephrine), mortality was lower in the vasopressin group (26.5% vs. 35.7%, $p = 0.05$).

Vasopressin may also be effective in the treatment of cardiac arrest unresponsive to epinephrine and defibrillation [40]. Revised guidelines for advanced cardiovascular life support recommend vasopressin as an alternative to epinephrine for the treatment of adult shock-refractory ventricular fibrillation, as well as an adjunctive agent in the treatment of patients with vasodilatory shock, such as septic shock or sepsis syndrome, refractory to standard therapy [5]. A meta-analysis of cardiac arrest trials demonstrated no significant differences between vasopressin and epinephrine groups in failure of return of spontaneous circulation, death within 24 hours, or death before hospital discharge [41]. In a randomized clinical trial of 2,894 patients with out-of-hospital cardiac arrest receiving advanced cardiac life support, the combination of vasopressin (40 IU) and epinephrine (1 mg) did not improve outcomes compared to epinephrine alone: return of spontaneous circulation, 28.6% versus 29.5%; survival to hospital admission, 20.7% versus

TABLE 32.2

SUMMARY OF ADVANCES IN THE MANAGEMENT OF HYPOTENSION

- Vasopressin improves blood pressure in patients with sepsis [37] or vasodilatory shock after cardiopulmonary bypass [38].
- Methylene blue is effective for refractory hypotension following cardiopulmonary bypass [53] and may be useful in preventing vasoplegia in high-risk patients [54].
- Recombinant human activated protein C (drotrecogin alfa activated) is indicated for severe sepsis (Apache II score >25) in the absence of bleeding [2,55–57].
- Stress-dose steroids improve hemodynamics and may reduce mortality in septic shock if adrenocortical insufficiency is present [62]. Doses of hydrocortisone should not exceed 200–300 mg/day [2].

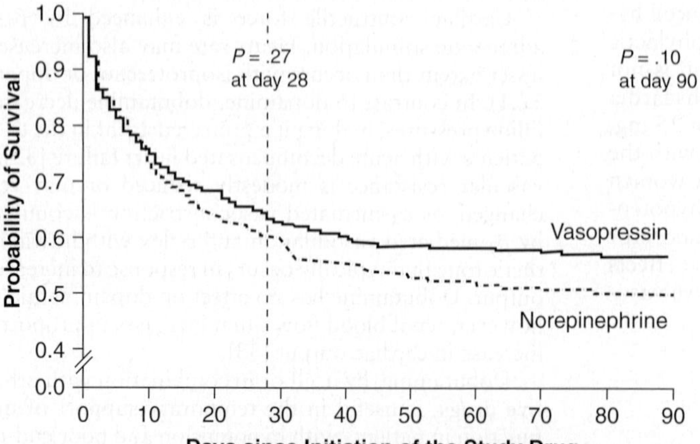

No. at Risk

Vasopressin	397	301	272	249	240	234	232	230	226	220
Norepinephrine	382	289	247	230	212	205	200	194	193	191

FIGURE 32.3. Kaplan–Meier survival curves for patients with septic shock randomized to vasopressin (*solid line*) or norepinephrine (*dashed line*). The dashed vertical line marks day 28. *P* values are calculated with use of the log rank test. [From Russell JA, Walley KR, Singer J, et al: Vasopressin versus norepinephrine infusion in patients with septic shock. *N Engl J Med* 358:877–887, 2008, with permission.]

21.3%; and survival to hospital discharge, 1.7% versus 2.3%; respectively [42]. In the setting of vasodilatory shock, vasopressin can be administered as a continuous infusion at 0.01 to 0.05 U per minute. Potential adverse effects of vasopressin include excess vasoconstriction causing end-organ ischemia including myocardial ischemia and hyponatremia. Cardiac output may also worsen owing to increased afterload.

Terlipressin is a synthetic long-acting analog of vasopressin that is currently undergoing clinical investigation [43]. In a recent pilot study of patients with septic shock despite adequate volume resuscitation, a continuous infusion of low-dose terlipressin (1.3 μg per kg per hour) was effective in reversing arterial hypotension and reducing catecholamine requirements [44]. Compared with vasopressin or norepinephrine, terlipressin was associated with less rebound hypotension upon discontinuation. Adverse effects associated with terlipressin include hypertension, bradycardia, skin pallor, and reduction in platelet count.

Adjunctive and Investigational Agents

In addition to the agents discussed previously, the phosphodiesterase inhibitor milrinone is commonly used in the management of acute decompensated heart failure. Milrinone increases cardiac contractility by directly inhibiting the breakdown of cyclic adenosine monophosphate, resulting in an increase in intracellular calcium [45]. In addition, phosphodiesterase inhibition in vascular smooth muscle causes systemic and pulmonary vasodilation [46]. Because milrinone does not require binding to adrenergic receptors to exert its effects, it is particularly useful in the treatment of patients taking β-adrenergic antagonists or those with advanced heart failure that may be resistant to β-agonist stimulation with dobutamine [35]. Milrinone is generally administered as an intravenous loading dose (50 μg per kg), followed by a continuous infusion at doses ranging from 0.25 to 0.75 μg per kg per minute. As it is renally excreted, milrinone should be dose-adjusted in renal failure; and in all patients, milrinone should be titrated cautiously, using invasive hemodynamic monitoring. Because it is a potent vasodilator, however, milrinone should be avoided in the treatment of patients with frank hypotension and is contraindicated in patients with severe aortic stenosis. Similarly, the use of levosimendan [47], a calcium sensitizer with phosphodiesterase and potassium channel inhibitor properties, may be limited by hypotension [48]. In a randomized, double-blind study of 1,327 patients with acute decompensated heart failure, intravenous levosimendan showed no benefit compared to dobutamine in reducing all-cause mortality at 180 days (26% vs. 28%, respectively; hazard ratio, 0.91; 95% confidence interval, 0.74 to 1.13; $p = 0.40$), and increased the incidence of atrial fibrillation [49]. Although approved for use in Europe, levosimendan remains investigational in the United States.

With the exception of vasopressin, all currently available vasopressors exert their action through stimulation of α-adrenergic receptors. This approach is often associated with worsening splanchnic perfusion, and in some patients may prove ineffective in restoring mean arterial pressure. Evidence of the central role of endothelium-derived nitric oxide (NO) in mediating vasodilation [50] led to the development of substances that interfere with NO production or activity. Several investigators have shown that analogs of L-arginine, the synthetic precursor of NO, can competitively inhibit the enzyme NO synthase, thereby decreasing NO production and increasing mean arterial pressure in patients with septic shock [51]. Others have shown that inhibition of guanylate cyclase, the target enzyme of NO, with methylene blue is effective in increasing mean arterial pressure, reducing the need for vasopressors and maintaining oxygen transport in septic shock [52]. Methylene blue has also been used successfully to treat refractory hypotension in patients with vasoplegia following cardiopulmonary bypass (Table 32.2) [53], and may be used to prevent vasoplegia in high-risk cardiac surgical patients [54]. However, the overall safety and efficacy of NO inhibition remains unproven. A large, randomized, placebo-controlled trial of the NO synthase inhibitor 546C88 in sepsis was stopped prematurely due to excess mortality at 28 days (59% vs. 49%, $p < 0.001$) in the active treatment arm [51]. As with adrenergic agents, lack of selectivity may have contributed to undesirable effects. More selective NO inhibitors are currently under investigation.

Another novel agent that has recently been approved for the treatment of patients with severe sepsis is recombinant human activated protein C (drotrecogin alfa activated) [55]. In the Recombinant Human Activated Protein C Worldwide Evaluation in Severe Sepsis study, 1,690 patients with systemic inflammation and organ failure owing to acute infection (71% of whom presented with shock) were randomized to receive drotrecogin alfa activated or placebo as a continuous infusion for 4 days [56]. Drotrecogin alfa activated reduced all-cause mortality by 19%, but tended to increase the risk of serious bleeding. Based on this study, drotrecogin alfa activated is recommended for the treatment of patients with severe sepsis and high risk of death (Apache II score greater than 25) (Table 32.2). The standard intravenous dosing is 24 μg per kg per hour for 96 hours, at a cost of approximately $6,000. In a subsequent study of patients with severe sepsis and low risk of death (Apache II score less than or equal to 25), there was no beneficial effect of drotrecogin alfa activated on either in-hospital or 28-day mortality [57]. The risk of serious bleeding was higher (2.4% vs. 1.2%, $p = 0.02$) in the drotrecogin alfa activated group. A randomized controlled study of drotrecogin alfa activated in children with severe sepsis also showed no benefit [58]. The 28-day mortality rates were 17.2% and 17.5% in the drotrecogin alfa activated and placebo groups, respectively ($p = 0.93$).

Several hormones including cortisol and thyroxine are known to play important roles in the maintenance of vascular tone, and their absolute or relative deficiency may contribute to hypotension in the critically ill patient. The adverse effects of hypothyroidism (see Chapter 103) and adrenal insufficiency (see Chapter 104) on central and peripheral hemodynamics have been well described. Although routine use of high-dose corticosteroids have not been shown to be beneficial in the treatment of sepsis, the administration of stress-dose steroids to patients suspected of having relative impairment of adrenocortical response may be helpful in restoring normal hemodynamics and improving outcomes.

In the 1990s, three small trials in patients with septic shock demonstrated decreased duration of shock with steroid treatment [59–61]. Subsequently, Annane et al. [62] randomized 300 patients with septic shock to receive hydrocortisone (50 mg intravenous bolus every 6 hours) and fludrocortisone (50 μg by mouth once daily) or matching placebos for 7 days. Patients were enrolled after undergoing a short corticotropin stimulation test. In the 229 nonresponders to corticotropin (i.e., with relative adrenal insufficiency), treatment with corticosteroids increased vasopressor withdrawal (57% vs. 40%, $p = 0.001$) and decreased mortality (53% vs. 63%, $p = 0.02$) at 28 days. There were no differences in outcomes between steroid and placebo groups in the corticotropin responders. Although this trial was criticized on both methodologic and clinical grounds, a subsequent meta-analysis (Fig. 32.4) showed that a 5- to 7-day course of physiologic hydrocortisone doses increased survival in patients with vasopressor-dependent septic shock [63].

In a more recent study, 499 patients with septic shock who remained hypotensive after fluid and vasopressor resuscitation were randomized to receive 50 mg of intravenous hydrocortisone or placebo every 6 hours for 5 days [64]. At 28 days, there was no significant difference in mortality between patients in

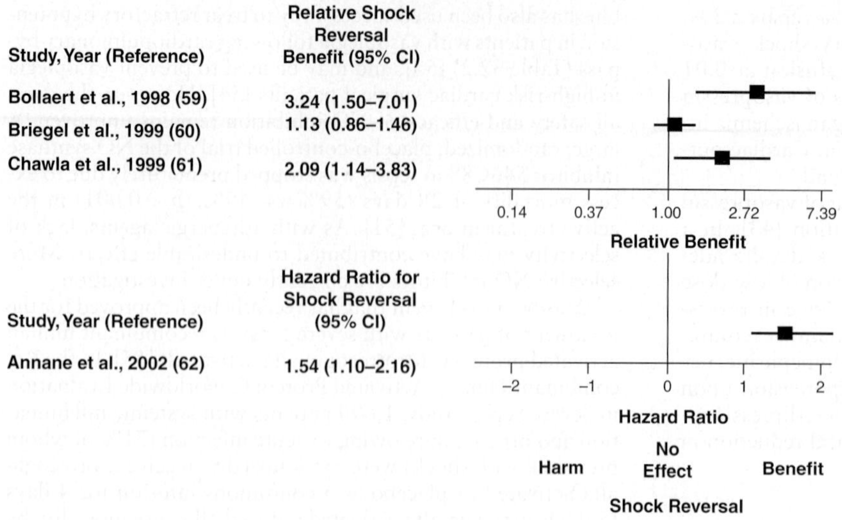

FIGURE 32.4. The relative benefit and hazard ratio (with 95% CI) of shock reversal for sepsis trials published after 1997. In three of the four trials, the discontinuation of vasopressor therapy with steroid treatment was significantly improved. [From Minneci PC, Deans KJ, Banks SM, et al: Meta-analysis: the effect of steroids on survival and shock during sepsis depends on the dose. *Ann Intern Med* 141:47–56, 2004, with permission.]

the two study groups whose plasma cortisol levels did not rise appropriately after administration of corticotropin (39.2% vs. 36.1% in the hydrocortisone and placebo groups, respectively; $p = 0.69$) or between those who had a response to corticotropin (28.8% vs. 28.7%, respectively; $p = 1.00$) (Fig. 32.5). As discussed previously, correction of relative vasopressin deficiency is an alternative or adjunctive therapeutic strategy in refractory shock.

Calcium

The routine use of intravenous calcium has been shown to have no benefit in the setting of cardiac arrest and may be detrimental by causing cellular injury [4]. Indications for acute calcium administration in the hypotensive patient include correction of clinically significant hyperkalemia (e.g., with acute kidney injury) or hypocalcemia (e.g., following multiple blood transfusions) and as an antidote to calcium channel blocker or beta-blocker overdose [65]. Calcium chloride (100 mg per mL in a 10-mL vial) is usually given as a slow intravenous push of 5 to 10 mL, and may be repeated as needed. Rapid intravenous administration of calcium may cause bradycardia or asystole particularly in patients receiving digoxin. In critically ill patients, ionized calcium rather than total calcium concentration should be followed.

CHOOSING AN AGENT

There are few large, randomized, well-controlled studies to guide the pharmacologic management of hypotension. The use of vasopressors and positive inotropes is generally based on data from animal studies and small, often poorly controlled clinical trials. Useful consensus recommendations can be found in the recently revised Advanced Cardiovascular Life Support guidelines [5] and the international guidelines for management of severe sepsis and septic shock updated in 2008 [2].

The selection of the appropriate vasoactive agent can be individualized with attention to the known or suspected underlying cause of hypotension (Table 32.3). However, the clinician is commonly faced with a patient who presents with life-threatening hypotension of unknown etiology. In this setting, it may be necessary to initiate a vasopressor as a temporizing measure even before the adequacy of intravascular volume repletion can be ensured. Consensus guidelines and expert panels recommend both dopamine and norepinephrine as first-line vasopressor agents. Although dopamine in moderate to high doses can provide both positive inotropic and vasopressor effects, arrhythmias may be provoked (see discussion of SOAP II later). For severe hypotension (systolic blood pressure less than 70 mm Hg), a more potent α_1-adrenergic agonist such as norepinephrine should be considered.

For the hypotensive patient with significant cardiac pump dysfunction (cardiac index less than 2.2 L per minute per m^2 associated with end-organ dysfunction), dobutamine should be considered. Milrinone is often not tolerated in this situation due to its vasodilating properties. With frank cardiogenic shock and concomitant vasoplegia, a drug with pressor action is usually needed. In this setting, vasopressin and norepinephrine can be used in combination with dobutamine. Rarely, epinephrine may be required. In patients with septic shock and related myocardial dysfunction, dobutamine can be added for additional inotropic support. Although dopamine is also often considered in such situations for its combined inotropic and pressor properties there has been recent concern of increased mortality when compared to norepinephrine in a subgroup of patients with cardiogenic shock in the recent SOAP II trial (see later).

Given the superior potency of norepinephrine and evidence of worsening splanchnic perfusion with high-dose dopamine, norepinephrine is emerging as the agent of choice for vasodilatory shock in sepsis [16]. Although in the landmark Sepsis Occurrence in Acutely Ill Patients (SOAP) II trial, there was no difference between the initial use of dopamine versus norepinephrine for shock in 28 day all-cause mortality, dopamine was associated with more adverse events, particularly atrial fibrillation [66]. Dopamine may be used as an alternate agent or in cases in which positive inotropic effects are desirable. Current experience with phenylephrine is insufficient to assess its efficacy relative to older agents, although its peripheral selectivity and lack of positive chronotropic effects make it a theoretically useful agent in cases in which tachycardia, tachyarrhythmias, or both limit the use of other drugs. Epinephrine is the least selective of the catecholamines and is occasionally added for refractory septic shock. Vasopressin is emerging as an alternative to adrenergic agents, but its use for hypotension may be limited to patients with hemodynamic collapse that is resistant to adequate fluid resuscitation and high-dose conventional vasopressors. For patients at high risk of death from sepsis (APACHE II score greater than 25) and low bleeding risk, recombinant human activated protein C is recommended [2,55]. For patients refractory to multiple pressors, including those status post cardiopulmonary bypass, a trial of methylene blue should be considered [52,53].

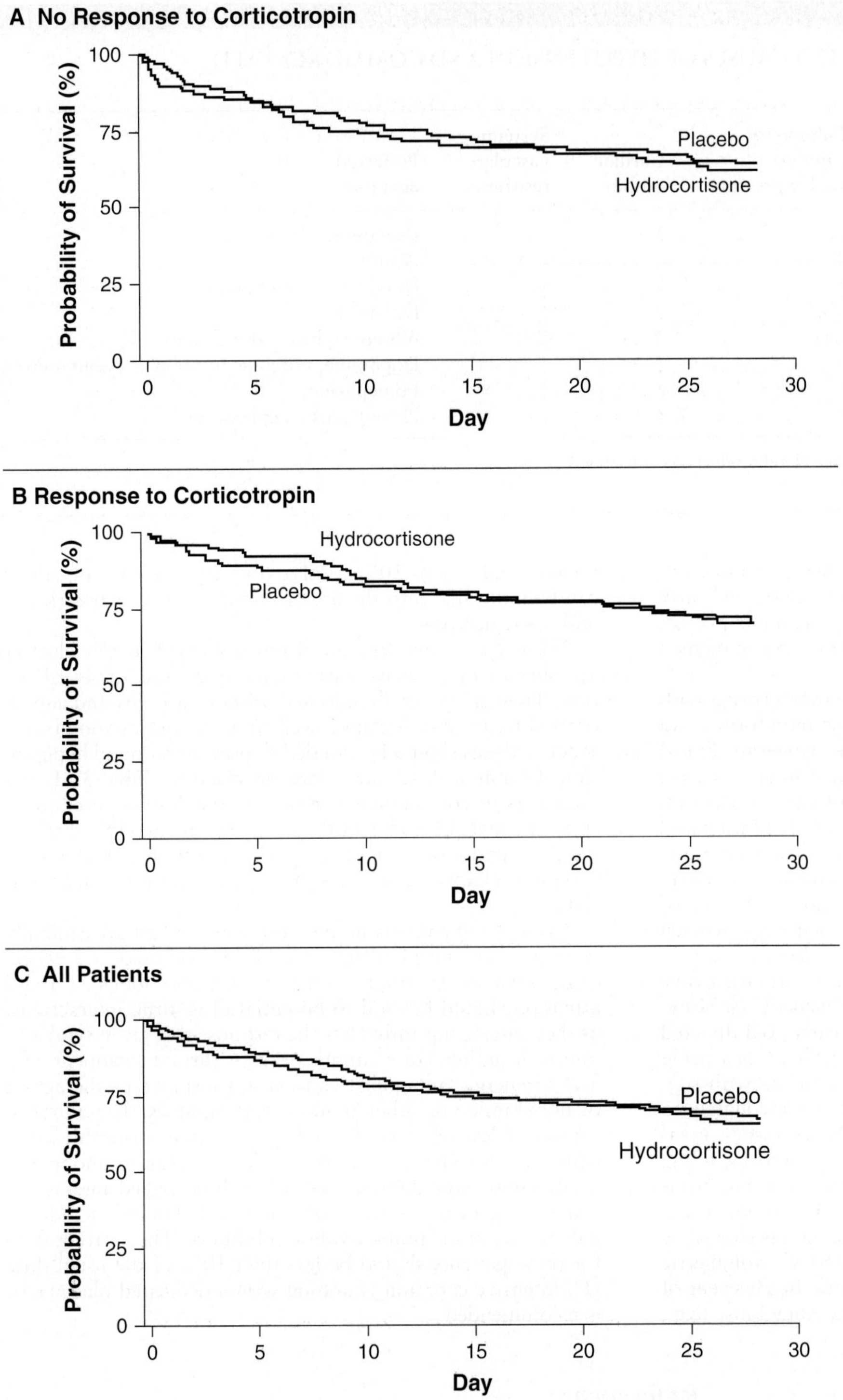

FIGURE 32.5. Shown are Kaplan–Meier curves for survival at 28 days comparing patients with septic shock who received hydrocortisone versus placebo. There was no difference among patients who did not have a response to a corticotropin test (*Panel A*), those who had a response to corticotropin (*Panel B*) and all patients randomized (*Panel C*). [From Sprung CL, Annane D, Keh D, et al: Hydrocortisone therapy for patients with septic shock. *N Engl J Med* 358: 111–124, 2008, with permission.]

CLINICAL USE OF VASOACTIVE DRUGS

In the volume-resuscitated patient with persistent hypotension, vasoactive medications are administered with the goal of improving arterial pressure while avoiding myocardial ischemia, arrhythmias, and excess vasoconstriction. Although a mean arterial blood pressure of greater than 60 mm Hg is usually adequate to maintain autoregulatory blood flow to vital organs [67], some patients may require considerably higher pressures. Therefore, it is essential to use other indicators of global and regional perfusion in addition to the mean arterial pressure to guide therapy. Altered mental status, oliguria, and cool skin are important clinical signs of poor perfusion, but are somewhat nonspecific. The clinical use of mixed venous oxygen saturation and serum lactate level, as well as intramucosal pH monitoring by gastric tonometry remains unproven [2]. Although some clinicians have advocated achieving "supranormal" levels of oxygen delivery in the treatment of critically ill patients, this approach is controversial [68], and adverse effects of hyperoxia have been demonstrated on coronary blood flow and myocardial function in patients with coronary artery disease [69] and heart failure [70], respectively. A meta-analysis in critically ill

TABLE 32.3

HEMODYNAMIC PROFILES OF SELECTED CAUSES OF HYPOTENSION AND COMMONLY USED FIRST-LINE AGENTS

Cause of hypotension	Pulmonary capillary wedge pressure	Cardiac output	Systemic vascular resistance	Preferred agent(s)
Unknown	?	?	?	Dopamine
Hypovolemia	↓	↓	↑	None[a]
Acute decompensated heart failure	↑	↓	↑	Dopamine, dobutamine
Cardiogenic shock	↑↔	↓	↑	Dopamine
Hyperdynamic sepsis	↓↔	↑	↓	Norepinephrine, dopamine
Sepsis with depressed cardiac function	?	↓	↓	Dopamine, norepinephrine plus dobutamine
Anaphylaxis	?	?	↓	Epinephrine
Anesthesia-induced hypotension	?	?	↓	Phenylephrine, ephedrine[b]

[a]Volume resuscitation with intravenous fluids and/or blood products recommended.
[b]For obstetric patients.

patients found that various approaches to hemodynamic optimization reduced mortality when patients were treated early to achieve hemodynamic goals before the development of organ failure and when therapy produced differences in oxygen delivery [71].

Vasopressors and positive inotropes are powerful drugs with considerable potential for toxicity. Diligent monitoring and careful adjustment of medications based on changes in clinical status are essential. Patients should be treated in an intensive care setting with continuous monitoring of cardiac rhythm, urine output, and arterial oxygenation. Fluid resuscitation and careful attention to intravascular volume are paramount, as up to 50% of patients with hypotension related to sepsis may stabilize with fluids alone [2]. Moreover, the administration of vasopressors to intravascularly depleted patients can worsen end-organ perfusion. The routine use of pulmonary artery catheters in this setting remains unproven, as overaggressive treatment may increase the risk of adverse events [72]. However, a randomized trial demonstrated that early goal-directed therapy, using a central venous catheter capable of measuring oxygen saturation, improved outcomes in patients with septic shock [73]. In patients who do not respond adequately to initial fluid boluses and brief infusion of vasopressors, invasive hemodynamic monitoring may aid in optimizing filling pressures and selecting the appropriate vasoactive agent. Intra-arterial cannulation and direct monitoring of blood pressure is suggested during prolonged vasopressor use. Drugs should be administered through central venous catheters via volumetric infusion pumps that deliver precise flow rates. In the event of vasopressor extravasation, an α_1-adrenergic antagonist (e.g., phentolamine, 5 to 10 mg, diluted in 10 to 15 mL of saline) can be infiltrated into the area to limit local vasoconstriction and tissue necrosis.

With few exceptions, the drugs discussed in this chapter are short-acting agents with rapid onset and offset of action. They are generally initiated without a bolus and can be titrated frequently. Abrupt lowering or discontinuation of vasoactive drugs should be avoided to prevent rebound hypotension. Common dose ranges are provided in Table 32.1, but there may be considerable variation in the dose required to restore adequate hemodynamics. Furthermore, an individual patient's response to an agent may diminish with time owing to several mechanisms, including adrenergic receptor desensitization.

Critically ill patients in the intensive care unit are generally treated with multiple drugs in addition to vasoactive agents (e.g., other cardiovascular medications, antibiotics). Careful attention should be paid to potential drug–drug interactions, as they can significantly alter the response to a given sympathomimetic amine. For example, prior or current treatment with a β-adrenergic antagonist can cause resistance to the action of dobutamine or other β-adrenergic agonists. The administration of less-selective drugs (e.g., norepinephrine) to a patient receiving chronic beta-blockade can result in unopposed α-adrenergic stimulation. Another well-described interaction is the exaggerated response to some catecholamines in individuals taking monoamine oxidase inhibitors. The starting dose for these patients should be less than 10% of the usual dose [1]. Intensive care unit rounding with a dedicated pharmacist is recommended.

References

1. Westfall TC, Westfall DP: Adrenergic agonists and antagonists, in Brunton LL (ed): *Goodman & Gilman's The Pharmacological Basis of Therapeutics.* 11th ed. New York, McGraw-Hill, 2005, pp 237–295.
2. Dellinger RP, Levy MM, Carlet JM, et al: Surviving Sepsis Campaign: international guidelines for management of severe sepsis and septic shock: 2008. *Crit Care Med* 36:296–327, 2008.
3. Elkayam U, NG TM, Hatamizadeh P, et al: Renal vasodilatory action of dopamine in patients with heart failure: magnitude of effect and site of action. *Circulation* 117:200–205, 2008.
4. Bellomo R, Chapman M, Finfer S, et al: Low-dose dopamine in patients with early renal dysfunction: a placebo-controlled randomised trial. Australian and New Zealand Intensive Care Society (ANZICS) Clinical Trials Group. *Lancet* 356:2139–2143, 2000.
5. Field JM, Hazinski MF, Sayre MR, et al: Part 1: executive summary: 2010 American Heart Association Guidelines for Cardiopulmonary Resuscitation and Emergency Cardiovascular Care. *Circulation* 122:S640–S656, 2010.
6. Loeb HS, Ostrenga JP, Gaul W, et al: Beneficial effects of dopamine combined with intravenous nitroglycerin on hemodynamics in patients with severe left ventricular failure. *Circulation* 68:813–820, 1983.
7. Leier CV, Heban PT, Huss P, et al: Comparative systemic and regional hemodynamic effects of dopamine and dobutamine in patients with cardiomyopathic heart failure. *Circulation* 58:466–475, 1978.
8. Brienza N, Malcangi V, Dalfino L, et al: A comparison between fenoldopam and low-dose dopamine in early renal dysfunction in critically ill patients. *Crit Care Med* 34:707–714, 2006.
9. Van de Borne P, Oren R, Somers VK: Dopamine depresses minute ventilation in patients with heart failure. *Circulation* 98:126–131, 1998.
10. Ruokonen E, Takala J, Kari A, et al: Regional blood flow and oxygen transport in septic shock. *Crit Care Med* 21:1296–1303, 1993.
11. Marik PE, Mohedin M: The contrasting effects of dopamine and norepinephrine on systemic and splanchnic oxygen utilization in hyperdynamic sepsis. *JAMA* 272:1354–1357, 1994.

12. McKinlay KH, Schinderle DB, Swaminathan M, et al: Predictors of inotrope use during separation from cardiopulmonary bypass. *J Cardiothorac Vasc Anesth* 18:404–408, 2004.
13. De Backer D, Creteur J, Silva E, et al: Effects of dopamine, norepinephrine, and epinephrine on the splanchnic circulation in septic shock: which is best? *Crit Care Med* 31:1659–1667, 2003.
14. Annane D, Vignon P, Renault A, et al: Norepinephrine plus dobutamine versus epinephrine alone for management of septic shock. *Lancet* 370:676–684, 2007.
15. Neumar RW, Otto CW, Link MS, et al: Part 8: adult advanced cardiovascular life support: 2010 American Heart Association Guidelines for Cardiopulmonary Resuscitation and Emergency Cardiovascular Care. *Circulation* 122:S729–S767, 2010.
16. Nasraway SA: Norepinephrine: no more "leave 'em dead"? *Crit Care Med* 28:3096–3098, 2000.
17. Martin C, Papazian L, Perrin G, et al: Norepinephrine or dopamine for the treatment of hyperdynamic septic shock? *Chest* 103:1826–1831, 1993.
18. Martin C, Viviand X, Leone M, et al: Effect of norepinephrine on the outcome of septic shock. *Crit Care Med* 28:2758–2765, 2000.
19. Bellomo R, Giantomasso DD: Noradrenaline and the kidney: friends or foes? *Crit Care* 5:294–298, 2001.
20. Ngan Kee WD, Lee A, Khaw KS, et al: A randomized double-blinded comparison of phenylephrine and ephedrine infusion combinations to maintain blood pressure during spinal anesthesia for cesarean delivery: the effects on fetal acid-base status and hemodynamic control. *Anesth Analg* 107:1295–1302, 2008.
21. Ngan Kee WD, Khaw KS, Ng FF: Prevention of hypotension during spinal anesthesia for cesarean delivery: an effective technique using combination phenylephrine infusion and crystalloid cohydration. *Anesthesiology* 103: 744–750, 2005.
22. Gregory JS, Bonfiglio MF, Dasta JF, et al: Experience with phenylephrine as a component of the pharmacologic support of septic shock. *Crit Care Med* 19:1395–1400, 1991.
23. Krejci V, Hiltebrand LB, Sigurdsson GH: Effects of epinephrine, norepinephrine, and phenylephrine on microcirculatory blood flow in the gastrointestinal tract in sepsis. *Crit Care Med* 34:1456–1463, 2006.
24. Chan WS, Irwin MG, Tong WN, et al: Prevention of hypotension during spinal anaesthesia for caesarean section: ephedrine infusion versus fluid preload. *Anaesthesia* 52:908–913, 1997.
25. Lee A, Ngan Kee WD, Gin T: A dose-response meta-analysis of prophylactic intravenous ephedrine for the prevention of hypotension during spinal anesthesia for elective cesarean delivery. *Anesth Analg* 98:483–490, 2004.
26. Smiley RM, Blouin J, Negron M, et al: Beta2-adrenoceptor genotype affects vasopressor requirements during spinal anesthesia for cesarean delivery. *Anesthesiology* 104:644–650, 2006.
27. Lowe MD, Rowland E, Brown MJ, et al: Beta(2) adrenergic receptors mediate important electrophysiological effects in human ventricular myocardium. *Heart* 86:45–51, 2001.
28. Roden DM: Drug-induced prolongation of the QT interval. *N Engl J Med* 350:1013–1022, 2004.
29. De Broux E, Lagace G, Chartrand C: Efficacy of isoproterenol on the failing transplanted heart during early acute rejection. *Ann Thorac Surg* 53:1062–1067, 1992.
30. Brembilla-Perrot B, Muhanna I, Nippert M, et al: Paradoxical effect of isoprenaline infusion. *Europace* 7:621–627, 2005.
31. Ruffolo RR Jr: The pharmacology of dobutamine. *Am J Med Sci* 294:244–248, 1987.
32. Givertz MM, Stevenson LW, Colucci WS: Strategies for management of decompensated heart failure, in Antman E (ed): *Cardiovascular Therapeutics*. 3rd ed. Philadelphia, PA, Elsevier, 2007 pp 385–409.
33. Wimmer A, Stanek B, Kubecova L, et al: Effects of prostaglandin E1, dobutamine and placebo on hemodynamic, renal and neurohumoral variables in patients with advanced heart failure. *Jpn Heart J* 40:321–334, 1999.
34. Abraham WT, Adams KF, Fonarow GC, et al: In-hospital mortality in patients with acute decompensated heart failure requiring intravenous vasoactive medications: an analysis from the Acute Decompensated Heart Failure National Registry (ADHERE). *J Am Coll Cardiol* 46:57–64, 2005.
35. Hare JM, Givertz MM, Creager MA, et al: Increased sensitivity to nitric oxide synthase inhibition in patients with heart failure: potentiation of beta-adrenergic inotropic responsiveness. *Circulation* 97:161–166, 1998.
36. Takkenberg JJ, Czer LS, Fishbein MC, et al: Eosinophilic myocarditis in patients awaiting heart transplantation. *Crit Care Med* 32:714–721, 2004.
37. Landry DW, Levin HR, Gallant EM, et al: Vasopressin pressor hypersensitivity in vasodilatory septic shock. *Crit Care Med* 25:1279–1282, 1997.
38. Argenziano M, Chen JM, Choudhri AF, et al: Management of vasodilatory shock after cardiac surgery: identification of predisposing factors and use of a novel pressor agent. *J Thorac Cardiovasc Surg* 116:973–980, 1998.
39. Russell JA, Walley KR, Singer J, et al: Vasopressin versus norepinephrine infusion in patients with septic shock. *N Engl J Med* 358:877–887, 2008.
40. Lindner KH, Prengel AW, Brinkmann A, et al: Vasopressin administration in refractory cardiac arrest. *Ann Intern Med* 124:1061–1064, 1996.
41. Aung K, Htay T: Vasopressin for cardiac arrest: a systematic review and meta-analysis. *Arch Intern Med* 165:17–24, 2005.
42. Gueugniaud PY, David JS, Chanzy E, et al: Vasopressin and epinephrine vs. Epinephrine alone in cardiopulmonary resuscitation. *N Engl J Med* 359:21–30, 2008.
43. Delmas A, Leone M, Rousseau S, et al: Clinical review: vasopressin and terlipressin in septic shock patients. *Crit Care* 9:212–222, 2005.
44. Morelli A, Ertmer C, Rehberg S, et al: Continuous terlipressin versus vasopressin infusion in septic shock (TERLIVAP): a randomized, controlled pilot study. *Crit Care* 13:R30, 2009.
45. DiBianco R: Acute positive inotropic intervention: the phosphodiesterase inhibitors. *Am Heart J* 121:1871–1875, 1991.
46. Givertz MM, Hare JM, Loh E, et al: Effect of bolus milrinone on hemodynamic variables and pulmonary vascular resistance in patients with severe left ventricular dysfunction: a rapid test for reversibility of pulmonary hypertension. *J Am Coll Cardiol* 28:1775–1780, 1996.
47. Slawsky MT, Colucci WS, Gottlieb SS, et al: Acute hemodynamic and clinical effects of levosimendan in patients with severe heart failure. *Circulation* 102:2222–2227, 2000.
48. Kivikko M, Lehtonen L, Colucci WS: Sustained hemodynamic effects of intravenous levosimendan. *Circulation* 107:81–86, 2003.
49. Mebazaa A, Nieminen MS, Packer M, et al: Levosimendan vs dobutamine for patients with acute decompensated heart failure: the SURVIVE Randomized Trial. *JAMA* 297:1883–1891, 2007.
50. Kelly RA, Balligand JL, Smith TW: Nitric oxide and cardiac function. *Circ Res* 79:363–380, 1996.
51. Lopez A, Lorente JA, Steingrub J, et al: Multiple-center, randomized, placebo-controlled, double-blind study of the nitric oxide synthase inhibitor 546C88: effect on survival in patients with septic shock. *Crit Care Med* 32:21–30, 2004.
52. Kirov MY, Evgenov OV, Evgenov NV, et al: Infusion of methylene blue in human septic shock: a pilot, randomized, controlled study. *Crit Care Med* 29:1860–1867, 2001.
53. Levin RL, Degrange MA, Bruno GF, et al: Methylene blue reduces mortality and morbidity in vasoplegic patients after cardiac surgery. *Ann Thorac Surg* 77:496–499, 2004.
54. Ozal E, Kuralay E, Yildirim V, et al: Preoperative methylene blue administration in patients at high risk for vasoplegic syndrome during cardiac surgery. *Ann Thorac Surg* 79:1615–1619, 2005.
55. Toussaint S, Gerlach H: Activated protein C for sepsis. *N Engl J Med* 361:2646–2652, 2009.
56. Bernard GR, Vincent JL, Laterre PF, et al: Efficacy and safety of recombinant human activated protein C for severe sepsis. *N Engl J Med* 344:699–709, 2001.
57. Abraham E, Laterre PF, Garg R, et al: Drotrecogin alfa (activated) for adults with severe sepsis and a low risk of death. *N Engl J Med* 353:1332–1341, 2005.
58. Nadel S, Goldstein B, Williams MD, et al: Drotrecogin alfa (activated) in children with severe sepsis: a multicentre phase III randomised controlled trial. *Lancet* 369:836–843, 2007.
59. Bollaert PE, Charpentier C, Levy B, et al: Reversal of late septic shock with supraphysiologic doses of hydrocortisone. *Crit Care Med* 26:645–650, 1998.
60. Briegel J, Forst H, Haller M, et al: Stress doses of hydrocortisone reverse hyperdynamic septic shock: a prospective randomized, double-blind, single-center study. *Crit Care Med* 27:723–732, 1999.
61. Chawla K, Kupfer Y, Goldma I: Hydrocortisone reverses refractory septic shock [Abstract], *Crit Care Med* 27:A23, 1997.
62. Annane D, Sebille V, Charpentier C, et al: Effect of treatment with low doses of hydrocortisone and fludrocortisone on mortality in patients with septic shock. *JAMA* 288:862–871, 2002.
63. Minneci PC, Deans KJ, Banks SM, et al: Meta-analysis: the effect of steroids on survival and shock during sepsis depends on the dose. *Ann Intern Med* 141:47–56, 2004.
64. Sprung CL, Annane D, Keh D, et al: Hydrocortisone therapy for patients with septic shock. *N Engl J Med* 358:111–124, 2008.
65. DeWitt CR, Waksman JC: Pharmacology, pathophysiology and management of calcium channel blocker and beta-blocker toxicity. *Toxicol Rev* 23:223–238, 2004.
66. De Backer D, Biston P, Devriendt J, et al: Comparison of Dopamine and Norepinephrine in the treatment of shock. *N Engl J Med* 362(9):779–789, 2010.
67. LeDoux D, Astiz ME, Carpati CM, et al: Effects of perfusion pressure on tissue perfusion in septic shock. *Crit Care Med* 28:2729–2732, 2000.
68. Huang YC: Monitoring oxygen delivery in the critically ill. *Chest* 128:554S–560S, 2005.
69. McNulty PH, King N, Scott S, et al: Effects of supplemental oxygen administration on coronary blood flow in patients undergoing cardiac catheterization. *Am J Physiol Heart Circ Physiol* 288:H1057–H1062, 2005.
70. Mak S, Azevedo ER, Liu PP, et al: Effect of hyperoxia on left ventricular function and filling pressures in patients with and without congestive heart failure. *Chest* 120:467–473, 2001.
71. Kern JW, Shoemaker WC: Meta-analysis of hemodynamic optimization in high-risk patients. *Crit Care Med* 31:1598–1599, 2003.
72. Shah MR, Hasselbland V, Stevenson LW, et al: Impact of the pulmonary artery catheter in critically ill patients: meta-analysis of randomized critical trials. *JAMA* 294:1664–1670, 2005.
73. Rivers E, Nguyen B, Havstad S, et al: Early goal-directed therapy in the treatment of severe sepsis and septic shock. *N Engl J Med* 345:1368–1377, 2001.

CHAPTER 33 ■ MANAGEMENT OF ADVANCED HEART FAILURE

G. WILLIAM DEC

Advanced heart failure accounts for a small minority (approximately 10%) of patients with chronic disease. It is generally defined as persistent New York Heart Association functional class IIIB or IV symptoms that limit daily activities and occur despite adequate pharmacologic treatment (see later) and is usually associated with a left ventricular ejection fraction below 30% [1]. Patients with advanced heart failure typically have experienced one or more hospitalizations for decompensated heart failure within the previous year.

PROGNOSTIC FEATURES

More than 50 variables have been examined in univariate and multivariate models and shown to predict prognosis in advanced heart failure populations. No single study has assessed all, or even most, of these predictors simultaneously and it is therefore impossible to rank prognostic features strictly based on their level of importance. Nonetheless, several features appear repeatedly in the published literature (Table 33.1). Eichhorn identified plasma norepinephrine level, B-type natriuretic peptide (BNP) level, left ventricular ejection fraction, peak oxygen uptake on cardiopulmonary exercise testing, advanced age, and a history of symptomatic ventricular arrhythmias or sudden cardiac death as the most important predictors of outcome [2].

Functional capacity, as assessed by the New York Heart classification remains among the most useful outcome predictors in advanced heart failure. One year mortality rates range from <5% for Class I, 10% to 15% for Class II, 20% to 30% for Class III, with Class IV patients experiencing rates of 30% to 70% depending on their response to therapy [2]. Although left ventricular ejection fraction (LVEF) is a consistent predictor of outcome in a heterogeneous population of patients whose left ventricular ejection fractions range from 10% to 50% [2], this parameter correlates very poorly with symptoms or day-to-day functional capacity and loses much of its predictive accuracy among patients with advanced symptoms [3]. In advanced heart failure, small variations in markedly depressed LVEF (i.e., between 10% and 20%) have little bearing on symptoms or prognosis [2,3].

Findings on physical examination also predict prognosis and should influence treatment during hospitalization. The presence of a chronic third heart sound or elevation in jugular venous pressure establishes more advanced disease and predict increased long-term mortality [4]. Both moderate-to-severe mitral or tricuspid regurgitation are also associated with increased symptoms, morbidity, and mortality [5].

Serum B-type natriuretic peptide (BNP) and N-terminal-pro-BNP are increasingly measured in patients with suspected heart failure. Recent data suggest that serial assessment of BNP during hospitalization is useful in predicting postdischarge prognosis and suggests that this approach may soon help guide heart failure inpatient management [6]. However, it should be recognized that a variety of etiologies including pulmonary embolism, acute coronary syndromes, and sepsis may also lead to markedly elevated BNP [7].

Renal dysfunction has recently been recognized as an extremely powerful predictor of heart failure outcome. Deterioration in renal function may result from diminished cardiac output and a corresponding reduction in glomerular filtration rate, alterations in the distribution of cardiac output, intrarenal vasoregulation, alterations in circulatory volume, more intense neurohormonal activation, and/or the nephrotoxic effects of medications administered during hospitalization [8]. The presence of chronic renal insufficiency, defined as a serum creatinine >1.4 mg/dL for women and >1.5 mg/dL for men, predicts an increased risk of death (risk ratio = 1.43) [8]. Unfortunately, approximately 25% of hospitalized patients with decompensated heart failure will exhibit deterioration in renal function despite appropriate medical therapy [9]. In these hospitalized patients, a rise in serum creatinine of only 0.1 to 0.5 mg/dL is associated with a longer length of hospital stay and increased in-hospital mortality [9]. This constellation of poorly understood physiologic mechanisms has been termed the "cardiorenal syndrome" and its optimal management remains to be defined.

Thus, a variety of demographic, clinical, hemodynamic and laboratory findings help to accurately characterize patients with advanced heart failure at increased risk of adverse events during hospitalization. Proper identification of these patients should lead to improved management strategies. Hernandez, et al. have reported that patients with heart failure undergoing major noncardiac surgical procedures experience substantially increased morbidity compared to patients with ischemic heart disease or an age-matched population [10]. After adjusting for demographic characteristics, type of surgery,

TABLE 33.1

PREDICTORS OF PROGNOSIS IN CHRONIC HEART FAILURE

Demographic	Advanced age, sex, ischemic etiology
Symptoms	NYHA class IV, syncope
Signs	Chronic S3, right heart failure
Laboratory	Na^+, creatinine, anemia, CTR, LVEDD
ECG	QRS or QTc prolongation, NSVT, VT
Hemodynamic	LVEF, PCW, CI
Exercise	6-min walk distance, peak VO_2
Neurohormonal	PNE, ANP, BNP

ANP, atrial natriuretic peptide; BNP, B-type natriuretic peptide; CI, cardiac index; CTR, cardiothoracic ratio on chest film; LVEDD, left ventricular end-diastolic dimension on echocardiogram; LVEF, left ventricular ejection fraction; NSVT, nonsustained ventricular tachycardia; PCW, pulmonary capillary wedge pressure; PNE, plasma norepinephrine; VO_2, oxygen consumption on cardiopulmonary exercise testing; VT, ventricular tachycardia.

and comorbid conditions, the risk-adjusted operative mortality (death before discharge or within 30 days of surgery) was 11.7% for heart failure patients, 6.6% for ischemic heart disease patients, and 6.2% for controls. Further, the risk-adjusted 30-day re-admission rates were 20% for the heart failure cohort compared with 14% for the ischemic population and 11% for age-match controls. The presence of a third heart sound or signs of overt heart failure clearly identifies patients at increased risk for adverse outcome during noncardiac surgical procedures [11]. Every effort must be made to detect unsuspected heart failure by careful evaluation and to optimize therapy before embarking on nonemergent procedures.

Fonarow et al., using the ADHERE registry data on over 33,000 hospitalizations has performed the most detailed risk stratification of in-hospital mortality in acute decompensated heart failure [12]. The best single predictor for morality was high admission level of blood urea nitrogen (>43 mg/dL), followed by an admission systolic blood pressure below 115 mm Hg, and a serum creatinine level >2.75 mg/dL. Using these three variables, patients could be readily stratified into groups at low, intermediate, and high risk for in-hospital mortality with rates ranging from 2.1% to 21.9% [12]. Additional predictive variables in other studies include troponin release, markedly elevated natriuretic peptide levels, and hyponatremia [13].

PHARMACOLOGICAL MANAGEMENT OF ADVANCED HEART FAILURE

Heart failure that persists after correction of potentially reversible causes (i.e., anemia, hyperthyroidism, valvular heart disease, myocardial ischemia) should be treated with dietary sodium restriction, diuretics for volume overload, vasodilator therapy (particularly angiotensin-converting enzyme (ACE) inhibitors or angiotensin receptor antagonists),and a beta-adrenergic blocker (Fig. 33.1). Sodium restriction (<4 g per day) is generally indicated for patients with advanced symptoms [14]. Likewise, most patients with advanced heart failure require a 1.5 to 2 L per day fluid restriction.

Diuretics

Diuretics remain the mainstay for "congestive symptoms" but have not been shown to improve survival. Neurohormonal activation (as measured by circulating renin, angiotensin, endothelin, and BNP) has been shown to acutely decrease during short-term diuretic therapy administered to lower markedly elevated filling pressures [15]. Two pharmacologic classes of agents are relevant to acute heart failure management: loop diuretics and distal tubular agents (Table 33.2). The loop diuretics (e.g., furosemide, torsemide, bumetanide, and ethacrynic acid) are the most potent. Some data suggest that torsemide and bumetanide may be more effective than furosemide in advanced heart failure, perhaps due to superior absorption from the gastrointestinal tract in the setting of elevated right-sided filling pressures [15]. Although once daily dosing of loop diuretic is usually effective for outpatient therapy, patients with persistent symptoms or those with marked hemodynamic instability during hospitalization often require dosing two or three times a day to adequately manage volume overload.

Thiazide diuretics such as hydrochlorothiazide and metolazone act mainly by inhibiting reabsorption of sodium and chloride in the distal convoluted tubule of the kidney. Used alone, thiazides produce a fairly modest diuresis; these agents are ineffective when glomerular filtration rate (GFR) falls below 40 ml per minute [15].

Diuretic tolerance is often encountered in patients with advanced heart failure. Lack of response to diuretic therapy may be caused by excessive sodium intake, use of agents that antagonize their effects (particularly nonsteroidal anti-inflammatory drugs), worsening renal dysfunction, addition of potentially nephrotoxic agents during hospitalization or compromised renal blood flow due to worsening cardiac function. Combined intravenous loop diuretic plus thiazide creates a synergistic response and should be considered for patients who fail to diurese despite optimal doses of an intravenous loop diuretic alone. Metolazone is particularly effective when administered with a loop diuretic. High-dose furosemide when administered as a continuous infusion (1 to 10 mg per hour) may also be more effective than bolus administration for hospitalized patients [16].

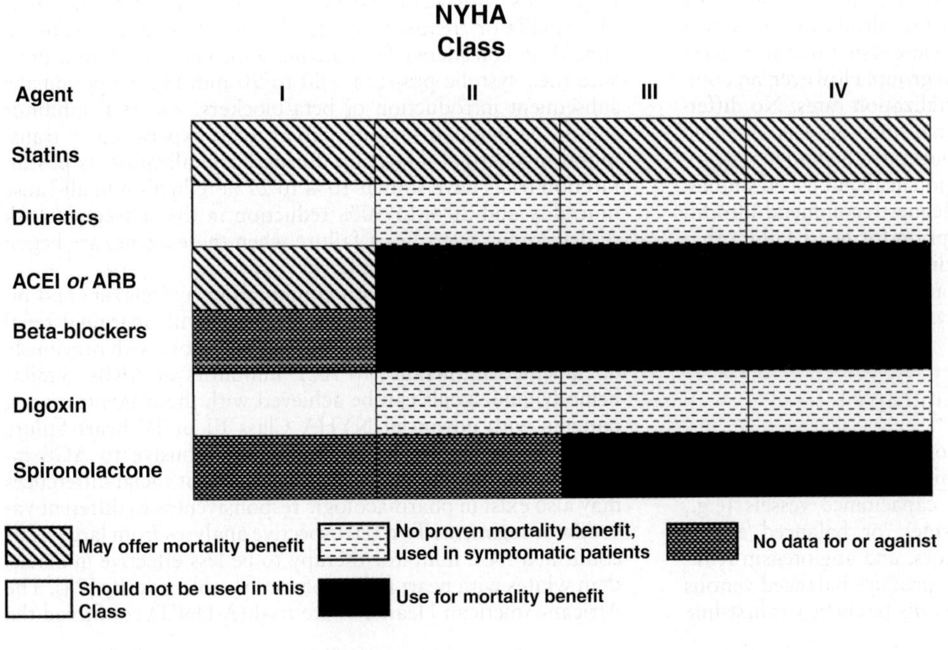

FIGURE 33.1. Standard pharmacological approach to heart failure based upon agent and severity of clinical heart failure symptoms [From Eichhorn E: Current pharmacologic treatment of heart failure. *Clin Cardiol* 22:V21–V29 (Figure 1), 1999, with permission.]

TABLE 33.2

INTRAVENOUS DIURETIC REGIMENS FOR TREATING DECOMPENSATED HEART FAILURE

Drug	Initial dose	Maximal single dose
Loop diuretics		
Furosemide	40 mg	200 mg
Bumetanide	1 mg	4–8 mg
Torsemide	10 mg	100–200 mg
Thiazide diuretics		
Chlorothiazide	500 mg	1,000 mg
Synergistic nephron blockade		
Chlorothiazide	500–1,000 mg + loop diuretics 1–4 × per day	
Metolazone	2.5–10 mg PO + loop diuretic 1–2 × per day	
Intravenous infusions		
Furosemide	40 mg IV loading dose; then 5–40 mg/hour infusion	
Bumetanide	1–2 mg IV loading dose; then 0.5–2 mg/hour infusion	
Torsemide	20 mg IV loading dose; then 5–20 mg/hour infusion	

IV, intravenous; PO, by mouth.

Elevated vasopressin levels play an important role in mediating fluid retention and contributing to hyponatremia. Short-term treatment with the V2-receptor antagonist, tolvaptan, has been shown to lower filling pressures, enhance diuresis, correct hyponatremia, and improve renal function [17]. However, tolvaptan had no effect on long-term mortality or heart-failure–related morbidity in a study of over 500 hospitalized with acute decompensated failure [17]. Thus, the role of this class of agents remains uncertain.

Ultrafiltration using a venovenous access approach is now feasible and potentially useful for acutely lowering elevated ventricular filling pressures when conventional high-dose combination diuretic therapy fails to produce adequate diuresis. Small, short-term observational studies suggest improvements in weight loss during hospitalization but have not demonstrated decreased length of stay or better preservation of renal function [18]. The UNLOAD trial randomized 200 patients with acute decompensated heart failure to standard intravenous diuretics versus ultrafiltration and demonstrated greater weight loss at 48 hours in the ultrafiltration cohort [19]. Readmissions for heart failure were also lower at 90 days (32% vs. 18%) for the ultrafiltration group. However, no comment was made on overall rehospitalization rates. No difference in in-hospital or outpatient renal function was observed between treatment groups [19]. Importantly, hemodynamic instability has been an exclusion criterion in all published studies. The latest ACC/AHA practice guidelines recommend ultrafiltration as a class IIA therapeutic option for heart failure that remains refractory to conventional diuretic therapy [14]. Additional prospective controlled trials are needed to establish the exact role of this new treat modality.

Vasodilator Therapy

Vasodilators remain a cornerstone of acute and chronic heart failure management [14]. Mechanisms of action vary and include a direct effect on venous capacitance vessels (e.g., nitrates), arterioles (e.g., hydralazine), or balanced effects (sodium nitroprusside, ACE inhibitors, and angiotensin II receptor blockers [ARBs]). Drugs that produce balanced venous and arteriolar dilatation should generally be chosen as first-line therapy since both preload and afterload are elevated in decompensated heart failure. However, in the ICU setting, it may sometimes be useful to use nitrates to reduce markedly elevated preload or hydralazine to treat elevated afterload for short periods of time. ACE inhibitors play a crucial role by altering the vicious cycle of hemodynamic abnormalities and neurohormonal activation that characterize advanced heart failure. Randomized, controlled clinical trials have demonstrated the beneficial effects of ACE inhibitors on functional capacity, neurohormonal activation, quality of life, and long-term survival in patients with chronic heart failure due to left ventricular systolic dysfunction (Table 33.3). There is compelling evidence that ACE inhibitor therapy should be prescribed whenever feasible in all symptomatic heart failure patients. Despite their unequivocal benefits, only 60% to 75% of all heart failure patients currently receive these agents [20]. The elderly and patients with advanced heart failure symptoms are least likely to receive this therapy [20]. It is especially important to recognize in patients with advanced heart failure that even low doses of vasodilator treatment confer benefit. Low-dose treatment should be considered for patients with marginal blood pressure (i.e., systolic pressure >80 to 90 mm Hg) to permit the subsequent introduction of beta-blockers. An ACE inhibitor should be initiated for any patient who experiences a transmural myocardial infarction during hospitalization as postinfarction trials have shown 10% to 27% reduction in all-cause mortality and 20% to 50% reduction in the subsequent risk of developing overt heart failure when these agents are begun following acute infarction [21].

Alternative therapy with combination hydralazine and nitrates should be considered for patients with marginal renal function (creatinine >2.5 mg per dL) and those with previously documented intolerance to ACE inhibitors or ARBs. Similar hemodynamic goals can be achieved with these agents among patients with advanced NYHA Class III or IV heart failure [22]. Women appear somewhat less responsive to ACE inhibitor therapy than do men [23]. Important racial differences may also exist in pharmacologic responsiveness to different vasodilator regimens. Two retrospective analyses from large trials confirmed ACE inhibitor therapy to be less effective in blacks than whites with heart failure of comparable severity [24]. The African-American Heart Failure trial (A-HeFT) confirmed the

TABLE 33.3

INHIBITORS OF THE RENIN–ANGIOTENSIN–ALDOSTERONE SYSTEM AND BETA-BLOCKERS USED FOR ADVANCED HEART FAILURE DUE TO SYSTOLIC DYSFUNCTION

Drug	Initial dose	Maximal dose
ACE inhibitors		
Captopril	6.25 mg three times daily	50 mg three times daily
Enalapril	2.5 mg twice daily	20 mg twice daily
Lisinopril	2.5 mg daily	40 mg daily
Fosinopril	5 mg daily	40 mg daily
Ramipril	1.25 mg daily	10 mg daily
Quinapril	5 mg twice daily	20 mg twice daily
Trandolapril	1 mg daily	4 mg daily
Angiotensin receptor blockers		
Losartan	25 mg daily	100 mg daily
Valsartan	20 mg twice daily	160 mg twice daily
Candesartan	4 mg daily	32 mg daily
Aldosterone antagonists		
Spironolactone	12.5 mg every other day	25 mg twice daily
Eplerenone	25 mg daily	50 mg daily
Beta-adrenergic blockers		
Metoprolol XL/CR[a]	12.5 mg daily	200 mg daily
Carvedilol	3.125 mg twice daily	50 mg twice daily
Bisoprolol	1.25 mg daily	10 mg daily

[a] Metoprolol succinate, extended release.

benefit of hydralazine and isosorbide dinitrate in this population; this combination should be considered when initiating therapy for hospitalized black patients [25].

ARBs are now also considered suitable first-line therapy for heart failure patients [14]. These drugs should be selected for ACE-inhibitor intolerant, non–African-American patients who experience rash or cough with an ACE inhibitor. They cannot be used for patients who experience ACE-inhibitor–related deterioration in renal function, hypotension, or hypokalemia [25]. Symptomatic and mortality benefits appear comparable between ACE inhibitors and ARBs [14]. For patients with advanced heart failure, the addition of a low-dose ARB to standard therapy with ACE inhibitor and beta-blocker provides significant morbidity benefit with reduction in recurrent hospitalizations but no mortality benefit [26]. A modest reduction in maintenance ACE inhibitor dose may be necessary to introduce an ARB in this population.

Digitalis

Digoxin continues to have an important role in the management of patients with advanced NYHA class III–IV symptoms [14]. The drug has mild positive inotropic effect on cardiac muscle, reduces activation of the sympathetic and renin angiotensin systems, and partially restores the favorable inhibitory effects of cardiac baroreceptor function. Short- and long-term controlled trials have provided unequivocal evidence that chronic digoxin administration increases left ventricular ejection fraction, improves exercise capacity, decreases advanced heart failure symptoms, and reduces heart failure associated hospitalizations [27]. Post hoc analysis has shown that patients most likely to demonstrate a favorable response had severe symptoms, greater degrees of left ventricular dysfunction, lower ejection fractions, and the presence of a third heart sound [27]. A prespecified subgroup analysis of patients enrolled in the Digitalis Investigation Group (DIG) trial provide confirmatory evidence that patients with severe heart failure (LVEF <25% or CT ratio >0.55) showed the greatest benefit [27]. The drug has neutral effects on all-cause and cardiovascular mortality [27]. As renal function may fluctuate considerably during hospitalization, measurement of serum digoxin levels is important [28]. Retrospective subgroup analysis has suggested an increased risk of all-cause mortality among both women and men who have digoxin levels >1.0 ng/dL [28]. Poor renal function, small lean body mass, and elderly patients are at greatest risk for developing digoxin toxicity during standard maintenance dosing. In addition, a number of commonly used drugs including verapamil, flecainide, spironolactone, and amiodarone will significantly increase serum digoxin levels. For adult patients with normal renal function, a dosage of 0.25 mg per day is appropriate. For patients at increased risk of toxicity, the initial starting dose should be 0.125 mg daily and up-titrated as necessary to achieve a trough level of 0.5 to 0.9 ng per dL.

Beta-Adrenergic Blockers

Three distinct classes of beta-blockers are now available for clinical use. Propranolol and other "first-generation" compounds such as timolol are nonselective agents with equal affinity for β_1 and β_2 receptors [29]. Metoprolol and bisoprolol are "cardioselective" second-generation compounds that block the β_1 receptor to a greater extent than the β_2 receptor. Metoprolol is approximately 75-fold more selective for β_1 than β_2 receptors while bisoprolol is 120-fold more selective [29]. Labetalol, carvedilol, and bucindolol are third-generation compounds that block β_1 and β_2 receptors with almost equal affinity. These agents also have ancillary properties including

α_1-blockade (labetalol and carvedilol), antioxidant properties (carvedilol), and intrinsic sympathomimetic activity (ISA) (bucindolol). Specific beta-blockers have been shown to lower all-cause mortality and decrease heart failure hospitalizations in a variety of randomized controlled trials in patients with NYHA class II–IV symptoms (Table 33.3) [30,31]. The mortality benefits of beta-blocker therapy in patients with advanced (NYHA class IV) heart failure symptoms have been established. The Carvedilol Perspective Randomized Cumulative Survival (COPERNICUS) trial evaluated patients with severe symptoms and LVEF <25% [32]. Carvedilol reduced all-cause mortality by 35%, the combined risk of death or cardiovascular hospitalization by 27%, and the risk of death or heart failure hospitalization by 31% [32]. Importantly, carvedilol-treated patients spent 40% fewer days in the hospital for acute heart failure decompensation [32]. It is appears that not all beta-blockers have equivalent benefits in heart failure. For example, bucindolol, a third-generation nonselective beta-blocker with ISA properties, was not associated with statistically significant reductions in overall mortality amongst patients with advanced heart failure. As such, unlike ACE inhibitors or ARBs, the specific beta-blockers validated in clinical trials should be prescribed. The effectiveness of these agents appears equal among men and women with advanced heart failure [33]. Clinicians should consider initiating carvedilol as first-line therapy, given its broader antiadrenergic effects whenever possible. However, for patients with marginal blood pressure in whom alpha blockade may be deleterious, metoprolol or bisoprolol may be suitable first-line agents.

A small minority of patients with advanced heart failure (<10%) are unable to tolerate even the lowest doses during initial attempts at drug introduction. Some investigators are now combining a phosphodiesterase inhibitor (enoximone or milrinone) with a beta-blocker [34]. Phosphodiesterase-III inhibitors improve hemodynamics and exercise performance but increase the risk of exacerbating myocardial ischemia and promoting ventricular arrhythmias. Theoretically, beta-blockers should counteract the ischemic and arrhythmic properties of these agents and provide synergistic benefits. Small uncontrolled short-term studies suggest that this approach may be beneficial in hospitalized patients with refractory heart failure [34]. Several randomized clinical trials are now evaluating the safety and efficacy of combination therapy.

Beta-blocker treatment should be attempted in all patients including those with advanced heart failure. For patients entering the intensive care unit who have not received such therapy, treatment should be initiated at very low doses and gradually up-titrated every few days or within 1 week. The usual starting doses are carvedilol 3.125 mg twice daily or metoprolol succinate 6.25 mg twice daily. Beta-blockers should not be initiated until optimal volume status and hemodynamic stability have been achieved.

The majority of chronic heart failure patients requiring hospitalization are already beta-blocker treated. In general, beta-blockers should not be withdrawn unless bradycardia or hemodynamic instability develops, due to the risk of rebound hypertension and tachycardia. Where necessary to facilitate management of acute decompensated heart failure, a 50% reduction in the ambulatory dose is often preferable to drug cessation. In a retrospective observational study of more than 2,300 patients eligible to receive beta-blocker during hospitalization, Fonarow et al. demonstrated that continuation of beta-blocker was associated with a significantly lower risk in propensity-adjusted postdischarge death and rehospitalization rates compared with the absence of beta-blocker [35]. Further, beta-blocker withdrawal was associated with a substantially higher adjusted risk for mortality (hazard ratio: 2:3) compared to continuation of beta-blockade.

Aldosterone Antagonists

Circulating aldosterone levels are elevated in relationship to heart failure severity, affect prognosis, and contribute to left ventricular remodeling following acute myocardial infarction. Potential deleterious effects include endothelial dysfunction, increased oxidative stress, enhanced platelet aggregation, activation of matrix metalloproteinase, and increased sympathetic activation. The mineralocorticoid receptor antagonist (MRA) spironolactone has been shown to reduce mortality in patients with severe heart failure by 30% [36]. Results of the EPHESUS trial confirm that eplerenone, a more selective MRA, can also reduce morbidity and mortality amongst patients with evidence of systolic dysfunction and heart failure following acute myocardial infarction [37]. The beneficial effects of MRAs appear to be independent of their diuretic actions, and likely relate to interruption of the downstream effects of aldosterone activation.

Spironolactone and eplerenone should not be initiated in the ICU setting. Both can be associated with serious hyperkalemia, particularly in the presence of impaired renal function or other medications which impair potassium excretion. They should be considered for addition to the patient's medical regimen prior to discharge following optimization of other heart failure therapies. Patients who have been receiving these agents should continue taking them during hospitalization unless marked hemodynamic instability, electrolyte disturbances, or worsening renal function ensue.

INTENSIVE CARE MANAGEMENT OF ADVANCED HEART FAILURE PATIENTS

Compensated Heart Failure States

A significant number of patients with advanced heart failure are hospitalized each year for management of noncardiac illnesses. Several principles apply to the in-hospital management of patients with compensated disease. Every attempt should be made to maintain the patient on the medical regimen that has provided optimal outpatient stability. Daily weights as well as a fluid restriction should be instituted for patients with advanced disease. Establishing a baseline weight and maintaining it through diuretic dosing adjustments is critical to prevent an acute decompensation. Diuretics should be switched to intravenous administration whenever questionable oral absorption (i.e., postoperative state) is expected. Once daily ACE inhibitor or ARB therapy is ideal for outpatient management to enhance compliance; however, if hemodynamic instability is anticipated during hospitalization, a temporary switch to a short-acting agent (e.g., captopril in place of lisinopril) should be considered. Among patients with deteriorating renal function, it may be necessary to withhold the ACE-inhibitor or ARB and transiently substitute hydralazine and nitrates, particularly when creatinine exceeds 3.0 mg per dL. Beta-blocker dosing should remain unchanged and may require a modest increase if atrial tachyarrhythmias are encountered in the postoperative state (see later). Serum electrolytes should be followed frequently, given the potential for electrolyte disarray (e.g., hypokalemia or hypomagnesemia) to potentiate atrial and ventricular arrhythmias in vulnerable patients. Despite marked reduction in LVEF, the majority of patients who require hospitalization for noncardiovascular illness will remain compensated with regard to their heart failure symptoms employing a continued maintenance regimen.

Decompensated Heart Failure States

Heart failure decompensation is the most common cause for hospitalization for patients over 65 years of age. Stevenson has popularized a 2-minute clinical assessment to ascertain the hemodynamic profiles for heart failure patients (Fig. 33.2) [23,38]. Patients are characterized in 2 × 2 fashion according to the presence or absence of congestion and low perfusion on physical examination [23]. The clinical profiles thus defined have been shown to correlate reasonably well with direct hemodynamic measurements of filling pressure and cardiac output and are correlated with prognosis following hospital discharge [23]. "Warm and dry" patients have normal resting hemodynamics and are well compensated. For these patients, other potential etiologies for dyspnea or fatigue should be considered. The majority (70% to 80%) of patients admitted with worsening symptoms fit the "warm and wet" profile. These individuals are volume overloaded but have adequate end-organ perfusion. The primary treatment goal is thus relief of "congestive" symptoms using intravenous loop diuretics alone or in combination with a thiazide. Those who fail to respond to escalating doses of intravenous loop diuretics may benefit from a continuous intravenous loop diuretic infusion. The small minority of patients with refractory volume overload may benefit from continuous venovenous hemofiltration (CVVH) or ultrafiltration [14,38]. Although neurohormonal antagonists including ACE-inhibitors, ARBs, and beta-blockers should ideally be maintained during periods of acute heart failure decompensation, for patients that are difficult to diurese or hypotensive, downward dose adjustment or temporary suspension (particularly of beta-blockers) should be considered. A very small minority of patients (<5%) fall into the "cold and dry" profile. These individuals have impaired cardiac output but do not adequately use the Starling mechanism to increase preload. Judicious hydration should be attempted. Patients who fail to demonstrate improvement in end-organ perfusion may require a short-term infusion of a positive inotropic agent such as dobutamine or milrinone.

Hemodynamically Guided Therapy

Approximately 10% to 15% of patients with advanced heart failure will demonstrate marked hemodynamic deterioration on admission ("cold and wet" profile). These patients have impending cardiogenic shock. Potential causes for acute decompensation such as recent myocardial infarction, rhythm change, worsening valvular disease, or medical/dietary nondiscretion should be sought. The ESCAPE trial randomized patients with acute decompensation without hemodynamic compromise to conventional medical management based on physical findings and symptoms versus tailored hemodynamic monitoring following insertion of a pulmonary artery catheter. Somewhat surprisingly, outcomes did not differ between the two management strategies [39]. Certain high-risk subgroups may, nonetheless, benefit from short-term hemodynamic monitoring for management of acute decompensated heart failure. Principal indications for hemodynamic monitoring with a pulmonary artery catheter include evidence of worsening end-organ dysfunction, need for withholding vasoactive medications due to hypotension, heart failure associated with other comorbidities (i.e., unstable angina or valvular heart disease) or inability to wean positive inotropic support (Table 33.4). "Tailored" hemodynamic treatment for refractory heart failure is outlined in Table 33.5. Following initial assessment of baseline hemodynamics, intravenous diuretics, vasodilators, or positive inotropes are administered to achieve desired hemodynamic

TABLE 33.4

INDICATIONS FOR HEMODYNAMIC MONITORING IN DECOMPENSATED HEART FAILURE

- Ongoing congestive symptoms and suspected end-organ hypoperfusion

• Narrow pulse pressure	Cool extremities
• Declining renal function	Hypotension on ACE or ARB
• Mental confusion	Progressive hyponatremia

- Heart failure and other medical comorbidities
  - Cardiac: unstable angina pectoris; stenotic valvular lesions, hypertrophic cardiomyopathy
  - Noncardiac: severe obstructive or restrictive pulmonary disease, advanced renal disease, sepsis
- Other situations
  - Perioperative monitoring to optimize status for high-risk procedure
  - Symptoms disproportionate to clinical assessment of degree of compensation
  - Uncertain volume status
  - Inability to wean inotropic support

ACE, angiotensin-converting enzyme; ARB, angiotensin receptor blocker.

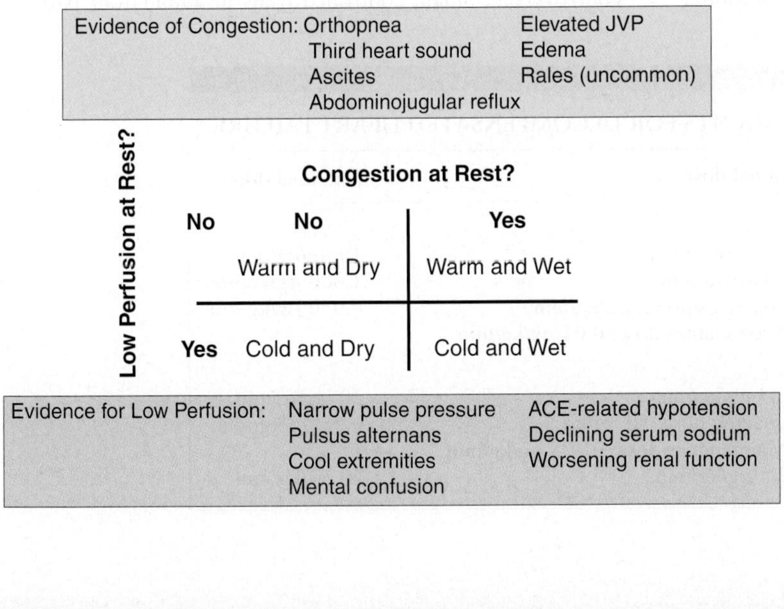

FIGURE 33.2. Diagram of hemodynamic profiles for patients presenting with heart failure symptoms. Most patients with advanced heart failure can be classified accurately in a 2-minute assessment of their physical findings and symptoms. [From Nohria J, Lewis E, Stevenson LW: Medical management of advanced heart failure. *JAMA* 287:639 (Figure 1), 2002, used with permission.]

TABLE 33.5

PRINCIPLES OF HEMODYNAMIC TAILORED HEART FAILURE THERAPY

Measure baseline resting hemodynamics (CVP, PAP, PCW, CI, SVR)
Administer intravenous diuretics, vasodilator (nitroprusside, nitroglycerin, or nesiritide) or inotropic agent (milrinone or dobutamine) dosed to achieve specific hemodynamic goals:
- Pulmonary capillary wedge pressure <16 mm Hg
- Right atrial pressure <8 mm Hg
- Cardiac index >2.2 L/min/m^2
- Systemic vascular resistance <1,000–1,200 dynes/sec/cm^5
- Systolic blood pressure >80 mm Hg

Maintain optimal hemodynamics for 24–48 hours
Up-titration of oral vasodilators as intravenous vasodilators are weaned
Adjust oral diuretics to keep optimal volume status

CI, cardiac index; CVP, central venous pressure; PAP, pulmonary artery pressure; PCW, pulmonary capillary wedge pressure; SVR, systemic vascular resistance.
Adapted from Stevenson LW: Tailored therapy to hemodynamic goals for advanced heart failure. *Eur J Heart Fail* 1:251–257, 1999 (Table 2, page 254), used with permission.

goals which generally include a pulmonary capillary wedge pressure below 15 mm Hg and a cardiac index above 2.2 L per minute per m^2. This intravenous program is maintained for 24 to 48 hours to effect desired diuresis and improve end-organ perfusion. Following this stage, oral vasodilators are up-titrated as intravenous agents are weaned. Further adjustment in diuretic dose and ambulation should be completed during the final 24 to 48 hours of hospitalization. This "tailored approach" produces sustained improvement in filling pressures, forward cardiac output, decreased mitral regurgitation, and decreased neurohormonal activation [23]. Oral vasodilator therapy and beta-blockers should be withheld during treatment with intravenous vasoactive agents.

Considerable controversy continues to exist regarding the relative roles of intravenous vasodilator drugs (i.e., nitroglycerin, nitroprusside, or nesiritide) versus positive inotropic agents (dobutamine, dopamine, or milrinone) in this population. Previously, inotropic infusions have been used for patients with moderate heart failure to promote brisk diuresis. These agents, however, are associated with an increased risk of ischemic events and tachyarrhythmias [40]. A second major limitation of short-term inotropic support is the additional complexity needed to readjust oral regimens as the infusions are weaned [23]. Although positive inotropes should not be routinely used for "warm and wet" patients, these agents can be life saving for patients with rapidly progressive hemodynamic collapse [38]. Patients who present or develop obtundation, anuria, persistent hypotension, or lactic acidosis may only respond to inotropic support, which should be continued until the cause of cardiac deterioration is determined and definitive therapy implemented. Brief inotropic treatment may also be appropriate for patients who develop the cardiorenal syndrome. It should be emphasized, however, that many patients with low cardiac output have high systemic vascular resistance that predictably improves with vasodilator therapy alone, obviating the need for inotropic support [23,38]. In-hospital mortality has also been shown to be lower for nonhemodynamically compromised patients treated with intravenous vasodilators compared to positive inotropes [41]. Intravenous nitroprusside, a direct nitrovasodilator, rapidly lowers filling pressures and improves cardiac output, which in turn, improves response to diuretic therapy. Hemodynamically monitored nitroprusside infusions rarely cause systematic hypotension but may be complicated by thiocyanate toxicity, particularly when high doses are required for prolonged periods of time in patients with preexisting hepatic or renal dysfunction. Intravenous nitroglycerin also produces arterial and venous dilatation but is less effective than nitroprusside. Nesiritide, a human recombinant form of endogenous BNP, rapidly improves symptoms. It has largely been used for patients demonstrating the "warm and wet" hemodynamic profile rather than those with more advanced "cool and wet" profiles. A small study suggested that short-term in-hospital nesiritide administration resulted in fewer rehospitalizations for heart failure and lower 6-month mortality following discharge compared with dobutamine [42]. However, the safety of nesiritide has been questioned and the hope that this agent would attenuate renal dysfunction during heart failure treatment has not been realized [43]. Two retrospective post hoc analyses have suggested short-term nesiritide treatment may be associated with worsening renal function and may increase short-term mortality risk. Further, it has not been studied extensively in patients with hypotension or hypoperfusion. The ongoing ASCEND-HF trial of 4,500 patients will address the safety and efficacy of short-term nesiritide therapy in acute decompensated heart failure. Table 33.6 summarizes vasaactive agents used to manage of acute decompensated heart failure.

Biomarker-Guided Therapy

The use of serial BNP or NT-pro-BNP to guide therapy remains controversial. Small, controlled trials in ambulatory patients

TABLE 33.6

INTRAVENOUS VASOACTIVE AGENTS FOR DECOMPENSATED HEART FAILURE

Drug	Initial dose	Maximal dose
Vasodilator		
Nitroprusside	0.20 μg/kg/min	10 μg/kg/min
Nitroglycerin	10 μg/kg/min	1,000 μg/kg/min
Nesiritide	Loading dose: 2 μg/kg/min Maintenance dose: 0.01 μg/kg/min	0.030 μg/kg/min
Positive inotropic agents		
Dobutamine	2.5 μg/kg/min	20 μg/kg/min
Milrinone	Loading dose: 50 μg/kg Maintenance dose: 0.375 μg/kg/min	0.75 μg/kg/min
Dopamine	2.5 μg/kg/min	20 μg/kg/min

with chronic heart failure demonstrated fewer heart failure rehospitalizations using BNP to adjust pharmacologic therapy. However, this approach recently failed to improve survival free of repeat hospitalizations or quality of life in a large cohort of patients [44]. A reasonable approach for inpatients with acute decompensated heart failure should include the measurement of BNP or NT-pro-BNP on admission and prior to discharge when the patient is euvolemic, both for prognostic purposes as well as to aid in tailoring postdischarge treatment [45]. Daily biomarker measurement does not add significant prognostic value. A fall of 30% or greater in BNP or NT-pro-BNP identifies patients at low risk at discharge. Conversely, a rise in either biomarker suggests worsening disease or inadequate therapy and should prompt a review of the patient's heart failure regimen.

PERIOPERATIVE MANAGEMENT OF ADVANCED HEART FAILURE PATIENTS

Nonemergent surgical procedures should be delayed until heart failure status has been optimized. Volume overload should be corrected and adequate oxygenation insured. Maintenance pharmacologic therapy including vasodilators, beta-blockers, and digitalis should be continued. A trough digoxin level should be checked and maintained below 1 ng per dL to minimize potential toxicity. Spironolactone should be withheld until stable hemodynamics and renal function have been achieved. Patients with refractory symptoms or deteriorating end-organ function should have a pulmonary catheter inserted to optimize their hemodynamics. Current evidence does not support the routine use of a pulmonary artery catheter for perioperative monitoring [11]. A single large-scale randomized clinical trial of pulmonary artery catheterization in high-risk surgical patients demonstrated no improvement in survival [46]. However, only 16% of patients enrolled in this trial had heart failure. Ejection fraction alone is insufficient to recommend the use of continuous hemodynamic monitoring. Many patients with markedly impaired ventricular function (LVEF <20%) may be well compensated on optimized pharmacologic therapy and undergo surgery without invasive monitoring. Conversely, some patients with only moderate impairment in LVEF may benefit from pulmonary artery monitoring when hemodynamic instability is anticipated. Practice guidelines for intraoperative hemodynamic monitoring published by the American Society of Anesthesiologists consider the severity of the patient's underlying cardiovascular disease, the type of surgical procedure, and the likelihood of major hemodynamic lability [47]. The extent of anticipated intraoperative and perioperative fluid shifts is another key factor. Current ACC/AHA guidelines recommend intraoperative pulmonary artery monitoring as a Class 2B indication as indicated for patients at risk for major hemodynamic disturbances that are easily detected by pulmonary artery catheter who are scheduled to undergo a procedure that is likely to cause these hemodynamic changes [11].

MANAGEMENT OF ARRHYTHMIAS

Atrial and ventricular arrhythmias are nearly ubiquitous in advanced heart failure patients and often contribute to clinical decompensation. Atrial fibrillation and flutter are the most commonly encountered supraventricular arrhythmias. The likelihood of atrial fibrillation increases with heart failure severity and approaches 40% for NYHA class III and IV patients. The potential adverse effects of atrial fibrillation include loss of atrioventricular synchrony, rapid or inappropriately slow ventricular response rates, variable diastolic filling times, and thromboembolic complications. Atrial fibrillation has been associated with increased mortality and more frequent hospitalizations in some, but not all, series [48]. Patients with a known history of chronic atrial fibrillation should have adequate heart rate control and anticoagulation whenever feasible (see later). Uncontrolled, sustained, rapid (>120 beats per minute) atrial fibrillation can result in a reversible dilated cardiomyopathy or, more typically, can worsen preexisting left ventricular systolic dysfunction. A heart rate below 100 beats per minute during modest ambulation is a reasonable goal. Beta-adrenergic blockers and digoxin remain first-line rate-controlled treatment options [4]. Calcium channel blockers (e.g., diltiazem and verapamil) should be avoided with advanced heart failure due to their negative inotropic effects. Amiodarone is a highly effective drug for rate control and is frequently useful for controlling persistent atrial arrhythmias in ICU patients [49].

Atrial fibrillation commonly occurs during hospitalization due to enhanced sympathetic stimulation. In all patients, thyroid function should be assessed to exclude hyperthyroidism as a contributor. For stable heart failure patients with atrial fibrillation initial therapy should focus on adequate rate control (HR <100 per minute) using digoxin or beta-blockers, with pharmacologic or electrical cardioversion reserved for those patients who in whom symptoms are refractory or those who are intolerant of conservative medical management. Patients who experience active angina pectoris or hemodynamic instability during new onset atrial fibrillation should undergo urgent synchronized cardioversion with initiation of an atrial-stabilizing agent to prevent recurrence. For heart failure patients in whom restoration or maintenance of sinus rhythm is desirable, amiodarone, dofetilide, and sotalol remain the most useful antiarrhythmic drugs [49]. In compensated heart failure, amiodarone is well tolerated from a hemodynamic standpoint. For patients with advanced heart failure symptoms or recent decompensation, the loading dose of amiodarone should be kept below 1,000 mg per day to prevent exacerbation of heart failure. Dronedarone, a new noniodinated derivative of amiodarone, has been shown to be effective for maintenance of sinus rhythm and rate-control in rapid atrial fibrillation [50]. However, increased mortality due to worsening heart failure has been reported in one recent controlled trial [1,49]. Until additional data are available, this agent should not be used for patients with severe systolic dysfunction or hemodynamic instability.

Dofetilide is a class III antiarrhythmic drug that blocks the repolarizing potassium current. It is highly effective in restoring sinus rhythm but is associated with torsades de pointes in up to 3% of patients [49]. Continuous ECG monitoring for the first 48 hours after initiation in the hospitalized patient is essential. Sotalol, an additional class III antiarrhythmic drug, may occasionally be substituted for other beta-blockers in heart failure patients, but carries with it a similar risk of torsades, and is generally less effective than amiodarone.

Asymptomatic nonsustained ventricular tachycardia (NSVT) occurs in over 50% of patients with NYHA class III/IV heart failure. Pharmacologic suppression of NSVT does not lower the risk of sudden death. Asymptomatic ventricular ectopy should be viewed as a marker of disease severity rather than a specific marker for sudden cardiac death risk [51]. Heart failure patients often develop frequent ventricular premature beats or short runs of NSVT during their ICU stay. Precipitating causes such as electrolyte disturbances (hypokalemia or hypomagnesemia), enhanced sympathetic tone, a decrease in beta-blocker dose, or withholding of prior antiarrhythmic therapy should be considered. The majority of patients have no symptoms and do not require pharmacologic

TABLE 33.7

RESULTS OF RANDOMIZED TRIALS OF PHARMACOLOGIC TREATMENT AND ULTRAFILTRATION IN ACUTE DECOMPENSATED HEART FAILURE

Intervention	Trial	Year	Study	No. of patients	Findings	Reference
Hydralazine-Nitrates	A-HeFT	2004	RCT	1,050	43% reduction in all-cause mortality in blacks	25
Carvedilol	COPERNICUS	2002	RCT	2,289	31% reduction in death or HF hospitalizations in NYHA class III/IV patients	32
Milrinone	OPTIME-CHF	2002	RCT	951	No reduction in hospitalizations for cardiac causes within 60 days of treatment with milrinone for ADHF	40
Ultrafiltration	UNLOAD	2007	RCT	200	UF resulted in greater weight loss and fewer rehospitalizations for heart failure	19
Pulmonary artery catheter (PAC) placement	ESCAPE	2005	RCT	433	PAC for tailoring of therapy did not lower mortality or rehospitalizations	39
Nesiritide vs. dobutamine	—	2002	Open label randomized	261	Nesiritide resulted in fewer readmissions and lower 6-month mortality than dobutamine	42
Nesiritide	NAPA	2007	RCT	279	Nesiritide improved renal function after CABG	

ADHF, acute decompensated heart failure; A-HeFT, African American Heart Failure Trial; CABG, coronary artery bypass grafting; COPERNICUS, Carvedilol Prospective Randomized Cumulative Survival Study; ESCAPE, Evaluation Study of Congestive Heart Failure and Pulmonary Artery Catheterization Effectiveness; NAPA, nesiritide-administered perianesthesia in patients undergoing cardiac surgery; RCT, randomized controlled trial; OPTIME-CHF, Outcomes of a Prospective Trial of Intravenous Milrinone for Exacerbation of Chronic Heart Failure.

suppression. Frequent runs of ventricular tachycardia or sustained monomorphic VT require antiarrhythmic treatment. Amiodarone (intravenous 0.50 to 1.0 mg/min) or lidocaine (0.5 to 2 mg per min) is generally most effective for acute management. Beta-blockers, sotalol, and amiodarone are effective long-term oral treatment options.

A growing percentage of advanced heart failure patients have implantable cardioverter defibrillators (ICDs) to treat symptomatic ventricular tachyarrhythmias or for primary prevention of sudden cardiac death. The ICD should be interrogated for any recent atrial or ventricular arrhythmias prior to admission and the device temporarily inactivated prior to surgical procedures that involve electrocautery. It should be reactivated and its function checked by an electrophysiologist in the early perioperative period.

Anticoagulation

Systemic anticoagulation is often a part of a heart failure patient's outpatient management. Studies have suggested that the risk of thromboembolic complications is lower than previously expected, averaging 1.5 to 3 episodes per 100 patient years when normal sinus rhythm is present. Current indications for systemic anticoagulation include paroxysmal or chronic atrial fibrillation, a history of thromboembolism, or echocardiographically documented left ventricular thrombus. Relative indications include a markedly dilated left ventricle (>75 mm) with severe systolic dysfunction and spontaneous echocardiographic contrast ("smoke") indicating sluggish intracavitary blood flow. The presence of a low ejection fraction alone is *insufficient* to warrant systemic anticoagulation. Warfarin should be continued with an INR goal of 2.0 to 3.0 if invasive procedures are not planned. If surgery or central venous catheter placement is required, warfarin can be reversed with vitamin K or fresh frozen plasma and transiently substituted with intravenous heparin or subcutaneous low-molecular weight heparin as feasible. For those patients who require anticoagulation but are unable to receive heparin (e.g., due to heparin-induced thrombocytopenia), alternative anticoagulants including the direct thrombin inhibitors argatroban and hirudin, or the pentasaccharide fondaparinux can be considered.

CONCLUSION

The patient with advanced heart failure requires special considerations. Meticulous attention to volume status and maintenance of appropriate vasodilator therapy and beta-adrenergic blockade form the cornerstones of acute management (Table 33.7). Negative inotropic drugs and agents that might further impair renal function should be avoided. Patients with refractory symptoms or recent decompensation may require hemodynamic monitoring via a pulmonary artery catheter and initiation of short-term vasoactive therapy including nitroprusside, nitroglycerin, nesiritide, milrinone, or dobutamine. Maintenance of sinus rhythm and suppression of recurrent ventricular tachyarrhythmias is mandatory. With careful management, hospital morbidity and mortality can be minimized despite the presence of severe ventricular systolic or diastolic dysfunction.

References

1. Adams K, Zannad F: Clinical definition and epidemiology of advanced heart failure. *Am Heart J* 135:S204–S215, 1998.
2. Eichhorn EJ: Prognosis determination in heart failure. *Am J Med* 110(7A): 14S–35S, 2001.
3. Kao W, Costanzo MR: Prognostic determination in patients with advanced heart failure. *J Heart Lung Transplant* 16:82–86, 1997.
4. Drazner MH, Rame JE, Stevenson LW, et al: Prognostic importance of elevated jugular venous pressure and a third heart sound in patients with heart failure. *NEJM* 345:574–581, 2001.
5. Koelling TM, Aaronson KD, Cody RJ, et al: Prognostic significance of mitral regurgitation and tricuspid regurgitation in patients with left ventricular systolic dysfunction. *Am Heart J* 144:373–376, 2002.
6. Valle R, Aspromonte N, Giovinazzo P, et al: B-type natriuretic peptide-guided treatment for predicting outcome in patients hospitalized in sub-intensive care unit with acute heart failure. *J Cardiac Fail* 14:219–224, 2008.
7. Daniels LB, Maisel AS: Natriuretic peptides. *J Am Coll Cardiol* 50:2357–2368, 2007.
8. Hillege HL, Nitsch D, Pfeffer MA, et al: Renal function as a predictor of outcome in a broad spectrum of patients with heart failure. *Circulation* 113:671–8.2006.
9. Damman K, Navis G, Voors AA, et al: Worsening renal function and prognosis in heart failure: systematic review and meta-analysis. *J Cardiac Fail* 13:599–608, 2007.
10. Hernandez AF, Whellan DJ, Htroud S, et al: Outcomes in heart failure patients after major non-cardiac surgery. *J Am Coll Cardiol* 44:1446–1453, 2004.
11. Fleisher LA, Beckman JA, Brown KA, et al: ACC/AHA 2007 guidelines on perioperative cardiovascular evaluation and care for non-cardiac surgery: executive summary. A report of the American College of Cardiology/American Heart Association Task Force on Practice Guidelines (Writing Committee to Update the 2002 Guidelines on Perioperative Cardiovascular Evaluation for Noncardiac Surgery). *J Am Coll Cardiol* 50:1707–1732, 2007.
12. Fonarow GC, Adams KF, Abraham WT, et al: for ADHERE Scientific Advisory Committee, Study Groups, and Investigators. Risk stratification for in-hospital mortality in acute decompensated heart failure. Classification and regression tree analysis. *JAMA* 293:572–580, 2005.
13. Gheorghiade M, Pang PS: Acute heart failure syndromes. *J Am Coll Cardiol* 53:557–573, 2009.
14. Jessup M, Abraham WT, Casey DE, et al: 2009 focused update: ACCF/AHA Guidelines for the Diagnosis and Management of Heart Failure in Adults: a report of the American College of Cardiology Foundation/American Heart Association Task Force on Practice Guidelines: developed in collaboration with the International Society for Heart and Lung Transplantation. *Circulation.* 119:1977–2016, 2009.
15. Johnson W, Omland T, Hall C, et al: Neurohormonal activation rapidly decreases after intravenous therapy with diuretics and vasodilators for class IV heart failure. *J Am Coll Cardiol* 39:1623–1629, 2002.
16. Dormans TPJ, ManMeyel JJM, Gerlag DDG, et al: Diuretic efficacy of high dose furosemide in severe heart failure: bolus infusion versus continuous infusion. *J Am Coll Cardiol* 28:376–382, 1996.
17. Konstam MA, Gheorghiade M, Burnett JC, et al: Effect of oral tolvaptan in patients hospitalized for worsening heart failure. The EVEREST outcome trial. *JAMA* 297:1319–1331, 2007.
18. Guglin M, Polavaram L: Ultrafiltration in heart failure. *Cardiol Rev* 15:226–230, 2007.
19. Costanzo MR, Guglin ME, Saltzberg MT, et al: Ultrafiltration versus intravenous diuretics for patients hospitalized for acute decompensated heart failure. *J Am Coll Cardiol* 49:675–683, 2007.
20. Stafford RS, Radley DC: The underutilization of cardiac medicines of proven benefit, 1990 to 2002. *J Am Coll Cardiol* 41:56–61, 2003.
21. ACE Inhibitor Myocardial Infarction Collaborative Group: Indications for ACE inhibitors in the early treatment of acute myocardial infarction: systematic overview of individual data from 100,000 patients in randomized trials. *Circulation* 97:2202–2212, 1991.
22. Fonarow GC, Chelimsky-Fallich C, Stevenson LW: Effect of direct vasodilation with hydralazine versus angiotensin-converting-enzyme inhibition with captopril on mortality in advanced heart failure. *J Am Coll Cardiol* 19:842–850, 1992.
23. Nohria A, Tsang SW, Fang JC, et al: Clinical assessment identifies hemodynamic profiles that predict outcomes in patients admitted with heart failure. *J Am Coll Cardiol* 41:1797–1804, 2003.
24. Exner DV, Dries DL, Domanski MJ, et al: Lesser response to angiotensin-converting enzyme inhibitor therapy in black compared to white patients with left ventricular dysfunction. *N Eng J Med* 344:1351–1357, 2001.
25. Taylor AL, Zieche S, Yancy C, et al: Combination of isosorbide dinitrate and hydralazine in blacks with heart failure. *N Eng J Med* 351:2049–2057, 2004.
26. Young JB, Dumlap ME, Pfeffer MA, et al: Mortality and morbidity reduction with candesartan in patients with chronic heart failure and left ventricular systolic dysfunction. Results of the CHARM low-left ventricular ejection fraction trials. *Circulation* 110:2618–2626, 2004.
27. The Digitalis Investigation Group: The effect of digoxin on mortality and morbidity in patients with heart failure. *N Eng J Med* 336:525–533, 1997.
28. Adams KF, Patterson JH, Gattis WA, et al: Relationship of serum digoxin concentration to mortality and morbidity in women in the Digoxin Investigation Group trial. A retrospective analysis. *J Am Coll Cardiol* 46:497–504, 2005.
29. Gheorghiade M, Colucci WS, Swedberg K: Beta-blockers in chronic heart failure. *Circulation* 107:1570–1575, 2003.
30. Domanski MJ, Krause-Steinrauf H, Massie BM, et al: A comparative analysis of the results from 4 trials of beta-blocker therapy for heart failure: BEST, CIBIS-II, MERIT-HF, and COPERNICUS. *J Cardiac Fail* 92:354–363, 2003.
31. Fonarow GC: A review of evidence-based beta-blockers in special populations with heart failure. *Rev Cardiovasc Med* 9:84–95, 2008.
32. Packer M, Coats AJ, Fowler MB, et al: Effect of carvedilol on survival in severe chronic heart failure. *N Eng J Med* 344:1651–1658, 2001.
33. Ghali JK, Pina IL, Gottlieb SS, et al: Metoprolol CR/XL in female patients with heart failure. Analysis of the experience in Metoprolol Extended-release Randomized Intervention Trial in Heart Failure (MERIT-HF). *Circulation* 105:1585–1591, 2002.
34. Metra M, Nodari S, D'Aloia A, et al: Beta-blocker therapy influences the hemodynamic response to inotropic agents in patients with heart failure: A randomized comparison of dobutamine and enoximone before and after chronic treatment with metoprolol or carvedilol. *J Am Coll Cardiol* 40:1248–1258, 2002.
35. Fonarow GC, Abraham WT, Albert NM, et al: Influence of beta-blocker continuation or withdrawal on outcomes in patients hospitalized with heart failure. Findings from the OPTIMIZE-HF Program. *J Am Coll Cardiol* 52:190–199, 2008.
36. Pitt B, Zannad F, Remme WJ, et al: The effect of spironolactone on morbidity and mortality in patients with severe heart failure. *NEJM* 341:709–717, 1999.
37. Pitt B, Remme W, Zannad F, et al: Eplerenone, a selective aldosterone blocker, in patients with left ventricular dysfunction after myocardial infarction. *NEJM* 348:1309–1321, 2003.
38. Nohria J, Lewis E, Stevenson LW: Medical management of advanced heart failure. *JAMA* 287:628–640, 2002.
39. The ESCAPE Investigators and Study Coordinators: Evaluation study of congestive heart failure and pulmonary artery catheterization effectiveness. The ESCAPE trial. *JAMA* 294:1625–1633, 2005.
40. Felker GM, Benza RL, Chandler AB, et al: for the OPTIME-CHF Investigators. Heart failure etiology and response to milrinone in decompensated heart failure. Results from the OPTIME-CHF study. *J Am Coll Cardiol* 41:997–1003, 2003.
41. Abraham WT, Adams KF, Fonarow GC, et al: In-hospital mortality in patients with acute decompensated heart failure requiring vasoactive medications. An analysis of the Acute Decompensated Heart Failure National Registry. *J Am Coll Cardiol* 46:57–64, 2005.
42. Silver MA, Horton DP, Ghali JK, et al: Effect of nesiritide versus dobutamine on short-term outcomes in the treatment of patients with acutely decompensated heart failure. *J Am Coll Cardiol* 39:798–803, 2002.
43. Witteles RM, Kao D, Christopherson D, et al: Impact of nesiritide on renal function in patients with acutely decompensated heart failure with pre-existing renal dysfunction. A randomized, double-blind, placebo-controlled clinical trial. *J Am Coll Cardiol* 50:1835–1840, 2007.
44. Pfisterer M, Buser P, Richli G, et al: BNP-guided vs. symptom-guided heart failure therapy. The trial of intensified vs. symptom-mediated therapy in elderly patients with congestive heart failure (TIME-CHF) randomized trial. *JAMA* 301:2183–2192, 2009.
45. Ahardwaj A, Januzzi JL: Natriuretic peptide-guided management of acutely decompensated heart failure. Rationale and treatment algorithm. *Crit Pathw Cardiol* 8:146–150, 2009.
46. Sandham JD, Hull RD, Brant RF, et al: for the Canadian Critical Care Clinical Trials Group. A randomized, controlled trial of the use of pulmonary-artery catheters in high risk surgical patients. *NEJM* 348:5–14, 2003.
47. Practice guidelines for pulmonary artery catheterization: A Updated Report by the American Society of Anesthesiologists Task Force on Pulmonary Artery Catheterization. *Anesthesiology* 99:988–1014, 2003.
48. Anter E, Jessup M, Callans DJ: Atrial fibrillation and heart failure. Treatment considerations for a dual epidemic. *Circulation* 119:2516–2525, 2009.
49. Efremidis M, Pappas L, Sideris A, et al: Management of atrial fibrillation in patients with heart failure. *J Cardiac Fail* 14:232–237, 2008.
50. Patel C, Yang GX, Kowey PR: Dronedarone. *Circulation* 120:636–644, 2009.
51. Huikuri HV, Makikallio RH, Raathkainen P, et al: Prediction of sudden cardiac death. Appraisal of studies and methods assessing the risk of sudden arrhythmic death. *Circulation* 108:110–115, 2003.
52. Mentzer RM, Oz MC, Sladen RN, et al: Effects of perioperative nesiritide in patients with left ventricular dysfunction undergoing cardiac surgery. The NAPA trial. *J Am Coll Cardiol* 49:716–726, 2007.

CHAPTER 34 ■ VALVULAR HEART DISEASE

GARRICK C. STEWART AND PATRICK T. O'GARA

The incidence of valvular heart disease continues to rise due to the increasing longevity of the population and remains a source of significant morbidity and mortality [1]. More than 5 million Americans are living with valvular heart disease and nearly 100,000 undergo valve surgery each year [2]. Patients with native or prosthetic valve disease constitute a significant proportion of intensive care unit (ICU) admissions. Many patients come to medical attention during an acute illness that triggers an abrupt change in cardiovascular physiology. While stabilization with medical management is possible for most patients with mild or moderate disease, surgery may be urgently required if severe disease is present. Prompt diagnosis often requires a high index of suspicion [3]. Timely cardiac imaging with transthoracic echocardiography (TTE) can define valve anatomy and lesion severity. Transesophageal echocardiography (TEE) may be required in select circumstances for better visualization and characterization. The need for an invasive hemodynamic assessment may follow. Early collaboration among intensivists, cardiologists, and cardiac surgeons is critical for optimizing patient outcome. This chapter will highlight an integrated approach to the diagnosis and treatment of the native and prosthetic valve diseases most commonly encountered in an ICU setting.

AORTIC STENOSIS

Aortic stenosis (AS) is a progressive disease for which there is no medical treatment. The ICU management of patients with AS may be quite challenging, particularly in the setting of concomitant medical illness. Characterizing the severity of stenosis is critical for determining the timing of surgical intervention and requires a careful history, physical examination, and initial imaging with TTE.

Etiology

AS accounts for one-quarter of all chronic valvular heart disease, with approximately 80% of symptomatic cases occurring in adult males (Fig. 34.1). Common etiologies of valvular AS include age-related calcific degeneration, stenosis of a congenitally bicuspid valve, and rheumatic heart disease. Age-related, degenerative calcific AS is the most common cause of AS among adults in the United States. More than 30% of adults older than 65 years exhibit aortic valve sclerosis, whereas only 2% have more significant valvular stenosis. The valve cusps are focally thickened or calcified in aortic sclerosis, with production of a systolic ejection murmur, but without significant outflow obstruction (peak jet velocity of <2.5 m per second). Recent studies suggest calcific AS is the end result of an active disease process rather than the inevitable consequence of aging [4]. There may also be a genetic predisposition to calcific degeneration of trileaflet valves [5]. The histologic appearance of a sclerotic valve is similar to atherosclerosis, with inflammation, calcification, and thickening. Both calcific AS and aortic sclerosis appear to be a marker for coronary heart disease events [6]. Older age, male sex, smoking, diabetes mellitus, hypertension, chronic kidney disease, and hypercholesterolemia are risk factors for calcific AS. Despite the compelling connection between atherosclerosis and calcific valve degeneration, high-dose lipid lowering therapy has thus far not been shown to retard the progression of AS in randomized trials [7,8].

Congenitally bicuspid aortic valves are present in 1% to 2% of the population, with a 4 to 1 male predominance, and seldom result in serious narrowing of the aortic orifice during childhood [9]. Abnormal valve architecture makes the two cusps susceptible to hemodynamic stresses, ultimately leading to thickening, calcification, and fusion of leaflets, and narrowing of the orifice. AS develops earlier in bicuspid valves, usually in the fifth or sixth decades, compared with trileaflet aortic valves, which usually do not exhibit calcific AS until the sixth or seventh decade of life [10]. Bicuspid aortic valves are also associated with aortic regurgitation (AR) and aortic root/ascending aortic dilatation and coarctation (Fig. 34.2). Up to 25% to 40% of patients with bicuspid aortic valve will have an ascending aortic aneurysm unrelated to the severity of the valve lesion. Patients with bicuspid aortic valves are susceptible to aortic dissection [11]. Medial degeneration similar to that seen in Marfan syndrome is responsible for aneurysm development in patients with a bicuspid aortic valve [12].

Rheumatic disease may affect the aortic leaflets leading to commissural fusion, fibrosis, and calcification, with narrowing of the valve orifice. Rheumatic AS is almost always accompanied by involvement of the mitral valve and concomitant AR. Radiation-induced AS as a sequela of cancer radiotherapy often occurs in conjunction with proximal coronary artery disease (CAD). Rare causes of valvular AS include Paget's disease of bone, rheumatoid arthritis, and ochronosis. By the time AS becomes severe, superimposed calcification may make it difficult to determine underlying valve architecture and the precise etiology.

In addition to valvular AS, other causes of left ventricular (LV) outflow obstruction include hypertrophic obstructive cardiomyopathy (HOCM), a congenitally unicuspid aortic valve, discrete congenital subvalvular AS resulting from a fibromuscular membrane, and supravalvular AS. The various causes of LV outflow obstruction can be differentiated by careful physical examination and TTE.

Pathophysiology

Obstruction to LV outflow produces a pressure gradient between the LV and the aorta (Fig. 34.3). The ventricle responds to this pressure overload with concentric hypertrophy, which is initially adaptive because it reduces wall stress and preserves ejection performance. The law of Laplace states that wall stress is directly proportional to the product of LV pressure and radius and inversely proportional to LV wall thickness. Compensatory hypertrophy may accommodate a large pressure gradient for years before it becomes maladaptive and LV function declines, with chamber dilatation and reduced cardiac output [13]. In the setting of AS with preserved ejection fraction (EF),

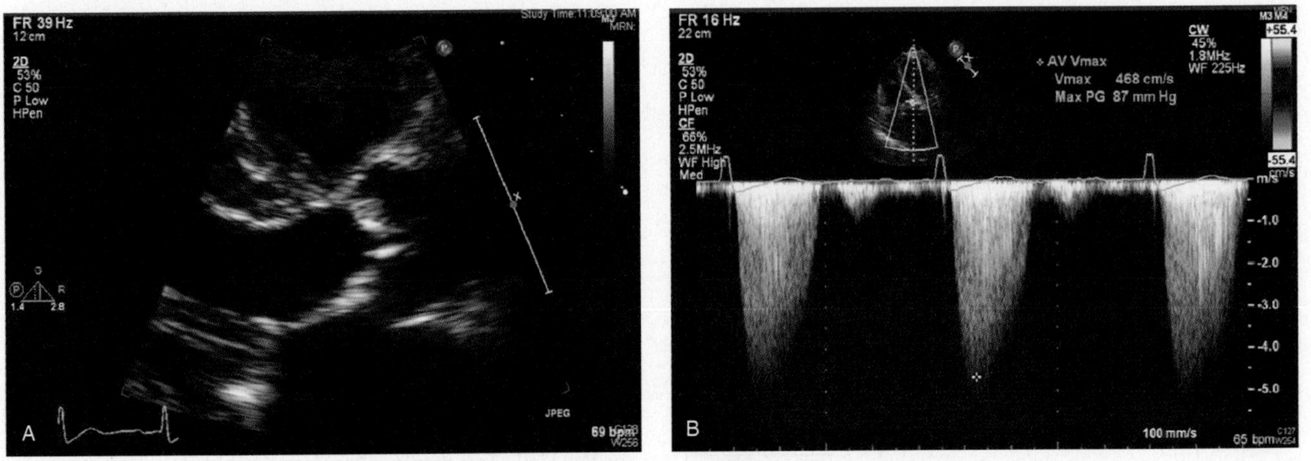

FIGURE 34.1. Transthoracic echocardiography of severe valvular aortic stenosis. **A:** Transthoracic echocardiogram parasternal long axis view of the aortic valve during systole. Aortic valve leaflets are thickened with severely restricted motion consistent with severe aortic stenosis. **B:** Transaortic continuous wave Doppler jet from the apical five-chamber view. Peak transaortic velocity is 4.68 m/sec, producing an estimated peak transaortic gradient of 87 mm Hg.

cardiac output may be normal at rest but fail to rise appropriately with exercise. Coronary flow reserve may be reduced because of the increased oxygen demand of the hypertrophied LV and increased transmural pressure gradient, and the longer distance blood must travel to reach the subendocardial layer. Taken together, these factors can contribute to subendocardial ischemia even in the absence of epicardial CAD [14]. The loss of appropriately timed atrial contraction, such as occurs with atrial fibrillation (AF), may cause rapid progression of symptoms because of the reliance on atrial systole to fill the stiff, hypertrophied LV.

No single parameter of valve structure or function is sufficient to define the severity of AS. Integration of the clinical history, physical examination, and TTE is required to place the lesion in context [15]. The physical examination of AS in the ICU may be particularly challenging, contributing to the greater importance of timely TTE. Echocardiographic criteria for severe AS in patients with normal underlying LV function include

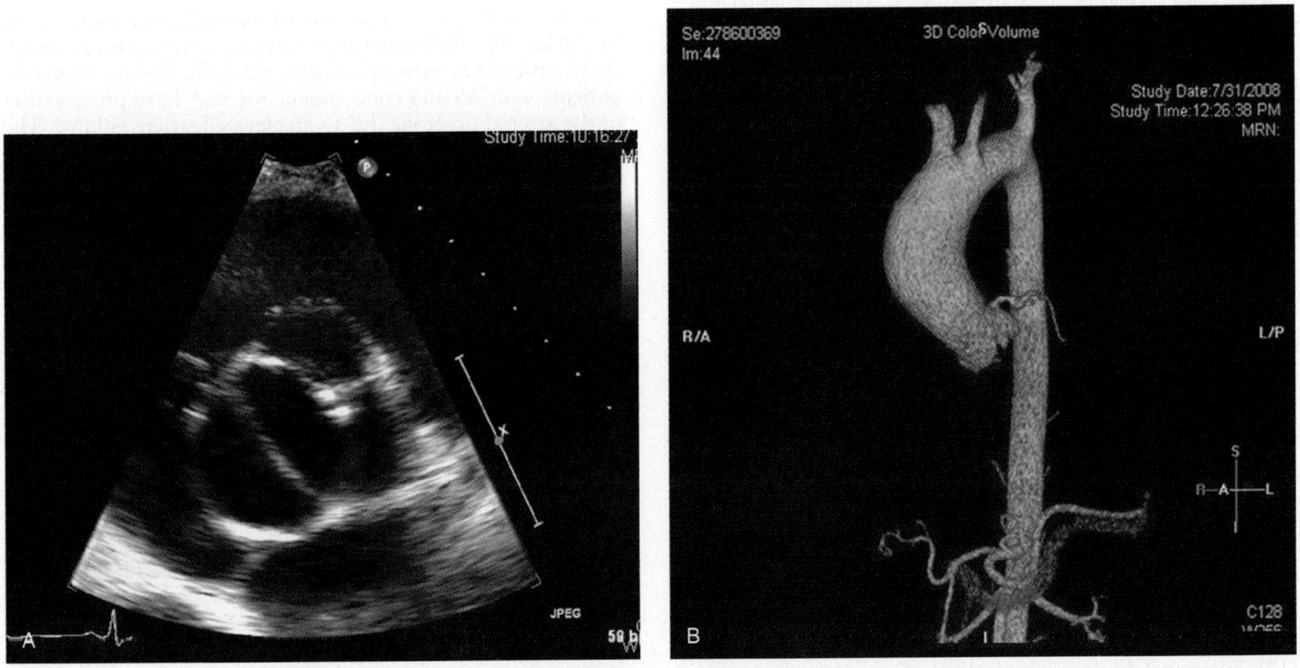

FIGURE 34.2. Bicuspid aortic valve and aortic root aneurysm. **A:** Transthoracic echocardiogram with parasternal short axis view at the level of the aortic valve reveals a bicuspid aortic valve with fusion of the left and noncoronary cusps. **B:** A 5.1-cm ascending aortic aneurysm in a 37-year-old man with bicuspid aortic valve disease and only moderate aortic stenosis (valve area, 1.2 cm^2). Patients with bicuspid disease frequently develop aneurysms of the ascending aorta independent of the severity of hemodynamic valvular impairment and are at risk for aortic dissection. Resection is indicated for maximal aneurysm size larger than 5.0 cm, an increase in aneurysm size of more than 0.5 cm/y, or at the time of aortic valve replacement if the aneurysm size exceeds 4.5 cm. [From Libby P (ed): *Essential Atlas of Cardiovascular Disease.* New York, NY, Springer, 2009, p 216, Figure 9–6, with permission.]

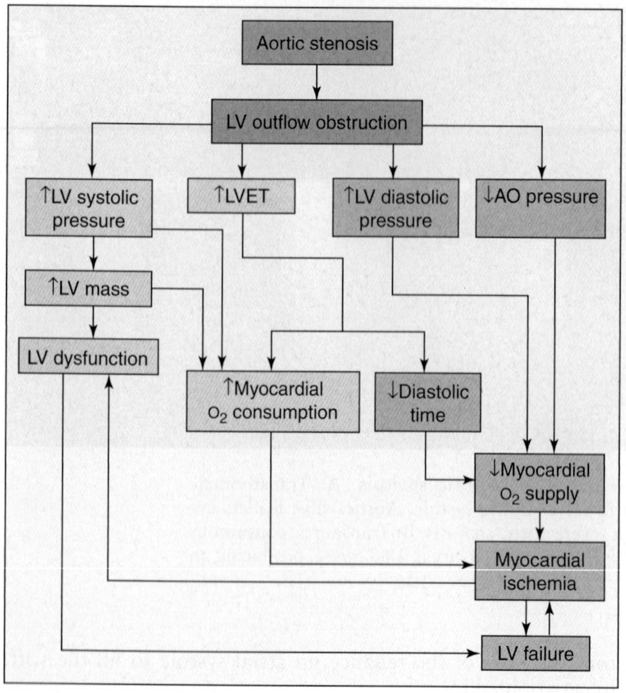

FIGURE 34.3. Pathophysiology of aortic stenosis. Left ventricular (LV) outflow obstruction results in a gradual increase in LV systolic pressure, an increase in LV ejection time (LVET), an increase in LV diastolic pressure, and a decrease in mean aortic (Ao) pressure. Increased LV systolic pressure results in compensatory LV hypertrophy (LVH), which may lead to LV dysfunction and failure. Increased LV systolic pressure, LVH, and prolonged LVET increase myocardial oxygen (O_2) consumption. Increased LVET results in a decrease in LV diastolic time (myocardial perfusion time). Increased LV diastolic pressure and decreased Ao diastolic pressure decrease coronary perfusion pressure, thereby decreasing myocardial supply. Increased myocardial O_2 consumption and decreased myocardial O_2 supply produce myocardial ischemia, which further compromises LV function. [Adapted from Bonow R, Braunwald E: Valvular heart disease, in Zipes D, et al. (eds): *Braunwald's Heart Disease*. Philadelphia, Elsevier, 2005, p 1585, with permission.]

calcified leaflets with reduced excursion, maximal transaortic jet velocity of more than 4 m per second, mean transaortic gradient of more than 40 mm Hg, or an effective aortic valve orifice of less than 1 cm^2 (Table 34.1). When there is underlying LV systolic dysfunction, severe AS may be present despite low transaortic velocity and mean gradient. Such patients are at particularly high risk for complications and require further evaluation to determine if true valvular AS is present or whether the reduced valve area relates to an underlying cardiomyopathy (pseudo-severe AS) [16].

Clinical Presentation

History

The cardinal symptoms of AS are dyspnea, angina, and syncope [17]. Exertional dyspnea is typically the first reported symptom and reflects an elevation in LV end-diastolic pressure transmitted to the pulmonary venous circulation. Some patients, particularly the elderly, may report generalized fatigue and weakness rather than dyspnea. Angina occurs in two thirds of patients with AS and is similar to that reported by patients with flow-limiting coronary atherosclerosis [18]. Syncope is effort related and due to cerebral hypoperfusion from a decrease in mean arterial pressure produced by the combination of peripheral

TABLE 34.1

SEVERITY OF AORTIC STENOSIS

Severity of stenosis	Valve area (cm^2)	Mean gradient (mm Hg)	Jet velocity (msec)
Mild	>1.5	<25	<3.0
Moderate	1.0–1.5	25–40	3.0–4.0
Severe	<1.0	>40	>4.0

vasodilatation in the presence of a fixed cardiac output or an inappropriate baroreceptor reflex. Severe AS is also rarely associated with acquired von Willebrand's disease related to sheering of von Willebrand multimers passing through the stenotic orifice [19]. As a result, gastrointestinal bleeding, epistaxis, or ecchymoses may be present in some patients.

Most patients with AS have gradually increasing LV obstruction over many years, producing a long latent phase. During this clinically silent period, there is a very low risk of sudden death (<1% per year) [20]. The rate of AS progression is variable, with an average increase in mean gradient of 7 mm Hg and reduction in valve area of 0.1 cm^2 per year [21]. Symptoms from valvular AS are rare until the valve orifice has narrowed to approximately less than 1 cm^2. The onset of symptoms is a critical turning point in the natural history of the disease, usually indicates severe AS, and heralds the need for surgical evaluation and treatment because of the markedly reduced survival [17] (Fig. 34.4). An abrupt change in the natural history of AS may occur with AF, endocarditis, or myocardial infarction (MI), each of which may trigger acute decompensation [22].

Physical Examination

The hallmark of AS is a carotid arterial pulse that rises slowly to a delayed peak, known as *pulsus parvus et tardus*. In the elderly, stiffened carotid arteries may mask this finding. Similarly, patients with AS and concomitant AR may have preservation of the arterial upstroke due to an elevated stroke volume. The LV apical impulse may be displaced laterally with a sustained contour due to LV hypertrophy (LVH) and prolonged systolic ejection.

The murmur of AS is a systolic ejection murmur commencing shortly after S1, rising in intensity with a peak in mid ejection, then ending just before aortic valve closure. It is

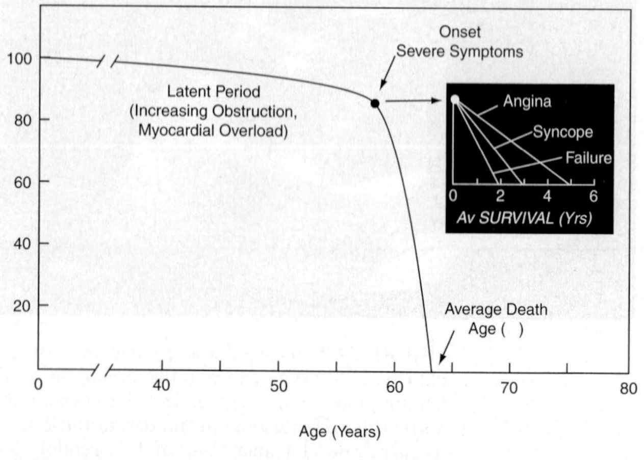

FIGURE 34.4. The onset of symptoms in patients with aortic stenosis initiates a rapid rise in the risk of mortality. Patients with angina have a better prognosis than those with syncope. [From Ross J Jr, Braunwald E: Aortic stenosis. *Circulation* 38(1S5):61–67, 1968, with permission.]

characteristically low-pitched, harsh, or rasping in character and best heard at the base of the heart in the second right intercostal space. The AS murmur radiates along the carotid arteries, though may sometimes be transmitted downward to the apex where it may be confused with the murmur of mitral regurgitation (MR) (Gallavardin effect). The murmur of AS is diminished with Valsalva maneuver and standing, in contrast to the murmur of hypertrophic cardiomyopathy which gets louder with these maneuvers. Often S2 becomes paradoxically split in severe AS because of prolonged LV ejection. An S4 is audible at the apex and reflects LVH with an elevated LV end-diastolic pressure. An S3 gallop generally occurs late in the course of AS when LV dilatation is present. Murmur intensity does not necessarily correspond to AS severity. The best predictors of AS severity on physical examination are a late peaking systolic murmur, a single S2 (absent aortic valve closure sound), and *pulsus parvus et tardus*. In patients with heart failure and a low cardiac output, the findings related to AS are less impressive.

Investigations

Electrocardiography

Most patients with severe AS will have evidence of LVH on electrocardiogram (ECG). Left atrial (LA) enlargement is common. Nonspecific ST and T wave abnormalities may be seen or evidence of LV strain may be apparent. Rarely, atrioventricular conduction defects may develop due to extension of perivalvular calcium into the adjacent conduction system. This finding is more common after aortic valve replacement (AVR). There is poor correlation between ECG findings and AS severity.

Chest Radiography

The chest radiograph may be normal in severe AS. There may be "poststenotic" dilation of the ascending aorta or a widened mediastinum if aortic aneurysmal dilatation is present in patients with a bicuspid aortic valve. LV chamber size is usually normal, though aortic valve calcification may be seen, especially on the lateral film. Valvular calcium deposits can be visualized using fluoroscopy during cardiac catheterization, chest computed tomography (CT), or TTE. A normal radiograph does not exclude severe AS. In the later stages of AS, the LV dilates leading to a widened cardiac silhouette, often accompanied by pulmonary congestion.

Echocardiography

TTE with Doppler is indicated for assessing the severity of AS. TTE visualizes aortic valve structure, including the number of cusps, degree of calcification, leaflet excursion, annular size, and supravalvular anatomy. Eccentric valve cusps are characteristic of congenitally bicuspid aortic valves, often accompanied by aneurysmal enlargement of the root or ascending aorta. TTE is also useful for identifying coexisting valvular disease, differentiating valvular AS from other forms of LV outflow tract obstruction, assessing pulmonary artery systolic pressure, and evaluating underlying biventricular function. The peak transvalvular jet velocity on continuous wave Doppler is critical for assessing AS severity. Peak and mean transvalvular gradients are derived from the jet velocity using the modified Bernoulli equation and the aortic valve area is estimated from the continuity equation. The dimensionless index, which is the ratio of LV outflow tract velocity to peak aortic velocity, can also be used to estimate AS severity when measurement of LV outflow tract diameter is difficult due to extensive calcification. A dimensionless index less than 0.25 is consistent with severe AS [15].

Cardiac Catheterization

Noninvasive assessment with TTE is now standard, but catheterization may be helpful if there is a discrepancy between the clinical and echocardiographic findings. Calculation of aortic valve area by invasive hemodynamic assessment requires accurate assessment of the transvalvular flow and mean transvalvular pressure gradient to calculate effective orifice area using the Gorlin formula [23]. Concerns have been raised about the risk of cerebral embolization during attempts to cross the aortic valve and directly measure the transaortic gradient. Angiography is indicated to detect CAD in patients older than 45 years who are being considered for operative treatment of severe AS [24]. Coronary CT angiography is likely to be performed more often for this indication in patients with a low pretest likelihood of CAD.

Special Case: Low-Output/Low-Gradient Aortic Stenosis

The evaluation and management of patients with AS and a depressed EF can be vexing. Patients with anatomically severe AS and reduced EF (<40%) often have a relatively low-pressure gradient (<30 mm Hg) due to a weakened ventricle and afterload mismatch. The true severity of AS can be difficult to determine when the cardiac output and transaortic gradient are low. If the ventricle itself is diseased and unable to generate sufficient systolic force to open the leaflets adequately, a reduced aortic valve area may be present at rest, overestimating AS severity. This condition is known as pseudo-severe AS [25]. In such cases, LV dysfunction is the predominant pathology and may be caused by prior MI or a primary cardiomyopathy. Patients either with true severe AS with reduced EF or pseudo-severe AS have a low-flow state with low transaortic gradients contributing to calculated aortic valve areas less than 1 cm^2. Pseudo-severe AS patients must be distinguished from those with true severe AS and poor LV function, since patients with true severe AS and contractile reserve will usually benefit from valve surgery, whereas patients with pseudo-severe AS are not operative candidates [26–28].

Dobutamine stress echocardiography has a well-defined diagnostic role in this setting [29] (Fig. 34.5). The inotropic effects of low-dose dobutamine will increase transvalvular flow in patients with a contractile reserve [30]. Contractile reserve is defined as an increase in stroke volume with inotropic infusion of more than 20%. Dobutamine infusion, particularly at doses $\leq$20 μg per kg per minute, is generally well tolerated but should only be performed in experienced centers with a cardiologist in attendance. In patients with true severe AS and LV dysfunction, dobutamine will increase cardiac output and mean transvalvular gradient, but the calculated aortic valve area will remain low (<1 cm^2). Patients with pseudo-severe AS will have an increase in aortic valve area into a range no longer considered severe (>1.2 cm^2) with little change in transvalvular gradient. Some patients will not show contractile reserve to dobutamine, signaling a poor prognosis [31]. Surgery is indicated in true severe AS with contractile reserve after dobutamine challenge, and generally contraindicated for patients with pseudo-severe AS or those without contractile reserve [32]. Patients with low-gradient AS undergoing AVR have a significantly higher perioperative and long-term mortality if multivessel CAD is present [27,33].

Intensive Care Unit Management

Surgery with AVR is the preferred treatment strategy for patients with symptomatic severe AS and for asymptomatic patients with severe AS who have a reduced EF (<50%). In

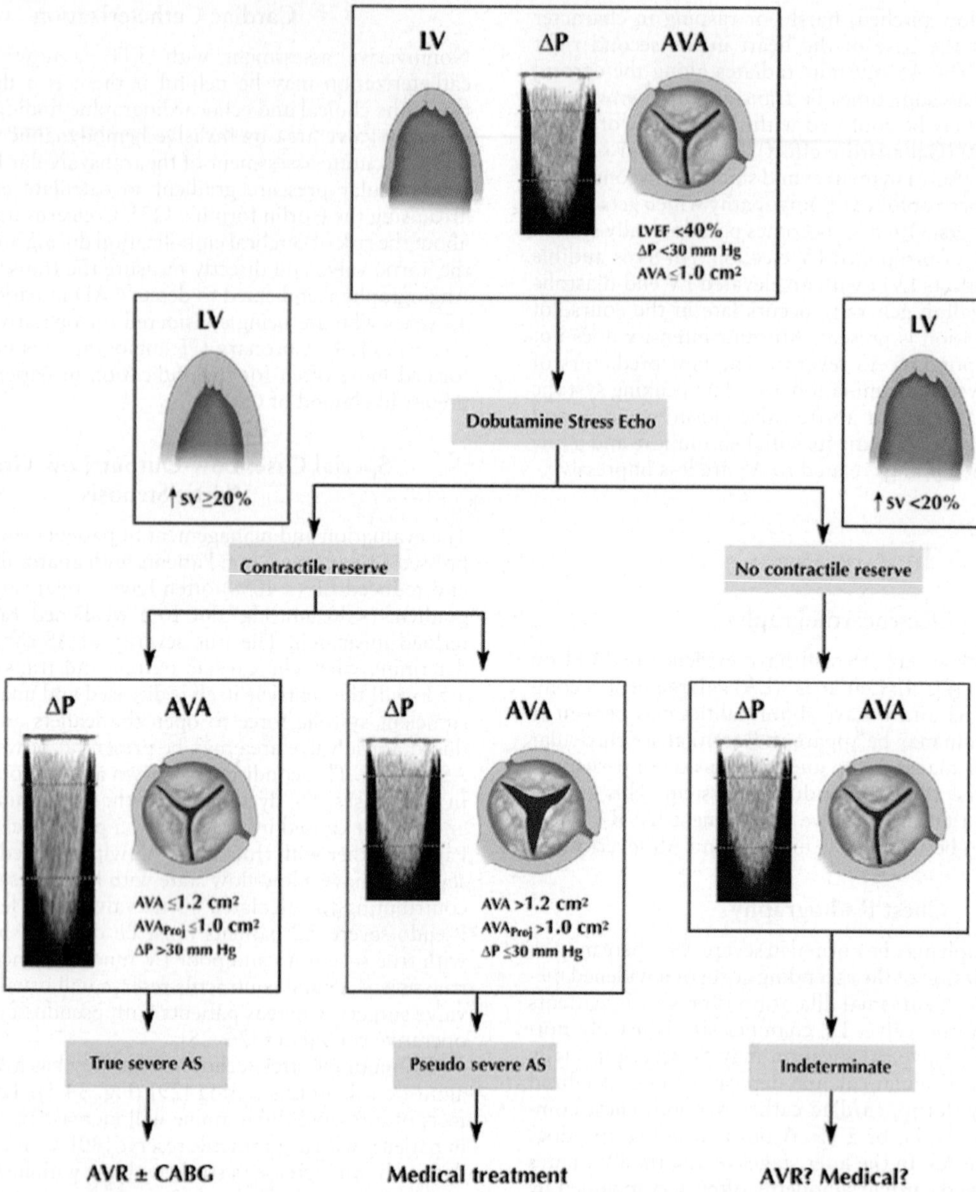

FIGURE 34.5. Decision making in low-flow, low-gradient aortic stenosis (AS). Dobutamine stress echocardiography aids decision making in low-flow AS. Contractile reserve is defined as an increase in stroke volume of >20%. When contractile reserve is elicited, patients with true severe AS have an increase in transvalvular gradient (ΔP) with a persistently low calculated valve area (AVA). One can also determine the projected AVA at a standardized normal flow rate (AVA_{proj}), with an AVA_{proj} ≤ 1 cm^2 consistent with true severe AS. Management decisions are more challenging if contractile reserve is absent. AVR, aortic valve replacement; CABG, coronary artery bypass grafting; LV, left ventricle. [From Picano E, Pibarot P, et al: The emerging role of exercise testing and stress echocardiography in valvular heart disease. *J Am Coll Cardiol* 54:2251–2260, 2009, with permission.]

contrast, surgery may be postponed in patients with severe, asymptomatic AS and normal LV function, as these patients may do well for years [34]. AVR is also indicated for patients with moderate AS who require other cardiac surgery, such as coronary artery bypass grafting (CABG) or aortic aneurysm repair. Patients with severe AS and cardiogenic shock may be considered for percutaneous aortic balloon valvuloplasty (PABV) as a bridge to AVR. Transcatheter aortic valve implantation (TAVI) has been performed in more than 5,000 patients worldwide and promises to be a viable treatment alternative for patients with severe AS who are considered too high risk for conventional surgery.

Medical Management

Medical interventions in severe AS are largely supportive until surgery is feasible. In patients with severe AS with heart failure or cardiogenic shock, management should be guided by invasive hemodynamic monitoring with a pulmonary artery catheter. Gentle diuresis may relieve pulmonary congestion, but patients with severe AS have a preload-dependent state, so overdiuresis can cause a severe drop in blood pressure. For patients in cardiogenic shock, arterial pressure should be supported with inotropes and/or vasopressors until valve surgery can be performed. Vasodilators are generally contraindicated, except in select patients with depressed EF [35]. In these select patients with EF less than 35%, severe AS and cardiogenic shock accompanied by high systemic vascular resistance, sodium nitroprusside infusion has been shown to modestly improve hemodynamics and can serve as a bridge to the operating room [36].

Surgical Treatment

AVR is the preferred treatment for severe symptomatic AS [32,37]. Choice of valve prosthesis depends on patient age, anticipated lifespan, and preference for and tolerance of anticoagulation [38]. The perioperative mortality for isolated AVR ranges from less than 1% in healthy, younger patients with normal LV systolic function to 10% or more in elderly patients with coexisting CAD and reduced EF. Age alone is not a contraindication to AVR. Other factors associated with reduced survival after AVR include chronic kidney disease, obstructive lung disease, reoperation, emergency operation, and age older than 65 years. The overall 10-year survival for patients with AVR is approximately 60%. Surgical risk for valve replacement can be estimated using one of several online calculators (Society for Thoracic Surgeons, EuroSCORE, or others) [39–41].

Percutaneous Aortic Balloon Valvuloplasty and Percutaneous Valve Replacement

PABV is often used instead of an operation in children and young adults with congenital, noncalcific AS. During the procedure in adults, a balloon is placed across the stenotic aortic valve and inflated to high pressure to fracture adherent calcium and increase effective orifice area [42]. A technically successful procedure can reduce the transaortic valve gradient to a mild degree but rarely increase valve area to more than 1 cm^2. Valvuloplasty is not widely used in adults with severe calcific AS because of high restenosis rates, frequent embolic complications (particularly stroke), and the development of AR [43]. In adults with acutely decompensated AS, PABV is particularly high risk and has no proven long-term benefits [44]. Given these risks, PABV is seldom used even in a palliative setting. In rare cases, it may be used as a bridge to AVR in patients with severe LV dysfunction and shock who are too ill to tolerate surgery without a period of metabolic recovery. PABV should not be considered as a substitute for AVR.

TAVI has generated considerable enthusiasm because it can eliminate the incremental risks conferred by sternotomy, cardiopulmonary bypass, and general anesthesia. TAVI can now be achieved in select patients and is undergoing active clinical investigation [45–48]. The procedure involve preparatory PABV followed by deployment of a balloon or self-expanding stented valve across the stenotic orifice. An antegrade, retrograde or LV transapical approach may be used. The retrograde approach is preferred but depends critically on whether relatively large diameter catheters can be successfully manipulated through the arterial system. Lower profile devices are under active development. There are several potential complications, though results with TAVI have been improving steadily and are quite promising [49]. TAVI will likely to have a major impact on management of AS in elderly, high-risk patients [50,51].

AORTIC REGURGITATION

Acute severe AR may occur in previously normal or only mildly diseased valves and often results in abrupt hemodynamic decompensation and respiratory compromise requiring ICU admission. Acute valvular regurgitation is a surgical emergency, but accurate diagnosis may be a challenge because examination findings may be subtle and the clinical presentation nonspecific [52]. Patients with acute AR appear gravely ill and have tachycardia, significant dyspnea, and often hypotension. The presentation of acute AR may even be mistaken for other acute conditions like sepsis, pneumonia, or nonvalvular heart failure. In marked contrast, chronic severe AR may be asymptomatic or minimally symptomatic and is rarely encountered in the ICU setting. In cases of acute valvular regurgitation, a high index of suspicion is required, along with timely TTE, and prompt surgical consultation.

Etiology

Most cases of acute severe AR are caused by infective endocarditis (IE), but other causes include aortic dissection and blunt chest trauma. Staphylococcus has emerged as the most important causative organism of native valve endocarditis [53,54]. Patients with antecedent aortic valve disease or a congenital bicuspid valve are at increased risk for IE, though organisms like *Staphylococcus aureus* can infect a normal trileaflet valve. IE is a particular problem among injection drug users, patients with indwelling catheters, and those on hemodialysis. Acute severe AR from IE is the consequence of tissue destruction, leaflet perforation, or bulky vegetations impairing leaflet coaptation [55].

AR is present in up to 65% of patients with Stanford Type A aortic dissection [56]. Ascending aortic dissection may be seen in Marfan syndrome, bicuspid aortic valve, or following CABG or AVR surgery. Retrograde extension of the dissection flap into the annulus may cause prolapse or eversion of the aortic valve leaflets. Type A aortic dissection with AR is a surgical emergency requiring prompt diagnosis and intervention [57]. Aneurysmal enlargement of the aortic root without dissection may also lead to AR. Although AR is usually chronic when produced by aortic root dilatation, an acute-on-chronic decompensation may occur if there is superimposed dissection or abrupt aneurysm enlargement [58]. Important causes of aortic root pathology producing AR include connective tissue disorders (Marfan syndrome and Ehlers-Danlos syndrome) and vasculitis (syphilis aortitis, giant cell arteritis, or Takayasu's arteritis). Aortic leaflets tears, perforation, or detachment producing AR may also follow blunt chest trauma or occur as a complication of PABV for AS [59].

Pathophysiology

Unlike in chronic AR, the LV in acute AR has not had time to develop compensatory eccentric hypertrophy in response to elevated afterload and preload (Fig. 34.6). The nondilated, noncompliant left ventricle receives a significant diastolic volume load from the regurgitant flow, resulting in an abrupt rise in LV end-diastolic pressure. This pressure may in turn be transmitted to the pulmonary bed resulting in pulmonary edema. Since the LV cannot dilate acutely in response to the volume load, forward stroke volume is decreased and tachycardia develops to maintain cardiac output. Impaired forward stroke volume leads to decreased systolic pressure and relatively narrow pulse pressure. Patients may present with signs of impending cardiogenic shock. LV diastolic pressure may equilibrate with aortic pressure during the latter half of diastole (diastasis), resulting in attenuation of the AR murmur in the acute setting. The elevation in end-diastolic pressure and tachycardia can increase myocardial oxygen demand and, when coupled with decreased diastolic coronary blood flow, can reduce myocardial perfusion and result in coronary ischemia. Ischemia from AR can be compounded by impairment in coronary flow from

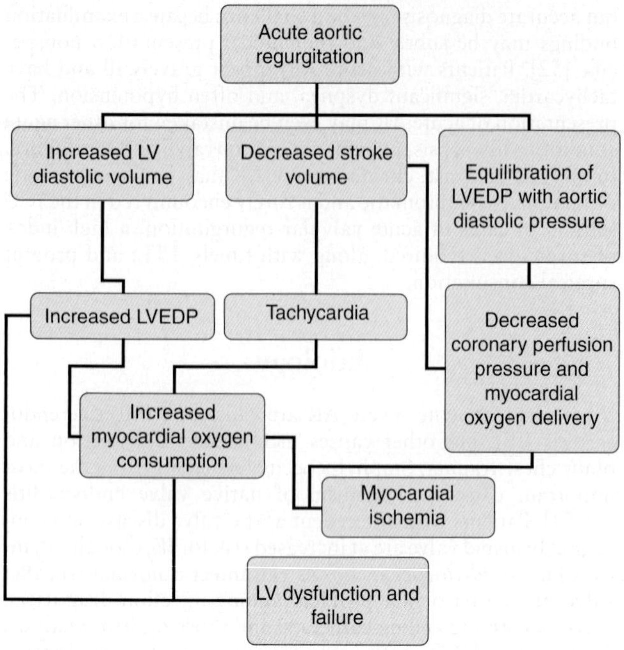

FIGURE 34.6. Pathophysiology of acute aortic regurgitation. LV, left ventricle; LVEDP, left ventricular end diastolic pressure. [Adapted from Bonow R, Braunwald E: Valvular heart disease, in Zipes D, et al. (eds): *Braunwald's Heart Disease*. Philadelphia, Elsevier, 2005, with permission.]

preexisting atherosclerosis or an aortic dissection flap. In acute severe AR, LV failure and cardiogenic shock develop if surgery is not promptly performed.

Clinical Presentation

History

Acute AR may present with little or no warning. Symptoms of weakness, profound dyspnea, angina, and presyncope are common. Antecedent valve disease, fever, and skin findings may suggest IE. Severe, ripping chest or back pain with hypertension may indicate aortic dissection. Signs of blunt chest trauma may be disarmingly subtle. The natural history of acute severe AR is one of LV failure and death in the absence of rapid intervention. Patients with chronic AR may present acutely with a sudden worsening of their underlying pathology.

Physical Examination

The classic eponymous signs observed in chronic AR are attenuated or absent in acute AR. Patients are often tachycardic with low or low-normal blood pressure. Pulse pressure may underestimate AR severity in the acute setting. Tachypnea, accessory muscle use, and hypoxemia are worrisome findings and pulmonary rales are common. LV apical impulse is not displaced unless prior LV dysfunction was present. The first heart sound (S1) is often soft due to premature closure of the mitral valve from the rapid LV diastolic pressure rise. There is often a low-pitched systolic ejection murmur from increased flow across the aortic valve, whereas the diastolic regurgitant murmur is of grade 1 or 2 intensity and of short duration. A pulse deficit or relative decrease may be appreciated in the setting of AR from aortic dissection.

Investigations

Electrocardiography

Sinus tachycardia is often present, though the ECG may be entirely normal in acute severe AR. In contrast, LVH is a feature of chronic AR. Nonspecific ST-segment and T-wave abnormalities or signs of LV strain are common. In IE, if there is paravalvular extension of the infection in the region of the atrioventricular node, heart block of varying degree may be present. In the setting of acute heart failure, supraventricular and ventricular tachycardias may occur.

Chest Radiography

The cardiac silhouette may be normal unless AR is chronic or there was preexisting heart disease. Pulmonary edema is common and characterized by cephalization of interstitial markings and Kerley B lines. A widened mediastinum may signify aortic dissection or thoracic aortic aneurysm.

Echocardiography

Urgent TTE is mandated whenever acute AR is suspected. Echocardiography can determine etiology and hemodynamic severity of AR while providing information on underlying LV function, aortic size, and coexisting valvular heart disease (Fig. 34.7). Severe AR is characterized by a wide regurgitant jet (vena contracta >6 mm) and holodiastolic flow reversal in the descending thoracic aorta [60]. The rapid rise in LV diastolic pressure with acute severe AR produces short pressure half time (<250 milliseconds) and premature mitral valve closure [61]. CT angiography has become the preferred imaging test to assess for acute dissection, but TEE may be indicated if the study is nondiagnostic and can be crucial for surgical planning [62,63].

Cardiac Catheterization

Establishing the hemodynamic severity of AR seldom requires catheterization, which can delay surgery [64]. Younger patients without coronary risk factors may proceed directly to emergency valve replacement without angiography. Patients with Type A dissection should proceed directly to surgical repair.

Intensive Care Unit Management

Medical Management

Acute severe AR has a high mortality rate. Medical management should not delay urgent or emergent surgery. Congestive heart failure and cardiogenic shock are the principle targets of acute medical therapies. Use of vasodilators, particularly sodium nitroprusside, and diuretics are the mainstays of medical therapy, if the systemic blood pressure allows [65]. Inotropes such as dopamine or dobutamine may be used to augment cardiac output. Pulmonary edema from acute AR frequently requires intubation and mechanical ventilation. Intra-aortic balloon counterpulsation (IABP) is strictly contraindicated. Beta-blockers should only be considered in cases of acute aortic dissection. Antibiotics are indicated for IE, but surgery must not be delayed once heart failure intervenes [24].

Surgical Treatment

Surgery is indicated for acute severe AR unless overwhelming patient comorbidities dictate otherwise. AVR is most commonly performed, but valve repair may be possible in

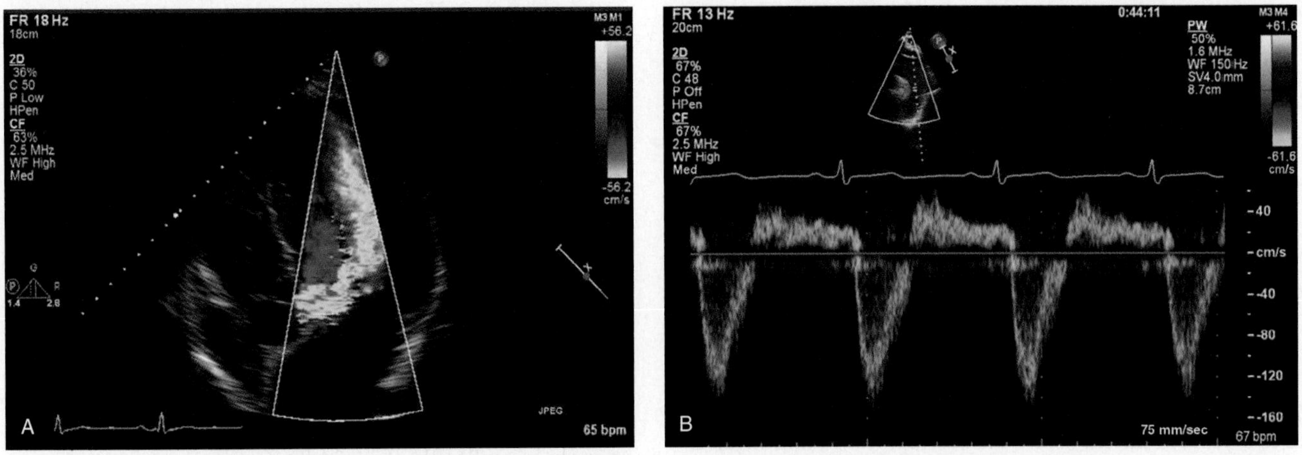

FIGURE 34.7. Echocardiographic appearance of severe aortic regurgitation. **A:** Transthoracic echocardiogram apical four-chamber view with severe aortic regurgitation from infective endocarditis. Color Doppler shows ventricular filling from the aorta during diastole. **B:** Pulse wave Doppler of the descending thoracic aortic reveals holodiastolic flow reversal consistent with severe aortic regurgitation.

cases of leaflet perforation. Most surgeons favor the use of homograft material for management of aortic valve/root IE given the low reinfection rates with cadaveric tissue. A composite valve-graft conduit may be used when disease dictates replacement of both the aortic root and valve [66]. Perioperative risk depends on age, preoperative LV function, etiology, and urgency of the surgery. Debridement of periaortic abscess or aortic root replacement compounds operative risk.

MITRAL STENOSIS

Widespread use of programs to detect and treat Group A streptococcal pharyngitis have reduced the incidence of rheumatic fever in the developed world, the leading cause of MS [67]. The burden of rheumatic valve disease in the developing world remains considerable and is a significant cause of premature death. Most cases of rheumatic MS in the United States are seen in patients who have recently emigrated from endemic areas [1]. Symptomatic MS requires mechanical relief of LV inflow obstruction. ICU management goals include treatment of heart failure, rate control of AF, and preparation for valvotomy or valve replacement surgery.

Etiology

Rheumatic fever produces valvular inflammation and scarring, though nearly half of patients may not recall history of acute rheumatic fever or chorea. Two thirds of patients with rheumatic MS are female and 40% of patients with rheumatic valvular disease will have isolated MS [68]. Screening TTE in endemic areas may detect up to 10 times as many cases of rheumatic valve disease compared with clinical screening alone [69]. By contrast, in developed countries, MS is more commonly produced by calcific degeneration of the annulus and mitral leaflets, congenital abnormalities, or collagen vascular diseases such as lupus or rheumatoid arthritis [70]. Atrial myxoma may mimic MS by causing obstruction to LV inflow. The natural history of MS is often dependent on the patient's nationality: in developing countries, patients tend to be younger with a more pliable valve, whereas in developed countries, patients are older with comorbid conditions [71].

Pathophysiology

Rheumatic fever leads to inflammation and scarring of the mitral valve, with fusion of the commissures and subvalvular apparatus [67]. Although the initial insult is rheumatic, altered flow patterns may lead to calcification and valve deformity, leading to a narrow funnel-shaped valve. Calcific degeneration of acquired mitral valve thickening may also produce MS. The mitral orifice is normally 4 to 6 cm^2. MS develops when the area is reduced to less than 2 cm^2 so that an elevated left atrioventricular pressure gradient is required to propel blood across the mitral valve. Severe MS is present when the valve area is less than 1 cm^2 and a mean transmitral gradient of more than 10 mm Hg is present (Table 34.2). An elevated LA pressure leads to pulmonary hypertension, exercise intolerance, and eventually right-sided heart failure. Adequate transit time is required to allow blood to flow across the stenotic mitral valve during diastole.

Clinical Manifestations

History

MS is a slowly progressive disease with a latent period of up to two decades between the episode of rheumatic carditis and symptom onset. Progression of MS in developing countries is more rapid and may be associated with recurrent episodes of rheumatic fever. The typical patient will have an asymptomatic period with an abnormal physical examination. As MS progresses, lesser stresses precipitate symptoms and the patient becomes limited in daily activities; orthopnea and paroxysmal

TABLE 34.2

SEVERITY OF MITRAL STENOSIS

Severity of stenosis	Valve area (cm^2)	Mean gradient (mm Hg)	PA systolic pressure (mm Hg)
Mild	>1.5	<5	<30
Moderate	1.0–1.5	5–10	30–50
Severe	<1.0	>10	>50

nocturnal dyspnea develop. Pulmonary edema in previously asymptomatic individuals may be triggered by tachyarrhythmias (AF), volume overload, fever, anemia, hyperthyroidism, or pregnancy [72]. Each of these circumstances shortens the diastolic filling period and elevates the LA–LV transvalvular gradient. Development of persistent AF marks a turning point in the patient's course, with an accelerated rate of symptom progression. Systemic embolization may be the first clue to the presence of MS, irrespective of underlying rhythm [73]. Patients may also suffer from hemoptysis due to shunting between the pulmonary and bronchial veins, leading to rupture. Underappreciated calcific MS may also be identified after failure to wean from mechanical ventilation.

The overall 10-year survival with untreated MS is 50% to 60% [74]. Asymptomatic patients have a survival of more than 80% at 10 years, whereas symptomatic MS led to death within 2 to 5 years in the era before the development of mitral valvotomy [75]. Once pulmonary hypertension develops, mean survival is less than 3 years. Common causes of death associated with MS are heart failure, systemic embolism, and infections, including endocarditis.

Physical Examination

MS produces signs of heart failure, including pulmonary rales, peripheral edema, ascites, an elevated jugular venous pressure, and congestive hepatomegaly. Patients with severe MS may also have a malar flush with pinched and blue facies. The first heart sound (S1) is usually accentuated in the early phases of the disease. The opening snap (OS) of MS is best appreciated in early diastole during expiration near the cardiac apex. The time interval between aortic valve closure (A2) and OS varies inversely with the severity of MS and the height of LA pressures. The OS is followed by a low-pitched rumbling diastolic murmur best heard at the apex with the patient in the left lateral decubitus position. Presystolic accentuation of the murmur may be present in sinus rhythm. In general, the duration of the murmur corresponds to the severity of stenosis. If the valve is heavily calcified and immobile, with low cardiac output or AF, it may be relatively "silent" with a soft S1, absent presystolic accentuation, and an inaudible diastolic rumble. Associated valvular lesions, including the murmurs of AR, pulmonic regurgitation (PR), and tricuspid regurgitation (TR), may be present, along with a loud P2 from pulmonary hypertension or a parasternal lift from right ventricle (RV) pressure or volume overload.

Investigations

Electrocardiogram

The ECG in sinus rhythm may reveal LA enlargement but AF can be present at any stage in the natural history. A vertical QRS axis may be present along with nonspecific ST-segment and T-wave abnormalities. Signs of RV hypertrophy signify advanced disease.

Chest Radiograph

Radiographic changes with MS include LA enlargement, dilation of the main pulmonary artery and its central branches, RV enlargement, and signs of pulmonary vascular congestion. Interstitial or alveolar edema signifies a marked and often acute elevation of pulmonary capillary wedge (PCW) pressure.

Echocardiography

Rheumatic MS is characterized by thickened mitral leaflet tips, immobility of the posterior leaflet, and restricted anterior leaflet motion. Calcific MS is marked by dense echogenic deposits throughout the mitral apparatus and turbulent LV diastolic inflow. Direct planimetry to measure valve area may be difficult in heavily calcified valves [76]. Continuous wave Doppler can be used to estimate the LA–LV pressure gradient. Estimates of mitral valve area can be made by the pressure half-time technique or the continuity equation [77]. Careful assessment of the degree and location of valvular calcification, thickening of the leaflet and subvalvular apparatus, and leaflet mobility can determine suitability for percutaneous mitral balloon valvuloplasty (PMBV) [78]. Routine assessment of chamber dimension and ventricular function should be performed. TEE is required to exclude LA thrombus in patients being considered for PMBV.

Cardiac Catheterization

Catheterization may be necessary to determine stenosis severity when noninvasive and clinical data are discordant or as a prelude to PMBV (Fig. 34.8). Cardiac output and mean transvalvular gradient measurements are used to calculate mitral valve area using the Gorlin formula [23].

Intensive Care Unit Management

Medical Therapy

Acute MS typically manifests as pulmonary edema. Reversible precipitants must be identified, such as rapid AF, anemia, sepsis, volume overload, or thyrotoxicosis. Medical therapy is directed at rate control of AF and alleviation of pulmonary and systemic congestion by loop diuretics. Nodal blocking agents such as beta-blockers or calcium-channel blockers are the preferred rate controlling agents and may be administered intravenously [79]. Cardioversion may be required in the acute setting to restore hemodynamic stability, though most patients respond to rate control. Anticoagulation should be initiated promptly. In patients with only mild-to-moderate MS, addressing one or more underlying precipitants will suffice without the need for mechanical intervention. Patients with severe MS have a poor prognosis without intervention, which may consist of PMBV, surgical commissurotomy, or mitral valve replacement (MVR) (Fig. 34.9).

Percutaneous Mitral Balloon Valvuloplasty

PMBV is the preferred treatment for symptomatic (NYHA Class II–IV) patients with isolated severe MS (valve area is <1 cm^2) and favorable valve morphology. Unlike PABV, PMBV has achieved durable results. Ideal patients for PMBV are younger (age <45 years), have better NYHA functional class, and have pliable mitral leaflets [80]. PMBV is performed by transseptal puncture, passing a guidewire across the mitral valve, and inflating a balloon (Inoue balloon) across the mitral orifice to split the commissures and widen the stenotic valve [43,81].

Successful PMBV doubles the mitral valve area, reduces mean transmitral gradient by half, and improves symptoms without development of significant MR [82]. Acute complications of PMBV include severe MR; residual atrial septal defect after transseptal puncture; and, less commonly, LV perforation, cardiac tamponade, and systemic emboli. Overall procedural morality is between 0.4% and 3.0% [83]. Patients have excellent event-free survival after PMBV with rates of 80% to 90% over 3 to 7 years when performed by a skilled operator in a high-volume center [84]. Short- and intermediate-term outcomes after PMBV are comparable with those after open surgical commissurotomy, but with reduced morbidity and at lower cost [85]. There is a significant rate of restenosis after both percutaneous and surgical commissurotomy with most patients requiring a repeat procedure within 10 to 15 years.

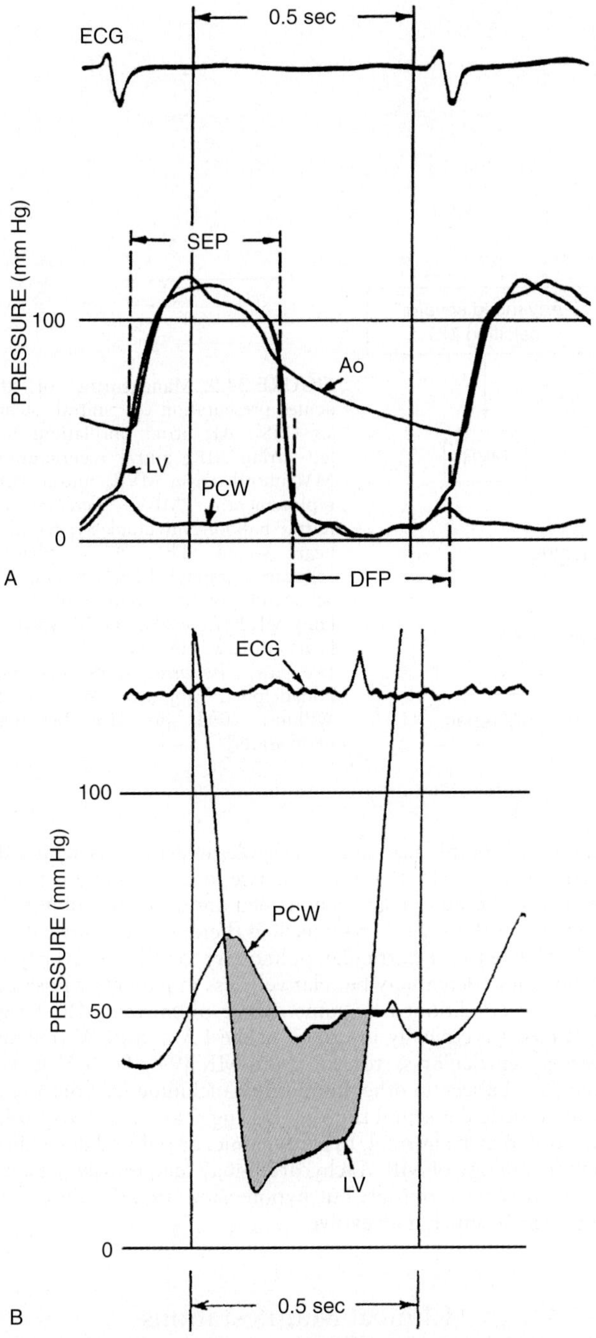

FIGURE 34.8. Hemodynamic measurements in mitral stenosis. **A:** Depicts normal left ventricle (LV), left atrial (LA), and aortic (Ao) pressure tracings. **B:** Depicts the pressure gradient between pulmonary capillary wedge (PCW) pressure and LV in a patient with MS (*shaded area*). DFP, diastolic filling period; SEP, systolic ejection period. [Adapted from Carabello BA: Modern management of mitral stenosis. *Circulation* 112(3):432–437, 2005, with permission.]

Surgical Treatment

If the anatomy is unfavorable for PMBV or the procedure is unsuccessful, open surgical valvotomy may be performed, which requires cardiopulmonary bypass [86]. MVR is necessary in patients with MS and significant MR and those in whom valve anatomy is too distorted to respond to commissurotomy alone. MVR is often performed with preservation of the chordal attachments to facilitate LV recovery. A surgical MAZE procedure or isolation of the pulmonary veins may also be performed to treat concomitant AF, though success rates are relatively lower in rheumatic MS patients. The average operative risk for MVR is 5%, with an overall 10-year survival in surgical survivors of 70%. Long-term prognosis is influenced by patient age, comorbid conditions, and the presence of concomitant pulmonary hypertension and RV dysfunction.

MITRAL REGURGITATION

Acute, severe MR presents with pulmonary edema and hemodynamic compromise because of the lack of time for the cardiopulmonary circuit to adapt to the additional volume load. Examination findings may be subtle and presentation may be mistaken for other acute conditions such as pneumonia or nonvalvular decompensated heart failure. A high clinical index of suspicion, timely evaluation by TTE, and prompt referral for surgical consultation are of critical value in the management of this condition [52]. Many patients in the ICU will have MR accompanied by reduced LV systolic function, from either MI or chronic cardiomyopathy. The management of patients with MR and advanced systolic heart failure remains controversial.

Etiology

MR may be caused by abnormalities of any component of the mitral apparatus: annulus, valve leaflets, chordae tendineae, papillary muscles, and adjacent LV free wall [87] (Table 34.3). Common causes of acute MR include chordal rupture from myxomatous degeneration, blunt trauma, or endocarditis; leaflet perforation from endocarditis or leaflet avulsion from trauma; papillary muscle infarction with rupture or displacement from acute or chronic ischemia and LV remodeling; acute rheumatic carditis or other acute condition like stress cardiomyopathy; and mitral prosthetic paravalvular leak [88–90]. Often, the causes of MR are divided into "organic" disorders involving the mitral valve leaflets and "functional" disorders due to tethering of the mitral apparatus from ventricular remodeling, LV dilatation, and increased sphericity. This classification emphasizes when attention should be directed toward mitral valve surgery (organic causes) or to addressing an underlying cardiomyopathy (functional causes).

Ischemic MR refers to MR produced after acute MI and, more commonly, in chronic ischemic cardiomyopathy. The most important mechanism of ischemic MR is mitral valve leaflet tethering due to chronic postinfarction remodeling, resulting in apical and lateral displacement of the papillary muscles. This shape change occurs after an inferior or posterior transmural MI leads to displacement of the posteromedial papillary muscle [91]. After MI, the presence of MR can augment postinfarction remodeling, further exacerbating the degree of functional MR [92]. Papillary rupture is a rare complication of acute MI (1% to 3%) with a bimodal peak at 1 day, then 3 to 5 days post-MI. The posteromedial papillary muscle has a single blood supply from the right coronary or left circumflex artery, and thus is 6 to 10 times more likely to rupture than the anterolateral papillary, which has a dual blood supply. Dynamic MR can occur during episodes of transient ischemia involving the papillary muscles but is not usually severe [93]. Dynamic MR is also a feature of HOCM and has been described in some patients with stress cardiomyopathy.

Pathophysiology

In acute MR, the LV ejects blood into a small, noncompliant LA leading to a rapid rise in LA pressure during systole. The difference in LA compliance explains why chronic MR

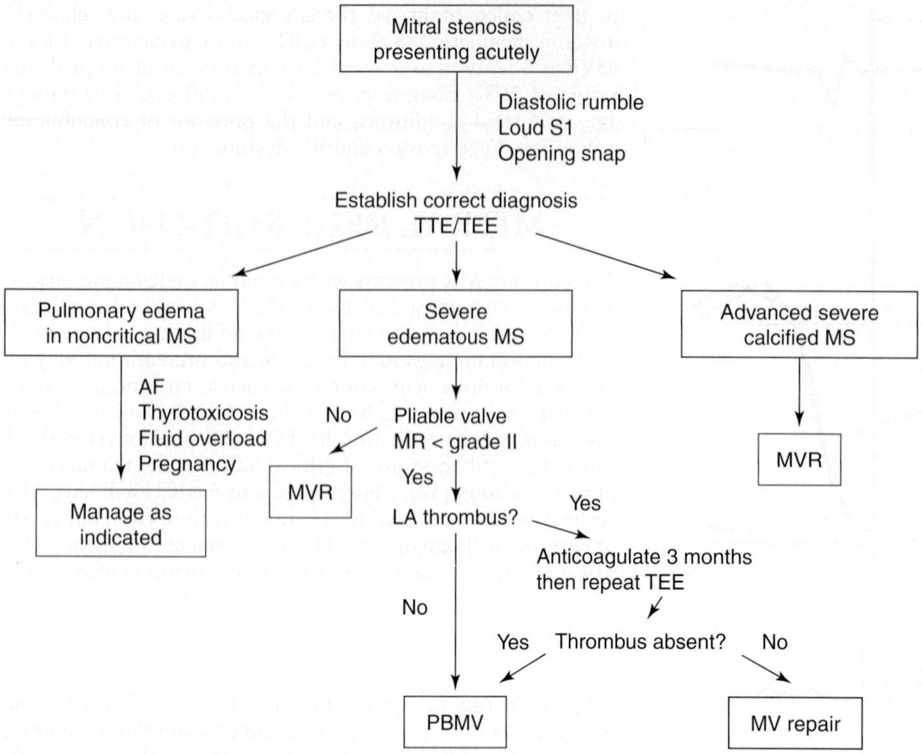

FIGURE 34.9. Management of the acute presentation of mitral stenosis (MS). AF, atrial fibrillation; LA, left atrial; MR, mitral regurgitation; MV, mitral valve; MVR, mitral valve replacement; PMBV, percutaneous mitral balloon valvuloplasty; S1, first heart sound; TEE, transesophageal echocardiography; TTE, transthoracic echocardiography. [Adapted from Bellamy MF, Enriquez-Sarano M: Valvular heart disease, in Irwin RS, Rippe JM (eds): *Intensive Care Medicine*. Philadelphia, Lippincott Williams & Wilkins, 2003, pp 313–328, with permission.]

TABLE 34.3

CAUSES OF ACUTE SEVERE NATIVE MITRAL REGURGITATION

Mitral annulus disorders
Infective endocarditis (abscess formation)
Trauma (valvular heart surgery)
Paravalvular leak due to suture interruption (surgical technical problems or infective endocarditis)
Mitral leaflet disorders
Infective endocarditis (perforation or interfering with valve closure by vegetation)
Trauma (tear during percutaneous balloon mitral valvuloplasty or penetrating chest injury)
Tumors (atrial myxoma)
Myxomatous degeneration
Systemic lupus erythematosus (Libman-Sacks lesion)
Rupture of chordae tendineae
Idiopathic (spontaneous)
Myxomatous degeneration (mitral valve prolapse, Marfan syndrome, Ehlers-Danlos syndrome)
Infective endocarditis
Acute rheumatic fever
Trauma (percutaneous balloon valvuloplasty, blunt chest trauma)
Papillary muscle disorders
Coronary artery disease (causing dysfunction and rarely rupture)
Acute global left ventricular dysfunction
Infiltrative diseases (amyloidosis, sarcoidosis)
Trauma

Bonow R, Braunwald E: Valvular heart disease, in Zipes D, et al. (eds): *Braunwald's Heart Disease*. Philadelphia, Elsevier Saunders, 2005, pp 1553–1621.

(increased compliance) can be well tolerated and why acute MR (reduced compliance) is not. The rise in LA pressure is transmitted to the pulmonary venous bed and leads to pulmonary edema, which may be asymmetric if there is an eccentric jet of MR directed to a particular pulmonary vein. The severity of pulmonary edema may be relatively less in patients whose LA has been conditioned by some degree of chronic MR. Large V waves are typically inscribed in the LA and PCW tracings during ventricular systole in acute MR [94]. Such V waves may also be seen in other conditions, including LV failure and acute ventricular septal rupture. During acute MR, LV systolic function may be normal, hyperdynamic, or reduced depending on the etiology of MR. Tachycardia may temporarily preserve forward cardiac output, but hypotension, organ failure, and cardiogenic shock may evolve.

Clinical Manifestations

History

In acute severe MR, symptoms of left heart failure predominate, including dyspnea, orthopnea, and cough. Patients with post-MI papillary muscle rupture or ischemic MR may have concurrent angina, dyspnea, and abrupt hemodynamic compromise. Spontaneous chordal rupture in myxomatous degeneration may be accompanied by chest pain in nearly half of patients. Symptoms of fevers, chills, malaise, and anorexia may be present in patients with endocarditis. Trauma is usually self-evident (Table 34.4).

Physical Examination

Patients with acute severe MR are tachycardic and tachypneic. Blood pressure is variable, though pulse pressure is often narrow due to reduced forward stroke volume. Jugular venous pressure may be normal or elevated. Rales or wheezes may be

TABLE 34.4

CLINICAL FINDINGS IN ACUTE SEVERE MITRAL REGURGITATION

	Acute organic MR	Papillary muscle rupture	Functional MR with CHF
Etiology	Ruptured chordae, endocarditis, trauma	1 or 3–5 d post-MI	Ischemic heart disease, dilated cardiomyopathy
Presentation	Acute pulmonary edema	Sudden onset pulmonary edema and cardiogenic shock	CHF and pulmonary edema
Clinical Examination			
Point of maximum impulse/apex beat	Normal or displaced thrill	Usually normal if no prior LV dysfunction	Displaced
Murmur	Holosystolic loud	May be very soft or absent	Early systolic, rarely holosystolic soft
Sounds	Third heart sound, second heart sound split	Decreased sounds	Third heart sound
Investigations			
Electrocardiogram	Normal	Acute MI	Left bundle branch block
Chest radiograph	Normal heart size	Usually normal	Cardiomegaly
Echocardiogram			
Two-dimensional	LV and LA size normal Ruptured chord	Normal LV Ruptured head of papillary muscle	LV and LA dilated Annular dilatation Tenting of mitral valve leaflets
Doppler	Pulmonary venous flow reversal	Unimpressive color	Restrictive filling
Quantitation	Large regurgitation volume Large effective regurgitation orifice	Free-flow MR	Variable regurgitation volume Dynamic effective regurgitation orifice

CHF, congestive heart failure; LA, left atrial; LV, left ventricular; MI, myocardial infarction; MR, mitral regurgitation.
From Parikh S, O'Gara PT: Valvular heart disease, in Rippe JM, Irwin RS (eds): *Intensive Care Medicine*. Philadelphia, Lippincott Williams & Wilkins, 2006.

audible over the lung fields and may be asymmetric. The precordium is often hyperdynamic with a palpable apical thrill. S1 is normal or decreased in intensity, whereas S2 may be widely split due to early closure of the aortic valve. A diastolic filling complex may be appreciated and consists of a third heart sound (S3) and a short mid-diastolic rumble from increased transmitral diastolic flow. The systolic murmur of acute MR may be highly variable, and even absent in up to half of cases of post-MI papillary muscle rupture. The murmur of acute MR is usually not holosystolic but rather early to mid-systolic in timing, with a crescendo–decrescendo configuration, and is coarse rather than high pitched. These features reflect the rapid LA pressure rise and diminution of the LV–LA pressure gradient throughout systole. The murmur of chronic MR, in contrast, is holosystolic (plateau) due to the persistent LV–LA gradient during systole. The murmur of acute MR is usually loudest at the left sternal border or apex, and the direction of radiation may provide a clue as to etiology. Anterior leaflet prolapse or flail produces a posterior-lateral regurgitant jet, so the murmur typically radiates to the axilla and back. With posterior leaflet involvement, the jet is anterior-medial in direction, so the murmur is transmitted to the base, where it may be confused with AS.

Investigations

Electrocardiogram

ECG may show sinus tachycardia or an atrial arrhythmia, such as AF. LA abnormality may be discernible if P waves are present, though signs of LV chamber enlargement are rare in the acute phase. With post-MI papillary muscle rupture, evidence of an evolving inferior-posterior or lateral MI may be seen.

Chest Radiograph

In acute MR, the cardiac silhouette is normal in size despite the present of alveolar pulmonary edema. Asymmetric edema may be present in patients with a flail leaflet producing an eccentric MR jet, particularly in the right upper lobe [95]. Decompensated chronic MR may have associated cardiomegaly, LA enlargement, and prominent pulmonary arteries.

Echocardiography

Prompt TTE is the most important study for patients with suspected acute MR (Fig. 34.10). TTE can delineate mitral anatomy, characterize severity, and document underlying LV function and coexisting valvular pathology. Flail leaflet may be diagnosed by rapid movement of a portion of leaflet/chordal tissue posteriorly in to the LA during systole. Chordal rupture, leaflet vegetations, and periannular abscess may be identified in endocarditis. In patients with functional MR, LV remodeling may be evident along with annular dilatation, papillary muscle displacement, and leaflet tethering. Semiquantitative assessment of MR severity can be performed with color flow and continuous wave Doppler interrogation. MR severity correlates with LA jet width area, pulmonary vein systolic flow reversal, effective regurgitant orifice area, and regurgitant fraction and volume [96,97]. These semiquantitative measures are less important as guides for acute decision making but remain important for longitudinal management (Table 34.5). TEE can

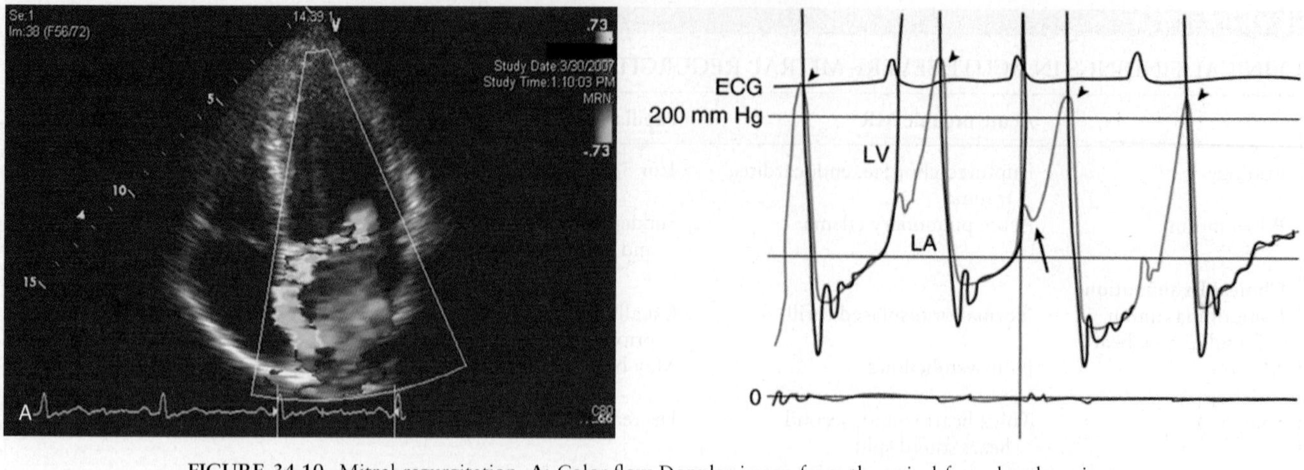

FIGURE 34.10. Mitral regurgitation. **A:** Color-flow Doppler image from the apical four-chamber view of a patient with myxomatous degeneration of the mitral valve with posterior leaflet prolapse producing an anteromedially directed jet of severe mitral regurgitation against the interatrial septum. Eccentric jets are common in prolapse and/or flail leaflet and are directed opposite the involved leaflet. **B:** The "V" wave of mitral regurgitation. This hemodynamic tracing shows a large left atrial "V" wave (arrowheads) occurring during ventricular systole in a patient with atrial fibrillation ("A" wave absent). Following the "V" wave, there is a rapid fall in left atrial (LA) pressure, along the course of the declining left ventricular (LV) pressure. In diastole, LA and LV pressures are equalized. The arrow indicated the "C" wave deflection. Giant "V" waves are defined by an increase in >10 mm Hg above mean pressure and are consistent with mitral regurgitation, but may be blunted in patients with large and compliant left atria. ECG, electrocardiogram. [From O'Gara PT: Valvular heart disease, in Libby P (ed): *Essential Atlas of Cardiovascular Disease*. New York, NY, Springer, 2009, p 216, Figures 9–20 and 9–22.]

further characterized mitral anatomy and MR severity if TTE images are suboptimal or complicated IE is suspected.

Cardiac Catheterization

Catheterization is rarely required to define MR etiology or severity. If there is a discrepancy between clinical findings and noninvasive imaging or when estimated pulmonary artery pressures are out of proportion to the degree of MR, then invasive hemodynamic assessment is indicated. MR severity may be qualitatively assessed by contrast ventriculography. Coronary angiography typically precedes surgery for patients with coronary risk factors and in those with suspected post-MI papillary rupture or dynamic, ischemic MR.

TABLE 34.5

ECHOCARDIOGRAPHIC FINDINGS CONSISTENT WITH SEVERE MITRAL REGURGITATION

Qualitative
Vena contracta width >0.7 cm with large central MR jet (area >40% left atrial area) or with a wall-impinging jet of any size, swirling in left atrium (Echo, Doppler)
Pulmonary vein systolic flow reversal (Doppler)
Dense contrast in left atrium (angiography)
Quantitative
Regurgitant volume ≥60 mL per beat
Regurgitant fraction ≥50%
Effective regurgitant orifice ≥0.40 cm^2

From Zoghbi WA, Enriquez-Sarano M, Foster E, et al: Recommendations for evaluation of the severity of native valvular regurgitation with two-dimensional and Doppler echocardiography. *J Am Soc Echocardiogr* 16:777–802, 2003, with permission.

Intensive Care Unit Management

Medical Therapy

The goal of medical therapy for acute severe MR is to stabilize the patient in anticipation of surgery for definitive treatment. Afterload reduction with intravenous vasodilators is the mainstay of acute medical therapy, as systolic blood pressure tolerates. Sodium nitroprusside infusion is preferred, though extended use requires monitoring of thiocyanate levels [65]. Inotropes such as dobutamine or dopamine may occasionally be required to support cardiac output and arterial pressure. IABP for mechanical afterload reduction may be particularly helpful in reducing regurgitant volume and decreasing LV end-diastolic pressure. If end-organ hypoperfusion or hypotension indicates that cardiogenic shock is present, IABP should be promptly initiated as a bridge to the operating room. Loop diuretics may help ameliorate pulmonary edema.

Adjunctive medical therapy is driven in part by suspected etiology. Antibiotics are indicated for IE and anti-ischemic therapy is required for post-MI papillary muscle rupture [98]. With medical therapy alone, the mortality after papillary rupture is 80% [99]. Although percutaneous coronary intervention (PCI) may help relieve MR in the setting of acute MI, severe MR will most often require surgical correction despite successful coronary reperfusion. Despite recent advances in percutaneous valve repair techniques, none has yet been tested in the setting of acute MR [100,101]. Similarly, cardiac resynchronization therapy (CRT) may help reduce chronic, functional MR related to contractile dyssynchrony but has no role in the acute setting [102]. Surgical planning should not be delayed, but an operation may have to await improvement in organ function after the measures described above are instituted.

Surgical Therapy

Surgery is indicated for the treatment of acute severe MR. In contrast to acute severe AR, many patients with acute severe

MR may be stabilized over the course of several days with IABP or inodilators to allow operation under less urgent circumstances [24]. Also unlike acute AR, acute severe MR may be treated with either repair or replacement. Valve repair is the preferred surgical therapy when possible [103]. Mitral repair involves valve reconstruction using a variety of valvuloplasty techniques and insertion of an annuloplasty ring. In addition to reducing the need for anticoagulation and the risk of late prosthetic valve failure, valve repair preserves the integrity of the subvalvular apparatus, which maintains LV function to a greater degree. Valve repair using an undersized annuloplasty ring is more likely to be used for ischemic MR [52]. Valve replacement with chordal sparing is needed when there is destruction, distortion, or infection of the native tissue that makes repair impossible. Surgical strategy is often guided by intraoperative TEE and direct visual inspection after the patients is placed on cardiopulmonary bypass.

Surgical outcome depends on age, underlying LV function, the presence of concomitant coronary disease, patient comorbidities, and the etiology of MR [104]. IE has a high mortality rate even with medical and surgical therapy, though mortality has decreased with improvements in operative technique and more widespread use of mitral repair [105,106]. With the addition of bypass grafting to mitral valve repair, operative mortality in patients with ischemic MR is now less than 10% [99,107].

The surgical approaches to patients with MR accompanied by advanced systolic heart failure continue to evolve and remain controversial [108]. There is broad consensus that patients with chronic MR and heart failure should be optimized on medical therapy, evaluated for revascularization if coronary disease is present, and provided with CRT if the EF is less than 35% and a wide QRS, left bundle branch block complex (>120 milliseconds) is present. After these steps, reconfirmation of MR severity is required before considering MV surgery. If severe MR is present, a careful integrated assessment of LV reverse remodeling viability (usually with cardiac magnetic resonance imaging), mitral apparatus geometry, and patient comorbidities must be made in consultation with cardiology and cardiac surgery colleagues [108]. As percutaneous and less invasive approaches to mitral valve disease in patients with heart failure continue to evolve, ongoing clinical trials will help refine the selection of candidates for mitral surgery and determine outcomes of mitral repair versus chord-sparing replacement.

TRICUSPID REGURGITATION

Most ICU patients with TR have functional regurgitation rather than a primary valvular abnormality. Functional TR is produced when the tricuspid annulus is dilated due to RV infarction, congenital heart disease, or pulmonary hypertension with RV dilatation, often secondary to chronic left heart failure. TR is often present in patients with chronic left-sided valve disorders that produce secondary pulmonary hypertension or with pathologic processes affecting multiple valves, such as rheumatic disease, endocarditis, or myxomatous degeneration [109]. The most important causes of primary valvular TR are trauma and IE, particularly in patients who abuse intravenous drugs. When severe, TR may contribute to symptoms of right heart failure, including fatigue, edema, and ascites. The murmur of TR usually increases in intensity with inspiration (Carvallo's sign). Examination of the neck veins reveals large V-waves. A pulsatile liver edge may also be felt in the right upper quadrant.

Despite the significant volume load imposed by severe TR, the RV tolerates TR remarkably well and operation is rarely indicated in the absence of other valve disease [32]. Therapy for TR is targeted at the underlying disease process and reversing secondary causes of pulmonary hypertension [110]. For example, with LV failure, appropriate management with diuresis and afterload reduction with vasodilators may reduce the degree of functional TR. When caused by left-sided heart disease, worsening TR can be a marker of underlying RV compromise and heralds a poor prognosis [111]. Secondary TR caused by mitral valve disease is increasingly addressed with annuloplasty repair at the time of mitral valve surgery, since functional TR occurring late after a left-sided valve operation is associated with high morbidity and mortality [112]. Tricuspid annuloplasty or valve replacement surgery may also be required for severe primary TR causing worsening RV systolic function or refractory right heart failure.

PROSTHETIC VALVE DYSFUNCTION

Valve replacement surgery has been a major breakthrough allowing patients with severe valvular heart disease to have better quality and length of life. Prosthetic valves may be either mechanical or bioprosthetic (Fig. 34.11). The choice of prosthesis is informed by patient age, the need for anticoagulation, hemodynamic profile, durability, and patient preference [113]. Mechanical valves have excellent durability and hemodynamic performance but require life-long anticoagulation to prevent thromboembolic complications [114]. In contrast, the principal advantage of bioprosthetic valves is the virtual absence of thromboembolic complication after 3 months, except when there are risk factors such as a hypercoagulable state or chronic AF with atrial enlargement [115]. Bioprosthetic valves are usually xenografts (porcine or cryopreserved, mounted bovine pericardium); homografts from human cadavers are used to treat aortic valve and root endocarditis. All bioprostheses are at risk for structural valve deterioration (SVD), which is mostly a function of age at implant. SVD occurs more rapidly among patients younger than 40 years compared with those older than 65 years. Rates of SVD may not differ between homograft and xenograft valves. Over the past 10 years, there has been a trend toward using bioprosthetic valves in relatively younger patients (ages 50 to 65 years) despite the inherent risk of SVD and need for reoperation, given the increased durability of the current generation xenograft valves, decreased risk at reoperation, aggregate risks of long-term anticoagulation, and patient lifestyle preferences.

All prosthetic valves are subject to dysfunction that can lead to significant hemodynamic compromise. Common prosthetic valve abnormalities include mechanical valve thrombosis, prosthetic valve endocarditis (PVE), structural deterioration and failure, and paravalvular regurgitation with or without hemolysis. For patients with a prosthetic valve admitted to the ICU, management focuses on appropriately excluding prosthetic valve dysfunction using TTE and TEE when required and maintaining optimal prosthetic valve function [116].

Prosthetic Valve Thrombosis

Prosthetic valve thrombosis (PVT) is any valve thrombus attached to or near an operated valve that occludes part of the blood flow path or interferes with the function of the valve [32]. PVT is a rare but life-threatening condition (Fig. 34.12). It is more common with older generation mechanical valves, particularly in the setting of inadequate anticoagulation. The incidence is estimated to be between 0.3% and 1.3% per year in patients with mechanical valves [117,118].

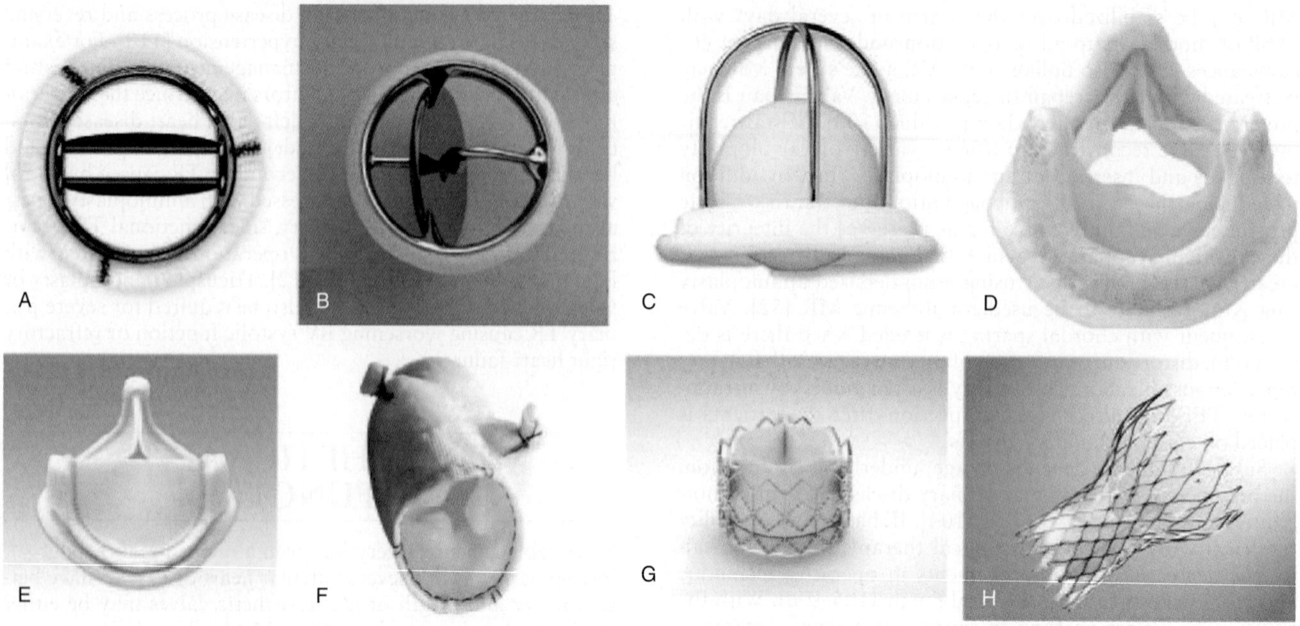

FIGURE 34.11. Different types of prosthetic heart valves. **A:** Bileaflet mechanical valve (St. Jude's); **B:** monoleaflet, tilting disk mechanical valve (Medtronic Hall); **C:** caged ball valve (Starr-Edwards); **D:** stented porcine bioprosthesis (Medtronic Mosaic); **E:** stented pericardial bioprosthesis (Carpentier-Edwards Magna); **F:** stentless porcine bioprosthesis (Medtronic Freestyle); **G:** percutaneous bioprosthesis expanded over a balloon (Edwards Sapien); **H:** self-expandable percutaneous bioprosthesis (CoreValve). [From Pibarot P, Dumesnil JG: Prosthetic heart valves: selection of the optimal prosthesis and long-term management. *Circulation* 119:1034–1048, 2009, with permission.]

Clinical Presentation and Investigations

PVT follows a rapid clinical course, unlike the in-growth of fibrous/pannus tissue within a prosthetic valve ring, which slowly gives rise to valve dysfunction and stenosis [119]. PVT manifests as abrupt onset of systemic embolization, congestive heart failure, or cardiogenic shock. The degree of hemodynamic compromise is determined by valve position and degree of resulting dysfunction. In general, the time course may be more insidious with caged-ball valves and more abrupt with tilting disk valves [120]. The physical examination may be unrevealing, though soft mechanical valve closure sounds or a pathologic murmur may be present.

A subtherapeutic international normalized ratio (INR) in a patient with a mechanical valve is a red flag for PVT [121]. Rapid diagnosis depends on prompt TTE or fluoroscopy, though both modalities may be complementary [122]. TTE can diagnose the presence of valve thrombus, its composition, and associated functional stenosis or regurgitation. TEE usually provides further risk stratification, particularly in cases of suspected mitral PVT and when TTE windows are inadequate [123]. Fluoroscopy can be useful to characterize caged-ball, tilting-disc, or bileaflet mobility. Excursion of tilting-disc mechanical valves is much better appreciated with fluoroscopy than with TTE.

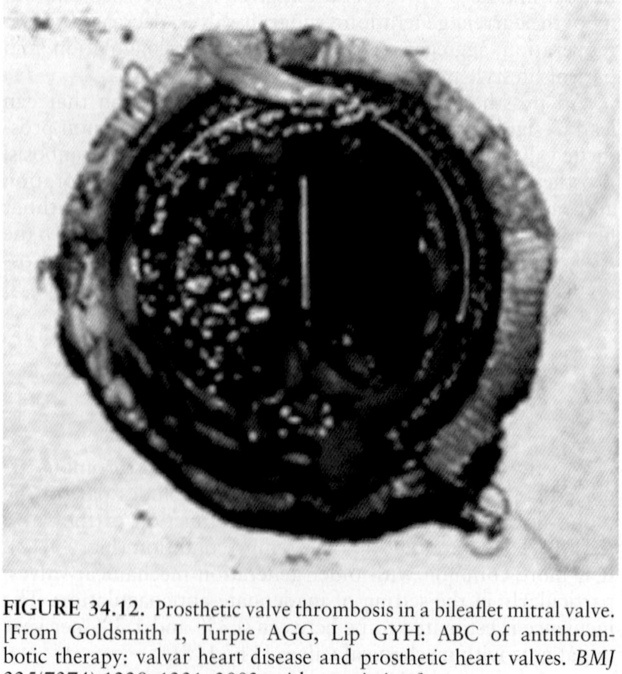

FIGURE 34.12. Prosthetic valve thrombosis in a bileaflet mitral valve. [From Goldsmith I, Turpie AGG, Lip GYH: ABC of antithrombotic therapy: valvar heart disease and prosthetic heart valves. *BMJ* 325(7374):1228–1231, 2002, with permission.]

Intensive Care Unit Management

Initial management should focus on systemic anticoagulation with intravenous heparin to prevent thrombus extension. Small thrombi without hemodynamic compromise are often treated with anticoagulation alone, whereas larger thrombi require either fibrinolytic therapy or surgery [24,37]. Fibrinolytic therapy is associated with risks of life-threatening hemorrhage and systemic embolization and thus is often delivered in the ICU for purposes of monitoring. The latter risk is low with right-sided PVT and higher with left-sided PVT, with a risk of cerebral embolism of 12% to 15% [124,125]. Fibrinolysis is considered first-line therapy for patients with right-sided PVT and for those with left-sided PVT, a small thrombus burden or NYHA Class I–II symptoms [32]. Fibrinolysis is less useful and potentially more harmful if LA thrombus is present, if the valve thrombus is older than 2 weeks, or if PVT is accompanied by shock. TTE after fibrinolysis can monitor for thrombus resolution and dictate the need for additional fibrinolysis for residual thrombus [126]. Alteplase is the most commonly used fibrinolytic for PVT, though urokinase and streptokinase have also been used. After successful fibrinolysis, unfractionated heparin should be initiated along with warfarin until an INR of 3.0 to 4.0 is achieved in patients with a prosthetic aortic valve or an INR of 3.5 to 4.5 for a prosthesis in the mitral position [24].

Emergency operation is recommended for patients with hemodynamic instability, NYHA Class III–IV symptoms, or a large clot burden as defined by TEE (>0.8 cm^2) [32,37]. Perioperative mortality rates approach 15% and are highest for PVT in the mitral position. A bioprosthesis is recommended after PVT to reduce future risk of valve thrombosis.

Prosthetic Valve Endocarditis

The incidence of PVE is 0.5% per year even with appropriate antibiotic prophylaxis and accounts for 7% to 25% of all cases of endocarditis in the developed world [54]. Endocarditis of a prosthetic valve is a devastating disease that carries a mortality rate of 30% to 50%. This high mortality reflects not only more serious infection but also the difficulty eradicating infection with antibiotics alone [127]. Infection may involve any part of the valve prosthesis, but the sewing ring may be particularly vulnerable. Sewing ring infection may result in abscess formation, paravalvular regurgitation, and further penetration into adjacent cardiac structures. The risk of PVE may be higher with mechanical valves in the first few months after implantation, but long-term risk is similar for mechanical and bioprosthetic valves [53]. Infection with coagulase-negative staphylococci is common within the first postoperative year; *S. aureus* and streptococci species dominate in later years [128–130].

Fever is the most common symptom and may be associated with other signs of prosthetic valve dysfunction including congestive heart failure, a new murmur, or embolic phenomena. Blood cultures are crucial and should be drawn prior to antibiotic therapy in any patient with a fever and a prosthetic valve. TEE is essential because of its greater sensitivity in detecting signs of PVE including vegetations, paraprosthetic abscess, or new paravalvular regurgitation [131].

Eradication of the infecting pathogen with antimicrobial therapy alone is often impossible and depends on the virulence of the organism and extent of infection. Medical therapy is more likely to be successful with late PVE or in nonstaphylococcal bacterial infections [132]. Surgical consultation should be sought early in the course of PVE. Indications for surgical therapy include failure of medical treatment marked by persistent bacteremia, hemodynamically significant prosthesis regurgitation with LV dysfunction, large vegetations, paravalvular extension with abscess or conduction defects, or development of intracardiac fistulas [32]. Surgery is almost always required in cases of *S. aureus* PVE. Infection with *S. aureus* is a marker for hospital mortality.

Structural Valve Deterioration

Failure of mechanical valves in the absence of infection is rare. Mechanical failure from strut fracture often presents with dyspnea, acute heart failure, and hemodynamic collapse with a physical examination marked by absent valve clicks. Death from mechanical valve strut fracture ensues rapidly if the valve is in the aortic position; patients with mitral valve failure can often be stabilized prior to surgery.

With conventional stented bioprostheses, freedom from SVD is 70% to 90% by 10 years, and 50% to 80% at 15 years [133,134]. SVD of bioprostheses is often related to tearing or rupture of one prosthetic valve cusp or progressive calcification and immobility [135]. Risk factors for SVD include younger age at implant, mitral valve position, renal insufficiency, and hyperparathyroidism [136]. Evaluation for SVD requires TTE and often TEE with care to exclude endocarditis as a complicating feature. SVD is the most common cause of reoperative valve replacement in patients with a bioprosthesis. Indications for reoperation are similar for those with native valve disease and are dominated by the development of heart failure.

TABLE 34.6

ADVANCES IN VALVULAR HEART DISEASE

- Transcatheter aortic valve implantation for advanced calcific AS has been safely performed in select centers and is being studied in multiple clinical trials [47–49]. It will likely become available for clinical use in high-risk AVR patients with severe AS.
- Given the incremental risk conferred by coronary artery bypass grafting along with valve surgery, hybrid surgical approaches combining percutaneous coronary intervention with primary or reoperative valve repair/replacement are now being used for high-risk patients [143].
- The natural history of bicuspid aortic valve disease is influenced by age at diagnosis, degree of valvular dysfunction, and aortic morphology [10]. In patients with bicuspid aortic valves who require valve surgery, careful elucidation of thoracic aortic morphology by CT angiography or MRI is required for optimal planning [144].
- In patients with low-flow, low-gradient AS, significant predictors of poor outcome are impaired functional capacity on 6-minute walk, severity of AS at a normalized transvalvular flow rate, reduced peak stress LV ejection fraction during dobutamine echocardiography, multivessel coronary artery disease, and low mean gradient (<20 mm Hg) [26,27,33].
- Despite the association between atherosclerosis and calcific valve degeneration, intensive lipid lower therapy has failed to halt the progression of calcific AS in multiple randomized clinical trials [7,8].
- In developing countries, systematic screening with echocardiography reveals a higher prevalence of rheumatic heart disease (approximately 10 times as great) compared with clinical screening, raising important public health implications [69].
- Endovascular edge-to-edge mitral valve clipping can reduce mitral regurgitation and stimulate reverse remodeling, offering an alternative to surgical repair for functional mitral valve disease [145].
- Novel oral anticoagulants have been developed (e.g., dabigatran, a direct thrombin inhibitor) for use in AF and are being studied for anticoagulation of mechanical valve prostheses [146].
- Transcatheter closure of prosthetic paravalvular leak is being used in select centers [141].
- Updated guidelines now recommend that routine antibiotic prophylaxis for infective endocarditis is no longer necessary except in patients at greatest risk for complications from endocarditis, including those with prosthetic valves or previous endocarditis [132,147].

AF, atrial fibrillation; AS, aortic stenosis; AVR, aortic valve replacement; CT, computerized tomography; LV, left ventricle; MRI, magnetic resonance imaging.

Development of percutaneous valve-in-valve bioprosthesis implantation is underway and may offer an alternative to reoperation in select high-risk patients [137].

Paravalvular Regurgitation

Paravalvular regurgitation is most often due to infection, suture dehiscence or fibrosis, and calcification of the native annulus leading to inadequate contact between the sewing ring and annulus. Mild paravalvular regurgitation on perioperative echocardiography has a benign course with reoperation required in less than 1% of patients at 2 years [138]. In patients with more severe paravalvular leak, close follow-up is required and surgical intervention is warranted for those who develop symptoms, progressive LV dysfunction, or hemolysis. A large proportion (>50%) of mechanical valve patients have some degree of mild intravascular hemolysis marked by anemia and an elevated lactate dehydrogenase. Paravalvular leaks, particularly small leaks, can lead to more severe anemia due to shearing of red blood cells. Severe, refractory anemia not responsive to iron, folate, and erythropoietin is an indication for repeat valve operation or closure of the paravalvular leak [139]. In high-risk patients not suitable for reoperation, percutaneous occlusion of the paravalvular leak may be achieved in select cases with the use of a septal or ductal occluder device [140,141].

PREVENTING INFECTIVE ENDOCARDITIS

Emerging data on the lifetime risk of IE, as well as trends in antibiotic resistance and antibiotic-associated adverse events, have led to changes in guideline recommendations for antibiotic prophylaxis [142]. IE is much more likely to occur from frequent exposure to random bacteremias associated with daily activities than from medical or dental procedures. Antibiotic prophylaxis for IE should only be provided to patients at greatest risk for complications from endocarditis, including patients with prosthetic valves, previous IE, complex congenital heart disease, or cardiac transplantation. Routine antibiotic prophylaxis for mitral valve prolapse is no longer recommended. In the ICU, antibiotic prophylaxis may be reasonable for procedures involving an infected respiratory, gastrointestinal, or genitourinary tract [32,132].

Advances in valvular heart disease are summarized in Table 34.6.

References

1. Nkomo VT, Gardin JM, Skelton TN, et al: Burden of valvular heart diseases: a population-based study. *Lancet* 368:1005–1011, 2006.
2. Lloyd-Jones D, Adams RJ, Brown TM, et al: Heart disease and stroke statistics–2010 update: a report from the American Heart Association. *Circulation* 121:e46–e215, 2010.
3. O'Gara PT, Braunwald E: Approach to the patient with a heart murmur, in Braunwald E, Fauci AS, Kasper DL, et al. (eds): *Harrison's Principles of Internal Medicine*. 15th ed. New York, NY, McGraw-Hill, 2001, pp 207–211.
4. Goldbarg SH, Elmariah S, Miller MA, et al: Insights into degenerative aortic valve disease. *J Am Coll Cardiol* 50:1205–1213, 2007.
5. Probst V, Le Scouarnec S, Legendre A, et al: Familial aggregation of calcific aortic valve stenosis in the western part of France. *Circulation* 113:856–860, 2006.
6. Otto CM, Lind BK, Kitzman DW, et al: Association of aortic-valve sclerosis with cardiovascular mortality and morbidity in the elderly. *N Engl J Med* 341:142–147, 1999.
7. Cowell SJ, Newby DE, Prescott RJ, et al: A randomized trial of intensive lipid-lowering therapy in calcific aortic stenosis. *N Engl J Med* 352:2389–2397, 2005.
8. Rossebo AB, Pedersen TR, Boman K, et al: Intensive lipid lowering with simvastatin and ezetimibe in aortic stenosis. *N Engl J Med* 359:1343–1356, 2008.
9. Hoffman JI, Kaplan S. The incidence of congenital heart disease. *J Am Coll Cardiol* 39:1890–1900, 2002.
10. Michelena HI, Desjardins VA, Avierinos JF, et al: Natural history of asymptomatic patients with normally functioning or minimally dysfunctional bicuspid aortic valve in the community. *Circulation* 117:2776–2784, 2008.
11. Tzemos N, Therrien J, Yip J, et al: Outcomes in adults with bicuspid aortic valves. *JAMA* 300:1317–1325, 2008.
12. Tadros TM, Klein MD, Shapira OM: Ascending aortic dilatation associated with bicuspid aortic valve: pathophysiology, molecular biology, and clinical implications. *Circulation* 119:880–890, 2009.
13. Spann JF, Bove AA, Natarajan G, et al: Ventricular performance, pump function and compensatory mechanisms in patients with aortic stenosis. *Circulation* 62:576–582, 1980.
14. Marcus ML, Doty DB, Hiratzka LF, et al: Decreased coronary reserve: a mechanism for angina pectoris in patients with aortic stenosis and normal coronary arteries. *N Engl J Med* 307:1362–1366, 1982.
15. Otto CM: Valvular aortic stenosis: disease severity and timing of intervention. *J Am Coll Cardiol* 47:2141–2151, 2006.
16. Carabello BA, Paulus WJ: Aortic stenosis. *Lancet* 373:956–966, 2009.
17. Ross J Jr, Braunwald E: Aortic stenosis. *Circulation* 38:61–67, 1968.
18. Hakki AH, Kimbiris D, Iskandrian AS, et al: Angina pectoris and coronary artery disease in patients with severe aortic valvular disease. *Am Heart J* 100:441–449, 1980.
19. Vincentelli A, Susen S, Le Tourneau T, et al: Acquired von Willebrand syndrome in aortic stenosis. *N Engl J Med* 349:343–349, 2003.
20. Rosenhek R, Binder T, Porenta G, et al: Predictors of outcome in severe, asymptomatic aortic stenosis. *N Engl J Med* 343:611–617, 2000.
21. Nassimiha D, Aronow WS, Ahn C, et al: Rate of progression of valvular aortic stenosis in patients > or = 60 years of age. *Am J Cardiol* 87:807–809, A9, 2001.
22. Ware LB, Matthay MA: Clinical practice. Acute pulmonary edema. *N Engl J Med* 353:2788–2796, 2005.
23. Gorlin R, Gorlin SG: Hydraulic formula for calculation of the area of the stenotic mitral valve, other cardiac valves, and central circulatory shunts. I. *Am Heart J* 41:1–29, 1951.
24. Bonow RO, Carabello BA, Kanu C, et al: ACC/AHA 2006 guidelines for the management of patients with valvular heart disease: a report of the American College of Cardiology/American Heart Association Task Force on Practice Guidelines (writing committee to revise the 1998 Guidelines for the Management of Patients With Valvular Heart Disease): developed in collaboration with the Society of Cardiovascular Anesthesiologists: endorsed by the Society for Cardiovascular Angiography and Interventions and the Society of Thoracic Surgeons. *Circulation* 114:e84–e231, 2006.
25. Carabello BA: Clinical practice. Aortic stenosis. *N Engl J Med* 346:677–682, 2002.
26. Tribouilloy C, Levy F, Rusinaru D, et al: Outcome after aortic valve replacement for low-flow/low-gradient aortic stenosis without contractile reserve on dobutamine stress echocardiography. *J Am Coll Cardiol* 53:1865–1873, 2009.
27. Clavel MA, Fuchs C, Burwash IG, et al: Predictors of outcomes in low-flow, low-gradient aortic stenosis: results of the multicenter TOPAS Study. *Circulation* 118:S234–S242, 2008.
28. Quere JP, Monin JL, Levy F, et al: Influence of preoperative left ventricular contractile reserve on postoperative ejection fraction in low-gradient aortic stenosis. *Circulation* 113:1738–1744, 2006.
29. Picano E, Pibarot P, Lancellotti P, et al: The emerging role of exercise testing and stress echocardiography in valvular heart disease. *J Am Coll Cardiol* 54:2251–2260, 2009.
30. Grayburn PA: Assessment of low-gradient aortic stenosis with dobutamine. *Circulation* 113:604–606, 2006.
31. Carabello BA: Is it ever too late to operate on the patient with valvular heart disease? *J Am Coll Cardiol* 44:376–383, 2004.
32. Bonow RO, Carabello BA, Chatterjee K, et al: 2008 Focused update incorporated into the ACC/AHA 2006 guidelines for the management of patients with valvular heart disease: a report of the American College of Cardiology/American Heart Association Task Force on Practice Guidelines (Writing Committee to Revise the 1998 Guidelines for the Management of Patients With Valvular Heart Disease): endorsed by the Society of Cardiovascular Anesthesiologists, Society for Cardiovascular Angiography and Interventions, and Society of Thoracic Surgeons. *Circulation* 118:e523–e661, 2008.
33. Levy F, Laurent M, Monin JL, et al: Aortic valve replacement for low-flow/low-gradient aortic stenosis operative risk stratification and long-term outcome: a European multicenter study. *J Am Coll Cardiol* 51:1466–1472, 2008.

34. Pellikka PA, Sarano ME, Nishimura RA, et al: Outcome of 622 adults with asymptomatic, hemodynamically significant aortic stenosis during prolonged follow-up. *Circulation* 111:3290–3295, 2005.
35. Khot UN, Novaro GM, Popovic ZB, et al: Nitroprusside in critically ill patients with left ventricular dysfunction and aortic stenosis. *N Engl J Med* 348:1756–1763, 2003.
36. Popovic ZB, Khot UN, Novaro GM, et al: Effects of sodium nitroprusside in aortic stenosis associated with severe heart failure: pressure-volume loop analysis using a numerical model. *Am J Physiol Heart Circ Physiol* 288:H416–H423, 2005.
37. Vahanian A, Baumgartner H, Bax J, et al: Guidelines on the management of valvular heart disease: the task force on the management of valvular heart disease of the European Society of Cardiology. *Eur Heart J* 28:230–268, 2007.
38. Rahimtoola SH: Choice of prosthetic heart valve for adult patients. *J Am Coll Cardiol* 41:893–904, 2003.
39. Ambler G, Omar RZ, Royston P, et al: Generic, simple risk stratification model for heart valve surgery. *Circulation* 112:224–231, 2005.
40. STS Adult Cardiovascular National Surgery Database–STS national database risk calculator. Available at: http://www.sts.org/sections/stsnationaldatabase/riskcalculator/. Accessed January 9, 2011.
41. Nashef SA, Roques F, Hammill BG, et al: Validation of European System for Cardiac Operative Risk Evaluation (EuroSCORE) in North American cardiac surgery. *Eur J Cardiothorac Surg* 22:101–105, 2002.
42. Safian RD, Berman AD, Diver DJ, et al: Balloon aortic valvuloplasty in 170 consecutive patients. *N Engl J Med* 319:125–130, 1988.
43. Vahanian A, Palacios IF: Percutaneous approaches to valvular disease. *Circulation* 109:1572–1579, 2004.
44. Kuntz RE, Tosteson AN, Berman AD, et al: Predictors of event-free survival after balloon aortic valvuloplasty. *N Engl J Med* 325:17–23, 1991.
45. Cribier A, Eltchaninoff H, Bash A, et al: Percutaneous transcatheter implantation of an aortic valve prosthesis for calcific aortic stenosis: first human case description. *Circulation* 106:3006–3008, 2002.
46. Webb JG, Pasupati S, Humphries K, et al: Percutaneous transarterial aortic valve replacement in selected high-risk patients with aortic stenosis. *Circulation* 116:755–763, 2007.
47. Webb JG, Altwegg L, Masson JB, et al: A new transcatheter aortic valve and percutaneous valve delivery system. *J Am Coll Cardiol* 53:1855–1858, 2009.
48. Grube E, Schuler G, Buellesfeld L, et al: Percutaneous aortic valve replacement for severe aortic stenosis in high-risk patients using the second- and current third-generation self-expanding CoreValve prosthesis: device success and 30-day clinical outcome. *J Am Coll Cardiol* 50:69–76, 2007.
49. Zajarias A, Cribier AG: Outcomes and safety of percutaneous aortic valve replacement. *J Am Coll Cardiol* 53:1829–1836, 2009.
50. Fann JI, Chronos N, Rowe SJ, et al: Evolving strategies for the treatment of valvular heart disease: preclinical and clinical pathways for percutaneous aortic valve replacement. *Catheter Cardiovasc Interv* 71:434–440, 2008.
51. Rosengart TK, Feldman T, Borger MA, et al: Percutaneous and minimally invasive valve procedures: a scientific statement from the American Heart Association Council on Cardiovascular Surgery and Anesthesia, Council on Clinical Cardiology, Functional Genomics and Translational Biology Interdisciplinary Working Group, and Quality of Care and Outcomes Research Interdisciplinary Working Group. *Circulation* 117:1750–1767, 2008.
52. Stout KK, Verrier ED: Acute valvular regurgitation. *Circulation* 119:3232–3241, 2009.
53. Baddour LM, Wilson WR, Bayer AS, et al: Infective endocarditis: diagnosis, antimicrobial therapy, and management of complications: a statement for healthcare professionals from the Committee on Rheumatic Fever, Endocarditis, and Kawasaki Disease, Council on Cardiovascular Disease in the Young, and the Councils on Clinical Cardiology, Stroke, and Cardiovascular Surgery and Anesthesia, American Heart Association: endorsed by the Infectious Diseases Society of America. *Circulation* 111:e394–e434, 2005.
54. Mylonakis E, Calderwood SB: Infective endocarditis in adults. *N Engl J Med* 345:1318–1330, 2001.
55. Haldar SM, O'Gara PT: Infective endocarditis: diagnosis and management. *Nat Clin Pract Cardiovasc Med* 3:310–317, 2006.
56. Mehta RH, Suzuki T, Hagan PG, et al: Predicting death in patients with acute type a aortic dissection. *Circulation* 105:200–206, 2002.
57. Januzzi JL, Eagle KA, Cooper JV, et al: Acute aortic dissection presenting with congestive heart failure: results from the International Registry of Acute Aortic Dissection. *J Am Coll Cardiol* 46:733–735, 2005.
58. Isselbacher EM: Thoracic and abdominal aortic aneurysms. *Circulation* 111:816–828, 2005.
59. Obadia JF, Tatou E, David M: Aortic valve regurgitation caused by blunt chest injury. *Br Heart J* 74:545–547, 1995.
60. Tribouilloy CM, Enriquez-Sarano M, Bailey KR, et al: Assessment of severity of aortic regurgitation using the width of the vena contracta: a clinical color Doppler imaging study. *Circulation* 102:558–564, 2000.
61. Bekeredjian R, Grayburn PA: Valvular heart disease: aortic regurgitation. *Circulation* 112:125–134, 2005.
62. Cigarroa JE, Isselbacher EM, DeSanctis RW, et al: Diagnostic imaging in the evaluation of suspected aortic dissection. Old standards and new directions. *N Engl J Med* 328:35–43, 1993.
63. Hagan PG, Nienaber CA, Isselbacher EM, et al: The International Registry of Acute Aortic Dissection (IRAD): new insights into an old disease. *JAMA* 283:897–903, 2000.
64. Penn MS, Smedira N, Lytle B, et al: Does coronary angiography before emergency aortic surgery affect in-hospital mortality? *J Am Coll Cardiol* 35:889–894, 2000.
65. Evangelista A, Tornos P, Sambola A, et al: Role of vasodilators in regurgitant valve disease. *Curr Treat Options Cardiovasc Med* 8:428–434, 2006.
66. Stevens LM, Madsen JC, Isselbacher EM, et al: Surgical management and long-term outcomes for acute ascending aortic dissection. *J Thorac Cardiovasc Surg* 138:1349–1357, e1, 2009.
67. Chandrashekhar Y, Westaby S, Narula J: Mitral stenosis. *Lancet* 374:1271–1283, 2009.
68. Waller BF, Howard J, Fess S: Pathology of mitral valve stenosis and pure mitral regurgitation—Part I. *Clin Cardiol* 17:330–336, 1994.
69. Marijon E, Ou P, Celermajer DS, et al: Prevalence of rheumatic heart disease detected by echocardiographic screening. *N Engl J Med* 357:470–476, 2007.
70. Carabello BA: Modern management of mitral stenosis. *Circulation* 112:432–437, 2005.
71. Iung B, Baron G, Butchart EG, et al: A prospective survey of patients with valvular heart disease in Europe: the Euro Heart Survey on Valvular Heart Disease. *Eur Heart J* 24:1231–1243, 2003.
72. Elkayam U, Bitar F: Valvular heart disease and pregnancy part I: native valves. *J Am Coll Cardiol* 46:223–230, 2005.
73. Chiang CW, Lo SK, Ko YS, et al: Predictors of systemic embolism in patients with mitral stenosis. A prospective study. *Ann Intern Med* 128:885–889, 1998.
74. Rowe JC, Bland EF, Sprague HB, et al: The course of mitral stenosis without surgery: ten- and twenty-year perspectives. *Ann Intern Med* 52:741–749, 1960.
75. Horstkotte D, Niehues R, Strauer BE: Pathomorphological aspects, aetiology and natural history of acquired mitral valve stenosis. *Eur Heart J* 12[Suppl B]:55–60, 1991.
76. Martin RP, Rakowski H, Kleiman JH, et al: Reliability and reproducibility of two dimensional echocardiograph measurement of the stenotic mitral valve orifice area. *Am J Cardiol* 43:560–568, 1979.
77. Hatle L, Brubakk A, Tromsdal A, et al: Noninvasive assessment of pressure drop in mitral stenosis by Doppler ultrasound. *Br Heart J* 40:131–140, 1978.
78. Wilkins GT, Weyman AE, Abascal VM, et al: Percutaneous balloon dilatation of the mitral valve: an analysis of echocardiographic variables related to outcome and the mechanism of dilatation. *Br Heart J* 60:299–308, 1988.
79. Alan S, Ulgen MS, Ozdemir K, et al: Reliability and efficacy of metoprolol and diltiazem in patients having mild to moderate mitral stenosis with sinus rhythm. *Angiology* 53:575–581, 2002.
80. Palacios IF, Sanchez PL, Harrell LC, et al: Which patients benefit from percutaneous mitral balloon valvuloplasty? Prevalvuloplasty and postvalvuloplasty variables that predict long-term outcome. *Circulation* 105:1465–1471, 2002.
81. Inoue K, Owaki T, Nakamura T, et al: Clinical application of transvenous mitral commissurotomy by a new balloon catheter. *J Thorac Cardiovasc Surg* 87:394–402, 1984.
82. Iung B, Cormier B, Ducimetiere P, et al: Immediate results of percutaneous mitral commissurotomy. A predictive model on a series of 1514 patients. *Circulation* 94:2124–2130, 1996.
83. Orrange SE, Kawanishi DT, Lopez BM, et al: Actuarial outcome after catheter balloon commissurotomy in patients with mitral stenosis. *Circulation* 95:382–389, 1997.
84. Palacios IF, Tuzcu ME, Weyman AE, et al: Clinical follow-up of patients undergoing percutaneous mitral balloon valvotomy. *Circulation* 91:671–676, 1995.
85. Reyes VP, Raju BS, Wynne J, et al: Percutaneous balloon valvuloplasty compared with open surgical commissurotomy for mitral stenosis. *N Engl J Med* 331:961–967, 1994.
86. Ben Farhat M, Ayari M, Maatouk F, et al: Percutaneous balloon versus surgical closed and open mitral commissurotomy: seven-year follow-up results of a randomized trial. *Circulation* 97:245–250, 1998.
87. Carabello BA: The current therapy for mitral regurgitation. *J Am Coll Cardiol* 52:319–326, 2008.
88. Chaput M, Handschumacher MD, Guerrero JL, et al: Mitral leaflet adaptation to ventricular remodeling: prospective changes in a model of ischemic mitral regurgitation. *Circulation* 120:S99–S103, 2009.
89. Simmers TA, Meijburg HW, de la Riviere AB: Traumatic papillary muscle rupture. *Ann Thorac Surg* 72:257–259, 2001.
90. Freed LA, Levy D, Levine RA, et al: Prevalence and clinical outcome of mitral-valve prolapse. *N Engl J Med* 341:1–7, 1999.
91. Levine RA, Schwammenthal E: Ischemic mitral regurgitation on the threshold of a solution: from paradoxes to unifying concepts. *Circulation* 112:745–758, 2005.
92. Beeri R, Yosefy C, Guerrero JL, et al: Mitral regurgitation augments post-myocardial infarction remodeling failure of hypertrophic compensation. *J Am Coll Cardiol* 51:476–486, 2008.
93. Kaul S, Spotnitz WD, Glasheen WP, et al: Mechanism of ischemic mitral regurgitation. An experimental evaluation. *Circulation* 84:2167–2180, 1991.

94. Grose R, Strain J, Cohen MV: Pulmonary arterial V waves in mitral regurgitation: clinical and experimental observations. *Circulation* 69:214–222, 1984.
95. Schnyder PA, Sarraj AM, Duvoisin BE, et al: Pulmonary edema associated with mitral regurgitation: prevalence of predominant involvement of the right upper lobe. *AJR Am J Roentgenol* 161:33–36, 1993.
96. Enriquez-Sarano M, Dujardin KS, Tribouilloy CM, et al: Determinants of pulmonary venous flow reversal in mitral regurgitation and its usefulness in determining the severity of regurgitation. *Am J Cardiol* 83:535–541, 1999.
97. Enriquez-Sarano M, Sinak LJ, Tajik AJ, et al: Changes in effective regurgitant orifice throughout systole in patients with mitral valve prolapse. A clinical study using the proximal isovelocity surface area method. *Circulation* 92:2951–2958, 1995.
98. Picard MH, Davidoff R, Sleeper LA, et al: Echocardiographic predictors of survival and response to early revascularization in cardiogenic shock. *Circulation* 107:279–284, 2003.
99. Kishon Y, Oh JK, Schaff HV, et al: Mitral valve operation in postinfarction rupture of a papillary muscle: immediate results and long-term follow-up of 22 patients. *Mayo Clin Proc* 67:1023–1030, 1992.
100. Feldman T, Wasserman HS, Herrmann HC, et al: Percutaneous mitral valve repair using the edge-to-edge technique: six-month results of the EVEREST Phase I Clinical Trial. *J Am Coll Cardiol* 46:2134–2140, 2005.
101. Babaliaros V, Cribier A, Agatiello C: Surgery insight: current advances in percutaneous heart valve replacement and repair. *Nat Clin Pract Cardiovasc Med* 3:256–264, 2006.
102. Solis J, McCarty D, Levine RA, et al: Mechanism of decrease in mitral regurgitation after cardiac resynchronization therapy: optimization of the force-balance relationship. *Circ Cardiovasc Imaging* 2:444–450, 2009.
103. Verma S, Mesana TG: Mitral-valve repair for mitral-valve prolapse. *N Engl J Med* 361:2261–2269, 2009.
104. Roques F, Nashef SA, Michel P: Risk factors for early mortality after valve surgery in Europe in the 1990s: lessons from the EuroSCORE pilot program. *J Heart Valve Dis* 10:572–577; discussion 577–578, 2001.
105. Iung B, Rousseau-Paziaud J, Cormier B, et al: Contemporary results of mitral valve repair for infective endocarditis. *J Am Coll Cardiol* 43:386–392, 2004.
106. Murdoch DR, Corey GR, Hoen B, et al: Clinical presentation, etiology, and outcome of infective endocarditis in the 21st century: the International Collaboration on Endocarditis-Prospective Cohort Study. *Arch Intern Med* 169:463–473, 2009.
107. Russo A, Suri RM, Grigioni F, et al: Clinical outcome after surgical correction of mitral regurgitation due to papillary muscle rupture. *Circulation* 118:1528–1534, 2008.
108. Di Salvo TG, Acker MA, Dec GW, et al: Mitral valve surgery in advanced heart failure. *J Am Coll Cardiol* 55:271–282, 2010.
109. Shiran A, Sagie A: Tricuspid regurgitation in mitral valve disease incidence, prognostic implications, mechanism, and management. *J Am Coll Cardiol* 53:401–408, 2009.
110. Rogers JH, Bolling SF: The tricuspid valve: current perspective and evolving management of tricuspid regurgitation. *Circulation* 119:2718–2725, 2009.
111. Bruce CJ, Connolly HM: Right-sided valve disease deserves a little more respect. *Circulation* 119:2726–2734, 2009.
112. Anyanwu AC, Chikwe J, Adams DH: Tricuspid valve repair for treatment and prevention of secondary tricuspid regurgitation in patients undergoing mitral valve surgery. *Curr Cardiol Rep* 10:110–117, 2008.
113. Vongpatanasin W, Hillis LD, Lange RA: Prosthetic heart valves. *N Engl J Med* 335:407–416, 1996.
114. Goldsmith I, Turpie AG, Lip GY: Valvar heart disease and prosthetic heart valves. *BMJ* 325:1228–1231, 2002.
115. Cannegieter SC, Rosendaal FR, Wintzen AR, et al: Optimal oral anticoagulant therapy in patients with mechanical heart valves. *N Engl J Med* 333:11–17, 1995.
116. Zoghbi WA, Chambers JB, Dumesnil JG, et al: Recommendations for evaluation of prosthetic valves with echocardiography and Doppler ultrasound: a report From the American Society of Echocardiography's Guidelines and Standards Committee and the Task Force on Prosthetic Valves, developed in conjunction with the American College of Cardiology Cardiovascular Imaging Committee, Cardiac Imaging Committee of the American Heart Association, the European Association of Echocardiography, a registered branch of the European Society of Cardiology, the Japanese Society of Echocardiography and the Canadian Society of Echocardiography, endorsed by the American College of Cardiology Foundation, American Heart Association, European Association of Echocardiography, a registered branch of the European Society of Cardiology, the Japanese Society of Echocardiography, and Canadian Society of Echocardiography. *J Am Soc Echocardiogr* 22:975–1014; quiz 1082–1084, 2009.
117. Grunkemeier GL, Li HH, Naftel DC, et al: Long-term performance of heart valve prostheses. *Curr Probl Cardiol* 25:73–154, 2000.
118. Roudaut R, Serri K, Lafitte S: Thrombosis of prosthetic heart valves: diagnosis and therapeutic considerations. *Heart* 93:137–142, 2007.
119. Barbetseas J, Nagueh SF, Pitsavos C, et al: Differentiating thrombus from pannus formation in obstructed mechanical prosthetic valves: an evaluation of clinical, transthoracic and transesophageal echocardiographic parameters. *J Am Coll Cardiol* 32:1410–1417, 1998.
120. Edmunds LH Jr: Thromboembolic complications of current cardiac valvular prostheses. *Ann Thorac Surg* 34:96–106, 1982.
121. Hering D, Piper C, Horstkotte D: Drug insight: an overview of current anticoagulation therapy after heart valve replacement. *Nat Clin Pract Cardiovasc Med* 2:415–422, 2005.
122. Shapira Y, Herz I, Sagie A: Fluoroscopy of prosthetic heart valves: does it have a place in the echocardiography era? *J Heart Valve Dis* 9:594–599, 2000.
123. Tong AT, Roudaut R, Ozkan M, et al: Transesophageal echocardiography improves risk assessment of thrombolysis of prosthetic valve thrombosis: results of the international PRO-TEE registry. *J Am Coll Cardiol* 43:77–84, 2004.
124. Roudaut R, Lafitte S, Roudaut MF, et al: Fibrinolysis of mechanical prosthetic valve thrombosis: a single-center study of 127 cases. *J Am Coll Cardiol* 41:653–658, 2003.
125. Piper C, Hering D, Langer C, et al: Etiology of stroke after mechanical heart valve replacement—results from a ten-year prospective study. *J Heart Valve Dis* 17:413–417, 2008.
126. Shapira Y, Herz I, Vaturi M, et al: Thrombolysis is an effective and safe therapy in stuck bileaflet mitral valves in the absence of high-risk thrombi. *J Am Coll Cardiol* 35:1874–1880, 2000.
127. Akowuah EF, Davies W, Oliver S, et al: Prosthetic valve endocarditis: early and late outcome following medical or surgical treatment. *Heart* 89:269–272, 2003.
128. Moreillon P, Que YA: Infective endocarditis. *Lancet* 363:139–149, 2004.
129. Hill EE, Herregods MC, Vanderschueren S, et al: Management of prosthetic valve infective endocarditis. *Am J Cardiol* 101:1174–1178, 2008.
130. Chu VH, Miro JM, Hoen B, et al: Coagulase-negative staphylococcal prosthetic valve endocarditis—a contemporary update based on the International Collaboration on Endocarditis: prospective cohort study. *Heart* 95:570–576, 2009.
131. Bach DS: Transesophageal echocardiographic (TEE) evaluation of prosthetic valves. *Cardiol Clin* 18:751–771, 2000.
132. Habib G, Hoen B, Tornos P, et al: Guidelines on the prevention, diagnosis, and treatment of infective endocarditis (new version 2009): the Task Force on the Prevention, Diagnosis, and Treatment of Infective Endocarditis of the European Society of Cardiology (ESC). *Eur Heart J* 30:2369–2413, 2009.
133. Pibarot P, Dumesnil JG: Prosthetic heart valves: selection of the optimal prosthesis and long-term management. *Circulation* 119:1034–1048, 2009.
134. Vesey JM, Otto CM: Complications of prosthetic heart valves. *Curr Cardiol Rep* 6:106–111, 2004.
135. Schoen FJ, Levy RJ: Calcification of tissue heart valve substitutes: progress toward understanding and prevention. *Ann Thorac Surg* 79:1072–1080, 2005.
136. Ruel M, Kulik A, Rubens FD, et al: Late incidence and determinants of reoperation in patients with prosthetic heart valves. *Eur J Cardiothorac Surg* 25:364–370, 2004.
137. Walther T, Falk V, Dewey T, et al: Valve-in-a-valve concept for transcatheter minimally invasive repeat xenograft implantation. *J Am Coll Cardiol* 50:56–60, 2007.
138. Davila-Roman VG, Waggoner AD, Kennard ED, et al: Prevalence and severity of paravalvular regurgitation in the Artificial Valve Endocarditis Reduction Trial (AVERT) echocardiography study. *J Am Coll Cardiol* 44:1467–1472, 2004.
139. Shapira Y, Vaturi M, Sagie A: Hemolysis associated with prosthetic heart valves: a review. *Cardiol Rev* 17:121–124, 2009.
140. Hourihan M, Perry SB, Mandell VS, et al: Transcatheter umbrella closure of valvular and paravalvular leaks. *J Am Coll Cardiol* 20:1371–1377, 1992.
141. Kim MS, Casserly IP, Garcia JA, et al: Percutaneous transcatheter closure of prosthetic mitral paravalvular leaks: are we there yet? *JACC Cardiovasc Interv* 2:81–90, 2009.
142. Wilson W, Taubert KA, Gewitz M, et al: Prevention of infective endocarditis: guidelines from the American Heart Association: a guideline from the American Heart Association Rheumatic Fever, Endocarditis, and Kawasaki Disease Committee, Council on Cardiovascular Disease in the Young, and the Council on Clinical Cardiology, Council on Cardiovascular Surgery and Anesthesia, and the Quality of Care and Outcomes Research Interdisciplinary Working Group. *Circulation* 116:1736–1754, 2007.
143. Byrne JG, Leacche M, Vaughan DE, et al: Hybrid cardiovascular procedures. *JACC Cardiovasc Interv* 1:459–468, 2008.
144. Fazel SS, Mallidi HR, Lee RS, et al: The aortopathy of bicuspid aortic valve disease has distinctive patterns and usually involves the transverse aortic arch. *J Thorac Cardiovasc Surg* 135:901–907, 907.e1–e2, 2008.
145. Feldman T, Kar S, Rinaldi M, et al: Percutaneous mitral repair with the MitraClip system: safety and midterm durability in the initial EVEREST (Endovascular Valve Edge-to-Edge REpair Study) cohort. *J Am Coll Cardiol* 54:686–694, 2009.
146. Connolly SJ, Ezekowitz MD, Yusuf S, et al: Dabigatran versus warfarin in patients with atrial fibrillation. *N Engl J Med* 361:1139–1151, 2009.
147. Nishimura RA, Carabello BA, Faxon DP, et al: ACC/AHA 2008 Guideline update on valvular heart disease: focused update on infective endocarditis: a report of the American College of Cardiology/American Heart Association Task Force on Practice Guidelines endorsed by the Society of Cardiovascular Anesthesiologists, Society for Cardiovascular Angiography and Interventions, and Society of Thoracic Surgeons. *J Am Coll Cardiol* 52:676–685, 2008.

CHAPTER 35 ■ CRITICAL CARE OF PERICARDIAL DISEASE

AKSHAY S. DESAI AND KENNETH L. BAUGHMAN†

PERICARDIAL ANATOMY

The pericardium consists of two layers: the inner layer (*visceral* pericardium) is a thin, elastic monolayer of mesothelial cells that is tightly adherent to the epicardial surface of the heart, whereas the outer layer (*parietal* pericardium) is a largely acellular network of collagen and elastin fibers that make up a thick, stiff fibrous envelope. The visceral pericardium reflects back near the origins of the great vessels and the junctions of the caval vessels with the right atrium, becoming continuous with the parietal pericardium and generating a potential space (pericardial *sac*) that is normally lubricated by up to 50 mL of serous fluid. Most of the heart (excepting a portion of the left atrium) and portions of the aorta, pulmonary trunk, pulmonary veins, and venae cavae are contained within this sac, which has ligamentous attachments to the diaphragm, sternum, and other structures in the anterior mediastinum. The main arterial blood supply of the pericardium is provided by the pericardiophrenic artery, a branch of the internal thoracic artery, whereas venous drainage occurs via pericardiophrenic veins that are tributaries of the brachiocephalic veins. Sensory enervation is provided by the phrenic nerves with vasomotor innervation from the sympathetic trunks [1,2].

NORMAL PHYSIOLOGY OF THE PERICARDIUM

Although an intact pericardium is not critical to the maintenance of cardiovascular function, the pericardium does have several physiologically relevant functions. First, it provides important structural support for the heart, limiting excessive cardiac motion within the thoracic cavity during respiration and changes in body position. In addition, it acts as a lubricant (minimizing friction between the cardiac chambers and the surrounding structures) and as an anatomic barrier to infection. Perhaps the best-characterized mechanical function of the normal pericardium, however, is as a restraint on cardiac filling and rapid chamber dilation [3]. At low applied stresses, approximating those at physiologic cardiac volumes, pericardial tissue is quite compliant. As the distending pressure increases, however, it abruptly becomes quite stiff and resistant to further stress. As a result, the pericardium passively restrains intracardiac volume and limits ventricular filling, with a component of intracavitary filling pressure reflecting transmitted pericardial pressure. In addition, this pericardial restraint defines a total compliance for the system, enhancing ventricular interdependence by accentuating the consequences of septum-mediated ventricular interactions during diastolic filling [4].

The pericardium itself has a small capacitance reserve (150 to 250 mL) that admits initial increments in intrapericardial volume with trivial increases in intrapericardial pressures. Once this capacitance is exceeded, rapid increases in intrapericardial volume result in steep increments in intrapericardial pressures, with potentially deleterious consequences for cardiac filling and ventricular performance [5,6]. By contrast, gradual changes in myocardial or pericardial volume (well in excess of the normal pericardial reserve) may be accommodated without invoking dramatic consequences of pericardial restraint. In experimental models of chronic volume overload, the pericardium exhibits the ability to undergo gradual stretch and hypertrophy, enhancing its compliance and diminishing its impact on the ventricular pressure–volume relationship [7]. Such chronic stretch is the primary mechanism permitting the accommodation of chronic cardiac dilation (as in dilated cardiomyopathy) or large, slowly accumulating pericardial effusions (as in malignant lymphoma), without hemodynamic embarrassment (Fig. 35.1).

†Deceased

PERICARDIAL PATHOPHYSIOLOGY

Pericardial manifestations are seen in a wide spectrum of medical and surgical conditions, including a host of infectious, immune/inflammatory, and neoplastic disorders (Table 35.1). Broadly speaking, from the vantage point of critical care, there are three conditions to be considered: (i) acute pericarditis, (ii) pericardial effusion and tamponade, and (iii) constrictive pericarditis. We consider the diagnosis, pathophysiology, and management of each of these in turn in the discussion to follow.

Acute Pericarditis

Pericardial inflammation presents in many clinical settings and has a wide range of causes. Although pericarditis is classically identified by the clinical triad of acute chest pain, pericardial friction rub, and characteristic electrocardiographic changes, subacute and chronic presentations are also possible. It may occur as an isolated entity or as the result of systemic disease; though most often a strictly inflammatory fibrinous lesion without clinically recognizable fluid, sequelae including pericardial effusion (occasionally progressing to tamponade), pericardial constriction, or recurrent (relapsing) pericarditis are often seen. A prevalence of around 1% in autopsy studies suggests that pericarditis may frequently be subclinical [8]. Pericarditis is thought to account for around 5% of presentations to emergency departments for nonischemic chest pain [9].

Causes

Despite an ever-expanding array of diagnostic techniques, the vast majority of cases of pericarditis remain idiopathic in etiology [10–12]. Even when pericardial fluid or tissue samples are obtained, the cause is undefined in up to 30% of patients.

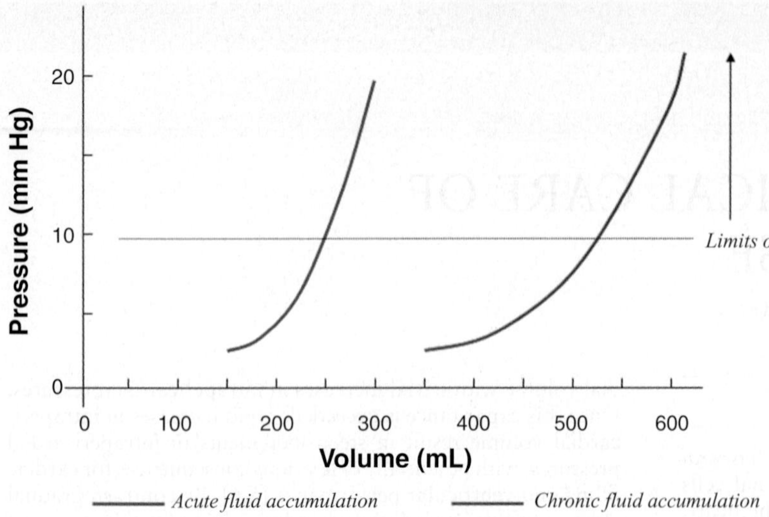

FIGURE 35.1. Pericardial pressure–volume relationship and relationship to development of pericardial tamponade. The ability of the pericardium to accommodate pericardial fluid without hemodynamic embarrassment depends heavily on the rate of fluid accumulation. Note the steepness of the relationship in normal pericardium and the marked flattening and shift to the right with chronic volume overload. [Adapted from Freeman G, LeWinter MM: Pericardial adaptations during chronic cardiac dilation in dogs. *Circ Res* 54:294–300, 1984.]

Broadly speaking, pericarditis is either infectious (two-thirds of cases) or noninfectious (one-third of cases) in etiology, with noninfectious cases attributable to one of a number of immune, neoplastic, traumatic, and metabolic conditions (see Table 35.1). A wide range of organisms cause infectious pericarditis, but viral infection remains the most common probable or identifiable cause. Organisms responsible for myocarditis are commonly implicated, particularly enteroviruses, adenoviruses, and influenza; herpes simplex and cytomegalovirus may also be important in immunocompromised individuals. Myopericarditis has also been reported after smallpox vaccination in US military personnel not previously exposed to vaccinia [13]. Although pericardial abnormalities are seen in up to 20% of patients with human immunodeficiency virus (HIV) infection, symptomatic pericarditis in these patients is commonly due to secondary infection (e.g., mycobacterial) or neoplasia (particularly lymphoma or Kaposi's sarcoma), and the frequency decreases with effective antiretroviral therapy [14]. Bacterial pathogens typically cause purulent pericarditis, but are implicated infrequently in pericardial disease, typically as a consequence of hematogenous seeding or direct extension from adjacent infected tissues (lungs or pleural space) [15]. *Mycobacterium tuberculosis* causes up to 4% of acute pericarditis cases and 7% of tamponade presentations in developed countries, and remains an important causal factor in developing nations and immunocompromised hosts [16,17]. Tuberculosis-related pericarditis can require pericardial biopsy for diagnosis and is complicated by pericardial effusion or constriction in up to 50% of cases [18].

In the remainder of patients, pericarditis occurs in conjunction with a dissecting aortic aneurysm (in which blood leaks into the pericardial space), after blunt or sharp trauma to the chest, as a result of neoplastic invasion of the pericardium, after chest irradiation, in association with uremia or dialysis, after cardiac or other thoracic surgery, in association with an inflammatory or autoimmune disorder, or as a result of certain pharmacologic agents. Iatrogenic cases are increasingly common, with postpericardiotomy syndrome reported in up to 20% of patients at a median of 4 weeks following cardiac surgery [19] and symptomatic pericarditis in up to 2% of patients undergoing percutaneous coronary intervention, catheter ablation procedures, or implantation of active fixation pacemaker or defibrillator leads [10]. Pericarditis associated with acute transmural myocardial infarction and the delayed immune-mediated postinfarction pericarditis of Dressler's syndrome used to be common, but the incidence has declined with the broader utilization of early reperfusion strategies for acute coronary syndromes (thrombolysis and primary angioplasty).

Presentation and Diagnosis

Although patients with acute pericarditis may be asymptomatic, the typical presentation is with chest pain that is retrosternal in location, sudden in onset, and exacerbated by inspiration (pleuritic). The pain may be made worse by lying supine and improved by sitting upright and leaning forward. Precordial distress may closely mimic angina, including a predominant pressure sensation with radiation to the neck, arms, or left shoulder. However, radiation of chest pain to one or both trapezius muscle ridges favors the diagnosis of pericarditis because the phrenic nerve, which innervates these muscles, traverses the pericardium. A prodrome of low-grade fever, malaise, and myalgia is common, but fever may be absent in elderly patients. Associated symptoms can include dyspnea, cough, anorexia, anxiety, and occasionally, odynophagia or hiccups.

Nearly 85% of patients with pericarditis have an audible friction rub during the course of their disease [12]. Typically, the rub is a high-pitched scratchy or squeaky sound best heard at the lower left sternal border or apex at end expiration with the patient leaning forward. Classically, it consists of three components corresponding to ventricular systole, early diastolic filling, and atrial contraction, and has been likened to the sound made when walking on crunchy snow. It is distinct from a pleural rub in that it is present throughout the respiratory cycle, whereas the pleural rub disappears when respirations are suspended. The pericardial friction rub is often a dynamic sound that can disappear and reappear over short periods of time. Because of this variable quality, frequent auscultation in the upright, supine, and left lateral decubitus positions is important for patients in whom a diagnosis of pericarditis is suspected.

Electrocardiogram

The electrocardiogram (ECG) is a key diagnostic test in suspected pericarditis, though typical changes are not always seen. The classic finding is widespread, concave ST-segment elevation, often with associated PR-segment depression (Fig. 35.2). Although the changes may appear regional and therefore mimic myocardial ischemia, reciprocal ST-segment depressions are absent, as are pathologic Q-waves. In addition, the ECG in pericarditis exhibits a typical pattern of evolution that is

TABLE 35.1

ETIOLOGIES OF ACUTE PERICARDIAL DISEASE

Etiology	Examples	Incidence	Treatment
Idiopathic[a]	—	85%–90%	Aspirin, NSAIDs
Infectious Viral[a] Bacterial[a] Mycobacterial[a] Fungal	Echovirus, coxsackievirus, adenovirus, cytomegalovirus, hepatitis B, Epstein–Barr virus (infectious mononucleosis), HIV/AIDS *Pneumococcus*, *Staphylococcus*, *Streptococcus*, *Mycoplasma*, *Borrelia* spp. (Lyme disease), *Haemophilus influenzae*, *Neisseria meningitidis*, *Mycobacterium tuberculosis*, *M. avium-intracellulare*, *Histoplasma*, *Coccidioides*	1%–2% 1%–2% 4%–5% Rare (<1%)	Aspirin, NSAIDs Antibiotics, surgical drainage Antimycobacterial therapy and prednisone Antifungal therapy, drainage
Immune/inflammatory	Connective tissue disease[a] (systemic lupus erythematosus, rheumatoid arthritis, scleroderma) Arteritis (polyarteritis nodosa, temporal arteritis) Drug induced[a] (e.g., procainamide, hydralazine, isoniazid, cyclosporine)	3%–5% Rare (<1%)	Aspirin, NSAIDs, glucocorticoids Discontinue drug; aspirin, NSAIDs
Neoplastic	Primary: mesothelioma, sarcoma, etc. Secondary[a]: breast carcinoma, lung carcinoma, lymphoma	5%–7%	NSAIDs, intrapericardial infusion of glucocorticoids
Myocardial infarction related Aortic dissection related	Early postmyocardial infarction (MI) Late postmyocardial infarction (Dressler's syndrome)[a] Proximal aortic dissection	5%–6% of patients with transmural MI Formerly 3%–4% of patients with MI, much less in the era of early reperfusion Rare (<1%)	Aspirin (avoid NSAIDs) Urgent surgery (do not drain)
Traumatic[a]	Blunt and penetrating trauma, postcardiopulmonary resuscitation	NA	NSAIDs (avoid aspirin)
Procedure and device related	Early postcardiac surgery Post-ICD/pacemaker,[a] postangioplasty,[a] late post cardiotomy or thoracotomy (Dressler's variant)[a]	Common Rare (<1%)	Aspirin, NSAIDs Aspirin, NSAIDs
Radiation induced[a]	Chest wall irradiation	Rare (<1%)	NSAIDs
Uremic or dialysis associated	—	~5% of patients with chronic kidney disease predialysis, ~13% after dialysis	Initiate or intensify dialysis, NSAIDs

[a]Conditions that manifest as acute pericarditis.

distinct from that of patients with evolving myocardial infarction. In patients with pericarditis, the ECG on presentation usually demonstrates diffuse ST-segment elevation and PR-segment depression (stage I) and evolves through three subsequent phases [20]. During the evolutionary phase (stage II), all ST-junctions return to baseline more or less "in phase," with little change in T-waves. (By contrast, in patients with ST-segment elevation due to acute myocardial injury, T-wave inversion begins to occur *before* the ST-segments return to baseline.) The T-waves subsequently flatten and invert (stage III) in all or most of the leads that showed ST-segment elevations. In stage IV, the T-waves return to their prepericarditic condition. The widespread T-wave inversions that appear in stage III are indistinguishable from those of diffuse myocardial injury, myocarditis, or biventricular injury. The entire ECG evolution occurs in a matter of days or weeks, but may not be seen in every patient. Often, the transition from stage III to stage IV is relatively slow, with some patients left with some degree of T-wave inversion for an indefinite period.

Although some 80% of patients with pericarditis exhibit a typical stage I ECG during their course [21], atypical variants (or even a normal ECG) may also be seen. An important ECG variant that can be quasidiagnostic is PR-segment (not PR-interval) depression in the absence of true ST-segment elevation, which though nonspecific, may be the only sign of pericarditis. This may occur as a consequence of superficial myocarditis affecting the atrium [22]. Although the ST-changes of pericarditis may occasionally resemble those of normal early

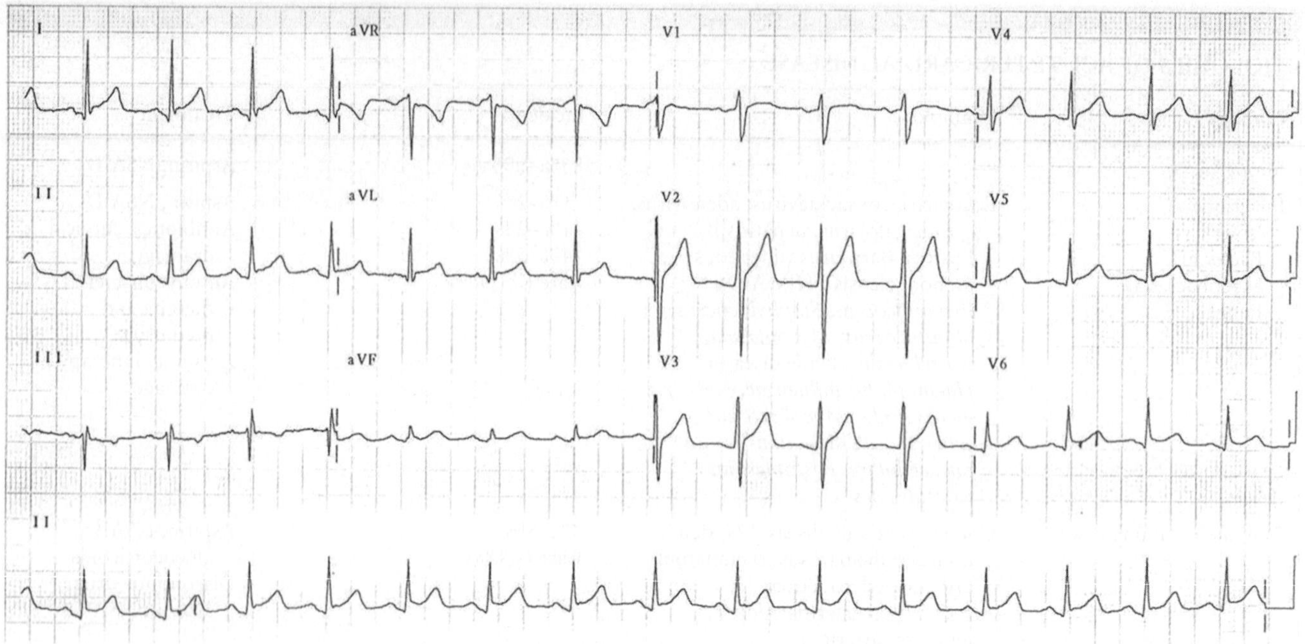

FIGURE 35.2. Electrocardiogram (ECG) in acute pericarditis. Note the diffuse, upward concave ST-segment elevation and PR-segment depression (lead II).

repolarization, a useful differentiating feature may be the ratio between the height of the ST-segment and the T-wave in lead V_6. A ratio exceeding 0.24 favors the diagnosis of pericarditis [23].

Imaging and Additional Laboratory Testing

Although laboratory findings in patients with suspected pericarditis are nonspecific, measurement of serum markers of inflammation (leukocyte count, erythrocyte sedimentation rate, C-reactive protein, and lactate dehydrogenase) and myocardial necrosis (creatine kinase, and troponins) may help to establish or confirm the diagnosis, define the extent of associated myocardial injury, and guide subsequent follow-up. The 2004 European Society of Cardiology guidelines on the management of pericardial diseases [24] therefore advise measurement of these parameters as part of the initial diagnostic evaluation in all patients, but this recommendation remains somewhat controversial. A markedly elevated white blood cell count, particularly in association with high fever, should raise suspicion for purulent pericarditis, and may prompt sampling of pericardial fluid (if present) for diagnosis. Cardiac enzymes including creatine kinase (creatine kinase, total and MB-fraction) and troponins are commonly elevated in patients with pericarditis due to associated epicardial inflammation or myocarditis [25]. Elevations in troponin I are seen more commonly than those in CK-MB and are frequently associated with male gender, ST-segment elevation, younger age at presentation, and pericardial effusion. The degree of troponin elevation is roughly related to the extent of myocardial inflammation and, distinct from acute coronary syndromes, does not appear to correlate with long-term prognosis [26]. Routine measurement of cardiac troponins in patients with suspected or definite pericarditis may therefore be unnecessary, unless there is suspicion for associated transmural myocardial infarction by ECG (due to the presence of pathologic Q-waves) [27]. Similarly, routine serologic testing for antinuclear antibodies or rheumatoid factor is rarely helpful, save in those patients in whom other clinical features suggest underlying connective tissue illness.

The chest radiograph is typically normal in acute pericarditis, but is often performed as a matter of course to assess for abnormalities in the mediastinum or lung fields, which may suggest an etiology, and to exclude cardiomegaly, which suggests the presence of a substantial pericardial effusion (>250 mL). Pericardial calcification is rarely seen, but may suggest constrictive pericarditis. Any suspicion for cardiomegaly should prompt a transthoracic echocardiogram to assess for hemodynamically significant pericardial effusion or tamponade. Routine echocardiography in patients with unequivocal evidence of pericarditis and normal hemodynamics by physical examination is probably unnecessary, though the detection of a pericardial effusion may help to support the diagnosis. In addition, detection of wall motion abnormalities or left ventricular dysfunction on echocardiography may be helpful in detecting associated myocardial infarction or in assessing the severity of associated myocarditis.

Natural History and Management

There are no large, randomized, controlled clinical trials to guide the therapy of patients with acute pericarditis. Initial management is directed at screening for specific etiologies and underlying conditions that may alter the treatment strategy (e.g., connective tissue disease, HIV infection, and tuberculosis) and control of symptoms. In the vast majority of patients, acute idiopathic pericarditis is a self-limited disease without significant complications or recurrence, and may be safely managed in the outpatient setting [28]. A subset of patients with high-risk features including fever greater than 38°C, subacute course (symptoms developing over days or weeks), large pericardial effusion (>20 mm in width in diastole by echocardiography), cardiac tamponade, or failure to respond to treatment with aspirin or nonsteroidal anti-inflammatory drugs (NSAIDs) should be considered for hospital admission to permit additional observation and a more extensive etiologic work-up [29]. Immunosuppressed patients and those with blunt or penetrating chest trauma, serologic evidence of myocarditis (based on elevated cardiac biomarkers), or need for oral anticoagulant therapy may also be at risk for complications and warrant closer observation [30].

Treatment of pericarditis may vary on the basis of etiology. For the minority of cases in which a specific diagnosis is identified, therapy should be tailored appropriately, as outlined in

Table 35.1. (Details of treatment for specific conditions are beyond the scope of this discussion.) In uncomplicated cases of idiopathic pericarditis, treatment with NSAIDs is the cornerstone of therapy. Across the board, these agents are effective in reducing inflammation and symptoms of pain, fever, and malaise associated with pericarditis. Limited observational data suggest that the various available NSAIDs have comparable efficacy [31]. As a first-line agent, many favor treatment with ibuprofen, which is well tolerated and can easily be titrated over a range of doses. The typical dose is 600 mg every 6 hours, which sometimes relieves pain within 15 minutes to 2 hours of the first dose. Depending on patient tolerance and therapeutic response, the individual dose can be reduced to 400 mg or raised to 800 mg or greater with continued observation for side effects. Should this fail, aspirin 600 to 900 mg four times per day may be given. Indomethacin may be used, always given on a full stomach and in divided doses from 100 to 200 mg per day, beginning with 25 mg every 6 hours. In patients with myocardial infarction–related pericarditis, indomethacin should probably be avoided in light of experimental work showing that it reduces coronary flow, increases experimental infarction size, and raises blood pressure. Aspirin is the agent of choice in these cases because among the NSAIDs, it least retards scar formation in the infracted heart [32]. In all patients receiving high-dose NSAIDs, gastrointestinal protection with an antacid or proton–pump inhibitor should be considered to reduce the risk of drug-induced gastritis or bleeding.

Pain is typically relieved within hours to days of initiation of anti-inflammatory medications. Occasionally, chest pain persists beyond 2 weeks of therapy with an NSAID, but responds to therapy with a different NSAID or to the addition of colchicine 0.6 mg twice daily. Recurrent pericarditis may complicate 15% to 32% of cases, and can be a particularly troublesome problem [33]. Colchicine has long been known to be effective in preventing relapses of polyserositis in familial Mediterranean fever [34]. A wealth of observational data now support the notion that colchicine as an adjunct to therapy with NSAIDs or corticosteroids is well tolerated and effective in the treatment and prevention of relapsing pericarditis [35]. A small, randomized, controlled trial seems to confirm this impression. In the Colchicine for Recurrent Pericarditis (CORE) [36] trial, 84 patients with a first episode of recurrent pericarditis were randomized to conventional therapy with aspirin alone or conventional treatment plus colchicine (1.0 to 2.0 mg the first day and then 0.5 to 1.0 mg day for 6 months). Treatment with colchicine significantly decreased the recurrence rate at 18 months from 50.6% to 24.0% ($p = 0.02$, 95% confidence interval 2.5 to 7.1) and simultaneously reduced symptom persistence at 72 hours.

Efficacy in recurrent pericarditis has spurred interest in the utilization of colchicine in the first episode of acute pericarditis for the prevention of recurrent pericarditis. In the Colchicine for Acute Pericarditis (COPE) [37] trial, 120 patients experiencing their first episode of acute pericarditis (idiopathic, viral, postpericardiotomy, and connective tissue disease related) were randomly assigned to conventional treatment with aspirin or conventional treatment plus colchicine (1.0 to 2.0 mg for the first day and then 0.5 to 1.0 mg per day for 3 months). Corticosteroid therapy was permitted but restricted to patients with aspirin contraindications or intolerance. During the 2,873 patient-months of follow-up, colchicine significantly reduced both the symptom persistence at 72 hours and the recurrence rate relative to conventional therapy alone (recurrence rates 10.7% vs. 32.3%, respectively, at 18 months, $p = 0.004$). Overall, the COPE trial provides evidence to support the use of colchicine as an adjunct to NSAIDs during a first episode of pericarditis to prevent recurrence, though routine use of this agent for this indication is not recommended.

Intractably symptomatic pericarditis occasionally calls for adjunctive treatment with narcotics or more aggressive immunosuppression with corticosteroids, azathioprine, or even cyclophosphamide, though there is limited clinical experience with many of these agents [38]. Caution should be exercised in particular with initiation of steroid therapy, given that many patients experience extreme difficulty in weaning once they are begun. Importantly, in both the CORE and COPE trials, prednisone therapy was a strong predictor of pericarditis relapse, confirming the empiric observation that glucocorticoid therapy is a major factor in recurrence [39]. Steroid therapy should therefore be reserved as a therapy of last resort for nontuberculous, nonconnective tissue disease–related pericarditis. When necessary, steroids should be utilized in the lowest effective dose and rapidly weaned. Intrapericardial instillation of steroids may be an alternative in refractory cases and may help to avert some of the side effects of systemic therapy [40]. Of note, pericardiectomy has occasionally been employed for recurrent pericarditis, but appears to be effective in the minority of patients, perhaps because complete removal of the pericardium is not possible, and residual pericardial or pleural surfaces may remain inflamed [41].

Pericardial Effusion and Tamponade

Pericardial effusion may appear as a complication of acute pericarditis or as an isolated entity. In 60% of cases, the etiology is related to a known systemic disease [42]. Effusions are common following cardiac surgery; as many as 10% may progress to late tamponade [43]. Severe circulatory congestion due to heart failure may result in transudative effusion as a consequence of markedly elevated intracardiac filling pressures or obstructed pericardial drainage. Hemopericardium is a potentially lethal complication of chest wall trauma, myocardial rupture, or proximal aortic dissection. In some cases of pericardial effusion, despite a thorough diagnostic evaluation, there may be no identifiable cause even when the effusion has been present for years; such idiopathic effusions generally have benign course, though tamponade can develop without warning over time [44]. Because of the high prevalence of idiopathic pericarditis, this disorder accounts for the bulk of pericardial tamponade; as noted, however, this condition typically has a benign, uncomplicated course. By contrast, effusions associated with bacterial, fungal, and HIV infection, those associated with neoplasia, and those associated with bleeding into the pericardial space have a high likelihood of progressing to tamponade [45].

Pericardial effusions may have a spectrum of hemodynamic effects ranging from the inconsequential to complete circulatory collapse. As noted previously, the pericardium has a limited reserve volume such that the rapid accumulation of even modest amounts of pericardial fluid may have important hemodynamic consequences for ventricular filling and overall cardiac performance. Slowly accumulating effusions may be accommodated by pericardial stretch over time and may therefore escape clinical diagnosis until they are quite large. Although computed tomography (CT) and magnetic resonance imaging (MRI) may be more sensitive for the identification of small amounts of pericardial fluid, echocardiography is the primary modality for evaluation of the functional consequences of any pericardial effusion.

Cardiac Tamponade

Cardiac tamponade is defined as hemodynamically significant cardiac compression due to accumulating pericardial contents that evoke and defeat compensatory mechanisms, resulting in a decline in cardiac output (Fig. 35.3) [46]. The severity of cardiac compression may vary widely depending on the quantity and rate of accumulation of fluid, blood, pus, or gas

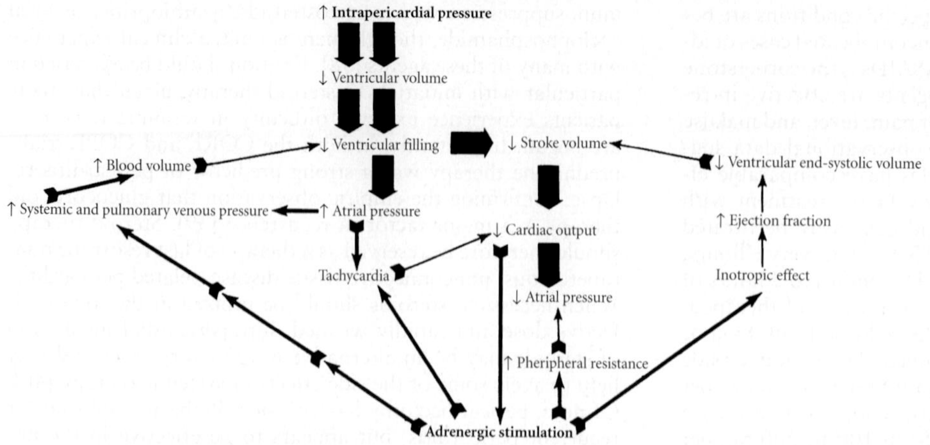

FIGURE 35.3. Cardiac tamponade (*heavy arrows without tails*) and compensatory mechanisms (*arrows with tails*). Thin-tailed arrows represent immediate mechanisms directed against tamponade changes; intermediate mechanisms are represented by heavier-tailed arrows. For example, decreased ventricular filling due to decreased ventricular volume is immediately supported by increased blood volume. Development of the latter is stimulated by the intermediate mechanism, increased venous pressures (see text).

(including air) in the pericardial space. Occasionally, pericardial effusion and tamponade are seen in combination with underlying constrictive physiology (constrictive–effusive pericarditis). Tamponade should be considered in the differential diagnosis of any patient with cardiogenic shock and systemic congestion.

Physiology

Understanding the physiology of cardiac tamponade is essential to diagnosis and treatment. The primary hemodynamic abnormality is an increase in pericardial pressure that affects the filling of one or more cardiac chambers; due to lower filling pressures in systole and diastole, right-heart performance is initially affected disproportionately to that of the left heart. For significant cardiac compression, the pericardial contents must increase at a rate exceeding the rate of stretch of the parietal pericardium (see Fig. 35.1) and, to some degree, the rate at which venous blood volume expands to maintain the small filling gradient to the right heart. As the chambers become progressively smaller and myocardial diastolic compliance is reduced, cardiac inflow becomes limited, ultimately equalizing mean diastolic pericardial and chamber pressures. Relentlessly increasing intrapericardial pressure progressively reduces ventricular volume to the point that even a high ejection fraction cannot avert critical reduction of stroke volume at any heart rate.

True filling pressure in the heart chambers is defined by the transmural pressure, which is equal to the difference between cavity pressure and pericardial pressure. Pericardial pressure is normally negative, and therefore augments transmural pressure (suction effect), facilitating cardiac filling. Increasing pericardial pressure due to accumulation of pericardial contents reduces and ultimately offsets transmural pressures, thereby compromising filling. In tamponade, both the ventricles fill against a common stiffness (pericardium plus fluid), evoking corresponding increases in left and right atrial pressures. Pericardial pressure quickly exceeds early diastolic pressure in the atria and right ventricle and rises further during ventricular diastolic expansion, causing early diastolic right ventricular collapse, which further impedes atrial emptying. Ultimately, there is elevation and near-complete equalization of pericardial and four-chamber pressures in diastole, abolishing the normal pressure gradient for filling; the ventricles may fill only during atrial systole, particularly at rapid heart rates. Because of reduced filling, ventricular systolic pressure ultimately falls, along with stroke volume, reducing cardiac output. As in heart failure, this fall in output triggers a cascade of compensatory neurohormonal mechanisms that generate tachycardia, increased contractility, enhanced circulating blood volume, and increased systemic vascular resistance in an attempt to defend end-organ perfusion (Fig. 35.3).

Presentation and Diagnosis

Cardiac tamponade may appear insidiously as the first sign of pericardial injury or intrapericardial bleeding, especially in conditions such as neoplasia, trauma, and connective tissue disorders. Commonly, however, it follows clinical acute pericarditis. The symptoms of tamponade are not specific, and may be similar to those of congestive heart failure (though frank pulmonary edema is uncommon). Dyspnea and fatigue are common presenting complaints, and patients may have other signs and symptoms of an associated systemic illness (e.g., malignancy or connective tissue disease). Those with advanced cardiac compression may exhibit signs of hypoperfusion, including pallor, cyanosis, confusion, diaphoresis, diminished urine output, and cold extremities. In patients with rapid tamponade due to hemorrhage, as in wounds and cardiac or aortic rupture, the dominant picture is one of shock, which if unchecked, can rapidly lead to electromechanical dissociation and death.

On physical examination, tachycardia and hypotension (relative or absolute) are the rule, though bradycardia may occasionally be seen in association with myxedema or uremia. Jugular venous distension is usually apparent, except in cases of rapid tamponade (e.g., acute hemopericardium), in which there has been insufficient time for the blood volume to increase. The venous contour typically exhibits an absent *y* descent due to loss of the gradient for passive ventricular filling in early diastole. The normal inspiratory fall in venous pressures is preserved in uncomplicated cardiac tamponade; a rise (or absence of fall) in the jugular venous pressure (Kussmaul's sign) is suggestive of associated constrictive physiology. When tamponade is due to inflammatory or neoplastic lesions, pericardial rubs frequently are present and can be quite loud, although the heart sounds may be distant due to insulating effects of the pericardial fluid and reduced ventricular function.

Excessive fluid in the pericardium often exaggerates the normal pericardial effects on ventricular interaction, heightening the normal inspiratory decrease in systemic blood pressure, leading to *pulsus paradoxus*. This is conventionally defined as a drop in systolic pressure of more than 10 mm Hg with normal inspiration, and may be palpable in muscular arteries (such as the femoral artery) [47]. The phenomenon occurs because in tamponade, increased right heart filling with inspiration can only be accommodated by bulging the atrial and ventricular septa toward the left atrium and ventricle (due to restraint by pericardial fluid). The decrease in left ventricular filling due to septal shift (enhanced by the normal decrease in left atrial filling on inspiration) diminishes left ventricular stroke volume and arterial pressure. Although pulsus paradoxus is the hallmark of tamponade, it may also be present in patients with obstructive lung disease (including severe asthma), pulmonary embolism, tense ascites, obesity, right heart failure due to mitral stenosis or right ventricular infarction, and hypovolemic and cardiogenic shock. Because pulsus paradoxus occurs when respiratory changes alternately favor right and left heart filling, it may be absent in conditions that balance or blunt the effects of inspiratory venous return on ventricular filling (e.g., pericardial adhesions, atrial septal defect, severe aortic insufficiency, or diminished left ventricular compliance due to severe hypertrophy, infiltrative myopathy, myocardial infarction, or advanced heart failure) or in cases of severe hypotension where respiratory blood pressure variations may be imperceptible.

Additional Diagnostic Testing

The ECG in tamponade is rarely diagnostic. Clinical signs of pericarditis (ST-segment elevations and PR-depressions) may persist, and frequently, there is some decrease in voltage of the QRS and T-waves (typically sparing the P-wave), reflecting insulation of the heart by surrounding fluid and the effects of cardiac compression [48]. Although common, however, low voltage is not a sensitive or specific finding for tamponade. By contrast, electric alternation (beat-to-beat variation in P- or QRS amplitude reflecting a shifting electrical axis as the heart swings within a large effusion) is fairly specific for tamponade and virtually pathognomonic when it affects the both the P-waves and the QRS complex (simultaneous alternation) [49]. Although an enlarged cardiac silhouette on chest radiography may suggest a pericardial effusion, the chest radiograph alone is rarely diagnostic because cardiomegaly, large pericardial cysts, and pericardial effusions may be difficult to distinguish.

Echocardiography has a high degree of sensitivity and specificity for recognizing pericardial fluid and is the key diagnostic test for assessing the hemodynamic significance of a pericardial collection. CT, spin-echo, and cine MRI can also be used to assess the size and extent of simple and complex pericardial effusions (and indeed may be more sensitive for small amounts of pericardial fluid), but measurements by CT and MRI tend to be larger than those by echocardiography, and neither radiographic technique is typically useful in the acute management of patients with suspected tamponade [50]. By echocardiography, a pericardial effusion typically appears as a lucent separation between visceral and parietal pericardium in the region of the posterior left ventricular wall. With larger effusions, the fluid is also demonstrated anterior to the right ventricle. As pericardial effusion increases, movement of the parietal pericardium decreases. When the amount of pericardial effusion is massive, the heart may have a "swinging" motion in the pericardial cavity, the echocardiographic correlate of electrical alternans seen on the ECG.

Several echocardiographic findings indicate that a pericardial effusion is large enough to cause hemodynamic compromise (tamponade physiology). Early diastolic collapse of the right ventricle and late diastolic right atrial inversion are seen when pericardial pressure transiently exceeds the intracavitary pressure and are characteristic, though not entirely specific signs of tamponade [51]. The inferior vena cava is typically dilated with blunted respiratory variation indicating elevated right-sided filling pressures. Inspiratory shift of the ventricular septum toward the left and respiratory variation in ventricular chamber size may also be seen, reflecting right ventricular filling at the expense of the left due to essentially fixed intrapericardial volume. Corresponding changes can be seen on Doppler echocardiography, which permits the detection of exaggerated respiratory variation in transmitral and transtricuspid flow velocities during diastole. During inspiration, intrapericardial pressure (and therefore left ventricular end-diastolic pressure) and intrathoracic pressure normally fall to the same degree, whereas in tamponade, intrapericardial pressure falls substantially less than intrathoracic pressure. This leads to discordant changes in pulmonary venous pressure and left ventricular end-diastolic pressure on inspiration that diminish the pressure gradient for left ventricular filling. As a result, mitral valve opening is delayed, isovolumic relaxation time is prolonged, and peak transmitral filling velocity decreases. Reciprocal changes occur on the right side of the heart, with a resultant inspiratory increase in peak transtricuspid filling velocity [52]. Corresponding changes are visible on Doppler interrogation of the pulmonary and hepatic venous flows and may enhance the sensitivity and specificity of echocardiography for diagnosis of tamponade [53].

Cardiac catheterization in patients with tamponade is often performed as a prelude to pericardiocentesis, but can also be diagnostic. Typically, the hemodynamics at catheterization are notable for elevation and equalization of average diastolic pressures across all four cardiac chambers in the range of 15 to 30 mm Hg. As with the jugular venous waveform, the right atrial pressure tracing displays an absent y descent and preserved x descent, corresponding to diminished atrial emptying during ventricular diastole as a consequence of elevated end-diastolic pressures. As with echocardiography, discordant inspiratory changes in right- and left-sided pressures are often seen, with a fall in left-sided filling pressures and stroke volume with inspiration corresponding to the pulsus paradoxus noted on physical examination and the diminished transmitral flow seen by Doppler. For reasons that remain unclear, despite comparable filling pressures to patients with advanced heart failure, patients with cardiac tamponade do not typically develop pulmonary edema [54].

Special Cases

Because tamponade physiology is merely the result of a pericardial pressure that exceeds intracavitary pressure, it may occur at lower diastolic pressures (6 to 12 mm Hg) in patients who have a decrease in circulating blood volume and cardiac filling pressures due to hypovolemia or hemorrhage. In these conditions, even a relatively modest elevation in pericardial pressure may lower the transmural filling pressure sufficiently to compromise stroke volume. Such "low-pressure" tamponade may lack the typical hemodynamic or clinical signature, and is typically observed in patients with preexisting effusions who undergo aggressive diuresis or hemodialysis [55]. In addition, regional tamponade, affecting only limited portions of the heart (or even a single cardiac chamber), may occur in the setting of pericardial adhesions and loculated fluid collections, as can be seen after cardiac bypass surgery (even after the pericardium is left open). In this case, the typical hemodynamic features may not be present on conventional imaging, and diagnosis may require transesophageal echocardiography [56].

Management

Although pericardial effusions that are small or resolve rapidly with anti-inflammatory treatment may not require invasive therapy, those associated with hemodynamic compromise should be promptly drained using either a percutaneous or surgical approach. Transient medical stabilization of patients with tamponade physiology can often be achieved through aggressive volume resuscitation (particularly in volume-depleted patients) and pressor support with inotropic agents (e.g., norepinephrine, isoproterenol, and dobutamine), but medical therapy alone is usually insufficient. Positive-pressure ventilation may precipitate hemodynamic collapse due to excessive preload reduction, and should be avoided where possible until pericardial drainage can be accomplished. Percutaneous needle pericardiocentesis may be performed by trained personnel in the cardiac catheterization laboratory or at the bedside with echocardiographic (or CT) guidance. Echocardiography is helpful in demonstrating the most accessible window for passage of a needle; typically, the subxiphoid approach is most effective, with insertion of a long needle underneath the xiphoid process at a 30-degree angle to the skin, directed gradually toward the left shoulder until pericardial fluid is aspirated. Attachment of an electrocardiographic lead to the needle may be useful for additional guidance in identifying the pericardial space because contact of the needle with myocardium generates an electrocardiographic current of injury. An apical approach (using a shorter needle inserted in the sixth or seventh rib space in the anterior axillary line) can also be considered if adequate fluid is visible in this region by echocardiography.

Once the pericardial space is reached, a soft-tipped guidewire is passed into the pericardial space and the needle removed. A multiholed catheter can then be introduced over the wire, sutured in place, and connected to a reservoir to allow complete drainage of the remaining pericardial fluid over the next several hours. Rapid reduction in intrapericardial pressures and associated hemodynamic improvement may be seen after the aspiration of only 100 to 200 mL of fluid. Fluid specimens should be sent for appropriate chemistry, cytology, and culture as appropriate for more definitive identification of etiology and direction of appropriate adjuvant therapy.

For patients with intrapericardial hemorrhage (e.g., due to proximal aortic dissection) or tamponade due to purulent pericarditis, surgical drainage may be optimal. A surgical approach may also be necessary in patients with rapid reaccumulation of pericardial fluid following pericardiocentesis (as is common in patients with malignant effusions), patients with loculated effusions causing regional tamponade (as following cardiac surgery), or in patients with large intrapericardial clots that are not amenable to catheter drainage. The two most commonly utilized surgical options are surgical subxiphoid incision and drainage and video-assisted thoracoscopic drainage [57] with creation of a pleuropericardial "window" to allow longer term egress of pericardial fluid into the pleural space. Thoracoscopic surgery provides the opportunity for concurrent performance of additional procedures such as biopsy of the lung, biopsy of pleural or mediastinal masses, or management of a concomitant pleural effusion, but requires single-lung ventilation and lateral decubitus positioning, which may preclude use of this approach in an emergency. Both the approaches may be accomplished with limited perioperative morbidity, and conversion to an open surgical approach (median sternotomy or anterolateral thoracotomy) is rarely necessary [58]. In patients who are poor candidates for surgical drainage, percutaneous balloon pericardiotomy may be an effective alternative [59].

Constrictive Pericarditis

Constrictive pericarditis is a rare, but severely disabling, consequence of chronic pericardial inflammation characterized by progressive fibrosis and dense adhesion of the pericardium that progressively impairs ventricular filling. Any patient with acute pericarditis may ultimately go on to develop constriction, but the syndrome appears particularly common in patients with pericardial disease due to tuberculosis, therapeutic chest irradiation, prior cardiac surgery, chest trauma, or uremia. The time course of development is variable, with constrictive physiology occasionally apparent acutely (constrictive–effusive pericarditis) but more commonly seen months to years following the initial inflammatory insult. The clinical presentation is that of marked venous congestion in the face of relatively preserved cardiac size and systolic function, and resembles that of right heart failure. Patients typically experience dyspnea, easy fatigability, and abdominal distension, and may exhibit dramatic physical findings including ascites, peripheral edema, and jugular venous distension with prominent *x* and *y* descents. The differential diagnosis is broad, and commonly includes restrictive cardiomyopathy, hepatic cirrhosis, or right heart failure due to any of a variety of causes including pulmonary embolism, right ventricular infarction, venous/valvular obstruction, or cor pulmonale.

Pathophysiology and Diagnosis

The fundamental physiologic abnormality in constrictive pericarditis is limited filling and enhanced interventricular dependence because of rigid encasement of the heart by thickened pericardium. Because the myocardium is intrinsically normal (unless there is a combined abnormality, as in patients with prior mediastinal irradiation), myocardial contractile function and relaxation may also be entirely normal (distinct from restrictive cardiomyopathy). Unlike cardiac tamponade, the heart is not compressed in early diastole and relaxes rapidly as filling proceeds until it reaches its pericardial limit (rubber-bulb effect). Early diastolic filling is rapid due to elevated right atrial pressures, but abruptly limited by the noncompliant pericardial shell, generating the classic "dip and plateau" or "square root" contour on intraventricular pressure recordings in diastole (Fig. 35.4). As the heart is effectively isolated from intrathoracic pressure variations by the stiff pericardial shell, jugular venous pressure increases during inspiration (Kussmaul's sign)

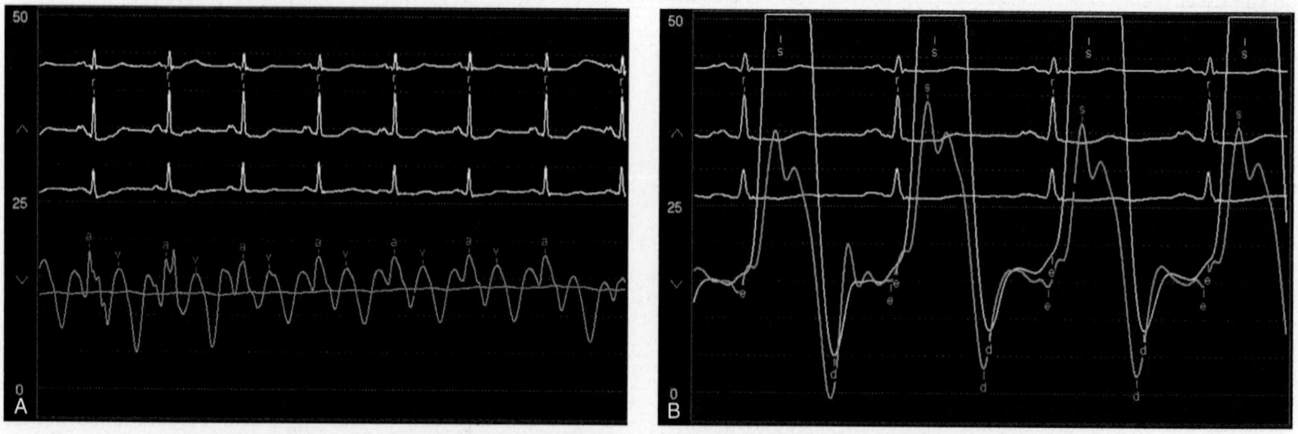

FIGURE 35.4. A: Right atrial pressure recording in a patient with constrictive pericarditis. Note the steep *x* and *y* descents, corresponding to the changes visible in the jugular venous contour. **B:** Simultaneous recording of LV (*yellow*) and RV (*green*) (pressure in the same patient). Note the near equalization of LV/RV pressures in diastole and the "square root" or "dip and plateau" sign reflecting abrupt cessation of ventricular filling due to pericardial constraint.

and pulsus paradoxus is typically absent, except in cases associated with pericardial fluid under pressure (constrictive–effusive pericarditis).

Like tamponade, constriction is characterized by elevation and equalization of left- and right-heart filling pressures, but there are important clinical differences. Distinct from tamponade, venous pressure contours show prominent *y* as well as *x* troughs. The *y* descent also tends to be deeper and more precipitous in constriction, as there is torrential filling in early diastole, with abrupt cessation of filling on reaching the pericardial limit. At this point, there may be an intense early diastolic third heart sound (sometimes called a "knock"). Clinical signs of right heart failure (due to elevated diastolic pressures) tend to dominate those of left heart failure, perhaps because cardiac output is relatively well preserved, and neurohormonal stimuli for salt and water retention may accordingly be less than that in systolic heart failure. The precordium is usually quiet to palpation, with no easily identifiable point of maximal impulse and the liver is often palpable and pulsatile. Laboratory findings are rarely diagnostic and are typically those of hepatic congestion and synthetic dysfunction. Hypoalbuminemia may occur as a consequence of liver impairment, malnutrition due to protein-losing enteropathy, or a proteinuric nephrotic syndrome, related to chronically high venous pressures [60]. ECG and chest radiograph findings are entirely nonspecific, though pericardial calcification may occasionally be seen (particularly in patients with tuberculous pericarditis).

Imaging with CT or MRI may support the diagnosis of constriction, and typically demonstrates tube-like ventricles, atrial enlargement, septal changes, and enlargement of the inferior vena cava as well as pericardial thickening. Any thickening greater than 3.5 mm (and more definitively >6 mm) is suggestive and helps to differentiate constrictive from restrictive cardiomyopathy. Although increased pericardial thickness has been considered an essential diagnostic feature of constrictive pericarditis, it should be remembered that in a large surgical series from the Mayo Clinic constriction was present in 18% of the patients with normal pericardial thickness [61]. In addition, constrictive pericarditis may rarely develop only in the epicardial layer in patients with previously removed parietal pericardium [62].

The most difficult pathophysiologic differential is typically between restrictive cardiomyopathy (due to primary myocardial disease such as amyloidosis or hemochromatosis) and constrictive pericarditis (see Table 35.2). Historical features often provide clues to systemic illness that suggest a diagnosis, but additional hemodynamic evaluation is often necessary. Typically, patients with restrictive cardiomyopathies tend to have higher left- than right-sided pressures and show greater inequalities during exercise and slower early- to midsystolic filling. Doppler echocardiography with tissue Doppler imaging or color M-mode imaging may be particularly helpful for distinction, showing marked respiratory variation in the peak early mitral inflow velocity (peak E-variation ≥25%), rapid mitral annular relaxation velocity (Ea ≥8 cm per second), and a slope of more than or equal to 100 cm per second for the first aliasing contour in the flow propagation velocity in patients with primary constrictive rather than restrictive disease [63,64]. Cardiac catheterization has traditionally been the gold standard for differentiation, though hemodynamic profiles may overlap

TABLE 35.2

DIFFERENTIATION OF CONSTRICTIVE PERICARDITIS AND RESTRICTIVE CARDIOMYOPATHY

Feature	Constrictive pericarditis	Restrictive cardiomyopathy
Prominent *y* descent in venous pressure	Present	Variable
Pulsus paradoxus	~1/3 of cases	Absent
Pericardial knock	Present	Absent
Cardiac catheterization		
Equalization of right/left heart filling pressures	Present	Left typically 3–5 mm Hg higher than right
Filling pressures >25 mm Hg	Rare	Common
Pulmonary artery systolic pressure >60 mm Hg	Rare	Common
"Square root" sign on RV/LV diastolic pressure waveform	Present	Present
Respiratory variation in left–right pressures/flows	Exaggerated	Normal
Echocardiography		
Ventricular wall thickness	Normal	Typically increased
Atrial size	Possible left atrial enlargement	Biatrial enlargement
Septal "bounce"	Present	Absent
Inspiratory variation in peak mitral inflow velocity (E)	Typically >25%	Typically varies by <10%
Blunting of pulmonary venous systolic flow (S-wave on PV Doppler)	Absent	Present
Mitral annular relaxation velocity on Doppler tissue imaging	Typically normal or mildly reduced	Diminished
Slope of flow propagation velocity on color M-mode	Increased, >100 cm/s	Diminished
Other		
Pericardial thickness (CT/MRI/TEE)	Increased	Normal
Endomyocardial biopsy	Usually normal or only mildly abnormal	May reveal infiltrative cardiomyopathy or extensive fibrosis, but may be normal

TABLE 35.3

EVIDENCED-BASED MANAGEMENT OF PERICARDIAL DISEASE

- Limited evidence from randomized trials is available to guide therapy of patients with pericardial disease
- The addition of colchicine to conventional medical therapy reduces the recurrence rate in patients presenting with recurrent pericarditis [36]
- The addition of colchicine to conventional medical therapy may also be useful in reducing the duration of symptoms and the recurrence rate in patients with a first episode of acute pericarditis [37]
- Treatment with nonsteroidal anti-inflammatory drugs is not useful in the management of persistent pericardial effusion following cardiac surgery [43]
- Two-dimensional echocardiography is preferable to CT or MRI for the initial evaluation of patients with pericardial effusion or suspected tamponade [50]
- In large observational studies of patients with constrictive pericarditis, older age, prior mediastinal radiation, and advanced heart failure predict poor outcomes following pericardiectomy [62,63]

considerably in the two states. Simultaneous left and right heart pressure recordings reveal equalization and elevation of pressures in the right atrium, right ventricle, left atrium pulmonary capillary wedge pressure (PCWP), and left ventricle during diastole. The right atrial (RA) pressure contour typically shows an "M"- or "W"-configuration with prominent x and y descents (Fig. 35.4). Systolic right ventricular pressure rises, but usually to less than 50 mm Hg, and the right ventricular end-diastolic pressure to systolic pressure ratio is usually greater than 0.3. Pulmonary hypertension is not a feature of constrictive pericarditis and indicates coexisting cardiac or pulmonary disease. Discordance or separation between right ventricular and left ventricular pressure contours with quiet inspiration or following fluid challenge is a marker of enhanced interventricular interdependence and is a highly specific marker of constriction [65]. Endomyocardial biopsy may also be useful in identifying primary myocardial disease when less invasive diagnostic modalities are inconclusive or ambiguous [66].

Management

Medical management of constrictive pericarditis resembles that of congestive heart failure because most signs and symptoms are related to systemic congestion. Diuretics are the mainstay of therapy and are useful in relieving volume overload and congestive symptoms, but do not alter the course of the disease. Definitive treatment requires surgical pericardiectomy. Access is typically obtained via either anterolateral thoracotomy or median sternotomy, with the target of removing as much pericardium as possible (ideally, from phrenic nerve to phrenic nerve). Areas of strong calcification or dense scaring may be left as islands to avoid major bleeding. Pericardiectomy for constrictive pericarditis carries a perioperative mortality rate of roughly 6%, and normalization of cardiac hemodynamics is reported in the minority of the patients, though most experience clinically relevant functional improvements [67]. Major complications include acute perioperative heart failure (likely due to underrecognized myocardial fibrosis or atrophy present prior to surgery) and ventricular wall rupture.

If an indication for surgery is established early, long-term survival after pericardiectomy may be good, though on average slightly inferior to that of age- and gender-matched controls (57% ± 8% at 10 years). In the reported Mayo Clinic experience, older age at presentation, poor preoperative New York Heart Association functional class, and prior radiation were the strongest predictors of early mortality [68]. A second series of 163 patients undergoing pericardiectomy over a 24-year period at the Cleveland Clinic suggested that in addition to age and prior radiation, poor renal function, elevated pulmonary artery systolic pressure, low serum sodium, and preoperative left ventricular (LV) dysfunction were important correlates of poor overall survival [69]. Seven-year survival in this experience ranged from 88% for patients with idiopathic constrictive pericarditis to 27% for patients with postradiation constrictive pericarditis, suggesting that the outcome of pericardiectomy is highly dependent on the specific cause, the degree of preoperative myocardial injury, and preoperative functional capacity. Early diagnosis and therapy are important because the anticipated postoperative outcome is heavily affected by preoperative heart failure severity. In addition, because pericardiectomy does not affect the course of underlying myocardial disease, careful exclusion of coincidence restrictive heart disease is important in selecting patients for surgery.

CONCLUSION

Pericardial manifestations are seen in a wide spectrum of infectious, inflammatory, and neoplastic disorders. Critical care of patients with pericardial disease depends on a basic understanding of pericardial physiology and thoughtful integration of data from physical examination, electrocardiography, noninvasive cardiovascular imaging, and invasive hemodynamic studies. Although limited data from randomized controlled trials are available to direct the optimal strategy for treatment of patients with acute pericarditis, pericardial effusion, and pericardial constriction, a wealth of observational experience provides important insights into the natural history and clinical management of these conditions.

Advances in critical care of pericardial disease, based on best available evidence, are summarized in Table 35.3.

References

1. Goldstein JA: Cardiac tamponade, constrictive pericarditis, and restrictive cardiomyopathy. *Curr Probl Cardiol* 29(9):503–567, 2004.
2. LeWinter MM, Kabbani S: Pericardial diseases, in Zipes DP, Libby P, Bonow RO, et al (eds.): *Braunwald's Heart Disease.* 8th ed. Philadelphia, Elsevier, 2008, pp 1829–1853.
3. Assanelli D, Lew WY, Shabetai R, et al: Influence of the pericardium on right and left ventricular filling in the dog. *J Appl Physiol* 63(3):1025–1032, 1987.
4. Santamore WP, Li KS, Nakamoto T, et al: Effects of increased pericardial pressure on the coupling between the ventricles. *Cardiovasc Res* 24:768–776, 1990.

5. Watkins MW, LeWinter MM: Physiologic role of the normal pericardium. *Annu Rev Med* 44:171–180, 1993.
6. Spodick DH: Threshold of pericardial constraint: the pericardial reserve volume and auxiliary pericardial functions. *J Am Coll Cardiol* 6:296–297, 1985.
7. Freeman G, LeWinter MM: Pericardial adaptations during chronic cardiac dilation in dogs. *Circ Res* 54:294–300, 1984.
8. Spodick DH: Acute pericarditis: current concepts and practice. *JAMA* 289:1150, 2003.
9. Troughton RW, Asher CR, Klein AL: Pericarditis. *Lancet* 363:717–727, 2004.
10. Zayas R, Anguita M, Torres F, et al: Incidence of specific etiology and role of methods for specific etiologic diagnosis of primary acute pericarditis. *Am J Cardiol* 75:378–382, 1995.
11. Imazio M, Brucato A, Trinchero R, et al: Diagnosis and management of pericardial diseases. *Nat Rev Cardiol* 6:743–751, 2009.
12. Maisch B, Ristic AD: The classification of pericardial disease in the age of modern medicine. *Curr Cardiol Rep* 4:13–21, 2002.
13. Halsell JS, Riddle JR, Atwood JE, et al: Myopericarditis following smallpox vaccination among vaccinia-naive US military personnel. *JAMA* 289:3283–3289, 2003.
14. Barbaro G, Klatt EC: HIV infection and the cardiovascular system. *AIDS Rev* 4:93–103, 2002.
15. Sagrista-Sauleda J, Barrabes JA, Permanyer-Miralda G, et al: Purulent pericarditis: review of a 20-year experience in a general hospital. *J Am Coll Cardiol* 22:1661–1665, 1993.
16. Sagrista-Sauleda J, Permanyer-Miralda G, Soler-Soler J: Tuberculous pericarditis: ten year experience with a prospective protocol for diagnosis and treatment. *J Am Coll Cardiol* 11:724–728, 1988.
17. Mayosi BM: Contemporary trends in the epidemiology and management of cardiomyopathy and pericarditis in sub-Saharan Africa. *Heart* 93:1176–1183, 2007.
18. Powler NO: Tuberculous pericarditis. *JAMA* 266:99–103, 1991.
19. Miller RH, Horneffer PJ, Gardner TJ, et al: The epidemiology of the post-pericardiotomy syndrome: a common complication of cardiac surgery. *Am Heart J* 116:1323–1329, 1988.
20. Spodick DH: The electrocardiogram in acute pericarditis: distributions of morphologic and axial changes by stages. *Am J Cardiol* 33:470, 1974.
21. Bruce MA, Spodick DH: Atypical electrocardiogram in acute pericarditis: characteristics and prevalence. *J Electrocardiol* 13:61, 1980.
22. Baljepally R, Spodick D: PR-segment deviation as the initial electrocardiographic response in acute pericarditis. *Am J Cardiol* 81(12):1505–1506, 1998.
23. Ginzton LE, Laks MM: The differential diagnosis of acute pericarditis from the normal variant: new electrocardiographic criteria. *Circulation* 65:1004–1009, 1982.
24. Maisch B, Seferovic PM, Ristic AD, et al: Guidelines on the diagnosis and management of pericardial diseases. Executive summary. The task force on the diagnosis and management of pericardial diseases of the European Society of Cardiology. *Eur Heart J* 25:58–610, 2004.
25. Bonnefoy E, Godon P, Kirkorian G, et al: Serum cardiac troponin I and ST-segment elevation in patients with acute pericarditis. *Eur Heart J* 21:832–836, 2000.
26. Imazio M, Demichelis B, Cecchi E, et al: Cardiac troponin I in acute pericarditis. *J Am Coll Cardiol* 42(12):2144–2148, 2003.
27. Newby LK, Ohman EM: Troponins in pericarditis: implications for diagnosis and management of chest pains patients. *Eur Heart J* 21(10):798–800, 2000.
28. Spodick DW: Pericardial diseases, in Braunwald E, Zipes D, Libby P (eds): *Heart Disease.* 6th ed. Philadelphia, WB Saunders, 2001, pp 1823–1876.
29. Imazio M, Spodick DH, Brucato A, et al: Controversial issues in the management of pericardial diseases. *Circulation* 121:916–928, 2010.
30. Imazio M, Cecchi E, Demichelis B, et al: Indicators of poor prognosis of acute pericarditis. *Circulation* 115:2739–2744, 2007.
31. Schifferdecker B, Spodick DH: Nonsteroidal anti-inflammatory drugs in the treatment of pericarditis. *Cardiol Rev* 11(4):211–217, 2003.
32. Lange RA, Hillis LD: Acute pericarditis. *N Engl J Med* 351(21):2195–2202, 2004.
33. Fowler NO: Recurrent pericarditis. *Cardiol Clin* 8(4):621–626, 1990.
34. Wright DG, Wolff SM, Fauci AS, et al: Efficacy of intermittent colchicine therapy in familial Mediterranean fever. *Ann Intern Med* 86:162–165, 1977.
35. Adler Y, Finkelstein Y, Guindo J, et al: Colchicine treatment for recurrent pericarditis: a decade of experience. *Circulation* 97:2183–2185, 1998.
36. Imazio M, Bobbio M, Cecchi E, et al: Colchicine as first-choice therapy for recurrent pericarditis: results of the CORE (COlchicine for REcurrent pericarditis) trial. *Arch Intern Med* 165(17):1987–1991, 2005.
37. Imazio M, Bobbio M, Cecchi E, et al: Colchicine in addition to conventional therapy for acute pericarditis: results of the COlchicine for acute PEricarditis (COPE) trial. *Circulation* 112(13):2012–2016, 2005.
38. Marcolongo R, Russo R, Laveder F, et al: Immunosuppressive therapy prevents recurrent pericarditis. *J Am Coll Cardiol* 26(5):1276–1279, 1995.
39. Imazio M, Demichelis B, Parrini I, et al: Management, risk factors, and outcomes in recurrent pericarditis. *Am J Cardiol* 96(5):736–739, 2005.
40. Maisch B, Ristic AD, Pankuweit S: Intrapericardial treatment of autoreactive pericardial effusion with triamcinolone: the way to avoid side effects of systemic corticosteroid therapy. *Eur Heart J* 23:1503–1508, 2002.
41. Fowler NO, Harbin AD, III: Recurrent acute pericarditis: follow-up study of 31 patients. *J Am Coll Cardiol* 7:300–305, 1986.
42. Sagrista-Sauleda J, Merce J, Permanyer-Miralda G, et al: Clinical clues to the causes of large pericardial effusions. *Am J Med* 109:95–101, 2000.
43. Meurin P, Tabet JY, Thabut G, et al: Nonsteroidal anti-inflammatory drug treatment for postoperative pericardial effusion: a multicenter, randomized, double-blind trial. *Ann Int Med* 152:137–143, 2010.
44. Sagrista-Sauleda J, Angel J, Permanyer-Miralda G, et al: Long-term follow up of idiopathic chronic pericardial effusion. *N Engl J Med* 341:2054–2059, 1999.
45. LeWinter MM, Kabbani S: Pericardial diseases, in Zipes DP, Libby P, Bonow RO, Braunwald E (eds): *Braunwald's Heart Disease.* 7th ed. Philadelphia, Elsevier, 2005, pp 1757–1780.
46. Spodick DH: Acute cardiac tamponade. *N Engl J Med* 349:684–690, 2003.
47. Shabetai R, Fowler NO, Fenton JC, et al: Pulsus paradoxus. *J Clin Invest* 44:1882, 1965.
48. Toney JC, Kolmen SN: Cardiac tamponade: fluid and pressure effects on electrocardiographic changes. *Proc Soc Exp Biol Med* 121:642, 1966.
49. Spodick DH: Electric alternation of the heart: its relation to the kinetics and physiology of the heart during cardiac tamponade. *Am J Cardiol* 10:155, 1962.
50. Mulvagh SL, Rokey R, Vick GW, et al: Usefulness of nuclear magnetic resonance imaging for evaluation of pericardial effusions, and comparison with two-dimensional echocardiography. *Am J Cardiol* 64:1002–1009, 1989.
51. Reydel B, Spodick DH: Frequency and significance of chamber collapses during cardiac tamponade. *Am Heart J* 119:1160–1163, 1990.
52. Burstow DJ, Oh JK, Bailey KR, et al: Cardiac tamponade: characteristic Doppler observations. *Mayo Clin Proc* 64(3):312–324, 1989.
53. Merce J, Sagrista-Sauleda J, Permanyer-Miralda G, et al: Correlation between clinical and Doppler echocardiographic findings in patients with moderate and large pericardial effusion: implications for the diagnosis of cardiac tamponade. *Am Heart J* 138[4, Pt 1]:759–764, 1999.
54. Spodick DH: Low atrial natriuretic factor levels and absent pulmonary edema in pericardial compression of the heart. *Am J Cardiol* 63:1271–1272, 1989.
55. Spodick DH: Acute cardiac tamponade. *N Engl J Med* 349:684–690, 2003.
56. Tsang TS, Barnes ME, Hayes SN: Clinical and echocardiographic characteristics of significant pericardial effusions following cardiothoracic surgery and outcomes of echo-guided pericardiocentesis for management: Mayo Clinic experience, 1979–1998. *Chest* 116(2):322–331, 1999.
57. Georghiou GP, Stamler A, Sharoni E, et al: Video-assisted thoracoscopic pericardial window for diagnosis and management of pericardial effusions. *Ann Thorac Surg* 80(2):607–610, 2005.
58. O'Brien PK, Kucharczuk JC, Marshall MB, et al: Comparative study of subxiphoid versus video-thoracoscopic pericardial "window." *Ann Thorac Surg* 80(6):2013–2019, 2005.
59. Galli M, Politi A, Pedretti F, et al: Percutaneous balloon pericardiotomy for malignant pericardial tamponade. *Chest* 108(6):1499–1501, 1995.
60. Nikolaidis N, Tziomalos K, Giouleme O, et al: Protein-losing enteropathy as the principal manifestation of constrictive pericarditis. *J Gen Intern Med* 20(10):958, 2005.
61. Talreja DR, Edwards WD, Danielson GK, et al: Constrictive pericarditis in 26 patients with histologically normal pericardial thickness. *Circulation* 108:1852–1857, 2003.
62. Byrne JG, Karavas AN, Colson YL, et al: Cardiac decortication (epicardiectomy) for occult constrictive cardiac physiology after left extrapleural pneumonectomy. *Chest* 122(6):2256–2259, 2002.
63. Rajagopalan N, Garcia MJ, Rodriguez L, et al: Comparison of new Doppler echocardiographic methods to differentiate constrictive pericardial heart disease and restrictive cardiomyopathy. *Am J Cardiol* 87(1):86–94, 2001.
64. Ha JW, Ommen SR, Tajik AJ, et al: Differentiation of constrictive pericarditis from restrictive cardiomyopathy using mitral annular velocity by tissue Doppler echocardiography. *Am J Cardiol* 94(3):316–319, 2004.
65. Hurrell DG, Nishimura RA, Higano ST, et al: Value of dynamic respiratory changes in left and right ventricular pressures for the diagnosis of constrictive pericarditis. *Circulation* 93:2007–2013, 1996.
66. Schenfeld MH: The differentiation of restrictive cardiomyopathy from constrictive pericarditis. *Cardiol Clin* 8:663–671, 1990.
67. Senni M, Redfield MM, Ling LH, et al: Left ventricular systolic and diastolic function after pericardiectomy in patients with constrictive pericarditis: Doppler echocardiographic findings and correlation with clinical status. *J Am Coll Cardiol* 33(5):1182–1188, 1999.
68. Ling LH, Oh JK, Schaff HV, et al: Constrictive pericarditis in the modern era: evolving clinical spectrum and impact on outcome after pericardiectomy. *Circulation* 100(13):1380–1386, 1999.
69. Bertog SC, Thambidorai SK, Parakh K, et al: Constrictive pericarditis: etiology and cause-specific survival after pericardiectomy. *J Am Coll Cardiol* 43(8):1445–1452, 2004.

CHAPTER 36 ■ ACUTE AORTIC SYNDROMES

LEON M. PTASZEK, ERIC M. ISSELBACHER AND AMY E. SPOONER

INTRODUCTION

Representing the most lethal conditions affecting the aorta, acute aortic syndromes are associated with a high mortality rate if not recognized and treated promptly. Although the classical presentation of "aortic agony" is characterized by severe, sudden-onset pain in the chest or back [1], this presentation, although quite recognizable, occurs only in a minority of cases. As the initial manifestations of acute aortic syndromes are frequently variable, arriving at the appropriate diagnosis in a timely manner may be quite challenging. Prompt recognition of the acute aortic syndromes may be the difference between life and death for the afflicted patient. Frequently, the clinician must depend on subtle findings gleaned from history, detailed physical examination, and imaging in order to decide on an appropriate treatment plan. Here, we review the commonly encountered aortic syndromes, with a focus on aortic aneurysm rupture, as well as acute aortic dissection and acute aortic intramural hematoma (IMH). We focus primarily on the means by which these syndromes can be recognized and treated. Attention is also given to etiology and pathophysiology of the specific disease processes to the extent that evaluation of these processes is relevant to diagnostic and treatment strategies. Because patients with suspected acute aortic syndromes are frequently critically ill and require rapid disposition to treatment, we offer a unified evaluation and treatment algorithm. Each individual section serves as a guide to a syndrome-specific evaluation. Key features of a focused history and physical examination are emphasized. In addition, critical laboratory and imaging tests are reviewed.

AORTIC DISSECTION

Definition and Classification

Dissection of the aortic wall involves longitudinal cleavage of the muscular media, leading to the formation of a second (or false) vessel lumen. The inciting event for a typical aortic dissection is thought to be a tear in the intima that leads to exposure of the underlying media, presumably weakened by medial degeneration. Once created, this cleavage front advances due to wall strain created by physiologic blood pressure. The cleavage front typically advances in the direction of blood flow, but dissection against the direction of flow is also observed [2].

There are multiple consequences of dissection. The native (or true) lumen is frequently compressed, leading to compromised downstream blood flow. The false lumen of the dissected aorta may also be less able to withstand physiologic blood pressure, due to changes in both its shape and its thinner external wall. The damaged aorta may therefore be more prone to rupture.

Aortic dissections are generally classified by location and extent. Dissections originate in the ascending aorta (65%) or in the descending aorta just distal to the origin of the left subclavian artery (20%). Dissection in the aortic arch (10%) and the abdominal aorta (5%) also occur [3]. Two classification systems for dissection location are in common use (Fig. 36.1). The DeBakey system includes three types of aortic dissection. Type I involves dissection of both the ascending and descending aorta, and/or the arch. Type II dissection involves only the ascending aorta proximal to the brachiocephalic artery, and type III involves only the descending aorta distal to the left subclavian artery [4]. The Stanford system includes two dissection types. All dissections involving the ascending aorta are included in type A: this includes types I and II in the DeBakey system. Stanford type B includes all dissections that do not involve the ascending aorta [5]. Classification of the location of a dissection carries prognostic and treatment importance. Surgery is indicated for dissection of the ascending aorta, whereas medical management is frequently the treatment of choice for descending dissection.

Chronicity of the dissection is defined as the time interval between onset of symptoms and evaluation. Dissections that are present for less than 2 weeks are defined as acute, whereas those that are present longer are defined as chronic [6]. It is noteworthy that the mortality associated with untreated ascending aortic dissection reaches 75% at 2 weeks [7].

Not all cases of aortic dissection are associated with an identified area of intimal tear. Several analyses have revealed that up to 13% of cases of apparent dissection turn out to be an IMH: a hemorrhage within the media that does not communicate with the intraluminal space [7–9]. In some cases, an atherosclerotic ulcer that penetrates from the intima beyond the internal elastic lamina is thought to precipitate intramural bleeding [10]. Classical aortic dissection and IMH are discussed separately later.

CLASSIC AORTIC DISSECTION

Epidemiology

Estimates of the incidence of aortic dissection range from 2 to 4 per 100,000 per year [11]. The highest incidence occurs in patients in their sixth and seventh decades of life. Incidence among men is double that for women [1,12]. Recent studies show that women tend to present later and with a more advanced disease state [12]. In addition, it has been shown that aortic dissection exhibits diurnal and seasonal rhythms. Dissections are most likely to occur in the morning or early afternoon, and more commonly in winter [13]. This seasonal difference does not appear to depend on climate [14].

Mortality rates associated with dissection are very high, and many patients do not survive to hospital admission. For those patients with aortic dissection who survive to admission, the early mortality rate is estimated to be as high at 1% per hour during the first day [7]. If left untreated, the associated mortality is estimated at 50% at 7 days and greater than 90% at 90 days [15]. Among patients who receive treatment, mortality during initial hospitalization ranges between 15% and 27.5%, as reported in several longitudinal studies [1,16,17].

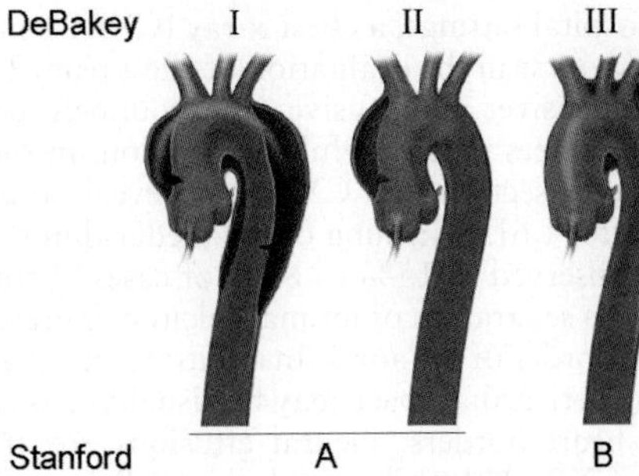

FIGURE 36.1. Dissection classification (DeBakey/Stanford). [© Massachusetts General Hospital Thoracic Aortic Center. Used with permission.]

Etiology and Pathophysiology

Any process that causes damage to the aortic tunica media, leading to medial degeneration, increases the risk for aneurysm or dissection. In the case of typical aortic dissection, the precipitating event is thought to be the creation of a tear in the intimal layer overlying a damaged area of the media. In the elderly patient with dissection, the presence of medial degeneration is correlated with the effects of aging, hypertension, and atherosclerotic disease [18–20]. Indeed, hypertension is found in 70% to 80% of patients with aortic dissection [1].

In the younger patient with aortic dissection, medial degeneration is still the culprit, but the constellation of correlated risk factors tends to differ [21]. Typically, young patients are more likely to have hereditary connective tissue disorders that compromise the integrity of the extracellular matrix in the tunica media, most notably Marfan syndrome, Ehlers–Danlos syndrome, bicuspid aortic valve, or familial thoracic aortic aneurysm syndrome (FTAAS) [1,6,21]. Young patients, defined in a recent study as being 40 years of age or younger, are also less likely to be hypertensive, and may have a larger aortic diameter on presentation. Paradoxically, mortality in this younger cohort does not appear to be lower than that in older patients [21]. All of these syndromes have been associated with breakdown of the fibrillin and collagen components of the extracellular matrix in the media, leading to medial degeneration. Aortic dissection risk is also increased in patients with Turner and Noonan syndromes [6]. Increased risk for dissection is found in a number of other conditions, including aortitis, especially in the context of giant cell arteritis and Takayasu arteritis [6,22,23]. Cocaine use has also been associated with dissection, ostensibly on the basis of increases in cardiac output, blood pressure, or as a consequence of direct vascular injury from cocaine itself (i.e., cocaine-induced vasculitis/endarteritis). In particular, crack cocaine has been identified as a potential precipitant of dissection [24,25].

As is the case for aortic aneurysm, the presence of certain structural abnormalities may be associated with an increased risk of dissection. In particular, a correlation has been described in patients with bicuspid aortic valve or, uncommonly, aortic coarctation. This association does not appear to be related to the hemodynamic effects of the abnormalities [26].

Notably, pregnancy is an independent risk factor for aortic dissection. The highest incidence of dissection is observed in the third trimester or early postpartum period. This risk is high particularly in pregnant women with a bicuspid aortic valve, Marfan, Ehlers–Danlos, or Turner syndrome [27,28]. In pregnant women with Turner syndrome, the risk of dissection or rupture exceeds 2%, and the risk of death is increased 100-fold [29]. Sporadic aortic dissections may occur in women without these predisposing conditions, possibly due to the elevated levels of relaxin and inhibin associated with pregnancy.

Iatrogenic injury to the aortic wall, sustained in the context of cardiac catheterization, intra-aortic balloon pump placement, or cardiac surgery, increases the risk of future aortic dissection [30–32]. Cardiac surgery involving the aortic valve appears to pose the greatest risk. Damage sustained by the aorta may take up to several years to develop into aneurysm and/or dissection [32,33].

Blunt trauma or rapid deceleration injury is frequently associated with injury to the aortic isthmus. Although this type of injury may be associated with tearing or transection of the aorta, a true dissection is uncommon [34,35].

Clinical Manifestations

There is no single physical examination finding that allows for positive identification of dissection: only imaging of the aorta verifies the diagnosis. Consequently, the initial evaluation and examination must incorporate a high index of suspicion and careful assessment.

The classic initial symptom of acute aortic dissection is severe chest or back pain. The severity of this pain is characteristically at its maximum at the point of inception. This is in sharp contrast with the typical crescendo onset of myocardial infarction pain [1]. The quality of the pain is often described as being "tearing" or "stabbing." Acute pain is present in 85% of the patients described in the International Registry of Aortic Diseases (IRAD) and is present in up to 96% of patients described in other studies [1,6,36]. Of the patients in the IRAD registry, 90% described this discomfort as being the worst pain they ever experienced. Indeed, patients may be prone to writhing or pacing because of the pain. The initial location of the pain is correlated to the location of the dissection: of the patients in reported clinical series who presented with anterior chest or neck pain, 65% to 90% were found to have dissection of the ascending aorta. Interscapular or back may also represent dissection of the descending aorta [6]. On occasion, the patient may report a migration of the pain in association with extension of the dissection. In a series reported by Spittell et al., 17% of patients reported pain migration [6]. Recently, it was noted that aortic dissection may, in some instances, present with abdominal pain [37].

A common finding at the time of presentation is hypertension. Of the patients in the IRAD series, 36% of patients with type A dissection had elevated blood pressure, whereas 70% of patients with type B dissection had hypertension. Conversely, hypotension may also be a presenting feature of aortic dissection. This is a particularly ominous finding, as it likely represents developing shock. Hypotension is seen more frequently in patients with type A than type B dissection (25% vs. 4%, respectively) [1]. It is also noteworthy that patients with dissections who present with a "deadly triad" of hypotension/shock, an absence of pain, and evidence of branch vessel involvement exhibit a markedly higher mortality [38].

Evidence of heart failure, most notably pulmonary edema and hypotension, is found in up to 7% of patients with aortic dissection [1,6]. This finding is most frequently due to aortic regurgitation caused by a type A dissection [39]. However, in a recent report, a surprisingly high percentage of patients with heart failure at the time of dissection actually had a type B syndrome, with heart failure presumably due to myocardial ischemia or diastolic dysfunction with hypertension.

Syncope is present in up to 9% of patients with dissection. In these patients, syncope that is associated with focal neurologic signs is usually the result of occlusion of a branch vessel. Syncope in the absence of any other neurologic findings, present in up to 5% of dissection patients, likely represents aortic rupture into the pericardial space with tamponade. This finding portends rapid decline and requires emergent surgery.

Pericardial tamponade in the context of type A aortic dissection is a surgical emergency, as it represents a tenuously compensated rupture of the aorta. Unless the patient is in extremis, pericardiocentesis should not be performed, as the release of pressure in the pericardial space may precipitate a rise in blood pressure, recurrent hemorrhage into the pericardium, and cardiovascular collapse [40]. Dissection into the pleural space may also lead to hypotension and syncope, and similarly requires immediate surgical intervention.

A number of other vascular complications of aortic dissection may be apparent on initial evaluation. In up to 20% of the cases reported in the IRAD series, subjects presented with signs and symptoms consistent with occlusion of branch vessels. These occlusion events are typically the result of the extension of the dissection into a branch vessel ("static" occlusion), occlusion of the ostium of the vessel due to migration of the intimal flap ("dynamic" occlusion), or impaired flow in the true lumen due to distention of the false lumen. The spectrum of clinical findings associated with aortic side-branch involvement ranges from no signs and symptoms, to subtle findings, to florid manifestations, including severe ischemia of the affected territories. The mass effect of the dissection may lead to focal neurologic defects in rare cases. Involvement of a subclavian artery may lead to a difference in measured blood pressure between the two arms or pulse deficit. Impaired flow in the mesenteric arteries leads to signs and symptoms consistent with mesenteric ischemia. Dissections may also lead to occlusion of the renal arteries, leading to acute renal failure or renal infarction. Rarely, dissection leads to spinal artery occlusion with resultant paraparesis or paraplegia [1,6]. Lower limb ischemia may also occur in type B dissection [41].

On occasion, type A dissection may extend proximally to the ostia of the coronary arteries, leading to myocardial infarction. Three percent of the patients in the IRAD series presented with dissection-related myocardial infarction, with attendant chest pain and biomarker elevation [1].

There is not yet a specific biomarker in common clinical use that allows the clinician to confirm the diagnosis. For example, the D-dimer is elevated in dissection, but has limited diagnostic utility [42,43]. Recent work has highlighted several specific biomarkers that are elevated in acute aortic dissection and may become diagnostically useful in the future. The most promising assay is an enzyme-linked immunosorbent assay (ELISA) for myosin heavy chain. The sensitivity and specificity of this test, when it is performed within 12 hours of the acute event, are 90% and 97%, respectively. The primary advantage of this test is its ability to distinguish dissection from other events, such as myocardial infarction. Assays for other compounds elevated in aortic dissection but not in other acute cardiac events, such as serum heart-type fatty acid–binding protein, elastin, and calponin, are also in development [44–47].

Imaging

Prompt imaging is critical in the evaluation of suspected aortic dissection. Multiple modalities are at the disposal of the clinician; however, the patient is best served by the modality that offers adequate image quality without delay or transport time. The specific technique of choice may differ among hospitals, as not all facilities have the same capabilities. Following is a discussion of the relative strengths and weaknesses of the commonly available imaging techniques in the diagnosis of aortic dissection. The decision regarding the optimal technique to be used in a specific context is left to the individual clinician. Frequently, multiple imaging modalities must be used in a single patient. In addition, a single patient may require serial studies if his/her signs or symptoms evolve [48].

In most hospital settings, a chest x-ray (CXR) is performed as a matter of course in the evaluation of chest pain. The CXR, which is noninvasive, inexpensive, and routinely performed at the bedside, offers much useful information. In the patient with an aortic dissection, the CXR may reveal an abnormal aortic silhouette [1,6]. Widening of the mediastinum is a variable finding, observed in 15% to 60% of cases. Another suggestive finding is separation of intimal calcium, if present, from the soft-tissue border of the aorta. In addition, extravasation of blood into the pericardial space may be visualized as expanded and blunted heart borders. Pleural effusions are also easily visualized on CXR. Although useful, the CXR cannot be considered a definitive study. Therefore, other modalities should be used, notably echocardiography, computerized tomography (CT) scanning, and magnetic resonance imaging (MRI) (Table 36.1).

Transthoracic echocardiography (TTE) is a readily available, noninvasive, and portable imaging modality that may be considered. A focused study can be performed within 15 minutes at the bedside. Dissected segments of aorta can be measured directly: this is typically restricted to the ascending aorta, as neither the aortic arch nor the descending aorta can be reliably visualized via an external approach. TTE is also a very reliable technique for the visualization of pericardial effusion. The intimal flap of aortic dissection may be seen as a "double" aortic wall. Direction of Doppler flow may also help the clinician distinguish between the "true" and "false" lumens of aortic dissection. It should be noted that sensitivity for type A dissection varies between 70% and 90%, and sensitivity for type B dissection is approximately 40% [49]. Given this suboptimal sensitivity, performing a TTE should not delay a more sensitive imaging study. Despite its convenience, TTE is limited in that it does not offer an unobstructed view of all portions of the aorta. Body habitus may also adversely affect the quality of TTE images.

A far more accurate ultrasound study for suspected aortic dissection is transesophageal echocardiography (TEE). By virtue of the close proximity of the aorta to the ultrasound probe in the esophagus, this technique offers clear views of most portions of the thoracic aorta and affords excellent information regarding aortic valve function. TEE may be useful to guide surgical intervention for type A aortic dissection. TEE, like TTE, is portable and can be performed easily at the bedside, which makes it the procedure of choice for evaluation of critically ill or medically unstable patients who may be at higher risk during transportation for radiographic examinations.

In aortic dissection, TEE is superior to TTE in visualization of the intimal flap; sensitivity varies between 90% and 100%, and specificity is approximately 90%. Color Doppler imaging may identify the blood flow between the true and false lumens. Perhaps the most important procedural drawback regarding TEE is the need for conscious sedation, which may be difficult to administer in a patient who is hemodynamically unstable.

CT scanning allows for a full view of the entire aorta. Consequently, the sensitivity (90% to 100%) and specificity (90%) for visualization of the intimal flap in aortic dissection are comparable to TEE [49]. Specific CT techniques, such as spiral CT, also allow for facile three-dimensional reconstruction. The "double barrel" produced by dissection can be quite distinct. In classic aortic dissection, an intimal flap can be seen, separating a true and false lumen. Pericardial and pleural effusions may be easily visualized, but blood flow and tamponade physiology cannot be assessed directly. A diagnostic CT scan requires intravenous contrast, and care must be taken to address the risks of allergic reaction and contrast nephropathy. Many patients presenting with the acute aortic syndromes may also have renal insufficiency or failure; however, in the critically ill patient in whom aneurysm rupture is suspected, definitive diagnosis and treatment of the aortic process should take priority.

TABLE 36.1

IMAGING MODALITIES FOR PATIENTS WITH SUSPECTED ACUTE AORTIC SYNDROMES

	Key findings	Advantages	Disadvantages
TTE	Intimal flap in ascending aorta Dilatation of aortic root Aortic valve regurgitation Pericardial effusion Color Doppler differentiation of flow in dissection-related "true" and "false" lumens	Readily available Noninvasive Quickly performed at bedside No ionizing radiation Intravenous contrast not required Aortic valve function can be directly assessed	Only aortic root and ascending aorta can be reliably assessed Image quality may be affected by body habitus Branch vessels and intramural hematomas are not reliably visualized
TEE	Intimal flap in aorta Dilatation of aorta Aortic valve regurgitation Pericardial effusion Color Doppler differentiation of flow in dissection-related "true" and "false" lumens	Readily available Noninvasive Quickly performed at bedside No ionizing radiation Intravenous contrast not required Image quality not affected by body habitus Ascending aorta, arch, and proximal descending aorta may be visualized Aortic valve function can be assessed directly	Distal thoracic and abdominal aorta cannot be visualized May only be performed by trained personnel Sedation required Branch vessels are not reliably visualized
CT	Intimal flap in aorta Dilatation of aorta in any segment Pericardial effusion Dissection-related "true" and "false" lumens or intramural hematoma accentuated with contrast	Readily available Noninvasive Quickly performed Image quality not affected by body habitus Full aorta may be assessed in single scan Most widely used first imaging test in suspected dissection	Requires use of ionizing radiation and intravenous contrast Transportation to scanner may be required in some centers Patient monitoring during scan may be difficult Aortic valve function cannot be assessed directly
MRI	Intimal flap in aorta Dilatation of aorta in any segment Pericardial effusion Dissection-related "true" and "false" lumens or intramural hematoma may be differentiated	Noninvasive No ionizing radiation Image quality not affected by body habitus Full aorta may be assessed in single scan Branch vessel visualization is excellent Contrast not required to visualize intramural hematoma or to differentiate between true and false lumen Aortic valve function can be directly assessed	Not readily available at many hospitals Transportation to scanner may be required in some centers Patient monitoring during scan may be difficult Scan time longer than other modalities
Aortogram	Intimal flap in aorta Dilatation of aorta in any segment True and false lumens may be differentiated with contrast	Best modality for branch vessel visualization Allows for assessment of full aorta	Invasive Study not as readily available due to required assembly of trained personnel Ionizing radiation and intravenous contrast required Intramural hematoma cannot be reliably assessed

CT scanning and MRI share several of the same advantages, such as high image resolution and the ability to scan the entire aorta. Overall, the sensitivity and specificity of intimal flap detection by MRI are nearly 100% [49]. MRI does not require the use of IV contrast, which represents an advantage over CT scanning; however, MRI is more expensive and not as readily available or as rapidly performed as CT scanning. The primary limitation of MRI is lack of availability: not all hospitals have MR scanners available for emergent use. Even when available, issues of transporting a potentially unstable patient are still present. MRI is also contraindicated in patients in whom vascular clips, implantable cardioverter-defibrillators (ICDs) or pacemakers are present.

In the past, retrograde aortography was considered the gold-standard technique for aortic imaging. Because aortography is an invasive test that requires the assembly of a catheterization laboratory team and the use of IV contrast and ionizing radiation, it is typically reserved for those cases where diagnostic uncertainty remains after one or more other imaging studies have been obtained. The ability of aortography to detect aortic dissection depends on the presence of blood flow between the true and false lumens; therefore, in cases where blood flow between these chambers is limited, the aortogram may be nondiagnostic. Overall, among patients with classic aortic dissection, the sensitivity and specificity for intimal flap visualization are 80% to 90% and 90% to 95%, respectively [49]. Aortography is still the study of choice for visualization of aortic branch vessels, which may not be visualized with other imaging modalities as well. In addition, aortography is particularly useful if endovascular treatment is contemplated.

Management

The primary goal of treatment in a patient with aortic dissection is to minimize the effects of the dissection while rapidly evaluating the patient's candidacy for surgical repair, if indicated (Figure 36.5). Initial medical management while waiting for possible surgery should focus on management of pain, decrease of blood pressure to a minimum acceptable level, and decrease in the force of left ventricular contraction (dP/dt). In general, long-acting agents are not favored, as such agents are difficult to titrate rapidly. Early observation should occur in an intensive care setting, with an arterial line in place. For patients presenting with evidence of heart failure, pulmonary artery catheter placement may be considered, but is usually not necessary.

Pain management is titrated aggressively in patients with dissection. The goals of pain treatment are patient comfort and decrease in adrenergic tone. Narcotic analgesics are effective in rapid reduction of symptom severity, especially when administered in intravenous form. Long-acting oral formulations of narcotics are not recommended.

Blood pressure and dP/dt can be simultaneously decreased with a beta-blocker. Noncardioselective agents such as propranolol, labetalol, and esmolol have been used extensively in this context. Beta-blockers should be considered even in patients who are not hypertensive at presentation, as the reduction in dP/dt is thought to be beneficial in reducing the advancement of dissection. The goal heart rate is 60 beats per minute, and the goal systolic blood pressure is no higher than 120 mm Hg. In the event that a patient's blood pressure is still elevated even after a goal heart rate has been reached with β-blockade, nitroprusside may also be administered as a constant intravenous infusion; however, intravenous nitroprusside should not be used without concomitant β-blockade, given the possibility of an increase in heart rate and dP/dt accompanying its potent vasodilatory effects.

In the event that a beta-blocker cannot be used, due to contraindications such as bronchospasm, nondihydropyridine calcium channel blockers are the second-line agents. Verapamil and diltiazem, both of which have vasodilator and negative inotropic/chronotropic effects, may be used. Some patients have hypertension that is resistant to blockade of both β-adrenergic receptors and calcium channels. In this case, dosing of an intravenous angiotensin converting enzyme inhibitor, such as enalaprilat, may be indicated.

Hypotension may be seen in conjunction with dissection. It should be noted that the mode of blood pressure measurement should be scrutinized before changing a treatment plan; "pseudohypotension" may occur if dissection propagates into the limb in which blood pressure is being measured. In such cases, it is recommended that hypotension be verified by measurement of blood pressure in other limbs prior to discontinuation of beta-blockers or calcium channel blockers (Tables 36.2 and 36.3).

Surgical Intervention

The primary concept that relates to the optimal choice of therapy has not changed for nearly 30 years. In most cases, the location of the dissection determines whether the patient should undergo immediate surgery. Type A dissection is treated with surgery in virtually all cases, as the outcomes associated with surgical repair are superior to outcomes with medical management: 26% versus 50% mortality at 30 days in the IRAD series [1]. The one relative contraindication to attempted surgical repair of type A dissection is stroke in evolution, due to high risk of hemorrhagic transformation of the stroke during surgery [50]. In aggregate, survival of patients with acute type A dissection who are treated with surgical repair has improved over the last 25 years [51]. Aortic dissection repair is

TABLE 36.2

COMMONLY USED MEDICATIONS WITH ROUTES/DOSES

Agents for heart rate and blood pressure reduction in acute aortic syndromes

Class	Medication	Dosing[a]
Beta-blockers	Metoprolol	2.5–5.0 mg IV q 5 min, up to three doses followed by 5–10 mg IV q 4–6 h
	Labetalol	20 mg IV administered over 2 min followed by 40–80 mg IV q 10 min with maximum initial dose 300 mg, to be followed by 2 mg/min IV infusion with 10 mg/min maximum rate
	Esmolol	500 μg/kg IV bolus dose, followed by 50 μg/kg/min IV infusion with 300 μg/kg/min maximum rate
Calcium channel blockers	Diltiazem	Bolus 5–10 mg IV, maximum dose 25 mg IV infusion 5–15 mg/h for up to 24 h 30–90 mg PO qid, maximum 360 mg/d
	Verapamil	80–120 mg PO tid–qid maximum 480 mg/d
	Nifedipine	10–20 mg PO tid, start with 10 mg dose, maximum 180 mg/d
	Nicardipine	20–40 mg PO tid, start with 20 mg dose, maximum 120 mg/d
	Nisoldipine	20–40 mg PO qd, start with 10 mg dose, maximum 60 mg/d
Vasodilators	Nitroprusside	0.3–10 μg/kg/min IV infusion up to 3 d

[a]Therapeutic goals include maintenance of systolic blood pressure 100–110 mm Hg, heart rate approximately 60 beats per minute.

TABLE 36.3

SUMMARY OF ADVANCES IN THE IDENTIFICATION AND MANAGEMENT OF ACUTE AORTIC SYNDROMES[a]

- Risk factors for aortic dissection in patients younger than 40 include familial thoracic aortic aneurysm syndrome (FTAAS); pregnancy; bicuspid aortic valve; and Marfan, Ehlers–Danlos, Turner, and Noonan syndromes [1,7,22,28,29]
- Risk factors for aortic dissection in older patients include cigarette smoking, hypertension, and atherosclerotic disease [1]
- Crack cocaine use has been recently identified as an independent risk factor for aortic dissection, especially in the descending aorta [25,26]
- Preferred treatment for type A dissection is typically urgent surgery, whereas medical management is preferred for type B aortic dissection, except for those cases involving aortic rupture or branch vessel compromise [1,38]
- β-Blockade for reduction of dP/dt is critical to the treatment of all the acute aortic syndromes, unless a clear contraindication is present [1,39,40]
- Pericardial tamponade in the context of type A aortic dissection should be treated with definitive surgical correction of the dissection rather than pericardiocentesis, unless hemodynamic collapse is present, in which case small-volume aspiration of pericardial fluid may be necessary [40]
- Endovascular stent grafting has been used successfully to treat type B dissections, as well as branch vessel disease associated with both type A and B dissections: this technique is an alternative to intimal flap fenestration [53–57]. The Investigation of Stent Grafts in Aortic Dissection (INSTEAD) study shows no advantage to use of endovascular stents for treatment of chronic type B dissection [58]
- Management strategy of intramural hematoma is informed by location in a manner that mirrors classic dissection: type A intramural hematoma should be treated surgically, whereas type B intramural hematoma should be treated medically unless another indication for surgical or endovascular management is present [10,62,74]
- The use of biomarkers to differentiate acute aortic syndromes from other etiologies of chest pain is not yet a validated component of standard clinical practice [42–47]

[a]Based on recent observational studies.

complex surgery, and each patient's medical comorbidities need to be addressed in detail before surgery as time allows. In the past, patients older than 80 were thought to have an operative survival rate too low to justify attempted repair. A recent multicenter study reported acceptable outcomes in aortic dissection repair performed in selected octogenarians. Although this study raises the possibility of aortic dissection repair in this age group, this approach remains controversial and each patient must be approached individually [52].

Patients with type B dissections are generally managed without urgent surgery, as mortality in patients undergoing surgical repair is roughly equal to the mortality in those patients treated medically [1,38,39]. Typically, patients with type B dissections are only treated surgically in the context of impending or established aortic rupture or branch vessel compromise, especially with malperfusion. Neither recurrent pain nor severe hypertension has been shown to predict adverse outcome in patients with type B dissection of the aorta, and neither alone should be considered a primary indication for urgent surgery [53,54].

Recent studies have investigated the use of percutaneous repair for managing type B dissection. Although percutaneous fenestration of the "false" lumen had previously been the therapeutic option of choice in this setting [1], this technique has been largely supplanted by the more definitive endovascular stent repair. It is thought that the minimally invasive nature of this technique may decrease perioperative mortality and thus improve outcomes. Initial results and short-term outcomes with endovascular therapy of acute type B dissections are promising [55–57]. A recently published randomized trial assessing the impact of endovascular stent grafting in addition to medical therapy in uncomplicated type B dissection revealed no advantage with stenting [58].

INTRAMURAL HEMATOMA

Not all cases of apparent aortic dissection involve communication between the true and false lumens via a tear in the intima. In 1988, the first cases of an "atypical" form of dissection without intimal rupture were described [59]. Intramural hematoma (IMH) is defined as a spontaneous collection of blood within the aortic media that does not apparently communicate with the lumen. The natural history of IMH is not fully understood. It is thought that it may represent a predecessor of aortic dissection with eventual intimal rupture [48,60].

Both classic aortic dissection and IMH are generally associated with the same set of risk factors [9,48] and may be indistinguishable clinically [9]. Diagnostic imaging studies, notably transesophageal echocardiography, CT angiography, or MRI, are required to distinguish them (Fig. 36.2). Consequences of untreated IMH suggest a similar risk for adverse outcome as in typical aortic dissection.

Epidemiology

IMH occurs in a minority of the patients presenting with an apparent aortic dissection. Acute dissection events included in the IRAD registry were found to be due to IMH 10% of the time [1]. Serial imaging of IRAD patients with IMH revealed that 16% evolved to dissection with intimal tear [48]. There was no statistically significant difference in mortality rate for typical dissection and IMH in this series. Other studies reveal that IMH can progress to typical dissection, as determined by serial scanning, in up to 45% of cases [61].

Although the risk factors [9,48] and clinical presentations of classic aortic dissection and IMH are indistinguishable, certain important differences are recognized. Compared to those with typical aortic dissection, patients with IMH tend to be older, tend to have more atherosclerotic disease, and are more likely to have a distal acute aortic syndrome; two-thirds of IMH cases are type B, in contrast with typical dissections, 65% of which are type A.

Long-term follow-up of patients with IMH reveals that the hematoma evolves most commonly into a true or false aortic aneurysm or especially when associated with penetrating atherosclerotic ulcer (PAU). Up to 45% of such aneurysms that are located in the ascending aorta lead to rupture [61]. Spontaneous regression occurs in up to one-third of cases. Regression is most likely with IMH not associated with increased aortic

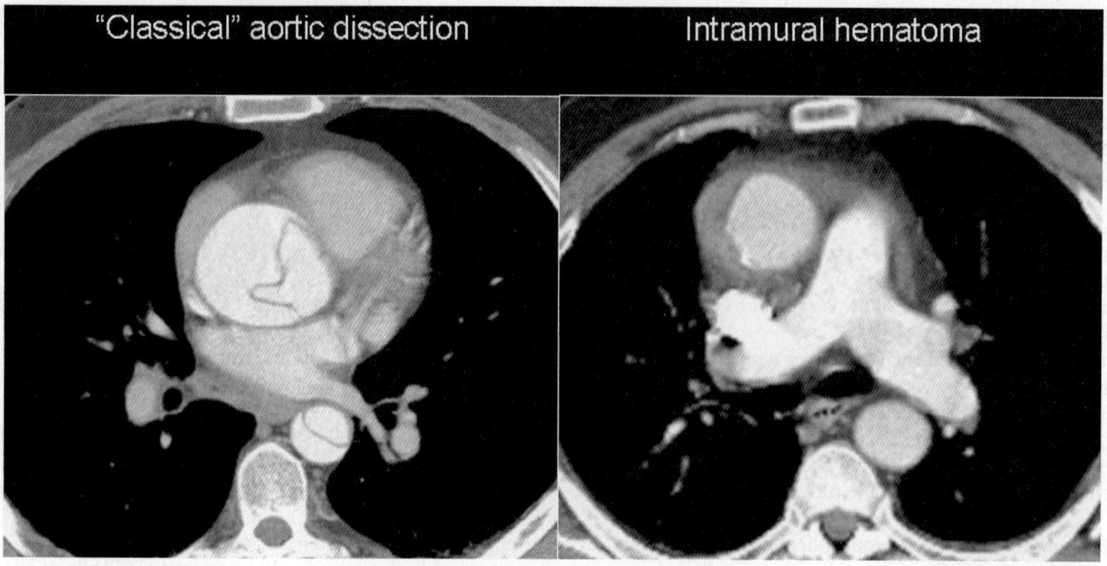

FIGURE 36.2. CT angiograms demonstrating the typical appearance of a "classical" aortic dissection, versus that of an aortic intramural hematoma. Note the smooth crescentic thickening of the wall of the ascending aorta in the patient with intramural hematoma and the obvious intimal flap seen in the patient with the acute dissection. [© Massachusetts General Hospital Thoracic Aortic Center. Used with permission.]

diameter at the time of presentation [62]. Clinical and radiographic progression of IMH is more likely when PAU is present (Fig. 36.3). IMH in the absence of PAU appears to follow a more stable course, especially when located in the descending thoracic aorta [63].

Etiology and Pathophysiology

There are two proposed mechanisms by which an IMH may form. The first is the rupture of the vasa vasorum in the aortic wall, which may be the result of medial degeneration. The other leading mechanism is the invasion of a PAU beyond the internal elastic lamina of the vessel, compromising the integrity of the media [64,65]. Once in the media, this ulceration can lead to hematoma formation. Both of these events could ostensibly be at work simultaneously.

Clinical Manifestations

The clinical presentation of IMH mirrors that of typical aortic dissection, and the two cannot be reliably distinguished on the basis of clinical criteria alone [48].

Imaging

Because the clinical presentation of IMH can overlap with that of classic dissection, prompt imaging is critical. The same set of imaging modalities used for classic aortic dissection is to be

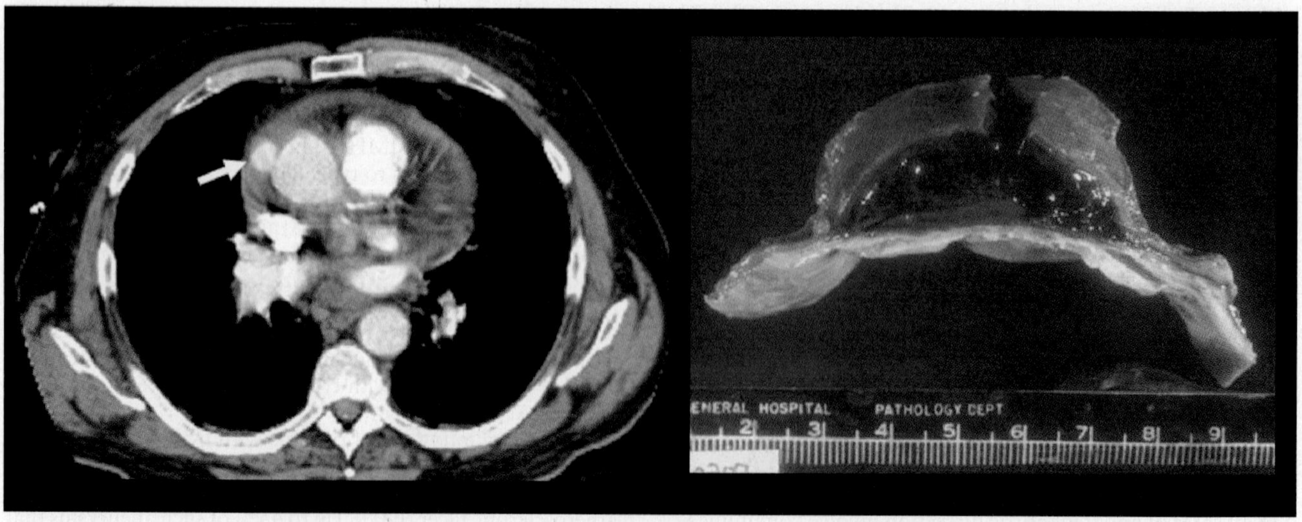

FIGURE 36.3. CT angiogram of an acute penetrating atherosclerotic ulcer, with corresponding pathologic specimen from the patient after ascending aortic repair.

used to image IMH. Some differences in utility exist, and are worthy of note. As with classic aortic dissection, it is frequently the case that multiple imaging modalities must be used in a single patient. As IMH frequently evolves, affected patients often require serial studies [48].

CXR findings associated with IMH mirror those for classic aortic dissection. Affected patients may exhibit an abnormal aortic silhouette or a widened mediastinum, but this finding is not as well validated as in classic dissection [1,6]. Separation of intimal calcium from the aortic border may also be visible. These are simply associated findings; differentiation of IMH from classic dissection requires other imaging modalities.

TTE does not allow for definitive, reliable diagnosis of IMH [9]. With TEE, IMH may appear as an echogenic, crescent-shaped segment of aortic wall. This is not a definitive modality, as in some cases, the thickened wall segment can be difficult to distinguish from atherosclerotic thickening [66].

With CT scanning, IMH appears as a crescent-shaped thickening of the aortic wall, but with a normal-appearing aortic lumen. A contrast study is required for a definitive diagnosis. The most important feature that distinguishes an IMH from a classic dissection is the absence of contrast within the aortic wall. MRI allows for diagnosis of IMH without the use of contrast. The intensity of the hematoma can be determined by the signal sequence. Aortography is not a useful method for evaluating IMH, as the sensitivity for identification of IMH is less than 20% [66].

Management

As is the case for management of typical dissection, early imaging and surgical consultation are the central components of the management of a patient with an IMH, which can be a rapidly progressive disease. Frequent reevaluation of the diseased aortic segment may also be warranted, especially if the patient presents with new hypotension or progressive symptoms. The most dangerous consequence of IMH is continued expansion and progression to typical dissection and/or aortic rupture. Given the high-risk nature of IMH in the ascending aorta, management is similar to typical aortic dissection: surgery for type A syndromes and medical management for type B syndromes [9]. The recent literature contains some controversy regarding the potential role for medical management of IMH in the ascending aorta, but at this time, there is no strong evidence to suggest that medical management is sufficient [48,67–72].

For type B IMH, medical management appears to be the consistently validated early treatment approach, unless a surgical indication is present. In-hospital mortality for patients in the IRAD series is less than 10% for patients receiving medical management [48].

There may be a role for prophylactic endovascular stent placement in patients with IMH who are thought to be in imminent danger of hematoma expansion and aortic rupture. Type B IMH should be frequently reassessed and reimaged as indicated, as these patients are at increased risk for evolution into classical dissection or rupture [73]. Several studies have suggested that a small proportion of IMH will resorb in short-term follow-up, and this appears to be correlated with smaller aneurysm size at presentation. However, a significant proportion of patients will go on to develop enlarging aortic aneurysm and/or pseudoaneurysm, classic aortic dissection, or rupture [62,74,75]. The role of endovascular stents in preventing these late outcomes is currently under investigation [76,77]. The use of endovascular stent grafting to manage a complication of a type B IMH with subsequent dissection is demonstrated in Figure 36.4. A summary of recommended management strategies for patients with acute aortic dissection or IMH is shown in Figure 36.5.

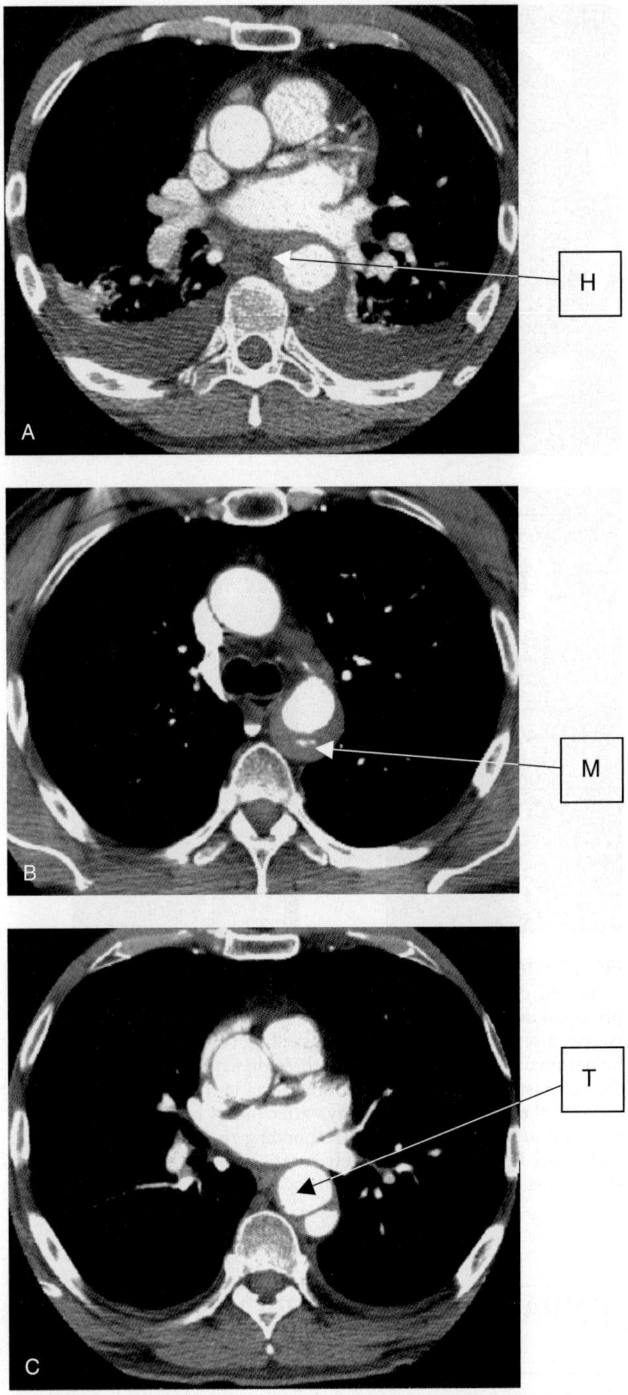

FIGURE 36.4. A–C: Endovascular aortic stent grafts for nonsurgical management of Stanford type B dissection. This patient initially presented with acute type B dissecting intramural hematoma. Panel A shows a contrast-enhanced (CT) scan of the chest demonstrating acute intramural hematoma just inferior to the pulmonary artery bifurcation with a circumferential, crescentic appearance (H). The IMH extended from just distal to the takeoff of the left subclavian artery down to the level of the celiac axis. Panel B shows evidence of active hemorrhage into the aortic media (M) at the proximal descending thoracic aorta. Panel C shows a follow-up contrast-enhanced chest CT of the same patient at 36 days after initial presentation, with evidence of evolution of the IMH into a classic dissection, with true lumen (T) and filling of the false lumen at the same level in the proximal descending aorta as shown in Panel A. (*continued*)

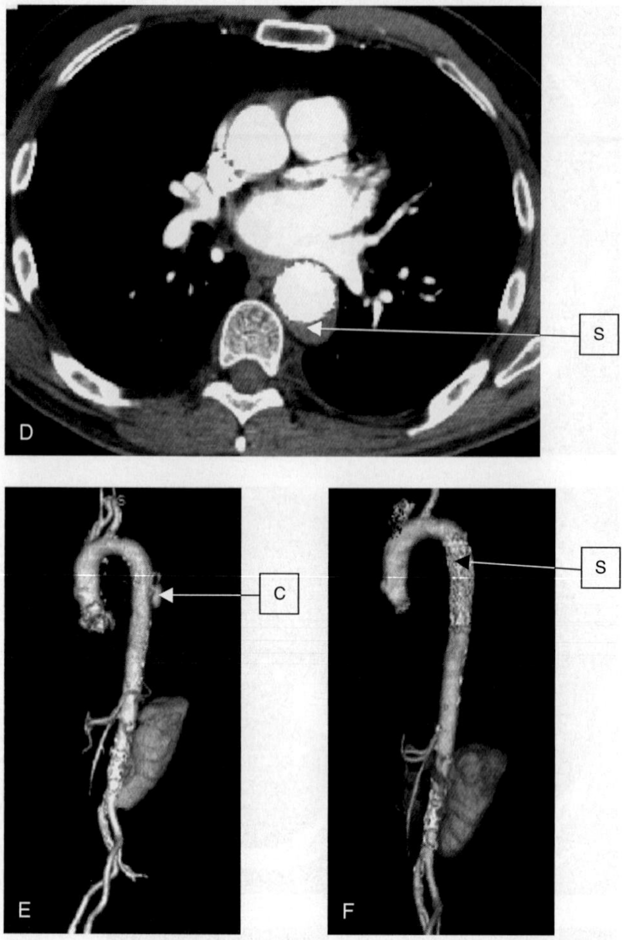

FIGURE 36.4. (*Continued*) **D–F:** Panel D shows the contrast-enhanced chest CT scan after placement of a stent graft (S) in the proximal descending aorta at the site of presumed communication between false and true lumen, demonstrating complete exclusion of the hematoma. Panel E demonstrates a three-dimensional reconstruction of the contrast-enhanced CT scan of the aorta in the left anterior oblique view of the same patient 36 days after initial presentation with extravasation of contrast (C) (corresponding to the image in Panel C), and Panel F shows the same left anterior oblique view of the aorta status-post endovascular stent grafting procedure (S, stent).

EXPANDING AORTIC ANEURYSM AND RUPTURE

Definition and Classification

An aortic aneurysm is broadly defined as a segment of the aortic lumen whose diameter exceeds 1.5 times the normal diameter for that segment [78]. The risk of aneurysm rupture increases as a function of diameter. In addition, rupture risk is thought to be higher in rapidly expanding aneurysms [79,80]. Aneurysms are also classified according to location (e.g., thoracic vs. abdominal), morphology, and etiology. All segments of the aorta can be affected and multiple aneurysms may be found in a single patient. Up to 13% of patients with an identified aortic aneurysm are found to have multiple aneurysm; as such, in patients in whom a single aneurysm has been detected, consideration should be given to scanning the entire aorta for additional aneurysms [81]. In the general population, abdominal aneurysms are more common than thoracic aneurysms [82].

The most commonly encountered aortic aneurysm morphology is fusiform—specifically, a symmetrical dilatation of an aortic segment, involving the entire circumference of the vessel wall (Fig. 36.6). Aneurysms may also be saccular, or may involve only a portion of the vessel, leading to an asymmetric dilatation. It is also important to distinguish between true and false aneurysms: a true aneurysm involves all three layers of the vessel wall, whereas a false aneurysm is typically a collection of blood underneath the adventitia or outside the vessel altogether. This collection is frequently the result of a defect in the aortic wall. The presence of a suspected saccular aneurysm deserves special note, as it may actually represent a false aneurysm caused by a partially contained rupture of the aortic wall.

Aortic aneurysms are frequently asymptomatic at the time of diagnosis, and tend to be detected with tests ordered for other reasons [83]. Indeed, an aortic aneurysm may not be associated with any symptoms until the time of rupture. As the clinical presentations of ruptured thoracic and abdominal aortic aneurysms (AAAs) frequently differ, they are discussed separately.

ANEURYSMS OF THE THORACIC AORTA

Epidemiology

The overall annual incidence of thoracic aortic aneurysm (TAA) is 6 per 100,000 [83], and up to 40% of all patients are asymptomatic at the time of diagnosis [84]. The risk of aneurysm rupture or dissection increases as a function of size. An abrupt increase in risk has been noted at a diameter of 6 cm: for aneurysms greater than 6 cm, the rupture rate has been observed to be 3.7% per year [79]. The most commonly affected segments are the aortic root and ascending aorta; 60% of observed cases involve these segments. Aneurysms of the descending aorta account for 40% of cases, and the aortic arch accounts for 10%.

The surgical treatment strategy for asymptomatic aortic aneurysms differ on the basis of location, size, and etiology: for an aneurysm in the aortic root or the ascending aorta, surgical repair is indicated for a diameter of 5.5 cm or more, although for patients who are at increased risk of rupture, such as patients with a bicuspid aortic valve (which is associated with an intrinsic defect in the medial smooth muscle layer) or Marfan syndrome, 5 cm (or less in certain cases, such as in patients with strong family histories for premature aortic dissection or rupture) is the recommended operative threshold [85,86]. In the descending aorta, surgery is recommended at a diameter of 6 cm or more [82].

For patients with large TAAs, survival without surgical repair is poor, with 5-year survival after initial identification at 20%. Rupture occurs in 32% to 68% of patients whose TAAs are not repaired surgically [87,88]. Of those patients whose rupture occurs outside a hospital setting, it is thought that less than half will arrive to a hospital alive. For those patients who survive until hospital admission, mortality at 6 hours is 54%. At 24 hours, mortality without surgery is 76% [89].

Etiology and Pathophysiology

Multiple factors have been implicated in the formation of TAAs, including atherosclerotic disease, specific gene defects, and infectious processes. In many cases, a central pathophysiologic process is medial degeneration, which leads

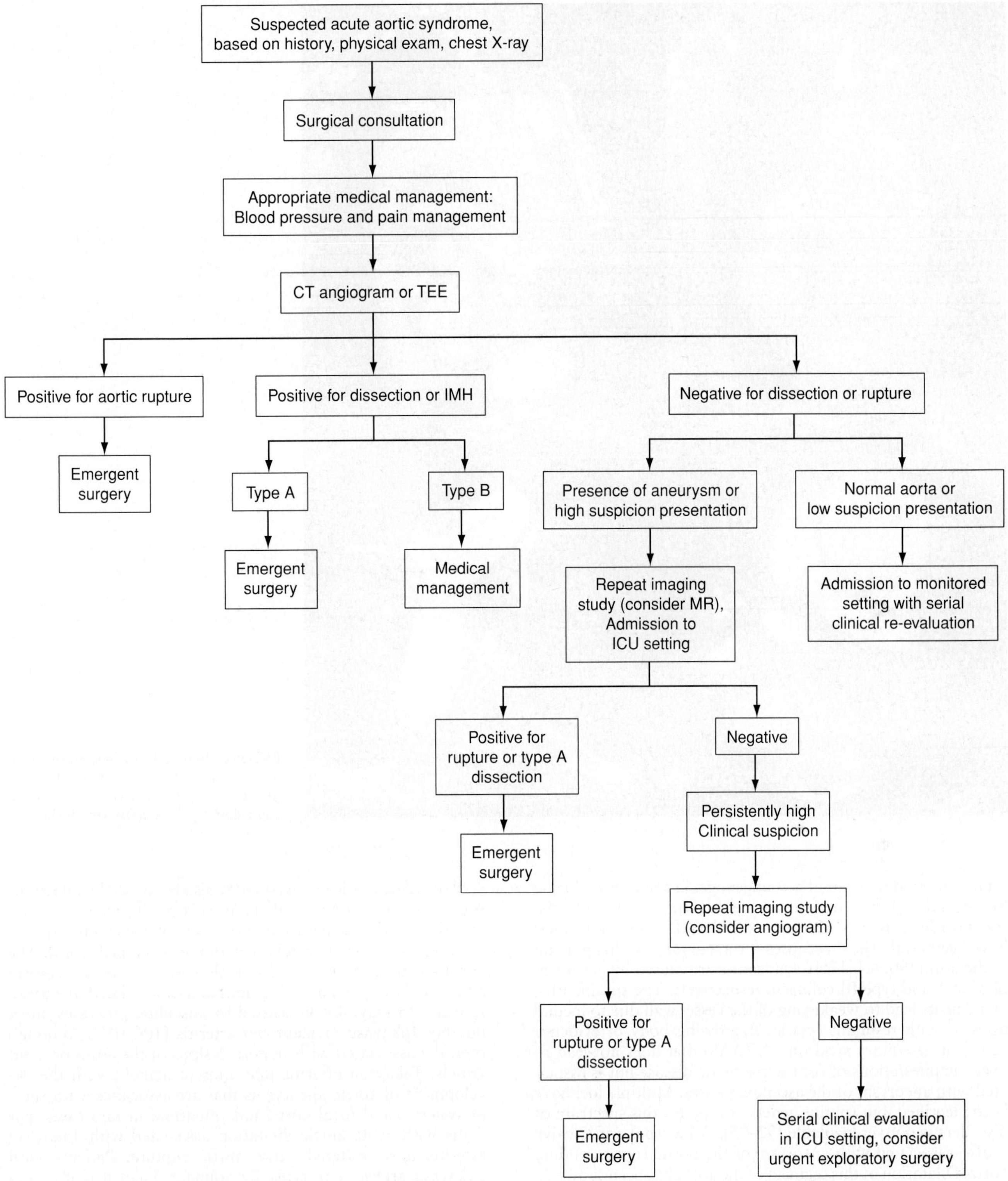

FIGURE 36.5. A suggested management strategy for patients with suspected acute aortic syndrome.

to the loss of elastic fibers and smooth muscle cells. This process, which is frequently correlated with aging, causes progressive stiffening and weakening of the vessel wall, leading to progressive dilatation. Hypertension accelerates dilatation due to the increase in wall strain [82,84,90]. The inciting factor that leads to aneurysm formation influences which portion of the aorta is affected and the age at which the abnormality tends to be diagnosed.

Aneurysms in the aortic root and ascending aorta are frequently associated with inherited defects in structural genes or with inflammation caused either by infection or by vasculitis. In general, aneurysms associated with structural genetic

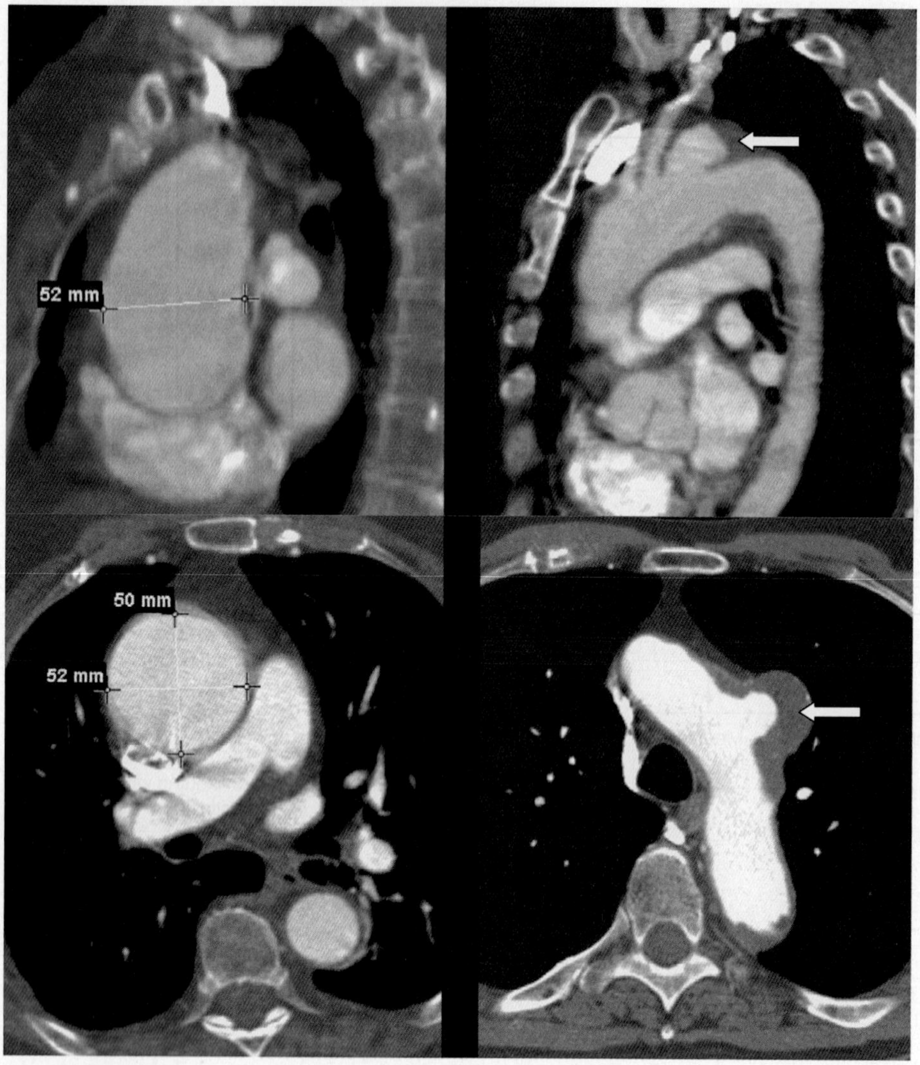

FIGURE 36.6. CT angiograms of a fusiform aneurysm (left-hand panels, with dimensions) and a saccular aneurysm (right-hand panels, *white arrows*).

mutations tend to occur at a younger age, in some cases during the second and third decades of life. Identified connective tissue disorders, such as Marfan and Ehlers–Danlos syndromes, have been established as causes for aneurysms in this portion of the aorta [90,91]. These syndromes are caused by deficits in fibrillin-1 and type III collagen, respectively. The specific protein deficits lead to weakening of the vessel wall due to medial necrosis with resultant ectasia. A growing body of evidence reveals a hereditary syndrome (FTAAS) that does not lead to overt manifestations of connective tissue disease but is associated with aneurysm of the ascending aorta. Multiple loci have been identified, but routine genetic testing for this spectrum of disorders is not yet available [92–95]. A bicuspid aortic valve is also associated with aneurysm of the aortic root/ascending aorta. Dilatation of this segment of the aorta has been shown to be due to medial degeneration that is independent of the potential hemodynamic effects of the abnormal valve. An acquired defect in the integrity of fibrillin-1 may also occur in some of these patients [96]. A growing body of evidence suggests that the enzymatic activity of several matrix metalloproteinases (MMPs) may play a central role in the loss of connective tissue integrity in patients with bicuspid aortic valve [97]. Turner syndrome is associated with an increased incidence of bicuspid aortic valve, as well as with aortic coarctation and aneurysm of the ascending aorta [98].

Ascending aortic aneurysm may also be caused by infectious processes, such as bacterial endaortitis or chronic spirochetal infection. Syphilis, once a common cause of aneurysm in the ascending aorta, is now rarely seen in the developed world. The aortitis caused by bacterial infection leads to both fusiform and saccular aneurysms [99]. Inflammation-related aneurysm in this area may also be caused by vasculitic processes, most notably Takayasu or giant cell arteritis [100,101]. Although typically associated with stenotic lesions of the aorta or great vessels, Takayasu arteritis may present acutely, with the development of aortic aneurysms that are associated with signs of systemic and focal aortic inflammation; in rare cases, patients with acute aortic dilatation associated with Takayasu arteritis have suffered acute aortic rupture. Patients with Takayasu arteritis are typically younger Asian females, who may show involvement of the pulmonary arteries as well. In contrast, aneurysms associated with giant cell arteritis are more frequently diagnosed in older Caucasian females with prior polymyalgia rheumatica and/or symptomatic temporal arteritis [100–102].

Aneurysms in the descending aorta are generally caused by atherosclerosis. As such, these aneurysms are more commonly found in men and are not frequently seen before the sixth decade of life. These aneurysms are found beyond the branch point of the left subclavian artery and are typically fusiform.

Saccular aneurysms may be found at the aortic isthmus, and are frequently the result of rapid deceleration trauma.

Clinical Manifestations

Expanding aneurysms of the ascending and descending thoracic aorta produce symptoms due to compression of neighboring thoracic structures and compromise of aortic valve function (see later in the chapter). Compression leads to chest and back pain in as many as 37% and 21% of cases, respectively [103]. Specific thoracic structures, when compressed by the aorta, lead to distinct signs and symptoms, including superior vena cava syndrome, pulmonary symptoms due to tracheal compression, or dysphagia due to esophageal compression. In addition, stretching of the recurrent laryngeal nerve may lead to unilateral vocal cord paralysis, with hoarseness (Ortner's syndrome).

Symptoms from rupture of a TAA are largely related to blood extending into adjoining thoracic spaces. The sudden onset of acute chest or back pain is a common feature of aneurysm rupture in all segments of the thoracic aorta. Perhaps the most salient feature of this pain is the fact that its maximal intensity occurs at onset. In patients whose aneurysms have produced prior symptoms, the pain at the time of rupture may be a more intense form of the same sensation, often at the same location. The quality of this pain does not necessarily have a tearing quality, as is often the case with dissection.

The most common area of blood flow from a rupture in the ascending aorta is the left pleural space, followed by the intrapericardial space. Blood flow into these areas lead to hemothorax and hemopericardium. Tamponade physiology may be present. Rupture of the descending aorta can lead to erosion into the esophagus: over time, an aortoesophageal fistula may form, leading to severe hematemesis. No matter where the point of blood egress is found, rapid loss of intravascular volume leads promptly to hypotension and shock if unrepaired. Ancillary warning signs include decreased urine output and altered mental status.

The heart examination may also exhibit distinct abnormalities with expanding aneurysm and rupture. Progressive dilatation of the aortic root may lead to dilatation of the valve annulus with consequent signs of aortic regurgitation. This phenomenon is associated with a diastolic murmur heard best over the left sternal border with the exception of aneurysms associated with ectasia of the aortic root, such as syphilitic aortitis, where the murmur of aortic regurgitation may be more noticeable along the right sternal border. Critical levels of regurgitation may be associated with left-sided heart failure. This murmur may be present in the absence of rupture. When rupture of one of the sinuses of Valsalva occurs, the murmur may be continuous; in this setting, the ruptured area may communicate with a cardiac chamber, such as the right atrium or ventricle.

In the context of acute rupture, the electrocardiography frequently shows evidence of ventricular "strain" or ischemia. Over time, markers of myocardial necrosis may be elevated as well. Several studies show an elevation in D-dimer in the context of aortic dissection, but elevation of this marker has not yet been validated in aneurysm progression or rupture [104]. There is currently no widely available biomarker in use to detect vascular injury in the context of aneurysm or rupture.

Imaging

Aortic aneurysm may be visualized as a widened mediastinum on anteroposterior views. Although this technique offers invaluable information, it cannot be considered a definitive study. TTE allows for the evaluation of the aortic root and ascending aorta. TEE is well suited to the evaluation of potentially aneurysmal segments in the aortic arch and descending aorta. As noted previously, perhaps the most important procedural drawback regarding TEE is the need for conscious sedation, which may be difficult to administer in a patient who is hemodynamically unstable.

CT scanning allows for evaluation of potentially aneurysmal segments in the entire aorta. Contrast CT imaging may also be helpful in identification of areas of blood extravasation in ruptured aortic aneurysms. MRI may be used for aortic measurement and identification of aneurysmal segments without contrast. Evaluation of blood extravasation with MRI is possible, but thought to be less sensitive than CT with contrast, especially for slow or low-volume extravasation. Aortography is a highly sensitive technique for assessing extravasation. The use of this technique in the acute setting is ordinarily reserved for those cases where neither CT scanning nor MRI is available.

Rupture of a Thoracic Aortic Aneurysm: Management

Rupture of a TAA is a surgical emergency. Open repair of the vessel is the most established repair technique. Typically, the procedure is performed with deep hypothermic circulatory arrest. The type of repair is determined by the location of the rupture and the presence or absence of aortic valve involvement. Dacron grafts are generally placed to replace the diseased vessel segment, with various strategies for aortic valve repair or replacement when necessary [105]. Recent work indicates that a less invasive form of repair, retrograde endovascular stent placement, may be useful in the repair of aneurysms in the descending aorta.

Patients with aneurysm of both ascending and descending segments present an additional challenge. Standard methods entail surgical replacement of diseased segments in a "staged" fashion; however, newer methods involving a hybrid approach of surgical replacement of the ascending aorta, with subsequent endovascular therapy of the distal segments, appear promising [106].

It may be that a particular patient presents with complaints raising concern for a ruptured aortic aneurysm. In the event that no rupture is found and the patient is hemodynamically stable, it is possible that expansion of the aneurysm is responsible for the symptoms. In such a case, the focus of immediate clinical treatment should be to decrease aortic wall strain and systemic blood pressure through the use of beta-blockers in the context of a critical care setting. Prompt surgical consultation plays a vital role in the continuing care of these patients.

ANEURYSMS OF THE ABDOMINAL AORTA

Epidemiology

AAAs are far more common than TAAs. The estimated prevalence of AAAs ranges between 1.3% and 8.9% in men and between 1.0% and 2.2% in women older than 60 years [107–110]. Most cases are observed in men older than 55 years and women older than 70 years. AAAs have been found to be correlated with smoking [111]. Overall prevalence of abdominal aneurysms has risen substantially over the past 30 years

[112]. This trend has been linked to the increased prevalence of atherosclerosis, which is thought to be the major etiology responsible for abdominal aneurysms. In addition, improvements in imaging technology have increased the rate of detection.

Rupture of AAAs is estimated to cause approximately 15,000 deaths per year in the United States [112,113]. The total mortality rate for patients with rupture ranges from 65% to 85% [107]. One prospective study revealed that 25% of patients with AAA rupture die before arriving at a hospital. Of those who arrived at the hospital alive, 51% died before surgery. Patients who did have surgery sustained a 46% operative mortality rate. Total 30-day survival rate for this population was 11% [80]. Given the poor prognosis associated with rupture, elective repair is recommended when possible. As is the case with TAAs, the risk of rupture increases as a function of aortic diameter. Recently published guidelines recommend elective surgery for AAA 5.5 cm or more in men and 5 cm in women [114].

Etiology and Pathophysiology

Incidence of AAA is closely correlated with the presence of atherosclerotic disease in the aorta. In general, the infrarenal segment of the aorta is most heavily affected by atherosclerosis, and this is also the segment where most abdominal aneurysms are observed. These aneurysms are typically fusiform, but saccular aneurysms may also be found.

The risk factor most closely associated with abdominal aneurysms is smoking, followed by age, hypertension, and hyperlipidemia [115]. There is also a strong association between gender and abdominal aneurysm formation [108]. Family history of AAA is associated with a 30% increase in risk for AAA formation, but there are not yet any specific genes linked with this finding [82,116].

Damage to the vessel wall, caused by atherosclerotic plaque, has been shown to cause local inflammation. This inflammatory process is thought to cause degradation of extracellular matrix proteins, notably elastin and collagen. In addition, it is thought that the proinflammatory cytokine milieu leads to cell death in the vessel wall. Weakening of the vessel wall follows, potentially accelerated by the action of multiple proteases, including MMP and cathepsin L [117,118]. There is some speculation that MMP polymorphisms may lead to a change in susceptibility to abdominal aneurysms, but there are no screening tests currently available to the clinician [119]. Hypertension increases the wall strain on the weakened vessel wall, leading to accelerated expansion. The full effects of smoking on aneurysm formation and expansion are not known, but increased atherosclerosis and hypertension are thought to be contributors.

Aneurysms in the descending thoracic aorta tend to be caused by atherosclerosis. These aneurysms often extend into the abdominal cavity, superior to the renal arteries. Such aneurysms are referred to as thoracoabdominal, and their management mirrors the management of aneurysms in the abdominal cavity.

Aneurysms in the descending thoracic or abdominal aorta may also be caused by acute bacterial infections. This is not a common finding, but tends to be found more often in patients who are intravenous drug users or who have traveled recently from a country where exposure to typical organisms (*Salmonella* and *Brucella*) is more likely to occur. Chronic tuberculosis is rarely associated with abdominal aneurysms. Syphilis may also be associated with abdominal aneurysms, but it is more commonly associated with the ascending aorta. Connective tissue disorders, such as Marfan and Ehlers–Danlos syndromes, do not typically affect the abdominal aorta; however, some systemic inflammatory disorders, notably Takayasu arteritis or Behcet's disease, may be associated with abdominal aneurysms [120,121].

Clinical Manifestations

As is the case with thoracic aneurysms, most abdominal aneurysms are asymptomatic and tend to be discovered with testing performed for other reasons. Those patients who do have aneurysm-related complaints tend to report pain in the hypogastric area and/or pain in the lower back. This pain is caused by the expansion of the aneurysm and tends to last for hours or days at a time, and is usually dull and steady. In the abdomen, fewer structures tend to be affected by the expanding aorta. The most common consequence of aortic expansion is compression of the ureter or kidney, leading to hydronephrosis or potentially renal failure.

An episode of rupture tends to be announced by a sudden onset or increase in abdominal and/or back pain. The most notable feature of this pain is that it is at its maximum at the time of onset. Rupture most frequently leads to blood leakage into the left retroperitoneal space. These patients may present with an initial episode of pain associated with the first rupture, followed by temporary tamponade of the retroperitoneal space. A larger, life-threatening bleed inevitably follows. Less frequently, the aneurysm may erode into surrounding structures, most notably the duodenum, leading to either formation of an aortoduodenal fistula or potentially massive gastrointestinal (GI) bleeding [113,122].

Physical examination of a patient with an AAA may reveal a palpable, pulsatile mass in the midline. This mass is easiest to palpate in the hypogastric or paraumbilical region. The sensitivity of the manual examination is suboptimal: 82% for aneurysms 5 cm or greater. Furthermore, a mass may be difficult to appreciate [123]. Consequently, the absence of a pulsatile mass on physical examination should not be interpreted as an absence of aneurysm. On rupture of an abdominal aneurysm, most patients become hypotensive, tachycardic, and diaphoretic. Patients may also exhibit signs of peritoneal irritation on examination. As noted, the patient may also present with evidence of GI bleeding. Laboratory analysis may reveal evidence of elevation in D-dimer or an elevation in cardiac biomarkers, due to demand-related myocardial ischemia.

Imaging

X-ray plain film is not an adequately sensitive technique for the assessment of AAAs. Echocardiography is not helpful for the evaluation for extrathoracic segments of the aorta. Transcutaneous ultrasound is a noninvasive and readily available technique for the evaluation of the abdominal aorta. This method is frequently used to track the size of abdominal aneurysms, though it is not the imaging modality of choice for the acute aortic syndromes. Like TTE, abdominal ultrasound is often limited by body habitus. As with thoracic aneurysms, the most definitive evaluations are provided by CT scanning and MRI. Aortography may provide useful information regarding aortic aneurysm, but it is not the modality of choice in the acute setting unless CT scanning and MRI are not available.

Rupture of an Abdominal Aortic Aneurysm: Management

Rupture of an AAA is a surgical emergency. Open repair, with replacement of the diseased segment with a Dacron graft, is the most established technique. Intraoperative mortality after rupture is very high, as noted previously. Retrograde endovascular stent placement is a promising technique [124–126], but it is not yet in common use in the acute setting [127,128]. Timely, but elective, surgical or endovascular intervention on the basis of size criteria, as assessed with longitudinal imaging, is the most effective means to prevent progression to rupture.

References

1. Hagan P, Nienaber CA, Isselbacher EM, et al: The International Registry of Acute Aortic Dissection (IRAD): new insights into an old disease. *JAMA* 283:897–903, 2000.
2. DeSanctis R, Doroghazi RM, Austen WG, et al: Aortic dissection. *N Engl J Med* 317:1060–1067, 1987.
3. Kitamura M, Hashimoto A, Akimoto T, et al: Operation for type A aortic dissection: introduction of retrograde cerebral perfusion. *Ann Thorac Surg* 59:1195–1199, 1995.
4. DeBakey M, McCollum CH, Crawford ES, et al: Dissection and dissecting aneurysms of the aorta: twenty-year follow-up of five hundred twenty-seven patients treated surgically. *Surgery* 92:1118–1134, 1982.
5. Daily P, Trueblood HW, Stinson EB, et al: Management of acute aortic dissections. *Ann Thorac Surg* 10:237–247, 1970.
6. Spittell P, Spittell JA Jr, Joyce JW, et al: Clinical features and differential diagnosis of aortic dissection: experience with 236 cases (1980 through 1990). *Mayo Clin Proc* 68:642–651, 1993.
7. Hirst A, Johns VJ, Kime SW Jr: Dissecting aneurysm of the aorta: a review of 505 cases. *Medicine* 37:217–279, 1958.
8. Wilson S, Hutchins GM: Aortic dissecting aneurysms: causative factors in 204 subjects. *Arch Pathol Lab Med* 106:175–180, 1982.
9. Nienaber C, von Kodolitsch Y, Petersen B, et al: Intramural hemorrhage of the thoracic aorta. Diagnostic and therapeutic implications. *Circulation* 92:1465–1472, 1995.
10. Kazerooni E, Bree RL, Williams DM: Penetrating atherosclerotic ulcers of the descending thoracic aorta: evaluation with CT and distinction from aortic dissection. *Radiology* 183:759–765, 1992.
11. Meszaros I, Morocz J, Szlavi J, et al: Epidemiology and clinicopathology of aortic dissection. *Chest* 117:1271–1278, 2000.
12. Nienaber C, Fattori R, Mehta RH, et al: International Registry of Acute Aortic Dissection. Gender-related differences in acute aortic dissection. *Circulation* 109:3014–3021, 2004.
13. Mehta R, Manfredini R, Hassan F, et al: International Registry of Acute Aortic Dissection (IRAD) Investigators. Chronobiological patterns of acute aortic dissection. *Circulation* 106:1110–1115, 2002.
14. Mehta R, Manfredini R, Bossone E, et al: International Registry of Acute Aortic Dissection (IRAD) Investigators. The winter peak in the occurrence of acute aortic dissection is independent of climate. *Chronobiol Int* 22:723–729, 2004.
15. Anagnostopoulos C, Prabhakar MJ, Kittle CF: Aortic dissections and dissecting aneurysms. *Am J Cardiol* 30:263–273, 1972.
16. Chirillo F, Marchiori MC, Andriolo L, et al: Outcome of 290 patients with aortic dissection. A 12-year multicentre experience. *Eur Heart J* 11:311–319, 1990.
17. Svensson L, Crawford ES, Hess KR, et al: Dissection of the aorta and dissecting aortic aneurysms. Improving early and long-term surgical results. *Circulation* 82[Suppl 5]:IV24–IV38, 1990.
18. Schlatmann T, Becker AE: Histologic changes in the normal aging aorta: implications for dissecting aortic aneurysm. *Am J Cardiol* 39:13–20, 1977.
19. Schlatmann T, Becker AE: Pathogenesis of dissecting aneurysm of aorta. Comparative histopathologic study of significance of medial changes. *Am J Cardiol* 39:21–26, 1977.
20. Mehta R, O'Gara PT, Bossone E, et al: International Registry of Acute Aortic Dissection (IRAD) Investigators. Acute type A aortic dissection in the elderly: clinical characteristics, management, and outcomes in the current era. *J Am Coll Cardiol* 40:685–692, 2002.
21. Januzzi J, Isselbacher EM, Fattori R, et al: International Registry of Aortic Dissection (IRAD). Characterizing the young patient with aortic dissection: results from the International Registry of Aortic Dissection (IRAD). *J Am Coll Cardiol* 43:665–669, 2004.
22. Nuenninghoff D, Hunder GG, Christianson TJ, et al: Mortality of large-artery complication (aortic aneurysm, aortic dissection, and/or large-artery stenosis) in patients with giant cell arteritis: a population-based study over 50 years. *Arthritis Rheum* 48:3532–3537, 2003.
23. Liu G, Shupak R, Chiu BK: Aortic dissection in giant-cell arteritis. *Semin Arthritis Rheum* 25:160–171, 1995.
24. Hsue P, Salinas CL, Bolger AF, et al: Acute aortic dissection related to crack cocaine. *Circulation* 105:1592–1595, 2002.
25. Palmiere C, Burkhardt S, Staub C, et al: Thoracic aortic dissection associated with cocaine abuse. *Forensic Sci Int* 141:137–142, 2004.
26. Larson E, Edwards WD: Risk factors for aortic dissection: a necropsy study of 161 cases. *Am J Cardiol* 53:849–855, 1984.
27. Immer F, Bansi AG, Immer-Bansi AS, et al: Aortic dissection in pregnancy: analysis of risk factors and outcome. *Ann Thorac Surg* 76:309–314, 2003.
28. Williams G, Gott VL, Brawley RK, et al: Aortic disease associated with pregnancy. *J Vasc Surg* 8:470–475, 1988.
29. Practice Committee ASfRM: Increased maternal cardiovascular mortality associated with pregnancy in women with Turner syndrome. *Fertil Steril* 83:1074–1075, 2005.
30. Ochi M, Yamauchi S, Yajima T, et al: Aortic dissection extending from the left coronary artery during percutaneous coronary angioplasty. *Ann Thorac Surg* 62:1180–1182, 1996.
31. Jacobs L, Fraifeld M, Kotler MN, et al: Aortic dissection following intraaortic balloon insertion: recognition by transesophageal echocardiography. *Am Heart J* 124:536–540, 1992.
32. Still R, Hilgenberg AD, Akins CW, et al: Intraoperative aortic dissection. *Ann Thorac Surg* 53:374–379, 1992.
33. Albat B, Thevenet A: Dissecting aneurysms of the ascending aorta occurring late after aortic valve replacement. *J Cardiovasc Surg* 33:272–275, 1992.
34. Fernandez A, Alvarez J, Martinez A, et al: Localized dissection of the descending thoracic aorta after blunt chest trauma. *Int J Cardiol* 105:227–228, 2005.
35. Rogers F, Osler TM, Shackford SR: Aortic dissection after trauma: case report and review of the literature. *J Trauma* 41:906–908, 1996.
36. Slater E, DeSanctis RW: The clinical recognition of dissecting aortic aneurysm. *Am J Med* 60:625–633, 1976.
37. Upchurch GJ, Nienaber C, Fattori R, et al: IRAD Investigators. Acute aortic dissection presenting with primarily abdominal pain: a rare manifestation of a deadly disease. *Ann Vasc Surg* 19:367–373, 2005.
38. Suzuki T, Mehta RH, Ince H, et al: International Registry of Aortic Dissection. Clinical profiles and outcomes of acute type B aortic dissection in the current era: lessons from the International Registry of Aortic Dissection (IRAD). *Circulation* 108[Suppl 1]:II312–II317, 2003.
39. Januzzi J, Eagle KA, Cooper JV, et al: Acute aortic dissection presenting with congestive heart failure: results from the International Registry of Acute Aortic Dissection. *J Am Coll Cardiol* 46:733–735, 2005.
40. Isselbacher E, Cigarroa JE, Eagle KA: Cardiac tamponade complicating proximal aortic dissection. Is pericardiocentesis harmful? *Circulation* 90:2375–2378, 1994.
41. Sandridge L, Kern JA: Acute descending aortic dissections: management of visceral, spinal cord, and extremity malperfusion. *Semin Thorac Cardiovasc Surg* 17:256–261, 2005.
42. Marill K: Serum D-dimer is a sensitive test for the detection of acute aortic dissection: a pooled meta-analysis. *J Emerg Med* 34:367–376, 2008.
43. Eggebrecht H, Naber CK, Bruch C, et al: Value of plasma fibrin D-dimers for detection of acute aortic dissection. *J Am Coll Cardiol* 44:804–809, 2004.
44. Suzuki T, Katoh H, Tsuchio Y, et al: Diagnostic implications of elevated levels of smooth-muscle myosin heavy-chain protein in acute aortic dissection. The smooth muscle myosin heavy chain study. *Ann Intern Med* 133:537–541, 2000.
45. Hazui H, Negoro N, Nishimoto M, et al: Serum heart-type fatty acid-binding protein concentration positively correlates with the length of aortic dissection. *Circ J* 69:958–961, 2005.
46. Shinohara T, Suzuki K, Okada M, et al: Soluble elastin fragments in serum are elevated in acute aortic dissection. *Arterioscler Thromb Vasc Biol* 23:1839–1844, 2003.
47. Suzuki T, Distante A, Zizza A, et al: Preliminary experience with the smooth muscle troponin-like protein, calponin, as a novel biomarker for diagnosing acute aortic dissection. *Eur Heart J* 29:1429–1435, 2008.
48. Evangelista A, Mukherjee D, Mehta RH, et al: International Registry of Aortic Dissection (IRAD) Investigators. Acute intramural hematoma of the aorta: a mystery in evolution. *Circulation* 111:1063–1070, 2005.
49. Moore A, Eagle KA, Bruckman D, et al: Choice of computed tomography, transesophageal echocardiography, magnetic resonance imaging, and aortography in acute aortic dissection: International Registry of Acute Aortic Dissection (IRAD). *Am J Cardiol* 89:1235–1238, 2002.
50. Appelbaum A, Karp RB, Kirklin JW: Ascending vs descending aortic dissections. *Ann Surg* 183:296–300, 1976.
51. Stevens L, Madsen J, Isselbacher E, et al: Surgical management and long-term outcomes for acute ascending aortic dissection. *J Thorac Cardiovasc Surg* 138:1349–1357, 2009.
52. Piccardo A, Regesta T, Zannis K, et al: Outcomes after surgical treatment for type A acute aortic dissection in octogenarians: a multicenter study. *Ann Thorac Surg* 88:491–497, 2009.
53. Januzzi JL, Movsowitz HD, Choi J, et al: Significance of recurrent pain in acute type B aortic dissection. *Am J Cardiol* 87:930–933, 2001.
54. Januzzi JL, Sabatine MS, Choi JC, et al: Refractory systemic hypertension following type B aortic dissection. *Am J Cardiol* 88:686–688, 2001.
55. Eggebrecht H, Lonn L, Herold U, et al: Endovascular stent-graft placement for complications of acute type B aortic dissection. *Curr Opin Cardiol* 20:477–483, 2005.

56. Dake M, Kato N, Mitchell RS, et al: Endovascular stent-graft placement for the treatment of acute aortic dissection. *N Engl J Med* 340:1546–1552, 1999.
57. Patel H, Williams D, Meekov M, et al: Long-term results of percutaneous management of malperfusion in acute type B aortic dissection: implications for thoracic aortic endovascular repair. *J Thorac Cardiovasc Surg* 138:300–308, 2009.
58. Nienaber C, Rousseau H, Eggebrecht H, et al: Trial. I. Randomized comparison of strategies for type B aortic dissection: the INvestigation of STEnt Grafts in Aortic Dissection (INSTEAD) trial. *Circulation* 120:2519–2528, 2009.
59. Yamada T, Tada S, Harada J: Aortic dissection without intimal rupture: diagnosis with MR imaging and CT. *Radiology* 168:347–352, 1988.
60. Ide K, Uchida H, Otsuji H, et al: Acute aortic dissection with intramural hematoma: possibility of transition to classic dissection or aneurysm. *J Thorac Imaging* 11:46–52, 1996.
61. Nienaber C, Eagle KA: Aortic dissection: new frontiers in diagnosis and management: Part I: from etiology to diagnostic strategies. *Circulation* 108:628–635, 2003.
62. Evangelista A, Dominguez R, Sebastia C, et al: Long-term follow-up of aortic intramural hematoma: predictors of outcome. *Circulation* 108:583–589, 2003.
63. Ganaha F, Miller DC, Sugimoto K, et al: Prognosis of aortic intramural hematoma with and without penetrating atherosclerotic ulcer: a clinical and radiological analysis. *Circulation* 106:342–348, 2002.
64. Stanson A, Kazmier FJ, Hollier LH, et al: Penetrating atherosclerotic ulcers of the thoracic aorta: natural history and clinicopathologic correlations. *Ann Vasc Surg* 1:15–23, 1986.
65. O'Gara P, DeSanctis RW: Acute aortic dissection and its variants. Toward a common diagnostic and therapeutic approach. *Circulation* 92:1376–1378, 1995.
66. Vilacosta I, San Roman JA, Ferreiros J, et al: Natural history and serial morphology of aortic intramural hematoma: a novel variant of aortic dissection. *Am Heart J* 134:495–507, 1997.
67. Song J, Kim HS, Song JK, et al: Usefulness of the initial noninvasive imaging study to predict the adverse outcomes in the medical treatment of acute type A aortic intramural hematoma. *Circulation* 108[Suppl 1]:II324–II328, 2003.
68. Kaji S, Nishigami K, Akasaka T, et al: Prediction of progression or regression of type A aortic intramural hematoma by computed tomography. *Circulation* 100[19, Suppl 2]:II281–II286, 1999.
69. Kaji S, Akasaka T, Horibata Y, et al: Long-term prognosis of patients with type a aortic intramural hematoma. *Circulation* 106[12, Suppl 1]:I248–I252, 2002.
70. Shimizu H, Yoshino H, Udagawa H, et al: Prognosis of aortic intramural hemorrhage compared with classic aortic dissection. *Am J Cardiol* 85:792–795, 2000.
71. Song J, Kim HS, Song JM, et al: Outcomes of medically treated patients with aortic intramural hematoma. *Am J Med* 113:181–187, 2002.
72. von Kodolitsch Y, Csosz SK, Koschyk DH, et al: Intramural hematoma of the aorta: predictors of progression to dissection and rupture. *Circulation* 107:1158–1163, 2003.
73. Moizumi Y, Komatsu T, Motoyoshi N, et al: Clinical features and long-term outcome of type A and type B intramural hematoma of the aorta. *J Thorac Cardiovasc Surg* 127:421–427, 2004.
74. Mohr-Kahaly S, Erbel R, Kearney P, et al: Aortic intramural hemorrhage visualized by transesophageal echocardiography: findings and prognostic implications. *J Am Coll Cardiol* 23:658–664, 1994.
75. Nishigami K, Tsuchiya T, Shono H, et al: Disappearance of aortic intramural hematoma and its significance to the prognosis *Circulation* 102[Suppl III]:III-243–III-247, 2000.
76. Monnin-Bares V, Thony F, Rodiere M, et al: Endovascular stent-graft management of aortic intramural hematomas. *J Vasc Interv Radiol* 20:713–721, 2009.
77. Manning B, Dias N, Manno M, et al: Endovascular treatment of acute complicated type B dissection: morphological changes at midterm follow-up. *J Endovasc Ther* 16:466–474, 2009.
78. Johnston KW, Rutherford RB, Tilson MD, et al: Suggested standards for reporting on arterial aneurysms. Subcommittee on reporting standards for arterial aneurysms, Ad Hoc committee on reporting standards, society for vascular surgery and North American chapter, International Society for Cardiovascular Surgery. *J Vasc Surg* 13:452–458, 1991.
79. Davies RR, Goldstein LJ, Coady MA, et al: Yearly rupture or dissection rates for thoracic aortic aneurysms: simple prediction based on size. *Ann Thorac Surg* 73:17–28, 2002.
80. Brown PM, Pattenden R, Vernooy C, et al: Selective Management of Abdominal Aortic Aneurysms in a Prospective Measurement Program. *J Vasc Surg* 23:213–220, 1996.
81. Crawford E, Cohen ES: Aortic aneurysm: a multifocal disease. Presidential address. *Arch Surg* 117:1393–1400, 1982.
82. Isselbacher E: Thoracic and abdominal aortic aneurysms. *Circulation* 111:816–828, 2005.
83. Bickerstaff LK, Pairolero PC, Hollier LH, et al: Thoracic aortic aneurysms: a population-based study. *Surgery* 92:1103–1108, 1982.
84. Coady M, Rizzo JA, Goldstein LJ, et al: Natural history, pathogenesis, and etiology of thoracic aortic aneurysms and dissections. *Cardiol Clin* 17:615–635, 1999.
85. Devereux R, Roman MJ: Aortic disease in Marfan's syndrome. *N Engl J Med* 340:1358–1359, 1999.
86. Gott V, Greene PS, Alejo DE, et al: Replacement of the aortic root in patients with Marfan's syndrome. *N Engl J Med* 340:1307–1313, 1999.
87. Pressler V, McNamara JJ: Thoracic aortic aneurysm: natural history and treatment. *J Thorac Cardiovasc Surg* 79:489–498, 1980.
88. Crawford E, DeNatale RW: Thoracoabdominal aortic aneurysm: observations regarding the natural course of the disease. *J Vasc Surg* 3:578–582, 1986.
89. Johansson G, Markstrom U, Swedenborg J: Ruptured thoracic aortic aneurysms: a study of incidence and mortality rates. *J Vasc Surg* 21:985–988, 1995.
90. Guo D, Hasham S, Kuang S-Q, et al: Familial thoracic aortic aneurysms and dissections: genetic heterogeneity with a major locus mapping to 5q13–14. *Circulation* 103:2461–2468, 2001.
91. Baxter B: Heritable diseases of the blood vessels. *Cardiovasc Pathol* 14:185–188, 2005.
92. Coady M, Davies RR, Roberts M, et al: Familial patterns of thoracic aortic aneurysms. *Arch Surg* 134:361–367, 1999.
93. Hasham S, Willing MC, Guo DC, et al: Mapping a locus for familial thoracic aortic aneurysms and dissections (TAAD2) to 3p24–25. *Circulation* 107:3184–3190, 2003.
94. Pannu H, Fadulu VT, Chang J, et al: Mutations in transforming growth factor-beta receptor type II cause familial thoracic aortic aneurysms and dissections. *Circulation* 112:513–520, 2005.
95. Vaughan C, Casey M, He J, et al: Identification of a chromosome 11q23.2-q24 locus for familial aortic aneurysm disease, a genetically heterogeneous disorder. *Circulation* 103:2469–2475, 2001.
96. de Sa M, Moshkovitz Y, Butany J, et al: Histologic abnormalities of the ascending aorta and pulmonary trunk in patients with bicuspid aortic valve disease: clinical relevance to the ross procedure. *J Thorac Cardiovasc Surg* 118:588–594, 1999.
97. LeMaire S, Wang X, Wilks JA, et al: Matrix metalloproteinases in ascending aortic aneurysms: bicuspid versus trileaflet aortic valves. *J Surg Res* 123:40–48, 2005.
98. Elsheikh M, Casadei B, Conway GS, et al: Hypertension is a major risk factor for aortic root dilatation in women with Turner's syndrome. *Clin Endocrinol* 45:69–73, 2001.
99. Lindsay JJ: Diagnosis and treatment of diseases of the aorta. *Curr Probl Cardiol* 22:485–542, 1997.
100. Procter C, Hollier LH: Takayasu's arteritis and temporal arteritis. *Ann Vasc Surg* 6:195–198, 1992.
101. Gelsomino S, Romagnoli S, Gori F, et al: Annuloaortic ectasia and giant cell arteritis. *Ann Thorac Surg* 80:101–105, 2005.
102. Kieffer E, Chiche L, Bertal A, et al: Descending thoracic and thoracoabdominal aortic aneurysm in patients with Takayasu's disease. *Ann Vasc Surg* 18:505–513, 2004.
103. Pressler V, McNamara JJ: Aneurysm of the thoracic aorta: review of 260 cases. *J Thorac Cardiovasc Surg* 89:50–54, 1985.
104. Hazui H, Fukumoto H, Negoro N, et al: Simple and useful tests for discriminating between acute aortic dissection of the ascending aorta and acute myocardial infarction in the emergency setting. *Circ J* 69:677–682, 2005.
105. Gott V, Gillinov AM, Pyeritz RE, et al: Aortic root replacement. Risk factor analysis of a seventeen-year experience with 270 patients. *J Thorac Cardiovasc Surg* 109:536–544, 1995.
106. Greenberg R, Haddad F, Svensson L, et al: Hybrid approaches to thoracic aortic aneurysms: the role of endovascular elephant trunk completion. *Circulation* 112:2619–2626, 2005.
107. Thompson M: Controlling the expansion of abdominal aortic aneurysms. *Br J Surg* 90:897–898, 2003.
108. Lederle F, Johnson GR, Wilson SE: Aneurysm Detection and Management Veterans Affairs Cooperative Study. Abdominal aortic aneurysm in women. *J Vasc Surg* 34:122–126, 2001.
109. Singh K, Bonaa KH, Jacobsen BK, et al: Prevalence of and risk factors for abdominal aortic aneurysms in a population-based study: the Tromso study. *Am J Epidemiol* 154:236–244, 2001.
110. Group MASS. Multicentre aneurysm screening study (MASS): cost effectiveness analysis of screening for abdominal aortic aneurysms based on four year results from randomised controlled trial. *BMJ* 325:1135–1141, 2002.
111. Vardulaki K, Walker NM, Day NE, et al: Quantifying the risks of hypertension, age, sex and smoking in patients with abdominal aortic aneurysm. *Br J Surg* 87:195–200, 2000.
112. Gillum R: Epidemiology of aortic aneurysm in the United States. *J Clin Epidemiol* 48:1289–1298, 1995.
113. Sakalihasan N, Limet R, Defawe OD: Abdominal aortic aneurysm. *Lancet* 365:1577–1589, 2005.
114. Brewster D, Cronenwett JL, Hallett JW Jr, et al: Joint council of the American Association for Vascular Surgery and Society for Vascular Surgery. Guidelines for the treatment of abdominal aortic aneurysms. Report of a subcommittee of the Joint Council of the American Association for Vascular Surgery and Society for Vascular Surgery. *J Vasc Surg* 37:1106–1117, 2003.

115. Lederle F, Johnson GR, Wilson SE, et al: Relationship of age, gender, race, and body size to infrarenal aortic diameter. The Aneurysm Detection and Management (ADAM) Veterans Affairs Cooperative Study Investigators. *J Vasc Surg* 26:595–601, 1997.
116. Frydman G, Walker PJ, Summers K, et al: The value of screening in siblings of patients with abdominal aortic aneurysm. *Eur J Vasc Endovasc Surg* 26:396–400, 2003.
117. Eriksson P, Jormsjo-Pettersson S, Brady AR, et al: Genotype-phenotype relationships in an investigation of the role of proteases in abdominal aortic aneurysm expansion. *Br J Surg* 92:1372–1376, 2005.
118. Liu J, Sukhova GK, Yang JT, et al: Cathepsin L expression and regulation in human abdominal aortic aneurysm, atherosclerosis, and vascular cells. *Atherosclerosis* 184:302–311, 2005.
119. Ye S: Influence of matrix metalloproteinase genotype on cardiovascular disease susceptibility and outcome. *Cardiovasc Res* 69:636–645, 2005.
120. Matsumura K, Hirano T, Takeda K, et al: Incidence of aneurysms in Takayasu's arteritis. *Angiology* 42:308–315, 1991.
121. Erentug V, Bozbuga N, Omeroglu SN, et al: Rupture of abdominal aortic aneurysms in Behcet's disease. *Ann Vasc Surg* 17:682–685, 2003.
122. Lemos D, Raffetto JD, Moore TC, et al: Primary aortoduodenal fistula: a case report and review of the literature. *J Vasc Surg* 37:686–689, 2003.
123. Fink H, Lederle FA, Roth CS, et al: The accuracy of physical examination to detect abdominal aortic aneurysm. *Arch Intern Med* 160:833–836, 2000.
124. Carrel T, Do DD, Triller J, et al: A less invasive approach to completely repair the aortic arch. *Ann Thorac Surg* 80:1475–1478, 2005.
125. Garzon G, Fernandez-Velilla M, Marti M, et al: Endovascular stent-graft treatment of thoracic aortic disease. *Radiographics* 25[Suppl 1]:S229–S244, 2005.
126. Larzon T, Lindgren R, Norgren L: Endovascular treatment of ruptured abdominal aortic aneurysms: a shift of the paradigm? *J Endovasc Ther* 12:548–555, 2005.
127. Criado F, Abul-Khoudoud OR, Domer GS, et al: Endovascular repair of the thoracic aorta: lessons learned. *Ann Thorac Surg* 80:857–863, 2005.
128. Katzen B, Dake MD, MacLean AA, et al: Endovascular repair of abdominal and thoracic aortic aneurysms. *Circulation* 112:1663–1675, 2005.

CHAPTER 37 ■ EVALUATION AND MANAGEMENT OF HYPERTENSION IN THE INTENSIVE CARE UNIT

BENJAMIN M. SCIRICA AND ROBERT J. HEYKA

HYPERTENSIVE URGENCIES AND EMERGENCIES

Patients with elevated blood pressure (BP) in the intensive care unit (ICU) present with either a BP that threatens to cause imminent target organ damage (TOD) to vascular beds or a transient, usually more benign elevation in BP without threat of TOD.

Definitions

Hypertensive syndromes have diverse etiologies and often have little in common besides a similar presentation. The terms used to describe these clinical syndromes are mostly of historic significance. In original usage, they applied to specific clinical findings often without an appreciation of their systemic abnormalities. They are often misapplied. *Hypertensive crisis* is loosely defined as any clinical situation with a severe elevation in BP [1]. Hypertensive emergencies and urgencies are categories of hypertensive crisis that may be life threatening and occur (a) against the background of worsening chronic essential hypertension, (b) with secondary forms of hypertension, or (c) in patients without previously known hypertensive disease.

There are not reliable data regarding the actual yearly number of hypertensive emergencies; however in the United States, hypertension is the primary diagnosis in more than 500,000 hospital admission [1]. Patients with essential hypertension who present to emergency rooms with hypertensive crises tend to be aware of their diagnosis of hypertension, on medication but noncompliant, are African-American or Hispanic, young males, and of lower socioeconomic status [2]. Other secondary forms of hypertension, including renovascular disease or endocrine causes [3] are found in a significant percentage of patients with hypertensive crisis.

In hypertensive crises, the elevation in BP tends to be severe with diastolic blood pressures (DBPs) greater than 120 mm Hg. However, the level of systolic blood pressure (SBP), DBP, or mean arterial pressure (MAP) does not distinguish them. Rather, it is the presence or absence of acute and progressive TOD [4,5].

Hypertensive emergency means the BP elevation is associated with ongoing neurologic, myocardial, vascular, hematologic, or renal TOD, whereas *hypertensive urgency* means that the potential for TOD is great and likely to occur if BP is not soon controlled. Examples of hypertensive emergencies are provided in Table 37.1. In many instances, a better term for urgencies is simply *uncontrolled BP* [4,5]. Many patients present to emergency rooms with inadequately treated BP and no evidence of TOD [6]. There is no evidence of benefit from rapid reduction in BP in these asymptomatic patients [7], and their difficult-to-control hypertension can be evaluated as outpatients [8].

Accelerated and *malignant hypertensions* are older terms named on the basis of ophthalmologic findings and refer to categories of hypertensive crises with exudative retinopathy, retinal hemorrhages, or papilledema. They probably represent a continuum of organ damage [9].

Accelerated hypertension may be an urgency or emergency with grade III Keith–Wagener–Barker retinopathy: that is, constriction and sclerosis (i.e., grades I or II) plus hemorrhages and exudates (grade III). The presence of exudate is more worrisome than hemorrhage alone. *Malignant hypertension* is grade IV Keith–Wagener–Barker retinopathy and with papilledema that signifies central nervous system (CNS) involvement, is a *hypertensive emergency*. It is frequently associated with diffuse TOD, such as hypertensive encephalopathy, left ventricular

TABLE 37.1

EXAMPLES OF HYPERTENSIVE EMERGENCIES

Severely elevated blood pressure and the presence of:
Acute ischemic stroke
Acute hemorrhagic stroke/subarachnoid hemorrhage
Acute myocardial infarction
Acute pulmonary edema
Acute aortic dissection
Encephalopathy
Perioperative hypertension
Postoperative bleeding
Severe epistaxis
Eclampsia
Pheochromocytoma crisis
Recreational drug abuse with cocaine, lysergic acid diethylamide (LSD), ecstasy, amphetamines
Acute renal failure
Hemolytic anemia
Monoamine–oxidase inhibitor interactions

failure, renal fibrinoid necrosis, or microangiopathic hemolytic anemia. In the 1930s, the term *malignant* was given to reflect the dismal survival among these patients, approximately 60% at 2 years after diagnosis and less than 7% at 10 years. With the introduction of effective hypertensive therapy, the prognosis has significantly improved, with a 5-year survival of 74%. The most common causes of death are renal failure (40%), stroke (24%), myocardial infarction (11%), and heart failure (10%) [10].

IMPORTANCE OF TARGET ORGAN DAMAGE

Most organ beds can regulate the amount of blood flow they receive over a wide range of systemic pressures by autoregulation: OBF = OPPr/OVR, where OBF is organ blood flow, OPPr is organ perfusion pressure, and OVR is organ vascular resistance [11]. Small arteries and arterioles constrict or dilate in response to local myogenic effectors acting on the endothelium that respond to transmural (perfusion) pressure gradients. A decrease in OPPr leads to vasodilation; an increase in OPPr leads to vasoconstriction and limits pressure-induced damage when systemic pressure rises. The cerebral circulation can maintain perfusion with changes in MAP from about 60 to 150 mm Hg [11]. When MAP exceeds the usual autoregulatory range, breakthrough or loss of autoregulation occurs.

Sustained BP greater than the usual autoregulatory range leads to damage of the endothelial lining of capillaries and arterioles, resulting in leakage of plasma into the vascular wall. Fibrin deposition reduces lumen diameters and precipitates local edema and sclerosis. In patients with chronic hypertension, the loss of autoregulation typically occurs only at extremely elevated BPs, whereas in patients without any significant hypertension, in whom the protective autoregulation has not developed, edema and the consequent organ-specific symptoms can be seen with DBPs greater than 100 mm Hg [12].

When OPPr falls to lesser than the lower limits of autoregulation, organ ischemia and infarction may occur. Limits of critical perfusion pressure and tolerance to variation in OPPr vary among individuals. The elderly or patients with chronic hypertension tolerate an elevated MAP because of an upward shift in their cerebral autoregulation curve but have a diminished tolerance to hypotension with vessel functional and structural changes [12]. Patients without antecedent hypertension may develop a hypertensive crisis with acute conditions such as acute vasculitis, subarachnoid hemorrhage (SAH), unstable angina, or eclampsia at lower systemic BP.

Cerebral circulation is the most sensitive vascular bed to breakthrough and ischemia [13]. Cardiac perfusion tolerates a more pronounced drop in BP, even with underlying atherosclerotic disease, because myocardial oxygen demands decrease dramatically when pressures decrease. In organ beds such as the kidneys with antecedent atherosclerotic, acute BP changes are less tolerated and may worsen renal perfusion [4,5].

In most patients with hypertensive crises, the pathophysiologic abnormality is an increase in systemic vascular resistance (SVR), not an increased cardiac output (CO) (MAP = CO × SVR). The increase in SVR elevates BP, overrides local autoregulation, and leads to organ ischemia.

APPROACH TO THE PATIENT

In the ICU, therapy must often begin before a comprehensive patient evaluation is completed. A systematic approach offers the opportunity to be expeditious and inclusive (Table 37.2).

A brief history and physical examination should assess the degree of TOD and rule out obvious secondary causes of hypertension. The history should include prior hypertension, other significant medical disease, medication use, compliance, recreational drugs use, and, most importantly, symptoms from TOD to neurologic, cardiac, or renal systems. Examination should verify BP readings in both arms, supine and standing, if possible and eliminate the rare but important finding of pseudohypertension due to extensive arterial calcification using Osler's maneuver, which is performed by inflating the BP cuff to greater than the brachial systolic BP. A palpable radial or brachial artery, despite being pulseless, signifies a significantly stiff artery and the likely overestimation of the true BP [14]. Intra-arterial monitoring may be necessary to verify readings and monitor treatment. Also include direct ophthalmologic examination looking for hemorrhages, exudates, or papilledema; auscultation of the lungs and heart; and evaluation of the abdomen for masses or bruits and the peripheral pulses for bruits, masses, or deficits. Signs of neurologic ischemia include altered

TABLE 37.2

INITIAL EVALUATION OF HYPERTENSIVE CRISIS IN THE INTENSIVE CARE UNIT

1. Continuous blood pressure monitoring
   a. Direct (intra-arterial)—preferred
   b. Indirect (cuff)
2. Brief initial evaluation, including history and physical examination with attention to
   a. Neurologic including funduscopic examination and cardiac, pulmonary, renal symptoms
   b. Assessment of organ perfusion and function (e.g., mental status, heart failure, urine output)
   c. Blood and urine studies—electrolytes, blood urea nitrogen, creatinine, complete blood cell count with differential, urinalysis with sediment; if indicated, serum catecholamines, cardiac enzymes
   d. Electrocardiogram (assess for strain or ischemia)
   e. Chest radiograph (assess size of aorta, cardiomegaly, or heart failure)
3. Initiation of therapy (within 1 h of presentation if TOD is identified)
4. Further evaluation of etiology once stabilized

TOD, target organ damage.

mental status, headaches, nausea, and vomiting in addition to focal neurologic deficits. Ancillary evaluation should include electrolytes, blood urea nitrogen and creatinine, complete blood cell count with differential, or echocardiogram (ECG), chest radiograph, and assessment of recent urine output. As the patient's condition stabilizes, further evaluation of unexplored reasons for the hypertensive crisis can be considered and pursued.

Patients with Neurologic Symptoms

In patients with neurologic symptoms, a noncontrast computed tomogram of the head is important to exclude intracerebral hemorrhages (ICHs) or mass effect. Magnetic resonance imaging is more sensitive for detecting early ischemic strokes, as well as the edema and white matter changes in the parieto-occipital region (posterior leukoencephalopathy syndrome) associated with hypertensive encephalopathy [15]. Early identification of acute vascular events such as ischemic strokes or ICHs is critical as early management and BP goals differ from hypertensive encephalopathy.

TREATMENT

Most studies of hypertensive emergencies are either nonrandomized or suffer from (a) tremendous variation and inconsistency in definitions and cutoffs, (b) absence of important and long-term outcomes such as mortality, (c) being underpowered with wide confidence intervals, and (d) inconsistent reporting of adverse effects. Thus, treatment recommendations for hypertensive emergencies are not based on a large body of randomized controlled studies. One systematic review of hypertensive urgencies and emergencies studies found no evidence supporting any one agent over another. For hypertensive emergencies, nitroprusside, captopril, and clonidine were acceptable choices. For urgencies, a number of agents were used and effective [16]. A systematic review for the Cochrane collaboration, which included more recent studies, again failed to detect any specific agent or strategy that was superior to another. There was well-documented efficacy for BP reduction with nitrates (including nitroprusside), angiotensin-converting enzyme (ACE) inhibitors, diuretics, α-adrenergic antagonist, calcium channel blockers, and dopamine agonists [17]. Given this lack of data to guide therapy, how should we proceed?

The intensity of intervention must be determined by the clinical situation. In many situations, intubation, seizure control, hemodynamic monitoring, and maintenance of urine output can be as important as control of BP. Initial therapy should terminate ongoing TOD, *not* return BP to normal. Because cerebral circulation is the most sensitive to ischemia, the lower limit of cerebral autoregulation for each patient determines the initial goal. This floor is approximately 25% lesser than the initial MAP or a DBP in the range of 100 to 110 mm Hg [11]. Reasonable initial therapy is to decrease MAP by 25% with an agent that decreases SVR, considering the medical history, initiating events, and ongoing TOD [5]. Patients with acute left ventricular failure, myocardial ischemia, or aortic dissection require more aggressive treatment [18–20].

The decision to use oral or parenteral therapy depends on several factors. Atherosclerotic disease puts the patient at higher risk if therapy overshoots the mark. The answers to the questions in Table 37.3 guides the decision of parenteral versus oral therapy. Table 37.4 lists recommendations and precautions for therapeutic agents, and Table 37.5 lists proper dosing for each agent.

Once the patient is stable, additional diagnostic studies may proceed. An oral regimen can be started as the situation stabilizes. Because the ICU is an artificial environment, physicians should avoid attempts to normalize BP especially if large doses of medications are required. Further fine-tuning of BP to levels suggested by Joint National Committee VII [6] or the European Society of Hypertension/European Society of Cardiology guidelines for the management of hypertension [21] should occur once the patient resumes his or her usual diet, activity, and compliance at home.

TABLE 37.3

PARENTERAL VERSUS ORAL THERAPY OF HYPERTENSION IN THE INTENSIVE CARE UNIT

Is this a hypertensive emergency?
Is rapid onset of effect needed?
Is rapid lowering of blood pressure needed?
Is a shorter duration of action important?
Is the patient at risk for overshoot hypotension?
Atherosclerotic heart disease
Renovascular hypertension
Cerebrovascular disease
Dehydration
Other recent antihypertensive therapy

SPECIFIC HYPERTENSIVE CRISES

Acute Left Ventricular Heart Failure

Decreases in SVR and MAP improve left ventricular function by decreasing cardiac work, left ventricular wall tension, and oxygen demand. Intravenous nitroglycerin or nitroprusside are the agents of choice in acute heart failure because they rapidly reduce preload and diminish pulmonary congestion [20]. Nitroprusside, a balanced vasodilation with a decrease in both preload and afterload, is usually administered with other acute therapy for pulmonary edema, such as diuretics. Nitroglycerin has greater effect on the venous (preload) side than on the arterial side. Nitroglycerin is preferred for management of ischemic heart failure [20]. Because of the fairly rapid development of tachyphylaxis to nitrates, alternative and more chronic therapy should be instituted within 24 hours of initiation of therapy. The use of an intravenous ACE inhibitor in this situation is contraindicated though oral agents can be resumed or initiated.

Myocardial Ischemia or Infarction

Treatment of elevated BP is only part of the overall therapy to preserve and restore cardiac perfusion with anti-ischemic medications, antithrombotic agents, thrombolytic therapy, percutaneous coronary intervention, or surgery. Therapy should maintain local coronary arterial flow and not induce a steal syndrome with differential relaxation of coronary vessels. Because nitroprusside may actually divert the flow away from poststenotic areas, nitroglycerin is preferred. Beta-blockers given intravenously also act to maintain coronary perfusion in the face of decreased systemic pressures and decrease myocardial oxygen demand by lowering heart rate and BP. The use of an intravenous ACE inhibitor in patients with an acute myocardial infarction and depressed left ventricular function should be avoided as it may precipitate symptomatic hypotension. Uncontrolled hypertension (SBP >180 mm Hg or DBP >110 mm Hg) is a relative contraindication to treatment with fibrinolytic treatment [18].

TABLE 37.4

TREATMENT OF HYPERTENSIVE EMERGENCIES

Type	Recommended drugs	Target of treatment
Neurologic		
Hypertensive encephalopathy	Nimodipine, labetalol	15%–25% decrease in MAP over 3–6 h
Intracerebral hemorrhage or subarachnoid hemorrhage	Nitroprusside, labetalol, nicardipine	Same (debated)
Cerebral infarction	Nitroprusside, labetalol, nimodipine, nicardipine	Same (debated)
Head injury	Nitroprusside	Same
Cardiovascular		
Myocardial ischemia, infarction	Nitroglycerin, beta-blockers, labetalol	Control of ischemia
Aortic dissection	Beta-blockers, nitroprusside, labetalol	Goal of SBP 120 mm Hg in 20–30 min
Acute left ventricular failure	Nitroprusside, nitroglycerin, loop diuretics, converting enzyme inhibitors	Improved Sx
Renal failure		
Acute renal failure	Fenoldopam, nitroprusside, labetalol	Decrease MAP 25%
Other		
Hemorrhagic	Nitroprusside, labetalol, others as needed	Control risk of bleeding
Malignant hypertension	As with encephalopathy; oral agents may be considered	
Obstetric	Hydralazine, methyldopa, $MgSO_4$	DBP <90 mm Hg

DBP, diastolic blood pressure; MAP, mean arterial pressure; SBP, systolic blood pressure; Sx, signs and symptoms.

Aortic Dissection

Aortic dissection is the most common acute aortic syndrome. It is imperative to begin therapy for aortic dissection immediately to prevent extension or rupture, regardless of the ultimate therapy. Uncomplicated acute type B dissection is usually treated with medication. Therapy is directed to lower BP and the rate of the rise of pressure (d*p*/d*t*). BP should be lowered rapidly to the lowest level, permitting continued good organ perfusion (i.e., no change in mental status or new neurologic symptoms and continued urine output). Intravenous beta-blockade is the initial therapy of choice, in particular with labetalol or esmolol. Any acute therapy that decreases BP without also decreasing d*p*/d*t* or induces reflex tachycardia can extend the dissection and should be avoided. Once beta-blockade is started, vasodilation with nitroprusside can be added if necessary [19,22].

Hypertensive Encephalopathy

Hypertensive encephalopathy occurs with severe BP elevation as cerebral autoregulation is overwhelmed and can lead to blindness, seizures, coma, and death. Pathologic findings include endothelial dysfunction, cerebral edema, petechial hemorrhages, and microinfarcts [11]. The typical patient has chronic untreated hypertension and the slow development of neurologic symptoms, especially headaches, over 48 to 72 hours. Hypertensive encephalopathy is much less common with better access to antihypertensive medication. Any degree of control of hypertension can dramatically decrease the likelihood of encephalopathy. As mentioned previously in the chapter, patients with severe hypertension and neurologic symptoms should have neuroimaging to exclude acute ischemic strokes or hemorrhages, in which the goals of hypertension management differ from hypertensive encephalopathy. Treatment with short-acting parenteral agents should lead to rapid resolution of symptoms. Continued symptoms suggest other CNS pathology [23].

Ischemic Stroke

Elevated BP is common in patients presenting with acute ischemic strokes. Both low and high BPs are associated with poor outcomes. For every increase in 10 mm Hg greater than 180, there is a 40% increase in the risk of worsening neurologic status [24]. Once ischemia occurs, a central core of dense ischemia of variable size is surrounded by less severe ischemia that can potentially be salvaged, termed the *ischemic penumbra* [25]. This area of stunned, but viable, tissue depends on continued blood flow and may need higher pressures for continued perfusion. Because of the concern about abrupt reduction in BP in patients presenting with acute strokes has led the American Heart Association and American Stoke Association guidelines for the early management of adults with ischemic stroke give a consensus recommendation that emergency use of BP-lowering agents should be withheld unless the DBP is greater than 120 mm Hg or the SBP is greater than 220 mm Hg. In patients who are potentially eligible for reperfusion therapy, it is recommended to consider therapy for levels greater than 185 mm Hg SBP or 110 mm Hg DBP with labetalol, nitroprusside, or nicardipine. Thrombolytic therapy should not be given if the BP remains elevated to greater than 185/110 mm Hg. After reperfusion therapy, labetalol or nicardipine is recommended for SBP levels greater than 180 mm Hg or DBP levels greater than 105 mm Hg and nitroprusside for SBP levels about 230 mm Hg [24]. If clinical deterioration is noted with BP reduction, higher BPs must be accepted.

Subarachnoid Hemorrhage

The treatment of SAH is complicated and unsettled. It is unclear if uncontrolled hypertension increases the risk of rebleeding [26,27]. A Cochrane review found that oral, but not intravenous, calcium channel blockers (CCB) reduce the risk of poor outcome and secondary ischemia [28], which is based primarily on studies using nimodipine. If vasospasm occurs later,

TABLE 37.5

PROPER DOSING FOR AGENTS TO TREAT HYPERTENSIVE CRISIS

Agent	Administration	Onset	Duration	Special indications
Direct vasodilators				
Nitroprusside	IV infusion: 0.25–10.0 μg/kg/min	Immediate	1–2 min	Hypertensive emergencies
Nitroglycerin	IV infusion: 5–200 μg/kg/min	2–5 min	5–10 min	Heart failure or cardiac ischemia
Fenoldopam	IV infusion: 0.1 μg/kg/min uptitrated by 0.05–0.1 μg/kg/min increments to maximum 1.6 μg/kg/min	5–15 min	30 min	Most hypertensive emergencies; avoid in glaucoma
Hydralazine	IV bolus: 10–20 mg	10–20 min	1–4 h	Eclampsia
Adrenergic blockers				
Phentolamine	IV 5–15 mg	1–2 min	10–20 min	Pheochromocytoma, catecholamine surge
Esmolol	IV bolus 250–500 μg /kg/min IV bolus—repeat after 5 min IV infusion 50–100 mg/kg/min; give new bolus when increase infusion	5–10 min	10–30 min	Most hypertensive emergencies
Labetalol	IV bolus: 20–80 mg q10 min IV infusion: 0.5–2 mg/min	5–10 min	3–6 h	Most hypertensive emergencies; not in decompensated heart failure
Calcium antagonists				
Nicardipine	IV infusion: 5–15 mg/h	5–10 min	1–2 h	Most hypertensive emergencies; not in heart failure
Nimodipine	IV infusion: 5–10 mg/h ↑ by mg/h, up to 15 mg q30 min, 60 mg q4h × 21 d; repeat	15–30 min	3–6 h	Subarachnoid hemorrhage
Clevidipine	IV infusion: 1–2 mg/h, double dose q90 s. As approach goal BP, ↑ by less than double and lengthen uptitration to q5–10 min. Typical goal is 4–6 mg/h	2–4 min	5–15 min	Most hypertensive emergencies
Angiotensin-converting enzyme inhibitors				
Captopril	PO 6.25–25 mg, repeat q30 min, if necessary	1 h	1–4 h	
Enalaprilat	IV bolus: 1.25–5.0 mg (over 5 min) q6h	15–30 min	6–8 h	Acute left ventricular failure; not in myocardial infarction
Central-acting agonists				
Clonidine	PO 0.2 mg initially; 0.2 mg/h (total 0.7 mg)		3 h	
Miscellaneous				
Trimethaphan	IV infusion: 0.5–5 mg/min	1–5 min	5–15 min	

IV, intravenous; PO, oral.

increases in BP with "triple-H" therapy (hypervolemia, hypertension, and hemodilution) is recommended but not proven [26].

Intracerebral Hemorrhage

Similar cautions apply to ICH. BP is often markedly elevated in patients with ICH. With severely elevated BP and neurologic symptoms, the differentiation of structural pathology from hypertensive encephalopathy can be difficult. The American Heart Association and American Stroke Association guidelines for the treatment of ICH acknowledge the lack of randomized trial data to guide therapy, but recommend initiation of therapy for (i) SBP levels greater than 200 mm Hg or MAP greater than 150 mm Hg and (ii) SBP levels greater than 180 mm Hg or MAP greater than 130 mm Hg, with evidence of increased intracerebral pressures to maintain a perfusing pressure of 60 mm Hg or more. In patients with SBP levels greater than 180 mm Hg or MAP greater than 130 mm Hg without any evidence of elevated intracerebral pressures, a target of an MAP of 110 mm Hg or BP of 160/90 mm Hg is likely beneficial [29].

ELEVATED BLOOD PRESSURE WITHOUT HYPERTENSIVE CRISIS

Elevated BP is seen in the ICU without TOD. Patients may require treatment of (a) chronic hypertension; (b) new, transient, and usually mild elevations in BP; or (c) elevated BP in the perioperative setting. The goal of treatment is not based solely on BP readings, but on an appreciation of the acute and chronic care of the patient [5].

Continued Therapy of Chronic Hypertension

Patients in the ICU often have a history of hypertension. BP levels may rise if the patient is unable to continue his or her usual antihypertensive regimen; therefore, alternative agents should be instituted. BP elevation in patients who have recently discontinued chronic therapy can be severe and present as rebound or *discontinuation syndrome*. The likelihood of rebound hypertension is proportional to the prior dose of medication.

TABLE 37.6

NEW ONSET OF HYPERTENSION IN THE INTENSIVE CARE UNIT

Situational
Pain
Anxiety
New-onset angina
Hypocarbia
Hypoxemia
Hypothermia with shivering
Rigors
Volume overload
Rebound or discontinuation syndrome
Prior, undiagnosed, untreated hypertension

Hypotension may develop in patients with chronic hypertension who were noncompliant with medication but have all medications given as prescribed on admission. BP may drop and require ICU admission for volume and pressor support. If noncompliance is suspected, it is better to start with lower doses and adjust upward.

New Onset of Hypertension

New and usually temporary increases in BP may occur in the ICU. Many factors may cause short-term elevations in BP (Table 37.6). Low doses of short-acting agents should be used to avoid sharp drops in BP in this usually self-limited situation. Undiagnosed essential or secondary hypertension should be considered especially if evidence of TOD is present.

Perioperative Hypertension

Uncontrolled BP can induce new TOD, can increase the risk of vascular suture breakdown or bleeding, and may worsen overall prognosis.

Preoperative Evaluation

Moderate chronic hypertension is not a major risk factor for surgery in otherwise stable patients, but it is a marker for potential coronary artery disease (CAD) [30]. Routine BP therapy should be continued as usual up to the morning of surgery and resumed either orally or intravenously as soon as possible postoperatively. Surgery should probably be delayed if BP is greater than 180/110 mm Hg in patient with CAD [31].

Perioperative Hypertension

A useful classification of hypertension associated with cardiovascular surgery considers the clinical situation and time of onset [32] (Table 37.7). Acute postoperative hypertension usually starts 2 to 6 hours after surgery and may persist for 24 to 48 hours. The immediate postoperative period (up to 2 hours) represents a time of significant patient instability, and BPs can vary widely mediated by increased catecholamines [33]. The goal is to avoid overshoot hypotension or TOD. Intravenous infusions or minibolus therapy allows the most controlled approach to BP regulation [34]. Nitroprusside or labetalol is effective in most situations; nitroglycerin is also beneficial [31].

TABLE 37.7

HYPERTENSION WITH CARDIOVASCULAR SURGERY

Preoperative period
Anxiety
Pain
Angina
Discontinuation of antihypertensive or cardiac therapy
Rebound hypertension
Intraoperative period
Induction of anesthesia
Drug effects—vasodilation, inotropic changes
Manipulation of viscera or trachea, urethra, and rectum
Sternotomy, chest retraction
With initiation of cardiopulmonary bypass
Postoperative period
Early (0–2 h)
Hypoxemia, hypercarbia, hypothermia with shivering, postanesthetic excitement or pain
After myocardial revascularization, valve replacement, repair of aortic coarctation
Intermediate (12–36 h)
As given previously
Fluid overload, mobilization
Reaction to endotracheal, nasogastric, chest, or bladder tube

PHARMACOLOGIC AGENTS

The choice between parenteral and oral therapy rests on the answers to several questions (Table 37.3). In a true hypertensive emergency, parenteral therapy with arterial BP monitoring offers a more controlled onset and offset of effect (Table 37.5).

The following are summary statements of available agents and are not meant to be inclusive. Additional information on the pharmacology of available agents can be found elsewhere [6,16,18,21,23,35–37].

Direct Vasodilators

Sodium Nitroprusside

Sodium nitroprusside has the longest track record for the treatment of severe hypertension. It dilates both arterioles and venules, reduces afterload and preload, and lowers myocardial oxygen demand. Its effects are mediated by intracellular cyclic guanosine monophosphate and nitric oxide in an endothelial-independent mechanism shared with other nitrosovasodilators. Nitroprusside has rapid onset and offset of action. Drug resistance is rarely observed. Nitroprusside is rapidly decomposed nonenzymatically in the blood to cyanide, which is then converted into thiocyanate in the liver. At high doses, acute toxicity occurs with cyanide accumulation (Table 37.8). The metabolite thiocyanate can accumulate with acute or chronic kidney injury, and thiocyanate levels should be monitored. Thiocyanate is removed with dialysis. Nitroprusside is light sensitive and must be wrapped in aluminum foil.

Nitroglycerin

Nitroglycerin preferentially dilates the venous system via cyclic guanosine monophosphate. Left ventricular diastolic pressure is reduced without any significant change in stroke volume or

TABLE 37.8

COMPLICATIONS OF TREATING HYPERTENSION

Complication	Causes
Overshoot hypotension	Infusion rate too rapid Prolonged duration of effect Additive drug effects New cardiac disease Volume depletion
Worsening neurologic status	Cerebral ischemia secondary to low blood pressure Hypertensive encephalopathy Increased intracranial pressure Medication side effect Thiocyanate toxicity Metabolic abnormality
Worsening of hypertension	Volume overload Pseudotolerance Unsuspected secondary hypertension Poor medical regimen Poor compliance
Metabolic acidosis	Cyanide toxicity Tissue hypoperfusion secondary
Worsening renal function	Hypoperfusion Volume depletion Acute tubular necrosis

CO, but MAP usually falls modestly. Nitroglycerin increases flow via collateral coronary blood vessels and can improve epicardial coronary blood flow. Nitroglycerin is useful after coronary bypass grafting, in coronary ischemia, and in heart failure. Nitroglycerin should be avoided in patients who have increased intracranial pressure, aortic stenosis, or hypertrophic obstructive cardiomyopathy.

Hydralazine

Parenteral hydralazine was removed from the market in 1993 and returned in 1994. It is a direct arterial vasodilator that increases CO and heart rate. Metabolism is by hepatic acetylation, the speed of which is genetically determined (slow vs. rapid acetylators). Excretion is renal. It is effective for eclampsia or left ventricular failure. Salt and water retention occur, requiring diuretics and beta-blockers in many cases. It is contraindicated with aortic dissection.

Beta-Blockers

Several beta-blockers, such as propranolol (nonselective), metoprolol (selective), and short-acting esmolol (selective), can be given parenterally. Labetalol is the beta-blocker most commonly used in the ICU.

Labetalol is a racemic mixture of a nonselective beta-blocker and a selective α_1-antagonist, and may be administered as minibolus or infusion, allowing titration of effect, rapid onset, and offset of action with prompt reduction in SVR and BP. The beta-blocker component prevents reflex tachycardia or significant changes in CO. Myocardial oxygen consumption is reduced, and coronary hemodynamics are improved in patients with CAD. Labetalol does not significantly affect cerebral blood flow. There is no dosage adjustment with renal failure, but some adjustment may be needed with severe hepatic disease.

Labetalol is a recommended agent with ischemic CVA or aortic dissection and hypertension [19,24]. It has been used with pheochromocytoma crisis because of its α_1-blocker properties and in aortic dissection because of its beta-blocker properties. The alpha-blocker effects of this agent can cause orthostatic hypotension. The ratio of beta-blockade to alpha-blockade is approximately 7 to 1. Any contraindication to beta-blockers applies to labetalol.

Calcium Antagonists

CCBs, particularly dihydropyridines, are widely used in the ICU. Calcium antagonists have been used for hypertensive urgencies and emergencies and are given via the parenteral or enteral routes.

Dihydropyridines

Nifedipine. It is administered orally, decreases peripheral vascular resistance, and increases collateral coronary blood flow. These effects result in decreased myocardial oxygen consumption, despite a tendency to reflex tachycardia and increased CO and stroke volume (in patients with preserved left ventricle function). Sublingual nifedipine should be abandoned because of safety concerns. The absorption is erratic; serious side effects from prolonged hypotension have been described, and the target BP is difficult to predict. Serious complications have included myocardial infarction or ischemia, worsening renal function, and cerebral ischemia [38].

Nicardipine. It is a rapid-acting systemic and coronary artery vasodilator. It has minimal effects on cardiac conduction and contractile function. Its advantages include potency, rapid onset, and ability to titrate in response to BP changes [39]. Disadvantages include tachycardia, hypotension, nausea, and vomiting. There is minimal cardiac depression, and continuous administration requires continuous monitoring.

Nimodipine. It crosses the blood–brain barrier and has recently been recommended for neurological emergencies [24,29]. A recent review of its use in SAH showed a statistically significant benefit on risk for severe disability, vegetative state, or death, but its putative effect on preventing vasospasm is less clear [28].

Clevidipine. It is a parenteral, short-acting calcium antagonist with a rapid onset that is a potent arterial dilator with little effect on venous capacitance or myocardial contraction. It may also prevent sequelae of ischemic damage through antioxidative properties [40].

Nondihydropyridines (Rate-Slowing Calcium Channel Blockers)

Verapamil. It is a phenylalkylamine CCB, which slows atrioventricular conduction and has a pronounced negative inotropic effect, with a rapid onset of action and a relatively low incidence of serious side effects. Verapamil can be given as repeated small boluses or a continuous intravenous infusion. The disadvantages include induction of various degrees of heart block and worsening heart failure because of its negative inotropic effects.

Diltiazem. It is a benzothiazepine calcium antagonist available as an intravenous preparation. It has effects intermediate between verapamil and dihydropyridines. It is widely used to slow the ventricular response to atrial fibrillation but not as a primary antihypertensive agent.

Angiotensin Converting Enzyme Inhibitors

Captopril

Captopril was the first ACE inhibitor available in the United States. It is rapidly absorbed, with peak blood levels reached 30 minutes after oral administration. Unlike some ACE inhibitors, captopril is not ingested as a prodrug and is therefore active as soon as it is absorbed. It is particularly effective in patients with heart failure or recent myocardial infarction with depressed ejection fraction. There is a risk of acute hypotension or worsening renal function in patients who are volume depleted, have bilateral high-grade renal artery stenoses, or high-grade stenosis in a solitary functioning kidney. Other acute side effects include bronchospasm, hyperkalemia, cough, angioedema, rash, and dysgeusia. It can accumulate with renal failure.

Enalaprilat

Enalaprilat is the only ACE inhibitor that can be administered parenterally. It is the active form of the oral agent, enalapril. A limited-dose titration response restricts the use of enalaprilat to lesser elevations in BP. Intravenous ACE inhibitor therapy is contraindicated in acute heart failure or acute myocardial infarction complicated by left ventricular dysfunction.

α-Agonists

Clonidine

Clonidine is a central α_2-agonist that decreases peripheral vascular resistance, venous return, and heart rate, and can contribute to reduction in CO. Clonidine is available orally and as a transdermal patch with an effectiveness of approximately 1 week. The patch should not be used to initiate therapy in the ICU, because it takes several days to achieve a steady state. However, patients previously on clonidine who are unable to take oral medications may be converted to a patch. Clonidine has been administered in an oral titration regimen to achieve gradual BP control in a period of 2 to 3 hours. Major disadvantages are sedation, dry mouth, and orthostatic hypotension. Caution should be used in patients requiring monitoring of mental status. Rebound hypertension may be observed if it is abruptly discontinued, particularly at higher doses.

α-Adrenergic Inhibitors

Phentolamine

Several α-adrenergic inhibitors are available for oral administration. The only available intravenous agent with α-adrenergic blocking properties is phentolamine, a nonselective α-receptor blocking agent. Its use is reserved for states associated with excess catecholamine levels, such as pheochromocytoma, rebound hypertension, or drug ingestion. The hypotensive effect of a single intravenous bolus lasts less than 15 minutes and is associated with significant reflex tachycardia. The advantage of phentolamine is its specific effect with pheochromocytoma. It is part of the anesthetic regimen in perioperative control of these patients. Disadvantages include abdominal cramping and pain, vomiting, diarrhea, tachycardia, dizziness, and arrhythmias.

TABLE 37.9

SUMMARY OF RECOMMENDATIONS BASED ON RANDOMIZED CONTROLLED TRIALS

- The best choice of antihypertensive agent in hypertensive urgency remains unclear [17]
- The best choice of antihypertensive agent in a hypertensive emergency remains unclear [17]
- There are no randomized trials comparing different treatment goals in hypertensive emergencies, but it is recommended that blood pressure not be lowered by more than 25% within the first hour and then to 160/100–110 mm Hg within the next 2–6 h [6]
- There is not enough evidence to evaluate the effect of altering blood pressure during acute stroke, though it is recommended to treat extremely elevated systolic (>220 mm Hg) or diastolic blood pressures (>120 mm Hg) [24]
- There is not enough evidence to recommend specific blood pressure management in acute intracerebral hemorrhage though it is recommended to treat extremely elevated systolic (>200 mm Hg) or diastolic blood pressures (>150 mm Hg) [29]

Fenoldopam

Fenoldopam is a specific dopamine I receptor agonist that is free of α- and β-adrenergic receptor effects. It reduces SVR, increases renal blood flow, increases fractional excretion of sodium, and increases water clearance. It is metabolized in the liver to multiple metabolites with uncertain clinical activity and may be particularly effective with impaired renal function, although a recent randomized controlled trial showed no difference compared to dopamine in renal protection [41].

Disadvantages are related to vasodilation, including flushing, headache, hypotension, nausea, and occasional ECG changes.

Diuretics

Many patients are actually hypovolemic from pressure natriuresis [5]. Patients with postoperative hypertension, cardiac dysfunction, or evidence of pulmonary edema may require diuresis. Many parenteral antihypertensive agents can cause fluid retention. Loop diuretics can help control intravascular volume, maintain urine output, and prevent resistance to antihypertensive therapy. They are given as a bolus or a slow infusion and have a threshold effect. Response—increased diuresis and natriuresis—is not seen unless sufficient drug reaches the renal tubules. Doses are titrated until increased urine output is seen or maximum doses are reached when other therapy must be initiated.

CONCLUSIONS

Advances in evaluation and management of hypertension in the ICU, based on randomized controlled trials or meta-analyses of such trials, are summarized in Table 37.9. Given the scarcity of data to support one particular hypertensive agent above another, the choice and goals of therapy are largely based on consensus recommendations and should be guided by the suspected etiology of the hypertension, the extent of TOD, and the individual hemodynamic profile of the patient.

References

1. Lloyd-Jones D, Adams RJ, Brown TM, et al: Heart disease and stroke statistics—2010 update: a report from the American Heart Association. *Circulation* 121:e46–e215, 2010.
2. Bennett NM, Shea S: Hypertensive emergency: case criteria, sociodemographic profile, and previous care of 100 cases. *Am J Public Health* 78:636–640, 1988.
3. Labinson PT, White WB, Tendler BE, et al: Primary hyperaldosteronism associated with hypertensive emergencies. *Am J Hypertens* 19:623–627, 2006.
4. Vaughan CJ, Delanty N: Hypertensive emergencies. *Lancet* 356:411–417, 2000.
5. Vidt DG: Hypertensive crises: emergencies and urgencies. *J Clin Hypertens (Greenwich)* 6:520–525, 2004.
6. Chobanian AV, Bakris GL, Black HR, et al: The Seventh Report of the Joint National Committee on Prevention, Detection, Evaluation, and Treatment of High Blood Pressure: the JNC 7 report. *JAMA* 289:2560–2572, 2003.
7. Elliott WJ: Clinical features in the management of selected hypertensive emergencies. *Prog Cardiovasc Dis* 48:316–325, 2006.
8. Moser M, Setaro JF: Clinical practice. Resistant or difficult-to-control hypertension. *N Engl J Med* 355:385–392, 2006.
9. Ahmed ME, Walker JM, Beevers DG, et al: Lack of difference between malignant and accelerated hypertension. *Br Med J (Clin Res Ed)* 292:235–237, 1986.
10. Lip GY, Beevers M, Beevers DG: Complications and survival of 315 patients with malignant-phase hypertension. *J Hypertens* 13:915–924, 1995.
11. Rose JC, Mayer SA: Optimizing blood pressure in neurological emergencies. *Neurocrit Care* 1:287–299, 2004.
12. Strandgaard S, Paulson OB: Cerebral blood flow and its pathophysiology in hypertension. *Am J Hypertens* 2:486–492, 1989.
13. Strandgaard S, Paulson OB. Cerebral autoregulation. *Stroke* 15:413–416, 1984.
14. Messerli FH, Ventura HO, Amodeo C: Osler's maneuver and pseudohypertension. *N Engl J Med* 312:1548–1551, 1985.
15. Hinchey J, Chaves C, Appignani B, et al: A reversible posterior leukoencephalopathy syndrome. *N Engl J Med* 334:494–500, 1996.
16. Cherney D, Straus S: Management of patients with hypertensive urgencies and emergencies: a systematic review of the literature. *J Gen Intern Med* 17:937–945, 2002.
17. Perez MI, Musini VM: Pharmacological interventions for hypertensive emergencies. *Cochrane Database Syst Rev* CD003653, 2008.
18. Antman EM, Anbe DT, Armstrong PW, et al: ACC/AHA guidelines for the management of patients with ST-elevation myocardial infarction—executive summary. A report of the American College of Cardiology/American Heart Association Task Force on Practice Guidelines (Writing Committee to revise the 1999 guidelines for the management of patients with acute myocardial infarction). *J Am Coll Cardiol* 44:671–719, 2004.
19. Hiratzka LF, Bakris GL, Beckman JA, et al: 2010 ACCF/AHA/AATS/ACR/ASA/SCA/SCAI/SIR/STS/SVM guidelines for the diagnosis and management of patients with thoracic aortic disease: a report of the American College of Cardiology Foundation/American Heart Association Task Force on Practice Guidelines, American Association for Thoracic Surgery, American College of Radiology, American Stroke Association, Society of Cardiovascular Anesthesiologists, Society for Cardiovascular Angiography and Interventions, Society of Interventional Radiology, Society of Thoracic Surgeons, and Society for Vascular Medicine. *Circulation* 121:e266–e369, 2010.
20. Jessup M, Abraham WT, Casey DE, et al: 2009 focused update: ACCF/AHA Guidelines for the Diagnosis and Management of Heart Failure in Adults: a report of the American College of Cardiology Foundation/American Heart Association Task Force on Practice Guidelines: developed in collaboration with the International Society for Heart and Lung Transplantation. *Circulation* 119:1977–2016, 2009.
21. Mancia G, De Backer G, Dominiczak A, et al: 2007 guidelines for the management of arterial hypertension: the Task Force for the Management of Arterial Hypertension of the European Society of Hypertension (ESH) and of the European Society of Cardiology (ESC). *Eur Heart J* 28:1462–1536, 2007.
22. Tsai TT, Nienaber CA, Eagle KA: Acute aortic syndromes. *Circulation* 112:3802–3813, 2005.
23. Rosei EA, Salvetti M, Farsang C: European Society of Hypertension Scientific Newsletter: treatment of hypertensive urgencies and emergencies. *J Hypertens* 24:2482–2485, 2006.
24. Adams HP Jr, del Zoppo G, Alberts MJ, et al: Guidelines for the early management of adults with ischemic stroke: a guideline from the American Heart Association/American Stroke Association Stroke Council, Clinical Cardiology Council, Cardiovascular Radiology and Intervention Council, and the Atherosclerotic Peripheral Vascular Disease and Quality of Care Outcomes in Research Interdisciplinary Working Groups: the American Academy of Neurology affirms the value of this guideline as an educational tool for neurologists. *Circulation* 115:e478–e534, 2007.
25. Bandera E, Botteri M, Minelli C, et al: Cerebral blood flow threshold of ischemic penumbra and infarct core in acute ischemic stroke: a systematic review. *Stroke* 37:1334–1339, 2006.
26. Bederson JB, Connolly ES Jr, Batjer HH, et al: Guidelines for the management of aneurysmal subarachnoid hemorrhage: a statement for healthcare professionals from a special writing group of the Stroke Council, American Heart Association. *Stroke* 40:994–1025, 2009.
27. Suarez JI, Tarr RW, Selman WR: Aneurysmal subarachnoid hemorrhage. *N Engl J Med* 354:387–396, 2006.
28. Rinkel GJ, Feigin VL, Algra A, et al: Calcium antagonists for aneurysmal subarachnoid haemorrhage. *Cochrane Database Syst Rev* CD000277, 2005.
29. Morgenstern LB, Hemphill JC, III, Anderson C, et al: Guidelines for the management of spontaneous intracerebral hemorrhage: a guideline for healthcare professionals from the American Heart Association/American Stroke Association. *Stroke* 41:2108–2129, 2010.
30. Fleisher LA, Beckman JA, Brown KA, et al: ACC/AHA 2007 guidelines on perioperative cardiovascular evaluation and care for noncardiac surgery: a report of the American College of Cardiology/American Heart Association Task Force on Practice Guidelines (Writing Committee to Revise the 2002 Guidelines on Perioperative Cardiovascular Evaluation for Noncardiac Surgery): developed in collaboration with the American Society of Echocardiography, American Society of Nuclear Cardiology, Heart Rhythm Society, Society of Cardiovascular Anesthesiologists, Society for Cardiovascular Angiography and Interventions, Society for Vascular Medicine and Biology, and Society for Vascular Surgery. *Circulation* 116:e418–e499, 2007.
31. Auerbach A, Goldman L: Assessing and reducing the cardiac risk of noncardiac surgery. *Circulation* 113:1361–1376, 2006.
32. Estafanous FG, Tarazi RC: Systemic arterial hypertension associated with cardiac surgery. *Am J Cardiol* 46:685–694, 1980.
33. St Andre AC, DelRossi A: Hemodynamic management of patients in the first 24 hours after cardiac surgery. *Crit Care Med* 33:2082–2093, 2005.
34. Haas CE, LeBlanc JM: Acute postoperative hypertension: a review of therapeutic options. *Am J Health Syst Pharm* 61:1661–1673, 2004; quiz 1674–1675.
35. Marik PE, Varon J: Hypertensive crises: challenges and management. *Chest* 131:1949–1962, 2007.
36. Perez M, Musini V, Wright J: Pharmacological interventions for hypertensive emergencies. *Cochrane Database Syst Rev* CD003653, 2008.
37. Varon J: Treatment of acute severe hypertension: current and newer agents. *Drugs* 68:283–297, 2008.
38. Grossman E, Messerli FH, Grodzicki T, et al: Should a moratorium be placed on sublingual nifedipine capsules given for hypertensive emergencies and pseudoemergencies? *JAMA* 276:1328–1331, 1996.
39. Neutel JM, Smith DH, Wallin D, et al: A comparison of intravenous nicardipine and sodium nitroprusside in the immediate treatment of severe hypertension. *Am J Hypertens* 7:623–628, 1994.
40. Aronson S, Dyke CM, Stierer KA, et al: The ECLIPSE trials: comparative studies of clevidipine to nitroglycerin, sodium nitroprusside, and nicardipine for acute hypertension treatment in cardiac surgery patients. *Anesth Analg* 107:1110–1121, 2008.
41. Bove T, Landoni G, Calabro MG, et al: Renoprotective action of fenoldopam in high-risk patients undergoing cardiac surgery: a prospective, double-blind, randomized clinical trial. *Circulation* 111:3230–3235, 2005.

CHAPTER 38 ■ UNSTABLE ANGINA/ NON–ST-SEGMENT ELEVATION MYOCARDIAL INFARCTION

SUZANNE J. BARON, CHRISTOPHER P. CANNON AND MARC S. SABATINE

The spectrum of acute coronary syndromes (ACS) ranges from unstable angina (UA) to non–ST-segment elevation myocardial infarction (NSTEMI) to ST-segment elevation myocardial infarction (STEMI) [1]. The latter condition is usually caused by acute total obstruction of a coronary artery [2,3], and urgent reperfusion is the mainstay of therapy. In contrast, the non–ST-segment elevation acute coronary syndromes (NSTEACS)—UA and NSTEMI—are usually associated with a severe, although nonocclusive, lesion in the culprit coronary artery [4].

Every year in the United States, approximately 1.3 million patients are admitted to the hospital with ACS; about 900,000 of these patients are suffering from UA/NSTEMI as compared with approximately 400,000 patients suffering from STEMI [5,6]. Worldwide, these numbers are each several times the totals in the United States. In the past few years, numerous advances have been made in the understanding of the pathophysiology, diagnosis, risk stratification, and management of UA/NSTEMI.

DEFINITION

The definition of UA is largely based on the clinical presentation. Angina pectoris is characterized by a poorly localized chest or arm discomfort or pressure (rarely described by patients as "pain") that is typically and reproducibly associated with physical exertion or emotional stress, and relieved by rest or sublingual nitroglycerin. UA is defined as angina pectoris (or equivalent type of ischemic discomfort) with one of three features: (a) occurring at rest (or with minimal exertion), usually lasting more than 20 minutes; (b) being severe and of new onset (i.e., within 1 month); or (c) occurring with a crescendo pattern (i.e., more severe, prolonged, or frequent) [7]. Some patients with this pattern of ischemic pain develop evidence of myocardial necrosis on the basis of serum biomarkers in the absence of ST-segment elevations on electrocardiogram (ECG) and thus have a diagnosis of NSTEMI. Previously, this diagnosis has been based on elevation of the creatine kinase (CK)-MB, but elevations in cardiac troponin T or I greater than the 99th percentile of the upper limit of normal now define MI on the basis of their higher sensitivity and specificity for myocardial necrosis and powerful prognostic capability [8].

PATHOPHYSIOLOGY

The development of UA/NSTEMI is due either to a reduction in the supply of blood flow and oxygen, or to an increase in myocardial oxygen demand, or both. The five broad etiologies are (a) plaque rupture with superimposed nonocclusive thrombus; (b) dynamic obstruction (i.e., coronary spasm); (c) progressive mechanical obstruction (i.e., restenosis); (d) inflammation and arteritis; and (e) conditions leading to increased myocardial oxygen demand, such as anemia, sepsis, or hypoxia [9]. Individual patients may have several of these processes contribute to the onset of their UA/NSTEMI.

Plaque Rupture

Atherosclerosis is a silent process that usually begins 20 to 30 years prior to a patient's clinical presentation [10,11]. Plaque rupture can be precipitated by multiple factors, including endothelial dysfunction [12], plaque lipid content [13], local inflammation [14], coronary artery tone at the site of irregular plaques and local shear stress forces, platelet function [15,16], and the status of the coagulation system (i.e., a potentially prothrombotic state) [17,18]. These processes culminate in formation of platelet-rich thrombi at the site of the plaque rupture or erosion and the resultant ACS [19–21].

Thrombosis

Coronary artery thrombosis plays a central role in the pathogenesis of UA/NSTEMI [4,19,20,22–26], as demonstrated in the Thrombolysis in Myocardial Infarction (TIMI) IIIA trial, in which 35% of patients had definite thrombus and an additional 40% had possible thrombus [4]. Thrombosis occurs in two interrelated stages: (a) primary hemostasis and (b) secondary hemostasis [27,28]. The first stage of hemostasis is initiated by platelets as they adhere to damaged vessels and form a platelet plug. With rupture or ulceration of an atherosclerotic plaque, the subendothelial matrix (e.g., collagen and tissue factor) is exposed to the circulating blood. Platelets then adhere to the subendothelial matrix via the glycoprotein (GP) Ib receptor and von Willebrand's factor (*platelet adhesion*). After adhering to the subendothelial matrix, the platelet undergoes a conformational change from a smooth discoid shape to a spiculated form, which increases the surface area on which thrombin generation can occur. This leads to degranulation of the alpha- and dense granules and the subsequent release of thromboxane A2, adenosine diphosphate (ADP), serotonin, and other platelet aggregatory and chemoattractant factors, as well as the expression and activation of GP IIb/IIIa receptors on the platelet surface such that it can bind fibrinogen. This process is called *platelet activation*. The final step is *platelet aggregation*, that is, the formation of the platelet plug. Fibrinogen (or von Willebrand's factor) binds to the activated GP IIb/IIIa receptors of two platelets, thereby creating a growing platelet aggregate. Antiplatelet therapy has been directed at decreasing the formation of thromboxane A2 (aspirin), inhibiting the ADP pathway of platelet activation (thienopyridines), and directly inhibiting platelet aggregation (GP IIb/IIIa inhibitors; Fig. 38.1).

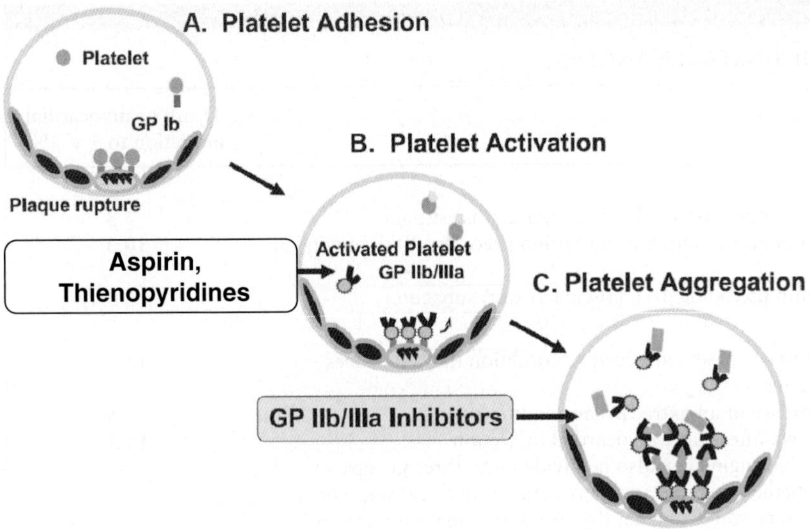

FIGURE 38.1. Primary hemostasis—process of platelet adhesion, activation, and aggregation. Platelets initiate thrombosis at the site of a ruptured plaque: the first step is *platelet adhesion* (**A**) via the glycoprotein (GP) Ib receptor in conjunction with von Willebrand's factor. This is followed by *platelet activation* (**B**), which leads to a shape change in the platelet, degranulation of the alpha and dense granules, and expression of GP IIb/IIIa receptors on the platelet surface with activation of the receptor, such that it can bind fibrinogen. The final step is *platelet aggregation* (**C**), in which fibrinogen (or von Willebrand's factor) binds to the activated GP IIb/IIIa receptors of two platelets. Aspirin (ASA) and clopidogrel act to decrease platelet activation (see text for details), whereas the GP IIb/IIIa inhibitors inhibit the final step of platelet aggregation. [Adapted from Cannon CP, Braunwald E: Unstable angina, in Braunwald E, Zipes DP, Libby P (eds): *Heart Disease: A Textbook of Cardiovascular Medicine*. 6th ed. Philadelphia, WB Saunders, 2001, pp 1232–1263, with permission.]

Secondary Hemostasis

Simultaneous with the formation of the platelet plug, the plasma coagulation system is activated (Fig. 38.2). Following plaque rupture, the injured endothelial cells on the vessel wall become activated and release *protein disulfide isomerase*, which acts to cause a conformational change in circulating tissue factor [29–32]. Tissue factor can then bind to factor VIIa and form a protein complex, leading to the activation of factor X. With the activation of factor X (to factor Xa), thrombin is generated and acts to cleave fibrinogen to form fibrin. Thrombin plays a central role in arterial thrombosis: (a) it converts fibrinogen to fibrin in the final common pathway for clot formation; (b) it is a powerful stimulus for platelet aggregation; and (c) it activates factor XIII, which leads to cross-linking and stabilization of the fibrin clot [27].

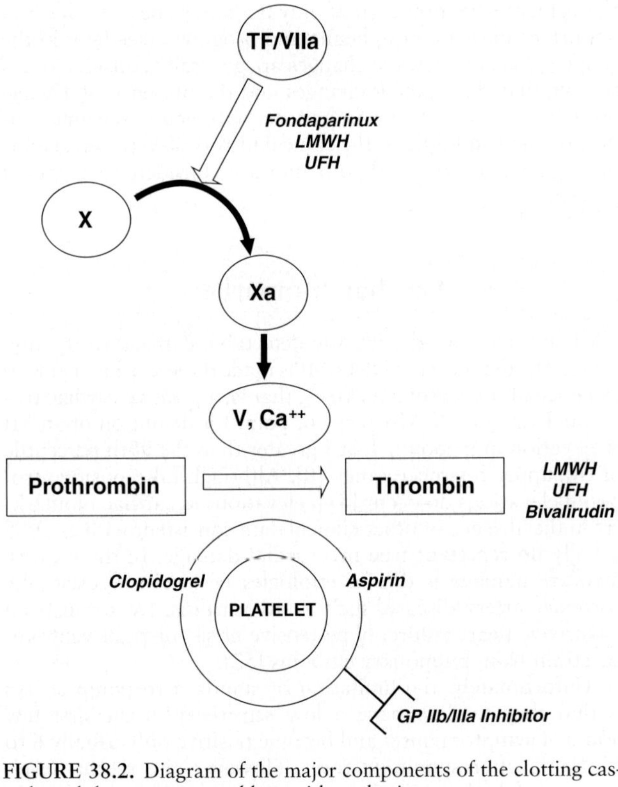

FIGURE 38.2. Diagram of the major components of the clotting cascade and the areas targeted by antithrombotic agents.

Coronary Vasoconstriction

Another etiologic factor in UA/NSTEMI is dynamic obstruction, that is, coronary vasoconstriction. The process is identified in three settings: (a) vasospasm in the absence of obstructive plaque, (b) vasoconstriction in the setting of atherosclerotic plaque, and (c) microcirculatory angina. Vasospasm can occur in patients without coronary atherosclerosis or in those with a nonobstructive atheromatous plaque. Vasospastic angina appears to be due to hypercontractility of vascular smooth muscle and endothelial dysfunction occurring in the region of spasm. Prinzmetal's variant angina, with intense focal spasm of a segment of an epicardial coronary artery, is the prototypic example [33]. Such patients have rest pain accompanied by transient ST-segment elevation. Vasoconstriction more commonly occurs in the setting of significant coronary atherosclerotic plaque, especially those with superimposed thrombus. Vasoconstriction can occur as the result of local vasoconstrictors released from platelets, such as serotonin and thromboxane A2 [34–36]. Vasoconstriction can also result from a dysfunctional coronary endothelium, which has reduced production of nitric oxide and increased release of endothelin. Adrenergic stimuli, cold immersion [37], cocaine [38,39], or mental stress [40] can also cause coronary vasoconstriction in susceptible vessels. A third setting in which vasoconstriction is identified is microcirculatory angina ("syndrome X"). In this condition, ischemia results from constriction of the small intramural coronary resistance vessels [41]. Although no epicardial coronary artery stenoses are present, coronary flow is usually slowed and does not increase appropriately in response to a variety of signals.

Progressive Mechanical Obstruction

Another etiology of UA/NSTEMI results from progressive luminal narrowing. This is most commonly seen in the setting of restenosis following percutaneous coronary intervention (PCI). However, angiographic [42] and atherectomy studies [43,44] have demonstrated that many patients without previous PCI show progressive luminal narrowing of the culprit vessel, likely related to rapid cellular proliferation, in the period preceding the onset of UA/NSTEMI.

TABLE 38.1

BRAUNWALD CLINICAL CLASSIFICATION OF UNSTABLE ANGINA

Class	Definition	Death or myocardial infarction to 1 y[a] (%)
Severity		
Class I	New onset of severe angina or accelerated angina; no rest pain	7.3
Class II	Angina at rest within past month but not within preceding 48 h (angina at rest, subacute)	10.3
Class III	Angina at rest within preceding 48 h (angina at rest, subacute)	10.8[b]
Clinical circumstances		
A (secondary angina)	Develops in the presence of an extracardiac condition that intensifies myocardial ischemia	14.1
B (primary angina)	Develops in the absence of an extracardiac condition	8.5
C (postinfarction angina)	Develops within 2 wk after acute myocardial infarction	18.5[c]
Intensity of treatment	Patients with unstable angina can also be divided into three groups depending on whether unstable angina occurs: (a) in the absence of treatment for chronic stable angina, (b) during treatment for chronic stable angina, or (c) despite maximal anti-ischemic drug therapy. These three groups can be designated subscripts 1, 2, or 3, respectively	—
Electrocardiographic changes	Patients with unstable angina can be further divided into those with or without transient ST-T–wave changes during pain	—

[a]Data from Scirica BM, Cannon CP, McCabe CH, et al: Prognosis in the thrombolysis in myocardial ischemia III registry according to the Braunwald unstable angina pectoris classification. *Am J Cardiol* 90(8):821, 2002.
[b]$p = 0.057$.
[c]$p < 0.001$.
Reprinted from Braunwald E: Unstable angina: a classification. *Circulation* 80:410, 1989, with permission.

Secondary Unstable Angina

Secondary UA is defined as UA precipitated by conditions extrinsic to the coronary arteries in patients with prior coronary stenosis and chronic stable angina. This change could occur either as a result of an increase in myocardial oxygen demand or as a decrease in coronary blood flow. Conditions that increase myocardial demand include tachycardia (e.g., a supraventricular tachycardia or new-onset atrial fibrillation with rapid ventricular response), fever, thyrotoxicosis, hyperadrenergic states, and elevations of left ventricular (LV) afterload, such as hypertension or aortic stenosis. Secondary UA can also occur as a result of impaired oxygen delivery, as in anemia, hypoxemia (e.g., due to pneumonia or congestive heart failure), hyperviscosity states, or hypotension. Although one might expect secondary angina to be associated with a more favorable prognosis, it appears to have a worse prognosis than primary UA [45] (Table 38.1), likely due to serious patient comorbidities.

CLINICAL PRESENTATION AND DIAGNOSIS

History and Physical Examination

A description of "ischemic pain" is the hallmark of UA/NSTEMI. Ischemic chest pain is usually described as a discomfort or pressure (rarely as a pain) that is brought on by exertion and relieved by rest. It is generally located in the retrosternal region but sometimes in the epigastrium and frequently radiates to the anterior neck, left shoulder, and left arm. The physical examination may be unremarkable or may support the diagnosis of cardiac ischemia [46]. Signs that suggest ischemia are sweatiness, pale cool skin, sinus tachycardia, a fourth heart sound, and basilar rales on lung examination.

Electrocardiogram

The ECG is the most widely used tool in the evaluation of ischemic heart disease. In UA/NSTEMI, ST-segment depression (or transient ST-segment elevation) and T-wave changes occur in up to 50% of patients [47–49]. Two analyses have shown ST-segment deviation even of only 0.5 mm to be a specific and important measure of ischemia and prognosis (see later in the chapter) [47,50]. T-wave changes are generally considered less specific than ST-segment changes and the presence of T-wave inversions of only 1 mm in patients with acute ischemic syndromes may add little to the clinical history. T-wave inversions of greater than or equal to 3 mm are considered significant [47,50].

Cardiac Biomarkers

UA is not associated with any detectable damage to the myocyte. The diagnosis of NSTEMI is made if there is biochemical evidence of myocardial necrosis, that is, a positive cardiac troponin T or I or CK-MB. The cut point for definition of an MI is elevation in troponin T or I greater than the 99th percentile of the upper reference range [8]. Although false-positive troponin elevations do occur [51], elevations in cardiac biomarkers in the absence of other clinical data consistent with an ACS usually do represent true myocardial damage. In these cases, myocyte damage is due to etiologies besides atherosclerotic coronary artery disease, such as myocarditis, LV strain from congestive heart failure, hypertensive crisis, or right ventricular strain from pulmonary embolus [52].

Unfortunately, the limitation of standard troponin assays is that they tend to have a low sensitivity in the first few hours of symptom onset and become positive only usually 6 to 12 hours after symptom onset. However, the recent development of high-sensitivity troponin assays has significantly improved the sensitivity of this test. Two recent studies have found that the use of high-sensitivity assays improve the early diagnosis of MI with sensitivity now exceeding 90% when tested in patients with chest pain at the time of presentation to the hospital [53,54]. Moreover, high-sensitivity assays can detect elevated levels of troponin in approximately 10% of outpatients with stable coronary disease, and these individuals are at a higher risk of subsequent cardiovascular death [55].

Ultrasensitive troponin assays, which have limits of detection lesser than the levels seen in a normal reference population, are also being developed. In a study looking at patients with NSTEACS, 72% of patients with NSTEMI were found to have circulating troponin levels at baseline greater than the 99th percentile (nano-cTnI >0.003 μg/L) when ultrasensitive troponin assays were utilized; yet all of these patients had an initially negative current-generation troponin assay. When these assays were used in patients presenting with UA (defined as lack of elevation of troponin using a current-generation commercial assay), 44% of patients had circulating troponin levels greater than the 99th percentile and 8 hours later, the percentage had risen to 82% [56]. Similarly, ultrasensitive assays have been used to detect rises in circulating troponin in proportion to the amount of ischemia experienced during exercise stress testing [57]. Thus, in the future, troponin may move from a semiquantitative assay ("negative" in most individuals and quantified in a subset) to quantifiable in all patients. The clinical implications of very low level values reported from ultrasensitive assays will need to be defined.

Cardiac Imaging

Currently, cardiac imaging is assuming increasing importance in the early diagnosis of patients presenting with suspected UA/NSTEMI, especially when the ECG is normal, nonspecific, or obscured by left bundle branch block or a paced rhythm. Myocardial perfusion imaging using technetium sestamibi has been useful for patients presenting with chest pain in the emergency department without a diagnostic ECG or positive biomarkers to discriminate patients with coronary artery disease from those with noncardiac chest pain [58,59]. Similarly, echocardiography is useful to screen for regional or global LV dysfunction, which may help in establishing (or excluding) the diagnosis of ischemic heart disease in patients who present to the emergency department with chest pain [60]. Coronary computed tomography angiogram (CTA) has also been shown to be effective in excluding coronary artery disease in patients presenting to the emergency department with a low-risk story of chest pain, nondiagnostic ECG, and negative biomarkers [61]. All of these modalities can also assess LV function, a powerful determinant of subsequent prognosis after MI (and presumably after UA) [62–64]. Coronary angiography is also used to establish the diagnosis of ACS and is considered the gold-standard modality to define the extent of coronary disease, and as a prelude to percutaneous revascularization (see later in the chapter) [4,48,65,66].

RISK STRATIFICATION

Given the multitude of treatment options for patients with UA/NSTEMI, risk stratification currently refers to two simultaneous processes (frequently carried out at the time of hospital presentation): (a) risk assessment (i.e., prediction of mortality/morbidity risk), and (b) selection of a management strategy (i.e., an early invasive vs. early conservative approach).

Risk assessment, using clinical and laboratory markers, identifies which patients are at highest risk for adverse outcomes. Moreover, data from several trials have demonstrated that early risk assessment (especially using troponins) has also been useful in predicting which patients will derive the greatest benefit from newer and more potent antithrombotic therapies, such as low-molecular-weight heparin (LMWH) and GP IIb/IIIa inhibitors. Risk assessment can similarly be used to determine the most appropriate level of care and monitoring (i.e., between the coronary intensive care unit or the step-down/telemetry unit). The "management strategy" refers to whether early angiography is performed with revascularization as appropriate directly following the index event or whether a conservative or ischemia-driven strategy is carried out, with noninvasive assessment of residual ischemia, and angiography and revascularization performed only if recurrent ischemia is documented (see later in the chapter).

Risk Assessment Using Clinical Predictors

The initial clinical evaluation can be used to risk-stratify patients quickly and assist in the triage [67,68]. As described in the ACC/AHA UA/NSTEMI guideline (Table 38.2), high-risk patients can be identified by the presence of prolonged, ongoing pain at rest, ST-segment depression of greater than or equal to 0.1 mV, positive troponin value, or the presence of hypotension or congestive heart failure on physical examination [67]. Such patients should be considered for the coronary care unit although the cardiac step-down (telemetry) unit may be adequate depending on the clinical situation. Lower risk patients can be adequately monitored and managed in a step-down unit.

Individual High-Risk Subgroups

Trials have identified several clinical subgroups that are at higher risk of adverse outcomes when they present with UA/NSTEMI. These groups derive greater benefit from more aggressive therapy.

Elderly Patients

Elderly patients comprise a subgroup for which outcomes are always worse compared with younger patients. In UA/NSTEMI, elderly patients appear to derive greater benefit from the newer, more potent antithrombotic therapies. In the Efficacy and Safety of Subcutaneous Enoxaparin in Non-Q-Wave Coronary Events (ESSENCE) trial, enoxaparin had greater benefit in patients 65 years or older as compared with younger patients [69]; a similar finding was noted in the TIMI 11B trial [70]. For the GP IIb/IIIa inhibitors, an equivalent relative benefit was observed in older versus younger patients, although the absolute benefit in number of events prevented is higher in elderly patients because they have higher baseline risk [49,71,72]. However, this increase in absolute benefit comes with the added price of an increased incidence of bleeding with GP IIb/IIIa inhibitors in elderly patients [71,72]. With regard to an invasive versus conservative management strategy, patients 65 years or older have better outcomes at 1 year when managed with an invasive strategy (12.5% vs. 19.5%; $p = 0.03$; age interaction $p = 0.04$) [73]. Similarly, in Fragmin and Fast Revascularization during Instability in Coronary Artery Disease (FRISC) II, and Treat Angina with Aggrastat and Determine Cost of Therapy with an Invasive or Conservative Strategy (TACTICS)-TIMI 18, there was a greater absolute benefit of an early invasive strategy in patients 65 years and older [74,75]. Thus, in UA/NSTEMI, elderly patients are at higher risk and derive particular benefit from more aggressive antithrombotic and interventional therapy.

TABLE 38.2

CLINICAL FEATURES ASSOCIATED WITH HIGHER LIKELIHOOD OF CORONARY ARTERY DISEASE AMONG PATIENTS PRESENTING WITH SYMPTOMS SUGGESTIVE OF UNSTABLE ANGINA

Feature	High likelihood (any below)	Intermediate likelihood (no high-likelihood features, but any below)	Low likelihood (no high- or intermediate-likelihood features, but may have any below)
History	History of crescendo symptoms in prior 48 h	Prior history of CAD, PAD, or CVA Prior aspirin use	
Character of pain	Ischemic chest pain that is prolonged (>20 min), ongoing, and occurring at rest	Ischemic, prolonged chest pain that is now resolved Nocturnal angina	Atypical chest pain not consistent with cardiac chest pain
Examination	Age >75 y Signs of CHF (pulmonary edema on CXR; rales and/or S3 on examination) Hypotension New or worsening MR murmur	Age >70 y	
ECG	Angina at rest with transient ST-segment changes >0.5 mm Sustained VT	T-wave changes Pathological Q-waves Resting ST-segment depressions <1 mm	Normal ECG
Cardiac markers	Positive	Normal	Normal

CAD, coronary artery disease; CHF, congestive heart failure; CVA, cardiovascular accident; CXR, chest X-ray; DM, diabetes mellitus; ECG, electrocardiogram; MR, mitral regurgitation; PAD, peripheral arterial disease; VT, ventricular tachycardia.
Adapted from Anderson JL, Adams CD, Antman EM, et al: ACC/AHA 2007 guidelines for the management of patients with unstable angina/non-ST-segment elevation myocardial infarction-2002: executive summary: a report of the American College of Cardiology/American Heart Association Task Force on Practice Guidelines (Writing Committee to Revise the 2002 Guidelines for Management of Patients With Unstable Angina/Non-ST-Segment Elevation Myocardial Infarction). *Circulation* 116:803–877, 2007.

Gender Differences

A patient's gender may factor into the decision regarding which treatment strategy to pursue in patients presenting with UA/NSTEMI. Subgroup analyses from some trials, including FRISC II [76], Randomized Intervention Treatment of Angina (RITA) 3 [77], and Organization to Assess Strategies for Ischemic Syndromes (OASIS) 5 [78], suggested that an early invasive strategy may be associated with a higher risk of death or MI in women, whereas other studies demonstrated that an early invasive strategy resulted in improved outcomes in women as well as men [79]. Because subgroup analyses may be insufficiently powered to address this question, a meta-analysis was performed using the data of eight large-scale trials. This meta-analysis demonstrated that high-risk women (classified as patients with positive biomarkers on presentation) had a 33% lower odds of death, MI or rehospitalization with ACS (OR 0.67) with an invasive strategy, whereas low-risk women (patients with normal biomarkers on presentation) did not have a significant benefit with invasive treatment [80]. These findings are reflected in the 2007 AHA/ACC guidelines for the management of patients with UA/NSTEMI, which recommend that women with high-risk features be considered for invasive treatment, whereas women with low-risk features be treated conservatively [67].

Patients with Diabetes

Patients with diabetes have long been known to be at higher risk than those without diabetes for adverse outcomes with ACS. In a large-scale meta-analysis, patients with diabetes were found to have a significantly higher mortality at 30 days (2.1% vs. 1.1%; $p < 0.001$). Furthermore, having diabetes at presentation with an NSTEMI was associated with a higher mortality at 1 year as well (hazard ratio [HR] 1.65; 95% confidence interval [CI] 1.3 to 2.1) [81].

Given the high risk of adverse cardiovascular outcomes associated with diabetes, researchers have looked to see if certain treatment strategies may be of more benefit in this particular subgroup. The relative benefit of early GP IIb/IIIa inhibition has been found to be significantly higher in patients with diabetes, with a 70% relative reduction in events ($p = 0.002$) [82], as compared with a 30% reduction in the overall population. More recently, a meta-analysis of all placebo-controlled, IIb/IIIa inhibitor trials found a mortality benefit of early IIb/IIIa inhibition in patients with diabetes, with no mortality difference in those without nondiabetes [83]. For an invasive versus conservative strategy, the relative benefit in patients with diabetes of an early invasive strategy was similar to that of those without diabetes, but the absolute benefit was higher among those with diabetes [84]. Similarly in the Trial to Assess Improvement in Therapeutic Outcomes by Optimizing Platelet Inhibition with Prasugrel - Thrombolysis in Myocardial Infarction (TRITON-TIMI) 38 trial, patients with diabetes had a 40% reduction in MI (8.2% vs. 13.2%; $p < 0.001$) with the use of more intensive antiplatelet therapy with prasugrel when compared to clopidogrel. Those without diabetes saw only an 18% reduction in MI with prasugrel (7.2% vs. 8.7%; $p = 0.009$) [85]. Thus, patients with diabetes represent a high-risk group that deserves aggressive pharmacologic and revascularization treatments.

Risk Assessment by Electrocardiography

The admission ECG is very useful in predicting long-term adverse outcomes. In the TIMI III registry of patients with

UA/NSTEMI, multivariable predictors of 1-year death or MI included left bundle branch block and ST-segment deviation of 0.5 mm or greater [47]. The presence of only 0.5-mm ST-segment depression on the admission ECG has also been found to be an independent determinant of 4-year survival [50]. In contrast, the presence of T-wave changes was associated with only a modest [50] or no increase in subsequent death or MI risk compared with no ECG changes [47]. Similar findings were observed in predicting 30-day and 6-month outcomes in the Global Use of Strategies to Open Occluded Coronary Arteries (GUSTO) IIb study, with the presence of ST-segment deviation of greater than 0.5 mm conferring a higher mortality than T-wave changes [86].

With regard to relative treatment benefit of particular therapies, in the ESSENCE trial, patients with ST-segment deviation treated with enoxaparin had a significant reduction in cardiac events compared with patients treated with unfractionated heparin (UFH; odds ratio [OR] 0:60; $p < 0.01$), whereas those without ST-segment deviation did not [87]. Similar findings were observed in the TIMI 11B trial [70]. In both the FRISC II and TACTICS-TIMI 18 trials, an invasive strategy had a particular benefit in patients with ST-segment depression at presentation [84,88]. Thus, not only ST-segment deviation is a marker of increased risk of adverse outcomes, but it also indicates those patients who may derive greater benefit from aggressive antithrombotic and interventional therapy.

Risk Assessment by Cardiac Markers

Creatine Kinase-MB and the Troponins

Patients with NSTEMI have a worse long-term prognosis than those with UA [73,89]. It has now been shown that patients with elevated troponins, even if their CK-MB is normal, also have a significantly worse prognosis, with a higher risk of subsequent cardiac complications, including mortality [90–92]. Beyond just a positive versus negative test result, there is a linear relationship between the level of troponin T or I in the blood and subsequent risk of death: the higher the troponin, the higher the mortality risk (Fig. 38.3). Furthermore, elevated markers (both troponin T and CK-MB) have been shown to correlate with a higher rate of thrombus at angiography [4,93–96]. Thus, cardiac biomarkers are very useful not only in diagnosing infarction [97] but also in assessing risk for patients who present with acute UA/NSTEMI.

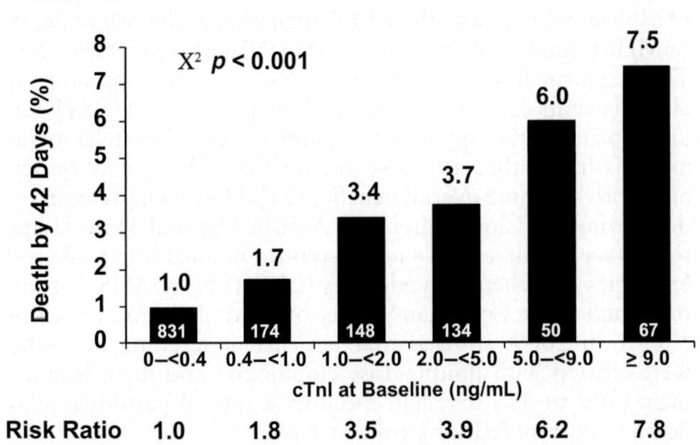

FIGURE 38.3. TIMI IIIB: a direct relationship was observed between increasing levels of troponin I and a higher 42-day mortality. cTnI, cardiac specific troponin I; Ng, negative. [Adapted from Antman EM, Tanasijevic MJ, Thompson B, et al: Cardiac-specific troponin I levels to predict the risk of mortality in patients with acute coronary syndromes. *N Engl J Med* 335:1342–1349, 1996, with permission.]

The presence of elevated biomarkers also correlates with the utility of particular therapies. In a trial examining the benefit of abciximab in patients with NSTEMI, the reduction in death or MI at 6 months was 70% in those who were troponin T positive, whereas there was no significant benefit for those who were troponin T negative ($p < 0.001$) [98] (Fig. 38.4, *left*). These findings have been duplicated with tirofiban versus heparin in the Platelet Receptor Inhibition for Ischemic Syndrome Management (PRISM) (Fig. 38.4, *right*) and PRISM in Patients Limited by Unstable Signs and Symptoms (PRISM-PLUS) trials [99,100] and more recently in the Intracoronary Stenting and Antithrombotic Regimen-Rapid Early Action for Coronary Treatment 2 (ISAR-REACT 2) trials [96]. In the TIMI 11B trial, even when looking at patients who were CK-MB negative, those who were troponin I positive derived a significantly greater benefit from the enoxaparin versus UFH, compared with those who had both markers negative [101]. Research has also demonstrated that biomarkers are useful when choosing an invasive versus conservative strategy in patients with UA/NSTEMI. In both the FRISC II and TACTICS-TIMI 18 trials, patients who had a positive troponin T or I (including those who had very low levels of troponin) had a dramatic reduction in cardiac events after allocation to an invasive strategy [91,102]. Thus, there is now evidence from multiple trials that the use of troponins can assist in both assessing the risk and determining which patients should be treated with newer antithrombotic agents and an invasive management strategy.

Other Biomarkers

Patients with an elevated C-reactive protein (CRP) have an increased risk of death and adverse cardiovascular events [103,104]. Even among patients with negative troponin I at baseline, CRP is able to discriminate high- and low-risk groups [105]. Recently, CRP levels have been shown to significantly add to low-density lipoprotein (LDL) levels in predicting recurrent adverse cardiovascular events in patients' post-ACS [106]. B-type natriuretic peptide (BNP) as well as N-terminal probrain natriuretic peptide (NT-proBNP), both biomarkers of LV wall stress, have also been shown to be a powerful predictor of mortality and heart failure in patients with NSTEMIs [107–110]. More recently, studies involving growth-differentiation factor 15 (GDF-15), a molecule that is induced by inflammation and cellular injury, have shown this molecule to be a similarly powerful predictor of adverse cardiovascular outcomes after NSTEMI [111]. Researchers have even suggested that GDF-15 may be able to direct treatment strategies after NSTEMI. A retrospective study looking at GDF-15 levels in patients with NSTEMI found that patients with markedly elevated GDF-15 levels had lower mortality when an invasive treatment strategy was used as opposed to conservative management [112]. Larger prospective studies are needed to see if GDF-15 will be a useful tool when deciding on the management of patients with NSTEMI. Multimarker strategies have also been employed to improve risk stratification. When using CRP and troponin T together, mortality is 0.4% for patients with both markers negative, 4.7% if either CRP or troponins are positive, and 9.1% if both are positive [105]. Similarly, the combination of troponin, CRP, and BNP can predict up to a 13-fold gradient in mortality post-ACS [113]. It should be noted that although CRP and BNP can be used as prognostic indicators, only troponin and potentially GDF-15 can identify patients who may derive greater benefit from specific interventions.

Combined Risk Assessment Scores

The TIMI risk score uses clinical factors, the ECG, and cardiac markers. It was developed using multivariate analysis, which identified seven risk factors: age 65 years or older, more than

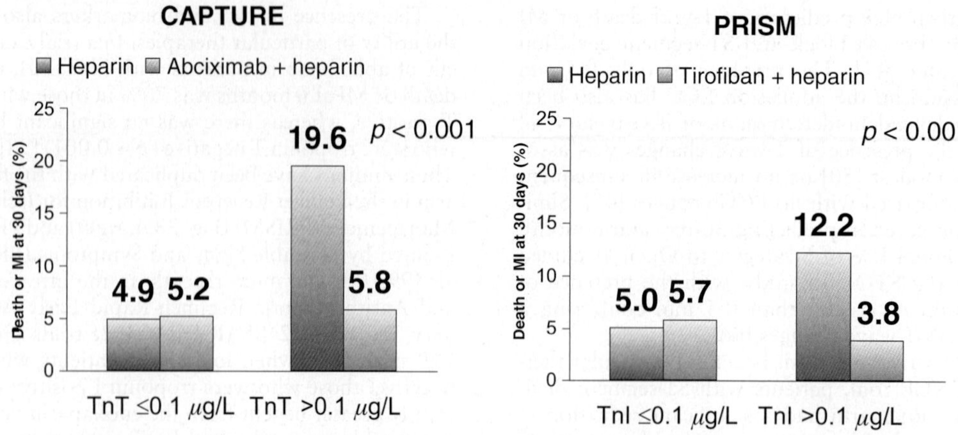

FIGURE 38.4. Use of troponin to determine benefit of GP IIb/IIIa inhibition. Benefit of abciximab in the CAPTURE trial of patients with refractory unstable angina treated with angioplasty in those with positive versus negative troponin T at study entry (*left panel*). Greater benefit of tirofiban versus heparin in patients with UA/NSTEMI was also seen in patients with positive troponin I values in the PRISM trial, with a nearly 70% reduction in death or MI at 30 days with the IIb/IIIa inhibitor (*right panel*). [Data from Hamm CW, Heeschen C, Goldmann B, et al: Benefit of abciximab in patients with refractory unstable angina in relation to serum troponin T levels. *N Engl J Med* 340(21):1623–1629, 1999; and Heeschen C, Hamm CW, Goldmann B, et al: Troponin concentrations for stratification of patients with acute coronary syndromes in relation to therapeutic efficacy of tirofiban. *Lancet* 354(9192):1757–1762, 1999, with permission.]

three risk factors for coronary artery disease, documented coronary artery disease at catheterization, ST-segment deviation of 0.5 mm or greater, more than two episodes of angina in the past 24 hours, aspirin use within prior week, or elevated serum cardiac markers. Use of this scoring system was able to risk-stratify patients across a 10-fold gradient of risk, from 4.7% to 40.9% ($p < 0.001$) [114]. Most importantly, this risk score identified patients who derived the greatest benefit from enoxaparin versus UFH [114], from use of a GP IIb/IIIa inhibitor [115], and from an early invasive management strategy [84].

The GRACE (Global Registry of Acute Coronary Events) risk score also utilized multiple variables to identify those patients who would be at greatest risk of death in the 6 months following an ACS. Those variables that conferred the greatest risk included older age, prior history of congestive heart failure or MI, elevated heart rate and relative hypotension at presentation, the presence of ST-segment depressions, elevated serum creatinine at presentation, elevated cardiac biomarkers, and lack of in-hospital PCI [116]. When applied to patients with NSTEMI, the GRACE risk score is also able to identify those patients who will benefit most from an early invasive strategy. In the Timing of Intervention in Patients with Acute Coronary Syndromes (TIMACS) trial, NSTEMI patients with a GRACE risk score of greater than 140 had a reduction of 35% in the primary end point (composite of death, MI, or stroke) with early coronary angiography when compared to delayed intervention of greater than 36 hours (13.9% vs. 21%; $p = 0.006$). In patients with a GRACE risk score of less than 140, there was no difference between the two groups (7.6% vs. 6.7%; $p = 0.48$) [117]. Therefore, combined risk assessment scores can not only identify those patients at the highest risk for an adverse cardiovascular event, but can also assist the clinician in management decisions regarding angiography and medication choices.

MEDICAL THERAPY

Treatment Goals

The treatment objectives for patients with UA/NSTEMI are focused on stabilizing and "passivating" the acute coronary lesion, treatment of residual ischemia, and long-term secondary prevention. Antithrombotic therapy (e.g., aspirin, P_2Y_{12} ADP receptor blockers such as clopidogrel, anticoagulants, and GP IIb/IIIa inhibitors) is used to prevent further clotting in the coronary artery and allow endogenous fibrinolysis to dissolve the thrombus and reduce the degree of coronary stenosis. Antithrombotic therapy is continued long term so that if future events occur, the degree of thrombosis is reduced. Anti-ischemic therapies (e.g., beta-blockers, nitrates, and calcium antagonists) are used to reduce myocardial oxygen demand. Coronary revascularization is frequently needed to treat recurrent or residual ischemia. After stabilization of the acute event, the many factors that led up to the event need to be reversed. Treatment of atherosclerotic risk factors such as hypercholesterolemia, hypertension, and cessation of smoking, which contributes to stabilization of the cholesterol-laden plaque and healing of the endothelium, is critical.

Aspirin

Several major studies have demonstrated clear beneficial effects of aspirin, with a more than 50% reduction in the risk of death or MI in patients who present with UA/NSTEMI [89,118–120]. Thus, aspirin has had a dramatic effect in reducing adverse clinical events early in the course of treatment of UA/NSTEMI, and is primary therapy for these patients. An antiplatelet meta-analysis found that any dose greater than 75 mg was associated with the same overall benefit [121]. However, preliminary data from the Clopidogrel and Aspirin Optimal Dose Usage to Reduce Recurrent Events - Seventh Organization to Assess Strategies in Ischemic Syndromes (CURRENT-OASIS 7) trial, presented at the European Society of Cardiology Annual Conference in 2009, showed that patients undergoing PCI who were treated with double-dose clopidogrel and high-dose aspirin (300 to 325 mg) had the lowest rate of cardiovascular death, recurrent MI, or stroke at 1 year.

Bleeding is the main side effect of aspirin, and the rate of gastrointestinal (GI) bleeding appears to be higher with higher doses [121]. Data from the Clopidogrel in Unstable Angina to Prevent Recurrent Events (CURE) trial have shown that doses of 75 to 100 mg have a 50% lower rate of major bleeding (2.0% at 1 year) compared with doses of 200 to 325 mg (4.0% at

1 year); thus, a dose of 75 to 81 mg per day could be the optimal dose for long-term therapy. For acute treatment peri-PCI, a dose of 325 mg is generally used. Absolute contraindications to aspirin include documented aspirin allergy (e.g., asthma or anaphylaxis), active bleeding, or a known platelet disorder. In patients with more minor intolerance to long-term aspirin therapy (e.g., dyspepsia), short-term use of aspirin is recommended on the basis of the large early benefit. However, clopidogrel is a recommended alternative to aspirin for patients who cannot tolerate aspirin [67].

P_2Y_{12} ADP Receptor Blockers

Clopidogrel is a thienopyridine derivative that inhibits platelet activation and aggregation by inhibiting the binding of ADP to the P_2Y_{12} receptor on the surface of the platelet. In the CURE trial, 12,562 patients with UA/NSTEMI were randomized to receive aspirin alone (75 to 325 mg per day) or aspirin plus clopidogrel (300-mg loading dose and then 75 mg per day) [122]. The primary end point of cardiovascular death, MI, or stroke was reduced by 20% (11.4% control vs. 9.3% clopidogrel; $p < 0.0001$) [122]. The reduction was seen in all subgroups, including patients with ST-segment depression, those without ST-segment changes, and those with positive or negative markers. Interestingly, patients with positive cardiac markers and those with negative markers had similar 20% reductions in the primary end point. The combination of clopidogrel plus aspirin was associated with a relative 35% increase in major bleeding (using the CURE trial definition), but the absolute increase was only 1% (from 2.7% to 3.7%). Furthermore, using the standard TIMI definition of bleeding, there was no significant increase in major bleeding risk and no increase in intracranial hemorrhage. In patients who went on to PCI, a significant 30% reduction was observed through follow-up [123]. The Kaplan–Meier event rates began to show a reduction in events starting just 2 hours after randomization. In addition, when analyzing the benefit in the first 30 days versus after 30 days, there was a similar 20% relative risk reduction during both time periods. Thus, it appears that clopidogrel afforded both an early and an ongoing benefit out to 1 year.

When to start clopidogrel in patients with UA/NSTEMI remains a matter of debate. Even with a loading dose, it takes several hours before significant antiplatelet effects emerge. For this reason, the notion of pretreatment with clopidogrel at least several hours prior to the PCI has emerged as a possible means to help ensure that sufficient platelet inhibition is in effect at the start of the PCI. Because clopidogrel, like aspirin, is an irreversible platelet inhibitor, its antiplatelet effect will last for several days after discontinuation. If a patient is found to require surgical revascularization, the procedure should then be put off for several days. The guidelines remained silent on the timing of clopidogrel. However, across the spectrum of ACS, data have emerged that pretreatment with clopidogrel before a patient undergoes PCI significantly reduces the risk of death and ischemic complications post-PCI [123–125]. Thus, the most recent PCI guidelines now recommend clopidogrel pretreatment before PCI, but they also continue to acknowledge that treatment before coronary anatomy is defined remains controversial [126].

Several pharmacogenetic and drug–drug interactions for clopidogrel are notable and can affect patient outcomes. Clopidogrel is a prodrug that requires hepatic biotransformation by CYP450 enzymes into an active metabolite. Approximately 25% to 30% of the population has a reduced-function genetic variant of *CYP2C19*, a member of the CYP450 enzyme family. When treated with clopidogrel, these individuals have lower circulating levels of the clopidogrel active metabolite, thereby leading to less platelet inhibition, and a higher rate of ischemic events including stent thrombosis [127–129].

Metabolism of clopidogrel may also be affected by certain drugs. Some studies had suggested an interaction between clopidogrel and proton pump inhibitors (PPIs), such as omeprazole. Initial data, gathered retrospectively from large registries, suggested that patients treated with both clopidogrel and a PPI had worse outcomes than did patients treated with clopidogrel alone [130]. On discovering this result, researchers began to investigate possible mechanisms to explain this interaction. Indeed, they found that some PPIs have been shown to be inhibitors of the enzyme, *CYP2C19*, and they subsequently hypothesized that simultaneous administration of PPIs and clopidogrel may lead to competitive metabolism by *CYP2C19*, thereby leading to decreased clopidogrel activity. This hypothesis was initially supported by a recent study, which demonstrated that dual administration of clopidogrel and a PPI resulted in reduced platelet inhibition when compared to just clopidogrel alone [131]. However, analysis of data from a clinical cohort of the TRITON-TIMI 38 trial demonstrated no association between PPI use and clinical outcomes in patients on clopidogrel [132]. The safety of the combination of clopidogrel and omeprazole was further demonstrated in the Clopidogrel and the Optimization of Gastrointestinal Events Trial (COGENT), which was recently presented at the 21st Annual Transcatheter Cardiovascular Therapeutics (TCT) Scientific Symposium in 2009. This study randomized patients to clopidogrel alone or a combination pill of clopidogrel plus omeprazole following PCI and they found no difference in cardiovascular outcomes over 4 months, although they did note a significant reduction in GI events in patients taking the PPI. Given the dependence of clopidogrel metabolism on the CYP450 system, certainly extravigilance should be taken when prescribing other drugs with clopidogrel.

Although clopidogrel is currently the most utilized P_2Y_{12} ADP receptor blocker, there are two newer generation drugs of the same class that have gained attention in recent years. Prasugrel is a third-generation P_2Y_{12} ADP receptor blocker. Although also an irreversible inhibitor, prasugrel has a quicker onset of action when compared to clopidogrel (30 to 90 minutes for prasugrel vs. 4 to 6 hours for clopidogrel) and has lower rates of variability in platelet inhibitory effects than clopidogrel, thereby resulting in greater platelet inhibition. The effectiveness of prasugrel in patients with ACS was evaluated in the TRITON-TIMI 38 trial, in which more than 13,000 patients, including 10,000 patients with moderate- to high-risk UA/NSTEMI and 3,000 patients with STEMI, who were scheduled to undergo PCI for treatment of their ACS, were randomized to receive aspirin and either prasugrel or clopidogrel. Patients receiving prasugrel had a 19% reduction in the rate of cardiovascular death, MI, and stroke (9.9% vs. 12.1%; $p < 0.001$) as well as a 52% reduction in stent thrombosis (1.1% vs. 2.4%; $p < 0.001$) [133,134] (Fig. 38.5). These positive effects come at the price of significantly increased rate of major bleeding with prasugrel after PCI (2.4% vs. 1.8%; $p < 0.001$) [133].

Ticagrelor is another P_2Y_{12} ADP inhibitor that has recently been evaluated. Like prasugrel, ticagrelor has a rapid onset of action of 1 to 2 hours and greater platelet inhibition than clopidogrel; however, in contrast to both prasugrel and clopidogrel, ticagrelor's actions are reversible. The Study of Platelet Inhibition and Patient Outcomes (PLATO) study directly compared clopidogrel and ticagrelor in 18,000 patients presenting with ACS, about 15,000 of whom were patients with UA/NSTEMIs. Ticagrelor significantly reduced the rate of death, MI, or stroke when compared to clopidogrel (9.8% vs. 11.7%; $p < 0.001$) (Fig. 38.6) and significantly reduced all-cause mortality by 22% [135]. Although there was no significant difference in the rate of total major bleeding between the two drugs (11.6% vs. 11.2%; $p = 0.43$), a higher occurrence of non-coronary artery bypass grafting surgery (CABG) major bleeding was observed with ticagrelor.

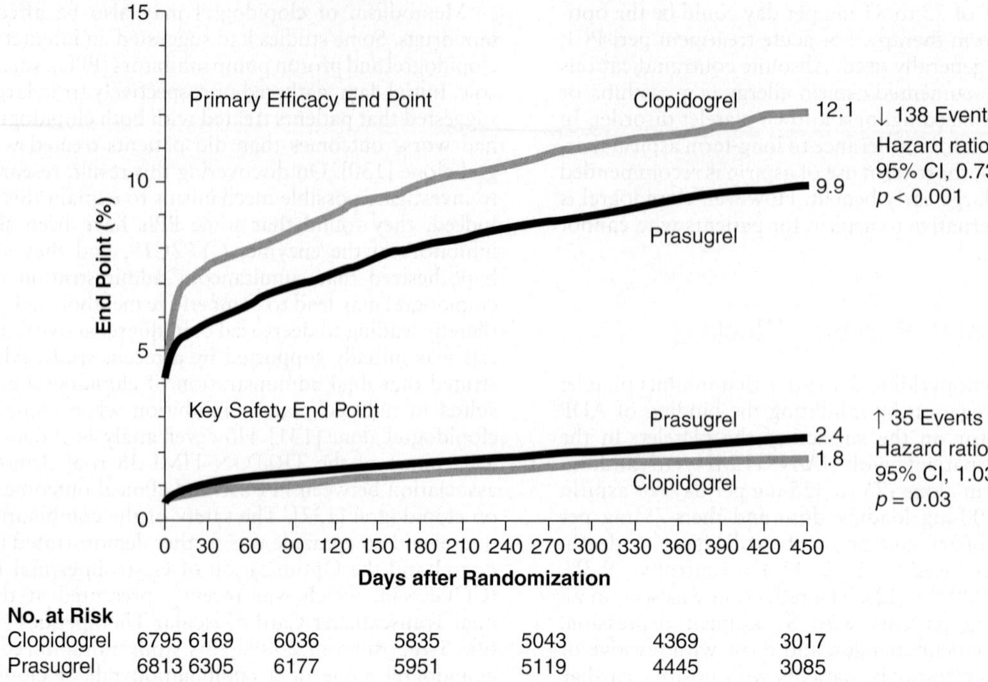

FIGURE 38.5. Kaplan–Meier curves demonstrating the superiority of prasugrel over clopidogrel in decreasing the incidence of the primary efficacy end point (composite of death from cardiovascular causes, nonfatal myocardial infarction, or nonfatal stroke) over 16 months. Also shown is the Kaplan–Meir curve comparing the incidence of the primary safety end point (TIMI major bleeding) between the two drugs—here, prasugrel was associated with an increased risk of TIMI-major bleeding. [From Wiviott SD, Braunwald E, McCabe CH, et al; for the TRITON-TIMI 38 Investigators: Prasugrel versus clopidogrel in patients with acute coronary syndromes. *New Engl J Med* 357:2001–2015, 2007, with permission.]

Heparin

Heparin appears to be beneficial in UA/NSTEMI [89,136]. A meta-analysis showed a 33% reduction in death or MI at 2 to 12 weeks' follow-up, when comparing heparin plus aspirin versus aspirin alone, 7.9% versus 10.4% (relative risk [RR] = 0.67; 95% CI 0.44 to 1.02; $p = 0.06$) [136] (Fig. 38.7). Although this reduction did not achieve statistical significance, these are the data cited to support the use of heparin plus aspirin in UA, as recommended in the 2007 ACC/AHA Updated Unstable Angina Guideline [67].

Using the available data, the current optimal regimen appears to be a weight-adjusted dosing (60 U per kg bolus with a maximum of 4,000 U and 12 U per kg per hour infusion with a maximum of 1,000 U per hour), frequent monitoring of the activated partial thromboplastin time (aPTT) (every 6 hours until in the target range and every 12 to 24 hours thereafter), and titration using a standardized normogram, with a target

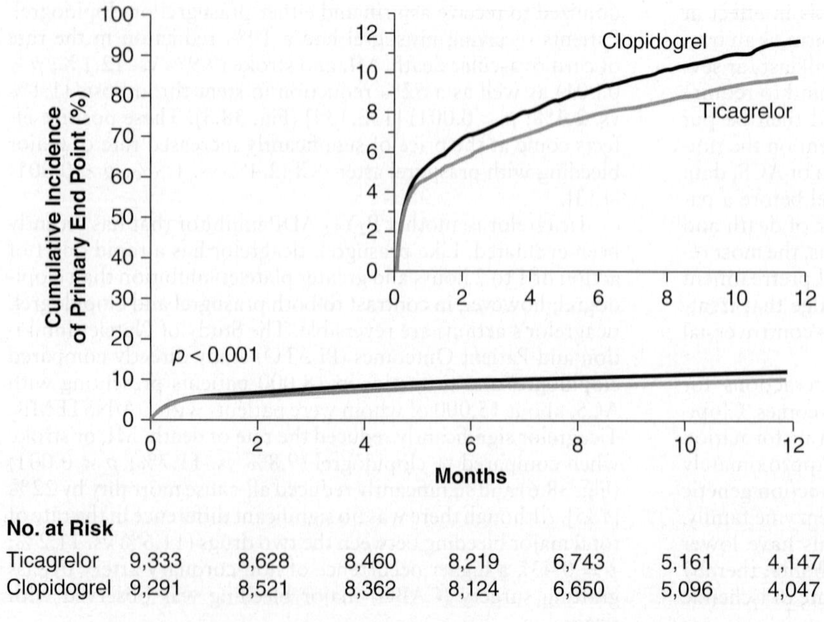

FIGURE 38.6. Kaplan–Meier curves demonstrating the superiority of ticagrelor over clopidogrel in decreasing the incidence of the primary efficacy end point (composite of death from vascular causes, myocardial infarction, or stroke) over 12 months. The primary end point occurred significantly less often with ticagrelor (9.8% vs. 11.7%; $p < 0.001$). [From Wallentin L, Becker RC, Budaj A, et al; for the PLATO Investigators: Ticagrelor versus clopidogrel in patients with acute coronary syndromes. *N Engl J Med* 361:1045–1057, 2009, with permission.]

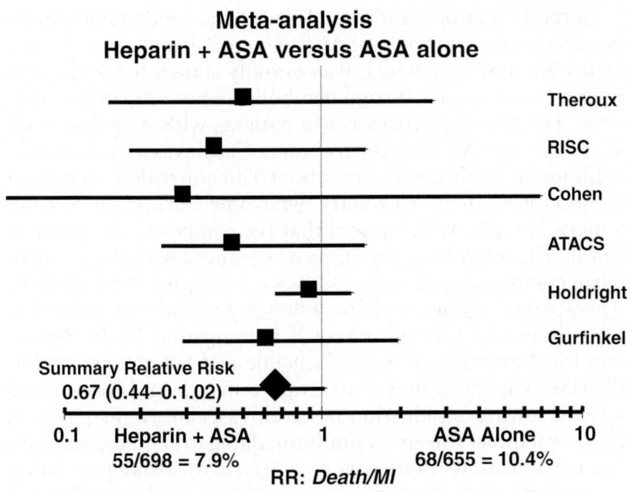

FIGURE 38.7. Meta-analysis of six randomized trials comparing unfractionated heparin plus aspirin versus aspirin alone, showing benefit of the combination therapy. [Adapted from Oler A, Whooley MA, Oler J, et al: Adding heparin to aspirin reduces the incidence of myocardial infarction and death in patients with unstable angina. A meta-analysis. *JAMA* 276:811–815, 1996, with permission.]

range of aPTT between 1.5 and 2.0 times control or approximately 50 to 70 seconds [67].

Low-Molecular-Weight Heparin

A major advance in the use of heparin has been the development of LMWHs, which are combined thrombin and factor Xa inhibitors. LMWHs are obtained by depolymerization of standard UFH and selection of those with lower molecular weight [137,138]. As compared with UFH with its nearly equal anti-IIa (thrombin) and anti-Xa activity, LMWHs have increased ratios of anti-Xa to anti-IIa activity of either 2:1 (e.g., dalteparin) or 3.8:1 (e.g., enoxaparin).

LMWH has several potential advantages over standard UFH. First, it inhibits thrombin as well as factor Xa, thereby inhibiting thrombin activity and its generation [138]. LMWH also induces a greater release of tissue factor pathway inhibitor than UFH and is not neutralized by platelet factor IV [137]. LMWH has been found to have a lower rate of thrombocytopenia than UFH [139]. Finally, the high bioavailability allows for subcutaneous administration.

Several trials have compared UFH with LMWH in patients with UA/NSTEMI, and in general, LMWH has been found to be superior [69,140]. In a meta-analysis of all trials of enoxaparin versus UFH in patients with UA/NSTEMI, treatment with enoxaparin significantly reduced the incidence of recurrent MI when compared to UFH (8% vs. 9.1%; $p = 0.005$), although there was no difference in mortality rates (3% vs. 3%; $p = 0.89$). Furthermore, treatment with enoxaparin in patients with NSTEMIs was not associated with an excess of major bleeding (6.3% vs. 5.4%; $p = 0.419$) [141] (Fig. 38.8). As might be expected, the benefit of enoxaparin appears greater in patients managed conservatively (who are typically on heparin for at least 48 hours) rather than in those managed invasively (who go to the catheterization laboratory within 48 hours and have their heparin discontinued thereafter) [142]. Given these results, the 2007 update of the ACC/AHA Unstable UA/NSTEMI Guideline offers a class IIa recommendation that enoxaparin be used over UFH, particularly for those patients who are managed conservatively [67].

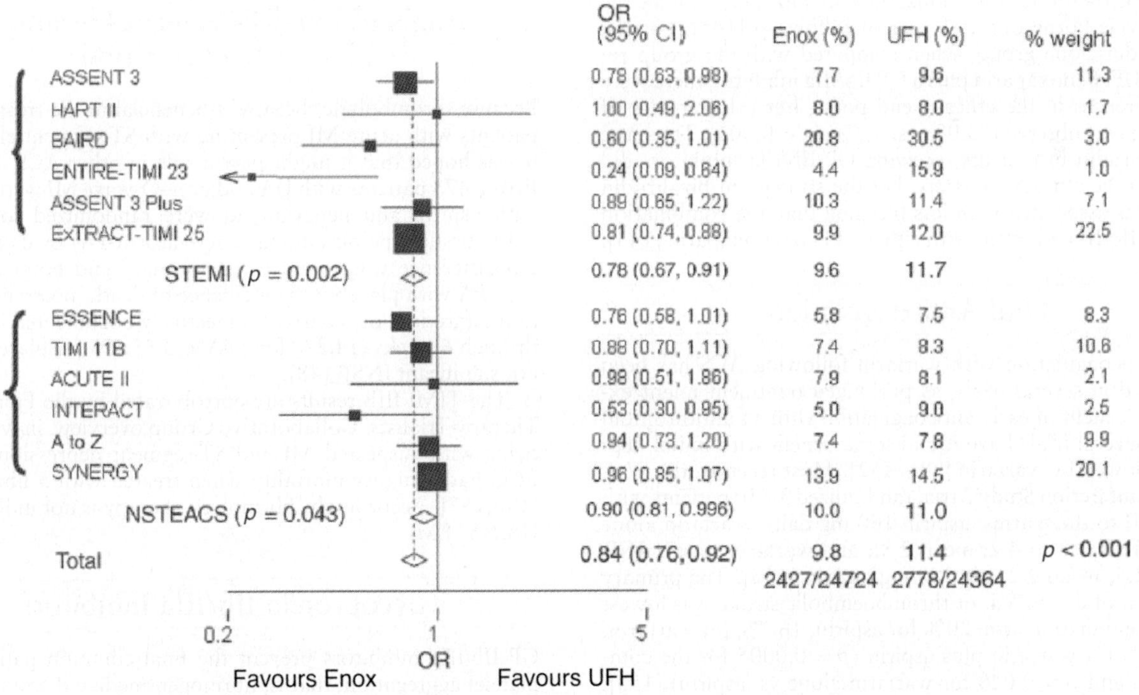

OR (95% CI)
Enox (%)
UFH (%)
% weight
ASSENT 3 0.78 (0.63, 0.98) 7.7 9.6 11.3
HART II 1.00 (0.49, 2.06) 8.0 8.0 1.7
BAIRD 0.60 (0.35, 1.01) 20.8 30.5 3.0
ENTIRE-TIMI 23 0.24 (0.09, 0.64) 4.4 15.9 1.0
ASSENT 3 Plus 0.89 (0.65, 1.22) 10.3 11.4 7.1
ExTRACT-TIMI 25 0.81 (0.74, 0.88) 9.9 12.0 22.5
STEMI (p = 0.002) 0.78 (0.67, 0.91) 9.6 11.7
ESSENCE 0.76 (0.58, 1.01) 5.8 7.5 8.3
TIMI 11B 0.88 (0.70, 1.11) 7.4 8.3 10.6
ACUTE II 0.98 (0.51, 1.86) 7.9 8.1 2.1
INTERACT 0.53 (0.30, 0.95) 5.0 9.0 2.5
A to Z 0.94 (0.73, 1.20) 7.4 7.8 9.9
SYNERGY 0.96 (0.85, 1.07) 13.9 14.5 20.1
NSTEACS (p = 0.043) 0.90 (0.81, 0.996) 10.0 11.0
Total 0.84 (0.76, 0.92) 9.8 11.4 p < 0.001
2427/24724 2778/24364
0.2
1
5
OR
Favours Enox
Favours UFH

FIGURE 38.8. Meta-analysis of 12 trials, 6 of which evaluated patients with UA/NSTEMI, which compared UFH with enoxaparin. Data from more than 49,000 patients demonstrated that enoxaparin was associated with a lower incidence of death of nonfatal MI. CI, confidence interval; ENOX, enoxaparin; OR, odds ratio; UFH, unfractionated heparin. [From Murphy SA, Gibson CM, Morrow DA, et al: Efficacy and safety of the low-molecular weight heparin enoxaparin compared with unfractionated heparin across the acute coronary syndrome spectrum: a meta-analysis. *Eur Heart J* 28:2077–2086, 2007, with permission.]

Fondaparinux

Fondaparinux is a synthetic pentasaccharide and a specific Xa inhibitor. When comparing fondaparinux and enoxaparin, researchers found that the rates of death, MI, or refractory ischemia throughout the first 9 days were virtually identical with either drug in patients with UA/NSTEMI [143]. The rate of major bleeding was nearly 50% lower in the fondaparinux arm. By 30 days, mortality was significantly lower in the fondaparinux arm. Notably, in the subset of patients undergoing PCI, fondaparinux was associated with more than a threefold increased risk of catheter-related thrombi. Supplemental UFH during PCI appeared to minimize this risk, and consequently, the ACC/AHA recommends that UFH and fondaparinux be used together during PCI. Thus, fondaparinux appears to be a new alternative in patients with UA/NSTEMI and is associated with a lower risk of bleeding; however, this medication needs to be used cautiously in patients undergoing PCI.

Bivalirudin

Bivalirudin is another antithrombotic drug used in the treatment of UA/NSTEMI, which acts by directly inhibiting thrombin and thus inhibiting clot formation. Bivalirudin was evaluated in the Acute Catheterization and Urgent Intervention Triage Strategy (ACUITY) trial, which randomized 13,820 patients with UA/NSTEMI, who were to be managed with an immediate invasive strategy, to one of three treatments: UFH or enoxaparin plus a GP IIb/IIIa inhibitor, bivalirudin plus a GP IIb/IIIa inhibitor, or bivalirudin alone. The study found no differences in the primary end point of death, MI, unplanned revascularization for ischemia, and major bleeding at 30 days between bivalirudin plus GP IIb/IIIa inhibitor and UFH/enoxaparin plus a GP IIb/IIIa inhibitor [144]. Furthermore, the similar rate of mortality among the groups was borne out at 1 year of follow-up [145]. For the bivalirudin-alone group, when compared with the group receiving UFH/enoxaparin plus a GP IIb/IIIa inhibitor, there were no differences in the efficacy end point, but a lower rate of bleeding was observed (3.0% vs. 5.7%; $p < 0.001$). Thus, use of bivalirudin in patients receiving GP IIb/IIIa inhibitors did not improve efficacy or safety, but the strategy of bivalirudin alone was associated with less bleeding than the combination of a GP IIb/IIIa inhibitor with either UFH or enoxaparin [144].

Oral Anticoagulation

Oral anticoagulation with warfarin following ACS has been examined in several trials, as prolonged treatment might extend the benefit of early anticoagulation with an antithrombin agent. Several trials have found some benefit with initial heparin followed by warfarin [146–152]. Most recently, the Warfarin Reinfarction Study 2 trial randomized 3,630 patients with acute MI to three arms: aspirin 160 mg daily; warfarin alone (target INR 2.8 to 4.2; mean 2.8); and warfarin (target INR 2.0 to 2.5; mean 2.2) plus 80 mg aspirin [153]. The primary end point of death, MI, or thromboembolic stroke was lowest in the combination arm: 20% for aspirin, 16.7% for warfarin, and 15% for warfarin plus aspirin ($p = 0.0005$ for the combination and $p = 0.028$ for warfarin alone vs. aspirin) [153]. The rate of major bleeding was low overall, but was increased from 0.15% per year for aspirin, to 0.58% for warfarin alone, and 0.52% for warfarin plus aspirin. Thus, the combination of warfarin plus aspirin appears to be an effective long-term treatment for secondary prevention of further cardiovascular events. However, the difficulty of maintaining warfarin within a narrow therapeutic window makes the routine use of this medication for this indication inconvenient.

Several other oral anticoagulants are currently under investigation for the treatment of ACS. Rivaroxaban is an oral direct factor Xa inhibitor, which was initially shown to be effective in preventing venous thromboembolism after orthopedic surgeries. The use of rivaroxaban in patients with ACS was studied in the Anti-Xa Therapy to Lower Cardiovascular Events in Addition to Aspirin with or without Thienopyridine therapy in Subjects with Acute Coronary Syndrome (ATLAS-ACS) trial, a phase II study, which found that the composite end point of death, MI, or stroke at 6 months was reduced with rivaroxaban when compared to placebo (3.9% vs. 5.5%; $p = 0.027$) [154]. Apixaban is another oral direct factor Xa inhibitor, which has recently passed through phase II investigation in the Apixaban for Prevention of Acute Ischemic and Safety Events (APPRAISE) trial and, similar to rivaroxaban, also demonstrated a trend toward a reduction in cardiovascular events [155]. A third oral direct thrombin inhibitor, dabigatran has gained notice recently as an alternative to warfarin in stroke prevention for patients with atrial fibrillation. However, this medication has also been evaluated for the prevention of recurrent ischemic events in patients with acute MI. Initial results from the phase II RE-DEEM (Randomized Dabigatran Etexilate Dose Finding Study in Patients with Acute Coronary Syndromes Post Index Event with Additional Risk Factors for Cardiovascular Complications Also Receiving Aspirin and Clopidogrel: Multicentre, Prospective, Placebo Controlled, Cohort Dose Escalation) study, which was presented at the American Heart Association Scientific Sessions in 2009, reported that dabigatran was associated with acceptable bleeding rates and would continue onto phase III studies to evaluate efficacy for use in patients with ACS. The clinical efficacy and utilization of these three oral antithrombin drugs will be borne out in the ongoing phase III trials over the next few years.

Thrombolytic Therapy for Unstable Angina/Non–ST-Segment Elevation Myocardial Infarction

Because thrombolytic therapy is beneficial in the treatment of patients with acute MI presenting with ST-segment elevation, it was hoped that it might play a role in other ACS. In TIMI IIIB, 1,473 patients with UA and non–Q-wave MI were treated with aspirin and heparin and were randomized to receive either tissue-type plasminogen activator (t-PA) or its placebo. No difference was found in the primary end point comparing t-PA with placebo: the incidence of death, postrandomization infarction, or recurrent, objectively documented ischemia through 6 weeks (54.2% for t-PA and 55.5% for placebo; $p =$ not significant [NS]) [48].

The TIMI IIIB results are corroborated by the Fibrinolytic Therapy Trialists' Collaborative Group overview, in which patients with suspected MI and ST-segment depression on the ECG had a higher mortality when treated with a fibrinolytic [156,157]. Accordingly, fibrinolytic therapy is not indicated in UA/NSTEMI.

Glycoprotein IIb/IIIa Inhibitors

GP IIb/IIIa inhibitors prevent the final common pathway of platelet aggregation, that is, fibrinogen-mediated cross-linkage of platelets via the GP IIb/IIIa receptor (see Fig. 38.2). Currently available GP IIb/IIIa inhibitors include abciximab, eptifibatide, and tirofiban. Abciximab is a monoclonal antibody Fab fragment directed at the GP IIb/IIIa receptor, whereas eptifibatide, a synthetic heptapeptide, and tirofiban, a nonpeptide molecule, are antagonists of the GP IIb/IIIa receptor whose structure mimics the arginine–glycine–aspartic acid amino acid sequence by which fibrinogen binds to the GP IIb/IIIa receptor.

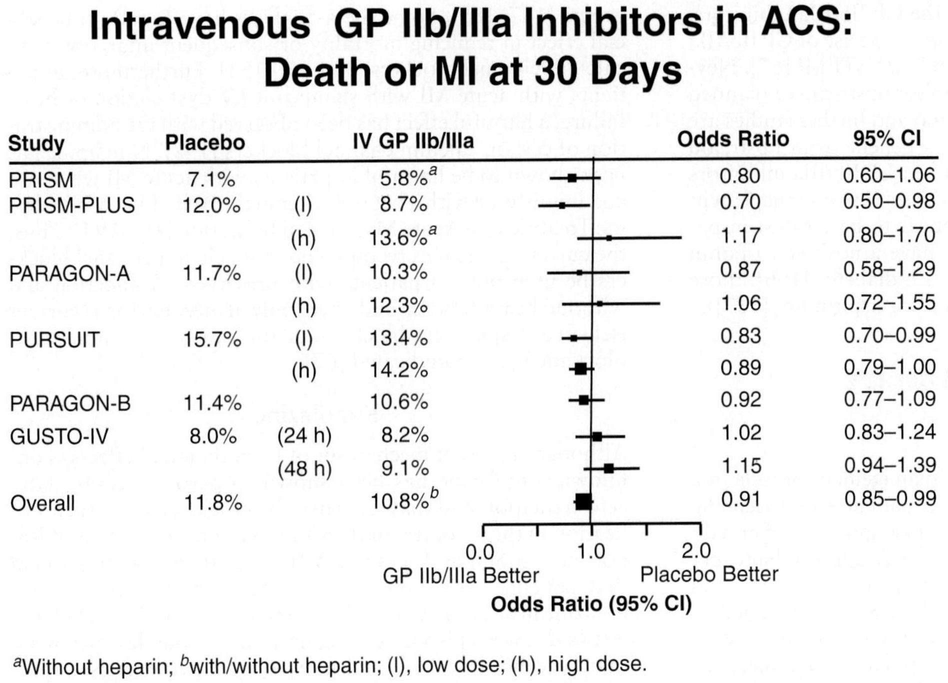
Intravenous GP IIb/IIIa Inhibitors in ACS:
Death or MI at 30 Days
Study
Placebo
IV GP IIb/IIIa
Odds Ratio
95% CI
PRISM 7.1% 5.8%a 0.80 0.60–1.06
PRISM-PLUS 12.0% (l) 8.7% 0.70 0.50–0.98
(h) 13.6%a 1.17 0.80–1.70
PARAGON-A 11.7% (l) 10.3% 0.87 0.58–1.29
(h) 12.3% 1.06 0.72–1.55
PURSUIT 15.7% (l) 13.4% 0.83 0.70–0.99
(h) 14.2% 0.89 0.79–1.00
PARAGON-B 11.4% 10.6% 0.92 0.77–1.09
GUSTO-IV 8.0% (24 h) 8.2% 1.02 0.83–1.24
(48 h) 9.1% 1.15 0.94–1.39
Overall 11.8% 10.8%b 0.91 0.85–0.99
0.0
1.0
2.0
GP IIb/IIIa Better
Placebo Better
Odds Ratio (95% CI)
aWithout heparin; bwith/without heparin; (l), low dose; (h), high dose.

FIGURE 38.9. Meta-analysis of the benefit of IV GP IIb/IIIa inhibitors in acute coronary syndrome (ACS): death or myocardial infarction (MI) at 30 days. [From Boersma E, Harrington RA, Molterno DJ, et al: Platelet glycoprotein IIb/IIIa inhibitors in acute coronary syndromes: a meta-analysis of all major randomized clinical trials. *Lancet* 359:189–198, 2002, with permission.]

The efficacy of the GP IIb/IIIa inhibitors in the treatment of NSTEMIs has been demonstrated in several studies. In the PRISM-PLUS trial involving 1,915 patients with UA/NSTEMI, tirofiban plus heparin and aspirin led to a significantly lower rate of death, MI, or refractory ischemia at 7 days than did placebo (i.e., heparin plus aspirin) (12.9% vs. 17.9%, a 32% risk reduction; $p = 0.004$). These results were borne out at 30 days as well [49]. (Death or MI was reduced by 30%, from 11.9% to 8.7%; $p = 0.03$.) In the PURSUIT (Platelet Glycoprotein IIb/IIIa in Unstable Angina: Receptor Suppression using Integrillin Therapy) trial, which involved 10,948 patients, eptifibatide reduced the rate of death or MI at 30 days by a relative 10% (from 15.7% to 14.2%; $p = 0.042$). A greater benefit was observed in patients who were treated with an early invasive strategy with early PCI plus eptifibatide (31% reduction in death or MI at 30 days; 16.7% vs. 11.6%; $p = 0.01$), whereas the relative benefit was less (7% reduction; $p = 0.23$) in those treated conservatively with delayed PCI or CABG as needed [71]. The benefit of GP IIb/IIIa inhibition appears to be restricted to troponin-positive patients (i.e., those patients with true NSTEMIs) as demonstrated in the ISAR-REACT 2 trial, which studied 2,022 patients and found that abciximab reduced the risk of adverse cardiovascular events by 25% only in patients with NSTEMIs being treated with PCI [96]. There was no difference in cardiovascular events in patients with UA and a normal troponin level.

Although GP IIb/IIIa drugs certainly appear to be useful in the management of patients with NSTEMIs, who are undergoing PCI, the question remains as to what the optimal time for administration of the drug is. Initial analyses of data suggested that perhaps early administration of a GP IIb/IIIa inhibitor was beneficial. A meta-analysis of three trials (PRISM-PLUS, PURSUIT, and CAPTURE [c7E3 antiplatelet therapy in unstable refractory angina]) involving 12,296 patients yielded a 34% relative reduction in death or MI with the early use of the GP IIb/IIIa antagonists, although the absolute difference in event rates was small (3.8% vs. 2.5%; $p = 0.001$) [158]. As was expected, an even greater benefit was seen when the agents were continued during PCI (8.0% vs. 4.9%; $p = 0.001$). These findings were confirmed, although less robustly, in a more recent meta-analysis involving six trials, which again found that the use of GP IIb/III antagonists resulted in a 9% relative reduction in death or MI when compared to placebo [159] (Fig. 38.9).

Later studies did not yield the same results. The GUSTO-IV ACS trial failed to show a benefit of abciximab when given upstream of PCI [160]. In addition, the ACUITY-Timing study found that early administration of GP IIb/IIIa inhibitors did not reduce recurrent ischemia when compared to selective administration of the medication in the catheterization laboratory during PCI (7.1% vs. 7.9%; $p = 0.44$), although bleeding was significantly increased with upstream administration (6.1% vs. 4.9%; $p < 0.001$) [161]. More recently, the EARLY ACS (Early Glycoprotein IIb/IIIa Inhibition in Non-ST-Segment Elevation Acute Coronary Syndrome) trial evaluated the use of routine use of upstream GP IIb/IIIa inhibitor eptifibatide versus delayed provisional use of the medication at the time of PCI [162]. In this trial, more than 9,000 patients with UA/NSTEMI, who were planned for an early invasive strategy with early PCI, were assigned to either receive upstream eptifibatide for the 12+ hours prior to catheterization or to the provisional use of eptifibatide after angiography. There was no significant difference in the composite rate of death, MI, urgent revascularization, or thrombotic complication during PCI between the two groups.

Although GP IIb/IIIa inhibitors may be efficacious in preventing adverse cardiovascular events, there are serious side effects associated with this class of drug. Several studies have demonstrated that the rate of major hemorrhage is slightly higher for patients treated with GP IIb/IIIa inhibitors. In PRISM-PLUS, major bleeding occurred in 4% of patients treated with tirofiban plus heparin plus aspirin versus 3.0% for heparin plus aspirin ($p = NS$) [49]. For eptifibatide, the rates of severe or moderate bleeding with eptifibatide versus placebo were 12.8% and 9.9%, respectively ($p < 0.001$) [71]. In EARLY ACS, patients who were given upstream eptifibatide had higher rates of non–life-threatening bleeding (5.8% vs. 3.4%; $p < 0.001$) and more blood transfusions (8.6 vs. 6.7; $p = 0.001$) [162].

Thrombocytopenia is also more common with GP IIb/IIIa inhibitors. For tirofiban in PRISM-PLUS, the rate of severe thrombocytopenia (<50,000 cells per mm^3) was 0.5%, versus 0.3% for heparin ($p = 0.44$). The latter event is associated with increased bleeding and in a smaller proportion of patients, recurrent thrombotic events [163,164]. This syndrome bears resemblance to heparin-induced thrombocytopenia and indicates a need to monitor platelet count daily during the GP IIb/IIIa infusion.

Despite the risks associated with the GP IIb/IIIa inhibitors, the current ACC/AHA guidelines support the use of GP IIb/IIIa inhibitors during PCI in patients with UA/NSTEMI [67]. Nevertheless, the use of a GP IIb/IIIa inhibitor upstream of planned PCI for UA/NSTEMI is now in question and further studies are needed to see if particular subgroups benefit from upstream administration of this medication. When GP IIb/IIIa inhibitors are used either during PCI or with conservative management of UA/NSTEMI, the benefit does appear to be greatest in patients at higher risk (i.e., those who have a positive troponin at baseline [96,98–100,165], those with diabetes [166], those with recurrent angina, or those with prior aspirin use [167]).

Anti-Ischemic Therapy

Nitrates

Nitrates are very useful in the acute management of ischemia and should be given sublingually if the patient is experiencing ischemic pain. Nitrates are provided for symptom relief and do not impart a mortality benefit. Both the Gruppo Italiano per lo Studio della Sopravvivenza nell'Infarto miocardico 3 and International Study of Infarct Survival (ISIS) 4 trials failed to demonstrate a survival benefit with nitrates in patients with suspected ACS, either in the overall population of subjects or in the subgroup of patients with NSTEMI [168,169]. If pain persists after three sublingual tablets and initiation of beta-blockade, intravenous nitroglycerin is recommended [67]. Because the goal of nitrate therapy is relief of pain, nitrates can frequently be tapered off during hospitalization.

Beta-Blockers

Several placebo-controlled trials in UA/NSTEMI have shown benefit of beta-blockers in reducing subsequent MI, recurrent ischemia, or both [170–174]. Early intravenous beta-blockade appears to provide early benefits in UA/NSTEMI [175]. In early studies performed in the prethrombolytic era that included patients with ST-segment elevation MI and NSTEMI, beta-blockers were shown to reduce infarct size, reinfarction, and mortality [176–179]. This beneficial effect of beta-blockers (intravenous followed by oral) has also been seen in subgroup analyses of patients with NSTEMI [179–181].

Beta-blockers are recommended for patients with UA/NSTEMI who do not have contraindications to their use (bradycardia, advanced atrioventricular block, persistent hypotension, pulmonary edema, and history of bronchospasm). If ischemia and chest pain are ongoing, early intravenous beta-blockade should be used, followed by oral beta-blockade. It should be noted that a reduced ejection fraction is no longer a contradiction to beta-blockade, and indeed, such patients may derive added benefit given the salutary effects seen with long-term beta-blockade in patients with heart failure [182–184]. However, beta-blockers should not be initiated in patients with evidence of decompensated heart failure until they have become hemodynamically stable [185].

Calcium Channel Blockers

Calcium channel blockers may be used in patients who have persistent or recurrent symptoms, but they are currently recommended only after nitrates and beta-blockade have been initiated [67]. In patients with contraindications to beta-blockade, improved heart rate control can be accomplished with some calcium channel blockers (e.g., diltiazem or verapamil). The Diltiazem Reinfarction Study, which involved 576 patients with non–Q-wave MI, showed that diltiazem reduced the rate of recurrent MI from 9.3% with placebo to 5.2% with diltiazem [186]. Furthermore, some studies have suggested that the use of amlodipine in stable patients with high-risk cardiovascular features can decrease the incidence of major cardiovascular events [187–189]. Some meta-analyses have found no beneficial effect in reducing mortality or subsequent infarction with calcium channel blockers [171,190,191]. Furthermore, in patients with acute MI with significant LV dysfunction or heart failure, a harmful effect has been observed with the administration of certain calcium channel blockers [192]. Nifedipine has been shown to be harmful in patients with acute MI when not coadministered with a beta-blocker in the trial of Early Nifedipine Treatment in Acute Myocardial Infarction [193,194]. Thus, the current guidelines recommend that calcium channel blockers be used only in patients with preserved LV function and without heart failure, and then only if needed for recurrent ischemia despite beta-blockade or for patients in whom beta-blockade is contraindicated [67].

Ranolazine

Although the exact mechanism of its antianginal effects is unknown, ranolazine has been shown to partially inhibit fatty acid oxidation and may improve the efficiency of oxygen utilization in the myocyte. In the Combination Assessment of Ranolazine in Stable Angina (CARISA) trial, researchers found that patients with stable angina, who were treated with ranolazine in addition to beta-blockers or calcium channel blockers, had fewer episodes of angina (one episode less per week than placebo; $p < 0.02$) and showed increased exercise capacity (115.6 seconds vs. 91.7 seconds; $p = 0.01$) [195]. Similar results reflecting the anti-anginal effects of ranolazine in patients with chronic stable angina were demonstrated in the MARISA (Monotherapy Assessment of Ranolazine in Stable Angina) trial [196]. The Metabolic Efficiency with Ranolazine for Less Ischemia in Non-ST Elevation Acute Coronary Syndrome (MERLIN)-TIMI 36 trial expanded the use of ranolazine to the NSTEMI population by evaluating 6,560 patients with NSTEMIs, 3,279 of whom were randomized to receive ranolazine and 3,281 of whom received placebo. Although there was no difference in the primary end point (a composite of cardiovascular death, MI, or recurrent ischemia) between the two groups (21.8% vs. 23.5%; $p = 0.11$), there was a significant reduction in the rates of recurrent ischemia with ranolazine (13.9% vs. 16.1%; $p = 0.03$) [197]. Follow-up analyses of the MERLIN-TIMI 36 trial confirmed the results of the CARISA and MARISA trials and demonstrated that anginal symptoms were improved with ranolazine (HR 0.77; 95% CI 0.59 to 1.00; $p = 0.048$) [198]. Hence, ranolazine remains an attractive addition to beta-blockers and nitrates for treatment of chronic, severe angina.

Angiotensin-Converting Enzyme Inhibitors

Angiotensin-converting enzyme (ACE) inhibitors have been shown to be beneficial in patients after MI, who have either LV systolic dysfunction (ejection fraction <40%) [199] or heart failure [200]. The Gruppo Italiano per lo Studio della Sopravvienza nell'Infarto miocardico-3, ISIS-4, and Chinese trials showed a 0.5% absolute mortality benefit of early (initiated within 24 hours) ACE inhibition in patients with acute MI [168,169]. However, in the ISIS-4 study, no benefit was observed in patients without ST-segment elevation. Thus, early routine ACE inhibition does not appear to confer survival benefit for patients with UA or NSTEMI.

On the other hand, long-term use of ACE inhibition is applicable to several groups of patients with cardiovascular disease, including those with LV systolic dysfunction [199]. Data based on evidence from the Heart Outcomes Prevention Evaluation trial suggests that ACE inhibition prevents recurrent cardiovascular events in patients with prior MI, peripheral arterial disease, or diabetes, even if ventricular function is preserved [201]. Similar results were also seen in the European Trial on Reduction of Cardiac Events with Perindopril in Stable Coronary Artery Disease (EUROPA) trial [202]. However, a third trial, the Prevention of Events with Angiotensin Converting Enzyme [ACE] inhibitor (PEACE) trial, did not show any benefit with routine use of trandolapril in this population of patients, perhaps because the patients in this study were relatively low risk and had been treated with more intensive statin therapy and more frequent coronary revascularization [203].

Angiotensin Receptor Blockers

Angiotensin receptor blockers (ARBs) provide an alternative to ACE inhibitors, and may block the renin–angiotensin system more completely than ACE inhibitors, because angiotensin II can be generated via pathways that are independent of ACE [204]. The Valsartan in Acute Myocardial Infarction Trial (VALIANT) was one of the first trials to directly compare ARBs and ACE inhibitors. In this study, about 15,000 patients with a history of MI that was complicated by heart failure were randomized to receive either an ARB (valsartan), an ACE inhibitor (captopril), or a combination of the two drugs [205]. Valsartan was found to be noninferior to captopril at 2 years with regard to mortality ($p = 0.004$) and with regard to recurrent cardiovascular events ($p < 0.001$). The VALIANT trial was subsequently followed by the On-going Telmisartan Alone and In Combination with Ramipril Global Endpoint Trial (ON-TARGET), which randomized patients with known vascular disease or diabetes to receive either telmisartan, an ARB, or ramipril, an ACE inhibitor, or both drugs together [206]. Again, the ARB was shown to be noninferior to the ACE inhibitor with similar rates of death, MI, stroke, or hospitalization for heart failure at 56 months (16.5% vs. 16.7%; RR 1.01; 95% CI 0.94 to 1.09). Furthermore, patients who received telmisartan had less complaints of cough (1.1% vs. 4.2%; $p < 0.001$) when compared to those receiving the ACE inhibitor. Hence, ARBs remain effective alternatives to ACE inhibitors and may even be better tolerated.

Lipid-Lowering Therapy

Long-term treatment with lipid-lowering therapy with statins has been shown to be beneficial in patients with a prior history of either MI or UA [207–209]. In individuals with UA in the Long-term Intervention with Pravastatin in Ischemic Disease Trial, pravastatin led to a 26% reduction in mortality ($p = 0.004$), as well as significant reductions in subsequent MI, coronary revascularization, and stroke [209].

An early benefit on overall clinical outcome has been found in the Myocardial Ischemia Reduction with Aggressive Cholesterol Lowering (MIRACL) trial. In 3,086 patients with UA/NSTEMI, atorvastatin 80 mg as compared to placebo was found to reduce the rate of the composite end point of death, MI, cardiac resuscitation, and angina, leading to rehospitalization by 4 months [210]. Further analysis demonstrated that this difference was mostly due to a reduction in the rate of rehospitalization for angina. In the Pravastatin or Atorvastatin Evaluation and Infection Therapy (PROVE-IT) TIMI 22 trial, intensive lipid-lowering therapy with atorvastatin 80 mg resulted in a 16% reduction in the primary end point and a 25% reduction in death, MI, or urgent revascularization, when compared with only moderate lipid-lowering therapy with pravastatin 40 mg [211]. The benefits emerged after only 30 days post-ACS [212], highlighting the importance of early initiation of intensive statin therapy post-ACS. When comparing the two arms of this study, it was noted that there was a significant difference in the LDLs achieved in each group. The average LDL achieved was 62 mg per dL in the atorvastatin 80 mg group and 95 mg per dL in the pravastatin 40 mg group. Based in part on these results, the adult treatment panel III of the National Cholesterol Education Program issued an update in which they recommended a new optional very low LDL goal of less than 70 mg per dL in patients with high-risk coronary heart disease [213].

TREATMENT STRATEGIES AND INTERVENTIONS

"Early Invasive" Versus "Ischemia-Guided" Strategy of Revascularization

Two general approaches to the use of coronary angiography and revascularization in UA/NSTEMI exist. The first is an "early invasive" strategy, involving routine angiography and revascularization with PCI or bypass surgery as appropriate. The other is a more conservative approach with initial medical management with angiography and revascularization only for recurrent ischemia, which could be termed an *ischemia-guided* strategy. Eight randomized trials have assessed these two general strategies [48,66,73,74,84,117,214] (Fig. 38.10).

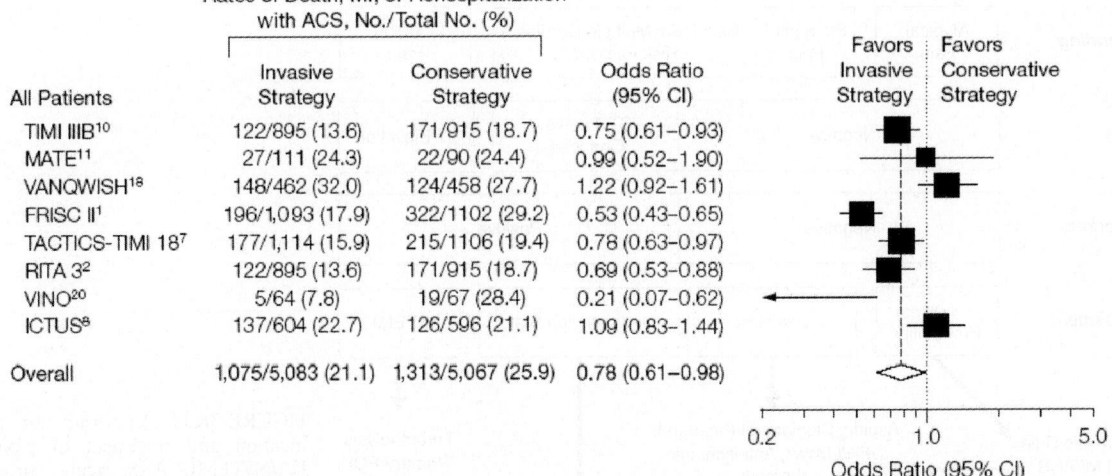

	Rates of Death, MI, or Rehospitalization with ACS, No./Total No. (%)		
All Patients	Invasive Strategy	Conservative Strategy	Odds Ratio (95% CI)
TIMI IIIB[10]	122/895 (13.6)	171/915 (18.7)	0.75 (0.61–0.93)
MATE[11]	27/111 (24.3)	22/90 (24.4)	0.99 (0.52–1.90)
VANQWISH[18]	148/462 (32.0)	124/458 (27.7)	1.22 (0.92–1.61)
FRISC II[1]	196/1,093 (17.9)	322/1102 (29.2)	0.53 (0.43–0.65)
TACTICS-TIMI 18[7]	177/1,114 (15.9)	215/1106 (19.4)	0.78 (0.63–0.97)
RITA 3[2]	122/895 (13.6)	171/915 (18.7)	0.69 (0.53–0.88)
VINO[20]	5/64 (7.8)	19/67 (28.4)	0.21 (0.07–0.62)
ICTUS[8]	137/604 (22.7)	126/596 (21.1)	1.09 (0.83–1.44)
Overall	1,075/5,083 (21.1)	1,313/5,067 (25.9)	0.78 (0.61–0.98)

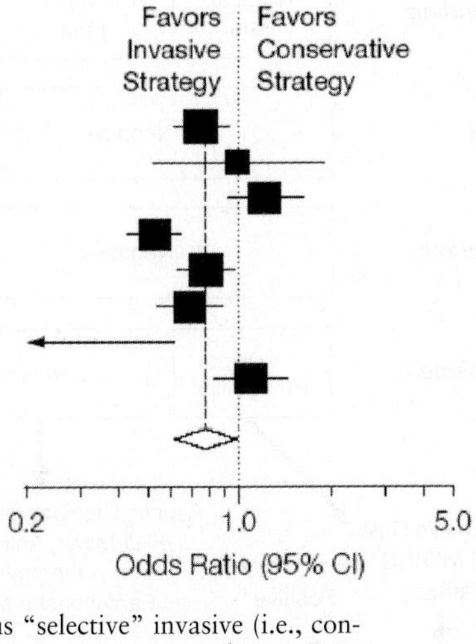

FIGURE 38.10. Meta-analysis of the benefit of a routine invasive versus "selective" invasive (i.e., conservative) strategy for patients with unstable angina or NSTEMI. ACS, acute coronary syndrome. Rate of death or MI or rehospitalization with ACS through follow-up. [From O'Donoghue M, Boden WE, Braunwald E, et al: Early invasive vs conservative treatment strategies in women and men with unstable angina and non-ST-segment elevation myocardial infarction: a meta-analysis. *JAMA* 300(1):71–80, 2008, with permission.]

The initial trials showed no benefit with an early invasive strategy. Subsequently, the FRISC II trial was conducted after coronary stenting had become available and found a significant benefit with an invasive strategy for the risk of death or MI at 6 months (9.4% vs. 12.1%; $p = 0.031$) [215]. At 1 year, there was a significant reduction in mortality in the invasive versus conservative groups (2.2% vs. 3.9%, respectively; $p = 0.016$) and in death or MI (10.4% vs. 14.1%, respectively; $p = 0.005$) [215]. Additional analyses showed greater benefit with the invasive strategy in higher risk groups identified by ST-segment depression on the admission ECG or troponin T greater than or equal to 0.01 ng per dL [216,217].

Subsequently, the TACTICS-TIMI 18 trial, wherein all patients were treated with an "upstream" GP IIb/IIIa inhibitor, found a significant reduction in death, MI, or rehospitalization for an ACS at 6 months with use of the early invasive strategy (from 19.4% in the conservative group to 15.9% in the early invasive strategy—OR, 0:78; $p = 0.025$) [84]. Similarly, death or nonfatal MI was significantly reduced at 30 days (7.0% to 4.7%, respectively; $p = 0.02$) and at 6 months ($p = 0.0498$). These effects were most magnified in patients with ST-segment changes, in those with positive troponin values compared with negative values, and in those with intermediate or high TIMI risk scores. In patients with a troponin I of greater than or equal to 0.1 ng per mL, there was a relative 39% risk reduction in the primary end point with the invasive versus conservative strategy ($p < 0.001$), whereas patients with a negative troponin had similar outcomes with either strategy [91]. Using the TIMI risk score, there was significant benefit of the early invasive strategy in intermediate- (score 3 to 4) and high-risk patients (5 to 7), whereas low-risk (0 to 2) patients had similar outcomes when managed with either strategy [84].

Randomized Intervention Treatment of Angina (RITA) 3 tested an early invasive versus conservative approach in 1,810 patients with UA/NSTEMI, all of whom were managed with enoxaparin [218]. An invasive strategy again proved superior, although the 34% reduction in the primary end point of death, MI, or refractory angina at 4 months was driven primarily by a reduction in refractory angina. Interestingly by 5 years, there was a significantly lower cardiovascular mortality rate in the early invasive arm [219].

The Invasive versus Conservative Treatment in Unstable Coronary Syndromes (ICTUS) trial also examined an invasive versus conservative approach in 1,200 patients. All patients received aspirin, enoxaparin, and abciximab at the time of PCI. At 1 year, there was no significant difference in the rate of the composite primary end point of death, MI, or rehospitalization for angina [220]. In fact, during the index hospitalization, there was a higher rate of MI in the invasive arm. In contrast, the risk of spontaneous MI tended to be lower (RR 0.80, 95% CI 0.46 to 1.34), and the risk of rehospitalization for angina was significantly lower in the invasive arm (RR 0.68, 95% CI 0.47 to 0.98).

Most recently, the TIMACS trial tackled the question of timing of an invasive management strategy in 3,031 patients presenting with UA/NSTEMI. Patients were randomized to undergo either early angiography within the first 24 hours of randomization or delayed angiography anytime after 36 hours after randomization. Similar to the ICTUS trial, at 6 months, there was no significant difference in the rate of the composite primary end point of death, MI, or stroke [117]. Nevertheless, subgroup analyses demonstrated that patients considered high risk did benefit from early invasive therapy with a significant reduction in the primary outcome of 13.9% versus 21% in the delayed intervention group (HR 0.65; 95% CI 0.48 to 0.89; $p = 0.006$). Furthermore, for patients of all risk groups, the secondary outcome of death, MI, and refractory ischemia was significantly reduced in the early invasive group (9.5%) as opposed to the delayed intervention group (12.9%) (HR 0.72; 95% CI 0.58 to 0.89; $p = 0.003$).

Using the available data, an early invasive strategy is likely superior to a conservative strategy in reducing cardiac events, in particular spontaneous MI after hospital discharge and refractory ischemia. This benefit appears greatest in patients at intermediate or high risk (especially those with positive troponin). In contrast, lower risk patients have similar outcomes

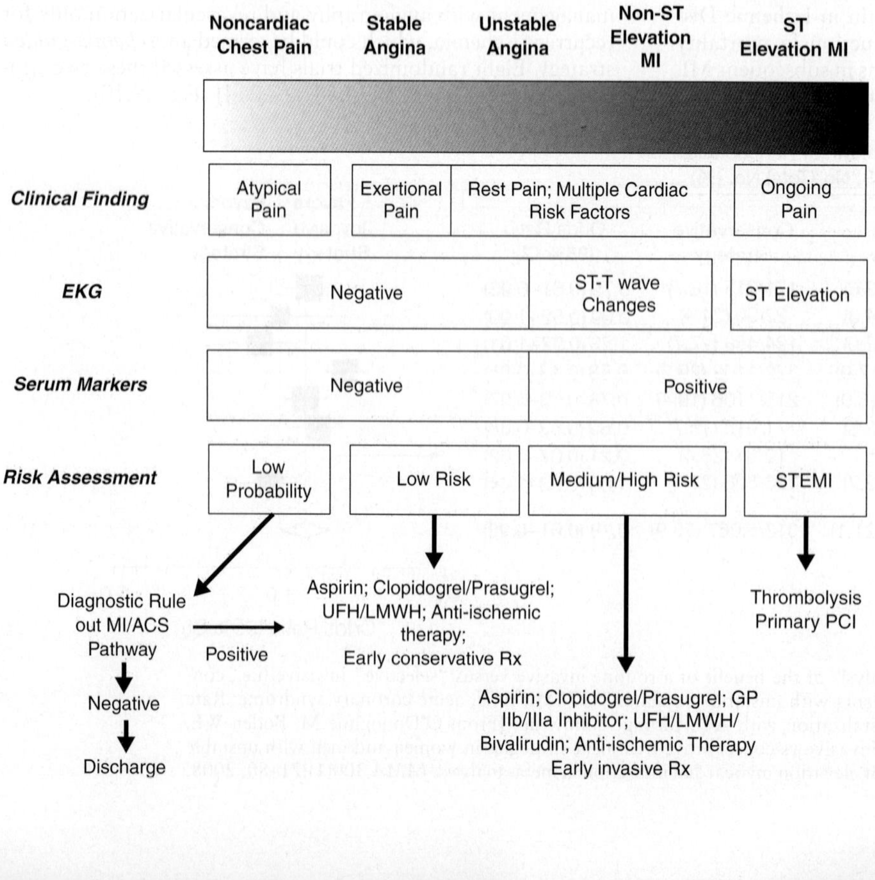

FIGURE 38.11. Algorithm for risk stratification and treatment of patients with UA/NSTEMI. ACS, acute coronary syndrome; DM, diabetes mellitus, ECG, electrocardiogram; LMWH, low-molecular-weight heparin; MI, myocardial infarction, Rx, treatment, STEMI, ST-segment elevation myocardial infarction; UFH, unfractionated heparin.

with either strategy, meaning that either a conservative or invasive strategy can be used in low-risk patients. These results have been incorporated into the update of the ACC/AHA and European Society of Cardiology guidelines for UA/NSTEMI, which recommend broader use of an early invasive strategy.

Percutaneous Coronary Intervention Versus Coronary Artery Bypass Graft

When revascularization is indicated, the choice between PCI versus surgery is faced. In the acute setting, PCI is undertaken much more frequently than CABG surgery. The presence of significant left main coronary artery disease leads to early surgery, with the expectation of improved survival relative to medical therapy alone [221,222]. Six comparative trials have compared PCI with CABG in the nonacute setting; both revascularization strategies resulted in similar rates of death, but a greater need for additional procedures was seen in those initially treated with PCI [223–228]. The SYNTAX (Synergy between Percutaneous Coronary Intervention with TAXUS and Cardiac Surgery) trial recently compared PCI with CABG in 1,800 patients with three-vessel or left main coronary artery disease and confirmed these prior findings—the rates of death were similar between the two groups, though the PCI group experienced relatively more major adverse cardiac or cerebrovascular events over the time course of the study (17.8% vs. 12.4% for CABG; $p = 0.002$) largely because of an increased rate of repeat revascularization with PCI (13.5% vs. 5.9% for CABG; $p < 0.001$) [228]. There was a higher rate of early stroke with CABG surgery. Differences in mortality with PCI and CABG were noted in certain subgroups. In the Bypass Angioplasty Revascularization Investigation trial, patients with diabetes who were treated surgically with a left internal thoracic artery graft were noted to have a significantly lower mortality compared with angioplasty [227]. This finding was further supported by a recent meta-analysis of ten randomized trials comparing PCI and CABG in patients with multivessel coronary disease in which mortality was shown to be lower with CABG in patients with diabetes or in those older than 65 years [229]. Using these data and those of previous trials of CABG versus medical therapy [221,222,230,231] and more recent observational data [232], CABG is recommended for patients with disease of the left main coronary artery, multivessel disease involving the proximal left anterior descending artery, multivessel disease, and impaired LV systolic function or multivessel disease and diabetes [229,233]. For other patients, either PCI or CABG is suitable. PCI has a lower initial morbidity and mortality than CABG but a higher rate of repeat procedures, whereas CABG is associated with more effective relief from angina and the need for fewer medications.

TABLE 38.3

ADVANCES IN MANAGING UA/NSTEMI

- Identification of high-risk patients is key to management of UA/NSTEMI [64,90,97–101]
- Aspirin leads to a more than 50% reduction in the risk of death or myocardial infarction [88,112–114]
- The addition of clopidogrel to aspirin further reduces risk by 20% [116], especially when given prior to percutaneous coronary intervention [117–119]. Prasugrel and ticagrelor are alternative P_2Y_{12} ADP receptor blockers that have been shown to be superior to clopidogrel in the treatment of NSTEMI
- Anticoagulation with one of four agents has been shown to be beneficial: heparin [121], low-molecular-weight heparin (dalteparin and enoxaparin) [128,129], fondaparinux [133], or bivalirudin [136]
- Glycoprotein IIb/IIIa inhibitors can be considered in troponin-positive patients [96–99]; however, the benefit of upstream administration in patients undergoing urgent percutaneous coronary intervention is questionable [162]
- Early, intensive statin therapy is beneficial [186,187]
- An early invasive strategy is beneficial in intermediate- and high-risk patients [76,117,198]

UA-NSTEMI, unstable angina/non–ST-segment elevation myocardial infarction.

CONCLUSIONS

An overall approach to patient management is shown in Figure 38.11. Using the medical history, ECG, and cardiac markers, one can identify patients who have a low likelihood of UA/NSTEMI, for whom a diagnostic "rule-out MI or ACS" is warranted. If this work-up is negative, the patient is discharged home; if positive, the patient is admitted and treated for UA/NSTEMI. These patients are treated with aspirin, a P_2Y_{12} ADP receptor blocker (either clopidogrel or prasugrel, or perhaps ticagrelor in the future), an anticoagulant (UFH or LMWH if at a low risk for bleeding, or bivalirudin if at high risk for bleeding), and anti-ischemic therapy with nitrates and beta-blockers. Risk stratification is used to identify patients at medium to high risk, for whom aggressive treatment with an early invasive strategy is warranted. For patients at low risk, standard treatment is likely sufficient, and a more conservative approach would be reasonable.

Advances in UA/NSTEMI, based on randomized controlled trials or meta-analyses of such trials, are summarized in Table 38.3.

References

1. Cannon CP, Braunwald E: The spectrum of myocardial ischemia. The paradigm of acute coronary syndromes, in Cannon CP (ed): *Contemporary Cardiology: Management of Acute Coronary Syndromes*. 2nd ed. Totowa, NJ, Humana Press, 2003, pp 3–18.
2. DeWood MA, Spores J, Notske R, et al: Prevalence of total coronary occlusion during the early hours of transmural myocardial infarction. *N Engl J Med* 303:897–902, 1980.
3. TIMI Study Group: The thrombolysis in myocardial infarction (TIMI) trial; phase I findings. *N Engl J Med* 312:932–936, 1985.
4. The TIMI IIIA Investigators: Early effects of tissue-type plasminogen activator added to conventional therapy on the culprit lesion in patients presenting with ischemic cardiac pain at rest. Results of the thrombolysis in myocardial ischemia (TIMI IIIA) trial. *Circulation* 87:38–52, 1993.
5. Lloyd-Jones D, Adams RJ, Brown TM, et al; on behalf of the American Heart Association Statistics Committee and Stroke Statistics subcommittee: Heart disease and stroke statistics 2010 update. A report from the American Heart Association. *Circulation*, published online on December 17, 2009.
6. Roe MT, Parsons LS, Pollack CV Jr, et al; for the National Registry of Myocardial Infarction Investigators: Quality of care by classification of myocardial infarction: treatment patterns for ST-segment elevation vs. non-ST-segment elevation myocardial infarction. *Arch Intern Med* 165:1630–1636, 2005.
7. Braunwald E, Antman EM, Beasley JW, et al: ACC/AHA guideline update for the management of patients with unstable angina and non-ST-segment elevation myocardial infarction-2002: summary article: a report of the American College of Cardiology/American Heart Association Task Force on Practice Guidelines (Committee on the Management of Patients With Unstable Angina). *Circulation* 106(14):1893–1900, 2002.

8. Thygesen K, Alpert JS, White HD, et al; on behalf of the Joint ESC/ACCF/AHA/WHF Task Force for the Redefinition of Myocardial Infarction: Universal definition of myocardial infarction. *J Am Coll Cardiol* 50:2173–2195, 2007.
9. Braunwald E: Unstable angina: an etiologic approach to management. *Circulation* 98(21):2219–2222, 1998.
10. Fuster V, Badimon L, Cohen M, et al: Insights into the pathogenesis of acute ischemic syndromes. *Circulation* 77:1213–1220, 1988.
11. Fuster V, Badimon L, Badimon JJ, et al: The pathophysiology of coronary artery disease and the acute coronary syndromes. *N Engl J Med* 326:242–250, 310–218, 1992.
12. Ludmer PL, Selwyn AP, Shook TL, et al: Paradoxical vasoconstriction induced by acetylcholine in atherosclerotic coronary arteries. *N Engl J Med* 315(17):1046–1051, 1986.
13. Lee RT, Libby P: The unstable atheroma. *Arterioscler Thromb Vasc Biol* 17(10):1859–1867, 1997.
14. Moreno PR, Bernardi VH, Lopez-Cuellar J, et al: Macrophages, smooth muscle cells, and tissue factor in unstable angina. Implications for cell-mediated thrombogenicity in acute coronary syndromes. *Circulation* 94:3090–3097, 1996.
15. Weiss EJ, Bray PF, Tayback M, et al: A polymorphism of a platelet glycoprotein receptor as an inherited risk factor for coronary thrombosis. *N Engl J Med* 334:1090–1094, 1996.
16. Ault K, Cannon CP, Mitchell J, et al: Platelet activation in patients after an acute coronary: results from the TIMI 12 trial. *J Am Coll Cardiol* 33:634–639, 1999.
17. Merlini PA, Bauer KA, Oltrona L, et al: Persistent activation of coagulation mechanism in unstable angina and myocardial infarction. *Circulation* 90:61–68, 1994.
18. Becker RC, Tracy RP, Bovill EG, et al: Surface 12-lead electrocardiogram findings and plasma markers of thrombin activity and generation in patients with myocardial ischemia at rest. *J Thromb Thrombolysis* 1:101–107, 1994.
19. Falk E: Unstable angina with fatal outcome: dynamic coronary thrombosis leading to infarction and/or sudden death. *Circulation* 71:699–708, 1985.
20. Davies MJ, Thomas A: Plaque fissuring—the cause of acute myocardial infarction, sudden ischemic death, and crescendo angina. *Br Heart J* 53:363–373, 1985.
21. Shah PK, Falk E, Badimon JJ, et al: Human monocyte-derived macrophages induce collagen breakdown in fibrous caps of atherosclerotic plaques. Potential role of matrix-degrading metalloproteinases and implications for plaque rupture. *Circulation* 92:1565–1569, 1998.
22. Sherman CT, Litvack F, Grundfest W, et al: Coronary angioscopy in patients with unstable angina pectoris. *N Engl J Med* 315:913–919, 1986.
23. Brunelli C, Spallarossa P, Ghigliotta G, et al: Thrombosis in refractory unstable angina. *Am J Cardiol* 68:110B–118B, 1991.
24. Mizuno K, Satumo K, Miyamoto A, et al: Angioscopic evaluation of coronary artery thrombi in acute coronary syndromes. *N Engl J Med* 326:287–291, 1992.
25. Sullivan E, Kearney M, Isner JM, et al: Pathology of unstable angina: analysis of biopsies obtained by directional coronary atherectomy. *J Thromb Thrombolysis* I:63–71, 1994.
26. Harrington RA, Califf RM, Holmes DR Jr, et al: Is all unstable angina the same? Insights from the coronary angioplasty versus excisional atherectomy trial (CAVEAT-I). *Am Heart J* 137(2):227–233, 1999.
27. Colman RW, Marder VJ, Salzman EW, et al: Overview of hemostasis, in Colman RW, Hirsh J, Marder VJ, et al (eds): *Hemostasis and Thrombosis: Basic Principles and Clinical Practice*. 3rd ed. Philadelphia, JB Lippincott Company, 1994, pp 3–18.
28. Handin RI, Loscalzo J: Hemostasis, thrombosis, fibrinolysis, and cardiovascular disease, in Braunwald E (ed): *Heart Disease*. 4th ed. Philadelphia, WB Saunders, 1992, pp 1767–1789.
29. Broze GJ Jr: The role of tissue factor pathway inhibitor in a revised coagulation cascade. *Semin Hematol* 29:159–169, 1992.
30. Furie B, Furie BC: Molecular and cellular biology of blood coagulation. *N Engl J Med* 326:800–806, 1992.
31. Badimon JJ, Lettino M, Toschi V, et al: Local inhibition of tissue factor reduces the thrombogenicity of disrupted human atherosclerotic plaques: effects of tissue factor pathway inhibitor on plaque thrombogenicity under flow conditions. *Circulation* 99(14):1780–1787, 1999.
32. Furie B, Furie BC: Mechanisms of thrombus formation. *N Engl J Med* 359(9):938–949, 2008.
33. Prinzmetal M, Kennamer R, Merliss R, et al: A variant form of angina pectoris. *Am J Med* 27:375–388, 1959.
34. Hirsch PD, Hillis LD, Campbell WB, et al: Release of prostaglandins and thromboxane into the coronary circulation in patients with ischemic heart disease. *N Engl J Med* 304:685–691, 1981.
35. Willerson JT, Golino P, Eidt J, et al: Specific platelet mediators and unstable coronary artery lesions. Experimental evidence and potential clinical implications. *Circulation* 80:198–205, 1989.
36. Eisenberg PR, Kenzora JL, Sobel BE, et al: Relation between ST segment shifts during ischemia and thrombin activity in patients with unstable angina. *J Am Coll Cardiol* 18(4):898–903, 1991.
37. Nabel EG, Ganz P, Gordon JB, et al: Dilation of normal and constriction of atherosclerotic coronary arteries caused by the cold pressor test. *Circulation* 77(1):43–52, 1988.
38. Daniel WC, Lange RA, Landau C, et al: Effects of the intracoronary infusion of cocaine on coronary arterial dimensions and blood flow in humans. *Am J Cardiol* 78(3):288–291, 1996.
39. Pitts WR, Lange RA, Cigarroa JE, et al: Cocaine-induced myocardial ischemia and infarction: pathophysiology, recognition, and management. *Prog Cardiovasc Dis* 40(1):65–76, 1997.
40. Yeung AC, Vekshtein VI, Krantz DS, et al: The effect of atherosclerosis on the vasomotor response of coronary arteries to mental stress. *N Engl J Med* 325(22):1551–1556, 1991.
41. Epstein SE, Cannon RO: Site of increased resistance to coronary flow in patients with angina pectoris and normal epicardial coronary arteries. *J Am Coll Cardiol* 8(2):459–461, 1986.
42. Kaski JC, Chester MR, Chen L, et al: Rapid angiographic progression of coronary artery disease in patients with angina pectoris. The role of complex stenosis morphology. *Circulation* 92(8):2058–2065, 1995.
43. Arbustini E, De Servi S, Bramucci E, et al: Comparison of coronary lesions obtained by directional coronary atherectomy in unstable angina, stable angina, and restenosis after either atherectomy or angioplasty. *Am J Cardiol* 75(10):675–682, 1995.
44. Flugelman MY, Virmani R, Correa R, et al: Smooth muscle cell abundance and fibroblast growth factors in coronary lesions of patients with nonfatal unstable angina. A clue to the mechanism of transformation from the stable to the unstable clinical state. *Circulation* 88(6):2493–2500, 1993.
45. Scirica BM, Cannon CP, McCabe CH, et al: Prognosis in the thrombolysis in myocardial ischemia III registry according to the Braunwald unstable angina pectoris classification. *Am J Cardiol* 90:821–826, 2002.
46. Braunwald E: The physical examination, in Braunwald E (ed): *Heart Disease*. 4th ed. Philadelphia, WB Saunders, 1992, pp 13–42.
47. Cannon CP, McCabe CH, Stone PH, et al: The electrocardiogram predicts one-year outcome of patients with unstable angina and non-Q wave myocardial infarction: results of the TIMI III registry ECG ancillary study. *J Am Coll Cardiol* 30:133–140, 1997.
48. The TIMI IIIB Investigators: Effects of tissue plasminogen activator and a comparison of early invasive and conservative strategies in unstable angina and non-Q-wave myocardial infarction: results of the TIMI IIIB trial. *Circulation* 89:1545–1556, 1994.
49. The platelet receptor inhibition for ischemic syndrome management in patients limited by unstable signs and symptoms (PRISM-PLUS) trial investigators: Inhibition of the platelet glycoprotein IIb/IIIa receptor with tirofiban in unstable angina and non-Q-wave myocardial infarction. *N Engl J Med* 338:1488–1497, 1998.
50. Hyde TA, French JK, Wong CK, et al: Four-year survival of patients with acute coronary syndromes without ST-segment elevation and prognostic significance of 0.5-mm ST-segment depression. *Am J Cardiol* 84(4):379–385, 1999.
51. Wright SA, Sawyer DB, Sacks DB, et al: Elevation of troponin I levels in patients without evidence of myocardial injury. *JAMA* 278(24):2144, 1997.
52. Jeremias A, Gibson M: Narrative review: alternative causes for elevated cardiac troponin levels when acute coronary syndromes are excluded. *Ann Intern Med* 142(9):786–791, 2005.
53. Reichlin T, Hochholzer W, Bassetti S, et al: Early diagnosis of myocardial infarction with sensitive cardiac troponin assays. *N Engl J Med* 361(9):858–867, 2009.
54. Keller T, Zeller T, Peetz D, et al: Sensitive troponin I assay in early diagnosis of acute myocardial infarction. *N Engl J Med* 361(9):868–877, 2009.
55. Omland T, deLemos JA, Sabatine MS, et al; for the Prevention of Events with Angiotensin Converting Enzyme Inhibition (PEACE) Trial Investigators: A sensitive cardiac troponin T assay in stable coronary artery disease. *N Engl J Med* 361(26):2538–2547, 2009.
56. Wilson SR, Sabatine MS, Braunwald E, et al: Detection of myocardial injury in patients with unstable angina using a novel nanoparticle cardiac troponin I assay: observations from the PROTECT-TIMI 30 trial. *Am Heart J* 158(3):386–391, 2009.
57. Sabatine MS, Morrow DA, deLemos JA, et al: Detection of acute changes in circulating troponin in the setting of transient stress test-induced myocardial ischaemia using an ultrasensitive assay: results from TIMI 35. *Eur Heart J* 30:162–169, 2009.
58. Veretto T, Cantalupi D, Altieri A, et al: Emergency room technetium-99 m sestamibi imaging to rule out acute myocardial ischemic events in patients with nondiagnostic electrocardiograms. *J Am Coll Cardiol* 22:1804–1808, 1993.
59. Tatum JL, Jesse RL, Kontos MC, et al: Comprehensive strategy for the evaluation and triage of the chest pain patient. *Ann Emerg Med* 29:116–125, 1997.
60. Berning J, Launbjerg J, Appleyard M: Echocardiographic algorithms for admission and predischarge prediction of mortality in acute myocardial infarction. *Am J Cardiol* 69:1538–1544, 1992.
61. Hoffmann U, Bamberg F, Chae CU, et al: Coronary computed tomography angiography for early triage of patients with acute chest pain: the ROMICAT (Rule Out Myocardial Infarction using Computer Assisted Tomography) trial. *J Am Coll Cardiol* 53:1642–1650, 2009.
62. Multicenter Postinfarction Research Group: Risk stratification and survival after myocardial infarction. *N Engl J Med* 309:331–336, 1983.
63. Zaret BL, Wackers FJT, Terrin ML, et al: Value of radionuclide rest and exercise left ventricular ejection fraction is assessing survival of patients after thrombolytic therapy for acute myocardial infarction: results of the

thrombolysis in myocardial infarction (TIMI) phase II study. *J Am Coll Cardiol* 26:73–79, 1995.
64. Nicod P, Gilpin E, Dittrich H, et al: Influence on prognosis and morbidity of left ventricular ejection fraction with and without signs of left ventricular failure after acute myocardial infarction. *Am J Cardiol* 61:1165–1171, 1988.
65. Diver DJ, Bier JD, Ferreira PE, et al: Clinical and arteriographic characterization of patients with unstable angina without critical coronary arterial narrowing (from the TIMI-IIIA trial). *Am J Cardiol* 74:531–537, 1994.
66. McCullough PA, O'Neill WW, Graham M, et al: A prospective randomized trial of triage angiography in acute coronary syndromes ineligible for thrombolytic therapy. Results of the medicine versus angiography in thrombolytic exclusion (MATE) trial. *J Am Coll Cardiol* 32(3):596–605, 1998.
67. Anderson JL, Adams CD, Antman EM, et al: ACC/AHA 2007 guidelines for the management of patients with unstable angina/non-ST-segment elevation myocardial infarction-2002: executive summary: a report of the American College of Cardiology/American Heart Association Task Force on Practice Guidelines (Writing Committee to Revise the 2002 Guidelines for Management of Patients With Unstable Angina/non-ST-segment Elevation Myocardial Infarction). *Circulation* 116:803–877, 2007.
68. Cannon CP, Thompson B, McCabe CH, et al: Predictors of non-Q-wave acute myocardial infarction in patients with acute ischemic syndromes: an analysis from the thrombolysis in myocardial ischemia (TIMI) III trials. *Am J Cardiol* 75:977–981, 1995.
69. Cohen M, Demers C, Gurfinkel EP, et al: A comparison of low-molecular-weight heparin with unfractionated heparin for unstable coronary artery disease. *N Engl J Med* 337:447–452, 1997.
70. Antman EM, McCabe CH, Gurfinkel EP, et al: Enoxaparin prevents death and cardiac ischemic events in unstable angina/non-Q-wave myocardial infarction: results of the thrombolysis in myocardial infarction (TIMI) 11B trial. *Circulation* 100(15):1593–1601, 1999.
71. The PURSUIT Trial Investigators: Inhibition of platelet glycoprotein IIb/IIIa with eptifibatide in patients with acute coronary syndromes. *N Engl J Med* 339:436–443, 1998.
72. The Platelet Receptor Inhibition for Ischemic Syndrome Management (PRISM) Study Investigators: A comparison of aspirin plus tirofiban with aspirin plus heparin for unstable angina. *N Engl J Med* 338:1498–1505, 1998.
73. Anderson HV, Cannon CP, Stone PH, et al: One-year results of the thrombolysis in myocardial infarction (TIMI) IIIB clinical trial. A randomized comparison of tissue-type plasminogen activator versus placebo and early invasive versus early conservative strategies in unstable angina and non-Q-wave myocardial infarction. *J Am Coll Cardiol* 26:1643–1650, 1995.
74. FRagmin and Fast Revascularisation during InStability in Coronary artery disease Investigators: Invasive compared with non-invasive treatment in unstable coronary-artery disease: FRISC II prospective randomised multicentre study. *Lancet* 354(9180):708–715, 1999.
75. Bach RG, Cannon CP, DiBattiste PM, et al: Enhanced benefit of early invasive management of acute coronary syndromes in the elderly: results from TACTICS-TIMI 18. *Circulation* 104[Suppl II]:II-548, 2001.
76. Lagerqvist B, Safstrom K, Stable E, et al: Is early invasive treatment of unstable coronary artery disease equally effective for both women and men? FRISC II Study Group Investigators. *J Am Coll Cardiol* 38(1):41–48, 2001.
77. Clayton TC, Pocock SJ, Henderson RA, et al: Do men benefit more than women from an interventional strategy in patients with unstable angina or non-ST-elevation myocardial infarction? The impact of gender in the RITA 3 trial. *Eur Heart J* 25(18):1641–1650, 2004.
78. Swahn E, Alfredsson H, Afzal R, et al: Early invasive compared with a selective invasive strategy in women with non-ST-elevation acute coronary syndromes: a substudy of the OASIS 5 trial and a meta-analysis of previous randomized trials. *Eur Heart J* 2009 (Epub ahead of print).
79. Glaser R, Hermann HC, Murphy SA, et al: Benefit of an early invasive management strategy in women with acute coronary syndromes. *JAMA* 288(24):3124–3129, 2002.
80. O'Donoghue M, Boden WE, Braunwald E, et al: Early invasive vs conservative treatment strategies in women and men with unstable angina and non-ST-segment elevation myocardial infarction: a meta-analysis. *JAMA* 300(1):71–80, 2008.
81. Donahoe SM, Stewart GC, McCabe CH, et al: Diabetes and mortality following acute coronary syndromes. *JAMA* 298(7):765–775, 2007.
82. Theroux P, Alexander J Jr, Pharand C, et al: Glycoprotein IIb/IIIa receptor blockade improves outcomes in diabetic patients presenting with unstable angina/non-ST-elevation myocardial infarction: results from the platelet receptor inhibition in ischemic syndrome management in patients limited by unstable signs and symptoms (PRISM-PLUS) study. *Circulation* 102(20):2466–2472, 2002.
83. Roffi M, Chew DP, Mukherjee D, et al: Platelet glycoprotein IIb/IIIa inhibitors reduce mortality in diabetic patients with non-ST-segment-elevation acute coronary syndromes. *Circulation* 104(23):2767–2771, 2001.
84. Cannon CP, Weintraub WS, Demopoulos LA, et al: Comparison of early invasive and conservative strategies in patients with unstable coronary syndromes treated with the glycoprotein IIb/IIIa inhibitor tirofiban. *N Engl J Med* 344(25):1879–1887, 2001.
85. Wiviott SD, Braunwald E, Angiolilo DJ, et al; for the TRITON-TIMI 38 Investigators: Greater clinical benefit of more intensive oral antiplatelet therapy with prasugrel in patients with diabetes mellitus in the trial to assess improvement in therapeutic outcomes by optimizing platelet inhibition with prasugrel thrombolysis in myocardial infarction 38. *Circulation* 118(16):1626–1636, 2008.
86. Savonitto S, Ardissino D, Granger CB, et al: Prognostic value of the admission electrocardiogram in acute coronary syndromes. *JAMA* 281(8):707–713, 1999.
87. Cohen M, Stinnett SS, Weatherley BD, et al: Predictors of recurrent ischemic events and death in unstable coronary artery disease after treatment with combination antithrombotic therapy. *Am Heart J* 139(6):962–970, 2000.
88. Diderholm E, Andren B, Frostfeldt G, et al: ST depression in ECG at entry identifies patients who benefit most from early revascularization in unstable coronary artery disease: a FRISC II substudy. *Circulation* 100[Suppl I]:I-497–I-498, 1999.
89. Theroux P, Ouimet H, McCans J, et al: Aspirin, heparin or both to treat unstable angina. *N Engl J Med* 319:1105–1111, 1988.
90. Antman EM, Tanasijevic MJ, Thompson B, et al: Cardiac-specific troponin I levels to predict the risk of mortality in patients with acute coronary syndromes. *N Engl J Med* 335:1342–1349, 1996.
91. Morrow DA, Cannon CP, Rifai N, et al: Ability of minor elevations of troponin I and T to predict benefit from an early invasive strategy in patients with unstable angina and non-ST elevation myocardial infarction: results from a randomized trial. *JAMA* 286:2405–2412, 2001.
92. Heidenreich PA, Alloggiamento T, Melsop K, et al: The prognostic value of troponin in patients with non-ST elevation acute coronary syndromes: a meta-analysis. *J Am Coll Cardiol* 38(2):478–485, 2001.
93. Zhao X-Q, Theroux P, Snapinn SM, et al: Intracoronary thrombus and platelet glycoprotein IIb/IIIa receptor blockade with tirofiban in unstable angina or non-Q-wave myocardial infarction. Angiographic results from the PRISM-PLUS trial (platelet receptor inhibition for ischemic syndrome management in patients limited by unstable signs and symptoms). *Circulation* 100:1609–1615, 1999.
94. Heeschen C, van Den Brand MJ, Hamm CW, et al: Angiographic findings in patients with refractory unstable angina according to troponin T status. *Circulation* 100(14):1509–1514, 1999.
95. Wong GC, Morrow DA, Murphy S, et al: Elevations in troponin T and I are associated with abnormal tissue level perfusion: a TACTICS-TIMI 18 substudy. *Circulation* 106(2):202–207, 2002.
96. Kastrati A, Mehilli J, Neumann FJ, et al: Abciximab in patients with acute coronary syndromes undergoing percutaneous coronary intervention after clopidogrel pretreatment: the ISAR-REACT 2 randomized trial. *JAMA* 295(13):1531–1538, 2006.
97. Antman EM, Grudzien C, Mitchell RN, et al: Detection of unsuspected myocardial necrosis by rapid bedside assay for cardiac troponin T. *Am Heart J* 133(5):596–598, 1997.
98. Hamm CW, Heeschen C, Goldmann B, et al: Benefit of abciximab in patients with refractory unstable angina in relation to serum troponin T levels. *N Engl J Med* 340(21):1623–1629, 1999.
99. Heeschen C, Hamm CW, Goldmann B, et al: Troponin concentrations for stratification of patients with acute coronary syndromes in relation to therapeutic efficacy of tirofiban. *Lancet* 354(9192):1757–1762, 1999.
100. Januzzi JL, Chai CU, Sabatine MS, et al: Elevation in serum troponin I predicts the benefit of tirofiban. *J Thromb Thrombolysis* 11:211–215, 2001.
101. Morrow DA, Antman EM, Tanasijevic M, et al: Cardiac troponin I for stratification of early outcomes and the efficacy of enoxaparin in unstable angina: a TIMI 11B substudy. *J Am Coll Cardiol* 36:1812–1817, 2000.
102. Laqerqvist B, Diderholm E, Lindahl B, et al: An early invasive treatment strategy reduces cardiac events regardless of troponin levels in unstable coronary artery (UCAD) with and without troponin-elevation: a FRISC II substudy. *Circulation* 100[Suppl I]:I-497, 1999.
103. Haverkate F, Thompson SG, Pyke SDM, et al: Production of C-reactive protein and risk of coronary events in stable and unstable angina. *Lancet* 349:462–466, 1997.
104. Toss H, Lindahl B, Siegbahn A, et al: Prognostic influence of increased fibrinogen and C-reactive protein levels in unstable coronary artery disease. *Circulation* 96(12):4204–4210, 1997.
105. Morrow DA, Rifai N, Antman EM, et al: C-reactive protein is a potent predictor of mortality independently and in combination with troponin T in acute coronary syndromes: a TIMI 11 A substudy. *J Am Coll Cardiol* 31:1460–1465, 1998.
106. Ridker PM, Cannon CP, Morrow D, et al: C-reactive protein levels and outcomes after statin therapy. *N Engl J Med* 352(1):20–28, 2005.
107. De Lemos JA, Morrow DA, Bentley JH, et al: The prognostic value of B-type natriuretic peptide in patients with acute coronary syndromes. *N Engl J Med* 345:1014–1021, 2001.
108. James SK, Lindahl B, Siegbahn A, et al: N-terminal pro-brain natriuretic peptide and other risk markers for the separate prediction of mortality and subsequent myocardial infarction in patients with unstable coronary artery disease: a global utilization of strategies to open occluded arteries (GUSTO)-IV substudy. *Circulation* 108(3):275–281, 2003.
109. Morrow DA, de Lemos JA, Blazing MA, et al: Prognostic value of serial B-type natriuretic peptide testing during follow-up of patients with unstable coronary artery disease. *JAMA* 294(22):2866–2871, 2005.
110. Eggers KM, Lagerqvist B, Venge P, et al: Prognostic value of biomarkers during and after non-ST-segment elevation acute coronary syndrome. *J Am Coll Cardiol* 54(4):357–364, 2009.

111. Wollert KC, Kempf T, Timo P, et al: Prognostic value of growth-differentiation factor-15 in patients with non-ST-elevation acute coronary syndrome. *Circulation* 115(8):962–971, 2007.
112. Wollert KC, Kemph T, Lagerqvist B, et al: Growth differentiation factor 15 for risk stratification and selection of an invasive treatment strategy in non-ST-elevation acute coronary syndrome. *Circulation* 116:1540–1548, 2007.
113. Sabatine MS, Morrow DA, de Lemos JA, et al: Multimarker approach to risk stratification in non-ST-elevation acute coronary syndromes: simultaneous assessment of troponin I, C-reactive protein, and B-type natriuretic peptide. *Circulation* 105(15):1760–1763, 2002.
114. Antman EM, Cohen M, Bernink PJ, et al: The TIMI risk score for unstable angina/non-ST elevation MI: a method for prognostication and therapeutic decision making. *JAMA* 284:835–842, 2000.
115. Morrow DA, Antman EM, Snapinn SM, et al: An integrated clinical approach to predicting the benefit of tirofiban in non-ST elevation acute coronary syndromes. Application of the TIMI risk score for UA/NSTEMI in PRISM-PLUS. *Eur Heart J* 23(3):223–229, 2002.
116. Eagle KA, Lim MJ, Dabbous OH, et al; for the GRACE investigators: A validated prediction model for all forms of acute coronary syndrome. Estimating the risk of 6-month postdischarge death in an international registry. *JAMA* 291(22):2727–2733, 2004.
117. Mehta S, Granger CB, Boden WE, et al; for the TIMACS Investigators: Early versus delayed invasive intervention in acute coronary syndromes. *N Engl J Med* 360(21):2165–2175, 2009.
118. Lewis HD, Davis JW, Archibald DG, et al: Protective effects of aspirin against acute myocardial infarction and death in men with unstable angina. *N Engl J Med* 309:396–403, 1983.
119. Cairns JA, Gent M, Singer J, et al: Aspirin, sulfinpyrazone, or both in unstable angina. *N Engl J Med* 313:1369–1375, 1985.
120. The RISC Group: Risk of myocardial infarction and death during treatment with low dose aspirin and intravenous heparin in men with unstable coronary artery disease. *Lancet* 336:827–830, 1990.
121. Antithrombotic Trialists' Collaboration: Collaborative meta-analysis of randomised trials of antiplatelet therapy for prevention of death, myocardial infarction, and stroke in high risk patients. *BMJ* 324(7329):71–86, 2002.
122. CURE Study Investigators: The clopidogrel in unstable angina to prevent recurrent events (CURE) trial programme; rationale, design and baseline characteristics including a meta-analysis of the effects of thienopyridines in vascular disease. *Eur Heart J* 21(24):2033–2041, 2000.
123. Mehta SR, Yusuf S, Peters RJ, et al: Effects of pretreatment with clopidogrel and aspirin followed by long-term therapy in patients undergoing percutaneous coronary intervention: the PCI-CURE study. *Lancet* 358(9281):527–533, 2001.
124. Steinhubl SR, Berger PB, Mann JT III, et al: Early and sustained dual oral antiplatelet therapy following percutaneous coronary intervention: a randomized controlled trial. *JAMA* 288(19):2411–2420, 2002.
125. Sabatine MS, Cannon CP, Gibson CM, et al: Effect of clopidogrel pretreatment before percutaneous coronary intervention in patients with ST-elevation myocardial infarction treated with fibrinolytics: the PCI-CLARITY study. *JAMA* 294(10):1224–1232, 2005.
126. King SB III, Smith SC Jr, Hirshfeld JW Jr, et al: 2007 focused update of the ACC/AHA/SCAI 2005 guideline update for percutaneous coronary intervention: a report of the American College of Cardiology/American Heart Association task force on practice guidelines: (2007 writing group to review new evidence and update the 2005 ACC/AHA/SCAI guideline update for percutaneous coronary intervention). *Circulation* 117:261–295, 2008.
127. Mega JL, Close SL, Wiviott SD, et al: Cytochrome P-450 polymorphisms and response to clopidogrel. *N Engl J Med* 360(4):354–362, 2009.
128. Simon T, Verstuyft C, Mary-Krause M, et al: Genetic determinants of response to clopidogrel and cardiovascular events. *N Engl J Med* 360(4):363–375, 2009.
129. Collet JP, Hulot JS, Pena A, et al: Cytochrome P450 2C19 polymorphism in young patients treated with clopidogrel after myocardial infarction: a cohort study. *Lancet* 373(9660):309–317, 2009.
130. Ho PM, Maddoz TM, Wang L, et al: Risk of adverse outcomes associated with concomitant use of clopidogrel and proton pump inhibitors following acute coronary syndrome. *JAMA* 301(9):937–944, 2009.
131. Gilard M, Arnaud B, Fornily JC, et al: Influence of omeprazole on the antiplatelet action of clopidogrel associated with aspirin: the randomized, double-blind OCLA (omeprazole clopidogrel aspirin) study. *J Am Coll Cardiol* 51:256–260, 2008.
132. O'Donoghue ML, Braunwald E, Antman EM, et al: Pharmacodynamic effect and clinical efficacy of clopidogrel and prasugrel with or without a proton-pump inhibitor: an analysis of two randomized trials. *Lancet* 374 (9694):989–997, 2009.
133. Wiviott SD, Braunwald E, McCabe CH, et al; for the TRITON-TIMI-38 Investigators: Prasugrel versus clopidogrel in patients with acute coronary syndromes. *N Engl J Med* 357(20):2001–2015, 2007.
134. Wiviott SD, Braunwald E, McCabe CH, et al: Intensive oral antiplatelet therapy for reduction of ischaemic events including stent thrombosis in patients with acute coronary syndromes treated with percutaneous coronary intervention and stenting in the TRITON-TIMI 38 trial: a subanalysis of a randomized trial. *Lancet* 371(9621):1353–1363, 2008.
135. Wallentin L, Becer RC, Budaj A, et al; for the PLATO Investigators: Ticagrelor versus clopidogrel in patients with acute coronary syndrome. *N Engl J Med* 361(11):1045–1057, 2009.
136. Oler A, Whooley MA, Oler J, et al: Adding heparin to aspirin reduces the incidence of myocardial infarction and death in patients with unstable angina. A meta-analysis. *JAMA* 276:811–815, 1996.
137. Hirsh J, Fuster V: Guide to anticoagulation therapy. Part 1: heparin. *Circulation* 89:1449–1468, 1994.
138. Hirsh J, Levine M: Low molecular weight heparin. *Blood* 79:1–17, 1993.
139. Warkentin TE, Levine MN, Hirsh J, et al: Heparin-induced thrombocytopenia in patients treated with low-molecular-weight heparin or unfractionated heparin. *N Engl J Med* 332:1330–1335, 1995.
140. Antman EM, Cohen M, Radley D, et al: Assessment of the treatment effect of enoxaparin for unstable angina/non-Q-wave myocardial infarction: TIMI 11B-ESSENCE meta-analysis. *Circulation* 100:1602–1608, 1999.
141. Murphy S, Gibson CM, Morrow DA, et al: Efficacy and safety of the low-molecular weight heparin enoxaparin compared with unfractionated heparin across the acute coronary syndrome spectrum: a meta-analysis. *Eur Heart J* (28):2077–2086, 2007.
142. De Lemos JA, Blazing MA, Wiviott SD, et al: Enoxaparin versus unfractionated heparin in patients treated with tirofiban, aspirin and an early conservative initial management strategy: results from the A phase of the A-to-Z trial. *Eur Heart J* 25(19):1688–1694, 2004.
143. Yusuf S, Mehta SR, Chrolavicius S, et al: Comparison of fondaparinux and enoxaparin in acute coronary syndromes. *N Engl J Med* 354(14):1464–1476, 2006.
144. Stone GW, McLaurin BT, Cox DA, et al: Bivalirudin for patients with acute coronary syndromes. *N Engl J Med* 355:2203–2216, 2006.
145. White HD, Ohman EM, Lincoff M, et al: Safety and efficacy of bivalirudin with and without glycoprotein IIb/IIIa inhibitors in patients with acute coronary syndromes undergoing percutaneous coronary intervention: 1-year results from the ACUITY (Acute Catheterization and Urgent Intervention Triage strategy) Trial. *J Am Coll Cardiol* 52(10):807–814, 2008.
146. Williams DO, Kirby MG, McPhearson K, et al: Anticoagulant treatment in unstable angina. *Br J Clin Pract* 40:114–116, 1986.
147. Cohen M, Adams PC, Parry G, et al: Combination antithrombotic therapy in unstable rest angina and non-Q-wave infarction in nonprior aspirin users. Primary end points analysis from the ATACS trial. *Circulation* 89:81–88, 1994.
148. Williams MJ, Morison IM, Parker JH, et al: Progression of the culprit lesion in unstable coronary artery disease with warfarin and aspirin versus aspirin alone: preliminary study. *J Am Coll Cardiol* 30(2):364–369, 1997.
149. Anand SS, Yusuf S, Pogue J, et al: Long-term oral anticoagulant therapy in patients with unstable angina or suspected non-Q-wave myocardial infarction: organization to assess strategies for ischemic syndromes (OASIS) pilot study results. *Circulation* 98(11):1064–1070, 1998.
150. The Organization to Assess Strategies for Ischemic Syndromes (OASIS) Investigators: Effects of long-term, moderate-intensity oral anticoagulation in addition to aspirin in unstable angina. *J Am Coll Cardiol* 37(2):475–484, 2001.
151. Brouwer MA, van den Bergh PJ, Aengevaeren WR, et al: Aspirin plus coumarin versus aspirin alone in the prevention of reocclusion after fibrinolysis for acute myocardial infarction: results of the antithrombotics in the prevention of reocclusion in coronary thrombolysis (APRICOT)-2 trial. *Circulation* 106(6):659–665, 2002.
152. Van Es RF, Jonker JJ, Verheugt FW, et al: Aspirin and Coumadin after acute coronary syndromes (the ASPECT-2 study): a randomised controlled trial. *Lancet* 360(9327):109–113, 2002.
153. Hurlen M, Abdelnoor M, Smith P, et al: Warfarin, aspirin, or both after myocardial infarction. *N Engl J Med* 347(13):969–974, 2002.
154. Mega JL, Braunwald E, Mohanavelu et al; for the ATLAS ACS-TIMI 46 study group: Rivaroxaban versus placebo in patients with acute coronary syndromes (ATLAS ACS-TIMI 46): a randomized, double-blind, phase II trial. *Lancet* 374(9683):29–38, 2009.
155. Alexander JH, Becker RC, Bhatt DL, et al; for the APPRAISE Steering Committee and Investigators: Apixaban, an oral, direct, selective factor Xa inhibitor, in combination with antiplatelet therapy after acute coronary syndrome: results of the apixaban for prevention of acute ischemic and safety events (APPRAISE) trial. *Circulation* 119(22):2877–2885, 2009.
156. Fibrinolytic Therapy Trialists' (FTT) Collaborative Group: Indications for fibrinolytic therapy in suspected acute myocardial infarction: collaborative overview of early mortality and major morbidity results from all randomised trials of more than 1000 patients. *Lancet* 343:311–322, 1994.
157. ISIS-2 (Second International Study of Infarct Survival) Collaborative Group: Randomised trial of intravenous streptokinase, oral aspirin, both, or neither among 17,187 cases of suspected acute myocardial infarction: ISIS-2. *Lancet* 2:349–360, 1988.
158. Boersma E, Akkerhuis KM, Theroux P, et al: Platelet glycoprotein IIb/IIIa receptor inhibition in non-ST-elevation acute coronary syndromes: early benefit during medical treatment only, with additional protection during percutaneous coronary intervention. *Circulation* 100(20):2045–2048, 1999.
159. Boersma E, Harrington RA, Molterno DJ, et al: Platelet glycoprotein IIb/IIIa inhibitors in acute coronary syndromes: a meta-analysis of all major randomized clinical trials. *Lancet* 359:189–198, 2002.
160. The GUSTO IV-ACS Investigators: Effect of glycoprotein IIb/IIIa receptor blocker abciximab on outcome in patients with acute coronary syndromes

without early coronary revascularization: the GUSTO IV-ACS randomized trial. *Lancet* 357(9272):1915–1924, 2001.
161. Stone GW, Bertrand ME, Moses JW, et al; for the ACUITY Investigators: Routine upstream initiation vs deferred selective use of glycoprotein IIb/IIIa inhibitors in acute coronary syndromes. The ACUITY timing trial. *JAMA* 297:591–602, 2007.
162. Giugliano RP, White JA, Bode C, et al; for the EARLY ACS Investigators: Early versus delayed provisional eptifibatide in acute coronary syndromes. *N Engl J Med* 360(21):2176–2190, 2009.
163. Mahaffey KW, Harrington RA, Simoons ML, et al: Stroke in patients with acute coronary syndromes: incidence and outcomes in the platelet glycoprotein IIb/IIIa in unstable angina receptor suppression using Integrilin therapy (PURSUIT) trial. *Circulation* 99(18):2371–2377, 1999.
164. Coulter SA, Cannon CP, Cooper RA, et al: Thrombocytopenia, bleeding, and thrombotic events with oral glycoprotein IIb/IIIa inhibition: results from OPUS-TIMI 16. *J Am Coll Cardiol* 35[Suppl A]:393A, 2000.
165. Newby LK, Ohman EM, Christenson RH, et al: Benefit of glycoprotein IIb/IIIa inhibition in patients with acute coronary syndromes and troponin t-positive status: the PARAGON-B troponin T substudy. *Circulation* 103(24):2891–2896, 2001.
166. Barr E, Thornton AR, Sax FL, et al: Benefit of tirofiban plus heparin therapy in unstable angina/non-Q wave myocardial infarction patients is observed regardless of interventional treatment. *Circulation* 98[Suppl I]:I-504, 1998.
167. Alexander JH, Harrington RA, Tuttle RH, et al: Prior aspirin use predicts worse outcomes in patients with non-ST-elevation acute coronary syndromes. PURSUIT investigators. Platelet IIb/IIIa in unstable angina: receptor suppression using integrilin therapy. *Am J Cardiol* 83(8):1147–1151, 1999.
168. Gruppo Italiano per lo Studio della Sopravvivenza nell'Infarto Miocardico: GISSI-3: effect of lisinopril and transdermal glyceryl trinitrate singly and together on 6-week mortality and ventricular function after acute myocardial infarction. *Lancet* 343:1115–1122, 1994.
169. ISIS-4 Collaborative Group: ISIS-4: randomized factorial trial assessing early oral captopril, oral mononitrate, and intravenous magnesium sulphate in 58,050 patients with suspected acute myocardial infarction. *Lancet* 345:669–685, 1995.
170. Gottlieb SO, Weisfeldt ML, Ouyang P, et al: Effect of the addition of propranolol to therapy with nifedipine for unstable angina: a randomized, double-blind, placebo-controlled trial. *Circulation* 73:331–337, 1986.
171. Yusuf S, Wittes J, Friedman L: Overview of results of randomized clinical trials in heart disease. II. Unstable angina, heart failure, primary prevention with aspirin and risk factor reduction. *JAMA* 260:2259–2263, 1988.
172. Muller JE, Turi ZG, Pearle DL, et al: Nifedipine and conventional therapy for unstable angina pectoris: a randomized, double-blind comparison. *Circulation* 69:728–739, 1984.
173. The Holland Interuniversity Nifedipine/Metoprolol Trial (HINT) Research Group: Early treatment of unstable angina in the coronary care unit: a randomised, double blind, placebo controlled comparison of recurrent ischaemia in patients treated with nifedipine or metoprolol or both. *Br Heart J* 56(5):400–413, 1986.
174. Theroux P, Taeymans Y, Morissette D, et al: A randomized study comparing propranolol and diltiazem in the treatment of unstable angina. *J Am Coll Cardiol* 5(3):717–722, 1985.
175. Rizik D, Timmis GC, Grines CL, et al: Immediate use of beta blockers, but not calcium blockers, improves prognosis in unstable angina. *Circulation* 84[Suppl II]:II-345, 1991.
176. The Norwegian Multicenter Study Group: Timolol-induced reduction in mortality and reinfarction in patients surviving acute myocardial infarction. *N Engl J Med* 304:801–807, 1981.
177. Hjalmarson A, Elmfeldt D, Herlitz J, et al: Effect on mortality of metoprolol in acute myocardial infarction, a double-blind randomized trial. *Lancet* 2:823–827, 1981.
178. Beta-Blocker Heart Attack Trial Research Group: A randomized trial of propranolol in patients with acute myocardial infarction. I. Mortality results. *JAMA* 247:1707–1714, 1982.
179. ISIS-1 (First International Study of Infarct Survival) Collaborative Group: Randomised trial of intravenous atenolol among 16,027 cases of suspected acute myocardial infarction. *Lancet* 2:57–66, 1986.
180. Hjalmarson A, Herlitz J, Holmberg S, et al: The Gotenborg metoprolol trial. Effects on mortality and morbidity in acute myocardial infarction. *Circulation* 67[Suppl I]:I-26–I-32, 1983.
181. Yusuf S, Sleight P, Rossi P, et al: Reduction in infarct size, arrhythmias and chest pain by early intravenous beta blockade in suspected myocardial infarction. *Circulation* 67[Suppl I]:I-32–I-41, 1983.
182. Packer M, Bristow MR, Cohn JN, et al: The effect of carvedilol on morbidity and mortality in patients with chronic heart failure. *N Engl J Med* 334:1349–1355, 1996.
183. The MERIT-HF Investigators: Effect of metoprolol CR/XL in chronic heart failure: metoprolol CR/XL randomised intervention trial in congestive heart failure (MERIT-HF). *Lancet* 353(9169):2001–2007, 1999.
184. The CIBIS-II Investigators: The cardiac insufficiency bisoprolol study II (CIBIS-II): a randomised trial. *Lancet* 353(9146):9–13, 1999.
185. Sabatine MS: Something old, something new: beta blockers and clopidogrel in acute myocardial infarction. *Lancet* 366(9497):1587–1589, 2005.
186. Gibson RS, Boden WE, Theroux P, et al: Diltiazem and reinfarction in patients with non-Q wave myocardial infarction. Results of a double-blind, randomized, multicenter trial. *N Engl J Med* 315:423–429, 1986.
187. Dahlof B, Sever PS, Pulter NR, et al; for the ASCOT Investigators: Prevention of cardiovascular events with an antihypertensive regimen of amlodipine adding perindopril as required versus atenolol adding bendroflumethiazide as required, in the Anglo-Scandinavian cardiac outcomes trial-blood pressure lowering arm (ASCOT-BPLA): a multicentre randomized controlled trial. *Lancet* 366:895–906, 2005.
188. Nissen SF, Tuzcu EM, Libby P, et al; for the CAMELOT Investigators: Effect of antihypertensive agents on cardiovascular events in patients with coronary disease and normal blood pressure. The CAMELOT study: a randomized controlled trial. *JAMA* 292:2217–2226, 2004.
189. Jamerson K, Weber MA, Bakris GL, et al; for the ACCOMPLISH Trial Investigators: Benazepril plus amlodipine or hydrochlorothiazide for hypertension in high-risk patients. *N Engl J Med* 359(23):2417–2418, 2008.
190. Teo KT, Yusuf S, Furberg CD: Effects of prophylactic antiarrhythmic drug therapy in acute myocardial infarction: an overview of results from randomized controlled trails. *JAMA* 270:1589–1595, 1993.
191. Hennekens CH, Albert CM, Godfried SL, et al: Adjunctive drug therapy of acute myocardial infarction—evidence from clinical trials. *N Engl J Med* 335:1660–1667, 1996.
192. The Multicenter Diltiazem Postinfarction Trial Research Group: The effect of diltiazem on mortality and reinfarction after myocardial infarction. *N Engl J Med* 319:385–392, 1988.
193. Wilcox RG, Hampton JR, Banks DC, et al: Trial of early Nifedipine in acute myocardial infarction: the TRENT study. *BMJ* 293:1204–1208, 1986.
194. The Israeli SPRINT Study Group: Secondary prevention reinfarction Israeli Nifedipine trial (SPRINT): a randomized intervention trial of nifedipine in patients with acute myocardial infarction. *Eur Heart J* 9:354–364, 1988.
195. Chaitman BR, Pepine CJ, Parker JO; for the Combination Assessment of Ranolazine in Stable Angina (CARISA) Investigators: Effects of ranolazine with atenolol, amlodipine, or diltiazem on exercise tolerance and angina frequency in patients with severe chronic angina: a randomized controlled trial. *JAMA* 291(3):309–316, 2004.
196. Chaitman BR, Skettino SL, Parker JO; for the MARISA Investigators: Anti-ischemic effects and long-term survival during ranolazine monotherapy in patients with chronic severe angina. *J Am Coll Cardiol* 43(8):1375–1382, 2004.
197. Morrow DA, Scirica BM, Karwatowska-Prokopszuk E, et al; for the MERLIN-TIMI 36 Trial Investigators: Effects of ranolazine on recurrent cardiovascular events in patients with non-ST-elevation acute coronary syndromes: the MERLIN-TIMI 36 randomized trial. *JAMA* 297(160):1775–1783, 2007.
198. Wilson SR, Scirica BM, Braunwald E, et al: Efficacy of ranolazine in patients with chronic angina observations from the randomized, double-blind, placebo-controlled MERLIN-TIMI (Metabolic Efficiency with Ranolazine for Less Ischemia in Non-ST-Segment Elevation Acute Coronary Syndromes) 36 trial. *J Am Coll Cardiol* 53(17):1510–1516, 2009.
199. Pfeffer MA, Braunwald E, Moye LA, et al: Effect of captopril on mortality and morbidity in patients with left ventricular dysfunction after myocardial infarction. *N Engl J Med* 327:669–677, 1992.
200. The Acute Infarction Ramipril Efficacy (AIRE) Study Investigators: Effect of ramipril on mortality and morbidity of survivors of acute myocardial infarction with clinical evidence of heart failure. *Lancet* 342:821–828, 1993.
201. Yusuf S, Sleight P, Pogue J, et al: Effects of an angiotensin-converting-enzyme inhibitor, ramipril, on cardiovascular events in high-risk patients. *N Engl J Med* 342:145–153, 2000. [Published erratum appears in *N Engl J Med* 342(10):748, 2000.]
202. Fox KM: Efficacy of perindopril in reduction of cardiovascular events among patients with stable coronary artery disease: randomised, double-blind, placebo-controlled, multicentre trial (the EUROPA study). *Lancet* 362(9386):782–788, 2003.
203. Braunwald E, Domanski MJ, Fowler SE, et al: Angiotensin-converting-enzyme inhibition in stable coronary artery disease. *N Engl J Med* 351(20):2058–2068, 2004.
204. Petrie MC, Padmanabhan N, McDonald JE, et al: Angiotensin converting enzyme (ACE) and non-ACE dependent angiotensin II generation in resistance arteries from patients with heart failure and coronary artery disease. *J Am Coll Cardiol* 37:1056–1061, 2001.
205. Pfeffer MA, McMurray JJV, Velazquez EJ, et al; for the Valsartan in Acute Myocardial Infarction Investigators: Valsartan, captopril, or both in myocardial infarction complicated by heart failure, left ventricular dysfunction or both. *N Engl J Med* 349(20):1893–1906, 2003.
206. The ONTARGET Investigators: Telmisartan, ramipril, or both in patients at high risk for vascular events. *N Engl J Med* 358:1547–1559, 2008.
207. Scandinavian Simvastatin Survival Study Group: Randomised trial of cholesterol lowering in 4444 patients with coronary heart disease: the Scandinavian simvastatin survival study (4S). *Lancet* 344:1383–1389, 1994.
208. Sacks RM, Pfeffer MA, Moye LA, et al: The effect of pravastatin on coronary events after myocardial infarction in patients with average cholesterol levels. *N Engl J Med* 335:1001–1009, 1996.
209. The Long-Term Intervention with Pravastatin in Ischaemic Disease (LIPID) Study Group: Prevention of cardiovascular events and death with pravastatin in patients with coronary heart disease and a broad range of initial cholesterol levels. *N Engl J Med* 339(19):1349–1357, 1998.

210. Schwartz GG, Olsson AG, Ezekowitz MD, et al: Effects of atorvastatin on early recurrent ischemic events in acute coronary syndromes: the MIRACL study: a randomized controlled trial. *JAMA* 285(13):1711–1718, 2001.
211. Cannon CP, Braunwald E, McCabe CH, et al: Intensive versus moderate lipid lowering with statins after acute coronary syndromes. *N Engl J Med* 350(15):1495–1504, 2004.
212. Ray KK, Cannon CP, McCabe C, et al: Early late benefits of high-dose Atorvastatin in patients with acute coronary syndromes: results from the PROVE-IT TIMI 22 trial. *J Am Coll Cardiol* 46:1405–1410, 2005.
213. Grundy SM, Cleeman JI, Merz CN, et al: Implications of recent clinical trials for the National Cholesterol Education Program Adult Treatment Panel III guidelines. *Arterioscler Thromb Vasc Biol Aug* 24(8):e149–e161, 2004.
214. Boden WE, O'Rourke RA, Crawford MH, et al: Outcomes in patients with acute non-Q-wave myocardial infarction randomly assigned to an invasive as compared with a conservative strategy. *N Engl J Med* 338:1785–1792, 1998.
215. Wallentin L, Lagerqvist B, Husted S, et al: Outcome at 1 year after an invasive compared with a non-invasive strategy in unstable coronary-artery disease: the FRISC II invasive randomised trial. FRISC II investigators. Fast revascularisation during instability in coronary artery disease. *Lancet* 356(9223):9–16, 2000.
216. Diderholm E, Andren B, Frostfeldt G, et al: ST depression in ECG at entry indicates severe coronary lesions and large benefits of an early invasive treatment strategy in unstable coronary artery disease; the FRISC II ECG substudy. *Eur Heart J* 23(1):41–49, 2002.
217. Lindahl B, Diderholm E, Lagerqvist B, et al: Mechanisms behind the prognostic value of troponin T in unstable coronary artery disease: a FRISC II substudy. *J Am Coll Cardiol* 38(4):979–986, 2001.
218. Fox KA, Poole-Wilson PA, Henderson RA, et al: Interventional versus conservative treatment for patients with unstable angina or non-ST-elevation myocardial infarction: the British Heart Foundation RITA 3 randomised trial. Randomized intervention trial of unstable angina. *Lancet* 360(9335):743–751, 2002.
219. Fox KA, Poole-Wilson P, Clayton TC, et al: 5-year outcome of an interventional strategy in non-ST-elevation acute coronary syndrome: the British Heart Foundation RITA 3 randomised trial. *Lancet* 366(9489):914–920, 2005.
220. De Winter RJ, Windhausen F, Cornel JH, et al: Early invasive versus selectively invasive management for acute coronary syndromes. *N Engl J Med* 353(11):1095–1104, 2005.
221. CASS Principal Investigators and Their Associates: Coronary artery surgery study (CASS): a randomized trial of coronary artery bypass surgery. Survival data. *Circulation* 68:939–950, 1983.
222. Chaitman BR, Fisher LD, Bourassa MD: Effect of coronary bypass surgery on survival patterns in subsets of patients with left main coronary artery disease. Report of the collaborative study in coronary artery surgery (SASS). *Am J Cardiol* 48:765–777, 1981.
223. RITA Trial Participants: Coronary angioplasty versus coronary artery bypass surgery: the randomized intervention treatment of angina (RITA) trial. *Lancet* 341:573–580, 1993.
224. Rodriquez A, Boullon F, Perez-Balino N, et al: Argentine randomized trial of percutaneous transluminal coronary angioplasty versus coronary artery bypass surgery in multivessel disease (ERACI): in-hospital results and 1-year follow-up. *J Am Coll Cardiol* 22:1060–1067, 1993.
225. Hamm CW, Reimers J, Ischinger T, et al: A randomized study of coronary angioplasty compared with bypass surgery in patients with symptomatic multivessel coronary disease. *N Engl J Med* 331:1037–1043, 1994.
226. King SB III, Lembo NJ, Weintraub WS, et al: A randomized trial comparing coronary angioplasty with coronary bypass surgery. *N Engl J Med* 331:1044–1050, 1994.
227. The Bypass Angioplasty Revascularization Investigation (BARI) Investigators: Comparison of coronary bypass surgery with angioplasty in patients with multivessel disease. *N Engl J Med* 335:217–225, 1996.
228. Serruys PW, Morice MC, Kappetein P, et al; for the SYNTAX Investigators: Percutaneous coronary intervention versus coronary-artery-bypass-grafting for severe coronary artery disease. *N Engl J Med* 360(10):961–972, 2009.
229. Hlatzky M, Boothroyd DB, Bravata DM, et al: Coronary artery bypass surgery compared with percutaneous coronary interventions for multivessel disease: a collaborative analysis of individual patient data from ten randomized trials. *Lancet* 373:1190–1197, 2009.
230. European Coronary Surgery Study Group: Long-term results of prospective randomized study of coronary artery bypass surgery in stable angina pectoris. *Lancet* 2:1173–1180, 1982.
231. The Veterans Administration Coronary Artery Bypass Surgery Collaborative Study Group: Eleven-year survival in the veterans administration randomized trial of coronary bypass surgery for stable angina. *N Engl J Med* 311:1333–1339, 1984.
232. Mark DB, Nelson CL, Califf RM, et al: Continuing evolution of therapy for coronary artery disease. Initial results from the era of coronary angioplasty. *Circulation* 89:2015–2025, 1994.
233. Hillis LD, Rutherford JD: Coronary angioplasty compared with bypass grafting. *N Engl J Med* 331:1086–1087, 1994.

CHAPTER 39 ■ ST-SEGMENT ELEVATION MYOCARDIAL INFARCTION

JAMES A. de LEMOS AND DAVID A. MORROW

Advances in the prevention, diagnosis, and management of patients with acute ST-segment elevation myocardial infarction (STEMI) have led to a reduction in mortality from this condition over the past few decades [1]. Rapid delivery of reperfusion therapy remains the cornerstone of management of STEMI. In recent years, substantial improvements in adjunctive therapies and processes of care delivery have been made, and these are expected to contribute to continued improvement in outcomes following STEMI.

PATHOPHYSIOLOGY

The initial pathophysiologic event leading to STEMI is rupture or erosion of a lipid-rich atherosclerotic plaque. The atherosclerotic plaque "vulnerable" to rupture tends to have a dense lipid-rich core and a thin protective fibrous cap, and is often not associated with critical narrowing of the arterial lumen. Molecular factors that regulate synthesis and dissolution of the extracellular matrix appear to modulate integrity of the protective fibrous cap. In unstable atherosclerotic lesions, inflammatory cells accumulate at the "shoulder" region of the plaque and release cytokines that degrade extracellular matrix and weaken the fibrous cap at this critical site [2].

Following plaque rupture, platelets adhere to subendothelial collagen, von Willebrand factor, or fibrinogen, and become activated by various local mediators such as adenosine diphosphate (ADP), collagen, and thrombin. Activated platelets undergo a conformational change and secrete the contents of their α-granules, promoting vasoconstriction and clot retraction. Activated platelets also express glycoprotein (GP) IIb/IIIa receptors in increased number and with greater binding affinity; fibrinogen-mediated cross-linking at this critical receptor leads to platelet aggregation. On the phospholipid surface of

TABLE 39.1

DIFFERENTIAL DIAGNOSIS OF ACUTE MI

Condition	Characterization of pain	Physical findings	ECG findings	Helpful diagnostic tests
Acute coronary syndrome	Pressure-type pain at rest, often radiating to neck or left arm	Examination often normal; check for signs of cardiogenic shock or CHF	ST-segment elevation, ST-segment depression, T-wave abnormalities, LBBB	Measurement of cardiac enzymes
Tako-Tsubo cardiomyopathy	Similar to AMI, but commonly precipitated by emotional stress	Examination often normal; may have signs of CHF	Anteroapical ST-segment elevation commonly with T-wave inversion	Cardiac enzymes only minimally elevated; anteroapical akinesis; normal coronary arteries
Aortic dissection	"Tearing" pain radiating to back	Diminished pulse or blood pressure in left arm	Nonspecific changes, LVH; ST-segment elevation if dissection involves coronary ostia	Chest x-ray, CT scan, or MRI; transesophageal echocardiography; aortogram
Pulmonary embolism	Pleuritic chest pain with dyspnea and cough	Tachypnea; tachycardia; pleural rub; right ventricular heave	Sinus tachycardia with nonspecific ST and T-wave changes; $S_1Q_3T_3$ pattern classic, but rarely seen	High-resolution chest CT; ventilation-perfusion lung scan; pulmonary angiogram
Pericarditis	Positional pain (worse lying flat)	Pericardial friction rub	Diffuse, concave ST-segment elevation with PR-segment depression	Echocardiogram

CT, computed tomography; CHF, congestive heart failure; LBBB, left bundle branch block; MRI, magnetic resonance imaging.

the platelet membrane prothrombin is converted to thrombin, catalyzing the conversion of fibrinogen to fibrin [3].

The distinguishing feature of the platelet–fibrin clot in STEMI is that it completely occludes the epicardial coronary artery, leading to transmural myocardial injury, manifested by ST-segment elevation on the electrocardiogram (ECG). Despite similar initial pathophysiologic features, unstable angina and non-STEMI (NSTEMI) are rarely associated with complete occlusion of the culprit coronary artery and do not benefit from fibrinolytic therapy. The distinction between Q-wave and non–Q wave MI can only be made retrospectively, and is not useful for early patient management. Accordingly, this terminology has been superseded by the terms STEMI and NSTEMI. Without reperfusion therapy, most patients with STEMI suffer transmural infarction and evolve Q-waves over the first few days after MI. Successful reperfusion therapy, however, may limit necrosis to the subendocardial regions and prevent development of Q-waves.

DIAGNOSIS AND RISK ASSESSMENT

History and Physical Examination

The pain of acute MI is qualitatively similar to angina and is classically described as a severe pressure-type pain in the midsternum, often radiating to the left arm, neck, or jaw. Associated symptoms include dyspnea, diaphoresis, nausea, vomiting, and weakness. In the elderly and those with diabetes, pain is often atypical, and may not be present at all [4]. Not uncommonly, inferior STEMI presents with nausea and vagal symptoms rather than chest pain. Silent infarction may occur in 25% or more cases. Characterization of the quality of the pain may help to distinguish MI from other conditions that cause chest discomfort, such as aortic dissection, pulmonary embolism, pericarditis, and gastrointestinal (GI) disorders such as cholecystitis and peptic ulcer (Table 39.1).

Patients with acute MI often appear pale and clammy; in many cases, they are in obvious distress. Elderly patients, in particular, may be agitated and incoherent. In contrast, patients with cardiogenic shock may be confused and listless. The objective of the initial examination should be to rapidly narrow the differential diagnosis and assess the stability of the patient. A focused examination can help to differentiate ischemia from conditions such as pneumothorax, pericarditis, aortic dissection, and cholecystitis (Table 39.1). Concomitant conditions, such as valvular heart disease, peripheral vascular disease, and cerebrovascular disease, may complicate patient management and can be rapidly detected by physical examination. A brief survey for signs of congestive heart failure should be performed. Cool extremities or impaired mental status suggests decreased tissue perfusion, whereas elevated jugular venous pressure and rales suggest elevated cardiac filling pressures. Finally, the hemodynamic and mechanical complications of acute MI can often be detected by careful attention to physical findings.

An increasingly recognized syndrome that may mimic acute MI is Tako-Tsubo cardiomyopathy, or the apical ballooning syndrome. This syndrome, more common among elderly women, is typically precipitated by an acute stress, including severe emotional distress or acute noncardiac medical illness. Chest pain associated with anteroapical ST-segment elevation and T-wave inversions is usually indistinguishable from an evolving anterior infarct. The diagnosis is typically made when normal coronary arteries and the distinctive anteroapical wall motion abnormality (Fig. 39.1) are seen at the time of

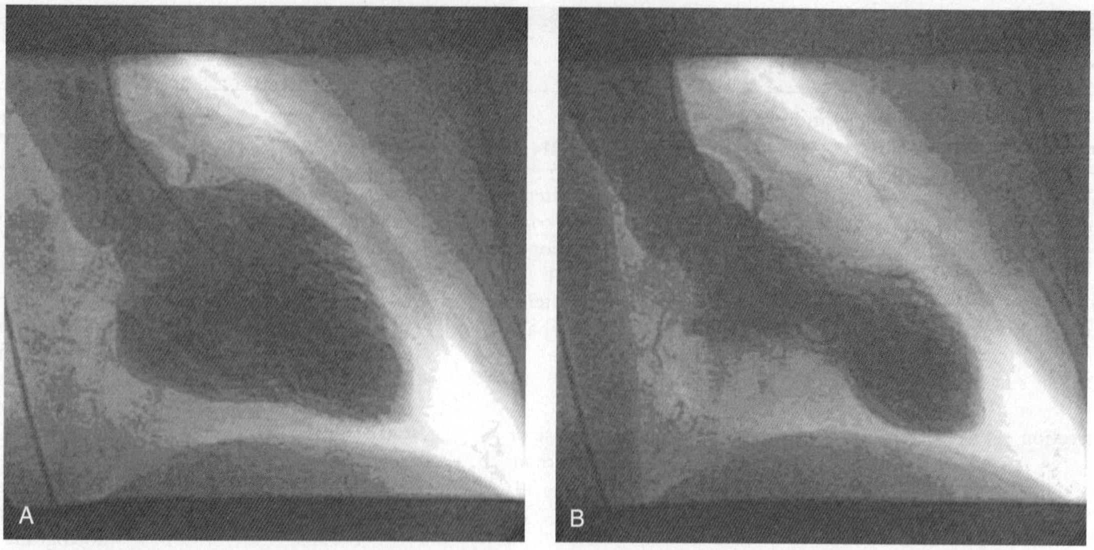

FIGURE 39.1. Representative contrast ventriculogram from a patient with Tako-Tsubo cardiomyopathy, demonstrating an anteroapical wall motion abnormality. The ventriculogram in Panel A was obtained at end diastole and in Panel B at end systole. [From the *Libyan J Med*, AOP: 070707, published July 19, 2007.]

emergent cardiac catheterization. In contrast to acute MI, cardiac enzymes usually elevate only modestly and the left ventricular (LV) functional abnormalities tend to be transient. The pathophysiology of this syndrome is thought to be due to catecholamine-mediated myocardial stunning.

Electrocardiogram

Performance of the 12-lead ECG in the prehospital setting significantly reduces time to reperfusion and shows a strong trend toward reducing mortality [5]. Because only about 25% of patients with STEMI transported by emergency medical services in the United States receive a prehospital ECG, this represents an important target for improvement [5]. The ability to transmit the 12-lead ECG and activate a STEMI care team prior to hospital arrival has provided an opportunity for a major enhancement in systems for STEMI care.

The ST-segment elevation of acute MI must be distinguished from that due to pericarditis or even the normal early repolarization variant. Ischemic ST-segment elevation typically has a convex configuration, is limited to selected ECG leads, and is often associated with reciprocal ST-segment depression (Fig. 39.2). Pericarditis, on the other hand, is typically associated with diffuse ST-segment elevation and depression of the PR segment (Fig. 39.3). The contour of the elevated ST segment in pericarditis and early repolarization variant is typically concave (upward sloping), in contrast to that seen with myocardial injury. Reversible ischemic ST-segment elevation is also seen with coronary vasospasm (Prinzmetal's variant angina).

A *new* (or presumed new) left bundle branch block (LBBB) in a patient with ischemic chest discomfort suggests a large

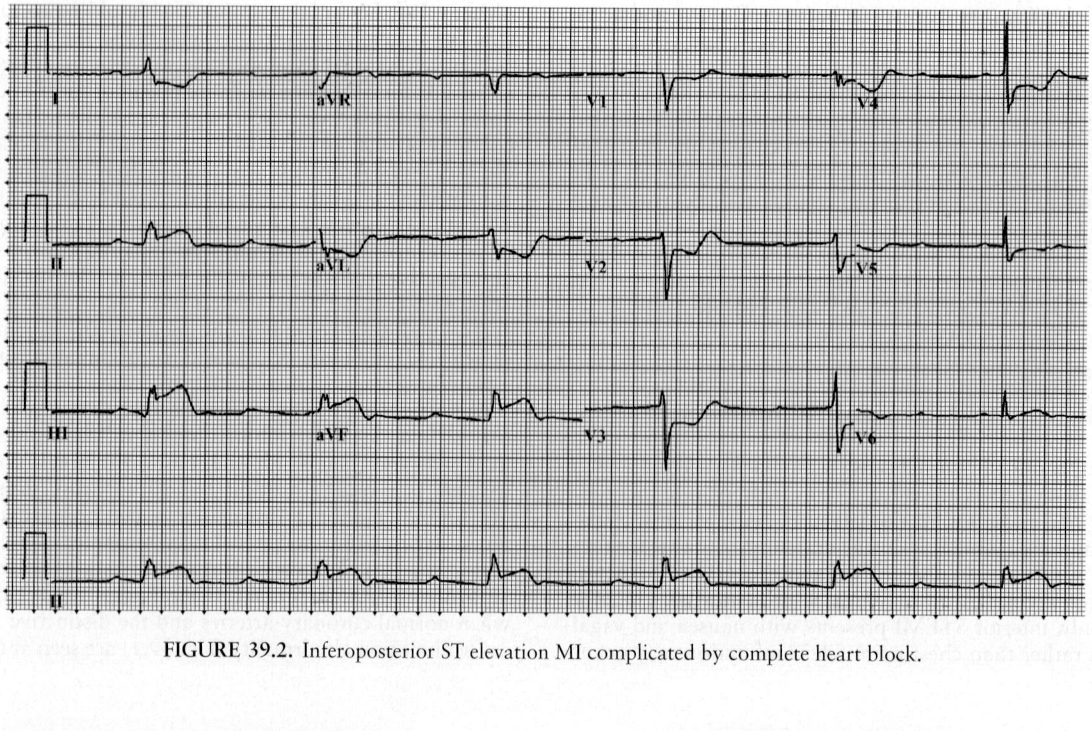

FIGURE 39.2. Inferoposterior ST elevation MI complicated by complete heart block.

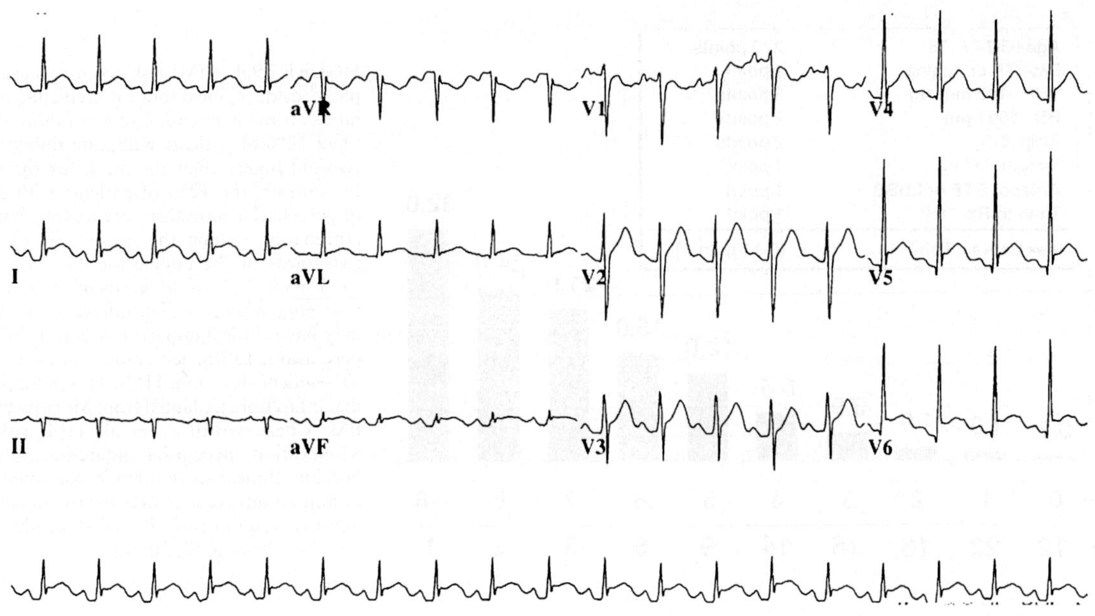

FIGURE 39.3. ECG changes characteristic of pericarditis. Concave (upsloping) ST-segment elevation is seen diffusely, together with PR-segment depression. Importantly, T-waves are essentially normal, another distinguishing feature from ST elevation MI.

anterior infarction, and is also an indication for reperfusion therapy. A LBBB of unknown age, however, presents a diagnostic dilemma, because many of these patients do not have ongoing transmural myocardial ischemia. Here, emergent echocardiography (to look for an anterior wall motion abnormality); bedside testing of serum cardiac markers, such as myoglobin, CKMB, or troponin; and even emergent cardiac catheterization should be considered. It should be emphasized that an acute STEMI leading to LBBB requires a very large ischemic territory, and would not be expected to be a subtle clinical event. In patients with a preexisting LBBB, no ECG criteria are sufficiently sensitive and specific to diagnose acute MI [6], so alternative methods are needed to make the diagnosis.

Cardiac Biomarkers and Other Tools for Risk Assessment

Cardiac biomarkers of necrosis are considerably more important in the initial diagnosis of NSTEMI than they are in the diagnosis of STEMI. For patients with STEMI, cardiac marker measurements are used to confirm the diagnosis in patients with equivocal electrocardiographic changes, to help gauge prognosis, and to estimate the likelihood of successful reperfusion therapy. Cardiac markers also provide prognostic information. Patients with an elevated myoglobin, troponin, or B-type natriuretic peptide level *prior* to initiation of reperfusion therapy are at higher risk for death and congestive heart failure (CHF), even after accounting for baseline variables such as infarct location and time to treatment [7–9]. When combined with subsequent measures of the efficacy of reperfusion therapy, such as the degree of ST-segment resolution, an accurate assessment of prognosis can be made [8]. Although the rate of rise of cardiac biomarkers (particularly myoglobin) can be used to help determine which patients have had successful or unsuccessful reperfusion [10], the clinical role of biomarker testing for reperfusion assessment is limited. The peak levels of troponin, CK, or CKMB provide a crude estimation of infarct size. It should be noted that with successful reperfusion, although the total amount of biomarker released is reduced, the peak value may actually increase, with an earlier peak and more rapid fall in biomarker levels.

Information from the patient's clinical presentation and physical examination are also very valuable for assessing the patient's prognosis. Evidence for heart failure or hemodynamic stress at the time of presentation is weighted heavily in this assessment. For example, it is possible to use the patient's age and vital signs at presentation to rapidly and accurately obtain a preliminary estimate of short-term survival [11]. Anterior infarct location, delays to therapy, and information regarding medical comorbidity all offer additional prognostic information [12]. As such, several tools that integrate age, the physical examination, the ECG, and other clinical parameters such as serum creatinine provide very strong discrimination of short- and long-term mortality risk, and may be implemented using either simple bedside calculation [12,13], handheld devices, or web-based tools [14,15] (Fig. 39.4).

REPERFUSION THERAPY

Rapid provision of reperfusion therapy is the primary treatment objective in patients presenting with STEMI. The managing clinician may choose between two principal reperfusion strategies: pharmacologic reperfusion versus primary percutaneous coronary intervention (PCI). This decision may be based on institutional resources, as well as patient factors as discussed in this section.

The Evolving Definition of "Optimal" Reperfusion

Early successful coronary reperfusion limits infarct size and improves LV dysfunction and survival. These benefits are due at least in part to the early restoration of antegrade flow in the infarct-related artery (IRA). In a retrospective analysis of six angiographic trials of different fibrinolytic regimens, patients who achieved normal (TIMI grade 3) antegrade flow in the IRA had a 30-day mortality rate of 3.6%, versus 6.6% in patients

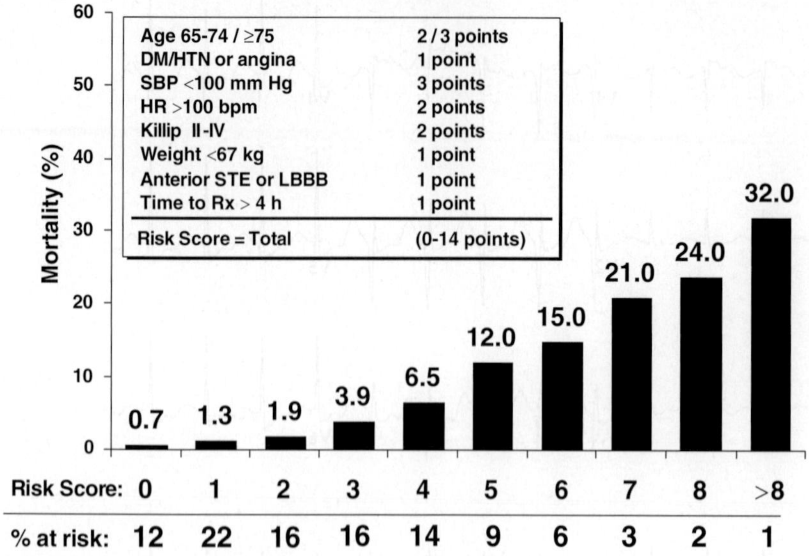

FIGURE 39.4. TIMI risk score for STEMI: a simple, bedside, clinical tool for predicting 30-day mortality. At the high end, a score of more than 5 identified 12% of patients with a mortality risk at least twofold higher than the mean for the population. In contrast, the 12% of patients with a risk score of zero had a mortality rate of less than 1%. Discriminating among the lower risk groups, nearly two-thirds of the population had risk scores of 0 to 3 with a 5.3-fold gradient in mortality over this range where smaller differences in absolute risk may have clinical impact. h/o, history of; HTN, hypertension; LBBB, left bundle branch block; STE, ST-segment elevation; TIMI, Thrombosis in Myocardial Infarction. [Adapted from Morrow DA, Antman EM, Charlesworth A, et al: TIMI risk score for ST-elevation myocardial infarction: a convenient, bedside, clinical score for risk assessment at presentation: an intravenous nPA for treatment of infarcting myocardium early II trial substudy. *Circulation* 102(17):2031–2037, 2000.]

with slow (TIMI grade 2) antegrade flow, and 9.5% in patients with an occluded artery (TIMI grade 0 or 1 flow) [16].

Even among patients who achieve normal (TIMI grade 3) epicardial blood flow in the IRA after reperfusion therapy, however, tissue-level perfusion may be inadequate. Using a number of different diagnostic tools (Table 39.2), investigators have demonstrated that measures of tissue and microvascular perfusion provide prognostic information that is independent of TIMI flow grade [17] (Fig. 39.5). For example, Ito and colleagues, using myocardial contrast echocardiography, found impaired tissue and microvascular perfusion in approximately one-third of patients with TIMI grade 3 blood flow after primary PCI: these patients were at increased risk for the development of CHF and death [18]. Impaired microvascular perfusion

TABLE 39.2

DIAGNOSTIC TOOLS USED TO EVALUATE TISSUE AND MICROVASCULAR PERFUSION IN PATIENTS WITH ST ELEVATION MI[a]

Technique	Finding suggestive of microvascular injury
Myocardial contrast echocardiography	Absence of microbubble contrast uptake in the infarct zone
Doppler flow wire	Abnormal coronary flow reserve; systolic reversal of coronary flow
PET scanning	Impaired regional myocardial blood flow as measured with $^{13}NH_3$
Nuclear SPECT imaging	Absence of tracer uptake into infarct zone
Contrast angiography	Abnormal myocardial "blush," with failure to opacify myocardium or prolonged dye washout from myocardium
MRI	Hypoenhancement of infarct zone following gadolinium contrast injection
ECG	Failure to resolve ST-segment elevation

[a] Assumes that the epicardial infarct artery is patent. These techniques can be presumed to reflect microvascular and tissue perfusion only when the infarct artery has been successfully recanalized.

assessed with cardiac magnetic resonance imaging also correlates with higher mortality risk. Microvascular dysfunction is thought to occur in the setting of MI as a result of distal embolization of microthrombi, tissue inflammation from myocyte necrosis, and arteriolar spasm caused by tissue injury.

Perhaps the most clinically relevant measure of tissue perfusion is a simple bedside assessment of the degree of resolution of ST-segment elevation on the 12-lead ECG. Greater degrees of ST-segment resolution are associated with a higher probability of achieving a patent IRA and TIMI grade 3 flow [19]. Furthermore, patients who have normal epicardial blood flow, but persistence of ST-segment elevation on the 12-lead ECG, have been shown to have abnormal tissue and microvascular perfusion using a variety of specific imaging modalities such as contrast echocardiography and nuclear SPECT perfusion imaging [20,21]. In addition, persistent ST-segment elevation has been shown to predict poor recovery of infarct zone wall motion and the clinical endpoints of death and heart failure [22]. As a result, ST-segment resolution appears to integrate epicardial and myocardial (microvascular) reperfusion, and as such may actually provide a more clinically useful assessment of reperfusion than coronary angiography [23].

Time to Reperfusion

Regardless of the choice of reperfusion strategy, several common themes are evident. First, the benefits of reperfusion therapy are time dependent. Patients who receive fibrinolytic therapy within 1 hour from the onset of chest pain have an approximately 50% reduction in mortality, whereas those presenting more than 12 hours after onset of symptoms derive little, if any, benefit. For each hour earlier that a patient is treated, there is an absolute 1% decrease in mortality [24]. Similarly, for primary PCI, the "door-to-balloon" time has been shown to be directly correlated with clinical benefit [25].

Fibrinolytic Therapy

The use of fibrinolytic therapy worldwide has decreased substantially. Nevertheless, fibrinolytic therapy remains the primary approach to reperfusion therapy in some countries and in some regions in the United States where there is no access to experienced centers for timely primary PCI.

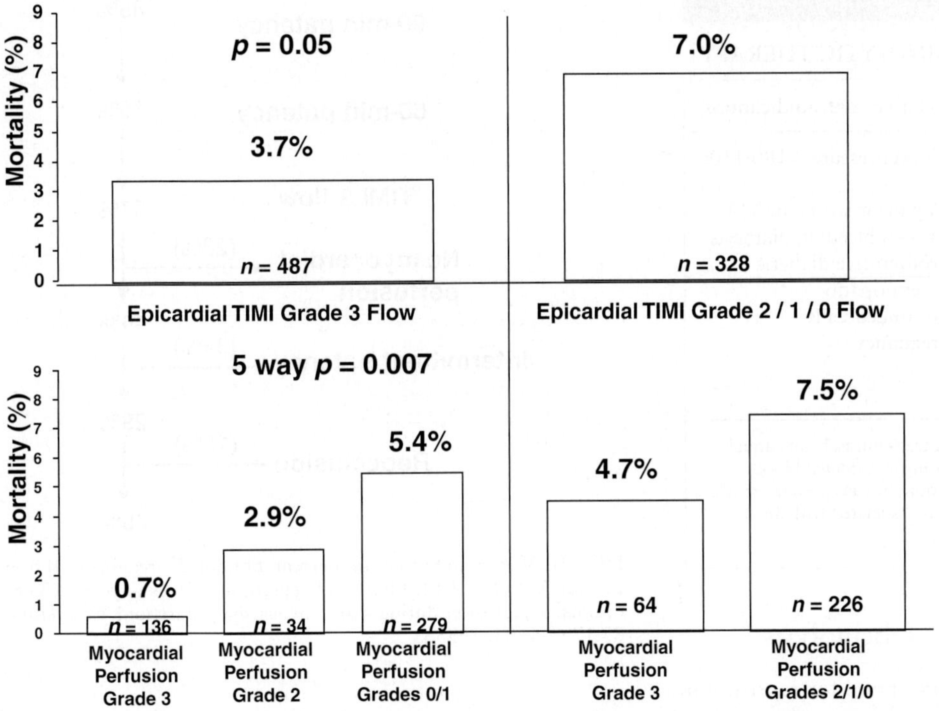

FIGURE 39.5. Relationship between epicardial perfusion, myocardial perfusion, and mortality after fibrinolytic therapy in the TIMI 10B trial. Myocardial perfusion was assessed using the TIMI Myocardial Perfusion Grade, which assesses the degree of microvascular "blush" seen on the routine coronary angiogram. This study found that myocardial perfusion was significantly associated with mortality independent of epicardial blood flow; using these two measures together provided incremental risk prediction. [Adapted from Gibson CM, Cannon CP, Murphy SA, et al; for the TIMI Study Group: The relationship of the TIMI Myocardial Perfusion Grade to mortality after thrombolytic administration. *Circulation* 101:125–130, 2000.]

Placebo-controlled trials using streptokinase, anistreplase (APSAC), and tissue plasminogen activator (tPA) established a clear benefit of fibrinolytic therapy for patients with STEMI. The Fibrinolytic Therapy Trialists' overview of all the large placebo-controlled studies reported a 2.6% absolute reduction in mortality for patients with STEMI treated within the first 12 hours after the onset of symptoms [24]. This benefit has been shown to persist through 10 years of follow-up. Highlights of differences in dosing, pharmacokinetics, recanalization rates, and cost between agents are shown in Table 39.3.

Several mutant forms of tPA have been developed that have a prolonged half-life (to allow bolus administration), as well as increased fibrin specificity and resistance to endogenous inhibitors of plasminogen, such as PAI-1. Bolus administration may minimize the risk for dosing errors, decrease "door to needle" time, and allow for prehospital administration. Reteplase (rPA) is a double-bolus agent that was shown to have similar efficacy and bleeding risk to accelerated tPA in the GUSTO III trial [26]. In the ASSENT II trial, tenecteplase (TNK-tPA)—a single-bolus agent—was shown to be equivalent to tPA in terms of mortality and intracranial hemorrhage (ICH), but was associated with a lower rate of noncerebral bleeding complications [27]. The safety advantage of this agent may be due to its increased fibrin specificity and the fact that the dose is adjusted for body weight.

Although the bolus fibrinolytic agents have not been demonstrated in placebo-controlled trials to reduce mortality or ICH, they are easier to use and have largely replaced tPA for this reason in the United States. Tenecteplase appears to offer a modest advantage in safety over other agents. Readministration of streptokinase or anistreplase should be avoided for at least 4 years (preferably indefinitely) because potentially neutralizing antibodies may develop and because anaphylaxis can occur on reexposure to these drugs.

TABLE 39.3

THROMBOLYTIC AGENTS IN CURRENT CLINICAL USE

	Alteplase	Reteplase	Tenecteplase	Streptokinase
Fibrin selective	+++	++	++++	–
Half-life	5 min	14 min	17 min	20 min
Dose	15 mg bolus; then 0.75 mg/kg over 30 min; then 0.5 mg/kg over 60 min (max 100 mg total dose)	Two 10 unit bolus doses given 30 min apart	0.53 mg/kg as a single bolus	1.5 million units over 30–60 min
Weight adjusted	Partial	No	Yes	No
Adjunctive heparin	Yes	Yes	Yes	Probably
Possible allergy	No	No	No	Yes
TIMI grade 2 or 3 flow (90 min)	80%	80%	80%	60%
TIMI grade 3 flow (90 min)	55%–60%	60%	55%–65%	32%
Efficacy vs. tPA	NA	Similar	Equivalent	1% ↑ mortality
Safety	NA	Similar	Similar ICH ↓ non-ICH bleeding	↓ ICH ↓ overall bleeding
Cost	+++	+++	+++	+

TABLE 39.4

CONTRAINDICATIONS TO FIBRINOLYTIC THERAPY

Absolute contraindications	Relative contraindications
Any prior intracranial hemorrhage	Blood pressure >180/110[a]
Stoke within past year	Any prior stroke or TIA
Recent head trauma	Known bleeding diathesis
Known brain tumor	Proliferative diabetic retinopathy
Active internal bleeding	Prolonged CPR
Suspected aortic dissection	Pregnancy
Major surgery or trauma within 2 wk	

CPR, cardiopulmonary resuscitation; TIA, transient ischemic attack.
[a]Prior recommendations have considered only a *sustained* blood pressure >180/110 a relative contraindication; however, even a single blood pressure greater than this threshold is associated with an increased risk for intracranial hemorrhage.

Current Guidelines for Fibrinolysis

Fibrinolytic therapy is indicated as an option for reperfusion therapy in patients presenting within 12 hours of symptom onset if they have ST-segment elevation or new LBBB and no contraindications to lytic therapy (Table 39.4). Patients who are older than 75 years of age, those who present more than 12 to 24 hours after the onset of acute MI, and those who are hypertensive but present with high-risk MI have a less favorable balance of risk and potential benefit, but may be considered for treatment with a fibrinolytic therapy when primary PCI is not available. Patients should not be given fibrinolytic therapy if the time to treatment is longer than 24 hours or if they present only with ST-segment depression [28].

Limitations of Fibrinolytic Therapy

Current fibrinolytic regimens achieve patency (TIMI grade 2 or 3 flow) in approximately 80% of patients, but complete reperfusion (TIMI grade 3 flow) in only 50% to 60% of cases. In addition, as noted previously in the chapter, approximately one-third of patients with successful epicardial reperfusion have inadequate myocardial and microvascular reperfusion [18]. Finally, even after successful fibrinolysis, a 10% to 20% risk of reocclusion is present. Reocclusion and reinfarction are associated with a two- to threefold increase in mortality [29,30] (Fig. 39.6).

Bleeding is the most common complication of fibrinolytic therapy. Major hemorrhage occurs in 5% to 15% of patients. ICH is the most devastating of the bleeding complications, causing death in the majority of patients affected and almost universal disability in survivors. In major clinical trials, ICH has occurred in 0.5% to 0.9% of patients, but in clinical practice, where patient selection is less rigorous, rates are higher. Patients at particularly high risk for ICH include the elderly (particularly elderly females), patients with low body weight, and those who receive excessive doses of heparin.

Combination Therapy with a GP IIb/IIIa Inhibitor and Reduced-Dose Fibrinolytic

Standard fibrinolytic therapy is directed at the fibrin-rich "red" portion of the coronary thrombus. Activated platelets are the critical component of the white portion of the arterial thrombus. Paradoxically, fibrinolytic agents directly and indirectly promote platelet activation [31], and activated platelets themselves contribute to fibrinolytic resistance by secreting PAI-1 and promoting clot retraction, thereby limiting penetration of the fibrinolytic agent into the thrombus. As a result of these observations, it was hypothesized that potent platelet inhibition with a GP IIb/IIIa inhibitor might augment the efficacy of fibrinolytic therapy.

Although a series of phase II studies comparing standard fibrinolytic therapy with various combinations of GP IIb/IIIa inhibitors and reduced doses of fibrinolytic agents suggested improved TIMI flow grade and ST-segment resolution with the combination regimens [32–35], definitive phase III trials revealed no convincing improvement in outcomes and an increase in ICH in the elderly with combination regimens [36,37]. Thus, despite initial promise, data do *not* support the use of GP IIb/IIIa inhibitor/fibrinolytic combinations as the primary reperfusion strategy for treatment of STEMI.

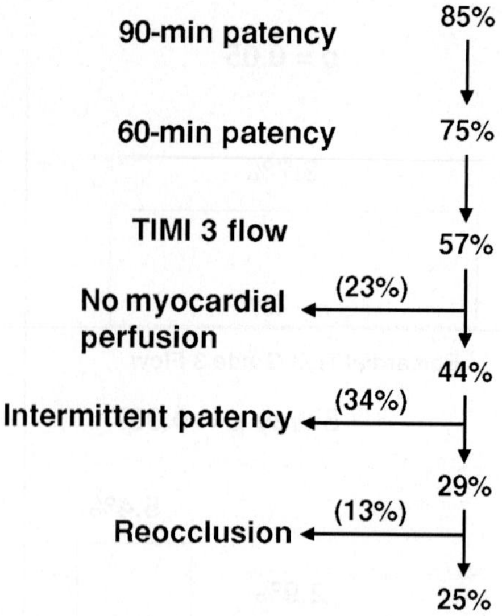

FIGURE 39.6. Limitations of current fibrinolytic regimens. [From Lincoff AM, Topol EJ: Illusion of reperfusion. Does anyone achieve optimal reperfusion during acute myocardial infarction? *Circulation* 87:1792–1805, 1993.]

Rescue Percutaneous Coronary Intervention

Because failure of fibrinolytic therapy is associated with high rates of morbidity and mortality, "rescue" PCI is frequently performed in such patients. Data to support rescue PCI in patients with an occluded infarct artery are limited, as tools to diagnose failed reperfusion are only modestly effective, and clinical trials evaluating rescue PCI have enrolled very slowly. In the MERLIN trial, 307 patients with ECG evidence of failed reperfusion (ST-segment resolution <50% measured 60 minutes after fibrinolytic therapy) were randomized to rescue PCI or conservative therapy. Rescue PCI was performed an average of approximately 90 minutes after the qualifying ECG and was associated with a 26% reduction in the composite endpoint of death, reinfarction, stroke, heart failure, and revascularization at 30 days. However, mortality was not significantly reduced. The most recent study performed was the REACT trial, in which 427 patients with ECG evidence of failed fibrinolysis at 90 minutes were randomized to repeat fibrinolysis, conservative treatment, or rescue PCI. No benefit was observed for repeat fibrinolysis, but rescue PCI reduced the primary endpoint of death, reinfarction, stroke, or severe heart failure at 6 months by 53%. Mortality was also reduced from 12.8% in the conservative therapy arm to 6.2% in the rescue PCI arm. We recommend urgent catheterization and PCI for all patients with persistent ST-segment elevation and ongoing chest pain 90 minutes after the administration of reperfusion therapy, unless they are at particularly low risk for complications (i.e., a young patient with an uncomplicated inferior MI). For patients who are pain free, but in whom the ST segments remain elevated, urgent catheterization should also be strongly considered, particularly if the patient has high-risk features, such as older age, anterior location of infarction, diabetes, or prior CAD.

Primary Percutaneous Coronary Intervention

In centers with adequate resources, experienced operators, and an institutional commitment to programmatic excellence, immediate or "primary" PCI has become the preferred reperfusion method for patients with STEMI. Randomized trials performed in both referral centers and experienced community hospitals have shown that primary PCI reduces the likelihood of death or MI when compared to fibrinolytic therapy [38]. Moreover, rates of major bleeding and stroke are also significantly lower with primary PCI than with fibrinolytic therapy (Fig. 39.7). The relative benefits of primary PCI are greatest in patients at highest risk, including those with cardiogenic shock, right ventricular infarction, large anterior MI, and increased age (due partly to an increased ICH rate with fibrinolytic therapy). However, as with fibrinolytic therapy, rapid time to treatment is paramount to success [25]. In addition, while operator and institutional experience are critical to realize the full benefit of primary PCI, excellent results with primary PCI have been demonstrated in well-trained community hospitals without on-site cardiac surgery [39]. Current ACC/AHA guidelines recommend primary PCI over fibrinolytic therapy when it can be performed by experienced operators in experienced centers within 90 minutes of presentation. When the door-to-balloon time is expected to be longer than 90 minutes, fibrinolysis is

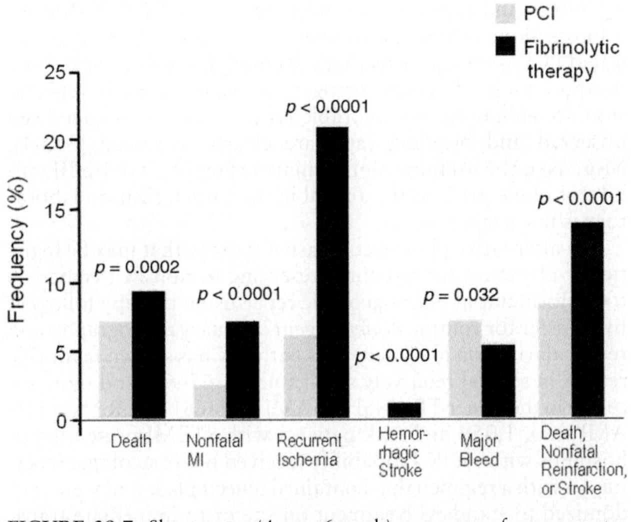

FIGURE 39.7. Short-term (4- to 6-week) outcomes from a meta-analysis of 23 randomized controlled trials comparing fibrinolytic therapy with primary PCI. [Adapted from Keeley EC, Boura JA, Grines CL: Primary angioplasty versus intravenous thrombolytic therapy for acute myocardial infarction: a quantitative review of 23 randomised trials. *Lancet* 361(9351):13–20, 2003.]

generally preferred for patients presenting within 12 hours of symptom onset unless contraindications are present [28].

Advances in PCI technology have been rapidly translated from elective to emergent PCI. Compared with primary PTCA, primary stenting is associated with similar rates of death and reinfarction, but lower subsequent target vessel revascularization rates [40,41]. Initial fears about stent thrombosis when drug-eluting stents (DES) were placed in the setting of STEMI have not been realized, and recent studies demonstrate that the advantages of DES over bare metal stents (BMS) with regard to in-stent restenosis and target vessel revascularization extend to patients with STEMI [42,43]. One logistical issue merits comment regarding stent choice. It may be difficult in the setting of an evolving STEMI to determine whether a patient is a good candidate for at least 1 year of uninterrupted aspirin and thienopyridine therapy; a BMS would be preferred in situations where the clinician cannot make this determination.

Because of the large thrombus burden in STEMI, distal embolization at the time of PCI is common and may cause additional tissue and microvascular injury. Strategies to prevent distal embolization using embolic protection devices, which are commonly used when PCI is performed in saphenous vein grafts, cause delays in reperfusion and do not appear to improve outcomes when STEMI is due to native vessel obstruction. In contrast, a simpler strategy of thrombus extraction has yielded very promising results. In a randomized trial of 1,071 patients with STEMI, manual thrombus aspiration before PCI was demonstrated to improve TIMI myocardial perfusion grade and ST-segment resolution ($p < 0.001$) [44], as well as 1-year mortality (3.6% vs. 6.7%; $p = 0.02$) [45]. Aspiration thrombectomy is a reasonable option for patients undergoing primary PCI, particularly in patients with large thrombus burden and shorter ischemic times [46].

Performance Improvement Measures to Improve Door-to-Balloon Times

Considerable attention has been focused on improving door-to-balloon times. A study by Bradley et al. [47] identified key strategies that discriminated hospitals with shorter versus longer door-to-balloon times (Table 39.5). Most of these strategies have been adopted by the Door-to-Balloon (D2B) Alliance, a quality improvement initiative aiming to achieve a door-to-balloon time of 90 minutes or shorter for 75% or more of nontransferred patients with STEMI [48].

TABLE 39.5

PROCESS MEASURES TO IMPROVE DOOR-TO-BALLOON TIMES

- Emergency medicine physician activates the catheterization laboratory
- A single call to a central page operator activates the catheterization laboratory
- A prehospital ECG is used to activate the catheterization laboratory activated while the patient is en route to the hospital
- Expectation that staff will arrive in the catheterization laboratory within 20–30 min (vs. >30 min) after being paged
- An attending cardiologist is always on site (sleeps in hospital)
- Real-time data feedback is provided to emergency department and the catheterization laboratory staff

Transfer for Primary Percutaneous Coronary Intervention

Although primary PCI is the preferred reperfusion option for most patients who present to dedicated centers that can perform interventional procedures quickly and expertly, most patients with STEMI present to centers without primary PCI readily available. In such cases, a decision must be made as to whether immediate pharmacologic reperfusion therapy or transfer for primary PCI (if possible) is the best alternative. For patients in whom a rapid transfer is possible (time from arrival at first hospital to balloon inflation <90 minutes or PCI-associated delay <1 hour), transfer for primary PCI is preferable. Unfortunately, data from the National Registry of Myocardial Infarction (NRMI) through 2002 suggested that only 4% of transferred patients underwent primary PCI with a door-to-balloon time shorter than 90 minutes [49]. More recently, several referral centers or metropolitan areas have initiated regional transfer networks that have achieved door-to-balloon times of 100 to 120 minutes [50–52]. For patients with contraindications to fibrinolytic therapy, evidence of failed fibrinolytic therapy, cardiogenic shock, or presentation more than 12 hours after symptom onset, transfer to a center that can perform emergent PCI is indicated, even if delay times are longer [53].

Several studies have compared strategies of routine transfer of patients eligible for fibrinolytic therapy for primary PCI versus immediate fibrinolysis with or without transfer. Although these studies have reported a lower incidence of adverse cardiac events among those randomized to transfer for primary PCI [54,55], generalizability of the results has been questioned as the very rapid transfer times in these studies are significantly shorter than those typically occur in the United States [49] and the rates of referral for rescue PCI were unusually low in these trials.

Subsequent analyses have helped to define the influence of symptom duration and transfer-related time delay on the benefits of transfer for primary PCI. For example, among the 850 patients enrolled in the PRAGUE-2 study, there was a significant and quantitatively large reduction in mortality (6.0% vs. 15.3%; $p < 0.02$) among those who were randomized more than 3 hours after symptom onset. In contrast, there was no reduction in mortality among patients presenting within 3 hours [56]. Similar findings were observed in the CAPTIM trial in which the control arm received prehospital fibrinolytic [57]. A meta-analysis of randomized studies has suggested that if the delay between immediate administration of a fibrinolytic and initiation of PCI is more than 1 hour, the pharmacologic therapy becomes favored with respect to survival [58] (Fig. 39.8). These data form the basis of the recommendation in the AHA/ACC guidelines that fibrinolysis is generally preferred in eligible patients who present within 3 hours of symptom onset, and more than a 1-hour delay between fibrinolytic and primary PCI is expected (Fig. 39.9).

Pharmacoinvasive Strategies

In light of the deleterious impact of delays to primary PCI on myocardial salvage, an approach in which reperfusion is initiated with a pharmacologic regimen and followed by angiography and PCI is attractive, particularly among patients being transferred for PCI. Nevertheless, there has been considerable controversy as to the role of PCI after apparently successful fibrinolytic therapy. In a series of trials performed in the late 1980s, the TIMI investigators reported no benefit from routine application of an immediate or delayed invasive strategy, compared to a more conservative strategy in which catheterization was reserved for patients with recurrent or provocable ischemia [59,60]. Because these trials were published, dramatic advances in interventional cardiology have taken place, including improvements in catheter and stent technology, careful attention to groin hemostasis, and improvements in adjunctive antiplatelet and antithrombotic regimens; as a result, PCI can be performed effectively and safely early after fibrinolytic therapy [61]. In addition, it is well known that patients who arrive in the catheterization laboratory with a patent IRA prior to "primary" PCI, either due to spontaneous lysis or due to pharmacologic reperfusion, have an extraordinarily low risk for mortality [62].

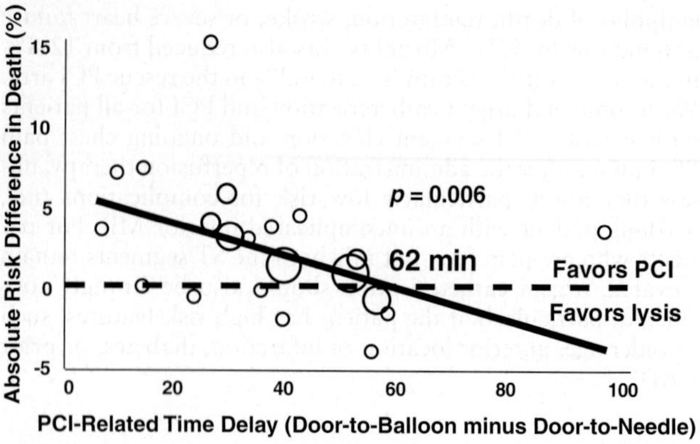

FIGURE 39.8. Metaregression evaluating the association between time delay associated with primary PCI and the absolute benefit of primary PCI over fibrinolytic therapy. Circle sizes represent the sample size of individual studies and the solid line represents the weighted metaregression. For every 10-minute delay to PCI, a 1% reduction in the mortality difference of primary PCI versus lytics was observed. [Adapted from Nallamothu BK, Bates ER: Percutaneous coronary intervention versus fibrinolytic therapy in acute myocardial infarction: is timing (almost) everything? *Am J Cardiol* 92(7):824–826, 2003.]

The term "facilitated" PCI has been coined to signify the administration of a pharmacologic reperfusion regimen en route to the cardiac catheterization laboratory for a planned "primary" PCI. A number of different pharmacologic pretreatment regimens have been proposed, including fibrinolytic agents alone (at full or reduced dose), combinations of GP IIb/IIIa inhibitors and reduced-dose fibrinolytics, and GP IIb/IIIa inhibitors alone. To date, the clinical trial results regarding facilitated PCI using regimens that contain a fibrinolytic have been disappointing: although surrogate measures of early reperfusion are enhanced, no favorable efficacy outcomes have been observed and bleeding rates are clearly increased [63,64]. Moreover, the usefulness of administration of a GP IIb/IIIa inhibitor alone prior to the arrival in the catheterization laboratory is uncertain [46,64].

An alternative pharmacoinvasive strategy that may be logistically attractive for patients presenting to non-PCI centers is to perform initial pharmacologic reperfusion therapy followed by transfer for routine *nonemergent* coronary angiography and revascularization if needed. This pathway has shown favorable results in several relatively small studies [65–67] and more recently in the larger TRANSFER-AMI trial [68]. In TRANSFER-AMI trial, 1,059 high-risk patients with STEMI presenting to hospitals without PCI capability received pharmacologic reperfusion with a regimen that contained tenecteplase and were randomized to standard treatment on site or to immediate transfer and PCI within 6 hours after fibrinolysis. Interestingly, most patients in the standard treatment arm underwent coronary angiography, but this was performed approximately 1 day later than in the transfer arm. The primary endpoint of death, MI, recurrent ischemia, CHF, or cardiogenic shock within 30 days

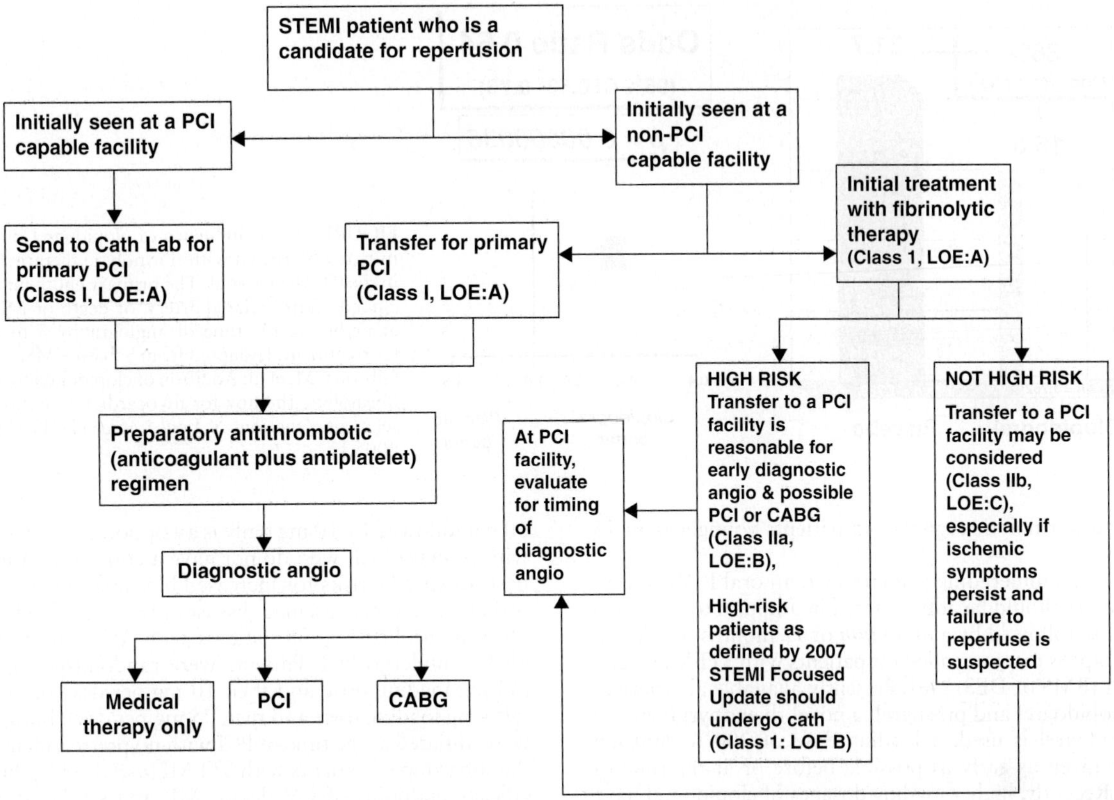

FIGURE 39.9. An algorithm for triage and transfer for primary PCI among patients with ST elevation MI. [Adapted from Kushner FG, Hand M, Smith SC Jr, et al: 2009 Focused Updates: ACC/AHA Guidelines for the Management of Patients With ST-Elevation Myocardial Infarction (updating the 2004 Guideline and 2007 Focused Update) and ACC/AHA/SCAI Guidelines on Percutaneous Coronary Intervention (updating the 2005 Guideline and 2007 Focused Update): a report of the American College of Cardiology Foundation/American Heart Association Task Force on Practice Guidelines. *Circulation* 120(22):2271–2306, 2009.]

was reduced from 17.2% in the standard treatment arm to 11.0% in the early PCI arm (HR 0.64; $p = 0.004$). For patients who present to hospitals without PCI capability and in whom the door-to-balloon time is expected to be longer than 90 minutes, these data support a strategy of "drip and ship," in which standard pharmacologic reperfusion therapy is administered and the patient transferred for subsequent catheterization and PCI. The timing of the catheterization and PCI remains controversial. Data from studies of facilitated PCI suggest that very early PCI (i.e., within 2 hours) is not helpful and may be harmful. However, the accumulated data described previously suggest favorable outcomes if the PCI is performed between 2 and 24 hours after successful fibrinolytic therapy. An important consideration may be the use of adequate anticoagulant and antiplatelet therapy in the setting of the transient prothrombotic state that may be initiated by the release of fibrin degradation products during fibrinolysis.

ADJUNCTIVE ANTIPLATELET AND ANTITHROMBOTIC THERAPY

Aspirin and Oral P_2Y_{12} Inhibitors

In patients with STEMI, aspirin decreases reocclusion and reinfarction rates by nearly 50% and mortality by approximately 25% [69]. The benefits of aspirin are comparable to those of fibrinolytic therapy, and when used together, aspirin and fibrinolytic therapy provide additive benefit [70]. Aspirin should be initiated at an oral dose of 162 to 325 mg (preferably chewed) at the time the patient is first encountered by medical personnel in the field or emergency department. Following MI, lifelong therapy with aspirin is indicated to prevent recurrent cardiac events. Efficacy appears to be similar at all doses greater than 75 mg, whereas bleeding risk clearly increases with higher aspirin dose. Thus, for most patients, an 81-mg dose of aspirin is preferred for long-term secondary prevention [71].

Clopidogrel is a thienopyridine derivative that inhibits the binding of ADP to the P_2Y_{12} receptor on the platelet surface, thereby decreasing platelet activation and aggregation. The CLARITY trial compared clopidogrel (300-mg loading dose followed by 75 mg per day) with placebo in 3,491 patients with STEMI who were treated with standard pharmacologic reperfusion including fibrinolytic therapy, aspirin, and heparin. The primary composite endpoint of death, MI, or an occluded IRA assessed at the time of protocol-mandated angiography (average 3 to 4 days) was reduced from 21.7% in the placebo arm to 15.0% in the clopidogrel arm ($p < 0.001$; Fig. 39.10). At 30 days, the clinical composite of death, MI, or urgent revascularization was reduced by 20% ($p = 0.03$) [72]. The much larger COMMIT trial was performed in more than 45,000 patients in China and was designed to evaluate the impact of adjunctive clopidogrel (administered at 75 mg per day without a loading dose) on death and major clinical events. Clopidogrel reduced death, reinfarction, or stroke by 9% and death alone by 7%, both of which were statistically significant [73]. In both these trials, the combination of clopidogrel and aspirin showed no excess in bleeding compared to aspirin alone. Using the results of these two trials, clopidogrel should now routinely be added

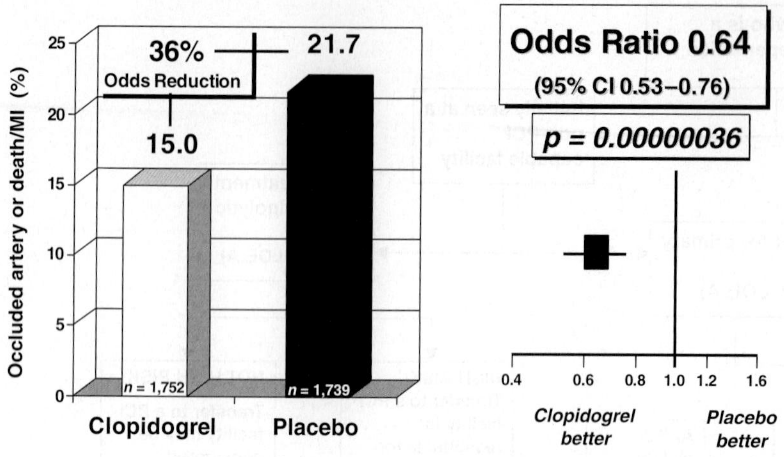

FIGURE 39.10. Influence of clopidogrel on outcomes in patients treated with fibrinolytic therapy for STEMI in the CLARITY trial. The primary endpoint was an occluded infarct-related artery, or death or MI occurring at or before the time of angiography 3 to 8 days after treatment. [Adapted from Sabatine MS, Cannon CP, Gibson CM, et al: Addition of clopidogrel to aspirin and fibrinolytic therapy for myocardial infarction with ST-segment elevation. *N Engl J Med* 352(12):1179–1189, 2005.]

to standard fibrinolytic regimens in patients younger than 75 years [28].

For patients undergoing primary PCI, an oral P_2Y_{12} receptor antagonist should be administered in addition to aspirin: a loading dose followed by a *minimum* of 12 months of maintenance therapy is recommended for patients with STEMI receiving a stent (BMS or DES) [46]. Presently available alternatives include clopidogrel and prasugrel, a novel thienopyridine.

If clopidogrel is used, a loading dose of 300 to 600 mg should be given as early as possible before or at the time of PCI [46]. Recently, higher loading dosages of clopidogrel have been evaluated in the CURRENT/OASIS 7 trial, which compared high-dose (600-mg loading dose, 150 mg per day for 7 days, and then 75 mg per day) with standard-dose (300-mg loading dose and then 75 mg per day) clopidogrel among 24,769 patients with ACS, 17,232 (70%) of whom underwent PCI. The overall result of the trial was neutral. However, in the subgroup of patients who underwent PCI, the higher dose clopidogrel strategy was associated with a lower rate of the primary endpoint of cardiovascular (CV) death, MI, or stroke at 30 days (4.5% vs. 3.9%; HR 0.85; $p = 0.036$). Risk reduction was similar in the STEMI ($n = 6{,}346$) and UA/NSTEMI ($n = 10{,}996$) subgroups; moreover, among patients with STEMI, high-dose clopidogrel was associated with a lower risk for stent thrombosis (4.0% vs. 2.8%). The higher dose clopidogrel regimen was also associated with a higher rate of major bleeding (1.1% vs. 1.6%; $p = 0.006$) [74].

Prasugrel is a novel thienopyridine that is more rapidly acting, more potent, and associated with less response variability than clopidogrel. Prasugrel administered as a loading dose of 60 mg followed by 10 mg daily is an option for patients treated with primary PCI, who do not have a contraindication on the basis of specific risks for increased bleeding (including history of known cerebrovascular disease) [46]. The TRITON-TIMI 38 trial enrolled 13,608 patients with ACS who were scheduled to undergo PCI. Patients were randomized to prasugrel (60-mg loading dose and then 10 mg per day) or clopidogrel (300-mg loading dose and then 75 mg per day): both the drugs were initiated at the time of PCI with no pretreatment given. In the subgroup of patients with STEMI ($n = 3{,}534$), the primary efficacy endpoint of CV death, MI, and stroke at a median of 14.5 months was reduced from 12.4% in the clopidogrel arm to 10.0% in the prasugrel arm (HR 0.79; $p = 0.02$). Stent thrombosis occurred in 2.4% patients randomized to clopidogrel versus 1.2% randomized to prasugrel ($p = 0.008$; Table 39.6). Importantly, in the STEMI subgroup, no significant differences were noted in non-CABG bleeding between treatment arms [75].

Although the absence of clopidogrel pretreatment in TRITON-TIMI 38 has important implications regarding the interpretation of the efficacy advantage of prasugrel in the overall trial, this issue is not relevant in patients with STEMI, who do not have time for pretreatment prior to primary PCI. Indeed, patients with STEMI, who tend to be younger and at lower risk for bleeding than those with UA/NSTEMI, and who may benefit from more rapid and intensive early antiplatelet therapy, may be particularly attractive candidates for prasugrel.

Ticagrelor is a novel direct acting and *reversible* oral antagonist of the P_2Y_{12} receptor. This agent, which as of 2010 was not commercially available, provides more rapid onset (and

TABLE 39.6

COMPARISON OF NOVEL ORAL ANTIPLATELET THERAPIES WITH CLOPIDOGREL: RESULTS FROM SUBGROUPS WITH STEMI

	TRITON-TIMI 38			PLATO		
	N = 3,534			N = 7,026		
Endpoint	Prasugrel	Clopidogrel	HR (95% CI)	Ticagrelor	Clopidogrel	HR (95% CI)
CV death, MI, stroke	10.0%	12.4%	0.79 (0.65–0.97)	8.5%	10.1%	0.84 (0.72–0.98)
Stent thrombosis[a]	1.6%	2.8%	0.58 (0.36–0.93)	2.2%	2.9%	0.75 (0.59–0.95)
Non-CABG TIMI major bleeding[a,b]	2.4%	2.1%	1.11 (0.70–1.77)	4.5%	3.8%	1.19 (1.02–1.38)

[a]The stent thrombosis and bleeding results from PLATO are from the entire study because the specific data for STEMI have not yet been reported.
[b]TIMI major bleeding (non-CABG) was the primary bleeding endpoint in TRITON-TIMI 38 and was an additional bleeding endpoint in PLATO.
Note that endpoint assessment was at 15 months in TRITON-TIMI 38 and 12 months in PLATO

offset) of action and a more potent and predictable antiplatelet response than clopidogrel. It does not require activation by the cytochrome p450 system. In the PLATO trial [76], ticagrelor (180-mg loading dose, 90 mg twice daily) was compared to clopidogrel (300- to 600-mg loading dose, 75 mg daily) in 18,624 patients with ACS, 38% of whom had STEMI. At the end of the 12-month follow-up period, the primary endpoint of CV death, MI, and stroke occurred in 11.7% of subjects in the clopidogrel arm versus 9.8% in the ticagrelor arm (HR 0.84; 95% CI 0.77 to 0.92; $p < 0.001$). The risk reduction was similar for UA/NSTEMI (HR 0.83; 95% CI 0.74 to 0.93) and STEMI (HR 0.84; 95% CI 0.72 to 0.98; Table 39.6). Similar to the CURRENT/OASIS 7 and TRITON-TIMI 38 trials, stent thrombosis was reduced significantly with the more potent oral antiplatelet regimen. Also consistent with prior studies, an increase in non-CABG major bleeding was observed in the ticagrelor arm (4.5% vs. 3.8%; $p = 0.03$); however, bleeding rates following CABG were lower with ticagrelor, likely because of the shorter half-life of the drug [76].

Several notable findings were observed with ticagrelor in the PLATO trial. First, a significant 21% relative risk reduction in vascular mortality and a 22% reduction in total mortality (5.9% vs. 4.5%; $p < 0.001$) were observed. This is notable as none of the thienopyridine trials demonstrated a mortality reduction. In addition, several unique side effects have been observed with ticagrelor, which are likely mediated by adenosine. These include transient dyspnea, which occurs in 10% to 15% of patients early after treatment initiation, but is not associated with heart failure and usually terminates within a week. Ventricular pauses may also be triggered by ticagrelor early after treatment initiation, but these also decrease in frequency over time, are rarely symptomatic, and have not required clinical intervention.

GP IIb/IIIa Inhibitors

Although use of GP IIb/IIIa inhibitors in elective PCI has been decreasing, these agents remain useful adjuncts to primary PCI in patients with STEMI when heparin is the anticoagulant used. In a meta-analysis involving 3,266 patients enrolled in four randomized trials comparing abciximab with placebo, patients receiving abciximab had a 46% reduction in 30-day death, reinfarction, and urgent target vessel revascularization compared to those who received placebo [77]. Fewer data are available for the other GP IIb/IIIa inhibitors (tirofiban and eptifibatide) in the primary PCI setting. Current ACC/AHA guidelines recommend selective use of any of these agents at the time of primary PCI (class IIa recommendation), for example, among patients with a large thrombus burden or those who have not received adequate thienopyridine loading [46].

Antithrombin Therapies in Patients Receiving Fibrinolytic Therapy

Using data from angiographic trials showing improved IRA patency rates 5 to 7 days after treatment with intravenous unfractionated heparin (UFH) and subsequent outcomes trials with alternative anticoagulants, the AHA/ACC guidelines recommend administration of an anticoagulant (UFH, enoxaparin, or fondaparinux) as adjunctive therapy in all patients receiving pharmacologic reperfusion therapy with the fibrin-specific agents alteplase, reteplase, or tenecteplase. For UFH, recommended dosing is a 60 U per kg bolus (maximum bolus of 4,000 U) plus an initial infusion of 12 U per kg per hour (with a maximum initial infusion rate of 1,000 U per hour) for up to 48 hours. Data to support antithrombin therapy for patients receiving streptokinase come from trials that evaluated the low-molecular-weight heparins (LMWHs) reviparin and enoxaparin among patients receiving streptokinase compared either to placebo (reviparin) or to UFH (enoxaparin) [78,79]. These trials provide both definitive evidence for the clinical benefit of administering an antithrombin in combination with a fibrinolytic and strong support for their use in conjunction with streptokinase as well as the fibrin-specific agents.

LMWHs represent an attractive alternative to UFH for patients receiving fibrinolytic therapy. Following a series of smaller studies that yielded promising results, the ExTRACT-TIMI 25 trial randomized 20,506 patients treated with standard fibrinolytic regimens to intravenous UFH for 48 hours or to enoxaparin. Enoxaparin was given as a 30-mg IV bolus followed by 1 mg per kg every 12 hours until hospital discharge [79]. The bolus dose was eliminated and the maintenance dose reduced to 0.75 mg per kg for patients older than 75 years, because previous trials had suggested a higher risk of ICH among elderly patients with STEMI who received full-dose enoxaparin [80]. The primary endpoint of death or reinfarction was reduced from 12.0% in the UFH arm to 9.9% in the enoxaparin arm (RR 0.83; $p < 0.001$). Major bleeding occurred in 1.4% of UFH-treated patients versus 2.1% of those treated with enoxaparin ($p < 0.001$), but there was no significant difference in ICH, and the net clinical benefit (death/MI/major bleeding) favored enoxaparin.

Fondaparinux, a novel factor Xa inhibitor, was evaluated in the OASIS 6 trial, a complex trial that included patients treated with both fibrinolytic therapy and primary PCI, and also included patients with and without indications for UFH. Although the rate of death or reinfarction was significantly reduced by 21% with fondaparinux compared with placebo, no difference was observed compared with UFH. No increase in bleeding risk was seen with fondaparinux. Notably, the OASIS 6 trial demonstrated a hazard associated with the use of fondaparinux to support primary PCI [81].

The direct antithrombin agents have also been extensively studied as adjuncts to fibrinolytic therapy, but appear to offer no significant advantage over UFH when given with any of the currently available fibrinolytic agents [82–84]. Thus, of the currently available antithrombin agents, LMWH administered for the duration of the hospitalization (up to 8 days) has been shown to be superior to guidelines-based use of UFH. Fondaparinux is superior to placebo and appears to provide similar efficacy and safety to UFH. Observations from both ExTRACT-TIMI 25 and OASIS 6 indicate that more prolonged administration of an anticoagulant for the duration of the index hospitalization is beneficial compared with administering UFH only for 48 hours. As such, present guidelines recommend that patients managed with fibrinolysis should receive anticoagulant therapy for a minimum of 48 hours and preferably for the duration of the hospitalization after STEMI, up to 8 days [53]. Enoxaparin or fondaparinux are preferred over UFH when administration of an anticoagulant for longer than 48 hours is planned in patients with STEMI treated with a fibrinolytic.

Antithrombin Therapy as an Adjunct to Primary PCI

Until recently, UFH—administered in combination with a GP IIb/IIIa receptor antagonist—has served as the preferred adjunctive regimen to support primary PCI for STEMI. In the HORIZONS-AMI trial [85], 3,602 patients undergoing primary PCI for STEMI were randomized to standard care with heparin plus a GP IIb/IIIa inhibitor or to bivalirudin (a direct-acting antithrombin) alone. The primary outcome, which was

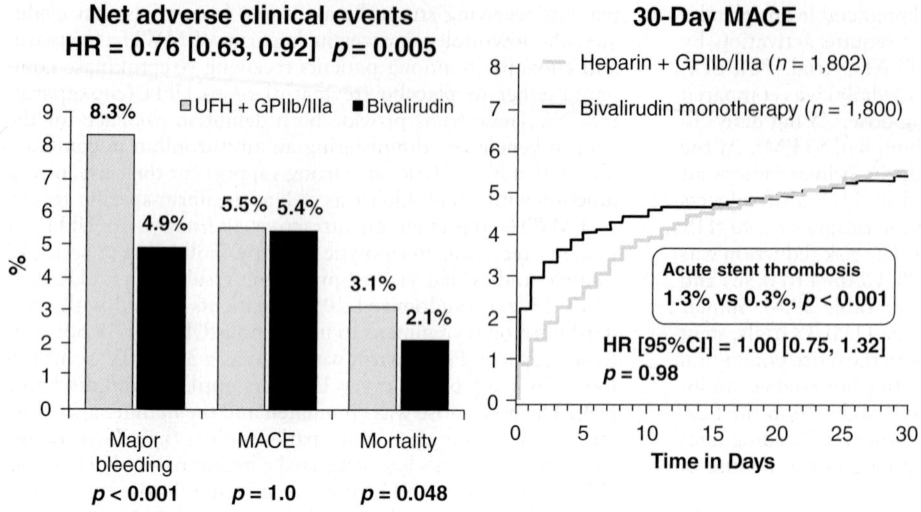

FIGURE 39.11. Results from the HORIZONS-AMI trial. Among patients receiving primary PCI for STEMI, randomization to bivalirudin, as compared to unfractionated heparin plus a GP IIb/IIIa inhibitor, reduced bleeding complications and mortality, but was associated with an increase in early stent thrombosis. [Adapted from Stone GW, Witzenbichler B, Guagliumi G, et al: Bivalirudin during primary PCI in acute myocardial infarction. *N Engl J Med* 358(21):2218–2230, 2008.]

a composite of efficacy and safety endpoints at 30 days, was significantly lower in the bivalirudin versus heparin/GP IIb/IIIa inhibitor arm (9.2% vs. 12.1%; RR 0.76; $p = 0.005$). This was mediated by lower rate of major bleeding with bivalirudin (4.9% vs. 8.3%; RR 0.60; $p < 0.001$) and similar rates of the ischemic outcomes. Total mortality (2.1% vs. 3.1%; $p = 0.05$) and cardiac mortality (1.8% vs. 2.9%; $p = 0.03$) trended lower in the bivalirudin arm (Fig. 39.11). One issue of some concern was an increased risk of stent thrombosis within the first 24 hours in the bivalirudin group. It is possible that this early risk for stent thrombosis may be mitigated by using higher loading doses of clopidogrel [86] or by using more potent novel P_2Y_{12} inhibitors, such as prasugrel. Bivalirudin is a useful alternative to heparin in patients undergoing primary PCI [46].

Warfarin/Oral Anticoagulation

Warfarin monotherapy appears to be at least as effective as aspirin for secondary prevention post-MI. There are several circumstances in which the benefit with warfarin therapy may exceed that of aspirin. First, warfarin is superior to aspirin in preventing systemic emboli in patients with atrial fibrillation. In addition, it reduces systemic emboli in patients with documented LV dysfunction following MI. Because there is a substantial risk of systemic embolization following a large anterior MI, even if thrombus is not visible on echocardiography, many experts recommend 3 to 6 months of warfarin therapy in these patients if they are suitable candidates for anticoagulation [53]. Studies have also evaluated the combination of warfarin and aspirin post-MI. Neither fixed-dose warfarin nor low-dose warfarin titrated to an INR of approximately 1.5 to 2.0 appears to be superior to monotherapy with either agent alone, and the combination is associated with excess bleeding risk [87]. Several studies have shown that the combination of aspirin and warfarin is effective in preventing reocclusion and clinical events when the INR is maintained at a higher level consistently [88–90]. However, these findings are of questionable significance in light of the results of the CLARITY and COMMIT trials, which have demonstrated similar benefit with a simpler regimen of aspirin and clopidogrel. Thus, warfarin plus low-dose aspirin may be a good choice in patients who have another indication for anticoagulation (such as atrial fibrillation or prosthetic valve), provided the bleeding risk is low and a warfarin clinic is available for very careful monitoring.

An increasingly challenging scenario relates to the combination of aspirin, clopidogrel, and warfarin. Emerging evidence suggests that "triple therapy" is associated with substantially increased risks for bleeding. It may be expected that risks will be even higher with combinations that include the newer and more potent antiplatelet agents such as prasugrel and ticagrelor. As such, we recommend attempting to avoid altogether or to minimize the duration of triple therapy. Consideration should be given to using BMS instead of DES, which would allow the duration of clopidogrel to be reduced to 1 month. For patients who require triple therapy, the INR should be maintained at the lowest end of the therapeutic range, aspirin dose should be reduced to 81 mg, and GI prophylaxis with an H_2 antagonist, such as ranitidine, should be considered. For patients with atrial fibrillation, a reevaluation of the risks of bleeding and stroke (using a tool such as the $CHADS_2$ score) should be performed and the threshold to initiate or continue warfarin should be higher among patients on aspirin and clopidogrel [91].

ANTI-ISCHEMIC THERAPY

Beta-Blockers

Beta-blockers were among the first therapeutic interventions used to limit the size of acute MI. Previous trials that excluded patients with heart failure, hypotension, or bradycardia demonstrated that very early administration of a beta-blocker decreases infarct size and prevents recurrent MI and death [92]. The fact that beta-blockers were particularly effective in reducing sudden death and reducing mortality among patients with complex ventricular ectopy at baseline suggests that beta-blockers exert much of their beneficial effect by reducing the frequency and severity of arrhythmias [93]. In addition, they appear to significantly decrease the risk of cardiac rupture. Data from the COMMIT trial in more than 45,000 patients, however, failed to demonstrate benefit from a strategy of immediate intravenous metoprolol followed by 200 mg metoprolol daily on in-hospital outcomes, including death and MI. Although early beta blockade reduced the risks of reinfarction and ventricular fibrillation (VF) compared to placebo, this was counterbalanced by an increased risk of cardiogenic shock during the first few days after admission [94]. Post-hoc analyses indicate that this increased risk was predominantly among patients with indicators of or risk factors for hemodynamic compromise. In addition, the outcome may have been influenced by the high dose of metoprolol used in this study. ACC/AHA guidelines now recommended that beta-blockers be initiated orally, within the first 24 hours, once it has been determined that the hemodynamic status is stable and there is no evidence of heart failure. Parenteral beta-blockers should be used only if there is a clear indication such as ongoing chest pain or an atrial tachyarrhythmia with normal or elevated blood pressure [28].

When given long term following MI, beta-blockers significantly reduce the incidence of nonfatal reinfarction and mortality, an effect that extends to most members of this class of agents [93]. The CAPRICORN trial examined the incremental effect of beta blockade to angiotensin-converting enzyme (ACE) inhibition in post-MI in patients with LV dysfunction but no clinical heart failure. Over a mean follow-up of 1.3 years, the composite of death and myocardial infarction was reduced from 20% in the placebo arm to 14% in the carvedilol arm, a 29% relative reduction. On the basis of robust clinical data and a very favorable cost-to-benefit ratio, long-term oral beta blockade should be continued indefinitely following MI.

Angiotensin-Converting Enzyme Inhibitors

ACE inhibitors are routinely used following STEMI to prevent adverse LV chamber remodeling, a gradual process by which the left ventricle assumes a more globular shape and dilates; remodeling is associated with an increased risk for CHF and death. A large overview of almost 100,000 patients found a 7% reduction in 30-day mortality when ACE inhibitors were given to all patients with acute MI, with most of the benefit observed in the first week. The benefit was greatest in high-risk groups, such as those in Killip class II or III, those with LV dysfunction, and those with an anterior MI [95]. In addition to preventing remodeling and CHF, ACE inhibitors also prevent recurrent ischemic events after MI [96]. As opposed to aspirin and reperfusion therapy, it is not crucial to introduce the ACE inhibitor in the hyperacute phase of acute MI.

Angiotensin receptor blockers (ARBs) are effective alternatives to ACE inhibitors in patients with LV dysfunction or heart failure following acute MI, and provide similar long-term outcomes [97]. However, combination therapy with ACE inhibitors and ARBs is not effective post-MI [97]. Because of the larger evidence base and lower cost of ACE inhibitors, they are preferred over ARBs unless side effects to ACE inhibitors develop.

Aldosterone antagonists should also be considered for use in appropriate high-risk patients following STEMI, who are receiving adequate doses of ACE inhibitors. In the EPHESUS trial, which included patients with an LV ejection fraction <40% following an MI and either heart failure symptoms or diabetes, eplerenone treatment (compared to placebo) was associated with a 15% reduction in the risk for mortality [98]. Because of its much lower cost, spironolactone may be considered as an alternative to eplerenone. Aldosterone antagonists should be avoided in patients with hyperkalemia or significant renal dysfunction.

Nitrates

Nitrates dilate large coronary arteries and arterioles, peripheral veins, and to a lesser extent, peripheral arterioles. Venodilation decreases preload, thus reducing both myocardial oxygen demand and symptoms of pulmonary congestion that may complicate MI. The GISSI-3 [99] and ISIS-4 [100] trials collectively enrolled almost 80,000 patients and evaluated the role of long-term (4- to 6-week) nitrate therapy post-MI. Neither study found a significant reduction in mortality with nitrates, although the power to detect such a difference may have been reduced because more than 50% of patients received off-protocol nitrates. Although evidence from randomized clinical trials does not support routine long-term nitrate therapy for patients with uncomplicated MI, it is reasonable to give intravenous nitroglycerin for the first 24 to 48 hours in patients with acute MI who have CHF, recurrent ischemia, or hypertension. Intravenous therapy is preferred in the early phases of MI due its immediate onset of action and ease of titration.

Calcium Channel Blockers

The calcium channel blockers in current use block the entry of calcium into cells via voltage-sensitive calcium channels. In vascular smooth muscle cells, this causes coronary and peripheral vasodilation, whereas in cardiac tissue, it leads to depression of myocardial contractility, sinus rate, and atrioventricular (AV) nodal conduction. The dihydropyridine calcium channel antagonists, of which nifedipine is the prototype, cause coronary and peripheral artery dilation without blocking sinus or AV nodal function. As a result, the potential benefit of these agents is counterbalanced by reflex tachycardia. The short-acting preparations of nifedipine, in particular, appear to be dangerous in the setting of acute MI, as they may cause rapid hemodynamic fluctuations. Sustained-release preparations of nifedipine, on the other hand, can be used safely in combination with a beta-blocker. Amlodipine is a third-generation agent that causes less reflex tachycardia than other dihydropyridines, but as with other calcium channel blockers, there is no documented benefit of this agent following MI, so it should only be used in patients who remain hypertensive after full-dose beta blockade and ACE inhibition.

Diltiazem and verapamil slow the heart rate and modestly reduce myocardial contractility, thereby decreasing myocardial oxygen demand. Of the two agents, verapamil has greater negative inotropic and chronotropic effects. These agents have been given to patients as secondary prevention after stabilization of an index MI. A pooled analysis indicated that verapamil and diltiazem had no effect on mortality following acute MI, but that they did significantly reduce the rate of reinfarction (6.0% vs. 7.5%; $p < 0.01$) [101]. Despite an overall neutral effect of these agents on mortality, among patients with depressed LV function or evidence of CHF, mortality is increased in patients treated with diltiazem or verapamil.

It should be emphasized that there have not been studies comparing the efficacy of verapamil or diltiazem to a beta-blocker. Beta-blockers consistently reduce both mortality and reinfarction and should be recommended for all patients who can tolerate them. Verapamil or diltiazem may be a reasonable alternative for patients who cannot tolerate a beta-blocker, provided LV function is normal, but they should not be given routinely following MI.

ARRHYTHMIAS COMPLICATING ST ELEVATION MYOCARDIAL INFARCTION (Table 39.7)

Ventricular Arrhythmias

Ventricular tachycardia (VT) occurs frequently during the first few days after MI, but does not appear to increase the risk for subsequent mortality if the arrhythmia is rapidly terminated. VT occurring after 24 to 48 hours, however, is associated with a marked increase in mortality. *Monomorphic* VT is usually due to a reentrant focus around a scar, whereas *polymorphic* VT is more commonly a function of underlying ischemia, electrolyte abnormalities, or drug effects.

TABLE 39.7

ELECTRICAL COMPLICATIONS OF ACUTE MI

Complication	Prognosis	Treatment
Ventricular tachycardia/fibrillation		
Within first 24–48 h	Good	Immediate cardioversion; amiodarone or lidocaine; beta-blockers
After 48 h	Poor	Immediate cardioversion; electrophysiology study/implantable defibrillator; amiodarone
Sinus bradycardia	Excellent	Atropine for hypotension or symptoms
Second-degree heart block		
Mobitz type I (Wenckebach)	Excellent	Atropine for hypotension or symptoms
Mobitz type II	Guarded	Temporary pacemaker
Complete heart block		
Inferior MI	Good	Temporary pacemaker
Anterior MI	Poor	Temporary pacemaker followed by permanent pacemaker

VF is the primary mechanism of arrhythmic sudden death. In patients with acute MI, most episodes of VF occur early (<4 to 12 hours) after infarction. As with sustained VT, *late* VF occurs more frequently in patients with severe LV dysfunction or CHF, and is a poor prognostic marker. Patients with VF, or sustained VT associated with symptoms or hemodynamic compromise, should be cardioverted emergently. Underlying metabolic and electrolyte abnormalities must be corrected, and ongoing ischemia should be addressed. We aim to maintain the serum potassium level to 4.5 mEq per L or greater and serum magnesium level 2 mEq per L or more. Intravenous amiodarone is a particularly effective antiarrhythmic agent in patients with acute MI, because it lowers heart rate. Lidocaine remains an effective alternative if amiodarone is not tolerated or is unsuccessful in controlling the arrhythmia. Prophylactic use of antiarrhythmic agents, other than beta-blockers, is not indicated.

Bradyarrhythmias

The usual cause of bradycardia is increased vagal tone or ischemia/infarction of conduction tissue. Sinus bradycardia is typically due to irritation of cardiac vagal receptors, which are located most prominently on the inferior surface of the left ventricle. Thus, this arrhythmia is usually seen with inferior MI. If the heart rate is extremely low (<40 to 50) and is associated with hypotension, intravenous atropine should be given.

Mobitz type I (Wenckebach) second-degree AV block is also very common in patients with inferior wall MI, and may be due to ischemia or infarction of the AV node or to increased vagal tone. The level of conduction block is usually located within the AV node, and therefore the QRS complex is narrow and the risk for progression to complete heart block is low. Atropine should be reserved for patients with hypotension or symptoms, and temporary pacing is rarely required. Mobitz type II block is observed much less often than Mobitz type I block in acute MI. As opposed to Mobitz type I block, Mobitz type II block is more frequently associated with anterior MI, an infranodal lesion, and a wide QRS complex. Because Mobitz type II block can progress suddenly to complete heart block, a temporary pacemaker is indicated.

Although compete heart block may occur with either inferior or anterior MI, the implications differ markedly depending on the location of the infarct. With inferior MI, heart block often progresses from first-(or Wenckebach) to third-degree AV block (see Fig. 39.2). The level of block is usually within or above the level of the AV node, the escape rhythm is often stable, and the effect is transient. Although temporary pacing is often indicated, a permanent pacemaker is rarely required.

TABLE 39.8

SUMMARY OF ADVANCES IN MANAGING STEMI BASED ON RANDOMIZED CONTROLLED CLINICAL TRIALS

- Performance of a prehospital ECG reduces reperfusion times in STEMI [5]
- Fibrinolytic therapy reduces mortality vs. placebo if administered within 12 h of symptom onset, but is associated with a small risk of intracranial hemorrhage [24]
- Aspirin reduces mortality to a similar extent as fibrinolytics [70]
- Primary PCI is superior to fibrinolytic therapy for patients who can be treated within 90 min of presentation in a high-volume center [38]
- Transfer to another facility for early nonemergent PCI should be considered following successful fibrinolytic therapy [68]
- The addition of clopidogrel to aspirin, antithrombins, and fibrinolytic therapy reduces recurrent MI and mortality [72,73]
- Prasugrel and ticagrelor represent alternatives to clopidogrel that reduce stent thrombosis and recurrent ischemic events, but at an increased risk for bleeding [75,76]
- Enoxaparin is superior to unfractionated heparin as an adjunct to fibrinolytic therapy, but is associated with slightly more bleeding [79]
- Beta-blockers improve long-term outcomes following STEMI, but may increase risk when given early to unstable patients [93,94]
- ACE inhibitors prevent adverse remodeling after STEMI and reduce death and heart failure events [95]
- Aldosterone antagonists reduce mortality in patients with LV dysfunction or heart failure following MI, but should be used in caution in individuals with renal dysfunction [98]
- Nitrates and calcium blockers are indicated in selected patients, but not routinely [100,101]

With anterior MI, complete heart block is usually a result of extensive infarction involving the bundle branches. The escape rhythm is usually unstable and the AV block permanent. Mortality is extremely high, and permanent pacing is almost always required in survivors.

Supraventricular Arrhythmias

Atrial fibrillation may occur in up to 15% of patients early after MI, but atrial flutter and paroxysmal supraventricular tachycardia are not commonly seen. Ischemia itself rarely causes atrial fibrillation, except in rare cases of atrial infarction: more common precipitants include heart failure and pericarditis. Although atrial fibrillation is usually transient, it is a marker for increased morbidity and mortality, probably because it is associated with other adverse risk predictors such as LV dysfunction and CHF. Management of supraventricular arrhythmias in the setting of acute MI is similar to management in other settings; however, there should be a lower threshold for cardioversion and ventricular rate should be more aggressively controlled (Table 39.8). Because of their beneficial effects in acute MI, beta-blockers are the agents of choice to control rate. Diltiazem or verapamil may serve as alternatives in patients without significant CHF or LV dysfunction, whereas digoxin should be reserved for patients with concomitant LV dysfunction. Of the antiarrhythmic agents available, amiodarone is safest in patients with recent MI, because it has a low risk for proarrhythmia.

References

1. Gibson CM, Pride YB, Frederick PD, et al: Trends in reperfusion strategies, door-to-needle and door-to-balloon times, and in-hospital mortality among patients with ST-segment elevation myocardial infarction enrolled in the National Registry of Myocardial Infarction from 1990 to 2006. *Am Heart J* 156(6):1035–1044, 2008.
2. Libby P: Molecular bases of the acute coronary syndromes. *Circulation* 91:2844–2850, 1995.
3. Theroux P, Fuster V: Acute coronary syndromes: unstable angina and non-Q-wave myocardial infarction. *Circulation* 97(12):1195–1206, 1998.
4. Canto JG, Shlipak MG, Rogers WJ, et al: Prevalence, clinical characteristics, and mortality among patients with myocardial infarction presenting without chest pain. *JAMA* 283(24):3223–3229, 2000.
5. Diercks DB, Kontos MC, Chen AY, et al: Utilization and impact of pre-hospital electrocardiograms for patients with acute ST-segment elevation myocardial infarction: data from the NCDR (National Cardiovascular Data Registry) ACTION (Acute Coronary Treatment and Intervention Outcomes Network) Registry. *J Am Coll Cardiol* 53(2):161–166, 2009.
6. Shlipak MG, Lyons WL, Go AS, et al: Should the electrocardiogram be used to guide therapy for patients with left bundle-branch block and suspected myocardial infarction? *JAMA* 281(8):714–719, 1999.
7. Ohman EM, Armstrong PW, White HD, et al; for the Gusto-III Investigators: Risk stratification with a point-of-care cardiac troponin T test in acute myocardial infarction. *Am J Cardiol* 84:1281–1286, 1999.
8. de Lemos JA, Antman EM, Giugliano RP, et al: Very early risk stratification after thrombolytic therapy with a bedside myoglobin assay and the 12-lead electrocardiogram. *Am Heart J* 140(3):373–378, 2000.
9. Mega JL, Morrow DA, De Lemos JA, et al: B-type natriuretic peptide at presentation and prognosis in patients with ST-segment elevation myocardial infarction: an ENTIRE-TIMI-23 substudy. *J Am Coll Cardiol* 44(2):335–339, 2004.
10. de Lemos JA, Morrow DA, Gibson CM, et al: Early noninvasive detection of failed epicardial reperfusion after fibrinolytic therapy. *Am J Cardiol* 88(4):353–358, 2001.
11. Morrow DA, Antman EM, Giugliano RP, et al: A simple risk index for rapid initial triage of patients with ST-elevation myocardial infarction: an InTIME II substudy. *Lancet* 358(9293):1571–1575, 2001.
12. Morrow DA, Antman EM, Charlesworth A, et al: TIMI risk score for ST-elevation myocardial infarction: a convenient, bedside, clinical score for risk assessment at presentation: an intravenous nPA for treatment of infarcting myocardium early II trial substudy. *Circulation* 102(17):2031–2037, 2000.
13. Morrow DA, Antman EM, Parsons L, et al: Application of the TIMI risk score for ST-elevation MI in the National Registry of Myocardial Infarction 3. *JAMA* 286(11):1356–1359, 2001.
14. Eagle KA, Lim MJ, Dabbous OH, et al: A validated prediction model for all forms of acute coronary syndrome: estimating the risk of 6-month post-discharge death in an international registry. *JAMA* 291(22):2727–2733, 2004.
15. Jacobs DR Jr, Kroenke C, Crow R, et al: PREDICT: A simple risk score for clinical severity and long-term prognosis after hospitalization for acute myocardial infarction or unstable angina: the Minnesota heart survey. *Circulation* 100(6):599–607, 1999.
16. Cannon CP, Braunwald E: GUSTO, TIMI and the case for rapid reperfusion. *Acta Cardiol* 49:1–8, 1994.
17. Gibson CM, Cannon CP, Murphy SA, et al; for the TIMI Study Group: The relationship of the TIMI Myocardial Perfusion Grade to mortality after thrombolytic administration. *Circulation* 101:125–130, 2000.
18. Ito H, Tomooka T, Sakai N, et al: Lack of myocardial perfusion immediately after successful thrombolysis: a predictor of poor recovery of left ventricular function in anterior myocardial infarction. *Circulation* 85:1699–1705, 1992.
19. de Lemos JA, Antman EM, Giugliano RP, et al: ST-segment resolution and infarct-related artery patency and flow after thrombolytic therapy. Thrombolysis in Myocardial Infarction (TIMI) 14 investigators. *Am J Cardiol* 85(3):299–304, 2000.
20. Santoro GM, Valenti R, Buonamici P, et al: Relation between ST-segment changes and myocardial perfusion evaluated by myocardial contrast echocardiography in patients with acute myocardial infarction treated with direct angioplasty. *Am J Cardiol* 82:932–937, 1998.
21. Angeja BG, Gunda M, Murphy SA, et al: TIMI myocardial perfusion grade and ST segment resolution: association with infarct size as assessed by single photon emission computed tomography imaging. *Circulation* 105(3):282–285, 2002.
22. Schröder R, Dissmann R, Bruggemann T, et al: Extent of early ST segment elevation resolution: a simple but strong predictor of outcome in patients with acute myocardial infarction. *J Am Coll Cardiol* 24:384–391, 1994.
23. de Lemos JA, Braunwald E: ST segment resolution as a tool for assessing the efficacy of reperfusion therapy. *J Am Coll Cardiol* 38(5):1283–1294, 2001.
24. Fibrinolytic Therapy Trialists' (FTT) Collaborative Group: Indications for fibrinolytic therapy in suspected acute myocardial infarction: collaborative overview of early mortality and major morbidity results from all randomised trials of more than 1000 patients. Fibrinolytic Therapy Trialists' (FTT) Collaborative Group. *Lancet* 343(8893):311–322, 1994.
25. Cannon CP, Gibson CM, Lambrew CT, et al: Relationship of symptom-onset-to-balloon time and door-to-balloon time with mortality in patients undergoing angioplasty for acute myocardial infarction. *JAMA* 283(22):2941–2947, 2000.
26. The Global Use of Strategies to Open Occluded Coronary Arteries (GUSTO III) Investigators: A comparison of reteplase with alteplase for acute myocardial infarction. *N Engl J Med* 337:1118–1123, 1997.
27. Assessment of the Safety and Efficacy of a New Thrombolytic (ASSENT-2) Investigators: Single-bolus tenecteplase compared with front-loaded alteplase in acute myocardial infarction: the ASSENT-2 double-blind randomised trial. *Lancet* 354:716–722, 1999.
28. Antman EM, Hand M, Armstrong PW, et al: 2007 Focused Update of the ACC/AHA 2004 Guidelines for the Management of Patients With ST-Elevation Myocardial Infarction: a report of the American College of Cardiology/American Heart Association Task Force on Practice Guidelines: developed in collaboration With the Canadian Cardiovascular Society endorsed by the American Academy of Family Physicians: 2007 Writing Group to Review New Evidence and Update the ACC/AHA 2004 Guidelines for the Management of Patients With ST-Elevation Myocardial Infarction, Writing on Behalf of the 2004 Writing Committee. *Circulation* 117(2):296–329, 2008.
29. Ohman EM, Califf RM, Topol EJ, et al; the TAMI Study Group: Consequences of reocclusion after successful reperfusion therapy in acute myocardial infarction. *Circulation* 82:781–791, 1990.
30. Gibson CM, Karha J, Murphy SA, et al: Early and long-term clinical outcomes associated with reinfarction following fibrinolytic administration in the Thrombolysis in Myocardial Infarction trials. *J Am Coll Cardiol* 42(1):7–16, 2003.
31. Coulter SA, Cannon CP, Ault KA, et al: High levels of platelet inhibition with abciximab despite heightened platelet activation and aggregation during thrombolysis for acute myocardial infarction: results from TIMI (thrombolysis in myocardial infarction) 14. *Circulation* 101(23):2690–2695, 2000.
32. Antman EM, Giugliano RP, Gibson CM, et al; for the Thrombolysis in Myocardial Infarction (TIMI) 14 Investigators: Abciximab facilitates the rate and extent of thrombolysis: results of TIMI 14 trial. *Circulation* 99:2720–2732, 1999.
33. de Lemos JA, Antman EM, Gibson CM, et al: Abciximab improves both epicardial flow and myocardial reperfusion in ST-elevation myocardial infarction. Observations from the TIMI 14 trial. *Circulation* 101(3):239–243, 2000.

34. Antman EM, Gibson CM, de Lemos JA, et al: Combination reperfusion therapy with abciximab and reduced dose reteplase: results from TIMI 14. *Eur Heart J* 21(23):1944–1953, 2000.
35. Strategies for Patency Enhancement in the Emergency Department (SPEED) Group: Trial of abciximab with and without low-dose reteplase for acute myocardial infarction. *Circulation* 101:2788–2794, 2000.
36. The GUSTO V Investigators: Reperfusion therapy for acute myocardial infarction with fibrinolytic therapy or combination reduced fibrinolytic therapy and platelet glycoprotein IIb/IIIa inhibition: the GUSTO V randomised trial. *Lancet* 357:1905–1914, 2001.
37. The Assessment of the Safety and Efficacy of a New Thrombolytic Regimen (ASSENT)-3 Investigators: Efficacy and safety of tenecteplase in combination with enoxaparin, abciximab, or unfractionated heparin: the ASSENT-3 randomised trial in acute myocardial infarction. *Lancet* 358:605–613, 2001.
38. Keeley EC, Boura JA, Grines CL: Primary angioplasty versus intravenous thrombolytic therapy for acute myocardial infarction: a quantitative review of 23 randomised trials. *Lancet* 361(9351):13–20, 2003.
39. Aversano T, Aversano LT, Passamani E, et al: Thrombolytic therapy vs primary percutaneous coronary intervention for myocardial infarction in patients presenting to hospitals without on-site cardiac surgery: a randomized controlled trial. *JAMA* 287(15):1943–1951, 2002.
40. Zhu MM, Feit A, Chadow H, et al: Primary stent implantation compared with primary balloon angioplasty for acute myocardial infarction: a meta-analysis of randomized clinical trials. *Am J Cardiol* 88(3):297–301, 2001.
41. Stone GW, Grines CL, Cox DA, et al: Comparison of angioplasty with stenting, with or without abciximab, in acute myocardial infarction. *N Engl J Med* 346(13):957–966, 2002.
42. Kastrati A, Dibra A, Spaulding C, et al: Meta-analysis of randomized trials on drug-eluting stents vs. bare-metal stents in patients with acute myocardial infarction. *Eur Heart J* 28(22):2706–2713, 2007.
43. Stone GW, Lansky AJ, Pocock SJ, et al: Paclitaxel-eluting stents versus bare-metal stents in acute myocardial infarction. *N Engl J Med* 360(19):1946–1959, 2009.
44. Svilaas T, Vlaar PJ, van der Horst IC, et al: Thrombus aspiration during primary percutaneous coronary intervention. *N Engl J Med* 358(6):557–567, 2008.
45. Vlaar PJ, Svilaas T, van der Horst IC, et al: Cardiac death and reinfarction after 1 year in the thrombus aspiration during percutaneous coronary intervention in Acute myocardial infarction Study (TAPAS): a 1-year follow-up study. *Lancet* 371(9628):1915–1920, 2008.
46. Kushner FG, Hand M, Smith SC Jr, et al: 2009 Focused Updates: ACC/AHA Guidelines for the Management of Patients With ST-Elevation Myocardial Infarction (updating the 2004 Guideline and 2007 Focused Update) and ACC/AHA/SCAI Guidelines on Percutaneous Coronary Intervention (updating the 2005 Guideline and 2007 Focused Update): a report of the American College of Cardiology Foundation/American Heart Association Task Force on Practice Guidelines. *Circulation* 120(22):2271–2306, 2009.
47. Bradley EH, Herrin J, Wang Y, et al: Strategies for reducing the door-to-balloon time in acute myocardial infarction. *N Engl J Med* 355(22):2308–2320, 2006.
48. Nallamothu BK, Krumholz HM, Peterson ED, et al: Door-to-balloon times in hospitals within the get-with-the-guidelines registry after initiation of the door-to-balloon (D2B) Alliance. *Am J Cardiol* 103(8):1051–1055, 2009.
49. Nallamothu BK, Bates ER, Herrin J, et al: Times to treatment in transfer patients undergoing primary percutaneous coronary intervention in the United States: National Registry of Myocardial Infarction (NRMI)-3/4 analysis. *Circulation* 111(6):761–767, 2005.
50. Ting HH, Rihal CS, Gersh BJ, et al: Regional systems of care to optimize timeliness of reperfusion therapy for ST-elevation myocardial infarction: the Mayo Clinic STEMI Protocol. *Circulation* 116(7):729–736, 2007.
51. Henry TD, Sharkey SW, Burke MN, et al: A regional system to provide timely access to percutaneous coronary intervention for ST-elevation myocardial infarction. *Circulation* 116(7):721–728, 2007.
52. Jollis JG, Roettig ML, Aluko AO, et al: Implementation of a statewide system for coronary reperfusion for ST-segment elevation myocardial infarction. *JAMA* 298(20):2371–2380, 2007.
53. Antman EM, Anbe DT, Armstrong PW, et al: ACC/AHA guidelines for the management of patients with ST-elevation myocardial infarction: a report of the American College of Cardiology/American Heart Association Task Force on Practice Guidelines (Committee to Revise the 1999 Guidelines for the Management of Patients with Acute Myocardial Infarction). *Circulation* 110(9):e82–e292, 2004.
54. Widimsky P, Groch L, Zelizko M, et al: Multicentre randomized trial comparing transport to primary angioplasty vs immediate thrombolysis vs combined strategy for patients with acute myocardial infarction presenting to a community hospital without a catheterization laboratory. The PRAGUE study. *Eur Heart J* 21(10):823–831, 2000.
55. Andersen HR, Nielsen TT, Rasmussen K, et al: A comparison of coronary angioplasty with fibrinolytic therapy in acute myocardial infarction. *N Engl J Med* 349(8):733–742, 2003.
56. Widimsky P, Budesinsky T, Vorac D, et al: Long distance transport for primary angioplasty vs immediate thrombolysis in acute myocardial infarction. Final results of the randomized national multicentre trial—PRAGUE-2. *Eur Heart J* 24(1):94–104, 2003.
57. Steg PG, Bonnefoy E, Chabaud S, et al: Impact of time to treatment on mortality after prehospital fibrinolysis or primary angioplasty: data from the CAPTIM randomized clinical trial. *Circulation* 108(23):2851–2856, 2003.
58. Nallamothu BK, Bates ER: Percutaneous coronary intervention versus fibrinolytic therapy in acute myocardial infarction: is timing (almost) everything? *Am J Cardiol* 92(7):824–826, 2003.
59. TIMI Study Group: Comparison of invasive and conservative strategies after treatment with intravenous tissue plasminogen activator in acute myocardial infarction. Results of the Thrombolysis in Myocardial Infarction (TIMI) Phase II Trial. *N Engl J Med* 320:618–627, 1989.
60. TIMI Research Group: Immediate vs delayed catheterization and angioplasty following thrombolytic therapy for acute myocardial infarction. TIMI II A results. *JAMA* 260:2849–2858, 1988.
61. Ross AM, Coyne KS, Reiner JS, et al: A randomized trial comparing primary angioplasty with a strategy of short-acting thrombolysis and immediate planned rescue angioplasty in acute myocardial infarction: the PACT trial. PACT investigators. Plasminogen-activator Angioplasty Compatibility Trial. *J Am Coll Cardiol* 34(7):1954–1962, 1999.
62. Brodie BR, Stuckey TD, Hansen C, et al: Benefit of coronary reperfusion before intervention on outcomes after primary angioplasty for acute myocardial infarction. *Am J Cardiol* 85(1):13–18, 2000.
63. Keeley EC, Boura JA, Grines CL: Comparison of primary and facilitated percutaneous coronary interventions for ST-elevation myocardial infarction: quantitative review of randomised trials. *Lancet* 367(9510):579–588, 2006.
64. Ellis SG, Tendera M, de Belder MA, et al: Facilitated PCI in patients with ST-elevation myocardial infarction. *N Engl J Med* 358(21):2205–2217, 2008.
65. Fernandez-Aviles F, Alonso JJ, Castro-Beiras A, et al: Routine invasive strategy within 24 hours of thrombolysis versus ischaemia-guided conservative approach for acute myocardial infarction with ST-segment elevation (GRACIA-1): a randomised controlled trial. *Lancet* 364(9439):1045–1053, 2004.
66. Zeymer U, Uebis R, Vogt A, et al: Randomized comparison of percutaneous transluminal coronary angioplasty and medical therapy in stable survivors of acute myocardial infarction with single vessel disease: a study of the Arbeitsgemeinschaft Leitende Kardiologische Krankenhausarzte. *Circulation* 108(11):1324–1328, 2003.
67. Armstrong PW: A comparison of pharmacologic therapy with/without timely coronary intervention vs. primary percutaneous intervention early after ST-elevation myocardial infarction: the WEST (Which Early ST-elevation myocardial infarction Therapy) study. *Eur Heart J* 27(13):1530–1538, 2006.
68. Cantor WJ, Fitchett D, Borgundvaag B, et al: Routine early angioplasty after fibrinolysis for acute myocardial infarction. *N Engl J Med* 360(26):2705–2718, 2009.
69. Roux S, Christeller S, Ludin E: Effects of aspirin on coronary reocclusion and recurrent ischemia after thrombolysis: a meta-analysis. *J Am Coll Cardiol* 19:671–677, 1992.
70. ISIS-2 (Second International Study of Infarct Survival) Collaborative Group: Randomised trial of intravenous streptokinase, oral aspirin, both, or neither among 17,187 cases of suspected acute myocardial infarction: ISIS-2. *Lancet* 2:349–360, 1988.
71. Antithrombotic Trialists' Collaboration: Collaborative meta-analysis of randomised trials of antiplatelet therapy for prevention of death, myocardial infarction, and stroke in high risk patients. *BMJ* 324(7329):71–86, 2002.
72. Sabatine MS, Cannon CP, Gibson CM, et al: Addition of clopidogrel to aspirin and fibrinolytic therapy for myocardial infarction with ST-segment elevation. *N Engl J Med* 352(12):1179–1189, 2005.
73. Chen ZM, Jiang LX, Chen YP, et al: Addition of clopidogrel to aspirin in 45,852 patients with acute myocardial infarction: randomised placebo-controlled trial. *Lancet* 366(9497):1607–1621, 2005.
74. Mehta SR: CURRENT OASIS 7: a 2×2 factorial randomized trial of optimal clopidogrel and aspirin dosing in patients with ACS undergoing an early invasive strategy with intent for PCI. Presented at the American Heart Association Meeting, November 2009.
75. Montalescot G, Wiviott SD, Braunwald E, et al: Prasugrel compared with clopidogrel in patients undergoing percutaneous coronary intervention for ST-elevation myocardial infarction (TRITON-TIMI 38): double-blind, randomised controlled trial. *Lancet* 373(9665):723–731, 2009.
76. Wallentin L, Becker RC, Budaj A, et al: Ticagrelor versus clopidogrel in patients with acute coronary syndromes. *N Engl J Med* 361(11):1045–1057, 2009.
77. Kandzari DE, Hasselblad V, Tcheng JE, et al: Improved clinical outcomes with abciximab therapy in acute myocardial infarction: a systematic overview of randomized clinical trials. *Am Heart J* 147(3):457–462, 2004.
78. Yusuf S, Mehta SR, Xie C, et al: Effects of reviparin, a low-molecular-weight heparin, on mortality, reinfarction, and strokes in patients with acute myocardial infarction presenting with ST-segment elevation. *JAMA* 293(4):427–435, 2005.
79. Antman EM, Morrow DA, McCabe CH, et al: Enoxaparin versus unfractionated heparin with fibrinolysis for ST-elevation myocardial infarction. *N Engl J Med* 354(14):1477–1488, 2006.
80. Wallentin L, Goldstein P, Armstrong PW, et al: Efficacy and safety of tenecteplase in combination with the low-molecular-weight heparin enoxaparin or unfractionated heparin in the prehospital setting: the Assessment of

the Safety and Efficacy of a New Thrombolytic Regimen (ASSENT)-3 PLUS randomized trial in acute myocardial infarction. *Circulation* 108(2):135–142, 2003.
81. Yusuf S, Mehta SR, Chrolavicius S, et al: Effects of fondaparinux on mortality and reinfarction in patients with acute ST-segment elevation myocardial infarction: the OASIS-6 randomized trial. *JAMA* 295(13):1519–1530, 2006.
82. The Global Use of Strategies to Open Occluded Coronary Arteries (GUSTO) IIb Investigators: A comparison of recombinant hirudin with heparin for the treatment of acute coronary syndromes. *N Engl J Med* 335:775–782, 1996.
83. Antman EM; for the TIMI 9B Investigators: Hirudin in acute myocardial infarction: thrombolysis and Thrombin Inhibition in Myocardial Infarction (TIMI) 9B trial. *Circulation* 94:911–921, 1996.
84. White H: Thrombin-specific anticoagulation with bivalirudin versus heparin in patients receiving fibrinolytic therapy for acute myocardial infarction: the HERO-2 randomised trial. *Lancet* 358(9296):1855–1863, 2001.
85. Stone GW, Witzenbichler B, Guagliumi G, et al: Bivalirudin during primary PCI in acute myocardial infarction. *N Engl J Med* 358(21):2218–2230, 2008.
86. Dangas G, Mehran R, Guagliumi G, et al: Role of clopidogrel loading dose in patients with ST-segment elevation myocardial infarction undergoing primary angioplasty: results from the HORIZONS-AMI (Harmonizing Outcomes with Revascularization and Stents in Acute Myocardial Infarction) trial. *J Am Coll Cardiol* 54(15):1438–1446, 2009.
87. Coumadin Aspirin Reinfarction Study (CARS) Investigators: Randomised double-blind trial of fixed low-dose warfarin with aspirin after myocardial infarction. *Lancet* 350:389–396, 1997.
88. van Es RF, Jonker JJ, Verheugt FW, et al: Aspirin and coumadin after acute coronary syndromes (the ASPECT-2 study): a randomised controlled trial. *Lancet* 360(9327):109–113, 2002.
89. Hurlen M, Abdelnoor M, Smith P, et al: Warfarin, aspirin, or both after myocardial infarction. *N Engl J Med* 347(13):969–974, 2002.
90. Brouwer MA, van den Bergh PJ, Aengevaeren WR, et al: Aspirin plus coumarin versus aspirin alone in the prevention of reocclusion after fibrinolysis for acute myocardial infarction: results of the Antithrombotics in the Prevention of Reocclusion in Coronary Thrombolysis (APRICOT)-2 Trial. *Circulation* 106(6):659–665, 2002.
91. Holmes DR Jr, Kereiakes DJ, Kleiman NS, et al: Combining antiplatelet and anticoagulant therapies. *J Am Coll Cardiol* 54(2):95–109, 2009.
92. The TIMI Study Group: Comparison of invasive and conservative strategies after treatment with intravenous tissue plasminogen activator in acute myocardial infarction: results of the Thrombolysis in Myocardial Infarction (TIMI) Phase II Trial. *N Engl J Med* 320:618–627, 1989.
93. Yusuf S, Peto R, Lewis J, et al: Beta-blockade during and after myocardial infarction: an overview of the randomized trials. *Prog Cardiovasc Dis* 27:335–371, 1985.
94. Chen ZM, Pan HC, Chen YP, et al: Early intravenous then oral metoprolol in 45,852 patients with acute myocardial infarction: randomised placebo-controlled trial. *Lancet* 366(9497):1622–1632, 2005.
95. ACE Inhibitor Myocardial Infarction Collaborative Group: Indications for ACE inhibitors in the early treatment of acute myocardial infarction: systematic overview of individual data from 100,000 patients in randomized trials. *Circulation* 97:2202–2212, 1998.
96. Rutherford JD, Pfeffer MA, Moye LA, et al; on behalf of the SAVE Investigators: Effects of captopril on ischemic events after myocardial infarction. Results of the Survival and Ventricular Enlargement Trial. *Circulation* 90:1731–1738, 1994.
97. Pfeffer MA, McMurray JJ, Velazquez EJ, et al: Valsartan, captopril, or both in myocardial infarction complicated by heart failure, left ventricular dysfunction, or both. *N Engl J Med* 349(20):1893–1906, 2003.
98. Pitt B, Remme W, Zannad F, et al; Efficacy tEP-AMIHF, Survival Study Investigators: Eplerenone, a selective aldosterone blocker, in patients with left ventricular dysfunction after myocardial infarction. *N Engl J Med* 348(14):1309–1321, 2003.
99. Gruppo Italiano per lo Studio della Sopravvivenza nell'infarto Miocardico: GISSI-3: effects of lisinopril and transdermal glyceryl trinitrate singly and together on 6-week mortality and ventricular function after acute myocardial infarction. *Lancet* 343(8906):1115–1122, 1994.
100. ISIS-4 Collaborative Group: ISIS-4: randomized factorial trial assessing early oral captopril, oral mononitrate, and intravenous magnesium sulphate in 58,050 patients with suspected acute myocardial infarction. *Lancet* 345:669–685, 1995.
101. Yusuf S, Held P, Furburg C: Update of effects of calcium antagonists in myocardial infarction or angina in light of the second Danish Verapamil Infarction Trial (DAVIT-II) and other recent studies. *Am J Cardiol* 67:1295–1297, 1991.

CHAPTER 40 ■ MECHANICAL COMPLICATIONS OF MYOCARDIAL INFARCTION

ANNABEL A. CHEN-TOURNOUX AND MICHAEL A. FIFER

PATHOPHYSIOLOGY UNDERLYING MYOCARDIAL STUNNING AND ITS TIME COURSE FOLLOWING ISCHEMIA AND REPERFUSION

Within 8 to 10 seconds after occlusion of an epicardial coronary artery, myocardial oxygen supply is exhausted, resulting in a shift from aerobic to anaerobic metabolism. High-energy phosphates (creatine phosphate and adenosine triphosphate [ATP]) become depleted, whereas hydrogen ions, lactate, and other metabolic products accumulate, causing intracellular pH to fall to 5.8 to 6.0 within 10 minutes of the onset of ischemia [1]. In addition, adenosine monophosphate (AMP) is degraded to adenosine, which diffuses into extracellular fluid, depleting the intracellular adenine nucleotide pool. The ischemic myocardium stretches instead of shortens during systole, corresponding to regional wall motion abnormalities observed with imaging modalities, such as echocardiography. Electrocardiogram (ECG) changes appear as well. Disruption of the cell membrane allows protein leakage out of the cell, producing serologic evidence of myocyte injury. If blood flow is restored within 15 minutes of coronary occlusion, myocyte injury is reversible. Glycolysis ceases after approximately 40 minutes of severe ischemia, after which time injury becomes irreversible and myocytes are not salvageable by reperfusion. Even with earlier restoration of blood flow, however, a phenomenon called myocardial stunning is observed.

First described in a dog model by Heyndrickx et al. [2] in 1975, stunning is defined as prolonged contractile dysfunction occurring after relief of a discrete episode or episodes of ischemia. Importantly, the dysfunction associated with stunning is completely reversible. By definition, myocardial perfusion must be restored to normal or near normal to distinguish stunning from myocardial dysfunction due to continued ischemia (hibernation). The severity and duration of stunning depend on multiple factors, such as the extent of the original ischemic insult, the adequacy of restored flow, the presence of preexisting collateral vessels, and prior ischemic preconditioning. In general, the myocardium is stunned for a period longer than that of the ischemic insult, often requiring hours to days to regain function [3].

Although early restoration of flow is necessary for myocardial survival, reperfusion is also thought to underlie the pathogenesis of stunning, through the development of oxidative stress and/or impaired calcium homeostasis [4]. In the first 5 minutes of reperfusion, there is marked hyperemia, with a 400% to 600% increase in flow, returning to the baseline level after 15 to 20 minutes. Because levels of oxygen-free radicals peak at 4 to 7 minutes, most of the free radical-induced injury responsible for stunning is thought to occur in the initial moments following reperfusion. Blunted calcium transients and dysfunction of the ryanodine receptor and the sarcoplasmic reticulum calcium ATPase (SERCA-2), which would lead to impaired myocyte excitation–contraction coupling, have also been described following ischemia–reperfusion. Other possible mechanisms of reperfusion injury involved in myocardial stunning include microvascular injury, endothelial cell dysfunction, and activation of neutrophils, platelets, and the complement system.

Stunning is observed in clinical scenarios in which the heart is reperfused after transient ischemia, whether it be global, as with cardioplegia during cardiac surgery or transplant harvest, or regional, as with acute coronary syndromes, percutaneous coronary interventions (PCI), or exercise-induced angina. In patients with coronary disease, stunning from repeated episodes of demand ischemia may lead to chronic left ventricular (LV) dysfunction.

Stunned, but viable, myocardium may be identified by echocardiographic, scintigraphic, and magnetic resonance imaging techniques [5]. Because ischemic myocytes have different rates of injury and recovery, the timing of improvement after acute myocardial infarction (MI) is variable and often unpredictable. The major clinical implication of stunning is that even brief periods of ischemia may be associated with prolonged contractile dysfunction. Moreover, because this dysfunction may be fully reversible, continued hemodynamic support, with intra-aortic balloon counterpulsation and/or inotropic agents such as catecholamines or phosphodiesterase inhibitors, may be indicated. Importantly, inotropic stimulation does not appear to worsen cell injury as long as the reperfused artery is patent. Finally, myocardial stunning has implications for the timing of evaluation of LV function to guide therapeutic decisions after MI. For example, LV ejection fraction assessment for implantable cardiac defibrillator implantation is generally deferred for at least 1 month following MI.

DIAGNOSIS, TREATMENT, AND OUTCOME OF SHOCK DUE TO LEFT VENTRICULAR PUMP FAILURE

Approximately 5% to 8% of patients with ST-segment elevation MI (STEMI) and 2.5% of patients with non–ST-segment elevation MI develop cardiogenic shock (CS), the leading cause of death in patients hospitalized with MI (Table 40.1). CS is broadly defined as a state of end-organ hypoperfusion due to cardiac failure. Clinical evidence of systemic hypoperfusion includes altered mental status, cold clammy skin, and oliguria. Hemodynamic parameters of CS include persistent ($\geq$1 hour) hypotension (systolic blood pressure <80 to 90 mm Hg or mean arterial pressure 30 mm Hg lower than baseline) not responsive to fluid or requiring inotropic or vasopressor support to be maintained; low cardiac index (<1.8 L per minute per m^2 without support or 2.0 to 2.2 L per minute per m^2 with support); and adequate or elevated filling pressures (LV end-diastolic pressure >15 mm Hg or right ventricular [RV] end-diastolic pressure >10 to 15 mm Hg).

In the absence of mechanical complications, the primary insult in CS associated with MI is LV dysfunction due to extensive infarction or ischemia. Although the magnitude of myocardial insult does not correlate perfectly with the development of CS [6], LV function nevertheless remains a prognostic factor in CS [7].

The observation of normal to low systemic vascular resistance among many patients with CS [8] suggests an important role for inappropriate vasodilation in CS. Indeed, neurohormonal and cytokine abnormalities consistent with the systemic inflammatory response syndrome (SIRS) have been observed (Fig. 40.1) [6]. For example, cytokines with myocardial depressant activity, such as tumor necrosis factor (TNF)-α and interleukin (IL)-6, increase over 24 to 72 hours after MI. MI is also associated with abnormal NO metabolism [9] and increased expression of inducible nitric oxide (NO) synthase; NO excess causes vasodilation, depressed myocardial contractility, and interference with catecholamine action in CS. Despite the

TABLE 40.1

NATIONAL REGISTRY OF MYOCARDIAL INFARCTION: ALL-CAUSE IN-HOSPITAL MORTALITY FOR PATIENTS WITH ACUTE MYOCARDIAL INFARCTION

Cause of death	All MI patients (359,755) (%, *n*)	No fibrinolytic therapy (228,512) (%, *n*)	Fibrinolytic therapy (91,218) (%, *n*)	*p*-value
Cardiogenic shock	3.5 (12,262)	4.1 (9,437)	2.3 (2,054)	<0.001
Sudden cardiac arrest	2.9 (10,217)	3.7 (8,435)	1.5 (1,282)	<0.001
Arrhythmias	1.5 (5,385)	1.9 (4,279)	0.9 (794)	<0.001
Recurrent MI	0.7 (2,511)	0.9 (1,993)	0.4 (384)	<0.001
EMD/myocardial rupture	0.8 (2,671)	0.8 (1,801)	0.7 (631)	<0.001
Other cardiac	1.2 (4,221)	1.6 (3,556)	0.5 (468)	<0.001
Overall mortality	10.4 (36,581)	12.9 (29,401)	5.9 (5,165)	<0.001

EMD, electromechanical dissociation; MI, myocardial infarction.
Adapted from Becker RC, Gore JM, Lambrew C, et al: A composite view of cardiac rupture in the United States National Registry of Myocardial Infarction. *J Am Coll Cardiol* 27:1321–1326, 1996, with permission.

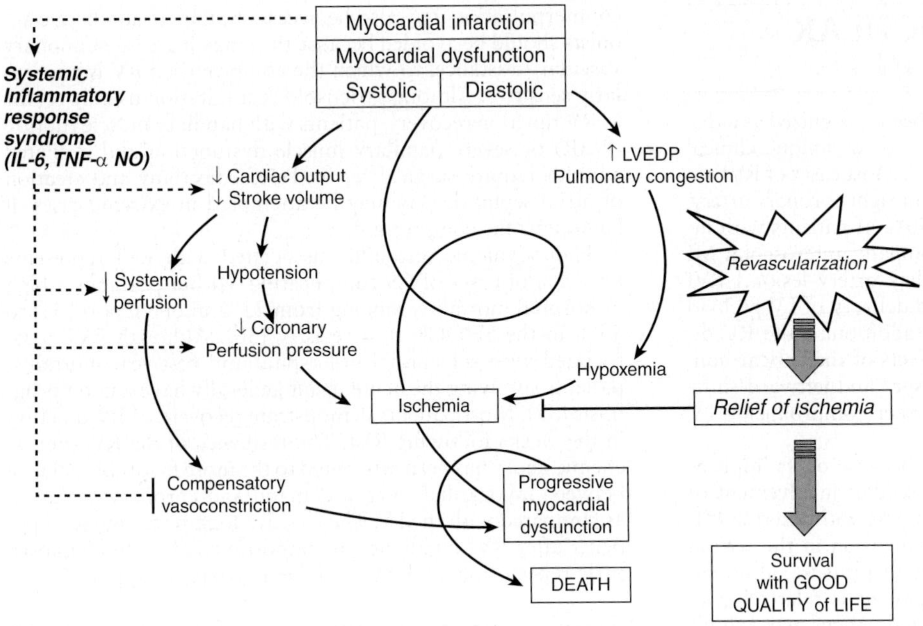

FIGURE 40.1. The cascade of physiologic events causing cardiogenic shock after MI. IL-6, interleukin-6; LVEDP, left ventricular end-diastolic pressure; NO, nitric oxide; TNF-α, tumor necrosis factor-α. [From Reynolds HR, Hochman JS: Cardiogenic shock: current concepts and improving outcomes. *Circulation* 117:686–697, 2008, with permission.]

growing recognition of SIRS associated with CS, therapies targeting it remain unproven at this time.

Most cases of CS after acute coronary syndrome develop after hospital presentation, with a median time of 10 to 11 hours (STEMI) and 76 hours (non–ST-segment elevation MI) [10]. Predictors for CS have varied among different studies over time and include older age; prior MI, heart failure, diabetes, hypertension, or cerebrovascular disease; failed reperfusion; lower blood pressure and glomerular filtration rate; and higher heart rate and serum glucose at presentation [6,11]. The only way to prevent CS appears to be very early reperfusion therapy for MI, whether through PCI or thrombolysis.

Outcome in CS is closely related to the patency of the infarct-related artery, in both retrospective analyses [12] and the prospective, randomized SHOCK (*sh*ould we emergently revascularize *o*ccluded *c*oronaries in cardiogenic shoc*k*) trial. In this multicenter study, patients with acute MI and CS were randomly assigned to early (within 6 hours) percutaneous or surgical revascularization (152 patients) or initial medical stabilization with subsequent revascularization permitted 54 hours after randomization (150 patients) [13,14]. Fibrinolysis was recommended in the initial medical stabilization group, and intra-aortic balloon counterpulsation was recommended in both treatment groups. Although there was an excess of death in the early revascularization group in the first 5 days, likely related to procedural complications, early revascularization improved survival at 6 months and 1 year (46.7% vs. 33.6%; $p < 0.03$), a benefit that remained stable at 3 and 6 years [15]. Although the benefit of revascularization increases the earlier it is achieved, there is a survival benefit as long as 48 hours after MI and 18 hours after shock onset. The benefit of early revascularization is similar for different subgroups (patients with diabetes, women, patients with prior MI, early vs. late shock) and whether revascularization is achieved with PCI or coronary artery bypass graft surgery [16]. Among patients undergoing PCI, registry data indicate that stenting and glycoprotein IIb/IIIa inhibitors are independently associated with improved outcomes [17]. On the basis of these results, emergency revascularization is recommended (class I) for patients younger than 75 years with MI and CS, who are determined to be suitable candidates [18]. If revascularization is not available, fibrinolysis and intra-aortic balloon pump placement followed by transfer to another facility is recommended.

In the SHOCK trial, lack of benefit with early revascularization was noted for patients 75 years and older, possibly due to imbalances in baseline ejection fraction. Later studies, including the SHOCK registry [19], have shown a consistent benefit of revascularization in elderly patients selected for it. Thus, an individualized approach weighing the risks and benefits of an aggressive revascularization strategy is warranted for elderly patients.

Multivessel or left main disease is extremely common in patients with MI and CS. Coronary bypass surgery is recommended for extensive disease [18], although PCI of the infarct-related artery may be initially necessary to stabilize the patient.

In addition to early revascularization, supportive therapy with inotropic agents and vasopressors (and avoidance of negative inotropes and vasodilators) is critical. Diuretics or intravenous fluids may be required, depending on the intravascular volume status. Routine antithrombotic therapy for MI includes aspirin, heparin, and if immediate surgery is unlikely, clopidogrel. Oxygen supplementation is standard and mechanical ventilation may be necessary. Intensive insulin therapy is also recommended in critically ill patients [18].

Hemodynamic management of CS may be guided by pulmonary artery catheter monitoring and echocardiography. Such monitoring also allows detection of mechanical complications such as papillary muscle or ventricular septal rupture (VSR).

The principal mechanical therapy for CS is intra-aortic balloon counterpulsation, which augments coronary perfusion and reduces cardiac afterload. For some patients who require a bridge to recovery or subsequent transplantation, short-term support may be offered in the form of LV assist device (LVAD) or extracorporeal life support [20]. Comparisons of percutaneous LVAD to intra-aortic balloon counterpulsation (IABP) have shown similar mortality rates [21–23].

Independent predictors of mortality in CS have varied in different studies over time, and include older age; history of hypertension, MI, or heart failure; lower blood pressure and worse renal function on presentation; failed reperfusion; and low LV ejection fraction [7,11,12,15]. Revascularization provides benefit at every level of risk, and registry studies in the United States and Europe have indicated significant decline (approximately 60% to 48%) in mortality from CS in recent years, in parallel with increasing revascularization with PCI [11,24,25].

RIGHT VENTRICULAR INFARCTION

Right ventricular infarction (RVI) has been recognized as a distinct entity since the initial description of its unique clinical and hemodynamic features in 1974 [26]. Most cases of RVI are due to proximal occlusion of a dominant right coronary artery, and RVI has been described in up to 50% of patients with inferior MI. (Very rarely, RVI may accompany anteroseptal MI due to a culprit left anterior descending artery lesion.) RVI leads to RV hypokinesis and decreased delivery of LV preload across the pulmonary vasculature. In addition, acute RV dilation in the face of the restraining effects of the pericardium leads to elevated intrapericardial pressure and leftward shifting of the interventricular septum, further compromising LV filling [27].

Early recognition of RVI is crucial because of its implications for management and prognosis, so that involvement of the RV should be considered in all patients with inferior MI. Clinical indicators of RVI include hypotension in the setting of clear lungs and elevated jugular venous pressure, although the latter may not be evident if the patient is relatively hypovolemic. Conversely, a volume-depleted patient may exhibit sensitivity to preload reduction, such as with the use of nitrates or diuretics. Patients may also display evidence of interventricular dependence, such as Kussmaul's sign (distention of jugular veins during inspiration), more classically associated with pericardial disease.

Several ECG signs indicate RV involvement: ST-segment elevation in lead 3 greater than in lead 2, ST-segment elevation in lead V_1, and ST-segment elevation in right-sided precordial lead V_{4R}, the latter being the most predictive [28] (Fig. 40.2). These ECG abnormalities may resolve quickly (50% within 10 hours) [29], underscoring the importance of obtaining a right-sided ECG on presentation for all patients with inferior MI. RVI may be associated with bradyarrhythmias (sinoatrial or atrioventricular [AV] block) and tachyarrhythmias (atrial fibrillation and ventricular tachyarrhythmias). Echocardiography reveals RV dilation and hypokinesis and abnormal septal motion, along with inferior LV hypokinesis, and possibly other complications of RVI, such as tricuspid regurgitation, VSR, RV mural thrombus and pulmonary embolism, and right-to-left shunting across a patent foramen ovale. A small study suggests that late-enhancement magnetic resonance imaging has superior sensitivity to detect RVI compared with physical examination, ECG, and echocardiography [30]. Finally, right heart catheterization demonstrating a right atrial pressure equal or greater than 10 mm Hg or greater than 80% of the pulmonary capillary wedge pressure supports the diagnosis of RVI [26].

Treatment of RVI should emphasize urgent reperfusion, whether by thrombolysis or PCI. Successful reperfusion is associated with significantly improved RV function and clinical outcome [31–33]. Supportive measures are critical as well. Intravenous fluid should be judiciously administered to maintain optimal RV preload. A cautious challenge of 1 to 2 L is a reasonable start. Central venous pressure (CVP) monitoring may be helpful in avoiding RV volume overload (CVP exceeding 10 to 14 mm Hg), which may compromise LV preload via ventricular interdependence [34]. Because right atrial contraction is an important contributor to right-sided output, AV synchrony should be maintained, with AV sequential pacing in the case of complete heart block or conversion to sinus rhythm in the case of atrial fibrillation. In cases where right coronary artery occlusion is proximal to the atrial branches, resulting in right atrial ischemia, the CVP tracing may demonstrate depressed A-waves and right atrial pacing may fail to capture. Inotropic support and LV afterload reduction with intra-aortic balloon counterpulsation may also be necessary. Pure α-adrenergic agonists should be avoided because they may increase pulmonary vascular resistance, to which the compromised RV is particularly sensitive. Although tricuspid regurgitation usually remits as RV function recovers, patients with papillary muscle rupture (PMR) or severe papillary muscle dysfunction and a dilated annulus require surgical repair. Pericardiectomy and creation of atrial septal defects may be attempted in extreme cases of hemodynamic compromise.

Hemodynamic instability associated with RVI represents only 5% of cases of CS complicating MI but portends a high in-hospital mortality, ranging from 23% in one report [35] to 53% in the SHOCK trial registry [36]. Although RVI is associated with substantial in-hospital and first-year mortality, patients surviving the acute insult generally have a good prognosis [37]. Most patients demonstrate recovery of RV function in the weeks following RVI. The resilience of the RV after ischemic injury has been attributed to the more favorable balance between myocardial oxygen demand and coronary perfusion as compared with the LV. The positive long-term course of patients after RVI highlights the importance of early diagnosis, early reperfusion, and intensive hemodynamic support.

MYOCARDIAL RUPTURE

Myocardial rupture is a rare, but immediately life-threatening, complication of MI, accounting for 10% to 15% of deaths. Transmural necrosis or myocardial hemorrhage is found at the site of rupture. In the National Registry of Myocardial Infarction, older age, female gender, and fibrinolysis were independent predictors of myocardial rupture [38].

Myocardial rupture may occur despite a limited infarct area and relatively preserved systolic function because of increased shear stress in the necrotic area or its ischemic boundaries. Rupture is possible at three sites: the ventricular free wall (85%), the ventricular septum (10%), or a papillary muscle (5%). The specific presentations and sequelae depend on the location of the defect(s) (Table 40.2), but in all cases, prompt diagnosis and definitive surgical therapy are critical.

Papillary Muscle Rupture

PMR involves the posteromedial papillary muscle (75%) more often than the anterolateral papillary muscle (25%) because of the single vascular supply of the former (right coronary or left circumflex artery, depending on dominance). In contrast, the anterolateral papillary muscle has a dual vascular supply, from the left anterior descending and circumflex arteries. The posteromedial papillary muscle consists of one or two trunks and multiple heads, all of which extend chordae to both mitral valve leaflets. Complete or partial rupture of a trunk or head leads to varying degrees of mitral regurgitation. (Severe mitral regurgitation may also occur with leaflet prolapse due to reduced tethering by an infarcted, but nonruptured, papillary muscle.)

Because PMR may occur despite a limited territory of infarction, it is not uncommon for patients to have relatively preserved LV function in comparison to the degree of heart failure and CS at presentation [39,40]. Patients present with acute dyspnea due to pulmonary congestion. Physical examination may include a systolic murmur, though this may be absent due to equalization of left atrial (LA) and LV pressures. Therefore, a heightened index of suspicion is necessary to distinguish PMR from pure LV dysfunction.

PMR is suggested by the presence of large V-waves in the pulmonary capillary wedge pressure tracing, although this

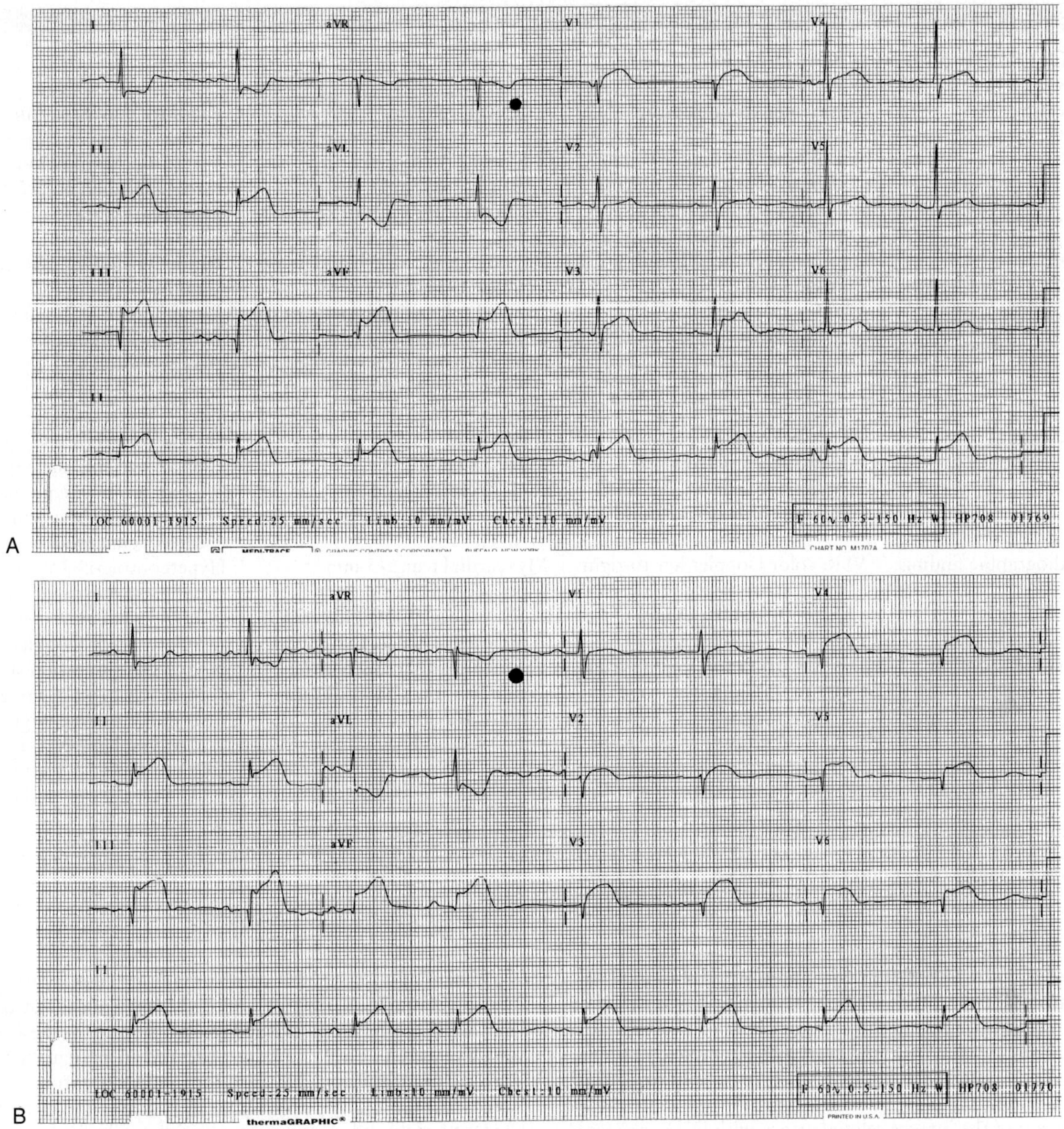

FIGURE 40.2. A: ECG of patient with inferior STEMI and sinus bradycardia showing ST-segment elevation in lead 3 greater than in lead 2 and ST-segment elevation in lead V_1, suggesting RV involvement. **B:** Right-sided placement of precordial leads demonstrates ST-segment elevation in lead V_{4R}, confirming RVI. In this figure, lead V_1 is V_{1R}, V_2 is V_{2R}, V_3 is V_{3R}, V_4 is V_{4R}, V_5 is V_{5R}, and V_6 is V_{6R}.

finding may also be seen with severe LV dysfunction, VSR, or other causes of mitral regurgitation. The diagnosis of PMR is made more definitively by echocardiography, on visualization of a flail portion of a mitral valve leaflet or a ruptured papillary muscle head prolapsing into the left atrium, along with color Doppler evidence of mitral regurgitation.

Stabilization may be accomplished with the use of inotropic agents, afterload reduction if possible, and insertion of an intra aortic balloon pump. However, with an in-hospital mortality of up to 80% and a long-term survival rate of approximately 6% with medical therapy alone [39,40], urgent surgical repair is indicated. This may consist of chordal-sparing mitral valve replacement or, if necrosis is limited, papillary muscle reimplantation with or without ring annuloplasty. Coronary angiography should be performed so that necessary revascularization may be performed at the time of surgery. Although perioperative mortality (10% to 24%) remains significant, it is reduced with concomitant coronary artery bypass grafting [41,42]. Long-term survival after surgery ranges from 60% to 80%, and is similar to that of matched patients with MI, but no PMR [42].

Ventricular Septal Rupture

The presentation of VSR has changed as treatment for acute MI has evolved to include fibrinolysis and primary PCI. Before the advent of fibrinolytic and percutaneous reperfusion therapies, VSR occurred in 1% to 2% of patients with acute MI, with a mean onset of 3 to 5 days after infarction. In the thrombolytic era, the incidence is approximately 0.2%, with a median onset in the first 24 hours after MI [38,43,44]. Approximately two thirds of VSR cases occur in the mid- to distal septum in association with anterior MI; the remainder occur in

TABLE 40.2

CHARACTERISTICS OF MYOCARDIAL RUPTURE

Characteristic	Ventricular septal rupture	Free wall rupture	Papillary muscle rupture
Incidence	1%–3% without reperfusion therapy; 0.2%–0.34% with fibrinolysis; 3.9% in patients with cardiogenic shock	0.8%–6.2%; primary angioplasty, but not fibrinolysis, appears to reduce risk	1%; posteromedial more frequent than anterolateral papillary muscle
Time course	Bimodal peak: <24 h and 3–5 d; range 1–14 d	Bimodal peak: <24 h and 3–5 d; range 1–14 d	Bimodal peak: <24 h and 3–5 d; range 1–14 d
Clinical manifestations	Chest pain, dyspnea, hypotension	Anginal, pleuritic, or pericardial chest pain; syncope, hypotension, arrhythmia, nausea, restlessness, hypotension, sudden death	Abrupt onset of dyspnea due to pulmonary edema; hypotension
Physical findings	Harsh holosystolic murmur, thrill, accentuated S_2, S_3, pulmonary edema, RV and LV failure, cardiogenic shock	Jugular venous distention, pulsus paradoxus, electromechanical dissociation, cardiogenic shock	Soft murmur in some cases, no thrill, variable signs of RV overload, severe pulmonary edema (may be asymmetric), cardiogenic shock
Echocardiographic findings	VSR, color Doppler left-to-right shunt across septum, RV dilation, and hypokinesis	Myocardial tear, >5 mm pericardial effusion not always visualized; clot within pericardial space, tamponade	Hypercontractile LV, torn papillary muscle or chordae tendineae, flail leaflet, severe MR by color Doppler
Cardiac catheterization	Oxygen saturation step up from RA to RV, large V-waves	Ventriculography insensitive; equalization of diastolic pressures	No oxygen saturation step up from RA to RV (may occur from RV to PA); large V-waves, high PCWP

LV, left ventricle; MR, mitral regurgitation; PA, pulmonary artery; PCWP, pulmonary capillary wedge pressure; RA, right atrial; RV, right ventricle; VSR, ventricular septal rupture.
Adapted from Antman EM, Anbe DT, Armstrong PW, et al: ACC/AHA guidelines for the management of patients with ST-elevation myocardial infarction: a report of the American College of Cardiology/American Heart Association Task Force on Practice Guidelines (Committee to Revise the 1999 Guidelines for the Management of Patients With Acute Myocardial Infarction). Available at www.acc.org/clinical/guidelines/stemi/index.pdf.

the basal septum in association with inferior MI. On the basis of the anatomy of the rupture track, VSR may be classified as simple (directly through and through) or complex (serpiginous, with an exit site remote from the entry site); complex VSRs are more frequently noted with inferior MI. Five percent to 10% of patients have multiple defects. VSR is typically associated with total occlusion of the infarct-related artery with little or no collateral flow. Risk factors for VSR include advanced age, female sex, anterior MI, and no previous smoking [44]. In addition, in patients with anterior MI, the presence of ST-segment elevation or Q-waves in the inferior leads, indicating a "wrap-around" left anterior descending artery supplying both the anterior and inferior LV walls, may identify patients at risk for VSR [45].

VSR causes sudden shunting of flow from the LV to the pulmonary circulation. This results in impaired forward cardiac output. There is acute pressure overload of the RV and volume overload of the pulmonary circulation and LV, which become evident clinically as right heart failure, pulmonary congestion, and CS. The degree of shunting depends on the rupture size, the relative resistance of the pulmonary and systemic circulations, and the relative function of the RV and LV. As the LV fails and systolic pressure decreases, left-to-right shunting decreases. If RV pressures exceed those on the left, right-to-left shunting occurs, resulting in hypoxemia.

Symptoms of VSR include chest pain and dyspnea. In contrast to patients with PMR, those with VSR have a harsh pansystolic murmur at the left sternal border, with a left parasternal thrill in 50%. Signs of RV failure are also present, including jugular venous distention and peripheral edema. ECG findings include persistent ST-segment elevation and AV nodal or infranodal conduction abnormalities.

The diagnosis of VSR can be made by right heart catheterization demonstrating a step up in the oxygen saturation (>8%) in the RV, to be distinguished from a step up in the pulmonary artery, which is occasionally observed in patients with severe mitral regurgitation. In addition, catheterization reveals increased pulmonary-to-systemic flow ratios ($\dot{Q}_p/\dot{Q}_s > 1.4$), increased right-sided pressures, and large V-waves in the pulmonary capillary wedge tracing; left ventriculography may identify the rupture site. Echocardiography with color Doppler imaging is commonly used for both diagnosis and surgical planning. A visible defect may be seen in association with the corresponding anterior or inferior wall motion abnormality. Continuous wave Doppler interrogation of flow at this site demonstrates dense, high-velocity flow from LV to RV. Echocardiography also provides information about LV and RV function and concomitant mitral valve pathology.

Nonsurgical therapy, such as afterload reduction, diuretics, and inotropic and intra-aortic balloon pump support, is purely temporizing and alone is associated with greater than 90% mortality. Surgical repair of the VSR, first performed in 1957, is definitive. Some have used biventricular mechanical support as a means to restore hemodynamic stability and avoid surgery on freshly infarcted tissue, before definitive surgical repair [46]. Surgical repair has improved 30-day mortality from VSR to 10% to 15% in cases of anterior MI and 30% to 35% in cases of inferior MI. As mortality is higher in patients with complex VSR and in those with RVI [47], the increased mortality with inferior VSRs has been attributed to the more challenging surgical repair due to complex anatomy and basal location and the possibility of concomitant RV infarction. CS at the time of surgical intervention and incomplete coronary revascularization have also been shown to be strong predictors of 30-day and long-term mortality [48]. Patients who survive the perioperative period have been reported to have a long-term survival rate of approximately 60% to 80%.

Recently, percutaneous transcatheter closure of VSR has been reported in a limited number of patients; appropriate patient selection, technical aspects of device selection and placement, durability of occlusion, and long-term outcome are unknown.

Free Wall Rupture

LV free wall rupture is by far the most common of all ruptures and usually results in sudden death. The temporal pattern of rupture has two peaks, the first within 24 hours and the second between 3 and 5 days after acute MI [49]. Risk factors for free wall rupture are similar to those for VSR, whereas successful early reperfusion and presence of collateral flow are important preventive factors. Pericardial tamponade and electromechanical dissociation often develop quickly, in which case death is inevitable without treatment.

LV pseudoaneurysm develops if free wall rupture is contained by adherent pericardium or clot formation, thus preventing immediate pericardial tamponade and death. Symptoms of contained rupture include recurrent chest pain or pleurisy, emesis without preceding nausea, unexplained restlessness, and syncope. Hypotension may be accompanied by "inappropriate" bradycardia. New ST-segment elevation or T-wave abnormalities may be evident. Pseudoaneurysms can be diagnosed by echocardiography, contrast or radionuclide ventriculography, or magnetic resonance imaging. Diagnostic pericardiocentesis may yield blood; therapeutic pericardiocentesis may destabilize a contained effusion and result in death. Surgical repair is usually necessary, although survival with pericardiocentesis and supportive medical therapy has been reported in selected patients [50].

LEFT VENTRICULAR REMODELING: PATHOPHYSIOLOGY, CONTEXT, PREVENTION, AND NATURAL HISTORY

Injuries to the LV that decrease systolic performance, such as acute MI, trigger a sequence of histopathologic events that lead to changes in LV size, shape, and function. This process of remodeling is initially compensatory but becomes maladaptive, with progressive hypertrophy, dilation, spherical distortion, and impairment of contractile function, and is associated with heart failure progression and poor clinical outcome.

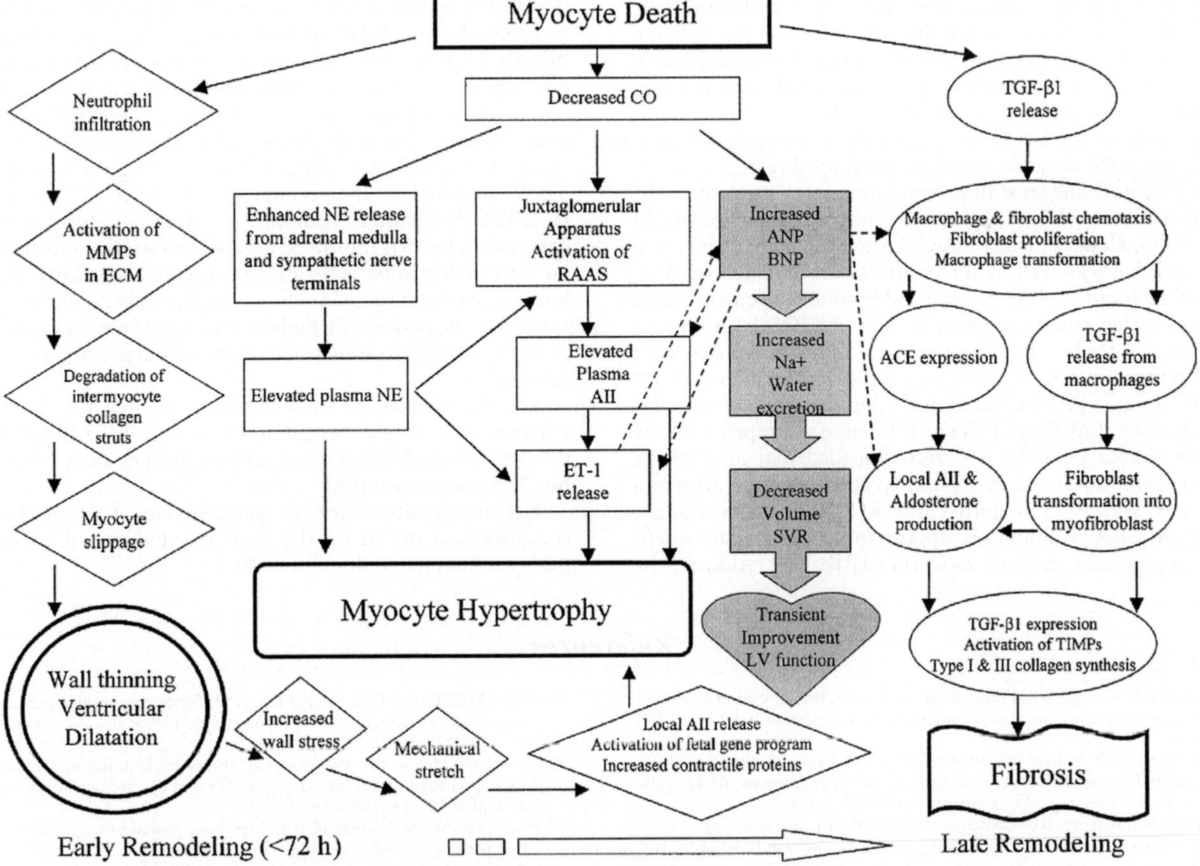

FIGURE 40.3. Ventricular remodeling after MI. AII, angiotensin II; ACE, angiotensin-converting enzyme; ANP, atrial natriuretic peptide; BNP, brain natriuretic peptide; CO, cardiac output; ECM, extracellular matrix; ET, endothelin; MMP, matrix metalloproteinase; NE, norepinephrine; RAAS, renin–angiotensin–aldosterone system; TGF, transforming growth factor; TIMP, tissue inhibitor of metalloproteinase. [From Sutton MG, Sharpe N: Left ventricular remodeling after myocardial infarction: pathophysiology and therapy. *Circulation* 101:2981–2988, 2000, with permission.]

Because LV remodeling is concordant with clinical outcomes over the natural history of heart failure, its prevention has been accepted as a reasonable therapeutic target.

The early phase of remodeling begins within 3 hours of MI and consists of infarct expansion due to collagen degradation by serine proteases and matrix metalloproteinases [51]. The resultant wall thinning and ventricular dilatation increase ventricular wall stress, thus promoting later remodeling, which includes collagen scar formation, fibrosis, and myocyte hypertrophy. The abnormal stresses related to mitral regurgitation [52] or ventricular mechanical dyssynchrony [53] resulting from the MI, if present, further promote remodeling.

The renin–angiotensin–aldosterone (RAAS) and sympathetic nervous systems are central mediators of remodeling [51,54] (Fig. 40.3). Myocyte stretch from increased wall stress stimulates the local production of angiotensin II, which in turn promotes myocyte hypertrophy, fibroblast proliferation, and collagen production. Adrenergic stimulation, in response to myocardial injury and/or hemodynamic compromise, leads to myocardial production of cytokines, such as TNF-α, IL-1β, and IL-6, which mediate myocyte hypertrophy, apoptosis, and changes in the extracellular matrix. Furthermore, adrenergic stimulation enhances the activity of the RAAS. Finally, there is growing evidence that oxidative stress after MI plays a role in the apoptosis, inflammation, fibrosis, and hypertrophy processes of myocardial remodeling.

Therapies to prevent or reduce postinfarction remodeling have focused on limiting infarct expansion and moderating the neurohormonal axes. Infarct expansion and remodeling are influenced by the size and location of the original infarct, patency of the infarct-related artery, presence of collateral flow, regional wall thickness, and radius of curvature. Reperfusion of the infarct-related artery restores stunned myocardium in the infarct border zone, reduces infarct size, and improves ventricular function and long-term prognosis.

Blockade of the RAAS and sympathetic nervous system is the cornerstone of pharmacologic therapy directed at interrupting remodeling and improving long-term outcome. The mechanisms of action of angiotensin-converting enzyme (ACE) inhibitors include beneficial effects on hemodynamics and loading conditions, as well as direct effects on remodeling. ACE inhibition attenuates the increase in LV volume occurring after MI and earlier commencement of ACE inhibition appears to produce greater benefit. This translates into a survival benefit in all patients with MI, including those with evidence of LV dysfunction, as demonstrated in the Survival and Ventricular Enlargement (SAVE) and Acute Infarction Ramipril Efficacy (AIRE) studies [55–57]. It is recommended that all patients without contraindications such as hyperkalemia or azotemia be treated with ACE inhibitors after STEMI. Patients who are intolerant of ACE inhibitors appear to derive similar benefit from angiotensin receptor blockers (ARB) [58]. Aldosterone blockade in patients without contraindication has also been shown to improve survival in patients with LV dysfunction after MI [59].

TABLE 40.3

SUMMARY OF RECOMMENDATIONS BASED ON RANDOMIZED CONTROLLED CLINICAL TRIALS

- Cardiogenic shock: Early revascularization by PCI or CABG in patients younger than 75 years who are otherwise suitable candidates reduces 1-year mortality. Patients older than 75 years may also benefit from early revascularization and an individualized treatment strategy is recommended [18]
- Remodeling: ACE inhibition or angiotensin-receptor blockade in patients with evidence of LV dysfunction after MI attenuates LV remodeling and improves survival [55–58]
- Remodeling: Beta-blockade in patients with evidence of LV dysfunction after MI attenuates LV remodeling and improves survival and LV remodeling [60,61]

ACE, angiotensin-converting enzyme; CABG, coronary artery bypass graft; LV, left ventricle; MI, myocardial infarction; PCI, percutaneous coronary intervention.

There are several potential mechanisms of benefit from beta-blockade. Beta-blockers reduce myocyte apoptosis, collagen deposition, and hypertrophy; they reduce myocardial oxygen demand by reducing heart rate and blood pressure, which may be especially beneficial for hibernating myocardium; and they directly oppose catecholamine stimulation of myocytes. Specific agents may have additional effects, such as the antioxidant and anti-inflammatory properties of carvedilol. Evidence of the benefit of beta-blockade includes early studies showing reduced remodeling in patients not receiving ACE inhibitors. The Carvedilol Post-Infarct Survival Control in LV Dysfunction (CAPRICORN) study demonstrated that beta-blockade with carvedilol after MI improved all-cause mortality and ventricular remodeling in patients already receiving standard ACE inhibitor treatment [60,61]. The survival benefit of beta-blockers is greatest in patients at highest risk for adverse events, such as those with LV dysfunction, ventricular arrhythmias, and no reperfusion.

Finally, patients with MI should be followed to determine whether they would benefit from cardiac resynchronization therapy for mechanical dyssynchrony [62] or intervention for mitral regurgitation [63].

Recommendations for the management of the mechanical complications of MI on the basis of randomized controlled trials are summarized in Table 40.3.

References

1. Kloner RA, Jennings RB: Consequences of brief ischemia: stunning, preconditioning, and their clinical implications: part 1. *Circulation* 104:2981–2989, 2001.
2. Heyndrickx GR, Millard RW, McRitchie RJ, et al: Regional myocardial functional and electrophysiological alterations after brief coronary artery occlusion in conscious dogs. *J Clin Invest* 56:978–985, 1975.
3. Kloner RA, Jennings RB: Consequences of brief ischemia: stunning, preconditioning, and their clinical implications: part 2. *Circulation* 104:3158–3167, 2001.
4. Moens AL, Claeys MJ, Timmermans JP, et al: Myocardial ischemia/reperfusion-injury, a clinical view on a complex pathophysiological process. *Int J Cardiol* 100:179–190, 2005.
5. Camici PG, Prasad SK, Rimoldi OE: Stunning, hibernation, and assessment of myocardial viability. *Circulation* 117(1):103–114, 2008.
6. Reynolds HR, Hochman JS: Cardiogenic shock: current concepts and improving outcomes. *Circulation* 117(5):686–697, 2008.
7. Picard MH, Davidoff R, Sleeper LA, et al: Echocardiographic predictors of survival and response to early revascularization in cardiogenic shock. *Circulation* 107:279–284, 2003.
8. Kohsaka S, Menon V, Lowe AM, et al: Systemic inflammatory response syndrome after myocardial infarction complicated by cardiogenic shock. *Arch Intern Med* 165(14):1643–1650, 2005.
9. Nicholls SJ, Wang Z, Koeth R, et al: Metabolic profiling of arginine and nitric oxide pathways predicts hemodynamic abnormalities and mortality in patients with cardiogenic shock after acute myocardial infarction. *Circulation* 116(20):2315–2324, 2007.
10. Holmes DR Jr, Berger PB, Hochman JS, et al: Cardiogenic shock in patients with acute ischemic syndromes with and without ST-segment elevation. *Circulation* 100:2067–2073, 1999.
11. Goldberg RJ, Spencer FA, Gore JM, et al: Thirty-year trends (1975–2005) in the magnitude of, management of, and hospital death rates associated with cardiogenic shock in patients with acute myocardial

infarction: a population-based perspective. *Circulation* 119(9):1211–1219, 2009.
12. Sutton AG, Finn P, Hall JA, et al: Predictors of outcome after percutaneous treatment for cardiogenic shock. *Heart* 91:339–344, 2005.
13. Hochman JS, Sleeper LA, Webb JG, et al: Early revascularization in acute myocardial infarction complicated by cardiogenic shock. SHOCK Investigators. Should We Emergently Revascularize Occluded Coronaries for Cardiogenic Shock. *N Engl J Med* 341:625–634, 1999.
14. Hochman JS, Sleeper LA, White HD, et al: One-year survival following early revascularization for cardiogenic shock. *JAMA* 285:190–192, 2001.
15. Hochman JS, Sleeper LA, Webb JG, et al: Early revascularization and long-term survival in cardiogenic shock complicating acute myocardial infarction. *JAMA* 295(21):2511–2515, 2006.
16. White HD, Assmann SF, Sanborn TA, et al: Comparison of percutaneous coronary intervention and coronary artery bypass grafting after acute myocardial infarction complicated by cardiogenic shock: results from the Should We Emergently Revascularize Occluded Coronaries for Cardiogenic Shock (SHOCK) trial. *Circulation* 112(13):1992–2001, 2005.
17. Klein LW, Shaw RE, Krone RJ, et al: Mortality after emergent percutaneous coronary intervention in cardiogenic shock secondary to acute myocardial infarction and usefulness of a mortality prediction model. *Am J Cardiol* 96(1):36–41, 2005.
18. Antman EM, Anbe DT, Armstrong PW, et al: ACC/AHA guidelines for the management of patients with ST-elevation myocardial infarction: a report of the American College of Cardiology/American Heart Association Task Force on Practice Guidelines (Committee to Revise the 1999 Guidelines for the Management of Patients With Acute Myocardial Infarction). Available at www.acc.org/qualityandscience/clinical/guidelines/stemi/Guideline1/index.pdf. Accessed December 11, 2006.
19. Dzavik V, Sleeper LA, Cocke TP, et al: Early revascularization is associated with improved survival in elderly patients with acute myocardial infarction complicated by cardiogenic shock: a report from the SHOCK trial registry. *Eur Heart J* 24:828–837, 2003.
20. Leshnower BG, Gleason TG, O'Hara ML, et al: Safety and efficacy of left ventricular assist device support in postmyocardial infarction cardiogenic shock. *Ann Thorac Surg* 81(4):1365–1370, 2006.
21. Burkhoff D, Cohen H, Brunckhorst C, et al: A randomized multicenter clinical study to evaluate the safety and efficacy of the Tandem Heart percutaneous ventricular assist device versus conventional therapy with intraaortic balloon pumping for treatment of cardiogenic shock. *Am Heart J* 152(3):469.e1–e8, 2006.
22. Thiele H, Sick P, Boudriot E, et al: Randomized comparison of intra-aortic balloon support with a percutaneous left ventricular assist device in patients with revascularized acute myocardial infarction complicated by cardiogenic shock. *Eur Heart J* 26(13):1276–1283, 2006.
23. Seyfarth M, Sibbing D, Bauer I, et al: A randomized clinical trial to evaluate the safety and efficacy of a percutaneous left ventricular assist device versus intra-aortic balloon pumping for treatment of cardiogenic shock caused by myocardial infarction. *J Am Coll Cardiol* 52(19):1584–1588, 2008.
24. Babaev A, Frederick PD, Pasta DJ, et al: Trends in management and outcomes of patients with acute myocardial infarction complicated by cardiogenic shock. *JAMA* 294(4):448–454, 2005.
25. Jeger RV, Radovanovic D, Hunziker PR, et al: Ten-year trends in the incidence and treatment of cardiogenic shock. *Ann Intern Med* 149(9):618–626, 2008.
26. Cohn JN, Guiha NH, Broder MI, et al: Right ventricular infarction. Clinical and hemodynamic features. *Am J Cardiol* 33:209–214, 1974.
27. Goldstein JA: Pathophysiology and management of right heart ischemia. *J Am Coll Cardiol* 40:841–853, 2002.
28. Robalino BD, Whitlow PL, Underwood DA, et al: Electrocardiographic manifestations of right ventricular infarction. *Am Heart J* 118:138–144, 1989.
29. Braat SH, Brugada P, de Zwaan C, et al: Value of electrocardiogram in diagnosing right ventricular involvement in patients with an acute inferior wall myocardial infarction. *Br Heart J* 49:368–372, 1983.
30. Kumar A, Abdel-Aty H, Kriedemann I, et al: Contrast-enhanced cardiovascular magnetic resonance imaging of right ventricular infarction. *J Am Coll Cardiol* 48(10):1969–1976, 2006.
31. Bowers TR, O'Neill WW, Grines C, et al: Effect of reperfusion on biventricular function and survival after right ventricular infarction. *N Engl J Med* 338:933–940, 1998.
32. Kinn JW, Ajluni SC, Samyn JG, et al: Rapid hemodynamic improvement after reperfusion during right ventricular infarction. *J Am Coll Cardiol* 26:1230–1234, 1995.
33. Pfisterer M: Right ventricular involvement in myocardial infarction and cardiogenic shock. *Lancet* 362:392–394, 2003.
34. Berisha S, Kastrati A, Goda A, et al: Optimal value of filling pressure in the right side of the heart in acute right ventricular infarction. *Br Heart J* 63:98–102, 1990.
35. Brodie BR, Stuckey TD, Hansen C, et al: Comparison of late survival in patients with cardiogenic shock due to right ventricular infarction versus left ventricular pump failure following primary percutaneous coronary intervention for ST-elevation acute myocardial infarction. *Am J Cardiol* 99(4):431–435, 2007.
36. Jacobs AK, Leopold JA, Bates E, et al: Cardiogenic shock caused by right ventricular infarction: a report from the SHOCK registry. *J Am Coll Cardiol* 41:1273–1279, 2003.
37. Gumina RJ, Murphy JG, Rihal CS, et al: Long-term survival after right ventricular infarction. *Am J Cardiol* 98(12):1571–1573, 2006.
38. Becker RC, Gore JM, Lambrew C, et al: A composite view of cardiac rupture in the United States National Registry of Myocardial Infarction. *J Am Coll Cardiol* 27:1321–1326, 1996.
39. Wei JY, Hutchins GM, Bulkley BH: Papillary muscle rupture in fatal acute myocardial infarction: a potentially treatable form of cardiogenic shock. *Ann Intern Med* 90:149–152, 1979.
40. Nishimura RA, Gersh BJ, Schaff HV: The case for an aggressive surgical approach to papillary muscle rupture following myocardial infarction: "From paradise lost to paradise regained." *Heart* 83:611–613, 2000.
41. Chevalier P, Burri H, Fahrat F, et al: Perioperative outcome and long-term survival of surgery for acute post-infarction mitral regurgitation. *Eur J Cardiothoracic Surg* 26(2):330–335, 2004.
42. Russo A, Suri RM, Grigioni F, et al: Clinical outcome after surgical correction of mitral regurgitation due to papillary muscle rupture. *Circulation* 118(15):1528–1534, 2008.
43. Birnbaum Y, Wagner GS, Gates KB, et al: Clinical and electrocardiographic variables associated with increased risk of ventricular septal defect in acute anterior myocardial infarction. *Am J Cardiol* 86:830–834, 2000.
44. Crenshaw BS, Granger CB, Birnbaum Y, et al: Risk factors angiographic patterns, and outcomes in patients with ventricular septal defect complicating acute myocardial infarction. *Circulation* 100(1):27–32, 2000.
45. Hayashi T, Hirano Y, Takai H, et al: Usefulness of ST-segment elevation in the inferior leads in predicting ventricular septal rupture in patients with anterior wall acute myocardial infarction. *Am J Cardiol* 96(8):1037–1041, 2005.
46. Conradi L, Treede H, Brickwedel J, et al: Use of initial biventricular mechanical support in a case of postinfarction ventricular septal rupture as a bridge to surgery. *Ann Thorac Surg* 87(5):e37–e39, 2009.
47. Vargas-Barrón J, Molina-Carrión M, Romero-Cárdenas A, et al: Risk factors, echocardiographic patterns, and outcomes in patients with acute ventricular septal rupture during myocardial infarction. *Am J Cardiol* 95(10):1153–1158, 2005.
48. Lundblad R, Abdelnoor M, Geiran OR, et al: Surgical repair of postinfarction ventricular septal rupture: risk factors of early and late death. *J Thorac Cardiovasc Surg* 137(4):862–868, 2009.
49. Oliva PB, Hammill SC, Edwards WD: Cardiac rupture, a clinically predictable complication of acute myocardial infarction: report of 70 cases with clinicopathologic correlations. *J Am Coll Cardiol* 22:720–726, 1993.
50. Figueras J, Cortadellas J, Evangelista A, et al: Medical management of selected patients with left ventricular free wall rupture during acute myocardial infarction. *J Am Coll Cardiol* 29:512–518, 1997.
51. Sutton MG, Sharpe N: Left ventricular remodeling after myocardial infarction: pathophysiology and therapy. *Circulation* 101:2981–2988, 2000.
52. Bursi F, Enriquez-Sarano M, Roger V, et al: Mitral regurgitation after myocardial infarction: a review. *Am J Med* 119(2):103–112, 2006.
53. Mollema SA, Liem SS, Suffoletto MS, et al: Left ventricular dyssynchrony acutely after myocardial infarction predicts left ventricular remodeling. *J Am Coll Cardiol* 50(16):1532–1540, 2007.
54. Udelson JE: Ventricular remodeling in heart failure and the effect of beta-blockade. *Am J Cardiol* 93:43B–48B, 2004.
55. Pfeffer MA, Lamas GA, Vaughan DE, et al: Effect of captopril on progressive ventricular dilatation after anterior myocardial infarction. *N Engl J Med* 319:80–86, 1988.
56. Pfeffer MA, Braunwald E, Moye LA, et al: Effect of captopril on mortality and morbidity in patients with left ventricular dysfunction after myocardial infarction. Results of the survival and ventricular enlargement trial. The SAVE Investigators. *N Engl J Med* 327:669–677, 1992.
57. Effect of ramipril on mortality and morbidity of survivors of acute myocardial infarction with clinical evidence of heart failure. The Acute Infarction Ramipril Efficacy (AIRE) Study Investigators. *Lancet* 342:821–828, 1993.
58. Pfeffer MA, McMurray JJ, Velazquez EJ, et al: Valsartan, captopril, or both in myocardial infarction complicated by heart failure, left ventricular dysfunction, or both. *N Engl J Med* 349:1893–1906, 2003.
59. Pitt B, Remme W, Zannad F, et al: Eplerenone, a selective aldosterone blocker, in patients with left ventricular dysfunction after myocardial infarction. *N Engl J Med* 348:1309–1321, 2003.
60. Dargie HJ: Effect of carvedilol on outcome after myocardial infarction in patients with left-ventricular dysfunction: the CAPRICORN randomised trial. *Lancet* 357:1385–1390, 2001.
61. Doughty RN, Whalley GA, Walsh HA, et al: Effects of carvedilol on left ventricular remodeling after acute myocardial infarction: the CAPRICORN echo substudy. *Circulation* 109:201–206, 2004.
62. St John Sutton MG, Plappert T, Abraham WT, et al: Effect of cardiac resynchronization therapy on left ventricular size and function in chronic heart failure. *Circulation* 107(15):1985–1990, 2003.
63. Carabello B: The current therapy for mitral regurgitation. *J Am Coll Cardiol* 52(5):319–326, 2008.

CHAPTER 41 ■ VENTRICULAR TACHYCARDIA

MELANIE MAYTIN AND BRUCE A. KOPLAN

INTRODUCTION

Ventricular tachycardia (VT) is defined as a wide QRS complex tachycardia (QRS width $\geq$0.12 second) of three or more consecutive beats at a rate faster than 100 per minute. VT arises from either reentry or automaticity in the ventricular myocardium or Purkinje system below the level of the His bundle. One of the common ways in which VT is classified is whether it is sustained or not. Nonsustained VT (NSVT) is that which terminates spontaneously within 30 seconds without causing severe symptoms. Spontaneous sustained VT requires an intervention, such as cardioversion or antiarrhythmic drug (AAD) administration for termination, or produces severe symptoms, such as syncope, prior to termination. VTs lasting longer than 30 seconds are usually designated as sustained.

Another way to classify VT is based on the QRS morphology (Fig. 41.1). Morphologic classifications include *monomorphic VT* (the same morphology from beat to beat), *polymorphic VT* (PMVT, varying morphologies from beat to beat), and *sinusoidal VT* (when the QRS has a duration similar to that of diastole). Torsades de pointes (TDP) is a unique subcategory of PMVT associated with QT prolongation.

VT can also be classified on the basis of its hemodynamic effects that are largely dependent on the rate of the tachycardia and the presence of underlying myocardial dysfunction. Indeed, for all sustained wide QRS tachycardias the first priority is to determine whether the patient is hemodynamically stable, with adequate blood pressure and perfusion. Pulseless VT is associated with no significant cardiac output and is approached in a similar manner as ventricular fibrillation (VF). VT can also be hemodynamically stable. This hemodynamic classification may be the most relevant classification system for initial management. Continuous electrocardiograph (ECG) monitoring should be implemented and a defibrillator should be at the patient's bedside for immediate use, even if the patient is hemodynamically stable. If the patient is pulseless and has impaired consciousness, angina, or severe pulmonary edema, prompt electrical cardioversion is warranted. Further therapy after cardioversion is determined by the type of tachycardia and underlying heart disease.

If the patient is hemodynamically stable, a brief history and a 12-lead ECG should be immediately obtained. The immediate history should include determination of known heart disease, in particular prior myocardial infarction, present medications, history of prior arrhythmias, whether the patient has an implanted defibrillator or pacemaker, and drug allergies. A limited initial physical examination should include the cardiovascular system and lungs. A 12-lead ECG should also be obtained following conversion of the tachycardia to compare the tachycardia QRS to that during sinus rhythm, as well as to evaluate underlying events, such as myocardial infarction, and QT interval prolongation, or other changes suggestive of electrolyte abnormalities. Previous ECGs are also helpful in this regard.

WIDE QRS MONOMORPHIC TACHYCARDIA

Monomorphic tachycardias have the same QRS configuration from beat to beat (Figs. 41.1A and 41.2). The differential diagnosis of this type of wide QRS complex tachycardia includes VT, supraventricular tachycardia (SVT) with aberrant interventricular conduction (bundle branch block; Fig. 41.3), and pre-excited SVT due to antegrade conduction from atrium to ventricle through an accessory pathway (Fig. 41.4B), or pre-excited QRS complexes during atrial fibrillation (AF) or atrial flutter (Fig. 41.3C). The differentiation is critical for prognosis and long-term management.

Initial Evaluation

Hemodynamic instability is an indication for electrical cardioversion. If the patient is hemodynamically stable, a limited history and physical examination should be performed and a 12-lead ECG obtained. The presence of hemodynamic stability does not indicate that the tachycardia is supraventricular. Hemodynamic stability is dependent on the rate of the tachycardia, underlying ventricular function, and the sympathetic nervous system response to tachycardia. VT can be hemodynamically stable, SVT may cause hemodynamic collapse, and vice versa. Wide QRS tachycardias should be managed as VT unless the diagnosis of SVT can be confirmed. Patients with a history of structural heart disease are more likely to have VT, whereas the absence of structural heart disease favors the diagnosis of SVT. Wide QRS tachycardia in patients with a history of myocardial infarction can be assumed to VT with greater than 95% certainty [1].

The physical examination is occasionally helpful in detecting the presence of dissociation between atrium and ventricle (AV dissociation) confirming VT as the diagnosis. Cannon "a"-waves in the jugular venous pulse occurring intermittently and irregularly during VT indicate periodic contraction of the right atrium against a closed tricuspid valve. AV dissociation may also cause variability in the intensity of the first heart sound and beat-to-beat variability in systolic blood pressure due to the variable contribution of atrial contraction to left ventricular filling. The absence of evidence of AV dissociation does not exclude the diagnosis of VT. Some patients have conduction from ventricle retrogradely over the His-Purkinje system and AV node to the atrium (VA conduction) during VT. Each ventricular beat is accompanied by a cannon "a-wave," a finding that is also seen in some SVTs (Table 41.1).

Electrocardiogram

VT can be somewhat irregular at its initiation, but persistence of an irregularly irregular wide QRS suggests AF with bundle

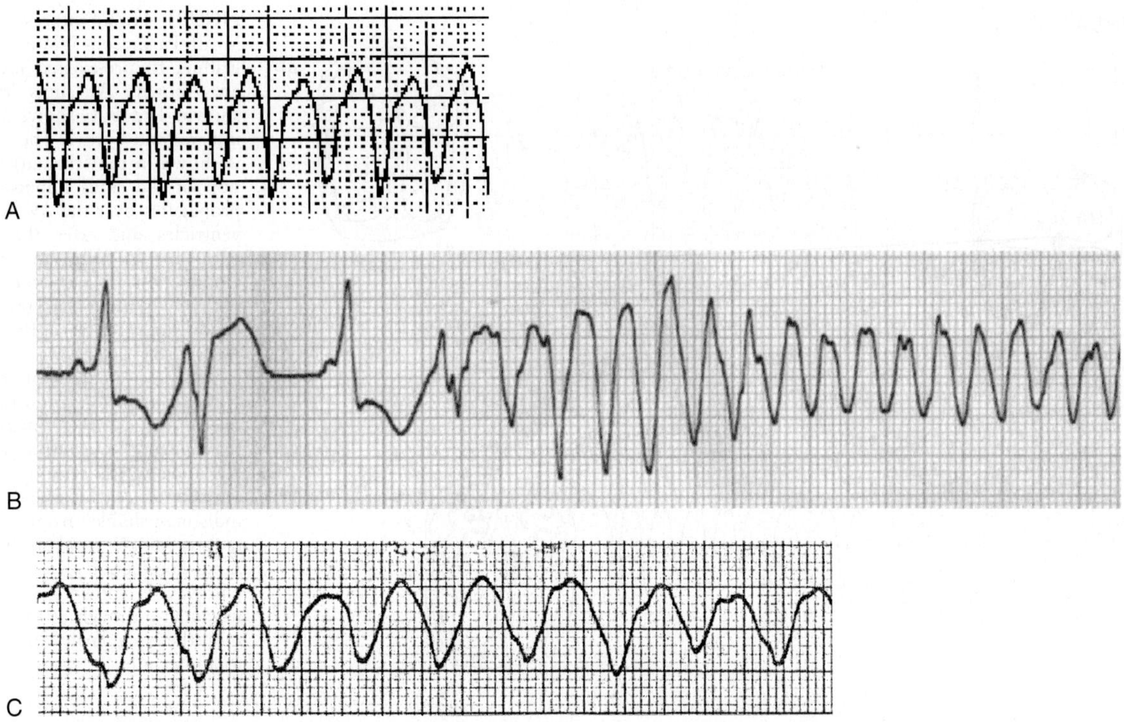

FIGURE 41.1. Three different wide QRS tachycardias are shown. **A:** monomorphic VT; **B:** polymorphic VT; and **C:** sinusoidal VT due to hyperkalemia. VT, ventricular tachycardia.

branch block or conduction over an accessory pathway rather than VT (Fig. 41.4). Comparing the QRS complex morphology during tachycardia with that of sinus rhythm on an old ECG or following cardioversion can be helpful. An identical QRS morphology during tachycardia and sinus rhythm suggests SVT [2] (with the uncommon exception of bundle branch reentry described later in the chapter). An old ECG may also reveal a short PR interval with δ-waves (Fig. 41.3A) that suggests Wolff–Parkinson–White (WPW) syndrome with an accessory pathway–mediated wide complex tachycardia (WCT; Fig. 41.3B). When the onset of tachycardia is recorded, initiation by a premature P-wave suggests SVT.

The following ECG criteria applied in a stepwise approach provide reasonable sensitivity and specificity to differentiate SVT from VT (Figs. 41.5 and 41.6) [3].

1. *AV dissociation:* Dissociation of P-waves (if identifiable) and QRS complexes suggests VT (Fig. 41.2). Because they may be partially buried in the QRS complex, or T-wave, the P-waves may be difficult to identify. Comparison of the contour of QRS and T-waves from beat to beat may be helpful; P-waves may be evident as a slight deflection occurring at regular intervals independent of QRS complexes. AV dissociation is probably the most reliable clue to the diagnosis of VT, especially if a nonsustained run of wide WCT is caught only on a telemetry rhythm strip.

AV dissociation is also indicated by QRS fusion or capture beats. *Fusion beats* occur when a supraventricular impulse conducts over the AV node and depolarizes a portion of the ventricle simultaneously with excitation from the tachycardia focus. They occur if AV dissociation is present

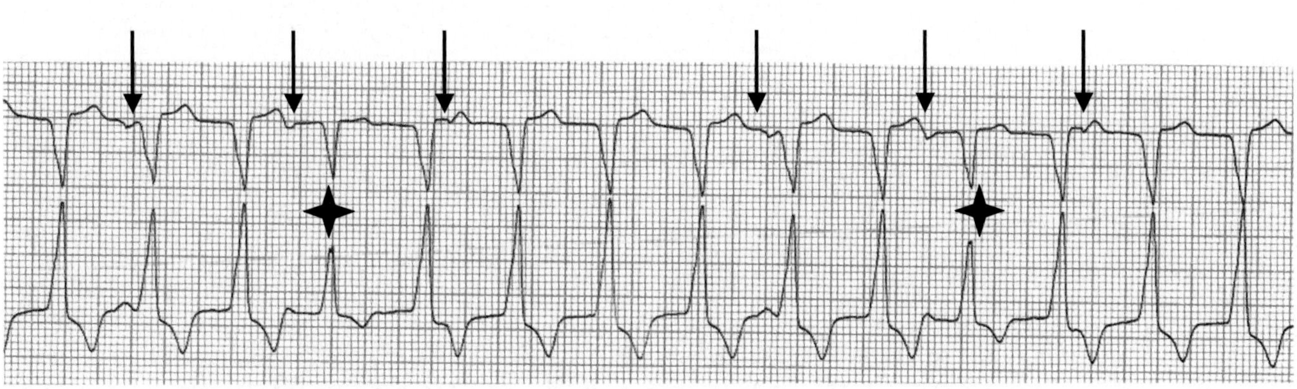

FIGURE 41.2. Sustained monomorphic ventricular tachycardia is present. Dissociated P-waves can be seen (*arrows*) with occasional fusion beats (*stars*) that occur when a sinus P-wave occurs with timing appropriate to conduct to the ventricle.

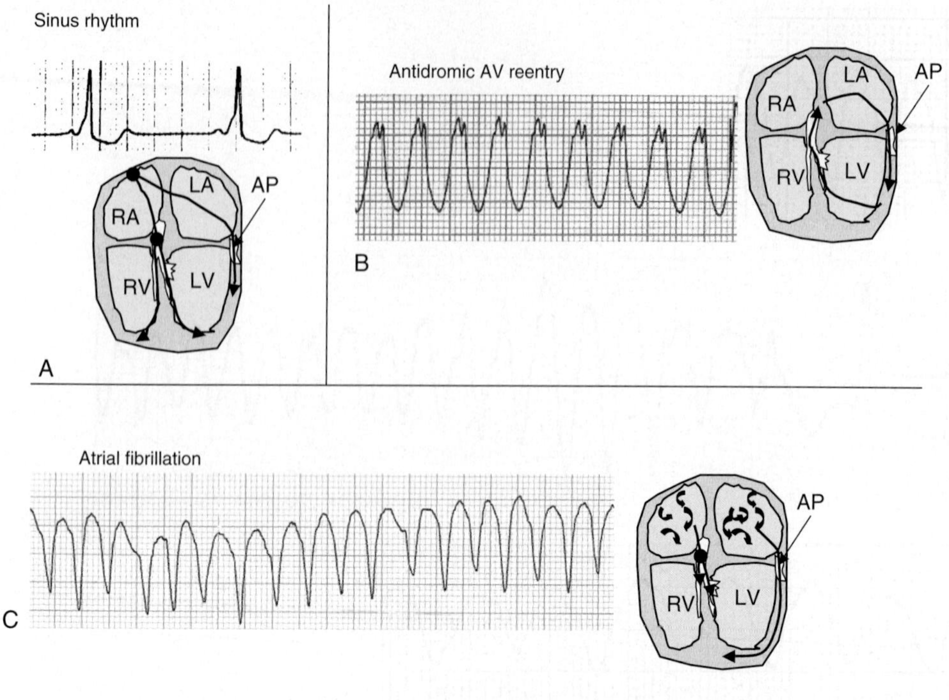

FIGURE 41.3. Features of the Wolff–Parkinson–White syndrome leading to pre-excited tachycardias are shown. **A:** sinus rhythm is shown. The ECG shows a short PR interval and δ-wave. The mechanism is shown in the schematic. Conduction of the sinus impulse (*arrows*) propagates over the AV node to the ventricles and over the accessory pathway (AP) to the ventricles. Conduction through the accessory pathway is faster than the AV node, producing the δ-wave. **B:** antidromic AV reentry is present. Tachycardia is due to circulation of the reentry wave front from atrium to ventricle over the accessory pathway, through the ventricle, and retrograde up the AV node to the atrium. Pre-excited antidromic tachycardia is often indistinguishable from ventricular tachycardia. **C:** atrial fibrillation with rapid conduction over an accessory pathway is shown. Tachycardia is irregular, although at the very rapid rate, the irregularity can be difficult to appreciate.

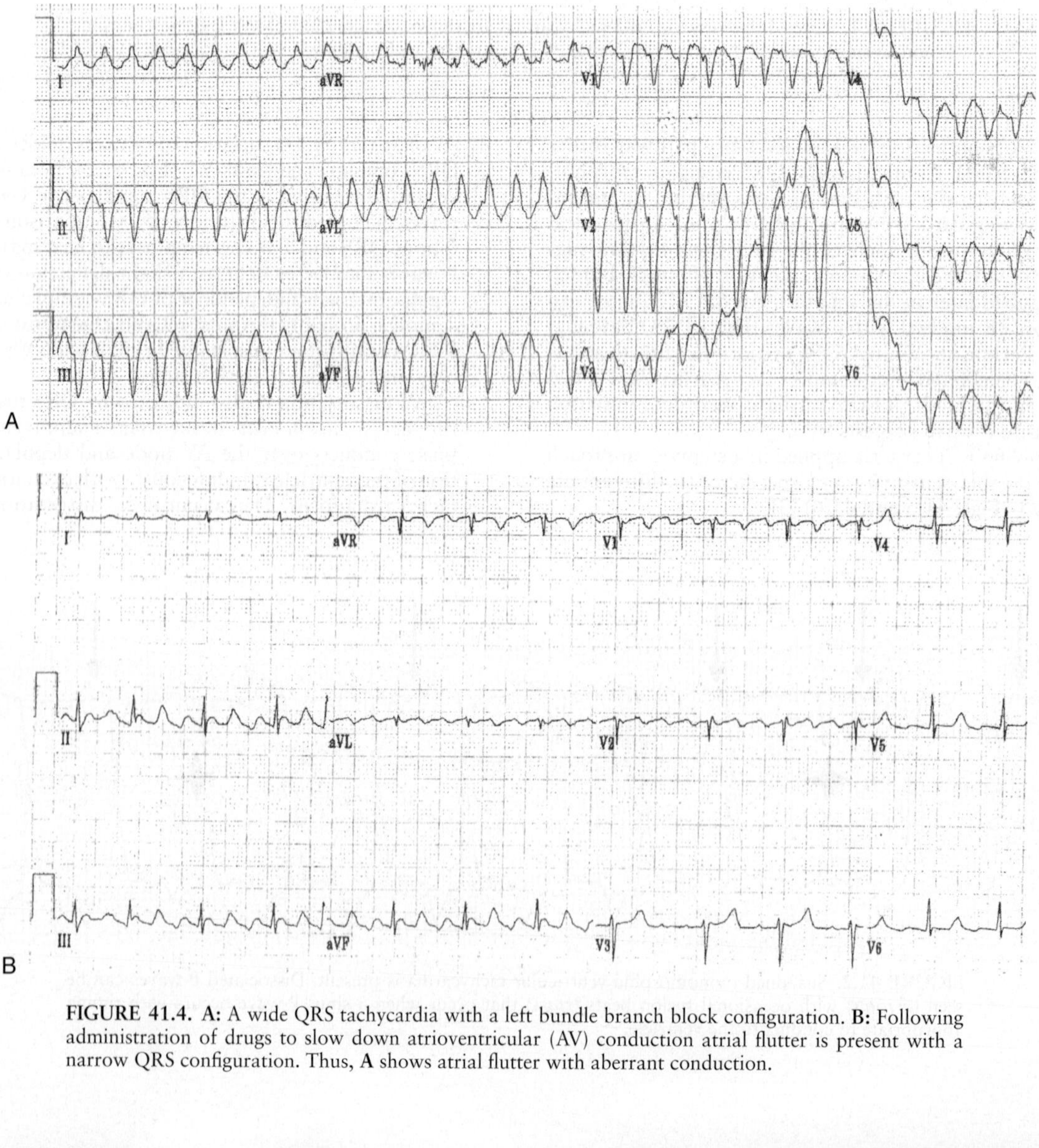

FIGURE 41.4. **A:** A wide QRS tachycardia with a left bundle branch block configuration. **B:** Following administration of drugs to slow down atrioventricular (AV) conduction atrial flutter is present with a narrow QRS configuration. Thus, **A** shows atrial flutter with aberrant conduction.

TABLE 41.1

SUPRAVENTRICULAR TACHYCARDIA VERSUS VENTRICULAR TACHYCARDIA

Findings suggesting ventricular tachycardia
AV dissociation
Electrocardiogram
Dissociated P-waves
Fusion beats, capture beats—indicate conduction of a fortuitously timed P-wave from atrium to ventricle before the ventricle is completely depolarized from the VT focus or circuit
AV dissociation on physical examination
Intermittent cannon *a*-waves in jugular venous pulse
Beat-to-beat variability in S_1 and systolic blood pressure
ECG leads V_1–V_6
QRS concordance: The absence of an rS or Rs complex in any precordial lead
RS >100 ms: An interval between the onset of the R and the nadir of the S-wave >100 ms in any precordial lead
Left bundle branch block VT
Initial R-wave in lead V_1 >30 ms in duration
Interval from onset of R to nadir of S in V_1 >60 ms
Notching in the downstroke of the S-wave in lead V_1
In V_6, a QS or QR pattern
Right bundle branch block VT
V_1: A monophasic R, QR, or RS pattern
V_6: An R to S <1 or a QS or a QR pattern

and the VT is not particularly fast. Fusion beats have a QRS morphology that is typically intermediate between that of a supraventricular beat and a ventricular beat. *Capture beats* have a similar significance to fusion beats. They occur when a supraventricular beat is able to conduct to the ventricles, depolarizing the ventricle in advance of the next tachycardia beat. These beats are morphologically identical to the QRS complex seen in sinus rhythm but occur in the midst of a wide QRS complex tachycardia.

2. *QRS concordance:* The absence of an rS or Rs complex in any precordial lead (V_1 to V_6) suggests VT.
3. *RS >100 ms:* An interval between the onset of the R and the nadir of the S-wave greater than 100 ms in any precordial lead (V_1 to V_6) favors VT.

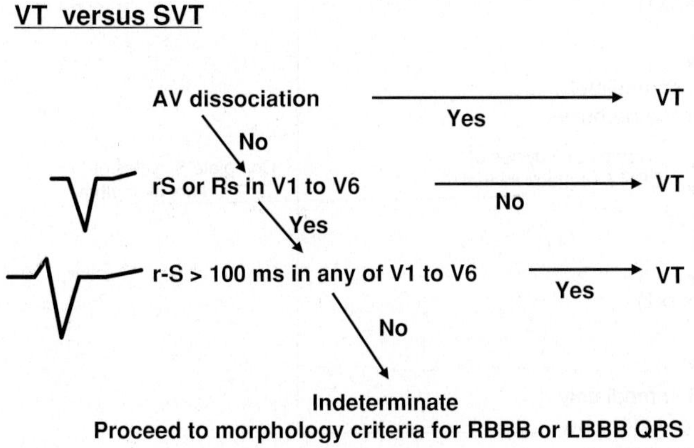

FIGURE 41.5. The schematic for an algorithm for ECG diagnosis of VT is shown. LBBB, left bundle branch block; RBBB, right bundle branch block; SVT, supraventricular tachycardia, VT, ventricular tachycardia.

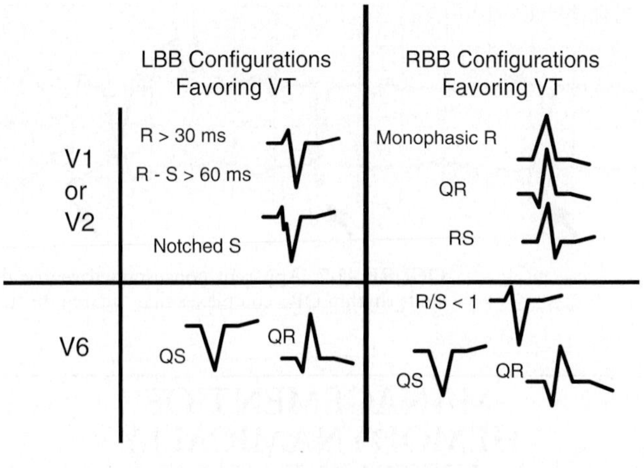

FIGURE 41.6. Electrocardiogram findings indicative of ventricular tachycardia (VT) or supraventricular tachycardia with aberrant conduction are shown. LBB, left bundle branch; RBB, right bundle branch.

If the diagnosis cannot be made after assessment for these features, a more thorough evaluation of the QRS morphology on the 12-lead ECG can be helpful (Fig. 41.6) [3]. For left bundle branch block morphology tachycardias, an initial R-wave in lead V_1 of greater than 30 ms in duration or a duration of greater than 60 ms from the onset of the R-wave to the nadir of the S-wave in V_1 suggests VT. Notching in the downstroke of the S-wave in lead V_1 also suggests VT. In V_6, a QS or QR pattern suggests VT. For right bundle branch block (RBBB) morphology tachycardias, a monophasic R, QR, or RS pattern in V_1 suggests VT. In V_6, an R-to-S amplitude ratio of less than 1 or QS or QR patterns suggests VT.

Electrocardiographic Artifacts that Mimic Wide Complex Tachycardia

Misinterpreting an electrocardiographic artifact, such as the one shown in Figure 41.7, as VT is a common error that has led to inappropriate and invasive procedures including cardiac catheterization, implantation of defibrillators, and even the occasional precordial thump [4]. Normal QRS complexes are often visible marching through the artifact at the sinus rate (arrows in Fig. 41.7). One author has referred to this as the "notches sign" because only small notches may be seen that march through the artifact at intervals that are the same as the RR intervals preceding the onset of tachycardia [5]. The history of the patient's activity at the time of the recording is often helpful in suggesting artifact. The recording in Figure 41.7 was performed during toothbrushing. Artifacts are also commonly caused by tremors, shivering, and electrical noise. The absence of symptoms or hemodynamic instability during the event (especially if the recording suggested a very fast heart rate) also suggests artifact.

ACUTE TREATMENT OF WIDE COMPLEX TACHYCARDIA

The misdiagnosis of VT as SVT followed by delivery of an inappropriate therapy is common in patients with wide QRS tachycardias [6]. As a general rule, wide QRS tachycardia should be treated as VT unless the diagnosis of SVT can be confirmed.

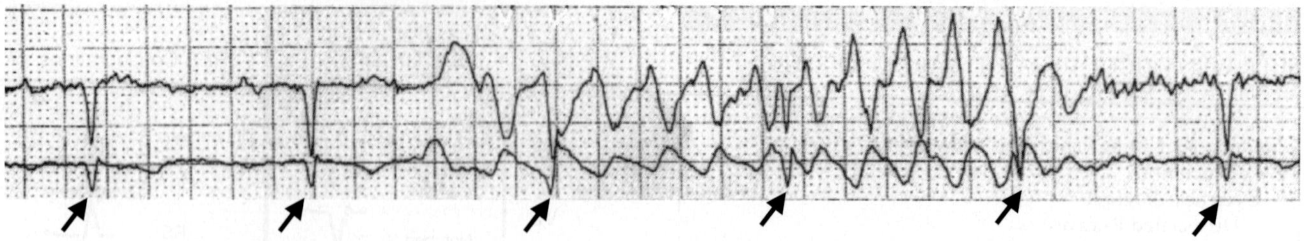

FIGURE 41.7. Apparent nonsustained ventricular tachycardia is actually artifact. Arrows indicate the sinus rhythm QRS complexes that "march through" the artifact.

MANAGEMENT OF HEMODYNAMICALLY UNSTABLE VT/VF

Figure 41.8 provides an algorithm for the management of hemodynamically unstable VT or VF. Hemodynamically unstable wide QRS tachycardia that is not due to sinus tachycardia with bundle branch block or artifact requires immediate electrical cardioversion. Both good basic life support (BLS) with prompt and efficient cardiopulmonary resuscitation (CPR) and rapid defibrillation are the most important measures to improve survival in unstable VT/VF [7]. Survival from VT/VF arrest diminishes by 7% to 10% per minute between collapse and defibrillation if CPR is not performed [8]. In fact, several studies have shown that survival from VT/VF arrest can be doubled or tripled if CPR is provided [9,10]. In keeping with these data, the most recent American Heart Association guidelines for cardiopulmonary resuscitation emphasize an integrated strategy of combined CPR and defibrillation [7]. If pulseless VT/VF persists after defibrillation, CPR should be promptly resumed and five cycles completed prior to additional therapy. When VT/VF is revealed during a rhythm check, CPR should be provided while the defibrillator is charging and resumed immediately following shock delivery. The algorithm for VF/pulseless VT should be followed (Fig. 41.8). Either epinephrine or vasopressin can be used as a first-line vasopressor agent if CPR continues to be required after two unsuccessful attempts at cardioversion [7]. If vasopressin is used, a one-time dose is appropriate as it has a half-life of 20 to 30 minutes. Epinephrine can be administered in 1-mg doses every 3 to 5 minutes.

Although definitive evidence of a long-term mortality benefit of any AADs for acute management of VT/VF is lacking, these agents should be used when initial attempts of electrical cardioversion are not successful [11,12]. When VF/pulseless VT persists after three shocks plus CPR and administration of a vasopressor, consider administering an antiarrhythmic, such as amiodarone. If amiodarone is unavailable, lidocaine may be considered. Magnesium should also be considered for TDP associated with a long QT interval [7]. In a trial of 504 patients

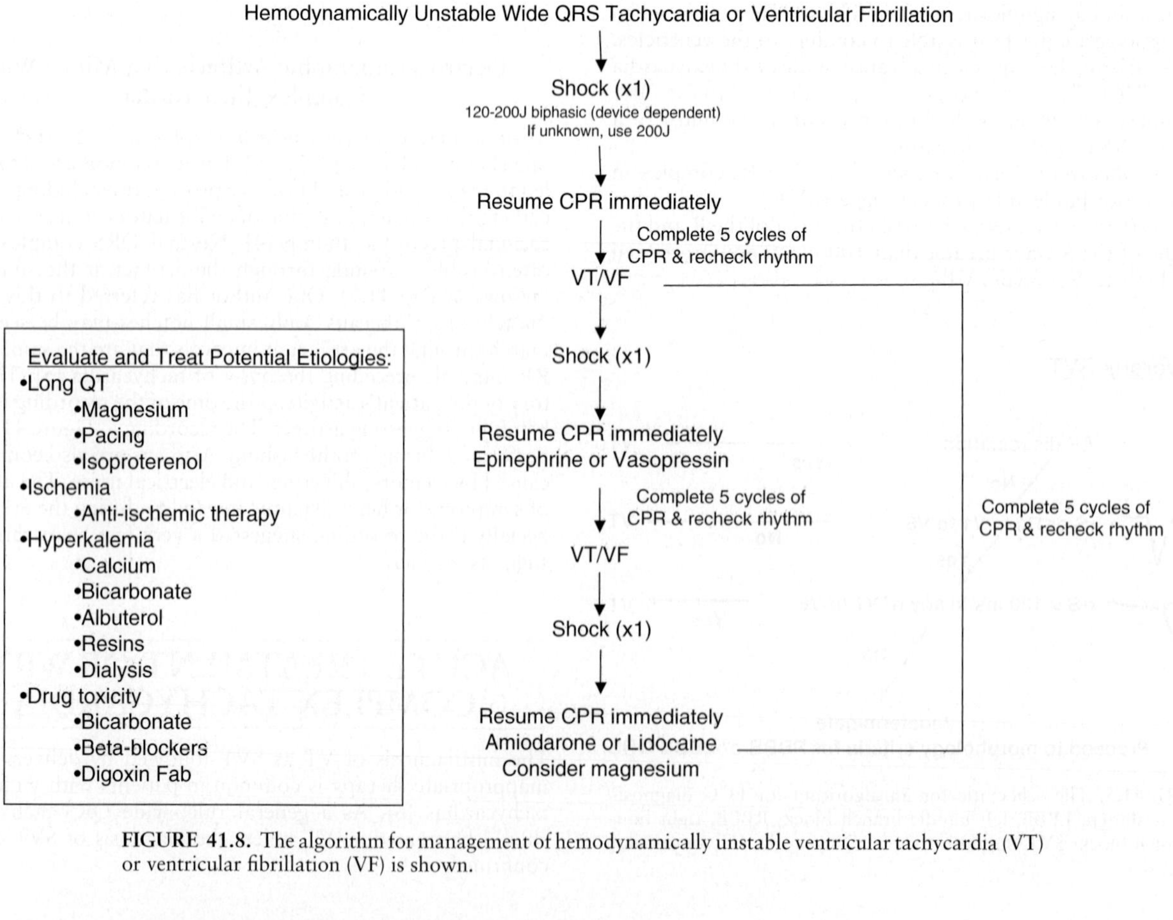

FIGURE 41.8. The algorithm for management of hemodynamically unstable ventricular tachycardia (VT) or ventricular fibrillation (VF) is shown.

with out-of-hospital VF or pulseless VT who failed three attempted cardioversions, administration of 300 mg of intravenous (IV) amiodarone was more effective than placebo for restoration of circulation and survival to hospital admission (44% of treated patients vs. 34% of untreated patients). Survival to hospital discharge was not improved and more patients who received amiodarone had hypotension (59% vs. 48%) or bradycardia (41% vs. 25%) [7,13,14]. Administration of IV procainamide can be considered as an alternative agent, but the data supporting its efficacy are limited [15]. Administration of IV lidocaine is most appropriate in the management of unstable VT/VF during suspected acute myocardial ischemia or infarct [16–18].

Although bretylium is an acceptable alternate antiarrhythmic agent for VT, it has been removed from advanced cardiac life support (ACLS) guidelines due to a combination of global supply shortage and lack of evidence showing its superiority over any of the previously mentioned AADs. Bretylium has similar efficacy to amiodarone for treatment of hemodynamically destabilizing VT that has failed cardioversion, but is associated with a greater incidence of hypotension compared to IV administration of amiodarone [7,18].

MANAGEMENT OF HEMODYNAMICALLY STABLE WIDE QRS TACHYCARDIA

In the absence of signs or symptoms of impaired consciousness or tissue hypoperfusion, a 12-lead ECG should be obtained to attempt to differentiate VT from SVT [7]. In patients in whom the diagnosis of SVT with aberrancy is suspected, the response to vagal maneuvers or adenosine administration while recording the ECG may also elucidate the diagnosis (Fig. 41.4). Vagotonic maneuvers and administration of IV adenosine often terminate or expose SVT and usually have no effect on VT. Close monitoring is required during these maneuvers; hypotension or precipitation of VF can rarely occur.

If the diagnosis remains unknown, the choice of initial antiarrhythmic agent should be influenced by the hemodynamic stability and rhythm analysis (Fig. 41.9). Administration of multiple antiarrhythmic agents should be avoided as polypharmacy increases the risk of precipitating incessant, although usually slower VT or new VTs, such as TDP (see later in the chapter). If the initial agent selected is ineffective, cardioversion is usually warranted.

First-line antiarrhythmic agents for stable wide QRS tachycardia of uncertain origin include procainamide, amiodarone, and in some circumstances, lidocaine. It is also appropriate to use electrical cardioversion as the initial therapy for stable tachycardia if appropriate sedation is available and can be safely achieved. Current ACLS guidelines state that IV administration of amiodarone, procainamide, sotalol (not available in IV form in the United States), and beta-blockers are preferable to lidocaine. Lidocaine is usually ineffective for treatment of sustained VT that is not due to acute myocardial ischemia or infarction [7,19]; procainamide and sotalol both have been shown to be more efficacious in this setting [20,21]. Procainamide and sotalol have negative inotropic effects and can induce hypotension. These agents should be avoided in patients with significantly impaired ventricular function (left ventricular ejection fraction <0.40) in favor of IV amiodarone [18,22,23]. Procainamide is acetylated to *n*-acetylprocainamide (NAPA). NAPA is a class III AAD that can cause TDP and is excreted entirely by the kidney; therefore, procainamide should also be avoided in patients with significant renal dysfunction. Each of these treatments (procainamide, amiodarone, or cardioversion) is also appropriate for SVT with aberrant conduction and therefore for wide QRS tachycardias of uncertain origin. If an accessory atrioventricular pathway with rapid repetitive conduction during AF or flutter is suspected (Fig. 41.3C), administration of IV procainamide or cardioversion are first-line therapies.

POLYMORPHIC VENTRICULAR TACHYCARDIA

VT with a continually changing QRS morphology is referred to as PMVT and is most often due to cardiac ischemia, metabolic disarray, or drug toxicity, often associated with QT prolongation. PMVT is often self-terminating, but likely to recur with a significant risk of hemodynamic instability and degeneration to VF.

The combination of PMVT and QT interval prolongation (usually a corrected QT interval [QTc]) greater than 500 ms is called torsades de pointes. The name is derived from the electrocardiographic appearance of twisting around the baseline as displayed in Figure 41.10. QT prolongation can be

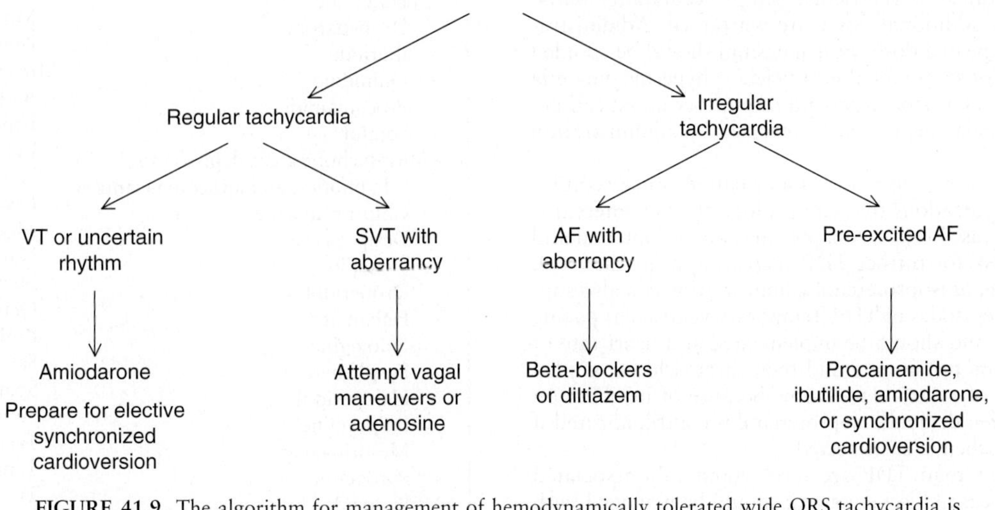

FIGURE 41.9. The algorithm for management of hemodynamically tolerated wide QRS tachycardia is shown. AF, atrial fibrillation; SVT, supraventricular tachycardia, VT, ventricular tachycardia.

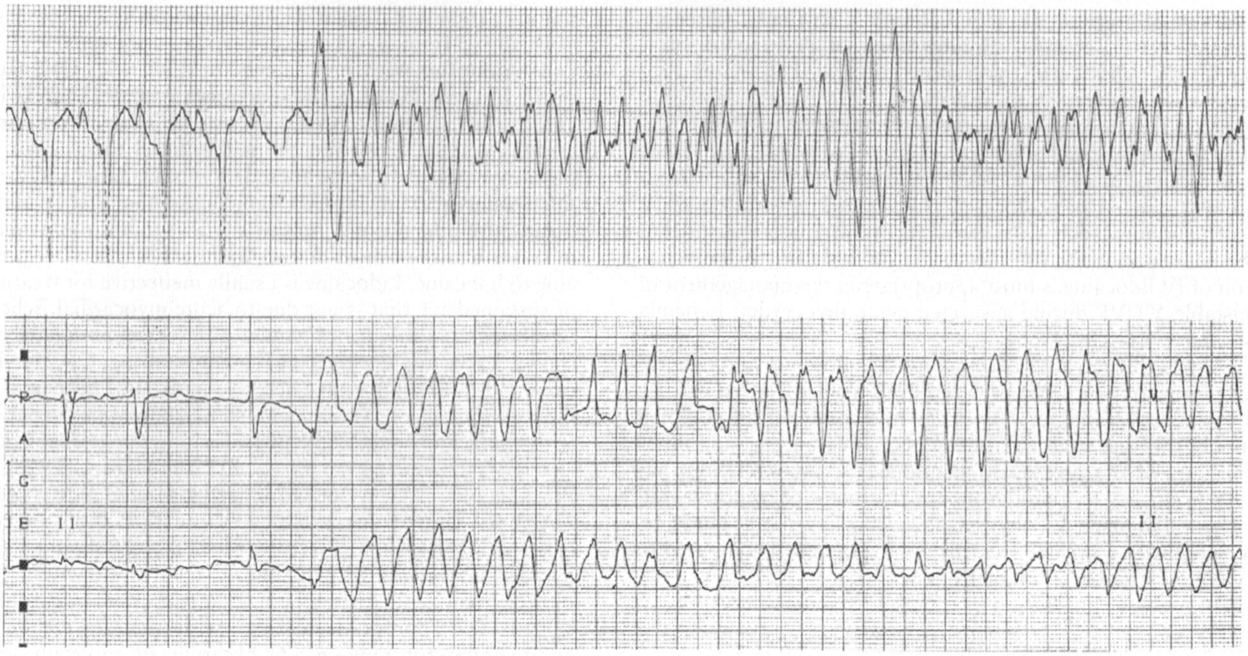
A
B

FIGURE 41.10. Two episodes of polymorphic ventricular tachycardia (VT) are shown. **A:** Polymorphic VT is due to acute myocardial infarction. The QT interval is normal prior to the onset of tachycardia. **B:** Torsades de pointes associated with QT prolongation prior to the onset of the tachycardia is present. A pause precedes onset of tachycardia.

acquired due to electrolyte abnormalities, QT-prolonging drugs, bradycardia, or a congenital ion channel disorder. A list of the acquired etiologies of TDP is provided in Table 41.2; a more extensive list is available at the QTdrugs.org Web site maintained and updated by the University of Georgetown, Department of Pharmacology. TDP often has a characteristic onset (Fig. 41.10B). A slowing of heart rate or pause produced by a premature ventricular contraction (PVC) further prolongs the QT interval. The T-wave of the longer QT interval is interrupted by the first beat of the PMVT. Thus, TDP is often referred to as "pause dependent."

TDP that leads to VF should immediately be defibrillated. Recurrent TDP is frequently suppressed by IV magnesium sulfate (1 to 2 g) that can be repeated in 5 to 15 minutes if no initial effect is seen [24]. Magnesium administration suppresses ventricular ectopy, but does not shorten the QT interval. It is often effective even if serum magnesium concentration is in the normal range. If ventricular ectopy recurs after initial administration, additional doses are warranted. Administration of large, repeated doses of magnesium should be avoided in the presence of severe renal insufficiency; hypermagnesemia with neuromuscular depression and respiratory arrest can occur. Neuromuscular depression is reversed by administration of IV calcium.

Correction of other electrolyte abnormalities and discontinuation of all medications that can prolong the QT interval is warranted. Because bradycardia prolongs the QT interval and increases the risk for further TDP, increasing heart rate with pacing, atropine, or isoproterenol administration can also suppress recurrent episodes of TDP. Temporary ventricular pacing is most reliable and should be implemented at a heart rate of 110 to 120 beats per minute and then titrated lower guided by suppression of ventricular ectopy. Because of its effect on increasing oxygen demand, isoproterenol is contraindicated if active cardiac ischemia is suspected.

PMVTs other than TDP are most commonly associated with acute myocardial ischemia and should be managed with anti-ischemic strategies including beta-blockers and revascularization. IV lidocaine and amiodarone can be considered for

TABLE 41.2

CAUSES OF TORSADES DE POINTES OR QT PROLONGATION

- **Congenital long QT syndrome**
- Bradycardia
- Electrolyte abnormalities
  - Hypokalemia
  - Hypomagnesemia
  - Hypocalcemia
- Central nervous system disorders
  - Subarachnoid hemorrhage
- Drugs
  - Antiarrhythmics
    - Amiodarone
    - Disopyramide
    - Dofetilide
    - Dronedarone
    - Ibutilide
    - Quinidine
    - Procainamide
    - Sotalol
  - Antipsychotics, antidepressants, hypnotics, and anticonvulsants
    - Chlorpromazine
    - Desipramine
    - Doxepin
    - Droperidol
    - Felbamate
    - Fluoxetine
    - Fosphenytoin
    - Haloperidol
    - Imipramine
    - Mesoridazine
    - Paroxetine
    - Pimozide
    - Quetiapine
    - Risperidone
    - Sertraline
    - Thioridazine
    - Venlafaxine
    - Ziprasidone
  - Antibiotics
    - Clarithromycin
    - Erythromycin
    - Foscarnet
    - Gatifloxacin
    - Halofantrine
    - Levofloxacin
    - Moxifloxacin
    - Pentamidine
  - Miscellaneous drugs
    - Arsenic trioxide
    - Bepridil
    - Indapamide
    - Isradipine
    - Levomethadyl
    - Moexipril/HCTZ
    - Naratriptan
    - Nicardipine
    - Octreotide
    - Probucol
    - Salmeterol
    - Sparfloxacin
    - Sumatriptan
    - Tacrolimus
    - Tamoxifen
    - Tizanidine
    - Zolmitriptan

recurrent episodes. If the cause of PMVT is unclear, such that both TDP and ischemia are possibilities, administration of IV magnesium and lidocaine are reasonable initial therapies, which are unlikely to aggravate arrhythmias from either cause.

SINUSOIDAL VENTRICULAR TACHYCARDIA

When the QRS has a similar duration to that of diastole, the tachycardia has a sinusoidal appearance (Fig. 41.1C). This is due to either very rapid monomorphic VT, also called ventricular flutter, which can occur due to any of the causes given previously in the chapter, or acute myocardial ischemia. Slow sinusoidal VT (Fig. 41.1C) occurs when the QRS is prolonged as a consequence of slowing of conduction through the myocardium. Such slow ventricular conduction is most commonly due to hyperkalemia or toxicity from a drug that blocks cardiac sodium channels, such as flecainide, propafenone, quinidine, procainamide, disopyramide, phenothiazines, or tricyclic antidepressants.

Hyperkalemia should be treated with administration of 1 g of IV calcium chloride or calcium gluconate, which promptly antagonizes the electrophysiologic effects of hyperkalemia. Administration of sodium bicarbonate intravenously also has almost-immediate effects. Calcium and $NaHCO_3$ should not be administered together in the same IV line, as they precipitate. Administration of hypertonic glucose and insulin has an effect in several minutes. The duration of action of these measures is transient, but does allow institution of measures to remove potassium with forced diuresis, potassium-binding resins (Kayexalate), or hemodialysis.

Slow sinusoidal VT due to toxicity from a sodium channel–blocking drug may respond to administration of hypertonic sodium in the form of sodium bicarbonate or sodium lactate [25,26]. Sodium bicarbonate administration is indicated for tricyclic antidepressant toxicity. Many of these drugs have a characteristic known as use-dependency, such that their electrophysiologic effect is greater at rapid heart rates. Slowing of the ventricular rate diminishes the toxicity. Thus, administration of β-adrenergic blockers can be helpful [27]. Supportive measures are required until the offending agent is excreted.

WIDE QRS TACHYCARDIAS DUE TO VENTRICULAR CONDUCTION OVER AN ACCESSORY PATHWAY

WCTs are also produced by conduction from atrium to ventricle over an accessory pathway in patients with the WPW syndrome (Fig. 41.3). These "pre-excited tachycardias" can be due to antidromic AV reentry (Fig. 41.3B) or AF or flutter conducting from atrium to ventricle over the accessory pathway (Fig. 41.3C). Clues that a wide QRS tachycardia may be a pre-excited tachycardia include: evidence of WPW on a prior ECG, with a short PR interval and a δ-wave (Fig. 41.3A); AF with a very fast ventricular response of 200 to 300 beats per minute (Fig. 41.3C); and irregularly irregular WCT with variation in beat-to-beat QRS morphology. Each QRS complex represents some degree of fusion between conduction over the accessory pathway and conduction through the AV node.

Pre-excited tachycardias should generally be managed as VT. Procainamide, which slows accessory pathway conduction, or electrical cardioversion are first-line therapies. IV lidocaine usually has little effect. Administration of medications that suppress AV nodal conduction without suppressing conduction over the accessory pathway can accelerate the ventricular response, precipitating VF or hemodynamic collapse. Thus, beta-blockers, diltiazem, verapamil, digoxin, and adenosine are contraindicated in this setting. IV amiodarone may also have this effect, because it suppresses AV conduction and should be administered with caution [28].

IMPLANTABLE CARDIOVERTER DEFIBRILLATORS

Implantable cardioverter defibrillators (ICDs) are a first-line therapy for many patients who have been resuscitated from a prior cardiac arrest or who are at high risk for arrhythmias and sudden cardiac death. An increasing number of patients with defibrillators are encountered in intensive care units (ICUs). Even when an ICD is present and programmed "on," its presence should not delay implementation of standard ACLS when VT or VF occurs. The ICD may deliver ineffective therapy or fail to detect the arrhythmia. External shocks, when required, should be delivered regardless of the presence of an ICD.

The ICD recognizes VT or VF largely by the presence of a heart rate that exceeds the programmed detection threshold. If an SVT exceeds the programmed rate threshold, the device will deliver an inappropriate therapy, either antitachycardia pacing or an electrical shock [29]. Recurrent episodes can lead to recurrent painful shocks. Occasionally antitachycardia pacing for an atrial arrhythmia initiates VT (Fig. 41.11). Recurrent inappropriate therapies can be managed by placing a magnet over the ICD pulse generator. This disables ICD arrhythmia detection. It is important to recognize that VT or VF will also not be detected with the magnet in place; external shocks will be required to treat these arrhythmias. Use of a magnet to suspend detection is a temporary maneuver until the inciting arrhythmia

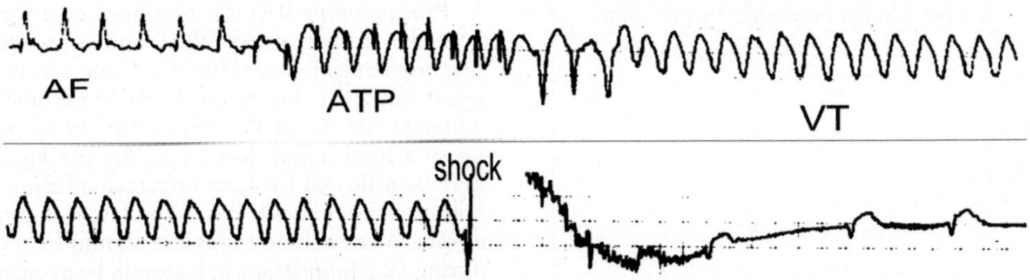

FIGURE 41.11. Tracings from a hospitalized patient who has an ICD are shown. From the *top left*, atrial fibrillation with a rapid ventricular response is present. The rapid ventricular response is incorrectly identified as ventricular tachycardia by the ICD and initiates a burst of antitachycardia pacing (ATP). ATP initiates sustained ventricular tachycardia (VT). The VT rate is faster than the previous rate, which falls into the programmed VF zone of the ICD, which then delivers a shock, restoring sinus rhythm. However, atrial fibrillation recurred (not shown) repeatedly. Recurrent ICD therapies were interrupted by placing a magnet over the ICD to suspend arrhythmia detection and treat the atrial fibrillation.

can be brought under control or the ICD can be reprogrammed to allow better arrhythmia discrimination.

Antiarrhythmic medications can have important interactions with ICDs [30]. These drugs can slow VT to a rate that it is lesser than the detect rate of the ICD. VT is then not detected or treated by the ICD. Antiarrhythmic drugs, particularly amiodarone, can increase the current required for defibrillation, such that the ICD no longer provides effective defibrillation; in this setting, external shocks are required.

NONSUSTAINED VT AND VENTRICULAR ECTOPY: "FIRST DO NO HARM"

PVCs and NSVT (more than three ventricular complexes) are common in the ICU particularly associated with myocardial ischemia, previous-healed myocardial infarction, and cardiomyopathies. Idiopathic PVCs also occur in some otherwise healthy patients, in whom they are of no consequence. The initial appearance of ventricular ectopy should prompt an evaluation for possible aggravating factors (Table 41.3). Increasingly frequent ectopy raises concern of increasing sympathetic tone possibly due to progression of the underlying illness. Treatment should be directed at the underlying condition. Therapy with β-adrenergic–blocking agents if not precluded due to hemodynamic or pulmonary impairment is reasonable. Other antiarrhythmic agents should, in general, be avoided.

NSVT is a marker for increased sudden death risk in patients who have had a prior myocardial infarction and in patients with left ventricular hypertrophy [31–33]. Patients with an ejection fraction 40% or lesser and NSVT should be considered for electrophysiologic study. Those with inducible VT have a 9% per year risk of sudden death; ICDs are protective, reducing total mortality from approximately 50% to 24% over 5 years [34,35].

TABLE 41.3

FACTORS AGGRAVATING VENTRICULAR ARRHYTHMIAS IN HOSPITALIZED PATIENTS

Acute myocardial ischemia and infarction
Transvenous catheter in the right ventricle mechanically inducing ectopic activity
Elevated sympathetic tone
Pain, anxiety
Acute illness
Sympathomimetic agents (dobutamine, dopamine, epinephrine, norepinephrine, milrinone, theophylline)
Hyperthyroidism
Hypoxemia
Acid/base disturbance
Electrolyte disturbance
Hypokalemia
Hyperkalemia
Hypocalcemia
Hypomagnesemia
Drugs
QT prolongation—torsades de pointes (see Table 41.2)
Digitalis toxicity

Patients with PVCs or NSVT who have relatively preserved left ventricular function do not usually need specific antiarrhythmic therapy. Therapy with beta-blockers can be considered for symptomatic patients. Rarely, other drugs are required to control symptoms. Aggravating factors, such as electrolyte abnormalities, should be sought and corrected. Therapy with class I AADs or sotalol is generally not indicated and may increase mortality [36,37].

Accelerated idioventricular rhythm (AIVR) is a wide-complex ventricular rhythm at a rate faster than 40 beats per minute and slower than 100 beats per minute and is usually hemodynamically stable. The mechanism is probably related to enhanced automaticity. This rhythm often occurs in the first 12 hours following reperfusion of an acute myocardial infarction during periods of elevated sympathetic tone, and its onset is typically preceded by sinus slowing [38]. AIVR usually resolves without specific therapy; AAD treatment is rarely necessary.

Digitalis-induced arrhythmias include ventricular ectopic activity, an accelerated junctional rhythm, monomorphic VT, or VF. Rarely, digitalis causes *bidirectional tachycardia*, in which the QRS morphology alternates between two different morphologies; mortality is high if left untreated [39]. Patients with digitalis-induced VT should receive digoxin immune Fab fragments (Digibind) [40].

OVERVIEW OF DRUGS COMMONLY USED FOR MANAGEMENT OF VT/VF IN THE ICU

AADs (Table 41.4) are commonly grouped according to the Vaughan Williams classification scheme on the basis of whether their predominant action is to block sodium channels (class I), β-adrenergic receptors (class II), potassium channels (class III), or L-type calcium channels (class IV) [41]. Although this classification scheme is imperfect (many of the drugs affect multiple channels or receptors), it remains in common use. The narrow toxic–therapeutic window and potential for proarrhythmia necessitate use of AADs only when the potential risks are justified by the need to suppress an arrhythmia. For most drugs, the initial dosing guidelines provide a starting point for drug administration. Titration to achieve the desired effect is often required.

Class I AADs block sodium channels with either intermediate (IA), fast (IB), or slow (IC) onset and recovery of channel block during diastole. Class IC AADs such as *flecainide* and *moricizine* increase long-term mortality in patients with coronary artery disease and depressed ventricular function [42,43]. Such agents are rarely used for VT in the ICU.

Procainamide (IA) is a first-line agent for the treatment of hemodynamically stable WCT, and as an alternative agent for hemodynamically unstable WCT and VF. It is also a first-line agent for WCT due to the WPW syndrome. Procainamide is administered as an IV infusion at 20 to 30 mg per minute up to a total initial dose of 17 mg per kg. The loading dose may be followed by a maintenance infusion of 1 to 4 mg per minute. Procainamide has vasodilatory and negative inotropic effects. Arterial blood pressure should be monitored carefully during IV administration. It should be avoided in patients with depressed ventricular function (left ventricular ejection fraction <0.40). In addition, NAPA, an active metabolite of the drug, exerts class III effects that can lead to prolongation of repolarization (increased QTc) and TDP. Serum levels of both procainamide and NAPA should be monitored if the drug is

TABLE 41.4

DRUGS COMMONLY USED FOR VT/VF IN THE ICU (GROUPED BY VAUGHAN WILLIAMS CLASS AND "OTHER")

Class	Antiarrhythmic drug	Common indications	IV dose: Load	IV dose: Maintenance	Contraindications	Side effects	Comments
IA	Procainamide	MVT, PMVT, WPW and AF, VF (second line)	20 mg/min until arrhythmia is suppressed or side effects occur up to 17 mg/kg total	1–4 mg/min	Hypotension, reduced EF, CHF (reduce dosage in renal failure), prolonged QT, previous TDP	Hypotension, negative inotropism, proarrhythmia, lupus-like syndrome	Active metabolite (NAPA) follow Proc and NAPA levels Discontinue if QRS widens by >50%
IB	Lidocaine	Monomorphic VT, polymorphic VT/VF	1.0–1.5 mg/kg (additional 0.75 mg/kg can be given as a second bolus)	1–4 mg/min	Seizure disorders, severe bradycardia or heart block, severe renal or hepatic dysfunction	Seizures, status asthmaticus, hypotension	Appears to be most effective during acute myocardial ischemia
II	β-adrenergic blockers	PMVT/MVT	Variable	Variable	Severe CHF; second- or third-degree heart block	Bradycardia, worsened CHF, AV delay, hypotension, bronchospasm	Proven mortality benefit in cardiac ischemia
III	Amiodarone	MVT, PMVT, VF	150 mg IV over 10 min (may be repeated multiple times up to ~2 g/24 h and 5–8 g total)	1 mg/min for 6 h and then 5 mg/min	Severe hepatic disease; second- or third-degree heart block	Hypotension, multiorgan toxicity (lung, liver, nervous system, eyes, skin, thyroid)	May be more effective than lidocaine for most ventricular arrhythmias
	Ibutilide	AF (cardioversion), WPW, and AF	1 mg IV (may repeat dose 10 min after initial dose)		Prolonged QT interval, electrolyte abnormalities (hypokalemia, hypomagnesemia), polymorphic VT	Torsades de pointes	
	Bretylium	VT/VF (second line)	5 mg/kg (may repeat)	1–2 mg/min	Severe renal failure	Frequent late hypotension	Removed from ACLS treatment algorithms due to limited supply
	Sotalol	*VT/VF	1.0–1.5 mg/kg at 10 mg/min*		Second- or third-degree heart block	Bradycardia, hypotension, TDP	*Not available intravenously in the United States
Other	Epinephrine	Cardiac arrest	1 mg IV (repeated as needed)	1–4 μg/min			
	Vasopressin	Pressor agent for cardiac arrest	40 U IV (not repeated)				Interchangeable with epinephrine
	Magnesium	Known low Mg^{+}, TDP	1–2 g (may be repeated)				

CHB, complete heart block; CHF, congestive heart failure; EF, ejection fraction; MVT, monomorphic VT; PMVT, polymorphic VT; TDP, torsades de pointes; VF, ventricular fibrillation; VT, ventricular tachycardia; AF, atrial fibrillation; WPW, Wolf–Parkinson–White.

continued for longer than 24 hours. In addition to the QTc interval, the width of the QRS complex should be monitored and the drug should be discontinued during initial loading or chronic therapy if the QRS widens by more than 50% of its baseline value.

Lidocaine (class IB) is indicated for the acute management of life-threatening ventricular arrhythmias, especially in patients suspected of having acute myocardial ischemia. It can be administered as 1.0 to 1.5 mg per kg IV bolus, which can be repeated to a maximum bolus of 3 mg per kg, followed by an infusion of 1 to 4 mg per minute. Unlike procainamide, lidocaine has few adverse hemodynamic side effects. Its toxicity is mainly due to neurologic side effects (seizures and tremors).

Beta-blockers (class II) antagonize the effects of β-adrenergic stimulation on the heart and have been shown to reduce mortality in patients with depressed ventricular function or ischemic heart disease during chronic therapy [44,45]. They can be considered for hemodynamically significant or symptomatic NSVT and PVCs, and for recurrent sustained ventricular tachyarrhythmias in which elevated sympathetic tone is felt to play a role. Negative inotropic effects, bradyarrhythmias, and aggravation of bronchospasm are major adverse effects. Metoprolol, propranolol, atenolol, and esmolol are all available for IV administration. *Metoprolol* can be given as a 5-mg slow IV push and can be repeated every 5 to 10 minutes up to a total of 20 mg IV or until the desired effect is obtained. Ongoing maintenance therapy can be administered as repeat IV boluses every 4 to 6 hours or through oral dosing. *Esmolol* has a short half-life (2 to 9 minutes), making it useful when there is concern that a beta-blocker may be poorly tolerated, such as in patients with hypotension or a history of bronchospasm. Termination of the infusion is followed by rapid dissipation of effect.

Class III AADs cause prolongation of repolarization primarily by potassium channel–blocking activity. This action is responsible for their antiarrhythmic and proarrhythmic (QTc prolongation and TDP) effects.

Amiodarone is usually classified as a class III agent, although it exhibits sodium, potassium, and calcium channel inhibition, as well as β-adrenergic–blocking effects. It has excellent efficacy in the management of ventricular arrhythmias and a low incidence of proarrhythmia [46]. Amiodarone is a first-line AAD option in the recently revised ACLS VF/pulseless VT algorithm [7]. Even though amiodarone causes QT prolongation, TDP is rare. IV amiodarone can be administered as 150 mg bolus over 10 minutes, followed by a continuous infusion at 1 mg per minute for 6 hours and then 0.5 mg per minute. Additional 150 mg boluses can be given for breakthrough arrhythmia up to a total load of approximately 2 g per 24 hours and 5 to 8 g total. Amiodarone has a large and variable volume of distribution (averaging 60 L per kg) and long half-life (averaging 53 days). Major complications during IV administration are hypotension and bradyarrhythmias. When administered through a peripheral IV line, amiodarone causes phlebitis; continuous infusions should be administered through a central venous catheter. During chronic long-term therapy, hepatic toxicity, hyper- or hypothyroidism, pneumonitis, pulmonary fibrosis, neuropathy, tremor, and skin toxicity are important concerns that require careful monitoring.

LONG-TERM MANAGEMENT AFTER RESUSCITATION FROM SUSTAINED VT/VF

Patients with ischemic heart disease and reduced ventricular function who are resuscitated from cardiac arrest or hemodynamically significant VT not attributable to acute myocardial infarction have a risk of recurrent cardiac arrest or VT that exceeds 30% to 40%. ICDs effectively terminate recurrent VT/VF and reduce mortality in these patients [47–49]. Thus, sudden cardiac arrest survivors warrant evaluation after resuscitation and management of any intercurrent illness to assess the need for placement of an ICD and other arrhythmia therapy. Catheter ablation of VT is a valuable treatment option for the control of recurrent arrhythmia. Therapeutic decisions are guided by the estimated risk of recurrence, underlying heart disease, functional status, and general prognosis.

Sustained Monomorphic VT

Sustained monomorphic VT is usually due to reentry through a region of myocardial scar, most commonly from an old myocardial infarction. Myocardial scars causing VT also occur in cardiomyopathies, cardiac sarcoidosis, arrhythmogenic right ventricular cardiomyopathy, and Chaga's disease. In all of these diseases, the substrate for the arrhythmia remains after resuscitation. The spontaneous recurrence rate exceeds 40% over the following 2 years. Patients who present with sustained monomorphic VT, but have elevated cardiac enzymes indicating infarction, should be presumed to remain at risk for VT from reentry from a prior infarct scar. An ICD or long-term therapy with amiodarone is generally considered after underlying myocardial ischemia and other aggravating factors are addressed. The underlying heart disease should be characterized; echocardiography and cardiac catheterization are often warranted.

Bundle Branch Reentry

Bundle branch reentry causes a unique form of monomorphic VT that results from a reentrant circuit utilizing the bundle branches as arms of the circuit. The reentry wave front typically circulates antegrade down the right bundle branch and up the left bundle branch, giving rise to a VT that has a left bundle branch block QRS configuration. In patients with left bundle branch block in sinus rhythm, the VT can have the same QRS morphology as sinus rhythm. This form of VT is most commonly seen in patients with nonischemic dilated cardiomyopathy [50]. Bundle branch reentry can be cured by radiofrequency ablation, but at least 25% of patients with this form of VT will have other VTs as well [51]. Therefore, an ICD is often recommended.

Rarely, sustained monomorphic VT occurs in a patient without structural heart disease. The most common of these idiopathic tachycardias originates from a focus in the right ventricular outflow tract, giving rise to VT that has a left bundle branch block, inferior axis QRS configuration. VT is often catecholamine sensitive and precipitated during exercise or physiologic stress, occasionally emerging during other illnesses. Idiopathic VT rarely causes cardiac arrest, although hypotension and syncope can occur [52]. Unlike other forms of VT, idiopathic VT is sometimes terminated with adenosine or vagal maneuvers [53]. Beta-blocker and verapamil (especially in IV form) can also be effective at terminating and suppressing idiopathic VT [54]. Long-term therapy focuses on suppression with beta-blockers or calcium channel blockers. Occasionally catheter ablation is required [55].

Polymorphic VTs

Patients who have had TDP should be viewed as having a susceptibility to the arrhythmia. All known precipitants of TDP or QT prolongation should be avoided (Table 41.3). Patient should be provided with a list of these medications. Following removal of aggravating factors, evaluation for possible congenital long QT syndrome should be conducted. The diagnosis is suggested by persistent QT prolongation and QT prolongation on prior ECGs when potential offending drugs were absent and/or a family history of unexplained sudden death. Long-term therapy and follow-up are required.

If the patient has a family history of sudden death and has been resuscitated from PMVT, but the QT interval is normal, other familial sudden death syndromes should be considered. The *Brugada syndrome* is a unique familial cause of sudden cardiac death that accounts for some cases of idiopathic VF [56]. Patients with this syndrome have a baseline ECG with RBBB, ST-segment elevation in leads V_1 to V_3 and no evidence of structural heart disease [57]. *Catecholaminergic polymorphic ventricular tachycardia* (CPVT) is an inherited primary electrical disorder of the heart associated with a high rate of sudden death [58,59]. Autosomal-dominant mutations of the ryanodine receptor account for the majority of cases, but autosomal-recessive mutations of calsequestrin have also been reported [59]. These patients frequently present at an early age with stress-induced syncope or sudden cardiac arrest. The resting ECG is usually unremarkable, and both invasive and noninvasive testing fail to reveal signs of structural heart disease. Exercise testing often demonstrates runs of PMVT during exercise frequently with a beat-to-beat 180-degree rotation of the QRS axis (bidirectional tachycardia) [58]. Genetic testing can aid in the diagnosis. Beta-blockers titrated to maximal doses are the mainstay of therapy for CPVT [58]. An ICD may be warranted for treatment of patients with these syndromes.

PMVT due to acute myocardial infarction usually occurs in the first hour of the infarction and is unusual after initial resuscitation. Recurrent episodes should prompt assessment for ongoing ischemia. The risk of recurrent cardiac arrest is similar to that for patients with a similar-size infarction without cardiac arrest.

TABLE 41.5

ADVANCES IN THE MANAGEMENT OF VENTRICULAR TACHYCARDIA

- Acute management involves assessment of hemodynamic status, ECG evaluation and diagnosis of ventricular tachycardia versus supraventricular tachycardia with aberrancy.
- Immediate cardioversion should be provided for hemodynamically unstable VT.
- Reversible causes of VT (e.g., ischemia, electrolyte abnormalites) should be identified and treated.
- Antiarrhythmic drugs should be considered when initial attempts at cardioversion are unsuccessful or when VT recurs.
- Long-term management may include consideration for an implantable defibrillator in appropriately selected patients.

Cardiac Arrest of Unclear Cause

Often the cause of a cardiac arrest cannot be determined with certainty. The patient resuscitated from VF who has enzymatic evidence of non–Q-wave myocardial infarction, but depressed ventricular function and evidence of a prior myocardial infarction might have suffered VT from reentry in the old infarct scar or an ischemic arrhythmia. Treatment for ischemia and an ICD is often considered.

A summary of advances in the management of VT, based on randomized controlled trials or meta-analyses of such trials, is given in Table 41.5.

References

1. Tchou P, Young P, Mahmud R, et al: Useful clinical criteria for the diagnosis of ventricular tachycardia. *Am J Med* 84:53–56, 1988.
2. Dongas J, Lehmann MH, Mahmud R, et al: Value of preexisting bundle branch block in the electrocardiographic differentiation of supraventricular from ventricular origin of wide QRS tachycardia. *Am J Cardiol* 55:717–721, 1985.
3. Brugada P, Brugada J, Mont L, et al: A new approach to the differential diagnosis of a regular tachycardia with a wide QRS complex. *Circulation* 83:1649–1659, 1991.
4. Knight BP, Pelosi F, Michaud GF, et al: Clinical consequences of electrocardiographic artifact mimicking ventricular tachycardia. *N Engl J Med* 341:1270–1274, 1999.
5. Littmann L, Monroe MH: Electrocardiographic artifact [Correspondence]. *N Engl J Med* 342:590–592, 2000.
6. Akhtar M, Shenasa M, Jazayeri M, et al: Wide QRS complex tachycardia. Reappraisal of a common clinical problem. *Ann Intern Med* 109:905–912, 1988.
7. ECC Committee, Subcommittees and Task Forces of the American Heart Association: 2005 American Heart Association Guidelines for Cardiopulmonary Resuscitation and Emergency Cardiovascular Care. *Circulation* 112[24, Suppl]:IV1–IV203, 2005.
8. Larsen MP, Eisenberg MS, Cummins RO, et al: Predicting survival from out-of-hospital cardiac arrest: a graphic model. *Ann Emerg Med* 22(11):1652–1658, 1993.
9. Valenzuela TD, Roe DJ, Cretin S, et al: Estimating effectiveness of cardiac arrest interventions: a logistic regression survival model. *Circulation* 96(10):3308–3313, 1997.
10. Holmberg M, Holmberg S, Herlitz J: Effect of bystander cardiopulmonary resuscitation in out-of-hospital cardiac arrest patients in Sweden. *Resuscitation* 47(1):59–70, 2000.
11. Levine JH, Massumi A, Scheinman MM, et al: Intravenous amiodarone for recurrent sustained hypotensive ventricular tachyarrhythmias. Intravenous Amiodarone Multicenter Trial Group. *J Am Coll Cardiol* 27(1):67–75, 1996.
12. Kowey PR, Levine JH, Herre JM, et al: Randomized, double-blind comparison of intravenous amiodarone and bretylium in the treatment of patients with recurrent, hemodynamically destabilizing ventricular tachycardia or fibrillation. The Intravenous Amiodarone Multicenter Investigators Group. *Circulation* 92:3255–3263, 1995.
13. Kudenchuk PJ, Cobb LA, Copass MK, et al: Amiodarone for resuscitation after out-of-hospital cardiac arrest due to ventricular fibrillation. *N Engl J Med* 341:871–878, 1999.
14. Helmy I, Herre JM, Gee G, et al: Use of intravenous amiodarone for emergency treatment of life-threatening ventricular arrhythmias. *J Am Coll Cardiol* 12:1015–1022. 1998.
15. Stiell IG, Wells GA, Hebert PC, et al: Association of drug therapy with survival in cardiac arrest: limited role of advanced cardiac life support drugs. *Acad Emerg Med* 2:264–273, 1995.
16. Lie KI, Wellens HJ, van Capelle FJ, et al: Lidocaine in the prevention of primary ventricular fibrillation. A double-blind, randomized study of 212 consecutive patients. *N Engl J Med* 291:1324–1326, 1974.
17. Davis J, Glassman R, Wit AL: Method for evaluating the effect of antiarrhythmic drugs on ventricular tachycardias in the infarcted canine heart. *Am J Cardiol* 49:1176–1184, 1982.
18. Cardinal R, Janse MJ, van Eeden J, et al: The effects of lidocaine on intracellular and extracellular potentials, activation and ventricular arrhythmias during acute regional ischemia in the isolated porcine heart. *Circ Res* 49:792–798, 1981.
19. Nasir N Jr, Taylor A, Doyle TK, et al: Evaluation of intravenous lidocaine for the termination of sustained monomorphic ventricular tachycardia in patients with coronary artery disease in patients with or without healed myocardial infarction. *Am J Cardiol* 74:1183–1186, 1994.
20. Gorgels AP, van den Dool A, Hofs A, et al: Comparison of procainamide and lidocaine in terminating sustained monomorphic ventricular tachycardia. *Am J Cardiol* 78(1):43–46, 1996.
21. Ho DS, Zecchin RP, Richards DA, et al: Double-blind trial of lignocaine versus sotalol for acute termination of spontaneous sustained ventricular tachycardia. *Lancet* 344:18–23, 1994.
22. Jawad-Kanber G, Sherrod TR: Effect of loading dose of procaine amide on left ventricular performance in man. *Chest* 66:269–272, 1974.
23. Nalos PC, Ismail Y, Pappas JM, et al: Intravenous amiodarone for short term treatment of refractory ventricular tachycardia or fibrillation. *Am Heart J* 122:1629–1632, 1991.

24. Tzivoni D, Banai S, Schuger C, et al: Treatment of torsades de pointes with magnesium sulfate. *Circulation* 77:392–397, 1988.
25. Bou-Abboud E, Nattel S: Relative role of alkalosis and sodium ions in reversal of class I antiarrhythmic drug-induced sodium channel blockade by sodium bicarbonate. *Circulation* 94:1954–1961, 1996.
26. Goldman MJ, Mowry JB, Kirk MA: Sodium bicarbonate to correct widened QRS in a case of flecainide overdose. *J Emerg Med* 15:183–186, 1997.
27. Myerburg RJ, Kessler KM, Cox MM, et al: Reversal of proarrhythmic effects of flecainide acetate and encainide hydrochloride by propranolol. *Circulation* 80:1571–1579, 1989.
28. Schutzenberger W, Leisch F, Gmeiner R: Enhanced accessory pathway conduction following intravenous amiodarone in atrial fibrillation. A case report. *Int J Cardiol* 16:93–95. 1987.
29. Schaumann A: Managing atrial tachyarrhythmias in patients with implantable cardioverter defibrillators. *Am J Cardiol* 83:214D–217D, 1999.
30. Krol RB, Saksena S, Prakash A: Interactions of antiarrhythmic drugs with implantable defibrillator therapy for atrial and ventricular tachyarrhythmias. *Curr Cardiol Rep* 1:282–288, 1999.
31. Bigger JT, Fleiss JL, Kleiger R, et al: The relationships among ventricular arrhythmias, left ventricular dysfunction, and mortality in the 2 years after myocardial infarction. *Circulation* 69:250–258, 1984.
32. Mukharji J, Rude RE, Poole WK, et al: Risk factors for sudden death after acute myocardial infarction: two-year follow-up. *Am J Cardiol* 54(1):31–36, 1984.
33. Bikkina M, Larson MG, Levy D: Asymptomatic ventricular arrhythmias and mortality risk in subjects with left ventricular hypertrophy. *J Am Coll Cardiol* 22:1111–1116, 1993.
34. Moss AJ, Hall WJ, Cannom DS, et al; for the MADIT Investigators: Improved survival with an implanted defibrillator in patients with coronary disease at high risk for ventricular arrhythmia. *N Engl J Med* 335:1933–1940, 1996.
35. Buxton AE, Lee KL, Fisher JD, et al: A randomized study of the prevention of sudden death in patients with coronary artery disease. Multicenter Unsustained Tachycardia Trial Investigators. *N Engl J Med* 341:1882–1890, 1999.
36. The Cardiac Arrhythmia Suppression Trial (CAST) Investigators. Preliminary report: effect of encainide and flecainide on mortality in a randomized trial of arrhythmia suppression after myocardial infarction. *N Engl J Med* 321(6):406–412, 1989.
37. MacMahon S, Collins R, Peto R, et al: Effects of prophylactic lidocaine in suspected acute myocardial infarction. An overview of results from the randomized, controlled trials. *JAMA* 1988;260:1910–1916.
38. Gorgels AP, Vos MA, Letsch IS, et al: Usefulness of AIVR as a marker for myocardial necrosis and reperfusion during thrombolysis in acute MI. *Am J Cardiol* 61:231, 1988.
39. Dreifus LS, McKnight EH, Katz M: Digitalis intolerance. *Geriatrics* 18:494–502, 1963.
40. Antman EM, Wenger TL, Butler VP, et al: Treatment of 150 cases of life-threatening digitalis intoxication with digoxin specific Fab antibody fragments: final report of a multicenter study. *Circulation* 81:1744–1752, 1990.
41. Vaughan Williams EM: The relevance of cellular to clinical electrophysiology in classifying antiarrhythmic actions. *J Cardiovasc Pharmacol* 20[Suppl 2]:S1, 1992.
42. Echt DS, Liebson PR, Mitchell LB, et al: Mortality and morbidity in patients receiving encainide, flecainide or placebo: the Cardiac Arrhythmia Suppression Trial. *N Engl J Med* 324:781–788, 1991.
43. The Cardiac Arrhythmia Suppression Trial II Investigators. Effect of the antiarrhythmic agent moricizine on survival after myocardial infarction. *N Engl J Med* 327:227–233, 1992.
44. ISIS I (First International Study of Infarct Survival) Collaborative Group. Randomized trial of intravenous atenolol among 16,027 cases of suspected acute myocardial infarction: ISIS-I. *Lancet* 2:57–65, 1986.
45. Heidenreich PA, Lee TT, Massie BM, et al: Effect of beta-blockade on mortality in patients with heart failure: a meta-analysis of randomized controlled trials. *J Am Coll Cardiol* 30:27–34, 1997.
46. Connoly SJ: Evidenced based analysis of amiodarone efficacy and safety. *Circulation* 100:2025–2034, 1999.
47. The Antiarrhythmics versus Implantable Defibrillators (AVID) Investigators. A comparison of antiarrhythmic-drug therapy with implantable defibrillators in patients resuscitated from near-fatal ventricular arrhythmias. *N Engl J Med* 337:1576–1583, 1997.
48. Kuck KH, Cappato R, Siebels J, et al: Randomized comparison of antiarrhythmic drug therapy with implantable defibrillators in patients resuscitated from cardiac arrest: the Cardiac Arrest Study Hamburg (CASH). *Circulation* 102(7):748–754, 2000.
49. Connolly SJ, Gent M, Roberts RS, et al: Canadian implantable defibrillator study (CIDS): a randomized trial of the implantable cardioverter defibrillator against amiodarone. *Circulation* 101:1297–1302, 2000.
50. Caceres J, Jazayeri M, McKinnie J, et al: Sustained bundle branch reentry as a mechanism of clinical tachycardia. *Circulation* 79:256–270, 1989.
51. Blanck Z, Dhala A, Deshpande S, et al: Bundle branch reentrant ventricular tachycardia: cumulative experience in 48 patients. *J Cardiovasc Electrophysiol* 4:253–262, 1993.
52. Rahilly GT, Prystowsky EN, Zipes DP, et al: Clinical and electrophysiologic findings in patients with repetitive monomorphic ventricular tachycardia and otherwise normal electrocardiogram. *Am J Cardiol* 50:459–468, 1982.
53. Lerman BB: Response of nonreentrant catecholamine-mediated ventricular tachycardia to endogenous adenosine and acetylcholine. Evidence for myocardial receptor-mediated effects. *Circulation* 87:382–390, 1993.
54. Gill JS, Mehta D, Ward DE, Camm AJ: Efficacy of flecainide, sotalol and verapamil in the treatment of right ventricular tachycardia in patients without overt cardiac abnormality. *Br Heart J* 68:392–397, 1992.
55. Wilber DJ, Baerman J, Olshansky B, et al: Adenosine-sensitive ventricular tachycardia. Clinical characteristics and response to catheter ablation. *Circulation* 87:126–134, 1993.
56. Chen Q, Kirsch GE, Zhang D, et al: Genetic basis and molecular mechanism for idiopathic ventricular fibrillation. *Nature* 392:293–296, 1998.
57. Brugada P, Brugada J: Right bundle branch block, persistent ST segment elevation and sudden cardiac death: a distinct clinical and electrocardiographic syndrome. A multicenter report. *J Am Coll Cardiol* 20:1391–1396, 1992.
58. Napolitano C, Priori SG: Diagnosis and treatment of catecholaminergic polymorphic ventricular tachycardia. *Heart Rhythm* 4(5):675–678, 2007.
59. Liu N, Ruan Y, Priori SG: Catecholaminergic polymorphic ventricular tachycardia. *Prog Cardiovasc Dis* 51(1):23–30, 2008.

CHAPTER 42 ■ SUPRAVENTRICULAR TACHYCARDIAS: RECOGNITION AND MANAGEMENT IN THE INTENSIVE CARE SETTING

AMMAR HABIB, JOSEPH J. GARD, TRACI L. BUESCHER AND SAMUEL J. ASIRVATHAM

OVERVIEW AND CLASSIFICATION

Supraventricular tachycardias (SVTs) are frequently encountered in the intensive care unit (ICU) setting [1]. Although generally considered benign, in the context of the critically ill patient, SVTs can be particularly problematic, complicating care and at times, contributing to patient morbidity and mortality.

Atrial fibrillation (AF) and macroreentrant atrial tachycardias are the most common SVTs observed in ICU practice. However, regular reentrant tachycardias such as atrioventricular node reentry (AVNRT) may be initiated or exacerbated by the stress of critical illness or the use of adrenergic agents.

The intensive care provider should be familiar with the common varieties of SVTs and have an approach developed to quickly diagnose the exact arrhythmia (Fig. 42.1). Such diagnosis is essential in the formulation of a management plan for the treatment of acute events as well as prevention of recurrence.

Although several approaches for the diagnosis of SVT have been described, in the context of the critically ill patient, the use of easily recognized parameters aids quick diagnosis and thus prompt institution of a management plan. In most situations, three criteria—regularity of the tachycardia (regular or irregular), QRS width (narrow complex or wide complex), and, when relevant, measurement of the RP interval (interval between the preceding QRS complex and a recognized P wave during tachycardia) provide sufficient data for accurate diagnosis.

In this chapter, regular narrow complex tachycardia is addressed first, followed by the more common irregular tachycardias. Each category includes a description of the pathogenesis, electrocardiographic recognition, and general principles of management of the common varieties. Because of the frequency of occurrence of AF, this arrhythmia is discussed in relatively more depth. For each section, emphasis is placed on points of interest designed to specifically assist the caregiver for critically ill patients.

REGULAR NARROW COMPLEX TACHYCARDIA

When a regular narrow complex tachycardia (QRS duration <120 milliseconds) is observed, several important arrhythmias should be considered in the differential diagnosis. These include sinus tachycardia, AVNRT, atrioventricular reentrant tachycardia (AVRT) using an accessory pathway (AP), and automatic atrial tachycardia. Each of these arrhythmias is discussed in more detail in the text to follow. Atrial flutter may present as a regular tachycardia, but often because of variable atrioventricular (AV) conduction block, it manifests as an irregular tachycardia and may be confused with AF. Junctional tachycardia is also a rare regular narrow complex tachycardia that is typically self limited and very unusual in the adult intensive care patient population.

These tachycardias may be of sudden onset and abrupt termination (AVNRT, AVRT) or may occur and dissipate gradually (sinus tachycardia, automatic atrial tachycardia). A useful further distinguishing electrocardiographic feature within this subset of SVTs is the RP interval. First, a careful search for the P wave should take place. If the P wave is recognized, it should be determined whether it occurs closer to the preceding QRS or to the succeeding QRS complex. If the P wave occurs closer to the succeeding QRS (long R–P tachycardia), sinus tachycardia and atrial tachycardia should be considered (Fig. 42.2). When the P wave is closer to the preceding QRS (short R–P tachycardia), AVNRT or AVRT are likely although important exceptions exist [2–4].

The P wave morphology may also be useful in determining the mechanism of arrhythmia. The P wave in sinus rhythm (upright in leads II, III, and aVF and biphasic in lead V_1) is easily recognized. When an abrupt change in the P wave morphology occurs regardless of the heart rate, a nonsinus mechanism including atrial tachycardia should be suspected (Fig. 42.3).

Sinus Tachycardia

Metabolic stress commonly encountered in the critically ill patient often causes increased automaticity of the sinus node, producing a regular narrow complex tachycardia. Other causes of sinus tachycardia in the critical care setting include administration of adrenergic medications, hypovolemia, and inflammation. Sinus tachycardia is characterized on ECG by regular PR interval and a uniform P wave morphology that is upright in leads II, III, and aVF. Ventricular rate typically ranges from 100 to 140 beats per minute with gradual variation in response to the underlying clinical condition or therapeutic intervention.

Sinus tachycardia is often a normal physiologic response to underlying systemic illness. Treatment of the underlying cause usually helps slow down the heart rate. At times, however, the increased heart rate (albeit a physiologic response to some other stress) may itself be detrimental. For example, in patients with critical coronary disease, rapid sinus rates may give rise to an acute ischemic syndrome and possible ventricular arrhythmia. Similarly, in conditions such as critical mitral stenosis and severe diastolic dysfunction, rapid rates are detrimental as diastolic filling times need to be maximized. In these circumstances, temporary use of beta-blockers or calcium channel blockers

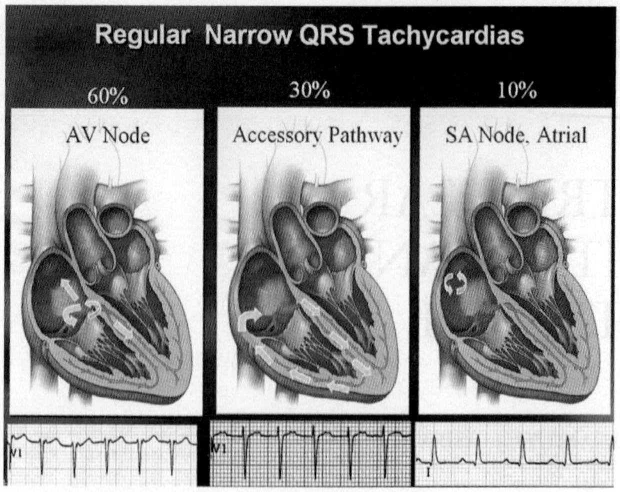

FIGURE 42.1. Narrow complex tachycardias in the intensive care unit. The most common regular narrow QRS tachycardias are atrioventricular node reentry, accessory-pathway related tachycardia, and automatic tachycardias such as sinus tachycardia and atrial tachycardia. These arrhythmias can be readily differentiated in most cases with careful analysis of the electrocardiogram. A long RP tachycardia (*right panel*) where each P wave is closer to the succeeding rather than the preceding QRS is characteristic of sinus tachycardia and atrial tachycardia. In tachycardias where an extranodal accessory pathway is used for retrograde conduction (orthodromic reciprocating tachycardia, ORT), a short RP interval is seen with an easily discernible retrograde P wave. With AV node reentry (*left panel*), because AV activation proceeds from a common turnaround point in or near the AV node, the R wave and P wave may be nearly simultaneous producing a very short RP interval and difficult to discern P wave (see text for details).

can decrease heart rates while the primary cause of the sinus tachycardia is being investigated.

Automatic *atrial tachycardias* are very similar in occurrence to sinus tachycardia in the intensive care setting. They are frequently seen in patients in shock, under stress, or on high doses of beta-adrenergic agents (epinephrine, high-dose dopamine). They can be readily distinguished from sinus tachycardia by close analysis of the P wave morphology. Unlike sinus tachycardia, however, these arrhythmias are not always a result of a persistent underlying abnormality (blood loss, hypoxia, etc.) and may be a primary cause of functional deterioration in a given patient [5,6]. Sodium channel blockers (class I antiarrhythmic agents) can be used for both acute termination and prevention of recurrences [7–9]. Typically, however, treatment of the underlying problem and decreasing the use of intravenous sympathomimetics is sufficient to prevent recurrence in patients who have developed atrial tachycardia in the setting of critical illness.

Specific Considerations in the Intensive Care Unit

In patients who are continuously monitored, sinus tachycardia can often be diagnosed by looking at the transition from normal heart rates to the present rate of tachycardia. For example, if the patient has a regular long R–P tachycardia at 170 beats per minute, all intervening rates from the baseline rate (100, 110, 130, 150 bpm, etc.) will be seen and demonstrate gradual onset of the tachycardia with progressively faster rates and a reverse pattern of resolution.

If an abrupt increase in heart rate is noted, a non-sinus mechanism should be suspected. However, some critically ill

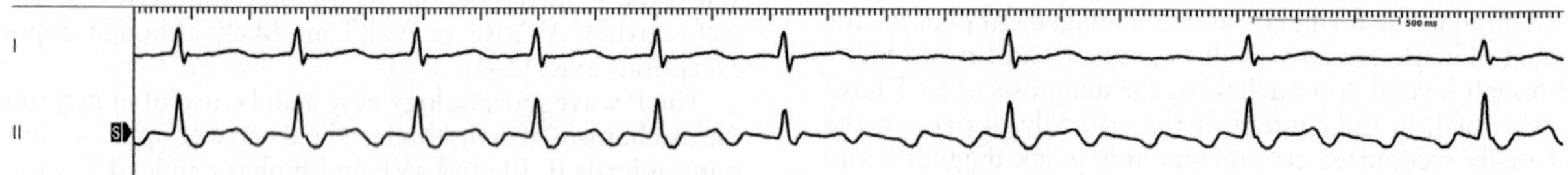

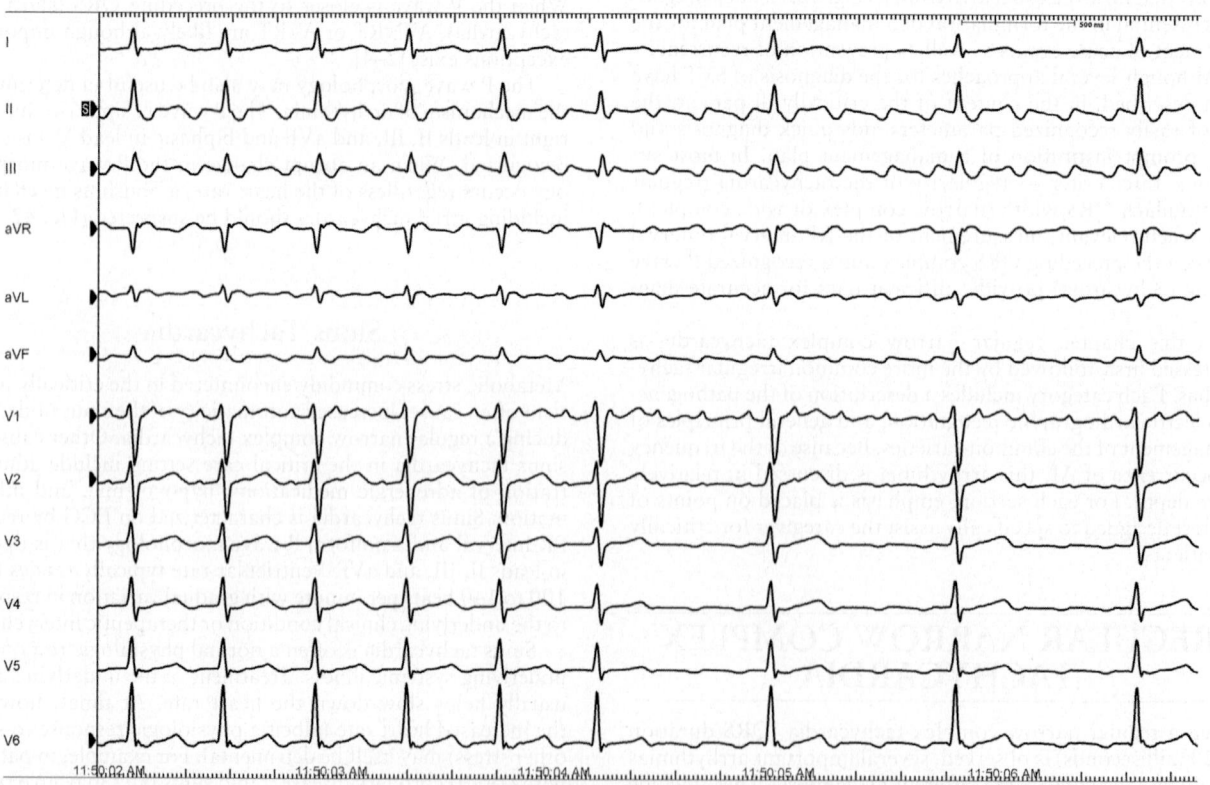

FIGURE 42.2. Patient with initially regular SVT than with a change in ventricular response rate. The underlying supraventricular arrhythmia is an atrial tachycardia (automatic or macroreentrant). Note the differences in P wave morphology to sinus rhythm with negative P waves in the inferior leads and all positive P wave (not biphasic) in lead V_1. The abrupt changes in ventricular responses may exacerbate symptoms especially in patients already compromised with critical illness.

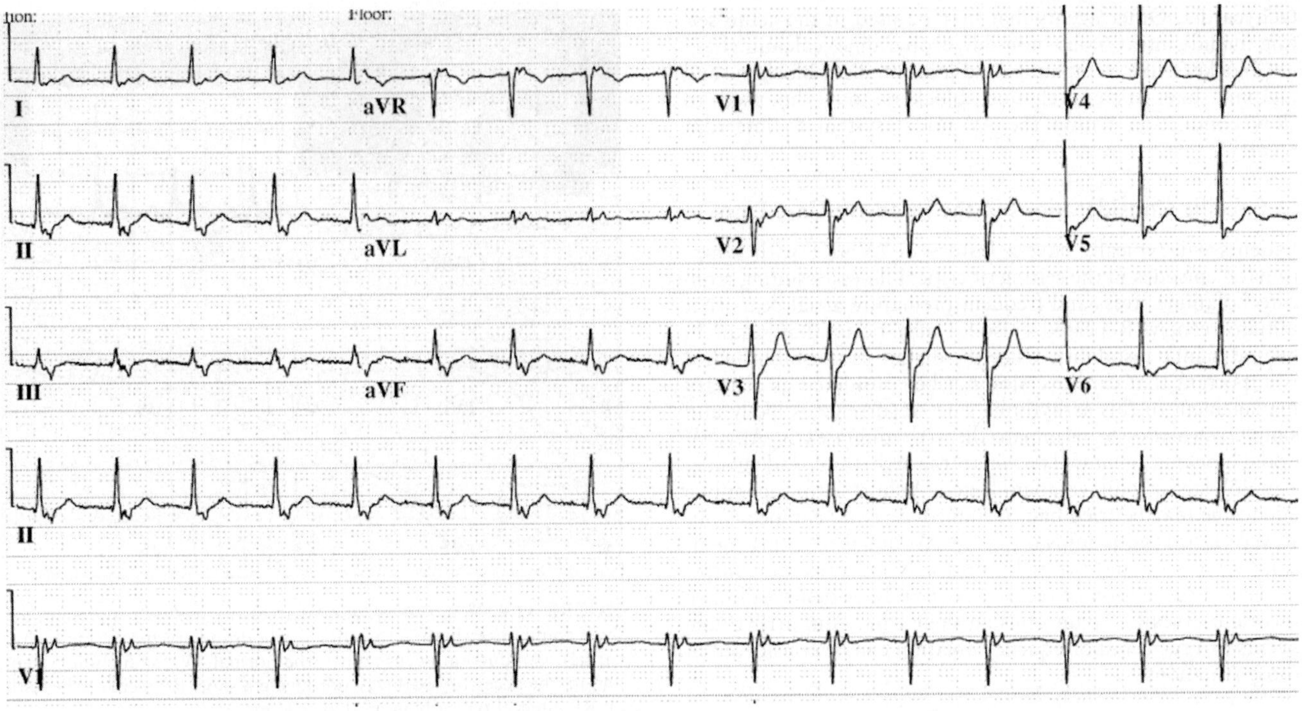

FIGURE 42.3. 12-Lead electrocardiogram of typical atrioventricular node reentry (AVNRT). The P waves are readily recognized just following the QRS complex. The regular tachycardia with short RP interval should raise suspicion for this arrhythmia. The P waves are typically very narrow in AVNRT as a result of the early septal activation during this tachycardia. AV nodal blockade will terminate the arrhythmia and likely prevent recurrence. This arrhythmia may be hemodynamically poorly tolerated even when relatively slow because of the near simultaneous atrioventricular activation. This results in atrial contraction against a closed atrioventricular valve producing increased back pressure in the venous beds (systemic and pulmonary).

patients develop inappropriate sinus tachycardia—a disorder of the autonomic control of the sinus node that results in P wave morphology identical to sinus rhythm but with abrupt and frequent increases in the heart rate for no apparent or definable reason [10–12]. Inappropriate sinus tachycardia may also be associated with other features of autonomic dysfunction and contribute to hypotension. Persistent tachycardia can be a feature of this condition, especially when patients recover from catastrophic illness.

Atrioventricular Nodal Reentry Tachycardia

AVNRT is a common arrhythmia in the ICU and the most common form of regular SVT, accounting for approximately 60% of cases [1,13]. It is more common in female patients between the ages of 20 and 40 years. Patients may complain of palpitations that occur with sudden onset and resolve spontaneously [14]. In addition, some patients may experience the urge to micturate either during or after termination of the rhythm. Older and debilitated patients may have severe symptoms in addition to the palpitations including angina and syncope.

AVNRT is a reentrant tachycardia that has a complex circuit. The atrial myocardial inputs to the AV node are discrete, involving an anterior input called the fast pathway and a posterior input in the region of the coronary sinus (CS) called the slow pathway. Because of these discrete inputs, in some patients, there is sufficient disparity in the conduction times and refractory periods of the two pathways, allowing initiation and maintenance of a reentrant tachycardia (AVNRT) [15–17].

In sinus rhythm, there is near simultaneous antegrade conduction through both the fast and slow pathway. Conduction proceeds more rapidly in the fast pathway and is responsible for the normal PR interval and conduction to the ventricle. Retrograde penetration of the slow pathway occurs and prevents the antegrade wave front through the slow pathway from reaching the AV node. Consequently, slow pathway activation remains electrically silent. When a premature atrial beat occurs, block in conduction down the fast pathway (relatively shorter refractory period) allows antegrade conduction with a long PR interval down the slow pathway. From this site, retrograde activation of the fast pathway may now occur and the reentrant arrhythmia ensues. Accordingly, the typical electrocardiographic feature of initiation of AVNRT is a premature atrial contraction with a long PR interval followed by the sudden onset of a regular narrow complex tachycardia with a very short RP interval.

AVNRT is characterized on ECG by a regular narrow complex tachycardia with P waves buried within or appearing either just before or after the QRS complex. The P wave is often closer to the preceding QRS complex, giving rise to a short RP tachycardia. The RP interval reflects the time from ventricular activation to atrial activation and is short in AVNRT because of the rapid conduction of the impulse retrograde to the atrium via the fast pathway. "Short RP" tachycardias signify fast retrograde activation that is characteristic of AVNRT. Ventricular rate is often noted to be between 150 and 250 beats per minute.

Acute management of symptomatic AVNRT often begins with attempts at Valsalva-like maneuvers which increase vagal tone and influence pathway refractoriness. If these are effective, no further therapy is usually required [18]. Medical therapy is indicated in patients with continued symptoms. Adenosine may be used as a first-line treatment and invariably terminates the tachycardia. Other agents that may be used in the acute setting include intravenous (non-dihydropyridine) calcium channel blockers like verapamil or diltiazem. Beta-blockers and digoxin, like calcium channel blockers, may be used to slow conduction within the AV nodal system to interrupt reentry.

Specific Considerations in the Intensive Care Unit

Patients will typically have a history of AVNRT with symptomatic episodes in the setting of critical illness resulting from catecholamine stress and frequent premature atrial beats that initiate reentry. Repeated episodes may occur that result in hemodynamic instability. Once the diagnosis is established, it is important that cardioversion not be considered as primary management of this arrhythmia since recurrence is likely and simpler measures to terminate the arrhythmia exist. Any AV nodal blocking agent will terminate the arrhythmia (adenosine, esmolol, metoprolol, verapamil, etc.). A short-acting agent like adenosine may be tried first. If immediate reappearance is observed, intravenous infusion of an AV nodal blocking agent can be initiated and titrated both for blood pressure control as well as prevention of recurrence. Rarely, patients will have incessant AVNRT compromising their care. Anti-arrhythmic agents or urgent radiofrequency ablation can be considered in those situations.

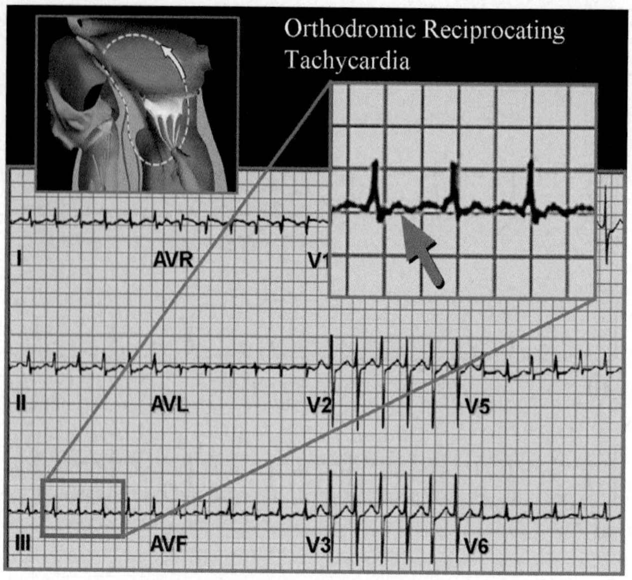

FIGURE 42.4. When an extranodal accessory pathway is present, the most common arrhythmia is ORT (orthodromic reciprocating tachycardia). Conduction occurs down the normal AV conduction system and up the accessory pathway producing a short RP tachycardia with an RP interval typically more than 100 ms.

Atrioventricular Reentry Tachycardia

AVRT is caused by a reentrant circuit that involves both the AV node and an extranodal AP. APs are typically muscular connections that traverse the AV annulus connecting atrial and ventricular myocardium directly, thus bypassing the AV node [19–21].

There are several manifestations with APs that may result in electrocardiographic changes and arrhythmia in the intensive care setting. In sinus rhythm, when the AP conducts in an antegrade direction, a typical constellation of electrocardiogram (ECG) findings result. The early part of the QRS is abnormal (δ wave) because of preexcitation of the ventricular myocardium rather than depolarization via the usual infrahisian conduction system. The combination of a short PR interval in addition to the δ wave enables ECG diagnosis of preexcitation. Wolff–Parkinson–White (WPW) syndrome results when reentrant tachycardia occurs in the presence of this pattern of preexcitation.

Reentrant tachycardias include those with antegrade conduction down the AV node and up the AP (orthodromic-reciprocating tachycardia) and the inverse circuit with antegrade conduction down the AP and retrograde conduction up the AV node (antidromic tachycardia). Finally, preexcited atrial fibrillation is a potentially life-threatening arrhythmia, the recognition and management of which is discussed in the text to follow (Figs. 42.4–42.6).

AVRT is a reentrant narrow complex tachycardia like AVNRT. Patients with AVRT have an AP that allows conduction to bypass the AV node. An impulse, either a premature atrial contraction or a premature ventricular contraction, travels to the AV node through the bundle of His, activating the ventricular system. Subsequently, the propagation travels up the AP causing retrograde conduction back to the atrium. This circuit is known as *orthodromic* AVRT because the antegrade pathway conducts the impulse to the ventricles via the normal AV node and His–Purkinje system. Orthodromic AVRT generally has a narrow QRS complex but may have a wide QRS complex when there is an underlying bundle-branch block. The ventricular rate continues to be controlled by the AV node during orthodromic AVRT. Because it is a regular narrow complex tachycardia, it may be difficult to distinguish this rhythm from AVNRT or atrial tachycardia (discussed later). Termination of this rhythm usually transpires secondary to AV nodal conduction fatigue, increased vagal tone, or a premature extrasystolic beat.

Antidromic tachycardia manifests as a regular *wide* complex tachycardia and can occur in patients with antegrade conducting APs [22,23] (Fig. 42.7). This variant is less common but important to recognize since it may be confused with ventricular tachycardia. Initiation typically occurs with a premature atrial contraction that blocks in the AV node. Antegrade conduction proceeds via the AP to the ventricle with the return

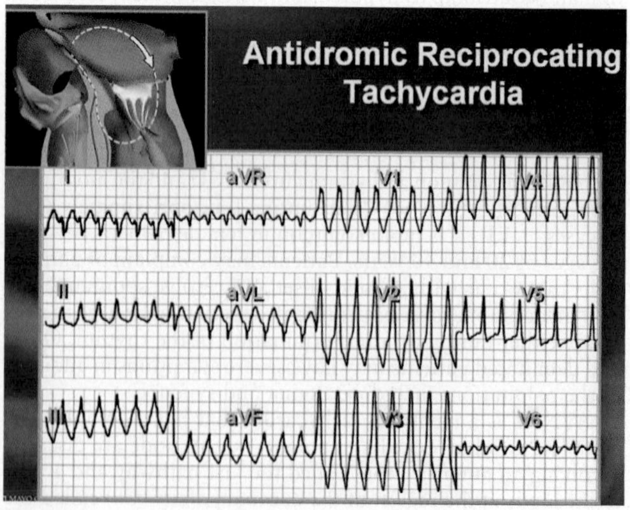

FIGURE 42.5. When an extranodal accessory pathway is present, a regular wide complex tachycardia may also result. Here, the tachycardia circuit proceeds antegrade down the accessory pathway and up through the AV nodal conduction system producing a regular wide QRS tachycardia with the QRS morphology dependent on the site of the accessory pathway. ART, antidromic-reciprocating tachycardia.

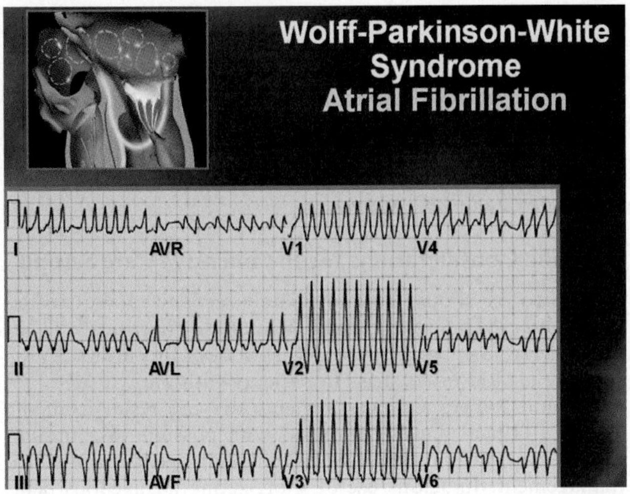

FIGURE 42.6. Potential life-threatening arrhythmia seen in patients when extranodal accessory pathway is preexcited atrial fibrillation. The AV node normally protects the ventricle from rapid ventricular rates during atrial fibrillation. However, when an accessory pathway is present, conduction may proceed down the accessory pathway as well as the AV node producing extremely rapid ventricular rates. The characteristics of a preexcited AF electrocardiogram include irregularly irregular R-R intervals along with rapid rates and importantly, irregular QRS duration and morphology as well (see text for details).

limb of the circuit through retrograde AV nodal conduction. Both orthodromic and antidromic AVRT are dependent on AV nodal conduction, and thus, AV nodal blockade (adenosine, beta-blockers, etc.) will terminate the arrhythmia and prevent recurrence. In contrast, a *preexcited* tachycardia occurs when another SVT (independent of the pathway) such as sinus tachycardia, AF, atrial flutter, etc., arises, but because of the presence of the antegrade conducting AP, rapid conduction to the ventricle takes place, bypassing the AV node. For these arrhythmias, AV nodal blockade would be contraindicated as there would be promotion of rapid aberrant conduction via the AP predisposing to ventricular arrhythmias. This is particularly problematic during AF when direct conduction through the antegrade AP may lead to ventricular fibrillation. The 2003 American College of Cardiology/American Heart Association (ACC/AHA) SVT management guidelines indicated that the incidence of sudden death with WPW is increased in patients with a minimum R-R interval <250 milliseconds during AF (regardless of whether AF is spontaneous or induced), a history of symptomatic tachycardia, multiple APs, and Ebstein's anomaly [24].

The acute management of regular tachycardia in patients with APs (orthodromic or antidromic AVRT) is similar and consists of AV nodal blockade to terminate the arrhythmia and the use of longer-term beta-blockers or calcium channel blockers to prevent recurrence. AV nodal blocking therapy is often sufficient as a temporizing maneuver until the patient's critical illness subsides and definitive ablation therapy can be offered [25,26].

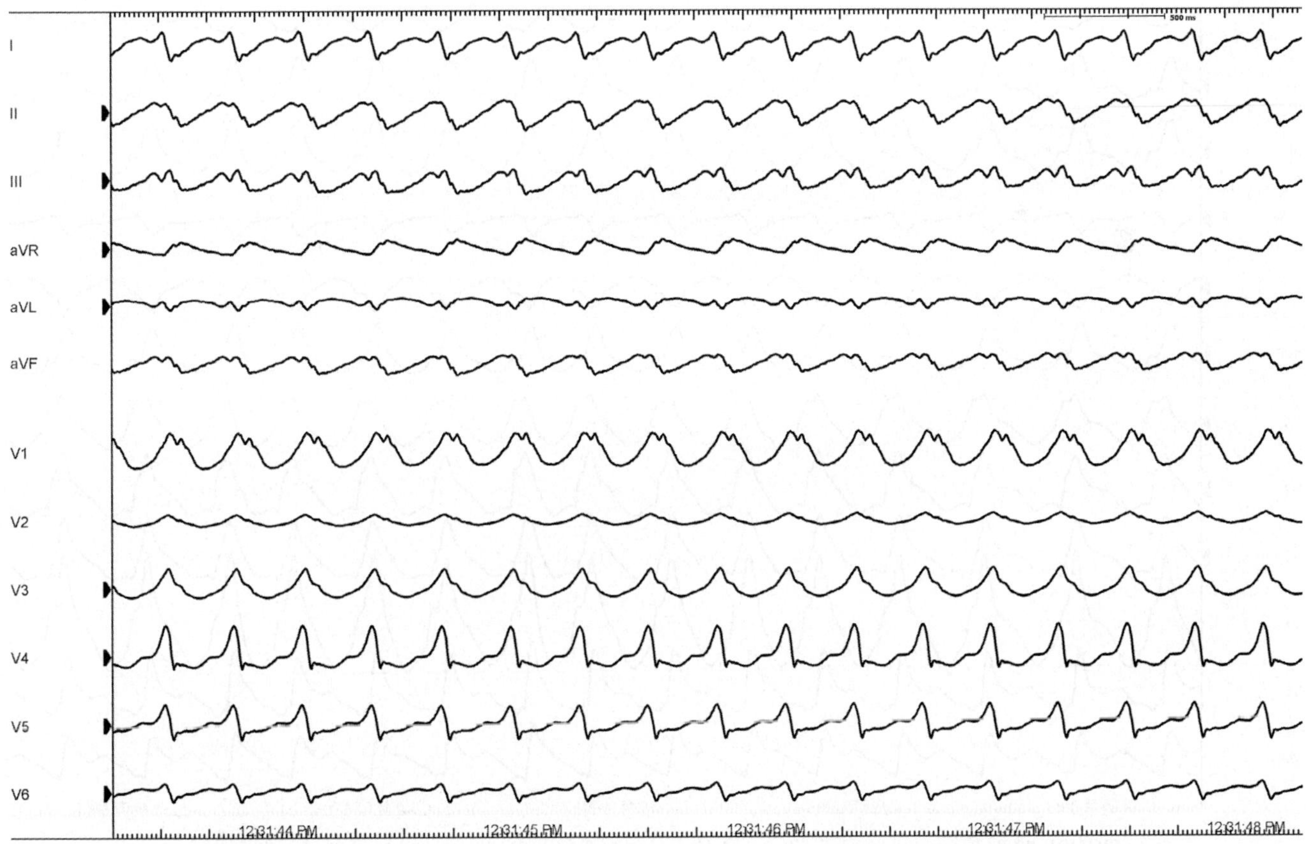

FIGURE 42.7. Regular wide complex tachycardia. When a regular wide complex tachycardia is seen in the critical care setting, ventricular tachycardia should always be considered. However, if the baseline electrocardiogram shows preexcitation, an *antidromic* tachycardia can be diagnosed and easily terminated with any AV nodal blocking agent. If the baseline electrocardiogram is not available, wide QRS tachycardia with consistent 1:1 R–P association in the absence of structural heart disease should raise suspicion for an accessory pathway-mediated mechanism.

Acute Management of Hemodynamically Significant AVRT

Valsalva-like maneuvers that increase vagal tone may be attempted initially. As with acute treatment of AVNRT, adenosine may be used as a first-line agent for medical management. Because of its very short half-life, a trial of adenosine may be attempted in patients with tenuous hemodynamics prior to emergent cardioversion. However, adenosine may potentially cause increased atrial vulnerability, a serious proarrhythmic side affect [27,28]. An alternative category of drugs often administered in the acute setting for treatment of orthodromic AVRT includes intravenous calcium channel blockers. Intravenous verapamil may be used and repeated every 2 to 3 minutes for acute termination of orthodromic AVRT but may be relatively contraindicated in patients with significant hypotension or depressed ventricular function or heart failure. Additional agents that may be used and often considered second-line treatment include intravenous beta-blockers (like metoprolol and propranolol) and procainamide. Rather than having a direct effect on AV nodal conduction, procainamide acts on the atrial and ventricular myocardium, causing decreased conduction and increase refractoriness of APs and the His–Purkinje system.

In contrast, when an irregular wide complex tachycardia is noted in a patient with known WPW, urgent intervention is required [29–31]. Preexcited AF once recognized, should be immediately terminated (Fig. 42.8). If the patient is hemodynamically unstable, urgent cardioversion is required. If not, an antiarrhythmic agent such as procainamide can be used. Procainamide may chemically convert the patient from AF to sinus rhythm and in addition, suppress conduction via the AP.

Patients with AVRT should be referred to a cardiac electrophysiologist for possible radiofrequency catheter ablation. Catheter ablation is highly successful, is associated with low risk, and eliminates the need for long-term drug therapy [32]. Ablation is often considered first-line therapy in young patients who prefer a curative approach.

Specific Considerations for the Intensive Care Setting

Preexcited AF should be immediately recognized and treated when observed but is an unusual presentation in critically ill patients. More commonly, repeated episodes of reentrant AVRT (usually orthodromic) arise in patients with known APs. Frequent and sometimes incessant episodes can result from the stress of critical illness combined with possible discontinuation of previously used AV nodal blocking agents for medical management. Judicious use of short-acting intravenous beta-blockers will help prevent recurrences of arrhythmia without major untoward hemodynamic consequences.

Caregivers of the critically ill patient must also be aware that the presence of a WPW pattern on the EKG by itself is not a contraindication to use beta-blockers or other AV nodal blocking agents if clinically required for comorbid illnesses such as coronary disease. If, however, a patient with WPW has AF, AV nodal blocking agents should be avoided or used in conjunction with antiarrhythmic agents like procainamide to suppress AP conduction (Fig. 42.9).

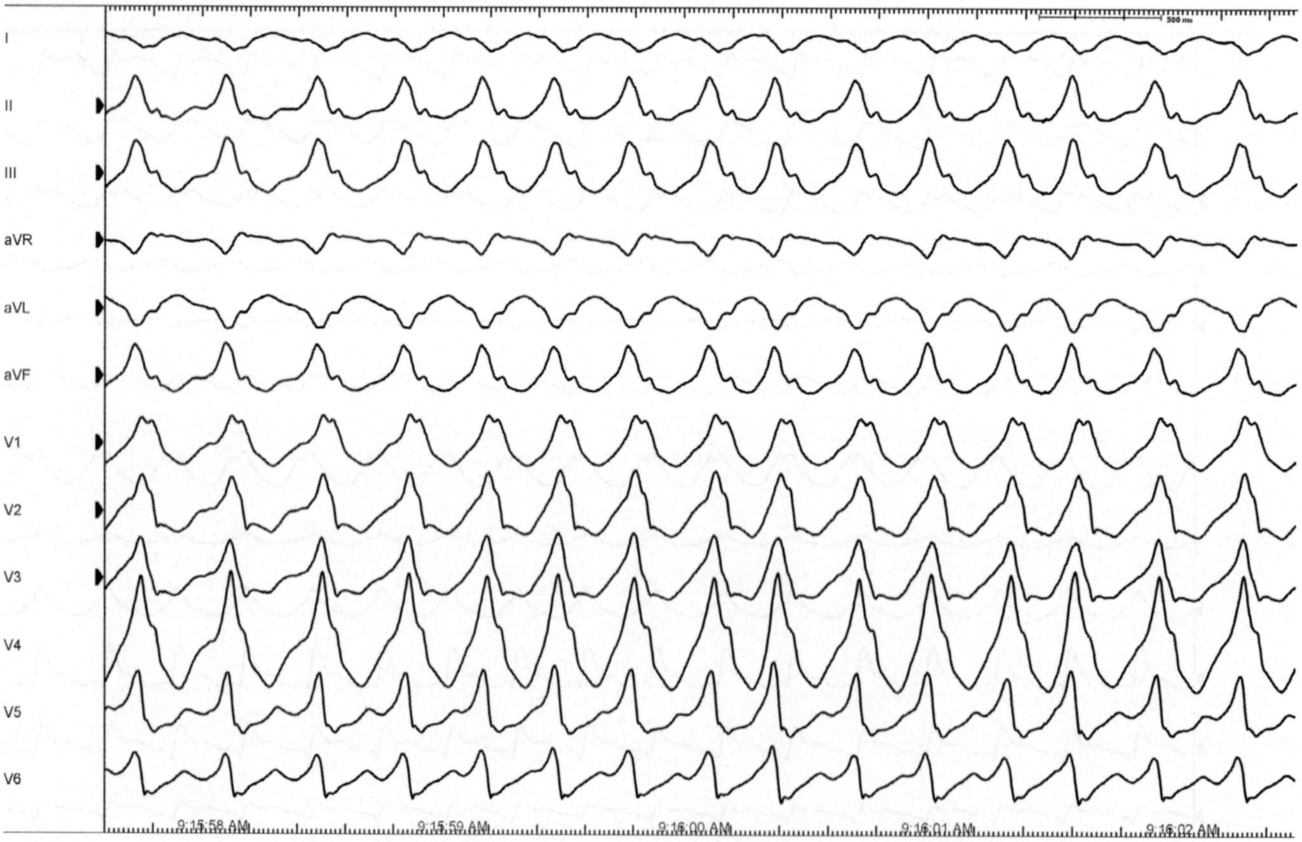

FIGURE 42.8. Preexcited atrial fibrillation. All caregivers for critically ill patients should be familiar with this pattern. An irregular wide complex tachycardia is noted. Importantly, the ventricular rates are fast, and each QRS morphology is slightly different. Especially if the baseline electrocardiogram had shown preexcitation (WPW) pattern, this urgent condition of preexcited atrial fibrillation should be immediately recognized. Regardless of present symptoms, cardioversion should be considered if the patient is relatively unstable; chemical cardioversion with an agent such as procainamide that may convert the atrial fibrillation to sinus rhythm and simultaneously slow conduction to the accessory pathway can be tried.

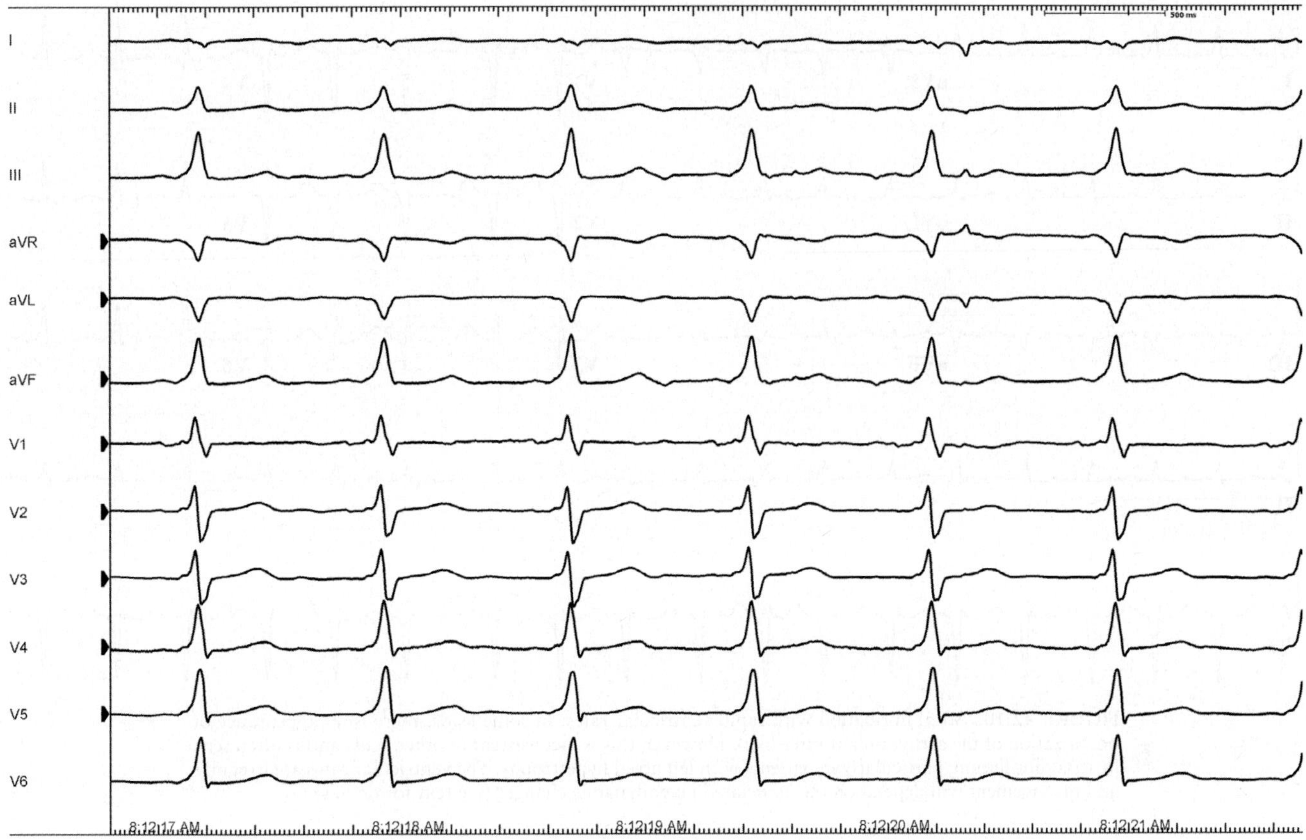

FIGURE 42.9. Characteristic electrocardiogram in patient with antegrade preexcitation. Note the short PR interval and the δ wave clearly seen in the lateral precordial leads and lead II. The R wave seen in lead V_1 and negative δ wave in lead I is consistent with the left-sided accessory pathway. If a patient with this baseline electrocardiogram develops atrial fibrillation, this should be treated as a medical emergency because of risk of ventricular fibrillation from the atrial fibrillatory waves conducting to the ventricle via this pathway without the intervening protective effects of the AV node.

IRREGULAR NARROW COMPLEX TACHYCARDIA

Several of the regular narrow complex tachycardias already discussed may occasionally present with irregular R-R intervals. However, by far, the most common irregular narrow complex tachycardia occurring in an ICU setting is AF. In this section, we discuss this common arrhythmia in detail, presenting information on pathogenesis, recognition of variants, and acute management in the critically ill patient. Although less common, atrial flutter with variable conduction block and multifocal atrial tachycardia should be distinguished from AF since management differs significantly.

Atrial Fibrillation

AF is the most common type of arrhythmia, and the most common SVT seen in the ICU. Incidence increases with age; it is found in less than 0.1% of adults younger than 55 years but in more than 9% of the population age 80 years or older [33,34]. AF is characterized by the presence of chaotic appearing multiple shifting reentrant atrial wavelets that may appear flat or irregular. Classification of AF usually depends on the duration and frequency of occurrence. Paroxysmal AF makes up about 40% of cases and may last up to 7 days, terminating spontaneously. Nonparoxysmal AF lasts more than 7 days and requires cardioversion for termination. Identification of AF is important clinically because of the increased risk of hemodynamic instability and mortality associated with this arrhythmia in the intensive care setting. AF is characterized by irregular atrial contractions, as demonstrated on ECG by irregularly irregular f waves that may manifest as continuous irregular variation in the baseline (Fig. 42.10).

AF may become problematic to patients in the intensive care setting due to hemodynamic instability. Hemodynamic compromise is likely in cases of AF associated with rapid ventricular response, especially when associated with diastolic dysfunction. In addition, hemodynamic instability is common in AF with rapid ventricular response in patients in whom a more prolonged diastolic filling period would be desirable, such as mitral stenosis, hypertrophic obstructive cardiomyopathy, restrictive cardiomyopathy, or constrictive pericardial disease. Patients with underlying WPW syndrome who develop AF can have hemodynamic instability due to a rapidly conducting antegrade AP as previously mentioned. If antegrade AP conduction is present during AF, ECG findings show an irregular wide complex tachycardia with varying degrees of ventricular preexcitation. As mentioned previously in the discussion of AVRT management, AV nodal blocking agents are contraindicated in this instance as they may enhance antegrade AP conduction and increase risk of ventricular fibrillation.

Another important complication of AF is thrombus formation in the left atrium that may embolize to the cerebral circulation and ultimately result in ischemic stroke. Therefore, early recognition of AF, its risk factors, and proper treatment is prudent in the management of the critically ill patient.

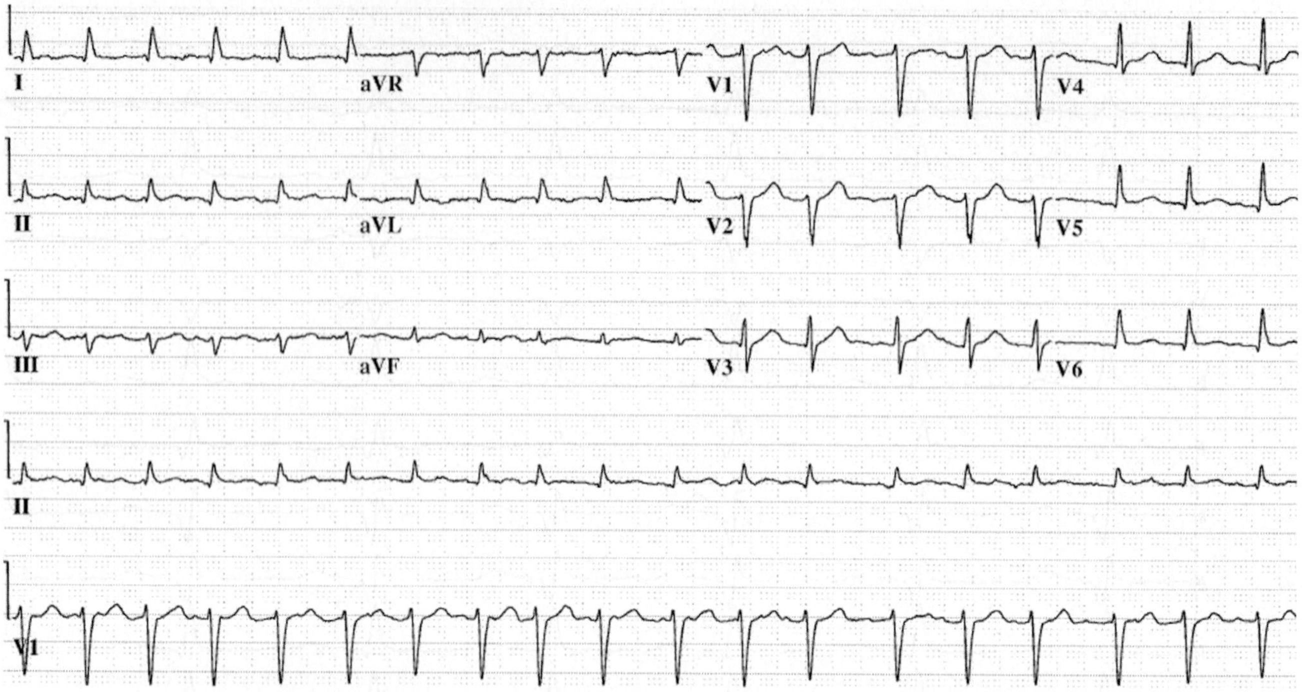

FIGURE 42.10. Atrial fibrillation with rapid ventricular rates. In some leads, there is an appearance of organization of the arrhythmia (flutter-like). However, this is inconsistent in other leads and is often seen in atrial fibrillation, particularly in patients with left atrial hypertrophy. The ventricular rates are irregular and management will depend on the associated hemodynamic changes (see text for details).

Causes of Atrial Fibrillation

Initiation and maintenance of AF varies and often is multifactorial. The three main initiating causes include rapidly discharging triggers or foci, the autonomic nervous system that triggers activity, and substrate abnormalities that permit and promote wavelet reentry [35–37]. The pulmonary veins are lined with myocardium that has a shorter effective refractory period and is capable of more rapid discharge than the endocardium. The muscular lining of the pulmonary veins is the most common site of rapid discharge leading to the initiation and maintenance of AF. The autonomic nervous system is also an important source in initiating AF. Sympathetic stimulation may facilitate altered automaticity and result in focal discharge. In addition, enhanced vagal tone may shorten the refractory period and increase heterogeneity. Patients with conditions like myocarditis, congestive heart failure, valvular heart disease, coronary artery disease, hypertension, and other diseases leading to atrial stretch and interstitial fibrosis may develop AF due to these substrate abnormalities. Substrate abnormalities cause heterogeneity in electrophysiologic cellular properties leading to breakdown in waveform propagation and multiple wavelet reentry. Because of electrical remodeling, the more frequent AF occurs, the greater the likelihood of further AF episodes [38,39].

In addition, several reversible risk factors have been identified to be associated with AF, and these should be recognized by the practitioner to aid in proper management. The most common underlying disease that may lead to AF is hypertension [40]. Studies have shown that treatment of hypertension with ACE inhibitors or ARBs may reduce the incidence of AF, especially in patients with altered left ventricular function [41]. The utilization of beta-blockers is also effective in controlling ventricular response. AF has been associated with up to 10% of patients suffering from an acute myocardial infarction. The underlying mechanism is thought to be secondary to atrial stretch or remodeling due to cardiomyopathy [42]. Other cardiac risk factors include pericarditis, myocarditis, congenital heart disease, and valvular heart disease. Obesity and metabolic syndrome have also been linked to AF [43]. Pulmonary embolism is also a risk factor for AF and should never be overlooked in the intensive care or postoperative setting. Consumption of excessive amounts of alcohol is a well-known risk factor for AF. Binge drinkers have a significantly increased risk of developing AF, a phenomenon referred to as *holiday heart syndrome* [44]. Moderate use of alcohol, in contrast, has not been consistently shown to be associated with AF [45]. Surgery, both cardiac and noncardiac is also associated with the development of AF. Cardiac surgeries, especially coronary artery bypass grafting and valvular repair or replacement, have a greater association with the development of AF than noncardiac surgeries. Perioperative administration of beta-blockers for prophylactic treatment has been shown to significantly reduce the incidence of AF in this setting [46,47]. Additional noncardiac risks factors associated with AF include obstructive sleep apnea, thyrotoxicosis, and inflammatory states.

AF is common in the surgical perioperative period (predominantly in the first 4 postoperative days), and as previously mentioned, most often observed in patients undergoing cardiac surgery. Studies have reported that AF may occur in up to 40% of patients undergoing coronary artery bypass grafting and up to 60% in those undergoing combined coronary grafting and valve surgery [48–50]. Postoperative AF may be reduced by administration of prophylactic doses of beta-blockers, calcium channel blockers, amiodarone, corticosteroids, or even lipid-lowering agents [51–54]. The increased incidence of AF in the perioperative setting is unknown but thought to be secondary to atrial ischemia, atrial incisions, pericarditis, inflammation, changes in autonomic tone, and large fluid shifts. Important risk factors for the development of AF postoperatively include cessation of beta-blocker therapy, chronic obstructive pulmonary disease, left atrial enlargement, advanced age, heart failure, and a previous history of AF. Atrial fibrillation in this setting is self-limited and usually resolves completely within 8 weeks.

Management of Atrial Fibrillation

The goal of AF treatment is to minimize symptoms (palpitations, shortness of breath, lightheadedness, dizziness, and fatigue), prevent or reduce tachycardia-induced cardiomyopathy, and prevent thromboembolic complications like stroke. Whether treatment of AF results in favorable outcomes is unknown. Although the Framingham study showed increased incidence of mortality in patients with AF after adjustment for common confounders, other, more recent studies have not shown that treatment contributes to improved survival rates [55]. However, as with all other arrhythmias, it is prudent to evaluate and assess the hemodynamic stability of a patient with AF. As mentioned previously, critically ill patients may develop hemodynamic instability in association with AF, especially those for whom a shortened diastolic filling period would be detrimental (e.g. mitral stenosis, hypertrophic obstructive cardiomyopathy, restrictive cardiomyopathy, constrictive pericarditis) or WPW. In these instances, synchronized direct current (DC) cardioversion is indicated. Premedication with an anxiolytic, opiates, or generalized anesthesia is appropriate. DC cardioversion usually results in successful conversion to normal sinus rhythm in a majority of cases. Treatment with intravenous procainamide or ibutilide may also be used in patients with AF and a wide-complex tachycardia associated with hemodynamic instability as these patients may have underlying WPW. Eventually, patients with AF in the setting of underlying WPW should undergo radiofrequency ablation of the AP once deemed clinically suitable.

In hemodynamically stable patients, a more conservative management approach is taken. Once the patient is considered to be hemodynamically stable, a history and physical examination focusing on delineating a possible reversible cause of AF should be undertaken. Common, reversible causes of AF in the critically ill patient include myocardial infarction, pericarditis, infection or inflammation, pulmonary embolism, hyperthyroidism, recent cardiac surgery, and stroke. In addition, a review of possible iatrogenic causes including administration of proarrhythmic medications like common sympathomimetics should be made. Special attention to electrolyte abnormalities and correction should also be done. The ultimate goal of therapy for otherwise hemodynamically stable patients who develop acute onset AF is improvement of quality of life by controlling rate, rhythm, or both, and providing anticoagulation when indicated.

Strategies that focus on either rate control or rhythm control in hemodynamically stable patients may be used. Rate control refers to an approach that uses AV nodal blocking agents to decrease ventricular rate and improve hemodynamics. Calcium channel blockers, beta-blockers, or even AV nodal ablation may be used to control the ventricular rate. Conversely, rhythm control is an attempt to keep the patient in sinus rhythm. Strategies include cardioversion, antiarrhythmic drug treatment, percutaneous ablation, and various surgical procedures. As discussed previously, the ultimate goal of treatment of AF is to improve the quality of life. Therefore, management with both rate control and rhythm control provides the greatest improvement in symptoms. However, the AFFIRM (Atrial Fibrillation Follow-up Investigation of Rhythm Management) trial, a study of 4,060 patients older than 65 years with a history of AF and additional risk factors for stroke and death who were randomly assigned to receive either rate control or rhythm control therapy showed no significant difference in improvement of quality of life between rate control strategies and rhythm control strategies [56]. As a result, individualizing treatment strategies to the patient's needs is important in management of AF. Although treatment strategies may vary, elderly patients who have minimal symptoms are often managed with rate control, whereas younger patients with significant symptoms and structural heart disease are often managed with rhythm control.

Specific Considerations for the Intensive Care Setting. In all patients with AF, systematic consideration to whether rate or rhythm control strategies should be adopted, and a decision as to which anticoagulation strategy is most appropriate should be made. In the critically ill patient, timely judgment regarding treatment with either urgent control of rate or rhythm becomes more crucial. In addition, a careful analysis of the potential risks associated with slowing of the heart rate or the development of proarrhythmic complications from antiarrhythmic therapy is needed.

Atrial fibrillation with obvious hemodynamic collapse requires urgent cardioversion regardless of anticoagulation status, attempts at rate control, etc. This situation is quite rare. Whenever significant hemodynamic compromise is noted in a patient with AF (particularly with reasonably controlled rates), another cause for hypotension or shock should be investigated. However, in patients with significant valvular disease (critical aortic stenosis) or with severe diastolic ventricular dysfunction (longstanding hypertension, hypertrophic cardiomyopathy), the onset of AF can be very symptomatic and occasionally lead to hypotension, pulmonary edema, and findings consistent with cardiogenic shock.

Nevertheless, in most situations, the clinician should assess systematically for optimal methods to control rate, and if symptoms continue despite rate control, methods to restore sinus rhythm and assess for anticoagulation are needed.

Rate Control

Rate control for patients with AF is often pursued not only to help alleviate symptomatic palpitations, but also to prevent hemodynamic compromise and prevent tachycardia-induced cardiomyopathy that may occur with prolonged rapid ventricular rates. Rate control provides adequate ventricular filling and reduces rate-related ischemia, thus, improving symptoms. On the basis of parameters used in the AFFIRM trial, rate control can be defined as having a resting heart rate of less than 80 beats per minute and a maximal heart rate less than 110 beats per minute during a 6-minute walk [57]. AV nodal blocking agents like beta-blockers and calcium channel blockers are the most commonly used agents in this setting. These agents have predominantly safe profiles. Conversely, awareness of calcium channel blockers' association with heart failure exacerbation must be recognized in patients with low left ventricular ejection fractions. Amiodarone may also be used to achieve rate control. In patients with labile blood pressures, digoxin is often used to provide rate control but may prove insufficient as a single agent.

Alternatively, in chronic settings beyond the scope of the ICU, AV node ablation combined with permanent pacemaker implantation may be considered when pharmacologic rate control therapy is either unsuccessful or not tolerated [58,59]. It is important to note that although AV node ablation decreases symptoms and improves quality of life, studies have shown no impact on overall survival [60,61].

Rate Control Issues in the Intensive Care Setting. Rate control can be particularly difficult when patients are hypotensive in AF as a result of coexisting critical illness. Digitalization is sometimes effective; however, in states of high circulating catecholamines, digoxin is not useful. Administering intravenous calcium just prior to initiating an intravenous calcium channel blocker (diltiazem, verapamil) may sometimes minimize hypotension while achieving reasonable rate control. Careful scrutiny of the utilization of intravenous sympathomimetic agents and titration of dose to decrease AV nodal conduction should be considered. For example, changing from high-dose dopamine or epinephrine to phenylephrine in a patient with septic shock may be sufficient to support the blood pressure without necessarily increasing AV nodal conduction and thus rapid ventricular rates.

Rhythm Control

Management of AF in stable patients may be geared toward restoration of sinus rhythm. DC or chemical cardioversion strategies can be employed. This may be a good option for young patients, but older patients with cardiomegaly and left atrial enlargement are less likely to have successful results. Hemodynamically stable patients who have documented development of acute AF for duration of 48 hours or less may proceed with early cardioversion. Alternatively, hemodynamically stable patients with AF that has lasted for more than 48 hours or have an unknown duration of AF may still undergo cardioversion. It is important to rule out intracardiac thrombus that may be associated with AF and can subsequently embolize with cardioversion and return to normal sinus rhythm. Therefore, two different strategies may be undertaken. First, transesophageal echocardiogram (TEE) can be utilized to rule out intracardiac thrombus formation. Once thrombus is excluded by TEE, cardioversion may proceed using the aforementioned strategies. Subsequent anticoagulation with warfarin is prudent, with an INR goal of 2 to 3 for at least 4 weeks [62]. Another strategy that may be used in patients with AF that has lasted for more than 48 hours or unknown duration is to anticoagulate with a goal INR of 2 to 3 for 3 weeks prior to cardioversion. Patients are subsequently instructed to continue anticoagulation therapy for an additional 4 weeks after cardioversion to prevent thromboembolic events that may result from delayed atrial mechanical recovery in this setting.

Concomitant use of antiarrhythmic medications with DC cardioversion increases the probability not only of successful cardioversion, but also maintenance of sinus rhythm for longer periods of time. Because antiarrhythmic drugs have many proarrhythmic side effects, the particular regimen chosen depends on the clinical setting and the underlying cardiovascular disease. Flecainide, propafenone, or sotalol are often used for patients without underlying structural heart disease. Amiodarone and dofetilide are often recommended in patients with underlying heart failure, while sotalol or dofetilide may be used in patients with coronary artery disease. Consultation with a cardiologist is recommended.

Drugs often used for chemical cardioversion in the acute setting include procainamide, flecainide, propafenone, dofetilide, and ibutilide. Although this is often an appropriate strategy, studies have shown pharmacologic cardioversion to be less effective than DC cardioversion in combination with antiarrhythmic drugs [63]. Studies have demonstrated a better outcome and safety profile with ibutilide compared with propafenone [64,65]. AV nodal blocking agents like beta-blockers or calcium channel blockers should be used with class Ia and Ic antiarrhythmics to prevent conversion of AF to a slow atrial flutter with 1:1 AV conduction.

Rhythm Control Issues in the Intensive Care Setting. A frequent clinical scenario in which AF is encountered in the ICU is the postcardiac surgical patient. The incidence of AF in these patients is high (8% to 34%) [33,49,66]. Because of this, unless a contraindication is present, many ICUs use amiodarone prophylactically in the postoperative period. When AF occurs in other situations and rate control is suboptimal, the choice of antiarrhythmic agent depends primarily on whether structural heart disease is present or not. In patients with structural heart disease, intravenous amiodarone is preferred with attempt at cardioversion either for hemodynamic instability or following initial amiodarone loading. In the absence of structural heart disease, when oral medication can be administered, rate control with a beta-blocker and initiation of a class Ic agent is a common management strategy. In addition, the temporary use of IV amiodarone can be considered until the medical illness subsides and long-term rhythm control with less toxic antiarrhythmic agents or with nonpharmacologic treatment options can be considered [33,51,53,67,68].

Prevention of Thromboembolic Complications

An important aspect in the management of AF is implementation of risk-appropriate anticoagulation. Studies have consistently shown an increase in cardioembolic stroke rates in patients with AF [69–71]. In addition to causing a hypercoagulable state, AF impairs proper atrial contraction leading to blood stasis in the left atrium and ultimately a physiologic state promoting thrombus formation [72,73]. Therefore, an understanding of risk factors for stroke in patients with AF is essential. Risk factors may be easily remembered by using the mnemonic *CHADS2*, which stands for *c*ardiac failure (recent heart failure), history of *h*ypertension, *a*ge greater or equal to 75 years, history of *d*iabetes, and a history of *s*troke or a transient ischemic attack [74]. The number 2 stands for the fact that a history of stroke counts as 2 risk factors points. The CHADS2 mnemonic is also used as a risk stratifying score to help predict patients at significantly increased risk of developing an ischemic stroke from a cardioembolic event in the setting of AF [74]. Based on these scores, the annual predicted stroke risk can be calculated. The adjusted annual stroke rate increases from 1.9% in patients with a CHADS2 score of 0% to 18.2% in patients with a CHADS2 score of 6.

Once the CHADS2 score and the risk for stroke are estimated for patients with AF, the decision on the type of prophylactic antithrombotic therapy, if any, needs to be determined. On the basis of the 2006 ACC/AHA/ESC guidelines for the management of AF, aspirin 81 mg to 325 mg daily is recommended for patients with no risk factors for thromboembolism (CHADS2 score of 0) [75]. Patients with a single risk factor or a CHADS2 score of 1 may be managed with either aspirin 81 to 325 mg daily or an adjusted-dose warfarin regimen with an INR goal of 2.0 to 3.0 [75]. For patients with risks that confer a high-risk score (a previous stroke or TIA, rheumatic mitral stenosis, or a CHADS2 score of 2 or higher), warfarin is recommended with an INR goal of 2.0 to 3.0 [75]. Anticoagulation with other agents like unfractionated or low-molecular-weight heparin may be used as alternative bridging therapy in patients requiring certain procedures or surgeries.

Anticoagulation Issues Relevant in the Intensive Care Unit. Appropriate anticoagulation in the critically ill patient is particularly problematic even when following present guidelines and using the CHADS2 scoring system [76,77]. Postsurgical patients, patients at risk for intracranial bleeding, patients with closed head or closed chest trauma, etc., frequently have a contraindication for systemic anticoagulation. If the patient has chronic AF and the CHADS2 score is ≤ 2, in general, anticoagulation can be safely discontinued for the period of the acute illness. In patients with CHADS2 >2, anticoagulation free intervals should be minimized and aspirin provided if not also contraindicated.

For patients who are hemodynamically compromised with new onset AF, urgent cardioversion can be performed regardless of anticoagulation status. When less urgent, TEE may first be performed to exclude evidence of an intra-atrial thrombus prior to cardioversion and reinitiation of anticoagulation when the risk of bleeding is minimal [78,79]. Atrial appendage occlusion devices, exclusion devices, or minimally invasive surgical techniques may be particularly useful in these situations and are being investigated for clinical efficacy and safety [80,81].

Atrial Flutter

Atrial flutter, like AF, is one of the most common arrhythmias encountered in the critically ill patient. It is identified by a characteristic sawtooth pattern of atrial activity at an atrial rate of 240 to 320 beats per minute. Although variable ventricular conduction may occur, a 2:1 transmission commonly transpires, resulting in a ventricular response rate of about 150 beats per minute. The mechanism of common atrial flutter is a macroreentry loop around the tricuspid annulus. The loop often runs in a counterclockwise direction, causing negative flutter waves in the inferior leads (II, III, aVF). Other reentry patterns may also be encountered but are beyond the scope of this chapter. Occasionally the ventricular rate may be greater than 150 beats per minute, making identification of the flutter waves difficult. Vagal maneuvers like carotid sinus massage or adenosine, a medication that briefly blocks AV nodal conduction, may be used in these instances to slow down the rate and allow for more accurate identification of the arrhythmia.

Patients with an acute onset of atrial flutter often present with symptoms of palpitations, dyspnea, chest discomfort, and worsening symptoms of heart failure. As with AF, prompt assessment of hemodynamic status is critical in this setting. Management of atrial flutter is similar to AF, and the same guidelines for rate control, rhythm control, and anticoagulation apply [82]. Rate control in atrial flutter often proves more difficult than in AF. Unlike AF, which has multiple reentrant wavelets, typical atrial flutter is composed of a single, fixed reentrant pathway that provides a target amenable to cure by radiofrequency catheter ablation. Ablation is usually performed within the right atrium between the tricuspid annulus and the inferior vena cava to interrupt the atrial flutter circuit [83]. Atrial flutter not associated with a typical reentrant circuit has less successful ablation outcomes [84]. Ablation of the AV node with subsequent permanent pacemaker implantation, a method used in management of AF, may be an option in certain circumstances.

Managing Atrial Flutter in the Intensive Care Unit

Atrial flutter is frequently an unstable arrhythmia in terms of ventricular rate response. Specific caution is necessary when instituting β-adrenergic agents in patients with otherwise well-controlled response rates. Rapid change from 2:1, 3:1 AV conduction to 1:1 conduction and ventricular rates of 300 beats per minute or more can occur. Such abrupt changes in ventricular rate are uncommon with AF but should be expected with atrial flutter. Cardioversion to sinus rhythm prior to initiating pharmacological agents that enhance AV nodal conduction should be considered. Unlike with AF, immediate recurrence of atrial flutter is uncommon, and therefore, routine administration of an antiarrhythmic agent to prevent return may not be required.

Urgent radiofrequency ablation for atrial arrhythmia is rare in the critically ill patient. However, if atrial flutter with rapid rates and recurrence following cardioversion is seen, the procedure can be considered. Procedural success for atrial flutter ablation is highest for cavotricuspid isthmus dependent flutter. This specific arrhythmia can be recognized by the flutter wave morphology wherein the terminal segment of the flutter wave in lead V_1 is positive [85,86]. The use of antiarrhythmic agents like procainamide or flecainide may further organize an atrial flutter and decrease the *atrial* rate of the flutter. This may, however, paradoxically result in more rapid ventricular conduction which can be consequential in critically ill patients. Low dose AV nodal blocking agents should be instituted simultaneously when membrane active drugs, such as type Ic agents, are started for atrial flutter in the ICU setting.

Patients with persistent atrial flutter, especially of more than a year's duration may have significant underlying sinus node dysfunction. When cardioversion or pace termination of the flutter is planned, prolonged sinus node pauses may occur, and standby external or endocardial temporary pacing should be considered [87] (Fig. 42.11).

Multifocal Atrial Tachycardia

Another commonly encountered irregular narrow complex tachycardia in the ICU is multifocal atrial tachycardia (MAT). This SVT is caused by several abnormal atrial foci. Thus, MAT is characterized by at least three different P wave morphologies in a single lead with variable PR intervals. The atrial rate often varies between 100 and 180 beats per minute with no single, dominant pacemaker. MAT is highly associated with underlying pathologic processes that increase atrial pressures. Common etiologies for the development of MAT include chronic obstructive pulmonary disease, pneumonia, pulmonary embolism, mitral stenosis, and congestive heart failure. Other common causes include various electrolyte and acid–base disturbances. Management of MAT involves aggressive treatment of the underlying disease. Acute measures aimed at ventricular rate control include calcium channel blockers or beta-blockers with varying degrees of success [88–90]. It is important to note that because this particular population is more prone to bronchospastic disease, calcium channel blockers may be preferred. Digoxin should not be used in this setting, as it shortens atrial refractoriness which may worsen the rhythm.

Multifocal Atrial Tachycardia in the Intensive Care Setting

Rate control can be extremely difficult with this arrhythmia. Unless underlying theophylline toxicity or hypoxia is corrected, managing rapid ventricular rates and symptoms resulting from deleterious hemodynamic effects are often futile. Consideration for AV node ablation in refractory patients even in the setting of critical illness can be considered, especially if rapid rates compromise attempts to manage the patient's hypotension and other complicating medical illnesses. Intravenous magnesium as hypoxia is being addressed may also help temporize patient compromise until hypoxia is corrected or a definitive procedure is performed [91].

SUMMARY

Management of SVT in critically ill patients can be challenging. To maximize results, quick and accurate diagnosis of the exact arrhythmia mechanism is required. The caregiver should have an approach to analyzing the electrocardiogram during SVT. If a *regular* narrow complex tachycardia is noted, then a careful search for the P wave should be made. An abrupt onset arrhythmia with a short RP interval is likely a reentrant SVT either AVNRT or AVRT. In both arrhythmias, adenosine for immediate conversion of the arrhythmia and intravenous AV nodal blocking therapy for prevention of recurrence is highly effective. Cardioversion is of little value in this situation because of the likelihood of recurrence and the almost certain conversion of the arrhythmia with pharmacological agents. When the P wave is difficult to identify, examine the terminal portion of the QRS complex to look for pseudo R′ waves (lead V_1) or pseudo S waves (leads II, III, and aVF) (Fig. 42.12).

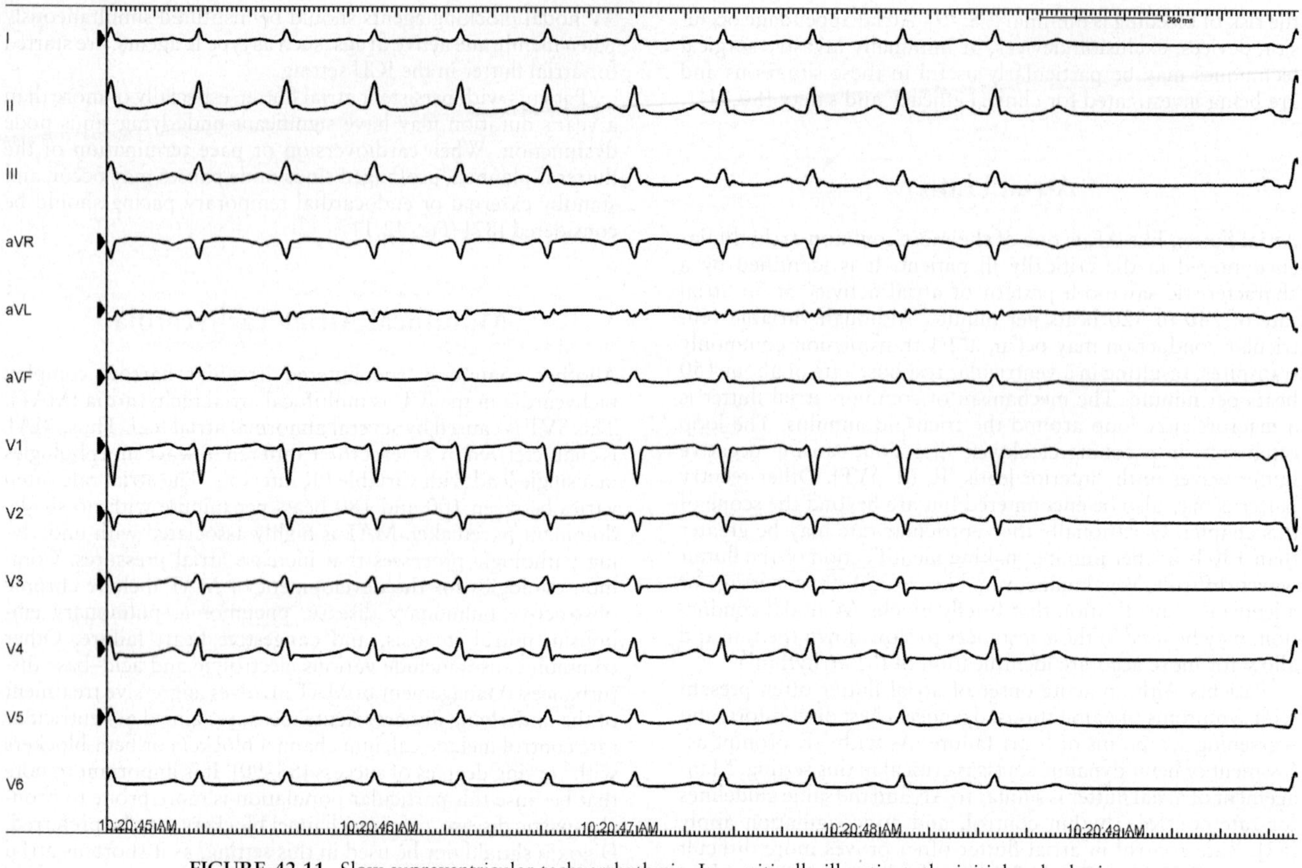

FIGURE 42.11. Slow supraventricular tachyarrhythmia. In a critically ill patient, the initial arrhythmia may be mistaken for sinus tachycardia. However, closer scrutiny of the P wave morphology defines a non-sinus mechanism (absence of terminal negative portion in the P wave in lead V_1). Note the abrupt termination that would essentially exclude a sinus mechanism. If recurrences are seen and associated with hemodynamic changes, intravenous antiarrhythmic agents can be considered. Automatic atrial tachycardias are often catecholamine sensitive, and when possible, the use of these agents for therapy should be minimized when the arrhythmia is seen. Note also the significant pause on termination of the arrhythmia suggesting underlying sinus node dysfunction.

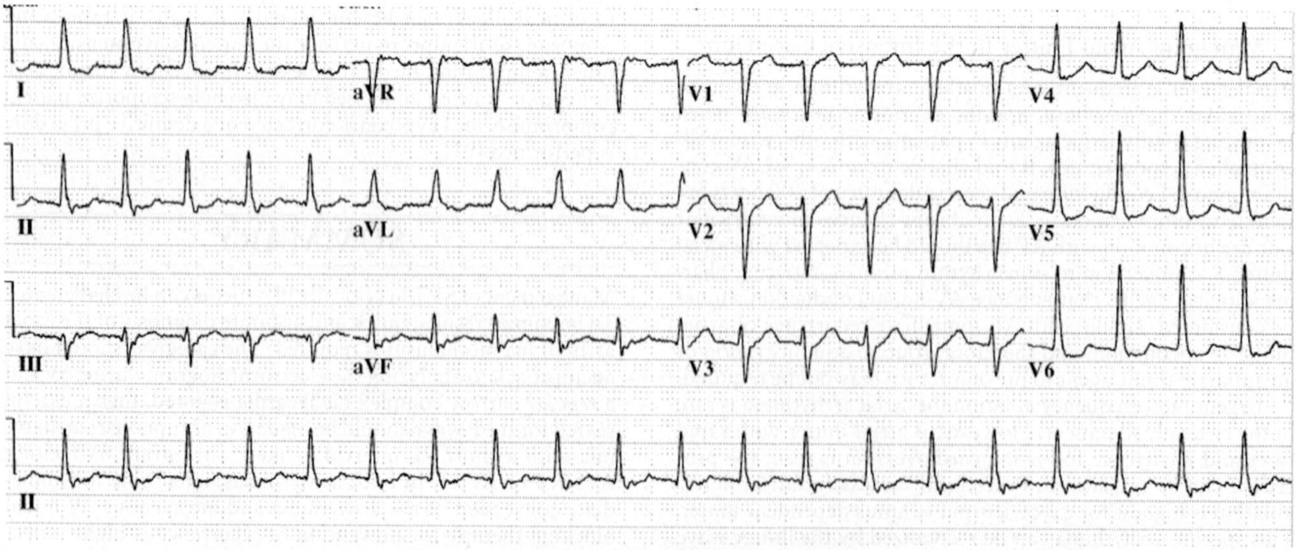

FIGURE 42.12. 12-Lead electrocardiogram in a patient with symptomatic atrioventricular node reentry during hospitalization. Note the P waves are difficult to define; however, the late "S" waves easily recognized in leads II, III, and aVF (pseudo S wave) are characteristic of this arrhythmia.

TABLE 42.1

SUMMARY OF EVIDENCE-BASED RECOMMENDATIONS FOR TREATMENT OF VARIOUS SUPRAVENTRICULAR TACHYCARDIAS

Disease	Treatment
Atrioventricular nodal reentrant tachycardia (AVNRT)	Adenosine Calcium channel blockers Beta-blockers
Atrioventricular reentry tachycardia (AVRT)—*hemodynamically stable*	Adenosine Calcium channel blockers Beta-blockers Procainamide Refer for possible ablation therapy
AVRT with underlying atrial fibrillation/atrial flutter	AV node blocking agents contraindicated
AVRT with wide complex (WPW)—*hemodynamically unstable*	Urgent cardioversion
AVRT with wide complex (WPW)—*hemodynamically stable*	Procainamide
Atrial fibrillation Hemodynamically stable	*See text regarding anticoagulation* *Rate control*: Beta-blockers, calcium channel blockers, amiodarone, digoxin, AV junction ablation *Rhythm control*: Cardioversion, antiarrhythmic drug treatment, ablation, various surgical procedures
Hemodynamically unstable	DC cardioversion Procainamide or ibutilide may be used in cases of wide-complex tachycardia (underlying WPW)
Atrial flutter	Management approach similar to atrial fibrillation
Multifocal atrial tachycardia	Calcium channel blockers Beta-blockers

Note: **Identifying an underlying cause of arrhythmia should always be attempted.**

For a gradual onset tachycardia with a long RP interval, either sinus tachycardia, inappropriate sinus tachycardia, or atrial tachycardia is likely. If the P wave morphology is not consistent with sinus rhythm, then an atrial tachycardia is present, and antiarrhythmic therapy with rate control is likely effective. If the P wave morphology is consistent with sinus rhythm, sinus tachycardia is most likely, and treatment directed to the underlying mechanism (blood loss, fever, hypotension, etc.) will likely result in eventual decrease in the sinus rates. No specific rhythm-based therapy is required. Inappropriate sinus tachycardia should be considered when no underlying cause for rapid sinus rates is noted and is often seen in the critically ill patient following the period of stress.

If an irregular SVT is noted, AF is most likely, but a search for regular flutter waves or multiple P wave morphologies (multifocal atrial tachycardia) is needed since these latter arrhythmias require a different management approach as detailed in the text.

Atrial fibrillation is by far the most common SVT arrhythmia encountered in the critical care setting. For each patient, rate control should be optimized, anticoagulation issues addressed, and when symptoms continue despite these measures, restoration of sinus rhythm strongly considered.

A summary of evidence-based management of supraventricular tachycardia is given in Table 42.1.

References

1. Artucio H, Pereira M: Cardiac arrhythmias in critically ill patients: epidemiologic study. *Crit Care Med* 18:1383–1388, 1990.
2. Olgin JE, Zipes DP: Specific arrhythmias: diagnosis and treatment, in Libby P, Bonow R, Mahn D, Zipes D (eds): *Braunwald's Heart Disease: A Textbook of Cardiovascular Medicine*. St. Louis, MO, WB Saunders, 2007, Chapter 35.
3. Delacretaz E. Clinical practice. Supraventricular tachycardia. *N Engl J Med* 354:1039–1051, 2006.
4. Asirvatham S: Supraventricular tachycardia: diagnosis and treatment, in Murphy J, Lloyd M (eds): *Mayo Clinic Cardiology: Concise Textbook*. 3rd ed. Rochester, Mayo Clinic Scientific Press: Informa Healthcare, 2007 pp 379–387.
5. Scheiman M, Basu D, Hollemberg M: Electrophysiological studies in patients with persistent atrial tachycardia. *Circulation* 50:266–269, 1976.
6. Pappone C, Stabile G, De Simone A, et al: Role of catheter-induced mechanical trauma in localization of target sites of radiofrequency ablation in automatic atrial tachycardia. *J Am Coll Cardiol* 27:1090–1097, 1996.
7. Vignati G, Mauri L, Figini A: The use of propafenone in the treatment of tachyarrhythmias in children. *Eur Heart J* 14:546–550, 1993.
8. Gillette PC, Garson A Jr: Electrophysiologic and pharmacologic characteristics of automatic ectopic atrial tachycardia. *Circulation* 56:571–575, 1977.
9. Creamer JE, Nathan AW, Camm AJ: Successful treatment of atrial tachycardias with flecainide acetate. *Br Heart J* 53:164–166, 1985.
10. Shen WK: How to manage patients with inappropriate sinus tachycardia. *Heart Rhythm* 2:1015–1019, 2005.
11. Richards K, Cohen A: Cardiac arrhythmias in the critically ill. *Anaesth Intensive Care Med* 7:289–293, 2006.
12. Krahn AD, Yee R, Klein GJ, et al: Inappropriate sinus tachycardia: evaluation and therapy. *J Cardiovasc Electrophysiol* 6:1124–1128, 1995.
13. Josephson ME: Paroxysmal supraventricular tachycardia: an electrophysiologic approach. *Am J Cardiol* 41:1123–1126, 1978.
14. Wood KA, Drew BJ, Scheinman MM: Frequency of disabling symptoms in supraventricular tachycardia. *Am J Cardiol* 79:145–149, 1997.
15. Srivathsan K, Gami AS, Barrett R, et al: Differentiating atrioventricular nodal reentrant tachycardia from junctional tachycardia: novel application of the delta H-A interval. *J Cardiovasc Electrophysiol* 19:1–6, 2008.
16. Jackman WM, Beckman KJ, McClelland JH, et al: Treatment of supraventricular tachycardia due to atrioventricular nodal reentry, by radiofrequency

catheter ablation of slow-pathway conduction. *N Eng J Med* 327:313–318, 1992.
17. Gimbel JR: A novel streamlined "anchored" anatomical approach to ablation of AVNRT. *Heart (British Cardiac Society)* 90:803, 2004.
18. Wen ZC, Chen SA, Tai CT, et al: Electrophysiological mechanisms and determinants of vagal maneuvers for termination of paroxysmal supraventricular tachycardia. *Circulation* 98:2716–2723, 1998.
19. Triedman JK: Management of asymptomatic Wolff-Parkinson-White syndrome. *Heart (British Cardiac Society)* 95:1628–1634, 2009.
20. Pietersen AH, Andersen ED, Sandoe E: Atrial fibrillation in the Wolff-Parkinson-White syndrome. *Am J Cardiol* 1992; 70:38A–43A.
21. Kinoshita S, Katoh T, Hagisawa K, et al: Accessory-pathway block on alternate beats in the Wolff-Parkinson-White syndrome: supernormal conduction as the mechanism. *J Electrocardiol* 40:442–447, 2007.
22. Goldberger JJ, Pederson DN, Damle RS, et al: Antidromic tachycardia utilizing decremental, latent accessory atrioventricular fibers: differentiation from adenosine-sensitive ventricular tachycardia. *J Am Coll Cardiol* 24:732–738, 1994.
23. Packer DL, Gallagher JJ, Prystowsky EN: Physiological substrate for antidromic reciprocating tachycardia. Prerequisite characteristics of the accessory pathway and atrioventricular conduction system. *Circulation* 85:574–588, 1992.
24. Blomstrom-Lundqvist C, Scheinman MM, et al: ACC/AHA/ESC guidelines for the management of patients with supraventricular arrhythmias–executive summary. a report of the American college of cardiology/American heart association task force on practice guidelines and the European society of cardiology committee for practice guidelines (writing committee to develop guidelines for the management of patients with supraventricular arrhythmias) developed in collaboration with NASPE-Heart Rhythm Society. *J Am Coll Cardiol* 42:1493–1531, 2003.
25. Goy JJ, Fromer M: Antiarrhythmic treatment of atrioventricular tachycardias. *J Cardiovasc Pharmacol* 17[Suppl 6]:S36–S40, 1991.
26. Obel OA, Camm AJ: Accessory pathway reciprocating tachycardia. *Eur Heart J* 19[Suppl E]:E13–E24, E50–E11, 1998.
27. Dougherty AH, Gilman JK, Wiggins S, et al: Provocation of atrioventricular reentry tachycardia: a paradoxical effect of adenosine. *Pacing Clin Electrophysiol* 16:8–12, 1993.
28. Exner DV, Muzyka T, Gillis AM: Proarrhythmia in patients with the Wolff-Parkinson-White syndrome after standard doses of intravenous adenosine. *Ann Intern Med* 122:351–352, 1995.
29. Gulamhusein S, Ko P, Klein GJ: Ventricular fibrillation following verapamil in the Wolff-Parkinson-White syndrome. *Am Heart J* 106:145–147, 1983.
30. Klein GJ, Gulamhusein S, Prystowsky EN, et al: Comparison of the electrophysiologic effects of intravenous and oral verapamil in patients with paroxysmal supraventricular tachycardia. *Am J Cardiol* 49:117–124, 1982.
31. Rinkenberger RL, Prystowsky EN, Heger JJ, et al: Effects of intravenous and chronic oral verapamil administration in patients with supraventricular tachyarrhythmias. *Circulation* 62:996–1010, 1980.
32. Jackman WM, Wang XZ, Friday KJ, et al: Catheter ablation of accessory atrioventricular pathways (Wolff-Parkinson-White syndrome) by radiofrequency current. *N Eng J Med* 324:1605–1611, 1991.
33. Crandall MA, Bradley DJ, Packer DL, et al: Contemporary management of atrial fibrillation: update on anticoagulation and invasive management strategies. *Mayo Clin Proc* 84:643–662, 2009.
34. Israel CW, Gronefeld G, Ehrlich JR, et al: Long-term risk of recurrent atrial fibrillation as documented by an implantable monitoring device: implications for optimal patient care. *J Am Coll Cardiol* 43:47–52, 2004.
35. Dixon BJ, Bracha Y, Loecke SW, et al: Principal atrial fibrillation discharges by the new ACC/AHA/ESC classification. *Arch Intern Med* 165:1877–1881, 2005.
36. Haissaguerre M, Jais P, Shah DC, et al: Spontaneous initiation of atrial fibrillation by ectopic beats originating in the pulmonary veins. *N Eng J Med* 339:659–666, 1998.
37. Jalife J, Berenfeld O, Mansour M: Mother rotors and fibrillatory conduction: a mechanism of atrial fibrillation. *Cardiovasc Res* 54:204–216, 2002.
38. Wijffels MC, Kirchhof CJ, Dorland R, et al: Atrial fibrillation begets atrial fibrillation. A study in awake chronically instrumented goats. *Circulation* 92:1954–1968, 1995.
39. Zipes DP: Electrophysiological remodeling of the heart owing to rate. *Circulation* 95:1745–1748, 1997.
40. Kannel WB, Abbott RD, Savage DD, et al: Epidemiologic features of chronic atrial fibrillation: the Framingham study. *N Eng J Med* 306:1018–1022, 1982.
41. Healey JS, Baranchuk A, Crystal E, et al: Prevention of atrial fibrillation with angiotensin-converting enzyme inhibitors and angiotensin receptor blockers: a meta-analysis. *J Am Coll Cardiol* 45:1832–1839, 2005.
42. Crenshaw BS, Ward SR, Granger CB, et al: Atrial fibrillation in the setting of acute myocardial infarction: the GUSTO-I experience. Global Utilization of Streptokinase and TPA for Occluded Coronary Arteries. *J Am Coll Cardiol* 30:406–413, 1997.
43. Watanabe H, Tanabe N, Watanabe T, et al: Metabolic syndrome and risk of development of atrial fibrillation: the Niigata preventive medicine study. *Circulation* 117:1255–1260, 2008.
44. Ettinger PO, Wu CF, De La Cruz C Jr, et al: Arrhythmias and the "Holiday Heart": alcohol-associated cardiac rhythm disorders. *Am Heart J* 95:555–562, 1978.
45. Benjamin EJ, Levy D, Vaziri SM, et al: Independent risk factors for atrial fibrillation in a population-based cohort. The Framingham Heart Study. *JAMA* 271:840–844, 1994.
46. Vaziri SM, Larson MG, Benjamin EJ, et al: Echocardiographic predictors of nonrheumatic atrial fibrillation. The Framingham Heart Study. *Circulation* 89:724–730, 1994.
47. Pires LA, Wagshal AB, Lancey R, et al: Arrhythmias and conduction disturbances after coronary artery bypass graft surgery: epidemiology, management, and prognosis. *Am Heart J* 129:799–808, 1995.
48. Hravnak M, Hoffman LA, Saul MI, et al: Predictors and impact of atrial fibrillation after isolated coronary artery bypass grafting. *Crit Care Med* 30:330–337, 2002.
49. Jongnarangsin K, Oral H: Postoperative atrial fibrillation. *Cardiol Clin* 27:69–78, viii, 2009.
50. Orlowska-Baranowska E, Baranowski R, Michalek P, et al: Prediction of paroxysmal atrial fibrillation after aortic valve replacement in patients with aortic stenosis: identification of potential risk factors. *J Heart Valve Dis* 12:136–141, 2003.
51. Burgess DC, Kilborn MJ, Keech AC: Interventions for prevention of post-operative atrial fibrillation and its complications after cardiac surgery: a meta-analysis. *Eur Heart J* 27:2846–2857, 2006.
52. Crystal E, Healey J, Connolly SJ: Atrial fibrillation after cardiac surgery: update on the evidence on the available prophylactic interventions. *Card Electrophysiol Rev* 7:189–192, 2003.
53. Halonen J, Halonen P, Jarvinen O, et al: Corticosteroids for the prevention of atrial fibrillation after cardiac surgery: a randomized controlled trial. *JAMA* 297:1562–1567, 2007.
54. Liu T, Li L, Korantzopoulos P, et al: Statin use and development of atrial fibrillation: a systematic review and meta-analysis of randomized clinical trials and observational studies. *Int J Cardiol* 126:160–170, 2008.
55. Benjamin EJ, Wolf PA, D'Agostino RB, et al: Impact of atrial fibrillation on the risk of death: the Framingham Heart Study. *Circulation* 98:946–952, 1998.
56. Jenkins LS, Brodsky M, Schron E, et al: Quality of life in atrial fibrillation: the Atrial Fibrillation Follow-up Investigation of Rhythm Management (AFFIRM) study. *Am Heart J* 149:112–120, 2005.
57. Reimold SC, Chalmers TC, Berlin JA, et al: Assessment of the efficacy and safety of antiarrhythmic therapy for chronic atrial fibrillation: observations on the role of trial design and implications of drug-related mortality. *Am Heart J* 124:924–932, 1992.
58. Kay GN, Ellenbogen KA, Giudici M, et al: The Ablate and Pace Trial: a prospective study of catheter ablation of the AV conduction system and permanent pacemaker implantation for treatment of atrial fibrillation. APT Investigators. *J Interv Card Electrophysiol* 2:121–135, 1998.
59. Rosenquvist M, Lee MA, Moulinier L, et al: Long-term follow-up of patients after transcatheter direct current ablation of the atrioventricular junction. *J Am Coll Cardiol* 16:1467–1474, 1990.
60. Ozcan C, Jahangir A, Friedman PA, et al: Long-term survival after ablation of the atrioventricular node and implantation of a permanent pacemaker in patients with atrial fibrillation. *N Eng J Med* 344:1043–1051, 2001.
61. Wood MA, Brown-Mahoney C, Kay GN, et al: Clinical outcomes after ablation and pacing therapy for atrial fibrillation: a meta-analysis. *Circulation* 101:1138–1144, 2000.
62. Hylek EM, Go AS, Chang Y, et al: Effect of intensity of oral anticoagulation on stroke severity and mortality in atrial fibrillation. *N Eng J Med* 349:1019–1026, 2003.
63. Kim SS, Knight BP: Electrical and pharmacologic cardioversion for atrial fibrillation. *Cardiol Clin* 27:95–107, ix, 2009.
64. Zhang N, Guo JH, Zhang H, et al: Comparison of intravenous ibutilide vs. propafenone for rapid termination of recent onset atrial fibrillation. *Int J Clin Pract* 59:1395–1400, 2005.
65. Fragakis N, Papadopoulos N, Papanastasiou S, et al: Efficacy and safety of ibutilide for cardioversion of atrial flutter and fibrillation in patients receiving amiodarone or propafenone. *Pacing Clin Electrophysiol* 28:954–961, 2005.
66. Hravnak M, Hoffman LA, Saul MI, et al: Atrial fibrillation: prevalence after minimally invasive direct and standard coronary artery bypass. *Ann Thorac Surg* 71:1491–1495, 2001.
67. Goodman S, Weiss Y, Weissman C: Update on cardiac arrhythmias in the ICU. *Curr Opin Crit Care* 14:549–554, 2008.
68. Heidt MC, Vician M, Stracke SK, et al: Beneficial effects of intravenously administered N-3 fatty acids for the prevention of atrial fibrillation after coronary artery bypass surgery: a prospective randomized study. *Thorac Cardiovasc Surg* 57:276–280, 2009.
69. Wolf PA, D'Agostino RB, Belanger AJ, et al: Probability of stroke: a risk profile from the Framingham Study. *Stroke* 22:312–318, 1991.
70. Wolf PA, Mitchell JB, Baker CS, et al: Impact of atrial fibrillation on mortality, stroke, and medical costs. *Arch Intern Med* 158:229–234, 1998.
71. Lin HJ, Wolf PA, Kelly-Hayes M, et al: Stroke severity in atrial fibrillation. The Framingham Study. *Stroke* 27:1760–1764, 1996.
72. Echocardiographic predictors of stroke in patients with atrial fibrillation: a prospective study of 1066 patients from 3 clinical trials. *Arch Intern Med* 158:1316–1320, 1998.
73. Mitusch R, Siemens HJ, Garbe M, et al: Detection of a hypercoagulable state in nonvalvular atrial fibrillation and the effect of anticoagulant therapy. *Thromb Haemost* 75:219–223, 1996.

74. Gage BF, Waterman AD, Shannon W, et al: Validation of clinical classification schemes for predicting stroke: results from the National Registry of Atrial Fibrillation. *JAMA* 285:2864–2870, 2001.
75. Fuster V, Ryden LE, Cannom DS, et al: ACC/AHA/ESC 2006 Guidelines for the Management of Patients with Atrial Fibrillation: a report of the American College of Cardiology/American Heart Association Task Force on Practice Guidelines and the European Society of Cardiology Committee for Practice Guidelines (Writing Committee to Revise the 2001 Guidelines for the Management of Patients With Atrial Fibrillation): developed in collaboration with the European Heart Rhythm Association and the Heart Rhythm Society. *Circulation* 114:e257–e354, 2006.
76. Fuster V, Ryden LE, Cannom DS, et al: ACC/AHA/ESC 2006 guidelines for the management of patients with atrial fibrillation–executive summary: a report of the American College of Cardiology/American Heart Association Task Force on Practice Guidelines and the European Society of Cardiology Committee for Practice Guidelines (Writing Committee to Revise the 2001 Guidelines for the Management of Patients With Atrial Fibrillation). *J Am Coll Cardiol* 48:854–906, 2006.
77. Henriksson KM, Farahmand B, Johansson S, et al: Survival after stroke—the impact of CHADS(2) score and atrial fibrillation. *Int J Cardiol* 141(1):18–23, 2010.
78. Mathew JP, Fontes ML, Tudor IC, et al: A multicenter risk index for atrial fibrillation after cardiac surgery. *JAMA* 291:1720–1729, 2004.
79. Villareal RP, Hariharan R, Liu BC, et al: Postoperative atrial fibrillation and mortality after coronary artery bypass surgery. *J Am Coll Cardiol* 43:742–748, 2004.
80. Friedman PA, Asirvatham SJ, Dalegrave C, et al: Percutaneous epicardial left atrial appendage closure: preliminary results of an electrogram guided approach. *J Cardiovasc Electrophysiol* 20:908–915, 2009.
81. Sick PB, Schuler G, Hauptmann KE, et al: Initial worldwide experience with the WATCHMAN left atrial appendage system for stroke prevention in atrial fibrillation. *J Am Coll Cardiol* 49:1490–1495, 2007.
82. Biblo LA, Yuan Z, Quan KJ, et al: Risk of stroke in patients with atrial flutter. *Am J Cardiol* 87:346–349, A349, 2001.
83. Lesh MD, Van Hare GF, Epstein LM, et al: Radiofrequency catheter ablation of atrial arrhythmias. Results and mechanisms. *Circulation* 89:1074–1089, 1994.
84. Yang Y, Cheng J, Bochoeyer A, et al: Atypical right atrial flutter patterns. *Circulation* 103:3092–3098, 2001.
85. Cosio FG, Arribas F, Palacios J, et al: Fragmented electrograms and continuous electrical activity in atrial flutter. *Am J Cardiol* 57:1309–1314, 1986.
86. Friedman PA, Luria D, Munger TM, et al: Progressive isthmus delay during atrial flutter ablation: the critical importance of isthmus spanning electrodes for distinguishing pseudoblock from block. *Pacing Clin Electrophysiol* 25:308–315, 2002.
87. de Groot NM, Schalij MJ: The relationship between sinus node dysfunction, bradycardia-mediated atrial remodelling, and post-operative atrial flutter in patients with congenital heart defects. *Eur Heart J* 27:2036–2037, 2006.
88. Arsura E, Lefkin AS, Scher DL, et al: A randomized, double-blind, placebo-controlled study of verapamil and metoprolol in treatment of multifocal atrial tachycardia. *Am J Med* 85:519–524, 1988.
89. Kastor JA: Multifocal atrial tachycardia. *N Eng J Med* 322:1713–1717, 1990.
90. McCord J, Borzak S: Multifocal atrial tachycardia. *Chest* 113:203–209, 1998.
91. Iseri LT, Fairshter RD, Hardemann JL, et al: Magnesium and potassium therapy in multifocal atrial tachycardia. *Am Heart J* 110:789–794, 1985.

CHAPTER 43 ■ BRADYARRHYTHMIAS AND TEMPORARY PACING

GAURAV A. UPADHYAY AND JAGMEET P. SINGH

INTRODUCTION

Implicated in over 40% of sudden cardiac deaths in the hospital, bradyarrhythmias are an important and heterogeneous group of cardiac rhythm disturbances [1]. Broadly classified, bradyarrhythmias are the manifestations of either a failure of cardiac impulse generation or impulse conduction leading to heart rates slower than normal sinus rhythm. By historical convention, normal sinus rhythm is defined between 60 and 100 beats per minute. Normal sinus rhythm is spontaneously generated by depolarizing pacemaker cells in the high right atrium within the sinoatrial (SA) node, and conducted through the atrium across internodal pathways to the atrioventricular (AV) node and subsequently to the bundle of His and to the left and right bundle branches of the Purkinje system [2,3]. Bradyarrhythmias may either be physiologic and benign, as in sinus bradycardia in athletes, or pathologic and warranting intervention, as in symptomatic bradycardia from either sinus node dysfunction or ventricular asystole from high-grade AV block.

Bradyarrhythmias may arise through several distinct mechanisms. Reduced automaticity in the SA node may be driven by hypoxia, hypothermia, or increased parasympathetic influence from gastrointestinal distress or genitourinary dysfunction. Periatrioventricular inflammation may reduce impulse propagation, as in Lyme's disease, myocarditis, or systemic lupus erythematosus. Significant AV and even infranodal block can occur in the setting of myocardial ischemia, drug toxicity or overdose, and severe electrolyte disturbance. Management begins by identifying the etiology of bradyarrhythmia and then attempting to restore normal sinus rhythm by correction or elimination of the identified precipitant. In situations where the bradyarrhythmia causes acute hemodynamic instability, the need for either pharmacologic intervention or electrical support through temporary cardiac pacing must be evaluated.

The purpose of this chapter is to review the pathophysiology of various bradyarrhythmias and to review treatment options available. Particular attention is placed on transcutaneous and transvenous pacing, as these advanced modalities are commonly employed in the medical and cardiac intensive care settings.

PATHOPHYSIOLOGY

Disorders of Impulse Generation

The most commonly encountered bradyarrhythmias of the normal conduction system include sinus bradycardia and sinus arrhythmia, both of which can be manifestations of normal physiologic states. Arbitrarily defined as a sinus node impulse rate of less than 60 beats per minute, sinus bradycardia may be a manifestation of an enhanced vagal tone seen commonly in athletes. Increased parasympathetic and decreased sympathetic tone during sleep also leads to bradycardic resting heart rates in nonathletes. Sinus arrhythmia is characterized as phasic changes observed in heart rate, secondary to autonomic influences on the sinus node triggered by normal respiration.

Sinus Arrhythmia

Thought to be due to reflex inhibition of vagal nerve tone during inspiration, sinus arrhythmia is the reduction in time from one P wave to another (P-P interval) between sinus discharges, leading to an increase in heart rate during inspiration and slowing during expiration, which is thought to help improve and synchronize alveolar gas exchange [4]. As such, respiratory sinus arrhythmia is considered the sign of a healthy conduction system. Marked sinus arrhythmia may even manifest with sinus pauses for 2 seconds or longer, but is rarely pathologic by itself. Small changes in P-wave morphology and PR interval can be attributed to variation in the pacemaking site within the SA node due to differential vagal stimulation. This periodicity in the heart rate is most pronounced in the young and decreases with age. The direct impact of the autonomic nervous system on the sinus node and sinus arrhythmia is confirmed by the fact vagal tone can be abolished through parasympathetic blockade by atropine or through anatomic denervation of hearts after cardiac transplant. Autonomic system dysregulation due to microvascular disease (as in diabetes) or degeneration (as in Shy–Drager syndrome) also reduces sinus arrhythmia. Indeed, depression of respiratory sinus arrhythmia after myocardial infarction is associated with an increased risk of sudden cardiac death [5]. In contrast to respiratory sinus arrhythmia, nonrespiratory sinus arrhythmia is the change of P-P intervals varying at random and may reflect drug toxicity from digitalis, intracranial hemorrhage, or ischemic heart disease [6].

Sinus Bradycardia

Symptomatic sinus bradycardia or sinus pauses causing reduced cardiac output or hemodynamic instability may be due to extracardiac disorders which profoundly increase vagal tone such as bowel obstruction, urinary retention, nausea and vomiting, or intracranial mass. Pharmacologic agents such as parasympathomimetic drugs, digitalis, beta-adrenergic-blocking drugs, and calcium antagonists can also exacerbate sinus bradycardia. Other disorders, such as carotid sinus hypersensitivity may also increase vagal tone and lead to transient ventricular asystole due to sinus arrest lasting up to 3 seconds or longer. Although some patients may require permanent pacemaker implantation due to recurrent, activity-related symptomatic pauses, they rarely require temporary pacemaker support as the negative chronotropic effect is relieved once pressure is removed from the carotid.

Sinus Node Dysfunction

Inappropriate SA node automaticity and disordered impulse generation is called sinus node dysfunction (also described as *sick sinus syndrome* by Ferrer [7]). It is commonly a disorder of senescence, although can occur at any age due to destruction of sinus node cells through infiltration, collagen vascular disease, trauma, ischemia, infection, or idiopathic degeneration [8]. Sinus node dysfunction affects men and women equally, commonly in the age range of 65 to 75 years, and is the primary indication for over 50% of permanent pacemaker implants in the United States [9,10]. Indeed, sinus node dysfunction comprises of a constellation of abnormalities of the sinus node characterized by inappropriate sinus bradycardia (in the absence of drugs), sinus arrest and chronotropic incompetence. Subsidiary and latent pacemakers further downstream become active in states of such dysfunction, and can give rise to bradyarrhythmias and tachyarrhythmias. These may originate in the atrium (e.g., atrial tachycardias, multifocal atrial rhythms, paroxysmal atrial fibrillation) or ventricles (e.g., idioventricular rhythms, ventricular tachycardias [VTs]). Coexisting AV nodal disturbance and block are also common, and intermittent periods of bradycardia punctuated by tachycardia have given rise to the term "tachy–brady syndrome." Many of these patients go on to need permanent pacemakers for effective rate control. The presentation in the intensive care setting is often due to an exacerbation of the underlying sinus node dysfunction through the use of cardioactive medications (see Table 43.1), which may result in a reduced cardiac output from diminished heart rate or unstable tachyarrhythmias. Given the diversity of potential etiologies and manifestations of sinus node dysfunction, it is often more useful to distinguish temporary or reversible causes of the syndrome (e.g., drug toxicity) from permanent etiologies (e.g., idiopathic fibrosis, degenerative changes of the conductive system) to identify the appropriate management strategy.

TABLE 43.1

CARDIOACTIVE DRUGS THAT MAY INDUCE OR WORSEN SINUS NODE DYSFUNCTION

Beta-blockers
Calcium channel blockers (e.g., verapamil, diltiazem)
Sympatholytic antihypertensives (e.g., α-methyldopa, clonidine, guanabenz, reserpine)
Cimetidine
Lithium
Phenothiazines (rarely)
Antihistamines
Antidepressants
Antiarrhythmic agents
May cause sinus node dysfunction (SND) in normal subjects: amiodarone
Frequently worsens *mild* SND: flecainide, propafenone, sotalol
Infrequently worsens *mild* SND: digitalis, quinidine, procainamide, disopyramide, moricizine
Rarely worsens *mild* SND: lidocaine, phenytoin, mexiletine, tocainide
Opioid blockers

Adapted from Podrid, Kowey: *Cardiac Arrhythmia*. Philadelphia, PA, Lippincott Williams and Wilkins, 2001 (Permission needed).

Disorders of Impulse Conduction

Conduction block may occur at any point in the conduction system and represents a failure of impulse propagation. This can occur at the level of the SA node, as in SA exit block, or further downstream, as in AV block or interventricular block. Importantly, conduction block is distinct from the normal physiologic phenomenon of interference, in which a preceding impulse causes a period of refractoriness due to inactivation of ion channels. Common terminology also differentiates between first-degree block, in which an impulse is delayed; second-degree block, in which impulses are intermittently transmitted; and third-degree block, in which impulses are not transmitted and dissociation may ensue. Bradyarrhythmias usually result from a combination of conduction block and disordered automaticity, for example, as in sinus rhythm with third-degree heart block and bradycardic junctional escape rhythm. Common types of conduction block are briefly reviewed here.

Sinoatrial Block

SA block, also called SA exit block, manifests as sinus arrest of variable length on the surface ECG. On the basis of a study of U.S. Air Force personnel, the prevalence is approximately 1% in otherwise normal subjects [11]. Considered by some to be a manifestation of sinus node dysfunction, the pathophysiology of SA block is a defect of impulse generation or propagation within the SA node. First-degree SA block cannot be detected on surface ECG as sinus node depolarization is not inscribed separately from atrial depolarization (the P wave). Type I second-degree SA block is the progressive prolongation of conduction block within the sinus node until complete exit block occurs. This manifests on surface ECG as progressive shortening of P-P intervals till a pause occurs. Type II second-degree SA block is the spontaneous block of a sinus impulse which leads to a sinus pause whose duration is an exact multiple of the preceding P-P interval. Third-degree SA block simply manifests as sinus arrest, usually with the eventual appearance of a subsidiary pacemaker rhythm such as a junctional escape. Sinus node dysfunction can be studied in the electrophysiology laboratory and quantified by techniques to specifically examine the sinus node electrograms, sinus node recovery time, and SA conduction studies. In the intensive care setting, diagnosis can be challenging, and it is usually sufficient to simply be able to recognize third-degree SA block which may necessitate temporary pacing if subsidiary pacemakers are not active or do not provide sufficient cardiac output.

Atrioventricular Block

AV block is frequently observed on surface electrocardiography, and may anatomically occur anywhere in the conduction system outside of the SA node. It is clinically important to attempt to distinguish AV block at the level of the AV node with block within or below the level of the His bundle, as infranodal block may be associated with instability and a worse clinical outcome. First-degree AV block is defined as a prolongation of the PR interval greater than 0.20 seconds, and is generally felt to be due to a block of impulse conduction at the level of the AV node, although when associated with bundle-branch block, may occur further down in the His–Purkinje system. In a study of over one hundred thousand airmen, the prevalence of first-degree AV block was found to be 0.65% [12]. In a 30-year longitudinal study, the association of first-degree AV block with a narrow QRS complex was thought to be largely benign [13]. More recent data from the Framingham cohort, however, suggest that significant PR prolongation may be associated with increased risks of atrial fibrillation, pacemaker implantation, and all-cause mortality over time [14]. Marked first-degree AV block may lead to hemodynamic derangement when atrial systole occurs in close proximity to the preceding ventricular systole, manifesting with symptoms similar to the pacemaker syndrome, although this is rare [15]. In the intensive care setting, second- and third-degree AV block are of greater significance.

Second-degree AV block was classified into two types by Mobitz in 1924 [16]. Mobtiz type-I second-degree AV block, or Wenckebach-type block, is characterized by progressive prolongation of the PR interval before nonconduction. Analogous to type I SA block which demonstrates shortening of P-P intervals, there is progressive shortening of the R-R intervals prior to a dropped beat in Mobitz type-I block. Irrespective of QRS width, Mobitz type-I block, or Wenckebach phenomenon, usually represents an appropriate physiologic response to increasing heart rate through decremental conduction in the AV node, and rarely requires intervention. Mobitz type-II block, on the other hand, usually represents infranodal disease, particularly when associated with a wide complex QRS. On the surface ECG, Mobitz type-II block manifests as a sudden nonconduction of an atrial impulse without change in preceding PR interval. Attention should be taken to distinguish Mobitz type-II block from block of a premature atrial complex, which is due to physiologic interference and not due to pathological involvement of the AV node. Mobitz type-II block is of significance in the clinical setting, as it may herald impending complete heart block, particularly when multiple consecutive impulses are nonconducted (often referred to as "advanced" or "high-grade" heart block). Third-degree AV block, or complete heart block, occurs with the absence of atrial impulse propagation to the ventricles and will manifest with ventricular standstill in the absence of an escape rhythm. When reversible etiologies are present, temporary pacing is critical toward providing electrical support, especially in the setting of ventricular asystole due to complete heart block. Temporary pacing is indicated when the subsidiary escape rhythm is unstable and cannot maintain hemodynamic stability, leading to cerebral hypoperfusion or further cardiac instability

Similar to sinus node dysfunction, there are myriad etiologies which may lead to AV block. In the intensive care setting, common etiologies include electrolyte disturbance, notably hyperkalemia or hypermagnesemia; drug toxicity, particularly from cardioactive drugs such as beta-adrenergic-blocking agents, nondihydropyridine calcium-channel blockers, digitalis derivatives, and antiarrhythmics; myocardial ischemia from inferior or anteroseptal infarction; infection from myocarditis or endocarditis, particularly involving the aortic valve; and trauma from cardiac surgery, catheter trauma, or radiation. Clinical history obtained from the patient is critical in determining the potential duration of the block and also prioritizing appropriate treatment modalities.

Intraventricular Block

Failure in ventricular activation due to block in the His–Purkinje system may also be the cause of complete heart block. The left and right bundle branches are commonly divided into a trifascicular system, consisting of the right bundle branch and the left anterior and posterior fascicles [17]. Although a septal fascicle has also been identified in anatomic studies, ECG manifestations of septal conduction block are debated and remain to be defined [18]. Bifascicular block is present when either left anterior or left posterior fascicular block is associated with right bundle branch block. Clinically, complete heart block is most often preceded by chronic bifascicular block, although the progression is often slow [19]. However, when first-degree AV block is associated with chronic bifascicular block and symptomatic bradycardia, there is an increased risk of sudden cardiac death (this combination is sometimes erroneously referred to as "trifascicular block"). Alternating bundle branch block seen on successive ECG tracings, either manifesting with sequential right and left bundle branch block, or right bundle branch block with left anterior and left posterior fascicular block, is also associated with increased mortality and can be correctly identified as representing intermittent trifascicular block.

Similar to other forms of conduction block, there are numerous potential etiologies which may lead to intraventricular block, although ischemia in the setting of a myocardial infarction (MI) is the most common in the intensive care setting. The SA nodal artery receives its blood supply from the proximal right coronary artery in 55% of the population, from the circumflex in 35%, and from both in approximately 10%. The AV nodal artery, on the other hand, arises from the posterior descending artery in 80% of cases, 10% from the circumflex, and approximately 10% from both arteries. Although, an inferior MI may lead to varying degrees of AV block from AV nodal artery ischemia or enhanced vagal tone from exaggeration of the Bezold–Jarisch reflex, intraventricular block is uncommon. An anterior MI, on the other hand, may cause ischemia of the fascicles directly and is associated with greater extent of left ventricular dysfunction. In the prethrombolytic era, new fascicular or bundle branch blocks were common after an MI and were associated with a significantly increased risk of mortality [20]. A simple scoring model characterizing the risk of progression to complete heart block after MI was developed by Lamas based on ECG criteria [21]. Patients with evidence of conduction block on ECG, including first or second-degree block (both type I and type II), left anterior and posterior fascicular block, right bundle branch block, or left bundle branch block had a linear relationship between their score (number of characteristics on presenting ECG) and the development of complete heart block. Patients without ECG evidence of any conduction block on presentation had a less than 4% risk of subsequent complete heart block, in contrast to those with scores of two, in whom the risk of developing complete heart block was 45%. Because of the relatively common incidence of bradycardia after MI, the American College of Cardiology (ACC) and the American Heart Association (AHA) have clear guidelines on intervention, including the use of temporary pacing, for AV and intraventricular disturbance (Table 43.2), which will also be further discussed later.

TABLE 43.2

ACC/AHA GUIDELINES FOR TREATMENT OF ATRIOVENTRICULAR AND INTRAVENTRICULAR CONDUCTION DISTURBANCES DURING STEMI[a]

Application of transcutaneous patches and standby transcutaneous pacing
Class I
Normal AV conduction *or* first-degree AV block *or* Mobitz type-I second-degree AV block with new bundle branch block
Normal AV conduction *or* first-degree AV block *or* Mobitz type-I second-degree AV block with fascicular block + RBBB
First-degree AV block with old or new fascicular block (LAFB or LPFB) *in anterior MI only*
First-degree AV block *or* Mobitz type-I *or* type-II second-degree AV block with old bundle branch black
Mobitz type-I *or* type-II second-degree AV block with normal intraventricular conduction
Mobitz type-I *or* type-II second-degree AV block with old or new fascicular block (LAFB or LPFB)
Class IIa
First-degree AV block with old or new fascicular block (LAFB or LPFB) *in nonanterior MI only*
Class IIb
Alternating left and right bundle branch block
Normal AV conduction with old bundle branch block
Normal AV conduction with new fascicular block (LAFB or LPFB)
First-degree AV block with normal intraventricular conduction
Mobitz type-II second-degree AV block with new bundle branch block
Mobitz type-II second-degree AV block with fascicular block + RBBB
Class III
Normal AV conduction with normal intraventricular conduction
Temporary transvenous pacing
Class I
Alternating left and right bundle branch block
Mobitz type-II second-degree AV block with new bundle branch block
Mobitz type-II second-degree AV block with fascicular block + RBBB
Class IIa
First-degree AV block *or* Mobitz type-I second-degree AV block with new bundle branch block
First-degree AV block *or* Mobitz type-I second-degree AV block with fascicular block + RBBB
Mobitz type-II second-degree AV block with old bundle branch block
Mobitz type-II second-degree AV block with normal intraventricular conduction
Mobitz type-II second-degree AV block with old or new fascicular block (LAFB or LPFB) *in anterior MI only*
Class IIb
Normal AV conduction with new bundle branch block
Normal AV conduction with fascicular block + RBBB
Mobitz type-I *or* type-II second-degree AV block with old bundle branch block
Mobitz type II second-degree AV block with old or new fascicular block (LAFB or LPFB) *in nonanterior MI only*
Class III
Normal AV conduction *or* first-degree AV block *or* Mobitz type-I second-degree AV block with normal intraventricular conduction
Normal AV conduction *or* first-degree AV block *or* Mobitz type-I second-degree AV block with old or new fascicular block (LAFB or LPFB)
Normal AV conduction with old bundle branch block

[a]Except where specified, all indications include anterior *and* nonanterior MI.
AV, atrioventricular; BBB, bundle branch block; BP, blood pressure; LAFB, left anterior fascicular block; LBBB, left bundle branch block; LPFB, left posterior fascicular block; MI, myocardial infarction; RBBB, right bundle branch block.
Adapted from the 2004 ACC/AHA Guidelines for the management of patients with ST-elevation myocardial infarction. *Circulation* 110:e82–e293, 2004 (Permission needed).

TREATMENT

Appropriate management of bradyarrhythmia is predicated upon identification of potential etiologies, selection of appropriate medical therapy, and assessment requirement for temporary cardiac pacing to maintain hemodynamic stability. Given the heterogeneous causes for bradyarrhythmias, in the acute setting it is critical to (1) identify and correct potential precipitants, (2) define a period for which medical or device therapy will be tried in the short term, and (3) identify the need for permanent pacing if it exists.

Medical Therapy

Upon initial presentation to the hospital emergency department, compromising bradycardia (or bradyarrhythmia leading to hemodynamic insufficiency) may be successfully resolved by conservative measures such as making the patient lie flat and bed rest in up to 40% of patients. Approximately 60%, however, require some form of pharmacologic therapy and 20% of these will go on to require advanced intervention with temporary pacing [22]. Conservative medical therapy is an effective measure for treating symptomatic bradycardia when applied with attention to potential etiology. Atropine (0.6 to 1.0 mg IV repeated every 5 minutes until desired effect or maximum dose of 0.04 mg per kg), is an anticholinergic whose well-documented vagolytic properties lead to increase in heart rate as well as blood pressure in settings of enhanced parasympathetic tone [23]. It has also been studied extensively in the setting of MI, and although may be associated with a small risk of worsening ischemia, is the drug of choice for treatment of AV block after inferior MI [24,25]. However, care should be taken to begin with doses of 0.6 mg or greater, as lower doses may cause a paradoxical increase in bradycardia. Aminophylline infusion (50 to 250 mg administered over 60 seconds, repeating as necessary) has also been studied in atropine-resistant AV block after inferior myocardial infarction [26]. Aminophylline has been shown to be effective in humans, and its mechanism of action is via the antagonism of locally accumulating adenosine during ischemia [27,28]. According to the 2005 AHA Guidelines regarding cardiopulmonary resuscitation, epinephrine (1 to 2 mg IV bolus along with 2 to 10 μg per min infusion) may also be considered for symptomatic bradycardias that are nonresponsive to atropine [29].

Isoproterenol infusions (5 to 20 μg per minute) or dopamine (5 to 20 μg per kg per minute) may also be used in an attempt to stimulate chronotropy during nonischemic bradyarrhythmias. These infusions should particularly be used cautiously in the setting of cardiogenic shock since they reduce coronary perfusion pressure and substantially increase the risk of worsening myocardial ischemia. Pharmacologic overdose is a common etiology of bradyarrhythmia. Glucagon (initial dose of 0.05 mg per kg or 3 to 5 mg followed by continuous infusion of 1 to 5 mg per hour) may also be of significant benefit in bradycardias due to beta-adrenergic or calcium antagonist toxicity [30]. By activating adenyl cyclase, glucagon increases cyclic AMP and increases intracellular calcium ion flux independently from the adrenergic receptor [31].

Other common causes of bradyarrhythmia include electrolyte disturbance and acidosis. When bradycardia is thought to be driven by acidosis, temporizing measures may include administration of sodium bicarbonate (1 mEq per kg) prior to initiation of hemodialysis or continuous venovenous hemofiltration. Similarly, the treatment of hyperkalemia often involves immediate steps to shift potassium to the intracellular compartment (e.g., calcium, glucose, insulin), along with initiation of longer-acting agents to stimulate potassium excretion (e.g., loop diuretic, sodium polystyrene sulfonate). These types of medical interventions must be tailored with attention to the underlying etiology of the bradyarrhythmia, along with concurrent assessment of whether advanced support through temporary cardiac pacing is indicated.

Device Therapy

Temporary cardiac pacing involves the application of electrical stimulation to the heart in order to override intrinsic rhythm and provide an exogenous source of pacemaking function. Whereas guidelines for permanent pacing have been clearly summarized by the ACC, the AHA, and the Heart Rhythm Society (see Table 43.3), indications for temporary cardiac pacing outside of acute MI remain undefined and up to individual clinical assessment [32]. The most frequent use of temporary cardiac pacing is to improve circulatory hemodynamics by improving cardiac output through increased heart rate in the setting of symptomatic bradycardia (i.e., bradycardia resulting in hypotension, cerebral hypoperfusion, or resulting systemic effects). Overdrive pacing of the heart may also be used to terminate some types of tachyarrhythmias, including sinus node reentry, AV node reentry, and AV reciprocating tachycardia with accessory bypass tract, although is rarely used for this purpose in clinical practice given the efficacy of medications and cardioversion [33]. There is still a role, however, for suppression of pause-dependent polymorphic VT (*torsades de pointes*) in limited situations while concurrent treatment of the underlying metabolic disturbance or proarrhythmic trigger is underway [34].

The decision to employ temporary cardiac pacing is made with attention to the temporality of the inciting arrhythmia. If the bradyarrhythmia is thought to be due to a transient precipitant which can be managed pharmacologically (as described earlier), medications are generally preferred due to their lower infectious and mechanical complication rates. Nearly 50% of patients in whom temporary pacing is used, however, ultimately require permanent pacemakers before discharge (see also Table 43.3) [35]. In these patients, delay in use of temporary pacing may expose patients to adverse outcomes.

Modalities which are available to deliver electrical stimulation include transcutaneous patches, transvenous endocardial leads, epicardial leads (usually placed at the time of surgery), transthoracic pacing through percutaneous needle insertion through the chest wall, or pacing through esophageal electrodes (which is primarily used for atrial pacing). Cardiac stimulation has also been demonstrated in humans through transcutaneous ultrasound energy delivery, although this approach remains largely investigational [36]. Although epicardial lead placement is common after cardiac surgery, the most commonly used modalities in medical and intensive care units are transcutaneous and transvenous pacing.

Transcutaneous Pacing

Temporary pacing has been used for the management of bradyarrhythmias since 1952, when the technique of transcutaneous pacing was initially described by Paul Zoll, who delivered a pulsating current through two electrodes attached via hypodermic needles to the chest walls of two patients with ventricular standstill [37]. Since that time, transcutaneous pacing has emerged as the first-line nonpharmacologic therapy for symptomatic bradycardia. Transcutaneous pacing systems consist of a pulse generator attached to high impedance external patch electrode pads (see Fig. 43.1). Most newer systems also incorporate defibrillator function in a stand-alone unit that provides combined antibradycardia, antitachycardia, and defibrillation capacity [38]. Pacing parameters have not changed over the past three decades, and include output, sensitivity, and

TABLE 43.3

ACC/AHA/HRS CLASS I RECOMMENDATIONS FOR PERMANENT PACING

Recommendations for permanent pacing in sinus node dysfunction
SND with documented symptomatic bradycardia, including frequent sinus pauses that produce symptoms
Symptomatic chronotropic incompetence
Symptomatic sinus bradycardia that results from required drug therapy for medical conditions
Recommendations for permanent pacing in acquired atrioventricular block in adults
Third-degree and advanced second-degree AV block at any anatomic level associated with bradycardia and symptoms (including heart failure) or ventricular arrhythmias presumed to be due to AV block
Third-degree and advanced second-degree AV block at any anatomic level associated with arrhythmias and other medical conditions that require drug therapy that results in symptomatic bradycardia
Third-degree and advanced second-degree AV block at any anatomic level in awake, symptom-free patients in sinus rhythm, with documented periods of asystole $\geq$3.0 sec or any escape rate less than 40 bpm, or with an escape rhythm that is below the AV node
Third-degree and advanced second-degree AV block at any anatomic level in awake, symptom-free patients with AF and bradycardia with 1 or more pauses of at least 5 sec or longer
Third-degree and advanced second-degree AV block at any anatomic level after catheter ablation of the AV junction
Third-degree and advanced second-degree AV block at any anatomic level with postoperative AV block that is not expected to resolve after cardiac surgery
Third-degree and advanced second-degree AV block at any anatomic level associated with neuromuscular diseases with AV block, such as myotonic muscular dystrophy, Kearns–Sayre syndrome, Erb dystrophy (limb-girdle muscular dystrophy), and peroneal muscular atrophy, with or without symptoms
Second-degree AV block with associated symptomatic bradycardia regardless of type or site of block
Asymptomatic persistent third-degree AV block at any anatomic site with average awake ventricular rates of 40 bpm or faster if cardiomegaly or LV dysfunction is present or if the site of block is below the AV node
Second- or third-degree AV block during exercise in the absence of myocardial ischemia
Recommendations for permanent pacing in chronic bifascicular block
Advanced second-degree AV block or intermittent third-degree AV block
Type II second-degree AV block
Alternating bundle-branch block
Recommendations for permanent pacing after the acute phase of myocardial infarction
Persistent second-degree AV block in the His–Purkinje system with alternating bundle-branch block or third-degree AV block within or below the His–Purkinje system after ST-segment elevation MI
Transient advanced second- or third-degree infranodal AV block and associated bundle-branch block. If the site of block is uncertain, an electrophysiological study may be necessary
Persistent and symptomatic second- or third-degree AV block
Recommendations for permanent pacing in hypersensitive carotid sinus syndrome and neurocardiogenic syncope
Recurrent syncope caused by spontaneously occurring carotid sinus stimulation and carotid sinus pressure that induces ventricular asystole of more than 3 sec
Recommendations for permanent pacing after cardiac transplantation
Persistent inappropriate or symptomatic bradycardia not expected to resolve and for other Class I indications for permanent pacing
Recommendations for permanent pacemakers that automatically detect and pace to terminate tachycardias
Reasonable for symptomatic recurrent SVT that is reproducibly terminated by pacing when catheter ablation and/or drugs fail to control the arrhythmia or produce intolerable side effects
Recommendations for permanent pacing to prevent tachycardia
Sustained pause-dependent VT, with or without QT prolongation

SND, sinus node dysfunction; AV, atrioventricular; SVT, supraventricular tachycardia; VT, ventricular tachycardia; MI, myocardial infarction.
Adapted from the 2008 ACC/AHA/HRS guidelines for device-based therapy of cardiac rhythm abnormalities. *Circulation* 117:2820–2840, 2008 (Permission needed).

rate, all of which can be manipulated in order to optimize capture and patient comfort [39].

Initiation of transcutaneous pacing begins with placement of electrode pads. Modern systems usually employ self-adhesive large-area (>80 cm^2) electrode pads which are impregnated with a conducting gel. Polymer-based electrode pads of low impedance are generally now preferred. Although the anteroposterior position is sometimes employed in hospital settings, most commercial machines suggest anterolateral positioning of pads to improve speed of application (see Fig. 43.2) and allow for continuous cardiopulmonary resuscitation with chest compressions if necessary. When possible, removal of chest hair with shaving reduces impedance [40]. Pulling away of hair follicles with extra pads is also effective and can be performed quickly in emergency situations. To synchronize pacing, most systems also require the placement of one to three additional electrodes to sense native QRS discharge.

A square-wave impulse is delivered over 20 to 40 milliseconds by the generator and is seen as a "spike" on its display. The relatively long pulse width attempts to reduce skeletal muscle and cutaneous nerve stimulation while still maximizing threshold of cardiac myocyte capture. Capture is achieved when each pacing discharge is immediately followed by a wide QRS complex of uniform morphology. Although most impulse generators can produce output of up to 200 mA, most healthy subjects will capture between 40 and 80 mA [41]. The patient threshold is defined as the lowest output that yields consistent electrical ventricular capture. In hospital settings, higher thresholds (up

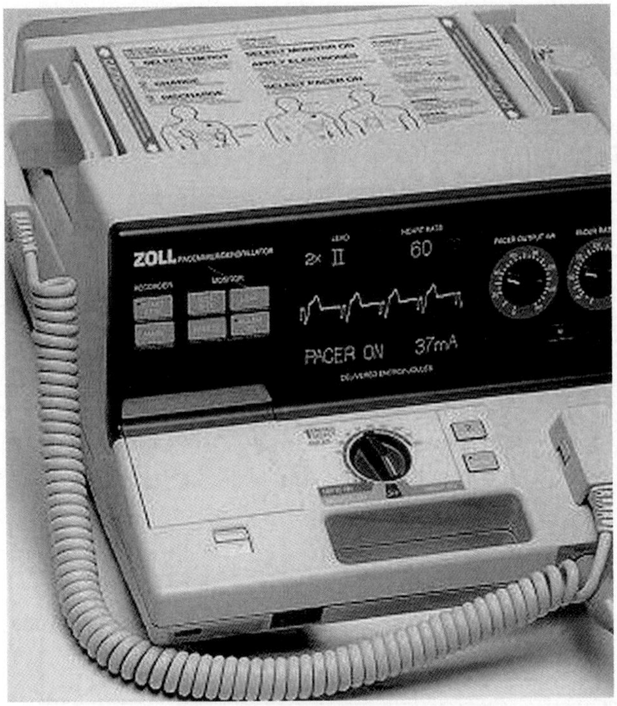

FIGURE 43.1. External pacemaker/defibrillator (pulse generator). (Courtesy of ZOLL Medical Corporation.)

to 140 mA output or more) are commonplace and may due to multiple etiologies. Suboptimal lead positioning—particularly over bone—as in the scapula, sternum, or spine, is an avoidable cause of increased pacing threshold. Other factors which may elevate thresholds that are beyond operator control include patient body habitus or obesity, transient myocardial ischemia, trapped pericardial fluid, mediastinal air, significant emphysema, use of positive pressure ventilation, or anoxia from prolonged resuscitation efforts [41,42].

By default, pacing mode in most machines is set at ventricular sensing, pacing, and inhibition in response to native ventricular conduction. Asynchronous pacing is usually only used during brady asystolic arrest, when cardiopulmonary resuscitation may cause artifact, particularly during chest compressions. Pacing rates of up to 180 bpm can also be achieved by most machines, allowing for overdrive pacing in the treatment of tachycardia or shortening of QT interval as needed. Hemodynamic response, as measured by cardiac output and blood pressure augmentation, is comparable with or better than right ventricular endocardial transvenous pacing [43].

Widespread use over the past three decades has established the overall efficacy of transcutaneous pacing in the treatment of bradyarrhythmia. In the largest single retrospective review of clinical trials in 1985, Zoll reported an overall success rate that approached 80% [41]. The use of newer electrode pads with improved capture yield a performance rate of nearly 100% when used in the very early and prophylactic treatment of bradyarrhythmias [44]. Timing is, of course, critical, and transcutaneous pacing for out of hospital asystolic arrest has been shown to be of no benefit [45].

Complications

The safety profile of transcutaneous devices has been well established over the past five decades, and suggests that its use is remarkably well tolerated. The primary limitation in its use is patient discomfort, and skin injury at contact site is the most commonly reported complication [41]. Prolonged animal pacing models have variably shown very small areas of focal myocardial injury, although no such injury has been shown in humans postmortem [41,42]. In normal individuals, transcutaneous pacing produces no measurable release of myoglobin, myocardial creatine kinase, or lactate dehydrogenase [42]. Also importantly, transcutaneous pacing has never been shown to induce arrhythmia, even in patients in whom MI or transvenous pacing precipitated ventricular tachycardia or ventricular fibrillation previously [41]. Taken together, transcutaneous pacing has supplanted transvenous pacing as the initial modality for bradyarrhythmic treatment in the emergency setting, particularly when pacing is only needed for short durations and patient comfort is not a primary consideration.

Transvenous Pacing

Furman and Robinson first described placement of an electrode catheter into the right ventricle for the management of high-grade conduction block in 1958 [46]. Transvenous electrodes circumvent patient discomfort and offer a reliable means of temporary pacemaker support in acute settings. Commonly used catheters are either bipolar electrodes, usually steel or platinum-tipped, embodied in plastic which may be flexible and associated with an inflatable balloon, or semirigid catheters which are deployed alone or with stylets. Most catheters have relied upon passive-fixation, although active-fixation, screw-in catheters with externalized pacemakers have also been recently employed for more prolonged temporary pacing requirements [47,48]. Preformed "J"-shaped catheters are also used for placement into the atrial appendage, but are not usually used in temporary pacemaking applications (see Fig. 43.3). Leads are attached to temporary pacemaker generators, which are generally constant-current output devices (see Fig. 43.4),

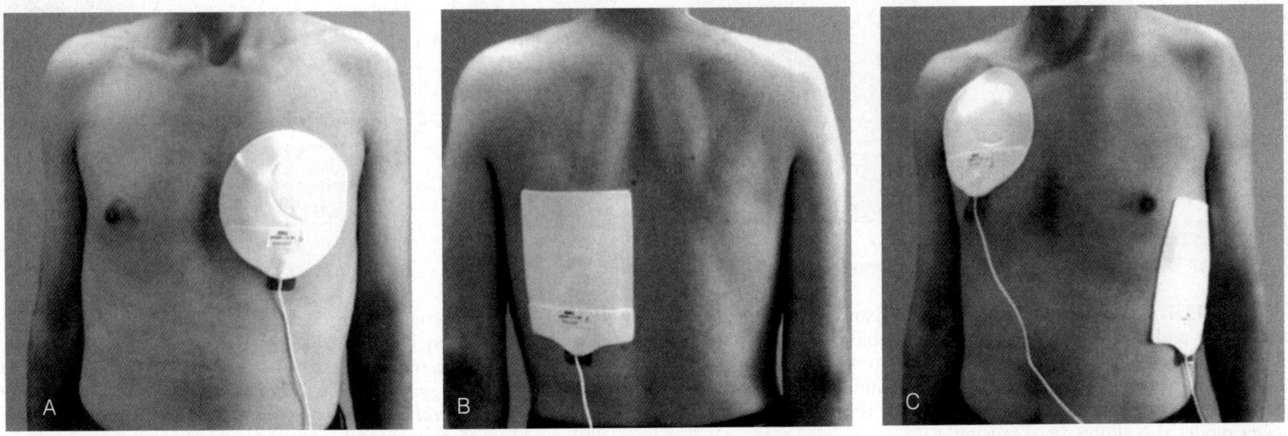

FIGURE 43.2. A, B: Positioning of transcutaneous electrode pads anteroposterior. C: Anterolateral positioning.

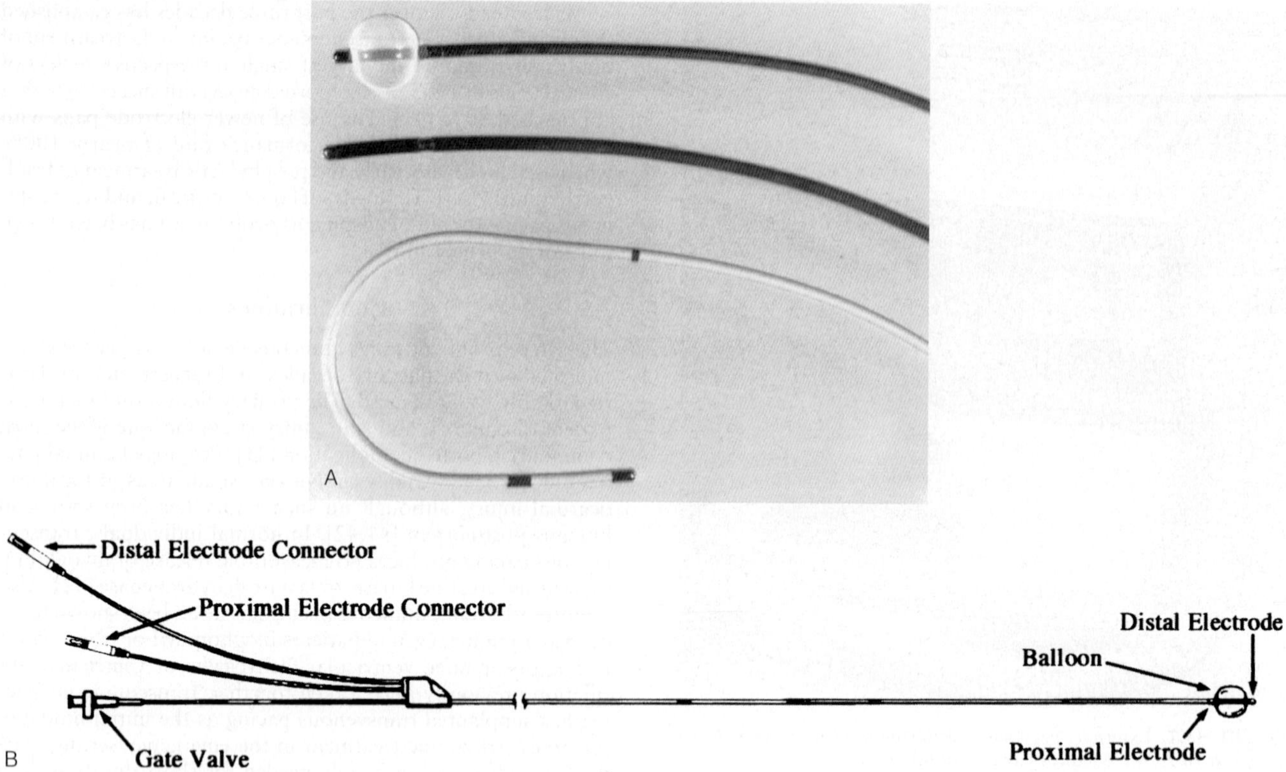

FIGURE 43.3. **A:** Cardiac pacing catheters. *Top*: Balloon tipped, flow-directed wire. *Middle*: Standard 5-Fr pacing wire. *Bottom*: Atrial J-shaped wire. **B:** Example of a balloon-tipped lumened pacing catheter with distal and proximal electrodes. [Swan-Ganz bipolar pacing catheter, courtesy of Edwards Lifesciences LLC.]

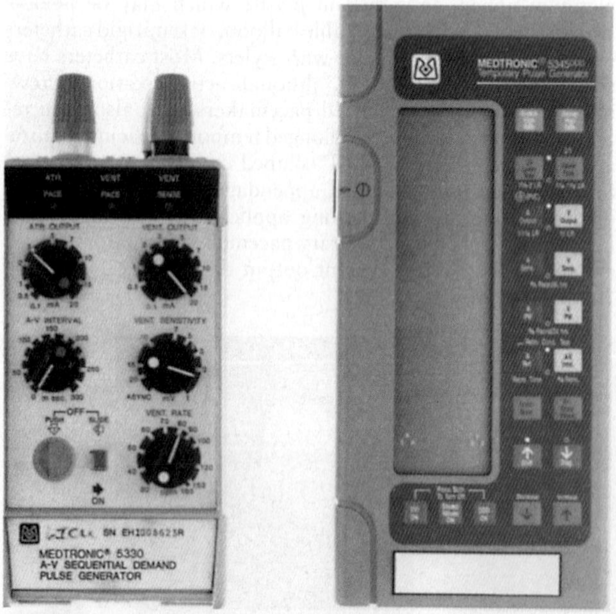

FIGURE 43.4. Temporary atrioventricular demand pulse generators, older (*left*) and recent (*right*) models. Adjustable parameters on the older model include pacing mode (synchronous or asynchronous), ventricular rate, ventricular current output (in milliamperes), atrial output (in milliamperes), and atrioventricular interval (in milliseconds). The newer model also allows atrial sensing.

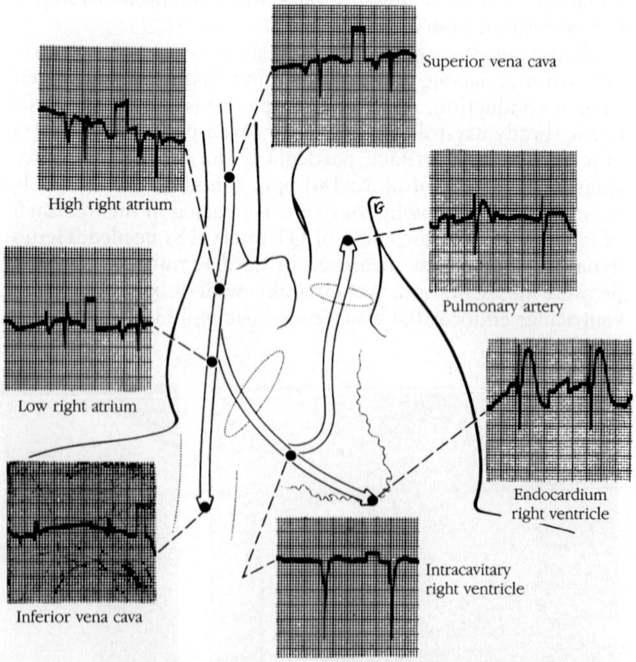

FIGURE 43.5. Pattern of recorded electrogram at various locations in the venous circulation. [From Harthorne JW, Eisenhauer AC, Steinhaus DM: Cardiac pacing, in Eagle KA, Haber E, De Sanctis RW (eds): *The Practice of Cardiology: The Medical and Surgical Cardiac Units at the Massachusetts General Hospital*. Boston, Little, Brown and Company, 1989, p 313, with permission.]

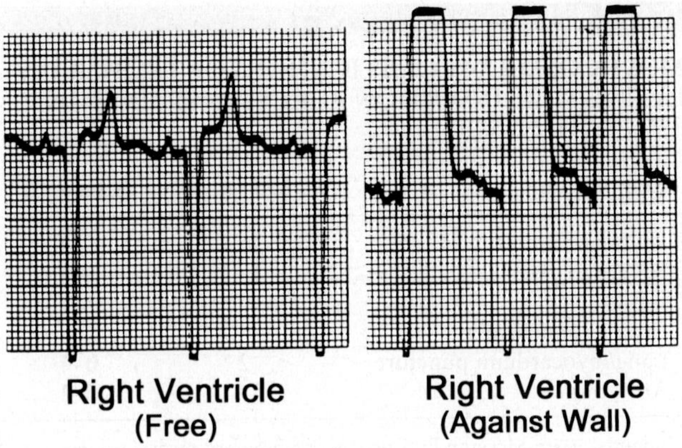

FIGURE 43.6. Injury current indicating positioning of electrode against right ventricular wall. [Reproduced with permission of OHL Bing, MD.]

although externalized pacemakers have been used for longer periods of electrical support in the setting of systemic infection [47,48]. Standard pulse generators deliver output ranging from 0 to 20 mA at a pulse width of 1 to 2 milliseconds. Optimal pacing thresholds are considered less than 1 mA, as thresholds usually escalate with patient movement or catheter dislodgement. In addition, thresholds may be affected by medications, electrolyte disturbances and ischemia; therefore, devices are usually set to discharge at an output of three to five times threshold.

Multiple approaches for placement have been described, including internal jugular, subclavian, femoral, and antecubital fossa vein routes [35,49–54]. Of these, the right internal jugular vein is preferred for ease as well as the lowest rate of complication [55]. A stereotypic transition of ECG recordings has been observed when advancing the catheter from the internal jugular or subclavian vein to the superior vena cava (see Fig. 43.5) [56]. Atrial- (or P wave) dominated ECG recordings are seen in the high and low right atrium. The QRS is readily seen

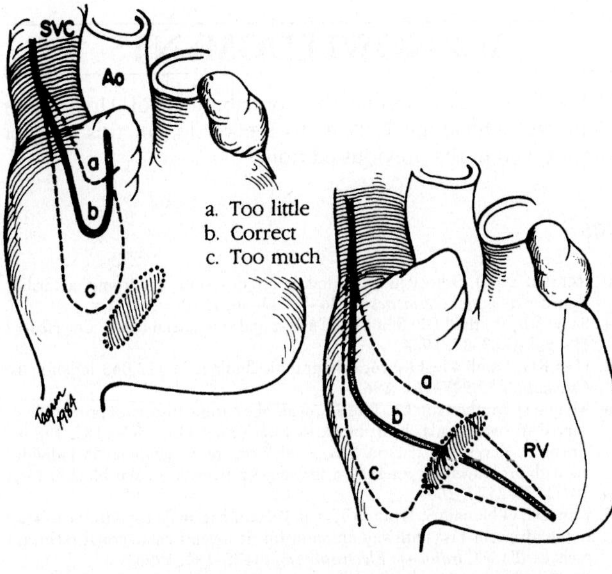

FIGURE 43.7. Sketch of fluoroscopic projection of catheter position. Ao, aorta; RV, right ventricle; SVC, superior vena cava [From Harthorne JW, Eisenhauer AC, Steinhaus DM: Cardiac pacing, in Eagle KA, Haber E, De Sanctis RW (eds): *The Practice of Cardiology: The Medical and Surgical Cardiac Units at the Massachusetts General Hospital*. Boston, Little, Brown and Company, 1989, p 315, with permission.]

from within the right ventricle. The catheter is then advanced to the right ventricular apex. After contacting the myocardium, a characteristic pseudo-"injury current" appearance is seen (see Fig. 43.6), representing catheter pressure against the ventricular wall and not actual injury to muscle. Figure 43.7 shows a sketch of a right anterior oblique fluoroscopic projection of proper positioning of both ventricular and atrial catheters. Table 43.4 provides a summary outline for bedside positioning of an electrode catheter in the right ventricle.

Complications

Transvenous pacing offers a reliable and stable means of cardiac pacing, which is generally easier for patients to tolerate, but associated with a greater risk of complications because of its invasive procedural placement. Multiple studies have reported on complications associated with transvenous pacing, although there has been marked variability in defining and measuring what constitutes a complication [35,49–54]. In a representative group of three studies, the overall complication rate ranged from 13% to 18% (see Table 43.5) [49,50,54]. Of these, induction of ventricular arrhythmia is the most immediately

TABLE 43.4

BEDSIDE POSITIONING OF A TEMPORARY ELECTRODE CATHETER

Setup
Sterile preparation (gowns, gloves, masks, drape, hat)
Equipment (pacing electrode catheter, pulse generator, surface electrodes, sheath)
Connections
V1 surface electrode connects to distal electrode
Proximal electrode catheter connects to positive pole of pulse generator
Testing components
Inflate balloon to test integrity
Document V1 recordings when inserting electrode catheter into the sheath
Procedure
Carefully advance electrode catheter 15 cm and inflate balloon
Observe V1 transition with advancement of catheter (see Fig. 43.5)
Atrial (P wave) dominant
Ventricular (QRS) dominant
Injury current
Stop advancing once injury current is detected
Pacing preparation
Confirm proximal electrode is connected to positive pole of pulse generator
Disconnect distal electrode from V1 surface lead and connect to the negative pole of the pulse generator
Pacing
Attempt pacing at 10 mA with the highest sensitivity
Observe capture
Determine thresholds and set output two to three times threshold (generally 5 mA)
Postprocedure
Document distance electrode is within the sheath
Confirm position with a chest radiograph
Routine care of pacemaker and site, including:
Pacing parameters (threshold, rate, sensitivity, output)
Skin site (observing for infection)

TABLE 43.5

COMPLICATIONS OF TEMPORARY TRANSVENOUS PACING[a]

Complication	Donovan [50]	Lumia [49]	Austin [54]
Ventricular tachycardia/ fibrillation	4.8	8.5	6.0
Other arrhythmias	NR	2.8	NR
Phlebitis	NR	4.2	5.0
Pulmonary embolism	NR	1.4	3.0
Hematoma/bleeding or arterial puncture	4.8	1.4	4.0
Perforation	1.9	2.1	4.0
Abscess at site	NR	0.7	3.0
Pneumothorax	1.0	NR	NR
Pacing failure with ventricular asystole	1.0	NR	NR
Diaphragm pacing	2.9	NR	NR

[a] All numbers are percentages.
NR, not reported.

TABLE 43.6

MOST COMMON COMPLICATIONS OF TEMPORARY PACING WIRE INSERTION ACROSS 15 STUDIES AND 3,747 PATIENTS [55]

Complication	Average rate (%)	Range (%)
Failure of access	15	6–40
Failure to place lead	10	5–25
Sepsis	9	2–18
Arterial puncture	4	0–6
Lung/myocardium puncture	2	0–4
Arrhythmias	1	0–2

Adapted from: McCann P: A review of temporary cardiac pacing wires. *Indian Pacing Electrophysiol J* 7:40–49, 2006.

life threatening, with myocardial puncture, pneumothorax, arterial bleeding and induction of infection leading to sepsis also being potentially deadly. Lead dislodgment can occur in a substantial number of patients within the first 48 hours of use, requiring replacement or re-positioning of the temporary pacemaker wire.

In a recent exhaustive narrative review, average rates of complications were compiled for 3,747 patients across 15 studies of cardiac pacing (see Table 43.6) [55]. Rates of infection were complications in as high as half of all procedures reported in some studies. In addition, older patients were at higher risk for suffering a complication, but that risks were lower when temporary pacemaker placement was performed by a specialist rather than a general practitioner. Given these findings, fluoroscopic placement of transvenous catheters by experienced personnel is preferred. In addition, prophylactic antibiotics should be considered for all temporary cardiac pacemakers, as these measures have already been shown to reduce the risk of infections after permanent pacemaker insertion [57].

With these concerns in mind, temporary transvenous pacing may still be required to definitively treat bradyarrhythmia and support patients through hemodynamic collapse. Attention to potential complications and meticulous technique can lower risks for what may be a lifesaving procedure.

SUMMARY

Cardiac bradyarrhythmias represent a heterogeneous group of rhythm disturbances of impulse generation or conduction. These may include potentially reversible etiologies such medication overdose and electrolyte disturbance, to progressive conduction system defect and irreversible ischemia. Appropriate treatment hinges upon the identification of the etiology of bradyarrhythmia in order to identify and eliminate precipitants if possible while initiating appropriate medical therapy. In situations of hemodynamic embarrassment, a concurrent assessment is made of whether temporary cardiac pacing may be required to bridge patients through acute instability and recovery or to permanent pacemaker placement. In the intensive care unit, commonly used modalities include transcutaneous pacing and transvenous pacing, which should be selected based on balance of patient comfort, potential for complication, and duration of use.

ACKNOWLEDGMENTS

The authors acknowledge the contributions of Drs. Glenn Meininger and Hugh Calkins to the version of this chapter as published in the previous edition.

References

1. Sanders P, Kistler PM, Morton JB, et al: Remodeling of sinus node function in patients with congestive heart failure: reduction in sinus node reserve. *Circulation* 110:897–903, 2004.
2. Anderson RH, Yanni J, Boyett MR, et al: The anatomy of the cardiac conduction system. *Clin Anat* 22:99–113, 2009.
3. James TN: Structure and function of the sinus node, AV node and his bundle of the human heart: part I-structure. *Prog Cardiovasc Dis* 45:235–267, 2002.
4. Yasuma F, Hayano J: Respiratory sinus arrhythmia: why does the heartbeat synchronize with respiratory rhythm? *Chest* 125:683–690, 2004.
5. Peltola M, Tulppo MP, Kiviniemi A, et al: Respiratory sinus arrhythmia as a predictor of sudden cardiac death after myocardial infarction. *Ann Med* 40:376–382, 2008.
6. Deboor SS, Pelter MM, Adams MG: Nonrespiratory sinus arrhythmia. *Am J Crit Care* 14:161–162, 2005.
7. Ferrer MI: The sick sinus syndrome. *Circulation* 47:635–641, 1973.
8. Dobrzynski H, Boyett MR, Anderson RH: New insights into pacemaker activity: promoting understanding of sick sinus syndrome. *Circulation* 115:1921–1932, 2007.
9. Lamas GA, Lee K, Sweeney M, et al: The mode selection trial (MOST) in sinus node dysfunction: design, rationale, and baseline characteristics of the first 1000 patients. *Am Heart J* 140:541–551, 2000.
10. Rodriguez RD, Schocken DD: Update on sick sinus syndrome, a cardiac disorder of aging. *Geriatrics* 45:26–30, 33–36, 1990.
11. Shaw DB, Southall DP: Sinus node arrest and sino–atrial block. *Eur Heart J* 5[Suppl A]:83–87, 1984.
12. Hiss RG, Lamb LE: Electrocardiographic findings in 122,043 individuals. *Circulation* 25:947–961, 1962.
13. Mymin D, Mathewson FA, Tate RB, et al: The natural history of primary first-degree atrioventricular heart block. *N Engl J Med* 315:1183–1187, 1986.
14. Cheng S, Keyes MJ, Larson MG, et al: Long-term outcomes in individuals with prolonged PR interval or first-degree atrioventricular block. *JAMA* 301:2571–2577, 2009.
15. Kim YH, O'Nunain S, Trouton T, et al: Pseudo-pacemaker syndrome following inadvertent fast pathway ablation for atrioventricular nodal reentrant tachycardia. *J Cardiovasc Electrophysiol* 4:178–182, 1993.
16. Mobitz W: Über die unvollständige störung der erregungsüberleitung zwischen vorhof und kammer des menschlichen herzens. *Z Gesamte Exp Med* 41:180–237, 1924.
17. Rosenbaum MB, Elizari MV, Lazzari JO, et al: Intraventricular trifascicular blocks. The syndrome of right bundle branch block with intermittent left anterior and posterior hemiblock. *Am Heart J* 78:306–317, 1969.
18. MacAlpin RN: In search of left septal fascicular block. *Am Heart J* 144:948–956, 2002.

19. Fisch GR, Zipes DP, Fisch C: Bundle branch block and sudden death. *Prog Cardiovasc Dis* 23:187–224, 1980.
20. Hindman MC, Wagner GS, JaRo M, et al: The clinical significance of bundle branch block complicating acute myocardial infarction. 1. Clinical characteristics, hospital mortality, and one-year follow-up. *Circulation* 58:679–688, 1978.
21. Lamas GA, Muller JE, Turi ZG, et al: A simplified method to predict occurrence of complete heart block during acute myocardial infarction. *Am J Cardiol* 57:1213–1219, 1986.
22. Sodeck GH, Domanovits H, Meron G, et al: Compromising bradycardia: management in the emergency department. *Resuscitation* 73:96–102, 2007.
23. Lonnerholm G, Widerlov E: Effect of intravenous atropine and methylatropine on heart rate and secretion of saliva in man. *Eur J Clin Pharmacol* 8:233–240, 1975.
24. Brady WJ Jr, Harrigan RA: Diagnosis and management of bradycardia and atrioventricular block associated with acute coronary ischemia. *Emerg Med Clin North Am* 19:371–384, 2001, xi–xii.
25. Antman EM, Anbe DT, Armstrong PW, et al: ACC/AHA guidelines for the management of patients with ST-elevation myocardial infarction; A report of the American College of Cardiology/American Heart Association Task Force on Practice Guidelines (Committee to Revise the 1999 Guidelines for the Management of patients with acute myocardial infarction). *J Am Coll Cardiol* 44:E1–E211, 2004.
26. Wesley RC Jr, Lerman BB, DiMarco JP, et al: Mechanism of atropine-resistant atrioventricular block during inferior myocardial infarction: possible role of adenosine. *J Am Coll Cardiol* 8:1232–1234, 1986.
27. Altun A, Kirdar C, Ozbay G: Effect of aminophylline in patients with atropine-resistant late advanced atrioventricular block during acute inferior myocardial infarction. *Clin Cardiol* 21:759–762, 1998.
28. Goodfellow J, Walker PR: Reversal of atropine-resistant atrioventricular block with intravenous aminophylline in the early phase of inferior wall acute myocardial infarction following treatment with streptokinase. *Eur Heart J* 16:862–865, 1995.
29. ECC Committee, Subcommittees and Task Forces of the American Heart Association: 2005 American Heart Association guidelines for cardiopulmonary resuscitation and emergency cardiovascular care. *Circulation* 112:IV1–IV203, 2005.
30. Love JN, Sachdeva DK, Bessman ES, et al: A potential role for glucagon in the treatment of drug-induced symptomatic bradycardia. *Chest* 114:323–326, 1998.
31. Entman ML, Levey GS, Epstein SE: Mechanism of action of epinephrine and glucagon on the canine heart. Evidence for increase in sarcotubular calcium stores mediated by cyclic 3′,5′-AMP. *Circ Res* 25:429–438, 1969.
32. Epstein AE, DiMarco JP, Ellenbogen KA, et al: ACC/AHA/HRS 2008 guidelines for device-based therapy of cardiac rhythm abnormalities: a report of the American College of Cardiology/American Heart Association Task Force on Practice Guidelines (Writing Committee to Revise the ACC/AHA/NASPE 2002 guideline update for implantation of cardiac pacemakers and antiarrhythmia devices) developed in collaboration with the American Association for Thoracic Surgery and Society of Thoracic Surgeons. *J Am Coll Cardiol* 51:e1–e62, 2008.
33. Batchelder JE, Zipes DP: Treatment of tachyarrhythmias by pacing. *Arch Intern Med* 135:1115–1124, 1975.
34. Roden DM: A practical approach to torsade de pointes. *Clin Cardiol* 20:285–290, 1997.
35. Hynes JK, Holmes DR Jr, Harrison CE: Five-year experience with temporary pacemaker therapy in the coronary care unit. *Mayo Clin Proc* 58:122–126, 1983.
36. Lee KL, Lau CP, Tse HF, et al: First human demonstration of cardiac stimulation with transcutaneous ultrasound energy delivery: implications for wireless pacing with implantable devices. *J Am Coll Cardiol* 50:877–883, 2007.
37. Zoll PM: Resuscitation of the heart in ventricular standstill by external electric stimulation. *N Engl J Med* 247:768–771, 1952.
38. Trigano JA, Birkui PJ, Mugica J: Noninvasive transcutaneous cardiac pacing: modern instrumentation and new perspectives. *Pacing Clin Electrophysiol* 15:1937–1943, 1992.
39. Zoll PM, Zoll RH, Belgard AH: External noninvasive electric stimulation of the heart. *Crit Care Med* 9:393–394, 1981.
40. Sado DM, Deakin CD, Petley GW, et al: Comparison of the effects of removal of chest hair with not doing so before external defibrillation on transthoracic impedance. *Am J Cardiol* 93:98–100, 2004.
41. Zoll PM, Zoll RH, Falk RH, et al: External noninvasive temporary cardiac pacing: clinical trials. *Circulation* 71:937–944, 1985.
42. Hedges JR, Syverud SA, Dalsey WC, et al: Threshold, enzymatic, and pathologic changes associated with prolonged transcutaneous pacing in a chronic heart block model. *J Emerg Med* 7:1–4, 1989.
43. Feldman MD, Zoll PM, Aroesty JM, et al: Hemodynamic responses to noninvasive external cardiac pacing. *Am J Med* 84:395–400, 1988.
44. Chapman PD, Stratbucker RA, Schlageter DP, et al: Efficacy and safety of transcutaneous low-impedance cardiac pacing in human volunteers using conventional polymeric defibrillation pads. *Ann Emerg Med* 21:1451–1453, 1992.
45. Cummins RO, Graves JR, Larsen MP, et al: Out-of-hospital transcutaneous pacing by emergency medical technicians in patients with asystolic cardiac arrest. *N Engl J Med* 328:1377–1382, 1993.
46. Furman S, Robinson G: The use of an intracardiac pacemaker in the correction of total heart block. *Surg Forum* 9:245–248, 1958.
47. Zei PC, Eckart RE, Epstein LM: Modified temporary cardiac pacing using transvenous active fixation leads and external re-sterilized pulse generators. *J Am Coll Cardiol* 47:1487–1489, 2006.
48. Braun MU, Rauwolf T, Bock M, et al: Percutaneous lead implantation connected to an external device in stimulation-dependent patients with systemic infection–a prospective and controlled study. *Pacing Clin Electrophysiol* 29:875–879, 2006.
49. Lumia FJ, Rios JC: Temporary transvenous pacemaker therapy: an analysis of complications. *Chest* 64:604–608, 1973.
50. Donovan KD, Lee KY: Indications for and complications of temporary transvenous cardiac pacing. *Anaesth Intensive Care* 13:63–70, 1985.
51. Abinader EG, Sharif D, Malouf S, et al: Temporary transvenous pacing: analysis of indications, complications and malfunctions in acute myocardial infarction versus noninfarction settings. *Isr J Med Sci* 23:877–880, 1987.
52. Murphy JJ: Current practice and complications of temporary transvenous cardiac pacing. *BMJ* 312:1134, 1996.
53. Betts TR: Regional survey of temporary transvenous pacing procedures and complications. *Postgrad Med J* 79:463–465, 2003.
54. Austin JL, Preis LK, Crampton RS, et al: Analysis of pacemaker malfunction and complications of temporary pacing in the coronary care unit. *Am J Cardiol* 49:301–306, 1982.
55. McCann P: A review of temporary cardiac pacing wires. *Indian Pacing Electrophysiol J* 7:40–49, 2006.
56. Bing OH, McDowell JW, Hantman J, et al: Pacemaker placement by electrocardiographic monitoring. *N Engl J Med* 287:651, 1972.
57. Da Costa A, Kirkorian G, Cucherat M, et al: Antibiotic prophylaxis for permanent pacemaker implantation: a meta-analysis. *Circulation* 97:1796–801, 1998.

CHAPTER 44 ■ HOW TO MANAGE CARDIAC PACEMAKERS AND IMPLANTABLE DEFIBRILLATORS IN THE INTENSIVE CARE UNIT

MELANIE MAYTIN AND USHA B. TEDROW

INTRODUCTION

Cardiac device technology has made great advancements since the introduction of the first implantable pacemaker in 1958. Since then, the number of cardiac device implants continues to increase annually as a result of the aging of the general population, expanding indications for device therapy, and ongoing innovation in the technology of cardiac pacing and defibrillation. As a result, many patients presenting to the intensive care unit (ICU) with noncardiac illness may have implanted cardiac devices. This chapter aims to briefly review basic cardiac device function and programming with emphasis on device malfunction and troubleshooting. A discussion of the indications for permanent pacing, defibrillator or resynchronization therapy is outside the scope of this text; for additional information regarding these topics, the reader is referred to the American College of Cardiology/American Heart Association/Heart Rhythm Society 2008 Guidelines for Device-Based Therapy of Cardiac Rhythm Abnormalities [1].

GENERAL DEVICE MANAGEMENT

Normal Device Function and Special Considerations

Identification of the type of device is critical in interpretation of its function. Although the patients would ideally be able to provide information regarding the type of device that has been implanted (pacemaker, implantable cardioverter defibrillator (ICD), cardiac resynchronization device, etc.) or carry a device identification card with them at all times, this is frequently not the case in hospitalized patients. Substantial device information can be gleaned from a chest radiograph, including the lead configuration, the type of device, abnormalities in lead position or integrity, and even the device manufacturer (Fig. 44.1A–C). Identification of the device manufacturer is essential if formal device interrogation or reprogramming is planned as each device company uses different software and programmers to communicate with their respective devices (Fig. 44.2). The overwhelming majority of devices implanted are manufactured by one of three companies, and patient device information and technical support are available 24 hours a day (Table 44.1).

The device system consists of a pulse generator or battery, logic circuits, and pacing or defibrillator lead(s). All implantable cardiac devices have programmable pacemaker functions. These devices can both sense intrinsic electrical depolarization and excite myocardial tissue through an artificial electrical stimulus delivered near the lead tip. Electrical stimuli can be delivered in many ways depending on how the device is programmed. Pacing nomenclature is standardized to easily communicate information regarding the device and the pacing mode (Table 44.2). Pacing algorithms are best understood as a function of timing cycles. A pacemaker operates like a timer with programmable intervals to coordinate all sensed and paced events. Nontracking modes of pacing (AAI, VVI, DDI) deliver electrical impulses at set intervals (*lower rate limit*) unless a sensed electrophysiologic cardiac event occurs in the appropriate chamber before the end of the programmed interval (in which case the timer resets, Fig. 44.3). Dual-chamber devices programmed to a tracking mode can provide pacing at the programmed lower rate or track-sensed intrinsic conduction up to a programmed *upper rate limit*. There is no sensing in asynchronous pacing modes (AOO, VOO, DOO) and electrical stimuli are produced at programmed intervals unaffected by intrinsic conduction.

Magnets

The placement of a magnet over a device affects pacemakers and defibrillators differently. Application of a magnet to a pacemaker will cause the reed switch to close and result in asynchronous pacing. The pacing rate is company-specific with a different rate once battery depletion has occurred. Thus, placement of a magnet over the device can assist with the determination of battery status and device identification. If exposure to electromagnetic interference (EMI) is anticipated, positioning a magnet over the device can prevent inappropriate pacing inhibition. On removal of the magnet, the pacing mode will revert to the originally programmed settings, and, in general, formal device interrogation is not required. In contrast, application of a magnet to a defibrillator will disable all antitachycardia therapies but will *not* affect the pacing mode. Therefore, magnets can be used to prevent inappropriate therapies due to supraventricular tachycardia (SVT), lead fracture, or EMI. On removal of the magnet, defibrillator therapies will be restored, and, in general, formal device interrogation is not required.

Electromagnetic Interference

In hospitals, many potential sources of EMI exist. Sources of electromagnetic energy that could possibly interfere with device function include magnetic resonance imaging (MRI), electrocautery, defibrillation, radiation therapy, neurostimulators, TENS units, radiofrequency ablation, electroconvulsive therapy, video capsule endoscopy, extracorporeal shock wave lithotripsy and therapeutic diathermy [2,3]. EMI exposure most commonly results in inappropriate inhibition or triggering of pacing stimuli, inappropriate ICD tachyarrhythmia

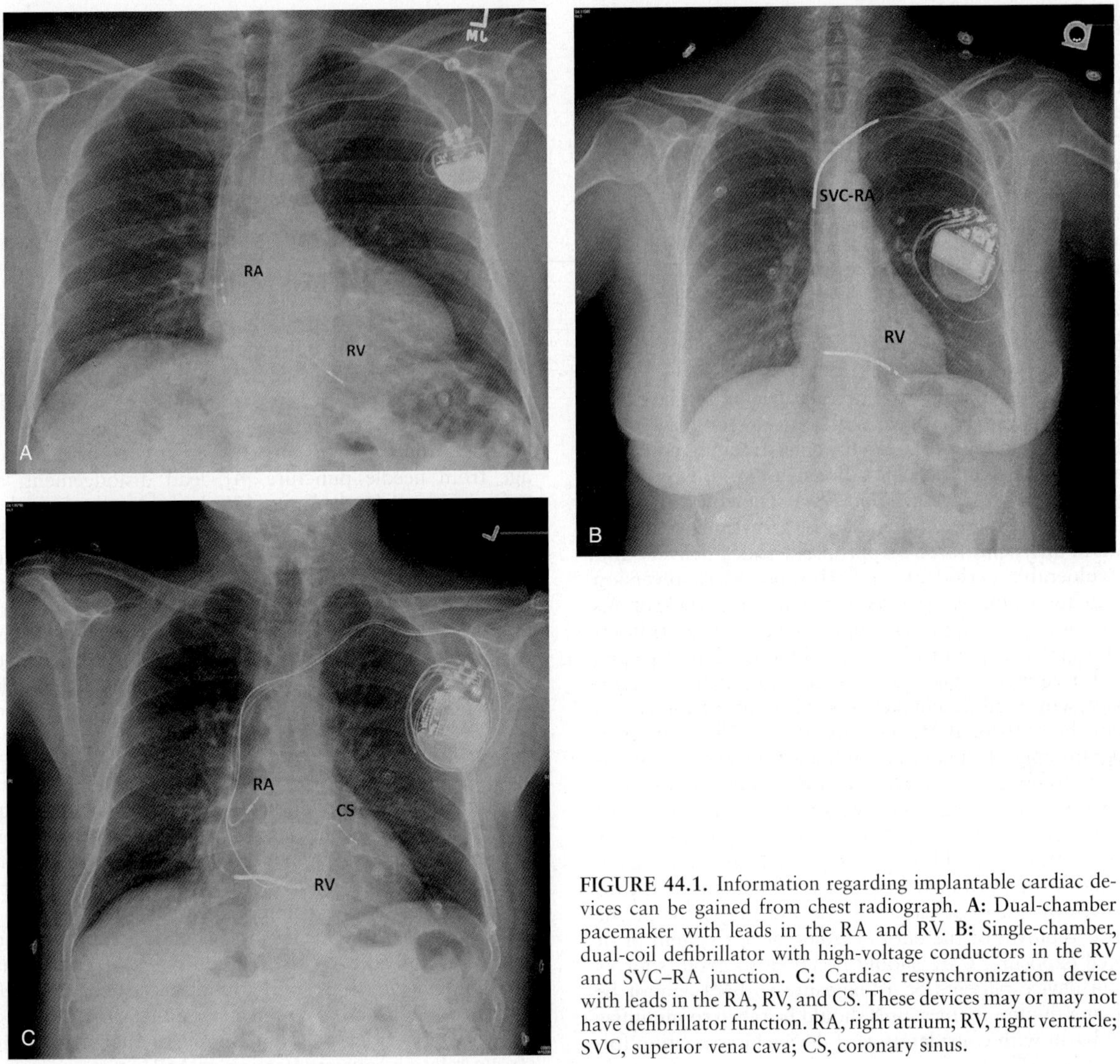

FIGURE 44.1. Information regarding implantable cardiac devices can be gained from chest radiograph. **A:** Dual-chamber pacemaker with leads in the RA and RV. **B:** Single-chamber, dual-coil defibrillator with high-voltage conductors in the RV and SVC–RA junction. **C:** Cardiac resynchronization device with leads in the RA, RV, and CS. These devices may or may not have defibrillator function. RA, right atrium; RV, right ventricle; SVC, superior vena cava; CS, coronary sinus.

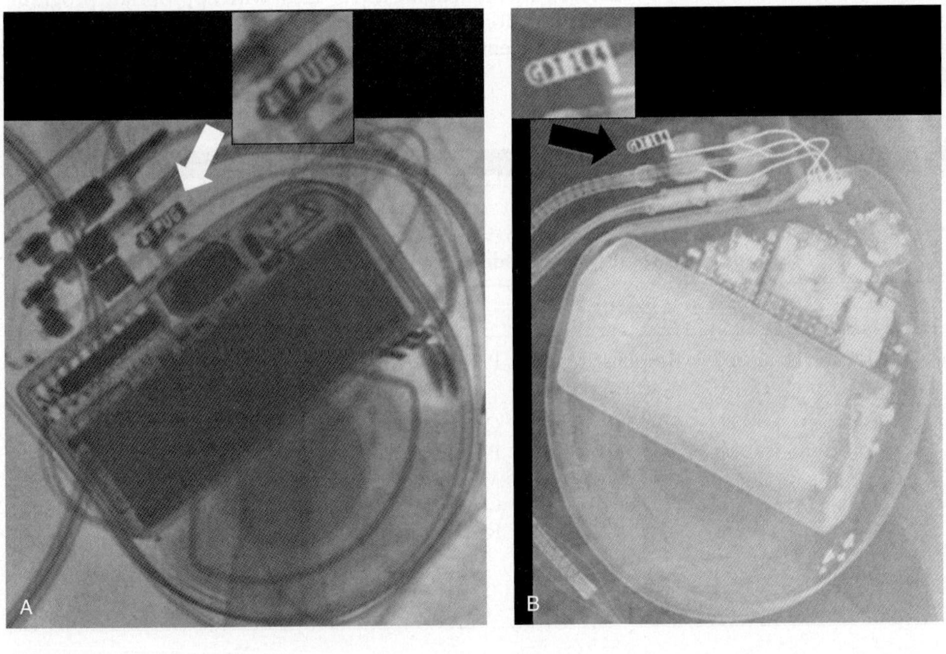

FIGURE 44.2. Many cardiac devices are marked with a radiopaque code that specifically identifies the manufacturer and model of the device. **A:** Medtronic ICD with magnified view of radiopaque code (inset). The manufacturer is identified by the Medtronic logo at the extreme left of the code and the model by the three letter code that represents the engineering series number. **B:** Boston Scientific ICD with magnified view of radiopaque code (inset). The manufacturer and model are identified by the radiopaque codes "GDT" and "104", respectively.

TABLE 44.1

DEVICE MANUFACTURERS' CONTACT INFORMATION

Medtronic	1.800.MEDTRONIC
Boston Scientific	1.800.CARDIAC
St. Jude Medical	1.800.PACEICD
Biotronik	1.800.547.0394
Sorin Group	1.800.352.6466

detection and therapy and reversion to an asynchronous pacing mode (*noise-reversion mode*).

Inappropriate inhibition of ventricular pacing can be catastrophic in the pacemaker-dependent patient; similarly atrial oversensing with inappropriate ventricular tracking could result in a myriad of symptoms including heart failure exacerbation, hypotension, or angina. Improper ICD tachyarrhythmia detection due to EMI could potentially be arrhythmia-inducing as a result of unsynchronized inappropriate shock delivery during the vulnerable period of repolarization. Noise-reversion mode is an algorithm that reverts transiently to asynchronous pacing in response to rapid frequency signals. The algorithm is designed to protect against inappropriate inhibition of pacing when high-frequency signals are sensed. Although this algorithm is present in all pacemakers regardless of manufacturer, this is not the case for ICDs. Less frequently, EMI can result in reprogramming of the device parameters or permanent circuitry or lead damage. When EMI exposure is unavoidable, certain measures can be taken to minimize the potential risk. For example, pacemaker or defibrillator patients requiring surgery with electrocautery should have a magnet placed over the device during the operation. Other forms of EMI (e.g. MRI, radiation therapy) carry substantial risk and may prompt the revision or removal of the entire cardiac device system prior to planned exposure. Care should be taken to avoid sources of EMI in device patients or, if exposure to EMI cannot be avoided, at a minimum, measures should be taken to minimize potential harm with consideration of device interrogation following exposure.

Mode Switch

Mode switch is a programmable pacing algorithm that automatically changes the pacing mode to a nontracking mode in response to a sensed atrial arrhythmia. The purpose of this algorithm is to prevent inappropriately fast ventricular tracking at the upper rate limit in response to a rapid atrial tachyarrhythmia. Once the device has mode switched, it will remain in a nontracking mode until the atrial rate has fallen below the mode switch threshold for a specific number of intervals. This algorithm is very useful for patients with paroxysmal atrial arrhythmias (e.g. SVT, atrial fibrillation or atrial flutter). The atrial rate at which mode switch occurs is programmable in most devices and the feature can even be programmed "off."

Line Management

The placement of central venous catheters in cardiac device patients warrants special consideration. Depending on the location and age of the device and the planned location of central venous access, a number of potential complications can occur. Reported complications associated with central venous catheters in cardiac device patients include lead damage from needle puncture [4], lead dislodgement, and inappropriate ICD therapies [5]. In addition, central venous stenosis as a consequence of prior cardiac device implantation may present a challenge to central venous catheter placement ipsilateral to the device [6]. Cardiac device infections and device-related endocarditis represent a particularly serious hazard of indwelling central venous catheters necessitating removal of the entire device system [7]. Central venous access should be performed contralateral to the device whenever possible.

Magnetic Resonance Imaging

The likelihood that patients with cardiac devices will require an MRI is high [8] but this imaging modality is not without risks in these patients. The potential hazards of magnetic resonance imaging in cardiac device patients include movement of the device, programming changes, asynchronous pacing, activation of tachyarrhythmia therapies, inhibition of pacing output, and induced lead currents that could lead to heating and cardiac stimulation [9], resulting in altered pacing and defibrillation thresholds, device damage, asystole, arrhythmias, or even death [10]. Although an implantable cardiac device remains a strong relative contraindication to MRI, certain centers have developed protocols for performing MRIs in cardiac device patients [11] and MRI-safe pacemakers are being developed. If an MRI is the only diagnostic imaging option in a cardiac device patient, imaging at 1.5 Tesla with appropriate programming and monitoring can likely be undertaken safely with careful assessment of the risk–benefit ratio on a case-by-case basis [11–14].

TABLE 44.2

PACING DESIGNATION

NASPE/BPEG Generic (NBG) Code					
Position	I	II	III	IV	V
Category	Chamber(s) pace	Chamber(s) sensed	Response to sensing	Programmability, rate modulation	Antitachy-arrhythmia function(s)
Letters used	O-None A-Atrium V-Ventricle D-Dual (A + V)	O-None A-Atrium V-Ventricle D-Dual (A + V)	O-None T-Triggered I-Inhibited D-Dual (T + I)	O-None P-Simple Programmable M-Multiprogrammable C-Communicating R-Rate modulation	O-None P-Pacing (antitachy-arrhythmia) S-Shock D-Dual (P + S)
Manufacturer's designation only	S-Single (A or V)	S-Single (A or V)			

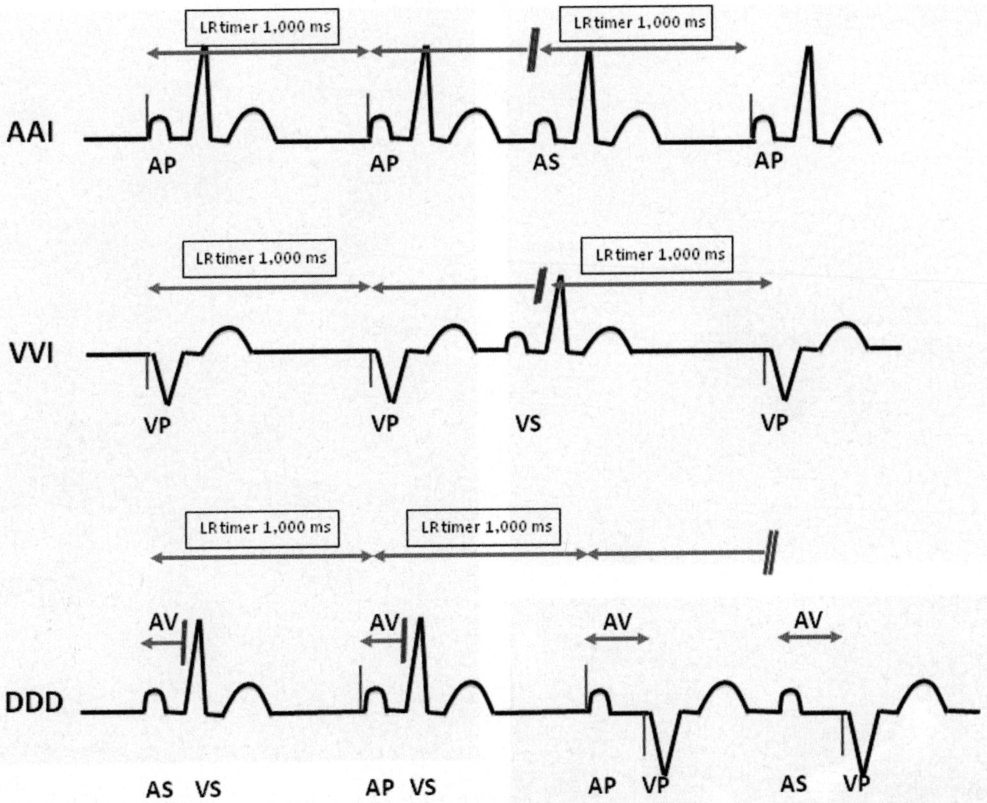

FIGURE 44.3. Timing of events in various pacing modes. AAI is an atrial nontracking mode of pacing that provides backup atrial pacing at the programmed lower rate limit. Similarly, VVI is a ventricular nontracking mode of pacing that provides backup ventricular pacing at the programmed lower rate limit. DDD is a dual-chamber mode of pacing that can both inhibit and trigger events in both the atrium and the ventricle. AS, atrial-sensed event; AP, atrial-paced event; VS, ventricular-sensed event; VP, ventricular-paced event; LR, lower rate limit.

External Defibrillation

In the event of a cardiac arrest or hemodynamically unstable arrhythmia in a patient with an implantable cardiac device, resuscitative efforts should proceed as per guidelines without deviation. Defibrillation or cardioversion can result in permanent damage to the cardiac device; to minimize these risks, the defibrillation pads should be placed at least 10 cm from the pulse generator [15]. Other potential risks of external defibrillation include device reprogramming [16] and myocardial damage at the interface with the lead resulting in an acute rise in threshold [17]. Following defibrillation or cardioversion, cardiac devices should be interrogated formally to insure proper function and programming. Again, the low potential risk of damage to the device should *not* impede usual and necessary resuscitative efforts for the patient.

Infection

Cardiac device related infection encompasses a disease spectrum from pocket infection to device-related endocarditis. The clinical manifestations of cardiac device-related infection are protean and can range from pain at the implant site without cutaneous manifestations to minor erythema or swelling of the device pocket (Fig. 44.4A) to overt erosion of the system (Fig. 44.4B) to device-related endocarditis (Fig. 44.4C) [18,19]. In the absence of bacteremia, systemic manifestations and leukocytosis are rare. Cultures of the device leads yield the highest results and, *Staphylococci* are the primary pathogen identified [20]. A high index of suspicion is warranted in a patient with implanted pacemaker or ICD and signs and symptoms of infection. Cardiac device-related infection requires prompt removal of the entire device system for complete treatment unless significant comorbidities preclude extraction [7,18]. Although no specific vegetation size has been established as a contraindication to transvenous extraction, most experts agree that vegetations greater than 3 cm in size are better treated surgically [7]. Patients with device-related endocarditis require a minimum of six weeks of intravenous antibiotics and pose a particular problem with respect to the timing of re-implant in pacemaker-dependent patients.

Pacemaker Malfunction

Oversensing

Sensing problems are one of the most common causes of pacemaker malfunction (Table 44.3). Oversensing is defined as the sensing of physiologic or nonphysiologic events that should not be sensed. Consequently, oversensing can lead to inappropriate inhibition of pacemaker output (Fig. 44.5). Physiologic events that can be the cause of oversensing include far-field P waves, wide QRS complexes, T waves, and myopotentials, either pectoral or diaphragmatic. Typically, oversensing due to physiologic events can be overcome by decreasing the programmed sensitivity. Nonphysiologic oversensing may be the result of EMI or hardware problems such as loose setscrew or lead dislodgement or fracture and will likely require device revision to correct. Oversensing and failure to pace in a pacemaker-dependent patient can be catastrophic. Application of a magnet over the device will change the device to an asynchronous

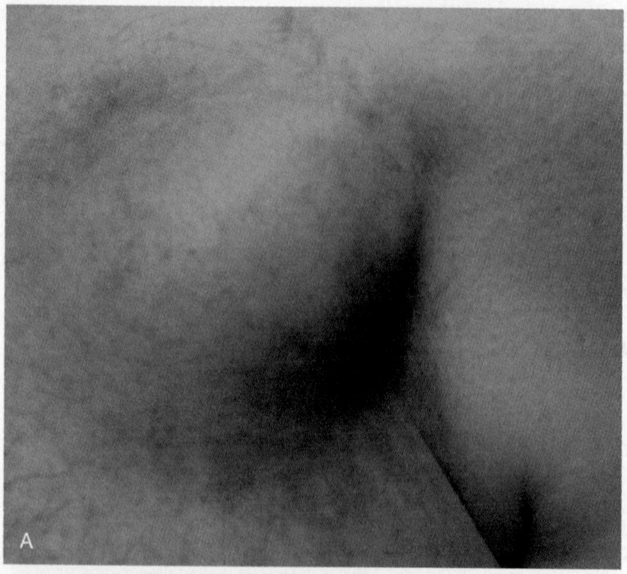

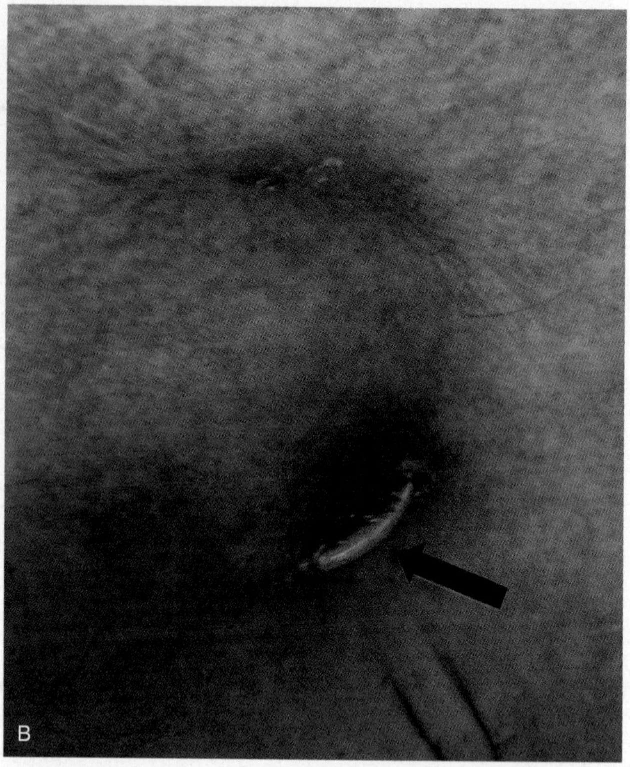

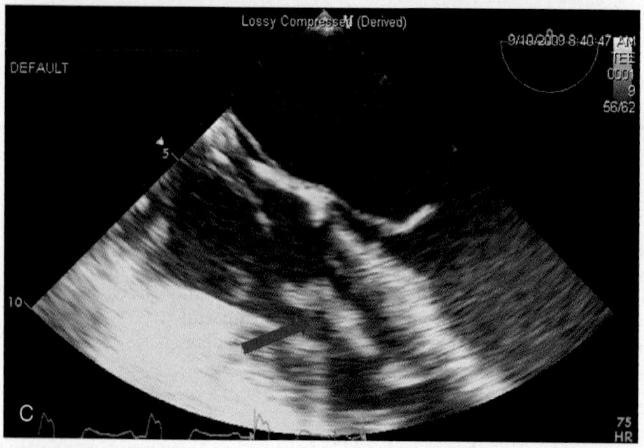

FIGURE 44.4. Different manifestations of device-related infections. **A:** Swelling and erythema suggest pocket infection although local signs of inflammation may be absent. **B:** Erosion of either the lead(s) or the device by definition is a manifestation of infection. In this example, the pocket appears swollen with areas of erythema and a pacing electrode (*arrow*) is seen eroding through the skin at the inferior margin of the pocket. **C:** Device-related infection could result in bacteria, vegetations and sepsis. Here, transesophageal echocardiography demonstrated a large vegetation (*arrow*) adherent to the atrial pacing lead and seen to prolapse across the tricuspid valve.

pacing mode and insure more reliable delivery of pacing until a formal evaluation can be performed.

Undersensing

In contrast, undersensing occurs when the device fails to sense intrinsic events. This results in the generation of unnecessary pacemaker impulses and "overpacing." Undersensing may be a result of alterations in electrogram amplitude of physiologic events or may represent hardware failure. Antiarrhythmic drug therapy, myocardial infarction, and metabolic derangements can alter electrogram amplitude transiently or permanently. Undersensing may be potentially corrected by changing the programmed sensitivity. Other etiologies of undersensing are similar to those of noncapture (lead dislodgement, perforation, or fracture). Asynchronous pacing modes, due to EMI or battery depletion, can mimic undersensing on surface electrocardiogram.

Noncapture

Noncapture occurs when electrical impulses emitted from the device fail to capture myocardium. The surface electrocardiogram will demonstrate pacing stimuli without evidence of capture (Fig. 44.6). Loss of capture can be intermittent or permanent, but often necessitates device revision. Causes of noncapture can be divided into changes in capture threshold and hardware malfunction. The capture threshold can rise in the first 4 to 6 weeks following lead implant due to inflammatory changes at the lead-myocardial border although this has become less relevant clinically with the advent and widespread use of steroid-eluting leads. A rise in capture threshold can be overcome by increasing the pacemaker output. Other causes of elevated capture thresholds include myocardial fibrosis or infarction near the exit of the pacing stimulus, metabolic derangements (specifically, hyperkalemia, acidemia and hyperglycemia), and certain medications. Class Ia, Ic, and III antiarrhythmic drugs [21–27] can increase capture thresholds as can mineralocorticoids and hypertonic saline [28]. If the capture threshold exceeds the maximal programmable output, this is termed *exit block*. Primary hardware problems such as lead dislodgement, perforation or fracture, and battery depletion can all result in noncapture. A chest radiograph can help diagnose specific lead issues (Fig. 44.7A–C). Formal pacemaker interrogation or magnet application can identify battery depletion.

No Output

The complete absence of pacemaker stimuli despite magnet application suggests complete battery depletion or generator damage. Damage to the generator can occur rarely as a result of direct trauma [29] or external defibrillation [15].

Pacemaker-Mediated Tachycardia

Pacemaker-mediated tachycardia (PMT) refers to any sustained tachyarrhythmia that is dependent on continued pacemaker participation in the circuit. Classically, the term PMT is used to

TABLE 44.3

TROUBLESHOOTING PACEMAKER MALFUNCTION

Problem	Etiology	Causes	Management
Failure to pace, no PPM stimuli	Oversensing	Physiologic events P, R, or T waves Myopotentials Nonphysiologic events EMI Lead fracture Loose setscrew	Reprogram. Avoid EMI sources. Device revision.
Failure to pace with PPM stimuli	Noncapture	Elevated threshold Exit block MI, fibrosis Medications Electrolytes Hardware failure Lead dislodgement Lead fracture Lead perforation Battery depletion	Reprogram, if possible. Correct reversible causes. May require device revision. Device revision.
Inappropriate pacing	Undersensing	Low EGM amplitude Low at implant MI, fibrosis Medications Electrolytes Lead dislodgement Lead fracture ERI Noise reversion	Reprogram, if possible. Correct reversible causes. May require device revision. Lead revision Lead revision Replace PPM Reprogram

EMI, electromagnetic interference; EGM, electrogram; ERI, elective replacement interval; PPM, pacemaker.

describe an endless loop tachycardia in dual-chamber devices consisting of ventricular pacing, retrograde atrial activation, appropriate sensing and triggered ventricular pacing perpetuating the tachycardia (Fig. 44.8). PMT should be suspected when ventricular pacing occurs at the programmed maximum tracking rate of the device. The PMT circuit can be interrupted with magnet application and the arrhythmia terminated.

DEVICE-SPECIFIC CONSIDERATIONS

Implantable Cardioverter Defibrillator

Electrical Storm

Electrical or ventricular tachycardia (VT) storm is defined as three or more episodes of VT or ventricular fibrillation within a 24-hour period. When a patient presents with electrical storm, suppression of the arrhythmias are of paramount importance. Identifying the trigger can be difficult [30] but attempts should be made to identify and correct potentially treatable causes (Table 44.4). Repeated defibrillator therapy is painful and highly stressful, can cause heightened sympathetic tone and result in early battery depletion, myocardial ischemia/stunning, and recurrent ventricular arrhythmias [31,32]. Thus, initial treatment should consist primarily of sympathetic blockade with beta-blockers and anxiolysis with benzodiazepines. Amiodarone is often the antiarrhythmic agent of choice [33,34]. Refractory cases may require intubation and deep anesthesia [35]; stellate ganglion blockade can be considered in extreme cases [36]. Catheter ablation is effective in the treatment of electrical storm and can be considered for electrical storm despite chronic antiarrhythmic therapy and for refractory cases [37].

Ineffective Defibrillation

Successful defibrillation occurs when a critical mass of myocardium is successfully depolarized and depends on shock vector, lead position, and the electrical milieu. The optimal three-dimensional orientation of the ICD shock vector should deliver energy uniformly throughout the left ventricle. The vector is dependent on the position of the high-voltage coils in the right ventricle (RV) and superior vena cava (SVC)-right atrial (RA) junction and the active can in relation to the left ventricle. Typically, the RV coil is the cathode and the SVC–RA coil and ICD can form the anode with current traveling from cathode to anode.

Implantable defibrillators can fail to deliver effective defibrillation therapy in certain situations. Elevated defibrillation thresholds (DFT) can occur as a result of metabolic derangements, myocardial ischemia, pneumothorax, hypoxia, multiple defibrillations, drug therapy, delays in arrhythmia detection, and device hardware malfunction (Table 44.5). Immediate management should consist of external defibrillation and treatment of potential reversible causes. Long-term management may require device revision or cessation/addition of specific antiarrhythmic medications.

Inappropriate Therapies

Inappropriate therapies are common in patients with implantable defibrillators regardless of indication [38] and are

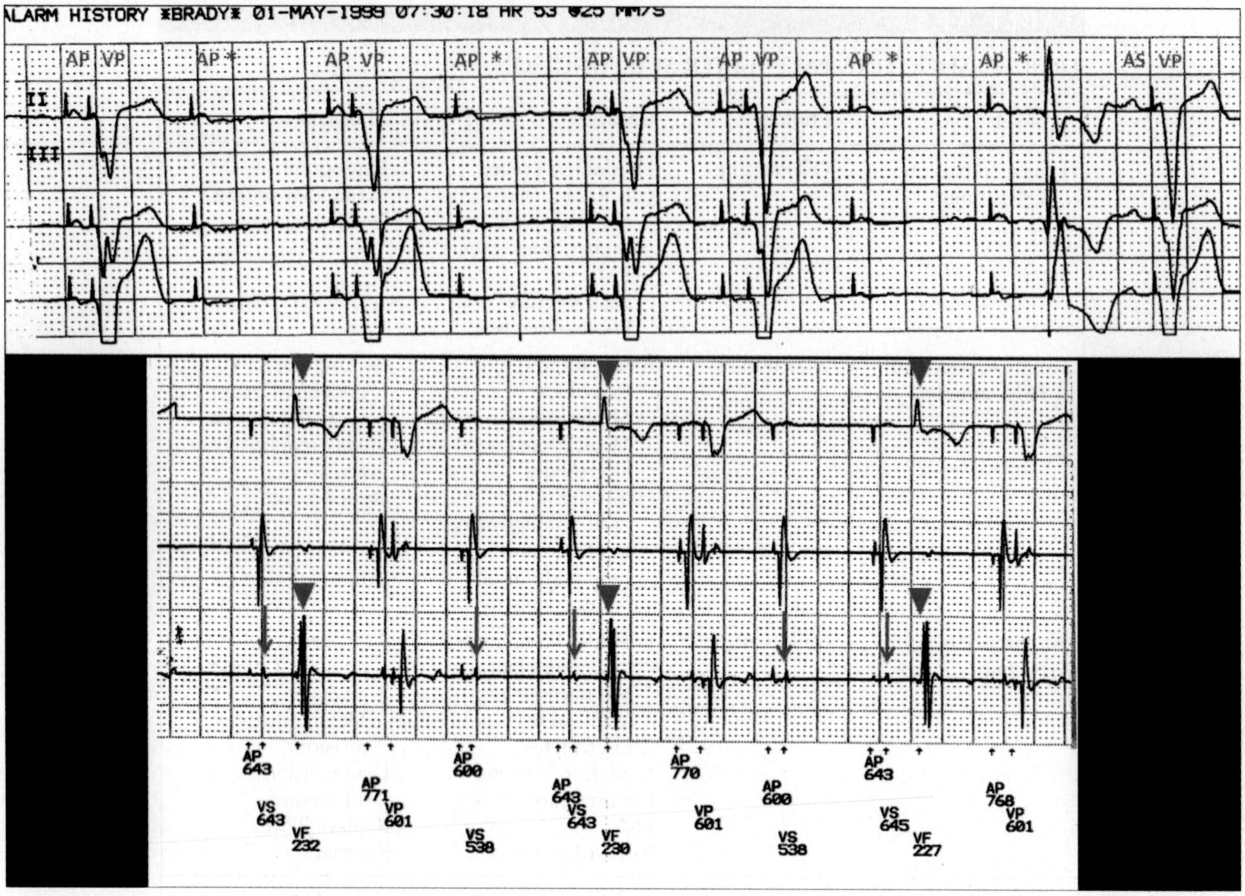

FIGURE 44.5. Dual-chamber defibrillator with evidence of ventricular oversensing. The top panel demonstrates atrial (AP) and ventricular (VP) sequential pacing with the intermittent absence of ventricular pacing stimuli (*asterisks*) following atrial paced events. The bottom panel represents the intracardiac electrograms from the same device with ventricular oversensing of atrial events (*arrows*). When intrinsic ventricular conduction does occur (*arrowheads*), the device incorrectly labels the event as "VF" (*arrowheads*) or a ventricular event that because of timing falls into the programmed ventricular fibrillation detection zone.

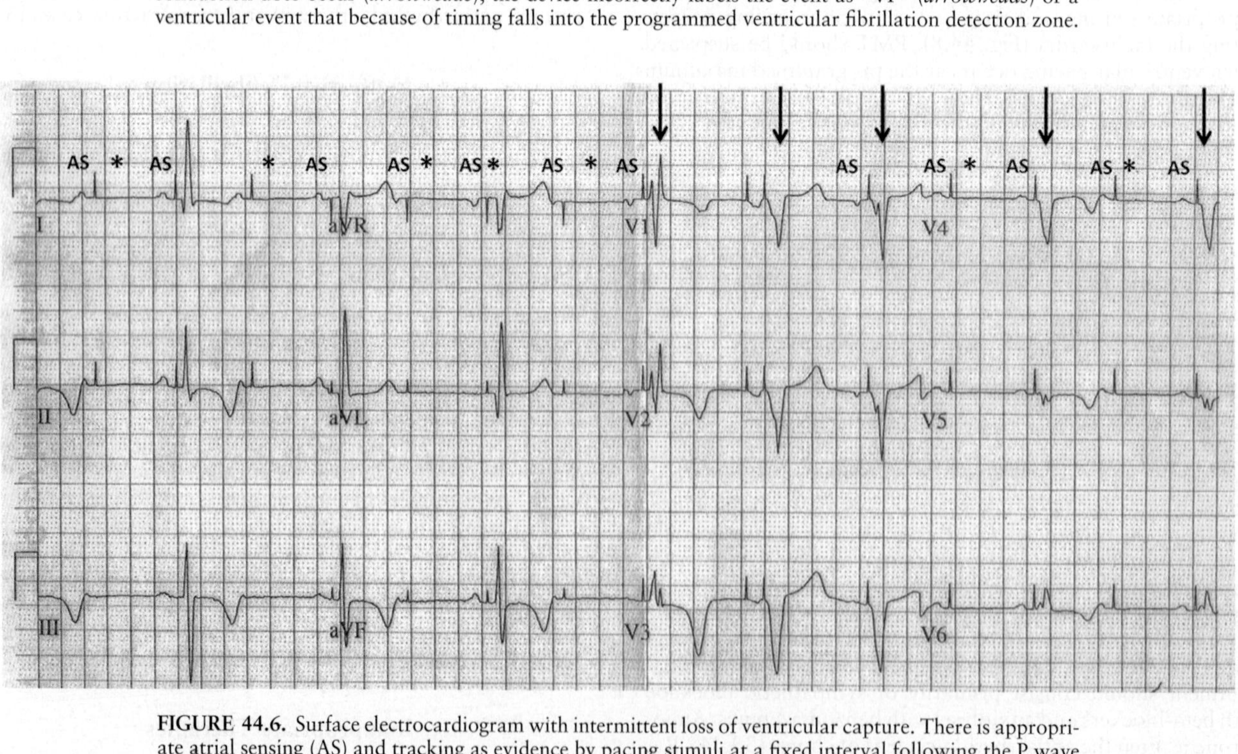

FIGURE 44.6. Surface electrocardiogram with intermittent loss of ventricular capture. There is appropriate atrial sensing (AS) and tracking as evidence by pacing stimuli at a fixed interval following the P wave but intermittent failure of ventricular output to capture the myocardium (*asterisks*). Evidence of varying degrees of fusion between intrinsic conduction and ventricular pacing is also observed (*arrows*).

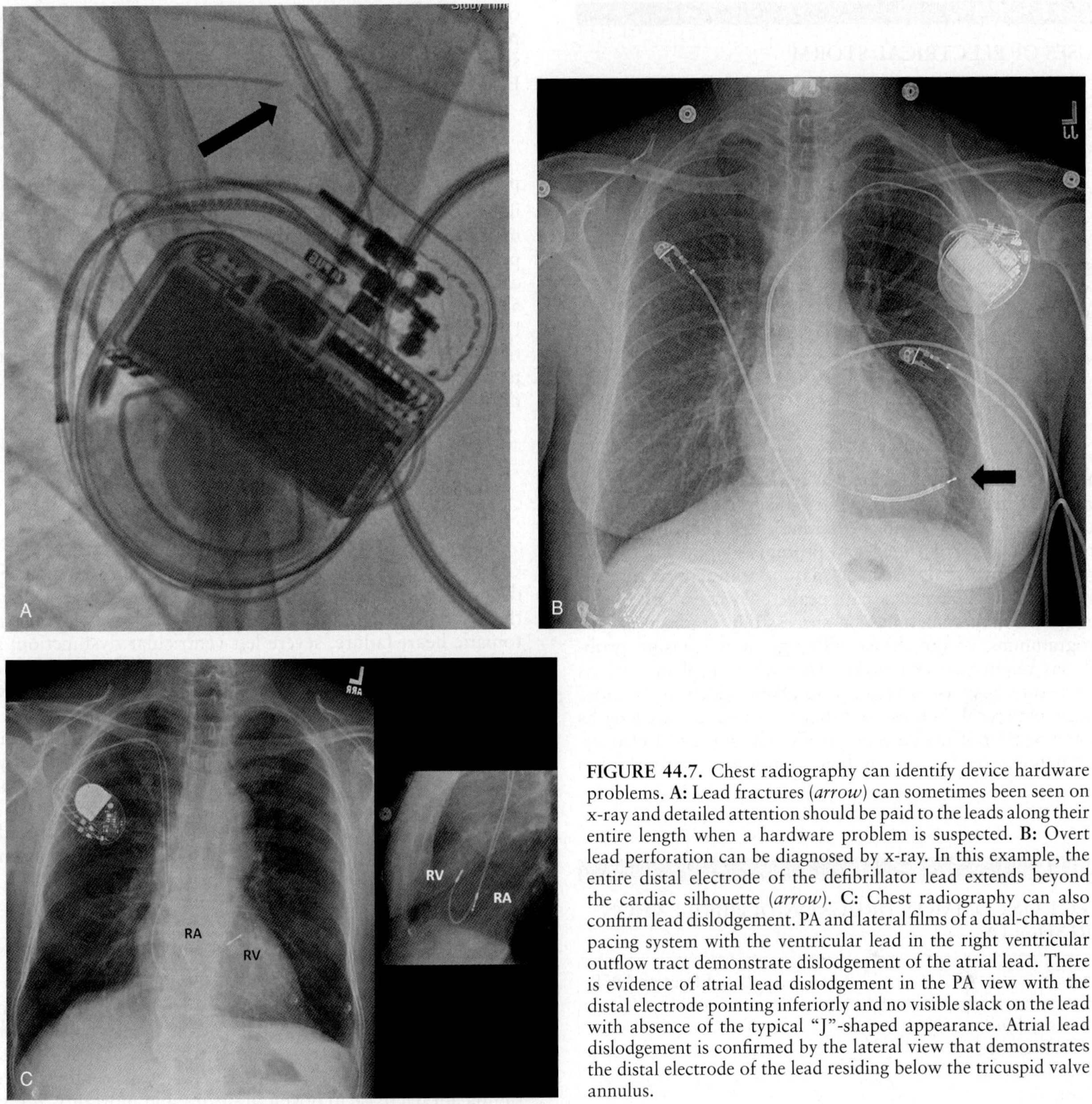

FIGURE 44.7. Chest radiography can identify device hardware problems. **A:** Lead fractures (*arrow*) can sometimes been seen on x-ray and detailed attention should be paid to the leads along their entire length when a hardware problem is suspected. **B:** Overt lead perforation can be diagnosed by x-ray. In this example, the entire distal electrode of the defibrillator lead extends beyond the cardiac silhouette (*arrow*). **C:** Chest radiography can also confirm lead dislodgement. PA and lateral films of a dual-chamber pacing system with the ventricular lead in the right ventricular outflow tract demonstrate dislodgement of the atrial lead. There is evidence of atrial lead dislodgement in the PA view with the distal electrode pointing inferiorly and no visible slack on the lead with absence of the typical "J"-shaped appearance. Atrial lead dislodgement is confirmed by the lateral view that demonstrates the distal electrode of the lead residing below the tricuspid valve annulus.

associated with significant morbidity and mortality [39,40]. Common causes of inappropriate therapies include SVT, ventricular sensing problems, lead failure, and EMI. The detection algorithms of ICDs are based primarily on heart rate, and any ventricular-sensed event that exceeds the programmed detection rate will trigger ICD therapy. Supraventricular discriminators related to arrhythmia onset, cycle length stability and electrogram morphology are also programmable but reduce inappropriate therapies only slightly [41,42]. Repeated inappropriate ICD therapies in hemodynamically stable patients should prompt magnet application or device deactivation with back-up external defibrillation available and definitive treatment directed at the underlying rhythm or problem.

The most common cause of inappropriate defibrillator therapy is atrial fibrillation although sinus tachycardia and other SVTs can result in inappropriate therapies. Surface electrocardiogram and clinical status may aid with the diagnosis if formal interrogation is not immediately available. The device should be inactivated and treatment directed at the underlying atrial arrhythmia. Ventricular sensing problems also

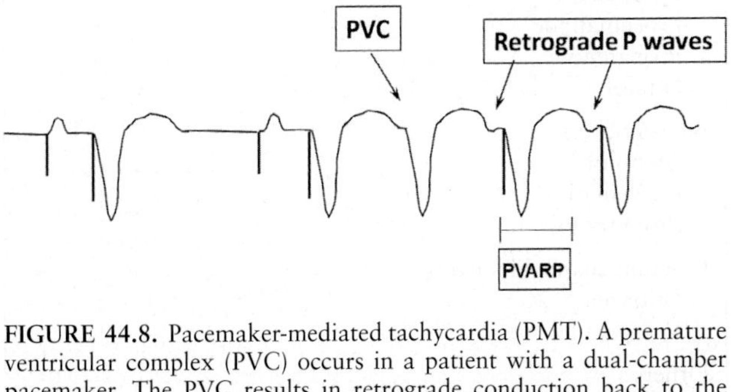

FIGURE 44.8. Pacemaker-mediated tachycardia (PMT). A premature ventricular complex (PVC) occurs in a patient with a dual-chamber pacemaker. The PVC results in retrograde conduction back to the atrium that is subsequently tracked by the ventricular lead and incessant tachycardia ensues. Retrograde atrial activation is sensed by the pacemaker because it falls outside the postventricular atrial refractory period (PVARP). One means of eliminating PMT is to extend the PVARP.

TABLE 44.4

CAUSES OF ELECTRICAL STORM

Acquired long QT
Decompensated heart failure
Electrolyte disturbances
Fever/sepsis
Hyperthyroidism
Lead dislodgement/position
Medication noncompliance
Myocardial ischemia
Myocarditis
Psychologic stressors
Substance abuse
Sympathomimetics

result in inappropriate therapies when other electrical events (P waves, T waves, wide QRS) are misinterpreted as a ventricular event. This "double counting" is erroneously interpreted as a tachyarrhythmia and prompts inappropriate ICD therapy. Ventricular oversensing may be transient as a result of metabolic derangements (e.g., peaked T waves with hyperkalemia) or may sometimes be successfully eradicated with reprogramming of the device although some sensing problems may require device revision. Hardware problems such as lead fracture, insulation break, lead dislodgement, or a loose setscrew may result in noise and short ventricular cycle lengths that can be mistakenly detected as VT. The surface electrocardiogram is extremely useful and will demonstrate sinus rhythm or tachycardia at the time of defibrillation. Device hardware problems cannot be overcome with reprogramming. The ICD should be deactivated until the system can be revised. Similarly, EMI can produce noise and result in inappropriate therapies.

TABLE 44.5

EFFECT OF COMMON DRUGS ON DEFIBRILLATION THRESHOLDS

Drug	Effect on DFT
Antiarrhythmics	
Amiodarone	↑
Disopyramide	↔
Dofetilide	↓
Ibutilide	↓
Flecainide	↑↔
Lidocaine	↑
Mexilitine	↑
Quinidine	↑↔
Procainamide	↑↔
Propafenone	↔
Sotalol	↓
Beta-blockers	
Atenolol	↔↓
Carvedilol	↑
Propranolol	↑
Calcium channel blockers	
Diltiazem	↑
Verapamil	↑
Others	
Digoxin	↔
Fentanyl	↑
Ranolazine	↔
Sildenafil	↑

Withdrawal of Care

Patients with ICDs and end-stage heart failure or other fatal illness warrant special consideration. Successful defibrillation may prolong life but it cannot prevent death. In addition, repeated ICD shocks in a patient with end-stage disease may cause unnecessary pain and anxiety. Defibrillation can be deactivated in ICDs without deactivating pacemaking functions. Discussions regarding ICD deactivation occur rarely even in patients with do-not-resuscitate orders [43]. It is important that patients and their families understand that deactivation of defibrillator therapies is always an option [44].

Cardiac Resynchronization Therapy (Biventricular Pacing)

Cardiac resynchronization therapy (CRT) improves symptoms, decreases hospitalizations, assists with reverse remodeling of the left ventricle, and reduces mortality in patients with symptomatic heart failure, severe left ventricular dysfunction, and mechanical dyssynchrony (QRS >120 ms) [45–48]. Ventricular resynchronization aims to achieve myocardial coordination through left ventricular preexcitation ideally at the site of latest activation. This can be achieved through an endovascular approach with left ventricular lead placement via coronary sinus cannulation or epicardially with a direct surgical approach (typically via left lateral thoracotomy). Approximately 70% of CRT patients demonstrate clinical improvement with reduction in symptoms [49,50] and even fewer show improvement in left ventricular function [51].

Loss of Resynchronization

Achieving resynchronization appears dependent not only on stimulating the ventricle at the site of latest activation but also providing reliable biventricular pacing. There appears to be a threshold effect of CRT related to frequency of biventricular pacing. A recent retrospective analysis demonstrated a significant decrease in hospitalizations and mortality at biventricular pacing above 92% [52]. Among CRT responders, loss of resynchronization can result in recurrent symptoms, diminished functional capacity, repeat hospitalization, and significant hemodynamic alterations. Although formal device interrogation is necessary to assess the degree of biventricular pacing over the long-term, careful observation of the telemetry monitor often can provide significant insight. Similarly, the 12-lead electrocardiogram can identify the site of ventricular stimulation and can be used to detect loss of biventricular pacing (Fig. 44.9A, B). Atrial arrhythmias with intact ventricular conduction exceeding the programmed lower rate of the CRT device are the most common reason for failure to achieve sufficient resynchronization. Other potential reasons for suboptimal biventricular pacing include elevated pacing threshold, lead fracture, or lead migration to an unfavorable location. Common reasons for a lack of response to CRT are lead location, suboptimal programming and underlying narrow QRS [53]. If the left ventricular pacing lead is not stimulating a late activation site in the basal posterolateral left ventricle, the degree of biventricular pacing is irrelevant. The electrocardiogram and chest radiograph are useful in identifying issues with left ventricular lead placement.

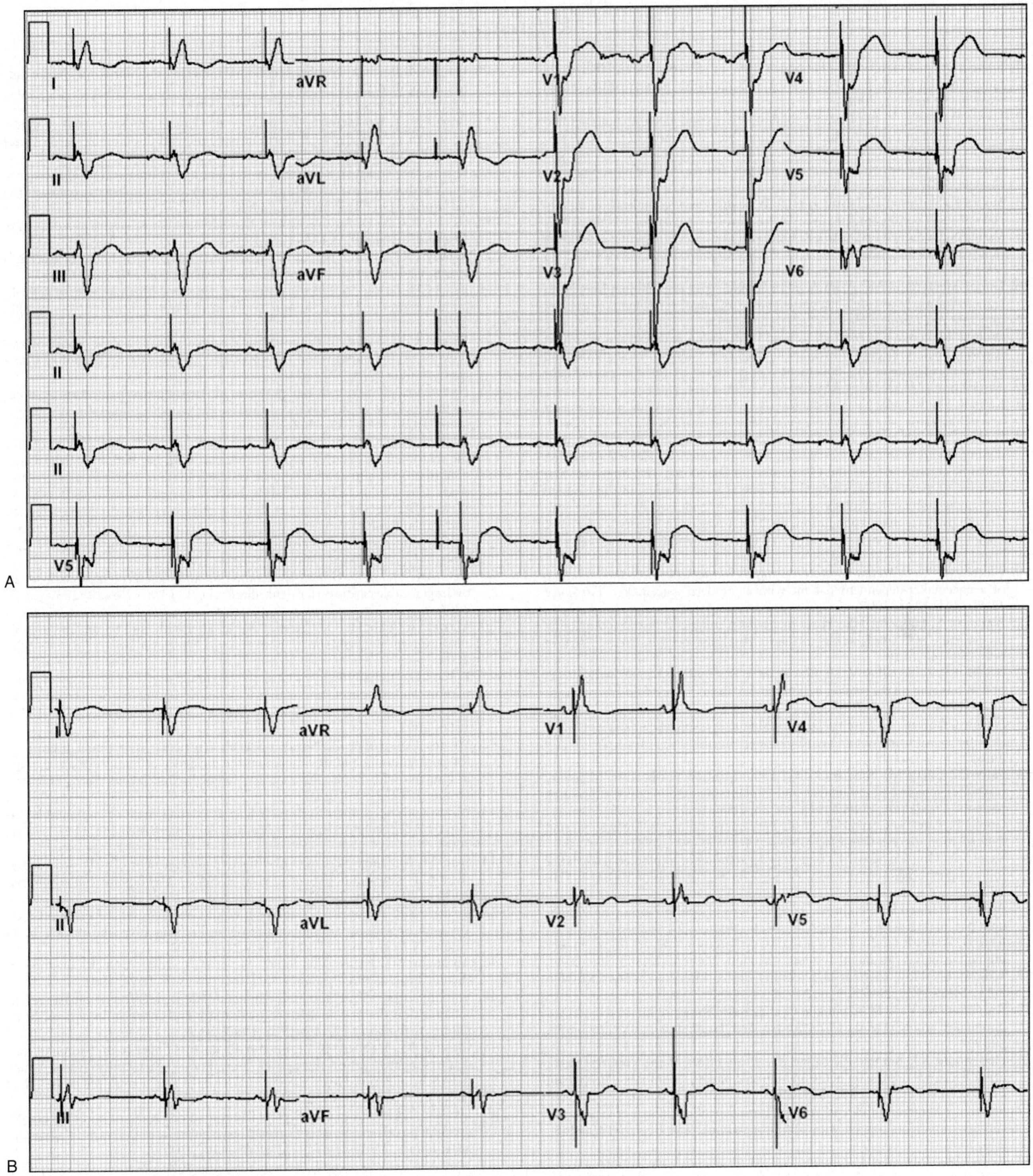

FIGURE 44.9. A, B: Electrocardiographic assessment of pacing site. A: Right ventricular apical pacing with left bundle branch morphology and superior frontal plane axis. B: In contrast, biventricular stimulation with right bundle morphology in V1 and QS waves in leads I and avL.

Summary

In the modern era, patients with implantable pacemakers, defibrillators and cardiac resynchronization devices are increasingly commonly admitted to the care of an intensivist. Attention to and understanding of the implanted device as a critical portion of the patient's acute care is warranted. Early involvement of electrophysiologist colleagues in the care of critically ill patients especially with device malfunction or infection is prudent.

References

1. Epstein AE, Dimarco JP, Ellenbogen KA, et al: ACC/AHA/HRS 2008 Guidelines for device-based therapy of cardiac rhythm abnormalities. *Heart Rhythm* 5(6):e1–62, 2008.
2. Dyrda K, Khairy P: Implantable rhythm devices and electromagnetic interference: myth or reality? *Expert Rev Cardiovasc Ther* 6(6):823–832, 2008.
3. Ellenbogen K, Kay GN, Lau CP, et al: (eds): *Clinical Cardiac Pacing, Defibrillation, and Resynchronization Therapy.* 3rd ed. Philadelphia, Saunders Elsevier, 2007.
4. Stokes K, Staffeson D, Lessar J, et al: A possible new complication of subclavian stick: conductor fracture. *Pacing Clin Electrophysiol* 10:748, 1987.
5. Varma N, Cunningham D, Falk R: Central venous access resulting in selective failure of ICD defibrillation capacity. *Pacing Clin Electrophysiol* 24(3):394–395, 2001.
6. Gurjar M, Baronia AK, Azim A, et al: Should blind internal jugular venous catheterization be avoided in a patient with ipsilateral permanent pacemaker implant? *Am J Emerg Med* 24(4):501–502, 2006.
7. Wilkoff BL, Love CJ, Byrd CL, et al: Transvenous lead extraction: Heart Rhythm Society Expert consensus on facilities, training, indications, and patient management: this document was endorsed by the American Heart Association (AHA). *Heart Rhythm* 6(7):1085–1104, 2009.
8. Kalin R, Stanton MS: Current clinical issues for MRI scanning of pacemaker and defibrillator patients. *Pacing Clin Electrophysiol* 28(4):326–328, 2005.
9. Levine GN, Gomes AS, Arai AE, et al: Safety of magnetic resonance imaging in patients with cardiovascular devices: an American Heart Association scientific statement from the Committee on Diagnostic and Interventional Cardiac Catheterization, Council on Clinical Cardiology, and the Council on Cardiovascular Radiology and Intervention: endorsed by the American College of Cardiology Foundation, the North American Society for Cardiac Imaging, and the Society for Cardiovascular Magnetic Resonance. *Circulation* 116(24):2878–2891, 2007.
10. Gimbel JR: Unexpected asystole during 3 T magnetic resonance imaging of a pacemaker-dependent patient with a 'modern' pacemaker. *Europace* 11(9):1241–1242, 2009.
11. Nazarian S, Halperin HR: How to perform magnetic resonance imaging on patients with implantable cardiac arrhythmia devices. *Heart Rhythm* 6(1):138–143, 2009.
12. Naehle CP, Zeijlemaker V, Thomas D, et al: Evaluation of cumulative effects of MR imaging on pacemaker systems at 1.5 Tesla. *Pacing Clin Electrophysiol* 32(12):1526–1535, 2009.
13. Naehle CP, Strach K, Thomas D, et al: Magnetic resonance imaging at 1.5-T in patients with implantable cardioverter-defibrillators. *J Am Coll Cardiol* 54(6):549–555, 2009.
14. Faris OP, Shein M: Food and drug administration perspective: Magnetic resonance imaging of pacemaker and implantable cardioverter-defibrillator patients. *Circulation* 114(12):1232–1233, 2006.
15. Gould L, Patel S, Gomes GI, et al: Pacemaker failure following external defibrillation. *Pacing Clin Electrophysiol* 4(5):575–577, 1981.
16. Barold SS, Ong LS, Scovil J, et al: Reprogramming of implanted pacemaker following external defibrillation. *Pacing Clin Electrophysiol* 1(4):514–520, 1978.
17. Aylward P, Blood R, Tonkin A: Complications of defibrillation with permanent pacemaker in situ. *Pacing Clin Electrophysiol* 2(4):462–464, 1979.
18. Klug D, Wallet F, Lacroix D, et al: Local symptoms at the site of pacemaker implantation indicate latent systemic infection. *Heart* 90(8):882–886, 2004.
19. Wilkoff BL: How to treat and identify device infections. *Heart Rhythm* 4(11):1467–1470, 2007.
20. Anselmino M, Vinci M, Comoglio C, et al: Bacteriology of infected extracted pacemaker and ICD leads. *J Cardiovasc Med (Hagerstown)* 10(9):693–698, 2009.
21. Hellestrand KJ, Burnett PJ, Milne JR, et al: Effect of the antiarrhythmic agent flecainide acetate on acute and chronic pacing thresholds. *Pacing Clin Electrophysiol* 6(5 Pt 1):892–899, 1983.
22. Soriano J, Almendral J, Arenal A, et al: Rate-dependent failure of ventricular capture in patients treated with oral propafenone. *Eur Heart J* 13(2):269–274, 1992.
23. Reiffel JA, Coromilas J, Zimmerman JM, et al: Drug-device interactions: clinical considerations. *Pacing Clin Electrophysiol* 8(3 Pt 1):369–373, 1985.
24. Dorian P, Fain ES, Davy JM, et al: Lidocaine causes a reversible, concentration-dependent increase in defibrillation energy requirements. *J Am Coll Cardiol* 8(2):327–332, 1986.
25. Dorian P, Fain ES, Davy JM, et al: Effect of quinidine and bretylium on defibrillation energy requirements. *Am Heart J* 112(1):19–25, 1986.
26. Marinchak RA, Friehling TD, Kline RA, et al: Effect of antiarrhythmic drugs on defibrillation threshold: case report of an adverse effect of mexiletine and review of the literature. *Pacing Clin Electrophysiol* 11(1):7–12, 1988.
27. Jung W, Manz M, Luderitz B: Effects of antiarrhythmic drugs on defibrillation threshold in patients with the implantable cardioverter defibrillator. *Pacing Clin Electrophysiol* 15(4 Pt 3):645–648, 1992.
28. Preston TA, Judge RD: Alteration of pacemaker threshold by drug and physiological factors. *Ann N Y Acad Sci* 167(2):686–692, 1969.
29. Hai AA, Kalinchak DM, Schoenfeld MH: Increased defibrillator charge time following direct trauma to an ICD generator: blunt consequences. *Pacing Clin Electrophysiol* 32(12):1587–1590, 2009.
30. Brigadeau F, Kouakam C, Klug D, et al: Clinical predictors and prognostic significance of electrical storm in patients with implantable cardioverter defibrillators. *Eur Heart J* 27(6):700–707, 2006.
31. Huang DT, Traub D: Recurrent ventricular arrhythmia storms in the age of implantable cardioverter defibrillator therapy: a comprehensive review. *Prog Cardiovasc Dis* 51(3):229–236, 2008.
32. Dorian P, Cass D: An overview of the management of electrical storm. *Can J Cardiol* 13(Suppl A):13A–17A, 1997.
33. Kowey PR: An overview of antiarrhythmic drug management of electrical storm. *Can J Cardiol* 12(Suppl B):3B–8B; discussion 27B–28B, 1996.
34. Israel CW, Barold SS: Electrical storm in patients with an implanted defibrillator: a matter of definition. *Ann Noninvasive Electrocardiol* 12(4):375–382, 2007.
35. Burjorjee JE, Milne B: Propofol for electrical storm; a case report of cardioversion and suppression of ventricular tachycardia by propofol. *Can J Anaesth* 49(9):973–977, 2002.
36. Nademanee K, Taylor R, Bailey WE, et al: Treating electrical storm : sympathetic blockade versus advanced cardiac life support-guided therapy. *Circulation* 102(7):742–747, 2000.
37. Carbucicchio C, Santamaria M, Trevisi N, et al: Catheter ablation for the treatment of electrical storm in patients with implantable cardioverter-defibrillators: short- and long-term outcomes in a prospective single-center study. *Circulation* 117(4):462–469, 2008.
38. Wilkoff BL, Hess M, Young J, et al: Differences in tachyarrhythmia detection and implantable cardioverter defibrillator therapy by primary or secondary prevention indication in cardiac resynchronization therapy patients. *J Cardiovasc Electrophysiol* 15(9):1002–1009, 2004.
39. Gehi AK, Mehta D, Gomes JA: Evaluation and management of patients after implantable cardioverter-defibrillator shock. *JAMA* 296(23):2839–2847, 2006.
40. Messali A, Thomas O, Chauvin M, et al: Death due to an implantable cardioverter defibrillator. *J Cardiovasc Electrophysiol* 15(8):953–956, 2004.
41. Boriani G, Occhetta E, Pistis G, et al: Combined use of morphology discrimination, sudden onset, and stability as discriminating algorithms in single chamber cardioverter defibrillators. *Pacing Clin Electrophysiol* 25(9):1357–1366, 2002.
42. Srivatsa UN, Hoppe BL, Narayan S, et al: Ventricular arrhythmia discriminator programming and the impact on the incidence of inappropriate therapy in patients with implantable cardiac defibrillators. *Indian Pacing Electrophysiol J* 7(2):77–84, 2007.
43. Goldstein NE, Lampert R, Bradley E, et al: Management of implantable cardioverter defibrillators in end-of-life care. *Ann Intern Med* 141(11):835–838, 2004.
44. Sears SF, Matchett M, Conti JB: Effective management of ICD patient psychosocial issues and patient critical events. *J Cardiovasc Electrophysiol* 20(11):1297–1304, 2009.
45. Bristow MR, Saxon LA, Boehmer J, et al: Cardiac-resynchronization therapy with or without an implantable defibrillator in advanced chronic heart failure. *N Engl J Med* 350(21):2140–2150, 2004.
46. Abraham WT, Fisher WG, Smith AL, et al: Cardiac resynchronization in chronic heart failure. *N Engl J Med* 346(24):1845–1853, 2002.
47. St John Sutton MG, Plappert T, Abraham WT, et al: Effect of cardiac resynchronization therapy on left ventricular size and function in chronic heart failure. *Circulation* 107(15):1985–1990, 2003.
48. Cleland JG, Daubert JC, Erdmann E, et al: Longer-term effects of cardiac resynchronization therapy on mortality in heart failure [the CArdiac REsynchronization-Heart Failure (CARE-HF) trial extension phase]. *Eur Heart J* 27(16):1928–1932, 2006.
49. Lecoq G, Leclercq C, Leray E, et al: Clinical and electrocardiographic predictors of a positive response to cardiac resynchronization therapy in advanced heart failure. *Eur Heart J* 26(11):1094–1100, 2005.
50. Molhoek SG, van Erven L, Bootsma M, et al: QRS duration and shortening to predict clinical response to cardiac resynchronization therapy in patients with end-stage heart failure. *Pacing Clin Electrophysiol* 27(3):308–313, 2004.
51. Nelson GS, Curry CW, Wyman BT, et al: Predictors of systolic augmentation from left ventricular preexcitation in patients with dilated cardiomyopathy and intraventricular conduction delay. *Circulation* 101(23):2703–2709, 2000.
52. Koplan BA, Kaplan AJ, Weiner S, et al: Heart failure decompensation and all-cause mortality in relation to percent biventricular pacing in patients with heart failure: is a goal of 100% biventricular pacing necessary? *J Am Coll Cardiol* 53(4):355–360, 2009.
53. Mullens W, Grimm RA, Verga T, et al: Insights from a cardiac resynchronization optimization clinic as part of a heart failure disease management program. *J Am Coll Cardiol* 53(9):765–773, 2009.

CHAPTER 45 ■ MECHANICAL SUPPORT FOR HEART FAILURE

JEFFREY J. TEUTEBERG AND FIRAS E. ZAHR

During the past two decades the incidence of cardiogenic shock has not significantly declined despite important progress in the management of patients with acute myocardial infarction and advanced heart failure [1,2]. Cardiogenic shock is characterized by persistent hypotension with systolic arterial pressures typically less than 80 mm Hg and marked reduction of cardiac index (<2 L per minute per m^2) in conjunction with elevated left ventricular (LV) filling pressures and evidence of end-organ hypoperfusion. Patients may present in shock as a complication of acute myocardial infarction, cardiac surgery, acute myocarditis, or an acute decompensation of chronic heart failure. Although the mortality of patients presenting with acute myocardial infarction and cardiogenic shock declined during the 1990s, the 1-month mortality remains nearly 50% despite aggressive efforts at reperfusion therapy [2–5]. In many cases of cardiogenic shock, medical therapy alone may be inadequate, and the patient may require temporary or even permanent mechanical support. The proper application of mechanical circulatory support (MCS) requires knowledge of the underlying mechanism of heart failure, understanding of the potential benefits and limitations of both medical and device therapy, familiarity with the full range of devices available for support, and perhaps most critically, careful selection of the appropriate timing for intervention.

MECHANICAL CIRCULATORY SUPPORT

Over the past five decades, mechanical circulatory support technology has evolved substantially from partial temporary support with intra-aortic balloon counterpulsation to a broad array of ventricular assist devices (VADs) capable of providing long-term complete support for one or both ventricles. In the 1990s, extensive experience with bridging patients to transplantation spurred the evolution from bulky extracorporeal devices to smaller, implantable designs, which allowed patients to be discharged from the hospital and have substantial improvements in functional status and quality of life. More recently, the prior generations of larger pulsatile pumps have been superseded by the introduction of smaller, more durable continuous flow devices with superior survival and fewer adverse events.

BENEFITS OF MECHANICAL CIRCULATORY SUPPORT

Hemodynamic

As the left ventricle begins to fail, cardiac output falls and intracardiac filling pressures rise. The main goals of MCS are to decompress the failing ventricle and augment systemic perfusion [6]. Mechanical unloading of the left ventricle leads to a decrease in the severity of mitral regurgitation, less pulmonary congestion, and a reduction in pulmonary arterial hypertension, all of which, in turn, can result in improved right ventricular (RV) function. Partial support pumps provide several liters of flow to augment the reduced native ventricular contribution to the total output, whereas full support pumps provide upwards of 6 to 7 L of flow with the native heart contributing little to the total output. Restoration of forward flow and the normalization of filling pressures also reduces neurohormonal activation, with attendant benefits on cardiorenal function; as a result, temporary VAD support may allow reverse ventricular remodeling and sufficient recovery of ventricular function to permit explantation in selected patients [7].

Biologic

The hemodynamic benefits of mechanical circulatory support with a LV assist device (LVAD) are also associated with favorable structural changes within the cardiac myocytes and extracellular matrix. In studies of isolated human cardiac myocytes, LVAD support increased the magnitude of contraction, shortened the time of peak contraction, and reduced the time to 50% relaxation. In addition, responses to beta-adrenergic stimulation were greater in isolated myocytes after LVAD support. This suggests that mechanical unloading might reverse the downregulation of beta-adrenergic receptors and improve cardiac responsiveness to inotropic stimulation [8–15]. In vivo, mechanical unloading with an LVAD is known to be associated with alteration of gene and protein expression within the cardiac myocyte [16,17], a reduction in nuclear size and DNA content, and a reduction in fibrosis and collagen content within the cardiac extracellular matrix [10,11].

SELECTION OF APPROPRIATE MECHANICAL SUPPORT

The clinical application of MCS grew from early experience with its application as temporary support in the operating room to supporting patients for months until transplant. A broad array of different ventricular support devices is now available (Table 45.1). Broadly speaking, the devices may be configured for isolated right ventricular (RVAD), left ventricular (LVAD), or biventricular (BiVAD) support and for short-term (bridge to recovery or bridge to decision), short-term (bridge to transplant), or long-term (destination therapy) support [18]. Some devices are extracorporeal or paracorporeal in location, with cannulae traversing the skin allowing for inflow and outflow of blood, whereas others are totally implantable with the pump and the cannulae housed in the thoracic and/or abdominal cavity with only a single percutaneous line supplying the power

TABLE 45.1

APPROVED MECHANICAL CIRCULATORY SUPPORT DEVICES

	Description	Approved devices	Advantages	Disadvantages
Temporary—LV support				
Extracorporeal pulsatile	Cannulated from LV apex to ascending aorta	• Abiomed BVS 5000	• Relatively easy to implant	• Unable to ambulate
Continuous flow	Catheter-based axial flow Centrifugal Often used emergently with resuscitation	• Impella 2.5 • TandemHeart System • Centrimag • ECMO	• Percutaneous placement in cath lab • Rapid placement • Place in catheterization lab without • Rapid surgical placement • Used with oxygenator when pulmonary concomitant pulmonary support required	• Partial support device • Current indication for high-risk PCI • Unable to ambulate • Leg ischemia from large bore cannula • Requires familiarity with transseptal cannula placement • Unable to ambulate • Usually surgically placed
Permanent—LV support				
	Description	**Approved devices**	**Advantages**	**Disadvantages**
Extracorporeal pulsatile	Inflow cannula from LV and outflow cannula to ascending aorta	• Thoratec PVAD • Abiomed AB5000	• Ease of implantation	• Total of two large cannula traversing skin • External pumps
Implantable pulsatile	Pump implanted in the abdomen or preperitoneally, allowing increased mobility and ability to discharge	• HeartMate XVE • Thoratec IVAD	• Requires only an aspirin, no Coumadin • Approved as DT • Durable	• Less durable if duration of support >9–12 months • BSA ≥1.5 m^2 • INR 2.5–3.5 • Less portable peripherals
Continuous flow	Pump implanted in the thoracic cavity with only one moving part.	• HeartMate II and MicroMed DeBakey	• Reduced size and noise • Much greater durability than pulsatile devices • Better adverse event profile than pulsatile pumps	• Difficult to assess BP and pulse due to lack of pulsatility • "Suck-down" caused by over unloading ventricle
Permanent—biventricular support/TAH				
Extracorporeal	Two pumps—one supporting the RV and one supporting the LV, but native heart remains in place	• Thoratec PVAD	• Easy to insert for unstable patients	• Two pumps with a total of four cannula transversing the skin • External pumps
Intracorporeal	Native heart removed completely	• AbioCor and SynCardia CardioWest	• Removes cardiac tissues which may contribute to inflammation and be susceptible to clots, arrhythmias or interference with pump	• Available only in select centers • Not applicable to most patients

LV, left ventricle; PCI, percutaneous coronary intervention; ECMO, extracorporeal membrane oxygenation; TAH, total artificial heart; BSA, body surface area; BP, blood pressure; RV, right ventricle.

and providing the connections to the external control systems. Early generation devices were volume displacement pumps, which had a volume chamber sequentially filled and emptied of blood, mimicking the native heart and providing pulsatile flow. However, the need for a volume displacement chamber resulted in a larger pump size and also required more moving parts resulting in mechanical wear and shorter pump life. The current generation of devices no longer has a displacement chamber, but rather has a continuously rotating impeller. This results in a continuous flow of blood and thus limited pulsatility, but allows for substantially smaller pump profiles and longer pump life.

Cannulation

VADs are typically implanted in parallel with the native right- or left-sided circulation. For long-term LVADs, the pump inflow is from a cannula placed directly into the LV apex and the pump outflow is a cannula that is anastomosed to the

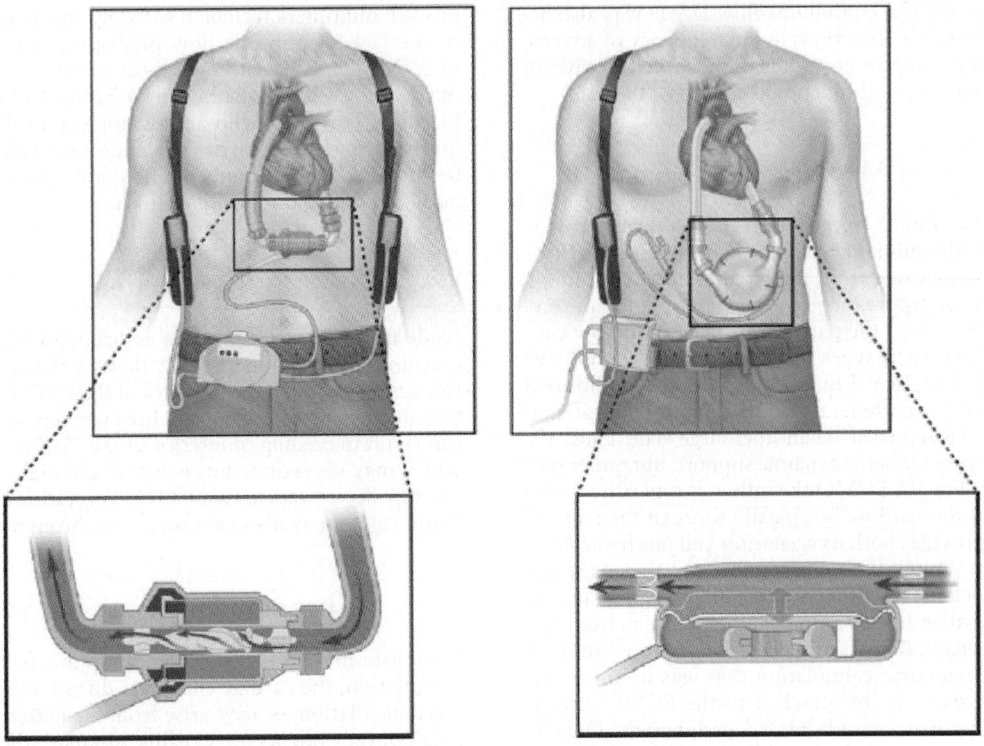

FIGURE 45.1. Representative left ventricular assist devices. (*Right*) Continuous flow LVAD (HeartMate II). Cardiac output is maintained by the continuous rotation of an impeller. (*Left*) Pulsatile flow LVAD (HeartMate XVE). Cardiac output is maintained by the sequential filling and emptying of a volume displacement chamber and unidirectional blood flow is provided with the use of valves before and after the displacement chamber. [From Wilson SR, Givertz MM, Stewart GC, et al: *J Am Coll Cardiol* 54:1647–1659, 2009, with permission.]

ascending aorta just distal to the aortic valve. Pulsatile systems typically have valves in the inflow and outflow cannulae, whereas continuous flow devices do not. For percutaneous systems, the pumps may be placed across the aortic valve and into the left ventricle or into the left atrium via transcatheter puncture of the interatrial septum. RVADs typically have inflow from the right atrium rather than the RV apex as RV apical cannulation typically provides less reliable flow. The venous blood may also be accessed from the cavae or femoral veins. Outflow is directed to the main pulmonary artery just distal to the pulmonic valve through either direct or transvenous cannulation.

Pulsatile Flow

Early-generation VADs are volume displacement pumps which fill and empty asynchronously with the cardiac cycle creating pulsatile arterial flow. The pulsatile pumps mostly fill passively or have limited ability to augment their filling; thus, the beat-to-beat filling of the pump depends partially on the cardiac cycle. Although most of the blood volume entering the left ventricle is diverted into the pump, the left ventricle does occasionally fill enough to eject and contribute to the total cardiac output. In settings of hypovolemia, the pump will fill less quickly and thus the pump rate will slow down, the converse is true in the setting of hypervolemia, thus maintaining a relatively constant state of decompression of the left ventricle.

Continuous Flow

In contrast to pulsatile flow pumps, continuous flow pumps have a continuously rotating impeller which produces forward flow. The left ventricle is continuously and actively unloaded and therefore the left ventricle rarely can fill to the point where it can eject blood during systole. Thus, the patient has little pulsatile contribution from their native ventricles and hence has little to no pulse pressure, but rather have a mean blood pressure. Patients supported with continuous flow LVADs therefore require Doppler ultrasound to assess their blood pressure. Continuous flow pumps are generally one of two major types: axial or centrifugal flow. Axial flow pumps have the impeller rotating in the same plane as the blood flow, whereas centrifugal pumps accelerate the blood perpendicularly to the axis of inflow. They typically have only one moving part (the impeller) which is magnetically or hydrodynamically suspended resulting in little wear over time. Given the size and wear considerations, among others, continuous flow pumps are now the pump of choice for long-term support. The internal and external components of representative pulsatile and continuous flow pumps are as seen in Figure 45.1.

Most recent data suggests that implantation of a continuous-flow LVAD, as compared with a pulsatile-flow device, significantly improved the probability of survival free of stroke and reoperation for device repair or replacement at 2 years in patients with advanced heart failure in whom medical therapy had failed and who were ineligible for transplantation. In addition, the 2 year actuarial survival with an LVAD was significantly better with a continuous-flow device than with a pulsatile-flow device. The continuous-flow LVAD was also associated with significant reductions in the frequency of adverse events and the rate of repeat hospitalization, as well as with an improved quality of life and functional capacity [19–22].

Extracorporeal Membrane Oxygenation

Extracorporeal membrane oxygenation (ECMO) can provide pulmonary or cardiopulmonary support for up to a week or more. Blood is withdrawn from the circulation via an inflow cannula to an extracorporeal continuous flow pump, an oxygenator, and then back to the patient through an outflow cannula. There are two basic types of ECMO: venovenous (VV) and venoarterial (VA). In VV ECMO, the blood is withdrawn from a large central or peripheral vein (jugular or femoral) and oxygenated blood is returned via another large vein. Thus, VV ECMO does not provide hemodynamic support, but rather pulmonary support. For VA ECMO the inflow is typically via the femoral vein and the outflow is typically through the femoral artery and thus provides both oxygenation and mechanical circulatory support. VA ECMO is most commonly used in the setting of severe shock in the setting of acute infarction, fulminant myocarditis or cardiac arrest or after a failure to wean from cardiopulmonary bypass. In the setting of a failure to wean from bypass, the intraoperative cannulation that was used for cardiopulmonary bypass can be attached to the ECMO circuit, rather than having new cannula placed peripherally. Outside the setting of the operating room, both VV and VA EMCO can be rapidly instituted even at the bedside, as either configuration can be achieved through peripheral access, but should only be performed by experienced personnel.

COMPLICATIONS

Although the focus of this chapter is the preoperative assessment and management of patients being considered for MCS, knowledge of some of the common postoperative complications of MCS are necessary to understand the implications of some of these preoperative considerations. The three most common are bleeding, infection, and thromboembolism.

Bleeding

Placement of an intracorporeal pump requires a sternotomy and cardiopulmonary bypass. The degree of perioperative bleeding can be affected by preexisting coagulopathy, liver congestion, and prior sternotomies or other concomitant corrective surgeries at the time of MCS. Most current-generation devices, whether temporary or permanent, require anticoagulation with heparin after post-operative bleeding subsides and then chronically with warfarin and, depending on the center, an antiplatelet agent(s). Most pulsatile devices have mechanical prosthetic valves requiring an INR of 2.5 to 3.5, whereas some of the current generation continuous flow devices may only require an INR of 1.5 to 2 [23]. Thus, there is a risk of continued or new onset bleeding throughout the duration of support, but current devices have a risk of bleeding requiring transfusion of about 0.85 per patient year beyond 30 days, which is a substantial improvement in comparison to previous generation pulsatile devices [24,25]. However, the continuous flow pumps present a unique risk for gastrointestinal bleeding. The high shear stress on the blood from the impeller can cause destruction of large multimers of von Willebrand factor (vWF), which results in a picture of acquired von Willebrand's disease [26,27]. Bleeding risk is mostly manifest from gastrointestinal arteriovenous malformation (AVMs), it is unknown if the loss of vWF multimers results in bleeding from pre-existing AVMs or the lack of pulsatile flow predisposes to the development of AVMs [27–29]. Although most patients have a demonstrable loss of vWF multimers, only a minority of patients develop bleeding. For those who are awaiting transplant, bleeding requiring transfusion carries the additional risk of sensitization to human leukocyte anitgen (HLA) antigens that may limit the pool of suitable donor organs [30].

Infection

Aside from the infection risks associated with surgery and indwelling lines postoperatively, there is the additional chronic risk associated with the presence of the VAD itself and the associated driveline or cannulae. However, sepsis from any source can result in seeding of interior of the VAD or its components, which may necessitate more urgent and higher risk transplant or even device replacement [31]. Vegetations on LVAD prosthetic valves may also be a source of thromboembolism [32].

Thromboembolism and Stroke

Embolism may result from the pump due to inadequate anticoagulation, the cardiac chambers due to arrhythmias such as atrial fibrillation, or may arise from the native vasculature as a result of the patients' preexisting vascular atherosclerosis. The overall incidence of ischemic stroke varies greatly with type of device, however with the current generation devices the rate is 0.09 per patient-year overall and 0.05 per patient-year after 30 days [33]. Maintenance of goal INR is critical to minimize the risk of thromboembolism.

INDICATIONS

MCS may be appropriate for either short-term (<1 week) or long-term support of patients with heart failure and shock. In the majority of cases, long-term MCS is intended as a hemodynamic 'bridge' to subsequent cardiac transplantation (BTT) [34]. For patients who are not candidates for transplant, an LVAD may be used for long-term support (destination therapy, DT) [19]. The only two devices that have been approved for DT in the United States are the HeartMate XVE, and more recently Thoratec's HeartMate II LVAD [19,22]. Occasionally, patients are placed on MCS in anticipation of ventricular recovery and device explantation (bridge-to-recovery), as in selected patients with postcardiotomy shock or acute heart failure due to potentially reversible causes (e.g., fulminant myocarditis) [34].

UNIVENTRICULAR VERSUS BIVENTRICULAR SUPPORT

Selection of the appropriate device for MCS depends initially on the type of support that is required. Most patients presenting with acute heart failure or shock predominantly have LV failure and may be candidates for isolated LV support with an LVAD. Successful LVAD implantation, however, relies heavily on confirmation of adequate native RV function, since RV function is required for LVAD filling [35]. For patients with concomitant, severe RV dysfunction, biventricular support may be necessary. Although recent experience suggests that selected BiVAD patients can be successfully discharged to home, outcomes are generally poorer than with LVAD alone, perhaps in part due to greater severity of illness and end-organ dysfunction amongst patients presenting initially with biventricular failure [36]. Since BiVAD treatment is currently available only for patients who are candidates for eventual cardiac transplantation, up-front BiVAD support should only be considered in transplant-eligible patients with prolonged shock, giant cell-myocarditis, refractory ventricular tachyarrhythmias, or a high likelihood of postoperative RV failure. Even with the current generation of continuous flow LVADs, there is an approximately 7% incidence of RV failure requiring an RVAD postoperatively, highlighting the need for careful assessment of RV function prior to VAD implantation [37–42]. In select centers, explant of the native heart and implantation of a total artificial heart (TAH) may provide an alternative to the use of BiVADs [43].

URGENT VERSUS ELECTIVE SUPPORT

Urgent MCS

Urgent mechanical support may be necessary in a subgroup of patients presenting with acute, medically refractory cardiogenic shock (e.g., acute myocardial infarction, fulminant myocarditis, acute valvular incompetence). In these subjects, time for comprehensive medical and surgical evaluation is limited, and the focus is on rapid hemodynamic stabilization and restoration of end-organ perfusion. Historically, because of widespread availability and ease of implantation, the IABP has been a cornerstone of therapy; however, for many patients an IABP may be inappropriate (e.g., those with severe peripheral arterial disease or aortic insufficiency (AI)) or inadequate in the setting of profound cardiac dysfunction. Increasingly, stabilization for such patients may be accomplished with temporary or percutaneous VADs (e.g., TandemHeart, Impella, CentriMag) or with urgent institution of extracorporeal membrane oxygenation (ECMO) [44]. Particularly for those patients with cardiogenic shock complicated by progressive hypoxemia despite adequate ventilation, ECMO, if instituted early, can be a lifesaving measure [45,46]. As such, transfer to a specialized medical center with experience in cardiac transplantation or MCS should be considered as soon as medically feasible. Once stabilized with MCS, patients can be either weaned gradually over time or, as appropriate, be transitioned to more permanent devices for long-term support (if irreversible end-organ damage has not already occurred). In general, critically ill patients have better outcomes if they are stabilized and undergo implantation of long-term MCS on an urgent rather than emergent basis, largely due to the extremely high rate of perioperative complications amongst patients presenting multisystem organ failure [24].

Elective MCS

For patients with advanced heart failure, MCS on a more elective basis is becoming the preferred strategy for optimizing outcomes for patients whether they are BTT or DT. End-stage heart failure is characterized by progressive functional decline and repeated heart failure hospitalizations which significantly impacts both resource utilization and quality of life [47,48]. Although support with intravenous inotropic agents (in hospital or at home) may provide temporary relief, these agents are associated with an increased risk of adverse outcomes including arrhythmia and sudden death [20]. Furthermore, patients may still experience progressive functional decline and end-organ dysfunction during long-term inotropic support. Since elective VAD implantation is most successful when instituted prior to the onset of irreversible end-organ (e.g., liver or kidney) dysfunction, early referral and implantation of patients with accelerating heart failure symptoms despite medical therapy for evaluation is especially important.

SELECTION OF CHRONIC HEART FAILURE PATIENTS FOR LONG-TERM MCS

Cardiac

RV Function

Assessment of RV function is critical when considering MCS particularly in those who are being implanted with the intent of long-term support. An LVAD alone is preferred for long-term support and only LVADs are approved for DT, but it is not a viable strategy if the RV cannot adequately fill the LVAD [36]. RV function can be acutely affected by the primary etiology of the myopathy such as with ischemia in the presence of acute infarction, inflammation in the setting of myocarditis, or persistent ventricular arrhythmias. The RV can also become dysfunctional as a result of chronic elevations of LV filling pressures and/or mitral valve pathology, which results in pulmonary hypertension and thus increased RV afterload. Lastly, other processes that may exacerbate pulmonary hypertension, such as hypoxic lung disease, sleep apnea, chronic thromboembolic disease, or pulmonary vasculopathy, can also contribute to RV dysfunction. Chronic severe RV dysfunction with concomitant increases in right atrial pressures and tricuspid regurgitation further exacerbates liver and renal dysfunction, leads to gut edema with poor absorption of medications and nutrients, and results in hypotension and an inability to tolerate diuresis, beta-blockade, and ACE inhibition [49].

LV mechanical support is generally beneficial to RV function, with chronic unloading of the left ventricle resulting in a reduction in pulmonary pressures and thus, RV afterload. However there may be deleterious effects of an LVAD on RV function, particularly when RV function is marginal. Profound unloading of the LV, particularly with continuous flow devices, can result in shift of the septum away from the RV and thus decrease the septal contribution to RV output. The RV may also struggle to accommodate the increased venous return as a result of the improved cardiac output from the LVAD [50,51].

Echocardiography provides valuable information about overall RV size and function, the degree of tricuspid regurgitation and can give estimates of pulmonary arterial systolic pressures. However, functional assessments of RVEF are quite subjective and even a fairly normal appearing RV on echocardiography may have little functional reserve [52]. Invasive hemodynamic assessment with a pulmonary arterial catheter is therefore essential to decision making regarding the adequacy of RV function. The degree of elevation in the right atrial pressure (RA), especially in relation to the wedge (W) pressure can be quite revealing. One would expect high RA and W pressures in the setting of heart failure, but with a normally functioning RV, the RA pressures are relatively lower than the W and thus the RA/W ratio typically remains less than 0.5. With the onset of RV dysfunction, the RA pressures increase out of proportion to the left-sided pressures and the RA/W ratio increases. A high right atrial pressure in the setting of low pulmonary arterial pressures and low RV stroke work index are also concerning for the presence of severe RV failure [53].

Given the morbidity associated with RV failure post-LVAD, a number of investigators have sought risk factors for postimplantation RV dysfunction. Univariate predictors for RV failure include RV stroke work index, small BSA, and mechanical ventilation [40,41]. Multivariate predictors include the need for preoperative circulatory support, female gender, and a nonischemic etiology of heart failure [40]. Researchers at the University of Michigan developed a risk score for RV failure based on vasopressor requirement, an AST ≥80 IU, total bilirubin ≥2 mg per dL, creatinine ≥2.3 mg per dL that is predictive of RV failure as well as overall survival [54]. However, there are many limitations to these studies including being based on single-center studies, small sample sizes, and are mostly based on prior generation pulsatile devices.

A recent study of 484 patients examined the predictors of RV dysfunction in patients receiving a current generation continuous flow device (HeartMate II) across multiple centers as a bridge to transplantation. Multivariate predictors of RV failure were preoperative ventilator support (OR 5.5), CVP/W > 0.63 (OR 2.3), and BUN > 39 (OR 2.1). Patients without RV failure also had significantly better survival at 6 months (89% vs. 67%, $p < 0.001$) and shorter lengths of stay (22 vs. 32 days, $p < 0.001$). This study, unlike other prior studies, also investigated the effects of intraoperative factors which might impact RV function. Those who required an RVAD required more units of packed red blood cells (14.3 vs. 5.6, $p < 0.03$) and had twice the incidence of reoperation for bleeding (40% vs. 19%, $p < 0.04$) [55].

Management of RV failure is similar to that of LV failure, decreasing excess preload, inotropy, and reducing afterload. RV preload should be reduced with aggressive diuresis and, if needed, mechanical volume removal if there is a renal limitation to diuresis. The dysfunctional RV may need slightly more preload to maintain output, but a goal should be to reduce the RA pressure to less than 13 mm Hg. Inotropy is often needed for LV support as well, but is often equally important to maintaining RV output [50]. Milrinone is typically the inotrope of choice for RV support in the setting of concomitant pulmonary hypertension due to its vasodilatory properties. Afterload is addressed through strategies to reduce elevated pulmonary pressures. Reducing the left sided filling pressures is the first and most important therapeutic targets and can be accomplished through a combination of diuresis, inotropy, IABP, and even a temporary LVAD. Patients must have adequate oxygenation to avoid hypoxic pulmonary vasoconstriction and if intubated positive end expiratory pressure should be minimized [56]. Nitric oxide may be considered in the intubated patient, but such patients may be too ill to consider LV support alone. There is little evidence for the use of other vasodilators such as prostaglandins and some evidence that such therapies may be deleterious in the setting of LV failure [57]. A summary of the management of RV function and the various organ systems discussed below is as seen in Table 45.2.

Arrhythmias

Ventricular tachyarrhythmias are reasonably common in the setting of acutely decompensated heart failure. Many patients with chronic heart failure will have a history of ventricular tachycardia or have an implantable cardioverter defibrillator (ICD) with or without resynchronization therapy [58]. Aside from their impact on the patient's stability in the acute phase of their presentation, the persistence of ventricular tachyarrhythmias has implications for outcomes on mechanical support. The presence of sustained ventricular tachycardia or ventricular fibrillation during LVAD support can substantially affect RV function, particularly in the setting of borderline RV function. Although ventricular tachyarrhythmias are not typically lethal in the setting of LVAD support alone, they will fairly routinely result in lower pump output, hypotension, and recurrent symptoms. For patients with an ICD they may also result in frequent ICD discharges. Preoperative ventricular tachyarrhythmias in the setting of substantially elevated filling pressures or acute ischemia often resolve after MCS as the heart failure state resolves. However, patients with persistent ventricular dysrhythmias despite reasonable filling pressures are at potentially higher risk of recurrence or persistence of these arrhythmias post-MCS and thus are more likely to need biventricular support.

Aortic Valve

The cardiac assessment of patients being considered for MCS should focus on other morphologic features of the heart other than the LV and RV function. The presence and quantification of AI is particularly important. Blood from the left ventricle empties into the device and is then pumped into the ascending aorta just distal to the aortic valve. The presence of significant AI will result in ineffectual forward flow as the blood that was pumped into the aorta is regurgitated back into the ventricle only to reenter the device, be pumped into the aorta, and regurgitate into the ventricle once again in a blind loop. Moderate or worse AI should prompt aortic valve repair, replacement with a tissue valve, or oversewing of the aortic valve. With adequate decompression by the LVAD, the left ventricle generates very little effective forward flow and hence rarely opens the aortic valve. In patients with mechanical aortic prostheses, this lack of flow across the valve may result in the formation of thrombosis and subsequent embolism [59]. Thus, mechanical aortic valves are either replaced with tissue valves at the time of surgery or are oversewn.

Other Cardiac Abnormalities

The presence of large atrial or ventricular septal defects should be ruled out as these will need to be addressed during the time of implantation. Mitral regurgitation essentially resolves post-MCS with adequate LV decompression, but significant mitral stenosis can impede LVAD filling and should be addressed at the time of implantation [60]. The degree of tricuspid regurgitation should be quantified as severe tricuspid regurgitation is a predictor of poor outcomes with LVAD alone [61]. LV thrombus can form in the setting of acute ischemia or with chronic LV dysfunction. Such thrombi are usually located in the LV apex, which is the site of cannulation for the LVAD. Although the ventricle is routinely inspected before insertion of the cannula, knowledge of the presence of thrombus preoperatively is nevertheless important as retained thrombus may systemically embolize or, more ominously, be sucked into the impeller of a continuous flow pump resulting pump dysfunction or failure. For patients with congenital heart disease it is important to establish the anatomical position of the systemic ventricle and aorta as well as the type and location of any previous corrective surgeries. Complex congenital heart disease may necessitate placement of the pump or inflow/outflow cannulae in atypical positions.

Noncardiac

Other chronic medical conditions, many of which are exacerbated by acute heart failure, should be optimized if possible prior to implantation of long-term MCS. Patients must be assessed for signs of infection and if found treated aggressively prior to implant. Active infection at the time of implantation can be catastrophic as septicemia can result in device infection which may be chronically suppressed but rarely cured with antibiotic therapy. If the pump or the pocket in which it sits becomes infected, the only recourse is urgent transplant, if indicated, as device exchanges in these situations often result in recurrent infection [62]. Renal dysfunction at the time of presentation is common from a variety of causes: poor renal perfusion, high right atrial pressures, preexisting renal dysfunction, high doses of diuretics, and the adverse neurohormonal milieu of heart failure. It is certainly advantageous if the

TABLE 45.2

ORGAN SYSTEM REVIEW OF CANDIDATES FOR MECHANICAL CIRCULATORY SUPPORT

Organ system	Review
LV dysfunction	
Preload	• Diuresis • Mechanical volume removal
Cardiac output	• Support with inotropy • IABP or temporary support as needed
After load	• Treat hypertension, if present • IABP
RV dysfunction	• Assess with invasive hemodynamics
Preload	• Diuresis • Mechanical volume removal
Inotropy	• Milrinone if concomitant pulmonary hypertension
Afterload	• Decreasing left-sided filling pressures • Milrinone • Avoiding hypoxia
Arrhythmias	• Rate control • Antiarrhythmics • Cardioversion if hemodynamically tenuous. • Persistent ventricular tachyarrhythmia despite adequate treatment of left heart failure may need consideration for BiVADs
Aortic valve	• Assess for AI • Presence of mechanical valve?
Noncardiac	
Infection	• Aggressive assessment and treatment
Renal dysfunction	• Decrease high right atrial pressures • Inotropy or IABP • Avoid nephrotoxic agents, contrast

Organ system	Review
Pulmonary disease	• Avoid hypoxia • Attempt to quantify extent/severity of lung disease
Liver disease	• Occult liver disease in the presence of persistently high right atrial pressures • Ultrasound/CT scan to assess for cirrhosis
Coagulation	• Stop any unneeded anticoagulants/antiplatelets • Review for history of hypercoagulable state
Vascular disease	• Review history • Confirmatory ultrasound/CT scanning
Nutrition	• Screen with prealbumin • Nutritional support
Surgical	
Identify	• ASD/VSD • Number of prior sternotomies • Location and number of prior bypass grafts • Congenital abnormalities • Prior cardiac surgeries • Intracardiac thrombus • Mitral stenosis
Other limitations	
Emotional	• Careful assessment and support
Physical	• Ability to care for and utilize device
Cognitive	• Understanding device
Social	• Support system available
Financial	• Adequate resources as both inpatient and outpatient

patient can be stabilized with inotropy, IABP, or even temporary mechanical support to allow for renal recovery. Improvement of renal function is often seen with restoration of cardiac output and resolution of the heart failure state after MCS, but is not the rule, especially when the patients are implanted in the setting of significant renal dysfunction [63,64]. Renal failure requiring dialysis after MCS remains a highly morbid event, likely reflecting the level of illness entering the surgery as well as an additional, persistent nidus of infection due to the need for vascular access [65].

Intrinsic pulmonary disease also has a number of implications for long-term MCS. Advanced lung disease impacts mortality and morbidity from the implantation surgery itself as well as the ability to rehabilitate and post-operative functional status. Hypoxic pulmonary vasoconstriction from intrinsic lung disease may also exacerbate preexisting pulmonary hypertension. Severe chronic pulmonary disease with an FEV1 of less than 1 L is should raise concerns about a patient's suitability for MCS [60]. Intubation and mechanical ventilation prior to implantation is also a strong predictor of poor outcomes [38]. Hepatic dysfunction is occasionally a result of shock from acute decompensation, but chronic occult hepatic dysfunction is not uncommon with chronic heart failure, especially in the setting of poor RV function with persistently high right atrial pressures or those with Fontan circulation [60]. These patients may have significant hepatic dysfunction without substantial baseline abnormalities of AST, ALT, or total bilirubin. There should be a low threshold to screen such patients with ultrasonography or CT or even liver biopsy to assess hepatic architecture for signs of cirrhosis. If there is evidence of cirrhosis then early involvement of hepatologists is essential. Patients with marginal hepatic function frequently have massive transfusion requirements during implantation and not infrequently have acute hepatic failure postoperatively. Careful management of antiplatelet and anticoagulant therapy around the time of VAD implant may be critical to minimizing the risk of perioperative bleeding. Extensive carotid or peripheral vascular disease may increase the risk of extracardiac vascular events following MCS, and must be evaluated appropriately with preoperative noninvasive testing [60]. In patients who present acutely, nutrition is not often a pressing issue, but nutritional impairment in patients with chronic heart failure can be quite profound and low BMI is a risk factor for poor outcomes [66]. Poor nutrition impacts T-cell function and is another risk factor for infection and poor wound healing postoperatively. For patients at nutritional risk supplemental feeding may be of some use, but should not delay implantation when MCS is indicated.

SURGICAL

Whenever patients are being considered for MCS the surgical team should be involved, not only to help assess a patient's suitability for support, but also allow them time to properly survey the patient for additional factors which may impact outcomes. The number of prior sternotomies will impact the ease of surgical approach, the operative time, the risk of postoperative bleeding, and perhaps even the overall candidacy for MCS. The presence and degree of AI, the presence of mechanical valves, the number and location of prior bypass grafts, the presence of intraventricular thrombus, and the details of congenital abnormalities and subsequent surgical corrections should be determined and communicated to the surgical team as previously noted. The details of past surgical ventricular reconstruction should be sought, as these surgeries usually involve the LV apex, the site of inflow cannulation for all long-term LVADs, and may present significant technical challenges.

OTHER CONSIDERATIONS

Aside from the many and varied medical and surgical considerations are emotional, physical, and social considerations. The acute nature of many patients' illness often precludes a detailed assessment of such issues, but for nonemergent situations addressing these issues prior to implantation is ideal. Physical limitations that may impact the patient's ability to care for the device such as the manual dexterity to change batteries or hear alarms are a critical part of such a review. Adequate cognitive ability is needed to understand the importance of the device and its components, the ability to troubleshoot problems, and recognize when to ask for assistance. The emotional wherewithal to adapt to the device, its implications, potential limitations, and adverse events is also important to maximizing long-term outcomes and quality of life. Lastly, patients must have an adequate social support network; although having an implanted VAD does not typically involve around the clock supervision, there must be a background of reliable support for assistance in an emergency and for long-term emotional support.

TIMING

When patients present to the intensive care unit with shock and are subsequently stabilized with aggressive medical therapy the decision to transition to MCS rests on the expectation of improvement in the patient's condition. For those who received an intervention, such as revascularization, waiting to see the impact of this intervention on the patient's clinical status is reasonable in the absence of further clinical deterioration. Many patients, however, will not have a readily identifiable or treatable proximate cause of their deterioration. For those who are eligible or are already listed for transplantation, the risk of continued medical therapy awaiting transplantation must be weighed against the risk of proceeding with MCS [67]. The advantages of waiting for transplantation in the setting of stable, yet critical illness are an increased likelihood of receiving an organ due to a higher status, avoiding a second surgery, and the potential morbidity and mortality of MCS itself. Disadvantages to delaying MCS include the high-risk nature of transplant during acute illness, further decompensation prior

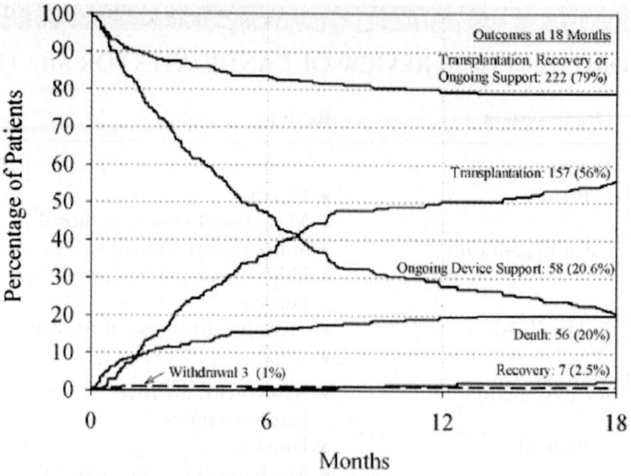

FIGURE 45.2. Competing outcomes analysis of patients with a continuous flow left ventricular assist device as a bridge to transplant. [From Pagani FD, Miller LW, Russell SD, et al: Extended mechanical circulatory support with a continuous-flow rotary left ventricular assist device. *J Am Coll Cardiol* 54:312–321, 2009, with permission.]

to transplant that may require a higher risk, emergent LVAD or biventricular support, becoming too ill for either transplant or mechanical support, or death. Proceeding with MCS early allows for surgery to be performed when the patient is less ill followed by a lower risk transplant once the patient is rehabilitated. Certain patients may be expected to have a short wait for transplantation based on their size, blood type, and level of sensitization and therefore the disadvantages of waiting for transplant may be minimized. Others may have clear indications for early MCS such as persistent pulmonary hypertension not responsive to medical therapy [68]. Unfortunately most patients do not have such a clear delineation of risk and determining the optimal timing of MCS can be quite difficult. However, there is an emerging evidence base that supports the earlier institution of MCS.

Prior reticence to institute MCS was based upon results using the prior generation of pulsatile LVADs with 6- and 12-month survival of approximately 75% and 60%, respectively. In contrast, the newer generation nonpulsatile pumps have 6- and 12-month survival of 82% and 73%, respectively [33] (Fig. 45.2). Furthermore, these devices are also associated with a much more favorable adverse event profiles and given their smaller size are applicable to almost the entire cohort of transplant eligible patients. When examining the survival of patients supported with MCS much of the mortality is early and attributable to patient selection, with the sickest patients preimplantation having the worst outcomes [36]. This has lead researchers to attempt to quantify this operative risk to improve patient selection.

Several risk prediction models are available for patients with chronic systolic heart failure. The Heart Failure Survival Score is comprised of clinical, laboratory data, and exercise data [69]. The Seattle Heart Failure Model incorporates a much wider array of clinical and laboratory variables and does not require an exercise test. However, these models were derived from a much less critically ill population and have not been validated in patients who are being considered for mechanical circulatory support [70]. Risk prediction models for patients undergoing LVAD exist, but are limited in that they describe risk attributable to device that is no longer used [71], are from a previous era of MCS support [72], or only examined patients implanted as destination therapy with a pulsatile device [73]. However, the factors associated with higher risk in these studies such as signs of RV failure, mechanical ventilation, infection,

TABLE 45.3

INTERMACS PROFILES

Profile	Description
1	Acutely decompensating
2	Failing inotropes
3	Inotrope dependent, stable
4	Recurrent, but not refractory advanced heart failure
5	Exertion intolerant, but no dyspnea at rest
6	Exertion limited, dyspnea with only mild activity
7	Advanced NYHA class III

NYHA, New York Heart Association.

and renal and hepatic dysfunction are also generally seen in patients who are more ill at the time of implantation.

The Interagency Registry for Mechanically Assisted Circulatory Support (INTERMACS) is large national registry of approved support devices that was recently established and has provided a means by which to risk assess patients undergoing MCS by their preimplant acuity of illness. INTERMACS has established seven different profiles for patients being implanted with MCS from advanced NYHA class III patients, through inotrope dependence, to acute shock despite maximal medical management (Table 45.3) [74]. Data from INTERMACS have shown that risk stratification based solely upon the preimplant profiles does indeed predict outcomes when applied to both pulsatile and continuous flow devices (Fig. 45.3) [33]. There is a substantial difference in survival at 1 year between even those who were profiles 1 and 2. A recent study of 101 patients who received current generation continuous flow devices stratified patients based on their preimplant INTERMACS category: group 1 was profile 1; group 2 was profiles 2 to 3; and group 3 was profiles 4 to 7. Survival at 18 months was 50% versus 73% versus 96% ($p < 0.01$) for groups 1, 2, and 3 respectively [75]. The implication for patients in the ICU who are stabilized and are being considered for long-term support is that there is an emerging consensus that earlier institution of mechanical support is preferable to waiting, as further decompensation will yield worse outcomes with both MCS and transplantation.

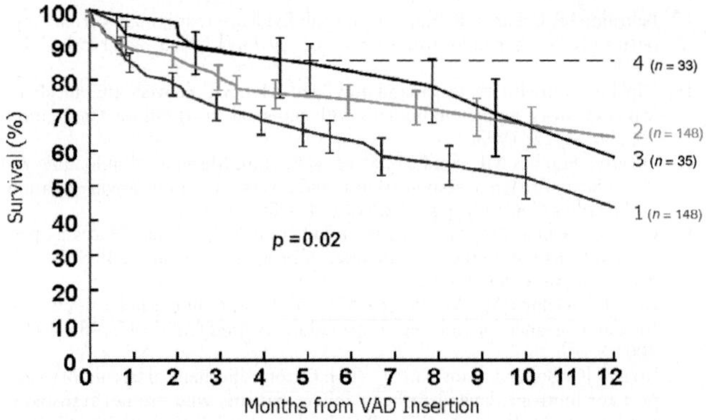

FIGURE 45.3. Survival after VAD stratified by INTERMACS profile. 1—Profile 1; 2—Profile 2; 3—Profile 3; 4—Profile 4. [From Kirklin JK, Naftel DC, Stevenson LW, et al: INTERMACS database for durable devices for circulatory support: first annual report. *J Heart Lung Transplant* 27:1065–1072, 2008, with permission.]

FUTURE DIRECTIONS

Mechanical circulatory support has evolved over the past 25 years from an investigational strategy reserved only for the moribund to a standard therapy supporting patients with stable advanced heart failure. Today, a wide variety of devices are available for short-term, medium-term, and long-term support at numerous centers worldwide.

A number of newer MCS devices are now in clinical use or clinical trials. Advances in pump technology are moving toward smaller pumps that still allow for full support, pumps that can be either implanted percutaneously or through minimally invasive surgeries, increased durability, totally implantable systems with transcutaneous energy transfer, and an improved device-patient interface. Research is also focused on improving biocompatibility, lowering risk of thrombosis, and better responsiveness to physiologic demands.

The role of MCS as an alternative to transplantation, that is, destination therapy, is likely to increase in the future. It is hoped that with advances in device design, patient selection, and medical management, MCS will be applicable to a greater proportion of patients with advanced heart failure, result in continued improvement in outcomes, and a reduction in adverse events and cost.

References

1. Rogers WJ, Canto JG, Lambrew CT, et al: Temporal trends in the treatment of over 1.5 million patients with myocardial infarction in the US from 1990 through 1999: the National Registry of Myocardial Infarction 1, 2 and 3. *J Am Coll Cardiol* 36:2056–2063, 2000.
2. Holmes DR Jr, Berger PB, Hochman JS, et al: Cardiogenic shock in patients with acute ischemic syndromes with and without ST-segment elevation. *Circulation* 100:2067–2073, 1999.
3. Hasdai D, Harrington RA, Hochman JS, et al: Platelet glycoprotein IIb/IIIa blockade and outcome of cardiogenic shock complicating acute coronary syndromes without persistent ST-segment elevation. *J Am Coll Cardiol* 36:685–692, 2000.
4. Hochman JS, Sleeper LA, Webb JG, et al: Early revascularization and long-term survival in cardiogenic shock complicating acute myocardial infarction. *JAMA* 295:2511–2515, 2006.
5. Hochman JS, Sleeper LA, Webb JG, et al: Early revascularization in acute myocardial infarction complicated by cardiogenic shock. SHOCK Investigators. Should We Emergently Revascularize Occluded Coronaries for Cardiogenic Shock. *N Engl J Med* 341:625–634, 1999.
6. Dandel M, Weng Y, Siniawski H, et al: Prediction of cardiac stability after weaning from left ventricular assist devices in patients with idiopathic dilated cardiomyopathy. *Circulation* 118:S94–S105, 2008.
7. James KB, McCarthy PM, Thomas JD, et al: Effect of the implantable left ventricular assist device on neuroendocrine activation in heart failure. *Circulation* 92:II191–II195, 1995.
8. Latif N, Yacoub MH, George R, et al: Changes in sarcomeric and non-sarcomeric cytoskeletal proteins and focal adhesion molecules during clinical myocardial recovery after left ventricular assist device support. *J Heart Lung Transplant* 26:230–235, 2007.
9. Rodrigue-Way A, Burkhoff D, Geesaman BJ, et al: Sarcomeric genes involved in reverse remodeling of the heart during left ventricular assist device support. *J Heart Lung Transplant* 24:73–80, 2005.
10. Li YY, Feng Y, McTiernan CF, et al: Downregulation of matrix metalloproteinases and reduction in collagen damage in the failing human heart after support with left ventricular assist devices. *Circulation* 104:1147–1152, 2001.
11. Bruggink AH, van Oosterhout MF, de Jonge N, et al: Reverse remodeling of the myocardial extracellular matrix after prolonged left ventricular assist device support follows a biphasic pattern. *J Heart Lung Transplant* 25:1091–1098, 2006.
12. Rivello HG, Meckert PC, Vigliano C, et al: Cardiac myocyte nuclear size and ploidy status decrease after mechanical support. *Cardiovasc Pathol* 10:53–57, 2001.
13. Scheinin SA, Capek P, Radovancevic B, et al: The effect of prolonged left ventricular support on myocardial histopathology in patients with end-stage cardiomyopathy. *ASAIO J* 38:M271–M274, 1992.
14. Bruckner BA, Stetson SJ, Perez-Verdia A, et al: Regression of fibrosis and hypertrophy in failing myocardium following mechanical circulatory support. *J Heart Lung Transplant* 20:457–464, 2001.

15. Beltrami AP, Urbanek K, Kajstura J, et al: Evidence that human cardiac myocytes divide after myocardial infarction. *N Engl J Med* 344:1750–1757, 2001.
16. Dipla K, Mattiello JA, Jeevanandam V, et al: Myocyte recovery after mechanical circulatory support in humans with end-stage heart failure. *Circulation* 97:2316–2322, 1998.
17. Ogletree-Hughes ML, Stull LB, Sweet WE, et al: Mechanical unloading restores beta-adrenergic responsiveness and reverses receptor downregulation in the failing human heart. *Circulation* 104:881–886, 2001.
18. Oz MC, Gelijns AC, Miller L, et al: Left ventricular assist devices as permanent heart failure therapy: the price of progress. *Ann Surg* 238:577–583; discussion 583–585, 2003.
19. Rose EA, Gelijns AC, Moskowitz AJ, et al: Long-term mechanical left ventricular assistance for end-stage heart failure. *N Engl J Med* 345:1435–1443, 2001.
20. Rogers JG, Butler J, Lansman SL, et al: Chronic mechanical circulatory support for inotrope-dependent heart failure patients who are not transplant candidates: results of the INTrEPID Trial. *J Am Coll Cardiol* 50:741–747, 2007.
21. Allen JG, Weiss ES, Schaffer JM, et al: Quality of life and functional status in patients surviving 12 months after left ventricular assist device implantation. *J Heart Lung Transplant* 29:278–285, 2010.
22. Slaughter MS, Rogers JG, Milano CA, et al: Advanced heart failure treated with continuous-flow left ventricular assist device. *N Engl J Med* 361:2241–2251, 2009.
23. Boyle AJ, Russell SD, Teuteberg JJ, et al: Low thromboembolism and pump thrombosis with the HeartMate II left ventricular assist device: analysis of outpatient anti-coagulation. *J Heart Lung Transplant* 28:881–887, 2009.
24. Kirklin JK, Naftel DC, Stevenson LW, et al: INTERMACS database for durable devices for circulatory support: first annual report. *J Heart Lung Transplant* 27:1065–1072, 2008.
25. Miller LW, Pagani FD, Russell SD, et al: Use of a continuous-flow device in patients awaiting heart transplantation. *N Engl J Med* 357:885–896, 2007.
26. Klovaite J, Gustafsson F, Mortensen SA, et al: Severely impaired von Willebrand factor-dependent platelet aggregation in patients with a continuous-flow left ventricular assist device (HeartMate II). *J Am Coll Cardiol* 53:2162–2167, 2009.
27. Geisen U, Heilmann C, Beyersdorf F, et al: Non-surgical bleeding in patients with ventricular assist devices could be explained by acquired von Willebrand disease. *Eur J Cardiothorac Surg* 33:679–684, 2008.
28. Crow S, John R, Boyle A, et al: Gastrointestinal bleeding rates in recipients of nonpulsatile and pulsatile left ventricular assist devices. *J Thorac Cardiovasc Surg* 137:208–215, 2009.
29. Letsou GV, Shah N, Gregoric ID, et al: Gastrointestinal bleeding from arteriovenous malformations in patients supported by the Jarvik 2000 axial-flow left ventricular assist device. *J Heart Lung Transplant* 24:105–109, 2005.
30. Mehra MR, Uber PA, Uber WE, et al: Allosensitization in heart transplantation: implications and management strategies. *Curr Opin Cardiol* 18:153–158, 2003.
31. Holman WL, Park SJ, Long JW, et al: Infection in permanent circulatory support: experience from the REMATCH trial. *J Heart Lung Transplant* 23:1359–1365, 2004.
32. Fischer SA, Trenholme GM, Costanzo MR, et al: Infectious complications in left ventricular assist device recipients. *Clin Infect Dis* 24:18–23, 1997.
33. Pagani FD, Miller LW, Russell SD, et al: Extended mechanical circulatory support with a continuous-flow rotary left ventricular assist device. *J Am Coll Cardiol* 54:312–321, 2009.
34. Stevenson LW, Rose EA: Left ventricular assist devices: bridges to transplantation, recovery, and destination for whom? *Circulation* 108:3059–3063, 2003.
35. Fukamachi K, McCarthy PM, Smedira NG, et al: Preoperative risk factors for right ventricular failure after implantable left ventricular assist device insertion. *Ann Thorac Surg* 68:2181–2184, 1999.
36. Farrar DJ, Hill JD, Pennington DG, et al: Preoperative and postoperative comparison of patients with univentricular and biventricular support with the thoratec ventricular assist device as a bridge to cardiac transplantation. *J Thorac Cardiovasc Surg* 113:202–209, 1997.
37. Bhama JK, Kormos RL, Toyoda Y, et al: Clinical experience using the Levitronix CentriMag system for temporary right ventricular mechanical circulatory support. *J Heart Lung Transplant* 28:971–976, 2009.
38. Ochiai Y, McCarthy PM, Smedira NG, et al: Predictors of severe right ventricular failure after implantable left ventricular assist device insertion: analysis of 245 patients. *Circulation* 106:I198–I202, 2002.
39. Kavarana MN, Pessin-Minsley MS, Urtecho J, et al: Right ventricular dysfunction and organ failure in left ventricular assist device recipients: a continuing problem. *Ann Thorac Surg* 73:745–750, 2002.
40. Tsukui H, Teuteberg JJ, Murali S, et al: Biventricular assist device utilization for patients with morbid congestive heart failure: a justifiable strategy. *Circulation* 112:I65–I72, 2005.
41. Fitzpatrick JR III, Frederick JR, Hiesinger W, et al: Early planned institution of biventricular mechanical circulatory support results in improved outcomes compared with delayed conversion of a left ventricular assist device to a biventricular assist device. *J Thorac Cardiovasc Surg* 137:971–977, 2009.
42. Zahr F, Ootaki Y, Starling RC, et al: Preoperative risk factors for mortality after biventricular assist device implantation. *J Card Fail* 14:844–849, 2008.
43. Morris RJ: Total artificial heart—concepts and clinical use. *Semin Thorac Cardiovasc Surg* 20:247–254, 2008.
44. Okuda M: A multidisciplinary overview of cardiogenic shock. *Shock* 25:557–570, 2006.
45. Chen YS, Yu HY, Huang SC, et al: Experience and result of extracorporeal membrane oxygenation in treating fulminant myocarditis with shock: what mechanical support should be considered first? *J Heart Lung Transplant* 24:81–87, 2005.
46. Peek GJ, Mugford M, Tiruvoipati R, et al: Efficacy and economic assessment of conventional ventilatory support versus extracorporeal membrane oxygenation for severe adult respiratory failure (CESAR): a multicentre randomised controlled trial. *Lancet* 374:1351–1363, 2009.
47. De Luca L, Fonarow GC, Adams KF Jr, et al: Acute heart failure syndromes: clinical scenarios and pathophysiologic targets for therapy. *Heart Fail Rev* 12:97–104, 2007.
48. Yancy CW, Lopatin M, Stevenson LW, et al: Clinical presentation, management, and in-hospital outcomes of patients admitted with acute decompensated heart failure with preserved systolic function: a report from the Acute Decompensated Heart Failure National Registry (ADHERE) Database. *J Am Coll Cardiol* 47:76–84, 2006.
49. Uretsky BF, Thygesen K, Daubert JC, et al: Predictors of mortality from pump failure and sudden cardiac death in patients with systolic heart failure and left ventricular dyssynchrony: results of the CARE-HF trial. *J Card Fail* 14:670–675, 2008.
50. Haddad F, Doyle R, Murphy DJ, et al: Right ventricular function in cardiovascular disease, part II: pathophysiology, clinical importance, and management of right ventricular failure. *Circulation* 117:1717–1731, 2008.
51. Farrar DJ: Ventricular interactions during mechanical circulatory support. *Semin Thorac Cardiovasc Surg* 6:163–168, 1994.
52. Farrar DJ, Compton PG, Hershon JJ, et al: Right heart interaction with the mechanically assisted left heart. *World J Surg* 9:89–102, 1985.
53. Mandarino WA, Winowich S, Gorcsan J III, et al: Right ventricular performance and left ventricular assist device filling. *Ann Thorac Surg* 63:1044–1049, 1997.
54. Matthews JC, Koelling TM, Pagani FD, et al: The right ventricular failure risk score a pre-operative tool for assessing the risk of right ventricular failure in left ventricular assist device candidates. *J Am Coll Cardiol* 51:2163–2172, 2008.
55. Kormos RL, Teuteberg JJ, Russell SD, et al: Right ventricular failure (RVF) in patients with continuous flow left ventricular assist devices (LVAD). *J Heart Lung Transplant* 27:S134, 2008.
56. Vieillard-Baron A, Jardin F: Why protect the right ventricle in patients with acute respiratory distress syndrome? *Curr Opin Crit Care* 9:15–21, 2003.
57. McLaughlin VV, McGoon MD: Pulmonary arterial hypertension. *Circulation* 114:1417–1431, 2006.
58. Deng MC, Tjan TD, Asfour B, et al: Combining nonpharmacologic therapies for advanced heart failure: the Munster experience with the assist device-defibrillator combination. *Am J Cardiol* 83:158D–160D, 1999.
59. Wilson SR, Mudge GH Jr, Stewart GC, et al: Evaluation for a ventricular assist device: selecting the appropriate candidate. *Circulation* 119:2225–2232, 2009.
60. Holman WL, Kormos RL, Naftel DC, et al: Predictors of death and transplant in patients with a mechanical circulatory support device: a multi-institutional study. *J Heart Lung Transplant* 28:44–50, 2009.
61. Potapov EV, Stepanenko A, Dandel M, et al: Tricuspid incompetence and geometry of the right ventricle as predictors of right ventricular function after implantation of a left ventricular assist device. *J Heart Lung Transplant* 27:1275–1281, 2008.
62. Schulman AR, Martens TP, Russo MJ, et al: Effect of left ventricular assist device infection on post-transplant outcomes. *J Heart Lung Transplant* 28:237–242, 2009.
63. Sandner SE, Zimpfer D, Zrunek P, et al: Renal function and outcome after continuous flow left ventricular assist device implantation. *Ann Thorac Surg* 87:1072–1078, 2009.
64. Butler J, Geisberg C, Howser R, et al: Relationship between renal function and left ventricular assist device use. *Ann Thorac Surg* 81:1745–1751, 2006.
65. Topkara VK, Dang NC, Barili F, et al: Predictors and outcomes of continuous veno-venous hemodialysis use after implantation of a left ventricular assist device. *J Heart Lung Transplant* 25:404–408, 2006.
66. Mano A, Fujita K, Uenomachi K, et al: Body mass index is a useful predictor of prognosis after left ventricular assist system implantation. *J Heart Lung Transplant* 28:428–433, 2009.
67. Taylor DO, Edwards LB, Aurora P, et al: Registry of the International Society for Heart and Lung Transplantation: twenty-fifth official adult heart transplant report–2008. *J Heart Lung Transplant* 27:943–956, 2008.
68. Torre-Amione G, Southard RE, Loebe MM, et al: Reversal of secondary pulmonary hypertension by axial and pulsatile mechanical circulatory support. *J Heart Lung Transplant* 29(2):195–200, 2010.
69. Aaronson KD, Schwartz JS, Chen TM, et al: Development and prospective validation of a clinical index to predict survival in ambulatory patients referred for cardiac transplant evaluation. *Circulation* 95:2660–2667, 1997.

70. Levy WC, Mozaffarian D, Linker DT, et al: Can the Seattle heart failure model be used to risk-stratify heart failure patients for potential left ventricular assist device therapy? *J Heart Lung Transplant* 28:231–236, 2009.
71. Deng MC, Loebe M, El-Banayosy A, et al: Mechanical circulatory support for advanced heart failure: effect of patient selection on outcome. *Circulation* 103:231–237, 2001.
72. Oz MC, Goldstein DJ, Pepino P, et al: Screening scale predicts patients successfully receiving long-term implantable left ventricular assist devices. *Circulation* 92:II169–II173, 1995.
73. Lietz K, Long JW, Kfoury AG, et al: Outcomes of left ventricular assist device implantation as destination therapy in the post-REMATCH era: implications for patient selection. *Circulation* 116:497–505, 2007.
74. Stevenson LW, Pagani FD, Young JB, et al: INTERMACS profiles of advanced heart failure: the current picture. *J Heart Lung Transplant* 28:535–541, 2009.
75. Boyle AJ, Ascheim DD, Russo MJ, et al: Clinical outcomes for continuous-flow left ventricular assist device patients stratified by pre-operative INTERMACS classification. *J Heart Lung Transplant* 2011, epublished.

SECTION IV ■ PULMONARY PROBLEMS IN THE INTENSIVE CARE UNIT

J. MARK MADISON • RICHARD S. IRWIN

CHAPTER 46 ■ RESPIRATORY FAILURE PART I: A PHYSIOLOGIC APPROACH TO RESPIRATORY FAILURE

THADDEUS C. BARTTER, MELVIN R. PRATTER, WISSAM ABOUZGHEIB AND RICHARD S. IRWIN

OVERVIEW

Respiration serves to oxygenate blood and to remove the volatile waste product of metabolism, carbon dioxide and results in hypoxemia, hypercapnia, or both combined. Although it is traditional to define respiratory failure with abrupt boundaries [i.e., arterial carbon dioxide tension ($PaCO_2$) greater than 49 mm Hg or arterial oxygen tension (PaO_2) less than 50 to 60 mm Hg] [1,2], this is too simplistic for the understanding and management of respiratory insufficiency. This chapter discusses the physiologies leading to the different presentations of respiratory failure and briefly discusses management.

The alveolar PO_2 and PCO_2 are determined by the relationship between alveolar ventilation and perfusion ($\dot{V}/\dot{Q}$ ratio). The ratio of $\dot{V}$ to $\dot{Q}$ is approximately 0.8 under normal resting conditions. In $\dot{V}/\dot{Q}$ mismatch, the ratio is altered and the exchange of gaseous O_2 and CO_2 becomes inefficient. There are two $\dot{V}/\dot{Q}$ mismatch scenarios, termed "high $\dot{V}/\dot{Q}$ mismatch" and "low $\dot{V}/\dot{Q}$ mismatch." High-$\dot{V}/\dot{Q}$ mismatch occurs in a lung region that receives a disproportionate increase in ventilation or decrease in blood flow. Low $\dot{V}/\dot{Q}$ mismatch occurs in a lung region that receives a disproportionate decrease in ventilation or increase in blood flow. As will be seen, low $\dot{V}/\dot{Q}$ mismatch plays a major physiologic role in respiratory failure.

In many cases of respiratory failure, a low PaO_2 is coupled with an elevated $PaCO_2$, but the physiology of oxygenation is different from that of CO_2 removal. The differences stem in part from the differences in the capacity of blood to carry each of the two gases. Oxygen must bind to hemoglobin for effective transport. Saturated hemoglobin can carry 1.39 mL of O_2 per gram, whereas plasma can carry only 0.003 times the PaO_2; only approximately 1% of oxygen transport is independent of hemoglobin. The amount of O_2 that blood can carry is thus limited by hemoglobin concentration (and function). Once hemoglobin is saturated, a doubling of the alveolar oxygen concentration has no meaningful impact on oxygen transport. For this reason, alveoli with high $\dot{V}/\dot{Q}$ mismatch cannot add extra oxygen to the pulmonary capillary blood to compensate for alveoli with low $\dot{V}/\dot{Q}$ mismatch in which the hemoglobin of the associated pulmonary capillary blood is not fully saturated [3].

The biochemistry of CO_2 is very different. CO_2 diffuses readily into blood; its quantity increases almost linearly as the $PaCO_2$ increases. The mechanisms for CO_2 transport include a buffering system mediated by carbonic anhydrase and the formation of carbonyl compounds. The net result is that a doubling of alveolar ventilation essentially doubles CO_2 elimination. For this reason, unlike the physiology of O_2 transport, lung units with normal or high $\dot{V}/\dot{Q}$ relationships can compensate for areas with low $\dot{V}/\dot{Q}$ relationships. Because of these differences between the two gases, abnormalities in their values are not always linked, and it is useful to approach the factors that can cause each to be abnormal.

Normal Blood Gas Values

"Normal" PaO_2 can be shown to decrease with age and with the supine position [4]. There is significant standard deviation, and in clinical practice the normal range for most laboratories, 80 to 100 mg Hg, suffices.

In normal human homeostasis, the $PaCO_2$ is tightly regulated by respiration at or close to 40 mm Hg. Unlike the PaO_2, the normal $PaCO_2$ remains at 40 mm Hg throughout life. It is unaffected by age [4] or position [5].

The normal pH of human arterial blood is at or close to 7.40. Like the $PaCO_2$, there is no predicted change with age.

HYPOXEMIA AND HYPERCAPNIA

There are six basic pathophysiologic mechanisms that can lead to hypoxemia. Some also cause hypercapnia [1,6,7]:

1. Low partial pressure of inspired O_2 (PIO_2)
2. Diffusion impairment
3. Right-to-left shunt
4. Low $\dot{V}/\dot{Q}$ mismatch
5. Hypoventilation
6. High partial pressure of inspired CO_2

Only three are clinically important: low $\dot{V}/\dot{Q}$ mismatch, right-to-left shunt, and hypoventilation. $\dot{V}/\dot{Q}$ mismatch and hypoventilation can cause both hypoxemia and hypercapnia.

Low Partial Pressure of Inspired Oxygen

Low PIO_2 is a potential cause of hypoxemia. A low PIO_2 occurs only at high altitudes and in conditions when other gases are present; it is not in the differential diagnosis of normal clinical management.

Diffusion Impairment

It was once thought that thickening of alveolar walls could lead to an increase in the diffusion distance great enough to prevent equilibrium of the partial pressure of oxygen between the alveoli and the associated pulmonary capillary blood. This physiologic concept is known as "alveolar–capillary block syndrome," [8]. Subsequent data, however, indicated that even radiographically "homogeneous" pulmonary disease rarely alters alveolar–capillary membranes uniformly throughout the lung. In addition, the efficiency of gas exchange within any single alveolus is such that even with a barrier to diffusion, diffusion impairment is not a factor; by the time blood leaves the alveolar capillaries, alveolar and capillary gas partial pressures are equal. Thus, hypoxemia at rest in patients with pathologies such as interstitial disease is due not to "alveolar–capillary block" but rather to areas of low $\dot{V}/\dot{Q}$ mismatch. In contrast, there may be a component of "alveolar–capillary block" in exercise; as the transit time of blood through alveolar capillaries decreases, there may be some true physiologic impairment of capillary/alveolar gas equilibrium that could result in hypoxemia [9].

Right-to-Left Shunt

In right-to-left shunt, blood from the right heart does not come into contact with oxygenated air before reaching the left heart; ventilation and perfusion are uncoupled [5]. Three kinds of shunt are recognized: cardiac, pulmonary vascular, and pulmonary parenchymal [10]. In a cardiac shunt, a defect allows blood to pass directly from the right atrium or ventricle into the left-sided chamber. For cardiac shunt to occur, there must be some relative increase in right-sided pressures. In a pulmonary vascular shunt, the shunting of blood occurs through arteriovenous malformations within the pulmonary vascular bed. These arteriovenous malformations can be small and not visible on chest imaging (as in some cases of cirrhosis), or large and visible as parenchymal densities (as with hereditary hemorrhagic telangiectasia) [11]. In pulmonary parenchymal shunt, alveolar consolidation or atelectasis prevents gases from reaching alveoli while blood flow continues through their capillary beds. Examples of conditions that cause parenchymal shunt are pneumonia, lobar collapse, and acute respiratory distress syndrome.

Note that right-to-left shunt is listed as a cause of hypoxemia but not of hypercapnia because of the capacity of alveoli with normal or high $\dot{V}/\dot{Q}$ ratios to compensate for the lack of clearance of CO_2 from shunted blood [6]. If the only gas exchange defect present is shunt, increased ventilation to the perfused alveoli leads to a normal $PaCO_2$ [6]. This increased ventilation has no effect on the PaO_2; as already noted, the dependency on hemoglobin for blood to carry oxygen results in an inability of areas with normal or elevated $\dot{V}/\dot{Q}$ ratios to compensate for areas with low $\dot{V}/\dot{Q}$ ratios. Thus, shunt is a cause of nonhypercapnic hypoxemic respiratory failure.

$\dot{V}/\dot{Q}$ Mismatch

Low $\dot{V}/\dot{Q}$ mismatch is the dominant physiology in abnormalities of gas exchange. Mild to moderate degrees of low $\dot{V}/\dot{Q}$ mismatch can cause hypoxemia alone, whereas more severe $\dot{V}/\dot{Q}$ mismatching leads to hypoxemia with hypercapnia. (For a patient breathing room air, $\dot{V}/\dot{Q}$ mismatch never causes hypercapnia in the absence of hypoxemia.) There are two reasons why a substantially greater amount of low $\dot{V}/\dot{Q}$ mismatch must be present to cause hypercapnia than to cause hypoxemia. The first reason is the higher solubility of CO_2 in blood as discussed earlier [6]; there is no saturation limit for CO_2. Thus while normal alveoli cannot increase oxygen uptake significantly after hemoglobin saturation, they can increase CO_2 removal as venous CO_2 content rises. The second reason is that, just as with shunt, patients with low $\dot{V}/\dot{Q}$ mismatch increase their minute ventilation to compensate for the potential elevation in CO_2 that the low $\dot{V}/\dot{Q}$ areas would otherwise generate [6]. With severe $\dot{V}/\dot{Q}$ mismatch, there are not enough normal and high $\dot{V}/\dot{Q}$ alveoli to compensate for the hypercarbia of those with low $\dot{V}/\dot{Q}$ mismatch; hypercapnia occurs in addition to hypoxemia.

Hypoventilation

Hypoventilation refers to conditions in which minute ventilation is reduced relative to the metabolic demand present for oxygen uptake and CO_2 production. By necessity, when minute ventilation is reduced alveolar ventilation must also be abnormally low, resulting in decreased gas exchange between the external environment and the alveoli [6]. Hypoventilation by definition causes both arterial hypoxemia and a raised arterial PCO_2. Some physicians use the terms "hypoventilation" and "carbon dioxide retention" interchangeably, a usage that confuses physiologies. Pure hypoventilation represents decreased minute ventilation with normal lungs. In contrast, other conditions that cause carbon dioxide retention (low $\dot{V}/\dot{Q}$ mismatch) are caused by airway or parenchymal lung disease and usually are associated with increased minute ventilation.

In hypoventilation as defined earlier, the alveolar PCO_2 can rise to the point that the partial pressure of O_2 is significantly reduced. The disorders that cause hypoventilation are called the *extrapulmonary* causes of respiratory failure because they do not involve abnormality of the pulmonary gas exchange mechanisms [7,12,13]. A defect leading to hypoventilation can occur anywhere in the normal physiologic linkages that affect minute ventilation; the differential diagnosis of extrapulmonary respiratory failure is listed in Table 46.1. Note that in this categorization, obstruction at or above the trachea and other large airways is classified as an extrapulmonary disorder because of the fact that the gas exchange mechanisms of the lung remain intact.

High Partial Pressure of Inspired Carbon Dioxide

The inhalation of a gas containing CO_2 can cause hypercapnia although it is not usually part of the differential diagnosis in clinical medicine. It does occur occasionally in iatrogenic situations; patients on a t-piece with extended tubing attached to the expiratory port may be forced to re-breathe exhaled CO_2 to the point of hypercapnia.

TABLE 46.1

DIFFERENTIAL DIAGNOSIS OF EXTRAPULMONARY RESPIRATORY FAILURE[a]

Site of abnormality	Disease
Central nervous system	Respiratory center depression owing to overdose, primary alveolar hypoventilation, myxedema
Peripheral nervous system	Spinal cord disease, amyotrophic lateral sclerosis, Guillain–Barré syndrome
Respiratory muscles	Muscle fatigue, myasthenia gravis, polymyositis, hypophosphatemia
Chest wall	Ankylosing spondylitis, flail chest, thoracoplasty
Pleura	Restrictive pleuritis
Upper airway obstruction	Tracheal stenosis, vocal cord tumor

[a]This table is not an exhaustive listing; it includes the more common causes for each involved compartment of the respiratory system.

Overlapping Factors

Several comments are in order. First, more than one mechanism may be operant in any individual case. For example, a high ventilatory requirement needed to compensate for areas of low $\dot{V}/\dot{Q}$ mismatch in a patient with chronic obstructive pulmonary disease may lead to muscle overload with fatigue and therefore add an extrapulmonary etiology of hypercapnia to primary pulmonary disease. Another common coupling would be the coexistence of $\dot{V}/\dot{Q}$ mismatch and pulmonary parenchymal shunt in a patient with pneumonia and underlying chronic obstructive pulmonary disease (COPD).

Second, a decrease in cardiac output may worsen hypoxemia primarily due to marked $\dot{V}/\dot{Q}$ abnormalities, a large right-to-left shunt, or both. A decrease in cardiac output forces a compensatory increase in oxygen extraction at the tissue level, leading to a decreased mixed-venous oxygen content. Isolated reduction in the mixed-venous oxygen content is not a cause of hypoxemia, but it can exacerbate the hypoxemia generated by any of the primary mechanisms described above.

Third, as mentioned, shunt alone is not a cause of hypercapnia, but if a significant shunt is present in conjunction with one of the primary causes of hypercapnia, then the capacity to compensate for the shunt is reduced and hypercapnia is worsened.

Finally, the $PaCO_2$ represents a balance between CO_2 production and CO_2 clearance; in patients with an impaired capacity to clear CO_2, increases in production may gain clinical relevance [14]. Fever increases CO_2 production by 13% for each 1°C temperature elevation above normal. Thus, lowering temperature to normal may have an impact on $PaCO_2$ in a febrile patient with a large amount of $\dot{V}/\dot{Q}$ mismatch. Nutritional support with excessive total calories or proportionally high-carbohydrate loads also increases CO_2 production [15]. It follows that decreasing total caloric load may influence the degree of hypercapnia in patients with limited ventilatory reserve.

ANALYTICAL TOOLS FOR HYPOXEMIA AND HYPERCAPNIA

Several tools can be used to categorize type and severity of the different causes of hypercapnia and hypoxemia. Simple calculation, maneuvers, and tests can give the clinician a better understanding of the underlying physiology.

Calculation of Alveolar–Arterial PO_2 Gradient and PaO_2/FIO_2 Ratio

The A–a PO_2 gradient, although a conceptual simplification, is clinically useful. It allows separation of extrapulmonary from pulmonary causes of respiratory failure [16,17]. It presents a mathematical model as though the lung were one large alveolus and the entire blood flow of the right heart passed around that alveolus. Rules of partial pressure and the respiratory exchange ratio, R, are used to calculate the theoretical alveolar PO_2 (PAO_2). The PIO_2 is reduced first by water pressure in the airways and then at the alveolar level by the alveolar $PaCO_2$. Exchange of oxygen and CO_2 at the alveolar level is reflected in the respiratory exchange ratio, R. This is the basis for the alveolar air equation [18],

$$PAO_2 = PIO_2 - PaCO_2/R$$

Ambient air at sea level has a total pressure of 760 mm Hg, 21% of which is oxygen. As air is inhaled it is humidified by water vapor, which has a partial pressure of approximately 47 at normal body temperature. The partial pressure of O_2 after inhaled air is humidified is therefore 0.21 (760 – 47), or 150. In a steady state, *R* can be assumed to be 0.8, even in patients with significant lung disease [18]. Given the previous assumptions and a normal $PaCO_2$ of 40 mm Hg, one gets an idealized PAO_2 of 100:

$$PAO_2 = 150 - 40/0.8 = 100$$

The A–a gradient is then obtained by subtracting the measured arterial PO_2 from the calculated PAO_2. $PCO_2/0.8$ is the same as the $PCO_2 \times 1.25$. Thus, for a person breathing room air at sea level,

$$\text{A–a gradient is equal to} = 150 - (1.25 \times PaCO_2) - PaO_2$$

In reality, the lung is not a single large alveolus, and there is not an oxygen gradient between the alveolus and the capillary. The calculated "gradient" represents a mixture of blood from alveoli with ideal characteristics with blood from alveoli that have low $\dot{V}/\dot{Q}$ mismatch and with shunted blood. The greater the contribution from alveoli with low $\dot{V}/\dot{Q}$ mismatch and from shunt, the greater the A–a "gradient."

One value of the concept of the A–a gradient is that it can be used to separate the extrapulmonary causes of respiratory failure from those that involve parenchymal lung disease [12] as long as the patient is breathing room air. With extrapulmonary failure, the A–a gradient remains normal. With shunt or $\dot{V}/\dot{Q}$ mismatch, the gradient is usually elevated. $\dot{V}/\dot{Q}$ mismatch and extrapulmonary respiratory failure are the two causes of hypercapnia encountered in clinical practice, and the A–a gradient is a useful tool for distinguishing between them. Gray and Blalock have noted that the A–a gradient is an imperfect tool; with very high $PaCO_2$, the gradient can narrow [19]. This is rarely an issue in clinical management. At any age, an A–a gradient exceeding 20 mm Hg on room air should be considered abnormal and indicative of pulmonary dysfunction [16].

When the FIO_2 is above 0.21, the A–a gradient becomes a less accurate measure of the efficiency of gas exchange and therefore a less valuable tool for the measurement of shunt, $\dot{V}/\dot{Q}$ mismatch, or the lack thereof. The PaO_2 divided by the FIO_2 (PaO_2/FIO_2 ratio) can be used to assess the severity of the gas exchange defect. For calculation, the FIO_2 is expressed as a decimal ranging from 0.21 to 1.00. The normal PaO_2/FIO_2 is 300 to 500. A value of <300 is indicative of gas exchange derangement and a value below 200 is indicative of severe impairment. Although the PaO_2/FIO_2 is felt to be a more reliable measure of degree of gas exchange impairment at higher FIO_2s, it too has the potential to be unreliable, particularly in the presence of a large shunt or a low FIO_2 [20–22].

100% Oxygen Inhalation Challenge

A trial of 100% oxygen inhalation can be used to separate low $\dot{V}/\dot{Q}$ mismatch from shunt as the cause of respiratory failure. In areas of low $\dot{V}/\dot{Q}$ mismatch, the alveolar PO_2 is low. If 100% oxygen is delivered via a closed system, even a poorly ventilated alveolus in theory soon contains 100% oxygen diluted only by the partial pressures of water and CO_2 [1]. Thus, with low $\dot{V}/\dot{Q}$ mismatch, the PaO_2 rises dramatically if the FIO_2 is increased. In contrast, areas of shunt are never exposed to O_2, and there is no response to an increase in FIO_2. If the PaO_2 with the patient breathing 100% O_2 is greater than 500 mm Hg, then prior hypoxemia is largely due to $\dot{V}/\dot{Q}$ mismatch [1]. If the PO_2 on 100% O_2 is less than 350 mm Hg, then major shunting is present.

Nuclear Scanning and Echocardiography

Nuclear scanning and echocardiography can be used to determine the etiology of a shunt. As previously stated, a right-to-left shunt can be pulmonary parenchymal, pulmonary vascular, or intracardiac. Nuclear perfusion scanning for evaluation of shunt takes advantage of the fact that the technetium-labeled macroaggregated albumin used for the scan is a relatively large particle that does not pass through capillaries. This characteristic can help to separate shunt with normal vasculature from shunt due to abnormal vascular connections. If vascular anatomy is normal (and shunt is produced by blood flow through normal capillaries traversing consolidated lung), the technetium-labeled molecules of the nuclear scan are filtered by the pulmonary capillaries and remain in the lung. In contrast, with abnormal connection(s) between the right and left heart vasculatures, significant amounts of technetium-labeled particles bypass pulmonary capillaries and are then filtered by systemic capillaries (e.g. brain and kidneys). Thus, a nuclear scan obtained to classify and quantify shunt shows immediate renal and cerebral uptake if the shunt is cardiac or pulmonary vascular and only pulmonary uptake if the shunt is of pulmonary parenchymal origin [10]. If the shunt is not pulmonary parenchymal, the final step to differentiate intracardiac from pulmonary parenchymal is contrast echocardiography. Contrast echocardiography can document right-to-left cardiac shunting if present [17,23,24]; immediate transit (within four cardiac cycles) to the left heart can be seen with intracardiac shunt. If there is no cardiac shunt or if contrast appears after five cardiac cycles, then the abnormal vascular connection is in the pulmonary circulation.

RESPIRATORY ACID–BASE DISORDERS

Acid–base analysis can be used to understand the nature and acuity of a respiratory disturbance, both essential for clinical management. Relationships between $PaCO_2$, pH, and bicarbonate concentration (HCO_3^-) can be used first to determine whether there is a primary respiratory or metabolic process, whether it is simple (one acid–base disturbance) or complicated (more than one), and whether it is acute or chronic [25]. A respiratory disturbance is defined by a primary change in $PaCO_2$, whereas a metabolic disorder involves a primary change in the HCO_3^- (see Chapter 72). An acute process is one occurring in minutes to hours, whereas a chronic process has persisted for several days or longer. This chapter concentrates on acute and chronic simple respiratory disorders.

Acid–base balance is assessed clinically from the arterial hydrogen ion (H^+) concentration and may be expressed either in nanoequivalents per liter or as the negative logarithm of that number, pH_a. H^+ concentration can be assessed with knowledge of the concentration of any of many potential hydrogen donors and the dissociation constant for that donor. The mass action equation that demonstrates the capacity of CO_2 to act as an acid ($CO_2 + H_2O \Leftrightarrow H_2CO_3 \Leftrightarrow H^+ + HCO_3^-$), is of clinical relevance and also convenient, given that $PaCO_2$ and HCO_3^- are easily measured. An increase in CO_2 drives the equation to the right, increasing H^+ concentration. An increase in HCO_3^- drives the equation to the left, decreasing the H^+ concentration. The Henderson version of the Henderson–Hasselbalch equation [3], $H^+ = 24\ (PaCO_2/HCO_3^-)$, calculates actual H^+ concentration using those measurements. Clinically, all acid–base disorders can be evaluated using this basic equation [4].

Calculation of H^+ Concentration

In clinical practice, the pH is the value reported, but knowledge of the H^+ concentration can often facilitate the diagnosis of respiratory acid–base disturbances. The relationship between H^+ and pH and how to predict H^+ from pH, essential to the following discussion, is covered in Chapter 11.

TABLE 46.2

THE DIFFERENTIAL DIAGNOSIS OF HYPERCAPNIA

Hypercapnia with elevated A–a gradient	Hypercapnia with normal A–a gradient
Low $\dot{V}/\dot{Q}$ mismatch COPD	Extrapulmonary respiratory failure (see Table 46.1) Obesity/hypoventilation syndrome Rebreathing CO_2

$\Delta H^+/\Delta PCO_2$ Ratio

Ability to calculate the H^+ concentration allows calculation of the $\Delta H^+/\Delta PCO_2$ ratio that is of value in understanding respiratory acid-base disorders. The $\Delta H^+/\Delta PCO_2$ is calculated as the change in H^+ from baseline (baseline assumed usually to be 40 nanoequivalents per liter that corresponds to a pH of 7.40) divided by the change in $PaCO_2$ from baseline (baseline again 40). For example, for the theoretical blood gas (pH, $PaCO_2$, PaO_2), 7.32/50/60, the change in PCO_2 is 10 and the change in H^+ concentration is 8 (48 − 40); the ratio is therefore 0.8.

An acute change of PCO_2 in either direction causes an immediate and predictable change in H^+ and thus a predictable $\Delta H^+/\Delta PCO_2$ [25,26]. If a respiratory alteration persists, however, renal mechanisms increase or decrease serum HCO_3^- in a direction that pushes the H^+ back toward normal; maintenance of H^+ homeostasis is a primal physiologic function. Thus, after renal compensation occurs, the $\Delta H^+/\Delta PCO_2$ ratio is altered. This alteration represents the chronic state.

Respiratory Acidosis/Respiratory Alkalosis

Respiratory acidosis is defined as an acidosis associated with and caused by an elevation of the $PaCO_2$. By definition therefore, respiratory acidosis is a product of hypercapnia (See Table 46.2). Knowledge of the H^+ concentration in addition to the $PaCO_2$, however, allows for calculation of the $\Delta H^+/\Delta PCO_2$ ratio. A ratio of 0.8 (as in the earlier example) implies an acute respiratory acidosis [26]. A ratio of 0.3 implies a chronic (and compensated) respiratory acidosis [26]. Values for the $\Delta H^+/\Delta PCO_2$ ratio between 0.3 and 0.8 correspond to an acute-on-chronic respiratory acidosis (as often occurs with an exacerbation of chronic obstructive pulmonary disease) [26].

Respiratory alkalosis is defined as an alkalosis caused by a decrease in $PaCO_2$ that drives the CO_2 in the mass action equation to the left: H^+ and HCO_3^- concentrations decrease. The differential diagnosis for respiratory alkalosis is listed in Table 46.3. When the $\Delta H^+/\Delta PCO_2$ ratio is used to analyze a pure respiratory alkalosis, a ratio of 0.8 corresponds to an acute respiratory alkalosis and a ratio of 0.17 corresponds to a chronic respiratory alkalosis [26].

CLINICAL APPROACH TO RESPIRATORY FAILURE

Respiratory failure occurs when gas exchange becomes significantly impaired. It is impossible to accurately predict PaO_2 and $PaCO_2$ using clinical criteria [27,28]; the diagnosis of respiratory failure depends on arterial blood gas (ABG) analysis. Various clinical signs and symptoms, including those reflecting the effects of hypoxemia or hypercapnia, or both, on the

TABLE 46.3

CAUSES OF RESPIRATORY ALKALOSIS[a]

Elevated A–a gradient	Normal A–a gradient
Sepsis and capillary leak syndrome	Central nervous system disorder
Hepatic failure with hepatopulmonary syndrome	Hepatic failure with normal lungs
Chronic interstitial lung diseases	Analeptic overdose drugs
Pulmonary edema	Salicylates
Cardiogenic	Catecholamines
Noncardiogenic (acute respiratory distress syndrome)	Progesterone
Pulmonary embolism	Thyroid hormone excess
Pneumonia	Pregnancy
Asthma	High altitude
Right-to-left shunt	Severe anemia (approximately 3 g/dL hemoglobin)
	Psychogenic hyperventilation
	Endotoxemia
	Mechanical hyperventilation with normal lungs
	During menses after ovulation

$P(A–a)O_2$, alveolar–arterial oxygen tension gradient.
[a]The differential diagnosis of respiratory alkalosis with an elevated $P(A–a)O_2$ gradient is the same as that of nonhypercapnic, hypoxemic respiratory failure.

central nervous system and cardiovascular system, may lead to suspicion of the diagnosis, but the ABG must be obtained for confirmation. A clinical approach to respiratory failure begins with analysis of the ABG for the severity, type, and acuity of the gas exchange disturbance. These factors and the expected duration of the process guide interventions.

Acute hypercapnia should be evaluated for reversible causes. If none is found, mechanical ventilatory support, invasive or noninvasive, is needed. This can take the form of intubation, but other options such as continuous positive airway pressure and noninvasive positive-pressure ventilation now have a documented role in the management of acute respiratory compromise [29]. Hypercapnia with a $\Delta H^+/\Delta PCO_2$ ratio of 0.3, indicating chronicity, uncommonly requires urgent ventilatory support.

CLINICAL EXAMPLES

Scenario 1

A 29-year-old man is brought to the emergency department in a stuporous state. ABGs drawn on room air at the time of arrival demonstrate a PaO_2 of 52, $PaCO_2$ of 68, and pH of 7.21. On calculation, the A–a gradient is 13 and the $\Delta H^+/\Delta PCO_2$ ratio is 0.8. You therefore know that you are dealing with an acute respiratory acidosis of extrapulmonary origin. The narcotic antagonist naloxone is administered, and the patient wakes up, with normalization of blood gases.

Scenario 2

The same patient, given naloxone and flumazenil, has no change in blood gases or mental status. Your differential diagnosis is now acute extrapulmonary respiratory failure other than narcotic or benzodiazepine respiratory suppression. You intubate and start mechanical ventilation.

Scenario 3

The patient arrives with a PaO_2 of 42, $PaCO_2$ of 68, and pH of 7.21. Calculation of the A–a gradient yields a value of 23. You administer naloxone and the patient does awaken, but he remains hypoxemic. This was anticipated owing to the elevated A–a gradient; you evaluate for an additional process such as aspiration of gastric contents.

In an acute-on-chronic situation, the trend of the acidosis is most crucial in deciding whether mechanical ventilatory support is necessary [7]. Although these ratios are strictly correct only for simple respiratory acid–base disturbances, the authors believe they should be applied therapeutically even in a complicated disturbance. If the ratio is consistent with an acute respiratory acidosis, the patient who fails to improve with treatment should receive ventilatory support (see Chapters 58, 59).

Fear of causing greater hypercapnia should not be a deterrent to the use of supplemental oxygen in an acutely ill hypoxemic patient. Although $PaCO_2$ predictably increases with the use of supplemental oxygen in patients with hypercapnia due to $\dot{V}/\dot{Q}$ mismatch, CO_2 narcosis is very uncommon. It does, however, make sense to start supplemental oxygen at a low concentration and then to slowly increase the FIO_2 until adequate oxygenation is achieved. The uncommon case of resultant severe hypercapnia can be treated with mechanical ventilatory support.

Respiratory alkalosis is not itself a cause of respiratory failure unless the increased work of breathing cannot be sustained by the respiratory muscles. Management therefore depends on diagnosis of the underlying stimulus for hyperventilation and on treatment specific to that condition (e.g., heparin for pulmonary embolism). When respiratory alkalosis continues to worsen in critically ill patients on mechanical ventilatory support, however, it may become necessary to treat the respiratory alkalosis directly. In such a setting, sedation with or without paralysis of skeletal muscles can be useful.

Hypoxemia that responds only minimally to large increases in FIO_2 involves significant shunt. (In many clinical situations, such as chronic obstructive pulmonary disease with pneumonia, the physiology involves a coupling of shunt and $\dot{V}/\dot{Q}$ mismatch.) Cardiac shunt or large pulmonary arteriovenous shunts may require an invasive intervention to correct them. Diffuse pulmonary parenchymal shunt, as can occur in acute respiratory distress syndrome, may be amenable to positive end-expiratory pressure.

Noninvasive ventilation has been studied extensively. In clinical scenarios in which reversal or amelioration of the underlying process may be possible within the short term, noninvasive ventilation may provide a therapeutic bridge that allows avoidance of the possible disadvantages of intubation and mechanical ventilation [29].

CONCLUSION

The basic physiologic mechanisms underlying all abnormalities of gas exchange have been delineated. Of these, the most clinically relevant are low $\dot{V}/\dot{Q}$ mismatch, hypoventilation, and shunt. A series of tools that can be used to analyze and differentiate these physiologic possibilities has been presented along with an analysis of how $H^+/PaCO_2$ relationships can help to define the acuity of a disorder. Analysis of the type and acuity of a process should lead to an attempt to define the responsible disease process(es) and to intervene specifically. The decision of when or whether to institute mechanical ventilatory support, especially with intubation, is not always clear from numbers alone; this decision involves the art as well as the science of medicine.

References

1. West JB: *Pulmonary Pathophysiology: The Essentials*. Baltimore, Williams & Wilkins, 1982.
2. Pontoppidan H, Geffin B, Lowenstein E: Acute respiratory failure in the adult. 1. *N Engl J Med* 287:690, 1972.
3. Murray JF: *The Normal Lung: The Basis for Diagnosis and Treatment of Pulmonary Disease*. Philadelphia, PA, WB Saunders, 1976.
4. Cerveri I, Zoia MC, Fanfulla F, et al: Reference values of arterial oxygen tension in the middle-aged and elderly. *Am J Respir Crit Care Med* 152:934, 1995.
5. Bates DV: *Respiratory Function in Disease*. Toronto, WB Saunders, 1989.
6. West JB: Causes of carbon dioxide retention in lung disease. *N Engl J Med* 284:1232, 1971.
7. Demers RR, Irwin RS: Management of hypercapnic respiratory failure: a systematic approach. *Respir Care* 24:328, 1979.
8. Finley TN, Swenson EW, Comroe JH Jr: The cause of arterial hypoxemia at rest in patients with "alveolar capillary block syndrome". *J Clin Invest* 41:618, 1962.
9. Murray JF: Pathophysiology of acute respiratory failure. *Respir Care* 28:531, 1983.
10. Robin ED, Laman PD, Goris ML, et al: A shunt is (not) a shunt is (not) a shunt. *Am Rev Respir Dis* 115:553, 1977.
11. Bartter T, Irwin RS, Nash G: Aneurysms of the pulmonary arteries. *Chest* 94:1065, 1988.
12. Pratter MR, Irwin RS: Extrapulmonary causes of respiratory failure. *J Int Care Med* 1:197, 1986.
13. Pratter MR, Corwin RW, Irwin RS: An integrated analysis of lung and respiratory muscle dysfunction in the pathogenesis of hypercapnic respiratory failure. *Respir Care* 27:55, 1982.
14. Weinberger SE, Schwartzstein RM, Weiss JW: Hypercapnia. *N Engl J Med* 321:1223, 1989.
15. Talpers SS, Romberger DJ, Bunce SB, et al: Nutritionally associated increased carbon dioxide production. Excess total calories vs high proportion of carbohydrate calories. *Chest* 102:551, 1992.
16. Mellemgaard K: The alveolar-arterial oxygen difference: its size and components in normal man. *Acta Physiol Scand* 67:10, 1966.
17. Chen WJ, Kuan P, Lien WP, et al: Detection of patent foramen ovale by contrast transesophageal echocardiography. *Chest* 101:1515, 1992.
18. Begin R, Renzetti AO Jr: Alveolar-arterial oxygen pressure gradient. I. Comparison between and assumed and actual respiratory quotient in stable chronic pulmonary disease. II. Relationship to aging and closing volume in normal subjects. *Respir Care* 22:491, 1977.
19. Gray BA, Blalock JM: Interpretation of the alveolar-arterial oxygen difference in patients with hypercapnia. *Am Rev Respir Dis* 143:4, 1991.
20. Bernard GR, Artigas A, Brigham KL, et al: The American-European Consensus Conference on ARDS. Definitions, mechanisms, relevant outcomes, and clinical trial coordination. *Am J Respir Crit Care Med* 149:818, 1994.
21. Whiteley JP, Gavaghan DJ, Hahn CE: Variation of venous admixture, SF6 shunt, PaO_2, and the PaO_2/FIO_2 ratio with FIO_2. *Br J Anaesth* 88:771, 2002.
22. Gowda MS, Klocke RA: Variability of indices of hypoxemia in adult respiratory distress syndrome. *Crit Care Med* 25:41, 1997.
23. Cox D, Taylor J, Nanda NC: Refractory hypoxemia in right ventricular infarction from right-to-left shunting via a patent foramen ovale: efficacy of contrast transesophageal echocardiography. *Am J Med* 91:653, 1991.
24. Suzuki Y, Kambara H, Kadota K, et al: Detection of intracardiac shunt flow in atrial septal defect using a real-time two-dimensional color-coded Doppler flow imaging system and comparison with contrast two-dimensional echocardiography. *Am J Cardiol* 56:347, 1985.
25. Narins RG, Emmett M: Simple and mixed acid-base disorders: a practical approach. *Medicine (Baltimore)* 59:161, 1980.
26. Bear RA, Gribik M: Assessing acid-base imbalances through laboratory parameters. *Hosp Practice* 157, 1974.
27. Mithoefer JC, Bossman OG, Thibeault DW, et al: The clinical estimation of alveolar ventilation. *Am Rev Respir Dis* 98:868, 1968.
28. Comroe JH Jr, Botelho S: The unreliability of cyanosis in the recognition of arterial anoxemia. *Am J Med Sci* 214:1, 1947.
29. Mehta S, Hill NS: Noninvasive ventilation. *Am J Respir Crit Care Med* 163:540, 2001.

CHAPTER 47 ■ RESPIRATORY FAILURE PART II: ACUTE RESPIRATORY DISTRESS SYNDROME

GILMAN B. ALLEN AND POLLY E. PARSONS

INTRODUCTION

Acute lung injury (ALI) and the acute respiratory distress syndrome (ARDS) represent a continuum of severity for the same pathologic condition, both being defined by noncardiogenic pulmonary edema and hypoxemia in the setting of direct or indirect lung injury. Because ARDS, by definition, simply represents a more severely advanced form of ALI, the term "ALI" can be used as a comprehensive term for both conditions. ALI represents a common pathologic endpoint of various potential insults to the lung that almost invariably lead to hypoxemic respiratory failure requiring support with mechanical ventilation. Despite the confirmed success of protective mechanical ventilation strategies in lowering mortality [1,2] and ongoing efforts to discover other effective interventions [3–6], treatment of this condition remains largely supportive, and ALI continues to be a major source of morbidity and mortality in the intensive care unit [7,8]. Fortunately, an enormous body of research already exists on the pathogenesis of this condition, and advances continue to develop with regard to our understanding of ALI, its prognostic implications, and how to best manage the condition medically.

DEFINITION

ALI is defined as a diminished arterial oxygen pressure (PaO_2) to fractional inspired oxygen (FiO_2) ratio (P to F (P:F) ratio less than 300), bilateral airspace disease on chest radiograph, and pulmonary edema from increased permeability, the latter defined by evidence of normal cardiac function [9]. ARDS is simply a subset of ALI having a more severely diminished P:F ratio (less than 200). However, because the P:F ratio can be affected by arbitrary ventilator settings [10], and because many

TABLE 47.1

RECOMMENDED CRITERIA FOR ACUTE LUNG INJURY (ALI) AND ACUTE RESPIRATORY DISTRESS SYNDROME (ARDS)

	Timing	Oxygenation	Chest radiograph	Pulmonary artery wedge pressure
ALI Criteria	Acute onest	$PaO_2/FiO_2 \leq 300$ mm Hg (regardless of PEEP)	Bilateral infiltrates seen on frontal chest radiograph	≤ 18 mm Hg when measured OR no clinical evidence of left atrial hypertension
ARDS Criteria	Acute onset	$PaO_2/FiO_2 \leq 200$ mm Hg (regardless of PEEP)	Bilateral infiltrates seen on frontal chest radiograph	≤ 18 mm Hg when measured OR no clinical evidence of left atrial hypertension

From Bernard GR, Artigas A, Brigham KL, et al: The American-European Consensus Conference on ARDS. Definitions, mechanisms, relevant outcomes, and clinical trial coordination. *Am J Respir Crit Care Med* 149:818–824, 1994.

studies have shown that indices of oxygenation are not strongly predictive of outcome [11–13], this differentiation may be of limited clinical relevance. Furthermore, the definition of ALI and ARDS has undergone significant evolution over the years, and limitations of this definition still exist [14], which can confound the interpretation of older research results and contribute added challenges to the design of new studies.

In response to the recognized limitations in determining the incidence and outcomes of ALI, a committee of leading investigators in the field met in 1994 to develop a consensus between the American Thoracic Society and the European Society of Intensive Care Medicine. The most current definition of ALI derives from this consensus [9] and defines the condition as the acute onset of hypoxemia and noncardiogenic pulmonary edema (see Table 47.1). Although the source of hypoxemia in ALI is multifactorial, it is one of the most easily gauged markers of "lung injury" in the intensive care unit and thus an important component of the definition. Despite its limited prognostic value, the more inclusive P:F ratio of less than 300 can serve to identify patients earlier in their course [11], thus expediting delivery of critical life saving interventions before progression to ARDS. In ALI, the pulmonary edema is the result of capillary leak, a parameter that is difficult to measure in the clinical setting. Accordingly, noncardiogenic pulmonary edema is defined using clinical parameters, which include the presence of "bilateral infiltrates" consistent with pulmonary edema on chest radiograph and either a pulmonary artery wedge pressure (PAWP) less than 18 mm Hg (when measured) or no clinical evidence of left atrial hypertension [9]. However, because the group recognized that ALI does not always exist exclusively without heart failure, the consensus more explicitly defines ALI as "a syndrome of inflammation and increased permeability that is associated with a constellation of clinical, radiologic, and physiologic abnormalities that cannot be explained by, but may coexist with, left atrial or pulmonary capillary hypertension"[9].

Despite the great lengths taken to clarify the current definition of ALI, it is not without its shortcomings, particularly because it does not delineate the cause of hypoxemia (i.e., alveolar damage) or clearly establish the presence of increased permeability [14]. Unfortunately, easily employed tests for microvascular permeability are not yet available, and what degree of permeability is needed to reliably predict the presence of alveolar damage is not known [14]. The boundaries for the P:F ratio are also arbitrary. The consensus committee recognized the difficulty in interpreting this ratio in the setting of different levels of positive end-expiratory pressure (PEEP) [15], and thus decided to not include this parameter in their definition. It would also be impractical to base the clinical definition of ALI upon histologic findings given the often critical condition of patients and their poor candidacy for biopsy by the time of clinical diagnosis. Nevertheless, the histopathology of ALI has been well characterized and is, in many ways, descriptive of its pathogenesis.

HISTOPATHOLOGY

Despite having many different potential etiologies [16–18], the histologic findings of ALI are fundamentally uniform and are collectively described by the term, *diffuse alveolar damage* (DAD) [19]. DAD represents a continuum of changes that can be temporally divided into *exudative*, *proliferative*, and *fibrotic* phases [19,20], between which considerable overlap exists. The *exudative* phase of DAD is the earliest phase, during which clinical symptoms first develop and lung mechanical changes become manifest [21]. This phase typically occupies the first week and is characterized by epithelial and endothelial cell death, neutrophil sequestration, platelet–fibrin thrombi, interstitial edema, and exudates within the airspaces, which consist of fluid, protein, and cellular debris [19]. These exudates compact into dense, protein-rich hyaline membranes that stain strongly with eosin and line the alveoli and alveolar ducts (Fig. 47.1A). During the second week of injury, the *proliferative* phase ensues, which is characterized by organization of the intra-alveolar exudates and proliferation of type II alveolar cells, fibroblasts, and myofibroblasts. During this phase, it is common to find areas of squamous metaplasia and granulation tissue occluding alveolar ducts in a manner similar to that of organizing pneumonia (Fig. 47.1B) [22].

The *fibrotic* phase has classically been considered the later phase of remodeling that occurs in patients who survive past 3 or 4 weeks [19]. However, studies suggest an increase in the *fibrotic* response to ALI as early as 24 hours from presentation [23], and histologic evidence can be seen within the first 2 weeks of diagnosis [24]. Because such overlap exists between the fibrotic and proliferative phases, the two are often described together as the *fibroproliferative* phase. On histology, alveolar septa are expanded and airspaces filled with sparsely cellular connective tissue [19]. Such airspace connective tissue formation can either resolve or progress to the point of complete airspace obliteration [24], fibrosis, and even honeycombing [22]. Regardless of severity, there is evidence that increased fibroproliferative signaling [23] and fibrosis [24] predict worse outcomes.

RADIOGRAPHIC FINDINGS

The diagnostic criteria of ALI require bilateral infiltrates on frontal chest radiograph [9]. These infiltrates will often initially appear as heterogeneous opacities, but later become more homogenous over hours to days [25] (see Fig. 47.2A). Although some have recommended using criteria such as cardiac

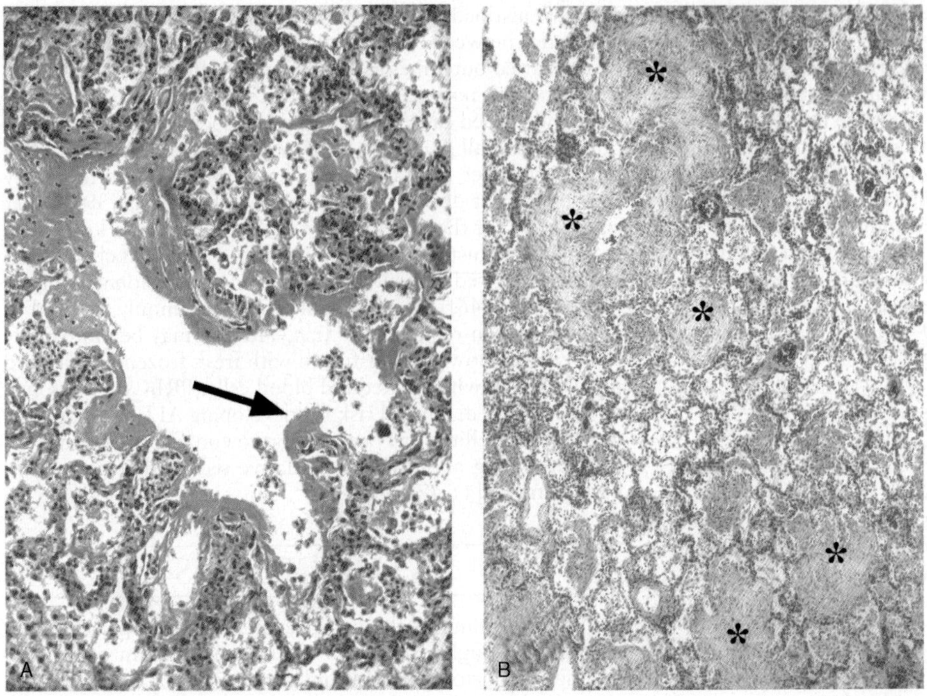

FIGURE 47.1. **A:** Histologic lung specimen from ARDS patient, showing red blood cells and neutrophils within the alveolar space and characteristic hyaline membranes (*arrow*) consistent with diagnosis of diffuse alveolar damage (DAD). **B:** Hematoxylin and eosin stained, 60×; demonstrates distal airspace granulation tissue (*asterisks*) consistent with organizing pneumonia. [Images were graciously provided by Dr. Martha Warnock.]

silhouette size and vascular pedicle width to differentiate cardiogenic from noncardiogenic edema, this differentiation has proven difficult [26]. Furthermore, the seemingly straightforward interpretation of bilateral infiltrates can be obscured by factors such as atelectasis, effusions, or isolated lower lobe involvement, all of which contribute to low interobserver agreement [27].

Prior to computed tomography (CT) scanning, the pulmonary edema seen on chest radiograph was widely believed to be a diffuse process. However, CT imaging has demonstrated

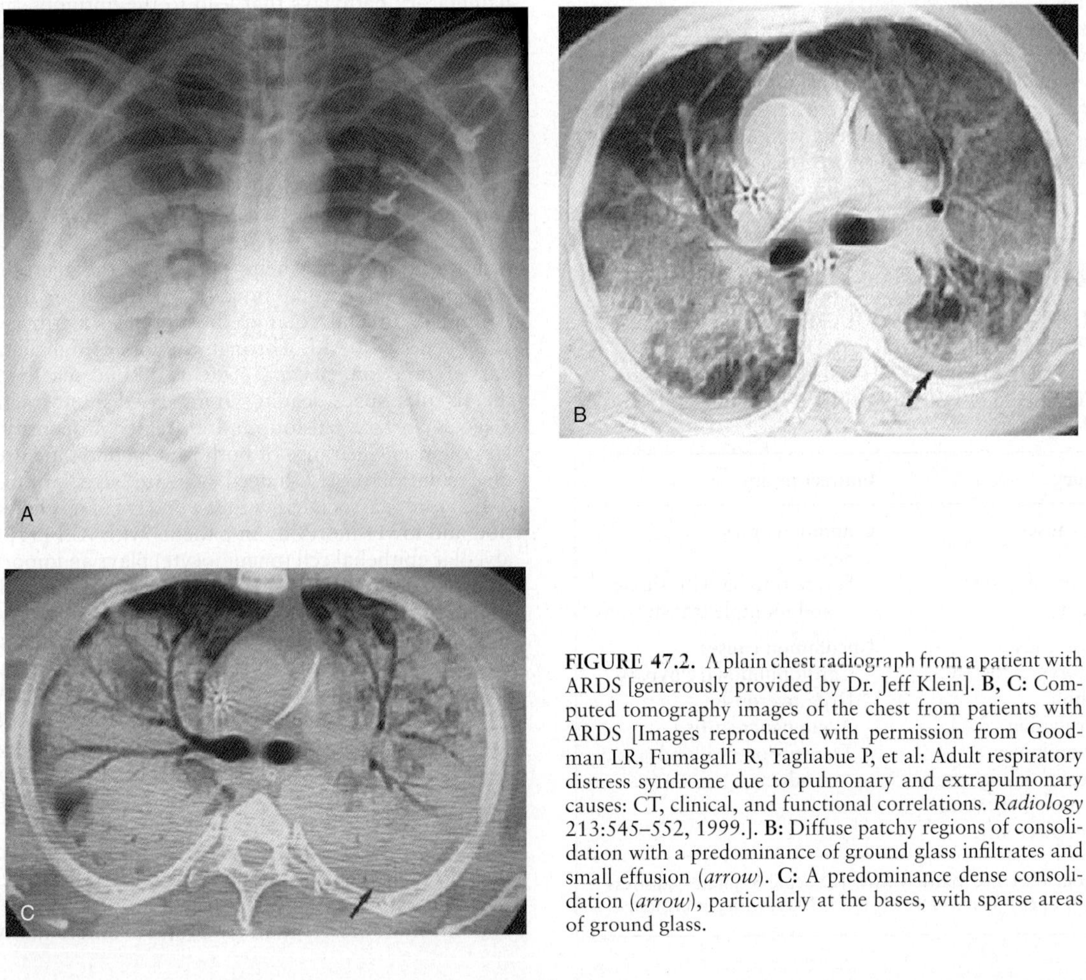

FIGURE 47.2. A plain chest radiograph from a patient with ARDS [generously provided by Dr. Jeff Klein]. **B, C:** Computed tomography images of the chest from patients with ARDS [Images reproduced with permission from Goodman LR, Fumagalli R, Tagliabue P, et al: Adult respiratory distress syndrome due to pulmonary and extrapulmonary causes: CT, clinical, and functional correlations. *Radiology* 213:545–552, 1999.]. **B:** Diffuse patchy regions of consolidation with a predominance of ground glass infiltrates and small effusion (*arrow*). **C:** A predominance dense consolidation (*arrow*), particularly at the bases, with sparse areas of ground glass.

the distribution of ALI to oftentimes be heterogeneous and patchy, with areas of normal-appearing, aerated lung interspersed among areas of mixed ground glass opacity and consolidation, the latter being concentrated in the more gravitationally dependent regions of the lung [28] (see Fig. 47.2B, C). Despite this pattern, a recent study using positron emission tomography (PET) to map cellular metabolic activity demonstrated that diffuse inflammatory change can be detected even in areas of the lung that appear spared radiographically [29]. Some investigators have also used PET imaging and magnetic resonance imaging (MRI) to estimate pulmonary microvascular leak and assist in the differentiation between high permeability and hydrostatic pulmonary edema [30–32], but these methods have yet to be adopted in clinical practice.

EPIDEMIOLOGY

The estimated incidence of ALI worldwide has been variable in the past due to its wide range of causes and previously nonuniform definition. The first estimate by the National Institutes of Health (NIH) projected an annual incidence of 75 cases per 100,000 in the United States [33]. Two subsequent cohort studies in Scandinavia and Australia, respectively, estimated an annual incidence of 18 and 34 cases per 100,000 [34,35], but these studies were limited in size and case inclusion. A much lager pool of prospective cases from the NHLBI-sponsored ARDS Network yielded a conservative estimate of 64.2 cases per 100,000 person-years [36]. A more recent and significantly larger prospective cohort study from King County in Washington State estimates an annual incidence of 78.9 cases per 100,000 person-years [7], which is more in accordance with the ARDS Network and original NIH estimates, and is likely to be the most accurate estimate to date for incidence in the United States.

In patients at risk of developing ALI, the onset of ALI is typically swift, with a median duration of 1 day (interquartile range 0 to 4 days) from the time of risk factor development to the time of diagnosis [37]. The known causes and risk factors for the development of ALI have been well characterized [16–18] (see Table 47.2), and can be categorized as ensuing from either direct or indirect injury to the lung [16,38]. This differentiation is justified by the demonstration of differing physiologic properties between ALI of a direct or indirect nature [38], and by the varied outcomes associated with different causes of ALI [7,11,13]. It is now well established that sepsis is the most commonly identified cause of ALI, and is associated with the worst outcome overall [7,13,18], while trauma-related ALI has a significantly lower mortality [7]. These differences in mortality may be in part due to differences in pathogenesis [39]. Other risk factors for the development of ALI following a known insult include a history of alcoholism [40–42], recent chemotherapy [41], delayed resuscitation [41], and transfusion with blood products [43–46]. The latter condition, commonly referred to as "transfusion-related ALI" (i.e., TRALI), may be more likely to develop following transfusion with fresh frozen plasma and platelets than with packed red blood cells (PRBCs) [44]. Curiously, in those at clinical risk for developing ALI, the diagnosis of diabetes mellitus has been shown to confer protection from ALI, providing about half the relative risk as that of nondiabetic patients [41,47].

TABLE 47.2

CLINICAL DISORDERS ASSOCIATED WITH THE DEVELOPMENT OF ALI AND ARDS, SUBCATEGORIZED INTO THOSE COMMONLY ASSOCIATED WITH DIRECT AND INDIRECT INJURY TO THE LUNG

Direct injury	Indirect injury
Common causes	**Common causes**
Pneumonia	Sepsis
Aspiration of gastric contents	Severe trauma with shock and multiple transfusions
Uncommon causes	**Uncommon causes**
Pulmonary contusion	Cardiopulmonary bypass
Fat emboli	Drug overdose
Near drowning	Acute pancreatitis
Inhalation injury	Transfusion of blood products
Reperfusion injury after lung transplantation or embolectomy	

Adapted from Ware LB, Matthay MA: The acute respiratory distress syndrome. *N Engl J Med* 342:1334–1349, 2000, with permission.

PATHOGENESIS

An understanding of the pathogenesis of ALI is perhaps best imparted through a reflection on the predominant pathologic findings on histology. First and foremost, ALI is a condition triggered by injury to the alveolar epithelium and capillary endothelium. The insult can be initially isolated to either the epithelium, as in the case of aspiration, or to the endothelium, as in most forms of indirect ALI such as sepsis. However, injury is generally detected in both the endothelium and epithelium by the time of diagnosis [19,48]. This injury invariably leads to a leakage of plasma proteins into the alveolar space. Many of these plasma proteins in turn activate procoagulant and proinflammatory pathways that lead to the fibrinous and purulent exudates seen on histology. Through increased transcription and release of proinflammatory cytokines, and an increased expression of cell surface adhesion molecules, a profound acute inflammatory response ensues. This is heralded by epithelial cell apoptosis and necrosis [49], further activation of inflammatory cascades, and a robust recruitment of neutrophils [50]. The increased expression of tissue factor and other procoagulant factors ultimately leads to coagulation within the microvasculature and airspaces, accompanied by a suppression of fibrinolysis, which helps perpetuate the microthrombi and fibrinous exudates that are pathognomonic for ALI.

Injury to the alveolar epithelium plays a critical role in the pathogenesis of ALI. Through the loss of tight junctions and barrier function, plasma proteins and edema fluid seep into the alveolar space, leading to increased shunt fraction, higher alveolar surface tension, and a greater propensity for alveolar collapse. Clearance of both protein and fluid are crucial to the resolution of ALI. Indeed, a greater alveolar fluid clearance (AFC) rate is associated with fewer days of mechanical ventilation and lower mortality in patients with ALI [51]. The type I alveolar epithelial cell (pneumocyte) plays an important role in barrier function, while the type II pneumocyte is the primary source of surfactant production and is known to participate in AFC. Although type I pneumocytes comprise 99% of the alveolar surface area and are presumed to participate in AFC, their exact role in this process remains undefined [52]. AFC occurs by fluid following a sodium concentration gradient established by active sodium transport at the basolateral membrane via Na, K-ATPase activity [53]. Despite the demonstrated impairment of AFC in the setting of lung injury [54], areas of preserved AFC can coexist with injury and epithelial barrier disruption [55], making AFC a potential target for interventional therapy (see "Management" section).

The resorption of protein from the alveolar space is believed to occur more slowly than AFC, and is differentially regulated depending on the burden of protein present. Alveolar albumin transport occurs primarily via receptor-mediated endocytosis at low concentrations, but occurs primarily via passive paracellular diffusion when present in higher concentrations, as in the case of ALI [56]. Removal of larger insoluble proteins such as fibrin can take much longer and require degradation [56].

On the other side of the alveolar capillary interface, injury to the endothelium results in increased permeability, release of inflammatory molecules, expression of cell adhesion molecules, and activation of procoagulant pathways. Although endothelial injury is detectable under electron microscopy [19], gross endothelial damage may be seen only sparingly [48,57]. Increased microvascular permeability has been widely demonstrated in ALI [32,58,59], but this may be more due to a functional alteration or activation of intact endothelium than due to actual cell lysis or necrosis. Endothelial cells can be activated by factors such as thrombin or endotoxin to increase surface expression of the potent neutrophil-tethering molecules called selectins [60] or to release preformed von Willebrand factor (vWF) [61] and potent neutrophil activating factors [62]. Endothelial cell activation of binding molecules on neutrophils can in turn promote their binding to the endothelium and transmigration into areas of injury. Furthermore, when endothelial cells are tethered to activated neutrophils, such interaction can promote neutrophil degranulation [63], further contributing to local injury and inflammation. The important role of endothelial activation in ALI is highlighted by the finding that elevated plasma levels of vWF have been shown to predict the development of ALI in patients at risk [64] and are associated with worse outcomes [65] and fewer organ failure-free days in established ALI [65].

Although widely accepted to play a key role in the pathogenesis of ALI [50,66,67], the neutrophil is not essential for the development of ALI, as evidenced by the development of ALI in the setting of neutropenia [68]. However, ALI can worsen during the recovery from neutropenia and after administration of the neutrophil growth and releasing factor, G-CSF [69]. Furthermore, neutrophil recruitment to the lung has been shown to be a crucial factor in experimentally induced ALI as demonstrated by attenuated pathology under neutrophil-depleted conditions [70,71].

Activated leukocytes and endothelial cells can also contribute to another recognized pathologic manifestation of ALI: dysregulated intravascular and extravascular coagulation [72,73]. Surface expression of tissue factor by alveolar macrophages and endothelial cells can activate the extrinsic coagulation cascade through factor VII [73], activating thrombin and generating fibrin [72]. Extravascular alveolar fibrin arising from increased procoagulant activity and impaired fibrinolysis [74,75] has been well described in ALI [48]. Fibrin formation and clearance in the lung is in part governed by the differential activity of fibrinolysis promoters and inhibitors [74–76]. Plasminogen activators enzymatically convert plasminogen to active plasmin, the key protease involved in fibrinolysis. Plasminogen activator inhibitor-1 (PAI-1) can prevent fibrinolysis via direct binding and inhibition of plasminogen activators [77]. PAI-1 inhibition of fibrinolysis in the BAL fluid of ALI patients was first recognized in 1990 [75]. Since then the importance of PAI-1 in ALI has been further recognized in that elevated plasma and edema fluid levels of PAI-1 are associated with higher mortality in ALI patients [78]. However, studies examining the direct role of PAI-1 in animal models of ALI have yielded mixed results [79,80]. With respect to the initial process of coagulation and fibrin generation, the activation and expression of tissue factor (TF) has received notable attention due to its known interaction with factor VIIa and downstream generation of thrombin. TF expression has been shown to be increased on the surface of alveolar epithelial cells and macrophages in patients with ALI, and is accompanied by increased procoagulant activity in the edema fluid [81].

Numerous additional pathways have been implicated in the pathogenesis of ALI, but an attempt to cover each in depth would extend beyond the intended breadth of this chapter. In brief, lipopolysaccharide (i.e., endotoxin) has long been recognized as a reliable initiator of ALI [82], particularly in the settings of sepsis and pneumonia, and the mechanisms of its action have been extensively elaborated [83]. Oxidant-mediated injury through the generation of reactive oxidant species is also a well-recognized pathway for injury in ALI [84]. The cytoprotective role of the heat-shock response in ALI, particularly through heat shock protein 70, is also widely acknowledged [85,86]. Dysregulated cell death and apoptosis through the release and accumulation of soluble Fas ligand is also thought to contribute to ALI and may also become a potential future target for therapeutic intervention [49,87]. The role of mechanical ventilation in contributing to the development and worsening of ALI is now also widely recognized and its mechanisms extensively researched [88,89].

PATHOPHYSIOLOGY

Because of the accumulation of extravascular lung water (i.e., pulmonary edema), the physiologic derangements of ALI invariably manifest as refractory hypoxemia [90], decreased respiratory compliance [91], and a propensity for alveolar closure [92]. As alveolar edema fluid and protein accumulate within the alveoli, physiologic shunt develops as blood flows through capillary units and perfuses alveoli that are either filled with fluid, or have collapsed from the resulting increase in surface tension (see Fig. 47.3A). Hypoxic vasoconstriction, the normal autoregulatory reflex that helps match ventilation and perfusion by shunting capillary blood flow away from poorly ventilated regions of the lung, is severely impaired within the diseased regions of the lung [93]. Hence, physiologic shunt is accentuated by an imbalance of flow to the poorly ventilated lung regions [93]. Increased vasoconstriction and scattered microthrombi within well-ventilated lung regions contribute to physiologic dead space or "wasted ventilation" via diminished blood flow to aerated lung [93] (see Fig. 47.3B). The combined effects of these derangements result in refractory hypoxemia and increased minute ventilation requirements, which explain the often challenging demands of managing these patients in the intensive care unit.

Overall, the average pulmonary vascular resistance is commonly elevated in patients with ALI [94,95], likely the result of a reduction in total luminal diameter of the vascular bed, stemming from hypoxia and thrombotic obstruction [95,96]. This in turn leads to the common finding of pulmonary

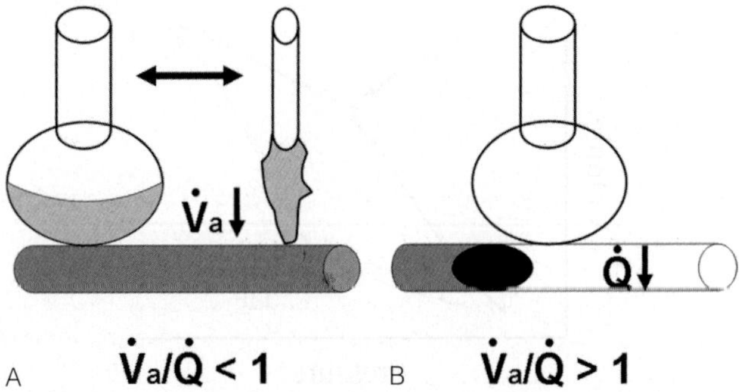

FIGURE 47.3. **A:** The edema fluid-filled alveolus and a neighboring collapsed alveolus, both with unrestricted blood flow, contributing to physiologic shunt. Double-headed (*arrow*) represents potential for fluid-filled alveolus to collapse and re-expand during normal tidal ventilation. **B:** The effect of a microthrombus (*black oval*) obstructing blood flow to a functioning alveolus, contributing to physiologic dead space.

hypertension in these patients, which can alter right ventricular loading and function [94,97], and predicts higher mortality in afflicted patients [97]. Because elevated pulmonary artery pressures could in theory contribute to increased pulmonary edema [94,98] and right heart strain, it is unclear whether pulmonary hypertension is directly contributing to mortality or simply a marker of disease severity [95].

The mechanical manifestations of ALI present mainly as a decrease in respiratory compliance. This is primarily due to a decrease in lung compliance, particularly in the more direct forms of ALI such as pneumonia. However, contribution from the chest wall and abdominal compartment can be significant under conditions such as trauma and peritonitis [38]. The reduction in lung compliance reflects the collective contribution of changes in the intrinsic elastic properties of the remaining aerated lung and a reduction in resting lung volume via alveolar flooding and collapse. The increased elastic properties of the aerated lung result from increased tissue stiffness due to interstitial edema and increased alveolar surface tension, but the contribution from interstitial edema is thought to be negligible relative to that from alveolar edema [99]. The increase in alveolar surface tension is thought to develop from the increased surface forces generated by a greater abundance of alveolar lining fluid and a decrease in surfactant activity [100]. This loss in surfactant activity is believed to result from inhibitory binding of surfactant by plasma proteins [101] and cholesterol [102], and decreased production of functionally active surfactant by type II pneumocytes [3,103]. To further complicate matters, the biomechanical effects of mechanical ventilation alone can alter the structure and biophysical properties of surfactant [104,105], an unfortunate consequence of a typically mandatory intervention for this condition.

Lower resting lung volumes in ALI result from persistently fluid filled or collapsed alveoli, leading to what has been colloquially referred to as "baby lung" [106]. The affected regions of the lungs are often so diseased that they may remain fluid-filled or collapsed throughout each tidal inflation [107] and hence contribute negligibly to compliance. In fact, CT imaging has demonstrated respiratory compliance to be more closely linked to the amount of aerated lung [108], lending some to assert that compliance is more of a direct measure of aerated lung volume than tissue stiffness [106]. As a result, tidal volumes delivered to the heterogeneously fluid-filled and atelectatic lung are shunted preferentially to more compliant, aerated regions of the lung [109]. This is one of the main postulated mechanisms through which mechanical ventilation can overdistend and injure the remaining regions of "normal lung" and lead to ventilator-induced lung injury (VILI) [88].

At the bedside, the reduction in compliance is typically observed as an increase in peak and plateau airway pressures but can also be seen as an expansion in the hysteresis of pressure–volume (PV) curves obtained during graded inflation of the lung (see Fig. 47.4). The decrease in slope of the inspiratory limb of the PV curve represents a decrease in volume obtained for any given change in pressure, and hence a decrease in compliance.

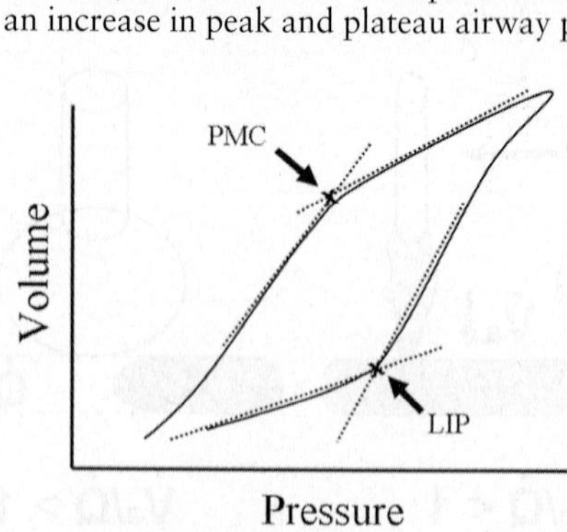

FIGURE 47.4. Simulated pressure volume curve obtained from typical acute lung injury patient, with pressure recorded during slow inflation to total lung volume. Lower inflection point (LIP) marked at point of sudden change in slope of inflation curve. Point of maximal curvature (PMC) also marked at point of maximal change in slope of deflation curve.

MANAGEMENT

Mechanical Ventilation

Mechanical Ventilation and Low Tidal Volumes

The early presentation of ALI is chiefly characterized by hypoxemic respiratory failure and the almost invariable need for support with mechanical ventilation. Because the greatest danger posed to patients with ALI is the development of multiorgan failure [110], establishing supportive ventilation modes that optimize hemodynamic function and oxygen delivery remain important objectives in the management of these patients. Prior to the late 1960s, endotracheal intubation and positive pressure mechanical ventilation were primarily used for supporting patients during general anesthesia. It was during this time that investigators first noted that larger tidal volumes could reduce the shunt associated with atelectasis during general anesthesia [111]. Soon afterward, the benefits of a larger tidal volume on shunt were demonstrated in animal models of ALI [112]. Because many of the techniques used for the support of patients with acute respiratory failure were originally adopted from general anesthesia practice, employing tidal volumes of 10 to 15 mg per kg became the standard for improving oxygenation and ventilation in patients with ALI [113,114].

We now know that idealized oxygenation and normal physiologic pH and $PaCO_2$ can come at a cost when employing higher tidal volumes in patients with ALI. After VILI was induced with higher tidal volumes in animal models [88,115], small retrospective and prospective uncontrolled trials suggested a benefit from limiting tidal volume and peak airway pressures in patients with ALI [116,117]. Numerous larger, randomized trials comparing traditional and lower tidal volumes have since been conducted, each trial differing in its methodology and results [1,2,118–120]. The largest randomized, multicenter trial to date, conducted by the ARDS Network, ultimately demonstrated a significant reduction in mortality when using a tidal volume of 6 mL per kg of predicted ideal body weight and a target plateau pressure of 30 cm H_2O or less (mortality 31.0%) as opposed to a tidal volume of 12 mL per kg and a target plateau pressure less than 50 cm H_2O (mortality 39.8%) [1].

In an effort to better understand the protection conferred by low tidal volumes, investigators have studied how this strategy modulates the inflammatory cascades associated with ALI and VILI. Evidence now exists to support the theory that low tidal volume ventilation improves outcomes at least in part through reduced activation of the inflammatory cascades associated with VILI and multiorgan failure. For instance, among patients enrolled in the ARDS Network trial of low tidal volume, it was found that higher plasma levels of soluble receptors for tumor necrosis factor-α (TNF-α) were associated with higher mortality and fewer organ-failure free days [121]. Furthermore, the lower tidal volume strategy was associated with lower levels of soluble TNF-α receptor I [121]. In another study from the same patient population, elevated plasma levels of interleukin (IL)-6, 8, and 10 were also linked to increased mortality while lower tidal volume was associated with a greater drop in IL-6 and IL-8 by day 3 of enrollment [122].

Many studies of low tidal volume ventilation adopted a strategy of permissive hypercapnia, in which investigators tolerated a reduction in minute volume and an ensuing increase in $PaCO_2$ to achieve lower target tidal volumes and airway pressures [117,118,120]. Most studies suggest that this strategy is safe [117,118], but the actual safety of this practice is not yet entirely known. Although some animal studies have demonstrated a potential protection by hypercapnic acidosis [123,124], others suggest that hypercapnic acidosis may worsen ALI and VILI [125,126]. Some guidelines acknowledge permissive hypercapnia as an acceptable practice when necessary to limit tidal volumes, but also stress that its use is limited in patients with preexistent metabolic acidosis, and contraindicated in patients with increased intracranial pressure [127]. Because no firm guidelines have been established, current options range from a allowing for an arterial pH as low as 6.8 [117], to increasing respiratory rate up to 35 and buffering with intravenous bicarbonate when pH drops below 7.3 [1]. Despite ongoing controversy [128] and the delayed adoption low tidal volume strategy in clinical practice [129,130], the current evidence has led professional societies to recommend the use of lower tidal volumes at goal plateau pressures less than 30 cm H_2O in patients with established ALI [127]. Because calculations based on total body weight may be partly responsible for the documented underuse of lower tidal volumes for patients with ALI [129], the importance of using predicted ideal body weight (IBW), based upon measured height and sex, cannot be overstressed. IBW (in kg) for males is calculated as 50 + 0.91 ((height in cm)—152.4), and for females as 45.5 + 0.91 ((height in cm)—152.4) [1]. Although no firm guidelines exist regarding patients without established ALI, there is clinical evidence that a low tidal volume strategy may help prevent progression to ALI in patients at risk [131,132]. Yet to be determined is whether a more optimal or "best" strategy exists beyond that employed in the ARDS Network sponsored study. Although data suggest that tidal volumes lower than 6 mL per kg may confer even greater protection from VILI [133], there is no general consensus on this practice. However, the authors note that in the original ARDS Network trial, the lower tidal volume assignment started with a goal of 6 mL per kg, but patients in this arm were oftentimes adjusted to as low as 4 mL per kg as needed to maintain plateau pressures less than 30 cm H_2O [1].

Recruitment

The physiologic abnormalities in ALI can, in some patients, be reversed by a recruitment maneuver (RM), typically delivered as a sustained deep inflation with the intention of reopening collapsed regions of the lung. However, because of the unusually high surface tension within affected alveoli, the benefit is often transient [134,135], especially if not followed by sufficiently high levels of PEEP [136]. The potential impact of RMs on morbidity and mortality is not trivial. In fact, because derecruitment leads to an effectively smaller ventilated lung, investigators have proposed the use of "open lung" strategies [137] with periodic delivery of RMs to limit regional overdistention and minimize injury from atelectasis and cyclic alveolar reexpansion [88]. The long-term effect of atelectasis in humans is unclear, but prolonged periods of atelectasis have been shown to promote vascular leak and right ventricular failure in rodents [138]. On the other hand, periodic RMs also have the potential to worsen oxygenation by shunting blood flow to poorly aerated regions [139] and impair cardiac output by limiting venous return and cardiac preload [140,141]. Furthermore, RMs could conceivably contribute to lung injury through excessive overdistention [142] or repeated opening of collapsed lung.

Despite encouraging findings from animal studies [143, 144], clinical studies have yielded mixed results regarding beneficial effects of RMs on oxygenation and lung function [134,141,145]. Although earlier clinical studies demonstrated the benefits of recruitment to be negligible or short-lived [134,140], recent larger trials have demonstrated more promising improvements in lung function and oxygenation but still failed to demonstrate any reduction in mortality [146,147]. Although no guidelines currently exist, it is important to note that patients with ALI of differing origin [38,136,148] and stages of injury [141] vary in their response to RM, and it may help to first differentiate responders from nonresponders [141,148]. When performed, RMs are traditionally delivered as sustained inflations with peak inflation pressures limited to between 30 and 40 cm H_2O, and held for a period ranging from 15 to 40 seconds [2,141,144].

Positive End-Expiratory Pressure

PEEP is another widely employed strategy shown to retard alveolar derecruitment in the injured lung. Several studies have demonstrated the ability of PEEP to prevent or delay alveolar derecruitment [149,150] and attenuate VILI [115,151]. However the protective effect of higher PEEP was called into doubt after a multicenter randomized trial failed to demonstrate an improvement in outcomes using a higher PEEP strategy during low tidal volume ventilation in ALI patients [152]. In this NHLBI-sponsored trial, higher levels of PEEP were arbitrarily coupled to each step-wise increment in FiO_2 requirement during low tidal volume ventilation [152]. The study failed to demonstrate any benefit in mortality or ventilator-free days with higher PEEP [152], but potential underpowering of this study has left room for continued debate [153]. In addition, since the amount of recruitable lung varies significantly among ALI patients [154], some have suggested that setting PEEP levels without first determining the level of recruitable lung may offset the potential benefits of PEEP. In a recent randomized trial, the selection of PEEP was more patient-directed and set at a level required to maintain plateau pressures of 28 to 30 cm H_2O [147]. This higher PEEP strategy again failed to demonstrate a reduction in mortality, but did demonstrate lasting improvements in oxygenation and compliance and an increase in ventilator-free and organ failure-free days [147]. Others have shown that more directly targeting PEEP to transpulmonary pressure by measuring esophageal pressures may be a safer and more effective means of determining optimal PEEP [155].

This raises the question of how one determines the "optimal" setting of PEEP. The often observed lower inflection point (LIP) on the inspiratory limb of the PV curve obtained from ALI patients is the point beyond which the slope of the curve dramatically increases (see Fig. 47.4). This dramatic increase in compliance at the LIP was initially believed to represent a sudden increase in lung volume and hence maximal alveolar recruitment. Thus, many have advocated using the LIP to guide the setting of "optimal" PEEP [2,156]. However, several studies have demonstrated significant recruitment beyond the LIP [157,158], a concept supported by mathematical models [159] and CT imaging [108,160]. Data from CT imaging in ALI patients has recently lent strong support to setting "optimal PEEP" at the point of maximal curvature (PMC) along the deflation limb of the PV curve [160] (see Fig. 47.4). Nevertheless, the concept of "optimal PEEP" has likely been oversimplified and controversy remains over how alveolar recruitment is best served by PEEP.

High-Frequency Ventilation and Extracorporal Membrane Oxygenation

With the data demonstrating a reduction of mortality with a low tidal volume strategy in humans and animal studies showing that even lower tidal volumes offer additional protection [133], high-frequency oscillation ventilation (HFOV), with very small tidal volumes equal to or less than dead space and delivered at a very high rate, would seem to be an ideal ventilatory strategy in ALI. How adequate ventilation is achieved with tidal volumes less than or equal to dead space is unknown. Proposed mechanisms include a pendelluft effect of mixing gases between lung regions of differing impedances, coaxial flow with net center inflow and net peripheral outflow, mixing of fresh and residual air along the leading edge of gas flow, and simple molecular diffusion through relatively still air [161]. HFOV first demonstrated clinical benefits among infants with respiratory distress syndrome [162,163]. Although early smaller studies of HFOV in adult ALI were promising [164,165], a larger multicenter-controlled trail failed to demonstrate any reduction in mortality from HFOV over conventional ventilation [166]. Nevertheless, newly developing strategies and equipment allow room for ongoing investigation of HFOV for adult ALI.

Extracorporeal membrane oxygenation (ECMO), used alone or in combination with HFOV, uses cardiopulmonary bypass to facilitate gas exchange while minimizing ventilation of the lung to limit barriers to healing. Despite demonstrated efficacy in neonates with severe respiratory distress syndrome [167], ECMO had until recently failed to demonstrate any reduction in adult mortality [168,169]. The largest controlled trial to date in ECHO for severe adult ARDS recently demonstrated an improvement in 6-month survival without disability when compared to conventional ventilatory support [170]. Despite noted strengths in study design, the lack of protocolized ventilator and critical care management in the control group, along with prohibitive issues of cost and availability has led experts to predict negligible resulting change in clinical use of this still controversial intervention [171].

Noninvasive and Partial Support Ventilation

As described earlier, the physiologic shunt responsible for refractory hypoxemia in ALI is attributed in part to alveolar collapse without adequate compensatory decrement in perfusion within the gravitationally dependent lung [172]. Noninvasive ventilation (NIV) and partial support ventilation modes such as pressure support ventilation, allow for patient triggering and cycling of breaths, resulting in more spontaneous breathing. The potential advantages of spontaneous breathing over controlled mechanical ventilation include improved patient–ventilator synchrony, lower sedation requirements, and improved hemodynamics and ventilation/perfusion ($\dot{V}a/\dot{Q}$) matching [173,174]. Partial assist modes of ventilation can still effectively help unload respiratory workload while allowing for variable degrees of spontaneous breathing [175,176]. These modes have also been shown to improve aeration and ventilation/perfusion matching within dependent lung regions [177], presumably due to more pronounced transpulmonary pressures generated within these regions by an actively moving diaphragm [178].

When these modes are applied noninvasively by face mask, an added benefit is the potential reduction in infectious complications, namely nosocomial pneumonia [179]. Studies have shown that NIV can be used safely for the treatment of ALI [180,181]. In a recent multicenter nonrandomized trial, the use of NIV as first line treatment for ALI helped to avoid intubation in 54% of cases and led to a reduction in the incidence of VAP [182]. However, authors could not recommend NIV in patients with a SAPS (Simplified Acute Physiology Score) II of greater than 34 due to a high rate of failure in this group.

Prone Positioning

Prone positioning was shown to improve oxygenation in patients with hypoxic respiratory failure as early as the mid-1970s [183], but how prone positioning improves oxygenation is still not entirely clear. Proposed mechanisms have centered around the potential reversal of gravitationally distributed perfusion to the better ventilated ventral lung regions [184] and improved ventilation of previously dependent dorsal lung [185], both of which would improve ventilation/perfusion matching. Curiously, however, prone positioning exerts limited gravitational effects on regional perfusion in either normal or injured lung [186] but can sufficiently increase dorsal transpulmonary pressures to improve ventilation within previously dependent dorsal regions of the lung [185]. Proposed mechanisms for this improvement in dorsal ventilation include a reduction in dependent lung compression by the heart and mediastinum [187] and regional changes in chest wall mechanics [188].

In animal models, prone positioning reduces physiologic shunt [187], protects against VILI [189], reduces PEEP requirements [190], and attenuates perfusion imbalances imposed by added PEEP [191]. Despite these known physiologic benefits, the first large randomized clinical trial of prone positioning demonstrated a significant improvement in oxygenation but no improvement in survival [192]. Post hoc analysis suggested an early survival advantage in the most severe subgroup of patients, which has also been suggested by subsequent studies [193]. The largest randomized clinical trial to date also demonstrated an improvement in oxygenation and a reduced incidence of ventilator-associated pneumonia with prone positioning, but again no benefit in survival [194]. This study, however, brought greater attention to safety concerns by demonstrating a higher incidence in pressure sores and inadvertent endotracheal tube displacement. Some experts still advocate an investigation of prone positioning in patients with severe ARDS [195], but the indiscriminant use of prone positioning for the general ALI population is not well supported by the current literature [192,194].

Fluid Management

Fluid management in ALI is an ongoing topic of controversy. Because pulmonary edema is the hallmark of ALI, it seems reasonable to aspire to keep patients relatively "dry." However, because the development of multiple organ dysfunction syndrome (MODS) increases mortality from ALI, the critical maintenance of adequate peripheral perfusion may require liberal administration of intravenous fluid. The type of fluid to administer is also controversial. As pulmonary edema is dependent on both hydrostatic and oncotic forces, the issues of optimal fluid balance and replacement of plasma colloid are not trivial. Diuretic therapy with combined albumin and furosemide has been shown to improve oxygenation and hemodynamics in hypoproteinemic ALI patients but does not reduce mortality [196]. In another study comparing the administration of albumin and furosemide with furosemide alone, a greater improvement in oxygenation was seen with albumin plus furosemide [197]. This suggests that albumin may either potentiate the effects of furosemide, allow for better tolerance of diuresis, or confer other favorable effects on oxidant balance [198] or endothelial permeability [199]. The NHLBI ARDS Network trial of conservative versus liberal fluid management demonstrated no difference in 60-day mortality between the two different strategies [200]. However, the patients in the conservative strategy group had a lower 7-day cumulative fluid balance with improved lung function and a reduced duration of mechanical ventilation without an increase in nonpulmonary organ failure [200].

An additional controversy is what parameter should be used to guide fluid management. Whether the indwelling pulmonary artery (PA) catheter is vital to the management of ALI depends upon two important considerations. First, optimal fluid balance must be crucial to preventing the progression of lung injury. Although this seems defensible in theory, it has yet to be proven. Second, these indwelling catheters must provide a critical and unique understanding of this balance that sufficiently and appropriately modifies clinical practice. This has also yet to be proven. The use of PA catheters came into question after a large observational study of 5,700 critically ill patients actually suggested a higher mortality rate associated with PA catheter use [201]. However, subsequent prospective trials have contradicted these findings [202,203]. Unfortunately, the lack of any clear protocol regarding when to place these lines, and how to interpret and adjust management according to the information provided, leaves ongoing uncertainty regarding their use in patients with ALI [204]. Results from the ARDS Network trial suggest that PA catheter-guided therapy does not improve survival in ALI patients and is associated with more complications than the use of central venous catheters alone [205].

Pharmacologic Intervention

As in any other medical disease or syndrome, it would seem that the "Holy Grail" among clinicians is the discovery of some novel agent that can either break the cycle of disease pathogenesis or help restore physiologic homeostasis and reduce disease severity and morbidity. The field of pharmacologic intervention has been exhaustively explored in the field of ALI, often yielding promising results in animal models and periodically demonstrating modest improvements in lung function and oxygenation in patients, but rarely translating into improved outcomes.

Pulmonary Vasodilators

Given the advanced endothelial injury, physiologic shunt, and commonly observed pulmonary hypertension in ALI, there has been extensive investigation into the therapeutic benefit of pharmacologic pulmonary vasodilatation. Initial studies examined the use of intravenously administered vasodilators such as nitroglycerin and prostacyclin [98,206], but simultaneous and nonselective reductions in systemic and pulmonary vascular resistance led to systemic arterial hypotension with increases in cardiac output and shunt. After the once described "endothelial-derived relaxing factor" was discovered to be nitric oxide (NO) [207], it was found that inhaled NO (iNO) could selectively dilate the pulmonary vasculature within well-ventilated regions of the lung [208], helping reverse both hypoxic vasoconstriction and physiologic shunt. Subsequently, two small-randomized controlled trials demonstrated a significant but transient improvement in oxygenation and shunt in ALI patients in response to iNO, but these benefits did not last past 24 hours, and there was no improvement in outcomes [209,210]. A larger multicenter trial failed to demonstrate a reduction in mortality or ventilator-free days when pooled data from all iNO dosing groups were compared with placebo [211], but the subgroup receiving 5 ppm iNO showed improvement in these parameters. A larger European trial of iNO has since demonstrated a reduction in the development of severe respiratory failure but no reduction in mortality [212].

Most studies have demonstrated minimal adverse effects of iNO other than dose-dependent methemoglobinemia [211]. At the present time, iNO has been approved by the Food and Drug Administration for use in neonates with hypoxic respiratory failure accompanied by pulmonary hypertension but is not approved for use in adult ALI. Experts have concluded that iNO can improve oxygenation in the early phase of its application with minimal adverse effects and is a feasible rescue therapy in severe and refractory ARDS [93]. Given the demonstrated benefits at lower doses, experts recommend using iNO at doses less than 10 ppm when used as rescue therapy.

Surfactant Replacement

Not long after ALI was first described [213] investigators demonstrated a reduction in the amount of surfactant retrieved from the lung and a derangement in the retrieved surfactant's biophysical properties [100]. Since then, numerous studies have supported these findings. The chief surface-tension lowering components of surfactant are phospholipids that align their hydrophilic polar heads along the surface of the alveolar lining fluid and reduce surface tension by interfering with the lateral forces imposed upon the alveolus by water tension. Phosphatidylcholine (PC) makes up the majority of the phospholipid fraction, followed in abundance by phosphatidylglycerol (PG) [214]. The large aggregate fractions consist of large lamellar structures, tubular myelin, and surfactant-associated proteins, and possess the primary surface-tension lowering properties, while the smaller aggregates contain smaller lipids, less surfactant protein, and have limited surface activity [215,216]. In ALI, the relative amount of large-to-small aggregates is reduced [215], as are amounts of bioactive PC and PG [215].

Surfactant-associated proteins also play varied and important roles in surfactant function. Surfactant protein A (SP-A) has been implicated in formation of tubular myelin and antimicrobial defense [217]. SP-B helps to enhance the distribution and stability of phospholipids within the air–liquid interface [218]. SP-C is hydrophobic and believed to closely interact with the surfactant film [219]. Bronchoalveolar lavage fluid (BAL) levels of SP-A and SP-B are reduced in patients with established ALI and those at risk [220]. At the same time, serum levels of SP-A and SP-D are typically elevated in these patients [220] and such elevations are associated with more severe disease and increased risk of mortality [221].

The fundamental rationale for surfactant replacement is to help restore the natural surfactant film and reduce surface tension at the air–liquid interface, thus reducing the tendency for alveolar collapse and improving oxygenation through a reduction in shunt. The evidence in support of surfactant replacement therapy for neonatal RDS is abundant [222,223]. Results from its investigated use in adult ALI patients have been less promising [3,224,225]. Some have speculated that the failure to demonstrate an improvement in mortality is due to the lack of a direct relationship between mortality and severity of respiratory failure alone [110,226]. However, under the assumption that alveolar collapse promotes progression of ALI during mechanical ventilation, many believe that restoring surfactant function holds promise in reducing morbidity and mortality by attenuating VILI. In fact, there is evidence from animal models that surfactant replacement therapy may help prevent VILI [227,228]. Current obstacles to demonstrating this benefit in patients are imposed by intricacies of surfactant administration and its potential inactivation by plasma proteins following delivery. For example, although there is improvement in lung function following surfactant replacement [229], the response is transient. This has been, at least in part, attributed to the tendency for the administered surfactant to be inactivated by plasma proteins in the airspace following [230,231]. This obstacle has been addressed, with mixed results, by adding surfactant proteins [231,232] or polyethylene glycol [233] to block serum protein binding of surfactant.

Despite ostensibly warranted enthusiasm, the largest multicenter randomized clinical trial in adult ALI failed to demonstrate any improvement in mortality with continuous aerosol delivery of the synthetic surfactant, Exosurf [224]. Another large-scale, randomized investigation of intratracheally delivered, recombinant SP-C in ALI patients demonstrated improvement in oxygenation but again no reduction in mortality or duration of mechanical ventilation [3]. Nevertheless, many investigators believe that a strong case can still be made for further research in surfactant replacement strategies [226].

Corticosteroids

Given the well-characterized acute inflammatory response of ALI and evidence that a fibroproliferative response can predict worse outcomes [23,24], considerable effort has been spent determining the therapeutic role of corticosteroid therapy for this condition. The use of steroids for ALI dates back to the original report of this condition in 1967, when Ashbaugh and Petty suggested a potential role for corticosteroids in fat-embolism and viral-related ALI [213]. Ashbaugh later drew parallels between the features of persistent ALI and idiopathic pulmonary fibrosis, and noted the potential for treating these patients with corticosteroids [234]. Numerous uncontrolled trials had initially suggested a potential benefit of corticosteroids for late or persistent ARDS [235–237]. However, treatment with corticosteroids during the acute phase of ALI has since been proven ineffective [238,239]. The first randomized controlled trial of corticosteroids for late ARDS demonstrated improved lung injury scores and oxygenation, decreased multiorgan dysfunction scores, and reduced ICU and in-hospital mortality in the group receiving steroids [240], but this study drew criticism for its small size and baseline differences between the treatment groups [241]. Since then, a significantly larger NHLBI sponsored multicenter trial completed by the ARDS Network exploring the use of corticosteroids for late persistent ARDS demonstrated more ventilator-free days and improved oxygenation in the group treated with methylprednisolone compared with placebo, but no reduction in 60-day mortality [242]. Furthermore, a higher 60- and 180-day mortality was observed when steroid therapy was initiated after 14 days of onset, suggesting a serious risk from this therapy for late ARDS.

Anticoagulation/Fibrinolysis

The importance of microvascular coagulation and thrombosis in ALI is underscored by the physiologic dead space, or "wasted ventilation," observed in ALI patients [243]. Minimizing microvascular thrombosis could conceivably improve oxygenation through improved ventilation–perfusion matching [244] and increase survival through prevention of multiorgan failure [245]. Thus, the importance of coagulation in the pathogenesis of ALI has become widely appreciated [72], and the use of anticoagulant therapy in ALI has in turn gained attention [246]. Although it has been shown that fibrin and its degradation products can promote inflammation [247], vascular leak, and wound remodeling [72], the detriment imposed by alveolar fibrin has also been accredited to its recognized in vitro capacity to bind with and inhibit the surface-tension lowering capacity of surfactant [248,249]. This has led to considerable interest in limiting in situ fibrin deposition as a means of preserving lung function [246]. As a result, several different anticoagulating agents have been investigated in animal models, some of which have been shown to attenuate lung injury and improve survival [244,250,251].

The most encouraging clinical evidence to support this therapeutic target initially came from a multicenter trial demonstrating a mortality benefit from activated protein C (APC) in severe sepsis [245]. However, because randomized trials of other potent anticoagulants, such as antithrombin III and tissue factor pathway inhibitor (TFPI), yielded no mortality benefit in sepsis [252,253], the postulated benefits from APC may be unrelated to its anticoagulant activity. Consequently, investigators have focused on the use of APC for ALI that is not accompanied by sepsis. Despite promising results in a rat model [251], the most recent phase II clinical trial failed to demonstrate a reduction in ventilator-free days with the use of APC [254]. Critics expressed concern about the study's statistical power and a priori likelihood of success [255], but in a similar vein, despite a promising animal studies [244,250], a recent multicenter Phase II trial of Tissue Factor inhibitor (site-inactivated VIIa) in ALI was terminated prematurely due to higher projected mortality rates in the high-dose treatment arm [256]. There was also an increased risk of adverse bleeding events with escalating doses of this drug [256]. Thus, it seems that the benefits of potent anticoagulation in ALI may ultimately be outweighed by risks of adverse bleeding, but further investigation is warranted.

β-Agonists

As discussed in the pathogenesis section, AFC often remains intact in the setting of injury. AFC can be directly increased by β-agonists in animal models [6,257], presumably through upregulated activity of Na, K-ATPase at the basolateral membrane [258]. In human subjects, the use of exogenous catecholamines has been retrospectively linked to increased AFC [51], but, until recently, the greatest support for pharmacologic AFC modulation in ALI came indirectly from findings of lower mortality in ALI patients having preserved/maximal AFC [51]. An early study demonstrated reduced extravascular lung water in patients receiving intravenous salbutamol, but treatment was complicated by supraventricular tachyarrhythmias [259]. A large multicenter randomized trial investigating the use of the aerosolized β-agonist, albuterol, for the treatment of ALI, was recently halted on the basis of projected futility [260]. In the wake of findings, there is currently no support for the use of β-agonists in the treatment of ALI.

Nutritional Supplementation

Over the past decade, enthusiasm has arisen over the use of nutritional supplements in sepsis and ALI, particularly with the use of omega-3 fatty acids and other natural antioxidants such as vitamin E. The rationale for supplementing patients with omega-3 fatty acids, such as eicosapentaenoic acid (EPA), in the setting of inflammatory disorders comes from the notion they can directly suppress monocyte production of inflammatory cytokines and incorporate into cell membrane phospholipids to compete with omega-6 fatty acids to promote the production of more favorable prostaglandins and leukotrienes [261]. Perhaps the most encouraging earlier data supporting omega-3 fatty acids in ALI came initially from small randomized trials comparing a standard isonitrogenous, isocaloric enteral diet with one supplemented with a proprietary mixture of EPA, gamma-linolenic acid (borage oil), and other antioxidants [262–264]. These studies demonstrated an improvement in gas exchange and lung function [262,264], a reduction in BALF levels of IL-8, leukotriene B_4, and neutrophils [263], and a reduction in ICU stay and mechanical ventilation days [262] with the EPA-rich supplement.

An effort was made to better clarify the effects of omega-3 fatty acids alone in a randomized controlled trial comparing the use of EPA and docosahexanoic acid with a nonnutrient saline supplement. This study failed to demonstrate any associated benefit in their a priori primary outcome (BALF IL-8 and LTB_4 levels), but it did show a yet unexplained trend toward a reduction in ICU length of stay and days on mechanical ventilation [265]. The largest trial of supplemental omega-3 fatty acids to date, conducted by the ARDS Network, was recently halted early due to projected futility [266], but the other component of this study investigating early versus delayed enteral feeding in ALI remains ongoing. Reasons for these negative findings are not yet well understood.

PROSPECTIVE FUTURE THERAPIES

Airway Pressure Release Ventilation

"Airway pressure release ventilation" (APRV) is a mode of ventilation that uses sustained high airway pressures and spontaneous breathing to maximize lung recruitment, with brief periods of "pressure release" to facilitate ventilation while minimizing derecruitment during exhalation [267]. Proponents assume that the periods of pressure release are brief enough to avoid alveolar closure and reexpansion [268], and efficacy relies heavily on the presence of spontaneous ventilation [269], which is believed to generate regionally variable transpulmonary pressures that favor recruitment of dependent lung regions [174]. Although APRV can be equally efficacious and safe when compared with SIMV and pressure support modes [174,270], most published experience in ALI with this mode has been in the surgical and trauma population [174,271,272], and the same findings may not hold true for more unstable forms of ALI resulting from direct pulmonary injury, such as pneumonia and aspiration.Fortunately, two studies comparing APRV with conventional low tidal volume ventilation in ALI are currently enrolling patients (ClinicalTrials.gov Identifiers NCT00750204 and NCT00793013).

Stem Cell Therapy

Recent attention has been given to use of bone marrow derived and circulating stem cells in an effort to expedite tissue regeneration through engraftment and suppress inflammation through immunomodulation [273]. Enthusiasm first came from findings suggesting a favorable rate of engraftment and epithelial differentiation of infused bone marrow derived stem cells in the injured lungs of mice [274]. Important clinical findings followed with the discovery that circulating epithelial progenitor cells (EPCs) are elevated in the plasma of patients with ALI, and that increased circulating EPCs are associated with reduced ALI mortality [275]. Newer studies suggest that the rates of stem cell engraftment and differentiation are not as robust as initially hoped, but many are examining ways of promoting engraftment [273]. This field has found added momentum in the discovery that infused bone marrow derived stem cells may also down regulate inflammation and dampen ALI progression, independent of engraftment [276].

HMG-CoA Reductase Inhibitors (The "Statins")

Recent animal experiments and observational human studies have provoked interest in the treatment of ALI with HMG-CoA Reductase Inhibitors (also called "statins"), a class of drugs originally developed for the treatment of dyslipidemia. In addition to reducing atherosclerotic inflammation, these drugs may also reduce morbidity in other inflammatory conditions such as rheumatoid arthritis [277], influenza [278], sepsis [279], and ALI [280]. The mechanisms through which statins are believed to provide benefit [281] include reduced expression of leukocyte and endothelial adhesion molecules [282,283], reduced production of acute phase reactants (C-reactive protein) and inflammatory cytokines (IL-6, IL-8 and TNF-α) [284,285], and impaired coagulation via platelet stabilization [286], reduced TF and thrombin activity [287,288], and suppressed PAI-1 expression [289]. These drugs have also been shown to promote the mobilization of circulating EPCs [290]. There is experimental data from animal models of ALI arising from ischemia-reperfusion [291] and endotoxemia [280] demonstrating an amelioration of lung inflammation and vascular permeability associated with statin therapy. To date, the only clinical data supporting statin use in ALI comes from a retrospective study of patients on statin therapy at the time of ALI diagnosis that demonstrated a 73% reduction in odds of death, but this did not reach statistical significance [292]. A large, randomized placebo-controlled trial is currently being conducted by the NHLBI ARDS Clinical Trials Network (ClinicalTrials.gov Identifier: NCT00979121).

Preemptive Intervention Protocols

The search for an effective pharmacologic intervention or management algorithm in ALI has thus been extensive and has now spanned decades. Despite this effort, with the exception of low tidal volume ventilation, the reward from most interventions has been limited to improvements in oxygenation [3,192] or fewer days of mechanical ventilation [147,200] (see Table 47.3). One important lesson from the work to date is that much of what we once thought was critical to the management of these patients, although grounded in sound rationale, is not only often ineffective, but can also be potentially harmful. We have become more aware of how sound basic and simple principles of ICU care, such as hand hygiene and protocols for ventilator-associated pneumonia prevention can substantially reduce overall morbidity in the ICU [293,294]. In keeping with this philosophy of preemptive intervention, two studies have recently demonstrated that something as simple as early intervention with physical therapy in mechanically ventilated patients is not only safe and cost-effective, but can also reduce the duration of delirium, mechanical ventilation, ICU and hospital length of stay, and promote greater functional independence by the time of discharge [295,296]. Investigators have also discovered reductions in ALI incidence following the enforcement of conservative transfusion policies (prevention of TRALI) and preemptive low tidal volume ventilation (prevention of VILI) in the care of patients "at risk" for the development of ALI [131,132]. Such practice seems compatible with an emerging theme that if clinicians are still limited to supportive care for ALI patients, then they should at least be doing "less harm" by delivering lower tidal volumes [1], limiting transfusion of blood products, [132,297], conservatively limiting fluids in stable resuscitated patients [298], and fastidiously preventing iatrogenic infections [299].

PROGNOSIS AND OUTCOMES

Prognosis

Numerous clinical factors have been shown to predict a higher mortality rate in ALI patients. These include male sex, African American race, advanced age, alcoholism, malignancy, liver disease, chronic steroid use, infection with human immunodeficiency virus, and ALI secondary to sepsis or aspiration [13,310]. Curiously, although patients of advanced age, particularly older than 70 years, are at a significantly higher risk of death from ALI, those who survive recover at the same rate as their younger counterparts [311,312]. Chronic alcoholism has been shown to not only increase the risk of developing ALI in patient at risk [42], but to also increase the risk of developing multiorgan dysfunction after the development of ALI [40]. Plasma granulocyte colony stimulating factor (G-CSF) levels [313] and body-mass index (BMI) [314] both exhibit a U-shaped distribution of relative risk for mortality in ALI, with higher risk falling on both the low and high ends of the curve. In the case of BMI, although it is somewhat intuitive that patients with either an exceedingly low or excessively high BMI would be at greater risk of death, investigators were somewhat surprised to find the lowest risk belonging to those considered "obese," with a BMI between 30 and 40 [314]. Investigators

TABLE 47.3

TABLE SUMMARIZING ALL RANDOMIZED TRIALS OF PHARMACOLOGIC TREATMENTS AND VENTILATION STRATEGIES FOR ACUTE LUNG INJURY AND ACUTE RESPIRATORY DISTRESS SYNDROME[a]

Intervention	Year	Study	No. of patients	Findings	Reference
High levels of positive end-expiratory pressure	1975	Observational	28	High incidence of pneumothorax	[300]
Extracorporeal membrane oxygenation	1979	Phase 3 multicenter	90	No benefit	[169]
High frequency ventilation	1983	Phase 3 multicenter	309	No benefit	[301]
Preventative PEEP (8 cm H_2O)	1984	Phase 3 single center	92	No benefit in patients at risk of ALI	[302]
Glucocorticoids (during acute phase)	1987	Phase 3	87	No benefit	[239]
Glucocorticoids (during acute phase)	1988	Phase 3	59	No benefit	[238]
Alprostadil: Intravenous	1989	Phase 3	100	No benefit	[303]
Liposomal	1999	Phase 3	350	Stopped for lack of efficacy	[304]
Extracorporeal membrane oxygenation	1994	Phase 3 single center	40	No benefit	[168]
Surfactant (aerosolized)	1996	Phase 3	725	No benefit	[224]
"Open-lung" approach (recruitment maneuver and "ideal PEEP")	1998	Phase 3 single center	53	Decreased 28-day but not in-hospital mortality	[2]
Low tidal volume ventilation (7 vs. 11 ml/kg)	1998	Phase 3	120	No benefit in patients at risk for ALI/ARDS	[120]
Low tidal volume ventilation (7 vs. 10 mL/kg)	1998	Phase 3	116	No benefit	[118]
Glucocorticoids during late fibrosing alveolitis	1998	Phase 3	24	Decreased mortality, but study small	[240]
Inhaled nitric oxide	1998	Phase 2	177	No benefit	[211]
Inhaled nitric oxide	1999	Phase 3	203	No benefit	[305]
Ketoconazole	2000	Phase 2	234	No benefit	[306]
Low tidal volumes (6 vs. 12 mL/kg)	2000	Phase 3, multicenter	861	Decreased mortality from 40% to 30%	[1]
Prone positioning during mechanical ventilation	2001	Phase 3, multicenter	304	Improved oxygenation, but no benefit in mortality	[192]
Partial liquid ventilation	2002	Phase 3, multicenter	90	Lower progression to ARDS, but no benefit in mortality	[307]
Recombinant surfactant protein C-based surfactant	2004	Phase 3, multicenter	448	Improved oxygenation at 24 hours but no benefit in mortality	[3]
Prone positioning for hypoxemic acute respiratory failure	2004	Phase 3, multicenter	791	No benefit in 28 or 90 day mortality and some safety concerns	[194]
Higher versus lower PEEP during low tidal volume ventilation	2004	Phase 3, multicenter	549	No benefit in mortality or days on the ventilator	[152]
Low and high dose partial liquid ventilation	2006	Phase 3, multicenter	311	No benefit in mortality and some safety concerns	[308]
Glucocorticoids for late/persistent ARDS	2006	Phase 3, multicenter	180	No benefit in mortality; increased mortality if started after 2 weeks	[242]
Conservative versus Liberal Fluid Management in ALI	2006	Phase 3, multicenter	1,000	No benefit in mortality; conservative strategy improved lung function and reduced ventilator days	[200]
Prolonged prone positioning for severe ALI	2006	Phase 3, multicenter	136	Nonsignificant reduction in mortality (43% vs. 58%, $p = 0.12$)	[193]
Low tidal volumes, recruitment maneuvers and high PEEP	2008	Phase 3, multicenter	983	No mortality benefit; less refractory hypoxemia and rescue therapy	[146]
Low tidal volumes with plateau pressure directed, high PEEP	2008	Phase 3, multicenter	767	No mortality benefit; higher organ failure free and ventilator free days and improved lung function	[293]
Activated Protein C	2008	Phase 2, multicenter	75	No benefit in ventilator-free days or mortality; reduced dead space	[254]

(*continued*)

TABLE 47.3

CONTINUED

Intervention	Year	Study	No. of patients	Findings	Reference
L-2-oxothiazolidine-4-carboxylic acid	2008	Phase 2, multicenter	215	Terminated early due to higher 30 day mortality & reduced vent-free days	[309]
Early mobilization in ICU for patients with respiratory failure	2008	Multicenter prospective	330	Decreased intensive care unit and hospital length of stay in survivors	[296]
Early physical therapy in ICU for patients with respiratory failure	2009	Randomized, two centers	104	Decreased days on mechanical ventilation and ICU length of stay; increased functional independence at time of discharge	[297]
Site-inactivated factor VIIa	2009	Phase 2, multicenter	46	Terminated early due to higher 28 day mortality in high dose group and trend toward increased bleeding	[256]
ECMO vs. conventional ventilatory support for severe adult respiratory failure (CESAR)	2009	Randomized multicenter	180	Reduced death or severe disability at 6 months	[170]
Albuterol to treat acute lung injury (ALTA)	2009	Phase 2 and 3, multicenter	282	Terminated early due to projected futility by DSMB	[260]
Fish oil in patients with ALI	2009	Phase 2 multicenter	90	No difference in BALF IL-8 or LTB_4; trend toward reduced ICU stay	[265]
Omega-3 fatty acids supplementation for ALI (EDEN-Omega)	2009	Phase 3, multicenter	272	"Omega" arm terminated early due to project futility	[266]
Neuromuscular blockade in early severe ARDS	2010	Phase 3, multicenter		48 hours cisartacurium reduced mortality and increased ventilator-free days without prolonged weakness	[338]

[a]Results of randomized clinical trials of pharmacologic treatments and ventilatory strategies for acute lung injury and acute respiratory distress syndrome.

Table partially adapted from Ware LB, Matthay MA: The acute respiratory distress syndrome. *N Engl J Med* 342:1334–1349, 2000, with updated additions.

are also uncovering genetic polymorphisms and phenotypes among ALI patients that lead to an increased risk of mortality. Individuals carrying specific haplotypes for IL-6 [315] or an endogenous inhibitor of NF-kB [316] have an increased susceptibility to ALI and mortality is increased in patients with ALI, with specific polymorphisms for surfactant protein B [317], pre-B-cell colony enhancing factor [318], or VEGF [319].

Outcomes

Estimates of mortality from ALI once ranged as high as 70% [110,320]. Despite a documented decline between the early 1980s and late 1990s [110,320], mortality from ALI appears to have now plateaued between 30% and 40% for all patients, [1,7,110,320]. As mortality has slowly improved for ALI, there has been growing interest in the long range consequences of this condition. In particular, ALI survivors have been shown to suffer from a prolonged disturbance in lung function [321,322], an impairment in neurocognitive skills [323,324], and a perception of poor quality of life [324,325]. By as far out as one year from recovery, although many have recovered spirometric lung function [326], the majority of ALI survivors have a diminished diffusing capacity and exercise tolerance [321,326]. One report noted less than half of all ALI survivors returning to work after 1 year [326], and many survivors suffer from depression and anxiety as far as 2 years out from recovery [324]. In a recently published study, symptoms of moderate to severe depression were reported by 41% of survivors within 6 to 48 months following discharge [327]. Posttraumatic stress disorder (PTSD) has been another growing concern among survivors [328] and delusional memories of ICU stay have been shown to correlate with the development of PTSD symptoms [329].

A regimented sedation protocol designed to promote daily awakenings and lower overall sedation in critically ill patients was associated with decreased days in the ICU and fewer days on mechanical ventilation [330]. Furthermore, to help raze the myth that daily awakening be traumatic for patients, this strategy has since been found to actually reduce PTSD-related symptoms following recovery [331]. The feasibility and importance of establishing clear sedation goals and using validated tools for sedation assessment in critically ill patients has been firmly established [332,333], and this standard of care is now a part of established professional society guidelines for sedation in the ICU [334]. It remains to be seen whether these guidelines will be adapted to accommodate recent findings showing a reduction in ARDS mortality with 48 hours of early neuromuscular blockade [338].

CONCLUSION

Since its first published description in 1967 [213], our understanding of the pathogenesis and pathophysiology of ALI has grown appreciably, and ongoing research efforts continue to provide hope for exciting new therapies in the future. Our improved understanding of this condition has already translated into improved outcomes for patients suffering from ALI [320], but it's still ominous prognosis for those acutely afflicted in the hospital [7], and those fortunate enough to survive [324], leaves room for ongoing progress in the management of these patients. Aside from the obvious importance of reducing mortality from this condition, a reduction in days on the ventilator and subsequent stay in the intensive care unit represent some of the other tangible and intangible benefits to both patients and society in general [335,336].

References

1. ARDS-Network: Ventilation with lower tidal volumes as compared with traditional tidal volumes for acute lung injury and the acute respiratory distress syndrome. The Acute Respiratory Distress Syndrome Network. *N Engl J Med* 342:1301–1308, 2000.
2. Amato MB, Barbas CS, Medeiros DM, et al: Effect of a protective-ventilation strategy on mortality in the acute respiratory distress syndrome. *N Engl J Med* 338:347–354, 1998.
3. Spragg RG, Lewis JF, Walmrath HD, et al: Effect of recombinant surfactant protein C-based surfactant on the acute respiratory distress syndrome. *N Engl J Med* 351:884–892, 2004.
4. Steinberg KP, Hudson LD, Goodman RB, et al: Efficacy and safety of corticosteroids for persistent acute respiratory distress syndrome [see comment]. *N Engl J Med* 354:1671–1684, 2006.
5. Pontes-Arruda A, Aragao AMA, Albuquerque JD: Effects of enteral feeding with eicosapentaenoic acid, gamma-linolenic acid, and antioxidants in mechanically ventilated patients with severe sepsis and septic shock [see comment]. *Crit Care Med* 34:2325–2333, 2006.
6. McAuley DF, Frank JA, Fang X, et al: Clinically relevant concentrations of beta2-adrenergic agonists stimulate maximal cyclic adenosine monophosphate-dependent airspace fluid clearance and decrease pulmonary edema in experimental acid-induced lung injury. *Crit Care Med* 32:1470–1476, 2004.
7. Rubenfeld GD, Caldwell E, Peabody E, et al: Incidence and outcomes of acute lung injury. *N Engl J Med* 353:1685–1693, 2005.
8. Shah CV, Localio AR, Lanken PN, et al: The impact of development of acute lung injury on hospital mortality in critically ill trauma patients. *Crit Care Med* 36:2309–2315, 2008.
9. Bernard GR, Artigas A, Brigham KL, et al: The American-European Consensus Conference on ARDS. Definitions, mechanisms, relevant outcomes, and clinical trial coordination. *Am J Respir Crit Care Med* 149:818–824, 1994.
10. Allardet-Servent J, Forel JM, Roch A, et al: FIO_2 and acute respiratory distress syndrome definition during lung protective ventilation [see comment]. *Crit Care Med* 37:202–207, 2009.
11. Doyle RL, Szaflarski N, Modin GW, et al: Identification of patients with acute lung injury. Predictors of mortality. *Am J Respir Crit Care Med* 152:1818–1824, 1995.
12. Monchi M, Bellenfant F, Cariou A, et al: Early predictive factors of survival in the acute respiratory distress syndrome. A multivariate analysis. *Am J Respir Crit Care Med* 158:1076–1081, 1998.
13. Zilberberg MD, Epstein SK: Acute lung injury in the medical ICU: comorbid conditions, age, etiology, and hospital outcome. *Am J Respir Crit Care Med* 157:1159–1164, 1998.
14. Schuster DP: What is acute lung injury? What is ARDS? *Chest* 107:1721–1726, 1995.
15. Schreiter D, Reske A, Stichert B, et al: Alveolar recruitment in combination with sufficient positive end-expiratory pressure increases oxygenation and lung aeration in patients with severe chest trauma. *Crit Care Med* 32:968–975, 2004.
16. Ware LB, Matthay MA: The acute respiratory distress syndrome. *N Engl J Med* 342:1334–1349, 2000.
17. TenHoor T, Mannino DM, Moss M: Risk factors for ARDS in the United States: analysis of the 1993 National Mortality Followback Study. *Chest* 119:1179–1184, 2001.
18. Hudson LD, Milberg JA, Anardi D, et al: Clinical risks for development of the acute respiratory distress syndrome. *Am J Respir Crit Care Med* 151:293–301, 1995.
19. Tomashefski JF Jr: Pulmonary pathology of acute respiratory distress syndrome. *Clin Chest Med* 21:435–466, 2000.
20. Blennerhassett JB: Shock lung and diffuse alveolar damage pathological and pathogenetic considerations. *Pathology* 17:239–247, 1985.
21. Byrne K, Cooper KR, Carey PD, et al: Pulmonary compliance: early assessment of evolving lung injury after onset of sepsis. *J Appl Physiol* 69:2290–2295, 1990.
22. Cheung O, Leslie KO: Acute Lung Injury, in Leslie KO, Wick MW (eds): *Practical Pulmonary Pathology*. Philadelphia, Churchill Livingstone, 2005 pp 71–95.
23. Marshall RP, Bellingan G, Webb S, et al: Fibroproliferation occurs early in the acute respiratory distress syndrome and impacts on outcome. *Am J Respir Crit Care Med* 162:1783–1788, 2000.
24. Martin C, Papazian L, Payan MJ, et al: Pulmonary fibrosis correlates with outcome in adult respiratory distress syndrome. A study in mechanically ventilated patients. *Chest* 107:196–200, 1995.
25. Goodman PC, Quinones Maymi DM: Radiographic findings in ARDS, in Matthay MA (ed): *Acute Respiratory Distress Syndrome*. New York, Marcel Dekker, Inc, 55–73, 2003.
26. Thomason JW, Ely EW, Chiles C, et al: Appraising pulmonary edema using supine chest roentgenograms in ventilated patients. *Am J Respir Crit Care Med* 157:1600–1608, 1998.
27. Rubenfeld GD, Caldwell E, Granton J, et al: Interobserver variability in applying a radiographic definition for ARDS. *Chest* 116:1347–1353, 1999.
28. Tagliabue M, Casella TC, Zincone GE, et al: CT and chest radiography in the evaluation of adult respiratory distress syndrome. *Acta Radiol* 35:230–234, 1994.
29. Bellani G, Messa C, Guerra L, et al: Lungs of patients with acute respiratory distress syndrome show diffuse inflammation in normally aerated regions: a [18F]-fluoro-2-deoxy-D-glucose PET/CT study. *Crit Care Med* 37:2216–2222, 2009.
30. Kaplan JD, Calandrino FS, Schuster DP: A positron emission tomographic comparison of pulmonary vascular permeability during the adult respiratory distress syndrome and pneumonia. *Am Rev Respir Dis* 143:150–154, 1991.
31. Berthezene Y, Vexler V, Jerome H, et al: Differentiation of capillary leak and hydrostatic pulmonary edema with a macromolecular MR imaging contrast agent. *Radiology* 181:773–777, 1991.
32. Raijmakers PG, Groeneveld AB, Teule GJ, et al: Diagnostic value of the gallium-67 pulmonary leak index in pulmonary edema. *J Nucl Med* 37:1316–1322, 1996.
33. Conference Report: Mechanisms of acute respiratory failure. *Am Rev Respir Dis* 115:1071–1078, 1977.
34. Bersten AD, Edibam C, Hunt T, et al: Incidence and mortality of acute lung injury and the acute respiratory distress syndrome in three Australian States. *Am J Respir Crit Care Med* 165:443–448, 2002.
35. Luhr OR, Antonsen K, Karlsson M, et al: Incidence and mortality after acute respiratory failure and acute respiratory distress syndrome in Sweden, Denmark, and Iceland. The ARF Study Group. *Am J Respir Crit Care Med* 159:1849–1861, 1999.
36. Goss CH, Brower RG, Hudson LD, et al: Incidence of acute lung injury in the United States. *Crit Care Med* 31:1607–1611, 2003.
37. Ferguson ND, Frutos-Vivar F, Esteban A, et al: Clinical risk conditions for acute lung injury in the intensive care unit and hospital ward: a prospective observational study. *Crit care (London, England)* 11:R96, 2007.
38. Gattinoni L, Pelosi P, Suter PM, et al: Acute respiratory distress syndrome caused by pulmonary and extrapulmonary disease. Different syndromes? *Am J Respir Crit Care Med* 158:3–11, 1998.
39. Calfee CS, Eisner MD, Ware LB, et al: Trauma-associated lung injury differs clinically and biologically from acute lung injury due to other clinical disorders [see comment]. *Crit Care Med* 35:2243–2250, 2007.
40. Moss M, Parsons PE, Steinberg KP, et al: Chronic alcohol abuse is associated with an increased incidence of acute respiratory distress syndrome and severity of multiple organ dysfunction in patients with septic shock. *Crit Care Med* 31:869–877, 2003.
41. Iscimen R, Cartin-Ceba R, Yilmaz M, et al: Risk factors for the development of acute lung injury in patients with septic shock: an observational cohort study [see comment]. *Crit Care Med* 36:1518–1522, 2008.
42. Moss M, Bucher B, Moore FA, et al: The role of chronic alcohol abuse in the development of acute respiratory distress syndrome in adults. *JAMA* 275:50–54, 1996.
43. Gajic O, Rana R, Winters JL, et al: Transfusion-related acute lung injury in the critically ill: prospective nested case-control study [see comment]. *Am J Respir Crit Care Med* 176:886–891, 2007.
44. Khan H, Belsher J, Yilmaz M, et al: Fresh-frozen plasma and platelet transfusions are associated with development of acute lung injury in critically ill medical patients. *Chest* 131:1308–1314, 2007.
45. Netzer G, Shah CV, Iwashyna TJ, et al: Association of RBC transfusion with mortality in patients with acute lung injury [see comment]. *Chest* 132:1116–1123, 2007.
46. Chaiwat O, Lang JD, Vavilala MS, et al: Early packed red blood cell transfusion and acute respiratory distress syndrome after trauma [see comment]. *Anesthesiology* 110:351–360, 2009.
47. Moss M, Guidot DM, Steinberg KP, et al: Diabetic patients have a decreased incidence of acute respiratory distress syndrome. *Crit Care Med* 28:2187–2192, 2000.
48. Bachofen M, Weibel ER: Structural alterations of lung parenchyma in the adult respiratory distress syndrome. *Clin Chest Med* 3:35–56, 1982.
49. Martin TR, Nakamura M, Matute-Bello G: The role of apoptosis in acute lung injury. *Crit Care Med* 31:S184–S188, 2003.
50. Abraham E: Neutrophils and acute lung injury. *Crit Care Med* 31:S195–S199, 2003.
51. Ware LB, Matthay MA: Alveolar fluid clearance is impaired in the majority of patients with acute lung injury and the acute respiratory distress syndrome. *Am J Respir Crit Care Med* 163:1376–1383, 2001.
52. Matthay MA, Fang X, Sakuma T, et al: Resolution of alveolar edema. Mechanisms and relationship to clinical acute lung injury, in Matthay MA (ed). *Acute Respiratory Distress Syndrome*. New York, Marcel Dekker, Inc, 2003 pp 409–438.
53. Matthay MA, Clerici C, Saumon G: Invited review: active fluid clearance from the distal air spaces of the lung. *J Appl Physiol* 93:1533–1541, 2002.
54. Lecuona E, Saldias F, Comellas A, et al: Ventilator-associated lung injury decreases lung ability to clear edema in rats. *Am J Respir Crit Care Med* 159:603–609, 1999.

55. Garat C, Meignan M, Matthay MA, et al: Alveolar epithelial fluid clearance mechanisms are intact after moderate hyperoxic lung injury in rats. *Chest* 111:1381–1388, 1997.
56. Hastings RH, Folkesson HG, Matthay MA: Mechanisms of alveolar protein clearance in the intact lung. *Am J Physiol* 286:L679–L689, 2004.
57. Bachofen M, Weibel ER: Alterations of the gas exchange apparatus in adult respiratory insufficiency associated with septicemia. *Am Rev Respir Dis* 116:589–615, 1977.
58. Wiener-Kronish JP, Albertine KH, Matthay MA: Differential responses of the endothelial and epithelial barriers of the lung in sheep to Escherichia coli endotoxin. *J Clin Invest* 88:864–875, 1991.
59. Mintun MA, Dennis DR, Welch MJ, et al: Measurements of pulmonary vascular permeability with PET and gallium-68 transferrin. *J Nucl Med* 28:1704–1716, 1987.
60. Zimmerman GA, Prescott SM, McIntyre TM: Endothelial cell interactions with granulocytes: tethering and signaling molecules. *Immunol Today* 13:93–100, 1992.
61. Ribes JA, Francis CW, Wagner DD: Fibrin induces release of von Willebrand factor from endothelial cells. *J Clin Invest* 79:117–123, 1987.
62. Strieter RM, Kunkel SL, Showell HJ, et al: Endothelial cell gene expression of a neutrophil chemotactic factor by TNF-alpha, LPS, and IL-1 beta. *Science* 243:1467–1469, 1989.
63. Topham MK, Carveth HJ, McIntyre TM, et al: Human endothelial cells regulate polymorphonuclear leukocyte degranulation. *FASEB J* 12:733–746, 1998.
64. Rubin DB, Wiener-Kronish JP, Murray JF, et al: Elevated von Willebrand factor antigen is an early plasma predictor of acute lung injury in nonpulmonary sepsis syndrome. *J Clin Invest* 86:474–480, 1990.
65. Ware LB, Eisner MD, Thompson BT, et al: Significance of von Willebrand factor in septic and nonseptic patients with acute lung injury. *Am J Respir Crit Care Med* 170:766–772, 2004.
66. Doerschuk CM, Mizgerd JP, Kubo H, et al: Adhesion molecules and cellular biomechanical changes in acute lung injury: Giles F. Filley Lecture. *Chest* 116:37S–43S, 1999.
67. Fujishima S, Aikawa N: Neutrophil-mediated tissue injury and its modulation. *Intensive Care Med* 21:277–285, 1995.
68. Laufe MD, Simon RH, Flint A, et al: Adult respiratory distress syndrome in neutropenic patients. *Am J Med* 80:1022–1026, 1986.
69. Azoulay E, Attalah H, Yang K, et al: Exacerbation with granulocyte colony-stimulating factor of prior acute lung injury during neutropenia recovery in rats. *Crit Care Med* 31:157–165, 2003.
70. Folkesson HG, Matthay MA, Hebert CA, et al: Acid aspiration-induced lung injury in rabbits is mediated by interleukin-8-dependent mechanisms. *J Clin Invest* 96:107–116, 1995.
71. Chignard M, Balloy V: Neutrophil recruitment and increased permeability during acute lung injury induced by lipopolysaccharide. *Am J Physiol* 279:L1083–L1090, 2000.
72. Idell S: Coagulation, fibrinolysis, and fibrin deposition in acute lung injury. *Crit Care Med* 31:S213–S220, 2003.
73. Abraham E: Coagulation abnormalities in acute lung injury and sepsis. *Am J Respir Cell Mol Biol* 22:401–404, 2000.
74. Idell S, Gonzalez K, Bradford H, et al: Procoagulant activity in bronchoalveolar lavage in the adult respiratory distress syndrome. Contribution of tissue factor associated with factor VII. *Am Rev Respir Dis* 136:1466–1474, 1987.
75. Bertozzi P, Astedt B, Zenzius L, et al: Depressed bronchoalveolar urokinase activity in patients with adult respiratory distress syndrome. *N Engl J Med* 322:890–897, 1990.
76. Idell S, James KK, Levin EG, et al: Local abnormalities in coagulation and fibrinolytic pathways predispose to alveolar fibrin deposition in the adult respiratory distress syndrome. *J Clin Invest* 84:695–705, 1989.
77. Vassalli JD, Sappino AP, Belin D: The plasminogen activator/plasmin system. *J Clin Invest* 88:1067–1072, 1991.
78. Prabhakaran P, Ware LB, White KE, et al: Elevated levels of plasminogen activator inhibitor-1 in pulmonary edema fluid are associated with mortality in acute lung injury. *Am J Physiol* 285:L20–L28, 2003.
79. Barazzone C, Belin D, Piguet PF, et al: Plasminogen activator inhibitor-1 in acute hyperoxic mouse lung injury. *J Clin Invest* 98:2666–2673, 1996.
80. Allen GB, Cloutier ME, Larrabee YC, et al: Neither fibrin nor plasminogen activator inhibitor-1 deficiency protects lung function in a mouse model of acute lung injury. *Am J Physiol* 296:L277–L285, 2009.
81. Bastarache JA, Wang L, Geiser T, et al: The alveolar epithelium can initiate the extrinsic coagulation cascade through expression of tissue factor. *Thorax* 62:608–616, 2007.
82. Brigham KL, Meyrick B: Endotoxin and lung injury. *Am Rev Respir Dis* 133:913–927, 1986.
83. Martin TR: Recognition of bacterial endotoxin in the lungs. *Am J Respir Cell Mol Biol* 23:128–132, 2000.
84. Brigham KL: Oxidant stress and adult respiratory distress syndrome. *Eur Respir J Suppl* 11:482S–484S, 1990.
85. Weiss YG, Maloyan A, Tazelaar J, et al: Adenoviral transfer of HSP-70 into pulmonary epithelium ameliorates experimental acute respiratory distress syndrome. *J Clin Invest* 110:801–806, 2002.
86. Bromberg Z, Deutschman CS, Weiss YG: Heat shock protein 70 and the acute respiratory distress syndrome. *J Anesth* 19:236–242, 2005.
87. Imai Y, Parodo J, Kajikawa O, et al: Injurious mechanical ventilation and end-organ epithelial cell apoptosis and organ dysfunction in an experimental model of acute respiratory distress syndrome. *JAMA* 289:2104–2112, 2003.
88. Dreyfuss D, Saumon G: Ventilator-induced lung injury: lessons from experimental studies. *Am J Respir Crit Care Med* 157:294–323, 1998.
89. Matthay MA, Bhattacharya S, Gaver D, et al: Ventilator-induced lung injury: in vivo and in vitro mechanisms. *Am J Physiol* 283:L678–L682, 2002.
90. Piantadosi CA, Schwartz DA: The acute respiratory distress syndrome. *Ann Intern Med* 141:460–470, 2004.
91. Matamis D, Lemaire F, Harf A, et al: Total respiratory pressure-volume curves in the adult respiratory distress syndrome. *Chest* 86:58–66, 1984.
92. Schiller HJ, McCann UG II, Carney DE, et al: Altered alveolar mechanics in the acutely injured lung. *Crit Care Med* 29:1049–1055, 2001.
93. Kaisers U, Busch T, Deja M, et al: Selective pulmonary vasodilation in acute respiratory distress syndrome. *Crit Care Med* 31:S337–S342, 2003.
94. Zapol WM, Snider MT: Pulmonary hypertension in severe acute respiratory failure. *N Engl J Med* 296:476–480, 1977.
95. Villar J, Blazquez MA, Lubillo S, et al: Pulmonary hypertension in acute respiratory failure. *Crit Care Med* 17:523–526, 1989.
96. Zapol WM, Kobayashi K, Snider MT, et al: Vascular obstruction causes pulmonary hypertension in severe acute respiratory failure. *Chest* 71:306–307, 1977.
97. Steltzer H, Krafft P, Fridrich P, et al: Right ventricular function and oxygen transport patterns in patients with acute respiratory distress syndrome. *Anaesthesia* 49:1039–1045, 1994.
98. Radermacher P, Santak B, Becker H, et al: Prostaglandin E1 and nitroglycerin reduce pulmonary capillary pressure but worsen ventilation-perfusion distributions in patients with adult respiratory distress syndrome. *Anesthesiology* 70:601–606, 1989.
99. Horie T, Hildebrandt J: Dynamic compliance, limit cycles, and static equilibria of excised cat lung. *J Appl Physiol* 31:423–430, 1971.
100. Petty TL, Reiss OK, Paul GW, et al: Characteristics of pulmonary surfactant in adult respiratory distress syndrome associated with trauma and shock. *Am Rev Respir Dis* 115:531–536, 1977.
101. Seeger W, Grube C, Gunther A, et al: Surfactant inhibition by plasma proteins: differential sensitivity of various surfactant preparations. *Eur Respir J* 6:971–977, 1993.
102. Gunasekara L, Schurch S, Schoel WM, et al: Pulmonary surfactant function is abolished by an elevated proportion of cholesterol. Biochim Biophys Acta 1737:27–35, 2005.
103. Hallman M, Spragg R, Harrell JH, et al: Evidence of lung surfactant abnormality in respiratory failure. Study of bronchoalveolar lavage phospholipids, surface activity, phospholipase activity, and plasma myoinositol. *J Clin Invest* 70:673–683, 1982.
104. Veldhuizen RA, Welk B, Harbottle R, et al: Mechanical ventilation of isolated rat lungs changes the structure and biophysical properties of surfactant. *J Appl Physiol* 92:1169–1175, 2002.
105. Veldhuizen RA, Tremblay LN, Govindarajan A, et al: Pulmonary surfactant is altered during mechanical ventilation of isolated rat lung. *Crit Care Med* 28:2545–2551, 2000.
106. Gattinoni L, Caironi P, Pelosi P, et al: What has computed tomography taught us about the acute respiratory distress syndrome? *Am J Respir Crit Care Med* 164:1701–1711, 2001.
107. Hubmayr RD: Perspective on lung injury and recruitment: a skeptical look at the opening and collapse story. *Am J Respir Crit Care Med* 165:1647–1653, 2002.
108. Gattinoni L, Pesenti A, Avalli L, et al: Pressure-volume curve of total respiratory system in acute respiratory failure. Computed tomographic scan study. *Am Rev Respir Dis* 136:730–736, 1987.
109. Gattinoni L, Pelosi P, Crotti S, et al: Effects of positive end-expiratory pressure on regional distribution of tidal volume and recruitment in adult respiratory distress syndrome. *Am J Respir Crit Care Med* 151:1807–1814, 1995.
110. Stapleton RD, Wang BM, Hudson LD, et al: Causes and timing of death in patients with ARDS. *Chest* 128:525–532, 2005.
111. Bendixen HH, Hedley-Whyte J, Laver MB: Impaired oxygenation in surgical patients during general anesthesia with controlled ventilation. *N Engl J Med* 269:991–996, 1963.
112. Hedley-Wyte J, Laver MB, Bendixen HH: Effects of changes in tidal ventilation on physiologic shunting. *Am J Physiol* 206:891–895, 1964.
113. Petty TL, Ashbaugh DG: The adult respiratory distress syndrome. Clinical features, factors influencing prognosis and principles of management. *Chest* 60:233–239, 1971.
114. Petty TL: Acute respiratory distress syndrome (ARDS). *Dis Mon* 36:1–58, 1990.
115. Webb HH, Tierney DF: Experimental pulmonary edema due to intermittent positive pressure ventilation with high inflation pressures. Protection by positive end-expiratory pressure. *Am Rev Respir Dis* 110:556–565, 1974.
116. Hickling KG, Henderson SJ, Jackson R: Low mortality associated with low volume pressure limited ventilation with permissive hypercapnia in severe adult respiratory distress syndrome. *Intensive Care Med* 16:372–377, 1990.

117. Hickling KG, Walsh J, Henderson S, et al: Low mortality rate in adult respiratory distress syndrome using low-volume, pressure-limited ventilation with permissive hypercapnia: a prospective study. *Crit Care Med* 22:1568–1578, 1994.
118. Brochard L, Roudot-Thoraval F, Roupie E, et al: Tidal volume reduction for prevention of ventilator-induced lung injury in acute respiratory distress syndrome. The Multicenter Trail Group on Tidal Volume reduction in ARDS. *Am J Respir Crit Care Med* 158:1831–1838, 1998.
119. Brower RG, Shanholtz CB, Fessler HE, et al: Prospective, randomized, controlled clinical trial comparing traditional versus reduced tidal volume ventilation in acute respiratory distress syndrome patients. *Crit Care Med* 27:1492–1498, 1999.
120. Stewart TE, Meade MO, Cook DJ, et al: Evaluation of a ventilation strategy to prevent barotrauma in patients at high risk for acute respiratory distress syndrome. Pressure- and Volume-Limited Ventilation Strategy Group. *N Engl J Med* 338:355–361, 1998.
121. Parsons PE, Matthay MA, Ware LB, et al: Elevated plasma levels of soluble TNF receptors are associated with morbidity and mortality in patients with acute lung injury. *Am J Physiol Lung Cell Mol Physiol* 288:L426–L431, 2004.
122. Parsons PE, Eisner MD, Thompson BT, et al: Lower tidal volume ventilation and plasma cytokine markers of inflammation in patients with acute lung injury. *Crit Care Med* 33:1–6; discussion 230–232, 2005.
123. Sinclair SE, Kregenow DA, Lamm WJ, et al: Hypercapnic acidosis is protective in an in vivo model of ventilator-induced lung injury. *Am J Respir Crit Care Med* 166:403–408, 2002.
124. Laffey JG, Tanaka M, Engelberts D, et al: Therapeutic hypercapnia reduces pulmonary and systemic injury following in vivo lung reperfusion. *Am J Respir Crit Care Med* 162:2287–2294, 2000.
125. Lang JD, Figueroa M, Sanders KD, et al: Hypercapnia via reduced rate and tidal volume contributes to lipopolysaccharide-induced lung injury. *Am J Respir Crit Care Med* 171:147–157, 2005.
126. Doerr CH, Gajic O, Berrios JC, et al: Hypercapnic acidosis impairs plasma membrane wound resealing in ventilator-injured lungs. *Am J Respir Crit Care Med* 171:1371–1377, 2005.
127. Dellinger RP, Carlet JM, Masur H, et al: Surviving Sepsis Campaign guidelines for management of severe sepsis and septic shock. *Crit Care Med* 32:858–873, 2004.
128. Eichacker PQ, Gerstenberger EP, Banks SM, et al: Meta-analysis of acute lung injury and acute respiratory distress syndrome trials testing low tidal volumes. *Am J Respir Crit Care Med* 166:1510–1514, 2002.
129. Young MP, Manning HL, Wilson DL, et al: Ventilation of patients with acute lung injury and acute respiratory distress syndrome: has new evidence changed clinical practice? *Crit Care Med* 32:1260–1265, 2004.
130. Kalhan R, Mikkelsen M, Dedhiya P, et al: Underuse of lung protective ventilation: analysis of potential factors to explain physician behavior. *Crit Care Med* 34:300–306, 2006.
131. Gajic O, Dara SI, Mendez JL, et al: Ventilator-associated lung injury in patients without acute lung injury at the onset of mechanical ventilation. *Crit Care Med* 32:1817–1824, 2004.
132. Yilmaz M, Keegan MT, Iscimen R, et al: Toward the prevention of acute lung injury: protocol-guided limitation of large tidal volume ventilation and inappropriate transfusion [see comment]. *Crit Care Med* 35:1660–1666; quiz 1667, 2007.
133. Frank JA, Gutierrez JA, Jones KD, et al: Low tidal volume reduces epithelial and endothelial injury in acid-injured rat lungs. *Am J Respir Crit Care Med* 165:242–249, 2002.
134. Oczenski W, Hormann C, Keller C, et al: Recruitment maneuvers after a positive end-expiratory pressure trial do not induce sustained effects in early adult respiratory distress syndrome. *Anesthesiology* 101:620–625, 2004.
135. Allen G, Lundblad LK, Parsons P, et al: Transient mechanical benefits of a deep inflation in the injured mouse lung. *J Appl Physiol* 93:1709–1715, 2002.
136. Lim CM, Jung H, Koh Y, et al: Effect of alveolar recruitment maneuver in early acute respiratory distress syndrome according to antiderecruitment strategy, etiological category of diffuse lung injury, and body position of the patient. *Crit Care Med* 31:411–418, 2003.
137. Lachmann B: Open up the lung and keep the lung open. *Intensive Care Med* 18:319–321, 1992.
138. Duggan M, McCaul CL, McNamara PJ, et al: Atelectasis causes vascular leak and lethal right ventricular failure in uninjured rat lungs. *Am J Respir Crit Care Med* 167:1633–1640, 2003.
139. Musch G, Harris RS, Vidal Melo MF, et al: Mechanism by which a sustained inflation can worsen oxygenation in acute lung injury. *Anesthesiology* 100:323–330, 2004.
140. Brower RG, Morris A, MacIntyre N, et al: Effects of recruitment maneuvers in patients with acute lung injury and acute respiratory distress syndrome ventilated with high positive end-expiratory pressure. *Crit Care Med* 31:2592–2597, 2003.
141. Grasso S, Mascia L, Del Turco M, et al: Effects of recruiting maneuvers in patients with acute respiratory distress syndrome ventilated with protective ventilatory strategy. *Anesthesiology* 96:795–802, 2002.
142. Lim CM, Soon Lee S, Seoung Lee J, et al: Morphometric effects of the recruitment maneuver on saline-lavaged canine lungs. A computed tomographic analysis. *Anesthesiology* 99:71–80, 2003.
143. Bond DM, Froese AB: Volume recruitment maneuvers are less deleterious than persistent low lung volumes in the atelectasis-prone rabbit lung during high-frequency oscillation. *Crit Care Med* 21:402–412, 1993.
144. Fujino Y, Goddon S, Dolhnikoff M, et al: Repetitive high-pressure recruitment maneuvers required to maximally recruit lung in a sheep model of acute respiratory distress syndrome. *Crit Care Med* 29:1579–1586, 2001.
145. Foti G, Cereda M, Sparacino ME, et al: Effects of periodic lung recruitment maneuvers on gas exchange and respiratory mechanics in mechanically ventilated acute respiratory distress syndrome (ARDS) patients. *Intensive Care Med* 26:501–507, 2000.
146. Meade MO, Cook DJ, Guyatt GH, et al: Ventilation strategy using low tidal volumes, recruitment maneuvers, and high positive end-expiratory pressure for acute lung injury and acute respiratory distress syndrome: a randomized controlled trial [see comment]. *JAMA* 299:637–645, 2008.
147. Mercat A, Richard JC, Vielle B, et al: Positive end-expiratory pressure setting in adults with acute lung injury and acute respiratory distress syndrome: a randomized controlled trial [see comment]. *JAMA* 299:646–655, 2008.
148. Pelosi P, Cadringher P, Bottino N, et al: Sigh in acute respiratory distress syndrome. *Am J Respir Crit Care Med* 159:872–880, 1999.
149. Halter JM, Steinberg JM, Schiller HJ, et al: Positive end-expiratory pressure after a recruitment maneuver prevents both alveolar collapse and recruitment/derecruitment. *Am J Respir Crit Care Med* 167:1620–1626, 2003.
150. Gattinoni L, D'Andrea L, Pelosi P, et al: Regional effects and mechanism of positive end-expiratory pressure in early adult respiratory distress syndrome. *JAMA* 269:2122–2127, 1993.
151. Tremblay L, Valenza F, Ribeiro SP, et al: Injurious Ventilatory Strategies Increase Cytokines and c-fos m-RNA Expression in an Isolated Rat Lung Model. *J Clin Invest* 99:944–952, 1997.
152. Brower RG, Lanken PN, MacIntyre N, et al: Higher versus lower positive end-expiratory pressures in patients with the acute respiratory distress syndrome. *N Engl J Med* 351:327–336, 2004.
153. Levy MM: PEEP in ARDS—How Much Is Enough? *N Engl J Med* 351:389–391, 2004.
154. Gattinoni L, Caironi P, Cressoni M, et al: Lung Recruitment in Patients with the Acute Respiratory Distress Syndrome 10.1056/NEJMoa052052. *N Engl J Med* 354:1775–1786, 2006.
155. Talmor D, Sarge T, Malhotra A, et al: Mechanical ventilation guided by esophageal pressure in acute lung injury. *N Engl J Med* 359:2095–2104, 2008.
156. Amato MB, Barbas CS, Medeiros DM, et al: Beneficial effects of the "open lung approach" with low distending pressures in acute respiratory distress syndrome. A prospective randomized study on mechanical ventilation. *Am J Respir Crit Care Med* 152:1835–1846, 1995.
157. Maggiore SM, Jonson B, Richard JC, et al: Alveolar derecruitment at decremental positive end-expiratory pressure levels in acute lung injury: comparison with the lower inflection point, oxygenation, and compliance. *Am J Respir Crit Care Med* 164:795–801, 2001.
158. Jonson B, Richard JC, Straus C, et al: Pressure-volume curves and compliance in acute lung injury. Evidence of recruitment above the lower inflection point. *Am J Respir Crit Care Med* 159:1172–1178, 1999.
159. Hickling KG: The pressure-volume curve is greatly modified by recruitment. A mathematical model of ARDS lungs. *Am J Respir Crit Care Med* 158:194–202, 1998.
160. Albaiceta GM, Taboada F, Parra D, et al: Tomographic study of the inflection points of the pressure-volume curve in acute lung injury. *Am J Respir Crit Care Med* 170:1066–1072, 2004.
161. Moss M, Parsons PE: Mechanical ventilation and the adult respiratory distress syndrome. *Semin Respir Crit Care Med* 15:289–299, 1994.
162. Gerstmann DR, Minton SD, Stoddard RA, et al: The Provo multicenter early high-frequency oscillatory ventilation trial: improved pulmonary and clinical outcome in respiratory distress syndrome. *Pediatrics* 98:1044–1057, 1996.
163. Group HS: High-frequency oscillatory ventilation compared with conventional mechanical ventilation in the treatment of respiratory failure in preterm infants. The HIFI Study Group. *N Engl J Med* 320:88–93, 1989.
164. Mehta S, Lapinsky SE, Hallett DC, et al: Prospective trial of high-frequency oscillation in adults with acute respiratory distress syndrome. *Crit Care Med* 29:1360–1369, 2001.
165. Fort P, Farmer C, Westerman J, et al: High-frequency oscillatory ventilation for adult respiratory distress syndrome–a pilot study. *Crit Care Med* 25:937–947, 1997.
166. Derdak S, Mehta S, Stewart TE, et al: High-frequency oscillatory ventilation for acute respiratory distress syndrome in adults: a randomized, controlled trial. *Am J Respir Crit Care Med* 166:801–808, 2002.
167. UK collaborative randomised trial of neonatal extracorporeal membrane oxygenation. UK Collaborative ECMO Trail Group. *Lancet* 348:75–82, 1996.
168. Morris AH, Wallace CJ, Menlove RL, et al: Randomized clinical trial of pressure-controlled inverse ratio ventilation and extracorporeal CO_2 removal for adult respiratory distress syndrome. *Am J Respir Crit Care Med* 149:295–305, 1994.
169. Zapol WM, Snider MT, Hill JD, et al: Extracorporeal membrane oxygenation in severe acute respiratory failure. A randomized prospective study. *JAMA* 242:2193–2196, 1979.
170. Peek GJ, Mugford M, Tiruvoipati R, et al: Efficacy and economic assessment of conventional ventilatory support versus extracorporeal membrane

oxygenation for severe adult respiratory failure (CESAR): a multicentre randomised controlled trial. *Lancet* 374:1351–1363, 2009.
171. Zwischenberger JB, Lynch JE: Will CESAR answer the adult ECMO debate? *Lancet* 374:1307–1308, 2009.
172. Pelosi P, D'Andrea L, Vitale G, et al: Vertical gradient of regional lung inflation in adult respiratory distress syndrome. *Am J Respir Crit Care Med* 149:8–13, 1994.
173. Putensen C, Zech S, Wrigge H, et al: Long-term effects of spontaneous breathing during ventilatory support in patients with acute lung injury. *Am J Respir Crit Care Med* 164:43–49, 2001.
174. Putensen C, Mutz NJ, Putensen-Himmer G, et al: Spontaneous breathing during ventilatory support improves ventilation-perfusion distributions in patients with acute respiratory distress syndrome. *Am J Respir Crit care Med* 159:1241–1248, 1999.
175. Brochard L, Rua F, Lorino H, et al: Inspiratory pressure support compensates for the additional work of breathing caused by the endotracheal tube. *Anesthesiology* 75:739–745, 1991.
176. Brochard L, Harf A, Lorino H, et al: Inspiratory pressure support prevents diaphragmatic fatigue during weaning from mechanical ventilation. *Am Rev Respir Dis* 139:513–521, 1989.
177. Neumann P, Wrigge H, Zinserling J, et al: Spontaneous breathing affects the spatial ventilation and perfusion distribution during mechanical ventilatory support. *Crit Care Med* 33:1090–1095, 2005.
178. Jousela I, Makelainen A, Tahvanainen J, et al: Diaphragmatic movement using ultrasound during spontaneous and mechanical ventilation: effect of tidal volume. *Acta Anaesthesiol Belg* 43:165–171, 1992.
179. Girou E, Schortgen F, Delclaux C, et al: Association of noninvasive ventilation with nosocomial infections and survival in critically ill patients. *JAMA* 284:2361–2367, 2000.
180. Rocker GM, Mackenzie MG, Williams B, et al: Noninvasive positive pressure ventilation: successful outcome in patients with acute lung injury/ARDS. *Chest* 115:173–177, 1999.
181. Antonelli M, Conti G, Rocco M, et al: A comparison of noninvasive positive-pressure ventilation and conventional mechanical ventilation in patients with acute respiratory failure. *N Engl J Med* 339:429–435, 1998.
182. Antonelli M, Conti G, Esquinas A, et al: A multiple-center survey on the use in clinical practice of noninvasive ventilation as a first-line intervention for acute respiratory distress syndrome. *Crit Care Med* 35:18–25, 2007.
183. Douglas WW, Rehder K, Beynen FM, et al: Improved oxygenation in patients with acute respiratory failure: the prone position. *Am Rev Respir Dis* 115:559–566, 1977.
184. Wiener CM, Kirk W, Albert RK: Prone position reverses gravitational distribution of perfusion in dog lungs with oleic acid-induced injury. *J Appl Physiol* 68:1386–1392, 1990.
185. Lamm WJ, Graham MM, Albert RK: Mechanism by which the prone position improves oxygenation in acute lung injury. *Am J Respir Crit Care Med* 150:184–193, 1994.
186. Glenny RW, Lamm WJ, Albert RK, et al: Gravity is a minor determinant of pulmonary blood flow distribution. *J Appl Physiol* 71:620–629, 1991.
187. Albert RK, Leasa D, Sanderson M, et al: The prone position improves arterial oxygenation and reduces shunt in oleic-acid-induced acute lung injury. *Am Rev Respir Dis* 135:628–633, 1987.
188. Pelosi P, Tubiolo D, Mascheroni D, et al: Effects of the prone position on respiratory mechanics and gas exchange during acute lung injury. *Am J Respir Crit Care Med* 157:387–393, 1998.
189. Broccard A, Shapiro RS, Schmitz LL, et al: Prone positioning attenuates and redistributes ventilator-induced lung injury in dogs. *Crit Care Med* 28:295–303, 2000.
190. Cakar N, der Kloot TV, Youngblood M, et al: Oxygenation response to a recruitment maneuver during supine and prone positions in an oleic acid-induced lung injury model. *Am J Respir Crit Care Med* 161:1949–1956, 2000.
191. Walther SM, Domino KB, Glenny RW, et al: Positive end-expiratory pressure redistributes perfusion to dependent lung regions in supine but not in prone lambs. *Crit Care Med* 27:37–45, 1999.
192. Gattinoni L, Tognoni G, Pesenti A, et al: Effect of prone positioning on the survival of patients with acute respiratory failure. *N Engl J Med* 345:568–573, 2001.
193. Mancebo J, Fernandez R, Blanch L, et al: A multicenter trial of prolonged prone ventilation in severe acute respiratory distress syndrome. *Am J Respir Crit care Med* 173:1233–1239, 2006.
194. Guerin C, Gaillard S, Lemasson S, et al: Effects of systematic prone positioning in hypoxemic acute respiratory failure: a randomized controlled trial. *JAMA* 292:2379–2387, 2004.
195. Slutsky AS: The acute respiratory distress syndrome, mechanical ventilation, and the prone position. *N Engl J Med* 345:610–612, 2001.
196. Martin GS, Mangialardi RJ, Wheeler AP, et al: Albumin and furosemide therapy in hypoproteinemic patients with acute lung injury. *Crit Care Med* 30:2175–2182, 2002.
197. Martin GS, Moss M, Wheeler AP, et al: A randomized, controlled trial of furosemide with or without albumin in hypoproteinemic patients with acute lung injury. *Crit Care Med* 33:1681–1687, 2005.
198. Quinlan GJ, Mumby S, Martin GS, et al: Albumin influences total plasma antioxidant capacity favorably in patients with acute lung injury. *Crit Care Med* 32:755–759, 2004.
199. Qiao RL, Ying X, Bhattacharya J: Effects of hyperoncotic albumin on endothelial barrier properties of rat lung. *Am J Physiol* 265:H198–H204, 1993.
200. The National Heart, Lung, and Blood Institute Acute Respiratory Distress Syndrome (ARDS) Clinical Trials Network: Comparison of two fluid-management strategies in acute lung injury. *N Engl J Med* 354(24):2564–2575, 2006.
201. Connors AF Jr, Speroff T, Dawson NV, et al: The effectiveness of right heart catheterization in the initial care of critically ill patients. SUPPORT Investigators. *JAMA* 276:889–897, 1996.
202. Harvey S, Harrison DA, Singer M, et al: Assessment of the clinical effectiveness of pulmonary artery catheters in management of patients in intensive care (PAC-Man): a randomised controlled trial. *Lancet* 366:472–477, 2005.
203. Rhodes A, Cusack RJ, Newman PJ, et al: A randomised, controlled trial of the pulmonary artery catheter in critically ill patients. *Intensive Care Med* 28:256–264, 2002.
204. Vincent JL, Dhainaut JF, Perret C, et al: Is the pulmonary artery catheter misused? A European view. *Crit Care Med* 26:1283–1287, 1998.
205. The National Heart L, and Blood Institute Acute Respiratory Distress Syndrome (ARDS) Clinical Trials Network,. Pulmonary-Artery versus Central Venous Catheter to Guide Treatment of Acute Lung Injury 10.1056/NEJMoa061895. *N Engl J Med* 354:2213–2224, 2006.
206. Colley PS, Cheney FW Jr, Hlastala MP: Pulmonary gas exchange effects of nitroglycerin in canine edematous lungs. *Anesthesiology* 55:114–119, 1981.
207. Palmer RM, Ferrige AG, Moncada S: Nitric oxide release accounts for the biological activity of endothelium-derived relaxing factor. *Nature* 327:524–526, 1987.
208. Pepke-Zaba J, Higenbottam TW, Dinh-Xuan AT, et al: Inhaled nitric oxide as a cause of selective pulmonary vasodilatation in pulmonary hypertension. *Lancet* 338:1173–1174, 1991.
209. Troncy E, Collet JP, Shapiro S, et al: Inhaled nitric oxide in acute respiratory distress syndrome: a pilot randomized controlled study. *Am J Respir Crit Care Med* 157:1483–1488, 1998.
210. Michael JR, Barton RG, Saffle JR, et al: Inhaled nitric oxide versus conventional therapy: effect on oxygenation in ARDS. *Am J Respir Crit Care Med* 157:1372–1380, 1998.
211. Dellinger RP, Zimmerman JL, Taylor RW, et al: Effects of inhaled nitric oxide in patients with acute respiratory distress syndrome: results of a randomized phase II trial. Inhaled Nitric Oxide in ARDS Study Group. *Crit Care Med* 26:15–23, 1998.
212. Lundin S, Mang H, Smithies M, et al: Inhalation of nitric oxide in acute lung injury: results of a European multicentre study. The European Study Group of Inhaled Nitric Oxide. *Intensive Care Med* 25:911–919, 1999.
213. Ashbaugh DG, Bigelow DB, Petty TL, et al: Acute respiratory distress in adults. *Lancet* 2:319–323, 1967.
214. Hallman M, Maasilta P, Sipila I, et al: Composition and function of pulmonary surfactant in adult respiratory distress syndrome. *Eur Respir J Suppl* 3:104S–108S, 1989.
215. Veldhuizen RA, McCaig LA, Akino T, et al: Pulmonary surfactant subfractions in patients with the acute respiratory distress syndrome. *Am J Respir Crit Care Med* 152:1867–1871, 1995.
216. Veldhuizen RA, Ito Y, Marcou J, et al: Effects of lung injury on pulmonary surfactant aggregate conversion in vivo and in vitro. *Am J Physiol* 272:L872–L878, 1997.
217. Korfhagen TR, LeVine AM, Whitsett JA: Surfactant protein A (SP-A) gene targeted mice. *Biochim Biophys Acta* 1408:296–302, 1998.
218. Clark JC, Wert SE, Bachurski CJ, et al: Targeted disruption of the surfactant protein B gene disrupts surfactant homeostasis, causing respiratory failure in newborn mice. *Proc Natl Acad Sci U S A* 92:7794–7798, 1995.
219. Spragg RG, Smith RM, Harris K, et al: Effect of recombinant SP-C surfactant in a porcine lavage model of acute lung injury. *J Appl Physiol* 88:674–681, 2000.
220. Greene KE, Wright JR, Steinberg KP, et al: Serial changes in surfactant-associated proteins in lung and serum before and after onset of ARDS. *Am J Respir Crit Care Med* 160:1843–1850, 1999.
221. Eisner MD, Parsons P, Matthay MA, et al: Plasma surfactant protein levels and clinical outcomes in patients with acute lung injury. *Thorax* 58:983–988, 2003.
222. Group TOC: Early versus delayed neonatal administration of a synthetic surfactant–the judgment of OSIRIS. The OSIRIS Collaborative Group (open study of infants at high risk of or with respiratory insufficiency—the role of surfactant. *Lancet* 340:1363–1369, 1992.
223. Schwartz RM, Luby AM, Scanlon JW, et al: Effect of surfactant on morbidity, mortality, and resource use in newborn infants weighing 500 to 1500 g. *N Engl J Med* 330:1476–1480, 1994.
224. Anzueto A, Baughman RP, Guntupalli KK, et al: Aerosolized surfactant in adults with sepsis-induced acute respiratory distress syndrome. Exosurf Acute Respiratory Distress Syndrome Sepsis Study Group. *N Engl J Med* 334:1417–1421, 1996.
225. Spragg RG, Richman P, Gilliard N, et al: The use of exogenous surfactant to treat patients with acute high-permeability lung edema. *Prog Clin Biol Res* 308:791–796, 1989.
226. Baudouin SV: Exogenous surfactant replacement in ARDS—one day, someday, or never? *N Engl J Med* 351:853–855, 2004.

227. Vazquez de Anda GF, Lachmann RA, Gommers D, et al: Treatment of ventilation-induced lung injury with exogenous surfactant. *Intensive Care Med* 27:559–565, 2001.
228. Welk B, Malloy JL, Joseph M, et al: Surfactant treatment for ventilation-induced lung injury in rats: effects on lung compliance and cytokines. *Exp Lung Res* 27:505–520, 2001.
229. Lutz C, Carney D, Finck C, et al: Aerosolized surfactant improves pulmonary function in endotoxin-induced lung injury. *Am J Respir Crit Care Med* 158:840–845, 1998.
230. Holm BA, Enhorning G, Notter RH: A biophysical mechanism by which plasma proteins inhibit lung surfactant activity. *Chem Phys Lipids* 49:49–55, 1988.
231. Seeger W, Gunther A, Thede C: Differential sensitivity to fibrinogen inhibition of SP-C- vs. SP-B-based surfactants. *Am J Physiol* 262:L286–L291, 1992.
232. Amirkhanian JD, Bruni R, Waring AJ, et al: Full length synthetic surfactant proteins, SP-B and SP-C, reduce surfactant inactivation by serum. *Biochim Biophys Acta* 1168:315–320, 1993.
233. Lu KW, Taeusch HW, Robertson B, et al: Polyethylene glycol/surfactant mixtures improve lung function after HCl and endotoxin lung injuries. *Am J Respir Crit Care Med* 164:1531–1536, 2001.
234. Ashbaugh DG, Maier RV: Idiopathic pulmonary fibrosis in adult respiratory distress syndrome. Diagnosis and treatment. *Arch Surg* 120:530–535, 1985.
235. Meduri GU, Chinn AJ, Leeper KV, et al: Corticosteroid rescue treatment of progressive fibroproliferation in late ARDS. Patterns of response and predictors of outcome. *Chest* 105:1516–1527, 1994.
236. Meduri GU, Belenchia JM, Estes RJ, et al: Fibroproliferative phase of ARDS. Clinical findings and effects of corticosteroids. *Chest* 100:943–952, 1991.
237. Hooper RG, Kearl RA: Established ARDS treated with a sustained course of adrenocortical steroids. *Chest* 97:138–143, 1990.
238. Luce JM, Montgomery AB, Marks JD, et al: Ineffectiveness of high-dose methylprednisolone in preventing parenchymal lung injury and improving mortality in patients with septic shock. *Am Rev Respir Dis* 138:62–68, 1988.
239. Bernard GR, Luce JM, Sprung CL, et al: High-dose corticosteroids in patients with the adult respiratory distress syndrome. *N Engl J Med* 317:1565–1570, 1987.
240. Meduri GU, Headley AS, Golden E, et al: Effect of prolonged methylprednisolone therapy in unresolving acute respiratory distress syndrome: a randomized controlled trial. *JAMA* 280:159–165, 1998.
241. Brun-Buisson C, Brochard L: Corticosteroid therapy in acute respiratory distress syndrome: better late than never? *JAMA* 280:182–183, 1998.
242. The National Heart L, and Blood Institute Acute Respiratory Distress Syndrome (ARDS) Clinical Trials Network,. Efficacy and Safety of Corticosteroids for Persistent Acute Respiratory Distress Syndrome. *N Engl J Med* 354:1671–1684, 2006.
243. Nuckton TJ, Alonso JA, Kallet RH, et al: Pulmonary dead-space fraction as a risk factor for death in the acute respiratory distress syndrome. *N Engl J Med* 346:1281–1286, 2002.
244. Welty-Wolf KE, Carraway MS, Miller DL, et al: Coagulation blockade prevents sepsis-induced respiratory and renal failure in baboons. *Am J Respir Crit Care Med* 164:1988–1996, 2001.
245. Bernard GR, Vincent JL, Laterre PF, et al: Efficacy and safety of recombinant human activated protein C for severe sepsis. *N Engl J Med* 344:699–709, 2001.
246. Laterre PF, Wittebole X, Dhainaut JF: Anticoagulant therapy in acute lung injury. *Crit Care Med* 31:S329–S336, 2003.
247. Leavell KJ, Peterson MW, Gross TJ: The role of fibrin degradation products in neutrophil recruitment to the lung. *Am J Respir Cell Mol Biol* 14:53–60, 1996.
248. Seeger W, Stohr G, Wolf HR, et al: Alteration of surfactant function due to protein leakage: special interaction with fibrin monomer. *J Appl Physiol* 58:326–338, 1985.
249. Seeger W, Elssner A, Gunther A, et al: Lung surfactant phospholipids associate with polymerizing fibrin: loss of surface activity. *Am J Respir Cell Mol Biol* 9:213–220, 1993.
250. Miller DL, Welty-Wolf K, Carraway MS, et al: Extrinsic coagulation blockade attenuates lung injury and proinflammatory cytokine release after intratracheal lipopolysaccharide. *Am J Respir Cell Mol Biol* 26:650–658, 2002.
251. Jian MY, Koizumi T, Tsushima K, et al: Activated protein C attenuates acid-aspiration lung injury in rats. *Pulm Pharmacol Ther* 18:291–296, 2005.
252. Abraham E, Reinhart K, Opal S, et al: Efficacy and safety of tifacogin (recombinant tissue factor pathway inhibitor) in severe sepsis: a randomized controlled trial. *JAMA* 290:238–247, 2003.
253. Warren BL, Eid A, Singer P, et al: Caring for the critically ill patient. High-dose antithrombin III in severe sepsis: a randomized controlled trial. *JAMA* 286:1869–1878, 2001.
254. Liu KD, Levitt J, Zhuo H, et al: Randomized clinical trial of activated protein C for the treatment of acute lung injury [see comment]. *Am J Respir Crit Care Med* 178:618–623, 2008.
255. Rubenfeld GD, Abraham E: When is a negative phase II trial truly negative? *Am J Respir Crit Care Med* 178:554–555, 2008.
256. Vincent JL, Artigas A, Petersen LC, et al: A multicenter, randomized, double-blind, placebo-controlled, dose-escalation trial assessing safety and efficacy of active site inactivated recombinant factor VIIa in subjects with acute lung injury or acute respiratory distress syndrome. *Crit Care Med* 37:1874–1880, 2009.
257. Frank JA, Wang Y, Osorio O, et al: Beta-adrenergic agonist therapy accelerates the resolution of hydrostatic pulmonary edema in sheep and rats. *J Appl Physiol* 89:1255–1265, 2000.
258. Barnard ML, Olivera WG, Rutschman DM, et al: Dopamine stimulates sodium transport and liquid clearance in rat lung epithelium. *Am J Respir Crit Care Med* 156:709–714, 1997.
259. Perkins GD, McAuley DF, Thickett DR, et al: The beta-agonist lung injury trial (BALTI): a randomized placebo-controlled clinical trial [see comment]. *Am J Respir Crit Care Med* 173:281–287, 2006.
260. Matthay MA, Brower R, Thompson BT, et al: Randomized, Placebo-Controlled Trial of an Aerosolized Beta-2 Adrenergic Agonist (Albuterol) for the Treatment of Acute Lung Injury. *Am J Respir Crit Care Med* 179 (abstract):A2166, 2009.
261. Simopoulos AP: Omega-3 fatty acids in inflammation and autoimmune diseases. *J Am Coll Nutr* 21:495–505, 2002.
262. Gadek JE, DeMichele SJ, Karlstad MD, et al: Effect of enteral feeding with eicosapentaenoic acid, gamma-linolenic acid, and antioxidants in patients with acute respiratory distress syndrome. Enteral Nutrition in ARDS Study Group. *Crit Care Med* 27:1409–1420, 1999.
263. Pacht ER, DeMichele SJ, Nelson JL, et al: Enteral nutrition with eicosapentaenoic acid, gamma-linolenic acid, and antioxidants reduces alveolar inflammatory mediators and protein influx in patients with acute respiratory distress syndrome. *Crit Care Med* 31:491–500, 2003.
264. Singer P, Theilla M, Fisher H, et al: Benefit of an enteral diet enriched with eicosapentaenoic acid and gamma-linolenic acid in ventilated patients with acute lung injury [comment, erratum appears in Crit Care Med 34(6):1861, 2006]. *Crit Care Med* 34:1033–1038, 2006.
265. Stapleton RD, Martin TR, Weiss NS, et al: A Phase II Randomized Placebo-Controlled Trial of Omega-3 Fatty Acids for the Treatment of Acute Lung Injury. *Crit Care Med* 2011 (In Press).
266. NHLBI. Versus Delayed Enteral Feeding and Omega-3 Fatty Acid/Antioxidant Supplementation for Treating People with Acute Lung Injury or Acute Respiratory Distress Syndrome (The EDEN-Omega Study) http://clinicaltrials.gov/ct2/show/NCT00609180.
267. Rasanen J, Cane RD, Downs JB, et al: Airway pressure release ventilation during acute lung injury: a prospective multicenter trial. *Crit Care Med* 19:1234–1241, 1991.
268. Habashi NM: Other approaches to open-lung ventilation: airway pressure release ventilation. *Crit Care Med* 33:S228–S240, 2005.
269. Putensen C, Rasanen J, Lopez FA, et al: Effect of interfacing between spontaneous breathing and mechanical cycles on the ventilation-perfusion distribution in canine lung injury. *Anesthesiology* 81:921–930, 1994.
270. Varpula T, Valta P, Niemi R, et al: Airway pressure release ventilation as a primary ventilatory mode in acute respiratory distress syndrome. *Acta Anaesthesiol Scand* 48:722–731, 2004.
271. Dart BWt, Maxwell RA, Richart CM, et al: Preliminary experience with airway pressure release ventilation in a trauma/surgical intensive care unit. *J Trauma* 59:71–76, 2005.
272. McCunn M, Habashi NM: Airway pressure release ventilation in the acute respiratory distress syndrome following traumatic injury. *Int Anesthesiol Clin* 40:89–102, 2002.
273. Weiss DJ, Kolls JK, Ortiz LA, et al: Stem Cells and Cell Therapies in Lung Biology and Lung Diseases. *Proc Am Thorac Soc* 5:637–667, 2008.
274. Krause DS, Theise ND, Collector MI, et al: Multi-organ, multi-lineage engraftment by a single bone marrow-derived stem cell. *Cell* 105:369–377, 2001.
275. Burnham EL, Taylor WR, Quyyumi AA, et al: Increased circulating endothelial progenitor cells are associated with survival in acute lung injury. *Am J Respir Crit Care Med* 172:854–860, 2005.
276. Gupta N, Su X, Popov B, et al: Intrapulmonary delivery of bone marrow-derived mesenchymal stem cells improves survival and attenuates endotoxin-induced acute lung injury in mice. *J Immunol* 179:1855–1863, 2007.
277. McCarey DW, McInnes IB, Madhok R, et al: Trial of Atorvastatin in Rheumatoid Arthritis (TARA): double-blind, randomised placebo-controlled trial. *Lancet* 363:2015–2021, 2004.
278. Frost FJ, Petersen H, Tollestrup K, et al: Influenza and COPD mortality protection as pleiotropic, dose-dependent effects of statins. *Chest* 131:1006–1012, 2007.
279. Gupta R, Plantinga LC, Fink NE, et al: Statin use and sepsis events [corrected] in patients with chronic kidney disease. *JAMA* 297:1455–1464, 2007.
280. Jacobson JR, Barnard JW, Grigoryev DN, et al: Simvastatin attenuates vascular leak and inflammation in murine inflammatory lung injury. *Am J Physiol* 288:L1026–L1032, 2005.
281. Gao F, Linhartova L, Johnston AM, et al: Statins and sepsis. *Br J Anaesthesia* 100:288–298, 2008.
282. Weber C, Erl W, Weber KS, et al: HMG-CoA reductase inhibitors decrease CD11b expression and CD11b-dependent adhesion of monocytes to endothelium and reduce increased adhesiveness of monocytes isolated from patients with hypercholesterolemia. *J Am Coll Cardiol* 30:1212–1217, 1997.

283. Yoshida M, Sawada T, Ishii H, et al: Hmg-CoA reductase inhibitor modulates monocyte-endothelial cell interaction under physiological flow conditions in vitro: involvement of Rho GTPase-dependent mechanism. *Arterioscler Thromb Vasc Biol* 21:1165–1171, 2001.
284. Albert MA, Danielson E, Rifai N, et al: Effect of statin therapy on C-reactive protein levels: the pravastatin inflammation/CRP evaluation (PRINCE): a randomized trial and cohort study. *JAMA* 286:64–70, 2001.
285. Inoue I, Goto S, Mizotani K, et al: Lipophilic HMG-CoA reductase inhibitor has an anti-inflammatory effect: reduction of MRNA levels for interleukin-1beta, interleukin-6, cyclooxygenase-2, and p22phox by regulation of peroxisome proliferator-activated receptor alpha (PPARalpha) in primary endothelial cells. *Life Sci* 67:863–876, 2000.
286. Huhle G, Abletshauser C, Mayer N, et al: Reduction of platelet activity markers in type II hypercholesterolemic patients by a HMG-CoA-reductase inhibitor. *Thromb Res* 95:229–234, 1999.
287. Solovey A, Kollander R, Shet A, et al: Endothelial cell expression of tissue factor in sickle mice is augmented by hypoxia/reoxygenation and inhibited by lovastatin. *Blood* 104:840–846, 2004.
288. Steiner S, Speidl WS, Pleiner J, et al: Simvastatin blunts endotoxin-induced tissue factor in vivo. *Circulation* 111:1841–1846, 2005.
289. Bourcier T, Libby P: HMG CoA reductase inhibitors reduce plasminogen activator inhibitor-1 expression by human vascular smooth muscle and endothelial cells. *Arterioscler Thromb Vasc Biol* 20:556–562, 2000.
290. Landmesser U, Engberding N, Bahlmann FH, et al: Statin-induced improvement of endothelial progenitor cell mobilization, myocardial neovascularization, left ventricular function, and survival after experimental myocardial infarction requires endothelial nitric oxide synthase. *Circulation* 110:1933–1939, 2004.
291. Naidu BV, Woolley SM, Farivar AS, et al: Simvastatin ameliorates injury in an experimental model of lung ischemia-reperfusion. *J Thorac Cardiovasc Surg* 126:482–489, 2003.
292. The Irish Critical Care Trials G: Acute lung injury and the acute respiratory distress syndrome in Ireland: a prospective audit of epidemiology and management. *Crit Care* 12:R30, 2008.
293. Pittet D, Hugonnet S, Harbarth S, et al: Effectiveness of a hospital-wide programme to improve compliance with hand hygiene. *Lancet* 356:1307–1312, 2000.
294. Rello J, Ollendorf DA, Oster G, et al: Epidemiology and outcomes of ventilator-associated pneumonia in a large US database. *Chest* 122:2115–2121, 2002.
295. Morris PE, Goad A, Thompson C, et al: Early intensive care unit mobility therapy in the treatment of acute respiratory failure. *Crit Care Med* 36:2238–2243, 2008.
296. Schweickert WD, Pohlman MC, Pohlman AS, et al: Early physical and occupational therapy in mechanically ventilated, critically ill patients: a randomised controlled trial. *Lancet* 373:1874–1882, 2009.
297. Silliman CC, Ambruso DR, Boshkov LK: Transfusion-related acute lung injury. *Blood* 105:2266–2273, 2005.
298. The National Heart LaBIARDSCTN: Comparison of two fluid-management strategies in acute lung injury. *N Engl J Med* 354:2564–2575, 2006.
299. Tablan OC, Anderson LJ, Besser R, et al: Guidelines for preventing health-care–associated pneumonia, 2003: recommendations of CDC and the Healthcare Infection Control Practices Advisory Committee. *MMWR Recomm Rep* 53:1–36, 2004.
300. Kirby RR, Downs JB, Civetta JM, et al: High level positive end expiratory pressure (PEEP) in acute respiratory insufficiency. *Chest* 67:156–163, 1975.
301. Carlon GC, Howland WS, Ray C, et al: High-frequency jet ventilation. A prospective randomized evaluation. *Chest* 84:551–559, 1983.
302. Pepe PE, Hudson LD, Carrico CJ: Early application of positive end-expiratory pressure in patients at risk for the adult respiratory-distress syndrome. *N Engl J Med* 311:281–286, 1984.
303. Bone RC, Slotman G, Maunder R, et al: Randomized double-blind, multicenter study of prostaglandin E1 in patients with the adult respiratory distress syndrome. Prostaglandin E1 Study Group. *Chest* 96:114–119, 1989.
304. Abraham E, Baughman R, Fletcher E, et al: Liposomal prostaglandin E1 (TLC C-53) in acute respiratory distress syndrome: a controlled, randomized, double-blind, multicenter clinical trial. TLC C-53 ARDS Study Group. *Crit Care Med* 27:1478–1485, 1999.
305. Payen D, Vallet B, Group G: Results of the French prospective multicenter randomized double-blind placebo-controlled trial on inhaled nitric oxide in ARDS. *Intensive Care Med* 25:S166, 1999.
306. The ARDS Network Authors for the ARDS Network: Ketoconazole for early treatment of acute lung injury and acute respiratory distress syndrome: a randomized controlled trial. *JAMA* 283:1995–2002, 2000.
307. Hirschl RB, Croche M, Gore D, et al: Prospective, randomized, controlled pilot study of partial liquid ventilation in adult acute respiratory distress syndrome. *Am J Respir Crit Care Med* 165:781–787, 2002.
308. Kacmarek RM, Wiedemann HP, Lavin PT, et al: Partial liquid ventilation in adult patients with acute respiratory distress syndrome. *Am J Respir Crit Care Med* 173:882–889, 2006.
309. Morris PE, Papadakos P, Russell JA, et al: A double-blind placebo-controlled study to evaluate the safety and efficacy of L-2-oxothiazolidine-4-carboxylic acid in the treatment of patients with acute respiratory distress syndrome. *Crit Care Med* 36:782–788, 2008.
310. Moss M, Mannino DM: Race and gender differences in acute respiratory distress syndrome deaths in the United States: an analysis of multiple-cause mortality data (1979–1996). *Crit Care Med* 30:1679–1685, 2002.
311. Esteban A, Anzueto A, Frutos-Vivar F, et al: Outcome of older patients receiving mechanical ventilation. *Intensive Care Med* 30:639–646, 2004.
312. Ely EW, Wheeler AP, Thompson BT, et al: Recovery rate and prognosis in older persons who develop acute lung injury and the acute respiratory distress syndrome. *Ann Intern Med* 136:25–36, 2002.
313. Suratt BT, Eisner MD, Calfee CS, et al: Plasma granulocyte colony-stimulating factor levels correlate with clinical outcomes in patients with acute lung injury. *Crit Care Med* 37:1322–1328, 2009.
314. O'Brien JM Jr, Phillips GS, Ali NA, et al: Body mass index is independently associated with hospital mortality in mechanically ventilated adults with acute lung injury. *Crit Care Med* 34:738–744, 2006.
315. Flores C, Ma SF, Maresso K, et al: IL6 gene-wide haplotype is associated with susceptibility to acute lung injury. *Transl Res* 152:11–17, 2008.
316. Zhai R, Zhou W, Gong MN, et al: Inhibitor kappaB-alpha haplotype GTC is associated with susceptibility to acute respiratory distress syndrome in Caucasians. *Crit Care Med* 35:893–898, 2007.
317. Currier PF, Gong MN, Zhai R, et al: Surfactant protein-B polymorphisms and mortality in the acute respiratory distress syndrome. *Crit Care Med* 36:2511–2516, 2008.
318. Bajwa EK, Yu CL, Gong MN, et al: Pre-B-cell colony-enhancing factor gene polymorphisms and risk of acute respiratory distress syndrome. *Crit Care Med* 35:1290–1295, 2007.
319. Zhai R, Gong MN, Zhou W, et al: Genotypes and haplotypes of the VEGF gene are associated with higher mortality and lower VEGF plasma levels in patients with ARDS. *Thorax* 62:718–722, 2007.
320. Milberg JA, Davis DR, Steinberg KP, et al: Improved survival of patients with acute respiratory distress syndrome (ARDS): 1983–1993. *JAMA* 273:306–309, 1995.
321. Orme J Jr, Romney JS, Hopkins RO, et al: Pulmonary function and health-related quality of life in survivors of acute respiratory distress syndrome. *Am J Respir Crit Care Med* 167:690–694, 2003.
322. McHugh LG, Milberg JA, Whitcomb ME, et al: Recovery of function in survivors of the acute respiratory distress syndrome. *Am J Respir Crit Care Med* 150:90–94, 1994.
323. Hopkins RO, Weaver LK, Pope D, et al: Neuropsychological sequelae and impaired health status in survivors of severe acute respiratory distress syndrome. *Am J Respir Crit Care Med* 160:50–56, 1999.
324. Hopkins RO, Weaver LK, Collingridge D, et al: Two-year cognitive, emotional, and quality-of-life outcomes in acute respiratory distress syndrome. *Am J Respir Crit Care Med* 171:340–347, 2005.
325. Schelling G, Stoll C, Vogelmeier C, et al: Pulmonary function and health-related quality of life in a sample of long-term survivors of the acute respiratory distress syndrome. *Intensive Care Med* 26:1304–1311, 2000.
326. Herridge MS, Cheung AM, Tansey CM, et al: One-year outcomes in survivors of the acute respiratory distress syndrome. *N Engl J Med* 348:683–693, 2003.
327. Adhikari NK, McAndrews MP, Tansey CM, et al: Self-reported symptoms of depression and memory dysfunction in survivors of ARDS. *Chest* 135:678–687, 2009.
328. Schelling G, Stoll C, Haller M, et al: Health-related quality of life and posttraumatic stress disorder in survivors of the acute respiratory distress syndrome. *Crit Care Med* 26:651–659, 1998.
329. Jones C, Griffiths RD, Humphris G, et al: Memory, delusions, and the development of acute posttraumatic stress disorder-related symptoms after intensive care. *Crit Care Med* 29:573–580, 2001.
330. Kress JP, Pohlman AS, O'Connor MF, et al: Daily interruption of sedative infusions in critically ill patients undergoing mechanical ventilation. *N Engl J Med* 342:1471–1477, 2000.
331. Kress JP, Gehlbach B, Lacy M, et al: The long-term psychological effects of daily sedative interruption on critically ill patients. *Am J Respir Crit Care Med* 168:1457–1461, 2003.
332. Ely EW, Truman B, Shintani A, et al: Monitoring sedation status over time in ICU patients: reliability and validity of the Richmond Agitation-Sedation Scale (RASS). *JAMA* 289:2983–2991, 2003.
333. Pun BT, Gordon SM, Peterson JF, et al: Large-scale implementation of sedation and delirium monitoring in the intensive care unit: a report from two medical centers. *Crit Care Med* 33:1199–1205, 2005.
334. Jacobi J, Fraser GL, Coursin DB, et al: Clinical practice guidelines for the sustained use of sedatives and analgesics in the critically ill adult. *Crit Care Med* 30:119–141, 2002.
335. Valta P, Uusaro A, Nunes S, et al: Acute respiratory distress syndrome: frequency, clinical course, and costs of care. *Crit Care Med* 27:2367–2374, 1999.
336. Navarrete-Navarro P, Rodriguez A, Reynolds N, et al: Acute respiratory distress syndrome among trauma patients: trends in ICU mortality, risk factors, complications and resource utilization. *Intensive Care Med* 27:1133–1140, 2001.
337. Goodman LR, Fumagalli R, Tagliabue P, et al: Adult respiratory distress syndrome due to pulmonary and extrapulmonary causes: CT, clinical, and functional correlations. *Radiology* 213:545–552, 1999.
338. Papazian L, Forel JM, Gacouin A, et al: Neuromuscular blockers in early acute respiratory distress syndrome. *N Engl J Med* 363:1107–1116, 2010.

CHAPTER 48 ■ RESPIRATORY FAILURE PART III: ASTHMA

J. MARK MADISON AND RICHARD S. IRWIN

Asthma is an inflammatory disease of the airways characterized by reversible airway obstruction [1,2]. Inflammation causes airway obstruction by making airway smooth muscle more sensitive to contractile stimuli [3], by thickening the airway wall with edema and inflammatory cell infiltration, by stimulating glands to secrete mucus into the airway lumen, by damaging the airway epithelium [4], and by remodeling the architecture of the airways [5]. Typically, intermittent worsening or exacerbation of asthma is triggered by exposure to environmental factors such as inhaled allergens, irritants, or viral infections of the respiratory tract. These exacerbations represent acute or subacute episodes of increased airflow obstruction that may be mild to life threatening in severity. Assessment, management, and prevention of exacerbations of asthma, especially those leading to respiratory failure, are the critical challenges of caring for adult patients with asthma [6,7], the focus of this chapter.

EPIDEMIOLOGY

Worldwide, asthma ranks among the most common chronic diseases, with a prevalence ranging from a low of 0.7% in Macau, 6.7% in Japan, 10.9% in the United States, and a high of 18.4% in Scotland [8]. In general, asthma prevalence increases with urbanization and westernization of societies. In the United States, from 1980 to 1996, self-reported asthma prevalence increased 73.9% but then stabilized from 1997 to 2004 [9].

Asthma exacerbation rates vary by season with peaks in emergency room visits and hospitalizations coinciding with respiratory viral infections, especially rhinovirus, in late summer and early autumn [10]. In 2002, annual rates of hospitalization for asthma in the United States were 27 per 10,000 population-age 0–17 years and 13 per 10,000 population-age 18 and over. Although there remain important racial and gender differences in the rates of hospitalization, this represents an overall decline in hospitalizations from 1995 to 2002 and this suggests the possibility of better management and prevention of asthma exacerbations in ambulatory settings over these years [11].

In 2002 there were 4,261 deaths due to asthma in the United States indicating a death rate of 1.5 per 100,000 population of all ages [9]. Asthma mortality rates also have an annual cycle, but do not strictly parallel the cycle for exacerbations. In children, mortality peaks in the summer months, but, with increasing age, asthma mortality becomes more common in winter months [10]. In 2002, the death rate for ages 18 years and older was 1.9 deaths per 100,000 population, but it is notable that there are very large racial differences in the risk of death due to asthma. Blacks aged 25 to 34 years are six times more likely to die from asthma than whites of the same age group [9]. Deaths among patients hospitalized for asthma do account for one third of asthma related mortality, but potential differences in hospital care do not appear to account for the striking racial disparities and this suggests that prehospitalization factors are more important [12].

PATHOPHYSIOLOGY

Pathology

Bronchial biopsy specimens of patients with asthma are pathologically abnormal [13–15], with collagen deposition beneath the epithelial basement membranes, mucosal infiltration by eosinophils and neutrophils, mast cell degranulation, and epithelial damage. These findings occur in both severe and mild asthma, suggesting that airway inflammation is of primary importance in the pathogenesis of asthma.

Asthma exacerbations show variable pathology, reflecting at least two recognized subtypes of exacerbation—slow onset and rapid onset. Slow onset exacerbations are the most common (approximately 80% of exacerbations) and the patient presents with more than 2 to 6 hours of symptoms—often days or weeks of symptoms [16–18]. This suggests that most such patients should have sufficient time to seek medical attention for worsening shortness of breath [19]. At autopsy, the lungs of patients who die of "slow-onset" asthma exacerbations are hyperinflated with thick tenacious mucus filling and obstructing the lumens of the airways [4]. Microscopically, there is an eosinophilic bronchitis, with pronounced areas of mucosal edema and desquamation of the epithelium. Typically, hypertrophy and hyperplasia of smooth muscle are present and the muscle appears contracted [4].

The patient with the rapid-onset type of exacerbation presents with severe symptoms that have rapidly progressed over 2 to 6 hours [16–18]. These rapid-onset exacerbations may represent 8% to 14% of asthma exacerbations in general and can be fatal, leading to death in only a few hours after symptom onset [16,18]. Pathologically, airway obstruction by mucus is not prominent, and there is a neutrophil, rather than eosinophil, predominance of inflammatory cells in the airway submucosa [20]. There are no specific clinical characteristics that reliably predict which patients are prone to these rapid-onset asthma exacerbations. However, patients with rapid onset asthma exacerbations may more commonly report sensitivity to nonsteroidal anti-inflammatory drugs (NSAIDs) [18].

Pathogenesis

Asthma is a disease or group of diseases with complex underlying genetics [21]. Why airway inflammation develops in the asthmatic patient is not understood entirely, but much evidence suggests an important role for Th2 cytokines [22]. Inhaled allergens, pollutants, smoke, and viral infections all may play a role in augmenting the baseline airway inflammation present in the asthmatic airway [1,23]. When these environmental triggers interact with the asthmatic airway, the inflammation is intensified and the released mediators have potent effects on smooth muscle cell function, epithelium and microvascular integrity, neural function, and mucus gland secretion. All these factors contribute to increased narrowing of the asthmatic airway with smooth muscle contraction, mucus secretion, epithelial cell sloughing into the lumen, and edema and inflammatory cell infiltration of the airway wall. The resulting acute increase in airway obstruction is commonly referred to as an *acute exacerbation of asthma*.

Physiology

The major physiologic consequences of airway obstruction are hypoxemia and increased work of breathing. Understanding these physiologic disturbances is important for management of severe exacerbations of asthma.

Narrowing the caliber of airway lumens causes hypoxemia by two mechanisms. First, increases in the resistance to flow in the conducting airways result in uneven distribution of ventilation to the alveoli. Hypoxic vasoconstriction of vessels that supply underventilated alveoli partially compensates for this uneven ventilation, but overall ventilation–perfusion ($\dot{V}/\dot{Q}$) ratios remain abnormal and are the principal cause of hypoxemia in asthma [24]. Consequently, even patients with severe exacerbations of asthma usually respond well to supplemental oxygen. A second, less common cause of hypoxemia in asthma is right-to-left shunt due to atelectasis of lung distal to airways that are completely occluded by mucus or due to interatrial shunt [25–27].

The second physiologic consequence of severe airway obstruction is increased work of breathing. During acute exacerbations, respiratory muscles must expend increased energy, generating large changes in pleural pressure to overcome high airway resistance [28]. The resulting discordance between respiratory effort and the change in thoracic volume also plays a role in the patient's sensation of dyspnea and central drive to increase minute ventilation. The ensuing rapid respirations further increase the work of breathing and worsen air trapping behind narrowed airways that prematurely close during expiration. The dynamic hyperinflation of the lung itself leads to increased respiratory muscle energy costs because it restricts vital capacity to high thoracic volumes where alveolar dead space is increased, the respiratory muscles are at suboptimal mechanical advantage, and the lung is less compliant. All of these factors contribute to the enormous increase in the work of breathing. Thus, the respiratory muscles must expend more energy to achieve the same alveolar ventilation. Initially, the respiratory muscles may be able to exert the force needed to maintain alveolar ventilation but the muscles may fatigue if airway resistance increases rapidly, is sustained, or if there is inadequate oxygen delivery to theses muscles [29,30]. Dynamic hyperinflation due to severe airway obstruction also may impair cardiac performance by increasing afterload, decreasing venous return to the heart, and causing diastolic dysfunction [7,27].

DIFFERENTIAL DIAGNOSIS

Not all wheezing is due to asthma (Table 48.1). Obstruction of the airway at any level can produce wheezing and dyspnea that can be confused with asthma. For example, vocal cord dysfunction syndrome [31–35] is an extrathoracic cause of upper airway obstruction that can be confused with acute asthma. This diagnosis is suggested by the presence of stridor and wheeze in the absence of increased alveolar-arterial oxygen tension difference, extrathoracic variable obstruction on flow-volume loop, and observing paradoxic closure of vocal cords during inspiration on laryngoscopy.

Furthermore, many disease processes other than asthma can obstruct the lower airways to produce wheezing and dyspnea (Table 48.1). Systemic anaphylaxis can cause wheezing and should be considered in the differential diagnosis especially when respiratory symptoms have been of rapid onset and progress [36]. A diagnosis of anaphylaxis is suggested by acute-onset wheezing, stridor, urticaria, nausea, diarrhea, and hypotension (especially after insect bites, drug administration, or intravenous contrast). Exacerbations of chronic obstructive pulmonary disease (COPD) present similarly to acute asthma, but chronic bronchitis or emphysema, or both, can usually be distinguished from asthma historically. Pulmonary thromboembolism can masquerade as an exacerbation of asthma because the mediators released by platelets in thromboemboli sometimes cause bronchoconstriction and wheezing. However, hemoptysis, pleuritic pain, and pleural effusions rarely are seen in acute exacerbations of asthma.

Pulmonary edema, either cardiogenic or noncardiogenic, can obstruct small airways with mucosal swelling to produce acute wheezing. However, in these cases the clinical history, physical examination, and chest radiograph changes that show

TABLE 48.1

DIFFERENTIAL DIAGNOSIS OF WHEEZING

Upper airway obstruction
Extrathoracic
Anaphylaxis
Arytenoid dysfunction
Bilateral vocal cord paralysis
Laryngeal edema
Laryngostenosis
Laryngocele
Mobile supraglottic soft tissue
Neoplasms
Postextubation granuloma
Postnasal drip syndrome
Relapsing polychondritis
Retropharyngeal abscess
Supraglottitis
Vocal cord dysfunction syndrome
Wegener granulomatosis
Intrathoracic
Acquired tracheomalacia
Airway neoplasms
Foreign body aspiration
Goiter
Herpetic tracheobronchitis
Right-side aortic arch
Tracheal stenosis due to intubation
Tracheobronchomegaly
Lower airway obstruction
Aspiration
Asthma
Bronchiectasis
Bronchiolitis
Carcinoid syndrome
Chronic obstructive pulmonary disease
Cystic fibrosis
Lymphangitic carcinomatosis
Pulmonary edema
Parasitic infections
Pulmonary embolism

vascular redistribution of blood flow and alveolar filling help exclude asthma as a diagnosis. Notably, however, acute, reversible left ventricular dysfunction has been described as a possible complication of severe exacerbations of asthma; the underlying mechanism for this is unclear [37]. Aspiration can present with acute dyspnea and wheezing. In this case, a history of impaired consciousness or inability to protect the airway suggests that the diagnosis and chest radiograph may show pulmonary infiltration.

ASSESSMENT

Physician failure to appreciate the severity of airway obstruction in acute asthma is not uncommon and contributes to mortality [1]. The cornerstone of evaluation of patients with asthma exacerbations is the objective measurement of airflow. However, because some patients, especially those with severe exacerbations, may be unable to perform the necessary testing maneuvers, the physician also must be adept at recognizing certain historical features and physical findings that strongly suggest high risk for severe airway obstruction.

History

Baseline pulmonary function tests that show persistent decreases in the forced expired volume of air in 1 second (FEV_1), loss of lung elastic recoil, and hyperinflation at total lung capacity are associated with increased risk of near-fatal asthma [38]. A recent history of poorly controlled asthma (increases in dyspnea and wheezing, frequent nocturnal awakenings due to shortness of breath, increased use of beta-adrenergic rescue medications, increased diurnal variability in peak expiratory flow, and recent hospitalizations or emergency department visits) and any history of a prior near-fatal asthma exacerbation (prior admission to an intensive care unit or intubation for asthma) are the two most important predictors of a patient's propensity for severe life-threatening asthma exacerbations [39–44]. Patient complaints of severe breathlessness or chest tightness or difficulty walking more than 100 feet (30.48 m) also suggest severe airway obstruction. Cigarette smoking also has been associated with higher in-hospital and posthospitalization mortality [43]. In general, patients are somewhat better judges of the severity of their airway obstruction during an attack of asthma than are physicians who elicit their history at the bedside [45]. However, the patient's own assessment of airway obstruction should never be the exclusive means of assessing the severity of airway obstruction. Notably, patients with a history of severe asthma often have a blunted perception of dyspnea [46–49]. In assessing risk for fatal asthma, other important historical details include identification of current medications and coexisting illnesses, such as psychiatric disease, that interfere with medical follow-up and cardiopulmonary disease. A history of known coronary artery disease is important because the patient may be more sensitive to the stimulatory effects of β_2-adrenergic agonists and to the cardiac complications of hypoxemia [50]. These patients may also be receiving β_2-adrenergic antagonists that are making control of their asthma worse.

Physical Examination

Physical examination is important for excluding other causes of dyspnea (see Differential Diagnosis section) and assessing the degree of airway obstruction [44]. Tachycardia (greater than 120 beats per minute), tachypnea (greater than 30 breaths per minute), diaphoresis [51], bolt-upright posture in bed, pulsus paradoxus greater than 10 mm Hg, and accessory respiratory muscle use all should be regarded as signs of severe airway obstruction [52]. However, because the absence of these signs does not rule out severe obstruction, physical examination cannot be relied on exclusively to estimate the severity of airway obstruction. The amount of wheezing heard on auscultation of the chest is a notoriously poor method of assessing the severity of airway obstruction [53]. Cyanosis is a late, insensitive finding of severe hypoxemia. Abnormal thoracoabdominal motion (e.g., respiratory muscle alternans, abdominal paradox) and depressed mental status due to hypoxemia and hypercapnia are ominous indicators and can herald the necessity for mechanical ventilation [54].

Pulmonary Function Tests

To evaluate patients who are having an acute exacerbation of asthma, an objective measure of maximal expiratory airflow should be performed. An exception to this is the patient who is unable to perform a testing maneuver due to a severe, life-threatening exacerbation with obvious airway compromise and cyanosis [44]. Peak expiratory airflow rate (PEFR) and FEV_1 are equally good bedside measures to quantify the degree of airway obstruction [55]. These tests are invaluable for the initial assessment and for following responses to therapy [44,56]. In general, a PEFR or FEV_1 of less than 40% of baseline (either the predicted value or the patient's best-known value) indicates severe obstruction and a severe exacerbation of asthma (Table 48.2).

Arterial Blood Gas Analysis

Analysis of arterial blood gases (ABGs) have a role in assessing and managing severe asthma exacerbations (see Chapter 11) and should be performed for suspected hypoventilation, severe respiratory distress, or when spirometric test results are less than 25% predicted [44]. Also, any patient who fails to respond to the first 30 to 60 minutes of intensive bronchodilator therapy should have an ABG analysis performed. Although ABG values are not predictive of overall patient outcome [55], there is some correlation between hypoxemia and hypercapnia and the degree of airway obstruction measured by FEV_1 [57]. A partial pressure of arterial oxygen (PaO_2) less than 60 mm Hg or a pulse oximeter oxygen saturation value less than 90% on room air should be regarded as additional evidence of severe airway obstruction. Therefore, although ABG analysis is not recommended as routine in the initial evaluation of asthma, it should be done for the evaluation of severe cases. One study found that the frequency of ABG analysis in cases of severe asthma actually decreased from 1997 to 2000, a trend needing improvement [58].

TABLE 48.2

OBJECTIVE ASSESSMENT OF AIRWAY OBSTRUCTION AFTER INITIAL INTENSIVE THERAPY

PEFR or FEV_1	Interpretation
$\geq$70% predicted	Good response
$\geq$40% but $\leq$69% predicted	Incomplete response
<40% predicted	Poor response

FEV_1, forced expired volume in 1 second; PEFR, peak expiratory flow rate.

Understanding the expected changes in the partial pressure of arterial carbon dioxide ($PaCO_2$) during an asthma exacerbation is important for recognition of a rapidly deteriorating course. With modest airway obstruction, the patient's mild dyspnea stimulates an increase in minute ventilation that meets or exceeds the level required to maintain normal alveolar ventilation. Thus, patients with modest obstruction have a normal or slightly below normal $PaCO_2$. As airway obstruction worsens, dyspnea becomes more severe and the central nervous system drive to increase minute ventilation becomes intense. Typically, the increase in minute ventilation exceeds the level required to maintain constant alveolar ventilation; consequently, patients with moderate-to-severe obstruction have lower than normal $PaCO_2$ and respiratory alkalosis. As the airway obstruction becomes more severe and prolonged, high minute ventilation can no longer be maintained by the respiratory musculature and alveolar ventilation decreases. As a result, the $PaCO_2$ rises toward normal and then continues to climb, resulting in hypercapnia and respiratory acidosis. Thus, a normal or high $PaCO_2$ (greater than 40 mm Hg) during a severe exacerbation of asthma is a potentially ominous finding, often signifying the impending need for mechanical ventilation. Any coexisting conditions (malnutrition, advanced age) or medications (sedatives) that weaken respiratory muscle function or depress respiratory drive should be expected to accelerate the onset of hypercapnic ventilatory failure during acute exacerbations of asthma.

Other Laboratory Studies

For acute exacerbations of asthma, routine chest radiographs reveal few abnormalities other than hyperinflation [59]. However, although not recommended for routine assessment, for severe exacerbations chest radiography can be helpful when there is clinical suspicion of other causes of dyspnea and wheezing (see Differential Diagnosis section) or complications of severe airway obstruction [44]. Chest radiographs should be examined for evidence of enlarged cardiac silhouette, upper lung zone redistribution of blood flow, pleural effusions, and alveolar or interstitial infiltrates because any one of these findings suggests a diagnosis other than or in addition to acute asthma. In addition, chest radiography allows the early detection of common complications of severe airway obstruction, including pneumothorax, pneumomediastinum, and atelectasis. Also, lung infiltrates on chest radiographs can be compatible with a diagnosis of asthma complicated by either allergic bronchopulmonary aspergillosis or Churg–Strauss syndrome.

In the elderly, in patients with severe hypoxemia, and in individuals with suspected cardiac ischemia or arrhythmia, an electrocardiogram should be performed. Sinus tachycardia is common during acute exacerbations of asthma, but less common and transient findings include right-axis deviation, right ventricular hypertrophy and strain, P pulmonale, ST- and T-wave abnormalities, right bundle-branch block, and ventricular ectopic beats [60].

THERAPEUTIC AGENTS

Optimal management of an acute exacerbation of asthma begins with a careful assessment of the degree of airway obstruction. This initial assessment and repeated objective measures of airway obstruction guide treatment that combines supportive measures, bronchodilator therapy, and anti-inflammatory therapy (Table 48.3).

Because the dominant causes of airway obstruction during an acute exacerbation of asthma are the result of airway inflammation, the cornerstone of treatment is anti-inflammatory therapy with systemic corticosteroids [61]. Because corticosteroids take at least 4 to 6 hours to begin to have a beneficial effect and the inflammatory causes of airway obstruction may take days to resolve, the medical challenge is to support patients until the inflammatory processes have responded to corticosteroids.

TABLE 48.3

TREATMENT OF SEVERE ACUTE EXACERBATIONS OF ASTHMA

Pharmacologic agents
Anti-inflammatory agents
Systemic corticosteroids (oral preferred unless impaired intestinal absorption)
Bronchodilators
Inhaled β_2-adrenergic agonists
Inhaled cholinergic antagonists
$MgSO_4$ (not routine; consider in severe, refractory cases)
Oral or intravenous methylxanthines (not routine or recommended)
Systemic β_2-adrenergic agonists (not routine or recommended)
General anesthetics (not routine)
Supportive measures
Frequent reassessment
Supplemental oxygen
Fluid management
Invasive mechanical ventilation if needed (controlled hypoventilation)
Helium-oxygen mixtures to drive nebulizer (not routine; consider in severe, refractory cases)
Lavage by bronchoscopy (not routine, intubated patients only)
Education
Avoidance of asthma triggers
Medication use
Access to medical follow-up
Home monitoring of airway obstruction

β_2-Adrenergic agonists relieve airway obstruction due to airway smooth muscle contraction, and this is an important therapeutic maneuver in initial treatment. Although these bronchodilators relieve only one component of the airway obstruction during severe exacerbations of asthma, even small improvements in airflow can lead to important clinical benefits in the acute setting. Of the available bronchodilators, β_2-adrenergic agonists are the most effective and rapidly acting and, therefore, most useful during that critical time before the onset of corticosteroid action [62]. Other measures that support the patient until the inflammatory processes in the airways have resolved include supplemental oxygen, judicious fluid administration, and, when indicated, mechanical ventilation.

β_2-Adrenergic Agonists

β_2-Adrenergic agonists bind to β_2-adrenergic receptors on airway smooth muscle cells and cause relaxation of the muscle cell. Although the primary cellular target of β_2-adrenergic agonists is airway smooth muscle, other cell types in the airways also express β_2-adrenergic receptors that may regulate mediator release by mast cells, epithelial cells, and nerves.

There are two general classes of β_2-adrenergic agonists. Short-acting β_2-adrenergic agonists (SABA) have bronchodilatory effects that last for 3 to 5 hours. They include epinephrine, isoproterenol, terbutaline, metaproterenol, albuterol, and fenoterol. These short-acting agents have an onset of action less than 5 minutes and are the mainstay of bronchodilator therapy for acute asthma. These agents differ in their selectivity for β_2-adrenergic receptors, the rank order of selectivity being epinephrine < isoproterenol < metaproterenol < fenoterol, terbutaline, and albuterol [63]. However, all of these agents have approximately equal efficacy in the treatment of asthma. Another class of drugs, the long-acting β_2-adrenergic agonists (LABA), have bronchodilatory effects for at least 12 hours, but these agents are not currently recommended in the treatment of acute exacerbations [1,2,44]. There has been significant controversy on whether chronic use of these long-acting agents predisposes patients to increased severe, life-threatening, or fatal asthma exacerbations [64].

Among the short-acting β_2-adrenergic agonists, a single-isomer preparation (i.e., R-albuterol or levalbuterol) is available. The potential advantage of this preparation is that the S-enantiomer present in racemic albuterol, does not contribute to bronchodilation and might have deleterious effects in the airways. However, although some studies of levalbuterol (R-albuterol) in the emergency department setting have suggested that levalbuterol is a more efficacious bronchodilator than racemic preparations, there have been no large, randomized, double-blind and controlled trials in adults to confirm these findings [65–67].

The major side effects of β_2-adrenergic agonists during the treatment of severe asthma exacerbations are tremor, cardiac stimulation, and hypokalemia [68]. Case reports have associated lactic acidosis with the use of β_2-adrenergic agonists as well [69]. These side effects are potentially serious, especially in the elderly, who frequently have underlying cardiac disease. Cardiac toxicity can be minimized by using agonists with high β_2-adrenergic receptor selectivity, by avoiding systemic administration of β_2-adrenergic agonists, and by maintaining adequate oxygenation [50,70].

β_2-Adrenergic agonists can be administered to patients by inhaled, subcutaneous, or intravenous routes. Numerous studies have shown that the bronchodilator effects of inhaled β_2-adrenergic agonists are rapid in onset and equal to the effect achieved by systemic delivery [71]. Because the inhaled route allows administration of comparatively small doses directly to the airways with minimal systemic toxicity, this route is almost always preferable to systemic delivery [1,2].

Several options exist for the delivery of inhaled β_2-adrenergic agonists (see Chapter 62). A small-volume nebulizer is widely used. However, studies have shown that metered-dose inhalers (MDIs) equipped with spacer devices are as effective as small-volume nebulizers in the treatment of acute asthma, although some patients may have difficulty coordinating MDI use, especially during an acute exacerbation with severe respiratory distress [1,72,73]. Frequent, multiple inhalations of the medication may allow for progressively deeper penetration of the drug into peripheral airways [74]. In fact, continuous administration by nebulizer may be more effective in severely obstructed patients [75,76]. For administration of inhaled albuterol in the treatment of severe exacerbations of asthma, National Institutes of Health guidelines recommend treatment with MDI (90 μg per puff; four to eight puffs every 20 minutes up to 4 hours, then every 1 to 4 hours as needed) or nebulizer treatments, either intermittent (2.5 to 5.0 mg every 20 minutes for 3 doses, then every 1 to 4 hours as needed) or continuous (10 to 15 mg per hour) [1] (see Management section).

Intermittent positive-pressure breathing devices to deliver aerosols were once popular but are not used today because many patients with severe asthma cannot tolerate the device and because the devices are no more effective than small-volume nebulizers [77]. Furthermore, the risk of barotrauma is significantly increased with intermittent positive-pressure breathing devices, and pneumothorax resulting in death has been reported [78].

Because of its lower density than oxygen, heliox-powered nebulizer treatments have the potential to improve penetration of aerosols into the lungs. Adult patients with severe asthma exacerbations had greater improvements in peak expiratory flow rates and dyspnea scores when albuterol was delivered using heliox, rather than oxygen, driven nebulization [79,80]. Current National Institute of Health Guidelines suggest that heliox-driven albuterol nebulization be considered for patients with life-threatening exacerbations or for those with severe exacerbations even after 1 hour of intensive conventional therapy [1].

Theoretically, systemic administration of beta-adrenergic agonists could deliver drugs via the bloodstream to obstructed airways that are poorly accessible to inhaled aerosols. However, this theoretical advantage has not been supported by most studies [71]. Subcutaneous epinephrine (adults, 0.3 mL of a 1 to 1,000 solution every 20 minutes for three doses) was a traditional therapy for acute asthma in emergency departments, but it is not more effective than aerosol delivery of β_2-adrenergic agonists [81]. A major concern with the use of subcutaneous epinephrine in adults has been cardiac toxicity [82]. More selective β_2-adrenergic agonists, such as terbutaline, are available for subcutaneous use, but cardiac toxicity in elderly individuals is still a significant concern even with these more selective agents. Formerly, intravenous isoproterenol (0.05 to 1.50 μg per kg per minute) was often used to treat severe exacerbations of asthma [83]. However, intravenous delivery of β_2-adrenergic agonists is no longer recommended for the routine treatment of even severe exacerbations of asthma [1,2]. No convincing evidence has shown intravenous administration to be superior to inhaled delivery of β_2-adrenergic agonists. The lack of enhanced efficacy and the potential cardiac toxicity of intravenous β_2-adrenergic agonists have led most authorities to reserve intravenous delivery for those rare patients who continue to deteriorate on mechanical ventilation despite maximal routine therapy with inhaled β_2-adrenergic agonists [83]. Intravenous β_2-adrenergic agonists should be used only in closely monitored adults because myocardial ischemia can occur [84]. It is important to emphasize again that intravenous β_2-adrenergic agonists are not recommended in current NIH guidelines and are unlikely to be any more effective than inhaled β_2-adrenergic agonists such as albuterol [1].

Cholinergic Antagonists

The muscarinic cholinergic antagonists (e.g., atropine, ipratropium and tiotropium) are less effective and more slowly acting bronchodilators than β_2-adrenergic agonists [85–87]. In general, these agents should not be used as the sole bronchodilator therapy for acute asthma. Exceptions may be bronchospasm induced by acetylcholinesterase inhibitors or β_2-adrenergic antagonists and patients with severe cardiac disease who are unable to tolerate β_2-adrenergic agonists.

However, inhaled cholinergic antagonists have a low incidence of side effects and are a recommended adjunct to β_2-adrenergic agonists in the initial emergency department treatment of severe exacerbations of asthma [1,88]. Because even small improvements in airflow could prove clinically significant in the severely obstructed and deteriorating patient, it is recommended that ipratropium be routinely added to β_2-adrenergic agonist therapy during the initial treatment of severe asthma exacerbations in the emergency department [1] (see Management section). However, although comparable trials for adults do not exist, controlled trials in children have not shown a benefit of continuing ipratropium treatment once the patient is hospitalized [89,90]. Therefore, inhaled ipratropium bromide currently is not recommended for hospitalized patients with severe exacerbations of asthma [1]. The long-acting anticholinergic, tiotropium, has a role in treating outpatients with difficult to control asthma, but whether it has a role in treating hospitalized patients with acute exacerbations of asthma is not yet known [91].

Methylxanthines

Because the literature does not demonstrate a benefit to adding methylxanthines to β_2-adrenergic agonists in the acute setting [92,93] and because they increase toxicity [92], methylxanthines are no longer recommended in the treatment of asthma exacerbations [1]. Whether newer, less toxic, subtype selective phosphodiesterase inhibitors have a role in the management of acute asthma exacerbations remains to be studied.

For rare patients whose condition is deteriorating despite maximal routine recommended therapy with bronchodilators, corticosteroids and other adjuncts [1], the use of methylxanthines might be considered by some physicians. For patients not already taking methylxanthines, a loading dose of aminophylline (6 mg per kg lean body weight) can be administered during 20 to 30 minutes, followed by an intravenous infusion at the rate of 0.6 mg per kg per hour. This infusion rate should be decreased if conditions are present that decrease methylxanthine clearance, especially congestive heart failure, cirrhosis, and the use of cimetidine, ranitidine, allopurinol, oral contraceptives, erythromycin, ciprofloxacin, or norfloxacin. Six hours after initiation of the infusion, the serum theophylline level should be checked and the infusion rate adjusted accordingly, with 10 to 15 μg per mL being therapeutic. Serum concentrations greater than 20 μg per mL are toxic.

Corticosteroids

Numerous studies have documented the safety and effectiveness of short courses of corticosteroids in the treatment of acute exacerbations of asthma [1,2,61,94–96]. Their beneficial effects are attributed to their many potent anti-inflammatory effects on multiple cell types [97]. Corticosteroids inhibit inflammatory cytokine release by macrophages and T cells; decrease expression of endothelial cell adhesion molecules to inhibit migration of inflammatory cells into the airway; increase neutral endopeptidase expression to enhance degradation of neuropeptides that regulate inflammation; decrease mast cells, eosinophils, and CD4+ T lymphocytes in the airway submucosa; and decrease secretions from gland cells [97].

Systemic corticosteroids are the principal therapy for acute exacerbations of asthma [1,2,61]. Prednisone, prednisolone, and methylprednisolone are the preferred agents. Compared with betamethasone and dexamethasone, neither prednisone nor methylprednisolone contain metabisulfites and both have shorter half-lives. Although hydrocortisone has the shortest half-life, it has greater mineralocorticoid effect and may cause idiosyncratic bronchospasm in some aspirin-sensitive individuals [98].

The optimal route of corticosteroid administration in the treatment of acute asthma is not well established by double-blind, placebo-controlled clinical studies. For initial treatment of an acute exacerbation of asthma, several studies suggest that oral administration of corticosteroids is as effective as intravenous therapy [1,2,61,99,100]. The oral route is preferred unless there is the possibility of impaired gastrointestinal tract transit time or absorption [1,2].

Currently, inhaled corticosteroids do not have a well-established role in the treatment of acute exacerbations of asthma in hospitalized patients [1,2,61,101]. However, mounting evidence suggests that inhaled corticosteroids are an effective addition to albuterol in the acute setting and they effectively prevent relapses of asthma after discharge from the emergency room [1,2,102,103]. Inhaled corticosteroids may have topical effects that rapidly (less than 3 hours) vasoconstrict bronchial mucosal blood vessels and this could be one rapid mechanism of relieving airway obstruction, at least partially [104].

The optimum dosages of corticosteroids for the treatment of acute asthma are not well established by randomized controlled clinical trials either [1,2,61,105]. One study compared 15, 40, and 125 mg methylprednisolone every 6 hours and suggested that patients improved most rapidly with the 125-mg dose [106]. However, most studies have failed to show a dose-response relationship for doses this high [105]. For example, one study showed no difference between 100 and 500 mg methylprednisolone in the emergency department treatment of asthma [107].

For adults, NIH guidelines recommend that prednisone, methylprednisolone or prednisolone all be given at 40 to 80 mg per day in one or two divided doses until PEFR is 70% of predicted or personal best [1]. GINA guidelines describe appropriate dosing as the equivalent of 60–80 mg of methylprednisolone as a single daily dose, with 40 mg of methylprednisolone being adequate in most cases [2]. According to NIH guidelines the duration of systemic corticosteroid treatment for a patient requiring an emergency department visit or a hospitalization is usually 3 to 10 days [1]. GINA guidelines recommend a 7-day course for adults [2]. For courses lasting less than 1 week and for treatment courses lasting up to 10 days, there is no established benefit to slowly tapering the daily oral corticosteroid dose, especially if the patient is also using inhaled corticosteroids [1,2,61].

Oxygen

Supplemental oxygen therapy should be the initial intervention in the emergency department [1,2]. Because $\dot{V}/\dot{Q}$ mismatch is the dominant cause of hypoxemia in asthma, the PaO_2 usually increases readily in response to low levels (2 to 4 L per minute oxygen by nasal prongs) of supplemental oxygen therapy. In addition to mitigating the cardiac and neurologic complications of severe hypoxemia, low-flow supplemental oxygen minimizes potential episodes of hypoxemia due to the acute administration of β_2-adrenergic agonists, decreases elevated pulmonary vascular pressures due to hypoxic vasoconstriction, decreases bronchospasm due to hypoxia, and improves oxygen delivery to respiratory muscles. Although low-flow oxygen is beneficial, the routine use of 100% oxygen to treat acute asthma should be avoided because this is usually not necessary and some evidence suggests that it may cause carbon dioxide retention [108].

Fluids

No convincing evidence has shown that fluid administration in excess of euvolemia hastens mobilization of inspissated secretions in the airways [1]. Fluid therapy should be used conservatively unless significant dehydration is present.

Other Agents

Intravenous magnesium sulfate (for adults, 2 g $MgSO_4$ in 50 mL saline during 20 minutes) has bronchodilator properties and it has been recommended that emergency department physicians consider its use in the treatment of severe asthma exacerbations [1,2]. The NIH guidelines recommend that it be used as adjunct treatment only in life-threatening exacerbations and in cases refractory to initial intensive conventional therapy because it may sometimes help to avoid intubation. Although no major adverse events have been associated with $MgSO_4$ in this setting, guidelines do not recommend its routine use in the treatment of severe acute asthma exacerbations in general because results of meta-analyses remain mixed [1,2,109–111]. Additional study is needed, but some evidence suggests that its use may reduce hospitalization rates in the most severely obstructed patients who have an FEV_1 less than 25% of predicted [112]. Inhaled, rather than intravenous, magnesium sulfate may also have a role in the treatment of acute asthma. That is, there is some evidence to suggest that albuterol nebulized in magnesium sulfate solution may be a more effective bronchodilator than albuterol nebulized in normal saline [113].

Neither GINA nor NIH asthma guidelines recommend helium–oxygen therapy for routine treatment of acute asthma exacerbations [1,2]. Some improvement in airway resistance may be achieved by delivering a mixture of helium and oxygen gases (heliox) to patients, but its role in the routine treatment of acute asthma remains unestablished [114,115]. However, other evidence does support a different role for heliox in the treatment of acute asthma and that is to improve the delivery of inhaled beta-adrenergic agonists, such as albuterol [79,80]. Current NIH guidelines suggest that heliox-driven albuterol nebulization be considered for life-threatening exacerbations or those exacerbations refractory to intensive conventional therapy [1].

Some therapeutic agents that are used in the treatment of stable asthma have no established role in the treatment of severe exacerbations of asthma in hospitalized patients. These include aerosolized corticosteroids and sodium cromolyn as well as oral β_2-adrenergic agonists, which may cause significant systemic toxicities. Although there is as yet no established role for the use of leukotriene antagonists in the treatment of acute asthma exacerbations, some evidence suggests a possible role and need for further study [116]. Mucus is an important cause of airway obstruction in acute exacerbations of asthma, but the routine use of mucolytics, such as acetylcysteine, potassium iodide, or human recombinant deoxyribonuclease (DNase), has not been shown to be effective in treating severe exacerbations of asthma, and at least one of these agents, acetylcysteine, may worsen cough and bronchospasm [117]. However, it is notable that acetylcysteine and DNase may be helpful during therapeutic bronchoscopy (see Additional and Unconventional Management Measures section).

Bacterial infections appear to play, at most, a minor role in the precipitation of severe asthma exacerbations [1,2,118]; for this reason, antibiotics are not routinely administered unless an active bacterial infectious process, particularly pneumonia and bacterial sinusitis, is suspected. However, intriguing evidence suggests that infections due to *Mycoplasma pneumoniae* [119] or *Chlamydia pneumoniae* [120] might play an important role in the pathogenesis of asthma and could be a precipitant of asthma exacerbations. Further work is needed to resolve this important issue.

Unless a patient is mechanically ventilated, sedatives and narcotics have no role in the treatment of severe exacerbations of asthma [1,2]. These agents depress the respiratory central drive to breathe that is critical for adequate minute ventilation. Theoretically, narcotics also may cause mast cell degranulation and worsen bronchospasm.

MANAGEMENT

Emergency Department

The National Asthma Education and Prevention Program, conducted under the auspices of the National Institutes of Health, published guidelines for the assessment and management of patients with acute exacerbations of asthma [1]. These guidelines have been widely accepted and we recommend them. Initial management of a patient with an acute exacerbation of asthma is based on the physician's assessment of the degree of airway obstruction and the patient's response to initial bronchodilator therapy using β_2-adrenergic agonists. If, in the initial assessment, the patient is in extreme distress and has evidence of fatigue, impaired consciousness, or hypercapnia such that respiratory arrest is judged imminent, endotracheal intubation and mechanical ventilation should be the first priorities and then systemic corticosteroids and nebulized β_2-adrenergic agonists and ipratropium should be started immediately. On the other hand, if respiratory arrest is not impending within minutes, 2 to 4 L per minute of supplemental oxygen should be initiated to keep oxygen saturation greater than 90%; β_2-adrenergic agonists should be delivered by aerosol for three doses over 60 to 90 minutes (e.g., albuterol, 2.5 to 5.0 mg, every 20 minutes by small-volume nebulizer for 3 doses, then 2.5 to 10 mg every 1 to 4 hours as needed, or 10 to 15 mg per hour continuously or, alternatively, albuterol, 90 μg per puff, four to eight puffs by MDI with spacer every 20 minutes up to 4 hours, then every 1 to 4 hours as needed). If the PEFR is less than 50% of the predicted value, an oral systemic corticosteroid should be started immediately and an inhaled anticholinergic as well (e.g., ipratropium bromide, 0.5 mg by nebulizer every 20 minutes for three doses and then every 2 to 4 hours as needed). After these treatments are initiated, a more detailed history and physical and laboratory examination can be completed. Close monitoring and repeated airflow measurements are critical for detecting further deterioration during this initial period of treatment.

After the initial treatment with a bronchodilator, patients are reassessed. Those who do not respond substantially (FEV_1 or PEFR greater than 70% of predicted) within 1 hour to initial treatment with β_2-adrenergic agonists should be given systemic corticosteroids (if not already given). Oral prednisone is generally recommended unless there is concern that gastrointestinal tract absorption will be less than optimal [1,2].

In addition to corticosteroids, treatment with β_2-adrenergic agonists and inhaled anticholinergics is continued for 1 to 3 hours with frequent reassessment. Patients who achieve an FEV_1 or PEFR of greater than 70% during this 1- to 3-hour period should be observed for at least 1 additional hour to ensure stability of the improvement. In one study, two thirds of patients who presented to the emergency department responded to albuterol, with the FEV_1 increasing to at least 60% of predicted [121]. Most patients with such a good response do not require hospitalization. Exceptions are patients with a history that is suggestive of high risk for mortality from asthma (e.g., history of intubation and mechanical ventilation; Table 48.4). Patients discharged from the emergency department should be continued on systemic corticosteroids and β_2-adrenergic agonists, considered for initiation of inhaled corticosteroids, given instructions on medication use, given an action plan in case symptoms worsen, and given specific instructions on medical follow-up [1,2,44,122].

Patients who have an FEV_1 or PEFR that is greater than 40% but less than 70% after 4 hours of treatment have an incomplete response and require a careful triage decision. Some patients do well if discharged with detailed instructions, close medical follow-up, and continued systemic corticosteroids. However, other patients do poorly if discharged. It has been recommended that patients with incomplete responses be hospitalized when there is any clinical feature to suggest high risk for asthma mortality (Table 48.4). Patients with an FEV_1 or PEFR of less than 40% of predicted after 4 hours of intensive bronchodilator therapy (poor response) should be hospitalized, often in an intensive care unit (ICU) setting.

TABLE 48.4

FACTORS FAVORING HOSPITALIZATION AFTER INITIAL BRONCHODILATOR THERAPY

Poor response to initial therapy
OR
Incomplete response to initial therapy and one or more of the following:
History of endotracheal intubation or ICU admission for asthma
Recent emergency department visit for asthma
Recent hospitalization for asthma
Multiple emergency department visits for asthma in last year
Duration of current exacerbation >1 wk
Current use of oral corticosteroids
Home situation inadequate for follow-up
Psychiatric conditions that may interfere with medical compliance
History of syncope or seizures during prior exacerbations

Treatment During Pregnancy

Pregnancy should not alter treatment of an uncomplicated acute exacerbation of asthma. Because severe asthma exacerbations have been associated with increased perinatal mortality, probably due to maternal hypoxia and respiratory alkalosis [123,124], the excellent control of asthma should be a main priority [125–127] (see Chapter 51). However, unfortunately, many pregnant women are suboptimally treated for asthma in the acute setting [128]. This is unfortunate because, in both the chronic and the acute setting, abundant evidence supports the safety of β_2-adrenergic agonist use during pregnancy [125]. Also, although chronic administration of systemic corticosteroids throughout pregnancy appears to carry some risk to the fetus [129], short courses of corticosteroids are considered safe for the fetus compared with the serious risks associated with poorly controlled asthma. Therefore, corticosteroids should not be withheld from pregnant women who present with an acute asthma exacerbation. Treatment of chronic asthma during pregnancy should include inhaled corticosteroids [130,131], which is important for preventing development of acute asthma exacerbations [132].

Routine Inpatient Management

Most patients with severe exacerbations of asthma who are admitted to the hospital can be monitored and managed safely on a hospital ward that is well staffed by physicians, experienced nursing personnel, and respiratory therapists. However, patients with severe airway obstruction who are at high risk for mortality from asthma, especially those with an elevated $PaCO_2$ (greater than 42 mm Hg) or changes in mental status despite initial intensive bronchodilator therapy, need the close monitoring of an ICU setting for possible intubation and mechanical ventilation.

Pharmacotherapy for hospitalized patients includes a continuation of the inhaled β_2-adrenergic agonists and systemic corticosteroids begun in the emergency department [1,2]. Specifically, it is not recommended that ipratropium bromide be routinely continued once a patient is hospitalized [1]. For patients with severe airway obstruction and only transient relief from treatment, inhaled β_2-adrenergic agonists can be administered frequently as needed (e.g., every 20 minutes). For patients with less severe obstruction or those with intolerable side effects, frequency can be reduced accordingly. Most patients require β_2-adrenergic agonists a minimum of every 4 hours; however, a recent study has shown that ad libitum administration of albuterol every 4 hours is as effective as regularly timed administration of albuterol [133]. Evidence indicates that delivery of β_2-adrenergic agonists by small-volume nebulizer and delivery by MDI with spacer give equivalent results [1,2,72].

Most hospitalized patients begin to show improvement in expiratory airflow after 6 to 12 hours of systemic corticosteroid therapy, but improvement sufficient for hospital discharge frequently takes 2 to 7 days [134]. In one series, mean length of hospital stay was 4 days, with a range of 0.5 to 17.0 days [135]. Expiratory airflow should be measured at least twice a day to assess the patient's progress. Patient exercise tolerance and PEFR usually improve incrementally during hospitalization, but it is common for patients recovering from exacerbations to have a hospital course punctuated by periods of worsening dyspnea, especially at night. These episodes of nocturnal worsening require patient assessment but generally respond well to inhaled β_2-adrenergic agonists. When the expiratory flow rate does not improve during the initial days of hospitalization, additional or alternative diagnoses, especially laryngeal dysfunction, congestive heart failure, and pulmonary thromboembolism, as well as gastroesophageal reflux disease and sinusitis, should be considered.

As the hospitalized patient recovers, the intensity of therapy is decreased gradually. When the patient has minimal or no wheezing, is no longer awakened by dyspnea at night, can tolerate activity without oxygen desaturation of hemoglobin, and has expiratory flow rates that have substantially improved, he or she is ready for hospital discharge. Patients generally should have a PEFR at least 70% of baseline at the time of discharge. Other patients with an incomplete response to therapy (50% to 70% of baseline) should be assessed individually.

Discharge planning is important for preventing future exacerbations (Table 48.5) [1,2,122]. Patients must be educated about asthma and the importance of seeking medical advice early in the course of exacerbations. Particularly important are detailed instructions on MDI use, routine measurement of PEFR, and keeping a symptom diary at home [136]. On discharge, the patient is given medication instructions with particular attention to oral and inhaled corticosteroids (see Corticosteroids section) [61,105]. This is important, because bronchial hyperresponsiveness remains high for at least 10 days after discharge from an ICU for severe asthma [137]. Patients who have recovered from an exacerbation of asthma should be instructed to use short-acting inhaled β_2-adrenergic agonists on an as-needed basis only.

TABLE 48.5

DISCHARGE PLANNING

Medications
Inhaled β_2-adrenergic agonists
Inhaled corticosteroids
Oral corticosteroids (with plan for cessation)
Education
Avoidance of asthma triggers
Home monitoring of peak expiratory flow rates
Metered-dose inhaler techniques
Action plan if relapse starts
Appointment for medical follow-up
Asthma comanagement program

MANAGEMENT OF RESPIRATORY FAILURE

Assessment

When severe hypoxemic or hypercapnic respiratory failure is present, mechanical ventilation is potentially life-saving. Even patients with severe obstruction can be supported with mechanical ventilation for the vital hours needed for corticosteroid action. However, mechanical ventilation for a severe asthma exacerbation can be complicated by morbidity and mortality, with mortality ranging from 0% to 38% in the literature [138–140].

The decision to initiate mechanical ventilation for a severe asthma exacerbation should be based on a number of considerations individualized for each patient [140]. For patients in severe distress in whom respiratory arrest has already occurred or is imminent, the need for intubation and mechanical ventilation is obvious. The possibility of pneumothorax should be promptly addressed in these patients. Patients who are not *in extremis* should be monitored closely during initial bronchodilator therapy, and the physician should be prepared to perform intubation in case of substantial deterioration. The decision to intubate during a severe asthma exacerbation is a clinical judgment. In severely obstructed patients with decreasing objective measures of airflow, worsening mental status, or signs of respiratory muscle fatigue despite bronchodilator therapy, urgent intubation and mechanical ventilation should be strongly considered. In general, any patient who responds poorly to initial bronchodilator therapy and has an initial $PaCO_2$ of 40 mm Hg or more in association with moderately severe hypoxemia should have close serial ABG monitoring. In patients with a $PaCO_2$ of greater than 55 to 70 mm Hg, increasing $PaCO_2$ (greater than 5 mm Hg per hour) in association with a PaO_2 of less than 60 mm Hg or the presence of metabolic acidosis, intubation and mechanical ventilation should be very strongly considered [52,138]. However, it is emphasized that when clinical signs indicate a need for intubation, the decision to intubate should be made immediately and never delayed, waiting for an ABG result. The role of noninvasive positive-pressure ventilation in managing patients with acute asthma is not established and NIH asthma guidelines do not make recommendations on its application, considering it experimental at this time [1,141–143] (see Chapter 59).

Endotracheal Intubation

Airway control should be established by the most experienced personnel available because even minor manipulation of the larynx and trachea can precipitate vagal reflexes that elicit laryngospasm and bronchospasm [140]. Atropine can be given before intubation to attenuate these vagally mediated reflexes. Lidocaine can be used to achieve topical anesthesia of the hypopharynx and larynx, but even lidocaine has been associated with bronchospasm [144]. Administration of a short- and rapid-acting intravenous benzodiazepine often can facilitate patient relaxation and preoxygenation, allowing time for a controlled intubation that minimally irritates the larynx and trachea. Opiates are not used for intubation or sedation in asthmatic patients because narcotics can provoke nausea and vomiting and theoretically can provoke histamine release that worsens bronchospasm.

Oral, rather than nasal, intubation is preferred in patients with a severe asthma exacerbation because nasal polyps and sinusitis are common in asthma and because the oral route allows placement of a larger endotracheal tube (internal diameter, 8 mm). A large endotracheal tube facilitates the option of therapeutic bronchoscopy at a later time.

TABLE 48.6

GOALS OF MECHANICAL VENTILATION

Maintain oxygen saturation of hemoglobin (>90%; 95% during pregnancy)
Minimize dynamic hyperinflation
Decrease minute ventilation
Increase expiratory time
Accept hypercarbia
Monitor closely for complications of mechanical ventilation

Invasive Mechanical Ventilation

The guiding principle for mechanical ventilation during a severe exacerbation of asthma is to provide adequate oxygenation while minimizing the risk of barotrauma (Table 48.6). Because the risk of barotrauma is related to dynamic hyperinflation of the lungs and high plateau airway pressures, a ventilatory strategy that minimizes lung volumes and airway pressures should be used [1,2,6,7,140]. (See Chapter 58 for a discussion of initiating mechanical ventilation.)

With outmoded mechanical ventilation strategies that aimed to normalize the $PaCO_2$, high tidal volumes and rapid frequencies of ventilation were required, and this promoted increased air trapping and high airway pressures. Most authorities now believe that high airway pressures are to be avoided because they are a major cause of serious morbidity and mortality during mechanical ventilation of asthmatic patients [140,145–147].

The modern strategy for mechanical ventilation for a severe exacerbation of asthma is controlled hypoventilation with permissive hypercapnia [6,7,140,145–148] (see Chapter 58). This strategy does not attempt to establish a normal $PaCO_2$ as long as the minute ventilation and fraction of inspired oxygen maintain adequate tissue oxygenation. Physician acceptance of hypercapnia in this setting is termed *permissive hypercapnia* [145–147]. When possible, measurement of volume at end inspiration should be part of the management plan to monitor for the development of dynamic hyperinflation [149] (see Chapter 58).

Although the use of sodium bicarbonate to treat acidosis is controversial, advocates for its use in severe acute respiratory acidosis have regarded a pH of 7.20 to be the minimum safe level [150]. This impression and the practice of infusing sodium bicarbonate to maintain a pH of more than 7.2 is based on two uncontrolled studies in which stuporous and comatose patients with acute respiratory acidosis markedly and quickly improved when infusion of sodium bicarbonate increased the pH to greater than 7.2 [151,152]. However, no controlled studies of respiratory acidosis support the use of sodium bicarbonate to maintain a specific pH value.

The physiologic responses to metabolic and respiratory acidosis include increases in cardiac output, pulmonary arterial pressure, and heart rate, whereas systemic vascular resistance decreases and mean systemic arterial pressure remains unchanged [153–155]. In diseased lungs, PaO_2 improves [153]. The hemodynamic changes are mediated directly by endogenous secretion of catecholamines, primarily norepinephrine, stimulated by decreases in pH. The effects of sodium bicarbonate infusions on these hemodynamic responses and gas exchange have been studied. As the acidosis lessens, cardiac output and PaO_2 worsen [154,155]. Moreover, sodium bicarbonate infusions have been shown neither to improve survival nor to enhance bronchodilation. Although studies from the 1950s and 1960s suggested that endogenous epinephrine release was depressed in acidosis, more recent studies have conclusively shown that it is either unchanged or augmented [155]. Because carbon dioxide is generated when infused sodium bicarbonate buffers hydrogen ions, infusion of sodium bicarbonate predictably raises carbon dioxide tensions in blood [156]. Because carbon dioxide readily diffuses across cell membranes, sodium bicarbonate therapy may cause paradoxic intracellular acidosis [157], and this may adversely affect survival. For these reasons, we suggest use of sodium bicarbonate only when the acidosis appears to be adversely affecting the patient's hemodynamic status.

In managing patients during mechanical controlled hypoventilation with permissive hypercapnia, the minimum safe pH is not known. In three uncontrolled studies, pH values were not maintained at greater than 7.2, and outcomes did not appear to be adversely affected. Sodium bicarbonate was not given in one study unless pH was less than 7.15 [149]; in the other two studies, it was not given to any patient even when pH was 7.02 and less than 7.00 [145,158].

Neuromuscular blocking agents, such as pancuronium, vecuronium, and atracurium, can be used to help maintain low airway pressures during delivery of mechanical ventilation (see Chapter 25). Paralyzing skeletal muscles prevents the development of high airway pressures due to the patient bucking or fighting the ventilator. Notably, a side effect of neuromuscular blocking agents can be severe bronchospasm. Vecuronium is often reported to be unlikely to cause bronchospasm, but case reports suggest that vecuronium too can rarely cause bronchospasm [159]. Another adverse effect of these agents is that patients who undergo even brief neuromuscular blockade in conjunction with corticosteroid administration have a risk of developing a prolonged and sometimes severe myopathy [160]. Because all patients with severe exacerbations of asthma are treated with corticosteroids, paralyzing agents should be avoided whenever possible. For patients who cannot be managed without neuromuscular blockade, continuous infusions of neuromuscular blocking agents should be avoided and muscle function should be allowed to recover partially between repetitive boluses.

Mechanical ventilation accomplishes the work of breathing while the severely obstructed patient is treated intensively with inhaled bronchodilators and glucocorticoids. With this intensive pharmacologic therapy, mechanical ventilation usually can be discontinued in 1 to 3 days once discontinuation guidelines are met [140,161–163] (see Chapter 60). Some patients may require 2 to 4 weeks of mechanical ventilation, especially when pneumonia complicates an acute exacerbation of asthma.

Complications of Mechanical Ventilation

Serious complications have been reported as a result of mechanical ventilation for severe exacerbations of asthma [138,139,140,148]. Most of these are preventable or treatable if detected early. Problems with airway control, including traumatic and esophageal intubation, should always be anticipated. Intubation of the right mainstem bronchus is a serious problem of airway control because delivery of tidal volumes to one lung increases the risk of barotrauma. Once an airway is established and mechanical ventilation initiated, hypotension may occur because high intrathoracic pressures that occur during mechanical ventilation in severe asthma exacerbations impede venous return to the right ventricle of the heart. This is treated by administering intravenous fluids and adjusting tidal volumes, respiratory frequency, and inspiratory flow to decrease hyperinflation and intrinsic positive end-expiratory pressure [164].

Barotrauma is a major cause of morbidity and mortality among patients receiving mechanical ventilation for severe exacerbations of asthma [140,148,164]. High plateau airway pressures are associated with overdistended alveoli that rupture. Air may dissect along the bronchovascular interstitium and sometimes is evident on chest radiograph as parenchymal air cysts, linear air streaks emanating from the hila, and perivascular air halos [165,166]. As the air dissects centrally, mediastinal and subcutaneous emphysema develop. As an alternative, air from ruptured alveoli may dissect through the pleural surfaces into the pleural space to create a pneumothorax [167]. For patients on mechanical ventilation, pneumothorax progresses to tension pneumothorax rapidly and always should be treated immediately with tube thoracostomy. It must be presumed, emergently, that any pneumothorax during mechanical ventilation is under tension [168]. (See Chapter 58 for the discussion of minimizing barotrauma during mechanical ventilation.)

Mucous plugging commonly occurs during acute exacerbations of asthma. Large mucous plugs occluding the endotracheal tube should be considered when there is insurmountable difficulty in ventilating a patient. Large mucous plugs also may cause lobar or lung atelectasis that impairs gas exchange and increases airway pressures. Therapeutic bronchoscopy may be considered to relieve large mucous plugs if conservative measures, corticosteroids, and bronchodilators are not effective. Retained secretions and atelectasis also contribute to the significant risk of nosocomial pneumonia during mechanical ventilation [169].

Other complications are indirectly related to mechanical ventilation. Thromboembolism and gastric stress ulcers may occur with greater frequency in patients with severe exacerbations of asthma [170]. Arrhythmias and hypokalemia may occur during treatment for acute asthma because of therapy with sympathomimetic drugs. Hypophosphatemia may develop secondary to alkalosis [171].

Additional and Unconventional Management Measures

Even after using bronchodilators, corticosteroids, sodium bicarbonate, and mechanical ventilation, airway obstruction sometimes is sufficiently severe to prevent maintenance of an acceptable arterial pH or adequate tissue oxygenation. In these rare cases, additional, sometimes unconventional, measures can be used to support the patient until corticosteroids have had time to suppress the underlying inflammatory process. Some of these measures are based on anecdotal experience (Table 48.7).

If airway pressures remain high on mechanical ventilation despite the proper application of controlled hypoventilation with permissive hypercapnia, delivering heliox by mechanical ventilation has been suggested to allow adequate ventilation

TABLE 48.7

SPECIAL OR UNCONVENTIONAL THERAPEUTIC MEASURES

Intravenous β_2-adrenergic agonists
Methylxanthines
Helium–oxygen mixtures delivered through the ventilator
General anesthetics
Bronchoscopy with therapeutic lavage (intubated patients only)
Hypothermia
Extracorporeal life support

of the patient at reduced airway pressures [172]. Caution is necessary when using heliox in this setting because the low density of the gas mixture makes ventilator settings inaccurate (e.g., tidal volume) [173].

Bronchospasm usually is not the major factor limiting airflow in patients who are already being maximally treated for an acute exacerbation of asthma. However, for those who fail to respond to maximal conventional therapy, a variety of strategies have been advocated to maximize bronchodilation. Some reports suggest that intravenous β_2-adrenergic agonists may significantly improve airway obstruction in select patients but this treatment is not established and not recommended in current NIH asthma guidelines because of danger of cardiac toxicity [1,83,84]. General anesthetics are excellent bronchodilators and an important option for patients whose conditions are refractory to maximal routine therapy. Anecdotally, halothane [174,175], thiopental [176], ketamine [177,178], and isoflurane [179] all have been used successfully to treat patients with severe asthma exacerbations. If general anesthetics are used, an anesthesiologist should be consulted.

Because a major cause of airway obstruction during an acute exacerbation of asthma is mucous plugging, therapeutic bronchoscopy with lavage has been used as an additional supportive measure in patients who are extremely difficult to ventilate adequately [180–182]. While therapeutic bronchoscopy is not performed routinely in asthma because worsening bronchospasm is a recognized complication of bronchoscopy in asthmatics, should the need arise, a flexible bronchoscope with a large suction channel should be used, and the mechanically ventilated patient should be sedated. *N*-acetylcysteine, a mucolytic agent, is associated with bronchospasm in asthmatic patients but, anecdotally, has been used successfully during therapeutic bronchoscopy by delivering a dilute solution (less than 1%) through the bronchoscope to dissolve mucous plugs [180]. DNase (2.5 mg in 10 mL of sterile normal saline) has been administered through a bronchoscope to relieve mucous plugging causing atelectasis in a child with asthma [183].

Case reports describe unconventional measures that might be considered for the management of rare, exceedingly difficult cases. For example, hypothermia and extracorporeal life support have been methods used to support critically ill patients whose conditions are refractory to conventional therapy [184,185].

Advances in asthma, based on randomized, controlled trials or meta-analyses of such trials, are summarized in Table 48.8 [186].

TABLE 48.8

TREATMENT OF ACUTE ASTHMA: RANDOMIZED CONTROLLED TRIALS AND META-ANALYSES

- β-Adrenergic agonists are first-line therapy for acute asthma because they are rapidly acting and provide more bronchodilation than methylxanthines and cholinergic antagonists [62].
- Metered-dose inhalers with a holding chamber are at least as effective as wet nebulization for the delivery of β-adrenergic agonists in the treatment of acute asthma [72,73].
- Adding inhaled ipratropium bromide to treatment with β-adrenergic agonists provides benefit to adults with acute asthma in the emergency department [88].
- In hospitalized adult patients with acute asthma, systemic glucocorticoids speed improvement of symptoms and lung function [96].
- In addition to a short course of oral corticosteroids, initiate or continue daily inhaled corticosteroids on emergency room discharge of patients with persistent asthma [186].

References

1. National Asthma Education and Prevention Program. Expert Panel Report 3: *Guidelines for the Diagnosis and Management of Asthma*. Publication No. 08-4051. Bethesda, MD, National Institutes of Health, 2007.
2. Global Strategy for Asthma Management and Prevention. Global Initiative for Asthma (GINA), 2009. Available from www.ginasthma.org. Date last updated, 2009.
3. Boushey HA, Holtzman MJ, Sheller JR, et al: Bronchial hyperreactivity. *Am Rev Respir Dis* 121:389, 1980.
4. Dunnill MS: The pathology of asthma, with special reference to changes in the bronchial mucosa. *J Clin Pathol* 13:27, 1960.
5. Pascual R, Peters S: Airway remodeling contributes to the progressive loss of lung function in asthma: An overview. *J Allergy Clin Immunol* 116:477, 2005.
6. McFadden ER: Acute severe asthma. *Am J Respir Crit Care Med* 168:740, 2003.
7. Rodrigo GJ, Rodrigo C, Hall JB: Acute asthma in adults: a review. *Chest* 125:1081, 2004.
8. Masoli M, Fabian D, Holt S, et al: The global burden of asthma: executive summary of the GINA dissemination committee report. *Allergy* 59:469, 2004.
9. Lugogo NL, Kraft M: Epidemiology of asthma. *Clin Chest Med* 27:1, 2006.
10. Johnston NW, Sears MR: Asthma exacerbations 1: Epidemiology. *Thorax* 61:722, 2006.
11. Getahun D, Demissie K, Rhoads GG: Recent trends in asthma hospitalization and mortality in the United States. *J Asthma* 42:373, 2005.
12. Krishnan V, Diette GB, Rand CS, et al: Mortality in patients hospitalized for asthma exacerbations in the United States. *Am J Respir Crit Care Med* 174:633, 2006.
13. Bousquet J, Chanez P, Lacoste JY, et al: Eosinophilic inflammation in asthma. *N Engl J Med* 323:1033, 1990.
14. Kay AB: Pathology of mild, severe, and fatal asthma. *Am J Respir Crit Care Med* 154:566, 1996.
15. Wenzel S: Severe asthma in adults. *Am J Respir Crit Care Med* 172:149, 2005.
16. Kolbe J, Fergusson W, Garrett J: Rapid onset asthma: a severe but uncommon manifestation. *Thorax* 53:241, 1998.
17. Rodrigo GJ, Rodrigo C: Rapid-onset asthma attack: a prospective cohort study about characteristics and response to emergency department treatment. *Chest* 118:1547, 2000.
18. Plaza V, Serrano J, Picado C, et al. Frequency and clinical characteristics of rapid-onset fatal and near-fatal asthma. *Eur Respir J* 19:846, 2002.
19. McFadden ER Jr, Warren EL: Observations on asthma mortality. *Ann Intern Med* 127:142, 1997.
20. Sur S, Crotty TB, Kephart GM, et al: Sudden-onset fatal asthma: a distinct entity with few eosinophils and relatively more neutrophils in the airway submucosa? *Am Rev Respir Dis* 148:713, 1993.
21. Ober C, Hoffjan S: Asthma genetics 2006: the long and winding road to gene discovery. *Genes and Immunity* 7:95, 2006.
22. Barnes PJ: Immunology of asthma and chronic obstructive pulmonary disease. *Nat Rev Immunol* 8:183, 2008.
23. Lemanske RF, Busse WW: Asthma. *New England J Med* 344:350, 2001.
24. Rubinfield AR, Wagner PD, West JB: Gas exchange during acute experimental canine asthma. *Am Rev Respir Dis* 118:525, 1978.
25. Rodriguez-Roisin R, Ballester E, Roca J, et al: Mechanisms of hypoxemia in patients with status asthmaticus requiring mechanical ventilation. *Am Rev Respir Dis* 139:732, 1989.
26. Robert R, Ferrandis J, Malin F, et al: Enhancement of hypoxemia by right-to-left atrial shunting in severe asthma. *Intensive Care Med* 20:585, 1994.
27. Rossi A, Ganassini A, Brusasco V: Airflow obstruction and dynamic pulmonary hyperinflation, in Hall JB, Corbridge T, Rodrigo C, et al (eds): *Acute Asthma: Assessment and Management*. New York, McGraw-Hill, 2000, p 57.
28. Freedman AR, Lavietes MH: Energy requirements of the respiratory musculature in asthma. *Am J Med* 80:215, 1986.
29. Martin JG, Powell E, Shore S, et al: The role of the respiratory muscles in the hyperinflation of bronchial asthma. *Am Rev Respir Dis* 121:441, 1980.
30. Bellemare F, Grassino A: Evaluation of human diaphragm fatigue. *J Appl Physiol* 53:1196, 1982.
31. Christopher KL, Wood RP, Eckert RC, et al: Vocal-cord dysfunction presenting as asthma. *N Engl J Med* 308:1566, 1983.
32. Newman KB, Mason UG III, Schmaling KB: Clinical features of vocal cord dysfunction. *Am J Respir Crit Care Med* 152:1382, 1995.

33. Elshami AA, Tino G: Coexistent asthma and functional upper airway obstruction. *Chest* 110:1358, 1996.
34. Bahrainwala AH, Simon MR: Wheezing and vocal cord dysfunction mimicking asthma. *Curr Opin Pulm Med* 7:8, 2001.
35. O'Connell MA, Sklarew PR, Goodman DL: Spectrum of presentation of paradoxical vocal cord motion in ambulatory patients. *Ann Allergy Asthma Immunol* 74:341, 1995.
36. Perskvist N, Edston E: Differential accumulation of pulmonary and cardiac mast cell-subsets and eosinophils between fatal anaphylaxis and asthma death: a postmortem comparative study. *Forensic Sci Int* 169:43, 2007.
37. Levine GN, Powell C, Bernard SA, et al: Acute, reversible left ventricular dysfunction in status asthmaticus. *Chest* 107:1469, 1995.
38. Gelb AF, Schein A, Nussbaum E, et al: Risk factors for near-fatal asthma. *Chest* 126:1138, 2004.
39. Eisner MD, Lieu TA, Chi F, et al: Beta agonists, inhaled steroids, and the risk of intensive care unit admission for asthma. *Eur Respir J* 17:233, 2001.
40. Malmstrom K, Kaila M, Kajosaari M, et al: Fatal asthma in Finnish children and adolescents 1976-1998: validity of death certificates and a clinical description. *Pediatr Pulmonol* 42:210, 2007.
41. Dhuper S, Maggiore D, Chung V, et al: Profile of near-fatal asthma in an inner-city hospital. *Chest* 124:1880, 2003.
42. Mitchell I, Tough SC, Semple LK, et al: Near-fatal asthma: a population-based study of risk factors. *Chest* 121:1407, 2002.
43. Marquette CH, Saulnier F, Leroy O, et al: Long-term prognosis of near-fatal asthma: a 6-year follow-up study of 145 asthmatic patients who underwent mechanical ventilation for a near-fatal attack of asthma. *Am Rev Respir Dis* 146:76, 1992.
44. Camargo CA, Rachelefsky G, Schatz M: Managing asthma exacerbations in the emergency department. *Proc Am Throac Soc* 6:357, 2009.
45. Shim CS, Williams MH: Evaluation of the severity of asthma: patients versus physicians. *Am J Med* 68:11, 1980.
46. Kikuchi Y, Okabe S, Tamura G, et al: Chemosensitivity and perception of dyspnea in patients with a history of near-fatal asthma. *N Engl J Med* 330:1329, 1994.
47. Magadle R, Berar-Yanay N, Weiner P: The risk of hospitalization and near-fatal and fatal asthma in relation to the perception of dyspnea. *Chest* 121:329, 2002.
48. Barreiro E, Gea J, Sanjuś C, et al: Dyspnoea at rest and at the end of different exercises in patients with near-fatal asthma. *Eur Respir J* 24:219, 2004.
49. Eckert DJ, Catcheside PG, McEvoy RD: Blunted sensation of dyspnoea and near fatal asthma. *Eur Respir J* 24:197, 2004.
50. Suissa S, Hemmelgam B, Blais L, et al: Bronchodilators and acute cardiac death. *Am J Respir Crit Care Med* 154:1598, 1996.
51. Brenner BE, Abraham E, Simon RR: Position and diaphoresis in acute asthma. *Am J Med* 74:1005, 1983.
52. Sahn SA, Mountain RD: Clinical features and outcome in patients with acute asthma presenting with hypercapnia. *Am Rev Respir Dis* 138:535, 1988.
53. Shim CS, Williams MH: Relationship of wheezing to the severity of obstruction in asthma. *Arch Intern Med* 143:890, 1983.
54. Cohen CA, Zagelbaum G, Gross D, et al: Clinical manifestations of inspiratory muscle fatigue. *Am J Med* 73:308, 1982.
55. Nowak RM, Pensler MJ, Sarkar DD, et al: Comparison of peak expiratory flow and FEV_1 admission criteria for acute bronchial asthma. *Ann Emerg Med* 11:64, 1982.
56. Fanta CH, Rossing TH, McFadden ER: Emergency room treatment of asthma. *Am J Med* 72:416, 1982.
57. McFadden ER, Lyons HA: Arterial blood gas tensions in asthma. *N Engl J Med* 278:1027, 1968.
58. Lenhardt R, Malone A, Grant EN, et al: Trends in emergency department asthma care in metropolitan Chicago. *Chest* 124:1774, 2003.
59. Findley LJ, Sahn SA: The value of chest roentgenograms in acute asthma in adults. *Chest* 80:535, 1981.
60. Siegler D: Reversible electrocardiographic changes in severe acute asthma. *Thorax* 32:328, 1977.
61. Krishnan JA, Davis SQ, Naureckas ET, et al: An umbrella review: corticosteroid therapy for adults with acute asthma. *A J Med* 122:977, 2009.
62. Rossing T, Fanta CH, Goldstein DH, et al: Emergency therapy of asthma: comparison of the acute effects of parenteral and inhaled sympathomimetics and infused aminophylline. *Am Rev Respir Dis* 122:365, 1980.
63. Tashkin DP, Jenne JW: Alpha and beta adrenergic agents, in Weiss EB, Segal MS, Stein M (eds): *Bronchial Asthma*. Boston, Little, Brown, 604, 1985.
64. Salpeter SR, Buckley NS, Ormiston TM, et al: Meta-analysis: effect of long-acting b-agonists on severe asthma exacerbations and asthma-related deaths. *Ann Intern Med* 144:904, 2006.
65. Nowak RM, Emerman CL, Schaefer K, et al: Levalbuterol compared with racemic albuterol in the treatment of acute asthma: results of a pilot study. *Am J Emerg Med* 22:29, 2004.
66. Nowak R: Single-isomer levalbuterol: a review of the acute data. *Curr Allergy Asthma Rep* 3:172, 2003.
67. Carl JC, Myers TR, Kirchner HL, et al: Comparison of racemic albuterol and levalbuterol for treatment of acute asthma. *J Pediatr* 143:731, 2003.
68. Nogrady SG, Hartley JPR, Seaton A: Metabolic effects of intravenous salbutamol in the course of acute severe asthma. *Thorax* 32:559, 1977.
69. Maury E, Ioos V, Lepecq B, et al: A paradoxical effect of bronchodilators. *Chest* 111:1766, 1997.
70. Newhouse MT, Chapman KR, McCallum AL, et al: Cardiovascular safety of high doses of inhaled fenoterol and albuterol in acute severe asthma. *Chest* 110:595, 1996.
71. Williams SJ, Winner SJ, Clark TJH: Comparison of inhaled and intravenous terbutaline in acute severe asthma. *Thorax* 36:629, 1981.
72. Rodrigo C, Rodrigo G: Salbutamol treatment of acute severe asthma in the ED: MDI versus hand-held nebulizer. *Am J Emerg Med* 18:637, 1998.
73. Turner MO, Patel A, Ginsburg S, et al: Bronchodilator delivery in acute airflow obstruction. *Arch Intern Med* 157:1736, 1997.
74. Brittan J, Tattersfield NA: Comparison of cumulative and noncumulative techniques to measure dose-response curves for β-agonist in patients with asthma. *Thorax* 39:597, 1984.
75. Camargo CA, Spooner CH, Rowe BH: Continuous versus intermittent beta-agonists for acute asthma, The Cochrane Database of Systematic Reviews (2003) Issue 4, Art. No.: CD001115. DOI:10.1002/14651858.CD001115/.
76. Rodrigo GJ, Rodrigo C: Continuous vs intermittent β-agonists in the treatment of acute adult asthma: a systematic review with meta-analysis. *Chest* 122:160, 2002.
77. Cherniack RM, Goldberg I: The effect of nebulized bronchodilator delivered with and without IPPB on ventilatory function in chronic obstructive emphysema. *Am Rev Respir Dis* 91:13, 1965.
78. Karetsky MS: Asthma mortality associated with pneumothorax and intermittent positive-pressure breathing. *Lancet* 1:828, 1975.
79. Lee DL, Hsu CW, Lee H, et al: Beneficial effects of albuterol therapy driven by heliox versus by oxygen in severe asthma exacerbation. *Acad Emerg Med* 12:820, 2005.
80. Kim K, Saville AL, Sikes KL, et al: Heliox-driven albuterol nebulization for asthma exacerbations: An overview. *Respir Care* 51:613, 2006.
81. Fanta CH, Rossing TH, McFadden ER: Treatment of acute asthma: is combination therapy with sympathomimetics and methylxanthines indicated? *Am J Med* 80:5, 1986.
82. Bendkowski B: Effects of adrenaline injections on ECG in elderly asthmatics. *J Coll Gen Pract* 8:66, 1964.
83. Parry WH, Martorano F, Colton EK: Management of life-threatening asthma with intravenous isoproterenol infusion. *Am J Dis Child* 130:39, 1976.
84. Kurland G, Williams J, Lewiston NJ: Fatal myocardial toxicity during continuous infusion intravenous isoproterenol therapy of asthma. *J Allergy Clin Immunol* 63:407, 1979.
85. Karpel JP, Appel D, Breidbart D, et al: A comparison of atropine sulfate and metaproterenol sulfate in the emergency treatment of asthma. *Am Rev Respir Dis* 133:727, 1986.
86. Gross NJ, Skorodin MS: Anticholinergic, antimuscarinic bronchodilators: state of the art. *Am Rev Respir Dis* 129:856, 1984.
87. Storms WW, Bodman SF, Nathan RA, et al: Use of ipratropium bromide in asthma. *Am J Med* 81:61, 1986.
88. Rodrigo GJ, Castro-Rodriguez JA: Anticholinergics in the treatment of children and adults with acute asthma: a systematic review with meta-analysis. *Thorax* 60:740, 2005.
89. Craven D, Kercsmar CM, Myers TR, et al. Ipratropium bromide plus nebulized albuterol for the treatment of hospitalized children with acute asthma. *J Pediatr* 138:51–58, 2001.
90. Goggin N, Macarthur C, Parkin PC: Randomized trial of the addition of ipratropium bromide to albuterol and corticosteroid therapy in children hospitalized because of an acute asthma exacerbation. *Arch Pediatr Adolesc Med* 155:1329, 2001.
91. Peters SP, Kunselman SJ, Icitovic N, et al: Tiotropium bromide step-up therapy for adults with uncontrolled asthma. *N Engl J Med* 363:1715, 2010 (10.1056/NEJMoa1008770).
92. Siegal D, Sheppard D, Gelb A, et al: Aminophylline increases the toxicity but not the efficacy of an inhaled beta-adrenergic agonist in the treatment of acute exacerbations of asthma. *Am Rev Respir Dis* 132:283, 1985.
93. Rossing T, Fanta CH, McFadden ER, et al: A controlled trial of the use of single versus combined-drug therapy in the treatment of acute episodes of asthma. *Am Rev Respir Dis* 123:190, 1981.
94. Manser R, Reid D, Abramson M: Corticosteroids for acute severe asthma in hospitalised patients. *Cochrane Database Syst Rev* (1):CD001740, 2001.
95. Rowe BH, Spooner CH, Ducharme FM, et al: Corticosteroids for preventing relapse following acute exacerbations of asthma. *Cochrane Database Syst Rev* CD00095, 2001.
96. Fanta CH, Rossing TH, McFadden ER: Glucocorticoids in acute asthma. *Am J Med* 74:845, 1983.
97. Barnes PJ: Mechanisms of action of glucocorticoids in asthma. *Am J Respir Crit Care Med* 154:S21, 1996.
98. Partridge MR, Gibson GJ: Adverse bronchial reactions to intravenous hydrocortisone in two aspirin-sensitive asthmatic patients. *BMJ* 1:1521, 1978.
99. Ratto D, Alfaro C, Sipsey J, et al: Are intravenous corticosteroids required in status asthmaticus? *JAMA* 260:527, 1988.
100. Harrison BDW, Hart GJ, Ali NJ, et al: Need for intravenous hydrocortisone in addition to oral prednisolone in patients admitted to hospital with severe asthma without ventilatory failure. *Lancet* 1:181, 1986.
101. Edmonds ML, Camargo CA, Pollack CV, et al: The effectiveness of inhaled corticosteroids in the emergency department treatment of acute asthma: a meta-analysis. *Ann Emerg Med* 40:145, 2002.

102. Rodrigo GJ: Comparison of inhaled fluticasone with intravenous hydrocortisone in the treatment of adult acute asthma. *Am Rev Respir Crit Care Med* 171:1231, 2005.
103. Lee-Wong M, Dayrit FM, Kohli AR, et al: Comparison of high-dose inhaled flunisolide to systemic corticosteroids in severe adult asthma. *Chest* 122:1208, 2002.
104. Kumar SD, Brieva JL, Danta I, et al: Transient effect of inhaled fluticasone on airway mucosal blood flow in subjects with and without asthma. *Am J Respir Crit Care Med* 161:918, 2000.
105. McFadden ER: Dosages of corticosteroids in asthma. *Am Rev Respir Dis* 147:1306, 1993.
106. Haskell RJ, Wang BM, Hansen JE: A double-blind, randomized trial of methylprednisolone in status asthmaticus. *Arch Intern Med* 143:1324, 1983.
107. Emerman CL, Cydulka RK: A randomized comparison of 100-mg vs 500-mg dose of methylprednisolone in the treatment of acute asthma. *Chest* 107:1559, 1995.
108. Chien JW, Ciufo R, Novak R, et al: Uncontrolled oxygen administration and respiratory failure in acute asthma. *Chest* 117:728, 2000.
109. Rodrigo G, Rodrigo C, Burschtin O: Efficacy of magnesium sulfate in acute adult asthma: a meta-analysis of randomized trials. *Am J Emerg Med* 18:216, 2000.
110. Porter RS, Nester X, Braitman LE, et al: Intravenous magnesium is ineffective in adult asthma, a randomized trial. *Eur J Emerg Med* 8:9, 2001.
111. Rowe BH, Bretzlaff JA, Bourdon C, et al: Intravenous magnesium sulfate treatment for acute asthma in the emergency department: a systematic review of the literature. *Ann Emerg Med* 36:181, 2000.
112. Silverman RA, Osborn H, Runge J, et al: Acute Asthma/Magnesium Study Group. IV magnesium sulfate in the treatment of acute severe asthma: a multicenter randomized controlled trial. *Chest* 122:489, 2002.
113. Blitz M, Blitz S, Beasely R, et al: Aerosolized magnesium sulfate for acute asthma: a systematic review. *Chest* 128:337, 2005.
114. Ho AMH, Lee A, Karmakar MK, et al: Heliox vs air-oxygen mixtures for the treatment of patients with acute asthma. *Chest* 123:882, 2003.
115. Rodrigo GJ, Rodrigo C, Pollack CV, et al: Use of helium-oxygen mixtures in the treatment of acute asthma. *Chest* 123:891, 2003.
116. Camargo CA, Smithline HA, Malice MP, et al: A randomized controlled trial of intravenous montelukast in acute asthma. *Am J Respir Crit Care Med* 166:528, 2003.
117. Bernstein IL, Ausdenmoore RW: Iatrogenic bronchospasm occurring during clinical trials of a new mucolytic agent, acetylcysteine. *Dis Chest* 46:469, 1964.
118. Graham VAL, Milton AF, Knowles GK, et al: Routine antibiotics in hospital management of acute asthma. *Lancet* 2:418, 1982.
119. Martin RJ, Kraft M, Chu HW, et al: A link between chronic asthma and chronic infection. *J Allergy Clin Immunol* 107:595, 2001.
120. Allegra L, Blasi F, Centanni S, et al: Acute exacerbations of asthma in adults: role of Chlamydia pneumoniae infection. *Eur Respir J* 7:2165, 1994.
121. Strauss L, Hejal R, McFadden ER Jr, et al: Observations on the effects of aerosolized albuterol in acute asthma. *Am J Respir Crit Care Med* 155:454, 1997.
122. Schatz M, Rachelefsky G, Krishnan JA: Follow-up after acute asthma episodes. *Proc Am Thorac Soc* 6:386, 2009.
123. Gordon M, Wiswander KR, Berendes H, et al: Fetal morbidity following potentially anoxic obstetric conditions. VII: Bronchial asthma. *Am J Obstet Gynecol* 106:421, 1970.
124. Motoyama EK, Acheson F, Rivard G, et al: Adverse effects of maternal hyperventilation on the fetus. *Lancet* 1:286, 1966.
125. Schatz M, Zeiger RS, Harden KM, et al: The safety of inhaled beta-agonist bronchodilators during pregnancy. *J Allergy Clin Immunol* 82:686, 1988.
126. Schatz M, Dobrowski MP: Asthma in pregnancy. *New Engl J Med* 360: 1862, 2009.
127. Nelson-Piercy C: Asthma in pregnancy. *Thorax* 56:325, 2001.
128. Cydulka RK, Emerman CL, Schreiber D, et al: Acute asthma among pregnant women presenting to the emergency department. *Am J Respir Crit Care Med* 160:887, 1999.
129. Reinisch JM, Simon NG, Karow WG, et al: Prenatal exposure to prednisone in humans and animals retards intrauterine growth. *Science* 202:436, 1978.
130. Greenberger PA, Patterson R: Beclomethasone dipropionate for severe asthma during pregnancy. *Ann Intern Med* 98:478, 1983.
131. Joint Committee for American College of Obstetricians and Gynecologists and the American College of Allergy, Asthma and Immunology: The use of newer asthma and allergy medications during pregnancy. *Ann Allergy Asthma Immunol* 84:475, 2000.
132. Wendel PJ, Ramin SM, Barnett-Hamm C, et al: Asthma treatment in pregnancy: a randomized controlled study. *Int J Gynecol Obstet* 56:99, 1997.
133. Chandra A, Shim C, Cohen H, et al: Regular vs ad-lib albuterol for patients hospitalized with acute asthma. *Chest* 128:1115, 2005.
134. Benfield GFA, Smith AP: Predicting rapid and slow response to treatment in acute severe asthma. *Br J Dis Chest* 77:249, 1983.
135. McFadden ER Jr, Elsanadi N, Dixon L, et al: Protocol therapy for acute asthma: therapeutic benefits and cost savings. *Am J Med* 99:651, 1995.
136. Chan-Yeung M, Chang JH, Manfreda J, et al: Changes in peak flow, symptom score, and the use of medications during acute exacerbations of asthma. *Am J Respir Crit Care Med* 154:889, 1996.
137. Rabbat A, Laaban JP, Orvoen-Frija E, et al: Bronchial hyperresponsiveness following acute severe asthma. *Intensive Care Med* 22:530, 1996.
138. Dales RE, Munt PW: Use of mechanical ventilation in adults with severe asthma. *Can Med Assoc J* 130:391, 1984.
139. Darioli R, Perret C: Mechanical controlled hypoventilation in status asthmaticus. *Am Rev Respir Dis* 129:385, 1984.
140. Brenner B, Corbridge T, Kazzi A: Intubation and mechanical ventilation of the asthmatic patient in respiratory failure. *Proc Am Thorac Soc* 6:371, 2009.
141. Ram FSF, Wellington SR, Rowe BH, et al: Non-invasive positive pressure ventilation for treatment of respiratory failure due to severe acute exacerbations of asthma. Cochrane Database of Systematic Reviews 2005, Issue 3. Art. No.: CD004360. DOI: 10.1002/14651858.CD004360.pub3.
142. Mehta S, Hill NS: Noninvasive ventilation. *Am J Respir Critical Care Med* 163:540, 2001.
143. Liesching T, Kwok H, Hill NS: Acute applications of noninvasive positive pressure ventilation. *Chest* 124:699, 2003.
144. Weiss EB, Patwardham AV: The response of lidocaine in bronchial asthma. *Chest* 72:429, 1977.
145. Bellomo R, McLaughlin P, Tai E, et al: Asthma requiring mechanical ventilation: a low morbidity approach. *Chest* 105:891, 1994.
146. Feihl F, Perret C: Permissive hypercapnia. *Am J Respir Crit Care Med* 150:1722, 1994.
147. Wilmoth DF, Carpenter RM: Preventing complications of mechanical ventilation: permissive hypercapnia. *AACN Clin Issues* 7:473, 1996.
148. Lazarus SC: Emergency treatment of asthma. *N Engl J Med* 363:755, 2010.
149. Williams TJ, Tuxen DV, Scheinkestel CD, et al: Risk factors for morbidity in mechanically ventilated patients with acute severe asthma. *Am Rev Respir Dis* 146:607, 1992.
150. Menitove SM, Goldring RM: Combined ventilator and bicarbonate strategy in the management of status asthmaticus. *Am J Med* 74:898, 1983.
151. Westlake EK, Simpson T, Kaye M: Carbon dioxide narcosis in emphysema. *Q J Med* 24:155, 1955.
152. Addis GJ: Bicarbonate buffering in acute exacerbation of chronic respiratory failure. *Thorax* 20:337, 1965.
153. Brimioulle S, Vachiery J-L, Lejeune P, et al: Acid-base status affects gas exchange in canine oleic acid pulmonary edema. *Am J Physiol* 260:H1080, 1991.
154. Brofman JD, Leff AR, Munoz NM, et al: Sympathetic secretory response to hypercapnic acidosis in swine. *J Appl Physiol* 69:710, 1990.
155. Ebata T, Watanabe Y, Amaha K, et al: Haemodynamic changes during the apnoea test for diagnosis of brain death. *Can J Anaesth* 38:436, 1991.
156. Cooper DJ, Walley KR, Wiggs BR, et al: Bicarbonate does not improve hemodynamics in critically ill patients who have lactic acidosis. *Ann Intern Med* 112:492, 1990.
157. Shapiro JI, Whalen M, Kucera R, et al: Brain pH responses to sodium bicarbonate and carbicarb during systemic acidosis. *Am J Physiol* 69:710, 1990.
158. Hickling KG, Henderson SJ, Jackson R: Low mortality associated with low volume pressure limited ventilation with permissive hypercapnia in severe adult respiratory distress syndrome. *Intensive Care Med* 16:372, 1990.
159. Uratsuji Y, Konishi M, Ikegaki N, et al: Possible bronchospasm after administration of vecuronium. *Masui* 40:109, 1991.
160. Hansen-Flaschen J, Cowen J, Raps EC: Neuromuscular blockade in the intensive care unit. *Am Rev Respir Dis* 147:234, 1993.
161. Higgins B, Greening AP, Crompton GK: Assisted ventilation in severe asthma. *Thorax* 41:464, 1986.
162. Braman SS, Kaemmerlen JT: Intensive care of status asthmaticus: a 10-year experience. *JAMA* 264:366, 1990.
163. Mansel JK, Stogner SW, Petrini MF, et al: Mechanical ventilation in patients with acute severe asthma. *Am J Med* 89:42, 1986.
164. Pepe PE, Marini JJ: Occult positive end-expiratory pressure in mechanically ventilated patients with airflow obstruction: the auto-PEEP effect. *Am Rev Respir Dis* 126:166, 1982.
165. Johnson TH, Altman AR: Pulmonary interstitial gas: first sign of barotrauma due to PEEP therapy. *Crit Care Med* 7:532, 1979.
166. Jamadar DA, Kazerooni EA, Hirschl RB: Pneumomediastinum: elucidation of the anatomic pathway by liquid ventilation. *J Comput Assist Tomogr* 20:309, 1996.
167. Haake R, Schlichtig R, Ulstad DR, et al: Barotrauma. *Chest* 91:608, 1987.
168. Albelda SM, Giefter WB, Kelley MA, et al: Ventilator-induced subpleural air cysts: clinical, radiographic, and pathologic significance. *Am Rev Respir Dis* 127:360, 1983.
169. Zwillich CW: Complications of assisted ventilation: a prospective study of 354 consecutive episodes. *Am J Med* 57:161, 1974.
170. Pingleton SK, Bone RC, Pingleton WW, et al: The efficacy of low-dose heparin in prevention of pulmonary emboli in a respiratory intensive care unit. *Chest* 79:647, 1981.
171. Laaban J-P, Waked M, Laromiguiere M, et al: Hypophosphatemia complicating management of acute severe asthma. *Ann Intern Med* 112:68, 1990.
172. Gluck EH, Onorato DJ, Castriotta R: Helium-oxygen mixtures in intubated patients with status asthmaticus and respiratory acidosis. *Chest* 98:693, 1990.
173. Tassaux D, Jolliet P, Thouret JM, et al: Calibration of seven ICU ventilators for mechanical ventilation with helium-oxygen mixtures. *Am J Respir Crit Care Med* 160:22, 1999.

174. O Rourke PP, Crone RK: Halothane in status asthmaticus. *Crit Care Med* 10:341, 1982.
175. Schwartz SH: Treatment of status asthmaticus with halothane. *JAMA* 251:2688, 1984.
176. Grunberg G, Cohen JD, Keslin J, et al: Facilitation of mechanical ventilation in status asthmaticus with continuous intravenous thiopental. *Chest* 99:1216, 1991.
177. Sarma VJ: Use of ketamine in acute severe asthma. *Acta Anaesthesiol Scand* 36:106, 1992.
178. Hemming A, MacKenzie I, Finfer S: Response to ketamine in status asthmaticus resistant to maximal medical treatment. *Thorax* 49:90, 1994.
179. Maltais F, Sovilj M, Goldberg P, et al: Respiratory mechanics in status asthmaticus: effects of inhalational anesthesia. *Chest* 106:1401, 1994.
180. Millman M, Goldman AH, Goldstein IM: Status asthmaticus: use of acetylcysteine during bronchoscopy and lavage to remove mucus plugs. *Ann Allergy* 50:85, 1983.
181. Smith DL, Deshazo RD: Bronchoalveolar lavage in asthma. *Am Rev Respir Dis* 148:523, 1993.
182. Henke CA, Hertz M, Gustafson P: Combined bronchoscopy and mucolytic therapy for patients with severe refractory status asthmaticus on mechanical ventilation: a case report and review of the literature. *Crit Care Med* 22:1880, 1994.
183. Greally P: Human recombinant DNase for mucus plugging in status asthmaticus. *Lancet* 346:1423, 1995.
184. Browning D, Goodrum DT: Treatment of acute severe asthma assisted by hypothermia. *Anaesthesia* 47:223, 1992.
185. Shapiro MB, Kleaveland AC, Bartlett RH: Extracorporeal life support for status asthmaticus. *Chest* 103:1651, 1993.
186. Krishnan JA, Nowak R, Davis SQ, et al: Anti-inflammatory treatment after discharge home from the emergency department in adults with acute asthma. *Proc Am Thorac Soc* 6:380, 2009.

CHAPTER 49 ■ RESPIRATORY FAILURE PART IV: CHRONIC OBSTRUCTIVE PULMONARY DISEASE

MEYER S. BALTER AND RONALD F. GROSSMAN

Chronic obstructive pulmonary disease (COPD) is defined in the National Heart, Lung, and Blood Institute/World Health Organization Global Initiative for Chronic Obstructive Lung Disease as a disease state characterized by airflow limitation that is not fully reversible [1]. The airflow limitation is usually both progressive and associated with an abnormal inflammatory response of the lungs to noxious particles or gases. Any patient presenting with symptoms of cough, sputum production, or dyspnea, and/or a history of exposure to risk factors should be considered as having the diagnosis of COPD. The diagnosis can be confirmed by spirometry especially if the forced expired volume of air in 1 second (FEV_1) measured after inhaled bronchodilator (postbronchodilator FEV_1) is less than 80% of the predicted value in combination with an FEV_1 to forced vital capacity ratio less than 70%.

Although a variety of conditions characterized by chronic airflow obstruction have been termed "COPD," the presence of largely irreversible chronic airflow obstruction predominantly in current or former cigarette smokers is the meaning commonly used in the subsequent discussion. Emphysema is the underlying disease process that is mainly responsible for severe airflow obstruction. The distinction between chronic obstructive bronchitis, bronchiolitis, and emphysema is difficult to make with precision and is usually clinically unimportant.

COPD affects more than 5% of the adult population and is associated with increasing morbidity and mortality in the United States and other countries [2]. Mortality rates in the United States have increased from 25.6 per 100,000 population in 1979 to 40.5 per 100,000 population in 2006 [3]. Approximately 750,000 admissions to hospital annually in the United States can be directly attributed to COPD, and the costs associated with the care of all COPD patients has been estimated to be around $24 billion [4]. The World Health Organization has predicted that COPD will be the third leading cause of death and fifth leading cause of disability worldwide by 2020 [5].

ETIOLOGY

The major risk factor associated with the development of COPD is cigarette smoking [6]. The total number of pack-years of smoking correlates best with development of COPD [7,8], although the total length of time spent smoking probably contributes as well [8]. Significant COPD develops in only a minority of even heavy cigarette smokers [9], suggesting that some cofactor(s) (e.g., host susceptibility) must be important. Homozygous α_1-antitrypsin deficiency (a relatively rare condition) is a risk factor for the development of COPD [10] even in the absence of cigarette smoking. It has been estimated that approximately 60,000 patients in the United States have this condition but only a minority are treated [10]. COPD does not necessarily develop in nonsmoking patients with α_1-antitrypsin deficiency, which may explain why only a minority of patients with this condition are treated. Various other factors may increase the risk of COPD, including childhood respiratory illnesses, adenovirus infection, air pollution, the presence of increased airway reactivity, and occupational exposures [11].

PATHOPHYSIOLOGY

Pathogenesis

Respiratory bronchiolitis is the initial lesion seen in smokers [12]. The inflammatory process may progress in susceptible people to glandular enlargement in bronchi, goblet cell metaplasia, smooth muscle hypertrophy, inflammation in membranous bronchioles, worsening respiratory bronchiolitis, and parenchymal involvement with emphysema [13]. The progression of COPD is strongly associated with an increase in the volume of tissue in the wall and the accumulation of inflammatory mucous exudates in the lumen of small airways [14]. Normally, a relative balance exists between destructive proteolytic enzymes, which are released in the lung as a result of inflammation, and various inhibitory, antiproteolytic substances, which act to dampen the response and limit the damage [15]. In some cigarette smokers, there may be a genetic tendency favoring a greater inflammatory and destructive response to certain elements of cigarette smoke. Population studies show a definite familial tendency toward COPD [16], and pulmonary function comparison studies of identical twins suggest a genetic susceptibility [17].

COPD is characterized by chronic inflammation throughout the airways, parenchyma, and pulmonary vasculature. Macrophages, T lymphocytes (predominately CD8+), and neutrophils are increased in various parts of the lung [18]. Activated inflammatory cells release a variety of mediators—including leukotriene B4, interleukin-8, tumor necrosis factor-α, and others—capable of damaging lung structures and/or sustaining neutrophilic inflammation [5]. There is a relationship between the extent of airway occlusion by inflammatory mucus exudates and the severity of COPD [14].

Physiologic Derangements

Expiratory airflow obstruction results from structural airway narrowing as well as functional narrowing due to loss of radial distending forces on the airways. Inflammatory edema, excessive mucus, and glandular hypertrophy are responsible for intrinsic obstruction of airways. Destruction of alveolar walls causes loss of elastic recoil and airflow obstruction, which increases in a dynamic fashion with expiratory effort.

The pathophysiologic consequences of severe, chronic airflow obstruction in the lung include (a) reduced flow rates that limit minute ventilation; (b) maldistributed ventilation, resulting in wasted ventilation (high ventilation-perfusion [$\dot{V}/\dot{Q}$] mismatch) and impaired gas exchange (low $\dot{V}/\dot{Q}$ mismatch) [19]; (c) increased airway resistance, which causes increased work of breathing [19]; and (d) air trapping and hyperinflation, which alter the geometry of the respiratory muscles and place them at a mechanical disadvantage. The maximum force that they are capable of generating is decreased, which may predispose them to fatigue [20]. In addition to these factors, some patients with COPD may have a blunted respiratory center drive, which further predisposes them to carbon dioxide retention [21].

DIAGNOSIS

The diagnosis of COPD is based on clinical grounds but confirmed by pulmonary function tests (PFTs). Arterial blood gas (ABG) values determine the diagnosis of respiratory failure. Clinical findings are used primarily to suggest the diagnosis, which then must be confirmed on the basis of laboratory findings.

History and Physical Examination

A chronic productive cough and dyspnea on exertion are the two symptoms most commonly associated with COPD. However, a history of a chronic productive cough is nonspecific and may result from a variety of other conditions. Previous studies indicated that there was little correlation found between a chronic productive cough (reflecting large-airway mucus hypersecretion) and the development of significant airflow limitation (predominantly a manifestation of disease of small airways less than 2 mm in diameter) [22]. However, recent studies have shown a consistent association between chronic mucus hypersecretion and both an accelerated decline in FEV_1 and an increased risk of subsequent hospitalization [23]. A history of dyspnea on exertion in a heavy cigarette smoker should always raise the possibility of COPD, which can then be confirmed by objective investigations.

The physical examination can distinguish patients who should undergo objective laboratory testing, but it is less accurate than PFTs in detecting and quantifying the severity of COPD [24]. The most useful physical finding is a definite decrease in breath sound intensity [25,26]. Other suggestive clinical signs include hyperinflation, prolonged forced expiratory time, and wheezing.

A combative, confused, or obtunded patient should alert the physician to the possibility of hypercapnia or hypoxia. Respiratory muscle fatigue is heralded by new onset of paradoxical respiratory motion or respiratory alternans [27]. During normal inspiration, the rib cage moves upward and outward, and the anterior abdominal wall moves outward. With diaphragmatic fatigue, the anterior abdominal wall may move inward during inspiration and outward during expiration. *Respiratory alternans* describes alternate abdominal (diaphragmatic) breathing and rib cage (intercostal) breathing. When overt, this condition can be detected clinically by observing dramatic shifts in relative movement of the abdomen and rib cage every few breaths.

Radiology

Radiographic findings may include (a) hyperinflation with flattened diaphragmatic domes and increased retrosternal and retrocardiac air space; (b) one of two distinctly different bronchovascular patterns, vascular attenuation or prominence of lung markings; (c) enlarged hilar pulmonary arteries and right ventricular enlargement; and (d) regional hyperlucency and bullae [28]. Radiographic studies have low sensitivity for the diagnosis of mild COPD [29].

Computed tomography scanning of the chest is superior to the chest radiograph in diagnosing emphysema and determining the nature and the extent of the disease [29]. Centrilobular emphysema is characterized by the upper lobe distribution of focal areas of low attenuation usually less than 1 cm in diameter. Panlobular emphysema is frequently more recognized in the lower lobes and there is a generalized decrease in lung markings with few blood vessels.

In patients presenting with acute deterioration in respiratory status, a chest radiograph may exclude reversible conditions such as pneumonia, pleural effusion, pneumothorax, atelectasis, and pulmonary edema. However, the diagnostic yield of routine radiographs is low [30]. In the intensive care unit (ICU), technical factors limit the quality of the chest films, making interpretation of a portable anteroposterior film even more difficult. Nevertheless, these studies provide valuable information, particularly in patients receiving mechanical ventilation.

Pulmonary Function Tests

A decrease in the ratio of FEV_1 to forced vital capacity is the hallmark of obstructive airways disease and is useful in the diagnosis of mild disease. However, it is the FEV_1 that is correlated with clinical outcome and mortality [23]. Hypercapnic respiratory failure from COPD is extremely unlikely unless FEV_1 is less than 1.3 L [31] and is usually not observed unless FEV_1 is less than 1 L. COPD is also associated with an increase in total lung capacity and residual volume and a reduction in carbon monoxide diffusing capacity [32].

PFTs are essential for the diagnosis and estimating the severity of COPD; on the other hand, ABG values provide the data necessary to diagnose and quantitate the severity of respiratory failure. The patient with severe COPD typically presents with an elevated arterial carbon dioxide tension ($PaCO_2$), substantially decreased arterial oxygen tension (PaO_2), and an alveolar–arterial oxygen tension gradient that is significantly increased [33].

DIFFERENTIAL DIAGNOSIS

Asthma, cystic fibrosis, bronchiectasis, and bronchiolitis obliterans all can cause expiratory airflow obstruction. A previous PFT demonstrating reversibility of the airflow obstruction, younger age, presence of blood or sputum eosinophilia, absence of cigarette smoking, and presence of expiratory and inspiratory monophonic wheezing are all suggestive of asthma. Cystic fibrosis is diagnosed on the basis of a positive sweat chloride test in a patient with obstructive lung disease, positive family history for cystic fibrosis, or pancreatic insufficiency. Bronchiectasis may be suggested by a history of copious sputum production, by recurrent chest infections or hemoptysis, or from the chest radiograph.

FACTORS CAUSING AN EXACERBATION OF CHRONIC OBSTRUCTIVE PULMONARY DISEASE

According to WHO/NHLBI Global Initiative for Chronic Obstructive Lung Disease (GOLD) document an acute exacerbation is defined as "an event in the natural course of the disease characterized by a change in the patient's baseline dyspnea, cough, and/or sputum that is beyond normal day-to-day variations, is acute in onset, and may warrant a change in regular medications in a patient with underlying COPD" [34]. This can be accompanied by a change in the color and consistency of the expectorated sputum, a feature that is predictive of bacterial infection [35]. Expiratory airflow obstruction is worsened, the work of breathing increases, and mucus production or mucociliary clearance, or both, are altered. Although many factors may be associated with an acute exacerbation (Table 49.1), the most commonly identified cause is an acute upper or lower respiratory tract infection that may be viral or bacterial in etiology [36]. Spirometry shows worsened expiratory airflow obstruction, whereas ABGs usually demonstrate an additional decrease in the PaO_2 and, in patients with severe COPD, development or worsening of arterial hypercapnia. Systemic effects such as fever and neutrophilia are uncommon, and the chest radiograph typically shows no new abnormality.

Some of the other factors listed in Table 49.1 may be easily recognizable, such as a large pneumothorax or pneumonia, but others may be subtle, such as an electrolyte abnormality or unrecognized use of drugs that can cause respiratory center depression. Furthermore, events such as pulmonary embolism may go totally unrecognized because clinical findings such as dyspnea or tachypnea may be attributed to the underlying COPD itself [37] and may be more common than previously thought [38].

TREATMENT

Treatment of the patient with COPD involves chronic management of the stable patient, treatment of acute exacerbations (Table 49.1), and treatment of respiratory failure.

TABLE 49.1

DIFFERENTIAL DIAGNOSIS OF ACUTE DECOMPENSATION IN CHRONIC OBSTRUCTIVE PULMONARY DISEASE

Air pollution
Aspiration
Bronchiolitis
Carcinoid syndrome
Cardiac arrhythmia
Chest wall injury (e.g., rib fracture)
Cigarette smoking
Cystic fibrosis
Lymphangitic carcinomatosis
Metabolic derangements (e.g., hypophosphatemia)
Parasitic infections
Pleural effusion
Pneumonia
Pneumothorax
Pulmonary edema
Pulmonary embolism
Sedation
Surgery
Systemic illness
Tracheobronchial infection
Upper respiratory tract infection

Chronic Management

Once COPD is diagnosed, smoking cessation is the most important and obvious first step in management. The annual decline in FEV_1 has been demonstrated to be less in ex-smokers than in current smokers [6]. The success of smoking cessation programs is limited, with a 70% to 80% relapse rate in the first year. However, nicotine replacement therapy, the antidepressant bupropion, and repeated counseling are effective in increasing quit rates [39]. The addition of varenicline, an $\alpha_4\beta_2$ nicotinic receptor partial agonist, has improved cigarette-smoking quit rates [40]. Annual influenza vaccination is a useful, cost-effective preventive measure and has been shown to decrease morbidity and mortality related to influenza even among patients with chronic respiratory disease [41,42]. Data regarding the benefit of pneumococcal vaccination are limited to bacteremic pneumococcal infection, but a decrease in hospitalizations and deaths among vaccinated patients with COPD has been observed in observational studies [43].

Inhaled bronchodilators improve airflow obstruction, although to a less marked degree than in asthmatic patients, and improve exercise capacity and quality of life [44]. Although β-agonists and the anticholinergic agent ipratropium bromide are efficacious, the combination is more effective than either of the two agents alone [45]. Long-acting β_2-adrenergic agonists in combination with ipratropium or theophylline are superior to either agent alone, and a long-acting β_2-adrenergic agonist combined with ipratropium is more effective than the short-acting β_2-adrenergic agonist plus ipratropium [46,47]. A long-acting β_2-adrenergic agonist appears to offer the additional benefit of extending the time to an exacerbation [47]. Long-acting anticholinergics have been demonstrated to improve lung function, reduce exacerbations, and improve health-related quality of life [48,49]. In addition to some bronchodilator effects, theophylline may have beneficial effects on diaphragmatic strength, resistance to fatigue, and central nervous system (CNS) respiratory drive [50,51]. This agent produces a clinical benefit in some patients with COPD [52] but, with its narrow therapeutic window, the potential for toxicity must be recognized. All categories of bronchodilators have been shown to increase exercise capacity in COPD without necessarily producing significant changes in FEV_1 probably by decreasing dynamic hyperinflation. Regular treatment with long-acting bronchodilators is more effective and convenient than treatment with short-acting bronchodilators, but more expensive. They safely attenuate airflow obstruction, decrease the frequency and severity of symptoms by reducing the amount of dynamic hyperinflation, and improve quality of life [53].

Although oral corticosteroids are not routinely recommended in the chronic management of patients with COPD, a small subgroup of patients does benefit [54]. A corticosteroid trial, with PFTs before and after a 2-week course of 20 to 40 mg prednisone daily, has been recommended in the past to identify these patients. More recent studies suggest, however, that this is a poor predictor of long-term response to inhaled corticosteroids [55]. Several studies have documented little effect on the rate of lung function decline with inhaled corticosteroid therapy, but the severity and number of exacerbations may be reduced, especially among patients with frequent exacerbations [56,57]. Short-term treatment with a combined inhaled glucocorticosteroid and long-acting β-agonist resulted in greater control of lung function and symptoms than combined anticholinergic and short-acting β-agonist [58]. Analysis of a number of placebo-controlled trials of inhaled corticosteroids has demonstrated a reduction in all-cause mortality by about 25% relative to placebo [59]. Stratification by individual trials and adjustments for age, sex, baseline postbronchodilator percentage predicted FEV_1, smoking status, and body mass index do not materially change the results. Former smokers and women seem to benefit the most.

There is a growing body of evidence to suggest that the use of a combination of inhaled corticosteroids and long-acting β_2-agonists improves lung function, symptoms, and health status and reduces exacerbations in patients with moderate-to-severe COPD [60]. There may also be a survival benefit. A subsequent post hoc analysis of the Toward a Revolution in COPD Health (TORCH) study indicated that pharmacotherapy with salmeterol plus fluticasone propionate, or the components, reduced the rate of decline of FEV_1 in patients with moderate-to-severe COPD, thus slowing disease progression [61].

The addition of a combination of inhaled corticosteroid and long-acting β_2-agonist (salmeterol plus fluticasone) to a long-acting anticholinergic (tiotropium) improved lung function, health status and reduced hospitalizations compared with the use of a long-acting anticholinergics alone [62]. Therapy with tiotropium added to other respiratory medication (mainly a combination of inhaled corticosteroid and long-acting β_2-agonist) was associated with improvements in lung function, quality of life, and exacerbations during a 4-year period but did not significantly reduce the rate of decline in FEV_1 [63].

Long-term oxygen therapy used for at least 15 hours per day in patients with severe COPD and hypoxia when breathing room air is associated with prolonged survival and improved quality of life, increasing life span by 6 to 7 years [64,65]. Oxygen therapy is recommended for patients with a PaO_2 of less than 55 mm Hg and those with a PaO_2 of 55 to 59 mm Hg who have polycythemia or right-sided heart failure. Significant increases in $PaCO_2$ usually do not occur as a result of this therapy [66].

Pulmonary rehabilitation programs have been demonstrated to improve exercise tolerance and reduce dyspnea and should be part of routine management for patients with significant COPD [67–69]. Nocturnal negative-pressure ventilatory assistance has been used to rest respiratory muscles [70]. Whether this intervention is beneficial is unclear, as a large controlled trial failed to demonstrate improvement in exercise tolerance, ABG values, or quality of life [71]. Successful therapeutic results with nocturnal noninvasive positive-pressure assistance in COPD patients have not been uniformly reported, but there may be a role for selected patients [72].

Acute Exacerbation

Treatment of acute exacerbation can be divided into two primary methods: supportive and specific.

Supportive Therapy

Oxygen Therapy. Supplemental oxygen therapy should be administered to all hypoxemic patients who present with an acute exacerbation. The $PaCO_2$ commonly rises somewhat when a patient with COPD receives supplemental oxygen, but carbon dioxide narcosis due to oxygen therapy is uncommon [73]. Patients should not be kept hypoxemic for fear that oxygen therapy will aggravate carbon dioxide retention, but ABG values should be closely monitored. Supplemental oxygen therapy is discussed later in this chapter (see Respiratory Failure section) and in Chapter 62.

Bronchodilators. Although COPD is characterized by poorly reversible airflow obstruction, there is frequently a significant reversible component, particularly in the setting of an acute exacerbation. Many patients with acute exacerbations of COPD respond to these agents with some improvement in airflow obstruction [74]. Inhaled β-agonists and ipratropium appear to be equally effective bronchodilators in patients with acute exacerbations [75]. These agents can be administered by nebulizer or, with equal efficacy, by metered-dose inhaler using a spacer device [76]. A metered-dose inhaler with an aerosol holding chamber also can be used effectively for patients on mechanical ventilation and is as effective as a nebulizer [77]. For specific details on the use of these agents, see Chapter 62.

The role of theophylline in acute exacerbations is less well accepted than in chronic management. A double-blind, placebo-controlled trial demonstrated no additional benefit of aminophylline over standard therapy, but increased adverse effects were noted [78].

Antibiotics. Although there is no evidence that antibiotics given routinely are beneficial in all exacerbations of COPD, antibiotic therapy is appropriate, particularly in more severe exacerbations (i.e., patients experiencing increased dyspnea and cough with increased sputum volume or purulence) [79]. Frequently, bacteria can be isolated from lower airway samples of patients who have COPD in the stable state. This is known as lower airway bacterial colonization and the presence of these organisms is associated with increased frequency and severity of exacerbations and a more rapid decline in FEV1 [80]. Microbiologic surveys in patients with severe exacerbations requiring mechanical ventilation reveal that potentially pathogenic organisms can be found in 72% [81]. The rate of Gram-negative enteric bacilli and Pseudomonas was high (30%) and could not be predicted clinically. Although the results of a number of earlier, poorly designed studies are inconclusive (Table 49.2), a double-blind, placebo-controlled study on the effects of broad-spectrum antibiotics on exacerbations of COPD demonstrated significant benefit [35]. Antibiotic treatment produced significantly earlier resolution of symptoms and prevented clinical deterioration [35]. A meta-analysis confirmed these observations, suggesting that antibiotics are useful, particularly in patients with significant impairment of lung function [82]. Another meta-analysis suggested antibiotics reduced the risk of short-term mortality by 77%, decreased the risk of treatment failure by 53% and the risk of sputum purulence by 44%; with a small increase in the risk of diarrhea [83]. Clinical benefits from antibiotic therapy are most likely to occur in patients

TABLE 49.2

SUMMARY OF PLACEBO-CONTROLLED TRIALS OF ANTIBIOTIC USE IN EXACERBATIONS OF CHRONIC OBSTRUCTIVE PULMONARY DISEASE

No. of patients	Antibiotic	Regimen	Outcome	Reference
71	TMP-SMX or amoxicillin	14-d course	No accelerated recovery	[132]
173	TMP-SMX, amoxicillin, or doxycycline	Ambulatory, 10-d course	Earlier resolution of symptoms; prevented deterioration	[35]
40	Tetracycline	Hospitalized, 7-d course	No benefit over placebo	[133]
259	Tetracycline or chloramphenicol	Ambulatory, 12-d course	Earlier recovery; no difference at 1 mo	[134]
30	Penicillin + streptomycin	Hospitalized, parenteral therapy	Prevented deterioration	[135]
56	Ampicillin	Hospitalized, 7-d course	No benefit over placebo	[136]

TMP-SMX, trimethoprim-sulfamethoxazole.

with more serious exacerbations, particularly those with fever and grossly purulent sputum [84]. The organisms that are usually responsible for bacterial infection in acute exacerbations include *Haemophilus influenzae*, *Streptococcus pneumoniae*, and *Moraxella catarrhalis*. Between 20% and 40% of strains of *H. influenzae* and 80% to 90% of strains of *M. catarrhalis* are β-lactamase-producing and are resistant to β-lactam antibiotics such as amoxicillin, although the rate of resistance of *H. influenzae* seems to be declining [85]. There is evidence to suggest that more potent, broad-spectrum antibiotics such as amoxicillin-clavulanate or respiratory fluoroquinolones may be associated with better outcomes [86].

Corticosteroids. Short-term use of corticosteroids has been generally advocated in acute exacerbations, although it is only recently that this has been supported by randomized clinical trials (Table 49.3). A short course (2 weeks) of prednisone results in a more rapid improvement in FEV_1, reduced rate of deterioration, and shortened hospital stay and prevents relapses [87–90]. The optimal dose and duration are unclear, but no benefit was noted with an 8-week course compared with 2 weeks [89]. The major adverse effect is hyperglycemia.

Other Interventions. In stable patients with COPD, chest percussion and postural drainage produce no significant improvement in airflow or gas exchange [91]. Moreover, there is no evidence to suggest that these modalities are effective in the COPD patient in exacerbation in the absence of bronchiectasis or bronchorrhea, or both (expectoration of sputum greater than 30 mL per 24 hours).

Patients with severe COPD are frequently nutritionally depleted, contributing to their overall poor status and decreased respiratory muscle strength [92,93]. Nutritional support should be instituted early in the course of hospitalization [94]. A high carbohydrate load via parenteral alimentation may, however, result in increased carbon dioxide production [95]. In a patient with a limited ability to increase ventilation, significant worsening of arterial hypercapnia can result, even requiring the institution of mechanical ventilatory support. Nonprotein calories in the form of fat cause a lower production of carbon dioxide compared with isocaloric amounts of carbohydrate, and a higher fat and reduced carbohydrate supplement may lessen the degree of hypercapnia in selected patients [96]. Such a modification in nutritional support is only necessary when excessive calories are given [97]. A recent systematic overview in patients with COPD suggested that patients with marginal ventilatory reserve might benefit from a dietary regimen in which a high percentage of calories are supplied by fat [98]. Although there are reports of the benefits of nutritional repletion, trials of more than 2 weeks failed to show consistent benefit on body weight.

TABLE 49.3

SUMMARY OF CLINICAL TRIALS OF CORTICOSTEROID USE IN EXACERBATIONS OF CHRONIC OBSTRUCTIVE PULMONARY DISEASE

Patients	Study design	Therapeutic regimen	Outcome	Reference
271	Randomized controlled	Methylprednisolone 125 mg every 6 h for 72 h IV followed by a tapering oral course of prednisone (2 or 8 wk)	Improved FEV_1, shorter hospital stay	[89]
56	Randomized controlled	30 mg prednisolone orally for 14 d	Improved FEV_1, shorter hospital stay	[88]
30[a]	Retrospective	IV in ED (mean dose 365 mg hydrocortisone) followed by oral (mean dose 42 mg)	Decreased relapse rate at 48 h	[90]
96	Randomized controlled	100 mg methylprednisolone as a single dose IV in ED	No difference in FEV_1 at 5 h or relapse at 48 h	[137]

[a]Thirty patients with 90 acute exacerbations treated with or without steroids.
ED, emergency department; FEV_1, forced expiratory volume in 1 second; IV, intravenously.

Patients with acute respiratory failure may have elevated levels of antidiuretic hormone, decreased renal blood flow, and right heart failure [99]. Diuretics are helpful in correcting these problems [99], but a complicating metabolic alkalosis may follow. In patients with COPD, digitalis preparations are of little benefit in the routine treatment of cor pulmonale unless concomitant left ventricular dysfunction is found [100]. Furthermore, because patients with acute decompensation of COPD tend to be at increased risk of digitalis toxicity [101], digitalis should be avoided in this setting.

Respiratory stimulants such as doxapram and nikethamide have not been shown to be beneficial, using clinically relevant end points [73,102], and are associated with substantial toxicity [73]. Almitrine may increase ventilation and improve $\dot{V}/\dot{Q}$ relationships in patients with COPD [103], but there is a high incidence of significant side effects [104].

Specific Therapy

Exacerbations of COPD are usually due to upper or lower airway infections (e.g., viral or bacterial, or both). However, should a specific condition among those listed in Table 49.1 be determined to be the cause of deterioration in respiratory status and specific treatment exists (e.g., anticoagulation for pulmonary embolism), it should be instituted.

Respiratory Failure

Administration of controlled oxygen therapy is probably the single most useful treatment in COPD-induced hypercapnic respiratory failure. The increasing availability and evidence for the benefits of noninvasive ventilation has decreased the need for invasive ventilation and led to improved outcomes. The decision to intubate the trachea and mechanically ventilate the lungs is often complicated by concerns that it may not be easy to wean the patient from the ventilator but most individuals with an acute reversible process are successfully liberated from the ventilator [105–107]. Those with significant comorbidity and high severity of illness scores are more likely not to survive an episode of acute respiratory failure [108,109]. Patients with progressive end-stage lung disease should be identified and carefully assessed to determine whether a reversible component exists.

Supplemental Oxygen

Patients with exacerbations of COPD may present with profound hypoxemia. A PaO_2 below 34 mm Hg in otherwise normal animals is associated with the development of lactic acidosis [110]. Any concomitant decrease in cardiac output leads to the development of lactic acidosis at even higher levels of PaO_2 [110]. A low PaO_2 leads to pulmonary arterial vasoconstriction and pulmonary hypertension [111]. Renal function, particularly the excretion of a free water load, may be significantly impaired when PaO_2 falls below 40 mm Hg [112]. The mechanism appears to be CNS release of antidiuretic hormone in response to severe hypoxemia [113]. Other consequences include CNS dysfunction [114] and cardiac arrhythmias or ischemia [115].

The use of supplemental oxygen leads to (a) a decrease in anaerobic metabolism and lactic acid production; (b) an improvement in brain function; (c) a decrease in cardiac arrhythmias and ischemia; (d) a decrease in pulmonary hypertension; (e) an improvement in right-sided heart function with improvement in right-sided heart failure; (f) a decrease in the release of antidiuretic hormone and an increase in the kidneys' ability to clear free water; (g) a decrease in the formation of extravascular lung water (i.e., pulmonary edema); (h) an improvement in survival; and (i) a decrease in red blood cell mass and hematocrit [116].

A simple relation between PaO_2 and oxygen delivery often does not exist in these patients. In individuals with an acute exacerbation of COPD with severe arterial hypoxemia, the administration of supplemental oxygen results in a direct increase in oxygen delivery with no change in cardiac output [117]. On the other hand, in patients with acute exacerbations of COPD and moderate degrees of arterial hypoxemia, the result of supplemental oxygen is no change in oxygen delivery but a decrease in previously elevated cardiac output [117].

Administration of supplemental oxygen is often associated with an additional rise in the $PaCO_2$. This is probably due to a change in dead space or shift of the hemoglobin–oxygen binding curve rather than decreased respiratory drive [118]. This rise is expected and should not be specifically treated unless it is excessive, resulting in a trend toward acute respiratory acidosis on serial ABG determinations, with CNS or cardiovascular side effects. Should this occur, the supplemental oxygen should not be discontinued abruptly but rather decreased slowly until the $PaCO_2$ returns to a more acceptable level [73] and the situation is stabilized. Because abrupt discontinuation of supplemental oxygen may not be associated with a prompt increase in ventilation, the $PaCO_2$ may not fall. Therefore, abrupt withdrawal of supplemental oxygen may additionally depress the already low PaO_2, causing more profound arterial hypoxemia [73]. Carbon dioxide narcosis may occur with excessive oxygen therapy but is much less likely with low-flow–controlled oxygen therapy [73]. It occurs more commonly in patients with more marked hypoxemia [79]. Clinically significant hypercapnia is less likely to occur with oxygen therapy administered to maintain oxygen saturation at 91% to 92% [119]. Oxygen therapy is more effective with a prescription chart [120]

Mechanical Ventilation

Whether to institute mechanical ventilatory support is often a difficult decision in hypercapnic respiratory failure associated with COPD. This decision reflects a continuous reassessment of the patient's status, including the trend of ABG values and determining whether the patient is strong and alert enough to clear his or her secretions and protect the airway. The presence of worsening acute respiratory acidosis with a low arterial pH (e.g., less than 7.2) and inadequate PaO_2 (e.g., less than 55 mm Hg) or CNS and cardiovascular dysfunction dictates the need for assisted ventilation. Difficulty arises when the data are not as definitive. An alternative to endotracheal intubation is noninvasive mask ventilation, and early institution of this mode of ventilatory support is associated with a significant outcome benefit.

Noninvasive Ventilation. Numerous randomized trials and recent systematic reviews have clearly shown that the use of noninvasive ventilation (NIV) markedly improves in-hospital outcomes in acute exacerbations of COPD [121–123] (Table 49.4). See Chapter 59 for a comprehensive discussion of this topic in general and in COPD patients.

Invasive Mechanical Ventilation. Although it is prudent to avoid intubating the trachea in a patient with COPD whenever possible, the development of stupor or coma may necessitate emergency intubation, a potentially disastrous complication. The decision to institute mechanical ventilatory support is a clinical one and supported by lack of response or intolerance to NIV or progressive acidosis or respiratory rate. See Chapter 58 for a comprehensive discussion of this topic in general and in patients with COPD.

TABLE 49.4

RECOMMENDATIONS BASED ON RANDOMIZED CONTROLLED CLINICAL TRIALS

Recommendation	References
1. Give bronchodilators	[44–49]
2. Give inhaled corticosteroids for people with an FEV1 less then 50%–60% predicted	[55–60]
3. Give antibiotics for purulent exacerbations of COPD	[35,82–84]
4. Use oxygen	[64,65]
5. Use noninvasive ventilation for patients with severe exacerbations and respiratory failure	[121–123]

PROGNOSIS

The prognosis for patients admitted to hospital for an acute exacerbation of COPD is variable and is related to the severity of the underlying disease and whether an ICU admission or ventilation was required. In-hospital mortality rates of 8% to 25% [124] are generally quoted with 1-year mortality ranging from 21% to 43% [125,126]. The prognosis for patients treated in the ICU is significantly worse with in-hospital mortality as high as 25% and 1-year mortality approaching 39% [127,128]. Although a dismal outcome is often quoted for patients with COPD who require prolonged ventilation (more than 21 days), half of these patients can ultimately be weaned [107]. Systemic markers of health such as APACHE II scores and serum albumin are the best predictors of ICU survival.

Readmission rates following hospitalization range from 61% to 80% in the year following discharge. Risk factors for readmission include a low FEV_1, number of days in hospital in the previous year, low physical activity scale, and poor overall quality of life scores [129].

The major predictors of hospital mortality in patients with acute exacerbations of COPD appear to be indices of nonrespiratory organ dysfunction (e.g., serum albumin, body mass index) and severity of illness [108], whereas the severity of respiratory disease predicts 1-year mortality [130]. Age older than 65 years is an important prognostic indicator [130,131]. Of note, parameters of cardiac dysfunction (cor pulmonale, arrhythmias) are important determinants of poor outcome [106,130].

References

1. Pauwels RA, Buist AS, Calverley PM, et al: Global strategy for the diagnosis, management, and prevention of chronic obstructive pulmonary disease. NHLBI/WHO Global Initiative for Chronic Obstructive Lung Disease (GOLD) Workshop summary. *Am J Respir Crit Care Med* 163:1256, 2001.
2. Chen JC, Mannino DM: Worldwide epidemiology of chronic obstructive pulmonary disease. *Curr Opin Pulm Med* 5:93, 1999.
3. Heron MP, Hoyert DL, Murphy SL, et al: *Deaths: Final Data for 2006. National Vital Statistics Reports.* Vol 57, No. 14. Hyattsville, MD, National Center for Health Statistics, 2009.
4. Sullivan SD, Ramsey SD, Lee TA: The economic burden of COPD. *Chest* 117:5S, 2000.
5. Barnes PJ: Chronic obstructive pulmonary disease. *N Engl J Med* 343:269–280, 2000.
6. Fletcher C, Peto R: The natural history of chronic airflow obstruction. *BMJ* 1:1645, 1977.
7. Burrows B, Knudson RJ, Cline MG, et al: Quantitative relationships between cigarette smoking and ventilatory function. *Am Rev Respir Dis* 115:195, 1977.
8. Beck GJ, Doyle CA, Schacter EN: Smoking and lung function. *Am Rev Respir Dis* 123:149, 1981.
9. Bates DV: The fate of the chronic bronchitic: a report of the ten-year follow-up in the Canadian Department of Veterans Affairs coordinated study of chronic bronchitis. *Am Rev Respir Dis* 108:1043, 1973.
10. Stoller JK, Aboussouan LS: α_1-Antitrypsin deficiency. *Lancet* 365:2225, 2005.
11. Madison R, Mittman C, Afifi AA, et al: Risk factors for obstructive lung disease. *Am Rev Respir Dis* 124:149, 1981.
12. Niewoehner DE, Kleinerman J, Rice DB: Pathologic changes in the peripheral airways of young cigarette smokers. *N Engl J Med* 291:755, 1974.
13. Hogg JC, Macklem PT, Thurlbeck WM: Site and nature of airway obstruction in chronic obstructive lung disease. *N Engl J Med* 278:1355, 1968.
14. Hogg JC, Chu F, Utokaparch S, et al: The nature of small-airway obstruction in chronic obstructive lung disease. *N Engl J Med* 350:2645, 2004.
15. Lam S, Chan-Yeung M, Abboud R, et al: Interrelationships between serum chemotactic factor inactivator, $alpha_1$-antitrypsin deficiency, and chronic obstructive lung disease. *Am Rev Respir Dis* 121:507, 1980.
16. Tager IB, Rosner B, Tishler PV, et al: Household aggregation of pulmonary function and chronic bronchitis. *Am Rev Respir Dis* 114:485, 1976.
17. Webster PM, Lorimer EG, Man SFP, et al: Pulmonary function in identical twins: comparison of nonsmokers and smokers. *Am Rev Respir Dis* 119:223, 1979.
18. Saetta M, Di Stefano A, Turato G, et al: CD8+ T-lymphocytes in peripheral airways of smokers with chronic obstructive pulmonary disease. *Am J Respir Crit Care Med* 157:822, 1998.
19. West JB: *Pulmonary Pathophysiology: The Essentials.* 2nd ed. Baltimore, Williams & Wilkins, 1982.
20. Roussos C, Macklem PT: The respiratory muscles. *N Engl J Med* 307:786, 1982.
21. Gelb AF, Klein E, Schiffman P, et al: Ventilatory response and drive in acute and chronic obstructive pulmonary disease. *Am Rev Respir Dis* 116:9, 1977.
22. Peto R, Speizer FE, Cochrane AL, et al: The relevance in adults of airflow obstruction, but not of mucus hypersecretion, to mortality from chronic lung disease: results from 20 years of prospective observation. *Am Rev Respir Dis* 128:491, 1983.
23. Vestbo J, Prescott E, Lange P: Association of chronic mucus hypersecretion with FEV1 decline and chronic obstructive pulmonary disease morbidity. Copenhagen City Heart Study Group. *Am J Respir Crit Care Med* 153(5):1530, 1996.
24. Pardee NE, Winterbauer RH, Morgan EH, et al: Combinations of four physical signs as indicators of ventilatory abnormality in obstructive pulmonary syndromes. *Chest* 77:354, 1980.
25. Badgett RG, Tanaka DJ, Hunt DK, et al: Can moderate chronic obstructive pulmonary disease be diagnosed by historical and physical findings alone? *Am J Med* 94:188, 1993.
26. Pardee NE, Martin CJ, Morgan EH: A test of the practical value of estimating breath sound intensity: breath sounds related to measured ventilatory function. *Chest* 70:341, 1976.
27. Cohen CA, Zagelbaum G, Gross D, et al: Clinical manifestations of inspiratory muscle fatigue. *Am J Med* 73:308, 1982.
28. Fraser RG, Pare JAP: *Diagnosis of Diseases of the Chest.* Vol 3. 2nd ed. Philadelphia, WB Saunders, 1979.
29. Cleverley JR, Muller NL: Advances in radiologic assessment of chronic obstructive pulmonary disease. *Clin Chest Med* 21:653, 2000.
30. Sherman S, Skoney JA, Ravikrishnan KP: Routine chest radiographs in exacerbations of chronic obstructive pulmonary disease: diagnostic value. *Arch Intern Med* 149:2493, 1989.
31. Gilbert R, Keighley J, Auchincloss JH Jr: Mechanisms of chronic carbon dioxide retention in patients with obstructive pulmonary disease. *Am J Med* 38:217, 1965.
32. Morrison NJ, Abboud RT, Ramadan F, et al: Comparison of single breath carbon monoxide diffusing capacity and pressure-volume curves in detecting emphysema. *Am Rev Respir Dis* 139:1179, 1989.
33. Parot S, Miara B, Milic-Emili J, et al: Hypoxemia, hypercapnia, and breathing pattern in patients with chronic obstructive pulmonary disease. *Am Rev Respir Dis* 126:882, 1982.
34. GOLD Executive committee: Global strategy for diagnosis, management, and prevention of COPD (Revised 2006). Available at: http://www.goldcopd.com/).
35. Anthonisen NR, Monfreda J, Warren CPW, et al: Antibiotic therapy in exacerbations of chronic obstructive pulmonary disease. *Ann Intern Med* 106:196, 1987.
36. Sethi S, Evans N, Grant BJB, et al: New strains of bacteria and exacerbations of chronic obstructive pulmonary disease. *N Engl J Med* 347:465, 2002.

37. Lippman M, Fein A: Pulmonary embolism in the patient with chronic obstructive pulmonary disease. *Chest* 79:39, 1981.
38. Rizkallah J, Man SFP, Sin DD: Prevalence of pulmonary embolism in acute exacerbations of COPD. *Chest* 135:786, 2009.
39. The Tobacco Use and Dependence Clinical Practice Guideline Panel, Staff, and Consortium Representatives: A clinical practice guideline for treating tobacco use and dependence. A US Public Health Service Report. *JAMA* 283:3244, 2000.
40. Tonstad S, Tonnesen P, Hajek P, et al: Effect of maintenance therapy with Varenicline on smoking cessation: a randomized, controlled trial. *JAMA* 296:64, 2006.
41. Nichol KL, Nordin J, Mullooly J, et al: Influenza vaccination and reduction in hospitalizations for cardiac disease and stroke among the elderly. *N Engl J Med* 348:1322, 2003.
42. Wongsurakiat P, Maranetra KN, Wasi C, et al: Acute respiratory illness in patients with COPD and the effectiveness of influenza vaccination: a randomized controlled study. *Chest* 125:2011, 2004.
43. Nichol KL, Baken L, Wuorenma J, et al: The health and economic benefits associated with pneumococcal vaccination of elderly persons with chronic lung disease. *Arch Intern Med* 159:2437, 1999.
44. Guyatt GH, Townsend M, Pugsley SO, et al: Bronchodilators in chronic airflow limitation: effects on airway function, exercise capacity and quality of life. *Am Rev Respir Dis* 135:1069, 1987.
45. Combivent Inhalation Aerosol Study Group: In chronic obstructive pulmonary disease, a combination of ipratropium and albuterol is more effective than either agent alone. An 85-day multicenter trial. *Chest* 105:1411, 1994.
46. Rennard SI, Anderson W, ZuWallack R, et al: Use of a long-acting inhaled $beta_2$-adrenergic agonist, salmeterol xinafoate, in patients with chronic obstructive pulmonary disease. *Am J Respir Crit Care Med* 63:1087, 2001.
47. D'Urzo AD, De Salvo MC, Ramirez-Rivera A, et al: In patients with COPD, treatment with a combination of formoterol and ipratropium is more effective than a combination of salbutamol and ipratropium: a 3-week, randomized, double-blind, within-patient, multicenter study. *Chest* 119:1347, 2001.
48. Littner MR, Ilowite JS, Tashkin DP, et al: Long-acting bronchodilation with once-daily dosing of tiotropium (Spiriva) in stable chronic obstructive pulmonary disease. *Am J Respir Crit Care Med* 161:1136, 2000.
49. Brusasco V, Hodder R, Miravitlles M, et al: Health outcomes following treatment for six months with once daily tiotropium compared with twice daily salmeterol in patients with COPD. *Thorax* 58:399, 2003.
50. Eaton ML, Green BA, Church TR, et al: Efficacy of theophylline in irreversible airflow obstruction. *Ann Intern Med* 92:758, 1980.
51. Aubier M, DeTroyer A, Sampson M, et al: Aminophylline improves diaphragmatic contractility. *N Engl J Med* 305:249, 1981.
52. Murciano D, Auclair M-H, Pariente R, et al: A randomized, controlled trial of theophylline in patients with severe chronic obstructive pulmonary disease. *N Engl J Med* 320:1521, 1989.
53. O'Donnell DE, Flüge T, Gerken F, et al: Effects of tiotropium on lung hyperinflation, dyspnoea and exercise tolerance in COPD. *Eur Respir J* 23:832, 2004.
54. Mendella LA, Manfreda J, Warren CPW, et al: Steroid response in stable chronic obstructive pulmonary disease. *Ann Intern Med* 96:17, 1982.
55. Burge PS, Claverley PM, Jones PW, et al: Randomised, double blind, placebo controlled study of fluticasone propionate in patients with moderate to severe chronic obstructive pulmonary disease: the ISOLDE trial. *BMJ* 320:1297, 2000.
56. Soriano JB, Sin DD, Zhang X, et al: A pooled analysis of FEV1 decline in COPD patients randomized to inhaled corticosteroids or placebo. *Chest* 131:682, 2007.
57. Agarwal R, Aggarwal AN, Gupta D, et al: Inhaled corticosteroids vs. placebo for preventing COPD exacerbations: a systematic review and metaregression of randomized controlled trials. *Chest* 137:318, 2010.
58. Donohue JF, Kalberg C, Emmett A, et al: A short-term comparison of fluticasone propionate/salmeterol with ipratropium bromide/albuterol for the treatment of COPD. *Treat Respir Med* 3:173, 2004.
59. Sin DD, Wu L, Anderson JA, et al: Inhaled corticosteroids and mortality in chronic obstructive pulmonary disease. *Thorax* 60:992, 2005.
60. Calverley PMA, Anderson JA, Celli B, et al: Salmeterol and fluticasone propionate and survival in chronic obstructive pulmonary disease. *N Engl J Med* 356:775, 2007.
61. Celli BR, Thomas NE, Anderson JA, et al: Effect of pharmacotherapy on rate of decline of lung function in chronic obstructive pulmonary disease: results from the Torch study. *Am J Respir Crit Care Med* 178:332, 2008.
62. Aaron SD, Vandemheen KL, Fergusson D, et al: Tiotropium in combination with placebo, salmeterol, or fluticasone–salmeterol for treatment of chronic obstructive pulmonary disease: a randomized trial. *Ann Intern Med* 146:545, 2007.
63. Tashkin DP, Celli B, Senn S, et al: A 4-year trial of tiotropium in chronic obstructive pulmonary disease. *N Engl J Med* 359:1543, 2008.
64. Nocturnal Oxygen Therapy Trial Group: Continuous or nocturnal oxygen therapy in hypoxemic chronic obstructive lung disease: a clinical trial. *Ann Intern Med* 93:391, 1980.
65. Stuart-Harris C, Bishop JM, Clark TJH, et al: Long-term domiciliary oxygen therapy in chronic hypoxemic cor pulmonale complicating chronic bronchitis and emphysema: report of the Medical Research Council Working Party. *Lancet* 1:681, 1981.
66. Goldstein RS, Ramcharan V, Bowes G, et al: Effect of supplemental nocturnal oxygen on gas exchange in patients with severe obstructive lung disease. *N Engl J Med* 310:425, 1984.
67. Goldstein RS, Gort EH, Stubbing D, et al: Randomised controlled trial of respiratory rehabilitation. *Lancet* 344:1394, 1994.
68. Finnerty JP, Keeping I, Bullough I, et al: The effectiveness of outpatient pulmonary rehabilitation in chronic lung disease: a randomized controlled trial. *Chest* 119:1705, 2001.
69. Troosters T, Casaburi R, Gosselink R, et al: Pulmonary rehabilitation in chronic obstructive pulmonary disease. *Am J Respir Crit Care Med* 172:19, 2005.
70. Cropp A, Dimarco AF: Effects of intermittent negative pressure ventilation on respiratory muscle function in patients with severe chronic obstructive lung disease. *Am Rev Respir Dis* 135:1056, 1987.
71. Shapiro SH, Ernst P, Gray-Donald K, et al: Effect of negative pressure ventilation in severe chronic obstructive pulmonary disease. *Lancet* 340:1425, 1992.
72. Hill NS: Noninvasive ventilation in chronic obstructive pulmonary disease. *Clin Chest Med* 21:783, 2000.
73. Bone RC: Treatment of respiratory failure due to advanced chronic obstructive lung disease. *Arch Intern Med* 140:1018, 1980.
74. Schmidt GA, Hall JB: Acute on chronic respiratory failure: assessment and management of patients with COPD in the emergency setting. *JAMA* 261:3444, 1989.
75. Karpel JP, Pesin J, Greenberg D, et al: A comparison of the effects of ipratropium bromide and metaproterenol sulfate in acute exacerbations of COPD. *Chest* 98:835, 1990.
76. Berry RB, Shinto RA, Wong FH, et al: Nebulizer vs spacer for bronchodilator delivery in patients hospitalized for acute exacerbations of COPD. *Chest* 96:1241, 1989.
77. Duarte AG, Momii K, Bidani A: Bronchodilator therapy with metered-dose inhaler and spacer versus nebulizer in mechanically ventilated patients: comparison of magnitude and duration of response. *Respir Care* 45:817, 2000.
78. Rice KL, Leatherman JW, Duane PG, et al: Aminophylline for acute exacerbations of chronic obstructive pulmonary disease: a controlled trial. *Ann Intern Med* 107:305, 1987.
79. Bach PB, Brown C, Gelfand SE, et al: Management of acute exacerbations of chronic obstructive pulmonary disease: a summary and appraisal of published evidence. *Ann Intern Med* 134:600, 2001.
80. Patel IS, Seemungal TAR, Wilks M, et al: Relationships between bacterial colonization and the frequency, character and severity of COPD exacerbations. *Thorax* 57:759, 2002.
81. Soler N, Torres A, Ewig S, et al: Bronchial microbial patterns in severe exacerbations of chronic obstructive pulmonary disease (COPD) requiring mechanical ventilation. *Am J Respir Crit Care Med* 157:1498, 1998.
82. Saint S, Bent S, Vittinghoff E, et al: Antibiotics in chronic obstructive pulmonary disease exacerbations. A meta-analysis. *JAMA* 273:957, 1995.
83. Ram FSF, Rogriguez-Roisin R, Granados-Navarrete A, et al: Antibiotics for exacerbations of chronic obstructive pulmonary disease. *Cochrane Database Syst Rev* (2):CD004403, 2006. DOI:10.1002/14651858.CD004403.pub2.
84. Nouira S, Marghli S, Belghith M, et al: Once daily oral ofloxacin in chronic obstructive pulmonary disease exacerbation requiring mechanical ventilation: a randomised placebo-controlled trial. *Lancet* 358:2020, 2001.
85. Heilmann KP, Rice CL, Miller AL, et al: Decreasing prevalence of β-lactamase production among respiratory tract isolates of Haemophilus influenzae in the United States. *Antimicrob Agents Chemother* 49:2561, 2005.
86. Dimopoulos G, Siempos II, Korbila IP, et al: Comparison of first-line with second-line antibiotics for acute exacerbations of chronic bronchitis. *Chest* 132:447, 2007.
87. Aaron SD, Vandemheen KL, Hebert P, et al: Outpatient oral prednisone after emergency treatment of chronic obstructive pulmonary disease. *N Engl J Med* 348:2618, 2003.
88. Davies L, Angus RM, Calverley PM: Oral corticosteroids in patients admitted to hospital with exacerbations of chronic obstructive pulmonary disease: a prospective randomised controlled trial. *Lancet* 354:456, 1999.
89. Niewoehner DE, Erbland ML, Deupree RH, et al: Effect of systemic glucocorticoids on exacerbations of chronic obstructive pulmonary disease. Department of Veterans Affairs Cooperative Study Group. *N Engl J Med* 340:1941, 1999.
90. Murata GH, Gorby MS, Chick TW, et al: Intravenous and oral corticosteroids for the prevention of relapse after treatment of decompensated COPD: effect on patients with a history of multiple relapses. *Chest* 98:845, 1990.
91. May DB, Munt PW: Physiologic effects of chest percussion and postural drainage in patients with stable chronic bronchitis. *Chest* 75:29, 1979.
92. Hunter AMB, Carey MA, Larsh HW: The nutritional status of patients with chronic obstructive pulmonary disease. *Am Rev Respir Dis* 124:376, 1981.
93. Arora NS, Rochester DF: Respiratory muscle strength and maximal voluntary ventilation in undernourished patients. *Am Rev Respir Dis* 126:5, 1982.

94. Driver AG, LeBrun M: Iatrogenic malnutrition in patients receiving ventilatory support. *JAMA* 244:2195, 1980.
95. Covelli HD, Black JW, Olsen MS, et al: Respiratory failure precipitated by high carbohydrate loads. *Ann Intern Med* 95:579, 1981.
96. Weinberger SE, Schwartzstein RM, Weiss JW: Hypercapnia. *N Engl J Med* 321:1223, 1989.
97. Taplers SS, Romberger DJ, Bunce SB, et al: Nutritionally associated increased carbon dioxide production: excess total calories vs high proportion of carbohydrate calories. *Chest* 102:551, 1992.
98. Ferreira IM, Brooks D, Lacasse Y, et al: Nutritional intervention in COPD: a systematic overview. *Chest* 119:353, 2001.
99. Heinemann HO: Right-sided heart failure and the use of diuretics. *Am J Med* 64:367, 1978.
100. Mathur PN, Powles ACP, Pugsley SO, et al: Effect of digoxin on right ventricular function in severe chronic airflow obstruction: a controlled clinical trial. *Ann Intern Med* 95:283, 1981.
101. Green LH, Smith TW: The use of digitalis in patients with pulmonary disease. *Ann Intern Med* 87:459, 1977.
102. Derenne J-P, Fleury B, Pariente R: Acute respiratory failure of chronic obstructive pulmonary disease. *Am Rev Respir Dis* 138:1006, 1988.
103. Powles ACP, Tuxen DV, Mahood CB, et al: The effect of intravenously administered almitrine, a peripheral chemoreceptor agonist, on patients with chronic air-flow obstruction. *Am Rev Respir Dis* 127:284, 1983.
104. Bardsley PA, Howard P, DeBacker W, et al: Two years treatment with almitrine bismesylate in patients with hypoxic chronic obstructive airways disease. *Eur Respir J* 4:308, 1991.
105. Kaelin RM, Assimacopoulos A, Chevrolet JC: Failure to predict six-month survival with COPD requiring mechanical ventilation by analysis of simple indices: a prospective study. *Chest* 92:971, 1987.
106. Menzies R, Gibbons W, Goldberg P: Determinants of weaning and survival among patients with COPD who require mechanical ventilation for acute respiratory failure. *Chest* 95:398, 1989.
107. Nava S, Rubini F, Zanotti E, et al: Survival and prediction of successful ventilator weaning in COPD patients requiring mechanical ventilation for more than 21 days. *Eur Respir J* 7:1645, 1994.
108. Nevins ML, Epstein SK: Predictors of outcome for patients with COPD requiring invasive mechanical ventilation. *Chest* 119:1840, 2001.
109. Putinati S, Ballerin L, Piatella M, et al: Is it possible to predict the success of non-invasive positive pressure ventilation in acute respiratory failure due to COPD? *Respir Med* 94:997, 2000.
110. Simmons DH, Alpas AP, Tashkin DP, et al: Hyperlactacidemia due to arterial hypoxemia or reduced cardiac output, or both. *J Appl Physiol* 45:195, 1978.
111. Harvey RM, Enson Y, Ferrer MI: A reconsideration of the origins of pulmonary hypertension. *Chest* 59:82, 1971.
112. Kilburn KH, Dowell AR: Renal function in respiratory failure: effects of hypoxia, hyperoxia, and hypercapnia. *Arch Intern Med* 127:754, 1971.
113. Anderson RJ, Pluss RG, Berns AS, et al: Mechanism of effect of hypoxemia on renal water excretion. *J Clin Invest* 62:769, 1978.
114. Gibson GE, Pulsinelli W, Blass JP, et al: Brain dysfunction in mild to moderate hypoxia. *Am J Med* 70:1247, 1981.
115. Tirlapur VG: Nocturnal hypoxemia and associated electrocardiographic changes in patients with chronic obstructive airways disease. *N Engl J Med* 306:125, 1982.
116. Findley LJ, Whelan DM, Moser KM: Long-term oxygen therapy in COPD. *Chest* 83:671, 1983.
117. Degaute JP, Domenighetti G, Naeije R, et al: Oxygen delivery in acute exacerbation of chronic obstructive lung disease: effects of controlled oxygen therapy. *Am Rev Respir Dis* 124:26, 1981.
118. Aubier M, Murciano D, Fournier M, et al: Effects of the administration of O_2 on ventilation and blood gases in patients with chronic obstructive pulmonary disease during acute respiratory failure. *Am Rev Respir Dis* 122:747, 1980.
119. Moloney ED, Kiely JL, McNicholas WT: Controlled oxygen therapy and carbon dioxide retention during exacerbations of chronic obstructive pulmonary disease. *Lancet* 357:526, 2001.
120. Dodd ME, Kellet F, Davis A, et al: Audit of oxygen prescribing before and after the introduction of a prescription chart. *BMJ* 321:864, 2000.
121. Ram FS, Picot J, Lightowler J, et al: Non-invasive positive pressure ventilation for treatment of ventilatory failure due to exacerbations of chronic obstructive pulmonary disease. *Cochrane Database Syst Rev* (3):CD004104, 2004.
122. Lightowler JV, Wedzicha JA, Elliott MW, et al: Non-invasive positive pressure ventilation to treat respiratory failure resulting from exacerbations of chronic obstructive pulmonary disease: Cochrane systematic review and meta-analysis. *BMJ* 326:185, 2003.
123. Keenan SP, Sinuff T, Cook DJ, et al: Which patients with acute exacerbation of chronic obstructive pulmonary disease benefit from non-invasive positive-pressure ventilation? A systematic review of the literature. *Ann Intern Med* 138:861, 2003.
124. Groenewegen KH, Schols AM, Wouters EF: Mortality and mortality-related factors after hospitalization for acute exacerbations of COPD. *Chest* 124:459, 2003.
125. Quinnell TG, Pilsworth S, Shneerson JM, et al: Prolonged invasive ventilation following acute ventilatory failure in COPD: weaning results, survival, and the role of noninvasive ventilation. *Chest* 129:133, 2006.
126. Mcghan R, Radcliff T, Fish R, et al: Predictors of rehospitalization and death after a severe exacerbation of COPD. *Chest* 132:1748, 2007.
127. Ai-Ping C, Lee K-H, Lim T-K: In-hospital and 5-year mortality of patients treated in the ICU for acute exacerbation of COPD: a retrospective study. *Chest* 128:518, 2005.
128. Uegun I, Metintas M, Moral H, et al: Predictors of hospital outcome and intubation in COPD patients admitted to the respiratory ICU for acute hypercapnic respiratory failure. *Respir Med* 100:66, 2006.
129. Gudmundsson G, Gislason T, Janson C, et al: Risk factors for rehospitalization in COPD: role of health status, anxiety, and depression. *Eur Respir J* 26:414, 2005.
130. Seneff MG, Wagner DP, Wagner RP, et al: Hospital and 1-year survival of patients admitted to intensive care units with acute exacerbation of chronic obstructive pulmonary disease. *JAMA* 274:1852, 1995.
131. Fuso L, Incalzi RA, Pistelli R, et al: Predicting mortality of patients hospitalized for acutely exacerbated chronic obstructive pulmonary disease. *Am J Med* 98:272, 1995.
132. Sachs AP, Koeter GH, Groenier KH, et al: Changes in symptoms, peak expiratory flow, and sputum flora during treatment with antibiotics of exacerbations in patients with chronic obstructive pulmonary disease in general practice. *Thorax* 50:758, 1995.
133. Nicotra MB, Rivera M, Awe RJ: Antibiotic therapy of acute exacerbations of chronic bronchitis: a controlled study using tetracycline. *Ann Intern Med* 97:18, 1982.
134. Pines A, Raafat H, Greenfield JSB, et al: Antibiotic regimens in moderately ill patients with purulent exacerbations of chronic bronchitis. *Br J Dis Chest* 66:107, 1972.
135. Pines A, Raafat H, Plucinski K, et al: Antibiotic regimens in severe and acute purulent exacerbations of chronic bronchitis. *BMJ* 2:735, 1968.
136. Elmes PC, King TKC, Langlands JHM, et al: Value of ampicillin in the hospital treatment of exacerbations of chronic bronchitis. *BMJ* 2:904, 1965.
137. Emerman CL, Connors AF, Lukens TW, et al: A randomized controlled trial of methylprednisolone in the emergency treatment of acute exacerbations of COPD. *Chest* 95:563, 1989.

CHAPTER 50 ■ RESPIRATORY FAILURE PART V: EXTRAPULMONARY CAUSES OF RESPIRATORY FAILURE

HELEN M. HOLLINGSWORTH, MELVIN R. PRATTER AND RICHARD S. IRWIN

The conditions that cause respiratory failure primarily by their effect on structures other than the lungs are discussed in this chapter. Severe impairment of the extrapulmonary compartment produces respiratory failure through the mechanism of hypoventilation (see Chapter 46), so the resultant respiratory failure is always hypercapnic. Extrapulmonary causes account for up to 17% of all cases of hypercapnic respiratory failure [1]. This chapter is organized to follow sequential sections of pathophysiology, diagnosis, differential diagnosis, and treatment.

PATHOPHYSIOLOGY

The extrapulmonary compartment includes the (a) central nervous system (CNS), (b) peripheral nervous system, (c) respiratory muscles, (d) chest wall, (e) pleura, and (f) upper airway [2]. Because many conditions can cause extrapulmonary respiratory failure, it is helpful to categorize them according to the specific component affected by the disease process (Fig. 50.1). We have limited the discussion that follows to descriptions of the individual diseases and conditions that are most important to the topic of respiratory failure. They are summarized in Tables 50.1 through 50.4.

The pathophysiology of extrapulmonary respiratory failure is described in Chapter 45. Functionally, extrapulmonary disorders can lead to hypercapnic respiratory failure due to a decrease in normal force generation (e.g., CNS dysfunction, peripheral nervous system abnormalities, or respiratory muscle dysfunction) or an increase in impedance to bulk flow ventilation (e.g., chest wall and pleural disorders or upper airway obstruction) [3].

DIAGNOSIS

General Considerations

Arterial hypercapnia in the presence of a normal alveolar–arterial oxygen tension [$P(A–a)O_2$] gradient on room air is the sine qua non of extrapulmonary respiratory failure [4]. The normal gradient reflects the fact that in pure extrapulmonary failure distal gas exchange is normal, and the decrease in the partial pressure of arterial oxygen (PaO_2) directly reflects the decrease in the partial pressure of alveolar oxygen (PAO_2). A $P(A–a)O_2$ gradient of less than 20 mm Hg in the presence of an elevated partial pressure of carbon dioxide ($PaCO_2$) is, with few exceptions, diagnostic of extrapulmonary respiratory failure [5–11]. The main exception occurs in patients with chronic obstructive pulmonary disease (COPD) who have increasing hypercapnia [12]. Their $P(A–a)O_2$ gradient can occasionally narrow to normal, probably related to substantial changes in the position of the alveolar and arterial points on the oxyhemoglobin dissociation curve related to ventilation–perfusion inequalities [12]. Thus, arterial hypercapnia with a normal $P(A–a)O_2$ gradient is consistent with pure extrapulmonary respiratory failure, but a normal $P(A–a)O_2$ cannot, by itself, rule out severe COPD.

Pulmonary parenchymal disease can also exist concomitantly with extrapulmonary dysfunction. For example, a patient with polymyositis can have respiratory muscle weakness in addition to interstitial pulmonary fibrosis. This may be suggested by the combination of hypercapnia and only mild-to-moderate widening of the $P(A–a)O_2$ gradient. A gradient between 20 and 30 mm Hg in the presence of arterial hypercapnia should raise the suspicion that a significant element of extrapulmonary dysfunction may be present. It is also important to realize that even when the $P(A–a)O_2$ gradient exceeds 30 mm Hg, some degree of extrapulmonary dysfunction can also be present in association with significant pulmonary impairment. For example, when hypercapnic respiratory failure results from an acute exacerbation of COPD, respiratory muscle fatigue often contributes to the development of carbon dioxide retention [13]. A less common example is the presence of a large abdominal ventral hernia in a patient with COPD. The resultant paradoxic breathing pattern can contribute significantly to abnormal gas exchange and increased dyspnea [14].

Decrease in Normal Force Generation

Because the inspiratory muscles generate the force that results in ventilation, any condition that directly or indirectly impairs respiratory muscle function can result in decreased force generation [3]. Dysfunction of the respiratory center, peripheral nervous system pathways, or the respiratory muscles themselves decreases the force available to produce ventilation. If this impairment is severe enough, the level of minute ventilation will be insufficient to clear the amount of carbon dioxide produced by ongoing metabolic processes, and hypercapnic respiratory failure results.

An acute decrease in CNS output sufficient to result in hypercapnic respiratory failure (e.g., acute narcotic overdose) is usually accompanied by obvious evidence of generalized CNS depression. In contrast, a chronic (e.g., primary alveolar hypoventilation) or episodic (e.g., central sleep apnea) cause of decreased impulse formation may present a much more difficult diagnostic dilemma. Tests to evaluate respiratory center drive, such as voluntary hyperventilation, carbon dioxide stimulation, or polysomnography, may be necessary to define the problem.

Peripheral nervous system dysfunction or primary weakness of the respiratory muscles is often indicated by the presence of certain suggestive clinical findings that vary depending on the

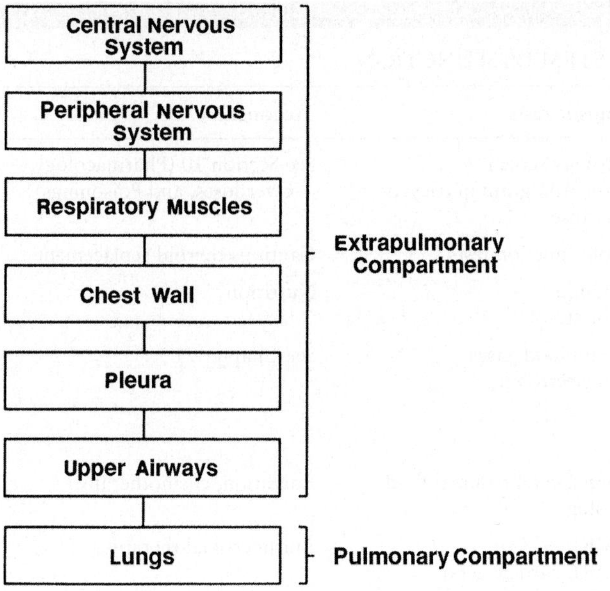

FIGURE 50.1. Schematic representation of the anatomy of the respiratory system.

specific entity present (see following discussion). Respiratory muscle fatigue or weakness may be suspected clinically and documented using a number of tests designed to evaluate respiratory muscle function.

Symptoms are usually nonspecific; patients may report dyspnea on exertion, either when supine (bilateral diaphragmatic paralysis) or when upright (C5–6 quadriplegia). Reports of weakness in other muscle groups, difficulty swallowing, and change in voice volume or tone may be other clues. Physical findings of changes in the rate, depth, and pattern of breathing suggest stressed, fatigued, or weakened respiratory muscles. For example, an increased respiratory rate, a decreased tidal volume, and paradoxic inward motion of the anterior abdominal wall during inspiration may be observed. The latter finding indicates a failure of the diaphragm to contract sufficiently to descend and move the abdominal contents downward and the abdominal wall outward during inspiration. A breathing pattern that cycles between predominantly chest wall or predominantly abdominal wall motion, called *respiratory alternans*, represents the alternating contraction of intercostal and accessory muscles, on the one hand, and the diaphragm, on the other. The assumption is that these two muscle groups alternate in their contribution to the work of breathing, allowing one another to rest during periods of muscle overload or fatigue.

Two readily available tests can be useful diagnostically to help assess respiratory muscle function. First, measurement of maximal inspiratory and expiratory pressures at the mouth is easy to perform, noninvasive, and can accurately predict the development of hypercapnic respiratory failure due to decreased respiratory muscle force generation [15,16]. Arterial hypercapnia due to respiratory muscle weakness is generally not seen until the maximal inspiratory pressure is reduced to 30% or less of normal [15,16]. Although normal predicted values vary (primarily on the basis of age and gender [17,18]), a maximal inspiratory pressure less negative than −30 cm H_2O is likely to be associated with arterial hypercapnia [16,19]. Maximal expiratory pressures are also reduced when there is respiratory muscle weakness, and in some neuromuscular disorders, the decrease may be even greater than that of the corresponding inspiratory pressure [16]. A maximal expiratory pressure of less than 40 cm H_2O is generally associated with a poor cough and difficulty clearing secretions [19].

A second measurement that is valuable in predicting the development of arterial hypercapnia due to neuromuscular weakness is the vital capacity. It can be performed either in the pulmonary function laboratory or at the bedside. [15,19]. Although a vital capacity of less than 1 L, or less than 15 mL per kg of body weight is commonly associated with arterial hypercapnia [1,19], the vital capacity is a less sensitive predictor of arterial hypercapnia than is the maximal inspiratory pressure, particularly in patients with chest wall disorders such as kyphoscoliosis [16]. Significant arterial hypercapnia is unlikely to occur with an inspiratory pressure more negative than −30 cm H_2O; however, arterial hypercapnia may be present with a vital capacity as high as 55% or as low as 20% of the predicted value [15,16].

The measurement of transdiaphragmatic pressures (P_{di}) and diaphragmatic electromyograms (EMGs), although not commonly used clinically, may be helpful. An inspiratory effort associated with a P_{di} consistently more than 40% of maximum predictably results in diaphragmatic fatigue [20]. Therefore, it follows that patients with diaphragmatic weakness and a reduced maximum P_{di} are at risk for developing diaphragmatic fatigue and respiratory failure, even in the face of normal inspiratory pressure [20]. Similarly, a decrease of more than 20% from baseline in the high- to low-frequency ratio as measured by the diaphragmatic EMG indicates diaphragmatic fatigue and portends the development of hypercapnic failure [21,22].

Central Nervous System Dysfunction

The respiratory center, located in the brainstem, is composed of two main parts, the medullary center and the pneumotaxic center [23,24]: The medullary center is responsible for initiation and maintenance of spontaneous respiration, and the pneumotaxic center in the pons helps coordinate cyclic respiration. A decrease in central drive can occur due to a direct central loss of sensitivity to changes in $PaCO_2$ and pH or a peripheral chemoreceptor loss of sensitivity to hypoxia as a result of CNS depressants, metabolic abnormalities, structural lesions, primary alveolar hypoventilation, and central sleep apnea (Table 50.1) [25–43].

Peripheral Nervous System Dysfunction

Disruption in impulse transmission from the respiratory center to the respiratory muscles can eventuate in respiratory failure. This disruption can be caused by spinal cord disease [44], anterior horn cell disease [45,46], peripheral neuropathy, or neuromuscular junction blockade [19] (Table 50.2) [5,25,44–88]. Denervation of the inspiratory muscles may occur as part of a generalized process (e.g., Guillain–Barré syndrome, myasthenia gravis [19]) or as an isolated abnormality (e.g., phrenic nerve palsy secondary to hypothermic cardioplegia during cardiac surgery [67,89]).

Peripheral nervous system dysfunction severe enough to produce hypercapnic respiratory failure is always associated with pulmonary function test findings of a reduced vital capacity (usually less than 50% of the predicted value [15,19]) and markedly decreased maximal inspiratory and expiratory pressures (usually 30% of the predicted pressures [15,19,55]). This type of respiratory failure is characterized by an ineffective cough and a high incidence of aspiration, atelectasis, and pneumonia [5].

The effect on the respiratory system of interruption of CNS impulse transmission due to spinal cord abnormalities is highly dependent on the level of the injury [44,47]. A lesion at the C3

TABLE 50.1

RESPIRATORY FAILURE CAUSED BY CENTRAL NERVOUS SYSTEM DYSFUNCTION

Causes [Reference]	Salient clinical features	Diagnostic tests	Treatment
Central nervous system depressant drugs [25–27]	Pupillary changes Needle marks	Toxicology screen Electrocardiogram in tricyclic overdose	See Section 10 (Pharmacology, Overdoses, and Poisonings)
Hypothyroidism [28]	Myxedema	Thyroid function tests	Cautious thyroid replacement
Starvation [29]	Cachexia Diarrhea	↓ Albumin ↓ Cholesterol	Nutrition
Metabolic alkalosis [30]	Lethargy Confusion	Arterial blood gases Serum electrolytes	See Chapter 71
Structural brainstem damage [27,31,32]	Localizing neurologic findings		
Neoplasm	Headache	CT, MRI, cerebrospinal fluid cytology	Radiation, chemotherapy
Infection	Headache, fever	CT, MRI CT, MRI, cardiac echo	Antimicrobial therapy
Primary alveolar hypoventilation (Ondine's curse) [33–41]	Daytime hypersomnolence Headache Rarely dyspneic Polycythemia Cor pulmonale	Blunted or absent ventilatory response to ↑ CO_2, ↓ O_2 in inspired gas Normal pulmonary function tests	Nighttime ventilatory support Electrophrenic pacing Medroxyprogesterone acetate Supplemental oxygen
Central sleep apnea [31,41–43]	Same as primary alveolar hypoventilation	Polysomnography: apnea without respiratory effort Normal CO_2, O_2 response curves while awake	Nighttime ventilatory support Electrophrenic pacing Supplemental oxygen

↓, decreased; ↑ increased; CT, computed tomography; MRI, magnetic resonance imaging.

vertebral level or above abolishes both diaphragmatic and intercostal activity, leaving only some residual accessory muscle function [47]. The result is severe hypercapnic respiratory failure. Acute spinal cord lesions at the C5 and C6 levels produce an immediate fall in the vital capacity to 30% of the predicted value, due to loss of intercostal and abdominal muscle function [44]. This is associated with a limitation of both inspiratory capacity and active expiration. Within approximately 3 months of injury, however, the denervated muscles become stiff, which enables improved diaphragmatic efficiency. This improvement usually leads to an increase in the vital capacity to 50% to 60% of normal. Midthoracic spinal cord lesions have relatively little impact on respiratory muscle function because they principally affect the abdominal muscles, resulting in only a limitation of active expiration and cough [5,47].

Most spinal cord diseases interrupt impulse transmission, resulting in respiratory muscle weakness, but two notable exceptions exist: tetanus and strychnine poisoning. In both conditions, inhibitory influences at the spinal cord and anterior horn cell level decrease [51–52], causing a simultaneous increase in motor activity to groups of muscles that are normally antagonistic to one another. This results in intense muscle spasms, including involvement of the upper airway muscles, diaphragm, and intercostal muscles. The repetitive spasms and episodes of apnea, result in severe arterial hypoxemia, hypercapnia, and metabolic acidosis [51,52].

Diseases that involve the anterior horn cells of the spinal cord interrupt efferent impulse transmission. Amyotrophic lateral sclerosis (ALS) is the most common anterior horn cell disease causing respiratory failure [5,45,47]. In most cases of ALS, the patient develops segmental muscular atrophy, weakness of the distal extremities, hyperreflexia, fasciculations, and bulbar paralysis [45]. Although respiratory failure usually develops late in the course of the disease, it may rarely be the presenting manifestation [45]. Repetitive episodes of aspiration secondary to bulbar dysfunction may contribute to respiratory impairment [5]. It has been speculated that antecedent poliomyelitis may be involved in some cases of amyotrophic lateral sclerosis [53]. A postpolio syndrome, characterized by new, slowly progressive muscle weakness, may develop years after recovery from acute poliomyelitis [57].

Polyneuropathies with prominent motor neuron involvement, (e.g. Guillain–Barré syndrome) can affect the respiratory nerves and lead to respiratory failure (see Chapter 175) [25]. Symmetric, predominantly distal muscle weakness with absent tendon reflexes is the typical presentation [25]. In one series of patients with Guillain–Barré syndrome, 28% required mechanical ventilatory assistance. The average duration of mechanical ventilation was 9 weeks (range, 3 weeks to 7 months). Although the mortality rate is generally low, 21% of hospitalized patients died in one series [90]. Guillain–Barré syndrome may be associated with autonomic dysfunction including new-onset hypertension (57%), sinus tachycardia (50%), postural hypotension (43%), or facial flushing (25%) [90].

Dinoflagellate toxin poisoning, from red tide-contaminated shellfish and ciguatera-contaminated reef and other fish, is a dramatic but uncommon cause of peripheral neuropathy resulting that can produce respiratory failure [61–66]. The responsible agents are heat-stable neurotoxins that interfere with action potential propagation along peripheral nerves. During the warm summer months, the dinoflagellates that produce the toxins proliferate and are ingested by shellfish and fish. The

TABLE 50.2

RESPIRATORY FAILURE CAUSED BY PERIPHERAL NERVOUS SYSTEM DYSFUNCTION

Causes [Reference]	Salient features	Diagnostic tests	Supportive
Spinal cord disease [5,25,44,47–50]	Above C5, diaphragm, intercostal and abdominal activity abolished	Spinal X-ray film, CT, MRI	Supportive, vital capacity tends to improve more than 3 mo in traumatic lesions C5 and below
Traumatic	Below C5, diaphragm preserved, intercostal and abdominal activity abolished		Phrenic nerve pacing for high cervical cord lesions with intact phrenic nerve
Neoplasm	Below T5, abdominal activity diminished, impaired force expiration		
Hemorrhage Syrinx Infarct Transverse myelitis			
Tetanus [51]	Intense muscle spasms Trismus Apnea Metabolic acidosis History of penetrating wound	Clinical setting Gram's stain, anaerobic culture of wound History of inadequate immunization	Human antitetanus antiglobulin Wound debridement Penicillin, high dose Tetanus toxoid vaccination to prevent recurrence
Strychnine [52]	Intense muscle spasms Apnea Metabolic acidosis	Toxicology screen Clinical picture	Supportive Gastric lavage, charcoal
Anterior horn cell disease Amyotrophic lateral sclerosis [5,45,46,53,54] Poliomyelitis [55,57]	Segmental muscle atrophy Hyperreflexia Fasciculations Distal extremity weakness	EMG	Supportive
Polyneuropathy [25]	Viral illness, symmetric ascending distal muscle weakness	Elevated CSF protein without pleocytosis	Prevention with vaccine
Guillain–Barré syndrome [25,58–60]	Ascending paralysis Areflexia Autonomic dysfunction	Demyelination by electrophysiology tests	See Chapter 175
Dinoflagellate poisoning	Paresthesias of face, progressive muscle weakness starting 30 min after ingestion of shellfish	History of contaminated shellfish ingestion	Supportive
Shellfish poisoning (red tide) [61–63]			
Ciguatera poisoning [64–66]	Gastrointestinal symptoms Paresthesias, abnormal temperature differentiation	Mouse bioassay, monoclonal antibody to ciguatoxin	Early gastric lavage, mannitol, avoid caffeine
Bilateral phrenic nerve palsy [67,69]	Severe orthopnea Abdominal paradoxic respiration	Fluoroscopy of diaphragm Surface EMG of diaphragm, transdiaphragmatic pressure	Diaphragmatic pacing
Charcot–Marie–Tooth disease [70]	Peripheral muscle weakness and wasting, hereditary pes cavus, hammertoes	EMG	Supportive
Diphtheria [25]	Numbness of lips, paralysis of pharyngeal and laryngeal muscles	Throat culture	Diphtheria antitoxin Penicillin G or Erythromycin
Tick paralysis [25]	Tick exposure Age <10 y	Find tick Normal sensation	Remove tick

(*continued*)

TABLE 50.2

CONTINUED

Causes [Reference]	Salient features	Diagnostic tests	Supportive
Acute intermittent porphyria [25]	Acute polyneuropathy-like Guillain–Barré syndrome Mental disturbance Abdominal pain	Urine for porphobilinogen, δ-aminolevulinic acid	Hemin chloride, cimetidine Avoid exacerbating drugs such as phenytoin, barbiturates, ethosuximide
Myasthenia gravis (autoimmune and drug-induced) [25,71–76]	Muscle weakness Rapid fatigability Antecedent surgery, glucocorticoid, or aminoglycoside	EMG Tensilon test Antibodies to acetylcholine receptors	Anticholinesterase/calcium gluconate/thymectomy/ glucocorticoids/ immunosuppressants See Chapter 176 Plasmapheresis
Eaton-Lambert syndrome [56,77]	Muscle wasting, hyporeflexia Associated cancer (e.g., small cell of lung)	Incremental pattern on EMG chest film	Treatment of associated cancer 3, 4-Diaminopyridine Anticholinesterase
Critical illness polyneuropathy [78–81]	Sepsis, multiorgan failure, generalized weakness, areflexia	Normal CSF, axonal degeneration by NCS	Supportive
Persistent drug-induced neuromuscular blockade [78,82,83]	Renal insufficiency Glucocorticoids	Creatinine phosphokinase, EMG, NCS, repetitive nerve stimulation	Limit use of neuromuscular blocking agents
Pseudocholinesterase deficiency [25]	Prolonged paralysis after succinylcholine Family history	Serum pseudocholinesterase EMG	Avoid succinylcholine
Botulism [85,86]	Wound infection, fever Ingestion of contaminated food: nausea and vomiting	Gram's stain and culture of stool, wound, or suspected food Demonstrate toxin in stool, serum, or food by mouse neutralization test	Trivalent antitoxin Wound debridement, penicillin G (or metronidazole if penicillin allergy) Nasogastric lavage
Organophosphates [87,88]	Dysphagia, diplopia, ptosis, dysarthria Use of insecticides Cholinergic toxicity (vomiting, diarrhea, weakness, cramps, sweating, ataxia, mental status changes)	History of exposure RBC Acetyl cholinesterase level Atropine 1 mg challenge	Atropine Pralidoxime Benzodiazepine Cutaneous decontamination
Neuralgic amyotrophy [68]	Shoulder and neck pain, upper extremity weakness, breathlessness, orthopnea	Fluoroscopy of diaphragm, chest film, EMG	Analgesics, possible glucocorticoids

CSF, cerebrospinal fluid; CT, computed tomography; EMG, electromyogram; MRI, magnetic resonance imaging; NCS, nerve conduction study; RBC, red blood cell.

clinical picture is virtually pathognomonic. Within 30 minutes of ingesting contaminated shellfish, tingling and numbness of the face, lips, and tongue develop. Paresthesias and muscle weakness follow, with rapid progression to limb and respiratory muscle paralysis [62,63]. Multiple-case presentations from one source of exposure are common.

Peripheral phrenic nerve palsies can contribute to or cause hypercapnic respiratory failure, particularly if they are bilateral [91]. Bilateral phrenic nerve palsies have been described as an uncommon complication of hypothermia used for cardioplegia during cardiac surgery (particularly when ice slush is used) [67], trauma [67,91], a variety of neurologic diseases (e.g., poliomyelitis and Guillain–Barré syndrome) [67,68,91], Charcot–Marie–Tooth disease [70], intrathoracic malignancies [92], and as a part of a paraneoplastic syndrome [93]. Bilateral diaphragmatic paralysis can also be idiopathic [94]. The characteristic clinical findings of bilateral diaphragmatic paralysis are severe orthopnea and marked abdominal paradoxic in the supine position [69,89,91,95]. Fluoroscopy during a sniff test is more helpful in identifying unilateral than bilateral diaphragm paralysis, as upward motion of the ribs during inspiration can make the diaphragm appear to descend. The diagnosis of diaphragmatic paralysis is usually confirmed by transdiaphragmatic pressure measurements that reveal a minimal or absent P_{di} gradient [91]. Electromyography of the diaphragm and phrenic nerve conduction velocity studies may also be helpful.

Several other causes of peripheral neuropathy can involve the efferent pathways to the respiratory muscles including diphtheria, herpes zoster infection, tick paralysis, acute intermittent porphyria, beriberi, and a variety of metabolic disorders [25]. Respiratory failure associated with diphtheria is of delayed onset, usually occurring 4 to 6 weeks after the onset of illness [25]. Tick paralysis is seen mainly in children in whom the presence of the tick goes unnoticed for 5 to 6 days [25]. In acute intermittent porphyria, respiratory involvement may be a slowly progressive process or may cause an abrupt deterioration in respiratory function due to bilateral phrenic nerve paralysis [37]. Myasthenia gravis [19], botulism [84–86], organophosphate poisoning [25], and a variety of drugs can produce neuromuscular blockade that results in respiratory failure [76]. Although patients with myasthenia gravis typically show signs of obvious muscle weakness and rapid fatigability, particularly of the cranial muscles, before the development of respiratory failure, acute respiratory failure is occasionally a presenting manifestation [25,72]. More commonly, respiratory failure complicates myasthenia gravis after surgical procedures, following the institution of glucocorticoid therapy, or, as a result of under- or overtreatment with anticholinesterase medications [19].

Although the diagnosis of myasthenia gravis is suspected on clinical grounds and a positive response to edrophonium chloride (Tensilon) is supportive, the diagnosis is confirmed by a typical EMG (decremental responses on repetitive nerve stimulation) and an elevated serum level of antibodies to acetylcholine receptors [71] (see Chapter 176). Part of the management of a patient with myasthenia gravis includes serial measurement of the, maximum inspiratory pressure and vital capacity to assess the risk for respiratory failure [25]. A decrease in maximum inspiratory pressure to a value less negative than −30 cm H_2O or a decrease in vital capacity to a liter or less is a warning sign of impending respiratory failure [19].

Eaton–Lambert syndrome, a form of neuromuscular blockade similar to myasthenia gravis, occurs in association with certain carcinomas, particularly small cell carcinoma of the lung [55,56]. The neuromuscular blockade in most cases precedes other evidence of the carcinoma, and the EMG shows an incremental pattern unlike that in true myasthenia.

Critical illness polyneuropathy occurs in the setting of sepsis and multiorgan failure in up to 30% of patients by clinical examination and up to 70% by electrophysiologic testing [78,81]. Profound generalized muscle weakness due to critical illness polyneuropathy is a major reason why these patients often require prolonged mechanical ventilatory support. Similar to patients with Guillain–Barré Syndrome, patients with critical illness polyneuropathy also have areflexia, but in contrast, they also may have prominent sensory nerve findings and a normal cerebrospinal fluid examination. Electrophysiologic testing helps to distinguish critical illness polyneuropathy from Guillain–Barré syndrome; in critical illness, polyneuropathy nerve conduction studies show axon degeneration rather than demyelination. Although the etiology of critical illness polyneuropathy is not known, it is predominantly a disease of older patients who stay in the intensive care unit for more than 28 days and who have elevated serum glucose and decreased albumin levels at the time of diagnosis. Approximately half of patients with sepsis, multiorgan system failure, and critical illness polyneuropathy survive and the prognosis of survivors for significant improvement from the neuropathy is good [79] (see Chapter 180 for additional details).

Prolonged administration (longer than 2 days) of neuromuscular blocking agents, such as pancuronium and vecuronium, has been associated with two distinct patterns of neuromuscular dysfunction [82]: (a) persistent neuromuscular junction blockade in patients with renal insufficiency who accumulate the parent drug and its active metabolites, and (b) an acute noninflammatory myopathy that becomes apparent as neuromuscular transmission improves. The myopathy appears to be a consequence of an interaction between neuromuscular blocking agents and glucocorticoids and seems to be related to the total dose of the neuromuscular blocking agent [83]. This has been particularly dramatic in previously healthy asthmatic patients who became quadriparetic for days to weeks after concomitant treatment with high-dose glucocorticoids and a neuromuscular-blocking agent [82].

Neuromuscular blockade also may occur as a result of administration of a variety of drugs [76]. Certain cardiovascular drugs (e.g., Xylocaine, quinidine, procainamide, and propranolol), anticonvulsants (e.g., phenytoin and trimethadione), D-penicillamine, and a number of antibiotics (most notably the aminoglycosides) can prolong postoperative respiratory depression, unmask underlying myasthenia gravis, or cause a drug-induced form of myasthenia gravis [76]. The definitive diagnosis of drug-induced neuromuscular blockade is usually made in retrospect if the abnormality reverses after elimination of the offending agent. In some cases, the administration of calcium gluconate has been reported to result in prompt improvement in neuromuscular transmission [76].

Prolonged neuromuscular blockade is occasionally seen after the administration of succinylcholine in individuals with pseudocholinesterase deficiency [25]. In contrast to the usual duration of paralysis of approximately 3 minutes, the effect in these individuals usually lasts 4 to 6 hours, during which time they require mechanical ventilatory support [25].

In botulism, neuromuscular blockade develops as a result of a neurotoxin produced by the bacteria *Clostridium botulinum*. Most cases are caused by neurotoxin-contaminated food [84–86], but occasionally botulism develops as a result of a wound infected with *C. botulinum* [51] (see Chapter 88). Certain findings help to predict whether respiratory failure requiring mechanical ventilation will develop. A vital capacity of 30% or less of the predicted value is generally associated with hypercapnic failure [50]. Other clues are the presence of nausea, vomiting, diarrhea, dyspnea, ptosis, or extremity weakness on initial examination.

Organophosphates, commonly used in insecticides, inhibit the enzyme cholinesterase, resulting in accumulation of acetylcholine at neurosynaptic junctions. The symptoms of organophosphate poisoning are those of cholinergic toxicity, including blurred vision, weakness, vomiting, diarrhea, cramps, sweating, increased secretions, incoordination, twitching, ataxia, mental status changes, and, if severe enough, respiratory failure and death [87,88]. Respiratory muscle paralysis combines with respiratory center depression, excessive secretions, and, possibly, bronchoconstriction to cause respiratory failure [87,88] (see Chapter 128). Neuralgic amyotrophy, a disorder of the peripheral nervous system affecting the brachial plexus, has recently been associated with diaphragmatic dysfunction and dyspnea [68]. It usually presents with acute severe shoulder pain that may extend to the neck, back, and arm. Motor weakness of the ipsilateral shoulder and arm usually develops within 1 month of the onset of pain. A sensory defect may be present in one fourth of patients. In one study [68], 12 of 16 patients had bilateral diaphragm paralysis, and 4 of 16 had unilateral diaphragm paralysis. Mild nocturnal desaturation, hypopneas, and obstructive sleep apneas (OSAs) were found in some patients, but alveolar hypoventilation was not found.

Respiratory Muscle Dysfunction

A number of systemic myopathies feature prominent respiratory muscle involvement, including muscular dystrophies, myotonic disorders, inflammatory myopathies, periodic paralyses, metabolic storage diseases, endocrine myopathies, infectious myopathies, toxic myopathies, rhabdomyolysis, and electrolyte disturbances (Table 50.3) [16,25,82,83,96–126].

TABLE 50.3

RESPIRATORY FAILURE CAUSED BY RESPIRATORY MUSCLE DYSFUNCTION

Causes [Reference]	Salient features	Diagnostic tests	Specific treatment
Muscle dystrophies [101–105]	Proximal muscle weakness and atrophy Hereditary	Muscle biopsy Elevated CPK Genetic analysis	Supportive Duchenne: prednisone
Myotonic dystrophies [106–109]	Myotonia, ptosis Distal and facial muscle weakness and atrophy Hereditary	Muscle biopsy EMG genetic analysis	Supportive Possibly mexiletine and acetazolamide
Periodic paralyses [25,109,110]	Hypokalemic, hyperkalemic, or normokalemic Genetic Muscle weakness associated with exercise, emotional upset, cold, alcohol	Serum potassium Family history	Avoid precipitating factors Carbonic anhydrase inhibitor
Glycogen storage diseases [25,97,97,111] (Pompe and McArdle diseases)	Exercise-related muscle cramping; slowly progressive muscle weakness and atrophy	CPK, muscle biopsy with assay for acid maltase, muscle phosphorylase levels	Supportive
Dermatomyositis/ polymyositis [16,112–114]	Proximal muscle weakness Rash in dermatomyositis Difficulty swallowing	Elevated CPK, aldolase EMG Muscle biopsy	Glucocorticoids Immunosuppressants
Hyperthyroidism [115]	Thyrotoxicosis heat intolerance, tachycardia, hyperreflexia	TSH, TFTs	Propylthiouracil, methimazole See Chapter 102
Hypothyroidism [25]	Myxedema, cold intolerance Hyporeflexia, bradycardia	TSH, TFTs	Replace thyroid hormone See Chapter 103
Hyperadrenocorticalism [25,116]	Cushingoid appearance	Serum cortisol Dexamethasone suppression test, adrenal CT scan	Depends on cause
Rhabdomyolysis secondary to colchicine [117] or chloroquine toxicity [25]	Muscle pain, swelling, myoglobulinuria	↑ CPK	Supportive
Infectious myositis Trichinosis [25,118] Viral [25]	Muscle tenderness, weakness, fever	Serology Muscle biopsy	Rest Glucocorticoids, thiabendazole or mebendazole
Hypophosphatemia [99,100,119,120]	Weakness Difficulty weaning	↓ Phosphate	Replete See Chapter 105
Hypermagnesemia or hypomagnesemia [100,121,122]	Weakness Difficulty weaning	↑ or ↓ Mg^{++}	
Hypokalemia [100]	Weakness	↓ K^{+}	Replete
Hypercalcemia [100,122]	Lethargy, confusion	↑ Ca^{++}	See Chapters 72, 105, and 116
Eosinophilia-myalgia [123–125]	L-tryptophan ingestion Muscle tenderness and weakness, fasciitis Fasciitis	Eosinophilia Muscle biopsy	Discontinue L-tryptophan Supportive
Procainamide-induced myopathy [126]	Weakness Respiratory failure	Muscle biopsy, ↑ CPK	Discontinue procainamide
Acute myopathy secondary to neuromuscular blocking agents [82,83]	Neuromuscular blocking agents Glucocorticoids Rapid onset weakness	EMG Muscle biopsy	Supportive

↓, decreased; ↑, increased; CPK, creatinine phosphokinase; CT, computed tomography; EMG, electromyography; TFT, thyroid function test; TSH, thyroid-stimulating hormone.

The clinical presentation generally is widespread skeletal muscle weakness. Muscle weakness is the inability of a muscle to generate the normal expected level of force and should be distinguished from muscle fatigue, which is the inability to generate the preexistent maximum force prior to putting the muscle under load or stress. Fatigue is reversible with rest; weakness may be reversible with reconditioning or the reversal or elimination of the causative factor (e.g. malnutrition, disuse atrophy). Respiratory muscle involvement and respiratory failure usually develop as the disease progresses. On occasion, however, respiratory failure may be the presenting manifestation of a generalized myopathy [97].

Myopathy-induced hypercapnic respiratory failure is almost invariably accompanied by a severely impaired cough mechanism and an inability to clear respiratory tract secretions [5]. Typical pulmonary function findings of respiratory muscle weakness are a decrease in maximum inspiratory and expiratory pressures and, as the disease progresses, a decrease in lung volumes [127].

The muscular dystrophies are inherited disorders that present with evidence of progressive proximal muscle weakness and atrophy [25,101]. Duchenne and Becker muscular dystrophies are caused by mutations in the dystrophin gene, located on the X chromosome [102]. Duchenne dystrophy usually presents at approximately 2 to 3 years of age and Becker dystrophy at approximately 15 to 20 years of age. The limb-girdle muscular dystrophies are a more heterogeneous group of disorders that show both autosomal recessive and autosomal dominant inheritance and include mutations in different members of the sarcoglycan complex including motilin, dysferlin, caveolin, and sarcoglycan. Myofibrillar myopathy is also associated with mutations in the motilin gene and both of these may eventuate in respiratory failure [103]. They frequently present later in adulthood than do the dystrophin-related muscular dystrophies [104]. The myotonic dystrophies are autosomal dominant disorders linked to two chromosome loci: 19q13, where a CTG repeat has been found in the intron of a serine threonine protein kinase gene, and 3q21, where a CCTG repeat has been found in the intron of zinc finger protein 9 [106,107]. The most prominent clinical features are myotonia (i.e., sustained contraction of muscles in response to direct stimulation), ptosis, prominent distal and facial muscle weakness, and atrophy [25,104,108].

The periodic paralyses are genetic disorders characterized by attacks of muscle weakness in response to a variety of precipitating factors such as exercise, emotional upset, exposure to cold, and, in some cases, exposure to alcohol [25]. Patients may exhibit hypokalemia, hyperkalemia, or normokalemia. In some patients, the disease is unmasked when they become hyperthyroid.

Glycogen storage diseases result from defects in muscle glycogenolysis or glycogen storage. Examples include acid maltase deficiency (type II) and McArdle disease (type V). Patients exhibit exercise-induced muscle cramping and slowly progressive muscle weakness, with or without atrophy [25,97,98,111]. On occasion, respiratory failure may be the presenting manifestation [97,111]. The diagnosis is confirmed by muscle biopsy and chemical assay for muscle acid maltase or phosphorylase levels [97,98].

Polymyositis and dermatomyositis are collagen vascular diseases that cause skeletal muscle inflammation. Proximal muscle weakness is prominent and usually develops over a period of weeks to months. Patients may have difficulty swallowing secondary to pharyngeal muscle involvement. Serum muscle enzyme levels are elevated. Typical EMG and muscle biopsy findings confirm the diagnosis [112]. Respiratory muscle failure is an uncommon, but not rare complication of inflammatory myositis [16,112]. Patients with polymyositis may also develop interstitial pulmonary fibrosis, bronchiolitis obliterans organizing pneumonia, and alveolar hemorrhage [113,114].

Procainamide has been reported to cause a necrotizing myopathy with diaphragm involvement and respiratory failure [126]. Although anti–double-stranded DNA and antihistone antibodies were positive, antinuclear antibodies were absent, and the muscle biopsy did not reveal an inflammatory infiltrate. Neuromuscular junction transmission was normal, suggesting that this was not a drug-induced myasthenic syndrome. Slow improvement in muscle strength followed discontinuation of procainamide in this study.

Increased Impedance to Bulk Flow

In a number of pulmonary disorders, the development of hypercapnic respiratory failure is the result of a marked increase in impedance to ventilation (e.g., increased airflow resistance in COPD or asthma or increased elastic recoil in interstitial fibrosis) that even normal respiratory muscle force generation cannot overcome [3]. It may be less widely appreciated that increases in extrapulmonary impedance to ventilation also can result in hypercapnic respiratory failure. These disorders can be divided into those involving a decrease in chest wall or pleural compliance (e.g., kyphoscoliosis or pleural fibrosis) and those involving an increase in airflow resistance, resulting from upper airway obstruction (e.g., tracheal stenosis or laryngeal edema) (Table 50.4) [5,42,43,128–189].

Chest Wall and Pleural Disorders

Kyphoscoliosis is a common cause of extrapulmonary respiratory failure [5]. The severity of the scoliosis (i.e., lateral curvature of the spine) is usually the more important factor in the development of respiratory failure than is the kyphosis (i.e., dorsal curvature of the spine) [5]. In idiopathic kyphoscoliosis, chronic hypercapnic respiratory failure generally occurs when the angle of curvature is 120 degrees or greater [5]. In contrast, in paralytic kyphoscoliosis (e.g., as a result of poliomyelitis), the angle of curvature does not reliably predict either vital capacity or hypercapnic respiratory failure [128]. This appears to be due to a greater element of muscle weakness in paralytic kyphoscoliosis [128]. Even in idiopathic kyphoscoliosis, however, the presence of markedly decreased chest wall compliance is further complicated by inspiratory muscle weakness [129] that contributes to the development of hypercapnic respiratory failure [94]. In addition, a modest element of pulmonary gas exchange abnormality is usually present [5].

Patients with kyphoscoliosis usually report progressive dyspnea on exertion and exercise limitation for a period of years before actual arterial hypercapnia develops [5]. In patients with moderately advanced kyphoscoliosis, acute hypercapnic respiratory failure may result from acute reversible complications such as pulmonary congestion, retained secretions, or pulmonary infection [130].

Massive chest wall obesity may be associated with significant hypoventilation and the development of hypercapnic respiratory failure [133]. This is termed the *obesity-hypoventilation syndrome*. The pathogenesis of respiratory failure appears to be multifactorial and includes significant reduction in chest wall compliance, decreased respiratory muscle efficiency, reduced or blunted respiratory center drive, and impaired pulmonary gas exchange as a result of pulmonary congestion [133–135].

TABLE 50.4

RESPIRATORY FAILURE CAUSED BY CHEST WALL, PLEURAL, AND UPPER AIRWAY DISEASES

Causes [Reference]	Salient features	Diagnostic tests	Specific treatment
Chest wall and pleural disorders			
Kyphoscoliosis [5,128–132]	Spinal curvature ≥120 degrees Progressive dyspnea on exertion over several years	Spinal X-ray films Restriction on PFTs	Nighttime ventilatory support
Obesity-hypoventilation [133–135]	Massive chest wall obesity ± sleep apnea	Polysomnography ↓CO_2 response curve ↓Chest wall compliance	Weight loss Nasal CPAP or BPAP
Flail chest [136]	Multiple rib fractures, paradoxic respiration ± pleuritic chest pain	Chest film	Mechanical positive-pressure ventilation
Fibrothorax [5,137–139]	Asbestos exposure, pleural infection, pleural hemorrhage, uremia, collagen vascular disease	Observation of chest wall Restriction on PFTs Decreased maximum static elastic recoil pressure	Decortication
Thoracoplasty [5]	Chest wall deformity secondary to resection of ribs	Restriction on PFTs Chest film	Supportive
Ankylosing spondylitis [5]	Limited chest expansion Apical pulmonary fibrosis Limited lumbar mobility Chronic lower back pain	PFTs (↑functional residual capacity, ↓total lung capacity) HLA-B27 Spine and sacroiliac X-ray films	Anti-inflammatory agents Flexibility exercises
Upper airway obstruction			
Acute epiglottis [140–143]	Fever, sore throat, stridor, dysphagia	Soft tissue films of neck	See Chapter 67
Acute laryngeal edema			
Angioedema/anaphylaxis [142,144–148]	Stridor in setting of *Hymenoptera* sting, contrast media, or drug administration	Other evidence of angioedema/anaphylaxis; complement levels	Epinephrine parenterally Cricothyroidotomy
Traumatic [149,150]	Stridor after endotracheal extubation	History	Inhaled racemic epinephrine Reintubation Helium–oxygen mixture
Foreign body aspiration [151–156]	Unable to speak Stridor or apnea	X-ray film helpful when foreign body below cords	Heimlich maneuver Bronchoscopy Cricothyroidotomy
Retropharyngeal hemorrhage [157]	Associated with anticoagulation or head and neck surgery Sore throat	Soft tissue film of neck CT scan or tomography	Reverse anticoagulation
Bilateral vocal cord paralysis [158–165]	Stridor Aspiration	Flow–volume loop Laryngoscopy	See text
Laryngeal and tracheal tumors [142,166–170]	Dyspnea Hoarseness; dysphonia Stridor	Flow–volume loop Tomography Laryngotracheoscopy	Laser or surgical resection, radiation
Tracheal stenosis [150,162,171–173]	Progressive dyspnea History of endotracheal intubation	Flow–volume loop Tomography	Tracheostomy Stent, resection of stenosis
Tracheomalacia [171,172]		Laryngotracheoscopy	Stent
Idiopathic obstructive sleep apnea [42,43,174–188,132]	Snoring Daytime hypersomnolence Pulmonary hypertension Cor pulmonale	Polysomnography	Nasal CPAP, bilevel CPAP Protriptyline Uvulopalatopharyngoplasty Tracheostomy Nocturnal oxygen Weight loss
Adenotonsillar hypertrophy [180]	Daytime hypersomnolence Obstructive sleep apnea stridor	Direct visualization Lateral X-ray film	Resection
Obstructive goiter [189]	Enlarged thyroid	Tomography CT scan	Suppression with exogenous thyroid hormone Resection

↓, decreased; ↑, increased; CPAP, continuous positive airway pressure; CT, computed tomography; PFT, pulmonary function test.

Upper Airway Obstruction

A variety of causes of upper airway obstruction involving the extrathoracic upper airway or intrathoracic trachea can result in the development of respiratory failure (Table 50.4).

Significant upper airway obstruction should be considered in the patient who reports dyspnea in association with inspiratory stridor (extrathoracic obstruction) or expiratory wheezing (intrathoracic obstruction), particularly if other symptoms suggest an upper airway process (e.g., dysphagia in epiglottitis). Unless the patient is acutely ill, the diagnosis can usually be confirmed by flow–volume loop analysis [190]. This technique not only demonstrates the presence of an upper airway obstruction but usually also helps determine whether it is extrathoracic or intrathoracic and variable or fixed [190]. Studies such as soft tissue neck radiographs, laryngoscopy, and bronchoscopy can identify the exact nature of the structural abnormality.

Upper airway obstruction from bilateral vocal cord paresis or paralysis may result from a variety of causes. The most common cause is trauma, particularly related to thyroid surgery [161] and, occasionally, after endotracheal intubation [162]. Other causes include tumors [142,166–170]; cricoarytenoid arthritis [160]; herpes simplex viral infection [163]; and neurologic conditions, including Guillain–Barré syndrome [160], extrapyramidal disorders such as Parkinson's disease [164], and myasthenia gravis [159]. Bilateral vocal cord paralysis should be considered when one of these conditions is present and the patient reports aspiration, dyspnea, or stridor [161]. Hoarseness is usually absent during normal speech in bilateral adductor paralysis. The results of flow–volume loop analysis can help confirm the presence of the typical extrathoracic variable obstruction associated with bilateral vocal cord paralysis [165].

Obstructive sleep apnea (OSA) is increasingly recognized as a cause of intermittent functional upper airway obstruction [3,175,176]. Although obesity is a significant risk factor, OSA can occur in its absence [175,176]. Episodic loss of pharyngeal muscle tone caused by decreased respiratory center motor output, usually during rapid eye movement sleep, results in intermittent airway obstruction [175,177]. This disturbance in respiratory center control also accounts for the mixed apneas (i.e., combination obstructive and central apneas) frequently seen in these patients [175,177].

Approximately 10% to 20% of patients with OSA have chronic alveolar hypoventilation with elevation in $PaCO_2$ even while awake. These patients frequently have concomitant COPD or morbid obesity. Hypoxemia, whether just at night or all day, eventually causes cardiac arrhythmias, pulmonary hypertension, and cor pulmonale [3,175,178,179].

The diagnosis of OSA can be established by a sleep study (polysomnography) [174,175]. Other conditions that can cause or exacerbate OSA should be excluded, including adenotonsillar hypertrophy [180]; deviated nasal septum [176]; retrognathia or micrognathia [3]; macroglossia from acromegaly [183]; endocrine and metabolic abnormalities such as hypothyroidism [67,184,185]; CNS depression from ethanol, barbiturates, and benzodiazepines [175,186]; and exogenous androgen administration [187,188] (see Chapter 69).

DIFFERENTIAL DIAGNOSIS

The major differential diagnosis of extrapulmonary respiratory failure is hypercapnic respiratory failure from intrinsic lung diseases (e.g., COPD) (Fig. 50.1). These conditions usually can be readily distinguished because they are almost always associated with a markedly elevated $P(A-a)O_2$ gradient when calculated on room air, reflecting a severe derangement of distal gas exchange. Hypercapnic respiratory failure may also result from a combination of pulmonary and extrapulmonary abnormalities. This combined diagnosis is suggested by a $P(A-a)O_2$ gradient in the range of 25 to 30 mm Hg. If the extrapulmonary abnormality is predominant, the gradient, although abnormal, is generally less than 25 mm Hg [5]. When primary pulmonary disease is severe enough to cause hypercapnia, the gradient is generally above 30 mm Hg.

TREATMENT

The treatment of extrapulmonary respiratory failure can be divided into specific and supportive therapy. Supportive therapy involves the use of noninvasive or invasive mechanical ventilatory assistance (see Chapters 58 and 59), supplemental oxygen, and techniques of airway hygiene (see Chapter 62). In addition, regardless of the primary cause of respiratory muscle weakness, malnutrition exacerbates it and nutritional replacement can increase respiratory muscle strength and function [191,192]. In selected circumstances, inspiratory resistive training of the respiratory muscles and the use of theophylline as a positive respiratory muscle inotrope have been reported to improve respiratory muscle function and associated hypercapnic respiratory failure [193–196]. Only specific forms of therapy are discussed here and in Tables 50.1 through 50.4.

Central Nervous System Depression

A description of specific treatment modalities for CNS depression is given in Table 50.1.

Peripheral Nervous System Dysfunction

Treatment for peripheral nervous system disorders is outlined in Table 50.2. In general, there is little in the way of specific therapy for established spinal cord or anterior horn cell disease. The use of phrenic nerve pacemakers for high-level cervical cord transection may help treat the resultant respiratory failure when nerve conduction studies have determined that the phrenic nerves are intact and functioning [48–50,91]. If pacing brings on OSA, tracheostomy or noninvasive positive airway pressure may be necessary.

The availability and value of specific therapy for peripheral neuropathy depend on the cause. In the case of acute Guillain–Barré syndrome, plasmapheresis or intravenous infusion of pooled gamma-globulin may be helpful when administered promptly for patients who reach or appear to be approaching the inability to walk without help or who have substantial decrease in ventilatory capacity or bulbar insufficiency (see Chapter 175 for more details on treating Guillain–Barré syndrome).

Patients with severe respiratory muscle weakness due to Guillain–Barré syndrome require supportive mechanical ventilatory assistance, usually for weeks to months, and occasionally for longer than 1 year [59]. If cranial nerve involvement is prominent, intubation for airway protection should be considered, even in the absence of overt respiratory failure. Management is complicated by autonomic nervous system dysfunction, which is commonly present and a leading cause of death in this syndrome [90]. Abnormalities of increased or decreased sympathetic and parasympathetic nervous system activity, such as hypertension, hypotension, bradyarrhythmias, tachyarrhythmias, flushing, diaphoresis, and ileus, frequently occur [90]. Because these events are often transient, minor fluctuations in heart rate or blood pressure should not be treated. When intervention is deemed necessary, short-acting and easily titratable drugs should be used [90]. Because patients are at increased risk for deep venous thrombosis and pulmonary embolism, prophylactic anticoagulation should be administered, according to guidelines for critically-ill patients (see Chapter 52 for more details on anticoagulation in critically ill patients). Treatment of respiratory failure caused by myasthenia gravis is directed primarily at the myasthenia (see Chapter 176).

Drug-induced neuromuscular blockade often improves simply by discontinuing the offending agent [57]. Intravenous calcium gluconate may help to shorten the recovery time by reversing the presynaptic component of the neuromuscular blockade [76]. If this fails and the patient improves after an edrophonium chloride test, neostigmine bromide may be effective by reversing the postsynaptic component [52]. When myasthenia gravis is exacerbated or made manifest by a drug, therapy directed specifically at the myasthenic symptoms may be required [76].

Treatment of botulism is directed at minimizing further binding of toxin to nerve endings while supporting the patient until bound toxin dissipates [85] (see Chapter 88). Recovery of ventilatory and upper airway muscle strength in type A botulism occurs slowly; patients recover most of their strength in the first 12 weeks, but full recovery may take up to a year [86].

Respiratory Muscle Dysfunction

The treatment of myopathy depends on the cause (Table 50.3). Although the mechanism is not known, glucocorticoid therapy has resulted in some improvement in muscle strength in Duchenne muscular dystrophy [102,105]. Mexiletine and acetazolamide may be helpful in myotonic dystrophy [109].

Some patients with each of the different subtypes of periodic paralysis have responded well to acetazolamide, a carbonic anhydrase inhibitor that is kaliuretic [111]. Acetazolamide is often dramatically effective in preventing acute attacks of hypokalemic periodic paralysis, perhaps by causing a metabolic acidosis that, in turn, protects against the sudden decreases in potassium that provoke attacks. Certain patients benefit from low-carbohydrate or low-sodium diets in addition to acetazolamide. Inhalation of the β-adrenergic agonist albuterol alleviates acute attacks of weakness in some patients [111].

Polymyositis-induced muscle weakness often responds to glucocorticoids or other immunosuppressants [112,114]. Muscle weakness from hypothyroidism, hypophosphatemia, hypomagnesemia, or hypokalemia responds to replacement therapy [25,115,116,119,121,122].

The specific treatment of trichinosis is less than satisfactory [118]. Thiabendazole may eliminate intestinal worms, but only if initiated within 1 day of ingestion of larvae. Thiabendazole has no effect on the larvae that have reached the muscle and also does not appear to alter the course of established infections. The mainstays of treatment are bed rest, glucocorticoids, and anti-inflammatory analgesic agents.

Chest Wall and Pleural Disorders

Treatment for chest wall and pleural disorders is largely supportive (Table 50.4). If acute respiratory failure develops in kyphoscoliosis, reversible factors such as pulmonary congestion, infection, retained secretions, and other intercurrent illnesses should be sought and treated [130]. Episodes of acute respiratory failure in patients with kyphoscoliosis can often be managed with noninvasive positive pressure ventilation (see Chapter 59 for details of noninvasive ventilation for acute respiratory failure).

When severe kyphoscoliosis is associated with significant chronic hypercapnic respiratory failure, nocturnal noninvasive positive pressure ventilation often results in marked improvement in daytime function and gas exchange [131,197].

Upper Airway Obstruction

The first step in treating acute upper airway obstruction is to establish an adequate airway. Specific definitive therapy can then be used. In acute bacterial epiglottitis associated with significant respiratory distress, immediate steps are mandatory to prevent development of total obstruction [140]. Chapter 67 provides a complete discussion of this and other treatment issues.

Treatment of OSA is indicated when significant sleep-related apneas or hypopneas are noted in the setting of signs and symptoms such as morning headaches, daytime functional impairment, peripheral edema, cor pulmonale, and elevated hematocrit. In general, nasal continuous or bilevel positive pressure devices (continuous positive airway pressure or bilevel continuous positive airway pressure) are effective [198–200] (see Chapters 59 and 62). In OSA complicated by life-threatening arrhythmias, severe arterial hypoxemia, or severe functional impairment [3,176], tracheostomy may rarely be necessary [3,42,176]. Other treatment modalities for OSA include weight loss [201], avoidance of alcohol and sedative drugs [175,186], mandibular and tongue repositioning appliances [202], and upper airway surgery other than tracheostomy (uvulopalatopharyngoplasty, tonsillectomy, adenoidectomy, deviated septum repair), as appropriate [180,203]. When an identifiable cause of OSA is present (e.g., hypothyroidism), correction of the problem may be curative [184,185].

A summary of advances in the treatment of extrapulmonary respiratory failure is given in Table 50.5.

TABLE 50.5

ADVANCES IN THE TREATMENT OF EXTRAPULMONARY RESPIRATORY FAILURE

Disease	Treatment
Duchenne muscular dystrophy	Glucocorticoids improve pulmonary function and slow disease progression [105].
Guillain–Barré syndrome	Both plasmapheresis and IVIG are effective when started within 4 weeks of onset of symptoms [60].
Myasthenia gravis	Plasmapheresis is effective in short-term management of myasthenic crisis [74].
Trichinosis	Thiabendazole and mebendazole are effective in reducing muscle weakness in trichinosis [118].
Obstructive sleep apnea	Nasal continuous positive airway pressure is effective in the treatment of obstructive sleep apnea [200].

IVIG, intravenous immunoglobulin.

References

1. Williams MH Jr, Shim CS: Ventilatory failure. *Am J Med* 48:477, 1970.
2. Pontoppidan H, Geffin B, Lowenstein E: Acute respiratory failure in the adult. *N Engl J Med* 287:690, 1972.
3. Pratter MR, Irwin RS: Extrapulmonary causes of respiratory failure. *J Intensive Care Med* 1:197, 1986.
4. Demers RR, Irwin RS: Management of hypercapnic respiratory failure: a systematic approach. *Respir Care* 24:328, 1979.
5. Bergofsky EH: Respiratory failure in disorders of the thoracic cage. *Am Rev Respir Dis* 119:643, 1979.
6. Aubier M, Murciano D, Fournier M, et al: Central respiratory drive in acute respiratory failure of patients with chronic obstructive pulmonary disease. *Am Rev Respir Dis* 122:191, 1980.
7. Bone RC, Pierce AK, Johnson RL Jr: Controlled oxygen administration in acute respiratory failure in chronic obstructive pulmonary disease. *Am J Med* 65:896, 1978.
8. Degaute JP, Domenighetti G, Naeije R, et al: Oxygen delivery in acute exacerbation of chronic obstructive pulmonary disease. *Am Rev Respir Dis* 124:26, 1981.
9. Weitzenblum E, Sautegeau A, Ehrhart M, et al: Long-term oxygen therapy can reverse the progression of pulmonary hypertension in patients with chronic obstructive pulmonary disease. *Am Rev Respir Dis* 131:493, 1985.
10. Marthan R, Castaing Y, Manier G, et al: Gas exchange alterations in patients with chronic obstructive lung disease. *Chest* 87:470, 1985.
11. Lejeune P, Mols P, Naeije R, et al: Acute hemodynamic effects of controlled oxygen therapy in decompensated chronic obstructive pulmonary disease. *Crit Care Med* 12:1032, 1984.
12. Gray BA, Blalock JM: Interpretation of the alveolar-arterial oxygen difference in patients with hypercapnia. *Am Rev Respir Dis* 143:4, 1991.
13. Braun NMT, Rochester DF: Respiratory muscle strength in obstructive lung disease. *Am Rev Respir Dis* 115:91, 1977.
14. Celli BR, Rassulo J, Berman JS, et al: Respiratory consequences of abdominal hernia in a patient with severe chronic obstructive pulmonary disease. *Am Rev Respir Dis* 131:178, 1985.
15. O'Donohue WJ Jr, Baker JP, Bell GM, et al: Respiratory failure in neuromuscular disease: management in a respiratory intensive care unit. *JAMA* 235:733, 1976.
16. Braun NMT, Arora NS, Rochester DF: Respiratory muscle and pulmonary function in polymyositis and other proximal myopathies. *Thorax* 38:616, 1983.
17. Smyth RJ, Chapman KR, Rebuck AS: Maximal inspiratory and expiratory pressures in adolescents: normal values. *Chest* 86:568, 1984.
18. Black LF, Hyatt RE: Maximal respiratory pressures: normal values and relationship to age and sex. *Am Rev Respir Dis* 99:696, 1969.
19. Gracey DR, Divertie MB, Howard FM Jr: Mechanical ventilation for respiratory failure in myasthenia gravis. *Mayo Clin Proc* 58:597, 1983.
20. Roussos CS, Macklem PT: Diaphragmatic fatigue in man. *J Appl Physiol* 43:189, 1977.
21. Gross D, Grassino A, Ross WR, et al: Electromyogram pattern of diaphragmatic fatigue. *J Appl Physiol* 46:1, 1979.
22. Cohen CA, Zabelbaum G, Gross D, et al: Clinical manifestations of inspiratory muscle fatigue. *Am J Med* 73:308, 1982.
23. Mitchell RA, Berger AJ: Neural regulation of respiration. *Am Rev Respir Dis* 111:206, 1975.
24. Berger AJ, Mitchell RA, Severinghaus JW: Regulation of respiration. *N Engl J Med* 297:138, 1977.
25. Ringel SP, Carroll JE: Respiratory complications of neuromuscular disease, in Weiner WJ (ed): *Respiratory Dysfunction in Neurologic Disease*. Mt. Kisco, NY, Futura, 1980, p 113.
26. Weil JV, McCullough RE, Kline JS, et al: Diminished ventilatory response to hypoxia and hypercapnia after morphine in normal man. *N Engl J Med* 292:1103, 1975.
27. Santiago TV, Pugliese AC, Edelman NH: Control of breathing during methadone addiction. *Am J Med* 62:347, 1977.
28. Skatrud J, Iber C, Ewart R, et al: Disordered breathing during sleep in hypothyroidism. *Am Rev Respir Dis* 124:325, 1981.
29. Doekel RC Jr, Zwillich CW, Scoggin CH, et al: Clinical semi-starvation depression of hypoxic ventilatory response. *N Engl J Med* 295:358, 1976.
30. Tuller MA, Mehdi F: Compensatory hypoventilation and hypercapnia in primary metabolic alkalosis. *Am J Med* 50:281, 1971.
31. Onders RP, Dimarco AF, Ignagni AR, et al: Mapping the phrenic nerve motor point: the key to a successful laparoscopic diaphragm pacing system in the first human series. *Surgery* 136:819, 2004.
32. Phillipson EA: Control of breathing during sleep. *Am Rev Respir Dis* 118:909, 1978.
33. Strohl KP, Hensley MJ, Saunders NA, et al: Progesterone administration and progressive sleep apneas. *JAMA* 245:1230, 1981.
34. Comroe JH Jr: Frankenstein, Pickwick and Ondine. *Am Rev Respir Dis* 111:689, 1975.
35. Hunt CE, Matalon SV, Thompson TR, et al: Central hypoventilation syndrome: experience with bilateral phrenic nerve pacing in 3 neonates. *Am Rev Respir Dis* 118:23, 1978.
36. Wolkove N, Altose MD, Kelsen SG, et al: Respiratory control abnormalities in alveolar hypoventilation. *Am Rev Respir Dis* 122:163, 1980.
37. Sugar O: In search of Ondine's curse. *JAMA* 240:236, 1978.
38. Butler J: Clinical problems of disordered respiratory control. *Am Rev Respir Dis* 110:695, 1974.
39. Skatrud JB, Dempsey JA, Kaiser DG: Ventilatory response to medroxyprogesterone acetate in normal subjects: time course and mechanism. *J Appl Physiol* 44:939, 1978.
40. Hyland RH, Jones NL, Powles AC, et al: Primary alveolar hypoventilation treated with nocturnal electrophrenic respiration. *Am Rev Respir Dis* 117:165, 1978.
41. Bubis MJ, Anthonisen NR: Primary alveolar hypoventilation treated by nocturnal administration of O_2. *Am Rev Respir Dis* 118:947, 1978.
42. Martin TJ, Sanders MH: Chronic alveolar hypoventilation: a review for the clinician. *Sleep* 18:617, 1995.
43. Shepard JWJ: Cardiorespiratory changes in obstructive sleep apnea, in Kryger MH, Roth T, Dement WC (eds): *Principles and Practice of Sleep Medicine*. 2nd ed. Philadelphia, WB Saunders, 1994, p 657.
44. Ledsom JR, Sharp JM: Pulmonary function in acute cervical cord injury. *Am Rev Respir Dis* 124:41, 1981.
45. Fromm GB, Wisdom PJ, Block AJ: Amyotrophic lateral sclerosis presenting with respiratory failure. *Chest* 71:612, 1977.
46. Brooks BR: Natural history of ALS: symptoms, strength, pulmonary function and disability. *Neurology* 47:S71, 1996.
47. Mansel JK, Norman JR: Respiratory complications and management of spinal cord injuries. *Chest* 97:1446, 1990.
48. Glenn WW, Hogan JF, Loke JS, et al: Ventilatory support by pacing of the conditioned diaphragm in quadriplegia. *N Engl J Med* 310:1150, 1984.
49. McMichan JC, Piepgras DG, Gracey DR, et al: Electrophrenic respiration. *Mayo Clin Proc* 54:662, 1979.
50. Gibson G: Diaphragmatic paresis: pathophysiology, clinical features and investigation. *Thorax* 44:960, 1989.
51. Thwaites CL, Farrar JJ: Preventing and treating tetanus. *BMJ* 326:117, 2003.
52. Boyd RE, Brennan PT, Deng JF, et al: Strychnine poisoning. *Am J Med* 74:507, 1983.
53. Mulder DW, Rosenbaum RA, Layton DD Jr: Late progression of poliomyelitis or forme fruste amyotrophic lateral sclerosis? *Mayo Clin Proc* 47:756, 1972.
54. Hopkins LC, Tatarian GT, Pianta TF: Management of ALS. respiratory care. *Neurology* 47:S123, 1996.
55. Hill R, Martin J, Hakim A: Acute respiratory failure in motor neuron disease. *Arch Neurol* 40:30, 1983.
56. Oh SJ, Claussen GG, Hatanaka Y, et al: 3,4-Diaminopyridine is more effective than placebo in a randomized, double-blind, cross-over drug study in LEMS. *Muscle Nerve* 40:795, 2009
57. Dalakas MC, Elder G, Hallett M, et al: A long-term follow-up study of patients with post-poliomyelitis neuromuscular symptoms. *N Engl J Med* 314:959, 1986.
58. Ropper AH: The Guillain-Barré syndrome. *N Engl J Med* 326:1130, 1992.
59. Chevrolet J, Deleamont P: Repeated vital capacity measurements as predictive parameters for mechanical ventilation need and weaning in the GB syndrome. *Am Rev Respir Dis* 144:814, 1991.
60. Hughes RA, Wijdicks EF, Barohn R, et al: Quality Standards Subcommittee of the American Academy of Neurology. Practice parameter: immunotherapy for Guillain-Barre syndrome: report of the Quality Standards Subcommittee of the American Academy of Neurology. *Neurology* 61:736, 2003.
61. Massachusetts Department of Public Health: The red tide: a public health emergency. *N Engl J Med* 288:1126, 1973.
62. Ahles MD: Red tide: a recurrent health hazard. *Am J Public Health* 64:807, 1974.
63. Isbister GK, Kiernan MC: Neurotoxic marine poisoning. *Lancet Neurol* 4:219, 2005.
64. Eastaugh JA: Delayed use of mannitol in ciguatera (fish poisoning). *Ann Emerg Med* 28:105, 1996.
65. Dinubile MJ, Hokama Y: The ciguatera poisoning syndrome from farm-raised salmon. *Ann Intern Med* 122:113, 1995.
66. Defusco DJ, O'Dowd P, Hokama Y, et al: Coma due to ciguatera poisoning in Rhode Island. *Am J Med* 95:240, 1993.
67. Chandler KW, Rozas CJ, Kory RC, et al: Bilateral diaphragmatic paralysis complicating local cardiac hypothermia during open heart surgery. *Am J Med* 77:243, 1984.
68. Mulvey DA, Aquilina RJ, Elliot MW, et al: Diaphragmatic dysfunction in neuralgic amyotrophy: an electrophysiologic evaluation of 16 patients presenting with dyspnea. *Am Rev Respir Dis* 147:66, 1993.
69. LaRoche C, Carroll N, Moxham J, et al: Clinical significance of severe diaphragm weakness. *Am Rev Respir Dis* 138:862, 1988.
70. Chan CK, Mohsenin V, Loke J, et al: Diaphragmatic dysfunction in siblings with hereditary motor and sensory neuropathy (Charcot-Marie-Tooth disease). *Chest* 91:567, 1987.
71. Drachman DB: Myasthenia gravis. *N Engl J Med* 298:186, 1978.
72. Dushay KM, Zibrak JD, Jensen WA: Myasthenia gravis presenting as isolated respiratory failure. *Chest* 97:232, 1990.
73. Zulueta J, Fanburg B: Respiratory dysfunction in myasthenia gravis. *Clin Chest Med* 15:683, 1994.

74. Gracey DR, Howard FM Jr, Divertie MB: Plasmapheresis in the treatment of ventilator-dependent myasthenia gravis patients. *Chest* 85:739, 1984.
75. Stricker RB, Kwiatkowska BJ, Habis JA, et al: Myasthenic crisis: response to plasma pheresis following failure of intravenous γ-globulin. *Arch Neurol* 50:837, 1993.
76. Argov Z, Mastaglia FL: Disorders of neuromuscular transmission caused by drugs. *N Engl J Med* 301:409, 1979.
77. McEvoy KM, Windebank AJ, Daube JR, et al: 3,4-Diaminopyridine in the treatment of Lambert-Eaton myasthenic syndrome. *N Engl J Med* 321:1567, 1989.
78. Raps EC, Bird SJ, Hansen-Flaschen J: Prolonged muscle weakness after neuromuscular blockade in the intensive care unit. *Crit Care Clin* 10:799, 1994.
79. De Jonghe B, Sharshar T, Lefaucheur JP, et al: Paresis acquired in the intensive care unit: a prospective multicenter study. *JAMA* 288:2859, 2002.
80. Witt NJ, Zochodne DW, Bolton CR, et al: Peripheral nerve function in sepsis and multiple organ failure. *Chest* 99:176, 1991.
81. Gorson KC, Ropper AH: Acute respiratory failure neuropathy: a variant of critical illness polyneuropathy. *Crit Care Med* 21:267, 1993.
82. Hansen-Flaschen J, Cowen J, Raps EC: Neuromuscular blockade in the intensive care unit: more than we bargained for. *Am Rev Respir Dis* 147:234, 1993.
83. Douglass JA, Tuxen DV, Horne M, et al: Myopathy in severe asthma. *Am Rev Respir Dis* 146:517, 1992.
84. Schmidt-Nowara WW, Samet JM, et al: Early and late pulmonary complications of botulism. *Arch Intern Med* 143:451, 1983.
85. Gupta A, Sumner CJ, Castor M, et al: Adult botulism type F in the United States, 1981–2002. *Neurology* 65:1694, 2005.
86. Wilcox PC, Morrison NJ, Pardy RL: Recovery of the ventilatory and upper airway muscles and exercise performance after type A botulism. *Chest* 98:620, 1990.
87. Guven M, Sungur M, Eser B, et al: The effects of fresh frozen plasma on cholinesterase levels and outcomes in patients with organophosphate poisoning. *J Toxicol Clin Toxicol* 42(5):617, 2004.
88. Newmark J: Therapy for nerve agent poisoning. *Arch Neurol* 61:649, 2004.
89. DeLisser J, Grippi M: Phrenic nerve injury following cardiac surgery, with emphasis on the role of topical hypothermia. *J Intensive Care Med* 6:195, 1991.
90. Zochodne DW: Autonomic involvement in Guillain-Barre syndrome: a review. *Muscle Nerve* 17:1145, 1994.
91. Moorthy SS, Markand ON, Mahomed Y, et al: Electrophysiologic evaluation of phrenic nerves in severe respiratory insufficiency requiring mechanical ventilation. *Chest* 88:211, 1985.
92. Piehler JM, Pairolero PC, Gracey DR, et al: Unexplained diaphragmatic paralysis: a harbinger of malignant disease? *J Thorac Cardiovasc Surg* 84:861, 1982.
93. Thomas NE, Passamonte PM, Sunderrajan EV, et al: Bilateral diaphragmatic paralysis as a possible paraneoplastic syndrome from renal cell carcinoma. *Am Rev Respir Dis* 129:507, 1984.
94. Spitzer SA, Korczyn AD, Kalaci J: Transient bilateral diaphragmatic paralysis. *Chest* 64:355, 1973.
95. Kreitzer SM, Feldman NT, Saunders NA, et al: Bilateral diaphragmatic paralysis with hypercapnic respiratory failure. *Am J Med* 65:89, 1978.
96. Chausow AM, Kane T, Levinson D, et al: Reversible hypercapnic respiratory insufficiency in scleroderma caused by respiratory muscle weakness. *Am Rev Respir Dis* 130:142, 1984.
97. Rosenow RC III, Engel AG: Acid maltase deficiency in adults presenting as respiratory failure. *Am J Med* 64:485, 1978.
98. Wokke JH, Ausems MG, Van den Boogaard MJ, et al: Genotype–phenotype correlation in adult-onset acid maltase deficiency. *Ann Neurol* 38:450, 1995.
99. Newman JH, Neff TA, Ziporin P: Acute respiratory failure associated with hypophosphatemia. *N Engl J Med* 296:1101, 1977.
100. Knochel JP: Neuromuscular manifestations of electrolyte disorders. *Am J Med* 72:521, 1982.
101. Lynn D, Woda R, Mendell J: Respiratory dysfunction in muscular dystrophy and other myopathies. *Clin Chest Med* 15:661, 1994.
102. Hoffman EP, Fischbeck KH, Brown RH, et al: Characterization of dystrophin in muscle. *N Engl J Med* 318:1363, 1988.
103. Olive M, Goldfarb LG, Shatunov A, et al: Myotilinopathy: refining the clinical and myopathological phenotype. *Brain* 128[Pt 10]:2315, 2005.
104. ATS Consensus Statement: Respiratory care of the patient with Duchenne muscular dystrophy. *Am J Respir Crit Care Med* 170:456, 2004.
105. Moxley RT III, Ashwal S, Pandya S, et al: Quality Standards Subcommittee of the American Academy of Neurology. Practice Committee of the Child Neurology Society. Practice parameter: corticosteroid treatment of Duchenne dystrophy: report of the Quality Standards Subcommittee of the American Academy of Neurology and the Practice Committee of the Child Neurology Society. *Neurology* 64:13, 2005.
106. Brook JD, McCurrach ME, Harley HG, et al: Molecular basis of myotonic dystrophy: expansion of a trinucleotide (CTG) repeat at the 3′ end of a transcript encoding a protein kinase family member [published erratum appears in *Cell* 69:385, 1992]. *Cell* 68:799, 1992.
107. Liquori CL, Ricker K, Moseley ML, et al: Myotonic dystrophy type 2 caused by a CCTG expansion in intron 1 of ZNF9. *Science* 293:864, 2001.
108. Begin R, Bureau MA, Lupien L, et al: Pathogenesis of respiratory insufficiency in myotonic dystrophy. *Am Rev Respir Dis* 125:312, 1982.
109. Platt D, Griggs R: Skeletal muscle channelopathies: new insights into the periodic paralyses and nondystrophic myotonias. *Curr Opin Neurol* 22:524, 2009.
110. Rojas CV, Wang JZ, Schwartz LS, et al: A Met-to-Val mutation in the skeletal muscle Na+ channel alpha-subunit in hyperkalaemic periodic paralysis. *Nature* 354:387, 1991.
111. Mellies U, Ragette R, Schwake C, et al: Sleep-disordered breathing and respiratory failure in acid maltase deficiency. *Neurology* 57:1290, 2001.
112. Troyanov Y, Targoff IN, Tremblay JL, et al: Novel classification of idiopathic inflammatory myopathies based on overlap syndrome features and autoantibodies: analysis of 100 French Canadian patients. *Medicine (Baltimore)* 84:231, 2005.
113. Schwarz MI, Sutarik JM, Nick JA, et al: Pulmonary capillaritis and diffuse alveolar hemorrhage: a primary manifestation of polymyositis. *Am J Respir Crit Care Med* 151:2037, 1995.
114. NIH Conference: Myositis: immunologic contributions to understanding the cause, pathogenesis and therapy. *Ann Intern Med* 122:715, 1995.
115. Siafakas NM, Milona I, Salesiotou V, et al: Respiratory muscle strength in hyperthyroidism before and after treatment. *Am Rev Respir Dis* 146:1025, 1992.
116. Nieman LK, Ilias I: Evaluation and treatment of Cushing's syndrome. *Am J Med* 118:1340, 2005.
117. Kunci RW: Colchicine myopathy and neuropathy. *N Engl J Med* 316:1562, 1987.
118. Watt G, Saisorn S, Jongsakul K, et al: Blinded, placebo-controlled trial of antiparasitic drugs for trichinosis myositis. *J Infect Dis* 182:371, 2000.
119. Varsano S, Shapiro M, Taragan R, et al: Hypophosphatemia as a reversible cause of refractory ventilatory failure. *Crit Care Med* 11:908, 1983.
120. Aubier M, Murciano D, Lecocguic Y, et al: Effect of hypophosphatemia on diaphragmatic contractility in patients with acute respiratory failure. *N Engl J Med* 313:420, 1985.
121. Dhingra S, Solven F, Wilson A, et al: Hypomagnesemia and respiratory muscle power. *Am Rev Respir Dis* 129:497, 1984.
122. Agus ZS, Wasserstein A, Goldfarb S: Disorders of calcium and magnesium homeostasis. *Am J Med* 72:473, 1982.
123. Hertzman PA, Blevins WL, Mayer J, et al: Association of the eosinophilia-myalgia syndrome with the ingestion of tryptophan. *N Engl J Med* 322:869, 1990.
124. Silver RM, Heyes MP, Maize JC, et al: Scleroderma, fasciitis, and eosinophilia associated with the ingestion of tryptophan. *N Engl J Med* 322:874, 1990.
125. Medsger TA Jr: Tryptophan-induced eosinophilia-myalgia syndrome. *N Engl J Med* 322:926, 1990.
126. Ventayya RV, Poole RM, Pentz WH: Respiratory failure from procainamide-induced myopathy. *Ann Intern Med* 119:345, 1993.
127. Black LF, Hyatt RE: Maximal static respiratory pressures in generalized neuromuscular disease. *Am Rev Respir Dis* 103:641, 1971.
128. Kafer ER: Respiratory failure in paralytic scoliosis. *Am Rev Respir Dis* 110:450, 1974.
129. Lisboa C, Moreno R, Fava M, et al: Inspiratory muscle function in patients with severe kyphoscoliosis. *Am Rev Respir Dis* 132:48, 1985.
130. Libby DM, Briscoe WA, Boyce B, et al: Acute respiratory failure in scoliosis or kyphosis. *Am J Med* 73:532, 1982.
131. Garay SM, Turino GM, Goldring RM: Sustained reversal of chronic hypercapnia in patients with alveolar hypoventilation syndromes: long-term maintenance with noninvasive nocturnal mechanical ventilation. *Am J Med* 70:269, 1981.
132. Meyer TJ, Hill NS: Noninvasive positive pressure ventilation to treat respiratory failure. *Ann Intern Med* 120:760, 1994.
133. Rochester DF, Enson Y: Current concepts in the pathogenesis of the obesity-hypoventilation syndrome. *Am J Med* 57:402, 1974.
134. Sampson MG, Grassino A: Neuromechanical properties in obese patients during carbon dioxide rebreathing. *Am J Med* 75:81, 1983.
135. Mokhlesi B, Kryger MH, Grunstein RR: Assessment and management of patients with obesity hypoventilation syndrome. *Proc Am Thorac Soc* 5:218, 2008.
136. Trinkle JK, Richardson JD, Franz JL, et al: Management of flail chest without mechanical ventilation. *Ann Thorac Surg* 19:355, 1975.
137. Colp C, Reichel J, Park SS: Severe pleural restriction: the maximum static pulmonary recoil pressure as an aid in diagnosis. *Chest* 67:658, 1975.
138. Miller A, Teirstein AS, Selikoff IJ: Ventilatory failure due to asbestos pleurisy. *Am J Med* 75:911, 1983.
139. Gilbert L, Ribot S, Frankel H, et al: Fibrinous uremic pleuritis: a surgical entity. *Chest* 67:53, 1975.
140. Black MJ, Harbour J, Remsen KA, et al: Acute epiglottitis in adults. *J Otolaryngol* 10:23, 1981.
141. Lederman MM, Lowder J, Lerner PI: Bacteremic pneumococcal epiglottitis in adults with malignancy. *Am Rev Respir Dis* 125:117, 1982.
142. Schecter WP, Wilson RS: Management of upper airway obstruction in the intensive care unit. *Crit Care Med* 9:577, 1981.
143. Phelan DM, Love JB: Adult epiglottitis: is there a role for the fiberoptic bronchoscope? *Chest* 86:783, 1984.
144. Hunt KJ, Valentine MD, Sobotka AK, et al: A controlled trial of immunotherapy in insect hypersensitivity. *N Engl J Med* 299:157, 1978.

145. Valentine MD: Anaphylaxis and stinging insect hypersensitivity. *JAMA* 268:2830, 1992.
146. Greaves M, Lawlor F: Angioedema: manifestations and management. *J Am Acad Dermatol* 25:155, 1991.
147. Chevailler A, Arland G, Ponard D, et al: CI-inhibitor binding monoclonal immunoglobulins in three patients with acquired angioneurotic edema. *J Allergy Clin Immunol* 97:998, 1996.
148. Israiliz H, Hall WD: Cough and angioneurotic edema associated with angiotensin-converting enzyme inhibitor therapy. *Ann Intern Med* 117:234, 1992.
149. Stauffer JL, Olson DE, Petty TL: Complications and consequences of endotracheal intubation and tracheotomy: a prospective study of 150 critically ill adult patients. *Am J Med* 70:65, 1981.
150. Harley HR: Laryngotracheal obstruction complicating tracheostomy or endotracheal intubation with assisted respiration. *Thorax* 26:493, 1971.
151. Mittleman RE, Wetli CV: The fatal cafe coronary. *JAMA* 247:1285, 1982.
152. Irwin RS, Ashba JK, Braman SS, et al: Food asphyxiation in hospitalized patients. *JAMA* 237:2744, 1977.
153. Gelperin A: Sudden death in an elderly population from aspiration of food. *J Am Geriatr Soc* 22:135, 1974.
154. Haugen RK: The cafe coronary. *JAMA* 186:142, 1963.
155. Heimlich HJ: A life-saving maneuver to prevent food choking. *JAMA* 234:398, 1975.
156. Abdulmajid OA, Ebeid AM, Motaweh MM, et al: Aspirated foreign bodies in the tracheobronchial tree: report of 250 cases. *Thorax* 31:635, 1976.
157. Rosenbaum L, Thurman P, Krantz SB: Upper airway obstruction as a complication of oral anticoagulation therapy. *Arch Intern Med* 139:1151, 1979.
158. Rodrigues JF, York EL, Nair CP: Upper airway obstruction in Guillain-Barré syndrome. *Chest* 86:147, 1984.
159. Schmidt-Nowara WW, Marder EJ, Feil PA: Respiratory failure in myasthenia gravis due to vocal cord paresis. *Arch Neurol* 41:567, 1984.
160. Libby DM, Schley WS, Smith JP: Cricoarytenoid arthritis in ankylosing spondylitis. *Chest* 80:641, 1981.
161. Proctor DF: The upper airways. II. The larynx and trachea. *Am Rev Respir Dis* 115:315, 1977.
162. Kastanos N, Miro RE, Perez AM, et al: Laryngotracheal injury due to endotracheal intubation: incidence, evolution, and predisposing factors—a prospective long-term study. *Crit Care Med* 11:362, 1983.
163. Magnussen CR, Patanella HP: Herpes simplex virus and recurrent laryngeal nerve paralysis. *Arch Intern Med* 139:1423, 1979.
164. Vincken WG, Gauthier SG, Dollfuss RE, et al: Involvement of upper-airway muscles in extrapyramidal disorders: a cause of airflow limitation. *N Engl J Med* 311:438, 1984.
165. Cormier Y, Kashima H, Summer W, et al: Upper airway obstruction with bilateral vocal cord paralysis. *Chest* 75:423, 1979.
166. Fleetham JA, Lynn RB, Munt PW: Tracheal leiomyosarcoma: a unique cause of stridor. *Am Rev Respir Dis* 116:1109, 1977.
167. Olmedo G, Rosenberg M, Fonseca R: Primary tumors of the trachea. *Chest* 81:701, 1982.
168. Braman SS, Whitcomb ME: Endobronchial metastasis. *Arch Intern Med* 135:543, 175.
169. Weber AL, Grillo HC: Tracheal tumors: a radiological clinical and pathological evaluation of 84 cases. *Radiol Clin North Am* 16:227, 1976.
170. Kvale PA, Eichenhorn MS, Radke JR, et al: YAG laser photoresection of lesions obstructing the central airways. *Chest* 87:283, 1985.
171. Gamsu G, Borson DB, Webb WR, et al: Structure and function in tracheal stenosis. *Am Rev Respir Dis* 121:519, 1980.
172. Feist JH, Johnson TH, Wilson RJ: Acquired tracheomalacia: etiology and differential diagnosis. *Chest* 68:340, 1975.
173. Bergstrom B, Ollman B, Lindholm CE: Endotracheal excision of fibrous tracheal stenosis and subsequent prolonged stenting: an alternative method in selected cases. *Chest* 71:6, 1977.
174. Epstein LJ, Kristo D, Strollo PJ, et al: Clinical guideline for the evaluation, management, and long-term care of obstructive sleep apnea in adults. *J Clin Sleep Med* 5:263, 2009.
175. Flemons WW: Clinical practice. Obstructive sleep apnea. *N Engl J Med* 347:498, 2002.
176. Walsh RE, Michaelson ED, Harkleroad LE, et al: Upper airway obstruction in obese patients with sleep disturbance and somnolence. *Ann Intern Med* 76:185, 1972.
177. Onal E, Lopata M, O'Connor T: Pathogenesis of apneas in hypersomnia: sleep apnea syndrome. *Am Rev Respir Dis* 125:167, 1982.
178. Motta J, Guilleminault C, Schroeder JS, et al: Tracheostomy and hemodynamic changes in sleep-induced apnea. *Ann Intern Med* 89:454, 1978.
179. Shepard JW Jr, Garrison MW, Grither DA, et al: Relationship of ventricular ectopy to oxyhemoglobin desaturation in patients with obstructive sleep apnea. *Chest* 88:335, 1985.
180. Orr WC, Martin RJ: Obstructive sleep apnea associated with tonsillar hypertrophy in adults. *Arch Intern Med* 141:990, 1981.
181. Heimer D, Scharf SM, Lieberman A, et al: Sleep apnea syndrome treated by repair of deviated nasal septum. *Chest* 84:184, 1983.
182. Davies SF, Iber C: Obstructive sleep apnea associated with adult-acquired micrognathia from rheumatoid arthritis. *Am Rev Respir Dis* 127:245, 1983.
183. Mezon BJ, West P, Maclean JP, et al: Sleep apnea in acromegaly. *Am J Med* 69:615, 1980.
184. Rajagopal KR, Abbrecht PH, Derderian SS, et al: Obstructive sleep apnea in hypothyroidism. *Ann Intern Med* 101:491, 1984.
185. Orr WC, Males JL, Imes NK: Myxedema and obstructive sleep apnea. *Am J Med* 70:1061, 1981.
186. Remmers JE: Obstructive sleep apnea: a common disorder exacerbated by alcohol. *Am Rev Respir Dis* 130:153, 1984.
187. Sandblom RE, Matsumoto AM, Schoene RB, et al: Obstructive sleep apnea syndrome induced by testosterone administration. *N Engl J Med* 308:508, 1983.
188. Johnson MW, Anch AM, Remmers JE: Induction of the obstructive sleep apnea syndrome in a woman by exogenous androgen administration. *Am Rev Respir Dis* 129:1023, 1984.
189. Torres A, Arroyo J, Kastanos N, et al: Acute respiratory failure and tracheal obstruction in patients with intrathoracic goiter. *Crit Care Med* 11:265, 1983.
190. Acres JC, Kryger MH: Clinical significance of pulmonary function tests: upper airway obstruction. *Chest* 80:207, 1981.
191. Rochester DF, Esau SA: Malnutrition and the respiratory system. *Chest* 85:411, 1984.
192. Kelly SM, Rosa A, Field S, et al: Inspiratory muscle strength and body composition in patients receiving total parenteral nutrition therapy. *Am Rev Respir Dis* 130:33, 1984.
193. Aldrich TK, Karpel JP: Inspiratory muscle resistive training in respiratory failure. *Am Rev Respir Dis* 131:461, 1985.
194. Gross D, Ladd HW, Riley EJ, et al: The effect of training on strength and endurance of the diaphragm in quadriplegia. *Am J Med* 68:27, 1980.
195. Howell S, Fitzgerald RS, Roussos CH: Effects of aminophylline, isoproterenol, and neostigmine on hypercapnic depression of diaphragmatic contractility. *Am Rev Respir Dis* 132:241, 1985.
196. Vires N, Aubier M, Murciano D, et al: Effects of aminophylline on diaphragmatic fatigue during acute respiratory failure. *Am Rev Respir Dis* 129:396, 1984.
197. Gonzalez C, Ferris G, Diaz J, et al: Kyphoscoliotic ventilatory insufficiency: effects of long-term intermittent positive-pressure ventilation. *Chest* 124:857, 2003.
198. Remmers JE, Sterling JA, Thorarinsson B, et al: Nasal airway positive pressure in patients with occlusive sleep apnea. *Am Rev Respir Dis* 130:1152, 1984.
199. Sanders MH: Nasal CPAP effect on patterns of sleep apnea. *Chest* 86:839, 1984.
200. Kushida CA, Littner MR, Hirshkowitz M, et al: American Academy of Sleep Medicine. Practice parameters for the use of continuous and bilevel positive airway pressure devices to treat adult patients with sleep-related breathing disorders. *Sleep* 29:375, 2006.
201. Browman CP, Sampson MG, Yolles SF, et al: Obstructive sleep apnea and body weight. *Chest* 85:435, 1984.
202. American Sleep Disorders Association: Practice parameters for the treatment of snoring and obstructive sleep apnea with oral appliances. *Sleep* 18:511, 1995.
203. Conway W, Fugita S, Zorick F, et al: Uvulopalato-pharyngoplasty. *Chest* 88:385, 1985.

CHAPTER 51 ■ RESPIRATORY FAILURE PART VI: ACUTE RESPIRATORY FAILURE IN PREGNANCY

CHRISTINE CAMPBELL-REARDON AND HELEN M. HOLLINGSWORTH

The overall pregnancy-related maternal mortality ratio in the United States during 1991 to 1999 was 11.8 deaths per 100,000 live births [1]. Acute respiratory failure remains an important cause of maternal and fetal morbidity and mortality. Thromboembolism, amniotic fluid embolism (AFE), and venous air embolism together account for approximately 20% of maternal deaths [2], and other causes of respiratory failure probably account for another 11% [1].

This chapter focuses on the causes of acute respiratory failure that are increased in frequency during pregnancy, are unique to pregnancy, or present special management requirements during pregnancy. The spectrum of problems associated with eclampsia is discussed in Chapter 156. Management of the acute respiratory distress syndrome (ARDS) caused by sepsis, trauma, or other etiologies unrelated to pregnancy is discussed in Chapter 47. Table 51.1 lists causes of acute respiratory failure in pregnancy.

NORMAL ALTERATIONS IN CARDIOPULMONARY PHYSIOLOGY DURING PREGNANCY

Pregnancy alters respiratory physiology by causing changes in lung volumes, mechanics of ventilation, and control of respiration. Despite mucosal changes to the airway of edema and hyperemia, spirometry studies reveal no significant changes in measurements of the forced expiratory volume in 1 second (FEV_1) during pregnancy, suggesting that airway function is maintained during pregnancy. Changes in lung volume associated with gestation are relatively small: total lung capacity decreases 4% to 6%, functional residual capacity (FRC) decreases approximately 15% to 25%, and residual volume remains constant. Despite the decrease in FRC, early airway closure has not been demonstrated and specific airway conductance remains constant [3]. Diffusing capacity is elevated in the first trimester but then declines, despite continued increases in cardiac output and plasma volume.

As gestation progresses, the resting level of the diaphragm rises, but diaphragmatic excursion with tidal breathing increases. An increased tidal volume (25% to 35%) accounts for much of the 20% to 40% increase in minute ventilation and the mild respiratory alkalosis that are characteristic of early-to-middle pregnancy. An increased respiratory rate also contributes to the increased minute ventilation late in pregnancy (Fig. 51.1).

Normal carbon dioxide tension ($PaCO_2$) during pregnancy is 27 to 34 mm Hg, suggesting chronic mild hyperventilation. The degree of hyperventilation has been found to be in excess of the amount needed to compensate for increased oxygen consumption; in fact, hyperventilation develops early in gestation, before any significant increase in oxygen consumption occurs. This has been attributed to elevation in levels of progesterone, which has a known respiratory stimulating effect. The exact mechanism by which it produces this effect is not known, but it is thought to include an increase in the central chemoreflex drive to breathe and to changes in acid–base balance such that central and plasma hydrogen ion concentration is increased for any given PCO_2. In addition, pregnancy is associated with increased sensitivity to CO_2 as measured by CO_2 ventilatory response curves, reflecting the new, lower set point in $PaCO_2$, possibly mediated by estrogen and progesterone. The respiratory alkalosis seen during pregnancy causes a compensatory renal excretion of bicarbonate to maintain an arterial pH between 7.40 and 7.45.

The normal arterial oxygen tension (PaO_2) in pregnant women ranges from 100 to 110 mm Hg. Oxygen consumption increases by 20% to 33% by the third trimester, secondary to both fetal and maternal demands. This increased rate of oxygen consumption and low oxygen reserve secondary to a reduced FRC place pregnant patients at risk for the rapid onset of hypoxia.

Circulatory changes occur during gestation to supply oxygen-rich blood to the placenta and to accommodate the stress of labor and delivery. Cardiac output begins to rise in the first trimester and peaks around the 20th week of gestation at 30% to 45% above resting, nonpregnant levels (Fig. 51.2). Thus, measured cardiac output during gestation that is in the normal range for a nonpregnant patient would represent significant hemodynamic compromise for the pregnant patient and, potentially, decreased oxygen delivery for the fetus. As pregnancy progresses, cardiac output becomes dependent on body position. In the supine position, cardiac output can be reduced by 25% to 30% due to compression of the inferior vena cava by the gravid uterus and a resultant decrease in venous return. Cardiac output is higher when the pregnant woman is in the left lateral decubitus position. Estimates of expected cardiac output during gestation should be revised upward for intercurrent stresses such as fever, infection, and pain.

The gestation-related increase in cardiac output reflects a combination of increases in heart rate and stroke volume. Heart rate increases progressively throughout gestation, reaching a 20% or 15 beats per minute increase over nonpregnant levels. Stroke volume increases more rapidly at first and then stabilizes. Left ventricular compliance must increase in pregnancy because the increased stroke volume appears to be related more to left ventricular enlargement than to increased emptying. The cardiac silhouette on chest radiography may appear enlarged as a result of mild normal left ventricular enlargement and lateral and upward displacement by the gravid uterus.

Further increases in cardiac output occur during labor; cardiac output increases up to 45% over third trimester values,

TABLE 51.1

CAUSES OF ACUTE RESPIRATORY FAILURE IN PREGNANCY

Thromboembolism
Amniotic fluid embolism
Venous air embolism
Aspiration of gastric contents
Respiratory infections
Asthma
HELLP syndrome
β-Adrenergic tocolytic therapy
Pneumomediastinum and pneumothorax
Acute respiratory distress syndrome (see Chapter 47)
Cardiomyopathy

HELLP, *h*emolytic anemia, *e*levated *l*iver function tests, *l*ow *p*latelets.

and during uterine contraction, cardiac output transiently increases another 10% to 15% because of increased venous return. Another factor that may be important in patients who are sensitive to left ventricular afterload is inhibition of blood flow to the uterus during labor contractions. Because uterine blood flow at term accounts for a significant proportion of the cardiac output, marked increases in afterload during contractions and immediately postpartum may occur. During labor, contractions are associated with increased blood return from the uterus. These "autotransfusions" may reach 500 mL when the uterus contracts after parturition. This effect, however, may be offset by blood loss. In the first few minutes postpartum, cardiac output may increase as much as 80% over prelabor levels, then decrease to 40% to 50% over prelabor values by 1 hour postpartum, and finally return to nearly pre-pregnant levels by 1 to 2 weeks postpartum.

Systemic vascular resistance is reduced in pregnancy due to vasodilatation and the low resistance of the uteroplacental vascular circuit. Possible factors leading to vasodilatation

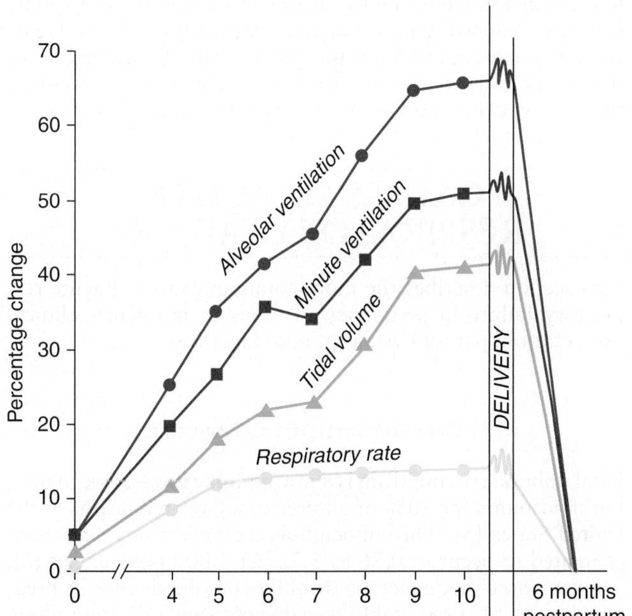

FIGURE 51.1. Changes in respiratory function during pregnancy. [Reprinted from Leontic EA: Respiratory disease in pregnancy. *Med Clin North Am* 61:111, 1977, with permission.]

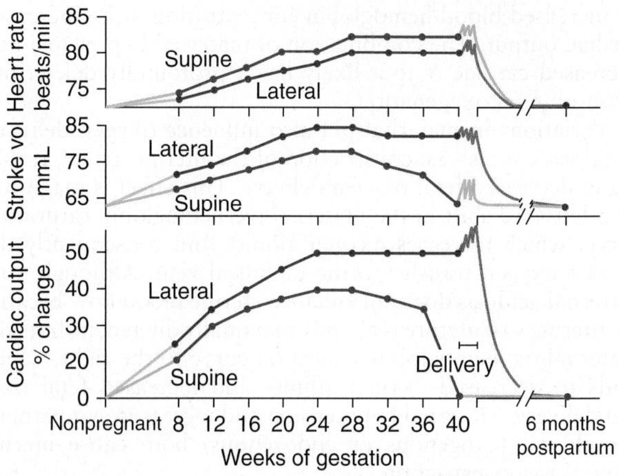

FIGURE 51.2. Changes in maternal heart rate, stroke volume, and output during pregnancy with the gravida in the supine and lateral positions. [Reprinted from Cheek TG, Gutsche BB: Maternal physiologic alterations during pregnancy, in Shnider SM, Levinson G (eds): *Anesthesia for Obstetrics*. Baltimore, MD, Williams & Wilkins, 1987, p 3, with permission.]

include a reduction in vascular responsiveness to norepinephrine and angiotensin II, increased endothelial prostacyclin production, and increased nitric oxide production. The mean blood pressure remains relatively constant despite increases in cardiac output. Pressures in the right ventricle, pulmonary artery, and pulmonary capillaries are no different from nonpregnant values.

During pregnancy, there is expansion of the extracellular fluid volume, with the plasma fluid volume increasing more than the interstitial volume. Maternal blood volume reaches its peak at 32 weeks and is 25% to 52% above prepregnancy levels. The erythrocyte mass increases by 20% to 30%. However, the plasma volume increases more than the erythrocyte volume, resulting in the physiologic anemia of pregnancy.

Colloid osmotic pressure measurements during gestation reveal a mean decrease of 5 mm Hg, which reaches a plateau at 26 weeks. This parallels a decrease in serum albumin concentrations from approximately 4.0 to 3.4 g per dL. A further decline in colloid osmotic pressure of roughly 4 mm Hg occurs immediately postpartum, probably as a result of a combination of factors, such as recumbency, crystalloid administration, and blood loss. These changes may be even more marked in patients with pregnancy-induced hypertension. Neither the absolute value of colloid osmotic pressure nor the colloid osmotic pressure–pulmonary capillary wedge pressure gradient is an accurate predictor of pulmonary edema because of the multiplicity of contributing variables. However, these trends in colloid osmotic pressure should be considered when interpreting pulmonary capillary wedge pressures, especially in patients who have received large amounts of crystalloid.

DETERMINANTS OF FETAL OXYGEN DELIVERY

Oxygen delivery to fetal tissues can be affected at many levels: maternal oxygen delivery to the placenta, placental transfer, and fetal oxygen transport from the placenta to fetal tissues. The major determinants of oxygen delivery to the placenta are the oxygen content of uterine artery blood, which is determined by maternal PaO_2; hemoglobin concentration and saturation; and uterine artery blood flow, which depends on maternal cardiac output. Thus, a decreased PaO_2 can be offset somewhat by increased blood hemoglobin concentration or by increased cardiac output. The combination of maternal hypoxemia and decreased cardiac output likely has a profoundly deleterious effect on fetal oxygenation.

Variations in maternal pH also influence oxygen delivery. Alkalosis causes vasoconstriction of the uterine artery, resulting in decreased fetal oxygen delivery. This effect is magnified by a leftward shift in the maternal oxyhemoglobin saturation curve, which increases oxygen affinity and consequently decreases oxygen transfer to the umbilical vein. Although mild maternal acidosis does not enhance uterine blood flow because the uterine vasculature is already maximally dilated, it shifts the maternal oxyhemoglobin saturation curve to the right, which leads to decreased oxygen affinity and increased fetal oxygen delivery. Maternal hypotension and increased sympathetic stimulation (exogenous or endogenous) both cause uterine arterial vasoconstriction.

The importance of maternal cardiac output is supported by the observation that women with left ventricular outflow obstruction have an increased incidence of fetal death and surviving infants have an increased incidence of congenital heart disease. Data from a sheep model, however, suggest that a decrease in uterine blood flow up to 50% for brief periods does not appreciably decrease fetal and placental oxygen uptake. Chronically decreased maternal cardiac output may have other effects, perhaps on placental development, that explain the results in women with left ventricular outflow obstruction.

The interaction of maternal and fetal circulations in the placenta most likely follows a concurrent exchange mechanism. This is less efficient than a countercurrent exchange mechanism and partly explains why the PaO_2 in the fetal umbilical vein, which carries oxygenated blood to fetus, is in the range of 32 mm Hg, far lower than uterine vein PaO_2, and why increased maternal inspired oxygen increases uterine artery oxygen tension but does not cause major increases in umbilical vein PaO_2. Despite low umbilical vein PaO_2, fetal oxygen content is actually quite close to maternal oxygen content because of the shape of the oxyhemoglobin saturation curve for fetal hemoglobin (Fig. 51.3). This is one of the major protective mechanisms for

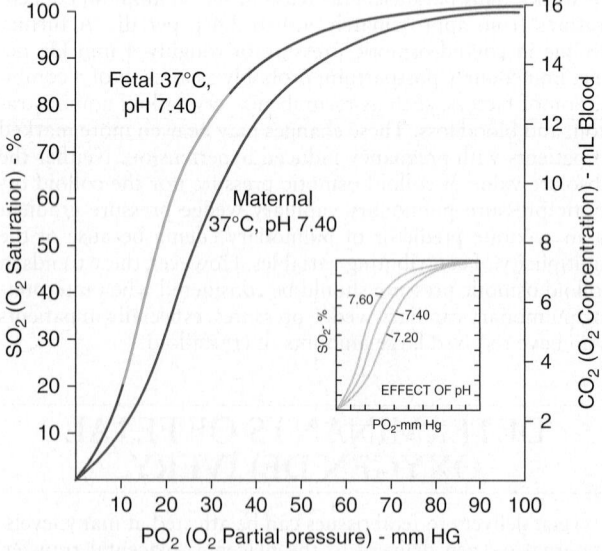

FIGURE 51.3. Oxygen dissociation (equilibrium) curves of human fetal and maternal blood. The effect of pH on the position of the curve (Bohr effect) is shown on the inset. The oxygen capacity of 16 mL per 100 mL blood on the right-hand ordinate refers to maternal blood. [Reprinted from Novy MJ, Edwards MJ: Respiratory problems in pregnancy. *Am J Obstet Gynecol* 99:1024, 1967, with permission.]

fetal oxygenation. The fetal oxyhemoglobin saturation curve is relatively unaffected by changes in pH; although acidosis may decrease maternal oxygen affinity, fetal oxygen affinity is unchanged.

Other placental factors that determine fetal oxygenation are the amount of intraplacental shunt, degree of matching of maternal and fetal blood flows, and the presence of any placental abnormalities, such as placental infarcts. There seem to be no placental autoregulatory mechanisms that increase blood flow in response to decreased maternal PaO_2.

Mathematical models predicting the optimal apportionment of fetal cardiac output between umbilical (to collect oxygen) and systemic (to deliver oxygen) circulations have yielded values surprisingly close to those measured under normal physiologic conditions. This appears to be another compensation mechanism for the apparent inefficiency (concurrent exchange mechanism) of the placenta. One disadvantage in terms of oxygen delivery to fetal tissues is that oxygenated umbilical vein blood is mixed in the fetal inferior vena cava with deoxygenated systemic venous blood before delivery to the systemic circulation. Thus, fetal arterial blood has an even lower PaO_2 than umbilical vein blood. This is compensated for in part by a high fetal cardiac output relative to oxygen consumption, thus enhancing oxygen delivery to fetal tissues. The fetal circulation appears to have the ability to autoregulate in the face of hypoxemia to protect the brain, adrenal glands, and heart. How long this adaptation can be depended on safely before organ damage occurs is not known.

How well do the compensatory mechanisms that provide adequate oxygen supply to the fetus under normal conditions manage during maternal hypoxia? Calculation of oxygen stores in the term infant with 60% hemoglobin saturation yields a total oxygen content of 40 mL. Given an oxygen consumption of 6 mL per kg per minute, or approximately 18 mL per minute at term, this reserve lasts barely 2 minutes when the maternal oxygen supply is completely interrupted. The shape of the fetal oxyhemoglobin dissociation curve places umbilical vein PaO_2 values below 30 mm Hg on the steep part of the curve, so small changes in maternal PaO_2 may cause significant changes in fetal oxygen content. A maternal PaO_2 greater than 70 mm Hg should be maintained to prevent adverse consequences to the fetus. Concern regarding the adequacy of fetal oxygen supply is further reduced if a normal maternal PaO_2 of 90 mm Hg or greater is achieved without too great a risk of maternal barotrauma or oxygen toxicity. Extensive referencing supporting this section can be found in Chapter 50 of sixth edition [4].

CAUSES OF ACUTE RESPIRATORY FAILURE

This section describes the more common causes of acute respiratory failure in pregnancy in terms of frequency, clinical presentation, pathophysiology, and diagnosis.

Thromboembolic Disease

Fatal pulmonary embolism is a rare complication in pregnancy, but it accounts for 20% of all pregnancy-related deaths in the United States [5]. Thromboembolic complications have been estimated to occur in 0.76 to 1.72 per 1,000 pregnancies [6]. The increased frequency of thromboembolic disease in pregnancy may be attributable to a hypercoagulable state along with venous stasis. During pregnancy, there is a progressive increase in coagulation factors I, II, VII, VIII, IX, and X. There is a decrease in protein S and a progressively increased resistance to activated protein C [6]. The activity of plasminogen activator inhibitor types 1 and 2, which are inhibitors of fibrinolysis, also increases [7]. Venous stasis may occur because of a hormonally induced dilation of capacitance veins and uterine pressure on the inferior vena cava [8]. Factors that further increase the risk of thromboembolic disease during pregnancy and the puerperium include (a) cesarean section, which has a 10 times greater risk of fatal pulmonary embolism than does vaginal delivery; (b) increased maternal age; (c) multiparity; (d) obesity, especially in association with bed rest; (e) personal or family history of thromboembolism; (f) suppression of lactation with estrogen; (g) surgical procedures during pregnancy and early puerperium; and (g) inherited thrombophilias such as deficiencies of proteins C or S, the presence of antiphospholipid antibodies, the presence of factor V Leiden, and prothrombin gene mutations [8–10].

The appropriate diagnostic steps and treatment of venous thrombosis and pulmonary embolism in nonpregnant patients are reviewed in Chapter 52. This chapter focuses on the diagnosis and management of massive pulmonary embolism associated with severe respiratory and hemodynamic compromise during pregnancy. Respiratory failure may ensue in pulmonary embolism when extensive occlusion of the pulmonary vasculature or concomitant pulmonary edema occurs. Pulmonary edema has been associated with pulmonary embolism in areas of intact blood flow and has been attributed to increased hydrostatic forces in nonoccluded vessels, vigorous crystalloid resuscitation, and increased microvascular permeability caused by platelet-derived mediators [11,12].

Although none of the symptoms, physical signs, or results of laboratory, radiographic, or electrocardiographic studies are specific for pulmonary embolism, these investigations can help rule out other diseases in the differential diagnosis. The usefulness of the serum D-dimer levels in diagnosing thromboembolic disease in pregnancy is limited because D-dimer levels are increased during normal pregnancy, with levels increasing as gestation progresses and peaking at delivery and in the early postpartum period [13,14]. Likewise, hemodynamic data obtained at pulmonary artery catheterization are more helpful in excluding other processes and in guiding hemodynamic management than in making a definitive diagnosis of pulmonary embolism.

The typical hemodynamic findings in nonpregnant patients with massive pulmonary embolism are delineated in Chapter 52. Although there are no data for pregnant patients with massive pulmonary embolism, similar findings would be anticipated because pregnancy does not significantly alter right heart and pulmonary artery pressures. Thus, in a pregnant patient with massive pulmonary embolism, pulmonary artery balloon occlusion pressure (i.e., pulmonary capillary wedge pressure) would be expected to be normal or low, mean pulmonary artery pressure moderately elevated ($\geq$35 mm Hg), and right atrial pressure moderately elevated (>8 mm Hg).

Doppler ultrasound of the lower extremities to assess for lower extremity deep venous thrombosis (DVT) may be chosen as the initial test in the evaluation for a pulmonary embolism. Further diagnostic evaluation is not required when a DVT is found in the legs, as the treatment for DVT and pulmonary embolism is the same. A negative Doppler ultrasound of the lower extremities does not rule out the presence of pulmonary embolism, so further diagnostic investigation is required. In the nonpregnant patient population, helical CT scanning with intravenous contrast has become the study of choice for pulmonary embolism. Data from PIOPED 2 determined the sensitivity and specificity of CT angiography for detecting pulmonary embolism to be 83% and 96%, respectively [15]. Pregnancy was an exclusion criteria in this study, so there is a lack of prospective data assessing CT angiography in pregnancy. However, CT angiography is now being used more commonly as the first screening examination for pulmonary embolism during pregnancy [16]. This trend is based on evidence that the dose of ionizing radiation from a helical CT scan is safe in all trimesters. The radiation dose to the fetus ranged from 0.00033 rad in the first trimester to 0.01308 rad in the third trimester. This radiation dose is comparable with the dose exposure during ventilation–perfusion scanning [17]. CT angiography also provides the opportunity of diagnosing other abnormalities that may be causing the patient's symptoms even if the scan is negative for thromboembolic disease.

Ventilation–perfusion lung scanning remains a useful diagnostic test for pulmonary embolism during pregnancy in patients who have a contraindication to radiocontrast. Pulmonary angiography may still be required for definitive diagnosis of a pulmonary embolism in some patients. Fetal exposure to radiation during imaging studies can be minimized by abdominal shielding and using brachial access.

Amniotic Fluid Embolism

AFE, also known as anaphylactoid syndrome of pregnancy, is a rare, but usually catastrophic, complication of pregnancy and delivery [18–20]. The incidence of AFE is approximately 1 in every 8,000 to 80,000 deliveries [21–23]. A retrospective, population-based cohort study of 3 million birth records in the United States reported an incidence of 7.7 cases per 100,000 births [23]. The mortality rates reported in the literature have been reported to be from 22% to 86% [21–23]. Of the women who survive AFE, only 15% of them are neurologically intact [21].

It is unknown why amniotic fluid enters the maternal circulation in some patients, although certain potential predisposing clinical factors have been suggested based on registry and cohort studies. These factors include older maternal age (mean, 32 years), multiparity (88% of cases), amniotomy, cesarean section, abruptio placentae, insertion of intrauterine fetal or pressure monitoring devices, and term pregnancy in the presence of an intrauterine device [23]. Amniotic fluid enters the maternal circulation through one of three ports: endocervical veins; uterine tears (small tears may occur in the lower uterine segment as a part of normal labor); and uterine injury secondary to iatrogenic manipulation, such as cesarean section, insertion of monitoring devices, or membrane rupture [18].

The two life-threatening consequences of AFE are cardiopulmonary collapse and disseminated intravascular coagulation (DIC). These may occur simultaneously or in sequence. The pathophysiologic process of cardiopulmonary collapse remains controversial. It is possible that amniotic fluid contains vasoactive substances or fetal antigens that provoke an abnormal hemodynamic and immunologic response in the mother that results in the AFE syndrome [24]. There may be a biphasic response to AFE with initial hypoxemia and acute pulmonary hypertension, followed by left ventricular failure. Elevation of the pulmonary balloon occlusion pressure and reduction in cardiac output and left ventricular stroke work index have been documented [25–27].

Although Morgan [28] described only a 24% incidence of pulmonary edema, an autopsy review demonstrated that most lungs exhibited pulmonary edema (10% severe, 60% moderate) [29]. Most cases are rapidly fatal, so radiographs have been infrequently obtained, which may explain the low incidence of pulmonary edema reported by Morgan [28]. The cause of pulmonary edema has variably been ascribed to vigorous fluid resuscitation, increased permeability pulmonary edema, and cardiac decompensation caused by hypoxia and tachycardia [26].

The other major consequence of AFE is coagulation failure. In 10% to 15% of patients, excessive bleeding, particularly uterine bleeding, may be the first sign of AFE. Up to 50% of patients who survive the first 30 to 60 minutes have clinical evidence of coagulopathy, and most of the remaining patients have laboratory evidence of DIC [28]. The initiating factors precipitating DIC are not known.

The abrupt onset of severe dyspnea, tachypnea, and cyanosis during labor or the early puerperium is the classic presentation of AFE, characterizing more than one half of cases. Shock, which is out of proportion to blood loss, is the first manifestation in another 10% to 15%. Seizure activity may be the presenting sign in 30% of cases. In addition, fetal bradycardia is seen in 17% of U.S. registry cases. Bleeding is the forerunning sign in 10% to 15% of patients, and the longer the survival, the greater the likelihood that the patient will manifest respiratory failure, cardiovascular collapse, and DIC. Whatever the presenting symptom complex, 90% of cases occur before or during labor [28]. Other complications, such as acute renal failure and signs of central nervous system injury, are probably secondary to hypotension and hypoxemia. Prodromal symptoms, such as vomiting and shivering, are nonspecific and frequently associated with otherwise uneventful deliveries.

Diagnostic criteria for AFE previously rested on demonstration of fetal elements such as epithelial squamous cells from fetal skin, lanugo hairs, fat from the vernix caseosa, mucin from fetal gut, and bile-containing meconium in the maternal circulation. These elements are not pathognomonic for AFE, as these amniotic fluid components are found in the maternal circulation of healthy pregnant women without AFE [30,31]. Therefore, the antemortem diagnosis of AFE still rests predominantly on the clinical setting and the exclusion of other causes of acute respiratory failure. The role of echocardiography in the diagnosis of AFE is not yet known. Cardiac echo may show decreased left ventricular function or echodense material in the right atrium or right ventricular outflow tract [32]. A serologic assay has been developed using a monoclonal antibody TKH-2 to detect a meconium and amniotic fluid-derived mucin-type glycoprotein. This assay is reported to have a high sensitivity for detecting AFE, but it is not yet recommended for routine clinical practice [33,34].

Fetal outcome is also poor in AFE. The perinatal mortality from the national registry was 21%, with 50% of the survivors experiencing permanent neurologic injury [21].

Venous Air Embolism

Venous air embolism has been described during normal labor, delivery of patients with placenta previa, criminal abortions using air, and insufflation of the vagina during gynecologic procedures [35,36]. There are also cases reported in the literature of venous embolism occurring following orogenital sex and after the use of a birth training device designed to stretch the peritoneum to prevent perineal injury by inflating and deflating a balloon [37,38]. Venous air embolism may account for as many as 1% of maternal deaths [35]. Presumably, the subplacental venous sinuses are the sites of air entry when antepartum or peripartum air embolism occurs [35].

Sudden, profound hypotension is the most common presenting sign of venous air embolism. Cough, dyspnea, dizziness, tachypnea, tachycardia, and diaphoresis also may be noted. Hypotension is usually followed quickly by respiratory arrest. The classic sign associated with air embolism is the mill wheel murmur, which is audible over the precordium [39]; a drum-like or bubbling sound may also be heard. Electrocardiographic evidence of ischemia, right heart strain, and arrhythmias have been described, and metabolic acidosis, presumably caused by lactic acid production, may be present [39] (see Chapter 61). Transesophageal echocardiography and transthoracic echocardiography have been utilized to identify air embolism, the route of the embolism, and the severity of the air embolism [40]. Precordial Doppler ultrasound may also be used for surveillance of air embolism by detection of alterations in the ultrasonic pattern caused by the embolism [41].

The volume of air that is likely to be lethal seems to vary with the rate of infusion and patient position. Any amount greater than 100 mL may cause death, but some patients have survived after infusion of up to 1,600 mL [42]. The mechanism by which air embolism leads to noncardiogenic pulmonary edema is not known. It is thought that entrapment of air bubbles in the pulmonary circulation leads to activation of complement, neutrophil, and platelets, resulting in mediator release and then endothelial injury [43]. This inflammatory response would then precipitate noncardiogenic pulmonary edema [44].

Aspiration of Gastric Contents

Aspiration of acidic gastric contents into the tracheobronchial tree was first described in 1946 by Mendelson [45] in women during labor and delivery. Maternal deaths from pulmonary aspiration have been steadily declining as a result of changing anesthesia practices including a shift to regional anesthesia from general anesthesia for delivery [46].

At term, several factors contribute to an increased risk of aspiration of stomach contents: (a) increased intragastric pressure caused by external compression by the gravid uterus, (b) progesterone-induced relaxation of the lower esophageal sphincter, (c) delayed gastric emptying during labor, (d) supine position, and (e) analgesia-induced decreased mental status and decreased vocal cord closure [47]. The pulmonary pathophysiologic consequences of gastric aspiration are a consequence of the acidity and the particulate content of the gastric contents and the risk of bacterial superinfection. Acid aspiration causes a direct injury to the airway resulting in desquamation and loss of ciliated and nonciliated cells including the alveolar type II cells. An inflammatory response is also triggered by the acid aspiration leading to an increase in alveolar permeability with a loss in lung compliance and a decrease in ventilation–perfusion matching [47]. Inhaled particulate matter may cause acute airway obstruction and immediate death.

The volume of acid aspiration determines, in part, the rapidity of symptom onset. Aspiration of smaller volumes may go unnoticed clinically until 6 to 8 hours later, when tachypnea, tachycardia, hypoxemia, hypotension, bronchospasm, and production of frothy, pink sputum are noted in association with diffuse infiltrates on chest radiography. Progression of chest radiographic findings may continue for up to 36 hours. The clinical course may follow one of three patterns: (a) rapid improvement during 4 to 5 days; (b) initial improvement followed by deterioration caused by supervening bacterial pneumonia, with a fatal outcome in up to 60%; and (c) early death as a result of intractable hypoxia [46]. Predictors of poor outcome include low pH, large volume, and a greater amount of particulate content of the aspirate. The bacterial pathogens in this setting are usually oropharyngeal anaerobes, although the longer the patient is in the hospital before clinical development of pneumonia, the greater the likelihood of facultative, Gram-negative bacillary and *Staphylococcus aureus* infections [48].

Respiratory Infections

The prevalence of pneumonia in pregnancy ranges from 0.78 to 2.7 cases per 1,000 deliveries. The maternal mortality rate from pneumonia has decreased from 20% to 3% since the advent of antibiotics [49]. The major factors in improving fetal and maternal outcome seem to have been earlier presentation and prompt institution of antibiotic therapy. Although pneumonia rarely progresses to respiratory failure, it is advisable to assess maternal oxygenation in all cases of maternal pneumonia. The spectrum of organisms to consider is similar to that in the nonpregnant population; the most common organisms are *Streptococcus pneumoniae*, *Haemophilus influenzae*, and *Mycoplasma pneumoniae*. *Legionella* pneumonia accounts for up to 22% of community-acquired pneumonia [50] and has been reported to cause respiratory failure in pregnancy [51].

Certain other respiratory infections (e.g., influenza, varicella, coccidioidomycosis, tuberculosis, listeriosis, and severe acute respiratory syndrome [SARS]) have been associated with increased maternal and fetal morbidity and mortality. These particular infections can be virulent in the pregnant patient because of alterations in the immune status. Specifically, during pregnancy there is a decreased lymphocyte proliferative response, a decrease in the natural killer cell activity, and a decrease in the number of helper T4 cells [52]. Fortunately, the impairment in maternal immune response is mild and the increase in maternal morbidity is small.

In the influenza pandemics of 1918 and 1957, an excess incidence of influenza pneumonia was noted among pregnant women. A 50% incidence of influenza pneumonia and an overall mortality of 27% for influenza in pregnancy were found in 1918 [53]. In the 1957 pandemic, several studies noted that 50% of deaths from influenza in women of childbearing age were in pregnant patients [53]. Autopsy reports noted that the cause of death in pregnant women was respiratory insufficiency caused by fulminant influenza pneumonia, rather than secondary bacterial infection, the more common cause of death in nonpregnant influenza patients. Similarly, the new strain of influenza A (novel influenza A H1N1), identified in 2009, has been associated with increased morbidity in pregnant women [54]. During the first weeks of this outbreak, 20 cases were identified in pregnant women; three were hospitalized and one died. These women presented with the typical symptoms of cough, fever, sore pharyngitis, rhinorrhea, diarrhea, headache, and myalgias [54].

Primary varicella-zoster infections progress to pneumonia more commonly in adults than in children, although only 20% of varicella cases occur in adults [55]. Cigarette smoking appears to be an important risk factor in the progression of varicella into pneumonia [56]. Progression to pneumonia has also been noted more frequently in pregnant women in their second and third trimesters; 10% of reported cases of varicella pneumonia have occurred in pregnant women. Historically, the maternal mortality rate for varicella pneumonia in pregnancy was 41%. Utilization of antiviral therapy has led to a decline in maternal mortality now in the range of 11% to 35% [49,56]. Respiratory failure requiring mechanical ventilation may occur in 40% to 57% of pregnant patients with varicella pneumonia, with a mortality rate of 25% [49,56].

Respiratory symptoms usually develop 2 days after the onset of fever, rash, and malaise. Typical symptoms are cough, dyspnea, hemoptysis, and chest pain [56]. Generalized varicella-zoster infections may also be associated with hepatitis, myocarditis, nephritis, thrombocytopenia, and adrenal hemorrhage [56]. Varicella during pregnancy can lead to intrauterine infection, which may result in prematurity, spontaneous abortion, and stillbirth [56]. In the absence of dissemination, herpes zoster does not appear to be associated with significant maternal morbidity or evidence of fetal infection [57].

SARS is an atypical pneumonia first described in 2002 that is caused by a coronavirus [58]. Symptoms of fever, chills, rigors, headache, malaise, and myalgias develop 2 to 7 days after exposure. A nonproductive cough or dyspnea may develop over 3 to 7 days. This may progress to hypoxemia and respiratory failure. The chest radiograph may show bilateral patchy interstitial infiltrates. The overall mortality rate for SARS is 3% [58]. One review of 12 cases of SARS during pregnancy demonstrated that 33% of pregnant women required mechanical ventilation, and the maternal mortality rate was 25% [59]. Pregnant patients with suspected or probable SARS should be placed on airborne precautions in a negative pressure isolation room [60].

Maternal *Coccidioidomycosis immitis* infections are rare, with less than 1 case in every 1,000 pregnancies. Historically, *Coccidioidomycosis* infection during pregnancy has been reported as having a 20.0% dissemination rate, compared with 0.2% in nonpregnant patients; infections contracted in the second or third trimester have a higher rate of dissemination [61]. Maternal mortality and fetal loss are preventable with appropriate treatment [61]. Case reports of cryptococcosis, blastomycosis, and sporotrichosis in pregnancy are rare enough to suggest that there is no increased susceptibility to these infections [61].

Disseminated coccidioidal infection should be suspected in patients with primary or chronic progressive coccidioidal pneumonia in whom rapidly progressive respiratory failure and a clinical picture resembling miliary tuberculosis develop. Diagnosis is sometimes difficult because sputum is positive in less than 40% of cases, and complement fixation titers may be low [61,62]. Evaluation of these patients should include a careful search for extrapulmonary disease (e.g., lumbar puncture, urinalysis, culture of skin lesions) [61,62].

Respiratory failure due to infection with *Mycobacterium tuberculosis* is rare, although before the advent of effective chemotherapy, maternal and infant mortality in cases of advanced disease approached 40% [63]. Pregnancy does not alter the pathogenesis of tuberculous infection or increase the likelihood of latent tuberculosis infection progressing to active disease [64]. In addition, pregnancy does not alter the response to purified protein derivative skin testing, so all pregnant women from populations recommended for screening should have a skin test performed if one has not been done previously [65].

In 2004, 27% of acquired immunodeficiency syndrome (AIDS) cases in the United States were in adult women [66]. As the number of women infected with the human immunodeficiency virus grows, the spectrum of respiratory disease in pregnancy will include an increasing proportion of opportunistic infections and other respiratory complications related to AIDS. *Pneumocystis jirovecii* (formerly *Pneumocystis carinii*) is the most common cause of AIDS-related death in pregnant patients [67]. A review of 22 cases of *Pneumocystis jirovecci* in pregnancy found a 59% rate of mechanical ventilation and a maternal mortality rate of 50%, compared with a mortality rate of 1% to 16% in nonpregnant patients [67]. Diagnostic evaluation follows the same protocol as in a nonpregnant patient with suspected PCP. Induced sputum should be examined for the presence of *P. jirovecii*; if this is negative, fiberoptic bronchoscopy with bronchoalveolar lavage should be performed.

Listeria monocytogenes, a cause of meningitis and sepsis in immunocompromised hosts, also has a predilection for pregnant women, most commonly resulting in abortion or neonatal sepsis. The incidence of Listeria infection among pregnant women is estimated at 12 per 100,000 compared with 0.7 per 100,000 in the general population [68]. The usual sporadic incidence is two to three cases for every 1 million of the population each year, but local outbreaks may occur as a result of ingestion of contaminated cheese, cabbage, or milk [68]. In an outbreak that caused 29 fetal and neonatal deaths, maternal morbidity was limited to fever and gastrointestinal symptoms [68]. However, in a few reported cases of maternal sepsis caused by *L. monocytogenes*, ARDS has developed [69]. In these cases, the fetal outcome was excellent despite *L. monocytogenes* sepsis. Diagnosis may be problematic because of difficulties in isolating the organism from respiratory tract secretions. When *L. monocytogenes* sepsis is suspected, cultures should be obtained from the blood, sputum, rectum, cervix, and amniotic fluid [68].

Asthma

Asthma affects between 3.7% and 8.4% of pregnant women in the United States [70]. The scope of this section is limited to asthmatic exacerbations during pregnancy that lead to respiratory failure. Studies have shown that poor asthma control during pregnancy is associated with adverse fetal and maternal outcomes. Pregnant women with frequent or severe asthma attacks were more likely to have fetal complications including growth retardation, preterm birth, low birth weight, neonatal hypoxia, and perinatal mortality. The maternal complications included preeclampsia, gestational hypertension, vaginal hemorrhage, hyperemesis, and complicated labor [71]. One study reported on the pregnancy outcomes of 486 asthmatic women who were enrolled in an active asthma management program compared with nonasthmatic, pregnant controls. There were no significant differences in either the fetal or maternal outcomes between the two groups. When active management of asthma during pregnancy is provided, maternal and fetal outcomes are no different than those of healthy, nonasthmatic women [70].

The initial clinical assessment of a pregnant woman with asthma should include personal history (detailing etiologic factors and prior therapy), physical examination, and either peak expiratory flow rate or spirometric pulmonary function testing (see Chapter 48). Peak expiratory flow rates and spirometry do not change with pregnancy and advancing gestation. Therefore, peak expiratory flow rates can be used as diagnostic and monitoring tools in the care of pregnant asthmatic women [72]. Although asthma may be the most common cause of airway obstruction during pregnancy, wheezing, shortness of breath, coughing, and sensation of chest tightness are nonspecific, and several other entities may mimic asthma (see Chapter 48).

Assuming the diagnosis of asthma is secure, certain findings taken together can be used to predict which patients are likely to require hospitalization [73]. These include diaphoresis, use of accessory muscles, assumption of upright posture, altered level of consciousness, pulse rate greater than 120 beats per minute, respiratory rate greater than 30 breaths per minute, pulsus paradoxus greater than 18 mm Hg, and peak expiratory flow rate less than 120 L per minute. When the FEV_1 is no more than 15% of predicted or is less than 0.5 L, both a pulsus paradoxus of 10 mm Hg or greater and use of accessory muscles of respiration are almost always found [74,75]. Conversely, the absence of both an elevated pulsus paradoxus and use of accessory muscles usually correlates with an FEV_1 greater than 40% of predicted or greater than 1.25 L [74,75]. Peak flows have been used in the evaluation of nonpregnant patients with asthma to predict the need for arterial blood gas determination. Flows greater than 200 L per minute (50% of predicted) are virtually never associated with significant hypoxemia or hypercapnia (see Chapter 48). However, as alveolar-arterial oxygen tension gradients are known to be widened in pregnancy [3], it seems prudent to obtain arterial blood gas measurements in pregnant women with asthma who do not show a significant improvement (>20%) in peak expiratory flow rate after an initial inhaled bronchodilator treatment. Continuous oxygen saturation monitoring is also appropriate.

During acute asthma attacks, arterial blood gas measurements typically reveal mild hypocapnia ($PaCO_2$ of 35 mm Hg) and moderate hypoxemia. In pregnancy, as noted previously, the baseline $PaCO_2$ is usually already depressed [3] and probably decreases further with an acute asthma attack. The importance of this is twofold: (a) a $PaCO_2$ of 35 mm Hg during an acute attack may actually represent "pseudonormalization" caused by fatigue, inability to meet the increased work of breathing, and impending respiratory failure and (b) persistent hypocapnia with associated respiratory alkalosis (pH greater than 7.48) may result in uterine artery vasoconstriction and decreased fetal perfusion [76].

β-Adrenergic Tocolytic Therapy

β-Adrenergic agents have been used therapeutically for inhibition of preterm labor [77]. The use of relatively β_2-selective agents, such as ritodrine and terbutaline, has diminished the frequency of unacceptable maternal tachycardia, but maternal pulmonary edema has remained a serious side effect. Pulmonary edema associated with tocolytic therapy appears to be unique to pregnancy because it has not been reported when these medications are used to treat asthma. Pulmonary edema occurs in approximately 1 in 400 women who are treated with β-agonists to control premature labor [78]. Calcium-channel blockers such as nifedipine and nicardipine have also been used for tocolysis, and cases of pulmonary edema induced by calcium-channel blockers when used for tocolysis have been reported [79,80]. Other tocolytics in clinical practice include cyclooxygenase-2 inhibitors and oxytocin antagonists. These are generally more specific for inhibition of preterm labor and less toxic than the β-adrenergic agents used for tocolysis [81]. A comparative study of atosiban, a selective oxytocin antagonist, versus β-agonists found atosiban to be as effective as the β-agonists as a tocolytic agent but significantly less likely to result in maternal cardiovascular side effects [82]. Atosiban is not approved for use in the United States because of concerns regarding drug safety when used in fetuses less than 28 weeks of gestation but is available in other countries [83].

The typical symptoms and signs of β-adrenergic tocolytic-induced pulmonary edema are chest discomfort, dyspnea, tachypnea (24 to 40 breaths per minute), crackles, and pulmonary edema on chest radiography. Evidence of pulmonary edema develops relatively acutely, occasionally after only 24 hours but usually after 48 hours of β-adrenergic tocolytic therapy. A nonproductive cough is occasionally present. Wheezes, in addition to crackles, were noted in one case [80]. The size of the heart has been difficult to assess on radiographs because of the normal increase in cardiac diameter with pregnancy. The relatively rapid improvement that occurs with discontinuation of β-adrenergic tocolytic therapy (usually in less than 24 hours), the absence of hypotension and clotting abnormalities, and the lack of need for mechanical ventilation support the possibility that these cases represent a separate syndrome related to β-adrenergic tocolytic therapy.

The pathophysiologic mechanisms leading to the development of tocolytic-induced pulmonary edema are not well defined. Fluid overload is an important factor contributing to the pathogenesis. Augmented aldosterone secretion secondary to pregnancy and β-agonist stimulation causes salt and water retention [81]. Tocolytic agents also stimulate antidiuretic hormone secretion, which increases water retention [82]. There are no compelling data to support the hypothesis of cardiac failure as the etiology of tocolytic-induced pulmonary edema. Echocardiography and hemodynamic assessment of affected patients have not revealed cardiac dysfunction [81]. The rapidity of improvement after diuresis is consistent with pulmonary edema caused by increased hydrostatic pressure, rather than an increase in capillary permeability [81].

Pneumomediastinum and Pneumothorax

Pneumomediastinum is another rare complication of pregnancy. Estimates of incidence range from 1 in 2,000 to 1 in 100,000 patients [84]. It occurs most commonly in the second stage of labor and is associated with chest or shoulder pain that radiates to the neck and arms, mild dyspnea, and subcutaneous emphysema of face and neck. Prolonged, dysfunctional labor, coughing, and severe emesis seem to be predisposing factors. Air from ruptured alveoli tracks centrally along the perivascular sheath into the mediastinum and along fascial planes into the subcutaneous tissues. Of the reported cases in pregnancy, only one patient required decompression of the mediastinum for treatment of venous obstruction [85].

Spontaneous pneumothorax with tension may occur with or without associated pneumomediastinum. It occurs rarely during pregnancy with an incidence estimated at 1 per 10,000 deliveries, but it should be considered in the differential diagnosis of respiratory failure during pregnancy [86]. Risk factors for pneumothorax include asthma, cigarette smoking, crack cocaine use, and history of pneumothorax. Pneumothoraces usually occur during labor or in the immediate postpartum period. Occurrence of pneumothorax may be caused by rupture of subpleural blebs by the changes in intrapleural pressure caused by Valsalva maneuvers during labor [86]. Symptoms of pneumothorax include sudden pleuritic chest pain, dyspnea, and cough. Hypotension may develop if a tension pneumothorax develops. The clinical significance of pneumothorax during pregnancy relates to impaired ventilation and hypoxemia, which can lead to fetal hypoxemia.

Acute Respiratory Distress Syndrome

ARDS is a type of respiratory failure caused by an inflammatory injury to the alveolar–capillary interface that leads to alveolar edema and resultant hypoxemia. The diagnosis of ARDS in pregnant patients is the same for nonobstetric patients. The criteria defined by the American-European Consensus Conference include (i) acute onset, (ii) a PaO_2/FiO_2 ratio of less than 200 mm Hg regardless of positive end-expiratory pressure (PEEP) level, (iii) bilateral infiltrates on chest x-ray, and (iv) a pulmonary artery wedge pressure of less than 18 mm Hg or the absence of clinical evidence of left atrial hypertension [87]. The pathogenesis of ARDS during pregnancy includes the same etiologies seen in the general population such as sepsis, aspiration, pancreatitis, trauma, inhalational injury, drowning, and pneumonia. Unique entities of pregnancy that may lead to ARDS include amniotic fluid embolism, eclampsia, HELLP syndrome, chorioamnionitis, and endometritis [88–91].

Published case series data report maternal mortality rates between 23% and 39%, with multisystem organ failure as the most common cause of death [90,91]. Neonatal outcomes are not well studied, but in one study of 13 women with ARDS, the perinatal fetal death rate was 23% [91]. In another published series of 10 women treated for ARDS, only 5 of the babies survived intact [91].

DIAGNOSTIC TESTING

Radiology

Evaluation of patients with respiratory failure usually requires at least one, if not sequential, chest radiographs. Potential adverse fetal effects include congenital malformation, intrauterine growth retardation, and increased risk of leukemia and other malignancies [92–94]. There is no evidence that there is an increased fetal risk of anomalies, growth retardation, or intellectual disability from radiation doses less than 0.05 Gy [93]. There may be a small increased risk of childhood leukemia, 1 in every 2,000 compared with a background rate of 1 in every 3,000 [94,95].

TABLE 51.2

FETAL RADIATION DOSE

Diagnostic test	Dose: mrad	Dose: μGy
Posterior-to-anterior and lateral chest radiograph	<1	10
Helical chest CT scan	0.33–13	3–131
Abdominal CT scan	250	2,500
Lung perfusion scan	6–12	60–120
Lung ventilation scan	1–19	10–190
Brachial pulmonary arteriogram	<50	<500
Femoral pulmonary arteriogram	221–374	2,210–3,740

CT, computed tomography.
Adapted from Ginsberg JS, Hirsch J, Rainbow AJ, et al: Risks to the fetus of radiologic procedures used in the diagnosis of maternal venous thromboembolic disease. *Thromb Haemost* 61:189, 1989; Bentur Y, Horlatsch N, Koren G: Exposure to ionizing radiation during pregnancy: perception of teratogenic risk and outcome. *Teratology* 43:163, 1991; Winer-Muram HT, Boone JM, Brown HL, et al: Pulmonary embolism in pregnant patients: fetal radiation does with helical CT. *Radiology* 224:487, 2002.

The National Council on Radiation Protection Handbook 54 established 5 rad (0.05 Gy or 5 cGy) as the embryonic exposure level not to exceed [94]. The estimated radiation exposures of selected procedures used in the evaluation of pregnant patients with respiratory failure are shown in Table 51.2 [95]. Portable chest radiographs performed daily for 2 weeks to assess location of endotracheal tubes and central venous catheters, as well as response of the underlying illness to treatment, would expose the fetus to approximately 7 mrad (0.07 Gy). A pregnant woman being evaluated for thromboembolic disease with a chest radiograph and helical chest CT-pulmonary angiogram would have a fetal exposure of less than 500 mrad (0.005 Gy or 0.5 cGy) [93,96].

Magnetic resonance imaging (MRI) and ultrasonography are not known to be associated with adverse fetal outcomes [96,97]. Previously, the National Radiological Protection Board had advised that MRI be avoided during the first trimester because its safety during organogenesis was unknown [98]. The American College of Radiology has subsequently published guidelines in which MRI may be considered as a nonionizing imaging study during any trimester if the risk–benefit ratio to the patient is favorable [99]. Gadolinium crosses the placenta to the fetus, so the use of gadolinium-based contrast is not recommended at any time in pregnant patients [99].

Hemodynamic Monitoring

Cardiopulmonary monitoring in critically ill patients has advanced rapidly since the introduction of flow-directed pulmonary artery catheters in 1970 [100,101]. There are no reports of specific complications of pulmonary artery catheterization pertaining to obstetric patients, who are at equal risk as nonobstetric patients for complications such as hematoma or pneumothorax at the time of insertion, balloon rupture, catheter knotting, pulmonary infarct, pulmonary artery rupture, thrombosis, embolism, arrhythmias, right bundle-branch block, valvular damage, and infection (see Chapter 4).

The changes that occur in maternal hemodynamics during pregnancy, labor, and delivery have been described. Pulmonary artery catheterization of 10 healthy pregnant patients was done at term and repeated during the nonpregnant state to determine the hemodynamic changes in normal pregnancy. There were significant reductions in systemic and pulmonary vascular resistances, colloid oncotic pressure, and the gradient between colloid oncotic pressure and pulmonary balloon occlusion pressure in the late third trimester. There was a significant increase in heart rate and cardiac output in all pregnant patients. There was no significant change in central venous pressure, pulmonary balloon occlusion pressure, mean arterial pressure, or left ventricular stroke work index [101,102].

Potential indications for pulmonary artery catheterization in obstetric patients include the diagnosis or management of septic shock, class III and IV cardiac patients in labor, severe preeclampsia or eclampsia during labor, pulmonary edema that does not quickly respond to diuretic therapy, pulmonary hypertension, and ARDS with PEEP of more than 15 mm Hg [103].

Because of the complications that may accompany pulmonary artery catheterization, the expense of the procedure, and the lack of formal demonstration of improved morbidity or mortality related to the technique, it has been suggested that caution be exercised when choosing to proceed with pulmonary artery catheterization [103]. Clinical assessment may be inadequate in obstetric patients to differentiate between cardiogenic and noncardiogenic pulmonary edema. Both increased-permeability pulmonary edema and pulmonary edema caused by volume overload are common causes of respiratory failure in pregnancy. In addition, careful hemodynamic management is needed to maintain adequate uterine blood flow in compromised patients. Maintaining a good risk-to-benefit ratio depends on obtaining accurate information, interpreting this information in the context of the stage of pregnancy or labor, and determining the specific situations in which the information will contribute significantly to patient management.

Noninvasive hemodynamic monitoring techniques such as Doppler echocardiography, esophageal Doppler monitoring, thoracic electrical bioimpedance, arterial pressure wave form algorithms, pulse pressure variation, and stroke volume variation require further study in critically ill obstetric patients [104–107].

Fetal Monitoring

When respiratory failure occurs early in gestation, before fetal viability is ensured, and when early delivery is not an option, the best course is to focus on optimizing care for the mother and not on minute-to-minute variations in fetal heart rate. However, it is reasonable to measure and record a daily fetal heart rate to document that the fetus is alive. When she is able, the mother can report whether fetal movement is present. If respiratory failure persists for several weeks, fetal growth measurement by ultrasound may be indicated. When gestation has progressed enough for delivery by cesarean section, amniocentesis may be helpful to determine fetal maturity [108]. Continuous external fetal heart rate monitoring may be helpful during surgical procedures to alert the anesthesiologist to problems with maternal ventilation or cardiac output [109,110].

TREATMENT

Supportive Therapy

Mechanical ventilation, nutritional support, and maintaining an adequate blood pressure are important considerations in respiratory insufficiency during pregnancy.

Mechanical Ventilation

The guidelines for intubation and mechanical ventilation are essentially the same for pregnant patients as for nonpregnant patients: (a) inability to maintain a minimal PaO_2 of 60 to 65 mm Hg with supplemental oxygen, (b) uncompensated respiratory acidosis, and (c) inability to clear secretions or need to protect the airway because of altered mental status (see Chapters 1 and 58).

Pregnancy is associated with alterations in physiology that may make airway management more difficult compared with that of nonpregnant patients. Elevated estrogen levels and an increase in blood volume seen in pregnancy may contribute to mucosal edema [111,112]. Smaller endotracheal tubes sized 6 to 7 mm may be required to minimize the risk of upper airway trauma during intubation [3]. The decreased FRC in pregnancy may lower the oxygen reserve such that, at the time of intubation, a short period of apnea may be associated with a precipitous decrease in PaO_2 [3]. Therefore, before any attempt at endotracheal intubation, 100% oxygen should be administered, either by mask when the patient is able to ventilate spontaneously or by hand resuscitation bag when the patient requires assisted ventilation. However, hyperventilation to increase the PaO_2 before intubation should be avoided because the associated respiratory alkalosis may actually decrease uterine blood flow. Multiple factors place a pregnant patient at an increase risk of aspiration during intubation. These include incompetence of the gastroesophageal junction caused by the position of the gravid uterus, delayed gastric emptying during labor, progesterone-mediated smooth muscle relaxation of the gastrointestinal mucosa, and decreased lower esophageal sphincter tone [112]. During assisted ventilation and intubation, cricoid pressure with the head and neck extended can help decrease gastric inflation and prevent regurgitation into the hypopharynx [113].

Initiating mechanical ventilation follows the same general principles for pregnant patients as for nonpregnant patients, although arterial blood gas goals are different in the pregnant patient [114]. In general, the minute ventilation should be adjusted to aim for a $PaCO_2$ of 30 to 32 mm Hg, the normal level in pregnancy; marked respiratory alkalosis should be avoided because of the resultant decrease in uterine blood flow. Maternal permissive hypercapnia may also be deleterious to the fetus because of resultant fetal respiratory acidosis. The transfer of carbon dioxide across the placenta depends on the difference of 10 mm Hg between the fetal and maternal umbilical veins [115]. Plateau pressure, which reflects transalveolar pressure, should be kept under 30 cm H_2O to minimize the risk of barotrauma. Adequate fetal oxygenation requires a maternal PaO_2 of 70 mm Hg or more which corresponds to an oxygen saturation of 95% [89].

Mechanical ventilation of a pregnant patient with ARDS should follow the guidelines of the ARDS Network Study using nonpregnant predicted body weight [116]. This study has shown the efficacy of delivering tidal volumes based on ideal body weight. This strategy avoids overdistention of the lung and maintains a plateau pressure less than 30 cm H_2O. The target value for tidal volume is 6 mL per kg of ideal body weight. The respiratory rate is increased to maintain a maternal PCO_2 between 28 and 32 mm Hg while monitoring for the development of intrinsic PEEP or dynamic hyperinflation. If the pregnant patient continues to have a respiratory acidosis despite a high respiratory rate, the tidal volume may be increased as long as the plateau pressure remains less than 30 cm H_2O. In patients with ARDS who require a fraction of inspired oxygen greater than 50% to maintain a PaO_2 of 65 mm Hg or greater, or an oxygen saturation greater than 90%, consideration should be given to adding PEEP. As in nonpregnant patients, the goals are to reduce the maternal inspired oxygen concentration to less than 50%, if possible, and to maintain adequate oxygen delivery without compromising cardiac output or risking further lung damage caused by excess intra-alveolar pressure [117]. Strict monitoring of fluid status is necessary because the hypervolemia of pregnancy may contribute to the progression of respiratory failure.

Alternative ventilation strategies for patients failing conventional ventilation modes in ARDS have not been studied in pregnancy. The routine use of airway pressure-release ventilation, high-frequency oscillatory ventilation, lung recruitment maneuvers, prone positioning, and inhaled vasodilators during pregnancy need further study before they can be recommended.

In patients with asthma, respiratory rate and tidal volume should be no greater than necessary to maintain oxygenation. Lower respiratory rates and tidal volumes help reduce airway pressures, thereby reducing volutrauma and barotrauma [116]. Inspiratory flow rates can be increased to allow adequate time for expiration. Increasing the inspiratory flow rate during volume-cycled mechanical ventilation decreases the inspiratory to expiratory ratio and mitigates air trapping. (See Chapters 47 and 58 for further discussion of mechanical ventilatory support of the patient with asthma.) Permissive hypercapnia is often necessary in patients with severe asthma to prevent volutrauma and hemodynamic compromise. There have been no reported cases of controlled hypoventilation during pregnancy, and the potential risk of fetal respiratory acidosis must be considered before instituting this therapy.

Lowering oxygen consumption by treating fever and suppressing spontaneous respiration is also helpful. Temperature regulation may be particularly important during gestation; an increased rate of congenital malformations has been associated with maternal fever, especially during the first few months of pregnancy [118]. Sedation and muscle paralysis, when indicated, are best accomplished with morphine sulfate and pancuronium bromide [119], which appear to be without adverse fetal effects except when used at the time of delivery or when used excessively, as in narcotic addiction [120]. Whether benzodiazepine use results in an increased risk of congenital malformations remains unclear, although the majority of studies are reassuring; this class of drugs is best avoided in the first trimester and used sparingly thereafter (see www.reprotox.org) [121]. Although sitting is usually the most advantageous position for weaning nonpregnant patients from mechanical ventilation, it may result in inferior vena cava compression in patients near term, in which case the lateral decubitus position is preferable. Weaning parameters for pregnant patients are not well established, but it seems reasonable to follow the same guidelines as for nonpregnant patients (see Chapter 59) [122].

Reversal of Hypotension

Supine recumbency may cause a significant decrease in venous return in women in their second or third trimesters. To counteract this, the right hip should be elevated 10 to 15 cm (15 degrees) to move the uterus off the inferior vena cava, or the lateral decubitus position should be used. As a corollary to this, if patients in the second or third trimester become hypotensive, placing them in the Trendelenburg position is unlikely to help and may actually decrease venous return because of vena cava compression.

When hypotension does not respond to reduction in uterine pressure on the vena cava, the fluid status of the patient should be assessed. If fluid boluses with 250 to 500 mL of saline do not resolve hypotension and the patient appears to be euvolemic, vasopressors should be considered. The ideal vasopressor would restore maternal blood pressure without compromising uterine blood flow. Ephedrine, which has both α- and β-stimulating effects, tends to preserve uterine blood flow while reversing systemic hypotension [3]. Phenylephrine has been used alone and in combination with ephedrine to reverse maternal hypotension associated with epidural anesthesia [123,124]. Predominantly α-adrenergic agents, such as norepinephrine, improve maternal blood pressure but decrease uterine blood flow because of uterine artery vasoconstriction. If maternal hypotension remains refractory, drugs with more α-adrenergic activity, such as epinephrine, norepinephrine, and dopamine, which do not preserve uterine blood flow, may be tried [3]. Dobutamine may also be added for life-threatening maternal hypotension when pulmonary artery pressure and cardiac output values indicate it is appropriate.

Nutrition

The importance of adequate nutrition during gestation is well recognized in that maternal weight gain correlates with fetal weight gain and a successful outcome. Maternal body stores are generally protected at the expense of fetal growth during semistarvation [125]. The duration of starvation or semistarvation that can be tolerated without ill effects on the fetus is unknown. In addition, maternal malnutrition has been shown to correlate in certain cases with intrauterine growth retardation and development of preeclampsia [126]. It is also well recognized that hospitalized patients who have experienced prolonged starvation have greater problems with wound healing and that diminished protein stores are associated with increased susceptibility to infection.

In critically ill obstetric patients, nutritional support is thought to be important for both maternal and fetal outcomes. As with nonobstetric patients, enteral nutrition is preferred over parenteral nutrition to avoid the risk of complications associated with central venous catheters, to reduce expense, and to minimize gastric mucosal atrophy [126]. Pregnancy is associated with decreased lower esophageal sphincter tone and decreased gastric motility; therefore, nasoduodenal tubes are preferred over nasogastric tubes to decrease the likelihood of reflux and aspiration, although scientific evidence for this is lacking.

Total parenteral nutrition (TPN) can provide complete nutritional support during pregnancy [127]. Given the stress of respiratory failure and its underlying causes, it seems reasonable to extend this experience with TPN to patients with respiratory failure who are unable to eat for more than 48 hours and whose gastrointestinal system cannot be used. Blood glucose levels should be measured, along with serum electrolyte concentrations, acid–base status, and renal and hepatic function. Measurement of trace element concentrations is needed for prolonged TPN. Periodic nutritional assessment should include evaluation of nitrogen balance, lymphocyte counts, transferrin, maternal weight, and fetal growth by ultrasound. If delivery occurs while the woman is receiving TPN, the neonate should be observed closely for hypoglycemia [127,128]. Vitamins should probably be replaced according to the recommended dietary allowances for pregnancy [128].

Specific Therapy

Thromboembolism

Recommendations for the treatment of venous thromboembolic disease in pregnancy have been published by the American College of Chest Physicians (ACCP) [129]. When massive pulmonary embolism is strongly suspected (>50% occlusion of pulmonary vascular bed or systemic hypotension), the major immediate goals of therapy are to (a) provide adequate oxygenation as dictated by arterial blood gas analysis, (b) treat hypotension and organ hypoperfusion by elevating right

TABLE 51.3

GUIDELINES FOR ANTICOAGULATION REGIMENS

Prophylactic LMWH: Dalteparin 5,000 units subcutaneously every 24 hours or Enoxaparin 40 mg subcutaneously every 24 hours
Intermediate-dose LMWH: Dalteparin 5,000 units subcutaneously every 12 hours or Enoxaparin 40 mg subcutaneously every 12 hours
Prophylactic UFH: Unfractionated heparin 5,000 units subcutaneously every 12 hours
Intermediate-dose UFH: Unfractionated heparin subcutaneously every 12 hours adjusted to target an anti-Xa level of 0.1–0.3 U/mL

LMWH, low-molecular-weight heparin.
Adapted from Bates SM, Greer IA, Pabinger I, et al: Venous thromboembolism, thrombophilia, antithrombotic therapy and pregnancy. American College of Chest Physicians Evidence-Based Clinical Practice Guidelines (8th ed). *Chest* 133;844S, 2008.

ventricular preload with colloid or crystalloid administration and vasopressor therapy if necessary, and (c) interrupt clot propagation by immediate anticoagulation with intravenous heparin. Anticoagulation should be instituted immediately in all patients without clear contraindications, such as active bleeding, rather than delay therapy pending conclusive diagnostic studies. The therapeutic options available include subcutaneous low-molecular-weight heparin (LMWH), intravenous unfractionated heparin (UFH), or subcutaneous UFH. Heparin is not teratogenic because it does not cross the placenta. Subcutaneous LMWH is preferred because of its safety profile, ease of administration, and efficacy [129]. Meta-analysis data in nonpregnant patients has shown that patients treated with subcutaneous LMWH for pulmonary embolism had decreased mortality, a reduction in thrombus size, and were less likely to experience a major hemorrhage [130].

Intravenous UFH is recommended in pregnant patients who have persistent hypotension due to pulmonary embolism or who are considered to be at a high risk of bleeding. Intravenous UFH has a short half-life and can be reversed quickly upon discontinuation and administration of protamine [129]. UFH would also be recommended in pregnant patients with severe renal failure rather than LMWH [129]. The half-life of LMWH is decreased in pregnancy, which may lead to subtherapeutic anticoagulation levels [129]. Twice-daily regimens should be titrated to antifactor Xa levels of 0.6 to 1.0 U per mL 4 hours postinjection [129]. Measurements of antifactor Xa levels can be made every 4 to 6 weeks to verify adequate dosing [129].

When hemodynamic and angiographic information confirms massive pulmonary embolism, placement of a retrievable inferior vena filter is usually indicated to provide immediate and reliable prophylaxis against recurrent thromboembolism. In addition, thrombolytic therapy, catheter-directed thrombolysis, or surgical embolectomy may be indicated [131,132]. Thrombolysis is not indicated for submassive pulmonary embolism, because large studies have failed to document that thrombolytic therapy results in any significant improvement in mortality or morbidity compared with heparinization [131]. Specific circumstances for which thrombolytic therapy might be preferable include (a) lack of immediate availability of surgery and cardiopulmonary bypass, (b) emboli that are inaccessible to the surgeon without dissection of the lung parenchyma, and (c) the absence of large vessel puncture sites or recent surgery that would increase the risk of bleeding (see Chapter 52). One problem with instituting thrombolytic therapy is that if it is unsuccessful in achieving clot lysis sufficient to improve the hemodynamic function, subsequent endarterectomy may be impossible because of the lytic state.

Pregnancy and the immediate postpartum state are relative contraindications to thrombolytic therapy because of the risk of hemorrhage during labor, delivery, and the first several days postpartum [133]. No controlled trials of the use of thrombolytics in pregnancy have been reported, but a review of the reported cases reveals 172 women who received thrombolytics during pregnancy for various indications, including 10 cases of pulmonary embolism [134]. The intrapartum or immediate postpartum risk of hemorrhage was 8.1% if thrombolysis was performed at the time of delivery. This compares with a 2% risk of hemorrhage for pregnant patients on full-dose subcutaneous heparin for DVT. The maternal and fetal mortality rates in pregnant patients treated with thrombolytics are each 1.2%, which is similar to the 1.1% and 2.5% of heparin-treated pregnant patients. There was no increased risk of premature labor or premature rupture of membranes in pregnant patients treated with thrombolytics compared with the baseline incidence of preterm labor in the United States. In a review of 13 patients who received thrombolytic therapy for pulmonary embolism during pregnancy, there were no maternal deaths, 4 nonfatal maternal major bleeding complications, 2 fetal deaths, and 5 preterm deliveries. The authors concluded that the fetal deaths and preterm deliveries were a consequence primarily related to the pulmonary embolism rather than thrombolytic therapy [135].

Recombinant tissue plasminogen activator is the recommended agent for thrombolysis. Streptokinase does not cross the human placenta, but streptokinase antibodies do cross [134]. Tissue plasminogen activator does not cross the placenta, and the risk of allergic reactions is lower than that of streptokinase. If thrombolytic therapy is used during pregnancy, it seems reasonable to limit the duration of therapy to the time needed for restoration of acceptable hemodynamic function and to discontinue therapy at least 4 to 6 hours antepartum. Continuous uterine massage and methylergonovine maleate should be used postpartum if thrombolytic therapy was only recently discontinued. Because aminocaproic acid crosses the placenta readily and is teratogenic, aprotinin (Trasylol), which does not cross the placenta, should be used when rapid reversal of the lytic state is needed before delivery [136]. Cryoprecipitate can also be used and is preferred over fresh-frozen plasma [133].

Laboratory monitoring of the lytic state during thrombolytic infusion is not recommended, because clot lysis and risk of bleeding do not correlate well with laboratory measurement of the lytic state [131]. Following completion of thrombolysis, heparin is administered once the activated partial thromboplastin time (aPTT) and thrombin time are less than twice the normal value [131]. If delivery is anticipated in the next 6 hours, initiation of heparin is delayed until after delivery.

Surgical embolectomy may be a treatment option for massive pulmonary embolism when conventional therapy or thrombolytic therapy has failed, or if there is a contraindication for thrombolysis. There have been eight published cases in which pregnant women underwent surgical embolectomy for pulmonary embolism. There were no maternal deaths, although fetal death was reported in six cases and preterm delivery in four cases [135]. Surgical embolectomy should be reserved as a lifesaving measure for the mother due to the high incidence of fetal loss [135]. Catheter-directed therapy may include catheter-directed mechanical embolectomy and/or catheter-directed thrombolytic therapy. Among four cases using these techniques during pregnancy, one fetal death and one preterm delivery were reported [135].

Once the patient has stabilized, continuous intravenous heparin can be transitioned to subcutaneous therapy. This can be done with either LMWH or adjusted dose UFH to prolong the aPTT 1.5 to 2.5 times control. The patient should be anticoagulated for the remainder of the pregnancy and for at least 6 weeks postpartum [129]. If the pulmonary embolism occurs late in pregnancy or in the postpartum period, anticoagulant therapy should be continued for at least 6 months and possibly longer, if persistent risk factors for a hypercoagulable state exist [129].

It is recommended that pregnant patients being treated with LMWH or UFH discontinue anticoagulation 24 hours prior to elective induction of labor [129]. If spontaneous labor occurs in a woman receiving adjusted doses of UFH, the aPTT should be monitored and corrected with protamine sulfate if delivery is near. Patients at high risk for recurrent thromboembolism during pregnancy should be placed on intravenous UFH, and this can be discontinued 4 to 6 hours prior to expected delivery. This approach minimizes the period of time without therapeutic anticoagulation [129]. The timing of reinstitution of anticoagulation following delivery will vary depending upon the type of delivery, the presence of bleeding, and the presence of a neuroaxial anesthesia catheter. As long as significant bleeding has not occurred, anticoagulation with a heparin may be resumed 6 hours after a vaginal birth or 12 hours after a cesarean section. However, after neuroaxial anesthesia, therapeutic LMWH should be administered no earlier than 24 hours postoperatively [137].

Amniotic Fluid Embolism

Treatment of AFE is limited to supportive measures aimed at providing adequate ventilation and oxygenation, maintenance of left ventricular output, blood pressure support, and management of bleeding. Most patients require intubation and mechanical ventilation. PEEP is helpful for oxygenation in some patients. No particular drug regimen has been used with any clear success to reverse pulmonary hypertension. If pulmonary capillary wedge pressures are elevated, it seems reasonable to use a diuretic to reduce hydrostatic pressures across the injured capillary endothelium. Measurement of changes in cardiac output can be used to guide this. In addition to fluid resuscitation to reverse hypotension, vasopressor therapy is frequently required with ephedrine as the first-line choice (see "Supportive Therapy" section).

Treatment of coagulopathy is likewise nonspecific. For active bleeding, transfusion with fresh-frozen plasma, cryoprecipitate, platelets, and factor replacement is indicated. Manual massage and uterotonic medications are used to reduce uterine bleeding. When uterine bleeding is refractory to these interventions, exploration for uterine tears or retained placenta should be considered. Hysterectomy may be required to control bleeding if all other medical interventions fail. There are case reports describing maternal survival from AFE following treatment with intra-aortic balloon counterpulsation, extracorporeal membrane oxygenation, and cardiopulmonary bypass [138]. In addition, one patient was treated successfully with inhaled nitric oxide, recombinant human factor VIIa, and a right ventricular assist device [139].

Venous Air Embolism

The goals of treatment are to identify the source of air entry, prevent further air entrainment, restore circulation, and remove embolized air. Placing the patient in the left lateral decubitus position may restore forward blood flow by causing the bubble of air to migrate away from the right ventricular outflow tract to a nonobstructing position [39]. Closed-chest cardiac compression has also been reported to be helpful [39]. Aspiration of air from the right atrium, right ventricle, or pulmonary outflow tract can be attempted with a central venous or pulmonary artery catheter [39]. Air bubble resorption may be accelerated by ventilating the patient with 100% oxygen to facilitate diffusion of nitrogen from the embolus. When air embolism occurs during general anesthesia, nitrous oxide should be discontinued because it has a high solubility and tends to increase the size of air bubbles in the pulmonary vasculature [39].

Patients with continued evidence of neurologic deficits or cardiopulmonary compromise because of air embolism should be considered for hyperbaric oxygen therapy. Hyperbaric oxygen accelerates nitrogen resorption, decreases air bubble size, and increases the arterial oxygen content [140]. Use of anticoagulation with heparin has been suggested to treat fibrin microemboli [39].

Aspiration of Gastric Contents

For patients with permeability pulmonary edema due to aspiration of gastric contents during labor and delivery, the main treatment is supportive care. Prophylactic antibiotics have not been found to be beneficial in aspiration pneumonitis [141]; therefore, antibiotics should be prescribed only when infection complicates the initial chemical pneumonitis. If the patient's clinical course suggests development of bacterial pneumonia, the choice of antibiotic should be guided by appropriate bacteriologic evaluation of respiratory secretions, pleural fluid (if present), and blood cultures. For patients who have been in the hospital for 48 hours or less, clindamycin or a beta lactam–beta-lactamase inhibitor combination is reasonable empiric choice to treat anaerobic organisms. Most studies have not supported an ameliorative role for glucocorticoids, despite early anecdotal suggestions of success [142–145]. Lung lavage with normal saline or alkaline solutions is not helpful and may worsen the patient's condition [145].

Respiratory Infections

Antibacterial agents to treat pneumonia during pregnancy should be selected according to the same principles used for nonpregnant patients [50]. Drugs with the least risk to fetus and mother should be chosen whenever possible. The following comments about antibiotic safety are derived from a review [146].

For community-acquired pneumonia in pregnancy, penicillins, ceftriaxone, azithromycin, and erythromycin (excluding the estolate, which is associated with an increased risk of cholestatic jaundice in pregnancy) are probably safe. Tetracycline is contraindicated because it is teratogenic and causes hepatic toxicity when administered intravenously in pregnancy. The aminoglycosides have the potential of causing eighth nerve toxicity in the fetus and should be used only when strong clinical indications exist. Serum drug levels should then be monitored closely. Sulfonamides are considered contraindicated at term because of the risk of neonatal kernicterus. Clindamycin has no reported adverse fetal effects, but experience is limited and it should be used with caution. Vancomycin hydrochloride may cause fetal renal and auditory toxicity and should be used with caution, with close monitoring of serum drug levels. Clarithromycin and levofloxacin are pregnancy risk factor class C and, therefore, should be used judiciously, weighing potential risks and benefits.

The predominant treatment of influenza pneumonia is supportive care, following the same practices as outlined for other causes of respiratory failure in pregnancy. For pregnant women who present with presumed or documented influenza pneumonia, the neuraminidase inhibitors, zanamivir and oseltamivir, are the usual first line of specific antiviral therapy [147]. These agents are active against both influenza A and B [147]. Either agent may be used, unless oseltamivir resistance is suspected, in which case zanamivir is preferred. When oseltamivir resistance is suspected, but the patient has a contraindication to zanamivir (e.g., asthma or COPD), a combination of oseltamivir and adamantine may be used. Fetal side effects have not been reported with either neuraminidase inhibitor, although experience with them is limited.

The adamantines (amantadine and rimantadine) are considered second-line therapy after the neuraminidase inhibitors, due to the rate of resistance in influenza isolates and drug-related side effects [53]. The main indication for use of an adamantine medication is infection with an influenza A strain that is resistant to oseltamivir in a patient with a contraindication to zanamivir [53]. Amantadine hydrochloride interferes with replication and shedding of influenza A virions, thus limiting spread of the virus within the respiratory tract and has also been shown to hasten resolution of symptoms and small airway dysfunction [53]. Only a few case reports have documented amantadine use in human pregnancy [53]. The usual dosage is 200 mg per day; mild central nervous system toxicity can be limited by using a split-dosage schedule [53]. Rimantadine (pregnancy risk factor class C) is also effective for influenza A prophylaxis and treatment and is given in 100-mg doses twice daily.

The novel influenza A (H1N1) virus that appeared in 2009 is sensitive to the neuraminidase inhibitor antiviral medications such as zanamivir and oseltamivir, but it is resistant to the adamantine antiviral agents. The Centers for Disease Control and Prevention (CDC) interim guidance indicates that pregnant women with a confirmed, probable, or suspected case of influenza A (H1N1) receive empiric institution of oseltamivir for a period of 5 or more days. Treatment should be started while results from testing are pending, as the maximal clinical benefit is seen when antiviral therapy is begun within 48 hours of the onset of symptoms [54].

Intravenous acyclovir has been shown to decrease maternal mortality from varicella pneumonia from 35% to 17% [56]. Acyclovir has not been shown to be teratogenic when used during human pregnancy [148]. The recommended dosing is 10 mg per kg every 8 hours intravenously, with adjustments made for renal insufficiency. The recommended length of therapy is 7 days. Maintenance of a euvolemic fluid status minimizes renal impairment secondary to acyclovir. Initiation of acyclovir at the first evidence of respiratory system involvement in pregnant patients with cutaneous varicella infection optimizes the chances of a favorable outcome [148]. Infants born to women in whom varicella infection developed within 4 days of delivery should receive varicella-zoster immune globulin within 72 hours of birth [148].

Amphotericin B is the drug of choice for severe disseminated coccidioidal infection during pregnancy [149]. Azoles are contraindicated during pregnancy; fluconazole exposure is teratogenic in the first trimester; and voriconazole is category D due to documented fetal harm and teratogenicity. There is not enough safety data to recommend caspofungin during pregnancy [149]. Amphotericin has been used with success in disseminated coccidioidal infection during pregnancy. It crosses the placenta and is present in umbilical cord serum at a concentration one third that of the maternal serum concentration. However, it does not appear to have an adverse effect on fetal development; normal, full-term infants have been born to women who received amphotericin B during the first trimester, as well as later in gestation. Because anemia often occurs during the course of amphotericin B therapy, blood cell counts and renal function should be monitored closely [61].

Active tuberculosis has been treated with modern chemotherapeutic agents with excellent maternal and fetal outcome. The initial treatment regimen should consist of isoniazid, rifampin, and ethambutol for a minimum of 9 months [150]. In the United States, pyrazinamide is not recommended for use during pregnancy [150]. Streptomycin has been associated with fetal hearing loss and vestibular dysfunction and should be avoided [151]. Ethionamide has been identified as a teratogen [150].

Treatment of *Pneumocystis jirovecci* during pregnancy includes trimethoprim–sulfamethoxazole, with the addition of glucocorticoids for severe disease characterized by a PaO_2 less than 70 mm Hg or an alveolar-arterial oxygen gradient of more than 35 mm Hg [152]. For *L. monocytogenes*–associated pneumonia in pregnancy, high-dose ampicillin is the treatment of choice (2 g intravenously every 4 hours) [153].

Asthma

The Working Group on Asthma and Pregnancy of the National Asthma Education Program has published a report summarizing the available data on asthma medications and management during pregnancy [71]. The first priority of therapy for pregnant women with asthma is to prevent or reverse the hypoxemia that, to some degree, accompanies virtually every exacerbation of asthma. Oxygen should be used in all asthmatic patients who present to the hospital with an exacerbation; the goal oxygen saturation is 95% or higher because hypoxemia may worsen initially with bronchodilator therapy, as a result of worsening ventilation–perfusion mismatching [154]. Other therapies are directed at the rapid reversal of bronchoconstriction and airways inflammation (see Chapter 48).

Bronchoconstriction is managed with inhalation of selective β_2-agonist and anticholinergic agents, given at 20-minute intervals or continuously. Typically, nebulized medication is given prior to intubation and then switched to metered dose inhaler (MDI) after intubation. The doses of albuterol and ipratropium are the same for obstetric and nonobstetric patients presenting with status asthmaticus [71]. The effects of inhaled agents are predominantly local, which should decrease the amount of fetal exposure, and selective β_2-agonists do not adversely affect uterine blood flow. There has been no evidence of fetal injury from the use of either systemic or inhaled β-adrenergic agonists [71,155], although neonates exposed to systemic β-agonists just prior to delivery have demonstrated tachycardia, hypoglycemia, and tremor [156]. These effects do not constitute a contraindication to the use of β-adrenergic agents.

Systemic glucocorticoids should be initiated promptly in all pregnant patients presenting with an acute asthma exacerbation who are not responding to one or two inhalational treatments with a β_2-agonist [71]. Institution of glucocorticoids helps to reverse airflow obstruction and, thereby, decrease the amount of high-dose β-adrenergic agonist therapy needed. The optimal dose of systemic glucocorticoid in this setting is not known. However, the same dose ranges are used in both obstetric and nonobstetric adults, prednisone or methylprednisolone 120 to 180 mg/day in 3 or 4 divided doses for the first 48 hours and then 60 to 80 mg a day until clinical improvement is significant and the peak expiratory flow has increased to 70% of predicted or personal best [71]. Further tapering is based on the response to treatment.

Prednisone and prednisolone cross the placenta poorly [71]. In rodents that were given glucocorticoids during gestation, an increased prevalence of spontaneous abortions, placental insufficiency, and cleft palate were found; it remains controversial whether a slight increase in risk of cleft palate pertains in humans [71]. Chronic maternal ingestion of systemic glucocorticoids has been associated with lower birth weight and increased incidence of premature deliveries [157–159].

In general, intravenous theophylline is not used during treatment of acute asthma exacerbations because of the lack of evidence of benefit. The use of aminophylline in the acute treatment of asthma during pregnancy does not shorten the length of stay or the response time [71]. However, for patients who normally take theophylline, the medication is normally continued during the hospitalization. If the patient is unable to take oral medication, intravenous theophylline is usually substituted. Because theophylline toxicity can develop in the fetus when theophylline is administered at the time of delivery [71], serum levels should be kept below 15 mg per mL. No loading dose is needed. Maintenance infusion is usually 0.5 mg per kg per hour, although concurrent cimetidine, viral infection, liver disease, heart disease, or erythromycin dictates a downward adjustment to 0.3 mg per kg per hour, and smoking or adolescence dictates an upward adjustment to 0.7 mg per kg per hour. Serum levels should be closely followed.

In patients with severe bronchoconstriction, who are refractory to inhaled nebulized albuterol sulfate, parenteral agents such as terbutaline sulfate, 0.3 mg, or epinephrine, 0.3 mL of a 1 to 1,000 solution, may rarely be given subcutaneously [71,160]. A major concern is that epinephrine may cause uterine artery vasoconstriction through its α-adrenergic effects; this potential risk would have to be balanced against the need to reverse refractory bronchoconstriction [161].

For patients who are extremely difficult to manage even with therapeutic levels of bronchodilators, high-dose glucocorticoids, and mechanical ventilation, a few less-studied therapeutic interventions such as intravenous magnesium sulfate [162] and inhaled isoflurane [163] can be considered. None of these interventions have been studied in pregnancy, so their use should be limited to situations in which the woman's life is in danger and all other forms of therapy have failed. For a full discussion, see Chapter 48.

Once a pregnant woman reaches the point of life-threatening refractory asthma, emergent delivery of the fetus by cesarean section should be considered. There have been anecdotal reports of significant maternal improvement after delivery of the fetus. The decision for urgent delivery is complicated and depends in part on the gestational age of the fetus and the clinical status of the mother [76].

Pneumomediastinum and Pneumothorax

The natural history of pneumomediastinum is spontaneous resolution within 3 to 14 days without permanent sequelae. Pneumomediastinum does not usually require drainage in adults because the air usually dissects out of the mediastinum into the subcutaneous tissues of the neck. Thus, treatment should be directed at improving any underlying predisposing cause, such as asthma, if present. Supplemental oxygen may promote reabsorption of the mediastinal air.

A spontaneous pneumothorax occupying less than 20% of the hemithorax in an asymptomatic patient not on mechanical ventilation can be monitored closely without immediate insertion of a chest tube. Supplemental oxygen should be administered to accelerate the resolution of the pneumothorax. In patients who are symptomatic, on mechanical ventilation, or have an enlarging pneumothorax, chest tube placement is mandatory. Patients whose pneumothorax develops as a complication of barotrauma during mechanical ventilation may also require adjustments in the ventilator settings to reduce airway pressures and further barotrauma.

Patients with an existing pneumothorax or history of one in the past are at increased risk of worsening or recurrence of pneumothorax during labor and delivery, particularly during the Valsalva maneuvers at parturition. Although formal evidence is lacking, use of epidural analgesia and assisted vaginal delivery is suggested to avoid prolonged Valsalva maneuvers [86]. For patients requiring cesarean section, analgesia with epidural anesthetic is preferred to general anesthesia with positive pressure ventilation.

The recurrence rate of ipsilateral spontaneous pneumothorax is 30% to 50% within 5 years without pleurodesis [164]. Pleurodesis with any tetracycline derivative through a chest tube is contraindicated in pregnancy because of possible fetal exposure. It is recommended that a minimally invasive elective video-assisted thoracoscopic surgery (VATS) with bleb resection and mechanical pleurodesis be considered in the subsequent convalescent period to prevent a recurrent pneumothoraces [86]. Thoracotomy or VATS with bleb resection and pleurodesis is indicated for pregnant patients with continued air leak and incomplete lung expansion [86]. Tocolytic therapy may be required to prevent preterm labor during this surgical intervention.

PREVENTION

Thromboembolic Disease

Preventing DVT is probably the most important intervention to reduce maternal mortality caused by pulmonary embolism. Patients who require bed rest or surgery during pregnancy should be treated prophylactically with a LMWH regimen such as dalteparin 5,000 U subcutaneously every 24 hours or enoxaparin 40 mg subcutaneously every 24 hours. In the setting of impaired creatinine clearance, UFH 5,000 U subcutaneously every 12 hours may be used [129]. Warfarin crosses the placenta and is teratogenic, so its use is contraindicated in pregnancy [165]. Patients who are receiving ongoing warfarin therapy for prior thromboembolic disease should be changed to subcutaneous heparin therapy before conception or at least before the sixth week of pregnancy. LMWH is recommended for prophylaxis and treatment because of the reduced risk of bone loss and heparin-induced thrombocytopenia as compared with UFH [129].

Pregnant women with a history of thromboembolic disease and/or hypercoagulable state should receive thromboembolic prophylaxis throughout pregnancy and for 4 to 6 weeks postpartum [129]. The ACCP guidelines recommend either prophylactic or intermediate-dose regimens of LMWH or UFH for these particular subgroups of pregnant patients (Table 51.3) [129]. Once adequate hemostasis has been accomplished postpartum, subcutaneous anticoagulation therapy can be resumed and continued until 6 weeks postpartum. Alternatively, warfarin can be added to subcutaneous heparin and the heparin stopped when therapeutic prolongation of the International Normalized Ratio (INR) is achieved.

Aspiration of Gastric Contents

Based on national surveys of obstetric practice, antacid administration, H_2 blockade, or proton pump inhibitors have been used for aspiration prophylaxis in pregnant women who require general anesthesia or analgesic therapy other than local or epidural anesthetics [47]. This is done despite the lack of complete protection achieved with gastric pH values greater than 2.5 and a recent meta-analysis that showed no evidence that any of these medications reduced the incidence of gastric aspiration [166]. Some authors recommend that all women in labor receive nothing by mouth except medications. This should probably be individualized, in view of the low risk of aspiration during spontaneous vaginal delivery in nonsedated patients and the small proportion of patients who require emergent general anesthesia. Other preventive measures that have been proposed are the use of regional anesthesia when possible, cuffed endotracheal tube, and application of cricoid pressure during intubation [46].

RESPIRATORY INFECTIONS

Immunization is the most effective method to prevent influenza pneumonia. The parenteral influenza vaccine contains inactivated virus and is not associated with adverse pregnancy outcomes. However, it should not be given to patients with egg allergy without prior skin testing to assess safety. Influenza vaccination is recommended for all women who will be pregnant during the influenza season [53]. The parenteral vaccination should be administered between October and mid-November regardless of their trimester of pregnancy [167]. The intranasal flu vaccine should not be given to pregnant women because it is a live-attenuated virus [53,167].

β-Adrenergic Tocolytic Therapy

The epidemiologic factors that place patients at increased risk for tocolytic-induced pulmonary edema include longer duration of intravenous β-adrenergic tocolytic therapy (24 to 48 hours), large volume of crystalloid infusion, multiple gestation, concomitant sepsis, and, possibly, preeclampsia [81]. If a β-adrenergic tocolytic agent must be used, limiting the intravenous phase of β-adrenergic therapy to less than 24 to 48 hours and adjusting the dose to keep the maternal heart rate under 120 beats per minute may reduce complications. The β-adrenergic agent should be discontinued immediately at the earliest sign of respiratory distress, such as chest pain, tachypnea, dyspnea, or reduced oxygen saturation. Careful fluid balance records should be maintained, and fluid restriction and possibly diuresis should be considered when intake exceeds output by greater than 500 mL. Sodium intake should be restricted to 4 to 6 g per day. If glucocorticoids are required to enhance fetal lung development, a formulation with the lowest mineralocorticoid potency should be used. If supplemental oxygenation, discontinuation of the drug, and gentle diuresis do not result in improvement after 1 hour, insertion of a pulmonary artery catheter to guide fluid management should be considered. Clinical improvement in tocolytic-induced pulmonary edema usually occurs within 12 hours after the drug is discontinued and diuresis is begun [168].

Patients with underlying cardiac disease, particularly structural defects causing outflow obstruction, should be excluded from β-adrenergic tocolytic therapy. Patients with multiple gestation should either be excluded or undergo prophylactic pulmonary artery catheterization. Patients with severe preeclampsia would likely benefit more from early delivery than from combining the increased risks of tocolytic therapy with those of continuing pregnancy-induced hypertension.

Advances in management of pregnancy based upon randomized, controlled clinical trials are summarized in Table 51.4.

TABLE 51.4

ADVANCES IN MANAGEMENT OF ACUTE RESPIRATORY FAILURE IN PREGNANCY BASED UPON CLINICAL TRIALS

- Mechanical ventilation of a pregnant patient with ARDS should follow the guidelines of the ARDS Network Study [116]. B
- Unfractionated heparin remains the drug of choice for massive pulmonary embolism during pregnancy [129]. D
- Low-molecular-weight heparin is safe and effective in pregnancy, and may be used for anticoagulation for pulmonary embolism during pregnancy once the patient is stabilized [129]. D
- Pregnancy is a relative contraindication for thrombolytic therapy. Thrombolysis has been used safely in life-threatening pulmonary embolism during pregnancy with maternal mortality of 1% and fetal loss 6%. Recombinant tissue plasminogen activator and streptokinase are the recommended thrombolytics during pregnancy [134]. D
- Systemic glucocorticoids should be instituted in all pregnant patients with an acute asthma exacerbation who are not quickly responsive to inhaled β_2-agonist therapy [71]. D

ARDS, acute respiratory distress syndrome; B, 1 RCT trial; D, nonrandomized, contemporaneous control group.

References

1. Chang J, Elam-Evans LD, Berg CJ, et al: Pregnancy-related mortality surveillance—United States, 1991–1999. *MMWR Morb Mortal Wkly Rep* 52(SS02):1, 2003.
2. Berg CJ, Atrash HK, Koonin LM, et al: Pregnancy-related mortality in the United States, 1991–1997. *Obstet Gynecol* 101:289, 2003.
3. Bobrowski RA: Pulmonary physiology in pregnancy. *Clin Obstet Gynecol* 53(2):285, 2010.
4. Campbell Reardon C, Hollingsworth H: Respiratory failure part VI: acute respiratory failure, in Irwin RS, Rippe JM (eds): *Pregnancy in Intensive Care Medicine.* 6th ed. Philadelphia, PA, Lippincott Williams & Wilkins 556–574, 2008.
5. Chang J, Elam-Evans LD, Berg CJ, et al: Pregnancy-related mortality surveillance—United States, 1991–1999. *MMWR Surveill Summ* 52:1, 2003.
6. Marik PE, Plante LA: Venous thromboembolic disease and pregnancy. *N Eng J Med* 359:2025, 2008.
7. Kruithof EK, Tran-Thang C, Guidinchet A, et al: Fibrinolysis in pregnancy: a study of plasminogen activator inhibitors. *Blood* 69:460, 1987.
8. Macklon NS, Greer IA, Bowman A: An ultrasound study of gestational and postural changes in the deep venous system of the leg in pregnancy. *Br J Obstet Gynaecol* 104:191, 1997.
9. Robertson L, Wu O, Langhorne P, et al: Thrombophilia in pregnancy: a systematic review. *Br J Haematol* 132:171, 2006.
10. Gerhardt A, Scharf RE, Beckmann MW, et al: Prothrombin and factor V mutations in women with a history of thrombosis during pregnancy and the puerperium. *N Engl J Med* 342:374, 2000.
11. Jobe RL, Forman MB: Focal pulmonary embolism presenting as diffuse pulmonary edema. *Chest* 103:644, 1993.
12. Famularo G, Minisola G, Nicotra GC: Massive pulmonary embolism masquerading as pulmonary edema. *Am J Emerg Med* 25:1086, 2007.
13. Kline JA, Williams GW, Hernandez-Nino J: D-dimer concentrations in normal pregnancy: new diagnostic thresholds are needed. *Clin Chem* 51:825, 2005.
14. Chan WS, Chunilal S, Lee A, et al: A red blood cell agglutination D-dimer test to exclude deep venous thrombosis in pregnancy. *Ann Intern Med* 147:165, 2007.
15. Stein PD, Fowler SE, Goodman LR, et al: Multidetector computed tomography for acute pulmonary embolism. *N Engl J Med* 354:2317, 2006.
16. Schuster ME, Fishman JE, Copeland JF, et al: Pulmonary embolism in pregnant patients: a survey of practices and policies for CT pulmonary angiography. *AJR Am J Roentgenol* 181:1495, 2003.
17. Winer-Muram HT, Boone JM, Brown HL, et al: Pulmonary embolism in pregnant patients: fetal radiation dose with helical CT. *Radiology* 224:487, 2002.
18. Moore J, Baldisseri MR: Amniotic fluid embolism. *Crit Care Med* 33:10S, S279, 2005.
19. Gilmore DA, Wakim J, Secrest J, et al: Anaphylactoid syndrome of pregnancy: a review of the literature with latest management and outcome data. *AANA J* 71:120, 2003.
20. Gist RS, Stafford IP, Leibowitz AB, et al: Amniotic fluid embolism. *Anesth Analg* 108:1599, 2009.
21. Clark SL, Hankins GDV, Dudley DA, et al: Amniotic fluid embolism: analysis of a national registry. *Am J Obstet Gynecol* 172:1158, 1995.
22. Tuffnell DJ: United Kingdom amniotic fluid embolism register. *BJOG* 112:1625, 2005.
23. Abenhaim HA, Azoulay L, Kramer MS, et al: Incidence and risk factors of amniotic fluid embolisms: a population-based study on 3 million births in the United States. *Am J Obstet Gynecol* 199:49, 2008.
24. Benson MD: A hypothesis regarding complement activation and amniotic fluid embolism. *Med Hypotheses* 68:1019, 2007.
25. Clark SL, Cotton DB, Gonik B, et al: Central hemodynamic alterations in amniotic fluid embolism. *Am J Obstet Gynecol* 158:1124, 1988.
26. Schechtman M, Ziser A, Markovits R, et al: Amniotic fluid embolism: early findings of transesophageal echocardiography. *Anesth Analg* 89:1456, 1999.

27. Stanten RD, Iverson LI, Daugharty TM, et al: Amniotic fluid embolism causing catastrophic pulmonary vasoconstriction: diagnosis by transesophageal echocardiogram and treatment by cardiopulmonary bypass. *Obstet Gynecol* 102:496, 2003.
28. Morgan M: Amniotic fluid embolism. *Anaesthesia* 34:20, 1979.
29. Peterson EP, Taylor HB: Amniotic fluid embolism. *Obstet Gynecol* 35:787, 1970.
30. Lee W, Ginsburg KA, Cotton DB, et al: Squamous and trophoblastic cells in the maternal pulmonary circulation identified by invasive hemodynamic monitoring during the peripartum period. *Am J Obstet Gynecol* 155:999, 1986.
31. Clark SL, Pavlova A, Horenstein J: Squamous cells in the maternal pulmonary artery circulation. *Am J Obstet Gynecol* 154:104, 1986.
32. Porat S, Leibowitz D, Milwidsky A, et al: Transient intracardiac thrombi in amniotic fluid embolism. *Br J Obstet Gynaecol* 111:506, 2004.
33. Oi H, Kobayashi H, Hirashima Y, et al: Serological and immunohistochemical diagnosis of amniotic fluid embolism. *Semin Thromb Hemost* 24:479, 1998.
34. Kobayashi H, Oi H, Hayakawa H, et al: Histological diagnosis of amniotic fluid embolism by monoclonal antibody TKH-2 that recognizes NeuAc alpha-2–6GalNAc epitope. *Hum Pathol* 28:428, 1997.
35. Kim CS, Liu J, Kwon JY, et al: Venous air embolism during surgery, especially cesarean delivery. *J Korean Med Sci* 23:753, 2008.
36. Kostash MA, Mensink F: Lethal air embolism during cesarean delivery for placenta previa. *Anesthesiology* 96:753, 2002.
37. Hill BR, Jones FS: Venous air embolism following orogenital sex during pregnancy. *Am J Emerg Med* 11:155, 1993.
38. Nicoll LM, Skupski DW: Venous air embolism after using a birth-training device. *Obstet Gynecol* 111:489, 2008.
39. O'Quinn RJ, Lakshminarayan S: Venous air embolism. *Arch Intern Med* 142:2173, 1982.
40. Milani RV, Lavi CJ, Gilliland YE, et al: Overview of transesophageal echocardiography for the chest physician. *Chest* 124:1081, 2003.
41. Furuya H, Suzuki T, Okumura F, et al: Detection of air embolism by transesophageal echocardiography. *Anesthesiology* 58;124, 1983.
42. Toung TJK, Rossberg MI, Hutchins GM: Volume of air in a lethal air embolism. *Anesthesiology* 94:360, 2001.
43. van Hulst RA, Klein J, Lachmann B: Gas embolism: pathophysiology and treatment. *Clin Physiol Funct Imaging* 23:237, 2003.
44. Orebaugh SL: Venous air emboli: clinical and experimental considerations. *Crit Care Med* 20;1169, 1992.
45. Mendelson CL: The aspiration of stomach contents into the lungs during obstetric anesthesia. *Am J Obstet Gynecol* 52:191, 1946.
46. Ng A, Smith G: Gastroesophageal reflux and aspiration of gastric contents in anesthetic practice. *Anesth Analg* 93:494, 2001.
47. Engelhardt T, Webster NR: Pulmonary aspiration of gastric contents in anesthesia. *Br J Anaesth* 83:453, 1999.
48. Lorber B, Swenson RM: Bacteriology of aspiration pneumonia. *Ann Intern Med* 81:329, 1974.
49. Goodnight WH, Soper DE: Pneumonia in pregnancy. *Crit Care Med* 33:S390, 2005.
50. Mandell LA, Wunderlink RG, Anzueto A, et al: Infectious Diseases Society of America/American Thoracic Society Consensus Guidelines on the management of community-acquired pneumonia in adults. *Clin Inf Dis* 44 (S2):527–572, 2007.
51. Soper DE, Melone PJ, Conover WB: Legionnaire disease complicating pregnancy. *Obstet Gynecol* 67:10S, 1986.
52. Goodrum LA: Pneumonia in pregnancy. *Semin Perinatol* 21:276–283, 1997.
53. Centers for Disease Control: Prevention and control of influenza: recommendations of the Advisory Committee on Immunization Practices (ACIP), 2008. *MMWR Recomm Rep* 57(7):1–60, 2008.
54. Centers for Disease Control: Novel Influenza A (H1N1) virus infections in three pregnant women-United States, April-May 2009. *MMWR Morb Mortal Wkly Rep* 58(18):497, 2009.
55. Harger JH, Ernest JM, Thurnau GR, et al: Risk factors and outcome of varicella-zoster virus pneumonia in pregnant women. *J Infect Dis* 185:422, 2002.
56. Daley AJ, Thorpe S, Garland SM: Varicella and the pregnant woman: prevention and management. *Austr N Z J Obstet Gynecol* 48:26, 2008.
57. Enders G, Miller E, Cradock-Watson J, et al: Consequences of varicella and herpes zoster in pregnancy: prospective study of 1739 cases. *Lancet* 343;1548, 1994.
58. Case definitions for surveillance of severe acute respiratory syndrome (SARS): Available at: World Health Organization Web site http://www.who.int/csr/sars/casedefinition. Accessed September 11, 2009.
59. Wong SF, Chow KM, Leung TN, et al: Pregnancy and perinatal outcomes of women with severe acute respiratory syndrome. *Am J Obstet Gynecol* 191:292, 2004.
60. Maxwell C, McGeer A, Young Tai KF, et al: Management guidelines for obstetric patients and neonates born to mothers with suspected or probable severe acute respiratory syndrome (SARS). *J Obstet Gynaecol Can* 31(4):358, 2009.
61. Wack EE, Ampel NM, Gagliani JN, et al: Coccidioidomycosis during pregnancy: an analysis of ten cases among 47,120 pregnancies. *Chest* 94:376, 1988.
62. Caldwell JW, Arsura EL, Kilgore WB, et al: Coccidioidomycosis in pregnancy during an epidemic in California. *Obstet Gynecol* 95:236, 2000.
63. Snider D: Pregnancy and tuberculosis. *Chest* 86:10S, 1984.
64. Starke JR: Tuberculosis in childhood and pregnancy, in Friedman LN (Ed): Tuberculosis: Current Concepts and Treatment. 2nd ed. Boca Raton, FL, CRC Press, 2000.
65. Diagnostic standards and classification of tuberculosis in adults and children. Official statement of the American Thoracic Society and the Centers for Disease Control and Prevention. *Am J Respir Crit Care Med* 161:1376, 2000.
66. Centers for Disease Control and Prevention: Epidemiology of HIV/AIDS-United States, 1981–2005. *MMWR Morb Mortal Wkly Rep* 55(21):589, 2006.
67. Ahmad H, Mehta NJ, Manikal VM, et al: *Pneumocystis carinii* pneumonia in pregnancy. *Chest* 120:666, 2001.
68. Mylonakis E, Paliou M, Hohmann EL, et al: Listeriosis during pregnancy. *Medicine* 81(4):260, 2002.
69. Boucher M, Yonekura ML, Wallace RJ, et al: Adult respiratory distress syndrome: a rare manifestation of *Listeria monocytogenes* infection in pregnancy. *Am J Obstet Gynecol* 149:686, 1984.
70. Kwon HL, Belanger K, Bracken MB: Effect of pregnancy and stage of pregnancy on asthma severity: a systematic review. *Am J Obstet Gynecol* 190:1201, 2004.
71. National Asthma Education and Prevention Program: Quick reference NAEPP expert panel report. *Managing asthma during pregnancy*. Recommendations for pharmacologic treatment, Update 2004. Bethesda, MD, National Institutes of Health, National Heart, Lung and Blood Institute, 2004. Publication 04–5246.
72. Brancazio LR, Laifer SN, Schwartz T: Peak expiratory flow rate in normal pregnancy. *Obstet Gynecol* 89:383, 1997.
73. Fischl MA, Pitchenik A, Gardner LB: An index predicting relapse and hospitalization in patients with acute bronchial asthma. *N Engl J Med* 305:783, 1981.
74. Rebuck AS, Read J: Assessment and management of severe asthma. *Am J Med* 51:788, 1971.
75. McFadden ER Jr, Kiser R, DeGroot WJ: Acute bronchial asthma: relations between clinical and physiologic manifestations. *N Engl J Med* 288:221, 1973.
76. Hanania NA, Belfort MA: Acute asthma in pregnancy. *Crit Care Med* 33:S319, 2005.
77. Caughey AP, Parere JT: Tocolysis with beta-adrenergic receptor agonists. *Semin Perinatol* 25:248, 2001.
78. Lamont RF: The pathophysiology of pulmonary oedema with the use of beta agonists. *BJOG* 107:439, 2000.
79. Dudenhausen J: 'Normal' pregnancy with adverse events on initial tocolytic treatment. *BJOG* 113[Suppl 3]:116, 2006.
80. Bal L, Thierry S, Brocas E, et al: Pulmonary edema induced by calcium-channel blockade for tocolysis. *Anesth Analg* 99:910, 2004.
81. Chandrahan E, Arulkumaran S: Acute tocolysis. *Curr Opin Obstet Gynecol* 17:151, 2005.
82. The Worldwide Atosiban versus Beta-agonists Study Group: Effectiveness and safety of the oxytocin antagonist atosiban versus beta-adrenergic agonists in the treatment of preterm labour. *BJOG* 108:133, 2001.
83. www.fda.gov/ohrms/dockets/ac/98/transcpt/3407t1.rtf, accessed August 9, 2009.
84. Balkan ME, Alver G: Spontaneous pneumomediastinum in 3rd trimester of pregnancy. *Ann Thorac Cardiovasc Surg* 12;362, 2006.
85. Karson EM, Saltzman D, David MR: Pneumomediastinum in pregnancy: two case reports and a review of the literature, pathophysiology and management. *Obstet Gynecol* 64:39S, 1984.
86. Lal A, Anderson G, Cowen M, et al: Pneumothorax and pregnancy. *Chest* 132;1044, 2007.
87. Bernard GR, Artigas A, Brigham KL, et al: The American-European Consensus Conference on ARDS: Definitions, mechanisms, relevant outcomes, and clinical trial coordination. *Am J Respir Crit Care Med* 149:818, 1994.
88. Cole DE, Taylor TL, McCullough DM, et al: Acute respiratory distress syndrome in pregnancy. *Crit Care Med* 33(10S):S269, 2005.
89. Catanzarie VA, Willms D. Adult respiratory distress syndrome in pregnancy: report of three cases and a review of the literature. *Obstet Gynecol Surv* 52:381, 1997.
90. Mabie WC, Barton JR, Sibai BM. Adult respiratory distress syndrome in pregnancy. *Am J Obstet Gynecol* 167(4, Pt 1):950, 1992.
91. Catanzarite V, Willms D, Wong D, et al: Acute respiratory distress syndrome in pregnancy and the puerperium: causes, courses, and outcomes. *Obstet Gynecol* 97(5, Pt 1):760, 2001.
92. ACOG Committee Opinion no. 299, September 2004 (replaces no. 158, September 1995). Guidelines for diagnostic imaging during pregnancy. *Obstet Gynecol* 104(3): 647–651, 2004.
93. Brent RL: Saving lives and changing family histories: appropriate counseling of pregnant women and men of reproductive age, concerning the risk of diagnostic radiation exposures during and before pregnancy. *Am J Obstet Gynecol* 200:4, 2009.
94. Preston DL, Cullings H, Suyama A, et al: Solid cancer incidence in atomic bomb survivors exposed in utero or as young children. *J Natl Cancer Inst* 100:428, 2008.

95. Bentur Y, Horlatsch N, Koren G: Exposure to ionizing radiation during pregnancy: perception of teratogenic risk and outcome. *Teratology* 43:163, 1991.
96. Shellock FG, Crues JV: MR procedures: biologic effects, safety, and patient care. *Radiology* 232:635, 2004.
97. Nagayama M, Watanabe Y, Okumura A, et al: Fast MR imaging in obstetrics. *Radiographics* 22:563, 2002.
98. National Radiation Protection Board: Advice on acceptable limits of exposure to nuclear magnetic resonance in clinical imaging. *Radiography* 50:220, 1984.
99. Kanal E, Barkovich AJ, Bell C, et al: ACR blue ribbon panel on MR safety. ACR guidance document for safe MR practices. *AJR* 188:1447, 2007.
100. Swan HJ, Ganz W, Forrester J, et al: Catheterization of the heart in man with use of flow-directed balloon-tipped catheter. *N Engl J Med* 283:447, 1970.
101. Clark SL, Cotton DB, Lee W, et al: Central hemodynamic assessment of normal term pregnancy. *Am J Obstet Gynecol* 161:1439, 1989.
102. Fujitani S, Baldisseri MR: Hemodynamic assessment in a pregnant and peripartum patient. *Crit Care Med* 33:10S, 354S, 2005.
103. Connor AF Jr, Speroff T, Dawson NV, et al: The effectiveness of right heart catheterization in the initial care of critically ill patients. *JAMA* 276:889, 1996.
104. Dyer RA, James MF: Maternal hemodynamic monitoring in obstetric anesthesia. *Anesthesiology* 109:765, 2008.
105. Langesaeter R, Rosseland LA, Subhaug A: Continuous invasive blood pressure and cardiac output monitoring during cesarean delivery: a randomized, double-blind comparison of low-dose versus high-dose spinal anesthesia with intravenous phenylephrine or placebo infusion. *Anesthesiology* 109:856, 2008.
106. McGee WT, Horswell JT, Calderon J, et al: Validation of a continuous, arterial pressure-based cardiac output measurement: a multicenter, prospective clinical trial. *Crit Care Med* 11:R105, 2007.
107. Compton FD, Zukunft B, Hoffmann C, et al: Performance of a minimally invasive uncalibrated cardiac output monitoring system (Flotrac^{tm}/Vigileo^{tm}) in haemodynamically unstable patients. *Br J Anaesth* 100:451, 2008.
108. Parer JT, King TL: Electronic fetal monitoring and diagnosis of fetal asphyxia, in Hughes SC, Levinson G, Rosen MA (eds): Shnider and Levinson's Anesthesia for Obstetrics. Philadelphia, Lippincott Williams & Wilkins, 2002, p 623.
109. Liu PL, Warren TM, Ostheimer GW, et al: Foetal monitoring in parturients undergoing surgery unrelated to pregnancy. *Can Anaesth Soc J* 32:525, 1985.
110. Biehl DR: Foetal monitoring during surgery unrelated to pregnancy. *Can Anaesth Soc J* 32:455, 1985.
111. Norwitz ER, Robinson JN, Maline FD: Pregnancy-induced physiologic alterations, in Dildy GA, Belfort MA, Saade GR, et al (eds): Critical Care Obstetrics. 4th ed. Malden, MA, Blackwell Science, 2004, p 1942.
112. Munnur U, Boisblanc B, Suresh MS: Airway problems in pregnancy. *Crit Care Med* 33[10, Suppl]:S259, 2005.
113. Sellick BA: Cricoid pressure to control regurgitation of stomach contents during induction of anesthesia. *Lancet* 2:404, 1961.
114. Grum CM, Morganroth ML: Initiating mechanical ventilation. *J Intensive Care Med* 3:6, 1988.
115. Meschia G: Placental respiratory gas exchange and fetal oxygenation, in Creasy RK, Resnik R (eds): *Maternal-Fetal Medicine*. Philadelphia, WB Saunders, 1999, p 260.
116. Acute Respiratory Distress Syndrome Network: Ventilation using low tidal volumes as compared with traditional tidal volumes in acute lung injury and the acute respiratory distress syndrome. *N Engl J Med* 342:1301, 2000.
117. Broddus VC, Berthiaume Y, Biondi JW, et al: Hemodynamic management of the adult respiratory distress syndrome. *J Intensive Care Med* 2:190, 1987.
118. Edwards MJ: Review: hyperthermia and fever during pregnancy. *Birth Defects Res* (Part A) 76:507, 2006.
119. Roizen MF, Feeley TW: Pancuronium bromide. *Ann Intern Med* 88:64, 1978.
120. Buhimschi CS, Weiner CP: Medications in pregnancy and lactation: Part 1. Teratology. *Obstet Gynecol* 113:166, 2009.
121. Buhimschi CS, Weiner CP: Medications in pregnancy and lactation: Part 2. Drugs with minimal or unknown human teratogenic potential. *Obstet Gynecol* 113(2, Pt 1):417, 2009.
122. Morganroth ML, Grum CM: Weaning from mechanical ventilation. *J Intensive Care Med* 3:109, 1988.
123. Mercier FJ, Riley ET, Frederickson WL, et al: Phenylephrine added to prophylactic ephedrine infusion during spinal anesthesia for elective cesarean section. *Anesthesiology* 95:668, 2001.
124. Ngan Kee WD, Khaw KS, Lau TK, et al: Randomised double-blinded comparison of phenylephrine vs ephedrine for maintaining blood pressure during spinal anaesthesia for non-elective Caesarean section. *Anaesthesia* 63:1319, 2008.
125. Martin R, Blackburn GL: Hyperalimentation during pregnancy, in Berkowitz RL (ed): *Critical Care of the Obstetric Patient*. New York, Churchill Livingstone, 1983, p 133.
126. Martindale RG, McClave SA, Vanek VW, et al: Guidelines for the provision and assessment of nutrition support therapy in the adult critically ill patient: Society of Critical Care Medicine and American Society for Parenteral and Enteral Nutrition: executive summary. *Crit Care Med* 37;5:1757, 2009.
127. Russo-Stieglitz KE, Levine AB, Wagner BA, et al: Pregnancy outcomes in patients requiring parenteral nutrition. *J Matern Fetal Med* 8(4):164, 1999.
128. Hamaoui E, Hamaoui M: Nutritional assessment and support during pregnancy. *Gastroenterol Clin North Am* 32:59, 2003.
129. Bates SM, Greer IA, Pabinger I, et al: Venous thromboembolism, thrombophilia, antithrombotic therapy, and pregnancy: American College of Chest Physicians Evidence-Based Clinical Practice Guidelines (8th edition). *Chest* 133:844S, 2008.
130. van Dongen DJ, van den BA, Prins MH, et al: Fixed dose subcutaneous low molecular weight heparins versus adjusted dose unfractionated heparin for venous thromboembolism. *Cochrane Database Syst Rev* CD001100, 2004.
131. Goldhaber SZ: Contemporary pulmonary embolism thrombolysis. *Chest* 107:45S, 1995.
132. Simonneau G, Azarian R, Brenot F, et al: Surgical management of unresolved pulmonary embolism: a personal series of 72 patients. *Chest* 107:52S, 1995.
133. Turrentine MA, Braems G, Ramirez MM: Use of thrombolytics for the treatment of thromboembolic disease during pregnancy. *Obstet Gynecol Surv* 24:1030, 1996.
134. Ahearn GS, Hadjiliadis D, Govert JA, et al: Massive pulmonary embolism during pregnancy successfully treated with recombinant tissue plasminogen activator. *Arch Intern Med* 162:1221, 2002.
135. te Raa GD, Ribbert LS, Snijder RJ, et al: Treatment options in massive pulmonary embolism during pregnancy: a case-report and review of literature. *Thromb Res* 124:1, 2009.
136. Hall RJC, Young C, Sutton GC, et al: Treatment of acute massive pulmonary embolism by streptokinase during labor and delivery. *BMJ* 4:647, 1972.
137. Horlocker TT, Wedel DJ, Benzon H, et al: Regional anesthesia in the anticoagulated patient: defining the risks (the second ASRA Consensus Conference on Neuroaxial Anesthesia and Anticoagulation). *Reg Anesth Pain Med* 28:172, 2003.
138. Hsieh YY, Chang CC, Li PC, et al: Successful application of extracorporeal membrane oxygenation and intraaortic balloon counterpulsation as lifesaving therapy for a patient with amniotic fluid embolism. *Am J Obstet Gynecol* 183:496, 2000.
139. Nagarsheth NP, Pinney S, Bassiy-Marcu A, et al: Successful placement of a right ventricular assist device for treatment of a presumed amniotic fluid embolism. *Anesth Analg* 107:962, 2008.
140. Leach RM, Rees PJ, Wilmshurst P: ABC of oxygen: hyperbaric oxygen therapy. *BMJ* 317:1140, 1998.
141. Mandell LA, Wunderink RG, Anzueto A, et al: Infectious Diseases Society of America/American Thoracic Society consensus guidelines on the management of community-acquired pneumonia in adults. *Clin Infect Dis* 2:S27, 2007.
142. Bernard GR, Luce JM, Spring CL, et al: High-dose corticosteroids in patients with the adult respiratory distress syndrome. *N Engl J Med* 317:1565, 1987.
143. Wolfe JE, Bone RC, Ruth WE: Effects of corticosteroids in the treatment of patients with gastric aspiration. *Am J Med* 63:719, 1977.
144. Downs JB, Chapman RL Jr, Modell JH, et al: An evaluation of steroid therapy in aspiration pneumonitis. *Anesthesiology* 40:129, 1974.
145. Taylor G, Pryse-Davies J: Evaluation of endotracheal steroid therapy in acid pulmonary aspiration syndrome (Mendelson's syndrome). *Anesthesiology* 29:17, 1968.
146. Niebyl JR: Antibiotics and other anti-infective agents in pregnancy and lactation. *Am J Perinatol* 20:405, 2003.
147. Moscona A: Neuraminidase inhibitors for influenza. *N Engl J Med* 353:1363, 2005.
148. Tan MP, Koren G: Chickenpox in pregnancy: revisited. *Reprod Toxicol* 21:410, 2006.
149. Spinello IM, Johnson RH, Baqi S: Coccidioidomycosis and pregnancy. *Ann NY Acad Sci* 1111:358, 2007.
150. ATS/CDC/IDSA guidelines: Treatment of tuberculosis and tuberculosis infection in adults and children. *Am J Respir Crit Care Med* 167:603, 2003.
151. Treatment of tuberculosis. *MMWR Recomm Rep* 52:1, 2003.
152. Benson CA, Kaplan JE, Masur H, et al: Treating opportunistic infections among HIV-exposed and infected children: recommendations from CDC, the National Institutes of Health, and the Infectious Diseases Society of America. *MMWR* 53(RR-15):1, 2004.
153. Armstrong D: *Listeria monocytogenes*, in Mandell GL, Douglas RG, Bennett JE (eds): *Principles and Practice of Infectious Diseases*. New York, John Wiley & Sons, 1985, p 1177.
154. Gazioglu K, Condemi JJ, Hyde RW, et al: Effect of isoproterenol on gas exchange during air and oxygen breathing in patients with asthma. *Am J Med* 50:185, 1971.
155. Schatz M, Zeiger RS, Harden KM, et al: The safety of inhaled β-agonist bronchodilators during pregnancy. *J Allergy Clin Immunol* 82:686, 1988.
156. Zilianti M, Aller J: Action of orciprenaline on uterine contractility during labor, maternal cardiovascular system, fetal heart rate, and acid–base balance. *Am J Obstet Gynecol* 109:1073, 1971.
157. Person Y, Van Lierde M, Ghysen J, et al: Retardation of fetal growth in patients receiving immunosuppressive therapy. *N Engl J Med* 313:328, 1985.

158. Reinisch JM, Simon Ng, Karow WG, et al: Prenatal exposure to prednisone in humans and animals retards intrauterine growth. *Science* 202:436, 1978.
159. Scott JR: Fetal growth retardation associated with maternal administration of immunosuppressive drugs. *Am J Obstet Gynecol* 128:668, 1977.
160. Appel D, Karpel JP, Sherman M: Epinephrine improves expiratory flow rates in patients with asthma who do not respond to inhaled metaproterenol sulfate. *J Allergy Clin Immunol* 84:90, 1989.
161. Briggs GG, Freeman RK, Yaffe SJ: *Drugs in Pregnancy and Lactation.* 3rd ed. Baltimore, MD, Williams & Wilkins, 1990, pp 237, 520.
162. Silverman RA, Osborn H, Runge J, et al: IV magnesium sulfate in the treatment of acute severe asthma: a multicenter randomized controlled trial. *Chest* 122:489, 2002.
163. Johnston RG, Noseworthy TW, Friesen EG, et al: Isoflurane therapy for status asthmaticus in children and adults. *Chest* 97:698, 1990.
164. Light RW: Management of spontaneous pneumothorax. *Am Rev Respir Dis* 148:245, 1993.
165. Chan WS, Anad S, Ginsberg JS: Anticoagulation of pregnant women with mechanical heart valves: a systematic review of the literature. *Arch Intern Med* 160:191, 2000.
166. Gyte GML, Richens Y: Routine prophylactic drugs in normal labour for reducing gastric aspiration and its effects. *Cochrane Database of Syst Rev* 3:CD005298, 2006.
167. American College of Obstetricians and Gynecologists: Influenza vaccination and treatment during pregnancy. ACOG Committee Opinion No 305. *Obstet Gynecol* 104:1125, 2004.
168. Canadian Preterm Labor Investigations Group: Treatment of preterm labor with the beta-adrenergic agonist ritodrine. *N Engl J Med* 327:308, 1992.

CHAPTER 52 ■ VENOUS THROMBOEMBOLISM: PULMONARY EMBOLISM AND DEEP VENOUS THROMBOSIS

CHARLES WILLIAM HARGETT, III AND VICTOR F. TAPSON

INCIDENCE AND NATURAL HISTORY

Venous thromboembolism (VTE) includes the spectrum of deep vein thrombosis (DVT) and pulmonary embolism (PE). Embolization of material into the pulmonary venous circulation may lead to marked cardiopulmonary dysfunction and is of particular interest to the critical care practitioner. Although VTE is extraordinarily common in hospitalized patients, estimating the frequency of VTE and PE is problematic. The nonspecific clinical findings and high rate of undiagnosed events likely underestimate the true incidence of disease, whereas autopsy data may overestimate meaningful events by detecting asymptomatic cases. That being considered, the incidence of VTE is thought to be in excess of 600,000 cases per year in the United States [1]. In one population-based study with autopsy data, the annual incidences (age and sex adjusted) of DVT and PE were 48 and 69 per 100,000, respectively [2]. In a study of critically ill patients, 10% to 30% of medical/surgical intensive care unit (ICU) patients experienced DVT within the first week of admission, and approximately 60% of trauma patients had DVT within the first 2 weeks, most of which were clinically silent [3]. The prevalence of VTE as a cause of critical illness is also uncertain, but approximately 15% to 20% of patients with diagnosed PE have significant hemodynamic and/or respiratory compromise [4,5]. Untreated symptomatic PE has a mortality rate of approximately 30%, but treatment reduces this risk considerably [6–13]. Adjusting for patients with concomitant terminal illnesses, acute PE likely account for more than 100,000 deaths per year in the United States in patients with an otherwise good prognosis [14,15].

RISK FACTORS

Recognizing the presence of risk factors for VTE is essential because more than 90% of deaths due to PE occur in patients who are not treated because the diagnosis was unsuspected and thus undetected [14,15]. Virtually every risk factor for VTE can be derived from Virchow's triad of stasis, venous injury, and hypercoagulability described nearly 150 years ago (Tables 52.1 and 52.2) [16]. Common major risk factors for VTE include increased age, malignancy, surgery, hospitalization with acute medical illness, and a history of prior VTE. Critically ill patients may be at especially high risk for VTE due to severe underlying disease, immobility, and venoinvasive catheters, and the incidence of VTE increases correspondingly with the number of risk factors present.

Inherited or acquired hypercoagulable states are now recognized in more than 20% of patients with VTE and occur at an even higher rate in patients with idiopathic or recurrent VTE (Table 52.3) [17,18]. Resistance to activated protein C due to the factor V Leiden mutation is one of the most common hypercoagulable states, with a prevalence of 5% in white individuals of European ancestry, and may be present in perhaps 20% of patients with PE [19–22]. Ethnicity is a risk factor, and whites and African Americans have a significantly higher incidence of VTE as compared with Hispanics and Asians [23].

Indwelling central venous catheters (CVCs), particularly common in critically ill patients, provide a constant nidus for clot formation. Thrombosis may occur in up to 67% of patients with invasive catheters [24]. Specific risk factors for thrombotic complications of CVCs may be related to technical or host factors and include femoral vein site, duration of cannulation (>days), nighttime placement, extremes of age, and multiple lines [25–28]. The frequency of clinically meaningful complications due to CVC-related thrombosis remains unclear.

PATHOPHYSIOLOGY

The sequence of events leading to venous thrombosis is not fully understood and likely varies based on the dynamic interactions between genetic and acquired risk factors. In one proposed scheme, endothelial stimulation results from either blood

TABLE 52.1

STRONG, MODERATE, AND WEAK RISK FACTORS FOR VENOUS THROMBOEMBOLISM (VTE)

Strong risk factors (odds ratio >10)
Hip or leg fracture
Hip or knee replacement
Major general surgery
Major trauma, including spinal cord injury
Moderate risk factors (odds ratio 2–9)
Arthroscopic knee surgery
Central venous catheterization
Congestive heart or respiratory failure
Hormone replacement and oral contraceptive therapy
Malignancy (active or recently treated)
Pregnancy[a]
Paralytic stroke
Prior VTE
Thrombophilia (inherited or acquired)
Weak risk factors (odds ratio <2)
Bed rest >3 d
Prolonged immobility due to sitting (e.g., car or air travel)
Increasing age
Laparoscopic surgery
Obesity
Pregnancy[a]
Varicose veins

[a]The risk associated with pregnancy is temporal (antepartum vs. postpartum) and specific for VTE subtype (deep venous thrombosis vs. pulmonary embolism). See section "Pregnancy" for further details.
Adapted from Anderson FA Jr, Spencer FA: Risk factors for venous thromboembolism. *Circulation* 107[23, Suppl 1]:I9, 2003.

stasis-induced hypoxia or direct vein wall injury, after which point tissue factor is transferred to the endothelial cell and initiates the enzymatic cascade of coagulation reactions, leading to thrombin generation and fibrin deposition [29]. Thus, it is not surprising that many venous thrombi arise in valve pockets, where blood flow tends to stagnate, or at a specific area of vascular disruption, such as an indwelling catheter site.

Lower extremity DVT is the most frequent source of PE and, in untreated patients with proximal DVT, approximately half will develop PE [30,31]. Other sources of PE include pelvic, renal, or upper extremity veins, as well as the right heart. After traveling to the lungs, a large thrombus may occlude a major pulmonary artery and cause significant cardiovascular symptoms, or it may break up into smaller clots and travel distally, where it is more likely to produce pleuritic chest pain. Thrombi are most frequently carried to the lower lobes due to the higher blood flow. Pulmonary infarction is relatively uncommon because of incomplete vessel occlusion by emboli and bronchial artery anastomoses.

Ventilation/perfusion ($\dot{V}/\dot{Q}$) mismatch is the principal physiologic effect of PE and leads to hypoxemia in most patients. $\dot{V}/\dot{Q}$ mismatch results from increased physiologic dead space and intrapulmonary shunting, which frequently produces an elevated alveolar-to-arteriolar oxygen gradient. Concomitant physiologic responses to PE include increased minute ventilation and airways resistance, as well as decreased vital and diffusion capacities [32–36]. In patients with a potentially patent foramen ovale, progressive pulmonary hypertension may lead to a right-to-left intra-atrial shunt, resulting in worsening hypoxemia and, rarely, paradoxical embolization.

The hemodynamic response to PE may vary depending on the degree of occlusion of the pulmonary arterial circulation and on the presence of underlying cardiopulmonary disease. Physiologically, PE causes a decrease in the cross-sectional area of the pulmonary arterial bed and leads to an increase in the pulmonary vascular resistance. This impedes right ventricular outflow, leading to reduced left ventricular preload and, ultimately, a diminished cardiac output. Progressive vascular obstruction and hypoxemia stimulates vasoconstriction and a further rise in pulmonary artery pressure. The normal right ventricle fails acutely when it cannot generate a systolic pressure to overcome a mean pulmonary artery pressure greater than 40 mm Hg needed to maintain pulmonary perfusion. The normal pulmonary circulation has a large reserve capacity and more than 50% obstruction is generally required for a substantial increase in the mean pulmonary artery pressure [37,38].

TABLE 52.2

THE PRESENCE OF RISK FACTORS IN PATIENTS TREATED FOR ACUTE VENOUS THROMBOEMBOLISM (VTE)

Risk factor	Patients (%)
Age ≥40 y[a]	88.5
Obesity	37.8
Prior VTE	26.0
Malignancy	22.3
Bed rest ≥5 d	12.0
Major surgery	11.2
Congestive heart failure	8.2
Varicose veins	5.8
Hip or leg fracture	3.7
Estrogen therapy	2.0
Stroke	1.8
Multiple trauma	1.1
Childbirth	1.1
Myocardial infarction	0.7
One or more risk factors	96.3
Two or more risk factors	76.0
Three or more risk factors	39.0

[a]Risk of VTE is particularly increased when age >70 years.
Adapted from Anderson FA Jr, Spencer FA: Risk factors for venous thromboembolism. *Circulation* 107[23, Suppl 1]:I9, 2003.

TABLE 52.3

INHERITED AND ACQUIRED RISK FACTORS FOR VENOUS THROMBOEMBOLISM

Inherited	Acquired
Factor V Leiden (APC resistance)	Antiphospholipid antibody syndrome
Antithrombin deficiency	Lupus anticoagulant
Protein C deficiency	Anticardiolipin antibodies
Protein S deficiency	Hyperhomocysteinemia
Prothrombin gene (G20210A) variant	
Heparin cofactor 2 deficiency	
Dysfibrinogenemia	
Disorders of plasminogen	
Elevated factor VIII levels	
Elevated factor XI levels	

APC, activated protein C.

Patients with underlying cardiopulmonary disease have less physiologic reserve as compared with healthy individuals, and it follows that they may suffer right heart failure with a lesser degree of pulmonary vascular occlusion [39,40].

CLINICAL MANIFESTATIONS

Recognizing the presence of VTE may be challenging as neither the signs nor symptoms associated with DVT and PE are sensitive or specific for the diagnoses [13,14,41,42]. Because DVT is usually asymptomatic and most cases of fatal PE are unsuspected prior to death, the most critical step in the diagnosis of VTE is the development of a clinical suspicion of the disease [6,43,44]. This suspicion is based on the constellation of risk factors, symptoms, signs, electrocardiography, blood tests, and chest radiographic findings. Although clinical assessment alone is inadequate in diagnosing and excluding DVT and PE, both clinical gestalt and clinical prediction rules are useful in establishing a pretest probability in which patients are typically classified into three groups based on the estimated prevalence of disease (Table 52.4) [45–49]. This clinical pretest probability serves as the root of algorithms for the diagnosis of DVT and PE [50–53].

The diagnosis of VTE in the critically ill patient may be particularly challenging. Underlying systemic illnesses or other superimposed acute illness may mimic or mask the common signs and symptoms of VTE. Also, common clinical likelihood models for predicting VTE may not be valid in the ICU setting [54]. Furthermore, definitive testing for VTE may be precluded by relative contraindications, such as mechanical ventilation, shock, and renal failure.

Symptoms and Signs

Although most DVT begins in the calf, the presenting symptoms and signs are often not noted until more proximal veins are involved [55]. The initial clinical manifestations of DVT may be acute, progressive, or resolve spontaneously and may include warmth, erythema, swelling, and pain or tenderness. Pain on forced dorsiflexion of the foot (Homans' sign) is neither sensitive nor specific for DVT [42]. The differential diagnosis of DVT should always be framed by the clinical presentation and consideration of risk factors for VTE. Cellulitis, trauma, Baker's cyst, musculoskeletal pain, or asymmetric edema unrelated to DVT may all result in signs and symptoms compatible with acute DVT.

Most patients with proven acute PE present with at least one of the following: dyspnea, pleuritic chest pain, or tachypnea (Table 52.5). Other findings may include tachycardia, a loud pulmonic component of the second heart sound, fever, crackles, pleural rub, wheezing, and/or leg tenderness or swelling. Pleuritic chest pain and hemoptysis occur more commonly with pulmonary infarction due to smaller, peripheral emboli. PE must always be considered in cases of unexplained dyspnea, syncope, or sudden hypotension. Symptoms and signs of PE are nonspecific and may frequently be seen in patients with concomitant cardiopulmonary disease; these findings may be due to a coexisting disease or a superimposed acute PE. Pulmonary embolism may be confused with many conditions including pneumonia, chronic obstructive lung disease exacerbation, pneumothorax, myocardial infarction, heart failure, pericarditis, musculoskeletal pain or trauma, pleuritis, malignancy, and, occasionally, intra-abdominal processes such as acute cholecystitis.

Given the kaleidoscopic presentation of VTE and the significant associated morbidity and mortality, there should be a low threshold for the clinical suspicion of PE in the ICU. Subtle signs such as worsening hypoxemia, a reduction in arterial carbon dioxide with spontaneous respirations (especially in a patient with chronic lung disease), increased central venous or pulmonary artery pressure, or unexplained fever should all be considered potential heralds of PE. Even in the presence of alternative diagnoses, the evaluation for possible VTE may still be appropriate when suggestive signs, symptoms, and risk factors are present.

TABLE 52.4

DETERMINING THE PRETEST PROBABILITY OF ACUTE PULMONARY EMBOLISM (PE) USING A STANDARDIZED POINT SYSTEM[a]

Variable	Points
Symptoms/signs of DVT	3.0
Alternative diagnosis deemed less likely than PE	3.0
Heart rate >100 beats/min	1.5
Immobilization/surgery in previous 4 wk	1.5
Previous VTE	1.5
Hemoptysis	1.0
Recent or current malignancy	1.0
Clinical Probability	**Total Points**
Low	<2.0
Intermediate	2.0–6.0
High	>6.0

[a]Note that this scoring system has not been prospectively evaluated in patients in whom PE is considered in the intensive care unit.
DVT, deep venous thrombosis; VTE, venous thrombosis.
Adapted from Wells PS, Anderson DR, Rodger M, et al: Derivation of a simple clinical model to categorize patients probability of pulmonary embolism: increasing the models utility with the SimpliRED D-dimer. *Thromb Haemost* 83:416, 2000.

DIAGNOSTIC TESTS

Chest Radiograph and Electrocardiogram

Under almost all circumstances, chest radiography cannot be used for the conclusive diagnosis or exclusion of PE. The chest radiograph is abnormal in more than 80% of patients with PE, but is nearly always nonspecific, with common findings including atelectasis, pleural effusion, pulmonary infiltrates, and mild elevation of a hemidiaphragm [41,56,57]. Classic findings such as Hampton's hump (juxtapleural wedge-shaped opacity at the costophrenic angle indicating pulmonary infarction) or Westermark's sign (focally decreased vascularity distal to the occlusion) are suggestive of the diagnosis of PE but are infrequently seen. These findings may be even more difficult to appreciate on portable anteroposterior films commonly employed in the ICU. A normal chest radiograph in a patient with severe dyspnea and hypoxemia and without bronchospasm or cardiac shunt strongly suggests the diagnosis of PE [56]. In young patients with acute pleuritic chest pain, the presence of a pleural effusion raises the probability of PE [58]. Although chest radiography may be useful in excluding other thoracic conditions (e.g., pneumothorax, rib fracture, pneumonia) that may produce signs and symptoms similar to PE, it is important to remember that PE may be present with other cardiopulmonary diseases.

The electrocardiogram is commonly abnormal but findings are nonspecific in most patients with acute PE. Tachycardia, T-wave and ST-segment changes, and right- or left-axis deviation are common electrocardiography findings [41,59]. The

TABLE 52.5

SYMPTOMS AND SIGNS IN PATIENTS WITH ACUTE PULMONARY EMBOLISM WITHOUT PREEXISTING CARDIOPULMONARY DISEASE

Symptoms	Patients (%)	Signs	Patients (%)
Dyspnea	73	Tachypnea (respiratory rate $\geq$20 breaths/min)	70
Pleuritic pain	66	Rales/crackles	51
Cough	37	Tachycardia (heart rate >100 beats/min)	30
Leg swelling	28	Fourth heart sound	24
Leg pain	26	Increased pulmonary component of second sound	23
Hemoptysis	13	DVT	11
Palpitations	10	Diaphoresis	11
Wheezing	9	Temperature >38.5°C	7
Angina-like pain	4	Wheezes	5
	4	Homans' sign	
	4	Right ventricular lift	
	3	Pleural friction rub	
	3	Third heart sound	
	1	Cyanosis	

DVT, deep venous thrombosis.
Adapted from Stein PD, Terrin ML, Hales CA, et al: Clinical, laboratory, roentgenographic, and electrocardiographic findings in patients with acute pulmonary embolism and no preexisting cardiac or pulmonary disease. *Chest* 100:598, 1991.

classic patterns of S1Q3T3; right ventricular strain; and new, incomplete, right bundle branch block are less commonly seen but may be more frequent with massive PE and cor pulmonale. A subepicardial ischemic pattern (T-wave inversion in the precordial leads) seems to correlate with the severity of PE and degree of right ventricular dysfunction [60].

Radiographic and electrocardiographic abnormalities are quite common in patients diagnosed with PE. Although these findings are nonspecific, it follows that a completely normal chest radiograph and electrocardiogram decrease the likelihood of PE.

Arterial Blood Gas and End-Tidal Carbon Dioxide

Arterial blood gas analysis is frequently used in assessing the severity of cardiopulmonary disease but is of limited value in diagnosing PE. Only about 85% to 90% of patients with proven PE have hypoxemia and an elevated alveolar–arterial difference [41,56,61,62]. Hypoxemia is almost uniformly present when there is a hemodynamically significant PE. Interestingly, however, in the Prospective Investigation of Pulmonary Embolism Diagnosis (PIOPED) study, there was no difference in either PaO_2 or $P(A\text{-}a)O_2$ between patients with or without PE, reflecting the common gas-exchange abnormalities present in multiple cardiopulmonary conditions. Due to increased ventilation, patients with PE will generally have a normal or reduced arterial carbon dioxide tension. Physiologic changes in PE may be particularly variable in young patients and those without underlying lung or heart disease. In any case, arterial blood gas values are of insufficient discriminant value to exclude the diagnosis of PE.

As a function of alveolar dead space, end-tidal CO_2 is a physiologically intuitive marker of pulmonary arterial blood flow that unfortunately has been of limited utility in identifying patients with PE [63–67]. End-tidal CO_2 may be physiologically insensitive for PE because of incomplete vessel occlusion by thrombus and also because of decreased ventilation at embolized areas due to local bronchoconstriction. Other cardiopulmonary conditions may alter the difference between the $PaCO_2$ and the end-tidal CO_2, decreasing the specificity for PE.

D-Dimer

Plasma measurements of D-dimer (a specific derivative of cross-linked fibrin) have been extensively studied in patients with acute DVT and PE [68–70]. Multiple inexpensive D-dimer tests are available, but rapid enzyme-linked immunosorbent assays are preferred. When used in the outpatient setting, D-dimer measurements are very sensitive and have shown a high negative predictive value in excluding the presence of VTE when used in concert with a low clinical pretest probability [51,71]. The low specificity of D-dimer testing for VTE (i.e., many conditions are associated with elevated levels) makes it less useful in unselected and hospitalized patients [72]. It follows that the positive predictive value of an elevated D-dimer for VTE is low and should not be used in isolation to initiate further evaluation.

Cardiac Troponin and Brain Natriuretic Peptide

Troponin is specific for cardiac myocyte damage, and patients with right ventricular strain due to acute PE may sometimes have elevated troponin T and I levels [73,74]. Patients with PE and elevated troponins are more likely to have elevated right ventricular systolic pressures, right ventricular dilation/hypokinesis, and are at increased risk for cardiogenic shock. Not surprisingly, a positive troponin is more common with large clot burdens and confers an increased risk of death [75,76]. Although an elevated troponin may hint at a potential diagnosis of PE in the appropriate clinical setting, a normal value is not sufficiently sensitive to rule out PE.

Plasma brain natriuretic peptide (BNP) is released in response to increased cardiac-filling pressure and can serve as a supplementary tool for evaluating right ventricular function in patients with acute PE. BNP appears elevated in the majority of cases of PE with right ventricular overload and may help in risk stratification [77–79]. However, because plasma BNP levels rise in a variety of cardiopulmonary conditions and are affected by several physiological factors, they are not diagnostic for PE.

Ventilation/Perfusion Scanning

Despite the increased use of contrast-enhanced spiral computed tomography (CT) of the chest, $\dot{V}/\dot{Q}$ scanning is still frequently used in suspected PE. $\dot{V}/\dot{Q}$ scans may be deemed normal or, when abnormal, are conventionally read as showing low, intermediate, or high probability of PE. A normal scan essentially excludes the diagnosis of PE. Otherwise, $\dot{V}/\dot{Q}$ scanning can be combined with clinical suspicion in a Bayesian fashion to improve the accuracy of diagnosis. In general, the predictive value of a $\dot{V}/\dot{Q}$ scan is highest with a concordant clinical likelihood assessment. In the PIOPED study, when the clinical suspicion of PE was high, PE was present in 96% of patients with high-probability lung scans [5]. However, in patients with a high clinical pretest probability for PE, 66% of patients with intermediate probability scans and 40% of patients with low probability scans were subsequently diagnosed with PE by pulmonary angiography. This emphasizes that low- and intermediate-probability $\dot{V}/\dot{Q}$ scans are nondiagnostic when there is a high clinical suspicion for PE. In the setting of a low clinical pretest probability for PE, a normal or low-probability $\dot{V}/\dot{Q}$ scan correctly excluded PE in more than 95% of cases. Because PE is commonly found in low- or intermediate-probability $\dot{V}/\dot{Q}$ scans, such findings are generally considered nondiagnostic and further evaluation is often appropriate.

Although $\dot{V}/\dot{Q}$ scanning can be successfully used in the intensive care setting, ventilation scans generally cannot be performed on mechanically ventilated patients, and the availability of bedside scintigraphic perfusion imaging has decreased [5,80,81]. The optimal scenario for the $\dot{V}/\dot{Q}$ scan is in the patient with a clear chest radiograph and without underlying cardiopulmonary disease. Large PE, however, are occasionally identified with portable perfusion scans based upon very large perfusion defects in ICU patients.

Chest Computed Tomographic Angiography

During the past decade, $\dot{V}/\dot{Q}$ scanning has decreased in favor of contrast-enhanced computed tomographic angiography (CTA) of the chest that may reveal emboli in the main, lobar, or segmental pulmonary arteries. The reported sensitivity and specificity of single-slice helical CTA has ranged from 53% to 100% and from 81% to 100%, respectively [82]. Visualization of segmental and subsegmental pulmonary arteries is substantially better with newer multidetector scanners as evidenced by the PIOPED II study, where the specificity of chest CTA was 95% and the sensitivity 83% [83]. As with $\dot{V}/\dot{Q}$ scanning, diagnostic testing with CTA is best used in the context of a pretest clinical assessment of probability of PE. In the PIOPED II, in patients with a high or intermediate clinical probability of PE as measured by the Wells score, abnormal findings on CTA had a positive predictive value of 96% and 92%, respectively. In patients with a low clinical likelihood of PE, normal findings on CTA had a 96% negative predictive value. PIOPED II generally supports the use of multidetector CTA as stand-alone imaging for suspected PE in the majority of patients. However, the 17% false-negative rate emphasizes that CTA still fails to detect emboli that may be better visualized by $\dot{V}/\dot{Q}$ scanning or traditional angiography. Many of these may be peripheral subsegmental PE, for which there is no consensus regarding treatment [84]. It nevertheless follows that a normal CTA in the context of a high clinical probability of PE is insufficient in excluding PE and such patients warrant further investigation.

A benefit of CTA for suspected PE over other diagnostic modalities is that it provides visualization of potential nonvascular pathology such as musculoskeletal or airway abnormalities, lymphadenopathy, pleural or pericardial disease, or parenchymal lesions such as consolidation or a lung tumor. CTA also has the advantage of rapid performance. Disadvantages of CTA include the risk of adverse reactions to contrast (such as anaphylaxis or nephrotoxicity) and lack of portability. ICU patients frequently have a prohibitive creatinine clearance.

Magnetic Resonance Imaging

Magnetic resonance imaging (MRI) has excellent sensitivity and specificity and may allow the simultaneous detection of DVT and PE [85–87]. Disadvantages of MRI include performance time and difficult utilization in the critically ill or ventilated patient.

Echocardiography

Although echocardiography (echo) is insensitive for the diagnosis of PE, it has several important roles in the evaluation of PE. The speed and portability of echo make it particularly useful in patients who are suspected of having PE and who are too unstable for further evaluation with CTA or $\dot{V}/\dot{Q}$ scan. In addition, echo has proven helpful for risk stratification in patients with proven PE, and serial examinations may demonstrate interval change in cardiac function [88–90]. Also, an initial diagnostic scan may be useful in identifying other causes of shock such as aortic dissection and cardiac tamponade.

Transthoracic echocardiographic signs of acute PE include dilatation and hypokinesis of the right ventricle, paradoxical motion of the interventricular septum, tricuspid regurgitation, and lack of collapse of the inferior vena cava (IVC) during inspiration [91]. McConnell's sign (free wall of the right ventricle hypokinesis that spares the apex) may be a more specific finding [92]. Rarely, direct visualization of thrombus may guarantee the diagnosis.

Pulmonary Angiography

Pulmonary artery angiography is extremely sensitive and specific in confirming or excluding acute PE and remains the "gold standard" diagnostic technique. Like many tests, however, angiography may be limited by interobserver agreement and tech nical factors [93]. In 1,111 cases from the PIOPED study, 3% of studies were nondiagnostic and 1% was incomplete, usually due to a complication. Although complications are more common in the ICU, angiography is generally deemed quite safe, with major morbidity and mortality rates of 1% and 0.5%, respectively [93]. Serious complications include respiratory failure (0.4%), renal failure (0.3%), and hemorrhage requiring blood transfusion.

Pulmonary angiography is frequently reserved for patients in whom preliminary noninvasive testing has been nondiagnostic. There is a growing consensus that clinically stable patients with nondiagnostic chest imaging may alternatively safely undergo further noninvasive study such as lower extremity evaluation in lieu of direct angiography [53,83,94–96]. For unstable patients in the ICU setting, angiography can be performed at the bedside using a pulmonary artery catheter and portable fluoroscopy in some centers [97].

Detection of Acute Deep Venous Thrombosis

In the critical care setting, the search for DVT can be especially useful in that it may establish a presumptive diagnosis of PE and direct therapy. The available technology used to pursue the diagnosis of DVT has expanded considerably, and each modality has advantages and limitations. Impedance plethysmography (IPG) is a portable test that employs electrical current to estimate venous outflow obstruction during sequential inflation and deflation of an occlusive thigh cuff. Although early studies were favorable, subsequent studies suggest that the sensitivity of IPG for proximal DVT is only about 65% [98–101]. Even in ideal hands, IPG may fail to detect nonocclusive or duplicated bilateral thrombi. It is essentially not used at all anymore.

Venous ultrasonography is the preferred noninvasive test for the diagnosis of symptomatic proximal DVT, where it has a weighted sensitivity and specificity of 95% and 98%, respectively [102]. For diagnosis of a first symptomatic proximal DVT, ultrasound has a positive predictive value of 97% and a negative predictive value of 98% [103]. Although it is generally appropriate to initiate or withhold treatment based on the result of the examination, an exception would be when the result is discordant with the clinical assessment. For instance, a negative compression ultrasound in the context of a high clinical suspicion for DVT would warrant further investigation such as venography, MRI, or CT venography (CTV). The combination of compression and Doppler ultrasonography is also accurate in detecting upper extremity DVT [104]. Limitations of venous ultrasonography include insensitivity for asymptomatic DVT and pelvic vein clots, operator dependence, and difficulty distinguishing acute from chronic DVT in symptomatic patients.

MRI and CTV are being increasingly employed to diagnose DVT. MRI is highly accurate and has multiple advantages, including excellent resolution of the IVC and pelvic veins, accuracy in diagnosing upper extremity DVT, concurrent thoracic as well as bilateral examination, differentiating acute from chronic disease, and lack of exposure to ionizing radiation [85–87,105]. However, MRI is expensive, time-consuming, not portable, and is restricted in patients with metallic devices or claustrophobia. As with MRI, CTA/CTV has the advantage of evaluating both PE and DVT in a single study. CTV is accurate in the detection of DVT and may be particularly useful in imaging the pelvis and upper thighs [106,107]. In the PIOPED II, concurrent leg evaluation with CTV increased the sensitivity of CTA from 83% to 90%, although the small improvement in overall diagnostic yield may not warrant the additional irradiation associated with CTV [83]. Contrast venography is rarely done anymore.

Special Diagnostic Considerations: Massive Pulmonary Embolism

Patients with suspected massive PE may present with severe hypoxemia and/or hypotension and a timely diagnosis is essential as perhaps two thirds of patients with ultimately fatal PE will die within 1 hour of presentation [108]. Diagnostic evaluation must be performed rapidly, but cardiopulmonary instability may limit the patient's ability to undergo transport or testing. In such cases, venous ultrasonography or echo in the acutely unstable patient may offer compelling evidence for VTE. Portable perfusion scans are more likely diagnostic (high probability) than when a less extensive clot burden is present. As noted, bedside angiography can sometimes be performed in the ICU using a pulmonary artery catheter and portable fluoroscopy. When obtainable, helical CTA is very unlikely to be negative in the setting of massive PE.

Diagnostic Algorithm

During the last 2 decades, considerable progress in technology and clinical research methods have led to marked improvements in the diagnosis of VTE [109,110]. The constellation of advances has decreased the complexity and uncertainty found in traditional diagnostic approaches. Despite this, however, the morbidity and mortality of VTE remains high. Although consensus guidelines exist for the standard diagnostic approach to VTE, there is no single, best approach that is always agreed on [95]. Also, not all of the new data regarding the evaluation of VTE may be applicable to patients in the ICU setting, and future studies will continue to define each modality in this context. Figures 52.1 and 52.2 illustrate the diagnostic algorithms for suspected PE in stable and unstable ICU patients, respectively.

TREATMENT

The primary goal of treatment of DVT is the prevention of thrombus extension and PE. Anticoagulation is the standard of care in patients with acute VTE, but other options in the treatment of PE include thrombolytic therapy, IVC filter placement, and surgical embolectomy. Each approach has specific indications as well as advantages and disadvantages. Table 52.6 lists the evidence-based advances in VTE management as they apply to critical care.

Anticoagulation

The anticoagulation regimens for the treatment of DVT and uncomplicated PE are generally similar. Although anticoagulants do not directly dissolve preexisting clot, they prevent thrombus extension and indirectly decrease clot burden by allowing the natural fibrinolytic system to proceed unopposed. When there is a strong clinical suspicion of PE, anticoagulation should be instituted immediately and before diagnostic confirmation, unless the risk of bleeding is deemed excessive.

Unfractionated Heparin

Therapy with unfractionated heparin (UFH) reduces the extension and recurrence of symptomatic proximal DVT as well as mortality in acute PE [111,112]. UFH is usually delivered by continuous intravenous infusion, and therapy is monitored by measurement of the activated partial thromboplastin time (aPTT) [113]. "Traditional" or physician-directed dosing of heparin often leads to subtherapeutic aPTT results, and validated dosing nomograms are generally favored [114,115]. Nomogram dosing reduces the time to achieve therapeutic anticoagulation that may be important in reducing the risk of recurrent VTE [116]. UFH should be administered as an intravenous bolus of 5,000 U followed by a continuous infusion maintenance dose of 30,000 to 40,000 U per 24 hours (the lower dose being used if the patient is considered at risk for bleeding) [117]. Two alternative dosing regimens include a 5,000-U bolus followed by 1,280 U per hour, or a bolus of 80 U

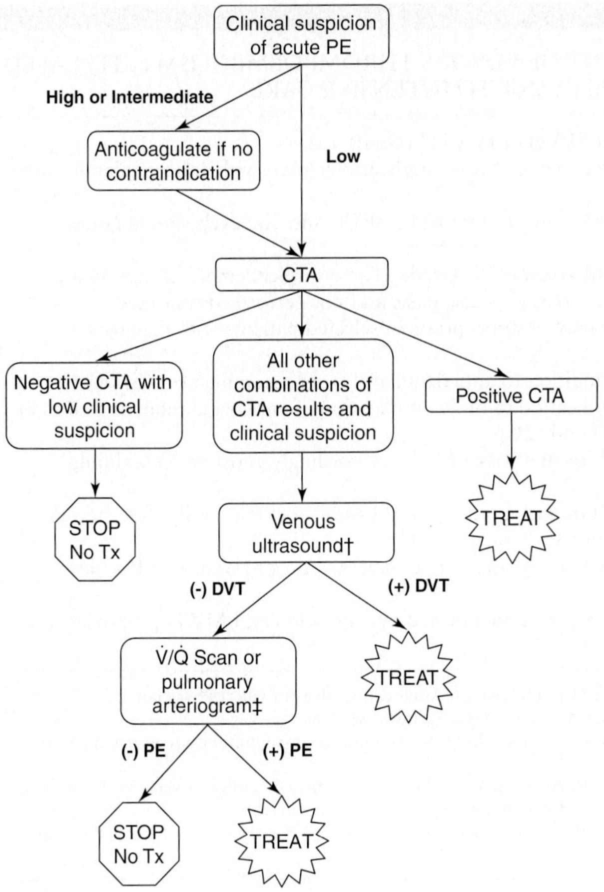

FIGURE 52.1. A contrast-enhanced computed tomographic angiography (CTA) of the chest-based algorithm for suspected acute pulmonary embolism (PE) in stable intensive care unit (ICU) patients. Contrast-enhanced CT scans may not be feasible in patients with significant kidney dysfunction or severe contrast allergy. Clinical probability scores and rapid enzyme-linked immunosorbent assay D-dimer testing are not included due to insufficient validation in the ICU setting. Appropriate supportive therapy is assumed. †Prior addition of CT venography during CTA would obviate the need for venous ultrasound. Ultrasound of the upper extremities should be considered in the presence of an invasive catheter or local symptoms of DVT. ‡The ventilation/perfusion V̇/Q̇ scan may be particularly useful when the chest radiograph is clear and when no underlying cardiopulmonary disease is present. Unfortunately, the V̇/Q̇ scan is often nondiagnostic, even when PE is present. DVT, deep venous thrombosis; Tx, treatment.

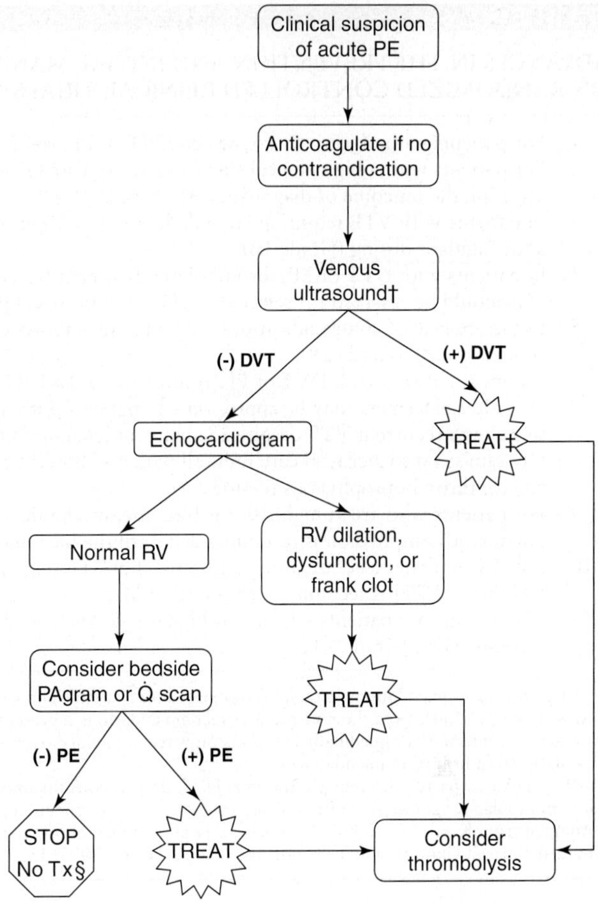

FIGURE 52.2. Diagnostic algorithm for suspected acute pulmonary embolism (PE) in unstable intensive care unit (ICU) patients. Unstable implies that the patient cannot be safely transported for testing such as chest computed tomography. Clinical probability scores and rapid enzyme-linked immunosorbent assay D-dimer testing are not included due to insufficient validation in the ICU setting. Appropriate supportive therapy is assumed. †Ultrasound of the upper extremities should be performed in the presence of an invasive catheter or local symptoms of deep venous thrombosis (DVT). ‡Consider inferior vena cava filter in the setting of massive PE with DVT when it is believed that any further emboli might be lethal and thrombolytic use is prohibited. §Stop anticoagulation after a negative pulmonary artery angiogram (PAgram) or a normal or low-probability perfusion Q̇ scan. RV, right ventricle; Tx, treatment.

per kg followed by 18 U per kg per hour [114,115]. Following initiation, the aPTT should be measured at 6-hour intervals until it is consistently in the therapeutic range of 1.5 to 2.0 times control values, which corresponds to a heparin level of 0.2 to 0.4 U per mL as measured by protamine sulfate titration [113]. Further adjusting of the UFH dose should be weight based. In patients deemed to have heparin resistance (requiring >35,000 U of UFH per day to achieve a therapeutic aPTT), antifactor Xa levels may be used to guide effective therapy [118].

Low-Molecular-Weight Heparin

Multiple clinical trials have demonstrated that low-molecular-weight heparin (LMWH) is at least as safe and effective as UFH for the treatment of acute VTE [119,120]. LMWH preparations offer several advantages over UFH, including greater bioavailability, longer half-life, lack of need for an intravenous infusion, and a more predictable anticoagulant response to weight-based dosing. LMWH can be administered subcutaneously once or twice per day and does not require monitoring of the aPTT. Monitoring antifactor Xa levels (typically 4 hours following injection) may be reasonable in certain settings such as morbid obesity, very small patients (<40 kg), pregnancy, renal insufficiency, or with unanticipated bleeding or recurrent VTE despite appropriate weight-based dosing [113,121–123]. Because the anticoagulant effect of UFH is short acting and can be rapidly reversed, it is often preferred over LMWH in the ICU, where patients are at increased risk for bleeding and may be undergoing fibrinolysis or need frequent procedures.

Fondaparinux is a highly bioavailable synthetic polysaccharide derived from heparin that is effective in the initial treatment and prophylaxis for VTE [124]. Fondaparinux does not appear to interact with platelet factor 4 so that heparin-induced thrombocytopenia (HIT), while it is possible, appears to be an exceedingly unlikely event. Its long half-life and renal clearance make it impractical for the ICU, and its anticoagulant effect is not reversible.

TABLE 52.6

ADVANCES IN THE PREVENTION AND INITIAL MANAGEMENT OF VENOUS THROMBOEMBOLISM (VTE) BASED ON RANDOMIZED CONTROLLED CLINICAL TRIALS AND RELEVANT TO INTENSIVE CARE

1. For patients with objectively confirmed DVT or PE, treat with SC LMWH or IV UFH (Grade 1 A).[a]
2. For patients with a high clinical suspicion of DVT or PE and in the absence of contraindications, treat with anticoagulants while awaiting the outcome of diagnostic tests (Grade 1C+).
3. In patients with VTE requiring large daily doses of UFH without achieving a therapeutic aPTT, anti-Xa levels should guide anticoagulant dosing (Grade 1B).
4. In patients with DVT or PE, thrombolytic treatment (Grade 2B) and mechanical (Grade 2C) or surgical embolectomy (Grade 2C) should be reserved for selected, highly compromised patients on a case-by-case basis and not performed routinely.
5. In the absence of contraindications, systemic thrombolytic therapy may be appropriate in selected patients with massive or submassive PE (Grade 2B).
6. For most patients with DVT or PE, routine use of an IVC filter in addition to anticoagulants is not recommended (Grade 1A).
7. IVC filter placement may be appropriate in patients with a contraindication to or a complication of anticoagulation, as well as in those with recurrent VTE despite adequate anticoagulant therapy (Grade 2C).
8. On admission to a critical care unit, all patients should be assessed for their risk of VTE. Accordingly, most patients should receive thromboprophylaxis (Grade 1A).
9. For patients who are at high risk for bleeding, mechanical prophylaxis with graded compression stockings and/or intermittent pneumatic compression is recommended until the bleeding risk decreases (Grade 1C+).[b]
10. For ICU patients who are at moderate risk for VTE (e.g., medically ill or postoperative patients), prophylaxis with low-dose UFH or LMWH is recommended (Grade 1A).
11. For critical care patients who are at higher risk, such as following major trauma or orthopaedic surgery, LMWH prophylaxis is recommended (Grade 1A).

[a]All graded recommendations in the table are based on available clinical trial data from the seventh American College of Chest Physicians consensus [143,154]. Even the non–grade A recommendations represent the standard of care in most clinical settings.
[b]In general, intermittent pneumatic compression is recommended over graded compression stockings in the intensive care unit, although few data are available for a firm recommendation.
aPTT, activated partial thromboplastin time; DVT, deep venous thrombosis; ICU, intensive care unit; IV, intravenous; IVC, inferior vena cava; LMWH, low-molecular-weight heparin; PE, pulmonary embolism; SC, subcutaneous; UFH, unfractionated heparin.
Adapted from Kearon C, Kahn SR, Agnelli G, et al. Antithrombotic therapy for venous thromboembolic disease. American College of Chest Physicians Evidence-Based Clinical Practice Guidelines (8th ed). *Chest* 2008; 133:454S–545.

Warfarin

For the same reasons as LMWH, warfarin therapy is less frequently used as therapeutic anticoagulation for ICU patients. Also, oral warfarin therapy must take into account many drug and food interactions, as well as genetic variations in drug metabolism. When warfarin is employed, administration should generally overlap with therapeutic heparin anticoagulation. In patients with thrombophilia (protein C or S deficiency), warfarin may cause a transient hypercoagulable state due to the abrupt decline in vitamin K-dependent coagulation inhibitors. With warfarin therapy, it is recommended that a heparin preparation be employed for at least 5 days and maintained at a therapeutic level until two consecutive international normalized ratio values of 2.0 to 3.0 have been documented at least 24 hours apart [125].

Novel Agents

Extraordinary advances in the understanding of thrombosis have led to the development of several novel anticoagulant therapies. Lepirudin (recombinant hirudin), argatroban, desirudin are direct thrombin inhibitors that make them unique in their ability to inactivate fibrin clot-bound thrombin. The first of these two drugs are Food and Drug Administration (FDA)-approved parenteral drugs used for the treatment of HIT [124]. A disadvantage of the direct thrombin inhibitors is lack of reversibility. Other agents, including oral direct factor Xa inhibitors such as rivaroxaban and apixaban and new direct thrombin inhibitors such as dabigatran, are currently being evaluated.

Special Case: Central Venous Catheter–Related Thrombosis

Upper extremity thrombosis is common in the critically ill patient and is most often related to a CVC. CVC-related thrombosis should generally be treated similarly to uncomplicated DVT, but with an additional emphasis on prompt catheter removal once the diagnosis is established. The risk of clot embolization that accompanies CVC extraction is outweighed by the risk for chronic thrombotic complications and potential infection.

Complications of Anticoagulation

Hemorrhage and HIT are the major complications of anticoagulation. A pooled analysis of 11 clinical trials involving approximately 15,000 patients treated with either UFH or LMWH reported the frequency of major bleeding at 1.9% and a fatal hemorrhage rate of 0.2% [119]. Protamine may rapidly neutralize the anticoagulant effect of UFH, although allergy, hypotension, and bradycardia are possible adverse reactions to administration. The anticoagulant effect of LMWH is partly but not completely reversed by protamine [113].

HIT is an antibody-mediated adverse drug reaction that may lead to venous and arterial thrombosis. The principal clinical feature of HIT syndrome is the development of an otherwise unexplained drop in platelet count (absolute thrombocytopenia or more than 50% decrease if the platelet nadir remains in the normal range) following exposure to heparin. HIT generally develops 5 to 10 days after the initiation of heparin but may occur earlier in the setting of prior heparin exposure [126]. Although relatively infrequent, HIT is one of the most serious causes of thrombocytopenia in the ICU, and careful evaluation and consideration is warranted in this setting [127,128].

Thrombolytic Therapy

Thrombolytic agents may accelerate thrombus resolution by activating plasminogen to form plasmin resulting in fibrinolysis as well as fibrinogenolysis. The case for thrombolysis is the strongest in patients with massive PE complicated by shock, where the mortality rate may be more than 30% [129–132]. A positive troponin may suggest the diagnosis of acute PE. In proven PE, it appears to portend a poor prognosis. In one large study, of 737 patients presenting to the emergency department with proven PE, troponin T was measured in 563 and was elevated in 27% [132]. In-hospital survival was 79% in troponin-positive patients compared with 94% in troponin-negative patients ($p < 0.001$). One-year survival was 71% in troponin-positive patients compared with 90% in troponin-negative patients ($p < 0.001$). Elevated troponin levels predicted a fourfold increased risk of in-hospital death and threefold higher risk of 1-year mortality, even after adjustment for the most important other risk factors for death in this population.

Without question, thrombolytic therapy has been shown to accelerate clot lysis in PE and lead to a more rapid resolution of abnormal right ventricular dysfunction [4,133–136]. Evidence of a survival benefit, however, has been generally lacking, primarily because large randomized studies have not included all important potential predictors of death such as severe hypoxemia, *severe* right ventricular dysfunction, and residual clot burden in the legs. Accepting the limitations of registry data, a recent analysis of the International Cooperative Pulmonary Embolism Registry (ICOPER) nonetheless showed that thrombolysis for massive PE did not reduce mortality or the rate of recurrent PE at 90 days [137]. Thrombolytic treatment in patients with acute submassive PE (echocardiographic evidence of right ventricular dysfunction without hypotension) may offer no survival benefit but may prevent clinical deterioration and the need for escalation of care [138]. The decision for thrombolysis should be made on a case-by-case basis. Even in the setting of a relative contraindication, thrombolytic therapy may be reasonable when a patient is extremely unstable from life-threatening PE.

Each of the FDA-approved thrombolytic agents is administered at a fixed dose, making measurements of coagulation unnecessary during infusion (Table 52.7). Tissue-type plasminogen activator (2-hour infusion) is most commonly used. Shorter regimens and even bolus dosing may be favored in cases of unstable patients with massive PE. Following infusion of thrombolytics, the aPTT should be measured and repeated at 4-hour intervals until the aPTT is less than twice the upper limit of normal, after which continuous intravenous UFH should be administered without a loading bolus dose. Although thrombolytics have been administered as local intrapulmonary arterial infusions, standard systemic intravenous therapy appears adequate in most cases [139–141].

Thrombolytic therapy is contraindicated in patients at high risk for bleeding (Table 52.8). Intracranial hemorrhage is the most devastating (and often fatal) complication of thrombolytic therapy and occurs in 1% to 3% of patients [11,142]. Invasive procedures should be minimized around the time of therapy to decrease the risk of bleeding. A vascular puncture above the inguinal ligament can lead to retroperitoneal hemorrhage that is often initially silent but may be life-threatening. Although there is some rationale for thrombolytic therapy in DVT, such use is controversial and current guidelines are generally not supportive [143]. Systemic thrombolysis decreases the incidence of postthrombotic syndrome and perhaps the risk of recurrent DVT, but at an unacceptable increase in the rate of major hemorrhage [144]. Catheter-directed thrombolysis is increasingly common and appears to be a safer alternative for the management of extensive, symptomatic DVT [145].

In summary, there has been increasing interest in risk-stratifying patients with acute PE to determine when a more aggressive approach should be undertaken [143].

TABLE 52.7

FOOD AND DRUG ADMINISTRATION–APPROVED THROMBOLYTIC THERAPY REGIMENS FOR ACUTE PULMONARY EMBOLISM

Drug	Protocol
Streptokinase	250,000 U IV (loading dose during 30 min); then 100,000 U/h for 24 h
Urokinase[a]	2,000 U/lb IV (loading dose during 10 min); then 2,000 U/lb/h for 12 to 24 h
tPA	100 mg IV during 2 h

[a]Limited availability.
IV, intravenous; tPA, tissue-type plasminogen activator.

TABLE 52.8

CONTRAINDICATIONS TO THROMBOLYTIC THERAPY IN PULMONARY EMBOLISM

Absolute	Relative
Previous hemorrhagic stroke	Bleeding diathesis/thrombocytopenia
Intracranial surgery or pathology, including trauma	Recent major trauma, internal bleeding, or nonhemorrhagic stroke
Active internal bleeding	Uncontrolled severe hypertension
	Cardiopulmonary resuscitation
	Recent major surgery[a]
	Pregnancy

[a]This time frame may depend on the type of surgery, associated bleeding risk, and the level of critical illness.

Inferior Vena Cava Interruption

Primary indications for IVC filter placement include contraindication to anticoagulation and failure of therapy as defined by recurrent VTE or significant bleeding [143]. Alternative rationales for use currently lack support from well-designed clinical trials. The Prévention du Risque d'Embolic Pulmonaire par Interruption Cave (PREPIC) study has validated the common thinking that, in patients with acute proximal DVT, IVC filter placement decreases the rate of PE (6.2% vs. 15.1%) [146]. Unsurprisingly, this benefit is countered by an increased risk of recurrent DVT in patients with IVC filters that arguably may cause as much morbidity as nonfatal PE. Filter placement appears to have no effect on mortality.

A number of IVC filter designs exist and they can be inserted via the jugular or femoral veins. As noted, thrombosis is a primary complication of filters, and all patients should receive extended anticoagulation when able to do so. Insertion-related complications and filter migration may also occur. More recently, temporary filters have been employed in patients in whom the risk of bleeding appears short term.

Pulmonary Embolectomy

Given its high morbidity and mortality, surgical embolectomy has traditionally been a treatment of last resort, often reserved for patients with documented central PE and refractory cardiogenic shock despite maximal therapy. Contemporary studies show improved outcomes and suggest that emergency surgical pulmonary embolectomy may be feasible in carefully selected patients and with an experienced surgical team [147]. Percutaneous embolectomy is a less well-studied method of improving hemodynamics by reducing the burden of central pulmonary artery thromboembolism.

Special Therapeutic Considerations: Massive Pulmonary Embolism

In cases of massive PE, therapy should progress as directed by clinical likelihood and the diagnostic results. The mere suspicion of massive PE warrants immediate supportive therapy. Cautious infusion of intravenous saline may augment preload and improve impaired right ventricular function. Dopamine and norepinephrine are favored if hypotension remains, and combination therapy with dobutamine may boost right ventricular output, although it may exacerbate hypotension [148]. Supplemental oxygen and mechanical ventilation may be instituted as needed to support respiratory failure. Anticoagulation, thrombolytic therapy, and pulmonary embolectomy should be considered and employed as previously described.

CLINICAL COURSE AND PREVENTION

Course

VTE is associated with several main sequelae: nonfatal recurrent VTE, postthrombotic syndrome, chronic PE with pulmonary hypertension, and the most feared event, fatal PE. Death occurs in approximately 6% of DVT cases and 12% of PE cases within 1 month of diagnosis [23]. The overall crude 3-month mortality rate for patients in the ICOPER was 17.4% [11]. In the PIOPED study, the overall 3-month mortality rate was approximately 15%, but only 10% of deaths during the first year of follow-up were attributed to PE [13].

Most patients who survive an acute episode of VTE suffer no long-term sequelae. During the initial 3 months of therapeutic anticoagulation for patients with proximal DVT, approximately 4% will have a recurrent episode of VTE, and about 1 in 250 will develop fatal PE [149]. The incidence of severe postthrombotic syndrome is about 3% after 1 year and 9% after 5 years, even with the use of graduated compression stockings [150]. About 3% to 4% of PE patients will develop chronic thromboembolic pulmonary hypertension [151].

Prevention

Although VTE prophylaxis unequivocally reduces the incidence of disease for those at risk, such measures appear to be grossly underused [152,153]. This may be particularly true in hospitalized medical patients; a heterogeneous group in whom the risk for VTE and the data for prophylaxis have traditionally lagged behind surgical practice [153]. Three well-designed, placebo-controlled studies in acutely ill medical patients have demonstrated a substantial decrease in asymptomatic DVT or symptomatic VTE with pharmacologic (LMWH, dalteparin, or fondaparinux) prophylaxis [154–156]. Combining all three trials, VTE prophylaxis reduced the frequency of asymptomatic DVT or symptomatic VTE by about 50%, and the risk of major bleeding was not increased. Intermittent pneumatic compression devices should be used when prophylactic anticoagulation is contraindicated, and it may be reasonable to employ both methods in patients deemed to be at exceptionally high risk for VTE. Essentially all critically ill patients require some form of VTE prophylaxis. Multiple regimens are FDA approved, and prophylactic therapy must be individualized to the patient and the clinical setting.

VENOUS THROMBOEMBOLISM IN PREGNANCY

VTE is a leading cause of death in pregnant women, in whom the age-adjusted risk of VTE is at least five times higher compared with nonpregnant women [1,157]. DVT is more common during the antepartum period and occurs with almost equal frequency in each of the three trimesters. In contrast, the incidence of PE is highest immediately postpartum.

In pregnancy, venous stasis arises due to increased venous distensibility and capacity as well as compression of large veins by a gravid uterus. Pregnancy is a hypercoagulable state, accompanied by changes in the coagulation and fibrinolytic systems. Obstetrical factors such as prolonged bed rest and instrument-assisted or cesarean delivery may also increase the risk of VTE.

The diagnosis of VTE during pregnancy is complicated by maternal physiologic changes and the reluctance of physicians to expose a fetus to ionizing radiation. As in nonpregnant patients, many symptoms, signs, and preliminary tests are nondiagnostic for VTE. In general, the evaluation for VTE in pregnancy should emphasize the early use of noninvasive studies of the legs. When ultrasonography does not demonstrate DVT, the diagnostic algorithm is similar to that described for nonpregnant patients. Although radiation exposure should be minimized to decrease the risk of fetal injury, a firm diagnosis is important because of the short- and long-term treatment implications.

Therapy for VTE in pregnancy is generally similar to that in nonpregnant women, except that warfarin should be avoided because it is teratogenic and can cross the placental barrier. LMWH has been shown to be safe in pregnancy and is often preferred as long-term therapy; warfarin may be employed postpartum [158]. Due to the risk of maternal hemorrhage and fetal demise, pregnancy is a relative contraindication for thrombolytic therapy. That being considered, controlled trials are lacking in this area, and thrombolysis may rarely be appropriate in cases of massive PE with hemodynamic instability. The indications for IVC filter placement in pregnant women are the same as in nonpregnant patients. Finally, VTE prophylactic therapy may be appropriate for pregnant women deemed at high risk for VTE, such as those with a history of prior VTE or in patients with an inherited or acquired thrombophilia.

NONTHROMBOTIC PULMONARY EMBOLI

Although thrombotic PE is the most common and important syndrome characterized by embolization of material into the pulmonary circulation, nonthrombotic pulmonary emboli may rarely occur in certain clinical settings. Fat embolism syndrome most commonly occurs after blunt trauma complicated by long-bone fractures. The characteristic findings of dyspnea, axillary and subconjunctival petechiae, and alterations in mental status generally occur between 12 and 48 hours after the primary event [159]. Cardiopulmonary derangement is likely due to venous obstruction by neutral fat and to a vasculitis and capillary leak syndrome caused by free fatty acids. The diagnosis of fat embolization syndrome is clinical; however, the identification of fat droplets within cells recovered by bronchoalveolar lavage may be helpful [160]. Therapy is generally prophylactic and supportive as more specific treatments have shown limited benefit. The syndrome is usually mild and the prognosis good.

Amniotic fluid embolism is uncommon, but it represents one of the leading causes of maternal death in the United States [161]. The condition may occur during or shortly after either spontaneous or cesarean delivery and there exist no consistent identifiable risk factors. Clinical hallmarks include hypoxemia, cardiogenic shock, altered mental status, and disseminated intravascular coagulation. The diagnosis is clinical and the therapy is primarily supportive. Amniotic fluid embolism is frequently fatal and permanent neurologic deficits are found in 85% of survivors [161].

Septic PE usually presents as multiple bilateral peripheral nodules that are often poorly marginated and may have cavitary changes. Right-sided endocarditis and septic thrombophlebitis are the most common source of septic pulmonary emboli [162]. Fever, rigors, and pleuritic chest pain may be more impressive in septic PE as compared with bland PE. Treatment centers on appropriate anti-infective therapy, but anticoagulation and surgical management may be appropriate in some circumstances. Intensive care is generally not necessary unless there is significant associated cardiopulmonary dysfunction.

Air embolism requires communication between the air and the venous circulation when venous blood pressure is below atmospheric pressure. Predisposing settings include invasive procedures, barotrauma, and the use of indwelling catheters. Air may gain entry into the arterial system by incomplete filtering of a large air embolus by the pulmonary capillaries or via paradoxical embolization through a patent foramen ovale [163]. The clinical picture is critical in raising the suspicion of disease as the signs and symptoms are generally nonspecific. Immediate Trendelenburg and left lateral decubitus positioning may open an obstructed right ventricular outflow tract, and air aspiration should be attempted if there is a CVC in the right atrium. Administration of 100% oxygen aids in bubble reabsorption via nitrogen washout, and hyperbaric oxygen therapy may also be beneficial.

Other miscellaneous nonthrombotic causes of pulmonary vascular obstruction include cancer cells, schistosomal disease, and inorganic material such as talc crystals or various fibers.

References

1. Prevention of venous thrombosis and pulmonary embolism. NIH Consensus Development. *JAMA* 256:744, 1986.
2. Silverstein MD, Heit JA, Mohr DN, et al: Trends in the incidence of deep vein thrombosis and pulmonary embolism: a 25-year population-based study. *Arch Intern Med* 158:585, 1998.
3. Attia J, Ray JG, Cook DJ, et al: Deep vein thrombosis and its prevention in critically ill adults. *Arch Intern Med* 161:1268, 2001.
4. The urokinase pulmonary embolism trial. A national cooperative study. *Circulation* 47[2, Suppl]:II1, 1973.
5. The PIOPED Investigators: Value of the ventilation/perfusion scan in acute pulmonary embolism. Results of the prospective investigation of pulmonary embolism diagnosis (PIOPED). *JAMA* 263:2753, 1990.
6. Stein PD, Henry JW: Prevalence of acute pulmonary embolism among patients in a general hospital and at autopsy. *Chest* 108:978, 1995.
7. Goldhaber SZ, Hennekens CH, Evans DA, et al: Factors associated with correct antemortem diagnosis of major pulmonary embolism. *Am J Med* 73:822, 1982.
8. The Columbus Investigators: Low-molecular-weight heparin in the treatment of patients with venous thromboembolism. *N Engl J Med* 337:657, 1997.
9. Simonneau G, Sors H, Charbonnier B, et al: A comparison of low-molecular-weight heparin with unfractionated heparin for acute pulmonary embolism. The THESEE Study Group. Tinzaparine ou Heparine Standard: Evaluations dans l' Embolie Pulmonaire. *N Engl J Med* 337:663, 1997.
10. Kasper W, Konstantinides S, Geibel A, et al: Management strategies and determinants of outcome in acute major pulmonary embolism: results of a multicenter registry. *J Am Coll Cardiol* 30:1165, 1997.
11. Goldhaber SZ, Visani L, De Rosa M: Acute pulmonary embolism: clinical outcomes in the International Cooperative Pulmonary Embolism Registry (ICOPER). *Lancet* 353:1386, 1999.
12. Alpert JS, Smith R, Carlson J, et al: Mortality in patients treated for pulmonary embolism. *JAMA* 236:1477, 1976.
13. Carson JL, Kelley MA, Duff A, et al: The clinical course of pulmonary embolism. *N Engl J Med* 326:1240, 1992.
14. Dalen JE: Pulmonary embolism: what have we learned since Virchow? Natural history, pathophysiology, and diagnosis. *Chest* 122:1440, 2002.
15. Dalen JE, Alpert JS: Natural history of pulmonary embolism. *Prog Cardiovasc Dis* 17:259, 1975.
16. Anderson FA Jr, Spencer FA: Risk factors for venous thromboembolism. *Circulation* 107[23, Suppl 1]:I9, 2003.
17. Greengard JS, Eichinger S, Griffin JH, et al: Brief report: variability of thrombosis among homozygous siblings with resistance to activated protein C due to an Arg → Gln mutation in the gene for factor V. *N Engl J Med* 331:1559, 1994.
18. Gerhardt A, Scharf RE, Beckmann MW, et al: Prothrombin and factor V mutations in women with a history of thrombosis during pregnancy and the puerperium. *N Engl J Med* 342:374, 2000.
19. Koster T, Rosendaal FR, de Ronde H, et al: Venous thrombosis due to poor anticoagulant response to activated protein C. Leiden Thrombophilia Study. *Lancet* 342:1503, 1993.
20. Ridker PM, Hennekens CH, Lindpaintner K, et al: Mutation in the gene coding for coagulation factor V and the risk of myocardial infarction, stroke, and venous thrombosis in apparently healthy men. *N Engl J Med* 332:912, 1995.
21. Price DT, Ridker PM: Factor V Leiden mutation and the risks for thromboembolic disease: a clinical perspective. *Ann Intern Med* 127:895, 1997.
22. Middeldorp S, Henkens CM, Koopman MM, et al: The incidence of venous thromboembolism in family members of patients with factor V Leiden mutation and venous thrombosis. *Ann Intern Med* 128:15, 1998.
23. White RH: The epidemiology of venous thromboembolism. *Circulation* 107[23, Suppl 1]:I4, 2003.
24. Chastre J, Cornud F, Bouchama A, et al: Thrombosis as a complication of pulmonary-artery catheterization via the internal jugular vein: prospective evaluation by phlebography. *N Engl J Med* 306:278, 1982.
25. Trottier SJ, Veremakis C, O'Brien J, et al: Femoral deep vein thrombosis associated with central venous catheterization: results from a prospective, randomized trial. *Crit Care Med* 23:52, 1995.
26. Martin C, Viviand X, Saux P, et al: Upper-extremity deep vein thrombosis after central venous catheterization via the axillary vein. *Crit Care Med* 27:2626, 1999.
27. Merrer J, De Jonghe B, Golliot F, et al: Complications of femoral and subclavian venous catheterization in critically ill patients: a randomized controlled trial. *JAMA* 286:700, 2001.
28. Timsit JF, Farkas JC, Boyer JM, et al: Central vein catheter-related thrombosis in intensive care patients: incidence, risks factors, and relationship with catheter-related sepsis. *Chest* 114:207, 1998.
29. Lopez JA, Kearon C, Lee AY: Deep venous thrombosis. *Hematology Am Soc Hematol Educ Program* 439, 2004.
30. Nicolaides AN, O'Connell JD: Origin and distribution of thrombi in patients presenting with clinical deep venous thrombosis, in Nicolaides AN (ed): *Thromboembolism; Aetiology: Advances in Prevention and Management*. Baltimore, MD, University Park Press, 1975, p 177.
31. Hull RD, Raskob GE, Hirsh J: Prophylaxis of venous thromboembolism. An overview. *Chest* 89[5, Suppl]:374S, 1986.
32. D'Alonzo GE, Bower JS, DeHart P, et al: The mechanisms of abnormal gas exchange in acute massive pulmonary embolism. *Am Rev Respir Dis* 128:170, 1983.
33. D'Alonzo GE, Dantzker DR: Gas exchange alterations following pulmonary thromboembolism. *Clin Chest Med* 5:411, 1984.
34. Riedel M, Stanek V, Widimsky J: Spirometry and gas exchange in chronic pulmonary thromboembolism. *Bull Eur Physiopathol Respir* 17:209, 1981.
35. Wilson JE III, Pierce AK, Johnson RL Jr, et al: Hypoxemia in pulmonary embolism, a clinical study. *J Clin Invest* 50:481, 1971.
36. Sasahara AA, Cannilla JE, Morse RL, et al: Clinical and physiologic studies in pulmonary thromboembolism. *Am J Cardiol* 20:10, 1967.
37. Benotti JR, Dalen JE: The natural history of pulmonary embolism. *Clin Chest Med* 5:403, 1984.
38. McIntyre KM, Sasahara AA: The hemodynamic response to pulmonary embolism in patients without prior cardiopulmonary disease. *Am J Cardiol* 28:288, 1971.

39. McIntyre KM, Sasahara AA: The ratio of pulmonary arterial pressure to pulmonary vascular obstruction: index of pre-embolic cardiopulmonary status. *Chest* 71:692, 1977.
40. McIntyre KM, Sasahara AA: Determinants of right ventricular function and hemodynamics after pulmonary embolism. *Chest* 65:534, 1974.
41. Stein PD, Terrin ML, Hales CA, et al: Clinical, laboratory, roentgenographic, and electrocardiographic findings in patients with acute pulmonary embolism and no pre-existing cardiac or pulmonary disease. *Chest* 100:598, 1991.
42. Cranley JJ, Canos AJ, Sull WJ: The diagnosis of deep venous thrombosis. Fallibility of clinical symptoms and signs. *Arch Surg* 111:34, 1976.
43. Tapson VF: Acute pulmonary embolism. *N Engl J Med* 2008;358:1037–1052.
44. Crowther MA, Cook DJ, Griffith LE, et al: Deep venous thrombosis: clinically silent in the intensive care unit. *J Crit Care* 20:334, 2005.
45. Miniati M, Monti S, Bottai M: A structured clinical model for predicting the probability of pulmonary embolism. *Am J Med* 114:173, 2003.
46. Wells PS, Anderson DR, Bormanis J, et al: Value of assessment of pretest probability of deep-vein thrombosis in clinical management. *Lancet* 350:1795, 1997.
47. Wells PS, Ginsberg JS, Anderson DR, et al: Use of a clinical model for safe management of patients with suspected pulmonary embolism. *Ann Intern Med* 129:997, 1998.
48. Wells PS, Anderson DR, Rodger M, et al: Derivation of a simple clinical model to categorize patients probability of pulmonary embolism: increasing the models utility with the SimpliRED D-dimer. *Thromb Haemost* 83:416, 2000.
49. Wicki J, Perneger TV, Junod AF, et al: Assessing clinical probability of pulmonary embolism in the emergency ward: a simple score. *Arch Intern Med* 161:92, 2001.
50. Anderson DR, Kovacs MJ, Kovacs G, et al: Combined use of clinical assessment and D-dimer to improve the management of patients presenting to the emergency department with suspected deep vein thrombosis (the EDITED Study). *J Thromb Haemost* 1:645, 2003.
51. Wells PS, Anderson DR, Rodger M, et al: Excluding pulmonary embolism at the bedside without diagnostic imaging: management of patients with suspected pulmonary embolism presenting to the emergency department by using a simple clinical model and D-dimer. *Ann Intern Med* 135:98, 2001.
52. Miniati M, Prediletto R, Formichi B, et al: Accuracy of clinical assessment in the diagnosis of pulmonary embolism. *Am J Respir Crit Care Med* 159:864, 1999.
53. van Belle A, Buller HR, Huisman MV, et al: Effectiveness of managing suspected pulmonary embolism using an algorithm combining clinical probability, D-dimer testing, and computed tomography. *JAMA* 295:172, 2006.
54. Ollenberger GP, Worsley DF: Effect of patient location on the performance of clinical models to predict pulmonary embolism. *Thromb Res* 118(6): 685–690, 2006.
55. Kearon C: Natural history of venous thromboembolism. *Circulation* 107[23, Suppl 1]:I22, 2003.
56. Stein PD, Alavi A, Gottschalk A, et al: Usefulness of noninvasive diagnostic tools for diagnosis of acute pulmonary embolism in patients with a normal chest radiograph. *Am J Cardiol* 67:1117, 1991.
57. Worsley DF, Alavi A, Aronchick JM, et al: Chest radiographic findings in patients with acute pulmonary embolism: observations from the PIOPED Study. *Radiology* 189:133, 1993.
58. McNeil BJ, Hessel SJ, Branch WT, et al: Measures of clinical efficacy. III. The value of the lung scan in the evaluation of young patients with pleuritic chest pain. *J Nucl Med* 17:163, 1976.
59. Rodger M, Makropoulos D, Turek M, et al: Diagnostic value of the electrocardiogram in suspected pulmonary embolism. *Am J Cardiol* 86:807, 2000.
60. Ferrari E, Imbert A, Chevalier T, et al: The ECG in pulmonary embolism. Predictive value of negative T waves in precordial leads—80 case reports. *Chest* 111:537, 1997.
61. Stein PD, Goldhaber SZ, Henry JW, et al: Arterial blood gas analysis in the assessment of suspected acute pulmonary embolism. *Chest* 109:78, 1996.
62. Rodger MA, Carrier M, Jones GN, et al: Diagnostic value of arterial blood gas measurement in suspected pulmonary embolism. *Am J Respir Crit Care Med* 162:2105, 2000.
63. Weg JG: A new niche for end-tidal CO_2 in pulmonary embolism. *Crit Care Med* 28:3752, 2000.
64. Robin ED, Forkner CE Jr, Bromberg PA, et al: Alveolar gas exchange in clinical pulmonary embolism. *N Engl J Med* 262:283, 1960.
65. Hatle L, Rokseth R: The arterial to end-expiratory carbon dioxide tension gradient in acute pulmonary embolism and other cardiopulmonary diseases. *Chest* 66:352, 1974.
66. Johanning JM, Veverka TJ, Bays RA, et al: Evaluation of suspected pulmonary embolism utilizing end-tidal CO_2 and D-dimer. *Am J Surg* 178:98, 1999.
67. Wiegand UK, Kurowski V, Giannitsis E, et al: Effectiveness of end-tidal carbon dioxide tension for monitoring thrombolytic therapy in acute pulmonary embolism. *Crit Care Med* 28:3588, 2000.
68. Wells PS, Brill-Edwards P, Stevens P, et al: A novel and rapid whole-blood assay for D-dimer in patients with clinically suspected deep vein thrombosis. *Circulation* 91:2184, 1995.
69. Wells PS, Anderson DR, Bormanis J, et al: SimpliRED D-dimer can reduce the diagnostic tests in suspected deep vein thrombosis. *Lancet* 351:1405, 1998.
70. Ginsberg JS, Kearon C, Douketis J, et al: The use of D-dimer testing and impedance plethysmographic examination in patients with clinical indications of deep vein thrombosis. *Arch Intern Med* 157:1077, 1997.
71. Wells PS, Anderson DR, Rodger M, et al: Evaluation of D-dimer in the diagnosis of suspected deep-vein thrombosis. *N Engl J Med* 349:1227, 2003.
72. Brotman DJ, Segal JB, Jani JT, et al: Limitations of D-dimer testing in unselected inpatients with suspected venous thromboembolism. *Am J Med* 114:276, 2003.
73. Tapson VF: Diagnosing and managing acute pulmonary embolism: role of cardiac troponins. *Am Heart J* 145:751, 2003.
74. Douketis JD, Crowther MA, Stanton EB, et al: Elevated cardiac troponin levels in patients with submassive pulmonary embolism. *Arch Intern Med* 162:79, 2002.
75. Giannitsis E, Muller-Bardorff M, Kurowski V, et al: Independent prognostic value of cardiac troponin T in patients with confirmed pulmonary embolism. *Circulation* 102:211, 2000.
76. Douketis JD, Leeuwenkamp O, Grobara P, et al: The incidence and prognostic significance of elevated cardiac troponins in patients with submassive pulmonary embolism. *J Thromb Haemost* 3:508, 2005.
77. Pruszczyk P, Kostrubiec M, Bochowicz A, et al: N-terminal pro-brain natriuretic peptide in patients with acute pulmonary embolism. *Eur Respir J* 22:649, 2003.
78. Binder L, Pieske B, Olschewski M, et al: N-terminal pro-brain natriuretic peptide or troponin testing followed by echocardiography for risk stratification of acute pulmonary embolism. *Circulation* 112:1573, 2005.
79. Wolde M, Tulevski II, Mulder JW, et al: Brain natriuretic peptide as a predictor of adverse outcome in patients with pulmonary embolism. *Circulation* 107:2082, 2003.
80. Henry JW, Stein PD, Gottschalk A, et al: Scintigraphic lung scans and clinical assessment in critically ill patients with suspected acute pulmonary embolism. *Chest* 109:462, 1996.
81. Miniati M, Pistolesi M, Marini C, et al: Value of perfusion lung scan in the diagnosis of pulmonary embolism: results of the Prospective Investigative Study of Acute Pulmonary Embolism Diagnosis (PISA-PED). *Am J Respir Crit Care Med* 154:1387, 1996.
82. Rathbun SW, Raskob GE, Whitsett TL: Sensitivity and specificity of helical computed tomography in the diagnosis of pulmonary embolism: a systematic review. *Ann Intern Med* 132:227, 2000.
83. Stein PD, Fowler SE, Goodman LR, et al: Multidetector computed tomography for acute pulmonary embolism. *N Engl J Med* 354:2317, 2006.
84. Le Gal G, Righini M, Parent F, et al: Diagnosis and management of subsegmental pulmonary embolism. *J Thromb Haemost* 4:724, 2006.
85. Evans AJ, Sostman HD, Knelson MH, et al: 1992 ARRS Executive Council Award. Detection of deep venous thrombosis: prospective comparison of MR imaging with contrast venography. *AJR Am J Roentgenol* 161:131, 1993.
86. Meaney JF, Weg JG, Chenevert TL, et al: Diagnosis of pulmonary embolism with magnetic resonance angiography. *N Engl J Med* 336:1422, 1997.
87. Fraser DG, Moody AR, Morgan PS, et al: Diagnosis of lower-limb deep venous thrombosis: a prospective blinded study of magnetic resonance direct thrombus imaging. *Ann Intern Med* 136:89, 2002.
88. Ribeiro A, Lindmarker P, Juhlin-Dannfelt A, et al: Echocardiography Doppler in pulmonary embolism: right ventricular dysfunction as a predictor of mortality rate. *Am Heart J* 134:479, 1997.
89. Grifoni S, Olivotto I, Cecchini P, et al: Short-term clinical outcome of patients with acute pulmonary embolism, normal blood pressure, and echocardiographic right ventricular dysfunction. *Circulation* 101:2817, 2000.
90. Kucher N, Rossi E, De Rosa M, et al: Prognostic role of echocardiography among patients with acute pulmonary embolism and a systolic arterial pressure of 90 mm Hg or higher. *Arch Intern Med* 165:1777, 2005.
91. Goldhaber SZ: Echocardiography in the management of pulmonary embolism. *Ann Intern Med* 136:691, 2002.
92. McConnell MV, Solomon SD, Rayan ME, et al: Regional right ventricular dysfunction detected by echocardiography in acute pulmonary embolism. *Am J Cardiol* 78:469, 1996.
93. Stein PD, Athanasoulis C, Alavi A, et al: Complications and validity of pulmonary angiography in acute pulmonary embolism. *Circulation* 85:462, 1992.
94. Hull RD, Raskob GE, Ginsberg JS, et al: A noninvasive strategy for the treatment of patients with suspected pulmonary embolism. *Arch Intern Med* 154:289, 1994.
95. Tapson VF, Carroll BA, Davidson BL, et al: The diagnostic approach to acute venous thromboembolism. Clinical practice guideline. American Thoracic Society. *Am J Respir Crit Care Med* 160:1043, 1999.
96. Fedullo PF, Tapson VF: Clinical practice. The evaluation of suspected pulmonary embolism. *N Engl J Med* 349:1247, 2003.
97. Rosengarten PL, Tuxen DV, Weeks AM: Whole lung pulmonary angiography in the intensive care unit with two portable chest x-rays. *Crit Care Med* 17:274, 1989.
98. Ginsberg JS, Wells PS, Hirsh J, et al: Reevaluation of the sensitivity of impedance plethysmography for the detection of proximal deep vein thrombosis. *Arch Intern Med* 154:1930, 1994.

99. Hull R, van Aken WG, Hirsh J, et al: Impedance plethysmography using the occlusive cuff technique in the diagnosis of venous thrombosis. *Circulation* 53:696, 1976.
100. Hull R, Taylor DW, Hirsh J, et al: Impedance plethysmography: the relationship between venous filling and sensitivity and specificity for proximal vein thrombosis. *Circulation* 58:898, 1978.
101. Anderson DR, Lensing AW, Wells PS, et al: Limitations of impedance plethysmography in the diagnosis of clinically suspected deep-vein thrombosis. *Ann Intern Med* 118:25, 1993.
102. Kearon C, Julian JA, Newman TE, et al: Noninvasive diagnosis of deep venous thrombosis. McMaster Diagnostic Imaging Practice Guidelines Initiative. *Ann Intern Med* 128:663, 1998.
103. Kearon C, Ginsberg JS, Hirsh J: The role of venous ultrasonography in the diagnosis of suspected deep venous thrombosis and pulmonary embolism. *Ann Intern Med* 129:1044, 1998.
104. Prandoni P, Polistena P, Bernardi E, et al: Upper-extremity deep vein thrombosis. Risk factors, diagnosis, and complications. *Arch Intern Med* 157:57, 1997.
105. Erdman WA, Jayson HT, Redman HC, et al: Deep venous thrombosis of extremities: role of MR imaging in the diagnosis. *Radiology* 174:425, 1990.
106. Cham MD, Yankelevitz DF, Shaham D, et al: Deep venous thrombosis: detection by using indirect CT venography. The Pulmonary Angiography–Indirect CT Venography Cooperative Group. *Radiology* 216:744, 2000.
107. Loud PA, Katz DS, Klippenstein DL, et al: Combined CT venography and pulmonary angiography in suspected thromboembolic disease: diagnostic accuracy for deep venous evaluation. *AJR Am J Roentgenol* 174:61, 2000.
108. Wood KE: Major pulmonary embolism: review of a pathophysiologic approach to the golden hour of hemodynamically significant pulmonary embolism. *Chest* 121:877, 2002.
109. Stein PD, Hull RD, Ghali WA, et al: Tracking the uptake of evidence: two decades of hospital practice trends for diagnosing deep vein thrombosis and pulmonary embolism. *Arch Intern Med* 163:1213, 2003.
110. Hull RD: Diagnosing pulmonary embolism with improved certainty and simplicity. *JAMA* 295:213, 2006.
111. Hull RD, Raskob GE, Hirsh J, et al: Continuous intravenous heparin compared with intermittent subcutaneous heparin in the initial treatment of proximal-vein thrombosis. *N Engl J Med* 315:1109, 1986.
112. Barritt DW, Jordan SC: Anticoagulant drugs in the treatment of pulmonary embolism. A controlled trial. *Lancet* 1:1309, 1960.
113. Hirsh J, Warkentin TE, Shaughnessy SG, et al: Heparin and low-molecular-weight heparin: mechanisms of action, pharmacokinetics, dosing, monitoring, efficacy, and safety. *Chest* 119[1, Suppl]:64S, 2001.
114. Cruickshank MK, Levine MN, Hirsh J, et al: A standard heparin nomogram for the management of heparin therapy. *Arch Intern Med* 151:333, 1991.
115. Raschke RA, Reilly BM, Guidry JR, et al: The weight-based heparin dosing nomogram compared with a "standard care" nomogram. A randomized controlled trial. *Ann Intern Med* 119:874, 1993.
116. Hull RD, Raskob GE, Brant RF, et al: Relation between the time to achieve the lower limit of the APTT therapeutic range and recurrent venous thromboembolism during heparin treatment for deep vein thrombosis. *Arch Intern Med* 157:2562, 1997.
117. Hull RD, Raskob GE, Rosenbloom D, et al: Optimal therapeutic level of heparin therapy in patients with venous thrombosis. *Arch Intern Med* 152:1589, 1992.
118. Levine MN, Hirsh J, Gent M, et al: A randomized trial comparing activated thromboplastin time with heparin assay in patients with acute venous thromboembolism requiring large daily doses of heparin. *Arch Intern Med* 154:49, 1994.
119. Gould MK, Dembitzer AD, Doyle RL, et al: Low-molecular-weight heparins compared with unfractionated heparin for treatment of acute deep venous thrombosis. A meta-analysis of randomized, controlled trials. *Ann Intern Med* 130:800, 1999.
120. Dolovich LR, Ginsberg JS, Douketis JD, et al: A meta-analysis comparing low-molecular-weight heparins with unfractionated heparin in the treatment of venous thromboembolism: examining some unanswered questions regarding location of treatment, product type, and dosing frequency. *Arch Intern Med* 160:181, 2000.
121. Weitz JI: Low-molecular-weight heparins. *N Engl J Med* 337:688, 1997.
122. Wilson SJ, Wilbur K, Burton E, et al: Effect of patient weight on the anticoagulant response to adjusted therapeutic dosage of low-molecular-weight heparin for the treatment of venous thromboembolism. *Haemostasis* 31:42, 2001.
123. Nagge J, Crowther M, Hirsh J: Is impaired renal function a contraindication to the use of low-molecular-weight heparin? *Arch Intern Med* 162:2605, 2002.
124. Weitz JI, Bates SM: New anticoagulants. *J Thromb Haemost* 3:1843, 2005.
125. Ansell J, Hirsh J, Poller L, et al: The pharmacology and management of the vitamin K antagonists: the Seventh ACCP Conference on Antithrombotic and Thrombolytic Therapy. *Chest* 126[3, Suppl]:204S, 2004.
126. Warkentin TE, Greinacher A: Heparin-induced thrombocytopenia: recognition, treatment, and prevention: the Seventh ACCP Conference on Antithrombotic and Thrombolytic Therapy. *Chest* 126[3, Suppl]:311S, 2004.
127. Crowther MA, Cook DJ, Meade MO, et al: Thrombocytopenia in medical-surgical critically ill patients: prevalence, incidence, and risk factors. *J Crit Care* 20:348, 2005.
128. Warkentin TE, Cook DJ: Heparin, low molecular weight heparin, and heparin-induced thrombocytopenia in the ICU. *Crit Care Clin* 21:513, 2005.
129. Agnelli G, Becattini C, Kirschstein T: Thrombolysis vs heparin in the treatment of pulmonary embolism: a clinical outcome-based meta-analysis. *Arch Intern Med* 162:2537, 2002.
130. Dalen JE: The uncertain role of thrombolytic therapy in the treatment of pulmonary embolism. *Arch Intern Med* 162:2521, 2002.
131. Wan S, Quinlan DJ, Agnelli G, et al: Thrombolysis compared with heparin for the initial treatment of pulmonary embolism: a meta-analysis of the randomized controlled trials. *Circulation* 110:744, 2004.
132. Janata KM, Leitner JM, Holzer-Richling N, et al: Troponin T predicts in hospital and one year mortality in patients with pulmonary embolism. *Eur Respir J 2009*; 34:1357–1363.
133. Levine M, Hirsh J, Weitz J, et al: A randomized trial of a single bolus dosage regimen of recombinant tissue plasminogen activator in patients with acute pulmonary embolism. *Chest* 98:1473, 1990.
134. Tissue plasminogen activator for the treatment of acute pulmonary embolism. A collaborative study by the PIOPED Investigators. *Chest* 97:528, 1990.
135. Dalla-Volta S, Palla A, Santolicandro A, et al: PAIMS 2: alteplase combined with heparin versus heparin in the treatment of acute pulmonary embolism. Plasminogen activator Italian multicenter study 2. *J Am Coll Cardiol* 20:520, 1992.
136. Goldhaber SZ, Haire WD, Feldstein ML, et al: Alteplase versus heparin in acute pulmonary embolism: randomised trial assessing right-ventricular function and pulmonary perfusion. *Lancet* 341:507, 1993.
137. Kucher N, Rossi E, De Rosa M, et al: Massive pulmonary embolism. *Circulation* 113:577, 2006.
138. Konstantinides S, Geibel A, Heusel G, et al: Heparin plus alteplase compared with heparin alone in patients with submassive pulmonary embolism. *N Engl J Med* 347:1143, 2002.
139. The UKEP study: multicentre clinical trial on two local regimens of urokinase in massive pulmonary embolism. The UKEP Study Research Group. *Eur Heart J* 8:2, 1987.
140. Leeper KV Jr, Popovich J Jr, Lesser BA, et al: Treatment of massive acute pulmonary embolism. The use of low doses of intrapulmonary arterial streptokinase combined with full doses of systemic heparin. *Chest* 93:234, 1988.
141. Verstraete M, Miller GA, Bounameaux H, et al: Intravenous and intrapulmonary recombinant tissue-type plasminogen activator in the treatment of acute massive pulmonary embolism. *Circulation* 77:353, 1988.
142. Kanter DS, Mikkola KM, Patel SR, et al: Thrombolytic therapy for pulmonary embolism. Frequency of intracranial hemorrhage and associated risk factors. *Chest* 111:1241, 1997.
143. Kearon C, Kahn SR, Agnelli G, et al: Antithrombotic therapy for venous thromboembolic disease. American College of Chest Physicians Evidence-Based Clinical Practice Guidelines (8th Edition). *Chest* 133:454S–545, 2008.
144. Forster AJ, Wells PS: The rationale and evidence for the treatment of lower-extremity deep venous thrombosis with thrombolytic agents. *Curr Opin Hematol* 9:437, 2002.
145. Mewissen MW, Seabrook GR, Meissner MH, et al: Catheter-directed thrombolysis for lower extremity deep venous thrombosis: report of a national multicenter registry. *Radiology* 211:39, 1999.
146. PREPIC Study Group: Eight-year follow-up of patients with permanent vena cava filters in the prevention of pulmonary embolism: the PREPIC (Prevention du Risque d'Embolie Pulmonaire par Interruption Cave) randomized study. *Circulation* 112:416, 2005.
147. Yalamanchili K, Fleisher AG, Lehrman SG, et al: Open pulmonary embolectomy for treatment of major pulmonary embolism. *Ann Thorac Surg* 77:819, 2004.
148. Tapson VF, Witty LA: Massive pulmonary embolism. Diagnostic and therapeutic strategies. *Clin Chest Med* 16:329, 1995.
149. Douketis JD, Kearon C, Bates S, et al: Risk of fatal pulmonary embolism in patients with treated venous thromboembolism. *JAMA* 279:458, 1998.
150. Prandoni P, Lensing AW, Cogo A, et al: The long-term clinical course of acute deep venous thrombosis. *Ann Intern Med* 125:1, 1996.
151. Becattini C, Agnelli G, Pesavento R, et al: Incidence of chronic thromboembolic pulmonary hypertension after a first episode of pulmonary embolism. *Chest* 130:172, 2006.
152. Goldhaber SZ: Venous thromboembolism in the intensive care unit: the last frontier for prophylaxis. *Chest* 113:5, 1998.
153. Geerts WH, Heit JA, Clagett GP, et al: Prevention of venous thromboembolism. *Chest* 126[3, Suppl]:338S, 2004.
154. Samama MM, Cohen AT, Darmon JY, et al: A comparison of enoxaparin with placebo for the prevention of venous thromboembolism in acutely ill medical patients. Prophylaxis in Medical Patients with Enoxaparin Study Group. *N Engl J Med* 341:793, 1999.
155. Leizorovicz A, Cohen AT, Turpie AG, et al: Randomized, placebo-controlled trial of dalteparin for the prevention of venous thromboembolism in acutely ill medical patients. *Circulation* 110:874, 2004.
156. Cohen AT, Davidson BL, Gallus AS, et al: Efficacy and safety of fondaparinux for the prevention of venous thromboembolism in older acute

medical patients: randomised placebo controlled trial. *BMJ* 332:325, 2006.
157. Toglia MR, Weg JG: Venous thromboembolism during pregnancy. *N Engl J Med* 335:108, 1996.
158. Bates SM, Greer IA, Hirsh J, et al: Use of antithrombotic agents during pregnancy: the Seventh ACCP Conference on Antithrombotic and Thrombolytic Therapy. *Chest* 126[3, Suppl]:627S, 2004.
159. Fabian TC: Unravelling the fat embolism syndrome. *N Engl J Med* 329:961, 1993.
160. Chastre J, Fagon JY, Soler P, et al: Bronchoalveolar lavage for rapid diagnosis of the fat embolism syndrome in trauma patients. *Ann Intern Med* 113:583, 1990.
161. Clark SL, Hankins GD, Dudley DA, et al: Amniotic fluid embolism: analysis of the national registry. *Am J Obstet Gynecol* 172(4, Pt 1):1158, 1995.
162. Fred HL, Harle TS: Septic pulmonary embolism. *Dis Chest* 55:483, 1969.
163. O'Quin RJ, Lakshminarayan S: Venous air embolism. *Arch Intern Med* 142:2173, 1982.

CHAPTER 53 ■ MANAGING HEMOPTYSIS

RICHARD S. IRWIN AND KIMBERLY A. ROBINSON

OVERVIEW

Hemoptysis is defined in *Stedman's Medical Dictionary* as "the spitting of blood derived from the lungs or bronchial tubes." This common symptom may be the primary reason for seeking consultation in approximately 8% to 15% of an average chest clinic population. It elicits great apprehension in the patient and is likely to prompt early medical attention. The basis for this fear is the presumption that the hemoptysis is caused by a serious disease (e.g., cancer) and that it signals impending massive bleeding. The patient may describe an associated burning pain, vague discomfort, or bubbling sensation in the chest and shortness of breath. Hemoptysis may be scant, producing the appearance of streaks of bright red blood in the sputum, or profuse, with expectoration of a large volume of blood.

Massive hemoptysis is defined as the expectoration of 600 mL of blood within 24 to 48 hours and occurs in 3% to 10% of all patients with hemoptysis [1]. *Nonmassive hemoptysis* produces a quantity smaller than massive hemoptysis and greater than blood streaking. Dark red clots may also be expectorated when blood has been present in the lungs for days.

Pseudohemoptysis, on the other hand, is the expectoration of blood from a source other than the lower respiratory tract. It may cause diagnostic confusion when patients cannot clearly describe the source of their bleeding. Pseudohemoptysis may occur when blood from the oral cavity, nares, pharynx, or tongue drains to the back of the throat and initiates the cough reflex; when blood is aspirated into the lower respiratory tract in patients who have hematemesis; and when the oropharynx is colonized with a red, pigment-producing, aerobic, Gram-negative rod, *Serratia marcescens* [2]. This colonization may occur in hospitalized or nursing home patients who have received broad-spectrum antimicrobial agents and/or mechanical ventilatory support. Other rare causes of pseudohemoptysis are self-inflicted injuries or other bizarre tactics in the malingering patient seeking hospitalization and rifampin overdose (red man syndrome). The causes and distinguishing features of pseudohemoptysis are listed in Table 53.1.

This chapter deals with managing hemoptysis in the intensive care unit (ICU) in the context of a general discussion of hemoptysis. The management of tracheoartery fistula, traumatic rupture of the pulmonary artery due to balloon flotation catheters, and diffuse intrapulmonary hemorrhage are highlighted.

ETIOLOGY

Hemoptysis can be caused by a wide variety of disorders (Table 53.2) [3]. Although the incidences of the causes of hemoptysis have been described in several populations of patients, we are not aware of any study that has reported the most frequent causes of hemoptysis in critically ill patients.

The etiology of hemoptysis is considered here in three general categories: nonmassive, massive, and idiopathic. Patients in the ICU frequently have nonmassive hemoptysis, and the spectrum of the causes of hemoptysis in these patients probably differs little from that reported in major series. Commonly, the causes include trauma (secondary to suctioning), overzealous anticoagulation, and infection. Unlike the general ICU patient, patients with massive hemoptysis are frequently in the ICU because of their hemoptysis and thereby constitute a different subgroup of patients.

Nonmassive Hemoptysis

Although bronchitis, bronchiectasis, pneumonia, lung carcinoma, and tuberculosis have always been among the most common causes of hemoptysis, their incidence has varied depending on the study population and era. For example, in the immunocompromised patient, *Pneumocystis jiroveci*, fungal disease, *Mycobacterium tuberculosis*, and *Mycobacterium avium intracellulare* may be at the top of the differential diagnosis [4–8].

Although bleeding from tracheoartery fistula complicating tracheostomy, rupture of pulmonary artery from a balloon flotation catheter, and diffuse intrapulmonary hemorrhage may be submassive, they are discussed in the following section.

Massive Hemoptysis

The more frequent causes of massive hemoptysis likely to be seen in the ICU are listed in Table 53.3. Virtually all causes of hemoptysis may result in massive hemoptysis, but it is most frequently caused by tuberculosis, bronchiectasis, lung abscess, and lung cancer [5,6]. Infection is also the cause of bleeding from aspergilloma [9] and cystic fibrosis [10]. Idiopathic hemoptysis is less frequent in patients with massive hemoptysis and usually constitutes less than 5% of cases [4].

TABLE 53.1

DIFFERENTIAL FEATURES OF PSEUDOHEMOPTYSIS

Cause	History	Physical examination	Laboratory tests
Upper respiratory tract	Little or no cough; epistaxis, bleeding from gums when brushing teeth	Gingivitis, telangiectasias, ulcerations, lacerations, or varices of the tongue, nose, or naso-, oro-, or hypopharynx	Observing actively bleeding lesion
Upper gastrointestinal tract	Coffee-ground appearance of blood due to mixture with HCl; usually lacks the bubbly, frothy appearance of bloody sputum; nausea, vomiting, or history of gastrointestinal disease	Epigastric tenderness; signs of chronic liver disease	Acid pH of blood; blood in nasogastric aspirate; barium swallow, esophagoscopy, and gastroscopy
Serratia marcescens	Previous hospitalization, broad-spectrum antibiotics, mechanical ventilation	Normal	No red blood cells in red sputum; culture of organism
Malingering	Psychiatric illness; unconfirmed history of massive hemoptysis at midnight	Normal unless self-induced lesions seen; patients unable to cough up blood on command (patients with true hemoptysis will)	True hemoptysis usually must be ruled out (see Table 53.4)

Rupture of a pulmonary artery complicates balloon flotation catheterizations in less than 0.2% of cases [11,12]. It is fortunate that it is uncommon because it carries a mortality rate approximating 40% [12]. With the less frequent use of this procedure, this complication will likely become even more rarely seen. *Tracheoartery fistula* is also an unusual but devastating condition, complicating approximately 0.7% of tracheostomies [13]. *Diffuse intrapulmonary hemorrhage*, usually due to an immunologically mediated disease, should also be considered in the differential diagnosis of massive hemoptysis in the ICU.

Idiopathic Hemoptysis

Using the systematic diagnostic approach outlined later and in Tables 53.4 and 53.5, the cause of hemoptysis can be found in most instances. In 2% to 32% of patients (average, 12%) [14], the cause cannot be determined. This condition, called *idiopathic* or *essential hemoptysis*, is seen most commonly in men between the ages of 30 and 50 years. Prolonged follow-up studies with rare exceptions usually fail to reveal the source of bleeding, even though 10% of patients continue to have occasional episodes of hemoptysis [15]. In a subset of patients, Dieulafoy disease of the bronchus (i.e., an abnormal superficial vessel contiguous to the epithelium of the bronchial mucosa) has been demonstrated at pathologic examination when surgery has been performed for massive bleeding [16].

PATHOGENESIS

To appreciate fully the pathogenesis of hemoptysis, it is necessary to review briefly the normal anatomy of the nutrient blood supply to the lungs [17]. The bronchial arteries are the chief source of blood of the airways (from mainstem bronchi to terminal bronchioles); the supporting framework of the lung that includes the pleura, intrapulmonary lymphoid tissue; and large branches of the pulmonary vessels and nerves in the hilar regions. The pulmonary arteries supply the pulmonary parenchymal tissue, including the respiratory bronchioles. Communications between these two blood supplies, bronchopulmonary arterial and venous anastomoses, occur near the junction of the terminal and respiratory bronchioles. These anastomoses allow the two blood supplies to complement each other. For instance, if flow through one system is increased or decreased, a reciprocal change occurs in the amount of blood supplied by the other system [18]. Arteriographic studies in patients with active hemoptysis have shown that the systemic circulation (bronchial arteries) is primarily responsible for the bleeding in approximately 92% of cases [19].

The pathogenesis of hemoptysis depends on the type and location of the disease [20]. In general, if the lesion is endobronchial, the bleeding is from the bronchial circulation, and if the lesion is parenchymal, the bleeding is from the pulmonary circulation. Moreover, in chronic diseases, repetitive episodes are most likely due to increased vascularity in the involved area [21].

In bronchogenic carcinoma, hemoptysis results from necrosis of the tumor, with its increased blood supply from bronchial arteries, or from local invasion of a large blood vessel. In bronchial adenomas, bleeding is usually from rupture of the prominent surface vessels. In bronchiectasis, granulation tissue often replaces the normal bronchial wall and, with infection, this area can become irritated and bleed. In acute bronchitis, bleeding results from irritation of the unusually friable and vascular mucosa [20].

The mechanism of hemoptysis in mitral stenosis is controversial, but the most likely explanation is rupture of the dilated varices of the bronchial veins in the submucosa of large bronchi [22] due to pulmonary venous hypertension. Pulmonary venous hypertension may also be responsible for the bleeding in congestive heart failure because it is associated with widening of the capillary anastomoses between bronchial and pulmonary arteries [21].

Hemoptysis in pulmonary embolism may be due to infarction, with necrosis of parenchymal tissue, or due to hemorrhagic consolidation secondary to increased bronchial artery blood flow, which forms collaterals with the pulmonary circulation to bypass the obstructing clot [23].

TABLE 53.2

CAUSES OF HEMOPTYSIS[a]

Tracheobronchial disorders	**Localized parenchymal diseases**
Acute tracheobronchitis	Acute and chronic nontuberculous pneumonia
Amyloidosis	Actinomycosis
Aspiration of gastric contents	Amebiasis
Bronchial adenoma	Ascariasis
Bronchial endometriosis	Aspergilloma
Bronchial telangiectasia	Bronchopulmonary sequestration
Bronchiectasis	Coccidioidomycosis
Bronchogenic carcinoma	Congenital and acquired cyst
Broncholithiasis	Cryptococcosis
Chronic bronchitis	Exogenous lipoid pneumonia
Cystic fibrosis	Histoplasmosis
Endobronchial hamartoma	Hydatid mole
Endobronchial metastases	Lung abscess
Endobronchial tuberculosis	Lung contusion
Foreign body aspiration	Metastatic cancer
Mucoid impaction of the bronchus	Mucormycosis
Thyroid cancer	Nocardiosis
Tracheobronchial trauma	Paragonimiasis
Tracheoesophageal fistula	Pulmonary endometriosis
Tracheoartery fistula	Pulmonary tuberculosis
Cardiovascular disorders	Sporotrichosis
Aortic aneurysm	Thoracic splenosis
Bronchial artery rupture	**Diffuse parenchymal disease**
Congenital heart disease	Disseminated angiosarcoma
Congestive heart failure	Drugs[b] (Alemtuzumab, abciximab, gemtuzumab, anti-CD 33 monoclonal antibody)
Coronary artery bypass graft	Farmer's lung
Fat embolization	Goodpasture's syndrome
Hughes-Stovin syndrome	Idiopathic pulmonary hemosiderosis
Mitral stenosis	Immunoglobulin A nephropathy
Neonatal intrapulmonary hemorrhage	Inhaled isocyanates
Postmyocardial infarction syndrome	Charcoal lighter fluid injection
Pulmonary arteriovenous fistula	Legionnaires' disease
Pulmonary artery aneurysm	Mixed connective tissue disease
Pulmonary embolism	Mixed cryoglobulinemia
Pulmonary venous varix	Polyarteritis nodosa
Schistosomiasis	Scleroderma
Subclavian artery aneurysm	Systemic lupus erythematosus
Superior vena cava syndrome	Trimellitic anhydride toxicity
Thoracic endometriosis	Viral pneumonitis
Tumor embolization	Wegener's granulomatosis
Hematologic disorders	Isolated pulmonary pauci-immune capillaritis
Antithrombotic therapy	Pulmonary capillaritis associated with systemic vasculitides
Disseminated intravascular coagulation	Bone marrow transplantation
Leukemia	Lysinuric protein intolerance
Thrombocytopenia	**Other**
Hemophilia	Idiopathic
	Iatrogenic
	Bronchoscopy
	Cardiac catheterization
	Needle biopsy of lung

[a]Common causes; For a complete list of references, see Robinson KA, Curley FJ, Irwin RS: Managing Hemoptysis, in Irwin RS, Rippe JM (eds): *Intensive Care Medicine.* 6th ed. Philadelphia, Lippincott Williams & Wilkins, 2008, pp 588–598.

[b]Sachdeva A, Matuschak M. Diffuse alveolar hemorrhage following alemtuzumab. *Chest* 133:133, 2008.

TABLE 53.3

COMMON CAUSES OF MASSIVE HEMOPTYSIS

Infectious
Bronchitis
Bronchiectasis
Tuberculosis
Cystic fibrosis
Aspergilloma
Sporotrichosis
Lung abscess
Pneumonia in human immunodeficiency virus–infected patients
Malignant
Bronchogenic cancer
Metastatic cancer
Leukemia
Cardiovascular
Arteriobronchial fistula
Congestive heart failure
Pulmonary arteriovenous fistula
Diffuse parenchymal disease
Diffuse intrapulmonary hemorrhage
Trauma
Iatrogenic
Pulmonary artery rupture
Malposition of chest tube
Tracheoartery fistula

In tuberculosis, bleeding can occur for a variety of reasons [24]. In the acute parenchymal exudative lesion, scant hemoptysis may result from necrosis of a small branch of a pulmonary artery or vein. In the chronic parenchymal fibroulcerative lesion, massive hemoptysis may result from rupture of a pulmonary artery aneurysm bulging into the lumen of a cavity [25]. The aneurysm occurs from tuberculous involvement of the adventitia and media of the vessel [26]. When a healed and calcified tuberculous lymph node erodes the wall of a bronchus because of pressure necrosis, the patient may cough up blood as well as the calcified node (broncholith). In endobronchial tuberculosis, hemoptysis may result from acute tuberculous ulceration of the bronchial mucosa. In healed and fibrotic parenchymal areas of tuberculosis, bleeding may arise from irritation of granulation tissue in the walls of bronchiectatic airways in the same areas.

TABLE 53.4

ROUTINE EVALUATION OF HEMOPTYSIS

History
Physical examination
Complete blood cell count
Urinalysis
Coagulation studies
Electrocardiogram
Chest radiographs
±Flexible bronchoscopy[a]

[a]Although flexible bronchoscopy should not be performed in patients with some conditions (e.g., pulmonary embolism, aortopulmonary fistula), it should be routinely considered (see text).

TABLE 53.5

SPECIAL EVALUATION OF HEMOPTYSIS

Tracheobronchial disorders
Expectorated sputa for tubercle bacilli, parasites, fungi, and routine cytologic testing
Bronchoscopy
High-resolution chest CT scan
Cardiovascular disorders
Echocardiogram
Arterial blood gases on 21% and 100% oxygen
Ventilation and perfusion lung scans, venous duplex scanning
Pulmonary angiogram, MRI, spiral chest CT scan with contrast
Aortogram, CT scan with contrast
Cardiac catheterization
Hematologic disorders
Coagulation studies
Bone marrow
Localized parenchymal diseases
Expectorated sputa for parasites, tubercle bacilli, fungi, and routine cytologic testing
Chest CT scan and MRI
Aspergillus precipitins in serum
Lung biopsy with special stains
Diffuse parenchymal diseases[a]
Expectorated sputa for cytologic testing
Blood urea nitrogen, creatinine, antinuclear antibody, rheumatoid factor, complement, cryoglobulins, lupus erythematosus preparation
Serum for circulating antiglomerular basement membrane antibody and antineutrophilic cytoplasmic antibody
Serum for precipitins for hypersensitivity pneumonitis screen
Acute and convalescent serum antibody studies for Legionnaires' disease and respiratory viruses
Lung or kidney biopsy with special stains, including immunofluorescence

[a]Diffuse implies involvement of all lobes.
CT, computed tomography; MRI, magnetic resonance imaging.

In traumatic *rupture of the pulmonary artery* by a balloon flotation catheter, risk factors include pulmonary hypertension, distal location of the catheter tip, excessive catheter manipulation in an attempt to obtain a pulmonary artery-occluded pressure measurement, a large catheter loop in the right ventricle, and advanced age [12].

In *tracheoartery fistula* complicating tracheostomy, bleeding is due to trauma from the tracheostomy cannula or balloon [13]. Bleeding usually is due to rupture of the innominate artery. The fistula can form at three tracheal locations: the stoma, the intratracheal cannula tip, and the balloon. Trauma at the stoma is caused by pressure necrosis, usually because the tracheostomy was created too low (below the fourth tracheal ring); at the cannula tip because of excessive angulation of the cannula; and at the balloon site due to pressure necrosis caused by use of excessive inflation pressures.

Diffuse intrapulmonary hemorrhage associated with immunologic diseases is due to an inflammatory lesion, usually of the capillaries [27–31].

DIAGNOSIS

General Considerations

The success rate in determining the cause of hemoptysis is excellent but variable. If one accepts the diagnosis of idiopathic (essential) hemoptysis as a distinct entity [15], the cause of hemoptysis can be determined in nearly 100% of cases [14]. The diagnostic work-up of hemoptysis involves routine (Table 53.4) as well as special evaluations (Table 53.5). Routine evaluations are initially performed in every patient, whereas special studies are ordered only when the clinical setting suggests they are indicated. In general, each category of disease (Table 53.2) has its special studies (Table 53.5).

Routine Evaluation

As in any diagnostic problem, a detailed history and physical examination must be performed. These should be performed in a systematic fashion to rule not only in the common causes of hemoptysis but also in the category of the cause (Table 53.2).

Although the amount of bleeding usually is not indicative of the seriousness of the underlying disease process, a history of the frequency, timing, and duration of hemoptysis may be helpful. For example, repeated episodes of hemoptysis occurring during months to years suggest bronchial adenoma and bronchiectasis [20], whereas small amounts of hemoptysis occurring every day for weeks are more likely to be caused by bronchogenic carcinoma [32], as hemoptysis is generally a late finding in these patients. Hemoptysis that coincides with the menses (catamenial) suggests the rare diagnostic possibility of pulmonary endometriosis [33,34], whereas bleeding associated with sexual intercourse [35] or other forms of exertion suggests passive congestion of the lungs.

Although hemoptysis may be a symptom at any age, it is distinctly uncommon in the young. When hemoptysis is present before the third decade of life, it suggests an acute tracheobronchitis, a congenital cardiac or lung defect, an unusual tumor, cystic fibrosis, a blood dyscrasia, or infectious pneumonia. No matter what the age, if a patient with pneumonia who is undergoing appropriate therapy has hemoptysis that persists for more than the usual 24 hours, an endobronchial lesion or coagulopathy should be suspected.

A travel history can often be helpful in bringing certain endemic diseases to mind. This is true of coccidioidomycosis and histoplasmosis in the United States; paragonimiasis and ascariasis in East Asia; and schistosomiasis in South America, Africa, and East Asia.

Chronic sputum production before hemoptysis suggests a diagnosis of chronic bronchitis, bronchiectasis, and cystic fibrosis. The presence of orthopnea and paroxysmal nocturnal dyspnea makes likely the diagnoses of passive congestion of the lungs from mitral stenosis and left ventricular failure. A history of antithrombotic therapy suggests an intrapulmonary bleed from too large a dose or recurrent pulmonary embolism from too small a dose. The possibility of pulmonary embolism should always be considered when a patient who presents with hemoptysis has been at increased risk for deep venous thrombosis [36].

The possibility of traumatic rupture of a pulmonary artery due to balloon flotation catheterization should always be considered when these catheters are used [11,12].

Although tracheoartery fistula must be considered in the differential diagnosis of hemoptysis in every patient with a tracheostomy, it is an infrequent cause in this setting. When it occurs, the onset is almost always at least 48 hours after the procedure [13]. Although the peak incidence is between the first and second week and 72% of fistulas bleed during the first 21 days after tracheostomy, hemorrhage from this complication can also occur as late as 18 months after the procedure [13]. There is a sentinel bleed in 34% to 50% of cases [13]. Before 48 hours, bleeding from the stoma is usually due to capillary bleeding from inadequate hemostasis. Whenever hemoptysis occurs in a patient with an endotracheal tube or tracheostomy in place, trauma from suctioning should be considered, especially when coagulation is abnormal.

Although patients with diffuse intrapulmonary hemorrhage typically have hemoptysis, they occasionally do not expectorate at all but just complain of dyspnea [37], fever, cough, and malaise. Therefore, lack of hemoptysis does not rule out a substantial intrapulmonary hemorrhage [37].

The diagnosis of trimellitic anhydride–induced pulmonary hemorrhage should be suspected in workers exposed to high-dose trimellitic anhydride fumes. Exposure occurs when heated metal surfaces are sprayed with corrosion-resistant epoxy resin coatings. The syndrome requires a latent period of exposure and appears to be antibody mediated [38,39]. Respiratory failure with pulmonary infiltrates and hemoptysis has also been reported in a patient with a documented exposure and antibodies to isocyanates [40].

In a patient with the triad of known upper airway disease, lower airway disease, and renal disease, systemic Wegener's granulomatosis should be suspected. Pulmonary hemorrhage can occur at any point during the course of the illness in the patient with systemic lupus erythematosus (SLE) and can also be the initial manifestation of the disease [41]. Goodpasture's syndrome (antibasement membrane antibody–mediated disease) typically occurs in young men [42], and it has been reported to be associated with influenza infection [43], inhalation of hydrocarbons [44], and penicillamine ingestion [45]. Therefore, it should be considered in these historical contexts.

Diffuse alveolar hemorrhage should be suspected in patients who have undergone recent hematopoietic stem cell transplantation when they present with cough, dyspnea, hypoxemia, and diffuse pulmonary infiltrates. This typically occurs with marrow recovery. It has been reported to occur in approximately 20% of patients during autologous bone marrow transplantation, and it was associated with an 80% mortality rate [46]. Lung tissue injury, inflammation, and cytokine release are implicated in the pathogenesis of diffuse alveolar hemorrhage in hematopoietic stem cell transplant patients.

Physical examination may be helpful in several ways. Inspection of the skin and mucous membranes may show telangiectasias, suggesting hereditary hemorrhagic telangiectasia, or ecchymoses and petechiae, suggesting a hematologic abnormality. Pulsations transmitted to a tracheostomy cannula should heighten suspicion, or risk, of a tracheoartery fistula. Inspection of the thorax may show evidence of recent or old chest trauma, and unilateral wheeze or rales may herald localized disease such as bronchial adenoma or carcinoma. Although pulmonary embolism is not definitively diagnosed on physical examination, tachypnea, phlebitis, and pleural friction rub suggest this disorder. If crackles are heard diffusely on chest examination, passive congestion as well as other diseases causing diffuse intrapulmonary hemorrhage should be considered (Table 53.2). Careful cardiovascular examination may rule in mitral stenosis, pulmonary artery stenosis, or pulmonary hypertension.

The routine laboratory studies listed in Table 53.4 are useful for the following reasons. The complete blood cell count results may suggest the presence of an infection, hematologic disorder, or chronic blood loss. Sputum should be sent for Gram stain and culture, including studies for acid-fast organisms. In addition, sputum should be sent for cytological evaluation if the patient is a smoker and older than 40 years [47]. Idiopathic hemosiderosis or other causes of diffuse intrapulmonary hemorrhage (Table 53.2) may present only with diffuse pulmonary infiltrates and iron deficiency anemia from chronic bleeding into the lungs. Urinalysis may reveal hematuria and suggest the presence of a systemic disease associated with diffuse parenchymal disease (e.g., pulmonary renal hemorrhage syndrome due to SLE, Goodpasture's syndrome, systemic Wegener's granulomatosis, and other systemic vasculitides; Table 53.2). Although there is simultaneous evidence of clinical involvement of the lungs and kidneys in 33% of cases of Goodpasture's syndrome, there can be clinical lung involvement without renal disease in 33% and clinical renal involvement without lung disease in 33% [48,49].

Coagulation studies may uncover a hematologic disorder that is primarily responsible for the hemoptysis or that contributes to excessive bleeding from another disease. The electrocardiogram may help suggest the presence of a cardiovascular disorder. Although as many as 30% of patients with hemoptysis have negative chest radiographs [3], routine posteroanterior and lateral films may be diagnostically valuable.

When pulmonary tumor or infection is not readily apparent, there are other radiographic signs that may help to elucidate the cause and source of bleeding. Radiopaque foreign bodies may give rise to hemoptysis even years after entry into the lungs. One may note the disappearance of a calcified mediastinal lymph node after it has eroded the bronchial wall and is expectorated as a broncholith. Aortic or pulmonary aneurysms may erode into the bronchial tree. Single or multiple pulmonary cavities may suggest pulmonary tuberculosis, fungal disease, parasitic disease, acute or chronic lung abscess, neoplasm, septic pulmonary emboli, or Wegener's granulomatosis. The finding of a mass within a cavitary lesion raises the possibility of a fungus ball (aspergilloma), whereas localized honeycombing may be indicative of bronchiectasis. The presence of a new infiltrate localized to the area subtending a balloon flotation catheter suggests a rupture of the pulmonary artery [11,12]. The appearance of a new air-fluid level in a preexisting cavity or cyst suggests the location of the source of bleeding, as does a nonsegmental alveolar pattern that clears within a few days. A solitary pulmonary nodule with vessels going toward it suggests an arteriovenous fistula. In patients with hemoptysis due to pulmonary embolism, a parenchymal density abutting a pleural surface with evidence of pleural reaction or effusion is usually present [36]. The cardiac silhouette, vascular or parenchymal patterns, and the presence of Kerley B lines may be useful in documenting cardiovascular disease.

When the chest radiograph shows diffuse pulmonary infiltrates, hemorrhage from bleeding disorders (e.g., thrombocytopenia in the compromised host), lung contusion from blunt chest trauma, freebase cocaine use, and passive congestion of the lungs should be considered, in addition to the diseases listed under "Diffuse Parenchymal Disease" in Table 53.2. In the earliest stages of diffuse intrapulmonary hemorrhage, chest radiographs may appear normal, but usually the hemorrhage first appears in a diffuse alveolar pattern. This progresses to a mixed alveolar–interstitial pattern and then, when bleeding ceases entirely, to an interstitial pattern, as hemosiderin deposition accumulates.

Bronchoscopy

Even if the history, physical examination, and chest radiograph are normal, or there is an "obvious" cause of hemoptysis on the chest radiograph, bronchoscopy is invaluable not only for accurate diagnosis but also for precise localization of the pulmonary hemorrhage. It is not uncommon for bronchoscopy to establish sites of bleeding different from those suggested by chest radiography [50,51]. Bronchoscopy may not be needed in patients with stable chronic bronchitis with one episode of blood streaking, particularly if associated with an exacerbation of acute tracheobronchitis, or in patients in whom the site of bleeding was recently documented by bronchoscopic examination. In addition, patients with acute lower respiratory tract infections, and patients with obvious cardiovascular causes of hemoptysis, such as congestive heart failure and pulmonary embolism, may not require bronchoscopic examination.

In localizing the bleeding site, the best results are obtained when bronchoscopy is performed during or within 24 hours of active bleeding. The bleeding site can be localized in up to 93% of patients with a flexible bronchoscope and in up to 86% with the rigid instrument [51,52]. When the procedure is done within 48 hours, localization of bleeding can drop to 51% [53]. When bronchoscopy is done after bleeding has ceased, accurate localization is likely to be reduced even further [52]. Although the flexible bronchoscope is usually the instrument of choice in diagnosing lower respiratory tract problems, rigid bronchoscopy is preferred in cases of massive, uncontrolled hemorrhage because patency of the airway is maintained more effectively during the procedure (see Chapter 9). There are data that show that obtaining high-resolution chest computed tomography scanning before bronchoscopy may enhance the yield of bronchoscopy [53]. With the exception of tracheoartery fistula, the tracheobronchial disorders that can be diagnosed by a bronchoscopic examination are listed in Table 53.2.

Bedside bronchoscopy should not be performed to rule in the diagnosis of tracheoartery fistula [13]. In tracheostomized patients with hemoptysis, bronchoscopy should be performed to rule out other causes, such as bleeding from suction ulcers, tracheitis, or lower respiratory tract disorders. If no other cause for hemoptysis can be found and bleeding has stopped, or anterior and downward pressure on the cannula on the stomal site or overinflation of the tracheostomy balloon slows down or stops the bleeding, a surgical consultation should be sought immediately and the patient brought to the operating room for examination in a more controlled environment. *As long as tracheoartery fistula remains a diagnostic possibility, the tracheostomy balloon should not be deflated, and the tracheostomy tube should not be removed without protecting the airway below the tracheostomy tube.*

When there is no active bleeding, bronchoscopy with bronchoalveolar lavage can be helpful in suggesting diffuse intrapulmonary hemorrhage. Return of bright red or blood-tinged lavage fluid from multiple lobes from both lungs and lack of change in the appearance of fluid during serial lavage processes suggests an active, diffuse intrapulmonary hemorrhage; hemosiderin-laden macrophages (i.e., siderophages) on cytologic analysis from these same specimens suggest bleeding that has been ongoing. Because healthy subjects may have siderophages in their alveoli, the diagnosis of diffuse alveolar hemorrhage requires a substantial number of siderophages to be recovered by bronchoalveolar lavage ($\geq$20% of total alveolar macrophages) [54]. Because carbon monoxide–diffusing capacity is increased due to binding of carbon monoxide by intra-alveolar red blood cells for 24 to 48 hours after bleeding stops, this test may be helpful in suggesting intra-alveolar hemorrhage in the stable patient without hemoptysis.

Although the definitive diagnosis of bronchiectasis can be made by high-resolution chest computed tomography scan, bronchiectasis is visible on routine chest radiographs in 80% to 88% of cases, and bronchoscopy can localize the bleeding to the corresponding abnormal areas [55].

Angiography

Angiography can determine the site of bleeding in 90% to 93% of cases. When performed routinely, diagnostic angiography establishes a diagnosis not identified by bronchoscopy in only 4% of patients [52]. Technetium-labeled colloid and red blood cell studies have rarely been shown to add any information that cannot be obtained by chest computed tomography scanning and bronchoscopy. Although angiography may not be initially helpful in confirming rupture of the pulmonary artery due to balloon flotation catheterization if the rent has sealed, it can be extremely helpful in detecting a pseudoaneurysm that has formed in the healing process [12]. Identification of an unstable lesion is important because it should be obliterated to prevent future rupture and death [12]. Angiography has not been useful in diagnosing tracheoartery fistula [13].

Special Evaluation

Depending on the results of the initial evaluation and the possible categories of cause of hemoptysis (Table 53.2), additional diagnostic evaluations should be systematically performed (Table 53.5).

The diagnosis of Goodpasture's syndrome is made by demonstrating linear deposition of immunoglobulin (Ig) G along the basement membrane of the lung or kidney and the presence of high titers of circulating anti–basement membrane antibody in the blood. Antibodies from patients with traditional Goodpasture's syndrome react with the α_3(IV) chain of type IV collagen. Although Goodpasture's syndrome is typically associated with IgG, there are also reports of a pulmonary-renal hemorrhagic syndrome associated with IgA [56]. The importance of this observation is that the immunoserologic testing must be designed to include both immunoglobulins [56]. Goodpasture's syndrome can also be mimicked by fibrillary glomerulonephritis [57].

Definitive diagnosis of the pulmonary vasculitides depends on histologic examination, including special stains and cultures that rule out tuberculosis and fungal diseases. Pulmonary capillaritis with hemorrhage has been reported in an ever-increasing number of conditions [27–31]. The diagnosis can sometimes be made on transbronchial biopsy, thus avoiding the need for open lung biopsy [30], but care must be taken to exclude infectious etiologies by using special stains. Antineutrophil cytoplasmic autoantibodies are helpful in diagnosing Wegener's granulomatosis and following disease activity [58]. The complete evaluation of Wegener's granulomatosis, SLE, and mixed cryoglobulinemia is reviewed in Chapters 193 and 196. The diagnostic features of polyarteritis nodosa, the hypersensitivity vasculitides, giant cell and Takayasu's arteritis, and Behçet's disease are also presented in detail in Chapter 196. In all of these, pulmonary involvement is rare. Several cases of Henoch-Schönlein syndrome, one of the hypersensitivity vasculitides, have been reported with severe alveolar hemorrhage, including one in which immunofluorescent stains of the lung revealed granular deposits of IgA consistent with an immune complex mediation [59]. Alveolar hemorrhage has also been reported with Behçet's syndrome [60]. Giant cell arteritis involvement of the lung is suggested by upper respiratory tract symptoms of sore throat and hoarseness [61].

Although high levels of IgG, IgA, and IgM antibody to trimellitic-coupled protein and trimellitic-conjugated erythrocytes have been found in patients with trimellitic anhydride-induced pulmonary disease [38,39], the diagnosis can be made clinically by obtaining a history of the exposure and ruling out other diseases (Table 53.2).

It is important to be aware that diseases may be considered and therefore evaluated in more than one category. For instance, a patient with hemoptysis due to overzealous antithrombotic therapy may be evaluated in three categories: (a) a hematologic disorder that may cause, (b) localized, and (c) diffuse parenchymal disease. A patient with chronic bleeding from the tracheobronchial disorder of diffuse bronchial telangiectasis could present with diffuse as well as localized parenchymal disease (aspiration hemosiderosis). A patient with long-standing passive congestion of the lungs, a cardiovascular disorder, might present with diffuse pulmonary hemosiderosis, whereas a patient with acute pulmonary edema usually presents with diffuse pulmonary infiltrates.

DIFFERENTIAL DIAGNOSIS

In evaluating patients with hemoptysis, it is necessary to rule out the causes of pseudohemoptysis. Features that can help to differentiate the causes of pseudohemoptysis from one another and pseudohemoptysis from true hemoptysis are found in Table 53.1 (see Chapter 146 for an in-depth discussion of epistaxis). In addition to history and routine physical examination, it is important to perform a meticulous examination of the nose and entire pharynx, preferably with a nasopharyngoscope. Unless the cause of pseudohemoptysis is definitively determined, the spitting up of blood must be assumed to be true hemoptysis. An upper-airway lesion must not be assumed to be the cause of the bleeding unless it is seen bleeding actively at the time of examination.

TREATMENT

The treatment of hemoptysis can be divided into supportive and definitive categories. In prescribing definitive therapy, it is important to consider the cause, the amount of bleeding, and the patient's underlying lung function.

Supportive Care

Supportive care usually includes bed rest and mild sedation. Drugs with antitussive effects (e.g., all narcotics) should not be used. An effective cough may be necessary to clear blood from the airways and avoid asphyxiation. Drugs with antiplatelet effects also should not be used. Depending on the results of pulse oximetry or arterial blood gas analysis, supplemental oxygen should be given. If bleeding continues and gas exchange becomes further compromised, endotracheal intubation and mechanical ventilation may become necessary. To facilitate flexible bronchoscopy with a sufficiently large suction port, an endotracheal tube with an internal diameter of 8 mm or greater should be used, if possible. Other respiratory adjunctive therapy, such as chest physiotherapy and postural drainage [62], should be avoided. Fluid and blood resuscitation should be given when indicated.

The amount of hemoptysis should be continuously quantitated until it stops. The amount helps determine the patient's subsequent care.

Definitive Care

Nonmassive Hemoptysis

In patients with scant or frank (submassive) hemoptysis, treatment is directed at the specific cause. For instance, suppurative bronchiectasis is treated with antibiotics plus a mucociliary escalator drug (e.g., theophylline [63], β-adrenergic agonists).

Chronic bronchitis associated with cigarette smoking is treated with a mucociliary escalator and cessation of cigarette smoking. Broad-spectrum antibiotic therapy should be considered if hemoptysis occurs in the context of an acute exacerbation of chronic bronchitis. In severe exacerbations in ICU patients, Gram-negative enteric rods, *Pseudomonas aeruginosa*, *Stenotrophomonas maltophilia*, and penicillin-resistant *Streptococcus pneumoniae* may be playing a role approximately 30% of the time [64]. Cystic fibrosis is treated with appropriate antibiotics to cover the likely pathogens [65], plus a mucociliary escalator. Bronchial adenoma and bronchogenic carcinoma should be resected whenever possible. Recently, radiofrequency ablation has been used in stages III and IV non–small cell lung cancer for palliation of hemoptysis, cough, and pain, as reduction in tumor volume can lead to symptomatic improvement. However, hemoptysis has been reported as a complication of radiofrequency ablation in 0% to 12% of cases [66]. Congestive heart failure is treated with combinations of drugs for preload and afterload reductions, mitral stenosis with diuretics, and pulmonary embolism with anticoagulation. There are no data showing that patients with hemoptysis due to pulmonary embolism bleed more with anticoagulation. Therefore, do not initially withhold treatment or undertreat these patients with nonmassive hemoptysis. The effects of overzealous anticoagulation are treated with cessation of blood thinning and perhaps fresh-frozen plasma and vitamin K. Tuberculosis is treated with antituberculous drugs (see Chapter 87). Appropriate antibiotic therapy is prescribed for acute infectious pneumonias (see Chapter 68).

Massive Hemoptysis

In patients with massive hemoptysis, treatment is directed not only at the specific cause but also at abrupt cessation of bleeding. Death from massive hemoptysis is predominantly due to asphyxiation, and the likelihood of death appears directly related to the rate of bleeding [1]. Urgent management in all cases of massive hemoptysis must emphasize protecting the uninvolved lung from aspiration of blood and tamponading the bleeding site.

When tracheoartery fistula may be present, the following steps should be considered. If bleeding is immediate and profuse, there may be time only to overinflate the balloon, tamponading the potential bleeding site at the balloon, and apply downward and forward pressure on the top of the tracheostomy tube, tamponading the potential bleeding site at the stoma. If the arterial rupture is at the cannula tip, these efforts are not helpful. If bleeding stops or slows down either by these efforts or spontaneously, an endotracheal tube should be placed distal to the tip of the tracheostomy tube and a surgical consultation requested immediately. Ideally, a surgeon should be present when the tracheostomy tube is removed; should crisp bleeding start again, the surgeon can attempt to finger-tamponade/compress the bleeding artery (usually the innominate) by bluntly dissecting down the anterior tracheal wall and behind the sternum to the vessel. The vessel, once reached, can be compressed against the back of the sternum [13]. When the situation has been stabilized, clots can be gently suctioned from the distal trachea and the patient taken to the operating room for definitive repair. A review of the definitive surgical options can be found elsewhere [13].

When bleeding originates from below the primary carina, the bleeding lung should be kept dependent to minimize aspiration of expectorated blood. Numerous techniques have been advocated to help minimize aspiration and have proved helpful. A bronchoscopically positioned endobronchial balloon may provide effective tamponade. Hemoptysis due to bleeding from all lobes except the right upper lobe, because of the acute angle takeoff, has been managed with balloon occlusion [67]. This technique involves positioning a balloon to completely occlude a bronchus, thus allowing the lung to collapse distally. Small-caliber catheters with balloons can be inserted in segmental airways with bronchoscopy. Placement of a double-lumen endotracheal tube, which intubates each mainstem bronchus separately, is helpful, but the tubes can be difficult to place, and once in position, their small diameter may prevent subsequent diagnostic flexible bronchoscopy. In cases of persistent massive hemoptysis, diagnostic considerations may need to be delayed because placement of a double-lumen endotracheal tube may be necessary to ensure patient survival.

Urgent treatment to stop massive hemoptysis may involve laser bronchoscopy, iced saline lavage, angiographic embolization, supportive treatment only, or surgical resection. Use of laser to stop hemoptysis can be successful in patients with cancer, but recurrence of bleeding within a few weeks is typical. No large studies of patients with massive hemoptysis have been reported. Because laser is useful only in patients with proximal airway lesions and is difficult to use during massive hemoptysis, laser therapy will probably not evolve into a common therapeutic tool for these patients [67].

Bronchoscopically directed iced-saline lavage of the bronchi leading to the site of hemorrhage has been reported to be successful in stopping hemorrhage in an uncontrolled series [67]. In addition, in a small number of patients, bronchoscopy-guided topical hemostatic therapy using oxidized regenerated cellulose has been successful in controlling life-threatening hemoptysis [68].

Angiography can identify the bleeding site in more than 90% of cases [19,52], and, when combined with an embolization procedure, has been successful in initially stopping bleeding in massive hemoptysis in 77% to 95% of cases [69]. Several angiographic sessions may be required, and systemic and pulmonary vessels may need to be studied. Approximately 16% of patients bleed again within 1 to 4 days, and multiple procedures are frequently necessary [19,70,71]. Once active bleeding ceases, 20% of patients bleed again during the next 6 months [72] and 22% of patients by 3 to 5 years [19]. More recent studies have shown similar results [69]. Angiographic embolization has been achieved with the use of polyurethane particles, polyvinyl alcohol particles, and steel coils. Sclerosing agents have led to subsequent massive lung necrosis and should be avoided [19]. Although early studies included several cases complicated by accidental embolization of the spinal artery, the prevalence is less than 1% and occurs when the spinal artery arises from the bronchial artery [70]. Other complications, such as pleurisy or hematoma formation, are infrequent and usually minor [19].

In patients with hemoptysis due to trauma, urgent thoracotomy has been advocated, with the recommendation that it is performed with the patient in the supine position to minimize aspiration, and that the bronchovascular trunk of the involved lung is clamped while the patient is stabilized to minimize the chance of air embolism while on positive-pressure ventilation [73].

Survival from iatrogenic rupture of the pulmonary artery has been reported. Several urgent maneuvers may prove helpful, and balloon tamponade and selective intubation should always be attempted. Balloon tamponade of the ruptured vessel with the Swan-Ganz balloon has been helpful [74]. With the balloon deflated, the catheter should be withdrawn 5 cm and the balloon inflated with 2 mL of air and allowed to float back into the hemorrhaging vessel to occlude it. Ideally, patients should immediately be intubated in the mainstem bronchus opposite the involved lung to minimize aspiration. In most patients, death from pulmonary artery rupture occurs before the bleeding lung can be identified. Because the catheter usually floats to the right pulmonary artery, when it is not known which pulmonary artery has been ruptured, selective intubation of the left mainstem bronchus or placement of a double-lumen endotracheal tube should be attempted. Selective intubation of the left mainstem bronchus can be facilitated by using a bronchoscope or suction catheter designed specifically to enter the left lung. All patients who stop bleeding require angiographic evaluation to help localize the arterial tear and check for the formation of a pseudoaneurysm [12]. At the time of angiography, embolization of the affected vessel should be performed if a pseudoaneurysm or a tear is found. Hemoptysis from a pseudoaneurysm usually occurs in the first day after formation but may occur weeks later [11,12].

The role of emergency surgery for hemoptysis has changed during the past 20 years since the first report of bronchial artery embolization. Bronchial artery embolization has increasingly become first-line treatment for control of massive hemoptysis [74]. Nonetheless, surgery remains the procedure of choice when massive hemoptysis is due to arteriovenous malformations, leaky aortic aneurysm, hydatid cyst, iatrogenic pulmonary rupture, chest trauma, bronchial adenoma, and fungal balls resistant to medical therapy [70].

In patients with cystic fibrosis, even with normal lung function, resection should be avoided because repeated episodes in other areas are likely to occur. A patient with a 1-second forced expiratory volume of less than 2 L or a maximum voluntary ventilation of less than 50% of predicted should not undergo surgery unless split-lung function studies reveal that the patient is not likely to be left a respiratory cripple due to disabling dyspnea.

With respect to surgery, it is clear that no treatment preference can be recommended for all patients on the basis of reported studies. The trials of therapy span different decades of practice, have widely differing causes of hemoptysis in their populations, and use several different definitions for massive hemoptysis. A review of the literature suggests the following strategy: (a) patients who are not candidates for surgery because of their pulmonary function, general medical condition, or diffuse nature of their lesions should be treated with selective embolization; (b) resectional surgery should be performed in operable patients when surgery is the definitive treatment for the underlying disease; and (c) all potentially operable patients who continue to bleed at rates of more than 1 L per day despite supportive, conservative care and subsequent embolization should undergo surgical resection. The correct therapy in a given patient depends on the cause of the bleeding, lung function, availability of resources, and local expertise.

In patients with diffuse intrapulmonary hemorrhage, selective arterial embolization and surgery are not options. Recombinant factor VIIa has been used successfully for treatment of diffuse alveolar hemorrhage due to disseminated aspergillosis, bone marrow transplantation, small-vessel vasculitis, and cystic fibrosis [75,76]. For immunologically mediated diseases, corticosteroids, cytotoxic agents, and other interventions (e.g., plasmapheresis in Goodpasture's syndrome) are available (see Chapter 196).

When corticosteroid therapy is given alone for critically ill patients with immunologic lung diseases, the dose is 1 mg per kg per day of intravenous methylprednisolone or the equivalent dose of another corticosteroid. Larger doses, on the order of 7 to 15 mg per kg per day for 1 to 3 days, have been recommended to control progressive pulmonary hemorrhage and hypoxemia of Goodpasture's syndrome, SLE, and the vasculitides (see Chapter 193 and 196) [42]. In general, corticosteroids should be administered initially in round-the-clock divided doses until substantial improvement has occurred. They can then be given once per day and tapered as the patient's condition dictates.

When combined corticosteroid and cytotoxic drug therapy is given, it is usually prescribed for immunologic lung diseases due to the vasculitides (e.g., Wegener's granulomatosis, rheumatoid vasculitis) and Goodpasture's syndrome. For details regarding specific therapy for these conditions, see Chapters 193 and 196.

References

1. Corey R, Hla KM: Major and massive hemoptysis: reassessment of conservative management. *Am J Med Sci* 294:301, 1987.
2. Gale D: Overgrowth of *Serratia marcescens* in respiratory tract, simulating hemoptysis. *JAMA* 164:1328, 1957.
3. Robinson KA, Curley FJ, Irwin RS: Managing Hemoptysis, in Irwin RS, Rippe JM (eds): *Intensive Care Medicine.* 6th ed. Philadelphia, Lippincott Williams & Wilkins, 2008, pp 588–598.
4. Johnston H, Reiza G: Changing spectrum of hemoptysis: underlying causes in 148 patients undergoing diagnostic flexible fiberoptic bronchoscopy. *Arch Intern Med* 149:1666, 1989.
5. Hirshberg B, Biran I, Glazer M, et al: Hemoptysis: etiology, evaluation, and outcome in a tertiary referral hospital. *Chest* 112:440, 1997.
6. Santiago S, Tobias J, Williams AJ: A reappraisal of the causes of hemoptysis. *Arch Intern Med* 151:2449, 1991.
7. Nelson JE, Forman M: Hemoptysis in HIV-infected patients. *Chest* 110:737, 1996.
8. Kallay N, Dunagan DP, Adair N, et al: Hemoptysis in patients with renal insufficiency: the role of flexible bronchoscopy. *Chest* 119:788, 2001.
9. Glimp RA, Bayer AS: Pulmonary aspergilloma: diagnostic and therapeutic considerations. *Arch Intern Med* 143:303, 1983.
10. Stern RC, Wood RE, Boat TF, et al: Treatment and prognosis of massive hemoptysis in cystic fibrosis. *Am Rev Respir Dis* 117:825, 1978.
11. Dieden JD, Friloux LA III, Renner JW: Pulmonary artery false aneurysms secondary to Swan-Ganz pulmonary artery catheters. *AJR Am J Roentgenol* 149:901, 1987.
12. Bartter T, Irwin RS, Phillips DA, et al: Pulmonary artery pseudoaneurysm: a potential complication of pulmonary artery catheterization. *Arch Intern Med* 148:471, 1988.
13. Schaefer OP, Irwin RS: Tracheo-artery fistula. *J Int Care Med* 10:64, 1995.
14. Rath GS, Schaff JT, Snider GL: Flexible fiberoptic bronchoscopy: techniques and review of 100 bronchoscopies. *Chest* 63:689, 1973.
15. Adelman M, Haponik EF, Bleeker ER, et al: Cryptogenic hemoptysis: clinical features, bronchoscopic findings, and natural history in 67 patients. *Ann Intern Med* 102:829, 1985.
16. Savale L, Parrot A, Khalil A, et al: Cryptogenic hemoptysis: from a benign to a life-threatening pathologic vascular condition. *Am J Respir Crit Care Med* 175:1181, 2007.
17. Murray JF: Postnatal growth and development of the lung, in Murray JF (ed): *The Normal Lung: The Basis for Diagnosis and Treatment of Pulmonary Disease.* Philadelphia, WB Saunders, 1976, p 42.
18. Auld PA, Rudolph AM, Golinko RJ: Factors affecting bronchial collateral flow in the dog. *Am J Physiol* 198:1166, 1960.
19. Rabkin JE, Astafjev VI, Gothman LN, et al: Transcatheter embolization in the management of pulmonary hemorrhage. *Radiology* 163:361, 1987.
20. Souders CR, Smith AT: The clinical significance of hemoptysis. *N Engl J Med* 247:791, 1952.
21. Wood DA, Miller M: Role of dual pulmonary circulation in various pathologic conditions of lungs. *J Thorac Surg* 7:649, 1938.
22. Ferguson FC, Kobilak RE, Deitrick JE: Varices of bronchial veins as source of hemoptysis in mitral stenosis. *Am Heart J* 28:445, 1944.
23. Dalen JE, Haffajee CI, Alpert JS, et al: Pulmonary embolism, pulmonary hemorrhage, and pulmonary infarction. *N Engl J Med* 296:1431, 1977.
24. Kneeling AN, Costello R, Lee MJ: Rasmussen's aneurysm: a forgotten entity? *Cardiovasc Intervent Radiol* 31:196, 2008.
25. Rasmussen V: On hemoptysis, especially when fatal, in its anatomical and clinical aspects. *Edinburgh Med J* 14:385, 1968.
26. Auerbach O: Pathology and pathogenesis of pulmonary arterial aneurysm in tuberculous cavities. *Am Rev Tuberculosis* 39:99, 1939.
27. Jennings CA, King TE Jr, Tuder R, et al: Diffuse alveolar hemorrhage with underlying isolated, pauciimmune pulmonary capillaritis. *Am J Respir Crit Care Med* 155:1101, 1997.
28. Green RJ, Ruoss SJ, Kraft SA, et al: Pulmonary capillaritis and alveolar hemorrhage: update on diagnosis and management. *Chest* 110:1305, 1996.
29. Schwarz MI, Sutarik JM, Nick JA, et al: Pulmonary capillaritis and diffuse alveolar hemorrhage: a primary manifestation of polymyositis. *Am J Respir Crit Care Med* 151:2037, 1995.
30. Imoto EM, Lombard CM, Sachs DPL: Pulmonary capillaritis and hemorrhage: a clue to the diagnosis of systemic necrotizing vasculitis. *Chest* 96:927, 1989.

31. Myers JL, Katzenstein AA: Microangiitis in lupus-induced pulmonary hemorrhage. *Am J Clin Pathol* 85:552, 1986.
32. Soll B, Selecky PA, Chang R, et al: The use of the fiberoptic bronchoscope in the evaluation of hemoptysis. *Am Rev Respir Dis* 115:165, 1977.
33. Rodman MH, Jones CW: Catamenial hemoptysis due to bronchial endometriosis. *N Engl J Med* 266:805, 1962.
34. Lattes R, Shepard F, Tovell H, et al: A clinical and pathologic study of endometriosis of the lung. *Surg Gynecol Obstet* 103:552, 1956.
35. Fagin ID: Hemoptysis with intercourse. *JAMA* 240:22, 1978.
36. Moser KM: Pulmonary embolism. *Am Rev Respir Dis* 115:829, 1977.
37. Thomas HM III, Irwin RS: Classification of diffuse intrapulmonary hemorrhage. *Chest* 68:483, 1975.
38. Ahmad D, Patterson R, Morgan WKC, et al: Pulmonary hemorrhage and haemolytic anemia due to trimellitic anhydride. *Lancet* 2:238, 1979.
39. Leach CL, Hatoum NS, Ratajczak HV, et al: Evidence of immunologic control of lung injury induced by trimellitic anhydride. *Am Rev Respir Dis* 137:186, 1988.
40. Patterson R, Nugent KM, Harris KE, et al: Immunologic hemorrhagic pneumonia caused by isocyanates. *Am Rev Respir Dis* 141:226, 1990.
41. Gould DB, Soriano RZ: Acute alveolar hemorrhage in lupus erythematosus. *Ann Intern Med* 83:836, 1975.
42. Briggs WA, Johnson JP, Teichman S, et al: Antiglomerular basement membrane antibody-mediated glomerulonephritis and Goodpasture's syndrome. *Medicine* 58:348, 1979.
43. Wilson CB, Smith RC: Goodpasture's syndrome associated with an influenza A2 virus infection. *Ann Intern Med* 76:91, 1972.
44. Kleinknecht D, Morel-Maroger L, Callard P, et al: Antiglomerular basement membrane nephritis after solvent exposure. *Arch Intern Med* 140:230, 1980.
45. Sternlieb I, Bennett B, Scheinberg H: D-Penicillamine–induced Goodpasture's syndrome in Wilson's disease. *Ann Intern Med* 82:673, 1975.
46. Sisson JH, Thompson AB, Anderson JR, et al: Airway inflammation predicts diffuse alveolar hemorrhage during bone marrow transplantation in patients with Hodgkin disease. *Am Rev Respir Dis* 146:439, 1992.
47. Lordan JL, Gascoigne A, Corris PA: The pulmonary physician in critical care. Illustrative case 7: Assessment and management of massive haemoptysis. *Thorax* 58:814, 2003.
48. Wilson CB, Dixon FJ: Anti-glomerular basement membrane antibody-induced glomerulonephritis. *Kidney Int* 3:74, 1973.
49. Zimmerman SW, Varanasi UR, Hoff B: Goodpasture's with normal renal function. *Am J Med* 66:163, 1979.
50. Kim JH, Follett JV, Rice JR, et al: Endobronchial telangiectasias and hemoptysis in scleroderma. *Am J Med* 84:173, 1988.
51. Smiddy JF, Elliott RC: The evaluation of hemoptysis with fiberoptic bronchoscopy. *Chest* 64:158, 1973.
52. Saumench J, Escarrabill J, Padro L, et al: Value of fiberoptic bronchoscopy and angiography for diagnosis of the bleeding site in hemoptysis. *Ann Thorac Surg* 48:272, 1989.
53. McGuinness G, Beacher JR, Harkin TJ, et al: Hemoptysis: prospective high-resolution CT/bronchoscopic correlation. *Chest* 105:1155, 1994.
54. De Lassence A, Fleury-Feith J, Escudier E, et al: Alveolar hemorrhage: diagnostic criteria and results in 194 immunocompromised hosts. *Am J Respir Crit Care Med* 151:157, 1995.
55. Ahya VN, Tino G: Bronchiectasis: new perspectives. *J Respir Dis* 22:252, 2001.
56. Border WA, Baehler RW, Bhathena D, et al: IgA anti-basement membrane nephritis with pulmonary hemorrhage. *Ann Intern Med* 191:21, 1979.
57. Masson RG, Rennke HG, Gottlieb MN: Pulmonary hemorrhage in a patient with fibrillary glomerulonephritis. *N Engl J Med* 326:36, 1992.
58. Nolle B, Specks U, Ludemann J, et al: Anticytoplasmic autoantibodies: their immunodiagnostic value in Wegener's granulomatosis. *Ann Intern Med* 111:28, 1989.
59. Kathuria S, Chejfec G: Fatal pulmonary Henoch-Schönlein syndrome. *Chest* 82:654, 1982.
60. Raz I, Okon E, Chajek-Shaul T: Pulmonary manifestations in Behçet's syndrome. *Chest* 95:585, 1989.
61. Fauci AS, Haynes BF, Katz P: The spectrum of vasculitis: clinical, pathologic, immunologic, and therapeutic considerations. *Ann Intern Med* 89:660, 1978.
62. Tyler ML: Complications of positioning and chest physiotherapy. *Respir Care* 27:458, 1982.
63. Sutton PP, Pavia D, Bateman JRM, et al: The effect of oral aminophylline on lung mucociliary clearance in man. *Chest* 80[Suppl]:889, 1981.
64. Ewig S, Soler N, Gonzalez J, et al: Evaluation of antimicrobial treatment in mechanically ventilated patients with severe chronic obstructive pulmonary disease exacerbations. *Crit Care Med* 28:692, 2000.
65. Sood N, Paradowski LJ, Yankaskas JR: Outcomes of intensive care unit care in adults with cystic fibrosis. *Am J Respir Crit Care Med* 163:335, 2001.
66. Rose SC, Thistlewaite PA, Sewell PE, et al: Lung cancer and radiofrequency ablation. *J Vasc Interv Radiol* 17:927, 2006.
67. Dweik RA, Stoller JK: Role of bronchoscopy in massive hemoptysis. *Clin Chest Med* 20:89, 1999.
68. Valipour A, Kreuzer A, Koller H, et al: Bronchoscopy-guided topical hemostatic tamponade therapy for the management of life-threatening hemoptysis. *Chest* 127:2113, 2005.
69. White RI Jr: Bronchial artery embolotherapy for control of acute hemoptysis: analysis of outcome. *Chest* 115:912, 1999.
70. Jean-Baptiste, E: Clinical assessment and management of massive hemoptysis. *Crit Care Med* 28:1642, 2000.
71. Yu-Tang GP, Lin M, Teo N, et al: Embolization for hemoptysis: a six -year review. *Cardiovasc Intervent Radiol* 25:17, 2002.
72. Stoll JF, Bettmann MA: Bronchial artery embolization to control hemoptysis: a review. *Cardiovasc Intervent Radiol* 11:263, 1988.
73. Wilson RF, Soullier GW, Wiencek RG: Hemoptysis in trauma. *J Trauma* 27:1123, 1987.
74. Remy T, Siproudhis L, Laurent JF, et al: Massive hemoptysis from iatrogenic balloon catheter rupture of pulmonary artery: successful early management by balloon tamponade. *Crit Care Med* 15:272, 1987.
75. Macdonald JA, Fraser JF, Foot CL, et al: Successful use of recombinant factor VII in massive hemoptysis due to community-acquired pneumonia. *Chest* 130:577, 2006.
76. Lau EMT, Yozghatlian V, Kosky C, et al: Recombinant activated Factor VII for massive hemoptysis in patients with cystic fibrosis. *Chest* 136:277–281, 2009.

CHAPTER 54 ■ ASPIRATION

KIMBERLY A. ROBINSON AND RICHARD S. IRWIN

Aspiration is defined in *Webster's New Universal Unabridged Dictionary* as inhaling fluid or a foreign body into the bronchi and lungs [1]. The foreign material may be particulate matter, irritating fluids (e.g., HCl, mineral oil, animal fat), or oropharyngeal secretions containing infectious agents. Although infectious pneumonias can be caused by inhaling air-containing organisms (e.g., infectious aerosols), aspiration of oropharyngeal contents or regurgitated gastric material is the primary manner in which bacterial pathogens are introduced into the lower respiratory tract. In fact, studies indicate that 5% to 15% of cases of community-acquired pneumonia are aspiration pneumonia [2]. The medical literature is not as precise, however, in defining aspiration-induced pulmonary injury or diagnosing its occurrence. For instance, the term *aspiration pneumonia* strongly denotes infectious sequelae to the aspiration event. However, there is a wide spectrum of conditions that result from aspirating foreign matter with varying clinical courses, not all of which are caused by infection [3–5]. It is difficult to predict exactly which course a patient will follow after an event. Although aspiration of a large volume of sterile gastric contents will likely lead to a chemical pneumonitis, aspiration of contaminated gastric contents will more likely

TABLE 54.1

ASPIRATION SYNDROMES

Mendelson syndrome
Foreign body aspiration
Bacterial pneumonia and lung abscess
Chemical pneumonitis
Exogenous lipoid pneumonia
Recurrent pneumonias
Chronic interstitial fibrosis
Bronchiectasis
Mycobacterium fortuitum or *chelonei* pneumonia
Diffuse aspiration bronchiolitis
Tracheobronchitis
Tracheoesophageal fistula
Chronic persistent cough
Bronchorrhea
Drowning

result in an infectious pneumonia. Although the frequency of all clinically significant aspirations in the intensive care unit (ICU) setting is not known, a review of Table 54.1 suggests that aspiration syndromes are common causes of pulmonary disease in the critically ill patient. An in-depth discussion of drowning can be found in Chapter 54.

NORMAL DEFENSES AGAINST ASPIRATION AND THE MANNER IN WHICH THEY MAY FAIL

Pathogenesis

Syndromes caused by aspiration are determined by (a) the material aspirated, (b) the amount aspirated, and (c) the state of the patient's defenses at the time of the event. An understanding of the normal defenses and how and when they become impaired is also the cornerstone for an understanding of the pathogenesis of the various aspiration syndromes.

Because gastric acid prevents bacterial growth, the gastric contents are sterile under normal conditions [6]. Nevertheless, it has long been thought that the pH of aspirated contents determined the clinical course, with lower pH aspirates portending a worse outcome. Elevation of gastric pH to protect the lung was cited as one reason to use prophylactic antacids in the critically ill patient. However, colonization of the stomach by pathogenic organisms may occur when the gastric pH is artificially elevated [7,8]. Therefore, routine intratracheal instillation of prophylactic antacids to minimize aspiration-related lung injury is not recommended. There is conflicting data as to whether or not proton pump inhibitors and H2 blockers increase the risk of pneumonia [9,10]. Continued use of prophylactic acid suppression to prevent gastric bleeding and ulceration is another issue entirely and is discussed in Chapter 92.

Upper Gastrointestinal Defenses

Gastrointestinal mechanisms normally work in a coordinated, synchronized fashion. The teeth break up large food particles, and the tongue propels fluid and masticated food into the hypopharynx. As the hypopharyngeal muscles prepare to move food into the esophagus, the epiglottis covers the laryngeal inlet and the vocal cords close and the upper esophageal sphincter (cricopharyngeus muscle) relaxes. Pharyngeal swallowing initiates primary peristaltic waves in the esophagus that carry fluid and food through a relaxed lower esophageal sphincter (LES) into the stomach. After the bolus enters the stomach, the LES then contracts and prevents, although not entirely, gastroesophageal reflux (GER).

Even in the absence of known trauma or neurologic insult that could affect the swallowing cascade, some of the previously mentioned defenses may become impaired with increasing age or during sleep leading to silent aspiration. The vocal cords close much more slowly after the age of 50 years and may not close at all during sleep or with sedation irrespective of age. Furthermore, the cough response to airway irritation is also decreased during sleep compared with the waking state and may be totally absent during rapid eye movement sleep. In fact, it has been estimated that half of all healthy adults aspirate oropharyngeal secretions during sleep [3].

The risk of aspirating fluid and food is increased when the normal swallowing and upper gastrointestinal mechanisms fail to work in a coordinated, synchronized manner. Failure to adequately masticate one's food, such as in the edentulous or sedated patient, establishes a high risk for aspiration [11]. Aspiration also may occur when the bolus cannot readily be cleared from the pharynx owing to neuromuscular disorders of any cause [12–15]. Structural abnormalities like Zenker's diverticulum places a patient at risk of aspiration because the diverticulum may empty "late" after the swallowing effort is completed, at the time when the vocal cords are abducted. Conditions in which vocal cord closure becomes excessively delayed (e.g., old age, debilitation, sedation, the presence of a tracheostomy, and after endotracheal extubation) place patients at high risk for aspiration.

Regurgitation and subsequent aspiration of stomach contents also occur in elderly, sedated, or sleeping patients, especially when their upper esophageal sphincter and LES have been rendered incompetent by an oral or nasogastric tube [16,17]. The risk of aspiration is enhanced when such a patient remains in the supine position [18], a scenario often encountered in the ICU setting.

Respiratory Defenses

For infectious agents to enter the lower respiratory tract (e.g., below the vocal cords), they must first escape aerodynamic filtration in the nose, mouth, and larynx. Particles larger than 10 μm in diameter never reach the lower respiratory tract because they are filtered out of the airstream in the upper airway. Particles between 2 and 10 μm in diameter can reach the airways, and those between 0.5 and 1.5 μm in diameter can reach the alveoli. This is particularly relevant as most bacteria are within this size range. Although mucociliary clearance removes the larger particles [19] from the larger airways, additional defense mechanisms are needed to clear the smaller particles. This is accomplished in respiratory bronchioles and alveoli primarily by the alveolar macrophages, aided by neutrophils [20]. Infectious agents are detoxified by lysozymes as part of the cellular clearance mechanism [21]. Enzymes secreted by alveolar macrophages, neutrophils, and proteases in mucus also contribute to the detoxification process.

The first line of defense is mucociliary clearance. The respiratory filtration system and mucociliary clearance may become overwhelmed with large-volume fluid and food aspiration or with large amounts of inhaled infectious agents. Respiratory defenses may also become ineffective in the following settings: inhalational or systemic general anesthesia, endotracheal intubation, endotracheal suctioning, hypercapnia and hyperoxia, smoking, asthma, chronic bronchitis, cystic fibrosis and bronchiectasis, and respiratory infections with viruses and *Mycoplasma pneumoniae*.

In the absence of mucociliary clearance, the airways can still be cleared of excessive secretions and foreign bodies if the patient has an effective cough [19]. However, cough is not a primary defense mechanism and only provides clearance when mucociliary clearance is inefficient or overwhelmed. An effective cough and rapid closure of the vocal cords might also limit the consequences of GER of gastric contents to a chemical laryngitis. Alternatively, an effective cough with slow closure of the vocal cords might limit the inhalational injury to a chemical tracheobronchitis. An effective cough is determined both by good expiratory flow rates and respiratory muscle strength [22]. Thus, cough may be ineffective in patients with severe asthma, chronic obstructive pulmonary disease, respiratory neuromuscular disorders, painful incisions, or in those receiving excessive sedation and analgesia with antitussive effects.

When the mechanical defenses are overwhelmed, alveolar macrophages represent the initial phagocytic response. These cells also trigger additional inflammatory and immune responses by secreting cytokines. This response is followed by the influx of neutrophils into the alveolar spaces. Neutrophils are critical for the eradication of bacterial agents and therefore any impairment in their function would be detrimental [20]. Aspirated bacteria cause infectious pneumonia when the alveolar phagocytes become impaired, such as in alcoholism, pH less than 7.2, acute alveolar hypoxia, alveolar hyperoxia, corticosteroid therapy, respiratory viral infections, hypothermia, starvation, and exposures to nitrogen dioxide, sulfur dioxide, ozone, and cigarette smoking on a long-term basis [3].

Immunologic defenses such as complement and immunoglobulins augment the nonimmunologic mechanisms previously mentioned by opsonizing bacteria for the alveolar phagocytes [23,24]. Although the role of immunologic defenses against infectious particles is sketchy, it is believed that they are important in augmenting and occasionally directing the alveolar phagocytes. For instance, patients with hereditary and acquired immunologic abnormalities, such as immunoglobulin G and complement deficiencies, are susceptible to frequent and often severe bacterial pneumonias. For a more complete list of references for this section, please refer to the previous edition of this chapter published in *Irwin and Rippe's Intensive Care Medicine*, sixth Edition [3].

PREVALENCE OF ASPIRATION IN THE CRITICALLY ILL

Aspiration should be considered in all ICU patients with a pulmonary problem. This is especially true for the elderly, debilitated, or sedated patient with unexplained deterioration in pulmonary status. Oral or nasal enteral feeding tubes that compromise the LES, anticholinergics that decrease gastric motility, history of dysphagia, and neck hyperextension increase the probability. The presence of an endotracheal tube or tracheostomy tube poses a high risk for aspiration and its consequences.

Translaryngeal Intubation

Clearly, no one to feed a patient with an oral or nasal endotracheal tube in place, given the obvious mechanical barrier and distortion of the swallowing structures. What is often less intuitive is that dysphagia may persist for a variable time after the endotracheal tube has been removed. It has been suggested that the swallowing reflex can be impaired for up to 48 hours after short-term extubation, but gradually improves within a week [25]. Recent data suggest that the addition of routine flexible endoscopic evaluation of swallowing (FEES) aids in the identification of patients who are at high risk of aspirating after endotracheal intubation [26–29]. Awake, postsurgical patients who were intubated for less than 28 hours for coronary artery bypass were evaluated for aspiration. Of the 24 patients examined immediately after extubation, 50% aspirated, whereas 25% and 5% aspirated when tested 4 and 8 hours, respectively, after extubation. Patients who were intubated for a longer duration of, on average, 6.3 ± 3.1 days also demonstrated a high incidence of aspiration when evaluated 2 to 3 days after extubation [30]. Twelve of the 22 patients aspirated when evaluated by modified barium swallow/video fluoroscopy (MBS/VF).

The basis of aspiration in patients who had translaryngeal intubation can be partially explained by well-documented changes of laryngeal and pharyngeal structure and function after extubation. Impaired laryngeal elevation, penetration, and pooling in the valleculae and pyriform sinuses can be witnessed on MBS/VF. Direct laryngoscopy revealed varying degrees of laryngeal edema in 94% of patients, in which 64% took up to 4 weeks to resolve [31]. Edema of the arytenoids, inflammation of the posterior aryepiglottic folds, and false vocal cords have also been described when evaluated 24 hours after decannulation [3]. Should aspiration occur, ciliary clearance and other respiratory defenses might not respond appropriately due to the physical insult of the endotracheal tube.

Tracheostomy Intubation

Patients with a tracheostomy tube, with or without dependence on mechanical ventilation, are also at high risk for aspiration. The tracheostomy tube interferes with proper laryngeal elevation that is necessary for effective glottic closure during swallowing [32], and an inflated cuff can compress neighboring swallowing structures, most notably the esophagus. Bronchoscopic evaluation of patients with chronic tracheostomy tubes often reveals laryngeal, pharyngeal, and subglottic edema, presumably owing to the irritation of pooled secretions. These anatomic changes may exacerbate dysphagia. In one study, despite a normal clinical bedside evaluation, a high clinical suspicion for aspiration prompted an MBS/VF examination, in which 63% of a selected group silently aspirated [33]. Another study evaluating the outcome of an MBS/VF examination of patients with chronic tracheostomies discovered that 50% aspirated, and 77% of the aspiration events were silent. These studies stress that bedside evaluation alone is insufficient to diagnose aspiration in these high-risk patients.

Enteral Feeding Catheters

Many patients in an ICU have nasal or oral gastric tubes for nutritional support. The mere presence of an oro- or nasogastric feeding tube increases the risk of reflux and aspiration by compromising the integrity and proper functioning of the LES by two mechanisms. First, the catheter prevents closure of the sphincter by direct mechanical interference. Second, the irritation of the pharynx by the tube promotes LES relaxation through vagally mediated pharyngeal mechanoreceptors [34]. In addition, the presence of a nasogastric feeding tube is associated with Gram-negative bacterial contamination of the oropharynx, which, when aspirated, can result in severe clinical deterioration [35].

Varying the size of the enteral feeding catheters and adjusting the location of the distal tip have been used in an attempt to minimize aspiration. However, decreasing the size of a nasal or oral tube for enteral feeding does not reduce GER or microaspiration events [36]. Small-bore feeding tubes appear to provide no added benefit with respect to reflux events, even when advanced to the postpylorus position [17,37]. Patients with long-standing swallowing defects or on prolonged mechanical ventilation may be candidates for percutaneous gastrostomy or jejunostomy tubes; however, even percutaneous enteral feeding tubes alter lower esophageal tone and allow for reflux [38]. This manner of enteral feeding is not completely protective against aspiration despite bypassing the LES. In fact, patients fed by gastrostomy tubes have the same incidence of pneumonia as those fed by nasogastric tubes [39,40]. However, early gastrostomy may reduce the frequency of ventilator-associated pneumonia as compared with nasogastric tubes in stroke or head injury patients [41]. Feeding tubes offer no protection against colonized oral secretion or aspiration of gastric contents that, in the presence of tube feeds, have an increased pH and are often colonized with bacteria. Furthermore, although a percutaneous jejunostomy tube may minimize the large-volume aspiration events, it is a misconception that it prevents aspiration or decreases its incidence relative to a percutaneous gastrostomy tube [42].

Although there is little agreement over what constitutes excessive gastric residual volumes that place a patient on enteral feeds at increased risk of aspiration, some authors cite 200 mL for nasogastric tubes and 100 mL with percutaneous gastrostomy tubes [43]. If life-threatening aspiration events continue to occur, it may become necessary to consider performing a tracheostomy and close off the laryngeal inlet with a purse-string suture in nonverbal patients who enjoy eating by mouth.

DIAGNOSIS OF AN ASPIRATION SYNDROME

Aspiration syndromes are underdiagnosed. Failure to make the diagnosis probably stems from the glut of articles in the 1970s, stressing the importance of anaerobic aspiration infections. In addition, diagnostic failures may be ascribed to a widespread tendency to consider only infectious pulmonary complications of aspiration, an overreliance on inaccurate sputum sampling techniques such as expectorated sputum, and the misconception that aspiration must be witnessed before it can be assumed to have occurred.

Bedside Evaluation

Table 54.2 outlines all the studies that may be necessary to diagnose aspiration syndromes accurately (see "Differential Diagnosis and Treatment" section). In addition to taking a history and performing a physical examination, the physician should watch the patient swallow from a glass of water, when appropriate, to uncover an obvious swallowing problem. Although the bedside evaluation is not sensitive, a pharyngeal problem may be evident by watching the patient cough, sputter, and tilt his or her neck and head in an unnatural posture.

Gag Reflex

Although the gag reflex is frequently assessed in clinical practice to predict the adequacy of swallowing and mental alertness, and by inference the potential risk of aspiration, theoretical considerations and the paucity of studies do not support this practice [44–46]. It should not be assumed that testing for an intact gag reflex helps assess swallowing for the following reasons: (a) the stimuli and the neuromuscular processes involved in gagging and swallowing are in opposite directions, (b) the normal stimulus for swallowing food does not normally stimulate gagging, (c) many healthy individuals who do not have a gag reflex can swallow normally, and (d) there are no studies

TABLE 54.2

MODALITIES FOR DIAGNOSING ASPIRATION SYNDROMES[a]

History
Physical examination
Baseline examination
Observation of patient drinking water
Chest radiographs
Lower respiratory studies
Expectorated samples
Bronchoscopy
Protected specimen brush with quantitative cultures
Bronchoalveolar lavage
Lung biopsy
Upper gastrointestinal studies
Contrast films
Endoscopy
Esophageal manometry
GE scintiscan
24-Hour esophageal pH/impedance monitoring
Speech and swallow evaluation
FEES or modified barium swallow/video fluoroscopy

[a]The order of when and in whom to order these tests will depend on the patient populations and their presentations.
FEES, flexible endoscopic evaluation of swallowing; GE, gastroesophageal.

that show that the presence or absence of a gag can predict adequacy of swallowing. In support of this viewpoint, 11 patents without prior neurologic disorders were examined for swallowing safety with an MBS/VF examination after prolonged translaryngeal intubation [47]. Although more than half had an intact gag, swallowing dysfunction was seen in all and frank aspiration in 25% of patents.

Modified Barium Swallow/Video Fluoroscopy

Although observing patients can be useful when there is obvious difficulty during swallowing, aspiration is often silent in the critically ill patient. The incidence of silent aspiration in stable patients receiving long-term mechanical ventilation via a tracheostomy is high, between 63% and 77%, as determined by MBS/VF [33,48]. Therefore, bedside evaluation alone, particularly in these high-risk populations, is insensitive; a negative bedside examination should be confirmed by a more objective method to evaluate aspiration.

Currently, the MBS/VF study remains the gold standard in the evaluation of possible aspiration because it defines the pharyngeal anatomy with swallowing of a radiopaque contrast material, and the swallowed bolus is followed in "real time" under fluoroscopy. Findings indicative of swallowing dysfunction that can be assessed by MBS/VF examination include premature leakage of oral contents into the pharynx, penetration of swallowed material into the nasopharynx during a swallow, retention of material in the valleculae and pyriform recesses, and laryngeal penetration and aspiration [49]. Also, the elevation and tilting of the larynx that accompanies a normal swallow can be observed easily. Lower esophageal diseases, such as reflux or obstruction, can also be observed with the MBS/VF study. Various consistencies of barium are used in this MBS/VF evaluation, such as thin liquids, paste consistency, and solid food.

The MBS/VF examination, however, has multiple limitations. MBS/VF is personnel-intensive, requires transporting patients to the radiology department, and exposes patients to radiation. In addition, patients must adhere to a defined body position to accommodate the fixed fluoroscopy setup, which may not be possible for all patients. MBS/VF requires the delivery of barium-covered food or liquid to evaluate proper swallowing function and cannot evaluate a "dry swallow." Thus, aspiration and resulting deterioration may occur as a consequence of the examination itself.

Ideally, a speech and swallowing evaluation should be ordered whenever a patient is undergoing an MBS/VF examination so that a speech pathologist can accompany the patient to the examination. Then, specific recommendations can be made to prevent or minimize aspiration. Recommendations may consist of eliminating oral feeding or instituting various swallowing strategies such as the chin tuck, multiple swallows, turning of the head, or changing the consistency of solids and liquids.

Flexible Endoscopic Evaluation of Swallowing

Evaluation of swallowing under flexible endoscopic visualization has been shown to be sensitive in discerning a delay in swallowing initiation, penetration, aspiration, and pharyngeal residue [29,50–53]. The potential advantages include reduced cost and decreasing waiting time as compared with an MBS/VF evaluation. Patients avoid radiation exposure, and the examination can be performed at the bedside in varying body positions. FEES also allows visualization of pharyngeal secretions as well as identifying the source of the secretions that cannot be seen during MBS/VF. Potential risks associated with the procedure include gagging, laryngospasm, vasovagal syncope, topical anesthetic adverse reactions, and epistaxis [50]. Furthermore, esophageal pathology and reflux cannot be concurrently evaluated as in MBS/VF.

FEES has now been extensively used in medical and surgical inpatients and, more specifically, in recently extubated ICU patients [26,54]. In 2001, the Evidence-Based Practice Center published data with regard to prevention of pneumonia in stroke patients [55]. In a long-term care facility, when FEES was used to evaluate for and manage dysphagia, there were no cases of aspiration pneumonia. There were 11 cases of pneumonia documented in those patients who did not undergo FEES during the 6-month study period [55]. Concurrent evaluation by FEES and MBS/VF has demonstrated that FEES is as sensitive, if not more so, as MBS/VF. Therefore, it may be a useful diagnostic adjunct in selected immobile ICU patients.

Culture Evaluation

Even when history or physical examination uncovers a swallowing defect, determining that an aspiration event has already occurred may also prove challenging. Furthermore, an infectious process is not always established with each aspiration event. It is often difficult to distinguish between an inflammatory or "chemical" pneumonitis and an infection because both may present with fever, cough, and an infiltrate on a chest radiograph. If an infection is suspected, identification of the responsible organism is oftentimes elusive because routine expectorated sputum smears and cultures are inaccurate. Specimens obtained from quantitative bronchoalveolar lavage or telescoping plugged catheters at bronchoscopy can help to identify the lower respiratory tract infectious agent more accurately and are used preferentially, although they require an invasive procedure and moderate sedation. When accurate lower respiratory sampling techniques are used and the culture and smear results are negative, in a patient who has not recently received antibiotics, an exogenous lipoid pneumonia or chemical pneumonitis must be considered [56].

Detection of Aspirated Enteral Feeds

With respect to bedside methods for detecting aspiration in tube-fed patients, two methods have predominated, neither test is sufficiently sensitive to be recommended and both are problematic. In the first, blue food coloring or methylene blue is added to enteral feeds and the tracheal secretions are assessed for blue discoloration. Potential problems with this method include tissue absorption of the dye as well as increased risk of infection if the dye is contaminated. The second method tests tracheal secretions with glucose oxidase reagent strips for aspirated carbohydrates. The glucose method is nonspecific because varying concentrations of glucose have been recovered from tracheal secretions in nonfed, parenterally fed, and enterally fed patients. [57]. Therefore, the glucose test lacks specificity.

DIFFERENTIAL DIAGNOSIS AND TREATMENT

Treatment of the various aspiration syndromes should be prophylactic as well as specific. As previously mentioned, a formal speech and swallowing evaluation should be obtained whenever a swallowing condition is suspected or diagnosed. Specific recommendations can often be made to mitigate or eliminate aspiration from dysphagia. Precautionary rather than reactionary measures are likely to be far more effective, with less associated morbidity and mortality. However, the only preventive interventions that have been proven effective in the acute care setting include withholding oral feeding in sedated patients to prevent aspiration [58] and elevating the head of the bed to at least 45 degrees to decrease GER and minimize subsequent aspiration [18].

A tracheoesophageal fistula is a rare complication resulting from injury to the posterior tracheal wall. This can occur from excessive endotracheal tube cuff pressure, direct injury during placement of a percutaneous tracheostomy, or erosion from the tip of a tracheostomy tube. In a mechanically ventilated patient, a tracheoesophageal fistula may present with increased secretions, evidence of aspiration of gastric contents, recurrent pneumonias, a persistent cuff leak, or severe gastric distention. Once a patient is extubated, the most frequent symptom is coughing after swallowing. The diagnosis can be made by bronchoscopy and esophagoscopy, or by computed tomography scan of the mediastinum. Although definitive repair often requires surgical intervention, aspiration can be minimized by placing the cuff of the tracheostomy tube distal to the fistula [59].

Although a cuffed endotracheal tube does not offer complete protection against aspiration, all patients with severely altered consciousness and enteral feeding tubes in place should be prophylactically intubated, whenever possible, for airway protection. Furthermore, once a patient is extubated, oral intake should not be resumed until an MBS/VF or FEES examination demonstrates swallowing competency [48]. Prophylactic antibiotics, corticosteroids [60], postpyloric feeding [42], gastric promotility agents, or gastric acid suppression cannot be routinely recommended at this time to prevent or minimize aspiration [5]. GER disease with aspiration can be treated with a variety of measures, including head-of-the-bed elevation; a high-protein, low-fat antireflux diet; nothing to eat or drink for

2 to 3 hours before recumbency; no snacking between meals; acid suppression; and prokinetic drugs. If these measures fail, surgery with fundoplication may become necessary [58].

Mendelson Syndrome

Mendelson syndrome is synonymous with the acute respiratory distress syndrome [3] owing to the parenchymal inflammatory reaction caused by a large volume of aspirated liquid gastric contents. After an aspiration event, clinical status and radiographic changes progress within the next 24 to 36 hours. Contrary to the general view that gastric aspirates with pH greater than 2.5 are benign, the same syndrome can occur at a pH of 5.9 [61]. Patients who develop this syndrome invariably have a marked disturbance of consciousness, such as sedative drug overdose or general anesthesia that interferes with vocal cord protection. The subsequent clinical course can include death in 30% to 62% of cases. Once liquid gastric content aspiration has occurred and the acute respiratory distress syndrome has supervened, ventilatory and medical strategies appropriate for treating the acute respiratory distress syndrome become the focus of care. Despite their frequent use, parenteral corticosteroids have not been shown to be helpful [3]. Antibiotics are indicated only when the syndrome is complicated by infection.

Foreign Body Aspiration

Aspiration of solid particles causes varying degrees of respiratory obstruction. Most cases occur in children. When foreign bodies are inhaled into the tracheobronchial tree, 38% of patients give a clear diagnostic history, 22% give a history of an acute choking and coughing episode, and 40% complain of cough and dyspnea and are heard to wheeze. Although the chest radiograph may demonstrate the foreign object, atelectasis, or obstructive emphysema, it is normal in 80% of the cases.

Food asphyxiation is obstruction by food of the upper respiratory tract, usually at the level of the hypopharynx. It may occur whenever and wherever people eat, including hospitalized patients. In restaurants, it is called the *café coronary* because it is often mistaken for a heart attack [62]. Food asphyxiation should be suspected in middle-aged or elderly patients with poor dentition or dentures that impair chewing adequately or in those sedated by alcohol or other drugs who attempt to swallow solid food. One key to a large foreign body aspiration that may obstruct the larynx or trachea is that the patient cannot speak. Particles that reach the lower respiratory tract and do not totally obstruct the trachea can be removed by coughing or bronchoscopy. Those that totally obstruct the trachea must be removed immediately by subdiaphragmatic abdominal thrusts and finger sweeps in the unconscious individual and chest thrusts in the markedly obese person and women in advanced stages of pregnancy [63].

Bacterial Pneumonia and Lung Abscess

Although not widely appreciated, most bacterial pneumonias are a consequence of aspiration of oropharyngeal infectious material in association with impairment of lower respiratory tract defenses [64]. Preexisting gingival disease is a prominent risk factor for anaerobic infections. The risk of aspiration pneumonia is lower in edentulous patients and in those who receive aggressive oral care [65]. Community-acquired pneumonia can occur when bacteria colonize the oropharynx prior to aspiration and are unable to be cleared by mucociliary clearance and detoxification by the alveolar phagocytes that have been rendered ineffective. Normal respiratory defenses and mucociliary clearance may be compromised by a preceding viral infection or underlying medical conditions that predispose to a bacterial "superinfection" [23]. Anaerobic pneumonia or lung abscess probably occurs in alcoholics with pyorrhea because an overwhelming number of anaerobes are aspirated [66]. Because cough is suppressed, the aspirate is not readily cleared and airways are temporarily obstructed. Distal to this obstruction, anaerobes may not be killed by alveolar phagocytes that are probably rendered ineffective owing to alcohol and acute local hypoxia. Community-acquired aspirational bacterial pneumonias are most commonly due to *Streptococcus pneumoniae* and other aerobic bacteria and anaerobes [67]. Nosocomial aspiration bacterial pneumonias, in contrast, are most commonly due to facultative, enteric Gram-negative bacilli and *Staphylococcus aureus* in 50% to 75% of cases [68,69]; anaerobes play little to no role at all. The intubated patient is particularly susceptible to aspiration pneumonia because the endotracheal or tracheostomy tube bypasses the aerodynamic filtration protection of the upper respiratory tract and physically hinders mucociliary clearance. The intubated patient who requires a narcotic is at even greater risk because cough is also suppressed.

Once a bacterial pneumonia or lung abscess is suspected, the causative organism(s) should be identified and appropriate antibiotic therapy given (see Chapters 68 and 77). To help prevent future anaerobic infections, periodontal disease must be definitively treated and the alcoholic persuaded to stop drinking.

Chemical Pneumonitis

Reminiscent of a chemical burn, airway and parenchymal injury may develop after an aspiration event that triggers a cascade of inflammatory mediators [5]. Fever, cough, rales, sputum production, hypoxemia, and infiltrates on chest radiograph may all be presenting signs and symptoms that are nonspecific. What distinguishes this syndrome from the other aspiration sequelae, however, is the rapid, self-limited course and clinical resolution over several days without the need for antimicrobial therapy. Infectious aspiration pneumonia may not be a primary event but may develop as a superinfection of aspiration-induced pulmonary injury, depending on the contents of the aspirated material and the patient's underlying clinical condition.

Exogenous Lipoid Pneumonia

Exogenous lipoid pneumonia is the result of aspirating any kind of oil- or fat-based substance. Examples of aspirated fatty substances that have led to an exogenous lipoid pneumonia include mineral oil, animal oil (e.g., cod liver oil, milk products), vegetable oil [70], and formula feedings [71]. Conditions more likely to be complicated by exogenous lipoid pneumonia include pharyngeal swallowing disorders, Zenker's diverticulum, cricopharyngeal achalasia, scleroderma involving the esophagus, epiphrenic diverticulum, esophageal carcinoma, esophageal achalasia, and GER disease [72]. Although patients with exogenous lipoid pneumonia usually do not appear toxic, the clinical presentation occasionally cannot be distinguished from that of acute bacterial pneumonia. The varying clinical presentation depends in part on the type of oil aspirated [70]. Aspiration of mineral oil is less likely to produce a toxic reaction than animal fat.

The important clues to the diagnosis must come from the history, physical examination, and upper gastrointestinal studies. The presence of food particles in a bronchoscopy specimen is diagnostic. Although fat stains performed on unfixed expectorated sputum, bronchoalveolar lavage specimens, or lung biopsy may reveal numerous lipid-laden alveolar macrophages, this finding only supports the diagnosis of exogenous lipoid pneumonia. Lipid-laden macrophages can also arise from an endogenous source or represent a nonspecific response of the lung to injury [56]. Quantitative cultures obtained with telescoping plugged catheters at bronchoscopy may be needed to rule out a bacterial infection, and lung biopsy may be needed to rule out cancer and to make the appropriate diagnosis. After the diagnosis is made, however, the inciting agent is usually identified with pointed questioning of patient practices.

If not diagnosed promptly, recurrent aspirations of lipid or small amounts of liquid gastric contents, or both, can present as recurrent hemoptysis, recurrent pneumonias, chronic interstitial fibrosis, bronchiolitis, or bronchiectasis [4,70]. Rarely, exogenous lipoid pneumonias are complicated by organisms of the *Mycobacterium fortuitum* complex [73]. Although corticosteroids may be helpful in cases of acute lipid aspiration, acute exogenous lipoid pneumonias usually resolve on their own. The key to therapy is to prevent recurrences. For example, the constipated patient must stop nocturnal mineral oil ingestion.

Tracheobronchitis

Tracheobronchitis must be considered, not only in outpatients with GER and chronic, persistent cough [74] but also in hospitalized patients. Examples of conditions that predispose to an aspiration tracheobronchitis include a debilitated state, the postoperative period, endotracheal intubation, recent extubation, and neuromuscular diseases [3]. Aspiration tracheobronchitis should be suspected in patients with cough, wheeze, and bronchorrhea, defined as expectoration of more than 30 mL of phlegm in 24 hours. Treatment is the same as described previously in "Exogenous Lipoid Pneumonia" section. In general, the bronchorrhea will disappear when oral intake is halted.

References

1. *Webster's New Universal Unabridged Dictionary*. New York, Barnes & Noble Books, 1996, p 124.
2. Moine P, Vercken JP, Chevret S, et al: Severe community-acquired pneumonia: etiology, epidemiology, and prognosis factors. *Chest* 105:1487, 1994.
3. Robinson KA, Markowitz DH, Irwin RS: Aspiration, in Irwin RS, Rippe JM (eds): *Intensive Care Medicine*. 6th ed. Philadelphia, Lippincott Williams & Wilkins, 2008 pp 599–606.
4. Matsuse T, Oka T, Kida K, et al: Importance of diffuse aspiration bronchiolitis caused by chronic occult aspiration in the elderly. *Chest* 110:1289, 1996.
5. Nelson J, Lesser M: Aspiration-induced pulmonary injury. *J Int Care Med* 12:279, 1997.
6. Marik, Paul E: Aspiration pneumonitis and aspiration pneumonia. *N Engl J Med* 344:665, 2001.
7. Garvey BM, McCambley JA, Tuxen DV: Effects of gastric alkalization on bacterial colonization in critically ill patients. *Crit Care Med* 17:211, 1989.
8. Bonten MJ, Gaillard CA, van der Geest S, et al: The role of intragastric acidity and stress ulcer prophylaxis on colonization and infection in mechanically ventilated ICU patients: a stratified, randomized, double-blind study of sucralfate versus antacids. *Am J Respir Crit Care Med* 152:1825, 1995.
9. Cook D, Guyatt G, Marshall J, et al: A comparison of sucralfate and ranitidine for the prevention of upper gastrointestinal bleeding in patients requiring mechanical ventilation. Canadian Critical Care Trials Group. *N Engl J Med* 338:791–797, 1998.
10. Gulmez SE, Holm A, Frederiksen H, et al: Use of proton pump inhibitors and the risk of community-acquired pneumonia. *Arch Intern Med* 167:950–955, 2007.
11. Mittleman R, Wetli C: The fatal cafe coronary: foreign-body airway obstruction. *JAMA* 247:1285, 1982.
12. Terzi N, Orlikowsi D, Aegerter P, et al: Breathing-swallowing interaction in neuromuscular patients. *Am J Respir Crit Care Med* 175:274–275, 2007.
13. Knochel J: Neuromuscular manifestations of electrolyte disorders. *Am J Med* 72:521, 1982.
14. Willard M, Gilsdorf R, Price R: Protein-calorie malnutrition in a community hospital. *JAMA* 243:1720, 1980.
15. Weber L, Nashel D, Mellow M: Pharyngeal dysphagia in alcoholic myopathy. *Ann Intern Med* 95:189, 1981.
16. Chernow B, Johnson L, Janowitz W: Pulmonary aspiration as a consequence of gastroesophageal reflux: a diagnostic approach. *Dig Dis Sci* 24:839, 1979.
17. Finucane T, Bynum J: Use of tube feeding to prevent aspiration pneumonia. *Lancet* 348:1421, 1996.
18. Torres A, Serra-Batlles J, Ross E, et al: Pulmonary aspiration of gastric contents in patients receiving mechanical ventilation: the effect of body position. *Ann Intern Med* 116:540, 1992.
19. Lastbom L, Camner P: Deposition and clearance of particles in the human lung. *Scand J Work Environ Health* 26[Suppl 1]:23, 2000.
20. Zhang P, Summer WR, Bagby GJ, et al: Innate immunity and pulmonary host defense. *Immunol Rev* 175:39, 2000.
21. Konstan M, Chen P, Sherman J, et al: Human lung lysozyme: sources and properties. *Am Rev Respir Dis* 123:120, 1981.
22. Synne J, Ramphal R, Hood C: Tracheal mucosal damage after aspiration: a scanning electron microscope study. *Am Rev Respir Dis* 124:728, 1981.
23. Hof D, Repine J, Peterson P, et al: Phagocytosis by human alveolar macrophages and neutrophils; qualitative differences in the opsonic requirements for uptake of *Staphylococcus aureus* and *Streptococcus pneumoniae* in vitro. *Am Rev Respir Dis* 121:65, 1980.
24. Heidbrink P, Toews G, Gross G, et al: Mechanisms of complement-mediated clearance of bacteria from the murine lung. *Am Rev Respir Dis* 125:517, 1982.
25. de Larminat V, Montravers P, Dureuil B, et al: Alteration in swallowing reflex after extubation in intensive care unit patients. *Crit Care Med* 23:486, 1995.
26. Ajemian MS, Nirmul GB, Anderson MT, et al: Routine fiberoptic endoscopic evaluation of swallowing following prolonged intubation: implications for management. *Arch Surg* 136:434, 2001.
27. Barquist E, Brown M, Cohn S, et al: Postextubation fiberoptic endoscopic evaluation of swallowing after prolonged endotracheal intubation: a randomized, prospective trial. *Crit Care Med* 29:1710, 2001.
28. Rees CJ: Flexible endoscopic evaluation of swallowing with sensory testing. *Curr Opin Otolaryngol Head Neck Surg* 14(6):425–430, 2006.
29. Smith Hammond CA, Goldstein LB: Cough and aspiration of food and liquids due to oral-pharyngeal dysphagia. ACCP evidence-based clinical practice guidelines. *Chest* 129:162S, 2006.
30. Curley F, Higgins D, Coolbaugh B, et al: Laryngeal dysfunction in critically ill patients post extubation: videofluoroscopic assessment [abstract]. *Am J Respir Crit Care Med* 163:A89, 2001.
31. Colice G: Resolution of laryngeal injury following translaryngeal intubation. *Am Rev Respir Dis* 145:361, 1992.
32. Nash M: Swallowing problems in the tracheotomized patient. *Otolaryngol Clin North Am* 21:701, 1988.
33. Tolep K, Getch C, Criner G: Swallowing dysfunction in patients receiving prolonged mechanical ventilation. *Chest* 109:167, 1996.
34. Mittal R, Stewart W, Schirmer B: Effect of a catheter in the pharynx on the frequency of transient lower esophageal sphincter relaxation. *Gastroenterology* 103:1236, 1992.
35. Gomes GF, Pisani JC, Macedo ED, et al: The nasogastric feeding tube as a risk factor for aspiration and aspiration pneumonia. *Curr Opin Clin Nutr Metab Care* 6:327, 2003.
36. Ferrer M, Bauer T, Torres A, et al: Effect of nasogastric tube size on gastroesophageal reflux and microaspiration in intubated patients. *Ann Intern Med* 130:991, 1999.
37. Strong R, Condon S, Solinger M, et al: Equal aspiration rates from postpylorus and intragastric-placed small-bore nasoenteric feeding tubes: a randomized, prospective study. *JPEN J Parenter Enteral Nutr* 16:59, 1992.
38. Kirby D, Craig R, Tsang T, et al: Percutaneous endoscopic gastrostomies: a prospective evaluation and review of the literature. *JPEN J Parenter Enteral Nutr* 10:155, 1986.
39. Park RH, Allison MC, Lang J, et al: Randomised comparison of percutaneous endoscopic gastrostomy and nasogastric tube feeding in patients with persisting neurological dysphagia. *BMJ* 304:1406, 1992.
40. Baeten C, Hoefnagels J: Feeding via nasogastric tube or percutaneous endoscopic gastrostomy: a comparison. *Scand J Gastroenterol Suppl* 194:95, 1992.
41. Kostadima E, Kaditis AG, Alexopoulos EI, et al: Early gastrostomy reduces the rate of ventilator-associated pneumonia in stroke or head injury patients. *Eur Res J* 26:106, 2005.
42. Montecalvo M, Steger K, Farber H, et al: Nutritional outcome and pneumonia in critical care patients randomized to gastric versus jejunal tube feedings. *Crit Care Med* 20:1377, 1992.
43. McClave S, Snider H, Lowen C, et al: Use of residual volume as a marker for enteral feeding intolerance: prospective blinded comparison with physical examination and radiographic findings. *JPEN J Parenter Enteral Nutr* 16:99, 1992.

44. Leder SB: Videofluoroscopic evaluation of aspiration with visual examination of the gag reflex and velar movement. *Dysphagia* 12:21, 1997.
45. Leder SB: Gag reflex and dysphagia. *Head Neck* 18:138, 1996.
46. Widdicombe JG: Reflexes from the upper respiratory tract, in Cherniack NS, Widdicombe JG (eds): *Handbook of Physiology: The Respiratory System: Control of Breathing*. Vol 2. Bethesda, MD, American Physiological Society, 1986, p 363.
47. DeVita M, Spierer-Rundback L: Swallowing disorders in patients with prolonged orotracheal intubation or tracheostomy tubes. *Crit Care Med* 18:1328, 1990.
48. Elpern E, Scott M, Petro L, et al: Pulmonary aspiration in mechanically ventilated patients with tracheostomies. *Chest* 105:563, 1994.
49. Sonies B, Baum B: Evaluation of swallowing pathophysiology. *Otolaryngol Clin North Am* 21:637, 1988.
50. Hiss SG, Postma GN: Fiberoptic endoscopic evaluation of swallowing. *Laryngoscope* 113:1386, 2003.
51. Langmore S, Schatz K, Olson N: Endoscopic and videofluoroscopic evaluations of swallowing and aspiration. *Ann Otol Rhinol Laryngol* 100:678, 1991.
52. Wu CH, Hsiao TY, Chen JC, et al: Evaluation of swallowing safety with fiberoptic endoscope: comparison with videofluoroscopic technique. *Laryngoscope* 107:396, 1997.
53. Leder S, Sasaki C, Burrell M: Fiberoptic endoscopic evaluation of dysphagia to identify silent aspiration. *Dysphagia* 13:19, 1998.
54. Leder S, Cohn S, Moller B: Fiberoptic endoscopic documentation of the high incidence of aspiration following extubation in critically ill trauma patients. *Dysphagia* 13:208, 1998.
55. Doggett DL, Tappe KA, Mitchel MD, et al: Prevention of pneumonia in elderly stroke patients by systematic diagnosis and treatment of dysphagia: an evidence-based comprehensive analysis of the literature. *Dysphagia* 16:275, 2001.
56. Corwin R, Irwin R: The lipid-laden alveolar macrophage as a marker of aspiration in parenchymal lung disease. *Am Rev Respir Dis* 132:576, 1985.
57. Metheny N, Clouse R: Bedside methods for detecting aspiration in tube-fed patients. *Chest* 111:724, 1997.
58. Richter J, Castell D: Gastroesophageal reflux: pathogenesis, diagnosis, and therapy. *Ann Intern Med* 97:93, 1982.
59. Reed MF, Mathisen DJ: Tracheoesophageal fistula. *Chest Surg Clin North Am* 13:271, 2003.
60. Sukumaran M, Grandada M, Berger H, et al: Evaluation of corticosteroid treatment in aspiration of gastric contents: a controlled clinical trial. *Mt Sinai J Med* 47:335, 1980.
61. Schwartz D, Wynne J, Gibbs C, et al: The pulmonary consequences of aspiration of gastric contents at pH values greater than 2.5. *Am Rev Respir Dis* 121:119, 1980.
62. Eller W, Haugen R: Food asphyxiation: restaurant rescue. *N Engl J Med* 289:81, 1975.
63. National Research Council: Standards and guidelines for cardiopulmonary resuscitation (CPR) and emergency cardiac care (ECC). *JAMA* 255:2905, 1986.
64. Bartlett J: Anaerobic bacterial infections of the lung and pleural space. *Clin Infect Dis* 16[Suppl 4]:S248, 1993.
65. Yoneyama T, Yoshida M, Matsui T, et al: Oral care and pneumonia. *Lancet* 354:515, 1999.
66. Kannangara D, Thadepalli H, Bach V, et al: Animal model for anaerobic lung abscess. *Infect Immun* 31:592, 1981.
67. Fick RJ, Reynolds H: Changing spectrum of pneumonia: news media creation or clinical reality? *Am J Med* 75:1, 1983.
68. LaForce F: Hospital-acquired gram-negative rod pneumonias: an overview. *Am J Med* 70:664, 1981.
69. Stamm W, Martin S, Bennett J: Epidemiology of nosocomial infections due to gram-negative bacilli: aspects relevant to development and use of vaccines. *J Infect Dis* 136[Suppl]:5151, 1977.
70. Spencer H. *Pathology of the Lung*. Elmsford, NY, Pergamon, 1977, p 468.
71. Winterbauer R, Durning R, Barron E, et al: Aspirated nasogastric feeding solution detected by glucose strips. *Ann Intern Med* 95:67, 1981.
72. Hughes R, Frelich R, Bytell D, et al: Aspiration and occult esophageal disorders. *Chest* 80:489, 1981.
73. Irwin R, Pratter M, Corwin R, et al: Pulmonary infection with *Mycobacterium chelonei*: successful treatment with one drug based on disk diffusion susceptibility data. *J Infect Dis* 145:772, 1982.
74. Irwin R, Corrao W, Pratter M: Chronic persistent cough in the adult: the spectrum and frequency of causes and successful outcome of specific therapy. *Am Rev Respir Dis* 123:413, 1981.

CHAPTER 55 ■ DROWNING

NICHOLAS A. SMYRNIOS AND RICHARD S. IRWIN

OVERVIEW

Drowning is the seventh most common cause of unintentional injury death in the United States [1]. In 2005, 3,582 people died from drowning in the United States [2]. The incidence of fatal drowning declined from 2.7 per 100,000 in 1983 to 1.21 per 100,000 in 2005. Drowning is most common in men, children younger than 14 years, Native Americans, and African Americans [2]. The states with the highest drowning rates are Alaska and Mississippi [3]. Statistics on nonfatal drowning are less exact because many nonfatal drowning victims do not seek medical attention. Estimates on the incidence of nonfatal drowning vary widely enough that a definitive statement cannot be made at this time.

The official nomenclature for submersion injuries has changed. Based on the results of a consensus conference held as part of the World Conference on Drowning in 2002, appropriate references to submersion injuries use the terms *fatal drowning* to describe death by submersion in water and *nonfatal drowning* to describe at least temporary survival after respiratory impairment from submersion in water [4]. However, some reports continue to use the terms *drowning* and *near-drowning* as synonyms for fatal drowning and nonfatal drowning, respectively. In addition, the terms *submersion* and *immersion* continue to be used to describe both fatal and nonfatal drowning together.

ETIOLOGY AND PATHOGENESIS

The following are considered risk factors for drowning.

Alcohol

Ethanol use is the major risk factor in submersion accidents. Thirty percent to 70% of drownings are associated with alcohol consumption [5–7]. Alcohol use seems to be an issue in drowned men in particular [8]. Alcoholic beverages reduce the ability to deal with emergency situations by depressing coordination, increasing response time, and decreasing awareness of stimuli. Furthermore, alcohol consumption by a potential rescuer or by the adult responsible for supervising a child in the water can destroy that person's ability to function effectively, often resulting in a double tragedy [7]. In addition, alcohol is frequently a factor in drownings that result from automobile accidents [9].

Inadequate Adult Supervision

Children die in water because adults do not supervise them well enough. The backyard pool and family bathtub are common sites of pediatric drowning [10–14]. Lack of appropriate precautions and supervision play a major role in most of these cases. Studies have shown lower rates of drowning in areas where swimming pools are required by law to be surrounded by a fence [15,16]. The fence must completely isolate the pool from unsupervised access by children to be effective. Appropriate sign posting in hazardous areas, effective educational programs on the dangers of water recreation, and the presence of lifeguards also minimize risk and improve survival [10,17,18].

Inattentive guardians also contribute to bathtub-related drownings. In one study, all bathtub-related submersions in children younger than 5 years occurred while the child was bathing unattended or with another young child [19]. The use of infant bath seats, while providing some sense of security to parents, may actually predispose to submersion accidents as the child may slip and become trapped by the seat, making it impossible to escape the water [20]. The practice of leaving infants to bathe in the custody of a toddler is inappropriate and should be discouraged [11,12]. Immersion in large industrial buckets used for home cleaning may also make up a substantial percentage of drownings of infants and toddlers [21].

Child Abuse

Unfortunately, submersion injuries in children are sometimes inflicted intentionally. One study indicated that 29% of all nonfatal pediatric drownings in bathtubs were purposely caused to inflict harm on the child. Another 38% of all nonfatal pediatric drownings revealed evidence of severe neglect [22]. In general, these children are younger than average for submersion injuries, and many have signs of previous abuse on close examination.

Seizures

Drowning is 15 to 19 times more common in people with epilepsy than in the general population [23]. In one study, a history of seizure disorder was found in 17 of the 293 cases of drowning that were reviewed [9]. This contrasts with the prevalence of seizures of 6 per 1,000 in the general population. Poor adherence to anticonvulsant regimens often plays a role. Many drownings of epileptic children occur in the bathtub [24]. Seizures that include a tonic component may be the most dangerous to victims. Tonic seizures include a forced exhalation component that increases body density and causes the victim to sink. When the tonic component relaxes, the negative intrathoracic pressure leads to an inhalation that will then be composed of water [25]. The intensity of supervision needed by epileptics in a water environment is frequently underestimated.

Boating Accidents

Of the 710 boating fatalities in the United States in 2006, 70% were due to drowning [2]. Both alcohol intake and failure to use personal flotation devices contributed to these deaths [9,26]. A blood alcohol level of 0.10 g per 100 mL is estimated to increase the risk of death associated with boating by a factor of 10 [6].

Aquatic Sports

Water-related activities produce approximately 140,000 injuries annually. Diving, surfing, and water skiing account for 77% of the 700 spinal cord injuries produced annually by aquatic sports. Diving and sliding headfirst produce the most serious injuries as a result of striking the bottom or side of a shallow body of water [10]. Patients who experience these injuries are at subsequent risk of drowning. In addition, injuries associated with the use of personal watercraft contribute to drowning incidence [27].

Drugs

Centrally acting drugs not only can cloud the sensorium, causing disorientation and inducing sleep, but also impair coordination and reduce the ability to swim. Existing data implicate both legal, therapeutic medications and illegal drugs [9,28].

PATHOPHYSIOLOGY

General Considerations

Two mechanisms produce the major pathologic changes responsible for morbidity in drowning: anoxia and hypothermia.

Anoxia

Most drownings are thought to follow a common pattern [29]. The drowning sequence begins with a period of breath holding because the victim's mouth and nose are below the level of the water. This voluntary breath holding is often followed by an intense laryngospasm that prevents breathing. This laryngospasm is usually due to water present in the pharynx or larynx. This prolonged inability to breathe renders the patient hypoxemic and hypercapnic. The laryngospasm eventually abates, followed by involuntary breaths with aspiration of varying amounts of water. In addition, water may be swallowed that is eventually regurgitated and aspirated. Eventually, the victim becomes unconscious and cardiac arrest occurs.

Hypothermia

The impact of hypothermia is complex. Survival after extremely long submersion is generally considered possible only when the victim has been submerged in icy water. There are reports of survival in children submerged up to 66 minutes [30–32]. Most authors believe that to achieve such spectacular survivals after long submersions, the core body temperature must be reduced quickly and the brain's metabolic activity slowed down in equally rapid fashion to prevent hypoxic damage to the brain. Factors that make this more likely in children include the increased relative body surface area, thin layer of subcutaneous fat, and smaller head size. In addition, children may ventilate water earlier in their submersion, and they may retain more water in the upper airway [33]. These factors may also play a role in rapid cooling.

On the other hand, humans tolerate hypothermia poorly. In the most well-known example, the deaths after the sinking of the *Titanic* occurred not because of inability to float in most cases but because of hypothermia caused by exposure to extremely cold water. Changes in human metabolism in response to hypothermia occur in two phases: the shivering phase and the nonshivering phase. Shivering occurs at a central temperature of 30°C to 35°C. The nonshivering phase occurs below 30°C, when muscle contractions nearly cease and oxygen consumption and metabolic rate decrease.

Shivering and voluntary muscular movements, which in a cold dry environment work together to increase heat production with minimal increase in heat loss, are ineffective in cold water [34]. Both shivering and voluntary muscular movements increase blood flow to the extremities, thereby increasing conductive heat loss. Voluntary movements of the extremities also stir the surrounding water and can increase heat loss from convection [35]. Body type may also play a major role. Obese men tolerate submersion in cold water longer than thin men due to increased insulation from body fat [36]. Water nearly eliminates the insulative function of clothing by replacing the air between the fibers, thereby increasing heat conductance.

Submersion in very cold water can acutely lead to death in three ways. First, a vagally mediated asystolic cardiac arrest may occur (immersion syndrome) [37]. Second, hypothermia produces an increased tendency toward malignant arrhythmias separate from this immediate response. Cardiac arrest from ventricular fibrillation is common at core temperatures below 25°C, and asystole occurs at less than 18°C [38]. These arrhythmias may be refractory to resuscitative efforts until the body temperature has been increased. Third, a decrease in core temperature can cause loss of consciousness and aspiration from the victim's inability to keep the head above water. This leads to aspiration of water and the sequence of events described previously.

Pulmonary Effects

The effects of aspiration of various water solutions on lung injury have been studied in animals [39,40]. Sterile water was found to be the most disruptive of pulmonary function. Normal and hypertonic saline solutions also cause significant increases in $(P_{A}\text{-}a)O_2$ gradient and shunt fraction, with a decrease in the PaO_2 to FIO_2 ratio. Decreases in arterial oxygen saturation and dynamic compliance as well as increases in minute ventilation, mean pulmonary artery pressure, and shunt fraction are seen in sheep after bilateral aspiration of either fresh- or seawater [40].

On a microscopic level, freshwater and saline solutions may cause their adverse pulmonary effects by different mechanisms. Atelectasis due to increased surface tension, bronchoconstriction, and noncardiogenic pulmonary edema all play a role in the development of hypoxemia at different times after freshwater aspiration [40,41]. Freshwater acts in part by inactivating surfactant in the alveoli and in part by damaging type-II pneumocytes, thereby preventing the production of surfactant for up to 24 hours [42,43]. The combination of these effects may damage the alveolar capillaries and interstitium and lead to the acute respiratory distress syndrome (ARDS). Hypertonic seawater may draw additional fluid from the plasma into the alveoli, thereby causing pulmonary edema despite a decreased intravascular volume [39]. The fluid-filled alveoli are then unavailable for efficient gas transfer, and a ventilation–perfusion mismatch occurs. This fluid may also damage the type-II pneumocytes by hypoxic and osmotic effects [41]. Aspiration of gastric contents and particles in the water complicates both fresh- and saltwater drowning. In clinical practice, the difference in the situation caused by freshwater and saltwater aspirations is small. In both cases, pulmonary edema causes decreased respiratory system compliance and hypoxemia. Unless specific therapies are developed that target the different mechanisms, there is probably little advantage in emphasizing the described differences.

Several other mechanisms of lung injury may occur with nonfatal drowning. Bacterial pneumonia, barotrauma, mechanical damage from cardiopulmonary resuscitation (CPR), chemical pneumonitis, centrally mediated apnea, and oxygen toxicity can cause respiratory deterioration in the postresuscitation period [41]. These must be considered along with ARDS in cases of respiratory distress occurring 1 to 48 hours after the event.

Neurologic Effects

The pathologic effects that most affect prognosis in drowning are related to the central nervous system (CNS). Cerebral injury is produced as a result of anoxia due to gas exchange impairment and subsequent cardiopulmonary arrest.

Anoxic damage begins 4 to 10 minutes after cessation of cerebral blood flow in most situations [44]. The actual time course and clinical significance of anoxia in a specific drowning victim is notoriously uncertain in cases of drowning because of the emotional condition of the witnesses and because the impact of hypothermia is difficult to judge [45].

Many drowning victims suffer neurologic impairment. Victims display pathologic features similar to those of patients with anoxic encephalopathy from other causes, including diffuse cerebral edema, focal areas of necrosis, mitochondrial swelling, and other ischemic changes [46]. These changes occur primarily in the cerebral cortex, hippocampus, and cerebellum.

In addition to death, severe anoxic encephalopathy with persistent coma, seizures, delayed language development, spastic quadriplegia, aphasia, and cortical blindness have been reported as sequelae of submersion accidents [47–50]. Therefore, a great deal of effort has gone into trying to establish a means to predict the ultimate neurologic outcome of drowning victims. Studies have proposed the following as means of predicting outcomes: (a) the presence of purposeful movements and normal brainstem function 24 hours after submersion [51]; (b) the Glasgow Coma Scale score and Pediatric Risk of Mortality index on admission to the intensive care unit [52]; (c) cardiovascular status on admission to the emergency department and neurologic status on admission to the intensive care unit [53]; and (d) shorter submersion and resuscitation times and recovery of cardiac and neurologic function in the field [54]. Despite this, it remains impossible to predict outcomes with uniform accuracy in individual patients [55].

Musculoskeletal Effects

Children who develop anoxic encephalopathy due to drowning frequently develop musculoskeletal problems [56]. These problems result from spasticity, which appears to be more aggressive in these children than in those with other forms of spastic disorder. The most common of these are lower extremity contractures, hip subluxation or dislocation, and scoliosis [56].

Serum Electrolytes

Experimental studies with animals reveal significant differences in serum electrolytes between fresh- and saltwater drowning [57,58]. In the clinical setting, swallowing large amounts of seawater over an extended period of repeated submersions has been reported to cause significant changes in serum sodium, potassium, chloride, and magnesium [59]. This happens rarely, however, and the body corrects most of the alterations that do occur [60]. Therefore, the actual clinical impact of electrolyte changes is minimal [61,62].

Hematologic Effects

Patients presenting with drowning episodes rarely require medical intervention for anemia. Several studies have demonstrated near-normal hemoglobin values in both sea- and freshwater [57,60]. Disseminated intravascular coagulation

(DIC) has been described as a complicating factor in freshwater drowning [63].

Renal Effects

Acute tubular necrosis, hemoglobinuria, and albuminuria all have been reported as consequences of submersion accidents [50,64,65]. Diuresis has traditionally been considered to be a result of changes in renal tubular function due to hypothermia [66]. However, diuresis is seen in experimental submersions at any temperature [67]. Drowning victims also frequently present with metabolic acidosis as a result of lactate accumulation [68].

Cardiac Effects

Submersion in water causes an increase in left atrial diameter and a decrease in heart rate [69]. Atrial fibrillation and sinus dysrhythmias are common but rarely require therapy [70]. PR, QRS, and QT interval prolongations as well as J point elevation (Osborn wave; see Chapter 65) can be seen as in other causes of hypothermia [71,72]. More severe cases may result in death due to ventricular fibrillation or asystole. Autopsy studies of drowned patients demonstrate focal myocardial necrosis that may be similar to findings in pheochromocytoma and other situations of high adrenergic output [73,74].

The anoxia caused by drowning can also have an effect on hemodynamics. Orlowski and colleagues [75] found transient increases in central venous and pulmonary artery balloon occlusion pressures after experimental drowning. In addition, there was a persistent decrease in cardiac output that lasted more than 4 hours. These findings were independent of the tonicity of the solutions used and no different from those of anoxic controls.

Infectious Complications

Although a variety of infections are reported to be associated with drowning, pneumonia is the predominant infection described. Aspiration of mouth contents, gastric contents, and contaminated water all play a role in the development of pneumonia after drowning. A wide variety of organisms, including aerobic Gram-negative bacteria, aerobic Gram-positive bacteria, and fungi, have been described. Combinations of infections, some with opportunistic organisms, have also been described [76]. Because organisms that can survive in very cold water usually cannot survive and proliferate at human body temperature, most pneumonia cases occur after warm-water drowning [77]. In addition to pneumonia, cases of brain abscess, meningoencephalitis, bacteremia, skin and soft tissue infections, and endophthalmitis are reported to occur.

DIAGNOSIS AND CLINICAL PRESENTATION

History

The minimum background historical information that must be obtained includes the patient's age; underlying cardiac, respiratory, or neurologic diseases; and medications used. It is also important to determine the activities precipitating the submersion, such as boating, diving, or ingestion of drugs or alcohol; the duration of submersion; and the temperature and type of water in which it occurred.

Physical Examination

The initial physical examination is often hurried, with more detailed assessment delayed until resuscitative efforts have been established. Tachypnea is the most frequent finding, and tachycardia is also common [60]. Patients may also be apneic and pulseless. Hypothermia is common and depends on the temperature of the water and duration of submersion. It is important that an appropriate thermometer be used that can accurately measure hypothermic temperatures because the duration of resuscitation may depend on this value. Other findings include fever and signs of pulmonary edema. Any physical findings seen in cases of cerebral anoxia or severe hypothermia also may be seen in drowning. In addition to revealing the consequences of hypoxia/anoxia and hypothermia, the major importance of the physical examination is to uncover coexisting injuries that may have caused or resulted from the submersion.

Victims of nonfatal drowning have traditionally been classified with a simple scale [78]. Category A patients are fully alert within 1 hour of presentation to the emergency department. These patients uniformly do well neurologically. Category B patients are obtunded and stuporous but arousable at the time of evaluation; 89% to 100% of these patients survive, and severe permanent neurologic is not usually seen [79]. Category C patients are comatose with abnormal respirations and abnormal response to pain. Category C may be further subdivided depending on the pain response: C1, decorticate posturing; C2, decerebrate posturing; and C3, flaccid [79]. Category C patients have a much higher mortality, and survivors, particularly children, have a higher rate of neurologic dysfunction.

Laboratory Studies

Hemoglobin, hematocrit, and serum electrolytes are usually normal on arrival in the emergency department whether the submersion occurred in freshwater or saltwater [80]. Arterial blood gas analysis frequently shows metabolic acidosis and hypoxemia. The blood alcohol level, prothrombin time, partial thromboplastin time, serum creatinine, urinalysis, and drug screen should also be obtained to help determine the cause of the accident and assess for complications of drowning. Cervical spine films should be performed whenever there is evidence of trauma. An electrocardiogram should be obtained and continuous monitoring performed whenever there is a significant chance of dysrhythmia.

Up to 20% of initial chest radiographs in drowning victims are normal [60,81–83]. The remaining 80% show evidence of varying degrees of pulmonary edema. Two patterns are commonly seen. Some films display confluent alveolar densities primarily in the perihilar regions, whereas others exhibit a diffuse, almost homogeneous nodular pattern bilaterally. Sand bronchograms have also been reported. These are associated with the aspiration of sand and its deposition in the airways [84].

THERAPY

The treatment of nonfatal drowning should be approached in four phases.

Initial Resuscitation

Resuscitation of apneic or pulseless drowning victims should be initiated immediately and continue as needed throughout the prehospital phase into the emergency department. Mouth-to-mouth resuscitation must be begun in the water and not delayed until the victim is brought to shore [85,86]. The rescuer should carefully support the victim's neck to prevent exacerbation of undiagnosed vertebral injuries. Full CPR with chest compressions should begin immediately on arrival on shore and proceed according to standard guidelines, and advanced life support should begin as soon as appropriate providers arrive [87]. The use of the Heimlich maneuver in the absence of a foreign body obstruction may exacerbate cervical spine injury and predispose to vomiting and aspiration [88]. Its routine use in resuscitation of drowning victims was strongly recommended against by an Institute of Medicine Report [88].

Resuscitation must be continued in victims of cold-water submersion at least until the patient has been rewarmed. Core temperature should be obtained immediately on arrival at the emergency department and monitored carefully during the first several hours. All drowning victims with cardiopulmonary arrest and hypothermia should be rewarmed rapidly only to a temperature between 32°C and 34°C and then maintained at that level (see following discussion) [89]. In the field, wet clothing should be removed and passive external rewarming plus inhalation of heated oxygen begun [90,91]. In the hospital, cardiopulmonary bypass should be used in cases of severe hypothermia from drowning, especially with circulatory collapse [30,90,92–94]. This method has the advantage of rapidly and directly rewarming the core. It can also correct the metabolic acidosis that commonly occurs. When this technique is not possible, rewarming with warmed peritoneal lavage, hemodialysis, or heated oxygen can be attempted. (See Chapter 65 for an in-depth discussion of rewarming techniques.)

A more difficult question is when and how long to resuscitate victims of warm-water submersion. As previously mentioned, there is no clearly established method of predicting ultimate neurologic recovery in individual patients. Therefore, until more information is available, the decision to terminate resuscitation must be based on a variety of factors particular to the individual case. On the other end of the clinical spectrum, most patients who are asymptomatic at or soon after presentation do very well. Victims who are asymptomatic and have normal oxygenation at 6 to 8 hours after presentation do not deteriorate during the subsequent 18 to 24 hours [95,96].

Therapy of the Underlying Cause

If there is any question of possible head or neck trauma, the neck should be immobilized in a brace until cervical spine films are available. Hypoglycemia and severe electrolyte abnormalities can be detected on routine serum testing and corrected rapidly in the emergency department. Serum alcohol levels and a drug screen can detect potential intoxicants and prompt administration of necessary antidotes or other measures. Anticonvulsant levels can help tailor therapy in known epileptic patients.

Treatment of Respiratory and Other Organ Failure

The initial management of all pulmonary edema states involves monitoring PaO_2 and providing appropriate supplemental oxygen. The use of nasal continuous positive airway pressure has been advocated for use in patients with pulmonary edema after drowning [97]. This technique has the advantage of being noninvasive and potentially less expensive than mechanical ventilation via endotracheal intubation. However, the literature supporting for this intervention is very limited and we cannot recommend its use. Mechanical ventilation with positive end-expiratory pressure should be instituted if refractory hypoxic or hypercapnic respiratory failure develops. The most important advance in the management of ARDS from any cause is the use of low tidal volume, low pressure ventilation [98] (Table 55.1). Use of such a strategy has been shown to have a major effect on survival of ARDS patients.

Other therapies for the respiratory complications of drowning have been proposed, but none of those has demonstrated improvements in outcomes. Examples of these types of therapies include exogenous surfactant in respiratory failure and prophylactic antibiotics. We do not advocate the use of either of these therapies.

Treatment of other end-organ damage must be approached systematically. Serum electrolytes rarely require therapy. The treatment of renal failure focuses on optimizing fluid status and renal blood flow. Severe cases may require temporary dialysis. Lactic acidosis should be corrected by restoration of adequate ventilation and circulation. The only clinically significant hematologic effect is DIC. The treatment of DIC is addressed in Chapter 108.

The cardiac dysrhythmogenic effects of hypothermia are corrected by rewarming. Sinus and atrial dysrhythmias as well as most interval prolongations rarely require additional therapy [70]. For a discussion of the treatment of hypothermia-related malignant ventricular dysrhythmias, see Chapter 65.

Musculoskeletal complications of nonfatal drowning are treated in standard fashion. Contractures are treated with casts or splints; subluxated or dislocated hips can be approached with various operative procedures; and scoliosis is treated with bracing or spinal instrumentation [56]. The relative success of these interventions in this population is unclear.

Neurologic Therapy

The recommendations of the World Congress on Drowning support the following interventions for patients following cardiopulmonary arrest from drowning:

TABLE 55.1

ADVANCES IN THE MANAGEMENT OF DROWNING BASED ON RANDOMIZED CLINICAL TRIALS

Intervention	Outcomes favorably affected	References
Small tidal volume ventilation for ARDS	Mortality, organ failure days, mechanical ventilation days	[98]
Therapeutic hypothermia for comatose survivors of cardiac arrest	Mortality	[100]
	Neurologic status	[99,100]

ARDS, acute respiratory distress syndrome.

- Restoration of spontaneous circulation is the highest priority goal.
- Core temperature should be monitored continuously.
- Therapeutic hypothermia to a core temperature of 32°C to 34°C should be maintained for a period of 12 to 24 hours. Hyperthermia should be prevented at all times in the acute recovery period.
- Seizures should be looked for and treated as necessary.
- Blood glucose concentrations should be monitored frequently and normoglycemia maintained.
- Hypoxemia should be avoided.
- Hypotension should be avoided.

The use of therapeutic hypothermia was substantiated in outpatient cardiac arrest victims in two randomized controlled trials published in 2002. In both studies, mortality and neurologic outcomes were improved by a treatment strategy including hypothermia when compared with conventional care and normothermia [99,100]. These findings are the basis for the strong recommendation given by the World Congress and other organizations.

CONCLUSIONS

The course of nonfatal drowning is variable. Patients who receive prompt CPR, are rapidly restored to a perfusing rhythm, and regain neurological function usually have dramatic and complete recoveries. On the other hand, patients with delayed resuscitation and those who do not rapidly recover neurological function often have a poor outcome. Although fresh- and seawater drownings cause different clinical pictures in experimental animals, they are difficult to distinguish in humans. In general, patients who aspirate water present with hypoxemia and metabolic acidosis. They usually do not aspirate enough fluid to produce changes in blood volume, electrolytes, hemoglobin, and hematocrit sufficient to be life-threatening.

The development of treatments specifically for drowning victims has been very slow. In general, most therapies are general treatments directed at cardiac arrest and ARDS. Treatment varies with the severity of the illness. In severely hypothermic patients, rewarming methods should be instituted immediately. These include removing wet clothing, covering with warm blankets, infusing warm fluids intravenously, and performing gastrointestinal irrigation with warm fluids. If the patient's temperature is less than 32°C, core rewarming may be most easily accomplished by cardiopulmonary bypass or peritoneal dialysis with a potassium-free dialysate warmed to 54°C. The desired core temperature for patients after cardiac arrest is 32°C to 34°C. Therapy for patients with severe hypoxemia includes institution of all the supportive modalities used in ARDS. Abnormalities of multiple organ systems must be addressed systematically. The most important ways for reducing deaths from drowning currently reside in the area of drowning prevention.

References

1. Centers for Disease Control and Prevention: Nonfatal and fatal drownings in recreational water settings—United States, 2001–2002. *MMWR Morb Mortal Wkly Rep* 53:447, 2004.
2. Centers for Disease Control and Prevention, National Center for Injury Prevention and Control: Web-Based Injury Statistics Query and Reporting System (WISQARS) [online]. Updated April 1, 2008. Quoted October 7, 2009.
3. Centers for Disease Control and Prevention, National Center for Injury Prevention and Control: *Drowning prevention* 2000.
4. Idris AH, Berg RA, Bierens J, et al: Recommended guidelines for uniform reporting of data from drowning—the "Utstein style." *Circulation* 108:2565, 2003.
5. Vyrostek SB, Annest JL, Ryan GL: Surveillance for fatal and nonfatal injuries—United States 2001. *MMWR* 53[SS07]:1, 2004.
6. Driscoll TR, Harrison JA, Steenkamp M: Review of the role of alcohol in drowning associated with recreational aquatic activity. *Inj Prev* 10:107, 2004.
7. Plueckhahn VD: Alcohol and accidental drowning: a 25-year study. *Med J Aust* 141:22, 1984.
8. Wintemute GJ, Kraus JF, Teret SP, et al: Drowning in childhood and adolescence: a population-based study. *Am J Public Health* 77:830, 1987.
9. Wintemute GJ, Kraus JF, Teret SP, et al: The epidemiology of drowning in adulthood: implications for prevention. *Am J Prev Med* 4:343, 1988.
10. Centers for Disease Control and Prevention: Aquatic deaths and injuries: United States. *MMWR Morb Mortal Wkly Rep* 31:417, 1982.
11. Pearn JH, Brown J, Wong R, et al: Bathtub drownings. Report of seven cases. *Pediatrics* 64:68, 1979.
12. Budnick LD, Ross DA: Bathtub-related drownings in the United States, 1979–1981. *Am J Public Health* 75:630, 1985.
13. Saluja G, Brenner RA, Trumble AC: Swimming pool drownings among US residents aged 5–24 years: understanding racial/ethnic disparities. *Am J Public Health* 96:728, 2006.
14. O'Carroll PW, Alkon E, Weiss B: Drowning mortality in Los Angeles County, 1976–1984. *JAMA* 260:380, 1988.
15. Pearn JH, Thompson J: Drowning and near-drowning in the Australian Capital Territory. A five-year total population study of immersion accidents. *Med J Aust* 1:130, 1988.
16. Pearn J, Wong RYK, Brown J: Drowning and near-drowning involving children. A 5-year total population study from the city and county of Honolulu. *Am J Public Health* 69:450, 1979.
17. Manolios N, Mackie I: Drowning and near-drowing on Australian beaches patrolled by life-savers: a 10-year study, 1973–1983. *Med J Aust* 148:165, 1988.
18. Pearn J: Drowning, the sea and life-savers: a clinical audit. *Med J Aust* 148:164, 1988.
19. Quan L, Gore EJ, Wentz K, et al: Ten-year study of pediatric drownings and near-drownings in Kings County, Washington: lessons in injury prevention. *Pediatrics* 83:1035, 1989.
20. Byard RW, Donald T: Infant bath seats and near-drowning. *J Paediatr Child Health* 40:305, 2004.
21. Jumbelic MI, Chambliss M: Accidental toddler drowning in 5-gallon buckets. *JAMA* 263:1952, 1990.
22. Lavelle JM, Shaw KN, Seidl T, et al: Ten-year review of pediatric bathtub near drownings: evaluation for child abuse and neglect. *Ann Emerg Med* 25:344, 1995.
23. Bell GS, Gaitatzis A, Bell CL, et al: Drowning in people with epilepsy. *Neurology* 71:578, 2008.
24. Pearn JH: Epilepsy and drowning in childhood. *BMJ* 1:1510, 1977.
25. Besag FMC: Tonic seizures are a particular risk factor for drowning in people with epilepsy. *BMJ* 321:975, 2000.
26. Centers for Disease Control (CDC): Aquatic deaths and injuries: United States. *MMWR Morb Mortal Wkly Rep* 31:417, 1982.
27. Branche CM, Conn JM, Annest JL: Personal watercraft related injuries: a growing public health concern. *JAMA* 278:663, 1997.
28. Gorniak JM, Jenkins AJ, Felo JA, et al: Drug prevalence in drowning deaths in Cuyahoga County, Ohio: a ten-year retrospective study. *Am J Foren Med Pathol* 26:240, 2005.
29. Layon AJ, Modell JH: Drowning update 2009. *Anesthesiology* 110:1211, 2009.
30. Bolte RG, Black PG, Bowers RS, et al: The use of extracorporeal rewarming in a child submerged for 66 minutes. *JAMA* 260:377, 1988.
31. Young RSK, Zalneraitis EL, Dooling EC: Neurologic outcome in cold water drowning. *JAMA* 244:1233, 1980.
32. Fritz KW, Kasperczyk W, Galaske R: Successful resuscitation in accidental hypothermia after drowning. *Anaesthetist* 37:331, 1988.
33. Xu X, Tikuisis P, Giesbrecht G: A mathematical model for human brain cooling during cold-water near-drowning. *J Appl Physiol* 86:265, 1999.
34. Reuler JB: Hypothermia: pathophysiology, clinical settings, and management. *Ann Intern Med* 89:519, 1978.
35. Keatinge WR: The effect of work and clothing on the maintenance of the body temperature in water. *Q J Exp Physiol* 46:69, 1961.
36. Pugh LGC: The physiology of channel swimmers. *Lancet* 2:761, 1955.
37. Goode RC, Duffin J, Miller R, et al: Sudden cold water immersion. *Respir Physiol* 23:301, 1975.
38. Hegnauer AH, Angelakos ET: Excitable properties of the hypothermic heart. *Ann N Y Acad Sci* 80:336, 1959.
39. Orlowski JP, Abulliel MM, Phillips JM: Effects of tonicities of saline solutions on pulmonary injury in drowning. *Crit Care Med* 15:126, 1987.
40. Halmagyi DFJ, Colebatch HJH: Ventilation and circulation after fluid aspiration. *J Appl Physiol* 116:35, 1961.
41. Pearn JH: Secondary drowning in children. *BMJ* 281:1103, 1980.

42. Giammona ST, Modell JH: Drowning by total immersion: effects on pulmonary surfactant of distilled water, isotonic saline, and sea water. *Am J Dis Child* 114:612, 1967.
43. Modell JH, Calderwood HW, Ruiz BC, et al: Effects of ventilatory patterns on arterial oxygenation after near-drowning in sea water. *Anesthesiology* 40:376, 1974.
44. Peterson B: Morbidity of childhood near-drowning. *Pediatrics* 59:364, 1977.
45. Conn AW, Edmonds JF, Barker GA: Cerebral resuscitation in near-drowning. *Pediatr Clin North Am* 26:691, 1979.
46. Griggs RC, Satran R: Metabolic encephalopathy, in Rosenberg RN (ed): *The Clinical Neurosciences*. New York, Churchill Livingstone, 1983.
47. Reilly K, Ozanne A, Murdoch BE, et al: Linguistic status subsequent to childhood immersion injury. *Med J Aust* 148:225, 1988.
48. Sibert JR, Webb E, Cooper S: Drowning and near-drowning in children. *Practitioner* 232:439, 1988.
49. King RB, Webster IW: A case of recovery from drowning and prolonged anoxia. *Med J Aust* 1:919, 1964.
50. Kvittingen TD, Naess A: Recovery from drowning in fresh water. *BMJ* 1:1315, 1963.
51. Bratton SL, Jardine DS, Morray JP: Serial neurologic examinations after drowning and outcome. *Arch Pediatr Adolesc Med* 148:167, 1994.
52. Spack L, Gedeit R, Splaingard M, et al: Failure of aggressive therapy to alter outcome in pediatric near-drowning. *Pediatr Emerg Care* 13:98, 1997.
53. Habib DM, Tecklenburg FW, Webb SA, et al: Prediction of childhood drowning and near-drowning morbidity and mortality. *Pediatr Emerg Care* 12:255, 1996.
54. Quan L, Kinder D: Pediatric submersions: prehospital predictors of outcome. *Pediatrics* 90:909, 1992.
55. Christensen DW, Jansen P, Perkin RM: Outcome and acute care hospital costs after warm water near drowning in children. *Pediatrics* 99:715, 1997.
56. Abrams RA, Mubarak S: Musculoskeletal consequences of near-drowning in children. *J Pediatr Orthop* 11:168, 1991.
57. Conn AW, Miyasaka K, Katayama M, et al: A canine study of cold water drowning in fresh versus salt water. *Crit Care Med* 23:2029, 1995.
58. Modell JH, Weibly TC, Ruiz BC, et al: Serum electrolyte concentrations after freshwater aspiration: a comparison of species. *Anesthesiology* 30:421, 1969.
59. Ellis RJ: Severe hypernatremia from sea water ingestion during near-drowning in a hurricane. *West J Med* 167:430, 1997.
60. Hasan S, Avery WG, Fabian C, et al: Near-drowning in humans: a report of 36 patients. *Chest* 59:191, 1971.
61. Modell JH, Moya F, Newby EJ, et al: The effects of fluid volume in seawater drowning. *Ann Intern Med* 67:68, 1967.
62. Modell JH, Davis JH: Electrolyte changes in human drowning victims. *Anesthesiology* 30:414, 1969.
63. Ports TA, Deuel TF: Intravascular coagulation in fresh-water submersion: report of three cases. *Ann Intern Med* 87:60, 1977.
64. Munroe WD: Hemoglobinuria from near-drowning. *J Pediatr* 64:57, 1964.
65. Grausz H, Amend WJC, Earley LE: Acute renal failure complicating submersion in seawater. *JAMA* 217:207, 1971.
66. Segar WE, Riley PA, Barila TG: Urinary composition during hypothermia. *Am J Physiol* 185:528, 1956.
67. Sramek P, Simeckova M, Jansky L, et al: Human physiological responses to immersion into water of different temperatures. *Eur J Appl Physiol* 81:436, 2000.
68. Opdahl H: Survival put to the acid test: extreme arterial blood acidosis (pH 6.33) after near drowning. *Crit Care Med* 25:1431, 1997.
69. Watenpaugh DE, Pump B, Bie P, et al: Does gender influence human cardiovascular and renal responses to water immersion? *J Appl Physiol* 89:621, 2000.
70. Gunton RW, Scott JW, Lougheed WM, et al: Changes in cardiac rhythm in the form of the electrocardiogram resulting from induced hypothermia in man. *Am Heart J* 52:419, 1956.
71. Trevino A, Razi B, Beller BM: The characteristic electrocardiogram of accidental hypothermia. *Arch Intern Med* 127:470, 1971.
72. Vandam LD, Burnap TK: Hypothermia. *N Engl J Med* 261:546, 1959.
73. Karch SB: Pathology of the heart in drowning. *Arch Pathol Lab Med* 109:176, 1985.
74. Lunt DWR, Rose AG: Pathology of the heart in drowning. *Arch Pathol Lab Med* 111:939, 1987.
75. Orlowski JP, Abulleil MM, Phillips JM: The hemodynamic and cardiovascular effects of near-drowning in hypotonic, isotonic, hypertonic solutions. *Ann Emerg Med* 18:1044, 1989.
76. Chaney S, Gopalan R, Berggren RE: Pulmonary *Pseudoallescheria boydii* infection with cutaneous zygomycosis after near-drowning. *South Med J* 97:683, 2004.
77. Ender PT, Dolan MJ: Pneumonia associated with near-drowning. *Clin Infect Dis* 25:896, 1997.
78. Modell JH, Conn AW: Current neurological considerations in near-drowning. *Can Anaesth Soc J* 3:197, 1980.
79. Conn AW, Montes JE, Barker GA, et al: Cerebral salvage in near-drowning following neurological classification by triage. *Can Anaesth Soc J* 27:201, 1980.
80. Sirik Z, Lev A, Ruach M, et al: Freshwater near-drowning: our experience in life-supportive treatment. *Israel J Med Sci* 20:523, 1984.
81. Wunderlich P, Rupprecht E, Trefftz F, et al: Chest radiographs of near-drowned children. *Pediatr Radiol* 15:297, 1985.
82. Hunter TB, Whitehouse WM: Fresh-water near-drowning: radiologic aspects. *Radiology* 112:51, 1974.
83. Rosenbaum HT, Thompson WL, Fuller RH: Radiographic pulmonary changes in near-drowning. *Radiology* 83:306, 1964.
84. Dunagan DP, Cox JE, Chang MC, et al: Sand aspiration with near drowning: radiographic and bronchoscopic findings. *Am J Respir Crit Care Med* 156:292, 1997.
85. Szpilman D, Soares M: In-water resuscitation—is it worthwhile? *Resuscitation* 63:25, 2004.
86. Orlowski JP: Drowning, near-drowning, and ice-water submersions. *Pediatr Clin North Am* 34:75, 1987.
87. American Heart Association: *ACLS Provider Manual*. Dallas, TX, American Heart Association, 2004.
88. Rosen P, Stoto M, Harley J: The use of the Heimlich maneuver in near drowning: Institute of Medicine Report. *J Emerg Med* 13:397, 1995.
89. van Dorp JC, Knape JTA, Bierens JJLM: Final Recommendations of the World Congress on Drowning. Amsterdam, the Netherlands, June 26–28, 2002.
90. Hayward JS, Steinman AM: Accidental hypothermia: an experimental study of inhalation rewarming. *Aviat Space Environ Med* 46:1236, 1975.
91. Wickstrom P, Ruiz E, Lilja GP, et al: Accidental hypothermia: core rewarming with partial bypass. *Am J Surg* 131:622, 1976.
92. Towne WD, Geiss P, Yanes HO, et al: Intractable ventricular fibrillation associated with profound accidental hypothermia. Successful treatment with cardiopulmonary bypass. *N Engl J Med* 287:1135, 1972.
93. Truscott DG, Firor WB, Clein LJ: Accidental profound hypothermia: successful resuscitation by core rewarming and assisted circulation. *Arch Surg* 106:216, 1973.
94. Husby P, Anderson KS, Owen-Falkenberg A, et al: Accidental hypothermia with cardiac arrest: complete recovery after prolonged resuscitation and rewarming by extracorporeal circulation. *Intensive Care Med* 16:69, 1990.
95. Causey AL, Titelli JA, Swanson ME: Predicting discharge in uncomplicated near-drowning. *Am J Emerg Med* 18:9, 2000.
96. Noonan L, Howrey R, Ginsburg CM: Freshwater submersion injuries in children: a retrospective review of seventy-five hospitalized patients. *Pediatrics* 98:368, 1996.
97. Dottorini M, Eslami A, Baglioni S, et al: Nasal-continuous positive airway pressure in the treatment of near-drowning in freshwater. *Chest* 110:1122, 1996.
98. The Acute Respiratory Distress Syndrome Network: Ventilation with lower tidal volumes as compared with traditional tidal volumes for acute lung injury and the acute respiratory distress syndrome. *N Engl J Med* 342:1301, 2000.
99. Bernard SA, Gray TW, Buist MD, et al: Treatment of comatose survivors of out-of-hospital cardiac arrest with induced hypothermia. *N Engl J Med* 346:612, 2002.
100. The Hypothermia After Cardiac Arrest Study Group: Mild therapeutic hypothermia to improve the neurologic outcome after cardiac arrest. *New Engl J Med* 346:549, 2002.

CHAPTER 56 ■ PULMONARY HYPERTENSION IN THE INTENSIVE CARE UNIT

KIMBERLY A. FISHER AND HARRISON W. FARBER

INTRODUCTION

Pulmonary hypertension, defined as a mean pulmonary artery pressure (mPAP) greater than 25 mm Hg, is a common finding in critically ill patients. It can be related to the underlying critical illness (respiratory failure, pulmonary embolism, decompensated heart failure), pre-existing conditions (left-sided heart disease, chronic obstructive pulmonary disease (COPD), interstitial lung disease), or may be the primary cause of critical illness, as in the case of decompensated right heart failure due to pulmonary arterial hypertension (PAH). Initiation of appropriate therapy requires differentiating among these possible etiologies.

CLASSIFICATION/ETIOLOGY

Pulmonary hypertension is classified into five groups based on similar pathology and response to treatment, according to the fourth World Symposium on Pulmonary Hypertension (Table 56.1) [1]. In this classification, groupings are based on whether the primary abnormality is in the precapillary arteries and arterioles (Group 1), postcapillary pulmonary veins and venules (Group 2), alveoli and capillary beds (Group 3), or due to chronic thromboemboli (Group 4). Group 5 comprises causes of pulmonary hypertension with multiple or unclear mechanisms.

PAH refers only to Group 1 and is distinct from other forms of pulmonary hypertension. PAH can be idiopathic (IPAH, formerly primary pulmonary hypertension or PPH), heritable (HPAH), or associated with underlying conditions such as collagen vascular disease, congenital heart disease, portal hypertension, HIV infection, and specific drugs (e.g., fenfluramine) or toxins (e.g., rapeseed oil). Pulmonary venous hypertension is the result of elevated pulmonary venous (e.g., sclerosing mediastinitis) or left-sided cardiac filling pressures that lead to passive elevation in pulmonary artery pressures (PAPs). This is typically caused by left ventricular (LV) systolic or diastolic heart failure, or valvular heart disease (mitral or aortic regurgitation or stenosis). Lung disease can cause pulmonary hypertension due to alveolar hypoxemia (hypoxic pulmonary vasoconstriction) and vascular destruction [2]. Chronic thromboembolic pulmonary hypertension (CTEPH) can be due to proximal and/or distal obstruction of the pulmonary vasculature by chronic thromboemboli.

Pulmonary hypertension related to critical illness can occur through multiple mechanisms, and therefore patients may fall into any of the above-described groups (Table 56.2). However, no matter the group, or the reason for admission to the intensive care unit (ICU), right heart failure in this setting is associated with a poor prognosis. Among patients with PAH or inoperable CTEPH admitted to the ICU with decompensated right heart failure, infection is the most commonly identified trigger (23% to 27%), with other causes including drug or dietary noncompliance, arrhythmia, pulmonary embolism, and pregnancy. In approximately 50% of cases of decompensated right heart failure, no precipitating etiology can be identified, suggesting it is due to underlying disease progression. Decompensated right heart failure requiring ICU admission is associated with a high mortality rate (32% to 41%) [3,4].

Decompensation of left heart disease can cause or worsen pulmonary venous hypertension. Exacerbations of chronic hypoxemic lung disease (chronic obstructive lung disease or interstitial lung disease) can be associated with pulmonary hypertension. Acute pulmonary embolism can cause pulmonary hypertension, depending on the degree of vascular obstruction. In a patient with normal pulmonary vasculature, greater than 50% obstruction of the pulmonary vasculature must occur before pulmonary hypertension occurs. Pulmonary hypertension may also occur following acute pulmonary embolism with lesser degree of pulmonary vascular obstruction in patients with underlying cardiopulmonary disease [5].

Pulmonary hypertension complicates most cases of acute respiratory distress syndrome (ARDS); for example, it has been reported in 93% to 100% of patients with severe ARDS [6,7]. When pulmonary hypertension occurs, it is almost always mild to moderate in severity; only 7% of patients have severe pulmonary hypertension [7]. The magnitude of pulmonary hypertension in ARDS correlates with severity of lung injury [8] and has adverse prognostic significance [9]. More recent data in the era of low tidal volume ventilation have demonstrated a significantly lower prevalence of echocardiographically detected acute cor pulmonale (25% vs. 61%) in patients with ARDS. The lack of direct hemodynamic data and differences in data acquisition in these studies (transesophageal vs. transthoracic echocardiograms) precludes definitive conclusion; however, these studies suggest that the incidence of pulmonary hypertension in ARDS may have decreased with changes in mechanical ventilation strategies [10,11]. Furthermore, a recent study has demonstrated a low rate of right ventricular (RV) failure among patients with ARDS [12].

PHYSIOLOGY OF THE PULMONARY CIRCULATION AND RIGHT VENTRICLE

The pulmonary circulation is the only vascular bed that accommodates the entire cardiac output while maintaining both low pressure and low vascular resistance. Normally, the pulmonary vasculature is able to accommodate increases in cardiac output without increases in pressure or resistance via dilation of pulmonary vessels and recruitment of previously closed vessels [13]. Pulmonary hypertension develops when abnormalities of the pulmonary vasculature lead to increases in pulmonary vascular resistance (PVR) and therefore increased RV afterload.

TABLE 56.1

UPDATED CLINICAL CLASSIFICATION OF PULMONARY HYPERTENSION (DANA POINT, 2008)

Group 1. Pulmonary arterial hypertension (PAH)
Idiopathic PAH
Heritable
Drug and toxin induced
Associated with connective tissues disease, HIV infection, portal hypertension, congenital heart diseases, schistosomiasis, chronic hemolytic anemia
Persistent pulmonary hypertension of the newborn
Pulmonary veno-occlusive disease and/or pulmonary capillary hemangiomatosis
Group 2. Pulmonary hypertension owing to left heart disease
Systolic dysfunction
Diastolic dysfunction
Valvular disease
Group 3. Pulmonary hypertension owing to lung disease and/or hypoxia
Chronic obstructive pulmonary disease
Interstitial lung disease
Other pulmonary diseases with mixed restrictive and obstructive pattern
Sleep-disordered breathing
Alveolar hypoventilation disorders
Chronic exposure to high altitude
Developmental abnormalities
Group 4. Chronic thromboembolic pulmonary hypertension
Group 5. Pulmonary hypertension with unclear multifactorial mechanisms
Hematologic disorders: myeloproliferative disorders, splenectomy
Systemic disorders: sarcoidosis, pulmonary Langerhans cell histiocytosis, lymphangioleiomyomatosis, neurofibromatosis, vasculitis
Metabolic disorders: glycogen storage disease, Gaucher disease, thyroid disorders
Others: tumoral obstruction, fibrosing mediastinitis, chronic renal failure on dialysis

Modified from Simonneau G, Robbins IM, Beghetti M, et al: Updated clinical classification of pulmonary hypertension. *J Am Coll Cardiol* 54:S43–S54, 2009.

TABLE 56.2

COMMON CAUSES OF PULMONARY HYPERTENSION IN THE INTENSIVE CARE UNIT

Hypoxemia/parenchymal lung disease
Acute respiratory distress syndrome
Pulmonary embolism
Interstitial lung disease
Obstructive sleep apnea
Chronic obstructive pulmonary disease
Left heart disease
Acute myocardial infarction
Valvular disease (mitral regurgitation/mitral stenosis)
Severe diastolic dysfunction
Cardiomyopathy
Postoperative states
Coronary artery bypass grafting
Cardiac transplantation
Lung/heart–lung transplantation
Pneumonectomy
Thromboembolic lung disease
Pulmonary embolism
Deterioration of chronic pulmonary arterial hypertension
Infection
Fluid overloaded state
Arrhythmias
Pulmonary embolism
Acute on chronic pulmonary hypertension
Medication withdrawal

Modified from Zamanian RT, Haddad F, Doyle RL, et al: Management strategies for patients with pulmonary hypertension in the intensive care unit. *Crit Care Med* 35:2037–2050, 2007.

Because the RV normally ejects blood against a significantly lower afterload than the LV, it has a thinner wall and is therefore more compliant. This allows it to accommodate large increases in volume (preload). However, increases in afterload result in proportionate decreases in RV stroke volume [14]. Decreased RV stroke volume reduces blood return to the LV, thereby decreasing cardiac output. In addition, RV pressure overload causes "ventricular interdependence," in which elevated right ventricular end-diastolic pressure (RVEDP) causes bowing of the interventricular septum toward the LV during diastole, preventing LV diastolic filling and further reducing cardiac output [15–17]. RV pressure overload can also open the foramen ovale, allowing the shunting of blood from right to left, with resultant hypoxemia [14].

PATHOLOGY AND PATHOGENESIS

Patients with PAH share common pathologic findings including intimal fibrosis, increased medial thickness, pulmonary arteriolar occlusion, and plexiform lesions [18]. Multiple molecular pathways involved in the pathogenesis of IPAH have been identified [19]. Patients with IPAH have an increase in mediators of vasoconstriction and vascular smooth muscle cell proliferation (thromboxane A2, Endothelin-1) [20–22] and a decrease in substances that promote pulmonary vasodilation and inhibition of vascular smooth muscle cell proliferation (prostacyclin, nitric oxide, vasoactive intestinal peptide) [23–25].

Pathologic findings of pulmonary hypertension associated with ARDS vary with the time course of illness. Micro- and macrothrombi have been demonstrated in most patients. Early in disease, there are findings of acute endothelial cell injury. In the intermediate phase, chronic capillary changes, fibrocellular obliteration of arteries, veins, and lymphatics can occur. Vascular remodeling with distorted, tortuous arteries and veins, arterial muscularization, and reduced capillary number are seen in late stages [26]. While hypoxia and hypoxic pulmonary vasoconstriction likely play a role in the pathogenesis of pulmonary hypertension seen in ARDS, both the pathologic findings and the persistence of pulmonary hypertension in ARDS even after correction of severe hypoxemia [27] suggest the presence of additional pathogenic mechanisms. Indeed, intravenous infusion of endotoxin increases PAP in sheep [28], suggesting that disease processes such as sepsis may contribute to the development of pulmonary hypertension associated with ARDS. Patients with ARDS have increased levels of the pulmonary vasoconstrictors thromboxane A2, LTC4, and LTD4 in bronchoalveolar lavage fluid [29,30]. Finally, circulating levels of endothelin-1 are elevated in patients with ARDS [31].

DIAGNOSIS

Signs and Symptoms

Patients with PAH typically present with exertional dyspnea. Other presenting symptoms may include fatigue, syncope or near syncope, palpitations, and chest pain. As the disease progresses, patients may develop symptoms referable to reduced cardiac output and RV failure including fatigue, abdominal bloating and distension, and lower extremity edema. The presence of orthopnea and paroxysmal nocturnal dyspnea is suggestive of pulmonary venous hypertension [32].

Signs of elevated PAP on physical examination include (a) prominent pulmonary component of the second heart sound or P2, (b) RV heave, (c) early systolic ejection click, (d) midsystolic ejection murmur, (e) RV S_4 gallop, and (f) prominent jugular "a" wave. With more advanced disease, patients may develop findings of tricuspid regurgitation, including a holosystolic murmur along the left lower sternal border, and elevated jugular venous pressure. Findings of RV failure include elevated jugular pressure, pulsatile hepatomegaly, peripheral edema, ascites, and hypotension [32,33]. Patients with non–Group 1 causes of pulmonary hypertension may also have findings related to the primary disease, such as wheezing, decreased breath sounds and prolonged expiratory phase in COPD, and crackles in interstitial lung disease. The presence of bruits over the lung fields is specific for CTEPH, although present in only 30% of patients [34].

Diagnostic Testing

Electrocardiography (ECG) findings suggestive of pulmonary hypertension include right axis deviation (RAD), right atrial enlargement (P-wave ≥2.5 mm), and right ventricular hypertrophy (RVH) (frontal plane QRS axis ≥80°, R-wave/S-wave ratio in lead V1 >1, R-wave in lead V1 >0.5 mV) [32,35]. RVH and RAD are seen in 87% and 79% of patients with IPAH, respectively [33]. In a study of 61 patients with IPAH or PAH related to connective tissue disease, 8 patients (13%) had completely normal ECGs; thus, ECG is not sufficiently sensitive to screen patients suspected of PAH. ECG findings in patients with IPAH have prognostic significance with findings of P-wave amplitude 2.5 MV or more in lead II, qR lead V1, and RVH by WHO criteria associated with significantly increased risk of death, even after controlling for hemodynamic parameters, functional class, and treatment [36].

Radiographic findings of pulmonary hypertension include enlarged main and hilar pulmonary arterial shadows (≥18 mm diameter in men, ≥16 mm diameter in women) with peripheral pulmonary vascular attenuation ("pruning") and RV enlargement as evidenced by decreased size of the retrosternal clear space [32,33]. Other radiographic findings may suggest an underlying cause for pulmonary hypertension such as hyperinflation (COPD), prominent interstitial markings and fibrosis (interstitial lung disease), or cephalization and Kerley B lines (left-sided congestive heart failure).

Computerized tomography may be helpful in further delineating underlying parenchymal lung disease. Ventilation/perfusion ($\dot{V}/\dot{Q}$) scanning is the test of choice for identifying CTEPH; however, this cannot be performed on intubated patients and may be difficult to obtain in unstable patients, limiting its utility in critically ill patients. A normal or low probability $\dot{V}/\dot{Q}$ scan virtually excludes the diagnosis of CTEPH. Computerized tomographic angiography can identify acute pulmonary emboli and often CTEPH as well, although the role of computerized tomographic angiography for diagnosing CTEPH remains poorly defined [34].

Laboratory evaluation may reveal underlying diseases associated with an increased risk of pulmonary hypertension, such as connective tissue disease positive anti-nuclear antibody (ANA), or HIV infection. Brain natriuretic peptide (BNP) may have prognostic value in patients with PAH [37]; however, BNP levels may be elevated in critically ill patients with shock, or cardiac dysfunction of any cause and is, therefore, a nonspecific finding of unclear clinical significance [14,38].

Pulmonary hypertension may be suggested in critically ill patients by echocardiography. Echocardiography can provide noninvasive estimates of pulmonary arterial pressures, assessment of right and LV function, and evaluation of valvular disease. Echocardiographic findings of pulmonary hypertension may include RV dilation and hypertrophy, D-shaped LV due to septal bowing in the LV during late systole, RV hypokinesis, tricuspid regurgitation, right atrial enlargement, and a dilated inferior vena cava (IVC) [17]. In patients with IPAH, right atrial enlargement and the presence of a pericardial effusion are associated with poor prognosis [39]. Although echocardiographic estimates of PAP correlate well with invasively measured PAP in patients with left-sided heart disease [40–42], multiple studies have demonstrated that echocardiographic estimates of PAPs in patients with suspected pulmonary hypertension or with underlying lung disease can be inaccurate; the false-positive rate is 30% to 40% under these circumstances [43–46].

Therefore, right heart catheterization remains the gold standard for diagnosis of pulmonary hypertension and must be performed to confirm the diagnosis, determine the appropriate etiology, and determine the treatment. As stated previously, pulmonary hypertension is defined as an mPAP of more than 25 mm Hg, measured by right heart catheterization. The finding of a pulmonary capillary wedge pressure (PCWP) greater than 15 mm Hg is indicative of pulmonary venous hypertension. Right heart catheter findings may include the following hemodynamic profiles: (a) elevated PAP, normal PCWP, elevated PVR, consistent with PAH or PH due to hypoxemic lung disease; (b) elevated PAP, elevated PCWP, normal pulmonary artery diastolic pressure (PAD)–PCWP gradient, consistent with pulmonary venous hypertension; (c) elevated PAP, elevated PCWP, elevated PAD–PCWP gradient, consistent with pulmonary venous hypertension with "active" component. In patients with IPAH, findings at right heart catheterization of mPAP greater than or equal to 85 mm Hg, right atrial pressure greater than or equal to 20 mm Hg, and cardiac index less than 2 L per minute per m^2 are associated with worsened survival [47].

Vasodilator testing may be performed at the time of right heart catheterization. This is done by measuring baseline hemodynamics, administering a short-acting pulmonary vasodilator (adenosine, inhaled nitric oxide [iNO], or prostacyclin), and then repeating the hemodynamic measurements. Vasodilator responsiveness is defined as a decrease in the mPAP by at least 10 mm Hg, to less than 40 mm Hg with no change or an increase in cardiac output [48]. Vasodilator responsiveness in patients with IPAH is predictive of response to treatment with high-dose calcium channel blockers and suggests a better prognosis. Of note, patients with IPAH who are not acutely vasodilator responsive respond to long-term treatment with pulmonary vasodilators [49]; therefore, the finding of vasodilator responsiveness should only be used to decide which patients might be treated with calcium channel blockers, not which patients should be treated in general. The clinical significance of vasodilator responsiveness in forms of pulmonary hypertension other than IPAH is unproven.

TREATMENT

Treatment of pulmonary hypertension is dictated by the underlying cause, according to the revised classification of pulmonary hypertension (Table 56.1). When treating pulmonary hypertension in the ICU, one must differentiate between patients with pulmonary hypertension associated with underlying critical illness and patients who are critically ill due to PAH with RV failure and hemodynamic compromise.

General Measures

Hypoxic pulmonary vasoconstriction may contribute to pulmonary hypertension in critically ill patients. Supplemental oxygen results in a small, but statistically significant, decrease in PVR and an increase in cardiac output in patients with pulmonary hypertension of diverse etiologies [50]. Therefore, maintaining adequate oxygenation in critically ill patients with pulmonary hypertension is an important therapeutic goal.

Optimal fluid management in critically ill patients with decompensated RV failure can be extremely challenging. Because the RV is preload dependent, hypovolemia can result in decreased preload and therefore decreased cardiac output. However, hypervolemia can exacerbate RV pressure overload and ventricular interdependence, leading to decreased LV filling, also reducing cardiac output. Finding the optimal fluid balance for any given patient may require invasive hemodynamic monitoring.

Patients with RV dysfunction are poorly tolerant of loss of atrioventricular (AV) synchrony as occurs with atrial fibrillation and complete AV block. Therefore, maintenance of sinus rhythm may have salutary hemodynamic effects [51].

Retrospective and nonrandomized prospective studies of anticoagulation in patients with IPAH have demonstrated survival benefit with anticoagulation [52–54]. In the absence of contraindication, anticoagulation is therefore recommended for patients with PAH. However, there are no studies of anticoagulation in critically ill patients with pulmonary hypertension and thus no proven role for anticoagulation in this patient population.

Pulmonary Vasodilators

Significant advances in the outpatient treatment of PAH have been made since 1996 when the first pulmonary specific vasodilator was approved by the Food and Drug Administration (FDA). Patients with PAH (Group 1) benefit from treatment with prostacyclins (epoprostenol, treprostinil, iloprost), endothelin-receptor antagonists (bosentan, ambrisentan), and phosphodiesterase-5 inhibitors (sildenafil, tadalafil). Table 56.3 summarizes the major randomized controlled trials that have demonstrated clinical benefit with each of these medications [55–61]. Choice of initial therapy in stable outpatients with PAH is dictated by patients' risk profile, as assessed by functional class, 6-minute walk distance, BNP level, hemodynamics, and echocardiographic findings [62]. Oral pulmonary vasodilators are reserved for stable outpatients with low-risk profiles.

Patients with PAH and decompensated RV failure requiring admission to an ICU generally require treatment with intravenous prostanoids, although the initiation of pulmonary vasodilators as "rescue therapy" in the setting of decompensated right heart failure has not been well studied. In one small, retrospective study of patients with PAH and decompensated right heart failure, treatment with iloprost (inhaled) or treprostinil (intravenous or subcutaneous) was associated with decreased mortality [3]. However, in another study, treatment with intravenous epoprostenol or continuous iNO did not influence survival in patients with PAH or inoperable CTEPH and acute RV failure [4]. Of note, neither study was designed to study or compare the effects of pulmonary vasodilators on mortality in decompensated RV failure; therefore, no conclusions regarding which treatment may be most efficacious in this setting can be made.

Intravenous epoprostenol is the only medication with proven survival benefit in patients with IPAH [55] and is therefore the drug of choice for patients with severe PAH and a high-risk profile [63]. Epoprostenol therapy is typically initiated in the ICU with a right heart catheter in place. It is started at a dose of 1 to 2 ng per kg per minute and uptitrated by 1 to

TABLE 56.3

RESULTS OF PROSPECTIVE, RANDOMIZED TRIALS OF PHARMACOLOGIC TREATMENTS FOR PAH

Medication	No. of patients	WHO functional class	Results	Reference
Epoprostenol	81	III, IV	Improved survival, 6MWD, hemodynamics, and quality of life	[55]
Treprostinil	470	II, III, IV	Improved 6MWD, signs and symptoms of PAH, hemodynamics; no difference in rates of death, transplantation, or clinical deterioration.	[56]
Iloprost	203	III, IV	Improved combined clinical endpoint of 10% increase in 6MWD, WHO functional class, and the absence of deterioration or death; improved individual endpoints of 6MWD, postinhalation hemodynamics, WHO functional class.	[57]
Bosentan	213	III, IV	Improved 6MWD, Borg dyspnea index, WHO functional class, delayed time to clinical worsening	[58]
Ambrisentan	394	I, II, III, IV	Improved 6MWD, and delayed time to clinical worsening.	[59]
Sildenafil	278	I, II, III, IV	Improved 6MWD, hemodynamics, WHO functional class; no delay in time to clinical worsening.	[60]
Tadalafil	405	I, II, III, IV	Improved 6MWD, delayed time to clinical worsening, decreased incidence of clinical worsening. No significant improvement in WHO functional class.	[61]

6MWD, 6-minute walk distance; clinical worsening defined as combined endpoint of death, lung transplantation, hospitalization for pulmonary hypertension, lack of clinical improvement or worsening leading to need for additional therapy for PAH, or atrial septostomy.

2 ng per kg per minute at intervals of 15 to 30 minutes, with the hemodynamic goal of increased cardiac output and decreased PAP and PVR. Dose escalation is limited by side effects, such as headache, jaw pain, nausea, diarrhea, and systemic hypotension [55].

Treatment with epoprostenol can be complicated by the development of pulmonary edema, due to increased delivery of blood to the left side of the heart with resultant increased left-sided filling pressures. The development of pulmonary edema following the initiation of epoprostenol therapy should prompt consideration of pulmonary venoocclusive disease or pulmonary capillary hemangiomatosis, but this can also be seen in more common conditions such as occult diastolic dysfunction [64,65]. Epoprostenol results in nonselective pulmonary vasodilation. This can worsen $\dot{V}/\dot{Q}$ matching and cause clinically significant oxygen desaturation [66]. For patients chronically treated with epoprostenol, this can cause severe hypoxemia if superimposed focal lung disease such as pneumonia occurs. Abrupt discontinuation of epoprostenol has been demonstrated to lead to severe rebound pulmonary hypertension and death.

Treatment of patients with non–Group 1 pulmonary hypertension is focused on treating the underlying disease. For patients with pulmonary venous hypertension, optimization of afterload reduction and fluid management is the mainstay of therapy. Ensuring adequate oxygenation of patients with pulmonary hypertension due to parenchymal lung disease (Group 3) and treating the underlying disease are the main goals of therapy.

Given the poor prognostic significance of pulmonary hypertension in patients with ARDS, much attention has been focused on treating this aspect of ARDS. Administration of intravenous pulmonary vasodilators (epoprostenol, prostaglandin E_1, diltiazem) to patients with ARDS and pulmonary hypertension increases intrapulmonary shunting with resultant deterioration in oxygenation without improving survival [67–69]. There is therefore no proven role for using these agents in patients with pulmonary hypertension related to ARDS.

Inhaled pulmonary vasodilators are only delivered to ventilated alveoli and therefore improve $\dot{V}/\dot{Q}$ matching and oxygenation in patients with ARDS, while reducing pulmonary pressures. Specifically, iNO improves oxygenation, reduces pulmonary shunting, and reduces PVR in patients with ARDS [68,70]. However, in two large, multicenter, randomized, controlled trials comparing treatment with iNO with conventional therapy in patients with ARDS, no mortality benefit was demonstrated [71,72]. Similarly, nebulized prostaglandin I_2 improves oxygenation and decreases PAPs in patients with ARDS, without improving survival [73,74].

Treatment of pulmonary hypertension in ARDS with oral medications such as endothelin-receptor antagonists and phosphodiesterase-5 inhibitors used for treatment of PAH has not been studied.

Vasopressors

Patients with pulmonary hypertension may develop hemodynamic instability requiring vasopressor support. This may be due to progression of pulmonary hypertension with the development of RV failure or due to the development of a superimposed process, such as sepsis. The main goals of vasopressor therapy in patients with pulmonary hypertension are to reduce PVR, preserve or improve cardiac output, and maintain systemic blood pressure. There are limited data to guide the choice of vasopressors in the setting of pulmonary hypertension and RV failure.

Dobutamine reduces PVR and increases cardiac output in animal models of pulmonary hypertension [14,75,76]. In humans with mild-to-moderate pulmonary hypertension, dobutamine decreased PVR and increased cardiac index; however, increased intrapulmonary shunting with resultant decrease in arterial oxygenation was also noted. Dobutamine administered in combination with iNO resulted in significant decreases in PVR with concomitant increases in cardiac index and improved oxygenation [77]. Of note, these studies were performed in patients with stable cardiopulmonary hemodynamics. The physiologic effects of dobutamine in critically ill patients with pulmonary hypertension have not been well characterized. In a prospective, observational study of patients with PAH or inoperable CTEPH with acute RV failure requiring treatment with catecholamines, increasing dobutamine dose was associated with increased mortality [4]. However, this more likely reflects patients with more severe disease, rather than a deleterious effect of dobutamine on survival.

Norepinephrine administration in patients with pulmonary venous hypertension and systemic hypotension following induction of anaesthesia resulted in increased mPAP and PVR, but with decreased ratio of PAP to SBP (i.e., systolic blood pressure [SBP] increased more than PAP) and no change in cardiac index (CI). By contrast, phenylephrine administration resulted in decreased CI, without a concomitant decrease in the ratio of PAP to SBP [78]. Norepinephrine may be beneficial in restoring systemic blood pressure in patients with persistent hypotension despite treatment with pulmonary vasodilators and dobutamine, but should otherwise be avoided due to its pulmonary vasoconstrictive effects. Similarly, phenylephrine increases mPAP and PVR, with evidence of worsened RV function in patients with chronic pulmonary hypertension [79]. It should therefore be avoided in patients with hemodynamic compromise due to pulmonary hypertension.

Dopamine decreases PVR and increases cardiac output in an animal model of acute pulmonary embolism [80]. Similar effects were noted in patients with pulmonary hypertension due to chronic obstructive lung disease [81]. In humans with pulmonary venous hypertension, dopamine infusions increased mPAP, but this effect was mediated through increased cardiac output, not by pulmonary vasoconstriction [82]. The effects of dopamine in patients with PAH have not been well studied. In a retrospective, single-center study of patients with PAH and decompensated RV failure, higher doses of dopamine were associated with increased mortality. However, patients requiring treatment with dopamine had significantly more severe disease, by both clinical and hemodynamic parameters [3].

The effects of vasopressin on cardiopulmonary hemodynamics have not been characterized in patients with pulmonary hypertension. In an animal model of pulmonary hypertension, high-dose vasopressin increased mPAP and PVR and decreased cardiac output [83]. However, the effects of lower dose vasopressin, as used in treatment of septic shock, have not been studied.

In an animal model of pulmonary hypertension, isoproterenol reduces PVR and improves cardiac output [84]. However, these beneficial effects are largely offset by induction of tachyarrhythmias [85]. Although isoproterenol reduces PVR in patients with IPAH, the chronotropic effects limit its role in patients with PAH [14].

There are no published studies of the hemodynamic effects of epinephrine in patients with pulmonary hypertension.

Mechanical Ventilation

Institution of mechanical ventilation has complex hemodynamic effects that can be of clinical significance, especially in patients with severe PAH and decompensated RV failure.

Mechanical ventilation increases RV afterload and decreases RV preload that can be of particular hemodynamic consequence in patients with pulmonary hypertension. The increased afterload effects appear mediated primarily through increased lung volume [86]. Many of the studies evaluating effects of mechanical ventilation on RV function were performed prior to the era of low tidal volume ventilation for ARDS; therefore, it is unknown whether these effects are as pronounced or clinically important at lower tidal volumes.

Permissive hypercapnia has become common with the widespread institution of low tidal volume ventilation. Hypercapnia increases pulmonary pressures, although it is unclear whether this is due simply to increased cardiac output or by a direct pulmonary vasoconstrictive effect [87–89]. In one study of hemodynamically stable patients following coronary artery bypass grafting, hypercarbia (mean $Paco_2$ 49.8 mm Hg) increased mPAP, PVR, and RVEDP and decreased right ventricular ejection fraction (RVEF) by 20% [87].

Similarly, elevations in positive end-expiratory pressure (PEEP) also increase pulmonary arterial pressure and PVR [90,91]. In one study of patients with ARDS, a mean increase in PEEP from 4 cm H_2O to 17 cm H_2O elevated mPAP from 27.7 mm Hg to 36.7 mm Hg [91].

Although the net effect of mechanical ventilation is to increase pulmonary arterial pressure, this is typically well tolerated in patients with mild-to-moderate pulmonary hypertension. These effects, however, may be of particular hemodynamic consequence in patients with PAH and RV failure. Mechanical ventilation in these patients should ideally be with low tidal volume and low PEEP, while avoiding permissive hypercapnia.

Surgical Management

Atrial septostomy, or the surgical creation of an atrial septal shunt, decompresses the RV by creating an alternative outflow tract for blood and increases left atrial filling. However, it is associated with very high morbidity and mortality in critically ill patients with RV failure [92–94]. It is complicated by oxygen desaturation through the creation of a right-to-left shunt. It is contraindicated in patients with mean right atrial pressure (RAP) greater than 20 mm Hg, significant hypoxemia, and PVR index greater than 4,400 dyne second per cm^5 per m^2 [93].

References

1. Simonneau G, Robbins IM, Beghetti M, et al: Updated clinical classification of pulmonary hypertension. *J Am Coll Cardiol* 54:S43–S54, 2009.
2. Weitzenblum E, Chaouat A: Pulmonary hypertension due to chronic hypoxic lung disease, in Peacock AJ, Rubin LJ (eds): *Pulmonary Circulation: Diseases and Their Treatment.* 2nd ed. New York, NY, Oxford University Press, 2004, p 376.
3. Kurzyna M, Zylkowska J, Fijatkowska A, et al: Characteristics and prognosis of patients with decompensated right ventricular failure during the course of pulmonary hypertension. *Kardiol Pol* 66:1033–1039, 2008.
4. Sztrymf B, Souza R, Bertoletti L, et al: Prognostic factors of acute heart failure in patients with pulmonary arterial hypertension [published online ahead of print November 6, 2009]. *Eur Respir J* 35:1286–1293, 2010.
5. Hargett CW, Tapson VF: Venous thromboembolism: pulmonary embolism and deep venous thrombosis, in *Irwin and Rippe's Intensive Care Medicine.* 6th ed. Philadelphia, PA, Lippincott Williams & Wilkins, 2008, p 576.
6. Zapol WM, Snider MT: Pulmonary hypertension in severe acute respiratory failure. *N Engl J Med* 296(9):476–480, 1977.
7. Beiderlinden M, Kuehl H, Boes T, et al: Prevalence of pulmonary hypertension associated with severe acute respiratory distress syndrome: predictive value of computed tomography. *Intensive care Med* 32:852–857, 2006.
8. Sibbald WJ, Paterson NAM, Holliday RL, et al: Pulmonary hypertension in sepsis. *Chest* 73:583–591, 1978.
9. Villar J, Blazquez MA, Lubillo S, et al: Pulmonary hypertension in acute respiratory failure. *Crit Care Med* 17:523–526, 1989.
10. Vieillard-Baron A, Schmitt JM, Augard R, et al: Acute cor pulmonale in acute respiratory distress syndrome submitted to protective ventilation: incidence, clinical implications, and prognosis. *Crit Care Med* 29:1551–1555, 2001.
11. Jardin F, Gueret P, Dubourg O, et al: Two-dimensional echocardiographic evaluation of right ventricular size and contractility in acute respiratory failure. *Crit Care Med* 13:952–956, 1985.
12. Osman D, Monnet X, Castelain V, et al: Incidence and prognostic value of right ventricular failure in acute respiratory distress syndrome. *Intensive Care Med* 35:69–76, 2009.
13. Rubin LJ: Pulmonary hypertension, in *Irwin & Rippe's Intensive Care Medicine.* 6th ed. Philadelphia, PA, Lippincott Williams & Wilkins, 2008, p 615.
14. Zamanian RT, Haddad F, Doyle RL, et al: Management strategies for patients with pulmonary hypertension in the intensive care unit. *Crit Care Med* 35:2037–2050, 2007.
15. Boxt LM, Katz FJ, Kolb T: Direct quantitation of right and left ventricular volumes with nuclear magnetic resonance imaging in patients with primary pulmonary hypertension. *J Am Coll Cardiol* 5:1326–1334, 1985.
16. Stone AC, Klinger JR: The right ventricle in pulmonary hypertension, in *Hill and Farber's Pulmonary Hypertension.* Totowa, NJ: Humana Press, 2008, p 96.
17. Vieillard-Baron A, Prin S, Chergui K, et al: Echo-Doppler demonstration of acute cor pulmonale at the bedside in the medical intensive care unit. *Am J Respir Crit Care Med* 166:1310–1319, 2002.
18. Rubin LJ: Primary pulmonary hypertension. *N Engl J Med* 336:111–117, 1997.
19. Farber HW, Loscalzo J: Mechanisms of disease: pulmonary arterial hypertension. *N Engl J Med* 351:1655–1665, 2004.
20. Christman BW, McPherson CD, Newman JH, et al: An imbalance between the excretion of thromboxane and prostacyclin metabolites in pulmonary hypertension. *N Engl J Med* 327:70–75, 1992.
21. Giaid A, Yanagisawa M, Langleben D, et al: Expression of endothelin-1 in the lungs of patients with pulmonary hypertension. *N Engl J Med* 328:1732–1739, 1993.
22. Vincent JA, Ross RD, Kassab J, et al: Relation of elevated plasma endothelin in congenital heart disease to increased pulmonary blood flow. *Am J Cardiol* 71:1204–1207, 1993.
23. Tuder RM, Cool CD, Geraci MW, et al: Prostacyclin synthase expression is decreased in lungs from patients with severe pulmonary hypertension. *Am J Respir Crit Care Med* 159:1925–1932, 1999.
24. Giaid A, Saleh D: Reduced expression of endothelial nitric oxide synthase in the lungs of patients with pulmonary hypertension. *N Engl J Med* 333:214–221, 1995.
25. Petkov V, Mosgoeller W, Ziesche R, et al: Vasoactive intestinal peptide as a new drug for treatment of primary pulmonary hypertension. *J Clin Invest* 111:1339–1346, 2003.
26. Tomashefski JF, Davies P, Boggis C, et al: The pulmonary vascular lesions of the adult respiratory distress syndrome. *Am J Pathol* 112:112–126, 1983.
27. Moloney ED, Evans TW: Pathophysiology and pharmacological treatment of pulmonary hypertension in acute respiratory distress syndrome. *Eur Respir J* 21:720–727, 2003.
28. Esbenshade AM, Newman JH, Lams PM, et al: Respiratory failure after endotoxin infusion in sheep: lung mechanics and lung fluid balance. *J Appl Physiol* 53:967–976, 1982.
29. Leeman M, Boeynaems JM, Degaute JP, et al: Administration of dazoxiben, a selective thromboxane synthetase inhibitor, in the adult respiratory distress syndrome. *Chest* 87:726–730, 1985.
30. Matthay MA, Eschenbacher WL, Goetzl EJ: Elevated concentrations of leukotriene D4 in pulmonary edema fluid of patients with the adult respiratory distress syndrome. *J Clin Immunol* 4:479–483, 1984.
31. Druml W, Steltzer H, Waldhausl W, et al: Endothelin-1 in adult respiratory distress syndrome. *Am Rev Respir Dis* 148:1169–1173, 1993.
32. McGoon M, Gutterman D, Steen V, et al: Screening, early detection, and diagnosis of pulmonary arterial hypertension: ACCP evidence-based clinical practice guidelines. *Chest* 126:14S–34S, 2004.
33. Rich S, Dantzker DR, Ayres SM, et al: Primary pulmonary hypertension. A national prospective study. *Ann Intern Med* 102:216–223, 1987.
34. Fedullo PF, Auger WR, Kerr KM, et al: Chronic thromboembolic pulmonary hypertension. *N Engl J Med* 345:1465–1472, 2001.
35. Ahearn GS, Tapson VF, Rebeiz A, et al: Electrocardiography to define clinical status in primary pulmonary hypertension and pulmonary arterial hypertension secondary to collagen vascular disease. *Chest* 122:524–527, 2002.
36. Bossone E, Paciocco G, Iarussi D, et al: The prognostic role of the ECG in primary pulmonary hypertension. *Chest* 121:513–518, 2002.
37. Nagaya N, Nishikimi T, Uematsu M, et al: Plasma brain natriuretic peptide as a prognostic indicator in patients with primary pulmonary hypertension. *Circulation* 102:865–870, 2000.
38. Maeder M, Fehr T, Rickli H, et al: Sepsis-associated myocardial dysfunction: diagnostic and prognostic impact of cardiac troponins and natriuretic peptides. *Chest* 129:1349–1366, 2006.

39. Raymond RJ, Hinderliter AL, Willis PW, et al: Echocardiographic predictors of adverse outcomes in primary pulmonary hypertension. *J Am Coll Cardiol* 39:1214–1219, 2002.
40. Yock PG, Popp RL: Noninvasive estimation of right ventricular systolic pressure by Doppler ultrasound in patients with tricuspid regurgitation. *Circulation* 70:657–662, 1984.
41. Currie PJ, Seward JB, Chan KL, et al: Continuous wave Doppler determination of right ventricular pressure: a simultaneous Doppler-catheterization study in 127 patients. *J Am Coll Cardiol* 6:750–756, 1985.
42. Skjaerpe T, Hatle L: Noninvasive estimation of systolic pressure in the right ventricle in patients with tricuspid regurgitation. *Eur Heart J* 7:704–710, 1986.
43. Colle IO, Moreau R, Godinho E, et al: Diagnosis of portopulmonary hypertension in candidates for liver transplantation: a prospective study. *Hepatology* 37:401–409, 2003.
44. Mukerjee D, St. George D, Knight C, et al: Echocardiography and pulmonary function as screening tests for pulmonary arterial hypertension in systemic sclerosis. *Rheumatology* 43:461–466, 2004.
45. Hachulla E, Gressin V, Guillevin L, et al: Early detection of pulmonary arterial hypertension in systemic sclerosis: a French nationwide prospective multicenter study. *Arthritis Rheum* 52:3792–3800, 2005.
46. Fisher MR, Forfia PR, Chamera E, et al: Accuracy of Doppler echocardiography in the hemodynamic assessment of pulmonary hypertension. *Am J Respir Crit Care Med* 179:615–621, 2009.
47. D'Alonzo GE, Barst RJ, Ayres SM, et al: Survival in patients with primary pulmonary hypertension. Results from a national prospective registry. *Ann Intern Med* 115:343–349, 1991.
48. Sitbon O, Humbert M, Jais X, et al: Long-term response to calcium channel blockers in idiopathic pulmonary arterial hypertension. *Circulation* 111:3105–3111, 2005.
49. McLaughlin VV, Genthner DE, Panella MM, et al: Reduction in pulmonary vascular resistance with long-term epoprostenol (prostacyclin) therapy in primary pulmonary hypertension. *N Engl J Med* 338:273–277, 1998.
50. Roberts DH, Lepore JJ, Maroo A, et al: Oxygen therapy improves cardiac index and pulmonary vascular resistance in patients with pulmonary hypertension. *Chest* 120:1547–1555, 2001.
51. Goldstein JA, Harada A, Yagi Y, et al: Hemodynamic importance of systolic ventricular interaction, augmented RA contractility, and AV synchrony in acute RV dysfunction. *J Am Coll Cardiol* 16:181–189, 1990.
52. Fuster V, Steele PM, Edwards WD, et al: Primary pulmonary hypertension: natural history and the importance of thrombosis. *Circulation* 70:580–587, 1984.
53. Rich S, Kaufmann E, Levy PS: The effect of high doses of calcium channel blockers on survival in primary pulmonary hypertension. *N Engl J Med* 327:76–81, 1992.
54. Kawut SM, Horn EM, Berekashvili KK, et al: New predictors of outcome in idiopathic pulmonary arterial hypertension. *Am J Cardiol* 95:199–203, 2005.
55. Barst RJ, Rubin LJ, Long WA, et al: A comparison of continuous intravenous epoprostenol (prostacyclin) with conventional therapy for primary pulmonary hypertension. *N Engl J Med* 334:296–302, 1996.
56. Simonneau G, Barst RJ, Galie N, et al: Continuous subcutaneous infusion of treprostinil, a prostacyclin analogue, in patients with pulmonary arterial hypertension. *Am J Respir Crit Care Med* 165:800–804, 2002.
57. Olschewski H, Simonneau G, Galie N, et al: Inhaled iloprost for severe pulmonary hypertension. *N Engl J Med* 347:322–329, 2002.
58. Rubin LJ, Badesch DB, Barst RJ, et al: Bosentan therapy for pulmonary arterial hypertension. *N Engl J Med* 346:896–903, 2002.
59. Galie N, Olschewski H, Oudiz RJ, et al: Ambrisentan for the treatment of pulmonary arterial hypertension. *Circulation* 117:3010–3019, 2008.
60. Galie N, Ghofrani HA, Torbicki A, et al: Sildenafil citrate therapy for pulmonary arterial hypertension. *N Engl J Med* 353:2148–2157, 2005.
61. Galie N, Brundage BH, Ghofrani HA, et al: Tadalafil therapy for pulmonary arterial hypertension. *Circulation* 119:2894–2903, 2009.
62. McLaughlin VV, Archer SL, Badesch DB, et al: ACCF/AHA 2009 expert consensus document on pulmonary hypertension. *J Am Coll Cardiol* 53:1573–1619, 2009.
63. Barst RJ, Gibbs SR, Ghofrani HA, et al: Updated evidence-based treatment algorithm in pulmonary arterial hypertension. *J Am Coll Cardiol* 54:S78–S84, 2009.
64. Gugnani MK, Pierson C, Vanderheide R, et al: Pulmonary edema complicating prostacyclin therapy in pulmonary hypertension associated with scleroderma: a case of pulmonary capillary hemangiomatosis. *Arthritis Rheum* 43:699–703, 2000.
65. Montani D, Achouh L, Dorfmuller P, et al: Pulmonary veno-occlusive disease: clinical, functional, radiologic, and hemodynamic characteristics and outcome of 24 cases confirmed by histology. *Medicine* 87:220–233, 2008.
66. Otulana B, Higenbottam T: The role of physiological deadspace and shunt in the gas exchange of patients with pulmonary hypertension: a study of exercise and prostacyclin infusion. *Eur Respir J* 1:732–737, 1988.
67. Bone RC, Slotman G, Maunder R, et al: Randomized double-blind, multicenter study of prostaglandin E_1 in patients with the adult respiratory distress syndrome. Prostaglandin E_1 Study Group. *Chest* 96:114–119, 1989.
68. Melot C, Lejeune P, Leeman M, et al: Prostaglandin E_1 in the adult respiratory distress syndrome. Benefit for pulmonary hypertension and cost for pulmonary gas exchange. *Am Rev Respir Dis* 139:106–110, 1989.
69. Rossaint R, Falke KJ, Lopez F, et al: Inhaled nitric oxide for the adult respiratory distress syndrome. *N Engl J Med* 328:399–405, 1993.
70. Zapol WM, Rimar S, Gillis N, et al: Nitric oxide and the lung. *Am J Respir Crit Care Med* 149:1375–1380, 1994.
71. Dellinger RP, Zimmerman JL, Taylor RW, et al: Effects of inhaled nitric oxide in patients with acute respiratory distress syndrome: results of a randomized phase 2 trial. Inhaled Nitric Oxide in ARDS Study Group. *Crit Care Med* 26:15–23, 1998.
72. Lundin S, Mang H, Smithies M, et al: Inhalation of nitric oxide in acute lung injury: results of a European multicentre study. The European Study Group of Inhaled Nitric Oxide. *Intensive Care Med* 25:911–999, 1999.
73. Walmrath D, Schneider T, Schermuly R, et al: Direct comparison of inhaled nitric oxide and aerosolized prostacyclin in acute respiratory distress syndrome. *Am J Respir Crit Care Med* 153:991–996, 1996.
74. Zwissler B, Kemming G, Habbler O, et al: Inhaled prostacyclin (PGI_2) versus inhaled nitric oxide in adult respiratory distress syndrome. *Am J Respir Crit Care Med* 154:1671–1677, 1996.
75. Bradford KK, Deb B, Pearl RG: Combination therapy with inhaled nitric oxide and intravenous dobutamine during pulmonary hypertension in the rabbit. *J Cardiovasc Pharmacol* 36:146–151, 2000.
76. Kerbaul F, Rondelet B, Motte S, et al: Effects of norepinephrine and dobutamine on pressure load-induced right ventricular failure. *Crit Care Med* 32:1035–1040, 2004.
77. Vizza CD, Rocca GD, Roma AD, et al: Acute hemodynamic effects of inhaled nitric oxide, dobutamine, and a combination of the two in patients with mild to moderate secondary pulmonary hypertension. *Crit Care* 5:355–361, 2001.
78. Kwak YL, Lee CS, Park YH, et al: The effect of phenylephrine and norepinephrine in patients with chronic pulmonary hypertension. *Anaesthesia* 57:9–14, 2002.
79. Rich S, Gubin S, Hart K: The effects of phenylephrine on right ventricular performance in patients with pulmonary hypertension. *Chest* 98:1102–1106, 1990.
80. Ducas J, Stitz M, Gu S, et al: Pulmonary vascular pressure-flow characteristics. Effects of dopamine before and after pulmonary embolism. *Am Rev Respir Dis* 146:307–312, 1992.
81. Philip-Joet F, Saadjian A, Vestri R, et al: Hemodynamic effects of a single dose of dopamine and L-dopa in pulmonary hypertension secondary to chronic obstructive lung disease. *Respiration* 53:146–152, 1988.
82. Holloway EL, Polumbo RA, Harrison DC: Acute circulatory effects of dopamine in patients with pulmonary hypertension. *Br Heart J* 37:482–485, 1975.
83. Leather HA, Segers P, Berends N, et al: Effects of vasopressin on right ventricular function in an experimental model of acute pulmonary hypertension. *Crit Care Med* 30:2548–2552, 2002.
84. Ducas J, Duval D, Dasilva H, et al: Treatment of canine pulmonary hypertension: effects of norepinephrine and isoproterenol on pulmonary vascular pressure-flow characteristics. *Circulation* 75:235–242, 1987.
85. Prielipp RC, McLean R, Rosenthal MH, et al: Hemodynamic profiles of prostaglandin E_1, isoproterenol, prostacyclin, and nifedipine in experimental porcine pulmonary hypertension. *Crit Care Med* 19:60–67, 1991.
86. Vieillard-Baron A, Loubieres Y, Schmitt J, et al: Cyclic changes in right ventricular output impedance during mechanical ventilation. *J Appl Physiol* 87:1644–1650, 1999.
87. Viitanen A, Salmenpera M, Heinonen J: Right ventricular response to hypercarbia after cardiac surgery. *Anesthesiology* 73:393–400, 1990.
88. Carvalho CRR, Barbas CSV, Medeiros DM, et al: Temporal hemodynamic effects of permissive hypercapnia associated with ideal PEEP in ARDS. *Am J Respir Crit Care Med* 156:1458–1466, 1997.
89. Balanos GM, Talbot NP, Dorrington KL, et al: Human pulmonary vascular response to 4 h of hypercapnia and hypocapnia measured using Doppler echocardiography. *J Appl Physiol* 94:1543–1551, 2003.
90. Jardin F, Farcot JC, Boisante L, et al: Influence of PEEP on LV performance. *N Engl J Med* 304:387–392, 1981.
91. Artucio H, Hurtado J, Zimet L, et al: PEEP-induced tricuspid regurgitation. *Intensive Care Med* 23:836–840, 1997.
92. Sandoval J, Gaspar J, Pulido T, et al: Graded balloon dilation atrial septostomy in severe primary pulmonary hypertension. A therapeutic alternative to vasodilator treatment. *J Am Coll Cardiol* 32:297–304, 1998.
93. Rothman A, Sklansky MS, Lucas VW, et al: Atrial septostomy as a bridge to lung transplantation in patients with severe pulmonary hypertension. *Am J Cardiol* 84:682–686, 1999.
94. Reichenberger F, Pepke-Zaba J, McNeil K, et al: Atrial septostomy in the treatment of severe pulmonary arterial hypertension. *Thorax* 58:797–800, 2003.

CHAPTER 57 ■ PLEURAL DISEASE IN THE CRITICALLY ILL PATIENT

PETER DOELKEN AND STEVEN A. SAHN

Pleural disease is an unusual cause for admission to the intensive care unit (ICU). Exceptions are a large hemothorax for monitoring bleeding rate and hemodynamic status and an unstable secondary spontaneous pneumothorax or large unilateral or bilateral pleural effusions that have caused acute respiratory failure.

Pleural disease can be overlooked in the critically ill patient because it may be overshadowed by the presenting illness that has resulted in ICU admission. Furthermore, it is often a subtle finding on the clinical examination and supine chest radiograph. A pleural effusion may not be seen on the supine chest radiograph because a diffuse alveolar filling process can mask the posterior layering of fluid or because bilateral effusions without parenchymal infiltrates are misinterpreted as an underexposed film or objects outside the chest. Pneumothorax may remain undetected in the supine patient because pleural air tends to be situated anteriorly and does not produce the diagnostic visceral pleural line seen on an upright radiograph. When the patient on mechanical ventilation support is at increased risk for barotrauma because airway pressures are high, the index of suspicion for pneumothorax should be heightened; if there is evidence of pulmonary interstitial gas (see following discussion) or subcutaneous emphysema, appropriate radiologic studies should be obtained.

RADIOLOGIC SIGNS OF PLEURAL DISEASE IN THE INTENSIVE CARE UNIT

Because the distribution of fluid and air in the normal pleural space tends to follow gravitational influences, and because the lung has a tendency to maintain its normal shape as it becomes smaller, fluid initially accumulates between the bottom of the lung and the diaphragm, and air accumulates between the top of the lung and the apex of the thorax in the upright position. When chest radiographs are obtained in other than the erect position, free pleural fluid and air change position and result in a different radiographic appearance.

PLEURAL FLUID

Standard Chest Radiograph

In healthy humans in the supine position, the radiolucency of the lung base is equal to or greater than that in the lung apex [1]. Furthermore, when in the supine position, breast and pectoral tissue tend to fall laterally away from the lung base. Thus, an effusion should be suspected if there is increased homogeneous density over the lower lung fields compared to the upper lung fields. As the pleural effusion increases, the increased radiodensity involves the upper hemithorax as well. However, failure of chest wall tissue to move laterally, cardiomegaly, prominent epicardial fat pad, and lung collapse or consolidation may obscure a pleural effusion on a supine radiograph. Patient rotation or an off-center X-ray beam can mimic a unilateral homogeneous density. An absent pectoral muscle, prior mastectomy, unilateral hyperlucent lung, scoliosis, previous lobectomy, hypoplastic pulmonary artery, or pleural or chest wall mass may lead to unilateral homogeneous increased density and mimic an effusion.

Approximately 175 to 525 mL of pleural fluid results in blunting of the costophrenic angle on an erect radiograph [2]. This quantity of effusion can be detected on a supine radiograph as an increased density over the lower lung zone. Failure to visualize the hemidiaphragm, absence of the costophrenic angle meniscus, and apical capping are less likely to be seen with effusions of less than 500 mL [1]. The major radiographic finding of a pleural effusion in a supine position is increased homogeneous density over the lower lung field that does not obliterate normal bronchovascular markings, does not show air bronchograms, and does not show hilar or mediastinal displacement until the effusion is massive. If a pleural effusion is suspected in the supine patient, ultrasonography (US) should be performed.

Other Radiographic Imaging

Sonography

US provides good characterization for pleural diseases and is a useful diagnostic modality for critically ill patients who cannot be transported for computed tomography (CT). US takes less time and is less expensive than CT, can be done at the bedside, and can be repeated serially. Disadvantages include hindrance of the ultrasonic wave by air, in either the lung or the pleural space, a restricted field of view, inferior evaluation of the lung parenchyma compared with CT, and operator dependence. US was helpful in diagnosis in 27 (66%) of 41 patients and treatment in 37 (90%) of 41 patients, and had an important influence on treatment planning in 17 (41%) of 41 critically ill patients [3].

US has also been demonstrated to be a useful modality to guide bedside thoracentesis in the mechanically ventilated patient, resulting in high success rate and excellent safety of the procedure [4].

Computed Tomography

CT is recognized as providing increased resolution compared with conventional imaging. Although moving a critically ill patient for CT has potential risks, the diagnostic advantage is justified in the stable patient when the clinical course is not congruent with the proposed diagnosis suggested by the portable chest radiograph. In selected patients with multisystem trauma, chest CT often provides additional diagnostic information and positively affects patient management and outcome.

PNEUMOTHORAX

When supine, pneumothorax gas migrates along the anterior surface of the lung, making detection on the anteroposterior radiograph problematic. The base, lateral chest wall, and juxtacardiac area should be carefully visualized for evidence of pneumothorax. Accumulation of air along the mediastinal parietal pleura may simulate pneumomediastinum [5]. An erect or decubitus (suspected hemithorax up) radiograph should be obtained to assess for the presence of a pneumothorax. US is sensitive for the detection of pneumothorax by determining the presence or absence of "lung sliding" [6]. In individuals without pneumothorax, the lung–chest wall interface, which represents a to-and-fro movement synchronized with respiration, can be identified. US visualization of lung sliding is correlated with the absence of pneumothorax, and from this sign alone, at least anterior pneumothorax can be excluded rapidly at the bedside of a mechanically ventilated patient. However, absence of lung sliding may be caused by the presence of large bullae or pleural symphysis caused by previous pleurodesis or pleural adhesions due to previous pleural disease. Hence, the absence of lung sliding is not specific for pneumothorax but detection of lung sliding reliably excludes the presence of pleural air in the examined area.

The most common radiographic signs of tension pneumothorax are contralateral mediastinal shift, ipsilateral diaphragmatic depression, and ipsilateral chest wall expansion. Underlying lung disease may prevent total lung collapse, even if tension is present; in patients on mechanical ventilation, little or no midline mediastinal shift may result from the tension [7]. In the latter, a depressed ipsilateral diaphragm is a more reliable sign of tension than mediastinal shift.

In patients with acute respiratory distress syndrome (ARDS), barotrauma can result in a localized tension pneumothorax with a subtle contralateral mediastinal shift, flattening of the cardiac contour, and depression of the ipsilateral hemidiaphragm [8]. Pleural adhesions and relative compressibility and mobility of surrounding structures, in addition to the supine position, probably account for these loculated tension pneumothoraces.

In a study of 88 critically ill patients with 112 pneumothoraces, the anteromedial and subpulmonic recesses were involved in 64% of patients in the supine and semierect position [9]. Furthermore, in 30% of the pneumothoraces in this study that were not initially detected by the clinician or radiologist, half of the patients progressed to tension pneumothorax. Therefore, a high index of suspicion is necessary to avoid catastrophic situations.

Factors that may contribute to an improved ability to diagnose this potentially lethal problem include (a) familiarity with atypical locations of pneumothoraces in critically ill patients, usually due to the supine or semierect position; (b) the consequence of underlying cardiopulmonary disease; and (c) knowledge of other risk factors contributing to misdiagnosis (e.g., mechanical ventilation, altered mental status, prolonged ICU stay, and development of pneumothorax after peak physician staffing hours) [10].

EVALUATIONS OF THE PATIENT WITH A PLEURAL EFFUSION IN THE INTENSIVE CARE UNIT

Diagnostic Thoracentesis

Indications

Patients with a pleural effusion provide the opportunity to diagnose, at least presumptively, the underlying process responsible for pleural fluid accumulation. Pleural effusions are most commonly caused by primary lung disease but may also result from disease in the gastrointestinal tract, liver, kidney, heart, or reticuloendothelial system.

Although disease of any organ system can cause a pleural effusion in critically ill patients, the diagnoses listed in Table 57.1 represent the majority of the causes seen in ICUs. The types of pleural effusions seen in medical and surgical ICUs are similar, but some causes related to surgical (coronary artery bypass grafting, chylothorax, abdominal surgery) and nonsurgical trauma (hemothorax) represent a substantial percentage of surgical ICU effusions.

When a pleural effusion is suspected on physical examination and confirmed radiologically, a diagnostic thoracentesis under ultrasonographic guidance should be performed in an attempt to establish the cause. Exceptions are patients with a secure clinical diagnosis and a small amount of pleural fluid, as in atelectasis, or patients with uncomplicated congestive heart failure (CHF) [11]. Observation may be warranted in these situations, but thoracentesis should be performed if there are adverse changes [12].

The indications for diagnostic thoracentesis do not change simply because the patient is in the ICU or on mechanical ventilation. In fact, establishing the diagnosis quickly in these critically ill patients may be more important and life-saving than in noncritically ill patients. It has been well documented that even in patients on mechanical ventilation, diagnostic thoracentesis is safe if there is strict adherence to the general principles of the procedure and US is used (see Chapter 10) [4,13]. Pneumothorax, the most clinically important complication of thoracentesis [11], is no more likely to occur in the patient on mechanical ventilation than in the patient who is not; however, if a

TABLE 57.1

CAUSES OF PLEURAL EFFUSIONS

In the medical ICU	In the surgical ICU
Atelectasis	Atelectasis
Congestive heart failure	Congestive heart failure
Pneumonia	Pneumonia
Hypoalbuminemia	Pancreatitis
Pancreatitis	Hypoalbuminemia
ARDS	Coronary artery bypass surgery
Pulmonary embolism	ARDS
Hepatic hydrothorax	Pulmonary embolism
Esophageal sclerotherapy	Esophageal rupture
Postmyocardial infarction	Hemothorax
Iatrogenic	Chylothorax
	Abdominal surgery
	Iatrogenic

ARDS, acute respiratory distress syndrome; ICU, intensive care unit.

pneumothorax does develop, the patient on mechanical ventilation is likely to develop a tension pneumothorax.

Contraindications

There are no absolute contraindications to diagnostic thoracentesis. If clinical judgment dictates that the information gained from the pleural fluid analysis may help in diagnosis and therapy, thoracentesis should be performed (see Chapter 10). Diagnostic thoracentesis with a small-bore needle can be performed safely in virtually any patient if meticulous technique is used. The major relative contraindications to thoracentesis are a bleeding diathesis or anticoagulation. A patient with a small amount of pleural fluid and a low benefit-to-risk ratio also represents a relative contraindication. Thoracentesis should not be attempted through an area of active skin infection.

Complications

Complications of diagnostic thoracentesis include pain at the needle insertion site, bleeding (local, intrapleural, or intra-abdominal), pneumothorax, empyema, and spleen or liver puncture (see Chapter 10). Pneumothorax has been reported in prospective studies to occur in 4% to 30% of patients [11,14–16]. However, when ultrasound-guided thoracentesis is performed by experienced physician sonographers, pneumothorax or other injuries due to organ puncture appear to be rare events [4]. Liver or spleen puncture tends to occur when the patient is not sitting absolutely upright because movement toward recumbency causes cephalad migration of the abdominal viscera. The upward displacement of abdominal organs is readily detected by US. However, even if the liver or spleen is punctured with a small-bore needle, generally the outcome is favorable if the patient is not receiving anticoagulants and does not have a bleeding diathesis.

Therapeutic Thoracentesis

Indications and Contraindications

The primary indication for therapeutic thoracentesis is relief of dyspnea. Contraindications to therapeutic thoracentesis are similar to those for diagnostic thoracentesis. However, there appears to be an increased risk of pneumothorax [11], thus making a therapeutic thoracentesis in patients on mechanical ventilation potentially hazardous.

The technique for therapeutic thoracentesis is essentially the same as for diagnostic thoracentesis, except that a blunt-tip needle or plastic catheter, rather than a sharp-tip needle, should be used (see Chapter 10). This reduces the risk of pneumothorax, which may occur as fluid is removed and the lung expands toward the chest wall. Again, the use of sonographic guidance is recommended [17].

The amount of fluid that can be removed safely from the pleural space at one session is controversial. Ideally, monitoring pleural pressure should dictate the amount of fluid that can be removed. As long as intrapleural pressure does not fall to less than −20 cm H_2O, fluid removal can continue [18]. However, intrapleural pressure monitoring is not done routinely. In the patient with contralateral mediastinal shift on chest radiograph who tolerates thoracentesis without chest tightness, cough, or light-headedness, probably several liters of pleural fluid can be removed safely. However, neither the patient nor the operator may be aware of a precipitous drop in pleural pressure. In patients without a contralateral mediastinal shift or with ipsilateral shift (suggesting an endobronchial obstruction), the likelihood of a precipitous drop in intrapleural pressure is increased, and pleural pressure should be monitored during thoracentesis. Alternatively, a small bore catheter connected to a standard thoracostomy pleural drainage system may be temporarily inserted, thus avoiding excessively negative pleural pressure development during drainage. Simple gravity drainage or drainage using any system incorporating a nonreturn valve do not reliably guard against the development of excessively negative pressure.

Physiologic Effects and Complications

Improvement in lung volumes up to 24 hours after therapeutic thoracentesis does not correlate with the amount of fluid removed, despite relief of dyspnea in those patients [19–21]. In some patients, however, maximum spirometric improvement may not occur for several days. Patients with initial negative pleural pressures and those with more precipitous falls in pleural pressure with thoracentesis tend to have the least improvement in pulmonary function after therapeutic thoracentesis because many have a trapped lung or endobronchial obstruction [18]. The mechanism of dyspnea from a large pleural effusion probably is related to the increase in chest wall resting volume resulting in shortening of the respiratory muscles resting length and consequent decrease in contractile efficiency [20]. Drainage of moderately sized pleural effusions (1,495 mL) does not appear to result in predictable changes in respiratory system compliance or resistances although a systematic decrease in work performed by the ventilator as a consequence of thoracentesis has been reported [22].

Complications of therapeutic thoracentesis are the same as those seen with diagnostic thoracentesis (see Chapter 10). Three complications that are unique to therapeutic thoracentesis are hypoxemia, unilateral pulmonary edema, and hypovolemia. After therapeutic thoracentesis, hypoxemia may occur despite relief of dyspnea [23,24] from worsening ventilation–perfusion relationships in the ipsilateral lung or clinically occult unilateral pulmonary edema.

Some investigators have concluded that the change in partial pressure of arterial oxygen (PaO_2) after therapeutic thoracentesis is unpredictable [24]; some have observed a characteristic increase in PaO_2 within minutes to hours [19], and others suggest a systematic decrease in PaO_2 that returns to prethoracentesis values by 24 hours [23] In the largest study, including 33 patients with various causes of unilateral pleural effusions, a significant increase in PaO_2 was found 20 minutes, 2 hours, and 24 hours after therapeutic thoracentesis [25]. This was in conjunction with a decrease in the alveolar–arterial oxygen gradient [$P(A–a)O_2$] and was accompanied by a small but significant decrease in shunt, without a change in V_D/V_T. Data suggest an improved ventilation-perfusion relationship after therapeutic thoracentesis, with an increase in ventilation of parts of the lung that were previously poorly ventilated but well perfused. The relief of dyspnea in these patients cannot be explained by improved arterial oxygen tension. The increases have been modest, and in some cases there has been a fall in PaO_2. Improvement in lung volumes is a constant finding after therapeutic thoracentesis but may take days or even weeks to maximize; immediate changes are usually modest and highly variable. Therefore, the relief of dyspnea cannot be adequately explained by changes in lung volume or in the mechanics of breathing but may be the result of decreased stimulation of lung or chest wall receptors, or both [20].

PLEURAL EFFUSIONS IN THE INTENSIVE CARE UNIT

The types of pleural effusions in critically ill patients are listed in Table 57.2.

TABLE 57.2

DIFFERENTIAL DIAGNOSIS OF PLEURAL EFFUSIONS IN CRITICALLY ILL PATIENTS

	Clinical presentation	Chest radiograph	Pleural fluid analysis	Diagnosis	Comments
Transudates					
Congestive heart failure	Usual signs and symptoms plus I > O, weight gain, worsening P(A–a)O_2, ↓ C_{ST}	Bilateral effusions, right > left, cardiomegaly, extravascular lung water	Serous, nucleated cells <1,000/μL, lymphocytes, mesothelial cells, pH 7.45–7.55	Presumptive	Associated with ↑ pulmonary capillary wedge pressure, acute diuresis may result in ↑ protein and LDH
Atelectasis	Asymptomatic or dyspnea, worsening P(A–a)O_2	Small unilateral or bilateral effusions, volume loss	Serous, nucleated cells <1,000/μL, lymphocytes, mesothelial cells, pH 7.45–7.55	Presumptive	Common after upper abdominal surgery, also with pulmonary embolism, mucous plug
Hepatic hydrothorax	Stigmata of liver disease, clinical ascites, asymptomatic or dyspnea, worsening P(A–a)O_2, poor response to low-flow O_2	Unilateral right or bilateral effusions, small to massive, normal heart size, no other CXR abnormalities	Serous-serosanguineous nucleated cells <1,000/μL, lymphocytes, mesothelial cells, pH 7.40–7.55	Presumptive, PF protein and LDH similar to ascitic fluid	6% of patients with clinical ascites, fluid movement from abdomen to chest via diaphragm defect
Hypoalbuminemia	Asymptomatic or dyspnea, anasarca	Small-to-moderate bilateral effusions, normal heart size, no other CXR abnormalities	Serous, nucleated cells <1,000/μL, lymphocytes, mesothelial cells, pH 7.45–7.55	Presumptive	Serum albumin <1.5 g/dL, never have isolated pleural effusion
Iatrogenic: extravascular migration of central venous catheter	Chest pain, dyspnea	Abnormal position of catheter, widening of mediastinum, small-to-large unilateral effusion	Serous-hemorrhagic or white, may contain PMNs, chemistries similar to infusate, PF/S glucose >1.0	Presumptive	Highest incidence with left external jugular vein placement, aspiration or retrograde flow of blood confirms intravascular placement
Exudates					
Parapneumonic effusions: uncomplicated	Fever, chest pain, ↑ WBC, purulent sputum	New alveolar infiltrate, minimal-to-moderate ipsilateral free-flowing effusion	Turbid, PMNs, glucose >60 mg/dL, LDH <700 IU/L, pH ≥7.30	Presumptive	Effusion resolves without sequelae on antibiotics only
Parapneumonic effusions: complicated	Fever, chest pain, ↑ WBC, purulent sputum	New alveolar infiltrate, moderate-to-large ipsilateral effusion with or without loculation	Pus, positive bacteriology, pH <7.10, glucose <40 mg/dL, LDH >1,000 IU/L	Based on PF acidosis, positive bacteriology, aspiration of pus, loculation	Putrid odor defines anaerobic empyema, requires pleural space drainage for resolution
Pancreatitis	Acute abdominal pain, nausea, vomiting, fever	Small, unilateral, left effusion (60%), atelectasis	Turbid, nucleated cells 10,000–50,000/μL, PMNs, pH 7.30–7.35, PF/S amylase >1.0	PF/S amylase >1.0 or >upper limits of normal for serum	Effusion resolves as pancreatitis resolves without need for pleural space drainage
Pulmonary embolism	Acute dyspnea, tachypnea, chest pain, ↑ P(A–a)O_2	Unilateral, small-to-moderate effusion, peripheral infiltrate, atelectasis	Serous-bloody nucleated cells 100–50,000/μL, PMNs or lymphocytes	Presumptive	20% transudates, effusion present on admission, 1/3 of hemithorax, reaches maximum volume by 72 h

(*continued*)

TABLE 57.2

CONTINUED

	Clinical presentation	Chest radiograph	Pleural fluid analysis	Diagnosis	Comments
Postcardiac injury syndrome	Chest pain, pericardial rub, fever, dyspnea 3 d to 3 wk after cardiac injury, ↑ WBC, ↑ erythrocyte sedimentation rate	Left or bilateral small-to-moderate effusion, left lower lobe infiltrates	Serosanguineous-bloody, nucleated cells 500–39,000/μL, PMNs or lymphocytes, pH >7.30	Presumptive	Effusion resolves in 1–3 wk, may require steroids
Esophageal sclerotherapy	Chest pain following sclerotherapy with large sclerosant volume, effusion appears by 48–72 h	Small, unilateral or bilateral effusion	Serosanguineous, nucleated cells 100–38,000/μL, PMNs or mononuclear, pH >7.30	Presumptive	Requires no specific therapy, resolves in days to weeks
ARDS	Depends on cause	Bilateral alveolar infiltrates tend to mask small bilateral effusions	Serous-serosanguineous, PMNs	Presumptive	Requires no specific therapy, effusions resolve as ARDS resolves
Spontaneous esophageal rupture	Severe retching or vomiting followed by thoracoabdominal pain, fever, subcutaneous air	Subcutaneous/mediastinal air; left pneumothorax, followed by left effusion	Early: serous, pH >7.30; later: turbid-purulent effusion, PMNs, pH approaches 6.00, ↑ amylase	Pleural fluid pH <7.00, with ↑ salivary amylase and positive bacteriology	With early diagnosis prognosis good with primary closure and drainage
Hemothorax	Following blunt and penetrating chest trauma, invasive procedures, malignancy, anticoagulation	Small-to-massive unilateral effusion, other abnormalities depending on cause of hemothorax	Gross blood, PF/blood Hct >50%	PF/blood Hct >50%	Often not appreciated on initial radiograph in setting of trauma; should be drained with chest tube
Coronary artery bypass graft	Asymptomatic, dyspnea	Small-to-moderate left effusion without parenchymal infiltrates, left lower lobe atelectasis, elevation of left hemidiaphragm	Hemorrhagic PF/blood Hct <5%, nucleated cells <10,000/μL, lymph predominant, pH >7.40	Presumptive	May require weeks for resolution, rarely results in trapped lung
Abdominal surgery	Asymptomatic 48–72 h after upper abdominal surgery	Small bilateral effusions, atelectasis	Serous nucleated cells <10,000/μL (75%), pH usually >7.40	Presumptive	Larger left effusions following splenectomy, most commonly found with atelectasis and diaphragmatic irritation, resolves spontaneously
Chylothorax (traumatic)	Asymptomatic or dyspnea following intrathoracic surgery, especially coarctation repair and esophagectomy	Small-to-massive left, right, or bilateral effusion	Milky fluid, nucleated cells <7,000/μL almost all lymphocytes, pH 7.40–7.80, ↑ triglycerides	Triglycerides >110 mg/dL, chylomicrons on lipoprotein electrophoresis	Defect in thoracic duct frequently closes spontaneously with tube drainage and minimizing chyle formation

ARDS, acute respiratory distress syndrome; CXR, chest radiograph; ↓, decreased; Hct, hematocrit; ↑, increased; I, input; LDH, lactate dehydrogenase; O, output; PF, pleural fluid; PF/S, pleural fluid/serum; PMN, polymorphonuclear leukocyte; WBC, white blood cell.

Atelectasis

Atelectasis is a common cause of small pleural effusions in comatose, immobile, pain-ridden patients in ICUs [26] and after upper abdominal surgery [27,28]. Other causes include major bronchial obstruction from lung cancer or a mucous plug. Atelectasis causes pleural fluid because of decreased pleural pressure. With alveolar collapse, the lung and chest wall separate further, creating local areas of increased negative pressure. This decrease in pleural pressure favors the movement of fluid into the pleural space, presumably from the parietal pleural surface. The fluid accumulates until the pleural or parietal-pleural interstitial pressure gradient reaches a steady state.

Pleural fluid from atelectasis is a serous transudate with a low number of mononuclear cells, a glucose concentration equivalent to serum, and pH in the range of 7.45 to 7.55. When atelectasis resolves, pleural fluid dissipates during several days.

Congestive Heart Failure

CHF is the most common cause of transudative pleural effusions and a common cause of pleural effusions in ICUs. Pleural effusions due to CHF are associated with increases in pulmonary venous pressure [29]. Most patients with subacute or chronic elevation in pulmonary venous pressure (pulmonary capillary wedge pressure of at least 24 mm Hg) have evidence of pleural effusion on US or lateral decubitus radiograph. Isolated increases in systemic venous pressure tend not to produce pleural effusions. Thus, patients with chronic obstructive pulmonary disease (COPD) and cor pulmonale rarely have pleural effusions, and the presence of pleural fluid implies another cause.

Most patients with pleural effusions secondary to CHF have the classic signs and symptoms. The chest radiograph shows cardiomegaly and bilateral small-to-moderate pleural effusions of similar size (right slightly greater than left). There is usually radiographic evidence of pulmonary congestion, with the severity of pulmonary edema correlating with the presence of pleural effusion [29].

The effusion is a transudate, with mesothelial cells and lymphocytes accounting for the majority of the less than 1,000 cells per μL [13]. Acute diuresis can raise the pleural fluid protein and lactate dehydrogenase into the range of an exudate [30,31]. In the patient with secure clinical diagnosis of CHF, observation is appropriate. Thoracentesis should be performed if the patient is febrile, has pleural effusions of disparate size, has a unilateral pleural effusion, does not have cardiomegaly, has pleuritic chest pain, or has a PaO_2 inappropriate for the degree of pulmonary edema.

Treatment consists of decreasing venous hypertension and improving cardiac output with diuretics, digitalis, and afterload reduction. In successfully managed heart failure, the effusions resolve during days to weeks after the pulmonary edema has cleared.

Hepatic Hydrothorax

Pleural effusions occur in approximately 6% of patients with cirrhosis of the liver and clinical ascites. The effusions result from movement of ascitic fluid through congenital or acquired diaphragmatic defects [32–34].

The patient usually has the classic stigmata of cirrhosis and clinically apparent ascites. The usual chest radiograph shows a normal cardiac silhouette and a right-sided pleural effusion, which can vary from small to massive; effusions are less likely isolated to the left pleural space or are bilateral [32–35]. Rarely, a massive pleural effusion may be found without clinical ascites (demonstrated only by US), implying the presence of a large diaphragmatic defect. The pleural fluid is a serous transudate with a low nucleated cell count and a predominance of mononuclear cells, pH greater than 7.40, and a glucose level similar to that of serum [13]. The fluid can be hemorrhagic due to an underlying coagulopathy or rupture of a diaphragmatic bleb. Demonstrating that pleural and ascitic fluids have similar protein and lactate dehydrogenase concentrations, substantiates the diagnosis [32]. If the diagnosis is problematic, injection of a radionuclide into the ascitic fluid with detection on chest imaging within 1 to 2 hours supports a pleuroperitoneal communication through a diaphragmatic defect [36]; delayed demonstration of the tracer suggests that the pathogenesis of the effusion is via convection through the mesothelium.

Hepatic hydrothorax may be complicated by spontaneous bacterial empyema (SBE), which is analogous to spontaneous bacterial peritonitis. The criteria for diagnosis of SBE are similar to those for the diagnosis of spontaneous bacterial peritonitis. SBE must be considered in the differential diagnosis of the infected cirrhotic patient, even in the absence of clinical ascites [37,38]. The pleural fluid culture and analysis may reveal positive culture, a total neutrophil count of more than 500 cells per μL, and a serum to pleural fluid albumin gradient greater than 1.1. The chest radiograph should not show a pneumonic process. Treatment of SBE is conservative with antibiotics unless purulence is present, in which case tube thoracostomy must be considered.

Treatment of hepatic hydrothorax is directed at resolution of the ascites, using sodium restriction and diuresis. The effusion frequently persists unchanged until all ascites is mobilized. If the patient is acutely dyspneic or in respiratory failure, therapeutic thoracentesis should be done as a temporizing measure. Care should be exercised with paracentesis or thoracentesis because hypovolemia can occur with rapid evacuation of fluid. Chest tube insertion should be avoided as it can cause infection of the fluid, and prolonged drainage can lead to protein and lymphocyte depletion and renal failure. Chemical pleurodesis via a chest tube is often unsuccessful due to rapid movement of ascitic fluid into the pleural space. Treatment options in hepatic hydrothorax refractory to medical management include transjugular intrahepatic portal systemic shunt and video-assisted thoracoscopy to patch the diaphragmatic defect, followed by pleural abrasion or talc poudrage in the properly selected patient [39,40].

Hypoalbuminemia

Many patients admitted to a medical ICU have a chronic illness and associated hypoalbuminemia. When the serum albumin level falls below 1.8 g per dL, pleural effusions may be observed [41]. Because the normal pleural space has an effective lymphatic drainage system, pleural fluid tends to be the last collection of extravascular fluid that occurs in patients with low oncotic pressure. Therefore, it is unusual to find a pleural effusion solely due to hypoalbuminemia in the absence of anasarca. Patients with hypoalbuminemic pleural effusions tend not to have pulmonary symptoms unless there is underlying lung disease, as the effusions are rarely large. Chest radiograph shows small-to-moderate bilateral effusions and a normal heart size. The pleural fluid is a serous transudate with less than 1,000 nucleated cells per μL, predominantly lymphocytes and mesothelial cells. The pleural fluid glucose level is similar to that of serum, and the pH is in the range of 7.45 to 7.55. Diagnosis is presumptive if other causes of transudative effusions can be excluded. The effusions resolve when hypoalbuminemia is corrected.

Iatrogenic

Extravascular migration of a central venous catheter can cause pneumothorax, hemothorax, chylothorax, or a transudative pleural effusion [42–44]. Its incidence is estimated at less than 1% but may be considerably higher. Malposition of the catheter on placement should be suspected if there is absence of blood return or questionable central venous pressure measurements. The immediate postprocedure chest radiograph should be assessed for proper catheter placement; a catheter placed from the right side should not cross the midline. If the catheter is not in the appropriate vessel, phlebitis, perforation of a vein or the heart, or instillation of fluid into the mediastinum or pleural space can occur. In the alert patient, acute infusion of intravenous fluid into the mediastinum usually results in new-onset chest discomfort and dyspnea. Depending on the volume and the rate at which it is introduced into the mediastinum, tachypnea, worsening respiratory status, and cardiac tamponade may ensue. The chest radiograph shows the catheter tip in an abnormal position [45,46], a widened mediastinum, and evidence of unilateral or bilateral pleural effusions. The effusion can have characteristics similar to those of the infusate (milky if lipid is being given) and may be hemorrhagic and neutrophil-predominant due to trauma and inflammation. The pleural fluid to serum glucose ratio is greater than 1.0 if glucose is being infused [43]. The pleural fluid glucose concentration can fall rapidly after glucose infusion into the pleural space, probably explaining the relatively low glucose concentrations in pleural fluid compared to the infusate [47]. Extravascular migration of a central venous catheter appears to be more common with placement in the external jugular vein, particularly on the left side. Left-sided catheters appear to put the patient at increased risk of perforation because of the horizontal orientation of the left compared to the right brachiocephalic vein. When catheters are introduced from the left side, they should be of adequate length for the tip to rest in the superior vena cava.

Free flow of fluid and proper fluctuation in central venous pressure during the respiratory cycle may not be reliable indicators of intravascular placement. This is probably because intrathoracic pressure changes are transmitted to the mediastinum and, thus, the venous pressure catheter. Aspiration of blood or retrograde flow of blood when the catheter is lowered below the patient's heart level should confirm intravascular catheter placement. If blood cannot be aspirated and the effusate is aspirated instead, extravascular migration is assured. The central venous catheter should be removed immediately. If there is a small effusion, observation is warranted. If the effusion is large, causing respiratory distress, or a hemothorax is discovered, thoracentesis or tube thoracostomy should be performed.

Parapneumonic Effusions

Community-acquired or nosocomial pneumonia is common in critically ill patients. The classic presentation is fever, chest pain, leukocytosis, purulent sputum, and a new alveolar infiltrate on chest radiograph. In the elderly, debilitated patient, however, many of these findings may not be present. The chest radiograph commonly shows a small-to-large ipsilateral pleural effusion [48–50]. When the effusion is free-flowing and anechoic on ultrasound, and thoracentesis shows a nonpurulent, polymorphonuclear (PMN) predominant exudate with a pH of 7.30 or greater, it is highly likely that the effusion will resolve during 7 to 14 days without sequelae with antibiotics alone (uncomplicated effusion). If the chest radiograph or CT demonstrates loculation and pus is aspirated, the diagnosis of empyema is established and immediate drainage is needed. In the free-flowing nonpurulent fluid, if Gram's stain or culture is positive or pH is less than 7.30, the likelihood of a poor outcome increases, and the pleural space should be drained.

Although a meta-analysis found that low risk patients with fluid pH between 7.20 and 7.30 may be managed without tube drainage, the patient admitted to the ICU typically cannot be considered low risk, and pH values of less than 7.30 should prompt drainage in most cases [51–53]. Drainage can be accomplished by standard chest tube or small-bore catheter. When loculations occur, pleural space drainage should be accomplished by placement of image-guided tubes or catheters with fibrinolytics or empyectomy and decortication [54,55]. Most thoracic surgeons routinely begin with thoracoscopy and, if not successful, proceed directly to a standard thoracotomy for empyectomy and decortication [56–59].

Pancreatitis

Pleuropulmonary abnormalities are commonly associated with pancreatitis, largely due to the close proximity of the pancreas to the diaphragm. Approximately half of patients with pancreatitis have an abnormal chest radiograph, with pleural effusions in 3% to 17% [60,61]. Mechanisms that may be involved in the pathogenesis of pancreatic pleural effusion include (a) direct contact of pancreatic enzymes with the diaphragm (sympathetic effusion), (b) transfer of ascitic fluid via diaphragmatic defects, (c) communication of a fistulous tract between a pseudocyst and the pleural space, and (d) retroperitoneal movement of fluid into the mediastinum with mediastinitis or rupture into the pleural space [60,62]. Ascitic amylase moves into the pleural space via the previously mentioned mechanisms. The pleural fluid-to-serum amylase ratio is greater than unity in pancreatitis because of slower lymphatic clearance from the pleural space compared with more rapid renal clearance.

The effusion associated with acute pancreatitis is usually small and left-sided (60%), but may be isolated to the right side (30%) or be bilateral (10%) [60]. The patient usually presents with abdominal symptoms of acute pancreatitis. The diagnosis is confirmed by an elevated pleural fluid amylase concentration that is greater than that in serum. A normal pleural fluid amylase may be found early in acute pancreatitis, but increases on serial measurements. The fluid is a PMN-predominant exudate with glucose values approximating those of serum. Leukocyte counts may reach 50,000 cells per μL. The pleural fluid pH is usually 7.30 to 7.35.

No specific treatment is necessary for the pleural effusion of acute pancreatitis; the effusion resolves as the pancreatic inflammation subsides. Drainage of the pleural space does not appear to affect residual pleural damage. If the pleural effusion does not resolve in 2 to 3 weeks, pancreatic abscess or pseudocyst should be excluded.

Pulmonary Embolism

The presence of a unilateral pleural effusion may suggest pulmonary embolism or obscure the diagnosis by directing attention to a primary lung or cardiac process. Pleural effusions occur in approximately 40% of patients with pulmonary embolism [63]. These effusions result from several different mechanisms including increased pleural capillary permeability, imbalance in microvascular and pleural space hydrostatic pressures, and pleuropulmonary hemorrhage [63,64]. Ischemia from pulmonary vascular obstruction, in addition to release of inflammatory mediators from platelet-rich thrombi, can cause capillary leak into the lung and, subsequently, the pleural space, explaining the usual finding of an exudative effusion.

Transudates, described in approximately 20% of patients with pulmonary embolism, result from atelectasis [64].

With pulmonary infarction, necrosis and hemorrhage into the lung and pleural space may result. More than 80% of patients with infarction have bloody pleural effusions, but more than 35% of patients with pulmonary embolism without radiographic infarction also have hemorrhagic fluid [63]. The presence of a pleural effusion does not alter the signs or symptoms in patients with pulmonary embolism. Chest pain, usually pleuritic, occurs in most patients with pleural effusions complicating pulmonary embolism, and is invariably ipsilateral [63]. The chest radiograph virtually always shows a unilateral effusion that occupies less than one third of the hemithorax [63]. An associated pulmonary infiltrate (infarction) is seen in approximately half of patients with pulmonary embolism and effusion.

Pleural fluid analysis is variable and nondiagnostic [64]. The pleural fluid is hemorrhagic in two thirds of patients, but the number of red blood cells exceeds 100,000 per μL in less than 20% [64]. The nucleated cell count ranges from less than 100 (atelectatic transudates) to greater than 50,000 per μL (pulmonary infarction) [64]. There is a predominance of PMNs when a thoracentesis is performed near the time of the acute injury and of lymphocytes with later thoracentesis. The effusion due to pulmonary embolism is usually (92%) apparent on the initial chest radiograph and reaches a maximum volume during the first 72 hours [63]. Patients with pleural effusions that progress with therapy should be evaluated for recurrent embolism, hemothorax secondary to anticoagulation, an infected infarction, or an alternate diagnosis. When consolidation is absent on chest radiograph, effusions usually resolve in 7 to 10 days; with consolidation, the resolution time is 2 to 3 weeks [64].

The association of pleural effusion with pulmonary embolism does not alter therapy. Furthermore, the presence of a bloody effusion is not a contraindication to full-dose anticoagulation because hemothorax is a rare complication of heparin therapy [65]. An enlarging pleural effusion on therapy necessitates thoracentesis to exclude hemothorax, empyema, or another cause. Active pleural space hemorrhage necessitates discontinuation of anticoagulation, tube thoracostomy, and placement of a vena cava filter.

Postcardiac Injury Syndrome

Postcardiac injury syndrome (PCIS) is characterized by fever, pleuropericarditis, and parenchymal infiltrates 3 weeks (2 to 86 days) after injury to the myocardium or pericardium [66–68]. PCIS has been described after myocardial infarction, cardiac surgery, blunt chest trauma, percutaneous left ventricular puncture, and pacemaker implantation. The incidence after myocardial infarction has been estimated at up to 4% of cases [66], but with more extensive myocardial and pericardial involvement, it may be higher. It occurs with greater frequency (up to 30%) after cardiac surgery [69]. The pathogenesis of PCIS remains obscure but is probably on an autoimmune basis in patients with myocardial or pericardial injury and, possibly, concomitant viral illness [70].

The diagnosis of PCIS remains one of exclusion, for no specific criteria exist. It is important to diagnose or exclude PCIS presumptively. Failure to diagnose accurately could lead to iatrogenic complications from inappropriate therapy, such as cardiac tamponade from anticoagulation for presumed pulmonary embolism and adverse effects related to antimicrobial therapy for presumed pneumonia.

Pleuropulmonary manifestations are the hallmark of PCIS. The most common presenting symptoms are pleuritic chest pain, found in virtually all patients, and fever, pericardial rub, dyspnea, and rales, which occur in half of patients [68]. Rarely, hemoptysis occurs, an important differential point when pulmonary embolism with infarction is in the differential diagnosis. Fifty percent of patients have leukocytosis, and almost all have an elevated erythrocyte sedimentation rate (average, 62 mm per hour) [68].

The chest radiograph is abnormal in virtually all patients, with the most common abnormality being left-sided and bilateral pleural effusions; a unilateral right effusion is unusual [68]. Pulmonary infiltrates are present in 75% of patients and are most commonly seen in the left lower lobe [66]. The pleural fluid is a serosanguineous or bloody exudate with a glucose level greater than 60 mg per dL and pleural fluid pH greater than 7.30. Nucleated cell counts range from 500 to 39,000 per μL, with a predominance of PMNs early in the course [68]. Pericardial fluid on echocardiogram is an important finding suggesting PCIS. The pleural fluid characteristics should help differentiate PCIS from a parapneumonic effusion and CHF, but do not exclude pulmonary embolism.

PCIS is usually self-limited and may not require therapy if symptoms are trivial. It usually responds to aspirin or nonsteroidal anti-inflammatory agents, but some patients require corticosteroid therapy for resolution. In those who respond, the pleural effusion resolves within 1 to 3 weeks.

Esophageal Sclerotherapy

Pleural effusions are found in approximately 50% of patients 48 to 72 hours after esophageal sclerotherapy with sodium morrhuate and in 19% of patients after absolute alcohol sclerotherapy [71–73]. Effusions may be unilateral or bilateral, with no predilection for side. Effusion appears more likely with larger total volumes of sclerosant injected and larger volume injected per site [71,72]. The effusions tend to be small, serous exudates with variable nucleated (90 to 38,000 per μL) and red cell counts (126 to 160,000 per μL) and glucose concentration similar to that of serum [71]. These effusions probably result from an intensive inflammatory reaction after extravasation of the sclerosant into the esophageal mucosa, resulting in mediastinal and pleural inflammation. The effusion not associated with fever, chest pain, or evidence of perforation is of little consequence, requires no specific therapy, and resolves during several days to weeks [71,72]. However, late perforation may evolve in patients with apparent innocuous effusions. In patients with symptomatic effusions for 24 to 48 hours, diagnostic thoracentesis should be done and an esophagram considered.

Acute Respiratory Distress Syndrome

The presence of pleural effusions in ARDS has not been well appreciated. In a retrospective study of 25 patients with ARDS, a 36% incidence of pleural effusions was found, a percentage similar to that found with hydrostatic pulmonary edema [74]. All patients had extensive alveolar pulmonary edema and endotracheal tube fluid that was compatible with increased permeability edema. Several experimental models of increased permeability pulmonary edema, including α-naphthyl thiourea, oleic acid, and ethchlorvynol, have been shown to produce pleural effusions. In the oleic acid and ethchlorvynol models, the development of pleural effusions lagged behind interstitial and alveolar edema by several hours. In the oleic acid model, 35% of the excess lung water collected in the pleural spaces. It appears that the pleura act as a reservoir for excess lung water in increased permeability and hydrostatic pulmonary edema. These effusions tend to be underdiagnosed clinically because the patient has bilateral alveolar infiltrates and the radiograph is taken with the patient in a supine position. Experimentally, the effusion is serous to serosanguineous, with a predominance of PMNs. These effusions usually require no specific therapy and resolve as ARDS resolves. However, in a series of positive end-expiratory pressure (PEEP)-unresponsive patients with ARDS, drainage of pleural effusion via tube thoracostomy has been shown to result in improved oxygenation [75]. The decision to proceed to pleural space drainage in ARDS should be approached on a case-by-case basis and is not generally recommended.

Spontaneous Esophageal Rupture

Esophageal rupture, a potentially life-threatening event, requires immediate diagnosis and therapy. The history in spontaneous esophageal rupture is usually severe retching or vomiting or a conscious effort to resist vomiting. In some patients, the perforation may be silent. Early recognition of spontaneous rupture depends on interpretation of the chest radiograph. Several factors influence chest radiograph findings: the time between perforation and chest radiograph examination, site of perforation, and mediastinal pleural integrity [76]. A chest radiograph taken within minutes of the acute injury is usually unremarkable. Mediastinal emphysema probably requires at least 1 to 2 hours to be demonstrated radiographically and is present in less than half of patients; mediastinal widening may take several hours [77]. Pneumothorax, present in 75% of patients with spontaneous rupture, indicates violation of the mediastinal pleura; 70% of pneumothoraces are on the left, 20% are on the right, and 10% are bilateral [77]. Mediastinal air is seen early if pleural integrity is maintained, whereas pleural effusion secondary to mediastinitis tends to occur later. Pleural fluid, with or without associated pneumothorax, occurs in 75% of patients. A presumptive diagnosis should immediately be confirmed radiographically. Esophagrams are positive in approximately 90% of patients [78]. In the upright patient, rapid passage of the contrast material may not demonstrate a small rent; therefore, the study should be done with the patient in the appropriate lateral decubitus position [79].

Pleural fluid findings depend on the degree of perforation and the timing of thoracentesis from injury. Early thoracentesis without mediastinal perforation shows a sterile, serous exudate with a predominance of PMNs, a pleural fluid amylase less than serum, and pH greater than 7.30 [80]. Once the mediastinal pleura tears, amylase of salivary origin appears in the fluid in high concentration [81]. As the pleural space is seeded with anaerobic organisms from the mouth, the pH falls rapidly and progressively to approach 6.00 [80,82]. Other pleural fluid findings suggestive of esophageal rupture include the presence of squamous epithelial cells and food particles. The diagnosis of spontaneous esophageal rupture dictates immediate operative intervention. If diagnosed and treated appropriately within the first 24 hours with primary closure and drainage, survival is greater than 90% [77]. Delay from the time of initial symptoms to diagnosis results in a reduced survival with any form of therapy.

Hemothorax

Hemothorax (blood in the pleural space) should be differentiated from a hemorrhagic pleural effusion, as the latter can be the result of only a few drops of blood in pleural fluid. An arbitrary, but practical, definition of a hemothorax with regard to therapy is a pleural fluid-to-blood hematocrit ratio greater than 30%. The majority of hemothoraces results from penetrating or blunt chest trauma [83]. Hemothorax can also result from invasive procedures, such as placement of central venous catheters, thoracentesis, and pleural biopsy, and pulmonary infarction, malignancy, or ruptured aortic aneurysm. Bleeding can occur from vessels of the chest wall, lung, diaphragm, or mediastinum. Blood that enters the pleural space clots, rapidly undergoes fibrinolysis, and becomes defibrinogenated; thus, it rarely causes significant pleural fibrosis.

Hemothorax should be suspected in any patient with blunt or penetrating chest trauma. If a pleural effusion is found on the admitting chest radiograph, thoracentesis should be performed immediately and the hematocrit measured on the fluid. The hemothorax may not be apparent on the initial chest radiograph, which may be due to the supine position of the patient. Because bleeding may be slow and not appear for several hours, it is imperative that serial radiographs be obtained in these patients. The incidence of concomitant pneumothorax is high (approximately 60%) [83]. Patients with traumatic hemothorax should be treated with immediate tube thoracostomy [83–85]. Large-diameter chest tube drainage evacuates the pleural space, may tamponade the bleeding (especially if the origin is from a pleural laceration), allows monitoring of the bleeding, and decreases the likelihood of subsequent fibrothorax [85,86]. If bleeding continues without signs of slowing, thoracotomy should be performed, depending on the individual circumstance [85]. Pleural effusions occasionally occur after removal of the chest tube from traumatic hemothoraces [87]. A diagnostic thoracentesis is indicated to exclude empyema. If empyema is excluded, the pleural effusion usually resolves without specific treatment and without residual pleural fibrosis.

Hemothorax is a rare complication of anticoagulation and has been reported in patients receiving heparin and warfarin. Coagulation studies are usually within the therapeutic range. The hemothorax tends to occur on the side of the pulmonary embolism. Anticoagulation should be discontinued immediately, a chest tube inserted to evacuate the blood, and a vena cava filter considered.

Coronary Artery Bypass Surgery

A small, left pleural effusion is virtually always present after coronary artery bypass surgery. This is associated with left lower lobe atelectasis and elevation of the left hemidiaphragm on chest radiograph. Left diaphragm dysfunction is secondary to intraoperative phrenic nerve injury from cold cardioplegia, stretch injury, or surgical trauma [88–90]. The larger and grossly bloody effusions tend to be associated with internal mammary artery grafting, which causes marked exudation from the bed where the internal mammary artery was harvested [91].

The pleural fluid is a hemorrhagic exudate with a low nucleated cell count, a glucose level similar to that of serum, and a pH greater than 7.40. Rarely, a loculated hemothorax may develop with trapped lung, resulting in clinically significant restriction [92]. If there is a large effusion that qualifies as a hemothorax (see previous section), the fluid should be drained by tube thoracostomy. It is also prudent to drain moderately large, bloody effusions to avoid later necessity for decortication.

Abdominal Surgery

Approximately half of the patients who undergo abdominal surgery develop small unilateral or bilateral pleural effusions within 48 to 72 hours of surgery [27,28]. The incidence is higher after upper abdominal surgery, in patients with postoperative atelectasis, and in patients who have free ascitic fluid at the time of surgery [27]. Larger left-sided pleural effusions are common after splenectomy [27]. The effusion is usually an exudate with less than 10,000 nucleated cells per μL. The glucose level is similar to that of serum, and pH is usually greater than 7.40 [27]. The effusion usually is related to diaphragmatic irritation or atelectasis. Small effusions generally do not require diagnostic thoracentesis, are of no clinical significance, and resolve spontaneously. Pleural effusion from subphrenic abscess or pulmonary embolism is unlikely to occur within 2 to 3 days of surgery. The only indication for diagnostic thoracentesis would be to exclude infection if the effusion is relatively large or loculated.

Chylothorax

Trauma from surgery accounts for approximately 25% of cases of chylothorax, second only to lymphoma. Most series estimate an incidence of chylothorax of less than 1% after thoracic surgery [93], but a 3% incidence has been reported after esophagectomy [94]. Virtually all intrathoracic procedures, including lobectomy, pneumonectomy, and coronary artery bypass grafting, have been reported to cause chylothorax. Other iatrogenic chylothoraces can be caused by complications of prolonged central vein catheterization. Nonsurgical trauma, such as penetrating and nonpenetrating neck, thoracic, and upper abdominal injuries, also has been associated with chylothorax.

When the thoracic duct is torn by stretching during surgery, chyle leaks into the mediastinum and subsequently ruptures through the mediastinal pleura. In the nonsurgical setting, penetrating injuries and fractures may directly tear the thoracic duct. Chylothorax from a central venous catheter usually involves venous thrombosis. Other rare causes of chylothorax include sclerotherapy of esophageal varices and translumbar aortography [95–97].

The patient may be asymptomatic if the effusion is small and unilateral, or may present with dyspnea with a large unilateral effusion or bilateral effusions. The pleural fluid is usually milky, but 12% can be serous or serosanguineous [98], with less than 7,000 nucleated cells per μL, virtually all lymphocytes. The pleural fluid pH is alkaline (7.40 to 7.80), and triglyceride levels are greater than plasma levels. Finding a pleural fluid triglyceride concentration of greater than 110 mg per dL makes the diagnosis of chylothorax highly likely [98]. If the triglyceride level is less than 50 mg per dL, chylothorax is highly unlikely. Triglyceride levels of 50 to 110 mg per dL indicate the need for lipoprotein electrophoresis [98]; the presence of chylomicrons confirms a chylothorax. The thoracic duct defect after trauma usually closes spontaneously within 10 to 14 days, with chest tube drainage as well as bed rest and total parenteral nutrition to minimize chyle formation. A pleuroperitoneal shunt relieves dyspnea, recirculates chyle, and prevents malnutrition and immunocompromise.

Duropleural Fistula

Disruption of the dura and parietal pleura by surgical and nonsurgical trauma may result in a duropleural fistula with subsequent development of a pleural effusion [99–102]. The pleural fluid characteristics depend on the severity of the trauma and the delay between the trauma and the pleural fluid analysis. Pleural fluid due to a chronic duropleural fistula is usually a colorless transudate with low mononuclear cell count; a duropleural fistula associated with recent trauma may be a transudate or an exudate [101,102]. The diagnosis may even be delayed because of a coexisting process such as hemothorax. The diagnosis of duropleural fistula is established by the detection of β_2-transferrin in the pleural fluid [103]. Confirmation of the fistula by conventional or radionuclide myelography is recommended if surgical management is contemplated.

PNEUMOTHORAX

Definition and Classification

Pneumothorax refers to air in the pleural space. Free air may also be found in the adventitial planes of the lung or the mediastinum (pneumomediastinum).

Spontaneous pneumothorax occurs without an obvious cause as a consequence of the natural course of a disease process. Primary spontaneous pneumothorax occurs without clinical findings of lung disease. Secondary spontaneous pneumothorax occurs as a consequence of clinically manifest lung disease, the most common being COPD. Traumatic pneumothorax results from penetrating or blunt chest injury. Iatrogenic pneumothorax occurs as an inadvertent consequence of diagnostic or therapeutic procedures.

Pathophysiology

Pressure in the pleural space is subatmospheric throughout the normal respiratory cycle, averaging approximately −9 mm Hg during inspiration and −5 mm Hg during expiration. Because of airways resistance, pressure in the airways is positive during expiration (+3 mm Hg) and negative (−2 mm Hg) during inspiration. Thus, in normal breathing, airway pressure is greater than pleural pressure throughout the respiratory cycle. Airway pressure may be increased markedly with coughing or strenuous exercise; however, pleural pressure rises concomitantly so that the transpulmonary pressure gradient is usually not substantially changed. When there are rapid fluctuations in intrathoracic pressure, however, a large transpulmonary pressure gradient occurs transiently. Bronchial and bronchiolar obstruction, resulting in air trapping, can significantly increase the transpulmonary pressure gradient. The alveolar walls and visceral pleura maintain the pressure gradient between the airways and pleural space. When the pressure gradient is transiently increased, alveolar rupture may occur; air enters the interstitial tissues of the lung and may enter the pleural space, resulting in a pneumothorax. If the visceral pleura remain intact, the interstitial air moves toward the hilum, resulting in pneumomediastinum [104,105]. Because mean pressure within the mediastinum is always less than in the periphery of the lung, air moves proximally along the bronchovascular sheaths to the hilum and mediastinal soft tissues. The development of pneumomediastinum after alveolar rupture requires continual cyclic respiratory efforts, which result in slow movement of air from the ruptured alveolus along a pressure gradient to the mediastinum [105]. Mediastinal air may decompress into the cervical and subcutaneous tissues or the retroperitoneum. With abrupt rise in mediastinal pressure or insufficient decompression to subcutaneous tissue, the mediastinal pleura may rupture, causing pneumothorax. Inadequate decompression of the mediastinum, rather than direct rupture of subpleural blebs into the pleural space, may be the major cause of pneumothorax [104].

When pneumothorax occurs, the elasticity of the lung causes it to collapse. Lung collapse continues until the pleural defect seals or pleural and alveolar pressures equalize. When a ball-valve effect occurs at the site of communication between the pleural space and the alveolus, permitting only egress of air from the lung, there is a progressive accumulation of air within the pleural space, which can result in markedly increased positive pleural pressure, producing a tension pneumothorax. Tension pneumothorax compresses mediastinal structures, resulting in impaired venous return to the heart, decreased cardiac output, and, at times, fatal cardiovascular collapse [106,107]. Rarely, tension along the bronchovascular sheaths and in the mediastinum can cause collapse of the pulmonary arteries and veins, resulting in cardiovascular collapse [104].

Patients with primary spontaneous pneumothorax have a decrease in vital capacity and an increase in the P(A–a)O_2 gradient, and usually present with hypoxemia due predominantly to the development of an intrapulmonary shunt and areas of low ventilation–perfusion in the atelectatic lung [108,109]. Hypercapnia does not occur because there is adequate function in the uninvolved lung to maintain necessary alveolar ventilation. Patients with secondary spontaneous pneumothorax, in contrast, commonly develop hypercapnia because the gas exchange abnormality caused by the pneumothorax is superimposed on lungs with preexisting abnormal pulmonary gas exchange.

Pneumothorax in the Intensive Care Unit

Patients with secondary spontaneous pneumothorax may be admitted to an ICU because they develop severe hypoxemic and, at times, hypercapnic respiratory failure. Patients with primary spontaneous pneumothorax rarely require ICU admission because the contralateral lung can maintain necessary alveolar ventilation and the hypoxemia can be managed with supplemental oxygen. The most common causes of pneumothoraces in ICU patients are invasive procedures and barotrauma.

Iatrogenic Pneumothorax

Central Venous Catheters. Central venous catheters are used routinely in critically ill patients for volume resuscitation, parenteral nutrition, and drug administration. Approximately 3 million central venous catheters are placed annually in the United States, and this procedure continues to be associated with clinically relevant morbidity and some mortality. The morbidity and mortality associated with central venous catheter use are most commonly physician-related [42]. Pleural complications of acquisition of venous access and the indwelling phase of central venous catheters include pneumothorax, hydrothorax, hemothorax, and chylothorax. In a recent study of mechanical complications of central venous catheters, 1.1% of 534 patients had pneumothorax [110]. This translates into approximately 33,000 pneumothoraces per year from central venous catheter insertions in critically ill patients in the United States. In the same study, none of the 405 patients developed pneumothorax when the central venous catheter was replaced over a guidewire.

The subclavian and internal jugular routes have been associated with pneumothorax, hemothorax, chylothorax, and catheter placement into the pleural space. Cannulation of the subclavian vein is associated with a higher risk of pneumothorax (less than 5%) [111] than cannulation of the internal jugular vein (less than 0.2%) [112]; with the external jugular venous approach, pneumothorax is avoided. There is a greater risk of pneumothorax with the infraclavicular compared to the supraclavicular approach to the subclavian vein. All complications of insertion, regardless of approach, can be reduced by appropriate physician training and experience. Operator inexperience appears to increase the number of complications with the internal jugular approach. It probably does not have as much impact on the incidence of pneumothorax with the subclavian vein approach, which accounts for 25% to 50% of all complications [113].

Most pneumothoraces occur at the time of the procedure from direct lung puncture, but delayed pneumothoraces have been noted; therefore, it is prudent to view a chest radiograph 12 to 24 hours after the procedure. Up to half of the patients with needle puncture pneumothorax may be managed expectantly without the need for tube drainage. Bilateral pneumothoraces have been reported to occur from unilateral attempts [113], and death can occur when there is a delay in the diagnosis of pneumothorax. As stated previously, a pneumothorax may be more difficult to detect while the patient is supine. Additional views should be taken, especially if the venous cannulation does not proceed as anticipated. With any newly placed central venous catheter, a postprocedure chest radiograph should be obtained, regardless of the site cannulated, to assure that the catheter tip is properly positioned. If a small pneumothorax is diagnosed by chest radiograph and the patient is asymptomatic and not on mechanical ventilation, the patient can be followed expectantly with repeat chest radiographs to assure that the leak has ceased. If the patient is on mechanical ventilation or the pneumothorax is large or has caused significant symptoms or gas exchange abnormalities, then tube thoracostomy should be performed as soon as possible.

Barotrauma. Pulmonary barotrauma is an important clinical problem because of the widespread use of mechanical ventilation. Barotrauma occurs in approximately 3% to 10% of patients on mechanical ventilation and includes parenchymal interstitial gas, pneumomediastinum, subcutaneous emphysema, pneumoperitoneum, and pneumothorax [7,114–118]. The most clinically important form is pneumothorax, occurring in 1% to 15% of all patients on mechanical ventilation. In patients with ARDS, rates of 6.5% to 87% have been reported [117,118]. The number of ventilation days, underlying disease (ARDS, COPD, necrotizing pneumonia), and use of PEEP have an impact on the incidence of pneumothorax [114–116,119,120]. When a pneumothorax develops in the setting of mechanical ventilation, 30% to 97% of patients develop tension [7,115,119,120]. The reported incidence of barotrauma varies widely between the studies with the lowest incidences reported in the most recent large series [118]. This may be partly explained by the adoption of less aggressive ventilation strategies over time.

The initial radiographic sign of barotrauma is often pulmonary interstitial gas or emphysema [117,121]. In the early stages, however, interstitial gas may be difficult to detect radiographically. This harbinger of pneumothorax may be detected as distinct subpleural air cysts, linear air streaks emanating from the hilum, and perivascular air halos. Subpleural air cysts, most commonly seen in ARDS, tend to appear abruptly on the chest radiograph as single or multiple thin-walled, round lucencies, and are most often visualized at the lung bases, medially or diaphragmatically [122]. The cysts, which may expand rapidly, are usually 3 to 5 cm in diameter. Differentiating between peripheral subpleural air cysts and a localized basilar pneumothorax may be problematic. Pleural air cysts appear to be more common in younger patients, possibly because connective tissue planes of the lung are looser in younger patients than in older patients [123]. The risk of tension pneumothorax is substantial in patients who have developed subpleural lung cysts with continued mechanical ventilation. When mechanical ventilation is discontinued, the cyst may resolve spontaneously or become secondarily infected.

US has emerged as a bedside modality for the detection of pneumothorax. The absence of lung sliding is the finding associated with pneumothorax [6]. False-positive results may occur and are due to bullous lung disease or preexisting pleural symphysis [6,124,125]. The disappearance of lung sliding that was present previously may be more specific for the development of pneumothorax; for example, after line placement. However, this subject awaits further study.

When evidence of barotrauma without pneumothorax is observed in any patient requiring continued mechanical ventilation, immediate attempts should be made to lower the plateau airway pressure. In ARDS, tidal volumes [126,127] and inspiratory flow rates should be lowered, an attempt should be made to reduce or remove PEEP, and neuromuscular blockers and sedation should be considered [128]. In status asthmaticus, in addition to the aforementioned maneuvers, controlled hypoventilation should be accomplished [129,130]. There is no evidence supporting the use of prophylactic chest tubes. However, the patient should be monitored closely for tension pneumothorax and provisions made for emergency bedside tube thoracostomy.

Tension Pneumothorax

Pneumothorax in the mechanically ventilated patient usually presents as an acute cardiopulmonary emergency, beginning with respiratory distress and, if unrecognized and untreated, progressing to cardiovascular collapse. In one report of 74 patients, the diagnosis of pneumothorax was made clinically in 45 (61%) patients based on hypotension, hyperresonance, diminished breath sounds, and tachycardia [120]. The mortality rate was 7% in these patients diagnosed clinically. In the remaining 29 patients, diagnosis was delayed between 30 minutes and 8 hours, and 31% of these patients died of pneumothorax. Other series of barotrauma in the setting of mechanical ventilation have reported mortality rates from 58% to 77% [7,116].

Tension pneumothorax is lethal if diagnosis and treatment are delayed. The diagnosis should be made clinically at the bedside for the patient on mechanical ventilation who develops a sudden deterioration characterized by apprehension, tachypnea, cyanosis, decreased ipsilateral breath sounds, subcutaneous emphysema, tachycardia, and hypotension. The diagnosis may be problematic in the unconscious patient, the elderly, and the patient with bilateral tension, which may be more protective of the mediastinal structures and lessen the impact on cardiac output.

In the unconscious or critically ill patient, hypoxemia may be one of the earlier signs of tension pneumothorax. In the patient on mechanical ventilation, increasing peak and plateau airway pressure, decreasing compliance, and auto-PEEP should raise the possibility of tension pneumothorax. Difficulty in bagging the patient and delivering adequate tidal volumes may be noted.

When the clinical signs and symptoms are noted in mechanically ventilated patients, treatment should not be delayed to obtain radiographic confirmation. If a chest tube is not immediately available, placement of a large-bore needle into the anterior second intercostal space on the suspected side is lifesaving and confirms the diagnosis, as a rush of air is noted on entering the pleural space. An appropriately large chest tube can then be placed and connected to an adequate drainage system that can accommodate the large air leak that may develop in mechanically ventilated patients [130].

On relief of the tension, there is a rapid improvement in oxygenation, increase in blood pressure, decrease in heart rate, and fall in airway pressures. In experimental tension pneumothorax, it has been observed that the inability to raise cardiac output in response to hypoxemia leads to a reduction in systemic oxygen transport and a decrease in mixed venous partial pressure of oxygen (PO_2), partially explaining the cardiovascular collapse seen in these patients [107]. In mechanically ventilated patients, a decrease in cardiac output is an inevitable consequence of tension pneumothorax.

BRONCHOPLEURAL FISTULA

Definition and Causes

Communication between the bronchial tree and the pleural space is a dreaded complication of mechanical ventilation [131,132]. There are three presentations of bronchopleural fistula (BPF): (a) failure to reinflate the lung despite chest tube drainage or continued air leak after evacuation of the pneumothorax in the setting of chest trauma; (b) complication of a diagnostic or therapeutic procedure, such as thoracic surgery; and (c) complication of mechanical ventilation, usually for ARDS [106]. In ARDS, often a pneumothorax occurs under tension and is later associated with empyema, multiple sites of leakage, and a poor prognosis. A large air leak through a BPF can result in failure of lung reexpansion, loss of a significant amount of each delivered tidal volume, loss of the ability to apply PEEP, inappropriate cycling of the ventilator [133], and inability to maintain alveolar ventilation (Table 57.3).

TABLE 57.3

CONSEQUENCES OF A LARGE BRONCHOPLEURAL FISTULA

Failure of lung reexpansion
Loss of delivered tidal volume
Inability to apply positive end-expiratory pressure
Inappropriate cycling of ventilator
Inability to maintain alveolar ventilation

If there is a continued air leak for longer than 24 hours after the development of pneumothorax, then a BPF exists. The main factors that perpetuate BPF are high airway pressures that increase the leak during inspiration, increased mean intrathoracic pressures throughout the respiratory cycle (PEEP, inflation hold, high inspiratory-to-expiratory ratio) that increase the leak throughout the breath, and high negative suction. In severe ARDS, all of these factors are present because they usually are necessary to support gas exchange and lung inflation.

Management

Given the frequency of barotrauma in BPF in mechanically ventilated patients, intensivists are called to give advice on the management of these difficult patients. Definitive therapy of BPF frequently involves invasive surgical approaches that include thoracoplasty, mobilization of the pectoralis or intercostal muscles, bronchial stump stapling, and decortication [134–139]. Although some of these techniques are still used today, there is a trend toward more conservative management of acute and chronic BPF, using innovations of standard techniques and new modalities that include chest tube management, drainage systems, ventilatory support, and definitive nonoperative therapy (Table 57.4). Even insertion of an endobronchial valve designed for the treatment of emphysema may be considered in selected patients [140]. Nonoperative therapy provides an alternative to the surgical approaches in patients who are poor operative candidates. Each patient with a BPF is unique and requires individual management based on the specific clinical setting. Attention to the basics of medical care of patients with BPF should not be neglected in the face of the potentially dramatic events related to the BPF. Nutritional status must be maintained, appropriate antibiotics used for the infected pleural space, and the space adequately drained.

Chest Tubes

The initial therapy for pneumothorax in a patient on mechanical ventilation is placement of a chest tube in an attempt to reexpand the lung (see Chapter 8). The chest tube is initially necessary, can be detrimental later, and may play a role more

TABLE 57.4

MANAGEMENT OF BRONCHOPLEURAL FISTULA IN PATIENTS REQUIRING MECHANICAL VENTILATION

Conservative
Adequate-size chest tube
Use of drainage system with adequate capabilities
Mechanical ventilation
Conventional (controlled, assist-control, intermittent mandatory ventilation)
High frequency
Independent lung
Flexible bronchoscopy
Direct application of sealant
Invasive
Mobilization of intercostal or pectoralis muscles
Thoracoplasty
Bronchial stump stapling
Pleural abrasion and decortication

important than that of a passive conduit. Air leaks in the setting of BPF range from less than 1 to 16 L per minute [141]; therefore, a chest tube that permits prompt and efficient drainage of this level of airflow is required. Gas moves through a tube in a laminar fashion and is governed by Poiseuille's law ($v = [\pi r^4 P/8lV]t$). In the clinical setting, the gas moving through a chest tube is moist; therefore, it is subject to turbulent flow and governed by the Fanning equation ($v = [\pi r^2 r^5 P/fl]$) [141–143]. Therefore, both the length (l) and, even more so, the radius (r) are important when choosing a chest tube and connecting tubing to evacuate a BPF adequately (as flow varies exponentially to the fifth power of the radius of the tube). The smallest internal diameter that allows a maximum flow of 15.1 L per minute at −10 cm H_2O suction is 6 mm [141,142] (a 32-Fr chest tube has an internal diameter of 9 mm). A chest tube with a diameter adequate to convey the potentially large airflow of the BPF must be considered. A chest tube with too small a diameter can lead to lung collapse and tension pneumothorax in the setting of a mobile mediastinum.

Not only can the chest tube be used to drain pleural air, it can also be used to limit the air leak in certain situations. One modality is the application of intrapleural pressure equivalent to the level of PEEP during the expiratory phase of ventilation [144–146]. With positive intrapleural pressure applied through the chest tube, the air leak persists during the inspiratory phase of ventilation but decreases during expiration, allowing maintenance of PEEP in patients in whom it is necessary for adequate oxygenation. Synchronized closure of the chest tube during the inspiratory phase has also been used to control the air leak [147,148]. A combination of these techniques has been suggested for patients with significant BPF air leaks during both the inspiratory and expiratory phases of mechanical ventilation [131,148]. These techniques pose potential hazards, including increased pneumothorax and tension pneumothorax [131,147], necessitating extremely close patient monitoring when such manipulations are used.

Instillation of chemical agents through the chest tube may potentially help close the BPF if the anatomic defect is small and single, but it is unlikely to be successful if the fistula is large or if there are multiple fistulas. Various agents have been successful in preventing recurrent pneumothoraces in patients who are not on mechanical ventilation [149–152] but BPF in the setting of mechanical ventilation is a different situation. One study compared the recurrence of pneumothorax in 39 patients with BPF randomized to intrapleural tetracycline or placebo groups [153]. There was no evidence that intrapleural tetracycline facilitated closure of the BPF. No adverse effects were encountered from the instillation of tetracycline in patients with persistent air leaks.

The chest tube may be associated with adverse effects in patients with BPF. The gas escaping through the chest tube represents part of the minute ventilation delivered to the patient and makes maintenance of an effective tidal volume problematic [154,155] Maintenance of a specific level of ventilation is not only affected by the amount of gas escaping through the fistula. The escaping gas does not passively flow from the airways into the BPF but is involved in physiologic gas exchange [154,155]. Approximately 25% of the minute ventilation has been found to escape via the BPF in patients with ARDS, with more than 20% of CO_2 excretion occurring by this route in half of the patients [155]. The role of the BPF in active CO_2 exchange is complex: Proposed mechanisms include drainage of gas from alveoli in the area of the BPF and removal of gas from remote alveolar areas by pressure gradients created by the BPF [156].

Carbon dioxide excretion and a reduction in minute ventilation occur to a lesser extent in BPF trauma victims [154]. In these patients, variable CO_2 excretion and loss of minute ventilation were dynamic and dependent on the level of chest tube suction. The difference between trauma and ARDS patients may have been due to the variability of lung compliance and the use of different ventilators [155]. Also, BPF may affect oxygen use, which generally decreases the use of inspired oxygen before it escapes through the fistula [154]. This relationship is variable but requires consideration in patients with oxygenation problems.

Negative pressure applied to the chest tube may be transmitted beyond the pleural space and into the airways, creating inappropriate cycling of the ventilator [133,156]. The increased flow through a BPF can occur with increased negative pleural pressure and may interfere with closure and healing of the fistulous site [131]. Therefore, the least amount of chest tube suction that keeps the lung inflated should be maintained in patients with BPF. The chest tube is a potential source of infection, both at the insertion site and within the pleural space.

Drainage Systems

As with the chest tube, the resistance of flow of gases is a consideration in the choice of the drainage system for the patient with a BPF [141]. The size of the air leak and the flow that the drainage system can accommodate are necessary considerations. In an experimental model of BPF that simulated the type of air leak seen clinically (mean maximal flow, 5 L per minute), four pleural drainage units (PDU) (Emerson Post-Operative Pump, Emerson; Pleur-Evac, Teleflex Medical; Sentinel Seal, Tyco; and Thora-Klex, Avilor) were tested at water seal, −20 cm H_2O, and −40 cm H_2O suction [141]. Compared with the water seal, −20 cm H_2O suction significantly increased the ability of all four PDUs to evacuate air via the chest tube, but an increase in suction to −40 cm H_2O did not significantly alter flow. When the air leak reached 4 to 5 L per minute, use of the Thora-Klex or Sentinel Seal became clinically impractical. The Pleur-Evac can handle flow rates up to 34 L per minute, but its use with rates greater than 28 L per minute is impractical due to intense bubbling in the suction control chamber [112]. Air leaks of this magnitude are infrequent clinically in BPF and are likely to be seen only with major airway disruption or diffuse parenchymal leak secondary to ARDS with severe barotraumas [156]. In the latter situations, the low-pressure, high-volume Emerson suction pump remains the only PDU capable of handling the air leak [141]. The choice of PDU should be influenced by its physiologic capabilities and the type of BPF air leak that is encountered.

Mechanical Ventilation

Conventional Ventilation. The dilemma with a BPF in a mechanically ventilated patient is achieving adequate ventilation and oxygenation while allowing repair of the BPF to occur. Because air flow escaping through a BPF theoretically delays healing of the fistulous site, reducing flow through the fistula has been a major goal in promoting repair. The BPF provides an area of low resistance to flow and acts as a conduit for the escape of a variable percentage of delivered tidal volume during conventional positive-pressure mechanical ventilation. Thus, the goal of management is to maintain adequate ventilation and oxygenation while reducing the fistula flow [131]. Using the lowest possible tidal volume, fewest mechanical breaths per minute, lowest level of PEEP, and shortest inspiratory time (see Chapter 58) can do this. Avoidance of expiratory retard also reduces airway pressures. Using the greatest number of spontaneous breaths per minute, thereby reducing use of positive pressure, may also be advantageous. Intermittent mandatory ventilation may have an advantage over assist-control ventilation in BPF.

In a retrospective study of 39 patients with BPF who were maintained on conventional ventilation, only two patients developed a pH less than 7.30 despite air leaks of up to 900 mL per breath [156]. Overall, mortality was higher when the BPF developed late in the illness and was higher with larger leaks (more than 500 mL per breath).

High-Frequency Ventilation. Despite anecdotal reports, experimental data, and clinical studies involving high-frequency ventilation (HFV) in the setting of BPF, controversy exists. However, there appear to be subgroups of patients with BPF in whom HFV may be beneficial. Both animal [157] and human [158] studies suggest that HFV is superior to conventional ventilation in controlling PO_2 and partial pressure of carbon dioxide (PCO_2) when there is a proximal (tracheal or bronchial) unilateral or bilateral fistula in the presence of normal lung parenchyma.

The use of HFV in BPF in patients with parenchymal lung disease, such as ARDS, is more controversial. Although some studies have shown that HFV improves or stabilizes gas exchange in patients with extensive parenchymal lung disease, others have not shown a beneficial effect on gas exchange or a reduction in fistula outflow [159,160]. A trial of HFV appears reasonable in the patient with a proximal BPF and normal lung parenchyma; however, it is unclear whether HFV should be considered the primary mode of ventilation in this setting. Despite discrepancies in clinical results, a trial of HFV in a critically ill patient with a BPF and diffuse parenchymal disease who fails conventional ventilation appears justified. Caution must be exercised, however, with close monitoring of gas exchange parameters and fistula flow whenever HFV is used.

Other Modes of Ventilation. Other maneuvers during both conventional ventilation and HFV can be potentially helpful in patients with BPF. Selective intubation and conventional ventilation of the unaffected lung in patients with unilateral BPF may be useful but predisposes to the collapse of the nonintubated lung [161–163]. The use of differential lung ventilation with conventional ventilation may be of benefit in some patients [159]. Positioning of the patient such that the BPF is dependent has been shown to decrease fistula flow [163].

Case reports and animal studies suggest other potential applications of HFV in BPF, including the use of independent lung ventilation with HFV applied to the BPF lung and conventional ventilation to the normal lung [164]. Another mode of HFV, ultra high-frequency jet ventilation, is being explored and has been used with some success in reducing BPF in humans [165] and animal models [166]. Independent lung ventilation with ultra high-frequency lung ventilation applied to the BPF lung and conventional ventilation to the normal lung led to rapid BPF closure in two of three patients [165].

Flexible Bronchoscopy

The flexible bronchoscope can be valuable in the diagnosis of BPF [167–169] Bronchoscopic therapy of BPF has several potential advantages, including low cost, shortened hospital stay, and relative noninvasiveness, particularly in poor operative candidates [167–169] (see Chapter 9). Proximal fistulas, such as those associated with lobectomy or pneumonectomy or stump breakdown, can be directly visualized through the bronchoscope. Distal fistulas cannot be visualized directly and require bronchoscopic passage of an occluding balloon to localize the bronchial segment leading to the fistula [170–172]. A balloon is systematically passed through the working channel of the bronchoscope and into each bronchial segment in question and then inflated; a reduction in air leak indicates localization of a bronchial segment communicating with the BPF. Once the fistula has been localized, various materials can be passed through a catheter in the working channel of the bronchoscope and into the area of the fistula [167–176]. Direct application of a sealant through the working-channel catheter onto the fistula site is the method generally used for directly visualized proximal fistulas. For distal fistulas, a multiple-lumen Swan–Ganz catheter has been used to localize the BPF and pass the occluding material of choice [170].

Several agents have been used through the bronchoscope in an attempt to occlude BPF. These include fibrin agents [169,170] cyanoacrylate-based agents [167], absorbable gelatin sponge (Gelfoam, Pfizer), blood-tetracycline [171], and lead shot [172]. The reports on all of these agents are limited to only a few patients. The cyanoacrylate-based and fibrin agents have received the most attention but still have had less than 20 total cases reported. These patients have had at least a 50% reduction of fistula flow, and most had closure of the fistula subsequent to sealant application, although multiple applications were necessary in some patients. These agents appear to work in two phases, with the agent initially sealing the leak by acting as a plug and subsequently inducing an inflammatory process with fibrosis and mucosal proliferation permanently sealing the area [167]. They are not useful with large proximal tracheal or bronchial ruptures or multiple distal parenchymal defects [170].

References

1. Woodring JH: Recognition of pleural effusion on supine radiographs: how much fluid is required? *AJR Am J Roentgenol* 142:59, 1984.
2. Collins JD, Burwell D, Furmanski S, et al: Minimum detectable pleural effusions: a roentgen pathology model. *Radiology* 105:51, 1975.
3. Yu C-J, Yang P-C, Chang D-B, et al: Diagnostic and therapeutic use of chest sonography: value in critically ill patients. *AJR Am J Roentgenol* 159:695, 1992.
4. Mayo PH, Goltz HR, Tafreshi M, et al: Safety of ultrasound-guided thoracentesis in patients receiving mechanical ventilation. *Chest* 125:1059, 2004.
5. Moskowitz PS, Griscom NT: The medial pneumothorax. *Radiology* 120:143, 1976.
6. Lichtenstein DA, Menu Y: A bedside ultrasound sign ruling out pneumothorax in the critically ill. Lung sliding. *Chest* 108:1345, 1995.
7. Rohlfing BM, Webb WR, Schlobohm RM: Ventilator-related extra-alveolar air in adults. *Radiology* 121:25, 1976.
8. Gobien RP, Reines HD, Schabel SI: Localized tension pneumothorax: unrecognized form of barotrauma in adult respiratory distress syndrome. *Radiology* 142:15, 1982.

9. Tocino IM, Miller MH, Fairfax WR: Distribution of pneumothorax in the supine and semirecumbent critically ill adult. *AJR Am J Roentgenol* 144:901, 1985.
10. Kollef MH: Risk factors for the misdiagnosis of pneumothorax in the intensive care unit. *Crit Care Med* 19:906, 1991.
11. Collins TR, Sahn SA: Thoracentesis: clinical value, complications, technical problems, and patient experience. *Chest* 91:817, 1987.
12. Lipscomb DJ, Flower CDR, Hadfield JW: Ultrasound of the pleura: an assessment of its clinical value. *Clin Radiol* 32:289, 1981.
13. Godwin JE, Sahn SA: Thoracentesis: a safe procedure in mechanically ventilated patients. *Ann Intern Med* 113:800, 1990.
14. Bartter T, Mayo PD, Pratter MR, et al: Lower risk and higher yield for thoracentesis when performed by experienced operators. *Chest* 103:1873, 1993.
15. Seneff MG, Corwin W, Gold LH, et al: Complications associated with thoracentesis. *Chest* 89:97, 1986.
16. Grogan DR, Irwin RS, Channick R, et al: Complications associated with thoracentesis. *Arch Intern Med* 150:873, 1990.
17. Heidecker J, Huggins JT, Sahn SA, et al: Pathophysiology of pneumothorax following ultrasound-guided thoracentesis. *Chest* 130:1173, 2006.
18. Light RW, Jenkinson SG, Minh V, et al: Observations on pleural pressures as fluid is withdrawn during thoracentesis. *Am Rev Respir Dis* 121:799, 1980.
19. Brown NE, Zamel N, Aberman A: Changes in pulmonary mechanics and gas exchange following thoracocentesis. *Chest* 74:540, 1978.
20. Estenne M, Yernault J-C, Detroyer A: Mechanism of relief of dyspnea after thoracentesis in patients with large effusions. *Am J Med* 74:813, 1983.
21. Light RW, Stansbury DW, Brown SE: Changes in pulmonary function following therapeutic thoracentesis. *Chest* 80:375, 1981.
22. Doelken P, Abreu R, Sahn SA: Effect of thoracentesis on respiratory mechanics and gas exchange in the patient receiving mechanical ventilation. *Chest* 130:1354, 2006.
23. Brandstetter RD, Cohen RP: Hypoxemia after thoracentesis: a predictable and treatable condition. *JAMA* 242:1060, 1979.
24. Karetzky M, Kothari GA, Fourre JA, et al: The effect of thoracentesis on arterial oxygen tension. *Respiration* 36:96, 1978.
25. Perpina M, Benlloch E, Marco V, et al: The effect of thoracentesis on pulmonary gas exchange. *Thorax* 38:747, 1983.
26. Mattison L, Coppage L, Alderman D, et al: Pleural effusions in the medical intensive care unit: prevalence, causes and clinical implications. *Chest* 111:1018, 1997.
27. Light RW, George RB: Incidence and significance of pleural effusion after abdominal surgery. *Chest* 69:621, 1976.
28. Nielsen PH, Jepsan SB, Olsen AD: Postoperative pleural effusion following upper abdominal surgery. *Chest* 96:1133, 1989.
29. Wiener-Kronish JP, Matthay MA, Callen PW, et al: Relationship of pleural effusions to pulmonary hemodynamics in patients with congestive heart failure. *Am Rev Respir Dis* 132:1253, 1987.
30. Shinto RA, Light RW: Effects of diuresis on the characteristics of pleural fluid in patients with congestive heart failure. *Am J Med* 88:230, 1990.
31. Chakko SC, Caldwell SH, Sforza PP: Treatment of congestive heart failure: its effect on pleural fluid chemistry. *Chest* 95:798, 1989.
32. Lieberman FL, Hidemura R, Peters RL, et al: Pathogenesis and treatment of hydrothorax complicating cirrhosis with ascites. *Ann Intern Med* 64:341, 1966.
33. Sadler TW: *Langman's Medical Embryology*. 7th ed. Baltimore, Williams & Wilkins, 1995, p 176.
34. Johnson RF, Loo RB: Hepatic hydrothorax: studies to determine the source of the fluid and report of 13 cases. *Ann Intern Med* 61:385, 1964.
35. Strauss RM, Boyer TD: Hepatic hydrothorax. *Semin Liver Dis* 17:227, 1997.
36. Frazer IH, Lichtenstein M, Andrews JT: Pleuroperitoneal effusion without ascites. *Med J Aust* 2:520, 1983.
37. Xiol X, Castellvi JM, Guardiola J, et al: Spontaneous bacterial empyema in cirrhotic patients: a prospective study. *Hepatology* 23:719, 1996.
38. Abba AA, Laajam MA, Zargar SA: Spontaneous neutrocytic hepatic hydrothorax without ascites. *Respir Med* 90:631, 1996.
39. Strauss RM, Martin LG, Kaufman SL, et al: Transjugular intrahepatic portal systemic shunt for the management of symptomatic cirrhotic hydrothorax. *Am J Gastroenterol* 89:1520, 1994.
40. Mouroux J, Perrin C, Venissac N, et al: Management of pleural effusion of cirrhotic origin. *Chest* 109:1093, 1996.
41. Eid AA, Keddissi JI, Kinasewitz GT: Hypoalbuminemia as a cause of pleural effusions. *Chest* 115:1066, 1999.
42. Scott WL: Complications associated with central venous catheters: a survey. *Chest* 94:1221, 1988.
43. Duntley P, Siever J, Korwes ML, et al: Vascular erosion by central venous catheters: clinical features and outcome. *Chest* 101:1633, 1992.
44. Ellis LM, Vogel SB 3rd, Copeland EM: Central venous catheter vascular erosions. *Ann Surg* 209:475, 1989.
45. Aslamy Z, Dewald LL, Heffner JE: MRI of central venous anatomy: Implications for central venous catheter insertion. *Chest* 114:820, 1998.
46. Wechsler RJ, Byrne KJ, Steiner RM: The misplaced thoracic venous catheter: detailed anatomical consideration. *Crit Rev Diagn Imaging* 21:289, 1982.
47. Ball GV, Whitfield CL: Studies on rheumatoid disease pleural fluid. *Arthritis Rheum* 9:846, 1966.
48. Heffner JE, McDonald J, Bareberi C, et al: Management of parapneumonic effusions: an analysis of physician practice patterns. *Arch Surg* 130:433, 1995.
49. Taryle DA, Potts DE, Sahn SA: The incidence and clinical correlates of parapneumonic effusions in pneumococcal pneumonia. *Chest* 74:170, 1978.
50. Light RW, Girard EM, Jenkinson SG, et al: Parapneumonic effusions. *Am J Med* 69:507, 1980.
51. Heffner JE: Indications for draining a parapneumonic effusion: an evidence-based approach. *Semin Respir Infect* 14:48, 1999.
52. Heffner JE, Brown LK, Barberi C, et al: Pleural fluid chemical analysis in parapneumonic effusions: a meta-analysis. *Am J Respir Crit Care Med* 151:1700, 1995.
53. Lesho EP, Roth BJ: Is pH paper an acceptable, low-cost alternate to the blood gas analyzer for determining pleural fluid pH? *Chest* 112:1291, 1997.
54. Ashbaugh DG: Empyema thoracis: factors influencing morbidity and mortality. *Chest* 99:1162, 1991.
55. Sahn SA: Use of fibrinolytic agents in the management of complicated parapneumonic effusions. *Thorax* 53[Suppl]:S65, 1998.
56. Ridley PD, Brainbridge MV: Thoracoscopic débridement and pleural irrigation in the management of empyema thoracis. *Ann Thorac Surg* 51:461, 1991.
57. Landreneau RJ, Keenan RJ, Hazelrigg SR, et al: Thoracoscopy for empyema and hemothorax. *Chest* 109:18, 1995.
58. Podbielski FJ, Maniar HS, Rodriguez HE, et al: Surgical strategy of complex empyema thoracis. *JSLS* 4:287, 2000.
59. Cunniffe MG, Maguire D, McAnena OJ, et al: Video-assisted thoracoscopic surgery in the management of loculated empyema. *Surg Endosc* 14:175, 2000.
60. Kaye MD: Pleuropulmonary complications of pancreatitis. *Thorax* 23:297, 1968.
61. Maringhini A, Ciambra M, Patti R, et al: Ascites, pleural, and pericardial effusions in acute pancreatitis: a prospective study of the incidence, natural history, and prognostic role. *Dig Dis Sci* 41:848, 1996.
62. Anderson WJ, Skinner DB, Zuidema GD, et al: Chronic pancreatic pleural effusions. *Surg Gynecol Obstet* 137:827, 1973.
63. Bynum LJ, Wilson JE III: Radiographic features of pleural effusions in pulmonary embolism. *Am Rev Respir Dis* 117:829, 1978.
64. Bynum LJ, Wilson JE 3rd: Characteristics of pleural effusions associated with pulmonary embolism. *Arch Intern Med* 136:159, 1976.
65. Simon HB, Daggett WN, DeSanctis RW: Hemothorax as a complication of anticoagulant therapy in the presence of pulmonary infarction. *JAMA* 208:1830, 1969.
66. Dressler W: The post-myocardial infarction syndrome: a report of 44 cases. *Arch Intern Med* 103:28, 1959.
67. Engle MA, Ito T: The post-pericardiotomy syndrome. *Am J Cardiol* 7:73, 1961.
68. Stelzner TJ, King TE Jr, Antony VB, et al: The pleuro-pulmonary manifestations of the postcardiac injury syndrome. *Chest* 84:383, 1983.
69. Kaminsky ME, Rodan BA, Osborne DR, et al: Post-pericardiotomy syndrome. *AJR Am J Roentgenol* 138:503, 1982.
70. Kim S, Sahn SA: Postcardiac injury syndrome: an immunologic pleural fluid analysis. *Chest* 109:570, 1996.
71. Bacon BR, Bailey-Newton RS, Connors AF Jr: Pleural effusions after endoscopic variceal sclerotherapy. *Gastroenterology* 88:1910, 1985.
72. Saks BJ, Kilby AE, Dietrich PA: Pleural and mediastinal changes following endoscopic injection sclerotherapy of esophageal varices. *Radiology* 149:639, 1983.
73. Parikh SS, Amarapurkar DN, Dhawan PS, et al: Development of pleural effusion after sclerotherapy with absolute alcohol. *Gastrointest Endosc* 39:404, 1993.
74. Aberle DR, Wiener-Kronish JP, Webb WR, et al: Hydrostatic versus increased permeability pulmonary edema: diagnosis based on radiographic criteria in critically ill patients. *Radiology* 168:73, 1988.
75. Talmor M, Hydo L, Gershenwald JG, et al: Beneficial effects of chest tube drainage of pleural effusion in acute respiratory failure refractory to positive end-expiratory pressure ventilation. *Surgery* 123:137, 1998.
76. Parkin GJS: The radiology of perforated esophagus. *Clin Radiol* 24:324, 1973.
77. O'Connell ND: Spontaneous rupture of the esophagus. *AJR Am J Roentgenol* 99:186, 1967.
78. Bladergroen MR, Lowe JE, Postlethwait RW: Diagnosis and recommended management of esophageal perforation and rupture. *Ann Thorac Surg* 42:235, 1986.
79. DeMeester TR: Perforation of the esophagus. *Ann Thorac Surg* 42:231, 1986.
80. Maulitz RM, Good JT Jr, Kaplan RL, et al: The pleuropulmonary consequences of esophageal rupture: an experimental model. *Am Rev Respir Dis* 120:363, 1979.
81. Sherr HP, Light RW, Merson MH, et al: Origin of pleural fluid amylase in esophageal rupture. *Ann Intern Med* 76:985, 1972.
82. Abbott OA, Mansour KA, Logan WD Jr, et al: Atraumatic so-called "spontaneous" rupture of the esophagus. *J Thorac Cardiovasc Surg* 59:67, 1970.
83. Graham JM, Mattox KL, Beall AC Jr: Penetrating trauma of the lung. *J Trauma* 19:665, 1979.

84. Beall AC Jr, Crawford HW, DeBakey ME: Considerations in the management of acute traumatic hemothorax. *J Thorac Cardiovasc Surg* 52:351, 1966.
85. Weil PH, Margolis IB: Systematic approach to traumatic hemothorax. *Am J Surg* 142:692, 1981.
86. Griffith GL, Todd EP, McMillin RD, et al: Acute traumatic hemothorax. *Ann Thorac Surg* 26:204, 1978.
87. Wilson JM, Boren CH, Peterson SR, et al: Traumatic hemothorax: is decortication necessary? *J Thorac Cardiovasc Surg* 77:489, 1979.
88. Iverson L, Mittal A, Dugan D, et al: Injuries to the phrenic nerve resulting in diaphragmatic paralysis with special reference to stretch trauma. *Am J Surg* 132:263, 1976.
89. Marco J, Hahn J, Barner H: Topical cardiac hypothermia and phrenic nerve injury. *Ann Thorac Surg* 23:235, 1977.
90. Wheeler W, Rubis L, Jones C, et al: Etiology and prevention of topical cardiac hypothermia-induced phrenic nerve injury and left lower lobe atelectasis during cardiac surgery. *Chest* 88:680, 1985.
91. Landymore RW, Howell F: Pulmonary complications following myocardial revascularization with the internal mammary artery graft. *Eur J Cardiothorac Surg* 4:156, 1990.
92. Kollef MH: Trapped-lung syndrome after cardiac surgery: a potentially preventable complication of pleural injury. *Heart Lung* 19:671, 1990.
93. Ferguson MK, Little AG, Skinner DB: Current concepts in the management of postoperative chylothorax. *Ann Thorac Surg* 45:542, 1985.
94. Orringer MB, Bluett M, Deeb GM: Aggressive treatment of chylothorax complicating transhiatal esophagectomy without thoracotomy. *Surgery* 104:720, 1988.
95. Hillerdal G: Chylothorax and pseudochylothorax. *Eur Respir J* 10:1157, 1997.
96. Nygaard SD, Berger HA, Fick RB: Chylothorax as a complication of oesophageal sclerotherapy. *Thorax* 47:134, 1992.
97. Weidner WA, Steiner RM: Roentgenographic demonstration of intrapulmonary and pleural lymphatics during lymphangiography. *Radiology* 100:533, 1971.
98. Staats BA, Ellefson RD, Budhan LL, et al: The lipoprotein profile of chylous and nonchylous pleural effusions. *Mayo Clin Proc* 55:700, 1980.
99. Monla-Hassan J, Eichenhorn M, Spickler E, et al: Duro-pleural fistula manifested as a large pleural transudate. *Chest* 114:1786, 1998.
100. D'Souza R, Doshi A, Bhojraj S, et al: Massive pleural effusion as the presenting feature of a subarachnoid-pleural fistula. *Respiration* 69:96, 2002.
101. Pollack II, Pang D, Hall W: Subarachnoid-pleural and subarachnoid mediastinal fistulae. *Neurosurgery* 26:519, 1990.
102. Assietti R, Kibble MB, Bakay R: Iatrogenic cerebrospinal fluid fistula to the pleural cavity: case report and literature review. *Neurosurgery* 33:1004, 1993.
103. Skedros DG, Cass SP, Hirsch BE, et al: Beta-2 transferrin assay in clinical management of cerebral spinal fluid and perilymphatic fluid leaks. *J Otolaryngol* 22:341, 1993.
104. Macklin MT, Macklin CC: Malignant interstitial emphysema of the lungs and mediastinum as an important occult complication in many respiratory diseases and other conditions: an interpretation of the clinical literature in the light of laboratory experiments. *Medicine* 23:281, 1944.
105. Macklin CC: Transport of air along sheaths of pulmonic blood vessels from alveoli to mediastinum: clinical implications. *Arch Intern Med* 64:913, 1939.
106. Gustman P, Yerger L, Wanner A: Immediate cardiovascular effects of tension pneumothorax. *Am Rev Respir Dis* 127:171, 1983.
107. Hurewitz AN, Sidhu U, Bergofsky B, et al: Cardiovascular and respiratory consequence of tension pneumothorax. *Bull Eur Physiopathol Respir* 22:545, 1986.
108. Norris RM, Jones JG, Bishop JM: Respiratory gas exchange in patients with spontaneous pneumothorax. *Thorax* 23:427, 1968.
109. Moran JF, Jones RH, Wolfe WG: Regional pulmonary function during experimental unilateral pneumothorax in the awake state. *J Thorac Cardiovasc Surg* 74:394, 1977.
110. Hagley MT, Martin B, Gast P, et al: Infectious and mechanical complications of central venous catheters placed by percutaneous venipuncture and over guide wires. *Crit Care Med* 20:1426, 1992.
111. Eerola R, Kaukinen L, Kaukinen S: Analysis of 13,800 subclavian catheterizations. *Acta Anesthesiol Scand* 29:193, 1985.
112. Tyden H: Cannulation of the internal jugular vein: 500 cases. *Acta Anesthesiol Scand* 26:485, 1982.
113. Weiner P, Sznajder I, Plavnick L, et al: Unusual complications of subclavian vein catheterization. *Crit Care Med* 12:538, 1984.
114. Kumar A, Pontoppidan H, Falke KJ, et al: Pulmonary barotrauma during mechanical ventilation. *Crit Care Med* 1:1, 1973.
115. Zimmerman JE, Dunbar BS, Klingenmaier CH: Management of subcutaneous emphysema, pneumomediastinum, and pneumothorax during respirator therapy. *Crit Care Med* 3:69, 1975.
116. Cullen DJ, Caldera DL: The incidence of ventilator-induced pulmonary barotrauma in critically ill patients. *Anesthesiology* 50:185, 1979.
117. Tocino I, Westcott JL: Barotrauma. *Radiol Clin North Am* 34:59, 1996.
118. Anzueto A, Frutos-Vivar F, Esteban A: Incidence, risk factors and outcome of barotrauma in mechanically ventilated patients. *Intensive Care Med* 30:612, 2004.
119. Zwillich CW, Pierson DJ, Creagh CE, et al: Complications of assisted ventilation: a prospective study of 354 consecutive episodes. *Am J Med* 57:161, 1974.
120. Steier M, Ching N, Roberts EB, et al: Pneumothorax complicating continuous ventilatory support. *J Thorac Cardiovasc Surg* 67:17, 1979.
121. Johnson TH, Altman AR: Pulmonary interstitial gas: first sign of barotrauma due to PEEP therapy. *Crit Care Med* 7:532, 1979.
122. Albelda SM, Gefter WB, Kelley MA, et al: Ventilator-induced subpleural air cysts: clinical, radiographic, and pathologic significance. *Am Rev Respir Dis* 127:360, 1983.
123. Westcott JL, Cole SR: Interstitial pulmonary emphysema in children and adults: roentgenographic features. *Radiology* 111:367, 1974.
124. Kirkpatrick AW, Ng AK, Dulchavsky SA, et al: Sonographic diagnosis of pneumothorax inapparent on plain radiography: confirmation by computed tomography. *J Trauma* 50:750, 2001.
125. Dulchavsky SA, Hamilton DR, Diebel LN, et al: Thoracic ultrasound diagnosis of pneumothorax. *J Trauma* 47:970, 1999.
126. Snyder J, Carrol G, Schuster DP, et al: Mechanical ventilation: physiology and application. *Curr Probl Surg* 21:1, 1984.
127. Suter PM, Fairley HP, Isenberg MD: Effect of tidal volume and positive end-expiratory pressure on compliance during mechanical ventilation. *Chest* 73:158, 1978.
128. Willetts SM: Paralysis of ventilated patients: yes or no? *Intensive Care Med* 11:2, 1985.
129. Darioli E, Perret C: Mechanical controlled hypoventilation in status asthmaticus. *Am Rev Respir Dis* 129:385, 1984.
130. Baumann MH, Sahn SA: Tension pneumothorax: diagnostic and therapeutic pitfalls. *Crit Care Med* 21:177, 1993.
131. Powner DJ, Grenvik A: Ventilatory management of life-threatening bronchopleural fistulae: a summary. *Crit Care Med* 9:54, 1981.
132. Ratliff JL, Hill JD, Fallat RJ, et al: Complications associated with membrane lung support by venoarterial perfusion. *Ann Thorac Surg* 19:537, 1975.
133. Tilles RB, Don HF: Complications of high pleural suction in bronchopleural fistulas. *Anesthesiology* 43:486, 1975.
134. Steiger Z, Wilson RF: Management of bronchopleural fistulas. *Surgery* 158:267, 1984.
135. Shenstone NS: The use of intercostal muscle in the closure of bronchopleural fistulae. *Ann Surg* 4:560, 1936.
136. Beltrami V: Surgical transsternal treatment of bronchopleural fistula postpneumonectomy. *Chest* 95:379, 1989.
137. Barker WL, Faber LP, Ostermiller WE, et al: Management of persistent bronchopleural fistulas. *J Thorac Cardiovasc Surg* 62:393, 1971.
138. Demos NJ, Timmes JJ: Myoplasty for closure of tracheobronchial fistula. *Ann Thorac Surg* 15:88, 1973.
139. Hankins JR, Miller JE, McLaughlin JS: The use of chest wall muscle flaps to close bronchopleural fistulas: experience with 21 patients. *Ann Thorac Surg* 6:491, 1978.
140. Ferguson JS, Sprenger K, VanNatta T: Closure of a bronchopleural fistula using bronchoscopic placement of an endobronchial valve designed for the treatment of emphysema. *Chest* 129:479, 2006.
141. Rusch VW, Capps JS, Tyler ML, et al: The performance of four pleural drainage systems in an animal model of bronchopleural fistula. *Chest* 4:859, 1988.
142. Batchelder TL, Morris KA: Critical factors in determining adequate pleural drainage in both the operated and nonoperated chest. *Am Surg* 28:296, 1962.
143. Swensen EW, Birath G, Ahbeck A: Resistance to airflow in bronchospirometric catheters. *J Thorac Surg* 33:275, 1957.
144. Downes JB, Chapman RL: Treatment of bronchopleural fistula during continuous positive pressure ventilation. *Chest* 69:363, 1976.
145. Phillips YY, Lonigan RM, Joyner LR: A simple technique for managing a bronchopleural fistula while maintaining positive pressure ventilation. *Crit Care Med* 7:351, 1979.
146. Weksler N, Ovadia L: The challenge of bilateral bronchopleural fistula. *Chest* 95:938, 1989.
147. Gallagher TJ, Smith RA, Kirby RR, et al: Intermittent inspiratory chest tube occlusion to limit bronchopleural cutaneous air leaks. *Crit Care Med* 4:328, 1976.
148. Bevelaqua FA, Kay S: A modified technique for the management of bronchopleural fistula in ventilator-dependent patients: a report of 2 cases. *Respir Care* 31:904, 1986.
149. Larrieu AJ, Tyers FO, Williams EH, et al: Intrapleural instillation of quinacrine for treatment of recurrent spontaneous pneumothorax. *Ann Thorac Surg* 28:146, 1979.
150. Goldszer RC, Bennett J, VanCampen J, et al: Intrapleural tetracycline for spontaneous pneumothorax. *JAMA* 241:724, 1979.
151. Macoviak JA, Stephenson LW, Ochs R, et al: Tetracycline pleurodesis during active pulmonary-pleural air leak for prevention of recurrent pneumothorax. *Chest* 81:78, 1982.
152. Verschoof AC, Vende T, Greve LH, et al: Thoracoscopic pleurodesis in the management of spontaneous pneumothorax. *Respiration* 53:197, 1988.
153. Light RW, O'Hara VS, Moritz TE, et al: Intrapleural tetracycline for the prevention of recurrent spontaneous pneumothorax. *JAMA* 264:2224, 1990.
154. Powner DJ, Cline CD, Rodman GH: Effect of chest-tube suction on gas flow through a bronchopleural fistula. *Crit Care Med* 13:99, 1985.

155. Bishop MJ, Benson MS, Pierson DJ: Carbon dioxide excretion via bronchopleural fistulas in adult respiratory distress syndrome. *Chest* 91:400, 1987.
156. Pierson DJ, Horton CA, Bates PW: Persistent bronchopleural air leak during mechanical ventilation: a review of 39 cases. *Chest* 90:321, 1986.
157. Kuwik RJ, Glass D, Coombs DW: Evaluation of high-frequency positive pressure ventilation for experimental bronchopleural fistula. *Crit Care Med* 9:164, 1981.
158. Turnbull AD, Carlon GC, Howland WS, et al: High-frequency jet ventilation in major airway or pulmonary disruption. *Ann Thorac Surg* 32:468, 1981.
159. Albeda SM, Hansen-Flaschen JH, Taylor E, et al: Evaluation of high-frequency jet ventilation in patients with bronchopleural fistulas by quantitation of the airleak. *Anesthesiology* 63:551, 1985.
160. Bishop MJ, Benson MS, Sato P, et al: Comparison of high-frequency jet ventilation with conventional mechanical ventilation for bronchopleural fistula. *Anesth Analg* 66:833, 1987.
161. Rafferty TD, Palma J, Motoyama EK, et al: Management of a bronchopleural fistula with differential lung ventilation and positive end-expiratory pressure. *Respir Care* 25:654, 1980.
162. Brown CR: Postpneumonectomy empyema and bronchopleural fistula: use of prolonged endobronchial intubation: a case report. *Anesth Analg* 52:439, 1973.
163. Lau K: Postural management of bronchopleural fistula. *Chest* 94:1122, 1988.
164. Feeley TW, Keating D, Nishimura T: Independent lung ventilation using high-frequency ventilation in the management of a bronchopleural fistula. *Anesthesiology* 69:420, 1988.
165. Crimi G, Candiani A, Conti G, et al: Clinical applications of independent lung ventilation with unilateral high-frequency jet ventilation (ILV-UHFJV). *Intensive Care Med* 12:90, 1986.
166. Orlando R, Gluck EH, Cohen M, et al: Ultra-high-frequency jet ventilation in a bronchopleural fistula model. *Arch Surg* 123:591, 1988.
167. Torre M, Chiesa G, Ravine M, et al: Endoscopic gluing of bronchopleural fistula. *Ann Thorac Surg* 43:295, 1987.
168. Hoier-Madsen K, Schulze S, Pedersen VM, et al: Management of bronchopleural fistula following pneumonectomy. *Scand J Thorac Cardiovasc Surg* 18:263, 1984.
169. Glover W, Chavis TV, Daniel TM, et al: Fibrin glue application through the flexible fiberoptic bronchoscope: closure of bronchopleural fistula. *J Thorac Cardiovasc Surg* 93:470, 1987.
170. Regel G, Sturm JA, Neumann C, et al: Occlusion of bronchopleural fistula after lung injury: a new treatment by bronchoscopy. *J Trauma* 29:223, 1989.
171. Lan R, Lee C, Tsai Y, et al: Fiberoptic bronchial blockade in a small bronchopleural fistula. *Chest* 92:944, 1987.
172. Ratliff JL, Hill JD, Tucker H, et al: Endobronchial control of bronchopleural fistulae. *Chest* 71:98, 1971.
173. Ellis JH, Sequeira FW, Weber TR, et al: Balloon catheter occlusion of bronchopleural fistulae. *AJR Am J Roentgenol* 138:157, 1982.
174. Roksvaag H, Skalleberg L, Nordberg C, et al: Endoscopic closure of bronchial fistula. *Thorax* 38:696, 1983.
175. Menard JW, Prejean CA, Tucker YW: Endoscopic closure of bronchopleural fistulas using a tissue adhesive. *Am J Surg* 155:415, 1980.
176. Jones DP, David I: Gelfoam occlusion of peripheral bronchopleural fistulas. *Ann Thorac Surg* 42:334, 1986.

CHAPTER 58 ■ MECHANICAL VENTILATION PART I: INVASIVE

RICHARD A. OECKLER, ROLF D. HUBMAYR AND RICHARD S. IRWIN

Mechanical ventilation refers to any method of breathing in which a mechanical apparatus is used to augment or satisfy the bulk flow requirements of a patient's breathing. Mechanical ventilation is indicated when the patient's spontaneous ventilation is not adequate to sustain life or when it is necessary to take control of the patient's ventilation to prevent impending collapse of other organ functions. At present, it is not known if mechanical ventilation should also be instituted to enable lung protection and prevent the potentially deleterious effects of hyperpnea in a spontaneously breathing patient with injured lungs. This chapter discusses the institution and maintenance of mechanical ventilation.

PRINCIPLES OF OPERATION

Negative-Pressure Ventilation

Until the mid-1950s, mechanical ventilators used for continuous ventilation were predominantly of the negative-pressure variety. The iron lung, or tank ventilator, was the most familiar of these. Bulk flow was mobilized into the patient's lungs by cyclically creating a subatmospheric pressure around the chest; actually, only the patient's head was not enclosed in the negative-pressure chamber. Subsequent ventilators applied negative external pressures to the rib cage only to induce inspiratory flow ($\dot{V}_i$) [1]. The original chest-enclosing ventilators of this type, called *cuirass ventilators*, incorporated a rigid shell that was applied to the chest. Later versions employed a much more flexible housing for the chest that was better tolerated by patients. The logistic problems encountered in providing routine nursing care for unstable patients resulted in an abandonment of negative-pressure ventilators in the acute care setting some 40 years ago. Interest in intermittent nocturnal mechanical ventilation as home therapy for chronic respiratory failure led to a minor resurgence in their use in the 1980s. However, because negative-pressure ventilators tend to be bulky, are poorly tolerated, may cause obstructive sleep apnea, and have not proved effective in the rehabilitation of patients with end-stage chronic obstructive pulmonary diseases (COPD), they have been largely replaced by positive-pressure ventilators for home use as well [2].

A recent experimental study in rabbits with injured lungs has rekindled interest in the use of negative pressure ventilators in the intensive care setting [3]. Rabbits ventilated with negative-body surface pressure had improved oxygenation and better lung recruitment than animals ventilated with equivalent amounts of positive pressure applied to the airway. The study was met with skepticism, because the results are not compatible with long established physical principles. Since the structures contained within the thorax are in essence incompressible, the findings suggest mode and instrumentation specific differences in respiratory impedance rather than inherent advantages of negative over positive pressure ventilation.

Positive-Pressure Ventilation

Positive-pressure ventilation is operative when a superatmospheric pressure is cyclically created at the upper airway. The resultant pressure gradient between the upper airway and the lungs pushes gases through the airways. In the acute care setting, positive-pressure ventilation is usually delivered through an endotracheal or tracheostomy tube. However, an increasing awareness of tube-related complications has contributed greatly to the emergence of noninvasive mechanical ventilation through a face mask, nasal mask, helmet, or mouth seal as a viable treatment option for some patients with respiratory failure (see Chapter 59 for a more complete discussion of noninvasive mechanical ventilation).

Conventional positive-pressure ventilation has come to be identified with respiratory rates up to 60 breaths per minute, even though rates above 30 breaths per minute are rarely used. Any mode of ventilation administered at higher respiratory rates is considered high-frequency positive-pressure ventilation. High-frequency oscillatory ventilation (HFOV) supports pulmonary gas exchange by entraining gas from a bias flow circuit and delivering subnormal tidal volumes (TVs) to the lungs at rates between 3 and 15 cycles per second (Hz) [4,5]. The technique was patented in the late 1950s, came to the attention of pulmonary physiologists in the 1970s, was then touted as promising treatment for babies with immature lungs, but was rejected after a large clinical trial (the HIFI study) found it to be inferior to conventional mechanical ventilation [6]. With the emergence of the "open lung concept" in the 1990s and the realization that ventilation with large TVs can injure susceptible lungs, HFOV attracted renewed interest in recent years [7,8]. In some centers, HFOV has emerged as a first-line treatment option in neonates with respiratory distress [9–14], and the MOAT trial showed a trend in favor of HFOV in adults with acute lung injury (ALI) [15]. A recent expert panel report provides detailed recommendations for HFOV [16]. Moreover, the panel identified areas for further study, such as the role of HFOV as first line treatment in adults with ALI and the choice of initial frequency settings [17]. The latter touches on unresolved issues of fundamental biologic significance: Is rate or the amplitude of lung deformation the more important risk factor for injury, and how does hypercapnia modify this risk?

Before discussing different categories and modes of positive-pressure ventilation, it is useful to review the basic mechanical determinants of patient–ventilator interactions.

Mechanical Determinants of Patient–Ventilator Interactions

Despite gross oversimplifications, linear models of the respiratory system have proved useful for the understanding of patient–ventilator interactions [18,19]. Figure 58.1 shows a simulation of volume preset (volume is the independent variable) mechanical ventilation in a linear respiratory system analogue. When ventilators are programmed to deliver a specific flow, the resulting inspiratory pressure profile contains information about the mechanical properties of the respiratory system. The pressure applied at time (t) to the tube inlet ($P_{i(t)}$, near the attachment to the ventilator) is equal to the sum of two pressures, an elastic pressure ($P_{el(t)}$) and a resistive pressure ($P_{res(t)}$).

$$P_{i(t)} = P_{el(t)} + P_{res(t)}$$

The tube outlet pressure at the junction with the balloon is equal to the pressure inside the balloon (P_{el}). P_{res} is the difference in pressure between the tube inlet and the tube outlet.

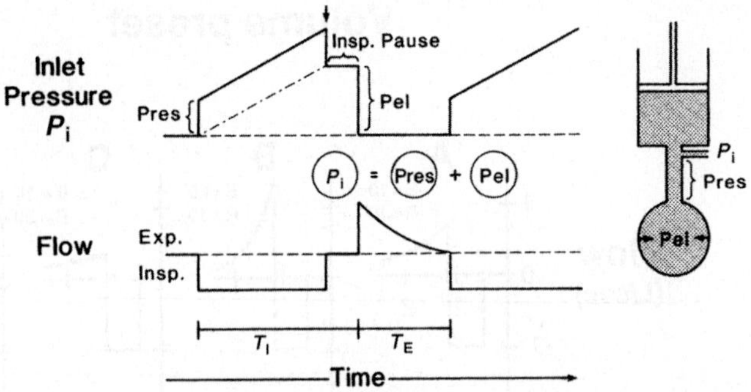

FIGURE 58.1. Components of inlet pressure. Model of the respiratory system consisting of a resistive element (straight tube) and an elastic element (balloon) connected to a ventilator (piston). During inflation of the model with constant flow (*bottom*), there is a stepwise increase in inlet pressure (P_i) that equals the loss of pressure across the resistive element (P_{res}) (*top*). Thereafter, P_i increases linearly and reflects the mechanical properties of the elastic element (P_{el}). P_i is the sum of P_{res} and P_{el}. At end inspiration, when flow has ceased (Insp. Pause), P_i decreases by an amount equal to P_{res}; P_i equals P_{el} during Insp. Pause. T_I, inspiratory time; T_E, expiratory time. [From Gay PC, Rodarte JR, Tayyab M, et al: The evaluation of bronchodilator responsiveness in mechanically ventilated patients. *Am Rev Respir Dis* 136:880, 1987, with permission.]

Assuming linear system behavior, the inlet pressure–time profile can be computed for any piston stroke volume (V_{stroke}) and flow ($\dot{V}$) setting, provided the resistive properties of the tube (R) and the elastic properties of the balloon (E) are known:

$$P_{i(t)} = E\,V_{(t)} + R\dot{V}_{(t)}$$

Elastance, E, is a measure of balloon stiffness and is equal to the ratio of P_{el} and V_{stroke} (assuming 0 volume and pressure at the beginning of balloon inflation). Therefore, $P_{el(t)}$ of the first equation can be substituted with $EV_{(t)}$ in the second equation. Applied to the respiratory system, E reflects the elastic properties of lungs and chest wall, whereas R reflects primarily the resistive properties of endotracheal tube and airways. Because Ohm's law states that the resistance R is equal to the ratio of pressure and flow, $P_{res(t)}$ of the first equation can be substituted with the product $R\dot{V}_{(t)}$ in the second equation.

During inflation with constant (square wave) flow, there is an initial step change in driving pressure measured at the inlet (P_i) that equals the pressure loss across the resistive element (P_{res}). Thereafter, P_i increases linearly with time and volume and attains a maximal value (P_{peak}) at the end of inflation. The linear rise in P_i with time (and volume) indicates that elastance of the respiratory system (E_{rs}) is constant over the tidal breathing range and suggests that the mechanical ventilator is the only source of pressure during inflation (i.e., the respiratory muscles are relaxed).

When the airway is occluded at end inspiration, flow ($\dot{V}_{insp}$) falls to zero and the airway pressure drops from P_{peak} to P_{ei} (the end inflation/static/plateau or pause pressure). P_{ei} represents the static elastic recoil pressure of the respiratory system at end-inflation volume (P_{el}). As long as P_{el} at end expiration is zero (absence of hyperinflation), E_{rs} can be calculated from the ratio of P_{ei} and tidal volume (TV).

Contrast the waveforms pertaining to volume preset mechanical ventilation in Figure 58.1 with the simulation of *pressure preset (pressure is the independent variable) mechanical ventilation* in Figure 58.2. When ventilators are programmed to generate a step change in pressure, the resulting inspiratory flow profile contains information about the mechanical properties of the respiratory system. Inspiratory flow rises to an early peak and then declines as the lungs fill with gas. The reason for the decline in flow with volume and time is the increase

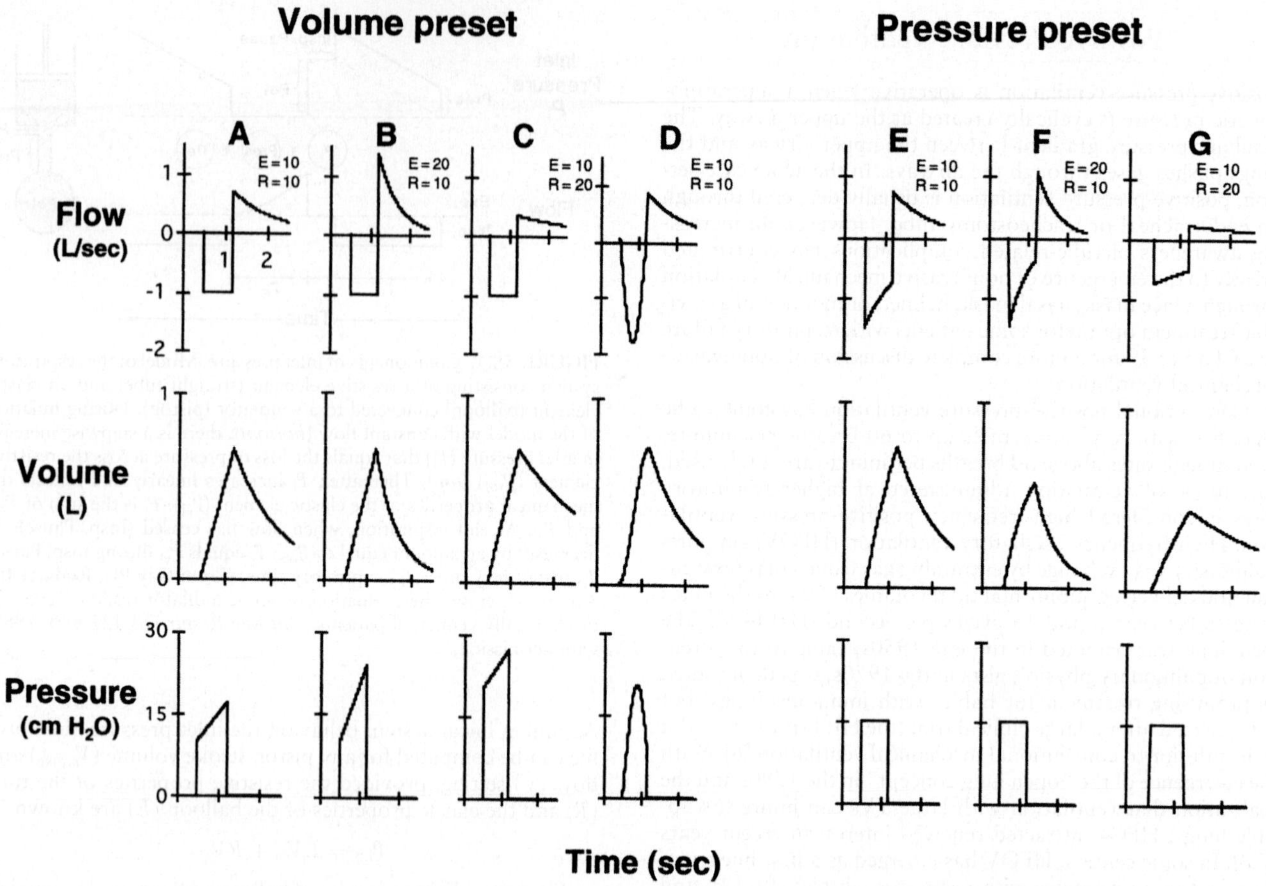

FIGURE 58.2. Schematic representation of the interdependence between pressure, volume, and flow during volume preset ventilation (A–D) and pressure preset ventilation (E–G). In the volume preset mode, increases in respiratory elastance (B) and resistance (C) as well as the choice of the inspiratory flow profile (D) affect airway pressure. In the pressure preset mode, the same changes in elastance (F) and resistance (G) compared to control (E) affect volume and flow profiles.

in elastic (balloon) pressure (*dashed line*) (see Fig. 58.1) with volume and time. The rise in balloon pressure (surrogate for alveolar pressure, P_{alv}) in the face of a constant P_i accounts for a progressive reduction in net driving pressure [$P_{i(t)} - P_{el(t)}$] during lung inflation. Because P_{res} varies with flow, P_{res} must also decline during lung inflation, reaching a minimum at end inflation. If inspiratory time is long enough to allow P_i and P_{alv} to equilibrate ($P_i = P_{el}$), as is the case in Figure 58.2, then inspiratory flow becomes 0 and E_{rs} may again be calculated from P_{ei} and TV.

The volume and flow profiles during pressure preset lung inflation are determined by the time constant of the respiratory system, which itself is a function of the respiratory system's mechanical properties. The time constant (τ) is a feature of linear systems and defines the time it takes an elastic element to fill to approximately 63% of its capacity or conversely to passively discharge 63% of its capacity when it is exposed to a step change in pressure.

$$\tau = R/E = R \times C$$

Notice from the third equation that τ is determined by the product of resistance and compliance. Because R is expressed in units of pressure × time × volume^{-1} and C in units of volume × pressure^{-1}, their product, τ, has the units of time. In the context of pressure preset mechanical ventilation, a low value for τ predicts that airway and alveolar pressure equilibrate rapidly and that TV depends largely on respiratory compliance. Alternatively, when τ is large, TV becomes sensitive to inspiratory time and to the resistance of the intubated respiratory system ($P_i > P_{alv}$ at t = end inflation).

Expiratory Mechanics of the Relaxed Respiratory System

Passive expiration is driven by the elastic recoil of the respiratory system (P_{el}). Assuming linear pressure–volume and pressure–flow relationships, the instantaneous expiratory flow $\dot{V}_{exp(t)}$) may be expressed as

$$\dot{V}_{exp(t)} = P_{el(t)}/R$$

$P_{el(t)}$ is a function of elastance (E) (1/Compliance) and of the instantaneous volume $V_{(t)}$; substituting for the previous equation:

$$\dot{V}_{exp(t)} = [E \times V_{(t)}]/R = V_{(t)}/[R \times C]$$

The product of R and C characterizes the time constant (τ) of single-compartment linear systems. As previously described, this represents the time at which approximately two thirds (63%) of the volume above relaxation volume (V_{rel}) has emptied passively.

CONVENTIONAL POSITIVE-PRESSURE VENTILATION

Modes

The mode of mechanical ventilation refers to the characteristics of the inspiratory pressure or flow program and determines whether a patient can augment TV or rate through his or her own efforts. Descriptors of ventilation mode are conveniently separated into determinants of amplitude, rate, and relative machine breath timing.

Amplitude of Machine Output

Volume Preset Ventilation

In this mode, the machine delivers a volume set on the control panel and, within limits, delivers that volume irrespective of the pressure generated within the system (Fig. 58.2A–D). Most ventilators offer several inspiratory flow profile options that range in shape from square wave (i.e., flow remains constant throughout the inspiratory cycle) to decreasing ramp and sine wave functions. For many years, physicians have considered volume preset ventilation to be the mode of choice in the treatment of adults with acute respiratory failure because a predefined minute volume delivery is guaranteed (for exceptions, see discussion of pop-off pressures in Inflation Pressure Setting section). Yet, proponents of pressure preset modes point to several drawbacks: (a) changes in the mechanical properties of the lungs from atelectasis, edema, or bronchoconstriction may cause high inflation pressures (perhaps increasing the risk of barotrauma); and (b) changes in inspiratory effort may not result in proportional changes in ventilation. Alternatively, those who consider the avoidance of high TVs imperative for lung protection will favor volume preset over pressure preset modes [20].

Pressure Preset Ventilation

During pressure preset ventilation, the ventilator applies a predefined target pressure to the airway during inspiration (Fig. 58.2E–G). The resulting TV and inspiratory flow profile vary with the impedance of the respiratory system and the strength of the patient's inspiratory efforts. Therefore, when either lungs or chest wall become stiff, when the airway resistance increases, or when the patient's own inspiratory efforts decline, TV decreases. An increase in respiratory system impedance can lead to a fall in minute ventilation ($\dot{V}_e$), hypoxemia, and CO_2 retention, but, in contrast to volume preset modes, pressure preset ventilation reduces the probability of lung injury from overdistention.

Means to Activate (Trigger) a Machine Breath

Controlled Mechanical Ventilation

Controlled mechanical ventilation is a mode during which rate, inspiratory-to-expiratory timing (I/E), and inspiratory flow (or pressure) profile are determined entirely by machine settings. Because there is never a reason to impose a rigidly set rate and breathing pattern, the term *controlled mechanical ventilation* usually refers to instances in which patients make no or ineffective inspiratory efforts.

Assist/Control Ventilation

The ventilator in assist/control (A/C) mode is sensitized to respond to the patient's inspiratory effort, if present; if such efforts are absent, the machine cycles automatically and delivers a controlled breath. Therefore, a patient might conceivably assist at a rate of 12 breaths per minute although the control rate is set at 10 breaths per minute. Because volume preset mechanical ventilation had been the most widely used mode of mechanical ventilation for many years, many providers associate the A/C mode with volume preset mechanical ventilation. Nevertheless, the A/C trigger algorithm is also associated with all pressure preset modes in which pressure amplitude and timing are defined by the provider. This is the case in pressure control ventilation but not pressure support ventilation or assisted pressure release ventilation (see following discussion).

Ventilators operating in A/C mode recognize patient efforts and switch from expiration to inspiration by one of two mechanisms. During pressure triggering, phase switching occurs whenever the airway pressure falls below a predetermined level (usually 1 to 2 cm H_2O below end-expiratory pressure). In this mode, a valve occludes the inspiratory port of the ventilator during expiration. An inspiratory effort against an occluded port lowers the airway opening pressure (P_{ao}), causes the demand valve to open, and initiates a machine breath. The flow-by-trigger mode, which is available on virtually all new-generation intensive care unit ventilators, is an alternative to conventional pressure-based machine trigger algorithms [21].

During flow-by, a continuous flow of gas is presented to the patient and is vented in through the expiratory tubing unless the patient makes an inspiratory effort. This so-called base flow can be set by the operator between limits of 5 to 20 L per minute. When the patient makes an inspiratory effort(s), he or she diverts flow into the lungs, resulting in a discrepancy between base flow and the flow of gas through the expiratory circuit. The minimal difference between inspiratory and expiratory flows, which results in a machine breath, is determined by the flow sensitivity setting and can vary from 1 to 3 L per minute. Most modern ventilators combine pressure and flow-triggering algorithms so that concerns about benefits of one over the other triggering mechanism are no longer relevant.

Short-lived inspiratory efforts that occur during early expiration are often insufficient to be recognized by either pressure or flow triggering algorithms. Careful inspection of airway pressure and flow profiles, of neck and chest wall motion, or intermittent flaring of the alae nasi should alert the physician to this phenomenon, which indicates a dissociation between machine rate and the patient's own intrinsic respiratory rate. Wasted inspiratory efforts are commonly seen in weak, sleeping, or heavily sedated patients and in patients unable to overcome intrinsic (or auto) positive end-expiratory pressure (PEEP) (see following discussion) [22].

The A/C feature has lured many physicians into the erroneous assumption that the machine backup rate setting is unimportant (see discussion on rate settings and troubleshooting in Minute Ventilation section). Although only a modest inspiratory effort is required to trigger the ventilator, many patients perform muscular work throughout the entire assisted breath in direct proportion to their ventilatory drive [23]. If the patient's work of breathing is deemed excessive and potentially fatiguing, the physician should lower the trigger sensitivity setting, consider raising $\dot{V}_i$, evaluate oxygenation and alveolar ventilation, assess the adequacy of machine backup rate and PEEP settings, and address sedation and pain control.

In years past, there had been a great reluctance to use of neuromuscular blocking agents (NMB) to prevent adverse patient–ventilator interactions. However for patients with ALI or the acute respiratory distress syndrome (ARDS), who frequently double their VT by breath stacking and are therefore at risk for ventilator associated lung injury, this reluctance may no longer be appropriate. In several randomized clinical trials, the group of Papazian has reported that patients with ALI, who were initially managed with NMB, had improved surrogate physiologic endpoints, spent fewer days requiring mechanical ventilation and were more likely to survive than those who were managed with sedatives and narcotics alone [24,25] However, the issue is far from settled, awaits independent confirmation, and importantly, the data do not apply to patient populations without acute lung injury, whose risk for ventilator induced injury is much lower.

Intermittent Mandatory Ventilation

Early versions of the intermittent mandatory ventilation (IMV) mode combined spontaneous breathing and volume preset-assisted ventilation [26]. For example, at an IMV rate of 6 breaths per minute, the ventilator would deliver a volume preset breath every 10 seconds. Between these mechanically controlled breaths, the patient would breathe spontaneously and the ventilator would serve as a source of warmed, humidified, potentially oxygen-enriched gas. During the years, IMV has become more complex. In modern ventilators, mandatory breaths may be volume or pressure preset and it has become commonplace to augment spontaneous breaths with positive airway pressure as well (e.g., by using the pressure support mode).

Virtually all modern ventilators use synchronized IMV algorithms that prevent the patient from getting a double breath with IMV (i.e., a machine breath is delivered at the end of a spontaneous inspiratory effort). At intervals determined by the IMV frequency setting, the machine becomes sensitized to the patient's inspiratory effort and responds by delivering a pressure or volume preset breath. Between these preset cycles, the patient breathes spontaneously (with or without pressure support) at a rate and depth of his or her own choosing. For example, at an IMV rate of 6 breaths per minute, the ventilator allows the patient to breathe spontaneously while the delivery of preset breaths is initially refractory to the patient's efforts. After 10 seconds elapse, the machine is rendered sensitive. When an effort occurs, the ventilator delivers a preset breath and the patient breathes spontaneously until 10 seconds after the end of the previous refractory period. If the patient does not make an inspiratory effort during the sensitive period, the ventilator delivers a controlled breath after sufficient time elapses. This time varies inversely with the IMV backup rate; it is equal to 60 seconds divided by the IMV rate. In the example given here, the period would be 10 seconds (60 divided by 6).

IMV is a very complex mode with numerous degrees of freedom. It was originally introduced as a weaning modality. However, in controlled clinical trials this mode has performed inferior to other weaning techniques (see Chapter 60) [27–29]. Nevertheless, in many institutions IMV remains the default mode for patients who are relatively easy to ventilate. Familiarity with this mode and the high incidence of ventilator-induced apneas in sleeping or comatose patients, who are supported in modes without mandatory backup rates, are likely reasons for the persistent popularity of IMVs [30–32].

Pressure Support Ventilation

Pressure support ventilation (PSV) is a form of pressure preset ventilation. It is intermittent positive-pressure breathing with a sensing device that delivers the breath at the time the patient makes an inspiratory effort. As the lungs inflate, $\dot{V}_i$ begins to decline because airway pressure and the pressure generated by inspiratory muscles are opposed by rising elastic recoil forces. When $\dot{V}_i$ reaches a threshold value (which differs among vendors), the machine switches to expiration. Inspiratory off-switch failure, that is, application of inspiratory pressure after cessation of inspiratory muscle activity, is common during PSV [31,33]. High inspiratory pressure settings, a low respiratory drive, airflow obstruction with dynamic hyperinflation, and air leaks predispose patients to this form of patient–ventilator asynchrony [31,34]. Asynchrony, in turn, is an underappreciated cause of sleep disruption [22,35].

PSV is a popular weaning mode for adults. A review of the weaning literature (see Chapter 60) suggests that this mode is as effective as intermittent T-piece trials of spontaneous breathing in liberating patients from mechanical ventilation [36–38]. It should also be noted that PSV is a useful alternative to volume preset mechanical ventilation, particularly in patients with increased rate demands and respiratory drive [39]. However, the risk of lung injury from sustained increases in TV probably applies to the PSV mode as well, because airway pressure despite being low does not inform about lung stress.

Pressure Control Ventilation

Pressure control ventilation (PCV) is a form of pressure preset ventilation. It differs from PSV in two important respects: The operator sets a machine backup rate and determines inspiratory time (T_i). The A/C feature assures ventilation of the lungs in patients who are prone to apneas. Cessation of inspiratory effort can be a problem in sleeping adults who are ventilated in the pressure support mode [30,40]. On the other hand, PCV does not offer the patient the same control over TV and breathing patterns as PSV. For this reason, PCV with long T_i, is usually reserved for hypoxic heavily sedated or paralyzed patients in whom the need to match ventilator rate and timing with intrinsic respiratory rhythms is not an issue.

Assisted Pressure Release Ventilation and Bilevel Support Modes

Although bilevel positive airway pressure ventilation (BiPAP) technically describes any mode in which the pressure applied to the airway cycles between two provider set levels, in practice most associate BiPAP with a PSV like mode that is often used in noninvasively mechanically ventilated patients. It is a pressure/time cycle mode which allows the patient's own breathing to supplement ventilator output. There are subtle differences in the cycling algorithms among devices of different vendors, somewhat clouding the literature on the topic. When bilevel pressure ventilation is delivered with an inverse inspiratory to expiratory time ratio, the mode becomes indistinguishable from assisted pressure release ventilation (APRV). Arguments in favor of bilevel pressure ventilation modes including APRV in patients with injured lungs center on improved gas exchange and maintenance of dependent lung aeration attributable to preserved diaphragm activity [41]. However, superiority of bilevel modes relative to volume preset modes has not been established. Detractors point out that it is more difficult to assure delivery of lung protective tidal volumes in pressure preset modes.

Noninvasive Mechanical Ventilation

Noninvasive mechanical ventilation (NMV) (see Chapter 59) encompasses all modes of ventilatory assistance that can be applied without an endotracheal tube. The realization that certain patients benefit from intermittent positive pressure breathing through a mask has fundamentally changed the initial management of many respiratory failure syndromes. The literature on NMV has grown exponentially, and the following comments focus on the use of NMV in the acute care setting.

Several randomized prospective clinical trials have shown NMV to be an effective initial therapy for patients with impending or overt respiratory failure [42–47]. The early application of NMV in the emergency department is particularly important in patients with exacerbation of airways obstruction as it may spare them the risks and discomfort associated with intubation and conventional mechanical ventilation. Other conditions in which NMV appears to be an effective initial rescue treatment include ventilatory insufficiency from chest wall disease, neuromuscular weakness, and sleep-related breathing disorders. The use of NMV in hypoxic forms of respiratory failure is increasing, but in comparison to COPD its efficacy is less well established [46,48–53], NMV is relatively contraindicated in patients who cannot protect their airway or who cannot clear their secretions, and in our experience NMV invariably fails in patients with shock or metabolic acidosis [54].

Less Commonly Used Modes of Mechanical Ventilation

Some new-generation mechanical ventilators feature modes with closed-loop feedback control of both pressure and volume [55,56]. Dual-control modes seek to provide a target ventilation while maintaining low inflation pressures. To this end, ventilator output is adjusted based on volume, flow, and pressure feedback within each machine cycle or gradually from one cycle to the next. Modes that adjust output within each cycle execute a predetermined pressure–time program as long as the desired TV is reached. When the TV target is not reached, inspiration continues at a preselected inspiratory flow rate (volume-limited) until the target volume is attained. Volume-assured pressure support and pressure augmentation are examples of such modes. Breath-to-breath dual control modes are pressure-limited and time or flow cycled. Ventilator output is derived from the pressure–volume relationship of the preceding breath and adjusted within predefined pressure limits to maintain the target TV. Pressure-regulated volume control, volume control plus, auto-flow, adaptive pressure ventilation, volume support, and variable pressure support are examples of breath-to-breath control modes.

Neurally adjusted ventilatory assistance (NAVA) and proportional assist ventilation (PAV) are the most complex and arguably the most promising closed-loop ventilation modes [57,58]. At the time of this writing, only PAV is commercially available in the United States. During PAV, the relaxation characteristics of the respiratory system are assessed on a breath-by-breath basis so the ventilator may provide a set fraction of the inspiratory elastic and flow resistive work [57–59]. Its applications in NMV will be discussed in Chapter 60. During NAVA, the diaphragm's electrical activity is recorded with an esophageal probe and the signal is conditioned and transposed into a positive airway pressure output. Preliminary observations on patients suggest that NAVA results in greater patient–ventilator synchrony than conventional modes [60]. Moreover, there is some evidence from animal models that NAVA affords greater lung protection from ventilator associated injury [61] by virtue of preserved coupling between respiratory control and motor output. At the time of this writing however, there is no evidence that either dual- or closed-loop modes are safer or more effective than conventional approaches.

Choice of Ventilation Mode

The therapeutic end points of mechanical ventilation vary considerably among different respiratory failure syndromes. For example, the ventilatory management of patients with ALI has little in common with that of patients suffering from exacerbation of COPD. However, the need for pathophysiology-based treatment objectives should not be confused with a need to find an optimal ventilation mode for each class of respiratory disorders. In general, the therapeutic goals of mechanical ventilation can be achieved with more than one mode [62].

Ventilator Settings

Fraction of Inspired Oxygen

The hazards of indiscriminate administration of oxygen to patients with CO_2 retention and the topic of pulmonary oxygen toxicity are discussed in Chapters 49 and 62. Notwithstanding these very real concerns, oxygen must never be withheld from a mechanically ventilated patient. If there is any suspicion that the patient may require oxygen, it should be given. Certain drugs, such as bleomycin, may sensitize the lungs to reactive oxygen species-mediated injury and it is advisable to minimize the fraction of inspired oxygen (FIO_2) in patients receiving them [63]. Adjustments in FIO_2 are usually guided by pulse oximetry and/or arterial blood gas analyses. Most caregivers dose FIO_2 to an arterial oxygen tension (PaO_2) more than 60 mm Hg and/or an oxygen saturation more than 90%. Although these targets are based on reasonable physiologic assumptions, they are nevertheless empiric. Some accept lower O_2 saturations in young patients with adequate end organ perfusion, when the treatment of hypoxemia seems risky. Ultimately, the risk associated with hypoxemia must be balanced against the risk of oxygen toxicity and the risks associated with raising PEEP and manipulating hemoglobin and cardiac output. It is currently believed that an FIO_2 below 0.6 is not injurious to the lungs even when used for days or weeks. Because the contribution of oxygen to lung injury cannot be separated from that of other insults (e.g., sepsis-related inflammatory mediator release, gastric acid, infectious agents, lung parenchymal stress), oxygen dosing recommendations remain open to debate.

Tidal Volume

When using a volume preset mode, TV is either set directly or follows from the minute volume and rate setting. When a pressure preset mode is used, TV is the consequence of the patient's respiratory effort, the mechanical properties of the respiratory system, the pressure amplitude setting, and the duration over which the inflation pressure is applied. TV is arguably the most important ventilator setting. Historically it had been common practice to scale TV to actual body weight. This practice is no longer acceptable because the high prevalence of obesity biases TV settings toward injurious levels, and because height and gender are much more powerful predictors of lung size than is body weight [64]. Height and gender are also used to estimate ideal or predicted body weight that by virtue of its use in the acute respiratory distress syndrome network (ARDS Net) trials has become the preferred TV scaling factor [65].

Predicted Body Weight (in kg):

$$\text{Men} = 50 + 2.3 \times (\text{height in inches} - 60)$$
$$\text{Women} = 45.5 + 2.3 \times (\text{height in inches} - 60)$$

Most experts suggest to target TV in patients with injured lungs between 6 ± 2 mL per kg predicted body weight. Although the evidence in support of lung protective TV settings in other patient population is less compelling, there is no reason to suspect that TV settings in excess of 8 ml/kg are of benefit. There is overwhelming evidence that inflating the lungs above total lung capacity (TLC) can damage normal lung units, particularly when this occurs in conjunction with large tidal excursions [66–68]. In patients with a normal body habitus (i.e., normal chest wall recoil and compliance), TLC corresponds to a plateau or end-inflation hold pressure between 30 and 35 cm H_2O [69]. For this reason most experts limit respiratory system inflation pressures to 30 cm H_2O or less, However, in light of recent data this guideline may have to be reevaluated (see discussion about inflation pressure setting later). Unless lung function is severely impaired, even large TVs are unlikely to distend the lungs beyond their structural limit (i.e., TLC). This has caused some experts to reason that reducing TV to values less than 8 mL per kg ideal body weight (as is custom in ARDS Net trials) is neither required nor beneficial in patients with plateau pressures less than 30 cm H_2O. We address this controversy in greater detail in the context of ventilator management of ARDS.

Sighing and Recruitment Maneuvers

Periodic hyperinflation (the "sigh" or "yawn" maneuver) is a spontaneous reflex in conscious humans. Periodic stretching of the lung stimulates surfactant production and release and therefore prevents atelectasis [70,71]. However, the effects of sighing on mechanics and gas exchange tend to be short lived and vary with disease state, posture, and ventilator mode and setting [72,73]. Some experts recommend that the lungs of patients with ARDS should be intermittently held at high volumes and pressures (e.g., 30 to 50 cm H_2O for 20 to 40 seconds) to recruit collapsed and/or flooded units [74–76]. The use of recruitment maneuvers has been associated with improved gas exchange, altered lung mechanics and less inflammation in experimental lung injury models [77–81]. By virtue of volume and time history, such maneuvers tend to potentiate the effects of PEEP on functional residual capacity [82]. Incorporating sighs into a lung-protective mechanical ventilation strategy in patients with early ALI/ARDS improved oxygenation and static compliance, but had no effect on survival [83]. This confirms that periodic lung inflation and recruitment maneuvers exert demonstrable effects on lung function, but are not appropriate surrogate markers of clinical efficacy. In fact, a post hoc analysis of the ARDS-Network low tidal volume trial revealed that patients, who had been randomized to the injurious high tidal volume arm had better oxygenation during the first 24 hours than those, who in hindsight, had received lung protection [65].

"Biologically variable mechanical ventilation" is an experimental mode of mechanical ventilation that seeks to maximize lung recruitment by preserving the normal breath-to-breath variability in TV and rate [84]. Biologically variable mechanical ventilation is superior to evenly timed sighs in improving gas exchange and lung function [85,86]. Moreover, biologically variable mechanical ventilation finds a strong mechanistic underpinning in the principle of stochastic resonance [87]. Stochastic resonance is a feature of nonlinear systems that explains why seemingly minor variability in input (e.g., TV) has major effects on output (e.g., number of recruited alveoli) [88]. At the time of this writing, this mode is not available for commercial use in North America.

Inflation Pressure Setting

Volume Preset Mode. Although pressure is a dependent variable during volume preset ventilation, generally the cycling pressure should not be allowed to increase without limit. Rather, a pressure limit or pop-off pressure should be imposed to guard against inadvertent overinflation and possible lung rupture [89]. This is set directly on the ventilator's control panel, and when and if it is reached, a visual and possibly audible alarm alerts the attendant to the fact that the machine has popped off. That particular cycled breath will have been partially aborted and the patient will have received only part of the volume set on the control panel. A random, infrequent pop-off cycle is most often caused by the patient's coughing or splinting, and need not be cause for concern. However, repeated popping off may be an indication that the patient is in acute respiratory distress and should prompt those in attendance to disconnect the patient from the ventilator to determine the cause of the problem. Although the patient is manually ventilated, a suction catheter should be passed through the endotracheal tube to determine whether it is patent, and the ventilator should be checked to ensure it is functioning properly. Other factors to consider are whether the patient is undersedated or anxious and in pain, whether the patient's airway resistance has increased (e.g., bronchospasm, excessive secretions, mucus plugging), whether the endotracheal tube has migrated beyond the carina, or whether a pneumothorax has developed.

Pop-off pressures should usually be set at a level slightly above P_{peak} observed during normal cycling and should not be higher than 40 cm H_2O, whereas PEEP and TV should generally be set to maintain plateau pressures 30 cm H_2O or less. Although no specific airway pressure is guaranteed to exclude the risk of barotrauma, higher airway pressures appear to impose an increased risk of alveolar overdistention that can lead to permeability pulmonary edema, alveolar hemorrhage, subcutaneous emphysema, pneumomediastinum, and pneumothorax. There is general agreement that the main determinant of alveolar overdistention is the end-inspiratory lung volume [67]. On the basis of this reasoning, Dreyfuss et al. [90] and Dreyfuss and Saumon [91] have coined the term *volutrauma* distinct from barotrauma. The term *barotrauma* refers to injury manifest as extra-alveolar air, whereas volutrauma denotes injury manifest as altered lung barrier function. Regardless, one should appreciate that lung stress (transpulmonary pressure) and lung volume cannot be uncoupled and that neither is routinely measured at the bedside. TV and plateau pressure, the variables that are being measured, inform only indirectly about lung volume and lung stress, and the provider must integrate them with estimates of chest wall compliance (or, more specifically, chest wall recoil) [92]. For these reasons, we believe that plateau pressure limits of 30 cm H_2O should be ignored in patients with obesity, ascites, or abdominal distention [93].

There is evidence that esophageal manometry guided PEEP management is associated with improved lung function compared to a conventional ARDS-Network based approach [94]. In a small clinical trial survival trends favored esophageal manometry guided PEEP management, even though a substantial number of patients were ventilated to plateau pressures in excess of 30 cm H_2O [95]. A subsequent report suggested that the majority of ARDS patients have substantially increased end-expiratory chest wall recoil pressures and that the corresponding implications for PEEP management may not be evident from airway pressure recordings alone [96]. The issue is far from settled, because of concerns for measurement bias in esophageal pressure derived estimates of transpulmonary pressure [97]. Nevertheless, a rigorous adherence to an absolute plateau pressure safety limit of 30 cm H_2O in patients with ALI seems no longer advisable. There is a healthy debate about the appropriate balance between maximizing lung recruitment (through the application of PEEP) and minimizing end-inspiratory parenchymal stress (by avoiding high inflation pressures). In following this debate, we conclude that there is neither a single safe inflation pressure nor safe tidal volume threshold. Rather both surrogates of injurious stress and strain are invariably intertwined. For example, inflating the lungs to near maximal capacity during HFOV seems quite safe provided tidal volumes are kept relatively low. Alternatively, a TV which would likely be injurious during HFOV is well tolerated provided lung inflation pressure is kept relatively low.

Because of the increasing risk of barotrauma with rising airway pressures, it is important to determine not only why peak airway pressures are increasing but also to try to reduce them. For instance, if agitation is responsible, the patient should be sedated and, as addressed earlier, at times even paralyzed [24,25]. Although lower $\dot{V}_i$ rates might help achieve the goal of decreasing peak airway pressure, it is not clear that this prevents susceptible lung units from overdistention injury. Reductions in flow without concomitant reductions in TV may simply reduce the resistive pressure that is dissipated across the endotracheal tube without lowering peak transpulmonary pressure or lung stress.

Pressure Preset Modes. In a pressure preset mode (see the previous discussion of PSV and PCV modes), ventilators require an inflation pressure amplitude setting as opposed to a pop-off pressure setting. The pressure amplitude setting (often referred to as "pressure control" or "pressure support" setting) determines the relative pressure increase during assisted inflation; it should be distinguished from peak airway pressure that is the sum of PEEP and the inflation pressure setting. Inflation pressure is an important determinant of peak lung volume as well as TV. For reasons previously outlined, inflating the respiratory system repeatedly to static (inflation hold) pressures in excess of 30 cm H_2O should be avoided unless concerns about lung recruitment and chest wall mechanics dictate otherwise.

Respiratory Rate, Flow, and Machine Cycle Timing

Volume Preset Mode. The choice of rate setting should be made after considering the patient's actual rate demand in conjunction with the T_i or I/E setting. Most ventilators are not smart enough to vary T_i in proportion to the spontaneous respiratory rate (fS) (as opposed to the set machine rate, fM). At an fM setting of 10 breaths per minute (A/C = 10), the total cycle time (TTOT; inspiration plus expiration) equals 6 seconds. If I/E is 1:2, T_i is 2 seconds and expiratory time (T_e) is 4 seconds. Imagine that the patient actually triggers at 20 breaths per minute (i.e., TTOT declines to 3 seconds). Inspiratory time remains fixed at 2 seconds because it is determined by the preset machine rate and I/E. The T_e must decrease from 4 seconds to 1 second and the actual I/E increases from 1:2 to 2:1. At a rate of 30 breaths per minute (TTOT = 2 seconds), T_e becomes 0 and fighting the ventilator results. For these reasons, the machine backup rate should always be set close to the patient's actual rate. If the actual rate is so high that effective ventilation cannot be achieved, the patient may need sedation alone or with paralysis.

All ventilators provide the option of maintaining lung volume at end inspiration for a predefined time. This time, also called *end inflation hold time* or *inspiratory pause time*, is usually expressed as a percentage of TTOT. For the purpose of defining I/E, the pause time is considered part of the expiratory machine cycle. Long pause times favor the recruitment of previously collapsed or flooded alveoli and offer a means of shortening expiration independent of rate and mean $\dot{V}_i$. Although alveolar recruitment is a desired therapeutic end point in the treatment of patients with edematous lungs, keeping the lungs expanded at high volumes (and pressures) for an extended period may damage relatively normal units [98–100].

Inspiratory Flow. Many ventilators require that $\dot{V}_i$, as opposed to I/E or TTOT, be specified. Because mean $\dot{V}_i$ is equal to the ratio of TV and T_i, flow cannot be changed without affecting at least one of the other timing variables. Under most clinical circumstances, $\dot{V}_i$ is 1 L per second or less during volume preset ventilation. Increasing flow always raises peak P_{ao}, but this need not be of concern if most of the added pressure is dissipated across the endotracheal tube. Although $\dot{V}_i$ is one factor that determines the regional distribution of inspired gas, in disease the effect of flow on pulmonary gas exchange and parenchymal stress is too unpredictable to warrant general guidelines. There is theoretical concern and some experimental evidence that the rate at which lung tissue is being stretched, which is a function of the flow setting, determines the probability of deformation injury [101,102]. It is also important to understand that the flow setting influences a patient's breathing rate and effort [32,103,104] and that the combined effects of flow, volume, and time settings determine the functional residual capacity (FRC) and degree of dynamic hyperinflation (see the following discussion) [105,106].

The $\dot{V}_i$ is rarely specified as part of the physician's orders. Rather, the respiratory therapist usually adjusts the $\dot{V}_i$ pattern and rate by observing patient–ventilator interactions. It has become common practice to deliver volume preset breaths with a decelerating flow pattern; that is, a profile in which flow declines with lung volume and time. In comparison to the traditional square wave flow pattern in which inspiratory flow is held constant throughout inflation, the use of decelerating flow patterns tends to promote alveolar recruitment and may reduce the risk of barotrauma. Although the reasoning seems mechanistically sound, this hypothesis has yet to find experimental support.

Mean Expiratory Flow. Mean expiratory flow is defined by the ratio of TV and T_e. Expiratory time is equal to TTOT minus T_i, and TTOT is equal to 60 per minute (60/f). Because the machine backup rate and actual frequency may differ in the A/C mode, assumed and actual TTOT may also differ. Recall from the discussion on rate and timing that T_i is defined by both the set machine backup rate (fM) and the set I/E, and that T_i remains constant irrespective of the actual rate. In contrast, T_e is affected by the actual breathing rate (fA) (i.e., $T_e = 60/fA - T_i$). Therefore, the choice of volume and timing settings, together with the patient's rate response, determine mean expiratory flow.

It is generally appreciated that end-expiratory alveolar pressure can remain positive during intermittent positive-pressure ventilation even when PEEP is not intentionally applied [107]; this is called auto-PEEP (or intrinsic PEEP [$PEEP_i$]) and is not readily apparent on the ventilator manometer. Mean expiratory flow, TV/T_e, is the principal ventilator setting-related determinant of dynamic hyperinflation. A patient with airways obstruction and a maximal forced expiratory flow of 0.2 L per second in the midvital capacity range ($FEF_{25\%-75\%}$) obviously cannot accommodate a TV/T_e of 0.3 L per second without an increase in end-expired lung volume. Dynamic hyperinflation will result.

Although $PEEP_i$ may be present in the majority of ventilated patients in intensive care units [108], it is likely to be worse in patients with COPD [109]. Intrinsic PEEP places the patient at risk for the same pulmonary and cardiovascular consequences as intentional external PEEP ($PEEP_e$). When disregarded, $PEEP_i$ effects can lead to serious errors in management. For instance, failure to recognize that $PEEP_i$ can elevate pulmonary artery balloon occlusion pressure or decrease cardiac output and blood pressure may lead to inappropriate fluid restriction or vasopressor therapy. At the bedside, $PEEP_i$ should be clinically suspected if exhalation has not ended before the next inhalation (Fig. 58.3). Intrinsic PEEP can be measured using

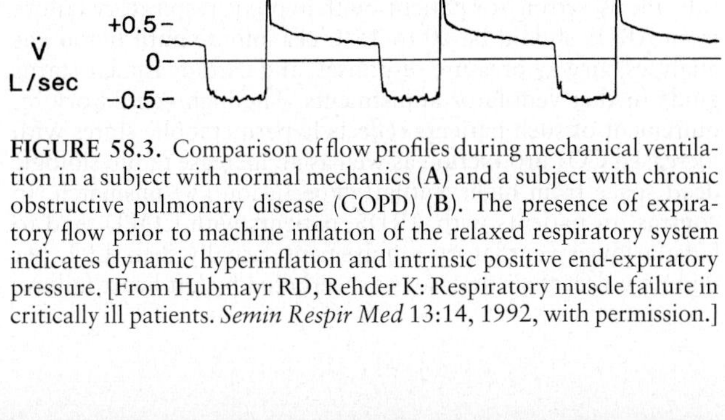

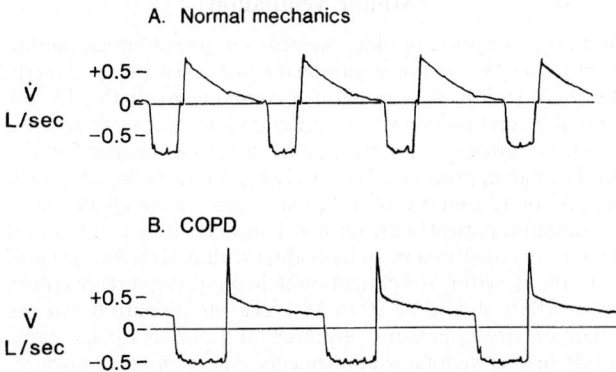

FIGURE 58.3. Comparison of flow profiles during mechanical ventilation in a subject with normal mechanics (A) and a subject with chronic obstructive pulmonary disease (COPD) (B). The presence of expiratory flow prior to machine inflation of the relaxed respiratory system indicates dynamic hyperinflation and intrinsic positive end-expiratory pressure. [From Hubmayr RD, Rehder K: Respiratory muscle failure in critically ill patients. *Semin Respir Med* 13:14, 1992, with permission.]

the expiratory port occlusion technique [107] or from the measurement of change of P_{ao} at the onset of $\dot{V}_i$ [108]. In many modern ventilators, the $PEEP_i$ measurement is automated, that is, individual machine-breaths can be delayed for appropriately timed airway occlusions. In patients with spontaneous respiratory efforts at end expiration, P_{ao} will not reach a plateau, and in these patients $PEEP_i$ cannot be estimated with this technique. It has been proposed that $PEEP_i$ be estimated from esophageal pressure measurements in spontaneously breathing patients. Because such estimates rely on subtle inflections in the esophageal pressure tracing and because the determinants of $PEEP_i$ in spontaneously breathing subjects are more complex than those during mechanical ventilation and include the contributions of expiratory muscles to intrathoracic pressure, such measurements should be interpreted with caution. Furthermore, the technique is invasive and subject to artifacts in recumbent individuals [110].

Intrinsic PEEP can be minimized by reducing mean expiratory flow requirement or increasing the patient's capacity to generate the required flow near V_{rel}. Examples of the former strategy are reductions in TV, increasing $\dot{V}_i$ and thereby increasing T_e, and reducing the actual ventilator rate through manipulations of the set backup rate, sedation, and pain control, or imposing neuromuscular blockade with sedation. Increasing the $\dot{V}_i$ setting can be counterproductive if it causes an increase in the respiratory rate [32,111]. Strategies for increasing the patient's flow-generating capacity include bronchodilators [105] and occasionally diuretics, when peribronchial edema contributes to obstruction. If subjects with $PEEP_i$ make inspiratory efforts while being ventilated in the A/C mode, it is crucial to use extrinsic PEEP to reduce inspiratory work requirements. As a general rule, PEEP settings approaching 75% of $PEEP_i$ are recommended [112,113].

Pressure Preset Mode. In contrast to volume preset ventilation, inspiratory flow is not a set variable, but is determined by patient mechanics and inspiratory effort as well as the PEEP, pressure amplitude, and T_i settings. During PSV, rate and T_i are largely patient-determined; during PCV, they are programmed. The importance of mean expiratory flow as a determinant of dynamic hyperinflation pertains to pressure as well as volume preset modes of ventilation. However, during pressure preset modes, mean expiratory flow and, hence, end-expiratory lung volumes are not as sensitive to changes in rate. This is because reductions in TTOT and, hence, T_i and T_e bring about reductions in TV.

Minute Ventilation

With the exception of older Siemens servo ventilators, minute ventilation ($\dot{V}_E$) is not a parameter that must be set directly by the operator. It is rather the consequence of the TV (or pressure amplitude) and rate settings. The A/C mode is not a foolproof safeguard for assuring a rate setting independent delivery of an appropriate $\dot{V}_E$. Therefore, a knee-jerk order, such as A/C of 12 and TV of 800, may cause severe alkalemia in a comatose patient with normal lungs, yet lead to profound respiratory acidemia in an individual with ARDS. As a general rule, the $\dot{V}_E$ setting for patients with hypoxic respiratory failure from ARDS should be 10 to 15 L per minute until blood gas analyses, airway pressure responses, and cardiovascular status guide further ventilator adjustments. The high ventilatory requirement of such patients reflects hypermetabolic states with increased CO_2 production as well as an increase in physiologic dead space from high ventilation/perfusion ($\dot{V}$) mismatch. In contrast to patients with ARDS, patients with COPD tend to have a lower ventilatory requirement, usually 8 to 12 L per minute unless their disease is exacerbated by left heart failure, sepsis, or pneumonia. Healthy individuals maintain normocapnia with a resting ventilation of approximately 5 L per minute.

Although normocapnia is a desired therapeutic end point, it is not essential. Increases in respiratory system impedance combined with increased ventilatory requirements and poor pulmonary gas exchange may necessitate a choice between permissive hypercapnia and risking lung injury [114,115]. Hypercapnic acidosis tends to be well tolerated provided patients are sedated and/or paralyzed [116]. Although there are no definitive clinical outcomes data that address the effectiveness of buffer solutions in patients with hypercapnic acidosis, many experts have abandoned their use even when the arterial pH is less than 7.2 [117–119]. Indeed, there is strong evidence that hypercapnia protects the lungs from certain forms of injury, including ventilator-induced lung injury [120,121]. Moreover, a post hoc analysis of patients enrolled in the low TV ARDS Net trial suggests a protective effect of hypercapnia in the usual care arm [122].

Positive End-Expiratory Pressure

The application of positive airway pressure during the expiratory phase of the respiratory cycle is commonly referred to as PEEP, continuous positive airway pressure (CPAP), or expiratory positive airway pressure (EPAP). Although there are subtle distinctions between these terms, they are largely technical and of historic interest. In patients with hypoxic respiratory failure, expiratory pressure is used to raise lung volume to recruit collapsed and flooded alveoli, to prevent cell abrasion in small conducting airways, and to improve oxygenation [123–126]. In contrast, the goal of PEEP/CPAP/EPAP therapy in patients with airways obstruction is to minimize inspiratory work [22,112,127].

Positive End-Expiratory Pressure in Hypoxic Respiratory Failure. PEEP is most useful in the treatment of patients with pulmonary edema resulting from increased alveolocapillary membrane permeability (ARDS) or increased hydrostatic pressure (cardiogenic pulmonary edema) [128,129]. It increases PaO_2 by diminishing intrapulmonary shunting of blood and improving the matching of ventilation and perfusion. Although it may work by redistributing intra-alveolar edema, it need not drive fluid out of the lungs [130].

In the 1970s and 1980s, most physicians considered the "best PEEP" to be the least amount of PEEP necessary to achieve adequate blood gas tensions (ordinarily this means arterial O_2 saturation 90% or more, or PO_2 60 mm Hg or more with FIO_2 values 0.6 or less). The emergence of the open lung approach and concerns about ventilator-induced lung injury have resulted in a revised PEEP management strategy [125,128,131–134]. Although many experts approach PEEP empirically, guided by arterial gas tensions, some advocate PEEP titration based on shape analyses of the respiratory system pressure/volume loop or on image analyses of the thorax [135–141]. Several physiology lessons may be drawn from related experimental literature: (a) the application of PEEP promotes aeration of previously flooded, closed, or atelectatic lung units (i.e., recruitment) and it increases the aeration of previously open or at least partially aerated units [135,136]; (b) in injured lungs there is no single volume or pressure at which all potentially recruitable units appear to be aerated [142]; and (c) even moderate amounts of PEEP may cause overdistension of some lung units [143]. The corresponding clinical lesson is that in the absence of efficacy studies, the pressure/volume curve cannot inform about best PEEP unless one is willing to make additional assumptions about the relative risks of low and high lung volume injury.

One approach that seeks to minimize these risks is the so-called stress–index-guided PEEP management [140,144]. The stress index is the exponent of the airway pressure–time relationship when it is measured during inflation of the relaxed respiratory system with constant (square wave) inspiratory flow. It is a measure of the linearity of the pressure ramp as shown in the schematic of Figure 58.1. A stress index more than 1 indicates that the tracing is convex to the time axis and that more pressure is required to inflate the lungs in the high as opposed to the low tidal range. This suggests that the lungs are being inflated to volumes near TLC; namely, above the upper inflection point of their inflation pressure/volume loop. At such high volumes, the lungs may be subjected to injurious stress. Conversely, a stress index less than 1 indicates that the pressure ramp is concave to the time axis and that it is easier to inflate the lungs in the high as opposed to the low tidal range. This suggests that the lungs are underrecruited and may be subjected to low volume injury from repeated opening and closure of unstable lung units. Proponents of the stress index concept argue that lungs should be ventilated over a volume range where the stress index is approximately 1, that is, over the linear portion of the inflation pressure/volume loop where the relative risks of high- and low-volume injury are minimal. Although there is some experimental support for this reasoning, the efficacy of this approach has not been tested in the clinical arena.

The volume of partially or nonaerated lung that may be recruited with PEEP varies considerably among patients with ALI and ARDS [142]. In general, patients with the most severe forms of alveolar edema have the largest absolute and relative volumes of recruitable lung. Some studies have suggested that patients with ARDS from extrapulmonary causes such as sepsis are more likely PEEP-responsive than patients with primary pulmonary insults, for example pneumonia [142,145,146]. However, this has not been a universal finding [142,146]. Three relatively large prospective randomized controlled clinical trials specifically designed to compare a high PEEP with a low PEEP management strategy have showed equivalence of the two approaches [147–149]. Those who advocate a high PEEP—open lung—strategy have been hesitant to embrace these results, in part because PEEP management decisions where not driven by patient-specific estimates of recruitable lung [150–152]. A much smaller trial of esophageal pressure guided PEEP management, in which outcomes favored high PEEP has rekindled this debate [95]. Furthermore, recent meta-analyses suggest a benefit from high PEEP strategies in patients with severe forms of ARDS [153,154]. Irrespective of one's interpretation of the PEEP literature adherence to low TVs and "safe" plateau pressures is paramount [65]. At the same time, most experts emphasize that patients with obesity, ascites, and abdominal distention (i.e., patients with high chest wall recoil and/or low chest wall compliance) should be ventilated with PEEP substantially greater than 5 cm H_2O [93].

There are two ways to raise lung volume in the hope of recruiting flooded or partially collapsed alveoli: the judicious use of extrinsic PEEP ($PEEP_e$) and dynamic hyperinflation. Because it is not uncommon for patients with ALI to be tachypneic, a component of dynamic hyperinflation is often present in mechanically ventilated ARDS patients [155]. Despite the short time constant for lung emptying, the use of PEEP values that often represent resistive as well as threshold loads and ventilator settings that require large mean expiratory flows (TV/T_e; see previous discussion) contribute to dynamic hyperinflation. Sedation and neuromuscular blockade are useful adjuncts to PEEP therapy insofar as they help raise lung volume by abolishing expiratory muscle activity. In general, the authors prefer to manipulate end-expired lung volume with extrinsic PEEP. There is at least a theoretical concern that the high respiratory rates required to achieve meaningful hyperinflation are in and of themselves injurious to the lungs [101].

In summary, there is general agreement that PEEP has beneficial effects on the function of injured lungs [91,131,134,156,157] so that in patients with ARDS a knee-jerk setting of 5 cm H_2O is inappropriately low. Unfortunately, this message has been slow to gain acceptance in clinical practice. A 2005 survey of ventilator practice around the world suggests that patients with ARDS are ventilated with a median PEEP setting of 8 cm H_2O (interquartile range, 5 to 10 cm H_2O). This means that 25% of ARDS patients still receive an inappropriately low PEEP setting of 5 cm H_2O or less (O. Gajic, personal communication, 2006).

Effects Of Positive End-Expiratory Pressure On Circulation. The major cardiovascular complication associated with PEEP is reduction in cardiac output. Although the effect of PEEP on cardiac output is complex, the decrease is caused predominantly by decreasing venous return (right ventricular filling) and direct heart-lung interactions [158,159]. It appears that PEEP affects apparent heart compliance rather than contractility. By increasing lung volume and intrathoracic pressure, PEEP (much like recruitment maneuvers) can increase pulmonary vascular resistance and thereby promote hypotension and right ventricular volume overload [160]. Associated changes in the position and shape of the interventricular septum, together with direct compression of the left ventricle by the expanding lungs, account for the fall in left ventricular compliance [161]. A reduction in cardiac output with hypotension should prompt the use of fluid-replacement therapy, vasopressor drugs, and a temporary reduction of PEEP until the former interventions take effect. Also, PEEP may lead to water retention in the lungs [162] by decreasing left atrial volume, thereby stimulating antidiuretic hormone secretion; may alter portal circulatory hemodynamics [163]; and may decrease perfusion to splanchnic organs that may lead to ischemia of the bowel [164]. All of the cardiovascular complications can be avoided or minimized by adhering to proper indications for use of PEEP and by careful monitoring during its use.

Changes in PEEP can introduce uncertainties in the measurement and interpretation of pulmonary artery pressures. Because left ventricular compliance can be affected by PEEP and because PEEP-induced changes in intrathoracic pressure are transmitted to the heart and the pulmonary vasculature, a change in the pulmonary artery occlusion pressure need not reflect a change in left ventricular end-diastolic volume. Indeed, it should be remembered that the pulmonary artery occlusion pressure is a very poor predictor of a patient's cardiac output response to fluid [165]. Although it is unlikely that Swan Ganz catheters will vanish from clinical practice, two prospective randomized controlled clinical trials, one in patients undergoing major cardiovascular surgery and the other in patients with ALI and ARDS, have failed to demonstrate efficacy of pulmonary artery catheter-guided management [166,167].

Positive End-Expiratory Pressure and the Obstructed Patient. Continuous positive airway pressure reduces the inspiratory work of breathing in dynamically hyperinflated patients by two mechanisms: (a) it helps oppose the expiratory action of P_{el} at end expiration (i.e., $PEEP_i$), and (b) it promotes active expiration below the predicted V_{rel} of the respiratory system [168]. As a result, CPAP can inflate the relaxed respiratory system to V_{rel} because of expiratory muscle derecruitment during inspi ration even if the inspiratory muscles were to remain inactive. It is crucial to oppose $PEEP_i$ with extrinsic PEEP in ventilator-dependent patients with COPD when they make inspiratory triggering efforts. If this is not done, the patient is forced to generate inspiratory pressures slightly above $PEEP_i$ before the machine can respond. Such efforts are potentially exhausting and could prevent successful weaning from mechanical ventilation.

Physiologic and Prophylactic Positive End-Expiratory Pressure. The term *physiologic PEEP* has been applied to the application of 5 cm H_2O of PEEP in intubated patients with healthy lungs. The term was coined because laryngeal breaking normally elevates tracheal pressure in the presence of expiratory flow by a few cm H_2O. Bypassing the larynx with an endotracheal tube is frequently associated with a decrease in end-expiratory lung volume [169]. This predisposes intubated patients to gas absorption atelectasis and may be prevented through the application of "physiologic" PEEP [170]. There is no conclusive data to show that prophylactic PEEP reduces the incidence of ARDS in predisposed patients [171] or that it prevents atelectasis after open heart surgery [172]. In fact, it may take more than 20 cm H_2O of pressure to reverse the atelectasis that accompanies inhalational anesthesia and neuromuscular blockade [173], and it takes as little as 6 cm H_2O of PEEP during induction of general anesthesia to prevent it [174,175]. This raises questions about the validity of older studies in which prophylactic PEEP may have been misapplied, mistimed, and underdosed. This is underscored by the demonstrated efficacy of mask CPAP in severely hypoxemic patients after abdominal surgery [176].

Considerations About Mode and Settings During Noninvasive Mechanical Ventilation

In the United States, NMV is most commonly delivered with a bilevel pressure device, that is, a ventilator that operates in a pressure preset mode. This is not to say that volume preset ventilators are inferior or ineffective. Indeed, the European trial that first established efficacy of NMV in the acute care setting used a volume preset mode to assist patients [44]. In addition, there are many patient–ventilator interfaces from which to choose, most notably nasal and full-face masks. This choice should be guided by patient preference. The debate as to the ideal mode for NMV hinges in part on one's bias if it is sufficient to acutely unload fatigued respiratory muscles or if immediate large reductions in arterial CO_2 tension are also required to gain long-term benefit. In practice, TV and pressure amplitude settings are usually limited by patient compliance, and facial pressures in excess of 15 cm H_2O are rarely tolerated. It is customary to set PEEP between 4 and 8 cm H_2O as a means of raising lung volume and promoting upper airway patency. Although most practitioners set the backup frequency between 8 and 12 breaths per minute (they operate the ventilator in a spontaneous/timed, i.e., A/C mode), machine breaths that do not coincide with a patient's inspiratory effort often meet a partially or completely obstructed upper airway. Inspired gas is generally supplemented with low levels of O_2. A need to raise FIO_2 above 0.5 to maintain a pulse oximetry reading above 90% should alert the care provider to the possibility of profound CO_2 retention. (For a more detailed discussion of NMV, see Chapter 59.)

DISEASE-ORIENTED MECHANICAL VENTILATION STRATEGIES

Mechanical Ventilation in Individuals with (Near) Normal Respiratory Mechanics and Pulmonary Gas Exchange

Most patients who require ventilation during anesthesia, neuromuscular blockade, and surgery; most patients with respiratory failure from central nervous system depressant drugs; and many patients with diseases of peripheral nerves and muscles have (near) normal respiratory mechanics and pulmonary gas exchange. The goal in these patients is to maintain or restore adequate alveolar ventilation and oxygenation; therefore, the single most important initial ventilator setting is minute volume ($\dot{V}_E$). Minute volume is the product of fM and TV and is an important determinant of the body's CO_2 stores and consequently of $PaCO_2$:

$$PaCO_2 = \dot{V}_{CO_2} \times k/\dot{V}_E\,(1 - V_D/TV)$$

$\dot{V}CO_2$ is the volume of CO_2 produced (in liters per minute); V_D/TV is the dead space-to-TV ratio, a variable with which the efficiency of the lung as a CO_2 eliminator can be approximated; k is a constant that equals 0.863 and that scales $\dot{V}_{CO_2}$ and $\dot{V}_E$ to the same temperature and humidity.

In resting patients with healthy lungs and metabolic rates, a $\dot{V}_E$ setting between 80 and 100 mL per kg usually results in normocapnia. Usual TV settings in a volume preset mode range between 6 and 10 mL per kg ideal body weight, with the occasional neuromuscular disease patient preferring higher TVs for comfort. Those who prefer to ventilate patients in a pressure preset mode can deliver similar volumes with pressure amplitudes of 10 to 15 cm H_2O applied for 0.75 to 1 second. If a subsequent blood gas analysis shows hypercapnia despite seemingly adequate $\dot{V}_E$ delivery, a hypermetabolic state (increased $\dot{V}_{CO_2}$) or $\dot{V}$ mismatch (abnormal V_D/TV) should be suspected. It may not be wise to normalize the $PaCO_2$ of patients with chronic CO_2 retention suddenly considering the adverse hemodynamic and metabolic effects of posthypercapnic alkalosis. Therefore, $\dot{V}_E$ settings of approximately 60 mL per kg should be used when the initial $PaCO_2$ and pH targets are approximately 55 mm Hg and 7.35, respectively. It remains unresolved whether patients with chronic CO_2 retention should be mechanically ventilated to normocapnia. Those who argue against this practice assume that a resetting of chemoresponsiveness toward normal elevates ventilatory requirement and prevents weaning. Proponents cite the adverse effects of hypercapnia on respiratory muscle contractility [177].

Mechanical Ventilation in Individuals with Airways Obstruction

Because of expiratory airflow limitation, patients with obstructive physiology are at risk of having mechanical ventilation cause or worsen dynamic hyperinflation (i.e., $PEEP_i$). This in turn increases the risk of barotrauma (e.g., pneumothorax), hypotension, and death. Therefore, the goal of therapy is to maintain adequate oxygenation while minimizing the thoracic volume about which the lungs are ventilated. The latter can be accomplished by (a) reducing airway inflammation and alleviating bronchoconstriction, (b) decreasing TV, (c) increasing inspiratory flow rate, and (d) accepting hypercapnia.

Status Asthmaticus

Insights into the determinants of gas trapping, barotrauma, and permissive hypercapnia have changed both indications and ventilator management principles in status asthmaticus [106,114,178,179]. In contrast to patients with chronic airflow obstruction from emphysema or bronchitis, patients with status asthmaticus suffer from airway closure and mucus plugging and have much more severe V/Q mismatch and a higher ventilatory requirement, and are therefore particularly prone to hyperinflation, barotrauma, cardiovascular collapse, and death (see Chapter 48). Intubation and mechanical ventilation should be viewed as measures of last resort and should be reserved for patients who have failed noninvasive mechanical ventilation and who require sedation, neuromuscular blockade, and ventilation with permissive hypercapnia.

Because the primary goal is to prevent overdistention of unobstructed lung units, relatively low initial TV settings (e.g., less than 8 mL per kg predicted body weight) should be used in conjunction with peak inspiratory flows of approximately 60 L per minute and rates of 12 to 16 breaths per minute. Higher rates should be used only if cardiovascular instability is attributed to severe respiratory acidemia rather than dynamic hyperinflation. In practice, it is rarely possible to make this distinction. Because peak airway pressure may not adequately reflect lung parenchymal stress in such patients, Tuxen et al. [178] proposed guiding ventilator adjustments on the basis of measurements of trapped gas volume.

The V_{EI} is the volume of air above FRC that is in the patient's lungs after delivery of TV. Although P_{peak} and P_{plat} are read directly off the ventilator manometer, V_{EI} is measured in a spirometer. For V_{EI} measurement, patients must be sedated, paralyzed, well oxygenated, and disconnected from the ventilator immediately after TV is delivered. Expired air must be collected in a spirometer until no more air escapes. In severely obstructed patients, this collection may take, on average, 40 to 60 seconds. Making ventilator changes aimed at keeping V_{EI} below 20 mL per kg has been shown to protect against barotrauma and hypotension in status asthmaticus [179].

To manage the most severely obstructed patients with status asthmaticus, we recommend making ventilatory changes as needed to stay below the V_{EI} threshold of 20 mL per kg. If V_{EI} is greater than 20 mL per kg after the patient has stabilized on the initial ventilator settings, the TV or rate should be decreased. If V_{EI} is greater than 20 mL per kg but gas exchange is marginal, ventilating the patient with a helium–oxygen mixture may be considered. Breathing helium has been associated with reduced lung inflation pressure, $PEEP_i$, and improved alveolar ventilation and oxygenation [180–183]. However, the use of helium–oxygen mixtures in conjunction with positive pressure ventilation is not a trivial undertaking.

Conventional mechanical ventilators are designed to operate safely with low-density and high-viscosity gas mixtures, so that local experience with this investigational intervention is critical. It must be stressed that there is no single upper $PaCO_2$ or lower pH threshold that has been associated with cardiovascular instability or poor outcome [116]. Therefore, concern for barotrauma must take precedence over maintenance of alveolar ventilation. (See Chapter 48 for the role of bicarbonate infusion.) The measurement of V_{EI} is cumbersome and can be accomplished only in paralyzed patients. We do not believe that it is appropriate to paralyze patients for the sole purpose of making a V_{EI} measurement. We also wish to remind the reader that large portions of the asthmatic lung may be completely obstructed, so that both V_{EI} and $PEEP_i$ often underestimate the degree of trapping [184].

Chronic Obstructive Pulmonary Disease

In general, the management principles for COPD are similar to those for asthmatic patients, except that patients with exacerbations of COPD rarely require neuromuscular blockade or permissive hypercapnia. Patients with COPD are prone to dynamic hyperinflation from expiratory flow limitation rather than airway closure and mucus plugging. The challenge is to minimize hyperinflation and inspiratory work despite limited control over respiratory rate (see Chapter 49). In a patient who is not paralyzed, the machine trigger rate, as opposed to the machine backup rate and I/E settings, determine T_e (see previous discussion). To the extent to which COPD patients remain tachypneic during mechanical ventilation, changing V_i and T_i settings may not be effective in reducing gas trapping. Increasing V_i under the assumption that it would prolong T_e may actually have the opposite effect because higher flows often increase respiratory rate [32,104]. Therefore, we initially choose a TV between 6 and 8 mL per kg predicted body weight, an intermediate inspiratory flow of 40 to 60 L per minute, and a rate close to the patient's spontaneous effort rate. We add up to 10 cm H_2O of CPAP to reduce machine trigger work (see previous discussion).

Because these patients are not paralyzed, it is not feasible to monitor trapped gas volume, as has been proposed for asthmatic patients. Rather, one should assure that end-inflation hold pressure remains below 30 cm H_2O. If the initial ventilator settings fail to reduce dyspnea and patient effort, we raise $PEEP_e$ until peak airway pressure starts to rise [112]. At that point, the difference between $PEEP_e$ and end-expiratory mean alveolar pressure is presumably at a minimum. If adjustments in $PEEP_e$ fail to reduce patient effort, as judged by symptoms or accessory muscle use, sedation must be increased and, rarely, neuromuscular blockade considered.

As pointed out in the section on minute volume settings and CO_2 homeostasis it is better to underestimate the minute volume requirement when initiating support during acute exacerbations. Otherwise one runs the risk of unmasking severe posthypercapnic metabolic alkalosis.

Acute Respiratory Distress Syndrome

Much of our treatment philosophy and its underpinnings for patients with ARDS are presented in the sections that discuss TV and rate settings and the use of PEEP. To summarize, we attempt to increase FRC and mean lung volume through the application of extrinsic PEEP, avoid end-inflation hold pressure in excess of 30 cm H_2O, and reduce TV as we raise PEEP to stay within safe volume boundaries. In practice, this means TV settings are between 4 and 8 mL per kg predicted body weight when we use volume preset modes or P_{peak} settings 30 cm H_2O or less when we use pressure preset modes. The rate is usually 20 to 30 breaths per minute unless the patient has been heavily sedated and paralyzed to tolerate hypercapnia. There is no upper limit to PEEP as long as the peak lung volume and recoil pressure guidelines are adhered to, but in practice it is rarely possible to deliver sufficient alveolar ventilation at cycling pressures between 20 (PEEP setting) and 30 cm H_2O (P_{plat}).

We should emphasize that overdistention is not the only mechanism by which large tidal excursions may injure the lungs. Large intermittent changes in alveolar surface area promote small aggregate conversion of surfactant, and with it lead to impairment in surface tension dynamics [185–187]. This mechanism has been invoked as an explanation for the development of noncardiogenic pulmonary edema in a sheep model with salicylate-induced spontaneous hyperventilation [188]. If this mechanism proves to be important, then the use of pressure-limited ventilation strategies such as bilevel pressure ventilation and assisted pressure release ventilation cannot be assumed protective unless the resulting TV remains between 4 and 8 mL per kg predicted body weight.

There is some suggestion that the use of lung protective ventilation with low TVs is also beneficial for patients without ALI and ARDS. In a retrospective review of patients with respiratory failure from causes other than ALI, Gajic et al. [189] identified TV as a risk factor for the subsequent development of noncardiogenic pulmonary edema. On the basis of this evidence and on mechanistic reasoning, the authors avoid TV in excess of 8 mL per kg predicted body weight in all patients, and in general adhere to the lung-protective ventilator management algorithms of the ARDS Net.

Patients who cannot be oxygenated at lung-protective settings need to be sedated and sometimes paralyzed and may be candidates for unconventional alternatives and investigational support modes. These include turning the patient to the prone posture, supplementing inspired gas with nitric oxide, and considering the use of high-frequency ventilators, extracorporeal membrane oxygenators, and extracorporeal CO_2 removal devices. To date, however, none of these interventions have proved efficacious in rigorously conducted clinical trials (see Chapter 47).

Despite several inconclusive or negative clinical efficacy trials there continued to be interest in prone positioning [190–192] as a lung protective intervention. However, the recent Prone Supine II study, a large randomized multicenter trial conducted in Spain and Italy, found no survival benefit in either patients with ARDS or in subgroups of patients with moderate and severe hypoxemia [193]. At this time, routine use of the prone position cannot be recommended.

The recent influenza pandemic has generated renewed interest in extracorporeal membrane oxygenation (ECMO) as rescue therapy for refractory hypoxemia [194–196]. Moreover, the recent publication of the CESAR trial [197] in which patients with severe ARDS were randomly assigned to either receive usual on site care or get transferred to a single ECMO center encouraged its use. Patients cared for at the ECMO center had a significantly better 6-month disability-free survival (63% vs. 47%; $p < 0.03$) than patients who were treated on site. Skeptics emphasize that conventional treatment was not standardized across the 103 study sites and that only 75% of patients transferred to the ECMO center actually received ECMO. Clearly ECMO remains a resource-intensive treatment modality reserved for major centers with a dedicated, highly trained, and multidisciplinary staff. At this time routine use of ECMO as rescue therapy is not recommended and the iatrogenic risks related to transport, vascular access and anticoagulation assessed on a case-by-case basis.

Head Trauma

The key to the ventilatory management of patients with head trauma is to avoid excessive intrathoracic pressures and at the same time provide sufficient ventilation to lower $PaCO_2$. It should be emphasized, however, that therapeutic hyperventilation and hypocapnia, when applied for more than 24 hours, have been associated with worse patient outcomes [198,199]. High intrathoracic pressures are transmitted to the subarachnoid space and may thereby reduce the perfusion pressure of a central nervous system that is already compromised by intracranial hypertension from bleeding or edema. However, measurements of PEEP effects on cerebrospinal fluid pressure and, more importantly, cerebral perfusion pressure in patients have generated conflicting results. This is because PEEP-related changes in systemic circulation and blood gas tensions have complex cerebrospinal fluid pressure-independent effects on cerebral blood flow [198]. As a general rule, raising PEEP is unlikely to lower cerebral perfusion pressure unless it is associated with a decrease in systemic blood pressure and cardiac output [200,201]. Because the assumption of the prone posture may also raise intracranial pressure [202], the patient's head must be raised appropriately.

Myocardial Ischemia and Congestive Heart Failure

In addition to the heart–lung interactions already discussed in the context of PEEP therapy, mechanical ventilation reduces systemic as well as myocardial oxygen demands. This may be critical in patients with ischemia and cardiogenic shock and is associated with a redistribution of blood from working respiratory muscles toward vital organs [203].

In principle, the ventilatory management of patients with ischemia and congestive heart failure is similar to that of patients with noncardiogenic forms of pulmonary edema. PEEP should be used to recruit flooded lung units and redistribute edema fluid from the alveolar to the interstitial spaces. When congestive heart failure complicates active ischemia, premature weaning attempts that focus only on maintenance of blood gas tension and ignore work of breathing and associated increases in myocardial oxygen demand are ill advised. Alternatively, it is important to recognize that weaning from mechanical ventilation may trigger congestive heart failure with or without myocardial ischemia [204–206]. Weaning-induced heart failure appears to be more prevalent in COPD (for further discussion, see Chapter 60).

Mechanical Ventilation in the Pregnant Patient

Pregnancy results in a number of physiologic changes that must be considered in the ventilatory management of patients in this condition. Changes include the reduction in chest wall compliance and increases in metabolic rate, minute volume, and respiratory drive. The consequent respiratory alkalosis is thought to aid fetal gas exchange. Alkalemia shifts the fetal oxyhemoglobin dissociation curve to the left, thereby increasing its ability to bind oxygen. Therefore, it stands to reason that in the pregnant mechanically ventilated patient, the minute volume setting should be adjusted to a PCO_2 target between 28 and 32 mm Hg [207]. However, in pregnant patients with ARDS or status asthmaticus, it might not be possible to reconcile this ventilation target with the principles of lung protection from mechanical injury. In the absence of clinical outcome data, it is impossible to offer strict management guidelines. All management decisions must balance benefits to the mother against possible risks to the fetus.

It is well established that gas tensions in maternal blood determine the acid or base status of the fetus. However, the risk of permissive hypercapnia to the unborn child is simply not known. Most experts agree that pregnant women with ARDS should be ventilated with TVs of 6 mL per kg ideal body weight. It is not known whether increasing respiratory rate to promote alkalemia is beneficial or whether associated changes in the rate of lung expansion offset the beneficial effects of low TVs. Because chest wall compliance is reduced, the application of PEEP (usually between 10 and 15 cm H_2O) might raise plateau pressure and predispose the pregnant patient to hypotension and decreased blood flow to the placenta.

Mechanical Ventilation in Individuals with a Bronchopleural Fistula

For discussion of the ventilatory strategy of this entity, see Chapter 57.

COMPLICATIONS ASSOCIATED WITH INTERMITTENT POSITIVE-PRESSURE VENTILATION

The hazards associated with mechanical ventilation can be divided into five major categories: (a) complications attributable to intubation and extubation [208–210], (b) complications associated with endotracheal or tracheostomy tubes [211], (c) complications attributable to operation of the ventilator, (d) medical complications occurring during assisted mechanical ventilation, and (e) psychologic effects.

Complications attributable to intubation and extubation and those associated with endotracheal or tracheostomy tubes include upper airway trauma, inadvertent placement or migration of the endotracheal tube into the right mainstem bronchus, vocal cord edema or granuloma, cuff-related damage to the trachea, accidental intubation of the esophagus, induction of vomiting with resultant aspiration, premature extubation, self-extubation, tube malfunction, nasal necrosis, and sinusitis. For a more complete discussion of these complications, see Chapters 1 and 12. Complications attributable to interfaces used during noninvasive forms of positive-pressure mechanical ventilation include nasal bridge ulcers, nasal congestion, and conjunctivitis from mask leaks directed to the eyes.

Complications attributable to operation of the ventilator include machine failure, alarm failure, alarm inadvertently turned off, inadequate nebulization or humidification, overheating of inspired air, ventilator asynchrony or noncapture, and bacterial contamination of various components of the mechanical ventilator. All of these can be minimized or eliminated if patients on ventilator support are not left unattended and infection-control methods are adhered to strictly. The implementation of ventilator-associated pneumonia (VAP) protection bundles, including head-of-bed elevation, chlorhexidine oral care, and daily sedation holidays have significantly reduced VAP across adult medical [212], surgical/trauma [213] and pediatric [214] ICUs.

Medical complications occurring during assisted ventilation include inadvertent alveolar hypoventilation and hyperventilation, bronchopulmonary dysplasia, hypotension caused by decreased cardiac output from a reduction in venous return, vascular insufficiency in patients with arteriosclerotic vascular disease caused by decreased cardiac output, water retention from increased circulating levels of antidiuretic hormone presumably stimulated when positive-pressure ventilation decreases left atrial volume [162], and lung barotrauma.

The classic manifestations of barotrauma are pulmonary interstitial emphysema with pneumomediastinum, subcutaneous emphysema, pneumoretroperitoneum, pneumoperitoneum, and pneumothorax with or without tension [89]. However, in the last two decades it has become abundantly clear that there are many more subtle manifestations of ventilator-induced lung injury originally attributed to intrinsic disease. These range from capillary leak and noncardiogenic edema to alveolar hemorrhage, inflammation, tissue remodeling, subpleural cyst formations, and fibrosis [67]. The clinical and experimental ventilator-associated lung injury literature has focused on TV and PEEP as major determinants of lung stress. There is no longer any doubt that these ventilator setting-dependent variables are important, but there remains considerable debate whether to apply specific numeric guidelines to individual patients, whether TV guidelines can be relaxed in spontaneously breathing patients who receive partial ventilator support, and what the TV-related injury mechanisms truly are. To understand these controversies, one needs to recall that there are four distinct injury mechanisms, namely (a) regional overexpansion caused by the application of a local stress or pressure that forces cells and tissues to assume shapes and dimensions that they do not assume during unassisted breathing; (b) so-called low-volume injury that is associated with the repeated recruitment and derecruitment of unstable lung units that causes the abrasion of the epithelial airspace lining by interfacial tension; (c) the inactivation of surfactant triggered by large alveolar surface area oscillations that stress surfactant adsorption and desorption kinetics, and that are associated with surfactant aggregate conversion; and (d) interdependence mechanisms that raise cell and tissue shear stress between neighboring structures with differing mechanical properties [215].

The older literature quotes an overall incidence of pneumothorax with intermittent positive-pressure ventilation of 3.5% [216], with values as high as 30% in the status asthmaticus subgroup [217]. It is hoped that an improved understanding of patient/ventilator interactions and lung biology will substantially reduce the incidence of barotrauma. Because 60% to 90% of pneumothoraces in patients on positive-pressure ventilation are under tension [218], and mortality increases from 7% to 31% when there is a delay from 30 minutes to 8 hours in diagnosing and treating pneumothoraces that occur on ventilators [219], there must be a high index of suspicion for this complication and it must be managed swiftly. For management of this problem, see Chapter 57.

Advances in initiation of mechanical ventilation, based on randomized, controlled trials or meta-analyses of such trials, are summarized in Table 58.1.

TABLE 58.1

ADVANCES IN VENTILATOR MANAGEMENT BASED ON RANDOMIZED CONTROLLED CLINICAL TRIALS

- Limiting tidal volume to 6 mL per kg predicted body weight reduces the probability of ventilator-associated lung injury and improves the survival of patients with ALI [20,131].
- For patients with ALI and ARDS who receive mechanical ventilation with a tidal volume goal of 6 mL per kg of predicted body weight and an end-inspiratory plateau-pressure limit of 30 cm of H_2O, clinical outcomes are similar whether lower or higher PEEP levels are used [148].
- Continuous positive airway pressure may decrease the incidence of endotracheal intubation and other severe complications in patients who develop hypoxemia after elective major abdominal surgery [176].
- The routine use of the prone posture in mechanically ventilated patients with ALI is not associated with a survival benefit [193].
- The use of high-frequency oscillatory ventilation should be considered as rescue treatment in patients with severe ARDS [15].
- Noninvasive mechanical ventilation enhances the survival of immunocompromised hosts with hypoxic respiratory failure [46] and is a viable alternative to invasive mechanical ventilation in patients with ALI [48,49].
- Pressure and volume preset modes result in similar outcomes in mechanically ventilated patients with acute respiratory failure [62].

ALI, acute lung injury; ARDS, acute respiratory distress syndrome; PEEP, positive end-expiratory pressure.

References

1. Hill NS: Clinical applications of body ventilators. *Chest* 90:897–905, 1986.
2. Shapiro SH, Ernst P, Gray-Donald K, et al: Effect of negative pressure ventilation in severe chronic obstructive pulmonary disease. *Lancet* 340:1425–1429, 1992.
3. Grasso F, Engelberts D, Helm E, et al: Negative-pressure ventilation: better oxygenation and less lung injury. *Am J Respir Crit Care Med* 177:412–418, 2008.
4. Ritacca FV, Stewart TE: Clinical review: high-frequency oscillatory ventilation in adults–a review of the literature and practical applications. *Crit Care* 7:385–390, 2003.
5. Venegas JG, Fredberg JJ: Understanding the pressure cost of ventilation: why does high-frequency ventilation work? *Crit Care Med* 22:S49–S57, 1994.
6. High-frequency oscillatory ventilation compared with conventional

mechanical ventilation in the treatment of respiratory failure in preterm infants. The HIFI Study Group. *N Engl J Med* 320:88–93, 1989.
7. Bryan AC: The oscillations of HFO. *Am J Respir Crit Care Med* 163:816–817, 2001.
8. Imai Y, Slutsky AS: High-frequency oscillatory ventilation and ventilator-induced lung injury. *Crit Care Med* 33:S129–S134, 2005.
9. Bollen CW, Uiterwaal CS, van Vught AJ: Cumulative metaanalysis of high-frequency versus conventional ventilation in premature neonates. *Am J Respir Crit Care Med* 168:1150–1155, 2003.
10. Courtney SE, Durand DJ, Asselin JM, et al: High-frequency oscillatory ventilation versus conventional mechanical ventilation for very-low-birth-weight infants. *N Engl J Med* 347:643–652, 2002.
11. Gerstmann DR, Minton SD, Stoddard RA, et al: The Provo multicenter early high-frequency oscillatory ventilation trial: improved pulmonary and clinical outcome in respiratory distress syndrome. *Pediatrics* 98:1044–1057, 1996.
12. Johnson AH, Peacock JL, Greenough A, et al: High-frequency oscillatory ventilation for the prevention of chronic lung disease of prematurity. *N Engl J Med* 347:633–642, 2002.
13. Rimensberger PC, Beghetti M, Hanquinet S, et al: First intention high-frequency oscillation with early lung volume optimization improves pulmonary outcome in very low birth weight infants with respiratory distress syndrome. *Pediatrics* 105:1202–1208, 2000.
14. Thomas MR, Rafferty GF, Limb ES, et al: Pulmonary function at follow-up of very preterm infants from the United Kingdom oscillation study. *Am J Respir Crit Care Med* 169:868–872, 2004.
15. Derdak S, Mehta S, Stewart TE, et al: High-frequency oscillatory ventilation for acute respiratory distress syndrome in adults: a randomized, controlled trial. *Am J Respir Crit Care Med* 166:801–808, 2002.
16. Fessler HE, Derdak S, Ferguson ND, et al: A protocol for high-frequency oscillatory ventilation in adults: results from a roundtable discussion. *Crit Care Med* 35:1649–1654, 2007.
17. Fessler HE, Hager DN, Brower RG: Feasibility of very high-frequency ventilation in adults with acute respiratory distress syndrome. *Crit Care Med* 36:1043–1048, 2008.
18. Bates JH, Rossi A, Milic-Emili J: Analysis of the behavior of the respiratory system with constant inspiratory flow. *J Appl Physiol* 58:1840–1848, 1985.
19. Hubmayr RD, Gay PC, Tayyab M: Respiratory system mechanics in ventilated patients: techniques and indications. *Mayo Clin Proc* 62:358–368, 1987.
20. Brower R, Thompson BT: Tidal volumes in acute respiratory distress syndrome–one size does not fit all. *Crit Care Med* 34:263–264, author reply 264–267, 2006.
21. Aslanian P, El Atrous S, Isabey D, et al: Effects of flow triggering on breathing effort during partial ventilatory support. *Am J Respir Crit Care Med* 157:135–143, 1998.
22. Tobin MJ, Jubran A, Laghi F: Patient-ventilator interaction. *Am J Respir Crit Care Med* 163:1059–1063, 2001.
23. Marini JJ, Rodriguez RM, Lamb V: The inspiratory workload of patient-initiated mechanical ventilation. *Am Rev Respir Dis* 134:902–909, 1986.
24. Forel JM, Roch A, Marin V, et al: Neuromuscular blocking agents decrease inflammatory response in patients presenting with acute respiratory distress syndrome. *Crit Care Med* 34:2749–2757, 2006.
25. Gainnier M, Roch A, Forel JM, et al: Effect of neuromuscular blocking agents on gas exchange in patients presenting with acute respiratory distress syndrome. *Crit Care Med* 32:113–119, 2004.
26. Weisman IM, Rinaldo JE, Rogers RM, et al: Intermittent mandatory ventilation. *Am Rev Respir Dis* 127:641–647, 1983.
27. Brochard L, Rauss A, Benito S, et al: Comparison of three methods of gradual withdrawal from ventilatory support during weaning from mechanical ventilation. *Am J Respir Crit Care Med* 150:896–903, 1994.
28. Esteban A, Frutos F, Tobin MJ, et al: A comparison of four methods of weaning patients from mechanical ventilation. Spanish Lung Failure Collaborative Group. *N Engl J Med* 332:345–350, 1995.
29. Trevisan CE, Vieira SR: Noninvasive mechanical ventilation may be useful in treating patients who fail weaning from invasive mechanical ventilation: a randomized clinical trial. *Crit Care* 12:R51, 2008.
30. Meza S, Mendez M, Ostrowski M, et al: Susceptibility to periodic breathing with assisted ventilation during sleep in normal subjects. *J Appl Physiol* 85:1929–1940, 1998.
31. Stroetz RW, Hubmayr RD: Patient-ventilator interactions. *Monaldi Arch Chest Dis* 53:331–336, 1998.
32. Tobert DG, Simon PM, Stroetz RW, et al: The determinants of respiratory rate during mechanical ventilation. *Am J Respir Crit Care Med* 155:485–492, 1997.
33. Giannouli E, Webster K, Roberts D, et al: Response of ventilator-dependent patients to different levels of pressure support and proportional assist. *Am J Respir Crit Care Med* 159:1716–1725, 1999.
34. Hotchkiss JR, Adams AB, Dries DJ, et al: Dynamic behavior during noninvasive ventilation: chaotic support? *Am J Respir Crit Care Med* 163:374–378, 2001.
35. Parthasarathy S, Tobin MJ: Effect of ventilator mode on sleep quality in critically ill patients. *Am J Respir Crit Care Med* 166:1423–1429, 2002.
36. Cook D, Meade M, Guyatt G, et al: Trials of miscellaneous interventions to wean from mechanical ventilation. *Chest* 120:438S–444S, 2001.
37. Esteban A, Alia I, Gordo F, et al: Extubation outcome after spontaneous breathing trials with T-tube or pressure support ventilation. The Spanish Lung Failure Collaborative Group. *Am J Respir Crit Care Med* 156:459–465, 1997.
38. MacIntyre NR, Cook DJ, Ely EW, Jr., et al: Evidence-based guidelines for weaning and discontinuing ventilatory support: a collective task force facilitated by the American College of Chest Physicians; the American Association for Respiratory Care; and the American College of Critical Care Medicine. *Chest* 120:375S–395S, 2001.
39. Ely EW, Baker AM, Dunagan DP, et al: Effect on the duration of mechanical ventilation of identifying patients capable of breathing spontaneously. *N Engl J Med* 335:1864–1869, 1996.
40. Morrell MJ, Shea SA, Adams L, et al: Effects of inspiratory support upon breathing in humans during wakefulness and sleep. *Respir Physiol* 93:57–70, 1993.
41. Hedenstierna G, Lattuada M: Gas exchange in the ventilated patient. *Curr Opin Crit Care* 8:39–44, 2002.
42. Azoulay E, Alberti C, Bornstain C, et al: Improved survival in cancer patients requiring mechanical ventilatory support: impact of noninvasive mechanical ventilatory support. *Crit Care Med* 29:519–525, 2001.
43. Brochard L: Non-invasive ventilation for acute exacerbations of COPD: a new standard of care. *Thorax* 55:817–818, 2000.
44. Brochard L, Mancebo J, Wysocki M, et al: Noninvasive ventilation for acute exacerbations of chronic obstructive pulmonary disease. *N Engl J Med* 333:817–822, 1995.
45. Girou E, Schortgen F, Delclaux C, et al: Association of noninvasive ventilation with nosocomial infections and survival in critically ill patients. *JAMA* 284:2361–2367, 2000.
46. Hilbert G, Gruson D, Vargas F, et al: Noninvasive ventilation in immunosuppressed patients with pulmonary infiltrates, fever, and acute respiratory failure. *N Engl J Med* 344:481–487, 2001.
47. Kramer N, Meyer TJ, Meharg J, et al: Randomized, prospective trial of noninvasive positive pressure ventilation in acute respiratory failure. *Am J Respir Crit Care Med* 151:1799–1806, 1995.
48. Antonelli M, Conti G, Bufi M, et al: Noninvasive ventilation for treatment of acute respiratory failure in patients undergoing solid organ transplantation: a randomized trial. *JAMA* 283:235–241, 2000.
49. Antonelli M, Conti G, Rocco M, et al: A comparison of noninvasive positive-pressure ventilation and conventional mechanical ventilation in patients with acute respiratory failure. *N Engl J Med* 339:429–435, 1998.
50. Ferrer M, Esquinas A, Leon M, et al: Noninvasive ventilation in severe hypoxemic respiratory failure: a randomized clinical trial. *Am J Respir Crit Care Med* 168:1438–1444, 2003.
51. Honrubia T, Garcia Lopez FJ, Franco N, et al: Noninvasive vs conventional mechanical ventilation in acute respiratory failure: a multicenter, randomized controlled trial. *Chest* 128:3916–3924, 2005.
52. Park M, Sangean MC, Volpe Mde S, et al: Randomized, prospective trial of oxygen, continuous positive airway pressure, and bilevel positive airway pressure by face mask in acute cardiogenic pulmonary edema. *Crit Care Med* 32:2407–2415, 2004.
53. Tomii K, Seo R, Tachikawa R, et al: Impact of noninvasive ventilation (NIV) trial for various types of acute respiratory failure in the emergency department; decreased mortality and use of the ICU. *Respir Med* 103:67–73, 2009.
54. Rana S, Jenad H, Gay PC, et al: Failure of non-invasive ventilation in patients with acute lung injury: observational cohort study. *Crit Care* 10:R79, 2006.
55. Branson RD, Johannigman JA, Campbell RS, et al: Closed-loop mechanical ventilation. *Respir Care* 47:427–451, discussion 451–423, 2002.
56. Brunner JX: Principles and history of closed-loop controlled ventilation. *Respir Care Clin N Am* 7:341–362, vii, 2001.
57. Sinderby C, Navalesi P, Beck J, et al: Neural control of mechanical ventilation in respiratory failure. *Nat Med* 5:1433–1436, 1999.
58. Younes M, Kun J, Masiowski B, et al: A method for noninvasive determination of inspiratory resistance during proportional assist ventilation. *Am J Respir Crit Care Med* 163:829–839, 2001.
59. Younes M, Webster K, Kun J, et al: A method for measuring passive elastance during proportional assist ventilation. *Am J Respir Crit Care Med* 164:50–60, 2001.
60. Laghi F: NAVA: brain over machine? *Intensive Care Med* 34:1966–1968, 2008.
61. Brander L, Sinderby C, Lecomte F, et al: Neurally adjusted ventilatory assist decreases ventilator-induced lung injury and non-pulmonary organ dysfunction in rabbits with acute lung injury. *Intensive Care Med* 35:1979–1989, 2009.
62. Esteban A, Alia I, Gordo F, et al: Prospective randomized trial comparing pressure-controlled ventilation and volume-controlled ventilation in ARDS. For the Spanish Lung Failure Collaborative Group. *Chest* 117:1690–1696, 2000.
63. Waid-Jones MI, Coursin DB: Perioperative considerations for patients treated with bleomycin. *Chest* 99:993–999, 1991.
64. Miller MR, Crapo R, Hankinson J, et al: General considerations for lung function testing. *Eur Respir J* 26:153–161, 2005.
65. Ventilation with lower tidal volumes as compared with traditional tidal volumes for acute lung injury and the acute respiratory distress syndrome. The

Acute Respiratory Distress Syndrome Network. *N Engl J Med* 342:1301–1308, 2000
66. dos Santos CC, Slutsky AS: The contribution of biophysical lung injury to the development of biotrauma. *Annu Rev Physiol* 68:585–618, 2006.
67. Dreyfuss D, Saumon G: Ventilator-induced lung injury: lessons from experimental studies. *Am J Respir Crit Care Med* 157:294–323, 1998.
68. Vlahakis NE, Hubmayr RD: Cellular stress failure in ventilator-injured lungs. *Am J Respir Crit Care Med* 171:1328–1342, 2005.
69. Agostoni E, Hyatt R, eds: *Static behavior of the respiratory system.* Bethesda, MD: American Physiological Society; 1986.
70. Davis K, Jr., Branson RD, Campbell RS, et al: The addition of sighs during pressure support ventilation. Is there a benefit? *Chest* 104:867–870, 1993.
71. Egbert LD, Laver MB, Bendixen HH: intermittent deep breaths and compliance during anesthesia in man. *Anesthesiology* 24:57, 1963.
72. Pelosi P, Bottino N, Chiumello D, et al: Sigh in supine and prone position during acute respiratory distress syndrome. *Am J Respir Crit Care Med* 167:521–527, 2003.
73. Pelosi P, Cadringher P, Bottino N, et al: Sigh in acute respiratory distress syndrome. *Am J Respir Crit Care Med* 159:872–880, 1999.
74. Johannigman JA, Miller SL, Davis BR, et al: Influence of low tidal volumes on gas exchange in acute respiratory distress syndrome and the role of recruitment maneuvers. *J Trauma* 54:320–325, 2003.
75. Lim CM, Jung H, Koh Y, et al: Effect of alveolar recruitment maneuver in early acute respiratory distress syndrome according to antiderecruitment strategy, etiological category of diffuse lung injury, and body position of the patient. *Crit Care Med* 31:411–418, 2003.
76. Medoff BD, Harris RS, Kesselman H, et al: Use of recruitment maneuvers and high-positive end-expiratory pressure in a patient with acute respiratory distress syndrome. *Crit Care Med* 28:1210–1216, 2000.
77. Chiumello D, Pristine G, Slutsky AS: Mechanical ventilation affects local and systemic cytokines in an animal model of acute respiratory distress syndrome. *Am J Respir Crit Care Med* 160:109–116, 1999.
78. Frank JA, McAuley DF, Gutierrez JA, et al: Differential effects of sustained inflation recruitment maneuvers on alveolar epithelial and lung endothelial injury. *Crit Care Med* 33:181–188, discussion 254–185, 2005.
79. Koh WJ, Suh GY, Han J, et al: Recruitment maneuvers attenuate repeated derecruitment-associated lung injury. *Crit Care Med* 33:1070–1076, 2005.
80. Lim SC, Adams AB, Simonson DA, et al: Intercomparison of recruitment maneuver efficacy in three models of acute lung injury. *Crit Care Med* 32:2371–2377, 2004.
81. Rimensberger PC, Pristine G, Mullen BM, et al: Lung recruitment during small tidal volume ventilation allows minimal positive end-expiratory pressure without augmenting lung injury. *Crit Care Med* 27:1940–1945, 1999.
82. Halter JM, Steinberg JM, Schiller HJ, et al: Positive end-expiratory pressure after a recruitment maneuver prevents both alveolar collapse and recruitment/derecruitment. *Am J Respir Crit Care Med* 167:1620–1626, 2003.
83. Badet M, Bayle F, Richard JC, et al: Comparison of optimal positive end-expiratory pressure and recruitment maneuvers during lung-protective mechanical ventilation in patients with acute lung injury/acute respiratory distress syndrome. *Respir Care* 54:847–854, 2009.
84. Lefevre GR, Kowalski SE, Girling LG, et al: Improved arterial oxygenation after oleic acid lung injury in the pig using a computer-controlled mechanical ventilator. *Am J Respir Crit Care Med* 154:1567–1572, 1996.
85. Mutch WA, Harms S, Lefevre GR, et al: Biologically variable ventilation increases arterial oxygenation over that seen with positive end-expiratory pressure alone in a porcine model of acute respiratory distress syndrome. *Crit Care Med* 28:2457–2464, 2000.
86. Mutch WA, Harms S, Ruth Graham M, et al: Biologically variable or naturally noisy mechanical ventilation recruits atelectatic lung. *Am J Respir Crit Care Med* 162:319–323, 2000.
87. Arold SP, Mora R, Lutchen KR, et al: Variable tidal volume ventilation improves lung mechanics and gas exchange in a rodent model of acute lung injury. *Am J Respir Crit Care Med* 165:366–371, 2002.
88. Suki B: Fluctuations and power laws in pulmonary physiology. *Am J Respir Crit Care Med* 166:133–137, 2002.
89. Macklin MT, Macklin CC: Malignant interstitial emphysema of the lungs and mediastinum as an important occult complication in many respiratory diseases and other conditions: an interpretation of the clinical literature in the light of laboratory experiment. *Medicine* 23:281, 1944.
90. Dreyfuss D, Soler P, Basset G, et al: High inflation pressure pulmonary edema. Respective effects of high airway pressure, high tidal volume, and positive end-expiratory pressure. *Am Rev Respir Dis* 137:1159–1164, 1988:
91. Dreyfuss D, Saumon G: Role of tidal volume, FRC, and end-inspiratory volume in the development of pulmonary edema following mechanical ventilation. *Am Rev Respir Dis* 148:1194–1203, 1993.
92. Talmor D, Sarge T, O'Donnell CR, et al: Esophageal and transpulmonary pressures in acute respiratory failure. *Crit Care Med* 34:1389–1394, 2006.
93. Gattinoni L, Chiumello D, Carlesso E, et al: Bench-to-bedside review: chest wall elastance in acute lung injury/acute respiratory distress syndrome patients. *Crit Care* 8:350–355, 2004.
94. Talmor D, Greenberg D, Howell MD, et al: The costs and cost-effectiveness of an integrated sepsis treatment protocol. *Crit Care Med* 36:1168–1174, 2008.
95. Talmor D, Sarge T, Malhotra A, et al: Mechanical ventilation guided by esophageal pressure in acute lung injury. *N Engl J Med* 359:2095–2104, 2008.
96. Loring SH, O'Donnell CR, Behazin N, et al: Esophageal pressures in acute lung injury-do they represent artifact or useful information about transpulmonary pressure, chest wall mechanics, and lung stress? *J Appl Physiol* 108(3):515–522, 2010.
97. Hubmayr RD: Is there a place for esophageal manometry in the care of patients with injured lungs? *J Appl Physiol* 108(3):481–482, 2010.
98. Kamlin CO, Davis PG. Long versus short inspiratory times in neonates receiving mechanical ventilation. *Cochrane Database Syst Rev* CD004503, 2004.
99. Nieszkowska A, Lu Q, Vieira S, et al: Incidence and regional distribution of lung overinflation during mechanical ventilation with positive end-expiratory pressure. *Crit Care Med* 32:1496–1503, 2004.
100. Tsuchida S, Engelberts D, Roth M, et al: Continuous positive airway pressure causes lung injury in a model of sepsis. *Am J Physiol Lung Cell Mol Physiol* 289:L554–564, 2005.
101. Hotchkiss JR Jr, Blanch L, Murias G, et al: Effects of decreased respiratory frequency on ventilator-induced lung injury. *Am J Respir Crit Care Med* 161:463–468, 2000.
102. Vlahakis NE, Schroeder MA, Pagano RE, et al: Role of deformation-induced lipid trafficking in the prevention of plasma membrane stress failure. *Am J Respir Crit Care Med* 166:1282–1289, 2002.
103. Georgopoulos D, Mitrouska I, Bshouty Z, et al: Effects of breathing route, temperature and volume of inspired gas, and airway anesthesia on the response of respiratory output to varying inspiratory flow. *Am J Respir Crit Care Med* 153:168–175, 1996.
104. Puddy A, Younes M. Effect of inspiratory flow rate on respiratory output in normal subjects. *Am Rev Respir Dis* 146:787–789, 1992.
105. Gay PC, Rodarte JR, Tayyab M, et al: Evaluation of bronchodilator responsiveness in mechanically ventilated patients. *Am Rev Respir Dis* 136:880–885, 1987.
106. Tuxen DV, Lane S. The effects of ventilatory pattern on hyperinflation, airway pressures, and circulation in mechanical ventilation of patients with severe air-flow obstruction. *Am Rev Respir Dis* 136:872–879, 1987.
107. Pepe PE, Marini JJ. Occult positive end-expiratory pressure in mechanically ventilated patients with airflow obstruction: the auto-PEEP effect. *Am Rev Respir Dis* 126:166–170, 1982.
108. Rossi A, Gottfried SB, Zocchi L, et al: Measurement of static compliance of the total respiratory system in patients with acute respiratory failure during mechanical ventilation. The effect of intrinsic positive end-expiratory pressure. *Am Rev Respir Dis* 131:672–677, 1985.
109. Reinoso MA, Gracey DR, Hubmayr RD: Interrupter mechanics of patients admitted to a chronic ventilator dependency unit. *Am Rev Respir Dis* 148:127–131, 1993.
110. Mead J, Gaensler EA: Esophageal and pleural pressures in man, upright and supine. *J Appl Physiol* 14:81–83, 1959.
111. Fernandez R, Mendez M, Younes M: Effect of ventilator flow rate on respiratory timing in normal humans. *Am J Respir Crit Care Med* 159:710–719, 1999.
112. Gay PC, Rodarte JR, Hubmayr RD: The effects of positive expiratory pressure on isovolume flow and dynamic hyperinflation in patients receiving mechanical ventilation. *Am Rev Respir Dis* 139:621–626, 1989.
113. Ranieri VM, Giuliani R, Cinnella G, et al: Physiologic effects of positive end-expiratory pressure in patients with chronic obstructive pulmonary disease during acute ventilatory failure and controlled mechanical ventilation. *Am Rev Respir Dis* 147:5–13, 1993.
114. Darioli R, Perret C: Mechanical controlled hypoventilation in status asthmaticus. *Am Rev Respir Dis* 129:385–387, 1984.
115. Hickling KG, Henderson SJ, Jackson R: Low mortality associated with low volume pressure limited ventilation with permissive hypercapnia in severe adult respiratory distress syndrome. *Intensive Care Med* 16:372–377, 1990.
116. Carvalho CR, Barbas CS, Medeiros DM, et al: Temporal hemodynamic effects of permissive hypercapnia associated with ideal PEEP in ARDS. *Am J Respir Crit Care Med* 156:1458–1466, 1997.
117. Kallet RH, Jasmer RM, Luce JM, et al: The treatment of acidosis in acute lung injury with tris-hydroxymethyl aminomethane (THAM). *Am J Respir Crit Care Med* 161:1149–1153, 2000.
118. Laffey JG, Engelberts D, Kavanagh BP: Buffering hypercapnic acidosis worsens acute lung injury. *Am J Respir Crit Care Med* 161:141–146, 2000.
119. O'Croinin D, Ni Chonghaile M, Higgins B, et al: Bench-to-bedside review: permissive hypercapnia. *Crit Care* 9:51–59, 2005.
120. Sinclair SE, Kregenow DA, Lamm WJ, et al: Hypercapnic acidosis is protective in an in vivo model of ventilator-induced lung injury. *Am J Respir Crit Care Med* 166:403–408, 2002.
121. Laffey JG, Tanaka M, Engelberts D, et al: Therapeutic hypercapnia reduces pulmonary and systemic injury following in vivo lung reperfusion. *Am J Respir Crit Care Med* 162:2287–2294, 2000.
122. Kregenow DA, Rubenfeld GD, Hudson LD, et al: Hypercapnic acidosis and mortality in acute lung injury. *Crit Care Med* 34:1–7, 2006.
123. Bilek AM, Dee KC, Gaver DP III: Mechanisms of surface-tension-induced epithelial cell damage in a model of pulmonary airway reopening. *J Appl Physiol* 94:770–783, 2003.
124. Hubmayr RD, ed: *Pulmonary micromechanics of injured lungs.* New York: Taylor & Francis; 2006.

125. Lachmann B: Open up the lung and keep the lung open. *Intensive Care Med* 18:319–321, 1992.
126. Muscedere JG, Mullen JB, Gan K, et al: Tidal ventilation at low airway pressures can augment lung injury. *Am J Respir Crit Care Med* 149:1327–1334, 1994.
127. Petrof BJ, Legare M, Goldberg P, et al: Continuous positive airway pressure reduces work of breathing and dyspnea during weaning from mechanical ventilation in severe chronic obstructive pulmonary disease. *Am Rev Respir Dis* 141:281–289, 1990.
128. Barbas CS, de Matos GF, Pincelli MP, et al: Mechanical ventilation in acute respiratory failure: recruitment and high positive end-expiratory pressure are necessary. *Curr Opin Crit Care* 11:18–28, 2005.
129. Masip J, Roque M, Sanchez B, et al: Noninvasive ventilation in acute cardiogenic pulmonary edema: systematic review and meta-analysis. *JAMA* 294:3124–3130, 2005.
130. Malo J, Ali J, Wood LD: How does positive end-expiratory pressure reduce intrapulmonary shunt in canine pulmonary edema? *J Appl Physiol* 57:1002–1010, 1984.
131. Amato MB, Barbas CS, Medeiros DM, et al: Effect of a protective-ventilation strategy on mortality in the acute respiratory distress syndrome. *N Engl J Med* 338:347–354, 1998.
132. Marini JJ: Ventilator-induced airway dysfunction? *Am J Respir Crit Care Med* 163:806–807, 2001.
133. Ranieri VM, Suter PM, Tortorella C, et al: Effect of mechanical ventilation on inflammatory mediators in patients with acute respiratory distress syndrome: a randomized controlled trial. *JAMA* 282:54–61, 1999.
134. Tremblay L, Valenza F, Ribeiro SP, et al: Injurious ventilatory strategies increase cytokines and c-fos m-RNA expression in an isolated rat lung model. *J Clin Invest* 99:944–952, 1997.
135. Gattinoni L, D'Andrea L, Pelosi P, et al: Regional effects and mechanism of positive end-expiratory pressure in early adult respiratory distress syndrome. *JAMA* 269:2122–2127, 1993.
136. Gattinoni L, Pelosi P, Crotti S, et al: Effects of positive end-expiratory pressure on regional distribution of tidal volume and recruitment in adult respiratory distress syndrome. *Am J Respir Crit Care Med* 151:1807–1814, 1995.
137. Gattinoni L, Pesenti A, Avalli L, et al: Pressure-volume curve of total respiratory system in acute respiratory failure. Computed tomographic scan study. *Am Rev Respir Dis* 136:730–736, 1987.
138. Hickling KG: The pressure-volume curve is greatly modified by recruitment. A mathematical model of ARDS lungs. *Am J Respir Crit Care Med* 158:194–202, 1998.
139. Matamis D, Lemaire F, Harf A, et al: Total respiratory pressure-volume curves in the adult respiratory distress syndrome. *Chest* 86:58–66, 1984.
140. Ranieri VM, Zhang H, Mascia L, et al: Pressure-time curve predicts minimally injurious ventilatory strategy in an isolated rat lung model. *Anesthesiology* 93:1320–1328, 2000.
141. Victorino JA, Borges JB, Okamoto VN, et al: Imbalances in regional lung ventilation: a validation study on electrical impedance tomography. *Am J Respir Crit Care Med* 169:791–800, 2004.
142. Gattinoni L, Caironi P, Cressoni M, et al: Lung recruitment in patients with the acute respiratory distress syndrome. *N Engl J Med* 354:1775–1786, 2006.
143. Vieira SR, Puybasset L, Richecoeur J, et al: A lung computed tomographic assessment of positive end-expiratory pressure-induced lung overdistension. *Am J Respir Crit Care Med* 158:1571–1577, 1998.
144. Grasso S, Terragni P, Mascia L, et al: Airway pressure-time curve profile (stress index) detects tidal recruitment/hyperinflation in experimental acute lung injury. *Crit Care Med* 32:1018–1027, 2004.
145. Gattinoni L, Pelosi P, Suter PM, et al: Acute respiratory distress syndrome caused by pulmonary and extrapulmonary disease. Different syndromes? *Am J Respir Crit Care Med* 158:3–11, 1998.
146. Thille AW, Richard JC, Maggiore SM, et al: Alveolar recruitment in pulmonary and extrapulmonary acute respiratory distress syndrome: comparison using pressure-volume curve or static compliance. *Anesthesiology* 106:212–217, 2007.
147. Mercat A, Richard JC, Vielle B, et al: Positive end-expiratory pressure setting in adults with acute lung injury and acute respiratory distress syndrome: a randomized controlled trial. *JAMA* 299:646–655, 2008.
148. Brower RG, Lanken PN, MacIntyre N, et al: Higher versus lower positive end-expiratory pressures in patients with the acute respiratory distress syndrome. *N Engl J Med* 351:327–336, 2004.
149. Meade MO, Cook DJ, Guyatt GH, et al: Ventilation strategy using low tidal volumes, recruitment maneuvers, and high positive end-expiratory pressure for acute lung injury and acute respiratory distress syndrome: a randomized controlled trial. *JAMA* 299:637–645, 2008.
150. Marini JJ: Lessons learned: the conditional importance of high positive end-expiratory pressure in acute respiratory distress syndrome. *Crit Care Med* 34:1540–1542, 2006.
151. Parshuram CS, Kavanagh BP: Positive clinical trials: understand the control group before implementing the result. *Am J Respir Crit Care Med* 170:223–226, 2004.
152. Caironi P, Cressoni M, Chiumello D, et al: Lung opening and closing during ventilation of acute respiratory distress syndrome. *Am J Respir Crit Care Med* 181(6):528–530, 2010.
153. Putensen C, Theuerkauf N, Zinserling J, et al: Meta-analysis: ventilation strategies and outcomes of the acute respiratory distress syndrome and acute lung injury. *Ann Intern Med* 151:566–576, 2009.
154. Oba Y, Thameem DM, Zaza T: High levels of PEEP may improve survival in acute respiratory distress syndrome: a meta-analysis. *Respir Med* 103:1174–1181, 2009.
155. Broseghini C, Brandolese R, Poggi R, et al: Respiratory resistance and intrinsic positive end-expiratory pressure (PEEPi) in patients with the adult respiratory distress syndrome (ARDS). *Eur Respir J* 1:726–731, 1988.
156. Argiras EP, Blakeley CR, Dunnill MS, et al: High PEEP decreases hyaline membrane formation in surfactant deficient lungs. *Br J Anaesth* 59:1278–1285, 1987.
157. Webb HH, Tierney DF: Experimental pulmonary edema due to intermittent positive pressure ventilation with high inflation pressures. Protection by positive end-expiratory pressure. *Am Rev Respir Dis* 110:556–565, 1974.
158. Fessler HE: Heart-lung interactions: applications in the critically ill. *Eur Respir J* 10:226–237, 1997.
159. Jardin F, Vieillard-Baron A. Monitoring of right-sided heart function. *Curr Opin Crit Care* 11:271–279, 2005.
160. Nielsen J, Ostergaard M, Kjaergaard J, et al: Lung recruitment maneuver depresses central hemodynamics in patients following cardiac surgery. *Intensive Care Med* 31:1189–1194, 2005.
161. Jardin F, Vieillard-Baron A: Right ventricular function and positive pressure ventilation in clinical practice: from hemodynamic subsets to respirator settings. *Intensive Care Med* 29:1426–1434, 2003.
162. Sladen A, Laver MB, Pontoppidan H: Pulmonary complications and water retention in prolonged mechanical ventilation. *N Engl J Med* 279:448–453, 1968.
163. Johnson EE, Hedley-Whyte J: Continuous positive-pressure ventilation and portal flow in dogs with pulmonary edema. *J Appl Physiol* 33:385–389, 1972.
164. Dorinsky PM, Hamlin RL, Gadek JE: Alterations in regional blood flow during positive end-expiratory pressure ventilation. *Crit Care Med* 15:106–113, 1987.
165. Michard F, Boussat S, Chemla D, et al: Relation between respiratory changes in arterial pulse pressure and fluid responsiveness in septic patients with acute circulatory failure. *Am J Respir Crit Care Med* 162:134–138, 2000.
166. Sandham JD, Hull RD, Brant RF, et al: A randomized, controlled trial of the use of pulmonary-artery catheters in high-risk surgical patients. *N Engl J Med* 348:5–14, 2003.
167. Wiedemann HP, Wheeler AP, Bernard GR, et al: Comparison of two fluid-management strategies in acute lung injury. *N Engl J Med* 354:2564–2575, 2006.
168. Martin JG, Shore S, Engel LA: Effect of continuous positive airway pressure on respiratory mechanics and pattern of breathing in induced asthma. *Am Rev Respir Dis* 126:812–817, 1982.
169. Quan SF, Falltrick RT, Schlobohm RM: Extubation from ambient or expiratory positive airway pressure in adults. *Anesthesiology* 55:53–56, 1981.
170. Dammann JF, McAslan TC: PEEP: its use in young patients with apparently normal lungs. *Crit Care Med* 7:14–19, 1979.
171. Weisman IM, Rinaldo JE, Rogers RM: Current concepts: positive end-expiratory pressure in adult respiratory failure. *N Engl J Med* 307:1381–1384, 1982.
172. Good JT Jr, Wolz JF, Anderson JT, et al: The routine use of positive end-expiratory pressure after open heart surgery. *Chest* 76:397–400, 1979.
173. Svantesson C, Sigurdsson S, Larsson A, et al: Effects of recruitment of collapsed lung units on the elastic pressure-volume relationship in anaesthetised healthy adults. *Acta Anaesthesiol Scand* 42:1149–1156, 1998.
174. Hedenstierna G, Rothen HU: Atelectasis formation during anesthesia: causes and measures to prevent it. *J Clin Monit Comput* 16:329–335, 2000.
175. Rusca M, Proietti S, Schnyder P, et al: Prevention of atelectasis formation during induction of general anesthesia. *Anesth Analg* 97:1835–1839, 2003.
176. Squadrone V, Coha M, Cerutti E, et al: Continuous positive airway pressure for treatment of postoperative hypoxemia: a randomized controlled trial. *JAMA* 293:589–595, 2005.
177. Juan G, Calverley P, Talamo C, et al: Effect of carbon dioxide on diaphragmatic function in human beings. *N Engl J Med* 310:874–879, 1984.
178. Tuxen DV, Williams TJ, Scheinkestel CD, et al: Use of a measurement of pulmonary hyperinflation to control the level of mechanical ventilation in patients with acute severe asthma. *Am Rev Respir Dis* 146:1136–1142, 1992.
179. Williams TJ, Tuxen DV, Scheinkestel CD, et al: Risk factors for morbidity in mechanically ventilated patients with acute severe asthma. *Am Rev Respir Dis* 146:607–615, 1992.
180. Gluck EH, Onorato DJ, Castriotta R: Helium-oxygen mixtures in intubated patients with status asthmaticus and respiratory acidosis. *Chest* 98:693–698, 1990.
181. Jaber S, Fodil R, Carlucci A, et al: Noninvasive ventilation with helium-oxygen in acute exacerbations of chronic obstructive pulmonary disease. *Am J Respir Crit Care Med* 161:1191–1200, 2000.
182. Marini JJ: Heliox in chronic obstructive pulmonary disease . . . time to lighten up? *Crit Care Med* 28:3086–3088, 2000.
183. Tassaux D, Jolliet P, Roeseler J, et al: Effects of helium-oxygen on intrinsic positive end-expiratory pressure in intubated and mechanically ventilated patients with severe chronic obstructive pulmonary disease. *Crit Care Med* 28:2721–2728, 2000.

184. Leatherman JW, Ravenscraft SA: Low measured auto-positive end-expiratory pressure during mechanical ventilation of patients with severe asthma: hidden auto-positive end-expiratory pressure. *Crit Care Med* 24:541–546, 1996.
185. Veldhuizen RA, Welk B, Harbottle R, et al: Mechanical ventilation of isolated rat lungs changes the structure and biophysical properties of surfactant. *J Appl Physiol* 92:1169–1175, 2002.
186. Veldhuizen RA, Yao LJ, Lewis JF: An examination of the different variables affecting surfactant aggregate conversion in vitro. *Exp Lung Res* 25:127–141, 1999.
187. Wyszogrodski I, Kyei-Aboagye K, Taeusch HW Jr, et al: Surfactant inactivation by hyperventilation: conservation by end-expiratory pressure. *J Appl Physiol* 38:461–466, 1975.
188. Mascheroni D, Kolobow T, Fumagalli R, et al: Acute respiratory failure following pharmacologically induced hyperventilation: an experimental animal study. *Intensive Care Med* 15:8–14, 1988.
189. Gajic O, Dara SI, Mendez JL, et al: Ventilator-associated lung injury in patients without acute lung injury at the onset of mechanical ventilation. *Crit Care Med* 32:1817–1824, 2004.
190. Gattinoni L, Tognoni G, Pesenti A, et al: Effect of prone positioning on the survival of patients with acute respiratory failure. *N Engl J Med* 345:568–573, 2001.
191. Guerin C, Gaillard S, Lemasson S, et al: Effects of systematic prone positioning in hypoxemic acute respiratory failure: a randomized controlled trial. *JAMA* 292:2379–2387, 2004.
192. Mancebo J, Fernandez R, Blanch L, et al: A multicenter trial of prolonged prone ventilation in severe acute respiratory distress syndrome. *Am J Respir Crit Care Med* 173:1233–1239, 2006.
193. Taccone P, Pesenti A, Latini R, et al: Prone positioning in patients with moderate and severe acute respiratory distress syndrome: a randomized controlled trial. *JAMA* 302:1977–1984, 2009.
194. Davies A, Jones D, Bailey M, et al: Extracorporeal Membrane Oxygenation for 2009 Influenza A (H1N1) Acute Respiratory Distress Syndrome. *JAMA* 302:1888–1895, 2009.
195. Dominguez-Cherit G, Lapinsky SE, Macias AE, et al: Critically Ill patients with 2009 influenza A(H1N1) in Mexico. *JAMA* 302:1880–1887, 2009.
196. Jain S, Kamimoto L, Bramley AM, et al: Hospitalized patients with 2009 H1N1 influenza in the United States, April-June 2009. *N Engl J Med* 361:1935–1944, 2009.
197. Peek GJ, Mugford M, Tiruvoipati R, et al: Efficacy and economic assessment of conventional ventilatory support versus extracorporeal membrane oxygenation for severe adult respiratory failure (CESAR): a multicentre randomised controlled trial. *Lancet* 374:1351–1363, 2009.
198. Stocchetti N, Maas AI, Chieregato A, et al: Hyperventilation in head injury: a review. *Chest* 127:1812–1827, 2005.
199. Muizelaar JP, Marmarou A, Ward JD, et al: Adverse effects of prolonged hyperventilation in patients with severe head injury: a randomized clinical trial. *J Neurosurg* 75:731–739, 1991.
200. McGuire G, Crossley D, Richards J, et al: Effects of varying levels of positive end-expiratory pressure on intracranial pressure and cerebral perfusion pressure. *Crit Care Med* 25:1059–1062, 1997.
201. Muench E, Bauhuf C, Roth H, et al: Effects of positive end-expiratory pressure on regional cerebral blood flow, intracranial pressure, and brain tissue oxygenation. *Crit Care Med* 33:2367–2372, 2005.
202. Lee ST: Intracranial pressure changes during positioning of patients with severe head injury. *Heart Lung* 18:411–414, 1989.
203. Aubier M, Trippenbach T, Roussos C: Respiratory muscle fatigue during cardiogenic shock. *J Appl Physiol* 51:499–508, 1981.
204. Richard C, Teboul JL, Archambaud F, et al: Left ventricular function during weaning of patients with chronic obstructive pulmonary disease. *Intensive Care Med* 20:181–186, 1994.
205. Srivastava S, Chatila W, Amoateng-Adjepong Y, et al: Myocardial ischemia and weaning failure in patients with coronary artery disease: an update. *Crit Care Med* 27:2109–2112, 1999.
206. Lemaire F, Teboul JL, Cinotti L, et al: Acute left ventricular dysfunction during unsuccessful weaning from mechanical ventilation. *Anesthesiology* 69:171–179, 1988.
207. Campbell LA, Klocke RA: Implications for the pregnant patient. *Am J Respir Crit Care Med* 163:1051–1054, 2001.
208. Carrion MI, Ayuso D, Marcos M, et al: Accidental removal of endotracheal and nasogastric tubes and intravascular catheters. *Crit Care Med* 28:63–66, 2000.
209. Epstein SK, Ciubotaru RL: Independent effects of etiology of failure and time to reintubation on outcome for patients failing extubation. *Am J Respir Crit Care Med* 158:489–493, 1998.
210. Epstein SK, Nevins ML, Chung J: Effect of unplanned extubation on outcome of mechanical ventilation. *Am J Respir Crit Care Med* 161:1912–1916, 2000.
211. Rana S, Pendem S, Pogodzinski MS, et al: Tracheostomy in critically ill patients. *Mayo Clin Proc* 80:1632–1638, 2005.
212. Hawe CS, Ellis KS, Cairns CJ, et al: Reduction of ventilator-associated pneumonia: active versus passive guideline implementation. *Intensive Care Med* 35:1180–1186, 2009.
213. Miller RS, Norris PR, Jenkins JM, et al: Systems initiatives reduce healthcare-associated infections: a study of 22,928 device days in a single trauma unit. *J Trauma* 68(1):23–31, 2010.
214. Bigham MT, Amato R, Bondurrant P, et al: Ventilator-associated pneumonia in the pediatric intensive care unit: characterizing the problem and implementing a sustainable solution. *J Pediatr* 154:582–587, e582, 2009.
215. Mead J, Takishima T, Leith D: Stress distribution in lungs: a model of pulmonary elasticity. *J Appl Physiol* 28:596–608, 1970.
216. Zwillich CW, Pierson DJ, Creagh CE, et al: Complications of assisted ventilation. A prospective study of 354 consecutive episodes. *Am J Med* 57:161–170, 1974.
217. Menitove SM, Goldring RM: Combined ventilator and bicarbonate strategy in the management of status asthmaticus. *Am J Med* 74:898–901, 1983.
218. Albelda SM, Gefter WB, Kelley MA, et al: Ventilator-induced subpleural air cysts: clinical, radiographic, and pathologic significance. *Am Rev Respir Dis* 127:360–365, 1983.
219. Haake R, Schlichtig R, Ulstad DR, et al: Barotrauma. Pathophysiology, risk factors, and prevention. *Chest* 91:608–613, 1987.

CHAPTER 59 ■ MECHANICAL VENTILATION PART II: NON-INVASIVE MECHANICAL VENTILATION FOR THE ADULT HOSPITALIZED PATIENT

SAMY S. SIDHOM AND NICHOLAS HILL

INTRODUCTION

Noninvasive ventilation (NIV) is the provision of mechanical ventilation without the need for an invasive artificial airway. NIV can be subdivided into a number of modalities with different mechanisms of action, including negative pressure ventilation that assists lung expansion by applying an intermittent negative pressure over the chest and abdomen, positive pressure ventilation that applies continuous or intermittent positive pressure to the upper airway, and abdominal displacement ventilators like pneumobelts and rocking beds that assist ventilation at least partly via the force of gravity on the abdominal contents [1–3]. Over the past two decades, noninvasive positive pressure ventilation (NPPV) [4] via the nose, mouth, or combination has become the predominant mode of NIV in both the outpatient and hospital settings.

In this chapter, we focus on acute applications, comparing and contrasting noninvasive and invasive approaches and describing epidemiologic trends of NIV. Next, we describe the equipment used for NPPV and discuss indications and selection of patients for NPPV in the acute care setting. We then make recommendation regarding the practical and safe application of NPPV, including selecting the proper location, appropriate monitoring, and avoiding complications. Finally, we consider the impact on global patient outcomes as well as health care and hospital quality measures.

TERMINOLOGY

As used in this chapter, NIV is a generic term for a number of different noninvasive approaches to assisting ventilation, whereas NPPV refers specifically to the form that facilitates ventilation by applying a positive pressure to the upper airway. This can be continuous positive airway pressure (CPAP) that can be used to successfully treat certain forms of respiratory failure or intermittent, combining a positive end-expiratory pressure (PEEP) with pressure support (PS), the latter used to actively assist inspiration. Some ventilators are derived from portable positive pressure devices to treat sleep apnea and are commonly referred to as bilevel positive airway pressure (BPAP) devices. With these, the term expiratory positive airway pressure (EPAP) is used rather than PEEP and inspiratory positive airway pressure (IPAP) refers to the total inspiratory pressure. Thus, the difference between IPAP and EPAP equals the level of pressure support.

WHY NONINVASIVE MECHANICAL VENTILATION

NIV has seen increasing popularity in acute care settings throughout Europe and the United States over the past two decades [5,6]. This trend is related to a number of advantages of NPPV over invasive mechanical ventilation, but only in select patients. By averting invasion of the upper airway, NIV avoids a number of well-known complications of intubation, including aspiration of gastric contents, dental trauma, trauma to the hypopharynx, larynx, and trachea including tracheal rupture [7], hypoglossal nerve paralysis, autonomic stimulation leading to arrhythmias, and hypotension [8].

Ongoing use of invasive ventilation increases the risk of ventilator-associated pneumonia (VAP) related to disruption of airway protective mechanisms, pooling of secretions above the tube cuff that leak into the lower airways, and formation of a bacterial biofilm within the tube that is distributed peripherally with suctioning. In addition, irritation from the tube stimulates mucus secretion and interferes with normal ciliary function. The need for repeated suctioning further traumatizes the airway and promotes bleeding and mucus secretion. Following extubation, immediate complications include upper airway obstruction due to glottic swelling, negative pressure pulmonary edema, tracheal hemorrhage, and laryngospasm [9,10]. Complications of prolonged invasive ventilation (in association with tracheostomy) include a spectrum of repeated airway and parenchymal infections, vocal cord dysfunction, and tracheal stenosis and malacia [4,11–14].

In addition, NPPV is usually better tolerated than invasive ventilation, requiring less or no sedation. It usually permits short breaks that help to enhance tolerance. The avoidance of intubation-associated complications and sedation promotes more rapid weaning compared to invasive ventilation, shortening ICU stays and potentially reducing resource utilization and costs.

On the other hand, NPPV should not be considered as a replacement for invasive mechanical ventilation. When used appropriately, NPPV serves as a way to avoid intubation and its attendant complications, but it must be used selectively, avoiding patients who have contraindications (see "Selection Guidelines for NPPV in Acute Respiratory Failure" section). Appropriate candidates must be able to protect their airways and cooperate. Sometimes, NPPV is initiated in inappropriate or marginal candidates who fail to respond favorably. In this situation, it is important to intubate promptly, avoiding delays that can lead to cardiopulmonary arrest, necessitating emergency intubation and increased morbidity and mortality [15].

UTILIZATION AND EPIDEMIOLOGY

Rates of NPPV utilization in acute care settings are increasing in Europe and North America [16,17]. An observational study of NIV utilization for chronic obstructive pulmonary disease (COPD) and cardiogenic pulmonary edema (CPE) patients in acute respiratory failure (ARF) in a single 26-bed French intensive care unit (ICU) revealed an increase from 20% of ventilator starts in 1994 to nearly 90% in 2001 [17]. In association with this increase, the occurrence of healthcare-acquired pneumonias and ICU mortality fell from 20% and 21% to 8% and 7%, respectively. The authors speculated that increasing experience and skill with NPPV in their units contributed to the improved outcomes. In an Italian study examining outcomes of NPPV in two different time periods during the 1990s, success rates remained steady despite an increase in acuity of illness scores, suggesting sicker patients in the later time period were being managed as successfully as less ill patients in the earlier period, a trend the authors attributed to increased skill of the caregivers [16].

Sequential surveys of European (mainly French) ICUs demonstrated an increase in the use of NIV as a percentage of total ventilator starts from 16% to 23% in 1997 and 2002, respectively, with utilization in patients with COPD and CPE increasing from 50% to 66% and from 38% to 47%, respectively [6]. Esteban et al. conducted a worldwide survey in more than 20 countries that compared the trends of mechanical ventilation use and demographics between 1998 and 2004, enrolling more than 1,600 patients and showing an overall increase of about 6% (11.1% from 4.4%) in NIV use [15]. In Italy, Confalonieri et al. reported high utilization rates of NIV in specialized respiratory intensive care units (RICUs) which are similar to "intermediate" or "step-down" units in the United States, where a large proportion of patients have COPD either as an etiology of ARF or as a comorbidity. In that setting, 425 out of 586 (72.5%) patients requiring mechanical ventilation were treated initially with NIV (374 using NPPV and 51 using an "iron lung") [18].

However, in a 2003 national audit of COPD exacerbations in the United Kingdom, NIV was unavailable in 19 of 233 hospitals and 39% of ICUs, 36% of "high-dependency units," and 34% of hospital wards [19]. Similar results were seen in a North American survey of NIV use in 71 hospitals in Massachusetts and Rhode Island [20]. Overall use of NPPV was estimated to be 20% of all ventilator starts, but 30% of hospitals had estimated rates <15%. Reasons for low utilization were mostly attributed to lack of physician knowledge of NPPV, inadequate equipment, and lack of staff training. Most disturbingly, estimated use of NIV for COPD exacerbations and CPE was only 29% and 39% of ventilator starts, respectively

[20]. A follow-up study in Massachusetts using data collected prospectively from 2005 to 2007 revealed an overall 38.7% NIV utilization rate, with 80% and 69% of COPD and CPE patients, respectively, receiving NIV as the initial mode [21].

A national survey of U.S. Department of Veterans Affairs hospitals showed that despite wide availability of NIV, its perceived use was low. Almost two-thirds of respiratory therapists responding to the survey felt that NIV was used less than half the time when it was indicated. The survey also revealed wide variations in the perception of NIV use depending on the size of the ICUs, larger ones reporting more frequent use [22]. Along these lines, a Canadian study reported that between 1998 and 2003, only 66% of patients meeting criteria for NPPV actually received it [23].

Suboptimal utilization has been reported in non-Western countries as well. A Korean survey reported that NIV was used in just 2 of 24 university hospitals and comprised only 4% of ventilator starts. A majority of the physician staff (62%) and 42% of the nurses expressed a desire for additional educational programs on NIV [24]. In an Indian survey of 648 physicians, perceived NIV use was mostly limited to the ICU (68.4%) while COPD was the most common indication for its use [25]. Findings of this survey were similar to those of the Korean, European, and North American surveys in that rates of NIV use varied widely between centers, with a substantial portion reporting low rates. These findings underline the need for NIV educational programs at individual hospitals that permit caregivers to develop the requisite expertise in administering NIV.

INDICATIONS FOR ACUTE APPLICATIONS OF NPPV

Indications for NPPV depend on the etiology of ARF and specific settings in which ARF occurs [i.e., do-not-intubate (DNI) patients]. As much as possible, our analysis is based on available evidence. We recommend application of NPPV for those diagnoses that are those supported by multiple randomized trials. We consider NPPV as an "option" when the application is supported by a single randomized trial, multiple historically controlled or cohort series, or sometimes conflicting evidence. Successful application of NPPV has been reported for all of these indications if applied in appropriately selected and monitored patients (Table 59.1).

Recommended Indications

Chronic Obstructive Pulmonary Disease

COPD Exacerbations. The best established acute indication for NPPV is to treat ARF due to COPD exacerbations. This is supported by a strong physiologic rationale. Studies demonstrate that the combinations of extrinsic PEEP and PS alone reduce diaphragmatic work of breathing more than either modality alone, because the expiratory pressure counterbalances intrinsic PEEP and the higher inspiratory pressure (pressure support) actively assists the inspiratory muscles [26]. In the setting of COPD exacerbations, NPPV thereby serves as a "crutch" to assist ventilation while medical therapy is given time to work.

Multiple randomized controlled trials (RCTs) and meta-analyses on COPD patients with ARF have established that NIV more rapidly reduces respiratory rate, improves dyspnea and gas exchange, reduces intubations from an average rate of 50% to 20%, and lowers mortality compared to standard therapy [5,27–32]. This evidence justifies the early use of NPPV for COPD exacerbations as a standard of care unless there are

TABLE 59.1

INDICATIONS FOR NONINVASIVE POSITIVE PRESSURE VENTILATION AS DETERMINED BY STRENGTH OF EVIDENCE

Recommended (supported by strong evidence[a])
COPD exacerbations
COPD—failure to wean from invasive mechanical ventilation
Acute cardiogenic pulmonary edema
Immunosuppressed patients with acute respiratory failure
Option (supported by weaker evidence[b])
Other obstructive airway diseases with acute respiratory failure
Asthma exacerbation
Cystic fibrosis
Hypoxemic respiratory failure[c]
ALI/ARDS
Community-acquired pneumonia
Trauma
Extubation failure
Mainly patients with COPD or congestive heart failure (CHF)
Postoperative respiratory failure
Prophylactic use of CPAP or "bilevel" after high-risk surgeries
Treatment of acute respiratory failure—mainly COPD or CHF
Do-not-intubate patients
To treat acute respiratory failure (COPD or CHF)
To palliate for relief of dyspnea or extend survival to settle affairs
Obesity hypoventilation
Neuromuscular disease
Partial upper airway obstruction (postextubation)
Not recommended
ALI/ARDS with multiorgan system dysfunction or hypotensive shock
End-stage pulmonary fibrosis with exacerbation
Total or near total upper airway obstruction

[a]Strong evidence refers to multiple randomized controlled trials and meta-analyses.
[b]Weaker evidence refers to mainly case series, case-matched series, single randomized trials, or some conflicting data.
[c]Must be monitored very carefully—not a routine indication.
ALI/ARDS, acute lung injury/acute respiratory distress syndrome.

contraindications. COPD exacerbations also respond well to NPPV when complicated by pneumonia [33] or occurring in the setting of a DNI status [34–36], or postoperative or postextubation respiratory failure [37,38].

Facilitation of Weaning in COPD Patients. Some patients with COPD exacerbations require intubation because they are not candidates for NPPV initially or fail a trial of NPPV. Multiple controlled trials have demonstrated that NIV permits earlier extubation in such patients, even if they have failed multiple "T" piece weaning trials [39–41]. Early extubation to NIV increases eventual weaning rates, shortens the duration of ventilator use and hospital length of stay (LOS), reduces the occurrence of nosocomial pneumonia, and reduces mortality. This approach should be considered whenever intubated COPD patients are failing spontaneous breathing trials, but it should be used with caution—only in a patient who is otherwise an excellent candidate for NIV, can breathe without any assistance for at least 5 minutes, can tolerate levels of pressure support deliverable by mask (i.e., inspiratory pressure <20 cm H_2O), and is not a "difficult intubation."

Cardiogenic Pulmonary Edema

Positive airway pressure has well-known therapeutic effects in patients with acute pulmonary edema. The increased functional residual capacity opens collapsed alveoli and rapidly improves compliance and oxygenation. The increased intrathoracic pressure reduces transmyocardial pressure and has preload and afterload reducing effects, thus enhancing cardiac function in patients with left ventricular dysfunction who are afterload-dependent.

Multiple RCTs have demonstrated that noninvasive CPAP (10 to 12.5 cm H_2O) alone dramatically improves dyspnea and oxygenation and lowers intubation rates in patients with acute pulmonary edema compared with standard O_2 therapy [17,42,43]. Subsequent studies evaluating the efficacy of NPPV (i.e., pressure support plus PEEP or BPAP) either compared with O_2 therapy or CPAP alone [44–46] have shown benefits similar to those previously demonstrated for CPAP. In one large RCT [47], CPAP and NPPV performed similarly, both improving dyspnea scores and pH more rapidly than oxygen alone, but neither lowered intubation nor mortality rate (the major outcome variable) compared to controls. However, the intubation rate in this study was slightly below 3% in all of the groups, including controls, suggesting that the enrolled patients were too mildly ill to manifest a significant mortality benefit.

Meta-analyses of the RCTs on CPAP or NPPV compared with O_2 therapy alone have confirmed the benefits described above, even showing a significant reduction in mortality with CPAP [48,49]. Meta-analyses comparing the two modalities show equivalency of NPPV and CPAP with regard to reduction of intubation, lengths of stay, and mortality, and with no increase in the myocardial infarction rate attributable to NPPV use [50]. However, some studies have found that NPPV reduces dyspnea and improves gas exchange more rapidly than CPAP alone [44,51]. Therefore, by virtue of its greater simplicity and potentially lower cost, CPAP alone is generally regarded as the initial noninvasive modality of choice for cardiogenic edema patients, but NPPV is substituted if patients treated initially with CPAP remain dyspneic or hypercapnic. The strong evidence favoring the use of CPAP or NPPV to treat CPE establishes either one as standard therapy for initial ventilatory assistance of appropriately selected CPE patients.

The success of noninvasive positive pressure to treat CPE has encouraged its extension into the prehospital setting. An emerging trend is to provide CPAP devices on ambulances for initial therapy of CPE. The experience thus far with this practice has been favorable. Plaisance et al. [52] observed a strong trend for reduced intubation and mortality rates among 124 CPE patients randomized to "early" (started immediately on site) versus "late" (delayed by 15 minutes) CPAP (7.5 cm H_2O). In another RCT, Thompson et al. observed an absolute reduction of 30% in intubation rate (17 out of 34 patients, or 50% vs. 7/35 or 20%, unadjusted OR = 0.25 and CI = 0.09 to 0.73) and 21% in mortality (OR 0.3; 95% CI 0.09 to 0.99) among CPE patients treated with CPAP compared to usual therapy with oxygen, including intubation and bag-valve-mask-ventilation if needed [53].

A pilot study by Duchateau et al. reported an improved respiratory status in 12 "do not intubate" (DNI) patients when offered NPPV out-of-hospital by emergency medical services (EMS). Respiratory rate decreased from 34 to 27 per minute, $p = 0.009$, and pulse oximetry improved from 86% to 94%, $p < 0.01$, with only one intolerant patient [54]. These studies suggest that outcomes of CPE patients can be improved by very early initiation of noninvasive positive pressure therapy in the field and adoption of this as a routine practice for EMS seems likely.

Immunodeficient Patients with Acute Respiratory Failure

Patients developing ARF with underlying immunodeficiency states such as human immunodeficiency virus and Pneumocystis pneumonia or following solid organ or bone marrow transplantation have poor outcomes when treated with invasive mechanical ventilation [55]. Nosocomial infections and fatal septicemia are common complications, and those with hematologic malignancies may encounter fatal airway hemorrhages due to upper airway trauma occurring with intubation in patients with thrombocytopenia and platelet dysfunction. NIV offers a way to avoid such complications and improve outcomes.

Randomized trials of NIV in patients with ARF who have undergone solid organ transplantation or bone marrow transplant for hematologic malignancy have demonstrated reduced intubation and mortality rates compared with controls [56–59]. NIV was begun in these patients before respiratory failure became severe, and even then the mortality rate in the NIV group in one study was 50% compared with 80% in the conventionally treated group [58]. Thus, NIV should be considered early during the development of respiratory failure in immunodeficient patients as a way to avoid intubation and its attendant morbidity and mortality [57].

WEAKER INDICATIONS—NPPV IS AN OPTION

NPPV can be used to treat ARF of other etiologies and in other settings, but the evidence to support these applications is weaker and use is optional but not necessarily recommended (Table 59.1).

Other Obstructive Diseases

Asthma Exacerbations

Retrospective cohort studies suggest that NPPV improves gas exchange and avoids intubation in patients with respiratory failure caused by asthma exacerbations [60,61]. However, there are only two randomized trials supporting the use of NPPV for this indication. In one RCT, NPPV improved FEV_1 more rapidly and reduced the hospitalization rate compared with sham controls [62]. The second study [63] reported similar findings with "high" inflation pressures compared to lower pressures (IPAP and EPAP 8 and 6 cm H_2O and 6 and 4 cm H_2O, respectively—all lower than most other studies) or standard medical therapy. Neither study was powered to examine intubation rates or mortality.

Pollack et al. demonstrated that NPPV is an acceptable way to deliver bronchodilator aerosol, showing a greater improvement in peak expiratory flow 1 hour after administration via a "bilevel" device than a standard nebulizer [64]. These studies suggest that when NPPV is used as an early treatment for asthma exacerbations, it can potentiate the bronchodilator effect of beta-agonists. However, in most clinical situations, NPPV is reserved for patients with "status asthmaticus," that is, those with severe airway obstruction who are not responding adequately to initial bronchodilator therapy, an application that is not yet supported by RCTs.

Cystic Fibrosis

Ideally, NPPV is initiated in patients with cystic fibrosis when they develop chronic respiratory failure before an acute crisis arises. For patients with acute exacerbations of cystic fibrosis, NPPV has been used mainly as a bridge to transplantation [65].

These patients may remain severely hypercapnic and require aggressive management of secretion retention, but NPPV permits avoidance of intubation and can sustain them for months while they await availability of donor organs.

Hypoxemic Respiratory Failure

Hypoxemic respiratory failure consists of severe hypoxemia (PaO_2/FIO_2 <200), severe respiratory distress, tachypnea (>30 per minute), and a non-COPD cause of ARF such as ARDS, acute pneumonia, trauma, or acute pulmonary edema [66]. Some RCTs on hypoxemic respiratory failure have observed reductions in the need for intubation, shortened ICU lengths of stay, and even mortality in the NIV group as opposed to controls [66,67], but it is difficult to draw firm conclusions about individual diagnostic groups within this very broad category. One concern is that favorable responses in one subgroup, such as those with CPE, could obscure unfavorable responses in another, such as ARDS or pneumonia patients.

Among studies examining subcategories specifically, Jolliet et al. found very high NPPV failure rates (>60%) in a cohort series of patients with severe community-acquired pneumonia [68]. Confalonieri et al. [33] found that NPPV reduced the need for intubation, shortened ICU LOS, and improved 90-day mortality in a RCT of patients with severe community-acquired pneumonia. However, these benefits were seen only in the COPD subgroup—not in non-COPD patients. Thus, no convincing evidence supports the use of NPPV over invasive ventilation in patients with severe community-acquired pneumonia lacking COPD, and although NPPV remains an option in such patients, it should be used only in carefully selected and monitored patients, with preparedness to intubate promptly if they are not responding well within an hour of NPPV initiation.

The situation with ARDS (which overlaps with severe community-acquired pneumonia) is quite similar, but no RCTs have been performed on the use of NPPV for ARDS per se. Small case series have suggested benefit [69], and in one interesting study that used NPPV as a "first-line" therapy for ARDS, the successful use of NPPV was associated with much lower ventilator-associated pneumonia and mortality rates than in NPPV failures [70]. The authors suggested that an initial simplified acute physiology score (SAPS) II of 34 or less and an improvement of PaO_2/FIO_2 to greater than 176 during the first hour of NPPV therapy could be used to identify patients likely to succeed. However, it is good to remember that this was not an RCT and that only 15% of the patients with ARDS admitted to the ICU (two thirds were intubated prior to ICU admission) actually succeeded with NPPV. Also, in a previous study on risk factors for NPPV failure in patients with hypoxemic respiratory failure, Antonelli et al. observed an odds ratio of 3.75 for ARDS and severe pneumonia [71]. Thus, as with severe pneumonia, NPPV should be used very selectively and cautiously in ARDS patients—only for those with lower acute physiology scores, hemodynamic stability, and good initial improvements in their oxygenation.

Posttrauma Respiratory Failure

Flail chest or mild acute lung injury (ALI) are conditions that are posited to respond favorably to NPPV after traumatic chest wall injuries. Support for this view comes from retrospective studies such as that by Beltrame et al. [72], in which 46 trauma patients with respiratory insufficiency were treated with NPPV and experienced rapid improvements in gas exchange and a 72% success rate, but burn patients responded poorly. More recently, a study that randomized thoracic trauma patients with PAO_2/FIO_2 <200 to NPPV or high flow oxygen was stopped early after enrollment of 50 patients because of significant reductions in intubation rate (12% vs. 40%) and hospital LOS (14 vs. 21 days) in the NPPV group [73]. These results support the use of NPPV for hypoxemic respiratory failure in postthoracic trauma cases, but it is good to remember that these were carefully selected patients.

Extubation Failure

The recurrence of respiratory failure after extubation of patients initially intubated for a bout of ARF is referred to as *extubation failure* and is associated with a high risk of morbidity and mortality (rates exceeding 40% in some studies [74,75]). NPPV has been proposed as a way to avoid extubation failure if begun early in patients at risk for extubation failure, reducing the need for reintubation and improving outcomes. However, some earlier randomized studies [76] comparing NPPV to standard O_2 therapy found no reduction in reintubation attributable to NPPV. In fact, Esteban et al. even found a significantly increased ICU mortality in the NIV group [77]. These studies were limited by low enrollment of COPD patients (only about 10% of patients), and the increased mortality was thought to be related to a 10-hour delay in reintubations in the NIV group compared with controls.

Two subsequent randomized trials [78,79] on patients deemed to be at "high risk" for extubation failure found that NIV reduced the need for reintubation and ICU mortality. Forty to fifty percent of patients in these trials had COPD or CHF and in one of the trials [78], most of the benefit was attributable to the COPD subgroup. Another recent trial focusing on patients with postextubation hypercapnia showed a significant reduction in the occurrence of postextubation respiratory failure as well as 90-day mortality in the group randomized to NPPV compared to oxygen-treated controls [80]. These studies support the use of NIV in patients at *high risk* of extubation failure, particularly if they have COPD, CHF, and/or hypercapnia. However, based on the Esteban study, NPPV to prevent extubation failure should be used very cautiously in at-risk patients who do not have these favorable characteristics because of the higher risk of NPPV failure and its attendant morbidity and mortality. Patients failing to improve promptly with NPPV should be reintubated without delay.

Postoperative Respiratory Failure/Insufficiency

Noninvasive positive pressure techniques, both CPAP and NPPV, have been used in postoperative patients in either of two ways: to prevent complications after high-risk surgeries or to treat frank postoperative respiratory failure. When used prophylactically after major abdominal surgery [81–83] or thoracoabdominal aneurysm repair [84], CPAP (10 cm H_2O) reduces the incidence of hypoxemia, pneumonia, atelectasis, and intubations compared with standard treatment. In the only randomized study of NPPV in patients with postoperative respiratory failure, post–lung resection patients had reduced intubation and mortality rates if treated with NPPV compared with standard management [85]. These studies strongly support the idea that both CPAP and NPPV should be considered to prevent and treat postoperative respiratory complications and failure, but because of the variety of surgeries and positive pressure techniques evaluated, more specific recommendations cannot be made.

Patients with a Do Not Intubate Status

NIV to treat DNI and palliative care patients has been controversial. Some argue that when patients are dying of respiratory failure, there is little to lose by trying NIV. Contrariwise, others counter that this is apt to add to patient discomfort and prolong suffering in a patient's final hours. Prospective cohort series demonstrate that many DNI patients treated with NIV actually survive the hospitalization, depending on the diagnosis [36,86]. In one series, 43% of 114 such patients survived to hospital discharge, 75% of CHF patients, and 53% of COPD patients, whereas hospital survivals for patients with pneumonia or an underlying malignancy had hospital survivals in the range of 25% [36]. The presence of cough, awake mental status, and hypercapnia also imparted a favorable prognosis.

Thus, it is possible to identify, on the basis of the diagnosis and some simple clinical observations, patients with a better than even chance of surviving the hospitalization, and NIV could be used in these patients as a form of life support with the hope of "bridging" them through their acute illness. NIV can also be used for palliation of patients with a poor prognosis for survival of the hospitalization, with the possible aims of alleviating dyspnea or to prolong survival slightly so that the patient has time to settle affairs or say goodbye to loved ones. As recommended by a consensus statement by a Society of Critical Care Medicine task force on NIV, it is necessary for the patient, family, and caregivers to agree on these goals and to cease promptly if NPPV seems to be adding to suffering (via mask discomfort, for example) rather than alleviating it [87].

Other Acute Applications of NPPV

Endoscopic Procedures

In separate randomized trials, CPAP alone (up to 7.5 cm H_2O) or NPPV both improved oxygenation and reduced postprocedure respiratory failure in patients with severe hypoxemia undergoing bronchoscopy compared with those receiving conventional O_2 supplementation [88,89]. The evidence supports the use of NIV to improve gas exchange and reduce potential complications during fiber-optic bronchoscopy, especially when the risk of intubation is deemed high such as in immunocompromised patients or in those with bleeding diatheses. However, patients must be monitored closely and the caregiver team must try to minimize the risk of aspiration and be prepared for the possible need for emergent intubation.

NPPV is also being used for other endoscopic procedures, such as placement of percutaneous gastrostomy tubes in patients with respiratory compromise due to neuromuscular disease and performance of transesophageal echocardiography [90,91].

Preoxygenation Before Intubation

A randomized trial in critically ill patients with hypoxemic respiratory failure showed that preoxygenation with NIV before intubation improved O_2 saturation during and after intubation and decreased the incidence of O_2 desaturations below 80% during intubation [92]. This approach is promising but needs further evaluation before routine use can be recommended. This also begs the question whether, if NIV improves oxygenation substantially, intubation could be avoided in some of these patients.

SELECTION GUIDELINES FOR NPPV IN ACUTE RESPIRATORY FAILURE

Determinants of Success/Failure

Selection of appropriate patients for NPPV is critical for optimizing success and providing benefit. Knowledge of factors that predict success or failure is helpful in selecting good candidates for NPPV. Such factors, compiled from previous studies, are shown in Table 59.2. In effect, the predictors indicate that patients who are most likely to succeed with NIV have incipient, milder respiratory failure than those who fail. This suggests that there is a "window of opportunity" for implementation of NIV when success is most likely. NIV should be started when patients have evidence of acute respiratory distress and increased acute physiology and chronic health evaluation II (APACHE II) scores, but not when patients are approaching respiratory arrest, have severe acidemia, high APACHE II scores, or are unable to cooperate.

TABLE 59.2

PREDICTORS OF NIV FAILURE

Inability to cooperate with therapy or GCS <12
RR >30 and hypoxemia
Severe dyspnea
Excessive accessory muscle or paradoxical breathing
Paradoxical breathing
Hypercapnic respiratory failure with acidemia, pH <7.10
Acute hypoxemic respiratory failure with PaO_2/FIO_2 <100
SAPS II score ≥34 or APACHE II score >29
Age >40 but <70 y
Serum HCO_3 <22
Multiorgan dysfunction
ARDS, pneumonia
Lack of improvement in respiratory rate within 1–2 h
Lack of increase in PaO_2/FIO_2 to >175 within 1 h

Predictors of success differ slightly between patients with hypercapnic and hypoxemic forms of respiratory failure. A chart to predict NPPV failure of COPD patients identified pH <7.25, respiratory rate ≥35, APACHE II score >29, and Glasgow Coma score ≤11 as independent predictors of NPPV failure [93], whereas a recent prospective multicenter study on NIV to treat patients with ARDS identified a SAPS II score of ≥34 and a PaO_2/FIO_2 ratio <175 after the first hour as independent predictors of NPPV failure [70]. In both analyses, the response to NPPV after the first hour or two had more predictive value than baseline values.

In hypercapnic respiratory failure, a rise in pH and improving mental status within an hour or two of initiating NPPV (presumably reflecting a drop in $PaCO_2$) predict success, whereas, not surprisingly, a substantial early improvement in oxygenation bodes well in patients with hypoxemic respiratory failure. These observations highlight the importance of a "1- to 2-hour checkpoint" after which if the patient is not improving sufficiently, prompt intubation should be contemplated rather than risk further deterioration and the need for a riskier emergent intubation.

Selection Process

The selection of patients with ARF to receive NPPV is based on criteria used in RCTs, and these are listed in Table 59.3. This is a simple three-step process, the first of which is to establish that the patient has a favorable diagnosis, ideally a condition like CPE or COPD, which is likely to respond to medical therapy fairly rapidly (a few days or less). Patients with weaker indications (i.e., acute asthma or pneumonia) can be tried on NPPV but must be monitored very closely in an ICU, especially if they have risk factors for NPV failure. Patients at very high risk for NPPV failure, such as those with sepsis and evolving multiorgan dysfunction, are generally best managed invasively rather than to delay needed intubation.

Step two is to identify patients who need ventilatory assistance so that the modality is not wasted on patients who are too mildly ill to warrant ventilatory assistance. This is done on the basis of simple bedside observations of dyspnea, vital signs, and evidence of increased work of breathing (such

TABLE 59.3

CRITERIA TO SELECT PATIENTS TO RECEIVE NPPV FOR ACUTE RESPIRATORY FAILURE[a]

Hypercapnic respiratory failure	Hypoxemic respiratory failure
Subjective	
Moderate to severe dyspnea	Moderate to severe dyspnea
Physiologic	
Respiratory rate >24/min	Respiratory rate >30/min
Increased accessory muscle use	Increased accessory muscle use
Abdominal paradox	Abdominal paradox
Gas exchange	
pH <7.35, >7.10	pH >7.20
$PaCO_2$ >45 mm Hg, <98 mm Hg	PaO_2/FIO_2 >100, <300

[a]From a composite of initiation criteria for randomized controlled trials.

as vigorous accessory muscle use). Arterial blood gas results showing acute-on-chronic CO_2 retention may be helpful, but needed ventilatory assistance should not be delayed pending availability of blood gas results.

The third step is to exclude patients who have contraindications to NPPV and should be managed invasively (Table 59.4). Most of the contraindications are relative and judgment must be exercised when deciding whether patients have excessive secretions, medical instability, or uncooperativeness. Coma and severe obtundation are no longer considered absolute contraindications as long as they are related to hypercapnia. Patients with hypercapnic coma (Glasgow Coma Scale <8) have success and survival rates with NPPV that are equivalent to those of similar noncomatose patients [94].

TECHNIQUES AND EQUIPMENT FOR NPPV

Interfaces

Nasal Masks

Nasal masks are the most commonly used interfaces for outpatients with chronic respiratory failure because they are more comfortable than nasal prongs or oronasal masks, even if they are less efficient than oronasal masks at eliminating CO_2 [95]. In addition, they permit speech and expectoration and, with some practice, eating during use. Manufacturers offer numerous modifications of the nasal mask that fit into several basic categories.

TABLE 59.4

CONTRAINDICATIONS TO NPPV IN ACUTE RESPIRATORY FAILURE

Cardiac/respiratory arrest
Medically unstable (hypotensive shock, uncontrolled cardiac ischemia, or arrhythmias)
Severe upper gastrointestinal bleeding
Unable to protect airway (impaired cough or swallowing)
Excessive secretions
Unable to apply mask due to facial surgery, trauma, burns, or facial deformity
Agitated or uncooperative
Undrained pneumothorax
Multiorgan system failure

Standard Nasal Masks

Standard nasal masks were first designed during the early 1980s to provide CPAP for obstructive sleep apnea (OSA) and consist of triangular clear plastic domes that fit over the nose (Fig. 59.1A). A soft, usually silicon cuff makes contact with the skin around the perimeter of the nose to form an air seal. These masks must be fit properly to minimize pressure over the bridge of the nose, which may induce redness, skin irritation, and occasionally ulceration. Forehead "spacers" or an adjustable joint are also often used to minimize pressure on the bridge of the nose. Strap systems that hold the masks in place are important for patient comfort. Various approaches have been used to enhance patient comfort, including an additional thin plastic flap or a baffle system to further reduce the strap tension necessary to maintain an air seal. Gel-containing seals, some that have heat-molding capabilities, may help to evenly distribute the pressure of the seal on the face.

Nasal Pillows

Nasal "pillows" consist of small rubber cones that are inserted directly into the nostrils. By removing the sealing surface from the eyes, these reduce claustrophobia and permit use of eyeglasses. They also eliminate contact with the nasal bridge and are helpful for patients with nasal bridge irritation or ulceration caused by standard nasal masks. However, they can cause irritation of the nostrils, and some patients alternate between different types of masks as a way of minimizing discomfort. These are less often used in the acute care setting.

Oronasal or Full-Face Masks

The main advantage of oronasal over nasal masks is that they reduce air leaking through the mouth because they cover both the nose and mouth. Mainly because of this advantage, Kwok et al. found that the oronasal was significantly better tolerated than the nasal mask in the acute setting [96]. Air seals of oronasal masks are similar to those of nasal masks, using a thin membrane of soft silicon to enhance comfort and minimize air leaks. Oronasal masks have built-in valves to prevent rebreathing or asphyxiation in the event of ventilator malfunction, especially for "bilevel"-type ventilators. Because of concerns that vomiting into an oronasal mask could cause aspiration, these masks have straps that allow rapid removal. Some oronasal masks incorporate a "shelf" that fits under the chin to stabilize it, aiming to minimize air leaking under the seal (Fig. 59.1B). Compared with nasal masks, oronasal masks interfere more with speech and eating, have more dead space, and are less comfortable. However, because of their better initial tolerability and more efficient CO_2 removal than nasal masks, they are usually preferred to treat ARF.

The Total Face Mask (Respironics, Inc.) is a larger version of an oronasal mask that seals around the perimeter of the face [97]. It relocates the sealing surface from the nose and mouth to the perimeter of the face. It easily accommodates most facial shapes and sizes and can be rapidly applied by fastening just two Velcro straps behind the head. Although some patients find it frightening and refuse to try it, most find it comfortable and no more claustrophobic than standard oronasal masks. A more recently introduced version of an oronasal mask is smaller than the Total Face Mask, resembling a snorkeling mask (Fig. 59.1C) and serves as an alternative if patients are intolerant of standard masks.

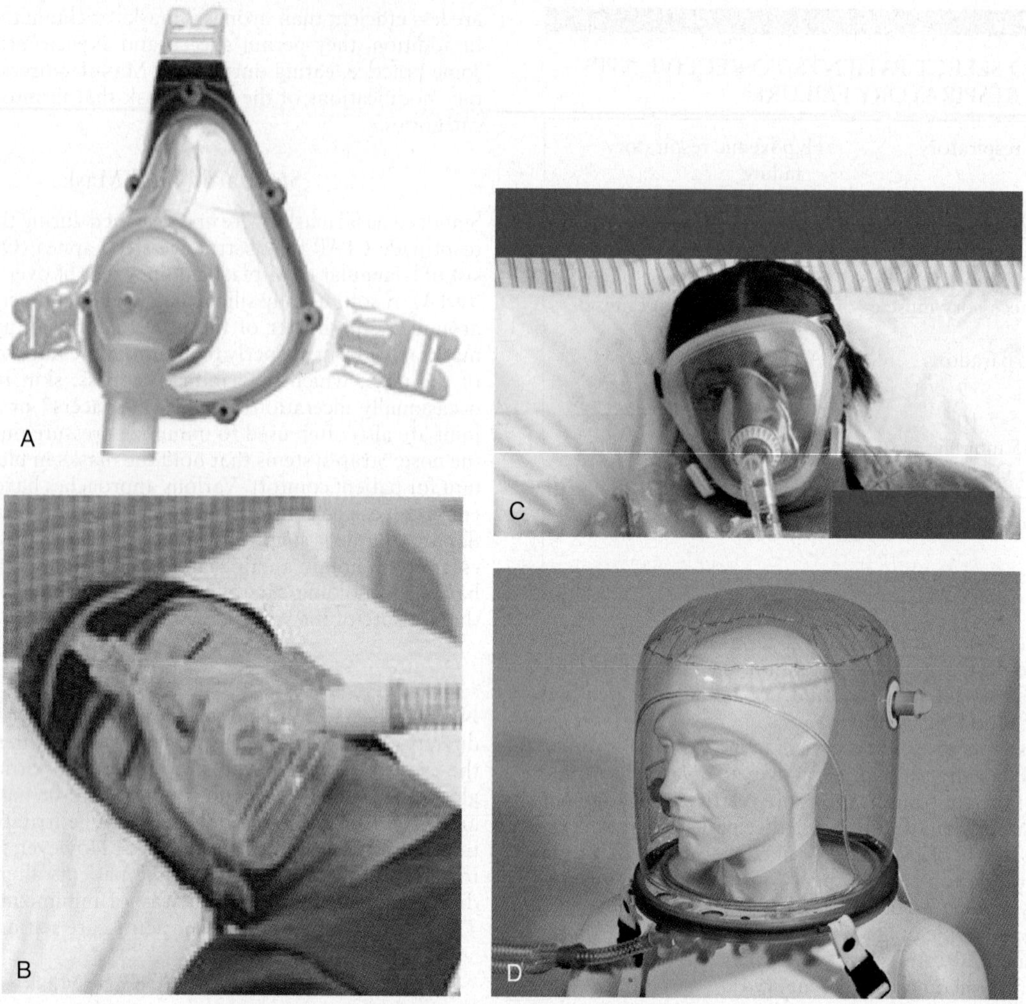

FIGURE 59.1. Examples of interfaces used in the acute care setting. **A:** Standard disposable nasal mask for use with "bilevel" ventilator. The single circuit of these ventilators necessitates an in-line exhaust valve shown by arrow (Mirage Quattro mask, ResMed, San Diego, CA). **B:** Disposable full-face mask with chin "shelf" to keep mandible in position and reduce air leaking under the seal (Model RT040, Fischer Paykel, Wellington, NZ). **C:** Larger full-face mask that resembles snorkel mask and removes mask seal farther from nose and mouth (Performax, Respironics, Inc. Murrysville, PA). **D:** "Helmet" interface that consists of clear plastic cylinder that fits over entire head and fits with strap under axillae.

Helmet

The helmet (Fig. 59.1D) has been used primarily in Italy and has not yet been approved for use with NIV in the United States. It consists of an inflatable plastic cylinder that fits over the head and seals around the neck and shoulders with straps under the axillae. Studies evaluating its use in COPD patients [98,99] show that it is more comfortable and reduces facial ulcerations compared with an oronasal mask. However, it is less efficient at CO_2 removal and can cause problems with triggering and cycling during pressure support ventilation [100]. It appears to be best suited for applying CPAP in patients with acute cardiogenic edema. To prevent rebreathing, high airflow rates are necessary, which render the helmet much noisier than oronasal masks (100 dB vs. 70 dB, respectively) [101]. Although the helmet has some advantages over the full-face mask, it is limited by less-efficient CO_2 removal, excessive noisiness, higher cost, and is unavailable in many countries.

Oral Interfaces

Oral interfaces consisting of a mouthpiece inserted into a lip seal that is strapped tautly around the head to minimize air leakage have been used to treat patients with chronic neuromuscular conditions for many decades. A commercially available oral interface was introduced more recently for the treatment of occasional patients with sleep apnea. These interfaces are not often used in the acute care setting, although some studies have had patients hold interfaces in their mouths to enhance their sense of control when initiating NIV [102].

Headgear

The straps used to hold interfaces in place are important for interface comfort and stability as well as for control of air leaks. The number of strap connections varies from two to five, depending on the mask. In general, the more connections, the more stable the interface, but discomfort and claustrophobia become concerns. Most straps use soft, elastic material fastened with Velcro, but abrasions can occur if the edges are too rough. Minimizing strap tension just to the point of controlling air leaks is important to optimize comfort.

Ventilators for NPPV

The specific ventilator chosen is probably not as important to NPPV success as the settings selected or the skill of the

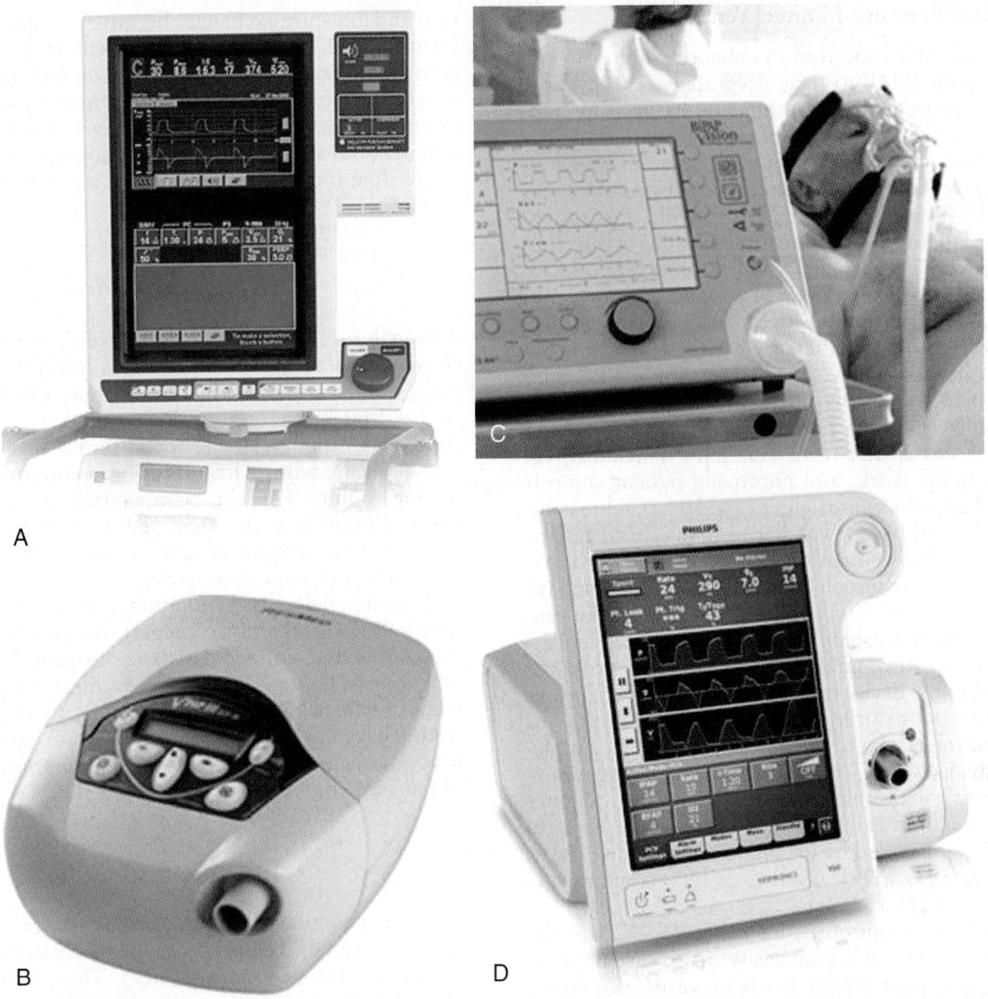

FIGURE 59.2. Examples of ventilators commonly used to deliver NPPV. A: "Critical care" ventilator that offers an "NIV" mode that permits multiple adjustments. May have trouble adapting to large leaks (Puritan Bennett 840, Covidien, Mansfield, MA). B: Typical "bilevel" ventilator designed mainly for home use but is capable of assisting ventilation in patients with acute respiratory failure (VPAP III STA, ResMed, Inc). C: Ventilator designed specifically for acute applications of NIV. Has oxygen blender and graphic monitoring screen (BiPAP Vision, Respironics, Inc). D: Updated version of ventilator in (C). Offers internal battery for portability and improved graphic screen (V60, Philips Respironics, Inc, Andover, MA).

care team. Many ventilator options are available, including critical care ventilators (designed mainly for invasive ventilation in the acute setting), ventilators designed especially for acute applications of NIV in the acute care setting, or portable positive-pressure ventilators designed mainly for use in the home. The choice of ventilator depends mainly on availability, patient needs, and practitioner preferences. For example, patients with hypoxemic respiratory failure may be very difficult to manage noninvasively and the sophisticated monitoring and oxygen delivery capabilities of a critical care ventilator may be preferred, whereas a patient with an exacerbation of COPD who is oxygenating adequately might do just as well with a small, portable, inexpensive bilevel device.

Critical Care Ventilators

The microprocessor-controlled ventilators currently used mainly for invasive mechanical ventilation in critical care units can be adapted for NPPV. These offer an array of volume-limited or pressure-limited modes and sophisticated monitoring and alarm capabilities. Advantages over "bilevel" positive pressure devices include the universal presence of O_2 blenders, accurate tracking of tidal and minute volumes, and a dual-limb circuit with an active exhalation valve that minimizes rebreathing (Fig. 59.2A). Most practitioners use the pressure support mode for NPPV with these ventilators because of enhanced comfort, combining it with PEEP [103,104]. Shortcomings of these ventilators when used to deliver NPPV include intolerance of air leaks that inevitably occur with NPPV, causing difficulty with triggering and cycling which sets off annoying alarms.

Many critical care ventilators now incorporate NIV modes that automatically improve leak tolerance and compensating abilities, disable nuisance alarms, and permit multiple adjustments including those to limit inspiratory time, thus enabling improved expiratory synchrony. These modes have undergone little evaluation in clinical settings, but a recent bench study demonstrated that most NIV modes on critical care ventilators work well to deliver set pressures or volumes unless there are large air leaks, in which case most of them require additional adjustments to maintain delivery [105]. Masks and circuitry for the application of NIV via critical care ventilators should not have the built-in exhalation valves designed for use with bilevel devices because these will increase air leaking and interfere with proper function. Some mask manufacturers use blue coloration for plastic parts of masks meant for use with critical ventilators so that they can be easily identified.

Bilevel Pressure-Limited Ventilators

These devices were first conceived to enhance comfort in patients requiring high CPAP to treat sleep apnea [106], but it rapidly became apparent that they function as pressure support ventilators as well [107]. Portable bilevel ventilators that deliver pressure assist or pressure support ventilation have seen increasing use in recent years. The prototype bilevel device was the "BiPAP S/T" (Respironics, Inc., Murrysville, PA), introduced during the late 1980s, but numerous versions of this technique are now available from many manufacturers (Fig. 59.2B).

Bilevel devices deliver two levels of positive pressure; preset inspiratory and expiratory positive airway pressures (IPAP and EPAP, respectively). The difference between the two is the level of inspiratory assistance, or pressure support. Pressure support modes provide sensitive inspiratory triggering and expiratory cycling mechanisms (usually by sensing changes in flow), permitting excellent patient–ventilator synchrony, reducing diaphragmatic work, and improving patient comfort [108]. Because these devices are lighter (5 to 10 kg), more compact (<0.025 m^3), and have fewer alarms than critical care or portable volume-limited ventilators, they are preferred for patients requiring only nocturnal use in the home. Most have limited IPAP (up to 20 to 35 cm H_2O, depending on the ventilator) and oxygenation capabilities and lack alarms or battery backup systems. Also, unlike volume-limited ventilators, bilevel pressure-limited devices are able to increase inspiratory airflow to compensate for air leaks, thereby potentially providing better support of gas exchange during leakage. O_2 supplementation is provided via a T-connector in the ventilator tubing or connector directly in the mask, the latter providing a slightly higher FIO_2. Even at flow rates of 15 liters per minute, though, the maximum recommended by the manufacturer, the FIO_2 is still only 45% to 50% [109], insufficient for many patients with hypoxemic respiratory failure.

The BiPAP Vision (Respironics, Inc.) (Fig. 59.2C) was designed for both invasive and noninvasive acute care applications, although it is used mainly for noninvasive. Equipped with an O_2 blender, it provides high FIO_2s and has more sophisticated alarm and monitoring systems than the traditional bilevels (including a graphic screen). It also features an adjustable rise time (the time taken to reach target inspiratory pressure) and inspiratory time limits that can help with comfort and synchrony during NIV. Because of these features, the Vision has been well-received as a device for the administration of NIV in acute care hospitals. Two new versions of the BiPAP are now available for acute applications of NIV: the V60 (Fig. 59.2D), which incorporates a battery backup, improved graphics, and some additional modes; and the Focus, a less expensive version that lacks a backup battery or oxygen blender.

Because they have a single ventilator circuit, rebreathing can occur during use of bilevel ventilators and can interfere with the ability to enhance CO_2 elimination [110]. The rebreathing can be minimized by using masks with in-mask exhalation ports, which are associated with less rebreathing than in-circuit valves [111], use of nonrebreathing valves, or EPAP pressures of 4 cm H_2O or greater, which ensure higher bias flows during exhalation [110]. In one study of patients receiving long-term nasal ventilation, a valve designed to minimize rebreathing (Plateau valve, Respironics, Inc.) did not lower nocturnal transcutaneous PCO_2 or daytime $PaCO_2$ compared with a standard in-tubing exhalation valve, probably because of CO_2 elimination during air leaking through the mouth which occurred frequently with both valves [112].

Adjuncts to NPPV

Humidification may enhance comfort during NPPV and is advised if NPPV is to be used for more than a few hours. For the acute care setting, a heated humidifier is preferred over a heat and moisture exchanger because the latter adds to work of breathing [113] and may interfere with triggering and cycling. Also, with excessive air leaking, a heated humidifier lowers nasal resistance [114]. Nasogastric tubes are not routinely recommended as adjuncts to NPPV, even when oronasal masks are used, but small bore flexible nasogastric tubes can be used for feeding if necessary and do not interfere much with mask sealing.

Ventilator Modes

Although pressure support (or bilevel) is the most commonly chosen mode to deliver NIV, others might be considered. Average volume-assured pressure support (AVAPS) is available on the V60 bilevel device (Respironics, Inc). It tracks delivered tidal volumes during the previous several minutes and automatically adjusts inspiratory pressure to achieve a target minute volume. This can be advantageous in hypoventilating patients as has been shown in obesity-hypoventilation patients [115], but no efficacy advantages over standard BiPAP have been shown in acute care settings.

Proportional assist ventilation, a mode that uses the inspiratory flow signal and its integral, volume, to determine how much flow and volume assistance to provide to the patient, functions well as a NPPV mode. It offers the potential advantages of enhanced comfort and synchrony [116]. Once again, studies have not been able to demonstrate improvements in efficacy over standard bilevel or pressure support modes in terms of reducing intubation or mortality rates.

Initiation of NPPV

NPPV is most often begun in the emergency department (ED) or ICU in acutely dyspneic patients who become panicky when masks are strapped to their faces. Thus, unlike initiation of invasive ventilation that consists of a sedated or even paralyzed patient, initiation of NPPV requires skill on the part of the caregiver to rapidly gain the confidence of the patient and help them cooperate so that they can benefit from the technique. Explaining clearly what is happening and what to expect, using verbal cues like "try to let the ventilator breathe for you" and giving patients control by allowing them to hold the mask on their face can be quite helpful.

Proper mask fit should be assured and the mask attached to the ventilator via tubing. Most practitioners start with relatively low ventilator pressures (i.e., 8 to 10 cm H_2O for IPAP and 4 to 5 cm H_2O for EPAP) for at least several minutes to allow the patient to become familiar with the mask and airflow. It is then extremely important to increase the inspiratory pressure (and thereby the level of pressure support) to reduce respiratory distress and effort, targeting a reduction of respiratory rate into the low 20 seconds per minute and an increase in tidal volume to 6 to 7 mL per kg. Patients are often intolerant of higher pressures, especially initially, because of the sensation of burning in the sinuses or pressure in the ears, or because of the perceived effort of breathing against an elevated pressure during expiration. Thus, the adjustment of inspiratory pressure becomes a titration, tailored for individual patients, balancing relief of respiratory distress and achievement of ventilatory targets against intolerance due to excessive pressures.

Expiratory pressure is usually kept at 4 to 5 cm H_2O, but can be adjusted upward if patients are having difficulty triggering due to intrinsic PEEP, upper airway obstructions due to sleep apnea, or are hypoxemic despite increases in FIO_2 to above 50% to 60%. L'Her et al. demonstrated in patients with ALI that increases in PEEP during NPPV were quite effective at improving oxygenation and pressure support in relieving dyspnea [117]. However, it is well to recall that if EPAP is increased during NPPV, IPAP must also be increased by the same amount to maintain the level of pressure support.

MONITORING

Location for NPPV

Because of the importance of prompt initiation to avoid further patient deterioration that could necessitate intubation, NPPV should be started wherever the patient comes to medical attention, as long as appropriate equipment and personnel are available. Once initiated, transfer to an appropriately monitored location becomes important. This depends on the patient's need for monitoring as well as the unit's monitoring capabilities and skills of the staff in managing NPPV. Assessment of a patient's need for monitoring includes consideration of the severity of the respiratory failure as well as any comorbidities. If in doubt, a brief trial of NPPV withdrawal may be helpful. In one study of patients treated with NPPV in the ED for acute pulmonary edema or COPD, patients who remained stable during a 15-minute discontinuation trial were transferred to a regular ward and none subsequently required intubation [118].

NPPV is used on regular wards in many hospitals because of the scarcity of ICU beds, but some guidelines have recommended that NPPV be applied only in the ICU because of concerns about patient safety [119]. Farha et al. [120] reported on their experience with 76 patients treated on a regular ward with NPPV. Of the 62 patients without a DNI status, 31% required intubation and were transferred to the ICU. The authors considered this comparable to the experience with patients treated in more closely monitored settings, concluding that NPPV can be administered safely on regular floors. But unless the ward has considerable experience administering NPPV, only stable patients should be treated there.

What to Monitor

Monitoring of NPPV shares similarities with that of invasive mechanical ventilation but also fundamental differences. Most importantly, subjective responses are critical to the success of NIV (Table 59.5). Alleviation of respiratory distress and good tolerance of the technique must be achieved without using large doses of analgesia and sedation as is commonly done with invasive ventilation. Thus, caregivers must observe patients closely for these responses and be prepared to make prompt adjustments as needed to maintain patient cooperation.

Physical signs of increased respiratory effort should also respond promptly when NPPV is administered properly, including reductions in accessory muscle use and respiratory rate. Air leaks should be sought. These are universal with NPPV, and with bilevel devices, the continuous leak through the exhalation device is intentional, of course. But leaks under the seal of the mask can be large and interfere with synchronization and efficacy and should be sought.

Poor synchrony between the patient and ventilator, sometimes caused by excessive air leaking, patient agitation, ventilator maladjustment, or other factors, is another factor contributing to failure and must be monitored. Oximetry should be monitored continuously until the patient has stabilized and arterial blood gases should be drawn at baseline and after 1 to 2 hours of therapy to assure the desired gas exchange response. One important aspect of NPPV monitoring is to determine early when patients are responding poorly to NPPV so that the reasons can be reversed or failing that, the patient can be intubated promptly, avoiding undue delay and possible respiratory arrest with the emergent intubation and attendant morbidity and mortality that may entail.

TABLE 59.5

WHAT TO MONITOR DURING NPPV

Subjective responses
Comfort
Mask related
Air pressure and flow related
Dyspnea
Claustrophobia
Agitation
Delirium
Vital signs
Respiratory rate
Heart rate
Blood pressure
Breathing effort
Accessory muscle use
Paradoxical breathing
Gas exchange
Continuous oximetry
Baseline and 1–2 h arterial blood gases, then as indicated
Synchrony
Triggering
Expiratory asynchrony
Air leaks
Mask seal
Through mouth with nasal masks
Secretion clearance
Cough effectiveness
Quantity of secretions
Development of complications (see Table 59.6)

Complications and Side Effects of NPPV and Possible Remedies

NPPV is successful in most patients and most adverse side effects are minor, but failure rates in studies representing "real-life" applications of NIV still approach 40% [6,75,121] and a knowledge of potential complications and ways of managing them can be helpful in minimizing NPPV failure rates. There are many possible adverse effects and complications, a variety of possible ways of categorizing them, and inevitable areas of overlap between the categories. For practical purposes, we distinguish between side effects related to the interface and those attributable to ventilator airflow and pressure, caregiver inexperience, and patient factors (Table 59.6).

Adverse Effects and Complications Associated with the Interface

Mask Discomfort

Mask discomfort is one of the most common reasons cited for NPPV failure. It may reflect a poorly fit mask, a patient's difficulty accepting the interface chosen, excessively tight head-straps, a dyspneic patient's discomfort at having foreign material strapped to their face, or other factors. The clinician faced with a patient tolerating NPPV poorly because of mask discomfort should quickly attempt to decipher the specific problem and correct it if possible. Often, inexperienced practitioners select masks that are too large and a trial with a smaller mask or a different mask type may help. If it does not lead to excessive air leaking, reseating the mask or loosening the straps often helps.

TABLE 59.6

ADVERSE EFFECTS AND COMPLICATIONS OF NPPV AND POSSIBLE REMEDIES

Adverse effect	Possible remedy
Interface related	
Mask discomfort	Check size and fit. Readjust headgear. Try different type.
Skin ulceration, irritation	Readjust mask. Loosen straps. Artificial skin prophylactically.
Air pressure and flow related	
Nasal, sinus pain, dryness	Lower pressure temporarily. Humidify gas. Nasal saline.
Conjunctivitis	Reseat mask. Check seal on nasal bridge. Artificial skin. Consider new mask type.
Gastric distension	Lower pressure if possible. Simethicone. Observe or distension, consider nasogastric drainage.
Patient–ventilator asynchrony	Eliminate leaks, treat agitation, assess for discomfort. Try lowering pressure support or limiting inspiratory time.
Rebreathing	Use mask with in-mask exhalation valve. Use adequate EPAP (≥4 cm H_2O). Use ventilator with active exhalation valve.
Air leaks	Reseat, readjust strap. Try different mask type. Chin strap if nasal mask. Lower pressure if possible.
Caregiver related	
Inadequate or excessive pressures	Monitor more carefully. Adjust upward as tolerated. Assure adequate training.
Inadequate equipment	Initiate NPPV program, with full selection of masks.
Patient related	
Agitation, anxiety	Assure proper mask fit, ventilator settings. Reassure, consider sedation.
Major complications	
NPPV failure	Optimal monitoring to detect and address problems before they lead to failure. If failure not responding to appropriate measures, intubate promptly to avoid delay.
Respiratory arrest	Monitor at-risk patients in ICU or closely in stepdown unit. Intubate before arrest occurs to avoid attendant morbidity and mortality.

As discussed earlier, an oronasal mask is usually the best initial mask choice, but some patients who are claustrophobic or expectorating frequently fare better with a nasal mask. Masks used in the acute setting are usually disposable after one use but some are reusable. They are relatively inexpensive compared to masks used for long-term applications of NPPV, but it is still desirable to check that the mask selected is likely to fit (using a fitting gauge, for example) to minimize the need to dispose of multiple masks for each patient application. Noisiness can contribute to intolerance with some mask types such as the helmet, with measured levels reaching upward of 90 dB in the CPAP mode [122].

Skin Irritation and Ulceration

Skin irritation and ulceration, mainly over the nasal bridge, is a common complication of NIV. Contributors to NIV-related skin breakdown include excessive strap tension, mask type, poor mask fit, prolonged ventilation, high inspiratory pressure necessitating more strap tension to control leaks, hypersensitivity to mask material, and patient factors such as age and comorbidities such as congestive heart failure that limit skin perfusion [123–126]. Facial structure and anatomical variation between patients also play a role. Skin complication rates vary considerably between studies ranging from less than 5% to as high as 43% [126–128]. A recent study by Dellweg et al. showed that a larger mask cushion size distributes contact pressure to the skin over a larger contact area [123], but the study did not show that cutaneous complications were lowered as a consequence.

Prevention rather than treatment of skin breakdown is the best management strategy. This can be accomplished by optimizing mask fit while using the lowest effective positive pressures and strap tension and applying artificial skin to the affected area at the first sign of redness. Also, newer mask model types have softer, larger silicon sealing surfaces that minimize trauma to the facial skin. With these interventions, a significant nasal bridge ulcer should now be a rare event during NPPV therapy.

Adverse Effects and Complications Associated with Airflow and Pressure

Nasal, Sinus and Ear Pain and Burning

Initiation of NPPV is commonly associated with the sensation of nasal, sinus and ear pain and burning. This is related to the patient's lack of familiarity with the sensation of air pressure and flow and usually subsides as the patient accommodates to the sensations. Using lower initial pressures and raising them gradually can help to minimize this problem as can making sure that leak is minimized. Use of routine humidification can help with these side effects too.

Conjunctivitis

Conjunctivitis is another common adverse consequence of airflow during NPPV. In this case, air leaks into the eye due to a combination of high inspiratory pressure and incomplete mask sealing along the steep sides of the nose related to suboptimal mask fit and, possibly, patient anatomic variations. This causes dryness, irritation, erythema, and discomfort after a period of hours and may respond to lowered inspiratory pressure (if possible), reseating the mask or tightening the straps, or trying a new mask type.

Gastric Distension

Gastric distension in patients receiving NPPV is common but is usually well tolerated. However, some recent cases were reported of extreme complications such as gastric perforation and abdominal compartment syndrome [129,130]. A study on obese patients found that those receiving NPPV with an inspiratory pressure of 16 cm H_2O had more gastric distension than those breathing spontaneously [131]. The authors cautioned that the increased gastric air might raise the risk of aspiration. As stated earlier, the amount of gastric distension during NPPV is usually clinically insignificant, but if it causes excessive abdominal distension, discomfort, nausea, bowel distension on a KUB exam, or a compartment syndrome, then drainage with a naso- or orogastric tube is the next logical step. Gas dispersing agents like simethicone can be tried but are usually unsuccessful. Lowering the inspiratory pressure as much as possible may also help. But if there is a high risk of vomiting and aspiration or if nasogastric suctioning is unsuccessful, then intubation and other methods to decompress the bowel should be considered.

Patient–Ventilator Asynchrony

Patient–ventilator asynchrony is the lack of coordination between a patient's own respiratory effort and the ventilator's output. The consequences of this phenomenon can include inefficient gas exchange, muscle fatigue, and ultimately, failure of NPPV [132]. Asynchrony occurs frequently during NIV, mostly because of air leaks, rendering it difficult for the ventilator to sense the onset of patient inspiration and expiration, altered patient respiratory drive or agitation, ventilator mode, and inappropriately high inspiratory pressure in patients with COPD, contributing to ineffective triggering and cycling [133–135]. An observational study in three teaching hospital ICUs used an asynchrony index [the number of asynchrony events/ventilator cycles + wasted respiratory effort) × 100] [132]. This study found that discomfort and air leaks were independent risk factors for asynchrony indices >10%. The study, however, was limited because it used only critical care ventilators.

The type of interface also is important considering that when used to deliver pressure support, helmets have high rates of asynchrony compared to other NIV interfaces, mostly due to their high structural compliance [136,137]. Strategies to deal with asynchrony include minimizing air leaks, changing to timed modes (such as pressure control) to reduce the persistence of ventilator inspiration into patient expiration that occurs with bilevel modes [134], lowering pressure support if tidal volumes are large and breathing efforts fail to trigger, and giving sedation to control agitation.

Rebreathing

Rebreathing of CO_2 is a concern with bilevel ventilators because of their single circuit design. Earlier bench and clinical studies demonstrated rebreathing during use of NPPV [138]. However, more recent studies have not demonstrated CO_2 rebreathing at levels deemed detrimental to patients, and rebreathing during NPPV has not been implicated in adverse patient outcomes [139–143]. The routine use of expiratory pressures of 4 cm H_2O or greater was shown in earlier studies to minimize rebreathing along with modifications in ventilator circuitry, and the placement of exhaust vents in masks themselves has also been shown to curb rebreathing [110,139,144,145]. Helmet masks are associated with high levels of rebreathing, especially in the CPAP mode, necessitating use of high flow rates to flush out the CO_2 and thereby generating high noise levels [98,146,147]. However, newer helmet designs with expiratory ports, as well as use in conjunction with open-circuit ventilators, have been shown to decrease rebreathing [136,147,148]. Thus, although concerns regarding rebreathing during NPPV continue to draw attention in the medical literature, the modifications to ventilators and interfaces over the past decade have largely eliminated the concern.

Air Leaks

Air leaks are universal during NPPV because of its open circuit design. Some leaks are intentional as with bilevel ventilators, but air also leaks under the mask seal through the mouth and even into the gastrointestinal tract. Small leaks (<30 to 40 L per minute) are generally well tolerated as most ventilators compensate quite easily for them. However, large leaks (>60 L per minute) can have deleterious effects by interfering with ventilator assistance and synchrony, leading to increased work of breathing, fatigue, oxygen desaturations, and NIV failure. Leaks also contribute to patient discomfort, contributing to conjunctivitis, sleep disruption, and dry mouth [144,149–152].

Air leaks are associated with improperly sized or sealed masks, loose or excessively tightened headstraps, the presence of facial hair, unusual facial anatomy variability, high inspiratory pressure settings, and the presence of surgical dressings or catheters that disrupt the seal. Nasal masks are commonly associated with mouth leaks, reported to occur in as many as 94% of patients receiving NPPV for hypercapnic ARF and contributing to the majority of mask failures [153]. In a comparison study of four different NPPV interfaces in patients with ARF, the mouthpiece had the largest leak, while there was no significant difference between the Total Face Mask, oronasal mask, or nasal mask [154].

Measures that can be undertaken by the clinician to minimize leaks include careful mask selection and fitting, proper strapping to the face, removal of facial hair, use of chin straps with nasal masks, and chin supports (built into certain mask types) for patients using oronasal masks. Reduction of inspiratory pressure usually helps, as well, if feasible. Leak-compensating ability of the ventilator is another consideration in patients having frequent large leaks. Most bilevel ventilators compensate quite well, but older critical care ventilators in the pressure support mode may have difficulty dealing with intermittent variable leaks. Many newer critical care ventilators have NIV modes that enhance leak-compensating abilities, but most need additional adjustments in the face of large leaks [105].

Caregiver-Related Factors

Complications of NPPV are sometimes related to caregiver decisions that inadvertently predispose to NPPV failure. Most commonly, these include selection of inappropriate candidates with excessively high risk of failure, such as ALI/ARDS patients who are septic and developing multiorgan failure or elderly pneumonia patients with poor cough and excessive secretions. Inadequate attention to detail during initiation predisposes to failure, including neglecting to spend time with the patient to instruct and win confidence or to properly fit or attach the mask.

Failure to increase the inspiratory pressure after initiation is a common cause of NPPV failure because the patient never receives adequate ventilator assistance. Inadequate monitoring, either because an unstable patient is never sent from a regular ward to the ICU or because caregivers neglect the early signs of deterioration, permitting a respiratory crisis to occur, are other common reasons for NPPV failure. Caregivers need to know when to intubate patients who are not responding adequately to NPPV before an emergency or respiratory arrest occurs, avoiding delays of needed intubation.

There is no substitute for having a skilled and experienced multidisciplinary team if NPPV success rates are to be optimized. Evidence from several studies indicates that as caregivers gain experience with NPPV, patient outcomes improve, or they can sustain the same favorable outcomes in sicker patients [16].

Multidisciplinary Approach

NPPV works best if administered as part of a team effort. Ideally, this is achieved in a specialized unit such as an ICU or step-down unit where members can gain experience by working together over time. Although team members may have different roles depending on the country they work in, the roles must be adopted by one team member or another in order for optimization of NPPV delivery. In North America, physicians must be skilled at selecting appropriate patients for NPPV and writing proper orders for its initiation. The respiratory therapist then fits and applies the interface and makes initial ventilator adjustments. Nurses then monitor the patient, notifying the physician and therapist if problems arise.

Physicians and therapists should also participate in monitoring so that they can intervene with timely adjustments to the mask or ventilator settings or with intubation, if needed. Pharmacologists assist in choosing the type and dose of sedation or analgesia if deemed indicated, and nutritionists assist in assuring that nutritional needs are met. Physical therapists may also become involved to help with secretion removal or early mobilization. In other countries such as in the United Kingdom, physiotherapists assume many of the roles of the respiratory therapist, and in many countries in the developing world, physicians are responsible for initiation and application of equipment in addition to their other duties. Regardless of how the responsibilities are distributed, most programs favor using protocols and having periodic training in-services for their team members.

Patient-Related Factors

Patients vary enormously in their ability to tolerate NPPV, and this is reflected in success rates. Patients who are cognitively impaired due to congenital or acquired processes, such as strokes, dementia, or delirium, are unlikely to tolerate NPPV because they cannot comprehend the purpose and become agitated. Other patients panic when a mask is strapped to their face, either because of claustrophobia or because of their already heightened anxiety and distress due to their respiratory condition. These factors must be kept in mind when selecting patients or when deciding that the modality has failed. Some anxious patients respond to reassurance and being given control of the mask and others require sedation. Patients with dementia or delirium can sometimes be managed successfully with anti-psychotics like haloperidol or risperidone.

Sedation and Analgesia During NPPV

Judicious use of sedation may help to calm patients having difficulty cooperating with NPPV, but most clinicians are very cautious, using smaller doses, mainly by intermittent bolus, than they use in invasively ventilated patients. Most respondents to a survey of critical care physicians from North America and Europe indicated that they used sedation or analgesia in less than 25% of patients [155]. They registered concerns about blunting the drive to breathe in spontaneously breathing patients. North Americans were more apt to use benzodiazepines alone and Europeans opioids alone as their preferred initial choice. More information from clinical studies is needed before specific recommendations on specific medications and doses can be made, but use of sedation or analgesia should be considered in patients at risk of failing NPPV because of agitation, apprehension, or discomfort.

Impact of NPPV on Quality Measures

The aging population in developed countries will place increasing stress on healthcare resources over the next couple of decades, so efficient utilization of resources while enhancing quality of care will become paramount goals [156]. Projections in the United States are an annual 2 million increase in prolonged (>96 hours) mechanical ventilation days through the year 2020 compared to the year 2000 and an annual increase of 3 million ICU days during the same time period [157]. In this context, appropriate use of NIV becomes even more necessary as it has the capability of improving outcomes as well as the efficiency of resource utilization.

Effects of NPPV on ICU and Hospital Lengths of Stay

A number of studies have demonstrated reduced ICU and hospital lengths of stay in association with NPPV use in COPD patients with respiratory failure. In a systematic analysis, Keenan et al. [158] derived an absolute reduction in hospital LOS of 4.49 days (CI 3.66–7.52 days). A meta-analysis of randomized trials in 2003 confirmed the positive effect of early NPPV use on hospital LOS for COPD patients [159]. When used to treat COPD patients with an infectious exacerbation or severe hypercapnic neurological dysfunction in the emergency room, Briones et al., in a case control study, found a significant reduction in hospital LOS with NPPV (11.1 ± 4.7 days for IMV vs. 6.5 ± 1.9 for NPPV, $p = 0.001$) [160]. Thus, the preponderance of evidence indicates that NPPV reduces ICU and hospital LOS compared to standard therapy in COPD patients with ARF.

The effects are not as robust in patients with other diagnoses, though. Although one recent study suggests that NPPV reduces ICU LOS as well as in-hospital mortality in patients with ARF due to a host of etiologies other than COPD [161], a Cochrane analysis of 21 studies comparing NPPV plus standard therapy to standard therapy alone in the treatment of ARF due to CPE found that NPPV reduced ICU LOS by 1 day but did not significantly reduce hospital LOS [162].

In patients with acute hypoxemic respiratory failure and ALI/ARDS, Agarwal et al. found no difference in ICU or hospital LOS between those treated with NPPV versus invasive mechanical ventilation [163,164]. A Swiss observational case-control study with a small number of subjects reported a reduction in ICU LOS along with an improvement in oxygenation in ARDS patients treated with NPPV compared to matched controls treated invasively. The study, however, showed a trend for a higher ICU mortality rate for the NIV patients [5].

The use of NIV for treatment of postoperative respiratory failure has also been shown to be advantageous in reducing ICU LOS. Michelet et al. reported an average reduction in ICU LOS of 8 days ($p = 0.034$) in patients who were treated with NPPV compared to conventional treatment for postoperative ARF after esophagectomy [165]. The impact of NIV on ICU LOS was also shown with great success in patients with persistent weaning failure who were immediately tried on NIV post extubation and were found to have shorter ICU LOS compared to those undergoing conventional weaning (14.1 ± 9.2 vs. 25.0 ± 12.5 days, $p = 0.002$) [38].

In summary, NPPV reduces resource consumption in COPD patients with ARF as well as in COPD patients with weaning and postsurgical respiratory failure. Most of the studies have been performed in Europe where average hospital and ICU LOS tend to be longer than in North America. The LOS shortening effect appears to be less potent for patients with other diagnoses such as CPE or ALI/ARDS. Nonetheless, NPPV is a modality that will likely have an expanding role in the therapy of ARF in the future, not only to improve patient outcomes, but also to improve efficiency of resource utilization, and thereby contribute to a reduction in healthcare costs.

SUMMARY AND RECOMMENDATIONS

NPPV has assumed an important role in the management of patients with ARF in critical care settings. Epidemiologic studies indicate that use of NPPV has increased substantially over the past decade throughout the world. Current evidence indicates that NPPV is well supported for therapy of ARF associated with COPD exacerbations, acute pulmonary edema, and immunocompromised states. Use is sensible in a number of other settings, including facilitation of weaning in intubated COPD patients and COPD or acute pulmonary edema patients in other settings, such as postoperative, postextubation, and patients with a DNI status. Less evidence supports use in acute asthma, obesity hypoventilation with an exacerbation, cystic fibrosis, or neuromuscular disease, but NPPV would be a consideration to treat these.

Most patients with ARDS or severe community-acquired pneumonia should not be treated with NPPV, but exceptions include those with minimal secretions, stable otherwise and with only one or at most two organ failures, and in a closely monitored setting. Initiation of NPPV requires a properly fit and tolerable interface and a ventilator that is appropriately set. Patients should be placed in a location that permits adequate monitoring for their state of acuity, and monitoring should pay particular attention to subjective adaptation including mask tolerance and adaptation to the ventilator. Administration should be by a skilled and experienced multidisciplinary team. Achievement of these goals should lead to appropriate and safe administration of NPPV with better overall patient outcomes and more efficient utilization of scarce ICU resources.

Summary of Major Recommendations

- NPPV should be considered the ventilator mode of first choice for respiratory failure associated with COPD exacerbations [31,159], acute CPE [50], and immunocompromised states [37].
- NPPV can be considered to treat other patients with ARF such as those with asthma, exacerbations of cystic fibrosis, or obesity hypoventilation [13].
- In patients with a DNI order, NPPV can be used as a form of life support or to palliate, but should be discontinued if goals are not being achieved [87].
- NPPV should not be used routinely but very selectively and with close monitoring in patients with ARDS or pneumonia [70].
- NPPV should be administered in an ICU or stepdown unit under close and continuous monitoring until stabilization has occurred [118].
- The full-face mask is the preferred initial interface for acute applications of NPPV [96].
- Increases in expiratory pressure can be used to treat hypoxemia and increases in pressure support reduce work of breathing [117].
- Patient/ventilator asynchrony and air leaks can contribute to NPPV failure and should be minimized [133].
- When NPPV is failing, intubation should not be delayed [77].

References

1. Corrado A, Ginanni R, Villella G, et al: Iron lung versus conventional mechanical ventilation in acute exacerbation of COPD. *Eur Respir J* 23(3):419–424, 2004.
2. Hill NS: Use of negative pressure ventilation, rocking beds, and pneumobelts. *Respir Care* 39(5):532–545, 1994; discussion 545–539.
3. Tobin MJ: Mechanical ventilation. *N Engl J Med* 330(15):1056–1061, 1994.
4. Make BJ, Hill NS, Goldberg AI, et al; Mechanical ventilation beyond the intensive care unit. Report of a consensus conference of the American College of Chest Physicians. *Chest* 113[Suppl 5]:289S–344S, 1998.
5. Domenighetti G, Moccia A, Gayer R: Observational case-control study of non-invasive ventilation in patients with ARDS. *Monaldi Arch Chest Dis* 69(1):5–10, 2008.
6. Demoule A, Girou E, Richard JC, et al: Increased use of noninvasive ventilation in French intensive care units. *Intensive Care Med* 32(11):1747–1755, 2006.
7. Alagoz A, Ulus F, Sazak H, et al: Two cases of tracheal rupture after endotracheal intubation. *J Cardiothorac Vasc Anesth* 23(2):271–272, 2009.
8. Anzueto A, Frutos-Vivar F, Esteban A, et al: Incidence, risk factors and outcome of barotrauma in mechanically ventilated patients. *Intensive Care Med* 30(4):612–619, 2004.
9. Papaioannou V, Terzi I, Dragoumanis C, et al: Negative-pressure acute tracheobronchial hemorrhage and pulmonary edema. *J Anesth.* 23(3):417–420, 2009.
10. Chuang YC, Wang CH, Lin YS: Negative pressure pulmonary edema: report of three cases and review of the literature. *Eur Arch Otorhinolaryngol* 264(9):1113–1116, 2007.
11. Elpern EH, Larson R, Douglass P, et al: Long-term outcomes for elderly survivors of prolonged ventilator assistance. *Chest* 96(5):1120–1124, 1989.
12. Rumbak MJ, Walsh FW, Anderson WM, et al: Significant tracheal obstruction causing failure to wean in patients requiring prolonged mechanical ventilation: a forgotten complication of long-term mechanical ventilation. *Chest* 115(4):1092–1095, 1999.
13. Nava S, Hill N: Non-invasive ventilation in acute respiratory failure. *Lancet* 374(9685):250–259, 2009.
14. Griesdale DE, Bosma TL, Kurth T, et al: Complications of endotracheal intubation in the critically ill. *Intensive Care Med* 34(10):1835–1842, 2008.
15. Esteban A, Ferguson ND, Meade MO, et al: Evolution of mechanical ventilation in response to clinical research. *Am J Respir Crit Care Med* 177(2):170–177, 2008.
16. Carlucci A, Delmastro M, Rubini F, et al: Changes in the practice of non-invasive ventilation in treating COPD patients over 8 years. *Intensive Care Med* 29(3):419–425, 2003.
17. Girou E, Brun-Buisson C, Taille S, et al: Secular trends in nosocomial infections and mortality associated with noninvasive ventilation in patients with exacerbation of COPD and pulmonary edema. *JAMA* 290(22):2985–2991, 2003.
18. Confalonieri M, Gorini M, Ambrosino N, et al: Respiratory intensive care units in Italy: a national census and prospective cohort study. *Thorax* 56(5):373–378, 2001.
19. Kaul S, Pearson M, Coutts I, et al: Non-invasive ventilation (NIV) in the clinical management of acute COPD in 233 UK hospitals: results from the RCP/BTS 2003 National COPD Audit. *COPD* 6(3):171–176, 2009.
20. Maheshwari V, Paioli D, Rothaar R, et al: Utilization of noninvasive ventilation in acute care hospitals: a regional survey. *Chest* 129(5):1226–1233, 2006.
21. Ozsancak A, Alkana P, Khodabandeh A, et al: Increasing utilization of non-invasive positive pressure ventilation in acute care hospitals in Massachusetts and Rhode Island. *Am J Respir Crit Care Med* 177:A283, 2008.
22. Bierer GB, Soo Hoo GW: Noninvasive ventilation for acute respiratory failure: a national survey of Veterans Affairs hospitals. *Respir Care* 54(10):1313–1320, 2009.
23. Sweet DD, Naismith A, Keenan SP, et al: Missed opportunities for noninvasive positive pressure ventilation: a utilization review. *J Crit Care* 23(1):111–117, 2008.
24. Hong SB, Oh BJ, Kim YS, et al: Characteristics of mechanical ventilation employed in intensive care units: a multicenter survey of hospitals. *J Korean Med Sci* 23(6):948–953, 2008.
25. Chawla R, Sidhu US, Kumar V, et al: Noninvasive ventilation: a survey of practice patterns of its use in India. *Indian J Crit Care Med* 12(4):163–169, 2008.
26. Appendini L, Patessio A, Zanaboni S, et al; Physiologic effects of positive end-expiratory pressure and mask pressure support during exacerbations of chronic obstructive pulmonary disease. *Am J Respir Crit Care Med* 149(5):1069–1076, 1994.
27. Domenighetti G, Gayer R, Gentilini R: Noninvasive pressure support ventilation in non-COPD patients with acute cardiogenic pulmonary edema and severe community-acquired pneumonia: acute effects and outcome. *Intensive Care Med* 28(9):1226–1232, 2002.

28. Keenan SP, Mehta S: Noninvasive ventilation for patients presenting with acute respiratory failure: the randomized controlled trials. *Respir Care* 54(1):116–126, 2009.
29. Quon BS, Gan WQ, Sin DD: Contemporary management of acute exacerbations of COPD: a systematic review and metaanalysis. *Chest* 133(3):756–766, 2008.
30. Pastaka C, Kostikas K, Karetsi E, et al: Non-invasive ventilation in chronic hypercapnic COPD patients with exacerbation and a pH of 7.35 or higher. *Eur J Intern Med* 18(7):524–530, 2007.
31. Brochard L, Mancebo J, Wysocki M, et al: Noninvasive ventilation for acute exacerbations of chronic obstructive pulmonary disease. *N Engl J Med* 333(13):817–822, 1995.
32. Kramer N, Meyer TJ, Meharg J, et al: Randomized, prospective trial of noninvasive positive pressure ventilation in acute respiratory failure. *Am J Respir Crit Care Med* 151(6):1799–1806, 1995.
33. Confalonieri M, Potena A, Carbone G, et al: Acute respiratory failure in patients with severe community-acquired pneumonia. A prospective randomized evaluation of noninvasive ventilation. *Am J Respir Crit Care Med* 160(5 Pt 1):1585–1591, 1999.
34. Bulow HH, Thorsager B: Non-invasive ventilation in do-not-intubate patients: five-year follow-up on a two-year prospective, consecutive cohort study. *Acta Anaesthesiol Scand* 53(9):1153–1157, 2009.
35. Fernandez R, Baigorri F, Artigas A: Noninvasive ventilation in patients with "do-not-intubate" orders: medium-term efficacy depends critically on patient selection. *Intensive Care Med* 33(2):350–354, 2007.
36. Levy M, Tanios MA, Nelson D, et al: Outcomes of patients with do-not-intubate orders treated with noninvasive ventilation. *Crit Care Med* 32(10):2002–2007, 2004.
37. Hilbert G, Gruson D, Portel L, et al: Noninvasive pressure support ventilation in COPD patients with postextubation hypercapnic respiratory insufficiency. *Eur Respir J* 11(6):1349–1353, 1998.
38. Ferrer M, Esquinas A, Arancibia F, et al: Noninvasive ventilation during persistent weaning failure: a randomized controlled trial. *Am J Respir Crit Care Med* 168(1):70–76, 2003.
39. Nava S, Ambrosino N, Clini E, et al: Noninvasive mechanical ventilation in the weaning of patients with respiratory failure due to chronic obstructive pulmonary disease. A randomized, controlled trial. *Ann Intern Med* 128(9):721–728, 1998.
40. Kilger E, Briegel J, Haller M, et al: Effects of noninvasive positive pressure ventilatory support in non-COPD patients with acute respiratory insufficiency after early extubation. *Intensive Care Med* 25(12):1374–1380, 1999.
41. Girault C, Daudenthun I, Chevron V, et al: Noninvasive ventilation as a systematic extubation and weaning technique in acute-on-chronic respiratory failure: a prospective, randomized controlled study. *Am J Respir Crit Care Med* 160(1):86–92, 1999.
42. Bersten AD, Holt AW, Vedig AE, et al: Treatment of severe cardiogenic pulmonary edema with continuous positive airway pressure delivered by face mask. *N Engl J Med* 325(26):1825–1830, 1991.
43. Ferrari G, Milan A, Groff P, et al: Continuous positive airway pressure vs. pressure support ventilation in acute cardiogenic pulmonary edema: a randomized trial. *J Emerg Med* 39:676–684, 2010.
44. Mehta S, Jay GD, Woolard RH, et al: Randomized, prospective trial of bilevel versus continuous positive airway pressure in acute pulmonary edema. *Crit Care Med* 25(4):620–628, 1997.
45. Rusterholtz T, Bollaert PE, Feissel M, et al: Continuous positive airway pressure vs. proportional assist ventilation for noninvasive ventilation in acute cardiogenic pulmonary edema. *Intensive Care Med* 34(5):840–846, 2008.
46. Park M, Sangean MC, Volpe Mde S, et al: Randomized, prospective trial of oxygen, continuous positive airway pressure, and bilevel positive airway pressure by face mask in acute cardiogenic pulmonary edema. *Crit Care Med* 32(12):2407–2415, 2004.
47. Gray A, Goodacre S, Newby DE, et al: Noninvasive ventilation in acute cardiogenic pulmonary edema. *N Engl J Med* 359(2):142–151, 2008.
48. Masip J, Roque M, Sanchez B, et al: Noninvasive ventilation in acute cardiogenic pulmonary edema: systematic review and meta-analysis. *JAMA* 294(24):3124–3130, 2005.
49. Peter JV, Moran JL, Phillips-Hughes J, et al: Effect of non-invasive positive pressure ventilation (NIPPV) on mortality in patients with acute cardiogenic pulmonary oedema: a meta-analysis. *Lancet* 367(9517):1155–1163, 2006.
50. Winck JC, Azevedo LF, Costa-Pereira A, et al: Efficacy and safety of non-invasive ventilation in the treatment of acute cardiogenic pulmonary edema—a systematic review and meta-analysis. *Crit Care* 10(2):R69, 2006.
51. Chadda K, Annane D, Hart N, et al: Cardiac and respiratory effects of continuous positive airway pressure and noninvasive ventilation in acute cardiac pulmonary edema. *Crit Care Med* 30(11):2457–2461, 2002.
52. Plaisance P, Pirracchio R, Berton C, et al: A randomized study of out-of-hospital continuous positive airway pressure for acute cardiogenic pulmonary oedema: physiological and clinical effects. *Eur Heart J* 28(23):2895–2901, 2007.
53. Thompson J, Petrie DA, Ackroyd-Stolarz S, et al: Out-of-hospital continuous positive airway pressure ventilation versus usual care in acute respiratory failure: a randomized controlled trial. *Ann Emerg Med* 52(3):232–241, 241.e231, 2008.
54. Duchateau FX, Beaune S, Ricard-Hibon A, et al: Prehospital noninvasive ventilation can help in management of patients with limitations of life-sustaining treatments. *Eur J Emerg Med* 17(1):7–9, 2010.
55. Ewig S, Torres A, Riquelme R, et al: Pulmonary complications in patients with haematological malignancies treated at a respiratory ICU. *Eur Respir J* 12(1):116–122, 1998.
56. Hilbert G, Gruson D, Vargas F, et al: Noninvasive ventilation in immunosuppressed patients with pulmonary infiltrates, fever, and acute respiratory failure. *N Engl J Med* 344(7):481–487, 2001.
57. Antonelli M, Conti G, Bufi M, et al: Noninvasive ventilation for treatment of acute respiratory failure in patients undergoing solid organ transplantation: a randomized trial. *JAMA* 283(2):235–241, 2000.
58. Depuydt PO, Benoit DD, Vandewoude KH, et al: Outcome in noninvasively and invasively ventilated hematologic patients with acute respiratory failure. *Chest* 126(4):1299–1306, 2004.
59. Azoulay E, Alberti C, Bornstain C, et al: Improved survival in cancer patients requiring mechanical ventilatory support: impact of noninvasive mechanical ventilatory support. *Crit Care Med* 29(3):519–525, 2001.
60. Meduri GU, Cook TR, Turner RE, et al: Noninvasive positive pressure ventilation in status asthmaticus. *Chest* 110(3):767–774, 1996.
61. Fernandez MM, Villagra A, Blanch L, et al: Non-invasive mechanical ventilation in status asthmaticus. *Intensive Care Med* 27(3):486–492, 2001.
62. Soroksky A, Stav D, Shpirer I: A pilot prospective, randomized, placebo-controlled trial of bilevel positive airway pressure in acute asthmatic attack. *Chest* 123(4):1018–1025, 2003.
63. Soma T, Hino M, Kida K, et al: A prospective and randomized study for improvement of acute asthma by non-invasive positive pressure ventilation (NPPV). *Intern Med* 47(6):493–501, 2008.
64. Pollack CV Jr, Fleisch KB, Dowsey K: Treatment of acute bronchospasm with beta-adrenergic agonist aerosols delivered by a nasal bilevel positive airway pressure circuit. *Ann Emerg Med* 26(5):552–557, 1995.
65. Hill AT, Edenborough FP, Cayton RM, et al: Long-term nasal intermittent positive pressure ventilation in patients with cystic fibrosis and hypercapnic respiratory failure (1991-1996). *Respir Med* 92(3):523–526, 1998.
66. Ferrer M, Esquinas A, Leon M, et al: Noninvasive ventilation in severe hypoxemic respiratory failure: a randomized clinical trial. *Am J Respir Crit Care Med* 168(12):1438–1444, 2003.
67. Antonelli M, Conti G, Rocco M, et al: A comparison of noninvasive positive-pressure ventilation and conventional mechanical ventilation in patients with acute respiratory failure. *N Engl J Med* 339(7):429–435, 1998.
68. Jolliet P, Abajo B, Pasquina P, et al: Non-invasive pressure support ventilation in severe community-acquired pneumonia. *Intensive Care Med* 27(5):812–821, 2001.
69. Rocker GM, Mackenzie MG, Williams B, et al: Noninvasive positive pressure ventilation: successful outcome in patients with acute lung injury/ARDS. *Chest* 115(1):173–177, 1999.
70. Antonelli M, Conti G, Esquinas A, et al: A multiple-center survey on the use in clinical practice of noninvasive ventilation as a first-line intervention for acute respiratory distress syndrome. *Crit Care Med* 35(1):18–25, 2007.
71. Antonelli M, Conti G, Moro ML, et al: Predictors of failure of noninvasive positive pressure ventilation in patients with acute hypoxemic respiratory failure: a multi-center study. *Intensive Care Med* 27(11):1718–1728, 2001.
72. Beltrame F, Lucangelo U, Gregori D, et al: Noninvasive positive pressure ventilation in trauma patients with acute respiratory failure. *Monaldi Arch Chest Dis* 54(2):109–114, 1999.
73. Hernandez G, Fernandez R, Lopez-Reina P, et al: Noninvasive ventilation reduces intubation in chest trauma-related hypoxemia: a randomized clinical trial. *Chest* 137(1):74–80, 2010.
74. Epstein SK: Etiology of extubation failure and the predictive value of the rapid shallow breathing index. *Am J Respir Crit Care Med* 152(2):545–549, 1995.
75. Boles JM, Bion J, Connors A, et al: Weaning from mechanical ventilation. *Eur Respir J* 29(5):1033–1056, 2007.
76. Keenan SP, Powers C, McCormack DG, et al: Noninvasive positive-pressure ventilation for postextubation respiratory distress: a randomized controlled trial. *JAMA* 287(24):3238–3244, 2002.
77. Esteban A, Frutos-Vivar F, Ferguson ND, et al: Noninvasive positive-pressure ventilation for respiratory failure after extubation. *N Engl J Med* 350(24):2452–2460, 2004.
78. Nava S, Gregoretti C, Fanfulla F, et al: Noninvasive ventilation to prevent respiratory failure after extubation in high-risk patients. *Crit Care Med* 33(11):2465–2470, 2005.
79. Ferrer M, Valencia M, Nicolas JM, et al: Early noninvasive ventilation averts extubation failure in patients at risk: a randomized trial. *Am J Respir Crit Care Med* 173(2):164–170, 2006.
80. Ferrer M, Sellares J, Valencia M, et al: Non-invasive ventilation after extubation in hypercapnic patients with chronic respiratory disorders: randomised controlled trial. *Lancet* 374(9695):1082–1088, 2009.
81. Ferreyra GP, Baussano I, Squadrone V, et al: Continuous positive airway pressure for treatment of respiratory complications after abdominal surgery: a systematic review and meta-analysis. *Ann Surg* 247(4):617–626, 2008.
82. Conti G, Cavaliere F, Costa R, et al: Noninvasive positive-pressure ventilation with different interfaces in patients with respiratory failure after abdominal surgery: a matched-control study. *Respir Care* 52(11):1463–1471, 2007.

83. Squadrone V, Coha M, Cerutti E, et al: Continuous positive airway pressure for treatment of postoperative hypoxemia: a randomized controlled trial. *JAMA* 293(5):589–595, 2005.
84. Kindgen-Milles D, Muller E, Buhl R, et al: Nasal-continuous positive airway pressure reduces pulmonary morbidity and length of hospital stay following thoracoabdominal aortic surgery. *Chest* 128(2):821–828, 2005.
85. Auriant I, Jallot A, Herve P, et al: Noninvasive ventilation reduces mortality in acute respiratory failure following lung resection. *Am J Respir Crit Care Med* 164(7):1231–1235, 2001.
86. Schettino G, Altobelli N, Kacmarek RM: Noninvasive positive pressure ventilation reverses acute respiratory failure in select "do-not-intubate" patients. *Crit Care Med* 33(9):1976–1982, 2005.
87. Curtis JR, Cook DJ, Sinuff T, et al: Noninvasive positive pressure ventilation in critical and palliative care settings: understanding the goals of therapy. *Crit Care Med* 35(3):932–939, 2007.
88. Antonelli M, Conti G, Riccioni L, et al: Noninvasive positive-pressure ventilation via face mask during bronchoscopy with BAL in high-risk hypoxemic patients. *Chest* 110(3):724–728, 1996.
89. Antonelli M, Conti G, Rocco M, et al: Noninvasive positive-pressure ventilation vs. conventional oxygen supplementation in hypoxemic patients undergoing diagnostic bronchoscopy. *Chest* 121(4):1149–1154, 2002.
90. Pope JF, Birnkrant DJ, Martin JE, et al: Noninvasive ventilation during percutaneous gastrostomy placement in Duchenne muscular dystrophy. *Pediatr Pulmonol* 23(6):468–471, 1997.
91. Guarracino F, Cabrini L, Baldassarri R, et al: Non-invasive ventilation-aided transoesophageal echocardiography in high-risk patients: a pilot study. *Eur J Echocardiogr* 11:554–556, 2010.
92. Baillard C, Fosse JP, Sebbane M, et al: Noninvasive ventilation improves preoxygenation before intubation of hypoxic patients. *Am J Respir Crit Care Med* 174(2):171–177, 2006.
93. Confalonieri M, Garuti G, Cattaruzza MS, et al: A chart of failure risk for noninvasive ventilation in patients with COPD exacerbation. *Eur Respir J* 25(2):348–355, 2005.
94. Diaz GG, Alcaraz AC, Talavera JC, et al: Noninvasive positive-pressure ventilation to treat hypercapnic coma secondary to respiratory failure. *Chest* 127(3):952–960, 2005.
95. Navalesi P, Fanfulla F, Frigerio P, et al: Physiologic evaluation of noninvasive mechanical ventilation delivered with three types of masks in patients with chronic hypercapnic respiratory failure. *Crit Care Med* 28(6):1785–1790, 2000.
96. Kwok H, McCormack J, Cece R, et al: Controlled trial of oronasal versus nasal mask ventilation in the treatment of acute respiratory failure. *Crit Care Med* 31(2):468–473, 2003.
97. Criner GJ, Travaline JM, Brennan KJ, et al: Efficacy of a new full face mask for noninvasive positive pressure ventilation. *Chest* 106(4):1109–1115, 1994.
98. Antonelli M, Pennisi MA, Pelosi P, et al: Noninvasive positive pressure ventilation using a helmet in patients with acute exacerbation of chronic obstructive pulmonary disease: a feasibility study. *Anesthesiology* 100(1):16–24, 2004.
99. Antonelli M, Conti G, Pelosi P, et al: New treatment of acute hypoxemic respiratory failure: noninvasive pressure support ventilation delivered by helmet—a pilot controlled trial. *Crit Care Med* 30(3):602–608, 2002.
100. Navalesi P, Costa R, Ceriana P, et al: Non-invasive ventilation in chronic obstructive pulmonary disease patients: helmet versus facial mask. *Intensive Care Med* 33(1):74–81, 2007.
101. Cavaliere F, Conti G, Costa R, et al: Noise exposure during noninvasive ventilation with a helmet, a nasal mask, and a facial mask. *Intensive Care Med* 30(9):1755–1760, 2004.
102. Patrick W, Webster K, Ludwig L, et al: Noninvasive positive-pressure ventilation in acute respiratory distress without prior chronic respiratory failure. *Am J Respir Crit Care Med* 153(3):1005–1011, 1996.
103. Fernandez R, Blanch L, Valles J, et al: Pressure support ventilation via face mask in acute respiratory failure in hypercapnic COPD patients. *Intensive Care Med* 19(8):456–461, 1993.
104. Ambrosino N, Nava S, Bertone P, et al: Physiologic evaluation of pressure support ventilation by nasal mask in patients with stable COPD. *Chest* 101(2):385–391, 1992.
105. Ferreira JC, Chipman DW, Hill NS, et al: Bilevel vs ICU ventilators providing noninvasive ventilation: effect of system leaks: a COPD lung model comparison. *Chest* 136(2):448–456, 2009.
106. Sanders MH, Moore SE, Eveslage J: CPAP via nasal mask: a treatment for occlusive sleep apnea. *Chest* 83(1):144–145, 1983.
107. Strumpf DC, Carlisle CC, Millman RP, et al: An evaluation of the Respironics BiPAP Bi-level CPAP device for delivery of assisted ventilation. *Respir Care* 35:415–422, 1990.
108. Fernandez-Vivas M, Caturla-Such J, Gonzalez de la Rosa J, et al: Noninvasive pressure support versus proportional assist ventilation in acute respiratory failure. *Intensive Care Med* 29(7):1126–1133, 2003.
109. Schwartz AR, Kacmarek RM, Hess DR: Factors affecting oxygen delivery with bi-level positive airway pressure. *Respir Care* 49(3):270–275, 2004.
110. Samolski D, Calaf N, Guell R, et al: Carbon dioxide rebreathing in non-invasive ventilation. Analysis of masks, expiratory ports and ventilatory modes. *Monaldi Arch Chest Dis* 69(3):114–118, 2008.
111. Schettino GP, Chatmongkolchart S, Hess DR, et al: Position of exhalation port and mask design affect CO_2 rebreathing during noninvasive positive pressure ventilation. *Crit Care Med* 31(8):2178–2182, 2003.
112. Hill NS, Carlisle C, Kramer NR: Effect of a nonrebreathing exhalation valve on long-term nasal ventilation using a bilevel device. *Chest* 122(1):84–91, 2002.
113. Lellouche F, Maggiore SM, Deye N, et al: Effect of the humidification device on the work of breathing during noninvasive ventilation. *Intensive Care Med* 28(11):1582–1589, 2002.
114. Richards GN, Cistulli PA, Ungar RG, et al: Mouth leak with nasal continuous positive airway pressure increases nasal airway resistance. *Am J Respir Crit Care Med* 154(1):182–186, 1996.
115. Storre JH, Seuthe B, Fiechter R, et al: Average volume-assured pressure support in obesity hypoventilation: a randomized crossover trial. *Chest* 130(3):815–821, 2006.
116. Gay PC, Hess DR, Hill NS: Noninvasive proportional assist ventilation for acute respiratory insufficiency. Comparison with pressure support ventilation. *Am J Respir Crit Care Med* 164(9):1606–1611, 2001.
117. L'Her E, Deye N, Lellouche F, et al: Physiologic effects of noninvasive ventilation during acute lung injury. *Am J Respir Crit Care Med* 172(9):1112–1118, 2005.
118. Thys F, Roeseler J, Reynaert M, et al: Noninvasive ventilation for acute respiratory failure: a prospective randomised placebo-controlled trial. *Eur Respir J* 20(3):545–555, 2002.
119. Sinuff T, Cook DJ, Randall J, et al: Evaluation of a practice guideline for noninvasive positive-pressure ventilation for acute respiratory failure. *Chest* 123(6):2062–2073, 2003.
120. Farha S, Ghamra ZW, Hoisington ER, et al: Use of noninvasive positive-pressure ventilation on the regular hospital ward: experience and correlates of success. *Respir Care* 51(11):1237–1243, 2006.
121. Seneviratne J, Mandrekar J, Wijdicks EF, et al: Predictors of extubation failure in myasthenic crisis. *Arch Neurol* 65(7):929–933, 2008.
122. Cavaliere F, Conti G, Costa R, et al: Exposure to noise during continuous positive airway pressure: influence of interfaces and delivery systems. *Acta Anaesthesiol Scand* 52(1):52–56, 2008.
123. Dellweg D, Hochrainer D, Klauke M, et al: Determinants of skin contact pressure formation during non-invasive ventilation. *J Biomech* 43(4):652–657, 2010.
124. Jones DJ, Braid GM, Wedzicha JA: Nasal masks for domiciliary positive pressure ventilation: patient usage and complications. *Thorax* 49(8):811–812, 1994.
125. Smurthwaite GJ, Ford P: Skin necrosis following continuous positive airway pressure with a face mask. *Anaesthesia* 48(2):147–148, 1993.
126. Gregoretti C, Confalonieri M, Navalesi P, et al: Evaluation of patient skin breakdown and comfort with a new face mask for non-invasive ventilation: a multi-center study. *Intensive Care Med* 28(3):278–284, 2002.
127. Meduri GU, Abou-Shala N, Fox RC, et al: Noninvasive face mask mechanical ventilation in patients with acute hypercapnic respiratory failure. *Chest* 100(2):445–454, 1991.
128. Criner GJ, Brennan K, Travaline JM, et al: Efficacy and compliance with noninvasive positive pressure ventilation in patients with chronic respiratory failure. *Chest* 116(3):667–675, 1999.
129. De Keulenaer BL, De Backer A, Schepens DR, et al: Abdominal compartment syndrome related to noninvasive ventilation. *Intensive Care Med* 29(7):1177–1181, 2003.
130. Jean-Lavaleur M, Perrier V, Roze H, et al: Stomach rupture associated with noninvasive ventilation. *Ann Fr Anesth Reanim* 28(6):588–591, 2009.
131. Delay JM, Sebbane M, Jung B, et al: The effectiveness of noninvasive positive pressure ventilation to enhance preoxygenation in morbidly obese patients: a randomized controlled study. *Anesth Analg* 107(5):1707–1713, 2008.
132. Thille AW, Rodriguez P, Cabello B, et al: Patient-ventilator asynchrony during assisted mechanical ventilation. *Intensive Care Med* 32(10):1515–1522, 2006.
133. Hubmayr RD: The importance of patient/ventilator interactions during non-invasive mechanical ventilation. *Acta Anaesthesiol Scand Suppl* 109:46–47, 1996.
134. Calderini E, Confalonieri M, Puccio PG, et al: Patient-ventilator asynchrony during noninvasive ventilation: the role of expiratory trigger. *Intensive Care Med* 25(7):662–667, 1999.
135. Achour L, Letellier C, Cuvelier A, et al: Asynchrony and cyclic variability in pressure support noninvasive ventilation. *Comput Biol Med* 37(9):1308–1320, 2007.
136. Racca F, Appendini L, Gregoretti C, et al: Effectiveness of mask and helmet interfaces to deliver noninvasive ventilation in a human model of resistive breathing. *J Appl Physiol* 99(4):1262–1271, 2005.
137. Moerer O, Herrmann P, Hinz J, et al: High flow biphasic positive airway pressure by helmet—effects on pressurization, tidal volume, carbon dioxide accumulation and noise exposure. *Crit Care* 13(3):R85, 2009.
138. Ferguson GT, Gilmartin M: CO_2 rebreathing during BiPAP ventilatory assistance. *Am J Respir Crit Care Med* 151(4):1126–1135, 1995.
139. Scala R, Naldi M: Ventilators for noninvasive ventilation to treat acute respiratory failure. *Respir Care* 53(8):1054–1080, 2008.
140. Szkulmowski Z, Belkhouja K, Le QH, et al: Bilevel positive airway pressure ventilation: factors influencing carbon dioxide rebreathing. *Intensive Care Med* 36:688–691, 2010.

141. Lofaso F, Brochard L, Hang T, et al: Home versus intensive care pressure support devices. Experimental and clinical comparison. *Am J Respir Crit Care Med* 153(5):1591–1599, 1996.
142. Lofaso F, Brochard L, Touchard D, et al: Evaluation of carbon dioxide rebreathing during pressure support ventilation with airway management system (BiPAP) devices. *Chest* 108(3):772–778, 1995.
143. Patel RG, Petrini MF: Respiratory muscle performance, pulmonary mechanics, and gas exchange between the BiPAP S/T-D system and the Servo Ventilator 900C with bilevel positive airway pressure ventilation following gradual pressure support weaning. *Chest* 114(5):1390–1396, 1998.
144. Louis B, Leroux K, Isabey D, et al: Effect of manufacturer-inserted mask leaks on ventilator performance. *Eur Respir J* 35(3):627–636, 2010.
145. Holanda MA, Reis RC, Winkeler GF, et al: Influence of total face, facial and nasal masks on short-term adverse effects during noninvasive ventilation. *J Bras Pneumol* 35(2):164–173, 2009.
146. Tonnelier JM, Prat G, Nowak E, et al: Noninvasive continuous positive airway pressure ventilation using a new helmet interface: a case-control prospective pilot study. *Intensive Care Med* 29(11):2077–2080, 2003.
147. Taccone P, Hess D, Caironi P, et al: Continuous positive airway pressure delivered with a "helmet": effects on carbon dioxide rebreathing. *Crit Care Med* 32(10):2090–2096, 2004.
148. Racca F, Appendini L, Gregoretti C, et al: Helmet ventilation and carbon dioxide rebreathing: effects of adding a leak at the helmet ports. *Intensive Care Med* 34(8):1461–1468, 2008.
149. Vignaux L, Vargas F, Roeseler J, et al: Patient-ventilator asynchrony during non-invasive ventilation for acute respiratory failure: a multicenter study. *Intensive Care Med* 35(5):840–846, 2009.
150. Storre JH, Bohm P, Dreher M, et al: Clinical impact of leak compensation during non-invasive ventilation. *Respir Med* 103(10):1477–1483, 2009.
151. Sopkova Z, Dorkova Z, Tkacova R: Predictors of compliance with continuous positive airway pressure treatment in patients with obstructive sleep apnea and metabolic syndrome. *Wien Klin Wochenschr* 121(11–12):398–404, 2009.
152. Rabec C, Georges M, Kabeya NK, et al: Evaluating noninvasive ventilation using a monitoring system coupled to a ventilator: a bench-to-bedside study. *Eur Respir J* 34(4):902–913, 2009.
153. Girault C, Briel A, Benichou J, et al: Interface strategy during noninvasive positive pressure ventilation for hypercapnic acute respiratory failure. *Crit Care Med* 37(1):124–131, 2009.
154. Fraticelli AT, Lellouche F, L'Her E, et al: Physiological effects of different interfaces during noninvasive ventilation for acute respiratory failure. *Crit Care Med* 37(3):939–945, 2009.
155. Devlin JW, Nava S, Fong JJ, et al: Survey of sedation practices during noninvasive positive-pressure ventilation to treat acute respiratory failure. *Crit Care Med* 35(10):2298–2302, 2007.
156. Cooksley CD, Avritscher EB, Rolston KV, et al: Hospitalizations for infection in cancer patients: impact of an aging population. *Support Care Cancer* 17(5):547–554, 2009.
157. Zilberberg MD, Shorr AF: Prolonged acute mechanical ventilation and hospital bed utilization in 2020 in the United States: implications for budgets, plant and personnel planning. *BMC Health Serv Res* 8:242, 2008.
158. Keenan SP, Sinuff T, Cook DJ, et al: Which patients with acute exacerbation of chronic obstructive pulmonary disease benefit from noninvasive positive-pressure ventilation? A systematic review of the literature. *Ann Intern Med* 138(11):861–870, 2003.
159. Lightowler JV, Wedzicha JA, Elliott MW, et al: Non-invasive positive pressure ventilation to treat respiratory failure resulting from exacerbations of chronic obstructive pulmonary disease: Cochrane systematic review and meta-analysis. *BMJ* 326(7382):185, 2003.
160. Briones Claudett KH, Briones Claudett MH, Chung Sang Wong MA, et al: Noninvasive mechanical ventilation in patients with chronic obstructive pulmonary disease and severe hypercapnic neurological deterioration in the emergency room. *Eur J Emerg Med* 15(3):127–133, 2008.
161. Tomii K, Seo R, Tachikawa R, et al: Impact of noninvasive ventilation (NIV) trial for various types of acute respiratory failure in the emergency department; decreased mortality and use of the ICU. *Respir Med* 103(1):67–73, 2009.
162. Vital FM, Saconato H, Ladeira MT, et al: Non-invasive positive pressure ventilation (CPAP or bilevel NPPV) for cardiogenic pulmonary edema. *Cochrane Database Syst Rev* (3):CD005351, 2008.
163. Agarwal R, Handa A, Aggarwal AN, et al: Outcomes of noninvasive ventilation in acute hypoxemic respiratory failure in a respiratory intensive care unit in north India. *Respir Care* 54(12):1679–1687, 2009.
164. Agarwal R, Aggarwal AN, Gupta D, et al: Etiology and outcomes of pulmonary and extrapulmonary acute lung injury/ARDS in a respiratory ICU in North India. *Chest* 130(3):724–729, 2006.
165. Michelet P, D'Journo XB, Seinaye F, et al: Non-invasive ventilation for treatment of postoperative respiratory failure after oesophagectomy. *Br J Surg* 96(1):54–60, 2009.

CHAPTER 60 ■ MECHANICAL VENTILATION PART III: DISCONTINUATION

RICHARD S. IRWIN, NICHOLAS A. SMYRNIOS AND ROLF D. HUBMAYR

A great deal of effort has been devoted to developing scientifically based strategies to more consistently achieve successful discontinuation of mechanical ventilation (MV). This chapter reviews the advances made in four general areas: (a) understanding the problem, (b) the value of criteria for reliably predicting discontinuation success, (c) identifying the most useful modes, and (d) managing discontinuation failure.

UNDERSTANDING THE DISCONTINUATION PROBLEM

Who Are the Patients and What Are Their Outcomes?

Patients with, or likely to develop, respiratory failure are the individuals who require MV support. Although there is overlap, respiratory failure can be generally categorized into lung failure and pump failure. *Lung failure* is pure gas-exchange failure and is manifested by hypoxemia. It is commonly due to the acute respiratory distress syndrome or cardiogenic pulmonary edema. *Pump failure* is synonymous with ventilatory failure and is manifested by hypercapnia and hypoxemia. It is commonly due to central nervous system depression (e.g., overdose, anesthesia) or respiratory muscle fatigue or weakness.

For those who recover from the insult that necessitated MV, most (80% to 90%) [1–4] can have MV easily discontinued and be extubated. In this group, MV can be discontinued in 77% of patients within 72 hours of the initiation of MV [4]. This group is composed predominantly of postoperative patients, patients with overdoses, and patients whose conditions cause pure lung failure that reverses rapidly. In the minority of patients, probably 10% to 20% overall, MV is more difficult to discontinue. Data suggest that duration of MV does not necessarily have an impact on long-term survival. For example, 1-year survival for patients on MV for more than 21 days can

TABLE 60.1

POTENTIALLY REVERSIBLE REASONS FOR PROLONGED MECHANICAL VENTILATION

Inadequate respiratory drive
Inability of the lungs to carry out gas exchange effectively
Inspiratory respiratory muscle fatigue/weakness
Psychological dependency
Combinations of these items

be as high as 93% [5]. Although it may take 3 months or longer to be able to discontinue MV in these patients in long-term facilities, the ultimate quality of life of the survivors ranges from being minimally to moderately impaired [6,7].

What Is Wrong with Patients on Prolonged Ventilator Support?

There are potentially four separate and reversible reasons for prolonged MV [8] (Table 60.1).

1. *Inadequate respiratory drive* may be due to nutritional deficiencies [9], sedatives, central nervous system abnormality, or sleep deprivation [10].
2. *Inability of the lungs to carry out gas exchange effectively* may continue if the underlying cause of respiratory failure has not sufficiently improved.
3. There may be profound *inspiratory respiratory muscle weakness* and possibly *fatigue.*
4. *Psychological dependency* may be an additional factor [11].

Although no studies have been performed to determine systematically the relative importance of these factors, and combinations of these factors may be responsible for prolonged MV, the literature suggests that pump failure due to inspiratory respiratory muscle fatigue/weakness [12] is primarily responsible for failure of discontinuation of MV in these patients [3,13,14]. *Muscle fatigue* is "a condition in which there is loss in the capacity for developing force and/or velocity of a muscle, resulting from muscle activity under load and which is reversible by rest" [15,16]. *Muscle weakness* is "a condition in which the capacity of a rested muscle to generate force is impaired" [15,16]. Although fatigue and weakness can be experimentally distinguished, this is not usually possible in the clinical setting. Therefore, the term muscle fatigue, when used clinically and by us in this chapter, may actually encompass fatigue or weakness, or both. Contributors to respiratory *muscle fatigue* may be (a) central nervous system depression, (b) mechanical defects (e.g., flail chest and kyphoscoliosis) that increase the work of breathing, (c) lung disease that increases the work of breathing, and (d) mediators of ongoing active diseases (e.g., sepsis, ventilator-induced diaphragmatic dysfunction) that adversely affect the respiratory muscles.

What Factors Impact upon Respiratory Muscle Fatigue and Weakness?

The cause of inspiratory respiratory muscle fatigue is likely to be multifactorial [17–36]. The major factors that compromise muscle strength and endurance are listed in Table 60.2. A few items deserve additional explanation.

TABLE 60.2

POSSIBLE CAUSES OF INSPIRATORY RESPIRATORY MUSCLE FATIGUE

Nutritional and metabolic deficiencies [18]
Hypokalemia [19]
Hypomagnesemia [20]
Hypocalcemia [21]
Hypophosphatemia [22]
Hypothyroidism [23]
Corticosteroids [24]
Chronic renal failure [25]
Systemic diseases
Decreased protein synthesis and increased degradation [26]
Decreased glycogen stores [27]
Hypoxemia and hypercapnia [28,29]
Persistently increased work of breathing (e.g., underlying disease, mechanical ventilator, airway humidification devices) [30–32]
Failure of the cardiovascular system (e.g., disease, ventilator) [33,34]
Neuromuscular dysfunction/disease
Drugs [35]
Critical illness polyneuropathy/myopathy [36]
Combinations of the items in this table

Mechanical Ventilation

Although it is assumed that one of the benefits of MV is that it rests the respiratory muscles, this may not actually occur [37]. The response of mechanical ventilators to rapid changes in patient effort is often inadequate. This is particularly true for older-generation ventilators. Positive pressure MV may increase minute volume without decreasing respiratory muscle work. In part, this is because ventilators used in either the assist control or synchronized intermittent mandatory ventilation (SIMV) mode do not synchronize their output with that of the patient's respiratory system. In extreme cases, the lack of synchronization causes patient effort to exceed that observed during unassisted breathing. Both SIMV and assist ventilation modes may cause problems in this regard. Also, SIMV systems expose patients to increases in airway resistance during spontaneous efforts that occur between machine breaths.

Continuous flow and demand valve systems have the potential for increasing the work of breathing. For instance, the continuous flow may not satisfy the patient's inspiratory flow demands. Demand valve SIMV systems may increase the work of breathing because they require substantial effort by the patient to breathe spontaneously. Moreover, in assist mode, the patient's inspiratory muscles might work throughout the entire inspiratory cycle if tidal volume and inspiratory flow rate do not meet the patient's inspiratory requirements. If auto–positive end-expiratory pressure (auto-PEEP) is present (see Chapter 58), the patient may not be able to trigger the ventilator or may be able to capture it only intermittently while performing a prohibitively large amount of work during assist ventilation, because he or she must drop airway pressure below the amount of auto-PEEP before triggering the ventilator. If there is an increased work of breathing due to the patient's ventilator that provokes respiratory distress, the patient's diaphragm may develop an inflammatory injury that may not appear clinically for days afterward [31,37–39]. Although it is important to minimize the work of strenuous muscle activity while patients are receiving MV, it is also important to avoid prolonged muscle unloading because neuromuscular inactivity ("rest") can lead to ventilator-induced diaphragmatic dysfunction [30].

Cardiovascular Disease

Failure of the cardiovascular system may prolong MV for a variety of reasons. Gas exchange may be impaired by passive congestion of the lungs, and this may contribute to an increased work of breathing during spontaneous breaths. Poor cardiac performance may contribute to an inadequate supply of oxygen to the respiratory muscles, while an increased work of breathing conversely may provoke myocardial ischemia [33]. Although MV may adversely affect cardiac output by increasing intrathoracic pressure, thereby decreasing venous return and cardiac output, it is also possible that some cardiovascular patients cannot have MV discontinued because the ventilator exerts a beneficial influence on cardiac function (i.e., unloading the left ventricle in left ventricular failure) [40]. Prematurely withdrawing MV from these patients may lead to deterioration in cardiac function.

Nutritional Factors

Nutritional deficiencies may prolong the discontinuation process from MV by leading to myocardial as well as respiratory muscle dysfunction [41]. Older studies have suggested that an appropriate amount of nutritional support may improve the success rate of discontinuation of MV [42,43], but these were not definitive. More recent randomized controlled trials comparing high-fat/low-carbohydrate feeds versus conventional feeds and growth hormone versus placebo showed no change in duration of MV or discontinuation success. These trials have been summarized elsewhere [44].

CRITERIA FOR PREDICTING SUCCESSFUL DISCONTINUATION

When Is It Appropriate to Begin the Discontinuation Process?

Because there are no objective, rigorously generated data to determine the appropriate time to initiate weaning, physicians must rely on their clinical judgment. Therefore, the authors recommend that clinicians consider a carefully monitored spontaneous breathing trial (SBT) of discontinuation when the following criteria, set forth in a national clinical practice guideline, have been met: (a) The underlying reason(s) for MV has been stabilized and the patient is improving, (b) the patient is hemodynamically stable on minimal-to-no pressors, (c) oxygenation is adequate (e.g., PaO_2/FIO_2 greater than 200, PEEP no more than 7.5 cm H_2O, FIO_2 less than 0.5), and (d) the patient is able to initiate spontaneous inspiratory efforts [45]. Because potentially harmful effects of suddenly having to take on the work of breathing occur early (albeit infrequently) during SBTs [46], patients should be closely monitored during the first 5 minutes. Basing weaning decisions on the rapid shallow breathing index (RSBI) in effect enforces this (see section Predictive Indices for Total Discontinuation of Mechanical Ventilation). SBTs, variably performed with a T-piece, with low-level pressure support ventilation, or with just a predetermined amount of continuous positive airway pressure (CPAP) in ventilators equipped with "flow-by" internal circuits, should be timed to coincide with the daily sedation holiday to maximize the opportunity for success and to allow assessment of patient comfort and behavioral effects on breathing.

If the patient deteriorates or becomes distressed during this brief period of observation, MV should be reinstituted. The authors caution against assuming that anxiety is causing the failure of a breathing trial. Although anxiety can mimic respiratory failure, in the authors' experience anxiety is not usually the cause of failure but rather a consequence of it. In fact, the "art of weaning" centers on the judgment whether weaning-induced distress is a manifestation of agitated delirium, sedative and narcotic withdrawal, pain and tube discomfort, or respiratory failure. When in doubt, the provider should assume the latter. We know of no validated test capable of distinguishing between these entities. To help decide in these situations, we sometimes observe patients who are difficult to wean while keeping them heavily sedated. If under these circumstances, unassisted breathing can be sustained without hypercapnia, hypoxemia, tachypnea, and tachycardia, we conclude that respiratory failure is no longer present, that agitation may be related to pain, anxiety, or sedative/hypnotic withdrawal, and proceed with a trial of extubation if and when we believe that the patient is able to protect his or her airway against the possibility of aspiration.

There are no data to show that attempts at starting the discontinuation of MV in this context lead to adverse consequences. On the contrary, screening patients daily to identify those who can breathe spontaneously can reduce the duration of MV and the cost of intensive care [47]. Because the authors' recommendations are guidelines and not rigorously tested criteria, it may also be appropriate to start the carefully monitored process in an individual patient who has not met all of the previously mentioned guidelines.

Predictive Indices for Total Discontinuation of Mechanical Ventilation

Studies have evaluated a wide variety of physiologic indices to predict a patient's ability to breathe spontaneously without MV [48]. These studies yield conflicting data due in large part to differences in methods and experimental design, such as population studied, choice of physiologic index threshold value, measurement techniques, definitions of success and failure, and perhaps because of selection bias in choosing patients for weaning studies [48].

A collective task force of clinician investigators co-facilitated by the American College of Chest Physicians, the American Association for Respiratory Care, and the American College of Critical Care Medicine developed evidence-based guidelines for weaning and discontinuing ventilatory support [45]. In their report, they evaluated the evidence for predicting success in weaning from MV [48]. A summary of their findings is as follows:

1. A large number of predictors have been found to be of no use in predicting the results of weaning.
2. A few predictors have been shown to be of some use, albeit inconsistent, in predicting discontinuation of the ventilator and successful extubation. Those include respiratory rate (RR) of less than 38 breaths per minute (sensitivity, 88%; specificity, 47%), a RSBI less than 100 breaths per minute per L (sensitivity, 65% to 96%; specificity, 0% to 73%), and an inspiratory pressure/maximal inspiratory pressure ratio less than 0.3. In addition, the combination of a RR of more than 38 breaths per minute and a RSBI more than 100 breaths per minute per L appears to reduce the probability of successful extubation.
3. Likelihood ratios (LRs) appear to provide the best format for presenting the results of weaning predictors.
   a. LR positive = the odds that a patient with weaning success will have a positive test result (RSBI <100), compared to the odds that a patient with weaning failure will demonstrate a positive test.
   b. LR negative = the odds that a patient with weaning success will have a negative test result (RSBI >100),

compared to the odds that a patient with weaning failure will have a negative test.

c. LRs greater than 10 or less than 0.1 imply large, clinically significant outcomes. LRs between 5 and 10 imply moderate, probably clinically significant outcomes. LRs between 2 and 5 imply small, possibly clinically significant outcomes. LRs between 0.5 and 2 are insignificant.
d. The Task Force found LRs greater than 10 or less than 0.1 only twice, and only when data from all trials were pooled. The ratio of airway pressure 0.1 second after the occlusion of the inspiratory port of unidirectional balloon occlusion valve ($P_{0.1}$) to maximal inspiratory pressure (PI_{max}) of 0.09 to 0.14 was highly predictive of successful extubation in two studies with a pooled LR of 16.3. No LRs between 5 and 10 were found.
e. When LRs were calculated for RSBI, pooled results for a test predicting successful discontinuation of ventilation and extubation showed a LR of 2.8; results for a test predicting failure of discontinuation and extubation showed a LR of 0.22. These results suggest mediocre accuracy.
f. The reliability of the RSBI will be diminished when it is measured during the first minute of SB when respiratory drive may still be suppressed, when it is measured in the presence of a small endotracheal tube (internal diameter of 7 mm or less), particularly in women [49], and as patients have the measurement made while receiving pressure support (PS) and/or CPAP [50,51]. It is recommended that RSBI measurements be made while patients are spontaneously breathing, as the test was originally described [52].

Although clinical observation of the respiratory muscles during spontaneous breaths was initially thought to be reliable in predicting subsequent discontinuation failure, respiratory-inductive plethysmographic studies [53] have shown this to be not necessarily the case. Any time there is a substantial increase in load on the respiratory muscles, a change in the rate, depth, and pattern of breathing may be observed. Because these signs may also be manifestations of fatigue, it is useful to note them. If these signs never appear, successful discontinuation is likely. If they do appear, patients must be observed closely for further deterioration because discontinuation inevitably fails if these signs are owing to fatigue.

When Is It Appropriate to Extubate the Patient?

Once MV has been discontinued, consider whether the patient is likely to fail extubation. The most common causes of extubation failure are upper-airway obstruction and inability to protect the airway and clear secretions. Patients at the highest risk of postextubation upper-airway obstruction are those who have been on prolonged MV, are female, and who have had repeated or traumatic intubations [54]. One method of assessing for the presence of upper airway obstruction during MV is the cuff-leak test. It is performed by comparing the exhaled volumes before and after the balloon of the endotracheal tube has been deflated. Although one study [55] showed that a cuff leak of less than 110 mL measured during assist-control ventilation within 24 hours of extubation identified patients at high risk of postextubation stridor, other studies have not [56]. Although the concept of measuring cuff leak is intuitively appealing, the benefits are not clearly identified, and the process and even the actual values for decision making are not broadly agreed upon. Values of 110, 130, and 140 mL are all used in recent studies. Other studies use an approach of auscultation to detect leak. In addition, the appropriate course of action to take for an abnormal test is not defined. Some authors suggest treatment with steroids, some delay of extubation, and some advocate having persons with advanced airway skills present for the extubation. Therefore, because we are unable to scientifically determine which patients should have a test, how we would conduct the test, and what we would do with an abnormal value if we had one, we do not advocate routinely performing or basing decisions on the results of a cuff-leak test. A provider may consider using a cuff-leak test in specific patients to gain a general appreciation of the airway status in a high-risk patient [57–59].

Patients may also fail extubation because they are unable to protect their airways or clear their secretions. A prospective observational study [60] showed that the strongest predictors of extubation failure in patients who passed a SB trial were (a) poor cough defined as a cough peak flow measurement of less than 60 L per minute, (b) secretion volume of 2.5 mL per hour or greater, and (c) poor mentation as determined by the inability to complete any of the four following tasks on command: open eyes, follow observer with eyes, grasp hand, and stick out tongue. In this series, reintubation took place in 12% of patients when one of these predictors was present and 80% when all three were present. (See Chapter 62 for an in-depth discussion of cough effectiveness and how to assess for it.)

Once extubation has taken place, the authors proceed cautiously before instituting feedings by mouth. Because there is no clinically reliable way of assessing the adequacy of swallowing at the bedside, a formal swallowing evaluation (e.g., speech pathology consult and videofluoroscopic evaluation of swallow) should be considered in patients at increased risk of aspiration before resuming oral feedings. Although it is commonly appreciated that older age, debilitation, sedation, oral or nasal enteral feeding tubes, history of dysphagia, acute stroke, cervical spine surgery, muscle weakness, and/or tracheostomy are risk factors for aspiration, it is less commonly known that endotracheal intubation carries the same risk [61,62]. After extubation, swallowing difficulties may exist in up to 50% of patients for up to 1 week, even when endotracheal intubation has been of short duration, and the patient is awake and not seriously ill. In awake, postsurgical patients evaluated for aspiration following extubation, 50% of those who aspirated did so immediately when fed, whereas 25% and 5% aspirated when tested 4 and 8 hours later, respectively. (See Chapter 54 for an in-depth discussion of this subject.)

Perspective

When the patient's clinical condition has been stabilized, it is reasonable to consider starting the discontinuation process even if predictive index thresholds for success have not been met. Valuable time may be lost in liberating patients from the ventilator if one relies solely on these indices because they are not powerful predictors of success or failure. Furthermore, there is no evidence that shows that unsuccessful discontinuation trials have long-term adverse consequences, provided patients are monitored closely and certain pitfalls are avoided. For example, it is unwise to attempt SBTs on patients with active ischemic heart disease because systemic oxygen demand and cardiac output can increase substantially during transition from controlled MV to SB [63,64]. Patients must be prepared psychologically to understand that failing a discontinuation trial has no bearing on their ultimate prognosis. Finally, it is prudent to guarantee sufficient respiratory muscle rest after a failed attempt at SB. With few exceptions, such as patients recovering from general anesthesia or sedation with or without muscle paralysis, the authors usually do not have their patients undergo more than one (failed) discontinuation trial in any 24-hour period. This practice is supported by the work of Esteban et al. [65], who showed that twice-daily SB trials offered no advantage over once-daily trials. Moreover, the inspiratory effort associated with a failed weaning trial may be sufficient to induce muscle fatigue that may not recover [65], unless it is followed by an extended period of rest.

With respect to extubation, it is reasonable to proceed when the patient's ability to protect the airway suggests that extubation will be successful. We do not routinely administer systemic steroids to prevent postextubation stridor because of the inconsistent benefit seen in studies, and the uncertain timing of extubation encountered in clinical practice, which could potentially lead to extended courses of steroids with their associated side effects [66].

PRINCIPLES AND MODES OF DISCONTINUING MECHANICAL VENTILATION

Principles of Weaning

Discontinuing MV is a time when the load associated with breathing is returned from the ventilator to the patient's respiratory muscles. Because breathing is a form of continuous muscular exercise, discontinuation should incorporate the appropriate principles of muscle training. Training stimuli for weaning must be of the appropriate type, intensity, and timing. These vary depending on where patients are in the continuum of inspiratory muscle fatigue.

There are no consistently reliable predictors of early fatigue. Therefore, the physician must rely on clinical findings (e.g., appearance of new dysrhythmia, worsening tachypnea, tachycardia, hypertension/hypotension, diaphoresis, asynchronous breathing patterns), judgment (e.g., patient complains of worsening shortness of breath and has a poor appearance), desaturation, and acute or acute-on-chronic respiratory acidosis. On the other hand, it is important not to terminate a discontinuation trial before making the patient's muscles work hard enough because this can markedly prolong the total duration of MV support.

How Long Should Discontinuation Trials Last?

The question regarding length of discontinuation trials has not been definitively answered. Therefore, the duration depends on the patient population, the weaning mode, and local practice. With respect to trials of unassisted SB, a number of authors have arbitrarily set a maximum limit of 2 hours per trial [46,63,67–71] and extubated patients who were deemed stable by clinical, respiratory, and hemodynamic parameters. With respect to trials of SIMV and PS modes, some have recommended that stable patients need only be on a SIMV rate of 5 per minute and a PS at a setting of 5 to 7 cm H_2O for 2 hours before extubation. With these guidelines, reintubation rates can be as high as 13.8% for SIMV, 18.9% for PS, and 22.6% for trials of SB [67]. With respect to SB trials, other authors have found no difference in success of discontinuing MV when 30-minute and 2-hour trial intervals have been compared [70,71]. Nevertheless, because reintubation has been prospectively shown to be associated with a significantly greater (a) risk of in-hospital mortality, (b) ICU and hospital length of stay, and (c) transfer rate to a long-term care or rehabilitation facility [68], and because it is prudent to minimize the need for reintubation, we recommend the following:

- The authors prefer SB trials over other modes because they are the most direct way to assess the patient's performance without ventilatory support.
- It is reasonable to consider extubation in patients who have well-tolerated SB trials of 30 to 120 minutes, with the following exceptions [72,73]: (a) patients with a tracheostomy who meet the definition of being on prolonged MV (i.e., at least 21 days for at least 6 hours per day), (b) neurologic patients who are predicted to have difficulty clearing their respiratory secretions, and (c) patients who have had to be reintubated after the recent discontinuation of MV. In the context of these exceptions, it is our practice to observe these patients breathing spontaneously for a period longer than 2 hours (e.g., up to 24 hours) before considering extubation.
- Weaning should be performed using a protocol or clinical practice guideline that allows responsibilities to be clearly defined and empowers nurses and respiratory therapists to act within the scope of their practice.

Conventional Modes of Discontinuing Mechanical Ventilation

Four modes of discontinuing patients from MV are in general use: (a) trials of SB with or without the addition of CPAP, (b) SIMV, (c) PS, and (d) noninvasive positive-pressure ventilation (NIPPV) [74]. Results of randomized controlled trials comparing methods for weaning subjects from MV suggest that both SB and PS trials are superior to SIMV trials [67,75,76]. Therefore, we strongly discourage the use of SIMV for weaning. There are no convincing data to support the superiority of SBTs or PS compared to each other, and no data to support the practice of changing modes in patients who are not weaning successfully. The use of NIPPV should be limited to use in patients with CO_2 retention [77]. In other situations, NIPPV has not been shown to avoid reintubation in comparison to standard modes and can be potentially dangerous by delaying reintubation time [74]. Because we do not recommend SIMV trials, we only provide examples of SB, PS, and NIPPV protocols.

Spontaneous Breathing Discontinuation Trial

SBTs consist of the sudden, complete withdrawal of machine support. Patients are closely observed as they breathe humidified gas mixtures delivered by the T-shaped tube that is connected to the endotracheal or tracheostomy tube; alternatively, they can remain connected to the ventilator and be allowed to breathe spontaneously in the CPAP mode. In contrast to techniques that involve the gradual withdrawal of machine support, such as SIMV and PS, during SBTs the patient's cardiorespiratory response patterns can be assessed without the confounding influence of machine settings. Although there is no generally agreed on standard of applying this method of discontinuation, most practitioners begin SBTs from assisted, not controlled, MV and assess the patient's tolerance.

Although CPAP is not universally used, the authors believe it is physiologically sound to undertake SBTs in conjunction with CPAP irrespective of the underlying disease process. The addition of 5 cm H_2O of CPAP mitigates the fall in end-expired lung volume that results from having eliminated glottic regulation of upper-airway resistance and flow with an endotracheal tube [78]. Furthermore, in patients with airflow obstruction, CPAP can substantially lower the work of breathing by counterbalancing end-expiratory system recoil pressures (i.e., intrinsic PEEP) and by shifting loads from inspiratory to expiratory muscles [79–81]. It is not likely that the 5 cm H_2O of external PEEP will provoke hyperinflation by exceeding intrinsic PEEP. Nevertheless, to guard against hyperinflation, the physician can monitor the effect of increasing levels of external PEEP on peak or end-inflation hold pressure on the ventilator before beginning weaning. When too much external PEEP has been applied and hyperinflation worsens, these pressures rise.

An alternative mechanism by which CPAP can reduce inspiratory elastic work in airflow obstruction is by recruiting expiratory muscles during SB. CPAP may result in exhalation below the new static equilibrium volume through the recruitment of expiratory muscles. Subsequent relaxation of the expiratory muscles inflates the lungs passively back to the new equilibrium volume. This may have the effect of unloading inspiratory muscles because the expiratory muscles do part of the inspiratory work. However, this mechanism is of limited value in patients with severe obstruction because low maximal flows prevent significant reductions in lung volume below static equilibrium volume.

In patients who continue to require MV only for oxygenation, CPAP may help maintain the benefits of improved oxygenation provided by PEEP without exposing the patient to the hazards of MV. It may also augment cardiac function during weaning.

Spontaneous Breathing Discontinuation Protocol. General guidelines for SB discontinuation are as follows:

1. When it has been decided that the patient is improving and stable, inform the patient that an attempt to remove MV will be made, why you believe he or she is ready, and what to expect. It is important to allow the patient to express fears whenever possible and to try to alleviate them [82].
2. Obtain baseline values and begin monitoring clinical parameters, such as pulse rate, respiratory rate, blood pressure, and subjective distress (e.g., have patients rate their dyspnea from 0 to 10), gas exchange (e.g., by pulse oximetry), and cardiac rhythm (e.g., by electrocardiographic monitoring). Record these values on a flow sheet that should be maintained and kept at the patient's bedside. The authors are unaware of any studies that support the need for frequent arterial blood gas analyses during discontinuation trials.
3. Ensure a calm atmosphere by having the nurse, respiratory therapist, or physician remain at the bedside to offer encouragement and support.
4. Avoid sedation to ensure maximal patient cooperation and effort.
5. Whenever possible, sit the patient upright in bed or in a chair.
6. Fit the patient's endotracheal tube with a T-tube connected to a heated nebulizer with an inspired oxygen concentration 10% greater than that prevailing during the previous course of MV. Ensure that the T-tube flow exceeds the patient's peak inspiratory flow and that the inhaled gas is constantly humidified. If CPAP is being used, the T-tube setup becomes unnecessary and the ventilator system tubing is used. Establishing the SB mode is done via commands on the ventilator.
7. Continue the trial to completion unless the following conditions develop:
   a. New onset diaphoresis
   b. New onset arrhythmias
   c. Systolic BP >180 mm Hg *or* a change (increase or decrease) of ≥20% of the original systolic value *or* a new requirement for vasopressors.
   d. Heart rate >120 *or* a change (increase or decrease) of >30 beats per minute
   e. SaO_2 <90%, FIO_2 >0.6
   f. If a blood gas is obtained, pH <7.30; PaO_2 <60 mm Hg; SaO_2 <90%; rise in $PaCO_2$ of more than 10 mm Hg
   g. Unstable pattern of ventilation
   h. Respiratory rate <8 breaths per minute, >35 breaths per minute for >5 minutes, change of >50% of original respiratory rate, or a RSBI (f/V_T) >100
   i. New onset altered mental status
   j. Signs of respiratory muscle failure including new onset use of accessory muscles of breathing or thoracoabdominal paradox
   k. Subjective discomfort of patient with dyspnea or pain rated as greater than 5/10
   l. Failure as determined by the subjective assessment of nurse, physician, or respiratory therapist

If the trial is terminated, place the patient back on the previous MV settings. The authors do not subject patients to more than one trial in a 24-hour period [75]. If a patient has no underlying lung disease, has been on an MV for only a short time (e.g., less than 1 week), appears to be tolerating SB without dyspnea for 2 hours, and maintains an adequate level of oxygenation, extubation may be performed after considering whether the patient is at risk of postextubation upper-airway obstruction or not being able to protect the airway or clear secretions. See the earlier discussion for additional information on duration of trials.

Pressure-Support Ventilation Discontinuation Trial

PS discontinuation decreases MV gradually, making the patient responsible for a progressively increasing amount of ventilation. Although it is commonly assumed that PS can be decreased to a low level (e.g., 5 to 7 cm H_2O) that compensates for endotracheal tube and circuit resistance, and patients can be safely extubated at that level, there is no simple way of predicting the level of PS that compensates for this resistance.

PS has become a popular mode of discontinuing MV for adults. In the PS mode, a target pressure is applied to the endotracheal tube that augments the inflation pressure exerted by the inspiratory muscles on the respiratory system [83]. As the lungs inflate, inspiratory flow begins to decline because airway pressure and the inflation pressure exerted by the inspiratory muscles are opposed by rising elastic recoil forces. When inspiratory flow reaches a threshold value (that differs among vendors), the machine switches to expiration [84]. Compared to the SIMV mode of discontinuation, during which spontaneous breaths are occasionally augmented by a volume-preset machine breath, PS is thought to offer greater patient autonomy over inspiratory flow, tidal volume, and inspiration time [85]. The popularity of PS is based on the premise that discontinuation from MV should be a gradual process. In addition, proponents of PS over SBTs argue that the work of unassisted breathing through an endotracheal tube is unreasonably high and could lead to inspiratory muscle failure in susceptible patients [86]. For example, it has become popular to assume that PS is an effective means to overcome the resistance of endotracheal tubes. However, this is conceptually incorrect because airway pressure during PS does not vary with flow. Furthermore, a reduction in pulmonary resistance is not demonstrated after extubation [87], and the work of breathing may actually increase [88]. This suggests that, at least immediately after extubation, most patients manifest upper-airway resistance that is, in effect, equal to or greater than that of an 8-mm internal diameter endotracheal tube.

Enthusiasm for using PS in all patients should be tempered by knowledge of its potential adverse patient–ventilator interactions. For example, elderly patients and even healthy individuals [89] are susceptible to PS setting–induced central apneas. The mechanism appears to be intermittent hypocapnia, resulting from the uncoupling of tidal volume from inspiratory effort. Problems may arise when the physician feels compelled to rest susceptible subjects with PS at night. Unless sufficiently high intermittent mandatory ventilation backup rates are used in combination with PS, the mechanical inhibition of inspiratory drive may result in apneas that trigger ventilator alarms and cause arousals and sleep fragmentation that can prolong the discontinuation process.

Dyssynchrony between patient and machine breaths is common in the ICU, particularly during PS. This is true for patients with high intrinsic respiratory rates, reduced inspiratory pressure output from low drive or respiratory muscle weakness, or airway obstruction, and when ventilator support results in greater than normal tidal volumes. However, the diagnostic and prognostic significance of this dyssynchrony is uncertain. When it impairs ventilatory assistance or causes patient discomfort, sedation and adjustments in CPAP, rate, flow, or trigger mode are required. On the other hand, when wasted inspiratory efforts are not perceived as uncomfortable, it is not clear that adjustments in ventilator settings are warranted. Increases in machine rate to match the rate of patient efforts may cause worsening dynamic hyperinflation in patients with airflow obstruction, and compromise circulation.

Pressure Support Discontinuation Protocol. General guidelines for PS discontinuation are as follows:

1. Repeat steps 1 through 5 of the SB protocol.
2. Switch the MV mode from volume-cycled breathing with assist or SIMV modes to PS, or, if the patient is already on PS as a ventilatory mode, decrease the amount of PS.
3. For patients who have received prolonged ventilator support (e.g., greater than 21 days) for whatever reason, patients with neurologic diseases, or patients who have recently failed extubation, begin PS at a pressure of 25 cm H_2O if switching from another ventilatory mode, or less than the amount previously used during PS ventilation, and increase the fraction of inspired oxygen by 10%. Decrease airway inflation pressure slowly. If the patient fails to assume the increased work of breathing at a lower pressure, increase the pressure to the previously tolerated level and then higher, if necessary, until the patient is stable again. Then, wait 24 hours and begin the process again.
4. In patients who have no underlying lung disease and who have been on MV for only a short time (e.g., less than 1 week), PS can be set at 7 cm H_2O. If this pressure is well tolerated for 2 hours, the patient should be assessed for extubation [69].

Noninvasive Positive-Pressure Ventilation as a Mode of Discontinuing Mechanical Ventilation

A comprehensive description of NIPPV can be found in Chapter 59. Patients can receive this form of ventilation using either a ventilator specifically designed for noninvasive positive-pressure or an ICU ventilator, using PS mode plus PEEP. Ventilation can be delivered with a nose or face mask or, outside the United States, a helmet. Current literature indicates that the use of noninvasive ventilation as a "rescue" therapy for patients who are experiencing respiratory failure following extubation is ineffective in preventing reintubation [90]. Noninvasive ventilation may be an effective strategy in reducing reintubations and mortality among patients with chronic CO_2 retention when used routinely early after extubation [91].

Noninvasive Positive-Pressure Ventilation. General guidelines for NIPPV discontinuation are as follows [92]:

1. Repeat steps 1 through 5 of the SB protocol.
2. Extubate the patient, apply a nose or face mask designed for NIPPV, and begin assisted breathing. Continuously adjust the ventilator settings (see Chapter 59) according to patient comfort, the presence of air leaks, and monitoring.
3. In between periods of 1 to 2 hours of SB with supplemental oxygen, intersperse intermittent periods of ventilation for 2 to 4 hours at a time. Then, gradually increase the duration of the SB periods as tolerated by the patient (e.g., monitor RR, gas-exchange, and cardiorespiratory parameters and dyspnea).
4. When the period of SB spans the entire day and the patient is only receiving nocturnal ventilation, consideration should be given for discontinuing NIPPV.

Unconventional Modes of Discontinuing Mechanical Ventilation

A variety of unconventional techniques have been tried for discontinuing MV. These include inspiratory strength training [93], adaptive support ventilation [94], biofeedback [95,96], automatic tube compensation [97,98], and proportional assist ventilation. None of these techniques are supported by adequate evidence to justify recommendation as routine care.

Uncontrolled reports suggest that inspiratory muscle strength training [93] may be useful in preparing patients who are on prolonged ventilatory support for discontinuation. This method is thought to serve as a means of respiratory muscle endurance training; it is implemented by having patients perform low-repetition, high-resistance SB exercises.

During adaptive support ventilation [94], an automatic microprocessor-controlled mode of MV ensures the delivery of preset minute ventilation. It does this by continuously adapting to the patient's respiratory activity. Adaptive-support ventilation was developed in an attempt to automatically discontinue patients from MV by feedback from one or more ventilator-measured parameters.

Biofeedback, the detection and transmission back to the patient of some biologic function that he or she cannot detect, may be helpful in certain patients [95,96]. For instance, by displaying respiratory volumes on bedside oscilloscopes and having patients make voluntary efforts to push volume tracings beyond limits taped on the screen, Corson et al. [95] allowed two patients with spinal cord lesions—one with a sensory level at C6 who lacked proprioceptive afferents from the chest wall—to gain control over their breathing. These authors assumed that the repeated practice of reaching the criteria of feedback increased the strength of the diaphragm and inspiratory muscles and may have had the net effect of enabling the medullary center to reinstate automatic breathing.

Automatic tube compensation (i.e., a means of resistive unloading during ventilator-assisted SB by compensating for the pressure drop across the endotracheal tube) has been best studied. Compared with SBT in a randomized controlled trial, there was no clear difference in clinically significant outcomes [99].

Proportional assist ventilation (PAV) is a mode of partial ventilatory support in which the ventilator applies pressure in proportion to the inspiratory effort [100]. This has potential value in liberating patients from MV. The theoretical advantage is that the support applied seems to coordinate well with the patient's own respiratory effort, thereby simulating SB but with less respiratory work. No studies have demonstrated a clinical advantage of this method over conventional methods.

MANAGING DISCONTINUATION FAILURE

The authors' general approach to managing patients who have failed to have MV discontinued is based on three tenets: (a) protocol-based weaning yields superior outcomes when compared to nonprotocolized weaning; (b) SBTs or PS trials should be performed once daily; and (c) barriers to weaning are clinical conditions that promote muscle fatigue and weakness. Interventions that address and reverse these barriers are keys to successfully liberate patients from mechanical ventilation.

Protocol-Based Weaning

Multiple randomized controlled clinical trials [46,101,102] and nonrandomized controlled trials [103–105] have shown overwhelming advantages in clinically significant outcomes (e.g., decreased duration of MV, reintubation rates, ICU and hospital LOS) generated by the use of protocol-directed weaning implemented by nonphysician healthcare providers. The only study to dispute those advantages employed a care model in the control group that mimicked many aspects of protocol-directed care such as a closed staffing model and system-based structured rounds [106]. Therefore, the authors recommend that institutions develop protocols or employ existing protocols developed elsewhere to direct interdisciplinary weaning efforts rather than wean by individual physician discretion.

Once-Daily Attempts at Liberation from Mechanical Ventilation

On the basis of multiple randomized controlled trials of methods for weaning subjects from MV [76], the authors recommend that once-daily SB or PS trials be used as the discontinuation mode of choice. Because duration of MV is primarily determined by admitting diagnosis and degree of physiologic derangement [107], there does not appear to be anything to be gained by switching from one mode to another if the discontinuation process is prolonged. Our experience suggests that switching to another mode and waiting to see the response directs the attention of clinicians away from addressing the most important reason why patients are on prolonged MV—the persistence of inspiratory muscle fatigue/weakness.

Addressing Factors That Perpetuate Respiratory Muscle Fatigue

The respiratory muscles play a pivotal role in the onset and perpetuation of respiratory failure. Respiratory muscle fatigue is almost always multifactorial in etiology (Table 60.2). Therefore, clinicians should systematically consider ways to increase muscle strength and decrease muscle demand.

The following measures should be considered to increase respiratory muscle strength:

1. Reverse malnutrition [18,42,43] and deficiencies in phosphorus [22], calcium [21], potassium [19], and magnesium [20].
2. Consider correcting or improving (by correcting metabolic alkalosis) chronic hypercapnia during MV because hypercapnia may adversely affect muscle strength and endurance [28,29,108,109].
3. Reverse hypothyroidism [23].
4. Improve cardiovascular function [40] and minimize cardiac ischemia. Poor cardiac performance may contribute to an inadequate supply of oxygen to the respiratory muscles.
5. Attempt to minimize the use of sedative drugs whenever possible. In randomized controlled clinical trials, daily interruption of sedation compared to continuous infusions significantly decreased duration of MV and length of stay in a medical ICU [110]. Less intense anesthetic/sedative regimens have led to earlier extubation in postcardiac surgery patients [111–114]. The use of a protocol to manage sedation that was paired with a protocol to manage weaning improved on the outcomes achieved with the use of a weaning protocol alone and also led to a mortality benefit [115]. To assist in managing sedation, clinicians are encouraged to use validated and reliable monitoring scales such as the Richmond Agitation-Sedation Scale [116].
6. Attempt to reduce the incidence of delirium. Some authors have advocated for the use of dexmedetomidine in ventilated patients to reduce the incidence of delirium that leads to increase sedation. Dexmedetomidine is used in place of medications, such as benzodiazepines, that are thought to be a cause of delirium in ICU patients. These arguments are supported by the results of a randomized trial that demonstrated reductions in the incidence of delirium and time on the ventilator seen with dexmedetomidine in comparison to midazolam [117].
7. Paradoxically, because sleep deprivation may suppress ventilatory drive [10] and contribute to central fatigue, short-acting sedatives may occasionally be used in selected, sleep-deprived individuals [118].
8. Progesterone may serve as a respiratory center stimulant [119,120] in patients who take few or no spontaneous breaths despite a lack of sedative drugs. The effect of 20 mg of medroxyprogesterone acetate three times per day should begin within 2 days and be maximal within 7 days. This is a controversial therapy because many believe the additional respiratory center stimulation may just be "whipping a tired horse" and precipitate worsening muscle fatigue.
9. Consider and evaluate for the possibilities of myopathy and polyneuropathy [36] and drug-induced neuromuscular dysfunction (e.g., neuromuscular blocking agents and antibiotics, especially aminoglycosides) [35,121]. Critical illness polyneuropathy and myopathy are major causes of persistent respiratory failure [122].
10. By taking advantage of gravity and having the patient sit up, the diaphragm may function better.
11. Consider administering theophylline. Theophylline may act as a direct respiratory center and diaphragm stimulant and can increase the strength of contraction and suppress fatigue of the diaphragm [123,124]. However, its role in MV discontinuation has yet to be determined in randomized, prospective studies. Calcium-channel antagonists were shown in an animal model to inhibit the beneficial effects of theophylline on diaphragm function [125].
12. Mobilize patients to the maximum of their tolerance and initiate physical and occupational therapy early in their course. A protocol of early physical and occupational therapy combined with daily interruption of sedation demonstrated significant improvements in return to baseline functional status at hospital discharge and in number of ventilator free days in the first 28 days of hospital stay [126].

The following measures should be considered to decrease respiratory muscle demand:

1. Maximize treatment of systemic disease (e.g., infection, acute and chronic uremia) to decrease metabolic requirements and mitigate production of chemical mediators with adverse effects on muscle [25–27,127].
2. Give bronchodilators for conditions associated with increased airway resistance (see Chapters 48 and 49); discontinue beta-blockers in asthmatic patients.
3. Assess for adrenal insufficiency because identification of this condition and supplementation with systemic corticosteroids can increase the success of ventilator weaning and shorten the weaning period [128]. Moreover, a course of systemic glucocorticoids is helpful in exacerbations of chronic obstructive pulmonary disease [129,130] and asthma. Conversely, systemic steroids may contribute to the development of myopathy and perpetuate muscle weakness.

4. Use diuretics to reduce lung water in patients with pulmonary edema; this makes the lungs more compliant. Closely monitor renal function and serum sodium to avoid precipitating renal failure and hypernatremia.
5. Routinely evaluate for compromised cardiac function. Echocardiography and assessments for myocardial ischemia can diagnose and facilitate improvement of underlying cardiac disorders. The increased work of breathing during discontinuation may steal oxygen from the heart as well as other organs and precipitate ischemia and heart failure in susceptible patients [40,131,132].
6. In average-size adults, endotracheal tubes less than 8 mm in internal diameter significantly increase airway resistance [133,134], although it is unlikely that tube size adversely affects the discontinuation process unless the tube is prohibitively small (i.e., <6 mm). If an effect on weaning success is suspected, replace the smaller tube with one with a larger internal diameter.
7. Consider CPAP in patients with marginal cardiac function. It may provide support for a failing heart by decreasing left ventricular preload [40,131].
8. Consider that the ventilator is increasing the work of breathing and make adjustments [32,37,135]. Potential factors include (a) the appropriateness of the sensitivity/responsivity of the ventilator triggering system, (b) whether the ventilator flow pattern is synchronized with the patient's demand, (c) the appropriateness of the ventilator settings to avoid dynamic hyperinflation, (d) considering usage of extrinsic PEEP to overcome an increased trigger-ing threshold load from $PEEP_i$, and (e) changing a heat and moisture exchanger to a heated humidifier to overcome the increased dead space and resistance of the exchanger [32,136].
9. Evaluate for overfeeding as the cause of increased CO_2 production. Excess total caloric intake, but not disproportionate carbohydrate intake, may precipitate respiratory acidosis in patients unable to increase their alveolar ventilation adequately when compensating for increased CO_2 production [137]. The treatment for this is to reduce the calorie intake.
10. Consider performing tracheostomy when patients are predicted to require prolonged MV. Tracheostomy may improve patient comfort and mitigate the need for more sedation, decrease airway resistance, decrease ventilator-associated pneumonia, and decrease duration of MV. While the best time to perform tracheostomy is not known, a randomized, controlled clinical trial showed that early tracheostomy (after 6–8 days of laryngeal intubation) compared with later tracheostomy (after 13–15 days of laryngeal intubation) did not result in significant improvement in incidence of ventilator-associated pneumonia [138]. Moreover, long-term outcome between the 2 groups did not differ.
11. Before extubating weak patients, assess whether they are at increased risk of developing postextubation stridor and whether they are able to protect their airway and clear their respiratory secretions (see section When Is It Appropriate to Extubate the Patient?).

TABLE 60.3

SUMMARY OF ADVANCES IN MANAGING DISCONTINUATION FROM MECHANICAL VENTILATION BASED ON RANDOMIZED CONTROLLED CLINICAL TRIALS

- Protocol-directed, ventilator management teams lead to favorable outcomes [46,101,102].
- Spontaneous breathing or pressure support trials are superior to SIMV trials [76].
- 30- and 120-min trials are equally successful [70,71].
- Twice-daily spontaneous trials offer no advantage over once-daily trials [75,76].
- Daily interruption of sedation leads to better outcomes than continuous infusions [110].
- A combination of a daily sedation holiday with once-daily spontaneous breathing trials improves outcomes [115].
- Early physical and occupational therapy reduces ventilator time [126].
- Early identification and treatment of adrenal insufficiency lead to increased weaning success and shorter weaning times [128].

SIMV, synchronized intermittent mandatory ventilation.

CONCLUSIONS

When managing patients with discontinuation failure, it is not likely that they fail for technologic reasons or the discontinuation mode but rather because of their diseases and causes of inspiratory muscle fatigue and how well these are managed. Advances in managing discontinuation from MV, based on randomized, controlled trials or meta-analyses of such trials, are summarized in Table 60.3. A number of studies have now been published that show that the most favorable discontinuation outcomes are most likely achieved by protocol-directed weaning. Such programs can improve the quality of care of patients on MV and decrease their length of ICU stay and hospital costs, especially when the protocol includes a search for and correction of medical barriers that perpetuate inspiratory muscle fatigue. In our protocol, we focus on a daily basis on minimizing or eliminating sedation, keeping the lungs dry without hurting the kidneys, improving nutrition, and maximizing cardiac function.

Although the optimum rate of reintubation is not known, it is the authors' perspective that it should be in the 10% to 15% range and it should be monitored as a quality indicator in ICUs. For example, if the reintubation rate is lower than 10%, it could be argued that too many patients are being "parked" on MV who should be extubated, placing them at risk of unnecessary endotracheal tube complications such as pneumonia. On the other hand, if the rate is much higher than 15%, it could be argued that patients are being prematurely extubated, placing them at risk of harm during the stress of recurrent respiratory failure and reintubation.

References

1. Elpern EH, Larson R, Douglass P, et al: Long-term outcomes for elderly survivors of prolonged ventilator assistance. *Chest* 96:1120, 1989.
2. Swinburne AJ, Fedullo AJ, Shayne DS: Mechanical ventilation: analysis of increasing use and patient survival. *J Intensive Care Med* 3:315, 1988.
3. Tobin MJ, Perez W, Guenther SM, et al: The pattern of breathing during successful and unsuccessful trials of weaning from mechanical ventilation. *Am Rev Respir Dis* 134:1111, 1986.
4. Morganroth ML, Grum CM: Weaning from mechanical ventilation. *J Intensive Care Med* 3:109, 1988.
5. Kurek CK, Cohen IL, Lamrinos J, et al: Clinical and economic outcome of patients undergoing tracheostomy for prolonged mechanical ventilation in New York State during 1993; analysis of 6,353 cases under diagnostic related group 483. *Crit Care Med* 25:983, 1997.
6. Chatila W, Kreimer DT, Criner GJ: Quality of life in survivors of prolonged mechanical ventilatory support. *Crit Care Med* 29:737, 2001.

7. Combes A, Costa M-A, Trouillet J-L, et al: Morbidity, mortality, and quality-of-life outcomes of patients requiring ≥14 days of mechanical ventilation. *Crit Care Med* 31:1373, 2003.
8. Laghi F, Tobin MJ: Disorders of the respiratory muscles. *Am J Respir Crit Care Med* 168:10, 2003.
9. Doekel RC, Zwillich CW, Scoggin CH, et al: Clinical semistarvation: depression of hypoxic ventilatory response. *N Engl J Med* 295:358, 1976.
10. Schiffman PL, Trontell MC, Mazar MF, et al: Sleep deprivation decreases ventilatory response to CO_2 but not load compensation. *Chest* 84:695, 1983.
11. Arslanian-Engoren C, Scott LD: The lived experience of survivors of prolonged mechanical ventilation: a phenomenological study. *Heart Lung* 32:328, 2003.
12. Laghi F, Cattapan SE, Jubran A, et al: Is weaning failure caused by low-frequency fatigue of the diaphragm? *Am J Respir Crit Care Med* 167:120, 2003.
13. Polkey MI, Moxham J: Clinical aspects of respiratory muscle dysfunction in the critically ill. *Chest* 119:926, 2001.
14. Manthous CA, Schmidt GA, Hall JB: Liberation from mechanical ventilation: a decade of progress. *Chest* 114:886, 1998.
15. NHLBI Workshop Summary: Respiratory muscle fatigue: report of the Respiratory Muscle Fatigue Workshop Group. *Am Rev Respir Dis* 142:474, 1990.
16. Mador MJ: Respiratory muscle fatigue and breathing pattern. *Chest* 100:1430, 1991.
17. Sassoon CSH, Te TT, Mahutee CK, et al: Airway occlusion pressure: an important indicator for successful weaning in patients with chronic obstructive pulmonary disease. *Am Rev Respir Dis* 135:107, 1987.
18. Wilson DO, Rogers RM: The role of nutrition in weaning from mechanical ventilation. *J Intensive Care Med* 4:124, 1989.
19. Knochel JP: Neuromuscular manifestations of electrolyte disorders. *Am J Med* 72:521, 1982.
20. Johnson D, Gallagher C, Cavanaugh M, et al: The lack of effect of routine magnesium administration on respiratory function in mechanically ventilated patients. *Chest* 104:536, 1993.
21. Aubier M, Viires N, Piquet J, et al: Effects of hypocalcemia on diaphragmatic strength generation. *J Appl Physiol* 58:2054, 1985.
22. Aubier M, Murciano D, Lecocguic Y, et al: Effect of hypophosphatemia on diaphragmatic contractility in patients with acute respiratory failure. *N Engl J Med* 313:420, 1985.
23. Datta D, Scalise P: Hypothyroidism and failure to wean in patients receiving prolonged mechanical ventilation at a regional weaning center. *Chest* 126:1307, 2004.
24. Shapiro JM, Condos R, Cole RP: Myopathy in status asthmaticus: relation to neuromuscular blockade and corticosteroid administration. *J Intensive Care Med* 8:144, 1993.
25. Tarasuik A, Heimer D, Bark H: Effect of chronic renal failure on skeletal and diaphragmatic muscle contraction. *Am Rev Respir Dis* 146:1383, 1992.
26. Mitch WE, Goldberg AL: Mechanisms of muscle wasting and the role of the ubiquitin-proteasome pathway. *N Engl J Med* 25:1897, 1996.
27. Gertz I, Hedenstierna G, Hellers G, et al: Muscle metabolism in patients with chronic obstructive lung disease and acute respiratory failure. *Clin Sci Mol Med* 52:395, 1977.
28. Juan G, Calverley P, Talamo C, et al: Effect of carbon dioxide on diaphragmatic function in human beings. *N Engl J Med* 310:874, 1984.
29. Esau SA: Hypoxic, hypercapnic acidosis decreases tension and increases fatigue in hamster diaphragm muscle in vitro. *Am Rev Respir Dis* 139:1410, 1989.
30. Vassilakopoulos T, Petrof BJ: Ventilator-induced diaphragmatic dysfunction. *Am J Respir Crit Care Med* 169:336, 2004.
31. Vassilakopoulos T, Katsaounou P, Karatza M-H, et al: Strenuous resistive breathing induces plasma cytokines: role of antioxidants and monocytes. *Am J Respir Crit Care Med* 166:1572, 2002.
32. Girault C, Breton L, Richard JC, et al: Mechanical effects of airway humidification devices in difficult to wean patients. *Crit Care Med* 31:1306, 2003.
33. Lemaire F, Teboul J-L, Cinotti L, et al: Acute left ventricular dysfunction during unsuccessful weaning from mechanical ventilation. *Anesthesiology* 69:171, 1988.
34. Srivastava S, Chatila W, Amoateng-Adjepong Y, et al: Myocardial ischemia and weaning failure in patients with coronary artery disease: an update. *Crit Care Med* 27:2109, 1999.
35. Arroliga A, Frutos-Vivar F, Hall J, et al: Use of sedatives and neuromuscular blockers in a cohort of patients receiving mechanical ventilation. *Chest* 128:496, 2005.
36. Bolton CF: Neuromuscular manifestations of critical illness. *Muscle Nerve* 32:140, 2005.
37. Tobin MJ, Jubran A, Laghi F: Patient-ventilator interaction. *Am J Respir Crit Care Med* 163:1059, 2001.
38. Jiang T-X, Reid WD, Belcastro A, et al: Load dependence of secondary diaphragm inflammation and injury after acute inspiratory loading. *Am J Respir Crit Care Med* 157:230, 1998.
39. van Gammeren D, Falk DJ, DeRuisseau KC, et al: Reloading the diaphragm following mechanical ventilation does not promote injury. *Chest* 127:2204, 2005.
40. Bradley TD, Holloway RM, McLaughlin PR, et al: Cardiac output response to continuous positive airway pressure in congestive heart failure. *Am Rev Respir Dis* 145:377, 1992.
41. Ulicny KS, Hiratzka LR: Nutrition and the cardiac surgical patient. *Chest* 101:836, 1992.
42. Bassili HR, Deitel M: Effect of nutritional support on weaning patients off mechanical ventilation. *JPEN J Parenter Enteral Nutr* 5:161, 1981.
43. Larca L, Greenbaum DM: Effectiveness of intensive nutritional regimes in patients who fail to wean from mechanical ventilation. *Crit Care Med* 10:297, 1982.
44. Cook D, Mende M, Guyatt G, et al: Trials of miscellaneous interventions to wean from mechanical ventilation. *Chest* 120[Suppl]:438S, 2001.
45. MacIntyre NR, Cook DJ, Ely EW Jr, et al: Evidence-based guidelines for weaning and discontinuing ventilatory support. *Chest* 120[Suppl]:375S, 2001.
46. Ely EW, Baker AM, Dunagan DP, et al: Effect on the duration of mechanical ventilation of identifying patients capable of breathing spontaneously. *N Engl J Med* 335:1864, 1996.
47. Jubran A, Grant BJ, Laghi F, et al: Weaning prediction: esophageal pressure monitoring complements readiness testing. *Am J Respir Crit Care Med* 171:1252, 2005.
48. Meade M, Guyatt G, Cook D, et al: Predicting success in weaning from mechanical ventilation. *Chest* 120[Suppl]:400S, 2001.
49. Epstein SK, Ciubotaru RL: Influence of gender and endotracheal tube size on preextubation breathing pattern. *Am J Respir Crit Care Med* 154:1647, 1996.
50. Krieger BP: Weaning parameters: read the methodology before proceeding. *Chest* 122:1873, 2002.
51. Jaeschke RZ, Meade MO, Guyatt UH, et al: How to use diagnostic test articles in the intensive care unit: diagnosing weanability using f/V_T. *Crit Care Med* 25:1514, 1997.
52. Yang KL, Tobin MJ: A prospective study of indexes predicting the outcome of trials of weaning from mechanical ventilation. *N Engl J Med* 324:1445, 1991.
53. Tobin MJ, Guenther SM, Perez W, et al: Konno-Mead analysis of ribcage-abdominal motion during successful and unsuccessful trials of weaning from mechanical ventilation. *Am Rev Respir Dis* 135:1320, 1987.
54. Epstein SK, Ciubotaru RL: Independent effects of etiology of failure and time to reintubation on outcome for patients failing extubation. *Am J Respir Crit Care Med* 158:489, 1998.
55. Miller R, Cole R: Association between reduced cuff leak volume and postextubation stridor. *Chest* 110:1035, 1996.
56. Engoren M: Evaluation of the cuff leak test in cardiac surgery patients. *Chest* 116:1029, 1999.
57. Chung YH, Chao TY, Chiu CT. The cuff leak test is a simple tool to verify severe laryngeal edema in patients undergoing long-term mechanical ventilation. *Crit Care Med* 34:409–414, 2006.
58. Jaber S, Chanques G, Matecki S, et al: Post extubation stridor in intensive care unit patients-risk factors evaluation and the importance of the cuff leak test. *Intensive Care Med* 29:69–74, 2003.
59. Wang CL, Tsai YH, Huang CC, et al: The role of the cuff leak test in predicting the effects of corticosteroid treatment on postextubation stridor. *Chang Gung Med J* 30:53–61, 2007.
60. Salam A, Tilluckdharry L, Amoateng-Adjepong Y, et al: Neurologic status, cough, secretions and extubation outcomes. *Intensive Care Med* 30:1334, 2004.
61. De Larminat V, Mongravers P, Dureuil B, et al: Alteration in swallowing reflex after extubation in intensive care patients. *Crit Care Med* 23:486, 1995.
62. Barquist E, Brown M, Cohn S, et al: Postextubation fiberoptic endoscopic evaluation of swallowing after prolonged endotracheal intubation: a randomized, prospective trial. *Crit Care Med* 29:1710, 2001.
63. Hubmayr RD, Loosbrock LM, Gillespie DJ, et al: Oxygen uptake during weaning from mechanical ventilation. *Chest* 94:1148, 1988.
64. Field S, Sanci S, Grassino A: Respiratory muscle oxygen consumption estimated by the diaphragm pressure-time index. *J Appl Physiol* 57:44, 1984.
65. Esteban A, Frutos F, Tobin MJ, et al: A comparison of four methods of weaning patients from mechanical ventilation. Spanish Lung Failure Collaborative Group. *N Engl J Med* 332:345, 1995.
66. Jubran A, Tobin MJ: Pathophysiologic basis of acute respiratory distress in patients who fail a trial of weaning from mechanical ventilation. *Am J Respir Crit Care Med* 155:906, 1997.
67. Khemani RG, Randolph A, Markovitz B: Corticosteroids for the prevention and treatment of post-extubation stridor in neonates, children and adults. *Cochrane Database Syst Rev* (3):CD001000, 2009.
68. Brochard L, Rauss A, Benito S, et al: Comparison of three methods of gradual withdrawal from ventilatory support during weaning from mechanical ventilation. *Am J Respir Crit Care Med* 150:896, 1994.
69. Epstein SK, Ciubotaru RL, Wong JB: Effect of failed extubation on the outcome of mechanical ventilation. *Chest* 112:186, 1997.
70. Esteban A, Alia I, Gordo F, et al: Extubation outcome after spontaneous breathing trials with T-tube or pressure support ventilation. The Spanish Lung Failure Collaborative Group [published erratum appears in *Am J Respir Crit Care Med* 156:2028, 1997]. *Am J Respir Crit Care Med* 156:459, 1997.

71. Esteban A, Alia I, Tobin MJ, et al: Effect of spontaneous breathing trial duration on outcome of attempts to discontinue mechanical ventilation. Spanish Lung Failure Collaborative Group. *Am J Respir Crit Care Med* 159:512, 1999.
72. Perren A, Domenighetti G, Mauri S, et al: Protocol-directed weaning from mechanical ventilation: clinical outcome in patients randomized for a 30-min or 120-min trial with pressure support ventilation. *Intensive Care Med* 28:1058, 2002.
73. MacIntyre NR, Epstein SK, Carson S, et al: Management of patients requiring prolonged mechanical ventilation: report of a NAMDRC Consensus Conference. *Chest* 128:3937, 2005.
74. Vallverdu I, Calaf N, Subirana M, et al: Clinical characteristics, respiratory functional parameters, and outcome of a two-hour T-piece trial in patients weaning from mechanical ventilation. *Am J Respir Crit Care Med* 158:1855, 1998.
75. Girault C: Noninvasive ventilation for postextubation respiratory failure: perhaps not to treat but at least to prevent. *Crit Care Med* 33:2685, 2005.
76. Meade M, Guyatt G, Stinuff T, et al: Trials comparing alternative weaning modes and discontinuation assessments. *Chest* 120[Suppl]:425S, 2001.
77. Burns KE, Adhikari NK, Meade MO: Noninvasive positive pressure ventilation as a weaning strategy for intubated adults with respiratory failure. *Cochrane Database Syst Rev* CD004127, 2003.
78. Quan SF, Falltrick RT, Schlobohm RM: Extubation from ambient or expiratory positive airway pressure in adults. *Anesthesiology* 55:53, 1981.
79. Martin JG, Shore S, Engel LA: Effect of continuous positive airway pressure on respiratory mechanics and pattern of breathing in induced asthma. *Am Rev Respir Dis* 126:812, 1982.
80. Milic-Emili J, Gottfried SB, Rossi A: Dynamic hyperinflation: intrinsic PEEP and its ramifications in patients with respiratory failure, in Vincent JL (ed): *Update in Intensive Care and Emergency Medicine*. New York, Springer-Verlag, 1987, p 192.
81. Petrof BJ, Legare M, Goldberg P, et al: Continuous positive airway pressure reduced work of breathing and dyspnea during weaning from mechanical ventilation in severe chronic obstructive pulmonary disease. *Am Rev Respir Dis* 141:281, 1990.
82. Bergbom-Engberg I, Haljamae J: Assessment of patients' experience of discomforts during respiratory therapy. *Crit Care Med* 17:1068, 1989.
83. MacIntyre NR: Respiratory function during pressure support ventilation. *Chest* 89:677, 1986.
84. MacIntyre NR, Ho L-I: Effects of initial flow rate and breath termination criteria on pressure support ventilation. *Chest* 99:134, 1991.
85. Brochard L, Pluskwa F, Lemaire F: Improved efficacy of spontaneous breathing with inspiratory pressure support. *Am Rev Respir Dis* 136:411, 1987.
86. Fiastro JF, Habib MP, Quan SF: Pressure support compensation for inspiratory work due to endotracheal tubes and demand continuous positive airway pressure. *Chest* 93:499, 1988.
87. Brochard L, Rua F, Lorino H, et al: Inspiratory pressure support compensates for the additional work of breathing caused by the endotracheal tube. *Anesthesiology* 75:739, 1991.
88. Nathan SN, Ishaaya AM, Koerner, SK, et al: Prediction of pressure support during weaning from mechanical ventilation. *Chest* 103:1215, 1993.
89. Morrell MJ, Shea SA, Adams L, et al: Effects of inspiratory support upon breathing in humans during wakefulness and sleep. *Respir Physiol* 93:57, 1993.
90. Esteban A., Frutos-Vivar F, Ferguson N, et al: Noninvasive positive-pressure ventilation for respiratory failure after extubation. *N Engl J Med* 350:2452–2460, 2004.
91. Ferrer M, Sellares J, Valencia M, et al: Non-invasive ventilation after extubation in hypercapnic patients with chronic respiratory disorders: randomized controlled trial. *Lancet* 374:1044–1045, 2009.
92. Girault C, Daudenthun I, Chevron V, et al: Noninvasive ventilation as a systematic extubation and weaning technique in acute-on-chronic respiratory failure: a prospective, randomized controlled study. *Am J Respir Crit Care Med* 160:86, 1999.
93. Sprague SS, Hopkins PD: Use of inspiratory strength training to wean six patients who were ventilator-dependent. *Phys Ther* 83:171, 2003.
94. Cassina T, Chiolero R, Mauri R, et al: Clinical experience with adaptive supportive ventilation for fast-tracking cardiac surgery. *J Cardiovasc Vasc Anesth* 17:571, 2003.
95. Corson JA, Grant JL, Moulton DP, et al: Use of biofeedback in weaning paralyzed patients from respirators. *Chest* 76:543, 1979.
96. Holliday JE, Hyers TM: The reduction of weaning time from mechanical ventilation using tidal volume and relaxation biofeedback. *Am Rev Respir Dis* 141:1214, 1990.
97. Haberthur C, Mols G, Elsasser S, et al: Extubation after breathing trials with automatic tube compensation, T-tube, or pressure support ventilation. *Acta Anaesthesiol Scand* 46:973, 2002.
98. Oczenski W, Kapka A, Krenn H, et al: Automatic tube compensation in patients after cardiac surgery. *Crit Care Med* 30:1467, 2002.
99. Cohen JD, Shapiro M, Grozovski E, et al: Extubation outcome following a spontaneous breathing trial with automatic tube compensation versus continuous positive airway pressure. *Crit Care Med* 34:682–686, 2006.
100. Bosma K, Ferreyra G, Ambrogio G, et al: Patient-ventilator interaction and sleep in mechanically ventilated patients: Pressure support versus proportional assist ventilation. *Crit Care Med* 35:1048, 2007.
101. Kollef MH, Shapiro SD, Silver P, et al: A randomized controlled trial of protocol-directed versus physician-directed weaning from mechanical ventilation. *Crit Care Med* 25:567, 1997.
102. Marelich GP, Murin S, Battistella F, et al: Protocol weaning of mechanical ventilation in medical and surgical patients by respiratory care practitioners and nurses. Effect on weaning time and incidence of ventilator-associated pneumonia. *Chest* 118:459, 2000.
103. Smyrnios NA, Connolly A, Wilson MM, et al: Effects of a multifaceted, multidisciplinary, hospital-wide quality improvement program on weaning from mechanical ventilation. *Crit Care Med* 30:1224, 2002.
104. Burns SM, Earven S, Fisher C, et al: Implementation of an institutional program to improve clinical and financial outcomes of mechanically ventilated patients: one-year outcomes and lessons learned. *Crit Care Med* 31:2752, 2003.
105. Dries DJ, McGonigal MD, Malian MS, et al: Protocol-driven ventilator weaning reduces use of mechanical ventilation, rate of early reintubation, and ventilator-associated pneumonia. *J Trauma-Injury Infect Crit Care* 56:943, 2004.
106. Krishnan JA, Moore D, Robeson C, et al: A prospective, controlled trial of a protocol-based strategy to discontinue mechanical ventilation. *Am J Respir Crit Care Med* 169:673, 2004.
107. Seneff MG, Zimmerman JE, Knaus WA, et al: Predicting the duration of mechanical ventilation: the importance of disease and patient characteristics. *Chest* 110:469, 1996.
108. Howell S, Fitzgerald RS, Roussos C: Effects of aminophylline, isoproterenol, and neostigmine on hypercapnic depression of diaphragmatic contractility. *Am Rev Respir Dis* 132:241, 1985.
109. Yanos J, Wood LDH, Davis K, et al: The effect of respiratory and lactic acidosis on diaphragm function. *Am Rev Respir Dis* 147:616, 1992.
110. Kress JP, Pohlman AS, O'Connor MF, et al: Daily interruption of sedative infusions in critically ill patients undergoing mechanical ventilation. *N Engl J Med* 342:1471, 2000.
111. Berry PD, Thomas SD, Mahon SP, et al: Myocardial ischaemia after coronary artery bypass grafting: early vs. late extubation. *Br J Anaesth* 80:20, 1998.
112. Michalopoulos A, Nikolaides A, Antzaka C, et al: Change in anaesthesia practice and postoperative sedation shortens ICU and hospital length of stay following coronary artery bypass surgery. *Respir Med* 92:1066, 1998.
113. Silbert BS, Santamaria JD, O'Brien JL, et al: Early extubation following coronary artery bypass surgery: a prospective, randomized, controlled trial. The Fast Track Cardiac Care Team. *Chest* 113:1481, 1998.
114. Engoren MC, Kraras C, Garzia F: Propofol-based versus fentanyl-isoflurane-based anesthesia for cardiac surgery. *J Cardiothorac Vasc Anesth* 12:177, 1998.
115. Girard TD, Kress JP, Fuchs BD, et al: Efficacy and safety of a paired sedation and ventilator weaning protocol for mechanically ventilated patients in intensive care (Awakening and breathing controlled trial): a randomised controlled trial. *Lancet* 371:126–134, 2008.
116. Ely EW, Truman B, Shintani A, et al: Monitoring sedation status over time in ICU patients: reliability and validity of the Richmond Agitation-Sedation Scale (RASS). *JAMA* 289:2983, 2003.
117. Riker RR, Shehabi Y, Bokessch PM, et al: Dexmedetomidine vs. midazolam for sedation of critically ill patients—a randomized trial. *JAMA* 301:489–499, 2009.
118. Barrientos-Vega R, Sanchez-Soria MM, Morales-Garcia C, et al: Prolonged sedation of critically ill patients with midazolam or propofol: impact on weaning and costs. *Crit Care Med* 25:33, 1997.
119. Skatrud JB, Dempsey JA, Kaiser DG: Ventilatory response to medroxyprogesterone acetate in normal subjects: time course and mechanism. *J Appl Physiol* 44:939, 1978.
120. Goldman AL, Morrison D, Foster LJ: Oral progesterone therapy: oxygen in a pill. *Arch Intern Med* 141:574, 1981.
121. Argov Z, Mastaglia FL: Disorders of neuromuscular transmission caused by drugs. *N Engl J Med* 301:409, 1979.
122. Leitjen FSS, Harinck-de Ward JE, Poortvliet DCJ, et al: The role of polyneuropathy in Motor Convalescence after prolonged mechanical ventilation. *JAMA* 274:1221–1225, 1995.
123. Murciano D, Aubier M, Lecocguic Y, et al: Effects of theophylline on diaphragmatic strength and fatigue in patients with chronic obstructive pulmonary disease. *N Engl J Med* 311:349, 1984.
124. Murciano D, Auclair M-H, Pariente R, et al: A randomized, controlled trial of theophylline in patients with severe chronic obstructive pulmonary disease. *N Engl J Med* 320:1521, 1989.
125. Kolbeck RC, Speir WA: Diltiazem, verapamil, and nifedipine inhibit theophylline-enhanced diaphragmatic contractility. *Am Rev Respir Dis* 139:139, 1989.
126. Schweickert WD, Pohlman MC, Pohlman AS, et al: Early physical and occupational therapy in mechanically ventilated, critically ill patients: a randomized controlled trial. *Lancet* 373:1874–1882, 2009.
127. Boczkowski J, Dureuil B, Branger C, et al: Effects of sepsis on diaphragmatic function in rats. *Am Rev Respir Dis* 138:260, 1988.
128. Huang C-J, Lin H-C: Association between adrenal insufficiency and ventilator weaning. *Am J Respir Crit Care Med* 173:276, 2006.
129. Niewoehner DE, Erbland ML, Deuphree RH, et al: Effect of systemic glucocorticoids on exacerbations of chronic obstructive pulmonary disease. *N Engl J Med* 340:1941, 1999.

130. Stanbrook MB, Goldstein RS: Steroids for acute exacerbations of COPD: how long is enough? *Chest* 119:675, 2001.
131. Rasanen J, Vaisanen IT, Heikkila J, et al: Acute myocardial infarction complicated left ventricular dysfunction and respiratory failure: the effects of continuous positive airway pressure. *Chest* 87:158, 1985.
132. Rasanen J, Nikki P, Heikkila J: Acute myocardial infarction complicated by respiratory failure: the effects of mechanical ventilation. *Chest* 85:21, 1984.
133. Sullivan M, Paliotta J, Saklad M: Endotracheal tube as a factor in measurement of respiratory mechanics. *J Appl Physiol* 41:590, 1976.
134. Demers RR, Sullivan MJ, Paliotta J: Airflow resistances of endotracheal tubes. *JAMA* 237:1362, 1977.
135. Hess D, Branson RD: Ventilators and weaning modes. *Respir Clin North Am* 6:407, 2000.
136. Le Bourdelles G, Mier L, Fiquet B, et al: Comparison of the effects of heat and moisture exchangers and heated humidifiers on ventilation and gas exchange during weaning trials from mechanical ventilation. *Chest* 110:1294, 1996.
137. Talpers SS, Romberger DJ, Bunce SB, et al: Nutritionally associated increased carbon dioxide production: excess total calories vs. high proportion of carbohydrate calories. *Chest* 102:551, 1992.
138. Terragni PP, Antonelli M, Fumagalli R, et al. Early vs late tracheotomy for prevention of pneumonia in mechanically ventilated adult ICU patients: a randomized controlled trial. *JAMA* 2010; 303: 1483–1489.

CHAPTER 61 ■ GAS EMBOLISM SYNDROMES: VENOUS GAS EMBOLI, ARTERIAL GAS EMBOLI, AND DECOMPRESSION SICKNESS

MARK M. WILSON

The gas embolism syndromes are known to occur in many different settings and may result in life-threatening emergencies. The clinical manifestations of these disorders are varied and the final pathophysiologic consequences depend on where the gas bubbles obstruct the circulation and how they impact the surrounding tissue. The nervous system, heart, lungs, and skin are the primary organ systems involved. The diagnosis of a gas embolism syndrome can be very difficult to establish. Clinicians must depend on a high level of suspicion in the appropriate settings to rapidly identify the problem, prevent further gas entry into the circulation, and begin effective treatment. Each of these entities is discussed in more detail based on the predominant location of the gas collections, although they are not always separate and distinct.

VENOUS GAS EMBOLISM

Although the actual incidence of venous gas embolism (VGE) in the United States is unknown, it has been estimated conservatively that at least 20,000 cases of "air" embolism occur annually [1]. The consequences of VGE range from clinically undetectable to being rapidly fatal.

Etiology

Clinical reports emphasize the high incidence of VGE in association with traumatic injuries and invasive procedures involving the head, neck, and chest (Table 61.1) [1]. Only the most common causes are discussed in detail here.

Surgical

Virtually any surgical procedure that transiently exposes an open vein to a relative negative pressure may be associated with VGE. The best-studied surgical procedure known to be commonly associated with VGE is craniotomy performed in the Fowler's (sitting) position. When monitors for VGE are prospectively used [1], VGE has been documented in 21% to 32% of all craniotomies and up to 58% of occipital craniotomies. Air may also enter the venous system via the occipital emissary veins, the dural sinuses, the diploic veins, the veins of tumors, or through burr holes.

Childbirth, hysterectomy, and abortion have been associated with an increased incidence of VGE [1]. It has been estimated that VGE causes 1% of maternal deaths. The incidence of VGE during cesarean section has been reported to be on the order of 39% to 71% overall, and the majority of episodes occur during uterine repair and placenta removal. During pregnancy, the veins of the uterus are exposed and fixed; when traumatized, they remain open and may serve as a portal of entry for gaseous emboli.

Prospective Doppler monitoring studies have documented a 31% to 83% incidence of VGE during total hip replacement [1]. The presumptive mechanism of embolization involves the forcible entry of air into the venous circulation through vascular openings in the bony medulla of the femur as a result of the high pressures generated in the distal shaft when the prosthesis is inserted.

Sinus lavage and dental surgical procedures have resulted in fatal cases of VGE [1]. Emboli are the result of intraosseous irrigation with water or air under pressure (at least 80 cm H_2O). There are no data available in the literature to suggest just how often VGE occurs during these procedures.

Trauma

Open or penetrating wounds—especially of the chest, neck, head, heart, spine, abdomen, and pelvis—may result in VGE due to the exposure of an open vein to a relative positive pressure gradient (i.e., atmospheric pressure as compared with

TABLE 61.1

CAUSES OF VENOUS GAS EMBOLISM

Surgical
Any head/neck/cardiothoracic surgery
Orthopedic surgery (arthroscopy, endoprosthesis placement)
Hysterectomy, caesarian section
Transurethral resection of the prostate
Abortion, uterine curettage
Normal childbirth, childbirth with placenta previa or extraction procedure
Liver transplantation/resection
Traumatic
Open/penetrating wounds
Vena cava lacerations
Positive-pressure mechanical ventilation
Self-contained underwater breathing apparatus diving
Decompression sickness
Pneumothorax/pneumoperitoneum
Cunnilingus/intercourse during pregnancy
Self-induced
Diagnostic and therapeutic procedures
Central venous catheterization
Pulmonary artery catheterization
Thoracoscopy, thoracentesis
Pleurodesis, percutaneous lung biopsy
Gravity infusion of blood/intravenous products
Pressurized injections/infusions (including contrast media)
Any involving gas insufflation
Hemodialysis
Pericardiocentesis
Pacemaker/defibrillator placement
Radiofrequency cardiac ablation
Endoscopic retrograde cholangiopancreatography
Epidural catheter insertion
Neodymium:yttrium-aluminum-garnet laser therapy
Liquid nitrogen cryosurgery
Hydrogen peroxide irrigation/ingestion
Blood donation

central venous pressure) [1]. Pneumothorax or pneumoperitoneum may result in VGE by the inadvertent puncture of intraabdominal or intrathoracic blood vessels during the mechanism of injury.

Some of the more unusual cases of traumatic embolization include reports of self-induced VGE due to urethral insufflation with an atomizer bulb, scrotal injection of air with a bicycle pump, and attempted suicide in hospital by forcible breathing into an intravenous line [1].

Diagnostic and Therapeutic Procedures

Air embolism in the setting of central venous catheterization has an unknown overall incidence, probably because the diagnosis is made only with large emboli. This fact also impacts the reported mortality rate in the literature of 29% to 43%, and it is possibly as high as 50% [1]. Morbidity is also significant because 42% of all survivors of recognized VGE were left with neurologic deficits. Air can enter the central venous system in several different ways: (a) during needle/wire/catheter insertion; (b) with fracture of the catheter, malfunction of a self-sealing diaphragm, or detachment of external connections; (c) after removal of a catheter that has been in place for several days, such that air is "sucked" into an open subcutaneous tissue tunnel that has formed a skin tract; and (d) as a result of a piggyback infusion running dry [2].

Thoracoscopy may produce VGE presumably due to the associated pneumothorax. Lung biopsy by percutaneous or bronchoscopic techniques creates a direct traumatic opening at the blood–air interface. Significant embolization might result whenever a medium-sized vein is exposed [1].

Gas insufflation procedures have been associated with gaseous embolization [1]. Diagnostic procedures involving the female genital tract, urethra, urinary bladder, kidney, retroperitoneal and perirenal spaces, peritoneal and pleural cavities, joints, cerebral ventricles, epidural space, and paranasal sinuses all carry a risk for VGE. To minimize this risk, the volume of gas introduced, the pressure resulting within the cavity, and the rate of injection should always be as low as possible. It has been suggested that carbon dioxide (CO_2) should be used as the insufflating agent whenever possible due to its high blood solubility and rapid clearance. This last recommendation begs a word of caution, however, because VGE-associated deaths have been reported even with the use of CO_2 [1].

Placement of epidural catheters for anesthesia has been noted prospectively to be associated with Doppler-detectable VGE [1]. In pregnant women placed in the left lateral decubitus position, VGE was noted to occur in 43%, almost half of whom were at least briefly symptomatic. The underlying mechanism relates to the rich plexus of veins of the epidural space, mostly anterior and lateral to the spinal cord. These veins are susceptible to trauma from a needle if the puncture is not directly in the midline or if the needle is rotated once in the epidural space. Because there are no valves in this plexus of veins, the intravascular pressure likely closely follows the central venous pressure. In the left lateral decubitus position, the site of puncture is above the level of the right atrium (RA), and, in pregnant women, uterine compression of the inferior vena cava is relieved, both of which serve to create a subatmospheric pressure in the epidural venous plexus.

Thermal tissue-ablation procedures using application of heat or cold have been associated with VGE [1]. Laser ablation/coagulation of tissues requires a continuous method for cooling of the laser tip. In general, these methods have involved using liquid (saline) or gas [air, nitrogen (N_2), CO_2]. Reports exist in the literature of the entry of these compressed gases into the venous circulation due to opening of vascular channels during the ablative procedure [1]. At the other temperature extreme, cryosurgery with instillation of liquid N_2 is used to extend the surgical margin of excision in many cancer operations. Direct contact between the tissues and the liquid N_2 may lead to entry of N_2 into the circulation in the gaseous state [1]. N_2 gas expands as it is warmed to a volume of greater than 500 times that it occupied in the liquid state. Gas emboli of this magnitude could be rapidly fatal.

Use of hydrogen peroxide (H_2O_2) in closed spaces or body cavities has been shown to result in VGE [1]. Animal and human studies have shown that H_2O_2 is readily absorbed from the intestines and the peritoneum. Oxygen (O_2) emboli arise from the systemic absorption of H_2O_2 as catalase-induced decomposition causes release of water and molecular O_2. One milliliter of a 3% H_2O_2 solution releases an estimated 10 mL of O_2 on contact with catalase [1], which is abundant in human blood.

Case reports of VGE during blood donation and insertion of peripheral intravenous catheters illustrate that there are no circumstances in which a vein is exposed to atmospheric pressure that the hazard of embolization is nonexistent [1].

Pathophysiology

Entry of Gas into the Circulation

VGE has been shown to occur with patients in essentially any position [1]. The critical factor common to all VGE lies in the pressure gradient created between the right side of the heart and the level of the open vessel. Any increase in the distance of the open vessel above the level of the heart or any decrease in intrathoracic pressure would increase the likelihood of air entering the venous circulation and traveling to the heart. For each 5 in. in vertical height above the level of the RA, there is an approximately 9.3 mm Hg decrease in local blood pressure. Any decrease in mean intrathoracic pressure or mechanisms resulting in a contracted blood volume or low central venous pressure will tend to enhance any existing venous pressure gradient.

Large amounts of gas can rapidly pass into the venous system under the proper conditions. Calculations indicate that approximately 100 mL of air per second would enter a vessel via a No. 14-gauge needle with only a 5 cm H_2O pressure gradient across it.

Travel of Gas to the Heart

Once gas has entered the venous circulation, it travels toward the point of lower pressure until it reaches an obstruction. Animal studies have found that passage of air emboli through the superior vena cava can be retarded or the air even retained at sites proximal to the superior vena cava for an indefinite period [1].

Large venous gas emboli are capable of lodging and then obstructing blood flow in the heart and the pulmonary vasculature [1]. Grossly, these events have been observed to cause immediate dilation of the RA, the right ventricle (RV), and the pulmonary outflow tract. A rapidly expanding zone of RV ischemia follows soon thereafter. Functional obstruction of the RV outflow tract may result due to an "air lock" phenomenon. A blood-froth mixture results from systolic compression of the compressible gas phase with the noncompressible whole-blood phase. This concoction is then able to expand during diastole, the net result being an inadequate pumping action of the RV. It has been postulated that turbulent blood flow results from this "whipping" type of action or from vortex flow around partially obstructing collections of air bubbles. This whipping subsequently enhances fibrin formation, platelet aggregation, and coalescence of intravascular fat.

Smaller collections of air may not impair the heart and they may pass directly to the pulmonary arteries. Larger collections enter the pulmonary arteries with associated collections of fat and fibrin emboli.

Fate of Gas Emboli

Bubbles with the smallest initial radii have the shortest life span and are occasionally seen to pass directly through a capillary bed after attaining a radius of approximately 5 μm [1]. The bulk of excretion of gaseous emboli is accounted for by molecular diffusion across the arteriolar wall into the alveolar spaces. The rate of washout is related to RV performance and mean pulmonary artery (PA) pressure [1].

Surface-tension relationships, vascular pressures, and the size range of the bubbles are several additional interacting factors that may influence passage of emboli across the lungs. Also, the composition of the gas influences the size of the bubbles and the rate of dissolution in the blood. Bubbles of air or N_2 are expected to remain in the blood for longer periods of time than O_2 or CO_2, especially if the ventilatory gases resemble room air composition. This relationship is due to the similarity in the partial pressures of the gases inside the bubbles with those of the surrounding blood, as well as to the different solubilities of the gases. Tonic factors affecting the diameter of pulmonary vessels (e.g., anesthetic agents, neurogenic or hypoxic pulmonary vasoconstriction, arterial tension of CO_2, endogenous mediators) may also influence the passage of bubbles across the lungs.

Cardiopulmonary Consequences of Embolization

Pulmonary vascular obstruction is a major consequence of VGE and can lead to death. Obstruction to blood flow through the RV and through the pulmonary vascular system results from pulmonary vasoconstriction and from the mechanical impediment to flow imposed by the gas bubbles [1]. The change in PA pressures depends on whether the gas emboli are the result of a slow continuous infusion or a rapid bolus injection. In the first instance, a brisk increase in PA pressure to a level of up to 300% of baseline is seen [1]. This rapid increase phase is believed to be due to pulmonary vascular vasoconstriction and is followed by a plateau phase. The plateau response likely represents the opening of anatomic intrapulmonary shunts or a balance between the rate of gas infusion and rate of elimination. In contrast, when approximately 100 mL of air is injected as a bolus, PA pressure declines by as much as 20%, as the right heart is acutely stressed beyond its capabilities. Larger bolus injections (125 to 200 mL) are consistently fatal.

Pulmonary edema from VGE has been described anecdotally in humans [1]. Increased hydrostatic pulmonary vascular pressures (from mechanical occlusion of the PA and from induced vasoconstriction) and increased capillary permeability have been suggested as mechanisms for edema formation [1]. Regardless, the edema proves to be transient and reverses as the gas emboli are rapidly absorbed.

Maldistribution in ventilation–perfusion ($\dot{V}/\dot{Q}$) matching is the major factor leading to hypoxemia and changes in CO_2 concentrations. With small amounts of continuous gas bubble infusion (0.2 mL per minute per kg) into the venous circulation, there is an increase in high $\dot{V}/\dot{Q}$ areas in the lung. With larger volume gas emboli (0.75 to 2 mL per kg), however, shunting and an increase in the physiologic dead space have been shown to occur and to increase proportionally as the volume of embolic gas increases. This effect can involve as much as 35% of the total cardiac output, and it may be severe enough to cause CO_2 retention in addition to hypoxemia.

The end-tidal CO_2 concentration ($ETCO_2$) decreases during VGE as a result of the increase in dead space caused by vascular obstruction. More simply, $ETCO_2$ decreases as CO_2 is "washed out" of alveoli that are ventilated but not perfused adequately. Inadequate $\dot{V}/\dot{Q}$ matching may further worsen in the setting of a reduced cardiac output, resulting directly from VGE or indirectly as a consequence of non–embolic-related events (e.g., blood loss, myocardial ischemia, vasoactive medications). Any reduction in pulmonary blood flow decreases the delivery of air in the venous blood to the alveoli, thereby further decreasing the $ETCO_2$.

Paradoxic Embolism

A paradoxic embolism may occur in the presence or absence of an anatomic intracardiac shunt. A gas embolism may elevate right-sided heart pressures, thus facilitating right-to-left shunting through a patent foramen ovale (PFO). Autopsy studies of patients with no history of cardiac disease document the presence of a probe-patent PFO in 25% to 35% of the general population [1].

Considered an anatomic variant, a probe-patent PFO is generally 1 to 10 mm in diameter and it remains functionally closed as long as left atrial pressure exceeds RA pressure. A reversal of the normal interatrial pressure gradient might be expected to increase the risk of paradoxic embolization. RA pressure has been demonstrated to be higher than left atrial pressure in the seated position in up to 54% of adult humans monitored during neurosurgical procedures [1]. The critical pressure necessary for gas bubbles to be forced through a probe PFO is not known, but it is likely to be small. After cardiac surgery, it has been shown that as little as a 4 mm Hg gradient can produce a 50% right-to-left intracardiac shunt [1].

Clinically, it may be important to distinguish between an anatomic PFO and functional PFO because it is the latter that has an impact on any morbidity and mortality experienced. It has been reported that paradoxic embolization occurs in only 15% to 25% of patients with a PFO [1]. Contrast echocardiography using agitated sterile saline given as a rapid intravenous bolus has documented a lower prevalence of functional PFO (i.e., 10% to 20%) [1], as compared to the known prevalence of 25% to 35% for anatomic PFO. The amount of contrast material crossing from the right heart to the left heart does not correlate with the magnitude of shunt flow, nor does the Valsalva maneuver provoke shunting in all patients with PFO [1]. The question remains as to whether this finding represents a low sensitivity of this method for detecting PFO or whether there are some anatomic PFOs that have no functional role. Consensus opinion is that all PFOs should be considered to have the potential for allowing paradoxic embolization. Multiple reports have documented that the absence of any agitated saline or color flow through the interatrial septum by echocardiography does not exclude the presence of a PFO; it only excludes the presence of a right-to-left interatrial shunt at that moment in time [1].

Bubble passage through the pulmonary circulation has been shown to occur in the absence of intracardiac communications when the rate of venous air infusion exceeds the rate of pulmonary filtration and excretion [1]. Paradoxic air embolization during cardiopulmonary bypass has been reported to occur in the absence of an intracardiac defect when the mean PA pressure exceeds approximately 30 mm Hg [1]. Animal research suggests the existence of this same "critical value" of PA pressure that, once exceeded, dramatically increases the tendency for paradoxic embolization [1]. This increase occurs presumably on the basis of direct arteriovenous anastomoses in the lung (seen only rarely, but may be as large as 500 μm in diameter), bronchopulmonary anastomoses (i.e., flow is from the PA to the bronchial veins and then to the pulmonary veins), or by routine transpulmonary passage of the gas across the capillary beds.

Factors Affecting Mortality

The size of the embolus, its rate of delivery, and the final destinations of the gaseous emboli are the most important factors influencing the severity of injury produced by VGE. In humans, accidental bolus injections of 100 and 300 mL of air have been reported to be fatal [1]. In critically ill patients with minimal cardiopulmonary reserve, smaller emboli could be expected to have a greater morbidity.

In the context of equal volumes, mortality is decreased if the embolism is of CO_2 rather than air or O_2. Animal work indicates that CO_2 may be injected to 5 times the volume of O_2 before symptoms of embolism appear, presumably due to its greater solubility in blood [1]. Although tolerated to a larger extent, it must be remembered that CO_2 emboli are not entirely benign and may lead to similar clinical consequences as air embolization.

When nitrous oxide (N_2O) is used for anesthesia, mortality is increased in the setting of VGE [1]. N_2O attains a high blood concentration because of its high solubility (approximately 20-fold that of O_2 and 34-fold that of N_2). Because a large concentration gradient would exist between this blood and any air embolus, N_2O would be expected to diffuse from the blood into the embolus. As a result, the embolus increases geometrically in size in direct relation to the partial pressure of N_2O because the N_2O molecules can diffuse from the blood into the air embolus much more rapidly than the N_2 can be removed. The end result is a potential worsening of any generated physiologic abnormalities or delay in the ultimate resolution of the embolus. The presence of N_2O in the anesthetic mixture has been shown to reduce the median lethal dose of a given volume of air by a factor of 3.4 [1].

Diagnosis

Clinical Manifestations

The symptoms of VGE are generally nonspecific. Patients may report feeling faint or dizzy, express a fear of impending doom, or even complain of dyspnea or substernal chest pain. This presentation, with or without paradoxic embolism, may mimic an acute cardiopulmonary or central nervous system (CNS) event. Severe VGE may present dramatically with elevated neck veins, "clear lungs," and hypotension, and it may be rapidly followed by altered mental status and death. Because signs and symptoms are nonspecific, the importance of a detailed history, familiarity with the clinical situations in which VGE occurs, and a high degree of clinical suspicion cannot be overemphasized if one is to make an accurate diagnosis.

Physical Examination

Physical examination is usually not helpful in making the diagnosis. The only "specific" sign attributed to VGE is the classic mill-wheel murmur, otherwise reported only to occur in the rare syndrome of hydropneumopericardium. This murmur has been described as the rhythmic splashing or churning sound generated by the agitation of gas trapped with fluid in a closed space. Most often, it is only audible transiently and is heard infrequently at best, even in severe VGE. With large emboli and resultant cardiovascular collapse, a sound resembling the "squeezing of a wet sponge" has been described over the precordium [1].

VGE may occur without any change in vital signs. Wheezing as a result of acute bronchospasm may occasionally be heard. In a prospective study of seated neurosurgical patients, marked hypotension was noted in 78%, respiratory changes in 61%, and ventricular ectopy in 50% [1].

Laboratory Data

Abnormal results may include electrocardiogram (ECG) changes consistent with myocardial ischemia or acute cor pulmonale, premature ventricular contractions, and/or arterial blood gas findings of hypoxemia and hypercapnia.

Radiographic Findings

Chest radiography may verify the presence of VGE, but it should not be relied on for the diagnosis, especially in emergent situations. Air in the main PA is pathognomonic of pulmonary VGE, and it is recognized as a characteristic bell-shaped lucency in the distal main PA. This sign is seen very infrequently, especially in supine patients. Other patterns seen are focal upper-lung zone oligemia, central PA dilation, and air in the systemic veins or the arterial circulation [1]. Pulmonary edema ranging from hilar haziness to generalized vascular redistribution may occur soon after VGE, and it usually persists for at least 16 to 24 hours [1]. Noncardiogenic pulmonary edema has been reported [1], is usually self-limited, and resolves over several days. Progression of noncardiogenic pulmonary edema to full-blown acute respiratory distress syndrome has also been described [1].

Ventilation–Perfusion Lung Scans

VGE may produce patterns consistent with "high probability" for pulmonary venous thromboembolism interpretations. Prompt and complete resolution of these scintigraphic perfusion defects within 24 hours has been documented [1], and it is probably characteristic for VGE. In contrast, perfusion defects produced by venous thromboembolism are known to resolve more slowly over a period of weeks to months and they may not ever resolve completely. Areas of $\dot{V}/\dot{Q}$ matching (i.e., "indeterminate probability") may coexist with $\dot{V}/\dot{Q}$ mismatches, and they are believed to represent reflex bronchoconstriction in conjunction with occlusion of the PA or its branches. The decreased ventilation is apparently due to the release of bronchoconstricting agents, such as serotonin, from the occluded segments of the PA. This phenomenon is readily reversible within several hours if the PA occlusion is transient, and it is related to rapid resolution of the gaseous emboli.

Detection and Monitoring Method

Precordial Doppler monitoring is generally considered one of the more sensitive techniques for detecting emboli. Because a gas–blood interface is an excellent acoustic reflector, when an ultrasonographic beam strikes a moving gas bubble, a distinctive and characteristic artifact is heard above the background flow signal.

VGE may be missed by this technique due to changes in the position of the detector or blood pressure. False-positive reports of VGE may arise due to arrhythmia. The sound pattern induced by a junctional rhythm may easily mimic changes produced by VGE. With a junctional rhythm, cannon A-waves may be present due to contraction of the RA against a closed tricuspid valve. The resultant turbulence in the RA is detected and confused for VGE.

Serial measurements of PA pressure should be a useful monitoring technique due to the fact that even small emboli may produce significant increases in PA pressures, major increases in PA pressure do not occur unless at least 10% of the vasculature is obstructed, the rise in PA pressure is roughly proportional to embolus size, and the likelihood of paradoxic embolism increases above a mean PA pressure of 30 mm Hg [1].

$ETCO_2$ and N_2 levels fluctuate with VGE. Because these changes probably result primarily from significant mismatch, it would be anticipated that they would detect emboli later than Doppler techniques or changes in PA pressure and that they would be more likely to miss small emboli. Like PA pressure changes, however, variations in $ETCO_2$ stay abnormal longer, and they are more closely related to the volume of gas embolized [1]. Potential confounding factors exist that may also cause a reduction in $ETCO_2$ in the absence of a VGE-related event, and they include any set of circumstances that result in an acute decrease in cardiac output, increases in alveolar ventilation, or increases in alveolar dead space.

Consideration of the advantages and disadvantages of the available VGE detection technology suggests that a combination of transesophageal echocardiography or precordial Doppler ultrasonography with PA pressure, $ETCO_2$, or transcutaneous O_2 devices would provide the sensitivity, the quantitative determination, and the physiologic response monitoring necessary. Across the United States, use of $ETCO_2$ monitoring in combination with precordial Doppler ultrasonography has become the primary, if not the standard, approach for VGE detection perioperatively.

Treatment

Because a fatal outcome may occur long before any diagnostic confirming tests can be performed, treatment must be initiated promptly at the earliest suspicion of gas embolization. Although no systematic studies comparing treatment modalities have been reported, improved detection of VGE appears to have decreased its severity. In combined retrospective and prospective analyses of seated neurosurgical procedures, a significant beneficial role was found for the use of routine precordial Doppler monitoring [1]. Before the advent of routine Doppler monitoring, VGE was clinically detected less often (5.7% before vs. 32% after), but the episodes noted had more severe sequelae. Once precordial Doppler monitoring became standard, the morbidity and mortality directly related to venous or arterial emboli was documented to be 0.5%. This improvement in event detection and reduction in the severity of VGE was ascribed to earlier recognition, allowing for earlier institution of therapy and prevention of further occurrences.

Routine Treatment Measures

Immediate measures should include identification of the site of gas entry and prevention of further gas entry, cessation or correction of exacerbating factors, administration of 100% O_2, and changing position to the left lateral decubitus position. In most patients, the site of gas entry is readily apparent. Failure to stop gas entry in a timely fashion may be fatal. If there is suspicion of a low central blood volume, volume should be rapidly repleted. Immediate cessation of delivery of N_2O and ventilating with 100% O_2 facilitates resolution of any gas emboli experienced during anesthesia with this agent.

Because air emboli are composed of approximately 79% N_2 and 21% O_2, any maneuver that rapidly increases the elimination of dissolved N_2 should decrease the size of the embolus. Administration of 100% O_2 achieves this goal by washing N_2 out of the alveoli and by creating a favorable gradient for N_2 to cross into the alveolus from the blood.

Placing patients in the left lateral decubitus position may facilitate movement of any air obstructing the pulmonary outflow tract toward the apex of the RV, thereby relieving the obstruction and improving survival.

Aspiration and Dislodgement

In patients with witnessed gas embolism or in whom monitoring techniques suggest that the gas is still trapped in the heart, attempts can be made to aspirate or dislodge the gas. Gas may be aspirated from the heart by placing a central venous catheter into the RA or RV or pulling back a PA catheter and then aspirating serially from each successive heart chamber [1]. In unwitnessed gas embolism, this early phase has usually passed before the embolism is detected, and these interventions may result in more harm than benefit. Closed-chest compression may dislodge the embolus from the RV.

Hyperbaric Oxygen

When available, use of hyperbaric oxygen (HBO) may be helpful. HBO is the only therapy demonstrated to have any benefit well after VGE has been clinically established [1]. Even after emboli of 150 to 500 mL, HBO produced rapid improvement of all cardiopulmonary and neurologic abnormalities despite delays in initiating therapy of up to 20 hours. The most common HBO treatment protocols in use today are the U.S. Navy Treatment Tables 5, 6, and 6A [3]. Use of these Tables is discussed later in the Treatment section of Decompression Sickness. Although it is accepted that HBO should be instituted as early as possible, the literature supports that special consideration be given to this modality at late stages, even in a seemingly irrecoverable situation [1].

Managing Unwitnessed Venous Gas Embolism

Given that VGE may mimic or cause a clinical presentation that is difficult to distinguish from venous pulmonary thromboembolism (PE), RV infarct, myocardial infarction (MI), or stroke, clinicians may frequently feel reluctant to consider the difficult-to-establish diagnosis of VGE and to begin treatment until other causes are ruled out. The simple measures indicated for the immediate management of VGE outlined herein are not contraindicated in the management of any of the other conditions typically in the differential diagnosis.

Little has been published on the clinical management of cardiovascular consequences of VGE. Because myocardial and RV infarct may frequently accompany large VGE, urgent, routine evaluation with ECG and echocardiography would be indicated in most cases. Because myocardial ischemia and subsequent MI in VGE probably result from hypoxemia, the effects of massive overdistention of the ventricle, and perhaps direct embolization of coronary vessels, the value of traditional management techniques for MI is not clear. There are no theoretical contraindications to the use of nitrates, aspirin, beta-blockers, calcium-channel blockers, or vasodilators in patients with ECG changes. The role of thrombolytic therapy in VGE is unclear.

Discrimination between PE and VGE in patients with unwitnessed, unmonitored events can be difficult. Patients at risk for VGE are frequently at risk for PE as well. Once gas has left the RV, changes in PA pressures and $ETCO_2$ values may be similar in both conditions. As noted, the radiologic findings may be similar, but they may resolve within 24 hours with VGE. If the clinical suspicion of PE is high, there is no known contraindication to initiating appropriate anticoagulation in patients with VGE.

Prevention

Preventive measures are likely the most valuable management strategy for VGE. All patients undergoing the procedures listed in Table 61.1 [1] should be considered at high risk. In addition, hyperventilation, obstructive lung disease, and hypovolemia are common clinical conditions that increase the natural pressure gradient between atmospheric air and the central venous compartment; they may, therefore, also increase the chances of VGE during predisposing manipulations. Patients with a known PFO, pulmonary hypertension, previous MI with markedly reduced RV function, known right-to-left shunts, or congenital heart disease with any of the mentioned abnormalities should also be considered at high risk, not for experiencing an embolism per se, but for being susceptible for increased morbidity and mortality of a paradoxic embolism. A high false-negative rate (sensitivity, 64%) limits the usefulness of preoperative transthoracic echocardiography with Valsalva maneuver in predicting the presence of PFO and the risk of paradoxic emboli [1].

In general, patients should have procedures performed in a supine rather than upright position, and the point of potential air entry should be kept lower than the RA. Placement, manipulation, and removal of subclavian and internal jugular venous catheters are probably the most common clinical procedures during which specific measures can be performed to prevent substantial air embolization [2]. All patients should be placed in the Trendelenburg position, and they should be asked to perform the Valsalva maneuver or to hold their breath during needle/wire/catheter insertion. The operator should completely occlude the hub of the needle during manipulations to prevent open communication with atmospheric pressure. During removal of central catheters, patients should also be placed in the Trendelenburg position, the entry site should be compressed, and an occlusive dressing applied.

ARTERIAL GAS EMBOLISM

Arterial gas embolism (AGE) probably occurs daily in most hospitals due to the prevalence of the situations known to be associated with AGE (Table 61.2) [4]. Although the prevalence of AGE is likely not as high as VGE, the clinical significance is potentially much greater than VGE (Fig. 61.1). In the clinical setting, most causes of AGE are preventable, and prompt treatment is frequently effective.

TABLE 61.2

RISK FACTORS AND CAUSES OF ARTERIAL GAS EMBOLISM

All causes listed for venous gas embolism in Table 61.1, via paradoxic embolization
Cardiopulmonary bypass/coronary artery bypass graft/open-heart procedures
Coronary angiography/angioplasty
Cardioplegic solution infusion
Misuse/malfunction of pump oxygenator
Intraaortic balloon pump
Penetrating lung injury/resection
Bronchovenous fistula (due to trauma, mechanical ventilation, biopsy, thoracentesis)
Arterial line, arteriography
Self-contained underwater breathing apparatus diving
Decompression sickness
Carotid endarterectomy

Etiology

Cardiac Surgery and Bypass

AGE during cardiopulmonary bypass has an estimated incidence that ranges from 0.1% to 11.0% [4]. There is evidence that the use of in-line filters and preferential use of membrane oxygenators over bubble oxygenators may decrease this risk significantly.

The importance of trapped air in the left heart as a potential source of AGE after an open cardiotomy has been appreciated for years. Air may remain adherent to the endocardium, sutures, and prosthetic valves, and in cul-de-sacs in the atria, ventricles, or aorta even after the heart is closed and beating spontaneously again. Complete air evacuation, even after specific and meticulous venting techniques, is nearly impossible to achieve [4]. Residual air has been shown to be present in the heart after discontinuation of bypass in approximately two-thirds of patients undergoing open cardiotomies and in approximately 12% of patients undergoing coronary artery bypass grafting (CABG) only, for an overall incidence of approximately 45%. The source of intracardiac air resulting from CABG operations is thought to be due to the ascending aorta being cross-clamped and suction then being applied to the left heart or the aortic root for the purpose of venting. The resultant pressure decrease is transmitted to the coronary arterial circulation, thus allowing air entry via the coronary arteriotomy site, with subsequent passage into the aortic root or left ventricle. Any gases trapped in a proximal coronary artery or in a distally attached vein graft may also pass into the aortic root in the absence of venting if the graft is injected under pressure, as occurs commonly during the administration of cardioplegic hypothermia.

Transcranial Doppler monitoring of the middle cerebral artery during open-heart operations has confirmed the occurrence of cerebral gas embolization [4]. With refined surgical techniques, over time there has been a considerable reduction in the incidence of major neurologic injury after cardiac surgery and CABG, with a currently reported incidence of approximately 5% to 10% [4]. Detailed neuropsychiatric function testing, however, has shown persistent impairment of cerebral function in up to 70% of patients after CABG [4].

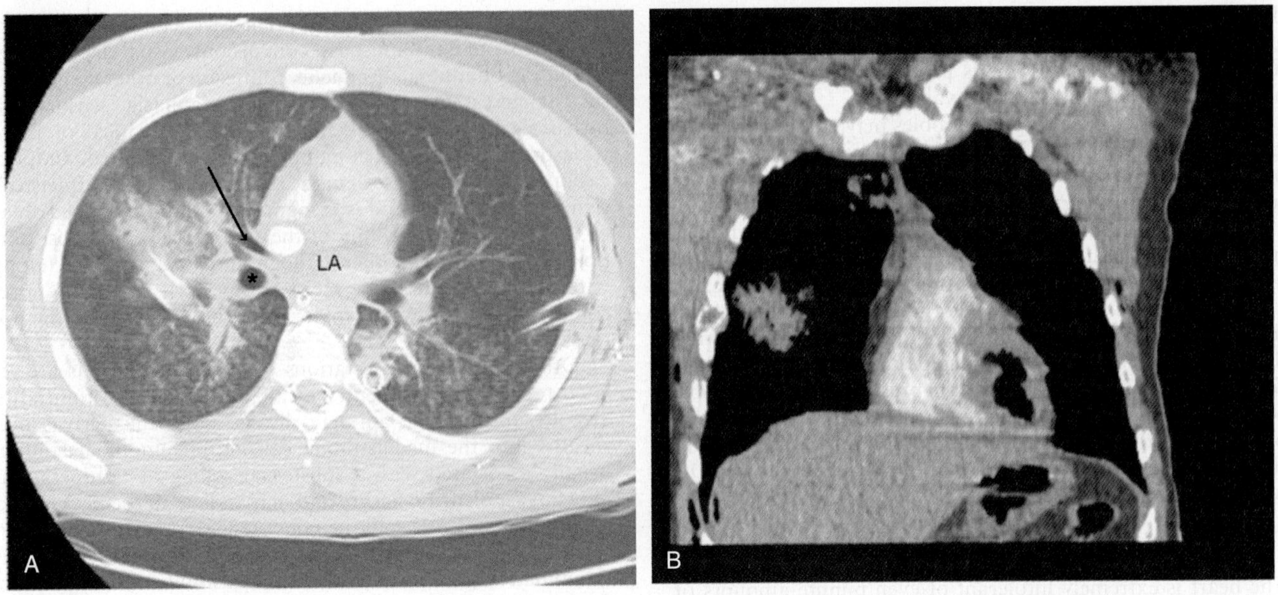

FIGURE 61.1. Fatal air embolism after massive facial trauma and prolonged extrication in an unbelted, backseat passenger in a car accident. **A:** Cross section of the chest showing air outlining the right superior pulmonary vein (*black arrow*) emptying into the left atrium (LA). Black* indicates the bronchus intermedius. **B:** Coronal reconstruction showing a massive air collection in the left ventricle.

Lung Trauma

Systemic AGE is a frequent and unrecognized cause of death in patients with blunt or penetrating lung trauma [4]. The mode of air entry after percutaneous lung puncture, penetrating or blunt lung trauma, or with positive-pressure mechanical ventilation is via creation of a bronchovenous fistula. Risk factors enhancing the chance of AGE include underlying emphysema, uncooperative patients, sneezing or coughing bouts, use of large-diameter needles, hypotension, hypovolemia, Valsalva maneuver, and site of involvement in close proximity to the hila. In patients with preexisting pulmonary fibrosis, one should expect an increased frequency and severity of systemic embolism due to the inability of the injured veins to retract and constrict. What has been referred to in the past as "pleural shock" (i.e., fainting, seizures, or even sudden death during a thoracentesis or therapeutic pneumothorax for treatment of tuberculosis) has since become recognized as a manifestation of AGE. Percutaneous procedures with needle calibers less than 20 gauge (0.9 mm) have generally been considered safe, despite a case report describing a cerebral AGE after transthoracic aspiration with a 23-gauge (0.6-mm) needle. The reported incidence for this complication for needles of 16 to 20 gauge (0.9 to 1.6 mm) has been variably estimated at 0.5 to 0.8 in 1,000 cases [4].

Arterial Lines

Cerebral AGE via retrograde flow from an indwelling radial arterial line has been reported as a case study and then followed up with a laboratory investigation [4]. Radioactive xenon mixed with 2 to 5 mL of air and injected at a rate of 0.6 to 2.5 mL per second into the radial artery resulted in demonstrable retrograde passage into the cerebral circulation. This low-flow rate is approximately fivefold to 25-fold less than the reported "safe range" of previous work [4]. Because the true "safe" amount of air that can remain in an arterial flush catheter without the risk of retrograde embolization remains unknown, medical personnel need to be vigilant and meticulous in ensuring removal of any entrapped air in arterial flush lines.

Percutaneous Transluminal Coronary Angioplasty

Most coronary artery gas emboli resulting from percutaneous transluminal coronary angioplasty are reportedly extremely small, and they do not result in symptoms or hemodynamic consequences [4]. Of the symptomatic episodes, most cause rapid onset of chest pain with ECG evidence of ischemia or infarction. The systemic blood pressure may be unaffected, or it may decrease mildly. In almost all patients, these effects clear spontaneously within 5 to 10 minutes, similar to experimental models. Only rarely does percutaneous transluminal coronary angioplasty–related AGE result in bradycardia, hypotension, ventricular fibrillation, MI, or asystole [4].

Pathophysiology

In AGE, gas enters the arterial system by the direct rupture of a blood–air interface, by direct passage from the PA to pulmonary venous system, or through a functional right-to-left cardiac shunt. Gas bubbles distribute themselves throughout the body primarily directed by the relative blood flow at the time. Bubble buoyancy is actually a minor factor unless there is a significant depression in forward systemic flow [4]. Because the heart, lung, and brain receive the greatest amount of blood flow, the consequences of embolization are most apparent in these organs. Pulmonary manifestations of AGE are uncommon, perhaps because the redundancy of the pulmonary vascular supply limits the consequences of bubble occlusion.

Systemic Mechanical and Biophysical Effects

Bubble formation results in two broad categories of effects: mechanical—physical obstruction to blood flow with distortion or tearing of tissues as the bubble forms and expands, and biophysical—where the blood–gas, blood–tissue or gas–endothelial interfaces stimulate a cascade of leukocyte, platelet, coagulation, fibrinolytic, and complement-mediated activations [4]. Research over the last two decades now recognizes the importance of oxidative stressors causing impairment of endothelium-dependent vasorelaxation (i.e., the endothelial dysfunction hypothesis). This is primarily caused by loss of nitric oxide activity in the vessel wall [5–7].

Similar to VGE, the trapped bubbles may pass through the circulation and exit in the lungs, or they may be slowly metabolized by body tissues. Unlike the situation when bubbles are trapped in a vein, an arterial occlusion may have an immediate clinical impact. Uptake and release of inert gas by a particular tissue depends on the rate of blood flow to that tissue, as well as the rate of gas diffusion out of the blood into the tissue.

When bubbles do form, the inert gas becomes isolated from the circulation, and it cannot be removed by blood flow until it diffuses back into tissues. The speed of diffusion is the result of the difference between the N_2 partial pressure in the air bubble compared with the N_2 partial pressure in the tissue. The partial pressure of the inert gas in the bubble also varies directly with the bubble's loss of O_2 through metabolic conversion into CO_2, which is 21 times more soluble than O_2.

Cardiovascular Effects

The heart is extremely intolerant of even minute amounts of arterial gas. AGE may produce MI, left ventricle compromise, dysrhythmia, hypotension, or hypertension. As little as 0.025 to 0.05 mL of air directly entering a coronary artery may result in transient impairment of ventricular function, focal MI, ventricular fibrillation, or death [4].

Central Nervous System Effects

Cerebral embolism produces stroke-like symptoms and cerebral edema. Injury is probably more a result of damage from endothelial mediators rather than being directly due to ischemia or edema. After 5 to 30 seconds of arrested cerebral blood flow, most gas bubbles easily pass through the pial arteries. Significant volumes of gas may subsequently be collected in "air traps" in the jugular veins [4]. Larger emboli (e.g., large enough to obstruct several generations of arteriolar branching) are also generally only temporarily obstructing, and they relocate to the cerebral and the jugular veins during the period of reactive hyperemia that follows periods of arrested cerebral blood flow. It has been proposed, therefore, that the CNS dysfunction that follows cerebral AGE is not the result of bubble entrapment alone; it is instead due in large part to effects on vascular endothelium or blood components.

Diagnosis

AGE, whether traumatic, iatrogenic, or dysbaric (i.e., solely as a result of changes in ambient pressures) in origin, typically presents immediately after the insult occurs. A myriad array of dramatic manifestations is possible, typically with symptoms suggestive of coronary or CNS involvement. Two general clinical patterns have been recognized: fulminant collapse and isolated CNS injury. In the former, the initial presentation is apnea, coma, and cardiac arrest. This pattern is known to occur in 4% to 5% of patients with dysbaric air embolism but has an unknown incidence for other types of AGE. The responsible mechanism is believed to be direct coronary artery embolization with resultant MI or gaseous embolization of the cerebral circulation, resulting in hypertension and marked dysrhythmias. This subgroup is generally unresponsive to resuscitative efforts (Fig. 61.1).

In the latter group, the initial presentation is that of stable respiratory and heart rates, but with a wide spectrum of neurologic signs and symptoms. Usually, the symptoms are abrupt in onset, and they progress rapidly to overt signs. Patients may feel faint or dizzy or have an apprehensive fear of death. There may be loss of consciousness, convulsions, visual disturbances (including blindness), headache, confusion or other mental status changes, coma, vertigo, nystagmus, aphasia, sensory disturbances, weakness or hemiparesis, or even focal or more widespread paralysis. The pupils are usually dilated, and, occasionally, air may be seen in the retinal vessels. Liebermeister's sign may be present and is recognized as sharply defined areas of tongue pallor. Marbling of the skin of the uppermost portions of the body is another pathognomonic sign of AGE (along with retinal gas and Liebermeister's sign) [4]. With prompt recompression therapy, the majority of these cases have the potential for full recovery.

Other clinical manifestations of extra-alveolar gas are related to the traumatic entry of air into the interstitium after alveoli rupture. The air may dissect along the perivascular sheaths into the mediastinum, causing pneumomediastinum, usually associated with a substernal aching or tightness that may have a pleuritic nature and may radiate to the neck, back, or shoulders. There may be coexistent subcutaneous emphysema and a notable "crunching" sound with each heartbeat (Hamman's sign) due to air in the mediastinum. Air may dissect further to cause a pneumothorax in up to 10% of cases [4]. Tension pneumothorax may occur in patients on positive-pressure mechanical ventilation or during decompression. Pneumopericardium and air in the retroperitoneum and subcutaneous tissues of the neck, trunk, or limbs may also occur. This extra-alveolar gas also has access to torn pulmonary blood vessels when the intrathoracic pressure decreases during normal inspiration after barotrauma has occurred. Once egress into the pulmonary venous circulation has occurred, migration to the left side of the heart and then to the arterial circulation may follow. Hemoptysis has often been mentioned as a cardinal sign of dysbaric air embolism, but it actually occurs in a minority (approximately 5%) of patients [4].

Treatment

Management of AGE and decompression sickness is similar. Appropriate therapy involves prompt recognition, initial stabilization (with emphasis on preventing further damage), and definitive specific therapy (Table 61.3) [4]. All patients undergoing cardiopulmonary procedures or with recent lung trauma must be considered at high risk for AGE. Therefore, it cannot be emphasized strongly enough that a high index of suspicion for these diagnoses is one of the most important elements of care. Like many other true medical emergencies, therapeutic interventions should not be delayed to implement diagnostic testing. Details of therapy are found in the next section.

DECOMPRESSION SICKNESS

Decompression sickness (DCS) occurs only when a transition is made to an environment with a relatively lower ambient pressure. Any rapid lowering of ambient pressure, regardless of the initial pressure level or saturation of inert gas, results in the release of bubbles of inert gas into the blood and tissues. This is equally true for too quick a return to a normobaric state after a hyperbaric exposure (as in diving or compressed air mining), or for rapid progression from a normobaric state into a hypobaric exposure (as in aviators, astronauts, or mountain climbers). It is estimated that around 9 to 10 million divers are currently active worldwide, performing more than 250 million dives annually. Statistics compiled by the Divers Alert Network (www.diversalertnetwork.org) indicate

TABLE 61.3

TREATMENT SUMMARY OF ARTERIAL GAS EMBOLISM AND DECOMPRESSION SICKNESS

- Of time-tested benefit
  - Prevent further bubble formation and extension of other injuries
  - Cardiopulmonary life support as needed
  - 100% concentration of inspired oxygen
  - Maintain intravascular volume with isotonic fluids
  - Treat coexisting problems
  - Transport as soon as possible to recompression facility
  - Hyperbaric therapy
- Unproven benefit (but generally believed to be helpful)
  - Trendelenburg/Durant position if arterial gas embolism suspected or unconsciousness with vomiting (would not maintain >30–60 min due to possible increased cerebral edema)
  - Avoid glucose-containing infusions
  - Avoid hypertension, anxiety
  - Diazepam for seizures, severe agitation, intractable vomiting (not used prophylactically)
- Experimental or of questionable benefit
  - Consider aspirin
  - Corticosteroids (possible central nervous system toxicity)
  - Calcium channel blockers
  - Lidocaine
  - Combination nonsteroidal anti-inflammatory drug, heparin, and prostaglandin I_2
  - Perfluorochemicals and/or other surface-active agents
  - Induced hypothermia
  - Cerebral venoarterial perfusion
- Proven detrimental
  - Recompression while submerged
  - Alcohol/analgesics
  - Delayed transport to hyperbaric oxygen facility
  - Additional hypobaric exposures

that there are more than 1,000 diving-related injuries annually in the United States alone, of which nearly 10% are fatal. DCS is the most frequent serious complication of self-contained underwater breathing apparatus (scuba) diving with an overall incidence of 4 to 6 cases per 10,000 dives [4,8,9]. DCS ranks third, after drowning and barotrauma/AGE (estimated incidence of 7 cases per 100,000 dives), as a cause of death among divers [4]. Strict enforcement of work regulations for tunnel workers and pilots has greatly decreased the incidence of DCS in these two groups.

Etiology

Diving

The turn of the 20th century saw the origin of decompression tables, which define set depths and time limits of hyperbaric exposure to be used by divers to minimize the risk of DCS. Although derived empirically by J. S. Haldane, all common schedules since have been based on his original methods. Haldane's work demonstrated that the human body could tolerate a twofold reduction in ambient pressure without symptoms of DCS. Haldane also formulated the concept that the tissues of the body absorb nitrogen at varying rates, depending on the type of tissue and its vascularity. Experience has shown that modern scuba divers can surface with a significant net accumulation of inert gas and yet remain without symptoms [4,10,11]. There is an important inter- and intraindividual variation in the degree of bubbling after a dive, indicating a significant, but as yet poorly characterized, influence of personal factors affecting gas saturation and desaturation [12,13].

Flying

DCS due to rapid hypobaric exposures from altitudes higher than approximately 18,000 ft is a syndrome indistinguishable from that produced in divers, and it is usually the result of accidental loss of cabin pressure in a pressurized aircraft. The altitude threshold for DCS is generally reported to be approximately 18,000 ft, but unless a person has had a hyperbaric exposure within the past 24 hours, there are rarely any difficulties with exposure to altitudes of up to 25,000 ft [4]. Exposures above this level up to approximately 48,000 ft for durations of 30 minutes to 3 hours have resulted in a DCS incidence of 1.5% [4]. More prolonged exposures and even greater altitudes increase the severity of an episode of DCS. Modern airline transportation has minimized these risks by pressurizing aircraft to maintain cabin pressures equivalent to 8,000 ft while flying at actual altitudes of greater than 40,000 ft. DCS may also occur while flying after a diving trip, and it may be produced by exposure to altitudes of as little as 4,000 ft, even when "no-decompression" type of diving took place. Current recommendations are to avoid all flying for at least 12 hours after any dive. For flights exceeding a cabin pressure equivalent of approximately 8,000 ft, or in the case of divers requiring decompression stops, at least a 24-hour delay is recommended before flying.

At the extreme of human hypobaric exposures is the astronaut. Astronauts performing activities outside their space vehicles are decompressed from a cabin pressure equivalent to sea level, down to a suit pressure equivalent of approximately 30,000 ft [4]. To minimize the risk of DCS, astronauts breathe 100% O_2 before decompression ("prebreathing") to reduce the partial pressure of N_2 before entering the space-suit environment. Only time and further space exploration will elucidate the risks of DCS from these types of exposures [14].

Pathophysiology

Bubble Formation

In DCS, gas dissolved in the body is released into the tissues and the bloodstream by decompression. Boyle's law states that the volume of a gas varies inversely with its surrounding absolute pressure. At sea level, the weight of air that we breathe is equal to 14.7 pounds per square inch, 760 mm Hg, or 1 atmosphere absolute (ATA), depending on the choice of units. Table 61.4 indicates that for every 33 ft of seawater a diver descends, the ambient pressure increases by 1 ATA and the volume occupied by that same gas decreases proportionally. The same table also demonstrates the reduction in pressure and volume expansion that accompanies increases in altitude.

The gear divers use to allow them to breathe underwater is designed to deliver air at the ambient pressure of the surrounding water, allowing the diver's lungs to remain fully expanded. As a scuba diver ascends slowly from depth, pressure in the lungs equalizes with ambient pressure as long as proper exhalation is achieved. If, for some reason, these expanding gases are not allowed to escape from the lungs (e.g., breath holding, localized gas trapping), overdistention of the alveoli may occur, which results in pulmonary barotrauma. The fragility of alveoli is not generally appreciated, but it is highlighted by the

TABLE 61.4

PRESSURE–VOLUME RELATIONSHIPS

	Pressure equivalents			
Distance from sea level (ft)	Pounds per inch^2	mm Hg	Atmosphere absolute	Bubble volume (%)
+48,000	1.85	96	0.126	794
+40,000	2.72	141	0.185	541
+32,000	3.98	206	0.271	369
+24,000	5.70	295	0.388	258
+16,000	7.97	412	0.542	185
+8,000	10.92	565	0.743	135
Sea level	14.70	760	1	100
−33	29.40	1,520	2	50
−66	44.10	2,280	3	33
−99	58.80	3,040	4	25
−132	73.50	3,800	5	20
−165	88.20	4,560	6	17

fact that with the lungs fully expanded on compressed air, a pressure differential of only 95 to 110 cm H_2O (equivalent to an ascent from a depth of only 4 to 6 ft) may be sufficient to rupture alveolar architecture [4]. With very few exceptions, all scuba diving is done at pressures less than 7 ATA, and most is done in the 2 to 4 ATA range [4,9].

Dalton's law of partial pressures states that the total pressure exerted by a mixture of gases is equal to the sum of the partial pressures of its constituent gases. The composition of gases that make up our atmosphere remains essentially constant up through an altitude of approximately 70,000 ft: 78.08% N_2, 20.95% O_2, and the remaining fraction of CO_2, hydrogen, helium, argon, and neon [4]. In most settings, N_2 is the predominant constituent of any inhaled gas mixture. N_2 is inert (i.e., it is unused/unchanged by passage through the body). This fact is in contrast to CO_2 and O_2, which are actively transported and therefore do not depend entirely on purely physical laws for removal. N_2 is more soluble in fat than in water, which suggests that during decompression, bubbles more likely form in lipophilic tissues such as bone marrow, fat, and spinal cord.

Henry's law of gas solubility states that the amount of gas that dissolves in a fluid is directly proportional to the pressure of that gas on that fluid. The deeper one descends underground or in the ocean, the greater the driving pressure for the gas on the blood and the bodily fluids. The total accumulation of dissolved N_2 into the tissues of the body is, therefore, dependent on the depth achieved and the time spent at that depth. As ambient pressure decreases on ascent, solubility decreases and gas is released from body fluids.

Studies on bubble formation suggest that of the total absorption of inert gas that occurs during a dive, only 5% to 10% is released as bubbles after a rapid decompression [4]. The site of origin of intravascular bubbles is controversial, but overwhelming human and animal experimental evidence shows that gas bubbles are first detected in the venous circulation during decompression. It is most probable that AGE in DCS arises from the venous circulation or from pulmonary barotrauma with entry of gas bubbles into the pulmonary veins (i.e., dysbaric air embolism).

Biophysical effects result from the blood–gas, blood–tissue and gas–endothelial interfaces, where an enormous chemical and physical discontinuity activates and amplifies reactive systems that are usually quiescent during normal blood flow. Electrochemical forces also exist at any blood-damaged endothelial interfaces, and they activate coagulation, complement, kinin, and fibrinolytic systems and allow for the denaturation of proteins. In DCS, and presumably in AGE, a localized hypercoagulable state develops, with a coexistent reduction in platelet count due to aggregation at the blood–bubble interface with leukocytes, red blood cells, and formed fibrin strands. The end result of this diffuse activation is to amplify any existing mechanical obstruction to blood flow with progressive sludging and clotting [4]. Further tissue injury then results from a decrease in local blood flow, edema formation, leukocyte chemotaxis, and the release of toxic O_2 radicals. These effects are likely to be most important in cases of CNS involvement, in which small areas of reduced blood flow can produce severe disability or death. A disturbance in barrier function would best account for the well-established features of AGE and DCS which are otherwise difficult to reconcile with simple vascular occlusion as the sole explanatory mechanism.

It is important to emphasize that divers perform safe decompressions millions of times each year. For most, this process involves only a slow ascent after a short-duration dive. Others may require staged ascents, with one or more stops at intermediate depths to give more time for N_2 elimination. Still others require planned periods of chamber recompression after diving to prevent DCS. The overall safety of decompression exposures has withstood the test of time, and it has improved with experience and use of preventive measures. Safe decompression is by far the rule, rather than the exception.

Diagnosis

The clinical manifestations of DCS are protean, reflecting the effects of bubbles distorting tissues, obstructing blood flow, and perhaps most importantly by endothelial activation and initiation of an inflammatory response. Symptoms will occur within 1 hour of a decompression event in approximately 75%, and within 12 hours in over 90% of afflicted individuals. A gross classification system is in common use based on the perceived severity of the clinical situation and the anticipated response to therapy [4]. Type I DCS encompasses 75% to 90% of patients and includes those with musculoskeletal pain; skin or lymphatic manifestations; or nonspecific symptoms of anorexia, malaise, and fatigue. Generally, these patients require no treatment or only a brief period of repressurization. Caution is still in order because up to 20% to 30% of this group may progress to a type II illness. Type II DCS is characterized by those cases with CNS or peripheral nerve involvement or any cardiorespiratory dysfunction. Overall, 10% to 25% of patients have type II DCS, and it generally represents a more severe illness with the potential for greater difficulties in treatment. The presence of a PFO is associated with a four- to sixfold increase in the odds ratio of developing a type II DCS [15–18].

Type I Decompression Sickness

Type I DCS includes the most common and classic manifestations usually associated with DCS. The majority of patients report an "aching" pain in a limb during decompression or within the first 36 hours after surfacing (95% of patients experience onset within 6 hours of surfacing). Initially, there may be a vague feeling that "something is wrong," and the limb discomfort is dull and poorly localized. With time, this may progress to an intense throbbing pain within a more circumscribed and specific location. The affected area is generally nontender to palpation, and movement of any affected joints does not exacerbate the pain, except in severe cases.

The limbs are the most common sites of symptoms of DCS (in approximately 92% of cases of DCS overall and as the initial clinical manifestations of DCS in approximately 77%) [4,9,10]. Shoulders, elbows, hips, and knees are the most commonly affected joints. More than one site may be involved, but rarely is the distribution bilaterally symmetric. Heat, ice, immobilization, and potent analgesics do not relieve the pain, which is due to collections of gas in the periarticular and perivascular tissues. The most striking characteristic of this pain is its rapid relief with recompression. This rapid relief of discomfort with the application of pressure, and especially the tendency for this pain to return to the same site if recompression is inadequate, distinguishes the pain of "the bends" from any coexistent musculoskeletal strain or from the ischemic pain resulting from AGE.

Usually, there are no objective physical signs associated with limb DCS, except for a potential "peau d'orange" appearance of the skin from local lymphatic obstruction. The skin exhibits two distinct types of manifestations of DCS: (a) a transient pruritus involving ears, trunk, wrists, and hands (more common after exposure in hyperbaric chambers); and (b) a more intense itching, usually limited to the trunk, that begins as erythema (from dermal vasodilation) and progresses to a characteristic mottling with confluent rings of pallor surrounding areas of cyanosis. This lesion blanches to the touch and is known as *cutis marmorate*. These changes are thought to result from bubble obstruction of the skin's venous drainage or bubble-induced vasospasm [4]. These abnormalities generally resolve spontaneously over a few days.

Type II Decompression Sickness

Type II DCS may occur separately or in combination with the musculoskeletal pain of type I DCS in up to 30% of patients [4,9,10]. The primary organ systems affected in this category are pulmonary, nervous, and vestibular.

Pulmonary DCS, known as "the chokes," occurs rarely in diving (approximately 2% of the overall cases [4,10]), and it is generally the result of very rapid or emergency-type ascents. Aviators, astronauts, and submarine trainees are also in situations in which sudden dramatic decompression may occur, and pulmonary DCS has been noted in nearly 6% in these groups [4,10]. Clinically, this condition usually begins with a substernal discomfort that starts within minutes of reaching the surface. As it progresses, the discomfort may take on a respirophasic nature. The respiratory pattern becomes more rapid and shallow, with occasional paroxysms of a nonproductive cough. Evidence of right heart strain or failure may develop and may progress to full-blown cardiovascular collapse. The underlying mechanism involves direct and indirect effects of massive pulmonary gas embolization from VGE.

Neurologic DCS has a varied incidence among different populations [4,10]. A wide range of possible presenting signs and symptoms may be produced by neurologic DCS, and all must be taken seriously even when there are no objective findings on neurologic examination. The spectrum of neurologic dysfunction ranges from pruritus with skin rash or "pins and needles" sensation (15% of cases) to full paralysis (6%) or convulsions (1%) and death. Personality changes and agitation occur in 3%, but they are very rarely the presenting symptoms. Visual disturbances (7%) and difficulties with cerebellar function (18%) are also frequently seen. The pathogenesis underlying CNS injury from DCS is the subject of much debate and controversy. Most researchers would agree that the notion of CNS tissue ischemia arising from obstructing arterial gas bubbles is too simplistic. As mentioned previously, the endothelial dysfunction hypothesis is currently under investigation as a better candidate mechanism to explain the varied manifestations of DCS.

Vestibular DCS, "the staggers," occurs relatively commonly as the initial manifestation of DCS, and it comprises a syndrome of nausea, vomiting, dizziness, and nystagmus. Frequently, tinnitus or hearing loss may also be present. Typical onset is immediately after decompression, and it occurs in 13% to 72% of patients with type II DCS. The underlying pathology has been demonstrated in animals to be the result of rupture of the fragile membranes in the cochlea and semicircular canals.

Treatment

Prompt Recognition and Diagnosis

The most common problem in DCS and AGE is making the initial diagnosis. Particularly in the case of DCS, there is an early tendency by patients for denial of the existence of any problems. Any neurologic or cardiorespiratory symptoms after diving must be assumed to relate to DCS until proven otherwise.

Stabilization

Nonspecific therapy may help to stabilize the patient and prevent an extension of injury. Immediate institution of cardiopulmonary resuscitation may be needed, and it takes precedence over all other measures. Endotracheal intubation is sometimes necessary to ensure patency and protection of the airway. All balloon cuffs (endotracheal and Foley) should be inflated with sterile water rather than air to minimize the volume changes of these compartments during recompression therapy.

When AGE is suspected, most authorities recommend the flat, supine position initially. If the patient is unconscious or vomiting, the left lateral decubitus (Durant) position is also recommended. The benefits of the Trendelenburg position have been questioned with the realization that maintaining this body position for extended periods may worsen any associated cerebral edema, and that keeping the head lower than the heart does not prevent migration of bubbles into the cerebral circulation unless the patient is in total circulatory arrest or an extremely low-output state [4].

Once any life-threatening concerns have been addressed, maintenance of intravascular volume and the administration of 100% O_2 become the next most important features of treatment while arranging transport to a hyperbaric facility. The 100% O_2 can be delivered intermittently or continuously for extended periods (generally up to 16 to 18 hours) without any serious concern for any resulting significant pulmonary toxicity. The high fraction of inspired O_2 is used to alleviate any tissue hypoxia and to provide a strong concentration gradient that will wash out as much inert gas as rapidly as possible.

As a result of capillary endothelial injury, the more severe the DCS syndrome, the greater the magnitude of plasma leakage from the vascular space, the reduction in blood volume, and the resultant hemoconcentration [4]. Increased blood viscosity resulting from hemoconcentration may further impair any compromised microcirculation; therefore, normovolemia should be the goal of infusion therapy. Intravascular volume maintenance can be achieved with isotonic fluids given at a rate sufficient to keep the urine output at 1 to 2 mL per kg per hour or more, and it is recommended for patients who are vomiting, unconscious, or having any symptoms more severe than isolated limb bends. Glucose-containing solutions are probably best avoided in the first 12 hours after suspected cerebral embolization because an increased serum glucose levels is one of the major determinants of the brain's lactate production, which has been associated with increased neuronal damage in the ischemic state [4,10]. Conscious patients may be given judicious amounts of oral liquids, such as nonacidic fruit juices or balanced electrolyte solutions. Alcohol-containing beverages should be strictly avoided.

When the diagnosis of cerebral air embolism is evident on clinical grounds, comprehensive diagnostic testing is not necessary. Diagnostic testing should never delay transport to a facility equipped to provide hyperbaric therapy or initiation of this specific therapy. If hyperbaric therapy is not immediately available, a noncontrast head computed tomography scan, chest radiography, and an ECG should be obtained while awaiting transport. In coma due to AGE or DCS, the head computed tomography would typically reveal multiple, small, well-defined, low-density areas in the brain. Head computed tomography scanning is also useful in ruling out possible correctable causes of intracerebral bleeding. Magnetic resonance imaging and single-photon emission tomography techniques, where available, are likewise potentially useful to document the presence of cerebral gas collections. Because these tests are highly insensitive, negative studies alone should never deny patients' access to HBO therapy in the appropriate clinical situation.

Patient Transport

When air evacuation is necessary to transfer a patient to a recompression facility, it is of utmost importance that the patient not be exposed to any further decreases in barometric pressure, as occurs with travel at increasing altitudes. In general, unless the aircraft is capable of maintaining a cabin pressure equivalent to sea-level pressure, flight altitude should not exceed 500 to 1,000 ft above the departure point because deaths have resulted from exposure to altitudes of only 4,000 to 5,000 ft [4,19]. It is believed to be preferable to await the arrival of a pressurized transport than to risk exposing a patient with DCS or AGE to further hypobaric insult.

To obtain a listing of the nearest recompression facility as well as advice on treatment options from a medical diving specialist on a 24-hour emergency basis, contact the Divers Alert Network at Duke University at (919) 684-8111 or (919) 684-4DAN (4326), collect.

Drug Therapy

To date there are no drugs of proven benefit in treating DCS or AGE. There is an unfortunate paucity of randomized controlled trials to guide treatment options. Several agents are used frequently, but this therapy is primarily based on expert opinion and limited trials involving small numbers of animal and human subjects [4,20–22].

Many authorities still prescribe intravenous corticosteroids for patients with DCS (and sometimes AGE) who have any documentable neurologic impairment, in an effort to reduce the impact of any inflammatory components of these diseases. Usually, dexamethasone (10- to 30-mg intravenous bolus followed by 4 mg intravenously every 6 hours) or hydrocortisone (1-g intravenous bolus followed by dexamethasone every 6 hours) is given for a total of 2 to 3 days. There is no solid evidence of effectiveness for steroids [4,8]. On the contrary, there is evidence that steroid use may actually increase the risks for CNS O_2 toxicity during recompression therapy [4,8]. Corticosteroid use in cases of documented neurologic impairment should, therefore, be made on an individual basis in consultation with a medical diving specialist.

Intravenous diazepam is effective in the control of seizures, severe agitation, and the intractable vomiting resulting from "the staggers." The typical regimen is a 5-mg intravenous bolus given over 3 minutes and then repeated every 5 minutes as needed (maximum dose, 20 to 30 mg) to control seizures. If intravenous access is not available, the intravenous preparation may be given rectally to adults in a dose of 7.5 to 10 mg every 5 minutes as needed. Diazepam is not recommended for use prophylactically because of its sedative properties and its propensity to mask the onset of CNS toxicity, thus affecting the ability of physicians to assess response to hyperbaric treatment. Generalized seizures unresponsive to benzodiazepine therapy may be suppressed with barbiturates [4,8].

Analgesics should be avoided because they also tend to mask the progression or new onset of symptoms. Given its low-risk profile, some authorities recommend administration of 0.5 to 1 g of oral aspirin to reduce platelet aggregation. Prior animal experimentation had shown no benefit to nonsteroidal agents (indomethacin, aspirin) when given alone; however, a recent double-blind, randomized, controlled trial of a small number of human subjects raised the possibility that the nonsteroidal agent tenoxicam may reduce the number of recompression sessions required for symptom resolution [23].

Intravenous lidocaine may have potential use in DCS and AGE due to its anticonvulsant and antidysrhythmic effects. Lidocaine may be given as a 0.5 to 1 mg per kg intravenous bolus at a rate of 25 to 50 mg per minute, followed by 0.5 mg per kg intravenously every 5 to 10 minutes as needed, to a maximum total of 225 mg or 3 mg per kg, whichever is lower. Patients with hypotension, cardiac arrest, or biventricular heart failure should receive only a single loading dose of 100 mg. After the loading doses, a continuous intravenous infusion at 2 to 4 mg per minute may be used to achieve and maintain a blood level of 2 to 4 μg per mL. Although not corroborated by any studies in humans, animal studies have shown an increased rate of neuronal recovery when lidocaine is given after experimental cerebral AGE [4,11]. The exact mechanism by which this recovery is accomplished is unknown, but it does not appear to be due to any direct vasoactive effects of lidocaine. Instead, it is more likely that any efficacy of this agent may be due to an ability to reduce cerebral metabolism and to stabilize neural membranes by decreasing the flux of sodium and potassium levels [4,11]. There are case reports of the successful use of lidocaine as an adjunct to recompression in divers with neurologic DCS [4,11]. Some caution is warranted, however, because moderately high doses of lidocaine may precipitate seizures in some patients. Use of lidocaine is currently not standard in the care of patients with DCS.

Calcium channel blocking agents have had limited or no beneficial effects in the treatment of cerebral ischemia in numerous animal models, as well as several human trials [4]. Efficacy seems to vary with the drug used and with the subject population studied. Currently, no consensus exists on the use of calcium channel blockers in AGE or DCS.

Until further study is performed, discretionary therapy with these adjunctive agents should be considered the realm of "clinical judgment" and "expert opinion." Evidence-based recommendations await results from further controlled trials.

Hyperbaric Therapy

Hyperbaric therapy involves exposing the entire body to prolonged periods of higher-than-atmospheric pressure; it specifically treats AGE and DCS [24]. Anecdotal reports of success in isobarically occurring AGE lends credence to the recommendation for early consideration of hyperbaric therapy for any suspected cerebral gas embolism [4]. Many treatment protocols have been proposed [25,26], and no one of them would be expected to be fully efficacious and life sustaining in each individual. As of 2009, no randomized controlled human studies exist that compare these different treatment options. A review of the pertinent literature on humans since the 1960s reveals a decrease in cerebral air embolism mortality from 93% for those not receiving therapy to 28% to 33% with closed-chest massage and "conventional therapy," and then to 7% with addition of HBO [4], and would seem to argue strongly for this modality in AGE [4].

Fully 80% to 90% of all patients with DCS or AGE effectively respond to recompression therapy [8,9,26,27]. While there is generally an inverse relationship between any delay to treatment and complete symptom resolution, evidence supports the use of HBO for AGE and DCS even after delays of more than 24 hours. Delays in initiating recompression therapy of up to 10 days have been anecdotally reported in the literature to be successful in up to 90% of these patients [4]. Recompression treatments may be repeated as needed until symptoms resolve entirely or until improvement reaches a plateau and there is no further improvement [9]. Approximately 40% of injured divers show complete resolution after the first treatment and only 20% require more than three rounds of recompression therapy [9].

The mechanism of action of HBO therapy involves a decrease in volume of any gas-filled spaces and resorption of bubbles back into body fluids. This process presumably results in a diminution in tissue distortion, vascular compromise, and bubble–endothelial surface contact. HBO therapy should be undertaken for at least 4 hours because elimination of bubbles may be reduced in areas of poor flow where sludging and edema exist [8,24]. It must be remembered that recompression acts only on the primary cause of these syndromes and not necessarily on any of the secondary effects that may result (e.g., endothelial dysfunction, activation of the inflammatory cascade).

Hyperoxygenation results from a markedly enhanced arterial O_2 content, primarily from O_2 dissolving more readily into the plasma. Although the oxyhemoglobin dissociation curve remains unchanged, the arterial partial pressure of O_2 may reach 2,000 mm Hg on a fractional inspired oxygen concentration of 100% and an ambient pressure of 3 ATA [8,24]. In the clinical setting, however, these high plasma O_2 concentrations are never transmitted fully to the tissue level due to progressive arteriolar vasoconstriction from the disease process itself, as well as a direct effect from the increasing O_2 concentration. Local tissue perfusion, although reduced further by HBO, is still sufficient to cause supranormal tissue partial pressure of O_2 levels of approximately 500 mm Hg. HBO allows the delivery of nearly 60 mL per L of blood (vs. 3 mL per L at atmospheric pressure), a rate sufficient to support resting tissues just on the basis of the O_2 dissolved in solution alone. In practice, the physiologic effects of high concentrations of O_2 to induce generation of O_2 free radicals and pulmonary O_2 toxicity necessitates that periods of hyperoxygenation be alternated with periods of lower fraction of inspired O_2 breathing to avoid potentially severe complications [3,24,25,27].

Opinions regarding the optimal hyperbaric regimen for AGE (whether or not dysbaric in origin) have varied in terms of the simulated depth (i.e., pressure) required, recompression time necessary, and inspired gas concentrations used. The time-tested method used by military and commercial diving operations in the United States has been a rapid recompression to 6 ATA (equivalent to the pressure exerted at a depth of 165 ft seawater), followed by periods of intermittent 100% O_2 from a level of 2.8 ATA (pressure equivalent of 65 ft seawater) back to sea level. This treatment regimen is well known as the U.S. Navy Treatment Table 6A and is illustrated in Figure 61.2 and Table 61.5 [3,4,25,27]. Other popular recompression tables in use worldwide include COMEX Table 30 and Royal Navy Tables 71 and 72 [9].

Extensive clinical experience has found no objective benefits to starting recompression at levels greater than 2.8 ATA [4,24,25]. Consensus opinion now recommends that if chamber treatment can be begun within approximately 4 to 6 hours from the time of the incident, then these "early" cases of AGE should undergo therapy following U.S. Navy Table 6A beginning at 6 ATA. The basis for this recommendation is that there may be a benefit in achieving maximal recompression before the occurrence of any significant intravascular bubble–blood interactions, and thereby minimize activation or release of mediators or any arteriolar vasoactivity. In contrast, a delay in hyperbaric therapy of more than 6 hours may allow for maximum endothelial dysfunction and the formation of solid thrombi that would not be expected to respond to any amount of increased ambient pressure. In this latter situation, HBO beginning at 2.8 ATA and following U.S. Navy Treatment Table 6 guidelines (Fig. 61.2, Table 61.5), with extensions as needed, would appear more logical.

Hyperbaric treatment recommendations for DCS are loosely based on the general category of illness patterns described previously [3,4,25,27]. In general, those patients with type I "pain only" DCS are in a more stable medical condition on arrival to a recompression facility; therefore, more time is available to perform a thorough and detailed physical examination before chamber treatment. Particular emphasis should be placed on the neurologic examination so that serial examinations can document the presence of any subtle findings and progress with therapy can be monitored. U.S. Navy Treatment Table 5 (basically a shortened version of U.S. Navy Table 6) is appropriate in this group who presents within 6 hours of reaching the surface and would be expected to achieve resolution of symptoms within 10 minutes of beginning recompression.

It has been suggested that an inadequate response to U.S. Navy Table 5 or the presence of any neurologic abnormality, no matter how subtle, requires initial treatment according to at least U.S. Navy Treatment Table 6. This would allow for more optimal therapy of any developing neurologic deficits, and it would therefore be expected to decrease the overall occurrence of progression to type II DCS. Mild cases of type II DCS may also allow sufficient time for more detailed neurologic examinations to assess the degree of spinal cord or brain involvement. Although these patients are generally reported to respond well to standard therapy with U.S. Navy Treatment Table 6 treatment, severe life-threatening DCS is believed to require immediate treatment following U.S. Navy Treatment Table 6A. In patients who do not respond adequately to standard protocols, extension periods or change to other established protocols might be indicated and decided on an individual basis [3,4,25,27].

Prevention

There are a limited number of time-tested recommendations that can be made in an effort to minimize the occurrence of DCS. These would include (a) following prescribed "no-decompression" limit diving profiles that factor in the duration of time spent at specific depths and duration of surface intervals between repetitive dives; (b) limiting ascent rates from depth to speeds slower than the ascent rate of the diver's exhaled air bubbles; and (c) avoiding any hypobaric insults in the postdive period with no flying for at least 12 hours in all divers, delay

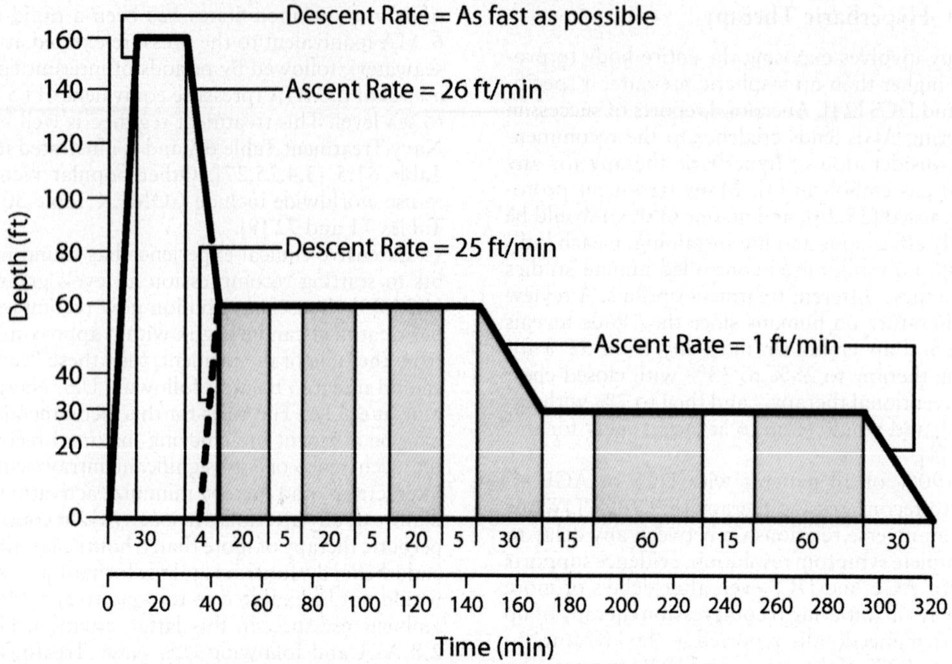

FIGURE 61.2. U.S. Navy Treatment Tables 6 and 6A. Treatment Table 6A is shown in its entirety and is used when symptoms are suspected to be due to arterial gas embolism or severe decompression sickness. Treatment Table 6 is superimposed (starting at *dotted line*) and is seen to begin with a simulated pressure descent on 100% fractional concentration of oxygen to 60 ft at a rate of 25 ft per minute. Thereafter, the tables are the same. Treatment Table 6 is recommended for treatment of type II or type I decompression sickness when symptoms are not relieved within 10 minutes at 60 ft. Nonshaded areas are periods of breathing room air. Shaded areas are periods of breathing 100% fractional concentration of oxygen. Individual time periods are shown first, with total elapsed time indicated underneath. [Adapted from U.S. Navy Diving Manual, Washington, DC, Department of the Navy, 2000, NAVSEA Technical Manual 5, 21–42. Revision 4; and Wilson MM, Curley FJ: Gas embolism: part II. Arterial gas embolism and decompression sickness. *J Intensive Care Med* 11:261, 1996, with permission.]

TABLE 61.5

DEPTH AND TIME PROFILES FOR U.S. NAVY TREATMENT TABLES 6 AND 6A

			Total elapsed time (h:min)	
Simulated depth (ft)	Time (min)	Breathing medium	6A	6
165	30	Air	0:30	—
165–60	4	Air	0:34	—
(0–60)[a]	(2.4)	(Oxygen)	(—)	0:02
60	20	Oxygen	0:54	0:22
60	5	Air	0:59	0:27
60	20	Oxygen	1:19	0:47
60	5	Air	1:24	0:52
60	20	Oxygen	1:44	1:12
60	5	Air	1:49	1:17
60–30	30	Oxygen	2:19	1:47
30	15	Air	2:34	2:02
30	60	Oxygen	3:34	3:02
30	15	Air	3:49	3:17
30	60	Oxygen	4:49	4:17
30–0	30	Oxygen	5:19	4:47

[a]Parentheses indicate profile when following the dotted line in Figure 61.2. This applies *only* to Table 6 profile and is not used when following Table 6A profile.

in flying for 24 hours or more if a dive profile included any mandatory decompression stops, and finally, flying should be prohibited for at least 72 hours after recompression therapy has been given to patients with DCS or AGE. As alluded to earlier, hypobaric stresses in these instances may result in new onset of one of these syndromes or in the recurrence of one of these previously treated disorders.

Extensive ongoing research is underway to evaluate the potential preventative roles of predive exercise [28,29], during-dive exercise [30,31], exogenous nitric oxide [29,32,33], predive normobaric O_2 [34], and predive hyperbaric O_2 [35,36]. These preconditioning agents are hypothesized to upregulate endogenous antioxidants, moderate inflammatory injury, and/or inhibit reperfusion injury.

References

1. Wilson MM, Curley FJ: Gas embolism: part I. Venous gas emboli. *J Intensive Care Med* 11:182–204, 1996.
2. Pronovost PJ, Wu AW, Sexton JB: Acute decompensation after removing a central line: practical approaches to increasing safety in the intensive care unit. *Ann Intern Med* 140:1025–1027, 2004.
3. *U.S. Navy Diving Manual.* Washington, DC, Department of the Navy, 2000. NAVSEA Technical Manual 5, 21–42. Revision 4.
4. Wilson MM, Curley FJ: Gas embolism: part II. Arterial gas embolism and decompression sickness. *J Intensive Care Med* 11:261–283, 1996.
5. Schulz E, Anter E, Keaney JF: Oxidative stress, antioxidants, and endothelial function. *Curr Med Chem* 11:1093–1104, 2004.
6. Duvall WL: Endothelial dysfunction and antioxidants. *Mt Sinai J Med* 72:71–80, 2005.
7. Madden LA, Laden G: Gas bubbles may not be the underlying cause of decompression illness—the at-depth endothelial dysfunction hypothesis. *Med Hypotheses* 72:389–392, 2009.
8. Tetzlaff K, Shank ES, Muth CM: Evaluation and management of decompression illness—an intensivist's perspective. *Intensive Care Med* 29:2128–2136, 2003.
9. Vann RD, Freiberger JJ, Caruso JL, et al: *DAN Report on Decompression Illness, Diving Fatalities and Project Dive Exploration*: 2005 Edition. Durham, NC, Divers Alert Network.
10. Tetzlaff K, Thorsen E: Breathing at depth: physiologic and clinical aspects of diving while breathing compressed gas. *Clin Chest Med* 26:355–380, 2005.
11. Levett DZH, Millar IL: Bubble trouble: a review of diving physiology and disease. *Postgrad Med J* 84:571–578, 2008.
12. Carturan D, Boussuges A, Vanuxem P, et al: Ascent rate, age, maximal oxygen uptake, adiposity, and circulating venous bubbles after diving. *J Appl Physiol* 93:1349–1356, 2002.
13. Marroni A, Bennet P, Cronje F, et al: A deep stop during decompression from 25 m significantly reduces bubble and fast tissue gas tensions. *Undersea Hyperbar Med* 31:233–243, 2004.
14. Foster PP, Butler BD: Decompression to altitude: assumptions, experimental evidence, and future directions. *J Appl Physiol* 106:678–690, 2009.
15. Cartoni D, De Castro S, Valente G, et al: Identification of professional scuba divers with patent foramen ovale at risk for decompression illness. *Am J Cardiol* 94:270, 2004.
16. Torti SR, Billinger M, Schwerzmann M, et al: Risk of decompression illness among 230 divers in relation to the presence and size of patent foramen ovale. *Eur Heart J* 25:1014, 2004.
17. Germonpre P: Patent foramen ovale and diving. *Cardiol Clin* 23:97–104, 2005.
18. Lairez O, Cournot M, Minville V, et al: Risk of neurological decompression sickness in the diver with right-to-left shunt: literature review and meta-analysis. *Clin J Sport Med* 19:231–235, 2009.
19. MacDonald RD, O'Donnell C, Allan GM: Interfacility transport of patients with decompression illness: literature review and consensus statement. *Prehosp Emerg Care* 10:482–487, 2006.
20. Bennett MH, Lehm JP, Mitchell SJ, et al: Recompression and adjunctive therapy for decompression illness. *Cochrane Database Syst Rev* (2):CD005277, 2007.
21. Montcalm-Smith EA, Fahlman A, Kayar SR: Pharmacological interventions to decompression sickness in rats: comparison of five agents. *Aviat Space Environ Med* 79:7–13, 2008.
22. Little T, Butler BD: Pharmacological intervention to the inflammatory response from decompression sickness in rats. *Aviat Space Environ Med* 79:87–93, 2008.
23. Bennett M, Mitchell S, Dominguez A: Adjunctive treatment of decompression illness with a non-steroidal anti-inflammatory drug (tenoxicam). *Undersea Hyperb Med* 30:195–205, 2003.
24. Gill AL, Bell CNA: Hyperbaric oxygen: its uses, mechanism of action and outcomes. *Q J Med* 97:385–395, 2004.
25. Antonelli C, Franchi E, Della Marta ME, et al: Guiding principles in choosing a therapeutic table for DCI hyperbaric therapy. *Minerva Anesthesiol* 75:151–161, 2009.
26. Cianci P, Slade JB Jr: Delayed treatment of decompression sickness with shunt, no-air-break tables: review of 140 cases. *Aviat Space Environ Med* 77:1003–1008, 2006.
27. Thalmann ED: Principles of US Navy recompression treatments for decompression sickness. 45th Workshop of the Undersea and Hyperbaric Medical Society, 1996. p 75–91.
28. Dujic Z, Duplancic D, Marinovic-Terzic I, et al: Aerobic exercise before diving reduces venous gas bubble formation in humans. *J Physiol* 555:637–642, 2004.
29. Wisloff U, Richardson RS, Brubakk AO: Exercise and nitric oxide prevent bubble formation: a novel approach to the prevention of decompression sickness? *J Physiol* 555:825–829, 2004.
30. Jankowski LW, Tikuisis P, Nishi RY: Exercise effects during diving and decompression on postdive venous gas emboli. *Aviat Space Environ Med* 75:489–495, 2004.
31. Dujic D, Palada I, Obad A, et al: Exercise during a 3-min decompression stop reduces postdive venous gas bubbles. *Med Sci Sports Exerc* 37:1319–1323, 2005.
32. Dujic D, Palada I, Zoran V, et al: Exogenous nitric oxide and bubble formation in divers. *Med Sci Sports Exerc* 38:1432–1435, 2006.
33. Duplessis CA, Fothergill D: Investigating the potential of statin medications as a nitric oxide (NO) release agent to decrease decompression sickness: a review article. *Med Hypothesis* 70:560–566, 2008.
34. Castagna O, Gempp E, Blatteau J-E: Pre-dive normobaric oxygen reduces bubble formation in scuba divers. *Eur J Appl Physiol* 106:167–172, 2009.
35. Butler BD, Little T, Cogan V, et al: Hyperbaric oxygen pre-breathe modifies the outcome of decompression sickness. *Undersea Hyperb Med* 33:407–417, 2006.
36. Katsenelson K, Arieli Y, Abramovich A, et al: Hyperbaric oxygen pretreatment reduces the incidence of decompression sickness in rats. *Eur J Appl Physiol* 101:571–576, 2007.

CHAPTER 62 ■ RESPIRATORY ADJUNCT THERAPY

SCOTT E. KOPEC AND RICHARD S. IRWIN

Various adjunct therapies are available to aid in the management of critically ill patients with existing or anticipated pulmonary dysfunction. In this chapter, we review several adjunct therapies, emphasizing any randomized trials determining efficacy and indications. We will specifically discuss the following: (a) aerosol therapy and humidification; (b) lung expansion techniques; (c) airway clearance techniques; (d) administration of medical gases; (e) nasal continuous positive airway pressure (CPAP) and bilevel positive airway pressure for sleep-related breathing disorders; and (f) communication alternatives for the patient with an artificial airway. A discussion of the use of bilevel positive airway pressure to provide noninvasive ventilatory support can be found in Chapter 59.

AEROSOL THERAPY

An *aerosol* is a stable suspension of solid or liquid particles dispersed in air as a fine mist. Bland aerosols are generally used to humidify inspired gases. Aerosol drug therapy represents the optimal modality for site-specific delivery of pharmacologic agents to the lungs in the treatment of a number of acute and chronic pulmonary diseases. Due to the cost and potential hazards of aerosol therapy, use should be limited to aerosols whose clinical value has been objectively shown [1].

Bland Aerosols

Bland aerosols include sterile water or hypotonic, normotonic, and hypertonic saline delivered with or without oxygen. These are typically delivered via an ultrasonic nebulizer in an effort to decrease or aid in the clearance of pulmonary secretions. The routine use of bland aerosols in the treatment of some specific diseases has demonstrated mixed results. An evidence-based recommendation for the use of bland aerosols has recently been released by the British Thoracic Society (BTS) [2]. The use of bland aerosols in the treatment of chronic obstructive pulmonary disease (COPD) and croup appears not to be of any benefit [2,3]. For patients with cystic fibrosis (CF), the use of 7% (hypertonic) saline, administered twice daily, may result in a significantly higher forced vital capacity (FVC) and forced expiratory volume in 1 second (FEV_1), and a decrease in the number of acute exacerbations when compared to the use of normotonic saline [4]. The use of nebulized saline or sterile water may improve sputum clearance in patients with non-CF bronchiectasis [2]. Delivery of bland aerosols is ineffective in liquefying secretions because sufficient volumes of water fail to reach the lower airways. Furthermore, bland aerosols may provoke bronchospasm and place patients at risk for nosocomial pneumonia [3,5].

Mist therapy, the delivery of a continuous aerosol of sterile water or saline, is frequently used to treat upper-airway infections in children, but has not been shown to be more effective than air humidification [3].

Humidity Therapy

Theoretic reasons for using humidified inspired gas are to prevent drying of the upper and lower airways, hydrate dry mucosal surfaces in patients with inflamed upper airways (vocal cords and above), enhance expectoration of lower-airway secretions, and induce sputum expectoration for diagnostic purposes [3]. Although adequate humidification is critical when dry medical gases are administered through an artificial airway (endotracheal or tracheostomy tube), there is little evidence to support the use of humidification in the nonintubated patient.

Humidity therapy is water vapor and, at times, heat added to inspired gas with the goal of achieving near-normal inspiratory conditions when the gas enters the airway [6]. Because adequate levels of humidity and heat are necessary to ensure proper function of the mucociliary transport system, humidification is imperative when the structures of the upper airway that normally warm and humidify inspired gases have been bypassed by an artificial airway. During mechanical ventilation, humidification is crucial to avoid hypothermia, atelectasis, inspissation of airway secretions, and destruction of airway epithelium because of heat loss, moisture loss, and altered pulmonary function [7]. Optimal humidification is the point at which normal conditions that prevail in the respiratory tract are simulated [8].

Several external devices are available to artificially deliver heat and moisture. Two such devices for mechanically ventilated patients are: (a) a heated waterbath humidifier, which is an external *active* source of heat and water, and (b) a heat and moisture exchanger filter (HMEF), which *passively* retains the heat and humidity, leaving the trachea during expiration and recycles it during the next inspiration. HMEFs are also known as *hygroscopic condenser humidifiers* or *artificial noses*. The HMEF is designed to combine air-conditioning and bacterial filtration. In a randomized controlled trial, both devices were shown to be equally safe [9]. Potential advantages of HMEFs over heated waterbath humidifiers include reduced cost and avoidance of airway burns and overhydration. A potential disadvantage is that resistance of airflow through an HMEF may progressively rise, increasing the work of breathing and conceivably impeding weaning from the ventilator [9].

Cold-water devices such as bubble humidifiers are frequently used to add humidity to supplemental oxygen administered to spontaneously breathing patients. Due to a lack of objective evidence to support the practice, the American College of Chest Physicians recommends elimination of the routine use of humidification of oxygen at flow rates of 1 to 4 L per minute when environmental humidity is sufficient [10], while the BTS does not recommend its use [2].

Patients requiring high flow rates of oxygen (>10 L per minute) frequently develop discomfort due to upper-airway dryness. There are several devices available to deliver humidification via nasal cannulae at high flow rates (high flow oxygen delivery), including Vapotherm (Vapotherm, Annapolis, MD) and the Fisher & Paykel 850 (Fisher and Paykel Healthcare Corp, Auckland, New Zealand). Although these devices have been shown to improve patients' comfort [11], we are not aware of any studies determining therapeutic benefits. Potential risk of exposure to *Ralstonia* spp in patients using Vapotherm has been reported [12], but by switching to disposable filters, the problem appears to have been addressed.

Pharmacologically Active Aerosols

Inhaled therapy has several well-recognized advantages over other drug delivery routes. The drug is delivered directly to its targeted site of action; therefore, when compared to other routes of administration, a therapeutic response usually requires fewer drugs, there are fewer side effects, and the onset of action is generally faster [13]. A broad range of drugs is available as aerosols to treat obstructive lung diseases. These include β-adrenergic agonists, anticholinergics, anti-inflammatory agents, and anti-infectives. Additionally, the inhaled route is used to deliver drugs that are not effective when delivered by the oral route (e.g., pentamidine) [14].

Although a variety of drugs are currently available in aerosolized form, dosing to the lung remains inexact because deposition is affected by several patient-, environment-, and equipment-related factors. Potential hazards of aerosol drug therapy include (a) a reaction to the drug being administered, (b) the risk of infection, (c) bronchospasm, and (d) the potential for delivering too much or too little of the drug [14]. With respect to the use of aerosolized ribavirin, there are potential hazards to healthcare providers administering the medication (see later).

Bronchodilators

There are two classes of inhaled bronchodilators: (a) β_2-adrenergic receptor agonists (short-acting and long-acting) and (b) anticholinergic agents.

Short-Acting β_2-Adrenergic Receptor Agonists. Although β_1- and β_2-adrenergic receptors are present in the lungs, β_2-adrenergic receptors appear to be entirely responsible for bronchodilation. Therefore, β_2-adrenergic receptor agonists (e.g., albuterol, pirbuterol, and terbutaline) are the agents commonly preferred for the relief of acute symptoms of bronchospasm. In addition to the bronchodilating properties of β_2-adrenergic receptor agonists, other actions include augmentation of mucociliary clearance; enhancement of vascular integrity; metabolic responses; and inhibition of mediator release from mast cells, basophils, and possibly other cells [3].

Inhalation of β_2-selective agonists is considered first-line therapy for the critically ill asthmatic [15] and COPD patient [5,16]. Although these agents can be administered orally, by inhalation, or parenterally, the inhaled route is generally preferred because fewer side effects occur for any degree of bronchodilation [3]. For most patients experiencing acute asthma attacks, inhalation is at least as effective as the parenteral route [3]. Inhaled β_2 agonists can be delivered as an aerosol from a jet or ultrasonic nebulizer or from a metered-dose inhaler (MDI). The relative efficacies of the nebulizer and MDI are dependent on the adequacy of technique. Although it was formerly a standard practice to deliver bronchodilators by nebulizer, several prospective, randomized controlled trials have challenged this practice. Delivering β_2 agonists by MDI with a spacer device (holding chamber) under the supervision of trained personnel is as effective in the emergency setting as delivery by nebulizer for adults and children [3]. In hospitalized patients, β_2 agonists delivered by MDI are as effective as therapy with a nebulizer and can result in a considerable cost savings [3]. An analysis of 16 trials (686 children and 375 adults) to assess the effects of MDIs with holding chambers compared to nebulizers for the administration of β_2 agonists for acute asthma concluded that MDI with a holding chamber produced at least equivalent outcomes as nebulizer delivery [17].

Ideal frequency of administration and dosing of β_2 agonists has not been determined. For emergency department and hospital-based care of asthma, the National Institutes of Health Expert Panel Report 2 [15] recommends up to three treatments in the first hour. Subsequent treatments should be titrated to the severity of symptoms and the occurrence of adverse side effects, ranging from hourly treatments for moderate severity to hourly or continuous treatments for severe exacerbations. Recommendations for initial treatment of severe acute exacerbations of COPD are for the administration of short-acting β_2 agonists every 2 to 4 hours if tolerated [5].

When given by jet nebulizer, the usual adult dose of albuterol is 0.5 mL of an 0.5% solution (2.5 mg) diluted in 2.5 mL of saline (or 3 mL of 0.083% unit-dose nebulizer solution). The frequency of dosing varies depending on the disease and the situation. It can range from every 4 to 6 hours in patients with COPD and stable asthma to every 20 to 30 minutes for six doses in patients with status asthmaticus [3]. In patients with acute asthma, albuterol solution has also been continuously nebulized for 2 hours [18]. In this randomized controlled trial of spontaneously breathing patients with FEV_1 less than 40% predicted, continuous delivery of high-dose (7.5 mg per hour) or standard-dose (2.5 mg per hour) albuterol were both superior to hourly intermittent treatments with 2.5 mg in increasing FEV_1. Although there was no difference in FEV_1 improvement between the two continuous doses, the standard dose had fewer side effects.

Although the usual dosage of bronchodilator by MDI is two puffs (90 μg per puff) every 4 to 6 hours in stable hospitalized and ambulatory adult patients, the dosage must be increased up to sixfold in acute severe asthma to achieve results equivalent to those achieved with small-volume nebulizers [3]. In an emergency department treatment study of severe asthma, four puffs of albuterol by MDI every 30 minutes for a total of six dosing intervals (24 puffs) was found to be safe and equivalent to 2.5 mg of albuterol diluted in 2 mL of saline given every 30 minutes for six doses [3]. Others have treated acute episodes of asthma in the emergency department in a dose-to-result fashion as follows: initially four puffs by MDI of bronchodilator of choice, followed by one additional puff every minute until the patient subjectively or objectively improved or side effects (e.g., tremor, tachycardia, arrhythmia) occurred [3]. In mechanically ventilated patients, the bronchodilator effect obtained with four puffs (0.4 mg) of albuterol from an MDI with holding chamber is comparable to that obtained with 6 to 12 times the same dose given by a nebulizer and is likely to be more cost-effective [19].

Tremor is the principal side effect of β_2 agonists, due to the direct stimulation of β_2-adrenergic receptors in skeletal muscle. Tachycardia and palpitations are less frequent with the selective β_2 agonists (e.g., albuterol) than with nonselective β_1-β_2 agonists such as isoproterenol. Although vasodilation, reflex tachycardia, and direct stimulation of the heart can occur even with the use of selective β_2 agonists, cardiac adverse occurrences are uncommon when usual doses of inhaled β_2 agonists are administered. A transient decrease in arterial oxygen tension may occur in patients with acute, severe asthma. This response is likely due to the relaxation of the compensatory vasoconstriction in areas of decreased ventilation together with increased blood flow due to increased cardiac output [3].

β_2-adrenergic agonists can cause acute metabolic responses including hyperglycemia, hypokalemia, and hypomagnesemia [3]. Although typically not seen in standard doses, if large and frequent doses of β agonists are given, electrocardiogram and serum potassium monitoring are indicated. After inhalation of 10- and 20-mg doses, the maximal decreases in potassium can be 0.62 ± 0.09 mmol per L and 0.98 ± 0.14 mmol per L, respectively [20].

Perinatal outcomes of 259 pregnant women with asthma who were treated with β_2-adrenergic agonists during pregnancy were compared to those of 101 women who were not treated with these agents, and 295 nonasthmatic women [3]. There were no differences in perinatal mortality rates, congenital abnormalities, preterm delivery, low birth weights, mean birth weights, or the number of small-for-gestational-age infants. In addition, there were no differences in Apgar scores, labor or delivery complications, or postpartum bleeding.

Levalbuterol (Xopenex, Sepracor Inc, Marlborough, MA) inhalation solution, the (R)-enantiomer of racemic albuterol, is a relatively selective, third-generation β_2-adrenergic receptor agonist approved for treatment of bronchospasm in adults and children aged 12 years or older. Levalbuterol appears to offer little benefit over albuterol in improving FEV_1 in patients with asthma, and is not associated with any fewer systemic side effects such as tachycardia and hypokalemia [21]. For further discussion of aerosolized β agonists in asthma and COPD, see Chapters 48 and 49.

Long-Acting Inhaled β_2 Agonists. Long-acting inhaled β_2 agonists (e.g., salmeterol and formoterol) are currently not recommended for use in acute exacerbations of asthma (Expert Panel Report 2) [15] or COPD [5]. One prospective, double-blind, randomized, placebo-controlled trial demonstrated a possible role for salmeterol as an adjunct to conventional therapy for hospitalized asthmatic patients [22], but larger studies are needed to clarify whether there is a potential benefit in the setting of acute asthma. If patients are using these agents as controller medications for asthma or COPD and are hospitalized for other reasons, consider continuing them for asthma maintenance during the hospitalization. These agents should be administered at regular intervals; additional doses to relieve symptoms should not be prescribed.

Anticholinergics. Anticholinergics appear to have a role in acute asthma when combined with sympathomimetic drugs [3], in exacerbations of COPD when combined with albuterol [5], in intubated patients to prevent bradycardia induced by suctioning [23], and in selected patients with severe bronchorrhea [24]. Ipratropium bromide is dosed at 500 μg in 2.5 mL normal saline (1 unit 0.02% unit-dose vial) or two to six puffs by MDI (18 μg per puff) every 6 to 8 hours. Ipratropium (18 μg per puff) and albuterol (103 μg per puff) are available as a combined MDI product (Combivent, Boehringer, Ingelheim; Ridgefield, CT). Ipratropium by MDI can be given to ventilated patients with the same spacer device used for β-agonist delivery. Tiotropium, a selective muscarinic antagonist, is available in a dry powdered form. Its use should be limited to the chronic management of patients with COPD. For further discussion of anticholinergic use in asthma and COPD, see Chapters 48 and 49.

Combined Bronchodilator Therapy. Although inhaled short-acting β-adrenergic receptor agonists remain first-line agents in the treatment of acute asthma, the addition of ipratropium bromide may result in an added benefit [25]. Anticholinergics may be of benefit as additive agents or as single agents in situations in which the patient cannot tolerate β-adrenergic side effects. Both agents appear effective in smoking-related chronic bronchitis.

Mucolytics

***N*-Acetylcysteine.** Theoretically, mucolytic agents facilitate expectoration of excessive lower-airway secretions and improve lung function [3]. Although *N*-acetylcysteine (Mucomyst, Apothecon, Princeton, NJ), the prototypic mucolytic agent, liquefies inspissated mucous plugs when administered by direct intratracheal instillation [26], it is of questionable clinical use when administered as an aerosol to nonintubated patients because very little of the drug is actually delivered to the lower respiratory tract. Inhaled *N*-acetylcysteine failed to prevent deterioration in lung function or exacerbations in patients with COPD [27], and failed to demonstrate any benefit of nebulized *N*-acetylcysteine in patients with CF [28]. However, a small randomized trial suggested that nebulized *N*-acetylcysteine in combination with aerosolized heparin reduced the incidence of acute lung injury (ALI) and decreased mortality in patients with acute smoke inhalational injuries [29]. Because mucolytic instillations or aerosols can induce bronchospasm in patients with airway disease [30] (especially asthma), mucolytics should be administered to these patients in combination with a bronchodilator [3]. However, given the lack of evidence from randomized trials supporting its benefits, we do not recommend the routine use of aerosolized *N*-acetylcysteine.

Recombinant Human DNase. Recombinant human DNase (Pulmozyme, Genentech, South San Francisco, CA), when given as an aerosol in a dose of 2.5 mg once or twice a day to patients with CF, led to a moderate but significant decrease in dyspnea, a reduction in costs related to exacerbations of respiratory symptoms, and a modest improvement in FEV_1 after 3 months [2]. However, there may not be any statistically significant therapeutic benefit of rhDNase when added to antibiotics and chest physical therapy [31].

Two double-blind, placebo-controlled clinical trials evaluated the safety and efficacy of nebulized rhDNase in the treatment of non-CF–related bronchiectasis [32,33]. In these studies, rhDNase was consistently found ineffective (and possibly harmful [32]) to patients with non-CF–related bronchiectasis.

In a randomized double-blind, placebo-controlled trial of patients with respiratory syncytial virus (RSV) bronchiolitis, significant improvement in chest radiographs occurred with the use of nebulized rhDNase compared to significant worsening in a placebo group. Although further investigation is needed, results of this trial indicate a possible future role for this therapy in the treatment of RSV in infants and young children [34].

Other Mucolytics. Studies to determine the efficacy of other mucolytic agents, including water, have produced conflicting results. Current evidence does not appear to justify their use in clinical practice. Consensus guidelines for asthma [15] and COPD [5] do not recommend the use of mucolytic agents in the treatment of acute exacerbations.

Anti-infectives

Aerosolization of antimicrobial solutions has been shown to be effective in CF patients with tracheobronchial infections and colonization [2]. In addition, inhaled antibiotics have also been used to treat tracheobronchial infections in patients with non-CF–related bronchiectasis, to treat and prevent ventilator-associated pneumonia, to treat chronic bronchitis in patients with COPD, to treat bronchiolitis in children, and to treat patients with multidrug-resistant tuberculosis (MDR-Tb) and mycobacterium avium complex (MAC) [13]. However, unlike their use in treating patients with CF, the benefits of using inhaled antibiotics for these other indications is less defined. Inhaled tobramycin has been demonstrated to decrease sputum bacteria counts, improve lung function, decrease the number of exacerbations, and improve quality of life in patients with pulmonary infections or colonization from CF [35]. For patients with non-CF–related bronchiectasis, inhaled antibiotics are not as well studied, but may decrease sputum bacteria counts and decrease the number of hospitalizations, but have no impact on lung function or survival [36]. Inhaled antibiotics have not been shown to provide any benefit in patients with chronic bronchitis or COPD [37]. Prophylactic use of inhaled antibiotics to decrease the risk of developing ventilator-associated pneumonia has not been shown to be of any benefit [37]. In addition, inhaled antibiotics appear to have no benefit over systemic antibiotics in treating ventilator-associated pneumonia [37]. A few small studies suggest that inhaled amikacin and rifampicin may be of some benefit in treating severe MDR-Tb and severe infections with MAC [38].

Only tobramycin is currently FDA approved for inhalational use. Other antibiotics occasionally administered via an aerosol include colistin, amikacin, gentamicin, aztreonam, azithromycin, vancomycin, ceftazidime, and imipenem. Inhaled colistin should be used with great caution. Colistin decomposes into several toxic compounds that, if inhaled, can result in acute lung injury and respiratory failure. Colistin suspension should be administered within 6 hours after it is prepared [39].

Inhaled tobramycin is approved for treatment of patients with CF who are (a) at least 6 years of age, (b) have FEV_1 greater than or equal to 25% and less than or equal to 75% predicted, (c) are colonized with *Pseudomonas aeruginosa*, and (d) are able to comply with the prescribed medical regimen [35]. When nebulizing tobramycin, it has been shown that different nebulizers and solutions and techniques may result in very different amounts of tobramycin being inhaled [40]. For example, the addition of albuterol lowered the surface tension of the solution in the nebulizer and resulted in a greater output of tobramycin. A prospective study [41] determined that antibiotics aerosolized by nebulizer could be effectively delivered to tracheostomized, mechanically ventilated patients. In this study, antibiotic concentrations similar to or greater than those achieved in spontaneously breathing individuals were "consistently demonstrated" in patients with a tracheostomy tube.

Aerosolized ribavirin has been used for patients with RSV infection and severe lower respiratory tract disease, or infants with chronic underlying conditions such as cardiac disease, pulmonary disease, or a history of prematurity [3]. However, proof of effectiveness in treating RSV infections is lacking. One study failed to establish the efficacy of inhaled ribavirin in immunocompromised adults with RSV infections [42]. Two prospective double-blind, randomized, placebo-controlled trials addressing the use of aerosolized ribavirin in treating children and adults with respiratory failure from RSV infections failed to show any improvement in length of time requiring mechanical ventilation, length of stay in the intensive care unit, and oxygen requirements or alter immediate outcome [3]. Aerosolized ribavirin has been suggested to be beneficial in treating infections due to influenza A and B [43]. However, a randomized double-blind, placebo-controlled trial found that aerosolized ribavirin only resulted in accelerating normalization of temperature in children with influenza, but had no effect on respiratory rate, pulse rate, cough, or level of consciousness [44].

Ribavirin, in combination with systemic corticosteroids, was used empirically for the treatment of severe acute respiratory syndrome (SARS). However, a review of 14 clinical reports failed to demonstrate that ribavirin decreased the need for mechanical ventilation, or mortality, in patients with SARS [45].

There are several potential hazardous effects of aerosolized ribavirin. It can cause nausea, headaches, and bronchospasm [46]. In addition, it poses potential risks to healthcare workers who administer the medication. It has been shown to cause conjunctivitis as it can precipitate on contact lenses, and bronchospasm in healthcare workers administering the medication [46]. In addition, ribavirin is highly teratogenic. Although studies suggest that absorption of ribavirin by healthcare workers administering the medication is minimal [3], the short-term and long-term risks to women remain unknown. Therefore, conservative safety practices must be followed [3,46]. Given the lack of evidence supporting its efficacy, its known and potential side effects, and the availability of more efficacious treatment options, we do not recommend the use of aerosolized ribavirin in treating infections with RSV. Further studies are needed to determine its efficacy in treating influenza.

Although studies in patients with acquired immunodeficiency syndrome suggest that aerosolized pentamidine can be effective and well tolerated in mild *Pneumocystis jiroveci* pneumonia, it is not recommended for routine clinical practice [47]. Although aerosolized pentamidine has been used with success for primary and secondary *P. jiroveci* pneumonia prophylaxis [47], trimethoprim-sulfamethoxazole has been recommended as the drug of choice for prophylaxis in both situations. Aerosolized pentamidine (300 mg reconstituted with sterile water, administered every 4 weeks), delivered by a Respirgard II nebulizer (Marquest, Englewood, CO), has been approved for *P. jiroveci* pneumonia prophylaxis [47]. A retrospective study suggested that a standard ultrasonic nebulizer (Fisoneb, Fisons, NY) would yield similar effects to Respirgard II, a jet nebulizer, in providing primary and secondary prophylaxis with aerosolized pentamidine [48]. Because toxicity studies on the secondhand effects of aerosolized pentamidine exposure on healthcare personnel are limited [49], conservative safety practices are necessary.

Corticosteroids

At present, there is no indication for the use of inhaled corticosteroids in the treatment of the critically ill with acute exacerbations of obstructive lung disease. Systemic corticosteroids (oral or intravenous) are the recommended first-line agents for the treatment of acute asthma [15] and COPD [5]. Because inhaled corticosteroids are an integral component of asthma therapy, on discharge, they should be used in all patients receiving tapering doses of oral prednisone. They are considered the most effective anti-inflammatory therapy for control of persistent asthma [15]. Inhaled corticosteroids are available as MDIs, dry-powder inhalers, or inhalation suspension (budesonide) for aerosolized use.

When patients are hospitalized for reasons other than acute airway obstruction, inhaled corticosteroids may be continued if patients have been taking these agents for asthma or COPD maintenance therapy. To reduce the risk of oral candidiasis, mouth rinsing and use of a spacer device with MDI are recommended.

Racemic Epinephrine

Racemic epinephrine is effective in decreasing laryngeal edema by causing vasoconstriction [3]. The usual adult dose is 0.5 mL of a 2.25% solution diluted in 3 mL of normal saline every 4 to 6 hours. Because rebound edema frequently occurs, patients must be observed closely. Tachycardia is common during treatment and may precipitate angina in patients with coronary artery disease [3]. The role of racemic epinephrine aerosol in epiglottitis is not known. Similarly, inhaled racemic epinephrine is used to treat postextubation stridor, but this use has not been rigorously studied. Nebulized racemic epinephrine appears to have no benefit over nebulized albuterol in the management of bronchiolitis [50]. Because racemic epinephrine aerosol is associated with potentially serious side effects in patients with coronary artery disease, administration of inhaled mixtures of helium and oxygen should be considered first to decrease airway resistance and, therefore, the work of breathing associated with laryngeal edema or other upper-airway diseases (see the section Helium-Oxygen [Heliox]).

Aerosolized Vasodilators. Iloprost is an approved inhaled prostacyclin analog used for the chronic treatment of primary pulmonary hypertension and pulmonary hypertension due to use of appetite suppressants, portopulmonary syndrome, connective tissue disease, and chronic thromboembolic disease. It has also been used in patients with acute pulmonary hypertension after coronary bypass surgery, and may be more effective than inhaled nitric oxide [51]. It is currently FDA approved for patients with primary pulmonary hypertension and New York Heart Association (NYHA) class III (symptoms with minimal activity) and class IV (symptoms at rest) symptoms. Iloprost is administered as 2.5 to 5 μg doses, six to nine times per day. It needs to be delivered via a specialized nebulizer system, the Prodose AAD system (Respironics, Murrysville, PA), to ensure proper dosing. A randomized double-blind, placebo-controlled trial demonstrated that iloprost produced improvements in 6-minute walk, hemodynamics, dyspnea, and quality of life after 12 weeks of therapy [52].

Inhaled Cyclosporin. A randomized double-blind, placebo-controlled trial demonstrated improvement in survival and longer periods free of chronic rejection in lung transplant patients treated with inhaled cyclosporin [53]. The patients in the treatment group received 300 mg of aerosolized cyclosporin (Novartis, East Hanover, NJ) three times a week for the first 2 years after lung transplantation, in addition to usual systemic immunosuppression. There was no increase risk of side effects or opportunistic infections in the treated group.

Modes of Delivery

In the critical care setting, there are generally two types of aerosol delivery devices in use: those that create and deliver wet particles (air-jet nebulizers) and those that deliver preformed particles (pressurized MDIs) with or without MDI auxiliary delivery systems (spacers). Patients on mechanical ventilation or patients breathing through a tracheostomy cannot use dry-powder inhalers. Successful aerosol therapy is dependent on the percentage of the drug that is delivered to the lungs. Factors that influence aerosol deposition and effectiveness, such as flow rate, breathing pattern, and incoordination, have been largely overcome with newer and more advanced designs.

Nebulizers

Air-jet nebulizers are a nonpropellant-based option for inhaled drug delivery. Jet nebulizers rely on a high gas flow (provided by a portable compressor, compressed gas cylinder, or 50-psi wall outlet), Venturi orifices, and baffles to generate respirable particles, generally in the range of 1 to 5 μm diameter [3]. Small-volume nebulizers, equipped with small fluid reservoirs, are used for drug delivery [3]. Factors that affect their performance include design, characteristics of the medication, and gas source. Large-volume nebulizers have reservoir volumes greater than 100 mL and can be used to deliver aerosolized solutions over an extended period. Large versions are used to deliver bland aerosols into mist tents.

Nebulizers are frequently used in pediatric and elderly populations as well as in the hospital setting. Nebulizer delivery of aerosolized drugs is indicated when a drug is not available in MDI form and when a patient cannot coordinate the use of an MDI. Disadvantages include the need for a gas flow source, lack of portability, cost, and the risk of bacterial contamination if not properly cleaned [54].

Metered-Dose Inhalers

An MDI is a pressurized canister that contains drug suspended in a propellant and combined with a dispersing agent. The canister is inverted, placed in a plastic actuator, and, when pressed, delivers a metered dose of drug. The MDI is capable of delivering a more concentrated drug aerosol, as a bolus, than the solutions commonly available for nebulizers [3]. Delivery of a therapeutic dose is dependent on the quality of the patient's technique, which requires a slow, deep inhalation followed by a breath hold (approximately 10 seconds). Because this maneuver can be difficult, especially if the patient is experiencing respiratory distress, it is essential that the technique be taught and supervised by trained personnel.

Older MDIs use chlorofluorocarbon propellants (CFCs). Their use has now been phased out after the United Nations passed the 1987 Montreal Protocol that called for the banning of substances that may adversely affect the ozone layer. Although medical devices were initially exempted, many pharmaceutical companies began to formulate alternative preparations and delivery systems. Hydrofluoroalkane-134a (HFA) has been found to be an effective alternative to chlorofluorocarbon propellants. In addition, dry-powder inhalers for long- and short-acting β agonists, corticosteroids, and tiotropium have been developed. Another advantage of the HFA-containing MDIs and the dry-powder inhalers is that lung deposition of the medication appears to be greater when compared to the CFC-containing MDIs.

Metered-Dose Inhaler Auxiliary Devices. To overcome problems such as incorrect administration, oropharyngeal deposition, and inconsistent dosing associated with MDI aerosol delivery, several auxiliary devices (i.e., spacer, holding chamber) were developed [3]. When used properly, these devices have the following advantages: (a) a smaller, more therapeutic particle size is achieved; (b) oropharyngeal impaction is decreased; (c) fewer systemic side effects are experienced due to less oropharyngeal deposition compared to MDI alone; and (d) the risk of oral thrush associated with inhaled corticosteroids is decreased. It has been shown that among patients who have difficulty with coordination—particularly the elderly, handicapped, infants, and children younger than 5 years of age—spacer devices improve the efficacy of MDIs [55].

Choice of Delivery System

Since the development of the first MDI in the 1960s, there has been continuing debate about which aerosol delivery system, nebulizers, or MDI is superior. In 1997, Turner et al. [56] published a meta-analysis of 12 studies that compared bronchodilator delivery via nebulizer to delivery via MDI. Studies included in the review were all randomized clinical trials of adults with acute asthma or COPD who were treated in the emergency department or hospital and measured FEV_1 or peak expiratory flow rate. In all but two of the trials, spacers were used with MDIs. Based on the results of these studies, the authors concluded that there was no difference in effectiveness between the two delivery methods.

A Cochrane Library meta-analysis by Cates et al. [17] compared the clinical outcomes of adults and children with acute asthma who received β_2 agonists by nebulizer or MDI with spacer. In this review that included 16 randomized controlled trials, the authors concluded that the outcomes (hospital admission, length of stay in the emergency department, respiratory rate, heart rate, arterial blood gases, tremor and lung function) of both groups were equivalent.

In the United States, MDIs are underused in the acute care setting [3]. Barriers to selection of these devices include reimbursement issues and the misconception of clinicians regarding efficacy. Many third-party payors reimburse for the nebulizer/drug package but not for the MDI. In the critical care setting, selection of an aerosol delivery system for the spontaneously breathing patients should be based on several factors. In general, because the MDI with or without spacer is the most convenient and cost-effective method of delivery, it should be chosen whenever possible. Its use may be limited by factors such as the patient's ability to actuate and coordinate the device, either of which can affect aerosol deposition to the lungs; patient preference; practice situations; and economic evaluations. Additionally, parenchymal dosing with drugs such as pentamidine and ribavirin requires the use of a nebulizer [3]. Cost considerations may determine which delivery system is chosen in different settings. Studies show that use of MDIs with spacers likely produce considerable reductions in hospital costs [57]. The cost of a disposable nebulizer system in a hospital setting may be lower than the cost of a MDI and spacer device if patients are discharged with a second spacer device [17].

Aerosols can be delivered to intubated and mechanically ventilated patients with small-volume side-stream nebulizers connected to the inspiratory tubing or MDIs with an aerosol holding chamber. Although both delivery systems are effective in delivering aerosolized medications to the ventilated patient [3], drug delivery can be significantly reduced if proper technique in setting up and using both devices is not followed.

LUNG-EXPANSION TECHNIQUES

A *lung-expansion technique* is any technique that increases lung volume or assists the patient in increasing lung volume above that reached at his or her usual unassisted or uncoached inspiration. Rationales for the use of various strategies to promote lung inflation include (a) increasing pulmonary compliance, (b) increasing partial arterial pressure of oxygen (PaO_2), (c) decreasing work of breathing, and (d) increasing removal of secretions [58]. Lung-expansion techniques are meant to duplicate a normal sigh maneuver. Theoretically, sighs or periodic hyperinflations to near-total lung capacity reverse microatelectasis [3].

Lung-expansion techniques are indicated to prevent atelectasis and pneumonia in patients who cannot or will not take periodic hyperinflations [3], such as postoperative upper-abdominal and thoracic surgical patients and patients with respiratory disorders due to neuromuscular and chest wall diseases. Adequately performed, maximum inspirations 10 times each hour while awake significantly decrease the incidence of pulmonary complications after laparotomy [59]. Whatever technique is used postoperatively (e.g., coached sustained maximal inspiration with cough, incentive spirometry, volume-oriented intermittent positive-pressure breathing, intermittent CPAP, or positive expiratory pressure [PEP] mask therapy [60]), it should be taught and practiced preoperatively. When properly used, coached sustained maximal inspiration with cough and incentive spirometry—the least expensive and safest techniques—are as effective as any other method [61]. Of the several commercially available incentive spirometers, the one chosen should combine accuracy, low price, and maximum patient accessibility [62]. Because there are no definitive studies comparing the relative efficacy of volume- and flow-oriented incentive spirometers, the choice of equipment must be based on empiric assessment of patient acceptance, ease of use, and cost. When chest percussion with postural drainage is added to the previously mentioned expansion techniques in patients without prior lung disease, it has failed to affect the incidence of postoperative pulmonary complications [63].

AIRWAY CLEARANCE

Efficient mucociliary clearance and effective cough are the two basic processes necessary for normal clearance of the airways. In abnormal situations, this system may be dysfunctional and lead to mucus retention. Recently both the ACCP [64] and the BTS [2] have published evidence-based guidelines reviewing both pharmacological and nonpharmacological methods of augmenting pulmonary clearance. Both guidelines are complete reviews on this topic. A summarized discussion of techniques aimed at enhancing airway clearance follows.

Augmentation of Mucociliary Clearance

Mucociliary clearance is one of the most important defense mechanisms of the respiratory system. Mucociliary dysfunction is any defect in the ciliary and secretory elements of mucociliary interaction that disturbs the normal defenses of the airway epithelium [65]. Ineffective mucociliary clearance leads to retention of tracheobronchial secretions. Mucociliary clearance may be ineffective because of depression of the clearance mechanisms or oversecretion in the face of normal mucous transport, or both. Mucus is ineffectively cleared and overproduced in smokers with or without chronic bronchitis and in asthmatic patients [3]. It is also ineffectively cleared in the following situations: (a) in patients with emphysema, bronchiectasis, and CF; (b) during and up to 4 to 6 weeks after viral upper respiratory tract infections; (c) during and for an unknown period after general anesthesia due to the inhalation of dry gas and cuffed endotracheal tubes used during surgery; and (d) during prolonged endotracheal intubation due to the presence of the cuffed tube, administration of elevated concentrations of inspired oxygen, and damage to the tracheobronchial tree from suctioning [3]. The most important consideration in improving mucociliary clearance is to remove the inciting cause(s) of ineffective clearance and overproduction of secretions.

Treatment

Mucociliary clearance can be enhanced pharmacologically and mechanically. Numerous drugs with potential mucociliary effect have been studied, but only a few are clinically useful. Pharmaceutical therapy is frequently used in conjunction with physical therapy.

Pharmacologic Augmentation. β agonists and aminophylline stimulate mucociliary clearance [3]. These drugs should be given in the same dose as given for bronchodilatation. Mucolytics and expectorants (e.g., potassium iodide, glyceryl guaiacolate, guaifenesin, ammonium chloride, creosote, and cocillana) have not been shown to increase mucociliary clearance [3]. There is no evidence to support the use of mucokinetic agents in COPD exacerbations [5]. In a randomized controlled trail, healthy volunteers and patients with mild asthma showed no improved mucociliary clearance when given inhaled furosemide [66].

In vitro studies have demonstrated that corticosteroids reduce mucous secretion from human airway cells [67], and the use of inhaled corticosteroids has been recommended in the management of bronchorrhea (i.e., mucus secretions of more than 100 mL per day) [68]. However, we know of no randomized controlled trials demonstrating the benefit of inhaled corticosteroids in the management of bronchorrhea.

Mechanical Augmentation

Chest physiotherapy (CPT). Usually, chest physiotherapy involves (a) gravity (therapeutic positioning), (b) percussion to the chest wall over the affected area, (c) vibration of the chest wall during expiration, and (d) coughing. Coughing appears to be the most important component of CPT (see the section Augmentation of Cough Effectiveness). It is felt to be beneficial in patients with CF and bronchiectasis, in the unusual COPD patient who expectorates more than 30 mL of sputum each day [64], and in patients with lobar atelectasis [2]. It is not indicated in asthmatic patients [64] or in those with uncomplicated pneumonias [2]. CPT does not improve FEV_1, provides only modest short-term effects, and long-term benefits are unproven [64]. In patients with COPD, alternative methods of airway clearance (see below) have not proven more effective than CPT, and the effects of CPT itself on patients with COPD may be minimal [69].

Complications of CPT are infrequent yet potentially severe [70]. They include massive pulmonary hemorrhage (perhaps caused by clots dislodged during percussion), decreased PaO_2 from positioning the "good" lung up in spontaneously breathing patients, rib fractures, increased intracranial pressure, decreased cardiac output, and decreased FEV_1.

Oscillatory devices. These devices include the flutter device (Varioraw SARL, Scandipharm Inc, Birmingham, AL), intrapulmonary percussive ventilation (Percussionator, IPV-1; Percussionaire, Sand Point, ID), and high-frequency chest wall oscillation. The flutter mucus clearance device is a small, handheld, pipe-like device used to facilitate the removal of mucus from the lungs. As patients exhale through the device, a steel ball rolls and bounces, producing vibrations that are transmitted throughout the airways. It is postulated that vibrations of the airways intermittently increase endobronchial pressure and accelerate expiratory airflow, thereby enhancing mucus clearance [71]. In a randomized controlled trial, the flutter device was compared to standard, manual chest therapy in hospitalized CF patients experiencing an acute exacerbation [72] and found to be a safe, efficacious, and cost-effective alternative to standard, manual chest percussion. Konstan et al. [71] compared periods of vigorous voluntary cough, postural drainage, and flutter-valve treatment. Among the therapies compared, the volume of sputum was three times greater with the flutter treatment. Although larger clinical trials are needed, it appears to be a useful device for self-administration of CPT and as an equal alternative to CPT [64].

Intrapulmonary percussive ventilation uses short bursts of air at 200 to 300 cycles per minute, along with entrained aerosols delivered via a mouthpiece [64]. In a study on patients with CF, this was found to be equal to chest physiotherapy [73]. A small study suggested that high-frequency chest well oscillation decreased breathlessness and fatigue in patients with ALS [74]. High-frequency chest wall oscillation delivered through an inflatable vest appears to offer no benefit over standard CPT [3].

PEP mask. In PEP therapy, a mask is applied tightly over the mouth and nose, and a variable-flow resistor is adjusted to achieve PEP during exhalation between 5 and 20 cm H_2O. This, combined with "huff" coughing, allows mobilization of peripherally located secretions upward into larger airways. A Cochrane review of 20 studies in patients with CF failed to demonstrate that PEP had any short-term benefits over CPT [75].

Mechanical insufflation–exsufflation. Mechanical insufflation–exsufflation (cough in-exsufflator) increases the volume inhaled during the inspiratory phase of cough, thereby increasing cough effectiveness [64]. Cough efficiency can be further enhanced by applying negative airway pressure for 1 to 3 seconds after the initial inspiration. This method appears to be most beneficial in patients with impaired cough due to neuromuscular disease [76].

In summary, the data available, although not abundant, indicate that in patients with copious secretions, clearance of secretions can be enhanced with selected physical therapy procedures. Although these modalities appear to increase expectoration of mucus, it is not clear what clinical benefit this achieves. There is no information about the influence of physical therapy maneuvers on healthcare outcomes, including frequency of hospitalization, hospital length of stay, longevity, and quality of life. It is clear that these techniques are well entrenched in the management of patients with mucus hypersecretion, especially those with CF; it is time for us to prove that they lead to clinically important outcomes. Evidence-based guidelines for the use of these modalities can be found elsewhere [2,64].

Suctioning. Although mechanical aspiration or suctioning is routine in most hospitals, many are unaware of the numerous potential complications associated with suctioning, such as tissue trauma, laryngospasm, bronchospasm, hypoxemia, cardiac arrhythmias, respiratory arrest, cardiac arrest, atelectasis, pneumonia, misdirection of catheter, and death [3]. Complications are generally avoidable or reversible if proper technique and indications are adhered to strictly.

Endotracheal. Endotracheal suctioning is performed in patients with an artificial tracheal airway in place. It should be used only when there is definite evidence of excessive retained secretions. Routine suctioning according to a predetermined schedule may cause excessive mucosal tissue damage, excessive impairment of mucociliary clearance, unnecessary exposure to the potential risks of hypoxemia associated with the procedure, arrhythmias, atelectasis, and bronchoconstriction [3]. Endotracheal suctioning is indicated when there is a need to (a) remove accumulated secretions, (b) obtain a sputum specimen for microbiological or cytologic examination, (c) maintain the patency and integrity of the artificial airway, and (d) stimulate cough in patients with ineffective cough [77].

Suction catheters are generally 22 in. long (adequate in length to reach the main stem bronchus) and sized in French units. Most have a side port to minimize mucosal damage. To avoid obstruction of the artificial airway, the outer diameter of the suction catheter should be less than half the size of the internal diameter of the endotracheal tube [rule of thumb: multiply the inner diameter of the endotracheal tube by 2 and use next smallest size (e.g., 8.0-mm endotracheal tube: $2 \times 8 = 16$, choose next smallest size = 14 French)] [78].

For patients receiving ventilatory support, closed, multiuse systems that are incorporated into the ventilator circuit are available. Because patients remain connected to the ventilator during suctioning, positive end-expiratory pressure (PEEP) and high fractional inspiration of oxygen (FIO_2) can be maintained, reducing the risk of hypoxemia. Preoxygenation with 100% O_2 is still necessary. The use of closed, multiuse systems may reduce cost and the risk of cross-contamination. However, these systems may increase tension on the tracheal tube and add resistance to the airway.

The practice of instilling normal saline into the airway before suctioning to aid secretion removal is common, but it is unclear whether it is effective and it may increase the risk of nosocomial pneumonia. The routine use of saline irrigation is not recommended [78].

Nasotracheal. While nasotracheal suctioning may be considered in patients who do not have an artificial tracheal airway, it is not recommended because of the potential side effects, and there are other, safer alternatives. It is rarely indicated because CPT can be used in conscious patients, and semicomatose or comatose patients with retained secretions can be intubated. Nasotracheal suctioning has been associated with fatal cardiac arrest, life-threatening arrhythmias presumably due to hypoxemia, and bacteremia [3]. Because quantitative cultures acquired with plugged telescoping catheters at bronchoscopy can be obtained more safely and are definitely more reliable than nasotracheal suction (see Chapter 9) in obtaining uncontaminated lower respiratory tract secretions for culture, nasotracheal suction is not recommended for this purpose.

Nasopharyngeal. Nasopharyngeal suctioning is indicated to clear the upper airway. Because the catheter does not reach the vocal cords or enter the trachea, nasopharyngeal suctioning is associated with fewer complications than nasotracheal suctioning [3]. The catheter should not touch or go beyond the vocal cords. This requires insertion to a depth that corresponds to the distance between the middle of the patient's chin and the angle of the jaw, just below the earlobe.

Endotracheal extubation. Before removal of the endotracheal tube, perform nasopharyngeal and oropharyngeal suctioning to clear secretions that have pooled above the vocal cords for the inflated cuff. Replace the catheter and perform endotracheal suctioning. In preparation for deflating the cuff, place the endotracheal suction catheter tip just distal to the endotracheal tube to aspirate any secretions that gravitate downward when the cuff is deflated. Deflate the cuff and intermittently suction while removing the tube and catheter as a unit.

Augmentation of Cough Effectiveness

Although mucociliary transport is the major method of clearing the airway in healthy subjects, cough is an important reserve mechanism, especially in lung disease [3]. All studies suggest that cough is effective in clearing secretions only if secretions are excessive.

Pathophysiology of Ineffective Cough

The effectiveness of cough in clearing an airway theoretically depends on the presence of secretions of sufficient thickness to be affected by two-phase, gas-liquid flow and the linear velocity of air moving through its lumen [3]. The ineffectiveness of voluntary coughing in normal subjects to clear tagged aerosol particles in the lower airways is probably due to the inability of the moving airstream to interact appropriately with the normally thin mucus layer on which the particles were deposited [3]. Once there is sufficiently thick material in the airways, the effectiveness of cough depends on achieving a high flow rate of air and a small cross-sectional area of the airway during the expiratory phase of cough to achieve a high linear velocity (velocity equals flow/cross-sectional area); therefore, any condition associated with decreased expiratory flow rates or reduced ability to compress airways dynamically places affected patients at risk of having an ineffective cough.

All conditions that may lead to an ineffective cough interfere with the inspiratory or expiratory phases of cough; most conditions affect both. Cough effectiveness is likely to be most impaired in patients with respiratory muscle weakness because their ability to take in a deep breath in (flow rates are highest at high lung volumes) and to compress their airways dynamically during expiration are impaired, placing them at double liability. The muscles of expiration appear to be the most important determinant in producing elevated intrathoracic pressures, and they are capable of doing so even with an endotracheal tube in place [3]. Therefore, tracheostomy should not be performed in the intubated patient just to increase cough effectiveness.

Assessment of Cough Effectiveness

Ideally, clinicians would like to predict clinically or physiologically when a patient is at risk of developing atelectasis, pneumonia, or gas-exchange abnormalities because of an ineffective cough. There are no such studies, however. The existing data that relate to assessment of cough effectiveness were generated in patients with muscular dystrophy and myasthenia gravis [3,79]. These studies suggested that mouth maximum expiratory pressure (MEP) measurements may be useful for assessing cough strength, but they did not correlate these measurements with any clinical outcomes. Using the absence of peak flow transients (i.e., a spike of flow with a cough to the otherwise sustained maximal expiratory flow) during cough flow–volume curves as an indication that expiratory muscle strength during coughing was not adequate to compress the airways dynamically, investigators found that MEP was the most sensitive predictor of flow transient production during coughing [3]. All patients who could produce cough transients had MEP values greater than 60 cm H_2O; those who could not produce transients had MEP values of 45 cm H_2O or less. This latter value is consistent with the clinical observations of Gracey et al. [79], who found in patients with myasthenia gravis that MEP values less than 40 cm H_2O were frequently associated with difficulty in raising secretions without suctioning.

Bach and Saporito [80] prospectively evaluated measurement of peak cough flows (PCF) (assisted and unassisted) as a predictor of successful extubation and decannulation in 49 patients with primary neuromuscular ventilatory insufficiency. In this study, the ability to generate at least 160 L per minute of PCF (measured with Peak Flow Meter, HealthScan Inc, Cedar Grove, NJ) resulted in successful extubation or decannulation, whereas no patients with PCFs under 160 L per minute were successfully extubated or decannulated. The authors concluded that the assisted PCF could be used to predict the ability to safely extubate or decannulate patients with neuromuscular disease regardless of the extent of ventilatory insufficiency.

Protussive Therapy

When cough is useful yet inadequate, protussive therapy is indicated (e.g., bronchiectasis, CF, pneumonia, postoperative atelectasis) [3]. The goal of protussive therapy is to increase cough effectiveness with or without increasing cough frequency. It can be of a pharmaceutical or mechanical nature.

Only a small number of pharmacologic agents have been adequately evaluated as protussive agents [81]. Of these, aerosolized hypertonic saline in patients with chronic bronchitis and amiloride aerosol in patients with CF have been shown to improve cough clearance [81,82]. Although aerosolized ipratropium bromide diminished the effectiveness of cough for clearing radiolabeled particles from the airways in COPD, aerosolized terbutaline after CPT significantly increased cough clearance in patients with bronchiectasis [3]. The conflicting results with these two types of bronchodilators suggest that terbutaline achieved its favorable effect by increasing hydration of mucus or enhancing ciliary beating, and these overcame any negative effects that bronchodilation had on cough clearance. If bronchodilators result in too much smooth muscle relaxation of large airways, flow rates can actually decrease even in healthy individuals when more compliant large airways narrow too much because they cannot withstand dynamic compression during forced expirations [3]. Although hypertonic saline, amiloride, and terbutaline by aerosol after CPT have been shown to increase cough clearance, their clinical use remains to be determined in future studies that assess short-term and long-term effects of these agents on the patient's condition.

Expiratory Muscle Training

Because expiratory muscle weakness diminishes cough, strengthening the muscles may improve cough effectiveness. In quadriplegic subjects, there was a 46% increase in expiratory reserve volume after a 6-week period of isometric training to increase the clavicular portion of the pectoralis major [83]. This technique may improve cough by allowing patients with neuromuscular weakness to generate higher intrathoracic pressures [3].

Mechanical Measures

A variety of mechanical measures have been advocated as possible therapies to improve cough effectiveness [3], including (a) positive mechanical insufflation, followed by (b) manual compression of the lower thorax and abdomen in quadriparetic patients (an abdominal push maneuver that assists expiratory efforts in patients with spinal cord injuries), (c) mechanical insufflation–exsufflation, (d) abdominal binding and muscle training of the clavicular portion of the pectoralis major in tetraplegic patients, and (e) CPT in patients with chronic bronchitis. The usefulness of the first four measures in improving clinical outcomes has yet to be studied, and in patients with CF, one technique does not appear to be superior to the others [3]. In patients with chronic bronchitis, the combination of short bouts of PEP breathing, forced expirations, and CPT resulted in reduced coughing, less mucus production, and fewer acute exacerbations compared with patients who received CPT alone. Except in patients with CF, there is no clear benefit of combining CPT with coughing over vigorous coughing alone [64].

The effect of deep lung insufflation on maximum insufflation capacities and peak cough flows for patients with neuromuscular disease was investigated [84]. In this study, the authors concluded that with training, the capacity to stack air to deep insufflations can be enhanced despite neuromuscular weakness, and this can result in increased cough effectiveness.

ADMINISTRATION OF MEDICAL GASES

Oxygen Therapy

Indications for Oxygen Therapy

In the acute setting, administration of supplemental oxygen is indicated for (a) acute respiratory failure (hypoxemic and hypercapnic), (b) acute myocardial infarction (MI), (c) acute asthma, (d) normoxemic hypoxia (states characterized by the potential or actual documentation of tissue hypoxia despite a normal PaO_2 such as carbon monoxide poisoning), (e) the perioperative and postoperative states, and (f) cluster headaches [3,85–87]. Additionally, oxygen should be administered empirically in cases of cardiac or respiratory arrest, respiratory distress, hypotension [88], shock, and severe trauma [85].

A dosage sufficient to correct the hypoxemia should be prescribed. The goal of oxygen therapy is to correct hypoxemia to a PaO_2 greater than 60 mm Hg or arterial oxygen saturation (SaO_2) greater than 90%. Due to the shape of the oxyhemoglobin dissociation curve, there is little benefit from increasing the PaO_2 to values much greater than 60 mm Hg, and in some cases, it may increase the risk, albeit small, of CO_2 retention [5].

Clinicians are cautioned regarding the haphazard use of oxygen, as there are potential complications associated with the administration of supplemental oxygen, particularly at high concentrations (i.e., $FIO_2 > 0.50$). Oxygen therapy should not be used in place of but in addition to mechanical ventilation when ventilatory support is indicated [85].

Respiratory Failure. Oxygen therapy is used in acute pulmonary conditions to prevent tissue hypoxia and the serious and often irreversible effects on vital organ function that can result from untreated hypoxemia. In the absence of hypercarbia, the risk of worsening alveolar hypoventilation with the administration of supplemental oxygen is essentially nonexistent. Even in patients with chronic hypercapnic respiratory failure, the administration of supplemental oxygen to achieve a PaO_2 of approximately 60 mm Hg is associated with only a small risk of worsening hypercapnia. The mechanism by which oxygen administration results in CO_2 elevation in patients with COPD is multifactorial. It cannot be explained solely by the effect of oxygen on ventilatory drives. It may also be due to an oxygen-induced increase in dead space resulting from relaxation of hypoxic vasoconstriction, and it also requires the presence of other respiratory abnormalities preventing compensatory hyperventilation [3]. Furthermore, in acute situations in which supplemental oxygen is necessary to maintain adequate tissue oxygenation, it should not be withheld even if there is a risk that ventilatory support may be required. Care should be taken, however, to avoid the administration of excessively rich oxygen mixtures. See Chapter 49 for further discussion of oxygen therapy in COPD.

Acute Myocardial Infarction Without Respiratory Failure. Based on studies demonstrating that breathing enriched oxygen mixtures limited infarct size in animals, it has become common practice to administer oxygen to patients suspected of experiencing ischemic-type chest discomfort [85]. Therefore, administration of supplemental oxygen, usually by nasal cannula, is recommended in the setting of acute ischemic-type chest discomfort. If SaO_2 is monitored, oxygen should be administered when the saturation is less than 90% [89]. The rationale for its use is based on the observation that even with uncomplicated MI, patients may be somewhat hypoxemic initially, probably due to ventilation-perfusion mismatch and excessive lung water [90].

Because nitroglycerin dilates the pulmonary vascular bed and increases ventilation-perfusion abnormalities, supplemental oxygen is recommended in the initial hours for all patients suspected of having an acute MI. Experimental studies have shown that supplemental oxygen may limit ischemic myocardial injury [91] and reduce ST-segment elevation in patients experiencing MI [92]. There appears to be little justification for continuing its routine use beyond 2 to 3 hours [89]. Whether it is of value to give concentrations greater than 40% is unclear. In the setting of MI complicated by left ventricular failure, arrhythmias, or pneumonia, the appropriate oxygen concentration should be determined by monitoring of the PaO_2 or SaO_2 [85].

Acute Asthma. Supplemental oxygen protects against hypoxemia resulting from pulmonary vasodilation induced by β agonists and minimizes hypoxemia-induced vasoconstriction [93]. Normal levels of oxygen (normoxia) may protect against cardiac arrhythmias and may also help oxygen delivery to peripheral tissues [3].

Supplemental oxygen is recommended for patients with hypoxemia and for patients with FEV_1 or peak expiratory flow less than 50% of the predicted value during an acute attack when arterial oxygen monitoring is not available. The Expert Panel Report 2 recommends oxygen administered via nasal cannula or mask to maintain an SaO_2 greater than 90% (greater than 95% in pregnant women and in patients with a history of heart disease) [15]. SaO_2 monitoring should continue until a definite response to bronchodilatory therapy occurs.

Normoxemic Hypoxia. *Normoxemic hypoxia* encompasses conditions that are characterized by the potential or actual documentation of tissue hypoxia but with a normal PaO_2 [85,94]. Tissue hypoxia occurs as a result of abnormalities in the function of hemoglobin or deficient delivery or use of oxygen by the tissues, or both. Examples of such conditions include acute anemia, carboxyhemoglobinemia (perhaps the most lethal), and homozygous sickle-cell crisis.

Recommendations for the use of supplemental oxygen for normoxemic hypoxic conditions are outlined as follows:

1. *Acute anemia*. Although the definitive treatment is sufficient blood replacement, supplemental oxygen is a reasonable temporizing measure.
2. *Carboxyhemoglobinemia* (carbon monoxide [CO] poisoning) [3]. Because a partial pressure of CO of less than 1 mm Hg can saturate 50% of hemoglobin and not interfere with lung function, measurements of oxygen tension are not useful in predicting the presence of CO poisoning or in directing oxygen therapy. Carboxyhemoglobin levels must be measured to detect CO poisoning. Administration of high concentrations of inspiratory oxygen is important in treating CO poisoning for two reasons: a higher amount of oxygen may be placed in the solution in the blood to supplement the oxygen already present, and a high PaO_2 accelerates the dissociation of CO from hemoglobin. In the absence of hyperbaric oxygen, a nonrebreathing mask driven by pure humidified oxygen is the treatment of choice. This should be given immediately and without interruption until it is verified that carboxyhemoglobinemia has fallen to less than 5%. Although hyperbaric oxygenation represents a potentially, albeit controversial, more effective alternative, it is not readily available to most patients. If it is available, patients with carboxyhemoglobin levels greater than 40% or with cardiac or neurologic symptoms should be considered for immediate transportation to the hyperbaric oxygen facility for treatment. (See Chapter 64 for further discussion of CO poisoning.)
3. *Sickle-cell crisis*. The role of oxygen therapy in sickle-cell crisis is unknown [95]. Because deoxygenation makes cells sickle, however, it seems reasonable to give supplemental oxygen in this setting. Because of the risk of oxygen toxicity, concentrations in excess of 50% should not be given for more than 48 hours.
4. *Cluster headache* [87,96]. A recent randomized placebo-controlled trial demonstrated that 100% oxygen delivered at a flow rate of 12 L per minute via a full-face mask can significantly reduce pain from cluster headaches within 15 minutes [87]. Oxygen inhalation's mechanism of action is unknown.

Prevention of Surgical Wound Infections. The perioperative administration of supplemental oxygen appears to be advantageous in reducing the incidence of postoperative surgical wound infections. In two randomized prospective, double-blind clinical trials of patients who underwent elective colorectal surgery, patients received either 80% or 30% supplemental oxygen during the perioperative period and for 2 hours or 6 hours postoperatively [97,98]. Supplemental oxygen was given regardless of the patient's SaO_2. The incidences of surgical wound infections were 5.2% [97] and 14.9% [98] in patients who received 80% oxygen, compared to 11.2% [97] and 24.4% [98] in the group who received 30% oxygen.

Postoperative State. An increase in the alveolar-arterial partial pressure of oxygen (PO_2) gradient and a decrease in the functional residual capacity are common perioperatively and postoperatively. Ventilation-perfusion abnormalities and intrapulmonary shunting may occur, and while generally corrected within the first few hours after most types of peripheral surgery, it may be more significant in the elderly, the obese, in patients with preexisting cardiopulmonary conditions, and after surgery of the upper abdomen and thorax. In these situations, PaO_2 may not normalize until postoperative day 2. Because the PaO_2 usually increases with the administration of supplemental oxygen, low concentrations of supplemental oxygen should be administered to those at risk of postoperative hypoxemia [99]. In some cases, lung-expansion maneuvers may be necessary if oxygen fails to correct the PaO_2 [84].

Oxygen Delivery Systems

In the acute setting, bulk supply systems are used as a relatively inexpensive means of oxygen delivery. When transporting hospitalized patients, gas cylinders and liquid tanks are used.

Oxygen Delivery Devices

A variety of devices are available to deliver supplemental oxygen. Selection should be based on the amount of oxygen the system can deliver and its clinical performance. Factors capable of affecting performance include the type of device chosen, flow rates used by the device, the fit of the device, respiratory rate, inspiratory flows, and tidal volumes. Types of devices are as follows:

1. Standard dual-prong nasal cannulas are the most commonly used oxygen delivery devices for administering low-flow oxygen. Flow rates of 0.5 to 1.0 L per minute by nasal prongs approximate an inspired oxygen concentration of 0.24, and a rate of 2 L per minute approximates 0.28. Nasal cannulas are easy to use, relatively comfortable, fairly unobtrusive, do not interfere with eating or talking, and relatively inexpensive. Generally, it is unnecessary to humidify oxygen administered by nasal cannulae at flow rates of 4 L per minute or less [85,86].
2. Simple oxygen masks deliver FIO_2 of approximately 0.35 to 0.50 oxygen with flow rates of 5 L per minute or greater. Because nasal cannulas and simple oxygen masks deliver an overlapping range of FIO_2, the nasal cannulas should be used unless the nares are unavailable or prone to irritation from the cannula. Face masks must be removed when eating and drinking, and caution should always be exercised in using oxygen face masks on sedated, obtunded, or restrained patients. Because these masks have a reservoir of 100 to 200 mL, there is a risk of rebreathing CO_2. For this reason, flow rates of at least 5 L per minute are recommended. Because relatively high flow rates are needed with simple masks, they are generally not appropriate for the delivery of a low FIO_2 (i.e., less than 0.30 to 0.35) [85].
3. Masks with reservoir bags, nonrebreathing and partial-rebreathing oxygen masks, can deliver a high FIO_2 (>0.50) with oxygen flowing into the reservoir at 8 to 10 L per minute to partially inflate the reservoir bag throughout inspiration. They are designed to deliver short-term high FIO_2 in situations when hypoxemia is suspected [100]. After the patient has been stabilized, if a high FIO_2 is required, a fixed performance device with a known FIO_2 should be substituted. Theoretically, the partial-rebreathing mask should deliver an FIO_2 of approximately 0.60, and the nonrebreathing mask should deliver 1.00. For the nonrebreathing mask to deliver an FIO_2 of 1.00, however, a tight-fitting mask is required so that, in clinical practice, both masks function similarly.

4. If an accurate FIO_2 is required, a Venturi-type mask can be used. Supplied by high oxygen flows, it maintains a fixed ratio of oxygen to room air so that the FIO_2 remains constant. These masks can deliver oxygen concentrations to the trachea of up to 0.50. FIO_2 settings are typically 0.24, 0.28, 0.31, 0.35, 0.40, and 0.50.

Oxygen-Conserving Devices

Several devices have been developed to improve the efficacy of oxygen delivery. Three such methods are reservoir cannulas [101], demand-pulse oxygen delivery, and transtracheal catheters [3].

1. The reservoir nasal cannula stores 20 mL of oxygen during exhalation and delivers this oxygen as a bolus at the start of inspiration.
2. Electronic demand devices deliver a pulse of oxygen during early inspiration rather than continuously throughout the ventilatory cycle.
3. Transtracheal catheters bypass the anatomic dead space, and oxygen is delivered directly into the trachea using the central airways as a reservoir for oxygen during end-expiration [3]. When caring for patients with transtracheal catheters in place before admission to the hospital, it is important to secure them with tape or sutures to prevent accidental dislodging. There is no need to remove the catheter before or during endotracheal intubation. While the patient is intubated, however, the transtracheal catheter should be capped.

Patients receiving transtracheal oxygen are at risk of developing inspissated secretions, mucus airway casts, and mucus balls, especially when the transtracheally delivered gas is not adequately humidified. Consequently, whenever a patient receiving transtracheal oxygen develops worsening hypoxemia or respiratory distress, mucus obstruction of the airway should be considered. In this setting, oxygen should be administered via nasal cannula and the transtracheal catheter removed. This maneuver can often shear off a mucus ball attached to the end of the catheter, allowing the patient to expectorate the accumulated mucus, and thereby improve the hypoxemia and eliminate the respiratory distress. The catheter can then be cleaned and reinserted with provision for adequate humidification of the transtracheally delivered gas. Transtracheal air and oxygen mixtures as therapy for obstructive sleep apnea [102] and as a nocturnal mechanical ventilation–assist device [3].

Choice of Oxygen Delivery Device

In the hypercapnic, hypoxemic patient, therapy can begin with 0.5 to 2.0 L per minute by nasal cannula or 0.24 to 0.28 FIO_2 by Venturi-type mask. If the PaO_2 remains less than 55 mm Hg 30 minutes later, administration of progressive increments of inspired oxygen is undertaken. Assessment of gas exchange is measured at frequent intervals, usually every 30 minutes [3] for the first 1 to 2 hours or until it is certain that the PaO_2 is 55 mm Hg or greater and CO_2 narcosis is not developing. In the hypercapnic patient, titration of supplemental oxygen is best assessed by arterial blood gas analysis rather than oximetry because the arterial blood gas provides $PaCO_2$ and oxygenation data. An initial modest increase in $PaCO_2$ (5 to 10 mm Hg) is expected in most hypercapnic patients given supplemental oxygen [103].

If a well-fitted Venturi-type mask delivering FIO_2 of 0.50 fails to achieve an oxygen saturation of at least 90% or a PaO_2 of 60 mm Hg or greater, the patient usually has severe cardiogenic pulmonary edema, acute respiratory distress syndrome (ARDS), overwhelming pneumonia, or a cardiac or pulmonary vascular shunt. In these settings, a nonrebreathing mask is recommended for two reasons. First, when properly worn, it has the potential to deliver the most predictable oxygen concentration (close to 1.00) of all the high-concentration delivery mask devices (e.g., aerosol masks, partial rebreathing masks, or face tents). Second, it can reveal the presence of a right-to-left shunt. If the PaO_2 is 60 mm Hg or less in the face of an inspired oxygen concentration of close to 1.00, a right-to-left shunt of approximately 40% of the cardiac output is present (see Chapter 46). If the chest radiograph in this setting demonstrates diffuse pulmonary infiltrates and the patient does not improve rapidly with diuretics, then generally it can be assumed that mechanical ventilation with PEEP is necessary.

Oxygen therapy should never be abruptly discontinued when hypercapnia has worsened and CO_2 narcosis is a possibility. This causes PaO_2 to fall to a level lower than it was before any oxygen was given [3] because the patient is breathing in a slower, shallower pattern.

Long-Term Continuous Oxygen Therapy

Continuous (24-hour) oxygen therapy significantly prolongs and improves the quality of life in hypoxemic patients with COPD [3]. If used for 15 hours per day or more, it decreases mortality 1.5 to 1.9 times for up to 3 years. Patients who should be given continuous oxygen during hospitalization and as outpatients include those with a PaO_2 of 55 mm Hg or less and those with a PaO_2 of 59 mm Hg or less plus peripheral edema, hematocrit of 55% or greater, or P pulmonale on electrocardiogram. Because many of these patients continue to improve as outpatients, the need for continuous oxygen therapy should be reassessed at 1 month [104].

Complications of Oxygen Therapy

In adults, decreased mucociliary clearance, tracheobronchitis, and pulmonary oxygen toxicity are the major complications of oxygen therapy. Mucociliary clearance is decreased by 40% when 75% oxygen is breathed for 9 hours and by 50% when 50% oxygen is breathed for 30 hours [3]. Symptomatic tracheobronchitis is caused consistently by the inhalation of high concentrations of oxygen (0.90 or higher) for 12 hours or more; it is manifested by substernal pain, cough, and dyspnea [105].

To avoid clinically significant pulmonary oxygen toxicity, prolonged administration of concentrations greater than 0.50 should be restricted, whenever possible, to 48 hours [3]. The pathology of oxygen toxicity is that of ARDS; it can lead to death from refractory and progressive hypoxemia due to interstitial fibrosis. It is best avoided by restricting delivery of oxygen to the lowest concentration and shortest duration absolutely necessary to achieve a satisfactory PaO_2. Therefore, prophylaxis consists of using any and all measures that allow a decrease in the concentration of inspired oxygen to a subtoxic level. PEEP has been shown to be useful in achieving this goal.

Mak et al. [106] studied the effects of hyperoxia on left ventricular function in patients with and without congestive heart failure and concluded that hyperoxia was associated with impairment of cardiac relaxation and increased left ventricular filling pressures in both groups. Based on these findings, the cautious use of high FIO_2 in normoxic patients, especially those with congestive heart failure, is advised.

For patients with previous bleomycin exposure, there appears to be a synergistic effect with subsequent exposure to high concentrations of inspired oxygen, resulting in the development of bleomycin pneumonitis [107]. Although it is unclear how long after bleomycin exposure that breathing high-inspired oxygen concentrations predisposes to pneumonitis, the risk appears highest within 6 months of bleomycin exposure.

A similar interaction can be seen in patients taking long-term amiodarone and exposure to high concentrations of inspired oxygen [108]. This risk appears higher in patients receiving high concentrations of inspired oxygen via mechanical ventilation. These patients can develop diffuse alveolar damage and ARDS, and mortality rates may be as high as 33% [109]. For patients with a history of either bleomycin or amiodarone exposure, we recommend using the lowest amounts of supplemental oxygen possible to maintain adequate oxygenation.

Although the complications of retrolental fibroplasia and bronchopulmonary dysplasia from oxygen toxicity have been limited in the past to pediatric patients, reports of adults with bronchopulmonary dysplasia, the eventual result of ARDS, have appeared [3]. Central nervous system dysfunction manifested by myoclonus, nausea, paresthesias, unconsciousness, and seizures is limited to hyperbaric oxygenation at pressures in excess of 2 atm [3].

Hyperbaric Oxygen Therapy

Hyperbaric therapy, 100% oxygen at 2 to 3 times the atmospheric pressure at sea level, is used as primary therapy in the treatment of patients with decompression sickness, arterial gas embolism, and severe CO poisoning [110]. In the case of CO poisoning, although hyperbaric therapy accelerates the resolution of symptoms, it does not appear to affect the rate of late sequelae [110] or long-term mortality in non–life-threatening cases [111]. It is used as adjunctive therapy in the treatment of osteoradionecrosis, clostridial myonecrosis/necrotizing fasciitis [112], and compromised skin grafts [113], although there is evidence to suggest that it does not improve outcomes in patients with necrotizing soft tissue infections [114]. Although hyperbaric oxygen therapy has been used for several other medical conditions, there is no current evidence demonstrating its benefits when used for treating traumatic brain injuries, acute ischemic cerebral accident, multiple sclerosis, or acute coronary syndrome [3,115–117].

Helium-Oxygen (Heliox)

Because helium is less dense than nitrogen, it has the potential to improve airflow where airflow is likely to be turbulent (i.e., density dependent). However, this primarily occurs in large airways when there is an upper airway–obstructing lesion. Heliox has successfully decreased airway resistance in patients with postextubation upper-airway obstruction [118], in children with severe croup who were refractory to inhaled racemic epinephrine [118], and in upper-airway obstruction due to tracheal tumors or extrinsic compression [119]. Although there have been favorable physiologic effects shown in a number of randomized controlled trials in spontaneously breathing patients with acute severe asthma [3], one large meta-analysis of seven studies [120] and an extensive review by the Cochrane Database [121] failed to show any benefit of using Heliox in the management of acute asthma patients. At this time, there is no definitive evidence to support the use of Heliox in the treatment of acute asthma. Heliox has been used with nebulized albuterol in the treatment of asthma, but any benefit is unclear as there are conflicting results in the literature [122,123]. In addition, Heliox has been shown to adversely impact the particle size of the medication [124], potentially limiting its delivery to the distal airways.

Heliox has not been shown to be beneficial in children with croup [125]. Heliox has been shown to improve oxygenation in patients undergoing fiberoptic bronchoscopy through endotracheal tubes with internal diameters less than 8 mm [126]. Therefore, if a bronchoscopy must be preformed in this setting, and changing the endotracheal tube to a larger size is not possible, performing the procedure with Heliox may be helpful.

The effect of increasing concentrations of helium in decreasing airway resistance is linear, but most reduction takes place when the concentration of helium reaches 40% [126]. Therefore, Heliox mixtures should contain a minimum of 40% helium, with the balance of the mixture being oxygen. For patients in respiratory distress with little hypoxemia due to laryngeal edema, a Heliox mixture of 80% helium and 20% oxygen would suffice. For patients in respiratory distress with profound hypoxemia due to pulmonary edema associated with laryngeal edema, however, a Heliox mixture of 40% helium and 60% oxygen would be most advantageous.

In an uncontrolled trial, intubated patients with status asthmaticus on mechanical ventilation [127] were successfully ventilated with a mixture of 60% helium and 40% oxygen and experienced a decrease in airway pressures and $PaCO_2$ with a resolution of acidosis. Because helium may affect how ventilators work, monitoring of ventilator outputs must be undertaken.

Jet nebulizers that are powered with Heliox rather than oxygen or air may be adversely affected. Heliox has been shown to alter the available inhaled mass and the particle size of albuterol if settings are not adjusted and flow rates changed. The clinical implications of this effect have not been determined [128]. Nebulizer performance with Heliox needs to be determined and correction factors derived before proceeding to clinical use.

Although Heliox may provide favorable short-term physiologic effects in patients with acute exacerbations of COPD [3], review of the literature has concluded that there is insufficient evidence to support the use of Heliox in the management of ventilated and nonventilated patients with acute exacerbations of COPD [129].

In summary, Heliox should only be considered a support modality that serves as a bridge, allowing specific therapies more time to work [130]. Only its use in the treatment of severe upper-airway obstruction can be supported at this time. Current studies do not support its routine use in the management of acute exacerbations of COPD and asthma, or croup and acute bronchiolitis in children. Nevertheless, in acute asthma and bronchiolitis, it is reasonable to consider the use of Heliox when conventional therapies have failed.

Nitric Oxide

Inhaled nitric oxide (NO) is a potent, selective pulmonary vasodilator. Early studies reported the clinical application of inhaled NO in adult patients with primary pulmonary hypertension and since then, hundreds of trials have been conducted to identify additional applications [131]. In a randomized controlled trial, inhaled NO reduced the need for extracorporeal membrane oxygenation (ECMO) in newborn infants with persistent pulmonary hypertension [132]. The results of a prospective, uncontrolled clinical trial [133] demonstrated that inhaled NO improved systemic oxygenation in infants with persistent pulmonary hypertension, reducing the need for more invasive treatments, such as ECMO. Although inhaled NO has been shown to improve oxygenation in newborns with persistent pulmonary hypertension and reduce the need for ECMO, it has not been shown to increase overall survival [131]. One- and 2-year follow-ups of infants with persistent pulmonary hypertension of the newborn who were treated with inhaled NO showed medical and neurological developmental outcomes to be similar to previous reports of patients treated with conventional therapy and ECMO [134].

Inhaled NO has been investigated in a variety of other areas, including (a) acute lung injury and ARDS, (b) status asthmaticus, (c) intestinal ischemia reperfusion, (d) thrombotic disorders, and (e) sickle-cell crisis [3]. An extensive review of the use of inhaled NO therapy in adults can be found elsewhere [135]. The benefits of using NO in these conditions are questionable. Inhaled NO appears to only transiently improve oxygenation and does not appear to decrease mortality in patients with severe lung injury [136]. In addition, a substantial number of patients are nonresponders to inhaled NO, showing no pulmonary vasodilation or improvement in oxygenation [3].

Delivery and monitoring systems for inhaled NO, as outlined by a workshop of the National Heart, Lung, and Blood Institute in 1993, have been summarized elsewhere [137]. The application of inhaled NO requires trained personnel with expertise and knowledge specific to the delivery systems, ventilator circuitry, and monitoring of patients.

Risks associated with the use of inhaled NO include vasodilation of the pulmonary circulation with increased blood flow to the left ventricle, causing an increase in left arterial pressure and pulmonary artery balloon occlusion pressure that may lead to pulmonary edema. Because rebound pulmonary arterial hypertension, increased intrapulmonary right to left shunting, and decreases in PaO_2 after abrupt discontinuation of inhaled NO have been described [138], gradual weaning is recommended. Before initiating inhaled NO, consideration should be given to the potential acute and long-term toxic effects. Acute inhaled NO overdose (>500 to 1,000 ppm) can result in the formation of nitrogen dioxide, methemoglobinemia, pulmonary alveolar edema and hemorrhage, hypoxemia, and death [139].

In summary, inhaled NO represents an experimental and costly therapy used to treat disease states characterized by pulmonary hypertension. Although it is useful in assessing potential pulmonary vasoresponsiveness to pharmacologic therapy, there is no evidence that the use of NO has any effects on survival [135,140].

NASAL CONTINUOUS POSITIVE AIRWAY PRESSURE FOR SLEEP-RELATED BREATHING DISORDERS

CPAP is an effective treatment for clinically significant obstructive sleep apnea/hypopnea syndrome, oxyhemoglobin desaturation, and respiratory event-related sleep arousals. This therapy is associated with improved morbidity due to reductions in daytime somnolence and improved cardiopulmonary function. Although further study of the long-term effects of CPAP is necessary, data suggest a possible reduction in mortality [141]. Since 1981, its efficacy has been repeatedly demonstrated [142]. Multiple controlled studies have shown that nasal CPAP can also be effective in patients with chronic left ventricular failure and Cheyne–Stokes respirations [3]. In these patients, nasal CPAP improved cardiac function and alleviated symptoms of heart failure and sleep-disordered breathing. Nasal CPAP has been shown to reverse central sleep apneas in some patients [143]. Simple snoring that is not associated with pauses in respiration or with clinical impairment is generally not treated with CPAP [141]. The use of CPAP and bilevel positive airways pressure (BiPAP) in the management of patients with acute respiratory failure is discussed in Chapter 59.

Application

Nasal CPAP acts as a pneumatic splint to prevent upper airway collapse. Patients usually respond rapidly to 3 to 15 cm H_2O. The optimal CPAP pressure is determined by a nocturnal polysomnogram in which pressure is titrated upward until sleep-related breathing events are eliminated [144]. Lack of response is often due to a poorly applied mask or patient intolerance [143]. Compliance rates can vary considerably (46% to 89%) [144].

Multiple nasal delivery devices are available that may improve patient comfort, including a variety of nasal and full-face masks. Rare serious complications [145] include bilateral bacterial conjunctivitis, massive epistaxis due to drying of nasal mucosa in a patient with coagulopathy, and worsening obstruction in a patient with a large lax epiglottis.

Because nasal CPAP is very effective, safe, and reasonably well tolerated, it has become the technique of choice in the treatment of idiopathic obstructive sleep apnea (i.e., no correctable anatomic abnormality identified). Relative contraindications include the presence of bullous lung disease and recurrent sinus or ear infections. There are no absolute contraindications [3]. It is important to realize that uvulopalatopharyngoplasty may compromise nasal CPAP therapy by increasing mouth air leak and reducing the maximal level of pressure that can be tolerated, and it benefits only some patients [146].

Alternative Modality

For patients with sleep apnea/hypopnea syndrome who cannot tolerate nasal CPAP because of the sensation of excessive pressure, nasal or full-face mask bilevel ventilation may be more tolerable. This permits independent adjustments of inspiratory positive airway pressure and expiratory positive airway pressure and has eliminated sleep-disordered breathing at lower levels of expiratory airway pressure compared with conventional nasal CPAP therapy in some patients [3].

COMMUNICATION ALTERNATIVES FOR THE PATIENT WITH AN ARTIFICIAL AIRWAY

Anxiety and fear are common emotions experienced by patients during mechanical ventilation. These emotions have been associated with the experience of agony/panic and insecurity related to the inability to communicate [147]. Patients with endotracheal and tracheostomy tubes in place experience these feelings because the tubes interfere with normal verbal communication. Providing a means of communication for patients undergoing mechanical ventilation has been shown to significantly increase patient satisfaction [148].

Intubation with cuffed, inflated intratracheal tubes impairs verbal communication because it blocks the normal airflow through the vocal cords. Deflated cuffed or cuffless tubes, generally reserved for spontaneously breathing patients, allow verbal communication, provided there is no pathologic obstruction (e.g., edema and granulation tissue or excessive secretions) blocking the passage of air through or above the vocal cords.

Communication Aids and Devices

A variety of communication aids are available depending on the situation [148]. A speech therapist can be indispensable in helping to select which aid is best for your patient.

Partial cuff deflation methods can be used in nonventilator- and ventilator-dependent patients. They are most commonly used in the nonventilator situation. Their use in the ventilator situation requires extremely close monitoring of the patient along with ventilator adjustments.

In the nonventilator-dependent patient, one can use deflation of the tracheostomy cuff with intermittent gloved finger occlusion of the tube or a device with a one-way valve (e.g., Passy-Muir Valve [PMV], Passy-Muir, Inc, Irvine, CA). The PMV is a one-way, positive-closure, no-leak valve that attaches to the hub of tracheostomy tubes (including cuffless fenestrated and nonfenestrated tubes, metal tubes, and cuffed tubes with the cuff fully deflated) [149]. It is indicated for awake and alert tracheostomized patients with sufficient air passage around the tracheostomy tube (or through a fenestrated tube) and through the upper airway. When the patient inhales, the PMV opens, allowing air to enter the lungs through the tracheostomy tube. As exhalation begins, the PMV closes, and remains closed through exhalation so that air is redirected around (or through) the tracheostomy tube, allowing for speech as the air passes through the vocal cords. Oxygen can be administered with the PMV in place at the tracheostomy tube site via oxygen mask, trach collar, or O_2 adapter. When using the PMV on tracheostomy tubes that have an inner cannula grasp ring that extends beyond the hub of the tube, the inner cannula should be removed when the PMV is in use to avoid obstruction of the valve's diaphragm movement.

In the ventilator-dependent patient, one can use partial deflation of the tracheostomy cuff alone or the one-way valve with *full* cuff deflation. During mechanical ventilation, both methods require close monitoring of the patient and the ventilator. Because use of the PMV with ventilator-dependent patients requires the cuff to be deflated, adjustments in tidal volume may be necessary to offset the volume loss caused by the air leak. Contraindications to the use of the one-way valve include the presence of an inflated cuff, absolute necessity for the cuff to remain fully inflated, tracheal/laryngeal obstruction or secretions preventing air from moving around or above the tube, laryngectomy, bilateral vocal cord paralysis, unconsciousness, and unstable medical condition [3]. Use of the valve with an inflated cuff can result in breath stacking with resultant intrinsic PEEP and barotrauma [150]. Because less-exhaled volume is returned to the ventilator with the deflated cuff methods, ventilator-exhaled volume alarms have to be adjusted [151]. Lack of intact oral and laryngeal musculature in some patients with neuromuscular diseases may preclude effective use of the valve [151].

For patients who cannot tolerate cuff deflation, a talking tracheostomy tube (Trach Talk, Portex, Inc, Keene, NH) is available to allow for whispered speech. A gas line is connected to air or oxygen, and when the thumb seal on the line is occluded, gas passes through the larynx, allowing the patient to speak.

The electronic larynx is a handheld mechanical device that can be used by patients who have undergone laryngectomy.

TABLE 62.1

ADVANCES IN RESPIRATORY ADJUNCT THERAPY

Topic	Reference	Findings
Aerosolized mist for croup	[2]	No benefit
Bland aerosols for CF	[2,4]	7% Saline improved FVC and FEV_1 vs. 0.9% saline
Humidification for ventilated patients	[9]	No difference in safety between heated water baths and HMEFs
Delivery of inhaled β agonist	[3]	No difference between MDI and nebulizer
NAC for COPD	[27]	No improvement on lung function or exacerbations vs. placebo
DNase of CF	[2]	Decrease in dyspnea and exacerbations vs. placebo
DNase for bronchiectasis	[32,33]	No benefit over placebo
DNase for RSV bronchiolitis	[34]	Improvement in chest radiographic findings vs. placebo
Aerosolized ribavirin for RSV	[3,42]	No effect vs. placebo
Iloprost for PPH	[52]	Improved 6-min walk, dyspnea, and hemodynamics vs. placebo
Inhaled cyclosporin for lung transplant	[53]	Improved survival and less rejection vs. placebo
Furosemide for mucociliary clearance	[66]	No improvement vs. placebo
Flutter valve for CF	[70]	As efficacious as CPT
High-frequency oscillation for CF	[72]	As efficacious as CPT
High-flow oxygen for cluster headaches	[87]	Significantly decreases pain within 15 min
Inhaled NO	[135,140]	No improvement in survival in ARDS/ALI
Iloprost for acute pulmonary hypertension after cardiac surgery	[51]	More effective than inhaled NO
Perioperative supplemental O_2	[96]	Decreases wound infections with 80% FIO_2 vs. 30% FIO_2

CF, cystic fibrosis; COPD, chronic obstructive pulmonary disease; DNase, recombinant human deoxyribonuclease; FEV_1, forced expiratory volume in 1 second; FIO_2, fractional inspiration of oxygen; FVC, forced vital capacity; HMEF, hydroscopic condenser humidifier; MDI, metered-dose inhaler; NAC, *N*-acetylcysteine; PPH, primary pulmonary hypertension; RSV, respiratory syncytial virus; NO, nitric oxide.

When pressed into the soft tissue of the neck, it generates a vibratory sound that escapes through the mouth and is articulated by the lips, tongue, and palate. Its disadvantage is the metallic-type sound that is produced [152]. The Blom–Singer tracheostoma valve (Forth Medical Ltd., Berkshire, UK) is available for prosthesis-assisted tracheoesophageal speech in postlaryngectomy voice rehabilitation [153]. Finally, a variety of computer-assisted communication devices and electric typewriters are available, but are usually considered for patients requiring long-term mechanical ventilation because of their complexity and expense [3].

Advances in respiratory adjunct therapy, based on randomized controlled trials or meta-analyses of such trials, are summarized in Table 62.1.

References

1. Brain J: Aerosol and humidity therapy. *Am Rev Respir Dis* 122:12, 1990.
2. Bott J, Blumenthal S, Buxton M, et al: Guidelines for the physiotherapy management of the adult, medical, spontaneously breathing patient. *Thorax* 64[Suppl 1]:i1, 2009.
3. Kopec SE, Connolly AE, Irwin RS: Respiratory adjunct therapy, in Irwin RS, Rippe JM (eds): *Intensive Care Medicine*. 6th ed. Philadelphia, PA, Lippincott Williams and Wilkins, 2007, p 705.
4. Elkins MR, Robinson M, Rose BR, et al: A controlled trial of long-term inhaled hypertonic saline in patients with cystic fibrosis. *N Engl J Med* 354:229, 2006.
5. American Thoracic Society/European Respiratory Society: Standards for the diagnosis and care of patients with chronic obstructive pulmonary disease. *Am J Respir Crit Care Med* 152:577, 1995.
6. Fink J: Humidity and bland aerosol therapy, in Wilkins RL, Stoller JK, Scanlan CL (eds): *Egan's Fundamentals of Respiratory Care*. 8th ed. St. Louis, Mosby, 2003, p 737.
7. AARC: Clinical practice guidelines. Humidification during mechanical ventilation. *Respir Care* 37:887, 1992.
8. Shelley MP, Lloyd GM, Park GR: A review of the mechanisms and the methods of humidification of inspired gas. *Intensive Care Med* 14:1, 1988.
9. Hurni J-M, Feihl F, Lazor R, et al: Safety of combined heat and moisture exchanger filters in long-term mechanical ventilation. *Chest* 111:686, 1997.
10. American College of Chest Physicians: NHLBI. National conference on oxygen therapy. *Respir Care* 29:922, 1984.
11. Chanques G, Constantin JM, Sauter M, et al: Discomfort associated with underhumidified high-flow oxygen therapy in critically ill patients. *Intens Care Med* 35:996, 2009.
12. Anonymous: Ralstonia associated with Vapotherm oxygen delivery devices. *MMWR Morb Mortal Wkly Rep* 54:1052, 2005.
13. Robinson BR, Athota KP, Branson RD: Inhalational therapies for the ICU. *Current Opin in Crit Care* 15:1, 2009.
14. Fink J: Aerosol drug therapy, in Wilkins RL, Stoller JK, Scanlan CL (eds): *Egan's Fundamentals of Respiratory Care*. 8th ed. St. Louis, Mosby, 2003, p 761.
15. National Asthma Education and Prevention Program. Expert Panel Report 2: Guidelines for the diagnosis and management of asthma. Bethesda. 2002 update: National Institutes of Health, NHLBI, NIH Publication no. 97–4051. Available at www.nhlbi.nih.gov/guidelines/asthma/asthgdln.htm.
16. GOLD Scientific Committee: Global strategy for the diagnosis, management, and prevention of chronic obstructive pulmonary disease. Bethesda, MD: National Heart, Lung, and Blood Institute/World Health Organization, National Institute of Health, 2005 update. Available at http://www.goldcopd.com.
17. Cates CJ, Crilly JA, Rowe BH: Holding chambers versus nebulizers for beta-agonist treatment of acute asthma. *Cochrane Database Syst Rev* 6, 2010.
18. Shrestha M, Bidadi K, Gourlay S, et al: Continuous vs. intermittent albuterol, at high and low doses, in the treatment of severe acute asthma in adults. *Chest* 110:42, 1996.
19. Dhand R, Tobin MJ: Inhaled bronchodilator therapy in mechanically ventilated patients. *Am J Respir Crit Care Med* 156:3, 1997.
20. Allon M, Dunlay R, Copkney C: Nebulized albuterol for acute hyperkalemia in patients on hemodialysis. *Ann Intern Med* 110:426, 1989.
21. Lotvall J, Palmqvist M, Arvidsson P, et al: The therapeutic ratio of R-albuterol is comparable with that of RS-albuterol in asthmatic patients. *J Allergy Clin Immunol* 108:726, 2001.
22. Peters JI, Shelledy, DC, Jones AP, et al: A randomized, placebo-controlled study to evaluate the role of salmeterol in the in-hospital management of asthma. *Chest* 118:313, 2000.
23. Winston SJ, Gravelyn TR, Sitrin RG: Prevention of bradycardic responses to endotracheal suctioning by prior administration of nebulized atropine. *Crit Care Med* 15:1009, 1987.
24. Wick MM, Ingram RH: Bronchorrhea responsive to aerosolized atropine. *JAMA* 235:1356, 1976.
25. Rodrigo G, Rodrigo C, Burschtin O: A meta-analysis of the effects of ipratropium bromide in adults with acute asthma. *Am J Med* 107:363, 1999.
26. Irwin RS, Thomas HM III: Mucoid impaction of the bronchus: diagnosis and treatment. *Am Rev Respir Dis* 108:955, 1973.
27. Decramer M, Rutten-van Molken M, Dekhuijzen PN, et al: Effects of N-acetylcysteine on outcome in chronic obstructive pulmonary disease. *Lancet* 365:1552, 2005.
28. Duijvestijn YC, Brand PL: Systemic review of N-acetylcysteine in cystic fibrosis. *Acta Paediatr* 88:38, 1999.
29. Miller AC, Rivero A, Ziad S, et al: Influence of nebulized unfractionated heparin and N-acetylcysteine in acute lung injury after smoke inhalation injury. *J Burn Care Res* 30:249, 2009.
30. Rao S, Wilson DB, Brooks RC, et al: Acute effects of nebulization of N-acetylcysteine on pulmonary mechanics and gas exchange. *Am Rev Respir Dis* 102:17, 1970.
31. Wilmott RW, Amin RS, Colin AA, et al: Aerosolized recombinant human DNase in hospitalized cystic fibrosis patients with acute pulmonary exacerbations. *Am J Respir Crit Care Med* 153:1914, 1996.
32. O'Donnell AE, Barker AF, Ilowite JS, et al: Treatment of idiopathic bronchiectasis with aerosolised recombinant human DNase 1. *Chest* 113:1329, 1998.
33. Wills PJ, Wodehouse T, Corkery K, et al: Short-term recombinant human DNase in bronchiectasis. *Am J Respir Crit Care Med* 154:413, 1996.
34. Nasr SZ, Strouse PJ, Soskolone E, et al: Efficacy of recombinant human deoxyribonuclease I in the hospital management of respiratory syncytial virus bronchiolitis. *Chest* 120:203, 2001.
35. Fiel SB: Aerosolized antibiotics in cystic fibrosis: current and future trends. *Expert Rev Respir Med* 2:479, 2008.
36. LoBue PA: Inhaled tobramycin: not just for cystic fibrosis anymore. *Chest* 127:1098, 2005.
37. MacIntyre NR, Rubin BK: Should aerosolized antibiotics be administered to prevent or treat ventilator-associated pneumonia in patients who do not have cystic fibrosis. *Respir Care* 52:416, 2007.
38. Mutti P, Wang C, Hickey AJ. Inhaled drug delivery for tuberculosis therapy. *Pharm Res* 26:2401, 2009.
39. FDA MedWatch: www.fda.gov/medwatch/report.htm; Accessed June 28, 2007.
40. Coates AL, MacNeish CF, Meisner D, et al: The choice of jet nebulizer, nebulizing flow, and addition of albuterol affects the output of tobramycin aerosols. *Chest* 111:1206, 1997.
41. Palmer LB, Smaldone GC, Simon SR, et al: Aerosolized antibiotics in mechanically ventilated patients: delivery and response. *Crit Care Med* 26(1):31, 1998.
42. Ebbert JO, Limper AH: Respiratory syncytial virus pneumonitis in immunocompromised adults: clinical features and outcome. *Respiration* 72:263, 2005.
43. Knight V, Gilbert BE: Ribavirin aerosol treatment for influenza. *Infect Dis Clinic North Am* 1:441, 1987.
44. Rodriguez WJ, Hall CB, Welliver R, et al: Efficacy and safety of aerosolized ribavirin in young children hospitalized with influenza. *J Pediatr* 125:129, 1994.
45. Fujii T, Nakamura T, Iwamoto A: Current concepts in SARS treatment. *J Infect Chemo* 10:1, 2004.
46. Krilov L: Safety issues related to the administration of ribavirin. *Pediatr Infect Dis J* 21:479, 2002.
47. Masur H: Prevention and treatment of *Pneumocystis* pneumonia. *N Engl J Med* 327:1853, 1992.
48. McIvor RA, Berger P, Pack LL, et al: An effectiveness community-based clinical trial of Respirgard II and Fisoneb nebulizers for *Pneumocystis carinii* prophylaxis with aerosol pentamidine in HIV-infected individuals. *Chest* 110:141, 1996.
49. McDiarmid MA, Fujikawa J, Schaefer J, et al: Health effects and exposure assessment of aerosolized pentamidine handlers. *Chest* 104:382, 1993.
50. Walsh P, Caldwell J, McQuillan KK, et al: Comparison of nebulized epinephrine to albuterol in bronchiolitis. *Acad Emerg Med* 15:305, 2008.
51. Winterhalter M, Simon A, Fischer S, et al: Comparison of inhaled iloprost and nitric oxide in patients with pulmonary hypertension during weaning from cardiopulmonary bypass in cardiac surgery: a prospective study. *J Cardiovasc Vasc Anesth* 22:406, 2008.
52. Olschewski H, Simonneau G, Galie N, et al: Inhaled iloprost for severe pulmonary hypertension. *N Engl J Med* 347:322, 2002.
53. Iacono AT, Johnson BA, Grgurich WF, et al: A randomized trial of inhaled cyclosporin in lung-transplant recipients. *N Engl J Med* 354:141, 2006.
54. Grossman J: The evolution of inhaler technology. *J Asthma* 31(1):55, 1994.
55. Tinkelman DG, Berkowitz RB, Cole WQ III: Aerosols in the treatment of asthma. *J Asthma* 28:243, 1991.

56. Turner MO, Patel A, Ginsburg S, et al: Bronchodilator delivery in acute airflow obstruction: a meta-analysis. *Arch Intern Med* 157(15):1736, 1997.
57. Jasper AC, Mohsenifar Z, Kahan S, et al: Cost-benefit comparison of aerosol bronchodilator delivery methods in hospitalized patients. *Chest* 91(4):614, 1987.
58. Murray JF: Indications for mechanical aids to assist lung inflation in medical patients. *Am Rev Respir Dis* 122(1):121, 1980.
59. Bartlett RH: Postoperative pulmonary prophylaxis: breathe deeply and read carefully. *Chest* 81:1, 1982.
60. Mahlmeister MJ, Fink JB, Hoffman GL, et al: Positive-expiratory pressure mask therapy: theoretical and practical considerations and a review of the literature. *Respir Care* 36:1218, 1991.
61. Indihar FJ, Forsberg DP, Adams AB: A prospective comparison of three procedures used in attempts to prevent postoperative pulmonary complications. *Respir Care* 27:564, 1982.
62. Demers RR, Irwin RS, Braman SS, et al: Variable accuracy of five commercially available incentive spirometers. *Am Rev Respir Dis* 117[Suppl]:108, 1978.
63. Torrington KG, Sorenson DE, Sherwood LM: Postoperative chest percussion with postural drainage in obese patients following gastric stapling. *Chest* 86:891, 1984.
64. McCool FD, Rosen MJ: Nonpharmacologic airway clearance therapies. *Chest* 129[Suppl 1]:250S, 2006.
65. Salathe M, O'Riordan TG, Wanner A: Treatment of mucociliary dysfunction. *Chest* 110:1048, 1996.
66. Hasani A, Pavia D, Spitery MA, et al: Inhaled furosemide does not affect lung mucociliary clearance in healthy and asthmatic subjects. *Eur Respir J* 7:1497, 1994.
67. Marom Z, Shelhamer J, Alling D, et al: The effects of corticosteroids on mucous glycoprotein secretion from human airways in vitro. *Am Rev Respir Dis* 129:62, 1984.
68. Kaliner M, Maron Z, Patow C, et al: Human respiratory mucus. *J Allergy Clin Immunol* 73:318, 1986.
69. van der Schans CP: Conventional chest physical therapy for obstructive lung disease. *Respir Care* 52:1198, 2007.
70. Tyler ML: Complications of positioning and chest physiotherapy. *Respir Care* 27:458, 1982.
71. Konstan MW, Stern RC, Doershuk CF: Efficacy of the flutter device for airway mucous clearance in patients with cystic fibrosis. *J Pediatr* 124:689, 1994.
72. Homnick DN, Anderson K, Marks JH: Comparison of the flutter device to standard therapy in hospitalized patients with cystic fibrosis: a pilot study. *Chest* 114(4):993, 1998.
73. Homnick DN, White F, deCastro C: Comparison of effects of an intrapulmonary percussive ventilator to standard aerosol and chest physiotherapy in treatment of cystic fibrosis. *Pediatr Pulmonol* 20:50, 1995.
74. Lange DJ, Lechtzin N, Davey C, et al: High-frequency chest wall oscillation in ALS. *Neurology* 67:991, 2006.
75. Elkins MR, Jones A, vander Schans C: Positive expiratory pressure physiotherapy for airway clearance in people with cystic fibrosis. *Cochrane Database Syst Rev* 2, 2004.
76. Tzeng AC, Bach RJ: Prevention of pulmonary mortality for patients with neuromuscular disease. *Chest* 118:1390, 2000.
77. Anonymous: Endotracheal suctioning of mechanically ventilated adults and children with artificial airways. AARC clinical practice guideline. *Respir Care* 38:500, 1993.
78. Rau JL: Airway management, in Wilkins RL, Stoller JK, Scanlan CL (eds): *Egan's Fundamentals of Respiratory Care*. 8th ed. St. Louis, Mosby, 2003, p 627.
79. Gracey DR, Divertie MB, Howard FM Jr: Mechanical ventilation for respiratory failure in myasthenia gravis: two-year experience with 22 patients. *Mayo Clin Proc* 58:597, 1983.
80. Bach JR, Saporito LR: Criteria for extubation and tracheostomy tube removal for patients with ventilatory failure: a different approach to weaning. *Chest* 110:1566, 1996.
81. Irwin RS, Curley FJ, Bennett FM: Appropriate use of antitussives and protussives: a practical review. *Drugs* 46:80, 1993.
82. Donaldson SH, Bennett WD, Zeman KL, et al: Mucus clearance and lung function in cystic fibrosis with hypertonic saline. *N Engl J Med* 354:241, 2006.
83. Estenne M, Knoop C, Vanvaierenber J, et al: The effect of pectoralis muscle training in tetraplegic subjects. *Am Rev Respir Dis* 112:22, 1989.
84. Lang SW, Back JR: Maximum insufflation capacity. *Chest* 118:61, 2000.
85. American Association for Respiratory Care: Clinical practice guideline: oxygen therapy in the acute care hospital. *Respir Care* 36:1410, 1991.
86. Fulmer JD, Snider GL: ACCP-NHLBI National Conference on Oxygen Therapy. *Chest* 86:234, 1984.
87. Cohen AS, Burns B, Goadsby PJ: High-flow oxygen for the treatment of cluster headaches: a randomized trial. *JAMA* 302:2451, 2009.
88. Bateman NT, Leach RM: ABC of oxygen: acute oxygen therapy. *BMJ* 317:798, 1998.
89. Antman EM, Anbe DT, Armstrong PE, et al: ACC/AHA guidelines for the management of patients with ST-elevation myocardial infarction: a report of the American College of Cardiology/American Heart Association Task Force on Practice Guidelines (Committee on Management of Acute Myocardial Infarction). *Circulation* 110:588, 2004.
90. Fillmore SJ, Shapiro M, Killip T: Arterial oxygen tension in acute myocardial infarction: serial analysis of clinical state and blood gas changes. *Am Heart J* 79:620, 1970.
91. Maroko PR, Radvany P, Braunwald E, et al: Reduction of infarct size by oxygen inhalation following acute coronary occlusion. *Circulation* 52:360, 1975.
92. Madias JE, Madias NE, Hood WB Jr: Precordial ST-segment mapping. 2. Effects of oxygen inhalation on ischemic injury in patients with acute myocardial infarction. *Circulation* 53[Suppl]:411, 1976.
93. Ballester E, Reyes A, Roca J, et al: Ventilation-perfusion mismatching in acute severe asthma: effects of salbutamol and 100% oxygen. *Thorax* 44:258, 1989.
94. Ilano AL, Raffin TA: Management of carbon monoxide poisoning. *Chest* 97:165, 1990.
95. Embury SH, Garcia JF, Mohandas N, et al: Effects of oxygen inhalation on endogenous erythropoietin kinetics, erythropoiesis, and properties of blood cells in sickle-cell anemia. *N Engl J Med* 311:291, 1984.
96. May A: Cluster headaches: pathogenesis, diagnosis, and management. *Lancet* 366:843, 2005.
97. Greif R, Ozan A, Horn EP, et al: Supplemental perioperative oxygen to reduce the incidence of surgical-wound infection. *N Engl J Med* 342:161, 2000.
98. Belda FJ, Aguilera L, Garcia da la Asuncion J, et al: Supplemental perioperative oxygen and the risk of surgical wound infection: a randomized controlled trial. *JAMA* 294:2035, 2005.
99. Fairley HB: Oxygen therapy for surgical patients. *Am Rev Respir Dis* 122:37, 1980.
100. Hunt G: Gas therapy, in Fink JB, Hunt GE (eds): *Clinical Practice in Respiratory Care*. Philadelphia, PA: Lippincott Williams & Wilkins, 1999, p 274.
101. Tiep BL, Burns M, Hererra J: A new pendant oxygen conserving cannula which allows pursed lips breathing. *Chest* 95:857, 1989.
102. Farney RJ, Walker JM, Elmer JC, et al: Transtracheal oxygen therapy for the treatment of obstructive sleep apnea. *Op Tech Otolaryngol Head Neck Surg* 2:132, 1991.
103. Woolf CR: Arterial blood gas levels after oxygen therapy. *Chest* 69:808, 1976.
104. Grant I, Heaton RK, McSweeney AJ, et al: Neuropsychologic findings in hypoxemic chronic obstructive pulmonary disease. *Arch Intern Med* 142:1470, 1982.
105. Sackner MA, Landa J, Hirsch J, et al: Pulmonary effects of oxygen breathing: a 6-hour study in normal man. *Ann Intern Med* 82:40, 1975.
106. Mak S, Azevoda E, Liu PP, et al: Effect of hyperoxia on left ventricular function and filling pressures in patients with and without congestive heart failure. *Chest* 120:467, 2001.
107. Ingrassia TS, Ryu JH, Trastek VF, et al: Oxygen exacerbated bleomycin pulmonary toxicity. *Mayo Clin Proc* 66:173, 1991.
108. Kay GN, Epstein AE, Kirklin JK, et al: Fatal postoperative amiodarone pulmonary toxicity. *Am J Cardiol* 62:490, 1988.
109. Camus P, Martin WJ, Rosenow EC: Amiodarone pulmonary toxicity. *Clin Chest Med* 25:65, 2005.
110. Ernest A, Zimrak JD: Current concepts: carbon monoxide poisoning. *N Engl J Med* 339(22):1603, 1998.
111. Hampson NB, Rugg RA, Hauff NM: Increased long-term mortality among survivors of acute carbon monoxide poisoning. *Crit Care Med* 37:1941, 2009.
112. Jallai N, Withey S, Butler PE: Hyperbaric oxygen as adjuvant therapy in the management of necrotizing fasciitis. *Am J Surg* 189:462, 2005.
113. Tibbles PM, Edelsberg JS: Medical progress: hyperbaric-oxygen therapy. *N Engl J Med* 334(25):1642, 1996.
114. George ME, Rueth NM, Skarda DE, et al: Hyperbaric oxygen does not improve outcome in patients with necrotizing soft tissue infection. *Surg Infect* 10:21, 2009.
115. Bennett MH, Trytko B, Jonker B: Hyperbaric oxygen therapy for the adjunctive treatment of traumatic brain injury. *Cochrane Database Syst Rev* 4, 2005.
116. Bennett MH, Wasiak J, Schnabel A, et al: Hyperbaric oxygen therapy for acute ischaemic stroke. *Cochrane Database Syst Rev* 4, 2005.
117. Bennett MH, Jepson N, Lehm J: Hyperbaric oxygen therapy for acute coronary syndrome. *Cochrane Database Syst Rev* 4, 2005.
118. Duncan PG: Efficacy of helium-oxygen mixtures in the management of severe viral and post-intubation croup. *Can Anesth Soc J* 26:206, 1979.
119. Lu TS, Ohmura A, Wong KC, et al: Helium-oxygen in treatment of upper airway obstruction. *Anesthesiology* 45:678, 1976.
120. Rodrigo GJ, Rodrigo C, Pollack CV, et al: Use of helium-oxygen mixtures in the treatment of acute asthma: a systematic review. *Chest* 123:676, 2003.
121. Rodrigo GJ, Pollack CV, Rodrigo C, et al: Heliox for non-intubated acute asthma patients. *Cochrane Database Syst Rev* 4, 2003.
122. Kim IK, Phrampus E, Venkataraman S, et al: Helium/oxygen-driven albuterol nebulization in the treatment of children with moderate to severe asthma exacerbations: a randomized controlled trial. *Pediatrics* 116:1127, 2005.
123. Rivers ML, Kim TY, Stewart GM, et al: Albuterol nebulized in heliox in the initial ED treatment of pediatric asthma: a blinded, randomized trial. *Am J Emerg Med* 24:38, 2006.

124. O'Callaghan C, White J, Jackson J, et al: The effects of heliox on the output and particle-size distribution of salbutamol using jet and vibrating mesh nebulizers. *J Aerosol Med* 20:434, 2007.
125. Vorwerk C, Coats TJ: Use of helium-oxygen mixtures in the treatment of croup: a systematic review. *Emerg Med* 25:547, 2008.
126. Pingleton SK, Bone RC, Ruth WC: Helium-oxygen mixtures during bronchoscopy. *Crit Care Med* 18:50, 1980.
127. Gluck EH, Onorato DJ, Castriotta R: Helium-oxygen mixtures in intubated patients with status asthmaticus and respiratory acidosis. *Chest* 98:693, 1990.
128. Hess DR, Acosta FL, Ritz RH, et al: The effect of heliox on nebulizer function using a beta-agonist bronchodilator. *Chest* 115:184, 1999.
129. Rodrigo R, Pollack CV, Rodrigo GJ, et al: Heliox for treatment of exacerbations of chronic obstructive pulmonary disease. *Cochrane Database Syst Rev* 3, 2002.
130. Madison JM, Irwin RS: Heliox for asthma: a trial balloon. *Chest* 107:597, 1995.
131. Steudel W, Hurford WE, Zapol M: Inhaled nitric oxide: basic biology and clinical applications. *Anesthesiology* 91:1090, 1999.
132. The Neonatal Inhaled Nitric Oxide Study Group: Inhaled nitric oxide in full-term and nearly full-term infants with hypoxic respiratory failure. *N Engl J Med* 333:597, 1997.
133. Roberts JD Jr, Fineman JR, Morin FC III, et al: Inhaled nitric oxide and persistent pulmonary hypertension of the newborn. The Inhaled Nitric Oxide Study Group. *N Engl J Med* 336:605, 1997.
134. Rosenberg AA, Kennaugh JM, Moreland SG, et al: Longitudinal follow-up of a cohort of newborn infants treated with inhaled nitric oxide for persistent pulmonary hypertension. *J Pediatr* 131:70, 1997.
135. Griffiths MJ, Evans TW: Inhaled nitric oxide therapy in adults. *N Engl J Med* 353:2683, 2005.
136. Sokol J, Jacobs SE, Bohn D: Inhaled nitric oxide for acute hypoxemic respiratory failure in children and adults. *Cochrane Database Syst Rev* 4, 2005.
137. Zapol WM, Rimar S, Gills N, et al: Nitric oxide and the lung. *Am J Respir Crit Care Med* 149:1375, 1994.
138. Roissaint R, Falke KJ, Lopez F, et al: Inhaled nitric oxide for the adult respiratory distress syndrome. *N Engl J Med* 328:399, 1993.
139. Greenbaum R, Bay J, Hargreaves MD, et al: Effects of higher oxides of nitrogen on the anesthetized dog. *Br J Anaesth* 39:393, 1967.
140. Hunt CM: Nitric oxide in adult lung disease. *Chest* 115:1407, 1999.
141. Anonymous: Indications and standards for use of nasal continuous positive airway pressure (CPAP) in sleep apnea syndromes. Official ATS Statement. *Am J Respir Crit Care Med* 150:1738, 1994.
142. Strohl KP, Cherniack NS, Gothe B: Physiologic basis of therapy for sleep apnea. *Am Rev Respir Dis* 134:791, 1986.
143. Issa FG, Sullivan CE: Reversal of central sleep apnea using nasal CPAP. *Chest* 90:165, 1986.
144. Piccirillo JF, Duntley S, Schotland H: Obstructive sleep apnea. *JAMA* 284(12):1492, 2000.
145. Hudgel DW: Treatment of obstructive sleep apnea: a review. *Chest* 109:1346, 1996.
146. Mortimore IL, Bradley PA, Murray JAM, et al: Uvulopalatopharyngoplasty may compromise nasal CPAP therapy in sleep apnea syndrome. *Am J Respir Crit Care Med* 154:1759, 1996.
147. Bergbom-Engberg I, Haljamae H: Assessment of patients' experience of discomfort during respirator therapy. *Crit Care Med* 17:1068, 1989.
148. Stovsky B, Rudy E, Dragonette P: Comparison of two types of communication methods used after cardiac surgery with patients with endotracheal tubes. *Heart Lung* 17:281, 1988.
149. Williams ML: An algorithm for selecting a communication technique with intubated patients. *Dimens Crit Care Nurs* 11:222, 1992.
150. Kaul K, Turcott JC, Lavery M: Passy-Muir speaking valve. *Dimens Crit Care Nurs* 15:298, 1996.
151. Manzano JL, Santiago L, Henriquez D, et al: Verbal communication of ventilator dependent patients. *Crit Care Med* 21:512, 1993.
152. Coltart L: Voice restoration after laryngectomy. *Nurs Standard* 13(12):36, 1998.
153. Vanden Hoogen FJ, Meevwic C, Oudes MJ, et al: The Blom-Singer tracheostoma valve as a valuable addition in the rehabilitation of the laryngectomized patient. *Eur Arch Otorhinolaryngol* 253:126, 1996.

CHAPTER 63 ■ CHEST RADIOGRAPHIC EXAMINATION

CYNTHIA B. UMALI* AND JERRY P. BALIKIAN

Radiographic examination of the critically ill patient in the intensive care unit (ICU) or coronary care unit (CCU) is often necessary to evaluate clinical status. In this setting, the basic role of radiology is to follow the patient's progress or changes in status after admission or after surgery; the primary diagnosis has been already established. Radiographic examinations are thus requested to evaluate the course of the primary disease and to diagnose complications that may ensue. Henscke et al. [1] studied the diagnostic efficacy of bedside chest radiographs and found that in 65% of the 1,132 consecutive radiographs analyzed, there were new findings or changes affecting patient management. Bekemeyer et al. [2], after analyzing 1,354 radiographs from a respiratory ICU, found a 34.5% incidence of new or increased abnormalities or tube or catheter malpositions. They concluded that routine morning radiographic examinations frequently demonstrated unexpected or changing abnormalities, many of which prompted changes in diagnostic management. The American College of Radiology established the appropriateness criteria for the need of ICU studies [3] and Trotman-Dickenson detailed the role of radiology in the ICU [4,5].

Critically ill patients in the ICU or CCU often cannot take advantage of numerous radiologic modalities that are readily available to mobile patients. Because these patients cannot be transported while their circulatory functions are labile and they are connected to electrocardiogram monitors, ventilators, catheters, and surgical appliances, usually one is left with the portable bedside radiographic examination. Most often, it is a chest examination that is needed; the chest film is especially important because physical examination to determine the presence of a complication such as atelectasis, pneumothorax, pneumonia, or pulmonary edema is difficult in the presence of a ventilator.

Until recently, portable radiographic examinations were restricted by inherent machine limitations in kilovoltage, milliamperage, and radiograph tube currents and by variations in battery charge. The need for adequate penetration to see line and catheter positions necessitated increasing normal exposure time (thereby increasing motion unsharpness) and using a higher kilovoltage (thereby increasing scatter radiation, which increases film fogging). A high kilovoltage also reduces subject contrast. These alterations and limitations cause deterioration of the image, often rendering the film of suboptimal quality for evaluation of subtle changes in the lung parenchyma. During the past few years, most of the above problems have been

*Deceased

practically eliminated with the use of state-of-the-art computed radiography.

Interpretation of portable examinations is fraught with pitfalls. Magnification of the cardiac silhouette cannot be eliminated because of the short tube-film distance and the often supine position of the patient. Signs used to evaluate postcapillary (pulmonary venous) hypertension are not valid on the supine film and may necessitate use of a horizontal beam (cross-table lateral view) to visualize the discrepancy between the dependent and nondependent vessels, which is far more difficult.

Films are often taken after a poor inspiratory effort because of the patient's inability to cooperate. Unless the type of respirator, phase of cycle, and pressure setting are indicated on the film, the appearance of parenchymal abnormalities is difficult to evaluate. Increased inflation of the lung may cause the opacities to appear less dense, but the apparent improvement secondary to increased aeration does not correspond to a true anatomic improvement. The reverse situation can occur as well.

A portable C-arm fluoroscope is often used at the bedside to monitor catheter placement (especially Swan–Ganz). The fluoroscope also can be used to evaluate alignment of fracture fragments during closed reduction and to visualize diaphragmatic motion. Portable ultrasound equipment is particularly useful for detecting fluid collections, including effusions (pericardial and pleural) and subdiaphragmatic abscesses. Portable gamma cameras are useful for evaluating possible pulmonary embolism in these patients.

With PACCS systems in many ICUs, digital images are now available on ICU monitors immediately after the images are taken.

EVALUATION OF TUBES AND CATHETERS

Endotracheal Tubes

The location of endotracheal tubes should be checked as soon as possible after insertion (see Chapter 1). To evaluate the position of the tube properly, Goodman et al. [6] showed that one must evaluate the head and neck position simultaneously because tube position can change with flexion and extension of the neck [7] by as much as 4 cm. Thus, to ensure that the tip of the tube is above the carina, one should follow these guidelines:

1. When the inferior border of the mandible is at or above C4, the tip should be 7 ± 2 cm from the carina.
2. When the inferior border of the mandible is at the C5-C6 level, the tip of the tube should be 5 ± 2 cm from the carina.
3. When the inferior border of the mandible is at T1 or below, the tip of the tube should be 3 ± 2 cm from the carina.

When the tube is too high, it may slip into the pharynx. If it is just below the vocal cords, its inflated cuff can cause glottic or subglottic edema, ulceration, and, ultimately, scarring. If it is too low, it can enter a bronchus and cause atelectasis of the lung supplied by the obstructed bronchus (Fig. 63.1).

Ideally, the tube should be one-half to two-thirds the width of the trachea, and the inflated cuff should fill the trachea without causing the lateral walls to bulge. When the ratio of the cuff diameter to the tracheal lumen exceeds 1.5%, tracheal damage is likely to result [8]. Ravin et al. [9] observed that repeated overdistention of the cuff on chest film, despite careful cuff inflation to the minimal leak level, should lead to suspicion of tracheomalacia (Fig. 63.2).

Immediately after intubation, and especially after difficult intubation, a film should be obtained to define the position of the tube. The radiologist should also look for signs of perforation of the pharynx, such as marked subcutaneous emphysema, pneumomediastinum, and pneumothorax. Dislodging of teeth, dental caps, and portions of dentures into the tracheobronchial tree has been reported after intubation. If this is suspected, a foreign body in the tracheobronchial tree should be carefully sought.

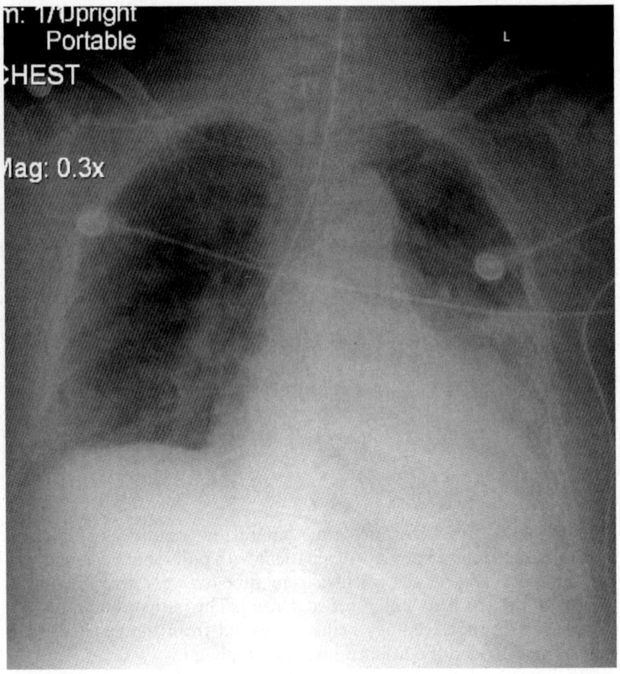

FIGURE 63.1. Endotracheal tube is 2 cm within the right main bronchus. As a result, there is partial obstruction of the orifice of the left main bronchus causing left lower lobe atelectasis. Recommend approximately 4 cm upward repositioning.

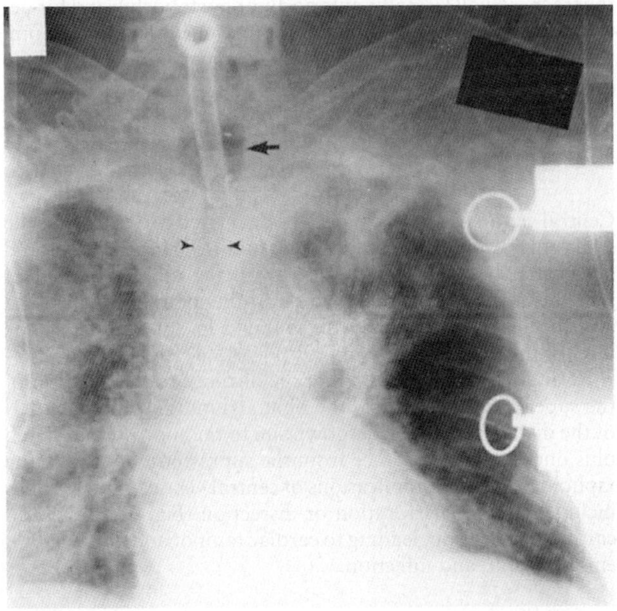

FIGURE 63.2. Overdistended tracheostomy tube cuff. Portable examination, anteroposterior view, in a patient with diffuse parenchymal infiltrates from acute respiratory distress syndrome with a tracheostomy tube. Lucent circular area (*arrow*) surrounding the tracheostomy tube is a distended cuff. It markedly exceeds normal tracheal diameter (*arrowheads*). This patient has tracheomalacia and has had the cuff reinflated to this size persistently after deflation and reinflation to the minimal leak level.

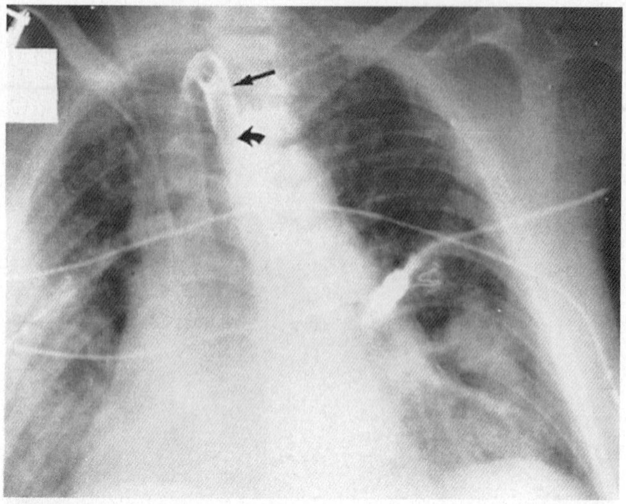

FIGURE 63.3. Tracheostomy tube lateral to shadow of trachea. Portable anteroposterior view of a patient with pulmonary edema, with the left lateral edge of the tracheostomy tube (*straight arrow*) lying to the left of the tracheal wall (*curved arrow*). The patient had a history of nasogastric tube feedings being recovered from the tracheostomy tube, which eroded the trachea into the esophagus.

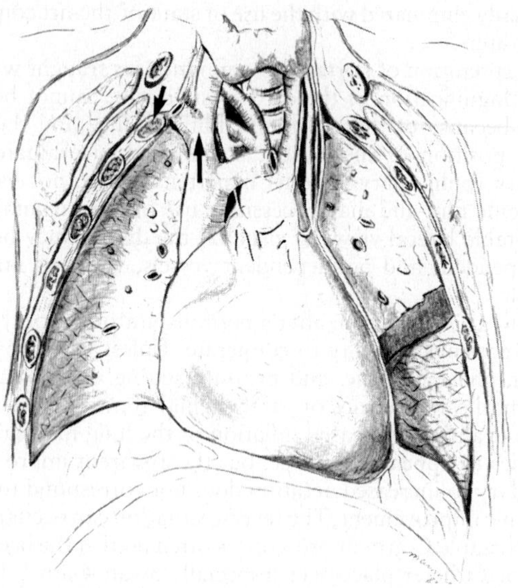

FIGURE 63.4. Junction of internal jugular vein and right subclavian vein. Veins shown in relation to the first rib. The junction of the internal jugular and right subclavian veins (*long arrow*) occurs at approximately the level of the first rib (*short arrow*). The central venous pressure line should be at or beyond this point to measure true venous pressure. (Drawing by Mary Cunnion.)

Tracheostomy Tubes

The tip of the tracheostomy tube should be located one-half to two-thirds of the way between the stoma and the carina. Unlike the endotracheal tube, the tracheostomy tube does not change position with flexion and extension of the neck. The tracheostomy tube should be evaluated to determine its inner diameter (which should be two-thirds that of the tracheal lumen); its long axis (which should parallel the tracheal lumen); the location of its distal end (Fig. 63.3) (which should not abut the tracheal wall laterally, anteriorly, or posteriorly); and for development of increasing pneumothorax, pneumomediastinum, or subcutaneous emphysema, which may require immediate attention.

Central Venous Catheters

Central venous catheters should be evaluated to ensure that the true central venous pressure is measured. The catheter should be located beyond the venous valves, the most proximal of which is just distal to the junction of the internal jugular vein and the subclavian veins. This is found at approximately the level of the first anterior rib [10] (Fig. 63.4) (see Chapter 2).

Brandt et al. [11] found that the distance to the junction of the superior vena cava and the right atrium is usually the total of the distance from the cutdown site to the suprasternal notch plus one-third the distance from the suprasternal notch to the xiphoid process. Complications of central venous catheter lines include vascular perforation or dissection (Fig. 63.5A,B) and cardiac perforation, leading to cardiac tamponade (Fig. 63.5C), embolization, and infection.

Swan–Ganz Catheters

Swan–Ganz catheters are used to perform right heart catheterizations [12]. Ideally, the tip of the Swan–Ganz catheter should be located in the right or left branch of the pulmonary artery. Occasionally, the tip may be malpositioned (Fig. 63.6); a film should be routinely taken to check its position. If it is more distal to the above location, the catheter may produce pulmonary infarction (Fig. 63.7) by blocking the artery directly or from a clot in or around the tip. Other rare complications include perforation of the pulmonary artery, the resulting focal hemorrhage leading to formation of "traumatic pseudoaneurysm" (Fig. 63.7D), balloon rupture, and pulmonary artery–bronchial tree fistulas.

Intra-Aortic Counterpulsation Balloons

The intra-aortic counterpulsation balloon (IACB) was designed to improve cardiac function in a setting of cardiogenic shock [13], and this remains the major indication for its use. Ideally, the tip of the IACB should be positioned at the level of the aortic arch just distal to the origin of the left subclavian artery to augment coronary perfusion maximally without occluding the subclavian and cerebral vessels (Fig. 63.8). Complications from IACBs are major vessel obstruction, embolization from a clot formed in or around the catheter, and aortic dissection with balloon rupture.

As with endotracheal tubes, the position of the IACB changes with a change in patient position, moving cephalad 1.0 to 4.5 cm when the patient moves from a recumbent to a sitting position [14]. The position, therefore, should be checked periodically.

Chest Tubes

Chest tubes (thoracostomy or pleural drainage tubes) are used to drain either fluid or air from the pleural space (see Chapter 8). If placed for a pneumothorax, the tube should be seen in the anterosuperior position as the air collects beneath the sternum; if placed to drain a pleural effusion, the tube should be seen in the posteroinferior position. To ascertain that the tube is in the pleural space, one must see opaque and nonopaque sides

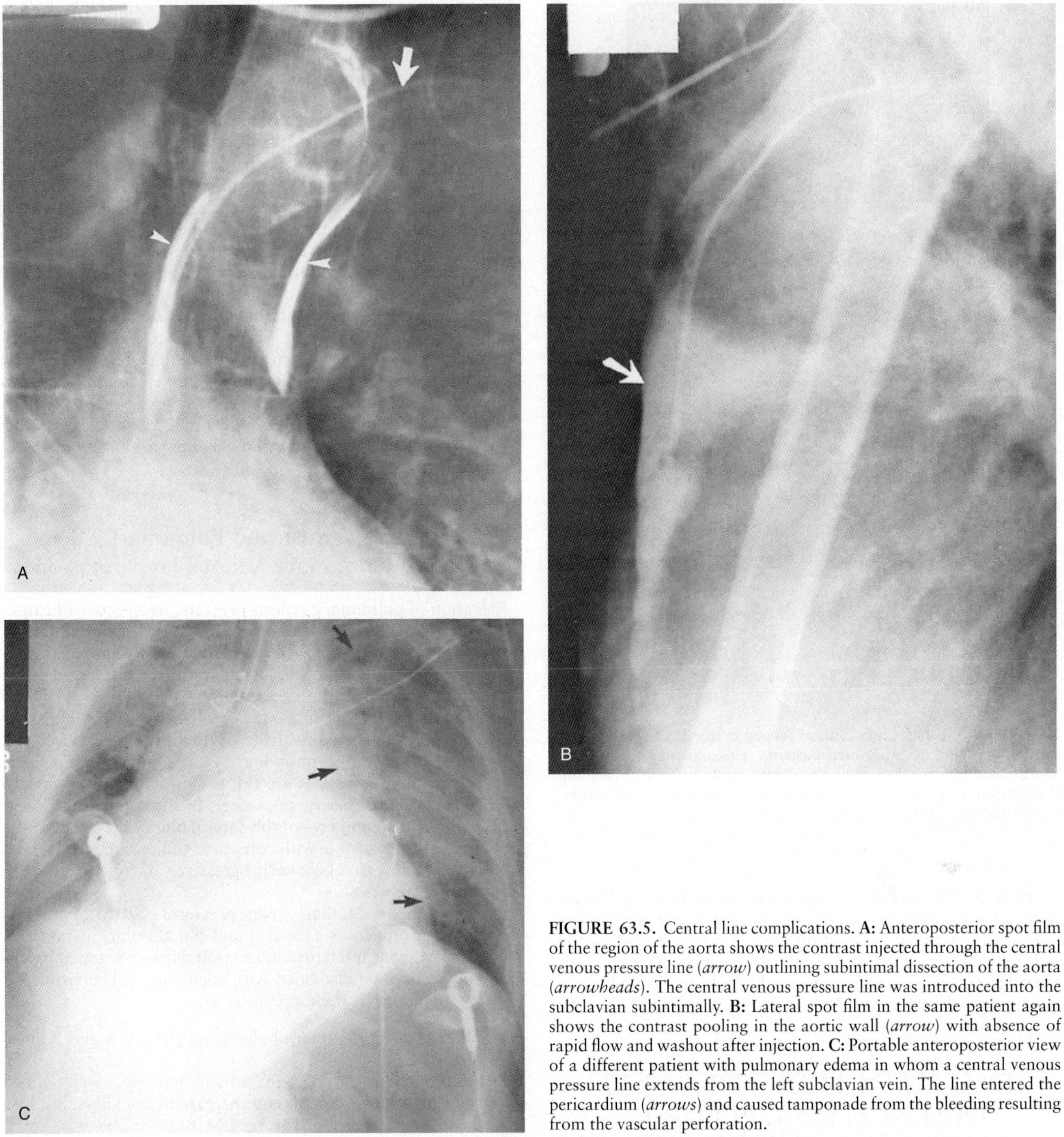

FIGURE 63.5. Central line complications. **A:** Anteroposterior spot film of the region of the aorta shows the contrast injected through the central venous pressure line (*arrow*) outlining subintimal dissection of the aorta (*arrowheads*). The central venous pressure line was introduced into the subclavian subintimally. **B:** Lateral spot film in the same patient again shows the contrast pooling in the aortic wall (*arrow*) with absence of rapid flow and washout after injection. **C:** Portable anteroposterior view of a different patient with pulmonary edema in whom a central venous pressure line extends from the left subclavian vein. The line entered the pericardium (*arrows*) and caused tamponade from the bleeding resulting from the vascular perforation.

of the tube. When the nonopaque side is not seen, it is because the subcutaneous tissue, which is similar to the tube in density, has silhouetted this nonopaque border and the tube is outside the pleural space [15]. The side hole of the tube (where there is a break in the opaque marker) also should be seen within the pleural space.

Nasogastric Tubes

The tip of the nasogastric tube and the side hole should be visible below the diaphragm within the gastric lumen. A malpositioned NG tube can be identified by its characteristic side hole (Fig. 63.9A,B).

Transvenous Pacemakers

The pacemaker is passed under fluoroscopic guidance to the apex of the right ventricle (see Chapter 5). Films should be checked for breaks or fractures in the wire (Fig. 63.10). A lateral view should be obtained to ascertain that the pacemaker tip is directed anteriorly 3 to 4 mm beneath the epicardial fat stripe [16]. A posteriorly directed tip in the lateral view, coupled with a cephalad direction in the anteroposterior (AP) view,

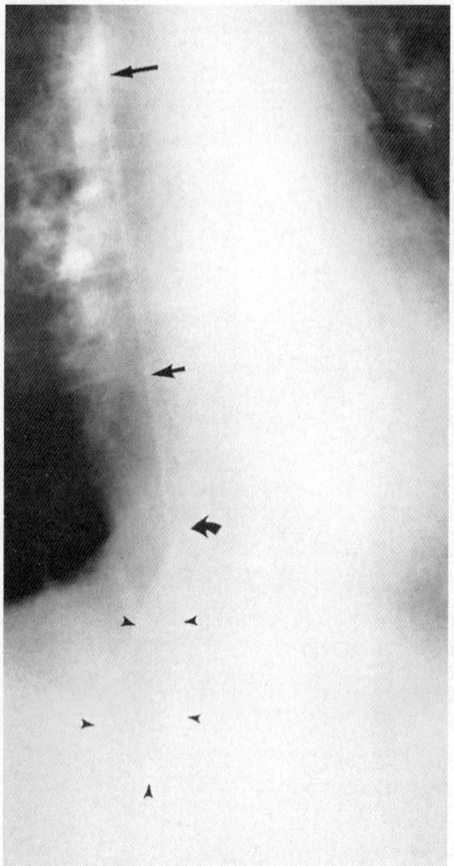

FIGURE 63.6. Swan–Ganz catheter looped in inferior vena cava and reentering right atrium. Anteroposterior close-up view shows the Swan–Ganz catheter through the superior vena cava (*long arrow*) and right atrium (*short arrow*), looping in the inferior vena cava (*arrowheads*) and reentering the right atrium (*curved arrow*).

suggests that the pacer is in the coronary sinus [17]. Projection of the pacemaker tip anterior to the epicardial fat stripe suggests myocardial perforation [16]. Air entrapment in the pulse generator pocket can produce a system malfunction with unipolar pulse generators; this should be kept in mind when examining patients with subcutaneous emphysema [18].

EVALUATION OF THE LUNG PARENCHYMA, PLEURA, MEDIASTINUM, AND DIAPHRAGM

Densities of the Lung Parenchyma

Pulmonary parenchymal densities in the critically ill patient may be caused either by infectious or noninfectious conditions, such as atelectasis, cardiogenic pulmonary edema, acute respiratory distress syndrome (ARDS), pulmonary infarction, or contusion. Radiologic evaluation to determine whether parenchymal densities are secondary to pulmonary edema, other causes, or a combination of edema and other causes is often necessary to complement or initiate a clinical search for pneumonia so that proper therapy can be started.

In 1973, Leeming [19] observed gravitational displacement of edema fluid to the dependent lung. He suggested that pulmonary edema could be differentiated from other causes by a positional shift in the infiltrate. In 1982, Zimmerman et al. [20] evaluated the gravitational shift test and concluded that it is a simple noninvasive method for detecting mobilizable lung water, useful even in the presence of pulmonary damage or an inflammatory process.

After baseline films are obtained, the gravitational shift test is performed, using bedside frontal films. The patient is maintained in a lateral decubitus position for 2 to 3 hours before the films are taken. The hemithorax with fewer parenchymal densities is placed in the dependent position. In 85% of their patients with pulmonary edema, Zimmerman et al. [20] found that the densities in the up lung shifted toward the dependent lung, whereas in 78% of patients with inflammatory disease, no shift was seen.

Evaluation of densities in the retrocardiac area may require an overpenetrated film (Fig. 63.11), a 15- to 30-degree left anterior oblique film, or a right lateral decubitus view. The latter position provides better aeration of the left lung and allows greater visualization of the retrocardiac area. In the presence of pleural effusion, a decubitus view may be necessary to displace the pleural fluid and allow better visualization of the parenchyma.

Congestive Failure and Pulmonary Edema Due to Pulmonary Venous Hypertension

Elevation of pulmonary venous pressure, irrespective of cause, produces a sequence of radiologic findings. When pulmonary venous pressures rise above normal, pulmonary vascular gravitational redistribution occurs [21], producing distention of the upper lobe vessels with a concomitant decrease in caliber of those in the lower lobe in the upright patient. In patients in the supine position, the equivalents of the upper lobe vessels are the anterior or ventral pulmonary vessels and the equivalents of the lower lobe vessels are the posterior or dorsal vessels. The change in caliber of the vessels in the supine position is discernible in a good cross-table lateral film of the chest. These changes are also visible with computed tomography (CT); on a CT, the dorsal vessels become progressively narrower as venous pressure increases.

At pulmonary capillary wedge pressures of 20 to 25 mm Hg, lymphatic drainage is exceeded and the alveolar interstitium, bronchovascular interstitium, interlobular septa, and subpleural tissues become distended with edema fluid. The visible radiologic changes at these pressures are:

1. Thickening of the interlobular septa (Kerley A and B lines) (Fig. 63.12)
2. Peribronchial cuffing, in which hairline, well-defined bronchial walls seen on end increase in thickness and lose their sharp definition (Fig. 63.13A,B)
3. Blurring or haziness of the perivascular outlines (Fig. 63.13A,B)
4. Thickening of the interlobular fissures (Fig. 63.13A,B)
5. Widening of the pleural layer over the convexity of the lungs secondary to the presence of fluid in the subpleural space
6. Pulmonary vascular redistribution (Fig. 63.13C)

Interstitial edema can clear rather rapidly after therapy (Fig. 63.13D). At pulmonary capillary wedge pressures of 25 to 40 mm Hg, edema fluid pours into the alveolar spaces and air space or alveolar edema is seen. The air space consolidation may extend to the subpleural zone, or the more characteristic butterfly or bat-wing edema pattern may be seen (Fig. 63.14).

Unilateral pulmonary edema is probably positional, related primarily to a gravitational shift of mobilizable fluids to the dependent lung [19]. It is postulated that asymmetric edema is often right sided because of cardiac enlargement that impedes

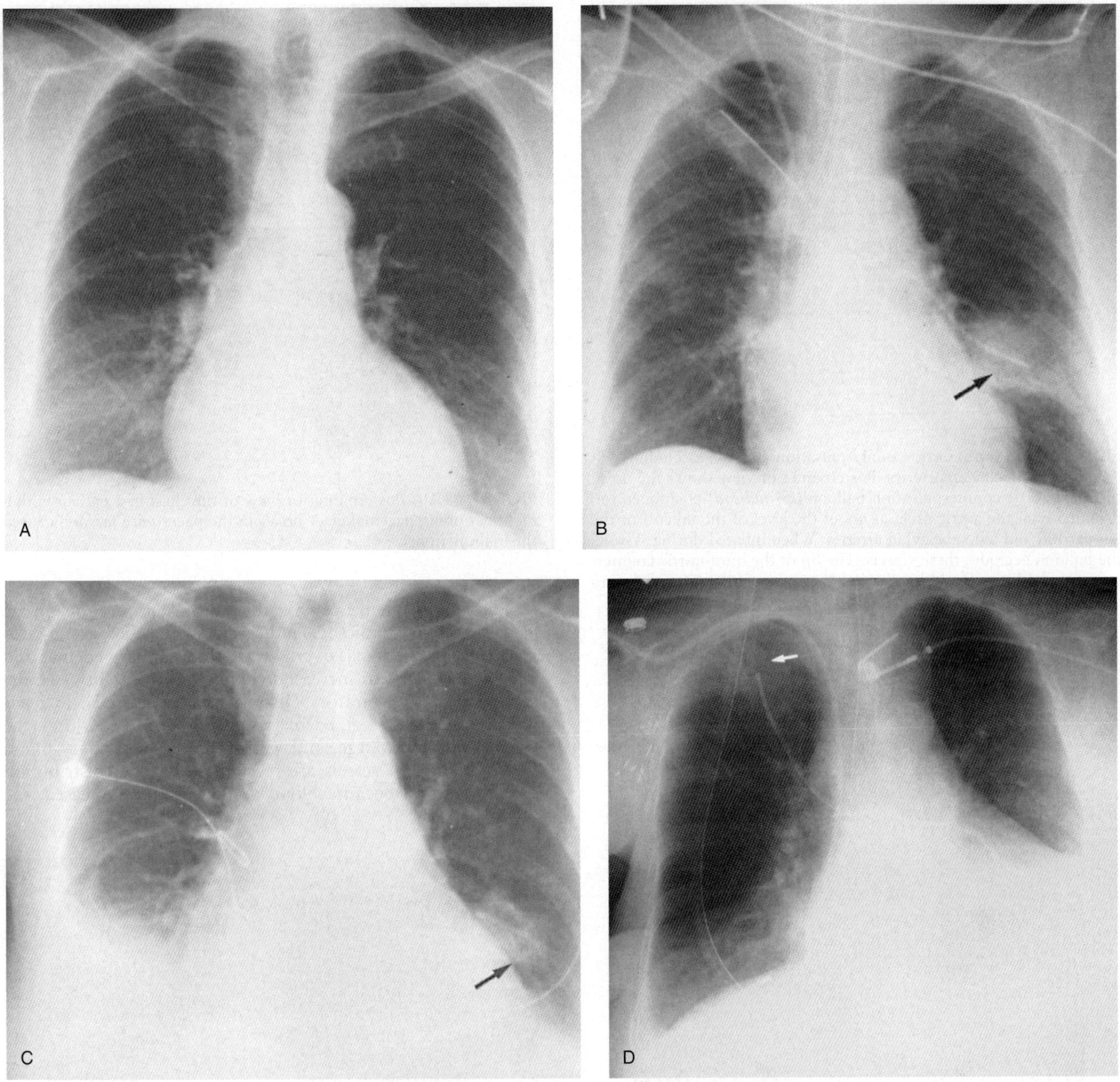

FIGURE 63.7. Infarction caused by Swan–Ganz catheter. **A:** Preoperative posteroanterior view of the chest shows bilaterally clear lung parenchyma. **B:** Postoperative posteroanterior view of the chest shows overly distal position of the Swan–Ganz catheter. An area of density (*arrow*) surrounds the tip of the catheter, representing a pulmonary infarct in the area supplied by the occluded artery. **C:** Posteroanterior film after 5 days shows a persistent left lower lobe density (*arrow*)—the resolving infarct. Right pleural effusion is also present. **D:** Note tip of Swan–Ganz catheter line at periphery of right upper lobe pulmonary artery and showing a round opacity representing "traumatic pseudoaneurysm" (*arrow*).

blood flow in the left pulmonary arterial system, thereby reducing capillary volume. Unilateral diminution in pulmonary blood flow, as seen in Swyer–James syndrome, right or left pulmonary artery thromboembolism, and surgical corrections of congenital heart disease (e.g., shunts for tetralogy of Fallot) are other causes of unilateral edema (Fig. 63.15).

Atypical patterns of congestive failure and pulmonary edema were described by Hublitz and Shapiro [22] in patients with chronic pulmonary disease. Of the four basic patterns they described, two differ in appearance from pulmonary edema in patients with normal lung compliance and vascularity. An asymmetric regional pattern, in which edema occurs only in zones with adequate vascularity, occurs in these patients. The extent of involvement varies greatly from one segment of the lung to another relative to the state of the vascular bed. Another pattern seen is the miliary nodular pattern. Hublitz and Shapiro [22] postulated that the thick-walled spaces in which thickened fibrous septa replace normal alveolar walls impair collateral ventilation and prevent dispersion of edema fluid throughout the lungs. Fluid is then trapped in relatively larger spaces that have replaced normal alveoli. Shadows produced do not coalesce, and the images are seen on radiographs as miliary nodular patterns. The other two patterns, interstitial and reticular, are also seen without chronic lung disease.

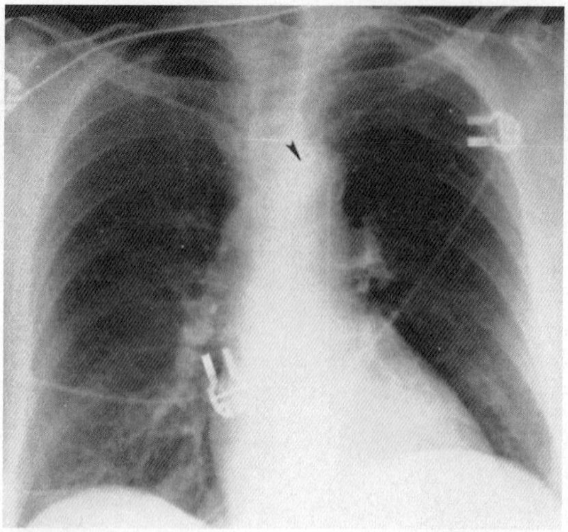

FIGURE 63.8. Intra-aortic counterpulsation balloon occluding left carotid and subclavian arteries. Posteroanterior view shows the tip of the intra-aortic counterpulsation balloon (*arrowhead*) positioned too proximally in the aortic arch, at about the level of the takeoff of the left carotid and left subclavian arteries. When inflated during systole, the balloon occludes these vessels. The tip of the intra-aortic counterpulsation balloon should be distal to the origin of the left subclavian artery.

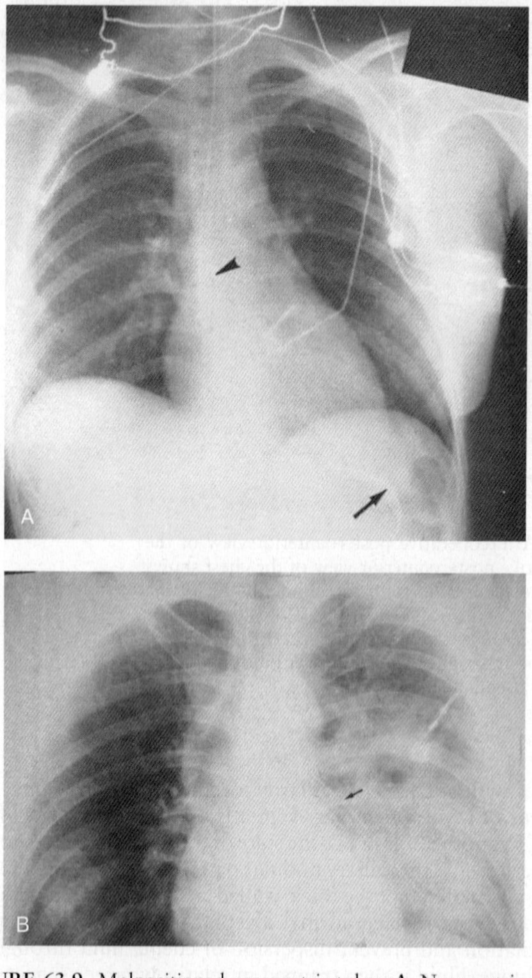

FIGURE 63.9. Malpositioned nasogastric tubes. **A:** Nasogastric tube tip in midesophagus (*arrowhead*) after looping in the stomach (*arrow*). **B:** Malpositioned nasogastric tube in left lower lobe with surrounding pulmonary hemorrhage. Note the side hole of the nasogastric tube (*arrow*).

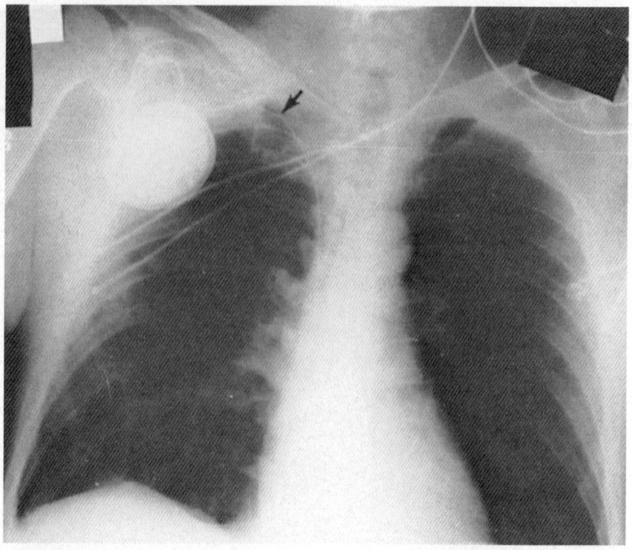

FIGURE 63.10. Posteroanterior view of the chest in a patient with a malfunctioning pacemaker. A break in the pacer wire (*arrow*) caused the malfunction.

Pulmonary edema can be due to cardiac or noncardiac causes. Different radiologic indices distinguish between hydrostatic (cardiac) edema, overhydration pulmonary edema, and edema secondary to increased capillary permeability (see the section Acute Respiratory Distress Syndrome) [23]. In overhydration edema (e.g., edema secondary to renal failure), the cardiac output is large, and, consequently, pulmonary blood flow is large. All vessels are recruited, and no redistribution of flow occurs. Because blood volume is also increased, the

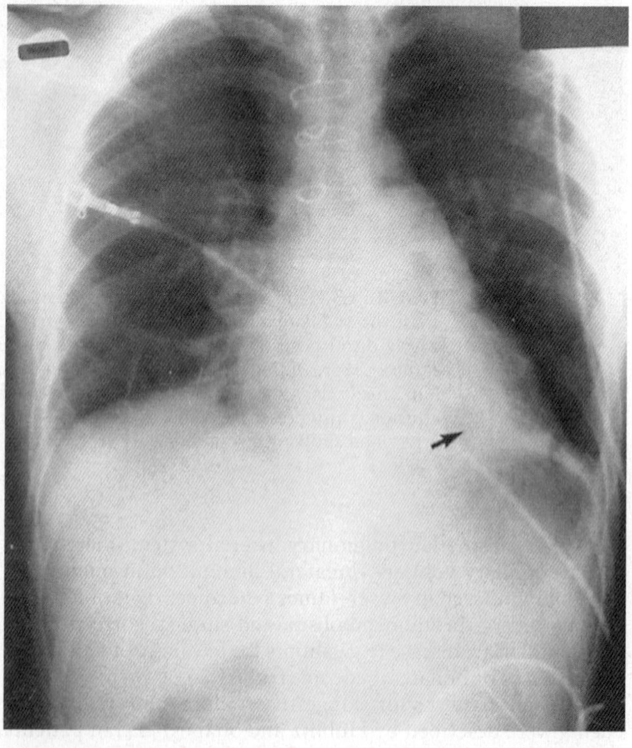

FIGURE 63.11. Left lower lobe atelectasis. Overpenetrated posteroanterior film demonstrates the presence of a retrocardiac density (*arrow*) secondary to atelectasis in a patient who had coronary artery bypass surgery.

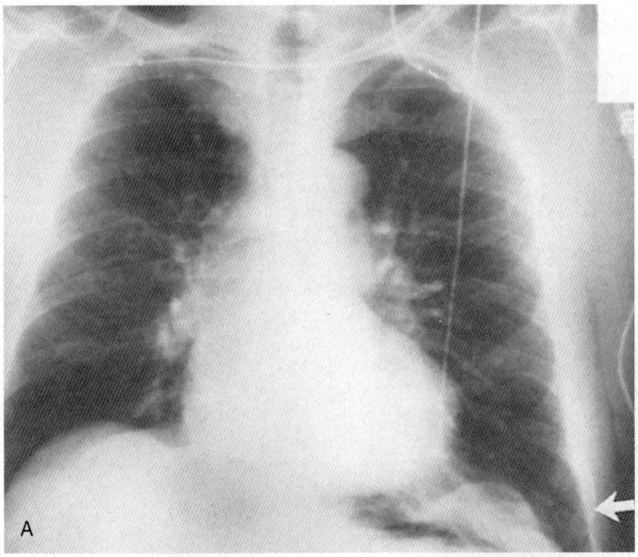

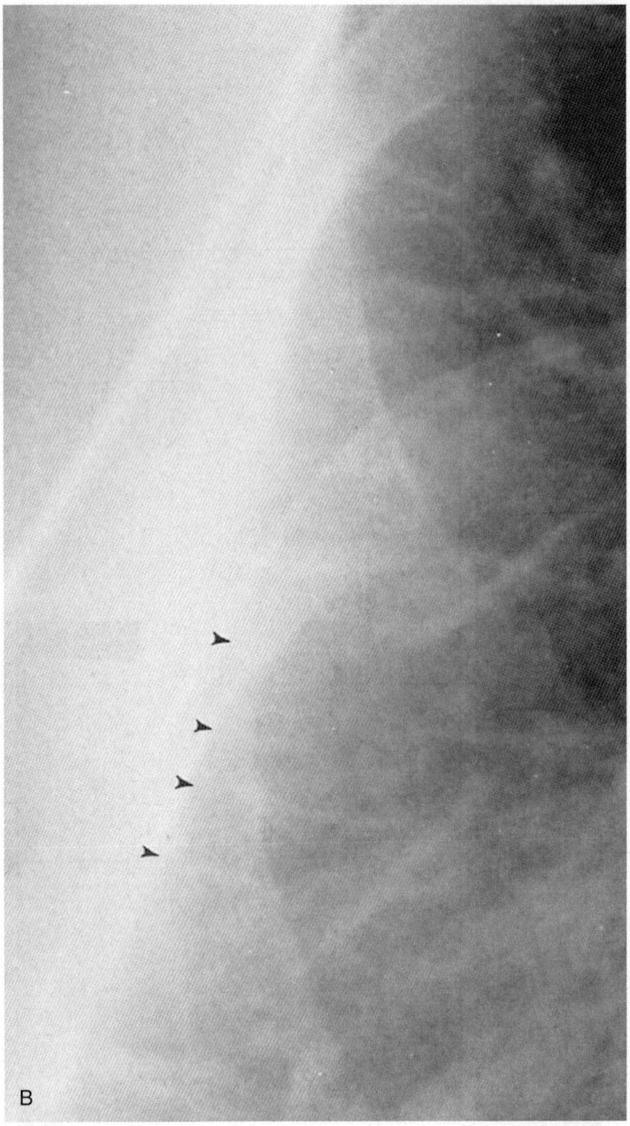

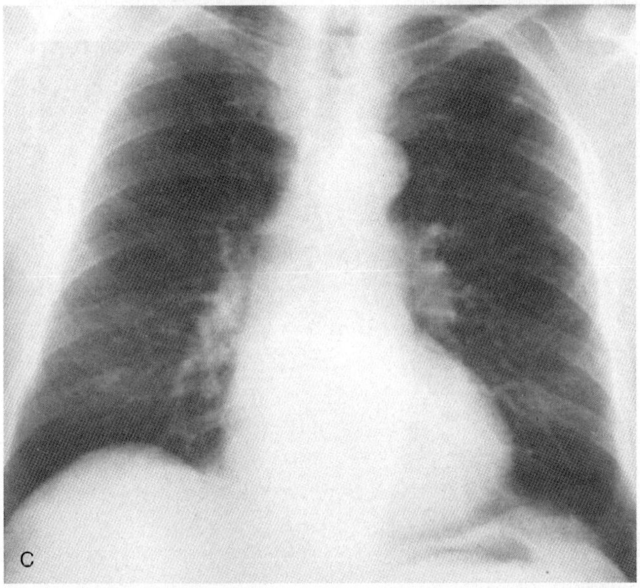

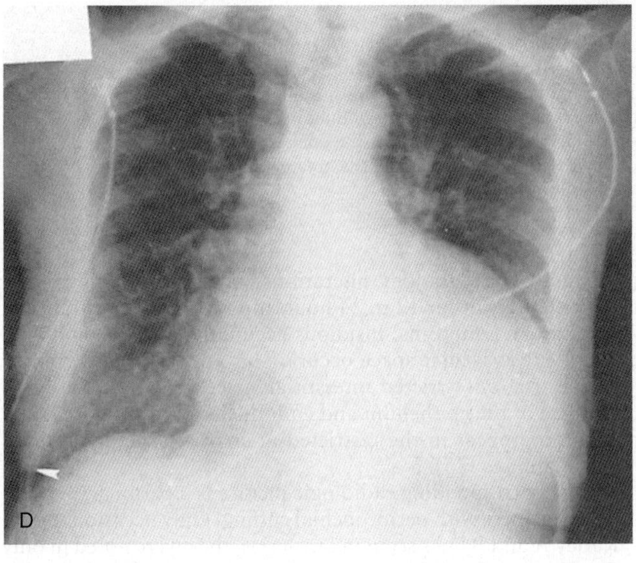

FIGURE 63.12. Congestive heart failure. **A:** Posteroanterior view of a patient in congestive heart failure. The heart size is at the upper limit of normal. Vascular redistribution and Kerley B lines (*arrow*) are present. **B:** Enlargement of a posteroanterior film of a different patient shows Kerley B lines (*arrowheads*) perpendicular to the lateral chest wall. **C:** Posteroanterior view of the first patient after therapy shows that pulmonary vascular redistribution is no longer present and Kerley B lines have disappeared. **D:** Posteroanterior view of a different patient in congestive failure shows cardiomegaly with left ventricular enlargement, numerous Kerley B lines on the right, and a pleural density (*arrowhead*), probably representing subpleural edema (density parallel to the right lower ribs).

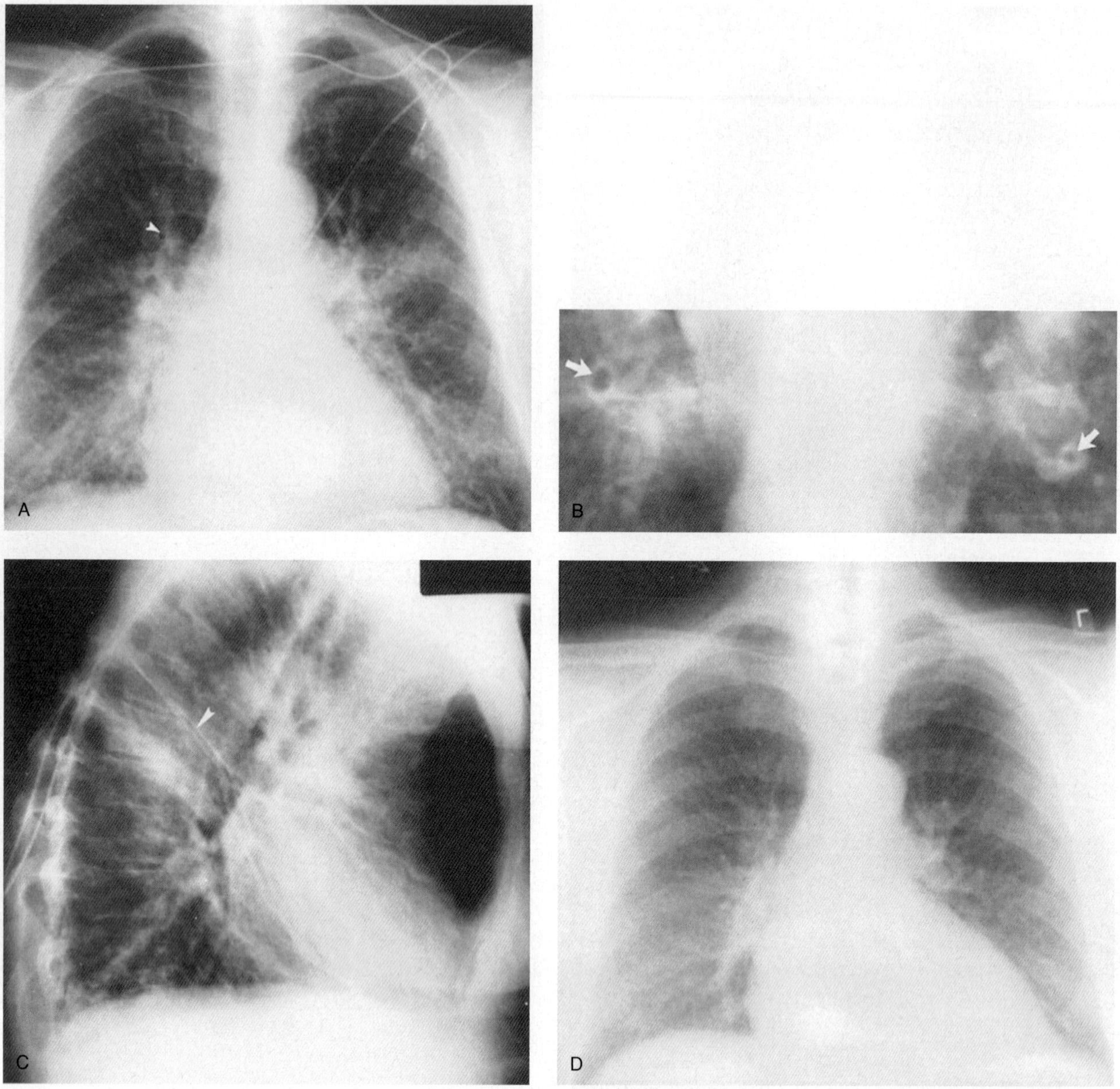

FIGURE 63.13. Interstitial edema. **A:** Posteroanterior film of a patient with congestive heart failure shows cardiomegaly, increased interstitial markings, and right-sided peribronchial cuffing (*arrowhead*) secondary to interstitial edema. **B:** Enlargement of a posteroanterior film of a different patient shows bilateral peribronchial cuffing (*arrows*). **C:** Lateral view of the first patient shows a small amount of fluid in the fissures (*arrowhead*). **D:** Follow-up film of the same patient after 6.5 weeks. Resolution of the congestive heart failure and interstitial edema has occurred. The size of the vessels in the upper lobes is greater than that of the vessels in the bases, suggesting that redistribution is still present.

vascular pedicle, azygos vein, and hilar vessels are large. In pure capillary permeability edema, there is no increase in blood volume, and therefore the vascular pedicle and azygos vein remain normal in size; no signs of pulmonary venous hypertension are present, and heart size is also normal. When different types of edema coexist, edema may occur at lower left atrial pressures, and wedge pressure readings may be low or only slightly elevated [24].

Acute Respiratory Distress Syndrome

Numerous factors can be responsible for ARDS, but the common denominator is always an acute injury to the alveolocapillary unit. The pathologic alterations with corresponding radiologic changes occur 12 to 24 hours after the first appearance of respiratory symptoms. Insidious accumulation of edema fluid in the extravascular space occurs. This appears to be confined to the true unrestricted interstitial space, in which the basal laminae of the epithelium and endothelium are separated, and does not appear in the restricted interstitial space with fused basal laminae [25].

The corresponding radiologic picture is a perihilar, perivascular haziness with peribronchial cuffing. Only occasionally are Kerley A and B lines seen; in one series, they were noted in only 5 of 75 cases [26]. During the acute stage, the alveoli also become nonhomogeneously filled with a proteinaceous and often hemorrhagic cell-containing fluid. Hyaline membranes form in

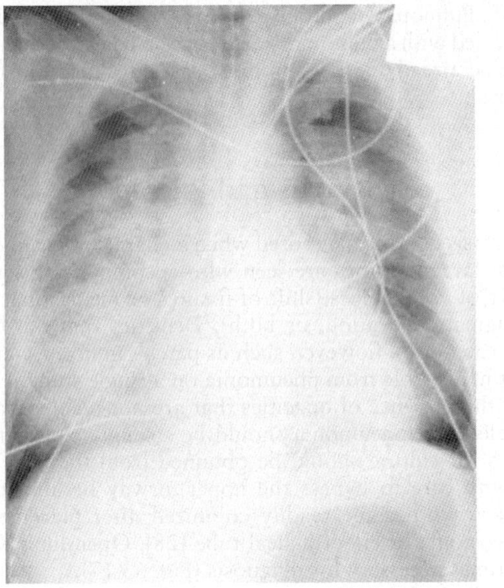

FIGURE 63.14. Alveolar pulmonary edema. Butterfly pattern of pulmonary edema can be seen in the perihilar areas.

the alveoli and sometimes in the alveolar ducts. The radiologic picture is one of patchy, ill-defined, confluent miliary nodular or alveolar densities that are not rapidly reversible (Fig. 63.16).

The course of ARDS is highly variable. In some patients, reabsorption of the exudates is complete within a few days, thereby producing radiologic clearing of the densities. In some, there is a delayed clearing of the exudates, with a corresponding delay in clearing of the radiologic picture. In a third group, progressive fibrosing alveolitis follows. The progression of fibrosis and the degree of tissue derangement do not correlate with the duration of the disease. Radiologically, this phase presents a diffuse, fibrotic pattern.

After the first week, the radiologist's main concern is the recognition of superimposed complications, such as pulmonary infections, oxygen toxicity, barotrauma, and pulmonary embolism with infarction. When clinical signs and symptoms of infection are present and the radiographic picture deteriorates, pneumonia should be suspected. Development of cavities and a change in the character of the densities should lead to suspicion of superimposed abscess, infarction, or cardiac failure. Unger et al. [27] showed that only direct hemodynamic measurements of the pulmonary capillary wedge pressure provide a dependable means of detecting superimposed failure in cases of

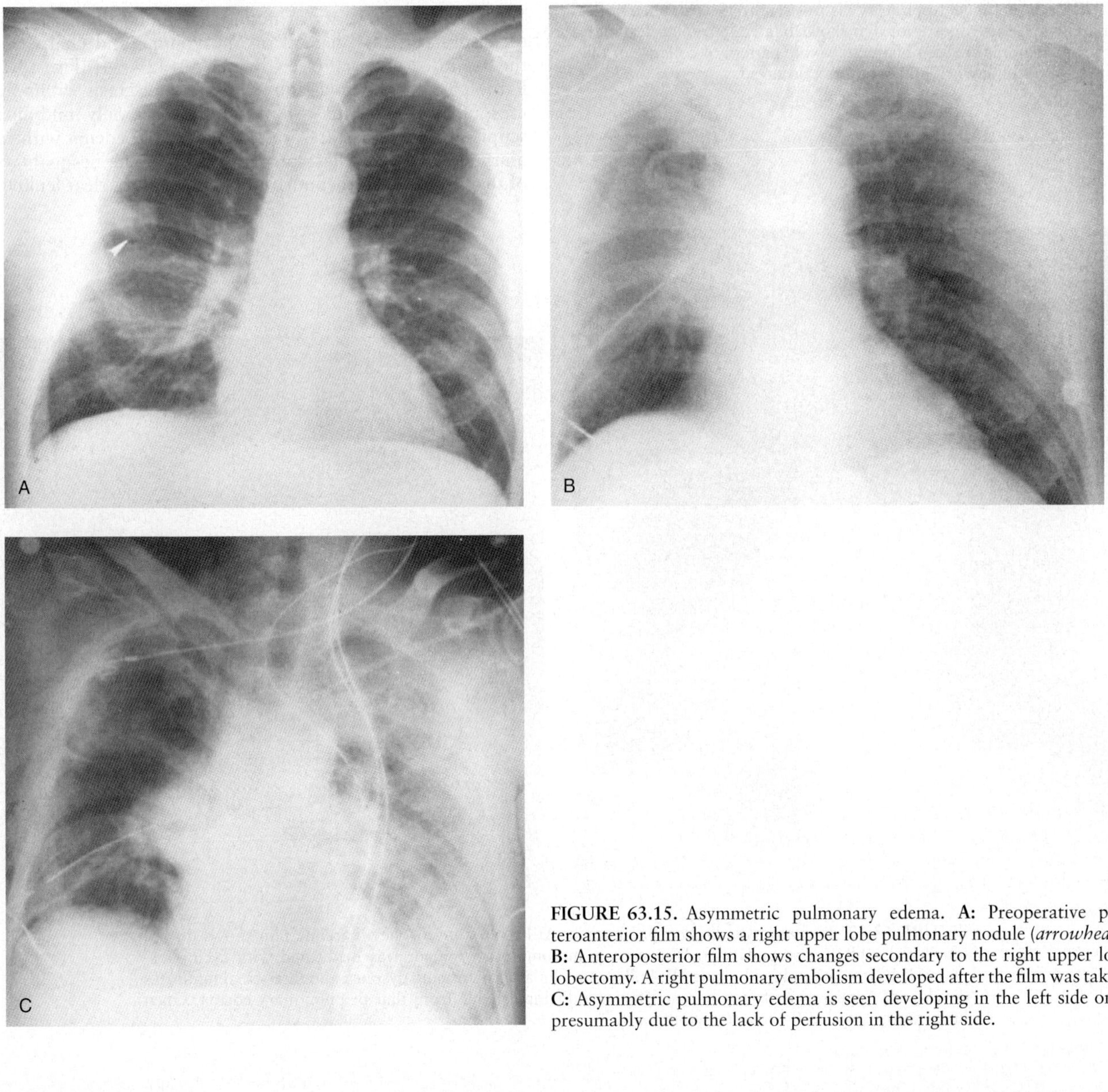

FIGURE 63.15. Asymmetric pulmonary edema. **A:** Preoperative posteroanterior film shows a right upper lobe pulmonary nodule (*arrowhead*). **B:** Anteroposterior film shows changes secondary to the right upper lobe lobectomy. A right pulmonary embolism developed after the film was taken. **C:** Asymmetric pulmonary edema is seen developing in the left side only, presumably due to the lack of perfusion in the right side.

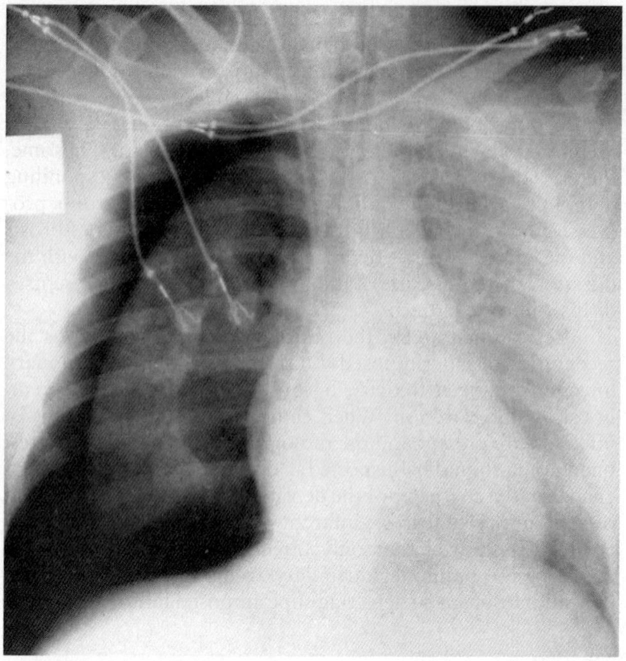

FIGURE 63.16. Acute respiratory distress syndrome with pneumothorax. Portable anteroposterior film shows bilateral alveolar densities. Air bronchograms are seen bilaterally. Note pattern of collapse of the relatively stiff lung when pneumothorax occurred.

ARDS. Pulmonary embolism, with or without infarction, can be verified with a pulmonary arteriogram using the Swan–Ganz catheter, already in place in most cases, to inject the contrast material.

Atelectasis and Pneumonia

Atelectasis is easily diagnosed when a characteristic linear density or large densities are seen with accompanying signs suggestive of volume loss (shift of fissures or mediastinal and diaphragmatic elevation, or both). Densities that fall between these categories, however, such as patchy infiltrates, are often indistinguishable from pneumonia on a single study.

In the presence of opacities that are not readily diagnosed as atelectasis, pneumonia should be strongly considered. Aspirates for culture should be obtained from the lung periphery, with care to bypass the upper airway because the central airways become readily colonized after placement of a tracheostomy or endotracheal tube [28]. Open lung biopsy is sometimes necessary for diagnosis (Fig. 63.17).

Chemical Aspiration Pneumonia

The extent and severity of pulmonary injury after aspiration of gastric contents depend on the volume and character of the aspirated material (see Chapter 54) [29–34] (Fig. 63.18). Pathologically, the lungs show areas of atelectasis within minutes; up to 1 hour after aspiration, however, only mild microscopic abnormalities are present (interstitial edema with capillary congestion). These progress to complete desquamation of the bronchial epithelium and polymorphonuclear leukocyte

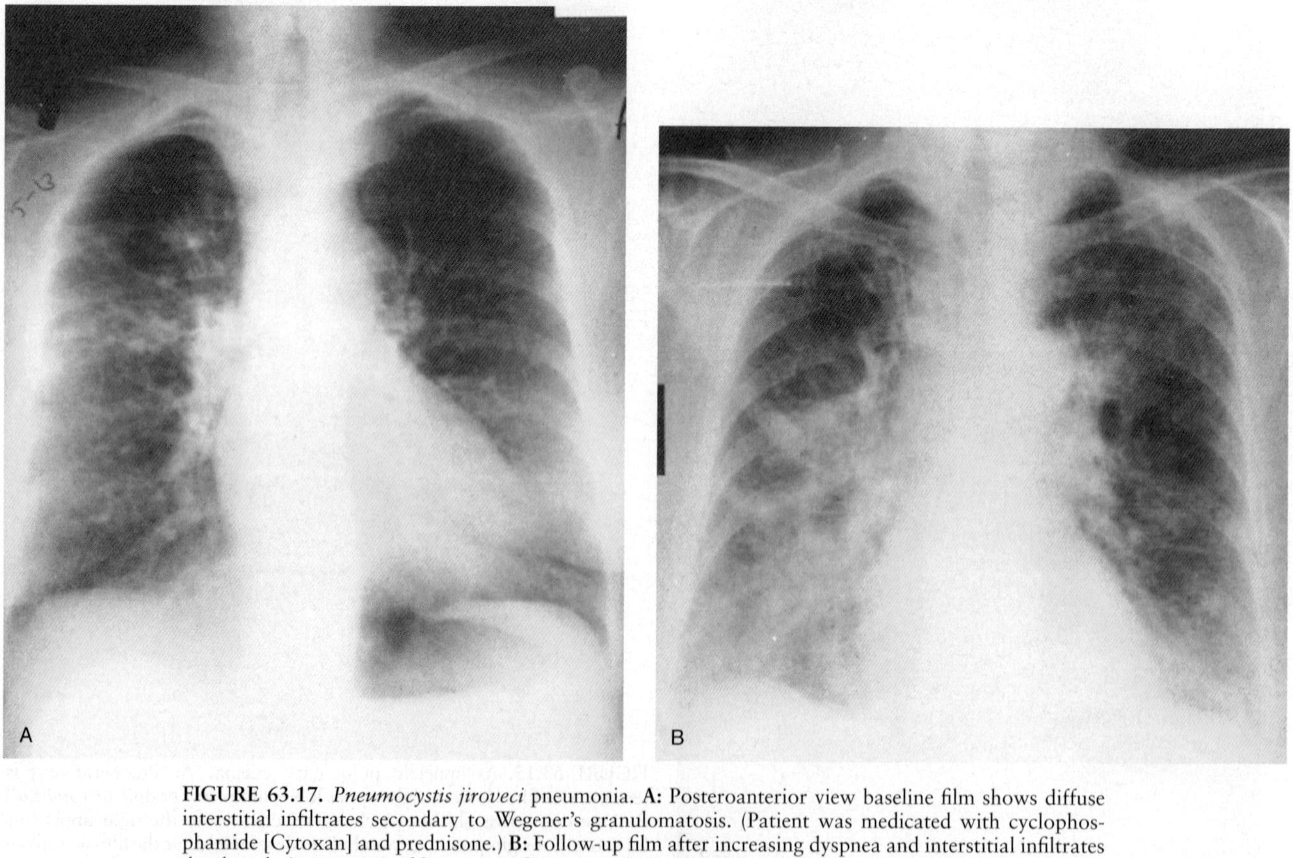

FIGURE 63.17. *Pneumocystis jiroveci* pneumonia. **A:** Posteroanterior view baseline film shows diffuse interstitial infiltrates secondary to Wegener's granulomatosis. (Patient was medicated with cyclophosphamide [Cytoxan] and prednisone.) **B:** Follow-up film after increasing dyspnea and interstitial infiltrates developed. Appearance of lung parenchyma is indistinguishable from that of pulmonary edema. Open lung biopsy revealed *P. jiroveci* pneumonia.

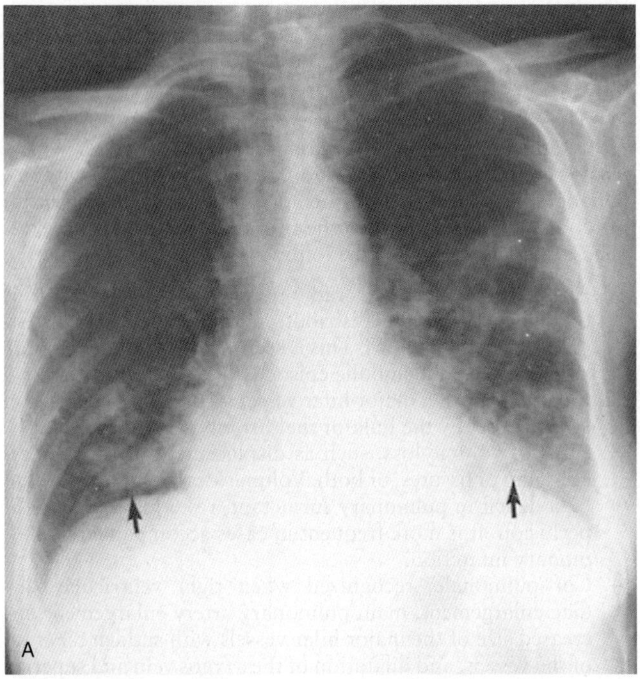

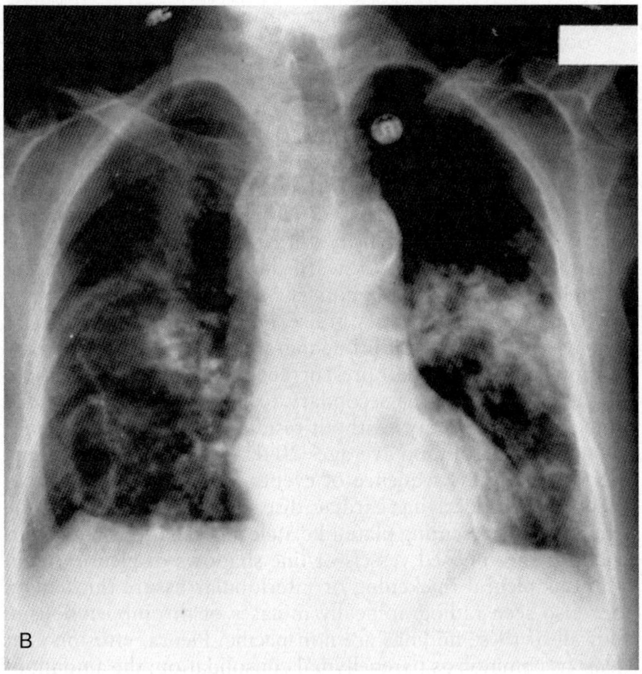

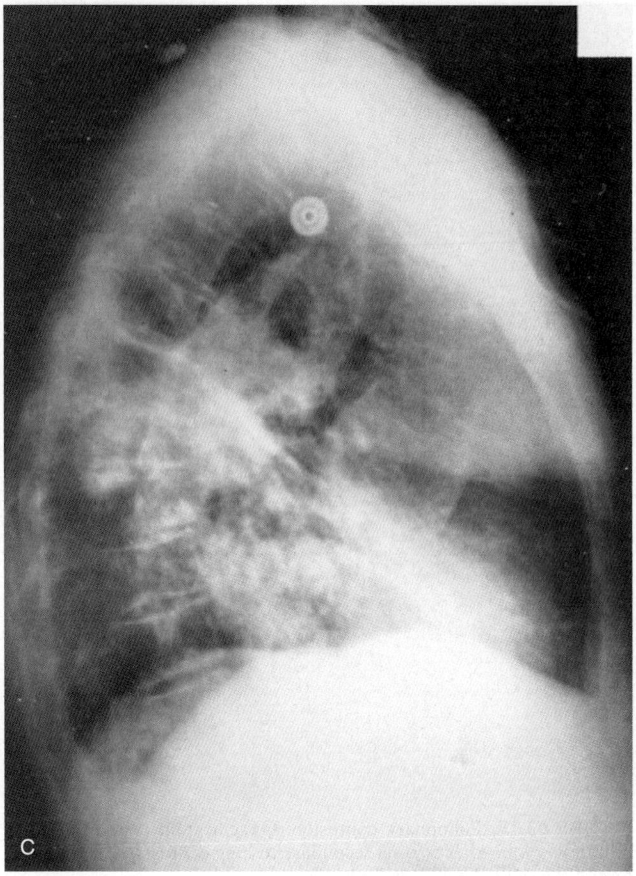

FIGURE 63.18. Aspiration pneumonia. **A:** Posteroanterior view of the chest shows bilateral basal densities (*arrows*) in a patient with aspiration pneumonia. **B,C:** Posteroanterior and lateral views in another patient show patchy densities scattered in both lungs from aspiration pneumonia.

infiltration of the area (bronchiolitis). Alveolar spaces fill with edema fluid, red blood cells, and polymorphonuclear leukocytes (alveolar infiltrates), progressing to consolidation in 24 to 48 hours. Formation of hyaline membranes occurs by 48 hours and organization or resolution within 72 hours. Complete resolution, focal parenchymal scars, or bronchiolitis obliterans may follow.

From the preceding discussion, it is clear that after aspiration, the chest film may show any finding or changes, ranging from interstitial edema or opacities simulating pneumonia to changes of ARDS. In ICU patients who aspirate, the incidence of complications is increased. In 75% of young patients without underlying medical disease, aspiration pneumonia follows an uncomplicated course, and the chest radiograph clears after 7 to 10 days. However, ICU patients are particularly prone to development of infectious complications, such as pneumonia, abscess formation, ARDS, and bronchiolitis, after aspiration of gastric contents.

Pulmonary Contusion, Hematoma, and Traumatic Lung Cyst

Pulmonary contusion is a frequent cause of posttraumatic pulmonary opacification (Fig. 63.19). It is often seen without evidence of rib or sternal fractures. Radiologically, it is seen as an area of increased density or a large area of consolidation with poorly defined margins that do not conform to the shape of the lobes or lung segments. The lack of sharp demarcation

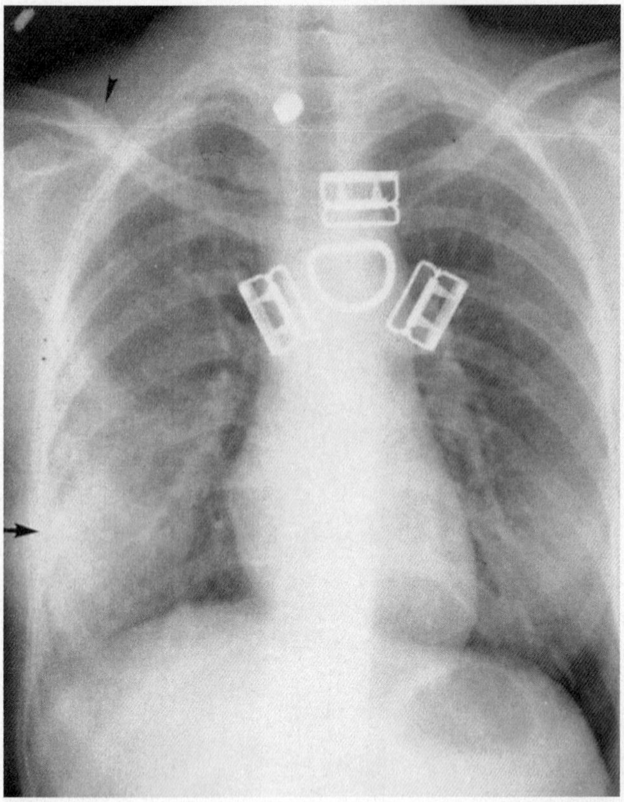

FIGURE 63.19. Pulmonary contusion. Opacification (*arrow*) of the right lower lobe after trauma secondary to lung contusion. Note fracture of the right clavicle (*arrowhead*).

of the margins is due to seepage of blood or edema fluid into the alveoli and probably into the interstitial tissues. The area of increased density or consolidation is usually seen within the first 6 hours. Improvement of the lesion is rapid, occurring within 24 to 48 hours. Complete clearing is usually seen in 3 to 10 days. Secondary infection leads to liquefaction of dead tissues and bronchial communication, producing an air-filled cavity with or without an associated fluid level.

When laceration or tearing of a lung occurs, commonly as a result of a penetrating injury or surgical resection, a pulmonary hematoma (a collection of blood within a space in the lung) forms. The cavity formed by retraction of the torn elastic tissues may be completely dense or partially air filled if bronchial communication occurs. The lesion may progressively increase in size in the next few days because of edema or seepage of blood. This is in contrast to a contusion, which regresses in size. The lesion may take weeks or months to clear. Occasionally, a clot may form and simulate an intracavitary fungus ball. Resolution may be incomplete, resulting in a pulmonary nodule.

Traumatic lung cysts also may occur after trauma. They may appear immediately after blunt trauma or may form after several hours or days. Single, multiple, or multilocular thin-walled, oval to spheric cystic spaces may be seen in the lung periphery or subpleurally. Bleeding into the cyst from ruptured capillaries may occur. The lung cysts persist for long periods, often more than 4 months, but progressively decrease in size during this period.

Pulmonary Thromboembolism and Infarction

Episodes of pulmonary thromboembolism usually show some changes on plain chest radiographs, such as linear atelectasis, elevation of a hemidiaphragm, or pleural effusion. Most embolic occlusions occur in the lower lobes, the right more often than the left, probably as a result of hemodynamic flow patterns (see Chapter 52).

The radiographic changes can be divided into two categories: those with increased radiographic density (with hemorrhagic consolidation or infarction, or both) and those without. Changes without associated hemorrhagic consolidation or infarction are seen only when the thromboembolism is massive. These changes consist of the following:

1. An area of increased radiolucency (local oligemia) of the lung within the distribution of the occluded artery (Westermark sign) [35]. This is seen within the first 36 hours after the thromboembolic episode.
2. Enlargement of a major hilar vessel secondary to distention of the vessel by the bulk of the thrombus.
3. Signs of volume loss, such as displacement of the hemidiaphragm or fissures, or both. Volume loss is probably caused by a deficit in pulmonary surfactant, resulting from loss of perfusion. It is more frequent in cases accompanied by pulmonary infarction.
4. Cor pulmonale, recognized when right ventricular cardiac enlargement, main pulmonary artery enlargement, increased size of the major hilar vessels with sudden tapering of the vessels, and dilatation of the azygos vein and superior vena cava are seen. These changes occur with widespread multiple peripheral embolism or massive central embolization.

Thromboembolism with increased density or infarction shows the same changes as thromboembolism without increased density, except for the sign of peripheral oligemia. The area of oligemia is replaced by parenchymal consolidation from tissue necrosis or hemorrhage and edema. The density is almost always pleurally based. Hampton's hump, a homogeneous, wedge-shaped density with its base contiguous to the pleural surface and apex toward the hilum, is rarely seen but is highly suggestive of pulmonary infarction.

The consolidations vary in size, but most are 3 to 5 cm in diameter (Fig. 63.20). Air bronchograms are rarely present; cavitation is unusual and, if present, suggests septic embolization. If the consolidation is secondary to hemorrhage and edema, it clears in 4 to 7 days without residua; if the infarction leads to necrosis, resolution averages 20 days and may take as long as 5 weeks. This sequence of events is more common in patients with underlying cardiac disease. Linear densities (line shadows) representing plate-like atelectasis, parenchymal scarring, or thrombosed vessels or line shadows of pleural origin (fibrous pleural thickening or interlobular fissure thickening) are also seen radiographically in cases of thromboembolism, but all of these findings are nonspecific. Pleural effusion is at least as common as parenchymal consolidation; the amount of fluid is frequently small, and the fluid is often unilateral.

The frequent presence of underlying chest disorders, such as ARDS, pulmonary edema, associated pneumonia, or chronic obstructive lung changes, often makes the radiologic diagnosis of pulmonary embolism virtually impossible on plain chest radiographs in the ICU patient. Radioisotopic scanning provides distinctive patterns for pulmonary embolism, congestive heart failure, and emphysema. Ventilation-perfusion scans should be performed whenever pulmonary embolism is suspected in patients with normal chest films. The clearest distinguishing feature of embolism is its focal segmental or local wedge-shaped configuration. An irregular, moth-eaten pattern, nonsegmental in nature, is seen in pulmonary congestion and chronic obstructive pulmonary disease. A nonmatched area on a scan (a combination of normal ventilation and abnormal perfusion) in the correct temporal setting is highly suggestive of embolism. Scans provide guidelines as to the probability of emboli and serve as

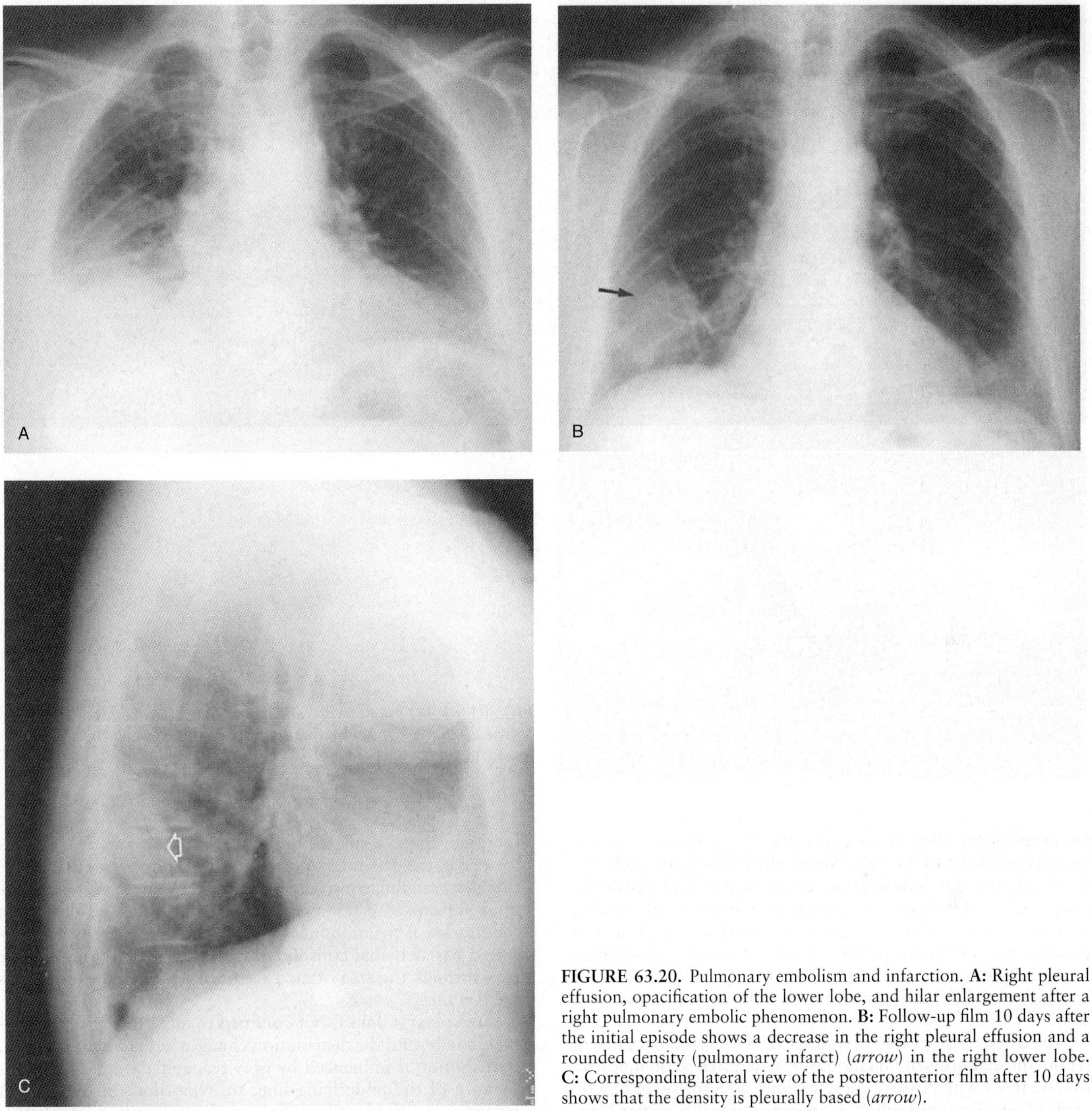

FIGURE 63.20. Pulmonary embolism and infarction. **A:** Right pleural effusion, opacification of the lower lobe, and hilar enlargement after a right pulmonary embolic phenomenon. **B:** Follow-up film 10 days after the initial episode shows a decrease in the right pleural effusion and a rounded density (pulmonary infarct) (*arrow*) in the right lower lobe. **C:** Corresponding lateral view of the posteroanterior film after 10 days shows that the density is pleurally based (*arrow*).

an excellent road map for pulmonary arteriography. They also serve as a baseline for future evaluation (see Chapter 52).

In patients with abnormalities on their chest films, multidetector CT angiography is the examination of choice [36]. And although there is a slight increase in diagnostic accuracy for pulmonary embolism by addition of CT venography, it does not appear to improve the diagnostic yield of CT pulmonary angiography enough to justify the additional radiation [37]. They can show intravascular filling defect(s) produced by the embolus/emboli up to the segmental artery level (Fig. 63.21). The gold standard for the diagnosis of thromboembolism is multidetector CT angiography.

Fat Embolism

Fat embolism usually follows trauma with associated fracture, but conditions such as severe burns, diabetes mellitus, fatty liver, pancreatitis, steroid therapy, sickle cell anemia, surgery for prosthetic hip placement, and acute osteomyelitis can also result in fat embolism. Most of the fat is believed to originate as neutral fats released from the marrow, entering the circulation via torn veins in the injured area and, to a lesser extent, through the lymphatic system. Fats are then transported to the lungs in the form of neutral triglycerides. Mechanical occlusion of small vessels occurs, but no significant physiologic abnormality results unless large amounts of fat embolize a great number of vessels. In the lungs, hydrolysis of fat occurs through the action of lipase, converting the triglycerides to unsaturated chemically toxic fatty acids. Congestion, edema, intra-alveolar hemorrhage, and loss of surfactant occur. The fat globules also appear to induce platelet and erythrocyte aggregation and stimulation of intravascular coagulation.

Another probable source of fat is the body fat deposits. Free fatty acids are mobilized and released into the blood after stress. Chylomicrons coalesce into larger fat globules; these

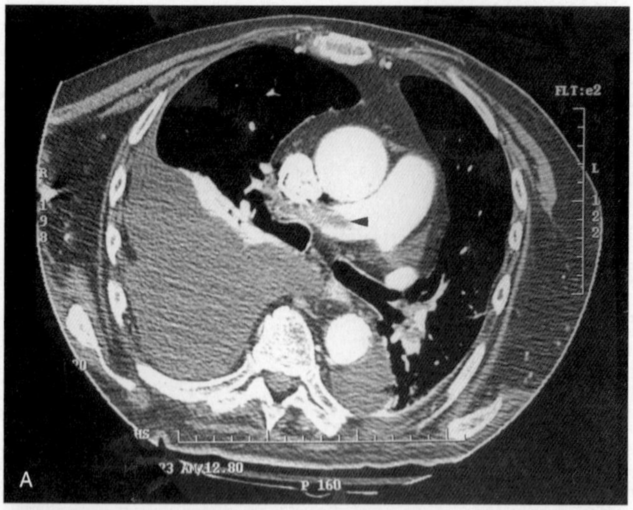

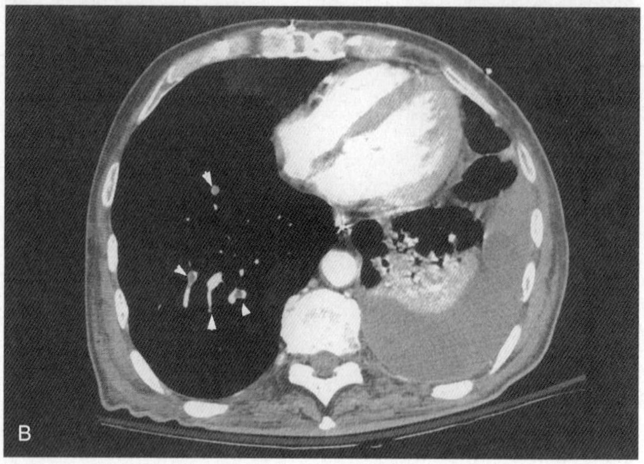

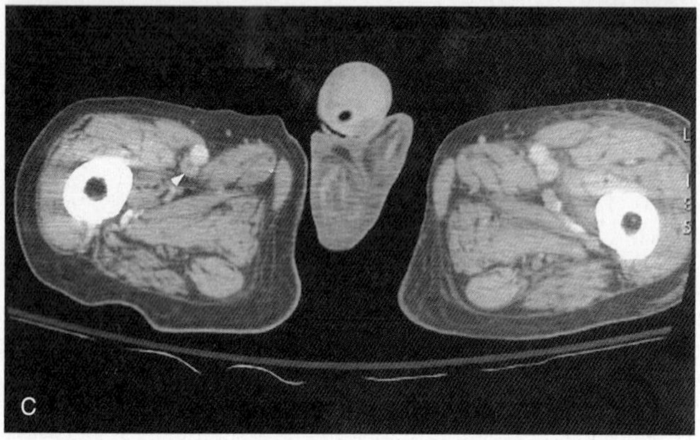

FIGURE 63.21. Pulmonary embolism. **A:** Intravascular filling defect (*arrowhead*) in the right pulmonary artery. **B:** Intravascular filling (*arrowheads*) in segmented branches. **C:** Intravascular filling defect (*arrowhead*) in the right femoral vein on computed tomographic venography.

fat droplets are then carried into the lungs, where they are hydrolyzed by lipase into the chemically active fatty acids.

Continuous fat embolization, conversion of triglycerides to fatty acids, and intravascular coagulation occur as an ongoing process. Usually within 1 to 3 days, the changes are sufficient to produce the full-blown picture of the syndrome. Emboli pass from the pulmonary circulation into the systemic circulation and lodge in different organs, notably the brain, kidney, and skin.

The chest radiograph is normal in 87.5% of patients in whom the diagnosis of fat embolism is made based on lipiduria [38]. In those with positive chest findings, widespread or patchy areas of air space consolidation are noted, due to alveolar hemorrhage and edema distributed predominantly in the peripheral and basal areas. The densities clear in 7 to 10 days but may take 4 weeks to resolve completely. Acute cor pulmonale with cardiac failure also may be seen.

ABNORMALITIES OF THE PLEURA, MEDIASTINUM, AND DIAPHRAGM

Pleural Effusion

The appearance of fluid in the pleural space is the same whether the fluid is serous, chylous, purulent, or sanguineous. The degree of opacity of the shadow depends on the amount of fluid and presence or absence of underlying pulmonary disease. Radiologically, pleural fluid is seen as a density that is free from lung markings, displaces the lung, and most often (if free) is located in the dependent portion of the thorax. It is easily identifiable when tangent to the radiograph beam; seen *en face*, the fluid appears as a homogeneous area of increased density in the thorax. If the amount is not too large or there is no associated parenchymal consolidation, vascular markings may be seen through the area of increased density when the effusion is seen *en face*.

Free pleural fluid is not confined to any portion of the thoracic cavity, and the distribution changes with patient position. Distribution is influenced by gravity, capillary action, and resistance of the underlying lung to expansion. In the upright position, the fluid collects first in the posterior costophrenic sulcus and subsequently in the lateral costophrenic sulcus. The typical meniscal configuration of pleural fluid (Fig. 63.22) is attributed to several factors, including capillary attraction drawing the fluid superiorly between the visceral and parietal pleural surfaces, the relation of the fluid collection to the radiograph beam, the greater retractility of the lung periphery, and the tendency of the lung to preserve its shape while recoiling from the chest.

Subpulmonary collection of pleural fluid is the typical pattern of free fluid collection in the upright position if no pleural adhesions are present [39]. Radiologically, the fluid presents as an opaque density, parallel to the diaphragm and simulating an elevated hemidiaphragm (Fig. 63.23). Subpulmonic effusion is recognized in the posteroanterior (PA) film when the apex of the pseudodiaphragmatic shadow peaks more laterally than usual. The pulmonary vessels in the lung posterior to the subpulmonic collection cannot be seen through the pseudodiaphragmatic contour because of the greater density of the fluid collection. On the left side, there is increased distance

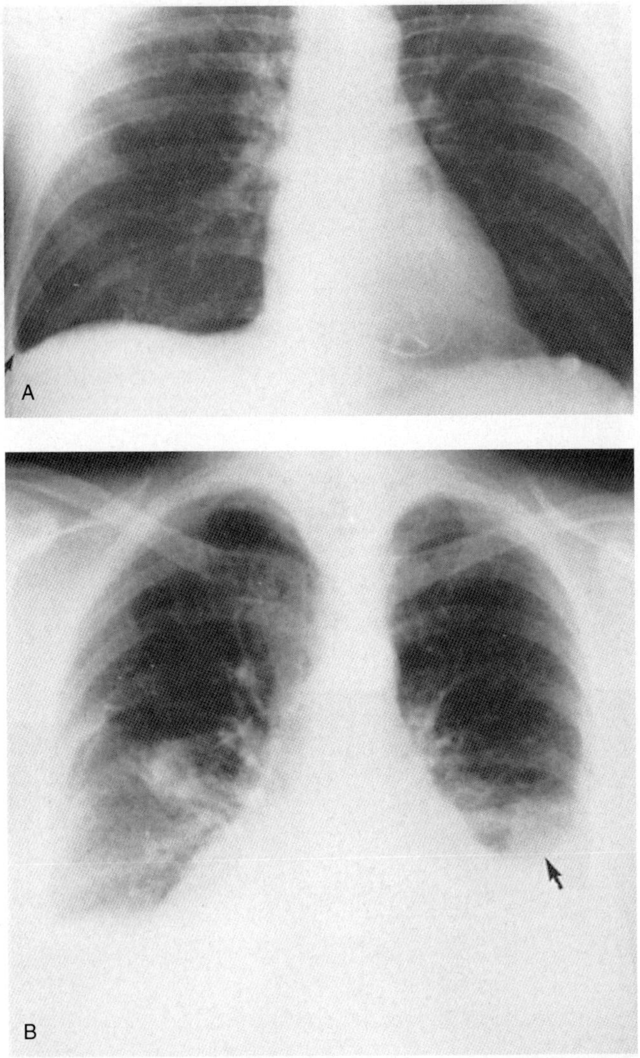

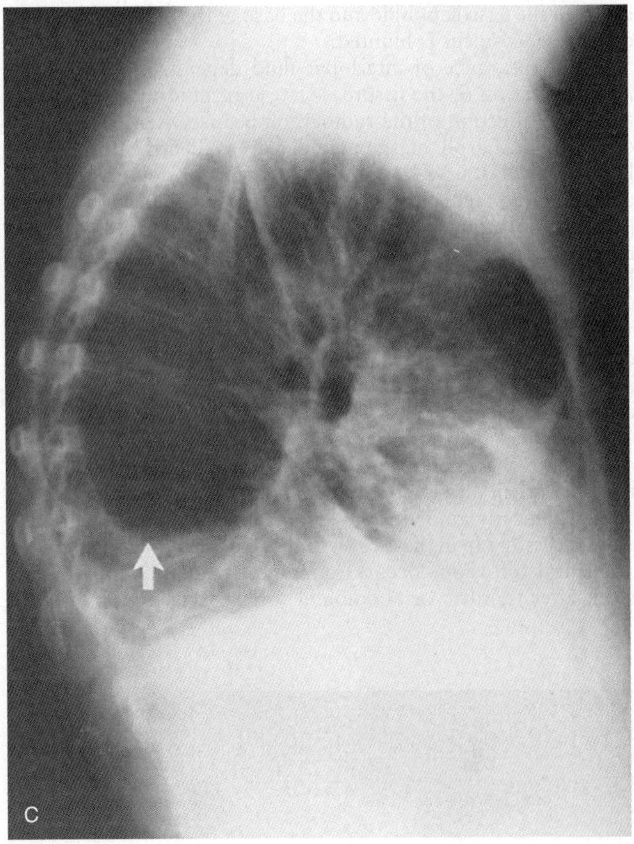

FIGURE 63.22. Pleural effusion meniscus. **A:** Anteroposterior film shows minimal blunting of the right costophrenic angle with meniscus. **B:** Anteroposterior view of a different patient shows meniscus level (*arrow*) in larger pleural effusion. **C:** Lateral view of meniscus level (*arrow*) in patient shown in (**B**).

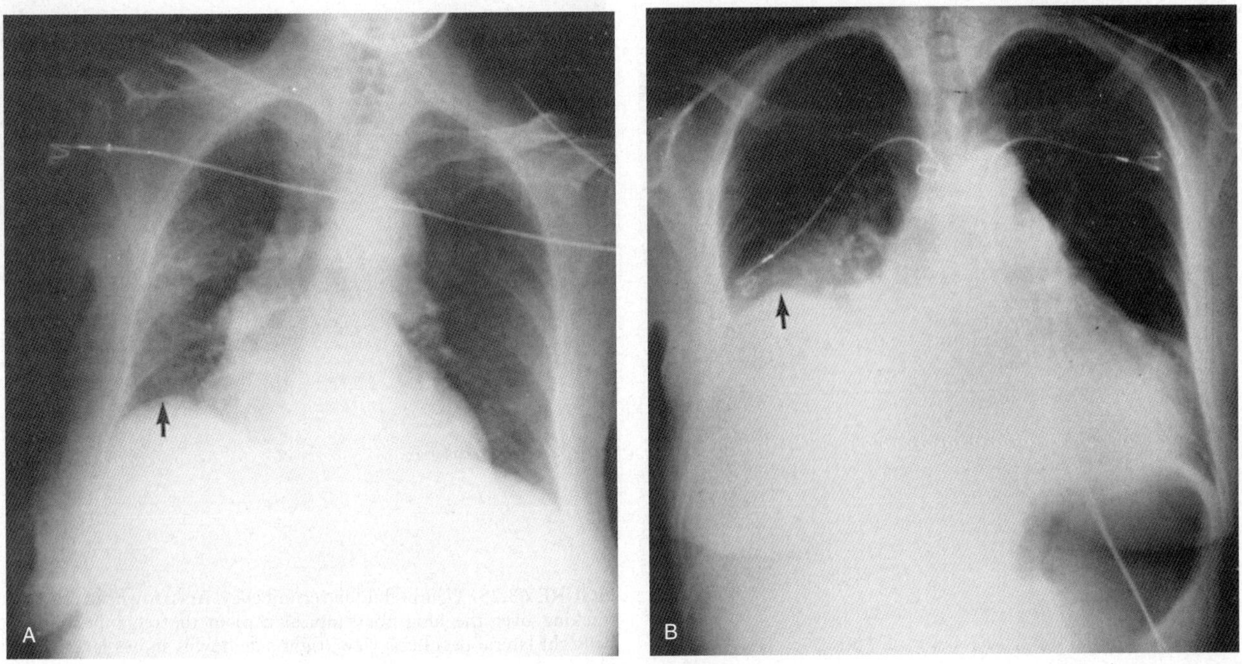

FIGURE 63.23. Subpulmonic effusion. Anteroposterior views of two different patients (**A,B**) with the subpulmonic effusion simulating elevated hemidiaphragms, with a more lateral than usual peak (*arrows*).

between the gastric bubble and the base of the lung. Often, the costophrenic sulcus is blunted.

The appearance of interlobar fluid depends on the shape and orientation of the fissure, location of fluid within the fissure, and direction of the radiograph beam. Often, an elliptic or rounded, sharply marginated density is identified on PA or lateral films (Fig. 63.24). A middle lobe step, or step-off appearance, may be seen when the fissures are incomplete laterally [40]. In the supine position, fluid layers may be seen posteriorly, producing a hazy density over the hemithorax. These layers also may produce an apical cap [41] (Fig. 63.25A) or widening of the paravertebral pleural line [42].

A lateral decubitus view can be obtained to confirm the presence of pleural effusion, rule out a parenchymal process coexisting with an effusion, or quantify grossly the amount of fluid in the pleural cavity. In the lateral decubitus view, fluid forms a shadow parallel to the thoracic wall (Fig. 63.25B,C). When a decubitus view cannot be obtained for a completely immobile patient, an ultrasonographic evaluation can be performed. Sonographically guided thoracentesis enhances the likelihood of a successful tap in these cases and when the fluid is loculated.

Pleural effusion occurs quite frequently in the first week after thoracic or abdominal surgery (Fig. 63.26). After

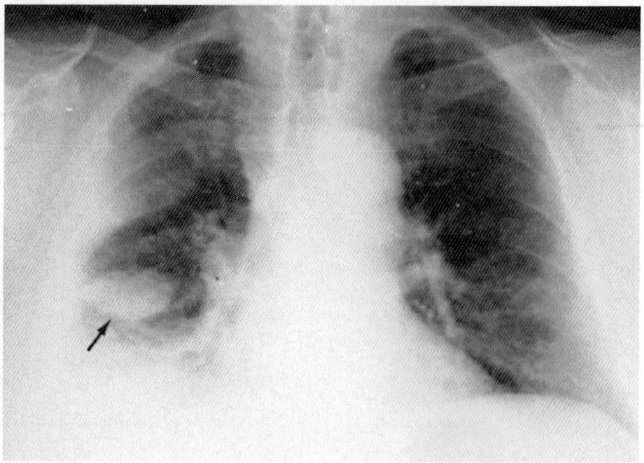

FIGURE 63.24. Interlobar effusion. Pseudotumor appearance of fluid (*arrow*) within the minor fissure.

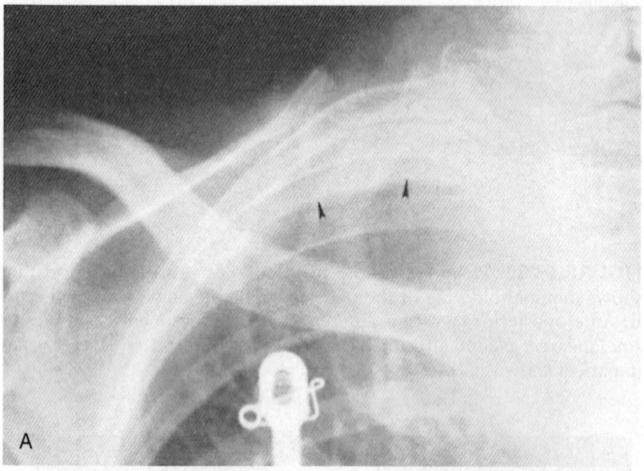

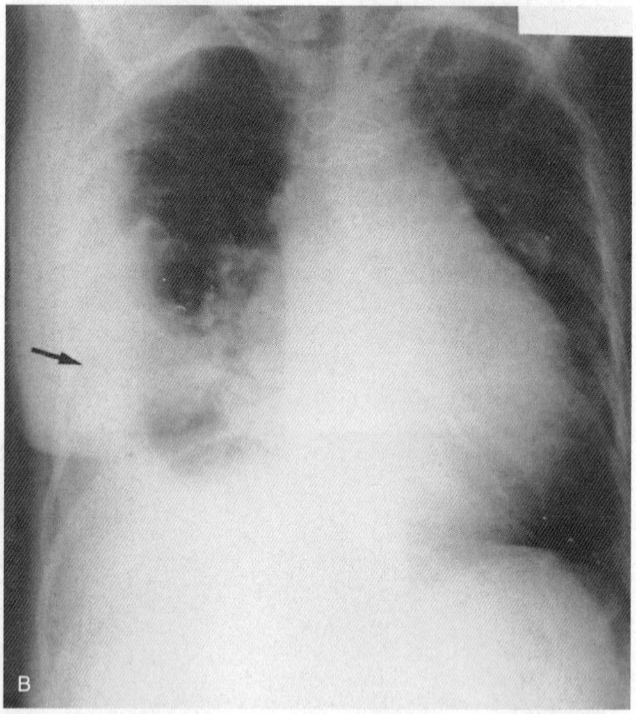

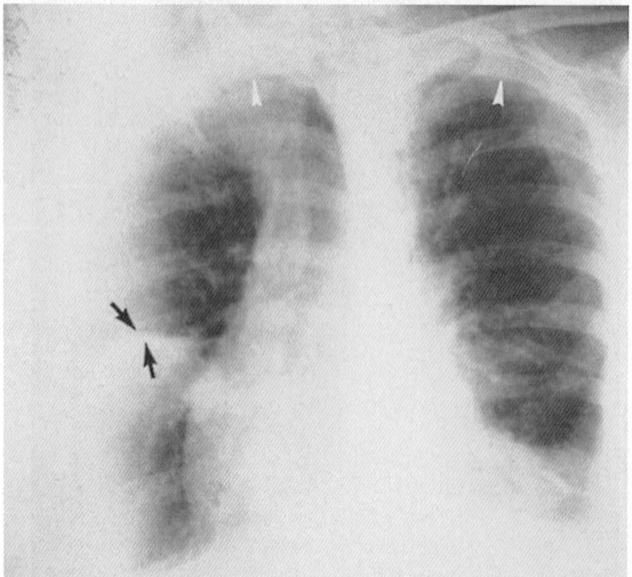

FIGURE 63.25. Pleural fluid in recumbency. **A:** Arrowheads show fluid tracking over the lung apex (apical cap) in the recumbent position. **B:** Right lateral decubitus view (right side down) shows layering of the pleural fluid (*arrow*). **C:** Right lateral decubitus view shows layering of pleural fluid and tracking into the minor fissure (*arrows*). Note bilateral apical caps (*arrowheads*).

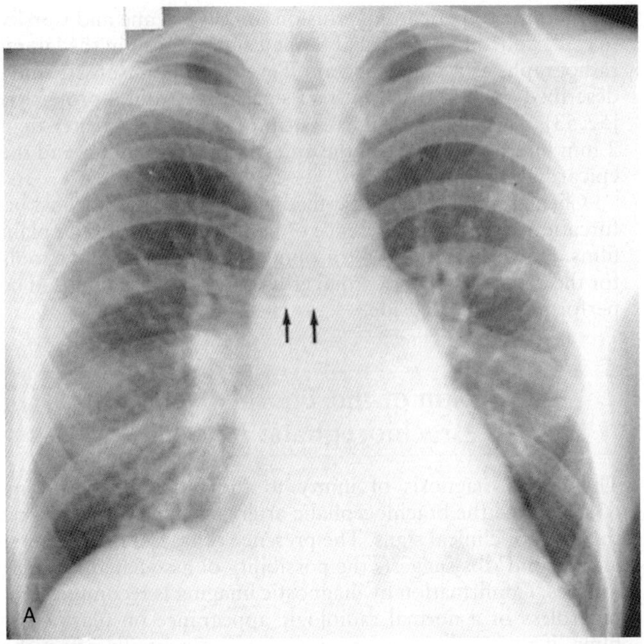

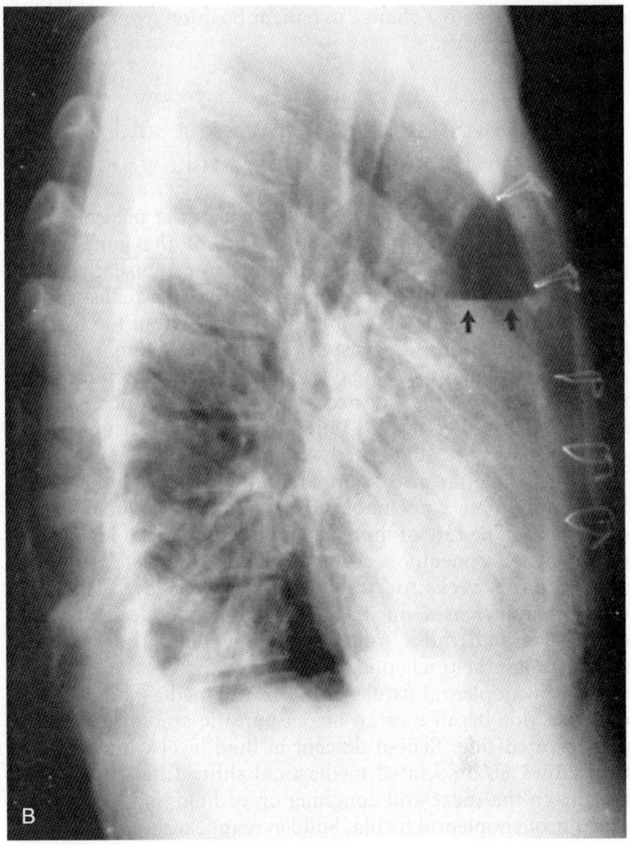

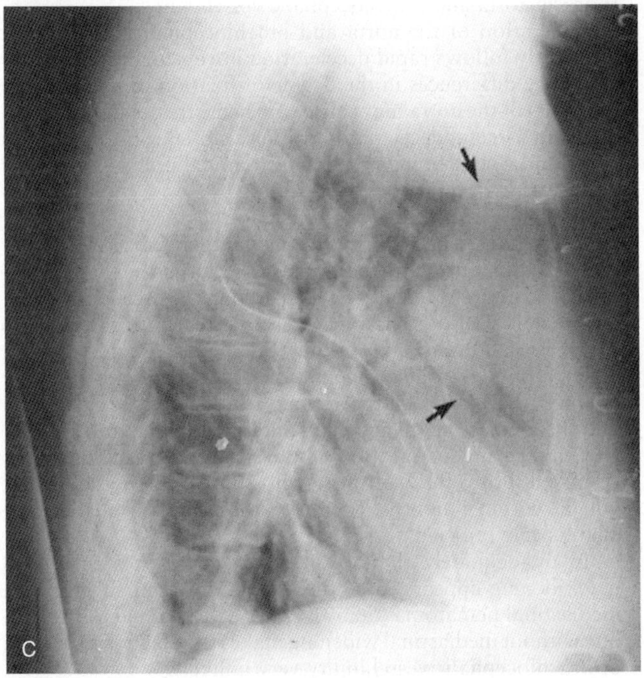

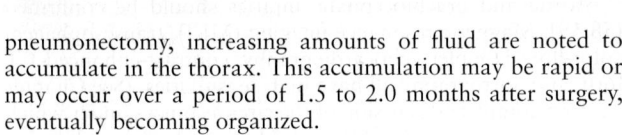

FIGURE 63.26. Fluid collections after surgery. **A:** Posteroanterior film of a patient several weeks after coronary artery bypass graft surgery shows an air-fluid level (*arrows*) superimposed on the shadow of the base of the heart. **B:** Lateral film of the same patient shows the air-fluid level (*arrows*) in the anterior mediastinum. **C:** Lateral film of a different patient outlines a semicircular soft tissue density (*arrows*) in the anterior mediastinum, representing a loculated fluid collection after surgery.

pneumonectomy, increasing amounts of fluid are noted to accumulate in the thorax. This accumulation may be rapid or may occur over a period of 1.5 to 2.0 months after surgery, eventually becoming organized.

Empyema and Peripheral Lung Abscess

An intrathoracic fluid-containing cavitary lesion adjacent to the chest wall may represent either a lung abscess (Fig. 63.26) or an empyema. By conventional radiography, visualization of the three-dimensional shape of the pleural lesion as oblong, flattened, and conforming to the shape of the thorax helps differentiate between the two lesions. A discrepancy in the width of the air-fluid levels between two 90-degree projections (i.e., when a wider level is apparent on AP than on lateral view, or vice versa) also suggests a pleural location. Abscesses are more spheric than empyemas and show no significant discrepancy in width on the two projections.

Often, however, one cannot distinguish between abscesses and empyemas by conventional radiography. In these cases, CT should be considered for adequate localization because there is a radical difference between the appropriate methods of treatment. Empyemas must be drained with a thoracostomy tube, whereas abscesses can be treated medically. Pugatch et al. [43] and Baber et al. [44] showed the usefulness of CT in differentiating between empyemas and abscesses. The former group showed that with CT, abscesses appear thick walled and irregular in shape, with an undulating or ragged inner wall. They often have multiple loculations, and their shape is unaltered by a change in patient position from supine or prone to decubitus. In contrast, empyemas appear more regular in shape and have smooth inner walls of uniform width. Their margins are sharply defined, with no loculi, and the shape of the cavity often changes with a change in patient position from supine or prone to decubitus.

Postpneumonectomy Space and Bronchopleural Fistula

After a pulmonary resection, air is seen in the pleural space from small air leaks in the cut surface of the lung. Small amounts of fluid also may be present. Air is usually reabsorbed gradually and continuously, followed by reabsorption of fluid, and both may be completely gone within the first 24 to 48 hours. Prolonged persistence of air and fluid may require drainage. Residual spaces may remain indefinitely without untoward effects and do not necessarily suggest bronchopleural fistula. Malamed et al. [45] stated that in 86% of cases, these residual spaces are obliterated within a year.

Air and fluid are always apparent in the basilar zone of the hemithorax after a pneumonectomy and may be loculated in some cases. The rate of fluid accumulation is variable, but the space left by a pneumonectomy is usually completely obliterated within 3 weeks to 7 months. If the fluid level decreases rather than increases, one must differentiate between a benign decrease in fluid and a bronchopleural fistula with loss of the fluid through the tracheobronchial tree.

A bronchopleural fistula displaces the mediastinum to the opposite side because of an increase in the amount of air on the operated side. Benign descent in fluid level without a fistula shows no associated mediastinal shift. Total clearing of fluid from the space and coughing up of fluid and blood suggest a bronchopleural fistula. Sudden reappearance of air in an obliterated space suggests either a bronchopleural fistula or a gas-forming infectious process.

A bronchopleural fistula can occur any time during the postoperative period but more often occurs within 8 to 12 days after surgery. If seen within the first 4 postoperative days, it is probably secondary to a mechanical failure of closure of the stump and requires reexploration and reclosure. A bronchopleural fistula also may occur after a suppurative pneumonia or massive pulmonary infarction, or even spontaneously.

Extremely rapid filling of a space with fluid suggests infection, hemorrhage, or malignant effusion. If secondary to infection, the rapid increase in height of the fluid level is usually associated with fever and leukocytosis. Empyema may occur alone or may be associated with a bronchopleural fistula. On the other hand, a bronchopleural fistula can occur without associated empyema, and the fluid in the pleural space in these cases is sterile.

Several methods have been used to diagnose bronchopleural fistulas, including the instillation of methylene blue into the pleural space [46], sinography, and bronchography [47]. Zelefsky et al. [48] demonstrated small leaks using xenon-133 in a gaseous state in a ventilation study. In the presence of a fistula, the xenon-133 activity accumulated in the pleural space and remained trapped within the pleural space on the washout study. The simplicity and reliability of this procedure make it a useful diagnostic tool.

Pericardial Effusion, Hemopericardium, and Tamponade

Fluid or blood in the pericardial cavity is suspected when an enlargement of the cardiac silhouette with a water-bottle configuration is noted; this typical configuration is not often seen. Fluoroscopy demonstrating diminished pulsations is frequently helpful but not diagnostic. In 1955, Kremens [49] and Torrance [50], using laminography, described the relation of the epicardial fat line to pericardial effusion. In 1968, Lane and Carsky [51,52] added the epicardial fat pad sign, as seen in the lateral radiograph, as a diagnostic aid. Several authors subsequently described the epicardial fat pad sign in the frontal projection [52,53]. This sign is seen as a strip of soft tissue greater than 2 mm interposed between the anterior mediastinal fat and the epicardial fat (Fig. 63.27).

Chen et al. [54] also described widening of the tracheal bifurcation angle in the presence of pericardial effusion on plain films. However, CT and ultrasound remain the definitive tools for the diagnosis of pericardial effusion, and ultrasound can be performed at the bedside.

Laceration of the Thoracic Aorta and Brachiocephalic Arteries

The initial diagnosis of injury to the thoracic aorta (Fig. 63.28A) and the brachiocephalic arteries may be suspected on the basis of clinical signs. The presence of fractures of the first and second ribs suggests the possibility of associated vascular injuries. Confirmation by diagnostic imaging is recommended, regardless of a normal radiologic appearance on plain chest films, if the mechanism of injury could potentially affect the thoracic aorta and brachiocephalic vessels.

Laceration of the aorta and brachiocephalic vessels most frequently follows rapid deceleration in vehicular accidents or falls. The differences in the degree of fixation of the different segments of the aorta may cause sufficient stresses between segments in forceful deceleration to cause closed rupture. Flexion stress and a sudden increase in intraluminal pressure also may be the cause of injury.

In 69% to 89% of cases, injury to the aorta occurs at the isthmus, the area between the origin of the left subclavian artery and the attachment of the ductus arteriosus. In the remaining cases, injury is equally divided among the ascending aorta, aortic arch, and descending aorta [55]. Tear is almost always transverse and may involve only one or all layers. When all layers are involved, exsanguination occurs; if the tear is only through the intima or the intima and media, the adventitia and the mediastinal pleura can contain the blood at least temporarily. Parmley et al. [47] emphasized that if the diagnosis is missed, up to 90% of those who survive the initial impact will die within 4 months. Therefore, the diagnosis must be very aggressively pursued.

In an adequately obtained plain film of the chest, mediastinal widening appears to be the most useful sign suggesting a mediastinal hematoma [56,57]. A perfectly normal aortic outline without mediastinal widening makes the diagnosis of aortic or brachiocephalic vessel injury very unlikely.

Aortic and brachiocephalic injuries should be confirmed [58,59]. Magnetic resonance imaging (MRI), transesophageal color-flow Doppler echocardiography, contrast-enhanced CT [60], and aortography all have high sensitivities. (See Chapter 36 for a complete discussion of the circumstances under which each method is preferred.) If static filming is performed during aortography, two angiographic series must be obtained, with the right posterior oblique projection as the acceptable standard and the frontal or AP projection as the second view (Fig. 63.28B,C).

Traumatic Diaphragmatic Hernia

Severe diaphragmatic injury after blunt or penetrating trauma to the thoracoabdominal area may allow escape of abdominal contents into the thorax. The presence of a gas-containing viscus within the thoracic cavity is the hallmark of traumatic

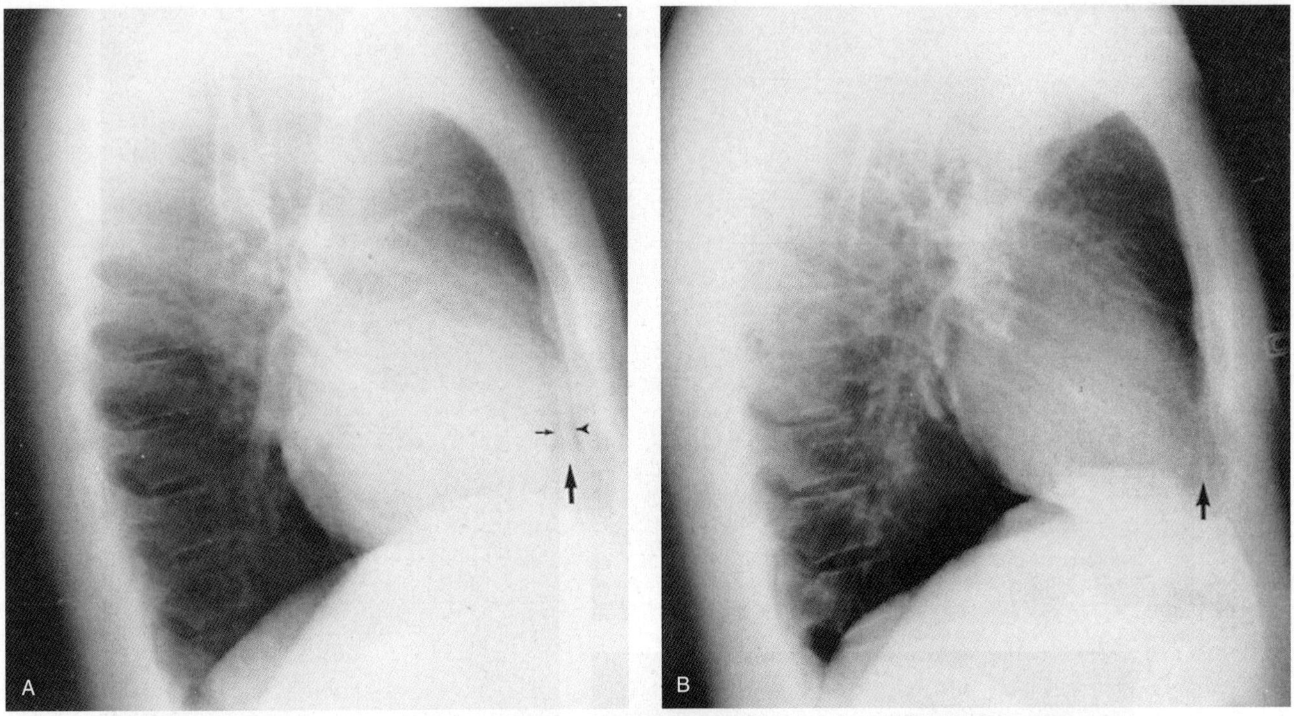

FIGURE 63.27. Pericardial effusion. **A:** Lateral view of the chest shows the pericardial effusion as a strip of density (*long arrow*) sandwiched between two strips of lucency. The posterior strip of lucency represents epicardial fat (*short arrow*), and the anterior strip represents mediastinal fat (*arrowhead*). An increase of the density to greater than 2 mm suggests pericardial fluid (effusion or hemopericardium). **B:** Follow-up lateral view of the same patient after resolution of the pericardial effusion. The cardiac size is smaller, and the width of the strip of density (*arrow*) has returned to normal.

diaphragmatic rupture with an associated hernia. Most hernias occur on the left side, because the liver acts as a buffer on the right. Very often, the condition may be overlooked during the initial phase (the first 14 days). During the latent period, which varies considerably, patients may have vague chronic symptoms or no symptoms at all. Symptomatic patients may be subjected to numerous diagnostic procedures in an attempt to unravel their vague abdominal complaints, which probably are due to intermittent incarceration of the herniated viscus. The obstructive phase may occur at any time, the obstruction being secondary to incarceration or strangulation.

Radiologic findings on plain chest films vary from what appears to be merely an arched or elevated diaphragm (with or without platelike atelectasis in the adjacent lung) to visualization of a hollow viscus above the diaphragm with a marked shift in the heart and mediastinum. Ball et al. [61] suggested that the chest film is the most reliable means of determining the correct diagnosis. Additional diagnostic aids include contrast studies with barium to demonstrate the presence of a viscus above the diaphragm, diagnostic pneumoperitoneum to outline the defect with free passage of air from the peritoneum into the pleural or pericardial cavity, and introduction of contrast into the pleural space to demonstrate free passage from the pleura into the peritoneal cavity. Lung and liver–spleen scans also have been used, as has ultrasound.

Toombs et al. [62] and Heiberg et al. [63] demonstrated the usefulness of CT in recognizing traumatic rupture of the diaphragm. CT identifies parts of the diaphragm as a separate structure, and a discontinuity in its contour can be recognized. The posterolateral portions of the diaphragm are well demonstrated, and tears are easy to see in these areas. Dynamic CT is particularly helpful. We found direct coronal sections (whenever the patient can be appropriately positioned in the CT gantry) to be extremely useful in diagnosing diaphragmatic tears with herniation. MRI is the definitive diagnostic imaging modality. It is able to image the muscles of the diaphragm, the defect or rent, and the bowel herniating through it.

EXTRA-ALVEOLAR AIR AND SIGNS OF BAROTRAUMA

Pneumothorax

The diagnosis of pneumothorax is made when air is seen superior, inferior, lateral, or anterior to the lung and the visceral pleural line is identified. The air creates a zone of radiolucency devoid of lung markings between the lung and the thoracic wall. The lung partially (Fig. 63.29A) or wholly (Fig. 63.29B) collapses and drops to the most dependent position, slung by its fixed attachment at the pulmonary ligament. The density of the partially collapsed lung may not increase when compared with the opposite side because blood flow through it diminishes correspondingly, the degree of diminution of flow progressing with increasing collapse. Thus, the ratio of air to blood is maintained and the lung density remains unaltered [64].

As air accumulates in the pleura, the mediastinum tends to shift to the opposite side. This is best seen in a film taken during the expiratory phase of respiration. For the mediastinum to shift, the intrapleural pressure must become merely less negative, not necessarily positive, on the side of the pneumothorax. If the mediastinum is not fixed, the diminished negative pressure on the side of the pneumothorax creates sufficient imbalance between the pleural pressures of the two sides to cause mediastinal displacement during the expiratory phase of

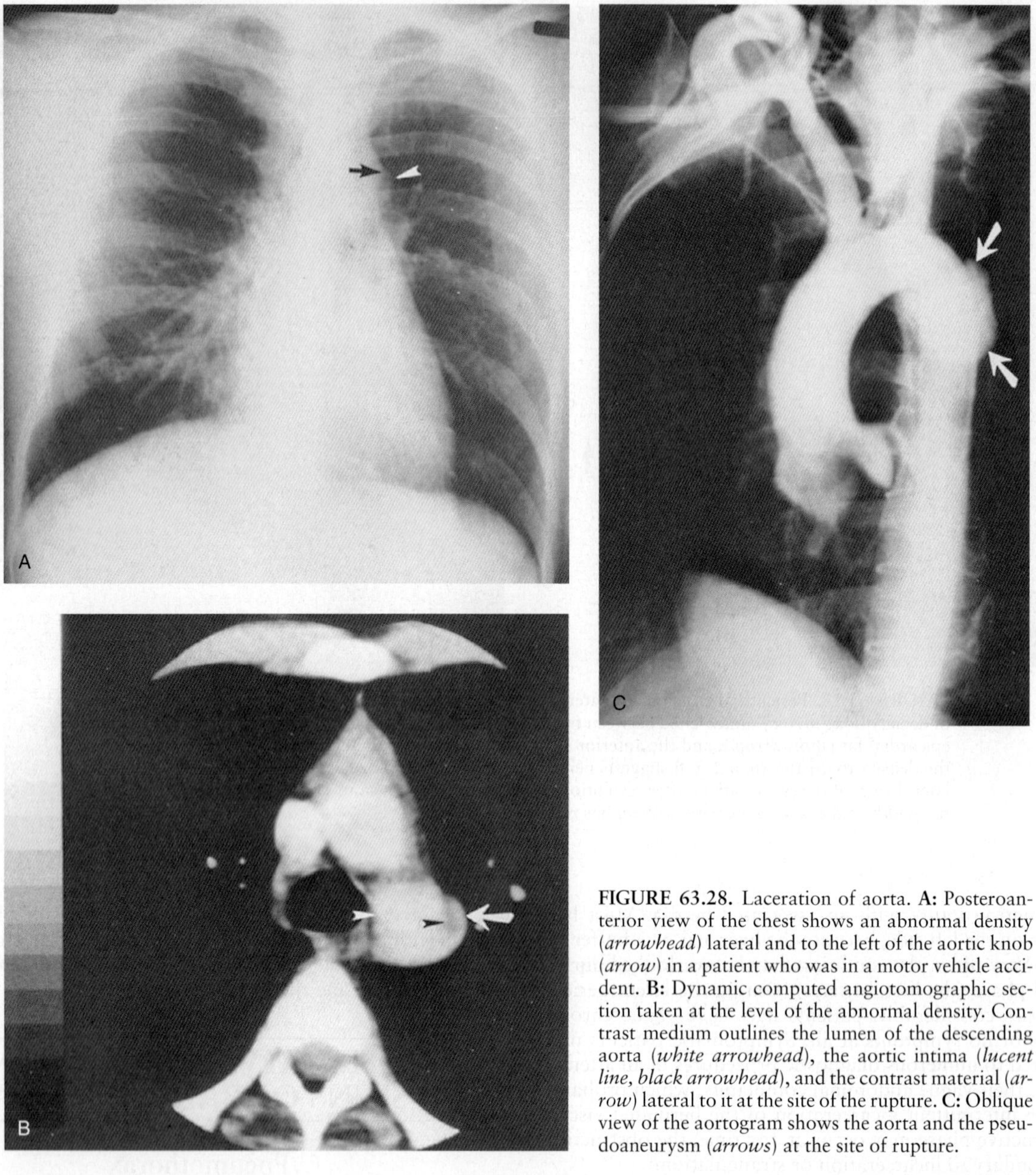

FIGURE 63.28. Laceration of aorta. **A:** Posteroanterior view of the chest shows an abnormal density (*arrowhead*) lateral and to the left of the aortic knob (*arrow*) in a patient who was in a motor vehicle accident. **B:** Dynamic computed angiotomographic section taken at the level of the abnormal density. Contrast medium outlines the lumen of the descending aorta (*white arrowhead*), the aortic intima (*lucent line, black arrowhead*), and the contrast material (*arrow*) lateral to it at the site of the rupture. **C:** Oblique view of the aortogram shows the aorta and the pseudoaneurysm (*arrows*) at the site of rupture.

respiration. If the mediastinum is not fixed, tension pneumothorax causes a shift of the mediastinum to the opposite side during inspiratory and expiratory phases of respiration. In addition, flattening, with progression to reversal of the normal curve of the hemidiaphragm, occurs in tension pneumothorax. Rhea et al. [65] described a simple reproducible means of measuring the percentage of pneumothorax present in upright PA and lateral films. The percentage of pneumothorax is calculated by means of an average interpleural distance, using the total lung volume of the partially collapsed lung and the total hemithoracic volume as parameters. Pneumothorax size can be predicted using a nomogram based on average interpleural distance.

The distribution of air in the pleural cavity is affected by pleural adhesions and by disease of the underlying lung. Adhesions prevent lung retraction; therefore, extensive adhesions may lead to a loculated pneumothorax. A diseased lung, especially one with scarring or atelectasis secondary to bronchial obstruction, tends to retract to a greater degree than the adjacent lung. Obstructive emphysema, consolidation, and interstitial emphysema make the lung rigid and interfere with retraction, keeping the lung or the involved segment expanded. The distribution of air is also influenced by patient position, because air rises to the nondependent portion of the thorax.

Early recognition of a pneumothorax is mandatory in ICU patients, especially those on respirators or those who are prone to barotrauma or rapid progression to tension pneumothorax. The presence of lower lobe disease, with the lobes resisting reaeration, causes air to collect in the subpulmonic region, simulating a pneumoperitoneum [66]. Thus, in ICU patients, the subpulmonic area must be carefully examined, even if the film is obtained in the upright position, because lower lobe disease, consolidation due to ARDS, and pneumonia are frequently present. In the supine patient, air collects in the anterior portion of the thorax, between the medial portion of the lung and the anterior mediastinum, or in the subpulmonic area (Fig. 63.30).

Subpulmonic pneumothorax is seen as a lucent area outlining the anterior costophrenic sulcus projected over the right or left upper quadrant [67] or only as a deep lateral costophrenic

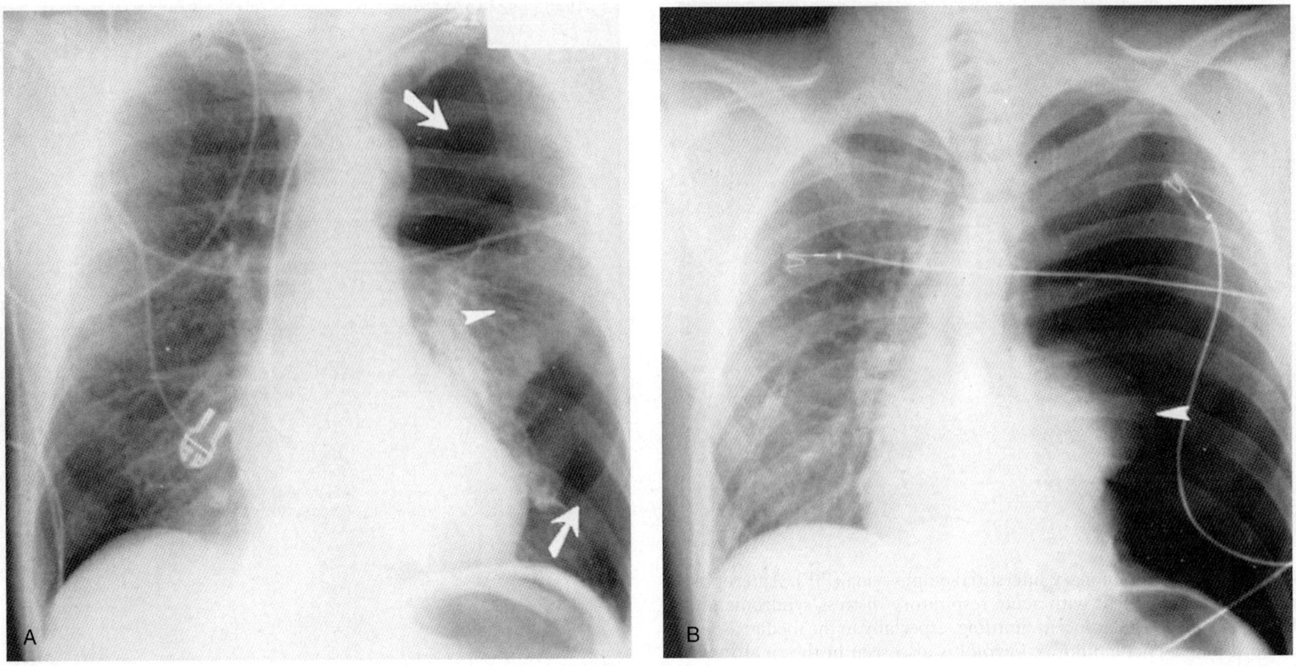

FIGURE 63.29. Pneumothorax. **A:** Posteroanterior film of a patient with left pneumothorax. Air in the pleural space (*arrows*) is differentiated from the aerated lung by the absence of bronchovascular markings. Note lack of increased density of the lateral aspect of the partially collapsed lung (*arrowhead*). **B:** Total collapse of the lung against the mediastinum (*arrowhead*) seen in another patient. Note increase in size of the left hemithorax and slight shift of the mediastinum to the contralateral side.

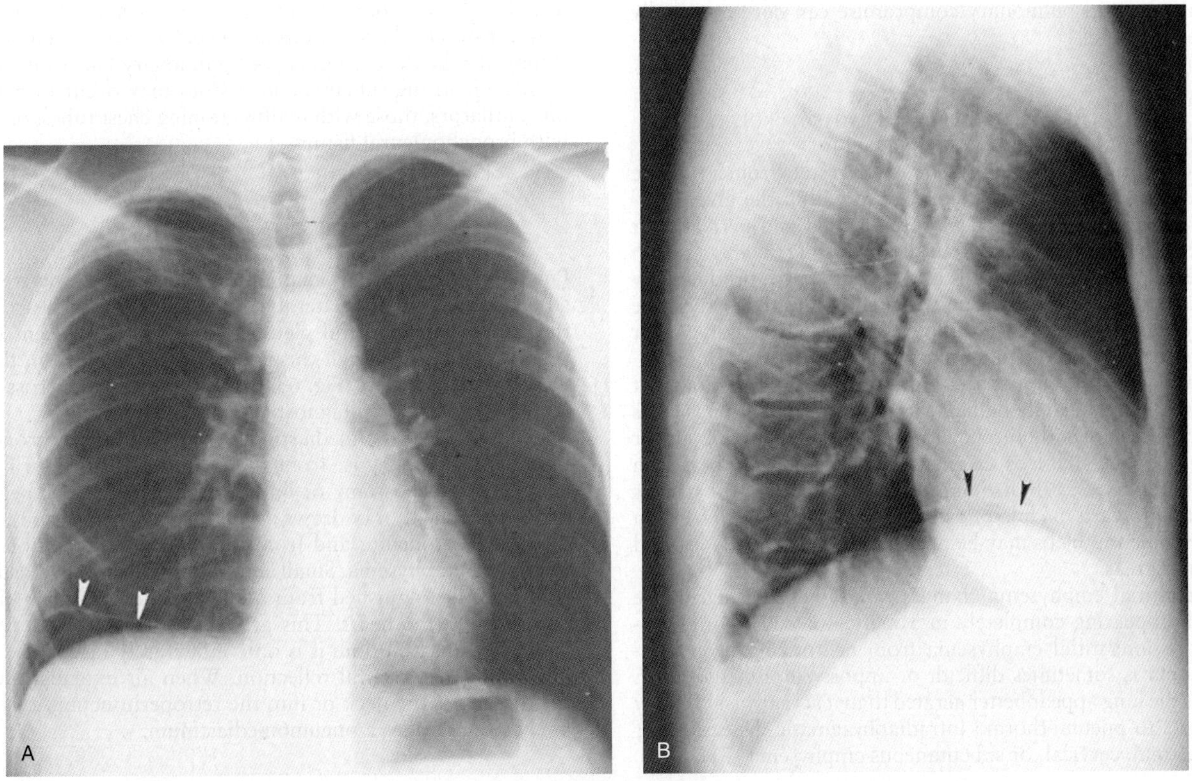

FIGURE 63.30. Subpulmonic pneumothorax. **A:** Posteroanterior view of the chest shows a linear density (*arrowheads*) representing the visceral pleura displaced superiorly by the collection of pleural air (subpulmonic pneumothorax) beneath it. **B:** Lateral view shows the same linear density (*arrowheads*) and subpulmonic pneumothorax.

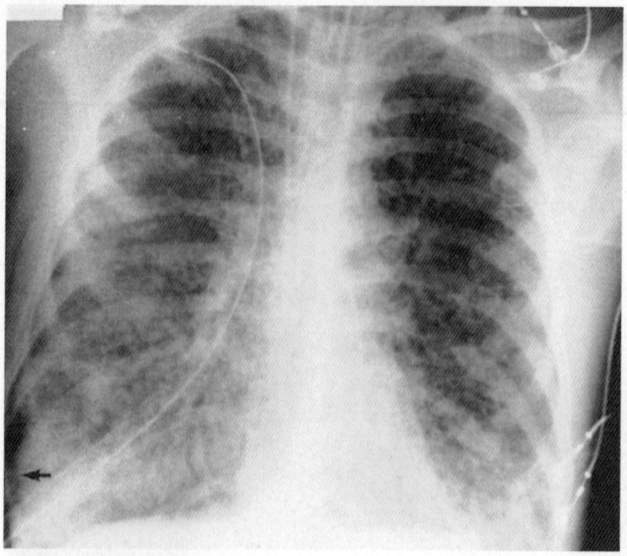

FIGURE 63.31. Pulmonary interstitial emphysema (PIE). Anteroposterior film of a patient with acute respiratory distress syndrome and PIE shows the irregular lucent mottling, especially in the medial aspect of both lungs. Pneumothorax (*arrow*) is also seen in the right lower hemithorax.

sulcus on the involved side [68]. Even with progression to a tension pneumothorax, in a patient with ARDS, it is possible for the only finding to be a flattening of the cardiac border or a lateral depression of the hemidiaphragm [69]. These findings should be recognized as signs of tension, because severe cardiovascular and pulmonary compromise can develop rapidly in these patients.

Pulmonary Interstitial Emphysema

Pulmonary interstitial emphysema (PIE) results from a rupture of the alveolar wall when the pressure within the alveoli exceeds that within the adjacent vascular bed and perivascular connective tissue. As a result, air dissects along the interstitium of the lungs. Histologically, PIE is seen as spaces produced by the dissection of air into the perivascular connective tissues, the interlobular septa, and the subpleural connective tissue, most extensively around the pulmonary veins [70].

Radiologically, these spaces are seen as irregular radiolucent mottling in the medial one-half to two-thirds of the lungs or as discrete areas of radiolucency (Fig. 63.31). They are 2 cm or more in diameter (blebs or pneumatoceles) and are best seen at the lung bases. PIE also may appear as radiolucent streaks radiating toward the hila or as a lucent halo around vessels on end. Subpleural blebs may be present, most frequently around the hilar areas.

Interstitial emphysema changes rapidly, decreasing in size and disappearing completely in a matter of days. Differentiation of interstitial emphysema from necrotizing bronchopneumonia is sometimes difficult or impossible. Extensive PIE makes the lung appear better aerated than it actually is. PIE may progress to pneumothorax; infradiaphragmatic dissection; or mediastinal, cervical, or subcutaneous emphysema [71].

Subcutaneous Emphysema

Air in the subcutaneous tissues is seen as linear streaks of lucency outlining tissue planes or as bubbles of lucency within the soft tissues (Fig. 63.32). Localized subcutaneous emphysema

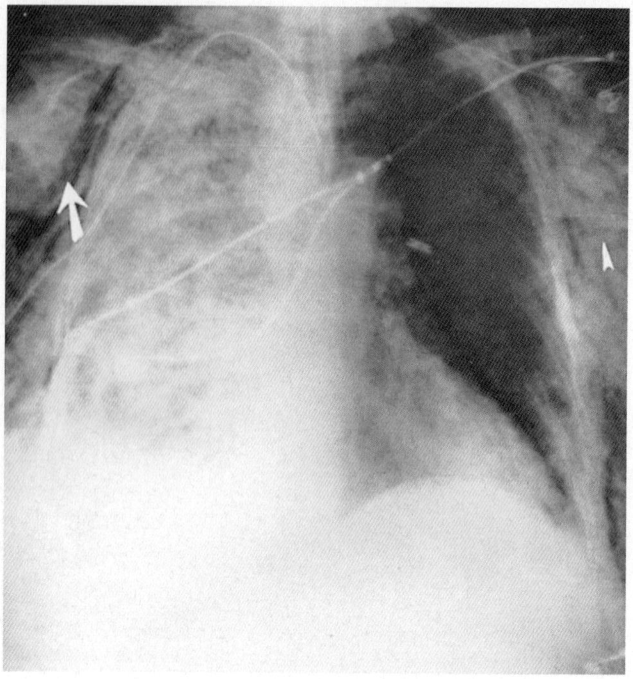

FIGURE 63.32. Subcutaneous emphysema. Anteroposterior film of a patient with right lung opacification from pneumonia with an endotracheal tube and right chest tube in place. The radiating lucencies in the left hemithorax (*arrowhead*) outline the pectoralis muscles. Other air collections (*arrow*) are in the subcutaneous tissues.

usually follows thoracostomy tube insertions, tracheostomies, and transtracheal aspirations and usually is of no significance. It may also be the earliest sign of pulmonary barotrauma. Extensive air in the subcutaneous tissues may occur in patients on ventilators, those with malfunctioning chest tubes, or those with bronchopleural fistulas.

Pneumomediastinum

Pneumomediastinum is manifested radiologically as vertical streaks of lucency just lateral to the borders of the heart, with the parietal and visceral pleura reflected by the lucent stripe (Fig. 63.33A). Although this condition can be seen in the PA view, the lateral view (Fig. 63.33B), specifically the cross-table lateral view, is more diagnostically useful.

Air can enter the mediastinum from a ruptured bronchus, trachea, or esophagus; from the neck (especially during the course of tracheostomy or line placement, when the negative pressure of the thorax draws air in through the incision); from the retroperitoneum; and from the lungs in association with interstitial emphysema. Small amounts of pneumomediastinum should be distinguished from the normal lucency of a kinetic halo around the heart. This artifactual halo is produced by normal cardiac motion; it is only moderately lucent and does not outline the pleural reflection. When air extends into the soft tissues of the neck or into the retroperitoneum, it is most likely secondary to a pneumomediastinum.

Pneumopericardium

Radiologic diagnosis of a pneumopericardium is made when a lucent stripe is seen around the heart extending to, but not beyond, the proximal pulmonary artery and outlining a thickened pericardium (Fig. 63.34). It may be difficult to differentiate

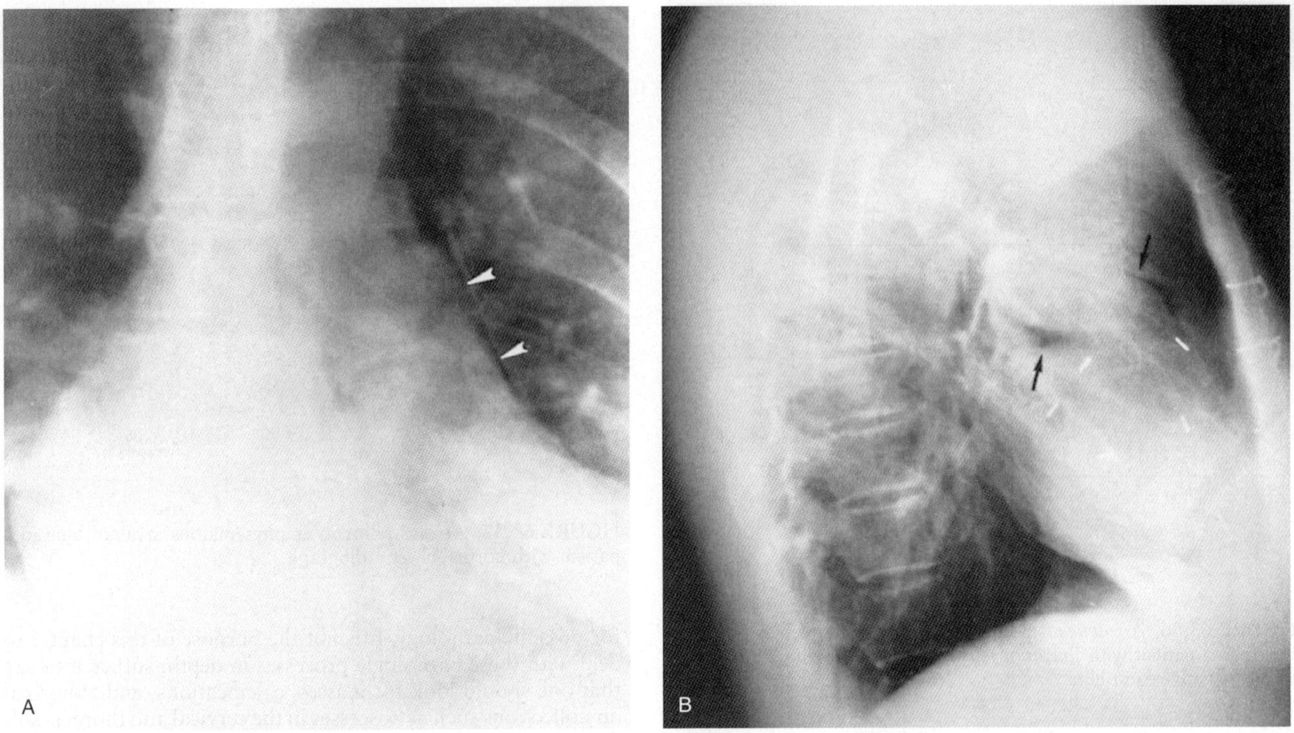

FIGURE 63.33. Pneumomediastinum. **A:** Posteroanterior view of the chest shows air in the mediastinum (*arrowheads*). **B:** Lateral view of chest in a different patient shows lucent areas (*arrows*) representing pneumomediastinum outlining the main pulmonary artery. The patient had previous coronary artery bypass surgery.

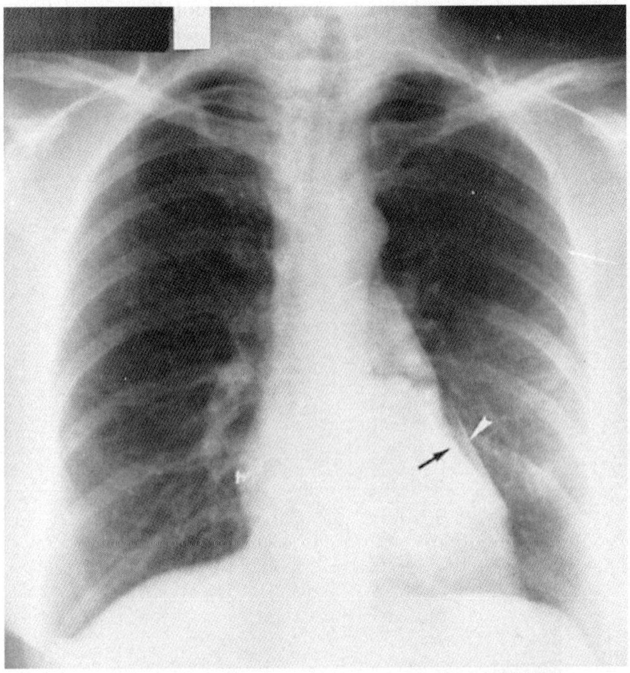

FIGURE 63.34. Pneumopericardium. Posteroanterior view of the chest shows a lucent area (pneumopericardium) lateral to the cardiac shadow (*arrow*) and medial to a strip of density of the pericardium (*arrowhead*). Slight blunting of the right costophrenic sulcus from a small pleural effusion is also present. The patient had previous coronary artery bypass surgery.

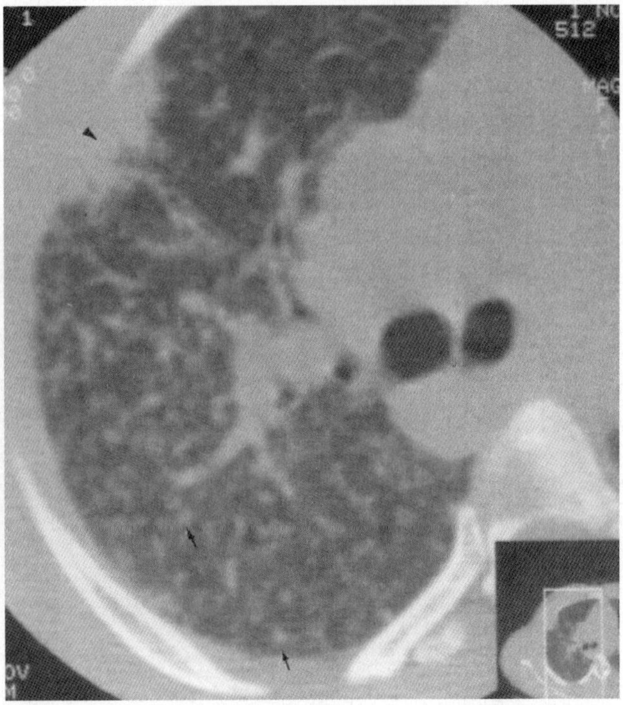

FIGURE 63.35. *Arrows* point to miliary nodules that are hardly visible on plain films but well seen by high-resolution computed tomography in a patient with miliary tuberculosis. *Arrowhead* points to an area of tuberculous consolidation.

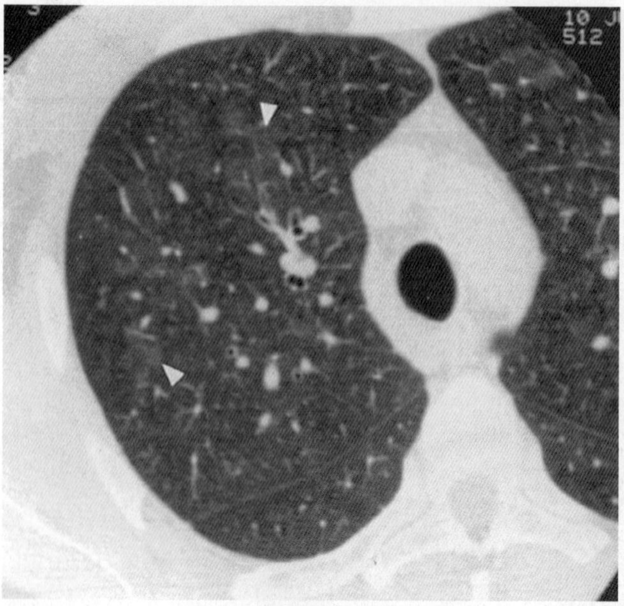

FIGURE 63.36. *Arrowheads* point to faint areas of alveolar opacification in a patient with *Pneumocystis jiroveci* pneumonia who had a totally negative chest film.

from a pneumothorax or pneumomediastinum; a cross-table lateral film may be necessary. Pneumopericardium is almost always the result of surgery but also may follow trauma or infection.

Extrapulmonary Structures

Evaluation of the chest radiograph is never complete unless the extrapulmonary, extrapleural, and extracardiac structures (extrathoracic soft tissues and bony thorax) are carefully assessed

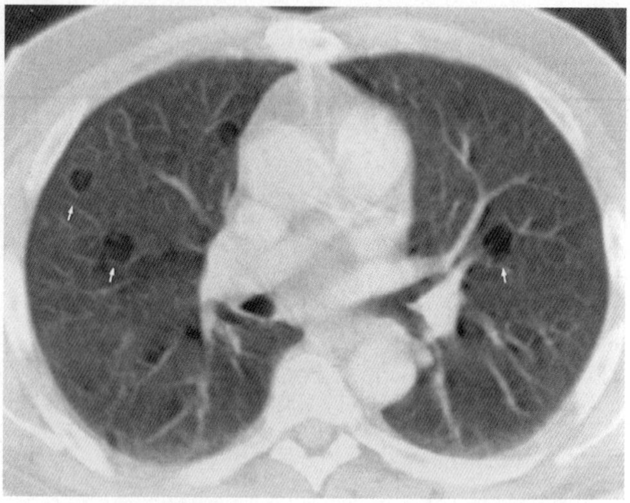

FIGURE 63.37. *Arrows* point to emphysematous areas of lung in a patient with normal chest radiograph.

for possible pathology. It is not the purpose of this chapter to deal with these pathologic processes in depth; suffice it to say that one should look for masses, calcifications, and abnormal air collections such as abscesses in the cervical and thoracic soft tissues and subphrenic areas. The bony structures also may provide clues to disease of a systemic nature (e.g., H-shaped vertebrae and bone infarcts in sickle cell anemia) or to metastases in the form of lytic or blastic bone lesions. Fractures after trauma, and occasionally rib fractures from resuscitation procedures after cardiac arrest, may be seen on the chest radiograph.

Additional Imaging

As previously stated, many patients cannot be moved from the ICU and CCU areas. For the patient who can be moved

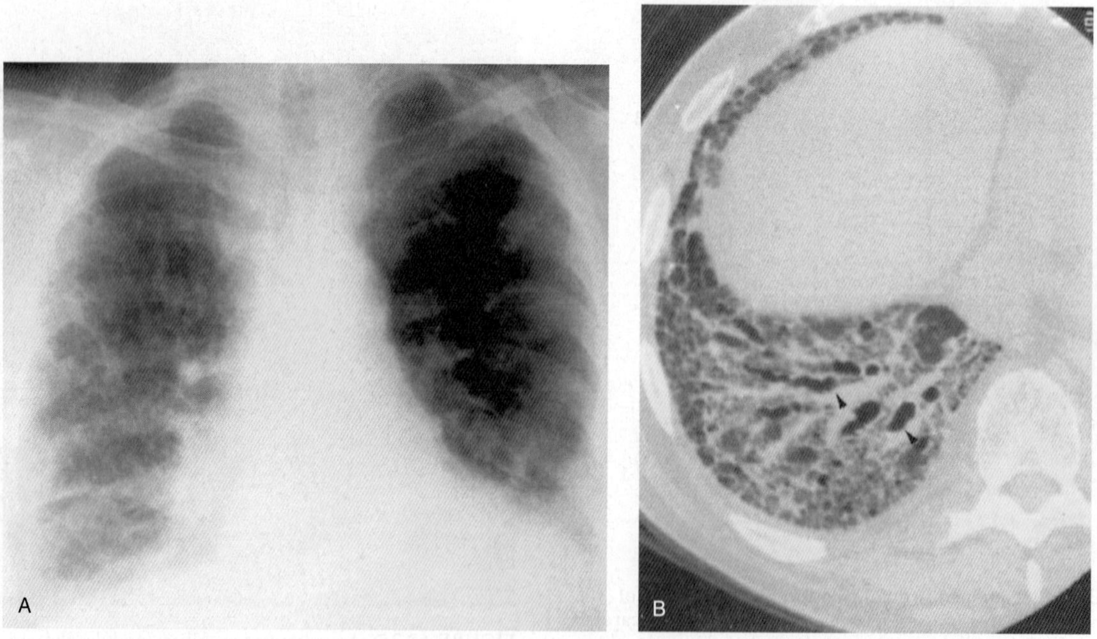

FIGURE 63.38. **A:** Patient with interstitial opacities in both lower lobes. **B:** High-resolution computed tomography shows extremely well the reticular interstitial opacities and the bronchiectasis (*arrowheads*) from the patient's idiopathic pulmonary fibrosis.

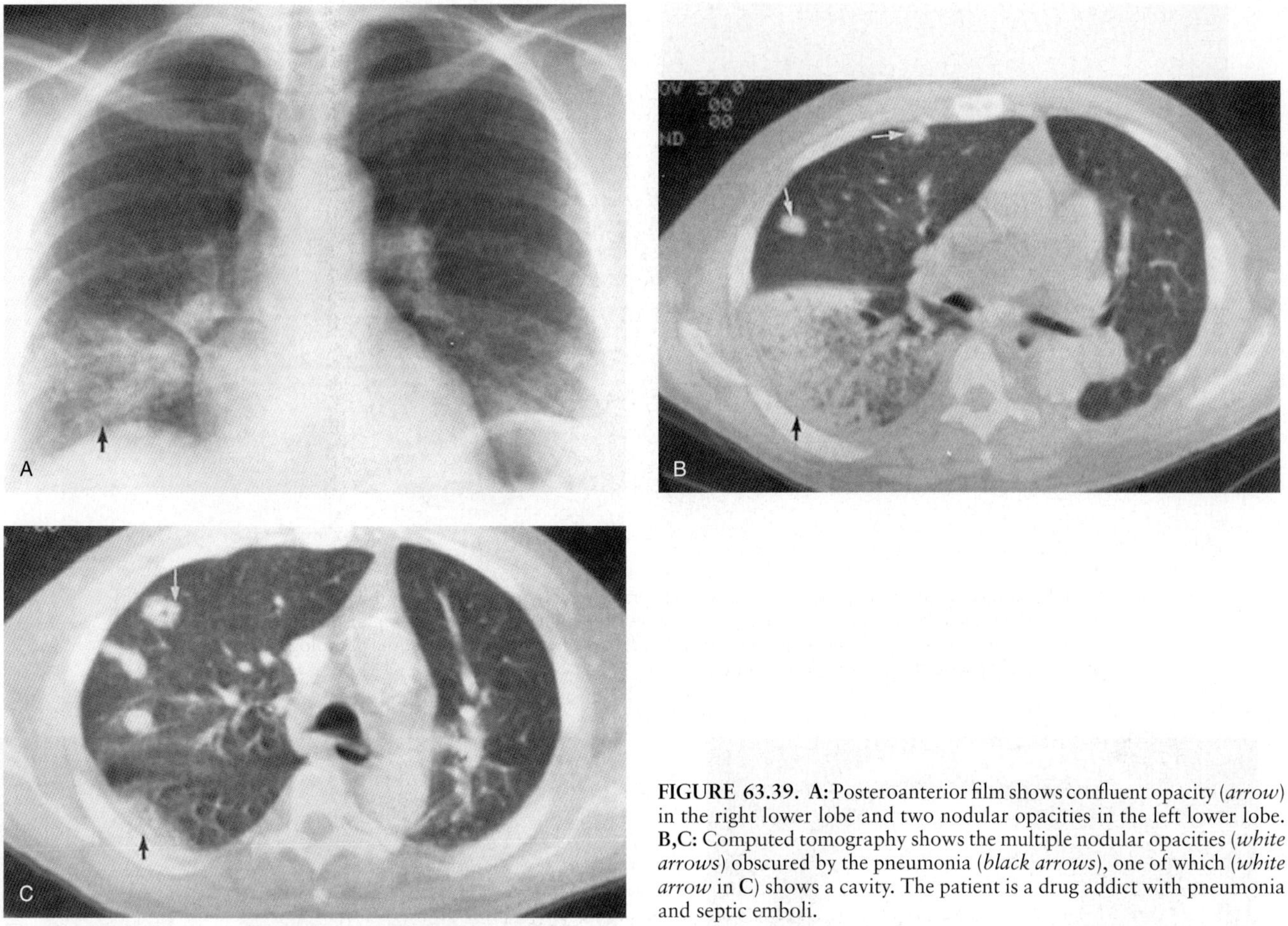

FIGURE 63.39. A: Posteroanterior film shows confluent opacity (*arrow*) in the right lower lobe and two nodular opacities in the left lower lobe. B,C: Computed tomography shows the multiple nodular opacities (*white arrows*) obscured by the pneumonia (*black arrows*), one of which (*white arrow* in C) shows a cavity. The patient is a drug addict with pneumonia and septic emboli.

and whose clinical conditions demand additional radiologic workup for diagnostic elucidation or therapeutic intervention, other modalities are available. CT pulmonary arteriography, CT venography, digital subtraction angiography, interventional procedures (e.g., catheter placement for pharmacotherapy and drainage of obstructed areas), ultrasonographically guided drainage of abscesses and pleural or pericardial effusions, positron emission tomography, and nuclear magnetic resonance are either available now or will be soon in the armamentarium of radiology departments.

CT, MRI, and ultrasound now form the armamentarium of imaging modalities in addition to plain films available to clinicians for thoracic imaging. The clinical problem to be solved dictates the modality to be used.

The modality of choice for imaging of the lung parenchyma is CT. High-resolution CT (1.5-mm sections at small fields of view and using edge-enhancement techniques) gives a very detailed look at the lung parenchyma, allowing early abnormalities of the lungs to be seen before they are visible on plain films (Figs. 63.35 and 63.36), assessment of the degree of emphysematous destruction of lung (Fig. 63.37), better characterization of parenchymal and interstitial abnormalities (Figs. 63.38 through 63.40), and even the ability to see through the diffuse opacification of the hemithoraces seen on plain films (Fig. 63.41).

The pleura is better assessed by CT than by plain film (Figs. 63.42 through 63.45). Differentiation between pleural and parenchymal abnormalities is easier using CT (Fig. 63.46). CT is the best modality to use when looking for calcification in a lesion, whether it be in lung, mediastinum, or pleura. Small amounts of air are also best seen using CT (Fig. 63.47).

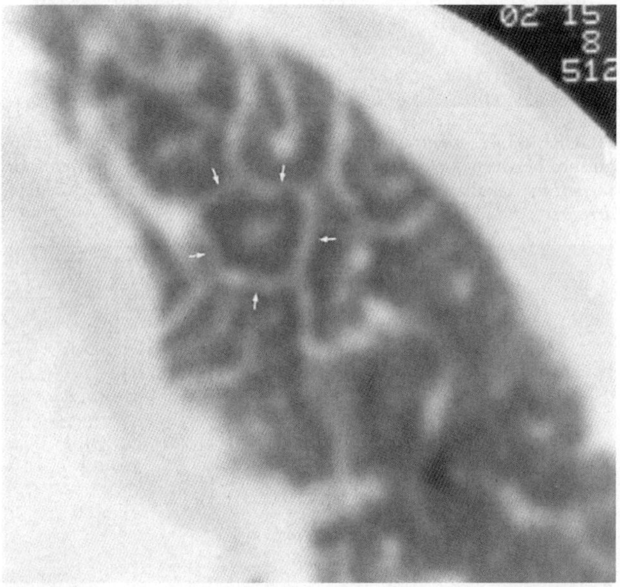

FIGURE 63.40. Enlargement of section of high-resolution computed tomography in a patient with lymphangitic metastasis from breast carcinoma. *Arrows* point to the distended interlobular septae forming the polygonal outline of a secondary lobule. Central density within the secondary lobule represents an arteriole.

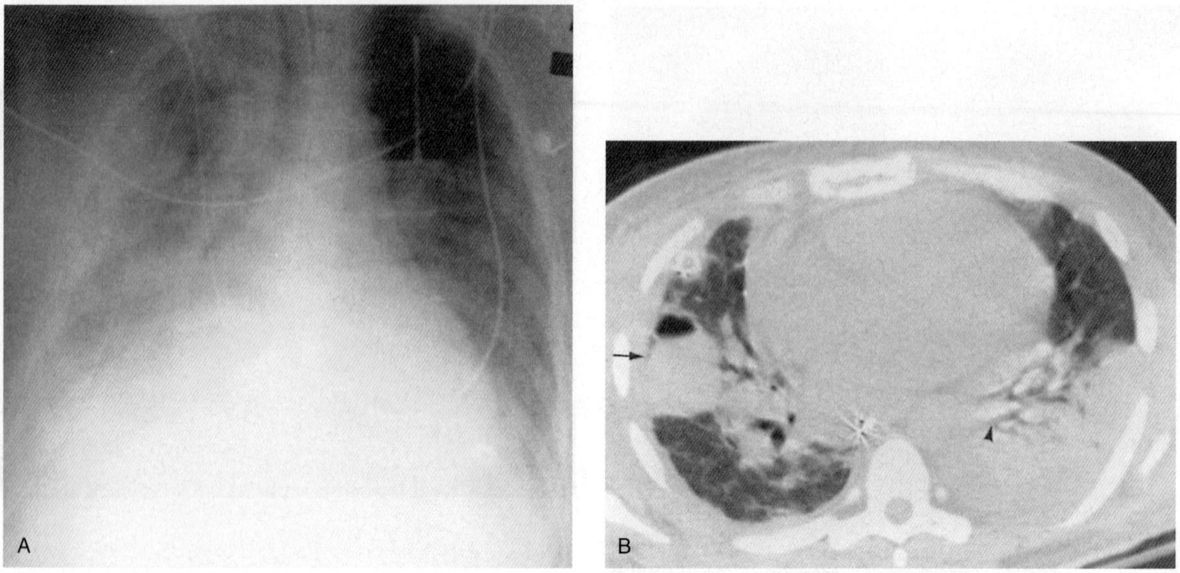

FIGURE 63.41. **A:** Posteroanterior film shows bilateral parenchymal opacification with greater involvement of the right side. **B:** Computed tomography shows the right lung abscess with air-fluid level (*arrow*) and the pneumonia with air bronchograms (*arrowhead*) in the left, defining better the pathology producing the areas of opacification in the posteroanterior film.

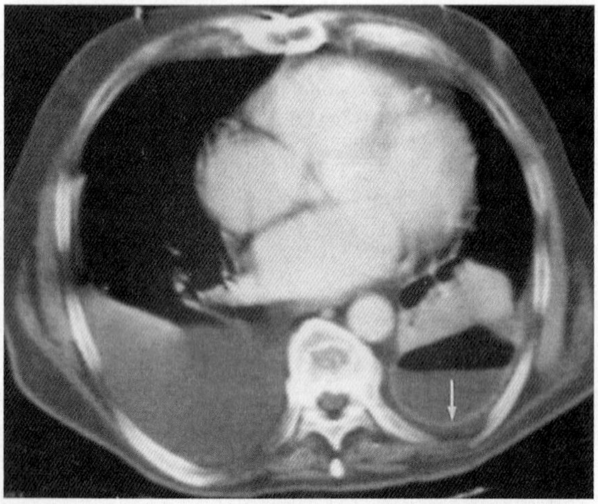

FIGURE 63.42. Contrast-enhanced computed tomography distinguishes between a pleural effusion on the right and an empyema on the left by visualization of an enhancing pleura (curvilinear white line, *arrow*).

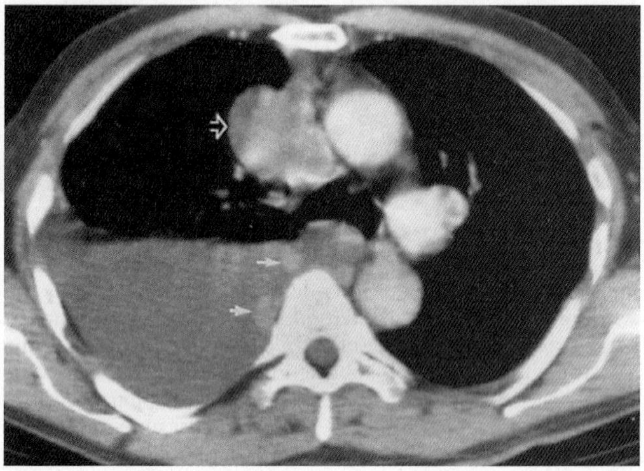

FIGURE 63.43. Patient with bronchogenic carcinoma (*open arrow*) with pleural effusion. White arrows point to metastatic pleural deposits that are not visible on plain films.

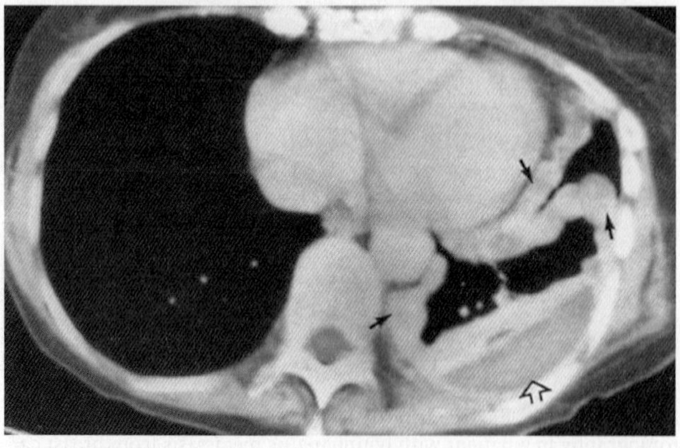

FIGURE 63.44. Patient with a densely opacified left hemithorax. Computed tomography shows the lobulated pleural thickening (*arrows*) and pleural effusion (*open arrow*) secondary to mesothelioma.

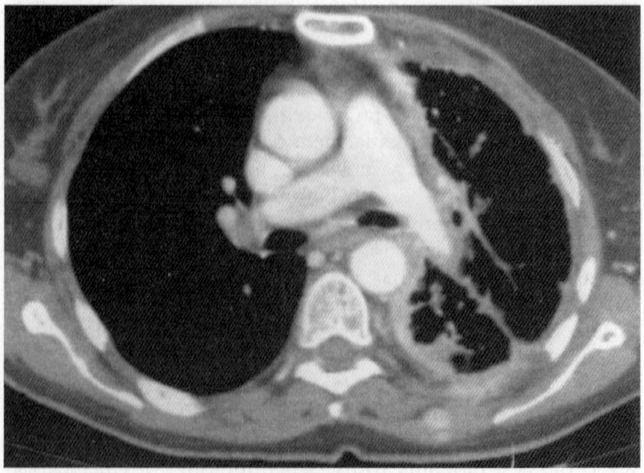

FIGURE 63.45. Irregular pleural opacity in the left pleural space from metastatic adenocarcinoma.

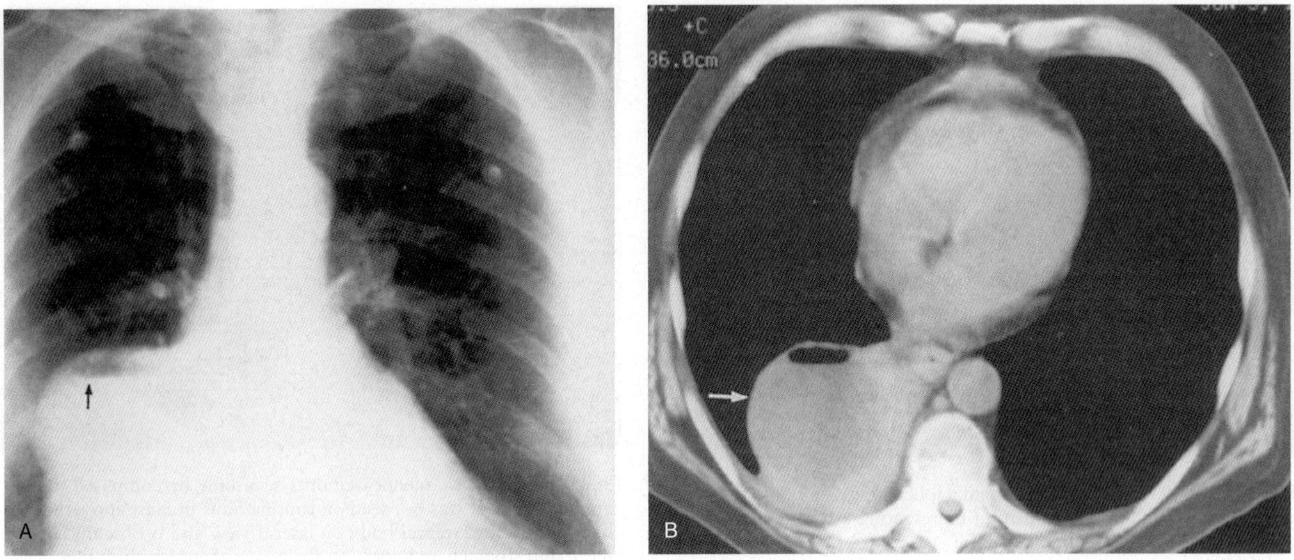

FIGURE 63.46. Mass opacity with air-fluid level on the posteroanterior view (*black arrow*) (**A**), clearly imaged by computed tomography (*white arrow*) (**B**), and shown to be a lung abscess.

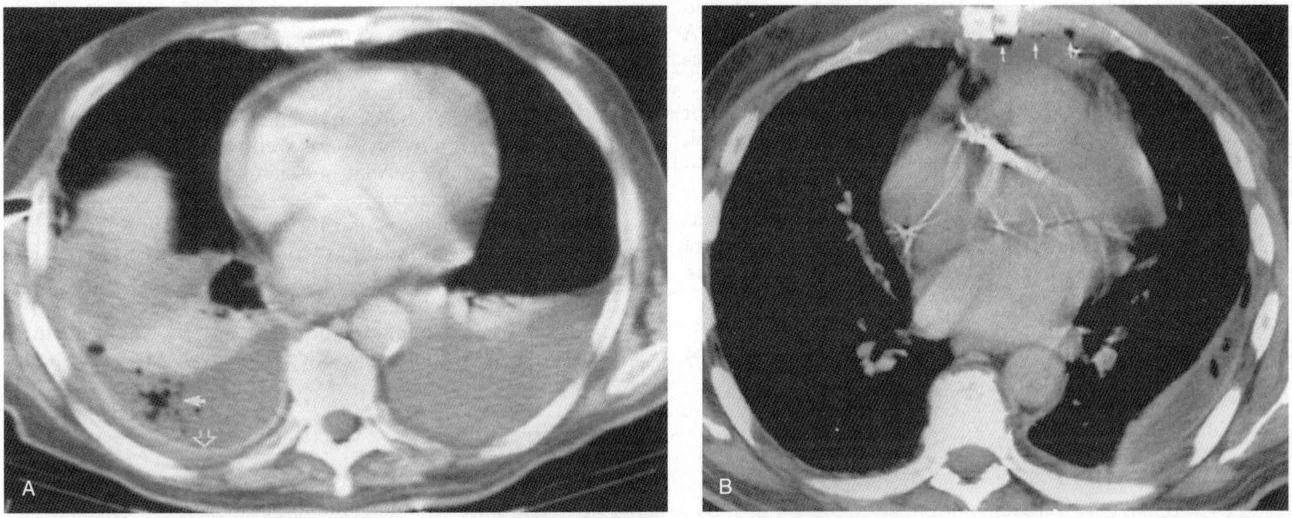

FIGURE 63.47. **A:** Patient with bilateral effusions. Computed tomography (CT) shows air within the effusion (*arrow*) and pleura enhancement (*open arrow*), allowing the diagnosis of an empyema. **B:** Patient who had coronary bypass surgery several weeks before this CT shows mediastinitis with air (*arrows*) in the retrosternal area. Empyema is also noted in the posterior left hemithorax.

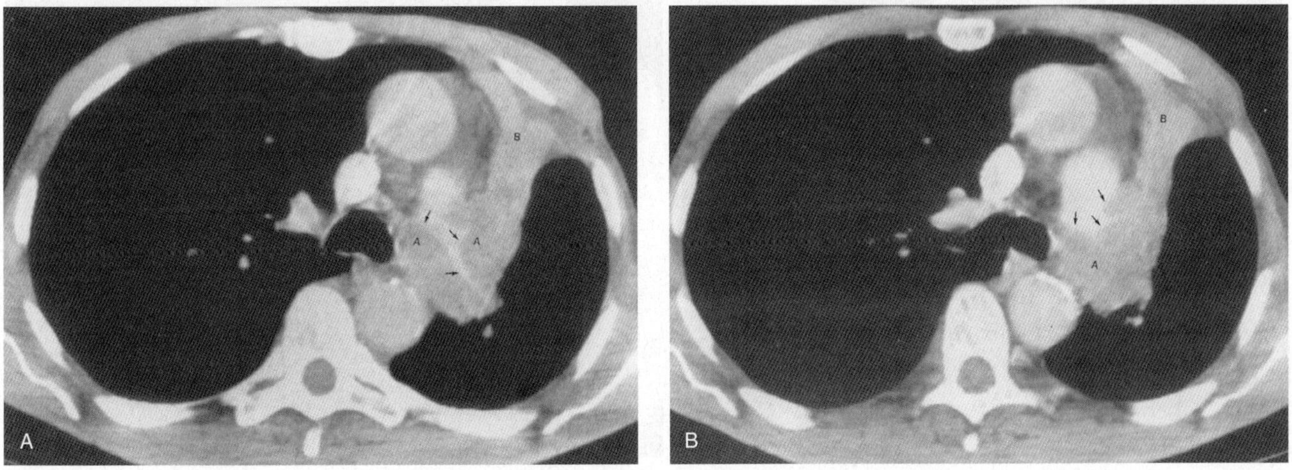

FIGURE 63.48. **A,B:** Contiguous computed tomography sections show the contrast-enhanced pulmonary artery (*arrows*) encased by and obstructed by the bronchogenic carcinoma (**A**), which has also produced postobstructive atelectasis (**B**). The mass and atelectasis, but not the pulmonary artery's involvement, could be seen on plain films.

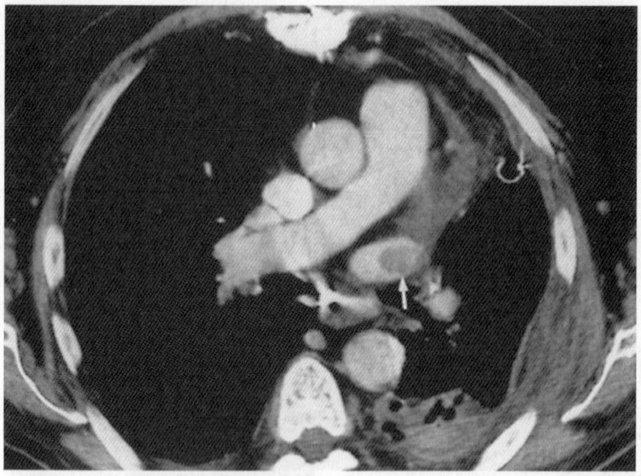

FIGURE 63.49. In a patient who had a lobectomy, computed tomography shows a filling defect (*arrow*) representing a thrombus within the contrast-enhanced pulmonary vein.

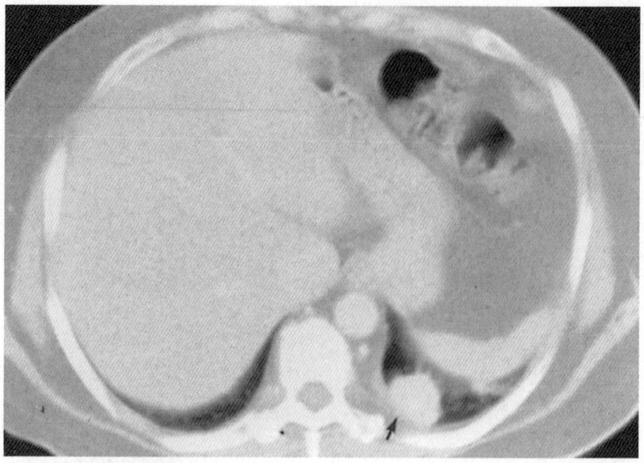

FIGURE 63.50. An adenocarcinoma seen only by computed tomography (*arrow*). It was not seen on routine films because it overlies the shadows of the vertebral body on lateral view and is obscured by the spleen and stomach and aorta on the posteroanterior chest film.

Involvement of the arteries and veins most often not identifiable on plain films can be seen using CT (Figs. 63.48 and 63.49). Abnormalities hidden by overlying structures in PA and lateral views can be seen in CT cross-sectional images (Fig. 63.50).

Mediastinal abnormalities can be imaged using CT, MRI, or ultrasonography. To determine the size of mediastinal nodes, CT's resolution would make it superior to MRI; CT can delineate the borders of small nodes lying close to each other or matted together, whereas MRI may make them appear as larger, pathologic-sized nodes. Posterior mediastinal lesions are probably best imaged using MRI to show their relation to an involvement of the spinal canal and spinal cord.

On the other hand, MRI is like CT in imaging vascular structures well. It is not within the scope of this chapter to discuss the principles and physics behind MRI. Suffice it to say that using spin-echo technique, flowing blood appears as a signal void (black) and as high-signal intensity (white) on gradient recall images. The latter provides an angiographic image similar to that achieved using angiography.

The cardiac chambers can be imaged equally well with MRI and ultrasonography but not as well with CT (Fig. 63.51). In the evaluation of the cardiac muscles, however, MRI is superior to CT or ultrasonography.

Aneurysms and dissecting aneurysms of the aorta can be imaged using all five modalities: contrast-enhanced CT, angiography, echocardiography for the root of the ascending aorta, transesophageal echocardiography for the descending aorta, and MRI. The advantage of ultrasonography is that it can be done at the bedside if necessary. However, MRI is superior

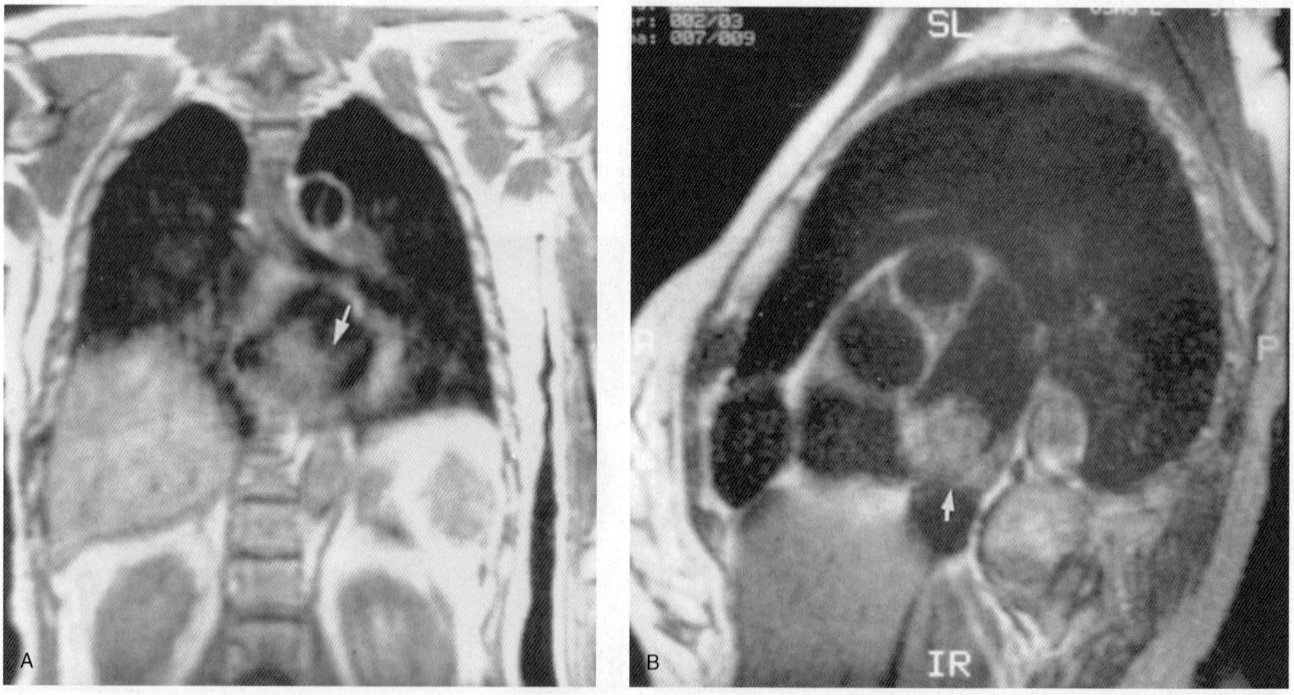

FIGURE 63.51. **A,B:** Coronal and sagittal plains on magnetic resonance imaging. *Arrows* point to an atrial myxoma. Echocardiography demonstrated this lesion also.

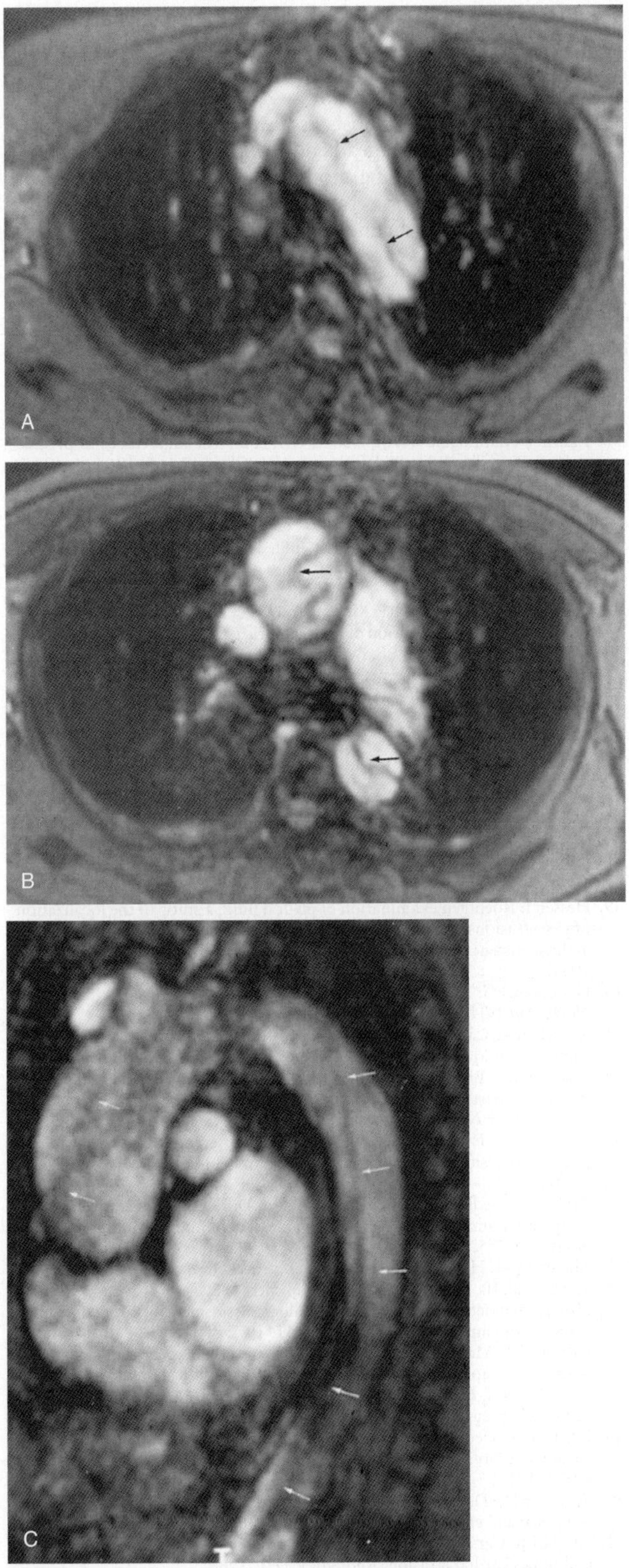

FIGURE 63.52. A–C: *Arrows* point to the flap in a dissecting aneurysm. Magnetic resonance images well the dissection and its extent in multiple planes.

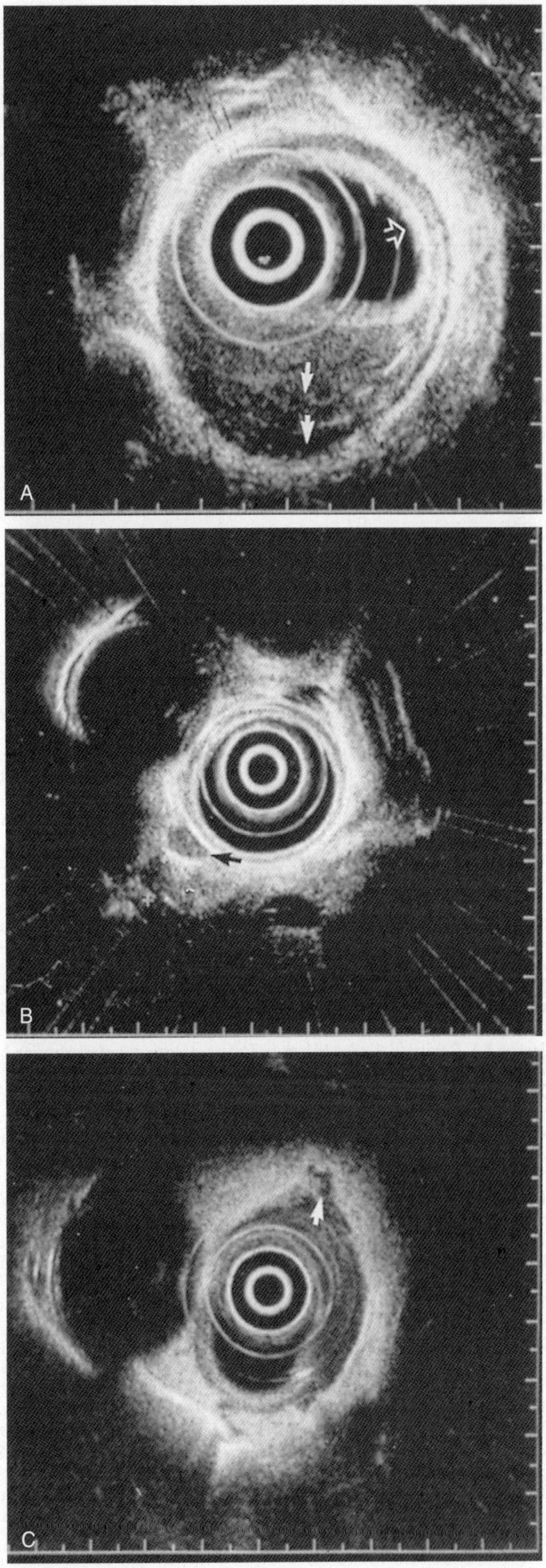

FIGURE 63.53. Esophageal endosonography in a patient with esophageal carcinoma. Open *arrow* shows normal thickness of the esophageal wall. White *arrows* in (**A**) and (**C**) show the extension of the lesion into the adventitia. Black *arrow* in (**B**) shows metastatic lymphadenopathy.

to either CT or ultrasonography because of the ability to do multiplane imaging and delineate the entire extent of the abnormality (Fig. 63.52) noninvasively.

Esophageal mucosal lesions are best assessed by barium swallow. Submucosal, mural, and serosal lesions and lesions extrinsic to the esophagus can be assessed using CT, ultrasonography, or MRI. Ultrasonography and MRI are probably superior to CT in delineating the layers of esophagus involved. Transesophageal ultrasonography is the least costly and most efficient modality to use, because the gastroenterologists would probably use a scope anyway in the presence of any esophageal problem. Transesophageal endosonography is superior to CT for staging a tumor and evaluating depth of tumor infiltration, especially in the early stages (Fig. 63.53). Severe stenosis is the main limiting factor to the use of transesophageal endosonography. The availability of the various imaging modalities provides clinicians with useful tools in addition to their clinical acumen and laboratory results for diagnostic problem solving in the ICU patient.

References

1. Henscke CI, Pasternak GS, Schroeder S, et al: Bedside chest radiography: diagnostic efficacy. *Radiology* 149:23, 1983.
2. Bekemeyer WB, Crapo RO, Calhoon S, et al: Efficacy of chest radiography in a respiratory intensive care unit. *Chest* 88:691, 1985.
3. Tocino I, Westcott J, Davis ST, et al: Routine daily portable x-ray. American College of Radiology. ACR Appropriateness Criteria. *Radiology* 215:621, 2000.
4. Trotman-Dickenson B: Radiology in the intensive care unit (part 1). *J Intensive Care Med* 18:198, 2003.
5. Trotman-Dickenson B. Radiology in the intensive care unit (part 2). *J Intensive Care Med* 18:239, 2003.
6. Goodman LR, Conrardy PA, Laing F, et al: Radiographic evaluation of endotracheal tube position. *AJR Am J Roentgenol* 127:433, 1976.
7. Conrardy PA, Goodman LR, Laing F, et al: Alteration of endotracheal tube position: extension and flexion of the neck. *Crit Care Med* 4:7, 1976.
8. Khan F, Reddy NC, Khan A: Cuff/trachea ratio as an indication of tracheal damage [abstract]. *Chest* 70:431, 1976.
9. Ravin CE, Handel DB, Kariman K: Persistent endotracheal tube cuff overdistension: a sign of tracheomalacia. *AJR Am J Roentgenol* 137:408, 1981.
10. Ravin CE, Putnam CE, McLoud TC: Hazards of the intensive care unit. *AJR Am J Roentgenol* 126:423, 1976.
11. Brandt RL, Foley WJ, Fink GH, et al: Mechanism of perforation of the heart with production of hydropericardium by a venous catheter and its prevention. *Am J Surg* 119:311, 1970.
12. Swan HJC, Ganz W, Forrester J, et al: Catheterization of the heart in man with use of a flow-directed balloon-tipped catheter. *N Engl J Med* 283:447, 1970.
13. Moulopoulos SD, Topaz SR, Kolff WJ: Diastolic balloon pumping (with carbon dioxide) in the aorta: a mechanical assistance to the failing circulation. *Am Heart J* 63:669, 1962.
14. Hyson EA, Ravin CE, Kelley MJ, et al: The intraaortic counterpulsation balloon: radiographic considerations. *AJR Am J Roentgenol* 128:915, 1977.
15. Webb WR, Godwin JD: The obscured outer edge: a sign of improperly placed pleural drainage tubes. *AJR Am J Roentgenol* 134:1062, 1980.
16. Ormond RS, Rubenfire M, Anbe DT, et al: Radiographic demonstration of myocardial penetration by permanent endocardial pacemakers. *Radiology* 98:35, 1971.
17. Hall WM, Rosenbaum HD: The radiology of cardiac pacemakers. *Radiol Clin North Am* 9:343, 1971.
18. Hearne SF, Maloney JD: Pacemaker system failure secondary to air entrapment within the pulse generator pocket: a complication of subclavian venipuncture for lead placement. *Chest* 82:651, 1982.
19. Leeming BWA: Gravitational edema of the lungs observed during assisted respiration. *Chest* 64:719, 1973.
20. Zimmerman JE, Goodman LR, St Andre AC, et al: Radiographic detection of mobilizable lung water: the gravitational shift test. *AJR Am J Roentgenol* 138:59, 1982.
21. Heitzman ER Jr, Fraser RG, Proto AV, et al: Radiologic physiologic correlations in pulmonary circulation, in Theros EG, Harris JH (eds): *Chest Disease Syllabus*. 3rd series. Chicago, American College of Radiology, 1981, p 375.
22. Hublitz UF, Shapiro JH: Atypical pulmonary patterns of congestive failure in chronic lung disease: influence of preexisting disease on appearance and distribution of pulmonary edema. *Radiology* 93:995, 1969.
23. Milne ENC: Some new concepts of pulmonary blood flow and volume. *Radiol Clin North Am* 16:515, 1978.
24. Milne ENC: Chest radiology in the surgical patient. *Surg Clin North Am* 60:1503, 1980.
25. Bachofen M, Weibel ER: Structural alterations of lung parenchyma in the adult respiratory distress syndrome. *Clin Chest Med* 3:35, 1982.
26. Joffe N: The adult respiratory distress syndrome. *Am J Roentgenol Radium Ther Nucl Med* 122:719, 1974.
27. Unger KM, Shibel EM, Moser KM: Detection of left ventricular failure in patients with adult respiratory distress syndrome. *Chest* 67:8, 1975.
28. Matthew EB, Holstrom FMG, Kaspar RL: A simple method for diagnosing pneumonia in intubated or tracheostomized patients. *Crit Care Med* 5:76, 1977.
29. Mendelsohn CL: The aspiration of stomach contents into the lungs during obstetric anesthesia. *Am J Obstet Gynecol* 52:191, 1946.
30. Exarhos ND, Logan WD Jr, Abbott OA, et al: The importance of pH and volume in tracheobronchial aspiration. *Dis Chest* 47:167, 1965.
31. Roberts RB, Shirley MA: The obstetrician's role in reducing the risk of aspiration pneumonitis: with particular reference to the use of oral antacids. *Am J Obstet Gynecol* 124:611, 1976.
32. Schwartz DJ, Wynne JW, Gibbs CP, et al: The pulmonary consequences of aspiration of gastric contents at pH values greater than 2.5. *Am Rev Respir Dis* 121:119, 1980.
33. Greenfield LJ, Singleton RP, McCaffree DR, et al: Pulmonary effects of experimental graded aspiration of hydrochloric acid. *Ann Surg* 170:74, 1969.
34. Landay MJ, Christensen EE, Bynum LJ: Pulmonary manifestations of acute aspiration of gastric contents. *AJR Am J Roentgenol* 131:587, 1978.
35. Westermark N. *Roentgen Studies of the Lungs and Heart.* Minneapolis, University of Minnesota, 1948.
36. Patel S, Kazerooni EA, Cascade PN. Pulmonary embolism: optimization of small pulmonary artery visualization at multidetector row CT. *Radiology* 227:455, 2003.
37. Rademeker J, Griesshaber V, Hidajat N, et al: Combined CT pulmonary angiography and venography for diagnosis of pulmonary embolism and deep vein thrombosis: radiation dose. *J Thoracic Imaging* 16:297, 2001.
38. Glas WW, Grekin TD, Musselman MM: Fat embolism. *Am J Surg* 85:363, 1953.
39. Hessen I: Roentgen examination of pleural fluid: a study of the localization of free effusions, the potentialities of diagnosing minimal quantities of fluid and its existence under physiological conditions. *Acta Radiol* 86[Suppl]:1, 1951.
40. Fleischner FG: Atypical arrangement of free pleural effusion. *Radiol Clin North Am* 1:347, 1963.
41. Raasch BN, Carsky EW, Lane EJ, et al: Pleural effusion: explanation of some typical appearances. *AJR Am J Roentgenol* 139:899, 1982.
42. Trackler RT, Brinker RA: Widening of the left paravertebral pleural line on supine chest roentgenograms in free pleural effusions. *Am J Roentgenol Radium Ther Nucl Med* 96:1027, 1966.
43. Pugatch RD, Faling LJ, Robbins AH, et al: Differentiation of pleural and pulmonary lesions using computed tomography. *J Comput Assist Tomogr* 2:601, 1978.
44. Baber CE, Hedlund LW, Oddson TA, et al: Differentiating empyemas and peripheral pulmonary abscesses: the value of computed tomography. *Radiology* 135:755, 1980.
45. Malamed M, Hipona FA, Reynes CJ, et al: *The Adult Postoperative Chest.* Springfield, IL, Charles C Thomas Publisher, 1977.
46. Hsu JT, Bennett GM, Wolff E: Radiologic assessment of bronchopleural fistula with empyema. *Radiology* 103:41, 1972.
47. Parmley LF, Mattingly TW, Manion WC, et al: Nonpenetrating traumatic injury of the aorta. *Circulation* 17:1086, 1958.
48. Zelefsky MN, Freeman LM, Stern H: A simple approach to the diagnosis of bronchopleural fistula. *Radiology* 124:843, 1977.
49. Kremens V: Demonstration of the pericardial shadow on the routine chest roentgenogram: a new roentgen finding: preliminary report. *Radiology* 64:72, 1955.
50. Torrance DJ: Demonstration of subpericardial fat as an aid in the diagnosis of pericardial effusion or thickening. *AJR Am J Roentgenol* 74:850, 1955.
51. Lane EJ Jr, Carsky EW: Epicardial fat: lateral plain film analysis in normals and in pericardial effusion. *Radiology* 91:1, 1968.
52. Carsky EW, Mauceri RA, Azimi F: The epicardial fat pad sign: analysis of frontal and lateral chest radiographs in patients with pericardial effusion. *Radiology* 137:303, 1980.
53. Spooner EW, Kuhns LR, Stern AM: Diagnosis of pericardial effusion in children: a new radiographic sign. *AJR Am J Roentgenol* 128:23, 1977.
54. Chen JTT, Putman CE, Hedlund LW, et al: Widening of the subcarinal angle by pericardial effusion. *AJR Am J Roentgenol* 139:883, 1982.
55. Davidson KG: Closed injuries to the aorta and great vessels, in Williams WJ, Smith RE (eds): *Trauma of the Chest*. Bristol, UK, John Wright, 1977, p. 69.
56. Barcia TC, Livoni JP: Indications for angiography in blunt thoracic trauma. *Radiology* 147:15, 1983.

57. Seltzer SE, D'Orsi C, Kirshner R, et al: Traumatic aortic rupture: plain radiographic findings. *AJR Am J Roentgenol* 137:1011, 1981.
58. Cigarroa JE, Isselbacher EM, DeSanctis RW, et al: Diagnostic imaging in the evaluation of suspected aortic dissection: old standards and new directions. *N Engl J Med* 328:35, 1993.
59. Nienaber CA, von Kodolitsch Y, Nicolas V, et al: The diagnosis of thoracic aortic dissection by noninvasive imaging procedures. *N Engl J Med* 328:1, 1993.
60. Fabian TM, Raptopoulos V, D'Orsi CJ, et al: Computed body angiotomography: dynamic scanning with table incrementation. *Radiology* 149:287, 1983.
61. Ball T, McCrory R, Smith JO, et al: Traumatic diaphragmatic hernia: errors in diagnosis. *AJR Am J Roentgenol* 138:633, 1982.
62. Toombs BD, Sandler CM, Lester RG: Computed tomography of chest trauma. *Radiology* 140:733, 1981.
63. Heiberg E, Wolverson MK, Hurd RN, et al: CT recognition of traumatic rupture of the diaphragm. *AJR Am J Roentgenol* 135:369, 1980.
64. Rabin CB, Baron MG: *Radiology of the Chest. Golden's Diagnostic Radiology Series*. Section 3. Baltimore, Williams & Wilkins, 1980.
65. Rhea JT, DeLuca SA, Greene RE: Determining the size of pneumothorax in the upright patient. *Radiology* 144:733, 1982.
66. Kurlander GJ, Helmen CH: Subpulmonary pneumothorax. *AJR Am J Roentgenol* 96:1019, 1966.
67. Rhea JT, van Sonnenberg E, McLoud TC: Basilar pneumothorax in the supine adult. *Radiology* 133:593, 1979.
68. Gordon R: The deep sulcus sign. *Radiology* 136:25, 1980.
69. Gobien RP, Reines HD, Schabel SI: Localized tension pneumothorax: unrecognized form of barotrauma in adult respiratory distress syndrome. *Radiology* 142:15, 1982.
70. Westcott JL, Cole SR: Interstitial pulmonary emphysema in children and adults: roentgenographic features. *Radiology* 111:367, 1974.
71. Johnson TH, Altman AR: Pulmonary interstitial gas: first sign of barotrauma due to PEEP therapy. *Crit Care Med* 7:532, 1979.

CHAPTER 64 ■ ACUTE INHALATION INJURY

DAVID J. PREZANT, DORSETT D. SMITH AND LAWRENCE C. MOHR JR

OVERVIEW

Chemicals with potential toxicity are regularly used and produced in a variety of industrial processes. If inhaled, many have the potential to cause asphyxiation or life-threatening acute lung injury. Although recent events have increased concern that toxic gases may be used as weapons of mass destruction, accidental exposures remain the greatest health threat [1]. Individuals may be exposed to the accidental release of toxic gases in the workplace [2] or in the general environment, including the home [1].

Smoke inhalation is another major cause of acute inhalation injury [3]. Thousands of individuals become smoke inhalation victims each year, having been exposed to toxic gases and airborne particulate matter from the burning of a variety of materials [4]. Smoke inhalation most commonly occurs as a result of industrial or residential fires, where large amounts of carbon monoxide, hydrogen cyanide (HCN), hydrogen chloride, acrolein, sulfur dioxide, phosgene, and other toxic, irritant gases are produced (Table 64.1). It remains the primary cause of death in approximately 80% of burn injury victims in the United States.

Toxic agents can be inhaled in several different physical states. A gas is a substance that, at standard temperature and pressure, has the ability for its molecules to diffuse freely and be distributed uniformly throughout any container. A gas in the atmosphere has the capability of infinite expansion. The density of a gas is expressed relative to air. The denser the gas, the heavier it is. Gases that are denser than air will typically gravitate to low areas. Cold gases are denser than the same gas at higher temperatures. A vapor is a substance in the gaseous state that normally exists as a liquid or solid and is formed when a substance is heated above its critical temperature, which is the temperature at which it cannot be liquefied regardless of the amount of pressure applied. A fog is a liquid aerosol formed by a condensation of a substance from a gaseous state to a liquid state. Dusts are fine particles of a solid organic or inorganic material that are small enough to be airborne, typically ranging from 0.1 to 25.0 μm in diameter. Fumes are extremely fine solid particles that are dispersed into the air by the combustion or melting of solid materials, particularly metals. Fumes usually consist of particles that range from 0.001 to 1.0 μm in diameter. Smoke consists of airborne particles resulting from the incomplete combustion of organic materials. These particles either contain or are coated with multiple chemical substances resulting from combustion and range in size from less than 0.3 μm to greater than 10 μm in diameter.

The nature of acute injury that an individual sustains after the inhalation of a toxic substance will depend on the chemical and physical properties of the inhaled toxicant, the pathophysiological mechanism by which the toxicant causes injury, the dose received, and whether prior pulmonary disease exists. This chapter will focus on the diagnosis and treatment of acute inhalation injury resulting from asphyxiant gases, toxic irritant gases, and smoke.

TABLE 64.1

TOXIC PRODUCTS OF COMBUSTION IN RESIDENTIAL FIRES

Acetaldehyde	Hydrogen fluoride
Acrolein	Hydrogen sulfide
Ammonia	Isocyanates
Carbon monoxide	Metals (Pb, Zn, Mn, Cd, Co)
Chlorine	Oxides of nitrogen
Hydrogen chloride	Phosgene
Hydrogen cyanide	Sulfur dioxide

ASPHYXIANT GASES

Background

Asphyxiants are gases that cause tissue hypoxia. They are classified as either *simple asphyxiants* or *chemical asphyxiants*

TABLE 64.2

SIMPLE ASPHYXIANTS

Heavier than air	Lighter than air
Argon	Acetylene
Butane	Ethylene
Carbon dioxide	Methane
Ethane	Neon
Natural gas	Nitrogen
Propane	

based on their mechanism of toxicity. Simple asphyxiants displace or dilute oxygen in the ambient atmospheric air causing a decrease in the fraction of oxygen in inspired air (FIO_2). Chemical asphyxiants, on the other hand, interfere with physiological processes associated with the uptake, transport, or utilization of oxygen. Simple asphyxiants include common gases such as carbon dioxide, natural gas, propane, methane, nitrogen, and acetylene. They may be lighter or heavier than air (Table 64.2). Simple asphyxiants that are lighter than air accumulate and displace oxygen in higher areas first, whereas those that are heavier than air accumulate and displace oxygen in low-lying areas first. Chemical asphyxiants can be further characterized as those that decrease oxygen-carrying capacity, such as carbon monoxide, and those that inhibit oxygen utilization by cells, such as HCN (Table 64.3). Medical problems related to the inhalation of the most common asphyxiants are discussed in the sections that follow.

Carbon Dioxide

Pathophysiology

Carbon dioxide (CO_2) is the most common simple asphyxiant. It is produced by aerobic metabolism and is exhaled into the atmosphere by humans and other animals. It is also a byproduct of carbohydrate fermentation, the combustion of carbonaceous material, and the oxidation of coal contaminants in coal mines. It exists in the frozen form as dry ice. CO_2 is heaver than air and reduces FIO_2 simply by diluting and displacing oxygen in ambient air. Most deaths from CO_2 asphyxiation result from the confinement of an individual in enclosed or poorly ventilated space. Such closed-space confinement prevents air with a normal FIO_2 from entering while exhaled CO_2 is accumulating and displacing oxygen inside. Simple asphyxiation from CO_2 has also been reported from environmental exposures. In 1986, for example, simple asphyxiation caused approximately 1,700 deaths from a cloudy mist of CO_2 and water droplets that rose suddenly from a lake in Cameroon [5]. Asphyxiation from CO_2 has also been reported by off-gassing from dry ice in a confined space [6].

In general, once the ambient CO_2 increases to the point where the FIO_2 has decreased to 0.15, acute signs and symptoms of hypoxia begin to appear within minutes. These include dyspnea, tachypnea, tachycardia, confusion, incoordination, and dizziness. As the FIO_2 decreases below 0.10, lethargy or coma may develop as a result of cerebral edema, and cardiopulmonary arrest may occur. Brain damage sustained as a result of extensive cerebral edema or prolonged hypoxia may be permanent in individuals with these conditions who are resuscitated and survive. It is unlikely that life can be sustained for more than several minutes with a FIO_2 less than 0.06 [7].

TABLE 64.3

CHEMICAL ASPHYXIANTS

Agents that decrease oxygen-carrying capacity
Carbon monoxide
Hydrogen sulfide
Oxides of nitrogen
Agents that inhibit cellular oxygen utilization
Acrylonitrile
Hydrogen cyanide
Hydrogen sulfide

Diagnosis and Management

CO_2 asphyxiation should be considered in any patient who presents with clinical signs of hypoxia, is unconscious, or is found to be in cardiopulmonary arrest after removal from an enclosed space or another source of potential CO_2 exposure. Clinical signs are nonspecific and related to the magnitude of hypoxia, as indicated earlier. Arterial blood gases, serum electrolytes, and measurement of the anion gap should be obtained. During and shortly after CO_2 asphyxiation, arterial blood gas analysis would be expected to show decreased arterial oxygen tension (PaO_2) and elevated carbon dioxide tension ($PaCO_2$). However, both PaO_2 and $PaCO_2$ typically return to normal shortly after the patient is removed from the source of CO_2 exposure. Once the patient breathes oxygenated air, CO_2 is rapidly excreted by hyperventilation. Most patients will be acidotic at the time of presentation as a result of respiratory acidosis from CO_2 retention and concurrent lactic acidosis from hypoxia. Lactic acidosis will cause an elevated anion gap. The respiratory acidosis typically resolves shortly after removal from the source of CO_2 exposure. The lactic acidosis will resolve once tissue oxygenation returns to normal but usually takes longer to resolve than the respiratory acidosis. The hypoxia caused by CO_2 asphyxiation can cause cardiac dysrhythmias and myocardial infarction, especially in individuals with underlying heart disease. Therefore, it is recommended that an electrocardiogram and serial cardiac biomarkers be obtained on all patients.

Removal from the source of exposure and administration of oxygen are the only specific therapies for CO_2 asphyxiation. If the patient is alert, has spontaneous respirations, and has a patent airway, it is recommended that high-flow oxygen be administered by a nonrebreather mask. Endotracheal intubation will be required if adequate oxygenation cannot be achieved by the use of a face mask or the patient has suffered mental status changes or cardiopulmonary arrest. Additional supportive care, such as cardiopulmonary resuscitation, hemodynamic support, manual ventilation, and mechanical ventilation should be used as required by the patient's overall condition. Cardiac dysrhythmias and myocardial infarction should be aggressively treated. Most victims of CO_2 asphyxiation will recover completely if removed from the source of CO_2 exposure prior to cardiopulmonary arrest and given medical treatment as soon as possible. Individuals who have experienced a prolonged period of hypoxia, however, may have irreversible brain damage and chronic neurological sequelae if they are successfully resuscitated.

Carbon Monoxide

Pathophysiology

Carbon monoxide (CO) is a colorless, odorless, tasteless, nonirritating gas. It is the most common chemical asphyxiant and the second most common atmospheric pollutant after carbon dioxide. CO is produced in a variety of ways, including incomplete combustion from fires, faulty heating systems, internal combustion engines (including gas-powered generators placed in poorly ventilated areas during electrical failures), wood stoves, charcoal grills, volcanic eruptions, and a variety of industrial processes. In vivo hepatic production of CO occurs in poisoning from methylene chloride that is commonly found in paint thinners and is easily absorbed through the skin.

More than 5,000 deaths are attributed to CO poisoning in the United States each year [8]. Most are intentional from exposures to motor vehicle exhaust. The minority are accidental and due to fires or the use of poorly ventilated generators following storms, blackouts, or other disasters [9]. CO poisoning is responsible for 80% of fatalities related to smoke inhalation [10,11]. Twenty-five percent of fatalities from CO poisoning occur in persons with underlying cardiopulmonary disease [11,12].

Upon inhalation, CO easily diffuses across alveolar-capillary membranes in the lung and is rapidly taken up by erythrocytes in the pulmonary capillary blood. It binds to the iron moiety of hemoglobin with an affinity that is approximately 240 times greater than the affinity of hemoglobin for oxygen. Thus, CO competes with oxygen for hemoglobin binding sites and, as a result of its greater affinity, displaces oxygen from hemoglobin. The binding of CO to the iron moiety also creates an allosteric change in the hemoglobin molecule that inhibits the off-loading of oxygen in the peripheral tissues and causes a shift of the oxyhemoglobin dissociation curve to the left. CO also interferes with intracellular oxygen utilization by inactivating intracellular respiratory enzymes, such as cytochrome oxidase [13]. Thus, the cumulative effect on peripheral oxygen delivery and utilization is greater than that expected from decreased oxygen transport alone [14]. Reoxygenation injury of the brain has also been described [15]. One mechanism for reoxygenation injury appears to be lipid peroxidation of the brain by xanthine oxidase that is generated by peroxidases and reactive oxygen species produced by activated neutrophils that become sequestered in the microvasculature of the brain following, but not during, CO poisoning [16]. In summary, CO toxicity involves four pathophysiological mechanisms: (a) a decrease in the oxygen-carrying capacity of blood; (b) decreased oxygen delivery to peripheral tissues as a result of the left shift in the oxyhemoglobin dissociation curve; (c) mitochondrial dysfunction and impairment of cellular respiration by inhibition of cytochrome oxidase activity; and (d) lipid peroxidation of the brain during reoxygenation. It has been suggested that an immunological response to myelin basic protein may also be involved in the delayed neurological dysfunction that is seen in over half of those with serious CO poisoning between 3 days and 4 weeks after exposure [17].

The clinical presentation of individuals with CO poisoning is highly variable with nonspecific symptoms and signs that are loosely correlated to carboxyhemoglobin levels (Table 64.4). Early symptoms of CO poisoning include headache, dizziness, sore throat, nausea, shortness of breath, and fatigue. These symptoms can mimic those of a nonspecific viral syndrome, especially when an entire family is affected from CO exposure related to a faulty home heating system during the winter months. Impaired ability to concentrate occurs in more than half of affected individuals, and 6% have been reported to experience loss of consciousness. The severity of symptoms appears to correlate better with duration of exposure than with carboxyhemoglobin levels [18]. The brain and heart are very sensitive to CO intoxication, and both neurologic and cardiovascular impairment predominate with prolonged exposures. Mental status changes, and seizures, loss of consciousness, tachypnea, tachycardia, cardiac dysrhythmias, hypotension, and myocardial ischemia are likely to occur when the carboxyhemoglobin concentration exceeds 20%. Loss of consciousness may then occur rapidly and without warning. Cardiovascular disorders may occur at lower concentrations in subjects with preexisting cardiopulmonary diseases. Evidence of myocardial ischemia has been observed in one third of individuals with moderate-to-severe CO intoxication, and it has recently been reported that myocardial injury, as determined by elevation of serial cardiac biomarkers, is an independent predictor of mortality from CO poisoning [12,19,20]. Metabolic acidosis, as a result of increased lactate production from anaerobic metabolism, is a common consequence of tissue hypoxia. Rhabdomyolysis can occur as a consequence of impaired aerobic metabolism in skeletal muscle cells. Renal failure can develop as a consequence of rhabdomyolysis, but this occurs infrequently [21]. Carbon monoxide poisoning is almost always fatal when the carboxyhemoglobin concentration exceeds 60% [10,22].

TABLE 64.4

CARBON MONOXIDE TOXICITY

HBCO level %	Clinical manifestations of carbon monoxide intoxication
0–5	Normal nonsmoker
5–10	Mild headache, shortness of breath with exertion, decreased exercise tolerance, decreased angina threshold
10–20	Moderate headache, fatigue, dizziness, blurred vision, nausea, decreasing threshold for exertional shortness of breath with possibly shortness of breath at rest
20–30	Severe headache, confusion and impaired judgment, vomiting, shortness of breath at rest, decreased cardiac arrhythmia threshold
30–40	Muscle weakness, incapacitation, cardiac arrhythmias, decreased seizure threshold
40–50	Seizures, syncope, cardiac arrest
50–60	Fatal

Fetal hemoglobin has a much greater affinity for CO than adult hemoglobin. Therefore, during pregnancy, the fetus may be more susceptible to CO poisoning than the mother. Once the mother is removed from the source of CO, clearance of carboxyhemoglobin may take four to five times longer in the fetus than it did in the mother [23]. Thus, the effective duration of CO exposure is considerably longer for the fetus than it is for the mother. It has been reported that severe CO toxicity in pregnant women can produce ischemic brain damage to the fetus and increase the risk of stillbirth [24,25].

Carbon monoxide poisoning can result in a delayed neuropsychiatric syndrome that may present at any time between 3 days and 4 months after apparent recovery from acute effects [10,26]. The syndrome has been reported to occur in 10% to 30% of individuals who survive CO poisoning. Symptoms include cognitive impairment, personality changes, parkinsonism, incontinence, focal neurological deficits, dementia, and psychosis. There is poor correlation between the development of the delayed neuropsychiatric syndrome and carboxyhemoglobin levels. Loss of consciousness during the acute illness phase, carboxyhemoglobin 25% or more, duration of exposure, and age appear to be significant risk factors (18). Brain imaging studies have shown that the areas most affected are the globus pallidus and deep white matter [10]. The exact mechanism for the development of this syndrome is unclear, but it is thought to be associated with reoxygenation brain injury, as discussed earlier. Most affected individuals recover within 1 year, although some may have chronic, long-term neurological or psychiatric impairment [10].

Diagnosis and Management

Because CO poisoning can present with a variety of nonspecific signs and symptoms, a high index of suspicion is needed to make the diagnosis. Cherry-red lips, cyanosis, and retinal hemorrhages have been reported in some cases of high-dose CO poisoning, but these signs occur infrequently and diagnosis depends on clinical history substantiated by increased levels of carboxyhemoglobin in arterial or venous blood [10]. Carboxyhemoglobin is most accurately measured by cooximetry because routine pulse oximetry cannot distinguish between carboxyhemoglobin and oxyhemoglobin. PaO_2 is also of little value, since in the absence of coexistent lung injury it is normal. This is due to the fact that a CO partial pressure of only 1 mm Hg in arterial blood can saturate more than 50% of hemoglobin without affecting gas exchange or the amount of dissolved oxygen.

Recently, noninvasive cooximetry has become commercially available. Studies show that it has a high degree of specificity but poor sensitivity [27,28]. Using a cutoff of 15% carboxyhemoglobin, noninvasive cooximetry had a poor sensitivity of 48% (correctly identified only 11 of 23 patients with elevated levels) but an excellent specificity of 99% (correctly identify 96 of 97 patients with levels below 15%) [28]. Until further studies are done, this would suggest that its primary value is ruling out the diagnosis when there are no symptoms. It is probably most useful in environments where it is difficult or not possible to obtain blood measurement such as by Emergency Medical Service (EMS) units in the prehospital environment [29].

The evaluation of patients with CO poisoning should also include a thorough examination for evidence of thermal injury to the skin or airways. If CO poisoning is the result of a suicide attempt, a drug screen and serum ethanol, salicylate, and acetaminophen levels should be obtained. Another advantage of measuring the arterial carboxyhemoglobin level is that it also allows for simultaneous measurement of arterial pH. The pH can be used in conjunction with the anion gap and the serum lactate level to assess the degree of metabolic acidosis which when elevated is an independent predictor of poor prognosis [10]. $PaCO_2$ is only helpful in assessing the ventilatory response to hypoxia and ventilatory compensation for lactic acidosis and should be obtained when mental status is abnormal or there is a prior history of chronic pulmonary disease. The serum creatine kinase level will be elevated if rhabdomyolysis has occurred. An electrocardiogram and serial cardiac biomarkers should be obtained in all patients to evaluate the possibility of myocardial ischemia or infarction. Because CO lowers the threshold for the development of ventricular dysrhythmias, patients should be carefully monitored until they are discharged from the emergency department or hospital [30]. The chest radiograph is usually normal, but signs of noncardiogenic pulmonary edema can rarely be seen in cases of severe CO poisoning [22], especially if there is coexistent smoke inhalation. Computed tomography (CT) of the head is useful if there is a need to rule out other causes of neurological impairment in this acute setting.

The initial treatment of CO poisoning is prompt removal from the source of exposure and administration of 100% oxygen via a nonrebreather mask to reduce the half-life of carboxyhemoglobin from 4 to 6 hours to 40 to 80 minutes [10,31]. Patients who are unconscious or have cardiopulmonary compromise should be intubated and receive 100% oxygen by mechanical ventilation and hyperbaric oxygen therapy (HBOT) be considered (see later). Oxygen should be administered until the carboxyhemoglobin level returns to normal. Pregnant women typically require oxygen for a longer period of time, because it takes longer for CO to be excreted from the fetus as a result of the greater affinity of fetal hemoglobin for CO [23].

Most patients with mild-to-moderate CO poisoning can be treated in the emergency department and discharged after the carboxyhemoglobin level has returned to normal and all abnormal signs and symptoms have resolved. Patients with severe CO poisoning, coexistent smoke inhalation, serious underlying diseases, neurologic or cardiopulmonary instability, or whose poisoning was an intentional suicide attempt should be admitted to the hospital for treatment and close observation.

HBOT has been used to treat patients with either extreme levels of CO poisoning ($\geq$25% carboxyhemoglobin) or end-organ sensitivity to CO at elevated but lower levels. Examples of this might include neurologic abnormalities or hemodynamic instability that was felt to be caused by CO poisoning. HBOT is performed by placing the patient in a chamber that is highly pressurized with 100% oxygen. HBOT produces a large increase in the amount of dissolved oxygen in blood that in turn greatly increases the partial pressure of oxygen in the blood. The half-life of carboxyhemoglobin decreases as the partial pressure of oxygen in the blood increases. HBOT with 100% oxygen at a pressure of 2.5 to 3.0 atmosphere will reduce the half-life of carboxyhemoglobin from 4 to 6 hours to approximately 20 minutes [10,22,31].

Several animal studies suggest that HBOT may attenuate the development of delayed neuropsychiatric symptoms following CO exposure [32]. Although, the efficacy of HBOT for preventing the development of the delayed neuropsychiatric syndrome in humans following CO poisoning has not been conclusively established [33], many experts argue for its use when levels exceed 20% to 25% [33,34]. HBOT will, however, hasten the resolution of symptoms and when available is currently recommended for patients with CO poisoning meeting any of the following criteria: any period of unconsciousness, coma, or persistent neurologic abnormalities; carboxyhemoglobin level of 25% or more; metabolic lactic acidosis; or cardiac dysrhythmias [10,12,18,26,35–37]. If myocardial ischemia is present, most experts believe cardiac catheterization with stenting of the blocked vessel to be the urgently required procedure. In a pregnant patient, fetal distress even at lower percentage of carboxyhemoglobin elevations would prompt consideration for HBOT if available.

The clearance of CO can also be accelerated by use of normocapnic hyperoxic hyperpnea. In this technique, the patient breathes a hyperoxic gas mixture that contains an FIO_2 of 95.2% to 95.5% and a small amount of CO_2, in the range of 4.5% to 4.8%, through a nonrebreathing circuit. The resulting increase in minute ventilation increases the partial pressure gradient for oxygen and CO between pulmonary capillary blood and alveolar gas but does not increase the partial pressure gradient for CO_2. In a clinical study, normocapnic hyperoxic hyperpnea reduced the half-life of carboxyhemoglobin to 31 minutes in comparison with 78 minutes in individuals treated with 100% oxygen at normal minute ventilation [38]. CO-poisoned patients in hospitals without access to hyperbaric chambers might benefit from this technique.

In addition to controversy concerning which patients with CO intoxication might benefit most from HBOT, there also exists controversy surrounding the need to treat for HCN toxicity (see later) in patients suffering severe CO poisoning from smoke inhalation. The likelihood for cyanide toxicity in smoke inhalation victims increases with increasing carboxyhemoglobin levels and increasing acidosis [39].

Hydrogen Cyanide

Pathophysiology

Hydrogen cyanide (HCN) is a chemical asphyxiant produced by the combustion of nitrogen-containing polymers during fires [39–41]. It is also part of jewelry making and various manufacturing processes (metal plating) and in the reclamation of silver from photographic and radiographic film. It has the potential to be used as a chemical agent in terrorist attacks [42]. It is a colorless, volatile liquid at room temperature but readily vaporizes into a gas. The gaseous form of HCN easily diffuses across the alveolar membrane after inhalation. Inhaled HCN is lethal in high doses, and its inhalation during a fire can contribute to the mortality of smoke inhalation victims [39–41]. The inhalation of lethal doses of HCN may also occur following accidental releases at industrial facilities or from its use in a terrorist attack.

After inhalation, HCN is rapidly distributed to tissues throughout the body. At the cellular level, HCN molecules bind to iron-containing sites on cytochrome a_3 in mitochondria that inhibits the enzyme's activity toxicity and decreases the cellular utilization of oxygen [39,42]. Cytochrome a_3 is a key enzyme in the cytochrome oxidase system that is important for carrying out and sustaining aerobic metabolism within cells. Inhibition of cytochrome a_3 by HCN will stop cellular respiration and oxidative phosphorylation, forcing affected cells into anaerobic metabolism. The binding of HCN to cytochrome a_3, and the resulting inhibition of cellular respiration, can occur very rapidly after HCN is inhaled, with clinical signs and symptoms typically occurring within 15 seconds after inhalation.

The clinical effects of HCN intoxication are directly related to its ability to stop cellular respiration. They are nonspecific and identical to the signs and symptoms typically seen during hypoxia. Hyperpnea, dyspnea, tachycardia, agitation, anxiety, dizziness, headache, confusion, nausea, muscle weakness, and trembling are common. Lactic acidosis occurs as a result of anaerobic metabolism and may be severe. Hypotension, flushing, seizures, and Parkinson-like symptoms may occur in cases of severe intoxication. Coma, apnea, and cardiac dysrhythmias are poor prognostic signs unless prompt treatment is given [42,43].

Diagnosis and Management

The diagnosis of HCN poisoning requires a high index of suspicion. It should be suspected in every individual with any of the above signs or symptoms for which there is no other obvious cause. It should routinely be suspected in smoke inhalation victims, victims of industrial accidents in which cyanide could have been released, and victims of terrorist attacks. Blood and urine cyanide concentrations can be obtained, but the results of these tests are usually confirmatory and because these tests are not routinely performed in most laboratories, results can only be used to confirm the diagnosis. Treatment for this potentially life-threatening poisoning must be initiated based on diagnostic suspicion alone.

There are several important clues that can be helpful in making a clinical diagnosis of HCN intoxication. In smoke inhalation victims, HCN toxicity should be suspected whenever CO intoxication occurs, and in fact, the likelihood increases with increasing carboxyhemoglobin levels [39]. Regardless of the etiology of HCN exposure, metabolic acidosis with an increased anion gap and an elevated serum lactate concentration should typically be present. Arterial and venous blood gases can provide potentially useful information. Arterial oxygen tension is usually above 90 mm Hg, whereas venous oxygen tension may be significantly elevated above the normal range of 35 to 45 mm Hg because of poor cellular extraction and utilization of oxygen. Similarly, arterial oxygen saturation is typically in the normal range of 95% to 100%, whereas the oxygen saturation of mixed venous blood may be in the vicinity of 85% or greater. Thus, the mixed venous oxygen saturation may be significantly higher than the normal range of 60% to 80%. This so called arteriolarization of venous blood can be a useful clue in considering the diagnosis of HCN intoxication [44].

Because HCN poisoning can rapidly progress, treatment must begin as soon as possible in patient presenting with seizures, coma, hypotension, or cardiac arrest in whom HCN toxicity is suspected [45,46]. The United States Food and Drug Administration has approved two forms of therapy for cyanide toxicity. The newest is the Cyanokit antidote consisting of Hydroxocobalamin, a precursor to vitamin B_{12}. It is a relatively benign substance with minimal side effects and rapid onset of action. For these reasons, it may be a superior antidote to the older more commonly available cyanide antidote kit (CAK) consisting of sodium nitrite and sodium thiosulfate [47,48]. Hydroxocobalamin has no adverse effect on the oxygen-carrying capacity of the red blood cells and no negative impact on the patient's blood pressure—significant benefits when treating victims of smoke inhalation. The mechanism of action is surprisingly simple: Hydroxocobalamin binds to cyanide forming vitamin B_{12} (cyanocobalamin), a nontoxic compound excreted in the urine. Patients tolerate the drug without hypotension or allergic reactions. Quickly passing side effects include reddish color to the skin, urine, and mucous membranes, which may interfere with some colorimetric laboratory tests (i.e., blood glucose, iron levels, creatinine, total hemoglobin concentration, carboxyhemoglobin, oxyhemoglobin, methemoglobin) [49,50]. Victims presenting with seizures, hypotension, or a coma in a setting consistent with cyanide toxicity should be considered candidates for empiric administration of Hydroxocobalamin 5 gm IV over 15 minutes through two intravenous or intraosseous lines. Consideration should be given to obtaining a blood sample for subsequent analysis for HCN and for baseline laboratory tests that could be interfered with by the presence of hydroxocobalamin.

Sodium nitrite and sodium thiosulfate can also be used for the treatment of HCN poisoning. These antidotes are found in the CAK, along with ampules of amyl nitrite inhalant. Sodium nitrite generates methemoglobin by changing the normal ferrous state of iron in the heme molecule of hemoglobin (Fe^{+2}) to the ferric state (Fe^{+3}). The ferric heme molecules in methemoglobin have a high affinity for HCN. Thus, HCN molecules preferentially bind to the methemoglobin generated by sodium nitrate, which in turn prevents HCN from entering cells and inhibiting cellular respiration. The adult dose of sodium nitrite is 300 mg in 10 mL of diluent (30 mg per mL) administered intravenously over 2 to 4 minutes and the pediatric dose is 0.33 mL per kg of a 3% solution, intravenously over 2 to 4 minutes, not to exceed 10 mL [42,43]. Following the administration of sodium nitrite, sodium thiosulfate should be administered intravenously. Sodium thiosulfate acts as a substrate for rhodanese, a detoxifying enzyme found in the liver. In the presence of sodium thiosulfate, rhodanese catalyzes the conversion of HCN cyanide to thiocyanate that is then excreted in the urine. The adult dose is 12.5 g of sodium thiosulfate in 50 mL of diluent (25% solution), administered intravenously at a rate of 3 to 5 mL per minute. The pediatric dose of sodium thiosulfate is 412.5 mg per kg (1.65 mL per kg) of a 25% solution, given intravenously at a rate of 3 to 5 mL per minute [42,44].

The inhalation of amyl nitrite from ampules can be used as a temporizing measure until venous access for the administration of sodium nitrite and sodium thiosulfate is obtained. The inhalation of amyl nitrite should never be considered a substitute for the administration of intravenous sodium nitrite and sodium thiosulfate. In fact, amyl nitrite can itself be associated with serious reactions such as hypotension, syncope, methemoglobinemia, and hemolysis in G6PD-deficient patients. These effects are more pronounced in children, the elderly, and in patients with cardiopulmonary diseases. Dose regimen is difficult to control and could even result in exposure of the healthcare provider to amyl nitrite's adverse effects. For these reasons, administration of amyl nitrite may be unwarranted, especially since hydroxocobalamin is now available [51].

One hundred percent oxygen should be administered to all patients with HCN poisoning to maximize the oxygen-carrying capacity of blood. Ventilatory support should be provided as needed. The administration of sodium bicarbonate should be considered for the treatment of severe lactic acidosis in patients who are unconscious or hemodynamically unstable. Arterial blood gas analysis should be used to guide the need for repeat doses of sodium bicarbonate to ensure that metabolic alkalosis does not develop.

Hydrogen Sulfide

Pathophysiology

Hydrogen sulfide (H_2S) is a colorless, highly flammable gas that has the characteristic odor of "rotten eggs." It is produced in a variety of settings, most commonly sewer systems, manure pits on farms, oil fields, and petroleum refining plants [52–54]. Its noxious, "rotten eggs" odor is detectable by smell at low concentrations but may not be detectable at high concentrations or after prolonged exposure because of olfactory fatigue. Inhaled H_2S is both a chemical asphyxiant and a respiratory tract irritant. As such, it can produce a variety of clinical effects, including central nervous system dysfunction [55], cardiac dysrhythmias, and pulmonary edema as a result of acute lung injury. The severity of symptoms and prognosis are dependent on the dose of H_2S inhaled.

As a chemical asphyxiant, H_2S blocks the cellular utilization of oxygen by inhibiting the activity of cytochrome a_3, a mitochondrial enzyme of the cytochrome oxidase system that is involved in aerobic metabolism. In this regard, the pathophysiologic mechanism of H_2S asphyxiation is identical to that of HCN. As with HCN intoxication, disruption of aerobic metabolism by H_2S causes a shift to anaerobic metabolism within affected cells that, in turn, leads to metabolic acidosis and an elevated anion gap due to increased lactate production. H_2S is lipid soluble and readily crosses the alveolar membrane after inhalation. Inhalation is the primary route of H_2S toxicity. After absorption through the lungs, H_2S easily dissolves in the blood and is rapidly distributed to tissues throughout the body. The respiratory system and organs with high oxygen demand, such as the brain and heart, are particularly vulnerable.

The severity of clinical signs and symptoms associated with H_2S toxicity depend on the exposure dose. Signs and symptoms of asphyxiation and mucosal irritation typically exist simultaneously. Local irritant effects dominate at low exposure doses, whereas pulmonary edema and life-threatening chemical asphyxiation dominate at higher exposure doses. Clinically detectable eye, mucous membrane, and respiratory tract irritation begin to occur at low exposure doses in the vicinity of 50 parts per million (ppm). Low-dose exposures in the range of 50 to 200 ppm are typically characterized by burning of the eyes, increased lacrimation, sore throat, nausea, cough, and occasional wheezing. Because olfactory function is lost at around 100 to 200 ppm, if exposed individuals can still smell the "rotten eggs" odor of H_2S, the concentration is usually not high enough to cause severe asphyxiation or irritant injury. At exposure concentrations of 200 to 250 ppm, H_2S produces intense irritation of mucous membranes, corneal ulceration, blepharospasm, and dyspnea. Pulmonary edema may occur at these concentrations as a result of irritant-induced acute lung injury. At concentrations greater than 500 ppm, chemical asphyxiation of the brain may produce headache, seizures, delirium, confusion, and lethargy. The central nervous system effects of H_2S toxicity may be exacerbated by hypoxemia secondary to severe pulmonary edema. In survivors, long-term neurologic sequelae, such as ataxia, intention tremor, sensorineural hearing loss, muscle spasticity, and memory impairment may occur [53].

Concentrations in the range of 750 to 1,000 ppm will cause severe inhibition of aerobic metabolism within the central nervous system and heart. Myocardial ischemia, arrhythmias, and dilated cardiomyopathy have all been reported after significant exposures [56,57]. As doses increase, loss of consciousness, cessation of brainstem function, and cardiopulmonary arrest will occur.

Diagnosis and Management

A high index of suspicion is the key to making the diagnosis of H_2S intoxication. Although blood levels of thiosulfate are helpful in confirming the diagnosis of H_2S poisoning [58], these tests are not readily available in most clinical laboratories. When available, atmospheric measures of H_2S concentration can be used to increase diagnostic suspicion and in classifying the expected severity of exposure and intoxication. In the absence of specific exposure information, signs of ocular irritation, inflammation of mucosal membranes, and the smell of "rotten eggs" on the clothing or breath of a patient should suggest the diagnosis of H_2S intoxication.

The inhibition of cytochrome a_3 by H_2S toxicity causes a decrease in the extraction and utilization of oxygen by affected cells. As a result, blood gas analyses typically show a PaO_2 in the normal range and an elevated mixed venous oxygen tension (PvO_2), typically in the range of 35 to 45 mm Hg. There may also be a "saturation gap" between the arterial saturation of oxygen (SaO_2) calculated from arterial blood gas data and the SaO_2 measured by cooximetry as a result of sulfide ions binding to some oxygen binding sites on hemoglobin molecules, forming molecules of sulfhemoglobin. In addition, both methemoglobin and sulfhemoglobin are produced during the treatment of H_2S poisoning with sodium nitrite and amyl nitrite, as discussed later. Therefore, if H_2S poisoning is known or suspected, SaO_2 should be measured by cooximetry. A rapid decline in either PaO_2 or SaO_2 could indicate the development or progression of pulmonary edema. Serum lactate concentration is typically elevated as a result of the inhibition of aerobic metabolism. The elevated lactate concentration causes a metabolic acidosis and elevation of the anion gap.

The treatment for H_2S intoxication is similar to that for HCN intoxication—100% oxygen, antidote, and possibly HBOT. One hundred percent oxygen should be given to all patients. Assisted ventilation should be provided as necessary. Sodium nitrite can be used as an antidote to generate methemoglobin by changing the normal ferrous state of iron in the heme molecule of hemoglobin (Fe^{+2}) to the ferric state (Fe^{+3}). The ferric heme molecules in methemoglobin have a high affinity for H_2S [59]. The preferential binding of H_2S molecules to methemoglobin results in the formation of sulfhemoglobin that prevents circulating H_2S from entering cells and inhibiting cellular respiration. Sodium nitrite should be administered as soon as possible after exposure. Inhalation of amyl nitrite from ampules contained in cyanide antidote kits can be administered as a temporizing measure until venous access is obtained for the administration of sodium nitrite. The detoxifying enzyme rhodanese is not involved in H_2S metabolism, as it is in HCN metabolism. Therefore, sodium thiosulfate or hydroxocobalamin should not be given for the treatment of H_2S intoxication. Several case reports argue for a beneficial effect of HBOT in H_2S intoxication [60,61]. Basic supportive measures should not be forgotten and include irrigation of the eyes with sterile saline and the treatment of irritant-induced bronchospasm with inhaled β_2-agonists. Consideration should be given to the administration of sodium bicarbonate for the treatment of severe metabolic acidosis in unconscious or hemodynamically unstable patients. A benzodiazepine, such as diazepam, or a barbiturate can be used to control seizures if present. If a benzodiazepine or barbiturate is given, patients should be carefully monitored for signs of respiratory insufficiency.

IRRITANT GASES

Irritant gases are those that cause chemical injury to the airways and lung tissue upon inhalation. The nature, location, and severity of respiratory tract injuries associated with the inhalation of an irritant gas are dependent on the physical and chemical properties of the gas, exposure dose, and host factors of exposed individuals. The most important physical and chemical properties are the water solubility and density of the gas. Exposure dose is determined by the concentration of the gas in the environment and the duration of exposure. Minute ventilation, age, and the presence of preexisting respiratory disease are the most important host factors (Table 64.5).

The sites of injury following inhalation of an irritant gas are dependent on the water solubility of the gas that determines where most of the gas will be deposited in the respiratory tract (Table 64.6). Highly soluble gases, such as ammonia and sulfur dioxide, generally cause irritant damage to exposed mucous membranes, such as the eyes and upper airway (nose, lips, pharynx, and larynx), while sparing the lower airways. At high concentrations, however, a highly soluble irritant gas can overwhelm the upper respiratory tract, and significant amounts may reach the upper and lower airways, thereby producing both mucous membrane and airway injury. Irritant gases of intermediate solubility, such as chlorine, may produce significant upper airway injury, especially in the pharynx and larynx, but the mucous membrane irritation is usually not as intense as that caused by highly soluble gases. Because of its intermediate solubility, the irritant effects of chlorine will extend more distally at higher concentrations. Thus, high concentrations of inhaled chlorine can produce both upper and lower airway injury, as well as pulmonary edema due to alveolar damage. The inhalation of low-solubility irritant gases, such as phosgene and oxides of nitrogen, typically produces minimal upper airway irritation but can cause intense lower airways and alveolar damage. As a result of lung tissue injury, the development of noncardiogenic pulmonary edema is more likely following inhalation of a low-solubility irritant gas or at high concentrations of gases with intermediate solubility. Irritant gases that are associated with the development of pulmonary edema are listed in Table 64.7. The inhalation of gases that are lipid soluble, but not water soluble, such as chloroform, ether, or other halogenated hydrocarbons, will produce central nervous system effects and little, if any, respiratory injury. Methylene chloride, found in paint remover and other solvents, is an exception to this rule in that high doses may cause pulmonary edema [62].

TABLE 64.5

DETERMINANTS OF SEVERITY OF LUNG INJURY

Duration of exposure
Minute ventilation
Age of victim
Proximity to source
Density of gas and height of victim
Temperature of gas
Toxicity of gas
Water solubility of gas
Particle size of mist, fog, or vapor
Breathing pattern-oronasal vs. mouth breathing
Host factors such as preexisting asthma, coronary disease, chronic obstructive pulmonary disease
Orthopedic problems that affect the ability to evacuate quickly

TABLE 64.6

IRRITANT GASES

High solubility gases
Ammonia
Methyl isocyanate
Sulfur dioxide
Intermediate solubility gas
Chlorine
Low solubility gases
Hydrogen sulfide
Oxides of nitrogen
Phosgene

Irritant gases cause damage to airways and lung tissues by direct cellular injury, cellular injury secondary to the production of free radicals, and production of an inflammatory response. Direct cellular injury is commonly produced by irritant gases that possess either a highly acidic or a highly alkaline pH. Chlorine and phosgene, for example, produce hydrochloric acid when they come in contact with water in mucous membranes. Ammonia forms a strong alkali, ammonium hydroxide, when it comes in contact with water in mucous membranes and airways. Ammonium hydroxide causes liquefaction damage to cells and tissues on contact, with the severity of damage directly related to the hydroxyl ion concentration. Damage to respiratory tract cells and tissues can also be caused by irritant gases that generate the production of free radicals. Oxides of nitrogen, for example, cause the production of free radicals that cause cellular damage by lipid peroxidation. Both direct cell damage and cell damage secondary to free radical formation result in the release of a variety of inflammatory mediators that elicit an inflammatory response, thereby causing further oxidant damage to respiratory tract cells. In the airways, the

TABLE 64.7

TOXIC GASES AND FUMES THAT CAN PRODUCE PULMONARY EDEMA

Acetaldehyde	Methylene chloride
Acrolein	Nickel carbonyl
Ammonia	Nitrogen dioxide
Antimony tri- or pentachloride	Osmium tetroxide
Beryllium	Ozone
Bismuth pentachloride	Paraquat
Boranes	Perchloroethylene
Cadmium and cadmium salts	Phosgene
Chloramine	Phosphine
Chlorine	Polytetrafluoroethylene
Cobalt metal	Selenium dioxide
Dichlorosilane	Silanes
Dimethyl sulfate	Silicone tetrachloride
Dioxane dimethyl sulfate	Silicone tetrafluoride
Fire smoke	Sulfur dioxide
Glyphosate herbicides	TDI in high concentrations
Hydrogen chloride	Titanium tetrachloride
Hydrogen fluoride	Trimellitic anhydride
Hydrogen selenide	Vanadium
Hydrogen sulfide	War gases
Lithium hydride	Zinc oxide and chloride
Mercury	Zirconium chloride
Methyl bromide	

damage caused by irritant gases is manifested by mucosal edema, mucus production, increased smooth muscle contraction, and airway obstruction. At the alveolar level, damage of type 1 pneumocytes occurs followed by capillary leakage due to epithelial cell damage, disruption of epithelial cell tight junctions, endothelial damage, and increased vascular permeability.

Specific Irritant Toxic Gases

Ammonia

Ammonia (NH_3) is a colorless, pungent, alkaline gas that is less dense than air and highly soluble. It forms ammonium hydroxide (NH_4OH) upon contact with water. Most inhalational injuries from NH_3 occur as a result of exposures occurring during fertilizer production [63], chemical manufacturing, and oil refining or the use of cleaning solutions [64]. Recently, exposures have occurred during the illicit production of methamphetamine [65]. The strong, pungent smell associated with NH_3 can be readily detected at a concentration as low as 50 ppm. Few individuals can tolerate a concentration greater than 100 ppm without experiencing nasal stuffiness and irritating cough.

As a highly soluble gas, NH_3 primarily causes irritation to the eyes, mucous membranes of the nasal–oral pharynx, and mucosa of the upper respiratory airways. The reaction of NH_3 with water in the conjunctivae, mucous membranes, and upper airway mucosa results in the formation of NH_4OH that causes liquefaction necrosis and intense pain in the eyes, mouth, nose, and throat. The voice is lost shortly after exposure, and patients typically experience sensations of choking and suffocation. The eyes are erythematous, swollen, and may show signs of corneal opacification or ulceration. Edema, ulceration, necrosis, and sloughing of the mucous membranes are typically seen. Airway obstruction due to laryngeal edema, bronchial inflammation, bronchoconstriction, and plugs of sloughed epithelium may cause dyspnea, wheezing, and hypoxemia [66]. Death from laryngospasm can occur within 1 minute after exposure to high concentrations ($\geq$1,500 ppm). With exposure to high concentrations, alveolar damage and pulmonary edema can occur within 24 hours [66]. Secondary bacterial bronchopneumonia may occur within days. Long-term sequelae of NH_3 inhalation include persistent airway obstruction from reactive airways dysfunction syndrome (RADS), asthma, bronchitis, bronchiectasis, and bronchiolitis obliterans [66,67].

Chlorine

Chlorine (Cl_2) is a dense, greenish-yellow gas under ambient conditions. It is highly reactive, has intermediate solubility, and has the characteristic pungent odor of bleach. Industrial uses of Cl_2 include the production of chemicals and bleaches, paper manufacturing, textile processing, and the production of polyvinyl chloride. Most Cl_2 exposures result from accidental releases at industrial sites, from ruptured tanks during its transportation or at swimming pools [68–70]. The relatively high density of Cl_2 causes it to accumulate in low-lying areas, which should be avoided following its accidental release.

Chlorine is detectable by smell at levels of 1 ppm. On contact with mucous membranes, chlorine reacts with water to produce hydrochloric acid (HCl), hypochlorous acid (HClO), and free oxygen radicals. Individuals exposed to low concentrations of Cl_2 typically experience burning of the eyes and mucous membranes, as well as choking and coughing due to inflammation of the nasal–oral pharynx and upper airway. At higher concentrations, laryngeal edema, lower airway inflammation, bronchoconstriction, and pulmonary edema can develop. The development of stridor reflects upper airway obstruction due to laryngeal edema and should be considered as a sign of impending respiratory failure. However, in some cases, slight wheezing and erythema of the conjunctivae and mucous membranes may be the only physical findings that are evident within the first hour after exposure. Unfortunately, the initial paucity of significant signs and symptoms may not reflect the true severity of the inhalational injury, and exposed individuals may be sent home from the emergency department prematurely. For example, an exposure concentration of 50 ppm may produce relatively mild signs and symptoms initially but can cause death from laryngospasm or massive pulmonary edema within 1 to 2 hours after exposure. The onset of pulmonary edema may also be delayed up to 24 hours after exposure. At any time within 2 days after Cl_2 exposure, airway inflammation and mucosal desquamation may cause plugging of medium and small bronchi, leading to airflow obstruction and atelectasis. Individuals with a history of asthma or airway hyperactivity may have particularly severe bronchospasm. Secondary bacterial bronchopneumonia may develop as a consequence of ulceration and desquamation of airway mucosa and/or alveolar damage. Fortunately, most exposed individuals will recover completely if they receive prompt medical treatment and survive the acute effects of Cl_2 exposure. However, chronic pulmonary problems may develop in some individuals, including RADS, asthma, bronchiectasis, and bronchiolitis obliterans [70–72].

Phosgene

Phosgene ($COCl_2$) is a heavy, poorly soluble, colorless gas that has the smell of freshly mown hay. Upon contact with water, it hydrolyzes to form CO_2 and HCl. $COCl_2$ has been used as a chemical warfare agent and was responsible for most gas fatalities during World War I [42]. It is currently use as a chlorinating agent in a variety of industrial processes, including the production of isocyanates, pesticides, dyes, and pharmaceutical agents. Fire fighters, welders, and paint strippers may be exposed to $COCl_2$ as a result of its release from heated chlorinated hydrocarbons, such as polyvinyl chloride [73]. Phosgene is approximately four times as dense as air and tends to accumulate close to the ground and in low-lying areas. Therefore, exposed individuals should avoid low-lying areas following an accidental release.

As a gas with low solubility, $COCl_2$ is less irritating to the eyes and mucous membranes than NH_3 or Cl_2 and causes mostly irritant damage in the lower airways and cellular damage at the alveolar level. Immediate symptoms include burning of the eyes, increased lacrimation, sore throat, rhinorrhea, coughing, choking, dyspnea, and chest tightness, which may be relatively mild and may resolve within several minutes after cessation of $COCl_2$ exposure. Laryngeal edema can occur shortly after high concentration exposures, with stridor and the potential for sudden death. As a result of its low solubility, the mucous membranes and upper airways are typically spared and there may be few, if any, additional symptoms for 2 to 24 hours following the acute inhalation of $COCl_2$. However, inhaled $COCl_2$ will eventually hydrolyze to form HCl in the lower airways and alveoli causing oxidative and inflammatory injury. As a result, bronchospasm and pulmonary edema typically develop between 2 and 6 hours following exposure, but pulmonary edema may be delayed for up to 24 hours. The pulmonary edema can progress to the acute respiratory distress syndrome (ARDS) and respiratory failure. Most victims survive without long-term sequelae if they receive prompt medical care. Those with ARDS have the worst prognosis and will require assisted ventilation and circulatory support as needed. Chronic problems may develop in some individuals with RADS, asthma, bronchiectasis, and bronchiolitis obliterans [74].

Nitrogen Oxides

The four stable oxides of nitrogen are nitrous oxide (N_2O), nitric oxide (NO), nitrogen dioxide (NO_2), and nitrogen tetroxide (N_2O_4). Oxides of nitrogen are used in the production of dyes, lacquer, and fertilizer. They are also generated in a variety of processes, including arc welding [73], chemical engraving, explosives, and the storage of fresh silage [75]. All oxides of nitrogen can produce serious acute respiratory tract injury upon inhalation. However, NO_2 is the most common and clinically important toxicant in this group. NO_2 is an irritating, low solubility, dense orange-brown gas. It forms nitric acid (HNO_3) and nitrous acid (HNO_2) upon contact with water.

NO_2 causes silo filler's disease, one of the best-characterized syndromes of toxic gas exposure. Silo filler's disease develops following exposure to NO_2 gas that accumulates just above the silage in recently filled, top-loading silos. During the first 2 weeks in the silo, carbohydrates in the silage ferment and produce organic acids. The organic acids then oxidize nitrates in the silage into NO_2. Within hours after it starts to be produced, NO_2 rapidly accumulates to toxic levels of 200 to 2,000 ppm. High concentrations of NO_2 typically persist for 1 to 2 weeks, then decrease. Entry into a silo without proper respiratory protection, especially within the first 2 weeks of the silo being filled with fresh silage, can cause a rapid loss of consciousness and sudden death. The incidence of this disorder is estimated to be 5 cases per 100,000 silo-associated farm workers per year [75].

The lower airways and lung are the primary sites of injury following acute inhalation of NO_2. The low water solubility of NO_2 results in a paucity of eye, mucous membrane, and upper airway irritant symptoms. The most significant effects occur in the lower airways and lungs as a result of the conversion of NO_2 to HNO_3 upon contact with water in bronchial mucosa and alveoli. The clinical response to inhaled NO_2 occurs in three phases [75,76]. The first phase is the *acute illness phase* that typically occurs within the first hour after exposure. The severity of symptoms in this first phase is dose related. At doses up to 100 ppm, cough, wheezing, dyspnea, and chest pain develop as a result of lower airway irritation and bronchospasm. Hypotension may occur in severe cases. At doses greater than 100 ppm, pulmonary edema may develop within 1 to 2 hours after exposure. The hypoxemia resulting from pulmonary edema is further exacerbated by NO_2-induced methemoglobinemia.

Without further NO_2 exposure, symptoms of the *acute illness phase* usually resolve over a period of 2 to 8 weeks. During this *latent phase*, the patient may have mild cough and wheezing, or may be totally asymptomatic. The patient may then develop a *delayed illness phase* that is characterized by the sudden onset of fever, chills, cough, dyspnea, and generalized lung crackles [75,76]. The *delayed illness phase* is characterized by bronchiolitis obliterans. Lung biopsies have shown that this is bronchiolitis of the proximal type without organizing pneumonia [75,76]. The bronchioles are typically packed with inflammatory exudate and fibrin that may obliterate the entire lumen. The bronchiolitis obliterans of the *delayed illness phase* may be extensive and cause severe, life-threatening hypoxemia. Symptom severity in the *acute illness phase* does not always correlate with the severity of bronchiolitis obliterans in the *delayed illness phase*. Therefore, patients with relatively mild symptoms in the days following acute NO_2 exposure may experience severe, life-threatening bronchiolitis obliterans in the *delayed illness phase*.

Sulfur Dioxide

Sulfur dioxide (SO_2) is a colorless, dense, irritating gas that is highly soluble in water. It has a readily identifiable, strong, pungent, odor. SO_2 is a common atmospheric pollutant from the combustion of coal and gasoline. It is used in a variety of industrial process, such as bleaching, refrigeration, and paper manufacturing [77]. SO_2 forms sulfuric acid (H_2SO_4) upon contact with water in human tissues. As a highly soluble gas, the predominant effects of SO_2 exposure are irritation of the eyes, nose, mucous membranes, pharynx, and upper respiratory tract. Exposure doses greater than 10 ppm typically cause bronchospasm with symptoms of cough, wheezing, dyspnea, and chest pain. Symptom severity increases with increasing exposure doses. Individuals with preexisting asthma or chronic obstructive lung disease are 10 times more likely to develop severe exacerbations [77]. These include RADS, asthma, bronchiolitis obliterans, and restrictive lung disease [77,78].

SMOKE

Smoke is a toxic, irritant mixture of gases, vapors, fumes, liquid droplets, and carbonaceous particles generated by the incomplete combustion or pyrolysis of multiple substances at very high temperatures. Approximately 80% of all fire-associated deaths are attributed to inhalation injury [79]. Smoke inhalation is the most common cause of death in fire victims without surface burns. Inhalation injury exerts a greater influence than burn size or age in determining burn mortality [80]. Patients being treated in burn centers have a mortality rate of 29% in the presence of inhalation injury, in comparison with a mortality rate of 2% in its absence [81].

Combustion occurs when oxygen reacts with fuel molecules under intense heat and the fuel molecules are oxidized to smaller compounds. Pyrolysis occurs as a result of heat alone, does not require oxygen, and consists of the melting or boiling of heated material. The toxic products of incomplete combustion or pyrolysis generated in a given setting are determined by multiple factors, including the type of fuel consumed, temperature, rate of heating, and distance from the source [79]. Black smoke results from particles of carbon or soot generated during the combustion or pyrolysis of carbon-containing materials. Common combustible materials in a fire include wood, paper, plastics, polyurethane, paints, and other polymers present in carpeting and upholstery.

Toxic gases are released during combustion and pyrolysis. These gases include both asphyxiants and irritants. CO and HCN are common asphyxiants found in smoke. Aldehydes, acrolein, NO_2, SO_2, and HCl are common irritants found in smoke. These irritant gases are more likely to be released during pyrolysis than combustion [82]. Particulates present in smoke adsorb these irritant chemicals to their surface, which can concentrate the chemicals and increase irritant damage to the respiratory tract upon inhalation [83].

Victims of smoke inhalation are exposed to multiple irritant gases [79,84], but several deserve special mention. Acrolein is an aldehyde released in fires involving polyethylene, polypropylene, vinyl materials, wood, and other organic fuels. At low concentrations, acrolein is intensely irritating to the upper respiratory tract and can cause significant upper airway edema. At high concentrations (>10 ppm), acrolein inhalation can cause severe, life-threatening pulmonary edema [85]. Isocyanate, a known cause of asthma, is also among the toxic products produced in fires. The inhalation of isocyanate contained in smoke can precipitate severe bronchospasm in individuals with or without a history of airway disease.

Smoke particles cause airway damage due to direct injury from heat and steam, irritation of the airway mucosa by the particles themselves, and from inflammation as a result of the irritant effects of toxic chemicals absorbed to their surface. Heat injury from hot gases and steam is usually limited to the upper respiratory tract as heat rapidly dissipates across the upper airways [85]. Smoke particles greater than 10 μm in diameter also contribute to upper airway injury (rhinosinusitis, pharyngitis, laryngitis, and upper airway edematous obstruction), as they do not penetrate into the lower airways unless present at high concentrations. Subglottic or supraglottic edema following smoke inhalation can lead to significant upper airway obstruction. Upper airway obstruction occurs in up to 30% of burn patients and may occur as early as 4 hours or as late as 24 hours after exposure [86]. The production of upper airway edema is due to a variety of factors, including direct mucosal damage and ulceration from heat and superheated steam, the release of inflammatory mediators from the damaged mucosa, and the production of oxygen free radicals from toxic chemicals on the surface of smoke particles. Acute upper airway edema following smoke inhalation usually resolves within 3 to 4 days. Rarely, thermal injury can produce circumferential, constricting eschars or scarring of the upper airway after the acute edema resolves. Such eschars can produce chronic upper airway obstruction.

In the large to medium size airways of the chest, tracheobronchitis can develop as a result of smoke inhalation. Severe cough and chest tightness without bronchoconstriction are common presenting symptoms. Tracheobronchitis is due to irritant chemical and/or particulate injury. Heat injury is rare and occurs only after the inhalation of superheated steam [85].

Particles less than 3 μm in diameter travel to the distal portions of the respiratory tract and can cause small airways and alveolar injury. Lower airway penetration by small smoke particulates can cause irritation, inflammation, and bronchoconstriction. Individuals with preexisting asthma or chronic obstructive pulmonary disease may experience exacerbations, but bronchoconstriction can also occur in individuals with no prior history of airway disease. Small smoke particles can also cause alveolar-capillary injury in the lung parenchyma by direct oxidative damage from adsorbed irritants and by oxygen free radicals and inflammatory mediators released by neutrophils that migrate to areas of irritant damage. Pulmonary edema can occur as a consequence of alveolar-capillary injury and may occur hours to days after smoke inhalation. Although pulmonary edema occurs in far less than 10% of smoke inhalation victims, it has a high mortality rate [87].

Airway injury, whether it is tracheobronchitis or small airway bronchoconstriction, can cause sloughing of necrotic tissue into the lower airways that can lead to mucous plugging, bronchial obstruction, atelectasis, hyperinflation, and altered mucociliary clearance. Secondary bacterial pneumonia can develop in obstructed lung segments or as the result of alveolar damage adversely affecting local immunodefenses.

Most smoke inhalation deaths are caused by asphyxiation as a result of CO or HCN in the inhaled smoke [14,39–41]. CO intoxication is responsible for 80% of smoke inhalation fatalities, and approximately one fourth of these occur in victims with underlying cardiac or pulmonary disease [10]. NO_2 may also be a component of inhaled smoke. In addition to being a potent irritant, NO_2 can cause the development of methemoglobinemia, which can further decrease the already impaired oxygen-carrying capacity of hemoglobin caused by carboxyhemoglobinemia. Coexisting HCN intoxication needs to be considered in all smoke inhalation victims with CO intoxication, especially those with clinical evidence of altered neurologic or cardiac status. In a study from Paris, a clear association was found between blood HCN levels and percent carboxyhemoglobin levels [39]. This association was strongest in patients with metabolic acidosis and elevated lactate levels [39]. In a study from the Dallas County Fire Department, an HCN blood level above 1.0 mg per L was a strong predictor of death, but the association between CO and HCN levels was not strong [88]. In this study [88], of the 144 patients that reached the emergency room alive, 12 had blood cyanide concentrations exceeding 1.0 mg per L and 8 of the 12 subsequently died. In these 12 patients, the relationship between percent carboxyhemoglobin levels and HCN blood levels was poor. For example, the highest percent carboxyhemoglobin level found was 40.0%, in a patient with a blood HCN level of 1.20 mg per L. The highest HCN level found was 11.50 mg per L in a patient with a percent carboxyhemoglobin level of 22.4%.

Diagnosis and Management of Irritant Toxic Gases, Including Smoke Inhalation

The most important factors in the diagnosis of toxic inhalational injury are a history of circumstances that caused the exposure, identification of the specific toxic gas to which an individual has been exposed, and an estimate of the exposure concentration. Exposure duration is based not only on exposure time but also on the patient's minute ventilation during that time. Chemical analyses of material at the site of exposure, if available, can be particularly helpful in identifying the offending toxicant and estimating its exposure concentration. The relative solubility of a toxic gas can be helpful in determining the areas of the respiratory tract where irritant injuries are most likely to occur, and obviously patients with preexisting pulmonary disease are most at risk. When the irritant toxic gases are in the setting of smoke inhalation, the exposure will be to multiple gases and particulates. Facial burns, singed eyebrows, soot in the upper airway, and carbonaceous sputum make smoke inhalation highly likely.

The management of acute inhalational injury from toxic irritants is at first supportive. All contaminated clothing should be removed to prevent further inhalation and percutaneous absorption of the toxic substance. Superficial burns should be treated conservatively with a topical antibiotic such as silver sulfadiazine. The eyes should be thoroughly flushed with sterile normal saline as soon as possible. Careful attention to the eyes is important because cataracts can occur following heavy exposures. Humidified oxygen should be given by face mask. Not everyone exposed to fire smoke warrants hospital admission. Victims with mild inhalation exposures may be treated and released if they are (i) asymptomatic with normal mental status and absent of confusion; (ii) no burns, carbon material, or edema in the upper airway; (iii) normal pulmonary examination without signs of respiratory distress, stridor, or wheeze; and (iv) if available a pulse oximeter and noninvasive carboxyhemoglobin reading that are normal or at baseline. Upon release, patients should be advised to seek medical attention if symptoms occur or reoccur, as the clinical manifestations of inhalation injury may take 4 to 24 hours to develop [87]. It is for this reason that borderline patients or patients with significant comorbidity should be observed rather than released whenever possible.

The medical evaluation after any exposure to potentially toxic irritant gases should focus on assessing the nature and extent of upper and lower respiratory tract injury, the adequacy of oxygenation, cardiac function, and the hemodynamic stability of the patient. Inhalation victims may be unconscious or have altered mental status at the time of presentation. Typical patient complaints include eye irritation, headaches, confusion, sore throat, chest tightness, and difficulty breathing. Common physical findings include irritation of the eyes, skin and other exposed mucosal surfaces, tachypnea, cough, stridor, wheezing, and rhonchi. Rales on presentation are unusual, as pulmonary edema is a later complication [87].

Arterial blood gases, oxygen saturation, should be obtained on all patients. The methemoglobin level should be measured in patients with suspected NO_2 exposure or after treatment with amyl or sodium nitrites for suspected HCN toxicity. Serum lactate concentration should be measured, and the magnitude of metabolic acidosis should be assessed. Although chest radiographs may be normal shortly after acute exposure, serial radiographs are useful for detecting the development of pulmonary edema and secondary bacterial pneumonia in hypoxemic individuals. An electrocardiogram should be obtained to detect the presence of myocardial ischemia and cardiac dysrhythmias. Hemodynamic monitoring may be necessary in complex, critically ill patients with pulmonary edema.

The carboxyhemoglobin level, a measure of CO intoxication, should be obtained in all patients with suspected exposure to smoke, fires, or other sources of combustion. If high levels of carboxyhemoglobin, methemoglobin, or HCN exist, the arterial oxygen tension (PaO_2) is not useful in assessing the adequacy of oxygen transport or tissue oxygenation. Arterial oxygen saturation should be measured by cooximetry because pulse oximetry and the calculation of SaO_2 from the PaO_2 will overestimate the actual oxygen saturation of hemoglobin.

All individuals with known or suspected inhalation injury should be given 100% humidified oxygen as soon as possible. This will help to improve the oxygen-carrying capacity of hemoglobin when high levels of carboxyhemoglobin or methemoglobin are present. High levels of methemoglobin are unusual but, if present, can be treated with intravenous methylene blue. The fraction of inspired oxygen can be titrated down to maintain a PaO_2 greater than 60 mm Hg once carboxyhemoglobin and methemoglobin levels have returned to normal. When available, HBOT should be considered for the treatment of CO intoxication according to the criteria for previously delineated in the section in this chapter. HBOT has been used to treat patients with extreme levels of CO poisoning ($\geq$25% carboxyhemoglobin) or end-organ sensitivity to CO at elevated but lower levels. Examples of this might include neurologic abnormalities or hemodynamic instability that was felt to be caused by CO poisoning.

Severely ill smoke inhalation patients presenting with seizures, coma, hemodynamic instability, and/or severe lactic acidosis should be suspected of having both CO and HCN intoxication [39–41,88]. Blood HCN levels can be measured, but results cannot be obtained in time to make therapeutic decisions and therefore the decision to treat for HCN toxicity should be based on the exposure characteristics and clinical presentation. NYC Fire Department protocol is to intubate such patients; provide hemodynamic support as needed; empirically treat for HCN poisoning with hydroxocobalamin; and, if noninvasive carboxyhemoglobin levels are elevated, to transport to a HBOT center. In addition, all smoke inhalation victims found in cardiac arrest receive hydroxocobalamin during cardiac resuscitation.

In smoke inhalation patients, with suspected HCN poisoning, hydroxocobalamin is preferable to sodium thiosulfate because of its rapid onset of action. Inhaled amyl nitrite and intravenous sodium nitrite should be avoided because they generate methemoglobin that can further impair the oxygen-carrying capacity of blood hemoglobin if high levels of carboxyhemoglobin or methemoglobin are already present. The Paris Fire Brigade routinely administers hydroxocobalamin to smoke inhalation patients and published their experience in 2006 [46]. Of the 29 patients in cardiac arrest, 18 (62%) recovered with cardiac resuscitation and hydroxocobalamin treatment. The average time between hydroxocobalamin administration and recovery of spontaneous cardiac activity was 19 minutes. In 15 hemodynamically unstable patients not in cardiac arrest, 12 (80%) showed hemodynamic improvement (blood pressure >90 mm Hg) after hydroxocobalamin. The average time for hemodynamic improvement was 49 minutes from the start of and 29 minutes from the end of hydroxocobalamin infusion. In a second study, 28 of 42 patients (67%) admitted to the ICU with smoke inhalation and confirmed a posteriori HCN poisoning survived after hydroxocobalamin administration [47].

Respiratory symptoms and distress are not only related to oxygen delivery/utilization problems. Irritant, toxic gases can also cause tachypnea, stridor, and hoarseness due to upper and lower airway disease. Patients are at high risk of developing progressive laryngeal edema with complete obstruction of the upper airway. Smoke inhalation further adds to this risk due to heat and particulate matter exposure. Patients with laryngeal edema can be extremely difficult to intubate and if intubation is delayed may require an emergency tracheostomy. However, not all patients require intubation [89]. Prompt inspection of the larynx with a laryngoscope is imperative [86]. Immediate intubation should be considered if there is evidence of significant upper airway edema or blisters. All patients with upper airway edema should be treated with nebulized racemic epinephrine and systemic corticosteroids. If edema is minimal and early intubation is not required, airflow can usually be maintained with positive pressure breathing administered by the use of continuous positive airway pressure (CPAP) or bilevel positive airway pressure (BiPAP). An inhaled mixture of helium and oxygen can also improve upper airway airflow by reducing turbulence as a result of its low density. If the clinical decision is not for immediate or early intubation [89], then patients with upper airway edema should be admitted to the hospital and closely monitored for signs of edema progression and the need for emergent intubation at a later time.

Lower airway involvement from irritant gas or smoke inhalation is typically diagnosed by history and physical examination. However, additional diagnostic evidence can be provided by laryngoscopic or bronchoscopic demonstration of edema, hemorrhage, or carbonaceous material distal to the vocal cords. Inhalation injury to the smaller airways and lung parenchyma can be confirmed by Xenon 133 ventilation scanning [90] or noncontrast chest CT scans [91,92]. Inhalation injury on chest CT should be suspected with findings of ground glass infiltrates (more central than peripheral). Sensitivity for both types of scans is high, but there are false positives, especially in patients with obstructive airway disease and their value in determining the need for intubation, treatment, and prognosis has not been determined [90–92].

Lower airway involvement should be suspected on physical examination when wheezing is present or when spirometry or challenge testing demonstrates acute reductions in lung function, bronchodilator responsiveness, or airway hyperreactivity [93–96]. Acute bronchospasm should be treated with β_2-agonists. Ipratropium can be added if significant improvement is not obtained with a β_2-agonist alone. In the presence of significant burn injuries, treatment with systemic corticosteroids is usually contraindicated, as their use is associated with increased mortality from sepsis [87,97]. Systemic corticosteroids should be reserved for severe upper airway obstruction, severe bronchospasm resistant to bronchodilator therapy, and failed extubation due to stridor or bronchospasm [87,97]. Low-dose inhaled corticosteroids have not been studied in large case series, but it is unlikely that they would negatively impact on mortality in burn patients. Animal studies have shown that inhaled corticosteroids improve oxygenation and attenuate the development of acute lung injury following chlorine exposure [98,99]. Although inhaled corticosteroids are often given following chlorine and phosgene inhalation, there are no controlled clinical trials regarding their efficacy. Chest physiotherapy and frequent suctioning may be helpful in those patients with mucus plugs and thick secretions. Intubation may be necessary if bronchial secretions are excessive and frequent bronchoscopic suctioning may be needed.

Noncardiogenic pulmonary edema from acute lung injury (ARDS) is far less common than airway injury but should be suspected in patients with worsening oxygenation and increasing dyspnea. A chest radiograph should be obtained if signs of respiratory distress, abnormal breath sounds, or worsening hypoxemia are noted. Pulmonary edema or ARDS from inhalation injury typically presents as scattered, nodular alveolar infiltrates on chest radiographs, although large, diffuse, confluent infiltrates may occur as the illness progresses. Careful attention to fluid and electrolyte balance is essential, especially if surface burns are present. If gas exchange abnormalities are severe, positive pressure ventilation with CPAP or BiPAP may help to support adequate oxygenation. If there is no response or secretions are burdensome, then intubation and assisted ventilation are required. Nasotracheal intubation should be avoided because of the severe nasal inflammation that typically occurs following the inhalation of chemical irritants and because the smaller endotracheal tube diameters needed for nasotracheal intubation do not allow for the repeated bronchoscopic suctioning that may be needed if secretions become a problem. Positive end-expiratory pressure in the range of 5 to 10 cm H_2O may help to improve oxygenation in mechanically ventilated patients [100–102]. The use of systemic corticosteroids for the treatment of pulmonary edema or ARDS following toxic irritant inhalation remains controversial [103]. Again, there are no controlled clinical trials evaluating the efficacy of corticosteroid treatment. Most experts believe that corticosteroids are not useful as pulmonary edema, or ARDS typically resolves 48 to 72 hours after inhalation exposure, with most patients surviving if appropriate supportive treatment is given. However, whether corticosteroids might be useful in preventing the few that develop pulmonary bronchiolitis obliterans or pulmonary fibrosis remain to be determined. Experimental studies suggest that treatment to block inflammatory mediators and free radicals may be effective in smoke inhalation victims [104–106]. Recent examples include retrospective analyses of mechanically ventilated smoke inhalation patients, adult [107] and pediatric [108] demonstrating successful treatment with nebulized unfractionated heparin and *N*-acetylcysteine. However, controlled clinical trials have not been conducted for any of the above experimental agents.

Secondary bacterial pneumonia can occur as a complication of irritant-induced airway or lung injury [109]. There is no evidence that the administration of prophylactic antibiotics reduces the incidence of secondary bacterial pneumonia. Antibiotics should be given only if pneumonia occurs, and the specific antibiotics chosen should be based on standard practice according to known community organisms and sensitivities until culture results return.

LONG-TERM COMPLICATIONS OF ACUTE INHALATION INJURY

Although most patients exposed to irritant gases or smoke will recover completely, others may develop chronic, long-term sequelae. The most common long-term complications are listed in Table 64.8. Some of these disorders may become evident in the

TABLE 64.8

LONG-TERM EFFECTS OF ACUTE INHALATION INJURY

Complete resolution of symptoms
Sinusitis/rhinitis
Gastroesophageal reflux
Asthma
Reactive airways dysfunction syndrome
Chronic bronchitis or chronic obstructive pulmonary disease
Bronchiectasis
Bronchiolitis obliterans
Bronchostenosis
Restrictive interstitial fibrosis

days or weeks following acute exposure, whereas others may take months, or even years, before clinical symptoms and signs become evident. Therefore, all patients with acute inhalational injury require medical follow-up for the potential development of these disorders, even if they are initially asymptomatic after resolution of acute signs and symptoms.

Some individuals may develop a chronic cough syndrome, dyspnea, and/or wheezing following recovery from acute inhalation injury. Pulmonary function tests, chest radiographs, and high resolution CT scans of the chest can be helpful in determining the etiology of chronic cough in such patients. When chest radiographs and chest CT scans are normal, the chronic cough is usually due to asthma, RADS, bronchitis, rhinosinusitis, and/or gastroesophageal reflux [110,111]. Pulmonary function tests may be normal. Such patients could have rhinosinusitis and/or gastroesophageal reflux disease and could also have RADS or irritant asthma. The diagnostic evaluation of such patients should be guided by a careful history and physical examination. RADS is characterized by immediate and persistent, nonspecific airway hyperreactivity following inhalation of a toxic substance in individuals with no prior history of cigarette smoking, allergen, or airway disease [112]. Irritant asthma is the more proper terminology if symptoms were not immediate or if there is a history of prior allergies, pulmonary disease, or smoking. When pulmonary function tests are normal, bronchial challenge testing (methacholine, histamine, mannitol, cold air, exercise) may be performed to evaluate airway hyperreactivity in patients suspected of having RADS or irritant asthma. Transient, self-limited bronchial hyperreactivity may occur in the weeks following irritant gas or smoke exposures, so the detection of early bronchial hyperreactivity may not always be predictive of RADS [93–96]. The evaluation of fire fighters with heavy exposure to dust and irritant gases during the first days after the World Trade Center collapse showed that bronchial hyperreactivity demonstrated by methacholine challenge testing after 1 month or 3 months postexposure was predictive of persistent airway hyperreactivity and RADS [96]. It can take months or years for the symptoms of RADS to resolve, and some patients may never have complete resolution. Treatment with an inhaled bronchodilator should be considered if a significant bronchodilator response is found. Even in the absence of a documented bronchodilator response, a trial should be considered if there is a history of symptoms with exercise, irritants, or change in temperature/humidity. Inhaled corticosteroids should be considered not only for symptom control but also for the possibility, albeit unproven concept, that early treatment may prevent progression or lead to resolution [113].

If symptoms persist, serial measurements of spirometry, lung volumes, and diffusion capacity should be assessed to determine if there is accelerated decline in lung function, hyperinflation, bronchiolitis obliterans, emphysema, or pulmonary fibrosis. A study of more than 12,000 firefighters and EMS workers exposed to dust and gases from the September 11, 2010, attack on the World Trade Center found that the decline in lung function in the first 6 to 12 months after the attack was 12 times the expected annual decline and even more important for the majority of those exposed to this decline persisted for the next 6 years [114]. Another study of firefighters exposed to World Trade Center dust and gases demonstrated that interstitial pulmonary fibrosis was exceedingly rare and that airway obstruction was probable cause of the persistent lung injury [115].

Bronchiolitis obliterans is a rare but particularly ominous complication following the inhalation of certain toxic gases, particularly NO_2, other oxides of nitrogen, SO_2, mustard gas, and/or smoke [116–119]. Inhaled toxicants that can produce bronchiolitis obliterans are listed in Table 64.9. Bronchiolitis obliterans can take two forms following acute inhalation injury. The first form is manifested by the acute onset of fever,

TABLE 64.9

AGENTS THAT CAN PRODUCE BRONCHIOLITIS OBLITERANS

Ammonia	Methyl isocyanate
Chlorine	Mustard gas
Cocaine free-base	Oxides of nitrogen
Fire smoke	Phosgene
Hydrogen selenide	Sulfur dioxide

chills, cough, dyspnea, and generalized lung crackles that develop 2 to 8 weeks after acute exposure to an offending gas, as discussed in "Nitrogen Oxides" section. Chest radiographs or high resolution CT scans typically show a diffuse "miliary" pattern of small nodules. Although lung biopsies are usually not necessary to make the diagnosis with a history of acute inhalation injury, they show a proximal bronchiolitis with occlusion of the bronchioles by inflammatory exudates and fibrin, but without organizing pneumonia [116]. This form of bronchiolitis obliterans can be life threatening if untreated, but typically resolves with systemic corticosteroid therapy [116]. It is recommended that patients with this form of bronchiolitis obliterans be treated with 40 to 60 mg of prednisone daily for at least 2 months, with the dose tapered after all symptoms and radiographic findings resolve. The second form of bronchiolitis obliterans occurs in patients who have persistent cough and dyspnea with an obstructive ventilatory impairment on pulmonary function tests that does not respond to inhaled corticosteroids or bronchodilators [116]. Chest radiographs may appear normal, but high-resolution CT scans of the chest often show areas of hyperinflation and air trapping. Lung biopsy may be necessary to make a definitive diagnosis and typically shows a pure constrictive bronchiolitis. This form of bronchiolitis obliterans is usually not responsive to corticosteroid therapy, and the prognosis for improvement is poor. Patients affected with this form of bronchiolitis obliterans may get progressively worse and suffer life-long disability. The administration of prophylactic corticosteroids to prevent bronchiolitis obliterans following inhalation injury is controversial with treatment effects in either direction [120,121].

References

1. Bronstein AC, Spyker DA, Cantilena LR Jr, et al: 2006 Annual Report of the American Association of Poison Control Centers' National Poison Data System (NPDS). *Clin Toxicol (Phila)* 45:815–917, 2007.
2. Worker Health Chartbook, Chapter 2, Poisonings, National Institute for Occupational Safety and Health, 2004. Available at: www.cdc.gov/niosh/docs/2004–146/ch2/ch2–9.asp.htm.
3. Pruitt BA Jr, Cioffi WG: Diagnosis and treatment of smoke inhalation. *J Intensive Care Med* 10:117–27, 1995.
4. Stefanidou M, Athanaselis S, Spiliopoulou C: Health impacts of fire smoke inhalation. *Inhal Toxicol* 20:761–766, 2008.
5. Baxter PJ, Kapila M, Mfonfu D: Lake Nyos disaster, Cameroon, 1986: the medical effects of large scale emission of carbon dioxide? *BMJ* 298(6685):1437, 1989.
6. Nelson L: Carbon dioxide poisoning. *Emerg Med* 32:36, 2000.
7. DeBehnke DJ: The hemodynamic and arterial blood gas response to asphyxiation: a canine model of pulseless electrical activity. *Resuscitation* 30:169, 1995.
8. Centers for Disease Control and Prevention: Nonfatal, unintentional, non-fire related carbon monoxide exposures—United States. 2004–2006. *MMWR Morb Mortal Wkly Rep* 57:896–899, 2008.
9. Centers for Disease Control and Prevention: Carbon monoxide exposures from hurricane-associated use of portable generators—Florida. *MMWR Morb Mortal Wkly Rep* 54:697–700, 2005.
10. Weaver LK: Clinical practice, carbon monoxide poisoning. *N Engl J Med.* 360:1217–1225, 2009.
11. Zawacki BE, Azen SP, Imbus SH, et al: Multifactorial probit analysis of mortality in burned patients. *Ann Surg* 189:1, 1979.
12. Henry CR, Satran D, Lindgren B, et al: Myocardial injury and long term mortality following moderate to severe carbon monoxide poisoning. *JAMA* 295:398, 2006.
13. Jaffe FA: Pathogenicity of carbon monoxide. *Am J Forensic Med Path* 18:406, 1997.
14. Douglas CG, Haldane JS, Haldane JBS: The laws of combination of hemoglobin with carbon monoxide and oxygen. *J Physiol* 44:275, 1912.
15. Zhang J, Piantadosi CA: Mitochondrial oxidative stress after carbon monoxide hypoxia in the rat brain. *J Clin Invest* 90:1193, 1992.
16. Thom SR: Leukocytes in carbon monoxide-mediated brain oxidative injury. *Tox Appl Pharmacol* 123:234, 1993.
17. Thom SR, Bhopale VM, Fisher D, et al: Delayed neuropathy after carbon monoxide poisoning is immune-mediated. *Proc Natl Acad Sci USA* 101:13660, 2004.
18. Weaver LK, Valentine KJ, Hopkins RO: Carbon monoxide poisoning: risk factors for cognitive sequelae and the role of hyperbaric oxygen. *Am J Respir Crit Care Med* 176:491–497, 2007.
19. Satron D, Henry CR, Adkinson C, et al: Cardiovascular manifestations of moderate to severe carbon monoxide poisoning. *J Am Coll Cardiol* 45:1513, 2005.
20. Kao HK, Lien TC, Kou YR, et al: Assessment of myocardial injury in the emergency department independently predicts the short-term poor outcome in patients with severe carbon monoxide poisoning receiving mechanical ventilation and hyperbaric oxygen therapy. *Pulm Pharmacol Ther* 22:473–477, 2009.
21. Wolff E: Carbon monoxide poisoning with severe myonecrosis and acute renal failure. *Am J Emerg Med* 12:347, 1994.
22. Kao LW, Nangas KA: Carbon monoxide poisoning. *Am Med Clin North Am* 22:985, 2004.
23. Hill EP, Hill JR, Power GG, et al: Carbon monoxide exchanges between the human fetus and mother: a mathematical model. *Am J Physiol* 232:H311, 1977.
24. Koren G, Sharav T, Pastuszak A, et al: A multicenter, prospective study of fetal outcome following accidental carbon monoxide poisoning in pregnancy. *Reprod Toxicol* 5:397, 1991.
25. Yildiz H, Aldemir E, Altuncu E, et al: A rare cause of perinatal asphyxia: maternal carbon monoxide poisoning. *Arch Gynecol Obstet* 281:251–254, 2010.
26. Thom SR, Taber RL, Mendiguren II, et al: Delayed neuropsychiatric sequelae after carbon monoxide poisoning: prevention by treatment with hyperbaric oxygen. *Ann Emerg Med* 25:474, 1995.
27. Suner S, Partridge R, Sucov A, et al: Non-invasive pulse co-oximetry screening in the emergency department identifies occult carbon monoxide toxicity. *J Emerg Med* 34:441–450, 2008.
28. Touger M, Birnbaum A, Wang J, et al: Performance of the RAD-57 pulse CO-oximeter compared with standard laboratory carboxyhemoglobin measurement. *Ann Emerg Med* 56(4):382–388, 2010.
29. Ben-Eli D, Peruggia J, McFarland J, et al: Detecting CO, Fire Department of New York (FDNY) studies prehospital assessment of COHb. *JEMS* 32:S36–S37, 2007.
30. DeBias DA, Banerjee CM, Birkhead WC, et al: Effects of carbon monoxide inhalation on ventricular fibrillation. *Arch Environ Health* 31:42, 1976.
31. Pace N, Stajman E, Walker EL: Acceleration of carbon monoxide elimination in man by high pressure oxygen. *Science* 111:652, 1950.
32. Thom SR: Functional inhibition of leukocyte B2 integrins in carbon monoxide-medicated brain injury in rats. *Toxicol Appl Pharmacol* 123:248, 1993.
33. Juurlink D, Buckley N, Stanbrook M, et al: Hyperbaric oxygen for carbon monoxide poisoning. *Cochrane Database Syst Rev* CD002041, 2005.
34. Weaver LK, Hopkins RO, Chen KJ, et al: Hyperbaric oxygen for acute carbon monoxide poisoning. *N Engl J Med* 347:1057, 2002.
35. Scheinkestal CD, Bailey M, Myles PS, et al: Hyperbaric or normobaric oxygen for acute carbon monoxide poisoning: a randomized controlled clinical trial. *Med J Aust* 170:203, 1999.
36. Piantodosi CA: Carbon monoxide poisoning. *N Engl J Med* 347:1054, 2002.
37. Isbister GK, McGettigan P, Harris I: Hyperbaric oxygen for acute carbon monoxide poisoning. *N Engl J Med* 348:557, 2003.
38. Takeuchi A, Vesely A, Rucker J, et al: A simple "new" method to accelerate clearance of carbon monoxide. *Am Rev Respir Crit Care Med* 161:1816, 2000.
39. Baud FJ, Barriot P, Toffis V, et al: Elevated blood cyanide concentrations in victims of smoke inhalation. *N Engl J Med* 325:1801, 1991.
40. Wetherell HR: The occurrence of cyanide in the blood of fire victims. *J Forensic Sci* 11:167, 1996.
41. Eckstein M, Maniscalco P: Focus on smoke inhalation—the most common cause of acute cyanide poisoning. *Prehosp Disaster Med* 21:49–55, 2006.

42. Baskin SI, Brewer TG: Cyanide poisoning, in Zajtchuk R, Bellamy RF (eds): *Medical Aspects of Chemical and Biological Warfare. Textbook of Military Medicine, Part I. Warfare, Weaponry and the Casualty*. Washington DC, United States Department of the Army, Office of the Surgeon General and Borden Institute, 1997, p 271.
43. Lazarus AA, Devereaux A: Potential agents of chemical warfare: worst case scenario and decontamination methods. *Postgrad Med* 112:133, 2002.
44. Johnson RP, Mellors JW: Arteriolarization of venous blood gasses: a clue to the diagnosis of cyanide poisoning. *J Emerg Med* 6:401, 1988.
45. Barillo DJ: Diagnosis and treatment of cyanide toxicity. *Burn Care Res* 30:148–152, 2009.
46. Fortin JL, Giocanti JP, Ruttimann M, et al: Prehospital administration of hydroxocobalamin for smoke inhalation-associated cyanide poisoning: 8 years of experience in the Paris Fire Brigade. *Clin Toxicol* 44:37–44, 2006.
47. Borron SW, Baud FJ, Imbert M, et al: Prospective study of hydroxocobalamin for acute cyanide poisoning in smoke inhalation. *Ann Emerg Med* 49:794–801, 2007.
48. Hall AH, Dart R, Bogdan G: Sodium thiosulfate or hydroxocobalamin for the empiric treatment of cyanide poisoning. *Ann Emerg Med* 49:806–813, 2007.
49. Beckerman N, Leikin SM, Aitchinson R, et al: Laboratory interferences with the newer cyanide antidote: hydroxocobalamin. *Semin Diagn Pathol* 26:49–52, 2009.
50. Lee J, Mukal D, Kreuter K, et al: Potential interference of hydroxocobalamin on cooximetry hemoglobin measurements during cyanide and smoke inhalation treatments. *Ann Emerg Med* 49:802–805, 2007.
51. Lavon O, Bentur Y: Does amyl nitrite have a role in the management of prehospital mass casualty cyanide poisoning? *Clin Toxicol (Phila)* 48(6):477–484, 2010.
52. Ballerino-Regan D, Longmire AW: Hydrogen sulfide exposure as a cause of sudden occupational death. *Arch Pathol Lab Med* 134:1105, 2010.
53. Poli D, Solarino B, Di Vella G, et al: Occupational asphyxiation by unknown compound(s): environmental and toxicological approach. *Forensic Sci Int* 197:19–26, 2010.
54. Yalamanchili C, Smith MD: Acute hydrogen sulfide toxicity due to sewer gas exposure. *Am J Emerg Med* 26:518, 2008.
55. Byungkuk N, Hyokyung K, Younghee C, et al: Neurological sequelae of hydrogen sulfide poisoning. *Ind Health* 42:83, 2004.
56. Amino M, Yoshioka K, Suzuki Y, et al: Improvement in a patient suffering from cardiac injury due to severe hydrogen sulfide poisoning: a long-term examination of the process of recovery of heart failure by performing nuclear medicine study. *Intern Med* 48:1745–1748, 2009.
57. Lee EC, Kwan J, Leem JH, et al: Hydrogen sulfide intoxication with dilated cardiomyopathy. *J Occup Health* 51:522–525, 2009.
58. Ago M, Ago K, Ogata M: Two fatalities by hydrogen sulfide poisoning: variation of pathological and toxicological findings. *Leg Med (Tokyo)* 10:148–152, 2008.
59. Ravizza AG, Carugo D, Cerchiari EC: The treatment of hydrogen sulfide intoxication, oxygen vs. nitrites. *Vet Hum Toxicol* 24:241, 1982.
60. Stine RJ, Slosberg B, Beacham BE: Hydrogen sulfide intoxication. A case report and discussion of treatment. *Ann Intern Med* 85:756–758, 1976.
61. Gunn B, Wong R: Noxious gas exposure in the outback: two cases of hydrogen sulfide toxicity. *Emerg Med (Fremantle)* 13:240–246, 2001.
62. Buie SE, Pratt DS, May JJ: Diffuse pulmonary injury following paint remover exposure. *Am J Med* 81:702, 1986.
63. Rahman MH, Bråtveit M, Moen BE: Exposure to ammonia and acute respiratory effects in a urea fertilizer factory. *Int J Occup Environ Health* 13:153–159, 2007.
64. Fedoruk MJ, Bronstein R, Kerger BD: Ammonia exposure and hazard assessment for selected household cleaning product uses. *J Expo Anal Environ Epidemiol* 15:534–544, 2005.
65. Bloom GR, Suhail F, Hopkins-Price P, et al: Acute anhydrous ammonia injury from accidents during illicit methamphetamine productions. *Burns* 34:713–738, 2008.
66. Leduc D, Gris P, Lheureux P, et al: Acute and long-term respiratory damage following inhalation of ammonia. *Thorax* 47:755, 1992.
67. Tonelli AR, Pham A: Bronchiectasis, a long-term sequela of ammonia inhalation: a case report and review of the literature. *Burns* 35:451–453, 2009.
68. Becker M, Forrester M: Pattern of chlorine gas exposures reported to Texas poison control centers, 2000 through 2005. *Tex Med* 104:52–57, 2008.
69. LoVecchio F, Blackwell S, Stevens D: Outcomes of chlorine exposure: a 5-year poison center experience in 598 patients. *Eur J Emerg Med* 12:109, 2005.
70. Babu RV, Cardenas V, Sharma G: Acute respiratory distress syndrome from chlorine inhalation during a swimming pool accident: a case report and review of the literature. *J Intensive Care Med* 23:275–280, 2008.
71. Schwartz DA, Smith DD, Lakshminarayan S: The pulmonary sequelae associated with accidental inhalation of chlorine gas. *Chest* 97:820, 1990.
72. Pariman T, Kanne JP, Pierson DJ: Acute inhalational injury with evidence of diffuse bronchiolitis following chlorine gas exposure. *Respir Care* 49:291, 2004.
73. Antonini JM, Lewis AB, Roberts JR, et al: Pulmonary effects of welding fumes: review of worker and experimental animal studies. *Am J Ind Med* 43:350–360, 2003.
74. Sciuto AM, Hurt HH: Therapeutic treatments of phosgene-induced lung injury. *Inhal Toxicol* 16:565–580, 2004.
75. Douglas WM, Hyzser NG, Colley TV: Silo-filler's disease. *Mayo Clin Proc* 64:291, 1989.
76. Schlesinger RB: Nitrogen oxides, in Rom WM, Markowitz SB (eds): *Environmental and Occupational Medicine*. 4th ed. Philadelphia, Lippincott Williams and Wilkins, 2007, pp 1466–1479.
77. Frampton MW, Utell MJ: Sulfur dioxide, in Rom WM, Markowitz SB (eds): *Environmental and Occupational Medicine*. 4th ed. Philadelphia, Lippincott Williams and Wilkins, 2007, pp 1480–1486.
78. Charan NB, Myers CG, Lakshminarayan S, et al: Pulmonary injuries associated with acute sulfur dioxide inhalation. *Am Rev Respir Dis* 119:555, 1979.
79. Haponik EF, Crapo RO, Herndon DN, et al: Smoke inhalation. *Am Rev Respir Dis* 138:1060, 1988.
80. Thompson PB, Herndon DN, Traper DL, et al: Effect on mortality of inhalation injury. *J Trauma* 26:163, 1986.
81. Saffle JR, Davis B, Williams P, et al: Recent outcomes in the treatment of burn injury in the United States: a report from the American Burn Association Patient Registry. *J Burn Care Rehabil* 16:219, 1995.
82. Levin BC, Paabo M, Fultz ML, et al: Generation of hydrogen cyanide from flexible polyurethane foam decomposed under different combustion conditions. *Fire Mater* 9:125, 1985.
83. Zikria BA, Ferrer JM, Floch HF: The chemical factors contributing to pulmonary damage in smoke poisoning. *Surgery* 71:704, 1972.
84. Treitman RO, Burgess WA, Gold A: Air contaminants encountered by fire fighters. *Am Ind Hyg Assoc J* 41:796, 1980.
85. Haponik EF, Summer WR: Respiratory complications in burned patients: pathogenesis and spectrum of injury. *J Crit Care* 2:49, 1987.
86. Haponik EF, Munster AM, Wise RA, et al: Upper airway function in burn patients: correlation of flow volume curves and nasopharyngoscopy. *Am Rev Respir Dis* 129:251, 1984.
87. Shirini KZ, Moylan JA, Pritt BA: Diagnosis and treatment of inhalation injury in burn patients, in Loke J (ed): *Pathophysiology and Treatment of Inhalation Injury*. New York, Marcel Dekker, 1988, p 239.
88. Silverman SH, Purdue GF, Hunt JL, et al: Cyanide toxicity in burned patients. *J Trauma* 28:171–176, 1988.
89. Cochran A: Inhalation injury and endotracheal intubation. *J Burn Care Res* 30:190–191, 2009.
90. Agee RN, Long JM, Hunt JL, et al: Use of Xenon133 in early diagnosis of inhalation injury. *J Trauma* 16:218, 1976.
91. Hsu HH, Tzao C, Chang WC, et al: Zinc chloride (smoke bomb) inhalation lung injury: clinical presentations, high-resolution CT findings, and pulmonary function test results. *Chest* 127:2064–2071, 2007.
92. Masaki Y, Sugiyama K, Tanaka H, et al: Effectiveness of CT for clinical stratification of occupational lung edema. *Ind Health* 45:78–84, 2007.
93. Sherman CB, Barnhart S, Miller MF, et al: Firefighting acutely increases airway responsiveness. *Am Rev Respir Dis* 140:185–190, 1989.
94. Chia KS, Jeyaratnam J, Chan TB, et al: Airway responsiveness of firefighters after smoke exposure. *Br J Ind Med* 47:524–527, 1990.
95. Kinsella J, Carter R, Reid W, et al: Increased airways reactivity after smoke inhalation. *Lancet* 337:595–597, 1991.
96. Banauch GI, Alleyne D, Sanchez R, et al: Persistent bronchial hyperreactivity in New York City firefighters and rescue workers following collapse of World Trade Center. *Am J Respir Crit Care Med* 168:54, 2003.
97. Mlcak RP, Suman OE, Herndon DN: Respiratory management of inhalation injury. *Burns* 33:2–13, 2007.
98. Gunnarsson M, Walther SM, Seidel T, et al: Effects of inhalation of corticosteroids immediately after experimental chlorine gas lung injury. *J Trauma* 48:101, 2004.
99. Wang J, Winskog E, Walther SM: Inhaled and intravenous corticosteroids both attenuate chlorine gas-induced lung injury in pigs. *Acta Anesthesiol Scan* 49:183, 2005.
100. Peck MD, Harrington D, Mlcak RP, et al: Potential studies of mode of ventilation in inhalation injury. *J Burn Care Res* 30:181–183, 2009.
101. Dries DJ: Key questions in ventilator management of the burn-injured patient (first of two parts). *J Burn Care Res* 30:128–138, 2009.
102. Dries DJ: Key questions in ventilator management of the burn-injured patient (second of two parts). *J Burn Care Res* 30:211–220, 2009.
103. Greenhalgh DG: Steroids in the treatment of smoke inhalation injury. *J Burn Care Res* 30:165–169, 2009.
104. Smith DD: Acute inhalation injury. *Clin Pulm Med* 6:224, 1999.
105. Sterner JB, Zanders TB, Morrise MJ, et al: Inflammatory mediators in smoke inhalation injury. *Inflamm Allergy Drug Targets* 8:63–69, 2009.
106. Toon MH, Maybauer MO, Greenwood JE, et al: Management of acute smoke inhalation injury. *Crit Care Resusc* 12:53–61, 2010.
107. Miller AC, Rivero A, Ziad S, et al: Influence of nebulized unfractionated heparin and N-acetylcysteine in acute lung injury after smoke inhalation injury. *J Burn Care Res* 30:249–256, 2009.
108. Desai MH, Mlcak R, Richardsson J, et al: Reduction in mortality in pediatric patients with inhalation injury with aerosolized heparin/N-acetylcysteine. *Burn Care Rehab* 19:210–212, 1998.

109. Edelman DA, Khan N, Kempf K, et al: Pneumonia after inhalation injury. *J Burn Care Res* 28:241–246, 2007.
110. Friedman S, Cone J, Eros-Sarnyai M, et al: Clinical guidelines for adults exposed to the World Trade Center Disaster. *City Health Information* 25:47, 2006.
111. Prezant DJ, Weiden M, Banauch GI, et al: Cough and bronchial responsiveness in firefighters at the World Trade Center site. *N Engl J Med* 347:806, 2002.
112. Brooks SM, Weiss MA, Bernstein IL: Reactive airways dysfunction syndrome. *Chest* 88:376, 1985.
113. Banauch GI, Izbicki G, Christodoulou V, et al: Trial of prophylactic inhaled steroids to prevent or reduce pulmonary function decline, pulmonary symptoms and airway hyperreactivity in firefighters at the World Trade Center Site. *Disaster Med Public Health Prep* 2:33–39, 2008.
114. Aldrich TK, Gustave J, Hall CB, et al: Long-term follow up of lung function in FDNY firefighters and EMS workers exposed to World Trade Center dust. *N Engl J Med* 362:1263–1272, 2010.
115. Weiden MD, Ferrier N, Nolan A, et al: Obstructive airways disease with air-trapping among firefighters exposed to World Trade Center dust. *Chest* 137:566–574, 2010.
116. Poletti V, Chilosi M, Zompatori M: Bronchiolitis, in Gibson JG, Geddes DM, Costabel U, et al (eds): *Respiratory Medicine*. 3rd ed. Edinburgh, Saunders, Elsevier Science Ltd, 2003, p 1526.
117. Pirjavec A, Kovic I, Lulic I, et al: Massive anhydrous injury leading to lung transplantation. *J Trauma* 67:E93–E97, 2009.
118. Beheshti J, Mark EJ, Akbaei HM, et al: Mustard lung secrets: long-term clinicopathological study following mustard gas exposure. *Pathol Res Pract* 202:739–744, 2006.
119. Ainslie G: Inhalational injuries produced by smoke and nitrogen dioxide. *Respir Med* 87:169, 1993.
120. Moylan JA: Supportive therapy in burn care smoke inhalation: diagnostic technique and steroids. *J Trauma* 19:917, 1979.
121. Moulick ND, Banavalli S, Abhyanker AD, et al: Acute accidental exposure to chlorine fumes: a study of 82 cases. *Indian J Chest Dis Allied Sci* 34:85, 1992.

CHAPTER 65 ■ DISORDERS OF TEMPERATURE CONTROL PART I: HYPOTHERMIA

M. KATHRYN STEINER, FREDERICK J. CURLEY AND RICHARD S. IRWIN

This chapter reviews the normal physiology of temperature regulation and the major hypothermic syndromes. Iatrogenic and intentional hypothermia are also reviewed. Three hyperthermic syndromes—heat stroke, malignant hyperthermia, and neuroleptic malignant syndrome—are reviewed in Chapter 66.

NORMAL PHYSIOLOGY OF TEMPERATURE REGULATION

The equilibrium between heat production and heat loss determines body temperature. In healthy, resting individuals, this equilibrium is tightly regulated, producing an average oral temperature of 36.60°C ± 0.38°C [1]. Table 65.1 is a conversion chart of temperatures in Celsius to Fahrenheit. Small shifts of this temperature set point occur, with a normal diurnal variation producing a peak temperature usually near 6:00 PM. Minute-to-minute changes in body temperature are quickly sensed, and appropriate changes are made in body heat production and loss to restore a normal balance.

Heat Production

In a neutral environment (28°C for humans), humans generate all net body heat from the energy released in the dissociation of high-energy bonds during the metabolism of dietary fats, proteins, and carbohydrates. At rest, the trunk and viscera supply 56% of the body heat, but during exercise up to 90% may be generated by the muscles. Although shivering or an increase in muscle tone may produce a fourfold rise in net heat production [2], vigorous exercise may cause a sixfold increase.

Heat Loss

Under usual environmental conditions, heat exchange with the environment takes the form of heat loss. Heat may be exchanged by radiation, conduction, convection, or evaporation [3–6]. Radiation exchange—the transfer of thermal energy between objects with no direct contact—accounts for 50% to 70% of heat lost by humans at rest in a neutral environment. Conduction involves the direct exchange of heat with objects in direct contact with the body. Large quantities of heat may be rapidly exchanged when the body is submerged in water; this is due to the much greater thermal conductivity of water as compared with air. Convection involves the exchange of heat with the warmer or cooler molecules of air that pass by the skin. Heat exchange by this mechanism increases rapidly with greater temperature differences between the skin and the air and with rapid airflow. Evaporative heat loss in humans occurs primarily through perspiration. Evaporation of sweat from the skin requires that energy be supplied by the skin, resulting in a net loss of heat from the body of 0.6 kcal per g of sweat absorbed. Unlike the other methods of heat exchange, evaporation can exchange heat loss even when a warmer environment surrounds the skin. Therefore, evaporation is the major means by which the body prevents hyperthermia in a warm environment.

Temperature Control Systems

The anatomy and regulation of the system that controls body temperature have been reviewed in depth by several

TABLE 65.1

FAHRENHEIT TO CELSIUS TEMPERATURE CONVERSIONS

°C	°F	°C	°F
45	113.0	32	89.6
44	111.2	31	87.8
43	109.4	30	86.0
42	107.6	29	84.2
41	105.8	28	82.4
40	104.0	27	80.6
39	102.2	26	78.8
38	100.4	25	77.0
37	98.6	24	75.2
36	96.8	23	73.4
35	95.0	22	71.6
34	93.2	21	69.8
33	91.4	20	68.0

investigators [2–6], as outlined in the previous edition and are only briefly described here. Neurons that are directly responsive to temperature ascend from the skin, the deep viscera, and the spinal cord through the lateral spinothalamic tract to the preoptic anterior hypothalamus. When the hypothalamus perceives a temperature increase, it modulates autonomic tone to produce (a) an increase in evaporative heat loss through increased sweat output by the body's 2.5 million sweat glands, (b) cutaneous vasodilation that allows direct flow of heat to the skin to increase convective and conductive heat losses, and (c) decreased muscle tone and activity to prevent any unnecessary heat production. When the hypothalamus perceives a temperature decrease, it modulates autonomic tone to cause (a) sweat production to cease or decrease, (b) cutaneous vasculature to constrict, and (c) muscle tone to increase involuntarily and shivering to begin.

The monoamines, baroreceptor data, hypothalamic calcium and sodium concentrations, and inflammatory cytokines (interleukin-1, interleukin-6, tumor necrosis factor-α [TNF-α]) are believed to be modulators of the anterior hypothalamic thermostat. They produce effects slowly and they have little to do with the regulation of acute temperature changes.

Voluntary responses play an important role in thermoregulation. Humans may respond to thermal stress by (a) adding or removing clothes (affecting evaporative, conductive, and radiant heat exchange), (b) moving to a warmer or cooler climate, (c) changing the level of activity, and (d) changing posture. Impairment of voluntary control places an unnecessary stress on autonomic control mechanisms and thereby predisposes to an imbalance in heat exchange and a change in body temperature.

The ability to regulate temperature effectively declines with age [7,8], probably as a result of deterioration in sensory afferents. Although younger individuals usually notice temperature changes as low as 0.8°C, older persons may not notice changes of up to 2.3°C. Moreover, because the sweat threshold increases and sweat volume decreases with age, an older individual may be more susceptible to hyperthermia than a younger person [9]. Old age may also be a liability for hypothermia because of (a) a lower basal metabolic rate, (b) a higher heat conductance due to a decline in body mass, (c) a decrease in the heat generated by shivering due to a smaller muscle mass, and (d) an inability to vasoconstrict cutaneous vessels in response to cold. In the elderly, restricted mobility or deterioration in cortical function can lead to a greater impact on the voluntary responses to temperature changes compared with the young.

UNINTENTIONAL HYPOTHERMIA

Hypothermia, defined as a core temperature less than 35°C, may occur at all ambient temperatures and in patients of all ages but more commonly in the elderly. Hypothermia often occurs within 24 hours of admission in more than 3% of intensive care unit admissions [10]. Hypothermia is a diagnosis that is frequently missed and underreported. When all data are reviewed, the overall mortality from hypothermia in the United States has been conservatively estimated at 30 deaths per 1 million population per year [11]. The mortality for treated hypothermia ranges from 12% [12] to 73% [13].

Causes and Pathogenesis

The most frequent causes of hypothermia appear to be exposure, use of depressant drugs, and hypoglycemia. Understanding the causes of hypothermia (Table 65.2) and their pathogenesis enables one to develop a rational approach to treatment.

Exposure to Cold

Wet, wind, and exhaustion contribute to increased loss of body heat. Wet clothing loses 90% of its insulating value [14], rendering soaked individuals effectively nude. Exposure to rain or snow contributed greatly to the development of hypothermia in 15 of 23 incidents in hikers discussed in one review [14]. Convective heat loss because of wind may increase to more than five times baseline values, increasing with wind velocity [15]. Hikers with poor selection of clothing, campers who fail to seek appropriate shelter, or skiing in unfavorable weather can result in fatal hypothermia [15]. Victims of hypothermia display inappropriate behavior that worsens hypothermia. Up to 25% may remove their clothing and burrow, hiding under a bed or on a shelf [16]. Many quickly experience loss of coordination and then stupor or collapse. Death may occur within an hour of the onset of symptoms [15]. Immersion in water at a temperature colder than 24°C leads to extremely rapid heat loss. Core temperature drops at a rate proportional to the temperature of the water [17]. Although survival times of 1 to 2 hours have been reported for individuals immersed in water at 0°C to 10°C, death may occur within minutes.

Drugs

Alcohol, phenothiazines, barbiturates, and paralytic agents frequently produce hypothermia by depressing sensory afferents, the hypothalamus, and effector responses. Alcohol impairs the perception of cold, clouds the sensorium, and acts as a direct vasodilator [18,19]. Alcoholics are also thought to be more susceptible to exposure because of a state of relative starvation, increased conductive losses from decreased subcutaneous

TABLE 65.2

CAUSES OF UNINTENTIONAL HYPOTHERMIA

Normal aging
Exposure to cold
Drugs (e.g., alcohol)
Endocrine dysfunction (e.g., hypoglycemia)
Central nervous system disorders
Spinal cord transection
Skin disorders
Debility
Trauma

fat, and high levels of blood alcohol that potentially impair the metabolic response to hypothermia by decreasing blood sugar and increasing acidosis. Most sedative–hypnotic drugs, such as barbiturates and phenothiazines, cause hypothermia by inhibiting shivering and impairing voluntary control. Phenothiazines increase the threshold necessary to produce shivering and lead to hypothalamic depression [10,20]; barbiturates decrease effective shivering [21]. Paralytic agents used to suppress ventilation prevent shivering and eliminate all voluntary control mechanisms [22,23]. Unexplained hypothermia has resulted from the administration of common antibiotics, such as penicillin [24] and erythromycin [25]. Bromocriptine may cause hypothermia by altering central dopaminergic tone [26].

Endocrine Dysfunction

Diabetic ketoacidosis, hyperosmolar coma, and hypoglycemia are frequently reported causes of hypothermia [18]. In one survey, 20% of patients with blood glucose levels less than 60 mg per dL had temperatures of less than 35°C. Hypoglycemia lowers cerebral intracellular glucose concentrations and impairs hypothalamic function [27]. In acute hypoglycemia (e.g., insulin administration), hypothermia occurs due to peripheral vasodilation and sweating. At glucose concentrations less than 2.5 mmol per L, subjects fail to perceive cold environments and fail to shiver [28]. This impairment appears transient because normal regulatory mechanisms and euthermia may be restored when normal serum glucose levels are restored.

The prevalence of hypothyroidism in patients ranges from 0% to 10%. Several patients with mild hypothyroidism have been safely rewarmed to euthermia without administration of exogenous thyroid hormone. In contrast, myxedema coma, a rare presentation of hypothyroidism, is associated with subnormal temperatures in 82% of cases [29]. It has a high mortality if not treated with exogenous thyroxine. Myxedema coma occurs most frequently in middle-aged to older women, and more than 90% of cases occur in winter [29]. Severe hypothermia with temperatures less than 30°C occurs in 15% of patients [29]. Coma arises because of a cerebral thyroxine deficiency. Hypothermia then results from a combination of loss of voluntary control mechanisms, from stupor or coma, decreased calorigenesis from thyroid deficiency, and decreased shivering, presumably from impaired hypothalamic regulation [29,30].

Panhypopituitarism and adrenal insufficiency are also rare causes of hypothermia. Unless profound insufficiency exists, these conditions rarely produce significant hypothermia in the absence of some other insult to the thermoregulatory system.

Central Nervous System Disorders

Diseases such as stroke, primary and metastatic brain tumors, luetic gliosis, and sarcoidosis may produce hypothermia by direct anatomic impingement on the hypothalamus [31,32]. Metabolic derangements from carbon monoxide poisoning or thiamine deficiency (Wernicke–Korsakoff syndrome) can also produce hypothermia, by affecting the hypothalamus [33–38]. Patients with anorexia nervosa have been shown to have multiple hypothalamic abnormalities resulting in the lack of shivering and vasoconstriction and a rapid drop in core temperature when they are exposed to cold [39]. Agenesis or lipoma of the corpus callosum has been reported to cause spontaneous periodic hypothermia by an unclear mechanism [21,40]. Several patients with multiple sclerosis have experienced transient hypothermia with flares of their neuropathy, suggesting the presence of hypothalamic plaques [41]. Drugs that are active on the central nervous system, such as neuroleptics or guanabenz, have resulted in hypothermia [42].

Spinal Cord Transection

Loss of skin and core temperature afferents, reduced body muscle mass, inability to shiver effectively, and, if mobility is compromised, inability to alter the environment make patients with spinal cord injury susceptible to thermal stress and hypothermia exposed to low ambient temperatures [43–45].

Skin Disorders

Skin disorders characterized by vasodilatation or increased transepithelial water loss may lead to hypothermia. Inappropriate conductive and convective heat losses in psoriasis, ichthyosis, and erythroderma have been shown to be associated with increased evaporative losses of up to 3 L per day; this computes to a potential loss of more than 1,700 kcal of heat per day [46,47]. Patients with extensive third-degree burns have been reported to have an even larger evaporative heat loss, losing up to 6 L fluid, or more than 3,400 kcal per day. When an additional cause of hypothermia is present, these patients may be in danger of severe drops in temperature. Heat loss and caloric requirements can be decreased dramatically by covering the skin with impermeable membranes to decrease evaporative losses [48–50].

Debility

Case reports suggest that hypothermia may occur in patients with debilitating illnesses such as Hodgkin's disease [51]; systemic lupus erythematosus [52,53]; and severe cardiac, renal, hepatic, or septic failure. In Israel, 29% of hypothermic elderly individuals had preexistent renal failure [54]. The exact causes are unclear, but many mechanisms are likely acting in concert to produce a drop in temperature. A decrease in cardiac index from 2.8 to 1.4 L per minute results in a drop in temperature from 37°C to 35°C [55]. Temperature promptly rises when cardiac index increases. Hypothermia in hepatic failure might result from intermittent hypoglycemia. Most debilitated patients are also compromised by some degree of immobility or decreased voluntary control.

Trauma

Trauma patients often are hypothermic [56,57], due to multiple insults to the thermoregulatory system, for example, loss of voluntary control in adverse environments, the presence of alcohol in up to 62% of cases in some series, and the rapid transfusion of unwarmed blood [57]. In patients with moderately elevated injury severity scores, during the first day of hospitalization, 42% experience hypothermia, with 13% having temperatures less than 32°C [56]. The presence of shock [56] and massive transfusion [57] significantly contributed to the development of hypothermia in these patients.

Pathophysiology

Profound metabolic alterations occur in every organ system in response to a core temperature less than 35°C. Beyond the immediate cardiovascular changes induced by vasoconstriction, metabolic changes that appear to be temperature dependent occur in two phases: shivering and nonshivering. The shivering phase, usually occurring in the range of 35°C to 30°C, is characterized by intense energy production from the breakdown of stored body fuels. In the nonshivering phase, which occurs approximately less than 30°C, the metabolism slows down dramatically, resulting at times in multiple organ failure.

Shivering involves an increase in muscle tone and rhythmic contraction of small and large muscle groups. The metabolic changes during the shivering phase parallel those seen during muscular exercise. In different patient populations with different measurement techniques, heat production has been shown to increase by four times the normal amount [58], oxygen consumption by two to five times [20], and metabolic rate by six times [59]. Central pooling of blood resulting from peripheral vasoconstriction may raise central venous pressure and slightly elevate cardiac output. Because cardiac output remains relatively close to normal and oxygen demand increases dramatically, mixed venous oxygen saturation decreases [60]. Although hepatic and muscular glycogenolysis may cause blood sugar levels to rise, this rise may not be seen in starved or exhausted patients or those with prolonged hypothermia [61,62]. The catabolism of fat increases the serum levels of glycerol, nonesterified fatty acids, and ketones. Anaerobic metabolism causes a rise in lactate levels; levels as high as 25.2 mmol per L have been reported [63]. The metabolic acidosis induced by this intense catabolism is compensated for the most part by the increased metabolism of lactate in the liver and increased minute ventilation [62]. Cortisol levels rise [13]. Most of these metabolic changes peak near 34°C or 35°C and become much less pronounced near a temperature of 30°C.

As core temperature falls toward 30°C, shivering nearly ceases and metabolism slows down dramatically. Near 30°C, metabolic rate approaches basal levels [64], and it may be half basal value by 28°C [59]. As shivering and metabolism slow down, oxygen consumption declines. At 30°C, oxygen consumption decreases to approximately 75% of basal value [64]; at 26°C to 35% to 53% [20]; and at 20°C to only 25% of basal value. This profound decrease in metabolism is reflected by changes in every organ system (Table 65.3).

Cardiovascular Function

Increasing degrees of hypothermia result in malignant arrhythmias, depressed cardiac function, and hypotension. A decrease in cardiac conductivity and automaticity [65–67] and an increase in refractory period [68,69] begin during the shivering phase and progress as core temperature decreases. The electrocardiogram (ECG) in mild hypothermia may show bradycardia with prolongation of the PR, QRS, and QT intervals. Below 30°C, first-degree block is usual, and at 20°C, third-degree block may be seen [61,70]. Below 33°C, the ECG commonly shows the characteristic J-point elevation (Fig. 65.1). As temperature drops below 25°C, the J wave increases [71,72], most prominent in the mid-precordial and lateral precordial leads [73]. J waves may persist 12 to 24 hours after restoration of normal temperature [74,75].

Atrial fibrillation is common at temperatures of 34°C to 25°C, and ventricular fibrillation frequently occurs at temperatures less than 28°C. The incidence of ventricular fibrillation increases with physical stimulation of the heart and is associated with intracardiac temperature gradients of greater than 2°C [76]. Purkinje cells show marked decreases in excitability in the range of 14°C to 15°C [67], and asystole is common when core temperatures drop below 20°C. Recovery of spontaneous electrical activity after hypothermic asystole may be related to protection from the calcium paradox afforded by hypothermia [77].

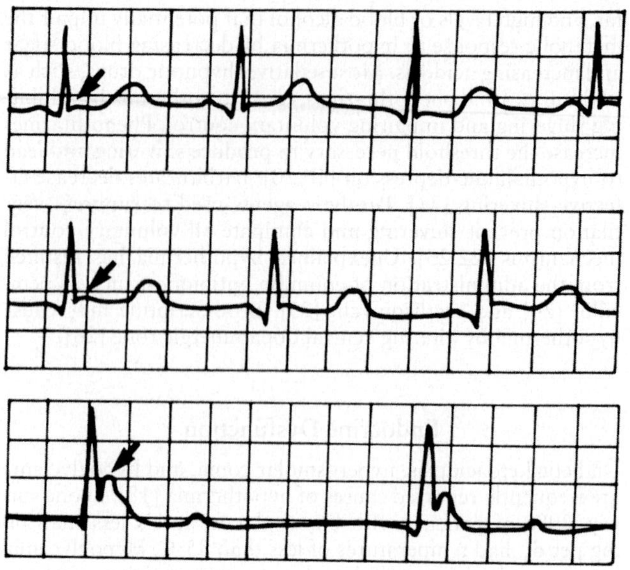

FIGURE 65.1. The electrocardiographic changes of hypothermia. As temperature decreases (*top to bottom*), the rate slows down and the PR and QT intervals become prolonged. J waves (*arrows*) appear at a temperature less than 35°C and become prominent by a temperature near 25°C. The J wave initially is seen (*top*) as a widened QRS interval with a slight ST elevation at the J point.

TABLE 65.3

COMMON EFFECTS OF HYPOTHERMIA

Metabolic depletion	Anemia, hemoconcentration
Cardiac arrhythmia	Thrombocytopenia
Hypotension	Ileus
Hypopnea	Pancreatitis
Dehydration	Hyperglycemia
Coma	Pneumonia
Granulocytopenia	Sepsis
Altered drug clearance	

Consequently, there is a gradual decrease in cardiac output. Systole may become extremely prolonged [78], greatly decreasing ejection fraction and aortic pressures. Ventricular compliance is severely reduced [79]. Output decreases to approximately 90% of normal at 30°C and may decrease rapidly at lower temperatures, with increasing bradycardia or arrhythmia. Regional blood flow is altered to preserve myocardial and cerebral perfusion [80]. Although blood pressure appears to be initially maintained by an increase in systemic vascular resistance (SVR) [81], systemic resistance decreases and hypotension is common [61] at temperatures less than 25°C. Oxygen demand usually decreases more rapidly than does cardiac output, causing mixed venous oxygen content to increase as the nonshivering phase begins.

Pulmonary Function

Pulmonary mechanics and gas exchange appear to change little with hypothermia [61,82–84]. Although the ventilatory response to an elevation in carbon dioxide tension (PCO_2) may be blunted [82], there is no clear decrease in hypoxic drive [61]. As the increased oxygen demand and acidosis of the shivering phase decline, minute ventilation decreases. Tidal volume and respiratory rate decline at lower temperatures [20]. At 25°C, respirations may be only 3 or 4 per minute [19]; at temperatures less than 24°C, respiration may cease [59]. Apnea is presumed to be secondary to failure of respiratory drive at a brainstem level.

Renal Function

As blood pressure decreases during the nonshivering phase, glomerular filtration rate (GFR) may decrease by 85% [61] and renal blood flow by 75% [20], without a significant change in urine production. Maintenance of a good urine output, despite decreases in blood pressure and GFR in hypothermia, has been termed *cold diuresis*. This results from a defect in tubular reabsorption. The urine may be extremely dilute, with an osmolarity of as low as 60 mOsm per L and a specific gravity of 1.002 [85]. The stimulus for this dilute diuresis may be the triggering of volume receptors as central volume increases with peripheral vasoconstriction [78], a relative insensitivity to antidiuretic hormone [75], or a direct suppression of antidiuretic hormone release [19]. Although kaliuresis and glycosuria may accompany the dilute diuresis, the net result for the patient is dehydration and a relatively hyperosmolar serum.

Neurologic Function

Hypothermic patients present with coma. Complete neurologic recovery has been described in hypothermic adults after 20 minutes of complete cardiac arrest [18] and after up to 3.5 hours of cardiopulmonary resuscitation (CPR) [85]. The mechanism by which hypothermia produces a seemingly protective effect is not well understood; it probably relates to a significant decrease in cerebral metabolism and a smaller injury by the no-reflow phenomenon [86], a mechanism whereby the brain is protected from injury until reperfusion.

Cerebral oxygen consumption decreases by approximately 55% for each 10°C decrease in temperature [87]. Cerebral blood flow decreases from 75% of normal at 30°C to only 20% of normal at 20°C [61]. The supply of nutrients and removal of wastes are adequate at these extremes given patient recovery and experimental evidence that the intracellular pH of brain tissue cooled to 20°C is unchanged even after 20 minutes of anoxia [88].

Visual [89,90] and auditory [91,92] evoked potentials demonstrate delayed latencies; latency increases as temperature decreases. The spectrum of electroencephalographic frequencies also changes with hypothermia. In healthy men cooled to 33°C by immersion, theta and beta activity increased by 17% and alpha activity decreased by 34% compared with control values [90]. Electromyography during hypothermia has been reported to be normal [93].

Hematologic Function

Hypothermia affects white blood cells (WBCs), red blood cells, platelets, and perhaps coagulation mechanisms. The WBC count in mild hypothermia remains normal to slightly elevated and drops severely at temperatures lower than 28°C [94,95]. The hematocrit usually rises in hypothermic patients at a temperature of 30°C in part due to hemoconcentration from dehydration caused by cold diuresis and in part due to splenic contraction [96]. The increase in blood viscosity in hypothermic patients appears to be due to decreased deformability of the red cell membrane [97]. After intravascular volume and euthermia have been restored, a mild anemia may last up to 6 weeks. Bone marrow aspirates obtained from these patients show erythroid hypoplasia and increased ringed sideroblasts, suggesting a maturation arrest [98]. Platelet counts drop as temperature decreases, and prolongation of the bleeding time has been noted at 20°C [94]; normal levels and function return on rewarming [99]. The decrease in platelet count is thought to be secondary to hepatic sequestration.

No clear evidence indicates that a coagulopathy is associated with hypothermia. Deep venous thrombosis (DVT) and disseminated intravascular coagulopathy (DIC) have been reported in hypothermic patients [34,100].

Gastrointestinal Tract Function

Ileus, pancreatitis, and hepatic dysfunction accompany hypothermia. Ileus is present at temperatures 30°C and lower. Subclinical pancreatitis appears to be common. Although patients usually lack symptoms of acute pancreatitis, more than half have amylase elevations greater than 550 Somogyi units and up to 80% of patients who die of hypothermia have evidence of pancreatitis at autopsy [101]. The relationship between alcohol use and pancreatitis in these patients is unclear. Hepatic dysfunction occurs commonly and involves synthetic and detoxification abilities [20]. Profoundly hypothermic patients in whom an acidosis develops are less able to clear lactate. Postmortem studies of patients who died from exposure-induced hypothermia have emphasized that gastric submucosal hemorrhage is common [102]. Duodenal ulceration and perforation may also be seen [103].

Endocrine Function

Hypothermia directly suppresses the release of insulin from the pancreas and increases resistance to insulin's action in the periphery [104,105]. The blood glucose level rises in early hypothermia, due to glycogenolysis and increased corticosteroid levels, and remains elevated because of a decreased concentration and the action of insulin. Elevations in blood glucose, however, are usually mild; only 9% of patients in one series had blood glucose levels higher than 200 mg per dL. Changes in thyroid and adrenal function occur, but they are less well defined. The responses to thyroid stimulating hormone (TSH) and adrenocorticotrophic hormone appear blunted [61]. In hypothyroid patients, TSH increases in response to cold [106]. Although corticosteroid levels vary a great deal among patients, they rarely appear to be severely depressed [62,107,108]. Urinary catecholamine levels are increased threefold to sevenfold on average in hypothermic deaths compared with death due to other causes [102].

Immune Function

Infection is a major cause of death in hypothermic patients. Hypoperfusion increases the risk of bacterial invasion in ischemic regions of the skin and intestine. Central nervous system depression reduces the cough reflex, leaving the patient more susceptible to aspiration pneumonia. A decrease in tidal volume and minute ventilation increases the risk of atelectasis, making subsequent infection possible. Survival in hypothermia varies directly with the severity of cold-induced granulocytopenia [95,109]. Evidence from hypothermic animals with induced sepsis indicates an impaired release of PMNs from the marrow [95], as well as delayed clearance of staphylococcal [110] and Gram-negative organisms from the blood. Ineffective clearance of organisms may permit a continued low-grade bacteremia [110]. Ineffective clearance probably relates to impaired phagocytosis, migration [111], and a decrease in the half-life of circulating PMNs in hypothermia [109]. Impaired killing of bacteria by pulmonary alveolar macrophages exposed to cold in vitro has been reported and presumably increases susceptibility to pneumonia. The role of changes in antigen–antibody interactions, known to be impaired by cold in vitro, has not been clearly defined in hypothermic patients. Wound healing is delayed in patients with mild perioperative hypothermia [112]. Cytokine production may be delayed and prolonged [113]. Few human data are available regarding the activation of inflammatory mediators in hypothermia. Interleukin-6 and TNF-α are assumed to play a role in modulating an inflammatory cascade that must occur with hypothermia. Interleukin-6 concentrations fall with rewarming [114]. Thus, the hypothermic host is more susceptible to invasion by pathogens and less equipped to defend itself if invasion occurs.

Drug Clearance

Little is known about the clearance of drugs in hypothermic adults. Complex interactions of reduced cardiac output, dehydration, slowed hepatic metabolism, decreased GFR, abnormal renal tubular filtration and reabsorption, and altered protein–drug dissociation constant alter the volume of distribution and total body clearance of many drugs [115]. The half-life of thiopental has been shown to increase 4 to 11 times at 24°C [20]. Because bile flow may be reduced by up to 75% at similar temperatures, excretion of toxins in the bile is also decreased [20].

Diagnosis

The diagnosis of hypothermia may be suggested by a history of exposure or immersion, clinical examination, and laboratory abnormalities. Elderly, alcoholic, diabetic, quadriparetic, or severely debilitated patients are at high risk of hypothermia. Signs of hypothermia vary with the patient's temperature. Cool skin, muscle rigidity, shivering, and acrocyanosis are present in most noncomatose patients. In obtunded patients, myxedema-type facies have been reported [101,116]. Although mental status changes vary widely among patients, they follow a typical pattern: between 35°C and 32°C, the patient may be stuporous or confused; between 32°C and 27°C, the patient may be verbally responsive but incoherent; and at temperatures less than 27°C, 83% of patients are comatose but able to respond purposefully to noxious stimuli [117]. Muscle tone remains increased after shivering stops. Reflexes remain normal until body temperature is lower than 27°C, when they become depressed and or absent. Plantar reflexes may be upgoing. The pupillary reflex may be sluggish below 30°C and may become fixed at temperatures less than 27°C. ECG changes are almost always present.

In the absence of an accurate temperature reading, the ECG can be used to gauge the degree of hypothermia [71,73]. J waves become prominent as temperature decreases and in the absence of a cerebrovascular accident appear to be pathognomonic for hypothermia. Prolonged PR or QT intervals in the presence of muscle tremor artifact and bradycardia strongly suggest the diagnosis. Because of the increased solubility of carbon dioxide and oxygen, blood gases reported at 37°C may show a value of partial pressure of oxygen (PO_2) + PCO_2 greater than 150 mm Hg on room air, a biochemical impossibility at euthermia. An elevated hematocrit, a good output of dilute urine with hypotension, ileus, and an elevated amylase are helpful but nonspecific indicators of hypothermia.

Because the symptoms of hypothermia frequently mimic those of other disorders, the diagnosis may be missed unless there is a clear history of exposure or an accurate temperature reading is taken. Thermometers calibrated to record temperatures less than 35°C must be used. Electronic temperature probes are accurate at low temperatures, can be used in several body sites, have a rapid response time, and can be left indwelling to provide online temperature readings during treatment. The lower temperature limit on individual probes must always be checked.

The site for recording the temperature is important (see Chapter 26). Oral or nasopharyngeal temperatures may not reflect core temperature because of the influence of surrounding airflow. Bladder, rectal, tympanic, esophageal, or great vessel temperatures are preferable. Bladder temperatures are accurate and convenient for initial measurements [118,119]. Great vessel temperature can be measured using the thermistor on a Swan-Ganz catheter. Esophageal temperature is mostly influenced by the inhalation of warmed air, great vessel temperature is highly affected by the infusion of heated fluids, and rectal temperature is greatly influenced by warmed peritoneal dialysis. During extracorporeal rewarming, bladder and pulmonary artery temperatures may increase faster than esophageal and rectal temperatures [119]. It may be helpful to monitor at least two core sites.

Differential Diagnosis

Clinical changes produced by hypothermia can mask and mimic other diseases. Rigidity of the cervical musculature may indicate meningitis. The abdomen is frequently boardlike, and absent bowel sounds simulate a state of intra-abdominal catastrophe. Because shock and coma have broad differential diagnoses, clinical judgment must guide the workup of these disorders.

Despite wide interpatient variation, deviation from the temperature–symptom relationship should suggest that the cause of a symptom may be other than hypothermia. For example, ventricular fibrillation or coma with a temperature higher than 30°C or shock with a low hematocrit or heme-positive stools should alert the physician to suspect another diagnosis and pursue further diagnostic evaluations. In a patient with hypothermia, especially after vigorous resuscitation attempts, establishing a diagnosis of myocardial infarction can be difficult. Creatine kinase, lactate dehydrogenase, and serum glutamic oxaloacetic acid transaminase values may be elevated because of hepatic hypoperfusion and presumed skeletal muscle damage. Elevations in MB and BB fractions of the creatine kinase have been reported in hypothermic patients with no evidence of myocardial or cerebral infarct [64]. The ECG changes in hypothermia do not mimic those seen in myocardial infarction. Therefore, an ECG is a more reliable indicator of myocardial damage than are enzyme elevations in hypothermic patients.

Treatment

With immediate appropriate treatment, mortality should be low. Accumulated statistics suggest that mortality varies with the severity of the underlying disease and the temperature at initial examination. The overall mortality in a series of city-dwelling hypothermic patients was 12%, but this increased to nearly 50% if a serious underlying disease was present [13]. In the same series of patients, mortality increased to 1.8% for each 1°C decrease in temperature on admission. Mortality is higher if hypothermia occurred indoors [120]. In healthy young mountain climbers, mortality was also found to vary with body core temperature on admission: Mortality was 25% for temperatures higher than 32°C versus 66% for temperatures lower than 27°C [59]. In patients in Ireland with hypothermia due to exposure, the overall mortality was 33%, and each 5°C drop in ambient temperature was estimated to double the mortality. In multivariate analysis, the strongest predictors of mortality were prehospital cardiac arrest, low or absent blood pressure, elevated blood urea nitrogen, and the need for tracheal intubation or nasogastric tube placement in the emergency department [121]. The Mount Hood tragedy suggests that serum potassium levels greater than 10 mEq per L, fibrinogen less than 50 mg per dL, and ammonia greater than 250 mmol per L at the time of diagnosis make survival unlikely [118]. Asphyxia due to submersion resulting in severe hypothermia may be associated with up to a 95% mortality rate [122]. The higher survival rates in city-dwelling patients are believed to represent the benefits of immediately accessible care. Many experts believe that without treatment, mortality in profound hypothermia may approach 100%.

Treatment should be aggressive. Functional survival in adults has been reported even after 6.5 hours of CPR [123]. Treatment includes initial field care and transport, stabilizing cardiopulmonary status, treating the cause of hypothermia, preventing the common complications of hypothermia, and rewarming.

Initial Field Care and Transport

The field management of hypothermia from exposure or immersion is important. Wet clothes should be removed and replaced with dry ones, if available. The victim should be insulated from cold and wind as much as possible with blankets or a sleeping bag. Sharing the body heat of another person in the same sleeping bag appears to offer no significant advantage [124]. Drinking hot drinks is no longer encouraged because it may increase hypothermia by producing peripheral vasodilation through a pharyngeal reflex [125]. Glucose drinks have been advocated, but recent work has shown that glycogen depletion does not impair shivering or rewarming [126].

A number of precautions should be taken to transport the victim. Patients should not be transported in the upright position because seizures may result, presumably from orthostatic hypotension [16]. Rough handling must be avoided because even minor manipulations can induce ventricular fibrillation [79,125,126]. Clothing should be cut off, and a team of many rescuers should carry the victim as gently as possible. A patient without a blood pressure or palpable pulse may already be in fibrillation and thus should be resuscitated in the usual fashion until adequate ECG and pressure monitoring are available (see Chapter 22) [127].

Stabilizing Cardiopulmonary Status

Because early death from hypothermia is due to hypotension and arrhythmia, the goal of initial in-hospital management of hypothermic patients should be to achieve a safe, stable cardiopulmonary status. Shock in mild hypothermia is usually due to the dehydration that results from cold diuresis; in more profound hypothermia, it may be cardiogenic. Fluid resuscitation should be attempted in all patients in hypothermic shock. Delivery of fluids through a central rather than a peripheral catheter is preferable for several reasons: vasoconstriction makes insertion of peripheral intravenous (IV) catheters difficult, vasoconstriction may impair delivery of peripherally injected medications, peripheral IV catheters may cause unnecessary damage to frostbitten extremities, and central catheter placement permits monitoring of central venous pressure and helps guide fluid management. Because most patients are hemoconcentrated and hyperosmolar, slightly hypotonic crystalloid fluids should be given. Whenever possible, all IV fluids should be warmed to at least room temperature before infusion. If fluid resuscitation fails, pressor agents should be administered. Although pressor agents increase the risk of ventricular fibrillation, they have been used safely in patients with hypothermia [127,128]. The use of arterial and central venous pressure monitors may help guide treatment. Swan-Ganz catheter monitoring can be performed safely and may aid in evaluation and treatment [129]. A low SVR in mild-to-moderate hypothermia strongly suggests infection or sepsis [81]. The increased risk of hemorrhage from hypothermia-induced thrombocytopenia and prolongation of bleeding times must, however, be considered when undertaking invasive procedures such as central venous catheter placement or intubation.

The management of arrhythmias must be approached in a nontraditional manner because many pharmacologic agents, pacing efforts, and defibrillation attempts do not work in the hypothermic patient [130–132]. Because supraventricular arrhythmias and heart block generally resolve spontaneously on rewarming [72,84], therapy is usually unnecessary. Digitalis should be avoided because the efficacy of the drug is unclear in hypothermia, and toxicity increases as the patient is warmed [68]. Little is known regarding the efficacy of calcium channel blockers in treating supraventricular tachyarrhythmias in hypothermic patients.

In hypothermic patients experiencing ventricular fibrillation, procainamide has been of little help [20] and lidocaine has been of only modest benefit [126]. Bretylium appears to be the drug of choice [125,133–135]. Electrical defibrillation should probably be attempted at least once, but it is unlikely to succeed until core temperature surpasses 30°C [18,76,136]. The role of pacing in patients with fibrillation and asystole is unclear [68,137]. If other avenues of support are unavailable, however, pacing should be tried [138].

Acid–base status and oxygenation should be assessed immediately. Accurate assessment of acid–base status in hypothermic patients is complicated by several issues. First, blood gases measured at 37°C produce different values of pH and PCO_2 than exist in a patient at a lower temperature. Second, normal values for pH and PCO_2 also change with temperature. Third, body buffer systems respond differently at colder temperatures. When blood is drawn from a hypothermic patient and then rewarmed to and measured at 37°C, the solubility of carbon dioxide decreases, resulting in higher PCO_2 and lower pH values than actually exist [139].

Normal values for pH and PCO_2 also change with temperature. At a temperature of 20°C, a pH of approximately 7.65 permits continued cellular function, and this value, not a pH of 7.40, should be regarded as normal. Normal values for $PaCO_2$ are altered because of the higher content of carbon dioxide in cooled blood, decreased rate of production of carbon dioxide, and slower rate of carbon dioxide elimination from relative alveolar hypoventilation. Respiratory exchange ratio values as low as 0.32 have been reported. On balance, these changes result in lower $PaCO_2$ values at colder temperatures.

Temperature changes the protein–drug dissociation constant of chemical reactions and reduces the ionization level of buffer proteins [139]. This produces a smaller effective protein buffer pool and places a greater reliance for buffering on the less efficient carbonic acid system. Because of this less effective buffering, acid–base disturbances that would be well tolerated at 37°C might be poorly tolerated at lower temperatures.

Despite these complex considerations, $PaCO_2$ and pH values that are uncorrected for temperature can be accurately used to assess the hypothermic patient's acid–base status, enhance the ease of interpretation, and morbidity or mortality does not change [140–145].

Because of a decrease in the solubility of oxygen on warming the blood to 37°C, arterial oxygen tension values reported at 37°C may be substantially higher than the actual value in colder patients. Therefore, PO_2 values must be corrected for temperature, or the presence of significant hypoxemia may be overlooked. Several nomograms to permit correction exist [140,146–148]. For clinical purposes, the following formula can be used to correct PO_2 for temperature: decrease the PO_2 measured at 37°C by 7.2% for each degree that the patient's temperature is less than 37°C.

Because acute respiratory distress syndrome may, and pneumonia [103] frequently does, accompany hypothermia, a chest radiograph should be obtained. Ninety percent to 100% oxygen should be administered until adequate oxygenation has been demonstrated. Oxygen saturation, after correction for temperature, should be maintained at greater than 90% to help prevent hypoxic damage. Stuporous or comatose patients should have prophylactic intubation to decrease the risk of aspiration pneumonia. Blind nasotracheal intubation may be required; orotracheal intubation may be difficult because the mandible may be unmovable as a result of muscle rigidity [130]. If respiratory failure is evident on blood gas analysis, the trachea should be intubated and the lungs mechanically ventilated.

Experiences during hypothermic surgery and in the treatment of unintentional hypothermia indicate that the initial ventilator settings should be similar to those normally used at temperatures of 37°C [140,141] (see Chapter 58).

Treating the Cause of Hypothermia

Diseases that are known to predispose to hypothermia should be diagnosed and treated early. Hypoglycemia is easily and rapidly detected by a glucose test strip and confirmed by blood glucose value. As a result of the ineffective action of insulin at low temperatures and the relatively high serum osmolarity from water diuresis, serious and difficult-to-treat hyperosmolarity may result from boluses of high concentrations of glucose [62,84]. Therefore, treatment with highly concentrated glucose solutions should be delayed until some measure of the blood glucose has been obtained. Once hypoglycemia has been documented, the patient should be given 25 to 50 g glucose as a 50% dextrose solution. Some patients have been reported to shiver on correction of hypoglycemia and to correct their hypothermia rapidly.

The possibility of alcohol or sedative drug use or overdose is usually indicated by history and confirmed by toxicologic screening. No reports indicate adverse effects of naloxone in hypothermia; it should routinely be given if coma is present.

A thorough neurologic examination may suggest central nervous system or peripheral nervous system disease. If the patient has a history of trauma, the neck should be stabilized until a cervical spine radiograph has been obtained. Flaccid extremities suggest a cord or peripheral nerve injury. Cerebral edema secondary to tumor may be seen on funduscopic examination. Treatment with thiamine is benign and should be given routinely in stuporous hypothermic patients until Wernicke–Korsakoff syndrome can be ruled out. Thiamine should be given with glucose if hyperglycemia is absent to decrease the chance of cerebral dysfunction. If the patient has Wernicke–Korsakoff encephalopathy, response to thiamine treatment may be seen within hours; if thiamine is not given, efforts to increase temperature may be futile [36,40]. Cyclic hypothermia is rarely fatal and responds to cyproheptadine, ephedrine, and naloxone [149,150].

Thyroid hormone should not be given routinely to every patient with hypothermia because such treatment is potentially harmful and hypothyroid coma is rare. In all cases of suspected myxedema, however, treatment with thyroid hormone is mandatory because it may be life saving. Conventional treatment of myxedema hypothermic coma begins with immediate IV administration of 0.2 to 0.5 mg thyroxine. If the patient has not clearly responded in 24 hours, this dose is repeated and the patient is maintained on 0.05 to 0.10 mg thyroxine IV daily until clinically stable (see Chapter 104).

Debilitating diseases such as congestive heart failure, sepsis, hepatic, or renal failure should be treated in a conventional manner. In diabetic patients, insulin resistance increases rapidly below 30°C; insulin administration should be delayed when possible until the patient's temperature is more than 30°C. If insulin is given during hypothermia, it must be administered intravenously because subcutaneous absorption is impaired by hypoperfusion. Also, insulin should be given in small doses, because its degradation may be delayed at low temperature and cumulative doses may produce hypoglycemia and rebound hypothermia as the patient is warmed.

Preventing Common Complications

Early attention to the prevention, diagnosis, and treatment of diseases that are commonly associated with hypothermia may significantly reduce morbidity and mortality [151]. Diabetic patients who have hypothermia and infection have a particularly grave prognosis. In patients with diabetic ketoacidosis, the prevalence of hypothermia was four times higher in those with underlying infection and mortality was three times higher [152]. The possibility of infection should be carefully evaluated in diabetic patients with hypothermia, and early intervention with antibiotics should be considered.

Pneumonia is a common complication in hypothermic patients who survive the rewarming period. The incidence of pneumonia can probably be reduced by early intubation in stuporous or comatose patients to protect the airway and thereby minimize aspiration. In addition, periodic hyperinflation [83], elevation of the head of the bed, and attention to pulmonary toilet may decrease the incidence of pneumonia in hypothermic patients. Antibiotics should only be given when infection is already likely to be present [151,153]. A study demonstrated that a low SVR in patients with mild-to-moderate hypothermia strongly indicates the presence of infection [81]. When SVR is low or diabetic ketoacidosis is present, we believe it is reasonable to give broad-spectrum antibiotic coverage for 24 to 48 hours pending results of the culture.

Because pancreatitis and ileus are both commonly associated with hypothermia, a nasogastric tube should be passed, a baseline amylase level should be obtained, and the patient should not be allowed to eat or drink until fully stable.

Prophylaxis of DVT in patients with hypothermia is a difficult issue. Subcutaneous heparin should not be used because it may be poorly absorbed for several days until skin function returns to normal. Pneumatic boots should not be placed on frostbitten extremities. Because of these concerns and because it is not clear that the risk of DVT from hypothermia outweighs that of systemic anticoagulation, we do not routinely recommend immediate prophylaxis for DVT. Because DIC has been reported, baseline clotting studies may be of value. DIC has occurred even in heparinized patients [154].

Acute tubular necrosis has been reported in hypothermia [70], but it is infrequent and probably results from shock and hypoxia, not as a direct action of hypothermia itself. Renal damage may be minimized by careful cardiovascular support. Hypermagnesemia reduces temperatures in hypothermic patients with renal failure and should be avoided [155]. Hypophosphatemia must be looked for because it may result from treatment [156]. Electrolyte levels must be carefully followed because serum potassium levels vary greatly during treatment.

In cases of exposure, frostbite frequently occurs on the ears, nose, face, penis, scrotum, and extremities. It may be painless and go unrecognized by the victim until he or she is rewarmed. Frostbite is detectable on physical examination because recently frozen tissue usually appears gray, white, or waxy. Soon after warming, the skin may become edematous, blister, or turn red or black because of hemorrhage or necrosis. The extent of damage and eschar formation is usually demarcated within 10 days. Limbs should be handled gently. Thawing frostbitten areas is best postponed until core temperatures have risen to normal and the patient's condition is otherwise stable. It is best accomplished by immersion for 30 to 60 minutes in water heated to 38°C to 43°C. After thawing, whirlpool débridement, intra-arterial reserpine, and anticoagulation with heparin or dextran may be helpful. Amputation may be necessary but should always be delayed as long as possible to allow a clear demarcation of viable tissue [125].

Because of the risk of relapse, hypothermic patients require prolonged monitoring. Elderly patients who have had one episode of hypothermia may experience relapse and, in addition, may be at greater risk for future hypothermic episodes [157]. Any patient who has sustained severe hypothermia under conditions other than extreme exposure should be monitored closely for recurrent episodes.

Rewarming

Rewarming methods can be divided into three categories: passive external rewarming, active external rewarming, and active central rewarming. These methods vary in level of invasiveness and the usual speed with which they provide rewarming.

Passive External Rewarming. Passive external rewarming is the least invasive and slowest rewarming technique. It requires that the patient be dry, sheltered from wind, and covered with blankets to decrease heat loss, thereby allowing thermogenesis to restore normal temperature. Temperature increase varies inversely with patient age; the average rate of temperature increase with this method is only 0.38°C per hour [64]. Passive rewarming is, therefore, appropriate only when hypothermia is not profound (i.e., when the patient's core temperature is >30°C).

Active External Rewarming. Active external rewarming is by far the most controversial method. It involves raising the core temperature by heating the skin with hot blankets, electric heating pads, and hot water bottles; circulating warmed air immediately adjacent to the skin [158,159]; or immersion in a tub of warm water. This method works [18,59,125,157,160] and has been successful in patients with temperatures as low as 17°C [161]. Initial reports [158,159] suggest that rewarming by covering the patient with a plastic blanket that contains tubes of circulating heated air is helpful for the mild hypothermia seen in the perioperative setting. Several studies have now documented that rewarming by the heated air method is safe and effective in moderate hypothermia of numerous etiologies [162]. Mortality with active external rewarming, however, appears to be higher than with passive or central rewarming methods [13]. This possible increase in mortality may be due to a (a) less accurate control over the rate of temperature increase, (b) increased risk of peripheral vasodilation and shock from warming the skin before the core, and (c) increased incidence of acidosis resulting from abrupt return of blood to the core from relatively hypoperfused areas. Treatment by immersion is extremely inconvenient and sometimes impossible in patients who require continuous ECG and temperature monitoring, central venous access, and artificial ventilation and who are in imminent danger of shock or arrest. Experience with patients undergoing external rewarming suggests that aggressive hydration and Swan-Ganz catheter monitoring are helpful [132]. Several studies have shown that the further drop in temperature experienced during the initial phase of active external rewarming is mostly independent of circulatory factors and merely reflects the natural physical laws of heat loss [162–164].

Active Central Rewarming. The fastest and most invasive warming methods are those designed to permit active central rewarming. Although commercial Food and Drug Administration–approved warmers limit fluid warming to 40°C, heated IV crystalloid to temperatures as high as 65°C have been shown to be safe in animal trials [165]. Oxygen that has been humidified and heated to 40°C to 46°C is a safe [13,166] and effective [161] rewarming technique; it can be delivered by face mask or an endotracheal tube. In the hospital, heated oxygen can be provided with a cascade humidifier, available in many ventilator systems. In other settings, portable systems that involve heat production by carbon dioxide and soda lime have been useful [167]. Temperature must be monitored orally to ensure that inspired air does not exceed 46°C, or mucosal damage or burns might occur. Temperature increase with heated oxygen is usually less than 1°C per hour.

Lavage by gastric or esophageal balloons also produces a slow temperature increase and has been shown to be effective [168]; however, this method involves risk of aspiration and ventricular fibrillation during balloon insertion. Peritoneal lavage can be performed conveniently at most hospitals, and it safely raises temperatures at a rate of up to 4°C per hour [85,100,169–171]. Average warming rates, however, are closer to 2°C per hour. Saline or dialysate fluid is heated to 38°C to 43°C and exchanged every 15 to 20 minutes. Alternatively, two peritoneal trocars can be placed and a continuous infusion and drainage circuit established. Pleural lavage with two chest tubes has also been reported and appears to be effective [172,173].

Insertion of femoral artery and vein catheters allows blood to be removed, heated, and returned to the body. This is usually performed with a hemodialysis machine [152] or pump oxygenator such as that used during cardiopulmonary bypass. Rewarming at a rate of 1°C to 2°C per hour has been reported by passing the blood from a surgically created arteriovenous fistula through a countercurrent fluid warmer with [174] or without [175,176] a roller pump. In patients with severe cardiopulmonary collapse, a pump oxygenator offers the advantage of hemodynamic support, rapid elevation of temperature, and nearly complete regulation of acid–base and oxygen disorders [70,79,118,126,134,177,178]. In one review of 68 patients presenting with a mean core temperature of 21°C and being treated with cardiopulmonary bypass primarily by the femoral route, there was a 60% survival, and 80% of survivors returned to their previous level of function [178]. No survival is reported in patients presenting with temperatures of less than 15°C. In cases of profound hypothermia, a median sternotomy approach may be preferable because of the possibilities of direct cardiac massage, improved blood flow, and easy access [118].

The desired rate of rewarming varies according to the patient's cardiopulmonary status and underlying disease. Results of experiments performed on hypothermic dogs suggest that if intramyocardial temperature gradients can be maintained at less than 2°C, the risk of fibrillation decreases [76]. This research argues that safe warming should be either slow enough to allow uniformity in tissue temperatures or fast enough to minimize the period of risk. Slower warming techniques allow a prolonged period of hypothermia and presumably should produce a higher risk of infection because of prolonged immune suppression and a higher incidence of acid–base and intravascular volume problems. A diagnosis of diabetes or myxedema may also influence the desired rate of rewarming. In diabetic ketoacidosis, for example, insulin resistance and the severity of the acidosis could be substantially improved by rapid rewarming, and a more active rewarming technique might therefore be preferred [101].

The rewarming method selected must be appropriate for the individual patient being rewarmed. In one study of 55 patients with accidental hypothermia, extracorporeal membrane oxygenation was used for those in cardiopulmonary arrest; peritoneal dialysis for those with unstable hemodynamics; and airway rewarming, insulation, and warmed fluids for those with stable hemodynamics. Survival was 100% [179].

IATROGENIC HYPOTHERMIA

Iatrogenic hypothermia occurs frequently in surgical recovery rooms and intensive care units [180–183], is associated with increased morbidity, and can be minimized with a systematic team approach. Although subnormal temperatures occur frequently during the postoperative period, frank hypothermia (temperature <35°C) is uncommon. In a series of 195 patients who underwent noncardiothoracic surgery, 60% had temperatures less than 36°C, 29% had less than 35.5°C, and 13% had less than 35°C [184]. Iatrogenic hypothermia results from the infusion of blood products or fluids at lower than body core temperatures [180,184], from continuous ultrafiltration at high flow rates in the intensive care unit [185], and from anesthesia and surgery performed in cool (<23°C) operating rooms [22,23,181,186,187]. In another series of 101 patients undergoing elective surgery under general anesthesia, 78% had temperatures less than 36°C. The average temperature decrease was 0.77°C, and maximal decrease was 2.5°C [187].

A detailed review of the evolution of anesthetic practices for hypothermic surgery or the management of specific classes of postoperative patients is beyond the scope of this chapter. Discussion is limited to those problems that are most pertinent to the intensive care physician.

Causes and Pathogenesis

Perioperative hypothermia results from increased heat loss, decreased heat production, and compromised thermoregulation [188]. Heat loss may be increased by loss of behavioral control mechanisms, decreased insulation because of exposure of larger skin surfaces, cutaneous vasodilation resulting from anesthetics, increased evaporative losses from serosal surfaces and volatile antiseptics applied to skin, and exposure to air-conditioned environments. Decreased heat production results from muscular paralysis. Impaired thermoregulation results from slowed or compromised afferent and efferent nerve impulses and hypothermic reflexes due to sedative anesthetics. Redistribution of heat from the core to the periphery is felt to be a primary factor in the cause of perioperative hypothermia. Temperature change may be abrupt with a 1°C core heat loss within 30 minutes of induction due to redistribution of heat from the core to the periphery [189].

The frequency and severity of heat loss increase with patient age [180,182,183], open chest or abdominal surgery [180,182,190], low operating room temperature [22,23], length of surgery [181], infusion of cool IV solutions, and certain types of anesthetics. Elderly patients experience a decrease in temperature, shiver less frequently, and take longer to rewarm than do younger patients [180,183]. Temperature decrease during surgery involving open body cavities may result in almost twice the decrease in temperature seen in extremity surgery [182]. Lightly anesthetized, paralyzed, draped patients who are not provided with active warming experience a temperature decrease of 0.3°C per hour at ambient temperatures less than 21°C [23]. Surgery involving muscle paralysis with curare-type agents produces twice the temperature decrease of nonparalyzing procedures [182]. Although halothane and epidural anesthesia may increase heat loss because of vasodilation, no major differences have been detected in the heat loss from most inhalational agents [182,183]. Laparoscopic procedures produce hypothermia that may be more severe than open laparotomy. Massive infusion of chilled solutions can induce hypothermia, as heat loss from infusion of room temperature solutions approximates 16 kcal per L [183]. Blood infused at its stored temperature of 4°C produces a heat loss of 32 kcal per L [184]. In an average human, infusion of 1 L of 4°C blood produces a 0.5°C decrease in temperature [180]. The mean temperature of patients given more than 20 units of blood in 24 hours has been reported to be 32.9°C ± 1.7°C [57]. Although most of these patients had multiple reasons for development of hypothermia, the rapid transfusion of blood not warmed to body temperature must be considered a risk factor for the development of mild hypothermia. The mean temperature of survivors and nonsurvivors after massive transfusion was no different.

Pathophysiology

Perioperative complications from mild hypothermia arise directly from the hypothermia and from the hypermetabolism triggered by the patient's efforts to restore body temperature. From the preceding in-depth discussion of patients with noniatrogenic, unintentional hypothermia, it is reasonable to suspect that an otherwise healthy individual with a temperature ranging from 34°C to 36°C should do well and should have (a) a slightly increased cardiac output, (b) an oxygen consumption up to five times basal levels, (c) an elevated SVR because of peripheral vasoconstriction, (d) a decrease in mixed venous oxygen saturation because of increased oxygen extraction, (e) shivering or muscle rigidity, and (f) a slightly depressed mental status. The alveolar-arterial oxygen gradient and even the arteriovenous oxygen difference [81] may be in the normal range [132]. Therefore, deviations from this pattern in the perioperative period and subsequent morbidity must reflect the additive effects of surgery and anesthesia on metabolism.

Alternatively, in critically ill postoperative patients with cardiac depression, one must be most concerned about the potential effects of mild hypothermia, because an increase in oxygen consumption could easily lead to acidosis and hypoxemia. Although acidosis results from an increase in anaerobic metabolism as metabolic demand outstrips oxygen delivery, minute ventilation is usually maintained to the degree necessary to preserve acid–base balance [191]. Hypoxemia may result from the combination of increased pulmonary parenchymal shunt (venous admixture) after surgery and lower mixed venous PO_2. In one study, shivering appeared to be accompanied by a drop in PO_2; arterial oxygen saturation fell below 90% in 53% of shivering patients and remained above 90% in all nonshivering patients [191]. However, the authors provided little information about inspired oxygen concentrations, raising the possibility that PO_2 may have been significantly improved by merely increasing the concentration of inspired oxygen. Although decreased temperature and shivering can elevate oxygen consumption and in some patients lower PO_2 [183,192], the clinical consequences of these physiologic changes remain obscure. Several studies have now demonstrated an increased morbidity due to hypothermia. Increased perioperative cardiac ischemia, ventricular tachycardia [193], delayed wound healing [112], perioperative bleeding requiring transfusion [113,194,195], increased length of stay in recovery, and increased length of stay in hospital [112] may occur with perioperative hypothermia. Patients with prolonged postoperative hypothermia have a higher mortality than those who return to normal temperatures in the first postoperative hour [196].

Prevention and Treatment

Numerous interventions have been attempted to minimize perioperative temperature decrease and shivering. The use of postoperative warming blankets alone does not prevent significant temperature loss because the body surface area exposed to heat is small [18,186,197]. The use of warming blankets plus heating of all infused liquids can maintain average temperature on arrival in the recovery room above 36°C [197]. Heating and humidifying the carbon dioxide used for laparoscopic insufflation to 30.0°C to 30.5°C decrease the heat loss associated with laparoscopic procedures [198]. Crystalloids can be easily warmed in a microwave oven to 39°C in 2 minutes [199]. The inhalation of heated, humidified air can be safely applied to most intubated patients and is effective in preventing temperature loss [192,200,201] and shivering [192]. Most publications clearly favor the use of preoperative, intraoperative, and postoperative forced air warmers [202–204]. Preliminary studies indicate that different manufacturers' products are not equally effective [205,206]. One hour of prewarming with an air warmer set to 43°C may minimize redistribution loss and decrease hypothermia for brief procedures. Vasodilators such as nitroprusside or nifedipine may be started hours preoperatively resulting in peripheral vasodilation and minimizing redistribution loss by prewarming the peripheral tissues. Cutaneous rewarming minimizes shivering. Meperidine may lower the shivering threshold and control pain in postoperative patients. Prewarming is felt to be the most effective strategy for high-risk patients [189].

All patients undergoing surgery should be observed closely for the development of hypothermia. Simple measures, such as minimizing preoperative and postoperative time in chilled rooms, covering the patient with drapes or blankets whenever possible, and infusing all solutions at least at room temperature, should be taken in all patients. Special measures should be taken in high-risk individuals. Groups of patients at high risk of hypothermia include those undergoing major abdominal or cardiothoracic surgery, surgery involving intentional hypothermia, or surgery with anesthesia times in excess of 4 hours; patients older than 60 years undergoing surgery; and patients with known or expected cardiac depression who are undergoing surgery. In these high-risk patients, preventive measures, including the use of preoperative [207–209] and intraoperative [203,210] forced warm air, heating of infused solutions to 37.5°C, and inhalation of heated humidified oxygen, should be beneficial. In any patient undergoing any type of extracorporeal bypass, the addition of a heat exchanger to the bypass circuit is simple and effective [211]. Blood and colloid solutions can be safely heated to 37.5°C [212]. These measures have been shown to be safe and effective in numerous clinical series and can provide the patient potential benefit at little cost or change in perioperative routine.

INTENTIONAL HYPOTHERMIA

Intentional hypothermia has been induced by partial immersion or surface or central cooling techniques to treat cancer, limit the toxicity of sepsis, help prevent the alopecia of chemotherapy, reduce carbon dioxide production in refractory status asthmaticus, assist in the amputation of limbs, and minimize the hypoperfusion injury associated with cardiothoracic surgery. Currently, mild-to-moderate hypothermia (32°C to 35°C) is the first treatment with proven efficacy for postischemic neurological injury, and employing intentional hypothermia to retard postcardiac arrest brain injury is now recommended by the American Heart Association.

Therapeutic Hypothermia after Cardiac Arrest

Therapeutic hypothermia improves survival and neurological outcomes after sudden cardiac arrest in several randomized controlled trials [213–215]. Adoption of this treatment has been slow, particularly in the United States, despite consensus recommendations by the liaison committee on resuscitation for the use of therapeutic hypothermia after sudden cardiac arrest [216]. Possible barriers to applying this therapeutic strategy include the complexity of implementing it, relative little published research in its use, and the need for improved cooling devices. A recent compilation of recent experiences, where implementation of therapeutic hypothermia within hospital systems outside clinical trials were compared, noted an increased survival with an odds ratio of 2.5 (95% confidence interval, 1.8 to 3.3) and favorable outcome with an odds ratio of 2.5 (95% confidence interval, 1.9 to 3.4) [216].

Cardiac arrest results in immediate termination of blood flow and loss of oxygen leading to neurological ischemic injury after only several minutes and permanent loss after 5 to 10 minutes. If resuscitation results in restoration of circulation, an additional reperfusion injury occurs. Several animal models including dogs showed that cooling after prolonged cardiac arrest (10 minutes no flow following 5 minutes low flow) provided considerable neurological benefit [217]. Subsequently, two pivotal, randomized, controlled trials were conducted and confirmed efficacy [214,215]. The first of these was a large, multicentered, randomized, controlled trial that enrolled 275 patients in nine European hospitals who had sustained a cardiac arrest with an initial rhythm of ventricular fibrillation. The second randomized, controlled trial enrolled 77 patients from four hospitals in Victoria, Australia, with similar inclusion criteria, however, did not exclude older patients or those who were hypoxic. The American Heart Association recommended, in review of these two studies, therapeutic hypothermia for 12 to 24 hours following resuscitation from out-of-hospital cardiac arrest for the treatment of neurological injury when the initial rhythm is ventricular fibrillation [218].

However, the role of therapeutic hypothermia is uncertain when the initial rhythm is asystole or pulseless electrical activity or when the cardiac arrest is in hospital or pediatric or due to a noncardiac cause such as asphyxia or drug overdose [219]. Also hemodynamically unstable patients were excluded from the European trial. In addition, the trials used therapeutic hypothermia several hours after resuscitation and therefore the role for earlier cooling or prolonged cooling was not evaluated. Given that survival rate in these other conditions is very low, it is unlikely that clinical trials will be undertaken to test the efficacy, as a very large sample size would be necessary to show a difference in outcomes. Given that the induction of hypothermia has become more feasible, the side effects are generally easily managed in the critical care setting, and there is a benefit for anoxic brain injury; consideration may be given to treat comatose post–cardiac arrest non–ventricular fibrillation patients with therapeutic hypothermia [219].

For Acute Myocardial Infarction

Timely myocardial reperfusion using thrombolytic therapy or angioplasty is the most effective therapy for patients with ST elevation myocardial infarction. Although mild hypothermia appears feasible and safe, its ability to limit infarct size or reduce rates of adverse cardiac events has not been proven [220].

For Spinal Cord Injury

Hypothermia strategies date back to the 1960s for the treatment of acute spinal cord injury, but no randomized phase III trials have been conducted to confirm efficacy and safety, let alone the appropriate therapeutic window. Hypothermia remains an experimental treatment with unknown clinical relevance for patients with acute spinal cord injury [221].

For Ischemic and Hemorrhagic Stroke

Hypothermia reduces brain edema and intracranial pressure (ICP) in patients with traumatic brain injury; however, only very few small pilot studies have investigated the role hypothermia may have in the treatment of acute ischemic stroke. There are no controlled trials performed for hypothermia in hemorrhagic stroke. Currently, barriers to its clinical use include critical care to start immediately in the emergency room, inability to induce hypothermia within 3 to 6 hours due to slow cooling rates, the necessity for proactive antishivering therapy for cooling, slow rewarming to prevent rebound brain edema, and increased risk for infectious and cardiovascular complications

TABLE 65.4

ADVANCES IN MANAGEMENT OF HYPOTHERMIA BASED ON RANDOMIZED CONTROLLED TRIALS

Induced hypothermia benefits survivors of cardiac arrest:
Unconscious adult patients with recovery of spontaneous circulation after out-of-hospital cardiac arrest should be cooled to 32°C to 34°C (89.6°F to 93.2°F) for 12 to 24 hours when the initial rhythm was VF
Similar therapy may be beneficial for patients with non-VF arrest out of hospital or for in-hospital arrest

VF, ventricular fibrillation.

[222]. On the contrary, the use of normothermia protocols is being actively studied.

For Acute Liver Toxicity

Patients with rapidly progressive acute liver failure, such as with acetaminophen overdose, are at high risk for developing cerebral edema, intracranial hypertension, brainstem herniation, and brain death or anoxic brain injury and permanent brain impairment. Techniques such as manipulating the body position, increasing sedation, and increasing osmolarity through medications can temporarily control this phenomenon. However, these steps often postpone but do not stop the development of brain herniation unless liver transplantation or spontaneous liver regeneration follows immediately. Using therapeutic hypothermia has been shown to effectively bridge patients to transplant by reducing cerebral edema and intracranial hypertension by decreasing splanchnic ammonia production, lowering oxidative metabolism within the brain, and restoring normal regulation of cerebral hemodynamics [223]. However, hypothermia has not been adequately studied for its safety, and concerns of increasing the risk of infection, cardiac arrhythmias, and bleeding may be accentuated. Multicenter, randomized, control trials are needed to determine if hypothermia protects the brain and improves survival without causing harm.

In Multisystem Trauma

Hypothermia may be helpful in attenuating the damage to tissues before adequate blood volume resuscitation can be restored in traumatic blood loss. Clinical trials to determine its efficacy are needed [224].

Advances in hypothermia, based on randomized, controlled trials or meta-analyses of such trials, are summarized in Table 65.4.

Methods of Cooling

Induction and maintenance of hypothermia requires blocking the body's normal thermoregulation mechanism as well as active heat exchange. Therapeutic hypothermia can be achieved through four mechanisms individually or in combination and include conduction, convection, radiation, and evaporation as previously described in this chapter. There are four phases of temperature modulation during therapeutic hypothermia: induction, maintenance, decooling, and normothermia [225]. Induction is typically initiated prehospital, especially in out-of-hospital cardiac arrests, but can occur in hospital for patients awaiting a liver transplant, with cerebral edema from acute liver failure and for control of refractory elevated ICP. Among cardiac arrest survivors, contraindications to perform therapeutic hypothermia would include if the patient can follow verbal commands, more than 8 hours have elapsed since return of spontaneous circulation, life-threatening bleeding or infection, cardiopulmonary collapse is imminent despite vasopressor or mechanical hemodynamic support, or an underlying terminal condition exists. It is commonly achieved by rapid bolus administration of 30 to 40 mL per kg cold (4°C) isotonic resuscitation fluid [225] targeting a goal temperature of 32°C to 34°C. Serum potassium will drop, and empirically repleting potassium for a goal of more than 3.8 mEq per dL is needed. Close monitoring and treatment for seizures is necessary. Simultaneous sedation, paralysis (for shivering), and use of commercial surface or intravascular cooling devices are concomitant therapeutic strategies [225].

Maintenance phase occurs in the intensive care unit and is a phase where both metabolic and hemodynamic homeostasis are maintained. The core temperature is kept at 33°C for 18 to 24 hours. Maintenance of brain perfusion by keeping mean arterial perfusion pressure at 65 mm Hg or more (cerebral perfusion pressure [CPP] may need to be monitored given cerebral autoregulatory failure [226]), normocarbia with volume-cycled mechanical ventilation to maintain a normal pH as hypercarbia is to be avoided; maintain a perfusing rhythm, antibiotic prophylaxis if pulmonary infiltrates present [225,227], maintenance of a blood glucose of 120 to 160 mg per dL [226], maintenance of normal electrolyte levels [225] and appropriate medication dosing given the reduction in drug metabolism and duration of action [225], skin care, and aggressive treatment of shivering with neuromuscular blockade [225].

After 24 hours of therapeutic hypothermia, the decooling phase starts and is associated with hemodynamic instability often referred to as the postresuscitation syndrome. It is characterized by an increase in inflammatory cytokine levels, vasodilatation, and hypotension [225]. The patient is also at increased risk for an elevation in the ICP and a decrease in the CPP [225]. Slow decooling at a goal rate of 0.2°C to 0.33°C per hour until the patient is at 36.5°C or 37°C is preferred to avoid large hemodynamic fluctuations. Supportive fluid boluses, inotropes, and vasopressors may be necessary to maintain CPP, especially if there are signs of elevated ICP. Use of neuromuscular blockade until the temperature reaches 35°C to avoid shivering and sedation is weaned once the body temperature reaches 36°C is recommended [225].

In patients who have undergone therapeutic hypothermia post–cardiac arrest, a rebound fever can occur and is harmful [228]. Brain injury may be attenuated by fever control [229]. Maintaining normothermia for at least 72 hours from return of circulation is thus common practice [225]. This is easily achieved by employing commercial cooling devices and resetting target temperature to 36.5°C to 37.5°C. Nursing attention to onset of fever spikes and frequent adjustments to the cooling device set points need to be closely observed.

A number of issues occur with induction, maintenance, and withdrawal of therapeutic hypothermia and require close attention. (i) Serum potassium needs to be aggressively replaced if levels are less than 3.8 mEq per dL as soon as therapeutic hypothermia is employed and the levels should be followed every 3 to 4 hours during the induction phase. (ii) One needs to be able to accurately measure the core temperature continuously and this is preferably achieved by bladder, rectal, central venous, or esophageal measurements. Bladder measurement may be inaccurate in oliguric patients and other monitoring sites are preferred. (iii) When using neuromuscular blockade to control shivering and or help in the induction phase of hypothermia, thorough neurology exam and adequate sedation a priori is important. (iv) None of the cooling devices currently used for therapeutic hypothermia post–cardiac arrest have been approved despite the fact that they have been routinely employed and thus the application of any of the cooling devices constitutes "off-label" use. (v) The incidence of pneumonia in post–cardiac arrest patients treated with hypothermia is 30% to 50% [215]. The etiology may be related to aspiration at the time of cardiac arrest or from the immunosuppressive effects from hypothermia. Preliminary data supports prophylactic antibiotics for presumed pneumonia [227]. (vi) Seizures can occur 19% to 34% of the time and go undetected with neuromuscular blockade [230]. Thus, continuous EEG monitoring in the paralyzed patient may be necessary. If continuous monitoring is not available, then empirically using antiepileptic sedatives to sedate the patient may be warranted [225]. (vii) Hemodynamic instability is common during the decooling phase due to cutaneous vasodilatation and the inflammatory state [225]. Close attention to monitoring adequate cardiac output, global tissue perfusion, and brain perfusion using intravenous isotonic fluids, inotropes, and/or vasopressor agents may be necessary. Hemodynamic monitoring may be achieved by using invasive or noninvasive cardiac output devices, urinary output if kidney function is normal, and central venous oxyhemoglobin saturation for tissue perfusion or direct invasive monitoring of brain metabolism [225]. To reduce shivering, focal counter rewarming [225] can be employed in which the face, neck, and extremities are actively warmed while the torso and central venous system are cooled. This paradoxically increases the cooling process by enhancing the cutaneous vasodilatation.

COOLING TECHNIQUES

The conventional method involves the use of cold saline or ringer's lactate solution at 4°C administered at 30 to 40 mL per kg and has been shown to decrease core temperature by 2°C to 4°C without left ventricular systolic dysfunction and a reduction in cardiac output [231]. This method is supported by multiple safety and efficacy trials [225] and should be the preferred method for induction in conventional cooling. Thereafter cooling can be maintained with ice packs applied to the neck, groin, and axilla and rubber cooling mats or blankets as used in the operating room. Ongoing infusion of cold fluid has not been shown to be an effective method to maintain hypothermia [232]. A number of issues associated with this method include the lack of an internal feedback loop making an accurate temperature maintenance difficult, a high incidence of overcooling, and the need for high level of nursing care. Nonetheless, it is widely available and cost-effective.

There are a number of commercial surface cooling devices of which the most widely available is the Arctic Sun device (Medivance, Louisville, CO) which uses proprietary heat exchange pads that adhere to the skin using a hydrophilic gel that conducts heat. The pads cover 40% of the body surface area and circulating water temperature is continually modulated by a servo mechanism to maintain a core body temperature at goal. This device was studied in the Hypothermia After Cardiac Arrest trial [233] and was noted to be relatively safe with infrequent overcooling and lack of vascular complications, sparing of the femoral and subclavian sites for catheterization, and allowing for defibrillator pads and compatibility with cardiac catheterization. However, it is not inexpensive with a potential for rare skin conditions [225].

Other devices such as CoolBlue (Innercool Therapies, San Diego, CA), Blanketroll III (Cincinnati SubZero Products, Cincinnati, OH), and Thermo wrap (MTRE Advanced Technologies, Rehovot, Israel) are less expensive and recently introduced but not as quick at reducing the temperature. They are without the gel-adhesion system, employ servo mechanisms and thus are safe and reduce nursing work, and cool by conduction as water circulates through pads that encircle the patient without adhering directly to the patient's skin. Experience with these devices is limited and efficacy has yet to be demonstrated in clinical trials [225]. The fastest cooling device is the Thermosuit System (Life Recovery Systems, Kinnelon, NJ), a cold immersion system that can cool human-sized swine to 33°C in 30 to 45 minutes [234]; however, safety data are awaited.

Methods using commercial intravascular cooling devices are dependent on central vascular catheters and its associated inherent risks [235]. Two devices include the Alsius temperature management system and the Celsius Control System (Inner cool Therapies) [225]. The Alsius system has a number of proprietary intravascular devices that serves as both a cooling device and central venous catheter, both of which are servo-controlled temperature modulation systems. In the Celsius system, water circulates through a metallic catheter with a textured surface in the inferior vena cava [236]. It is effective in providing precise temperature control, it may increase the patient's risk for thromboembolism, and it requires a separate catheter for the administration of supportive medications. Other less commonly used methods to cool include medications such as neurotensin, extracorporeal circuits, body cavity lavage, whole body ice water immersion, continuous venovenous hemoinfiltration, cooling helmets, and air conduction hypothermia devices.

Therapeutic hypothermia can be achieved by conventional modalities that are readily available in most hospitals or with one of the newer devices now commercially available. Temperature management can be complex and the circumstances highly variable, such as persistent neurogenic fever and uncontrollable shivering in patients with a traumatic brain injury despite normothermia with ice packs and cold fluid while other patients are uneventfully cooled and rewarmed. This variability requires close attention by a highly trained intensive care team.

References

1. Dinarello CA, Wolff SM: Pathogenesis of fever in man. *N Engl J Med* 298:607, 1978.
2. Iampietro PF, Vaughn JA, Goldman RF, et al: Heat production from shivering. *J Appl Physiol* 15:632, 1960.
3. Cabanac M: Regulation and modulation in biology. A reexamination of temperature regulation. *Ann N Y Acad Sci* 15:813, 1997.
4. Cabanac M: Temperature regulation. *Annu Rev Physiol* 37:415, 1975.
5. Kenney WL, Munce TA: Invited review: aging and human temperature regulation. *J Appl Physiol* 95(6):2598, 2003.
6. Nomoto S, Shibata M, Iriki M, et al: Role of afferent pathways of heat and cold in body temperature regulation. *Int J Biometeorol* 49(2):67, 2004.
7. Wagner JA, Robinson S, Marino RP: Age and temperature regulation of humans in neutral and cold environments. *J Appl Physiol* 37:562, 1974.
8. Collins KJ, Dore C, Exton-Smith AN, et al: Accidental hypothermia and impaired temperature homeostasis in the elderly. *BMJ* 1:353, 1977.
9. Ellis FP, Exton-Smith AN, Foster KG, et al: Eccrine sweating and mortality during heat waves in very young and very old persons. *Isr J Med Sci* 12:815, 1976.
10. Whittle JL, Bates JH: Thermoregulatory failure secondary to acute illness: complications and treatment. *Arch Intern Med* 139:418, 1979.
11. Centers for Disease Control: Hypothermia-related deaths, Georgia—January 1996–December 1997, and United States, 1979–1995. *MMWR Morb Mortal Wkly Rep* 47:1037, 1998.
12. Miller JW, Danzl DF, Thomas DM: Urban accidental hypothermia: 135 cases. *Ann Emerg Med* 9:456, 1980.
13. Mathews JA: Accidental hypothermia. *Postgrad Med* 43:662, 1967.
14. Pugh LG: Accidental hypothermia in walkers, climbers and campers: reports to the medical commission on accident prevention. *BMJ* 1:123, 1966.
15. Rothschield MA, Schneider V: Terminal burrowing behaviour: a phenomenon of lethal hypothermia. *Int J Legal Med* 108:116, 1995.
16. Milner JE: Hypothermia. *Ann Intern Med* 89:565, 1978.

17. Hayward JS, Eckerson JD, Collis ML: Thermal balance and survival time prediction of man in cold water. *Can J Physiol Pharmacol* 53:21, 1974.
18. Jessen K, Hagelsten JO: Search and rescue service in Denmark with special reference to accidental hypothermia. *Aerosp Med* 43:787, 1972.
19. Raheja R, Puri BK, Schaeffer RC: Shock due to profound hypothermia and alcohol ingestion. *Crit Care Med* 9:644, 1984.
20. Vandam LD, Burnap TK: Hypothermia. *N Engl J Med* 261:546, 1959.
21. Duff RS, Farrant PC, Leveaux VM, et al: Spontaneous periodic hypothermia. *Q J Med* 30:329, 1961.
22. Morris RH: Operating room temperature and the anesthetized, paralyzed patient. *Arch Surg* 102:95, 1971.
23. Morris RH, Wilkey BR: The effects of ambient temperature on patient temperature during surgery not involving body cavities. *Anesthesiology* 32:102, 1972.
24. Hassel B: Acute hypothermia due to penicillin. *BMJ* 304:882, 1992.
25. Hassel B: Hypothermia from erythromycin. *Ann Intern Med* 115:69, 1991.
26. Pfeiffer RF: Bromocriptine-induced hypothermia. *Neurology* 40:383, 1990.
27. Freinkel N, Metzger BE, Harris E, et al: The hypothermia of hypoglycemia: studies with 2-deoxy-D-glucose in normal human subjects and mice. *N Engl J Med* 287:841, 1972.
28. Gale EA, Bennett T, Green JH, et al: Hypoglycemia, hypothermia and shivering in man. *Clin Sci* 61:463, 1981.
29. Forrester CF: Coma in myxedema. *Arch Intern Med* 111:100, 1963.
30. Hamburger S, Collier RE: Myxedema coma. *Ann Emerg Med* 11:156, 1982.
31. Fitzgerald FT: Hypoglycemia and accidental hypothermia in an alcoholic population. *West J Med* 133:105, 1980.
32. Branch EF, Burger PC, Brewer DL: Hypothermia in a case of hypothalamic infarction and sarcoidosis. *Arch Neurol* 25:245, 1971.
33. Kearsley JH, Musso AF: Hypothermia and coma in the Wernicke-Korsakoff syndrome. *Med J Aust* 2:504, 1980.
34. Koeppen AH, Daniels JC, Baroron KD: Subnormal body temperatures in Wernicke's encephalopathy. *Arch Neurol* 21:493, 1969.
35. Hansen B, Larsson C, Wiren J, et al: Hypothermia and infection in Wernicke's encephalopathy. *Acta Med Scand* 215:185, 1984.
36. Ackerman WJ: Stupor, bradycardia, hypotension and hypothermia: a presentation of Wernicke's encephalopathy with rapid response to thiamine. *West J Med* 121:428, 1974.
37. Philip G, Smith JF: Hypothermia and Wernicke's encephalopathy. *Lancet* 2:122, 1973.
38. Donnan GA, Seeman E: Coma and hypothermia in Wernicke's encephalopathy. *Aust N Z J Med* 10:438, 1980.
39. Mechlenburg RS, Loriaux DL, Thompson RH, et al: Hypothalamic dysfunction in patients with anorexia nervosa. *Medicine* 53:147, 1974.
40. Shapir WR, Williams GH, Plum F: Spontaneous recurrent hypothermia accompany agenesis of the corpus callosum. *Brain* 92:423, 1969.
41. Lammens M, Lissoir F, Carton H: Hypothermia in three patients with multiple sclerosis. *Clin Neurol Neurosurg* 91:117, 1989.
42. Perroen J, Hoffman RS, Jones B, et al: Guanabenz induced hypothermia in a poisoned elderly female. *J Toxicol Clin Toxicol* 32:445, 1994.
43. Randall WC, Wurster RD, Lewin RJ: Responses of patients with high spinal transection to high ambient temperatures. *J Appl Physiol* 21:985, 1966.
44. Pledger HG: Disorders of temperature regulation in acute traumatic tetraplegia. *J Bone Joint Surg* 44B:110, 1962.
45. Altus P, Hickman JW, Nord J: Accidental hypothermia in a healthy quadriplegic patient. *Neurology* 35:427, 1985.
46. Krook G: Hypothermia in patients with exfoliative dermatitis. *Acta Derm Venereol* 40:142, 1960.
47. Grice KA, Bettley FR: Skin water loss and accidental hypothermia in psoriasis, ichthyosis, and erythroderma. *BMJ* 2:195, 1967.
48. Moncrief JA: Burns. *N Engl J Med* 288:444, 1973.
49. Roe CF, Kinney JM, Blair C: Water and heat exchange in third-degree burns. *Surgery* 56:212, 1964.
50. Stoner HB: Mechanism of body temperature changes after burns and other injuries. *Ann N Y Acad Sci* 150:722, 1968.
51. Buggini RV: Hypothermia in Hodgkin's disease. *N Engl J Med* 312:244, 1985.
52. Csuka ME, McCarty DJ: Transient hypothermia after corticosteroid treatment of subacute cutaneous lupus erythematosus. *J Rheumatol* 11:112, 1984.
53. Kugler SL, Costakos DT, Aron AM, et al: Hypothermia and systemic lupus erythematosus. *J Rheumatol* 17:680, 1990.
54. Bonneh DY, Shvartzman P: Hypothermia in the elderly in the Negev. *Harefuah* 127:509, 1994.
55. Doherty N, Ades A, Shah PK, et al: Hypothermia with acute myocardial infarction. *Ann Intern Med* 101:797, 1984.
56. Jurkovich GJ, Greiser WB, Luterman A: Hypothermia in trauma victims: an ominous predictor of survival. *J Trauma* 27:1019, 1987.
57. Wilson RF, Dulchavsky SA, Soullier G, et al: Problems with 20 or more blood transfusions in 24 hours. *Am Surg* 53:410, 1987.
58. Iampietro PF, Faughn JA, Goldman RF, et al: Heat production from shivering. *J Appl Physiol* 15:632, 1960.
59. Martyn JW: Diagnosing and treating hypothermia. *Can Med Assoc J* 125:1089, 1981.
60. Michenfelder JD, Uihlein A, Daw EF, et al: Moderate hypothermia in man: hemodynamic and metabolic effects. *Br J Anaesth* 37:738, 1965.
61. Hardy JD, Bard P: *Body Temperature Regulation in Medical Physiology*. St. Louis, MO, Mosby, 1974.
62. Stoner HB, Frayn KN, Little RA, et al: Metabolic aspects of hypothermia in the elderly. *Clin Sci* 59:19, 1980.
63. Cohen DJ, Cline JR, Lepinski SM, et al: Resuscitation of the hypothermic patient. *Am J Emerg Med* 6:475, 1988.
64. MacLean D, Griffiths PD, Browning MC, et al: Metabolic aspects of spontaneous rewarming in accidental hypothermia and hypothermic myxoedema. *Q J Med* 43:371, 1974.
65. Cooper KE: The circulation in hypothermia. *Br Med Bull* 17:48, 1961.
66. Trevino A, Rasi B, Beller BM: The characteristic electrocardiogram of accidental hypothermia. *Arch Intern Med* 127:470, 1971.
67. Southwick FS, Dalglish PH: Recovery after prolonged asystolic cardiac arrest in profound hypothermia. *JAMA* 243:1250, 1980.
68. Angelakos ET, Torres J, Driscoll R: Ouabain on the hypothermic dog heart. *Am Heart J* 56:458, 1958.
69. Bjornstad H, Tande PM, Refsum H: Cardiac electrophysiology during hypothermia and implications for medical treatment. *Arctic Med Res* 50[Suppl]:71, 1991.
70. Kugelberg J, Schuller H, Berg B, et al: Treatment of accidental hypothermia. *Scand J Thorac Cardiovasc Surg* 1:142, 1967.
71. Thompson R, Rich J, Chmelik F, et al: Evolutionary changes in the electrocardiogram of severe progressive hypothermia. *J Electrocardiol* 10:67, 1977.
72. Rankin AC, Rae AP: Cardiac arrhythmias during rewarming of patients with accidental hypothermia. *BMJ* 289:874, 1984.
73. Clements SD, Hurst JW: Diagnostic value of electrocardiographic abnormalities observed in subjects accidentally exposed to cold. *Am J Cardiol* 29:729, 1972.
74. Yan GX, Antxzelevitch C: Cellular basis of the electrocardiographic J wave. *Circulation* 93:372, 1996.
75. Van Mieghem C, Sabbe M, Knockaert D: The clinical value of the ECG in non cardiac conditions. *Chest* 125(4):1561, 2004.
76. Mouritzen CV, Andersen MN: Myocardial temperature gradients and ventricular fibrillation during hypothermia. *J Thorac Cardiovasc Surg* 49:937, 1965.
77. Lomsky M, Ekroth R, Poupa O: The calcium paradox and its protection by hypothermia in human myocardium. *Eur Heart J* 4[Suppl]:139, 1983.
78. Hervey GR: Hypothermia. *Proc R Soc Med* 66:1055, 1973.
79. Althaus U, Aeberhard T, Schupbach P, et al: Management of profound accidental hypothermia with cardiorespiratory arrest. *Ann Surg* 195:492, 1982.
80. Zarins CK, Skinner DB: Circulation in profound hypothermia. *J Surg Res* 14:97, 1973.
81. Morris DL, Chambers HF, Morris MG, et al: Hemodynamic characteristics of patients with hypothermia due to occult infection and other causes. *Ann Intern Med* 102:153, 1985.
82. Blair E, Esmond WG, Attar S, et al: The effect of hypothermia on lung function. *Ann Surg* 160:814, 1964.
83. Hedley-Whyte J, Pontoppidan H, Laver MB, et al: Arterial oxygenation during hypothermia. *Anesthesiology* 26:595, 1965.
84. Rosenfeld JB: Acid-base and electrolyte disturbances in hypothermia. *Am J Cardiol* 12:678, 1963.
85. Pickering BG, Bristow GK, Craig DB: Core rewarming by peritoneal irrigation in accidental hypothermia with cardiac arrest. *Anesth Analg* 56:574, 1977.
86. Norwood WI, Norwood CR: Influence of hypothermia on intracellular pH during anoxia. *Am J Physiol* 243:C62, 1982.
87. Michenfelder JD, Theye RA: Hypothermia: effect on canine brain and whole-body metabolism. *Anesthesiology* 29:1107, 1965.
88. Norwood WI, Norwood CR, Castaneda AR: Cerebral anoxia: effect of deep hypothermia and pH. *Surgery* 86:203, 1979.
89. Russ W, Kling D, Lofsevitz A, et al: Effect of hypothermia on visual evoked potentials (VEP) in humans. *Anesthesiology* 61:207, 1984.
90. FitzGibbon T, Hayward JS, Walker D: EEG and visual evoked potentials of conscious man during moderate hypothermia. *Electroencephalogr Clin Neurophysiol* 58:48, 1984.
91. Stockard JJ, Sharbrough FW, Tinker JA: Effects of hypothermia on the human brainstem auditory response. *Ann Neurol* 3:368, 1978.
92. Marshall NK, Donchin E: Circadian variation in the latency of brainstem responses and its relation to body temperature. *Science* 212:356, 1981.
93. Maclean D, Griffiths PD, Emslie-Smith D: Serum-enzymes in relation to electrocardiographic changes in accidental hypothermia. *Lancet* 2:1266, 1968.
94. Blair E: A physiologic classification of clinical hypothermia. *Surgery* 58:607, 1965.
95. Doherty P, Bohn D, Bigger D: Hyperthermia and neutrophil dysfunction: clinical and experimental observations. *Crit Care Med* 12:233, 1984.
96. Kanter GS: Hypothermic hemoconcentration. *Am J Physiol* 214:856, 1968.
97. Poulos ND, Mollitt DL: The nature and reversibility of hypothermia-induced alterations in blood viscosity. *J Trauma* 31:996, 1991.
98. O'Brien H, Ames JA, Mollin LD: Recurrent thrombocytopenia, erythroid hypoplasia and sideroblastic anaemia associated with hypothermia. *Br J Haematol* 51:451, 1982.
99. Thomas RT, Hessel EA, Harker LA, et al: Platelet function during and after deep surface hypothermia. *J Surg Res* 31:314, 1981.

100. Schissler P, Parker MA, Scott SJ: Profound hypothermia: value of prolonged cardiopulmonary resuscitation. *South Med J* 74:474, 1981.
101. Maclean D, Murison J, Griffiths PD: Acute pancreatitis and diabetic ketoacidosis in accidental hypothermia and hypothermic myxoedema. *BMJ* 4:757, 1973.
102. Hirvonen J, Huttunen P: Increased urinary concentration of catecholamines in hypothermia deaths. *J Forensic Sci* 27:264, 1982.
103. Mant AK: Autopsy diagnosis of accidental hypothermia. *J Forensic Med* 16:126, 1969.
104. Baum D, Dillard DH, Porte D: Inhibition of insulin release in infants undergoing deep hypothermic cardiovascular surgery. *N Engl J Med* 279:1309, 1968.
105. Curry DL, Curry KP: Hypothermia and insulin secretion. *Endocrinology* 87:750, 1970.
106. O'Malley BP, Davies TJ, Rosenthal FD: TSH responses to temperature in primary hypothyroidism. *Clin Endocrinol* 13:87, 1980.
107. Maclean D, Browning MC: Plasma 11-hydroxycorticosteroid concentrations and prognosis in accidental hypothermia. *Resuscitation* 52:249, 1974.
108. Woolff PD, Hollander CS, Mitsuma T, et al: Accidental hypothermia: endocrine function during recovery. *J Clin Endocrinol Metab* 34:460, 1972.
109. Bohn D, Baker C, Kent G, et al: Accidental and induced hypothermia: effects on neutrophil migration in vivo. *Crit Care Med* 129:A112, 1984.
110. DeGuzman VC, Webb WR, Grogan JB: The effect of hypothermia on clearance of staphylococcal bacteremia. *Clin Res* 10:58, 1962.
111. Biggar WD, Bohn DJ, Kent G, et al: Neutrophil migration in vitro and in vivo during hypothermia. *Infect Immun* 46:857, 1984.
112. Kurz A, Sessler DI, Lenhardt R: Perioperative normothermia to reduce the incidence of surgical wound infection and shorten hospitalization. Study of wound infection and temperature group. *N Engl J Med* 334:1209, 1996.
113. Fairchild KD, Viscardi RM, Hester L, et al: Effects of hypothermia on cytokine production by cultured mononuclear phagocytes from adults and newborns. *J Interferon Cytokine Res* 20(12):1049, 2000.
114. McInerney J, Breakell A, Madira W, et al: Accidental hypothermia and active rewarming: the metabolic and inflammatory changes observed below and above 32°C. *Emerg Med J* 19:219, 2002.
115. Koren G, Barker C, Bohn D, et al: Influence of hypothermia on the pharmacokinetics of gentamicin and theophylline in piglets. *Crit Care Med* 13:844, 1985.
116. Rosin AJ, Exton-Smith AN: Clinical features of accidental hypothermia, with some observations on thyroid function. *BMJ* 1:16, 1964.
117. Fischbeck KH, Simon RP: Neurological manifestations of accidental hypothermia. *Ann Neurol* 10:384, 1981.
118. Hauty MG, Esrig BC, Hill JG, et al: Prognostic factors in severe accidental hypothermia: experience from the Mt. Hood tragedy. *J Trauma* 27:1107, 1987.
119. Lilly JK, Boland JP, Zekan S: Urinary bladder temperature monitoring: a new index of body core temperature. *Crit Care Med* 8:742, 1980.
120. Megarbane B, Axler O, Chary I, et al: Hypothermia with indoor occurrence is associated with a worse outcome. *Intensive Care Med* 26(12):1843, 2000.
121. Danzl DF, Hedges JR, Pozos RS: Hypothermia outcome score: development and implications. *Crit Care Med* 17:227, 1989.
122. Farstad M, Anderson KS, Koller ME, et al: Rewarming from accidental hypothermia by extracorporeal circulation—a retrospective study. *Eur J Cardiothorac Surg* 20:58, 2001.
123. Lexow K: Severe accidental hypothermia: survival after 6 hours 30 minutes of cardiopulmonary resuscitation. *Arctic Med Res* 50[Suppl]:112, 1991.
124. Giesbrecht GG, Sessler DI, Mekjavic IB, et al: Treatment of mild immersion hypothermia with direct body to body contact. *J Appl Physiol* 76:2373, 1994.
125. Bangs C, Hamelt M: Out in the cold: management of hypothermia, immersion and frostbite. *Top Emerg Med* 2:19, 1980.
126. Neufer PD, Young AJ, Sawka MN, et al: Influence of skeletal muscle glycogen on passive rewarming after hypothermia. *J Appl Physiol* 65:805, 1988.
127. 2005 American Heart Association Guidelines for emergency resuscitation and emergency cardiovascular care. *Circulation* 112:24[Suppl]:136–138, 2005.
128. Towne WD, Geiss WP, Yanes HO, et al: Intractable ventricular fibrillation associated with profound accidental hypothermia: successful treatment with partial cardiopulmonary bypass. *N Engl J Med* 287:1135, 1972.
129. Steinman AM: Cardiopulmonary resuscitation and hypothermia. *Circulation* 74:IV29, 1986.
130. DaVee TS, Reineberg EJ: Extreme hypothermia and ventricular fibrillation. *Ann Emerg Med* 9:100, 1980.
131. Nicodemus HF, Chaney RD, Herold R: Hemodynamic effects of inotropes during hypothermia and rapid rewarming. *Crit Care Med* 9:325, 1981.
132. Harari A, Regnier B, Rapin M, et al: Haemodynamic study of prolonged deep accidental hypothermia. *Eur J Intensive Care Med* 1:65, 1975.
133. Danzl DF, Sowers MB, Vicario SJ, et al: Chemical ventricular defibrillation in severe accidental hypothermia. *Ann Emerg Med* 11:698, 1982.
134. Dronen S, Nowak RM, Tomlanovich MC: Bretylium tosylate and hypothermic ventricular fibrillation. *Ann Emerg Med* 9:335, 1980.
135. Buckley JJ, Bosch OK, Bacaner MB: Prevention of ventricular fibrillation during hypothermia with bretylium tosylate. *Anesth Analg* 50:587, 1971.
136. Alexander L: *The Treatment of Shock from Prolonged Exposure to Cold, Especially in Water.* London, Combined Intelligence Objectives Subcommittee, APO 413, CIOS Item 24, HMSO, 1945.
137. Truscott DG, Frior WB, Clein LJ: Accidental profound hypothermia: successful resuscitation by core rewarming and assisted circulation. *Arch Surg* 106:216, 1973.
138. Dixon RG, Dougherty JM, White LJ, et al: Transcutaneous pacing in a hypothermic dog model. *Ann Emerg Med* 29:602, 1997.
139. Reeves RB: Temperature-induced changes in blood acid-base status: pH and PCO_2 in a binary buffer. *J Appl Physiol* 40:752, 1976.
140. Severinghaus JW: Respiration and hypothermia. *Ann N Y Acad Sci* 80:384, 1959.
141. Rhan H, Reeves RB, Howell BJ: Hydrogen ion regulation, temperature, and evolution. *Am Rev Respir Dis* 112:165, 1975.
142. Blayo MC, Lecompte Y, Pocidalo JJ: Control of acid-base status during hypothermia in man. *Respir Physiol* 42:287, 1980.
143. Ream AK, Reitz BA, Silverberg G: Temperature correction of PCO_2 and pH in estimating acid-base status: an example of the emperor's new clothes? *Anesthesiology* 56:41, 1982.
144. Kroncke GM, Nichols RD, Mendenhall JT, et al: Ectothermic philosophy of acid-base balance to prevent fibrillation during hypothermia. *Arch Surg* 121:303, 1986.
145. Swain JA: Hypothermia and blood pH. *Arch Intern Med* 148:1643, 1988.
146. Malan A: Blood acid-base state at a variable temperature: a graphical representation. *Respir Physiol* 31:259, 1977.
147. Kelman GR, Nunn JF: Nomograms for correction of blood PO_2, PCO_2, pH, and base excess for time and temperature. *J Appl Physiol* 21:1484, 1966.
148. Brooks DK: The meaning of pH at low temperatures during extra-corporeal circulation. *Anaesthesia* 19:337, 1964.
149. Flynn MD, Mawson DM, Tooke JE, et al: Cyclical hypothermia: successful treatment with ephedrine. *J R Soc Med* 84:753, 1991.
150. Kloos RT: Spontaneous periodic hypothermia. *Medicine* 74:268, 1995.
151. Hudson LD, Conn RD: Accidental hypothermia: associated diagnoses and prognosis in a common problem. *JAMA* 227:37, 1974.
152. Guerin JM, Meyer P, Segrestaa JM: Hypothermia in diabetic ketoacidosis. *Diabetes Care* 10:801, 1987.
153. Lewis S, Brettman LR, Holzman RS: Infections in hypothermic patients. *Arch Intern Med* 141:920, 1981.
154. Carr ME Jr, Wolfert AI: Rewarming by hemodialysis for hypothermia: failure of heparin to prevent DIC. *J Emerg Med* 6:277, 1988.
155. Freeman RM: The role of magnesium in the pathogenesis of azotemic hypothermia. *Proc Soc Exp Biol Med* 137:1069, 1971.
156. Levy LA: Severe hypophosphatemia as a complication of the treatment of hypothermia. *Arch Intern Med* 140:128, 1980.
157. Ledingham IM, Mone JG: Treatment of accidental hypothermia: a prospective clinical study. *BMJ* 280:1102, 1980.
158. Sessler DI, Moayeri A: Skin surface warming: heat flux and central temperature. *Anesthesiology* 73:218, 1990.
159. Grange C, Clery G, Purcell G, et al: Evaluation of the Bair Hugger warming device. *Anaesth Intensive Care* 20:122, 1992.
160. Myers RA, Britten JS, Cowley RA: Quantitative aspects of therapy. *JACEP* 8:523, 1979.
161. Anderson S, Herbring BG, Widman B: Accidental profound hypothermia. *Br J Anaesth* 42:653, 1970.
162. Steele MT, Nelson MJ, Sessler DI, et al: Forced air speeds rewarming in accidental hypothermia. *Ann Emerg Med* 27(4):479, 1996.
163. Mittleman KD, Mekjavic IB: Effect of occluded venous return on core temperature during cold water immersion. *J Appl Physiol* 65:2709, 1988.
164. Hoskin RW, Melinyshyn MJ, Romet TT, et al: Bath rewarming from immersion hypothermia. *J Appl Physiol* 61:1518, 1986.
165. Sheaff CM, Fildes JJ, Keogh P, et al: Safety of 65°C intravenous fluid for the treatment of hypothermia. *Am J Surg* 172:52, 1996.
166. Hayward JS, Steinman AM: Accidental hypothermia: an experimental study of inhalation rewarming. *Aviat Space Environ Med* 46:1236, 1975.
167. Lloyd EL, Conliffe NA, Orgel H, et al: Accidental hypothermia: an apparatus for central rewarming as a first aid measure. *Scott Med J* 17:83, 1972.
168. Ledingham IM, Douglas IH, Rauth GS, et al: Central rewarming system for treatment of hypothermia. *Lancet* 1:1168, 1980.
169. Edwards HA, Benstead JG, Brown K, et al: Apparent death with accidental hypothermia. *Br J Anaesth* 42:906, 1970.
170. Johnson LA: Accidental hypothermia: peritoneal dialysis. *JACEP* 6:556, 1977.
171. Troelsen S, Rybro L, Knudsen F: Profound accidental hypothermia treated with peritoneal dialysis. *Scand J Urol Nephrol* 20:221, 1986.
172. Brunette DD, Sterner S, Robinson EP, et al: Comparison of gastric lavage and thoracic cavity lavage in the treatment of severe hypothermia in dogs. *Ann Emerg Med* 16:1222, 1987.
173. Winegard C: Successful treatment of severe hypothermia and prolonged cardiac arrest with closed thoracic cavity lavage. *J Emerg Med* 15(5):629, 1997.
174. Gregory JS, Bergstein JM, Aprahamian C, et al: Comparison of three methods of rewarming from hypothermia: advantages of extracorporeal blood warming. *J Trauma* 31:1247, 1991.
175. Gentilello LM, Cobean RA, Offner PJ, et al: Continuous arteriovenous rewarming: rapid reversal of hypothermia in critically ill patients. *J Trauma* 32:316, 1992.
176. Gentillello LM, Rifley WJ: Continuous arteriovenous rewarming: report of a new technique for treating hypothermia. *J Trauma* 31:1151, 1991.

177. Maresda L, Vasko JS: Treatment of hypothermia by extracorporeal circulation and internal rewarming. *J Trauma* 27:89, 1987.
178. Vretenar DF, Urschel JD, Parrot JC, et al: Cardiopulmonary bypass resuscitation for accidental hypothermia. *Ann Thorac Surg* 58:895, 1994.
179. Kornberger E, Mair P: Important aspects in the treatment of severe accidental hypothermia: the Innsbruck experience. *J Neurosurg Anesth* 8:83, 1996.
180. Roe CF, Goldberg MJ, Blair CS, et al: The influence of body temperature on early postoperative oxygen consumption. *Surgery* 60:85, 1966.
181. Jones HD, McLaren CA: Postoperative shivering and hypoxaemia after halothane, nitrous oxide and oxygen anesthesia. *Br J Anaesth* 37:35, 1965.
182. Goldberg MJ, Roe CF: Temperature changes during anesthesia and operations. *Arch Surg* 93:365, 1966.
183. Vaughn MS, Vaughn RW, Cork RC: Postoperative hypothermia in adults: relationship of age, anesthesia, and shivering to rewarming. *Anesth Analg* 60:746, 1981.
184. Flacke JW, Flacke WE: Inadvertent hypothermia: frequent, insidious, and often serious. *Anesthesia* 3:183, 1983.
185. Matamis D, Tsagourias M, Koletsos K, et al: Influence of continuous haemofiltration-related hypothermia on haemodynamic variables and gas exchange in septic patients. *Intensive Care Med* 20:43, 1994.
186. Morris RH, Kumar A: The effect of warming blankets on maintenance of body temperature of the anesthetized, paralyzed adult patient. *Anesthesiology* 36:408, 1972.
187. Kean M: A patient temperature audit within a theatre recovery unit. *Br J Nurs* 9(23):150, 2000.
188. Sessler DI: Mild perioperative hypothermia. *N Engl J Med* 336(24):1730, 1997.
189. Leslie K, Sessler DI: Perioperative hypothermia in the high risk surgical patient. *Best Pract Res Clin Anaesthesiol* 17(4):485, 2003.
190. Roe CF: Effect of bowel exposure on body temperature during surgical operations. *Am J Surg* 122:13, 1971.
191. Bay J, Nunn JF, Prys-Roberts C: Factors influencing arterial PO_2 during recovery from anesthesia. *Br J Anaesth* 40:398, 1968.
192. Pflug AE, Aasheim GM, Foster C, et al: Prevention of post-anaesthesia shivering. *Can Anaesth Soc J* 25:43, 1978.
193. Frank SM, Fleisher LA, Breslow MJ, et al: Perioperative maintenance of normothermia reduces the incidence of morbid cardiac events: a randomized clinical trial. *JAMA* 277:1127, 1997.
194. Schmied H, Kurz A, Sessler D, et al: Mild intraoperative hypothermia increases blood loss and allogeneic transfusion requirements following total hip arthroplasty. *Lancet* 347:289, 1996.
195. Kahn HA, Faust GR, Richard R, et al: Hypothermia and bleeding during abdominal aortic aneurysm repair. *Ann Vasc Surg* 8:6, 1994.
196. Slotman GJ, Jed EH, Burchard KW: Adverse effects of hypothermia in postoperative patients. *Am J Surg* 149:495, 1985.
197. Roizen MF, Sohn YJ, L'Hommedieu CS, et al: Operating room temperature prior to surgical draping: effect on patient temperature in recovery room. *Anesth Analg* 59:852, 1980.
198. Ott DE: Correction of laparoscopic insufflation hypothermia. *J Laparoendosc Surg* 1:183, 1991.
199. Leaman PL, Martyak GG: Microwave warming of resuscitation fluids. *Ann Emerg Med* 14:876, 1985.
200. Newton DE: The effect of anaesthetic gas humidification on body temperature. *Br J Anaesth* 47:1026, 1975.
201. Caldwell C, Crawford R, Sinclair I: Hypothermia after cardiopulmonary bypass in man. *Anesthesiology* 55:86, 1981.
202. Ciufo D, Dice S, Coles C: Rewarming hypothermic postanesthesia patients: a comparison between a water coil warming blanket and a forced-air warming blanket. *J Post Anesth Nurs* 10:309, 1995.
203. MacKenzie MA, Herman AR, Wollersheim HC, et al: Thermoregulation and afterdrop during hypothermia in patients with poikilothermia. *Q J Med* 86:205, 1993.
204. Taguchi A, Arkilic CF, Ahluwalia A, et al: Negative pressure rewarming vs. forced hot air warming in hypothermic postanaesthetic volunteers. *Anesth Analg* 92(1):261, 2001.
205. Geisbrecht GG, Ducharme MB, McGuire JP: Comparison of forced-air patient warming systems for perioperative use. *Anesthesiology* 80:671, 1994.
206. Ouellette RG: Comparison of four intraoperative warming devices. *AANA J* 61:394, 1993.
207. Glosten B, Hynson J, Sessler DI, et al: Preanesthetic skin-surface warming reduces redistribution hypothermia caused by epidural block. *Anesth Analg* 77:488, 1993.
208. Camus Y, Delva E, Sessler DI, et al: Pre-induction skin-surface warming minimizes intraoperative core hypothermia. *J Clin Anesth* 7:384, 1995.
209. Just B, Trevien V, Delva E, et al: Prevention of intraoperative hypothermia by preoperative skin-surface warming. *Anesthesiology* 79:214, 1993.
210. Russell SH, Freeman JW: Prevention of hypothermia during orthotopic liver transplantation: comparison of three different intraoperative warming methods. *Br J Anaesth* 74:415, 1995.
211. Ireland KW, Follette DM, Iguidbashian J, et al: Use of a heat exchanger to prevent hypothermia during thoracic and thoracoabdominal aneurysm repairs. *Ann Thorac Surg* 55:534, 1993.
212. Dalili H, Andriani J: Effects of various blood warmers on the components of bank blood. *Anesth Analg* 53:125, 1974.
213. Hachimi-Idrissi S, Corne L, Ebinger G, et al: Mild hypothermia induced by a helmet device: a clinical feasibility study. *Resuscitation* 51:275–281, 2001.
214. Bernard SA, Gray TW, Buist MD, et al: Treatment of comatose survivors of out of hospital cardiac arrest with induced hypothermia. *N Engl J Med* 346:557–563, 2002.
215. HACA Investigators: Mild therapeutic hypothermia to improve neurologic outcome after cardiac arrest. *N Engl J Med* 346:549–556, 2002.
216. Sagalyn E, Band RA, Gaieski DF, et al: Therapeutic hypothermia after cardiac arrest in clinical practice: review and compilation of recent experiences. *Crit Care Med* 37(7):S223–S226, 2009.
217. Stertz F, Safar P, Tisherman SA, et al: Mild hypothermic cardiopulmonary resuscitation improves outcome after cardiac arrest in dogs. *Crit Care Med* 19:379–389, 1991.
218. American Heart Association: 2005 Guidelines for cardiopulmonary resuscitation and emergency cardiovascular care. *Circulation* 112:IV1–IV203, 2005.
219. Bernard S: Hypothermia after cardiac arrest: expanding the therapeutic scope. *Crit Care Med* 37(7):S227–S233, 2009.
220. Parham W, Edelstein K, Unger B, et al: Therapeutic hypothermia for acute myocardial infarction: past, present, and future. *Crit Care Med* 37(7):S234–S237, 2009.
221. Dietrich WD: Therapeutic hypothermia for spinal cord injury. *Crit Care Med* 37(7):S238–S242, 2009.
222. Linares G, Mayer AS: Hypothermia for the treatment of ischemic and hemorrhagic stroke. *Crit Care Med* 37(7):S243–S249, 2009.
223. Stravitz RT, Larsen FS: Therapeutic hypothermia for acute liver failure. *Crit Care Med* 37(7):S258–S264, 2009.
224. Fukodome EY, Alam HB: Hypothermia in multisystem trauma. *Crit Care Med* 37(7):S265–S272, 2009.
225. Seder DB, Van der Kloot TE: Methods of cooling: practical aspects of therapeutic temperature management. *Crit Care Med* 37(7):S211–S222, 2009.
226. Sundgreen C, Larsen FS, Herzog TM, et al: Autoregulation of cerebral blood flow in patients resuscitated from cardiac arrest. *Stroke* 32:128–132, 2001.
227. Sirvent JM, Torres A, El-Ebiary M, et al: Protective effect of intravenously administered cefuroxime against nosocomial pneumonia in patients with structural coma. *Am J Respir Crit Care Med* 155:1729–1734, 1997.
228. Bergman R, Tjan DH, Adriaanse MW, et al: Unexpected fatal neurological deterioration after successful cardio-pulmonary resuscitation and therapeutic hypothermia. *Resuscitation* 76:142–145, 2008.
229. Oddo M, Frangos S, Milby A, et al: Induced normothermia attenuates cerebral metabolic distress in patients with aneurysmal subarachnoid hemorrhage and refractory fever. *Stroke* 40:1913–1916, 2009.
230. Jordan K: Nonconvulsive status epilepticus in acute brain injury. *J Clin Neurophysiol* 16:332–340, 1999.
231. Polderman KH, Rijnsburger ER, Peerdeman SM, et al: Induction of hypothermia in patients with various types of neurological injury with use of large volumes of ice cold intravenous fluid. *Crit Care Med* 33:2744–2751, 2005.
232. Kliegel A, Janata A, Wandaller C, et al: Cold infusions alone are effective for induction of therapeutic hypothermia but do not keep patients cool after cardiac arrest. *Resuscitation* 73:46–53, 2007.
233. The Hypothermia after Cardiac Arrest Study Group: Mild therapeutic hypothermia to improve the neurologic outcome after cardiac arrest. *N Engl J Med* 346:549, 2002.
234. Janata A, Weihs W, Bayegan K, et al: Thermosuit after prolonged cardiac arrest in pigs. *Resuscitation* 69:145, 2006.
235. Simosa HF, Peterson DJ, Agarwal SK, et al: Increased risk for deep vein thrombosis with endovascular cooling in patients with traumatic head injury. *Am Surg* 73:461–464, 2007.
236. Badjatia N: Celsius control system. *Neurocrit Care* 1:201–203, 2004.

CHAPTER 66 ■ DISORDERS OF TEMPERATURE CONTROL PART II: HYPERTHERMIA

M. KATHRYN STEINER, FREDERICK J. CURLEY AND RICHARD S. IRWIN

This chapter reviews the pathobiology, pathophysiology, diagnosis, differential diagnosis, and treatment of four major hyperthermic syndromes—heat stroke, malignant hyperthermia, neuroleptic malignant syndrome, and drug-induced hyperthermia. Establishing the correct diagnosis and promptly instituting specific therapy are essential to management as mortality rises with any delay in treatment.

HEAT STROKE

Heat stroke is a syndrome of acute thermoregulatory failure in warm environments characterized by central nervous system (CNS) depression, core temperatures usually above 40°C, and typical biochemical and physiologic abnormalities. Most cases of heat stroke occur in youths exercising in the sun, especially military recruits and athletes, or in elderly or ill patients during severe heat waves. Mortality in some series is as high as 70% [1]. During a warm summer in the United States, approximately 4,000 deaths may occur as a direct result of heat stroke [2–4].

Causes and Pathogenesis

Heat stroke may be subclassified by its two distinct clinical presentations: exertional and nonexertional (classic, heat stroke). Exertional heat stroke is typically seen in younger individuals exercising at higher than normal ambient temperatures. The thermoregulatory mechanisms are intact, but overwhelmed by the thermal challenge of the environment and the great increase in endogenous heat production. Nonexertional heat stroke occurs in the elderly or sick individuals during a heat wave. Patients frequently have some impairment of thermoregulatory control, and temperatures rise easily with increased thermal challenge.

The causes of heat stroke fall into two categories (Table 66.1): increased heat production and impaired heat loss.

Increased Heat Production

Endogenous heat production during exertion ranges from 300 to 900 kcal per hour. Even in conditions favoring the maximal evaporation of sweat, only 500 to 600 kcal per hour of heat may be lost. Endogenous heat production may also be increased by fever, thyrotoxicosis, or the hyperactivity associated with amphetamine and hallucinogen use. In these conditions of increased thermogenesis, especially during maximal exercise, a healthy individual with intact regulatory mechanisms may develop hyperthermia.

Impaired Heat Loss

Schizophrenic, comatose, senile, or mentally deficient patients are at increased risk of heat stroke when ambient temperatures are high, owing to impaired voluntary control [5,6]. These patients may fail to perceive a temperature rise and take appropriate action. Impermeable clothing in hot environments has a great reduction in evaporative heat loss and individuals may suffer heat stroke [7,8].

Acclimatization increases heat tolerance by increasing cardiac output; decreasing peak heart rate; and increasing stroke volume. This lowers the threshold necessary to induce sweating; increases the volume of sweating; and, via an increase in aldosterone, expands extracellular volume and minimizes sweat sodium loss [9,10]. However, unacclimatized individuals who do not mount an adaptive response are at increased risk of suffering exertional heat stroke [11].

Dehydration and impaired cardiovascular performance increases the risk of heat stroke due to a decrease in skin or muscle blood flow, thus decreasing the movement of heat from the core to the environment [10,12]. Hypokalemia increases the risk of heat stroke by decreasing muscle blood flow, impairing cardiovascular performance, and possibly decreasing sweat gland function [9,10]. Adequate fluid intake and maintenance of a normal vascular volume prevents heat stroke. Heat load places a stress on the cardiovascular system and produces hyperthermia in patients with cardiovascular dysfunction. In one report, 75% of patients with compensated cardiac failure developed overt heart failure and temperatures up to 38.0°C after as little as 4 hours' exposure to temperatures of 32.2°C. Respiratory rate, blood pressure, and central venous pressure (CVP) also tended to rise [13].

Many drugs are known to predispose to heat stroke. Anticholinergic drugs such as phenothiazines, butyrophenones, thiothixenes, and anti-Parkinson's medications reduce sweat activity [14]). Barbiturate overdose may produce sweat gland necrosis [10]. Diuretics promote dehydration and hypokalemia. Beta-blockers may increase the risk of heat stroke because of cardiodepression. Alcohol consumption may increase the risk of heat stroke 15-fold because of dehydration secondary to antidiuretic hormone inhibition and inappropriate vasodilation [6].

Skin disorders that impair sweat gland function, such as cystic fibrosis and chronic idiopathic anhydrosis, predispose to heat stroke [15]. Hypothalamic lesions impair thermoregulation. During the early stages of heat stroke, the hypothalamus regulates autonomic responses to limit hyperthermia to occur. In the later stages, after thermal toxicity has occurred, hypothalamic regulation is impaired [16]. Anhydrosis has been reported in up to 100% of heat stroke victims in some series [17]. The hypothalamic set point may be elevated. The exact cause of hypohidrosis remains unclear and may reflect hypothalamic dysfunction or only the secondary effects of dehydration and cardiovascular collapse. Electron microscopic studies of eccrine sweat glands in a patient with fatal exertional heat stroke show changes suggestive of sweat gland fatigue [18]. Heat stroke can, however, occur in individuals who perspire profusely, indicating that sweat gland malfunction is not the only factor contributing to the pathogenesis of the syndrome.

TABLE 66.1

CAUSES OF HEAT STROKE

Increased heat production	
	Exercise
	Fever
	Thyrotoxicosis
	Amphetamines
	Hallucinogens
Impaired heat loss	
	High ambient temperature or humidity
	Ineffective voluntary control
	Lack of acclimatization
	Dehydration
	Cardiovascular disease
	Hypokalemia
Drugs	
	Anticholinergics
	Phenothiazines
	Butyrophenones
	Thiothixenes
	Barbiturates
	Anti-Parkinson's agents
	Diuretics
	Beta-blockers
	Alcohol
Debilitating conditions	
	Skin diseases
	Cystic fibrosis
	Central nervous system lesions
	Older age

The increased risk of heat stroke in the elderly is predominantly due to a decreased ability to sweat and a compromised cardiovascular response to heat exposure when compared with younger individuals [8,19]. In one report, 84% of elderly patients showed no evidence of sweating at the time heat stroke was diagnosed [20]. Elderly patients are more likely to have deficient voluntary control, poor acclimatization, and they take drugs that adversely affect thermoregulation.

Pathophysiology

The primary injury in heat stroke is due to the direct cellular toxicity of temperatures above 42°C, the *critical thermal maximum* [21]. Cell function deteriorates owing to cessation of mitochondrial activity, alterations in chemical bonds involved in enzymatic reactions, and cell membrane instability. This toxic effect may account for the widespread organ damage seen in all three of the major hyperthermic syndromes [22].

Heat stress activates numerous cytokines that modulate the body's response to increased temperature [23]. In most cases, the inflammatory response in heat stroke parallels that seen in heat stress from exertion. Tumor necrosis factor α, interleukin-(IL)1β, IL-2, IL-6, IL-8, IL-10, IL-12, and interferon gamma are typically increased in heat stroke. IL-6 is activated in the muscles and modulates inflammatory response by controlling cytokine levels and hepatic production of acute phase proteins. Endotoxemia from bacterial translocation of an ischemic gut further exacerbates the inflammatory response. Endothelial injury activates the coagulation cascade, promoting a prothrombotic state. Heat shock proteins are transcribed in response to heat stress and act in the brain to induce tolerance to heat stress [24].

Dehydration, metabolic acidosis, and local hypoxia alter the pathophysiologic consequences and clinical presentation of each of the hyperthermic syndromes. For example, classic heat stroke may occur with relatively little metabolic acidosis because no exertion was involved in its onset; however, it may be associated with more pronounced dehydration due to the gradual rise in temperature and prolonged sweating. Exertional heat stroke, alternatively, may be accompanied by a severe metabolic acidosis and hypoxia due to muscular exercise. It is typically associated with a more normal volume status because the onset of temperature elevation is abrupt.

Muscle Effects

Muscle degeneration and necrosis occur as a direct result of high temperatures. Muscle damage is more severe in exertional heat stroke owing to the local increases in heat, hypoxia, and metabolic acidosis associated with exertion. Significant muscle enzyme elevation and severe rhabdomyolysis are extremely common in exertional heat stroke [12,25,26] but rare in classic heat stroke [27].

Cardiac Effects

Cardiac output is increased [28] due to increased demands and low peripheral vascular resistance secondary to vasodilation and dehydration. Dehydration frequently results from sweat rates that may easily reach 1.5 to 2.0 L per hour during episodes of heat stroke [29]. CVP is initially elevated [30].

Hypotension occurs commonly as a result of high-output failure or temperature-induced myocardial hemorrhage and necrosis with subsequent cardiac depression and failure [9,12,31]. Tachyarrhythmias are frequent. Postmortem specimens show focal myocytolysis, myocyte necrosis, and hemorrhage in subepicardial, intramuscular, subendocardial, or intravalvular tissues [32].

Central Nervous System Effects

Direct thermal toxicity to brain and spinal cord rapidly produces cell death, cerebral edema, and local hemorrhage. These may lead to profound stupor or coma, almost universal features of all the hyperthermic syndromes. Seizures secondary to edema and hemorrhage are not uncommon. Because Purkinje cells of the cerebellum are particularly sensitive to the toxic effects of high temperatures, ataxia, dysmetria, and dysarthria may be seen acutely and in survivors of hyperthermia [10,33]. Progressive cerebellar atrophy has been documented by computed tomography and magnetic resonance imaging [34]. Lumbar punctures in classic and exertional heat stroke may reveal increased protein levels, xanthochromia, and a slight lymphocytic pleocytosis [12,20]. Survivors of severe heat stroke may show premature cataract formation, considered to be secondary to dehydration [35]. Up to 33% of survivors of heat stroke have at least moderate neurologic impairment after discharge from the hospital [36].

Renal Effects

Renal damage occurs in nearly all hyperthermic patients; it is potentiated by dehydration, cardiovascular collapse, and rhabdomyolysis. In classic heat stroke, acute renal failure occurs on average in 5% of patients as a result of dehydration [9]. In exertional heat stroke, acute renal failure occurs in up to 35% of cases [9,31]. Dehydration, pigment load, hypoperfusion, and urate nephropathy are thought to contribute to a clinical picture of acute tubular necrosis [31]. Other features include low serum osmolarity, moderate proteinuria, active sediment, and characteristic machine-oil appearance of the urine. In one series, the incidence of acute tubular necrosis increased with survival time [32]. Hypocalcemia and creatine phosphokinase values above 10,000 U per L increase the risk of acute renal failure [37]. Respiratory alkalosis is common in mild hyperthermia with metabolic acidosis predominating at temperatures greater than 41°C [24].

Gastrointestinal Tract Effects

The combination of direct thermotoxicity and relative hypoperfusion of the intestines during hyperthermia leads to ischemic intestinal ulcerations that may result in frank bleeding [9]. Hepatic necrosis and cholestasis occurs 2 to 3 days after hyperthermic insult, and 5% to 10% of cases result in death [10].

Hematologic Effects

White blood cell counts are elevated owing to catecholamine release and hemoconcentration. Anemia and a bleeding diathesis [29] are present due to (a) direct inactivation of platelets and bleeding factors by the heat, (b) a decrease in coagulation factor synthesis owing to liver failure, (c) a decrease in platelet and megakaryocyte counts, (d) platelet aggregation [38], and (e) disseminated intravascular coagulation (DIC). Megakaryocyte counts are reduced in up to 50% of specimens, and surviving megakaryocytes are morphologically abnormal [32]. DIC is present in most cases of fatal hyperthermia [32,39], most frequently appearing on the 2nd or 3rd day after hyperthermic insult. It is thought to be due to activation of the clotting cascade by vascular endothelial damage and generalized cell necrosis [40]. In cases of DIC, cardiac, CNS, pulmonary, gastrointestinal (GI) tract, and renal complications are exacerbated. An increase in blood viscosity of up to 24% has been postulated to facilitate thromboses [41].

Endocrine Effects

Hypoglycemia may occur in severe exertional heat stroke due to metabolic exhaustion [26]. In milder heat stroke, hyperglycemia and elevations of serum cortisol have been reported [42]. Although in autopsies the adrenal glands frequently show pericortical hemorrhages, survivors show little evidence of adrenal dysfunction [22,31]. Growth hormone and aldosterone levels actually increase abruptly during severe, acute heat exposure and are thought to act to preserve volume.

Electrolyte Effects

Hyperthermia produces frequent imbalances in potassium, sodium, phosphate, and calcium levels [29,43]. In heat stroke, sweating involves the active excretion of potassium from the body, producing normal to low serum potassium levels and slightly decreased total body potassium concentrations. In cases of exertional heat stroke with severe cell injury, potassium levels may be extremely elevated owing to cell lysis. Although mild hypophosphatemia occurs frequently as a result of intracellular trapping and possible parathyroid hormone resistance, phosphate levels may decrease to less than 1 mg per 100 mL in cases of hyperthermia with severe rhabdomyolysis [43]. Calcium values may fall 2 to 3 days after cellular injury owing to intracellular precipitation. In patients with severe tissue injury rebound, hypercalcemia may occur 2 to 3 weeks after hyperthermia as a result of parathyroid hormone activation [43].

Pulmonary Effects

Direct thermal injury to the pulmonary vascular endothelium may lead to cor pulmonale or acute respiratory distress syndrome. This and the tendency toward myocardial dysfunction make pulmonary edema common. Increased oxygen demands and acidosis frequently produce a respiratory alkalosis. Metabolic acidosis is, however, the most common acid–base disorder [44].

Diagnosis

Heat stroke is usually readily suggested by history and physical examination, and the diagnosis confirmed by recording a rectal temperature above 40°C. The temperature of any individual found comatose during a heat wave should be taken. Any laborer or athlete displaying incoordination followed by stupor and collapse while exercising in the heat should be assumed to have heat stroke until proven otherwise. Because more than 6 million workers in the United States experience occupational heat stress [8], a history of the exact events precipitating collapse may be helpful.

Heat stroke should be expected in any patient exercising in hot weather or in susceptible individuals during heat waves (see Table 66.1). Coma or profound stupor is nearly always present, but the other traditional criteria of anhidrosis and core temperature above 41°C may be absent. Although anhidrosis occurs in 84% of elderly patients with classic heat stroke [20], profuse sweating is typically present in exertional heat stroke [10]. Thus, the presence of anhidrosis is helpful, but its absence is not. Likewise, by the time the patient receives medical care, the temperature may have fallen significantly owing to cessation of exertion, removal from a hot environment, or cooling measures undertaken during transport. Most patients do have a temperature above 40°C, however. Because the level of serum creatine kinase is almost always elevated, the authors believe diagnostic criteria for heat stroke should include (a) a core temperature above 40°C, (b) severely depressed mental status or coma, (c) elevated serum creatine kinase level, and (d) compatible historical setting.

Classic heat stroke occurs more frequently when ambient peak temperatures exceed 32°C and minimum temperatures do not fall below 27°C. The risk is greater in urban areas, where minimum temperatures may exceed that in surrounding communities by more than 5°C [3]. Death rates during these heat waves may exceed twice the normal rates, and heat stroke deaths usually lag behind peak temperatures by approximately 24 hours. More than 80% of heat stroke victims are older than 65 years [20,40]. Other major high-risk groups are schizophrenics, patients with parkinsonism, alcoholics, and paraplegics or quadriplegics [45,47].

Exertional heat stroke may be seen when ambient temperatures are in the 25°C range, but more frequently it occurs at higher temperatures. Exertional heat stroke is frequently seen in military recruits during basic training [11,26], amateur football players [10,48], and marathon runners [49–52]. Miners and others who labor in hot local environments are also at high risk [31]. Heat stroke remains the second leading cause of death in athletes, second only to injuries of the head and spinal cord [9].

Differential Diagnosis

Several publications outline an approach to fever in the critically ill patient [53,54]. Table 66.2 lists the common causes of hyperthermia. Hyperthermia and coma may occur with hypothalamic injury, severe infection, or endocrinopathy [55]. Hypothalamic tumors or hemorrhage may produce hyperthermia by elevating the regulated temperature set point and may be distinguished from heat stroke by the constancy of the temperature and associated defects, such as diabetes insipidus and

TABLE 66.2

DIFFERENTIAL DIAGNOSIS OF HYPERTHERMIA

Hyperthermic syndromes
Exertional heat stroke
Nonexertional heat stroke
Malignant hyperthermia
Neuroleptic malignant syndrome
Drug-induced hyperthermia/serotonin syndrome
Infection
Meningitis
Encephalitis
Sepsis
Endocrinopathy
Thyroid storm
Pheochromocytoma
Central nervous system
Hypothalamic bleed
Acute hydrocephalus

anhidrosis, which may be unilateral [56]. Meningitis and encephalitis usually lack the characteristic enzyme elevations and may be distinguished by lumbar puncture.

Treatment

Primary Therapy of Hyperthermia

Primary therapy includes cooling and decreasing thermogenesis. Some cooling may be achieved in the field by moving the victim to a shaded, cooler area; removing the clothes; constantly wetting the skin; and fanning or transport in an open vehicle to create a breeze. Once the victim reaches hospital, cooling and subsequent supportive care are best provided in an intensive care setting.

Cooling by evaporative or direct external methods has proved effective. Evaporative cooling methods involve placing a nude patient in a cool room, wetting the skin with water, and encouraging evaporation by using fans. In one specially designed evaporative cooling unit, patients were sprayed with 15°C water and their skin fanned at 30 times per minute with air heated to 45°C to 48°C. Temperature reduction was rapid and mortality was 11% [57]. There was no mortality in 25 patients with nonexertional heat stroke treated with cooling by covering with a cool, wet, 20°C sheet and fanning with two 35-cm electric fans. Fanning was adjusted to maintain skin temperature at 30°C to 32°C; skin temperature fell 1°C every 11 minutes [58]. In 14 patients with nonexertional heat stroke, there was one death when evaporative/convective cooling was employed. The median time to return to temperature less than 39.4°C was 60 minutes.

Direct external cooling involves immersing the patient in ice water or packing the patient in ice. Ice water immersion with massage has been effective with little complication [59]. Colder water cools more rapidly (up to 0.35°C per minute), with one study demonstrating that 2°C water cooled volunteers twice as rapidly than 8°C water [60]. Because cold skin temperatures produce vasoconstriction, however, constant massage may be necessary to allow circulation to carry heat from the core. Direct external cooling is highly effective but makes patient monitoring and management extremely inconvenient. Therefore, some authors advocate evaporative cooling as a safer cooling method in patients at high risk of cardiovascular collapse [52]. As comparative studies of cooling techniques use different water temperatures for immersion and different evaporative cooling protocols, there is no consensus on which technique is superior. In most cases, treatment will be determined by what resources are immediately available. The Israeli Defense Forces protocol involves moving the collapsed patient to the shade, removing clothing, splashing the skin with water while fanning, and transport to hospital in an open vehicle. These measures yielded a cooling rate of 0.11°C per minute [61]. The US Marine Corps protocol calls for covering the patient with sheets covered with ice and then fanning the patient. This has had no mortalities in 200 cases and has reduced temperatures to below 39°C in 10 to 40 minutes [62].

In rare instances in which evaporative and direct external cooling methods fail to reduce the temperature, peritoneal lavage with iced saline cooled to 20°C or 9°C, gastric lavage, or hemodialysis or cardiopulmonary bypass with external cooling of the blood may be necessary to reduce the temperature. Temperature should be continuously monitored and cooling stopped as it approaches 39°C. Although chlorpromazine in an intravenous (IV) dose of 10 to 25 mg has been advocated to prevent shivering during cooling, it is usually unnecessary. Cooling blankets, although commonly used, are extremely ineffective and are not recommended [63]. Dantrolene has been shown to be ineffective in reducing hospitalization rate in heat stroke [64], and although it may improve cooling rate, it did not alter mortality [65].

Therapy for Complications of Hyperthermia

Arrhythmias, metabolic acidosis, and cardiogenic failure complicate the early management of hyperthermic crises. Supraventricular tachyarrhythmias usually require no treatment because they respond to restoration of normal temperature and metabolism. Digitalis should be avoided owing to the likelihood of hyperkalemia.

Hypotension should be treated initially with normal saline and, if necessary, isoproterenol. Dopaminergic and α-agonists should be avoided because they tend to produce peripheral vasoconstriction. Volume expansion with dextran is contraindicated owing to its anticoagulating effect. Pulmonary artery and arterial catheter monitoring may be helpful in the management of hypotension because patients frequently have low peripheral resistance, dehydration, and impaired cardiac function and are at a high risk for congestive heart and renal failure. As 64% of patients may have a normal central venous pressure before resuscitation, volume expansion in most cases should be guided by intravascular pressure monitoring where available [66]. Seizures, quite common in heat stroke, usually respond to diazepam.

Blood gas status should be determined early in treatment. Blood gases drawn at temperatures above 39°C should be corrected for temperature, although to our knowledge no studies have demonstrated that this is clinically necessary. The solubility of oxygen and carbon dioxide increases as blood drawn from the patient is cooled to 37°C for analysis. This lowers the carbon dioxide and oxygen tensions and elevates the pH when compared with values present in the patient. Therefore, the patient is more acidotic and less hypoxic than the uncorrected values indicate. Normal values of intracellular pH and changes on the body's buffering system in hyperthermia have been poorly described. Because normal values for blood gases in hyperthermic patients are unavailable, by convention the blood gas values are corrected for temperature, using any reliable nomogram, and clinical decisions are made as if the patient were euthermic [67–69]. The following approximate corrections have been used: for each 1°C that the patient's temperature is above 37°C, the oxygen tension is increased by 7.2%, carbon dioxide (CO_2) tension increased by 4.4%, and pH is lowered by 0.015 units. More research is needed before definite conclusions can be made. Nevertheless, 100% oxygen should be delivered until adequate oxygenation is ensured. Bicarbonate should be administered, guided by frequently obtained arterial blood gas values. The base deficit is frequently large, and up to 30 g of bicarbonate has been required for correction. Comatose patients should have prophylactic intubation to protect their airways from aspiration.

Urine output should be closely monitored with an indwelling bladder catheter. Patients should be routinely given 1 to 2 mg per kg of mannitol over 15 to 20 minutes to promote continued urine flow and possibly decrease cerebral edema. Continuous urine output should then be maintained with intermittent doses of furosemide. In all cases of hyperthermia, serum potassium levels should be closely followed. In cases of oliguria or potential renal failure, polystyrene sulfonate should be given early because hyperkalemia frequently increases.

Moderate-to-severe liver failure is common, may prolong illness, and, in combination with renal failure, may make administration of several drugs difficult or impossible. Although no clinical data are yet available, histamine receptor type 2 (H_2)–blocking drugs or proton pump inhibitors given prophylactically may decrease the incidence of GI tract bleeding.

The occurrence of DIC greatly affects mortality: Most patients who die of heat stroke have evidence of DIC [70]. Coagulation parameters such as prothrombin time, partial thromboplastin time, platelet count, and fibrinogen should be carefully followed. Should DIC occur, traditional recommendations for treatment should be followed (see Chapter 108).

The use of steroids and prophylactic antibiotics are not recommended [20,26]. Steroids are of no known benefit in heat stroke. Infection has not been reported as a major cause of morbidity and mortality in hyperthermia, and antibiotics are associated with superinfections.

Prognosis

Morbidity and mortality are directly related to the peak temperature reached and time spent at elevated temperatures. A delay in treatment of only 2 hours may result in the likelihood of death up to 70% [11,52]. When heat stroke is swiftly recognized and aggressively treated, mortality should be minimal. For example, in one series of 15 patients with exertional heat stroke, all were successfully treated with no mortality and little morbidity [11]. Another study predicts mortality of only 5% when heat stroke patients are managed properly [10]. A recent review of 34 elderly patients with classic heat stroke revealed 18% mortality. Seventy-three percent recovered without sequelae, and 9% had some residual neurologic deficit.

Although patients with temperatures as high as 46.5°C have survived without sequelae [71], mortality is increased with premorbid debility and higher maximal temperatures [44]. When ventricular fibrillation, DIC, coma lasting more than 6 to 8 hours, or high lactate levels complicate hyperthermia, mortality is predictably increased. A continued rise in growth hormone levels despite therapy has been reported to be associated with a worse prognosis [72].

With respect to morbidity, neurologic function usually rapidly returns to normal after restoration of euthermia; however, some patients may be left with a mild cerebellar disorder [73]. Hepatic and renal failure in mild and moderate cases is usually completely resolved. Moderate muscle weakness may persist for several months in patients with severe muscle damage.

Although it has not been proven, patients who have experienced hyperthermic crises should be considered at high risk to develop a recurrence on exposure to similar heat stresses and should be advised accordingly.

MALIGNANT HYPERTHERMIA

Malignant hyperthermia is a drug- or stress-induced hypermetabolic syndrome characterized by vigorous muscle contractions, an abrupt increase in temperature, and subsequent cardiovascular collapse. Malignant hyperthermia occurs, on average, in 1 of every 50,000 to 150,000 adult patients given anesthesia [71,74]. With treatment, mortality is between 10% and 30% [75].

Cause and Pathogenesis

The cause of the temperature increase in malignant hyperthermia is similar to that of exertional heat stroke: Increased thermogenesis overwhelms the patient's ability to dissipate heat. When exposed to various drugs, muscles may develop sustained or repeated contractions (Table 66.3). Current evidence indicates that patients with malignant hyperthermia have a defect in calcium metabolism in skeletal muscle cell membranes [76–79]. In most cases, a defect in the ryanodine receptor (RYR1) results in release of calcium from the sarcoplasmic reticulum, resulting in muscle contraction and heat generation [80]. Heat production occurs due to sustained or repetitive muscular contractions with hydrolysis of adenosine triphosphate and the activation of catabolic pathways, hepatic and muscular glycogenolysis, and catecholamine-induced accelerated turnover of substrates and metabolism of lactate.

Although halothane and succinylcholine are involved in more than 80% of cases, malignant hyperthermia has developed after the use of many other agents as well (see Table 66.3). Stress, excitement, anoxia, viral infections, and lymphoma have also been reported to trigger malignant hyperthermia [81,82]. Some data suggest that conditions of ischemia or hypoxia are the common triggers to hyperthermia in susceptible individuals. It is generally assumed that the causes of heat stroke would also increase the likelihood of malignant hyperthermia in susceptible individuals (see Table 66.1).

TABLE 66.3

DRUGS AND MALIGNANT HYPERTHERMIA

Drugs known to trigger malignant hyperthermia
Halothane
Methoxyflurane
Enflurane
Succinylcholine
Decamethonium
Gallamine
Diethyl ether
Ethylene
Ethyl chloride
Trichloroethylene
Ketamine
Phencyclidine
Cyclopropane
Drugs generally considered safe for patients with malignant hyperthermia
Nitrous oxide
Barbiturates
Diazepam
Tubocurarine
Pancuronium, vecuronium
Opiates

The hyperthermic reaction to anesthetics is not allergic in nature; patients may have received the same anesthetic previously or may be exposed later without developing a reaction. There is little evidence that impaired heat dissipation or altered hypothalamic regulation is instrumental in producing acute hyperthermia in these patients. However, sympathetic activity and heat dissipation may be abnormal during exercise [83].

Pathophysiology

Direct thermal injury is the predominant cause of toxicity in malignant hyperthermia. Damage results from the metabolic consequences of a sudden increase in temperature to levels frequently above 42°C. Physiologic and pathologic changes parallel those described for patients with exertional heat stroke [84]. DIC, hepatic failure, seizures, ventricular dysrhythmias, and electrolyte abnormalities are more common and severe than in heat stroke.

Vigorous muscle contracture at the onset of malignant hyperthermia almost immediately precipitates a severe metabolic acidosis, with increased CO_2 production and compensatory hyperventilation. High elevations of creatine kinase, lactate dehydrogenase, and aldolase are present [65] and reflect ongoing rhabdomyolysis. Hyperkalemia follows within minutes to hours [76]. Renal failure frequently occurs in malignant hyperthermia, most likely secondary to pigment load. Dehydration and low cardiac output do not contribute until later. The degree of hypocalcemia, hypophosphatemia, and hyperkalemia varies with the duration and peak of hyperthermia and degree of secondary myonecrosis. All three are more severe in malignant hyperthermia than in heat stroke. Direct thermal injury producing cerebral edema and cerebral hemorrhage results in coma. Seizures occur in most uncontrolled cases. DIC is a nearly universal finding [85]. Initially, volume status is normal because little volume has been lost in sweat. Cardiac output increases to meet metabolic demands and in response to the vasodilation of muscle beds. Sinus tachycardia, supraventricular tachyarrhythmias, and ventricular fibrillation occur soon after temperature exceeds 40°C. Tissue hypoxia, acidosis, and hyperkalemia make ventricular arrhythmias common. Because higher maximal temperatures are usually seen in malignant hyperthermia, hepatic failure and GI tract bleeding are more prominent than in heat stroke [85]. In survivors, hepatic necrosis and cholestasis peak in 2 to 3 days and may be severe.

Diagnosis

The metabolic predisposition to malignant hyperthermia appears, in general, to be inherited in an autosomal dominant fashion, with variable penetrance and expressivity. Although multiple screening strategies have been attempted [76,86–89], tests using caffeine or halothane stimulation of excised muscle are the standard screening tests recommended by the Malignant Hyperthermia Association of the United States [90]. Their false-positive rate is near 10% and false-negative rate near zero [91]. Because there is no one noninvasive test suitable for screening the general population, screening of family members of proven cases remains the best method of identifying susceptible individuals before hyperthermic crisis occurs. RYR1 gene mutation analysis of cells from buccal samples may help identify high-risk individuals. Only 25% of those susceptible have an identified mutation. Although an identified mutation would suggest susceptibility, the absence of a mutation would not rule out susceptibility [92,93].

Although malignant hyperthermia may occur under any severe stress, it most commonly follows administration of an anesthetic agent. Malignant hyperthermia occurs at any age but is most frequent in young patients; the mean age is 22 years, 65% of patients are male, 21% have had previous uneventful anesthesia, and 76% have no family history of malignant hyperthermia [94,95]. Early signs of hyperthermic crisis vary with the anesthetic agent administered but include masseter muscle contracture after the administration of succinylcholine, muscle rigidity, sinus tachycardia, supraventricular tachyarrhythmias, mottling or cyanosis of the skin, increased CO_2 production, and hypertension. Hyperthermia is typically a late sign in an acute crisis, but it may be rapidly followed by hypotension, acidosis, peaked T-waves on the electrocardiogram owing to hyperkalemia, and malignant ventricular arrhythmias [85]. In one case report, desaturation measured by oximetry preceded temperature elevation by 40 minutes [96].

Two signs may be helpful in making a prehyperthermic diagnosis: increased end-tidal CO_2 and masseter spasm [97–103]. Monitoring of end-tidal CO_2 is recommended for all anesthetic procedures and is mandatory for patients at risk of malignant hyperthermia [91,94,95]. Severe masseter spasm after succinylcholine has been recognized as an early warning sign of malignant hyperthermia; however, the decision to discontinue anesthesia in patients with succinylcholine-induced spasm remains controversial [100–104]. If surgery must be continued, dangerous triggering anesthetics should be avoided, dantrolene should be given or at least be immediately accessible, and temperature and end-tidal CO_2 should be monitored online.

Differential Diagnosis

Because malignant hyperthermia occurs almost exclusively in the perioperative setting, the differential diagnosis is more limited than that for heat stroke (see Table 66.2) [104]. Endocrinopathies and drug reactions, not infection, are the most frequent diseases in the differential diagnosis. Thyroid storm and pheochromocytoma may be very difficult to distinguish from malignant hyperthermia in the anesthetized patient [105]. Thyroid storm is now infrequent, owing to ease and extent of preoperative thyroid function test screening and prophylaxis of patients at risk. Dantrolene in doses used for malignant hyperthermia has been shown to decrease temperature in perioperative thyroid storm [106]. The temperature rise in pheochromocytoma is typically much slower than that in malignant hyperthermia [107]. Hyperthermia, owing to narcotic administration in patients taking monoamine oxidase inhibitors, also must be considered.

Treatment

Dantrolene, a hydantoin derivative, acts by uncoupling the excitation–contraction mechanism in skeletal muscle and lowering myoplasmic calcium. This action is now known to take place directly at the RYR1 receptor [108]. Dantrolene used for less than 3 weeks rarely causes toxicity [109]. In an acute crisis, 1.0 to 2.5 mg per kg of fresh dantrolene should be administered intravenously every 5 to 10 minutes. Effects may be seen 2 to 3 minutes after injection. Although cases that required 42 mg per kg have been reported [110], most authorities advise not to exceed 10 mg per kg [75,76,110,111]. The half-life of action is approximately 5 hours [76], and because relapse may occur, oral or IV dosages of 1 mg per kg IV or 2 mg per kg by mouth every 6 hours should continue for at least 24 to 48 hours [76]. Oral dantrolene provides excellent blood levels and may be substituted once the patient is alert [112]. With dantrolene, temperatures often rapidly decrease; without it, they may increase 1°C to 2°C every 15 minutes [95,97,110]. The cost of dantrolene is currently approximately $35 per 20-mg IV dose vial. As the diluent for dantrolene contains mannitol, urine output should be carefully monitored. Because even minute quantities of the triggering agent may continue to produce the syndrome, anesthesia should be immediately stopped, and the anesthesia apparatus, tubing, and ventilation equipment should be immediately changed.

Direct external cooling by submersion in ice water is helpful, but management of associated problems such as arrhythmia, arrest, and renal failure then becomes almost impossible. As with heat stroke, iced saline, gastric or peritoneal lavage, evaporative cooling, and infusion of chilled electrolyte solutions may be helpful. Aggressive management with cardiopulmonary bypass with external cooling of the blood may be necessary when dantrolene fails to slow down thermogenesis promptly [113]. When patients respond to therapy quickly, before severe temperature elevation occurs, only minimal supportive measures may be necessary. Once temperature exceeds 41°C, complications are widespread and patients frequently require long-term intensive care unit (ICU) support.

Ventricular fibrillation with subsequent cardiac collapse is the most common cause of death in the early stages of the syndrome. Procainamide should be given to all patients prophylactically as soon as malignant hyperthermia is diagnosed [76]. Procainamide acts to increase the uptake of calcium from the myoplasm directly and in early stages may help reduce hyperthermia. Administration of digitalis should be avoided because of the increased likelihood of hyperkalemia. Hypotension should be treated with saline infusion and isoproterenol. Avoid dopaminergic and α-agonists, as they reduce heat dissipation due to peripheral vasoconstriction. Seizures often occur in malignant hyperthermia. Prophylactic treatment with phenobarbital is strongly recommended because seizures may increase heat production, metabolic acidosis, and hypoxia. Arterial blood gas values should be adjusted for temperature, as noted for heat stroke. Mannitol and furosemide may be needed to promote continued urine output and may reduce the likelihood of cerebral edema and acute tubular necrosis. The serum potassium level increases over several hours and is treated with polystyrene sulfonates. Hepatic failure and DIC require supportive treatment. With prolonged supportive care, hepatic, renal, and neurologic functions typically normalize. Muscle weakness, however, may last for months.

Prognosis

With current management techniques, mortality resulting from malignant hyperthermia should be less than 30%. In one review, prompt dantrolene therapy in cases of confirmed malignant hyperthermia resulted in a 100% survival rate [25].

NEUROLEPTIC MALIGNANT SYNDROME

Neuroleptic malignant syndrome results primarily from an imbalance of central neurotransmitters, usually owing to neuroleptic drug use, and is characterized by hyperthermia, muscular rigidity, and altered consciousness. Most current knowledge is derived from case reports rather than systematic study. Since the syndrome was first described in 1968 [114], fewer than 3,000 cases have appeared in the world's literature, and most are from the 1980s and 1990s.

Retrospective studies estimated the incidence of neuroleptic malignant syndrome to be as high as 1% of all patients taking neuroleptic agents [115]. Prospective studies conducted in inpatient psychiatric hospitals have found incidences as low as 0% [116], 0.07% [117], 0.2% [118], and 0.9% [119]. The highest recent estimate of incidence was 2.2% [120]. Early estimates of mortality were as high as 30% [121]. Incidence also appears to be declining [122]. Mortality rate since 1986 has fallen to less than 12% [123]. Two prospective series reported 24 and 68 cases with mortality rates of 0% [124] and 5% [125], respectively.

The syndrome may be diagnosed in any patient with (a) an unexplained elevation in temperature, (b) muscular rigidity and characteristic extrapyramidal signs, and (c) a history of recent neuroleptic drug use. This liberal definition is more appropriate in the intensive care setting so that cases may not be underdiagnosed. A strict definition would require mental status changes and autonomic instability. Mental status changes, coma, and catatonia are common.

Cause and Pathogenesis

In all reports of neuroleptic malignant syndrome, patients received agents that decrease dopaminergic hypothalamic tone, or the syndrome appeared after withdrawal of dopaminergic agents (Table 66.4). Butyrophenones [126–140], phenothiazines [126,128,131,134,141,142], thioxanthenes [143–145], and dibenzoxazepines [146] are believed to act as dopamine receptor–blocking agents. Atypical antipsychotics, such as risperidone [147], molindone [148], clozapine [149], and fluoxetine [150], and dopamine blockers used to treat GI tract disease, such as metoclopramide and domperidone [151], have also caused the syndrome. The incidence of the syndrome with the newer atypical antipsychotics has not changed [152]. Drugs acting at the D_2 dopamine–binding sites appear to have the greatest potential for causing the syndrome. Most cases occur in patients taking butyrophenones or piperazines, agents with a high incidence of extrapyramidal reactions. The rate of increase in dose appears more important than the maximal

TABLE 66.4

DRUGS ASSOCIATED WITH THE ONSET OF NEUROLEPTIC MALIGNANT SYNDROME

Butyrophenones
Haloperidol
Bromperidol
Phenothiazines
Chlorpromazine
Levomepromazine
Trifluoperazine
Fluphenazine
Thioxanthenes
Thiothixene
Dibenzoxazepines
Loxapine
Dihydroindolones
Molindone
Flurooxypropylamincs
Fluoxetine
Tricyclic-dibenzodiazepines
Clozapine
Dopamine-depleting agents
Tetrabenazine
α-Methyltyrosine
Withdrawal of levodopa, carbidopa, amantadine
Domperidone
Metoclopramide

dose achieved [123]. Dopamine-depleting agents such as tetrabenazine and α-methyltyrosine produced neuroleptic malignant syndrome in a patient with Huntington's disease [121]. Abrupt withdrawal of levodopa (L-dopa), dopa-carbidopa, or amantadine produced the syndrome in patients suspected of having Parkinson's disease [153–155]. Initiation of metoclopramide therapy has produced the syndrome, presumably owing to alteration in central dopaminergic tone [156–158].

The increase in muscular rigidity, akinesia, mutism, and tremor are considered to be due to hypothalamic dopaminergic imbalance. Motor abnormalities vary, but in general, they are typical of the parkinsonian type extrapyramidal reactions. Unlike typical neuroleptic-induced side effects, however, the muscular effects are frequently seen at low therapeutic doses soon after treatment begins. The central origin of the muscle spasm is further suggested by its resolution with the use of centrally acting dopaminergic agents such as bromocriptine, amantadine, and L-dopa. A role for peripheral muscle abnormality, however, has been suggested, in that sarcoplasmic calcium concentration is higher in patients who have had the syndrome [125], hypocalcemia accompanies 54% of cases [124], the syndrome may resolve with nifedipine use [159], and the syndrome has been reported to be triggered by hypoparathyroidism [160].

Hyperthermia results from an increase in endogenous heat production, impaired heat dissipation, loss of voluntary temperature regulation, and possibly an elevation of the hypothalamic set point. The fact that the degree of temperature increase varies directly with the severity of rigidity evident on examination strongly suggests that muscle contracture is responsible for increased thermogenesis [126]. A decrease in muscle rigidity by uncoupling contraction with dantrolene or by paralysis with succinylcholine results in a decrease in temperature [161]. Impaired heat dissipation from the anticholinergic-induced hypohidrosis of neuroleptics may also occur. The high prevalence of diaphoresis and presumed dehydration in patients with neuroleptic malignant syndrome suggests, however, that this effect may be minimal. The most likely hypothesis is that regulatory reflexes remain intact, but muscle rigidity from hypothalamic influences and subsequent increased thermogenesis exceed dissipative capacity. In this sense, the syndrome is similar to malignant hyperthermia, in which regulatory mechanisms appear intact, but muscle contracture initiated at the level of the muscle, not the hypothalamus, overwhelms dissipative capacity.

Although the development of neuroleptic malignant syndrome is usually described as idiosyncratic, age, sex, and systemic factors appear to be important predisposing factors. The mean and median age at the onset of the syndrome is 40 years [162]. This is surprising because impairment in temperature regulation and the prevalence of parkinsonian side effects of neuroleptics both increase with age. Onset at an early age suggests that neuroleptic drugs are more frequently used in this age group or young persons are unusually sensitive to dopaminergic agents. Neuroleptic malignant syndrome develops 1.8 times more frequently in men than in women [162,163]. The larger muscle mass in men may predispose to the development of hyperthermia. There is, however, no difference in mean maximal temperature between men and women. A case control study has shown that environmental temperature does not affect the incidence of the neuroleptic malignant syndrome but several factors do: total neuroleptic dose, mental retardation, intramuscular administration of a neuroleptic, psychomotor agitation, or increasing dose or recent introduction of a neuroleptic drug [164].

Complications

Because of the relatively low maximal temperatures—39.9°C, on average [163]—in patients with neuroleptic malignant syndrome compared with those of patients with heat stroke and malignant hyperthermia, it is not surprising that direct thermal injury occurs less often. Only 40% of patients have temperatures above 40°C [165]. The complications of neuroleptic malignant syndrome are summarized in Table 66.5. Cardiovascular collapse, renal failure, and electrolyte abnormalities are less common and less severe than in classic heat stroke.

TABLE 66.5

COMPLICATIONS OF NEUROLEPTIC MALIGNANT SYNDROME

Rhabdomyolysis
Renal failure
Seizure
Cardiovascular collapse
Disseminated intravascular coagulation
Hepatic failure
Aspiration pneumonia
Respiratory failure
Death

Rhabdomyolysis, most probably secondary to hyperthermia and muscle rigidity, is frequently seen, with typical creatine kinase elevations in the range of 1,000 to 5,000 IU. Although rhabdomyolysis is usually mild, creatine kinase elevations to greater than 10,000 IU have been reported [145,166,167] and may occur in up to one third of patients [124]. Prolonged muscle weakness or dysfunction in survivors is not described.

Renal failure occurs in 9% to 30% of patients [124,162]. Proteinuria occurs in up to 91% of patients [124]. Renal failure is owing to myoglobin-induced acute tubular necrosis and the dehydration that results from diaphoresis. Renal dysfunction in most patients is transient and mild and, even in cases of acute tubular necrosis, may return to premorbid values after brief periods of dialysis support [129]. Mortality in renal failure patients, however, may be as high as 56% [123].

Neuroleptic malignant syndrome has been associated with worsening of underlying psychiatric conditions, amnesia, cognitive impairments, and peripheral neuropathy [168,169]. Coma is not uncommon in severe cases. Grand mal seizure has rarely been reported [129,144]. The electroencephalogram typically is normal or shows nonspecific diffuse slowing [124]. Computed tomography scans are normal in 95% of patients. Cerebrospinal fluid analysis after lumbar puncture is normal in 97% of patients, showing an elevated protein level in the other 3% [162,170]. In one case, a magnetic resonance imaging scan revealed hyperintensity of the occipitoparietal white matter [171]. Pathologic examinations of patients at autopsy revealed no specific lesions [154].

Although death from cardiovascular collapse has been reported [126], specific cardiac abnormalities have been poorly described. There is no evidence that severe atrophy, heart block, or congestive heart failure occurs frequently in the syndrome.

Hematologic alterations are mild. The white blood cell count is elevated in 78% of cases [124,162], usually less than 20,000 cells per mm^3, and rarely exceeding 25,000 cells per mm^3. Elevation may be due to hemoconcentration and catecholamine release. Platelet count is elevated in 56% of patients [124]. A hemolytic coagulopathy, possibly DIC, has been reported rarely [132]. Deep venous thrombosis or antemortem embolic phenomena are not reported in the English literature. Thrombotic events, when they do occur, may be a result of the patient's immobility due to coma and muscle rigidity rather than to any temperature-mediated change.

Lactate dehydrogenase, serum glutamic oxaloacetic acid transaminase, serum glutamic pyruvic transaminase, and alkaline phosphatase frequently show mild elevations compatible with rhabdomyolysis and mild hepatic dysfunction. Other significant GI tract abnormalities have not been reported.

Pulmonary complications occur frequently but appear to be related not to hyperthermia but to the extrapyramidal actions of the neuroleptics. Muscle dysfunction produces frequent dysphagia [126]. Sialorrhea can be copious and necessitate intubation [140]. It is reported that several patients have clearly aspirated, presumably owing to muscle dysfunction, and subsequent pneumonias were most likely due to this aspiration. Pneumonia and respiratory distress [131,132,134,140,145, 153,161,163,166] requiring intubation occur in 13% to 21% of patients [124,162] and are probably the most serious frequent sequelae of the neuroleptic malignant syndrome.

Diagnosis

The neuroleptic malignant syndrome may occur after any one of the commonly prescribed neuroleptic agents is used and in any age group. Onset of symptoms may occur within hours after the initial neuroleptic treatment or up to 4 weeks later [162]. In the majority of cases, onset occurs within 1 week from initial neuroleptic drug use, and 88% occur within 2 weeks of a dosage increase of an already prescribed neuroleptic agent [162]. Most reported cases have occurred in patients with underlying neuropsychiatric disorders. Most cases have a slow progression of symptoms over at least 24 to 48 hours and last 2 weeks after stopping the inciting drug [171].

Early symptoms usually include dysphagia or dysarthria owing to diffuse muscular rigidity, pseudoparkinsonism, dystonia, or catatonic behavior. In one series, 96% of patients demonstrated rigidity, 92% of patients demonstrated tremor, and 96% of patients demonstrated muteness or hypophonia in the 48 hours before diagnosis [124]. Rigidity precedes hyperthermia in 59% of patients, is concurrent in 23%, and is subsequent in only 8%. Changes in mental status or rigidity are the presenting symptoms in 82% of patients [172]. Autonomic signs of hypermetabolism usually suggest the onset of hyperthermia. Diaphoresis, tachycardia, changes in blood pressure, and tachypnea reflect efforts to dissipate the thermogenesis of muscle contracture and to expel CO_2 effectively. Peak temperatures are reached within 48 hours after the onset of symptoms in 88% of patients [124]. Temperatures may reach as high as 42.2°C [132] but are typically lower: 53% are more than 40°C and 13% are higher than 41°C [124]. Because many patients may be tachypneic, rectal or core, rather than oral, temperatures may need to be followed to ensure accuracy (see Chapter 26). Elevations in creatine kinase and transaminase levels and leukocytosis parallel the body temperature. Creatine kinase level is elevated in 97% to 100% of patients, typically all MM isoenzyme, exceeds 10,000 IU in 33% of patients, and peaks 2 to 3 days after diagnosis in 64% of patients and by 1 week in 93% of patients [124,163].

Differential Diagnosis

A thorough examination and diagnostic evaluation for other causes of hyperthermia should be conducted (see Table 66.2). In one series, all patients referred to an ICU with a suspicion of neuroleptic malignant syndrome had another diagnosis that would explain fever [119]. Because many patients taking neuroleptic agents develop extrapyramidal side effects and relatively few cases of hyperthermia are a result of neuroleptic malignant syndrome, other more common causes of hyperthermia (e.g., meningitis or streptococcal pharyngitis) could easily be missed if a hasty diagnosis of neuroleptic malignant syndrome is made. Appropriate cultures, chest radiograph, lumbar puncture, and thorough physical examination are mandatory. Patients without classic symptoms are more likely to have another cause of hyperthermia [173].

Catatonia, heat stroke, malignant hyperthermia, and hyperthermic reactions to other drugs may occasionally be confused with the neuroleptic malignant syndrome. Acute lethal catatonia presents with psychotic excitement and automatisms for a few weeks before motor deficit. Thus, in lethal catatonia, hyperactivity and hyperthermia present before the administration of neuroleptics [174]. However, lethal catatonia with rigidity and fatal hyperthermia rarely occurs in patients not taking neuroleptic agents. The treatment and prognosis of these patients remain unclear [163,175,176]. If rigidity and hyperthermia subsequently develop in a catatonic patient, however, the development of neuroleptic malignant syndrome should be presumed and all neuroleptic agents should be stopped. If catatonia has been induced or exacerbated by neurolepsis, withdrawal of the neuroleptic drug should aid in clarifying the diagnosis.

Heat stroke must be considered when temperature elevation develops in a patient taking neuroleptics during periods of high ambient temperature or after vigorous exercise. Unlike neuroleptic malignant syndrome, however, heat stroke is usually accompanied by flaccid obtundation, and muscle rigidity is rare.

Malignant hyperthermia resembles neuroleptic malignant syndrome in that both conditions have increased thermogenesis secondary to muscular rigidity as well as similar laboratory findings, and both respond to dantrolene. In most cases, an adequate history should clearly separate the two syndromes; hyperthermia results from the use of entirely different agents (compare Tables 66.3 and 66.4). Moreover, the symptoms of malignant hyperthermia are much more rapid in onset and more severe. Extrapyramidal symptoms are also very unusual in malignant hyperthermia. In the rare circumstance in which the two syndromes cannot be distinguished, attempts at paralysis with curare or pancuronium may aid diagnosis. These agents produce a flaccid paralysis in neuroleptic malignant syndrome but should have no effect on the postsynaptically medicated muscle contracture of malignant hyperthermia.

Idiosyncratic drug reactions and anaphylaxis accompanying severe hyperthermia may usually be diagnosed by their distinct clinical presentations. Monoamine oxidase inhibitors may produce hyperthermia, especially when administered with meperidine, linezolid, or dextromethorphan [177–180]. In patients with neuropsychiatric disorders who are receiving neuroleptic agents and monoamine oxidase inhibitors, malignant hyperpyrexia may result from either agent. In these cases, both agents should be stopped. Therapies for neuroleptic malignant syndrome, such as bromocriptine or L-dopa, are, however, contraindicated in these patients because of their recent use of monoamine oxidase inhibitors.

Treatment

The goal of treatment for neuroleptic malignant syndrome is to reduce the temperature, reverse extrapyramidal side effects, and prevent sequelae such as renal failure and pneumonia.

Specific agents used to decrease thermogenesis by reducing muscle contracture include dantrolene, curare, pancuronium, amantadine, bromocriptine, and L-dopa (Table 66.6). One study, however, showed no difference between patients receiving active treatment and those receiving only supportive care [181]. The only other controlled study demonstrated a shortened duration of symptoms and more rapid reduction in temperature when methylprednisolone (1 g in 2 days) was administered to Parkinson's patients who developed the

TABLE 66.6

TREATMENTS FOR NEUROLEPTIC MALIGNANT SYNDROME

Dantrolene
Paralysis (curare, pancuronium)
Bromocriptine
Amantadine
Levodopa
Electroconvulsive therapy

syndrome after withdrawal of medications [182]. Dantrolene reduces thermogenesis by uncoupling muscle contracture at the membrane level and in doses as small as 1 mg per kg may result in a temperature decrease of 1°C to 2°C within hours [135,136,140,183]. Dantrolene may also favorably alter CNS dopaminergic metabolism [184]. Although doses of up to 10 mg per kg have been used, current practice would recommend doses of 1.0 to 2.5 mg per kg IV every 6 hours until a dose of 100 to 300 mg per day by mouth can be given [185,186]. Paralysis with curare or pancuronium should produce a similar prompt decrease in temperature, but this treatment necessitates mechanical ventilation and extensive support [161]. Bromocriptine, amantadine, and dopamine increase central dopaminergic tone; this decreases the central drive, reducing muscular rigidity and thermogenesis. These agents also are beneficial in that they act directly to reduce extrapyramidal side effects. Prompt decreases in temperature have been reported after the use of 2.5 mg of bromocriptine three times per day [134,138,167,187], 100 or 200 mg of amantadine twice per day [139,188], or 10 to 100 mg of carbidopa/L-dopa three times per day [127,155].

Failures of these therapies, however, have also been published [141,143,153,187]. The appropriate dosing remains an important question. Some authorities have advocated bromocriptine doses as high as 60 mg per day [185]. Use of a centrally acting dopamine agonist is clearly warranted when the neuroleptic malignant syndrome is believed to occur because of the withdrawal of anti-Parkinson's agents. The use of dantrolene, bromocriptine, and amantadine has yet to be shown to reduce mortality significantly [123]. Electroconvulsive therapy has been successful in several patients [131,132,189,190] and is the only therapeutic modality that may be used successfully to treat simultaneously hyperthermia, the extrapyramidal side effects, and the underlying neuropsychiatric disorder for which the neuroleptic drug was prescribed. Because of several reports of cardiovascular collapse in patients undergoing electroconvulsive therapy, this therapy should be given only to patients at low risk of cardiovascular disease who have failed other therapy.

Less-specific agents, such as diphenhydramine, benztropine, diazepam, and trihexyphenidyl, have been used successfully [127,130,134,137,139,146] but more typically have not been substantially helpful [121,134,140,141,161,187,188]. Little has been published on the use or efficacy of nonspecific measures, such as acetaminophen [191], cooling blankets, iced saline gastric lavage, and cooled peritoneal dialysis. The usefulness of these methods, however, would be restricted simply to lowering body temperature; they would not be expected to inhibit the underlying ongoing drive to thermogenesis or extrapyramidal reactions.

Reduction in core temperature and muscle rigidity should decrease the risk of renal failure and pneumonia. Decreases in temperature are accompanied by a decrease in creatine kinase levels [126]. By minimizing rhabdomyolysis and aggressive hydration and diuresis, acute tubular necrosis and renal failure might be avoided. Early reversal of coma, dysphagia, and sialorrhea when present should minimize the risk of aspiration and subsequent pneumonia. Prophylactic intubation should be strongly considered for patients with excessive sialorrhea, swallowing dysfunction, or coma. All obtunded patients or those with swallowing difficulty should take nothing by mouth.

The best treatment regimen for neuroleptic malignant syndrome remains to be determined [124,162,192–197]. Because many patients respond to symptomatic treatment after withdrawal of neuroleptic therapy [181], and because all current knowledge is derived from case reports, not clinical trials, treatment recommendations are difficult to make. The average time to recovery with supportive care only is 9.6 days [165]. Treatment should be guided by clinical judgment. Because of the frequency of coma, renal failure, respiratory insufficiency, and cardiovascular collapse, patients with temperatures greater than 39°C should be initially evaluated and observed in the ICU. Treatment and close observation should be continued for at least 1 week, longer when necessary. The duration of symptoms varies with the rate of excretion of neuroleptic metabolites. In patients receiving long-acting neuroleptic agents such as fluphenazine, symptoms may last for weeks. When therapy is withdrawn, symptoms may recur up to and after 11 days of drug abstinence [187]. Therefore, the duration of treatment must be adjusted according to the metabolism of the inciting agent, but in most cases, it can be tapered over 1 to 2 weeks. Acetaminophen and cooling of IV solutions during the acute period produce few side effects and may be beneficial. Bromocriptine therapy appears safe and effective in reducing temperature and minimizing extrapyramidal reactions. Dantrolene therapy does carry a risk of hepatotoxicity, but in patients with temperatures greater than 40°C, its use is specific and should be beneficial. Electroconvulsive therapy should be considered only for patients who do not respond properly to bromocriptine, dantrolene, and supportive therapy. More aggressive interventions, such as paralysis, use of cooled dialysate, or cardiopulmonary bypass cooling, should be reserved for refractory life-threatening cases.

Prognosis

Although mortality rates as high as 20% to 30% have been reported [115], this rate can probably be reduced to less than 10% with appropriate support and treatment. Age and sex do not appear to influence mortality greatly. Mortality rate does appear to be influenced by peak temperature, inciting neuroleptic drug, and renal failure. No death among patients with maximal temperatures lower than 40°C has been reported. Haloperidol is statistically less likely to result in death than other neuroleptics [123]. Death has been reported as a result of cardiovascular collapse [126], pneumonia [131,161], renal failure [129,145], and hepatic failure [145]. More than 57 cases of acute renal failure due to neuroleptic malignant syndrome have been reported [198]. The development of renal failure is particularly ominous; in some series, 46% of patients with myoglobinuria and 56% of those with renal failure died [123].

Typically, ICU stay is prolonged owing to the frequency of complications and slow response to therapy. Although dopaminergic therapy lowers the mean time to response from 6.8 to 1.1 days [199], the mean time to recovery is long—13 days when the syndrome results from nondepot neuroleptics and 26 days for depot neuroleptics [162]. One patient receiving haloperidol decanoate was symptomatic for months [200]. Rechallenge with neuroleptics may cause the syndrome to recur, but this occurs much more frequently during the first 2 weeks [201,202]. The prognosis among survivors appears to be excellent, and sequelae other than mild extrapyramidal symptoms compatible with prior neuroleptic treatment appear unusual [203].

DRUG-INDUCED HYPERTHERMIA

Most of our knowledge about drug-induced hyperthermia is derived from case reports. Numerous drugs have been suggested to cause hyperthermia. Drugs that blunt cardiovascular performance, such as beta-blockers, or alter heat dissipation, such as chlorpromazine, are widely used and clearly can contribute to temperature elevation. These drugs rarely result in clinically significant hyperthermia without some other precipitant. Patients on regimens of such agents typically present with heat stroke. This section focuses on drugs that independently produce significant elevations of temperature (Table 66.7).

Commonly abused street drugs may result in severe hyperthermia without other pharmacologic or environmental stimuli. Temperature elevation accompanies phencyclidine use in 2.6% of cases [204]. Temperatures as high as 41.9°C have been reported [205]. Amphetamine use may result in temperatures higher than 43°C [205,206]. Although ecstasy (MDMA, 3,4-methylenedioxymethamphetamine) has resulted in fatal hyperthermia, use is usually associated with a more mild temperature elevation [207]. Hyperthermia (temperatures greater than 37.5°C) was more prevalent (36%) in patients admitted to emergency departments due to overdose of paramethoxyamphetamine than MDMA [208]. Although all these drugs have a low incidence of producing severe hyperthermia, owing to the prevalence of their use, they may account for a large percentage of cases of hyperthermia presenting to an emergency room.

Common prescription drugs that alter central serotonin levels and lysergic acid diethylamine, a serotonin analog, may result in hyperthermia greater than 41°C [209]. These drugs may produce a characteristic constellation of symptoms now known as the *serotonin syndrome* [209–214]. Monoamine oxidase inhibitors and selective serotonin reuptake inhibitors may produce hyperthermia, especially when administered with meperidine or dextromethorphan [177–179], a tricyclic antidepressant [177,215], or each other. Severe hyperthermia is rare. Increasingly combinations of drugs, which independently would not cause serotonin toxicity, act in concert to result in hyperthermia and the serotonin syndrome [216]. For example, a postoperative patient who receives linezolid, a weak monoamine oxidase inhibitor, and tramadol, a weak serotonin reuptake inhibitor, may present with fever, confusion, and clonus. Tramadol, meperidine, fentanyl, dextromethorphan, dextropropoxyphene, pentazocine, brompheniramine, chlorpheniramine, and linezolid in combination with other drugs may cause fever and the serotonin syndrome [180]. In addition, abrupt withdrawal of baclofen, especially after intrathecal administration, has resulted in severe sequelae including hyperpyrexia and potential multiorgan failure and death [180].

Aspirin receives mention as a cause of hyperthermia secondary to increased metabolism, but few hard data are available [217].

TABLE 66.7

DRUGS THAT MAY CAUSE HYPERTHERMIA AND/OR SEROTONIN SYNDROME

Monoamine oxidase inhibitors	
Phenelzine = Nardil	
Tranylcypromine = Parnate	
Linezolid	
Serotonin releasers	
Amphetamines	
Ecstasy (MDMA, 3,4-methylenedioxymethamphetamine)	
LSD	
Serotonin reuptake inhibitors SRI:	
Citalopram = Celexa	
	Fluoxetine = Prozac
	Fluvoxamine = Luvox
	Paroxetine = Paxil
	Sertraline = Zoloft
Tricyclics:	Clomipramine = Anafranil
	Imipramine – Tofranil
	Venlafaxine = Effexor
Analgesics:	Tramadol
	Methadone
	Dextromethorphan
	Dextropropoxyphene
	Pentazocine
	Chlorpheniramine
Antihistamines:	Brompheniramine
Other	Withdrawal of baclofen

Pathogenesis

These drugs are assumed to cause hyperthermia as a result of muscular contracture or hypermetabolism. Virtually all cases of drug-induced hyperthermia mention increased muscle tone, rigidity, or tremor. Cocaine, amphetamine, phencyclidine, and hallucinogens appear to produce hyperthermia by centrally and perhaps peripherally inducing vigorous muscle contractions [218,219]. Repeated cocaine use may elevate temperature by depletion of postsynaptic dopamine [218].

Many drugs such as tricyclics, amphetamines (paramethoxyamphetamine, MDMA), monoamine oxidase inhibitors, and the serotonin reuptake inhibitors may elevate CNS serotonin, resulting in hyperthermia [177,179,219–221]. Buspirone, serotonin agonists, lithium, and carbamazepine stimulate postsynaptic serotonin receptors. Monoamine oxidase inhibitors increase serotonin release and inhibit serotonin metabolism [222]. Selective serotonin reuptake inhibitors, dextromethorphan, and meperidine are believed to inhibit serotonin reuptake and, in susceptible patients, may increase already high serotonin levels and trigger a hyperthermic crisis [200]. In many patients, combination drug therapy contributes to triggering the syndrome. In general, a 2-week, drug-free period after stopping a monoamine oxidase inhibitor before starting a selective serotonin reuptake inhibitor is indicated. Any opiate may trigger the syndrome when another drug already predisposes the patient.

Some patients may have a component of exertional heat stroke, in that they are frequently found running in an agitated or confused manner. Almost all suffer from some loss of voluntary control of temperature. Status epilepticus frequently accompanies drug-induced hyperthermia but is unlikely to contribute greatly to hyperthermia, in that status epilepticus is rarely associated with significant temperature elevation in the absence of drug use [223]. Reactions appear mostly idiosyncratic; they are infrequent in comparison with the total number of persons using the drug; occur by IV, enteral, and nasal insufflation usage; and occur after low-dose use and massive overdose [224].

Pathophysiology

The pathophysiology of drug-induced hyperthermia is most similar to that of exertional heat stroke or malignant hyperthermia. In the serotonin syndrome, direct stimulation of the 5-HT1A and 5-HT2 receptors in the raphe nuclei may directly result in hyperthermia. Rise in temperature is frequently rapid, and multiple organ failure may rapidly ensue with prolonged elevation of temperature. Patients, however, may also be affected by the direct toxic action of the drug, and it may be difficult to separate the sequelae of hyperthermia from those of direct drug toxicity. Amphetamine overdose, for example, may result in severe rhabdomyolysis, DIC, and renal failure at temperatures of less than 40°C. Hyperthermia can be assumed to have the same physiologic sequelae in these patients as others, but prompt correction of temperature may not be adequate to ensure survival.

Diagnosis

In most case reports, patients are described as agitated, hyperexcited, and diaphoretic and have increased muscle tone. Because nonexertional heat stroke is uncommon in youth, hyperthermia at a young age always suggests possible drug intoxication. The diagnosis of drug-induced hyperthermia should be considered mostly when the patient is young, is an outpatient, has not engaged in recent heavy exertion, has a history of drug abuse, or is on a drug or combination of drugs that may result in the serotonin syndrome.

Patients with the serotonin syndrome typically display tremor, hyperreflexia, myoclonus, tachycardia, diarrhea, confusion, and diaphoresis [210–214]. Serotonin syndrome should be suspected and treated whenever patients have spontaneous clonus and are on a serotonergic agent. Nausea and diarrhea are atypical of the neuroleptic malignant syndrome and may help suggest the serotonin syndrome in complicated cases [225]. The onset of symptoms is within 2 hours of medication ingestion in 50% of cases and within 24 hours in 75% of cases [222]. Myoclonus or rigidity is present in 50% of cases, and mental status changes in 40% of cases. Severe hyperthermia occurs in approximately one third of cases [211]. Diagnosis may be confirmed by toxicologic screen or history.

Treatment

In all cases, treatment should be directed at minimizing the toxicity of the causative drug. Suspected offending drugs should be discontinued. Treatment of hyperthermia should be symptomatic and directed at the underlying physiology. Treatment in general parallels that for exertional heat stroke and is extensively outlined in that section. Evaporative cooling and external cooling with ice are the preferred methods of cooling and should be instituted in any patient with a temperature above 39°C. Many patients may be dehydrated from diaphoresis and require volume replacement. As in malignant hyperthermia and exertional heat stroke, hyperkalemia, acidosis, and myoglobinuria demand careful attention. Because the temperature appears to be generated from muscular contraction, paralysis or use of dantrolene would appear to be useful therapy. Paralysis has been effective in several cases. Paralysis and support with mechanical ventilation should be considered in any patient with a temperature above 40°C not responding promptly to symptomatic cooling. If therapeutic drug levels persist, rebound hyperthermia may occur as paralysis resolves.

When the serotonin syndrome is suspected, therapy with benzodiazepines, propranolol, 50 mg chlorpromazine, cyproheptadine, or postsynaptic serotonin blockers such as methysergide has been advocated, but clinical experience is minimal [218–220,226]. No study to date reports a systematic trial of therapy. As hyperthermia may be mediated by central serotonin receptors, doses of cyproheptadine high enough to block central receptors, 20 to 50 mg, should be considered [227]. One regimen advises 12 mg by mouth or nasogastric tube then 4 to 8 mg every 4 to 6 hours [216].

Prognosis

Hyperthermia owing to amphetamine overdose appears to be well tolerated, with 10 of 11 patients reported in the literature surviving [205,206,228,229]. Hyperthermia in cocaine overdose is frequently accompanied by renal failure [224,230,231], DIC [231,232], and seizure [231,232] and several fatalities [224,231–233] have been reported. Survival despite high temperature has been recorded as well [224,230,234]. Phencyclidine with hyperthermia has resulted in renal failure [235], respiratory and liver failure with coma, and subsequent death [236].

Death and serious morbidity due to the serotonin syndrome appear to be rare [208]. No large series involving significant hyperthermia have been reported, and death and cure with

TABLE 66.8

DISTINGUISHING CHARACTERISTICS OF THE HYPERTHERMIC SYNDROMES

	Heat stroke	Malignant hyperthermia	Neuroleptic malignant syndrome	Acute lethal catatonia	Serotonin syndrome
Inciting factor	Ambient temperature: max >32°C, min >27°C	Triggering anesthetic	Triggering neuroleptic or withdrawal of dopaminergic agent	Excitement and automatisms prior to neuroleptic use	Serotonin active drug(s)
Time to fever	Hours to days	Minutes	Hours to days	Weeks	Minutes to hours
Mental status	Obtunded	Anesthetized	Mute, stuporous	Excited transitioning to catatonia	Confused, agitated
Muscle tone	Flaccid	Rigid, spasm	Extrapyramidal rigid	Variable	Clonus, hyperreflexia, tremor, pyramidal rigidity
Temperature	>40°C	>40°C	>40°C in 40%		>40°C only when late in syndrome

max, maximum; min, minimum.

TABLE 66.9

ADVANCES IN MANAGEMENT OF HYPERTHERMIA BASED ON RANDOMIZED CONTROLLED TRIALS

- No randomized clinical trials have been conducted comparing the effectiveness of different cooling methods for any hyperthermic syndrome [237].
- Dantrolene sodium is ineffective in heat stroke [64]. Dantrolene did not alter survival in heat stroke [65].
- There are no other randomized studies involving the treatment of heat stroke or malignant hyperthermia or drug-induced hyperthermia.
- In neuroleptic malignant syndrome, treatment with dantrolene and bromocriptine may offer no advantage over supportive care [176].
- Solu-Medrol may benefit patients with neuroleptic malignant syndrome due to withdrawal from Parkinson's medications [182].

appropriate treatment have been reported [179]. As severe hyperthermia would likely signify a much more severe case than usual, the physician should always consider the patient at risk of death and ICU level care would always be warranted.

Table 66.8 compares the distinguishing characteristics of the hyperthermic syndromes. Advances in hyperthermia based on randomized, controlled trials or meta-analyses of such trials are given in Table 66.9.

HYPERTHERMIA AND FEVER CONTROL IN BRAIN INJURY

Fever in the neurocritical care is frequent and often results in an adverse outcome for all disease states. Morbidity and mortality is increased among patients who have ischemic brain injury, intracerebral hemorrhage, and cardiac arrest. Fever appears to have a longer impact after subarachnoid hemorrhage and traumatic brain injury. New techniques (see hypothermia chapter 65) have made treatment of fever and maintaining normothermia possible. There are, however, no prospective randomized trials to prove benefit of fever control in these patient populations. In addition, the indication and timing remain unknown. Prospective randomized controlled trials are needed to determine the beneficial impact of secondary injury prevention compared with the potential risks of prolonged fever control [238].

References

1. Gauss H, Meyer KA: Heat stroke: a report of 158 cases from Cook County Hospital, Chicago. *Am J Med Sci* 154:554, 1917.
2. Clowes GHA, O'Donnell TF: Heat stroke. *N Engl J Med* 291:564, 1974.
3. Ellis EP: Mortality from heat illness and heat-aggravated illness in the United States. *Environ Res* 5:1, 1972.
4. Heat stroke: United States, 1980. *MMWR Morb Mortal Wkly Rep* 30:277, 1981.
5. Wise TN: Heat stroke in three chronic schizophrenics: case reports and clinical considerations. *Compr Psychiatry* 14:263, 1973.
6. Kilbourne EM, Choi K, Jones S, et al: Risk factors for heat stroke: a case control study. *JAMA* 247:3332, 1982.
7. Cole RD: Heat stroke during training with nuclear, biological, and chemical protective clothing. Case report. *Mil Med* 148:624, 1983.
8. Fatalities from occupational heat exposure. *MMWR Morb Mortal Wkly Rep* 33:410, 1984.
9. Stine FJ: Heat illness. *JACEP* 8:154, 1979.
10. Knochel JP: Environmental heat illness: an eclectic review. *Arch Intern Med* 133:841, 1974.
11. O'Donnell TF: Acute heat stroke: epidemiologic, biochemical, renal, and coagulation studies. *JAMA* 234:824, 1975.
12. Shibolet S, Coll R, Gilat T, et al: Heat stroke: its clinical picture and mechanism in 36 cases. *Q J Med* 36:525, 1967.
13. Ansari A, Burch GE: Influence of hot environments on the cardiovascular system. *Arch Intern Med* 123:371, 1969.
14. Adams BE, Manoguerra AS, Lilja GP, et al: Heat stroke: associated with medications having anticholinergic effects. *Minn Med* 60:103, 1977.
15. Dann EJ, Berkman N: Chronic idiopathic anhydrosis: a rare cause of heat stroke. *Postgrad Med J* 68:750, 1992.
16. Chun-Jen S, Mao-Tsun L, Shih-Han T: Experimental study on the pathogenesis of heat stroke. *J Neurosurg* 60:1246, 1984.
17. Attia M, Khogali M, El-Khatib G: Heat stroke: an upward shift of temperature regulation set point at an elevated body temperature. *Int Arch Occup Environ Health* 53:9, 1983.
18. Baba N, Ruppert RD: Alteration of eccrine sweat gland in fatal heat stroke. *Arch Pathol* 85:669, 1968.
19. Sprung CL: Hemodynamic alterations of heat stroke in the elderly. *Chest* 75:361, 1979.
20. Levine JA: Heat stroke in the aged. *Am J Med* 47:251, 1969.
21. McElroy CR: Update on heat illness. *Top Emerg Med* 2:1, 1980.
22. Fajardo LF: Pathologic effects of hyperthermia in normal tissues. *Cancer Res* 44[Suppl]:4826S, 1984.
23. Bouchama A, Knockel J: Heat stroke. *N Engl J Med* 346:1978, 2002.
24. Bouchama A, De Vol EB: Acid base alterations in heat stroke. *Intensive Care Med* 27:680, 2001.
25. Vertel RM, Knochel JP: Acute renal failure due to heat injury: an analysis of 10 cases associated with the high incidence of myoglobinuria. *Am J Med* 43:435, 1967.
26. Costrini AM, Pitt HA, Gustafson AB, et al: Cardiovascular and metabolic manifestations of heat stroke and severe heat exhaustion. *Am J Med* 66:296, 1979.
27. Hart GR, Anderson RJ, Crumpler CP, et al: Epidemic classical heat stroke: clinical characteristics and course of 28 patients. *Medicine (Baltimore)* 61:189, 1982.
28. Dahmash NS, Al Harthi SS, Akhtar J: Invasive evaluation of patients with heat stroke. *Chest* 103:1210, 1993.
29. Knochel JP: Heat stroke and related heat disorders. *Dis Mon* 35:306, 1989.
30. Atar S, Rozner E, Rosenfeld T: Transient cardiac dysfunction and pulmonary edema in exertional heat stroke. *Mil Med* 168:671, 2003.
31. Kew MC, Abrahams C, Levin NW, et al: The effects of heat stroke on the function and structure of the kidney. *Q J Med* 36:277, 1967.
32. Malamud N, Haymaker W, Custer RP: Heat stroke: a clinicopathologic study of 125 fatal cases. *Mil Surg* 97:397, 1946.
33. Manto MU: Isolated cerebellar dysarthria associated with a heat stroke. *Clin Neurol Neurosurg* 98:55, 1996.
34. Grohan H, Hopkins PM: Heat stroke: implications for clinical care. *Br J Anaesth* 88:700, 2002.
35. Minassian DC, Mehra V, Jones BR: Dehydrational crises from severe diarrhea or heat stroke and risk of cataract. *Lancet* 1:751, 1984.
36. Dematte JE, O'Mara K, Buescher J, et al: Near-fatal heat stroke during the 1995 heat wave in Chicago. *Ann Intern Med* 129:173, 1998.
37. Shieh SD, Lin YF, Lu KC, et al: Role of creatine phosphokinase in predicting acute renal failure in hypocalcemic exertional heat stroke. *Am J Nephrol* 12:252, 1992.
38. Gader AM, Al-Mashhadani SA, Al-Harthy SS: Direct activation of platelets by heat is the possible trigger of coagulopathy of heat stroke. *Br J Haematol* 74:86, 1990.
39. Jones TS, Liang AP, Kilbourne EM, et al: Morbidity and mortality associated with the July 1980 heat wave in St. Louis and Kansas City, MO. *JAMA* 247:3328, 1982.
40. Bouchamma A, Hammami MM, Haq A, et al: Evidence for endothelial cell activation/injury in heat stroke. *Crit Care Med* 24:1173, 1996.
41. Keatinge WR, Coleshaw SR, Easton JC, et al: Increased platelet and red cell counts, blood viscosity, and plasma cholesterol levels during heat stress, and mortality from coronary and cerebral thrombosis. *Am J Med* 81:795, 1986.
42. Al-Harthi SS, Karrar O, Al-Mashhadani SA: Metabolite and hormonal profiles in heat stroke patients at Mecca pilgrimage. *J Intern Med* 228:343, 1990.
43. Knochel JP, Caskey JH: The mechanism of hypophosphatemia in acute heat stroke. *JAMA* 238:425, 1977.
44. Tucker CE, Stanford J, Graves B, et al: Classic heat stroke: clinical and laboratory assessment. *South Med J* 78:20, 1985.
45. Buck CW, Carscallen HB, Hobbs GE: Temperature regulation in schizophrenia. *Arch Neurol Psych* 64:828, 1950.
46. Litman RE: Heat stroke in parkinsonism. *Arch Intern Med* 89:562, 1952.
47. Randall WC, Wurster RD, Lewin RJ: Responses of patients with high spinal transection to high ambient temperatures. *J Appl Physiol* 21:985, 1966.
48. McLeod RN: Heat illness in early season football practice. *J Ky Med Assoc* 70:613, 1972.
49. Hanson PG, Zimmerman SW: Exertional heat stroke in novice runners. *JAMA* 242:154, 1979.

50. Rose RC, Hughes RD, Yarbrough DR, et al: Heat injuries among recreational runners. *South Med J* 73:1038, 1980.
51. Whitworth JAG, Wolfman MJ: Fatal heat stroke in a long distance runner. *Lancet* 1:545, 1984.
52. Wyndham CH: Heat stroke and hyperthermia in marathon runners. *Ann N Y Acad Sci* 301:128, 1977.
53. O'Donnell J, Axelrod P, Fischer C, et al: Use and effectiveness of hypothermia blankets for febrile patients in the intensive care unit. *Clin Infect Dis* 24(6):1214, 1997.
54. Marik PE: Fever in the ICU. *Chest* 117(3):855, 2000.
55. Talman WT, Florek G, Bullard DE: A hyperthermic syndrome in two subjects with acute hydrocephalus. *Arch Neurol* 45:1037, 1988.
56. Chesanow RL: A 65-year-old woman with heat stroke. *Am J Med* 41:415, 1961.
57. Khogali M, Weiner JS: Heat stroke: report on 18 cases. *Lancet* 2:276, 1980.
58. Al-Aska AK, Abu-Aisha H, Yaqub B, et al: Simplified cooling bed for heatstroke. *Lancet* 1:381, 1987.
59. Costrini A: Emergency treatment of exertional heatstroke and comparison of whole body cooling techniques. *Med Sci Sports Exerc* 22(1):15, 1990.
60. Proulx CL, Ducharme MB, Kenny GP: Effect of water temperature on cooling efficiency during hypothermia in humans. *J Appl Physiol* 94(4):1317, 2003.
61. Haddad E, Moran DS, Epstein Y: Cooling heat stroke patients by available field measures. *Intensive Care Med* 30(2):338, 2004.
62. Gaffin SL, Garner JW, Flinn SD: Cooling methods for heatstroke victims. *Ann Intern Med* 132(8):678, 2000.
63. O'Grady NP, Barie PS, Bartlett J, et al: Practice parameters for evaluating new fever in critically ill adult patients. *Crit Care Med* 26:392, 1998.
64. Bouchama A, Cafege A, Devol EB, et al: Ineffectiveness of dantrolene sodium in the treatment of heat stroke. *Crit Care Med* 19:176, 1991.
65. Channa AB, Seraj MA, Saddique AA, et al: Is dantrolene effective in heat stroke patients? *Crit Care Med* 18(3):290; 19(2):176, 1990.
66. Seraj MA, Channa AB, Al Harthi SS, et al: Are heat stroke patients volume depleted? Importance of monitoring central venous pressure as a simple guideline to therapy. *Resuscitation* 21:33, 1991.
67. Severinghaus JW: Respiration and hypothermia. *Ann N Y Acad Sci* 80:384, 1959.
68. Malan A: Blood acid base state at variable temperature, a graphical representation. *Respir Physiol* 31:259, 1977.
69. Kelman GR, Nunn JF: Nomograms for correction of blood Po_2, PCO_2, pH, and base excess for time and temperature. *J Appl Physiol* 21:1484, 1966.
70. Chao TC, Simniah R, Pakiam JE: Acute heat stroke deaths. *Pathology* 13:145, 1981.
71. Slovis CM, Anderson GF, Casolaro A: Survival in a heat stroke victim with a core temperature in excess of 46.5°C. *Ann Emerg Med* 11:269, 1982.
72. Alzeer A, Arifi A, el-Hazmi M, et al: Thermal regulatory dysfunction of growth hormone in classic heat stroke. *Eur J Endocrinol* 134:727, 1996.
73. Lee S, Merriam A, Skim TS, et al: Cerebellar degeneration in neuroleptic malignant syndrome: neuropathologic findings and review of the literature concerning heat-related nervous system injury. *J Neurol Neurosurg Psychiatry* 52:387, 1989.
74. Ali SZ, Taguchi A, Rosenberg H: Malignant hyperthermia. *Best Pract Res Clin Anaesthesiol* 17(4):519, 2003.
75. Aldrete JA: Advances in the diagnosis and treatment of malignant hyperthermia. *Acta Anaesthesiol Scand* 25:477, 1981.
76. Gronert GA: Malignant hyperthermia. *Anesthesiology* 53:395, 1980.
77. Michelson JR, Gallant EM, Litterer LA, et al: Abnormal sarcoplasmic reticulum ryanodine receptor in malignant hyperthermia. *J Biol Chem* 263:9310, 1988.
78. Wallace AJ, Woolridge W, Kingston HM, et al: Malignant hyperthermia: a large kindred linked to the RYR1 gene. *Anaesthesia* 51:16, 1996.
79. McCarthy TV, Healy JM, Heffron JJ, et al: Localization of the malignant hyperthermia susceptibility locus to human chromosome 19q12–13.2. *Nature* 343:562, 1990.
80. Denborough M: Malignant hyperthermia. *Lancet* 352:1131, 1998.
81. Schiller HH: Chronic viral myopathy and malignant hyperthermia. *N Engl J Med* 292:1409, 1975.
82. Tsueda K, Dubick MN, Wright BD, et al: Intraoperative hyperthermic crisis in two children with undifferentiated lymphoma. *Anesth Analg* 57:511, 1978.
83. Campbell IT, Ellis FR, Evans RT, et al: Studies of body temperatures, blood lactate, cortisol and free fatty acid levels during exercise in human subjects susceptible to malignant hyperpyrexia. *Acta Anaesthesiol Scand* 27:349, 1983.
84. Denborough MA: Etiology and pathophysiology of malignant hyperthermia. *Int Anesthesiol Clin* 7:11, 1979.
85. Steward DJ: Malignant hyperthermia: the acute crisis. *Int Anesthesiol Clin* 17:1, 1979.
86. Kalow W, Britt BA, Chan F-Y: Epidemiology and inheritance of malignant hyperthermia. *Int Anesthesiol Clin* 17:119, 1979.
87. Lutsky I, Witkowski J, Henschel EO: HLA typing in a family prone to malignant hyperthermia. *Anesthesiology* 56:224, 1982.
88. Harriman DGF: Preanesthetic investigations of malignant hypothermia: microscopy. *Int Anesthesiol Clin* 17:97, 1979.
89. Payen JF, Bosson JL, Bourdon L, et al: Improved noninvasive diagnostic testing for malignant hyperthermia: susceptibility from a combination of metabolites determined in vivo with 31P-magnetic resonance spectroscopy. *Anesthesiology* 78:848, 1993.
90. Britt BA: Preanesthetic diagnosis of malignant hyperthermia. *Int Anesthesiol Clin* 17:63, 1979.
91. Glisson SN: Malignant hyperthermia. *Compr Ther* 14:33, 1988.
92. Litman RS, Rosenberg H: Malignant hyperthermia: update on susceptibility screening. *JAMA* 293(23):2918, 2005.
93. Sei Y, Sambuughin NN, Davis E, et al: Malignant hyperthermia in North America: genetic screening of the three hot spots in the type 1 ryanodine receptor gene. *Anesthesiology* 101(4):824, 2004.
94. Strazis KP, Fox AW: Malignant hyperthermia: a review of published cases. *Anesth Analg* 72:297, 1993.
95. Felice-Johnson J, Sudds T, Bennett G: Malignant hyperthermia: current perspectives. *Am J Hosp Pharm* 38:646, 1981.
96. Bacon AK: Pulse oximetry in malignant hyperthermia. *Anaesth Intensive Care* 17:208, 1989.
97. Baudendistel L, Goudsouzian N, Cote C, et al: End tidal CO_2 monitoring: its use in the diagnosis and management of malignant hyperthermia. *Anesthesia* 39:1000, 1984.
98. Liebenschutz F, Mai C, Pickerodt VW: Increased carbon dioxide production in two patients with malignant hyperpyrexia and its control by dantrolene. *Br J Anaesth* 51:899, 1979.
99. Triner L, Sherman J: Potential value of expiratory carbon dioxide measurement in patients considered to be susceptible to malignant hyperthermia. *Anesthesiology* 55:482, 1981.
100. Badgwell JM, Heaver JE: Masseter spasm heralds malignant hyperthermia or merely academia gone mad? *Anesthesiology* 61:230, 1984.
101. Schwartz L, Rockoff MA, Koka BV: Masseter spasm with anesthesia: incidence and implications. *Anesthesiology* 61:772, 1984.
102. Flewellen E, Nelson TE: Halothane-succinylcholine induced masseter spasm: indicative of malignant hyperthermia susceptibility? *Anesth Analg* 63:693, 1984.
103. Ellis FR, Halsall PJ: Suxamethonium spasm: a differential diagnostic conundrum. *Br J Anaesth* 56:381, 1984.
104. Larach MG, Rosenberg H, Larach DR, et al: Prediction of malignant hyperthermia susceptibility by clinical signs. *Anesthesiology* 66:547, 1987.
105. Peters KR, Nance P, Wingard DW: Malignant hyperthyroidism or malignant hyperthermia? *Anesth Analg* 60:613, 1981.
106. Bennett MH, Wainwright AP: Acute thyroid crisis on induction of anaesthesia. *Anaesthesia* 44:28, 1989.
107. Crowley KG, Cunningham AJ, Conroy B, et al: Phaeochromocytoma: a presentation mimicking malignant hyperthermia. *Anaesthesia* 43:1031, 1988.
108. Nelson TE, Lin M, Zapata-Sudo G, et al: Dantrolene sodium can increase or attenuate activity of skeletal muscle ryanodine receptor calcium release channel. Clinical implications. *Anesthesiology* 84:1368, 1996.
109. Gallant EM, Ahern CP: Malignant hyperthermia: responses of skeletal muscles to general anesthetics. *Mayo Clin Proc* 58:758, 1983.
110. Blank JW, Boggs SD: Successful treatment of an episode of malignant hyperthermia using a large dose of dantrolene. *J Clin Anesth* 5:69, 1993.
111. Kolb ME, Horne ML, Martz R: Dantrolene in human malignant hyperthermia: a multicenter study. *Anesthesiology* 56:254, 1982.
112. Allen GC, Cattran CB, Peterson RG, et al: Plasma levels of dantrolene following oral administration in malignant hyperthermia-susceptible patients. *Anesthesiology* 69:900, 1988.
113. Ryan JF, Donlon JV, Malt RA, et al: Cardiopulmonary bypass in the treatment of malignant hyperthermia. *N Engl J Med* 290:1121, 1974.
114. Delay J, Deniker P: Drug-induced extrapyramidal syndromes, in Vinken PJ, Bruyn GW (eds): *Diseases of the Basal Ganglia*. Amsterdam, the Netherlands, North Holland Publishing Company, 1968, p 248.
115. Caroff SN: The neuroleptic malignant syndrome. *J Clin Psychiatry* 41:79, 1980.
116. Modestin J, Toffler G, Drescher JP: Neuroleptic malignant syndrome: results of a prospective study. *Psychiatry Res* 44:251, 1992.
117. Gelenberg AJ, Bellinghausen B, Wojcik JD, et al: A prospective survey of neuroleptic malignant syndrome in a short-term psychiatric hospital. *Am J Psychiatry* 145:517, 1988.
118. Friedman JH, Davis R, Wagner RL: Neuroleptic malignant syndrome: the results of a 6-month prospective study of incidence in a state psychiatric hospital. *Clin Neuropharmacol* 11:373, 1988.
119. Keck PE Jr, Pope HG Jr, McElroy SL: Frequency and presentation of neuroleptic malignant syndrome: a prospective study. *Am J Psychiatry* 144:1344, 1987.
120. Hermesh H, Aizenber D, Weizman A, et al: Risk for definite neuroleptic malignant syndrome: a prospective study of 223 consecutive inpatients. *Br J Psychiatry* 161:254, 1992.
121. Burke RE, Fahn S, Mayeaux R, et al: Neuroleptic malignant syndrome caused by dopamine-depleting drugs in a patient with Huntington's disease. *Neurology (NY)* 31:1022, 1981.
122. Keck PE, Pope HG, McElroy SL: Declining frequency of neuroleptic malignant syndrome in a hospital population. *Am J Psychiatry* 148:880, 1991.
123. Shalev A, Hermesh H, Munitz H: Mortality from neuroleptic malignant syndrome. *J Clin Psychiatry* 50:18, 1989.
124. Rosebush PI, Stewart TD: A prospective analysis of 24 episodes of neuroleptic malignant syndrome. *Am J Psychiatry* 146:717, 1989.
125. Lopez JR, Sanchez V, Lopez MJ: Sarcoplasmic ionic calcium concentration in neuroleptic malignant syndrome. *Cell Calcium* 10:223, 1989.

126. Itoh H, Ohtsuka N, Ogita K, et al: Malignant neuroleptic syndrome: its present status in Japan and clinical problems. *Folia Psychiatr Neurol Jpn* 31:565, 1977.
127. Stoudemire A, Luther JS: Neuroleptic malignant syndrome and neuroleptic induced catatonia: differential diagnosis and treatment. *Int J Psychiatry Med* 14:57, 1984.
128. Oppenheim G: Mutism and hyperthermia in a patient treated with neuroleptics. *Med J Aust* 2:228, 1973.
129. Eiser AR, Neff MS, Slifkin RF: Acute myoglobinuric renal failure: a consequence of the neuroleptic malignant syndrome. *Arch Intern Med* 142:601, 1982.
130. Geller B, Greydanus DE: Haloperidol induced comatose state with hyperthermia and rigidity in adolescence: two case reports with a literature review. *J Clin Psychiatry* 40:102, 1979.
131. Jesse SS, Anderson GF: ECT in the neuroleptic malignant syndrome: case report. *J Clin Psychiatry* 44:186, 1983.
132. Eles GR, Songer JE, DiPette DJ: Neuroleptic malignant syndrome complicated by disseminated intravascular coagulation. *Arch Intern Med* 144:1296, 1984.
133. Liskow BI: Relationship between neuroleptic malignant syndrome and malignant hyperthermia. *Am J Psychiatry* 142:390, 1985.
134. Mueller PS, Vester JW, Fermaglich J: Neuroleptic malignant syndrome: successful treatment with bromocriptine. *JAMA* 249:386, 1983.
135. May DC, Morns SW, Stewart RM, et al: Neuroleptic malignant syndrome: response to dantrolene sodium. *Ann Intern Med* 98:183, 1983.
136. Coons DJ, Hillman FJ, Marshall RW: Treatment of neuroleptic malignant syndrome with dantrolene sodium: a case report. *Am J Psychiatry* 139:944, 1982.
137. Feibel JM, Schiffer RB: Sympathoadrenal medullary hyperactivity in the neuroleptic malignant syndrome: a case report. *Am J Psychiatry* 138:1115, 1981.
138. Dhib-Jalbut S, Messelbrock R, Brott T, et al: Treatment of the neuroleptic malignant syndrome with bromocriptine. *JAMA* 250:484, 1983.
139. Amdurski S, Radwan M, Levi A, et al: A therapeutic trial of amantadine in haloperidol-induced malignant neuroleptic syndrome. *Curr Ther Res* 33:225, 1983.
140. Goulon M, de Rohan-Chabot P, Elkharrat D, et al: Beneficial effects of dantrolene in the treatment of neuroleptic malignant syndrome: a report of two cases. *Neurology* 33:516, 1983.
141. Tollefson GD, Garvey MJ: The neuroleptic syndrome and central dopamine metabolites. *J Clin Psychopharmacol* 4:150, 1984.
142. Lew T, Tollefson G: Chlorpromazine-induced neuroleptic malignant syndrome and its response to diazepam. *Biol Psychiatry* 18:1441, 1983.
143. Downey GP, Rosenberg M, Carroff S, et al: Neuroleptic malignant syndrome patient with unique clinical and physiologic features. *Am J Med* 77:338, 1984.
144. McAllister RG: Fever, tachycardia and hypertension with acute catatonic schizophrenia. *Arch Intern Med* 138:1154, 1978.
145. Weinberg S, Twersky RS: Neuroleptic malignant syndrome. *Anesth Analg* 62:848, 1983.
146. Tollefson G: A case of neuroleptic malignant syndrome: in vitro muscle comparison with malignant hyperthermia. *J Clin Psychopharmacol* 2:266, 1982.
147. Bonwick RJ, Hopwood MJ, Morris PL: Neuroleptic malignant syndrome and risperidone: a case report. *Aust N Z J Psychiatry* 30:419, 1996.
148. Gradon JD: Neuroleptic malignant syndrome possibly caused by molindone hydrochloride. *Ann Pharmacother* 25:1071, 1991.
149. Anderson ES, Powers PS: Neuroleptic malignant syndrome associated with clozapine use. *J Clin Psychiatry* 52:102, 1991.
150. Halman M, Goldbloom DS: Fluoxetine and neuroleptic malignant syndrome. *Biol Psychiatry* 28:518, 1990.
151. Spirt MJ, Chan W, Thieberg M, et al: Neuroleptic malignant syndrome induced by domperidone. *Dig Dis Sci* 37:946, 1992.
152. Anath J, Parameswaran S, Gunatilake S, et al: Neuroleptic malignant syndrome and atypical antipsychotic drugs. *J Clin Psychiatry* 65:464, 2004.
153. Henderson VW, Wooten GF: Neuroleptic malignant syndrome: a pathogenetic role for dopamine receptor blockade? *Neurology (NY)* 31:132, 1981.
154. Sechi GP, Tanda F, Mutani R: Fatal hyperpyrexia after withdrawal of levodopa. *Neurology* 34:249, 1984.
155. Toru M, Matsuda O, Makiguchi K, et al: Neuroleptic malignant syndrome-like state following withdrawal of anti-parkinsonian drugs. *J Nerv Ment Dis* 1969:324, 1981.
156. Patterson JF: Neuroleptic malignant syndrome associated with metoclopramide. *South Med J* 81:674, 1988.
157. Samie MR: Neuroleptic malignant-like syndrome induced by metoclopramide. *Mov Disord* 2:57, 1987.
158. Friedman LS, Weinrauch LA, D'Elia JA: Metoclopramide-induced neuroleptic malignant syndrome. *Arch Intern Med* 147:1495, 1987.
159. Hermesh H, Molcho A, Aizenberg D, et al: The calcium antagonist nifedipine in recurrent neuroleptic malignant syndrome. *Clin Neuropharmacol* 11:552, 1988.
160. Lim R: Idiopathic hypoparathyroidism presenting as the neuroleptic malignant syndrome. *Br J Hosp Med* 41:182, 1989.
161. Morris HH, McCormick WF, Reinarz JA: Neuroleptic malignant syndrome. *Arch Neurol* 37:462, 1980.
162. Keck PE, Caroff SN, McElroy SL: Neuroleptic malignant syndrome and malignant hyperthermia: end of a controversy? *J Neuropsychiatry Clin Neurosci* 7:135, 1995.
163. Curley FJ, Irwin RS: Disorders of temperature control, Part I. Hyperthermia, Part 2. *J Intensive Care Med* 1:591, 1986.
164. Viejo LF, Morales V, Punal P, et al: Risk factors in neuroleptic malignant syndrome. A case-control study. *Acta Psychiatr Scand* 107:45, 2003.
165. Caroff SN, Mann SC: Neuroleptic malignant syndrome. *Med Clin North Am* 77:185, 1993.
166. Denborough MA, Collins SP, Hopkinson KC: Rhabdomyolysis and malignant hyperpyrexia. *BMJ* 288:1878, 1984.
167. Granato JE, Stern BJ, Ringel A, et al: Neuroleptic malignant syndrome: successful treatment with dantrolene and bromocriptine. *Ann Neurol* 4:89, 1983.
168. Adityanjee, Sajatovic M, Munshi K: Neuropsychiatric sequelae of the neuroleptic malignant syndrome. *Clin Neuropharmacol* 28(4):197, 2005.
169. Becker T, Kornhuber J, Hofmann E, et al: MRI white matter hyperintensity in neuroleptic malignant syndrome (NMS): a clue to pathogenesis? *J Neural Transm* 90:151, 1992.
170. Caroff SN, Mann SC: Neuroleptic malignant syndrome. *Psychopharmacol Bull* 24:25, 1988.
171. Susman VL: Clinical management of the neuroleptic malignant syndrome. *Psychiatr Q* 72(4):325, 2001.
172. Velamoor VR, Norman RM, Caroff, et al: Progression of symptoms in the neuroleptic malignant syndrome. *J Nerv Ment Dis* 182:168, 1994.
173. Sewell DD, Jeste DV: Distinguishing neuroleptic malignant syndrome (NMS) from NMS-like acute medical illnesses: a study of 34 cases. *J Neuropsychiatry Clin Neurosci* 4:265, 1992.
174. Banushali MJ, Tuite PJ: The evaluation and management of patients with the neuroleptic malignant syndrome. *Neurol Clin North Am* 23:389, 2004.
175. Anderson WH: Lethal catatonia and the neuroleptic malignant syndrome. *Crit Care Med* 19:1333, 1991.
176. Chiang WK, Herschman Z: Lethal catatonia and the neuroleptic malignant syndrome. *Crit Care Med* 20:1622, 1992.
177. Gong SNC, Rogers KJ: Role of brain monoamines in the fatal hyperthermia induced by pethidine or imipramine in rabbits pretreated with a monoamine oxidase inhibitor. *Br J Pharmacol* 48:12, 1978.
178. Browne B, Linter S: Monoamine oxidase inhibitors and narcotic analgesics: a critical review of the implications for treatment. *Br J Psychiatry* 151:210, 1987.
179. Meyer D, Halfin V: Toxicity secondary to meperidine in patients on monoamine oxidase inhibitors: a case report and critical review. *J Clin Psychopharmacol* 1:319, 1981.
180. McAllen, KJ, Schwartz DR. Adverse drug reactions resulting in hyperthermia in the intensive care unit. *Crit Care Med* 38[Suppl]:S244–S252, 2010.
181. Rosebush PI, Stewart T, Mazurek MF: The treatment of neuroleptic malignant syndrome: are dantrolene and bromocriptine useful adjuncts to supportive care? *Br J Psychiatry* 159:709, 1991.
182. Sato Y, Asoh T, Metoki N, et al: Efficacy of methylprednisolone pulse therapy on neuroleptic malignant syndrome in Parkinson's disease. *J Neurol Neurosurg Psychiatry* 74:574, 2003.
183. Goekoop JG, Carboat PA: Treatment of neuroleptic malignant syndrome with dantrolene. *Lancet* 2:49, 1982.
184. Nisijima K, Ishiguro T: Does dantrolene influence central dopamine and serotonin metabolism in the neuroleptic malignant syndrome? A retrospective study. *Biol Psychiatry* 33:45, 1993.
185. Olmsted TR: Neuroleptic malignant syndrome: guidelines for treatment and reinstitution of neuroleptics. *South Med J* 81:888, 1988.
186. Harpe C, Stondemire A: Aetiology and treatment of neuroleptic malignant syndrome. *Med Toxicol* 2:166, 1987.
187. Zubenko G, Pope MG: Management of a case of neuroleptic malignant syndrome with bromocriptine. *Am J Psychiatry* 40:1619, 1983.
188. McCarron MM, Boettger ML, Peck JJ: A case of neuroleptic malignant syndrome successfully treated with amantadine. *J Clin Psychiatry* 43:381, 1982.
189. Hermesh H, Aizenberg D, Weizman A: A successful electroconvulsive treatment of neuroleptic malignant syndrome. *Acta Psychiatr Scand* 75:237, 1987.
190. Addonizio G, Susman VL: ECT as a treatment alternative for patients with symptoms of neuroleptic malignant syndrome. *J Clin Psychiatry* 48:102, 1987.
191. Lotstra F, Linkowski P, Mendlewicz J: General anesthesia after neuroleptic malignant syndrome. *Biol Psychiatry* 18:243, 1983.
192. Maling TJB, MacDonald AD, Davis M, et al: Neuroleptic malignant syndrome: a review of the Wellington experience. *N Z Med J* 101:193, 1988.
193. Smego RA, Durack DT: The neuroleptic malignant syndrome. *Arch Intern Med* 142:1183, 1982.
194. Birkhimer LJ, DeVane CL: The neuroleptic malignant syndrome: presentation and treatment. *Drug Intell Clin Pharm* 18:462, 1984.
195. Conner CS: Therapy of syndrome malin. *Drug Intell Clin Pharm* 17:639, 1983.
196. Neuroleptic malignant syndrome. *Lancet* 1:545, 1984.
197. Dallman JH: Neuroleptic malignant syndrome: a review. *Mil Med* 149:471, 1984.
198. Nishioka Y, Miyazaki M, Kubo S, et al: Acute renal failure in neuroleptic malignant syndrome. *Ren Fail* 24(4):539, 2002.

199. Rosenberg MR, Green M: Neuroleptic malignant syndrome. *Arch Intern Med* 149:1927, 1989.
200. Legras A, Hurel D, Dabrowski G, et al: Protracted neuroleptic malignant syndrome complicating long-acting neuroleptic administration. *Am J Med* 85:875, 1988.
201. Wells AJ, Sommi RW, Crismon ML: Neuroleptic rechallenge after neuroleptic malignant syndrome: case report and literature review. *Drug Intell Clin Pharm* 22:475, 1988.
202. Rosebush PI, Stewart TD, Gelenberg AJ: Twenty neuroleptic rechallenges after neuroleptic malignant syndrome in 15 patients. *J Clin Psychiatry* 50:295, 1989.
203. Koponen H, Repo E, Lepola U: Long-term outcome after neuroleptic malignant syndrome. *Acta Psychiatr Scand* 84:550, 1991.
204. McCarron MM, Schulze BW, Thompson GA, et al: Acute phencyclidine intoxication: incidence of clinical findings in 1,000 cases. *Ann Emerg Med* 10:237, 1981.
205. Ginsberg MD, Hertzman M, Schmidt-Nowara WW: Amphetamine intoxication with coagulopathy, hyperthermia, and reversible renal failure: a syndrome resembling heatstroke. *Ann Intern Med* 73:81, 1970.
206. Krisko I, Lewis E, Johnson JE: Severe hyperpyrexia due to tranylcypromine-amphetamine toxicity. *Ann Intern Med* 70:559, 1969.
207. Ling LH, Marchant C, Buckley NA, et al: Poisoning with the recreational drug paramethoxyamphetamine (death). *Med J Aust* 174(9):453, 2001.
208. Dar KJ, McBrien ME: MDMA-induced hyperthermia: report of a fatality and review of current therapy. *Intensive Care Med* 22(9):995, 1996.
209. Friedman SA, Hirsch SE: Extreme hyperthermia after LSD ingestion. *JAMA* 217:1549, 1971.
210. Mills KC: Serotonin syndrome. *Crit Care Clin* 13(4):763, 1997.
211. Mason PJ, Morris VA, Balcezak TJ: Serotonin syndrome: presentation of 2 cases and review of the literature. *Medicine (Baltimore)* 79(4):201, 2000.
212. Sporer KA: The serotonin syndrome: implicated drugs, pathophysiology, and management. *Drug Saf* 13(2):94, 1995.
213. Brown TM, Skop BP, Mareth TR: Pathophysiology and management of the serotonin syndrome. *Ann Pharmacother* 30(5):527, 1996.
214. Martin TG: Serotonin syndrome. *Ann Emerg Med* 28(5):520, 1996.
215. Schuckit M, Robins E, Feighner J: Tricyclic antidepressants and monoamine oxidase inhibitors. *Arch Gen Psychiatry* 24:509, 1971.
216. Gillman PK: Monoamine oxidase inhibitors, opioid analgesics and serotonin toxicity. *Br J Anaesth* 95(4):431–441, 2005.
217. Leatherman JW, Schmitz PG: Fever, hyperdynamic shock, and multiple-system organ failure: a pseudo sepsis syndrome associated with chronic salicylate intoxication. *Chest* 100:1391, 1991.
218. Kosten TR, Kleber HD: Rapid death during cocaine abuse: a variant of the neuroleptic malignant syndrome? *Am J Drug Alcohol Abuse* 14:335, 1988.
219. Kline SS, Mauro LS, Scala-Barnett DM, et al: Serotonin syndrome versus neuroleptic malignant syndrome as a cause of death. *Clin Pharm* 8:510, 1989.
220. Nijhawan PK, Katz G, Winter S: Psychiatric illness and the serotonin syndrome: an emerging adverse drug effect leading to intensive care unit admission. *Crit Care Med* 24:1086, 1996.
221. Mueller PD, Korey WS: Death by ecstasy: the serotonin syndrome? *Ann Emerg Med* 32(3):377, 1998.
222. Ener RA, Meglathery SB, Van Decker WA, et al: Serotonin syndrome and other serotonergic disorders. *Pain Med* 4(1):63, 2003.
223. Rosenberg J, Pentel P, Pond S, et al: Hyperthermia associated with drug intoxication. *Crit Care Med* 14:964, 1986.
224. Merigian KS, Roberts JR: Cocaine intoxication: hyperpyrexia, rhabdomyolysis and acute renal failure. *Clin Toxicol* 25:135, 1987.
225. Carbone JR: The neuroleptic malignant and serotonin syndromes. *Emerg Med Clin North Am* 18(2):317, 2000.
226. Graudis A, Stearman A, Chan B: Treatment of the serotonin syndrome with cyproheptadine. *J Emerg Med* 16(4):615, 1998.
227. Gillman PK: The serotonin syndrome and its treatment. *J Psychopharmacol* 13(1):100, 1999.
228. Kendrick WC, Hull AR, Knochel JP: Rhabdomyolysis and shock after intravenous amphetamine administration. *Ann Intern Med* 86:381, 1977.
229. Zalis E, Parmley L Jr: Fatal amphetamine poisoning. *Arch Intern Med* 112:822, 1963.
230. Menashe PI, Gottlieb JE: Hyperthermia, rhabdomyolysis, and myoglobinuric renal failure after recreational use of cocaine. *South Med J* 81:379, 1988.
231. Campbell BG: Cocaine abuse with hyperthermia, seizures and fatal complications. *Med J Aust* 149:387, 1988.
232. Bauwens JE, Boggs JM, Hartwell PS: Fatal hyperthermia associated with cocaine use. *West J Med* 150:210, 1989.
233. Loghmanee F, Tobak M: Fatal malignant hyperthermia associated with recreational cocaine and ethanol abuse. *Am J Forensic Med Pathol* 7:246, 1986.
234. Bettinger J: Cocaine intoxication: massive oral overdose. *Ann Emerg Med* 9:429, 1980.
235. Patel R, Das M, Palazzolo M, et al: Myoglobinuric acute renal failure in phencyclidine overdose: report of observations in eight cases. *Ann Emerg Med* 9:549, 1980.
236. Armen R, Kanel G, Reynolds T: Phencyclidine-induced malignant hyperthermia causing submassive liver necrosis. *Am J Med* 77:167, 1984.
237. Yeo TP: Heat Stroke: a comprehensive review. *AACN Clin Issues* 15(2):280, 2004.
238. Badjatia N: Hyperthermia and fever control in brain injury. *Crit Care Med* 37(7):S250–S257, 2009.

CHAPTER 67 ■ SEVERE UPPER AIRWAY INFECTIONS

STEPHEN J. KRINZMAN, SUNIL RAJAN AND RICHARD S. IRWIN

The components of the upper airway include the nose, mouth, nasopharynx, oropharynx, and hypopharynx. It communicates with the paranasal sinuses and tympanic cavity. Although minor infections in these areas are commonly observed in the outpatient setting, occasionally, they may become severe and life threatening. This class of disease requires intense observation and aggressive management and is the focus of this chapter.

SINUSITIS

In patients on mechanical ventilatory support, sinusitis is one of four common causes of fever, along with pneumonia, catheter-related infection, and urinary tract infection [1–4]. Sinusitis is encountered in the intensive care unit (ICU) in two situations: as an uncommon, potentially fatal complication of a community-acquired sinus infection such as meningitis, osteomyelitis, orbital infection, or brain abscess and as a hospital-acquired sinus infection that may be a frequent cause of occult fever in a critically ill patient.

Incidence

The frequency of nosocomial sinusitis varies greatly from less than 5% to 100% [5,6], depending on the patient population studied and the diagnostic criteria used. In one series, 95% of nasotracheally intubated patients developed radiographic evidence of pansinusitis [7], as did 25% of patients who were orotracheally intubated. Only 40% of patients with "radiographic sinusitis" were found to have positive cultures, although some cultures may have been sterilized by prior use of broad-spectrum antibiotics. Using stringent diagnostic criteria based on antroscopy, histopathology, and microbiology, the rate of infectious sinusitis may be closer to 10% in patients on long-term mechanical ventilation [4,5].

Pathogenesis

Critically ill patients are predisposed to develop nosocomial sinusitis for several reasons. The diameter of the ostia, normally as small as 1 or 2 mm, has been shown to decrease with recumbency as much as 23% because of venous hydrostatic pressures [8]. In addition, the maxillary sinus ostia are poorly located for gravitational drainage [8]. Nasotracheal and nasogastric tubes strongly predispose patients to develop sinusitis. Patients with orotracheal tubes have a lower incidence of bacterial sinusitis than those with nasotracheal tubes [4,9]. In one series, 73% of mechanically ventilated patients developed culture-proven sinusitis within 7 days of placement of nasogastric or nasotracheal tubes [7]. Larger intranasal tubes (tracheal) will induce radiographic sinus changes more quickly than smaller tubes (gastric) [4]. Using multiple logistic regression analysis, risk factors for nosocomial sinusitis, of strongest association, are sedative use, nasogastric feeding tubes, Glasgow coma scale less than 8, and nasal colonization with enteric Gram-negative bacteria [10].

Etiology

The microbiology of nosocomial sinusitis is quite distinct from that of community-acquired sinusitis. *Haemophilus influenzae* and *Streptococcus pneumoniae* are rarely isolated in the nosocomial setting. Nosocomial sinusitis is polymicrobial in 44% to 58% of cases [11,12], with Gram-negative organisms being the causative agents in two thirds of cases, and Gram-positive organisms being implicated in one third [13]. Anaerobes are isolated in 0% to 15% of cases [11,14]. *Staphylococcus aureus* is the most common Gram-positive organism identified, and *Pseudomonas* species are the leading Gram-negative pathogens [4,13,15]. The organisms isolated in nosocomial sinusitis are the ones frequently identical to those cultured from the lower respiratory tract [3,14]. Such findings support the concept of general colonization of the airways in critically ill patients.

Specific situations warrant consideration of infection with more unusual pathogens. Rhinocerebral mucormycosis, an invasive infection usually caused by the branching fungus *Rhizopus*, a Zygomycetes, is seen most often in association with diabetes mellitus with ketoacidosis, burns, chronic renal disease, cirrhosis, and immunosuppression [16,17]. Other fungal infections, primarily with *Aspergillus* species, can be seen in normal hosts but are usually invasive diseases of immunocompromised patients [18]. *Cryptococcus neoformans* can cause sinusitis with a high relapse rate and significant mortality in immunocompetent and immunocompromised patients [19]. *Candida* species [20], *Pseudoallescheria boydii* and *Cytomegalovirus* species, and other unusual organisms have been isolated in patients with acquired immunodeficiency syndrome with sinusitis [21].

Complications

Complications of acute sinusitis are rare but can be rapidly fatal and are best managed in an ICU. Orbital complications include edema, predominantly of the eyelids, orbital cellulitis, orbital abscess, subperiosteal abscess, and cavernous sinus thrombosis [22,23]. The last one is the most severe, with a mortality of greater than 20% [24–26]. Intracranial complications have an overall mortality of 40% and include osteomyelitis, meningitis, epidural abscess, subdural empyema, and brain abscess [24–26]. In these cases, sinus drainage is imperative and antibiotics directed by culture result. Several investigators have examined the relationship between nosocomial sinusitis and ventilator-associated pneumonia. When *S. aureus* and *Pseudomonas aeruginosa* are isolated in patients with nosocomial sinusitis, the same organisms are identified in lower respiratory tract cultures in one third of cases [12]. Ventilator-associated pneumonia is more frequent in patients with confirmed nosocomial sinusitis [7]. In a prospective, randomized study of a strategy to systematically detect and treat nosocomial sinusitis, both radiographic evidence and bacteriologic evidence of sinusitis were found in 55% of febrile, mechanically ventilated patients [11]. All patients in the study were nasotracheally intubated. Seventy percent of patients with positive radiographs had positive quantitative cultures. Ventilator-associated pneumonia occurred in significantly fewer patients (34% vs. 47%, $p = 0.02$) in the group in which there was systematic screening for and treatment of sinusitis. Taken together, these findings suggest a causal relationship between nosocomial sinusitis and ventilator-associated pneumonia.

Nosocomial sinusitis may also cause fever of unknown origin (FUO) in mechanically ventilated patients. van Zanten and colleagues prospectively studied 351 orotracheally intubated patients with fever for more than 48 hours despite treatment with broad-spectrum antibiotics [3]. In 198 patients, the cause of the fever remained unknown despite initial investigations that included chest radiographs. Based on the results of sinus radiographs and subsequent sinus cultures, infectious sinusitis was confirmed in 105 of 198 (53%) patients with FUO and was found to be the sole cause of fever in 16% of cases.

Diagnosis

Computed Tomography Scans and Radiographs

Computed tomography (CT) scanning has become the imaging modality of choice for the diagnosis of nosocomial sinusitis. Compared with plan sinus radiographs, sinus CT scans can more accurately visualize the ethmoid and sphenoid sinuses and are also superior in differentiating mucosal thickening from air–fluid levels [27]. Portable sinus radiographs performed in the supine position have been recommended to identify sinus infections in critically ill patients who cannot travel for standard sinus films or a CT scan [28]. As discussed earlier, patients may have sterile cultures despite radiographic evidence of sinusitis.

Ultrasonography

With the increasing use of ultrasound in the ICU, there has been a renewed interest in this modality to diagnose nosocomial sinusitis. Although bone often presents obstacles to ultrasound imaging, the anterior walls of the maxillary sinuses are flat bones composed of compact tissue, allowing adequate ultrasound penetration. Prior investigations had demonstrated that ultrasound was 67% sensitive and 87% specific for maxillary sinusitis visualized on CT scans [29]. Accuracy is improved when the patient is in the semi-recumbent position, and not supine [30].

More recent investigations have shown further improvements in diagnostic accuracy. Vargas and coworkers used B-mode ultrasound in the semi-recumbent position in

120 patients with suspected sinusitis [30]. They found that in 36 patients with negative sinus ultrasounds, none had evidence of maxillary sinusitis on CT scan. Extensive maxillary sinus disease is indicated by hyperechogenic visualization of the posterior wall and extension to the internal and and external walls was, in one investigation, found to be 100% specific for total opacification of the sinus on CT scan [31]. On transnasal puncture, fluid could be aspirated from all such patients, and the cultures were positive in 67% of patients [30]. In patients where only the posterior wall of the maxillary sinus is hyperechogenic, 80% of transnasal punctures yield fluid, and cultures are positive in half of those where fluid is obtained.

Rhinoscopy and Antral Aspiration

As reviewed earlier, opacification of the paranasal sinuses in the critically ill patient does not necessarily indicate infectious sinusitis; in some series, a majority of such patients have sterile cultures. Endoscopically obtained cultures from the middle meatus do not correlate with the cultures from the antral lavage aspirate in the febrile ICU patient [32]. Rhinoscopy can add significantly to the diagnostic yield in patients with suspected sinusitis. In patients with both purulent secretions in the middle meatus by rhinoscopy and radiographic evidence of sinusitis, 92% have positive cultures by antral lavage. Although cultures obtained from the maxillary sinus by antral puncture have been considered the gold standard for diagnosis of nosocomial sinusitis, the high correlation between culture findings from the sinuses and those obtained from endotracheal specimens [14] suggests that performing antral puncture to obtain sinus secretions for culture may not be necessary in most cases.

Treatment

Nosocomial sinusitis is most often related to the presence of nasopharyngeal and oropharyngeal catheters and tubes [4,12,33]. Therefore, in addition to antibiotics and decongestants, treatment includes removal of all nasal tubes to eliminate the source of obstruction and irritation in addition to decongestants and antibiotics. Because the spectrum of bacteria causing nosocomial sinusitis is similar to that causing other nosocomial respiratory infections [4,13,15], broad-spectrum Gram-positive and Gram-negative coverage is indicated. With removal of nasal tubes and antibiotic therapy, 67% of patients become afebrile within 48 hours [34]. Because the majority of patients respond to these conservative measures, consideration of surgical drainage can be reserved for patients who fail to respond to medical therapy and in whom no other source of infection is identified.

SPHENOID SINUSITIS

Sphenoid sinusitis deserves separate mention because of its potentially fulminant nature and difficulty in diagnosis. Delay in its diagnosis has been associated with serious morbidity and mortality [35,36]. The typical presentation of acute infection is severe headache that interferes with sleep, often accompanied by fever and nasal discharge [35,36]. Neurologic deficits can be prominent features; trigeminal hyperesthesia or hypoesthesia occurs in one third of cases [36]. Gram-positive organisms have been isolated from the cultures of most patients with acute sinusitis, whereas equal numbers of Gram-positive and facultative Gram-negative pathogens have been cultured from those with chronic sphenoid sinusitis [35,36]. Serious sequelae including permanent neurologic deficits and death can result from the spread to nearby structures (e.g., cavernous sinus, pituitary gland, optic chiasm). When findings suggest extension of the infection, early CT scan of the sinuses is essential. Surgical drainage may be necessary if symptoms persist or neurologic signs develop while the patient is receiving appropriate antibiotic therapy.

OTOGENIC INFECTIONS

Serious complications of otologic infection occur rarely [37,38]. Anatomically, the external auditory canal is one-half cartilaginous, and the medial half tunnels through the temporal bone. The auditory tube (pharyngotympanic tube) passes into the nasopharynx along the superior border of the lateral pharyngeal space (LPS). Other structures that are accessible by infection include the mastoid air cells, the jugular foramen, cranial nerves (especially the facial nerve), the internal carotid artery, and the dura mater of the posterior cranial fossa.

Mastoiditis

Acute mastoiditis is an uncommon complication of otitis media, seen primarily in children and young adults. Inflammation spreads from the middle ear to the modified respiratory mucosa lining of the mastoid air cells. The closed space infection leads to accumulation of purulent exudate, increased pressure, and bony necrosis. Pain, typically postauricular, fever, and abnormal tympanic membranes are the most common findings on presentation [39]. In approximately 50% of patients with mastoiditis, acute otitis media was diagnosed within days to weeks of admission [40]. Radiographic abnormalities of the mastoid are common and demonstrate opacification or cloudiness of the mastoid air cells and, less frequently, evidence of bone destruction [40]. CT scan of the temporal bone can identify and confirm intracranial complications [40]. Up to 25% of patients have complications on presentation, including subperiosteal abscess with or without epidural abscess, meningitis, cranial nerve involvement, and sigmoid sinus thrombophlebitis [41]. Lateral sinus thrombosis secondary to mastoiditis [42] has also been associated with septic pulmonary emboli [43,44]. The most common bacterial organisms isolated include *S. pneumoniae*, group A streptococci, and *S. aureus; Pseudomonas* may be commonly isolated as well [39]. Treatment includes broad-spectrum antibiotics that can adequately penetrate cerebrospinal fluid and surgical intervention for those who fail to improve within 24 to 72 hours.

Chronic mastoiditis and chronic otitis media result from a progressive inflammatory process that usually leads to obstruction of the communication between the middle ear and mastoid (aditus) or the middle ear and nasopharynx (eustachian tube) [39]. Often a cholesteatoma or epidermal inclusion cyst within the tympanomastoid compartment may be involved and may become secondarily infected [39]. Presenting symptoms include hearing loss, painless otorrhea, and tympanic membrane perforation [39]. Other symptoms (e.g., facial nerve paresis, headache, ear pain, fever) may be present if complications have occurred. Uncomplicated chronic otitis media and mastoiditis are treated medically with local hygiene, topical antibiotics often including a corticosteroid, and oral, or infrequently parenteral, antibiotics [39]. Broad-spectrum antibiotics are required to cover a wide range of aerobic and anaerobic organisms. Surgery is usually reserved for recurrent disease, often associated with a cholesteatoma, which can be identified by CT scan of the temporal bone [39].

Malignant External Otitis

Malignant, or necrotizing, external otitis (MEO) most often affects elderly diabetic patients. Diabetic microangiopathy, an altered immune response, the biochemistry of diabetic cerumen, and characteristics of the usual etiologic organism have been implicated in the pathogenesis of MEO [45]. MEO most commonly presents with otalgia; granulation tissue in the external auditory canal, most prominently at the osteocartilaginous junction; and often purulent and fetid otorrhea [45]. Spread of infection is anteriorly toward the parotid compartment or downward into the temporal bone; spread to the mastoid is less common [37]. Extension leads to pain and tenderness of the tissues around the ear. In MEO, *P. aeruginosa* is the most commonly implicated pathogen [45]. Patients with acquired immunodeficiency syndrome may develop infection from a wider variety of organisms and may accumulate less granulation tissue in the external auditory canal [46]. *Aspergillus* species have been identified, primarily in immunocompromised patients [47,48]. Osteomyelitis [49], cranial nerve paralysis [50], and central nervous system (meningitis) and vascular (thrombophlebitis) spread [51] are potential severe and fatal complications of MEO.

CT and magnetic resonance imaging scanning, along with technetium-99 bone scans, are valuable components of the diagnostic evaluation of MEO [51]. The therapy for MEO includes prolonged antibiotics directed against *P. aeruginosa* unless the culture data suggest otherwise. This may include a semisynthetic penicillin or ceftazidime with an aminoglycoside. Oral fluoroquinolones have also been used successfully [51]. The duration of treatment is not clearly defined. Surgical intervention can be complementary and is based on the response to conservative treatment and the presence of complications.

SUPRAGLOTTITIS (EPIGLOTTITIS)

Acute supraglottitis is an uncommon infection of the structures located above the glottis. These structures include the epiglottis, aryepiglottic folds, arytenoids, pharynx, uvula, and tongue base. The true vocal cords are rarely involved. The infection may progress to abrupt and fatal airway obstruction. This entity is well described in children, in whom the presentation and course are usually fulminant. In the pediatric population, increased awareness and prophylactic airway control have reduced overall mortality to less than 1% [52,53]. In children, *H. influenzae* type B is the most identifiable causative organism. Since the introduction of a vaccine against *H. influenzae* type B in 1995, the incidence of pediatric epiglottitis has decreased substantially [54–56]. As a result, it appears supraglottitis is becoming a disease of adults, in whom the course is frequently indolent but with a mortality rate that may reach 5%, mostly because of misdiagnosis and unexpected airway obstruction [52,56–59].

Incidence

In the post–*H. influenzae* type B vaccine era, the annual incidence of acute supraglottitis is estimated between 0.6 and 0.78 cases per 100,000 immunized children [58]. In adults, the incidence of acute supraglottitis has increased from 0.79 cases per 100,000 adults in 1986 to 2.1 cases per 100,000 adults in 2005 [58]. Adults with acute supraglottitis usually present in their 40s and 50s, with a male preponderance, and children usually present between the ages of 2 and 5 years [58].

TABLE 67.1

ORGANISMS IMPLICATED IN ACUTE EPIGLOTTITIS

Organism	References
Haemophilus influenzae	[3,5,15,17]
Streptococcus pneumoniae	[18,19]
β-Hemolytic streptococci	[9,20,21]
Staphylococcus aureus	[21,23,24]
Klebsiella pneumoniae	[24,25]
Neisseria meningitides	[12]
Bacteroides species	[26]
Haemophilus parainfluenzae	[15,27]
Candida albicans[a]	[28–31]
Pasteurella multocida	[32,33]
Herpes simplex virus type 1[b]	[34,35]

[a]Cultured from epiglottic swab or seen on autopsy; all others recovered from blood.
[b]Epiglottis biopsy specimen histology and viral culture.

Pathogenesis and Pathophysiology

In children, the inflammation is mainly restricted to the epiglottis because of loose mucosa on its lingual aspect. This provides a readily available space for edema to collect within. Swelling reduces the airway aperture by curling the epiglottis posteriorly and inferiorly, accentuating the juvenile omega shape. When edema spreads to involve the aryepiglottic folds, respiratory distress can occur as inspiration draws these structures downward, further exacerbating the obstruction and resulting in stridor. The adult airway is relatively protected because the larynx is larger and the epiglottis is shaped more like a spatula.

Etiology

Although various bacteria, viruses, and *Candida* species have been recognized as causes of acute supraglottitis (Table 67.1) [60–68], *H. influenzae* type B is the most common cause identified in pediatric and adult cases [60,68]. Although vaccine failure has been reported in children who had received an early polysaccharide vaccine [61], significant declines in the incidence of this infection have been noted with the use of conjugated vaccines that can be administered to even younger children [60]. In adults, blood cultures are positive in less than 20% of cases, and *H. influenzae* is the isolate in one third of these cases [62,68].

Noninfectious causes of acute supraglottitis have been described and include thermal injuries related to inhalation drug use, ingestion of hot food, apparent caustic injury from aspiration, and posttransplant lymphoproliferative disorder [63,64]. McKinney and Grigg [66] described a case of epiglottitis after general anesthesia administered via a laryngeal mask.

Diagnosis

History and Physical Examination

In children, the classic presentation is of a 3-year-old child who initially complains of a sore throat followed by dysphagia and/or odynophagia, which then progresses within hours to stridor. The child prefers to sit, leaning forward, and usually appears pale and frightened. Breathing is slow and quiet with characteristic drooling noted. These symptoms may lead to sudden respiratory depression and arrest. The progression of symptoms can be remembered as the four "Ds": dysphagia, dysphonia, drooling, and distress.

In adults, the classic presentation is more the exception than the rule, and as such, the frequency of misdiagnosis has been reported as high as 60% to 75% [52,58,59]. More than 90% of adults seek medical attention complaining of sore throat with or without dysphagia [63,67]. Many patients report antecedent upper respiratory tract infections [60,68]. Other less common signs and symptoms are respiratory distress, muffled voice, drooling, fever, and stridor [52,53,63,67,68]. Hoarseness or true dysphonia is not observed because the process usually spares the true vocal cords. Children and adults often prefer an upright posture with the neck extended and mouth slightly open [69].

The duration of symptoms varies, ranging from hours to several days [70]. Patients presenting within 8 hours of the onset of symptoms are more likely to have signs of upper airway obstruction [71]. In general, patients who present early in their disease course have more severe symptoms, fever, and leukocytosis. They are also more likely to be infected with *H. influenzae* [70]. These patients are at increased risk of needing artificial airways and of dying [72].

Evaluation of patients with suspected supraglottitis depends, in part, on their age and the severity of their symptoms. In young children with a classic presentation, pharyngeal examination should not be attempted. An artificial airway should be established in the controlled setting of an operating room, where an examination can be performed with less risk of airway obstruction. When there is doubt about the diagnosis in a stable child, a lateral neck radiograph to look for the classic, "thumb sign" of a swollen epiglottis is the proper first step (Fig. 67.1).

In older children and adults, supraglottitis should be considered when sore throat and dysphagia seem to be out of proportion to visible signs of pharyngitis. In this situation, if the patient has no respiratory distress, examination of the larynx and supralaryngeal structures is recommended. The epiglottis may appear cherry red in color but more commonly is pale and edematous. Other supraglottic structures may be edematous as well, resulting in the inability to visualize the vocal cords [60].

Diagnostic Tests

A lateral soft tissue radiograph of the neck has frequently been used to diagnose acute supraglottitis [60]. The radiograph should be taken in the upright position to avoid pooling of secretions posteriorly and potentially increasing the obstruction. Because the disease is unpredictable, the patient must be observed at all times by someone skilled in airway management. Characteristic radiographic changes (see Fig. 67.1) have been detected in most endoscopically proven infections [72]. These changes include epiglottic thickening of more than 8 mm (producing the thumb sign) [73], swelling of the aryepiglottic folds of more than 7 mm [73], ballooning of the hypopharynx [74], and narrowing of the vallecula [74]. However, it is important to remember that a normal radiograph is inadequate to exclude the diagnosis of supraglottitis, and direct visualization of the structures should be performed if suspicion is high [75].

Few laboratory tests are helpful at the time of initial evaluation. An elevated white blood cell count and C-reactive protein level may identify a patient at higher risk. Throat cultures are positive in less than 33% of the cases and blood cultures detect a causative agent in less than 20% of the cases [58,63]. Direct visualization guided swab culture of the epiglottis may reflect more closely the causative agent and has been positive in up to 75% of the cases [59,63].

Differential Diagnosis

Supraglottitis in children is a clinical diagnosis. Since immediate airway control is a priority, recognizing other pediatric illnesses presenting with a sore throat and not requiring this intervention is important [76,77]. The most common infection is croup, a predominantly viral laryngotracheobronchitis that occurs up to 40 times more frequently than epiglottitis [77]. Typically, the child is younger than 3 years and has had an upper respiratory tract infection of at least 48 hours' duration. Hoarseness develops initially and is followed by a distinctive

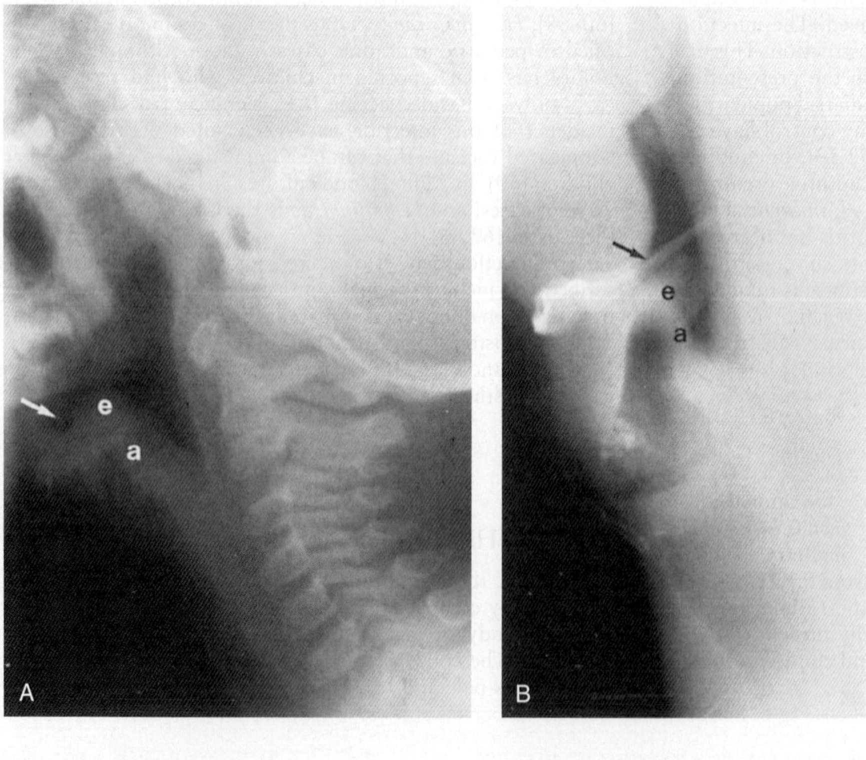

FIGURE 67.1. Acute supraglottitis. Lateral radiographs of the neck obtained with soft tissue technique in a 2-year-old child (**A**) and a 42-year-old adult (**B**). There is epiglottic (*e*) swelling (thumb sign), thickening of the aryepiglottic folds (*a*), and narrowing of the vallecula (*arrow*) in both patients. Compare with normal epiglottis in Figure 67.11(*a*).

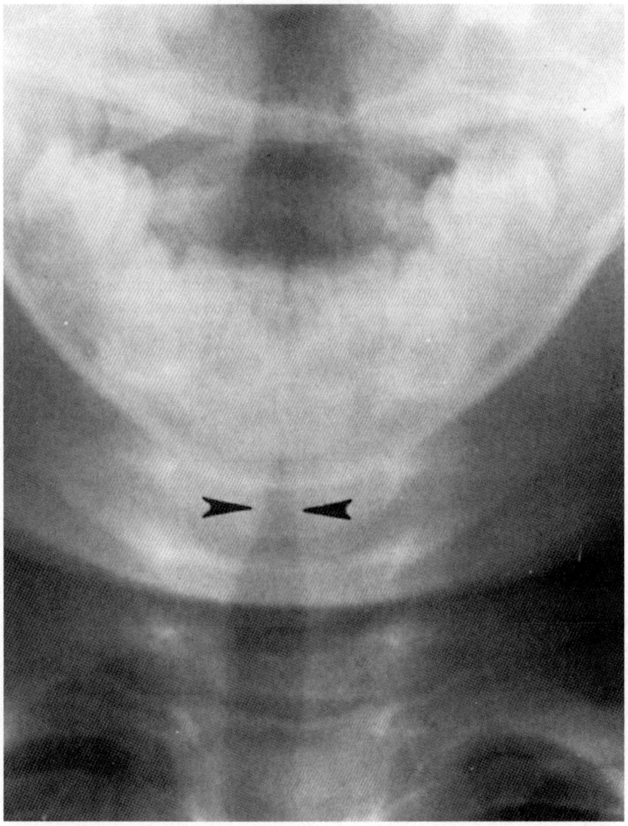

FIGURE 67.2. Croup. Anteroposterior radiograph of the neck in a 19-month-old child. Subglottic edema produces smooth tapering (*arrowheads*) of the tracheal air column (the steeple sign).

barking cough. Although respiratory distress with stridor is common, intubation is rarely needed [76,77]. Anteroposterior and lateral views of the neck may show the classic, "steeple sign" (Fig. 67.2), a gradual narrowing of the proximal tracheal air column secondary to subglottic edema. Other less common infectious considerations in children include pseudomembranous croup (bacterial laryngotracheobronchitis), retropharyngeal abscess, lingual tonsillitis, and diphtheria [76,77].

In adults, infectious mononucleosis, often with massive tonsillar hypertrophy leading to stridor, and a unilateral pharyngeal mass should be considered when patients complain of sore throat and dysphagia. Pharyngitis may present a picture indistinguishable from that of mild or early supraglottitis [72].

Bacterial tracheitis is a potentially life-threatening illness with features similar to those of supraglottitis and viral croup. Although more often seen in the pediatric population, adults can also be affected [78]. These patients present with a brief, progressive upper respiratory tract prodrome including a brassy cough, stridor, high fever, and toxicity but do not exhibit dysphagia or drooling [76,77]. Airway obstruction is due to subglottic mucosal edema and thick, inspissated, mucopurulent tracheal secretions [78]. Bacterial superinfection of a preceding viral tracheitis occurs most commonly with *S. aureus* and *H. influenzae* [77]. Rare cases of membranous tracheobronchitis due to a fungal agent have been described in immunocompromised hosts [79], but these infections have involved primarily the lower respiratory tract. Lateral neck radiographs demonstrate subglottic narrowing and may show mucosal irregularities or membranes in the tracheal air column [80]. Chest radiographs may show signs of atelectasis due to central bronchial obstruction by mucus or necrotic debris [81]. Management is similar to that for supraglottitis, and bronchoscopy should be performed for diagnosis [82]. Intubation or tracheostomy is usually necessary to relieve obstruction and provide adequate tracheal suctioning [78,82]. Antibiotic therapy should be directed against *S. aureus* and other common causative respiratory pathogens.

Rhinoscleroma should also be considered in the differential diagnosis. *Klebsiella rhinoscleromatis* is the etiologic agent of this chronic granulomatous disorder [83,84]. Although nasal and oral mucous membranes are the most common sites of infection, patients have presented acutely with upper airway obstruction due to indolent spread to the larynx and tracheobronchial tree. This condition may be seen in immigrants to the United States from endemic areas such as Central America, Central Europe, Africa, and Asia. The nodular and indurated endoscopic appearance is nondiagnostic, so multiple biopsy specimens for culture and histologic examination are required. Treatment is with a prolonged course of oral antibiotics. Repeated cultures of biopsy specimens may be needed to ascertain whether bacteriologic cure has been achieved [84].

Noninfectious causes of acute upper airway obstruction are usually suggested by the history obtained and by the patient's nontoxic appearance. These include foreign body aspiration, allergic edema, chemical laryngitis from gastroesophageal reflux, and necrotizing tracheobronchitis as a complication of mechanical ventilation [85]. Paraquat poisoning can cause a pharyngeal membrane similar to diphtheria that is accompanied by signs of shock and sepsis [86].

Treatment

The treatment of supraglottitis has two major components: airway management and medical therapy. The early placement of an artificial airway in children has significantly reduced mortality. Moreover, because airway obstruction is the most common cause of death in adults in whom airways are not secured when the diagnosis of supraglottitis is made, some authors favor establishing an artificial airway prophylactically, as is performed in children [53,58,69]. We tend to agree that intubation should be reserved for adult patients with early signs of airway obstruction [63,69,87]. Predictors of the need for an artificial airway in adults include drooling, diabetes mellitus, rapid onset of symptoms, and abscess formation [57]. All patients should be observed in an ICU with the immediate availability of equipment and personnel for emergent intubation.

Both tracheostomy and translaryngeal endotracheal intubation have been performed. No difference in mortality has been noted when comparing these two modalities [88,89]. Significant reductions in duration of airway control, incidence of upper airway complications, and length of hospital stay have been observed in patients with endotracheal intubation when compared with tracheostomy [89,90]. The acute complications of tracheostomy, including pneumothorax, hemorrhage, and subcutaneous or mediastinal emphysema, occur with increased frequency in patients younger than 12 years [88]. Accidental extubation, particularly in children, is the greatest risk of endotracheal intubation [88,89]. Much of the morbidity of the artificial airway is associated with its prolonged maintenance, which is unlikely to occur in supraglottitis. In one large series, 90% of children were extubated in less than 24 hours [91]. The choice of an artificial airway should be determined by the skill of available personnel in placing and maintaining the airway. Endotracheal intubation is preferred, with surgical backup, should the attempt fail.

The appropriate time for extubation in a patient recovering from acute supraglottitis varies. Some physicians remove the artificial airway when the patient's general toxic appearance and fever have subsided [91]. Others wait until repeat laryngoscopy or lateral neck radiographs show decreased edema of

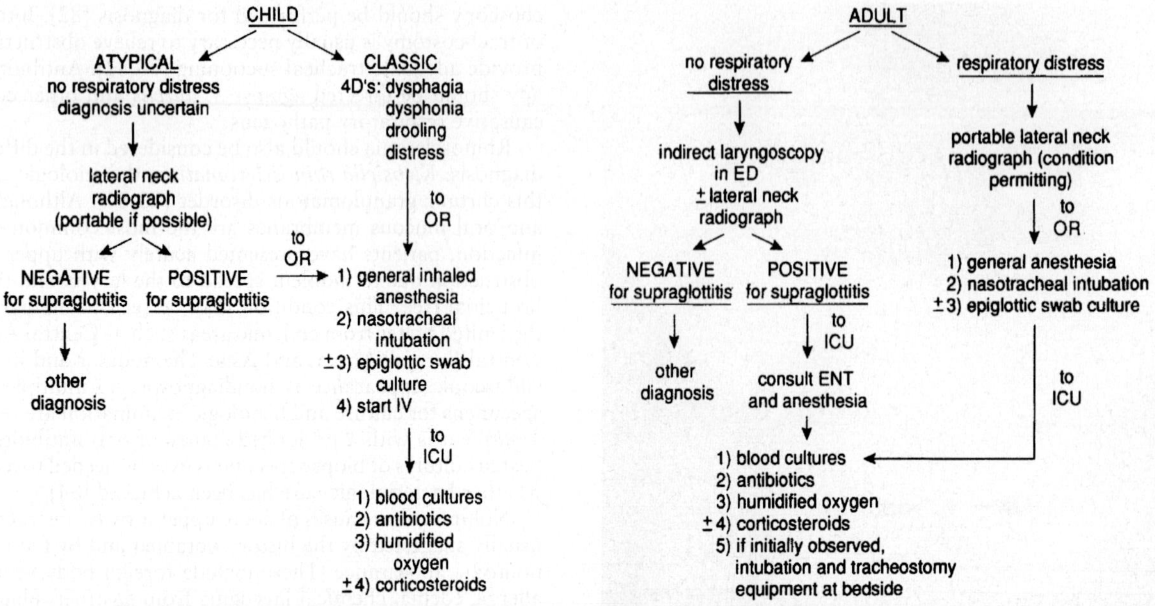

FIGURE 67.3. Management algorithm for acute supraglottitis; ± for epiglottic swab relates to questionable use; for corticosteroids reflects inconclusive study data. ED, emergency department; ENT, ear, nose, and throat specialist; ICU, intensive care unit; OR, operating room.

the involved structures [92]. One can deflate the cuff to test for an air leak around the tube or the patient's ability to breathe with the tube plugged for a brief moment [93]. It is important to remember that if the tube fills the trachea, the patient may not be able to breathe even if supraglottitis has completely resolved.

Medical therapy is crucial for rapid recovery from supraglottitis. All patients require close observation, humidification, and, often, mild sedation [60]. Many antibiotics are effective, and the regimens must cover *H. influenzae* infection. With the high frequency of β-lactamase–producing strains of *H. influenzae*, ampicillin is no longer adequate as an initial single agent. The initial drug of choice is a second- or third-generation cephalosporin that covers ampicillin-resistant *H. influenzae* as well as the other possible pathogens in adults: *S. aureus*, *S. pneumoniae*, and other streptococcal species [72]. Cefotaxime has been considered the antibiotic of choice; ceftriaxone and ampicillin/sulbactam have also been found to be effective [60]. Trimethoprim–sulfamethoxazole can be used as an alternative agent in penicillin-allergic patients. With the rising frequency of penicillin-resistance and multidrug-resistant *S. pneumoniae*, one may need to modify the initial antibiotic regimen based upon culture data. The antibiotics should be initially administered intravenously for several days, depending on the response, and then continued by mouth for 7 to 10 days [93].

Corticosteroid therapy is controversial in patients with infectious supraglottitis. Many authors, finding no contraindications, use steroids empirically [60,88]. There have been no randomized, controlled trials assessing the effectiveness of corticosteroids in patients with acute epiglottitis. Steroids have been noted to be effective in a large, randomized, controlled trial of children with moderate-to-severe croup, lending some support to the hypothesis that steroids may be beneficial in infectious upper airway disease [94]. The use of a helium–oxygen mixture (Heliox) could be considered to diminish the work of breathing and provide a bridge to avoid intubation while antibiotics take effect.

Complications of the disease differ between the pediatric and adult populations. The former has a higher incidence of pneumonia and accidental extubation [95]. Pulmonary edema immediately after intubation for severe stridor has been described in children [96]. In adults, an epiglottic abscess may be suggested by a persistent or deteriorating clinical condition [57,87]. CT scan of the neck may be helpful in making this diagnosis, particularly if direct visualization is not adequate [57,97]. Both groups face risks and complications associated with intubation and tracheostomy [90]. Treatment recommendations are outlined in Figure 67.3.

INFECTIONS OF THE DEEP SPACES OF THE NECK

Deep neck infections can be fatal extensions of upper airway infections. These potentially catastrophic infections are infrequently encountered today due to the prompt treatment of pharyngitis, tonsillitis, odontogenic, and otologic infections with antibiotics. Whenever a delay in diagnosis or treatment occurs, life-threatening complications such as airway compromise, jugular vein thrombosis, pneumonia, pericarditis, mediastinitis, and arterial erosion may develop [98]. Tonsillitis remains the most common cause of this disease in children, whereas poor dental hygiene and injection drug abuse are the most common causes in adults [99]. Some other causes include trauma, surgical trauma, esophageal perforation, laryngopyocele, infected branchial cleft, infected thyroglossal duct cysts, thyroiditis, and mastoiditis with Bezold's (mastoid tip) abscess [99]. An understanding of the complex interconnections between anatomic spaces is essential for early diagnosis and timely intervention of these conditions.

General Pathogenesis and Anatomy

Knowledge of the cervical fasciae is a prerequisite to understanding the etiology, manifestations, complications, and treatment of deep neck infections. The fascial planes separate and connect distant areas, thereby limiting and directing the spread of infection (Fig. 67.4). Suppurative processes in the submandibular, lateral pharyngeal, and retropharyngeal spaces (RPSs) are considered life threatening and are the focus of this discussion.

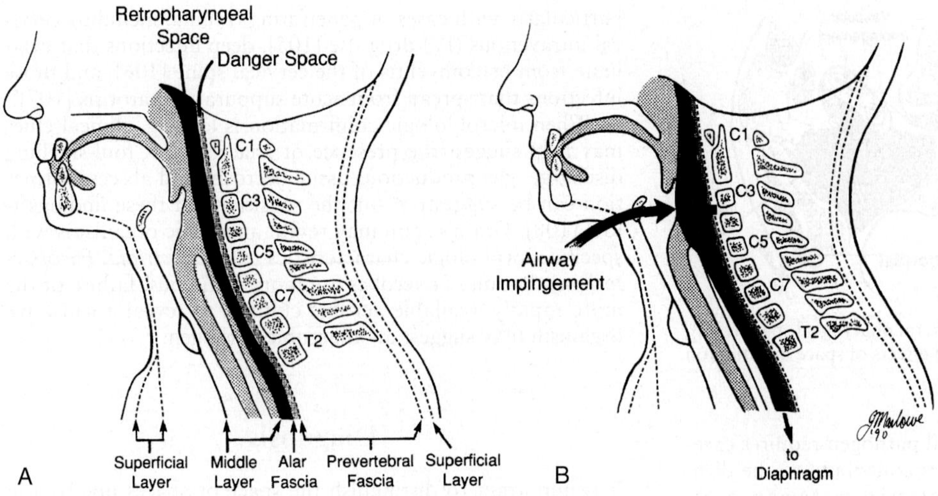

FIGURE 67.4. Schematic representation of cervical fascial planes and spaces. **A:** Normal. **B:** Retropharyngeal space abscess. [Adapted from Netter FH: *Atlas of Human Anatomy*. Summit, NJ, Ciba-Geigy, 1989.]

The submandibular space (SMS) (Fig. 67.5) consists of the sublingual and submylohyoid spaces, which communicate around the free posterior border of the mylohyoid muscle. It extends from the mucous membrane of the floor of the mouth above to the superficial layer of the deep cervical fascia below. It is bounded by the mandible both anteriorly and laterally. Superolaterally is the buccopharyngeal gap, an important opening behind the styloglossus muscle, which connects the SMS to the LPS.

The LPS (Fig. 67.6), also called the *pharyngomaxillary* or *parapharyngeal space*, is shaped like an inverted cone with its apex at the hyoid bone and its base at the base of the skull. The styloid process penetrates the space and divides it into two functional units: anterior (muscular) and posterior (neurovascular) compartments. The former lies lateral to the tonsillar fossa and connects inferomedially to the SMS. The latter contains the carotid sheath and its contents (internal carotid artery, internal jugular vein, vagus nerve, and lymph nodes), cranial nerves IX through XII, and the cervical sympathetic trunks. Both compartments abut the RPS.

The RPS, also called the *posterior visceral space*, (see Fig. 67.4) lies between the middle layer of the deep cervical fascia, which surrounds the pharynx and esophagus anteriorly, and the alar layer of the deep cervical fascia posteriorly. It extends from the base of the skull to the level of T1 or T2 in the superior mediastinum. Laterally, it abuts the LPS. Two chains of lymph nodes that drain many structures of the head are located on either side of midline.

Immediately posterior to the RPS is the *danger space* (see Fig. 67.4), so named because it is the pathway into the chest for all neck infections. It extends from the base of the skull to the diaphragms and is bounded posteriorly by the prevertebral layer of the deep cervical fascia. Involvement of this space by infection is a result of extension from the RPS or prevertebral space and can result in life-threatening complications.

The prevertebral space (see Fig. 67.4) lies between the vertebral bodies and the prevertebral layer of the deep cervical fascia. Infections in this location most often represent chronic processes arising from cervical spine injuries or infections.

Etiology

Bacteria found in normal oral flora are primarily responsible for deep cervical infections. When mucosal barriers are interrupted, bacteria can penetrate into the deeper spaces. Infections are typically polymicrobial with anaerobes predominating over aerobes. Fungi and mycobacteria are uncommon etiologic agents in these infections.

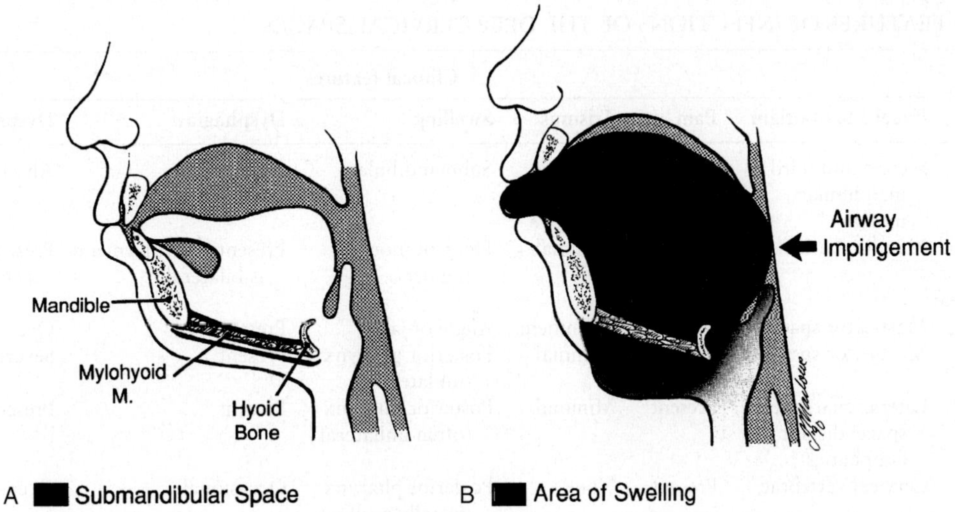

FIGURE 67.5. Schematic representation of submandibular space. **A:** Normal. **B:** Ludwig's angina. The submandibular space consists of sublingual and submylohyoid spaces. Area of swelling in **B** fills the submandibular space.

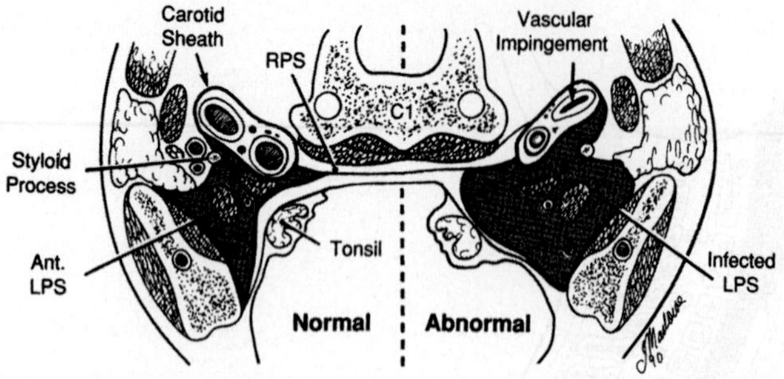

FIGURE 67.6. Cross-sectional view of lateral pharyngeal space (LPS), showing normal anatomic landmarks and effects of space infection on them. RPS, retropharyngeal space.

Correct identification of the causal pathogen requires careful culture techniques. Several factors contribute to the difficulty in obtaining meaningful bacteriologic data. Most patients receive antibiotics before hospitalization, many deep infections resolve with empiric antibiotic therapy without the need for aspiration procedures, and cultures obtained perorally are often contaminated by nonpathogenic organisms colonizing the oropharynx [98–102]. With proper anaerobic collection and transport techniques, three anaerobic isolates are most commonly identified: *Peptostreptococcus*, *Fusobacterium* (mostly *F. nucleatum*), and *Bacteroides* (mostly *B. melaninogenicus*) [98–101]. Although obligate anaerobes as a class are recovered most often, aerobic streptococci (mostly *Streptococcus viridans*) [100] and staphylococci are the most frequent individual isolates [100].

Facultative Gram-negative bacilli colonize the oropharynx in 6% to 18% of healthy adults [102] but are less common causes of deep neck infections. Rates of colonization may be as high as 60% in hospitalized and institutionalized patients and in individuals with diabetes and alcoholism [103]. *Escherichia coli*, *P. aeruginosa*, *Klebsiella pneumoniae*, *H. influenzae*, *Enterobacter*, *Proteus mirabilis*, *Citrobacter freundii*, and *Actinomyces* species have been isolated from deep cervical infections [98–103]. *Eikenella corrodens*, a facultative anaerobic Gram-negative rod, is an emerging pathogen in head and neck infections that is uniformly resistant to clindamycin [104]. Staphylococci should be considered in deep neck infections, particularly with cases of penetrating trauma, including cervical intravenous (IV) drug use [105], deep infections that originate from osteomyelitis of the cervical spine [106], and those infections that spread from acute suppurative parotitis [107].

When microbiologic confirmation is lacking, clinical clues may help suggest the presence of anaerobes. A foul-smelling discharge, gas production, tissue necrosis, and abscess formation can be suggestive, but the sensitivity of these findings is low [108]. Gram's stain may reveal anaerobic organisms with specific morphologic characteristics (e.g., *Clostridia*, *Fusobacterium*). Because anaerobes are more fastidious, failure of the more rapidly available aerobic cultures to reveal a causative organism may suggest an anaerobic pathogen.

Diagnosis

It is important to distinguish the space or spaces involved in deep neck infections to allow for early recognition and prevention of potentially devastating complications. The clinical picture may be confusing because of involvement of multiple spaces and interference with the physical examination by trismus. Fever and systemic toxicity are common early symptoms. Other signs and symptoms may be helpful to localize the primary site of infection (Table 67.2) [109]. Serologic testing contributes little to the diagnostic evaluation. Initial assessment should include a lateral neck radiograph.

Submandibular Space Infection

Infection in the SMS is exemplified by Ludwig's angina. This is a potentially life-threatening, bilateral cellulitis originating in the SMS. It spreads rapidly by direct extension, rather than via lymphatics, and can involve the submental and sublingual spaces [110]. Glandular structures are spared, and gangrene is produced without abscess formation. (see Fig. 67.5) [111]. Most patients are young, previously healthy adult men (male to female ratio, 2 to 3:1) [112]. The presenting symptoms are neck pain and swelling, tooth pain, and dysphagia [109,113]. Odontogenic infections are implicated in 70% to 90% of cases of Ludwig's angina [113]. Dyspnea, tachypnea, and stridor have been reported in as many as 27% of cases [113]. Other

TABLE 67.2

COMPARATIVE FEATURES OF INFECTIONS OF THE DEEP CERVICAL SPACES

		Clinical features				
Space infections	Usual site of origin	Pain	Trismus	Swelling	Dysphagia	Dyspnea
Submandibular	Second and third mandibular molars	Present	Minimal	Submandibular	Absent	Absent
Sublingual	Mandibular incisors	Present	Minimal	Floor of mouth (tender)	Present if involvement is bilateral	Present if involvement is bilateral
Lateral pharyngeal						
Anterior	Masticator spaces	Intense	Prominent	Angle of jaw	Present	Occasional
Posterior	Masticator spaces	Minimal	Minimal	Posterior pharynx (unilateral)	Present	Severe
Retropharyngeal (and danger)	Lateral pharyngeal space; distant via lymphatics	Present	Minimal	Posterior pharynx (often unilateral)	Present	Present
Prevertebral	Cervical vertebrae	Present	None	Posterior pharynx (usually midline)	Occasional	Occasional

Modified from Megran DW, Scheifele DW, Chow AW: Odontogenic infections. *Pediatr Infect Dis* 3:257, 1984.

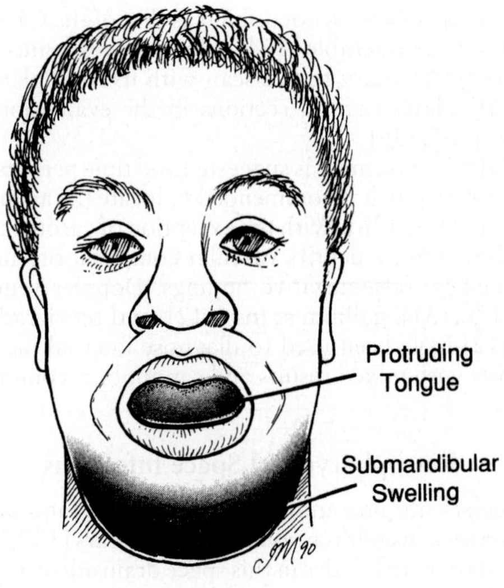

FIGURE 67.7. Schematic representation of salient clinical findings of Ludwig's angina.

symptoms include a muffled voice, drooling, and swelling of the tongue [109,113].

Ludwig's angina is essentially a clinical diagnosis. Physical examination (Fig. 67.7) reveals bilateral, firm submandibular swelling [111,113]; distortion of the mouth secondary to enlargement of the tongue, which is elevated and often protruding [112,114]; fever; and general toxicity [113]. Up to 51% of patients develop trismus, which indicates that the infection has spread to the LPS [113,114]. Airway obstruction can be a frequent and life-threatening complication of Ludwig's angina. Respiratory compromise can result from obstruction by the swollen, displaced tongue; edema of the neck and glottis; extension of edema to involve the epiglottis; and poor control of pharyngeal secretions [115,116]. Most patients with SMS involvement demonstrate soft tissue swelling (Fig. 67.8) [117]. Such a finding should prompt radiographic examination of the mandible in patients without a clear odontogenic source [118]. Mortality rates have decreased significantly due to more effective antibiotic therapy and early airway control [112,115].

Lateral Pharyngeal Space Infections

The signs and symptoms of LPS infections are determined by which of the two compartments is affected (see Fig. 67.6). The four major clinical signs of anterior compartment involvement include systemic toxicity with high fever and rigors; unilateral trismus due to irritation of the internal pterygoid muscle; induration and swelling along the angle of the jaw; and medial bulging of the lateral pharyngeal wall with the palatine tonsil protruding into the airway [113,114] (Fig. 67.9). Other symptoms may include dysphagia and pain involving the jaw or side of the neck. Pain may be referred to the ipsilateral ear and may worsen with turning the head to the unaffected side, which compresses the inflamed space by contraction of the sternocleidomastoid muscle. A history of recent upper respiratory tract infection is common [119]. Other sites of initial infection, especially in children, include the teeth, adenoids, parotid gland, middle ear with associated mastoiditis, and lymph nodes draining the nose and pharynx [113,114]. Extension from the SMS and RPS has also been implicated.

In infection of the posterior compartment, signs of sepsis—fever, leukocytosis, and often hypotension and respiratory alkalosis—are the cardinal features. Trismus and tonsillar prolapse are notably absent [120]. Dyspnea may be present as edema descends to involve the larynx and epiglottis [112]. External swelling may be visible when it spreads to the parotid space (see Fig. 67.9), but most patients have no localizing signs.

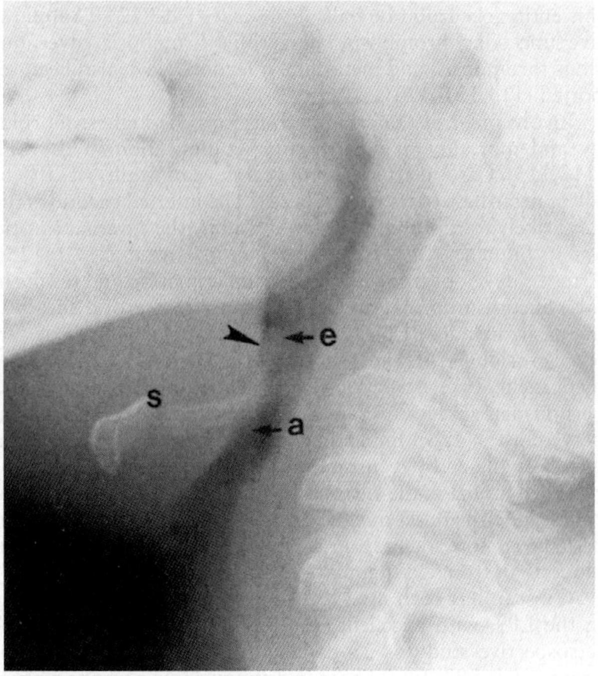

FIGURE 67.8. Ludwig's angina. Lateral radiographs of the neck obtained with soft tissue technique in a 7-year-old child. There is soft tissue swelling of the submandibular space (*s*), producing a smooth impression on the airway anteriorly, compressing and practically ablating the vallecula (*arrowhead*): the epiglottis (*e*) and aryepiglottic folds (*a*) are normal.

Many symptoms and signs in LPS infections are due to involvement of the neurovascular structures. Suppurative jugular venous thrombosis is the most common complication. Bacteremia and septic emboli, the most frequent consequences of

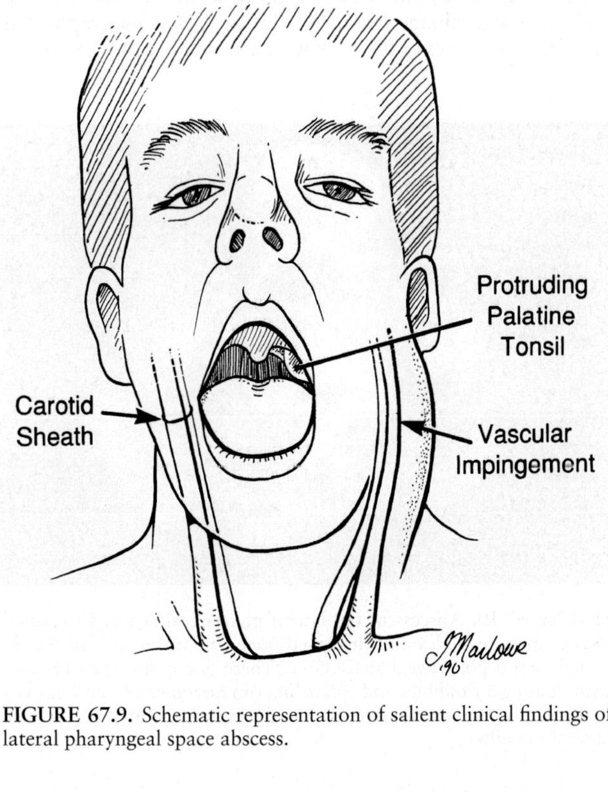

FIGURE 67.9. Schematic representation of salient clinical findings of lateral pharyngeal space abscess.

this entity, occur in one half of the cases [113,121]. Suppurative subclavian thrombosis, lateral sinus thrombosis, cavernous sinus thrombosis, and metastatic infections have also been reported [113,121–123].

Involvement of the carotid artery has the highest morbidity and mortality of any vascular complication in the LPS [112,113]. Carotid artery rupture carries a mortality of 20% to 40%, regardless of treatment [124]. The internal carotid is the most likely to rupture (62%), followed by the external carotid and its branches (25%) and the common carotid (13%) [125]. Arteritis develops from contiguous inflammation and results in false aneurysm formation [126]. Because the carotid sheath is not easily invaded, 1 or 2 weeks of illness usually precedes arterial erosion [124]. Signs suggestive of carotid sheath involvement include persistent tonsillar swelling after resolution of a peritonsillar abscess, ipsilateral Horner's syndrome, and cranial nerve palsies [126]. Impending rupture of a carotid aneurysm may be signaled by recurrent bleeds from the nose, mouth, or ears; hematoma in the surrounding tissue; a protracted clinical course; and the onset of shock [124]. Death after carotid hemorrhage is more likely from asphyxiation by the aspiration of blood than from exsanguination [124].

CT scan has been used to define neck masses, particularly in the LPS, with excellent results (Fig. 67.10) [127,128]. A retrospective study of 38 patients found a sensitivity of approximately 88% for CT scan in distinguishing parapharyngeal space (LPS) or RPS abscesses from cellulitis [129]. In another study, contrast-enhanced scans yielded an accuracy of 100% in separating abscess, cellulitis, and neoplastic lymphadenopathy [130]. Additional CT findings suggestive of an abscess are cystic or multiloculated masses with central air or fluid, soft tissue air, and surrounding edema [112,128]. Because the complications of deep neck abscesses are potentially fatal, CT scan of the neck is indicated in all cases, especially when surgical intervention is contemplated. The scan can be extended inferiorly to include the chest and mediastinum. IV contrast is helpful to enhance the abscess capsule and better evaluate the vascular structures of the LPS, but it may not specifically identify thrombosis of the internal jugular vein [131].

Ultrasonography of the neck has been used to identify fluid-filled masses and guide needle aspiration for culture material and surgical drainage techniques [132]. Ultrasonography has identified abscesses of the neck with a sensitivity of 95% [133], although its specificity is not as high as that of the CT scan, and therefore CT is preferable [134]. Magnetic resonance imaging can be complementary to CT scan with its multiplanar capability, particularly sagittal sections in the evaluation of RPS infections [135,136].

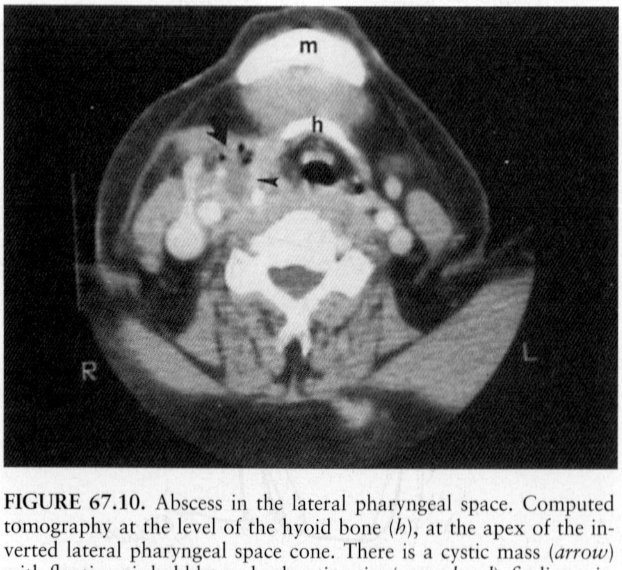

FIGURE 67.10. Abscess in the lateral pharyngeal space. Computed tomography at the level of the hyoid bone (*h*), at the apex of the inverted lateral pharyngeal space cone. There is a cystic mass (*arrow*) with floating air bubbles and enhancing rim (*arrowhead*), findings virtually pathognomonic of abscess caused by gas-forming organisms. *m*, base of mandible.

If arterial involvement is suggested and time permits, carotid artery angiography is recommended to locate the aneurysm before surgery [124,126]. With the exception of carotid angiography, studies used to identify vascular complications in the LPS are plagued by false-negative findings. Doppler venous flow studies [126,131], gallium scans [112], and retrograde venography [112] have been used to diagnose internal jugular vein thrombosis with mixed results and cannot be recommended at this time.

Retropharyngeal Space Infections

RPS abscesses are uncommon but potentially fatal infections, most often seen in children younger than 6 years [137,138]. The two chains of lymph nodes in this space drain adjacent muscles, nose, nasopharynx, pharynx, middle ear, eustachian tubes, and paranasal sinuses and are the source of most RPS abscesses. Their regression by approximately 4 years of age explains the higher frequency of this process in young children [113]. In children, the initial symptoms include fever, irritability, and refusal to eat [101]. The neck is often stiff and sometimes tilted away from the involved side [137]. Dyspnea and dysphagia occur as the swelling increases. Respiratory distress can occur as the abscess protrudes anteriorly (see Fig. 67.4). This may impair the child's ability to handle secretions [112].

In children, spontaneous rupture of a retropharyngeal abscess may result in aspiration and asphyxiation or upper airway obstruction from a combination of a child's high larynx and anterior displacement of the pharyngeal wall [101]. This can occur in adults as well, but the larger airway offers some protection from rapid airway occlusion. Uncommon complications include meningitis and epiglottitis [139].

Adults generally exhibit signs and symptoms directly referable to the pharynx. There may be a history of trauma to the posterior pharynx by intubation [113], ingestion of a foreign body [140], or an external penetrating injury [140]. Fever, sore throat, dysphagia, nasal obstruction, noisy breathing, stiff neck, and dyspnea are most common [112,113,137,138]. Pain originating in or radiating to the posterior neck that increases with swallowing is also most suggestive [137]. Severe respiratory distress, particularly if accompanied by chest pain or pleurisy, suggests mediastinal extension.

The lateral neck radiograph can aid in making the diagnosis by its ability to detect prevertebral soft tissue swelling (Fig. 67.11) [141]. The radiograph should be a true lateral view, with the neck in full extension, and should be made during inspiration. Exhalation, crying, and swallowing, especially in children, may cause thickening of the upper cervical soft tissues. Normal dimensions have been defined as less than 7 mm in all age groups at the C2 (retropharyngeal) level and less than 14 mm in children or 22 mm in adults at the C6 (retrotracheal) level [142]. Loss or reversal of the normal cervical lordosis secondary to inflammation-induced muscle spasm also suggests an RPS infection. CT scans can be valuable as well in the diagnosis of retropharyngeal abscess [135].

Descending Infections

Any deep neck infection can have access to the posterior mediastinum and diaphragms by the common pathways of the RPS and danger space [112,143,144]. Descending necrotizing mediastinitis can carry a mortality of greater than 40% [144]. The process can develop within 12 hours to as long as 2 weeks from the onset of the primary infection. An early diagnosis is difficult to make. Severe dyspnea and pleuritic or retrosternal chest

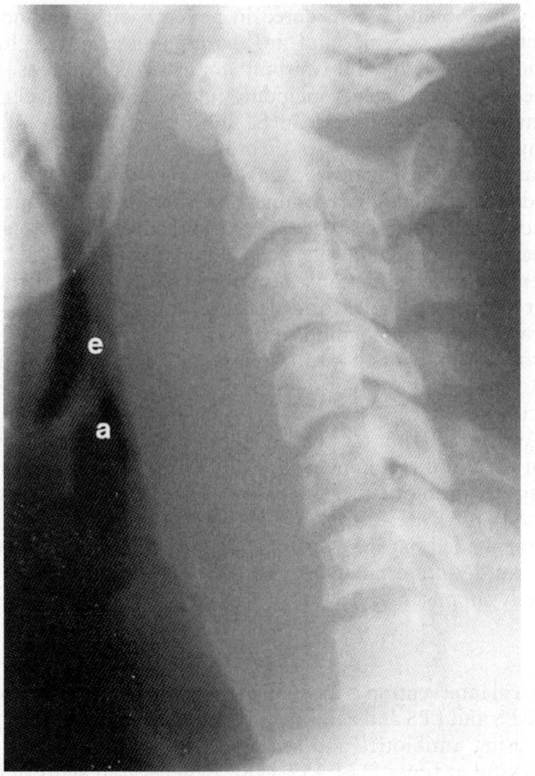

FIGURE 67.11. Retropharyngeal abscess. Lateral neck radiograph. There is marked swelling of the prevertebral soft tissues extending from the base of the skull to the base of the neck, with bulging and anterior displacement of the airway. There is mild reversal of the normal lordosis of the neck secondary to muscle spasm. The epiglottis (*e*) and aryepiglottic folds (*a*) are normal.

pain concomitant with or subsequent to the onset of symptoms of an oropharyngeal infection suggest this process. Manifestations include a widespread necrotizing process extending to the diaphragms and occasionally into the retroperitoneal space, a mediastinal abscess that may rupture into the pleural cavity, or purulent pleural and pericardial effusions [144]. Suggestive physical findings include diffuse, bulky induration of the neck and upper chest associated with pitting edema or crepitation [101,113].

Cervical necrotizing fasciitis, fascial infection with muscle necrosis, often without pus or abscess formation, can progress superficially along the fascial planes of the neck and chest wall [145–147]. Early in the course of this disease, the physical appearance may be deceptively benign. Skin erythema occurs initially and progresses to dusky skin discoloration, blisters, or bullae and eventually to visible skin necrosis [148]. Crepitation may be absent, but gas in the tissues can readily be seen using CT. Surgical exploration with wide excision is essential to determine the full extent of necrosis and to improve prognosis [145–147].

Differential Diagnosis

Few clinical entities must be distinguished from deep cervical infections. Common causes of submandibular swelling include cervical adenitis and submandibular sialoadenitis. In the proper settings, the differential diagnosis includes anticoagulant overdose with sublingual hematoma, tumor of the floor of the mouth, superior vena cava syndrome, and angioedema. None of these presents with the classic physical findings or respiratory symptoms of SMS infection due to Ludwig's angina.

The major entities from which LPS infection must be differentiated are peritonsillar abscess, anaerobic tonsillitis, and masticator space infections. In the latter, the patient presents with fever, trismus, pain, and swelling over the mandible, and the oropharyngeal examination is normal [112]. Peritonsillar abscess becomes evident with fever and tonsillar prolapse but without extreme toxicity, trismus, or parotid swelling [149]. Vincent's angina is an anaerobic tonsillitis due to *Fusobacterium necrophorum*, which produces a foul smelling discharge that forms a pseudomembrane and can be associated with bacteremia and metastatic abscesses [107].

Acute suppurative parotitis can occur as a complication of pharmacologic therapy (e.g., diuretics, anticholinergics) [149]. Reduced salivary flow allows normal oral flora to spread to Stensen's duct and into the gland. The most common pathogen is *S. aureus*, but infection is also seen with hemolytic streptococcus, Gram-negative bacilli, and anaerobes [114,149]. The mainstays of therapy are hydration, sialagogues, and often a broad-spectrum antibiotic with anti–β-lactamase activity. Despite appropriate treatment, complications may include spread to the mastoid, entrapment of the facial nerve, severe swelling of the pharynx and neck resulting in airway obstruction, and problems typical of involvement of the LPS [114,149]. Mortality may approach 25% [114,149].

The septic complications of LPS infection can mimic right-sided bacterial endocarditis [112] and be misdiagnosed as community-acquired pneumonia, pancreatic abscess, periorbital cellulitis, and temporomandibular joint pain [131]. Lemierre's syndrome, first described in 1900, but given its eponym in 1936, is the occurrence of suppurative thrombophlebitis, sepsis, and metastatic abscesses in the setting of an acute oropharyngeal infection [121,150]. With the widespread use of antibiotics for the treatment of tonsillitis/pharyngitis, there has been a dramatic decrease in the occurrence of the syndrome. As such, clinicians must be aware of its existence. The time of onset from the initial infection to sepsis is usually 1 week. Clinical evidence of internal jugular vein thrombophlebitis includes severe neck pain at the angle of the mandible and along the anterior border of the sternocleidomastoid muscle, trismus, and dysphagia [146]. Infectious emboli most commonly result in pleuropulmonary infection, although metastatic infections of the joints, bones, meninges, and liver have been reported [121,150]. *F. necrophorum* is the primary pathogen in the great majority of cases. Although penicillins had been the treatment of choice, the increasing frequency of β-lactamase–producing organisms may warrant the use of an antibiotic with β-lactamase resistance.

Retropharyngeal swelling might be due to tumors [151], hematomas [152], lymphadenopathy [153], enlargement of the prevertebral space as can occur with a cervical spine fracture [153], or tendinitis of the prevertebral muscles [151]. In children presenting with fever, sore throat, nuchal rigidity, drooling, or respiratory distress, all components of RPS abscess, severe croup, epiglottitis, and meningitis must also be considered.

Treatment

All patients with deep neck infections require hospitalization. Therapy has three components: airway management, IV antibiotics, and timely surgical exploration.

Airway Management

Establishment of an artificial airway is not universally required, but it should be done when evidence of airway obstruction exists, such as dyspnea and stridor or inability to handle secretions. The method of airway protection in patients with deep cervical infections must be individualized for the patient and to the expertise of the available personnel [154]. Upper airway obstruction is most often a complication of infections involving the SMS, for which the standard method of airway control has been tracheostomy [115,116]. Because of the proximity of the tracheostomy to submandibular wounds created for drainage, there is a potential risk of aspiration pneumonia and anterior mediastinitis [113]. Moreover, the surgical risks of tracheotomy may be increased by the distortion of the neck with edema. Because of these concerns, cricothyroidotomy has been recommended as an alternative, particularly in emergent situations [155], because of the low immediate and delayed complication rates and because it can be performed rapidly. Distortion of neck landmarks may equally complicate this procedure, but fewer critical structures are in proximity, which may reduce some procedure-related risks.

Endotracheal intubation can be difficult to achieve because of trismus and intraoral swelling. Trismus may be a more significant problem when infection has spread to the LPS. Blind intubation is unsafe because of the risk of trauma to the posterior pharyngeal wall, rupture of abscesses in the LPS or RPS, and possibly laryngospasm precipitating lower airway obstruction [115,116]. Intubation over a fiberoptic laryngoscope may be useful but requires a cooperative, stable patient and may therefore be useful only in certain cases [154]. Inhaled anesthesia to relieve trismus, along with an antisialagogue, may allow for intubation under direct vision [115,116]. If this is attempted, skilled personnel should be available to establish an emergent surgical airway if needed.

Antimicrobial Therapy

Antibiotic therapy should be given intravenously for all neck infections. Optimum empiric coverage is recommended with either penicillin in combination with a β-lactamase inhibitor (such as amoxicillin, ticarcillin with clavulanic acid, piperacillin/tazobactam) or a β-lactamase–resistant antibiotic (such as cefoxitin, cefuroxime, imipenem, or meropenem) in combination with a drug that is highly effective against most anaerobes (such as clindamycin or metronidazole) [101]. Vancomycin should be considered in patients with immune dysfunction, neutropenia, and in IV drug abusers at risk for infection with Methicillin-resistant Staphylococcus aureus [101]. If needed, other agents including linezolid, daptomycin, and quinupristin/dalfopristin can be substituted in place of vancomycin. The addition of gentamicin for effective Gram-negative coverage against *K. pneumoniae*, which is resistant to clindamycin, is highly recommended for diabetic patients with intact renal function [101]; an alternative for the seriously ill patient with penicillin allergy is chloramphenicol [112]. Parenteral antibiotic therapy should be continued until the patient has been afebrile for at least 48 hours, followed by oral therapy using amoxicillin with clavulanic acid, clindamycin, ciprofloxacin, trimethoprim–sulfamethoxazole, or metronidazole [101]. The antibiotic regimen can be de-escalated based on culture data.

Anticoagulation for septic internal jugular thrombosis has been used and recommended [124], but its efficacy as an adjuvant to antibiotic therapy has not been conclusively demonstrated [156]. Resection of a thrombosed vein is not widely recommended but may be unavoidable in a patient who deteriorates despite drainage of the LPS, or in one whose vein is frankly suppurative [131].

Surgery

Surgical intervention is most important when infections involve the RPS and LPS and can rarely be avoided. Conservative therapy using antibiotics and selective needle aspirates has been successful at times [127,157,158]. In general, if signs of clinical improvement are not observed after receiving IV antibiotics for 24 to 48 hours, then reimaging and surgical intervention are likely warranted [113]. Most recommendations are for broad-spectrum antibiotics and surgical treatments consisting of cervical drainage, thoracotomy with radical surgical debridement of the mediastinum and excision of necrotic tissue, decortication, and irrigation [159,160]. A less invasive thoracoscopic approach has also been described [161]. In contrast to LPS and RPS infections, up to one half of the cases of Ludwig's angina are cured without surgical drainage [120]. Dental extraction may be required [162]. Specific surgical approaches are reviewed elsewhere [159–161,163,164].

References

1. Meduri GU, Mauldin GL, Wunderink RG, et al: Causes of fever and pulmonary densities in patients with clinical manifestations of ventilator-associated pneumonia. *Chest* 106:221–235, 1994.
2. Marik PE: Fever in the ICU. *Chest* 117:855–869, 2000.
3. van Zanten ARH, Dixon JM, Nipshagen MD, et al: Hospital-acquired sinusitis is a common cause of fever of unknown origin in orotracheally intubated critically ill patients. *Crit Care* 9:R583–R590, 2005.
4. Westergren V, Lunblad L, Hellquist HB: Ventilator-associated sinusitis: a review. *Clin Infect Dis* 27:851–864, 1998.
5. Geiss HK: Nosocomial sinusitis. *Intensive Care Med* 25:1037–1039, 1999.
6. Talmor M, Li P, Barie PS: Acute paranasal sinusitis in critically ill patients: guidelines for prevention, diagnosis, and treatment. *Clin Infect Dis* 15:1441–1446, 1997.
7. Rouby JJ, Laurent P, Gosnach M, et al: Risk factors and clinical relevance of nosocomial maxillary sinusitis in the critically ill. *Am J Respir Crit Care Med* 150:776–783, 1994.
8. Rohr AS, Spector SL: Paranasal sinus anatomy and pathophysiology. *Clin Rev Allergy* 2:387–395, 1984.
9. Bach A, Boehrer H, Schmidt H, et al: Nosocomial sinusitis in ventilator patients: nasotracheal versus orotracheal intubation. *Anaesthesia* 47:335–339, 1992.
10. George DL, Falk PS, Meduri UG, et al: Nosocomial sinusitis in patients in the medical intensive care unit: a prospective epidemiological study. *Clin Infect Dis* 27:463–470, 1998.
11. Holzapfel L, Chastang C, Demigeon G, et al: A randomized study assessing the systematic search for maxillary sinusitis in nasotracheally mechanically ventilated patients. Influence of nosocomial maxillary sinusitis on the occurrence of ventilator-associated pneumonia. *Am J Respir Crit Care Med* 159:695–701, 1999.
12. Bert F, Lambert-Zechovsky N: Sinusitis in mechanically ventilated patients and its role in the pathogenesis of nosocomial pneumonia. *Eur J Clin Microb Infect Dis* 15:533–544, 1996.
13. Stein M, Caplan ES: Nosocomial sinusitis: a unique subset of sinusitis. *Curr Opin Infect Dis* 18:147–150, 2005.
14. Souweine B, Mom T, Traore O, et al: Ventilator-associated sinusitis: microbiological results of sinus aspirates in patients on antibiotics. *Anesthesiology* 93:1255–1260, 2000.
15. Bert F, Lambert-Zechhovsky N: Microbiology of nosocomial sinusitis in intensive care unit patients. *J Infect* 31:5–8, 1995.
16. Ferguson BJ: Mucormycosis of the nose and paranasal sinuses. *Otolaryngol Clin North Am* 33:349–365, 2000.
17. Strasser MD, Kennedy RJ, Adam RD: Rhinocerebral mucormycosis: therapy with amphotericin B lipid complex. *Arch Intern Med* 156:337–339, 1996.
18. Hunt SM, Miyamoto RC, Cornelius RS, et al: Invasive fungal sinusitis in the acquired immunodeficiency syndrome. *Otolaryngol Clin North Am* 33:335–347, 2000.
19. Choi SS, Lawson W, Bottone EJ, et al: Cryptococcal sinusitis: a case report and review of the literature. *Otolaryngol Head Neck Surg* 99:414–418, 1988.
20. Dooley DP, McAllister CK: Candidal sinusitis and diabetic ketoacidosis: a brief report. *Arch Intern Med* 149:962–964, 1989.
21. Marks SC, Upadhyay S, Crane L: Cytomegalovirus sinusitis: a new manifestation of AIDS. *Arch Otolaryngol Head Neck Surg* 122:789–791, 1996.
22. Shahin J, Gullane PJ, Dayal VS: Orbital complications of acute sinusitis. *J Otolaryngol* 16:23–27, 1987.
23. Gallagher RM, Gross CW, Phillips CD: Suppurative intracranial complications of sinusitis. *Laryngoscope* 108:1635–1642, 1998.

24. Dolan RW, Chowdhury K: Diagnosis and treatment of intracranial complications of paranasal sinus infections. *J Oral Maxillofac Surg* 53:1080–1087, 1995.
25. Parker GS, Tami TA, Wilson JF, et al: Intracranial complications of sinusitis. *South Med J* 82:563–569, 1989.
26. Singh B, Van Dellen J, Ramjettan S, et al: Sinogenic intracranial complications. *J Laryngol Otol* 109:945–950, 1995.
27. Witte RJ, Heurter JV, Orton DF, et al: Limited axial CT of the paranasal sinuses in screening for sinusitis. *Am J Radiol* 167:1313–1315, 1996.
28. Aebert H, Hunefeld G, Regel G: Paranasal sinusitis and sepsis in ICU patients with nasotracheal intubation. *Intensive Care Med* 15:27–30, 1988.
29. Hilbert G, Vargas F, Valentino R, et al: Comparison of B-mode ultrasound and computed tomography in the diagnosis of maxillary sinusitis in mechanically ventilated patients. *Crit Care Med* 29:1337–1342, 2001.
30. Vargas F, Bui HN, Boyer A: Transnasal puncture based on echographic sinusitis evidence in mechanically ventilated patients with suspicion of nosocomial maxillary sinusitis. *Intensive Care Med* 32:858–866, 2006.
31. Lichtenstein D, Biderman P, Meziere G, et al: The "sinusogram", a real-time ultrasound sign of maxillary sinusitis. *Intensive Care Med* 24:1057–1061, 1998.
32. Kountakis SE, Skoulas IG: Middle meatal vs. antral lavage cultures in intensive care patients. *Otolaryngol Head Neck Surg* 126:377–381, 2002.
33. Salord F, Gaussorgues P, Marti-Flich J, et al: Nosocomial maxillary sinusitis during mechanical ventilation: a prospective comparison of orotracheal versus the nasotracheal route for intubation. *Intensive Care Med* 16:390–393, 1990.
34. Deutschman CS, Wilton P, Sinow J, et al: Paranasal sinusitis associated with nasotracheal intubation: a frequently unrecognized and treatable source of sepsis. *Crit Care Med* 14:111–114, 1986.
35. Grillone GA, Kasznica P: Isolated sphenoid sinus disease. *Otolaryngol Clin North Am* 37:435–451, 2004.
36. Wang ZM, Kanoh N, Dai CF, et al: Isolated sphenoid sinus disease: an analysis of 122 cases. *Ann Otol Rhinol Laryngol* 111:323–327, 2002.
37. Leskinen K, Jero J: Acute complications of otitis media in adults. *Clin Otolaryngol* 30:511–516, 2005.
38. Agrawal S, Husein M, MacRae D: Complications of otitis media: an evolving state. *J Otolaryngol* 34[Suppl 1]:S33–S39, 2005.
39. Nadol JB Jr, Eavey RD: Acute and chronic mastoiditis: clinical presentation, diagnosis, and management. *Curr Clin Top Infect Dis* 15:204–229, 1995.
40. Luntz M, Keren G, Nusem S, et al: Acute mastoiditis: revisited. *Ear Nose Throat J* 73:648–654, 1994.
41. Shanley DJ, Murphy TF: Intracranial and extracranial complications of acute mastoiditis: evaluation with computed tomography. *J Am Osteopath Assoc* 92:131–134, 1992.
42. Grafstein E, Fernandes CM, Samoyloff S: Lateral sinus thrombosis complicating mastoiditis. *Ann Emerg Med* 25:420–423, 1995.
43. Hughes CE, Spear RK, Shinabarger CE, et al: Septic pulmonary emboli complicating mastoiditis: Lemierre's syndrome revisited. *Clin Infect Dis* 18:633–635, 1994.
44. Stokroos RJ, Manni JJ, de Kruijk Jr, et al: Lemierre syndrome and acute mastoiditis. *Arch Otolaryngol Head Neck Surg* 125:589–591, 1999.
45. Rubin Grandis J, Branstetter BF, Yu VL: The changing face of malignant (necrotising) external otitis: clinical, radiological, and anatomic correlations. *Lancet Infect Dis* 4:34–39, 2004.
46. Ress BD, Luntz M, Telischi FF, et al: Necrotizing external otitis in patients with AIDS. *Laryngoscope* 107:456–460, 1997.
47. Gordon G, Giddings NA: Invasive otitis externa due to *Aspergillus* species: case report and review. *Clin Infect Dis* 19:866–870, 1994.
48. Harley WB, Dummer JS, Anderson TL, et al: Malignant external otitis due to *Aspergillus flavus* with fulminant dissemination to the lungs. *Clin Infect Dis* 20:1052–1054, 1995.
49. Murray ME, Britton J: Osteomyelitis of the skull base: the role of high resolution CT in diagnosis. *Clin Radiol* 49:408–411, 1994.
50. Boringa JB, Hoekstra OS, Roos JW, et al: Multiple cranial nerve palsy after otitis externa: a case report. *Clin Neurol Neurosurg* 97:332–335, 1995.
51. Amorosa L, Modugno GC, Pirodda A: Malignant external otitis: review and personal experience. *Acta Ololaryngol Suppl (Stockh)* 521:3–16, 1996.
52. Guldfred LA, Lyhne D, Becker BC: Acute epiglottitis: epidemiology, clinical presentation, management and outcome: *J Laryngol Otol* 122, 818–823, 2008.
53. Nakamura H, Tanaka H, Matsuda A, et al: Acute epiglottitis: a review of 80 patients. *J Laryngol Otol* 115:31–34, 2001.
54. McVernon J, Slack MP, Ramsay ME: Changes in the epidemiology of epiglottitis following introduction of *Haemophilus influenzae* type b (Hib) conjugate vaccines in England: a comparison of two data sources. *Epidemiol Infect* 134:570–572, 2006.
55. Faden H: The dramatic change in the epidemiology of pediatric epiglottitis. *Pediatr Emerg Care* 22:443–444, 2006.
56. Hafidh MA, Sheahan P, Keogh I, et al: Acute epiglottitis in adults: a recent experience with 10 cases: *J Laryngol Otol* 120, 310–313, 2006.
57. Berger G, Landau T, Berger S, et al: The rising incidence of adult acute epiglottitis and epiglottic abscess. *Am J Otolaryngol* 24:374–383, 2003.
58. Ames WA, Ward VM, Tranter RM, et al: Adult epiglottitis: an under-recognized, life-threatening condition. *Br J Anaesth* 85:795–797, 2000.
59. Hebert PC, Ducic Y, Boisvert D, et al: Adult epiglottitis in a Canadian setting. *Laryngoscope* 108:64–69, 1998.
60. Glynn F, Fenton JE: Diagnosis and management of supraglottitis (epiglottitis). *Curr Infect Dis Rep* 10:200–204, 2008.
61. Hickerson SL, Kirby RS, Wheeler JG, et al: Epiglottitis: a 9-year case review. *South Med J* 89:487–490, 1996.
62. Trollfors B, Nylen O, Carenfelt C, et al: Aetiology of acute epiglottis in adults. *Scand J Infect Dis* 30:49–51, 1998.
63. Mayo-Smith MF, Spinale JW, Donskey CJ, et al: Acute epiglottitis: an 18-year experience in Rhode Island. *Chest* 108:1640–1647, 1995.
64. Kornak JM, Freije JE, Campbell BH: Caustic and thermal epiglottitis in the adult. *Otolaryngol Head Neck Surg* 114:310–312, 1996.
65. Lai SH, Wong KS, Liao SL, et al: Non-infectious epiglottitis in children: two cases report. *Int J Pediatr Otorhinolaryngol* 55:57–60, 2000.
66. McKinney B, Grigg R: Epiglottitis after anaesthesia with a laryngeal mask. *Anaesth Intensive Care* 23:618–619, 1995.
67. Frantz TD, Rasgon BM, Quesenberry CP Jr: Acute epiglottitis in adults: analysis of 129 cases. *JAMA* 272:1358–1360, 1994.
68. Shah RK, Roberson DW, Jones DT: Epiglottitis in the *Haemophilus influenzae* type B vaccine era: changing trends; *Laryngoscope*, 114:557–560, 2004.
69. Park KW, Darvish A, Lowenstein E: Airway management for adult patients with acute epiglottitis: a 12-year experience at an academic medical center (1984–1995). *Anesthesiology* 88:254–261, 1998
70. Mustoe T, Strome M: Adult epiglottitis. *Am J Otolaryngol* 4:393–399, 1983.
71. Deeb ZE, Yenson YC, DeFries HO: Acute epiglottitis in the adult. *Laryngoscope* 95:289–291, 1985.
72. MayoSmith MF, Hirsch PJ, Wodzinski SF, et al: Acute epiglottitis in adults: an eight-year experience in the state of Rhode Island. *N Engl J Med* 314:1133–1139, 1986.
73. Schumaker HM, Doris PE, Birnbaum G: Radiographic parameters in adult epiglottitis. *Ann Emerg Med* 13:588–590, 1984.
74. Schabel SI, Katzberg RW, Burgener FA: Acute inflammation of epiglottitis and supraglottic structures in adults. *Radiology* 122:601–604, 1977.
75. Schamp S, Pokiesser P, Danzer M, et al: Radiologic findings in acute epiglottitis. *Eur Radiol* 9:1629–1631, 1999.
76. Schroeder LL, Knapp JF: Recognition and emergency management of infectious causes of upper airway obstruction in children. *Semin Respir Infect* 10:21–30, 1995.
77. Stroud RH, Friedman NR: An update on inflammatory disorders of the pediatric airway: epiglottitis, croup, and tracheitis. *Am J Otolaryngol* 22:268–275, 2001.
78. Valor RR, Polnitsky CA, Tanis DJ, et al: Bacterial tracheitis with upper airway obstruction in a patient with the acquired immunodeficiency syndrome. *Am Rev Respir Dis* 146:1598–1599, 1992.
79. Edmonds LC, Prakash UB: Lymphoma, neutropenia, and wheezing in a 70-year-old man. *Chest* 103:585–587, 1993.
80. Nemzek WR, Katzenberg RW, Van Slyke MA, et al: A reappraisal of the radiologic findings of acute inflammation of the epiglottis and supraglottic structures in adults. *Am J Neuroradiol* 16:495–502, 1995.
81. Seigler RS: Bacterial tracheitis: an unusual radiographic presentation. *Clin Pediatr (Phila)* 33:374–377, 1994.
82. Donnelly BW, McMillan JA, Weiner LB: Bacterial tracheitis: report of eight new cases and review. *Rev Infect Dis* 12:729–735, 1990.
83. Yigla M, Ben-Izhak O, Oren I, et al: Laryngotracheobronchial involvement in a patient with nonendemic rhinoscleroma. *Chest* 117:1795–1798, 2000.
84. Amoils CP, Shindo ML: Laryngotracheal manifestations of rhinoscleroma. *Ann Otol Rhinol Laryngol* 105:336–340, 1996.
85. Chechani V, Vasudevan VP, Kamholz SL: Necrotizing tracheobronchitis: complication of mechanical ventilation in an adult. *South Med J* 84:271–273, 1991.
86. Bismuth C, Garnier R, Baud FJ, et al: Paraquat poisoning. An overview of the current status. *Drug Saf* 5:243–251, 1990.
87. Deeb ZE: Acute supraglottitis in adults: early indicators of airway obstruction. *Am J Otolaryngol* 18:112–115, 1997.
88. Cantrell RW, Bell RA, Morioka WT: Acute epiglottitis: intubation versus tracheostomy. *Laryngoscope* 88:994–1005, 1978.
89. Oh TH, Motoyama EK: Comparison of nasotracheal intubation and tracheostomy in management of acute epiglottitis. *Anesthesiology* 46:214–216, 1977.
90. Wood DE: Tracheostomy. *Chest Surg Clin North Am* 6:749–764, 1996.
91. Butt W, Shann F, Walker C, et al: Acute epiglottitis: a different approach to management. *Crit Care Med* 16:43–47, 1988.
92. Sheikh KH, Mostow SR: Epiglottitis—an increasing problem for adults. *West J Med* 151:520–524, 1989.
93. Cummings CW: Supraglottitis (Epiglottitis): *Cummings Otolaryngology: Head & Neck Surgery*. 4th ed. 2005.
94. Tibballs J, Shann FA, Landau LI: Placebo-controlled trial of prednisolone in children intubated for croup: *Lancet*: 340(8822):745–748, 1992.
95. Crockett DM, McGill TJ, Healy GB, et al: Airway management of acute supraglottitis at the Children's Hospital, Boston: 1980–1985. *Ann Otol Rhinol Laryngol* 97:114–119, 1988.
96. Bonadio WA, Losek JD: The characteristics of children with epiglottitis who develop the complication of pulmonary edema. *Arch Otolaryngol Head Neck Surg* 117:205–207, 1991.
97. Smith MM, Mukherji SK, Thompson JE, et al: CT in adult supraglottitis. *Am J Neuroradiol* 17:1355–1358, 1996.

98. Larawin V, Naipao J, Dubey SP: Head and neck space infections. *Otolaryngol Head Neck Surg* 135:889–893, 2006.
99. Eftekharian A, Roozbahany NA, Vaezeafshar R, et al: Deep neck infections: a retrospective review of 112 cases. *Eur Arch Otorhinolaryngol* 266:273–277, 2009.
100. Boscolo-Rizzo P, Marchiori C, Montolli F, et al: Deep neck infections: a constant challenge. *J Otorhinolaryngol Relat Spec* 68(5):259–265, 2006.
101. Vieira F, Allen SM, Stocks RMS, et al: Deep neck infection. *Otolaryngol Clin North Am* 41:459–483, 2008.
102. Greenberg RN, James RB, Marier RL, et al: Microbiologic and antibiotic aspects of infections in the oral and maxillofacial region. *J Oral Surg* 37:873–884, 1979.
103. Chen MK, Wen YS, Chang CC, et al: Deep neck infections in diabetic patients. *Am J Otolaryngol* 21:169–173, 2000.
104. Sheng WS, Hsueh PR, Hung CC, et al: Clinical features of patients with invasive *Eikenella corrodens* infections and microbiological characteristics of the causative isolates. *Eur J Clin Microbiol Infect Dis* 20:231–236, 2001.
105. Myers EM, Kirkland LS Jr, Mickey R: The head and neck sequelae of cervical intravenous drug abuse. *Laryngoscope* 98:213–218, 1988.
106. Singh G, Shetty RR, Ramdass MJ, et al: Cervical osteomyelitis associated with intravenous drug use. *Emerg Med J* 23(2):e16, 2006.
107. Brook I: Current management of upper respiratory tract and head and neck infections. *Eur Arch Otorhinolaryngol* 266(3):315–323, 2009.
108. Brook I: Microbiology and principles of antimicrobial therapy for head and neck infections. *Infect Dis Clin North Am* 21(2):355–391, vi., 2007.
109. Tovi F, Fliss DM, Zirkin HJ: Necrotizing soft-tissue infections in the head and neck: a clinicopathological study. *Laryngoscope* 101:619–625, 1991.
110. Chou YK, Lee CY, Chao HH, et al: An upper airway obstruction emergency: Ludwig angina. *Pediatr Emerg Care* 23(12):892–896, 2007.
111. Britt JC, Josephson GD, Gross CW: Ludwig's angina in the pediatric population: report of a case and review of the literature. *Int J Pediatr Otorhinolaryngol* 52:79–87, 2000.
112. Blomquist IK, Bayer AS: Life-threatening deep fascial space infections of the head and neck. *Infect Dis Clin North Am* 2:237–264, 1988.
113. Reynolds SC, Chow AW: Severe soft tissue infections of the head and neck: a primer for critical care physicians. *Lung* 187:271–279, 2009.
114. Lee CY, Herzog S: Infections in the lateral pharyngeal space: anatomy, diagnosis and management. *Ann Dent* 50:3–7, 1991.
115. Neff SP, Merry AF, Anderson B: Airway management in Ludwig's angina. *Anaesth Int Care* 27:659–661, 1999.
116. Marple BF: Ludwig angina: a review of current airway management. *Arch Otolaryngol Head Neck Surg* 125:596–599, 1999.
117. Chow AW, Roser SM, Brady FA: Orofacial odontogenic infections. *Ann Intern Med* 88:392–402, 1978.
118. Patterson HC, Kelly JH, Strome M: Ludwig's angina: an update. *Laryngoscope* 92:370–378, 1982.
119. Huang TT, Liu TC, Chen PR, et al: Deep neck infection: analysis of 185 cases. *Head Neck* 26:854–860, 2004.
120. Moreland LW, Corey J, McKenzie R: Ludwig's angina: report of a case and review of the literature. *Arch Intern Med* 148:461–466, 1988.
121. Chirinos JA, Lichtstein DM, Garcia J, et al: The evolution of Lemierre syndrome: report of 2 cases and review of the literature. *Medicine* 81:458–465, 2002.
122. Reynolds SC, Chow AW: Life-threatening infections of the peripharyngeal and deep fascial spaces of the head and neck. *Infect Dis Clin North Am* 21(2):557–576, 2007.
123. Bentham JR, Pollard AJ, Milford CA, et al: Cerebral infarct and meningitis secondary to Lemierre's syndrome. *Pediatr Neurol* 30:281–283, 2004.
124. Alexander DW, Leonard JR, Trail ML: Vascular complications of deep neck abscesses. *Laryngoscope* 78:361–370, 1968.
125. Salinger S, Pearlman SJ: Hemorrhage from pharyngeal and peritonsillar abscesses. *Arch Otolaryngol* 18:464, 1933.
126. Blum DJ, McCaffrey TV: Septic necrosis of the internal carotid artery: a complication of peritonsillar abscess. *Otolaryngol Head Neck Surg* 91:114–118, 1983.
127. Nagy M, Backstrom J: Comparison of the sensitivity of lateral neck radiographs and computed tomography scanning in pediatric deep-neck infections. *Laryngoscope* 109:775–779, 1999.
128. Wang LF, Kuo WR, Tsai SM, et al: Characterizations of life-threatening deep cervical space infections: a review of one hundred ninety-six cases. *Am J Otolaryngol* 24:111–117, 2003.
129. Lazor JB, Cunningham MJ, Eavey RD, et al: Comparison of computed tomography and surgical findings in deep neck infections. *Otolaryngol Head Neck Surg* 111:746–750, 1994.
130. Holt GR, McManus K, Newman RK, et al: Computed tomography in the diagnosis of deep-neck infections. *Arch Otolaryngol* 108:693–696, 1982.
131. Celikel TH, Muthuswamy PP: Septic pulmonary emboli secondary to internal jugular vein phlebitis (postanginal sepsis) caused by *Eikenella corrodens. Am Rev Respir Dis* 130:510–513, 1984.
132. Chao HC, Chiu CH, Lin SJ, et al: Colour Doppler ultrasonography of retropharyngeal abscess. *J Otolaryngol* 28:138–141, 1999.
133. Siegert R: Ultrasonography of inflammatory soft tissue swellings of the head and neck. *J Oral Maxillofac Surg* 45:842–846, 1987.
134. Vogel CC, Boyer KM: Metastatic complications of *Fusobacterium necrophorum* sepsis: two cases of Lemierre's postanginal septicemia. *Am J Dis Child* 134:356–358, 1980.
135. Munoz A, Castillo M, Melchor MA, et al: Acute neck infections: prospective comparison between CT and MRI in 47 patients. *J Comput Assist Tomogr* 25:733–741, 2001.
136. Weber AL, Siciliano A: CT and MR imaging evaluation of neck infections with clinical correlations. *Radiol Clin North Am* 38:941–968, 2000.
137. Lalakea M, Messner AH: Retropharyngeal abscess management in children: current practices. *Otolaryngol Head Neck Surg* 121:398–405, 1999.
138. Goldenberg D, Golz A, Joachims HZ: Retropharyngeal abscess: a clinical review. *J Laryngol Otol* 111:546–550, 1997.
139. Ramsey PG, Weymuller EA: Complications of bacterial infections of the ears, paranasal sinuses, and oropharynx in adults. *Emerg Med Clin North Am* 3:143–160, 1985.
140. Poluri A, Singh B, Sperling N, et al: Retropharyngeal abscess secondary to penetrating foreign bodies. *J Craniomaxillofac Surg* 28:243–246, 2000.
141. Chong V, Fan Y: Radiology of the retropharyngeal space. *Clin Radiol* 55:740–748, 2000.
142. Furst I, Ellis D, Winton T: Unusual complication of endotracheal intubation: retropharyngeal space abscess, mediastinitis, and empyema. *J Otolaryngol* 29:309–311, 2000.
143. Sancho LM, Minamoto H, Fernandez A, et al: Descending necrotizing mediastinitis: a retrospective surgical experience. *Eur J Cardiothorac Surg* 16:200–205, 1999.
144. Kiernan PD, Hernandez A, Byrne WD, et al: Descending cervical mediastinitis. *Ann Thorac Surg* 65:1483–1488, 1998.
145. Djupesland PG: Necrotizing fascitis of the head and neck—report of three cases and review of the literature. *Acta Otolaryngol Suppl* 543:186–189, 2000.
146. Whitesides L, Cotto-Cumba C, Myers R: Cervical necrotizing fasciitis of odontogenic origin: a case report and review of 12 cases. *J Oral Maxillofac Surg* 58:144–151, 2000.
147. Mohammedi I, Ceruse P, Duperret S, et al: Cervical necrotizing fasciitis: 10 years' experience at a single institution. *Intensive Care Med* 25:829–834, 1999.
148. Stoykewych AA, Beecroft WA, Cogan AG: Fatal necrotizing fasciitis of dental origin. *J Can Dent Assoc* 58:59–62, 1992.
149. Herzon FS, Nicklaus P: Pediatric peritonsillar abscess: management guidelines. *Curr Probl Pediatr* 26:270–278, 1996.
150. Lustig LR, Cusick BC, Cheung SW, et al: Lemierre's syndrome: two cases of postanginal sepsis. *Otolaryngol Head Neck Surg* 112:767–772, 1995.
151. Husaru AD, Nedzelski JM: Retropharyngeal abscess and upper airway obstruction. *J Otolaryngol* 8:443–447, 1979.
152. Owens DE, Calcaterra TC, Aarstad RA: Retropharyngeal hematoma: a complication of therapy with anticoagulants. *Arch Otolaryngol* 101:565–568, 1975.
153. Barratt GE, Koopman CF Jr, Coulthard SW: Retropharyngeal abscess: a ten-year experience. *Laryngoscope* 94:455–463, 1984.
154. Ovassapian A, Tuncbilek M, Weitzel EK, et al: Airway management in adult patients with deep neck infections: a case series and review of the literature. *Anesth Analg* 100:585–589, 2005.
155. Isaacs JH Jr, Pedersen AD: Emergency cricothyroidotomy. *Am Surg* 63:346–349, 1997.
156. Yau PC, Norante JD: Thrombophlebitis of the internal jugular vein secondary to pharyngitis. *Arch Otolaryngol Head Neck Surg* 106:507–508, 1980.
157. Lee KC, Tami TA, Echavez M, et al: Deep neck infections in patients at risk for acquired immunodeficiency syndrome. *Laryngoscope* 100:915–919, 1990.
158. Plaza Mayor G, Martinez-San Millan J, Martinez-Vidal A: Is conservative treatment of deep neck space infections appropriate? *Head Neck* 23:126–133, 2001.
159. Iwata T, Sekine Y, Shibuya K, et al: Early open thoracotomy and mediastinopleural irrigation for severe descending necrotizing mediastinitis. *Eur J Cardiothorac Surg* 28:384–388, 2005.
160. Hirai S, Hamanaka Y, Mitsui N, et al: Surgical treatment of virulent descending necrotizing mediastinitis. *Ann Thorac Cardiovasc Surg* 10:34–38, 2004.
161. Isowa N, Yamada T, Kijima T, et al: Successful thoracoscopic debridement of descending necrotizing mediastinitis. *Ann Thorac Surg* 77:1834–1837, 2004.
162. Juang YC, Cheng DL, Wang LS, et al: Ludwig's angina: an analysis of 14 cases. *Scand J Infect Dis* 21:121–125, 1989.
163. Mora R, Jankowska B, Catrambone U, et al: Descending necrotizing mediastinitis: ten years' experience. *Ear Nose Throat J* 83:774, 776–780, 2004.
164. Kirse DJ, Roberson DW: Surgical management of retropharyngeal space infections in children. *Laryngoscope* 111:1413–1422, 2001.

CHAPTER 68 ■ ACUTE INFECTIOUS PNEUMONIA

VERONICA BRITO AND MICHAEL S. NIEDERMAN

Pneumonia is a common community- and hospital-acquired infection that is managed in the intensive care unit (ICU) when it leads to acute respiratory failure or septic shock and complicates the course of an otherwise serious illness. Modern medical technology has not been able to eliminate this infection. Rather, it has promoted its emergence by the application of novel, life-sustaining therapies that lead to specific at-risk populations who have impairments in respiratory tract host defenses. This chapter reviews the scope of the problem in seriously ill patients.

Pneumonia occurs in up to 6 million outpatients annually (community-acquired pneumonia, CAP), with up to 1 million requiring hospitalization [1]. Pneumonia also develops in the hospital (nosocomial pneumonia or hospital-acquired pneumonia [HAP]), particularly in those patients with underlying serious illnesses, at the rate of approximately five to ten cases per one thousand hospital admissions [2]. In the hospital, the incidence of pneumonia is directly related to the degree of underlying systemic illness in a given patient, with the incidence being higher in medical than in surgical patients, and in those requiring prolonged mechanical ventilation than in those managed by short-term ventilatory support [2]. Recently, the distinction between CAP and HAP has become blurred, because patients with chronic illness often live in complex environments out of the hospital (nursing homes), or patients are repeatedly admitted to the hospital, or they receive treatments in healthcare settings such as dialysis centers. These individuals come in contact with the healthcare environment, even when they are not hospitalized, and can become infected with hospital-associated drug-resistant pathogens, and when they develop pneumonia, it is termed healthcare-associated pneumonia (HCAP) [2].

Certain patient populations are at increased risk for pneumonia, primarily as a result of disease-associated impairments in lung host defenses. These include the elderly and those with cardiac disease, alcoholism, chronic obstructive pulmonary disease (COPD), congestive heart failure (CHF), malnutrition, head injury, cystic fibrosis, bronchiectasis, malignancy, splenic dysfunction, renal failure, liver failure, diabetes mellitus, and any immunosuppressive illness or therapy [2,3]. In addition, hospitalized patients often receive therapeutic interventions that predispose them to pneumonia, including antibiotic therapy, enteral feeding, endotracheal intubation, tracheostomy, and the use of certain medications (such as corticosteroids, aspirin, digitalis, morphine, and pentobarbital) [3].

The mortality implications of pneumonia (along with influenza) rank it as the eighth leading cause of death in the United States, the sixth leading cause of death in those older than 65 years, and the number one cause of death from infectious diseases [4]. Although CAP can vary from a mild to a severe illness, those who enter the ICU with this infection have a mortality rate that can vary from 20% to greater than 50% [5]. Older studies questioned whether use of the ICU was even beneficial for severe CAP, but that was at a time when the ICU was only used when the disease was far advanced. In more recent studies, an effort has been made to identify patients with severe CAP at the earliest possible time point, and thus while as many as 90% of ICU admitted CAP patients in older studies were intubated and mechanically ventilated, more recently, only about 60% to 70% of CAP patients in the ICU receive this intervention. This means that the indications for ICU admission and the definitions of severe CAP are changing, and with good reason, since the later in the hospital course that the ICU is used, the higher the mortality [6]. Recently, Woodhead et al. [6] found that CAP accounted for 5.9% of all ICU admissions, but that early admission (within 2 days of hospitalization) appeared to be preferable and was associated with a lower mortality (46.3%) than late admission (>7 days in the hospital, 50.4% mortality). Thus, the mortality associated with severe CAP is a reflection of how accurately the ICU is used, what organisms are causing the infection, what complications develop in the hospital, and how effective is the initial empiric therapy [7] (Table 68.1).

In data from the National Nosocomial Pneumonia Infection Surveillance System, pneumonia is the most common, ICU-acquired infection, with 86% of episodes being associated with mechanical ventilation [8]. Patients usually develop HAP because of an underlying chronic illness, and thus the question arises, if they die, whether their death was due to the pneumonia itself or a result of the underlying, predisposing illness. This issue of "attributable mortality" has been studied, and as many as 60% of those who die do so as a direct result of their pneumonia [9]. Not all studies report attributable mortality, particularly those involving surgical and trauma patients, a group that seems to acquire pneumonia commonly but usually without a major direct effect on mortality [10]. In those with acute respiratory distress syndrome (ARDS), the mortality rate of pneumonia has been reported to be high, with only 12% of patients with pneumonia surviving in contrast to 67% survival in the absence of infection [11]; however, more recent data report lower death rates from pneumonia in patient with ARDS.

Bacteriology is another important factor adding to mortality in HAP, with Kollef et al. [12] reporting a high attributable mortality for late-onset ventilator-associated pneumonia (VAP) caused by potentially drug-resistant organisms such as *Pseudomonas aeruginosa*, *Acinetobacter* spp, and *Stenotrophomonas maltophilia*. Rello et al. [13] matched patients with VAP caused by methicillin-resistant *Staphylococcus aureus* (MRSA) with controls having caused by other organisms. They found that the mortality for MRSA VAP was 48%, compared with 25% for control patients ($p < 0.01$). Heyland et al. [14] compared 177 patients with VAP to a matched control group of critically ill ventilated patients without pneumonia and found that patients with pneumonia had a longer duration of mechanical ventilation, longer stay, and a trend toward increased mortality, particularly with the use of initially inappropriate empiric antibiotic therapy. Thus, similar to the data with severe CAP, mortality in HAP is also affected by patient characteristics, bacteriology, and the accuracy of therapy. In studies of HCAP, when patients are admitted to the ICU, mortality can also be high, and it is increased if patients do not receive appropriate initial antibiotic therapy [15].

TABLE 68.1

RISK FACTORS FOR PNEUMONIA MORTALITY IN PATIENTS WITH CAP

Physical findings
Abnormal vital signs
Respiratory rate >30/min
Hemodynamic compromise: systolic or diastolic hypotension
Tachycardia (>120/min)
Afebrile or high fever (>38°C)
Altered mental status or coma
Laboratory findings
Respiratory failure: hypoxemic or hypercarbic
Multilobar infiltrates
Rapidly progressive infiltrates
Positive blood culture
Multiple organ failure
Hypoalbuminemia
Renal insufficiency
Polymicrobial infection
Historical information
Serious comorbidity or advanced age
Poor functional status at presentation
Recent hospitalization
Immunosuppression (including systemic corticosteroids)
Nonrespiratory clinical presentation
Delayed or inappropriate therapy
Prolonged mechanical ventilation

TYPES OF PNEUMONIA ENCOUNTERED IN THE INTENSIVE CARE UNIT

Serious pneumonia occurs when a potential pathogen overwhelms a patient's host defenses, and then, because of either overwhelming infectious challenge or an excessive inflammatory response to infection, the patient develops respiratory failure or septic shock. Certain pathogens are so virulent that they can even overcome an intact, and normal, host defense system, as is the case with epidemic viral illness. Normal host defenses can also be overcome if the inoculum of the pathogen is large (as with massive aspiration), but smaller inocula can be pathogenic if disease-associated factors interfere with immune function. Certain patients seem to become ill because of an excessive inflammatory response to a localized infection, and genetic polymorphisms in the immune response are being identified to explain this phenomenon.

Community-Acquired Pneumonias Leading to Intensive Care Unit Admission

Although less than 20% of all patients with CAP require hospitalization, those patients ill enough to enter the hospital may have a substantial mortality rate. As classically described by Austrian and Gold [16], for certain patients with advanced illness, even penicillin therapy could not eliminate the mortality of pneumococcal pneumonia, because the disease process was too advanced at the time of presentation.

When CAP leads to ARDS, a complication that occurs in less than 5% of cases, the mortality rate can exceed 70% [17]. For a general ICU population, the mortality rate of CAP, reported in a meta-analysis of 788 patients, was just more than 35%, and other series have reported even lower rates [18]. Pneumonia caused by bacteria, viruses, fungi, and protozoa can occasionally be severe enough to prompt admission to the ICU. Pathogens that have been described as causing severe CAP include *Streptococcus pneumoniae* (pneumococcus), *Legionella pneumophila*, *Haemophilus influenzae*, enteric Gram-negative bacteria, *S. aureus* (including community-acquired methicillin-resistant strains), *Mycoplasma pneumoniae*, *Pneumocystis jiroveci*, *Mycobacterium tuberculosis*, *Chlamydophila pneumoniae*, endemic fungi (blastomycosis, histoplasmosis) influenza virus, respiratory syncytial virus, varicella, severe acute respiratory syndrome virus (SARS, caused by a coronavirus), and the bacteria associated with aspiration pneumonia [4].

Definition of Severe CAP and Prognostic Factors/Scoring Systems

Although "severe" CAP does not have a uniform definition, the term has been used to refer to patients with CAP who require ICU care, although, recently, some investigators have focused on defining patients with CAP who need invasive respiratory or vasopressor support (IRVS), independently of site of admission [4,5]. Torres et al. [19] estimated that CAP accounted for 10% of all admissions to an ICU over a 4-year period, and that these patients were admitted directly to the ICU 42% of the time, after admission to another ward 37% of the time, and in transfer from another hospital 21% of the time.

There are some patients in whom pneumonia is such a virulent infection that survival may have already been determined when they reach the ICU because the patient is already "too far gone." Some older studies questioned whether treating CAP patients in the ICU could even impact mortality, since as many as 75% of patients with pneumococcal pneumonia managed in the ICU died. However, in older series, most of these patients were mechanically ventilated when admitted to the ICU so that the ICU may have been used very late in the course of illness. In more recent studies, only about 60% to 70% of patients with CAP in the ICU receive mechanical ventilation [6]. In these series of severe CAP, the mortality rates have varied from 21% to 54%, with the lower mortality rates being found when not all patients were mechanically ventilated, and the higher mortality rates being seen when nearly 90% were being ventilated [5]. These findings suggest that there is value in defining the need for ICU care at the earliest possible time point, and not reserving the ICU for extreme circumstances such as overt respiratory failure and shock.

Poor prognostic factors in CAP are as follows: multilobar pneumonia, respiratory rate greater than 30 breaths per minute, severe hypoxemia, abnormal liver function, low serum albumin, signs of clinical sepsis, and delayed or inappropriate antibiotic therapy [4,18]. While sepsis increases CAP mortality, bacteremia by itself is not a mortality risk. In a recent study [20], bacteremia was not an independent mortality risk or a predictor of delayed clinical response, after controlling for other variables such as age, comorbidities, and abnormal vital signs at presentation.

Over the past decade, a number of studies have examined prognostic scoring systems for patients with CAP. In general, there are two widely used approaches, the Pneumonia Severity Index (PSI) and the British Thoracic Society approach (CURB-65). Each uses a point scoring system to predict a patient's mortality risk, with the CURB-65 being simpler and more focused on acute illness parameters, whereas the PSI is a more complex system that incorporates measurements of both chronic and acute disease factors [5]). While both tools predict mortality risk, neither is a direct measure of severity of illness. For example, as many as 37% of those admitted to the ICU in one study [21] were in PSI classes I–III, pointing out that even those with a low risk for death (which PSI can measure) may benefit from aggressive intensive care support [21]. Conversely, patients in higher PSI classes do not always need ICU care if they fall into these high mortality risk groups because of advanced age and comorbid illness in the absence of physiologic findings of severe pneumonia.

In one recent study [22], both tools were applied to the same patients, and each was similarly accurate for identifying low-risk patients. However, the CURB-65 was more discriminating in predicting mortality risk for patients with more severe illness. This approach gives one point for each of five abnormalities: confusion, elevated blood **u**rea nitrogen (BUN) (>19.6 mg per dL), respiratory rate 30 per minute or more, low **b**lood pressure (BP) (either systolic ≤90 mm Hg or diastolic ≤60 mm Hg), and whether the patient is at least **65** years old. If three of these five criteria are present, the predicted mortality rate is greater than 20%, and these patients are generally considered for ICU admission [23]. A similar approach has been developed by the Japanese Respiratory Society, the A-DROP scoring system, that assesses **A**ge (male ≥70 years, female ≥75 years); **D**ehydration (BUN ≥210 mg per L); **R**espiratory failure (Sao(2) ≤90% or Pao(2) ≤60 mm Hg); **O**rientation disturbance (confusion); and low blood **P**ressure (systolic BP ≤90 mm Hg) [24].

Another scoring system, developed by España et al., based on data from 1,057 patients in Spain, suggested that the need for ICU admission could be defined by the presence of one of two major criteria (arterial pH <7.39 or a systolic BP <90 mm Hg), or the presence of two of six minor criteria, which included confusion, BUN greater than 30 mg per dL, respiratory rate greater than 30 per minute, PaO_2/FiO_2 ratio less than 250, multilobar infiltrates, and age 80 years or older. This approach gave different point values to each abnormality, and when severity criteria were met, the tool was 92% sensitive for identifying those with severe CAP and was more accurate than the PSI or the CURB-65 [25]. Another tool, the SMART-COP approach [26], was developed in Australia to predict the need for IRVS using eight clinical features, in which the acronym referred to systolic BP less than 90 mm Hg, multilobar infiltrates, albumin less than 3.5, respiratory rate elevation (>25 for those younger than 50 years, and >30 for those older than 50 years), tachycardia (>125 per minute), confusion, low oxygen (<70 mm Hg if younger than 50 years or <60 mm Hg if older than 50 years), and arterial pH less than 7.35. The abnormalities in the systolic BP, oxygenation, and arterial pH each received 2 points, whereas the five other criteria received 1 point each, and with this system, the need for IRVS was predicted by a SMART-COP score of at least 3 points. Using this cutoff, the sensitivity for the need for IRVS was 92.3% and the specificity of 62.3%, with a positive and negative predictive value of 22% and 98.6%, respectively. Both PSI and CURB-65 did not perform as well overall.

The adverse prognostic factors discussed above are particularly applicable to the elderly, and those with nursing home–acquired pneumonia often have a higher mortality rate than those with simple CAP [5]. One factor that may explain this finding is that older patients often have atypical clinical presentations of pneumonia, which may lead to their being diagnosed at a later, more advanced stage of illness, resulting in an increased risk of death [5]. Older patients from nursing homes presenting with pneumonia are now included in a separate category, called HCAP.

Recently, the accuracy of prognostic scoring systems has been enhanced by biomarker measurements. Salluh et al. [27] and others have found that baseline cortisol levels showed a good correlation with CAP outcome. The most data have focused on procalcitonin (PCT), a "hormokine" that has increased plasma concentrations in the presence of severe bacterial infections, but not in viral illness. Masia et al. [28] found that PCT levels correlated well with the PSI score and the development of complications such as empyema, mechanical ventilation, and septic shock in a study of 185 patients. In another study performed in patients with severe CAP, a rise in PCT during hospitalization correlated with mortality. In other studies, PCT data have supplemented the information provided by prognostic scoring tools. Krüger et al. [29] found that PCT identified low-risk patients in all severity classes, and that the finding of a low PCT value had a 98.9% negative predictive value for mortality, regardless of the results of prognostic scoring tools. Similarly in a study of 1,651 patients admitted with CAP, there were 546 in high PSI classes (IV and V), but in the 126 of these who had low PCT levels, only 2 died [30], suggesting the advantage of combining serum markers with the commonly used prognostic indices.

Although there are no absolute criteria for severe pneumonia, or need for ICU admission, in the 2007 American Thoracic Society/Infectious Society Diseases of America (ATS/IDSA) guidelines, [4] severe CAP was defined as the presence of one of two major criteria (need for mechanical ventilation, or septic shock requiring pressors) or the presence of three of nine minor criteria. These minor criteria were a PaO_2/FiO_2 ratio of 250 or less, respiratory rate 30 per minute or more, confusion, multilobar infiltrates, systolic BP less than 90 mm Hg despite aggressive fluid resuscitation, BUN greater than 20 mg per dL, leukopenia (<4,000 cells per mm^3), thrombocytopenia (<100,000 cells per mm^3), and hypothermia (<36°C) [4]. This approach requires further validation, but in one study of 2,102 patients, of which 235 were admitted to the ICU, this predictive rule had a sensitivity of 71% and a specificity of 88% for determining need for ICU admission. This degree of accuracy was similar to the 2001 ATS guideline rule [31]. The use of only minor criteria to define need for ICU care is uncertain, since in that study, only 47 of 219 patients meeting only minor criteria needed ICU admission, and the presence of minor criteria alone did not increase mortality risk.

CAP Prognostic Factors Defined After Initial Management

The above discussion has focused on data available on admission that can be used to guide the site of care decision. However, after admission, the results of cultures become available, and therapy (accurate or not) is given, and these events can impact prognosis. Garau et al. [32] have found that late and overall CAP mortality are reduced if patients have negative blood cultures, and if antibiotic therapy is given according to guidelines. Among patients with severe CAP, the most important prognostic finding during therapy is radiographic progression [19]. Ineffective initial empiric therapy has also been identified as a potent predictor of death, being associated with a 60% mortality rate, compared with an 11% mortality rate when patients received initial effective therapy [33]. Similarly, in other studies of CAP, the use of a combination of a β-lactam and a macrolide antibiotic was associated with a lower mortality than if other therapies were given [4], and the use of guideline compliant therapy was associated with a reduced duration of mechanical ventilation [34]. In the setting of pneumococcal bacteremia, the use of combination therapy is associated with reduced mortality, compared with monotherapy, particularly for patients treated in the ICU [4]. Not only must initial therapy be accurate, it must be timely, and in patients with septic shock (from all sources, including pneumonia), mortality increases by 7% for each hour in the delay of initiating therapy [35]. Retrospective data have also shown a reduced mortality for admitted CAP patients who are treated within 4 hours of arrival to the hospital compared with those who are treated later [4].

The interaction between prognostic factors related to therapy and bacteriology is most evident when patients with CAP are infected with drug-resistant organisms, particularly drug-resistant pneumococcus. Pneumococcal resistance to penicillin is increasing and is present in more than 40% of all pneumococci by older definitions of in vitro resistance [4]. Studies have defined the clinical features of patients at risk for drug-resistant pneumococcus (drug-resistant *S. pneumoniae* [DRSP]) [4] and these include older than 65 years, β-lactam therapy in the past 3 months, multiple medical comorbidities, alcoholism, nosocomial acquisition, and contact with a child in day care. Recently, the criteria for resistance in nonbacteremic infection have changed, and fewer organisms are defined as resistant, compared with the past, since many available therapies are known to be effective [36]. Studies of bacteremic pneumococcal pneumonia have shown that the presence of resistance is not itself a predictor of a poor outcome or a risk factor for mortality. In the absence of meningitis, clinical failure with high-dose β-lactam therapy is currently unlikely [4,36]. Most investigators have found no difference in mortality for patients infected with resistant or sensitive organisms, after controlling for comorbid illness [36,37], although patients with resistant organisms may have a more prolonged hospital stay, and suppurative complications such as empyema [38], and in HIV infection, the presence of high-level penicillin resistance has been associated with increased mortality [39]. The breakpoint for clinically significant penicillin resistance is a minimum inhibitory concentration value of 4 μg per mL or more, with increased mortality in patients with invasive disease (bacteremia) and this degree of resistance, who do not die in the first 4 days of illness [40].

Nosocomial Pneumonia in the Intensive Care Unit: Hospital-Acquired Pneumonia

Risk Factors for HAP and VAP

As mentioned, pneumonia is the nosocomial infection most likely to contribute causally to the death of patients, particularly those treated with mechanical ventilation (VAP). Risk factors for this infection fall into four categories: the underlying primary critical illnesses leading to ICU admission; coexisting medical illness; factors associated with therapies that are frequently used in the ICU; and malnutrition. Thus, some of the common conditions associated with nosocomial pneumonia include risk factors present on admission such as immune-suppressive illness, risk of aspiration (coma, impaired consciousness), serious comorbid illnesses (chronic heart or lung disease, renal failure, malignancy, diabetes mellitus), ARDS, malnutrition (serum albumin <2.2 mg per dL), obesity, older than 60 years, smoking and drug abuse, need for major surgery, and recent major trauma or burns. Other nonmodifiable risk factors that increase the risk of nosocomial pneumonia are treatment related such as prior antibiotic therapy, immune suppressive therapy (including corticosteroids), need for multiple transfusions, transport out of the ICU, mechanical ventilation with PEEP, tracheostomy, nasogastric tube use, supine position in the first 24 hours after admission, and intestinal bleeding prophylaxis [2,41]. The most important risk factor for nosocomial pneumonia is probably mechanical ventilation, explained later in the chapter.

HAP is currently the second most common nosocomial infection in the United States and is associated with high mortality and morbidity [2]. HAP accounts for up to 25% of all ICU infections and for more than 50% of the antibiotics prescribed [2]. The presence of HAP increases hospital stay by an average of 7 to 9 days per patient and VAP leads to an excess cost of more than $40,000 per patient [2]. Available data suggest that it occurs at a rate of between five and ten cases per one thousand hospital admissions, and that critically ill patients who develop VAP appear to be twice as likely to die compared with similar patients without VAP (pooled odds ratio [OR], 2.03; 95% confidence interval, 1.16 to 3.56) [9].

In ICU patients, nearly 90% of episodes of HAP occur during mechanical ventilation, referred to as VAP, when the illness develops after 48 hours of endotracheal intubation and ventilation. Intubation increases the risk of acquiring pneumonia by as much as 6- to 20-fold [2]. Older studies estimated that the risk of nosocomial pneumonia was 1% per day of mechanical ventilation, but other data show a risk of 3% per day for the first 5 days, 2% per day for days 6 to 10 days, and 1% per day for days 11 through 15 [42]. Although VAP occurs in 9% to 27% of all intubated patients [2], since many patients are intubated for only a short time, up to half of all VAP episodes begin within the first 4 days of mechanical ventilation (early-onset pneumonia) [2]. In the past, mortality rates were high in mechanically ventilated patients, with Craven et al. [43] reporting a 55% mortality rate in 49 patients with nosocomial pneumonia treated with mechanical ventilation, and Bryan and Reynolds [44] finding a 58% mortality rate in patients with bacteremic nosocomial pneumonia.

Recently, in the United States, there has been a focus on prevention of VAP, through the use of "ventilator bundles," and there have been numerous reports of "zero VAP" as a consequence of these efforts [45]. These bundles, which include daily assessment for weaning, daily interruption of sedation, elevation of the head of the bed, prophylaxis of deep vein thrombosis, and gastrointestinal bleeding, have been quite successful, but most studies have reported a reduction in the frequency of VAP, without associated reductions in mortality or antibiotic use. Thus, it is unclear if VAP is really being prevented, or if the disease is being diagnosed less often, especially given the subjective nature of the VAP definition, and the possibility of treating patients for another diagnosis. If VAP does occur, proper management can impact outcome, with several studies showing that management with a guideline-concordant therapy can improve outcomes [46,47].

The relation between pneumonia and ARDS is particularly interesting. In older studies, as many as one third of all cases of ARDS were the result of pneumonia [48], but secondary pneumonia was the most common nosocomial infection acquired by patients with established ARDS [2,11]. When patients with ARDS develop pneumonia, it is generally a late event, occurring after at least 7 days of mechanical ventilation [2], and when it occurs [11], it can be the start of a progressive downhill course characterized by multiple organ failure. In a European collaborative study of 583 patients with ARDS, pneumonia was the cause in 33% of cases and a complication in 34% [49]. When quantitative diagnostic methods were used in ARDS patients, Chastre et al. [50] found an incidence of 55% of VAP in patients with ARDS; however, there were no significant changes in survival between ARDS patients with VAP and those without VAP. All patients who developed VAP had a significantly longer duration of mechanical ventilation, regardless of whether they had coexisting ARDS.

Healthcare-Associated Pneumonia

The other type of pneumonia that has been described recently and may require ICU admission is HCAP. This entity refers to patients who develop infection while having contact with the healthcare environment, such as those residing in nursing homes, those treated in dialysis units, patients who have been in the hospital in the past 90 days, and those getting home infusion therapy of home wound care (Table 68.2), and some of these patients are at risk for infection with multidrug resistant (MDR) organisms. This has also been addressed in the ATS/IDSA guidelines as a form of HAP [2]. However, recent studies have shown that patients who qualify has having HCAP are a heterogeneous population, and that when HCAP patients

TABLE 68.2

HOSPITAL-ACQUIRED PNEUMONIA AND HEALTHCARE-ASSOCIATED PNEUMONIA: RISK FACTORS FOR MULTIDRUG RESISTANT ORGANISMS

Current hospitalization of ≥5 d
Antibiotic treatment in prior 90 d
High frequency of antibiotic resistance in the community/specific hospital unit
Immunosuppressive disease/therapy
Presence of multiple risk factors for healthcare-associated pneumonia
Hospitalization for 2 d or more in the preceding 90 d
Residence in a nursing home or extended care facility
Home infusion therapy (including antibiotics)
Chronic dialysis within 30 d
Home wound care
Family member with multidrug-resistant pathogen

Adapted from Niederman MS, Craven DE, Bonten MJ, et al: Guidelines for the management of adults with hospital-acquired, ventilator-associated, and healthcare-associated pneumonia. *Am J Respir Crit Care Med* 171:388–416, 2005, with permission.

are managed in the ICU, the frequency of MDR pathogens is much greater than when they are not as ill and do not need ICU care [51].

PATHOGENESIS OF PNEUMONIA

Normal Host Defenses

When an organism enters the respiratory tract, it encounters a host defense system designed to repel and remove it from every anatomic site in the airway. Pneumonia develops when the size of the organism inoculum overcomes the host defense system, when the organism is so virulent that it cannot be repelled, or when the patient is so impaired that he or she is unable to resist an organism type or inoculum size that could ordinarily be handled by a fully functioning host defense system.

The oropharynx is ordinarily free of enteric Gram-negative bacilli because salivary proteases, secretions, and local immunoglobulin-A (IgA) antibody prevent these bacteria from establishing a foothold on the mucosal surface. The intrinsic ability of the oral epithelium to bind or adhere to Gram-negative bacteria is poor in healthy people [52]. With a variety of acute illnesses, such as malnutrition, uremia, and general surgery, Gram-negative bacteria can bind more avidly to the oral epithelium, and colonization can occur [52].

The lower respiratory tract (starting beneath the vocal cords) has a complex host defense system that keeps this site sterile in normal people [2,3]. For this area to become infected, organisms must overcome the physical barrier of the vocal cords and the tracheobronchial protective mechanisms of cough, bronchoconstriction, airway angulation, and the upward transport of the mucociliary blanket [3]. As in the oropharynx, bacterial adherence is necessary for Gram-negative bacteria to colonize the tracheobronchial tree. Protective substances in respiratory secretions include IgA, the predominant immunoglobulin of the upper airway; IgG, which dominates in the lower respiratory tract; complement; lysozymes; surfactant; and fibronectin [3]. The resident phagocytic cell of the lower respiratory tract is the alveolar macrophage, but its function can be augmented by the production of inflammatory cytokines which can promote the recruitment of blood neutrophils and the development of cell-mediated and humoral immunity.

In the setting of focal lung infection, the cytokine inflammatory response is normally localized to the site of initial infection [53]. Severe pneumonia occurs when the inflammatory response is unable to be localized (due to overwhelming infection or inappropriate bilateral inflammation) or if the inflammatory response extends to the systemic circulation (sepsis syndrome). The innate immune response of the lung is organized to recognize pathogens and once this occurs, a cytokine response follows. Pathogen recognition is mediated by toll-like receptors for Gram-negative bacteria or by pathogen-stimulated production of interleukin 1 (IL-1) or tumor necrosis factor (TNF). Once pathogens are recognized through these mechanisms, nuclear factor κB is produced by inflammatory cells, which in turn leads to cytokine production that can recruit more inflammatory cells. In addition, the lower airway handles individual pathogens in specific ways. For example, *S. aureus* is removed by resident alveolar macrophages, whereas certain enteric Gram-negative bacteria and the pneumococcus require the recruitment of neutrophils (presumably in response to interleukin-8) to be cleared [53]. Cell-mediated immunity is required to resist infection with *L. pneumophila* and *M. tuberculosis*. Viruses are handled somewhat differently from bacteria, and important factors in defense against these agents include the alveolar macrophage, neutralizing antibodies (IgG, IgA, IgM), cytotoxic T lymphocytes, and cytokines such as interferon. Specific genetic immune impairments or acquired immune dysfunction can cause specific aspects of the inflammatory response to malfunction and lead to infection with specific, predictable pathogens.

How Microorganisms Reach the Lung

Bacteria and other infectious agents can reach the lung by inhalation from ambient air, hematogenously from distal sites of infection, by direct extension or exogenous penetration, and by aspiration from a colonized oropharynx and nasopharynx [2,3]. Inhalation is an uncommon route of organism entry except for pathogens such as *L. pneumophila*, viruses, and *M. tuberculosis*. Hematogenous spread can occur with septic emboli from such sites as the valves of the right cardiac chambers. Exogenous penetration is an unlikely route of bacterial entry but can occur, for example, with extension of an abdominal infection into the pleural space and then the lung parenchyma. Most pneumonias result when microorganisms are aspirated from a previously colonized oropharynx [2]. Nosocomial pneumonia is frequently preceded by Gram-negative bacillary colonization of the oropharynx [2]. The source of bacteria that colonize the upper airway is most likely the patient's own lower intestinal flora, but the nasal sinuses and stomach can also harbor bacteria that can subsequently reach the lung. The coexistence of nosocomial sinusitis and pneumonia has been documented, often with the same organisms, and both infections can be promoted by the presence of a nasogastric or nasotracheal tube [2].

In addition to promoting sinusitis, the endotracheal tube and the nasogastric tube can also serve as additional pathways for bacterial entry to the lung. Insertion of an endotracheal tube allows organisms direct access to the lung from the hands of the ICU staff, thereby avoiding the defense mechanisms present above the vocal cords. Any organisms that reach the inside of the endotracheal tube can proliferate to large numbers because this site is free from host defenses, and a biofilm commonly lines the interior of the endotracheal tube and can contain as many as 10^6 organisms per cm of the tube surface [54]. These organisms can reach the lung every time an intubated patient is suctioned [2]. Recently, this problem has been addressed by developing new materials for endotracheal tubes that are antibacterial, one such device is a silver-coated endotracheal tube, which may be able to reduce the incidence of VAP, but has had no impact on mortality [55]. Another factor in VAP pathogenesis is the ventilator circuit tubing, which can easily be contaminated by large numbers of bacteria [2]. Interestingly, the ventilator circuits are usually not contaminated by the ventilator but rather by the patient, as the circuit becomes colonized in large numbers, as bacteria proliferate in the water condensate in the tubing. If handled carefully, the circuits are not a major source of pneumonia pathogens, and the incidence of pneumonia is not increased even if ventilator circuit tubing is never changed during the course of therapy [2]. The presence of an endotracheal tube can promote infection, and studies [2] have shown that when an endotracheal tube is present, some bacteria, particularly *P. aeruginosa*, can colonize the lower airway directly without first colonizing the oropharynx.

The gastrointestinal tract, particularly the stomach, can serve as a reservoir for bacteria, and several investigators have shown that Gram-negative bacilli can move retrograde from the stomach to the oropharynx and then antegrade into the lung [56]. The stomach can be the source of 20% to 40% of the enteric Gram-negative bacteria that colonize the trachea of intubated patients [56], but it is difficult to determine if these colonizing gastric bacteria also lead to pneumonia. One of the ways that the stomach can be an important source of pneumonic organisms is through the mechanism of reflux and aspiration. When a nasogastric tube is used for feeding, it can promote aspiration, especially if a large-bore tube is used with a bolus feeding method rather than with a continuous infusion of enteral nutrients, and if the patient is kept in a supine position [57]. When a nasogastric tube is present, it may promote pneumonia if the gastric contents have a pH above 4 to 6, as can occur with the use of antacids, H_2 blockers, and enteral feeding. An elevated pH can increase the number of Gram-negative bacteria in the stomach, increases to as many as 1 to 100 million per mL of gastric juice, and elevation of gastric pH has been reported as a risk factor for nosocomial pneumonia, although not in all studies [43,58]. The Canadian Critical Care Trials Group reported that acidified enteral feeds preserve gastric acidity and substantially reduce gastric colonization in critically ill patients; however, in this study, there was no impact on the incidence of pneumonia with this intervention [58]. Increases in gastric volume can be detrimental and promote aspiration, thus accounting for the observation that when continuous enteral feeding leads to an elevation of gastric pH (and presumably an elevation of gastric volume), the incidence of pneumonia is higher than when continuous feeding is used but does not raise pH [59]. Placing the feeding tube into the jejunum to avoid an elevation in gastric pH did not reduce the risk of pneumonia [60]. Another way to minimize the impact of the stomach and to avoid aspiration is to keep patients in a semierect position whenever possible, particularly because the supine position can favor aspiration when a nasogastric tube is in place [57].

Airway Colonization and Nosocomial Pneumonia

Colonization (the persistence of organisms in the absence of a host response and without an adverse effect to the host) of the respiratory tract by enteric Gram-negative bacilli is the first step toward the development of nosocomial pneumonia [2]. Risk factors for Gram-negative colonization of the upper and lower respiratory tract are similar and include antibiotic therapy, endotracheal intubation, smoking, malnutrition, general surgery, and therapies that raise gastric pH [3,52]. Additional risk factors for oropharyngeal colonization include azotemia, diabetes, coma, hypotension, advanced age, and underlying lung disease [52]. Additional risk factors for tracheobronchial colonization include chronic bronchitis, cystic fibrosis, ciliary dysfunction, tracheostomy, bronchiectasis, acute lung injury, and viral infection [52]. The distinction between colonization and infection in mechanically ventilated patients is less clear than in the past, with recognition and focus on ventilator-associated tracheobronchitis (VAT) [61]. Some patients who are mechanically ventilated can have high concentrations of pathogenic organisms in the tracheobronchial tree, in the absence of pneumonia, yet some may be clinically ill, and therapy could potentially prevent some from progressing to VAP.

One pathogenetic mechanism that links many of the clinical risk factors for upper and lower airway colonization is a cell–cell interaction termed bacterial mucosal adherence. Many clinical disease states can alter the oropharyngeal or tracheal epithelium, making the cell surface more receptive for binding by such bacteria as *P. aeruginosa* [52]. Diseases that result in an increased number of oropharyngeal and tracheal cell bacterial receptors are many of the same processes that promote colonization of these sites [52]. One study of intubated patients demonstrated the rapidity with which the endotracheal tube itself became colonized with enteric Gram-negatives and found that colonization took place despite the use of bacterial filters in the ventilator circuit [62]. Colonization is a common finding in intubated patients, and the presence of potential pathogens in the respiratory secretions of intubated patients is to be expected, and does not require therapy unless there are clinical signs of infection.

Host Defense Impairments in Acute and Chronic Illness that Predispose to Pneumonia

Many systemic diseases increase the risk of pneumonia as a result of disease-associated malfunctions in the respiratory host defense system, including ARDS, sepsis, CHF, malnutrition, renal failure, diabetes mellitus, chronic liver disease, alcoholism, cancer, and collagen vascular disease [63]. For example, sepsis can lead to a number of inflammatory events that interfere with respiratory tract immune defenses. In addition, many illnesses can be complicated by pneumonia because they require therapy with medications that interfere with immune function. Several studies have shown that acute and chronic malnutrition (Table 68.3) can increase the risk of bacterial and viral infections both in and out of the hospital. Genetic polymorphisms may explain why patients who have certain inherited patterns of immune response are more prone to severe forms of pneumonia than others, and even mortality. CAP severity is increased with genetic changes in the IL-10-1082 locus that are often present along with changes in the TNF-α-308 locus. Another genetic change associated with an increased risk of septic shock from CAP is a modification in heat shock protein 70-2

TABLE 68.3

LUNG HOST DEFENSE IMPAIRMENTS WITH MALNUTRITION

Increased tracheal and buccal cell adherence
Altered macrophage function and migration
Reduced recruitment of neutrophils
Impaired cell-mediated immunity and T-cell depletion
Diminished secretory immunoglobulin A
Complement deficiency

[64]. Currently, there are large number of genes that can affect the severity and outcome of CAP, but the clinical application of this is not defined. One recent observation about gender differences in the immune response was that men have a higher degree of systemic inflammation on admission for CAP (higher levels of TNF, IL-6, and IL-10), and that higher levels of these mediators increased pneumonia mortality risk [65].

ETIOLOGY OF PNEUMONIA

Community-Acquired Pneumonia

Even with extensive diagnostic testing, a specific etiologic agent can be identified in only approximately 50% of pneumonias that develop outside of the hospital, although the rate of pathogen recovery may be higher in intubated and mechanically ventilated patients [66,67]. Although the exact incidence of viral pneumonias is unknown, these agents may account for up to one third of all community-acquired cases. The most common pathogen identified in pneumonias arising out of the hospital is the pneumococcus, followed by *M. pneumoniae*, *L. pneumophila*, *H. influenzae*, *C. pneumoniae*, anaerobes, *S. aureus*, and enteric Gram-negative bacilli, although the exact incidence of each pathogen varies depending on a number of factors. These include the severity of the acute illness, the age of the patient, and the types of comorbidity present in a given patient population [4,67]. In the elderly, although pneumococci are still the most common pathogens, enteric Gram-negative organisms may be responsible for 20% to 40% of all cases of pneumonia, and anaerobes and *H. influenzae* are other common agents [68]. However, age alone has little impact on the bacterial etiology of CAP, but rather, the comorbid illnesses that become more common in the elderly affect bacteriology [69]. The most common CAP pathogens leading to ICU admission (severe pneumonia) are pneumococcus, *L. pneumophila*, epidemic viruses (influenza), *S. aureus* (including MRSA), and enteric Gram-negative bacilli, including, in some patients, *P. aeruginosa* [4,67,68]. The incidence of CAP caused by community-acquired MRSA (CA-MRSA) is on the rise, but the exact frequency and the impact on mortality and other outcomes remain to be defined [70]. Although Gram-negatives are more common in VAP and HCAP than in CAP, risk factors for Gram-negative pneumonia (in addition to nursing home residence, an HCAP risk factor) are cardiac disease, smoking history, and clinical features of severe illness including hyponatremia, septic shock, and severe tachypnea [71].

Other pathogens that can lead to respiratory failure include *H. influenzae*, pathogens associated with aspiration (such as anaerobes), *P. jiroveci*, *tuberculosis*, varicella, and respiratory syncytial virus. Mixed infection occurs in more than 10% of patients with CAP requiring hospitalization, and in one study, in patients with mixed CAP, *S. pneumoniae* was the most prevalent microorganism (44 out of 82; 54%) [72]. In that study, the most frequent combination was *S. pneumoniae* with *H. influenzae* (17 out of 82; 21%), and influenza A occurred with *S. pneumoniae* in 5 out of 28 (18%). Of note, patients with mixed pyogenic pneumonia more frequently developed shock when compared with patients with single pyogenic pneumonia (18% vs. 4%) [72].

When evaluating a patient with pneumonia, it is important to understand the status of each individual's respiratory host defense system to predict which possible pathogen is most likely (Table 68.4). Thus, CAP in a previously healthy person is most likely due to a pathogen of such intrinsic virulence that it can overcome even an intact host defense system. These pathogens include *S. pneumoniae*, *Legionella* sp, *S. aureus*, and *M. pneumoniae.* Certain agents should be suspected in specific clinical settings. If the patient has a serious underlying illness, then organisms of less intrinsic virulence that would ordinarily be eliminated by a normal host can be responsible. When an alcoholic has pneumonia, anaerobes and *Klebsiella pneumoniae* become more likely; those with chronic bronchitis may be infected with nontypeable *H. influenzae* and *Moraxella catarrhalis*; cardiac patients commonly have pneumococcal infection; those with cystic fibrosis are commonly infected by *S. aureus* and *P. aeruginosa*; and those with risk factors for aspiration can have enteric

TABLE 68.4

LIKELY PATHOGENS FOR PNEUMONIA IN THE CRITICALLY ILL

Database	Suspected pathogen
Alcoholism—acute or chronic	*Streptococcus pneumoniae* (including DRSP), anaerobes, Gram-negative bacilli, *Mycobacterium* sp
Chronic obstructive pulmonary disease	*S. pneumoniae, Haemophilus influenzae, Moraxella catarrhalis*
Recent viral infection	*S. pneumoniae, Staphylococcus aureus* (including MRSA), *H. influenzae*, Gram-negative bacilli
Nursing home (age >75 y)	Gram-negative bacilli (including resistant ones such as *Pseudomonas aeruginosa, Acinetobacter* spp), *S. pneumoniae, H. influenzae*, aspiration (anaerobes), *S. aureus, Chlamydophila, Mycobacterium tuberculosis*
AIDS (risk groups: intravenous drug abuser, hemophilia, homosexual)	*S. pneumoniae, Salmonella*, cytomegalovirus, *H. influenzae, Cryptococcus, P. jiroveci*, anaerobes, *M. tuberculosis*
Hospital acquired	Gram-negative bacilli (including *P. aeruginosa*), *S. aureus* (including MRSA)
High-risk aspiration	Anaerobes (if aspirate while not intubated), Gram-negative bacilli, chemical pneumonitis
Cardiac disease	*S. pneumoniae*, Gram-negative bacilli
Neutropenia	*P. aeruginosa, Aspergillus* sp, Gram-negative bacilli
Recent antibiotic therapy	DRSP, *P. aeruginosa*, MRSA (especially in HAP)
Postinfluenza	Pneumococcus, *S. aureus* (including MRSA), enteric Gram-negatives
Endobronchial obstruction	Anaerobes, Gram-negative bacilli
Structural lung disease (cystic fibrosis, bronchiectasis)	*P. aeruginosa, P. cepacia, S. aureus*

AIDS, acquired immunodeficiency syndrome; DRSP, drug-resistant *S. pneumoniae*; HAP, hospital-acquired pneumonia; MRSA, methicillin-resistant *S. aureus.*

TABLE 68.5

HISTORICAL AND PHYSICAL FEATURES USEFUL IN PNEUMONIA DIAGNOSIS

Clinical setting	Organisms
Environmental contact	
Birds, bats	*Chlamydophila psittaci, Cryptococcus neoformans, Histoplasma capsulatum*
Bird droppings	*C. psittaci, H. capsulatum* (histoplasmosis)
Ungulates	*Coxiella burnetii* (Q fever)
Hunting (animal and insect bites)	*Yersinia pestis* (plague), *Francisella tularensis* (tularemia)
Infected hides	Anthrax
Travel or location	
Southeast Asia	*Pseudomonas pseudomallei*, SARS (coronavirus)
Southwestern United States	*Coccidioides immitis* (coccidioidomycosis)
Midwestern United States	*H. capsulatum* (histoplasmosis)
Prison environment	*Mycobacterium* sp (tuberculosis)
Poor dental hygiene	Anaerobes

SARS, severe acute respiratory syndrome.

Gram-negative bacterial or anaerobic lung infection. Other associations are listed in Table 68.4. Certain historical information can be valuable, such as an appropriate travel or exposure history that suggests specific etiologic pathogens (Table 68.5).

Nosocomial Pneumonia

Both VAP and HCAP may be caused by a variety of Gram-positive and Gram-negative bacteria, many of which are multidrug resistant (MDR). These infections may be polymicrobial and are seen more often in patients with ARDS than in other ventilated patients [73]. Viral or fungal pathogens are rarely causative in immunocompetent hosts [74,75]. Nosocomial viral infections can occur if infected staff members come to work when their illness is incubating. Common pathogens include aerobic Gram-negative bacilli, such as *P. aeruginosa*, *Escherichia coli*, *K. pneumoniae*, and *Acinetobacter* species. Gram-positive infections include *S. aureus*, particularly MRSA, which has been increasing in the United States [76]. Pneumonia due to *S. aureus* is more common in patients with diabetes mellitus, head trauma, and ICU patients. In the National Nosocomial Infections Surveillance (NNIS) system data examining changes in the organisms from 1986 to 2003, Gram-negative aerobes persisted as being the most frequent organisms in HAP (65.9%), with little change in their distribution over this period, except for a rise in the proportion of *Acinetobacter* in 2003, from 1.5% in 1975 to 6.9% in 2003. The commonest Gram-negative organism reported was *Pseudomonas* (18.1%), and others included *Klebsiella* spp (7.2%), *Acinetobacter* spp (6.9%), and *E. coli* (5%). The Gram-positive organisms included *S. aureus* (included *Enterobacter* spp (10%), 27.8%), coagulase-negative *Staphylococcus* (1.8%), and *Enterococci* (1.3%) [77]. Among patients who have a prolonged hospital stay, therapy with corticosteroids or antibiotics, need for long-term mechanical ventilation, and in those with ARDS, the pathogen most likely to cause pneumonia is *P. aeruginosa*, but in many hospitals, *Acinetobacter* is becoming an increasing concern. Contamination with *Legionella* sp in the water system can lead to infection, especially if patients are being treated with corticosteroids. Another pathogen that should be considered when nosocomial pneumonia arises in the setting of corticosteroid therapy for COPD is *Aspergillus* sp. [78]. HAP involving anaerobic organisms may follow aspiration in nonintubated patients but is rare in patients with VAP [2]. Gram-negative organisms are more common with aspiration, especially in the healthcare environment, including the nursing home [51,68]. Oropharyngeal commensals such as viridans group streptococci, coagulase-negative staphylococci, *Neisseria* species, and *Corynebacterium* species can produce infection in immunocompromised hosts and some immunocompetent patients [2]. The identity of specific MDR pathogens causing HAP varies from one ICU to another, and depends on the patient population treated and the degree of prior antibiotic exposure, but the dominant organisms change over time [2,77]. Risk factors for infection with MDR pathogens are summarized in Table 68.2.

Elderly patients represent a diverse population of patients with pneumonia, particularly HCAP. Elderly residents of long-term care facilities have been found to have a spectrum of pathogens similar to late-onset HAP and VAP [2,51,79].

In patients aged 75 years and older with severe pneumonia, El-Solh et al. found *S. aureus* (29%), enteric Gram-negative rods (15%), *S. pneumoniae* (9%), and *Pseudomonas* species (4%) as the most frequent causes of nursing home–acquired pneumonia [74]. In this population, MDR organisms are most likely in patients with a history or prior antibiotic therapy and poor functional status. Scant data are available about HAP in patients who are not mechanically ventilated. In general, the bacteriology of nonventilated patients is similar to that of ventilated patients, including infection with MDR pathogens. The frequency of resistant Gram-negative bacilli is often high enough in nonventilated patients that they should be accounted for in designing an empiric therapy regimen. Sopena et al. [80] looked at a multicenter population of non–ICU admitted patients with HAP in Spain and described that the most common etiologies were *S. pneumoniae*, *L. pneumophila*, *Aspergillus* sp, *P. aeruginosa*, and several Enterobacteriaceae. Another study therapy for nonsevere HAP and HCAP [81] found among 303 patients, 53.5% had an identifiable etiology, with *Enterobacteriaceae* in 19.5%, followed by *S. pneumoniae* in 12.9% and *S. aureus* in 11.6%. In a study that examined both HAP and VAP in the same hospital, patients with VAP had infection with non-Enterobacteriaceae Gram-negatives (*P. aeruginosa* and *Acinetobacter* spp) more commonly than HAP patients, while *S. pneumoniae* was more common in HAP patients [82].

The bacteriology of HCAP is widely variable depending on which study is examined [51]. Current data show that HCAP is a heterogeneous disease, including a wide range of patients, some severely ill and others not. In the severely ill population, often treated in the ICU, MDR Gram-negatives and MRSA are common and must be considered when designing empiric therapy. These resistant organisms are a particular concern in severely ill patients with other risk factors, including poor functional status, prior antibiotic therapy, immune-suppressive therapy, and a history of recent hospitalization. In one study, focusing on HCAP with nearly half of the patients treated in the ICU [15], the most common pathogens were *S. aureus*, then *S. pneumoniae*, followed by *P. aeruginosa*.

CLINICAL FEATURES OF PNEUMONIA

General Features of Community-Acquired Pneumonia

The signs and symptoms of pneumonia depend on both host and bacterial factors, and in the past, the presentation was classified as being either "typical" or "atypical," but data have shown that this approach is not clinically useful [4]. In several studies, the clinical presentations of CAP (including severe CAP) have overlapped enough among all etiologies that clinical features could not be used to identify the likely etiologic pathogen or to guide initial antibiotic therapy [4,7,69]. The common clinical features of CAP include fever, cough, sputum production, dyspnea, and occasionally pleuritic chest pain. Gastrointestinal symptoms that may be seen include nausea, vomiting, and diarrhea, which were regarded previously as "atypical features." In the elderly patient, pneumonia can have a nonrespiratory presentation with symptoms of confusion, falling, failure to thrive, altered functional capacity, or deterioration in a preexisting medical illness, such as CHF.

Because many of the symptoms of pneumonia result from the host inflammatory response, patients who have altered immune function have less dramatic symptoms. Thus, those with advanced age, chronic lung disease, cardiac disease, renal failure, diabetes, immunosuppressive therapy, and other chronic illnesses have not only an increased incidence of pneumonia but also a less distinct and subtler clinical presentation. In this patient population, fever has been absent in up to 10% of those with bacteremic pneumonia [83].

General Features of Nosocomial Pneumonia

One of the major controversies in critical care medicine is how to determine when hospital-acquired (particularly ventilator-associated) pneumonia is present. On clinical grounds alone, the diagnosis is imprecise and is a particular problem in those with ARDS or lung contusion. Fagon et al. [84], using quantitative cultures collected with a protected specimen brush (PSB) to define this infection in mechanically ventilated patients, have reported that up to two thirds of cases that are diagnosed based on clinical criteria alone are not truly pneumonia. Most clinical definitions of nosocomial pneumonia require the patient to be hospitalized 48 to 72 hours before the onset of purulent sputum, leukocytosis, fever, and a new and persistent infiltrate. If these features exist along with isolation of a potential pathogen from the sputum, then this organism is deemed to be responsible for the infection. The findings of a positive blood culture or radiographic cavitation add to the likelihood of pneumonia being present. Positive blood cultures in nosocomial pneumonia can support the diagnosis, but if the organism present in the blood culture is different from the one in the respiratory tract, the bacteremia may be secondary to an extrapulmonary infection [2]. One approach to the clinical definition of VAP, developed by Pugin et al. [85], has been to use a scoring system that weights the likelihood of pneumonia using six clinical variables: fever, white blood cell count and differential, the presence of pathogens in the sputum, sputum purulence, radiographic patterns, and oxygenation changes. When this clinical pulmonary infection score (CPIS) has been used, the clinical and quantitative bacteriologic definitions of pneumonia have correlated very well. These observations suggest that there may still be a role for careful clinical judgment in the diagnosis of this confusing infection.

In the presence of diseases such as ARDS, atelectasis, pulmonary embolism, lung contusion, and CHF, all of which may be associated with lung infiltrates, pneumonia may be overlooked, or these processes may be incorrectly diagnosed as lung infection. In addition, the elderly and immunosuppressed may have few clinical findings when pneumonia develops in the hospital. Limited sputum production due to impaired immunologic status and mobilization of leukocytes compound the difficulties in diagnosis. Conversely, those on a mechanical ventilator with VAT may have purulent sputum, fever, and pathogens colonizing the sputum but not have invasive parenchymal lung infection. The use of biomarkers, both in the serum and in the respiratory secretions, may help in making this difficult diagnosis. In patients with VAP, the role of biomarkers to corroborate the clinical diagnosis is being studied. To date, studies have used PCT [86], C-reactive protein [87], soluble triggering receptors expressed on myeloid 1 (STREM) [88], and IL-6 [89], among others.

DIAGNOSTIC APPROACH TO THE PATIENT WITH SEVERE PNEUMONIA

Once the presence of severe pneumonia has been defined, the patient should be categorized by place of origin of infection, defining the illness as CAP, HCAP, or HAP (including VAP). Then the immune competence of the patient, the types of comorbid diseases present, and the existence of risk factors for specific pathogens should be defined to identify the most likely etiologic pathogens. Historical data, physical examination, and laboratory findings pertinent to diagnoses will also be helpful in determining which etiologic agent is responsible and what specific therapy should be instituted (see Tables 68.4 and 68.5). For example, contact with animals, especially birds, rats, and rabbits, can suggest the diagnosis of psittacosis, tularemia, and plague, respectively.

Historical Information

The history can be used to determine if the patient has pneumonia as the cause of his or her acute illness, recognizing that certain populations, such as the elderly, may have an altered, nonclassical presentation of pneumonia. In the elderly and compromised host, the infection may be heralded only by lethargy and confusion [69]. In the compromised host with malignancy or immunosuppressive therapy, the presentation may be so stunted that pneumonia may be discovered only serendipitously at autopsy.

Hemoptysis is an important historical feature, since it implies tissue necrosis and is most common with pyogenic streptococcal pneumonia (groups A to D), anaerobic lung abscess, *S. aureus*, necrotizing Gram-negative organisms, and invasive aspergillosis. Microaspiration of anaerobic organisms leading to pneumonia is more likely with a history of preexisting severe periodontal disease or with a history of seizure disorder,

TABLE 68.6

EXTRAPULMONARY FINDINGS IN PNEUMONIA

Findings	Organisms
Dermatologic findings	
Herpes labialis	*Streptococcus pneumoniae*
Erythema multiforme	*Mycoplasma* sp, *Chlamydophila psittaci*
Erythema nodosum	*Mycobacterium tuberculosis*, *Coccidioides immitis*
	Histoplasma capsulatum
Skin nodules	*Nocardia* sp
	Aspergillus sp
	Coccidioides immitis
	Blastomyces sp
Pharyngitis, bullous myringitis	*Mycoplasma* sp
Splenomegaly	*Francisella tularensis*
	C. psittaci
	Coxiella burnetii (Q fever)
Pleural effusion	*Haemophilus influenzae*
	S. pneumoniae
	Pyogenic streptococci
	Aspergillus sp
	F. tularensis

altered consciousness, or esophageal obstructive disease. Extrapulmonary symptoms may give clues to specific etiologic agents, with diarrhea and abdominal discomfort being seen in patients with *Legionella* sp and otitis media and pharyngitis with *M. pneumoniae* (Table 68.6).

In the patient with nosocomial pneumonia, the history should focus on whether the patient has recently received antibiotics and how long the patient has been in the hospital prior to the onset of infection. Both are risk factors for infection with MDR Gram-positive and Gram-negative bacteria. In addition, the specific antibiotics used in the past 2 weeks should be recorded, since the pathogens causing the current infection are likely to be resistant to those agents [2,4]. Other risk factors for MDR pathogens that can be present in those with HAP and HCAP include hospitalization in the past 90 days, poor functional status, and immunosuppressive therapy (including corticosteroid use).

Physical Examination

The physical examination is valuable for suggesting the presence of pneumonia and in grading its severity. Tachypnea (>20 breaths per minute) may be the earliest sign of pneumonia in the elderly, and findings of consolidation are more specific for pneumonia than crackles, especially in the ICU [90]. In patients with CAP, an admission respiratory rate greater than 30 breaths per minute is an important negative prognostic feature, and in some studies mortality increases dramatically when respiratory rate exceeds this level [91]. Signs of pleural effusion are particularly common in *H. influenzae*, pneumococcal, streptococcal, and aspergillus pneumonia, where pleural friction rubs may be detected. Pleural involvement can be seen, although less often, in *Legionella* and *Mycoplasma* pneumonia. Relative bradycardia is a frequent finding in many pneumonias caused by *Mycoplasma*, *Legionella*, and *Chlamydophila* organisms [92].

Dermatologic manifestations (erythema nodosum, erythema multiforme, and skin nodules) may be observed with *Mycoplasma*, fungal, *Nocardia*, and tuberculous infections. Horder's spots (pale macular rash), long considered part of the presentation of psittacosis, should lead the clinician to look for other evidence of this infection. Ecthyma gangrenosum, an indurated, round skin lesion with a central dark area surrounded by erythema, is characteristic of Gram-negative septicemia, especially with *P. aeruginosa.* Central nervous system abnormalities can be found in infections with pneumococcus, *M. tuberculosis*, *H. influenzae*, Gram-negative organisms, cryptococci, *Aspergillus* sp, *Legionella* sp, *Toxoplasma gondii*, varicella zoster, and cytomegalovirus (CMV). Other physical findings that narrow the differential diagnosis include splenomegaly in the case of psittacosis and tularemia, herpes labialis in pneumococcal infection, bullous myringitis with *M. pneumoniae* infection, and lymphadenopathy with tularemia. The predictive value of many of these observations has not been evaluated rigorously (Table 68.6).

Routine Diagnostic Testing

Routine Laboratory Testing

The IDSA/ATS guidelines for CAP recommend a relatively streamlined evaluation, including chest radiograph, routine blood chemistries and blood counts, blood cultures (in the critically ill), assessment of oxygenation (oximetry or blood gas), and a clinical evaluation of severity of illness. The routine use of sputum culture or Gram stain of sputum is not recommended, reserving these tests for the patient who is at risk for infection with unusual or drug-resistant organisms. If a sputum sample is obtained, it should be prior to therapy, rapidly transported to the lab, and of good quality with little evidence of oral contamination. For the critically ill, intubated patients should have an endotracheal aspirate sent for culture, and *Legionella* and pneumococcal urinary antigen testing should be considered. The routine use of serologic testing is not encouraged [4]. The impact of diagnostic testing in patients with severe CAP remains uncertain, and several studies have shown that even if the etiologic diagnosis is known, outcome may not be affected, whereas the use of early and effective empiric therapy has been associated with an improved outcome [4,33]. However, Rello et al. [92] have shown that knowing the etiologic pathogen can help to focus and simplify treatment in nearly one third of cases of severe CAP.

Most routine laboratory results are not specific for individual pathogens, and the focus of diagnostic testing is to assess disease severity. Extremes of white blood cell count (<4,000 or >30,000 per mm^3) may indicate overwhelming sepsis and may be a poor prognostic finding [4]. Elevated liver function tests are not a specific finding but can be seen in a variety of viral and bacterial pneumonias, including those associated with *Legionella* sp, *M. tuberculosis*, *Mycoplasma* sp, Q fever, tularemia, and psittacosis, as well as in pneumococcal infection. Similarly, electrolyte disturbances, including hypophosphatemia and hyponatremia, are not predictive of a specific pathogen in the individual patient with pneumonia, but hyponatremia (<130 mEq per L) on admission may predict a poor outcome [93].

Serology, Urinary Antigen, and PCR Testing

As mentioned earlier, routine serologic testing is not recommended because results are rarely positive at the time of presentation (i.e., convalescent serologic testing is usually needed), and even if positive, results are usually not available during the first 24 to 48 hours of critical illness [4]. Serologic responses are useful for retrospective epidemiologic purposes to document viral and so-called atypical pathogen infection and may be useful if the patient is not responding to appropriate empiric therapy (discussed later). Many patients with CAP have serologic evidence for recent atypical pathogen infection, but in the setting of an illness like *Legionella* pneumonia, convalescent titers are essential and less than 10% of those with acute illness have a positive serologic result. To make the diagnosis of *Legionella* pneumonia acutely, urinary antigen testing has the highest yield (approximately 50%), but is specific for serogroup I infection, and is the test that is most likely to be positive early in the disease [4]. The direct immunofluorescent stain of sputum for *L. pneumophila* has a sensitivity of between 25% and 50% and a specificity of more than 90% for this organism. The urinary antigen for the detection of pneumococcal pneumonia has also been described for patients with severe disease, asplenia, liver disease, alcoholism, or leukopenia. Genetic probes for specific viral DNA and RNA are available for CMV, varicella zoster, herpes simplex, influenza virus, and adenovirus. In one study, real-time polymerase chain reaction (PCR) for viruses and atypical pathogens was more sensitive than conventional methods, and results were obtained in a clinically relevant time period. Microbiological diagnoses were determined for 52 (49.5%) of 105 patients by conventional techniques and for 80 (76%) of 105 patients by real-time PCR, and the time to obtain the result of real-time PCR could be reduced to 6 hours. In addition, patients with more severe infection had mixed infection identified more commonly by PCR than by conventional techniques (10.2% with conventional techniques, compared with 35% with PCR diagnosis), and some of these mixed infections involved viral pneumonia [94]. Further development of this technology may change the diagnostic approach to CAP in the future.

Chest Radiographic Interpretation

The chest radiograph is essential for the diagnosis of pneumonia in the critically ill patient (Table 68.7), and the use of pattern reading can help to narrow the differential diagnosis of CAP and HAP, particularly when used in concert with other available information. For example, the rapid development of a diffuse alveolar pattern frequently implies a hematogenously disseminated infection such as varicella or CMV, or the development of ARDS as a pneumonic complication. Hyperinflation is characteristic of respiratory syncytial virus pneumonia. A more subacute presentation of diffuse alveolar infiltrates may represent hematogenous dissemination of tuberculosis. *P. jiroveci* must be considered in the setting of a diffuse alveolar or reticulonodular pattern in groups at risk for HIV infection. Noninfectious causes of pulmonary infiltrates such as heart failure, bronchiolitis obliterans and organizing pneumonia (BOOP), drug toxicity, and lymphangitic carcinomatosis can also frequently present in this fashion. Focal infiltrates (i.e., confined to single segments or lobes) are most likely to represent bacterial pneumonia related to microaspiration into a particular area of the lung.

Acute bacterial pneumonias generally progress more rapidly (hours to days) than fungal or mycobacterial infections (days to weeks). Pleural effusions occur commonly in *H. influenzae* pneumonia (>50%) and pneumococcal infection (25%) but can also be seen in patients with group A streptococcal pneumonia. Cavitation can occur in both infectious and noninfectious lung disease, but the finding of multiple cavitary nodules suggests septic embolization from right-sided endocarditis. Rapid cavitation is also common in Gram-negative pneumonias, whereas a subacute course with cavitation suggests anaerobic or mycobacterial infection. Cavitations and necrotizing pneumonia also are present in CA-MRSA pneumonia, and its presence is often used to guide initial empirical antibiotic treatment. Occasionally, ventilator-associated bacterial pneumonia can progress rapidly and fatally, emphasizing the need for timely recognition and therapy. Chronic cavitation (weeks to months) is more likely due to a noninfectious problem, such as carcinoma, lymphoma, or Wegener's granulomatosis, especially in the absence of the systemic signs of acute infection.

The limitation of the chest radiograph in the critically ill patient is considerable, especially for the detection of VAP, when the clinician must rely on a portable film, which may not show findings very clearly. Also, in the ICU, coexisting and preexisting lung disease may obscure the findings of pneumonia. A recent study showed that chest radiographs are of limited value in predicting the causative pathogen in CAP, but are useful in determining the extent of pneumonia and detecting complications such as parapneumonic effusion [95].

Sputum Examination and Evaluation of Other Respiratory Secretions

Although Gram stain of the sputum has been the traditional first step in the evaluation of patients with suspected

TABLE 68.7

RADIOGRAPHIC PATTERNS IN DIAGNOSIS OF PNEUMONIA

Diffuse infiltrates		
Acute	**Chronic**	
Pneumocystis jiroveci pneumonia	Tuberculosis (typical or atypical)	
Viral	Fungi	
Cardiogenic edema	Radiation injury	
Drug reaction	Drug reaction	
Alveolar hemorrhage	Lymphangitic cancer	
Focal infiltrates		
Acute	**Chronic**	**Cavitation**
Streptococcus pneumoniae	Fungi	Fungi/*Nocardia* sp
Staphylococcus aureus	Tuberculosis	Anaerobes
Legionella sp	Malignancy	Gram-negative bacilli
Gram-negative bacilli		*S. aureus*
Lung infarction		Tuberculosis
Bronchiolitis obliterans and organizing pneumonia		Malignancy
		Wegener's granulomatosis

pneumonia, this is problematic in the critically ill patient who is not intubated and may be unable to expectorate. When a specimen is obtained, interpretation depends on the quality of the sample and on the criteria used to define a "positive" sample. Although no studies correlate Gram stain findings to alveolar cultures in patients with pneumonia, the goal is to evaluate respiratory secretions from deep in the lower airway, and such a specimen from a nonintubated patient should have more than 25 polymorphonuclear cells and less than 10 epithelial cells per low-power field. When such criteria are met and intracellular organisms are identified, a bacterial density above 10^5 colony-forming units per mL of secretions is usually present [4]. The presence of elastin fibers on potassium hydroxide staining, along with a positive Gram stain, is more suggestive of pneumonia than airway infection or colonization. In addition to not always being able to distinguish airway colonization from pneumonia, the sputum Gram stain may be falsely negative up to 50% of the time compared with blood cultures. Some findings in sputum may suggest specific etiologies. For example, an inflammatory Gram stain (polymorphonuclear cells) without organisms in a patient with pneumonia is presumptive evidence of an atypical (*Legionella* or *Mycoplasma*) or viral cause. Gram stain may be best used to broaden initial empiric therapy, rather than to narrow it, especially if an unusual pathogen that is not routinely treated is thought to be present. For example, the finding of Gram-positive cocci in clusters in a patient with influenza would lead to empiric therapy for *S. aureus*. The use of special stains for tuberculosis and silver or Giemsa staining for *P. jiroveci* may provide definitive evidence for these organisms. With the use of rapid point-of-care diagnostic tests for influenza virus, treatment and chemoprevention can be offered. Rapid influenza can sometimes differentiate influenza A from influenza B and this can guide treatment decision. Other diseases caused by agents of bioterrorism and endemic diseases can be identified with the use of examination of respiratory secretions.

Culture

A definitive etiologic diagnosis of pneumonia can be made if cultures of blood, pleural fluid, or spinal fluid are positive in the presence of a lung infiltrate and a compatible clinical picture. Bacteremia is uncommon in most pneumonias, occurring in less than 15% of patients with CAP, in 20% of pneumococcal infections, and in only 8% to 15% of nosocomial pneumonias [44]. In nosocomial pneumonia, the presence of bacteremia may imply an extrapulmonary infection, especially if the organism present in the blood culture is different from the one in the respiratory tract. Blood cultures are indicated in all patients admitted to the ICU with a diagnosis of pneumonia but are most valuable if collected prior to antibiotic therapy. In patients without severe illness, the yield is lower, and findings can be misleading (false-positive rate may exceed the true positive rate) [96]. Sputum cultures can be difficult to interpret because of the problem in separating infection from colonization in the critically ill. In a study of bacteremic nosocomial pneumonia, sputum culture yielded both false-positive and false-negative findings compared with blood cultures, with only 49% of the cases having the same organism recovered from both blood and sputum [44]. Sputum cultures are sensitive but not specific and are often unable to distinguish colonizing from infecting pathogens. In intubated patients, colonization is present after several days, so the culture should be interpreted in the clinical context of the patient, and a sample should not be cultured in the absence of clinical signs of infection.

Viruses may be cultured from respiratory secretions, but this procedure may take up to 20 days, depending on the virus. Thus, cytologic evidence of viral infection that can be recognized sooner may provide helpful information. For example, inclusion bodies and multinucleated giant cells are suggestive of CMV or herpesvirus infection.

Invasive Diagnostic Sampling and Quantitative Cultures

Because of the inherent problems distinguishing colonizing from infecting pathogens in samples of lower respiratory tract secretions, investigators have advocated for the collection of deep respiratory secretions through invasive (bronchoscopic) or semi-invasive (catheter-lavage) means, combined with analysis of the results using quantitative cultures. Early efforts at invasive sampling involved transtracheal aspiration in a nonintubated patient, using a polyurethane catheter, but the technique was difficult and potentially dangerous and led to false-positive results more than 20% of the time.

Percutaneous needle aspiration of the lung in an area of infiltrate has also been studied, but it is limited by a high incidence of false-negative results and an unacceptable complication rate, including pneumothorax in up to 30% of patients and a 10% rate of hemoptysis. Although open lung biopsy is the unequivocal standard for the diagnosis of infection, it has been applied primarily in the immunocompromised host with rapidly advancing, life-threatening infections. *Aspergillus*, CMV, herpes simplex, and *T. gondii* infections are more readily diagnosed by open lung biopsy than by other described techniques. In patients with CAP, open lung biopsy is rarely needed, and its potential for demonstrating a treatable infection that will alter outcome is low, and similar findings have been reported when it is used in patients with HAP [97] (Table 68.8) (see Chapter 69).

Bronchoscopic sampling has been used in the critically ill, particularly in those who are immunosuppressed or who already have an endotracheal tube in place, such as patients with VAP and severe CAP [2,84,98]. Cultures are obtained by using the bronchoscopically directed PSB, or bronchoalveolar lavage (BAL), and the samples cultured quantitatively. When PSB samples are cultured quantitatively, patients with nosocomial pneumonia will have greater than 10^3 organisms per mL of respiratory secretions. When BAL is used, a threshold concentration of 10^4 to 10^5 organisms per mL is used to define pneumonia [98]. In some studies, lower airway cells recovered by lavage have been examined for the presence of intracellular organisms, and the finding of more than 5% to 25% of cells with intracellular bacteria may predict the diagnosis of pneumonia, confirmed by PSB. Quantitative endotracheal aspirates have also been used, particularly patients with severe nursing home pneumonia, and this technique has a very good correlation with results of BAL if a threshold of 10^4 colony-forming organisms per mL is used [2,99]. Although the role of bronchoscopy in patients with suspected VAP is still controversial, most investigators agree that BAL is valuable in establishing a nonbacterial cause of infection, especially in the immunocompromised host or the patient with HIV infection, where it can reliably diagnose *P. jiroveci* pneumonia and CMV infection [100].

Quantitative cultures have been proposed as the most accurate way to establish the presence of VAP and to define the etiologic pathogen. Although the clinical diagnosis of VAP has been much maligned, it may be very accurate, particularly if it is objectively defined by calculating the CPIS and if the score incorporates a Gram's stain of a lower respiratory tract sample [101]. Once the clinical diagnosis of VAP is made, a culture is needed to identify the etiologic pathogen, but this culture could be quantitative or semiquantitative (light, moderate, or heavy growth), and collected as an endotracheal aspirate or via bronchoscopy or catheter lavage. Quantitative culture-based diagnosis may not be more accurate than clinical diagnosis, and quantitative cultures have a number of methodologic

TABLE 68.8

DIAGNOSTIC TECHNIQUES IN PNEUMONIA

Test	Advantages	Disadvantages
Expectorated sputum Gram stain	Easy to perform; rapidly available; inexpensive	High false-positive and false-negative rates
Expectorated sputum culture	Easy to obtain	High false-positive and false-negative rates
Blood culture	High specificity	Low sensitivity, not always a lung source
Transtracheal aspiration	Less contamination than expectorated sputum	High false-positive rates in colonized patients; bleeding; impractical to do
Needle aspiration (percutaneous)	High specificity; useful for children and malignancy	High risk of pneumothorax especially in patients with chronic obstructive pulmonary disease and in ventilated patients; not widely done
Bronchoscopy (protected brush, bronchoalveolar lavage [BAL])	Low morbidity and mortality; useful in ventilated patients and for nonbacteriologic diagnosis and in compromised host	"Invasive"; requires special training; less useful if patient already on antibiotics; wide range of sensitivity; may bias against the treatment of early infection
Nonbronchoscopic BAL	May give quantitative culture data in ventilated patients; can be done any time of the day by respiratory therapists or physicians	Variable accuracy, assumes that random sampling is reflective of bacteriology throughout the lung; same benefits/ disadvantages of relying on other quantitative methods
Open lung biopsy	Excellent for nonbacterial diagnosis and in compromised host	Most invasive; critically ill may not be able to undergo procedure; may not change prognosis

limitations that can cause both false-positive and false-negative results. Some studies have reported false-positive results in patients on long-term ventilation, even in the absence of infection [102], and the reproducibility of the sampling technique is also questionable. False-negative results are also common, particularly with sampling errors, and in the presence of prior effective antibiotic therapy. Finally, a number of studies have suggested that clinical management without quantitative cultures may be accurate, and that outcomes such as mortality and change in antibiotics to a focused regimen are not improved by the use of quantitative cultures [103].

The impact of quantitative sampling on patient outcome is controversial. One study suggested that the data from bronchoscopy can lead to antibiotic changes, but these changes are made too late to affect mortality [2]. Another study concluded that bronchoscopic culture results are frequently associated with changes in antibiotic therapy, but there was increase in mortality as a result of inappropriate early antibiotic therapy despite a subsequent microbiologically guided change [104]. Other studies have demonstrated the importance of getting initial therapy correct, and the use of quantitative cultures has never been shown to aid in this goal [2].

Studies of the impact of quantitative culture methods on VAP outcome have been mixed, but a recent meta-analysis showed no effect on mortality [105]. An early study by Fagon et al. [106] reported that a bronchoscopic-based invasive management strategy, with quantitative cultures, compared with a clinical approach based on endotracheal aspirate cultures, led to improved mortality at 14 days, reduced organ failure at 7 days, and reduced antibiotic usage. However, another study by Singh et al. [107] used clinical diagnosis and management with the CPIS and showed that patients with suspected VAP and a low score could be safely managed with a short course of antibiotics, and that these patients did as well as those treated with standard regimens [107]. In a large multicenter trial, Heyland et al. [108] compared management of VAP using cultures obtained via endotracheal aspirates with those obtained by BAL. They found no difference in mortality between the two groups, and similar rates of adjusting antibiotic therapy after initial empiric management. Unlike the earlier study, in this investigation, all patients initially received antibiotic therapy, so cultures were used to adjust antibiotics but never to withhold them. One of the limitations on the applications of these data is that patients with known colonization with *Pseudomonas* sp and MRSA were initially excluded from the study so that less than 15% had MDR pathogen pneumonia. Fewer studies have been done to investigate the impact of quantitative lower respiratory secretion cultures in patients with severe CAP, but Rello et al. [92] have shown that information from bronchoscopic sampling can help to narrow and focus antibiotic therapy in patients with severe CAP. However, in patients with severe CAP, PSB and BAL only give an etiologic diagnosis in one quarter to one third of all patients (which is less than with sputum or endotracheal aspirate cultures), but in this group, antibiotics were changed in nearly 75%.

Reconciling these different views, the ATS/IDSA guidelines for nosocomial pneumonia have recommended that all patients have a lower respiratory tract sample collected prior to starting therapy, and that the technique and culture method be one that the clinician is expert at performing and interpreting. Lower respiratory tract cultures can be obtained bronchoscopically or nonbronchoscopically and can be cultured quantitatively or semiquantitatively. Quantitative cultures increase specificity of the diagnosis of HAP but may potentially delay the initiation of therapy in patients with early pneumonia. Nonquantitative cultures are sensitive but may lead to some colonizing organisms being treated. Regardless of which method is used, it should only be initiated once the clinician has made a clinical diagnosis of pneumonia and is ready to initiate therapy. Therapy should be prompt and not delayed for the purpose of collecting diagnostic sample, especially in patients who are clinically unstable or septic from pneumonia [2,106]. Extrapulmonary infection should be ruled out prior to the administration of antibiotic therapy.

Differential Diagnosis

In the evaluation of a patient with lung infiltrates, it is necessary to determine (a) if pneumonia, or another infiltrative or inflammatory process, is responsible for the constellation of symptoms and signs being evaluated and (b) if it is pneumonia, what is the etiologic pathogen. Since the features of pneumonia are nonspecific, it is necessary to consider such alternative noninfectious processes such as aspiration with chemical pneumonitis, acute pulmonary embolism, pulmonary infarction, pulmonary hemorrhage, ARDS, CHF, bronchiolitis obliterans organizing pneumonia, radiation pneumonitis, bronchoalveolar carcinoma, and atelectasis. An increasingly common problem is the differentiation of acute infectious pneumonia from drug-induced pneumonitis caused by agents such as amiodarone, bleomycin, busulfan, and methotrexate, and eosinophilia may be an important clue. Amiodarone pneumonitis may be indistinguishable from CAP, producing focal changes on chest radiography and occasionally pleural effusion; the illness generally occurs only in patients receiving more than 400 mg per day, and there is a subacute presentation, a low or declining diffusing capacity, and abnormal lipid-laden cells in BAL.

In immunocompromised patients, a new lung infiltrate may represent infection, progression of the underlying primary disease, or drug-induced lung disease. As in all patients, the nature of the immune impairment determines which pathogens are most likely. Although *P. jiroveci* pneumonia is a cause of rapidly progressive hypoxemic respiratory failure in the patient with HIV infection, a similar picture may be seen with tuberculosis, and pneumococcus is also a common respiratory pathogen in these patients [109]. Many have suggested that tuberculosis is poorly recognized in the intensive care setting and should be considered in patients with a history of inadequately treated tuberculosis or radiographic evidence of previous infection. The use of corticosteroid therapy in doses more than 20 mg per day increases the risk of opportunistic fungi, with reports stressing the occurrence of invasive aspergillosis in patients receiving high-dose steroid therapy for exacerbations of COPD [78]. Patients with B-cell–specific problems such as multiple myeloma are particularly prone to pneumonia with encapsulated organisms, including pneumococcus and *H. influenzae*. A similar organism profile can be seen in the splenectomized patient and in those with complement defects. Even in the setting of established pneumonia, patients may have a second infectious process such as extrapulmonary infection (catheter-associated bacteremia) or complications of antibiotic therapy, such as antibiotic-induced colitis.

THERAPY

Supportive Therapy

The role of supportive therapy in pneumonia in the critically ill is crucial because the use of antibiotics may not alter outcome during the first 24 to 72 hours of treatment. Many of the commonly applied measures are based on traditional practice, with little documentation of efficacy.

Nutritional Support

Evidence implicating malnutrition as a cofactor in pneumonia is substantial [69], but the evidence that nutritional intervention alters the outcome of severe pneumonia is lacking. Catabolic stress may be expected in the septic syndrome and has been related to progressive multiorgan failure if the patient survives the acute phase of critical illness. Enteral nutrition is preferred, if this can be practically accomplished, because data suggest better preservation of immune function using this route compared with total parenteral nutrition [110]. When enteral feedings are given, a small-bore tube, preferably placed in the small bowel, should be used along with a continuous infusion method to prevent aspiration and to optimize the delivery of calories [111]. The use of large-bore tubes placed in the stomach with bolus feeding has been associated with an increased risk of aspiration. All patients should be kept semierect and not supine as much as possible, to reduce the risk of reflux and aspiration [57]. The optimal time for initiating enteral feeding has not been determined.

Chest Physiotherapy

There is little support for the routine application of chest physiotherapy in patients who have an effective cough and scant amounts of respiratory secretions. Such maneuvers have the potential to worsen hypoxemia and mucociliary clearance when applied to routine pneumonia, and have not been demonstrated to affect duration of hospitalization [112,113]. Because of the labor-intensive nature of this intervention, techniques such as percussion, vibration, and postural drainage should be specifically targeted at patients with large volumes of purulent secretions (>30 mL per day) and an ineffective cough (see Chapter 62). In patients at bed rest in the ICU, the use of positioning and rotation may be helpful in clearing secretions [114]. In several studies, particularly in surgical trauma patients, the use of beds that rotate patients from side to side, and presumably accelerate mucus clearance, has led to a reduced incidence of nosocomial pneumonia [114].

Aerosols and Humidification

Humidification has been a traditional practice of respiratory therapy aimed at reducing sputum viscosity and promoting mucociliary clearance. Because the deposition of water vapor depends on particle size and the degree of airway obstruction, however, it is likely that most such aerosols are deposited above the glottis and act only to stimulate cough. Although mucolytic agents such as acetylcysteine offer the theoretic benefit of reducing the viscosity of purulent secretions, they may act as irritants that can provoke bronchospasm, and thus must be used selectively. Bronchodilator therapy with β_2 agents can enhance mucociliary clearance and ciliary beat frequency, but there have been no controlled trials that have demonstrated improved outcome with their use in pneumonia, in the absence of underlying bronchospasm. The greatest benefit of bronchodilator therapy may be expected in the patient with COPD in whom pneumonia develops (see Chapter 62).

Other Supportive Modalities

Other routine ICU care is applicable to the patient with severe pneumonia. Since many patients with severe pneumonia have signs of systemic sepsis, it is important to provide adequate early volume resuscitation. In addition, control of hyperglycemia may be beneficial, especially in surgical patients, and BP support with vasoactive medications may also be needed if the patient has septic shock. Other nonantibiotic, pharmacologic therapies for pneumonia patients with septic shock, including activated protein C and systemic corticosteroids, are discussed below.

Antibiotic and Other Pharmacologic Therapy

In the critically ill patient, the timely initiation of appropriate antimicrobial therapy has been shown to improve survival for patients with both severe CAP and VAP [2,4,33]. Because it is often impossible to identify a specific etiologic agent at the time that therapy is started, initial therapy is necessarily empiric but can be modified and focused (de-escalated) once the results of diagnostic testing become available. The ATS and IDSA have developed algorithms for initial empiric therapy of severe pneumonia arising in both the community and the hospital [2,4].

Community-Acquired Pneumonia

Because the use of clinical syndromes or sputum Gram stain to guide therapy is often inaccurate and not recommended, initial therapy is empiric, based on the likely etiologic pathogens. For patients treated in the ICU, monotherapy is not recommended, using any agent, and all patients require initial therapy directed at pneumococcus (including DRSP), atypical pathogens (especially *Legionella*), *H. influenzae*, and enteric Gram-negatives (including *P. aeruginosa* in some patients). In selected patients, particularly following influenza or other viral infections, empiric therapy for *S. aureus*, including MRSA, is necessary. Aspiration pneumonia, including anaerobic pathogens, can occasionally present as severe illness, needing ICU care. Endemic viruses can also cause severe CAP, and the use of antiviral agents depends on local epidemiology and whether influenza or another viral agent is prevalent at the time that the patient is being evaluated. In the ICU, initial therapy is determined by whether the patient has risks for *P. aeruginosa*, which include structural lung disease (bronchiectasis), therapy with broad-spectrum antibiotics for more than 7 days in the last month, use of corticosteroids (>10 mg of prednisone daily), malnutrition, or HIV infection [2,4].

For the patient with severe CAP, mixed infection, involving a bacterial pathogen and an atypical pathogen, is also common and should be accounted for in the initial empiric regimen. Every patient should receive therapy directed at these organisms, which can be either primary pathogens or copathogens, but studies have shown that the use of a macrolide may be of specific value. In patients with bacteremic pneumococcal pneumonia, particularly in those with severe illness, dual therapy including a macrolide has been associated with improved outcomes [115,116]. A quinolone can also be used to treat atypical pathogen infection and may have an advantage in the patient with suspected *Legionella* infection, where the outcomes using quinolones are exceptionally good [117].

If the patient has no risk factors for *Pseudomonas*, then therapy should be with an intravenous β-lactam (ceftriaxone, cefotaxime, or ertapenem) with activity against DRSP plus either intravenous azithromycin or an intravenous quinolone (levofloxacin 750 mg or moxifloxacin 400 mg). When the patient has risk factors for *Pseudomonas*, then therapy should involve two antipseudomonal agents, in addition to providing coverage for DRSP and *Legionella* [4]. For these patients, therapy can be a two-drug regimen, using a selected antipseudomonal β-lactam (cefepime, piperacillin/tazobactam, imipenem, meropenem, doripenem), in combination with an antipseudomonal quinolone (ciprofloxacin, high-dose levofloxacin 750 mg daily). Alternatively, the above-mentioned β-lactams can be combined with an aminoglycoside and either azithromycin or an antipneumococcal quinolone (levofloxacin 750 mg or moxifloxacin 400 mg). In the penicillin-allergic patient, aztreonam can be combined with an aminoglycoside and an antipneumococcal fluoroquinolone [4].

As mentioned earlier, no patient with severe CAP should receive monotherapy, even with a quinolone, since studies have not proven the efficacy of this approach [118]. Moxifloxacin is safe and efficacious for CAP, even in the elderly, but few patients with severe CAP have been studied. In the Community-Acquired Pneumonia Recovery in the Elderly (CAPRIE) study, comparing moxifloxacin with levofloxacin for CAP in the elderly who were hospitalized outside of the ICU, although the cure rate for moxifloxacin (94.7%) was greater than levofloxacin (84.6%) in the severe CAP subgroup, the difference was not statistically significant [119]. One study of nearly 400 patients with severe CAP compared monotherapy with high-dose levofloxacin (500 mg twice daily) with the combination of ceftriaxone/ofloxacin, and although an equivalent clinical response was observed in both treatment groups (79.1% with levofloxacin compared with 79.5% with combination therapy), patients with shock were excluded from the study, and in patients with mechanical ventilation, treatment with levofloxacin resulted in a lower clinical cure rate (63% compared with 72% with combination therapy) [118]. Therefore, quinolone monotherapy is not recommended in severe CAP, especially in the setting of septic shock and respiratory failure.

Although quinolones are acceptable as monotherapy for patients not admitted to the ICU, it is currently uncertain if the outcome is different if a quinolone is used in place of macrolide, as part of a combination regimen for patients in the ICU. In one report, the use of initial empiric therapy with a β-lactam plus a fluoroquinolone for severe CAP was associated with increased short-term mortality (OR, 2.71; 95% confidence interval, 1.2 to 6.1), in comparison with other guideline-recommended antimicrobial regimes [120]. On the other hand, a recent meta-analysis of 23 randomized trials of CAP therapy outside the ICU compared the use of fluoroquinolones with other antibiotics, including β-lactams, macrolides, or both. Although there was no mortality difference in favor of the fluoroquinolones, for patients with more severe pneumonia, those who required hospitalization and those requiring intravenous therapy, the quinolones were more effective [121].

Occasionally, these broad-empiric approaches should be modified, particularly if clinical or culture data suggest an organism that is not included in the initial regimen (e.g., *S. aureus* or MRSA). In addition, certain comorbidities predispose to specific pathogens, and these should be covered by any empiric regimen (see Table 68.4). Thus, those with recent influenza should be treated for *S. aureus*, including CA-MRSA, in addition to the other usual severe CAP pathogens. CA-MRSA is different from nosocomial MRSA, as it occurs in previously healthy people, carries the Panton-Valentine leukocidin gene (a virulence factor which causes tissue necrosis), and causes a necrotizing, often bilateral severe pneumonia [70]. The best therapy for CA-MRSA is unclear, but the options include vancomycin, linezolid, or the combination of vancomycin and clindamycin. The latter two regimens have the ability to inhibit bacterial toxin synthesis (by linezolid or clindamycin), which may be part of the pathogenesis of severe CA-MRSA infection, but current recommendations are not definitive about whether antitoxin therapy is needed [4]. Anecdotal reports suggest a benefit to this approach [122].

If DRSP is present, any of the recommended regimens will be effective. Although pneumococcal resistance to multiple agents is present at rates up to 40%, using older definitions of resistance, the outcome in CAP is generally not worsened by the presence of penicillin-resistant organisms, compared with penicillin-sensitive organisms, and that these resistant organisms can still be effectively treated by high doses of penicillin, amoxicillin, amoxicillin/clavulanate, the third-generation cephalosporins (ceftriaxone or cefotaxime), or the antipneumococcal fluoroquinolones [4]. If highly resistant pneumococcus (but not cephalosporin resistant) is documented and meningitis is present, therapy should be initiated with vancomycin, cefotaxime, or ceftriaxone. Discordant therapy of DRSP usually has no impact on outcome, but even in studies when it was independently associated with death (OR, 27.3), it was very unlikely that discordant therapy would be given with ceftriaxone or cefotaxime [123]. Ceftriaxone is usually used at doses of 1 to 2 mg per day, but if DRSP and severe infection are present, the dose can be increased to 2 g every 12 hours. A notable exception to using cephalosporins in severe CAP is cefuroxime. Yu et al. [124] studied the impact of concordant antibiotic therapy (using an antibiotic with in vitro activity against *S. pneumoniae*) versus discordant therapy (inactive in vitro) on mortality in bacteremic pneumococcal pneumonia. Discordant therapy with penicillins, cefotaxime, and ceftriaxone did not result in a higher mortality rate, but this did not apply to cefuroxime, which did increase mortality in the presence of in vitro resistance. *H. influenzae* is also becoming increasingly resistant to common antimicrobials because of the production of β-lactamases, and these organisms can be treated with second- or third-generation cephalosporins, quinolones, macrolides, or ampicillin/sulbactam.

Recent advances in the treatment of sepsis and septic shock, such as activated (activated drotrecogin α) and possibly steroids, are applicable to CAP as well. In severe CAP, patients treated with drotrecogin α had a relative risk reduction in mortality of 28% at 28 days, with a relative risk reduction in mortality of 14% observed at 90 days from the start of study drug infusion. The survival benefit was greatest in severe CAP patients with *S. pneumoniae* and in those at high risk of death as indicated by an Acute Physiology and Chronic Health Evaluation II score of 25 or more. Therefore, in addition to antibiotics, activated protein C could be considered as a potential therapeutic intervention, but its value was limited in patients already receiving appropriate therapy, and it was not useful in nosocomial pneumonia [125].

The role of low-dose (replacement) steroids in septic shock has been the topic of numerous studies, and relative adrenal insufficiency occurs in a high proportion of patients with severe CAP [27,126]. Salluh et al. [27] have shown that in patients with severe CAP, median cortisol levels were 15.5 μg per dL, and 65% of patients met the criteria for adrenal insufficiency (cortisol levels <20 μg per dL). When patients with septic shock were evaluated, 63% had adrenal insufficiency. Higher doses may also have value to modify the inflammatory response in patients with severe CAP. A recent placebo-controlled, randomized study of 46 patients used hydrocortisone as an intravenous 200-mg bolus followed by infusion at a rate of 10 mg per hour for 7 days. The treatment arm had a significant improvement in the PaO_2/FiO_2 ratio and chest radiograph score and a significant reduction in C-reactive protein levels, multiple-organ dysfunction syndrome score, and delayed septic shock, compared with the control group. Hydrocortisone treatment was associated with a significant reduction in length of hospital stay ($p = 0.03$) and mortality ($p = 0.009$) [127]. A recent systematic review of the use of systemic steroids in the treatment of CAP showed that in two studies, there was a significant clinical benefit [128], but two other trials failed to demonstrate a positive effect [129]. These results suggested that at least, steroid use in the setting of severe CAP does not appear to be harmful, but routine use in severe CAP is not recommended. One other setting in which corticosteroids may have benefit is when pneumococcal pneumonia is complicated by meningitis. In this setting, pretreatment with corticosteroids, prior to antibiotic therapy, may lead to more favorable neurologic outcomes [130].

Other new antibiotics may become available for the therapy of CAP. Tigecycline is a novel glycylcycline antibacterial agent, with an expanded broad spectrum of activity including proven utility against Gram-positive, Gram-negative, anaerobic, and atypical pathogens. It is effective in vitro against clinically important community- and hospital-acquired resistant organisms—*Acinetobacter*, MRSA, DRSP, vancomycin-resistant *Enterococcus* spp, *E. coli*, and *K. pneumoniae* expressing extended-spectrum β-lactamases (ESBLs). Currently, it is approved for CAP, but not nosocomial pneumonia [131]. New anti-Staphylococcal agents are also being developed, and may have utility in severe CAP, including telavancin, ceftaroline, and ceftobiprole [132].

Hospital-Acquired Pneumonia, Including VAP and HCAP

Although Gram-negative bacterial infection is the most common cause of nosocomial pneumonia, the frequency of Gram-positives, including MRSA, is rising, and in the impaired host, opportunistic fungi and mycobacterial infections are also possible. Defining the underlying disease and knowledge of patterns of bacterial infection and antibiotic resistance in a given ICU are important for selecting a therapy regimen that is likely to be active against the responsible pathogens.

In most patients, initial therapy is empiric, and if that therapy is "inappropriate" (i.e., not active against the etiologic pathogen), then mortality is higher than if the therapy was appropriate [2,4]. The approach to VAP in the 2005 ATS/IDSA guidelines [2] provides therapy recommendations for patients with HAP, VAP, and HCAP and focuses on multiple areas of management including the need for early diagnosis, prompt and accurate treatment, avoiding unnecessary antibiotics, and efforts to avoid future increases in antibiotic resistance. The key decision point in initial empiric therapy is to determine whether the patient has risk factors for MDR organisms, as outlined in Table 68.2. In the most recent guidelines, and unlike earlier guidelines, "early" onset of HAP, within the first 4 days of hospitalization, was only one factor to consider when defining whether the patient is at risk for MDR pathogen infection [2]. To be considered not at risk for MDR pathogens, the patient must have both early onset of infection, and no risks for HCAP such as recent hospitalization, treatment in a healthcare-associated facility (nursing home, dialysis center, etc.), and the patient should not have received antibiotic therapy in the past month. On the other hand, patients with either late-onset infection or the presence of any of the other MDR risk factors are treated empirically for infection with MDR Gram-negative and Gram-positive pathogens. Some patients with healthcare-associated infections are bacteriologically similar to hospital-acquired infections and also at risk for infection with MDR pathogens [51,79], but recent studies have shown that not all HCAP patients are at the same risk [51,133]. In the HCAP patient with severe pneumonia, the presence of any of the following risks should lead to the patient being treated for MDR pathogens: antibiotic therapy or hospitalization in the past 3 months, poor functional status, and immune suppression. In the absence of these risk factors, the HCAP patient in the ICU should be treated with a severe CAP regimen.

Initial empiric therapy is either with a narrow-spectrum, generally monotherapy regimen, or with a broad-spectrum, multidrug regime (see Table 68.2). In the 2005 guidelines [2], patients with HCAP fell into the second group, but this may not be necessary for those without MDR risk factors. The timing of accurate antimicrobial therapy is an important mortality predictor, and changing antimicrobial therapy once culture results are available may not reduce the excess risk of hospital mortality associated with initial inappropriate treatment [2]. This need to get initial therapy correct has led to many patients getting a broader spectrum regimen than may be needed, and thus it is necessary to obtain cultures prior to therapy and de-escalate after 2 to 3 days, once the culture data are available.

Guidelines make a distinction between appropriate therapy and adequate therapy, with both requiring the use of an agent to which the etiologic pathogen is sensitive. However, adequate therapy also requires that the drug penetrates to the site of infection, and that it is administered in the correct dose and with multiple agents if required. The regimens listed in Table 68.9 are directed at providing appropriate therapy that is targeted to the most likely pathogens. Therapy for those who are not at risk for MDR pathogen infection can be with a second- or third-generation cephalosporin, a β-lactam/β-lactamase inhibitor combination, ertapenem, a

TABLE 68.9

INITIAL EMPIRIC ANTIBIOTIC THERAPY FOR NOSOCOMIAL PNEUMONIA

Hospital-acquired pneumonia and ventilator-associated pneumonia: early onset, no known risk factors for multidrug resistant (MDR) pathogens, any disease severity	
Potential pathogen	**Recommended antibiotic for patient type; drugs listed are meant as a group to treat all listed pathogens**
Streptococcus pneumoniae *Haemophilus influenzae* or Methicillin-sensitive *Staphylococcus aureus*	Ceftriaxone OR Levofloxacin, moxifloxacin, or ciprofloxacin OR
Antibiotic-sensitive enteric Gram-negative bacilli *Escherichia coli* *Klebsiella pneumoniae* *Proteus* spp *Serratia marcescens* *Enterobacter* spp	Ampicillin/sulbactam OR Ertapenem
Hospital-acquired pneumonia, ventilator-associated pneumonia, and healthcare-associated pneumonia: late onset, or with risk factors for MDR pathogens, any disease severity	
Potential pathogens	**Combination antibiotic therapy (for patient type; drugs listed are meant as a group to treat all listed pathogens)**
Pathogens listed above PLUS MDR pathogens	Antipseudomonal cephalosporin (cefepime, ceftazidime) or
Pseudomonas aeruginosa *K. pneumoniae*	Antipseudomonal carbapenem (imipenem or meropenem) or
Acinetobacter spp	β-Lactam/β-lactamase inhibitor (piperacillin–tazobactam) PLUS
PLUS Consider[a]	Antipseudomonal fluoroquinolone (ciprofloxacin or levofloxacin)
Legionella pneumophila	OR Aminoglycoside (amikacin/gentamicin/tobramycin) PLUS
Methicillin-resistant *S. aureus*	Linezolid or vancomycin

[a]If an environmental source of Legionella is present, with a known nosocomial outbreak, use fluoroquinolone in the regimen.
Adapted from Niederman MS, Craven DE, Bonten MJ, et al: Guidelines for the management of adults with hospital-acquired, ventilator-associated, and healthcare-associated pneumonia. *Am J Respir Crit Care Med* 171:388–416, 2005, with permission.

quinolone (moxifloxacin or levofloxacin), or, for penicillin-allergic patients, the combination of clindamycin and aztreonam. Therapy for those at risk for MDR pathogens is directed at *P. aeruginosa*, *Acinetobacter* spp, ESBL producing *K. pneumonia and Enterobacter* spp, and MRSA [2]. Patients at risk for infection with these organisms should initially receive a combination an antipseudomonal β-lactam plus either an antipseudomonal quinolone (ciprofloxacin or levofloxacin) or an aminoglycoside (amikacin, gentamicin, or tobramycin). The antipseudomonal β-lactams include cefepime, doripenem, imipenem, meropenem, and piperacillin/tazobactam. Aztreonam can be used in penicillin-allergic patients. This combination regimen is generally supplemented with therapy for MRSA with either vancomycin or linezolid. In the future, telavancin may be another option for MRSA therapy.

To ensure adequate therapy, the right doses have to be used—typically, for critically ill patients with normal renal function, the correct doses of common antibiotics include cefepime 1 to 2 g every 8 to 12 hours; imipenem 500 mg every 6 hours or 1 g every 8 hours; meropenem 1 g every 8 hours; piperacillin-tazobactam 4.5 g every 6 hours; levofloxacin 750 mg daily or ciprofloxacin 400 mg every 8 hours; vancomycin 15 mg per kg every 12 hours leading to a trough level of 15 to 20 mg per L; linezolid 600 mg every 12 hours; and aminoglycosides of 7 mg per kg per day of gentamicin or tobramycin and 20 mg per kg of amikacin [2]. There is interest in optimizing dosing of antibiotics, and this means using continuous or prolonged infusions of β-lactams which are bactericidal in a time-dependent fashion, or giving once-daily high doses of aminoglycosides or quinolones, which are bactericidal in a concentration-dependent fashion. Doripenem is a new carbapenem and has been studied for the treatment of HAP and VAP, with similar efficacy to other antipseudomonal β-lactams and can be given as a 4-hour infusion to ICU patients, with some enhanced efficacy against *P. aeruginosa* when this dosing approach is used [134].

In the therapy of nosocomial pneumonia, in addition to *P. aeruginosa*, the other challenging Gram-negative organisms are *Acinetobacter* spp and ESBL-producing *Enterobacteriaceae*. For both groups of pathogens, a carbapenem is the most effective therapy, if the organisms are sensitive, but if not, then novel therapies may be needed. *Acinetobacter* can be treated with tigecycline but generally not as monotherapy, since it has not shown efficacy in clinical trials when utilized this way.

Colistin, a polymyxin, may be necessary in this setting, with some risk of nephrotoxicity. There are reports of using combinations of a carbapenem or colistin, with tigecycline, showing some efficacy against resistant *Acinetobacter* organisms [135]. Colistin has also been used to treat highly resistant ESBL-producing Gram-negatives, but if an institution has concern about these organisms, third-generation cephalosporins should not be used, since they can further induce the selection of ESBL-producing organisms and are generally not effective therapy [136].

The treatment options for suspected MRSA pneumonia have been expanded with the availability of agents such as the oxazolidinones (linezolid) and the streptogramins (quinupristin/dalfopristin). Still in development with efficacy in clinical trials is telavancin, while tigecycline, ceftobiprole, and ceftaroline are still being investigated for the therapy of MRSA pneumonia [132]. Linezolid is effective for nosocomial pneumonia, especially caused by MRSA, and is an alternative to vancomycin for the treatment of MRSA VAP. In a subset analysis of two prospective, randomized trials, linezolid had a clinical and microbiologic advantage over vancomycin for patients with documented MRSA VAP [137]. This advantage may be due to the higher penetration of linezolid into the epithelial lining fluid than with vancomycin [138]. This agent may also be preferred if patients have renal insufficiency or are receiving other nephrotoxic agents such as aminoglycosides, because of concerns of synergistic nephrotoxicity with vancomycin, but this is not conclusively proven. Linezolid is generally well tolerated, but patients must be monitored for drug-induced thrombocytopenia, especially after prolonged use (>14 days). Quinupristin/dalfopristin is an option but was less efficacious compared with vancomycin in treatment of nosocomial pneumonia caused by MRSA [139]. Teicoplanin is a glycopeptide antibiotic with antimicrobial activity similar to vancomycin and can be given once a day, but it is not available in the United States [140].

For patients at risk for infection with MDR pathogens, initial empiric therapy should involve a combination of agents, but the role of continued combination therapy is uncertain. One advantage of combination therapy is to provide synergy in the therapy of *P. aeruginosa*, which is only accomplished when an aminoglycoside is combined with a β-lactam. Synergy has only been proven to be of value in patients with neutropenia and pseudomonal bacteremia, both uncommon in the therapy of VAP [141]. Although combination therapy could theoretically prevent the emergence of resistance that is common with monotherapy, this has not been proven to be a benefit [142]. The major utility of combination therapy is to provide broader spectrum coverage than is possible with one agent alone, since most hospitals do not have a single agent that is able to cover all the likely pathogens with a high enough frequency. Adding a second agent increases the likelihood that initial empiric therapy will be appropriate, if MDR pathogens are present. In the Canadian Clinical Trials Group study of VAP, the use of combination therapy increased the likelihood of appropriate therapy for patients who had MDR pathogens from 11% to 84%, with an associated improvement in microbiologic eradication [143].

Combination therapy should include agents from different antibiotic classes to avoid antagonism of therapeutic mechanisms. For Gram-negatives, regimens usually involve the combination of a β-lactam with either a quinolone or an aminoglycoside. Although quinolones can penetrate into the lung better than aminoglycosides and have less potential for nephrotoxicity, a trend toward improved survival has been seen with aminoglycoside-containing, but not with quinolone-containing, combinations [144]. In some studies, combination therapy has been continued for less than the full course of therapy, with discontinuation of the aminoglycoside after 5 days if the patient is improving [145]. Monotherapy should be used when possible because combination therapy is often expensive and exposes patients to unnecessary antibiotics, thereby increasing the risk of drug toxicity and the selection of antibiotic resistant organisms. Once cultures are available, if the etiologic pathogen is susceptible, it is possible to change to monotherapy, using one of the agents that has proven to be effective in critically ill ventilated patients with pneumonia due to susceptible pathogens: ciprofloxacin, levofloxacin, doripenem, imipenem, meropenem, cefepime, and piperacillin/tazobactam [2]. Monotherapy with ciprofloxacin has been successful in patients with mild HAP (defined as a CPIS of 6 or less) but is less effective in severe HAP [107].

The choice of initial therapy should be based on local patterns of antimicrobial susceptibility and anticipated side effects, and should also take into account which therapies patients have recently received (within the past 2 weeks), striving not to repeat the same antimicrobial class, if possible. In addition, some studies have shown that recent therapy with quinolones promotes not only Gram-negative resistance to quinolones but also to β-lactams, and they can lead to the emergence of MRSA and MDR Gram-negatives [146]. Therefore, it may be better not to use quinolones for a first episode of hospital infection, because it may make both β-lactams and quinolones less effective if therapy is needed for a subsequent infection. Because many hospitalized patients do develop multiple infections, this strategy will preserve some therapeutic options for a second episode of infection [147]. In addition, in many hospitals, Gram-negative susceptibility to quinolones has declined and empiric coverage is improved only if an aminoglycoside is added to a β-lactam, but not if a quinolone is added [148].

For the initial antimicrobial therapy regimen to account for local bacteriologic patterns, each ICU should ideally have its own antibiogram that is updated as often as possible. Variability in the microorganisms associated with hospital-acquired infections among hospitals, as well as within the ICUs of large hospitals, has been demonstrated to occur [2]. In addition, changing temporal patterns of nosocomial pathogens and antimicrobial susceptibility have been described. Current and frequently updated knowledge of such data can increase the likelihood of prescribing appropriate initial antibiotic treatment. This is especially important for infection with MDR pathogens, as empiric therapy should be with agents that are known to be effective against these organisms. Each ICU should establish its own "go to" empiric antibiotic regimen, tailored to the antibiotic susceptibility patterns of the local flora. If patients develop HAP during or shortly after antibiotic treatment for a different infection, the empiric therapy should involve an agent from a different antibiotic class. Recent exposure to a class of antibiotics can predict subsequent resistance to a variety of agents, usually to the same class but occasionally to other classes of agents as well [149].

In the treatment of nosocomial pneumonia, the ATS/IDSA guideline emphasizes the need for a "de-escalation" strategy of usage [2]. After 2 to 3 days, the clinical course can be assessed and the culture data reviewed, and in responding patients, efforts can be made to change the initial broad-spectrum therapy. This de-escalation can involve focusing to a more narrow spectrum agent, reducing the number of antibiotics, stopping therapy altogether in patients not likely to have infection, and making efforts to reduce duration of therapy [150]. When this strategy has been used, outcomes such as the frequency of secondary infection, antimicrobial resistance, and mortality have improved [150]. De-escalation can only be accomplished if lower respiratory tract cultures are obtained prior to initiating therapy, although rates can be high with either a non-quantitative endotracheal aspirate or a quantitatively cultured bronchoscopic sample [108]. Negative lower respiratory tract cultures can be used to stop antibiotic therapy in a patient who has had cultures obtained in the absence of an antibiotic change in the past 72 hours and who is clinically doing well. In retrospect, such a patient may not have pneumonia but rather another diagnosis such as CHF or atelectasis. Combination therapy can be de-escalated to monotherapy once culture data are available, and aminoglycosides may be used for a short duration (5 days), when used in combination with a β-lactam to treat *P. aeruginosa* pneumonia. In clinical practice, physicians do not de-escalate often enough, even though data do not show adverse outcomes when this approach is applied to patients who are responding to initial empiric therapy [151].

The recommended duration of therapy for VAP has been the subject of recent studies. In earlier reports, significant improvements were observed for all clinical parameters generally within the first 6 days of the start of antibiotics [152]. Luna et al. [153] observed that patients who survived VAP after receiving appropriate therapy tended to have a clinical improvement by days 3 to 5, especially reflected by improved PaO_2/FiO_2 ratio, whereas nonresponding patients did not have such a response during the same time period. On the other hand, prolonged antibiotic therapy simply leads to colonization with resistant bacteria, which may be a risk factor for recurrent VAP. A multicenter, randomized, controlled trial demonstrated that patients who received appropriate, initial empiric therapy of VAP for 8 days had outcomes similar to those patients who received therapy for 14 days [154]. A trend to greater rates of relapse for short-duration therapy was seen if the etiologic agent was *P. aeruginosa* or *Acinetobacter* spp. Thus, for patients who receive initially appropriate antibiotics and have a good clinical response to therapy, the duration of therapy should be as short as 7 days, provided that the etiologic pathogen is not *P. aeruginosa*. The optimal duration of therapy for VAP due to MDR organisms such as *P. aeruginosa* or *Acinetobacter* spp is not known. Two recent, randomized, multicenter studies showed that PCT can help guide therapy discontinuation for VAP and help decrease number of days on antibiotic. Stolz et al. [86] compared a PCT-guided approach with the usual guideline approach in 101 patients. The use of the biomarker impacted significantly on a shorter duration of therapy, with a reduction of 27% in the number of antibiotic days, without showing an in-hospital mortality difference or a longer duration of mechanical ventilation between the two groups. Similar results were found by Bouadma et al. [155] when they compared 307 patients where the therapy was guided by the biomarker and the use of 314 controls. The number of antibiotic-free days was approximately 2.7 days less in the PCT group, with no differences in 28- or 60-day mortality between the two groups.

Although aminoglycosides are used in VAP, there is concern about nephrotoxicity (especially in the elderly) and these drugs being less active in areas of the lung that have a low pH levels, as may occur with pneumonia. Also, these antibiotics achieve only 40% of the serum concentration in respiratory secretions, when given intravenously. Although once-daily dosing has been proposed to take advantage of the postantibiotic effect of aminoglycosides to enhance efficacy, while reducing the need for monitoring serum levels and reducing the toxicity, a meta-analysis has shown neither enhanced efficacy nor reduced toxicity with once-daily dosing [2]. Another approach used by some investigators is the direct delivery of aminoglycosides into the airway in an effort to achieve high levels of antibiotic at the site of infection, with little risk of systemic absorption and toxicity. Clinical studies of aerosolized aminoglycosides have shown this approach to be effective in cystic fibrosis and severe Gram-negative pneumonia [156]. Small and uncontrolled series have shown that when patients have VAP due to MDR *P. aeruginosa* or *Acinetobacter* spp, aerosolized aminoglycosides, polymyxin, or colistin may be helpful as adjunctive therapy to systemic antibiotics [157,158]. One side effect of aerosolized antibiotics has been bronchospasm, which can be induced by the antibiotic or the associated diluents present in certain preparations. Pending further investigation, this therapy should be used as an adjunct to systemic antibiotics, only in patients with severe Gram-negative pneumonias who are not responding to intravenous therapy, or in patients infected by a relatively resistant organism that might be eliminated only with high local drug concentrations.

STRATEGIES FOR PREVENTION OF PNEUMONIA

Community-Acquired Pneumonia

Preventive strategies can be applied in the outpatient (prehospital) setting or in the hospital and ICU. Outpatient measures proven to reduce the incidence of severe lower respiratory tract infection are immunization against pneumococcal and influenza infection in susceptible populations [4,159]. The pneumococcal polyvalent vaccine (PPV) is directed at 23 strains of pneumococcus (accounting for 85% to 90% of all infections), and it is both cost-effective and potentially cost saving among individuals older than 65 years for the prevention of bacteremia. In a study of US hospitals, prior vaccination against pneumococcus was associated with improved survival (adjusted OR, 0.50; 95% confidence interval, 0.43 to 0.59), decreased chance of respiratory failure or other complications, and decreased length of stay among hospitalized patients with CAP [159]. With documented effectiveness of 75% in this age group, the recommendation is that all immune-competent patients aged 65 years or older should be immunized [4]. If prior history of vaccination is not available, revaccination is also safe, as there was no difference in the risk of adverse events following more than three doses of PPV, compared with one or two doses [160]. This may be relevant following vaccination with 23-valent PPV, because pneumococcal antibody levels decline to prevaccination levels within 6 to 10 years. More studies are needed before routine revaccination is advised. The current PPV is not maximally immunogenic, and a more immunogenic, 7-valent conjugate, vaccine has been developed for children, but is not yet available for adults.

Annual influenza vaccination has reduced the frequency and severity of influenza in the elderly and chronically ill patient, and vaccination of medical personnel may reduce nosocomial transmission of influenza from staff to patients [161]. Antiviral chemoprophylaxis (with oseltamivir, zanamivir, amantadine, or rimantadine) may be adjunctive to immunization and is 70% to 90% effective in avoiding infections with influenza A if it is started at the earliest recognition of an outbreak and if the circulating strain is sensitive to these agents (which has not always been the case in recent epidemics). Studies of amantadine prophylaxis demonstrated substantial reduction in nosocomial attack rates [162]. The new neuraminidase inhibitors, zanamivir and oseltamivir, are active against both influenza A and B, for prophylaxis and treatment if started within 36 hours of the onset of symptoms. They reduce clinical illness [163] and viral shedding by 2 days and prevent secondary complications of influenza, such as otitis media and sinusitis [162].

Nosocomial Pneumonia

In the ICU, several general strategies may be used to reduce the incidence of pneumonia [2] (Table 68.10). In recent years, some of these measures have been combined and applied to intubated patients as a "ventilator bundle," leading to dramatic reductions in the rate of VAP.

TABLE 68.10

PREVENTATIVE STRATEGIES AVAILABLE IN INTENSIVE CARE UNIT PNEUMONIA

To prevent tracheobronchial colonization
Infection control
Handwashing
Respiratory therapy equipment: careful handling
Maintain endotracheal tube cuff pressure to avoid aspiration
Change no more than every 48 h
Isolate patients with resistant organisms
Avoid endotracheal intubation (noninvasive ventilation)
Aspiration avoidance
Reduce use of nasogastric tubes (place orally, and if possible postpyloric)
Avoid central nervous system depressants
Daily interruption of sedation
Start enteral feeding only after >24–48 h after intubation
Keep patients semierect when possible
"Ventilator bundles"
Consider using subglottic secretion drainage
Host defense fortification
Nutritional support: consider site of feeding, pH of feeding, continuous or discontinuous enteral feeding
Avoid immunosuppressants
Restricted blood transfusion policy
Glycemic control
Influenza and pneumococcal vaccine: consider hospital-based programs
Provide antiviral prophylaxis (especially for influenza A)
Consider immunostimulation: cytokine infusion or blockade
Other potentially useful measures (multiple targets)
Topical aerosolized lower respiratory antibiotics
"Selective digestive decontamination"—oropharynx and GI tract
Selective oral decontamination
Careful consideration of GI bleeding prophylaxis in the context of enteral feeding
Antibiotic rotation/cycling
Active and passive immunization against groups of potential pathogens
Secretion mobilization: lateral rotational therapy

GI, gastrointestinal.

Infection Control and Ventilator Equipment Handling

A nationwide epidemiologic survey, the Study on the Efficacy of Nosocomial Infection control (SENIC) study, suggested that effective infection control and surveillance programs could potentially reduce the rate of nosocomial pneumonia by 20% [164]. Handwashing, although simple and effective in reducing the spread of resistant organisms, is frequently neglected in the ICU. Proper disinfection of nebulization equipment should be done after each use. Heat moisture exchangers in the ventilator circuit can eliminate the need for cascade humidification but have not been shown to reduce the incidence of nosocomial pneumonia. Ventilator circuit changes should be made no more often than every 48 hours, and more frequent changes and manipulations may add to the risk of infection [2,43]. In fact, there is no increased infection risk if tubing is never changed [165].

Prophylactic Antibiotics

Numerous studies have documented the efficacy of topical antibiotics applied to the lower airway in preventing nosocomial pneumonia in an ICU setting. However, these studies, done in the early 1970s, showed that this approach was associated with the emergence of resistant bacteria that could themselves cause fatal pneumonia, and thus the strategy was deemed unsafe and was abandoned [166].

Intense interest has been focused on "selective digestive decontamination (SDD)" as a means of preventing both nosocomial pneumonia and sepsis [167]. This approach attempts to sterilize the intestine and oral cavity of all Gram-negative organisms, assuming that the gastrointestinal tract is the source of the organisms that cause pneumonia.

Several large meta-analyses and four recent prospective trials have shown a benefit for SDD in preventing VAP and in reducing mortality [167]. The full regimen is usually a combination of topical (polymyxin, tobramycin, and amphotericin or related compounds) and systemic antibiotics (nonpseudomonal third-generation cephalosporin), but the use of only topical oral antibiotics (selective oral decontamination, SOD) or oral antiseptics (such as chlorhexidine) has also reduced the incidence of infection, but with generally no influence on overall mortality [168]. However, in a recent, large randomized trial, both SDD and SOD reduced ICU mortality rates [169]. In spite of these possible benefits, widespread use of SDD in all ICU patients should not be encouraged. In many studies, the benefits have applied only to selected populations such as surgical and trauma patients, with less benefit to medical patients. In addition, those at the extremes of disease severity (mild or severely ill) may not benefit. In addition, to be fully effective, SDD needs to be used in all patients in a given ICU, and this widespread use has been shown in some studies to promote the emergency of resistant bacteria, particularly Gram-positives such as MRSA. This is likely to be an even greater problem in ICUs with a high baseline rate of resistance. SDD may also lead to an increased rate of hospital-acquired infections in patients after they leave the ICU [170].

Control of Respiratory Secretions

Stagnation of respiratory secretions can lead to both pneumonia and atelectasis, and efforts to remove these secretions could reduce the incidence of pneumonia. One way to achieve this objective is through the use of continuous lateral rotation delivered by a rotating bed that is used in place of a traditional hospital bed to improve mucociliary clearance and help mobilize secretions. Another way to control respiratory secretions is to remove oropharyngeal contents before they can be aspirated into the lung. Continuous aspiration of subglottic secretions, through the use of a specially designed endotracheal tube, has significantly reduced the incidence of early-onset VAP in several studies [2]. Other measures to reduce the aspiration of oropharyngeal bacteria include limiting the use of sedative and paralytic agents that depress cough and other host-protective mechanisms and maintaining endotracheal cuff pressure greater than 20 cm H_2O [2].

Intestinal Bleeding Prophylaxis

Several clinical studies have documented that neutralization of gastric pH with antacids or H_2 blockers can add to the risk of nosocomial pneumonia (especially late-onset infection) in mechanically ventilated patients [2,43], because an increase in gastric pH can lead to Gram-negative overgrowth of the stomach contents, which can then be aspirated into the lung [56]. Although not all studies have shown that the gastric reservoir is an important source of infection, prevention strategies should take into account its potential influence by minimizing gastric volume and preventing aspiration of gastric contents; however, ventilator bundles have been able to reduce VAP rates, even if H_2 blockers are used. This is likely because gastric acid neutralization is combined with elevation of the head of the bed, which may prevent aspiration of gastric contents. Although some studies have suggested a benefit of performing intestinal bleeding prophylaxis with sucralfate, at least one large, double-blind, randomized trial comparing ranitidine with sucralfate, which demonstrated a trend toward lower rates of VAP with sucralfate, also reported that clinically significant gastrointestinal bleeding was 4% higher in the sucralfate group [171]. Another study of VAP in patients with ARDS showed that the use of sucralfate and the duration of exposure to sucralfate were associated with an increased risk of VAP [73].

Ventilator Bundles

Several simple prevention strategies have been incorporated into a "ventilator bundle" that can be routinely applied to all ventilated patients. The most widely used approach is to combine five measures: peptic ulcer disease prophylaxis, deep vein thrombosis prophylaxis, elevation of the head of the bed, daily interruption of sedation, and daily assessment of readiness to wean. Some centers also apply routine mouth care and oral chlorhexidine. When applied, this strategy has been reported to lead to a 44.5% reduction in the incidence of VAP in the 35 ICUs that used this approach, and the benefit was greatest when adherence to the protocol was high [172]. In the last several years, this approach has become so popular and apparently effective that many believe that it can lead to a "zero VAP" rate. However, there is concern that the benefits of ventilator bundles have been overstated, and that it is impossible to eliminate VAP in certain high-risk patients [41,173]. In addition, although studies have shown a reduction in VAP rates, secondary benefits such as reduction in mortality and antibiotic use have not generally been reported.

Other Measures

Blood Transfusions and Glucose Control

Multiple studies have identified exposure to allogeneic blood products as a risk factor for postoperative infection and postoperative pneumonia, and the length of time of blood storage as another contributing [2]. The use of leukocyte-depleted red blood cell transfusions resulted in a reduced incidence of postoperative infections and specifically a reduced incidence of pneumonia in patients undergoing colorectal surgery [174]. In another study, in less severely ill patients, mortality was improved with a restricted transfusion strategy (transfusion trigger 7 g per dL, instead of 9 g per dL), likely due to immunosuppressive effects of nonleukocyte-depleted red blood cell units, leading to an increased risk for infection [175]. Routine red blood cell transfusion should be conducted with a restricted transfusion trigger policy.

The role of hyperglycemia in ICU infections has received much attention. Hyperglycemia may directly or indirectly increase the risk of complications and poor outcomes in critically ill patients. Van den Berghe et al. [176] randomized surgical ICU patients to receive either intensive insulin therapy to maintain blood glucose levels between 80 and 110 mg per dL or to receive conventional treatment. The group receiving intensive insulin therapy had reduced mortality (4.6% vs. 8%). When compared with the control group, those treated with intensive insulin therapy had a 46% reduction of bloodstream infections, fewer antibiotic treatment days, and significantly shorter length of mechanical ventilation and ICU stay. In the medical ICU setting, the results were less promising. Intensive insulin therapy significantly reduced morbidity but not mortality in medical ICU patients, and this was seen more in patients treated for 3 or more days [177]. More recent data have suggested that very tight control of blood glucose in the ICU may not be beneficial and may lead to clinically relevant hypoglycemia [178].

Role of Noninvasive Ventilation

The role of invasive devices in breaching mucosal barriers has been discussed earlier. Noninvasive ventilation (NIV), instead of conventional mechanical ventilation in patients with acute respiratory failure due to COPD or acute cardiogenic pulmonary edema, led to a significantly lower risk of nosocomial pneumonia, less antibiotic use, shorter ICU stay, and lower mortality [2]. Improved outcomes with NIV were also shown

TABLE 68.11

RECENT ADVANCES IN PNEUMONIA MANAGEMENT BASED ON RANDOMIZED TRIALS, LARGE DATABASE ANALYSES, AND META-ANALYSIS

- Antibiotic duration in VAP should be as short as possible. In patients with a low clinical suspicion, based on serial clinical observations, therapy can be stopped after 3 days, while those with microbiologically confirmed VAP can be safely treated for 8 days, provided that initial therapy is appropriate and that a nonfermenting Gram-negative is not responsible [61,150].
- Activated protein C can reduce mortality in patients with severe CAP, especially if *Streptococcus pneumoniae* is the etiologic pathogen, and may have particular benefit if initial empiric therapy is inappropriate [4,125].
- Linezolid is associated with a lower mortality and higher bacteriologic eradication rate than vancomycin in patients with VAP that is proven to be caused by MRSA, but quinupristin/dalfopristin is not superior to vancomycin [122,137,139].
- Quinolone monotherapy should not be used for patients with severe CAP, since it has not been proven to be safe and effective for all of the types of patients admitted to the ICU [4,118].
- Mortality in CAP can be reduced by administering the first dose of antibiotics with 4 hours of a patient's arrival to the hospital [4].
- In patients with VAP, diagnosis can be made with either endotracheal aspirate culture or bronchoscopic culture, with no difference in mortality, comparing the two methods [2].
- Combination antimicrobial therapy in VAP increases the likelihood of initially effective empiric therapy for patients who are likely to have multidrug-resistant pathogen infection, but the use of combination therapy has not been definitively proven to reduce mortality [2].
- When cephalosporins are used for empiric therapy of severe CAP, and drug-resistant *S. pneumoniae* is suspected, ceftriaxone and cefotaxime are reliable choices, while cefuroxime is not [4].
- In the presence of CAP with pneumococcal bacteremia, use of dual antibiotic therapy is associated with reduced mortality, compared with monotherapy, especially for patients with severe pneumonia [115,116].

CAP, community-acquired pneumonia; ICU, intensive care unit; MRSA, methicillin-resistant *Staphylococcus aureus*; VAP, ventilator-associated pneumonia.

in immunosuppressed patients with pulmonary infiltrates and respiratory failure [179]. In addition, to reduce the duration of mechanical ventilation and the risk of VAP, specific strategies in ICU patients are needed, such as the use of protocols to facilitate and accelerate weaning and judicious use of sedation [2]. Accidental extubation and reintubation should be avoided, as they increase the risk of VAP [180].

Nutritional Support. Traditionally, early enteral feeding has been recommended in ICU patients over parenteral nutrition. However, in VAP, enteral nutrition has been considered a risk factor mainly because of an increased risk of aspiration of gastric contents [2]. In an attempt to define the timing of starting enteral nutrition, a strategy of early enteral feeding (day 1 of intubation) was associated with a higher risk for ICU-acquired VAP when compared with late administration (day 5 of intubation) [181]. In terms of site of feeding, a meta-analysis showed that postpyloric feeding compared with gastric feeding was associated with a significant reduction in ICU-acquired HAP (relative risk, 0.76; 95% confidence interval, 0.59 to 0.99) [58].

Role of Antibiotic Rotation

The concept of antibiotic rotation or cycling has also been investigated as a resistance control strategy, with potential benefits of reducing the incidence of VAP, especially due to resistant organisms. In theory, a class of antibiotics or a specific antibiotic is withdrawn from use for a defined time period and reintroduced at a later point in time in an attempt to limit bacterial resistance to the cycled antimicrobial agents [145,182]. Although there was initial enthusiasm for this approach, recent studies have been less supportive, and most ICUs focus on antimicrobial stewardship, focusing on monitoring local patterns of resistance and introducing heterogeneity into the choice of antibiotics [145,183].

Advances in managing acute infectious pneumonia, based on randomized, controlled trials or meta-analyses of such trials, are summarized in Table 68.11.

References

1. National Center for Health Statistics: *Health, United States, 2006*. Available at: http://www.cdc.gov/nchs/data/hus/hus06.pdf. Accessed January 17, 2007.
2. Niederman MS, Craven DE, Bonten MJ, et al: Guidelines for the management of adults with hospital-acquired, ventilator-associated, and healthcare-associated pneumonia. *Am J Respir Crit Care Med* 171:388–416, 2005.
3. Ahmed QA, Niederman MS: Respiratory infection in the chronically critically ill patient. Ventilator-associated pneumonia and tracheobronchitis. *Clin Chest Med* 22:71–85, 2001.
4. Mandell LA, Wunderink RG, Anzueto A, et al: Infectious Diseases Society of America/American Thoracic Society consensus guidelines on the management of community-acquired pneumonia in adults. *Clin Infect Dis* 44:S27–S72, 2007.
5. Niederman, MS: Making sense of scoring systems in community acquired pneumonia. *Respirology* 14:327–335, 2009.
6. Woodhead M, Welch CA, Harrison DA, et al: Community-acquired pneumonia on the intensive care unit: secondary analysis of 17,869 cases in the ICNARC Case Mix Programme Database. *Crit Care* 10[Suppl 2]:S1, 2006.
7. Ruiz M, Ewig S, Torres A, et al: Severe community-acquired pneumonia: risk factors and follow-up epidemiology. *Am J Respir Crit Care Med* 160: 923–929, 1999.
8. Richards MJ, Edwards JR, Culver DH, et al: Nosocomial infections in medical intensive care units in the United States. National Nosocomial Infections Surveillance System. *Crit Care Med* 27:887–892, 1999.
9. Safdar N, Dezfulian C, Collard HR, et al: Clinical and economic consequences of ventilator-associated pneumonia: a systematic review. *Crit Care Med* 33:2184–2193, 2005.
10. Papazian L, Bregeon F, Thirion X, et al: Effect of ventilator-associated pneumonia on mortality and morbidity. *Am J Respir Crit Care Med* 154:91–97, 1996.
11. Seidenfeld JJ, Pohl DF, Bell RD, et al: Incidence, site, and outcome of infections in patients with the adult respiratory distress syndrome. *Am Rev Respir Dis* 134:12–16, 1986.
12. Kollef MH, Silver P, Murphy DM, et al: The effect of late-onset ventilator associated pneumonia in determining patient mortality. *Chest* 108:1655–1662, 1995.
13. Rello J, Torres A, Ricart M, et al: Ventilator-associated pneumonia by *Staphylococcus aureus*. Comparison of methicillin-resistant and methicillin-sensitive episodes. *Am J Respir Crit Care Med* 150:1545–1549, 1994.
14. Heyland DK, Cook DJ, Griffith L, et al: The attributable morbidity and mortality of ventilator-associated pneumonia in the critically ill patient. The Canadian Critical Trials Group. *Am J Respir Crit Care Med* 159:1249–1256, 1999.
15. Micek ST, Kollef K, Reichley RM, et al: Health care-associated pneumonia and community-acquired pneumonia: a single-center experience. *Antimicrob Agents Chemother* 51:3568–3573, 2007.
16. Austrian R, Gold J: Pneumococcal bacteremia with especial reference to bacteremic pneumococcal pneumonia. *Ann Intern Med* 60:759–776, 1964.
17. Baumann WR, Jung RC, Koss M, et al: Incidence and mortality of adult respiratory distress syndrome: a prospective analysis from a large metropolitan hospital. *Crit Care Med* 14:1–4, 1986.
18. Fine MJ, Smith MA, Carson CA, et al: Prognosis and outcomes of patients with community-acquired pneumonia: a meta-analysis. *JAMA* 275:134–141, 1996.
19. Torres A, Serra-Batlles J, Ferrer A, et al: Severe community-acquired pneumonia. Epidemiology and prognostic factors. *Am Rev Respir Dis* 144:312–318, 1991.
20. Bordón J, Peyrani P, Brock GN, et al: The presence of pneumococcal bacteremia does not influence clinical outcomes in patients with community-acquired pneumonia: results from the Community-Acquired Pneumonia Organization (CAPO) International Cohort study. *Chest* 133:618–624, 2008.
21. Restrepo M, Motersen E, Velez J, et al: A comparative study of community-acquired pneumonia patients admitted to the ward and the ICU. *Chest* 133:610–617, 2008.
22. Aujesky D, Auble TE, Yealy DM, et al: Prospective comparison of three validated prediction rules for prognosis in community-acquired pneumonia. *Am J Med* 118:384–392, 2005.
23. Lim WS, van der Eerden MM, Laing R, et al: Defining community acquired pneumonia severity of presentation to hospital: an international derivation and validation study. *Thorax* 58:377–382, 2003.
24. Shindo Y, Sato S, Maruyama E, et al: Comparison of severity scoring systems A-DROP and CURB-65 for community-acquired pneumonia. *Respirology* 13:731–735, 2008.
25. España PP, Capelastegui A, Gorordo I, et al: Development and validation of a clinical prediction rule for severe community-acquired pneumonia. *Am J Respir Crit Care Med* 174:1249–1256, 2006.
26. Charles PG, Wolfe R, Whitby M, et al: SMART-COP: a tool for predicting the need for intensive respiratory or vasopressor support in community-acquired pneumonia. *Clin Infect Dis* 47:375–384, 2008.
27. Salluh JI, Bozza FA, Soares M, et al: Adrenal response in severe community-acquired pneumonia: impact on outcomes and disease severity. *Chest* 134:947–954, 2008.
28. Masiá M, Gutiérrez F, Shum C, et al: Usefulness of procalcitonin levels in community-acquired pneumonia according to the patients outcome research team pneumonia severity index. *Chest* 128:2223–2229, 2005.
29. Krüger S, Ewig S, Marre R, et al: Procalcitonin predicts patients at low risk of death from community-acquired pneumonia across all CRB-65 classes. *Eur Respir J* 31:349–355, 2008.
30. Huang DT, Weissfeld LA, Kellum JA, et al: Risk prediction with procalcitonin and clinical rules in community-acquired pneumonia. *Ann Emerg Med* 52:48–58, 2008.
31. Liapikou A, Ferrer M, Polverino E, et al: Severe community-acquired pneumonia: validation of the Infectious Diseases Society of America/American Thoracic Society guidelines to predict an intensive care unit admission. *Clin Infect Dis* 48:377–385, 2009.
32. Garau J, Baquero F, Pérez-Trallero E, et al: Factors impacting on length of stay and mortality of community-acquired pneumonia. *Clin Microbiol Infect* 14:322–329, 2008.
33. Leroy O, Santré C, Beuscart C, et al: A five-year study of severe community-acquired pneumonia with emphasis on prognosis in patients admitted to an intensive care unit. *Intensive Care Med* 21:24–31, 1995.
34. Shorr AF, Bodi M, Rodriguez A, et al: Impact of antibiotic guideline compliance on duration of mechanical ventilation in critically ill patients with community-acquired pneumonia. *Chest* 130:93–100, 2006.
35. Kumar A, Roberts D, Wood K, et al: Duration of hypotension before initiation of effective antimicrobial therapy is the critical determinant of survival in human septic shock. *Crit Care Med* 34:1589–1596, 2006.
36. Niederman MS: Recent advances in community-acquired pneumonia: inpatient and outpatient. *Chest* 131:1205–1215, 2007.

37. Moroney JF, Fiore AE, Harrison LH, et al: Clinical outcomes of bacteremic pneumococcal pneumonia in the era of antibiotic resistance. *Clin Infect Dis* 33:797–805, 2001.
38. Metlay JP, Hofmann J, Cetron MS, et al: Impact of penicillin susceptibility on medical outcomes for adult patients with bacteremic pneumococcal pneumonia. *Clin Infect Dis* 30:520–528, 2000.
39. Turett GS, Blum S, Fazal BA, et al: Penicillin resistance and other predictors of mortality in pneumococcal bacteremia in a population with high human immunodeficiency virus seroprevalence. *Clin Infect Dis* 29:321–327, 1999.
40. Feikin DR, Schuchat A, Kolczak M, et al: Mortality from invasive pneumococcal pneumonia in the era of antibiotic resistance, 1995–1997. *Am J Public Health* 90:223–229, 2000.
41. Uçkay I, Ahmed QA, Sax H, et al: Ventilator-associated pneumonia as a quality indicator for patient safety? *Clin Infect Dis* 16:557–563, 2008.
42. Cook DJ, Walter SD, Cook RJ: Incidence of and risk factors for ventilator-associated pneumonia in critically ill patients. *Ann Intern Med* 129:433–440, 1998.
43. Craven DE, Kunches LM, Kilinsky V, et al: Risk factors for pneumonia and fatality in patients receiving continuous mechanical ventilation. *Am Rev Respir Dis* 133:792–796, 1986.
44. Bryan CS, Reynolds KL: Bacteremic nosocomial pneumonia: analysis of 172 episodes from a single metropolitan area. *Am Rev Respir Dis* 129:668–671, 1984.
45. Zilberberg MD, Shorr AF, Kollef MH: Implementing quality improvements in the intensive care unit: ventilator bundle as an example. *Crit Care Med* 37:305–309, 2009.
46. Soo Hoo GW, Wen YE, Nguyen TV, et al: Impact of clinical guidelines in the management of severe hospital-acquired pneumonia. *Chest* 128:2778–2787, 2005.
47. Nachtigall I, Tamarkin A, Tafelski S, et al: Impact of adherence to standard operating procedures for pneumonia on outcome of intensive care unit patients. *Crit Care Med* 37:159–166, 2009.
48. Sloane PJ, Gee MH, Gottlieb JE, et al: A multicenter registry of patients with acute respiratory distress syndrome. *Am Rev Respir Dis* 146:419–426, 1992.
49. Carlet J, Hemmer M, Flandre P, et al: Infection and ARDS: a complex interaction: a prospective study of 583 patients. *Am Rev Respir Dis* 139:A270, 1989.
50. Chastre J, Trouillet JL, Vuagnat A, et al: Nosocomial pneumonia in patients with acute respiratory distress syndrome. *Am J Respir Crit Care Med* 157:1165–1172, 1998.
51. Brito V, Niederman MS: Healthcare-associated pneumonia is a heterogenous disease, and all patients do not need the same broad-spectrum antibiotic therapy as complex nosocomial pneumonia. *Curr Opin Infect Dis* 22:316–325, 2009.
52. Niederman MS: The pathogenesis of airway colonization: lessons learned from the study of bacterial adherence. *Eur Respir J* 7:1737–1740, 1994.
53. Boutten A, Dehoux MS, Seta N, et al: Compartmentalized IL-8 and elastase release within the human lung in unilateral pneumonia. *Am J Respir Crit Care Med* 153:336–342, 1996.
54. Inglis TJ, Millar MR, Jones G, et al: Tracheal tube biofilm as a source of bacterial colonization of the lung. *J Clin Microbiol* 27:2014–2018, 1989.
55. Kollef MH, Afessa B, Anzueto A, et al: Silver-coated endotracheal tubes and incidence of ventilator-associated pneumonia: the NASCENT randomized trial. *JAMA* 300:805–813, 2008.
56. Niederman MS, Craven DE: Devising strategies for preventing nosocomial pneumonia—should we ignore the stomach? *Clin Infect Dis* 24:320–323, 1997.
57. Torres A, Serra-Batlles J, Ros E, et al: Pulmonary aspiration of gastric contents in patients receiving mechanical ventilation: the effect of body position. *Ann Intern Med* 116:540–543, 1992.
58. Heyland DK, Cook DJ, Schoenfeld PS, et al: The effect of acidified enteral feeds on gastric colonization in critically ill patients: results of a multicenter randomized trial. Canadian Critical Care Trials Group. *Crit Care Med* 27:2399–2406, 1999.
59. Jacobs S, Chang RW, Lee B, et al: Continuous enteral feeding: a major cause of pneumonia among ventilated intensive care unit patients. *JPEN J Parenter Enteral Nutr* 14:353–356, 1990.
60. Montecalvo MA, Steger KA, Farber HW, et al: Nutritional outcome and pneumonia in critical care patients randomized to gastric versus jejunal tube feedings. *Crit Care Med* 20:1377–1387, 1992.
61. Craven DE, Chroneou A, Zias N, et al: Ventilator-associated tracheobronchitis: the impact of targeted antibiotic therapy on patient outcomes. *Chest* 135:521–528, 2009.
62. Feldman C, Kassel M, Cantrell J, et al: The presence and sequence of endotracheal tube colonization in patients undergoing mechanical ventilation. *Eur Respir J* 13:546–551, 1999.
63. Mason CM, Nelson S: Pulmonary host defenses and factors predisposing to lung infection. *Clin Chest Med* 26:11–17, 2005.
64. Waterer GW, Quasney MW, Cantor RM, et al: Septic shock and respiratory failure in community-acquired pneumonia have different TNF polymorphism associations. *Am J Respir Crit Care Med* 163:1599–1604, 2001.
65. Reade MC, Yende S, D'Angelo G, et al: Differences in immune response may explain lower survival among older men with pneumonia. *Crit Care Med* 37:1655–1662, 2009.
66. Marston BJ, Plouffe JF, File TM Jr, et al: Incidence of community-acquired pneumonia requiring hospitalization: results of a population based active surveillance study in Ohio. The Community-Based Pneumonia Incidence Study Group. *Arch Intern Med* 157:1709–1718, 1997.
67. Ruiz M, Ewig S, Marcos MA, et al: Etiology of community-acquired pneumonia: impact of age, comorbidity, and severity. *Am J Respir Crit Care Med* 160:397–405, 1999.
68. Arancibia F, Bauer TT, Ewig S, et al: Community-acquired pneumonia due to gram-negative bacteria and *Pseudomonas aeruginosa*: incidence, risk, and prognosis. *Arch Intern Med* 162:1849–1858, 2002.
69. Riquelme R, Torres A, el-Ebiary M, et al: Community-acquired pneumonia in the elderly: clinical and nutritional aspects. *Am J Respir Crit Care Med* 156:1908–1914, 1997.
70. Francis JS, Doherty MC, Lopatin U, et al: Severe community-onset pneumonia in healthy adults caused by methicillin-resistant *Staphylococcus aureus* carrying the Panton-Valentine leukocidin genes. *Clin Infect Dis* 40:100–107, 2005.
71. Kang CI, Song JH, Oh WS, et al: Clinical outcomes and risk factors of community-acquired pneumonia caused by gram-negative bacilli. *Eur J Clin Microbiol Infect Dis* 27:657–661, 2008.
72. de Roux A, Ewig S, Garcia E, et al: Mixed community-acquired pneumonia in hospitalised patients. *Eur Respir J* 27:795–800, 2006.
73. Markowicz P, Wolff M, Djedaïni K, et al: Multicenter prospective study of ventilator-associated pneumonia during acute respiratory distress syndrome. Incidence, prognosis, and risk factors. ARDS Study Group. *Am J Respir Crit Care Med* 161:1942–1948, 2000.
74. El-Solh AA, Pietrantoni C, Bhat A, et al: Microbiology of severe aspiration pneumonia in institutionalized elderly. *Am J Respir Crit Care Med* 167:1650–1654, 2003.
75. Chastre J, Fagon JY: Ventilator-associated pneumonia. *Am J Respir Crit Care Med* 165:867–903, 2002.
76. Fridkin, SK: Increasing prevalence of antimicrobial resistance in intensive care units. *Crit Care Med* 29:N64–N68, 2001.
77. Gaynes R, Edwards JR: Overview of nosocomial infections caused by gram-negative bacilli. *Clin Infect Dis* 41:848–854, 2005.
78. Rodrigues JM, Niederman MS, Fein AM, et al: Nonresolving pneumonia in steroid-treated patients with obstructive lung disease. *Am J Med* 93:29–34, 1992.
79. Kollef MH, Shorr A, Tabak YP, et al: Epidemiology and outcomes of health-care-associated pneumonia: results from a large US database of culture positive patients. *Chest* 128:3854–3862, 2005.
80. Sopena N, Sabria M, Neunos 2000 Study Group: Multicenter study of hospital-acquired pneumonia in non-ICU patients. *Chest* 127:213–219, 2005.
81. Yakovlev SV, Stratchounski LS, Woods GL, et al: Ertapenem versus cefepime for initial empirical treatment of pneumonia acquired in skilled-care facilities or in hospitals outside the intensive care unit. *Eur J Clin Microbiol Infect Dis* 25:633–641, 2006.
82. Weber DJ, Rutala WA, Sickbert-Bennett EE, et al: Microbiology of ventilator-associated pneumonia compared with that of hospital-acquired pneumonia. *Infect Control Hosp Epidemiol* 28:825–831, 2007.
83. Gleckman RA, Hibert D: Afebrile bacteremia. A phenomenon in geriatric patients. *JAMA* 248:1478–1481, 1982.
84. Fagon JY, Chastre J, Hance AJ, et al: Detection of nosocomial lung infection in ventilated patients. Use of a protected specimen brush and quantitative culture technique in 147 patients. *Am Rev Respir Dis* 138:110–116, 1988.
85. Pugin J, Auckenthaler R, Mili N, et al: Diagnosis of ventilator-associated pneumonia by bacteriology analysis of bronchoscopic and nonbronchoscopic "blind" bronchoalveolar lavage fluid. *Am Rev Respir Dis* 143:1121–1129, 1991.
86. Stolz D, Smyrnios N, Eggimann P, et al: Procalcitonin for reduced antibiotic exposure in ventilator-associated pneumonia: a randomised study. *Eur Respir J* 34:1364–1375, 2009.
87. Póvoa P, Coelho L, Almeida E, et al: C-reactive protein as a marker of ventilator-associated pneumonia resolution: a pilot study. *Eur Respir J* 25:804–812, 2005.
88. Gibot S, Cravoisy A, Levy B, et al: Soluble triggering receptor expressed on myeloid cells and the diagnosis of pneumonia. *N Engl J Med* 350:451–458, 2004.
89. Ramírez P, Ferrer M, Gimeno R, et al: Systemic inflammatory response and increased risk for ventilator-associated pneumonia: a preliminary study. *Crit Care Med* 37:1691–1695, 2009.
90. McFadden JP, Price RC, Eastwood HD, et al: Raised respiratory rate in elderly patients: a valuable physical sign. *Br Med J* 284:626–627, 1982.
91. Farr BM, Sloman AJ, Fisch MJ: Predicting death in patients hospitalized for community-acquired pneumonia. *Ann Intern Med* 115:428–436, 1991.
92. Rello J, Bodi M, Mariscal D, et al: Microbiological testing and outcome of patients with severe community-acquired pneumonia. *Chest* 123:174–180, 2003.
93. Nair V, Niederman MS, Masani N, et al: Hyponatremia in community-acquired pneumonia. *Am J Nephrol* 27:184–190, 2007.
94. Templeton KE, Scheltinga SA, van den Eeden WC, et al: Improved diagnosis of the etiology of community-acquired pneumonia with real-time polymerase chain reaction. *Clin Infect Dis* 41:345–351, 2005.

95. Boersma WG, Daniels JM, Lowenberg A, et al: Reliability of radiographic findings and the relation to etiologic agents in community-acquired pneumonia. *Respir Med* 100:926–932, 2006.
96. Metersky ML, Ma A, Bratzler DW, et al: Predicting bacteremia in patients with community-acquired pneumonia. *Am J Respir Crit Care Med* 169:342–347, 2004.
97. Dunn IJ, Marrie TJ, Mackeen AD, et al: The value of open lung biopsy in immunocompetent patients with community-acquired pneumonia requiring hospitalization. *Chest* 106:23–27, 1994.
98. Torres A, Ewig S: Diagnosing ventilator-associated pneumonia. *N Engl J Med* 350:433–435, 2004.
99. El Solh AA, Akinnusi ME, Pineda LA, et al: Diagnostic yield of quantitative endotracheal aspirates in patients with severe nursing home-acquired pneumonia. *Crit Care* 11:R57, 2007.
100. Feller-Kopman D, Ernst A: The role of bronchoalveolar lavage in the immunocompromised host. *Semin Respir Infect* 18:87–94, 2003.
101. Fartoukh M, Maitre B, Honoré S, et al: Diagnosing pneumonia during mechanical ventilation: the clinical pulmonary infection score revisited. *Am J Respir Crit Care Med* 168:173–179, 2003.
102. Baram D, Hulse G, Palmer LB: Stable patients receiving prolonged mechanical ventilation have a high alveolar burden of bacteria. *Chest* 127:1353–1357, 2005.
103. Niederman MS: The argument against using quantitative cultures in clinical trials and for the management of ventilator-associated pneumonia.. Clin Infect Dis 51[Suppl 1]:S93–S99, 2010.
104. Rello J, Gallego M, Mariscal D, et al: The value of routine microbial investigation in ventilator-associated pneumonia. *Am J Respir Crit Care Med* 156:196–200, 1997.
105. Berton DC, Kalil AC, Cavalcanti M, et al: Quantitative versus qualitative cultures of respiratory secretions for clinical outcomes in patients with ventilator-associated pneumonia. *Cochrane Database Syst Rev* 4:CD006482, 2009.
106. Fagon JY, Chastre J, Wolff M, et al: Invasive and noninvasive strategies for management of suspected ventilator-associated pneumonia. A randomized trial. *Ann Intern Med* 132:621–630, 2000.
107. Singh N, Rogers P, Atwood CW, et al: Short-course empiric antibiotic therapy for patients with pulmonary infiltrates in the intensive care unit. A proposed solution for indiscriminate antibiotic prescription. *Am J Respir Crit Care Med* 162:505–511, 2000.
108. Heyland DK, Dodek P, Muscedere J, et al: Randomized trial of combination versus monotherapy for the empiric treatment of suspected ventilator-associated pneumonia. *Crit Care Med* 36:737–744, 2008.
109. Noskin GA, Glassroth J: Bacterial pneumonia associated with HIV-1 infection. *Clin Chest Med* 17:713–723, 1996.
110. Moore FA, Moore EE, Jones TN, et al: TEN versus TPN following major abdominal trauma: reduced septic mortality. *J Trauma* 29:916–922, 1989.
111. Heyland DK, Drover JW, MacDonald S, et al: Effect of postpyloric feeding on gastroesophageal regurgitation and pulmonary microaspiration: results of a randomized controlled trial. *Crit Care Med* 29:1495–1501, 2001.
112. Graham WB, Bradley DA: Efficacy of chest physiotherapy and intermittent positive-pressure breathing in the resolution of pneumonia. *N Engl J Med* 299:624–627, 1978.
113. Britton S, Bejstedt M, Vedin L: Chest physiotherapy in primary pneumonia. *Br Med J* 290:1703–1704, 1985.
114. Sahn SA: Continuous lateral rotational therapy and nosocomial pneumonia. *Chest* 99:1263–1267, 1991.
115. Waterer GW, Somes GW, Wunderink RG: Monotherapy may be suboptimal for severe bacteremic pneumococcal pneumonia. *Arch Intern Med* 161:1837–1842, 2001.
116. Baddour LM, Yu VL, Klygkan KP, et al: Combination antibiotic therapy lowers mortality among severely ill patients with pneumococcal bacteremia. *Am J Respir Crit Care Med* 170:440–444, 2004.
117. Yu VL, Greenberg RN, Zadeikis N, et al: Levofloxacin efficacy in the treatment of community-acquired legionellosis. *Chest* 125:2135–2136, 2004.
118. Leroy O, Saux P, Bédos JP, et al: Comparison of levofloxacin and cefotaxime combined with ofloxacin for ICU patients with community-acquired pneumonia who do not require vasopressors. *Chest* 128:172–183, 2005.
119. Anzueto A, Niederman MS, Pearle J, et al: Community-acquired pneumonia recovery in the elderly (CAPRIE): efficacy and safety of moxifloxacin therapy versus that of levofloxacin therapy. *Clin Infect Dis* 41:73–81, 2006.
120. Mortensen EM, Restropo MI, Anzueto A, et al: The impact of empiric antimicrobial therapy with a beta-lactam and fluoroquinolone on mortality for patients hospitalized with severe pneumonia. *Crit Care* 10:R8, 2005.
121. Vardakas KZ, Siempos II, Grammatikos A, et al: Respiratory fluoroquinolones for the treatment of community-acquired pneumonia: a meta-analysis of randomized controlled trials. *CMAJ* 179:1269–1277, 2008.
122. Micek ST, Dunne M, Kollef MH: Pleuropulmonary complications of Panton-Valentine leukocidin-positive community-acquired methicillin-resistant *Staphylococcus aureus*: importance of treatment with antimicrobials inhibiting exotoxin production. *Chest* 128:2732–2738, 2005.
123. Lujan M, Gallego M, Fontanals D, et al: Prospective observational study of bacteremic pneumococcal pneumonia: effect of discordant therapy on mortality. *Crit Care Med* 32:625–631, 2004.
124. Yu VL, Chiou CC, Feldman C, et al: An international prospective study of pneumococcal bacteremia: correlation with in vitro resistance, antibiotics administered, and clinical outcome. *Clin Infect Dis* 37:230–237, 2003.
125. Laterre PF, Garber G, Levy H, et al: Severe community-acquired pneumonia as a cause of severe sepsis: data from the PROWESS study. *Crit Care Med* 33:952–961, 2005.
126. Dellinger RP, Carlet JM, Masur H, et al: Surviving Sepsis Campaign guidelines for management of severe sepsis and septic shock. *Crit Care Med* 32:858–873, 2004.
127. Confalonieri M, Urbino R, Potena A, et al: Hydrocortisone infusion for severe community-acquired pneumonia: a preliminary randomized study. *Am J Respir Crit Care Med* 171:242–248, 2005.
128. Garcia-Vidal C, Calbo E, Pascual V, et al: Effects of systemic steroids in patients with severe community-acquired pneumonia. *Eur Respir J* 30:951–956, 2007.
129. Salluh JI, Póvoa P, Soares M, et al: The role of corticosteroids in severe community-acquired pneumonia: a systematic review. *Crit Care* 12:R76, 2008.
130. de Gans J, van de Beek D: Dexamethasone in adults with bacterial meningitis. *N Engl J Med* 347:1549–1556, 2002.
131. Falagas ME, Metaxas EI: Tigecycline for the treatment of patients with community-acquired pneumonia requiring hospitalization. *Expert Rev Anti Infect Ther* 7:913–923, 2009.
132. Boucher HW, Talbot GH, Bradley JS, et al: Bad bugs, no drugs: no ESKAPE! An update from the Infectious Diseases Society of America. *Clin Infect Dis* 48:1–12, 2009.
133. Carratalà J, Mykietiuk A, Fernández-Sabé N, et al: Health care-associated pneumonia requiring hospital admission: epidemiology, antibiotic therapy, and clinical outcomes. *Arch Intern Med* 167:1393–1399, 2007.
134. Réa-Neto A, Niederman M, Lobo SM, et al: Efficacy and safety of doripenem versus piperacillin/tazobactam in nosocomial pneumonia: a randomized, open-label, multicenter study. *Curr Med Res Opin* 24:2113–2126, 2008.
135. Schafer JJ, Goff DA, Stevenson KB, et al: Early experience with tigecycline for ventilator-associated pneumonia and bacteremia caused by multidrug-resistant *Acinetobacter baumannii*. *Pharmacotherapy* 27:980–987, 2007.
136. Paterson DL, Ko WC, Von Gottberg A, et al: Antibiotic therapy for *Klebsiella pneumoniae* bacteremia: implications of production of extended-spectrum β-lactamases. *Clin Infect Dis* 39:31–37, 2004.
137. Wunderink RG, Rello J, Cammarata SK, et al: Linezolid vs vancomycin: analysis of two double-blind studies of patients with methicillin-resistant *Staphylococcus aureus* nosocomial pneumonia. *Chest* 124:1789–1797, 2003.
138. Conte JE Jr, Golden JA, Kipps J, et al: Intrapulmonary pharmacokinetics of linezolid. *Antimicrob Agents Chemother* 46:1475–1480, 2002.
139. Fagon JY, Patrick H, Haas DW, et al: Treatment of Gram-positive nosocomial pneumonia. Prospective randomized comparison of quinupristin/dalfopristin versus vancomycin. *Am J Respir Crit Care Med* 161: 753–762, 2000.
140. Greenwood D: Microbiologic properties of teicoplanin. *J Antimicrob Chemother* 21[Suppl A]:1–13, 1988.
141. Safdar N, Handelsman J, Maki DG: Does combination antimicrobial therapy reduce mortality in Gram-negative bacteraemia? A meta-analysis. *Lancet Infect Dis* 4:519–527, 2004.
142. Cometta A, Baumgartner JD, Lew D, et al: Prospective randomized comparison of imipenem monotherapy with imipenem plus netilmicin for treatment of severe infections in nonneutropenic patients. *Antimicrob Agents Chemother* 38:1309–1313, 1994.
143. Aarts MA, Hancock JN, Heyland D, et al: Empiric antibiotic therapy for suspected ventilator-associated pneumonia: a systematic review and meta-analysis of randomized trials. *Crit Care Med* 36:108–117, 2008.
144. Fowler RA, Flavin KE, Barr J, et al: Variability in antibiotic prescribing patterns and outcomes in patients with clinically suspected ventilator-associated pneumonia. *Chest* 123:835–844, 2003.
145. Gruson G, Gilles H, Vargas F, et al: Rotation and restricted use of antibiotics in a medical intensive care unit. Impact on the incidence of ventilator-associated pneumonia caused by antibiotic-resistant gram-negative bacteria. *Am J Respir Crit Care Med* 162:837–842, 2000.
146. Nseir S, Di Pompeo C, Soubrier S, et al: First-generation fluoroquinolone use and subsequent emergence of multiple drug-resistant bacteria in the intensive care unit. *Crit Care Med* 33:283–289, 2005.
147. Niederman MS: Reexamining quinolone use in the intensive care unit: use them right or lose the fight against resistant bacteria. *Crit Care Med* 33:443–444, 2005.
148. Beardsley JR, Williamson JC, Johnson JW, et al: Using local microbiologic data to develop institution-specific guidelines for the treatment of hospital-acquired pneumonia. *Chest* 130:787–793, 2006.
149. Trouillet JL, Vuagnat A, Combes A, et al: *Pseudomonas aeruginosa* ventilator-associated pneumonia: comparison of episodes due to piperacillin-resistant versus piperacillin-susceptible organisms. *Clin Infect Dis* 34:1047–1054, 2002.
150. Niederman MS: De-escalation therapy in ventilator-associated pneumonia. *Curr Opin Crit Care* 12:452–457, 2006.
151. Kollef MH, Morrow LE, Niederman MS, et al: Clinical characteristics and treatment patterns among patients with ventilator-associated pneumonia. *Chest* 129:1210–1218, 2006.
152. Dennesen PJ, van der Ven AJ, Kessels AG, et al: Resolution of infectious parameters after antimicrobial therapy in patients with ventilator-associated pneumonia. *Am J Respir Crit Care Med* 163:1371–1375, 2001.

153. Luna CM, Blanzaco D, Niederman MS, et al: Resolution of ventilator-associated pneumonia: prospective evaluation of the clinical pulmonary infection score as an early clinical predictor of outcome. *Crit Care Med* 31:676–682, 2003.
154. Chastre J, Wolff M, Fagon JY, et al: Comparison of 8 vs 15 days of antibiotic therapy for ventilator-associated pneumonia in adults: a randomized trial. *JAMA* 290:2588–2598, 2003.
155. Bouadma L, Luyt CE, Tubach F, et al: Use of procalcitonin to reduce patients' exposure to antibiotics in intensive care units. *Lancet* 375:463–474, 2010.
156. Palmer L, Smaldone G, Simon S, et al: Aerosolized antibiotics in mechanically ventilated patients: delivery and response. *Crit Care Med* 26:31–39, 1998.
157. Michalopoulos A, Kasiakou SK, Mastora Z, et al: Aerosolized colistin for the treatment of nosocomial pneumonia due to multidrug-resistant Gram-negative bacteria in patients without cystic fibrosis. *Crit Care* 9: R53–R59, 2005.
158. Goldstein I, Wallet F, Robin AN, et al: Lung deposition and efficiency of nebulized amikacin during *Escherichia coli* pneumonia in ventilated piglets. *Am J Respir Crit Care Med* 166:1375–1381, 2002.
159. Fisman DN, Abrutyn E, Spaude KA, et al: Prior pneumococcal vaccination is associated with reduced death, complications, and length of stay among hospitalized adults with community-acquired pneumonia. *Clin Infect Dis* 42:1093–1101, 2006.
160. Walker FJ, Singleton RJ, Bulkow LR, et al: Reactions after 3 or more doses of pneumococcal polysaccharide vaccine in adults in Alaska. *Clin Infect Dis* 40:1730–1735, 2005.
161. Fiore AE, Shay DK, Broder K, et al: Prevention and control of seasonal influenza with vaccines: recommendations of the Advisory Committee on Immunization Practices (ACIP), 2009. *MMWR Recomm Rep* 58:1–52, 2009.
162. Arden NH, Patriarca PA, Fasano MB, et al: The roles of vaccination and amantadine prophylaxis in controlling an outbreak of influenza A (H3N2) in a nursing home. *Arch Intern Med* 148:865, 1988.
163. Jefferson T, Jones M, Doshi P, et al: Neuraminidase inhibitors for preventing and treating influenza in healthy adults: systematic review and meta-analysis. *BMJ* 339:b5106, 2009.
164. Haley RW, Culver DH, White JW, et al: The nationwide nosocomial infection rate. A need for new vital statistics. *Am J Epidemiol* 21:159–167, 1985.
165. Dreyfuss D, Djedaini K, Weber P, et al: Prospective study of nosocomial pneumonia and of patient and circuit colonization during mechanical ventilation with circuit changes every 48 hours versus no change. *Am Rev Respir Dis* 143:738–743, 1991.
166. Feeley TW, Du Moulin GC, Hedley-Whyte J, et al: Aerosol polymyxin and pneumonia in seriously ill patients. *N Engl J Med* 293:471–475, 1975.
167. Brar NS, Niederman MS: Should all ICU patients receive systemic digestive decontamination? *Curr Respir Med Rev* 6:45–51, 2010.
168. Scannapieco FA, Yu J, Raghavendran K, et al: A randomized trial of chlorhexidine gluconate on oral bacterial pathogens in mechanically ventilated patients. *Crit Care* 13:R117, 2009.
169. de Smet AM, Kluytmans JA, Cooper BS, et al: Decontamination of the digestive tract and oropharynx in ICU patients. *N Engl J Med* 360:20–31, 2009.
170. de Smet AM, Hopmans TE, Minderhoud AL, et al: Decontamination of the digestive tract and oropharynx: hospital acquired infections after discharge from the intensive care unit. *Intensive Care Med* 35:1609–1613, 2009.
171. Cook D, Guyatt G, Marshall J, et al: Canadian Critical Care Trials Group. A comparison of sucralfate and ranitidine for the prevention of upper gastrointestinal bleeding in patients requiring mechanical ventilation. *N Engl J Med* 338:791, 1998.
172. Resar R, Pronovost P, Haraden C, et al: Using a bundle approach to improve ventilator care processes and reduce ventilator-associated pneumonia. *Jt Comm J Qual Patient Saf* 31:243, 2005.
173. Klompas M, Platt R: Ventilator-associated pneumonia—the wrong quality measure for benchmarking. *Ann Intern Med* 147:803–805, 2007.
174. Jensen LS, Kissmeyer-Nielsen P, Wolff B, et al: Randomised comparison of leukocyte-depleted versus buffy-coat-poor blood transfusion and complications after colorectal surgery. *Lancet* 348:841–845, 1996.
175. Hebert PC, Wells G, Blajchman MA, et al: Transfusion requirements in critical care investigators, Canadian Critical Care Trials Group. A multicenter, randomized, controlled clinical trial of transfusion requirements in critical care. *N Engl J Med* 340:409–417, 1999.
176. Van den Berghe G, Wouters P, Weekers F, et al: Intensive insulin therapy in the medical ICU. *N Engl J Med* 345:1359, 2001.
177. Van den Berghe G, Wilmer A, Hermans G, et al: Intensive insulin therapy in the medical ICU. *N Engl J Med* 354:449–461, 2006.
178. Finfer S, Chittock DR, Su SY, et al: NICE-SUGAR Study Investigators. Intensive versus conventional glucose control in critically ill patients. *N Engl J Med* 360:1283–1297, 2009.
179. Hilbert G, Gruson D, Vargas F, et al: Noninvasive ventilation in immunosuppressed patients with pulmonary infiltrates, fever, and acute respiratory failure. *N Engl J Med* 344:481–487, 2001.
180. Torres A, Gatell JM, Aznar E, et al: Re-intubation increases the risk of nosocomial pneumonia in patients needing mechanical ventilation. *Am J Respir Crit Care Med* 152:137–141, 1995.
181. Ibrahim EH, Mehringer L, Prentice D, et al: Early versus late enteral feeding of mechanically ventilated patients: results of a clinical trial. *J Parenter Enteral Nutr* 26:174–181, 2002.
182. Niederman MS: Is "crop rotation" of antibiotics the solution to a "resistant" problem in the ICU? *Am J Respir Crit Care Med* 156:1029–1031, 1997.
183. Dellit TH, Owens RC, McGowan JE Jr, et al: Infectious Diseases Society of America and the Society for Healthcare Epidemiology of America guidelines for developing an institutional program to enhance antimicrobial stewardship. *Clin Infect Dis* 44:159–177, 2007.

CHAPTER 69 ■ LUNG BIOPSY

SCOTT E. KOPEC AND RICHARD S. IRWIN

Lung biopsy is indicated whenever it is necessary to obtain a definitive diagnosis of a localized or diffuse pulmonary disease, usually after noninvasive diagnostic modalities have been used unsuccessfully.

Multiple lung biopsy techniques are available that have been well characterized with regard to tissue yield, diagnostic yield, complications, contraindications, and mortality rate. The relative usefulness of a particular biopsy technique depends not only on the availability of local expertise but also on the clinical situation. Each of the commonly used biopsy procedures is briefly described, and an approach to the lung biopsy procedure in the critically ill patient that focuses on the following questions is outlined: (a) When should a lung biopsy be considered in the critically ill patient? (b) Which biopsy technique should be chosen? (c) How should the specimens be handled?

BIOPSY PROCEDURES

General Considerations

Lung biopsy procedures can be grouped into two broad categories: open (i.e., surgical) and closed (i.e., nonsurgical). The major distinction between the two is that closed procedures avoid major surgical intervention and general anesthesia at the expense of a lower likelihood of obtaining a definitive

TABLE 69.1

CONTRAINDICATIONS AND RELATIVE CONTRAINDICATIONS TO LUNG BIOPSY [1–5]

Open thoracotomy biopsy
Contraindication
Too ill to undergo general anesthesia
Thorascopic lung biopsy
Contraindications
Too ill to undergo general anesthesia
Extensive pleural adhesions
Uncorrectable coagulopathy
Postpneumonectomy patient
Severe pulmonary hypertension
Relative contraindications
Inability to place a double-lumen endotracheal tube
Inability to tolerate single lung ventilation
Closed biopsy
Contraindications
Uncorrectable coagulopathy (including uremia)[a]
Unstable cardiovascular status
Severe hypoxia likely to worsen during bronchoscopy
Inadequately trained bronchoscopist
Poor patient cooperation
Relative Contraindications
Recent myocardial infarction or unstable angina
Adjacent vascular abnormalities
Positive-pressure ventilation
Cavitating lesions (especially with air-fluid levels or >10 cm diameter)
Severe pulmonary hypertension
Adjacent emphysematous lung disease
Suspected echinococcal disease
Uncontrollable cough

[a]Bronchoalveolar lavage can be performed safely in patients with severe thrombocytopenia.

diagnosis. Contraindications and relative contraindications for open and closed lung biopsy procedures are listed in Table 69.1 [1–5].

Open Biopsy Procedures

Open Thoracotomy Lung Biopsy

Because thoracotomy allows the surgeon to obtain relatively large specimens of lung tissue under direct observation, open lung biopsy is a consistently accurate lung biopsy technique. The procedure requires endotracheal intubation, general anesthesia, and pleural catheter drainage for at least 24 hours after the biopsy. A description of the technique used to perform an open lung biopsy can be found elsewhere [3,4]. The following interventions maximize diagnostic yield [4]. First, average, rather than normal or markedly abnormal, lung tissue should be preferentially sampled. Second, in cases of diffuse pulmonary disease, more than one site should be sampled, if possible. Third, areas corresponding to ground-glass appearance on high-resolution chest tomography should be biopsied, as they are more likely to reveal the inflammatory process [5]. Some authors believe that biopsies of the tip of the lingula or right middle lobe should be avoided because prior scarring, inflammation, and passive congestion of a nonspecific nature are likely to occur in these sites [6]. However, several studies refute this [4,7].

Thoracoscopic Lung Biopsy

Thoracoscopy is a percutaneous procedure that involves the endoscopic exploration and sampling of the contents of the thoracic cavity [1,8]. Unlike the other percutaneous procedures, thoracoscopic lung biopsy is considered a surgical procedure. Although there are a variety of potential uses for thoracoscopy, only lung biopsy is highlighted here. Thoracoscopic lung biopsy involves multiple small chest wall incisions and a controlled pneumothorax to collapse the lung. One incision allows the insertion of a sterile flexible endoscope to visualize the lung and pleural surfaces. A biopsy device is inserted through another incision and guided by direct endoscopic vision/video monitoring. Multiple points of entry may be necessary to determine the ideal endoscopic approach.

An advantage of thoracoscopy is that it can obtain a larger piece of lung tissue than bronchoscopy techniques, equal in size to that obtained at open lung biopsy. Where available, it is the open procedure of choice for patients in stable condition who are not requiring mechanical ventilation. Some authors caution that ventilator-dependent patients should not routinely undergo biopsy procedures by thoracoscopy because they typically cannot tolerate the change to a double-lumen endotracheal tube or the single-lung ventilation technique (see Table 69.1).

Although several studies of noncritically ill patients with interstitial lung disease demonstrated that thoracoscopy and open lung biopsy were identical in providing the diagnosis and complications [2], we are unaware of any study that compares open lung biopsy with thoracoscopic biopsy in critically ill patients. Due to the absolute and relative contraindications of thoracoscopic lung biopsy, critically ill patients on mechanical ventilation should preferentially undergo an open procedure.

Closed Biopsy Procedures

Percutaneous Transthoracic Needle Aspiration Biopsy

Percutaneous transthoracic needle aspiration biopsy involves the insertion, under guidance of fluoroscopy or computed tomography (CT), of a sterile needle through the chest wall into the area of the lung to be sampled [9]. Yields appear greatest if the procedure is performed under CT-guided fluoroscopy [10]. Needles of varying sizes (18-, 20-, 22-, and 24- to 25-gauge) can be used. In general, the thinner the needle, the fewer the complications [11]. A specimen is obtained by aspiration; it usually consists of cells (e.g., neoplastic, parenchymal, inflammatory), tissue fluids, or small tissue fragments. The major advantage of this procedure is that it can be easily performed with local anesthesia. The major disadvantages are that lung architectural integrity may not be maintained in the specimen, and the incidence of pneumothorax can be as high as 20% [12].

Bronchoscopic Procedures

A variety of techniques, including bronchial and transbronchial biopsy, bronchial brushing, transbronchial needle aspiration, and bronchoalveolar lavage (BAL), can be easily and safely performed with the flexible bronchoscope. A detailed discussion of flexible bronchoscopy is presented in Chapter 9.

Transbronchial Lung Biopsy. Transbronchial lung biopsy is performed by passing the bronchoscope to the segmental level, instilling a dilute solution of epinephrine, and then advancing flexible biopsy forceps into the radiographically abnormal area [13]. The forceps usually are advanced under fluoroscopic guidance. They are passed in the closed position until resistance is met or the patient signals that he or she has chest (pleural) pain. If pain is felt, the forceps are withdrawn in 1-cm increments until pain is no longer perceived. If no pain is felt, the forceps are opened, pressure is gently applied, and the forceps are closed. If no chest pain is felt, the forceps are then removed. Some authors recommend wedging the bronchoscope into the airway from which the biopsy was taken to tamponade any potential bleeding and to prevent any blood from spilling out into other airways. However, a technique of applying continuous suction while moving the bronchoscope back and forth in the airway has been shown to be effective at controlling bleeding [14]. Synchronization of the biopsy to a phase of respiration has affected neither the amount of alveolar tissue obtained nor the integrity of the specimen [15]. Because specimens are small (not greater than 3.9 mm^2 on average [15]), multiple specimens should be obtained to maximize the yield of this technique.

Bronchial Brush Biopsy. Using a flexible wire brush, the operator performs a bronchial brush biopsy in a manner similar to forceps biopsy [16,17]. Usually under fluoroscopic guidance, the brush is passed into the radiographically abnormal area. The usefulness of this method is limited by the fact that only cellular material can be obtained and, in general, only endobronchial processes are sampled. A nodule not in communication with the bronchial tree cannot be entered with the brush, although the nodule can be sampled with a needle passed transthoracically.

Transbronchial Needle Aspiration. The transbronchial needle aspiration technique allows the clinician to pierce the walls of airways and aspirate cellular contents and tissue fluid or processes not in communication with the tracheobronchial tree. Specially designed catheters with attached needles are passed through the suction channel of the bronchoscope to the abnormal area [2]. As long as the vascularity of the area to be aspirated is appreciated or has been defined, transbronchial puncture with aspiration can be safely performed [18]. The use of endobronchial ultrasound to locate the exact location of lymph nodes and blood vessels improves yield while decreasing complications [19]. This procedure has a role in the diagnosis and staging of lung cancer and in the diagnosis of some benign mediastinal diseases, such as bronchogenic cysts and sarcoidosis [20]. When appropriately applied and with good cytopathologic support, this procedure can eliminate the need for surgical staging in a substantial number of patients with inoperable lung cancer [21].

Bronchoalveolar Lavage. BAL is a safe diagnostic extension of routine flexible bronchoscopy [22]. The tip of the bronchoscope is wedged into a segmental or smaller airway, and physiologic saline is instilled and withdrawn through the suction channel. Using this technique, it is possible to sample cellular and soluble components from the distal airways and alveoli. A detailed discussion of the use of BAL analysis in a variety of lung diseases can be found elsewhere [23]. The usefulness of BAL and bronchoscopy-protected brush-catheter cultures in diagnosing lung infections is reviewed in Chapters 9 and 68. Because BAL is not really a biopsy procedure and little or no associated bleeding occurs, it may be performed in patients with bleeding abnormalities and pulmonary hypertension.

EXPECTED RESULTS FROM LUNG BIOPSY

General Considerations

To determine what type of lung biopsy procedure should be performed and when, it is important to appreciate the expected results. The yield of positive diagnoses and the complications incurred depend on the procedure performed, the disease process, and the clinical stability of the patient. Table 69.2 lists the usefulness of several procedures with respect to specific disease processes [2,24].

TABLE 69.2

POTENTIALLY HIGH YIELDING BIOPSY PROCEDURES FOR A VARIETY OF UNDERLYING DISEASE PROCESSES [2,24]

Bronchoalveolar lavage
Infections (PCP, mycobacteria, endemic fungal)
Alveolar proteinosis
Alveolar hemorrhage
Acute eosinophilic pneumonia
Lung cancer
Lymphoma
Exogenous lipoid pneumonia
Transbronchial needle aspiration
Lung cancer
Lymphoma
Infections (endemic fungi, mycobacteria, Nocardia)
Bronchial brush biopsy
Lung cancer
Metastatic cancers
Transbronchial lung biopsy
Sarcoidosis
Lymphangitic carcinomatosis
Alveolar proteinosis
Lung cancer
Chronic eosinophilic pneumonia
Amyloidosis
Lymphocytic interstitial pneumonia
Cryptogenic organizing pneumonitis
Hypersensitivity pneumonitis
Invasive aspergillosis
Open lung biopsy or video-assisted thoracoscopic biopsy
Pulmonary capillaritis
Diffuse alveolar damage
Idiopathic pulmonary fibrosis
Nonspecific interstitial pneumonitis
Inorganic pneumoconiosis

Diffuse Parenchymal Disease in Clinically Stable Patients

To maximize the diagnostic yield, the ideal biopsy procedure is one that maintains the architectural lung integrity in the specimen. The procedures that best meet this requirement are (a) open lung biopsy, (b) thoracoscopic biopsy, and (c) transbronchoscopic lung biopsy. A number of reports on stable patients with diffuse lung disease have documented average rates of mortality, complications, and diagnostic yield for these procedures (Table 69.3) [1,2]. The highest tissue and diagnostic yields with low morbidity and very low mortality rates are obtained with open and thoracoscopic lung biopsies. Transbronchoscopic lung biopsy has lower diagnostic yields but carries the lowest morbidity and mortality rates of any of these biopsy procedures.

Although open and thoracoscopic lung biopsies more consistently yield adequate tissue and an increased likelihood of definitive diagnosis than transbronchoscopic forceps lung

TABLE 69.3

REPRESENTATIVE RESULTS OF LUNG BIOPSY PROCEDURES IN DIFFUSE LUNG DISEASE

Procedure	Mortality (%)	Complications (%)	Diagnostic yield (%)
Open	0–4.7	5–7[a]	94–95
Thoracoscopy	0–8	0–15[b]	96–100
Transbronchial forceps	<0.12	<10[c]	84

[a]Includes pneumothorax, empyema, and bleeding.
[b]Includes subcutaneous emphysema, infection, persistent air leak, and hemorrhage with need to convert to an open thoracotomy.
[c]Includes pneumothorax and hemorrhage.

biopsy, the latter may be preferred as an initial procedure to avoid the morbidity of general anesthesia, postoperative chest tube drainage, residual parenchymal and pleural scarring, postoperative pain, and increased length of hospital stay. The potential morbidity of empyema that may complicate an open or thoracoscopic lung biopsy procedure is also avoided with transbronchoscopic lung biopsy. This closed procedure is much less expensive and less painful and carries less mortality than open lung biopsy.

The overall complication rate for transbronchoscopic lung biopsy is less than 10%. The most common complication is pneumothorax, which may require chest tube drainage in up to 50% of cases [2]. Although the definitive diagnostic accuracy of transbronchoscopic lung biopsy is less than that of open and thoracoscopic lung biopsy (the tissue is smaller in quantity, often crushed, usually only peribronchiolar in origin, and not obtained under direct vision), its diagnostic yield is sufficiently high under certain conditions to justify its use as the initial biopsy procedure. For instance, in diffuse diseases such as carcinomatosis, sarcoidosis, and *Pneumocystis jiroveci* infection, transbronchoscopic forceps lung biopsy yields a specific diagnosis in 80% to 90% of cases [24,25].

Percutaneous needle aspiration (lung tap) also has a role in patients with diffuse parenchymal disease due to infection. The diagnostic yield in this setting varies from 40% to 82% [2]. Although percutaneous needle aspiration rarely causes mortality or air embolism, pneumothorax is common, occurring in approximately 25% of cases [2]. Hemoptysis occurs in 1% to 11% of patients [2]. Complication rates can be reduced by using an ultrathin needle (24- or 25-gauge) [2].

Lung Mass in Clinically Stable Patients

Because solid or cavitary masses are most often due to malignant or infectious causes, and because these diagnoses can often be readily confirmed by analyzing cellular material and fluid, open lung biopsy is usually not the preferred initial procedure. When open or thoracoscopic biopsy is performed, however, tissue and diagnostic yields should consistently approach 100%. Because nodules are usually resected in their entirety, surgical mortality depends on the severity of illness and extent of the resection [26]. The operative mortality associated with wedge resections by open thoracotomy of benign nodules in otherwise healthy, young patients is less than 1%, whereas it may vary from 2% to 12% in older patients with bronchogenic carcinomas who undergo pneumonectomy [27]. Complications of thoracotomy for lung masses in clinically stable patients are similar to those in such patients with diffuse lung disease. In a report of 242 solitary pulmonary nodules excised by video-assisted thoracoscopic surgery, there was a complication rate of 3.6% and no mortality [6] in patients undergoing thoracoscopy alone.

Percutaneous needle aspiration is extremely useful in evaluating lung masses. It carries a high diagnostic yield. A definite diagnosis is obtained in 80% to 97% of all masses, and adequate samples are obtained in 82% to 98% of cases [28,29]. If the lesion is less than 2 cm in diameter, the likelihood of obtaining adequate material is significantly decreased [28,30]. The diagnostic yield in solid malignant nodules can approach 96% [29]; in malignant and infectious cavitary lesions, 90% to 100% [28]; and in "benign" inflammatory disease, such as sarcoid nodules, 72% [2]. Although percutaneous needle aspiration is rarely associated with fatalities, complications such as pneumothorax, hemoptysis, and intraparenchymal hemorrhage or hemothorax are not uncommon [28–31]. The risk of pneumothorax increases with smaller size lesions and the presence of surrounding emphysema [32]. Hemorrhage and pneumothorax occur much more frequently in cavitary lesions. It has been demonstrated that aspiration biopsy using smaller, ultrathin 24- to 25-gauge needles results in a significant decrease in complications without loss of excellent diagnostic yield [33]. Although some authors feel that the risk of needle-track implantation of cancer is remote and it should not be considered a contraindication to the procedure [34], the risk of spread of malignant cells may be as high as 60% [35].

Peripheral lung nodules and masses can also be sampled using the transbronchoscopic brush and forceps techniques. Complication rates are less than those for percutaneous needle aspiration biopsy. Although the diagnostic yield is also diminished and the procedures are more difficult and time consuming than percutaneous needle biopsy, transbronchial biopsies more frequently yield tissue with architectural integrity. This may allow the pathologist a better opportunity to diagnose benign conditions. In peripheral malignant lesions, the diagnostic yield of transbronchial forceps biopsy relates directly to the number of biopsies obtained under fluoroscopic guidance. With brushing alone, the diagnostic yield is approximately 40%; with brushing plus one transbronchoscopic forceps lung biopsy, diagnostic accuracy improves to 55%; with brushing plus four transbronchoscopic forceps lung biopsies, accuracy reaches 60%; and with brushing plus five transbronchoscopic forceps lung biopsies, diagnostic accuracy improves to 75% [36].

Diffuse and Localized Disease in Clinically Unstable Patients

Lung biopsy in critically ill, clinically unstable patients is most commonly considered in those who are immunocompromised hosts or who have acute respiratory distress syndrome (ARDS).

Numerous studies have considered the merits of various lung biopsy procedures in the immunocompromised host who do not have acquired immunodeficiency syndrome (AIDS). The choice of which biopsy procedure to perform depends on a number of factors, including the severity and rate of progression of the illness, differential diagnosis, underlying medical conditions, radiographic findings, and level of experience and expertise of the physician performing the procedure. The diagnostic yields of the different biopsy procedures also depend on a number of factors, including differential diagnosis, underlying medical conditions, and radiographic findings.

For critically ill patients with rapidly progressing hypoxemia and radiographic infiltrates, open lung biopsy is the procedure of choice because it is associated with the highest yield and can be surprisingly well tolerated in critically ill patients [37]. Mortality rates are probably less than 1%, with several studies reporting a mortality rate of 0% [37–39]. For less severely ill patients in whom progressive hypoxemia is not an immediate problem, less invasive procedures can be attempted first.

For all non-AIDS immunocompromised patients, the overall yield of BAL is around 40%, but the yield of making a specific diagnosis increases to 70% when a transbronchial biopsy is also performed [40]. However, studies have demonstrated different yields for specific groups of immunocompromised patients. For example, for solid-organ transplant patients with diffuse infiltrates, bronchoscopy with BAL can result in the correct diagnosis 59% to 85% of the time and is associated with little to no morbidity [41,42]. In neutropenic leukemic patients with diffuse infiltrates, however, BAL is of little value as it is associated with a very low yield for invasive aspergillosis, has a very high false-positive rate for bacterial pathogens, and does not aid in diagnosing drug-induced pulmonary processes [43]. In addition, in neutropenic patients, the bronchoscopic procedure itself can result in the development of pneumonia, bacteremia, and sepsis [43,44]. For patients who are immunocompromised due to a recent bone marrow transplant, BAL results in a 34% to 50% yield in determining the etiology of pulmonary infiltrates [45]. In patients with AIDS, the sensitivity of lavage alone for diagnosing *P. jiroveci* can be as high as 97% [46]. In nonneutropenic patients, BAL does not increase the already low complication rate of routine diagnostic flexible bronchoscopy (see Chapter 9).

Transbronchial biopsy in patients with diffuse pulmonary infiltrates and solid-organ transplants is associated with yields of 46% to 78% [47,48], and in patients with hematologic malignancies, a yield of 55% [47]. Transbronchial biopsy has the highest frequency in diagnosing tuberculosis, fungal pneumonia, and pulmonary involvement of hematological malignancies [47]. In non-AIDS patients, BAL in combination with transbronchial biopsy has a higher yield than BAL or transbronchial biopsy alone [40]. In this setting, the combination of BAL and transbronchial biopsy can increase yield to 70% [40]. In the bone marrow transplant population, transbronchial biopsy appears to have a low yield and adds little information while being associated with increased risks due to the frequency of thrombocytopenia [49].

Transthoracic needle aspiration biopsy has the highest yield in immunocompromised hosts with focal pulmonary processes, especially peripheral lung lesions. In these clinical settings, sensitivities of a transthoracic needle biopsy can be greater than 80% for infectious processes and greater than 90% for malignant processes [50]. Yields for fungi, tuberculosis, and *Nocardia* can be greater than 90% [50].

In critically ill patients requiring mechanical ventilation, lung biopsy may be considered to assist in diagnosis and management and to ensure that no treatable disease process is overlooked. Specific diagnosis may be made in up to 70% to 80% of the cases [38,50]. Other studies report lower yields, however, and suggest that the results of the biopsy may not alter management. While two studies demonstrated that open lung biopsy in this setting provided information that altered therapy only 47% to 60% of the time [39,51], one study demonstrated an alteration in therapy based on the biopsy results 81% of the time [38]. A second study demonstrated that altered therapy based on the open lung biopsy results lead to an improvement in survival in patients with suspected ARDS [37]. Open lung biopsy may also be helpful in the critically ill pediatric population. A study of 26 children demonstrated that open lung biopsy was diagnostic in 96% and associated with no mortalities [52]. Open lung biopsy is the recommended surgical procedure of choice in evaluating the etiology of diffuse pulmonary infiltrates in bone marrow patients with a nondiagnostic BAL [49]. Lung biopsy is particularly useful in diagnosing invasive aspergillosis in these patients [53]. However, a 20% false-negative rate for detecting fungal infections has been reported [49]. Overall, the results of open lung biopsy can change specific therapeutic interventions in 63% of bone marrow patients with diffuse pulmonary infiltrates [54].

There is no consensus about which biopsy technique is best and under which clinical circumstances in clinically unstable patients. A wide range of expected diagnostic yields exists for all procedures, and the etiology of lung disease in these patients may remain unknown in 19% to 45%, even when adequate tissue is obtained by open lung biopsy. Deciding who, when, and how to sample is further complicated by the occasionally excessive mortality rates associated with lung biopsy procedures, and by the knowledge that even with adequate biopsy material and appropriate therapy, the high mortality rates seen in this group of patients may not be altered [55]. Consequently, the clinician must adopt a practical approach to management that combines empiric therapy with available biopsy procedures.

In patients with AIDS, open lung biopsy is the most sensitive and specific procedure. However, open or thoracoscopic lung biopsy should not be the first procedure contemplated or attempted because diffuse infiltrates are most likely due to opportunistic infection, and bronchoscopic procedures accurately diagnose infection in 90% or more of the cases [46]. Open lung biopsy or thoracoscopic biopsy is appropriate when at least one bronchoscopic examination with BAL and transbronchial biopsy (unless contraindicated) has been nondiagnostic [50]. It is rarely useful in patients who worsen after treatment for a diagnosis established by bronchoscopy [46], and it should not be repeated often.

INDICATIONS FOR LUNG BIOPSY IN CRITICALLY ILL PATIENTS

General Considerations

A lung biopsy is indicated in critically ill patients when (a) the pulmonary disease process progresses and its etiology remains unknown, (b) an initial evaluation short of lung biopsy has failed to reveal the etiology and logical empiric therapy has failed to reverse the process, (c) no contraindications exist to performing the procedures, (d) the prognosis of the patient's underlying disease is good, and (e) the potential benefit from performing the procedure outweighs associated morbidity and mortality [55].

Management of Critically Ill Patients with Pulmonary Disease

The lung biopsy is part of an extensive evaluation of a pulmonary abnormality, yet in critically ill patients it is never the initial step. Any critically ill patient is, for clinical purposes, a compromised host and should be managed as such (Table 69.4).

Because of their altered defense mechanisms, critically ill patients are particularly susceptible to infection by opportunistic as well as pathogenic organisms. Nonimmunologic defenses (e.g., altered physical barriers, altered indigenous microbiologic flora) as well as immunologic defenses (e.g., altered humoral or cellular immunity) may be impaired. These impairments may be partial or transient (e.g., alcoholism, diabetes mellitus, sickle cell anemia, uremia, malnutrition) as well as prolonged or permanent (e.g., Hodgkin's disease, chronic lymphatic leukemia, acute myelogenous leukemia, multiple myeloma, inherited immune deficiency diseases, cytotoxic chemotherapy, corticosteroids, irradiation).

TABLE 69.4

MANAGEMENT OF THE COMPROMISED HOST WITH PULMONARY DISEASE

Identify the patient as a compromised host.
Construct a list of differential possibilities that remains constant from patient to patient.
Integrate the history, physical examination, and laboratory data with chest radiographic pattern to narrow the diagnostic possibilities.
Assess the urgency of the situation and the need for invasive diagnostic studies.

Four major differential diagnostic possibilities should be considered in every critically ill (compromised) patient with pulmonary disease (Table 69.5). After general diagnostic considerations, the diagnostic possibilities are narrowed by integrating the history, physical examination, and laboratory data (e.g., routine blood work; serologic studies; and smears and cultures of blood, urine, sputum, cerebrospinal fluid, ascites, and pleural effusion) with the chest radiographic pattern. A previous recent or remote chest radiograph may confirm or rule out the presence of another stable process. Although unilateral or focal infiltrates suggest bacterial infection, the presence of bilateral disease does not rule out infectious processes [52]. Unusual and opportunistic organisms such as *P. jiroveci* often present as bilateral infiltrates after administration of immunosuppressive drugs or chemotherapy [56].

The final step involves assessing clinical urgency to evaluate the need for invasive diagnostic studies such as lung biopsy. In some clinical cases, empiric therapy should be considered and invasive biopsy avoided. These cases include patients with underlying diseases that limit life expectancy, such as advanced AIDS or advanced cancer; leukemia before treatment, as the risk for opportunistic infection is low, and there is a high probability of successful treatment with antibacterial therapy; uncontrolled coagulopathies; severely impaired pulmonary function such that an invasive procedure would not be tolerated; and patient refusal to undergo an invasive procedure [50].

In other clinical settings, other less invasive treatment options should be attempted first. For example, in the thrombocytopenic, immunocompromised host who has diffuse pulmonary infiltrates and who is clinically stable with supplemental oxygen, platelet transfusions and observation may be adequate therapy. As many as 70% of infiltrates in these patients may be due to intrapulmonary bleeding [57].

Finally, in other clinical settings, lung biopsy (especially open lung biopsy) should be considered early on in the management plan. Solid-organ transplant patients and patients with other immunocompromised states (with life expectancies measured in years) who develop hypoxemia with fever and diffuse infiltrates are more likely to benefit from a biopsy [50].

TABLE 69.5

DIFFERENTIAL DIAGNOSIS OF PULMONARY DISEASE IN THE COMPROMISED HOST

Manifestation of basic disease
Complication of management
Lipid embolization
Pulmonary edema
Pulmonary hemorrhage
Leukoagglutinin reaction
Radiation pneumonitis
Drug-induced pneumonitis
The presence of another, unrelated basic disease
Infection
Bacterial
Viral
Fungal
Parasitic

SELECTION OF LUNG BIOPSY PROCEDURE

Three factors should be considered in choosing a particular lung biopsy procedure: (a) local expertise, (b) the patient's condition, and (c) the potential yield of the procedure.

Local Expertise

Local expertise includes the availability of personnel skilled in performing the procedure and laboratory personnel skilled in specimen processing and analysis. If local expertise is limited (e.g., a skilled cytopathologist is not available to read bronchial brush or percutaneous needle aspiration specimens, or the microbiology laboratory is not equipped to process reliably specimens for the variety of organisms seen in immunocompromised hosts), the patient should be transferred to another institution with expanded resources.

Patient Condition

Once it has been decided that the patient's prognosis is potentially good enough to justify a lung biopsy technique, the next decision is the choice of biopsy procedure. If it is determined that the patient's condition allows time for only one diagnostic procedure (i.e., the patient is rapidly deteriorating), then an open or thoracoscopic lung biopsy should be performed. If there are no contraindications to a closed procedure and the patient's condition is such that there will be time for another diagnostic procedure if necessary, then one of the closed procedures may be preferable. Mechanical ventilation with positive pressure should not be considered an absolute contraindication to transbronchial biopsy [2]. Useful information has been obtained with transbronchial lung biopsy with acceptable morbidity (e.g., pneumothorax, hemorrhage) in a limited number of hemodynamically stable, mechanically ventilated patients.

Potential Yield of the Procedure

The usefulness of several biopsy techniques is summarized in Table 69.2. The potential yield of a particular biopsy procedure depends on local expertise and the individual clinical setting. For example, in the elderly patient with a solitary pulmonary nodule and clinically obvious disseminated carcinomatosis, percutaneous needle aspiration biopsy, which has a high diagnostic yield and relatively low complication rate, should be the initial procedure of choice to document whether the nodule is malignant. When a patient with a solitary pulmonary nodule has a clinical picture of vasculitis, however, open lung biopsy (or thoracoscopy biopsy if the lesion is peripheral) might be considered first or performed after bronchial brushing and forceps biopsies and percutaneous needle aspirations yield nonspecific findings without evidence of malignancy or infection.

In patients with diffuse pulmonary disease, the clinical setting influences the choice of procedure. When a biopsy is performed to document the presence and type of inorganic pneumoconiosis, open lung biopsy and thoracoscopic biopsy [58] are the only procedures that yield a sufficient amount of tissue for all the requisite analyses (chemical analysis must be included). When diffuse pulmonary infiltrates suggesting sarcoidosis or carcinomatosis occur in the appropriate clinical setting, transbronchoscopic forceps lung biopsy should be initially considered because it has an extremely high yield in these situations [24,25]. In the non-AIDS immunocompromised host with diffuse pulmonary infiltrates, transbronchoscopic lung biopsy may yield a diagnosis overall up to 78% of the time [47]. In chronic interstitial pneumonias (e.g., idiopathic pulmonary fibrosis), open or thoracoscopic lung biopsy is diagnostically superior to transbronchoscopic lung biopsy [24]. If chronic eosinophilic pneumonia, desquamative interstitial pneumonitis, or bronchiolitis obliterans organizing pneumonia can be ruled in by transbronchoscopic forceps lung biopsy, however, open or thoracoscopic lung biopsy may not be necessary. If infection and malignancy can be ruled out by transbronchoscopic forceps lung biopsy and other nonbiopsy laboratory techniques, it also may be unnecessary to perform an open procedure. If the diffuse process worsens, corticosteroids can be empirically initiated, and the response to therapy can be assessed by noninvasive means (e.g., chest radiograph, gallium scan, pulmonary function studies).

HANDLING OF SPECIMENS

To maximize the diagnostic yield from any lung biopsy procedure, specimens must be rapidly transported to the appropriate laboratories by a person directly involved in the patient's management. All analyses should be planned in advance by the team involved in the case (e.g., pathologist, microbiologist, pulmonologist, infectious disease specialist).

Because large samples of tissue are obtained from open lung and thoracoscopy biopsies, multiple pieces should be processed for a variety of analyses. First, under sterile conditions, a piece of fresh tissue should be kept moist with physiologic saline and transported immediately to the microbiology laboratory to be minced, ground, and cultured for aerobic and anaerobic bacteria, fungi, and *Mycobacterium* and *Legionella* sp. A second piece should be snap frozen in liquid nitrogen and stored at −70°C to ensure that immunofluorescent studies (e.g., immunoglobulin deposition as well as T- and B-lymphocyte markers, direct fluorescent antibody staining for *Legionella* sp.), oil-red-O staining, and viral cultures can be performed if necessary. If pneumoconiosis is suspected, special studies can be performed on formalin-fixed, paraffin-embedded tissue. At this juncture, touch preparations of a freshly cut surface of the tissue can be made for cytologic analysis, and special stains can be used for rapid diagnosis of microorganisms. The pathologist should perform a frozen-section analysis to (a) advise the surgeon whether an adequate biopsy has been obtained (i.e., the tissue does or does not exhibit a pathologic lesion), (b) obtain information that could focus the workup of the specimen (e.g., order a lymphoma workup or specific viral culture), and (c) attempt to obtain a rapid definitive diagnosis. The remainder of the tissue should be placed in 10% formalin for routine histologic study and special stains.

Unlimited analysis on specimens from transbronchoscopic forceps lung biopsies cannot be performed because of the relatively small amount of tissue obtained. To maximize the diagnostic yield, four to six pieces should be obtained [36,59]. In immunocompromised patients, touch preparations of transbronchial biopsies should be obtained and stained for microorganisms. If an exogenous lipoid pneumonia, immunologic disease, or *Legionella* infection is suspected, one piece should be snap frozen for fat stains and immunofluorescent studies. One piece can be submitted to microbiology and the remaining pieces processed for routine and special pathologic stains. Once the slides have been made from bronchial brush biopsies, they can be stained in a manner similar to needle aspiration specimens.

A specimen obtained by percutaneous transthoracic needle aspiration should be sent for microbiologic as well as cytologic analyses unless infection is not even a remote possibility. For cytologic analysis, a few drops of the aspirate can first be smeared on to frosted glass slides that are immediately placed in 95% alcohol. Then, a portion can be injected into a test tube with physiologic saline so that it can be processed using the Millipore filter or cytocentrifuge, or into a vial containing a fluid preservative for use in one of the instruments capable of preparing cell monolayers [60]. Filters and slides can be stained routinely by the Papanicolaou technique and specifically by Gomori-methenamine silver (for fungi and *P. jiroveci*), periodic acid-Schiff (for fungi), and Ziehl–Neelsen stains (for acid-fast organisms). When evaluating for the possibility of *P. jiroveci*, immunofluorescent staining with monoclonal antibodies can increase the yield. Sensitivity and specificity of this test have been reported to be greater than 90% [61]. The portion for microbiology should be immediately injected into prereduced anaerobic transport medium and transported to the microbiology laboratory. In the laboratory, drops of the specimen are placed on several sterile slides and allowed to air dry for Gram's, Ziehl–Neelsen, and direct fluorescent antibody stains for *Legionella* organisms. The remaining specimen can be cultured for anaerobic and aerobic bacteria, fungi, and *Mycobacterium* and *Legionella* sp.

After submitting an aliquot of BAL fluid for microbiologic analysis, the specimen should be handled in the cytology laboratory in a manner similar to that of percutaneous aspiration specimens.

References

1. Fountain SW: Pulmonary wedge biopsy: technique and application in interstitial lung disease, in Walker WS (ed): *Video-Assisted Thoracic Surgery*. Oxford, Isis Medical Media, 1999, p 115.
2. Kopec SE, Irwin RS: Lung biopsy, in Irwin RS, Rippe JM (eds): *Intensive Care Medicine*. 6th ed. Philadelphia, PA, Lippincott Williams & Wilkins, 2007, p 848.
3. LoCicero J: Segmentectomy and lesser pulmonary resections, in Shields TW, LoCierco J, Ponn RB, et al (eds): *General Thoracic Surgery*. 6th ed. Philadelphia, PA, Lippincott Williams & Wilkins, 2005, p 496.
4. Knight H, Ponn RB: Diffuse lung disease, in Shields TW (ed): *General Thoracic Surgery*. 6th ed. Philadelphia, PA, Lippincott Williams & Wilkins, 2005, p 1373.
5. Chechani V, Landrenau RJ, Shaikh SS: Open lung biopsy for diffuse interstitial lung disease. *Ann Thorac Surg* 54:296, 1992.
6. Gaensler EA: Open and closed lung biopsy, in Sackner MA (ed): *The Human Lung in Biology: Techniques in Pulmonary Disease, Part 2*. New York, Marcel Dekker Inc, 1980, p 579.
7. Ayed AK: Video-assisted thoracoscopic lung biopsy in the diagnosis of diffuse interstitial lung disease. *J Cardiovasc Surg* 44:115, 2003.
8. McKenna RJ: Video-assisted thoracic surgery for wedge resection, lobectomy, and pneumonectomy, in Shields TW, LoCierco J, Ponn RB, Rusch V (eds): *General Thoracic Surgery*. 6th ed. Philadelphia, PA, Lippincott Williams & Wilkins, 2005, p 524.
9. Sinner WN: Technique of needle aspiration biopsy, in Sinner WN (ed):

Needle Biopsy and Transbronchial Biopsy. New York, Thieme-Stratton, 1982, p 35.
10. Froelich JJ, Ishaque N, Regn J, et al: Guidance of percutaneous pulmonary biopsy with real-time CT fluoroscopy. *Eur J Radiology* 42:74, 2002.
11. Zavala DC, Schoell JE: Ultrathin needle aspiration of the lung in infections and malignant diseases. *Am Rev Respir Dis* 123:125, 1981.
12. Richardson CM, Pointon KS, Manhire AR, et al: Percutaneous lung biopsy: a survey of UK practice based on 5,444 biopsies. *Brit J Radiology* 75:731, 2002.
13. McDonald JC, Cortese DA: Bronchoscopic lung biopsy, in Praskash UB (ed): *Bronchoscopy*. New York, Raven Press, 1994, p 141.
14. Chhajed PN, Aboyoun CL, Malouf MA, et al: Risk factors and management of bleeding associated with transbronchial biopsy in lung transplant recipients. *J Heart Lung Transplant* 22:195, 2003.
15. Schure D, Abraham JL, Konopka R: How should transbronchial biopsies be performed and processed? *Am Rev Respir Dis* 126:342, 1982.
16. Cortese DA, McDougall JC: Biopsy and brushing of peripheral lung cancer with fluoroscopic guidance. *Chest* 75:141, 1979.
17. Cortese DA, McDougall JC: Bronchoscopy in peripheral and central lesions, in Praskash UB (ed): *Bronchoscopy*. New York, Raven Press, 1994, p 135.
18. Wang KP, Terry PB: Transbronchial needle aspiration in the diagnosis and staging of bronchogenic carcinoma. *Am Rev Respir Dis* 127:344, 1983.
19. Herth FJ, Ernst A: Innovative bronchoscopic diagnostic techniques: endobronchial ultrasound and electromagnetic navigation. *Curr Opin Pulm Med* 11:278, 2005.
20. Trisolini R, Agli LL, Cancellieri A, et al: The value of flexible transbronchial needle biopsy in the diagnosis of stage 1 sarcoidosis. *Chest* 124:2126, 2003.
21. Shannon JJ, Bude RO, Orens JB, et al: Endobronchial ultrasound-guided needle aspiration of mediastinal adenopathy. *Am J Respir Crit Care Med* 153:1424, 1996.
22. Helmers RA, Pisani RJ: Bronchoalveolar lavage, in Praskash UB (ed): *Bronchoscopy*. New York, Raven Press, 1994, p 155.
23. Meyer KC: The role of bronchoalveolar lavage in interstitial lung disease. *Clinic Chest Med* 25:637, 2004.
24. Schwarz MI, King TE Jr, Raghu G: Approach to the evaluation and diagnosis of interstitial lung disease, in Schwarz MI, King TE Jr (eds): *Interstitial Lung Disease*. 4th Ed. Hamilton, Ontario, BC Decker Inc, 2003, p 21.
25. Gilman MJ, Wang KP: Transbronchial lung biopsy in sarcoidosis. *Am Rev Respir Dis* 122:721, 1980.
26. Lillington GA: The solitary pulmonary nodule—1974. *Am Rev Respir Dis* 110:699, 1974.
27. Kopec SE, Irwin RS, Umali-Torres CB, et al: The postpneumonectomy state. *Chest* 144:1158, 1998.
28. Berquist TH, Bailey PB, Cortese DA, et al: Transthoracic needle biopsy. *Mayo Clin Proc* 55:475, 1980.
29. Lopez Hanninen E, Vogl TJ, Ricke J, et al: CT-guided percutaneous core biopsies of pulmonary lesions. Diagnostic accuracy, complications, and therapeutic impact. *Acta Radiologica* 42:151, 2001.
30. Poe RH, Robin RE: Sensitivity and specificity of needle biopsy in lung malignancy. *Am Rev Respir Dis* 122:755, 1980.
31. Sinner WN: Material and results, in Sinner WN (ed): *Needle Biopsy and Transbronchial Biopsy*. New York, Thieme-Stratton, 1982, p 18.
32. Cox JE, Chiles C, McManus CM, et al: Transthoracic needle aspirate biopsy: variables that affect risk of pneumothorax. *Radiology* 212:165, 1999.
33. Zavala DC, Schoell JU: Ultrathin needle aspiration of the lung in infectious and malignant diseases. *Am Rev Respir Dis* 123:125, 1981.
34. Sinner WN: Complications, in Sinner WN (ed): *Needle Biopsy and Transbronchial Biopsy*. New York, Thieme-Stratton, 1982, p 44.
35. Sawabata N, Ohta M, Maeda H: Fine-needle aspiration cytologic technique for lung cancer has a high potential of malignant cell spread through the tract. *Chest* 118:936, 2000.
36. Popovich J Jr, Koace PA, Eichenhorn MS, et al: Diagnostic accuracy of multiple biopsies from flexible fiberoptic bronchoscopy. *Am Rev Respir Dis* 125:521, 1982.
37. Papazian L, Doddoli C, Chetaille B, et al: A contributive result of open-lung biopsy improves survival in acute respiratory distress syndrome patients. *Crit Care Med* 35:755, 2007.
38. Baumann HJ, Kluge S, Balke L, et al: Yield and safety of bedside open lung biopsy in mechanically ventilated patients with acute lung injury or acute respiratory distress syndrome. *Surgery* 143:426, 2008.
39. Patel SR, Karmpaliotis D, Ayas NT, et al: The role of open-lung biopsy in ARDS. *Chest* 125:197, 2004.
40. Jain P, Sandur S, Meli Y, et al: Role of flexible bronchoscopy in immunocompromised patients with lung infiltrates. *Chest* 125:712, 2004.
41. Chang GC, Wu CL, Pan SH, et al: The diagnosis of pneumonia in renal transplant recipients using invasive and noninvasive procedures. *Chest* 125:541, 2004.
42. Nusair S, Kramer MR: The role of fiber-optic bronchoscopy in solid organ, transplant patients with pulmonary infections. *Respir Med* 93:621, 1999.
43. Robbins H, Goldman AL: Failure of a prophylactic antimicrobial drug to prevent sepsis after fiberoptic bronchoscopy. *Am Rev Respir Dis* 116:325, 1977.
44. Beyt BE, King DK, Glew RH: Fatal pneumonitis and septicemia after fiberoptic bronchoscopy. *Chest* 72:105, 1977.
45. Patel NR, Lee PS, Kim JH, et al: The influence of diagnostic bronchoscopy on clinical outcomes comparing adult autologous and allogeneic bone marrow transplant patients. *Chest* 127:1388, 2005.
46. Narayanswami G, Salzman SH: Bronchoscopy in the human immunodeficiency virus-infected patients. *Semin Respir Infect* 18:80, 2003.
47. Cazzadori A, DiPerri G, Todeschini G, et al: Transbronchial biopsy in the diagnosis of pulmonary infiltrates in immunocompromised patients. *Chest* 107:101, 1995.
48. Lehto JT, Koskinen PK, Anttila VJ, et al: Bronchoscopy in the diagnosis and surveillance of respiratory infections in lung and heart-lung transplant recipients. *Transpl Int* 18:562, 2005.
49. Yen KT, Lee AS, Krowka MJ, et al: Pulmonary complications in bone marrow transplantation: a practical approach to diagnosis and treatment. *Clin Chest Med* 25:189, 2004.
50. Rubin RH, Greene R: Clinical approach to the compromised host with fever and pulmonary infiltrates, in Rubin RH, Young LS (eds): *Clinical Approach to Infections in the Compromised Host*. 3rd ed. New York, Plenum Publishing, 1994, p 121.
51. Soh LH, Chian CF, Su WL, et al: Role of open lung biopsy in patients with diffuse infiltrates and acute respiratory failure. *J Formosan Med Assoc* 104:17, 2005.
52. Steinberg R, Freud E, Ben-Ari J, et al: Open lung biopsy—successful diagnostic tool with therapeutic implications in the critically ill paediatric population. *Acta Paediatr* 87:945, 1998.
53. Kim K, Lee MH, Kim J, et al: Importance of open lung biopsy in the diagnosis of invasive pulmonary aspergillosis in patients with hematological malignancies. *Am J Hematol* 71:75, 2002.
54. Wang JY, Chang YL, Lee LN, et al: Diffuse pulmonary infiltrates after bone marrow transplantation: the role of open lung biopsy. *Ann Thorac Surg* 78:267, 2004.
55. Hiatt JR, Gong H, Mulder DG, et al: The value of open lung biopsy in the immunosuppressed patient. *Surgery* 92:285, 1982.
56. Tenholder MF, Hooper RG: Pulmonary infiltrates in leukemia. *Chest* 78:468, 1980.
57. Drew WL, Finley TH, Golde DW: Diagnostic lavage and occult pulmonary hemorrhage in thrombocytopenic immunocompromised patients. *Am Rev Respir Dis* 116:215, 1977.
58. Bensard DD, McIntyre RC Jr, Waring BJ, et al: Comparison of video thoracoscopic lung biopsy to open lung biopsy in the diagnosis of interstitial lung disease. *Chest* 103:765, 1993.
59. Roethe RA, Fuller PD, Byrd RB, et al: Transbronchoscopic lung biopsy in sarcoidosis. Optimal number and sites for diagnosis. *Chest* 77:400, 1980.
60. Hutchinson ML, Cassin CM, Ball HG III: The efficacy of an automated preparation device for cervical cytology. *Am J Clin Pathol* 96:300, 1991.
61. Kovacs JA, Ng JL, Masur H, et al: Diagnosis of *Pneumocystis carinii* pneumonia: improved detection in sputum with use of monoclonal antibodies. *N Engl J Med* 318:589, 1988.

CHAPTER 70 ■ SLEEP ISSUES IN THE INTENSIVE CARE UNIT SETTING

KIM L. GORING AND NANCY A. COLLOP

OVERVIEW OF NORMAL SLEEP

Adequate quantity and quality of sleep is necessary for normal physiologic function. The average adult is recommended to obtain 7.5 to 8.5 hours of consolidated sleep within a 24-hour cycle to sustain normal neurohormonal function. The ability to achieve a normal duration and pattern of sleep rests on several factors internal and external to the subject. The important internal factors include the homeostatic and circadian drive to sleep, volitional control of the length of sleep, age, drugs, and comorbid illness. External factors include ambient temperature, noise, and light exposure, all of which influence the quantity and sleep-stage distribution throughout the night [1].

Sleep is divided between non-rapid eye movement (NREM) and rapid eye movement (REM) cycles. The normal human adult begins sleep in NREM with REM sleep occurring approximately 90 to 120 minutes later. NREM sleep is composed of stages 1 (N1), 2 (N2), and 3 (N3). Slow-wave sleep (stage 3), a deeper and more restful sleep, predominates in the first third of the night and tends to occur soon after sleep onset. As noted, REM sleep (R) occurs after 90 to 120 minutes then alternates with NREM at a periodicity of approximately 90 minutes. In a young adult, the percentage of total sleep time is broken down into N1, 2% to 5%; N2, 45% to 55%; N3 (slow-wave sleep), 13% to 24%; and REM, 20% to 25%.

Sleep is regulated through both circadian and homeostatic mechanisms. The circadian rhythm, through a 24-hour cycle of internal pacemaker activity originating in the suprachiasmatic nucleus of the hypothalamus, helps to determine the sleep–wake cycle. This cycle tends to be synchronized to the 24-hour day predominantly by environmental stimuli, specifically light exposure, and can easily be disrupted in an environment devoid of light/dark shifts. Melatonin is a hormone involved in the regulation of the sleep–wake cycle. It is synthesized in the pineal gland and its secretion underlies a strong circadian periodicity designed to promote sleep at night. Maximum secretion tends to be associated with an absence of light, almost exclusively at night between 9 PM and 3 AM, with lowest baseline values between 7 AM and 9 AM [2], thereby increasing the drive to sleep at night. Hormone secretion (e.g., cortisol) and body temperature changes throughout the day are other examples of systems exhibiting circadian activity.

Homeostatic mechanisms also influence sleep–wake cycles. Homeostatic drive is similar to thirst: the longer you are without sleep, the sleepier you become. Voluntary control of sleep onset and prior sleep deprivation enhance the homeostatic drive to sleep, regardless of environmental cues, and also affects sleep regulation.

Sleep onset is associated with a loss of wakefulness stimuli that, even in normal, healthy people is associated with an initial instability in ventilation. N1 sleep is characterized by a decrease in respiratory drive with irregular breathing, decrease in muscle activity, and an increase in upper airway compliance. As sleep progresses through N2 and N3, respirations become stable with a regular rate and tidal volume but a fall in minute ventilation of 0.5 to 1.5 L per minute (approximately 13% decrease) occurs. This is thought to be secondary to resetting of the central chemoreceptor set point that controls the ventilatory drive [3]. The result is a gradual increase in $PaCO_2$ by 4 to 6 mm Hg and a decrease in pH by 0.03 to 0.05 units across the night (Fig. 70.1). On awakening, the central chemoreceptor set point returns to normal and minute ventilation increases.

Sleep is a necessary part of life. Sleep deprivation is associated with decreased or abnormal immune function [4,5], impaired motor and cognitive function [6,7], and has been shown to influence morbidity and mortality outcomes in critically ill patients [8]. Animal data show that extremes of sleep deprivation lead to failure to thrive and eventual death [9]. Metabolic consequences of fragmented sleep in humans are increasingly being recognized. The development of insulin resistance with increased blood pressure, heart rate, cortisol level, and sympathetic activity have been recognized to occur with short-term sleep deprivation. There is an abnormality in thermal regulation and an increase in inflammatory cytokines (tumor necrosis factor-α [TNF-α], interleukin 1 [IL-1], and IL-6) and C-reactive protein, which are known to cause vascular injury and increase insulin resistance [10,11]. This serves to highlight the necessity of good-quality sleep for normal metabolic and physiologic function, especially important in a critically ill population.

ABNORMALITIES OF SLEEP IN THE INTENSIVE CARE UNIT

Abnormal Quantity and Quality of Sleep

Sleep research in the ICU is a murky pond made cloudy by the multitude of confounding variables and questionable reliability of methods used to evaluate sleep during critical illness. The sleep architecture of ICU patients has been well documented to be abnormal. However, there is a great variation in reported abnormalities in both NREM and REM sleep amongst investigators. This may in part be due to the tools used to measure sleep which range from polysomnography (PSG) (the gold standard) to actigraphy, bedside observation, and patient recall. The PSG is expensive and time consuming resulting in the utilization of the other methods to detect sleep. The significant limitations of the other methods include an inability to describe sleep architecture and the occurrence of sleep state misperception. Their strengths include the ability to study large numbers and over extended periods [12]. PSG results using Rechtschaffen and Kales methodology for sleep staging may be unreliable because of discrepancies in analyzing electroencephalographic (EEG) waveforms in part due to distortion of waveforms from medication, underlying illness (e.g., sepsis, encephalopathy), and measurement artifact due to the ICU environment [13,14]. An observational methodologic study evaluating the reproducibility

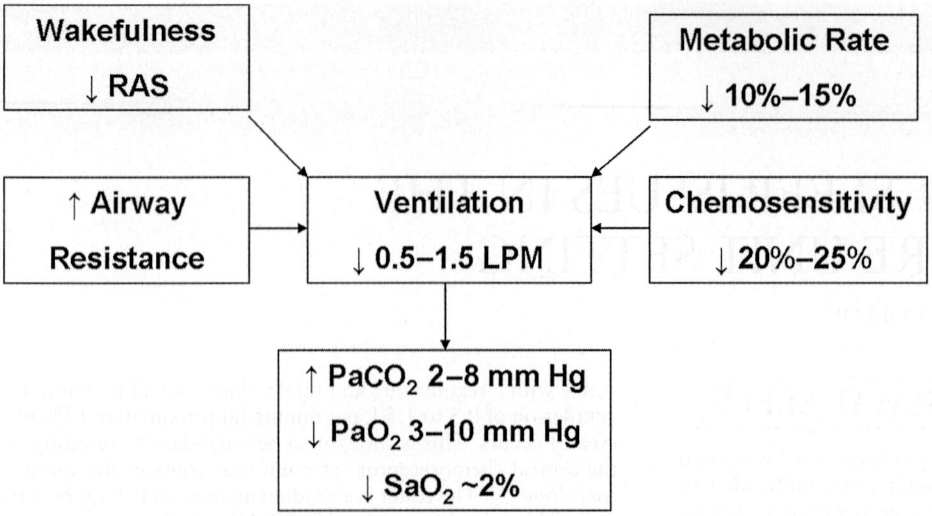

FIGURE 70.1. Changes in the respiratory system and blood gases during normal sleep. The decrease in reticular activating system (RAS), metabolic rate, and responsiveness to arterial PaO_2 and PCO_2 along with increased airway resistance would lead to decreased ventilation and arterial blood gases during sleep in normal individuals. LPM, liters per minute. [From Mohsenin V: Sleep in chronic obstructive pulmonary disease. *Semin Respir Crit Care Med* 26:110, 2005, with permission].

of manual versus computer-based sleep assessment concluded that more reproducible results of EEG analysis may be obtained with the use of computer-based spectral analysis as opposed to the manual method of scoring [15]. Notwithstanding the above discussion, sleep architecture in the ICU has generally been reported to have higher quantities of lighter N1 and N2 sleep and reduced slow wave and REM sleep. In addition, some patients have abnormal EEG characteristics of stage 2 sleep (absence of spindles and K complexes) [8]. Partial arousal states have been reported; the EEG shows slow-wave sleep but accompanied by movements typical of wakefulness [8]. Studies with 24-hour PSG recordings have found total sleep time to range between 3.6 and 6.2 hours a day in patients both with and without sedatives or hypnotics [16–18]. Other studies reveal average total sleep times of 7 to 10.4 hours per day, but with large variations in total sleep time among patients, with some sleeping for less than an hour and others for 12 to 15 hours [8,19,20]. Many studies highlight that patients spend almost equal amounts of time asleep during the day as at night [8,18]. Estimations of patient's total sleep time based on observation alone tend to overestimate the amount of sleep and have no way of detecting more subtle episodes of sleep disruption [17,21].

Critically ill patients were found to spend 6% or less of total sleep time in REM [8,20,22]. By contrast, Gabor and colleagues reported REM sleep to be as much as 14.3% of total sleep time [18]. It is unclear if this represented REM rebound from prior ICU-associated sleep deprivation or may have been a rebound from REM-suppressant medication. Patients were also found to experience frequent arousals and awakenings, with investigators reporting a range of 35 to 54 arousals per hour of total sleep time [8,23].

This highlights that not only is sleep in the ICU different from normal in terms of less time spent in deeper stages but the lighter stages of sleep have abnormal EEG patterns of uncertain clinical significance and more frequent arousals throughout total sleep time. Sleep patterns remain altered with continued ICU stay. It may take several days for sleep architecture to normalize after the patient is transferred to the general medical ward [18].

More recently, the effect of continuous versus intermittent sedation versus neuromuscular blocking agents on sleep in mechanically ventilated patients was evaluated. In all groups, there was an increase in total sleep time coupled with an increase in slow-wave sleep of low amplitude. The authors speculated that the increased delta activity may have been the result of a metabolic process or medication effect [24]. This highlights the fact that an elevated total sleep time in the ICU resulting from medication is not identical to physiologic sleep and cannot be assumed to deliver the same restorative function.

The sequelae of abnormal sleep in the ICU ranges from patient perception of excessive sleepiness while in the ICU coupled with an appreciation of poor-quality sleep as compared to home [25] to abnormalities in ventilation and even acute psychoses.

CAUSES OF SLEEP DISRUPTION

Noise and Hospital Staff

The environmental stimulus most reported in the literature as disturbing sleep is noise [25–29]. The level of noise in the ICU ranges from 50 to 85 decibels (dB) through a 24-hour period [26–29]. This level of noise is comparable with a busy office (70 dB) or a pneumatic drill heard 50 ft away (80 dB) [28–30]. These noise levels exceed that recommended by the US Environmental Protection Agency for hospital settings suggested to be 45 dB during the day and 35 dB at night [31]. The sources of noise as identified by ICU patients include equipment and conversation among staff [24]. Noise may disrupt sleep in two ways: either arouse/awaken the patient or produce a change to a lighter sleep stage. There is some debate, however, as to what degree the noise causes the arousal or whether noise may simply coincide with many of the frequent awakenings ICU patients experience.

Reports have suggested that the response to noise may vary based on the age and gender of the patient. Healthy men and women were monitored for changes in sleep stages with EEG in a controlled environment. The environmental noise in these studies included simulated sonic booms and jet aircraft flyover noise. Older individuals and women had lower sleep thresholds and were more likely to be awakened or shift to a different sleep stage [29]. However, findings in healthy subjects may not apply to critically ill patients whose sleep threshold is altered by sleep deprivation, drugs, or encephalopathic states. One study showed no difference in perceived ICU sleep quality or daytime sleepiness by way of gender nor were there significant correlations between perceived sleep quality and age or length of ICU stay. However, in this study, information was gained by way of a sleep questionnaire without EEG monitoring [25].

Freedman et al. [25], using a questionnaire distributed to ICU patients on the day of their discharge from the unit, showed perceived differences in individual environmental factors in terms of their degrees of ICU sleep disruption. Checking vital signs and phlebotomy were perceived as most disruptive. These were followed by noise, diagnostic tests, nursing interventions (e.g., bathing), ambient light, and medication administration. In terms of environmental noise, talking and telemetry alarms were perceived as significantly more disruptive to sleep than the phone or beepers. The investigators also compared perceived sleep disruption between patients discharged from medical, surgical, and cardiac ICUs and concluded that medical ICU patients perceived their sleep to be more disrupted by environmental factors than did patients in other units. The study's design was again limited by lack of EEG verification of sleep architecture and the lack of control for severity of illness and medications used. This study highlighted that environmental noise, although an important contributor to sleep disruption, is but one of many environmental factors causing poor sleep in the ICU.

Another study using a questionnaire administered to ICU patients within the first week of their stay reported that the physical stressors patients considered the most important included pain and inability to sleep due to noise and nasogastric and endotracheal tubes. Loss of self-control, autonomy, and lack of understanding about attitudes and procedures were the main psychological stressors [32].

Does reduction in noise levels result in better sleep in the ICU? Investigators evaluated sleep outcomes in 18 female patients in an acute obstetrics/gynecologic unit and found a statistically significant improvement in subjective outcome measures in those who wore earplugs as compared with those who did not [33]. A PSG study in healthy volunteers randomly exposed to either simulated ICU noise or earplugs during sleep showed an increase in sleep disruption associated with ICU noise as compared with use of earplugs. There was also an increase in REM sleep in those using earplugs [34]. Whether it is the peak noise level or a change in the noise level that causes sleep disruption is unclear. Investigators added white noise to the background noise and reported a decrease in arousal frequency from 48 per hour to the no noise baseline of 13 per hour [35]. This supports the thought that maintenance of a certain level of unobtrusive background noise in the ICU may be helpful in reducing arousal frequency.

Sleep in the ICU is poor in terms of quality and lack of continuity. Nursing care activities, phlebotomy, noise, the presence of invasive tubes, pain, and patients' lack of understanding of their medical care all contribute to the poor sleep. Despite this, the cause of 68% of arousals could not be identified by Gabor and coworkers [18] in a PSG study assessing noise as a cause of disrupted sleep in seven mechanically ventilated patients. Other potential culprits include underlying medical illness, mechanical ventilator mode, and medications.

Medications

The effect on sleep of the vast number of medications used in the ICU setting is not well established. Many drugs improve sleep and others have adverse effects, and often patients are on a number of medications that may have polarizing effects on sleep. Table 70.1 lists medications that are often used in the ICU and characterizes their known effects on sleep.

Sedative/hypnotics are frequently used in the ICU to control symptoms of anxiety and insomnia. They are also used as muscle relaxants and anticonvulsants. The most frequently used sedative/hypnotics are of the benzodiazepine class. Benzodiazepines exert their sedative/hypnotic effect through the γ-aminobutyric acid-benzodiazepine receptor complex. Equally popular are two nonbenzodiazepine drugs, zolpidem and zaleplon. Zolpidem is an imidazopyridine compound and zaleplon is a pyrazolopyrimidine compound. Both drugs also bind selectively to the γ-aminobutyric acid-benzodiazepine receptor complex. The neuroanatomic sites at which these drugs act is less well understood, but a number of findings suggest that the basal forebrain and anterior hypothalamus are the crucial areas [36,37]. The half-life of the benzodiazepines ranges from 48 to 120 hours (flurazepam) to 2 to 6 hours (triazolam). They are lipophilic, which may result in an increase in the volume of distribution, especially in the elderly or the obese. Metabolism is through the hepatic microsomal system, therefore limiting their safe use in hepatically impaired patients. Overall, these drugs are generally well tolerated and have much less respiratory depressant effect than barbiturates.

PSG studies of benzodiazepines reveal decreased sleep latency and increased total sleep time, consistent with their clinical effects. There is increased spindle activity and mild

TABLE 70.1

DRUGS COMMONLY USED IN INTENSIVE CARE UNITS AND THEIR EFFECTS ON SLEEP PATTERN

Drug class or individual drug	Sleep disorder, induced or reported	Possible mechanism
Benzodiazepines	↓ REM, ↓ SWS	γ-Aminobutyric acid type A receptor stimulation
Opioids	↓ REM, ↓ SWS	μ-Receptor stimulation
Clonidine	↓ REM	α_2-Receptor stimulation
Nonsteroidal anti-inflammatory drugs	↓ TST, ↓ SE	Prostaglandin synthesis inhibition
Norepinephrine/epinephrine	Insomnia, ↓ REM, ↓ SWS	α_1-Receptor stimulation
Dopamine	Insomnia, ↓ REM, ↓ SWS	D_2-Receptor stimulation/α_1-receptor stimulation
Beta-blockers	Insomnia, ↓ REM, nightmares	Central nervous system beta-blockade by lipophilic agents
Amiodarone	Nightmares	Unknown mechanism
Corticosteroids	Insomnia, ↓ REM, ↓ SWS	Reduced melatonin secretion
Aminophylline	Insomnia, ↓ REM, ↓ SWS, ↓ TST, ↓ SE	Adenosine receptor antagonism
Quinolones	Insomnia	γ-Aminobutyric acid type A receptor inhibition
Tricyclic antidepressants	↓ REM	Antimuscarinic activity and α_1-receptor stimulation
Selective serotonin reuptake inhibitors	↓ REM, ↓ TST, ↓ SE	Increased serotonergic activity
Phenytoin	↑ Sleep fragmentation	Inhibition of neuronal calcium influx
Phenobarbital	↓ REM	Increased γ-aminobutyric acid type A activity
Carbamazepine	↓ REM	Adenosine receptor stimulation and/or serotonergic activity

REM, rapid eye movement; SE, sleep efficiency; SWS, slow-wave sleep; TST, total sleep time.
From Bourne R, Mills G: Sleep disruption in critically ill patients: pharmacological considerations. *Anaesthesia* 59:376, 2004, with permission.

reduction of REM sleep. More striking is the reduction in slow-wave sleep. The clinical ramification of decreased slow-wave sleep is unclear. The nonbenzodiazepines, zolpidem and zaleplon, have minimal or no effect on slow-wave or REM sleep. These drugs, however, are thought to induce more normal sleep patterns than barbiturates (a once popular sedative/hypnotic choice) that caused a severe reduction in REM sleep. Clinical efficacy studies of short-term use of both the benzodiazepines and nonbenzodiazepines in an outpatient population show that patients have better subjective ratings of sleep with minimal chance of developing tolerance.

Perception of sleep quality in ICU patients on high doses of sedatives is less predictable. A questionnaire rating sleep quality with nocturnal propofol as opposed to midazolam was administered to a group of nonintubated critically ill patients. Although there was no difference in self-perception of sleep quality between the two drugs, there was a disparity in perceived sleep quality, with some patients reporting improved sleep quality and others rating extremely poor sleep, although all infusions had been titrated to achieve deep but arousable sleep to the observer [38]. Dexmedetomidine (Dex), a sedative with analgesic properties, was compared with Propofol in a randomized clinical trial in patients post-CABG evaluating the patient reported level of satisfaction in the 24-hour postoperative period. There was no statistically significant advantage of Dex over Propofol [40].

Although use of a sedative/hypnotic is a reasonable approach to promote a sleep state in an ICU patient, the quality of the sleep may not be in direct proportion to the quantity. This medicated sleep state while mimicking normal sleep has enough abnormal architecture to lead one to question whether the patient receives the necessary restorative, physiologic boost a good night's sleep should provide.

Psychoactive medications such as *antidepressants* and *antipsychotics* are not often prescribed in the acute setting in the ICU, but many patients may come into the unit taking these medications. PSG shows tricyclic depressants generally increase total sleep time and decrease wakefulness, especially the tertiary amines such as amitriptyline and imipramine. The secondary amines (e.g., nortriptyline, desipramine) are less sedating. Serotonin-selective reuptake inhibitors generally increase sleep latency and decrease REM sleep and total sleep time.

Sedation is a common side effect of the traditional antipsychotics, but the incidence and degree of sedation varies significantly among the drugs. Haldol is less sedating than the older chlorpromazine. Clozapine is a newer agent with significant sedating effects. Sedation is reported less frequently with risperidone and olanzapine.

ICU patients may need *antiseizure medication*. It is well known that sedation occurs across the classes of antiepileptics. A few well-known examples include phenobarbital, phenytoin, and valproic acid. The sedative effect is to some extent dose dependent, but generally, there is decreased sleep latency and increased total sleep time with impaired daytime function. The newer agents (e.g., lamotrigine and topiramate) also have subjective reports of increased sedation, but PSG data are lacking.

Several drugs used in the ICU for *hemodynamic support* are also psychomotor stimulants. They include norepinephrine, dopamine, and phenylephrine infusions. They are all direct sympathomimetics and serve to raise blood pressure either through chronotropic and inotropic effects on the heart or through vasoconstriction of peripheral vessels. There is an associated increase in arousal, motor activity, and alertness that is most likely masked in the ICU by the concomitant use of sedatives. There are no PSG studies to our knowledge examining the effect of these drugs on sleep. Kong and coworkers [39] studied the efficacy of midazolam and isoflurane in reducing plasma levels of catecholamines with similar levels of sedation. Although comparable levels of sedation were achieved with both drugs, isoflurane but not midazolam lowered plasma catecholamine levels. PSG data were not simultaneously recorded, but given the central nervous system stimulant effect of catecholamines, it is a reasonable assumption that high levels may produce sleep fragmentation in the ICU. In summary, patients receiving continuous infusions of sympathomimetics or drugs with sympathomimetic effects such as β-agonists may have fragmented, disrupted sleep architecture. Despite the concomitant use of sedatives leading to an unconscious state resembling sleep, these patients may derive little physiologic benefit associated with true sleep.

Other miscellaneous drugs that are commonly used in the ICU and have known sleep effects include beta-blockers, corticosteroids, and theophylline. Beta-blockers as a class are associated with insomnia, nightmares, decreased total sleep time, and REM sleep with increased daytime fatigue. These side effects are generally worse the more lipophilic the drug. Patients often note that corticosteroids disrupt sleep, although data are mainly through subjective patient reports. The results of objective studies are inconsistent. The most consistent PSG findings in healthy subjects is decreased REM. Theophylline is being used less because of better drugs with fewer side effects, although it is still occasionally used for its respiratory stimulant and bronchodilator effects. It is chemically related to caffeine and is frequently reported to disrupt sleep. The subjective reports are consistent with PSG data, which show fragmented sleep.

Other medications frequently used in the ICU include angiotensin-converting enzyme inhibitors, calcium antagonists, vasodilators, diuretics, and histamine$_2$-antagonists. There is little information about these drugs' effect on sleep, especially in the ICU patient. H_2-blockers likely do not cause sleep disturbance because they do not easily cross the blood–brain barrier. The manufacturers admit to a 2% incidence of insomnia, but there are no PSG data.

Underlying Medical Illness

The Effect of Sleep on Cardiopulmonary Syndromes

Sleep-disordered breathing in the form of obstructive sleep apnea–hypopnea (OSAH) syndromes is commonly encountered in the ICU. Many critically ill patients are admitted with an acute exacerbation of a chronic cardiopulmonary disorder, commonly congestive heart failure (CHF), and chronic obstructive pulmonary disease (COPD). Further destabilization of gas exchange may occur with sleep onset due to the following mechanisms.

1. Loss of respiratory muscle activity occurs with sleep onset due to sleep-induced muscle relaxation. The intercostals and accessory muscles of respiration play an important role in maintaining normal minute ventilation in those with abnormal ventilation perfusion matching, for example, parenchymal lung disease, chest wall deformity. A reduction in respiratory muscle activity can result in profound deterioration in gas exchange.
2. Autonomic nervous system changes with sleep onset as characterized by an increase in parasympathetic and concomitant decrease in sympathetic nervous system activity with the onset of NREM sleep results in a decrease in heart rate, stroke volume. This can lead to undesirable hemodynamic consequences in the compromised patient [41].
3. Upper airway collapse in those with underlying OSAH leads to high negative intrathoracic pressure swings in an attempt to end the apnea or hypopnea. The large intrathoracic pressure swings coupled with hypoxemia occurring from the obstructed upper airway results in an increase in afterload, preload, and ventricular dysfunction. In the patient with

cardiac dysfunction, this sleep-induced upper airway closure has been shown to exacerbate CHF [42,43].

4. Instability of the respiratory control mechanism occurs with sleep onset in the normal individual with an alteration in the central chemoreceptor set point. There is a decrease in minute ventilation by 20% coupled with a 4% to 6% increase in PCO_2 level across the night [44]. The response of the respiratory system to upper airway collapse, hypoxemia, may be exaggerated due to sleep-induced instability of the feedback loop [45]. An increase in respiratory rate beyond that necessary to correct the hypoxemia/hypercapnia may cause a decrease in PCO_2 levels below apnea threshold (the physiologic PCO_2 level above which ventilation is triggered, and below which apnea ensues). The exaggerated loop gain has been well documented to occur during circulatory delay as occurs in CHF with a low ejection fraction. The result often is a crescendo–decrescendo pattern of breathing known as Cheyne-Stokes respiration (CSR). CSR is rarely observed during REM sleep, more so occurring during NREM sleep. CSR-CSA is associated with nocturnal arousals, awakenings. Patients with severe CSR demonstrate frequent central apneas with frequent arousals, fragmented sleep, and increased sleep state changes [46–50].
5. The supine position in a normal individual is associated with a decrease in the functional residual capacity of the lung by approximately 20%. This change in posture with sleep onset coupled with sleep-induced decrease in respiratory muscle activity can lead to worsened ventilation perfusion mismatch especially in those with massive obesity, CHF, and diaphragmatic paralysis [51].
6. Patients suffering from severe COPD (forced expiratory volume in the first second less than 1.0 L) have been found to have more fragmented sleep with more wake time as documented by overnight PSG as compared with an age-matched control group [52]. Other investigators had similar findings in a hypercapnic COPD group without obstructive sleep apnea. A significant number of arousals lasting more than 1 minute were noted, along with a decrease in total sleep time and increases in sleep state changes [52,53].

It stands to reason that if patients with stable chronic disease have such disrupted sleep as a consequence of their underlying medical illness, the acute decompensation of their cardiorespiratory system as occurs with decompensated CHF or COPD will further add to reduced nocturnal total sleep time, sleep fragmentation, and increased daytime sleep.

Many hospitalized patients may attribute some of their fragmented sleep to pain. PSG data evaluating sleep stages after burn injury showed reduced total sleep time and increased fragmented sleep, with more than 63 arousals per hour. The abnormal sleep was attributed to their burn state [19]. Similarly, sleep in nine postabdominal surgery patients was analyzed. As with other reports, there was more lighter sleep and less slow-wave sleep, but the arousal index was not reported. The authors suggested that pain may have been part of the cause of the abnormal sleep architecture [17].

In summary, chronic cardiorespiratory illness, sleep-disordered breathing, and pain as a result of the underlying illness all may contribute to poor sleep in the ICU.

Mechanical Ventilation

Mechanical ventilation is commonly used in the ICU, where roughly 40% of patients require assistance with breathing [54]. Positive pressure ventilation improves gas exchange and helps with respiratory muscle rest [55]. Mechanically ventilated patients experience fragmented sleep, averaging 20 to 63 arousals per hour from a variety of internal and externally driven factors [8,18,19]. The sleep-disrupting factors external to the patient associated with the mechanical ventilation include discomfort from the endotracheal and nasogastric tubes, suctioning, physical restraints, and alarms, including ventilator alarms [56]. A specific factor internal to the patient promoting fragmented sleep is central apneas occurring during mechanical ventilation. Meza et al. [57] showed central apneas in healthy volunteers during sleep while on pressure support ventilation (PSV). The mechanism behind the central apneas could be either through a chemically mediated loss of respiratory drive by way of a ventilator-induced reduction of the PCO_2 below the apnea threshold or via a nonchemical mechanism. Other investigative work showed an inhibition of respiratory motor output in healthy volunteers on assist-control and controlled modes of ventilation whose respiratory rates or tidal volumes were increased while maintaining normocapnia [58]. The authors concluded that continuous mandatory ventilation at increased frequency, plus moderate elevations in tidal volume, reset respiratory rhythm and inhibited respiratory motor output to a greater extent than did increased tidal volume alone. In effect, central apneas may be caused either by ventilator-induced hypocapnia or ventilator-induced reset of respiratory drive with normocapnia.

Data also suggest that the mode of ventilation can influence sleep quality. A comparison was made between pressure support and assist-control mode of ventilation on sleep quality in 11 critically ill patients [55]. There was greater sleep fragmentation (79 vs. 54 arousals and awakenings per hour) and lower sleep efficiency during pressure support than during assist control ventilation. Central apneas occurred in 6 of the 11 patients during pressure support but not during assist control ventilation due to the backup rate in the assist-control mode (Fig. 70.2). These central apneas occurred predominately in heart failure patients and were secondary to a reduction of their PCO_2 below apnea thresholds. The central apneas and overall sleep efficiency in the pressure support group were improved by addition of dead space to the ventilator circuit, which caused an increase in CO_2 levels above the apnea threshold. The number of arousals and awakenings decreased from 83 to 44 events per hour in this group (Fig. 70.2). The conclusion was that pressure support mode may lead to hypocapnia that, when combined with the lack of a backup rate and wakefulness drive, can lead to central apneas with sleep fragmentation, especially in patients with heart failure. Other investigators report conflicting data—Hardin et al. failed to find any difference in arousal frequency with different ventilator modes. Of note, the small study size and patient sedation may have contributed to their findings [24]. Other investigators compared a low level PSV (6 cm H_2O) with the assist-control mode in patients with acute or chronic respiratory failure who were near extubation. Assist-control mode was associated with improved sleep architecture with increased slow-wave sleep and REM sleep [59]. Cabello and Thille [60] compared automatically adjusted PSV with clinician-adjusted PSV and assist-control in nonsedated patients. There was no appreciable difference in sleep between the groups. Proportional assist ventilation was compared with PSV in sedated patients; proportional assist was associated with better patient–ventilator synchrony, less arousals and awakenings, and improved sleep architecture than in the PSV group [61].

Melatonin

Melatonin secretion in healthy individuals follows a stable circadian rhythm promoting consolidated nocturnal sleep. The loss of adequate melatonin secretion could lead to sleep deprivation, especially deleterious in an already physiologically compromised group such as the critically ill patient. Measurement of a urinary metabolite of melatonin in 17 septic, sedated

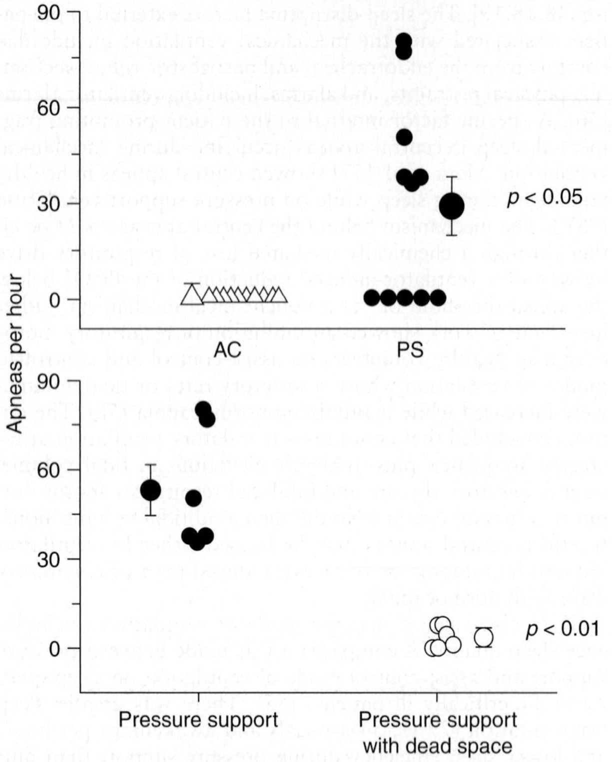

FIGURE 70.2. Number of apneas per hour during assist-control ventilation (AC; *open triangles*), pressure support (PS; *closed circles*), and pressure support with added dead space (*open circles*). Six of 11 patients developed apneas during pressure support as compared with none during assist-control ventilation (*top*). In the patients who developed apneas, the number of apneas decreased with the addition of dead space (*bottom*). Individual and group mean values are shown. Bars represent the standard error (SE). [From Parthasarathy S, Tobin M: Effect of ventilator mode on sleep quality in critically ill patients. *Am J Respir Crit Care Med* 166:1425, 2002, with permission.]

patients as compared with nonseptic patients and a normal control group suggested impaired melatonin secretion occurred in the septic group as compared with the nonseptic patients and the control group [62]. Other investigators have found a loss of circadian release of melatonin in mechanically ventilated, sedated patients with no relation of the level of sedation to the abnormality of melatonin secretion [63]. Beta-blockers are also known to impair melatonin secretion through blockade of central β-adrenoreceptors, which control secretion of melatonin from the pineal gland [64,65].

The impairment of melatonin secretion in critically ill patients, therefore, is most likely multifactorial, in which endogenous factors such as sepsis play a role, and exogenous factors including medications such as beta-blockers and the loss of the external zeitgeber (light/dark cycles) amplify the disruption.

There is one small pilot study and several anecdotal reports of melatonin use in critically ill patients that described improved sleep quality and efficiency, leading in some instances to quicker ventilator weaning [66,67]. The doses used varied from 5 to 10 mg according to clinician discretion. More recently, a larger randomized clinical trial evaluating melatonin in tracheostomized ICU patients failed to show a statistically significant difference in total sleep time or diurnal variation of sleep between the control and intervention groups despite confirmation of therapeutic serum drug levels in the intervention group [68]. At this point, the data on melatonin does not warrant its use in ICU patients as a sedative or to help reset circadian rhythm.

CONSEQUENCES OF SLEEP FRAGMENTATION AND DEPRIVATION

Sleep is essential for normal physiologic function. Animal studies showed multiorgan dysfunction leading to death in sleep-deprived rats as compared with a non–sleep-deprived control group [9]. Healthy human subjects with 24 to 48 hours of sleep deprivation and or fragmented sleep demonstrate impaired memory, labile moods, slower response times to controlled stimuli, and poor impulse control [6,7]. The lack of consolidated sleep may influence morbidity in critically ill patients.

Neurologic Consequences

Sleep deprivation has been associated with the development of mental status changes in ICU patients. These changes include delirium, agitation, and psychosis. This has been labeled the "ICU syndrome" and is typically seen after a week in the ICU. Helton and colleagues [69] were among the first to describe mental status changes in ICU patients. They studied 62 critically ill patients and found that delirium occurred in one third of patients with severe sleep deprivation (>50% sleep loss), 10% of those with moderate sleep deprivation (<50% sleep loss), and 3% of those with adequate sleep. The limitations of the study include the lack of PSG data; sleep was assessed by the staff and may have been underestimated, and a cause-and-effect relationship between sleep deprivation and delirium was inferred. Other authors have described delirium occurring in up to 60% of older hospitalized patients [70].

Wood et al. [71] reported 83% of a mechanically ventilated cohort developed delirium during an ICU stay and the delirium persisted in 10% of these patients at hospital discharge. Baseline dementia appears to be a risk factor for the development of delirium in the ICU.

The development of posttraumatic stress disorder is recognized as a significant problem occurring after a stay in the ICU. Jones and Griffiths [72] studied 45 patients discharged from the ICU and proposed that the development of posttraumatic stress disorder symptoms may have been related more to the recall of delusions as opposed to the memories of real adverse events that occurred during their ICU stay.

Cardiopulmonary Consequences

Sleep loss has been shown to impair respiratory muscle performance. A comparison of respiratory muscle strength and pulmonary function was made in healthy subjects after normal sleep and after 30 hours without sleep [73]. There was a decrease in inspiratory muscle endurance, but preservation of expiratory muscle strength. Other aspects of respiratory muscle control are compromised by sleep deprivation. Genioglossal muscle activity (important in upper-airway patency) deteriorates after sleep deprivation in healthy subjects [74–76], and other investigators have found decreased spirometric values in stable COPD patients after a period of sleep loss [74–77]. There are no data on respiratory muscle performance in sleep-deprived critically ill patients. Based on the data presented here, however, respiratory muscle response to increased mechanical loads either during or after mechanical ventilation in a sleep-deprived patient may be compromised, potentially interfering with recovery from an acute cardiorespiratory illness.

The effect of sleep deprivation on the ventilatory response to hypoxia or hypercapnia is controversial. Initial reports found an impaired hypoxic and hypercapnic ventilatory response in healthy young men after 24 hours without sleep, but with intact resting ventilation [77]. Subsequent reports refuted this finding; after strictly controlled environmental influences, healthy subjects without sleep for 24 hours were not found to have an alteration in chemoreceptor set points (i.e., no change in hypoxic or hypercapnic ventilatory response after sleep deprivation) [78]. There are no data in critically ill patients.

"REM rebound" is a well-recognized result of sleep deprivation. Once out of the ICU or in the recovery phase of their illness, previously sleep-deprived patients experience both increased REM and slow-wave sleep for repayment of their sleep debt [19]. Moreover, REM sleep is known for the accompanying autonomic variability in the form of irregular breathing, heart rate, and more profound hypoxemia in the susceptible patient. REM rebound therefore carries the inherent risk of hemodynamic instability in those with cardiorespiratory compromise and may play a role in ICU morbidity and mortality.

Immunologic and Metabolic Consequences

Sleep deprivation alters immune function. There is a decreased production of lymphocytes and reduced leukocyte phagocytic action [4,5]. Studies in young, healthy men showed an increase in urinary nitrogen after 48 hours of no sleep, suggesting sleep deprivation leads to a catabolic state [79]. Although there have been no studies in critically ill patients, the implication remains that sleep deprivation may play a role in impaired recovery from infection and poor tissue healing.

Activity of the corticotropic axis is circadian driven. Plasma levels of adrenocorticotropin and cortisol are highest in the morning and lowest in the evening, near the point of sleep onset in normal individuals. This axis is modulated by the sleep/wake condition. Sleep onset is associated with a short-term inhibition of cortisol secretion. Sleep deprivation is associated with an increase in evening cortisol the day following sleep loss. Sleep loss appears to delay the return to decreased evening activity of the corticotropic axis [80–82].

The thyroid axis is also affected by sleep deprivation. Plasma thyroid-stimulating hormone (TSH) levels are at their lowest in the day and highest in the night around the beginning of the sleep period. During sleep, there is a progressive decline in TSH levels. Sleep overall inhibits TSH secretion, and sleep deprivation relieves this inhibition; awakenings during nocturnal sleep are associated with short-term increases in plasma TSH and triiodothyronine (T_3) levels [83,84].

METHODS TO IMPROVE SLEEP IN THE INTENSIVE CARE UNIT

It is important to ensure an adequate amount of time for patients to sleep. Before improving quality, quantity must be guaranteed. Several hospitals have now put in place protocols allowing an uninterrupted period of sleep for critically ill patients [85]. Obtaining vital signs, laboratory draws, or other bedside care is deferred during this period.

As discussed previously, a noisy environment is responsible for an estimated 30% of fragmented sleep, and the use of earplugs, in combination with background white noise, may be of some benefit to improving patients' sleep.

Enhancing the drive to sleep at night is facilitated by different methods. Realignment of the intrinsic body clock to a normal day/night schedule is helped by introducing light/dark cycles into the ICU. Exposure to sunlight or overhead lights (10,000 lux or more) in the morning helps to reduce endogenous melatonin secretion and decreases the drive to sleep during the day. In addition, sitting the patient out of bed and avoiding sedatives during the day will decrease daytime sleep episodes and consequently increase the homeostatic and circadian drive to sleep at night. Administration of a short-acting sedative/hypnotic at night with reduction of ambient lights to less than 250 lux, or complete darkness, encourages endogenous melatonin secretion that may consolidate and improve sleep quality. There may be a role for exogenous melatonin in those with impaired melatonin secretion; however, further studies are needed to determine which patients may benefit.

An awareness of the effect of underlying medical illness on the quality of sleep is important and, as is practical, should be addressed, including screening for and initiation of noninvasive positive pressure ventilation for treatment of obstructive sleep apnea (OSA) and Central sleep apnea-Cheyne-Stokes Respiration (CSA-CSR) as indicated. There needs to be adequate treatment of pain syndromes.

Application of the principles presented here may improve overall sleep quality and quantity in the ICU and ultimately lead to improved morbidity and mortality. A multidisciplinary approach involving physicians, nurses, other hospital personnel, and the administration is needed to increase awareness and improve both the environment and the approach to enhanced sleep in the hospital setting. Further studies are needed on sleep in the ICU, but the challenge of controlling for confounding influences in the ICU still remains and makes such research difficult.

References

1. Kryger M, Roth T, Dement W, eds: *Principles and Practice of Sleep Medicine*. 3rd ed. Philadelphia, Elsevier, 2005.
2. Brzezinski A: Melatonin in humans. *N Engl J Med* 336:186, 1997.
3. Mohsenin V: Sleep in COPD. *Semin Respir Crit Care Med* 26:109, 2005.
4. Palmblad J, Pettrini B, Wasserman J, et al: Lymphocyte and granulocyte reactions during sleep deprivation. *Psychosom Med* 41:273, 1979.
5. Palmblad J, Cantell K, Strander H, et al: Stressor exposure and immunological response in man: interferon-producing capacity and phagocytosis. *Psychosom Res* 20:193, 1976.
6. Van Dongen HP: Brain activation patterns and individual differences in working memory impairment during sleep deprivation. *Sleep* 28:386, 2005.
7. Amedt JT, Owens J: Neurobehavioral performance of residents after heavy night call vs after alcohol ingestion. *JAMA* 294:1025, 2005.
8. Cooper AB, Thornley KS, Young GB, et al: Sleep in critically ill patients requiring mechanical ventilation. *Chest* 117:809, 2000.
9. Rechtschaffen A, Gilliland M: Physiological correlates of prolonged sleep deprivation in rats. *Science* 221:182, 1983.
10. Spiegel K, Sheridan JF, Van Cauter E: Effect of sleep deprivation on response to immunization. *JAMA* 288:1471–1472, 2002.
11. Osturk L, Pelin Z, Van Cauter E: Effects of 48 hours sleep deprivation on human immune profile. *Sleep Res Online* 2:107–111, 1999.
12. Bourne R, Minelli C: Clinical review: sleep measurements in critical care patients: research and clinical implications. *Crit Care* 11:226, 2007.
13. Danker-Hopfe H, Kunz D: Interrater reliability between scorers from eight European sleep laboratories in subjects with different sleep disorders. *J Sleep Res* 13:63–69, 2004.
14. Fanfulla F, Delmastro M: Effect of different ventilator settings on sleep and inspiratory effort in patients with neuromuscular disease. *Am J Respir Crit Care Med* 172:619–624, 2005.
15. Ambrogio C, Koebnick J: Assessment of sleep in ventilator-supported critically ill patients. *Sleep* 31(11):1559–1568, 2008.
16. Hilton BA: Quantity and quality of patients' sleep-disturbing factors in a respiratory intensive care unit. *J Adv Nurs* 1:453, 1976.
17. Aurell J, Elmqvist D: Sleep in the surgical intensive care unit: continuous polygraphic recording postoperative care. *BMJ* 290:1029, 1985.
18. Gabor JY, Cooper AB, Crombach SA, et al: Contribution of the intensive care unit environment to sleep disruption in mechanically ventilated patients and healthy subjects. *Am J Respir Crit Care Med* 167:708, 2003.
19. Gottschlich MM, Jenkins ME: The 1994 Clinical Research Award. A prospective clinical study of the polysomnographic stages of sleep after burn injury. *J Burn Care Rehabil* 15:486, 1994.

20. Freedman NS, Gazendam J, Levan L, et al: Abnormal sleep/wake cycles and the effect of environmental noise on sleep disruption in the intensive care unit. *Am J Respir Crit Care Med* 163:451, 2001.
21. Edwards GB, Schuring LM: Pilot study: validating staff nurses' observations of sleep and wake states among critical ill patients, using polysomnography. *Am J Crit Care* 2:125, 1993.
22. Knill RL, Moote CA, Skinner MI, et al: Anesthesia with abdominal surgery leads to intense REM sleep during the first postoperative week. *Anesthesiology* 73:52, 1990.
23. Parthasarathy S, Tobin MJ: Effect of ventilator mode on sleep quality in critically ill patient. *Am J Respir Crit Care Med* 166:1423, 2002.
24. Hardin K, Seyal M: Sleep in critically ill chemically paralyzed patients requiring mechanical ventilation. *Chest* 129:1468–1477, 2006.
25. Freedman N, Kotzer N, Schwab R: Patient perception of sleep quality and etiology of sleep disruption in the intensive care unit. *Am J Respir Crit Care Med* 159:1155, 1999.
26. Bentley S, Murphy F, Dudley H: Perceived noise in surgical wards and an intensive care area. *BMJ* 2:1503, 1977.
27. Meyer T, Eveloff S, Bauer M, et al: Adverse environment conditions in the respiratory and medical ICU settings. *Chest* 105:1211, 1994.
28. Redding JS, Hargest TS, Minsky SH: How noisy is intensive care? *Crit Care Med* 5(6):275, 1997.
29. Lukas JS: Noise and sleep: a literature review and a proposed criterion for assessing effect. *J Acoust Soc Am* 58:1232, 1996.
30. Falk S, Woods N: Hospital noise levels and potential health hazards. *N Engl J Med* 289:774, 1973.
31. Environmental Protection Agency: Information on levels of environmental noise requisite to protect public health and welfare with an adequate margin of safety (Report no. 550–9-74–004). Washington, DC, US Government Printing Office, 1974.
32. Novaes M, Aronovich A, Ferraz M, et al: Stressors in ICU: patients' evaluation. *Intensive Care Med* 23:1282, 1997.
33. Haddock J: Reducing the effects of noise in hospitals. *Nurs Stand* 8:25, 1994.
34. Wallace CJ, Robins J, Alvord LS, et al: The effect of earplugs on sleep measures during exposure to simulated intensive care unit noise. *Am J Crit Care* 8:210, 1999.
35. Stanchina ML, Abu-Hijleh M, Chaudhry BK: The influence of white noise on sleep in subjects exposed to ICU noise. *Sleep Med* 6:423–428, 2005.
36. Mendelson WB: Effects of microinjection of triazolam into the ventrolateral preoptic area on sleep in the rat. *Life Sci* 65(25):301, 1999.
37. Simerly RB, Swanson Lu: The organization of neural inputs to the medial preoptic nucleus of the rat. *J Comp Neurol* 246:12, 1985.
38. Treggiari-Venzi M, Borgeat A, Fuchs-Buder T, et al: Overnight sedation with midazolam or propofol in the ICU: effects on sleep quality, anxiety and depression. *Intensive Care Med* 22:1186, 1996.
39. Kong KL, Willatts SM, Prys-Roberts C, et al: Plasma catecholamine concentration during sedation in ventilated patients requiring intensive therapy. *Intensive Care Med* 16:171, 1990.
40. Corbett S, Rebuck J: Dexmedetomidine does not improve patient satisfaction when compared with propofol during mechanical ventilation. *Crit Care Med* 33(5):2005.
41. Somers VK, Dyken ME: Sympathetic activity neural mechanisms in obstructive sleep apnea. *J Clin Invest* 96:1897–1904, 1995.
42. Parker JD, Brooks D: Acute and chronic effects of airway obstruction on canine left ventricular performance. *Am J Respir Crit Care Med* 160:1888–1896, 1999.
43. Shahar E, Whitney CW: Sleep disordered breathing and cardiovascular disease: cross sectional results of the Sleep Heart Health Study. *Am J Respir Crit Care Med* 163:19–25, 2001.
44. Dempsey JA, Smith CA: The ventilatory responsiveness to CO_2 below eupnoea as a determinant of ventilatory stability in sleep. *J Physiol* 560:1–11, 2004.
45. Solin P, Roebuck T: Peripheral and central ventilator responses in central sleep apnea with and without heart failure. *Am J Respir Crit Care Med* 162:2194–2200, 2000.
46. Findley LJ, Zwillich CZ, Ancoli-Israel S, et al: Cheyne-Stokes breathing during sleep in patients with left ventricular heart failure. *South Med J* 78:11, 1985.
47. Hanly PJ, Millar TW, Stwljes DG, et al: Respiration and abnormal sleep in patients with congestive heart failure. *Chest* 96:480, 1989.
48. Dark DS, Pingleton SK, Kerby GR, et al: Breathing pattern abnormalities and arterial oxygen desaturation during sleep in the congestive heart failure syndrome. *Chest* 91:833, 1987.
49. Hanly PJ, Millar TW, Steljes DG, et al: The effect of oxygen on respiration and sleep in patients with congestive heart failure. *Ann Intern Med* 111:777, 1989.
50. Takaski Y, Orr D, Popkin J, et al: The effects of nasal continuous positive airway pressure on sleep apnea in congestive heart failure. *Am Rev Respir Dis* 140:1578, 1989.
51. Yap JCH, Moore DM: Effect of supine posture on respiratory mechanics in chronic left ventricular failure. *Am J Respir Crit Care Med* 162:1285–1291, 2000.
52. Brezinova V, Cantterall JR, Douglas NJ, et al: Night sleep of patients with chronic ventilatory failure and age matched controls: number and duration of the EEG episodes of intervening wakefulness and drowsiness. *Sleep* 5:123, 1982.
53. Fleetham J, West P, Mezon B, et al: Sleep, arousals, and oxygen desaturation in chronic obstructive pulmonary disease: the effects of therapy. *Am Rev Respir Dis* 126(3):429, 1982.
54. Esteban A, Anzueto A, Alia I, et al: How is mechanical ventilation employed in the intensive care unit? An international utilization review. *Am J Respir Crit Care Med* 161:1450, 2000.
55. Parthasarathy S, Tobin M: Effects of ventilator mode on sleep quality in critically ill patients. *Am J Respir Crit Care Med* 166:423, 2002.
56. Metha S, Hill NS: Noninvasive ventilation. *Am J Respir Crit Care Med* 163:540, 2001.
57. Meza S, Mendez M, Osrtrowski M, et al: Susceptibility to periodic breathing with assisted ventilation during sleep in normal subjects. *J Appl Physiol* 85:1929, 1998.
58. Rice A, Nakayama HC, Haverkamp HC, et al: Controlled versus assisted mechanical ventilation effects on respiratory motor output in sleeping humans. *Am J Respir Crit Care Med* 168:92, 2003.
59. Toulbanc B, Rose D: Assist-control ventilation vs. low levels of pressure support ventilation on sleep quality in intubated ICU patients. *Intensive Care Med* 33:1148–1154, 2007.
60. Cabello B, Thille A: Sleep quality in mechanically ventilated patients: comparison of three ventilatory modes. *Crit Care Med* 36:1749–1755, 2008.
61. Bosma K, Ferreyra G: Patient-ventilator interaction and sleep in mechanically ventilated patients: pressure support versus proportional assist ventilation. *Crit Care Med* 35:1048–1054, 2007.
62. Mundigler G, Delle-Karth G, Koreny M, et al: Impaired circadian rhythm of melatonin secretion in sedated critically ill patients with severe sepsis. *Crit Care Med* 30:536, 2002.
63. Olofsson K, Alling C, Lundberg D, et al: Abolished circadian rhythm of melatonin secretion in sedated and artificially ventilated intensive care patients. *Acta Anaesthesiol Scand* 48:679, 2004.
64. Sakotnik A, Lercher P: Influence of beta blockers on melatonin release. *Eur J Clin Pharmacol* 55:111, 1999.
65. Cowen PJ, Bevan JS: Treatment with beta adrenoceptor blockers reduces plasma melatonin concentration. *Br J Clin Pharmacol* 19:258, 1985.
66. Shilo H, Dagan Y: Effects of melatonin on sleep quality of COPD intensive care patients: a pilot study. *Chronobiol Int* 17:71, 2000.
67. Mohan S, Brunner H: Melatonin in critically ill patients [letter]. *Acta Anaesthesiol Scand* 49:1397, 2005.
68. Ibrahim I, Bellamo R: A double-blind placebo-controlled randomized pilot study of nocturnal melatonin in tracheostomised patients. *Crit Care Resusc* 8(3):187–191, 2006.
69. Helton MC, Gordon SH, Nunnery SL: The correlation between sleep deprivation and the intensive care unit syndrome. *Heart Lung* 9:464, 1989.
70. Heller SS, Frank KA, Malm JR, et al: Psychiatric complications of open-heart surgery. *N Engl J Med* 283:1015, 1970.
71. Wood G, Kelly S, Ely W: What does it mean to be critically ill and elderly. *Curr Opin Crit Care* 9:316, 2003.
72. Jones C, Griffiths RD: Memory, delusions and the development of acute posttraumatic stress disorder related symptoms after intensive care. *Crit Care Med* 29:73, 2001.
73. Chen H, Tang Y: Sleep loss impairs inspiratory muscle endurance. *Am Rev Respir Dis* 140:907, 1989.
74. Cooper KR, Phillips BA: Effect of short-term sleep loss on breathing. *J Appl Physiol* 53:855, 1982.
75. Leiter JC, Knuth SL, Bartlett D: The effect of sleep deprivation on activity of the genioglossal muscle. *Am Rev Respir Dis* 132:1242, 1985.
76. Phillips BA, Cooper KR, Burke TV: The effect of sleep loss on breathing in chronic obstructive pulmonary disease. *Chest* 91:29, 1987.
77. White DP, Douglas NJ, Pickett CK, et al: Sleep deprivation and the control of ventilation. *Am Rev Respir Dis* 128:984, 1983.
78. Spengler C, Shea S: Sleep deprivation per se does not decrease the hypercapnic ventilatory response in humans. *Am J Respir Crit Care Med* 161:1124, 2000.
79. Scrimshaw NS, Habicht JP, Pellet P, et al: Effects of sleep deprivation and reversal of diurnal activity on protein metabolism of young men. *Am J Clin Nutr* 19:313, 1966.
80. Van Cauter E, Blackman JD: Modulation of glucose regulation and insulin secretion by circadian rhythmicity and sleep. *J Clin Invest* 88:934, 1991.
81. Weitzman ED, Zimmerman JC: Cortisol secretion is inhibited during sleep in normal man. *J Clin Endocrinol Metab* 77:1170, 1993.
82. Leproult R, Copinschi G: Sleep loss results in an elevation of cortisol levels the next evening. *Sleep* 20:865, 1997.
83. Brabant G, Prank K: Physiologic regulation of circadian and pulsatile thyrotropin secretion in normal man and woman. *J Clin Endocrinol Metab* 70:403, 1990.
84. Parker DC, Rossman LG: Effect of 64 hr sleep deprivation on the circadian waveform of thyrotropin (TSH), further evidence of sleep related inhibition of TSH release. *J Clin Endocrinol Metab* 64:157, 1987.
85. Inouye S, Bogardus J: A multicomponent intervention to prevent delirium in hospitalized older patients. *N Engl J Med* 340:669, 1999.

SECTION V ■ RENAL PROBLEMS IN THE INTENSIVE CARE UNIT

PANG-YEN FAN

CHAPTER 71 ■ METABOLIC ACIDOSIS AND METABOLIC ALKALOSIS

ROBERT M. BLACK

NORMAL ACID–BASE PHYSIOLOGY

Acidemia and alkalemia denote, respectively, blood pHs below or above the normal value of 7.40. A simple (single) acid–base disturbance always causes the blood pH to change. In comparison, the coexistence of two opposing primary acid–base disturbances, such as a metabolic acidosis due to diarrhea with metabolic alkalosis due to vomiting, may result in little or no deviation of the blood pH from normal. Maintenance of blood pH at approximately 7.40 is necessary to stabilize intracellular pH at 7.20, a crucial chemical condition for optimal cell physiology.

Renal Regulation of H^+ Secretion

Maintenance of a normal plasma bicarbonate (HCO_3^-) concentration depends on reclamation of the 4,500 mEq of HCO_3^- filtered by the kidneys each day. Reabsorption of filtered HCO_3^- takes place almost entirely in the proximal tubule (Fig. 71.1). In this process, luminal HCO_3^- combines with H^+ secreted into the tubular lumen by an Na-H antiporter. The formation and subsequent dissociation of carbonic acid (H_2CO_3) to carbon dioxide (CO_2) and water (H_2O), catalyzed by carbonic anhydrase, permit CO_2 to enter the luminal membrane of the proximal tubular cell. Once inside the cell, CO_2 combines with OH^- to form HCO_3^-. An Na-3HCO_3 cotransporter then carries HCO_3^- across the peritubular membrane into the blood. As a result, filtered HCO_3^- is returned to the circulation without any net loss of H^+.

A fall in proximal tubular bicarbonate reabsorption causes urinary HCO_3^- loss and may lead to a fall in plasma HCO_3^- concentration and to metabolic acidosis. The carbonic anhydrase inhibitor acetazolamide, for example, reduces the activity of luminal carbonic anhydrase, thereby decreasing the entry of H_2O and CO_2 across the luminal membrane, which decreases HCO_3^- reabsorption by the tubular cell (Fig. 71.1).

The process of reclamation of all filtered HCO_3^- by itself is not sufficient to maintain a normal blood pH. The kidney must also excrete the 50 to 100 mEq per kg of H^+ generated each day from the metabolism of dietary proteins, particularly sulfur-containing amino acids (i.e., methionine, cystine), which are converted to sulfuric acid. This acid load is initially buffered in the body to minimize changes in blood pH, causing a clinically undetectable decrease in the plasma HCO_3^- concentration. The kidney must eventually excrete this daily acid increment to replete the HCO_3^- used in this process, however, or more severe acidemia will develop over time.

Energy requirements limit the ability of the kidney to excrete acid (H^+ ions) when the urine pH falls below 4.5. To offset this limitation, urinary buffers are present in the urine that maintain the urine pH above this critical value, permitting ongoing excretion of the daily acid load.

Two distinct urinary buffering systems enable continued H^+ secretion: titratable acids and ammonia. Titratable acids (primarily HPO_4)[1] are freely filtered through the glomerulus and can combine with H^+:

$$HPO_4^- + H^+ \rightarrow H_2PO_4$$

Approximately one-half of the daily acid load is excreted in this way.

By comparison, the most important urinary buffer is ammonia, as the abundance of this buffer can be varied according to physiologic needs. Ammonia synthesis occurs in the proximal tubule, derived principally from the breakdown of glutamine to α-ketoglutarate (Fig. 71.2) [1]. This process is stimulated by intracellular acidosis and by hypokalemia, both of which act by decreasing the intracellular pH (see following). Ammonia thus generated can combine with intracellular H^+, forming ammonium (NH_4^+). NH_4^+ is then secreted into the proximal tubule lumen by substituting for H^+ on the Na-H antiporter. Ammonia (NH_3) that forms by the dissociation of H^+ from NH_4^+ is largely reabsorbed, recycled, and then secreted into the collecting tubule. There, it is trapped in the tubular lumen as NH_4^+ by combining with secreted H^+ and excreted as ammonium chloride (NH_4Cl). For each molecule of buffered H^+ excreted in the urine, an HCO_3^- is regenerated (Fig. 71.2), thus replenishing the HCO_3^- used initially by the body to buffer daily metabolic acid load.

METABOLIC ACIDOSIS

Metabolic acidosis can be categorized by the presence or absence of an increased anion gap. The *anion gap* (AG) refers to the difference between measured cations (Na^+) and measured anions (chloride [Cl^-] and HCO_3^-):[2]

$$AG = Na^+ - (Cl^- + HCO_3^-)$$

The normal AG varies between 3 and 11 mEq per L and averages approximately 7 to 8 mEq per L [2]. These unmeasured anions consist of proteins (primarily albumin), sulfates, phosphates, and circulating organic acids. Uric acid is a large molecule and therefore does not contribute significantly to the AG even when hyperuricemia is present.

[1] *Titratable acidity is determined by adding alkali to the daily urine volume. It is equal to the number of milliequivalents of base required to return the urine pH to 7.4.*

[2] *Potassium (K^+) is usually not included in the calculation of the AG because changes large enough to alter the gap significantly are uncommon or incompatible with life.*

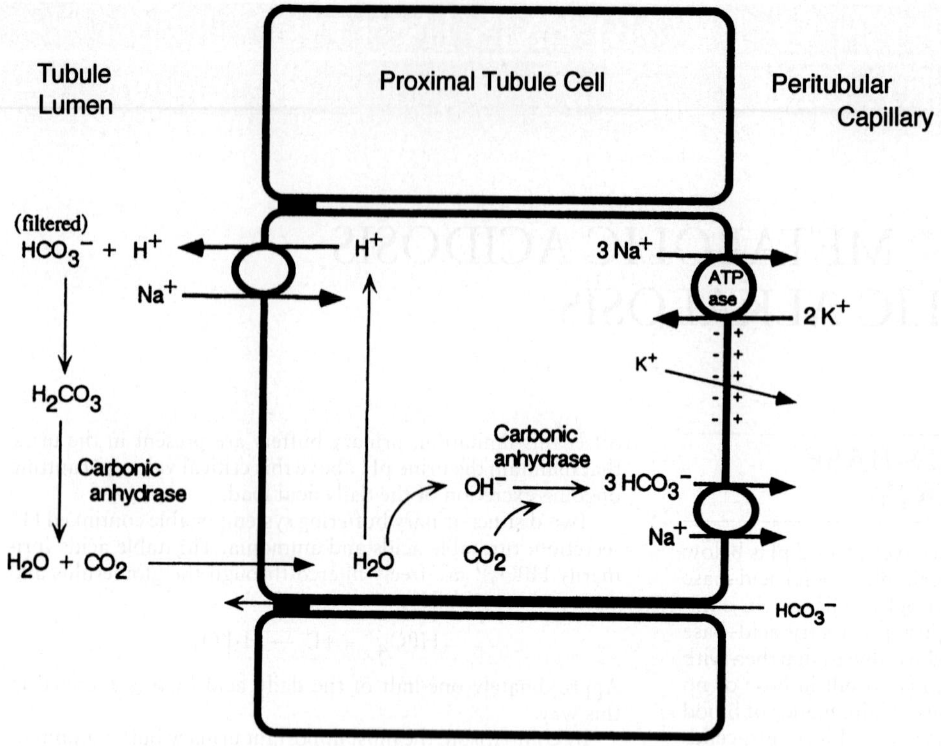

FIGURE 71.1. Proximal tubular reclamation of filtered bicarbonate (HCO_3). The first step in maintaining normal acid–base balance is the reabsorption of all filtered HCO_3. Inability to accomplish this results in metabolic acidosis (proximal, type 2, renal tubular acidosis). See text for details. ATPase, adenosine triphosphatase.

A reduction in the plasma albumin concentration can lower the baseline AG (approximately 2.5 mEq for every 1 g per dL fall in the albumin concentration) [3]. Thus, the hypoalbuminemic patient may not have a high AG even in the presence of a disorder that typically causes an elevation (e.g., lactic acidosis; see later).

Metabolic Acidosis with an Increased Anion Gap

The causes of metabolic acidosis associated with an increased AG are listed in Table 71.1. Lactic acidosis is the most frequent form in hospitalized patients, whereas chronic renal failure is the principal cause of an increased AG in ambulatory persons.

Chronic Kidney Disease (CKD)

Renal disease represents an interesting example of the potential overlap between normal and elevated AG acidosis. The high AG in patients with advanced chronic kidney disease is usually a late finding and reflects a severe reduction in glomerular filtration rate (GFR). As the GFR falls below 20 to 30 mL per minute (plasma creatinine >3 to 4 mg per dL), anions, such as sulfate and phosphate, that would normally be excreted by filtration are retained. With lesser degrees of renal dysfunction, however, metabolic acidosis appears primarily because H^+ (HCl) secretion is reduced, with little or no effect on the AG.

The metabolically generated daily acid load on a typical American diet approximates 50 to 100 mEq. This acid, mainly sulfuric, is immediately buffered by $NaHCO_3$:

$$H_2SO_4 + 2NaHCO_3 \rightarrow Na_2SO_4 + 2CO_2 + 2H_2O$$

The excess sulfate is excreted in the urine. If glomerular and tubular function decline in parallel, then the H^+ and the SO_4^{2-} are retained, producing metabolic acidosis with a high AG. If, however, there is more significant tubular dysfunction, the excretion of acid is diminished, but excretion of sulfate may be maintained due to reduced reabsorption. In the latter setting, the AG may not rise as the serum HCO_3^- concentration decreases.

Therefore, the decrease in plasma HCO_3^- (severity of acidemia) need not correlate with extent of the rise in AG in renal dysfunction. Typically, the plasma bicarbonate concentration is greater than 12 mEq per L in patients with uncomplicated CKD. A search for a second acid–base disorder is indicated when a lower HCO_3^- concentration is identified.

Lactic Acidosis

Lactic acidosis is probably the most common cause of severe metabolic acidosis encountered in the intensive care unit. The AG is always increased above baseline (normal lactate level

TABLE 71.1

CAUSES OF METABOLIC ACIDOSIS WITH AN INCREASED ANION GAP

Chronic kidney disease[a]
Lactic acidosis
Ketoacidosis (diabetic, alcoholic, starvation)[a]
Rhabdomyolysis
Ingestions
Salicylates
Methanol
Ethylene glycol
Pyroglutamic acid[b]
Toluene[c]

[a]May be associated with normal anion gap early in course or during therapy (ketoacidosis); see text for details.
[b]Usually due to acetaminophen.
[c]Toluene also may cause a non–anion gap acidosis (see Table 71.3).

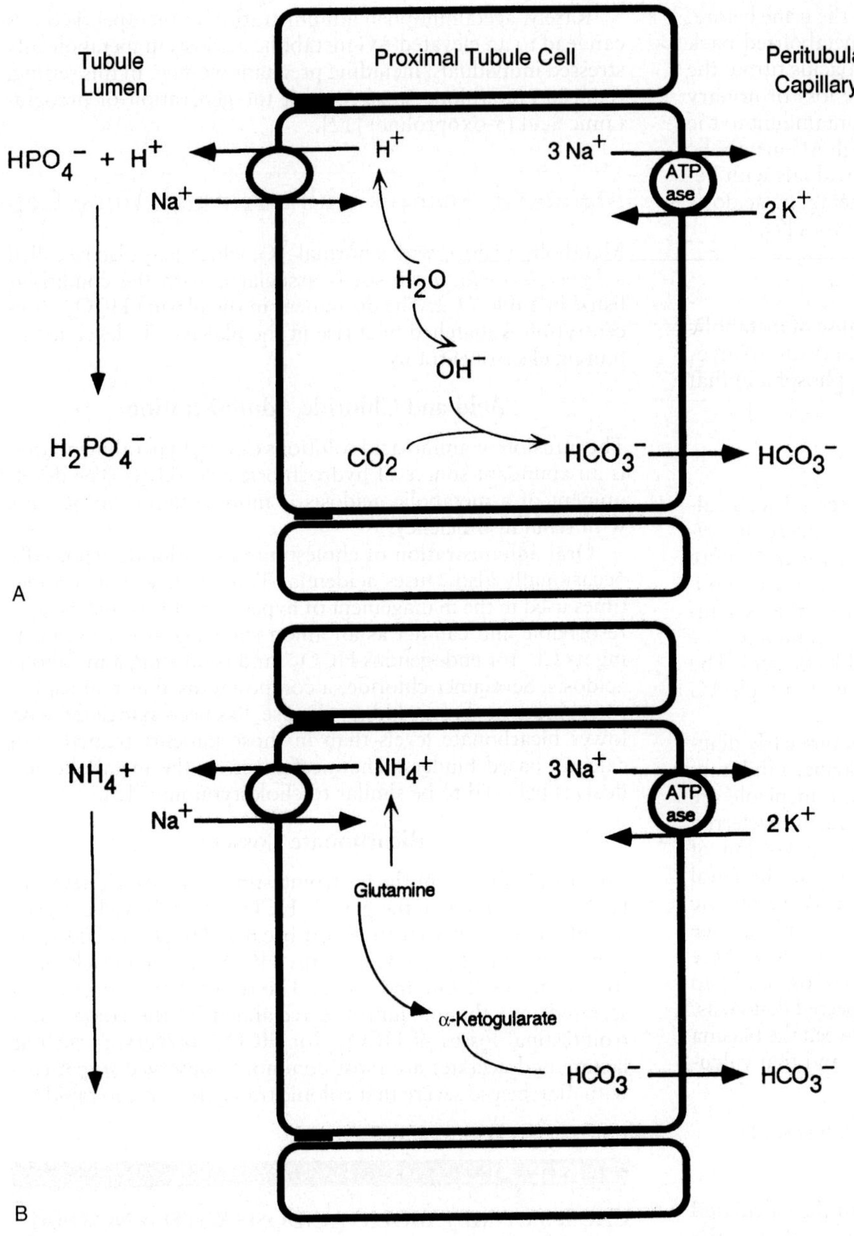

FIGURE 71.2. Excretion of the daily acid load permits the regeneration of bicarbonate (HCO_3) that was used as a buffer. Two processes are involved: the excretion of titratable acid (A) and the excretion of ammonium (NH_4^+) (B). The latter is particularly important because acidosis stimulates the breakdown of glutamine to ammonia. By comparison, hyperkalemia impairs the capacity of the proximal tubule to make ammonia, thus contributing to the metabolic acidosis observed in hyperkalemic disorders. ATPase, adenosine triphosphatase.

is <1.0 mmol per L)[3] because lactate does not appear in the urine until a higher plasma concentration (at least 6 to 8 mmol per L) is achieved. Lactate levels greater than 5 mmol per L are considered diagnostic of lactic acidosis, although levels between 2 and 5 mmol per L may be significant in the appropriate clinical circumstances [4]. Metformin, a biguanide commonly used in the treatment of type II diabetes mellitus, can cause lactic acidosis, particularly in patients who present with acute or chronic renal insufficiency. Hemodialysis has been used in the treatment of metformin-induced acidosis [5].

Most cases of lactic acidosis involve the L-isomer. By comparison, D-lactic acidosis, a disorder observed most commonly in patients with abnormal bowel anatomy, results in a rise in the AG, but the lactate level is normal [6]. D-Lactate is not detected by the usual lactate assay, which measures only L-lactate and a specific assay must be requested to diagnose this disorder.

Ketoacidosis

Ketoacidosis occurs when acetoacetic acid and β-hydroxybutyric acid are overproduced by the liver (see Chapter 101 for a complete discussion). Acetone, a breakdown product of acetoacetic acid, is not an acid; as such, it does not contribute to the acidemia or to the increased AG observed in this disorder.[4]

Although ketoacidosis is generally associated with an elevated AG, loss of ketoanions in the urine, particularly during intravenous fluid therapy, may attenuate the expansion of the

[3] *The more recently described condition of D-lactic acidosis requires a specific search for D-lactic acid, which is not routinely measured. This acid may be present in patients with short bowel syndrome or occasionally during antibiotic therapy, and is formed by intestinal bacteria [9,10]. Diagnosis requires a specific enzymatic assay because human lactate dehydrogenase metabolizes only L-lactate.*

[4] *Isopropyl alcohol is metabolized to acetone and can cause acute kidney injury. In this setting, ketonemia and ketonuria are characteristically present, whereas any increase in the AG is typically not due to ketoacidosis because acetoacetic acid and β-hydroxybutyric acid are not usually produced.*

AG. Once formed, ketones may be excreted in the urine before, under the influence of insulin, they can be metabolized back to HCO_3^-. Because the initially produced ketoacids titrate the plasma HCO_3^- concentration downward, the loss of urinary ketoanions (as sodium or potassium salts) is tantamount to the renal loss of HCO_3^-. The net effect is that a high AG metabolic acidosis is present before therapy in most individuals with ketoacidosis but may convert to a normal AG metabolic acidosis once saline repletion occurs and ketogenesis ceases [7].

Rhabdomyolysis

Massive muscle breakdown is an important cause of metabolic acidosis with an increased AG. Acute kidney injury due to myoglobinuria can cause retention of anions (e.g., phosphate) that have been released from damaged myocytes.

Ingestions

The most common acid–base abnormality observed with salicylate intoxication is a respiratory alkalosis caused by direct stimulation of the medullary respiratory center. A pure metabolic acidosis owing to aspirin toxicity is uncommon. With moderate-to-severe salicylate intoxication, the AG increases as salicylic acid, not simply due to accumulation of salicylate in the blood, promotes formation of lactic acid. The consequence is a mixed respiratory alkalosis with a high AG metabolic acidosis.

Methanol and ethylene glycol ingestions require early diagnosis because prompt treatment may be lifesaving. Inhibitors of alcohol dehydrogenase such as ethanol and fomepizole are used for this latter purpose, with fomepizole being the preferred agent, if available. Either agent can limit the conversion of the alcohols to their more toxic metabolic products. Methanol or ethylene glycol ingestion as a cause for high AG metabolic acidosis is suggested by the history and physical findings (see Chapter 119). The turnaround time for measurement of these toxins may delay treatment. The detection of an osmolal gap is a relatively quick way of supporting the suspected diagnosis.

The *osmolal gap* refers to the difference between the plasma osmolality (P_{Osm}) measured by the laboratory and that calculated using the following formula:

$$\text{Calculated } P_{Osm}(\text{mOsm/kg}) = 2 \times Na^+ + \text{glucose}/18 + \text{BUN}/2.8$$

Normally, the measured P_{Osm} is higher than the calculated value by 10 mOsm per kg. A larger osmolal gap indicates the presence of osmotically active substances not normally present. The most frequent causes of an increased osmolal gap are ethyl alcohol, isopropyl alcohol, ketones, lactate, mannitol, ethylene glycol, and methanol. If ethanol, lactate, or ketones cannot be identified in a patient with an AG metabolic acidosis with an osmolal gap, the diagnosis of ethylene glycol or methanol intoxication should be strongly suspected [8]. In the intensive care unit setting, a high osmolal gap acidosis has also been associated with the use of continuous high-dose infusions of lorazepam for more than 48 hours. Propylene glycol, which is used as a solvent for intravenous medications including lorazepam, has been implicated as the cause of the hyperosmolar metabolic acidosis in this scenario [9]. It is important to understand that the presence of an osmolal gap that results from an ingested alcohol may only be detected when P_{Osm} is measured in the laboratory by freezing-point depression [10]. Also, after the alcohol is metabolized, the osmolal gap may disappear.

Toluene (present in glue and metabolized to hippuric acid) is a rare cause of metabolic acidosis. The AG rises early and then returns toward normal, as hippurate is excreted by the kidneys, a process that is similar to the renal handling of ketones (see previous discussion) [11].

Rarely, acetaminophen administration in therapeutic doses can lead to an elevated AG metabolic acidosis in metabolically stressed individuals, including pregnant women. In this setting, reduced glutathione stores permit the generation of pyroglutamic acid (5-oxoproline) [12].

Metabolic Acidosis with a Normal Anion Gap

Metabolic acidosis with a normal AG, which may also be called a *hyperchloremic acidosis*, is associated with the conditions listed in Table 71.2. The decrement in the plasma HCO_3^- concentration is matched by a rise in the plasma Cl^- level, maintaining electroneutrality.

Acid and Chloride Administration

The infusion of amino acid solutions during hyperalimentation is an abundant source of hydrochloric acid (HCl). The development of a metabolic acidosis is more common in patients with renal insufficiency.

Oral administration of cholestyramine chloride reportedly occasionally also causes acidemia. This resin, which is sometimes used in the management of hypercholesterolemia, is nonresorbable and can act as an anion-exchange resin, exchanging its Cl^- for endogenous HCO_3^- and producing a metabolic acidosis. Sevelamer chloride, a compound used as a phosphorous binder in chronic kidney disease, has been associated with lower bicarbonate levels than in those patients treated with calcium-based binders. The mechanism of the metabolic acidosis is believed to be similar to cholestyramine [13].

Bicarbonate Losses

Loss of HCO_3^- from the gastrointestinal tract or kidneys can lead to a reduction in the plasma HCO_3^- level. Bowel contents are alkaline compared to blood because HCO_3^- is added by pancreatic and biliary secretions. HCO_3^- is later exchanged for Cl^- in the ileum and colon. The result is that most alkali secreted into the gut lumen is reclaimed by the colon. Gastrointestinal losses of HCO_3^- (or HCO_3^- precursors such as lactate and acetate) are most commonly observed in patients with diarrhea so severe that colonic transit time is too rapid for

TABLE 71.2

CAUSES OF METABOLIC ACIDOSIS WITH A NORMAL ANION GAP

Acid administration
Hyperalimentation with HCl-containing amino acid solutions
Bicarbonate losses
Gastrointestinal
Diarrhea
Pancreatic or biliary drainage
Cholestyramine and sevelamer chloride
Urinary diversions (ureterosigmoidostomy)
Renal
Proximal (type 2) renal tubular acidosis
Ketoacidosis (particularly during therapy)
Post–chronic hypocapnia
Impaired renal acid excretion
With hypokalemia
Classic distal (type 1) renal tubular acidosis
With hyperkalemia
Hyperkalemic distal renal tubular acidosis
Hypoaldosteronism (type 4 renal tubular acidosis)
Reduced renal perfusion

TABLE 71.3

SOME CAUSES OF TYPES 1 AND 2 RENAL TUBULAR ACIDOSIS (RTA)

Distal (type 1) RTA	Proximal (type 2) RTA
Idiopathic	Hereditary disorders
Genetic	Cystinosis
Familial	Wilson's disease[c]
Marfan's syndrome	Glycogen storage disease, type 1
Ehlers–Danlos syndrome	Acquired disorders
Disorders of calcium metabolism	Multiple myeloma[c]
Idiopathic hypercalciuria	Primary hyperparathyroidism
Hypergammaglobulinemic states	Toxins and drugs
Amyloidosis[a]	Lead
Cryoglobulinemia	Cadmium
Drugs and toxins	Mercury
Amphotericin B	Copper (Wilson's disease)[c]
Lithium carbonate	Carbonic anhydrase inhibitors
Toluene[b]	Topiramate
Autoimmune diseases	
Sjögren's syndrome[a]	
Thyroiditis	
Chronic active hepatitis	
Primary biliary cirrhosis	
Miscellaneous	
Cirrhosis	
Medullary sponge kidney	
Associated with hyperkalemia	
Urinary tract obstruction	
Sickle cell anemia	
Systemic lupus erythematosus	
Renal transplant rejection[a]	

[a] Also may cause proximal RTA.
[b] Metabolism to hippuric acid may cause the anion gap to increase.
[c] Also may cause distal RTA.

alkali reabsorption. At times, the resulting HCO_3^- losses can approach 40 mEq per L of stool. Less frequently, metabolic acidosis from HCO_3^- depletion is a result of pancreatic fistulae, biliary drainage, or a ureterosigmoidostomy. In the last circumstance, the excretion of acid (as NH_4Cl) urine directly into the colon permits the exchange of HCl for HCO_3^- because the colon is permeable to H^+ and Cl^-, unlike the urinary bladder [14]. This problem does not usually occur with an ileal bladder.

Pancreatic HCO_3^- losses are also observed in essentially all patients with a pancreatic allograft anastomosed directly to the urinary bladder. Bicarbonate secreted into the bladder cannot be reabsorbed.

Renal bicarbonate losses can cause or contribute to acidemia in type 2 (proximal) renal tubular acidosis (RTA; Table 71.2),[5] during recovery from ketoacidosis (see previous discussion), and in patients who are posthypercapnia. In patients with proximal RTA (Table 71.3), the normal reabsorptive threshold for HCO_3^- is reduced. As a result, HCO_3^- can no longer be reabsorbed at a rate adequate to maintain the normal plasma level of approximately 25 mEq per L. As a consequence, the urine pH is alkaline (>5.3), and the fractional excretion of HCO_3^- is elevated (>15% of the filtered load).[6] Normally, this value is less than 3% because more than 97% of HCO_3^- filtered through the glomerulus is reclaimed, primarily in the proximal tubule (Fig. 71.1). HCO_3^- wasting ceases, however, and the urine becomes acidic (pH <5.3) once the plasma HCO_3^- concentration has stabilized at the new (lower) level. This process explains why the urine pH may be high or low in proximal RTA.

Renal HCO_3^- losses also occur as compensation for chronic respiratory alkalosis (chronic hypocapnia). During chronic hyperventilation, the blood pH increases as the PCO_2 decreases. As can be seen in Figure 71.1, an increase in intracellular pH diminishes H^+ excretion, leading to a concomitant decrease in HCO_3^- reabsorption. These changes cause the plasma HCO_3^- concentration to fall, partially compensating for the alkalemia. If the stimulus for hyperventilation (e.g., hypoxemia) is suddenly eliminated, the PCO_2 rapidly returns to normal. Renal compensation, by comparison, continues for 1 to 2 more days, causing a persistent reduction in the plasma HCO_3^- concentration. The resulting posthypocapnic metabolic acidosis normally resolves spontaneously.

[5] *The RTAs can be classified as type 1 (distal), type 2 (proximal), and type 4 (hypoaldosteronism). Type 3 refers to what is now considered to be an infantile variant of type 1; therefore, type 3 RTA is a term not generally applied to adults.*

[6] *The fractional excretion of HCO_3^- is equal to the amount of HCO_3^- excreted divided by the filtered load:*

$$\text{Fractional excretion }(HCO_3) = \frac{\text{urine } HCO_3^- \times \text{plasma creatinine}}{\text{urine creatinine} \times \text{plasma } HCO_3^-} \times 100.$$

Reduced Renal H^+ Excretion

Reduced renal acid excretion can be observed in four conditions: chronic kidney disease, type 1 (distal) RTA (Table 71.3), type 4 RTA (hypoaldosteronism), and states of reduced renal perfusion. The acidosis of chronic kidney disease is primarily caused by a reduction in ammonia production. Patients with chronic renal insufficiency have a substantial drop in the number of functioning nephrons. Nephrons that continue to filter, however, characteristically have filtration rates and acid excretion rates per nephron that are above normal. Impaired acid excretion in these patients occurs because the number of hyperfiltering nephrons is inadequate to compensate for those that are nonfunctioning. The AG is frequently normal in mild-to-moderate kidney disease (plasma creatinine <3 mg per dL) because Cl^- replaces the HCO_3^- used to buffer the retained acid. At this time, the GFR is still high enough to permit the excretion of anions like phosphate, which contribute to the rise in AG as renal function declines further.

The classic form of type 1 (distal) RTA (Table 71.3) occurs when H^+ cannot be pumped into the tubule lumen by the intercalated cells of the collecting tubule. The result is that urine cannot be maximally acidified (urine pH is always ≥5.5). In addition to metabolic acidosis, hypokalemia is typically present. The K^+ deficit is caused in part by enhanced distal nephron Na-K exchange, a process that is necessary to maintain Na^+ balance because H^+ cannot be secreted in response to Na^+ reabsorption. Recent studies also report distal RTA resulting from a translocation of the bicarbonate–chloride exchanger from the peritubular to the luminal membrane. The net effect is secretion of bicarbonate into the collecting tubule lumen.

The most important clinical complication of distal RTA is the formation and deposition of calcium throughout the kidney (nephrocalcinosis). This process begins in the collecting tubules, where the urine is most concentrated, and is commonly accompanied by the formation of calcium phosphate calculi. The factors that may contribute to the renal stone disease in this disorder include hypercalciuria, because metabolic acidosis causes a release of bone calcium that can then be filtered and excreted; the alkaline urine pH, which predisposes to the precipitation of calcium phosphate crystals; and, most importantly, hypocitraturia. The reduction in urinary citrate is a direct result of the metabolic acidosis, which increases proximal tubular citrate reabsorption [15]. Since calcium citrate is significantly more soluble than calcium phosphate, hypocitraturia facilitates the precipitation of calcium phosphate crystals in the tubular lumen.[7] In comparison with distal RTA, stone formation is less common and less severe in patients with proximal RTA, possibly because a proportion of these patients may have the full Fanconi syndrome, in which proximal tubular reabsorption of HCO_3^- and many other substances, including citrate, is impaired [16].

In addition to the classic form of type 1 (distal) RTA, in which hypokalemia is characteristic, a hyperkalemic variety has also been described. This disorder, as well as type 4 (hypoaldosteronism) RTA, is discussed in Chapter 72.

Clinical Signs and Symptoms of Metabolic Acidosis

Kussmaul respirations on physical examination suggest the presence of metabolic acidosis. This unusual respiratory pattern reflects an increase in tidal volume rather than a rise in respiratory rate and is caused by stimulation of the respiratory center in the brainstem by the low blood pH. As acidemia becomes more severe, nausea and vomiting or mental status changes, including coma, may occur.

Secondary hypotension also may be observed in severely acidemic patients, the hypotension resulting from depressed myocardial contractility and arterial vasodilation. Although circulating catecholamines may initially counteract the adverse cardiovascular effects of acidemia, such compensation becomes insufficient as the blood pH falls below 7.20.

The plasma K^+ concentration may be altered by the degree of metabolic acidosis. Infusion of a mineral acid such as arginine HCl, for example, causes a prompt rise in the plasma K^+ concentration as K^+ moves out of cells in exchange for H^+. By comparison, a shift of K^+ is less likely to occur in those patients with metabolic acidosis caused by organic acids, such as lactic and ketoacidosis [17]. The reason for this apparent difference is uncertain, but it may relate to the release of insulin by organic substrates (e.g., lactate), which would drive K^+ into cells.

Diagnosis

The diagnosis of a simple metabolic acidosis is made relatively easy by the presence of a low blood pH and plasma bicarbonate concentration. The detection of a widened AG can then be used to identify a specific cause for the disorder. The likelihood of identifying a specific acid(s) in a patient with a high AG acidosis increases as the width of the AG increases.

In comparison with patients with a simple metabolic acidosis, many individuals have a concomitant respiratory or second metabolic acid–base disorder. Consequently, knowledge of the appropriate respiratory compensation as well as an understanding of the ratio of the increment in AG to decrement in plasma HCO_3^- concentration is useful.

Respiratory Compensation

Stimulation of the brainstem respiratory center by acidemia causes a fall in the PCO_2 that, in uncomplicated metabolic acidosis, can be estimated from the following equation:

$$\text{Expected } PCO_2 \text{ (mm Hg)} = [(1.5 \times HCO_3^-) + 8] \pm 2$$

A PCO_2 that is substantially different from the expected value indicates a superimposed respiratory acidosis or alkalosis. For example, if the plasma bicarbonate concentration were 10 mEq per L, the expected PCO_2 would be approximately 23 mm Hg [(1.5 × 10) + 8] = 23. A lower PCO_2 would indicate the presence of a concomitant respiratory alkalosis (as might be seen with a salicylate overdose), whereas a higher PCO_2 would signify a simultaneous respiratory acidosis. *This calculation is useful only in the evaluation of the respiratory response to metabolic acidosis and it is inaccurate when the plasma bicarbonate concentration is more than 20 mEq per L.*

There is a more rapid method to determine the appropriateness of respiratory compensation in patients with a primary metabolic acidosis. By a quirk of mathematics, the last two digits of the pH (27 in a patient with a pH of 7.27) should equal the PCO_2 if respiratory compensation is appropriate. A lower PCO_2 indicates a superimposed respiratory alkalosis, whereas a higher value signifies a primary respiratory acidosis.

Ratio of Change in Anion Gap to Change in Bicarbonate Concentration in Metabolic Acidosis and Its Use in Identifying a Second Metabolic Acidosis or a Metabolic Alkalosis

In patients with a high AG metabolic acidosis, the identification of a second metabolic acid–base disorder (normal AG acidosis)

[7] *Most renal calculi are composed of calcium oxalate. In comparison, the presence of a persistently alkaline urine pH predisposes to calcium phosphate stone formation.*

can be made by comparing the change in the AG to the change in the plasma HCO_3^- concentration.

The elevation in AG is due to the increase in the unmeasured anions. However, there is not always a 1-to-1 relationship between the increase in AG (ΔAG) and the fall in plasma bicarbonate (ΔHCO_3^-) because some of the excess hydrogen ions are buffered by nonbicarbonate buffers (including intracellular proteins and bone).

The magnitude of the increment in AG, therefore, generally exceeds that of the decrement in plasma HCO_3^- concentration. As the plasma HCO_3^- concentration falls, there is a progressive reduction in extracellular-buffering capacity (which almost entirely consists of HCO_3^-) [18]. The result is that the Δ/Δ ratio averages approximately 1.4 to 1.6:1 in lactic acidosis. Thus, a patient with a plasma HCO_3^- concentration of 14 mEq per L (10 mEq per L below normal) should have an AG that is approximately 24 mEq per L (16 mEq per L above normal), assuming that the baseline (normal) AG is 8 mEq per L.

Although the same principles apply to ketoacidosis, the Δ/Δ ratio averages approximately 1:1. In this disorder, the loss of ketoacid anions in the urine (as the sodium and potassium salts of β-hydroxybutyrate and acetoacetate) lowers the initially elevated AG without affecting the plasma HCO_3^- concentration. In contrast, urinary anion loss is minimal in lactic acidosis because shock is typically associated with reduced urinary flow rate, and most of the lactate that is filtered can be reabsorbed by a specific sodium-L-lactate cotransporter in the luminal membrane of the proximal tubular cells.

The amount of ketoacid anions excreted in ketoacidosis depends on the degree to which glomerular filtration is maintained. Patients with impaired renal function (owing to underlying diabetic nephropathy or volume depletion) retain the ketoacid anions and have a relatively high AG in relation to the fall in the plasma HCO_3^- concentration, similar to that in lactic acidosis. In comparison, patients with relatively normal renal function can lose large quantities of ketoacids in the urine and may have a Δ/Δ below 1. In fact, the loss of ketoacid anions in the urine causes the frequent development of a hyperchloremic (normal AG) metabolic acidosis during the treatment (recovery phase) of diabetic ketoacidosis [19].

Conversely, when the ΔAG is more than double the ΔHCO_3^-, a coexisting metabolic alkalosis and metabolic acidosis is likely. An example of this situation would be severe vomiting in a patient with ketoacidosis.

Changes in the concentration of other unmeasured cations or anions in the plasma can also lead to miscalculation of the AG. As an example, hypoalbuminemia (decreased unmeasured anions) and severe hypercalcemia (increased unmeasured cations) can lower the AG. Thus, a patient with one or both of these disorders may have a baseline AG of 4 rather than 8 or 9 mEq per L. In this setting, an AG of 13 mEq per L, which is only mildly above normal, represents a true elevation in the AG of 9 mEq per L. As a result, calculation of the Δ/Δ is most accurate when the preacidosis AG is known.

Urinary Anion Gap

Another useful tool in the evaluation of a metabolic acidosis is the urinary AG (UAG). The UAG is the difference between the sum of the urinary Na^+ and K^+ and the urinary Cl^-:

$$UAG = (Na^+ + K^+) - Cl^-$$

The most frequent use of the UAG is to identify the etiology of a normal AG metabolic acidosis with hypokalemia [20,21]. The most common nonrenal cause is diarrhea, which provokes an appropriate increase in renal H^+ secretion. These additional H^+ ions are buffered in the urine by ammonia and excreted primarily as NH_4Cl. Because NH_4^+ is not measured in the calculation of the UAG, but Cl^- is, an increased rate of renal H^+ secretion causes the UAG to become a negative number. Conversely, the presence of a positive UAG in an individual with a non-AG metabolic acidosis suggests that the disorder is due to impaired renal H^+ excretion (e.g., distal RTA). In this setting, impaired H^+ secretion leads to a fall in urinary Cl^- (which would be excreted as NH_4Cl) and a positive calculated UAG. It is important to note, however, that underlying renal insufficiency may also be associated with impaired NH_4Cl excretion owing to a limitation in ammonia synthesis; in these individuals, the UAG may remain positive even in the presence of diarrhea.

Treatment of Metabolic Acidosis

Treatment of metabolic acidosis must be directed at correction of acidemia as well as the cause of the acid–base disturbance. The likelihood that alkali administration is necessary and that it will be effective depends on the blood pH, compensatory mechanisms, and the underlying cause.

The degree of acidemia and hypobicarbonatemia should be evaluated before administering alkali. As a general rule, alkali therapy generally is not needed until the arterial blood pH drops below 7.15 to 7.20 [22]. An exception may occur when the plasma HCO_3^- concentration falls to less than 10 to 12 mEq per L, despite a blood pH of more than 7.15. Alkali administration is usually unnecessary if the acidosis is likely to resolve spontaneously (e.g., lactic acidosis after a grand mal seizure).

Alkali Administration

HCO_3^- therapy should be considered in patients with moderate-to-severe metabolic acidosis. However, depending on the etiology, the use of exogenous bicarbonate remains controversial [22]. The initial goal of alkali therapy is to raise the arterial blood pH to 7.20, a typically safe level at which the patient is at less risk of cardiovascular compromise. The pH does not need to be corrected back to normal because the potential risks of HCO_3^- therapy (e.g., hypernatremia, hypercapnia, fluid overload, cerebrospinal fluid acidosis, and "overshoot" alkalosis) are likely to outweigh the benefits, as long as renal function (and therefore acid-excretory ability) is relatively intact.

The quantity of exogenous bicarbonate required to produce a change in pH is determined by estimating the total body HCO_3^- deficit. The apparent HCO_3^- space is about 50% of lean body weight in healthy subjects. In patients with more severe metabolic acidosis (plasma HCO_3^- concentration <10 mEq per L), cellular and bone buffering become more prominent owing to the marked reduction in the quantity of available extracellular buffer (primarily HCO_3^-). This preferential entry of H^+ into cells causes the HCO_3^- space to expand to approximately 70% of the lean body weight.

These are only rough guidelines and cannot replace ongoing monitoring of serum bicarbonate level and arterial pH during the correction phase. Furthermore, if there is continuing alkali loss from diarrhea, then the HCO_3^- requirements are substantially increased because the apparent volume of distribution of HCO_3^- is much greater than 70% of body weight in this setting.

Treatment of Specific Causes of Metabolic Acidosis

Renal Disease. Treatment of the metabolic acidosis of renal dysfunction depends on the clinical manifestations and the severity of the acidosis. Most individuals with acute kidney injury can be managed with dialysis or using the guidelines for alkali administration listed previously. There is some recent data suggesting that alkali therapy can slow down the rate of decline in chronic kidney disease and reduce mortality in this setting [23].

Ketoacidosis. The plasma glucose concentration does not correlate with the degree of acidemia in ketoacidosis [24]. Moreover, the blood glucose level may normalize before ketoacid production has ceased.

The initial management of patients with diabetic ketoacidosis with very large fluid volumes has been challenged [7]. The advantages of intensive fluid administration may be limited after the intravascular volume has been restored because volume expansion then leads to the excretion of ketone anions in the urine. Moreover, excessive expansion of the plasma volume reduces proximal tubular HCO_3^- reabsorption, in part by reducing Na-H exchange. The net effect is normalization of the AG without a significant increase in the plasma HCO_3^- concentration. In this setting, spontaneous correction of the metabolic acidosis requires regeneration of new bicarbonate by the kidney (a process that may take several days), in contrast to the rapid increase in HCO_3^- that occurs when ketone anions are metabolized back to HCO_3^- in the liver as insulin is given. Consequently, fluid administration should be tempered after intravascular volume compromise has been corrected.

Alkali administration is not usually necessary for patients with ketoacidosis, There appears to be no difference in mortality between patients treated with $NaHCO_3$ versus controls [22]. Insulin therapy should raise the plasma HCO_3^- concentration as ketone anions are metabolized. Patients who may benefit from cautious alkali therapy include those with severe acidemia (in whom cardiovascular compromise is secondarily present) and those with a normal AG acidosis. As already discussed, the latter condition pertains to those who have sustained major urinary losses of ketones, rendering them depleted of potential bicarbonate substrate.

Lactic Acidosis. Correction of any predisposing disorder is the primary therapy for lactic acidosis. Reversal of circulatory failure, hypoxemia, or sepsis reduces the rate of lactate production and enhances its removal.

The benefit of $NaHCO_3$ in the treatment of lactic acidosis remains unproven [22]. The potential benefits of alkali administration principally involve the maintenance of normal cardiovascular homeostasis. This potential advantage must be weighed against possible deleterious effects such as volume overload, hypernatremia, and overshoot alkalosis after restoration of tissue perfusion. Recent data also suggest that HCO_3^- therapy may not improve the blood pH or survival in lactic acidosis. Alkali therapy may also have a direct negative effect on cardiac function by reducing coronary perfusion pressure, which could explain the fall in cardiac output observed in some patients treated with HCO_3^- in this setting [14].

As a result of these potential problems, no concrete recommendations can be made regarding alkali therapy in lactic acidosis. One approach might be to administer HCO_3^- to maintain the arterial blood pH above 7.15 to 7.20 and the plasma HCO_3^- concentration above 10 to 12 mEq per L, as suggested previously (see Alkali Administration section). However, if the lactate level increases without a significant improvement in clinical status or blood pH, the benefit of continuing alkali administration should be questioned. It appears that correction of the underlying cause of lactic acidosis is the most important goal, as measures raise the bicarbonate level without a fall in lactate have not been associated with a reduction in mortality [14]. These findings are consistent with the hypothesis that the high mortality in lactic acidosis results from the underlying disorder causing the acidosis, not from the acidemia per se.

Drug and Toxin Ingestions. The treatment of toxins and ingestions is discussed in Section 10.

Renal Tubular Acidosis. The acidemia of type 1 (distal) RTA can be corrected with HCO_3^- or a precursor such as citrate. The usual requirement is 1 to 3 mEq per kg per day, which should be sufficient to buffer that fraction of the daily acid load (50 to 100 mEq per day) that is not being excreted. In general, a potassium salt is administered (e.g., potassium citrate) because this repairs the K^+ deficit as well. Large doses of oral $NaHCO_3$ can cause gastrointestinal symptoms by generating CO_2 in the stomach. This problem can be minimized by the use of citrate, most of which is ultimately metabolized in the body to HCO_3^-. Solutions are available that contain 1 to 2 mEq per mL of sodium, potassium, or sodium and potassium citrate.

The initial step in the management of type 2 (proximal) RTA is to determine the presence of a treatable underlying disorder, such as vitamin D deficiency, multiple myeloma, or the use of a carbonic anhydrase inhibitor. Even if no specific therapy is available, correction of the acidemia may not be required in adults if the patient is asymptomatic and if there is only mild-to-moderate reduction in the plasma HCO_3^- concentration. In comparison, treatment is always indicated in young children because restoring acid–base balance can permit normal growth to resume.

The evaluation and treatment of the hyperkalemic form of distal RTA and of type 4 RTA (hypoaldosteronism), in which hyperkalemia is also present, can be found in Chapter 73.

METABOLIC ALKALOSIS

Primary metabolic alkalosis is characterized by an elevated plasma HCO_3^- concentration in the presence of an arterial pH above 7.40. When there is a concomitant metabolic acidosis, however, the blood pH may be increased, decreased, or normal. Because hyperbicarbonatemia may represent the appropriate response to chronic respiratory acidosis, by itself it is not diagnostic of metabolic alkalosis. These conditions can be easily distinguished by measurement of the arterial blood pH, which is reduced in respiratory acidosis.

Pathophysiology and Etiology

There are two steps involved in the development of metabolic alkalosis. The factors that mediate the *generation* phase may differ from those that enable its *maintenance*. For this reason, the evaluation and treatment of metabolic alkalosis are made easier by first reviewing the pathophysiology of these factors.

A primary rise in the plasma HCO_3^- concentration can be induced by one or more of three mechanisms: (a) loss of acid from the gastrointestinal tract or in the urine, (b) administration of HCO_3^- or a precursor such as citrate, or (c) loss of fluid with a Cl^--to-HCO_3^- ratio that is higher than that of plasma [25]. The third condition is sometimes referred to as *contraction alkalosis* because the total HCO_3^- content remains relatively unchanged while the extracellular fluid volume "contracts around it," thereby elevating the HCO_3^- concentration. In contrast to the first two mechanisms, contraction alkalosis is rarely responsible for more than a mild increase in the plasma HCO_3^- concentration. Loss of fluid with an electrolyte composition similar to that of plasma, as might occur with hemorrhage, does not result in a contraction alkalosis because HCO_3^- is lost proportionately to the other molecular components of plasma.

The excess in HCO_3^- generated by any of these processes should be rapidly excreted in the urine. The maintenance of a metabolic alkalosis, therefore, indicates an impairment of renal HCO_3^- excretion. The most common hindrances to renal disposal of bicarbonate are volume and potassium depletion.

Under ordinary conditions, HCO_3^- appears in the urine when the plasma level rises above the normal value of approximately 25 mEq per L. In the presence of volume depletion, however, the capacity of the proximal tubule to reabsorb HCO_3^- increases, allowing the plasma HCO_3^- level to rise without triggering bicarbonaturia. Several mechanisms account for these changes, including stimulation of luminal Na-H countertransport (Fig. 71.1) by angiotensin II, generated in response to volume contraction [26]. Most hypovolemic states are associated with Cl^- depletion. Because tubular luminal Cl^- appears to be important in distal nephron Cl^-–HCO_3^- exchange, it is not surprising that correction of the metabolic alkalosis usually requires Cl^- repletion as well [27]. In comparison, giving Cl^- may be ineffective when primary or secondary hyperaldosteronism, severe hypokalemia, or renal insufficiency is responsible for the defect in HCO_3^- excretion. The cause of a metabolic alkalosis can usually be identified by how readily it responds to administration of Cl^- (see Diagnosis section). The effect of hypokalemia in the maintenance of metabolic alkalosis is discussed later in this chapter.

Alkali Administration

Because administered HCO_3^- is normally excreted rapidly in the urine, alkali administration must be massive, or renal impairment must limit the excretion of HCO_3^- if metabolic alkalosis is to develop. Milk-alkali syndrome is an uncommon disorder characterized by hypercalcemia and metabolic alkalosis. It is now rarely seen, probably because nonabsorbable antacids, proton-pump inhibitors, and H_2-blockers have largely supplanted the use of large quantities of baking soda and milk as treatment of gastritis and peptic ulcer disease. The chronic ingestion of milk and calcium carbonate–containing antacids can lead to the development of metabolic alkalosis, however, because the increased HCO_3^- load cannot be excreted as a result of renal impairment from chronic hypercalcemia [28].

Chloride-Responsive Metabolic Alkalosis

Generation of Chloride-Responsive Metabolic Alkalosis. The two most common causes of metabolic alkalosis are diuretic therapy and loss of gastric secretions (resulting from nasogastric suction or vomiting) (Table 71.4). Thiazide and loop diuretics can generate a metabolic alkalosis, regardless of whether they are given to treat hypertension or states of volume overload such as congestive heart failure. H^+ loss results from increased distal Na^+ presentation in the presence of elevated aldosterone levels, which causes enhanced distal nephron Na-H exchange. Hydrogen secretion in this nephron segment is associated with increased HCO_3^- generation. The proximal tubule may also play an important role because stimulation of the renin–angiotensin system by volume depletion enhances the activity of the Na-H antiporter, thereby increasing H^+ secretion and HCO_3^- reabsorption. To the degree that the urinary anion losses represent primarily Cl^-, a component of contraction alkalosis may also occur.

Although volume contraction may contribute to the metabolic alkalosis caused by vomiting and nasogastric suction, and occasionally with intestinal Cl^- wasting [29], gastric H^+ losses are primarily responsible for the generation of metabolic alkalosis in this setting. Secretion of gastric acid results in the retention of 1 mEq of HCO_3^- for each milliequivalent of H^+ that is secreted because both of the ions are derived from the intracellular dissociation of carbonic acid:

$$H_2CO_3 \rightarrow HCO_3^- + H^+$$

This process does not normally lead to metabolic alkalosis because the 80 to 200 mEq of HCl secreted by the stomach each day enters the duodenum, where it stimulates an equivalent amount of HCO_3^- secretion from the pancreas. By comparison, when vomiting or nasogastric suctioning occurs, the H^+ secreted by the stomach never reaches the duodenum and therefore cannot induce pancreatic HCO_3^- secretion. Hence, there is a net retention of HCO_3^-. As in diuretic use, distal nephron Na-H exchange also contributes to the development of this disorder because aldosterone levels are stimulated by the loss of extracellular volume.

Renal H^+ and K^+ losses also contribute to the metabolic alkalosis and K^+ depletion observed in hypercalcemic states [30].

Metabolic alkalosis also may be observed after the rapid correction of chronic respiratory acidosis. This *posthypercapnic metabolic alkalosis* occurs because chronic respiratory acidosis activates compensatory renal mechanisms that induce HCl loss in the urine; the ensuing rise in the plasma HCO_3^- concentration is appropriate in that it returns the arterial pH toward normal. The plasma HCO_3^- generally increases by approximately 3.5 mEq per L for every 10 mm Hg rise in the arterial PCO_2. If hypercapnia is rapidly reversed, however (most frequently by artificial ventilation), because the excess HCO_3^- that has been generated may persist a while, alkalemia ensues.

TABLE 71.4

MAJOR CAUSES OF METABOLIC ALKALOSIS

Hydrogen loss
Gastrointestinal
Loss of gastric secretions (vomiting or nasogastric suction)[a]
Chloride-losing diarrheal states
Renal
Loop or thiazide-type diuretic[a]
Mineralocorticoid excess[a]
Postchronic hypercapnia
Hypercalcemia[b]
High-dose intravenous penicillins
Bartter's and Gitelman's syndromes
Bicarbonate retention
Massive blood transfusion
Administration of large amounts of $NaHCO_3$
Milk-alkali syndrome
Contraction alkalosis
Diuretics[a]
Loss of high chloride/low bicarbonate gastrointestinal secretions[a] (vomiting and some diarrheal states)
Hydrogen movement into cells
Hypokalemia
Refeeding

[a] Most common causes.
[b] Primary hyperparathyroidism is frequently associated with a mild metabolic acidosis (see text for details).

Maintenance of Chloride-Responsive Metabolic Alkalosis. As reviewed previously, renal excretion of HCO_3^- normally begins when the plasma level exceeds 25 mEq per L. The normal kidney can excrete large quantities (>1,000 mEq per L) without a substantial increase in the plasma HCO_3^- concentration. As a result, maintenance of a Cl^--responsive alkalosis implies a reduction in renal HCO_3^- excretion. Reduced GFR and, more importantly, enhanced proximal tubular $NaHCO_3$ reabsorption limit HCO_3^- excretion, allowing the increase in plasma HCO_3^- to persist. Normally, Cl^- is the major anion reabsorbed with Na^+. In states of Cl^- depletion, as occurs in Cl^--responsive metabolic alkalosis, however, Na^+ must be reabsorbed with the next most abundant anion, HCO_3^-.

Consequently, the need to preserve volume prevents correction of the alkalosis.

Hypokalemia also promotes renal HCO_3^- reabsorption and contributes to the maintenance of metabolic alkalosis. K^+ losses frequently occur with diuretic administration or gastric acid losses. If the plasma HCO_3^- concentration exceeds the reabsorptive capacity of the proximal renal tubule, the resultant bicarbonaturia obligates excretion of a cation (e.g., Na^+). Some of the Na^+ leaving the proximal tubule with HCO_3^- is then reabsorbed distally in exchange for K^+. These urinary K^+ losses are primarily responsible for the hypokalemia seen with vomiting; gastric K^+ losses are usually less important because these secretions have a K^+ concentration of less than 10 mEq per L. As a result of K^+ depletion, relative intracellular acidosis occurs as H^+ shifts into cells to maintain electroneutrality as K^+ moves extracellularly in response to hypokalemia.[8] Ultimately, this intracellular acidosis stimulates proximal tubular Na-H exchange, which further reduces renal HCO_3^- excretion (Fig. 71.1).

Chloride-Resistant Metabolic Alkalosis

Metabolic alkalosis in some individuals is not responsive to the administration of Cl^--containing solutions. In these disorders, a primary increase in mineralocorticoid activity, potassium depletion, or disorders of renal tubular Cl^- wasting (Bartter's and Gitelman's syndromes [31]) are usually responsible for the generation and maintenance of the alkalosis. In all of these circumstances, there is enhanced renal H^+ excretion and HCO_3^- reabsorption. Either there is no Cl^- depletion or there is an inability to reabsorb Cl^-explaining why NaCl and KCl do not correct the metabolic alkalosis in these individuals. Edematous states, such as congestive heart failure and cirrhosis, also are generally unresponsive to volume (and Cl^-) replacement, despite the reduction in effective arterial blood volume.

Mineralocorticoid Excess. Mineralocorticoids, such as aldosterone, act in the cortical collecting tubule (see Chapter 72), where they enhance Na-K exchange as well as H^+ secretion. As a result, overproduction of an endogenous mineralocorticoid (as occurs in primary aldosteronism) or with the ingestion of a substance that can increase the mineralocorticoid activity of cortisol (e.g., glycyrrhizic acid in licorice [32]) leads to hypokalemia and metabolic alkalosis. Hypertension is characteristically present in these disorders. In contrast to patients with secondary increases in mineralocorticoid activity (e.g., as in congestive heart failure), edema does not occur. This phenomenon, called *aldosterone escape*, results at least in part from the high renal interstitial pressures generated by the hypertension that limits further NaCl reabsorption; it is also possible that atrial natriuretic peptide, released in response to volume expansion, contributes to this phenomenon.

In addition to the direct effect of aldosterone on H^+ secretion, hypokalemia also appears to be necessary for the maintenance of a significant metabolic alkalosis in patients with primary mineralocorticoid excess. The mechanism of this effect involves the development of intracellular acidosis with increased H^+ secretion and HCO_3^- reabsorption by the proximal tubule and enhanced distal nephron Na-H exchange.

Severe Hypokalemia. The effect of mild-to-moderate hypokalemia on the generation and maintenance of metabolic alkalosis has been discussed. Severe hypokalemia (plasma K^+ <2 mEq per L) can additionally impair distal Cl^- reabsorption by an unknown mechanism. In this setting, some of the Na^+ that is normally reabsorbed with Cl^- must be reabsorbed in exchange for H^+.

Bartter's and Gitelman's Syndromes. Bartter's syndrome is a rare cause of metabolic alkalosis typically seen in children and young adults. The loop of Henle appears to be the site responsible for this disorder. Metabolic alkalosis is also present in patients with Gitelman's syndrome, in which the defect occurs in the thiazide-sensitive site of the distal tubule. In contrast to patients with primary aldosteronism, patients with Bartter's and Gitelman's syndromes are normotensive or slightly hypotensive. The associated volume depletion causes chronic activation of the renin–angiotensin–aldosterone system, increasing distal nephron K^+ and H^+ secretion, as in patients receiving to a loop or thiazide diuretic.

Clinical Manifestations

Most patients with metabolic alkalosis do not suffer clinically from the effects of alkalemia [33]. When symptoms are present, they are typically those associated with volume depletion (e.g., weakness, muscle cramps, postural dizziness) or hypokalemia (e.g., muscle weakness, polyuria, polydipsia). The usual symptoms of alkalemia are due to increased neuromuscular excitability and are exhibited as paresthesias, carpopedal spasm, or lightheadedness, although these findings are relatively more common in patients with acute respiratory alkalosis.

Diagnosis

The cause of metabolic alkalosis can usually be elicited from the history and physical examination. One of the most important aspects of the physical examination in identifying a cause is the determination of blood pressure. Except for the hypertensive individual taking a diuretic, hypokalemia in the presence of metabolic alkalosis and hypertension should suggest the presence of a primary mineralocorticoid-induced disease, such as hyperaldosteronism. Normotensive individuals with no obvious cause most often have surreptitious vomiting or diuretic ingestion (*pseudo-Bartter's syndrome*) as the precipitating event; Bartter's and Gitelman's syndromes are much rarer.

The urinary Cl^- concentration is important because urinary Na^+ wasting may occur in the presence of a high plasma HCO_3^- concentration even if volume depletion is present. $NaHCO_3^-$ losses develop when the plasma HCO_3^- level exceeds the renal reabsorptive threshold, a condition that obligates the excretion of HCO_3^- with a cation to maintain electroneutrality. The most abundant cation in the filtrate is Na^+, even in low perfusion states. As a result, the urine Na^+ concentration should not be used to infer the volume status of an individual with an increased plasma HCO_3^- concentration, unless it is less than 20 mEq per L. By comparison, the urinary Cl^- concentration characteristically is low in hypoperfusion states because Cl^- is not affected by bicarbonaturia.

[8] *The pathophysiology of this phenomenon is more complex and probably depends on a change in the membrane potential induced by hypokalemia. As can be seen in Figure 71.1, the interior of the tubular cell is electronegative compared with the outside. This potential difference is determined primarily by the difference between K^+ intracellular and K^+ extracellular. Because there is substantially more K^+ inside the cell (approximately 130 mEq per L) than in plasma (approximately 4 mEq per L), a fall in the plasma K^+ concentration causes the inside of the cell to become more electronegative as the membrane potential increases. It appears that this negative intracellular charge on the basolateral membrane is the driving force for Na-3HCO_3 reabsorption. Thus, the cell interior may become more acid in hypokalemic states because more HCO_3^- leaves the cell.*

TABLE 71.5

URINE CHLORIDE CONCENTRATION IN METABOLIC ALKALOSIS

Less than 15 mEq/L	Greater than 20 mEq/L
Vomiting	Mineralocorticoid excess
Nasogastric suction	Alkali loading
Postdiuretic administration	During diuretic administration
Posthypercapnia	Severe hypokalemia
High-dose penicillin therapy	Bartter's and Gitelman's syndromes
Alkali loading[a]	

[a] Since the maintenance of metabolic alkalosis requires impairment of renal bicarbonate excretion, the pathophysiology of the renal limitation determines the urinary chloride concentration. If, for example, there is underlying hypovolemia, the urinary chloride concentration is low (<15 mEq/L); in comparison, the urinary chloride concentration is >20 mEq/L when the cause of renal bicarbonate retention is a reduction in glomerular filtration rate, as in the milk-alkali syndrome, or in patients with acute tubular necrosis who received large alkali loads.

Measurement of the urinary Cl^- concentration is useful in differentiating these disorders (Table 71.5). The urinary Cl^- concentration is typically less than 15 mEq per L, with hypovolemia caused by vomiting or diuretic therapy (if the effect of the diuretic has worn off). Higher values are found if the diuretic is still in effect, if Bartter's or Gitelman's syndromes or severe hypokalemia are present, or if there is primary mineralocorticoid excess (e.g., primary aldosteronism). Diuretic abuse may be distinguished from Bartter's or Gitelman's syndromes in some cases by screening the urine for diuretics.

Mixed Acid–Base Disturbances with Metabolic Alkalosis

Respiratory Compensation. The increased arterial pH in metabolic alkalosis leads to a compensatory rise in the PCO_2. This decrease in respiration is due to direct suppression of the medullary respiratory center by alkalemia. In general, the PCO_2 rises approximately 0.7 mm Hg for every 1 mEq per L elevation in the plasma HCO_3^- concentration [34], a relationship that pertains up to a PCO_2 rises approximately 60 mm Hg (plasma HCO_3^- concentration = 53 mEq per L); values above this level are unusual because further hypoventilation is limited by the development of hypoxemia. The identification of a PCO_2 greater or less than predicted suggests the presence of a second primary acid–base disturbance, respiratory acidosis or respiratory alkalosis, respectively.

Metabolic Alkalosis with Metabolic Acidosis. The ratio of the increment in AG to decrement in the plasma HCO_3^- concentration (Δ/Δ) can be used to identify the presence of a metabolic alkalosis in a patient with metabolic acidosis. In such cases, the increment in the serum AG is greater in magnitude than the apparent fall in the bicarbonate level.

Treatment of Metabolic Alkalosis

Rapid correction of metabolic alkalosis is usually not necessary due to the general rarity of adverse effects directly related to the rise in pH. As a result, there is ordinarily time to identify the cause of the disorder and to institute specific therapy. Any exogenous sources of alkali (e.g., preparations containing HCO_3^-, acetate, lactate, or citrate) should be discontinued.

Because hypomagnesemia may be present in some patients with metabolic alkalosis, a serum magnesium level should be checked, particularly in patients with refractory hypokalemia, as hypomagnesemia predisposes to renal potassium wasting.

Chloride-Responsive Metabolic Alkalosis

Chloride replacement (as NaCl, KCl, or both) is appropriate for management of most individuals with a low urinary Cl^- concentration. Administration of Cl^--containing fluid with K^+ ameliorates the alkalosis by permitting renal excretion of the excess HCO_3^-. It allows more Na^+ to be reabsorbed with Cl^-, rather than in exchange for H^+; it reduces the volume stimulus for Na^+ retention, permitting HCO_3^- excretion in the urine; and it increases the plasma K^+ concentration, which raises the tubular cell pH and reduces renal H^+ secretion. Replacement of the volume deficit with non–Cl^--containing solutions of Na^+ or K^+ does not correct the alkalosis or hypokalemia because non-Cl^- anions obligate further K^+ and H^+ excretion. Patients with vomiting or nasogastric suction also may benefit from H_2-blockers or other medications that reduce gastric acid secretion. They are not, however, substitutes for Cl^- replacement, which is still necessary to correct the already present chloride deficit.

The therapy of metabolic alkalosis in edematous patients (e.g., those with congestive heart failure and advanced liver disease) is more difficult. Although renal perfusion is characteristically reduced, leading to a low urinary Cl^- concentration, Cl^- administration (e.g., as 0.9% saline) does not enhance HCO_3^- excretion because the reduced effective arterial blood volume is not corrected by this therapy. In this setting, the carbonic anhydrase inhibitor acetazolamide (at a dose of 250 to 375 mg once or twice daily orally or intravenously) may be useful because it permits fluid mobilization while decreasing HCO_3^- reabsorption in the proximal tubule. An adverse consequence of acetazolamide administration is the tendency for more K^+ wasting. Careful monitoring of the plasma K^+ concentration is necessary. When the plasma K^+ level is low, the use of a distally acting K^+-sparing diuretic (e.g., amiloride or spironolactone) can be considered.

In extremely rare instances, these maneuvers may be insufficient, or the metabolic alkalosis may be so severe that adverse neurologic symptoms of alkalemia are present. In such instances, HCl can be given intravenously to lower the plasma HCO_3^- concentration. HCl is usually given as a solution isotonic to plasma (150 mEq H^+ and 150 mEq Cl^- in each liter of distilled H_2O). The volume needed to reduce the plasma HCO_3^- concentration can be estimated from the HCO_3^- deficit. Because the volume of distribution of HCO_3^- is approximately 50% of the lean body weight, the amount of HCl needed to lower the plasma HCO_3^- concentration from 45 to 35 mEq per L in a 70-kg man can be calculated as follows (assuming there are no ongoing HCO_3^- losses):

$$HCO_3^- \text{ excess} = 0.5 \times 70 \times (45 - 35) = 350\,\text{mEq}$$

This would require administration of slightly more than 2 L of an isotonic HCl solution. Because the very low pH of this solution can injure small veins and tissues, particularly if extravasation occurs, administration should generally occur during at least 24 hours using a large (central) vein. As a result, the administration of HCl may outweigh the potential benefits.

Dialytic therapy may be helpful in the unusual patient presenting with metabolic alkalosis, volume overload, and renal failure. Peritoneal dialysis typically contains lactate as the HCO_3^- precursor at a concentration of approximately 40 mEq per L, an amount that may worsen the alkalosis. By comparison, the alkali level can be adjusted with most current hemodialysis machines. It is important to note that citrate used for anticoagulation in some continuous dialytic therapies can lead to metabolic alkalosis as well [35].

Chloride-Resistant Metabolic Alkalosis

Individuals with a urinary chloride concentration greater than 15 mEq per L are unlikely to respond to Cl^--containing solutions such as physiologic saline, with correction of the metabolic alkalosis. Since the effective renal blood flow is already normal or Cl^- reabsorption must be impaired, the administered Cl^- is rapidly excreted in the urine. Moreover, enhanced distal Na^+ presentation increases Na-K exchange, leading to a rise in urinary K^+ excretion with more severe hypokalemia in states of primary mineralocorticoid excess.

In a hypertensive patient, primary aldosteronism should be considered. Removing the source of aldosterone (by adrenalectomy when an aldosterone-secreting adenoma is present) or blocking its action (with a K^+-sparing diuretic, such as amiloride) is usually sufficient to correct the hypokalemia and metabolic alkalosis and to control hypertension in this disorder.

The abnormality in Bartter's and Gitelman's syndromes, impaired Cl^- reabsorption, cannot be corrected with treatment. Therapy is therefore directed at improving the laboratory abnormalities, particularly hypokalemia and metabolic alkalosis. Nonsteroidal anti-inflammatory drugs (including COX-2 inhibitors) reduce renin secretion (a prostaglandin-dependent process) and may be effective in reducing the plasma HCO_3^- and K^+ levels to or near normal, although K^+ supplementation also may be required. Angiotensin-converting enzyme inhibitors or K^+-sparing diuretics may be useful alone or in combination, but they have the potential risk of causing the already slightly low blood pressure to fall. It is important to exclude surreptitious diuretic use or forced vomiting in these individuals before assigning a diagnostic or therapeutic regimen used for Bartter's or Gitelman's syndromes because the former are far more common disorders.

References

1. Schoolwerth AC: Regulation of renal ammoniagenesis in metabolic acidosis. *Kidney Int* 40:961, 1991.
2. Winter SD, Pearson R, Gabow PA, et al: The fall of the serum anion gap. *Arch Intern Med* 150:311, 1990.
3. Kraut JA, Madias NE: Serum anion gap: its uses and limitations in clinical medicine. *Clin J Am Soc Nephrol* 2:162, 2007.
4. Gluck SL: Acid-base. *Lancet* 352:474, 1998.
5. Nyirenda MJ, Sandeep T, Grant I, et al: Sever acidosis in patients taking metformin-rapid reversal and survival despite high APACHE score. *Diabet Med* 23:432, 2006.
6. Uribarri J, Oh MS, Carroll, HJ: D-Lactic acidosis. A review of clinical presentation, biochemical features, and pathophysiologic mechanisms. *Medicine* 77:73, 1998.
7. Adrogue HJ, Madias ME: Management of life-threatening acid-base disorders (part 1). *N Engl J Med* 338:26, 1998.
8. Schelling JR, Howard RL, Winter SO, et al: Increased osmolal gap in alcoholic ketoacidosis and lactic acidosis. *Ann Intern Med* 113:580, 1990.
9. Arroliga AC, Shehab N, McCarthy K, et al: Relationship of continuous infusion lorazepam to serum propylene glycol concentration in critically ill adults. *Crit Care Med* 32:1709, 2004.
10. Sweeney TE, Beuchat CA: Limitations of methods of osmometry: measuring the osmolality of body fluids. *Am J Physiol* 264:R469, 1993.
11. Carlisle EJ, Donnelly SM, Vasuvattakul S, et al: Glue-sniffing and distal renal tubular acidosis: sticking to the facts. *J Am Soc Nephrol* 1:1019, 1991.
12. Fenves AZ, Kirkpatrick HM, Patel VV, et al: Increased anion gap metabolic acidosis as a result of 5-oxoproline (pyroglutamic acid): a role for acetaminophen. *Clin J Am Soc Nephrol* 1:441, 2006.
13. Brezina B, Qunibi W, Nolan CR: Acid loading during treatment with sevelamer hydrochloride: mechanisms and clinical implications. *Kidney Int* 66:S-39, 2004.
14. Kette F, Weil MH, Gazmuri RJ: Buffer solutions may compromise cardiac resuscitation by reducing coronary perfusion pressure. *JAMA* 266:2121, 1991.
15. Simpson D: Citrate excretion: a window on renal metabolism. *Am J Physiol* 244:F223, 1983.
16. Messiaen T, Deret S, Mougenot B, et al: Adult Fanconi syndrome secondary to light chain gammopathy. *Medicine* 79:135, 2000.
17. Adrogue HJ, Madias NE: Changes in plasma potassium concentration during acute acid-base disturbances. *Am J Med* 71:456, 1981.
18. Fernandez PC, Cohen RM, Feldman GM: The concept of bicarbonate distribution space: the crucial role of body buffers. *Kidney Int* 36:747, 1989.
19. Oh M, Carroll H, Goldstein D, et al: Hyperchloremic acidosis during the recovery phase of diabetic ketoacidosis. *Ann Intern Med* 89:925, 1978.
20. Halperin ML, Vasuvattakul S, Bayoumi A: A modified classification of metabolic acidosis. A pathophysiologic approach. *Nephron* 60:129, 1992.
21. Batlle D, Hizon M, Cohen E, et al: The use of the urinary anion gap in the diagnosis of hyperchloremic metabolic acidosis. *N Engl J Med* 318:594, 1988.
22. Kraut JA, Kurtz I: Use of base in the treatment of severe acidemic states. *Am J Kidney Dis* 38:703, 2001.
23. Kovesdy CP, Anderson JE, Kalantar-Zadeh K: Association of serum bicarbonate levels with mortality in patients with non-dialysis-dependent CKD. *Nephrol Dial Transplant* 24:1232, 2009.
24. Brandt K, Miles J: Relationship between severity of hyperglycemia and metabolic acidosis in diabetic ketoacidosis. *Mayo Clin Proc* 63:1071, 1988.
25. Adrogue HJ, Madias NE: Management of life-threatening acid-base disorders (part 2). *N Engl J Med* 338:107, 1998.
26. Liu F-Y, Cogan MG: Angiotensin II stimulates early proximal bicarbonate absorption in the rat by decreasing cAMP. *J Clin Invest* 84:83, 1989.
27. Wesson DE, Dolson GM: Enhanced HCO_3 secretion by distal tubule contributes to NaCl induced correction of chronic alkalosis. *Am J Physiol* 264:F899, 1993.
28. Beall DP, Scofield RH: Milk-alkali syndrome associated with calcium carbonate consumption. *Medicine (Baltimore)* 74:89, 1995.
29. Perez GO, Oster JR, Rogers TJ: Acid-base disturbances in gastrointestinal disease. *Dig Dis Sci* 32:1033, 1987.
30. Jaeger P, Tellier M, Fowler N, et al: Effect of parathyroid hormone related peptides on proximal tubular handling of HCO_3 [abstract]. *Kidney Int* 37:467, 1990.
31. Kurtz I: Molecular pathogenesis of Bartter's and Gitelman's syndromes. *Kidney Int* 54:1396, 1998.
32. Whorwood CB, Sheppard MC, Stewart PM: Licorice inhibits 11b-hydroxysteroid messenger ribonucleic acid levels and potentiates glucocorticoid hormone action. *Endocrinology* 132:2287, 1993.
33. Galla JH: Metabolic alkalosis. *J Am Soc Nephrol* 11:369, 2000.
34. Javaheri S, Shore N, Rose B, et al: Compensatory hypoventilation in metabolic alkalosis. *Chest* 81:296, 1982.
35. Gupta M, Wadhwa NK, Bukovsky R, et al: Regional citrate for continuous venovenous hemodiafiltration using calcium-containing dialysate. *Am J Kidney Dis* 43:67, 2004.

CHAPTER 72 ■ DISORDERS OF PLASMA SODIUM AND PLASMA POTASSIUM

ROBERT M. BLACK

DISORDERS OF PLASMA SODIUM

Hyponatremia and hypernatremia are conditions commonly observed in the intensive care unit. They are defined as plasma Na^+ concentration below 135 mEq per L and above 145 mEq per L, respectively. The correct management of patients with these disorders depends on an understanding of normal salt (NaCl) and water (H_2O) physiology.

It is important to appreciate that hyponatremia represents a disorder of water balance; the plasma sodium concentration reflects the ratio of water to sodium in the body. By itself, however, the presence of hypo- or hypernatremia cannot be used to assess the volume status of a patient. Furthermore, the plasma sodium concentration has little relationship to the urinary sodium concentration.

Hypothalamic osmoreceptors influence thirst and the release of antidiuretic hormone (ADH). The latter increases U_{Osm}, causing water retention by enhancing the permeability of the collecting tubules to water. ADH is also released in response to effective volume depletion (hypovolemia). Although water retention causes extracellular volume expansion, this is slight, as approximately two thirds of the water enters the cells. As a result, volume-mediated ADH release can occur even in states of hyponatremia (see following discussion).

Relationship Between Plasma Na^+ and Plasma Osmolality

The osmolality of plasma (P_{Osm}) is determined by the sum of the osmolar contributions of the individual osmotically active substances. In plasma, Na^+ salts, glucose, and urea (blood urea nitrogen [BUN]) are the major determinants of osmolality. Therefore, the P_{Osm} can be estimated by the following formula:

$$P_{Osm} \approx 2 \times \text{plasma Na}^+ + \text{glucose}/18.0 + \text{BUN}/2.8$$

Using this equation,[1] it is evident that the major determinant of the P_{Osm} in healthy individuals is the plasma Na^+ concentration.

The ability of a solute (such as sodium) to promote shifts of water between the intracellular and extracellular compartments depends not only on its capacity to increase the P_{Osm} but also on its exclusion from one of these compartments. Because urea can cross almost all cell membranes readily, it cannot promote the movement of water between the intracellular and extracellular spaces. As such, urea is referred to as an *ineffective osmole*. A rise in the BUN is detected as an increase in the measured (by the laboratory) and calculated P_{Osm}, but there is no change in the plasma Na^+ concentration because urea does not obligate water movement from the intracellular to the extracellular space. Because urea is an ineffective osmole and because glucose normally contributes less than 8 mOsm per kg, the effective P_{Osm} correlates best with the plasma Na^+. Thus, effective P_{Osm} can be described as follows:

$$P_{Osm}(\text{effective}) \approx 2 \times \text{plasma Na}^+\text{concentration}$$

Sodium is confined primarily to the extracellular fluid by the Na-K antiporter present in most cells. This pump also maintains a high (approximately 130 mEq per L) intracellular K^+ concentration; thus, potassium is the principal effective osmole inside cells. The ability of water to cross almost all cell membranes indicates that the P_{Osm} must be in equilibrium with the intracellular osmolality. In fact, osmolality is equal throughout all body compartments, explaining the need for only one osmoreceptor.

Because osmotic equilibrium exists throughout body water, calculation of water deficits or excesses, when dealing with a hyponatremic or hypernatremic individual, respectively, must be based on total body water (TBW) and not merely on the extracellular fluid volume. Moreover, loss of potassium from the body, as might occur with diuretic administration, affects the plasma Na^+ concentration.

Two processes participate in the reduction in plasma Na^+ concentration induced by potassium losses. Sodium movement into cells to maintain electroneutrality lowers the plasma Na^+, and loss of potassium from the gastrointestinal tract or kidneys causes a fall in the plasma potassium with a larger fall in the intracellular potassium. The result is a reduction in the intracellular osmolality that leads to water movement from cells to the extracellular compartment.

Finally, although plasma hypoosmolality is always associated with hyponatremia, a high P_{Osm} can occur in the absence of hypernatremia. Other ineffective osmoles (in addition to urea) have the ability to raise the measured P_{Osm} without affecting water shifts. The most important of these are the alcohols: ethanol, ethylene glycol, and methanol. By contrast, severe hyperglycemia can induce hyponatremia by pulling water out of cells, but the P_{Osm} will be elevated. This phenomenon, seen most often in diabetics, is referred to as *hyperosmolar hyponatremia*.

Regulation of Plasma Osmolality

Maintenance of the plasma Na^+ concentration within narrow limits (285 to 292 mOsm per kg) depends on the ability of the kidneys to excrete water (to prevent and on a normal thirst mechanism with access to water). Under normal conditions, the quantity of water that can be excreted in the urine far exceeds the amount ingested.

Renal water excretion is determined by two factors: urinary solute excretion and the ability to generate a maximally dilute

[1] *The molecular weights of glucose and nitrogen are 180 and 14, respectively. As a result, the osmotic effect of glucose is determined by dividing by 18 (because the concentration is in 100 mL of plasma and not 1 L), whereas that of BUN is obtained by dividing by 2.8 (there are two nitrogens on each molecule of urea).*

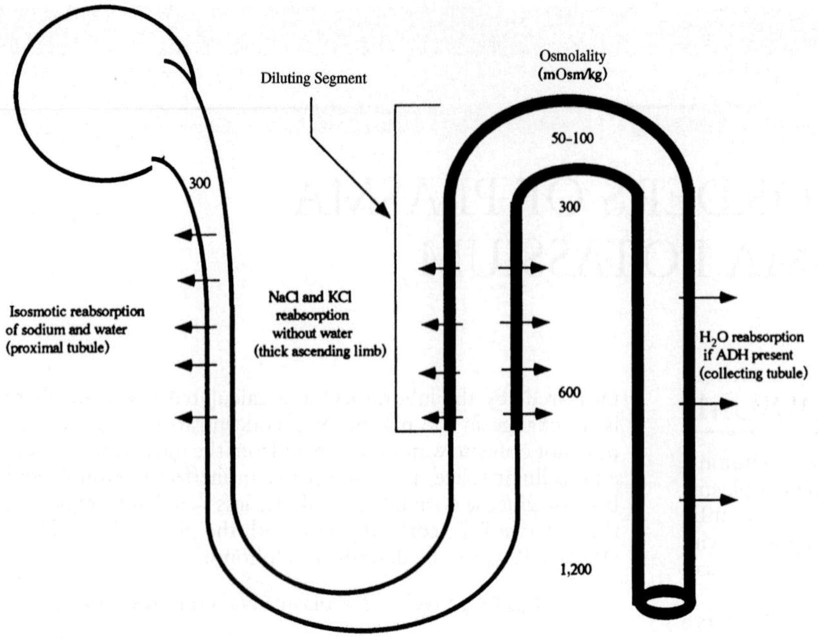

FIGURE 72.1. Excretion of a dilute urine. Solute entering the early proximal tubule has an osmolality identical to that of plasma; fluid is isotonically reabsorbed in this nephron segment. Separation of solute from water (H_2O) within the tubule begins in the thick ascending limb of Henle, which is impermeable to H_2O. Excretion of a urine with a minimum osmolality of 50 to 100 mOsm per L requires intact function of this nephron segment as well as suppression of antidiuretic hormone (ADH) release. [Adapted from Iwasaki Y, Oiso Y, Yamauchi K, et al: Osmoregulation of plasma vasopressin in myxedema. *J Clin Endocrinol Metab* 70:534, 1990.]

urine (U_{Osm} <100 mOsm per kg) [1]. The typical American diet affords a solute intake between 600 and 1,200 mOsm—average 900 mOsm—per day. Assuming an output that approximates intake, the daily urinary solute excretion of a typical adult would also average 900 mOsm. Dietary NaCl, KCl, and protein, which is broken down to urea, make up most of this solute load. The individual who excretes 900 mOsm of solute per day and who can dilute urine maximally (down to 50 mOsm per kg) has the capacity to excrete up to 18 of water in a 24-hour period:

$$900\,\text{mOsm}/50\,\text{mOsm/kg} = 18\,\text{L}$$

The capacity to dilute urine begins in the loop of Henle and continues to the collecting tubule. This portion of the nephron, which is impermeable to water, is often referred to as the *diluting segment* (Fig. 72.1). As filtrate passes through the loop of Henle, solute is removed by the Na-K-2Cl transporter located in the cells of thick ascending limb and by the NaCl carrier in the distal tubule. Filtrate leaving the diluting segment and entering the early collecting tubule characteristically is very dilute, with a urinary osmolality (U_{Osm}) of less than 100 mOsm per kg.

A maximally dilute urine cannot be excreted if the removal of salt by the pumps and carriers in the diluting segment is impaired or if the collecting tubule is rendered permeable to water by the presence of ADH (see following discussion). Inability to dilute the urine may have serious consequences. For example, for a patient unable to achieve urinary dilution below an osmolality of 300 mOsm per kg, the amount of water that can be excreted on a normal diet is reduced to 3 L:

$$900\,\text{mOsm}/300\,\text{mOsm/kg} = 3\,\text{L}$$

As discussed earlier, solute excretion is normally determined by dietary intake. A reduction in dietary sodium and protein intake, as is seen in the patient on a "tea-and-toast" diet, limits the capacity to excrete water. If solute intake falls to 150 mOsm per day, for instance, water excretion is limited to approximately 3 L even when urinary dilution is normal:

$$150\,\text{mOsm}/50\,\text{mOsm/kg} = 3\,\text{L}$$

It is easy to see that the combination of impaired diluting ability with a concomitant reduction in solute intake is more likely to impair water excretion and result in hyponatremia than either disturbance alone.

Regulation of Antidiuretic Hormone

Healthy adults are able to excrete very large or very small volumes of urine, the concentration of which varies according to the P_{Osm}. The primary hormone regulating water excretion in health is ADH. ADH (called *arginine vasopressin* in humans) is synthesized in the supraoptic and paraventricular nuclei of the hypothalamus. Hypothalamic osmoreceptors for ADH release are stimulated by hyperosmolality and inhibited by hypoosmolality. A change in osmoreceptor cell volume is probably the factor that modifies ADH secretion in response to changes in the P_{Osm}. The concentration of urea, an ineffective osmole incapable of altering cell volume, neither promotes nor inhibits ADH release.

A 1% to 2% reduction in P_{Osm} (P_{Osm} <280 mOsm per kg) maximally inhibits ADH release, leading to a U_{Osm} that is less than 100 mOsm per kg [2]. By contrast, a 1% to 2% increase in P_{Osm} above normal, or a 7% to 10% decrease in blood pressure or volume (even in the presence of plasma hypoosmolality), stimulates ADH release [1]. In the presence of ADH, the luminal membranes of the cortical and medullary collecting tubules become permeable as water channels (aquaporins) are generated. This change permits water reabsorption, increasing the final urine osmolality.

Hyponatremia

In most settings, the development of hyponatremia with hypoosmolality represents the retention of ingested or administered water. Thus, the causes of hyponatremia can be divided into those in which water excretion is abnormal and those in which water excretion is normal but water ingestion is considerably increased.

TABLE 72.1

CAUSES OF HYPONATREMIA

Impaired water excretion (U_{Osm} >100 mOsm/kg and usually >300 mOsm/kg)
Hypovolemic states
True volume depletion (by gastrointestinal, skin, or renal losses)
Edematous states with reduced effective arterial blood volume (advanced liver and heart disease)
Diuretics (particularly thiazides)
Advanced chronic kidney disease
Endocrine deficiencies (hypothyroidism and hypoadrenalism)
Syndrome of inappropriate antidiuretic hormone secretion
Cerebral salt wasting
Reduced solute intake (tea-and-toast diet, beer drinkers' hyponatremia)[a]
Normal water excretion (U_{Osm} >100 mOsm/kg)
Primary polydipsia
Psychiatric disorders (particularly with phenothiazines)
Hypothalamic disorders
Hyponatremia without hypoosmolality
Normal P_{Osm}
Pseudohyponatremia (hypertriglyceridemia, hyperproteinemia, genitourinary tract irrigation)
Increased P_{Osm}
Hyperosmolar hyponatremia (hyperglycemia, mannitol infusion in renal failure)
Azotemia (effective osmolality is reduced)

[a] U_{Osm} <100 mOsm/kg, but normal water excretion is impaired by the reduced solute load; see text for details.
P_{Osm}, osmolality of plasma; U_{Osm}, osmolality of urine.
Adapted from Iwasaki Y, Oiso Y, Yamauchi K, et al: Osmoregulation of plasma vasopressin in myxedema. *J Clin Endocrinol Metab* 70:534, 1990; and Stasior D, Kikeri D, Duel B, et al: Nephrogenic diabetes insipidus responsive to indomethacin plus dDAVP [letter]. *N Engl J Med* 324:850, 1991.

Hypoosmolar Disorders with Impaired Water Excretion

The U_{Osm} is typically greater than 100 mOsm per kg in patients with reduced water excretion (Table 72.1). An exception to this rule occurs when solute intake is markedly reduced, as in the patient subsisting on a solute-poor diet.

Hypovolemic Hyponatremia. A fall in effective perfusion pressure stimulates release of ADH [3]. Hypovolemic hyponatremia can occur in states of volume depletion or in edematous individuals with congestive heart failure (CHF) or advanced liver disease because each of these conditions is associated with a reduced effective arterial blood volume. As discussed previously, the resulting increase in the U_{Osm} (e.g., to 600 mOsm per kg) would limit renal water excretion on a 900 mOsm per day diet to 1.5 L, assuming all of the ingested solute were excreted (900 mOsm per kg 600). Solute excretion tends to be reduced in these settings, which are characterized by enhanced tubular salt reabsorption. In addition, most stimuli that activate angiotensin II release also stimulate thirst and lead to increased water ingestion, despite concurrent hypoosmolality.

Diuretic-Induced Hyponatremia. The ability to excrete a dilute urine is impaired by diuretics, whether they act in the thick ascending limb of Henle (loop diuretics) or in the distal tubule (thiazide-type diuretics) (Fig. 72.2). Each class reduces salt transport out of the diluting segment, thus raising the minimum achievable U_{Osm}. Raising the minimum U_{Osm}, however,

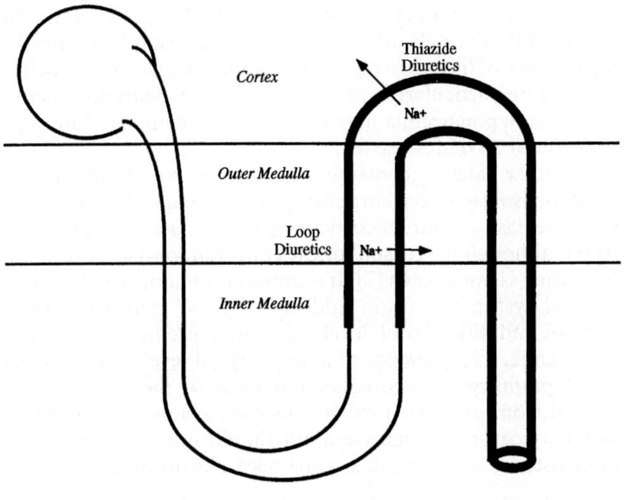

FIGURE 72.2. Site of action of loop and thiazide diuretics. Loop diuretics inhibit the Na-K-2Cl cotransporter in the medullary portion of the thick ascending limb of Henle, whereas thiazides block a simple NaCl carrier in the cortical portion of the distal tubule. These differences explain, in part, the susceptibility of individuals treated with thiazide-type diuretics to the development of hyponatremia. See text for details. [Adapted from Iwasaki Y, Oiso Y, Yamauchi K, et al: Osmoregulation of plasma vasopressin in myxedema. *J Clin Endocrinol Metab* 70:534, 1990.]

does not usually lead to hyponatremia because a large volume of urine can still be excreted by most patients.

Almost all cases of diuretic-induced hyponatremia in otherwise healthy individuals have been caused by thiazide-type, rather than loop, diuretics [4]. This observation is attributable, in part, to different sites of the action within the renal tubule (Fig. 72.2). Loop diuretics, which act in the outer medulla, reduce the solute concentration in the renal medullary interstitium. Although ADH *permits* water reabsorption from the collecting tubule, medullary osmolality *drives* the process. A fall in the interstitial osmolality from 1,200 to 300 mOsm per kg, for instance, would limit the maximum U_{Osm} that can be generated from 1,200 to 300 mOsm per kg. By comparison, thiazide diuretics, which act in the cortex, impair diluting capacity but have a lesser effect on concentrating ability. Thus, the U_{Osm} may be 600 mOsm per kg in the thiazide-treated individual; if the urinary osmoles are primarily NaCl and KCl, urinary electrolyte losses can exceed those contained in an equal volume of plasma. In these patients, therefore, the plasma Na^+ may actually fall in the absence of ongoing water intake. For reasons that are not well understood, however, most individuals with thiazide-induced hyponatremia gain weight, indicating that the hyponatremia is at least in part a result of increased water intake [4]. This disorder occurs more frequently in women, typically occurs early in therapy (within 1 to 4 weeks), and is more likely to be observed in elderly individuals [5]. As discussed previously, accompanying hypokalemia also may contribute to the fall in P_{Osm}.

Advanced Chronic Kidney Disease. The normal glomerular filtration rate (GFR) is approximately 180 L per day. As renal function decreases, the ability to excrete water also decreases. The limitation in water excretion occurs for two reasons: tubular dysfunction leads to an inability to dilute the urine maximally, even in the absence of ADH, and the drop in GFR, particularly when severe, reduces daily solute excretion.

Endocrine Deficiency. Hypothyroidism and hypocortisolism can impair water excretion. Both may reduce cardiac output or stroke volume, leading to increased ADH release. The resulting fall in GFR adversely affects free water excretion by diminishing delivery of filtrate to the diluting segments. Decreased delivery may be particularly important in patients with myxedema in whom hyponatremia may develop despite appropriate suppression of ADH release [6].

Another factor contributing to the hyponatremia of hypocortisolism is that corticotropin-releasing factor promotes the corelease of adrenocorticotropic hormone (ACTH) and ADH, although the reason for the concomitant release of these hormones is not known [7]. It is important to note that adrenocortical dysfunction (as in Addison's disease) leads to reduced cortisol and aldosterone levels, the latter predisposing to hyperkalemia. The presence of a low cortisol level alone, due to either pituitary or hypothalamic disease, or the abrupt withdrawal from prolonged exogenous corticosteroid administration may cause hyponatremia but should not alter potassium homeostasis, because aldosterone release is normal.

Syndrome of Inappropriate Antidiuretic Hormone Secretion. The syndrome of inappropriate ADH secretion (SIADH) is characterized by the following: plasma hypoosmolality; U_{Osm} more than 100 to 150 mOsm per kg (because ADH should be absent in the hypoosmolar state); urinary Na^+ concentration of more than 20 mEq per L, reflecting normal renal perfusion; normal adrenal, renal, and thyroid function; and normal potassium and acid–base balance. *The U_{Osm} does not need to exceed the P_{Osm} to make this diagnosis.* SIADH may be caused by enhanced hypothalamic ADH secretion, ectopic hormone production (usually by cancer), or administration of medications with ADH activity (Table 72.2).

In approximately one third of patients, the SIADH is associated with resetting of the hypothalamic osmostat. This disorder has been described in patients with hypovolemia, psychosis, and chronic malnutrition and in normal pregnancy (in which the plasma Na^+ concentration decreases by the second trimester from 140 to 135 mEq per L). ADH release is not suppressed until the P_{Osm} falls well below normal in this disorder. As a result, the P_{Osm} may vary between 240 and 250 mOsm per kg (plasma Na^+ approximately 120 to 125 mEq per L), compared with the normal value of approximately 285 to 292 mOsm per kg. In contrast to the classic form of the SIADH, in which nonsuppressible ADH release is seen, ADH secretion ceases when the P_{Osm} falls below this new, reset level. Because suppression of ADH prevents a further fall in the plasma Na^+ concentration, the severity of hyponatremia is limited in this condition.

An increasingly common cause of hyponatremia is symptomatic human immunodeficiency virus (HIV) infection [8]. Although hyponatremia in HIV-infected patients may result from volume deficiency or adrenal insufficiency, many patients have SIADH. Pneumonia due to *Pneumocystis jiroveci* or other organisms, central nervous system infections, and malignant disease are most often responsible in this setting.

Elevated ADH levels have been reported with the use of medications and various recreational drugs. The association of hyponatremia with the use of 3,4-methylenedioxymethamphetamine (Ecstasy) has been reported. The cause has been reported to be related to increased water drinking and the inappropriate presence of ADH [2]. Similar effects may be seen with the commonly prescribed selective serotonin reuptake inhibitors (SSRIs) used for the treatment of depression [9].

Cerebral Salt Wasting. Cerebral salt wasting is a rare disorder characterized by a low P_{Osm}, a U_{Osm} above 100 to 150 mOsm per kg, and a urine Na^+ concentration greater than 20 mEq per L [10]. Unlike SIADH, however, evidence of volume depletion (including low central filling pressures) is present. In affected individuals, therefore, the high urinary Na^+ represents inappropriate salt wasting rather than a response to normal tissue perfusion (as in SIADH patients).

TABLE 72.2

MAJOR CAUSES OF THE SYNDROME OF INAPPROPRIATE ANTIDIURETIC HORMONE (ADH) SECRETION

Disorders	Comments
Pulmonary diseases	Acute asthma, atelectasis, empyema, pneumothorax, acute respiratory failure, tuberculosis, carcinoma, pneumonia
Neurologic disorders	Meningitis, tumors, psychiatric disorders, subarachnoid hemorrhage, herpes zoster, Wernicke's encephalopathy
Ectopic production	Cancer (particularly oat-cell carcinoma of lung)
Drugs	Intravenous cyclophosphamide, carbamazepine, chlorpropamide, nonsteroidal anti-inflammatory drugs (because prostaglandins block ADH effect), cisplatin[a]
After major surgery	Pain afferents stimulate hypothalamic ADH release (lasts for 2–5 d), after mitral commissurotomy for mitral stenosis (acute decrease in left atrial pressure releases ADH)
Administration of exogenous ADH or oxytocin	Oxytocin can reduce plasma Na^+ concentration in mother and fetus
Symptomatic human immunodeficiency virus infection	See text for details
Idiopathic	Important to continue periodic monitoring for an underlying disorder, particularly carcinoma; vasculitis (such as temporal arteritis) should be considered in elderly patients when no other cause is apparent
Cerebral salt wasting	See text for details

[a] Hyponatremia induced by cisplatin may be due to renal salt wasting.

The cause of this putative syndrome is unclear. It has been proposed that there may be increased release of natriuretic peptide from hormone-producing neurons in the brain that are activated by central nervous system dysfunction [11]. Both hypouricemia and renal tubular dysfunction have been reported. Mineralocorticoid replacement therapy with fludrocortisone acetate has been effective in some patients.

Reduced Solute Intake. As discussed previously, a reduction in salt and protein intake can lead to hypoosmolality if water intake exceeds output. Severely reduced solute intake, as occurs with a tea-and-toast diet, can cause hyponatremia even with normal degrees of water intake. "Beer drinkers' hyponatremia" occurs for a similar reason; the limited amount of solute in beer relative to its water content may be inadequate to permit excretion of the ingested water. In both conditions, the U_{Osm} should be maximally dilute (U_{Osm} <100 mOsm per kg). The absence of polyuria and the development of hyponatremia with normal or slightly above normal fluid intake distinguish these individuals from those with primary polydipsia (see following discussion).

Hypoosmolar Disorders with Normal Water Excretion. Psychiatric patients, particularly those with schizophrenia, often have abnormalities in water balance. Evaluation of psychotic patients has revealed that a variety of defects in water handling can occur that affect thirst, the release of ADH, and the renal response to ADH. Depending on the abnormality that is present, the patient may present with polydipsia and polyuria or hyponatremia.

Hyponatremia has been reported in as many as 13% of marathon runners and may occasionally be fatal. Although the exact mechanism has not been elucidated, risk factors for developing low serum sodium levels include weight gain during the race, female sex, racing time, and lower body mass index [12].

Primary Polydipsia. These individuals may have psychiatric disorders or may intentionally drink large volumes of water for social (dietary) or health reasons. This may be manifested clinically by exaggerated weight gain during the day associated with a transient reduction in the plasma sodium concentration [13].

In some individuals, a central defect in thirst regulation plays an important role in the pathogenesis of polydipsia. For example, the osmotic threshold for thirst may be reduced below the threshold for the release of ADH [14]. These patients continue to drink until the P_{Osm} is less than the threshold level. This implies truly prodigious water intake, as ADH secretion is suppressed by the fall in P_{Osm}, resulting in rapid excretion of the excess water and continued stimulation of thirst. The osmotic regulation of thirst differs from that of healthy subjects, in whom the thirst threshold is roughly equal to or a few milliosmoles per kilogram higher than the threshold for ADH [15]. The mechanism responsible for abnormal thirst regulation in this setting is unclear [16]. Drug therapy may contribute to the increase in water intake if the medication induces the sensation of a dry mouth.

Because people with normally functioning kidneys and regulation of ADH secretion are capable of excreting more than 10 to 15 L of urine per day, hyponatremia due to polydipsia is unusual. Despite this, there are rare patients in whom severe, and potentially fatal, hyponatremia has developed even though the U_{Osm} was appropriately dilute. More commonly, however, polydipsic patients manifesting hyponatremia have a concurrent abnormality in ADH release or response [17]. Concurrent thiazide diuretic therapy for systemic hypertension can lead to a marked and symptomatic reduction in the plasma sodium concentration in these patients.

There is no proven specific therapy for primary polydipsia with or without hyponatremia in psychotic patients. Limiting water intake rapidly raises the plasma sodium concentration because the excess water is readily excreted in a dilute urine. The risk of inducing osmotic demyelination (see later) in this setting is unclear; it has been suggested that patients with primary polydipsia and repeated episodes of acute hyponatremia are generally resistant to neurologic injury induced by rapid correction (see following discussion).

Over time, limiting the use of drugs that cause dry mouth, restricting fluid intake, and frequent weighing (to detect water retention) may be helpful. Antagonists to ADH are not likely to be useful if the urine is already maximally dilute but may help in patients with primary polydipsia and concomitant SIADH.

Hyponatremia Without Hypoosmolality

Hyponatremia may occur without plasma hypoosmolality. An increase in the plasma concentration of proteins (as immunoglobulins in multiple myeloma) or lipids (primarily triglycerides in lipemic plasma) can reduce the plasma Na^+ concentration. Lipids and proteins displace water from a given volume of plasma but do not affect the Na^+ concentration in the water phase of plasma [18]. As a result, the measured P_{Osm} is normal in this condition, which is called *pseudohyponatremia*. Because the sodium concentration in the aqueous component of plasma is normal, this form of hyponatremia is not of pathophysiologic consequence. The methods of electrolyte determination currently used in many laboratories (ion-selective electrodes) are not affected by plasma lipids or proteins.

An unusual form of hyponatremia, sometimes associated with a normal P_{Osm} but occasionally with hypoosmolality, can be observed after lithotripsy, uterine irrigation after endometrial ablation, or with transurethral prostatectomy [19–21], which often requires the use of as much as 20 to 30 L of nonconductive flushing solutions containing glycine, sorbitol, or mannitol. Some patients absorb 3 L or more of fluid through the exposed mucosal vascular plexus, leading to a dilutional reduction in the plasma sodium concentration that may fall below 100 mEq per L. In one prospective study of 100 patients, the incidence of hyponatremia after transurethral prostatectomy was 7%; there was one death [22]. Even when P_{Osm} is not notably reduced, confusion, disorientation, twitching, seizures, and hypotension may occur. Several methods have been devised to attempt to monitor the amount of fluid absorbed so that patients at risk for severe hyponatremia can be detected. Frequent determinations of the plasma sodium concentration are important.

There are instances in which patients with plasma hyperosmolality may develop hyponatremia (*hyperosmolar hyponatremia*). This most commonly occurs with severe hyperglycemia or when mannitol is given to patients with renal failure, resulting in an osmotic shift of water from cells into the extracellular fluid, diluting the plasma Na^+ concentration. In contrast to hypoosmolar hyponatremia, treatment is directed at correcting the high glucose concentration with insulin and free water repletion because cellular dehydration is present. For every 100 mg per dL rise in the blood sugar, the plasma Na^+ concentration falls by approximately 1.6 mEq per L [23], although this estimate varies with body size, falling more in a smaller individual.

Symptoms of Hypoosmolality

The neurologic manifestations of hyponatremia appear to be entirely due to the consequences of plasma hypoosmolality. A fall in P_{Osm} causes water movement from the extracellular space into cells. The resulting increase in cell water, which is of particular importance in the central nervous system, can lead to brain swelling. A variety of symptoms may be found, including lethargy, confusion, nausea, vomiting, and, in severe cases, seizures and coma. Focal neurologic symptoms are uncommon. Hyponatremic encephalopathy is generally reversible, although permanent neurologic damage or death has been reported, chiefly in premenopausal women [24]. Hyponatremic women may progress rapidly from minimal symptoms (such as headache and nausea) to respiratory arrest. Cerebral edema and herniation have been found in those women who died, suggesting a possible hormonally mediated decrease in the efficiency of the osmotic adaptation (see following discussion). The reason for the higher morbidity in this patient population is not well understood.

The likelihood that symptoms will develop is related to the level of hyponatremia and the rapidity with which it develops [25]. For example, a rapid decline in the plasma Na^+ concentration during several hours or days (e.g., from 140 to 115 mEq per L) may be associated with severe neurologic findings.

In comparison, a similar fall in plasma sodium occurring during 1 week or more may not cause any symptoms. In the latter circumstance, the degree of cerebral edema is much less [26]. This protective response, which begins on the first day and is complete within several days, occurs in two major steps:

1. The initial cerebral edema elevates the interstitial hydraulic pressure, creating a gradient for extracellular fluid movement out of the brain into the cerebrospinal fluid.
2. The brain cells lose solutes, leading to the osmotic movement of water out of the cells and less brain swelling [27]. The volume regulatory response begins with the movement of potassium and sodium salts out of the cells, followed by organic solutes, particularly the amino acids glutamine, glutamate, and taurine, and, to a lesser degree, the carbohydrate inositol. Electrolyte movement occurs quickly because it is mediated by the activation of quiescent cation channels in the cell membrane; organic solute loss occurs later because it requires synthesis of new transporters.

The organic solutes (called *osmolytes*) account for approximately one third of the cellular solute loss in chronic hyponatremia. Changes in the concentration of these solutes offer the advantage of restoring cell volume without interfering with protein function; in comparison, a potentially deleterious effect on protein function would occur if the volume adaptation were mediated *entirely* by changes in the cell cation (potassium plus sodium) concentration.

This adaptation is so efficient that it is not uncommon to see patients with heart failure or SIADH who are asymptomatic despite a plasma sodium concentration of 115 to 120 mEq per L. The occurrence of symptoms in patients with chronic hyponatremia usually signifies a profoundly low serum sodium concentration, less than 110 to 115 mEq per L.

Diagnosis of Hyponatremia

Three laboratory findings provide important information in the differential diagnosis of hyponatremia: P_{Osm}, U_{Osm}, and urinary sodium concentration.

Plasma Osmolality

Because P_{Osm} is mainly determined by the plasma sodium concentration, it is reduced in most hyponatremic patients. In some cases, however, the P_{Osm} is either normal (as in pseudohyponatremia) or elevated (as in hyperosmolar hyponatremia) [18].

Urine Osmolality

In patients with hypoosmolar hyponatremia, the U_{Osm} can be used to distinguish between patients with impaired water excretion, accounting for most cases, and primary polydipsia, in which water excretion is normal but intake is so high that it exceeds excretory capacity. Hyponatremia caused by primary polydipsia should completely suppress ADH secretion, resulting in the excretion of a maximally dilute urine with an osmolality less than 100 mOsm per kg and a specific gravity less than 1.003. A higher U_{Osm} indicates an inability to excrete free water normally, which suggests continued secretion of ADH.

Urinary Sodium Concentration

The two major causes of hyponatremia are hypovolemia and SIADH. These disorders can usually be distinguished by measuring the urinary sodium concentration. The urinary sodium concentration of patients with hypovolemia is typically less than 20 mEq per L, assuming the patient is not receiving diuretics. Because patients with SIADH have normal renal perfusion, unless they are on a very low sodium intake, the urinary sodium concentration is greater than 40 mEq per L. Patients with the SIADH can conserve urinary sodium normally and raise the urine osmolality further if intravascular volume depletion occurs.

Evaluation of acid–base and potassium balance may aid in the diagnosis in some hyponatremic patients. As examples, metabolic alkalosis and hypokalemia suggest diuretic use or vomiting, metabolic acidosis and hypokalemia suggest diarrhea or laxative abuse, and metabolic acidosis and hyperkalemia suggest adrenal insufficiency. On the contrary, plasma bicarbonate and potassium concentrations are typically normal in patients with SIADH. Although water retention tends to lower these values by dilution, as it does the plasma sodium and chloride concentrations, normal levels are restored by the factors that normally regulate acid–base and potassium balance.

The initial water retention and volume expansion in patients with SIADH are typically associated with hypouricemia (plasma uric acid concentration of ≤ 3 mg per dL) due to increased uric acid excretion in urine [28]. Also, urinary urea losses may cause a fall in the BUN to less than 5 mg per dL. These findings are the opposite of what is typically seen in volume depletion and thiazide-induced hyponatremia.

All of the findings seen in SIADH also have been described in the controversial syndrome of *cerebral salt wasting*, a disorder in which the high urinary sodium concentration occurs as a result of defective tubular reabsorption, and the elevation in ADH and subsequent development of hyponatremia are due to the associated volume depletion. Hypouricemia also may be present, which presumably is another manifestation of impaired renal tubular function (see previous discussion).

Fractional Excretion of Sodium

The fractional excretion of sodium (FE_{Na}) is a more accurate assessment of volume status than the urinary sodium concentration in patients with acute kidney injury; an FE_{Na} less than 1% suggests effective volume depletion. This observation has led many physicians to use the FE_{Na} in any situation in which the urinary sodium concentration might be helpful. However, the FE_{Na} may be misleading in patients with relatively normal renal function because the expected value to differentiate volume depletion from euvolemia varies with the GFR. A value of less than 1% is not the correct dividing line in this setting because this value may occur in euvolemic patients (such as those with SIADH) who have a urinary sodium concentration above 50 mEq per L and who excrete more than 100 mEq of sodium per day. As a result, the random urinary sodium concentration is more accurate for assessing the volume status in patients with hyponatremia with a normal plasma creatinine concentration. The FE_{Na} should generally not be used in this setting.

Treatment of Hyponatremia

Saline or Water Restriction

In general, the plasma sodium concentration can be raised by giving patients salt (either as saline or salt tablets) or by restricting their water intake to below the level of excretion. The choice of therapy is primarily governed by the cause of the hyponatremia. The more recent additions of antagonists to the ADH receptor in the collecting tubule (vaptans) will also be discussed.

Salt administration, usually as isotonic saline, is appropriate in those with true volume depletion; diuretic therapy, provided the diuretic is no longer acting; or adrenal insufficiency, in which cortisol replacement is also indicated. Water restriction is used in patients without neurologic symptoms who have edematous states such as heart failure and hepatic cirrhosis and in those with SIADH, primary polydipsia, or advanced chronic kidney disease.

In a state of true volume depletion, isotonic saline corrects the hyponatremia by two mechanisms. Each liter of saline infused raises the plasma sodium by 1 to 2 mEq per L because saline has a higher sodium concentration (154 mEq per L) than plasma. By eventually causing volume repletion, it also removes the stimulus to ADH release, thereby allowing the water surfeit to be excreted. At this time, the plasma sodium concentration may return rapidly toward normal.

Isotonic saline should be considered in patients with mild-to-moderate or asymptomatic hyponatremia. In contrast, symptomatic patients or those with a plasma sodium less than 115 mEq per L usually require initial therapy with hypertonic saline. It must be emphasized, however, that careful monitoring is essential because overly rapid correction carries the risk of inducing iatrogenic neurologic complications (see following discussion) [3].

In primary polydipsia, the initiation of water restriction may result in a dramatic rise in the plasma sodium concentration. There is, however, some evidence suggesting that these patients may be less predisposed to osmotic demyelination because their hyponatremia often is of rapid onset, with less brain cell adaptation apt to occur [29].

The optimal rate of correction of hyponatremia varies with the clinical state of the patient. The following represents a reasonable approach, given the information currently available [3,30]. In asymptomatic patients, who are more likely to have chronic hyponatremia, the plasma sodium concentration should be raised at a maximum rate of approximately 0.5 mEq per L per hour and less than 12 mEq per L per day. A more rapid elevation can increase the risk of osmotic demyelination.

More rapid initial correction is indicated in patients with symptomatic hyponatremia, particularly those presenting with seizures or other severe neurologic manifestations, which primarily result from cerebral edema induced by acute (developing during 2 to 3 days) hyponatremia [30]. Here, the plasma sodium concentration can be raised at an initial rate of 1.5 to 2.0 mEq per L per hour for the first 3 to 4 hours (or longer, if the patient remains symptomatic) because the risk of persistent severe hyponatremia outweighs that of overly rapid correction. This appears to be particularly important in premenopausal women, who may progress from minimal symptoms (headache and nausea) to coma and respiratory arrest; furthermore, irreversible neurologic damage or death is relatively common in younger women with symptomatic hyponatremia, even if the hyponatremia is corrected at an appropriate rate. In comparison, men are at much less risk of symptomatic hyponatremia and of permanent neurologic injury. After the initial 3 to 4 hours of rapid correction, the rate should be slowed down so that the total rise in plasma sodium does not exceed approximately 12 mEq during the initial 24 hours.

The quantity of sodium required to achieve the desired elevation in the plasma sodium concentration *in patients with true volume depletion* can be estimated from the product of the plasma sodium deficit per liter and the TBW, which represents the osmotic space of distribution of the plasma sodium concentration. Normal values for the TBW are 0.5 and 0.6 times the lean body weight in women and men, respectively. If the initial aim in an asymptomatic hyponatremic 60-kg woman is to raise the plasma sodium concentration from 110 to 120 mEq per L, then

$$\text{Sodium deficit for initial therapy} = 0.5 \times 60 \times (120 - 110) = 300 \text{ mEq}$$

Thus, 600 mL of 3% hypertonic saline (which contains roughly 1 mEq of sodium per 2 mL, 500 mEq Na, and 500 mEq Cl per L) should be given during 20 hours at a rate of 30 mL per hour. This regimen should raise the plasma sodium concentration at the desired rate of 0.5 mEq per L per hour, and serial monitoring of the plasma sodium concentration (beginning at 2 to 3 hours) is still required.

The preceding formula may be less accurate in patients with SIADH [3]. In this setting, the administered salt in the hypertonic 3% saline is excreted because plasma volume expansion is present. Therefore, the rise in plasma sodium is not due to sodium retention. Because there are approximately 1,000 mEq of solute (Na and Cl) in a liter of 3% saline, the fluid in the renal collecting tubule is relatively hyperosmotic. This causes water to be retained in the urine and excreted simultaneously with the salt load. If, for example, the U_{Osm} were 500 mOsm per kg, the 1,000 mEq of salt excreted would obligate the elimination of 2 L of urine (a net loss of 1 L of free water, because 1 L of water was administered with the hypertonic saline). The result would be no change in total body sodium; the plasma sodium concentration would increase because of the loss of 1 L of water. Administration of the same hypertonic saline solution to an individual with SIADH and a U_{Osm} of 250 mOsm per kg would result in the loss of 4 L of urine (a net water loss of 3 L). The serum sodium would increase by a greater amount than it did in the person with the higher U_{Osm}. As a consequence of the excretion of the salt load and varying levels of U_{Osm} in patients with SIADH, the sodium replacement formula is frequently misleading in this setting.

Effect of Potassium

Potassium is as osmotically active as sodium, and giving potassium can raise the plasma sodium concentration and osmolality in a hyponatremic subject. As most of the excess potassium goes into the cells, electroneutrality is maintained in one of three ways, each of which raises the plasma sodium concentration: (a) intracellular sodium moves into the extracellular fluid; (b) extracellular chloride moves into the cells with potassium; the increase in cell osmolality promotes free water entry into the cells; and (c) intracellular hydrogen moves into the extracellular fluid. These hydrogen ions are buffered by extracellular bicarbonate and, to a much lesser degree, by plasma proteins. This buffering renders the hydrogen ions osmotically inactive; the ensuing fall in extracellular osmolality leads to water movement into the cells.

Thus, any administration of potassium must be taken into account when calculating the sodium deficit. This relationship becomes clinically important in the patient with severe diuretic or vomiting-induced hyponatremia who is also hypokalemic.

Risk of Osmotic Demyelination

Severe hyponatremia, especially if acute in onset, can lead to cerebral edema, potentially irreversible neurologic damage, and death [24]. This most often occurs when large volumes of hypotonic fluids are given to postoperative patients who have pain-induced ADH release that impairs the ability of the kidneys to excrete water or to patients with acute thiazide-induced hyponatremia. Within 24 hours, however, the brain begins to lose extracellular water into the cerebrospinal fluid and loses intracellular water by extruding sodium and potassium salts and osmolytes, thereby lowering the brain volume toward normal (see previous discussion).

The effect is that hyponatremia that develops slowly (i.e., during >2 to 3 days) is associated with a lesser likelihood of neurologic symptoms. In this setting, in which brain volume has fallen toward normal, rapid correction of severe hyponatremia may lead within 1 to several days to the development of a neurologic disorder called *osmotic demyelination* or *central pontine myelinolysis*. These lesions are detectable by cerebral computed tomography or magnetic resonance imaging. Results of these diagnostic tests may not become positive for as long as 4 weeks, however [31].

It has been suggested that there are differences in individual susceptibility to osmotic demyelination. For example, observations indicate that psychiatric patients with primary polydipsia are relatively resistant to osmotic demyelination despite having repeated episodes of hyponatremia and, due to normal water excretory capacity, rapid correction of the plasma sodium concentration [29]. The reasons for this are not known, but this resistance to demyelination may not characterize the polydipsia of chronic alcoholics [32].

The mechanisms responsible for osmotic demyelination are not completely understood. Rapid elevation in the plasma sodium concentration leads to water movement out of the brain, which can lower the brain volume below normal. Such osmotically induced shrinkage in axons could sever their connections with surrounding myelin sheaths. Alternatively, the initial brain cell response to brain shrinkage may be the uptake of potassium and sodium from the extracellular fluid; this elevation in cell cation concentration could be toxic to the cells.

The manifestations of osmotic demyelination, which may be irreversible, include mental status changes, dysarthria, dysphagia, paraparesis or quadriparesis, and coma; seizures may occur but are less common. Patients in whom the plasma sodium concentration is raised to more than 20 mEq per L in the first 24 hours or is overcorrected to greater than 140 mEq per L are at greatest risk. Other putative risk factors for osmotic demyelination include chronic alcoholism, malnutrition, prolonged diuretic use, liver failure and transplantation, and burns [33]. On the contrary, late neurologic deterioration is rare if the hyponatremia is corrected at an average rate equal to or less than 0.5 mEq per L per hour [3,30].

Studies in experimental animals indicate that the total rate of correction during the first 24 hours is more important than the maximum rate in any given hour [34]. Demyelinating lesions are most common when the plasma sodium concentration in severe hyponatremia is raised to more than 20 mEq per L per day and are rare at a rate less than 10 to 12 mEq per L per day. This is similar to the safe average rate of correction of 0.5 mEq per L per hour observed in humans.

Recommendations

The preferred rate at which the plasma sodium concentration should be elevated varies with the clinical presentation. Due to the cerebral adaptation previously described, patients with chronic asymptomatic hyponatremia are generally at little risk for neurologic symptoms. In this setting, rapid correction is not indicated and may be harmful. Although the optimal rate of correction is not clearly proven, the current recommendation in asymptomatic patients is that the plasma sodium concentration be raised at a maximum rate of 12 mEq per L per day (which represents an average correction of 0.5 mEq per L per hour). Although it may be safe to increase the plasma sodium concentration at a rate of more than 12 mEq per day, there is no reason to correct it more rapidly *in the absence of symptoms*.

It is not known whether there is a potential benefit to administering water to previously hypoosmolar patients whose hyponatremia has been corrected much too rapidly. In rodents, a marked reduction in the incidence and severity of brain lesions was demonstrated if overly rapid correction (30 mEq per L or more during several hours) was partially reversed so that the net daily elevation in the plasma sodium concentration was less than 20 mEq per L [35]. This improvement was seen if therapy was begun before the onset of neurologic symptoms; benefit was much less likely in animals with symptomatic demyelination. The applicability of these findings to humans is uncertain.

More aggressive initial correction, at a rate of 1.5 to 2.0 mEq per L per hour, is indicated for the first 3 to 4 hours (or until the symptoms resolve) in patients who present with seizures or other severe neurologic abnormalities due to untreated and usually acute hyponatremia. The primary problem in these patients is cerebral edema, and the risk of delayed therapy is greater than the potential risk of too rapid correction. Even in this setting, however, the plasma sodium concentration should probably not be raised by more than 12 mEq per L in the first 24 hours because partial cerebral adaptation has already occurred. It is usually not necessary to continue hypertonic saline once the plasma sodium concentration is greater than 120 mEq per L.

Treatment of Hyponatremia in the Syndrome of Inappropriate Antidiuretic Hormone Secretion. Hyponatremia in SIADH results primarily from ADH-induced retention of ingested water. Appropriate therapy in this disorder depends on the severity of the hyponatremia and on the fact that, although water excretion is impaired, sodium handling is intact because there is no abnormality in volume-regulating mechanisms such as the renin–angiotensin–aldosterone system. Water restriction is the mainstay of therapy in asymptomatic hyponatremia of chronic SIADH. The associated negative water balance raises the plasma sodium concentration toward normal.

Severe, symptomatic, or resistant hyponatremia often requires the administration of salt. If the plasma sodium concentration is to be elevated, the osmolality of the fluid given must exceed that of the urine. This can be illustrated by a simple example (Table 72.3). Suppose a patient with SIADH and hyponatremia has a U_{Osm} that cannot be reduced below 616 mOsm per kg. If 1,000 mL of isotonic saline is given (containing 154 mEq each of Na and Cl or 308 mOsm), all of the salt is excreted (because sodium handling is intact), but in only 500 mL of water (308 mOsm in 500 mL of water equals 616 mOsm per kg). The retention of half of the administered water leads to a further reduction in the plasma sodium concentration. As a result, correction of the hyponatremia in these cases requires the administration of hypertonic 3% saline intravenously or salt tablets orally, preferably in combination with a drug that lowers the U_{Osm} and increases water excretion by impairing the renal responsiveness to ADH. A loop diuretic is most often used for this purpose.

Demeclocycline and lithium act on the collecting tubule cell to diminish its responsiveness to ADH, thereby increasing water excretion. These drugs tend to be too toxic or ineffective in most patients. Specific antagonists to the ADH-V_2 (antidiuretic) receptor in the cortical collecting tubule have shown promise and two have now been approved for clinical use. Two of these have been approved by the Food and Drug Administration (FDA) at the time of this writing.

TABLE 72.3

MECHANISM OF NORMAL SALINE-INDUCED WORSENING OF HYPONATREMIA IN THE SYNDROME OF INAPPROPRIATE ANTIDIURETIC HORMONE SECRETION[a]

	Solute (mOsm)	Water (mL)
Input	308	1,000
Output	308	500
Net gain	0	+500

[a]This calculation assumes that the individual cannot dilute the urine below a urine osmolality of 616 mOsm/kg and that all the administered solute is excreted in the urine.

Conivaptan, an antagonist to both the V_1 (vascular) and V_2 (ADH) receptors, was the first. It must be given intravenously in the hospital and has the propensity to cause phlebitis. Recent data suggest that a single 20 mg bolus intravenously over 30 minutes results in a sustained water diuresis and may avoid vascular injury. It is not suitable for chronic use. Tolvaptan is an oral ADH antagonist which is specific for the V_2 receptor. It must also be initiated in the hospital but can be administered in the outpatient setting after that. Tolvaptan has been shown to decrease body weight in chronic heart failure patients in a single controlled study [36].

The choice of initial therapy in symptomatic patients is usually 3% saline and this is the preferred treatment with severe neuropathology (such as seizures). In less symptomatic individuals, a vaptan may be effective. However, as there are no controlled prospective studies comparing hypertonic saline with the vaptans, it is difficult to recommend the latter in the SIADH as first-line agents, particularly when cost is considered. When they are administered, it is important to relax fluid restriction during the initial titration with these agents to avoid an excessive rise in the serum sodium concentration.

Reset Osmostat. Hyponatremia due to a reset osmostat may occur in association with any of the causes of SIADH and accounts for between 25% and 30% of cases overall. Downward resetting of the osmostat can also occur in hypovolemic states in which the baroreceptor stimulus to ADH release is superimposed on osmoreceptor function; quadriplegia, in which effective volume depletion may result from venous pooling in the legs; psychosis; tuberculosis; and chronic malnutrition. The plasma sodium concentration also falls by approximately 5 mEq per L in normal pregnancy. How this occurs is incompletely understood, but human chorionic gonadotropin may play an important role [37].

The presence of a reset osmostat should be suspected in any patient with apparent SIADH who has mild hyponatremia (usually between 125 and 135 mEq per L) that is stable over many days despite variations in sodium and water intake. The diagnosis can be confirmed clinically by observing the response to a water load (10 to 15 mL per kg given orally or intravenously during 30 minutes). Healthy subjects and those with a reset osmostat should excrete more than 80% within 4 hours, whereas excretion is impaired in classic SIADH.

Identification of a reset osmostat is important because the therapeutic recommendations for SIADH discussed here do not apply in this setting. These patients generally have mild, asymptomatic hyponatremia due to downward resetting of the threshold for both ADH release and thirst. Because osmoregulatory function is normal around the new baseline, attempting to raise the plasma sodium concentration increases ADH levels and makes the patient very thirsty, a response that is similar to that seen with water restriction in healthy subjects. Thus, efforts to raise the plasma sodium concentration are both unnecessary and likely to be ineffective. Treatment should be primarily directed at the underlying disease.

Treatment of Hyponatremia in Edematous States. Raising the plasma sodium concentration in patients with edema may be more difficult than in those conditions described earlier. Most of these individuals have advanced CHF or liver disease. Consequently, sodium administration is generally contraindicated.

Congestive Heart Failure. Restricting water intake is the mainstay of therapy in hyponatremic patients with heart failure, although this is often not tolerable because of the intense stimulation of thirst. The combination of an angiotensin-converting enzyme (ACE) inhibitor (or angiotensin receptor blocker [ARB]) and a loop diuretic may induce an elevation in the plasma sodium concentration [38,39]. Tolvaptan may be useful in some patients (see above) but must be initiated in the hospital. Conivaptan is not indicated for treatment of hyponatremia in this setting.

Liver Disease. Hyponatremia in patients with hepatic cirrhosis usually develops slowly and produces no cerebral edema or symptoms. It is possible, however, that a low plasma sodium concentration can exacerbate hepatic encephalopathy. In view of the marked sodium and water retention, the mainstay of therapy in this setting is restricting water intake to a level sufficient to induce negative water balance and partial correction of the hyponatremia. Hypertonic saline or salt tablets are indicated only in patients with symptomatic hyponatremia. Diuretics can be given concurrently to prevent worsening of the edema, but overly rapid correction must be avoided to minimize the risk of central demyelinating lesions. As is the case with hyponatremic CHF patients, demeclocycline has been evaluated in this setting, but its use has been limited because of its nephrotoxicity [40].

Hypernatremia

Hypernatremia can be produced by the administration of hypertonic sodium solutions. However, in almost all cases, there is loss of free water. Persistent hypernatremia does not occur in healthy subjects because the ensuing rise in P_{Osm} stimulates both thirst and the release of ADH, which minimizes further water loss. The associated increase in water intake then lowers the plasma sodium concentration to normal. This regulatory system is so efficient that the P_{Osm} is maintained within a range of 1% to 2% despite wide variations in sodium and water intake. Even patients with diabetes insipidus, who often have marked polyuria due to diminished ADH effect, maintain a near-normal plasma sodium concentration by appropriately increasing water intake.

The result is that hypernatremia occurs primarily in those patients who cannot express thirst normally; most often, these patients are infants and adults with impaired mental status, and the elderly, who also appear to have diminished osmotic stimulation of thirst via an unknown mechanism [41]. A patient with a plasma sodium concentration of 150 mEq per L or more who is alert but not thirsty has, by definition, a *hypothalamic lesion* (either structural or functional) affecting the thirst center.

Etiology of Hypernatremia

The major causes of hypernatremia are listed in Table 72.4.

TABLE 72.4

MAJOR CAUSES OF HYPERNATREMIA

Unreplaced water loss
Insensible and sweat losses
Gastrointestinal losses
Central or nephrogenic diabetes insipidus
Hypothalamic lesions affecting thirst or osmoreceptor function
Primary hypodipsia
Essential hypernatremia
Reset osmostat in mineralocorticoid excess
Water loss into cells
Severe exercise or seizures
Sodium overload
Intake of hypertonic sodium solutions

Free Water Loss. The unreplaced loss of solute-free water leads to an elevation in the plasma sodium concentration. Because the plasma sodium concentration and P_{Osm} are determined by the ratio of total body solutes (i.e., *effective osmoles*, chiefly sodium and potassium salts) to TBW, the amounts of sodium and potassium in a fluid determine how loss of that fluid affects body osmolality [3]. The composition of diarrheal fluid can be used to illustrate this point. Many viral and osmotic diarrheas are associated with an isosmotic diarrheal fluid that has a sodium-plus-potassium concentration between 40 and 100 mEq per L; organic solutes, which do not affect the plasma sodium concentration, make up the remaining osmoles. Loss of this fluid tends to induce hypernatremia because water is being lost in excess of sodium plus potassium. Similar considerations apply to urinary losses during an osmotic diuresis induced by glucose, mannitol, or urea (see following discussion). Patients with secretory diarrheas such as cholera excrete a diarrheal fluid with a sodium–potassium concentration similar to that of plasma. Loss of this fluid causes volume and potassium depletion but does not directly affect the plasma sodium concentration.

With these considerations in mind, the sources of free water loss that can lead to hypernatremia if intake is not increased include the following:

- *Insensible and sweat losses.* Insensible water losses from the skin by evaporation and sweat are relatively dilute. The loss of this fluid is increased by fever, exercise, and exposure to high temperatures.
- *Gastrointestinal losses.* As mentioned previously, most gastrointestinal losses promote the development of hypernatremia because the sodium-plus-potassium concentration is less than that in the plasma. An elevation in the plasma sodium concentration with a diarrheal illness is particularly common in infants.
- *Central or nephrogenic diabetes insipidus.* Decreased release of ADH or renal resistance to its effect causes the excretion of a relatively dilute urine (see following discussion). Most affected patients have a normal thirst mechanism and, therefore, typically present with polyuria and polydipsia and, at most, a high-normal plasma sodium concentration. However, marked and symptomatic hypernatremia occurs if there is inadequate replacement (either oral or intravenous) of the urinary water losses.
- *Osmotic diuresis.* An osmotic diuresis due to glucose, mannitol, or urea causes an increase in urine output in which the sodium-plus-potassium concentration is well below that in the plasma because of the presence of the excreted organic solute. Patients with diabetic ketoacidosis or nonketotic hyperglycemia typically present with hyperosmolality, although the plasma sodium concentration may be kept normal or low by the hyperglycemia-induced water movement out of cells.
- *Hypothalamic lesions affecting thirst or osmoreceptor function.* Hypernatremia can occur in the absence of increased water losses if there is a primary hypothalamic disease impairing thirst (called *hypodipsia*). In patients with this problem, forced water intake is usually sufficient to maintain a normal plasma sodium concentration, although central diabetes insipidus (CDI), if present, should be treated.

Other hypodipsic patients do not respond to water loading, as the excess water is excreted in the urine with little change in the plasma sodium concentration. These patients have selective injury to the hypothalamic osmoreceptors, with ADH secretion being primarily governed by changes in blood volume (volume receptors remain intact). Thus, the suppression of ADH release by water loading in such patients is due to the associated mild volume expansion rather than to a fall in P_{Osm}. This disorder is termed *essential hypernatremia* [42]. Correction is difficult, since ADH release and suppression is driven by volume and not by the serum osmolality.

True upward resetting of the osmostat has been described only in patients with primary mineralocorticoid excess (such as in primary hyperaldosteronism). Presumably, the suppressive effect of chronic mild volume expansion on ADH release is responsible for this phenomenon. The plasma sodium concentration in these patients is frequently between 141 and 145 mEq per L and may be a clue to the diagnosis.

Water Loss into Cells. Transient hypernatremia, in which the plasma sodium concentration can rise by 10 to 15 mEq per L within a few minutes, can be induced by intense exercise or seizures, activities that are also associated with lactic acidosis. In this setting, the intracellular breakdown of glycogen into smaller, more osmotically active molecules, such as lactate, can increase water uptake into cells. The plasma sodium concentration returns to normal within 5 to 15 minutes after the cessation of exertion.

Sodium Overload. Acute and often marked hypernatremia, with plasma sodium concentrations even higher than 175 mEq per L, can be induced by administration of hypertonic sodium-containing solutions. Examples include salt poisoning in infants and young children, infusion of hypertonic sodium bicarbonate to treat metabolic acidosis, and massive salt ingestion, such as can occur when a highly concentrated saline emetic or gargle is swallowed [43].

This type of hypernatremia corrects spontaneously if renal function is normal because the excess sodium is rapidly excreted in the urine. Even with optimal therapy, however, the mortality rate is extremely high in adults with a plasma sodium concentration that has suddenly risen to more than 180 mEq per L [44]; for reasons that are poorly understood, severe hypernatremia is often better tolerated in young children.

Symptoms of Hypernatremia

Hypernatremia is basically a mirror image of hyponatremia. The rise in the plasma sodium concentration and osmolality causes rapid water movement out of the brain; this decrease in brain volume can cause tension leading to rupture of the cerebral veins with focal intracerebral and subarachnoid hemorrhages and possible irreversible neurologic damage. The clinical manifestations of this disorder begin with lethargy, weakness, and irritability and can progress to twitching, seizures, and coma. Severe symptoms usually require an acute elevation in the plasma sodium concentration to more than 158 mEq per L.

Despite the generalized reduction in cell volume with hypernatremia, brain volume is gradually restored due to both water movement from the cerebrospinal fluid into the brain (thereby increasing the interstitial volume) and to the uptake of solutes by the brain cells (thereby pulling water into the cells). The latter response involves an initial uptake of sodium and potassium salts, followed by the later accumulation of osmolytes such as inositol and the amino acids glutamine and glutamate [45]. The effect is that these osmolytes, which do not interfere with cell function, account for approximately 35% of the new cell solute.

As in hyponatremia, the cerebral adaptation in hypernatremia has two important clinical consequences:

1. Chronic hypernatremia is much less likely to induce neurologic symptoms. Assessment of symptoms attributable to hypernatremia is often difficult because most affected adults have underlying neurologic disease, which diminishes the protective thirst mechanism that normally prevents the

development of hypernatremia, even in patients with diabetes insipidus.

2. Correction of chronic hypernatremia must occur slowly to prevent rapid fluid movement into the brain leading to cerebral edema, which can cause seizures and coma. Although the brain cells can rapidly lose potassium and sodium in response to this cell swelling, the loss of accumulated osmolytes occurs more slowly, a phenomenon that acts to hold water within the cells. The loss of inositol, for example, requires both a reduction in synthesis of new sodium–inositol cotransporters and the activation of a specific inositol efflux mechanism in the cell membrane. The delayed clearance of osmolytes from the cell can predispose to cerebral edema if the plasma sodium concentration is corrected too rapidly.

Diagnosis of Hypernatremia and Polyuric Disorders

The cause of the hypernatremia is usually evident from the history. When the cause is unclear, the correct diagnosis can usually be established by evaluation of the integrity of the ADH-renal axis via measurement of the U_{Osm}. A rise in the plasma sodium concentration is a potent stimulus to ADH release as well as to thirst; furthermore, a P_{Osm} of more than 295 mOsm per kg (representing a plasma sodium concentration of approximately 145 to 147 mEq per L) generally leads to sufficient ADH secretion to maximally stimulate urinary concentration.

Thus, if both hypothalamic and renal functions are intact, the U_{Osm} of a person with hypernatremia should exceed 700 to 800 mOsm per kg. In this setting, unreplaced insensible or gastrointestinal losses, sodium overload, or, rarely, a primary defect in thirst is likely to be responsible for the hypernatremia. Exogenous ADH does not produce a further rise in the U_{Osm}.

The chemical composition of the urine is diagnostically useful. The urinary sodium concentration should be less than 20 mEq per L when water loss and volume depletion are the primary problems, but it is typically well above 100 mEq per L in a salt-overload state [43]. If the U_{Osm} is significantly lower than that of the hyperosmolar plasma, then either central (ADH-deficient) or nephrogenic (ADH-resistant) diabetes insipidus is present.

Diagnosis of Polyuric States and Diabetes Insipidus. *Polyuria* can be arbitrarily defined as urine output exceeding 3 L per day. It must be differentiated from the more common complaints of frequency and nocturia, which are usually not associated with an increase in the total urine output. Not counting the glucose-induced osmotic diuresis of uncontrolled diabetes mellitus, there are three major causes of polyuria in the outpatient setting. Each of these causes is due to dysregulation of water balance, leading to excessive excretion of dilute urine (U_{Osm} usually <250 mOsm per kg).

Primary Polydipsia. Primary polydipsia (also called *psychogenic polydipsia*) is characterized by a primary increase in water intake (see Hyponatremia section). This disorder is most often seen in anxious, middle-aged women and in patients with psychiatric illnesses, including those taking medications that can lead to the sensation of dry mouth. Primary polydipsia can also be induced by hypothalamic lesions that directly affect the thirst center, as may occur with an infiltrative disease such as sarcoidosis. As expected, polyuria resulting from primary polydipsia is not associated with hypernatremia.

Central Diabetes Insipidus. CDI is associated with deficient secretion of ADH. This condition is most often idiopathic (possibly due to autoimmune injury to the ADH-producing cells) or induced by trauma, pituitary surgery or infiltration, or hypoxic or ischemic encephalopathy. When CDI develops following trauma or surgery, a triphasic response may be observed [46]. In this condition, initial inhibition of ADH results in polyuria; this is followed by uncontrolled release of ADH from injured cells and, subsequently, by permanent CDI.

Nephrogenic Diabetes Insipidus. Nephrogenic diabetes insipidus (NDI) is characterized by normal ADH secretion but varying degrees of renal resistance to its water-retaining effect. In its mild form, NDI is relatively common because most patients who are elderly or who have underlying renal disease have a reduction in maximum concentrating ability. This defect, however, is not severe enough to produce a symptomatic increase in urine output. True polyuria due to ADH resistance occurs primarily in four settings: X-linked hereditary NDI in children, in which there is an abnormality in the renal V_2 receptors for ADH or in the ADH-sensitive water channel (*aquaporin 2*) [47]; chronic lithium use, which can lead to polyuria in approximately 20% of patients; hypercalcemia; and severe hypokalemia.

Each of these conditions is associated with an increase in water output and the excretion of a relatively dilute urine. With primary polydipsia, the polyuria is an appropriate response to excessive water intake. In comparison, the water loss is inappropriate with either form of diabetes insipidus. Thus, a low plasma sodium concentration at presentation (<137 mEq per L) due to water overload is usually indicative of primary polydipsia, whereas a high-normal plasma sodium concentration (>142 mEq per L) points toward diabetes insipidus. Marked hypernatremia is uncommon in diabetes insipidus because the initial loss of water stimulates the thirst mechanism, resulting in an increase in intake to match the urinary losses. An exception to this general rule is the patient with a central lesion impairing both ADH release and thirst whose plasma sodium concentration can exceed 160 mEq per L.

The correct diagnosis is often inferred from the plasma sodium concentration and from the history. The patient should be questioned about the causes of CDI or NDI and about the rate of onset of the polyuria; the polyuria is usually abrupt in CDI ("I suddenly began urinating excessively 2 days ago") but gradual in NDI or primary polydipsia.

Even if the diagnosis seems straightforward based on the history or plasma sodium concentration, it should be confirmed. This is accomplished by challenging the kidneys' ability to concentrate the urine in response to a high P_{Osm}. The P_{Osm} can be raised either by water restriction or, less commonly, by the administration of hypertonic saline (0.05 mL per kg per minute for no more than 2 hours). These maneuvers are unnecessary if the patient's P_{Osm} is already at or above 295 mOsm per kg. At this point, exogenous ADH is administered.

The water restriction test for the evaluation of polyuria involves measurement of the urine volume and osmolality every hour and plasma sodium concentration and P_{Osm} every 2 hours. The patient should stop drinking 2 to 3 hours before beginning the test; overnight fluid restriction should be avoided because potentially severe volume depletion and hypernatremia can be induced in patients with marked polyuria.

Interpretation of the water restriction test is based on the following observations: (a) raising the P_{Osm} leads to a progressive elevation in ADH release and, therefore, an increase in the U_{Osm} in normal individuals; and (b) once the P_{Osm} reaches 295 to 300 mOsm per kg (normal, 280 to 290 mOsm per kg), endogenous ADH effect on the kidney is maximal. At this point, administering ADH does not elevate the U_{Osm} unless endogenous ADH release is impaired (i.e., unless the patient has CDI).

The water restriction test is continued until the U_{Osm} reaches a clearly appropriate level of concentration (approximately 600 mOsm per kg, indicating that both ADH release and effect are intact), the U_{Osm} is stable on two or three successive measurements despite a rising P_{Osm}, more than 3% to 5% of body weight is lost, or the P_{Osm} exceeds 295 to 300 mOsm per kg. In the last two cases, exogenous ADH is then given, usually in the form of 10 μg of deamino-8-D-arginine vasopressin [DDAVP; also called desmopressin] by nasal insufflation, and the U_{Osm} and volume are monitored over every 30 minutes for 90 minutes. Measuring the serum ADH level at the start of the test and immediately before DDAVP is administered may be useful.

Each of the causes of polyuria produces a distinct pattern:

1. CDI is usually partial and, therefore, associated with a rise in the U_{Osm} as the P_{Osm} increases. The degree of urinary concentration is clearly submaximal, however, and because ADH release is inadequate, exogenous ADH leads to a rise in the U_{Osm} of 15% to 50% and a corresponding fall in urine output.
2. NDI also is associated with a submaximal rise in U_{Osm}, but there is no urinary response to exogenous ADH. It must be emphasized that NDI is a rare cause of true polyuria in adults in the absence of lithium use, hypercalcemia, hypokalemia, or, rarely, renal tubular disease.
3. Primary polydipsia is associated with a rise in U_{Osm}, usually to more than 500 mOsm per kg, and no response to exogenous ADH because endogenous release is intact. The chronic polyuria in this disorder can partially wash out the medullary interstitial solute gradient; as a result, maximal concentrating ability is impaired and the U_{Osm} may only reach 500 to 600 mOsm per kg, as compared with 800 mOsm per kg or more in healthy subjects.

A properly performed test in which ADH is not given until the P_{Osm} exceeds 295 mOsm per kg usually establishes the correct diagnosis. The different patterns of response are depicted in Figure 72.3. There is, however, one major potential source

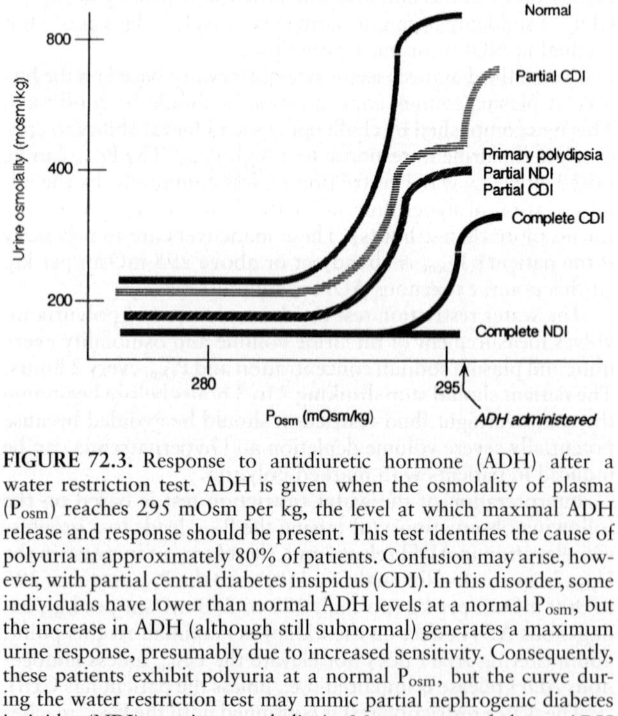

FIGURE 72.3. Response to antidiuretic hormone (ADH) after a water restriction test. ADH is given when the osmolality of plasma (P_{osm}) reaches 295 mOsm per kg, the level at which maximal ADH release and response should be present. This test identifies the cause of polyuria in approximately 80% of patients. Confusion may arise, however, with partial central diabetes insipidus (CDI). In this disorder, some individuals have lower than normal ADH levels at a normal P_{osm}, but the increase in ADH (although still subnormal) generates a maximum urine response, presumably due to increased sensitivity. Consequently, these patients exhibit polyuria at a normal P_{osm}, but the curve during the water restriction test may mimic partial nephrogenic diabetes insipidus (NDI) or primary polydipsia. Measurement of plasma ADH levels may be needed to distinguish these possibilities. [From Zerbe R, Robertson G: A comparison of plasma vasopressin measurements with a standard indirect test in the differential diagnosis of polyuria. *N Engl J Med* 305:1539, 1981, with permission.]

of error. Patients with partial CDI may be hyperresponsive to the submaximal rise in ADH induced by water restriction, perhaps because of receptor upregulation. As a result, they may be polyuric at the normal P_{Osm} of 285 to 290 mOsm per kg when ADH levels are very low, but they may have a maximally concentrated urine at a P_{Osm} of more than 295 mOsm per kg when ADH levels are somewhat higher. In such patients, exogenous ADH is without effect, resulting in a pattern suggestive of primary polydipsia or NDI. Therefore, measurement of plasma ADH levels may be useful. In this condition, the serum sodium concentration is normal or elevated, in contrast to primary polydipsia, where it is typically below 140 mEq per L.

The previous discussion has emphasized the diagnostic approach to a water diuresis. In some polyuric patients, however, the increase in urine output is due to a solute or to osmotic diuresis in which decreased solute reabsorption is the primary abnormality. Although glucosuria is the most common cause of osmotic diuresis in outpatients, other conditions may account for inpatient cases. These include high-protein feedings (in which urea acts as the osmotic agent) and volume expansion due to saline loading or the administration of mannitol. The U_{Osm} in these disorders is usually greater than 300 mOsm per kg, in contrast to the dilute urine typically found with a water diuresis. Total solute excretion, which is calculated from the product of the U_{Osm} and volume of a 24-hour urine sample, is normal with a water diuresis (600 to 900 mOsm per day) but markedly increased with an osmotic diuresis.

Although renal disease can impair sodium conservation in the presence of volume depletion, it rarely causes sufficient sodium wasting to induce true polyuria. The polyuria of postobstructive diuresis is often misunderstood. Physicians observing a urine output that may initially exceed 1,000 mL per hour may feel compelled to replace the urine output with intravenous fluids. This merely prolongs the polyuria by protracting the volume expansion. Optimal therapy of a postobstructive diuresis consists of fluid infusion at a maintenance level, such as 75 mL of one-half isotonic saline per hour. The development of volume depletion, as evidenced by hypotension or a rise in the BUN, is unusual with this regimen.

Treatment of Hypernatremia

The water deficit of a hypernatremic patient can be estimated from the following calculation. The quantity of osmoles in the body is equal to the osmolal space (the TBW) times the osmolality of the body fluids:

$$\text{Total body osmoles} = \text{TBW} \times P_{Osm}$$

$$\text{Water deficit} = \text{current body water (plasma Na}^{+}/140 - 1)$$

where current (observed) body water = 60% body mass.

This formula estimates the amount of positive water balance required to return the plasma sodium concentration to 140 mEq per L. It does not account for electrolyte losses that may occur conjointly with water losses in such settings as osmotic diuresis or diarrhea. In addition, hypernatremia itself may cause mild urinary sodium wasting in hypovolemic subjects, largely as a result of reduced aldosterone release. Both hypernatremia and concurrent hypokalemia (due to gastrointestinal or renal losses) may act directly on reducing aldosterone production by adrenal glands.

Rate of Correction. As in hyponatremia, overly rapid correction is potentially dangerous in hypernatremia [45]. Rapidly lowering the plasma sodium concentration once osmotic adaptation has occurred may cause cerebral edema and lead to seizures, permanent neurologic damage, or death. This adverse sequence has been described in children in whom hypernatremia was corrected at a rate exceeding 0.7 mEq per L per hour. In comparison, no neurologic sequelae were induced when the plasma sodium concentration was lowered at 0.5 mEq per L per hour [48].

The water deficit represents the existing amount of water loss that must be offset; ongoing free water losses, including insensible losses (approximately 40 mL per hour), must also be replaced. The replacement fluid can be administered orally or intravenously as dextrose in water. Sodium or potassium can be added if there are concurrent losses of these cations, but the addition of these solutes decreases the amount of free water that is being given. It should be emphasized that an isotonic saline solution should be used as initial therapy in the volume-depleted, hypotensive patient because restoration of tissue perfusion is of primary importance.

Treatment of Diabetes Insipidus. The major symptoms of both forms of diabetes insipidus are polyuria and polydipsia, related to the urinary concentrating defect (see previous discussion). Treatment for these disorders is aimed at decreasing the urine output.

Central Diabetes Insipidus. Because the primary problem is deficient secretion of ADH, control of the polyuria can be achieved by hormone replacement using DDAVP (desmopressin), a two–amino acid synthetic analogue of ADH. DDAVP is administered by nasal spray in a usual dose starting at 5 μg once a day. Since nocturia is often the most troubling symptom, the initial dose is usually given at night. Tablets of desmopressin are also available although their absorption may vary in different patients. Therefore, switching from one of the intranasal form to a tablet may require retitration and close monitoring. The starting dose of the tablet is 0.05 mg per day. The size and necessity for a daytime dose can be determined by the effectiveness of the evening dose. If, for example, polyuria does not recur until noon, then one-half of the evening doses may be sufficient at that time.

One important potential risk inherent in treating CDI with DDAVP is that of water retention leading to the development of hyponatremia. There are several reasons why this may occur. Patients are no longer polyuric once on therapy. Because they are on a fixed dose of DDAVP, their ADH activity is constant and not regulated. V_2 receptors may be upregulated as a result of prolonged deprivation of vasopressin. Finally, some patients may retain their habitually large consumption of water even after their polyuria ceases. Hyponatremia in this context can be avoided by giving the minimum dose that is required to control the polyuria.

Nephrogenic Diabetes Insipidus. NDI results from partial or complete resistance of the kidney to the effects of ADH. As a result, patients with this disorder are not likely to respond to either hormone administration (such as DDAVP) or to drugs such as chlorpropamide and carbamazepine that increase either the renal response to ADH or ADH secretion.

In adults, a concentrating defect severe enough to produce polyuria due to NDI is most often due to chronic lithium use or hypercalcemia. Less frequently, it is caused by other conditions that impair tubular function, such as Sjögren's syndrome (see previous discussion). Therapy targets correction of the underlying disorder or discontinuing a causative drug. In hypercalcemic patients, for example, normalization of the plasma calcium concentration usually leads to amelioration of polyuria. In contrast, lithium-induced NDI may be irreversible if the patient already has severe tubular injury and a marked concentrating defect.

Thiazide diuretics can diminish the degree of polyuria in patients with persistent and symptomatic NDI. The potassium-sparing diuretic amiloride may be helpful because of its additive effect with a thiazide diuretic and, in cases of reversible lithium-induced disease, may allow lithium to be continued (see following discussion) [49].

The combination of a low-sodium diet with a thiazide diuretic (such as hydrochlorothiazide, 25 mg once or twice daily) acts by inducing mild volume depletion. As little as a 1.0- to 1.5-kg weight loss reduced the urine output by more than 50%, from 10.0 L per day to less than 3.5 L per day, in one study of patients with NDI. This effect is presumably mediated by a hypovolemia-induced increase in proximal sodium and water reabsorption, thereby diminishing water delivery to the ADH-sensitive sites in the collecting tubules and reducing the urine output. The initial natriuresis and, therefore, the antipolyuric response can be enhanced by combination therapy with amiloride (or another potassium-sparing diuretic) [49]. This regimen has an additional benefit in that amiloride partially blocks the potassium wasting induced by the thiazide.

Thiazide diuretics also limit the ability to dilute the urine. As a result, the concentration of urine in a thiazide-treated individual with NDI typically increases, even in the absence of ADH. This contributes to the decrease in urine volume. As an example, in a patient with a normal solute excretion rate of 900 mOsm per kg per day and a maximum U_{Osm} of 150 mOsm per kg due to NDI, a urine output of at least 6 L per day is expected (900 ÷ 150). In contrast, if a thiazide diuretic limits the minimum U_{Osm} to 300 mOsm per day, daily urine output decreases to approximately 3 L each day (900 ÷ 300).

The efficacy of amiloride in patients with reversible lithium nephrotoxicity is directly related to its site and mechanism of action. This drug closes the sodium channels in the luminal membrane of the collecting tubule cells. These channels constitute the mechanism by which filtered lithium normally enters these cells and then interferes with their response to ADH. In contrast to amiloride, thiazide diuretics should be used cautiously, if at all, in patients with lithium-induced NDI *who are still taking lithium* because volume depletion can lead to increased proximal lithium reabsorption and potentially toxic plasma lithium levels.

Nonsteroidal anti-inflammatory drugs (NSAIDs) cause inhibition of renal prostaglandin synthesis. This has the effect of increasing concentrating ability because prostaglandins normally antagonize the urinary concentrating action of ADH. If, for example, healthy subjects are given a submaximal dose of ADH, the ensuing rise in U_{Osm} can be increased by more than 200 mOsm per kg if the patient has been pretreated with an NSAID. The result in patients with NDI may be a 25% to 50% reduction in urine output, a response that is partially additive to that of a thiazide diuretic. Not all NSAIDs are equally effective in a given patient. For example, some patients may have a good response to indomethacin but derive little, if any, benefit from ibuprofen. How this applies to cyclooxygenase-2 inhibitors remains to be determined. However, case reports have shown that cyclooxygenase-2 inhibitors can exacerbate CHF and have been associated with fluid overload, in a manner similar to that of traditional nonselective NSAIDS [50].

Dietary modification via the use of a low-sodium, low-protein diet can diminish the urine output in patients with NDI. The resultant decrease in net solute excretion (as sodium salts and urea) at any given U_{Osm} reduces the urine output.

Most patients with NDI have partial, rather than complete, resistance to ADH. It is therefore possible that administering exogenous ADH in doses sufficient to achieve supraphysiologic hormone levels can increase the renal effect of ADH. Although one case report of a patient with lithium-induced NDI suggested that this benefit is more likely to be achieved if DDAVP is combined with an NSAID, this has not been our experience, particularly in patients with more severe NDI.

DISORDERS OF PLASMA POTASSIUM

Potassium is the major intracellular cation. Only approximately 2% of body potassium is located in the extracellular space, where the concentration (3.5 to 5.0 mEq per L) is much lower than inside cells (125 to 140 mEq per L). This concentration difference is preserved by the Na^+/K^+–ATPase pump that actively transports sodium out of, and potassium into, most cells. Because such a small proportion of K^+ is extracellular, even a slight change in plasma potassium concentration can engender dramatic effects on myoneural cell physiology.

Normal Potassium Homeostasis

Daily potassium intake in the United States varies between 40 and 120 mEq. Most of this (approximately 90%) is eliminated by the kidney; the rest is excreted in stool. In chronic kidney disease, gastrointestinal potassium excretion increases, a process that depends, in part, on aldosterone.

Only approximately 50% of potassium ingested in the diet or administered parenterally appears in the urine during the first 4 hours. Consequently, more than half of an acute potassium load must be rapidly translocated into cells if life-threatening hyperkalemia to be averted.

Transcellular Potassium Shifts

The most important factors involved in transporting K^+ intracellularly are insulin and β-adrenergic stimulation. Insulin stimulates the Na^+/K^+–ATPase pump present in most cell membranes, accelerating the transfer process.

Activation of β-adrenergic receptors (specifically the β_2-receptor) also stimulates K^+ movement from the plasma into cells. The pathophysiology is due in part to direct stimulation of the Na^+/K^+–ATPase pump. The observation that the hypokalemic effect of terbutaline (a β-adrenergic agonist) can be blunted by somatostatin suggests that insulin may have a mediatory role in the hypokalemic response to β-adrenergic stimulation.

Aldosterone is the principal hormone stimulating K^+ secretion by the renal tubule (see following discussion). This effect is important in all epithelial cell surfaces, although its contribution to translocation of K^+ into nonepithelial cells is more controversial [51].

Renal Regulation of Potassium Excretion

Potassium is freely filtered at the glomerulus so that the concentration of K^+ entering the early proximal tubule is approximately 4 mEq per L. Ninety percent of the filtered potassium load has been reabsorbed by the time the glomerular filtrate reaches the distal tubule. Most renal K^+ excretion normally occurs as a result of secretion by the distal nephron. Potassium secretion occurs in the principal cells of the cortical collecting tubule (Fig. 72.4). Movement of potassium from the tubular cell into the lumen is controlled by the existing state of potassium balance, the rate of sodium reabsorption (a process driven by aldosterone) that generates a lumen-negative electrical gradient down which K^+ can move, and the rate of distal urine flow that maintains a high tubular cell–to–lumen potassium gradient by washing away secreted K^+.

Aldosterone enters the principal cell from the basolateral (antiluminal) side. Once inside, it binds to receptors, which increase the number of open luminal sodium channels and increase the number and activity of the Na^+/K^+–ATPase pumps

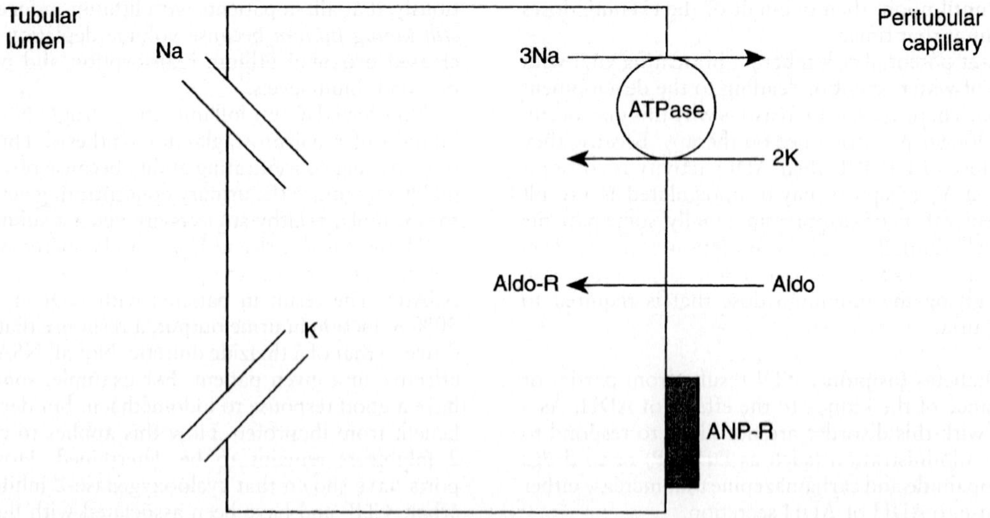

FIGURE 72.4. Schematic representation of sodium and potassium transport mechanisms in the sodium-reabsorbing cells in the collecting tubules. The entry of filtered sodium into the cells is mediated by selective sodium channels in the apical (luminal) membrane; the energy for this process is provided by the favorable electrochemical gradient for sodium (cell interior electronegative and low cell sodium concentration). Reabsorbed sodium is pumped out of the cell by the Na^+/K^+–adenosine triphosphatase (ATPase) pump in the basolateral (peritubular) membrane. The reabsorption of cationic sodium makes the lumen electronegative, thereby creating a favorable gradient for the secretion of potassium into the lumen via potassium channels in the apical membrane. Aldosterone (Aldo), after combining with the cytosolic mineralocorticoid receptor (Aldo-R), leads to enhanced sodium reabsorption and potassium secretion in the cortical collecting tubule by increasing both the number of open sodium channels and the number of Na^+/K^+–ATPase pumps. Atrial natriuretic peptide (ANP), on the contrary, acts primarily in the inner medullary collecting duct by combining with its basolateral membrane receptor (ANP-R) and activating guanylate cyclase. ANP inhibits sodium reabsorption by closing the sodium channels. The potassium-sparing diuretics amiloride and triamterene act by closing the sodium channels directly, and spironolactone acts by competing with aldosterone for binding to the mineralocorticoid receptor.

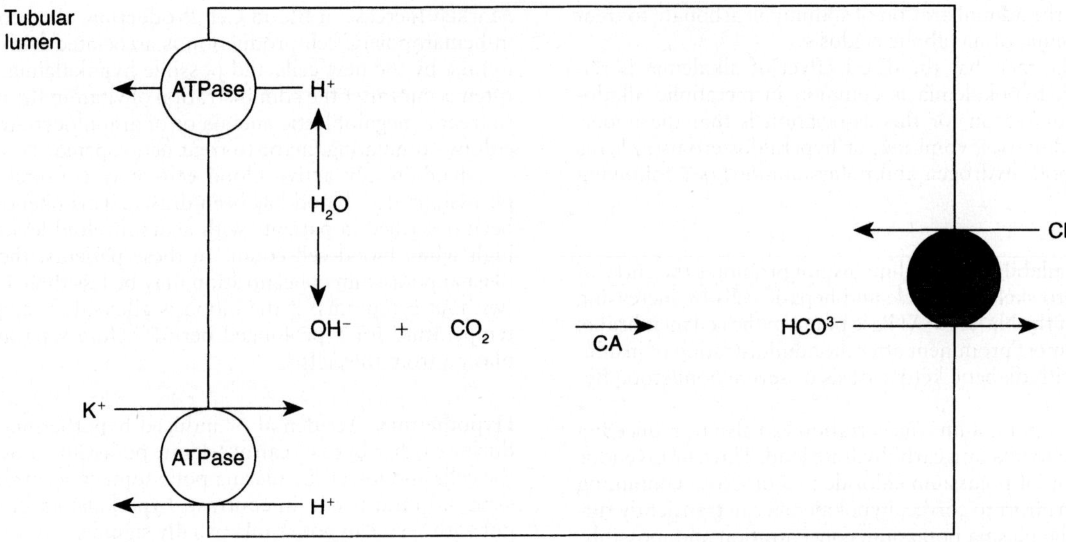

FIGURE 72.5. Transport mechanisms involved in hydrogen secretion and bicarbonate and potassium reabsorption in type-A intercalated cells in the cortical collecting tubule and in the outer medullary collecting tubule cells. Water (H_2O) within the cell dissociates into hydrogen and hydroxyl anions. The former are secreted into the lumen by H–adenosine triphosphatase (ATPase) pumps in the luminal membrane; chloride may be cosecreted with hydrogen to maintain electroneutrality. The hydroxyl anions in the cell combine with carbon dioxide to form bicarbonate in a reaction catalyzed by carbonic anhydrase (CA). Bicarbonate is then returned to the systemic circulation via chloride–bicarbonate exchangers in the basolateral membrane. The favorable inward concentration gradient for chloride (plasma and interstitial concentration greater than that in the cell) provides the energy for bicarbonate reabsorption. H-K–ATPase pumps, which lead to both hydrogen secretion and potassium reabsorption, may also be present in the luminal membrane. The number of these pumps increases with potassium depletion, suggesting that their main function is to promote potassium conservation.

in the basolateral membrane. The ensuing increase in cell potassium favors the secretion of K^+ into the lumen, down the electrochemical gradient provided by Na^+ reabsorption.

In states of potassium depletion, potassium secretion in the cortical collecting tubule is reduced, and potassium reabsorption stimulated. Reabsorption takes place in the intercalated (acid-secreting) cells of this nephron segment (Fig. 72.5).

Hypokalemia

Potassium entering the body is largely stored in the cells and then excreted in the urine. Thus, a reduction in the plasma potassium concentration can result from decreased intake, increased cellular uptake, or increased losses. These losses, which are the most common contributors to hypokalemia, can occur via the urine, the gastrointestinal tract, or, less commonly, through the skin (Table 72.5).

Causes of Hypokalemia

Decreased Potassium Intake. Because the kidney can lower potassium excretion to less than 25 mEq per day in response to potassium depletion [52], decreased intake alone rarely causes hypokalemia, but it can enhance the severity of other causes of potassium depletion such as diuretic therapy.

Increased Entry Into Cells. The markedly inequitable distribution of potassium between the cells and the extracellular fluid is maintained by the Na^+/K^+–ATPase pump in the cell membrane. Occasionally, increased potassium entry into cells may result in transient hypokalemia. Barium sulfide, used in pesticides, radiologic imaging, and depilatory agents, has been reported to cause severe transient hypokalemia when ingested [53].

Elevation in Extracellular pH. The transcellular hydrogen-ion shifts accompanying metabolic and respiratory alkalosis obligate increased sequestration of potassium in cells. In general, this direct effect is relatively small because the plasma potassium concentration falls to less than 0.4 mEq per L for every 0.1-unit rise in pH [54]. This phenomenon provides the

TABLE 72.5

MAJOR CAUSES OF HYPOKALEMIA

Decreased potassium intake
Increased entry into cells
Elevation in extracellular pH
Increased availability of insulin
Elevated β-adrenergic activity
Hypokalemic periodic paralysis
Marked increase in blood cell production
Increased gastrointestinal losses
Increased urinary losses
Diuretics
Primary mineralocorticoid excess
Loss of gastric secretions
Nonreabsorbable anions
Renal tubular acidosis
Hypomagnesemia
Amphotericin B
Aminoglycosides
Salt-wasting nephropathies, including Bartter's syndrome
Polyuria
Increased sweat losses
Dialysis

rationale for the administration of sodium bicarbonate to treat the hyperkalemia of metabolic acidosis.

Despite the fact that the direct effect of alkalemia is relatively small, hypokalemia is common in metabolic alkalosis. The major reason for this association is that the underlying cause (diuretics, vomiting, or hyperaldosteronism) leads to losses of both hydrogen and potassium ions (see following discussion).

Increased Availability of Insulin. Insulin promotes the entry of potassium into skeletal muscle and hepatic cells by increasing the activity of the Na^+/K^+–ATPase pump in the cell membrane. This effect is most prominent after the administration of insulin to patients with diabetic ketoacidosis or severe nonketotic hyperglycemia.

The plasma potassium concentration can also be reduced in nondiabetic patients by a carbohydrate load. Thus, intravenous administration of potassium chloride in a dextrose-containing solution in an effort to correct hypokalemia can transiently further reduce the plasma potassium concentration and, possibly, lead to cardiac arrhythmias [55].

Elevated β-Adrenergic Activity. Catecholamines, acting via β_2-adrenergic receptors, promote potassium entry into the cells by increasing Na^+/K^+–ATPase activity. As a result, transient hypokalemia can occur with stress-induced release of epinephrine, as in acute illness, coronary ischemia, theophylline intoxication, or alcohol withdrawal. A similar effect, in which the plasma potassium concentration can fall acutely by more than 0.5 to 1.0 mEq per L, can be achieved by the administration of a β-adrenergic agonist (such as albuterol, terbutaline, or epinephrine) [56]. This effect must be considered when diuretic therapy is used for the treatment of hypertension in patients receiving β-agonists for asthma or chronic lung disease. The hypokalemic response to epinephrine can be blocked by a nonselective beta-blocker (such as propranolol), but a β_1-selective agent (such as atenolol) offers no protection, at least at lower doses (<100 mg per day).

Hypokalemic Periodic Paralysis. Hypokalemic periodic paralysis is a rare disorder of uncertain cause characterized by potentially fatal episodes of muscle weakness or paralysis that can affect the respiratory muscles. Acute attacks—in which the sudden movement of potassium into the cells can lower the plasma potassium concentration to as low as 1.5 to 2.5 mEq per L—are often precipitated by rest after exercise, stress, or a carbohydrate meal, events that are often associated with increased release of epinephrine or insulin.

Hypokalemic periodic paralysis may be familial with autosomal dominant inheritance, or it may be acquired in patients (often, but not exclusively, Asian men) with thyrotoxicosis [57]. Recent studies indicate that the abnormal gene in patients with the inherited form of this disorder appears to code for part of the dihydropyridine calcium channel in skeletal muscle [58]. How this predisposes to hypokalemia is unclear. A recent article reported location of the gene to a locus on chromosome one [59].

Oral administration of 60 to 120 mEq of potassium chloride usually aborts acute attacks within 15 to 20 minutes. Another 60 mEq can be given if no improvement is noted. The presence of hypokalemia must be confirmed before therapy because potassium can worsen episodes caused by the normokalemic or hyperkalemic forms of periodic paralysis. Furthermore, excess potassium administration during an acute episode may lead to posttreatment hyperkalemia as potassium moves back out of the cells.

Marked Increase in Blood Cell Production. An acute increase in hematopoietic cell production is associated with potassium uptake by the new cells and possible hypokalemia. This most often occurs after the administration of vitamin B_{12} or folic acid to treat a megaloblastic anemia or of granulocyte-macrophage colony-stimulating factor to treat neutropenia.

Metabolically active blood cells may continue to absorb potassium after blood has been drawn. This phenomenon has been described in patients with acute myeloid leukemia and a high white blood cell count. In these patients, the measured plasma potassium concentration may be less than 1 mEq per L (without symptoms) if the blood is allowed to stand at room temperature for a prolonged period before separation of the plasma from the cells.

Hypothermia. Accidental or induced hypothermia (as occurs during cardiac bypass) can accelerate potassium movement into the cells and lower the plasma potassium concentration to less than 3.0 mEq per L. In contrast, hyperkalemia in an individual with severe hypothermia usually signifies irreversible tissue necrosis (including rhabdomyolysis) and is associated with a high mortality rate [60].

Acute Chloroquine Intoxication. Hypokalemia is a complication of severe chloroquine overdose [61].

Increased Gastrointestinal Losses. Loss of gastric or intestinal secretions from any cause (vomiting, diarrhea, laxatives, or tube drainage) is associated with potassium wasting and, possibly, hypokalemia. However, it should be emphasized that the concentration of potassium in gastric secretions is relatively low (5 to 10 mEq per L) and that the potassium depletion is primarily due to increased urinary losses [62]. The metabolic alkalosis that results from loss of gastric secretions raises the plasma bicarbonate concentration and, therefore, the filtered bicarbonate load above its proximal tubular reabsorptive threshold. More sodium bicarbonate and water are thus delivered to the distal potassium secretory site in the presence of hypovolemia-induced aldosterone release. Secreted potassium combines with the negatively charged bicarbonate and is excreted in the final urine, leading to hypokalemia.

The urinary potassium wasting seen with loss of gastric secretions is typically most prominent in the first few days; thereafter, proximal bicarbonate reabsorptive capacity increases, leading to a marked reduction in urinary sodium, bicarbonate, and potassium excretion. At this time, the urine pH falls from more than 7.0 to less than 5.5.

Increased Urinary Losses. Urinary potassium excretion is mostly derived from potassium secretion in the distal nephron, particularly by the principal cells in the cortical collecting tubule. This process is primarily influenced by two factors: aldosterone and the distal delivery of sodium and water. Urinary potassium wasting generally requires increases in aldosterone or in distal flow. Aldosterone acts partly by stimulating sodium reabsorption. The removal of cationic sodium makes the lumen relatively electronegative, thereby promoting passive potassium secretion from the tubular cell into the lumen through specific potassium channels in the luminal membrane.

Diuretics. Any diuretic that acts proximal to the potassium secretory site, including carbonic anhydrase inhibitors and loop and thiazide diuretics, increases distal delivery and, via the induction of volume depletion, activates the renin–angiotensin–aldosterone system. As a result, urinary potassium excretion increases, potentially leading to hypokalemia.

Primary Mineralocorticoid Excess. Urinary potassium wasting is characteristic of any condition associated with primary hypersecretion of a mineralocorticoid, as occurs with an aldosterone-producing adrenal adenoma. Affected patients are usually hypertensive, and the differential diagnosis includes diuretic therapy (which may be surreptitious) in a patient with underlying hypertension and renovascular disease, in which increased secretion of renin leads to enhanced aldosterone release. By comparison, plasma renin activity is suppressed in primary states of mineralocorticoid excess.

Nonreabsorbable Anions. The presence of nonreabsorbable anions in the filtrate draws increased amounts of sodium to the distal nephron where it is reabsorbed at the expense of potassium. Examples of nonreabsorbable anions include bicarbonate in vomiting-induced metabolic alkalosis, β-hydroxybutyrate in diabetic ketoacidosis, hippurate in toluene exposure (glue sniffing) [63], and penicillin in patients receiving high-dose penicillin therapy. The effect of nonreabsorbable anions is augmented when there is concurrent volume depletion. Both the resulting decrease in distal chloride delivery (limiting the ability of chloride reabsorption to dissipate the lumen-negative gradient) and the enhanced secretion of aldosterone promote potassium secretion [64].

Metabolic Acidosis. Increased urinary potassium losses can occur in several forms of metabolic acidosis by mechanisms similar to those already described. In diabetic ketoacidosis, for example, increased distal sodium and water delivery (due to the glucose-induced osmotic diuresis), hypovolemia-induced hyperaldosteronism, and β-hydroxybutyrate acting as a nonreabsorbable anion all can contribute to potassium wasting. Potassium wasting can also occur in both type-1 (distal) and type-2 (proximal) renal tubular acidosis (RTA) (see Chapter 73).

Hypomagnesemia. Hypomagnesemia is present in up to 40% of patients with hypokalemia [65]. In many cases, as with diuretic therapy, vomiting, or diarrhea, there are concurrent potassium and magnesium losses. Hypomagnesemia of any cause can lead to increased urinary potassium losses. Speculation surrounds the mechanism by which hypomagnesemia promotes kaliuresis; a direct effect of magnesium on tubular potassium transport is likely [66]. Moreover, in the cells of the thick ascending limb of Henle's loop, magnesium acts as a calcium channel blocker, limiting K losses from the cell into the tubule lumen. Magnesium deficiency enhances K losses from these cells. Documenting the presence of hypomagnesemia is particularly important because the hypokalemia often cannot be corrected until the magnesium deficit is repaired [65].

Salt-Wasting Nephropathies. Occasionally, renal diseases associated with decreased proximal, loop, or distal sodium reabsorption can lead to hypokalemia via a mechanism similar to that induced by diuretics. This problem may arise in patients with Bartter's or Gitelman's syndromes, tubulointerstitial diseases, such as interstitial nephritis due to Sjögren's syndrome or lupus, hypercalcemia, and tubular injury that may be induced by lysozyme in patients with acute monocytic or myelomonocytic leukemia [67]. Increased potassium uptake by the leukemic cells may also contribute to the fall in the plasma potassium concentration.

Polyuria. In the presence of potassium depletion, healthy subjects can lower their urinary potassium concentration to 5 to 10 mEq per L. If, however, the urine output is greater than 5 to 10 L per day, obligatory potassium losses can exceed to 50 to 100 mEq in this period. This problem is most likely to occur in primary polydipsia, in which the urine output may be elevated during a prolonged period [68]. An equivalent degree of polyuria can also occur in CDI, but patients with this disorder typically seek medical care soon after the polyuria has begun.

Transcutaneous Losses. Daily potassium loss through the skin is normally negligible because the volume of perspiration is low and the potassium concentration is only 5 to 10 mEq per L. However, subjects exercising in a hot climate can produce 10 L or more of sweat per day, leading to potassium depletion if these losses are not replaced. Urinary potassium excretion also may contribute because aldosterone release is enhanced by both exercise (via catecholamine-induced renin secretion) and volume loss.

Extensive burns are another situation in which potassium losses through the skin may cause hypokalemia. Although the concentration of potassium in sweat is low, the potassium concentration of fluid lost through the skin after burns may greatly exceed the plasma level because of local tissue breakdown, which leads to the release of potassium from cells.

Dialysis. Although patients with end-stage renal disease typically retain potassium and tend to be mildly hyperkalemic, hypokalemia can be induced in some patients by maintenance dialysis. This is more likely to occur in patients on chronic peritoneal dialysis, in whom dialysis is performed every day. By comparison, hemodialysis treatments are typically administered only three times per week. Nevertheless, transient hypokalemia often follows a hemodialysis treatment.

Clinical Manifestations

Most individuals with mild hypokalemia exhibit no symptoms referable to the low plasma K^+ concentration. The major disturbances seen with more severe K^+ deficiency are changes in cardiovascular, neuromuscular, and renal function. Cardiac toxicity may be manifested by serious arrhythmias due to hyperpolarization of the myocardial cell membrane, leading to a prolonged refractory period and increased susceptibility to reentrant arrhythmias. Earlier electrocardiographic changes of hypokalemia include T-wave depression with prominent U waves (Fig. 72.6).

Hyperpolarization also slows down nerve conduction and muscle contractions, which may contribute to symptoms such as muscle weakness, cramps, and paresthesias, although these are usually not observed until the plasma K^+ concentration is less than 2.5 mEq per L. Severe hypokalemia may promote rhabdomyolysis. Profound hypokalemia can also impair respiratory muscle function, leading to hypoventilation.

Polyuria due to stimulation of thirst and resistance to the action of ADH are the primary renal manifestations of hypokalemia. Increased thirst results from direct stimulation of the hypothalamic thirst center as well as from an appropriate response to polyuria. The mechanism of resistance to ADH appears to be due to reduced expression of the water channel (aquaporin-2) that fuses with the luminal membrane under the influence of ADH [69]. With potassium depletion, the fall in

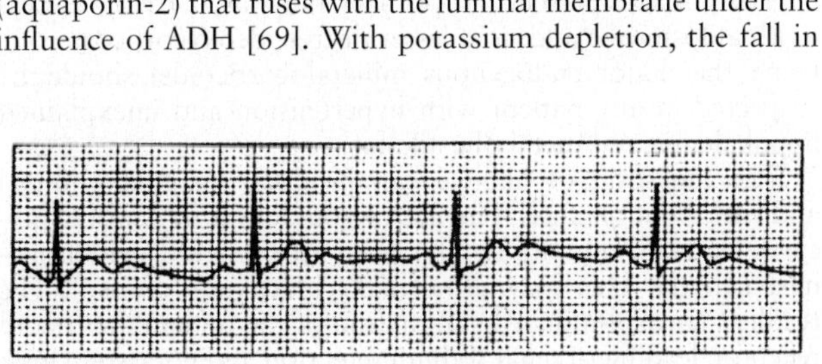

FIGURE 72.6. Both hypokalemia and hyperkalemia can cause changes in the patient's electrocardiogram. The electrocardiogram from a patient with moderate hypokalemia shows prominent U waves.

concentrating ability may occur before hypokalemia is present [70].

Diagnosis

The cause of hypokalemia can usually be determined from the history. In some cases, the diagnosis is not readily apparent. The surreptitious vomiting of bulimia or the diarrhea of laxative abuse may not be omitted from the patient's history. Measurement of blood pressure and urinary potassium excretion and assessment of acid–base balance are often helpful in such cases.

Urinary Response. In the presence of potassium depletion, a healthy subject should lower urinary potassium excretion to less than 30 mEq per day; values above this level reflect at least a contribution from urinary potassium wasting. Random measurement of the urine potassium concentration can be used but is less accurate than a 24-hour collection. Extrarenal losses probably are present if the urine potassium concentration is less than 15 mEq per L unless the patient is markedly polyuric. Higher values do not necessarily indicate potassium wasting if the urine volume is reduced. The response to potassium depletion is twofold: decreased potassium secretion by the collecting tubule principal cells and increased active potassium reabsorption by H/K–ATPase pumps in the luminal membrane of the adjacent type-A intercalated cells (Fig. 72.5) [71,72]. These pumps, which are activated by hypokalemia, reabsorb potassium and secrete hydrogen.

Once urinary potassium excretion is measured, the following diagnostic possibilities should be considered in the patient with hypokalemia of uncertain origin:

- Metabolic acidosis with a low rate of renal potassium excretion is suggestive of lower gastrointestinal losses due to diarrhea, laxative abuse, or a villous adenoma.
- Metabolic acidosis with renal potassium wasting is most often caused by diabetic ketoacidosis or by type-1 (distal) or type-2 (proximal) RTA. A salt-wasting nephropathy can produce similar findings, with the associated renal insufficiency responsible for the acidemia.
- Metabolic alkalosis with a low rate of urinary potassium excretion may be due to surreptitious vomiting or diuretic use if the urinary collection is obtained several days after the vomiting or diuretic use has been halted.
- Metabolic alkalosis with renal potassium wasting and a normal blood pressure most often results from ongoing vomiting, diuretic use, or, far less commonly, from Bartter's or Gitelman's syndromes. A low urine chloride concentration helps to distinguish the hypokalemia of vomiting from that of diuretics or Bartter's and Gitelman's syndromes.
- Metabolic alkalosis with potassium wasting and hypertension suggests surreptitious diuretic therapy in patients with underlying hypertension, renovascular disease, or one of the causes of primary mineralocorticoid excess.

The possible presence of primary mineralocorticoid excess (with aldosterone and, to a lesser degree, deoxycorticosterone being the major endogenous mineralocorticoids) should be suspected in any patient with hypertension and unexplained hypokalemia and metabolic alkalosis.

The ingestion of licorice can produce a similar clinical and metabolic picture. The active compound in licorice, glycyrrhizic acid, inhibits renal 11β-hydroxysteroid dehydrogenase activity. This enzyme normally inactivates cortisol. The result is cortisol-induced stimulation of the mineralocorticoid receptor, leading to renal sodium retention and potassium loss.

The other major cause of hypertension and hypokalemia is renovascular disease, in which the hypersecretion of renin leads sequentially to increased secretion of angiotensin II and then aldosterone. It is important to be aware that hypokalemia is characteristic of malignant hypertension, which is a high-renin, high-aldosterone state, regardless of the underlying cause.

Treatment

Although hypokalemia can be transiently induced by the entry of potassium into the cells, most cases are caused by unreplaced gastrointestinal or urinary losses. Optimal therapy depends on the severity of the potassium deficit; somewhat different considerations are required to minimize continued urinary losses due to diuretic therapy or, less often, to one of the causes of primary hyperaldosteronism.

Potassium Deficit. The total potassium deficit can only be approximated because there is no strict correlation between the plasma potassium concentration and total body potassium stores. In general, the loss of 200 to 400 mEq of potassium is required to lower the plasma potassium concentration from 4 to 3 mEq per L; the loss of an additional 200 to 400 mEq lowers the plasma potassium concentration to approximately 2 mEq per L [73]. Continued potassium losses do not as readily worsen the degree of hypokalemia because of the release of potassium from the intracellular pool.

These estimates assume a normal distribution of potassium between the cells and the extracellular fluid. The most common setting in which this does not apply is diabetic ketoacidosis, a disorder in which hyperosmolality and insulin deficiency favor the movement of potassium out of the cells. As a result, patients with this disorder may have a normal or even elevated plasma potassium concentration at presentation, despite having incurred a marked potassium deficit due to urinary or gastrointestinal losses, or both. Potassium supplementation for these patients should begin once the plasma potassium concentration is 4.5 mEq per L or less, provided that the patient is producing urine, because the administration of insulin and fluids may cause a precipitous drop in the plasma potassium concentration.

Potassium Preparations. Intravenous or oral potassium chloride generally is the preferred treatment for hypokalemia. Use of the chloride salt has two important advantages. First, potassium chloride more rapidly raises the plasma potassium concentration than does potassium bicarbonate or potassium citrate, the citrate being rapidly metabolized to bicarbonate. Bicarbonate enters cells more readily than does chloride. The retention of chloride in the extracellular fluid, obligated by the need to maintain electroneutrality, limits the initial entry of potassium into the cells, thereby maximizing the rise in the plasma potassium concentration. Second, most patients with hypokalemia also have metabolic alkalosis. For example, with diuretic therapy, vomiting, and hyperaldosteronism, hydrogen loss accompanies that of potassium. Potassium must be given with chloride to such patients if both the hypokalemia and the alkalosis are to be corrected optimally (see Chapter 71). In comparison, potassium bicarbonate or potassium citrate can be given to patients with hypokalemia and metabolic acidosis, such as occurs in RTA and chronic diarrheal states.

Oral potassium chloride can be given in crystalline form (salt substitutes), as a liquid, or in a slow-release tablet or capsule. Salt substitutes contain 50 to 65 mEq per level teaspoon; they may be the ideal form of oral therapy, as they are safe, well tolerated, and much cheaper than the other preparations. Potassium chloride solutions, on the other hand, are often unpalatable, and the slow-release preparations can, in rare cases, cause ulcerative or stenotic lesions in the gastrointestinal tract as a result of the local accumulation of high concentrations of potassium.

Merely increasing the intake of potassium-rich foods such as oranges and bananas is generally less effective in the absence of renal insufficiency. These foods contain phosphate and citrate rather than chloride and are, therefore, less likely to correct the hypokalemia and metabolic alkalosis.

Potassium chloride can be given intravenously to patients who are unable to eat or who have severe hypokalemia (see following discussion). It is usually added to a solution in which the concentration should generally not exceed 40 mEq of potassium per liter because higher concentrations can lead to pain and sclerosis of a peripheral vein. A saline solution is preferred to a dextrose solution for initial therapy because the administration of dextrose can lead to a transient 0.2 to 1.4 mEq per L reduction in the plasma potassium concentration because of glucose-induced insulin release [55].

Mild-to-Moderate Potassium Depletion. The majority of patients have a plasma potassium concentration between 3.0 and 3.5 mEq per L; this degree of potassium depletion usually produces no symptoms, except in patients with advanced liver disease or in patients with heart disease, particularly if they are taking digoxin. Treatment in this setting is directed toward replacing the lost potassium, usually beginning with 40 to 80 mEq of potassium chloride per day, and toward treating the disorder responsible for the loss of potassium.

Potassium replacement alone may be insufficient to treat patients with ongoing urinary losses due to chronic diuretic therapy, tubular dysfunction, or primary hyperaldosteronism. Potassium-sparing diuretics such as amiloride, triamterene, the aldosterone antagonists, spironolactone, and eplerenone are generally more effective than other agents, as they limit further urinary losses of both potassium and magnesium. It is frequently underappreciated, however, that, in the presence of high levels of aldosterone, greater than usual doses (up to 20 to 40 mg of amiloride and 150 to 300 mg of spironolactone) may be required to block potassium secretion. The combination of a potassium-sparing diuretic with potassium supplements should be used only with careful monitoring to prevent possible overcorrection with development of hyperkalemia and should be avoided in most patients with renal insufficiency.

Severe Hypokalemia. Potassium repletion is more urgent for patients with profound or symptomatic hypokalemia (i.e., arrhythmias, marked muscle weakness). This is most easily done orally. The plasma potassium concentration transiently rises by as much as 1.0 to 1.5 mEq per L after 40 to 60 mEq and by 2.5 to 3.5 mEq per L after 135 to 160 mEq and falls, as most of the exogenous potassium is taken up by the cells. In light of these fluxes, careful monitoring is required, and more potassium should be given as necessary. A patient with a plasma potassium concentration of 2.0 mEq per L, for example, *may* have a 400 to 800 mEq potassium deficit.

Some patients with severe hypokalemia must be treated intravenously because of medical instability or an inability to take medication orally. There are two potential limitations to intravenous therapy: A *maximum* concentration of 50 to 60 mEq per L can be administered via a peripheral vein without irritation, and, because saline solutions are preferable, volume overload is a potential risk in susceptible subjects.

The necessity for aggressive intravenous therapy occurs primarily in patients with diabetic ketoacidosis or nonketotic hyperglycemia with hypokalemia due to marked urinary potassium losses. As described previously, treatment with insulin and fluids exacerbates the hypokalemia. Because these patients are also quite volume depleted, the addition of 40 to 60 mEq of potassium chloride to each liter of half-isotonic saline can supply large quantities of potassium with less risk of pulmonary congestion.

In general, the maximum rate of intravenous potassium administration is 10 to 20 mEq per hour, although as much as 40 to 100 mEq per hour has been given to selected patients with paralysis or life-threatening arrhythmias [74]. In these cases, solutions containing as much as 200 mEq of potassium per L (20 mEq in 100 mL of isotonic saline) have been used. They should be infused into a large vein, such as the femoral vein; a central venous line has also been used, but a local increase in the potassium concentration could have a deleterious effect on cardiac conduction.

It must be emphasized that rapid intravenous administration of potassium is potentially dangerous, even in potassium-depleted patients. Thus, careful monitoring of the physiologic effects of hypokalemia (electrocardiogram [ECG] abnormalities, muscle weakness, or paralysis) is essential. Once these problems are no longer severe, the rate of potassium repletion should be slowed down to 10 to 20 mEq per hour, even though there may be persistent hypokalemia.

Hyperkalemia

Hyperkalemia is a relatively common laboratory abnormality in critically ill patients, particularly in those with oliguric acute or chronic kidney disease.

Etiology

Hyperkalemia is rare in healthy subjects because the transcellular and renal disposal adaptations prevent significant potassium accumulation in the extracellular fluid. Furthermore, the efficiency of potassium handling is increased if potassium intake is slowly enhanced, thereby allowing what might otherwise be a fatal potassium load to be tolerated. This phenomenon, called *potassium adaptation*, is mostly due to more rapid potassium excretion in the urine.

Therefore, increasing potassium intake is not commonly a cause of hyperkalemia, unless the patient has an impaired capacity for potassium excretion or the potassium loading occurs too rapidly for such adaptation to occur. As examples, acute hyperkalemia can be induced (primarily in infants because of their small size) by the administration of intravenous potassium penicillin as an intravenous bolus or by the ingestion of a potassium-containing salt substitute.

The net release of potassium from the cells, either due to enhanced release or decreased entry, can also cause hyperkalemia. As with exogenous potassium loading, the elevation is typically transient because the excess potassium is excreted in the urine. Because persistent hyperkalemia requires impairment in urinary potassium excretion, it may be inferred that this problem is generally associated with a reduction in either aldosterone effect or in the delivery of sodium and water to the distal secretory site. The causes of hyperkalemia are listed in Table 72.6.

Increased Potassium Release from Cells

Pseudohyperkalemia. *Pseudohyperkalemia* refers to conditions in which the elevation in the measured plasma potassium concentration is due to potassium movement out of the cells during or after the blood specimen has been drawn. The major cause of this problem is mechanical trauma during venipuncture, resulting in hemolysis. Because this is an in vitro phenomenon, the patient demonstrates no clinical signs and symptoms of hyperkalemia (see following discussion).

Potassium also moves out of white cells and platelets after clotting has occurred. Thus, the serum potassium concentration normally exceeds the true value in the plasma by as much as 0.5 mEq per L. This difference in normal levels is not clinically important. In contrast, a patient with marked leukocytosis or thrombocytosis (white cell or platelet count $>$100,000 per μL or 1,000,000 per μL, respectively) may have a measured serum potassium concentration as high as 9 mEq per L. This phenomenon is most often observed in patients with

TABLE 72.6

MAJOR CAUSES OF HYPERKALEMIA

Increased potassium release from cells
Pseudohyperkalemia
Metabolic acidosis
Insulin deficiency
Hyperglycemia and hyperosmolal states
Increased tissue catabolism
β-Adrenergic blockade
Exercise
Other
Digitalis overdose
Hyperkalemic periodic paralysis
Succinylcholine
Arginine hydrochloride
Reduced urinary potassium excretion
Hypoaldosteronism
Renal disease
Reduced effective circulatory volume
Selective impairment of potassium excretion
Medications
Dapsone
Trimethoprim
Nonsteroidal anti-inflammatory drugs
Angiotensin-converting enzyme inhibitors
Angiotensin receptor blockers
Heparin
Potassium-sparing diuretics

myeloproliferative diseases. With essential thrombocytosis, for example, the measured serum potassium concentration rises by approximately 0.15 mEq per L for every 100,000 per μL elevation in the platelet count.

Pseudohyperkalemia should be suspected whenever there is no apparent cause for an elevated plasma potassium concentration in an asymptomatic patient and particularly in patients with persistent hyperkalemia despite normal renal function. Comparing the serum potassium concentration with that in plasma (collected using a heparinized specimen tube) often establishes the diagnosis. Comparing the serum potassium levels drawn with and without a tourniquet also may be useful diagnostically if a significant difference is observed.

Metabolic Acidosis. The buffering of excess hydrogen ions in the cells can lead to potassium movement into the extracellular fluid; this transcellular shift is necessitated, in part, by the need to maintain electroneutrality. This phenomenon is less likely to occur in the organic acidoses, ketoacidosis, and lactic acidosis. Although the potassium level may be elevated in both of these conditions, hyperkalemia appears to result from insulin deficiency and tissue breakdown, with potassium leakage from cells rather than from the acidosis itself.

Insulin Deficiency, Hyperglycemia, and Hyperosmolality. Insulin promotes potassium entry into cells; thus, the ingestion of glucose (which stimulates endogenous insulin secretion) minimizes the rise in the plasma potassium concentration induced by concurrent potassium intake. On the contrary, in patients with uncontrolled diabetes mellitus, the combination of insulin deficiency and the hyperosmolality induced by hyperglycemia frequently leads to hyperkalemia, even though a patient may be markedly potassium depleted from previously incurred urinary potassium losses.

An elevation in P_{Osm} results in osmotic water movement from cells into the extracellular fluid. This is accompanied by potassium movement out of the cells. A similar rise in plasma potassium can occur with any solute that increases the effective P_{Osm}, such as mannitol, particularly in patients with renal failure [75].

Somatostatin, by inhibiting insulin release, can raise the plasma potassium concentration by an average of 0.6 mEq per L in healthy subjects but by more than 1.5 mEq per L to potentially dangerous levels in selected patients with end-stage renal disease [76].

Increased Tissue Breakdown. Any cause of increased tissue breakdown can result in the release of potassium into the extracellular fluid. Hyperkalemia is particularly likely to develop in this setting if renal impairment is also present. Clinical examples include breakdown of a large hematoma, as might occur in the wake of a gastrointestinal hemorrhage; rhabdomyolysis from any cause; cell breakdown in patients receiving cytotoxic or radiation therapy for lymphoma or leukemia (the tumorlysis syndrome); and in patients with severe hypothermia. Although hypothermia characteristically results in a fall in plasma potassium concentration, hyperkalemia occurs when the insult has been sufficient to cause tissue breakdown, and it carries an extremely high mortality rate [60].

β-Adrenergic Blockade. β-Adrenergic blockers interfere with the β_2-adrenergic facilitation of potassium uptake by the cells (Fig. 72.4). This effect is associated with only a minor elevation in the plasma potassium concentration in healthy subjects (<0.5 mEq per L) because the excess potassium can be easily excreted in the urine. True hyperkalemia is rare, except in conjunction with an additional defect in potassium handling, such as a large potassium load, marked exercise, hypoaldosteronism, or renal failure [77].

Exercise. Potassium is normally released from muscle cells during exercise. The release of potassium may have a physiologic function, because the local increase in the plasma potassium concentration has a vasodilatory effect, increasing blood flow and energy delivery to the exercising muscle [78].

The increment in the systemic plasma potassium concentration is less pronounced and is related to the degree of exercise: 0.3 to 0.4 mEq per L with slow walking; 0.7 to 1.2 mEq per L with moderate exertion (including prolonged aerobic exercise with marathon running); and as much as 2.0 mEq per L after exercise to exhaustion [79].

The rise in the plasma potassium concentration is reversed after several minutes of rest and is typically associated with mild-rebound hypokalemia (averaging 0.4 to 0.5 mEq per L below the baseline level) that may be arrhythmogenic in susceptible individuals. The degree of potassium release is attenuated by prior physical conditioning (perhaps due to increased Na^+/K^+–ATPase activity) but may be exacerbated by the administration of beta-blockers.

Exercise can interfere with accurate measurement of the plasma potassium concentration. Repeated fist clenching during blood drawing can acutely raise the plasma potassium concentration by more than 1 mEq per L in that forearm, thereby representing another form of pseudohyperkalemia. Careful drawing of the blood and comparison of the plasma to the serum potassium value should identify most cases [80].

Other. Rarer causes of hyperkalemia due to translocation of potassium from the cells into the extracellular fluid include (a) digitalis overdose from dose-dependent inhibition of membrane Na^+/K^+–ATPase and (b) the hyperkalemic form of periodic paralysis, an autosomal dominant disorder in which episodes of weakness or paralysis are usually precipitated by cold exposure, rest after exercise, or the ingestion of small amounts of potassium.

The primary abnormality in at least some families with hyperkalemic periodic paralysis appears to be a point mutation in the gene for the α-subunit of the skeletal muscle cell sodium channel [81]. How this abnormality accounts for episodic muscle weakness is not clear. One possibility is that the activity of the sodium channel is inappropriately increased by a slight elevation in the plasma potassium concentration. The consequent entry of sodium to the cell down a very favorable concentration gradient depolarizes the cell membrane. This favors potassium diffusion out of the cells (because the cell potassium concentration is so much higher than that in the extracellular fluid) and the development of hyperkalemia.

Administration of succinylcholine to patients with burns, extensive trauma, or neuromuscular disease can also cause hyperkalemia.

Reduced Urinary Potassium Excretion

Impaired urinary potassium excretion generally requires an abnormality in one or both of the two major factors required for adequate renal potassium handling: aldosterone and distal nephron sodium and water delivery.

Hypoaldosteronism. Any cause of decreased aldosterone release or effect diminishes the efficiency of potassium secretion and can lead to hyperkalemia (Table 72.7). The resulting rise in the plasma potassium concentration directly stimulates potassium secretion, partially overcoming the relative absence of aldosterone. As a consequence, the rise in the plasma potassium concentration is small in patients with normal renal function, but it can be clinically important in the presence of underlying renal insufficiency or a high potassium intake.

Hyperkalemia in hypoaldosteronism is usually associated with a mild metabolic acidosis. This condition has been called *type-4 RTA* and appears to be primarily due to decreased urinary ammonium excretion.

Although aldosterone also promotes sodium retention, decreased availability of aldosterone is not typically associated with prominent sodium wasting with type-4 RTA in adults because of the ability of other antinatriuretic factors such as angiotensin II and norepinephrine to compensate. Hyponatremia is also uncommon because there is no hypovolemic stimulation for ADH release. If hyponatremia is present, primary adrenal insufficiency should be suspected. In this disorder, the concurrent lack of cortisol is a potent stimulus to ADH secretion, leading to water retention and a fall in the plasma sodium concentration.

The causes of hypoaldosteronism include disorders that affect adrenal aldosterone synthesis, the renal response to aldosterone, or renal (and perhaps adrenal) renin release (Table 72.7).

TABLE 72.7

MAJOR CAUSES OF HYPOALDOSTERONISM

Hyporeninemic hypoaldosteronism
Renal disease, most often diabetic nephropathy
Nonsteroidal anti-inflammatory drugs
Angiotensin-converting enzyme inhibitors
Cyclosporine
Human immunodeficiency virus infection, including trimethoprim administration
Primary adrenal insufficiency
Potassium-sparing diuretics (trimethoprim may act similarly)
Heparin
Congenital adrenal hyperplasia, with 21-hydroxylase deficiency being most common
Isolated impairment in aldosterone synthesis
Pseudohypoaldosteronism (end-organ resistance)
Severe illness

Hyporeninemic Hypoaldosteronism. The syndrome of hyporeninemic hypoaldosteronism, a form of type-4 RTA, is characterized by coexisting defects in the release of renin by the kidney and aldosterone by the adrenal cortex. The adrenal dysfunction may involve a local renin–angiotensin system because there is evidence that angiotensin II produced within the adrenal gland may stimulate the release of aldosterone [82].

This relatively common disorder most often occurs in patients with mild-to-moderate renal insufficiency due to diabetic nephropathy or chronic interstitial nephritis. Low plasma renin levels are common in diabetic patients, partly due to a defect in the conversion of the precursor prorenin into active renin [83]. Volume expansion induced by diabetes and other chronic kidney diseases may play a contributory role; the increase in atrial natriuretic peptide release in this setting can suppress both the release of renin and the hyperkalemia-induced secretion of aldosterone [84].

Similar hemodynamic and humoral changes occur in the acute nephritic syndrome of postinfectious glomerulonephritis: volume expansion, leading to appropriate suppression of renin release and enhanced secretion of atrial natriuretic peptide [85]. In some patients, these changes can lead to hyperkalemia that responds to mineralocorticoid replacement [86]. Recovery of renal function within 1 to 2 weeks is associated with restoration of normal potassium balance.

Low renin and aldosterone levels may also occur in several other settings:

- *NSAIDs.* NSAIDs lower renal renin secretion, which is normally partially mediated by locally produced prostaglandins. The result is that the plasma potassium concentration rises approximately 0.2 mEq per L in subjects with normal renal function but can rise by more than 1.0 mEq per L when renal insufficiency is superimposed. This can occur with specific cyclooxygenase-2 inhibitors as well as nonselective NSAIDs.
- *ACE inhibitors, ARBs, and direct renin inhibitors.* Similar considerations apply to agents that block the production or action of angiotensin II, since angiotensin II is necessary for normal aldosterone release in response to volume depletion or hyperkalemia.
- *Other.* Other causes of hyporeninemic hypoaldosteronism include the use of cyclosporine, which can lead to hyperkalemia in 15% to 25% of renal transplant recipients [87], likely from diminished secretion of and responsiveness to aldosterone, and HIV infection. Adrenalitis is frequently present in HIV. The administrations of the antibiotics trimethoprim and pentamidine are other causes of hyperkalemia. Both agents appear to close sodium channels in the distal nephron in a manner similar to that of the potassium-sparing diuretic amiloride [88,89].

Primary Adrenal Insufficiency. Primary adrenal cortical failure (also called *Addison's disease*) is associated with lack of cortisol and aldosterone. Pituitary disease, in comparison, does not lead to hypoaldosteronism because ACTH does not have a major role in the regulation of aldosterone release. Primary adrenal insufficiency is frequently due to autoimmune destruction of the steroid-producing cells in the adrenal cortex.

Potassium-Sparing Diuretics. Potassium-sparing diuretics are probably the most common cause of hyperkalemia due to impairment of aldosterone function. These drugs antagonize the action of aldosterone on the collecting tubule cells: spironolactone and eplerenone by competing for the aldosterone receptor, and amiloride and triamterene by closing the sodium channels in the luminal membrane.

Heparin. Commercial heparin preparations exert a direct toxic effect on the zona glomerulosa cells of the adrenal cortex [90]. Even low-dose heparin can lead to a 75% reduction in plasma aldosterone levels. The mechanism appears to involve a reduction in the number and affinity of adrenal angiotensin II receptors involved in aldosterone synthesis and release. There are some reports of heparin causing hyponatremia by similar mechanisms of diminished aldosterone release [91].

Adrenal Enzyme Deficiency. In children, hypoaldosteronism can result from a deficiency of enzymes required for aldosterone synthesis, which may be associated with concurrent abnormalities in cortisol and androgen production.

Pseudohypoaldosteronism. Decreased aldosterone activity also occurs in the syndrome of pseudohypoaldosteronism. This disorder is associated with generalized resistance to the actions of aldosterone due to a marked reduction in the number of mineralocorticoid receptors in the kidney and in other target organs such as the colon and sweat glands [92].

Severe Illness. Hypoaldosteronism due to decreased adrenal production is common in critically ill patients. The stress-induced hypersecretion of ACTH in these patients may be responsible for this defect by inducing activity of 17α-hydroxylase in the zona glomerulosa. This enzyme enhances the synthesis of cortisol at the expense of aldosterone.

Chronic Kidney Disease. The ability to maintain potassium excretion at near-normal levels is generally maintained in patients with renal disease as long as both aldosterone secretion and distal tubular urine flow are maintained [93]. Patients who are oliguric or who have an additional problem such as a high-potassium intake, increased tissue breakdown, or hypoaldosteronism are more predisposed to hyperkalemia.

Effective Circulating Volume Depletion. Decreased distal tubular urine flow due to marked effective volume depletion, as might occur in heart failure or hepatic cirrhosis, can lead to hyperkalemia. In this setting, there is also a fall in the quantity of sodium presented to the potassium-secretory site in the collecting tubule. Hyperkalemia may occur even though aldosterone activity is high.

Hyperkalemic Type-1 Renal Tubular Acidosis. In some patients with type-1 (distal) RTA, the primary defect is impaired sodium reabsorption in the cortical collecting tubule. The movement of sodium from the lumen into the cell at this site makes the lumen electronegative, thereby promoting both hydrogen and potassium secretion. Inhibiting the transport of sodium, therefore, reduces both hydrogen and potassium secretion, leading to metabolic acidosis and hyperkalemia. This form of type-1 RTA is most often seen in patients with urinary tract obstruction or sickle cell disease. Patients with type-1 RTA have normal or even high aldosterone levels and are unable to acidify the urine normally (urine pH $\leq$5.0), in contrast to individuals with hypoaldosteronism and other forms of type-4 RTA who frequently exhibit a urine pH of less than 5.3.

Clinical Manifestations

The symptoms induced by hyperkalemia are related to impaired neuromuscular transmission. The ease of generating an action potential, called *membrane excitability*, is related both to the magnitude of the resting membrane potential and to the activation state of membrane sodium channels. Opening of these sodium channels, leading to the passive diffusion of extracellular sodium into the cells, is the primary step in this process. According to the Nernst equation, the resting membrane potential is related to the ratio of the intracellular to the extracellular potassium concentration. An elevation in the extracellular potassium concentration decreases this ratio and, therefore, partially depolarizes the cell membrane, making the resting potential less electronegative. This change initially increases membrane excitability because less of a depolarizing stimulus is required to generate an action potential. The later effect seen in patients is different. Persistent depolarization inactivates sodium channels in the cell membrane, thereby producing a net decrease in membrane excitability that may be manifested clinically by impaired cardiac conduction or muscle weakness, or both, or by paralysis.

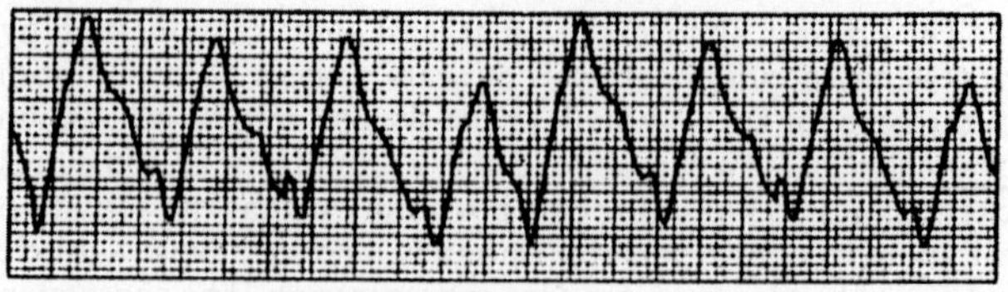

FIGURE 72.7. Marked hyperkalemia results in peaked T waves and widened QRS complexes in this electrocardiogram.

In general, severe symptoms of hyperkalemia do not occur until the plasma potassium concentration is more than 7.5 mEq per L. There is, however, substantial interpatient variability because factors such as hypocalcemia and metabolic acidosis can increase the toxicity of excess potassium. Thus, careful monitoring of the ECG and muscle strength is indicated to assess the functional consequences of the hyperkalemia. A plasma potassium concentration of more than 7.5 to 8.0 mEq per L, severe muscle weakness, or marked electrocardiographic changes are potentially life threatening and require immediate treatment using the modalities described here [94].

The earliest ECG abnormality is symmetric peaking of T waves, followed by reduced P-wave voltage and widening of QRS complexes (Fig. 72.7). If untreated, severe hyperkalemia can cause the normal QRS morphology to be lost altogether so that the ECG pattern deteriorates into a sinusoidal ECG form, with one oscillation representing a wide QRS complex and the complementary oscillation representing an abnormal T wave. ECG changes usually do not appear until the plasma K^+ concentration exceeds 6.5 mEq per L, and are more likely to develop when the rise in K^+ occurs rapidly. There is, however, no consistent relationship between the severity of the electrolyte disturbance and the ECG; in rare cases, the ECG can remain unchanged even with a plasma potassium concentration of more than 9 mEq per L [95].

The neuromuscular manifestations of hyperkalemia are nonspecific. The earliest findings are paresthesias and weakness, which can progress to paralysis affecting the respiratory muscles. These symptoms are similar to those seen with hypokalemia; cranial nerve function remains unaffected.

Diagnosis

Pseudohyperkalemia should be considered when there is evidence of hemolysis in the sample or when the platelet or white blood cell counts are markedly increased.

An asymptomatic patient with a plasma potassium concentration of 6.5 mEq per L and no ECG changes can be treated with a cation exchange resin (Kayexalate) alone, and patients with a level below 6.0 mEq per L can often be treated just with a low-potassium diet and diuretics. Any extra source of potassium intake (salt substitutes, potassium supplements, and foods with a high potassium content) should be eliminated, and any potentiating drugs (e.g., NSAIDs or ACE inhibitors) should be discontinued.

Treatment

Specific treatment of severe or symptomatic hyperkalemia is directed at antagonizing the membrane effects of potassium, driving extracellular potassium into the cells, or removing excess potassium from the body [96]. Although this can often be done in the outpatient setting, some patients should be hospitalized [97]. The following modalities, which are listed according to their rapidity of action, all may be beneficial.

Calcium. Calcium directly antagonizes the membrane actions of hyperkalemia. As mentioned previously, hyperkalemia-induced depolarization of the resting membrane potential leads to inactivation of sodium channels and decreased membrane excitability. Calcium antagonizes this membrane effect of hyperkalemia, although how this is achieved is not well understood.

The protective effect of calcium begins within minutes but is relatively short lived. As a result, calcium infusions are indicated only for severe hyperkalemia, when it is potentially dangerous to wait the 30 to 60 minutes required for insulin and glucose or sodium bicarbonate to act. The usual dose is 10 mL (1 ampule) of a 10% calcium gluconate solution infused slowly during 2 to 3 minutes with constant cardiac monitoring. This dose can be repeated after 5 minutes if the ECG changes persist.

Calcium should not be given in bicarbonate-containing solutions because this can lead to its precipitation as calcium carbonate. Because hypercalcemia can induce digitalis toxicity, calcium should be administered only when absolutely necessary to patients taking digoxin.

Insulin and Glucose. Increasing the availability of insulin lowers the plasma potassium concentration by driving potassium into the cells, apparently by enhancing the activity of the Na^+/K^+–ATPase pump in skeletal muscle. Hyperinsulinemia can be induced either by giving insulin with glucose to prevent hypoglycemia or by the intravenous administration of glucose (50 mL of a 50% glucose solution), which rapidly enhances endogenous insulin secretion in a nondiabetic patient. Glucose alone may produce a smaller rise in the plasma insulin concentration and a lesser reduction in plasma potassium concentration than does the insulin-plus-glucose regimen. Effective therapy usually produces a 0.5 to 1.5 mEq per L fall in the plasma potassium concentration. This effect begins in 15 minutes, peaks at 60 minutes, and lasts for several hours [98]. Although patients with chronic kidney disease are relatively resistant to the glycemic effect of insulin, they are not resistant to the hypokalemic effect because Na^+/K^+–ATPase activity is still enhanced.

Exogenous insulin can induce symptomatic hypoglycemia unless adequate glucose is given concurrently. If, for example, 10 units of regular insulin are given with 25 g of glucose, the plasma glucose concentration may fall to less than 55 mg per dL in as many as 75% of initially normoglycemic patients [98]. Increasing the initial glucose dose to 40 g, followed by a continuous dextrose infusion, generally prevents this problem.

Proper therapy in diabetic patients varies with the plasma glucose concentration. Both insulin and glucose should be given when the plasma glucose concentration is normal or mildly elevated because endogenous insulin release is impaired. Insulin in this case reduces the plasma potassium concentration directly by preventing a rise in the plasma glucose concentration that can exacerbate the hyperkalemia. The osmotic force generated by the high extracellular glucose concentration pulls water and, secondarily, potassium out of the cells. In comparison, insulin alone is sufficient if the patient is already hyperglycemic.

Sodium Bicarbonate. Raising the systemic pH with sodium bicarbonate promotes hydrogen ion release from the cells and a reciprocal movement of potassium into the cells. The elevation in the plasma bicarbonate concentration appears to have another direct, albeit not delineated, effect on lowering the plasma potassium concentration that is independent of pH [99].

The potassium-lowering action of sodium bicarbonate is most prominent in patients with metabolic acidosis, beginning within 30 to 60 minutes and persisting for several hours. Sodium bicarbonate appears to be less effective in correcting hyperkalemia in patients with renal failure. Insulin plus glucose or a β_2-agonist is more predictably effective in this setting.

The usual dose is 45 mEq (1 ampule of a 7.5% sodium bicarbonate solution) infused slowly during 5 minutes; this dose can be repeated in 30 minutes if necessary. Alternatively, sodium bicarbonate can be added to a glucose and saline solution. This regimen may have an additional advantage in hyponatremic patients because raising the plasma sodium concentration with this hypertonic solution can also reverse the electrocardiographic effects of hyperkalemia. Both an increase in the rate of membrane depolarization and a fall in the plasma potassium concentration by dilution may contribute to this effect. These sodium-containing solutions should be used with extreme caution in edematous patients with advanced heart failure or renal failure. Despite the physiologic rationale, bicarbonate administration appears to be less effective in lowering the serum potassium concentration in patients with end-stage renal disease who are receiving dialysis.

β_2-Adrenergic Agonists. Like insulin, β_2-adrenergic agonists drive potassium into the cells by increasing Na^+/K^+–ATPase activity. Albuterol (20.0 mg in 4 mL of saline by nasal inhalation for 10 minutes or 0.5 mg by intravenous infusion) can lower the plasma potassium concentration by 0.5 to 1.5 mEq per L within 30 to 60 minutes. Furthermore, the effect of these agents is additive to that of insulin plus glucose. The only common side effects of the β_2-agonists are mild tachycardia and the possible induction of angina in susceptible individuals. Thus, these agents should probably be avoided in patients with known active coronary disease.

Loop or Thiazide Diuretics. Loop and thiazide diuretics can be used when hyperkalemia is present in an individual with hypertension or volume overload. However, the effectiveness of diuretic therapy is frequently limited by moderate-to-severe renal insufficiency.

Cation Exchange Resin. The most readily available cation exchange resin is sodium polystyrene sulfonate (SPS). In the gut, this resin takes up potassium, and calcium and magnesium to lesser degrees, and releases sodium. Each gram of resin may bind as much as 1 mEq of potassium and release 1 to 2 mEq of sodium. Thus, a potential side effect is exacerbation of any preexisting degree of sodium overload.

The resin can be given either orally or as a retention enema. The oral dose is usually 20 g given with 100 mL of a 20% sorbitol solution to prevent constipation. However, preliminary data suggest that alternative vehicles may be safer and more effective than sorbitol [100,101]. This can be repeated every 4 to 6 hours as necessary. Lower doses (5 to 10 g with meals) are generally well tolerated (no nausea or constipation) and can be used to control chronic mild hyperkalemia in patients with renal insufficiency.

When given as an enema, 50 g of resin is mixed with 50 mL of 70% sorbitol plus 100 to 150 mL of tap water. This solution should be kept in the colon for at least 30 to 60 minutes, preferably for 2 to 3 hours. Each enema can lower the plasma potassium concentration by as much as 0.5 to 1.0 mEq per L and can be repeated every 2 to 4 hours.

Intestinal necrosis is an occasional occurrence, particularly when SPS is given orally with sorbitol within the first week after surgery [101]. Why this occurs is not clear; it is possible that a postoperative ileus plays an important role by increasing the duration of drug contact with the intestinal mucosa.

Recently, there have been reports questioning the effectiveness of SPS. This issue remains unresolved at this time, but anecdotal experience supports its effectiveness in lowering the serum potassium level in many patients. Still, with the possible, although uncommon, risk of bowel injury, other measure should be tried first.

Dialysis. Dialysis can be used if the conservative measures listed in the preceding sections are ineffective, if the hyperkalemia is severe, if the patient has marked tissue breakdown and is releasing large amounts of potassium from the injured cells, or, of course, if the patient has hyperkalemia in the setting of renal failure. The rate of potassium removal with hemodialysis is preferred in the last two settings because it is many times faster than with peritoneal dialysis.

References

1. Black R (ed): *Rose and Black's Clinical Problems in Nephrology*. New York, Little, Brown and Company, 1996, Chapter 1.
2. Budisavljevic MN, Stewart L, Sahn SA, et al: Hyponatremia associated with 3,4-methylenedioxymethamphetamine ("ectasy") abuse. *Am J Med Sci* 326:89, 2003.
3. Adrogue HJ, Madias NE: Hyponatremia. *N Engl J Med* 342:1581, 2000.
4. Friedman E, Shadel M, Halkin H, et al: Thiazide-induced hyponatremia. Reproducibility by a single dose rechallenge and an analysis of pathogenesis. *Ann Intern Med* 110:24, 1989.
5. Clark BA, Shannon RP, Rosa RM, et al: Increased susceptibility to thiazide-induced hyponatremia in the elderly. *J Am Soc Nephrol* 5:1106, 1994.
6. Iwasaki Y, Oiso Y, Yamauchi K, et al: Osmoregulation of plasma vasopressin in myxedema. *J Clin Endocrinol Metab* 70:534, 1990.
7. Kalogeral KT, Nieman LK, Friedman TC, et al: Inferior petrosal sampling in healthy human subjects reveals a unilateral corticotropin-releasing hormone-mediated arginine vasopressin release associated with ipsilateral adrenocorticotropin secretion. *J Clin Invest* 97:2045, 1996.
8. Vitting K, Gardenswartz M, Zabatekis P, et al: Frequency of hyponatremia and nonosmolar vasopressin release in the acquired immune deficiency syndrome. *JAMA* 263:973, 1990.
9. Fabian TJ, Amico AA, Kroboth PD, et al: Paroxetine-induced hyponatremia in older adults. *Arch Intern Med* 164:327, 2004.
10. Tanneau R, Pennec Y, Jouquan J, et al: Cerebral salt-wasting in elderly patients. *Ann Intern Med* 107:120, 1987.
11. Ganong C, Kappy M: Cerebral salt wasting in children. The need for recognition and treatment. *Am J Dis Child* 147:167, 1993.
12. Almond CS, Shin AY, Fortescue EB, et al: Hyponatremia among runners in the Boston marathon. *New Engl J Med* 352:1550, 2005.
13. Vieweg W, Hundley P, Godelski L, et al: Diurnal weight gain as a predictor of serum sodium concentration among patients with psychosis, intermittent hyponatremia, and polydipsia. *Psychiatry Res* 26:305, 1988.
14. Thompson C, Edwards C, Baylis P: Osmotic and non-osmotic regulation of thirst and vasopressin secretion in patients with compulsive water drinking. *Clin Endocrinol (Oxf)* 35:221, 1991.
15. Thompson C, Selby P, Baylis P: Reproducibility of osmotic and nonosmotic tests of vasopressin secretion in men. *Am J Physiol* 260:R533, 1991.
16. Goldman M, Blake L, Marks R, et al: Association of nonsuppression of cortisol on the DST with primary polydipsia in chronic schizophrenia. *Am J Psychiatry* 150:653, 1993.
17. Goldman MB, Robertson GL, Luckins DJ, et al: The influence of polydipsia on water excretion in hyponatremia, polydipsic, schizophrenic patients. *J Clin Endocrinol Metab* 81:1465, 1996.
18. Oster JR, Singer I: Hyponatremia, hyposmolality, and hypotonicity. Tables and fables. *Arch Intern Med* 159:333, 1999.
19. Monitoring TURP [editorial]. *Lancet* 338:606, 1991.
20. Gonzalez R, Brensilver JM, Rovinsky JJ: Posthysteroscopic hyponatremia. *Am J Kidney Dis* 23:735, 1994.
21. Silver SM, Kozlowski SA, Baer JE, et al: Glycine-induced hyponatremia in the rat: a model of post-prostatectomy syndrome. *Kidney Int* 47:262, 1995.
22. Hahn R: Relations between irrigant absorption rate and hyponatremia during transurethral resection of the prostate. *Acta Anaesthesiol Scand* 32:53, 1988.
23. Katz M: Hyperglycemia-induced hyponatremia: calculation of expected serum sodium depression. *N Engl J Med* 289:843, 1973.
24. Ayus J, Wheeler J, Arieff A: Postoperative hyponatremic encephalopathy in menstruant women. *Ann Intern Med* 117:891, 1992.
25. Ellis SJ: Severe hyponatraemia: complications and treatment. *QJM* 88:905, 1995.
26. Laureno R, Karp BI: Myelinolysis after correction of hyponatremia. *Ann Intern Med* 126:57, 1997.
27. Lien V, Shapiro J, Chan L: Study of brain electrolytes and osmolytes during correction of chronic hyponatremia. Implications for the pathogenesis of central pontine myelinolysis. *J Clin Invest* 88:303, 1991.
28. Decaux G, Namias B, Gulbis B, et al: Evidence in hyponatremia related to inappropriate secretion of ADH that V1 receptor stimulation contributes to the increase in renal uric acid clearance. *J Am Soc Nephrol* 7:805, 1996.
29. Cheng J, Zikos D, Skopicki H, et al: Long-term neurologic outcome in psychogenic water drinkers with severe symptomatic hyponatremia: the effect of rapid correction. *Am J Med* 88:561, 1990.
30. Sterns R: The treatment of hyponatremia: first, do no harm. *Am J Med* 88:557, 1990.
31. Brunner J, Redmond J, Haggar A, et al: Central pontine myelinolysis and pontine lesions after rapid correction of hyponatremia: a prospective magnetic resonance imaging study. *Ann Neurol* 27:61, 1990.
32. Tanneau R, Bourbigot B, Rouhart F, et al: High incidence of neurologic complications following rapid correction of severe hyponatremia in psychogenic water drinkers (abstract). *Kidney Int* 44:471, 1993.
33. Abbot R, Silber E, Felber J, et al: Osmotic demyelination syndrome. *BMJ* 331:829, 2005.
34. Soupart A, Penninckx R, Stenuit A, et al: Treatment of chronic hyponatremia in rats by intravenous saline: comparison of rate versus magnitude of correction. *Kidney Int* 41:1662, 1992.
35. Soupart A, Penninckx R, Stenuit A, et al: Prevention of brain demyelination after excessive correction of chronic hyponatremia in rats by excessive serum sodium lowering [abstract]. *J Am Soc Nephrol* 3:329, 1992.
36. Goldsmith SR, Gheorghiade M: Vasopressin antagonism in heart failure. *J Am Coll Cardiol* 46:1785, 2005.
37. Lindheimer MD, Barron WM, Davison JM: Osmoregulation of thirst and vasopressin release in pregnancy. *Am J Physiol* 257:F503, 1989.
38. Oster J, Materson B: Renal and electrolyte complications of congestive heart failure and effects of treatment with angiotensin-converting enzyme inhibitors. *Arch Intern Med* 152:704, 1992.
39. Leier CV, Dei Cas L, Metra M: Clinical relevance and management of the major electrolyte abnormalities in congestive heart failure: hyponatremia, hypokalemia, and hypomagnesemia. *Am Heart J* 128:562, 1994.
40. Papadakis M, Fraser C, Arieff A: Hyponatraemia in patients with cirrhosis. *Q J Med* 76:675, 1990.
41. Phillips P, Bretherton M, Johnston C, et al: Reduced osmotic thirst in healthy elderly men. *Am J Physiol* 261:R166, 1991.
42. DeRubertis F, Michelis M, Davis B: Essential hypernatremia. *Arch Intern Med* 134:889, 1974.
43. Meadow R: Non-accidental salt poisoning. *Arch Dis Child* 68:448, 1993.
44. Moder K, Hurley D: Fatal hypernatremia from exogenous salt intake: report of a case and review of the literature. *Mayo Clin Proc* 65:1587, 1990.
45. Lien Y, Shapiro J, Chan L: Effect of hypernatremia on organic brain osmoles. *J Clin Invest* 85:1427, 1990.
46. Hoorn EJ, Zietse R: Water balance disorders after neurosurgery: the triphasic response revisited. *NDT Plus* 3:42, 2010.
47. Nielsen S, Kwon TH, Christensen BM, et al: Physiology and pathophysiology of renal aquaporins. *J Am Soc Nephrol* 10:647, 1999.
48. Blum D, Brasseur D, Kahn A, et al: Safe oral rehydration of hypertonic dehydration. *J Pediatr Gastroenterol Nutr* 5:232, 1986.
49. Knores N, Monnens L: Amiloride-hydrochlorothiazide versus indomethacin-hydrochlorothiazide in the treatment of nephrogenic diabetes insipidus. *J Pediatr* 117:499, 1990.
50. Noroian G, Clive D: Cyclo-oxygenase-2 inhibitors and the kidney. *Drug Safety* 25:165, 2002.
51. Serra A, Uehlinger DE, Ferrari P, et al: Glycyrrhetinic acid decreases plasma potassium concentrations in patients with anuria. *J Am Soc Nephrol* 13:191, 2002.
52. Squires R, Huth E: Experimental potassium depletion in normal human subjects: I. Relation of ionic intakes to the renal conservation of potassium. *J Clin Invest* 38:1134, 1959.
53. Sigue G, Gamble L, Pelitre M, et al: From profound hypokalemia to life-threatening hyperkalemia: a case of barium sulfide poisoning. *Arch Intern Med* 160:548, 2000.
54. Adrogue H, Madias N: Changes in plasma potassium concentration during acute acid-base disturbances. *Am J Med* 71:456, 1981.
55. Kunin A, Surawicz B, Sims E: Decrease in serum potassium concentration and appearance of cardiac arrhythmias during infusion of potassium with glucose in potassium-depleted patients. *N Engl J Med* 266:228, 1962.
56. Braden GL, von Oeyen PT, Germain MJ, et al: Ritodrine- and terbutaline-induced hypokalemia in preterm labor: mechanisms and consequences. *Kidney Int* 51:1867, 1997.
57. Manoukian MA, Roote JA, Crapo LM: Clinical and metabolic features of thyrotoxic periodic paralysis in 24 episodes. *Arch Intern Med* 159:601, 1999.
58. Fontaine B, Lapie P, Plassart E, et al: Periodic paralysis and voltage-gated ion channels. *Kidney Int* 49:9, 1996.
59. Wang Q, Liu M, Xu C, et al: Novel CACNA1 S mutation causes autosomal dominant hypokalemic periodic paralysis in a Chinese family. *J Mol Med* 83:203, 2005.

60. Schaller M, Fischer A, Perret C: Hyperkalemia: a prognostic factor during acute severe hypothermia. *JAMA* 264:1842, 1990.
61. Clemessy JL, Favier C, Borron SW, et al: Hypokalaemia related to acute chloroquine ingestion. *Lancet* 346:877, 1995.
62. Argarwal R, Afzalpurkar R, Fordtran JS: Pathophysiology of potassium absorption and secretion by the human intestine. *Gastroenterology* 107:548, 1994.
63. Carlisle E, Donnelly S, Vasuvattakul S, et al: Glue-sniffing and distal renal tubular acidosis: sticking to the facts. *J Am Soc Nephrol* 1:1019, 1991.
64. Carlisle E, Donnelly S, Ethier J, et al: Modulation of the secretion of potassium by accompanying anions in humans. *Kidney Int* 39:1206, 1991.
65. Whang R, Whang D, Ryan M: Refractory potassium depletion. A consequence of magnesium deficiency. *Arch Intern Med* 152:40, 1992.
66. Nichols CG, Ho K, Hebert S: Mg$^{(2+)}$-dependent inward rectification of ROMK1 potassium channels expressed in Xenopus oocytes. *J Physiol* 476:399, 1994.
67. Perazella M, Eisen R, Frederick W, et al: Renal failure and severe hypokalemia associated with acute myelomonocytic leukemia. *Am J Kidney Dis* 22:462, 1993.
68. Decaux G, Prospert F, Penninckx R, et al: 5-Year treatment of the chronic syndrome of inappropriate secretion of antidiuretic hormone with oral urea. *Nephron* 63:468, 1993.
69. Gennari FJ: Hypokalemia. *N Engl J Med* 339:451, 1998.
70. Amlal H, Krane CM, Chen Q, et al: Early polyuria and urinary concentrating defect in potassium deprivation. *Am J Physiol* 279:F655, 2000.
71. Cheval L, Barlet-Bas C, Khadouri C, et al: K^+-ATPase-mediated Rb^+ transport in rat collecting tubule: modulation during K^+ deprivation. *Am J Physiol* 260:F800, 1991.
72. Okuso M, Unwin R, Velazquez H, et al: Active potassium absorption by the renal distal tubule. *Am J Physiol* 262:F488, 1992.
73. Sterns R, Cox M, Feig P, et al: Internal potassium balance and the control of the plasma potassium concentration. *Medicine (Balt)* 60:339, 1981.
74. Kruse J, Carlson R: Rapid correction of hypokalemia using concentration intravenous potassium chloride infusions. *Arch Intern Med* 150:613, 1990.
75. Conte G, Dal Canton A, Imperatore P, et al: Acute increase in plasma osmolality as a cause of hyperkalemia in patients with renal failure. *Kidney Int* 38:301, 1990.
76. Sharma A, Thiede H, Keller F: Somatostatin-induced hyperkalemia in a patient on maintenance hemodialysis. *Nephron* 59:445, 1991.
77. Arthur S, Greenberg A: Hyperkalemia associated with intravenous labetalol therapy for acute hypertension in renal transplant recipients. *Clin Nephrol* 33:269, 1990.
78. Daut J, Maiser-Rudolph W, von Beckerath N, et al: Hypoxic dilation of coronary arteries is mediated by ATP-sensitive potassium channels. *Science* 247:1341, 1990.
79. Lindinger M, Heigenhauser G, McKelvie R: Blood ion regulation during repeated maximal exercise and recovery in humans. *Am J Physiol* 262:R126, 1992.
80. Wiederkehr MR, Moe OW: Factitious hyperkalemia. *Am J Kidney Dis* 36:1049, 2000.
81. Rojas C, Wang J, Schwartz L, et al: A Met-to-Val mutation in the skeletal muscle Na^+ channel alpha-subunit in hyperkalemic periodic paralysis. *Nature* 354:387, 1991.
82. Kifor I, Moore T, Fallo F, et al: Potassium-stimulated angiotensin release from superfused adrenal capsules and enzymatically digested cells of the zona glomerulosa. *Endocrinology* 129:823, 1991.
83. Lush D, King J, Fray J: Pathophysiology of low renin syndromes: sites of renal secretory impairment and prorenin over expression. *Kidney Int* 43:983, 1993.
84. Clark B, Brown R, Epstein F: Effect of atrial natriuretic peptide on potassium-stimulated aldosterone secretion: potential relevance to hypoaldosteronism in man. *J Clin Endocrinol Metab* 75:399, 1992.
85. Rodriguez-Iturbe B, Colic D, Parra G, et al: Atrial natriuretic factor in the acute nephritic and nephrotic syndromes. *Kidney Int* 38:512, 1990.
86. Don B, Schambelan M: Hyperkalemia in acute glomerulonephritis due to transient hyporeninemic hypoaldosteronism. *Kidney Int* 38:1159, 1990.
87. Kamel K, Ethier J, Quaggin S, et al: Studies to determine the basis for hyperkalemia in recipients of a renal transplant who are treated with cyclosporine. *J Am Soc Nephrol* 2:1279, 1992.
88. Alappan R, Perazella MA, Buller GK: Hyperkalemia in hospitalized patients treated with trimethoprim-sulfamethoxazole. *Ann Intern Med* 124:316, 1996.
89. Kleyman TR, Roberts C, Ling BN: A mechanism for pentamidine-induced hyperkalemia: inhibition of distal nephron sodium transport. *Ann Intern Med* 122:103, 1995.
90. Oster JR, Singer I, Fishman LM: Heparin-induced aldosterone suppression and hyperkalemia. *Am J Med* 98:575, 1995.
91. Norman NE, Sneed AM, Brown C, et al: Heparin-induced hyponatremia. *Ann Pharmacother* 38:404, 2004.
92. Kuhnle U, Nielsen M, Teitze HU, et al: Pseudohypoaldosteronism in eight families: different forms in inheritance are evidence for various genetic defects. *J Clin Endocrinol Metab* 70:638, 1990.
93. Allon M: Hyperkalemia in end-stage renal disease: mechanisms and management. *J Am Soc Nephrol* 6:1134, 1995.
94. Wilson NS, Hudson JQ, Cox Z, et al: Hyperkalemia-induced paralysis. *Pharmacotherapy* 29:1270, 2009.
95. Szerlip H, Weiss J, Singer I: Profound hyperkalemia without electrocardiographic manifestations. *Am J Kidney Dis* 7:461, 1986.
96. Weiner ID, Wingo CS: Hyperkalemia: a potential silent killer. *J Am Soc Nephrol* 9:1535, 1998.
97. Charytan D, Goldfarb DS: Indications for hospitalization of patients with hyperkalemia. *Arch Intern Med* 160:1605, 2000.
98. Allon M, Copkney C: Albuterol and insulin for treatment of hyperkalemia in hemodialysis patients. *Kidney Int* 38:869, 1990.
99. Allon M, Shanklin N: Effect of bicarbonate administration on plasma potassium in dialysis patients: interactions with insulin and albuterol. *Am J Kidney Dis* 28:508, 1996.
100. Emmett M, Hootkins RE, Fine KD, et al: Effect of three laxatives and a cation exchange resin on fecal sodium and potassium excretion. *Gastroenterology* 108:752, 1995.
101. Gerstman B, Kirkman R, Platt R: Intestinal necrosis associated with postoperative orally administered sodium polystyrene sulfonate in sorbitol. *Am J Kidney Dis* 20:159, 1992.

CHAPTER 73 ■ ACUTE KIDNEY INJURY IN THE INTENSIVE CARE UNIT

JAHAN MONTAGUE AND KONSTANTIN ABRAMOV

OVERVIEW OF ACUTE KIDNEY INJURY

Sudden disruption of previously normal or stable kidney function, usually occurring over hours or days, is termed *acute kidney injury (AKI)*, formerly referred to as *acute renal failure*. The new term underscores the diverse clinical context in which patients with many forms and causes of AKI may present, while the term failure implies an end stage of this clinical spectrum. The pathogenesis of AKI differs from that of chronic kidney disease (CKD), in which nephron loss is more gradual. However, AKI can occur in the setting of antecedent CKD.

AKI is often diagnosed when a patient is noted to have azotemia. This elevation in the blood urea nitrogen (BUN) and serum creatinine typically represents a decline in glomerular filtration rate (GFR), but in certain cases may reflect increased production without any reduction in GFR (Table 73.1).

TABLE 73.1

CAUSES OF BLOOD UREA NITROGEN OR SERUM CREATININE ELEVATION WITHOUT REDUCTION OF GLOMERULAR FILTRATION RATE

Increased biosynthesis of urea
Gastrointestinal bleeding
Drug administration
Corticosteroids
Tetracycline
Increased protein intake
Amino acid administration
Hypercatabolism and febrile illness
Increased biosynthesis of creatinine
Increased release of creatine from muscle (rhabdomyolysis)
Drug interference with tubular creatinine secretion
Cimetidine
Trimethoprim
Spuriously elevated creatinine colorimetric assay
Ketoacids (diabetic ketoacidosis)
Cephalosporins

Oliguria, a reduction in urine output to less than 20 mL per hour, may be present, although many forms of AKI are nonoliguric. When tubular reabsorption of glomerular filtrate is reduced as a result of either tubular dysfunction or diuretic administration, patients may be polyuric even though GFR is markedly reduced.

AKI can occur prior to a significant increase in creatinine. Several recent studies reported that even a small rise in serum creatinine correlated with increased mortality [1,2]. Therefore, the Acute Dialysis Quality Initiative Group has proposed a new classification of AKI based not only on serum creatinine but also on the degree of urinary output reduction and the requirement for renal replacement therapy [3]. This classification is reflected in the RIFLE criteria (Table 73.2), which have been shown to predict renal outcome and mortality in a variety of critically ill and hospitalized patients [4,5].

AKI may stem from any of three general conditions: impaired renal perfusion without parenchymal injury, damage to the renal parenchyma, or obstruction of the urinary tract. These etiologies are referred to as *prerenal*, *renal*, or *postrenal* causes of AKI, respectively, and are summarized in Table 73.3. Although it is helpful to consider the complete array of renal diseases when evaluating AKI, in the inpatient setting two thirds of cases will be due to either acute tubular necrosis (ATN) or prerenal azotemia. Hence, an extensive search for other forms

TABLE 73.3

CAUSES OF ACUTE KIDNEY INJURY

Prerenal azotemia
Hypovolemia
Reduced effective circulating volume
Autoregulatory failure
Intrinsic renal disease
Glomerular diseases
Vascular diseases (main renal artery and microcirculation)
Tubulointerstitial disease
Acute tubular necrosis
Acute cortical necrosis
Postrenal failure
Ureteric obstruction (bilateral or solitary kidney)
Lower tract obstruction (bladder neck or urethra)

of renal disease is indicated in the intensive care unit (ICU) setting only when suggested by clinical signs or laboratory findings such as urinary abnormalities indicative of glomerular disease.

Prerenal Azotemia and Autoregulatory Failure

When renal perfusion pressure decreases to a point at which GFR falls, prerenal azotemia is said to be present. This is a functional condition that does not represent intrinsic renal disease as such, although it may be superimposed on preexisting renal disease. The causes of prerenal azotemia are listed in Table 73.4. Normalization of renal blood flow, if possible, promptly restores renal function.

Hypovolemia serious enough to cause prerenal azotemia may result from gastrointestinal losses, hemorrhage, venous pooling, sequestering of fluid in "third spaces," or excessive urinary or skin losses of sodium and water. Patients will usually exhibit signs of hypovolemia, including thirst, diminished skin turgor and mucous membrane moistness, and postural hypotension. Patients whose vascular volume is functionally reduced by the hemodynamic alterations of congestive heart failure, cirrhosis, or hypoalbuminemia may develop prerenal azotemia despite having a normal or even expanded extracellular fluid (ECF) volume. Because the *effective circulatory volume* is reduced, renal perfusion is impaired just as in true hypovolemia.

When glomerular perfusion is threatened, autoregulatory mechanisms help maintain glomerular capillary pressure. If autoregulatory mechanisms are inoperative, a given reduction

TABLE 73.2

RIFLE CRITERIA

	Serum creatinine (Cr)/glomerular filtration rate (GFR) criteria	Urinary output criteria
Risk	Cr increase ×1.5 above baseline or GFR decline >25%	<0.5 mL/kg/h × 6 h
Injury	Cr increase ×2 above baseline or GFR decline >50%	<0.3 mL/kg/h × 24 h
Failure	Cr increase ×3 above baseline or Cr ≥4 mg/dL or GFR decline >75%	<0.3 mL/kg/h 24 h or anuria × 12 h
Loss	Persistent AKI >4 wk	
End stage	End-stage renal disease (AKI >3 mo)	

Summary of RIFLE criteria of AKI. Sensitivity for AKI increases toward the top of the chart, while specificity increases toward the bottom of the chart. [Bellomo R, Ronco C, Kellum JA, et al; Acute Dialysis Quality Initiative Workgroup: Acute renal failure—definition, outcome measures, animal models, fluid therapy and information technology needs: the Second International Consensus Conference of the Acute Dialysis Quality Initiative (ADQI) Group. *Crit Care* 8:R204–R210, 2004.]

TABLE 73.4

CAUSES OF PRERENAL AZOTEMIA

Hypovolemia
Gastrointestinal losses
Vomiting
Diarrhea
Surgical drainage
Renal losses
Osmotic agents
Diuretics
Renal salt-wasting disease
Adrenal insufficiency
Skin losses
Burns
Excessive diaphoresis
Hemorrhage
Translocation of fluid ("third spacing")
Postoperative
Pancreatitis
Reduced effective circulating volume
Hypoalbuminemia
Hepatic cirrhosis
Left ventricular cardiac failure
Peripheral blood pooling (vasodilator therapy, anesthetics, anaphylaxis, sepsis, toxic shock syndrome)
Renal artery occlusion
Small vessel disease (malignant hypertension, toxemia, scleroderma)
Renal vasoconstriction (hypercalcemia, hepatorenal syndrome, cyclosporine, pressor agents)
Autoregulatory failure
Nonsteroidal anti-inflammatory drugs (preglomerular vasoconstriction)
Angiotensin-converting enzyme inhibitors (postglomerular vasodilation)

in renal blood flow provokes a sharper decline in GFR. The mechanisms of these processes are shown in Figure 73.1. Use of nonsteroidal anti-inflammatory drugs (NSAIDs) in patients with renal hypoperfusion, for example, can lead to severe AKI [6–8]. Likewise, administration of angiotensin-converting enzyme (ACE) inhibitors in patients whose renal blood flow is obstructed by bilateral renovascular renal artery stenoses can cause severe azotemia [9].

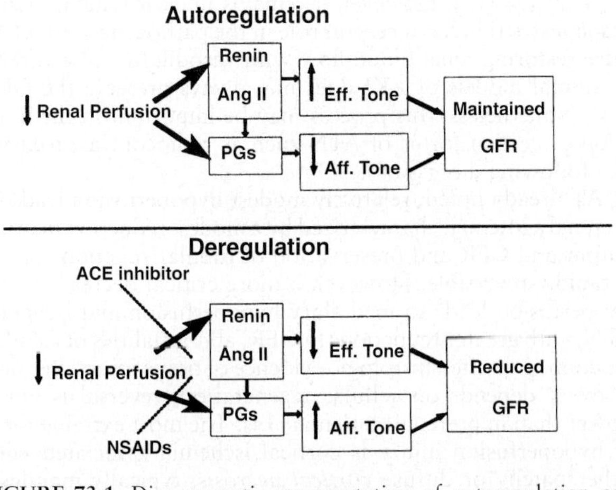

FIGURE 73.1. Diagrammatic representation of autoregulation and deregulation caused by use of either nonsteroidal anti-inflammatory drugs (NSAIDs), which lead to afferent (Aff.) vasoconstriction, or angiotensin-converting enzyme (ACE) inhibitors, which produce efferent (Eff.) vasodilation. Ang II, angiotensin II; GFR, glomerular filtration rate; PGs, prostaglandins.

Reduced renal perfusion slows down the flow of filtrate through the renal tubules, enhancing the reabsorption of urea. Because creatinine is not reabsorbed in the renal tubules, its clearance is unaffected by these nephronal factors. Thus, the clearance of urea is reduced disproportionately to that of creatinine, explaining the unusually high BUN–creatinine ratio that is often seen in prerenal states. In such situations, the BUN–creatinine ratio typically exceeds 20 to 1.

A high urea–creatinine ratio, however, is not pathognomonic of prerenal azotemia. When urea production is accelerated in catabolic states (as is seen in tetracycline and corticosteroid therapy) or by resorption of a large hematoma or gastrointestinal bleeding, BUN levels rise unless renal urea clearance can increase to meet the augmented urea burden. To establish whether a high BUN–creatinine ratio is due to increased urea production or reduced excretion, calculation of the fractional urea clearance may be useful.

The hallmark of prerenal conditions is the intense renal conservation of salt and water as reflected in the urine composition, which generally shows a low sodium concentration (U_{Na} <10 mEq per L; fractional excretion of sodium [FE_{Na}] <1%) and a high osmolality (U_{Osm} >500 mOsm per kg). Renal conservation of sodium involves both proximal and distal tubular mechanisms. A low urinary sodium concentration is expected in these states; its absence signifies a coexisting abnormality of tubular function, the effect of diuretics, or the presence of nonreabsorbable anionic substances in the urine, such as bicarbonate in patients with metabolic alkalosis, or certain penicillins, that obligate the excretion of cations like sodium. Impaired sodium reabsorption is also seen during osmotic diuresis and in certain forms of chronic renal disease.

Intrinsic Renal Disease

Reduced renal function may also result from renal parenchymal injury. Such injury may arise from glomerular, vascular, and tubulointerstitial disorders (Table 73.3) and may represent either primary kidney disease or the renal effects of an underlying systemic illness (e.g., systemic lupus erythematosus).

Glomerular and Vascular Diseases

The GFR may be abruptly reduced in acute glomerulonephritis. In poststreptococcal glomerulonephritis, the prototypic nephritic disorder, patients often present with AKI and oliguria.

Hypertension and edema result from their inability to excrete salt and water normally. The constellation of hypertension, edema, azotemia, and hematuria is known as the *acute nephritic syndrome*. Although the history of a previous sore throat or streptococcal infection may provide diagnostic clues, the urinalysis is particularly valuable. The urine may be grossly bloody or tea colored. The urinary sediment contains red blood cells (RBCs) and often RBC casts (Fig. 73.2). Similar findings are frequent in patients with other primary nephritic disorders as well as in secondary nephritides, such as those seen in systemic lupus, and bacterial endocarditis. The crescentic glomerulonephritides (rapidly progressive glomerulonephritis) can evoke the acute nephritic syndrome.

Diseases affecting either the main renal arteries or their branches may precipitate AKI. Renal artery occlusion by *acute thrombosis* or *thromboembolism* typically only causes AKI if it is bilateral or involves a solitary functioning kidney. These processes may be silent or may produce flank pain and hematuria, particularly if abrupt enough to cause renal infarction. Fever, moderate leukocytosis, and an elevated serum level of

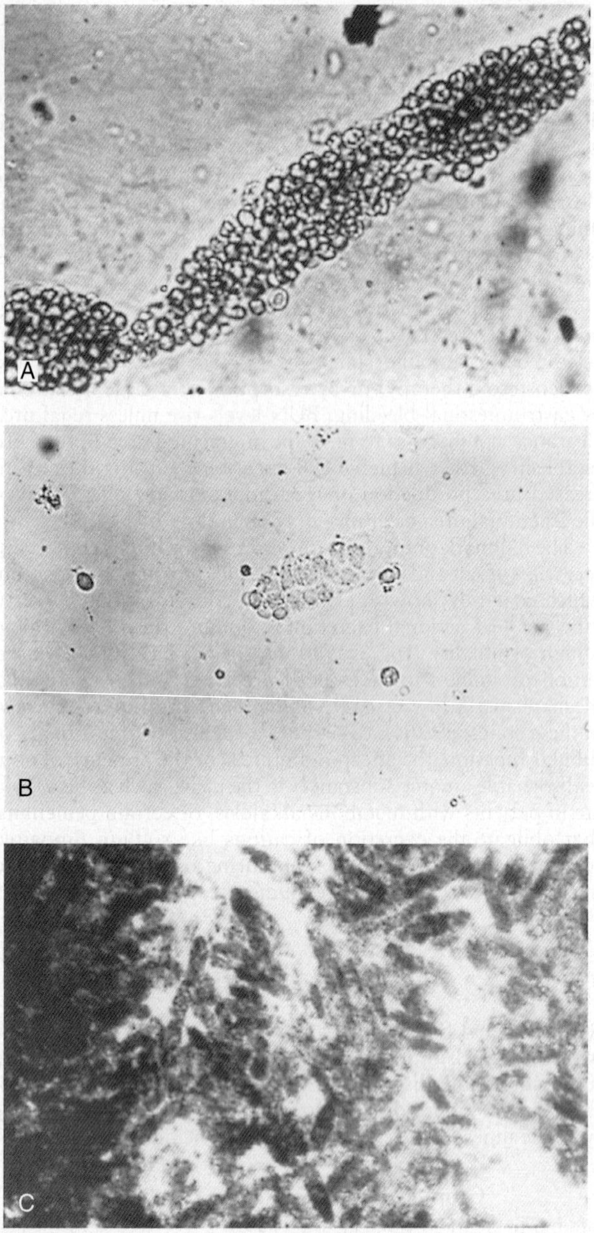

FIGURE 73.2. Typical urinary sediments from patients with parenchymal renal diseases. A: Sediment from patient with acute glomerulonephritis showing free red blood cells and red blood cell casts. B: Sediment from patient with acute interstitial nephritis demonstrating pyuria and white blood cell cast. C: Typical muddy brown, coarse, granular casts in a patient with acute tubular necrosis.

lactate dehydrogenase should raise the suspicion of infarction. With rare exceptions, renal arterial thromboembolism occurs only in the settings of acute myocardial infarction, atrial fibrillation, bacterial endocarditis, hypercoagulable disorders, or other cardiac valvular disease.

Acute renal vein thrombosis seldom causes renal failure unless both kidneys are simultaneously occluded. Acute flank pain and hematuria are the clinical hallmarks. Renal venous obstruction may occur as a complication of nephrotic syndrome and renal cell carcinoma.

Microscopic occlusion of smaller vessels occurs in a variety of disorders, including atheroembolic renal disease, thrombotic thrombocytopenic purpura (TTP) and hemolytic-uremic syndrome, scleroderma, postpartum kidney injury, and malignant hypertension. Scleroderma or malignant hypertension may appear as AKI, with severe blood pressure elevation due to activation of the renin–angiotensin system. These vascular disorders produce renal injury by reducing glomerular blood flow. Because the lesion is proximal to the glomerulus, the urine sediment is usually acellular and bland.

Vasculitis produces AKI either through direct involvement of the renal arterial system or by inducing glomerulonephritis. Often, microscopic polyarteritis or Wegener's granulomatosis may present with evident renal parenchymal disease, as suggested by urinary abnormalities such as microscopic hematuria, RBC casts, and proteinuria. These patients may present to the ICU when there is multiorgan involvement, such as the pulmonary disease that occurs in Wegener's granulomatosis. Fulminant presentations with severe hypoxemia and pulmonary hemorrhage may be accompanied by rapidly progressive renal dysfunction. In these cases, glomerular involvement may range from focal and segmental necrotizing glomerulitis to severe crescentic glomerulonephritis.

Tubulointerstitial Diseases

Two syndromes are responsible for most cases of parenchymal AKI in hospitalized populations: *ATN* and *acute interstitial nephritis (AIN)*.

Acute Tubular Necrosis. ATN is a syndrome that may result from renal ischemia or exposure to nephrotoxins such as aminoglycoside antibiotics, radiocontrast agents, heavy metals, and myoglobin. Although historically many other names have been applied to this syndrome, the term *acute tubular necrosis* prevails even though frank tubular cell necrosis does not appear in all cases. Historically, the pathophysiology of AKI in ATN has been attributed to three processes: (a) *obstruction of tubular lumens* by sloughed epithelial cells and cellular debris, (b) *back-leak* of filtered wastes into the circulation through the disrupted tubular epithelium, and (c) *sustained reduction in glomerular blood flow* following the inciting stimulus. Along these lines, severe cortical vasoconstriction has been noted early in the course of ATN [10], which is likely mediated by endothelial cell injury and locally acting vasoconstrictors, such as endothelin [11]. Afferent arteriolar vasoconstriction has also been described. In ATN, impaired proximal solute reabsorption increases distal chloride delivery to macular densa, which, in turn, mediates afferent constriction via the secretion of adenosine. This process is termed *tubuloglomerular feedback* [12]. However, it remains unclear whether renal vasoconstriction has a central role in the pathogenesis of ATN, since restoring renal blood flow with vasodilators in a variety of animal models of AKI does not always preserve the GFR [13]. Nonetheless, this process may be important in the initiation of certain forms of ATN such as radiocontrast toxicity (see following discussion).

As already noted, relatively modest hypoperfusion leads to prerenal azotemia, characterized by a modest reduction in urine output and GFR and preservation of tubular function, which is rapidly reversible. However, a more critical decrease in renal perfusion leads to medullary hypoperfusion and ischemic ATN, with greater reductions in GFR, abnormalities of tubular function, and often histologic evidence of tissue injury. Because recovery depends on cellular regeneration, reversal is much slower than in prerenal azotemia [14]. The most extreme form of hypoperfusion injury is cortical ischemia associated with either patchy or diffuse *cortical necrosis*, typically manifesting the most severe reduction in GFR and a much less certain prognosis for recovery of renal function. The medullary thick ascending limb segment of the loop of Henle is particularly vulnerable to ischemic and nephrotoxic insults because of a combination of low ambient partial pressure of oxygen and intense,

TABLE 73.5

PROTEIN BIOMARKERS FOR THE EARLY DETECTION OF ACUTE KIDNEY INJURY

Biomarker	Associated injury
Cystatin C	Proximal tubule injury
KIM-1	Ischemia and nephrotoxins
NGAL	
L-FABP	
Netrin-1	Sepsis, ischemia, nephrotoxins I
NHE3	Prerenal, ischemia, postrenal
α-GST	Acute rejection, proximal tubule injury
π-GST	Acute rejection, distal tubule injury
Cytokines (IL-6, IL-8, IL-18)	Delayed graft function
Actin–actin depolymerizing F	
Keratin-derived chemokine	

GST, glutathione S-transferase; IL, interleukin; KIM, kidney injury molecule; L-FABP, L-type fatty acid binding protein; NGAL, neutrophil gelatinase-associated lipocalin; NHE, sodium–hydrogen exchanger. From Ronco C, Haapio M, House AA, et al: Cardiorenal syndrome. *J Am Coll Cardiol.* 52:1527, 2008.

transport-driven oxygen consumption. Other factors, such as adenosine triphosphate depletion activation of phospholipases, cytosolic and mitochondrial calcium overload, and release of free radicals [15], may contribute to cellular damage. In experimental ATN, cytoskeletal reorganization can be demonstrated in proximal tubular cells, leading to loss of normal cell polarity. The sodium–potassium adenosine triphosphatase transport system may thus be translocated from its normal basolateral position to the apical surface of the cell, impairing reabsorptive function.

There is growing evidence that immune system plays a critical role in pathogenesis of ATN through recruitment of various inflammatory cells, cytokine release, complement activation, and induction of tubular cell apoptosis [16,17]. Adhesion molecules, such as intracellular adhesion molecule 1 (ICAM-1), appear to play a role in the development of postischemic ATN in experimental animal models. However, anti-ICAM antibody failed to protect against ischemic AKI in a clinical trial of kidney transplant patients [18]. Another regulatory molecule expressed in the kidney, the protein neutrophil gelatinase-associated lipocalin (NGAL), is released early in the course of ischemic ATN and appears to attenuate tubular cell injury and apoptosis [19]. There is considerable interest in using NGAL and other molecules as biomarkers of early kidney injury (Table 73.5) with the hope that timely diagnosis of AKI will allow clinicians to make therapeutic interventions that will ultimately improve outcomes (discussed further in "Diagnosis" section).

History of exposure to a predisposing factor, such as prolonged ischemia or toxin, can be elicited in approximately 80% of patients with ATN. Most individuals with this syndrome have the classic findings of sloughed renal tubular epithelial cells, epithelial cell casts, or muddy brown granular casts in the urinary sediment (Fig. 73.2). These findings are not seen in prerenal azotemia. In addition, calculating the fractional excretion of filtered sodium (FE_{Na}) may enable the clinician to differentiate between ATN and prerenal azotemia. The FE_{Na} expresses urinary sodium excretion as a percentage of filtered load. It provides a more precise representation of tubular sodium avidity than the urinary sodium concentration because it is not influenced by changes in urine concentration or flow rate. The FE_{Na} is very low in prerenal azotemia as a result of active sodium reabsorption by the renal tubules. When frank tubular damage has occurred, as in ATN, the tubules can no longer reclaim sodium efficiently, and the FE_{Na} is generally high (Fig. 73.3). See "Diagnosis" section for more detail on the FE_{Na}. Urinary concentration is also impaired in tubular necrosis; as a result, urinary osmolality approximates that of plasma, and the BUN–creatinine ratio is less than 20.

Acute Interstitial Nephritis. The term *acute interstitial* (or *tubulointerstitial*) *nephritis* encompasses a collection of disorders characterized by acute inflammation of the renal interstitium and tubules. Depending on the specific nature of the condition, the inflammatory infiltrate may consist of a combination of neutrophils, eosinophils, and lymphocytes or plasma cells. Most cases of AIN represent an allergic reaction with eosinophilia and skin eruptions, usually induced by medication. Interstitial disease can also occur as a result of infectious agents, including brucellosis, leptospirosis, legionella, toxoplasmosis, and Epstein–Barr virus.

These disorders are to be distinguished from the familiar entity *acute pyelonephritis*. Acute pyelonephritis is a suppurative

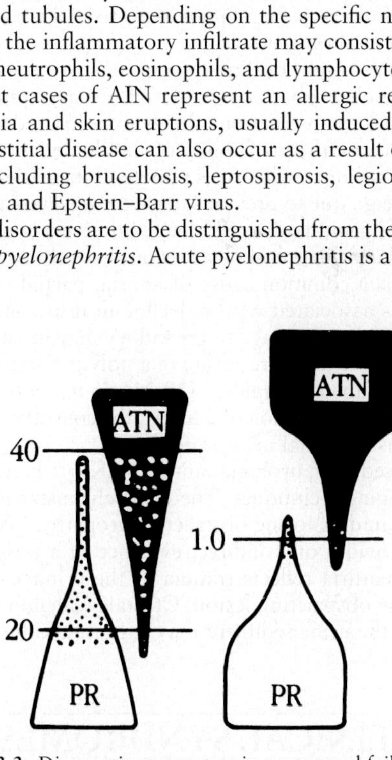

FIGURE 73.3. Diagnostic parameters in acute renal failure. Two laboratory tests used to distinguish prerenal (PR) azotemia from acute tubular necrosis (ATN) are shown. **Left:** Urinary sodium concentration (U_{Na}, mEq per L). **Right:** Fractional excretion of sodium (FE_{Na}, %). Area within each symbol denotes the proportion of patients with each condition correlated with the laboratory parameter. Note that although considerable numbers of patients with PR and ATN fall in an intermediate zone of U_{Na} (20 to 40 mEq per L), the FE_{Na} almost completely differentiates the two groups. [Adapted from Rudnick MR, Bastl CP, Elfinbein IB, et al: The differential diagnosis of acute renal failure, in Brenner BM, Lazarus JM (eds): *Acute Renal Failure*. New York, Churchill Livingstone, 1988, p 177.]

disease of the tubulointerstitium, usually caused by bacterial infection ascending from the urinary bladder. Acute pyelonephritis rarely causes renal dysfunction. AIN, however, is an important cause of AKI and is discussed in detail later.

Postrenal Azotemia

The term *postrenal azotemia*, or *obstructive uropathy*, refers to azotemia caused by obstruction of urine flow from the kidneys. Renal outflow obstruction has many causes, but the most common causes are prostatic enlargement, nephrolithiasis, and genitourinary tumors. For obstruction to produce azotemia, both kidneys must be involved because one normally functioning kidney is sufficient to maintain a near normal GFR. AKI may occur with unilateral obstruction in a patient who has one functioning kidney or in whom unilateral obstruction is superimposed on underlying CKD.

The clinical history often helps in the diagnosis of obstructive uropathy. Prior kidney stones should raise the index of suspicion for obstruction, particularly in the setting of symptoms of renal colic. AKI in an elderly man who has been experiencing urinary hesitancy most likely represents obstruction of the bladder outlet by an enlarged prostate. A history of genitourinary malignancy in an azotemic patient also makes obstruction the most likely diagnosis. AKI in the setting of painless gross hematuria and a history of NSAID use should prompt a suspicion of papillary necrosis, a condition in which sloughed-off renal papilla can cause bilateral ureteral obstruction. Finally, renal failure in a newborn infant is likely to be due to congenital anatomic ureteral obstruction.

When urine output declines precipitously or ceases entirely (anuria), complete obstruction of the urinary tract must be ruled out. Such an obstruction is likely to be located at the bladder outlet because the probability of simultaneous obstruction in both ureters from any cause is remote. If the patient has only one kidney (e.g., due to previous nephrectomy, unilateral renal disease, or congenital solitary kidney), however, anuria may occur with unilateral ureteral obstruction. Even though complete obstruction is a common cause of anuria, partial obstruction is not always associated with a decline in urine output. With partial obstruction, damage to the kidney may impair the ability to concentrate urine, resulting in a polyuric state (acquired nephrogenic diabetes insipidus) [20,21]. In patients with complete unilateral obstruction of a ureter, the contralateral kidney often sustains a normal urine output.

As discussed later, urologic causes of AKI are best diagnosed by renal imaging techniques. The urine chemistry is generally of little help in diagnosing obstructive uropathy. Likewise, the urinalysis provides only indirect evidence of a possible cause of AKI. Hematuria reflects trauma to the urinary epithelium caused by the obstructing lesion. Crystals (calcium oxalate or uric acid) in the urine sediment may suggest a kidney stone.

CLINICAL SYNDROMES ASSOCIATED WITH AKI IN THE INTENSIVE CARE SETTING

With the higher level of acuity of illness, and more radical approaches to surgical and pharmacologic therapeutics, the incidence of AKI is increasing. As with other areas of clinical medicine, patterns of presentation often can be recognized and can lead the physician to the most likely diagnoses. The following section explores in greater detail the specific AKI syndromes most commonly encountered in the ICU (listed in Table 73.6).

TABLE 73.6

INTENSIVE CARE SYNDROMES ASSOCIATED WITH ACUTE KIDNEY INJURY (AKI)

Ischemic AKI
Extracellular volume depletion
Postoperative (particularly cardiac surgery)
Severe ventricular dysfunction or cardiogenic shock
Sepsis
Pancreatitis
Trauma
Burns
Acute bilateral cortical necrosis
Nephrotoxicity and drug-induced AKI
Myoglobinuric AKI
Radiocontrast nephropathy
Drugs (see Table 73.13)
Renal vascular disease
Major vessel disease
Renal artery embolism or thrombosis
Renal vein thrombosis
Microvascular disease
Atheroembolism
Vasculitis
Scleroderma
Cancer related
Obstructive uropathy
Hypercalcemia
Tumor-lysis syndrome
ATN secondary to chemotherapy
Renal dysfunction with liver disease
Prerenal azotemia
ATN
Hepatorenal syndrome

ATN, acute tubular necrosis.

Ischemic Acute Kidney Injury

The most common forms of AKI in the ICU result from renal hypoperfusion. Because frank hypotension is documented in fewer than half of these cases, the causal events may often be overlooked or obscured by multiple factors. Frequently, more than one causal factor is necessary to provoke AKI. For example, the presence of hypovolemia enhances the risk for AKI due to nephrotoxic insults.

Extracellular Volume Depletion

Extracellular volume depletion accounted for approximately 17% of cases of AKI in a prospective study of AKI in a major hospital [14]. In most instances, urinary losses are the cause of hypovolemia. Injudicious use of diuretics and the osmotic diuresis that accompanies diabetic hyperglycemia are the most common etiologies. Cessation of diuretic therapy and volume repletion lead to rapid recovery; consequently, the mortality is quite low [14].

In rare instances, gastrointestinal losses of substantial magnitude may lead to AKI. (In the developing world, however, this is one of the most common causes of AKI and the major cause of morbidity and mortality in epidemic cholera.) In such cases, the source of the gastrointestinal losses, either gastric or intestinal, may lead to distinctive electrolyte abnormalities. In the former, metabolic alkalosis mandates repletion with chloride-rich replacement solutions (normal saline, usually with potassium chloride, as most patients are also hypokalemic). With intestinal losses of fluid, metabolic acidosis often ensues, and appropriate replacement may consist of a buffer solution of either isotonic bicarbonate or lactate-containing (Ringer's) solution in combination with saline. (This is more fully discussed in Chapter 71.)

Transdermal fluid losses usually occur in the setting of major burns, with the degree of hypovolemia and the severity of AKI corresponding to the extent of thermal injury (body surface-area involvement). Significant burns can lead to severe hypovolemia as a result of massive evaporative and exudative fluid loss across the damaged epidermis as well from redistribution of fluid due to edema in the injured tissues. This hypovolemia can stimulate a sympathetic nerve-mediated response with resultant renal vasoconstriction. In some instances, the severity of renal vasoconstriction, superimposed on hypovolemia, culminates in ATN. In addition, deeper thermal injury with skeletal muscle involvement may induce myoglobinuric AKI (see following discussion). Dermal losses of fluid are also seen in the setting of hyperthermia and heat stroke. The evaporative loss of sweat, which is hypotonic, leads to a hypertonic dehydration in these cases. Replacement with half-normal saline corrects free water and sodium deficits.

Postoperative

Postoperative AKI has long been recognized as a common complication of major vascular, abdominal, and open-heart surgery. The pathogenesis of postoperative renal dysfunction varies with the type of the surgery and the preoperative condition of the patient. AKI following abdominal surgery is often the result of translocation of fluid into the peritoneal cavity. In this phenomenon, third spacing causes intravascular hypovolemia and subsequent renal hypoperfusion. AKI is uncommon in patients undergoing routine abdominal surgery, but the risk is substantial in surgery for obstructive jaundice; this complication may develop in approximately 10% of patients [22]. Major vascular surgery, particularly aortic repairs, is also frequently complicated by AKI, especially in the setting of a ruptured aortic aneurysm [23]. Elective repair of an aortic aneurysm is seldom associated with AKI unless cross clamping is placed above the renal arteries. Although the definition of AKI and its incidence varies among studies, cardiac surgery appears to generate most of the cases in the acute care hospital. In a prospective study, cardiac surgery accounted for nearly two thirds of the postoperative AKI with an overall incidence of 15% [14]. Repeated episodes of AKI and sepsis complicating AKI are associated with substantially higher mortality (85%) after surgery.

Myers and Moran [10] have described three distinct clinical patterns of AKI following open-heart surgery. The abbreviated pattern, observed in 80% to 90% of patients, usually has an abrupt onset after surgery, followed by a brief and mild rise in the serum creatinine, peaking by 3 to 4 days, after which recovery is rapid. This form of AKI is frequently associated with the use of vasoconstrictors, such as norepinephrine and epinephrine, in the immediate postoperative period. The overt form is associated with a more severe reduction in GFR and rise in serum creatinine, which peaks 1 to 2 weeks after surgery. This is generally associated with poor cardiac performance following surgery, whereas recovery is associated with improved ventricular function. The protracted form of AKI generally follows a second insult after surgery, such as sepsis or pericardial tamponade, and is associated with prolonged AKI and a poor prognosis.

Several predisposing factors for the development of postoperative AKI have been identified, which can be used to stratify risk (Table 73.7). These include emergent surgery, an elevated preoperative serum creatinine, the use of an intra-aortic balloon pump, and combined coronary artery bypass graft and valvular surgery [24]. Still, it is often difficult to prospectively identify those patients at heightened risk for perioperative AKI, especially since 40% of patients who develop AKI do not have frank perioperative hypotension or evidence of shock. Other factors appear to be important in the development of AKI. For example, aprotinin, an antifibrinolytic agent used until recently to decrease perioperative blood loss in cardiac surgery patients, tends to increase AKI and postoperative mortality [25]. Prolonged cardiopulmonary bypass appears to induce oxidative stress, embolism, and systemic inflammation, thus contributing to AKI [26]. An improved mortality and reduced incidence of AKI is observed with the use of "off-pump" technology in one large observational study [27]. Prospective, randomized trials are underway to study the effects of the off pump cardiac surgery.

A number of methods have been used to try to protect kidney function in patients undergoing surgery. Administration of "low-dose" dopamine has long been advocated for the prevention of AKI but has fallen out of favor due to the lack of efficacy [28]. A meta-analysis of fenoldopam, a selective dopamine receptor agonist, demonstrated a reduction in mortality and the need for dialysis in cardiac surgery patients [29]. A large, randomized, prospective trial of preventive role of fenoldopam is underway. Nesiritide, a recombinant human B-type natriuretic peptide, which increases diuresis, natriuresis, and afterload reduction, was studied in a double-blind, randomized trial of 300 patients with mostly preserved renal function undergoing coronary artery bypass graft surgery [30]. The use of nesiritide was associated with improved postoperative serum creatinine and reduced length of hospital stay as compared with the placebo. Nevertheless, significant concerns remain regarding the safety of nesiritide, especially in patients with acute decompensated heart failure (ADHF) and reduced renal function (discussed later in the chapter). Several other strategies, including perioperative N-acetylcysteine and mannitol administration, have not been shown to be effective for the prevention of postoperative AKI [31,32]. The use of calcium channel blockers, ACE

TABLE 73.7

A CLINICAL SCORE TO PREDICT AKI REQUIRING DIALYSIS AFTER CARDIAC SURGERY

Risk factor	Points
Female gender	1
Congestive heart failure	1
Left ventricular ejection fraction <35%	1
Preoperative use of intra-aortic balloon pump	2
Chronic obstructive pulmonary disease	1
Diabetes requiring insulin	1
Previous cardiac surgery	1
Emergency surgery	2
Valvular surgery only	1
Coronary artery bypass graft surgery plus valvular surgery	2
Other cardiac surgeries	2
Preoperative serum creatinine 1.2 to <2.1 mg/dL	2
Preoperative serum creatinine ≥2.1 mg/dL	5

Minimum score, 0; maximum score, 17. Risk of development of AKI requiring dialysis increases with higher score. Frequency of AKI requiring dialysis for score of 0–2 point is 0.5%, 3–5 points is 2%, 6–8 points is 8%, 9–13 points is 22%.
From Thakar CV, Arrigain S, Worley S, et al: A clinical score to predict acute renal failure after cardiac surgery. *J Am Soc Nephrol* 6:162, 2005.

inhibitors, or diuretics has been disappointing in this context as well [33]. In fact, perioperative furosemide use has been associated with detrimental effect on renal function after cardiac surgery [34]. Furosemide should be used only in patients with definite volume overload.

Prevention of postoperative renal failure still hinges on withdrawal of vasopressors as early as safely possible and maintenance of adequate perioperative intravascular volume. Identification of modifiable risk factors for the prevention of postoperative AKI is paramount. A retrospective study of 3,500 patients identified three potentially modifiable risk factors associated with AKI after cardiac surgery, such as preoperative anemia, perioperative RBC transfusions, and the need for surgical reexploration [35].

Cardiogenic Shock and Acute Decompensated Heart Failure

Our understanding of "cardiorenal syndrome" is evolving beyond the concept of low cardiac output causing renal dysfunction. We know that approximately half of patients with ADHF have preserved left ventricular function [36]. In the Evaluation Study of Congestive Heart Failure and Pulmonary Artery Catheterization Effectiveness (ESCAPE), optimization of hemodynamics did not prevent AKI, further suggesting that reduction in cardiac output does not fully explain the development of impaired renal function [36].

A complex bidirectional relationship emerges, whereby heart failure and associated renal dysfunction affect each other. In addition to the traditional hemodynamically mediated AKI due to low cardiac output, the heart and the kidney are simultaneously affected by activation of the sympathetic nervous and renin–angiotensin–aldosterone systems. Such activation results in systemic vasoconstriction, salt and water retention, and volume overload, further exacerbating kidney dysfunction and heart failure. In addition, the immune system affects renal and cardiac function through monocyte-mediated endothelial activation, cytokine release, and apoptosis induction [16,17,37]. Furthermore, CKD, a risk factor for coronary artery disease [38], contributes to volume overload, diuretic resistance, and poor prognosis in CHF [39] and ADHF [36]. Here, we will focus on acute ADHF with AKI as a common clinical problem in the ICU setting.

ADHF is frequently complicated by AKI. The Acute Decompensated Heart Failure Registry (ADHERE) of more than 30,000 patients with ADHF suggests that AKI has poor prognostic implications and predicts mortality in this patient group [40]. In one study, more than a quarter of patients with ADHF developed AKI as defined by a rise in serum creatinine of 0.3 mg per dL. However, even this relatively small rise was associated with 7.5-fold increase in hospital mortality [41].

Traditional treatment strategies of ADHF include diuresis, afterload reduction, and administration of inotropic agents. However, these patients are frequently diuretic resistant and hypotensive. The use of ACE inhibitors is often limited by AKI and hyperkalemia. Recently, nesiritide, a recombinant B-type natriuretic peptide, was approved for management of symptomatic ADHF [42]. However, a meta-analysis of five randomized clinical trials in more than 1,200 patients with ADHF suggested nesiritide was associated with worsening of renal function [43]. New trials are ongoing to further investigate the risk and benefit of nesiritide. Tolvaptan, a vasopressin antagonist, has been studied in a large international randomized trial of more than 4,000 heart failure patients [44]. Tolvaptan was statistically better then placebo at improving dyspnea, edema, and weight loss but did not significantly improve the rate of death and rehospitalization for heart failure.

Inotropic agents such as dobutamine and milrinone are used in the treatment of ADHF. Dobutamine acts primarily on β_1-adrenergic receptors, with minimal effects on β_2 and α_1 receptors. Dobutamine increases cardiac output and stroke volume and decreases systemic vascular resistance and pulmonary capillary wedge pressure. The 2004 ACC/AHA STEMI guidelines suggest using dobutamine in patients with hypotension who do not have clinical evidence of shock [45]. Milrinone is a phosphodiesterase inhibitor that increases myocardial contractility, reduces systemic vascular resistance, and improves left ventricular diastolic relaxation. However, inotropes increase myocardial oxygen consumption and can worsen myocardial ischemia, and their use has been limited by arrhythmia development and adverse outcomes. In a large prospective, randomized trial, milrinone infusion was associated with increased hypotension and atrial arrhythmias as well as a trend toward increased mortality [46]. The use of inotropes is limited to patients with ADHF and low cardiac output who fail or cannot tolerate diuretic and vasodilator therapy. Additional information on the use of inotropes can be found in Chapter 33 of the "Cardiovascular Problems and Coronary Care" section.

Other strategies for diuretic-resistant patients with ADHF include mechanical fluid removal with ultrafiltration or paracentesis. The use of ultrafiltration in the ICU setting is discussed in "Renal Replacement Therapies" section of the text. Mullens et al. suggested that elevated intra-abdominal pressures in ADHF may play a role in the pathogenesis of renal dysfunction [47]. The reduction of intra-abdominal pressure from approximately 13 to 7 mm Hg by paracentesis was associated with a reduction in serum creatinine from 3.4 to 2.4 mg per dL in diuretic-resistant patients.

Sepsis

Sepsis is among the most common causes of AKI. In one large series of patients with ATN, sepsis was believed to be the cause in 15%, with a mortality rate of 40% [48]. The association between septicemia and AKI is confounded by the experience that renal dysfunction due to other causes is often complicated by infection. Although the incidence of sepsis in patients with AKI has been reported as high as 75% [49], only one third of patients have clinically apparent septicemia at the outset of renal dysfunction [50].

AKI may develop in a setting of sepsis through multiple mechanisms. As discussed previously, inflammation appears to play a significant role. In animal models, sepsis can cause renal impairment even in the absence of hypotension [51]. Clinically, it is likely that endotoxin causes a reduction in GFR through hemodynamic mechanisms, including vascular pooling and renal vasoconstriction, which are mediated by local vasoconstrictors such as thromboxane and endothelin. Although cardiac output is often elevated in patients with sepsis, systemic vasodilation coupled with renal vasoconstriction can shunt perfusion away from the kidneys. Vascular pooling and third spacing generally necessitate volume expansion with isotonic saline. Because myocardial suppression, oliguria, and capillary leakage may accompany sepsis, it is essential to monitor the administration of fluids closely.

Pancreatitis

Pancreatitis may occur in association with various causes of AKI but can itself induce ATN. This is a rare phenomenon and is generally seen in patients with severe or hemorrhagic pancreatitis with serum amylase values of more than 1,000 U per L. Mortality may approach 70% to 80% in this setting, especially in those with multiorgan failure.

Trauma

AKI associated with severe trauma generally reflects the combination of acute volume depletion, hemorrhage, and myoglobinuria (see following discussion). Survival after trauma is markedly reduced when complicated by AKI.

Acute Bilateral Cortical Necrosis

Acute bilateral cortical necrosis is rare. Unlike ATN, in which only tubular elements are involved, in acute cortical necrosis, glomeruli and tubules are destroyed by a process in which cortical vessels may be occluded with fibrin thrombi. Cortical necrosis usually occurs after profound hypotension. Approximately two thirds of cases are related to obstetric complications, including abruptio placentae, preeclampsia and eclampsia, septic abortion, and amniotic fluid embolism [52]. Nonobstetric cortical necrosis is most common in shock, sepsis, and disseminated intravascular coagulopathy, but isolated cases have been reported with snakebites [53], arsenic ingestion [54], and hyperacute renal allograft rejection [55]. The pathogenesis of AKI in these conditions involves the hemodynamic insults of hypoperfusion and renal vasoconstriction and formation of fibrin thrombi in the renal microvasculature.

Typically, patients with bilateral cortical necrosis have anuric AKI. Although the diagnosis may be suspected early in the course of renal injury, ATN remains far more likely. When renal function fails to recover after several weeks, cortical necrosis may be confirmed by a renal biopsy. Other diagnostic tests are less specific. Renal scintigraphy most often demonstrates complete absence of isotope in the region of the kidneys. Computed tomography (CT) with contrast enhancement may demonstrate similar findings, indicating absence of perfusion to the renal cortex. Renal angiography shows patency of the main renal arteries and either a complete absence of cortical filling or a mottled nephrogram. Given the severity of the inciting disorder, mortality is high in acute cortical necrosis, with fewer than 20% of patients surviving. At least 25% of survivors eventually require maintenance dialysis [50].

Nephrotoxicity and Drug-Induced Acute Kidney Injury

Many cases of AKI in the ICU can be linked to the effects of endogenous and exogenous nephrotoxins.

Myoglobinuria and Hemoglobinuria

Rhabdomyolysis is often associated with leakage of myocyte contents, particularly the pigment protein myoglobin, into the plasma. Myoglobin, with a molecular weight of approximately 17,000 daltons, is freely filtered by the glomerulus. In the distal nephron, myoglobin forms proteinaceous casts that obstruct urine flow. Myoglobin may also exert direct cytotoxic effects on tubular epithelium through the generation of reactive oxygen species.

Myoglobinuric AKI is a consequence of massive skeletal muscle injury of diverse causes. Traumatic rhabdomyolysis occurs in the setting of direct mechanical injury (crush syndrome), burns, or prolonged pressure. Myoglobinuric renal failure is an important cause of morbidity in virtually all wide-scale human catastrophes. Indeed, much of what is known about the syndrome derives from experiences with victims of wars and natural disasters. Crush injuries during the Armenian earthquake of 1988 necessitated emergent mobilization of dialysis resources on a massive scale [56].

Nontraumatic rhabdomyolysis can occur with toxic, metabolic, and inflammatory myopathies, vigorous exercise, severe potassium and phosphate depletion, and hyperthermic states such as the neuroleptic malignant syndrome and malignant hyperthermia. Lipid-lowering drugs currently represent one of the most common causes of rhabdomyolysis. The use of heroin and amphetamines [57,58] has been reported in association with rhabdomyolysis.

As with other forms of AKI, the prognosis depends largely on the gravity of the predisposing condition; AKI following massive trauma can be expected to run a longer course than that associated with nontraumatic causes, such as drugs. In particularly severe cases, oliguria and dialysis dependence may persist for weeks.

Clinical signs and symptoms of muscle injury, such as muscle tenderness, are absent in at least half of cases of significant nontraumatic rhabdomyolysis. The diagnosis is suggested by markedly elevated serum levels of muscle enzymes with serum creatine kinase levels usually higher than 5,000. The serum levels of phosphate and potassium are also typically elevated in rhabdomyolysis because lysis of muscle cells causes release of intracellular contents into the blood. A fall in the serum calcium is quite common. Rebound hypercalcemia often occurs during the recovery phase.

The therapy of myoglobinuria is similar to that of other forms of AKI, but there are several particular considerations. The tubular toxicity of myoglobin is enhanced when urine flow rates are low, urine is concentrated, and urinary acidification is maximal. It is therefore important in the early phases of the illness to ensure that the patient is in a volume-replete state and maintaining a rapid diuresis (i.e., urine output of at least 150 mL per hour). To this end, isotonic fluids may be administered. Most experts recommend the administration of bicarbonate-rich fluids to alkalinize the urine above a pH of 6.5 so as to improve the solubility of myoglobin. Diuresis may be enhanced with concurrent administration of loop diuretics. Some have argued that loop diuretics may introduce the potentially adverse effect of increasing urinary acid excretion and have advocated the use of osmotic diuretic agents such as mannitol [59]. Mannitol, however, has the potential drawback of causing intravascular volume overload in patients whose kidneys may already have impaired urine output.

Hemoglobinuria can also result in AKI. The pathophysiologic mechanisms are similar to those involved in myoglobinuric AKI. Hemoglobinuric renal failure is relatively rare. Hemoglobin, with a molecular weight almost four times that of myoglobin, is less readily filtered. Furthermore, when hemoglobin is released into the plasma, it binds to haptoglobin, forming a bulky, nonfilterable molecular complex. Only when the haptoglobin binding capacity is saturated (at plasma hemoglobin concentrations >100 mg per dL) does hemoglobin appear in the tubular fluid. Thus, only massive intravascular hemolysis, as may occur with fulminant transfusion reactions, autoimmune hemolytic crises, and mechanical hemolysis [60] from a dysfunctional prosthetic heart valve (Waring blender syndrome), can induce AKI.

Radiocontrast-Induced Nephropathy

The administration of intravascular radiocontrast agents leads to a syndrome of rapidly developing AKI. Contrast-induced nephropathy (CIN) is commonly defined as an absolute increase in serum creatinine of 0.5 mg per dL or a relative increase of 25% from the baseline within 48 to 72 hours of contrast exposure. The serum creatinine level begins to rise 12 to 24 hours and peaks approximately 4 days after the procedure [61]. Some patients develop a transient increase in urine output as a result of contrast-induced osmotic diuresis, followed by oliguria. The majority of patients are nonoliguric and do not require dialysis. Some, but not all, studies identified an increased mortality risk in patients with CIN [62–64]. In patients who have undergone endovascular procedures, CIN must be differentiated from atheroembolic disease, which has a significantly worse prognosis (discussed below).

TABLE 73.8

RISK FACTORS ASSOCIATED WITH RADIOCONTRAST NEPHROPATHY

Preexisting renal insufficiency
Diabetic nephropathy, with renal insufficiency
Volume depletion
Diuretic use
Large contrast dose (>2 mL/kg)
Age >60 y
CHF
Hepatic failure
Multiple myeloma (with high osmolar contrast agent)
Use of intra-aortic balloon pump

TABLE 73.9

PREVENTIVE MEASURES FOR RADIOCONTRAST NEPHROPATHY

Volume expansion with normal saline or isotonic bicarbonate (3 mL/kg bolus over 1 h prior to the procedure, followed by 1 mL/kg/h for 6 h postexposure)
Limit radiocontrast load to ≤1 mL/kg in high-risk patients
Avoid high osmolar contrast agents
Discontinue diuretics, ACE inhibitors, and nonsteroidal anti-inflammatory drugs for 24 h postprocedure
N-acetylcysteine (4 doses of 600–1,200 mg PO every 12 h with 2 doses before and 2 doses after procedure)

Prospective studies report that the incidence of radiocontrast-induced kidney injury ranges from 1% to more than 50%. Some of this variance in frequency can be attributed to the disparity in the definitions of AKI, the number of associated risk factors, and the type of procedure performed [65]. The incidence appears to be low in patients with normal renal function, even in the presence of diabetes. Preexisting CKD, however, particularly in patients with diabetes, confers a 6- to 10-fold increased likelihood of radiocontrast-induced AKI [66,67]. Contrast-enhanced CT is associated with a lower risk of CIN as compared with coronary angiography. Noncoronary angiography had the highest incidence of CIN in a study of 660 military veterans, reaching 15% in patients with GFR less than 60 mL per minute per 1.73 m^2 [68]. Other risk factors are listed in Table 73.8.

There are several mechanisms by which radiocontrast-induced renal injury may develop. Hemodynamic factors are believed important, as contrast exposure causes initial vasodilation followed by prolonged vasoconstriction of the renal circulation. The finding of a low FE_{Na} in some patients with contrast-induced AKI and the tendency toward rapid recovery suggest a role for reversible vasoconstriction. The intensity and duration of the vasoconstriction may be influenced by the underlying characteristics of the renal microcirculation. Endothelial factors that promote vasoconstriction of preglomerular vessels, such as endothelin, may participate in the pathogenesis of radiocontrast-induced nephropathy [11,69]. Tubular adenosine receptors appear to be stimulated by radiocontrast agents in animal models [70,71]. Adenosine induces afferent glomerular vasoconstriction and reduction in GFR. However, the protective effect of theophylline, an antagonist of adenosine receptors, was not statistically significant in the meta-analysis of available trials of CIN prevention [65]. Other postulated mechanisms of radiocontrast-induced nephropathy include the generation of reactive oxygen species and the direct cytotoxic effect of the contrast media, especially with highly osmolar agents [72].

Because there is no specific treatment for radiocontrast-induced nephropathy other than supportive measures, attention has focused on methods of prevention. The best preventive measure is avoidance of radiocontrast and use of an alternative noncontrast imaging procedure if at all possible.

A number of prophylactic measures (listed in Table 73.9) have been promoted. Experimental data and retrospective clinical studies suggest that radiocontrast injury is augmented by preexisting hypovolemia, particularly in the presence of prostaglandin inhibitors [73–76]. Therefore, modest hydration before the procedure and avoidance of diuretics and NSAIDs are justifiable.

Reports suggest that pharmacoprophylaxis of radiocontrast nephropathy may be possible. In a German study, *N*-acetylcysteine (NAC) was given to patients with CKD once before and once after they underwent angiography. The incidence of radiocontrast nephropathy in these patients was 2%, compared with 9% in an untreated control group. Both groups received concomitant hydration, and low-osmolality contrast medium was used [77]. Some, but not all, subsequent studies have confirmed these results [78,79]. Maranzi et al. [80] compared two different regimen of NAC in patient undergoing emergent angioplasty for STEMI. Patients receiving a high dose of NAC (1,200 mg IV prior to procedure, followed by 1,200 mg orally for four more doses) had a significantly lower incidence of CIN. The benefit of NAC remains controversial as conflicting results continue to emerge from other studies [65,81]. However, NAC appears to be a low risk intervention and is frequently used. We typically give NAC 1,200 mg orally for two doses before and two doses after the contrast exposure.

A nonpharmacologic prophylactic intervention of current interest is urinary alkalinization. In the study by Merten et al. [82], increases in serum creatinine of greater than 25% of the baseline level were significantly less likely to occur in patients receiving isotonic sodium bicarbonate (three 50-mEq ampules of sodium bicarbonate in 1 L of 5% dextrose in water administered at a rate of 3 mL per kg per hour for 1 hour before and at 1 mL per kg per hour for 6 hours after the radiocontrast exposure) than in control patients. A recent study of 326 patients at medium to high risk for CIN compared various strategies of prevention, including volume expansion with isotonic bicarbonate versus normal saline. This study suggested that isotonic bicarbonate may be more effective than normal saline [83]. Another randomized, controlled trial of 500 patients undergoing coronary angiography demonstrated no benefit of bicarbonate (3 mL per kg per bolus, followed by 6-hour infusion at 1 mL per kg per hour) over normal saline (1 mL per kg per hour for 12 hours before and after contrast exposure) [84]. There is no consensus on the best type of fluid for volume expansion due to conflicting data from other trials [85,86]. However, no clear risk of bicarbonate use has been demonstrated. We commonly use isotonic bicarbonate bolus, 3 mL per kg over 1 hour before administration of contrast agent, followed by 1 mL per kg per hour infusion for 6 hours after procedure.

Fenoldopam, a vasodilatory analog of dopamine initially thought to be protective against radiocontrast-induced nephropathy, has recently been shown to be without benefit [87].

Low-osmolality radiocontrast formulations (600 to 800 mOsm per kg) have been shown to be less nephrotoxic then high osmolar agents (>1,400 mOsm per kg) and are now commonly used in all patients [88]. However, iso-osmolar agents, such as iodixanol, have not been shown to have a clear additional benefit as compared with low-osmolar agents in three small, randomized, controlled trials [89–91] of patients undergoing contrast enhanced CT and coronary angiography.

Removal of contrast media by hemodialysis or hemofiltration to prevent CIN was studied in several small trials. A meta-analysis of these trials revealed no benefit and even suggested harm. The relative risk of CIN in that study was 1.35 (CI, 0.93 to 1.94) [92]. Three subsequent clinical trials yielded conflicting information [93–95]. Taken together, these data cannot justify the routine use of prophylactic extracorporeal modalities following radiocontrast exposure.

Acute Phosphate Nephropathy

Oral sodium phosphate (OSP) is a hyperosmolar laxative used in preparation for colonoscopies and bowel surgery. OSP causes severe hyperphosphatemia, especially in those with underlying reduced kidney function and volume depletion. A transient AKI occurring immediately after phosphate OSP administration is likely the result of hemodynamic alterations due to volume depletion and may not represent a true acute phosphate nephropathy (APN). AKI occurring days to weeks after OSP administration is likely caused by increased intratubular phosphate concentration, calcium phosphate precipitation, tubular obstruction, and direct tubular injury. Biopsy findings in these patients reveal calcium phosphate deposition in the tubules and interstitium, as well as interstitial inflammation and ATN [96].

The incidence of APN is uncertain due to heterogeneity of the study population, variability in the definition of AKI, and underrecognition of the condition. The largest observational study of almost 10,000 patients who underwent colonoscopy with OSP preparation revealed 114 cases of AKI, which was defined as 50% increase in serum creatinine within 1 year [97]. In another retrospective study, the incidence of AKI following OSP was 6.3%, which was associated with the use of ACEI and ARBs [98].

The prognosis of APN is poor, since kidney function rarely recovers completely. Most patients are left with CKD or progress to ESRD. In the study by Hurst et al. sited above, creatinine returned to baseline in 16 of 114 patients [97]. However, since no biopsies were performed, those who recovered may have had ATN without APN.

There is no specific treatment for APN. OSP should be avoided in patients with reduced kidney function for whom polyethylene glycol is the preferred bowel purgative. It is essential to maintain adequate intravascular volume prior to the procedure, particularly in the elderly, patients with diabetes, hypertension, or those who use medications that reduce renal perfusion such as NSAIDs or ACEI/ARBs [99].

Hydroxyethyl Starch

Hydroxyethyl starch (HES) is a colloid volume expander used in the ICU setting. The mechanism of HES-induced AKI is not completely understood. Most types of HES preparations have a molecular weight between 130 and 200 kDa which result in delayed renal clearance. HES administration is associated with an osmotic tubular injury, increased inflammation, and interstitial fibrosis in an isolated porcine renal perfusion model [100]. A multicenter, randomized trial by Schortgen et al. [101] compared HES with a gelatin-based colloid and found a higher incidence of AKI in the HES group. Although this trial was criticized for its methodology, another prospective trail of 537 patients with sepsis demonstrated a higher incidence of AKI and requirement for renal replacement therapy after HES treatment as compared with a group given lactated Ringer's solution [102]. Lower molecular weight HES may not have the same nephrotoxicity as the higher molecular weight compounds [103] but should be used with caution.

Abdominal Compartment Syndrome

A variety of critical illness can lead to the intra-abdominal hypertension (IAH) and abdominal compartment syndrome (ACS), such as intra-abdominal hemorrhage, peritonitis, or "third spacing" of fluid into the abdominal cavity associated with abdominal surgery, ileus, or pancreatitis, as well as overdistention with gas following laparoscopy. IAH is defined as an intra-abdominal pressure of more than 12 mm Hg measured by a bladder transducer on three separate occasions at least 4 hours apart. ACS is defined as an intra-abdominal pressure of more than 20 mm Hg, associated with one or more organ system failure [104]. The increase in intra-abdominal pressure leads to visceral ischemia, including AKI. The precise incidence of AKI resulting from ACS is unknown but appears underreported [105]. Treatment usually requires urgent surgical decompression of the abdomen.

Drug-Induced Syndromes

Hospitalized patients, particularly those in ICUs, are exposed to numerous pharmacologic agents. Since many drugs are capable of inducing abnormalities in renal function, the appearance of AKI in any patient should prompt the clinician to investigate a possible drug-related cause. Drug-induced AKI has four major syndromes (Table 73.10).

Acute Tubular Injury. Acute tubular injury syndrome is caused by drugs with direct nephrotoxic effects; the renal tubular epithelium is most often affected. Such agents include aminoglycoside antibiotics, heavy metals, certain cephalosporins, and amphotericin B [106]. The incidence of tubular injury varies among these drugs and ranges from 10% to 15% for tobramycin, from 20% to 30% for gentamicin, and as high as 50% for cisplatin. The new antiviral agent foscarnet has been found to have an incidence of nephrotoxicity of up to 65% [107]. Volume contraction, preexisting CKD, and liver disease enhance the risk of drug-induced tubular injury. Logically, the risk of nephrotoxicity is reduced by ensuring that patients are well hydrated before therapy. If possible, nonnephrotoxic therapeutic alternatives should be sought in patients with underlying renal and hepatic disease.

Tubular injury is almost always reversible after withdrawal of the inciting agent, although recovery may take several days to 2 weeks. Occasionally, specific renal tubular functional abnormalities may persist; these include magnesium and

TABLE 73.10

SYNDROMES OF DRUG-INDUCED KIDNEY INJURY

Acute tubular injury
Aminoglycoside antibiotics
Cephalosporin antibiotics
Antifungal agents (amphotericin)
Antiviral agents (foscarnet)
Heavy metals (cisplatin)
Intratubular microobstruction
Methotrexate
Acyclovir
Sulfamethoxazole
Dextran
Acute interstitial nephritis (see list in Table 73.13)
Autoregulatory failure
Angiotensin-converting enzyme inhibitors
Nonsteroidal anti-inflammatory drugs

potassium wasting, renal tubular acidosis, and mild impairment of renal-concentrating ability.

Intratubular Microobstruction. A second form of acute nephrotoxicity is caused by drugs that precipitate in and obstruct the nephrons. Such agents are generally poorly soluble at low pH, as characterizes the distal tubular fluid. This syndrome has been reported in patients receiving relatively high doses of intravenous methotrexate, acyclovir, low-molecular-weight dextran, and sulfamethoxazole. It has also been described in the setting of oral therapy with NSAIDs such as sulindac. Other NSAIDs, presumably because of their uricosuric properties, can precipitate tubular blockade with uric acid crystals, in a manner analogous to that of the tumor lysis syndrome (see following discussion).

Prevention of microobstructive AKI necessitates optimal hydration of the patient and maintenance of a high urine flow rate. Urinary alkalinization may be of benefit, depending on the nature of the obstructing agent. The syndrome is usually readily reversible and short lived.

Acute Interstitial Nephritis. An enlarging list of drugs has been associated with the syndrome of AKI accompanied by allergic manifestations such as skin rash, noninfectious fever, and eosinophilia (Table 73.11). As an allergic phenomenon, AIN has a more variable course than do syndromes of direct nephrotoxicity. Clear dose-risk relationships are lacking, and cases may vary widely in the time of onset following exposure to the inciting agent (days to years), the severity of the renal injury, and the time required for reversal following withdrawal of the drug (days to months). In addition to hematuria and pyuria, the urine sediment may show a preponderance of eosinophils [108,109]. White blood cell casts are a common finding (Fig. 73.2). The pathogenesis of AKI in this disorder is poorly understood. The renal histopathology early in the course of the disease shows mainly interstitial infiltration with inflammatory cells, often (but not always) eosinophils.

Although steroids have never been shown to reduce morbidity in a controlled trial, most experts use them in severe cases of AIN (i.e., those in which supportive dialysis may become necessary). See the Treatment section for more details on management of AIN.

A variant form of AIN is occasionally encountered in patients who take NSAIDs, particularly fenoprofen, meclofenamate, tolmetin, and indomethacin. The hallmarks of allergy, drug rash, eosinophilia, and eosinophiluria are absent. The urinalysis is nonspecific; some cases are marked by nephrotic range proteinuria. The renal pathology shows interstitial inflammation and normal-appearing glomeruli. As with classic allergic interstitial nephritis, this disorder regresses after cessation of therapy with the offending agent. Patients who have had this disorder should probably be considered at risk for recurrence with other NSAIDs [8].

TABLE 73.11

DRUGS MOST OFTEN IMPLICATED IN ACUTE INTERSTITIAL NEPHRITIS

Antibiotics
Penicillinase-resistant penicillins
Cephalosporins
Ampicillin
Amoxicillin
Penicillin G
Sulfonamides and sulfa-trimethoprim
Rifampin
Ethambutol
Tetracycline
Diuretics
Furosemide
Thiazides and related compounds
Nonsteroidal anti-inflammatory drugs
Ibuprofen
Indomethacin
Fenoprofen
Naproxen
Phenylbutazone
Mefenamic acid
Tolmetin
Miscellaneous drugs
Diphenylhydantoin
Cimetidine
Methyldopa
Allopurinol
Captopril

Hemodynamic or Autoregulatory Failure. The final form of drug-related AKI pertains to drugs that cause abnormalities of glomerular blood flow. Two pathophysiologic subsets of hemodynamically mediated AKI may be identified, depending on whether the main action of the drug is on the afferent or efferent glomerular arteriole. When the medication increases afferent vasoconstriction, autoregulation of renal blood flow is impaired, and prerenal azotemia develops. This effect may be seen in association with NSAIDs, which reduce the synthesis of vasodilatory prostaglandins [110], or drugs that directly constrict the preglomerular vessels (i.e., vasopressors and possibly radiocontrast agents). When preglomerular vasoconstriction is severe and prolonged, frank ischemic tubular necrosis may result. More often, a rapidly reversible, prerenal form of AKI occurs.

The other subset of hemodynamically mediated, drug-induced renal failure is seen in association with ACE inhibitors, which block the formation of angiotensin II from angiotensin I. In addition to their role as antihypertensives, these are commonly used as afterload reducers for the treatment of congestive heart failure. When used in this setting, they may engender an improvement of renal perfusion, as reduced peripheral vascular resistance leads to reduced left ventricular impedance. Under conditions of attenuated and fixed renal blood flow, however (as would occur with bilateral renal artery stenosis), ACE inhibitors may cause a sharp reduction in GFR [9,111].

These syndromes are encountered almost exclusively in patients with significant underlying impairment of renal perfusion or function. Unless severe renal ischemia has occurred, renal function should rapidly return to baseline levels after withdrawal of the responsible drug.

Renal Vascular Disease

Major Renal Vascular Disease

Renal vascular disease is divisible into major vascular and microvascular syndromes. Major renal vascular disease is an unusual cause of AKI. In a prospective series from a major teaching hospital, renal artery occlusion accounted for only 1 of 129 reported cases of AKI [14]. Renal artery occlusion does not produce AKI unless it is bilateral or occurs in a solitary functioning kidney. The sudden appearance of flank pain and a rising serum creatinine should lead the physician to consider acute renal artery embolism or thrombosis. The differential diagnoses in this scenario include nephrolithiasis, pyelonephritis (with or without urinary obstruction), and renal vein thrombosis (RVT). Pain, however, is not a sine qua non of renal artery occlusion. In a series of cases of renal artery embolism, 5 of 17 patients experienced no flank or abdominal pain [112].

Renal artery emboli occur most frequently in the setting of cardiac disease, particularly in patients with arrhythmias or mural cardiac thrombi. Frequently, multiple organs are involved, including brain, lung, and spleen. AKI is more likely to occur with a distribution of emboli to both kidneys, although azotemia has been reported with a unilateral embolus [112].

If the thrombus or embolus involves a solitary functioning kidney, oligoanuria and a rising level of azotemia can be expected. In a series of 17 cases of renal embolism, 15 patients experienced a rising serum creatinine. Seven of nine patients in whom urine volumes were recorded were either anuric or oliguric [112]. In addition to flank pain and diminished urine volume, at least 50% of patients experience nausea or fever, or both. The urinalysis is not specific. Leukocyturia, hematuria, and low-grade proteinuria have been found, as has a bland urine sediment. Radionuclide scanning often demonstrates patchy uptake of isotope or, in the case of total occlusion, no isotopic uptake. CT may demonstrate similar findings of diminished contrast uptake either by the whole kidney or localized wedge-shaped areas of nonperfusion.

Accurate diagnosis of renal arterial disease requires radiologic imaging. Renal artery duplex scan may reveal the absence of Doppler signal if total occlusion occurs, but provides only limited anatomical information if stenosis is present. The renal artery duplex is not as sensitive or specific for the diagnosis of stenosis as compared with angiography or magnetic resonance arteriography. Angiography provides the most accurate anatomic information, but it is also the most invasive test.

Occlusion of the renal artery does not inevitably lead to infarction. Particularly in patients with slowly developing atherosclerotic disease, collateral circulation via capsular or ureteric vessels may protect the kidney from infarction even though renal arterial blood flow is inadequate to maintain function. Surgery may be preferable in patients with renal artery thrombosis, although supportive care with anticoagulation has been the preferred treatment for renal arterial embolism. Recent reports of successful treatment with fibrinolytic agents (either urokinase or streptokinase) have led some to consider this the preferred treatment for renal artery occlusive disease, particularly in patients for whom surgery represents too great a risk.

Renal Vein Thrombosis

RVT is an uncommon cause of AKI. Bilateral renal vein occlusion occurs most commonly in severe dehydrated children. In adults, it usually accompanies nephrotic syndrome or may occur in patients with renal cell carcinoma. Hypercoagulable conditions, sickle cell disease, pregnancy, use of oral contraceptives, or trauma may also cause RVT. RVT generally does not cause AKI unless it is acute and bilateral or occurs in a solitary kidney. Flank pain and microscopic hematuria are the usual clinical manifestations in acute RVT. Duplex venography and CT scan can often establish the diagnosis and are less invasive than radiocontrast renal venography. Treatment usually consists of anticoagulation, although fibrinolytic therapy should be considered in patients with AKI and RVT.

Atheroembolic Renal Disease (Cholesterol Emboli)

Atheroembolic renal disease is increasingly recognized as a cause of AKI; it is probably still underdiagnosed. Atheroembolic disease is often found on postmortem examination. It is important to distinguish this syndrome from renal arterial thromboembolism.

Cholesterol embolization occurs only in patients with severe aortic atherosclerosis, usually after trauma to the wall of the aorta such as with aortography, major vascular surgery, or blunt trauma to the abdomen [113]. Atheroemboli may also occur spontaneously, particularly in patients with diabetic macrovascular disease and those receiving anticoagulant therapy. Diffuse occlusion of the microvasculature by atheroemboli leads to tissue damage in either a subacute or acute fashion. Patients may experience relatively minor abnormalities such as infarction of the tip of a single toe. Renal involvement is particularly common when diffuse embolization accompanies major arteriography or aortic surgery. Involvement of other visceral organs, including the pancreas, bowel, spleen, retina, and brain, may also occur. Typically, the cholesterol emboli form needlelike occlusions in small vessels, which then develop a chronic inflammatory response that can include the formation of a granulomatous reaction [113]. Extensive infarction of bowel or sudden neurologic abnormalities may bring the patient to the ICU, where, in addition to the presenting findings, AKI is noted. In the kidney, occlusion of a sufficient proportion of the microvasculature results in varying degrees of azotemia. The azotemia may be sudden, after the precipitating event, or may develop more slowly and may follow a stuttering course marked by acute deterioration with intervening periods of incomplete recovery. The latter course helps to distinguish this diagnosis from that of radiocontrast nephropathy, which typically occurs within 24 to 48 hours after arteriography.

The diagnosis is often missed unless there are peripheral signs of involvement such as blue distal digits or livedo reticularis of the lower extremities. A more subtle and less frequently observed physical manifestation is the finding of visible cholesterol emboli in the retinal vessels (Hollenhorst plaques). Less specific manifestations include peripheral eosinophilia and hypocomplementemia. The urine sediment is nonspecific.

Patients with atheroembolic renal disease experience the full spectrum of renal dysfunction, from minor degrees of azotemia to full-blown, irreversible renal failure. After an initial rise in serum creatinine, there may be an improvement in GFR over several weeks, probably attributable to nephron adaptation with hyperfiltration in remnant glomeruli. No specific management is available for atheroembolic renal disease. Management of renal failure, including dialytic therapy, may be indicated. Use of anticoagulants may worsen this condition.

Thrombotic Microangiopathies

Thrombotic microangiopathies are a group of disorders associated with AKI. These disorders can be seen in the ICU setting and include TTP, hemolytic uremic syndrome (HUS), scleroderma renal crisis, malignant hypertension, and antiphospholipid antibody syndrome. AKI, thrombocytopenia, and microangiopathic hemolytic anemia are common clinical features of these disorders. Histologically, occlusion of the preglomerular and glomerular microvasculature by platelet microthrombi is observed and accounts for the rapid deterioration in renal function. Clinical and histopathologic features of malignant hypertension are seen occasionally.

TTP and HUS, which were previously thought of as the same entity with different clinical presentation, are now considered separate diseases based on different pathogenesis [114]. TTP often presents with a pentad of fever, thrombocytopenia, microangiopathic hemolytic anemia, AKI, and neurological abnormalities. In TTP, an abnormally enlarged von Willebrand Factor (vWF) leads to platelet activation and aggregation, microthrombi formation, and ischemia. This disorder is linked to a diminished activity of a vWF cleaving protein belonging to a family of zinc metalloproteinases called ADAMTS (a disintegrin and metalloprotease with thrombospondin type 1 repeat). Decreased activity or mutations of ADAMTS13 protein are observed in recurrent and familial forms of TTP [115]. TTP can also be seen with certain infections, such as HIV. Several medications are associated with TTP, including clopidogrel, cyclosporine, and chemotherapeutic agents, such as cisplatinum, bleomycin, and others (for additional details, see Chapter 114).

In HUS, hematological and renal features predominate, and ADAMTS13 activity is normal. HUS is associated with a variety of infectious diseases, such as enteric infections, particularly with *Escherichia coli* 0157:H7, Mycoplasma, Legionella, and Coxsackie A and B viruses. Clinical presentation of HUS has a diarrheal and a nondiarrheal form. In the diarrheal form, a Shiga-like toxin is postulated to cause AKI by entering the circulation, binding to the proximal tubular cells as well as arteriolar and glomerular capillary endothelium and causing inflammation and platelet activation. The pathogenesis of the nondiarrheal form is not well understood. A rare familial form of nondiarrheal HUS exists, which is characterized by loss of activity of complement factor H. A deficiency in prostaglandin I2, abnormalities in coagulation cascade, and endothelial cell damage have been implicated in some forms of nondiarrheal HUS [116–118].

Treatment of thrombotic angiopathies varies greatly. TTP is a medical emergency, requiring prompt and aggressive plasmapheresis and plasma exchange to provide the missing enzyme and to remove vWF cleaving protein inhibitor. If untreated, mortality reaches to 90%. Treatment of HUS is largely supportive. There is no proven benefit to plasmapheresis, factor H replacement, or the use of fibrinolytics and antithrombotic agents in HUS [119,120]. See Chapter 114 of "Hematologic and Oncologic Problems in the Intensive Care Unit" section for further discussion of TTP and HUS and their treatment.

Autoimmune diseases associated with thrombotic microangiopathies are discussed in the Rheumatology section. Briefly, the mainstay of therapy for antiphospholipid antibody syndrome, which is frequently associated with SLE, is anticoagulation. Scleroderma renal crisis is treated with ACE inhibitors. See Hypertension chapter for the discussion of malignant hypertension.

Acute Kidney Injury in the Cancer Patient

AKI is a relatively common complication in patients with neoplastic diseases. Many malignancies cause hypercalcemia, a well-defined cause of AKI. Hypercalcemia may induce AKI through alterations in renal hemodynamics (afferent arteriolar vasoconstriction and diminished GFR) and by causing volume depletion. The pathogenesis and therapy of hypercalcemia of malignancy are described in greater detail in Chapters 106 and 118.

The term *tumor lysis syndrome* refers to the sudden release of tumor cell contents in response to induction chemotherapy. These intracellular products include phosphates, uric acid, and other purine metabolites. They may cause diffuse tubular microobstruction once they enter the nephron, which results in sudden onset of AKI. The syndrome occurs almost exclusively in patients with hematologic and lymphoproliferative malignancies, especially when the tumor cell mass is large and cell turnover high. Patients at risk for this syndrome should routinely receive prophylaxis before the initiation of chemotherapy, including volume expansion and pretreatment with allopurinol or rasburicase. Rasburicase, a recombinant uricolytic enzyme product, has been introduced to prevent severe hyperuricemia in this setting. The value of alkalinizing the urine by administration of bicarbonate is debatable. The increased urine pH achieved has the advantage of promoting the conversion of uric acid to urate which has increased solubility. However, alkalinization may promote the precipitation of calcium and phosphate in various soft tissues including the kidney. To date, there are no studies showing improved outcomes with alkalinization [121].

A reasonable approach would be to limit hydration with bicarbonate-based solutions to patients with tumor lysis syndrome who also have a significant metabolic acidosis [122]. Of note, once the tumor lysis syndrome becomes established, the resulting oliguria and AKI may further complicate therapy. This often requires a delicate balance between continued hydration and intermittent diuretics to maintain urine output and to avoid volume overload.

A number of commonly used antineoplastic agents have renal side effects and can cause AKI. Principal among these is cisplatin, which, like other heavy metals, can induce ATN [123]. The incidence of this complication is less with the newer analog carboplatin. Saline loading of patients who are about to receive platinum-containing chemotherapeutic agents helps reduce the risk of AKI. High-dose (>2 g per day) methotrexate therapy can cause AKI; the mechanism is believed to be tubular microobstruction from intraluminal crystallization of methotrexate metabolites. As is usually the case with renal injury syndromes that arise through this mechanism, maintenance of a forced diuresis is usually effective prophylaxis.

Many neoplasms involve the ureteric bed or periureteric lymph nodes. Obstructive uropathy must be considered in any case of unexplained AKI in an oncologic patient, particularly one with lymphoma or with prostatic, colorectal, or cervical carcinoma. Such obstructions are usually readily detectable by ultrasonographic examination. If the sonogram fails to detect hydronephrosis but obstruction is strongly suspected, further imaging can be completed to determine the patency of the ureters. These tests may include CT Urogram, MR Urogram, and retrograde cystoureterography. One must carefully consider the patient's GFR and their ability to receive various contrast solutions before selecting a test. In cases in which urethral obstruction is confirmed, nephrostomy drainage is often required. Ureteral stents can be considered but may fail if extrinsic compression remains present. Regardless, such drainage measures may only be needed temporarily in tumors that respond sufficiently to radiation or chemotherapy [124].

Multiple myeloma is a neoplasm that is especially frequently complicated by AKI. Patients with this disease may develop renal injury from several mechanisms. Hypercalcemia is very common in myeloma. In addition, the paraproteins, particularly light chains (Bence-Jones proteins), can be directly nephrotoxic. Finally, filtered paraproteins can form occlusive casts within the urinary space (cast nephropathy).

Tumor infiltration of the renal parenchyma is an unusual cause of AKI, despite the frequency of metastases to the kidneys. Imaging studies should reveal kidney enlargement. Successful reversal with radiation or chemotherapy is unusual. Decisions regarding the use of dialysis in patients with widespread metastatic disease must be based on a realistic appraisal of the prognosis of the underlying disease and on the patient's wishes.

Renal Dysfunction in Patients with Liver Disease

Renal dysfunction is extremely common in patients with advanced liver disease. The most common renal syndrome associated with liver disease is prerenal azotemia. Circulatory redistribution associated with portal hypertension, hypoalbuminemia, and neurohumoral influences that are active even in the incipient stages of liver disease combine to reduce renal perfusion. In addition, evidence has also been shown that the increase in intra-abdominal pressure due to ascites may exert an adverse effect on renal hemodynamics. The balance between control of ascites and peripheral edema and prevention of prerenal azotemia may be difficult. Patients with progressive prerenal azotemia are typically initially managed by holding diuretics. In patients who do not respond to this therapy or in individuals with more severe intravascular depletion, volume expansion with normal saline can be used. In patients with edema and ascites, albumin may be given to avoid further exacerbating volume overload. In patients with significant anemia, packed RBCs may be the ideal form of colloid. Despite adequate volume expansion, a subgroup of patients may not respond to this therapy and will go on to be diagnosed with hepatorenal syndrome (HRS).

Endless debate has centered around the proper definition of the HRS and its specific relationship to prerenal azotemia. In general, HRS can be considered a form of prerenal azotemia, associated with severe hepatic dysfunction, that is not responsive to an "adequate" volume challenge. It is usually seen in advanced cirrhosis, but it has also been reported in patients with acute hepatitis [125] or hepatic neoplasm [126,127]. Onset of the syndrome may be sudden or insidious. Type 1 HRS is defined as at least a 50% lowering of creatinine clearance to a value less than 20 mL per min or at least a twofold increase in serum creatinine to a level of greater than 2.5 mg per dL in less than a 2-week period [128]. In contrast, type 2 HRS is a chronic process that results in a slow decline in GFR over months to years. A more specific definition has been published by the International Ascites Club as detailed in Table 73.12 [129].

The pathogenesis of the HRS can be explained by a complex set of events that initially starts with the development of portal hypertension in a patient with liver injury. The increase in portal pressure causes the release of local vasodilators, which result in splanchnic arterial vasodilation. The decrease in vascular resistance in the splanchnic beds leads to a drop in systemic perfusion pressure. The body responds with compensatory activation of the sympathetic nervous system and the renin–angiotensin system that in turn results in severe vasoconstriction in the renal cortex and diminished GFR. This explanation is supported by the following findings: (i) The kidney's ability to retain salt and water suggests a hemodynamic alteration rather than parenchymal injury. (ii) Postmortem angiography of hepatorenal kidneys demonstrates severe vasoconstriction within the renal cortex (Fig. 73.4). (iii) Finally, the process can reverse when the involved kidney is transplanted into a recipient with normal liver function.

The vasodilatation in the splanchnic vascular beds that initiates HRS has been the target of several therapies including combined treatment with midodrine and octreotide. Midodrine (a selective α_1-adrenergic agonist) and octreotide (a somastatin analog) work together to increase vascular resistance in the

TABLE 73.12

DEFINITION OF HEPATORENAL SYNDROME [129]

- Cirrhosis with ascites
- Serum creatinine >1.5 mg/dL
- No improvement of serum creatinine after 2 d with diuretic withdrawal and volume expansion with albumin. The recommended dose of albumin is 1 g/kg of body weight per day up to a maximum of 100 g/d
- Absence of shock, ongoing bacterial infection, current or recent treatment with nephrotoxic drugs, gastrointestinal or renal fluid loss
- Absence of parenchymal disease as indicated by proteinuria <0.5 g/d, microhematuria (>50 red blood cells per high power field) no abnormalities on renal ultrasound.

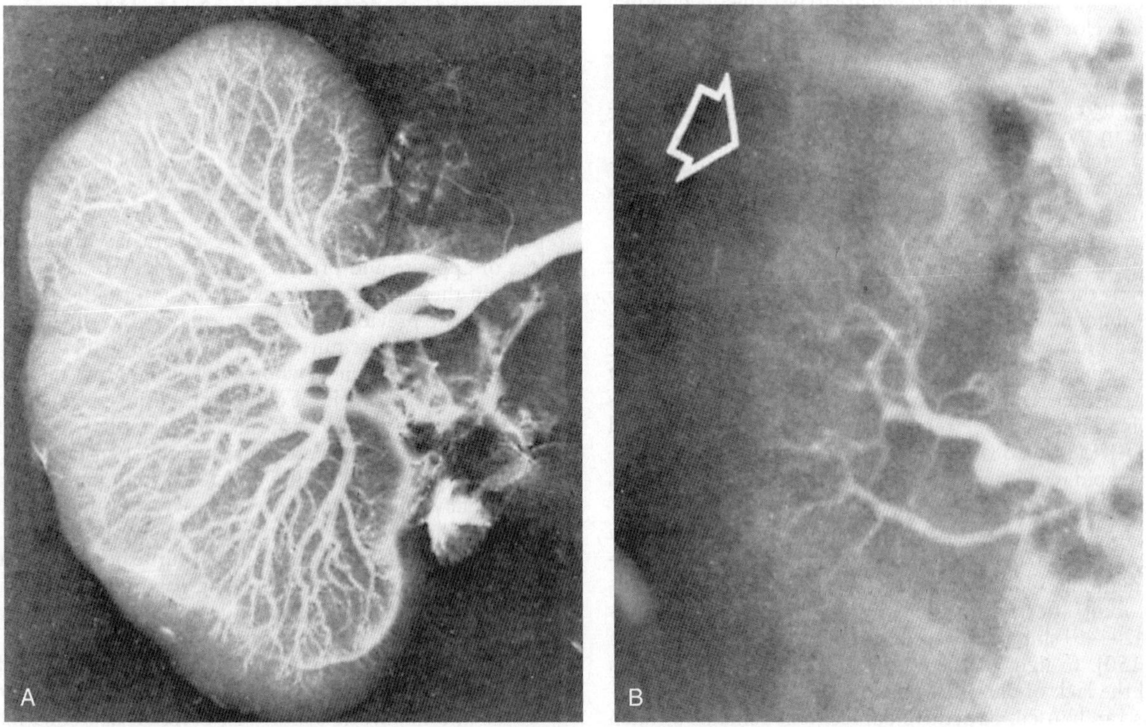

FIGURE 73.4. Angiographic pattern in hepatorenal syndrome with severe renal cortical vasoconstriction. Premortem (A) and postmortem (B) angiograms of a representative patient are shown. The arrow points to severe cortical vasoconstriction; it is a process that appears to reverse when the involved kidney is transplanted into a hepatically intact host. [Reprinted from Battle DC, Arruda JA, Kurtzman NA: Hyperkalemic distal renal tubular acidosis associated with obstructive uropathy. *N Engl J Med* 304:373, 1981, with permission].

splanchnic beds, which in turn decreases the ongoing renal vasoconstriction present in patients with HRS [130,131].

Midodrine (started at 10 mg orally three times a day) and octreotide (started at 100 μg subcutaneously three times a day) are often combined with albumin with the goal of increasing mean arterial blood pressure by 15 mm Hg. Other therapies such as epinephrine and vasopressin analogs, such as terlipressin, have been used. These therapies have not been evaluated in large clinical trials, and concerns regarding both safety (especially for ischemic complications) and effectiveness remain [132,133].

Hepatic disease predisposes patients to ATN of the other causes (i.e., nephrotoxic drug exposure, radiocontrast exposure, hypotension, and sepsis). Patients with severe hepatic disease often have one or more of these risk factors. Furthermore, hyperbilirubinemia may predispose to AKI through the actions of bile on renal tubules [134] and the renal and systemic hemodynamics [135]. Although the urinary sediment in most cases of ATN is distinctive, showing renal tubular epithelial cells and muddy brown granular casts, jaundiced patients without tubular necrosis may manifest pigmented granular casts simply as a direct result of the interaction of bilirubin with tubular cells [134]. The diagnosis of ATN can be further complicated by the finding of a low FE_{Na}. Patients with ATN typically have a FE_{Na} of greater than 2% as a result of tubular injury impairing sodium reabsorption. Because of the extreme nature of sodium avidity in the setting of cirrhosis, patients may have a FE_{Na} of less than 1% despite renal tubular injury.

Management of cirrhotic patients with sodium and volume overload is extremely challenging. Cirrhotic patients are in a tenuous physiologic state; they have little tolerance for small deviations, either positive or negative, from their optimal state of fluid balance. In both prerenal and hepatorenal states, urinary sodium excretion is reduced (usually <20 mEq per day). Sodium balance must be regulated with dietary restriction or diuretics, or both, if ascites and edema are to be controlled. When oliguria develops in patients with advanced cirrhosis, conventional therapy may fail to achieve adequate diuresis. High doses of intravenous diuretics, in combination or as continuous infusions, can be used. Since aldosterone appears to play a significant role in the sodium retention of cirrhosis, spironolactone may be a useful adjunct in diuretic therapy. Although patients with significant peripheral edema can often tolerate as much as a net diuresis of 3 L per day, those with ascites but no edema should be managed more cautiously to avoid AKI.

In patients with significant ascites that is refractory to diet and diuretic therapy, large volume paracentesis (LVP) can help alleviate abdominal pressure and reduce respiratory symptoms. Patients can have up to 4 L of peritoneal fluid removed safely with paracentesis, but simultaneous albumin infusions (8 g of albumin per liter removed) should be administered in patients undergoing larger volume removal to avoid hypotension and possible AKI [136–138]. Although LVP does offer the convenience of rapid resolution of ascites, it does lead to protein loss and carries the risk of procedural complications.

Peritoneovenous shunts, such as the Denver and LeVeen shunts, have been used to infuse ascitic fluid into the central circulation. While reversal of the HRS [139] and recovery can occur after portosystemic [140,141] or peritoneovenous [142–149] shunting procedures, overall results have been mixed [150]. In light of the high perioperative complication rate and the lack of data showing increased survival, the procedure is rarely used. Repetitive paracentesis remains a much more commonly employed method of palliating ascites.

The biochemical abnormalities that characterize AKI in the patient with hepatic disease are the same as those found in other settings, with a few special considerations. Azotemic patients with hepatic failure have increased metabolic substrate for ammonia production and therefore are at heightened risk for encephalopathy. Potassium depletion, a common electrolyte imbalance in cirrhosis, further enhances ammonia synthesis. Since cirrhosis is often associated with diminished perfusion pressure, hyponatremia may develop in response to increased antidiuretic hormone (ADH) levels and decreased capacity to excrete free water. Patients with significant hyponatremia should have their water intake restricted to less than 1,500 mL per day.

Acid–base disturbances are common and varied in patients with advanced hepatocellular disease. Respiratory alkalosis can occur as a result of increased progesterone levels stimulating hyperventilation. The use of diuretics as well as the presence of secondary hyperaldosteronism can cause a metabolic alkalosis that can aggravate hepatic encephalopathy. As plasma pH rises, ammonium ions lose protons to the plasma; the resulting ammonia penetrates the blood–brain barrier more readily.

Although the finding of metabolic alkalosis is common, acid–base disturbances can rapidly change in the cirrhotic patient. Patients with diarrhea may develop a nonanion gap acidosis. Or in patients with severe hypotension, a high anion gap metabolic acidosis related to lactic acid may develop. Lactic acidosis may be particularly severe in patients with liver disease because extraction and metabolism of lactic acid from the blood depend largely on hepatic function. In patients with a metabolic alkalosis, the subsequent development of a metabolic acidosis may be missed, as the bicarbonate may be in the normal range. This is a particularly treacherous combined acid–base disturbance because a near-normal serum pH may belie the true extent of the acidosis. As the acidosis worsens, the pH may plummet because of depletion of the bicarbonate buffer system, deficiencies of protein buffers, and inability to maintain adequate respiratory compensation.

DIAGNOSIS OF ACUTE KIDNEY INJURY

History and Physical Examination

Because the symptoms of renal injury are nonspecific, the history provided by the patient is not always of diagnostic help. In patients with CKD, the history may be useful in establishing whether renal dysfunction is truly a progressive, long-standing problem versus AKI. For example, a patient with long-standing loss of appetite and pruritus is more likely to have CKD than AKI. In these cases, the background information often elicits evidence of previous renal or urinary abnormalities such as hypertension, proteinuria, or a history of diabetes mellitus. A thirsty patient, or one in whom daily weight loss has been documented, may have volume depletion causing prerenal azotemia. The avenues of fluid loss are usually identifiable. Exposure to nephrotoxic agents or a recent episode of sustained hypotension suggests the possibility of ATN. Symptoms of renal colic, abnormal voiding pattern, or a history of genitourinary malignancy point toward an obstructive cause.

The physical examination often furnishes some diagnostic information, particularly regarding volume status. Diminished skin turgor, sunken eyes, dry mucous membranes, the absence of axillary sweat, or orthostatic hypotension supports a diagnosis of prerenal azotemia. In disorders characterized by reduced effective circulatory volume, such as congestive heart failure and nephrotic syndrome, prerenal azotemia may exist in the setting of an expanded extracellular volume. Hypertension in patients with AKI should raise suspicion of intrinsic renal disease. The clinician must be alert for signs of systemic disease that can cause acute renal injury, including vasculitis, endocarditis, and sepsis. Bladder distention and prostatic enlargement point to an obstructive cause. A full discussion of relevant history and physical findings for the different causes of AKI is beyond the scope of this chapter.

Urine Tests

The laboratory workup should commence with a urinalysis. The measurements of urine osmolality, electrolytes, and creatinine concentration are simple and useful, particularly in differentiating between ATN and prerenal azotemia. Urine specific gravity can be measured at the bedside while the results of the more accurate urine chemistry tests are pending. A high urine specific gravity generally correlates with a concentrated urine and is expected in prerenal azotemia, except in the presence of diuretics.

The familiar dipstick tests provide a readily available method for determining whether the urine contains protein or heme pigments. When positive, they should raise the suspicion of intrinsic renal pathology. As the dipstick test for protein measures only albuminuria, Bence-Jones proteins will not be detected. Light chains can be made to precipitate in urine by adding sulfosalicylic acid to the specimen and heating it to 60°C.

Formed elements in the urine sediment yield invaluable information about the nature of AKI, particularly in intrinsic renal disease. The significance of hematuria, pyuria, renal tubular epithelial cells, and casts in the urine has already been discussed. The presence of RBC casts distinguishes the hematuria associated with glomerulonephritis from that of postrenal or urologic causes. Broad and waxy casts suggest that renal disease is chronic. Virtually any lesion that can cause obstruction in the genitourinary tract can produce hematuria. Crystalluria often occurs in association with obstruction due to renal calculi or medications

The FE_{Na} can indicate the degree of renal sodium avidity, which generally reflects renal perfusion. A value of less than 1% typically indicates prerenal azotemia. However, this test can be confounded by concomitant diuretic therapy, common situation in critically ill patients. In these situations, the FEUrea can be used instead, since urea clearance is unaffected by diuretics. The FEUrea is calculated via the same formula, but substituting urea for sodium and a value of less than 35% is suggestive of renal hypoperfusion (see Table 73.13 for additional details [151–154]).

TABLE 73.13

FORMULAS FOR ESTIMATING RENAL FUNCTION

Fractional Excretion of Sodium (FE_{Na}) [151]

The FE_{Na} is the proportion of the filtered load of sodium excreted:

$$FE_{Na} = U_{Na}/P_{Na} \times P_{cr}/U_{cr} \times 100$$

Urine sodium (U_{Na}) and plasma sodium (P_{Na}) are expressed as millimoles and urine creatinine (U_{cr}) and plasma creatinine (P_{cr}) are expressed as milligrams per deciliter.

Cockcroft–Gault equation [152]

Creatinine clearance (CrCl) can be estimated by using the Cockcroft and Gault formula which uses the patient's age and body weight, where weight is expressed in kilograms and plasma creatinine (P_{cr}) is expressed as milligrams per deciliter:

$$C_{cr} = (140 - \text{age}) \times \text{weight}/(P_{cr} \times 72)$$

Abbreviated MDRD equation [153]

A series of derivations based on data from the MDRD study have yielded several equations that more accurately represent GFR serum creatinine concentration (SCr) measured in milligrams per deciliter.

$$\text{GFR, in mL/min per } 1.73\ m^2 = 186.3 \times \text{SCr}\ (\exp[-1.154]) \times \text{age}\ (\exp[-0.203]) \times (0.742 \text{ if female}) \times (1.21 \text{ if black})$$

CrCl determined by 24-h urine collection [154]

CrCl can be estimated by collecting a urine sample for 24 h. This formula tends to overestimate the true GFR by at least 10% and some cases significantly more, as some of the creatinine in the urine is derived from tubular secretion.

Urine creatinine (U_{cr}) and plasma creatinine (P_{cr}) are expressed as milligrams per deciliter. U_v is 24-h urine volume in mL.

$$\text{CrCl mL/min} = (U_{cr} \times U_v)/(P_{cr} \times 1{,}440)$$

GFR, glomerular filtration rate; MDRD, Modification of Diet in Renal Disease.

Blood Tests

Clearly, measurement of the BUN and creatinine is essential to identifying and monitoring AKI. As noted, the ratio of BUN to creatinine carries some diagnostic value, as a high value (>20:1) may indicate prerenal azotemia. Serial blood chemistries will help identify acid–base and electrolyte disturbances common with AKI (discussed later in the chapter). Anemia may suggest underlying CKD. Eosinophilia frequently accompanies AIN.

Specialized serologic tests may help answer specific diagnostic questions. The presence of antinuclear antibodies is consistent with autoimmune nephropathy such as lupus nephritis or scleroderma, both of which may cause AKI. The serum protein electrophoresis or immunoelectrophoresis may aid in the diagnosis of multiple myeloma, which may present as AKI of uncertain cause [155].

Estimates of GFR may be helpful in assessing the severity of AKI as well as for adjusting medication dosages. However, these formulas have limited utility in the early phases of AKI, since the calculations are based on the assumption that serum creatinine reflects a steady state. For example, the creatinine of a patient with AKI from complete loss of renal blood flow will take many days to rise to steady state even though the GFR is negligible from the outset. Estimates of GFR in the first few days will grossly overestimate the patient's residual renal function. See Table 73.13 for equations used to estimate GFR.

Radiography

Various radiographic techniques may contribute to the evaluation of AKI. The abdominal flat plate (kidneys and urinary bladder) is an easily obtained study that can help establish the presence and size of both kidneys. If both kidneys are small, azotemia may be of a chronic nature. Radiopaque stones may be identified on abdominal plain films.

Renal ultrasonography, a safe, quick, high-yield procedure, is probably the first radiologic test that should be ordered in the evaluation of any azotemic patient. It permits the identification and measurement of both kidneys and is very sensitive for detecting obstructive uropathy (Fig. 73.5). Helical CT, with or without contrast, is a versatile and high-yield technique for establishing the size of the kidneys and recognizing hydronephrosis (Fig. 73.6). The contrast agent administered during the test can itself produce severe impairment of renal function in patients with renal insufficiency, hypovolemia, or multiple myeloma. It should therefore be avoided when any of these conditions is suspected. Magnetic resonance imaging

TABLE 73.14

PREDIALYSIS MANAGEMENT OF ACUTE KIDNEY INJURY

Fluid balance
Weigh patient daily
Monitor input and output
In volume-depleted patients, replace extracellular fluid with isotonic saline (or bicarbonate)
In normovolemic or edematous patients, restrict fluid intake (~1,500 mL/d) and sodium intake (≤2 g/d)
Acid–base and electrolyte
Avoid water overload and hyponatremia (restrict free water intake, particularly in oliguric patients)
Restrict potassium intake (≤2 g/d) and treat hyperkalemia (see Chapters 73 and 74)
Maintain serum bicarbonate ≥12 and 15 mM
Use phosphate binders ($CaCO_3$) to maintain PO_4 ≤5.0 mg/dL
Treat symptomatic hypocalcemia (see text)
Drugs
Avoid nephrotoxins when possible
Adjust doses of all renally excreted drugs
Withhold nonsteroidal anti-inflammatory drugs and angiotensin-converting enzyme inhibitors in patients with prerenal conditions
Avoid magnesium-containing drugs (e.g., antacids, milk of magnesia)
Nutrition
Restrict protein intake to ≤0.5 g/kg/d
Caloric (carbohydrate) intake of ≥400 kcal/d
Reduction of infectious risks
Remove indwelling urinary catheter in oliguric, nonobstructed patients
Strict aseptic technique and rapid removal, when feasible, of vascular catheters

offers similar data as helical CT but is less commonly used because of cost and availability. The use of gadolinium contrast should be avoided, if possible, in the setting of AKI due to the risk of nephrogenic systemic fibrosis.

Retrograde pyelography is reserved for patients in whom urinary tract obstruction is strongly suspected despite the inability to confirm this finding on other imaging techniques. It is generally performed in anticipation of relieving such obstructions as soon as they are identified, usually by placement of ureteral stents.

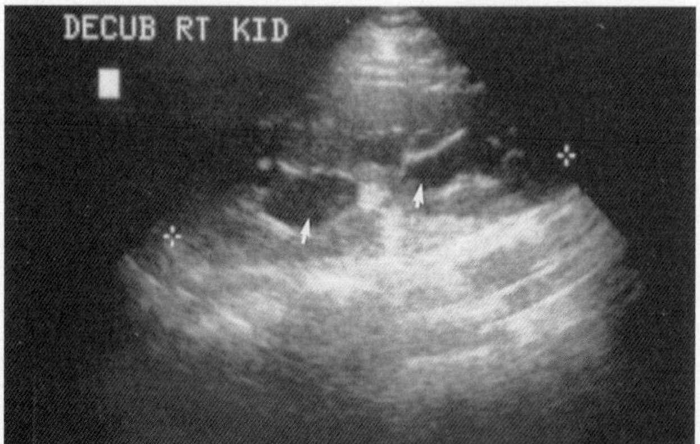

FIGURE 73.5. Sonogram with right hydronephrosis. Kidney poles are marked by crosses. Dark, echolucent areas (*arrows*) in the center represent dilated collecting system.

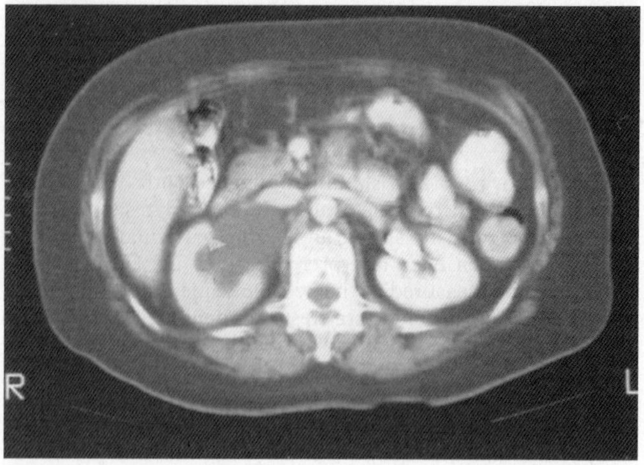

FIGURE 73.6. Computed tomographic scan with right hydronephrosis. **Left:** Unobstructed kidney is shown for comparison. Note enlarged pelvocaliceal system on right (*arrowhead*).

Isotopic renal scanning provides a safe means for locating the kidneys and allows estimation of their functional capacity. Radionuclide flow studies can be used to assess the rapidity of uptake of tracer by the kidneys. A delay in uptake helps to establish the diagnosis of impaired renal perfusion, whether due to structural renovascular disease or functionally impaired renal blood flow. Prolonged retention of radioisotope by the kidneys is suggestive of outflow obstruction. Radioisotopic scanning may be particularly helpful in assessing patients with prolonged AKI for the absence of blood flow and the possible diagnosis of cortical necrosis or renal infarction (Fig. 73.7).

Renal artery duplex scanning offers an alternative method of assessing renal arterial flow. Although noninvasive, the test requires significant operator expertise. In rare instances where a vascular lesion is strongly suspected, CT angiogram or even full renal arteriography may be necessary. Arteriography is more invasive but offers the opportunity for immediate therapeutic intervention such as angioplasty or vascular stenting.

Renal Biopsy

Renal biopsy is reserved for patients who are thought to have parenchymal renal disease. The indications for renal biopsy are a matter of some controversy, but the procedure should be considered when (a) azotemia is of recent onset and unknown cause; (b) there is a possibility that the patient has a renal disease that may require drug treatment (e.g., steroids or cytotoxic drugs) as with patients with probable glomerulonephritis, vasculitis, or AIN; (c) heavy proteinuria or nephrotic syndrome is present; or (d) the biopsy result might be of prognostic importance.

COMPLICATIONS AND TREATMENT OF ACUTE KIDNEY INJURY

General Principles of Treatment

The predialysis management of AKI is outlined in Table 73.14. These steps are applicable to any patient with AKI and are quite

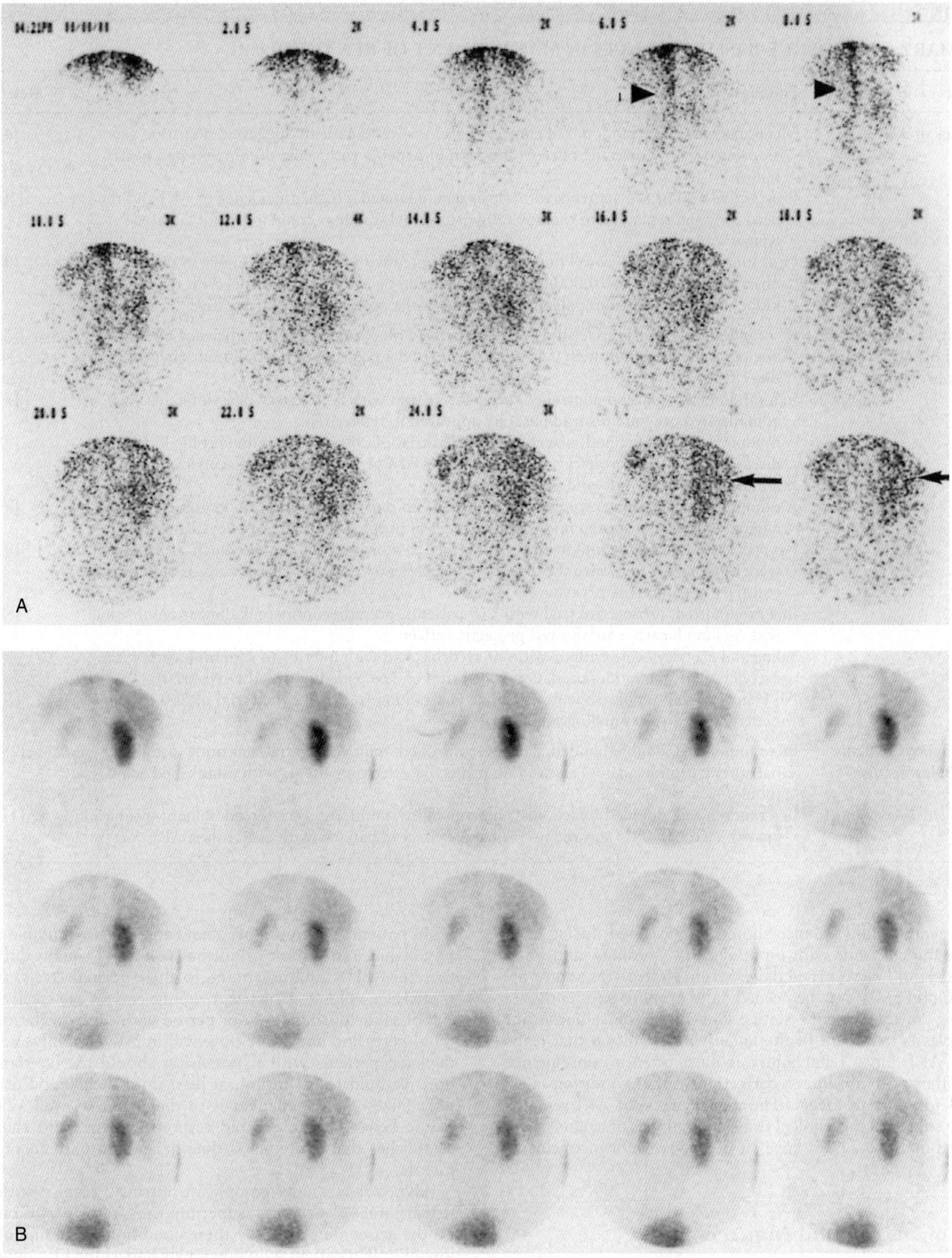

FIGURE 73.7. Renal radioisotopic scan with myelin-associated glycoprotein-3 demonstrating poor uptake of tracer in patient with left renal artery occlusion. **A:** Early flow phase in which each panel represents a 2-second interval. Scintigraphic activity is seen in proximal aorta (*arrowheads*) and right kidney (*arrows*). Note the absence of scintigraphic activity over the area of left kidney. **B:** Functional scan (1-minute intervals). Note marked diminution of scintigraphic activity over the area of the left kidney.

TABLE 73.15

SUMMARY OF EVIDENCE-BASED ADVANCES IN MANAGEMENT OF RENAL FAILURE

Topic	Findings	Reference
Causes of AKI	Meta-analysis of five randomized clinical trials in >1,200 patients suggested nesiritide was associated with worsening of renal function in patients with acute decompensated heart failure.	[43]
	Prospective trial of 537 patients with sepsis demonstrated a higher incidence of AKI and the need for renal replacement therapy in hydroxyethyl starch as compared with lactated Ringer's group.	[102]
	Oral sodium phosphate bowel purgative is associated with acute kidney injury in the observational study of 10,000 patients and should be avoided in patients with reduced kidney function in whom polyethylene glycol is the preferred bowel purgative.	[99]
Prophylaxis of radiocontrast nephropathy	In a randomized, prospective study of 78 patients with chronic renal insufficiency undergoing angiography, hydration with 0.45% saline exerted a protective effect; diuretics neutralized this effect	[76]
	In a randomized, placebo-controlled, prospective trial with 83 patients, acetylcysteine administered pre- and postradiography appeared to reduce risk.	[77]
	A randomized, double-blind, placebo-controlled trial of 200 patients with chronic kidney disease undergoing coronary angiography showed a protective effect of acetylcysteine administered orally pre- and postcontrast.	[78]
	A randomized, prospective study in 79 patients with renal insufficiency undergoing coronary angiography demonstrated no beneficial effect of prophylaxis with acetylcysteine.	[79]
	No protective effect of fenoldopam was observed in a prospective trial in which 157 patients were randomized to receive the drug and 158 patients received placebo prior to and during coronary angiographic procedures.	[82]
	In a randomized, prospective trial with 119 patients, preradiocontrast alkalinization of urine with sodium bicarbonate showed protective effect	[83]
	Saline and acetylcysteine with or without ascorbic acid with inferior to sodium bicarb with acetylcysteine in a randomized, controlled trial of 326 patients (REMEDIAL trial).	[84]
	No benefit of sodium bicarbonate vs. saline in a randomized, controlled trial of 500 patients undergoing coronary angiography.	[85]
Prophylaxis of acute tubular necrosis	In a randomized, double-blinded, placebo-controlled, multicenter trial, anaritide (atrial natriuretic peptide analog) showed no protective effect in patients with established acute tubular necrosis	[198]
	In a randomized, double-blinded, placebo-controlled, multicenter trial, recombinant insulin-like growth factor (IGF-1) showed no protective effect in patients with established ARF.	[173]

fundamental. Fluid balance should be measured during each 8 hour nursing shift with input/output recordings, and body weight should be recorded daily. Serum electrolytes and/or arterial blood gases may be needed daily or more frequently depending on the patient's status. One of the most important principles is treatment of the underlying condition that leads to the AKI. Since renal injury is most often a consequence of another primary illness, correction of that condition is essential for renal recovery. The management of AKI remains largely supportive as clinical trials of a number of agents (summarized in Table 73.15) have yielded negative or inconclusive results.

Fluid Management

Fluid management is crucial because sodium and water excretion may be limited, particularly in oliguric patients. It should not be assumed that because the patient has renal dysfunction, fluid intake must be restricted. Nonrenal losses of fluid must be carefully accounted for. While respiratory fluid losses are often minimal for patients on mechanical ventilation, insensible losses are significantly increased with high fever or dermal injury. Gastrointestinal fluid losses can be difficult to quantify. Daily weights are often the best means of assessing the net balance between intake and output.

In patients with pure prerenal azotemia attributable to hypovolemia, restoration of normal volume is usually sufficient to return BUN and creatinine to their normal levels. A normotensive, volume-depleted, azotemic patient can receive up to 1 L of saline during a 4-hour period with the expectation that renal perfusion and urine flow will improve rapidly. Volume-depleted patients with hypotension should receive more aggressive fluid resuscitation, at least until their blood pressure normalizes. This maneuver is of diagnostic as well as therapeutic benefit because rapid response to the fluid challenge establishes that azotemia is due, at least in part, to prerenal factors.

Hypovolemia may complicate intrinsic renal disease and urinary tract obstruction, superimposing a low perfusion state on the azotemia caused by these conditions. The finding of a low FE_{Na} in a patient who previously had a high FE_{Na} might indicate that, although tubular function has recovered, renal hypoperfusion persists [156]. Fluid replacement should be given using isotonic saline.

The estimate of isotonic fluid replacement should be based on the clinical findings. With orthostasis, it may be estimated that the patient is experiencing an ECF deficit of at least 10%. Fluid replacement in these circumstances should be administered regardless of the patient's urine output or the presumptive diagnosis of ATN. In either case, recovery of renal function can be hastened by rapid volume repletion.

In euvolemic patients, the following formula can be applied to estimate daily fluid requirement: daily fluid replacement (mL per day) = (urinary + extrarenal + insensible losses) − 250, where insensible losses = 500 mL per day. For febrile patients, add 500 mL per day for every degree Fahrenheit more than 101. In edematous patients requiring volume removal, the rate of diuresis should be limited to avoid exacerbating the AKI by inducing hypotension of intravascular volume depletion.

Diuretics are a mainstay of management in patients with volume overload and nonoliguric AKI. However, studies have shown no demonstrable improvement in patient survival when nonoliguric patients with AKI are treated with high-dose loop diuretics [157].

In addition, a meta-analysis of nine randomized furosemide studies to prevent or treat AKI failed to show a decreased need for dialysis or improved survival [158].

Despite the paucity of data regarding beneficial effects on renal recovery or survival, diuretics are essential for the maintenance of fluid balance in responsive patients. Loop diuretics are the principal agents and are given as intravenous bolus or through continuous infusion. However, diuretic administration may worsen renal perfusion in a patient with antecedent hypovolemia and may cause hearing loss and tinnitus in patients treated with high dosages [159]. Some data suggest that infusions are more effective and cause less toxicity [160]. Concomitant use of other diuretic agents that act at different segments of the nephron may enhance urine output. Patients with diuretic-resistant oliguria often require renal replacement therapy. This will be discussed in detail in Chapter 76.

Parenchymal Renal Disease

If renal damage occurs as a result of exposure to a drug with allergic or nephrotoxic potential, the offending agent should be withdrawn, if feasible (see Table 73.11). Although AIN usually responds to discontinuation of the culpable drug, the recovery may be protracted. The data on steroids in allergic drug-induced acute interstitial nephritis (DI-AIN) is mixed [161].

Nevertheless, the use of steroids appears to hasten recovery and reduce the likelihood of developing CKD [162]. Certainly, steroids should be considered in patients with DI-AIN associated with a significant reduction in GFR or in patients who do not promptly respond to withdrawal of the offending agent. These patients often require a renal biopsy to confirm the diagnosis. If steroids are used, the initial dose of prednisone is 1 mg per kg per day (maximum dose, 60 mg daily) for 1 to 2 weeks followed by a slow taper over 1 to 3 months, depending on the response.

The treatment of various forms of glomerulonephritis is beyond the scope of this text. Briefly, in patients with glomerulonephritis of unclear etiology, a renal biopsy may be helpful not only to aid in diagnosis but also as a means of predicting response to therapy. Specific treatment may not be required, such as in postinfectious glomerulonephritis or glomerulonephritis associated with bacterial endocarditis. In the former case, spontaneous remission usually occurs; in the latter, antibiotic treatment of the underlying condition may result in clearing of the immune complex induced renal lesion. AKI from lupus nephritis or one of the idiopathic forms of rapidly progressive glomerulonephritis may respond to high-dose intravenous corticosteroids (pulse therapy, consisting of 1 g of methylprednisolone per day for 3 to 5 days) or a combination of oral prednisone, a cytotoxic agent (cyclophosphamide or azathioprine), and plasmapheresis [163]. The latter approach is aimed at clearing the plasma of offending antibodies (e.g., antiglomerular basement membrane antibodies), cytokines, or immune complexes while simultaneously decreasing their formation [164]. Renal injury associated with necrotizing vasculitis can be treated with corticosteroid alone, cytotoxic agents alone, or a combination of both. Cyclophosphamide is generally accepted as the treatment of choice for Wegener's granulomatosis [165].

A number of different therapies have been proposed for the treatment of ATN. Some authors have advocated the use of low-dose dopamine infusion in the treatment of established ATN. Dopamine at low doses dilates the interlobular arteries, afferent and efferent arterioles resulting in increased renal blood flow. However, recent trials have not supported its efficacy, and it is generally no longer recommended by nephrologists [166–168].

It has been speculated that the use of selective dopamine-1 receptor antagonists, such as fenoldopam, which lack α- and β-adrenergic effects, may offer better protection and treatment for AKI [169,170]. Beyond its vasodilatory actions on the renal vasculature, fenoldopam has anti-inflammatory effects that may be of particular importance in the setting of AKI. A 2007 meta-analysis of 16 randomized trials of fenoldopam versus placebo or dopamine for prevention or treatment of AKI found that fenoldopam decreased the need for renal replacement and hospital death [171]. However, because of various limitations of the study, fenoldopam is not commonly used for treatment of AKI. A large randomized study will be required to fully clarify fenoldopam's role in AKI.

A number of biopharmacologic interventions are currently being examined as potential therapeutic agents in ATN, including atrial natriuretic peptide [172], insulin-like growth factor [173], epidermal growth factor [174], and hepatocyte growth factor [175]. It has been postulated that the pathogenesis of ATN may involve inflammatory processes. Experimental data indicate that intercellular adhesion molecules (ICAMs) enable leukocytes to adhere to vascular endothelium in the kidney, from which they gain entrance to renal tissue and mediate the pathogenesis of AKI [176]. In one study, antibodies to ICAM-1 reduced inflammation and intraluminal tubular pressure in experimental renal injury [177]. In a more recent investigation, although the anti–ICAM-1 antibody prevented infiltration of the kidney by leukocytes, the course of AKI was not altered [178]. These substances have proved capable of attenuating the course of experimental toxic and ischemic AKI in animal models. In clinical trials, atrial natriuretic peptide has been shown to produce modest improvements in outcome of oliguric patients; the results, although not striking, warrant further investigation [172]. A multicenter trial of human recombinant insulin-like growth factor I failed to demonstrate any benefit to patients with AKI [173].

Treatment of Postrenal Failure

Relief of urinary obstruction is the object of therapy in postrenal AKI. Acute intervention is mandatory in the presence of complete or bilateral urinary tract obstruction, severe azotemia, or any of the metabolic or hemodynamic complications of AKI. Coexisting fever or any other evidence that urinary infection lies proximal to the obstruction requires a rapid decompression procedure to avoid bacteremic shock.

When bladder outlet obstruction is suspected, insertion of a urethral catheter should be attempted. If this is not possible, as is occasionally the case in patients with prostatic enlargement or ureteral stricture, ureteral dilation or percutaneous cystostomy should be performed. AKI due to upper urinary tract obstruction can be relieved by either the retrograde insertion of a ureteral catheter or the percutaneous placement (under ultrasonic, fluoroscopic, or CT scan guidance) of a catheter in the renal pelvis.

Obstructive uropathy is associated with defects of the distal nephron, including hydrogen ion and potassium secretion, as well as urinary concentration. Consequently, the patient, particularly if there is prolonged high-grade obstruction, may display hyperkalemia, hyperchloremic metabolic acidosis, hypernatremia, or a combination of all three [179,180]. Water and bicarbonate replacement are often required and can be administered as a solution of 5% glucose and water to which sodium bicarbonate has been added. The patient's plasma volume and serum sodium should determine the tonicity of the administered fluid. If the patient is hypovolemic, an isotonic solution should be used. If the patient is hypernatremic, a hypotonic solution is needed. Hyperkalemia may respond to the institution of a diuresis that accompanies the relief of the obstruction and correction of the acidosis.

A diuresis often ensues after relief of urinary obstruction, particularly when prolonged. This usually reflects mobilization of urine sequestered within the dilated ureterovesicular system as well as excess ECF retained during the period of obstruction. As such, this postobstructive diuresis is considered appropriate to the preexisting volume expansion [181]. In some patients with correction of bilateral obstruction, a large diuresis and natriuresis may ensue, which result in hypovolemia and, sometimes, frank shock. The mechanism for this inappropriate diuresis is poorly understood but may involve release of a natriuretic substance [182]. These patients require fluid replacement, usually with hypotonic saline, to repair the deficit and match urinary losses. A useful technique is to measure the urinary sodium and potassium concentrations periodically to determine the composition of the replacement fluid.

Abnormal Drug Metabolism

A complete survey of all of the patient's medications should be made. Drugs, such as NSAIDs or ACE inhibitors, that may interfere with renal blood flow or GFR autoregulation should be discontinued. When possible, aminoglycoside antibiotics or other nephrotoxic drugs should be replaced with nonnephrotoxic agents. Contrast procedures should be avoided so as not to compound renal dysfunction in patients with acute or CKD. If this is not feasible, the risk should be minimized by taking prophylactic measures (see previous discussion). In addition, the dosage of drugs dependent on renal metabolism and excretion should be adjusted appropriately. Some drugs (e.g., aminoglycoside antibiotics, digoxin) are excreted almost entirely by the kidneys. If the dose or dosing interval is unchanged, reduced renal function leads to accumulation of the drug in body fluids and eventual drug toxicity. Other agents are hepatically metabolized, but the active metabolites are renally excreted (e.g., benzodiazepines). Phenytoin, independent of its excretion, may reach toxic concentrations because a larger proportion of the administered drug is displaced from albumin-binding sites in uremia. Drug doses need to be altered in most instances to account for residual renal function and the effect of dialysis on drug removal. It is important to remember that as the patient recovers renal function, upward adjustment of the dosage of renally excreted drugs is necessary. This subject is covered in detail in Chapter 75.

Nutritional Therapy

It is not our purpose to describe nutritional therapy here (see Section 15). The guidelines for nutritional therapy in AKI are similar to those in other ICU patients. Patients with AKI are often catabolic and increase their production of nitrogenous products that require excretion. The degree of catabolism reflects the level of the patient's metabolic stress and is, in turn, a function of the severity of the underlying illness. Protein and caloric requirements are much higher for patients with catastrophic illness and multiple organ system failure than for those with mild and moderate illness [183]. Although caloric replacement needs to be adequate to reduce tissue catabolism, prevent ketosis, and meet the patient's basal nutritional needs, the clinician must avoid providing excessive substrate for generation of metabolic wastes. This is particularly challenging in patients who are not yet being dialyzed; once patients are on dialysis, they are allowed a more liberal fluid intake and can receive a greater intake of carbohydrates, protein, and fat, limited only by the rate of dialytic fluid and solute removal (see Chapter 76). The use of nutritional therapy to enhance survival and recovery from AKI is controversial. Early studies suggested that recovery and survival were enhanced [184,185], but these were not confirmed by more recent controlled trials [186,187].

Hyperkalemia

Hyperkalemia is the most immediately life-threatening electrolyte imbalance encountered in patients with renal disease (see Chapter 72). In AKI, hyperkalemia arises from the inability of the kidneys to handle the excretory burden of potassium. Sources of potassium should be identified and regulated appropriately. Potassium loads may be endogenous (e.g., tissue breakdown, hematoma reabsorption) or exogenous (e.g., diet, intravenous fluids, medications). Even when the GFR is substantially reduced, the kidneys can excrete large amounts of potassium, provided that tubular secretion is intact. For this reason, hyperkalemia more often occurs in patients with parenchymal or postrenal AKI. Urine flow rate is an important determinant of tubular potassium secretion; therefore, oliguric patients are more prone to potassium imbalance than are nonoliguric patients. Many commonly used medications, including heparin, NSAIDs, and ACE inhibitors, can also inhibit tubular potassium secretion. These should be discontinued in hyperkalemic patients.

Metabolic Acidosis

The kidneys' ability to excrete metabolically produced acids may be reduced, particularly in parenchymal and obstructive disease. Because acid excretion is primarily a tubular function, the degree of acidosis may not always correlate with the degree of GFR impairment. Indeed, pure tubular acid excretion abnormalities may exist independently of azotemia (renal tubular acidosis). Metabolic acidosis that results from failure of the tubules to excrete hydrogen ions or conserve bicarbonate normally produces a hyperchloremic or low anion gap acidosis (see Chapter 71). When the GFR is severely impaired, retention of acid wastes may produce a high anion gap acidosis.

Abnormal Salt and Water Metabolism

Although most fluids administered to patients are hypotonic, plasma osmolality normally remains within tightly fixed limits. The process by which plasma tonicity is preserved depends on the suppression of vasopressin release and the formation of free water in the ascending limb of the loop of Henle. This latter function is impeded whenever GFR is reduced, which results in water retention and hyponatremia. Conversely, some renal disorders are characterized by failure to conserve water. This situation, referred to as *nephrogenic diabetes insipidus*, is most common in tubulointerstitial disease and in partial obstruction of the urinary tract. Patients with these disorders are prone to dehydration and hypernatremia. The subject is covered in more detail in Chapter 72.

Abnormal Calcium and Phosphorus Metabolism

The ability of the kidney to excrete phosphorus normally is impaired when the GFR falls to approximately one third of normal. High serum phosphorus levels lead to formation of insoluble calcium phosphate salts, which may precipitate in soft tissue. If the product of the serum calcium and phosphorus concentrations exceeds 70, precipitation in soft tissues becomes more likely. For this reason, administration of calcium to patients with AKI should be reserved for emergent situations, such as the appearance of tetany, seizures, or refractory hypotension. The tendency toward hypocalcemia with AKI may be additionally aggravated by the injured kidneys' failure to form 1,25-dihydroxycholecalciferol, although vitamin D therapy is rarely required in cases of AKI.

Hyperphosphatemia is common in patients with AKI, particularly in patients with rhabdomyolysis or tumor lysis syndrome. Phosphate binders are typically initiated when phosphate levels rise to more than 6.0 mg per dL. The main phosphate binders available include aluminum hydroxide, calcium salts (calcium acetate and calcium carbonate), sevelamer, and lanthanum hydroxide. Unless the patient is hypercalcemic, calcium carbonate can be administered (1.0 to 1.5 g with meals) as the phosphate-binding agent. Although potent, aluminum-based binders are limited to short-term use because of concerns with aluminum intoxication.

Uremia

Accumulation of endogenous toxins in the body eventually results in uremia. The uremic syndrome is a multisystemic symptom complex. The exact identities of the so-called uremic toxins are not known, although many possibilities have been suggested. Urea and creatinine are not uremic toxins but rather are markers of renal excretory capacity. One cannot deduce on the basis of urea nitrogen and creatinine levels exactly when a patient will become uremic. In general, the syndrome manifests itself at a GFR of less than 10 mL per minute.

Although uremia is considered an indication to initiate dialytic therapy, the syndrome may be insidious in onset and produce only vague symptoms. Lethargy, anorexia, nausea, and malaise, all of which may herald uremia, may well be attributed to extrarenal disease in the patient with AKI. Other, less subjective uremic manifestations constitute stronger indications for prompt initiation of dialysis, including bleeding diathesis, seizures, coma, and the appearance of a pericardial rub.

Dialysis

The use of renal replacement therapy in AKI is discussed in depth in Chapter 75. Briefly, the decision of when to initiate dialysis is historically controversial. Patients with intractable volume overload, hyperkalemia, metabolic acidosis, or frank uremia clearly meet criteria for dialysis. However, many patients with significant AKI do not meet one of these criteria. This has led to a discussion regarding the merits of early or even "prophylactic" dialysis. The rationale for forestalling dialysis includes the invasive nature of the procedure as well as concern that renal replacement therapy can exacerbate hemodynamic instability that might prolong the course of AKI. There is also significant labor and cost associated with performing the procedure in the ICU. Nevertheless, several observational studies appear to show decreased morbidity and mortality in patients initiated early on dialysis. It has been argued that early dialysis results in improved volume control as well as the clearance of a variety of cytokines and/or toxins that may be harmful. Unfortunately, at this time, there is still not adequate data to establish the optimal time to initiate dialysis. This issue is discussed in detail in Chapter 75.

Prognosis and Outcome of Acute Kidney Injury

Overall, the mortality from AKI ranges from 25% [14] to 64% [188]. The large disparity in mortality no doubt reflects the varied intensities of illness and case mixes in the reports. A large retrospective study by McMurray et al. [48] demonstrated 14% mortality in patients with nephrotoxic forms of AKI compared with 35% mortality for all other causes. Similarly, in the prospective study by Hou et al. [14], mortality ranged from a low of 6% in radiocontrast-induced nephropathy to 80% in cases of HRS. Even within the group of patients with AKI due to renal hypoperfusion, mortality varied between 9% in patients with volume depletion and 100% in patients with cardiogenic shock. An analysis of 618 critically ill patients with ATN found the following characteristics associated with mortality: age (odds ratio [OR], 1.13 per decade), sepsis (OR, 1.50), adult respiratory distress syndrome (OR, 1.79), liver failure (OR, 1.62), and creatinine of less than 2.0 mg per dL (OR, 1.99) [189]. Despite medical advances, mortality in AKI has not improved during the past 50 years [190].

Although patients with AKI clearly have increased mortality, there has been some debate about whether this is related to comorbid conditions versus AKI as an independent risk factor. A study by Hoa et al. looked at 843 patients' post–cardiac surgery of which 145 developed AKI. After completing a multivariate analysis, AKI was found to be an independent risk factor for mortality with a hazard ratio of 7.8. It is not entirely clear how AKI impacts the risk of death, but it is known that patients with significant AKI have compromised immune system and platelet function placing them at higher risk for complications. Indeed, in the series reported by Kleinknecht et al. [50], most deaths were the result of sepsis, gastrointestinal hemorrhage, or cardiac causes.

At least half of all cases of AKI are nonoliguric [191]. Nonoliguria is associated with an improved likelihood of recovery of renal function and approximately half the mortality (26%) of oliguric AKI (50%) [191]. AKI is more likely to have developed in nonoliguric patients as a result of exposure to a nephrotoxin than in oliguric patients [191]. Most of these individuals do not have multiorgan failure, and their improved survival may be the result of a less severe primary illness than those for oliguric patients.

The long-term prognosis of patients with AKI is impacted by several factors including the severity of the initial injury as well as baseline patient characteristics. Patients with a brief ischemic event, as may occur with suprarenal clamping of the aorta, typically develop a mild form of AKI that resolves within 72 hours [192]. Patients with prolonged episodes of ischemia or injury may have variable degrees of recovery. A study by Spurney at al. in ICU patients with AKI requiring dialysis found that the majority of the patients were left with some degree of CKD with the average creatinine remaining 1 to 2 mg per dL above their prior baselines [193]. In other studies, elderly individuals as well as patients with baseline CKD have been found to reduced probability of full recovery [194,195].

Delayed recovery can be anticipated in those patients with poor cardiac output [196] or in those with hypovolemia. Therefore, it is imperative that ECF volume be assessed, particularly in patients on hemodialysis or peritoneal dialysis in whom volume depletion may occur. Nevertheless, more than 80% of the patients who survive AKI will recover renal function and remain dialysis free [197].

References

1. Lassnigg A, Schmidlin D, Mouhieddine M, et al: Minimal changes of serum creatinine predict prognosis in patients after cardiothoracic surgery: a prospective cohort study. *J Am Soc Nephrol* 15:1597–1605, 2004.
2. Levy MM, Macias WL, Vincent JL, et al: Early changes in organ function predict eventual survival in severe sepsis. *Crit Care Med* 33(10):2194–2201, 2005.
3. Bellomo R, Ronco C, Kellum JA, et al; Acute Dialysis Quality Initiative Workgroup: Acute renal failure—definition, outcome measures, animal models, fluid therapy and information technology needs: the Second International Consensus Conference of the Acute Dialysis Quality Initiative (ADQI) Group. *Crit Care* 8:R204–R210, 2004.
4. Hoste EA, Clermont G, Kersten A, et al: RIFLE criteria for acute kidney injury are associated with hospital mortality in critically ill patients: a cohort analysis. *Crit Care* 10:R73–R83, 2006.
5. Uchino S, Bellomo R, Goldsmith D, et al: An assessment of the RIFLE criteria for acute renal failure in hospitalized patients. *Crit Care Med* 34:1913–1917, 2006.
6. Stoff JS, Clive DM: Role of arachidonic acid metabolites in acute renal failure, in Brenner BM, Lazarus JM (eds): *Acute Renal Failure*. 2nd ed. New York, Churchill Livingstone, 1988, p 143.
7. Francis GS: Neuroendocrine manifestations of congestive heart failure. *Am J Cardiol* 62:9A, 1988.
8. Clive DM, Stoff JS: Renal syndromes associated with nonsteroidal anti-inflammatory drugs. *N Engl J Med* 310:563, 1984.
9. Hricik DE, Browning PJ, Kopelman R, et al: Captopril-induced functional renal insufficiency in patients with bilateral renal-artery stenoses or renal-artery stenosis in a solitary kidney. *N Engl J Med* 308:373, 1983.
10. Myers BD, Moran SM: Hemodynamically mediated acute renal failure. *N Engl J Med* 314:97, 1986.
11. Tomita K, Ujiie K, Nakanishi T, et al: Plasma endothelin levels in patients with acute renal failure. *N Engl J Med* 321:1127, 1989.
12. Mason J, Takabatake T, Olbricht C, et al: The early phase of experimental acute renal failure. III. Tubuloglomerular feedback. *Pflugers Arch* 373(1):69–76, 1978.
13. Smolens P, Stein JH: Hemodynamic factors in acute renal failure: pathophysiologic and therapeutic implications, in Brenner BM, Stein JH (eds): *Acute Renal Failure (Contemporary Issues in Nephrology Series)*. New York, Churchill Livingstone, 1980, p 180.
14. Hou S, Bushinsky DA, Wish JB, et al: Hospital-acquired renal insufficiency: a prospective study. *Am J Med* 74:243, 1983.
15. Brezis M, Epstein FH: Cellular mechanisms of acute ischemic injury in the kidney. *Annu Rev Med* 44:27, 1993.
16. Friedewald JJ, Rabb H: Inflammatory cells in ischemic acute renal failure. *Kidney Int* 66(2):486–491, 2004.
17. Lieberthal W, Koh JS, Levine JS: Necrosis and apoptosis in acute renal failure. *Semin Nephrol* 18(5):505–518, 1998.
18. Salmela K, Wramner L, Ekberg H, et al: A randomized multicenter trial of the anti-ICAM-1 monoclonal antibody (enlimomab) for the prevention of acute rejection and delayed onset of graft function in cadaveric renal transplantation: a report of the European Anti-ICAM-1 Renal Transplant Study Group. *Transplantation* 67(5):729–736, 1999.
19. Mishra J, Dent C, Tarabishi R, et al: Neutrophil gelatinase-associated lipocalin (NGAL) as a biomarker for acute renal injury after cardiac surgery. *Lancet* 365:1241, 2005.
20. Badr KF, Brenner BM: Renal circulatory and nephron function in experimental obstruction of the urinary tract, in Brenner BM, Lazarus JM (eds): *Acute Renal Failure*. 2nd ed. New York, Churchill Livingstone, 1988, p 91.
21. Early LE: Extreme polyuria in obstructive uropathy. *N Engl J Med* 255:600, 1956.
22. Dawson JL: Acute post-operative renal failure in obstructive jaundice. *Ann R Coll Surg Engl* 42:163, 1968.
23. Berisa F, Beaman M, Adu D, et al: Prognostic factors in acute renal failure following aortic aneurysm surgery. *Q J Med* 76:689, 1990.
24. Thakar CV, Arrigain S, Worley S, et al: A clinical score to predict acute renal failure after cardiac surgery. *J Am Soc Nephrol* 16(1):162–168, 2005.
25. Fergusson DA, Hebert PC, Mazer CD, et at: A comparison of aprotinin and lysine analogues after a high-risk cardiac surgery. *N Engl J Med* 358:2319–2331, 2008.
26. Rosner MH, Okusa MD: Acute kidney injury associated with cardiac surgery. *Clin J Am Soc Nephrol* 1:19–32, 2006.
27. Hix JK, Thakar CV, Katz EM, et al: Effect of off-pump coronary artery bypass graft surgery on postoperative acute kidney injury and mortality. *Crit Care Med* 34:2979–2983, 2006.
28. Carcoana OV, Hines RL: Is renal dose dopamine protective or therapeutic? Yes. *Crit Care Clin* 12:677, 1996.
29. Landoni G, Biondi-Zoccai GG, Marino G: Fenoldopam reduces the need for renal replacement therapy and in-hospital death in cardiovascular surgery: a meta-analysis. *J Cardiothorac Vasc Anesth* 22(1):22–33, 2008.
30. Mentzer RM, Oz MC, Sladen RN, et al: Effects of perioperative nesiritide in patients with left ventricular dysfunction undergoing cardiac surgery: the NAPA trial. *J Am Coll Cardiol* 49(6):716–726, 2007.
31. Haase M, Haase-Fielitz A, Bagshaw SM, et al: Phase II, randomized, controlled trial of high-dose N-acetylcysteine in high-risk cardiac surgery patients. *Crit Care Med* 35:1324–1331, 2007.
32. Yallop KG, Sheppard SV, Smith DC: The effect of mannitol on renal function following cardiopulmonary bypass in patients with normal preoperative creatinine. *Anaesthesia* 63:576–582, 2008.
33. Zacharias M, Conlon NP, Herbison GP, et al: Interventions for protecting renal function in the perioperative period. *Cochrane Database Syst Rev* (4):CD003590, 2008.
34. Lassnigg A, Donner E, Grubhofer G, et al: Lack of renoprotective effects of dopamine and furosemide during cardiac surgery. *J Am Soc Nephrol* 11(1):97–104, 2000.
35. Karkouti K, Wijeysundera DN, Yau TM, et al: Acute kidney injury after cardiac surgery: focus on modifiable risk factors. *Circulation* 119(4):495–502, 2009.
36. Nohria A, Hasselblad V, Stebbins A, et al: Cardiorenal interaction: insights from the ESCAPE trial. *J Am Coll Cardiol* 51:1268–1274, 2008.
37. Ronco C, Haapio M, House AA, et al: Cardiorenal syndrome. *J Am Coll Cardio* 52(19):1527–1539, 2008.
38. Weiner DE, Tighiouart H, Amin MG, et al: Chronic kidney disease as a risk factor for cardiovascular disease and all-cause mortality: a pooled analysis of community-based studies. *J Am Soc Nephrol* 15:1307–1315, 2004.
39. Dries DL, Exner DV, Domanski MJ, et al: The prognostic implications of renal insufficiency in asymptomatic and symptomatic patient with left ventricular systolic dysfunction. *J Am Coll Cardiol* 35:681–689, 2000.
40. Abraham WT, Adams K, Fonarow GC, et al: In-hospital mortality in patients with acute decompensated heart failure requiring intravenous vasoactive medications. Analysis from the Acute Decompensated Heart Failure Registry (ADHERE). *J Am Coll Cardiol* 46:57–64, 2005.
41. Forman DF, Butler J, Wang Y, et al: Incidence, predictors at admission, and impact of worsening renal function among patients hospitalized with heart failure. *J Am Coll Cardiol* 43:61–67, 2004.
42. Adams KF, Lindenfield J, Arnold JMO, et al: Executive summary: HFSA 2006 comprehensive heart failure practice guideline. *J Card Fail* 12:29–32, 2006.
43. Sackner-Bernstein JD, Skopicki HA, Aaronson KD: Risk of worsening renal function with nesiritide in patients with acutely decompensated heart failure. *Circulation* 111(12):1487–1491, 2005.
44. Gheorghiade M, Konstam MA, Burnett JC Jr, et al: Short-term clinical effects of tolvaptan, an oral vasopressin antagonist, in patients hospitalized for heart failure: the EVEREST Clinical Status Trials. *JAMA* 297(12):1332–1343, 2007.
45. Antman EM, Anbe DT, Armstrong PW, et al: ACC/AHA guidelines for the management of patients with ST-elevation myocardial infarction—executive summary: a report of the American College of Cardiology/American Heart Association Task Force on Practice Guidelines (Writing Committee to Revise the 1999 Guidelines for the Management of Patients With Acute Myocardial Infarction). *Circulation* 110(5):588–636, 2004.
46. Cuffe MS, Califf RM, Adams KF Jr, et al: Short-term intravenous milrinone for acute exacerbation of chronic heart failure: a randomized controlled trial. *JAMA* 287(12):1541–1547, 2002.
47. Mullens W, Abrahams Z, Skouri HN, et al: Elevated intra-abdominal pressure in acute decompensated heart failure: a potential contributor to worsening renal function? *J Am Coll Cardiol* 51.300–306, 2008.
48. McMurray SD, Luft FC, Maxwell DR, et al: Prevailing patterns and predictor variables in patients with acute tubular necrosis. *Arch Intern Med* 136:950, 1978.
49. Schaefer JH, Jochimsen F, Keller F, et al: Outcome prediction of acute renal failure in medical intensive care. *Intensive Care Med* 17:19, 1991.
50. Kleinknecht D, Jungers P, Chanard J, et al: Uremic and non-uremic complications of acute renal failure: evaluation of early and frequent dialysis on prognosis. *Kidney Int* 1:190, 1972.
51. Wang W, Falk S, Jittikanont S, et al: Protective effect of renal denervation on normotensive endotoxemia-induced acute renal failure in mice. *Am J Physiol Renal Physiol* 283:F583–F587, 2002.
52. Kleinknecht D, Grunfeld JP, Cia Gomez P: Diagnostic procedures and long-term prognosis in bilateral renal cortical necrosis. *Kidney Int* 4:390, 1973.
53. Kaplinsky C, Frand M, Rubenstein ZJ: Disseminated intravascular clotting and renal cortical necrosis complicating snake bite. *Clin Pediatr* 19:229, 1980.
54. Gerhardt RE, Hudson JB, Rao RN, et al: Chronic renal insufficiency from cortical necrosis induced by arsenic poisoning. *Arch Intern Med* 138:1267, 1978.
55. Williams GM, Horne DM, Hudson KP Jr: Hyperacute renal homograft rejection in man. *N Engl J Med* 279:611, 1968.
56. Solez K, Bihari D, Collins AJ, et al: International dialysis aid in earthquake and other disasters. *Kidney Int* 44:479, 1993.
57. Honda N, Kurokawa K: Acute renal failure and rhabdomyolysis. *Kidney Int* 23:888, 1983.
58. Roth D, Alarcon FJ, Fernandez JA, et al: Acute rhabdomyolysis associated with cocaine intoxication. *N Engl J Med* 319:673, 1990.

59. Better OS, Stein JH: Early management of shock and prophylaxis of acute renal failure in traumatic rhabdomyolysis. *N Engl J Med* 322:825, 1990.
60. Dubrow A, Flamenbaum W: Acute renal failure associated with myoglobinuria and hemoglobinuria, in Brenner BM, Lazarus JM (eds): *Acute Renal Failure*. 2nd ed. New York, Churchill Livingstone, 1988, p 279.
61. Berns AS: Nephrotoxicity of contrast media [clinical conference]. *Kidney Int* 36:730, 1989.
62. Weisbord SD, Chen H, Stone RA, et al: Associations of increases in serum creatinine with mortality and length of hospital stay after coronary angiography. *J Am Soc Nephrol* 17:2871–2877, 2006.
63. From AM, Bartholmai BJ, Williams AW, et al: Mortality associated with nephropathy after radiographic contrast exposure. *Mayo Clin Proc* 83:1095–1100, 2008.
64. Wiesord SD, Mor MK, Resnick AL, et al: Incidence and outcomes of contrast-induced AKI following computed tomography. *Clin J Am Soc Nephrol* 3:1274–1281, 2008.
65. Kelly AM, Dwamena B, Cronin P, et al: Meta-analysis: effectiveness of drugs for preventing contrast-induced nephropathy. *Ann Intern Med* 148(4):284–294, 2008.
66. Rudnick MR, Goldfarb S, Wexler L, et al: Nephrotoxicity of ionic and nonionic contrast media in 1196 patients: a randomized trial. The Iohexol Cooperative Study. *Kidney Int* 47(1):254–261, 1995.
67. Barrett BJ: Contrast nephrotoxicity. *J Am Soc Nephrol* 5(2):125–137, 1994.
68. Weisbord SD, Mor MK, Resnick AL, et al: Prevention, incidence, and outcomes of contrast-induced acute kidney injury. *Arch Intern Med* 168:1325–1332, 2008.
69. Margulies KB, Hildebrand FL, Heublein DM, et al: Radiocontrast increases plasma and urinary endothelin. *J Am Soc Nephrol* 2:1041, 1991.
70. Lee HT, Jan M, Bae SC, et al: A1 adenosine receptor knockout mice are protected against acute radiocontrast nephropathy in vivo. *Am J Renal Physiol* 290(6):F1367–F1375, 2006.
71. Hansen PB, Schnermann J: Vasoconstrictor and vasodilator effects of adenosine in the kidney. *Am J Physiol Renal Physiol* 285(4):F590–F599, 2003.
72. Detrenis S, Meschi M, Musini S, et al: Lights and shadows on the pathogenesis of contrast-induced nephropathy: state of the art. *Nephrol Dial Transplant* 20(8):1542–1550, 2005.
73. Heyman SN, Brezis M, Greenfeld Z, et al: Protective role of furosemide and saline in radiocontrast-induced acute renal failure in the rat. *Am J Kidney Dis* 14:377, 1989.
74. Shusterman N, Strom BL, Murray TG, et al: Risk factors and outcome of hospital-acquired acute renal failure: clinical epidemiologic study. *Am J Med* 83:65, 1987.
75. Porter GA: Experimental contrast-associated nephropathy and its clinical implications. *Am J Cardiol* 66:18F, 1990.
76. Solomon R, Werner C, Mann D, et al: Effects of saline, mannitol, and furosemide to prevent acute decreases in renal function induced by radiocontrast agents. *N Engl J Med* 331:1416, 1994.
77. Tepel M, van der Giet M, Schwarzfeld C, et al: Prevention of radiographic-contrast agent–induced reductions in renal function by acetylcysteine. *N Engl J Med* 343:210, 2000.
78. Kay J, Chow WH, Chan TM, et al: Acetylcysteine for prevention of acute deterioration of renal function following elective coronary angiography and intervention. A randomized controlled trial. *JAMA* 289:553, 2003.
79. Durham JD, Caputo C, Dokko J, et al: A randomized controlled trial of N-acetylcysteine to prevent contrast nephropathy in cardiac angiography. *Kidney Int* 62:2202, 2002.
80. Meranzi G, Assanelli E, Marana I, et al: N-acetylcysteine and contrast-induced nephropathy in primary angioplasty. *N Engl J Med* 354:2773–2782, 2006.
81. Gonzalez DA, Norsworthy KJ, Kern SJ, et al: A meta-analysis of N-acetylcysteine in contrast-induced nephrotoxicity: unsupervised clustering to resolve heterogeneity. *BMC Med* 5:32, 2007.
82. Merten GJ, Burgess WP, Gray LV, et al: Prevention of contrast-induced nephropathy with sodium bicarbonate: a randomized controlled trial. *JAMA* 291:2328, 2004.
83. Briguori C, Airoldi F, F'Andrea D, et al: Renal Insufficiency Following Contrast Media Administration (REMEDIAL): a randomized comparison of 3 preventive strategies. *Circulation* 15:1211–1217, 2007.
84. Maioli M, Toso A, Leoncini M, et al: Sodium bicarbonate versus saline for the prevention of contrast-induced nephropathy in patients with renal dysfunction undergoing coronary angiography or intervention. *J Am Coll Cardiol* 52:599–604, 2008.
85. Brar SS, Shen AY, Jorgensen MB, et al: Sodium bicarbonate vs sodium chloride for the prevention of contrast medium-induced nephropathy in patients undergoing coronary angiography: a randomized trial. *JAMA* 300:1038–1046, 2008.
86. Adolph E, Holdt-Lehmann B, Chatterjee T, et al: Renal Insufficiency Following Radiocontrast Exposure Trial (REINFORCE): a randomized comparison of sodium bicarbonate versus sodium chloride hydration for the prevention of contrast-induced nephropathy. *Coron Artery Dis* 19:413–419, 2008.
87. Stone GW, McCullough PA, Tumlin JA, et al: CONTRAST Investigators: Fenoldopam mesylate for the prevention of contrast-induced nephropathy: a randomized controlled trial. *JAMA* 290:2284–2291, 2003.
88. Barrett BJ, Carlisle EJ: Metaanalysis of the relative nephrotoxicity of high- and low-osmolality iodinated contrast media. *Radiology* 188:171, 1993.
89. Solomon RJ, Natarajan MK, Doucet S, et al: Cardiac Angiography in Renally Impaired Patients (CARE) study: a randomized double-blind trial of contrast-induced nephropathy in patients with chronic kidney disease. *Circulation* 115:3189–3196, 2007.
90. Kuhn MJ, Chen N, Sahani DV, et al: The PREDICT study: a randomized double-blind comparison of contrast-induced nephropathy after low- or isoosmolar contrast agent exposure. *AJR AM J Roentgenol* 191:151–157, 2008.
91. Rudnick MR, Davidson C, Laskey W, et al: Nephrotoxicity of iodixanol versus ioversol in patient with chronic kidney disease: The Visipaque Angiography/Interventions with Laboratory Outcomes in Renal Insufficiency (VALOR) Trial. *Am Heart J* 156:776–782, 2008.
92. Cruz DN, Perazella MA, Bellomo R, et al: Extracorporeal blood purification therapies for prevention of radiocontrast-induced nephropathy: a systematic review. *Am J Kidney Dis* 48:361–371, 2006.
93. Lee PT, Chou KJ, Liu CP, et al: Renal protection for coronary angiography in advanced renal failure patients by prophylactic hemodialysis: a randomized controlled trial. *J Am Coll Cardiol* 50:1015–1020, 2007.
94. Reinecke H, Fobker M, Wellmann J, et al: A randomized controlled trial comparing hydration therapy to additional hemodialysis or N-acetylcysteine for the prevention of contrast medium-induced nephropathy: The Dialysis versus Diuresis (DVD) Trial. *Clin Res Cardiol* 96:130–139, 2007.
95. Shiragami K, Fujii Z, Sakumura T, et al: Effect of a contrast agent on long-term renal function and the efficacy of prophylactic hemodiafiltration. *Circ J* 72:427–433, 2008.
96. Markowitz GS, Nasr SH, Klein P, et al: Renal failure due to acute nephrocalcinosis following oral sodium phosphate bowel cleansing. *Hum Pathol* 35(6):675–684, 2004.
97. Hurst FP, Bohen EM, Osgard EM, et al: Association of oral sodium phosphate purgative use with acute kidney injury. *J Am Soc Nephrol* 18:3192–3198, 2007.
98. Brunelli SM, Lewis JD, Gupta M, et al: Risk of kidney injury following use of oral phosphosoda bowel preparations. *J Am Soc Nephrol* 18:3199–3205, 2007.
99. Wexner SD, Beck DE, Baron TH, et al: A consensus document on bowel preparation before colonoscopy: prepared by a Task Force from the American Society of Colon and Rectal Surgeons (ASCRS), the American Society for Gastrointestinal Endoscopy (ASGE), and the Society of American Gastrointestinal and Endoscopic Surgeons (SAGES). *Surg Endosc* 20:1161, 2006.
100. Hüter L, Simon TP, Weinmann L, et al: Hydroxyethyl starch impairs renal function and induces interstitial proliferation, macrophage infiltration and tubular damage in an isolated renal perfusion model. *Crit Care* 13(1):R23, 2009.
101. Schortgen F, Lacherade JC, Bruneel F, et al: Effects of hydroxyethylstarch and gelatin on renal function in severe sepsis: a multicentre randomized study. *Lancet* 357:911–916, 2001.
102. Brunkhorst FM, Engel C, Bloos F, et al: Intensive insulin therapy and pentastarch resuscitation in severe sepsis. *N Engl J Med* 358:125–139, 2008.
103. Blasco V, Leone M, Antonini F, et al: Comparison of the novel hydroxyethylstarch 130/0.4 and hydroxyethylstarch 200/0.6 in brain dead donor resuscitation on renal function after transplantation. *Br J Anaesth* 100:504–508, 2008.
104. Malbrain ML, Cheatham ML, Kirkpatrick A, et al: Results from the International Conference of Experts on Intra-abdominal Hypertension and Abdominal Compartment Syndrome: I. Definitions. *Intensive Care Med* 32:1722–1732, 2006.
105. Shibagaki Y, Tai C, Nayak A, et al: Intra-abdominal hypertension is an under-appreciated cause of acute renal failure. *Nephrol Dial Transplant* 21:3567–3570, 2006.
106. Humes HD: Aminoglycoside toxicity. *Kidney Int* 33:900, 1988.
107. Deray G, Martinez F, Katlama C: Foscarnet nephrotoxicity: mechanism, incidence, and prevention. *Am J Nephrol* 9:316, 1989.
108. Galpin JE, Shinaberger JH, Stanley TM: Acute interstitial nephritis due to methicillin. *Am J Med* 65:756, 1978.
109. van Ypersele de Strihou C: Acute oliguric interstitial nephritis. *Kidney Int* 16:751, 1979.
110. Walshe JJ, Venuto RC: Acute oliguric renal failure induced by indomethacin: possible mechanism. *Ann Intern Med* 91:47, 1979.
111. Hricik DE, Dunn MJ: Angiotensin-converting enzyme inhibitor-induced renal failure: causes, consequences, and diagnostic uses. *J Am Soc Nephrol* 1:845, 1990.
112. Lessman RK, Johnson SF, Coburn JW, et al: Renal artery embolism. *Ann Intern Med* 89:477, 1978.
113. Fraser I, Ihle B, Kincaid-Smith P: Renal failure due to cholesterol emboli. *Aust N Z J Med* 21:418, 1991.
114. Hosler GA, Cusumano AM, Hutchins GM: Thrombotic thrombocytopenic purpura and hemolytic uremic syndrome are distinct pathologic entities. *Arch Pathol Lab Med* 127:834–839, 2003.
115. Remuzzi G, Galbusera M, Noris M, et al, and the Italian Registry of Recurrent and Familial HUS/TTP: Von Willebrand factor cleaving protease

(ADAMTS13) is deficient in recurrent and familial thrombotic thrombocytopenic purpura and hemolytic uremic syndrome. *Blood* 100:779–785, 2002.
116. Andreoli SP, Trachtman H, Acheson DW, et al: Hemolytic uremic syndrome: epidemiology, pathophysiology, and therapy. *Pediatr Nephrol* 17:293–298, 2002.
117. Moake JL: Mechanism of disease: thrombotic microangiopathies. *N Engl J Med* 347:589–600, 2002.
118. King AJ: Acute inflammation in the pathogenesis of hemolytic uremic syndrome. *Kidney Int* 61:1553–1564, 2002.
119. Regenetti P, Noris M, Remussi G: Thrombotic microangiopathy, hemolytic uremic syndrome, and thrombotic thrombocytopenic purpura. *Kidney Int* 60:831–846, 2001.
120. Tsai H-M: Advances in the pathogenesis, diagnosis and treatment of thrombotic thrombocytopenic purpura. *J Am Soc Nephrol* 14:1072–1081, 2003.
121. Conger JD, Falk SA: Intrarenal dynamics in the pathogenesis and prevention of acute urate nephropathy. *J Clin Invest* 59:786, 1977.
122. Coiffier B, Altman A, Pui CH, et al: Guidelines for the management of pediatric and adult tumor lysis syndrome: an evidence-based review. *J Clin Oncol* 26:2767, 2008.
123. Blachley JD, Hill JB: Renal and electrolyte disturbances associated with cisplatin. *Ann Intern Med* 95:628, 1981.
124. Garnick MB, Mayer RJ: Management of acute renal failure associated with neoplastic disease, in Yarboro J, Bornstein R (eds): *Oncologic Emergencies*. New York, Grune & Stratton, 1981.
125. Ring Larsen H, Palazzo U: Renal failure in fulminant hepatic failure and terminal cirrhosis: a comparison between incidence, types, and prognosis. *Gut* 22:585, 1981.
126. Mas A, Arroyo V, Rodes J, et al: Ascites and renal failure in primary liver cell carcinoma. *Br Med J* 3:692, 1975.
127. Rosanasky SJ, Mullens CC: The hepatorenal syndrome associated with angiosarcoma of the gall bladder. *Ann Intern Med* 96:191, 1982.
128. Arroyo V, Gines P, Gerbes AL, et al: Definition and diagnostic criteria of refractory ascites and hepatorenal syndrome in cirrhosis. International Ascites Club. *Hepatology* 23:164, 1996.
129. Salerno F, Gerbes A, Gines P, et al: Diagnosis, prevention and treatment of hepatorenal syndrome in cirrhosis. *Gut* 56:1310, 2007.
130. Esrailian E, Pantangco ER, Kyulo NL, et al: Octreotide/midodrine therapy significantly improves renal function and 30-day survival in patients with type 1 hepatorenal syndrome. *Dig Dis Sci* 52:742–748, 2007.
131. Esrailian E, Runyon BA: Alcoholic cirrhosis-associated hepatorenal syndrome treated with vasoactive agents. *Nat Clin Pract Nephrol* 2:169–172, 2006.
132. Martín-Llahí M, Pépin MN, Guevara M, et al: TAHRS Investigators: Terlipressin and albumin vs albumin in patients with cirrhosis and hepatorenal syndrome: a randomized study. *Gastroenterology* 134:1352–1359, 2008.
133. Alessandria C, Ottobrelli A, Debernadrdi-Vernon W, et al: Noradrenalin vs terlipressin in patients with hepatorenal syndrome: a prospective, randomized, unblinded pilot study. *J Hepatol* 47:499–505, 2007.
134. Levinsky NG: Pathophysiology of acute renal failure. *N Engl J Med* 296:1453, 1977.
135. Green J, Better OS: Systemic hypotension and renal failure in obstructive jaundice—mechanistic and therapeutic aspects. *J Am Soc Nephrol* 5:1853, 1995.
136. Runyon BA: Management of adult patients with ascites due to cirrhosis: an update. *Hepatology* 49:2087, 2009.
137. Gines P, Tito L, Arroyo V, et al: Randomized study of therapeutic paracentesis with and without intravenous albumin in cirrhosis. *Gastroenterology* 94:1493, 1988.
138. Runyon BA: Patient selection is important in studying the impact of large-volume paracentesis on intravascular volume. *Am J Gastroenterol* 92:371, 1997.
139. Clark F, O'Leary JP: Survival associated with hepatorenal syndrome. *South Med J* 72:87, 1979.
140. Ariyan S, Sweeney T, Kerstein MD: The hepatorenal syndrome: recovery after portacaval shunt. *Ann Surg* 181:847, 1975.
141. Fischer JE, Foster GS: Survival from acute hepatorenal syndrome following splenorenal shunt. *Ann Surg* 814:22, 1976.
142. Kronborg IJ, Radvan G, Zipser RD: Urinary excretion of prostaglandins and thromboxanes in the hepatorenal syndrome, in Samuelsson P, Paoletti R, Ramwell P (eds): *Advances in Prostaglandin, Thromboxane, and Leukotriene Research*. New York, Raven Press, 1983.
143. Epstein M: Peritoneovenous shunt in the management of ascites and hepatorenal syndrome. *Gastroenterology* 82:790, 1982.
144. Fullen WD: Hepatorenal syndrome: reversal of peritoneovenous shunt. *Surgery* 82:337, 1977.
145. Kinney MJ, Schneider A, Sapnick S, et al: The hepatorenal syndrome and refractory ascites. *Nephron* 23:228, 1979.
146. Schroeder ET, Anderson GH, Smulyan H: Effects of portacaval or peritoneovenous shunt on renin in the hepatorenal syndrome. *Kidney Int* 15:54, 1979.
147. Schwartz ML, Vogel SG: Treatment of hepatorenal syndrome. *Am J Surg* 139:370, 1980.
148. Wapnick S, Grosberg A, Kinney M, et al: LeVeen continuous peritoneojugular shunt. *JAMA* 237:131, 1977.
149. Epstein M: The LeVeen shunt for ascites and hepatorenal syndrome. *N Engl J Med* 302:628, 1980.
150. Linas SL, Schaefer JW, Moore EE, et al: Peritoneovenous shunt in the management of the hepatorenal syndrome. *Kidney Int* 30:736, 1986.
151. Rose BD: Pathophysiology of renal disease. 2nd ed. McGraw-Hill, New York, 1987, pp 68–69.
152. Cockcroft DW, Gault MH: Prediction of creatinine clearance from serum creatinine. *Nephron* 16:31, 1976.
153. Levey AS, Greene T, Kusek JW, et al. A simplified equation to predict glomerular filtration rate from serum creatinine [abstract]. *J Am Soc Nephrol* 11:A0828, 2000.
154. Shemesh O, Golbetz H, Kriss JP, et al: Limitations of creatinine as a filtration marker in glomerulopathic patients. *Kidney Int* 28:830, 1985.
155. Border WA, Cohen AH: Renal biopsy diagnosis of clinically silent multiple myeloma. *Ann Intern Med* 93:43, 1980.
156. Rudnick MR, Bastl CP, Elfinbein IB, et al: The differential diagnosis of acute renal failure, in Brenner BM, Lazarus JM (eds): *Acute Renal Failure*. New York, Churchill Livingstone, 1988, p 177.
157. Cantarovich F, Rangoonwala B, Lorenz H, et al: High-dose furosemide for established ARF: a prospective, randomized, double-blind, placebo-controlled, multicenter trial. *Am J Kidney Dis* 44:402, 2004.
158. Ho KM, Sheridan DJ: Meta-analysis of frusemide to prevent or treat acute renal failure. *BMJ* 333:420, 2006.
159. Mehta RL, Pascual MT, Soroko S, et al: Diuretics, mortality, and nonrecovery of renal function in acute renal failure. *JAMA* 288:2547, 2002.
160. Salvador D, Rey N, Ramos G, et al: Continuous infusion versus bolus injection of loop diuretics in congestive heart failure. *Cochrane Database Syst Rev* 1:CD003178, 2004.
161. Clarkson MR, Giblin L, O'Connell FP, et al: Acute interstitial nephritis: clinical features and response to corticosteroid therapy. *Nephrol Dial Transplant* 19:2778, 2004.
162. Gonzalez E, Gutierrez E, Galeano C, et al: Early steroid treatment improves the recovery of renal function in patients with drug-induced acute interstitial nephritis. *Kidney Int* 73:940, 2008.
163. Lockwood CM, Pinching AJ, Swemy P, et al: Plasma-exchange and immunosuppression in the treatment of fulminating immune complex crescentic glomerulonephritis. *Lancet* 1:63, 1977.
164. Lockwood CM, Pearson TA, Rees AJ, et al: Immunosuppression and plasma-exchange in the treatment of Goodpasture's syndrome. *Lancet* 1:711, 1976.
165. Fauci AS, Haynes BF, Katz P, et al: Wegener's granulomatosis: prospective clinical and therapeutic experience with 85 patients for 21 years. *Ann Intern Med* 98:76, 1983.
166. Marik PE, Iglesias J: Low-dose dopamine does not prevent acute renal failure in patients with septic shock and oliguria. NORASEPT II Study Investigators. *Am J Med* 107:387, 1999.
167. Bellomo R, Chapman M, Finfer S, et al: Low-dose dopamine in patients with early renal dysfunction: a placebo-controlled randomised trial. *Lancet* 356:2139, 2000.
168. Lauschke A, Teichgraber UK, Frei U, et al: 'Low-dose' dopamine worsens renal perfusion in patients with acute renal failure. *Kidney Int* 69:1669, 2006.
169. Singer I, Epstein M: Potential of dopamine A-1 agonists in the management of acute renal failure. *Am J Kidney Dis* 31:743, 1998.
170. Halpeny M, Markos F, Snow HM, et al: Effects of prophylactic fenoldopam on renal blood flow adrenal tubular function during acute hypovolemia in anesthetized dogs. *Crit Care Med* 29:855, 2001.
171. Landoni G, Biondi-Zoccai GG, Tumlin JA, et al: Beneficial impact of fenoldopam in critically ill patients with or at risk for acute renal failure: a meta-analysis of randomized clinical trials. *Am J Kidney Dis* 49:56, 2007.
172. Sward K, Valsson F, Odencrants P, et al: Recombinant human atrial natriuretic peptide in ischemic acute renal failure: a randomized placebo-controlled trial. *Crit Care Med* 32:1310–1315, 2004.
173. Hirschberg R, Kopple J, Lipsett P, et al: Multicenter clinical trial of recombinant human insulin-like growth factor I in patients with acute renal failure. *Kidney Int* 56:2423, 1999.
174. Coimbra T, Cieslinski DA, Humes HD: Epidermal growth factor enhances renal tubule cell regeneration and repair and accelerates the recovery of renal function in postischemic acute renal failure. *J Clin Invest* 84:1757, 1989.
175. Miller SB, Martin DR, Kissane J, et al: Hepatocyte growth factor accelerates recovery from acute ischemic renal injury in rat. *Am J Physiol* 266:F129, 1994.
176. Goligorsky MS, Dibona GF: Pathogenetic role of Arg-Gly-Asp-recognizing integrins in acute renal failure. *Proc Natl Acad Sci U S A* 90:5700, 1993.
177. Kelly KJ, Williams WW Jr, Colvin RB, et al: Antibody to intercellular adhesion molecule 1 protects the kidney against ischemic injury. *Proc Natl Acad Sci U S A* 91:812, 1994.
178. Ghielli M, Verstrepen WA, De Greef KEJ, et al: Antibodies to both ICAM-1 and LFA-1 do not protect the kidney against toxic ($HgCl_2$) injury. *Kidney Int* 58:1121, 2000.
179. Battle DC, Arruda JAL, Kurtzman NA: Hyperkalemic distal renal tubular acidosis associated with obstructive uropathy. *N Engl J Med* 304:373, 1981.

180. DeFronzo RA: Hyperkalemia and hyporeninemic hypoaldosteronism. *Kidney Int* 17:118, 1980.
181. Rose BD: Urinary tract obstruction, in Rose BD (ed): *Pathophysiology of Renal Disease*. New York, McGraw-Hill, 1981, p 347.
182. Wilson DR, Honrath V: Cross circulation of natriuretic factors in post-obstructive diuresis. *J Clin Invest* 57:380, 1976.
183. Druml W: Nutritional management of acute renal failure. *Am J Kidney Dis* 37[Suppl 2]:S89, 2001.
184. Abel RM, Beck CH, Abbott WM, et al: Improved survival from acute renal failure after treatment with intravenous essential L-amino acids and glucose. Results of a prospective, double-blind study. *N Engl J Med* 288:695, 1973.
185. Back SM, Makabali GG, Bryan-Brown CW, et al: The influence of parenteral nutrition on the course of acute renal failure. *Surg Gynecol Obstet* 141:405, 1975.
186. Freund H, Harmian S, Fischer JE: Comparative studies of parenteral nutrition in renal failure using essential and non-essential amino acid containing solutions. *Surg Gynecol Obstet* 151:652, 1980.
187. Feinstein EI, Blumenkrantz MJ, Healy M, et al: Clinical and metabolic responses to parenteral nutrition in acute renal failure. *Medicine* 60:124, 1981.
188. Spiegel DM, Ullian ME, Zerbe GO, et al: Determinants of survival and recovery in acute renal failure patients dialyzed in intensive-care units. *Am J Nephrol* 11:44, 1991.
189. Chertow GM, Soroko SH, Paganini EP, et al: Mortality after acute renal failure: models for prognostic stratification and risk adjustment. *Kidney Int* 70:1120, 2006.
190. Ympa YP, Sakr Y, Reinhart K, et al: Has mortality from acute renal failure decreased? A systematic review of the literature. *Am J Med* 118:827, 2005.
191. Dixon BS, Anderson RJ: Nonoliguric acute renal failure. *Am J Kidney Dis* 6:71, 1985.
192. Myers BD, Miller C, Mehigan JT, et al: Nature of the renal injury following total renal ischemia in man. *J Clin Invest* 73:329, 1984.
193. Spurney RF, Fulkerson WJ, Schwab SJ: Acute renal failure in critically ill patients: prognosis for recovery of kidney function after prolonged dialysis support. *Crit Care Med* 19:8, 1991.
194. Hsu CY, Chertow GM, McCulloch CE, et al: Nonrecovery of kidney function and death after acute on chronic renal failure. *Clin J Am Soc Nephrol* 4:891, 2009.
195. Ishani A, Xue JL, Himmelfarb J, et al: Acute kidney injury increases risk of ESRD among elderly. *J Am Soc Nephrol* 20:223, 2009.
196. Moran SM, Myers BD: Pathophysiology of protracted acute renal failure in man. *J Clin Invest* 1440:1448, 1985.
197. Liano F, Felipe C, Tenorio MT, et al: Long term outcome of acute tubular necrosis: a contribution to its natural history. *Kidney Int* 71:679, 2007.
198. Allgren RL, Marbury TC, Rahman SN, et al: Anaritide in acute tubular necrosis. *N Engl J Med* 336:828, 1997.

CHAPTER 74 ■ DRUG DOSING IN RENAL AND HEPATIC FAILURE: A PHARMACOKINETIC APPROACH TO THE CRITICALLY ILL PATIENT

SONIA LIN, KEITH J. FOSTER, RONALD J. DEBELLIS AND BRIAN S. SMITH

Estimates of the incidence of preventable adverse drug events in the intensive care unit (ICU) range from 10 up to 40 per 1,000 patient-days [1,2]. Patients in an ICU are approximately twice as likely to experience an adverse drug event when compared with patients in a general medicine unit. This increased risk is likely a result of the greater number of medical problems faced by patients in the ICU plus their wider range of drug exposures. Critically ill patients are also at increased risk for developing renal dysfunction, with acute kidney injury (AKI) occurring in 7% to 25% of all patients admitted to the ICU. AKI in the ICU is associated with a severalfold increase in mortality [3,4]. Renal injury is also a risk factor for adverse drug events. As many as 45% of patients with an estimated creatinine clearance less than 40 mL per minute receive medications that are dosed as much as 2.5 times higher than the maximum recommended dose [5]. In addition, adverse drug reactions occur in approximately 9% of patients with blood urea nitrogen less than 20 mg per dL versus 24% of patients with blood urea nitrogen greater than 40 mg per dL [6]. Adverse drug events not only place patients at increased risk for morbidity and mortality but also have a tremendous impact financially. It has been estimated that each adverse drug event increases hospital costs by $2,000 to $4,600 [7–9]. For all of these reasons, appropriate drug dosing in critically ill patients with kidney or liver injury is essential. The following review uses pharmacokinetic principles to discuss key concepts of drug dosing in critically ill patients with renal and hepatic dysfunction and provides drug dosage tables to assist clinicians with dosage adjustments in the setting of renal or hepatic disease (Tables 74.1 and 74.2).

PHARMACOKINETIC AND PHARMACODYNAMIC PRINCIPLES

To design an effective and safe medication regimen, a clinician must have a general understanding of a drug's pharmacokinetic and pharmacodynamic characteristics and be able to adjust for changes in the drug's disposition that occur with critical illness, AKI, and hepatic dysfunction. *Pharmacokinetics* relates to the principles of drug absorption, distribution, metabolism, and excretion, whereas *pharmacodynamics* describes the pharmacologic response resulting from the drug at the site of action (receptor). Clinical pharmacokinetics is the application of knowledge of drug absorption, distribution, metabolism, and excretion to design patient-specific drug regimens with the goal of maximizing therapeutic outcomes and minimizing toxicity (Fig. 74.1).

Most drugs used in critically ill patients are metabolized with linear, or first-order, pharmacokinetics. This means that the drug is eliminated from plasma at a constant rate. As the plasma concentration increases or decreases, the amount of drug eliminated increases or decreases in a directly proportional relationship. Clinically, if a drug dose is increased, the plasma concentration increases proportionally, as does the amount eliminated (Fig. 74.2). If a drug's plasma concentration is plotted versus time using a logarithmic scale, two different slopes are evident (Fig. 74.3): The upper portion is known as the *alpha* (or *distribution*) *phase*, which represents the process

TABLE 74.1

GUIDELINES FOR DRUG DOSING IN CRITICALLY ILL EATIENTS WITH RENAL FAILURE

		Creatinine clearance			Extracorporeal drug removal		
Drug	Normal dose	30–50 mL/min	10–30 mL/min	<10 mL/min	HD	CVVHD, CVVHDF	Notes
Acyclovir [10,11]	5–10 mg/kg IV q8h (higher doses are used in CNS infections and immunocompromised patients) [12,13]	5–10 mg/kg IV q12h	5–10 mg/kg IV q24h	2.5–5.0 mg/kg IV q24h	2.5–5.0 mg/kg IV q24h; administer after HD	5–10 mg/kg IV q24h	To help avoid nephrotoxicity after IV acyclovir, it is recommended that the patient have 1 mL of urine for each 1.3 mg of acyclovir administered [14]
Amantadine [15,16]	100 mg PO q12h	100 mg PO q24h	100 mg PO q48h	200 mg q7 d	200 mg q7 d	100 mg PO q48h	
Amikacin [11,17,18]	7.5 mg/kg IV q12h	7.5 mg/kg IV q18–24h	7.5 mg/kg IV q24–48h	7.5 mg/kg IV q48h	7.5 mg/kg IV based on serum levels, re-dose with levels <5 μg/mL	7.5 mg/kg IV q24–48h	Trough levels should be <10 μg/mL
Amphotericin B (conventional) [17,19]	0.3–1.0 mg/kg IV q24h (maximum dose: 1.5 mg/kg)	0.3–1.0 mg/kg IV q24h	0.3–1.0 mg/kg IV q24h	0.3–1.0 mg/kg IV q48h	0.3–1.0 mg/kg IV q48h	0.3–1.0 mg/kg IV q24h	—
Amphotericin B (liposomal) [11,20,21]	3–5 mg/kg IV q24h (higher doses of 15 mg/kg/d have been used) [22]	3–5 mg/kg IV q24h	3–5 mg/kg IV q24h	3–5 mg/kg IV q48h	3–5 mg/kg IV q48h	3–5 mg/kg IV q24h	—
Ampicillin [23]	1–2 g IV q4–6h	1–2 g IV q6–8h	1–2 g IV q8–12h	1–2 g IV q12h	1–2 g IV q12h; supplemental doses are not needed if maintenance doses are scheduled after HD	1–2 g IV q8–12h	
Ampicillin/ sulbactam [11,23,24]	1.5–3.0 g IV q6h	1.5–3.0 g IV q8h	1.5–3.0 g IV q12h	1.5–3.0 g IV q24h	1.5–3.0 g IV q12–24h administered at the end of HD	CVVH: 1.5–3.0 g IV q8–12h CVVHD, CVVHDF: 1.5–3.0 g IV q6–8h	
Aztreonam [23,25]	1–2 g IV q6–8h	1–2 g IV q6–8h	Loading dose 1–2 g, then 1 g IV q6–8h	Loading dose 1–2 g, then 0.5 g IV q6–8h	Loading dose 1–2 g, then 0.5 g IV q6–8h; administer dose after HD	Loading dose 1–2 g, then 1–2 g IV q8–12h	Note that the dosing interval remains constant, and there is a reduction in dose with worsening renal function

Bivalirudin [26]	Coronary angioplasty: 0.75 mg/kg bolus, then 1.75 mg/kg/h × 4 h [27]: myocardial infarction undergoing PCI: 0.75 mg/kg/h, then 1.75 mg/kg/h during procedure [28]	No change	1 mg/kg/h; no bolus needed	1 mg/kg/h; no bolus needed	0.25 mg/kg/h, no bolus needed	—	Metabolic clearance may be the predominant route of elimination [29]
Capreomycin [10,30,31]	1 g/d (maximum: 20 mg/kg/d) for 60–120 d, followed by 1 g 2–3 times/wk or 15 mg/kg/d (maximum: 1 g/dose) for 2–4 mo, followed by 15 mg/kg (maximum: 1 g/dose) 2–3 times/wk	No change	12–15 mg/kg (maximum: 1 g/dose) 2–3 d/wk (**NOT** daily)	12–15 mg/kg (maximum: 1 g/dose) 2–3 d/wk (**NOT** daily)	12–15 mg/kg (maximum: 1 g/dose) 2–3 d/wk (**NOT** daily)	5 mg/kg IV q24h	
Cefazolin [11]	1–2 g IV q8h	1–2 g IV q8h	1–2 g IV q12h	1–2 g IV q24h	1–2 g IV q24h administered at the end of HD	CCVHD: 1–2 g IV q12h CVVHDF: 2 g IV q12h	—
Cefepime [11,32,33]	1–2 g IV q8–12h	1–2 g IV q12–24h	1–2 g IV q24h	0.5–1.0 g IV q24h	0.5–1.0 g IV q24h administered at the end of HD	CCVHD: 1–2 g IV q12h CVVHDF: 2 g IV q12h	Covers *Pseudomonas aeruginosa* as well as some Gram-positive organisms
Cefotaxime [11]	1–2 g IV q8h	1–2 g IV q8h	1–2 g IV q12h	1–2 g IV q24h	1–2 g IV q24h administered at the end of HD	CCVHD: 1–2 g IV q12h CVVHDF: 2 g IV q12h	—
Cefotetan [34]	1–2 g IV q12h	1–2 g IV q12h	1–2 g IV q24h	1–2 g IV q48h	1–2 g IV q48h administered at the end of HD	1–2 g IV q12h	—
Cefoxitin [35]	1–2 g IV q6–8h	1–2 g IV q8h	1–2 g IV q12h	1–2 g IV q24h	1–2 g IV q24h administered after HD	1–2 g IV q12h	
Ceftazidime [11,36,37]	2 g IV q8h	2 g IV q12h	Loading dose 2 g IV, then 0.5–1.0 g IV q24h	Loading dose 2 g IV, then 1 g IV q48h	Loading dose 2 g IV, then 1 g IV q48h administered at the end of HD	Loading dose 2 g IV, then 1–2 g IV q12h	Covers *P. aeruginosa*; has limited, if any, Gram-positive coverage
Ceftobiprole [38]	500 mg every 8–12 h	500 mg every 12 h	250 mg every 12 h	—	—	—	
Cefuroxime [10]	0.75–1.5 g IV q8h	0.75–1.5 g IV q8h	0.75–1.5 g IV q12h	0.75–1.5 g IV q24h	0.75–1.5 g IV q24h administered at the end of HD	0.75–1.5 g IV q12h	—
Chloramphenicol [10]	50–100 mg/kg/d IV in divided doses q6h (max: 4 g/d)	—	—	—	—	—	Use with caution in renal failure

(*continued*)

TABLE 74.1

CONTINUED

Drug	Normal dose	Creatinine clearance 30–50 mL/min	10–30 mL/min	<10 mL/min	Extracorporeal drug removal HD	CVVHD, CVVHDF	Notes
Cidofovir [39]	Induction: 5 mg/kg IV once weekly; Maintenance: 5 mg/kg q2 wk	Contraindicated	Contraindicated	Contraindicated	Contraindicated	Contraindicated	Administer probenecid and IV hydration with normal saline with each dose; if Scr increases by 0.3–0.4 mg/dL, decrease dose to 3 mg/kg; discontinue if Scr increases by >0.5 mg/dL
Ciprofloxacin [11,23,40,41]	400 mg IV q12h	400 mg IV q12h	400 mg IV q24h	250–500 mg PO q24h or 400 mg IV q24h	400 mg IV q24h administered at the end of HD	200–400 mg IV q12–24h	—
Clarithromycin [42]	250–500 mg PO q12h	No change	250–500 mg PO q24h	250–500 mg PO q24h	—	—	
Colistimethate [11,43]	2.5–5 mg/kg/d in 2–4 divided doses; 3–8 mg/kg/d in 3 divided doses for cystic fibrosis	Scr 1.3–1.5 mg/dL 2.5–3.8 mg/kg/d divided q12h	Scr 1.6–2.5 mg/d: 2.5 mg/kg/d divided q12–24h	Scr 2.6–4.0 mg/dL: 1.5 mg/kg/d divided q36h	1.5 mg/kg IV q24–48h	2.5 mg/kg IV q48h	CRRT dosing may be as frequent as q12h. [44]
Cycloserine [45,46]	250–500 mg PO q12h	250–500 mg PO q12h	250–500 mg PO q24h	250–500 mg PO q24h	—	—	
Daptomycin [11]	4–6 mg/kg IV q24h	4–6 mg/kg IV q24h	4–6 mg/kg IV q48h	4–6 mg/kg IV q48h	4–6 mg/kg IV q48h administered after HD	4–6 mg/kg IV q48h	
Demeclocycline [47]	150 mg PO q6h	Not recommended	Not recommended	Not recommended	Not recommended	Not recommended	
Diazepam	2–10 mg IV/IM q2–4h p.r.n.; 2–10 mg PO q6–12h p.r.n	No change	No change	No change	No change	No change	Active metabolites may accumulate in RF; doses should be titrated to patient response
Digoxin	IV 0.4–1.0 mg/d loading dose, 0.125–0.375 mg/d maintenance dose; PO 0.75–1.25 mg/d loading dose, 0.125–0.375 mg/d maintenance dose	Same loading dose IV/PO; maintenance dose 0.125–0.375 mg q24h	0.625 mg loading dose; IV/PO maintenance dose 0.125–0.375 mg q24–48h	0.625 mg loading dose; IV/PO maintenance dose 0.125–0.375 mg q48h	No supplement for HD	Normal loading dose, IV/PO maintenance dose 0.125–0.375 mg q36h	The volume of distribution of digoxin can decrease by up to 50% in patients with RF, necessitating dose adjustment

Dofetilide	500 μg PO b.i.d.; IV dose for atrial fibrillation/ flutter: 2.5–4.0 μg/kg bolus, repeat doses given 15 min later if conversion did not occur [48]	250 μg PO b.i.d. with CrCl from 40–60 mL/min	125 μg PO b.i.d. with CrCl from 20–40 mL/min	Contraindicated when CrCl <20 mL/min	Contraindicated when CrCl <20 mL/min	Contraindicated when CrCl <20 mL/min	Patients should be off amiodarone for at least 3 mo before using dofetilide; >50% of dose is excreted in urine, leading to an increased half-life in RF [49]
Doripenem [50]	500 mg IV q8h	250 mg IV q8h	250 mg IV 12 h	—	—	—	
Enoxaparin [51,52]	Prophylaxis: 30 mg SC q12h or 40 mg SC q24h; treatment: 1 mg/kg SC q12h or 1.5 mg/kg SC q24h	No change, use caution	Prophylaxis: 30 mg SC q24h; treatment: 1 mg/kg SC q24h	Prophylaxis: 30 mg SC q24h; treatment: 1 mg/kg SC q24h	No guidelines determined	No guidelines determined	Patients with renal failure are at increased risk for bleeding
Ertapenem	1 g IV q24h	1 g IV q24h	500 mg IV q24h	500 mg IV q24h	500 mg IV q24h		
Erythromycin [53]	0.5–1 g IV q6h	No change	No change	0.25–0.5 g IV q6h	0.25–0.5 g IV q6h		
Famotidine [54]	20–40 mg IV q12h	20 mg IV q12h	20 mg IV q12h	20 mg IV q24h or 40 mg IV q48h	20 mg IV q24h at the end of HD	20 mg IV q12h	—
Fluconazole [11,23,55,56]	400–800 mg IV/PO q24h	Loading dose 400–800 mg IV/PO, then 200–400 mg IV/PO q24h	Loading dose 400–800 mg IV/PO, then 100–200 mg IV/PO q24h	Loading dose 400–800 mg IV/PO, then 100–200 mg IV/PO q24h	100–400 mg IV/PO after each HD only	Loading dose 400–800 mg IV/PO, then 400–800 mg IV/PO q24h	—
Fondaparinux	DVT prophylaxis: 2.5 mg SC q24h	No change, use caution (clearance estimated to be reduced by 40%)	Contraindicated (clearance estimated to be reduced by 55%)	Contraindicated	No guidelines determined	No guidelines determined	Treatment dose not recommended for use in patients with CrCl <30 mL/min. Use of 2.5 mg SC after hemodialysis on dialysis days, with anti-Xa monitoring has been reported [57]
Foscarnet [58]	40–80 mg/kg/dose IV q8h	CrCL (mL/min/kg): >1–1.4: 30–45 mg IV q8h >0.8–1: 35–50 mg IV q12h >0.6–0.8: 25–40 mg IV q12h >0.5–0.6: 40–60 mg IV q24h >0.4–0.5: 35–50 mg IV q24h	Not recommended	Not recommended	45–60 mg/kg after each HD session	—	

(continued)

TABLE 74.1
CONTINUED

Drug	Normal dose	Creatinine clearance 30–50 mL/min	Creatinine clearance 10–30 mL/min	Creatinine clearance <10 mL/min	Extracorporeal drug removal HD	Extracorporeal drug removal CVVHD, CVVHDF	Notes
Ganciclovir [59]	Induction: 5 mg/kg IV q12h; maintenance: 5 mg/kg IV q24h	Induction: 2.5 mg/kg IV q24h; maintenance: 1.25 mg/kg IV q24h	Induction: 1.25 mg/kg IV q24h; maintenance: 0.625 mg/kg IV q24h	Induction: 1.25 mg IV 3 × wk; maintenance: 0.625 mg/kg IV 3 × wk	Induction: 1.25 mg IV 3 × wk; maintenance: 0.625 mg/kg IV 3 × wk	Induction: 1.25 mg/kg IV q24h; maintenance: 0.625 mg/kg IV q24h	Accumulation of ganciclovir occurs in renal tissue [60]
Gentamicin	Varied, depends on traditional versus large dose-extended interval dosing regimens; consult institution-specific guidelines	—	—	2 mg/kg based on lean body weight; follow levels once daily and re-dose when trough level is <2.0 μg/mL	2 mg/kg after each HD treatment	Dose based on CrCl of 25 mL/min	Trough aminoglycoside levels post-HD should be drawn 4 h after HD has stopped to allow for equilibrium
Imipenem and cilastatin [11,23,61]	500 mg IV q6h for ≥70 kg; subsequent dose adjustments are based on a total of 2 g/d (considered to be an average ICU dose); 500 mg IV q8h, 60–70 kg; 250 mg IV q6h, 50–60 kg; 250 mg IV q6h, 40–50 kg	500 mg IV q8h for ≥70 kg; 250 mg IV q6h, 60–70 kg; 250 mg IV q6h, 50–50 kg; 250 mg IV q8h, 40–50 kg	250 mg IV q6h for ≥70 kg; 250 mg IV q8h, 60–70 kg; 250 mg IV q8h, 50–60 kg; 250 mg IV q12h, 40–50 kg	250 mg IV q12h for all weights from 40 to ≥70 kg	500 mg IV q12h; administer dose after HD	500 mg IV q6–8h	Use cautiously in patients with renal impairment; adjusting dose may not be adequate to prevent seizure [62]; average time to seizure is 7 d
Lepirudin [63,64]	HIT: 0.4 mg/kg bolus, infuse at 0.15 mg/kg/h	0.2 mg/kg bolus, infuse at 0.045–0.075 mg/kg/h	0.2 mg/kg bolus, infuse at 0.0225 mg/kg/h	0.08–0.1 mg/kg bolus, monitor aPTT and rebolus when aPTT falls to 1.5 × standard	0.08–0.10 mg/kg bolus, monitor aPTT and rebolus when aPTT falls to 1.5 × standard	0.08–0.1 mg/kg bolus, follow aPTT and re-dose when aPTT falls to 1.5 × standard	Monitor aPTT closely, especially in patients with renal impairment; therapeutic range: aPTT 1.5–2.5 × normal
Levofloxacin [23,41]	500–750 mg IV/PO q24h	Loading dose 500–750 mg IV/PO × 1, then 250–500 mg IV/PO q24h	Loading dose 500–750 mg IV/PO × 1, then 250–500 mg IV/PO q48h	Loading dose 500–750 mg IV/PO × 1, then 250–500 mg IV/PO q48h	Loading dose 500–750 mg IV/PO × 1, then 250–500 mg IV/PO q48h administered at end of HD	Loading dose 500–750 mg IV/PO × 1, then 250–750 mg IV/PO q24–48h	—
Linezolid [11,23,65]	600 mg IV/PO q12h	No change	No change	No change	No change, time dose to occur after HD	No change	Metabolites may accumulate in renal failure but clinical significance is unknown [66,67]

Lorazepam	1–10 mg IV/IM q2–4h p.r.n.; 0.5–10 mg PO q4–6h p.r.n.	No change	No change	No change	No change	No change	Doses should be titrated to patient response. Use IV lorazepam with caution in patients with RF due to propylene glycol toxicity [68]
Mannitol	0.25–2 g/kg IV q4–6h	0.25 g/kg IV q6–12h	0.25 g/kg IV q8–12h	Avoid use	Avoid use	Avoid use	Maintain serum osmolarity of 290–310
Meperidine [69]	50–100 mg IV q3–4h, titrate for pain control	37.5–75 mg IV q3–4h, titrate for pain control	37.5–75 mg IV q3–4h, titrate for pain control	25–50 mg IV q3–4h, titrate for pain control	Avoid	37.5–75 mg IV q3–4h, titrate for pain control	Normeperidine, a toxic metabolite, affects the central nervous system and can lead to seizure when meperidine is used in patients with RF
Meropenem [11,23,70,71]	1 g IV q8h	1 g IV q12h	500 mg IV q12h	500 mg IV q24h	500 mg IV q24h; administer dose after HD	0.5–1 g IV q8–12h	Seizures have occurred only in patients with preexisting seizure disorder [72]
Metoclopramide	10–20 mg IV q6h	7.5–15 mg IV q6h	7.5–15 mg IV q6h	5–10 mg IV q6h	5–10 mg IV q6h, administered at the end of HD	7.5–15 mg IV q6h	—
Metronidazole [73]	250–500 mg IV/PO q8h	No change	No change	250 mg IV/PO q8h	Administer dose after HD	No change	Treatment for *Clostridium difficile* diarrhea; causes dark urine
Midazolam [17]	0.01–0.05 mg/kg (0.5–4 mg) IV load over 2–5 min, then 0.02–0.1 mg/kg/h titrated to response	No change	No change	0.5–4 mg/kg load over 2–5 min, then 0.01–0.05 mg/kg/h titrated to response	Guidelines not determined	Guidelines not determined	Prolonged infusions, especially in patients with RF, may result in prolonged sedation due to the accumulation of metabolites; doses should be titrated to patient response [74]
Milrinone [75]	50–75 μg/kg load over 10 min; 0.375–0.75 μg/kg/min infusion based on clinical response	Same load, 0.38–0.43 μg/kg/min infusion based on clinical response	Same load, 0.28–0.33 μg/kg/min infusion based on clinical response	25–50 μg/kg load over 10 min; 0.2–0.23 μg/kg/min infusion based on clinical response	No data	Use normal dose	85% of dose eliminated unchanged in urine within 24 h

(*continued*)

TABLE 74.1

CONTINUED

Drug	Normal dose	Creatinine clearance 30–50 mL/min	10–30 mL/min	<10 mL/min	Extracorporeal drug removal HD	CVVHD, CVVHDF	Notes
Morphine [76]	2–15 mg IV q2–4h, titrate for pain control	1.5–12 mg IV q2–4h, titrate for pain control	1.5–12 mg IV q2–4h, titrate for pain control	1–8 mg IV q2–4h, titrate for pain control	1–8 mg IV q2–4h, titrate for pain control	1.5–12 mg IV q2–4h, titrate for pain control	Although morphine is hepatically metabolized, dose adjustment in renal insufficiency is recommended to avoid accumulation of morphine-6-glucuronide, which may have narcotic activity [77,78]
Nadolol	40–320 mg PO qd in single or divided doses	20–160 mg PO daily in single or divided doses, or use normal dose and change interval to q24–36h	20–160 mg PO daily in single or divided doses, or use normal dose and change interval to q24–48h	10–80 mg PO daily in single or divided doses, or use normal dose and change interval to q48h	Supplement 40 mg after HD	20–160 mg q24h in single or divided doses, or use normal dose and change interval to q24–48h	Alteration of the interval instead of dose is an option [79]
Nesiritide	IV bolus of 2 μg/kg followed by a continuous infusion at a dose of 0.01 μg/kg/min; maximum dose 0.03 μg/kg/min	No change	No change	No change	No guidelines established	No guidelines established	Use if nesiritide in patients with renal insufficiency has been associated with elevations of Scr [80]
Nitroprusside [17]	0.25–10 μg/kg/min; titrate for BP control	No change	No change	No change	No change	No change	Thiocyanate, a toxic metabolite, accumulates in RF, causing seizure and coma; thiocyanate is removed via HD [81]
Norfloxacin [17]	400 mg PO q12h	No change	400 mg PO q24h	400 mg PO q24h	400 mg PO q24h	—	
Ofloxacin [82,83]	300 mg PO q12h	300 mg PO q24h	150–300 mg PO q24h	150 mg PO q24h		300 mg PO q24h	
Oseltamivir [84,85]	75–150 mg PO q12h	No change	75–150 mg PO q24h	—	30 mg after every other HD	—	Higher doses are recommended for treatment of H1N1 influenza infection [86]

Pancuronium	0.04–0.10 mg/kg load, then 0.01–0.06 mg/kg as needed to maintain paralysis	0.02–0.05 mg/kg load, then 0.01–0.03 mg/kg as needed to maintain paralysis	0.02–0.05 mg/kg load, then 0.01–0.03 mg/kg as needed to maintain paralysis	Avoid use	Guidelines not determined	Guidelines not determined	—
Penicillin G [17,23]	1–4 million units IV q4–6h; 1–2 million units for most uses, 4 million units in meningitis	0.75–3 million units IV q4–6h	0.75–3 million units IV q4–6h	0.5–2 million units IV q4–6h	0.5–2 million units IV q4–6h; supplemental doses are not needed if maintenance doses are scheduled after HD	2–4 million U IV q4–6h	—
Pentamidine [10,13]	3–4 mg/kg IV q24h	No change	No change	3–4 mg/kg IV q24–36h	3–4 mg IV q24–36h		No adjustment in renal failure has been reported [87]
Pentostatin [88]	4 mg/m² every 2 wk	2–3 mg/m² every 2 wk	2 mg/m² every 2 wk	Not recommended	—	—	
Phenobarbital	Status epilepticus: 10–20 mg/kg IV; 60–250 mg PO q24h	No change	No change	60–100 mg PO q24h	No change, dose after dialysis	—	Monitor levels closely; therapeutic range: 10–40 μg/mL
Phenytoin [89]	15 mg/kg IV load, then 200–400 mg PO/IV daily divided q8–12h	No change	No change	No change	No change	No change	Monitor levels closely. Phenytoin binding is altered in uremic patients and patients with low albumin; serum levels should be monitored accordingly
Piperacillin [90]	3–4 g IV q4–6h	3–4 g IV q6–8h	3–4 g IV q6–8h	3–4 g IV q8h	3–4 g IV q8h administered at the end of HD	3–4 g IV q6–8h	—
Piperacillin/ tazobactam [11,23,90,91]	Nosocomial pneumonia: 4.5 g IV q6h; moderate-to-severe infections: 3.375 g IV q6h	CrCl 20–40 mL/min: Nosocomial pneumonia: 3.375 g IV q6h; moderate-to-severe infections: 2.25 g IV q6h	CrCl <20 mL/min: Nosocomial pneumonia: 2.25 g IV q6h; moderate-to-severe infections: 2.25 g IV q8h	See CrCl <20 mL/min	Nosocomial pneumonia: 2.25 g IV q8h; moderate-to-severe infections: 2.25 g IV q12h	2.25–3.375 g IV q6–8h	Because HD removes 30%–40% of piperacillin/ tazobactam, give a supplementary dose of 0.75 g intravenously after dialysis
Polymyxin B [92]	15,000–25,000 units/kg/d IV divided q12h	11,250–18,750 units/kg/d IV divided q12h	7,500–12,500 units/kg/d IV divided q12h	2,250–3,750 units/kg/d divided q12h	2,250–3,750 units/kg/d divided q12h	—	
Posaconazole [93,94]	200–400 mg PO q12h	No change	No change	No change	No change	—	Monitor breakthrough fungal infections due to variability in drug exposure

(continued)

TABLE 74.1

CONTINUED

Drug	Normal dose	Creatinine clearance			Extracorporeal drug removal		Notes
		30–50 mL/min	10–30 mL/min	<10 mL/min	HD	CVVHD, CVVHDF	
Procainamide [17,95]	50–100 mg/min IV until arrhythmia is suppressed or dose reaches 500–1,000 mg, then infuse at 2–6 mg/min; oral: 500–1,000 mg PO q4–6h	500 mg PO q[illegible]h	500 mg PO q12h	500 mg PO q12–24h	500 mg PO q24h after dialysis	—	Monitor electrocardiogram, procainamide, and NAPA levels closely in renal dysfunction. Procainamide: 4–12 μg/mL; NAPA: 5–15 μg/mL [96]
Ranitidine [97]	50 mg IV q8h or 6.25 mg/h continuous infusion	50 mg IV q12–24h	50 mg IV q12–24h	50 mg IV q24h	50 mg IV q24h, administered at end of HD	50 mg IV q12h	—
Rifabutin [98,99]	300 mg PO q24h	No change	150 mg PO q24h	150 mg PO q24h	150–300 mg PO q24h	—	
Rifampin [13,77]	600 mg PO/IV q24h	300–600 mg PO/IV q24h	300–600 mg PO/IV q24h	300 mg PO/IV q24h	300–600 mg PO q24h	300–600 mg PO q24–48h	—
Sotalol [100]	80–320 mg PO q12h; start with 80 mg PO q12h	Lengthen dosing interval to q24h	Lengthen dosing interval to q36–48h, based on clinical response	Dose according to clinical response	Supplement 80 mg after HD	Lengthen dosing interval to q36–48h based on clinical response	Data suggest that HD patients need a decrease in dose and increase in interval [101]
Spironolactone [77]	25–200 mg PO q24h	12.5–100 mg PO q24h	12.5–100 mg PO q24h	Not effective	Not effective	Not effective	Use should be avoided in patients with GFRs <10 mL/min; monitor for hyperkalemia
Streptomycin [77]	1 g IM q12–24h	1 g IM q24–48h	1 g IM q48–72h	1 g IM q72–96h	1 g IM q72–96h, administer after HD	—	
Sulfamethoxazole and trimethoprim [102,103]	8–20 mg/kg/d; when IV, divided into q6h; when PO, divided q6–12h	No change	4–10 mg/kg/d; when IV or PO, divided q12h	4–10 mg/kg/d; when IV or PO, divided q12h	4–10 mg/kg/d; when IV or PO, divided q12h, administer dose after HD	4–10 mg/kg/d when IV or PO, divided q12h	Dosing values are based on the trimethoprim component
Ticarcillin/clavulanate potassium [11,23]	3.1 g IV q4–6h	2 g IV q4h	2 g IV q8h	2 g IV q12h	2 g IV q12h, administered at the end of HD	2–3.1 g IV q6–8h	Patients with CrCl <10 mL/min with hepatic dysfunction should receive 2 g IV q24h

Tinzaparin [51]	Deep venous thrombosis therapy: 175 anti-Xa IU/kg SC qd × 6 d or adequate warfarin anticoagulation is in place; deep venous thrombosis prophylaxis: 3,500 anti-Xa IU SC qd	Use with caution	Use with caution	—	—	—	Not recommended for use in patients with CrCl <30 mL/min unless monitoring anti-Xa levels [104]
Tobramycin	See gentamicin	—	—	—	—	—	—
Valacyclovir [105]	1 g PO q8h	1 g PO q12h	1 g PO q24h	500 mg PO q24h	500 mg PO q24h, administered after HD	—	—
Valganciclovir [13,59,106]	Induction: 900 mg PO q12; Maintenance: 900 mg PO q24h	I: 450 mg PO q12–24h M: 450 mg PO q24–48h	I: 450 mg PO q24–48h M: 450 mg PO q48h to 2×/wk	Not recommended	Not recommended	M: 450 mg PO q48h [107]	—
Valproic acid	10–15 mg/kg/d	No change	No change	May requite dosage adjustment; see comments	No change	No change	Do not infuse faster than 20 mg/min. With renal impairment, may see increase in free levels. Measurement of total concentration can therefore be misleading
Vancomycin [11,108,109]	Refer to institution-specific guidelines	—	—	—	1 g IV every wk, measure random vancomycin level on 4th day after dose to ensure blood levels, dose for level <10 μg/mL	7.5–15 mg/kg q12–48h	—
Voriconazole [110]	6 mg/kg IV q12h × 2 doses; follow with 4 mg/kg IV q12h	IV not recommended	IV not recommended	IV not recommended	IV not recommended	IV not recommended	IV formulation not recommended in CrCL <50 mL/min; accumulation of the intravenous vehicle (cyclodextrin) can occur
Ziprasidone [111]	40–80 mg PO q12h; 10 mg IM q24h	No change for PO. Caution with IM use	No change for PO. Caution with IM use	No change for PO. Caution with IM use	—	—	Injection form contains cyclodextrin sodium that is renally eliminated. Caution recommended with IM use in renal impairment

aPTT, activated partial thromboplastin time; b.i.d., twice daily; CrCl, creatine clearance; CVVDH, continuous venovenous hemodialysis; CVVHDF, continuous venovenous hemodiafiltration; DVT, deep vein thrombosis; ESRD, end-stage renal disease; GFR, glomerular filtration rate; HD, hemodialysis; ICU, intensive care unit; IM, intramuscularly; IV, intravenous; NAPA, *N*-acetyl procainamide; PO, by mouth; p.r.n., as needed; q, every, t.i.d., three times a day; RF, renal failure; SC, subcutaneously; Scr, serum creatinine.

TABLE 74.2

GUIDELINES FOR DRUG DOSING IN CRITICALLY ILL PATIENTS WITH HEPATIC FAILURE

Drug	Normal dose	Child-Pugh score A (mild)	Child-Pugh score B (moderate)	Child-Pugh score C (severe)	Special circumstances/notes
Abacavir [112]	300 mg PO q12h OR 600 mg PO q24h	200 mg PO q12h	Use is contraindicated	Use is contraindicated	
Alprazolam [113]	0.25–1 mg PO 2–3 times a d Max: 4 mg/d				Hepatic impairment: reduce dose by 50%–60%; avoid in cirrhosis
Amlodipine [114,115]	Usual dose: 5–10 mg PO q24h				Hypertension: initial dose 2.5 mg PO q24h; angina: initial dose 5 mg PO q24h
Argatroban [116]	HIT/HITTS: initial dose: 2 μg/kg/min; PCI: initial dose: 25 μg/kg/min and administer bolus dose of 350 μg/kg; Cerebral thrombus: 60 mg/d by continuous infusion for 2 d, followed by 10 mg IV twice daily for 5 d. Myocardial infarction: 100 μg/kg IV bolus followed by 2–3 μg/kg/min infusion for 6–72 h.		HIT/HITTS: initial dose: 0.5 mcg/kg/min		During PCI, avoid use in patients with elevations of ALT/AST (>3 times ULN); the use of argatroban in these patients has not been evaluated.
Aspirin [117,118]	81–325 mg PO q24h			Avoid use	
Carvedilol [119,120]	Hypertension: 6.25–25 mg PO q12h; heart failure: 3.125–50 mg PO q12h			Use is contraindicated	Extended release is contraindicated in hepatic impairment; liver impairment with cirrhosis: reduce dose by 20%
Caspofungin [121]	Candidiasis, Aspergillosis (invasive): initial dose: 70 mg IV on day 1; subsequent dosing: 50 mg IV q24h	No adjustment necessary	Initial: 70 mg IV loading dose, then 35 mg IV q24h	No clinical experience	
Colchicine [122]	Acute attacks: PO: 0.5–1.2 mg, followed by 0.6 mg PO every 1–2 h to a max of 6 mg; IV: 1–2 mg then 0.5 mg every 6 h to a max of 4 mg				Dosage adjustment should be considered in severe hepatic impairment. Treatment course should not be repeated more than once in a 2-wk period.
Cyclobenzaprine [123]	5–10 mg PO q8h	Initial: 5 mg PO; use with caution and consider less frequent dosing	Use not recommended	Use not recommended	Mild-severe impairment: not recommended for extended release formulation
Cytarabine [124–126]	Remission induction: *IV*: 100–200 mg/m²/d for 5–10 d or 100 mg/m²/d for 7 d or 100 mg/m²/dose every 12 h for 7 d; *IT*: 5–75 mg/m² q2–7 d until CNS findings normalize; Remission maintenance: *IV*: 70–200 mg/m²/d for 2–5 d at monthly intervals; *IM, SubQ*: 1–1.5 mg/kg single dose for maintenance at 1- to 4-wk intervals				AST/ALT (any elevation): administer 50% of dose; TBili >2 mg/dL: administer 50% of dose

Daunorubicin [124,127]	Range: 30–60 mg/m^2/d for 3 d, repeat dose in 3–4 wk; ALL combination therapy: 45 mg/m^2/d for 3 d; AML combination therapy (induction): adults <60 y: induction: 45 mg/m^2/d for 3 d of the first course of induction therapy; subsequent courses: 45 mg/m^2/d for 2 d				TBili 1.2–3 mg/dL: administer 75% of dose; serum TBili >3 mg/dL: administer 50% of dose; serum TBili >5 mg/dL: avoid use.
Diazepam [128,129]	2.5–10 mg PO 2–4 times a day ICU sedation: 0.05–0.1 mg/kg IV every 30 min to 6 h; Status epilepticus: IV 5–10 mg every 5–10 min, max of 30 mg				Patients with cirrhosis: reduce dose by 50%
Docetaxel [124,130]	Breast cancer: *locally advanced or metastatic:* 60–100 mg/m^2 every 3 wk; *operable, node-positive:* 75 mg/m^2 every 3 wk for 6 courses; non-small cell lung cancer: 75 mg/m^2 every 3 wk; prostate cancer: 75 mg/m^2 every 3 wk; Gastric adenocarcinoma: 75 mg/m^2 every 3 wk; head and neck cancer: 75 mg/m^2 every 3 wk for 3 or 4 cycles				TBili >ULN, or AST and/or ALT >1.5 times ULN concomitant with ALK >2.5 times ULN: should not be administered; hepatic impairment dosing adjustment specific for gastric adenocarcinoma: *AST/ALT >2.5 to ≤5 times ULN and alkaline phosphatase ≤2.5 times ULN:* administer 80% of dose *AST/ALT >1.5 to ≤5 times ULN and alkaline phosphatase >2.5 to ≤5 times ULN:* administer 80% of dose *AST/ALT >5 times ULN and/or alkaline phosphatase >5 times ULN:* discontinue docetaxel; AST/ALT 1.6–6 times ULN: administer 75% of dose; AST/ALT >6 times ULN: use clinical judgment
Doxorubicin [124,131]	60–75 mg/m^2/dose q21 d or 60 mg/m^2/dose q2 wk or 40–60 mg/m^2/dose q3–4 wk or 20–30 mg/m^2/d for 2–3 d every 4 wk or 20 mg/m^2/dose once weekly				TBili 1.2–3 mg/dL: administer 50% of dose; 3.1–5 mg/dL: administer 25% of dose; severe hepatic impairment: use is contraindicated; AST/ALT 2–3 times ULN: administer 75% of dose; AST/ALT >3 times ULN or TBili 1.2–3 mg/dL: administer 50% of dose; TBili 3.1–5 mg/dL: administer 25% of dose; TBili >5 mg/dL: do not administer
Epirubicin [132,133]	Breast cancer: *CEF-120:* 60 mg/m^2 on days 1 and 8 q28 d for 6 cycles; *FEC-100:* 100 mg/m^2 on day 1 q21 d for 6 cycles				TBili 1.2–3 mg/dL or AST 2–4 times the ULN: administer 50% of recommended starting dose; TBili >3 mg/dL or AST >4 times the ULN: administer 25% of recommended starting dose; severe hepatic impairment: use is contraindicated
Esomeprazole [134,135]	20–40 mg PO/IV 1–2 times a day	No adjustment necessary	No adjustment necessary	Do not exceed 20 mg IV/PO q24h	

(continued)

TABLE 74.2

CONTINUED

Drug	Normal dose	Child-Pugh score A (mild)	Child-Pugh score B (moderate)	Child-Pugh score C (severe)	Special circumstances/notes
Etoposide [124,125, 136,137]	Small cell lung cancer: IV: 35 $mg/m^2/d$ for 4 d or 50 $mg/m^2/d$ for 5 d every 3–4 wk; IVPB: 60–100 $mg/m^2/d$ for 3 d; CIV: 500 mg/m^2 over 24 h every 3 wk; Testicular cancer: IVPB: 50–100 $mg/m^2/d$ for 5 d repeated every 3–4 wk; IV: 100 mg/m^2 every other day for 3 doses repeated every 3–4 wk; BMT/relapsed leukemia: IV: 2.4–3.5 g/m^2 or 25–70 mg/kg administered over 4–36 h				TBili 1.5–3 mg/dL or AST >3 times ULN: administer 50% of dose; TBili 1.5–3 mg/dL or ALT or AST >180 units/L: administer 50% of dose; TBili 1.5–3 mg/dL or AST 60–180 units/L: administer 50% of dose; TBili >3 mg/dL or AST >180 units/L: avoid use
Ezetimibe [138]	10 mg PO q24h	No adjustments necessary	Not recommended	Not recommended	
Fluorouracil [124,125]	*IV bolus:* 500–600 mg/m^2 every 3–4 wk or 425 mg/m^2 on days 1–5 every 4 wk; *continuous IV infusion:* 1,000 $mg/m^2/d$ for 4–5 d every 3–4 wk or 2,300–2,600 mg/m^2 on day 1 every wk or 300–400 $mg/m^2/d$ or 225 $mg/m^2/d$ for 5–8 wk				TBili >5 mg/dL: avoid use; TBili <5 mg/dL: administer 100% of dose
Glipizide [139]	*Immediate release:* 2.5–20 mg PO 1–2 times a day; *Extended release:* 5–20 mg PO q24h				Initial: 2.5 mg PO q24h
Glyburide [140]	*Immediate release:* 1.25–20 mg PO 1–2 times a day. Max 20 mg/day; *Micronized tablets*: 0.75–12 mg PO q24h	No adjustments necessary	No adjustment necessary	Avoid use	
Idarubicin [141,142]	Leukemia: *IV:* induction: 12 $mg/m^2/d$ for 3 d consolidation: 10–12 $mg/m^2/d$ for 2 d; stem cell transplantation: *IV:* 20 $mg/m^2/24$ h continuous IV infusion or 21 $mg/m^2/24$ h continuous infusion for 48 h				TBili >5 mg/dL: should not be administered
Ifosfamide [124,143]	Antineoplastic: testicular cancer: 1,200 $mg/m^2/d$ for 5 d every 3 wk; Dose ranges used in other cancers: 4,000–5,000 $mg/m^2/d$ for 1 d every 14–28 d or 1,000–3,000 $mg/m^2/d$ for 2–5 d every 21–28 d				TBili >3 mg/dL: administer 25% of dose
Imatinib [144,145]	400–800 mg PO daily	No adjustments necessary	No adjustments necessary	Reduce dose by 25%	TBili >3 times ULN or AST/ALT >5 times ULN occur, withhold treatment until TBili <1.5 times ULN and AST/ALT <2.5 times ULN: resume treatment at a reduced dose as follows: Adults: if current dose 400 mg, reduce dose to 300 mg; if current dose 600 mg, reduce dose to 400 mg; if current dose 800 mg, reduce dose to 600 mg

Lamotrigine [146]	25–375 mg PO daily in 2 divided doses	No adjustment necessary	Without ascites: initial, escalation and maintenance: decrease by 25%; With ascites: initial, escalation and maintenance: decrease by 50%		
Losartan [147]	25–100 mg PO q24h				Reduce initial dose to 25 mg PO q24h
Methadone [148]	2.5–40 mg PO/IV q24h	No adjustment necessary	No adjustment necessary	Avoid use	
Naltrexone [149]	25–50 mg PO q24h	No adjustment necessary	No adjustment necessary	Use with caution	
Nicardipine [150]	*IV*: initial: 5 mg/h increased by 2.5 mg/h every 15 min to a maximum of 15 mg/h; consider reduction to 3 mg/h after response is achieved; *immediate release*: 20–40 PO q8h; *sustained release*: 30–60 mg PO q12h				*Immediate release:* starting dose: 20 mg PO q12h with titration; *sustained release:* no initial dose adjustment necessary
Nimodipine [151]	60 mg PO every 4 h				Liver failure: reduce dosage to 30 mg PO every 4 h.
Paclitaxel [152]	Ovarian carcinoma: *IV*: 135–175 mg/m^2 over 3 h every 3 wk or 135 mg/m^2 over 24 h every 3 wk or 50–80 mg/m^2 over 1–3 h weekly or 1.4–4 mg/m^2/d continuous infusion for 14 d every 4 wk; *intraperitoneal*: 60 mg/m^2 on d 8 of a 21-d treatment cycle for 6 cycles; metastatic breast cancer: 175–250 mg/m^2 over 3 h every 3 wk or 50–80 mg/m^2 weekly or 1.4–4 mg/m^2/d continuous infusion for 14 d every 4 wk; non-small cell lung carcinoma: 135 mg/m^2 over 24 h every 3 wk; AIDS-related Kaposi's sarcoma: 135 mg/m^2 over 3 h every 3 wk or 100 mg/m^2 over 3 h every 2 wk				24-h infusion: *AST/ALT <2 times ULN and TBili level ≤1.5 mg/dL:* 135 mg/m^2 *AST/ALT 2 to <10 times ULN and TBili level ≤1.5 mg/dL:* 100 mg/m^2 *AST/ALT <10 times ULN and TBili level 1.6–7.5 mg/dL:* 50 mg/m^2 *AST/ALT ≥10 times ULN or TBili level >7.5 mg/dL:* avoid use; 3-h infusion: *AST/ALT <10 times ULN and TBili level ≤1.25 times ULN:* 175 mg/m^2 *AST/ALT <10 times ULN and TBili level 1.26–2 times ULN:* 135 mg/m^2 *AST/ALT <10 times ULN and TBili level 2.01–5 times ULN:* 90 mg/m^2 *AST/ALT ≥10 times ULN or TBili level >5 times ULN:* avoid use
Paroxetine [153–156]	10–60 mg PO q24h				*Paxil®, Pexeva®:* initial: 10 mg PO q24h; maximum dose: 40 mg/day; *Paxil CR®:* initial: 12.5 mg PO q24h; maximum dose: 50 mg/d

(*continued*)

TABLE 74.2

CONTINUED

Drug	Normal dose	Child-Pugh score A (mild)	Child-Pugh score B (moderate)	Child-Pugh score C (severe)	Special circumstances/notes
Procainamide [157]	*Immediate release formulation:* 250–500 mg/dose PO every 3–6 h; *extended release formulation:* 500 mg to 1 g PO every 6 h; *Procanbid®:* 1,000–2,500 mg PO every 12 h; *IV*: loading dose: 15–18 mg/kg administered as slow infusion over 25–30 min or 100–200 mg/dose repeated every 5 min as needed to a total dose of 1 g. Maintenance dose: 1–4 mg/min by continuous infusion				Liver impairment: reduce dose by 50%
Quetiapine [158,159]	*Immediate release:* 25–50 mg PO 2–3 times a day. Max dose of 800 mg/d; *extended release*: 50–300 mg PO q24h. Max dose 800 mg/d				*Immediate release*: initial: 25 mg PO q24h; *extended release:* initial: 50 mg PO q24h
Risperidone [160]	1–6 mg PO q24h; 12.5–50 mg IM every 2 wk				Initial dose of 0.5 mg PO q12h; initial dose of 12.5 mg IM
Sirolimus [161,162]	Low-to-moderate immunologic risk renal transplant patients: *Oral:* <40 kg: loading dose: 3 mg/m^2 on day 1, followed by maintenance dosing of 1 mg/m^2 once daily ≥40 kg: loading dose: 6 mg on day 1; maintenance: 2 mg once daily; high immunologic risk renal transplant patients: *Oral:* loading dose: up to 15 mg on day 1; maintenance: 5 mg/d; obtain trough concentration between days 5 and 7 and adjust accordingly	Reduce dose by 33%	Reduce dose by 33%	Reduce dose by 50%	
Tigecycline [163]	Load: 100 mg IV followed by 50 mg IV every 12 h	No adjustment necessary	No adjustment necessary	Load: 100 mg IV followed by 25 mg IV every 12 h	
Tramadol [164,165]	*Immediate release formulation:* 50–100 mg PO every 4–6 h (not to exceed 400 mg/d) *Ultram® ER:* patients not currently on immediate release: 100 mg PO q24h (maximum: 300 mg/d)			*Extended release:* should not be administered	Hepatic impairment with cirrhosis: *Immediate release:* Recommended dose: 50 mg PO q12h; *Ryzolt*™ should not be used in any degree of hepatic impairment
Triazolam [166]	0.125–0.5 mg PO at bedtime	No adjustment necessary	No adjustment necessary	0.125 mg PO at bedtime	Avoid use in cirrhosis

Vinblastine [124,167]	Antineoplastic (typical dosages): *IV*: initial: 3.7 mg/m^2; adjust dose every 7 d up to 5.5 mg/m^2 (second dose); 7.4 mg/m^2 (third dose); 9.25 mg/m^2 (fourth dose); and 11.1 mg/m^2 (fifth dose). Usual range: 5.5–7.4 mg/m^2 every 7 d; maximum dose: 18.5 mg/m^2; Hodgkin's disease: usual dose: 6 mg/m^2 every 2 wk; testicular cancer: usual dose: 0.11 mg/kg daily for 2 d every 3 wk or 6 mg/m^2/d for 2 d every 3–4 wk; Bladder cancer: 3 mg/m^2 every 7 d for 3 out of 4 wk or 3 mg/m^2 days 2, 15, and 22 of a 28-d treatment cycle; melanoma: 2 mg/m^2 days 1–4 and 22–25 of a 6-wk treatment cycle; non-small cell lung cancer: 4 mg/m^2 d 1, 8, 15, 22, and 29, then every 2 wk; ovarian cancer: 0.11 mg/kg daily for 2 d every 3 wk; prostate cancer: 4 mg/m^2 every wk for 6 wk of an 8-wk treatment cycle				TBili >3 mg/dL: administer 50% of dose; TBili >3.1 or AST/ALT >3 times ULN: avoid use; TBili 1.5–3 mg/dL or AST 60–180 units: administer 50% of dose; TBili 3–5 mg/dL: administer 25% of dose; TBili >5 mg/dL or AST >180 units: avoid use
Vinorelbine [168]	Non-small cell lung cancer: Single-agent therapy: 30 mg/m^2/dose every 7 d Combination therapy with cisplatin: 25–30 mg/m^2/dose every 7 d; breast cancer: 25 mg/m^2/dose every 7 d; cervical cancer: 30 mg/m^2/dose days 1 and 8 of a 21-d treatment cycle; Ovarian cancer: 25 mg/m^2/dose every 7 d or 30 mg/m^2/dose days 1 and 8 of a 21-d treatment cycle				TBili ≤2 mg/dL: administer 100% of dose; TBili 2.1–3 mg/dL: administer 50% of dose; TBili >3 mg/dL: administer 25% of dose
Voriconazole [110]	100–200 mg PO every 12 h IV: Load: 6 mg/kg every 12 h for 2 doses followed by 3–4 mg/kg every 12 h	Reduce dose by 50%	Reduce dose by 50%	Should only use if benefits outweighs risks	
Zolpidem [169]	*Ambien®*: 10 mg PO immediately before bedtime; maximum dose: 10 mg; *Ambien CR®*: 12.5 mg PO immediately before bedtime				Hepatic impairment: Ambien®: 5 mg PO at bedtime; Ambien CR®: 6.25 mg PO at bedtime

b.i.d., twice daily; HIT, heparin-induced thrombocytopenia; HITTS, heparin-induced thrombotic thrombocytopenia syndrome; IM, intramuscularly; IV, intravenous; PCI, percutaneous coronary intervention; PO, by mouth; q, every; SC, subcutaneously; TBili, total bilirubin; t.i.d., three times a day; ULN, upper limits of normal.

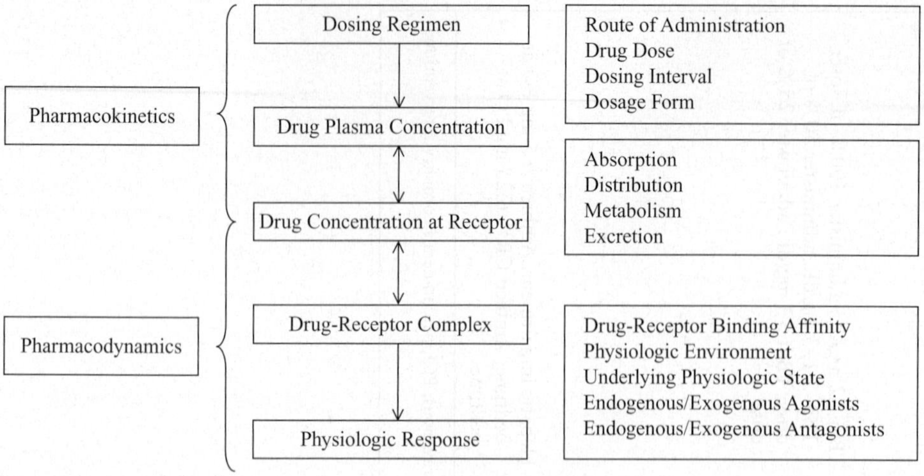

FIGURE 74.1. The relationship between pharmacokinetics and pharmacodynamics. [Adapted from Chernow B (ed): *Critical Care Pharmacotherapy*. Baltimore, MD, Williams & Wilkins, 1995, p 4.]

of achieving equilibrium between the central and peripheral compartments. When monitoring serum drug concentrations, it is important to sample after the distribution phase is complete to avoid making decisions based on falsely elevated drug levels. The *beta* (or *elimination*) *phase* describes the section of the graph once distribution is completed. This phase represents drug elimination from the central compartment. The elimination rate constant (K_{el}) is obtained by calculating the slope of the line during the elimination phase, and it can be used to calculate a drug's half-life ($t_{1/2}$).

Some drugs, such as phenytoin, follow zero-order or nonlinear kinetics. *Zero-order*, or *Michaelis-Menten pharmacokinetics*, refers to removal of a constant quantity of drug per unit of time. As the plasma concentration of the drug decreases or increases, the amount eliminated remains the same. This is the result of metabolism by a saturated enzyme system capable of eliminating drug only at a constant rate, regardless of the serum concentration. Clinically, this means small increases in the drug's dose can lead to large increases in the plasma concentration; hence, the term *nonlinear pharmacokinetics* (Fig. 74.2).

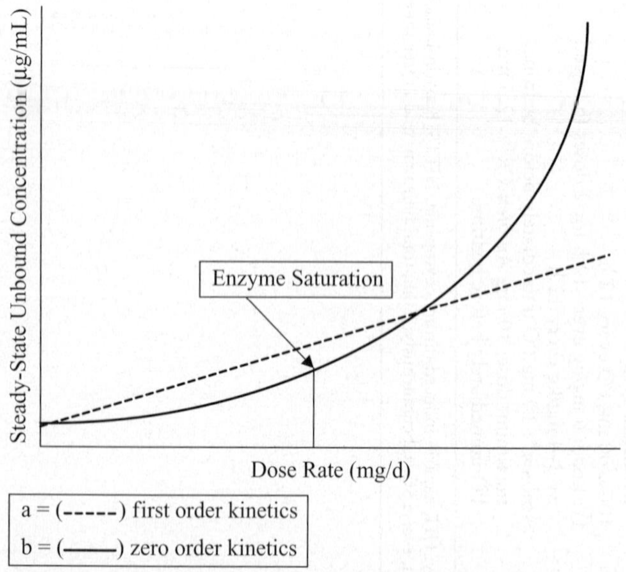

FIGURE 74.2. The effect of increasing daily dose on average steady-state drug concentrations for drugs undergoing nonlinear or zero-order pharmacokinetic modeling is shown in this figure by the *solid line*. The effect of increasing daily dose on average steady-state drug concentrations for drugs undergoing linear or first-order pharmacokinetic modeling is shown by the *dotted line*.

PHARMACOKINETIC TERMINOLOGY

The half-life of a medication is defined as the amount of time required for the concentration of the drug to decrease by 50% and is a function of drug metabolism and elimination. The half-life of a specific drug remains constant provided that the metabolizing and eliminating processes remain constant. If a patient's renal or hepatic function declines, the half-life of the drug can be significantly prolonged.

The half-life of a medication can be used to determine the time required for a drug to reach steady state. Steady state is achieved when the amount of drug entering the body equals the amount eliminated, so plasma drug levels no longer increase. Steady-state conditions are achieved at a time approximately equal to four half-lives. A clinician should generally wait for steady state to be achieved before obtaining a drug serum

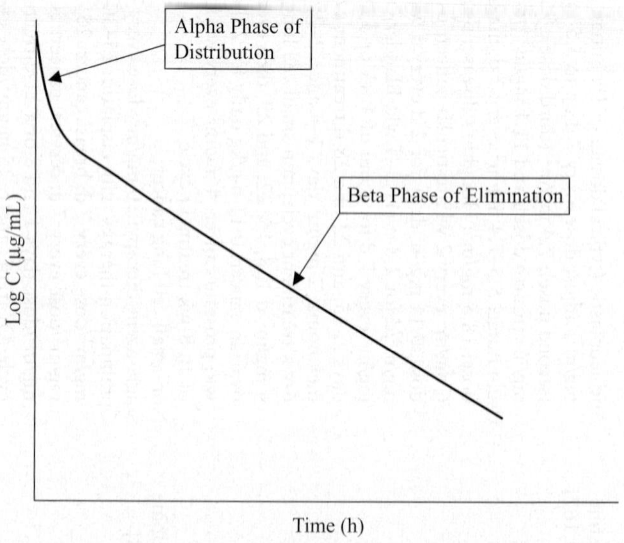

FIGURE 74.3. Logarithm of plasma concentration (Cp) versus time plot for a drug after rapid intravenous injection, delineating the alpha distribution and beta elimination phases.

concentration or changing medication dose. Knowledge of a drug's half-life may help estimate how long it should take for a pharmacologic or toxic effect to wear off. It is also important to be aware, however, that certain drugs (e.g., azithromycin) may be pharmacologically active longer than would be predicted from serum concentrations.

The rate of drug elimination from the body is described as the K_{el}. With first-order elimination, a constant percentage of drug is removed from the plasma per unit of time and is often expressed as minutes^{-1} or hours^{-1}. The K_{el} is also inversely proportional to the drug's half-life. A drug's K_{el} and half-life are constants and do not change unless the metabolizing or eliminating processes (or both) change.

Volume of distribution is not a physiologic volume but rather a theoretical volume that relates the plasma concentration to the administered dose. It is easiest to explain the concept of volume of distribution by providing an example. If a 700-mg dose of a drug administered as an intravenous bolus to 70-kg patient results in a calculated maximum plasma concentration of 7 mg per L, it appears as if the drug is dissolved in 100 L of fluid. The volume of distribution would be 100 L or 1.429 L per kg. Under normal physiologic conditions, however, a 70-kg adult does not have 100 L of body fluid. A large volume of distribution means that the amount of drug available to be measured in the plasma is reduced due to distribution among peripheral compartments or binding to plasma proteins. Medications that are hydrophilic and remain in the central (vascular) compartment, and without high affinity for plasma protein binding, tend to have a lower volume of distribution with a value that is closer to the intravascular volume. Drugs that are highly lipophilic and distribute to peripheral tissues, or are highly plasma protein bound, tend to have a very large volume of distribution.

Clearance describes the volume of fluid cleared of drug over time. Clearance through an organ is determined by the product of blood flow to the organ and the extraction ratio for the organ. The *extraction ratio* is the percentage of medication removed from the blood as it passes through the eliminating organ: It depends not only on the blood flow rate but also on the free fraction of drug and the intrinsic ability of the organ to eliminate drug.

Changes in blood flow to the organ responsible for clearing the drug or any factor altering the extraction ratio of a drug can alter a drug's clearance. For example, a patient experiencing septic or cardiogenic shock may have impaired blood flow to the liver or kidneys, hampering the clearance of a particular drug. In addition, if a pharmacologic vasopressor is added to the therapy, blood flow to the gastrointestinal tract may be compromised, resulting in a decreased absorption and transport of drug to the site of action.

RENAL DRUG EXCRETION

The primary organ of drug and drug metabolite clearance is the kidney. There are three major processes involved in renal drug clearance: glomerular filtration, tubular secretion, and tubular reabsorption. Both critical illness and renal dysfunction can alter any of these pathways individually or in combination. Studies evaluating the effect of renal impairment on drug elimination typically examine changes in total body clearance or serum concentration, since it is difficult to determine the specific impact on each pathway individually if multiple clearance routes are affected simultaneously.

Glomerular filtration is the most common pathway of renal medication excretion. The glomerular filtration rate (GFR) for an average healthy adult is between 100 and 125 mL per minute and represents approximately 20% of total plasma flow to the kidneys. Many physiologic factors affect glomerular filtration, including hydrostatic pressure and osmotic gradients. For drugs whose primary route of elimination is glomerular filtration, excretion occurs at a rate that is directly proportional to GFR (first-order process). The degree of plasma protein binding also affects filtration because only unbound drug is sufficiently small in size to be filtered across the glomerular capillaries. To estimate the possible impact of decreased filtration, it is important for the clinician to be aware of the fraction of renal drug elimination, in addition to the excretion method for any active or toxic metabolite.

Tubular secretion refers to the active process of drug transport from the interstitial fluid surrounding the proximal tubule into the tubule's lumen. The secretion rate depends on the intrinsic activity of the transporter, proximal tubule blood flow, and the percent of free or unbound drug. Tubular secretion can be an extremely efficient process with drug clearance rates exceeding filtration clearance [170]. Impaired renal function impacts tubular secretion because endogenous and exogenous organic acids and bases accumulate and compete for the transporters required for active secretion. It is difficult to predict if secretion will be increased or diminished, which may ultimately lead to drug toxicity or reduced efficacy [171].

Tubular reabsorption of drugs can be active or passive. Most of the ultrafiltrate passing through the nephron is reabsorbed. As the volume of fluid in the tubule decreases with this massive reabsorption, there can be a dramatic increase in drug concentration in the tubule, which promotes passive diffusion from inside the tubule into the plasma. Manipulation of urine pH can be used to decrease drug reabsorption and, therefore, increase excretion. Urine alkalization enhances the elimination of weak acids (e.g., barbiturates) by increasing the fraction of ionized drug.

PHARMACOKINETIC CHANGES IN CRITICALLY ILL PATIENTS WITH RENAL DYSFUNCTION

The pharmacokinetics of drugs used in critically ill patients can be altered as a function of the many dynamic physiologic changes that occur. Studies examining the pharmacokinetics of drugs used in the critically ill patient population are limited; most are performed in healthy volunteers or in relatively stable patients with a specific disease state. Patients with chronic kidney disease take multiple medications, and thus have an inherently increased risk of drug interactions, particularly in the context of altered pharmacokinetics associated with worsening renal dysfunction and critical illness. The next section of this chapter addresses some of the known pharmacokinetic changes and drug interactions that may occur in critically ill patients with renal impairment.

Absorption

Drug absorption in patients with renal dysfunction may be altered for many reasons. Gastrointestinal edema, nausea and vomiting due to uremia, and delayed gastric emptying all affect drug absorption in this patient population. In addition, patients may have comorbidities that contribute to changes in drug absorption, such as diabetic gastroparesis, diarrhea, and cardiovascular failure. Patients with chronic kidney disease and diabetic gastroparesis often are prescribed prokinetic agents (e.g., metoclopramide or erythromycin). The use of these agents may decrease enteral absorption of medications due to decreased gastric transit time, leading to decreased therapeutic effect or delayed onset of action [172]. Patients requiring phosphate-binding medications or antacids (aluminum or calcium salts) are at risk for having these medications chelate or bind to other medications and decrease their absorption. To minimize chelation, certain medications administered enterally, such as ciprofloxacin, need to be spaced around the dosing of antacid/phosphate binders by at least 2 hours [173]. Changes in gastric pH from antacids or other acid-suppressing medications may impair the dissolution process of other enteral medications, leading to incomplete drug absorption. Bioavailability studies are lacking in critically ill patients, as most are conducted in healthy adults. In a majority of medications, however, the bioavailability in patients with impaired renal function is unchanged or increased [174].

Distribution

The distribution of drugs with high affinity for plasma protein binding can be significantly altered in critically ill patients with renal failure. Highly protein-bound drugs exist in a state of equilibrium between unbound (free) and bound drug (not free). Only the unbound drug is pharmacologically active. This means that if binding decreases, the amount of free drug available to exert a pharmacologic and toxic effect increases. Drug–drug interactions can occur when two highly plasma protein–bound drugs (>90% bound to plasma proteins) compete for the same plasma protein. If drugs such as warfarin, phenytoin, valproic acid, and salicylates (all highly bound to albumin) are administered together, displacement-mediated drug interactions may occur [175]. Drug-binding interactions also occur in patients with poor renal function due to changes in the configuration of albumin [176,177]. For example, the pharmacodynamic effects of phenytoin and warfarin are increased in patients with renal failure due to changes in albumin.

Critically ill patients often have reduced albumin levels due to malnutrition or the metabolic stress of acute illness (or both), and this can lead to higher free fractions of drugs and potentially increase the risk of toxicity. If a patient taking warfarin rapidly develops hypoalbuminemia due to critical illness, the result is an increased availability of free drug, resulting in an elevated international normalized ratio and potential risk for bleeding.

The volume of distribution for drugs administered to critically ill patients with renal failure can fluctuate considerably as fluid status changes. This can affect the clearance of drugs, and also protein binding, by altering the amount of free drug available to be metabolized, eliminated, or both. Although it is very difficult, if not impossible, to predict these changes in drug distribution, it is important for the clinician to be aware of the risks and monitor for the signs of efficacy and toxicity so that the interactions are recognized and corrected.

Metabolism

The kidneys also actively metabolize medications, and impaired renal function can affect both renal and hepatic drug metabolism. Therefore, clinicians must potentially adjust drug dosages to account for diminished renal metabolism as well as decreased renal elimination [178,179]. Drugs that are oxidized by the cytochrome P450 2D6 isoenzyme are more likely affected than those metabolized by other isoenzymes [180]. The clinical significance of these effects in critically ill patients with renal disease remains to be determined and the true relevance is difficult to define, since critically ill patients often have impaired metabolic function from nonrenal causes, including hepatic damage, diminished hepatic blood flow (shock, elderly), and use of medications that act as enzyme inhibitors or inducers.

Elimination

Determining drug elimination in the critically ill patient population is challenging for many reasons. First, the majority of the studies to determine drug pharmacology and clearance are performed in critically ill patients undergoing anesthesia or in patients with chronic diseases limited to a single organ system. It is difficult to apply these data to a critically ill patient with unstable, multiple organ dysfunction. In addition, critically ill patients each have a unique combination of factors (i.e., liver failure, hemodynamic instability, malnutrition) that can affect renal drug clearance.

AKI is often accompanied by metabolic acidosis and respiratory alkalosis, which may affect the ionization of drug molecules and, therefore, affect tissue redistribution and clearance. A low serum albumin is often associated with AKI and can lead to an increase in filtration of free drug and increased clearance of drugs that are normally highly plasma protein bound.

Dysfunction of other organ systems can significantly alter renal drug clearance through various mechanisms. For example, low cardiac output from a cardiomyopathy or acute myocardial infarction or shunting of blood away from the kidney to the heart, brain, and muscle secondary to increased sympathetic nerve activity can lower renal perfusion. Both of these mechanisms decrease drug delivery to the glomeruli, thus reducing the clearance of drugs that are eliminated primarily by glomerular filtration. Retention of fluid may increase a drug's volume of distribution and further reduce drug clearance. States of profound vasodilation, such as sepsis, systemic inflammatory response syndrome, pancreatitis, and liver failure, may impair renal drug elimination by decreasing GFR. Patients with mechanical ventilation may have reduced cardiac output (due to increased mean intrathoracic pressure), volume of distribution changes, and acid–base imbalance, which can affect renal drug disposition.

ASSESSING RENAL FUNCTION

Assessment of kidney function in a critically ill patient is challenging but essential for appropriately dosing renally eliminated medications. There are many equations available to clinicians to estimate GFR. The Cockroft-Gault equation is the most commonly used in the clinical and research settings. The Cockroft-Gault equation generally overestimates the true GFR, thus appropriate clinical judgment should be exercised. The Modification of Diet in Renal Disease (MDRD) study equation is an alternative method and is the preferred equation for patients with chronic kidney disease [181]. Depending on the equation used to estimate GFR, discordance rates of between 12% and 36% of dose adjustment recommendations can be observed [182–184]. The clinician should be aware of the potential limitations of the currently available methods of GFR estimation and use clinical judgment to assess the level of renal function to use the medication dosage guidelines in Table 74.1 appropriately. A more detailed discussion regarding the assessment of renal function can be found in Chapter 73.

DIALYSIS

The clinician must often make decisions on medication dose adjustments for patients on renal replacement therapy despite a paucity of available information. It is therefore important to consider the dialysis system and drug characteristics that affect drug clearance, in addition to the degree, if any, of residual renal function. Detailed information regarding the many individual factors that must be considered to estimate dialysis drug clearance is discussed elsewhere [185,186]. Postdialysis replacement doses are usually necessary if clearance is particularly efficient, or residual renal function is significant. In Table 74.1, dosing information for hemodialysis, continuous venovenous hemofiltration, and continuous venovenous hemodiafiltration is provided. Drug dosing in peritoneal dialysis is not included because it is not commonly used in critically ill patients. Drug dosing recommendations with newer forms of dialysis such as slow low-efficiency dialysis, sustained low-efficiency daily dialysis, and extended daily dialysis are not included due to the limited availability of data.

Drug level monitoring may be useful for medications with established correlation between serum levels and drug efficacy or toxicity. Peak levels are usually drawn 1 to 2 hours after oral drug administration and approximately 30 minutes after parenteral administration to allow an appropriate period of time for tissue redistribution (alpha phase). Peak levels are usually monitored 4 hours postdialysis for drugs with a high volume of distribution (e.g., digoxin) because tissue penetration of these medications is more extensive and therefore less of these drugs are available in the blood to be cleared by dialysis. As a result, the intercompartmental re-equilibration postdialysis takes longer, so measurement of the level must be delayed to ensure an accurate result. Additional information regarding dialysis can be found in Chapter 75.

PHARMACOKINETIC CHANGES IN CRITICALLY ILL PATIENTS WITH HEPATIC FAILURE

Similar to renal disease, liver disease has the potential to significantly alter the pharmacokinetics of many drugs used in critically ill patients. Again, like renal dysfunction, liver dysfunction may alter the absorption, distribution, metabolism, and elimination of a drug. Unfortunately, there are limited data to help clinicians assess the impact of liver dysfunction on drug metabolism and facilitate appropriate dosage adjustments. For this reason, it is imperative for clinicians practicing in an ICU have an understanding of a drug's pharmacokinetic profile, understand potential mechanisms by which liver disease and critical illness may affect the kinetics and dynamics of drugs, and use the pharmacology of the drug to appropriately monitor for efficacy and toxicity.

Absorption

Drugs administered via the enteral route are absorbed through the gastrointestinal lining, enter the portal circulation, and pass through the liver before entering the systemic circulation. Some drugs are immediately metabolized during this initial transit through the liver, a phenomenon often called *first-pass metabolism* or the *first-pass effect*. Critically ill patients with hepatic dysfunction may have a reduced capacity to metabolize drugs which may limit the extent of first-pass metabolism. This will effectively increase the bioavailability of an enterally administered medication, resulting in higher serum levels of the drug. Medications such as morphine, midazolam, and labetalol all undergo significant first-pass metabolism and all may have increased bioavailability when given orally to patients with liver disease [187–189].

Distribution

Liver disease and critical illness may increase a medication's volume of distribution. This is often a result of a reduction in plasma proteins, development of ascites or edema, or a combination of these factors. The effects of reduced plasma protein binding on volume of distribution have been discussed earlier in this chapter. The role of plasma protein binding on hepatic metabolism and elimination will be discussed later in this chapter.

Metabolism and Elimination

Liver failure may directly alter the pharmacokinetics of a drug by a reduction in metabolism and elimination. There are many factors involved in the hepatic metabolism and eliminations of drugs. Three major factors include cellular metabolism, hepatic blood flow, and protein binding.

The two primary pathways for cellular hepatic metabolism of medications involve phase I and/or phase II metabolism. Phase I metabolism often involves the cytochrome P450 enzyme system, whereas phase II metabolism generally consists of conjugation reactions. It is important to note that liver dysfunction tends to reduce phase I metabolic pathways more than phase II metabolic pathways [190,191]. An example of this effect can be seen with midazolam and lorazepam. Midazolam undergoes phase I metabolism via CYP450 3A4 and lorazepam undergoes phase II metabolism via glucuronidation. Liver failure significantly reduces the metabolic clearance (phase I) of midazolam but does not have a significant effect on the metabolic clearance (phase II) of lorazepam [192]. Critical illness has the potential to alter both phase I and phase II metabolic activity. Data are limited, but there is some evidence to suggest the hepatic metabolism of phenytoin may be increased after severe head injury [193]. Clinicians must also be aware of changes that may influence CYP450 activity. Some patients may have genetic polymorphisms, which will result in increased or decreased drug metabolism, or patients may receive other drugs that inhibit or induce CYP450 activity. Detailed discussion of the CYP450 system and drug–drug interactions is beyond the scope of this chapter.

Hepatic Blood Flow

The clearance of drugs by the liver is determined primarily by the extraction ratio and hepatic blood flow. The hepatic extraction ratio is the fraction of drug removed after passing through the liver. The rate of hepatic metabolism of drugs with high extraction ratios (>0.7) tends to depend on hepatic blood flow and depend less on cellular metabolism. Drugs with high extraction ratios include morphine and fentanyl. For example, if a critically ill patient is receiving intravenous morphine and has a reduction in hepatic blood flow from septic shock, one might anticipate a reduction in morphine metabolism secondary to the reduction in hepatic blood flow. The rate of hepatic metabolism of drugs with a low extraction ratio (<0.3) tends to depend on cellular metabolism and depend less on hepatic blood flow. Medications with low extraction ratios include lorazepam, diazepam, and methadone [194,195].

Protein Binding

Plasma protein binding can be classified as nonrestrictive or restrictive. Medications that bind in a nonrestrictive fashion are easily dissociated from plasma proteins so that free drug is available for hepatic metabolism. Changes in protein binding for drugs exhibiting nonrestrictive binding have minimal impact on hepatic metabolism because free drug is readily available for metabolism. Drugs that display restrictive protein binding will have less free drug available for metabolism. If there is a reduction in plasma proteins during critical illness, there will be an increase in free drug available for metabolism and there may be a resulting increase in the extraction ratio.

Estimating Hepatic Drug Metabolism

Although creatinine clearance can be a useful estimate for renal function in critically ill patients, currently there are no readily available, accurate, inexpensive methods for a clinician to quantify hepatic drug metabolism. Some studies have used scoring systems such as the Child's Score or Child's Score with Pugh Modification. These scoring systems have been useful in assessing the severity of hepatic disease and predicting mortality, but they do not accurately quantify the ability of the liver to metabolize medications and should be used cautiously. To appropriately assess hepatic function as it relates to drug metabolism, a clinician must consider many factors including laboratory data (bilirubin, albumin, prothrombin time), clinical features (hepatic blood flow, protein binding, ascites), other medications (drug–drug interactions), a medication's pharmacokinetic profile (absorption, distribution, metabolism, elimination), and the pharmacologic properties of the medication (efficacy and toxicity). In Table 74.1, dosing guidelines for varying levels of hepatic function as assessed by the Child-Pugh Score or serum bilirubin level are summarized. It is important for the clinician to use judgment when applying these dosing recommendations in clinical practice so that drug efficacy and patient safety may be optimized.

References

1. Leape LL, Cullen DJ, Clapp MD, et al: Pharmacist participation on physician rounds and adverse drug events in the intensive care unit. *JAMA* 282(3):267–270, 1999.
2. Rothschild JM, Christianson A, Landrigan CP, et al: The critical care safety study: the incidence and nature of adverse events and serious medical errors in intensive care. *Crit Care Med* 33(8):1694–1700, 2005.
3. Thakar CV, Freyberg R, Almenoff P, et al: Incidence and outcomes of acute kidney injury in intensive care units: a Veterans Administration study. *Crit Care Med* 37(9):2552–2258, 2009.
4. Barrantes F, Tian J, Vasquez R, et al: Acute kidney injury criteria predict outcomes of critically ill patients. *Crit Care Med* 36(5):1397–1403, 2008.
5. Cantu TG, Ellerbeck EF, Yun SW, et al: Drug prescribing for patients with changing renal function. *Am J Hosp Pharm* 49(12):2944–2948, 1992.
6. Smith JW, Seidl LG, Cluff LE: Studies on the epidemiology of adverse drug reactions. V. Clinical factors influencing susceptibility. *Ann Intern Med* 65(4):629–640, 1966.
7. Bates DW, Spell N, Cullen DJ, et al: The costs of adverse drug events in hospitalized patients. *JAMA* 277(4):307–311, 1997.
8. Classen DC, Pestotnik SL, Evans RS, et al: Adverse drug events in hospitalized patients. Excess length of stay, extra costs, and attributable mortality. *JAMA* 277(4):301–306, 1997.
9. Bates DW, Leape LL, Cullen DJ, et al: Effect of computerized physician order entry and a team intervention on prevention of serious medication errors. *JAMA* 280(15):1311–1316, 1998.
10. Aronoff GR, Bennett WM, Berns JS, et al: *Drug Prescribing in Renal Failure: Dosing Guidelines for Adults and Children*. 5th ed. Philadelphia, PA, American College of Physicians, 2007.
11. Trotman RL, Williamson JC, Shoemaker DM, et al: Antibiotic dosing in critically ill adult patients receiving continuous renal replacement therapy. *Clin Infect Dis* 41(8):1159–1166, 2005.
12. Zovirax(R) Injection, Acyclovir [product information]. Research Triangle Park, NC, GlaxoSmithKline, 2002.
13. Gupta SK, Eustace JA, Winston JA, et al: Guidelines for the management of chronic kidney disease in HIV-infected patients: recommendations of the HIV Medicine Association of the Infectious Diseases Society of America. *Clin Infect Dis* 40(11):1559–1585, 2005.
14. Balfour HH, McMonigal KA, Bean B: Acyclovir therapy of varicella-zoster virus infections in immunocompromised patients. *J Antimicrob Chemother* 12[Suppl B]:169–179, 1983.
15. Symmetrel [package insert]. Endo Pharmaceuticals, Inc, 2009.
16. Horadam VW, Sharp JG, Smilack JD, et al: *Ann Intern Med* 94(4, Pt 1):454–458, 1981.
17. Bennett WM, Aronoff GR, Golper TA, et al: *Drug Prescribing in Renal Failure*. Philadelphia, PA, American College of Physicians, 1994.
18. Amikacin [package insert]. Sicor Pharmaceuticals, Inc, 2005.
19. Fungizone [prescribing information]. Apothecon, 2009.
20. AmBisome [prescribing information]. Gilead Sciences, Inc, 2008.
21. Lyman CA, Walsh TJ: Systemically administered antifungal agents. A review of their clinical pharmacology and therapeutic applications. *Drugs* 44(1):9–35, 1992.
22. Walsh TH, Goodman JL, Pappas P, et al: Safety, tolerability, and pharmacokinetics of high-dose liposomal amphotericin b (AmBisome) in patients infected with *aspergillus* species and other filamentous fungi: maximum tolerated dose study. *Antimicrob Agents Chemother* 45(12):3487–3496, 2001.
23. Heintz BH, Matzke GR, Dager WE: Antimicrobial dosing concepts and recommendations for critically ill adult patients receiving continuous renal replacement therapy or intermittent hemodialysis. *Pharmacotherapy* 29(5):562–572, 2009.
24. Blum RA, Kohli RK, Harrison NJ, et al: Pharmacokinetics of ampicillin (2.0 grams) and sulbactam (1.0 gram) coadministered to subjects with normal and abnormal renal function and with end-stage renal disease on hemodialysis. *Antimicrob Agents Chemother* 33(9):1470–1476, 1989.
25. AZACTAM [package insert]. Bristol-Myers Squibb Company, 2007.
26. Angiomax [prescribing information]. Ben Venue Laboratories, 2005.
27. Bittl JA, Strony J, Brinker JA, et al: Treatment with bivalirudin (Hirulog) as compared with heparin during coronary angioplasty for unstable or postinfarction angina. Hirulog Angioplasty Study Investigators. *N Engl J Med* 333(12):764, 1995.
28. Kushner FG, Hand M, Smith SC Jr, et al: 2009 Focused Updates: ACC/AHA guidelines for the management of patients with ST-elevation myocardial infarction (Updating the 2004 guideline and 2007 focused update) and ACC/AHA/SCAI guidelines on percutaneous coronary intervention (updating the 2005 guideline and 2007 focused update): a report of the American College of Cardiology Foundation/American Heart Association Task Force on Practice Guidelines. *J Am Coll Cardiol* 54(23):2205–2241, 2009.
29. Fox I, Dawson A, Loynds P, et al: Anticoagulant activity of Hirulog, a direct thrombin inhibitor, in humans. *Thromb Haemost* 69(2):157–163, 1993.
30. Lehmann CR, Garrett LE, Winn RE, et al: Capreomycin kinetics in renal impairment and clearance by hemodialysis. *Am Rev Respir Dis* 138(5):1312–1313, 1988.
31. Joint Statement of the American Thoracic Society, CDC, and Infectious Diseases Society of America: Treatment of tuberculosis. *MMWR Morb Mortal Wkly Rep* 52(RR11):1–77, 2003.
32. Allaouchiche B, Breilh D, Jaumain H, et al: Pharmacokinetics of cefepime during continuous veno-venous hemodiafiltration. *Antimicrob Agents Chemother* 41(11):2424–2427, 1997.
33. Malone RS, Fish DN, Abraham E, et al: Pharmacokinetics of cefepime during continuous renal replacement therapy in critically ill patients. *Antimicrob Agents Chemother* 45(11):3148–3155, 2001.
34. Martin C, Thomachot L, Albanese J: Clinical pharmacokinetics of cefotetan. *Clin Pharmacokinet* 26(4):248–258, 1994.
35. Marshall WF, Blair JE: The cephalosporins. *Mayo Clin Proc* 74(2):187–95, 1999.
36. Davies SP, Lacey LF, Kox WJ, et al: Pharmacokinetics of cefuroxime and ceftazidime in patients with acute renal failure treated by continuous arteriovenous haemodialysis. *Nephrol Dial Transplant* 6(12):971–976, 1991.
37. Slaker RA, Danielson B: Neurotoxicity associated with ceftazidime therapy in geriatric patients with renal dysfunction. *Pharmacotherapy* 11(4):351–352, 1991.
38. Murthy B, Schmitt-Hoffmann A: Pharmacokinetics and pharmacodynamics of ceftobiprole, an anti-MRSA cephalosporin with broad-spectrum activity. *Clin Pharmacokinet* 47(1):21–33, 2008.
39. Hitchcock MJ, Jaffe HS, Martin JC, et al: Cidofovir, a new agent with potent anti-herpesvirus activity. *Antivir Chem Chemother* 7:115–127, 1996.
40. Davies SP, Azadian BS, Kox WJ, et al: Pharmacokinetics of ciprofloxacin and vancomycin in patients with acute renal failure treated by continuous haemodialysis. *Nephrol Dial Transplant* 7(8):848–854, 1992.
41. Malone RS, Fish DN, Abraham E, et al: Pharmacokinetics of levofloxacin and ciprofloxacin during continuous renal replacement therapy in critically ill patients. *Antimicrob Agents Chemother* 45(10):2949–2954, 2001.
42. Peters DH, Clissold SP: Clarithromycin: a review of its antimicrobial activity, pharmacokinetic properties, and therapeutic potential. *Drugs* 44(1):117–164, 1992.
43. Colistimethate for Injection [prescribing information]. Paddock Laboratories, Inc, 2004.

44. Li J, Rayner CR, Nation RL, et al: Pharmacokinetics of colistin methanesulfonate and colistin in a critically ill patient receiving continuous venovenous hemodiafiltration. *Antimicrob Agents Chemother* 49(11):4814–4815, 2005.
45. Davidson PT, Le HQ: Drug treatment of tuberculosis—1992. *Drugs* 43(5):651–673, 1992.
46. Drugs for tuberculosis. *Med Lett Drugs Ther* 35(908):99–101, 1993.
47. Smilack JD, Wilson WR, Cockerill FR III: Tetracyclines, chloramphenicol, erythromycin, clindamycin, and metronidazole. *Mayo Clin Proc* 66(12):1270–1280, 1991.
48. Suttorp MJ, Polak PE, van't Hof A, et al: Efficacy and safety of a new selective class III antiarrhythmic agent dofetilide in paroxysmal atrial fibrillation or atrial flutter. *Am J Cardiol* 69(4):417–419, 1992.
49. Tham TC, MacLennan BA, Burke MT, et al: Pharmacodynamics and pharmacokinetics of the class III antiarrhythmic agent dofetilide (UK-68,798) in humans. *J Cardiovasc Pharmacol* 21(3):507–512, 1993.
50. Keam SJ: Doripenem: a review of its use in the treatment of bacterial infections. *Drugs* 68(14):2021–2057, 2008.
51. Hirsh J, Bauer KA, Donati MB, et al: Parenteral anticoagulants: American College of Chest Physicians Evidence-Based Clinical Practice Guidelines (8th Edition). *Chest* 133[6, Suppl]:141S–159S, 2008.
52. Lovenox [prescribing information]. Sanofi-Aventis US LLC, 2009.
53. Erythrocin Lactobionate [package insert]. Hospira, Inc, 2006.
54. Lin JH, Chremos AN, Yeh KC, et al: Effects of age and chronic renal failure on the urinary excretion kinetics of famotidine in man. *Eur J Clin Pharmacol* 34:41–46, 1988.
55. Toon S, Ross CE, Gokal R, et al: An assessment of the effects of impaired renal function and haemodialysis on the pharmacokinetics of fluconazole. *Br J Clin Pharmacol* 29:221–226, 1990.
56. Dudley MN: Clinical pharmacology of fluconazole. *Pharmacotherapy* 10(Suppl):141S–145S, 1990.
57. Haase M, Bellomo R, Rocktaeschel J, et al: Use of fondaparinux (ARIXTRA) in a dialysis patient with symptomatic heparin-induced thrombocytopaenia type II. *Nephrol Dial Transplant* 20(2):444–446, 2005.
58. Aweeka FT, Jacobson MA, Martin-Munley S, et al: Effect of renal disease and hemodialysis on foscarnet pharmacokinetics and dosing recommendations. *J Acquir Immune Defic Syndr Hum Retrovirol* 20(4):350–357, 1999.
59. Czock D, Scholle C, Rasche FM, et al: Pharmacokinetics of valganciclovir and ganciclovir in renal impairment. *Clin Pharmacol Ther* 72(2):142–150, 2002.
60. Shepp DH, Dandliker PS, de Miranda P, et al: Activity of 9-[2-hydroxy-1-(hydroxymethyl) ethoxymethyl]guanine in the treatment of cytomegalovirus pneumonia. *Ann Intern Med* 103(3):368–373, 1985.
61. Fish DN, Teitelbaum I, Abraham E: Pharmacokinetics and pharmacodynamics of imipenem during continuous renal replacement therapy in critically ill patients. *Antimicrob Agents Chemother* 49(6):2421–2428, 2005.
62. Leo RJ, Ballow CH: Seizure activity associated with imipenem use: clinical case reports and review of the literature. *DICP* 25(4):351–354, 1991.
63. Warkentin TE, Greinacher A, Koster A, et al: Treatment and prevention of heparin-induced thrombocytopenia: American College of Chest Physicians Evidence-Based Clinical Practice Guidelines (8th Edition). *Chest* 133[6, Suppl]:340S–380S, 2008.
64. Refludan [prescribing information]. Bayer HealthCare Pharmaceuticals Inc, 2006.
65. Mauro LS, Peloquin CA, Schmude K, et al: Clearance of linezolid via continuous venovenous hemodiafiltration. *Am J Kidney Dis* 47(6):e83–e86, 2006.
66. Brier ME, Stalker DJ, Aronoff GR, et al: Pharmacokinetics of linezolid in subjects with renal dysfunction. *Antimicrob Agents Chemother* 47(9):2775–2780, 2003.
67. Tsuji Y, Hiraki Y, Mizoguchi A, et al: Pharmacokinetics of repeated dosing of linezolid in a hemodialysis patient with chronic renal failure. *J Infect Chemother* 14(2):156–160, 2008.
68. Arroliga AC, Shehab N, McCarthy K, et al: Relationship of continuous infusion lorazepam to serum propylene glycol concentration in critically ill adults. *Crit Care Med* 32(8):1709–1714, 2004.
69. American Pain Society: *Principles of Analgesic Use in the Treatment of Acute Pain and Cancer Pain*. 5th ed. American Pain Society, 2003.
70. Leroy A, Fillastre JP, Etienne I, et al: Pharmacokinetics of meropenem in subjects with renal insufficiency. *Eur J Clin Pharmacol* 42(5):535–538, 1992.
71. Ververs TF, van Dijk A, Vinks SA, et al: Pharmacokinetics and dosing regimen of meropenem in critically ill patients receiving continuous venovenous hemofiltration. *Crit Care Med* 28(10):3412–3416, 2000.
72. Merrem [prescribing information]. AstraZeneca Pharmaceuticals LP, 2009.
73. Lau AH, Chang CW, Sabatini S: Hemodialysis clearance of metronidazole and its metabolites. *Antimicrob Agents Chemother* 29(2):235–238, 1986.
74. Bauer TM, Ritz R, Haberthur C, et al: Prolonged sedation due to accumulation of conjugated metabolites of midazolam. *Lancet* 346(8968):145–147, 1995.
75. Woolfrey SG, Hegbrant J, Thysell H, et al: Dose regimen adjustment for milrinone in congestive heart failure patients with moderate and severe renal failure. *J Pharm Pharmacol* 47(8):651–655, 1995.
76. Aronoff GR, Berns JS, Brier ME, et al (eds): *Drug Prescribing in Renal Failure*. 4th ed. Philadelphia, PA, American College of Physicians, 1999.
77. Mazoit JX, Butscher K, Samii K: Morphine in postoperative patients: pharmacokinteric and pharmcodynamic of metabolites. *Anesth Analog* 105(1):70–78, 2007.
78. Portenoy RK, Foley KM, Stulman J, et al: Plasma morphine and morphine-6-glucuronide during chronic morphine therapy for cancer pain: plasma profiles, steady-state concentrations and the consequences of renal failure. *Pain* 47(1):13–19, 1991.
79. Corgard [Product Information]. King Pharmaceuticals, Inc, 2006.
80. Sackner-Bernstein JD, Skopicki HA, Aaronson KD: Risk of worsening renal function with nesiritide in patients with acutely decompensated heart failure. *Circulation* 111(12):1487–1491, 2005.
81. Rindone JP, Sloane EP: Cyanide toxicity from sodium nitroprusside: risks and management. *Ann Pharmacother* 26(4):515–519, 1992.
82. Thalhammer F, Kletzmayr J, El Menyawi I, et al: Ofloxacin clearance during hemodialysis: a comparison of polysulfone and cellulose acetate hemodialyzers. *Am J Kidney Dis* 32(4):642–645, 1998.
83. FLOXIN [prescribing information]. Ortho-McNeil-Janssen Pharmaceuticals, Inc, 2008.
84. Tamiflu. Roche Pharmaceuticals, Inc, 2008.
85. Robson R, Buttimore A, Lynn K, et al: The pharmacokinetics and tolerability of oseltamivir suspension in patients on haemodialysis and continuous ambulatory peritoneal dialysis. *Nephrol Dial Transplant* 21(9):2556–2562, 2006.
86. Centers for Disease Control and Prevention (CDC): Antiviral treatment options, including intravenous peramivir, for treatment of influenza in hospitalized patients for the 2001–2010 season. Available at: http://www.cdc.gov/h1n1flu/EUA/peramivir_recommendations.htm. Accessed January 26, 2010.
87. Conte JE Jr: Pharmacokinetics of intravenous pentamidine in patients with normal renal function or receiving hemodialysis. *J Infect Dis* 163(1):169–175, 1991.
88. Lathia C, Fleming GF, Meyer M, et al: Pentostatin pharmacokinetics and dosing recommendations in patients with mild renal impairment. *Cancer Chemother Pharmacol* 50(2):121–126, 2002.
89. Dilantin [prescribing information]. Pfizer Inc, 2009.
90. Dowell JA, Korth-Bradley J, Milisci M, et al: Evaluating possible pharmacokinetic interactions between tobramycin, piperacillin, and a combination of piperacillin and tazobactam in patients with various degrees of renal impairment. *J Clin Pharmacol* 41:979–986, 2001.
91. Valtonen M, Tiula E, Takkunen O, et al: Elimination of the piperacillin/tazobactam combination during continuous venovenous haemofiltration and haemodiafiltration in patients with acute renal failure. *J Antimicrob Chemother* 48(6):881–885, 2001.
92. Zavascki AP, Goldani LZ, Cao G, et al: Pharmacokinetics of intravenous polymyxin B in critically ill patients. *Clin Infect Dis* 47(10):1298–1304, 2008.
93. Herbrecht R: Posaconazole: a potent, extended-spectrum triazole antifungal for the treatment of serious fungal infections. *Int J Clin Pract* 58(6):612–624, 2004.
94. Courtney R, Sansone A, Smith W, et al: Posaconazole pharmacokinetics, safety, and tolerability in subjects with varying degrees of chronic renal disease. *J Clin Pharmacol* 45(2):185–192, 2005.
95. Gibson TP, Atkinson AJ Jr, Matusik E, et al: Kinetics of procainamide and N-acetylprocainamide in renal failure. *Kidney Int* 12(6):422–429, 1977.
96. Campbell TJ, Williams KM: Therapeutic drug monitoring: antiarrhythmic drugs. *Br J Clin Pharmacol* 46(4):307–319, 1998.
97. Zantac Injection [prescribing information]. GlaxoSmithKline, 2009.
98. Bassilios N, Launay-Vacher V, Mahani AA, et al: Pharmacokinetics and dosage adjustment of rifabutin in a haemodialysis patient [letter]. *Nephrol Dial Transplant* 17(3):531–532, 2002.
99. Mycobutin [prescribing information]. Pfizer Inc, 2007.
100. Betapace [prescribing information]. Bayer HealthCare Pharmaceuticals Inc, 2007.
101. Dumas M, d'Athis P, Besancenot JF, et al: Variations of sotalol kinetics in renal insufficiency. *Int J Clin Pharmacol Ther Toxicol* 27(10):486–489, 1989.
102. Varoquaux O, Lajoie D, Gobert C, et al: Pharmacokinetics of the trimethoprim-sulfamethoxazole combination in the elderly. *Br J Clin Pharmacol* 20(6):575–581, 1985.
103. Mofenson LM, Oleske J, Serchuck L, et al: Treating opportunistic infections among HIV-exposed and infected children: recommendations from CDC, the National Institutes of Health, and the Infectious Diseases Society of America. *MMWR Recomm Rep* 53(RR-14):1–92, 2004.
104. Smith BS, Gandhi PJ: Pharmacokinetics and pharmacodynamics of low-molecular-weight heparins and glycoprotein IIb/IIIa receptor antagonists in renal failure. *J Thromb Thrombolysis* 11(1):39–48, 2001.
105. Perry CM, Faulds D: Valacyclovir. A review of its antiviral activity, pharmacokinetic properties and therapeutic efficacy in herpesvirus infections. *Drugs* 52(5):754–772, 1996.
106. VALCYTE [prescribing information]. Genentech, Inc, 2009.
107. Perrottet N, Robatel C, Meylan P, et al: Disposition of valganciclovir during continuous renal replacement therapy in two lung transplant recipients. *J Antimicrob Chemother* 61(6):1332–1335, 2008.
108. Rodvold KA, Blum RA, Fischer JH, et al: Vancomycin pharmacokinetics in patients with various degrees of renal function. *Antimicrob Agents Chemother* 32(6):848–852, 1988.
109. Joy MS, Matzke GR, Frye RF, et al: Determinants of vancomycin clearance by continuous veno-venous hemofiltration and continuous veno-venous hemodialysis. *Am J Kidney Dis* 31(6):1019–1027, 1998.

110. VFEND [prescribing information]. Pfizer Inc, 2008.
111. Geodon [prescribing information]. Pfizer Inc, 2009.
112. ZIAGEN [prescribing information]. Research Triangle Park, NC, GlaxoSmithKline, 2002.
113. Xanax [prescribing information]. Kalamazoo, MI, Pharmacia & Upjohn Company, 1997.
114. Abernethy DR: Amlodipine: pharmacokinetic profile of a low-clearance calcium antagonist. *J Cardiovasc Pharmacol* 17[Suppl 1]:S4–S7, 1991.
115. NORVASC [prescribing information]. New York, NY, Pfizer Inc, 2005.
116. Argatroban [prescribing information]. Research Triangle Park, NC, GlaxoSmithKline, 2005.
117. Gilman AG, Rall TW, Nies AS, et al (eds): *Goodman and Gilman's The Pharmacological Basis of Therapeutics*. 8th ed. New York, NY, Macmillan Publishing Co, 1990.
118. Tainter ML: *Aspirin in Modern Therapy: A Review*. New York, NY, Bayer Co of Sterling Drugs Inc, 1969, p 85.
119. Neugebauer G, Gabor M, Reiff K: Pharmacokinetics and bioavailability of carvedilol in patients with liver cirrhosis. *Drugs* 36[Suppl 6]:148–154, 1988.
120. COREG [prescribing information]. Research Triangle Park, NC, GlaxoSmithKline, 2005.
121. CANCIDAS [prescribing information]. Whitehouse Station, NJ, Merck & Co., Inc., 2005.
122. Colchicine [prescribing information]. Corona, CA, Watson Laboratories, Inc., 2001.
123. Flexeril [prescribing information]. West Point, PA, Merck & Co., Inc, 2001.
124. Floyd J, Mirza I, Sachs B, et al: Hepatotoxicity of chemotherapy. *Semin Oncol* 33(1):50–67, 2006.
125. Koren G, Beatty K, Seto A, et al: The effects of impaired liver function on the elimination of antineoplastic agents. *Ann Pharmacother* 26(3):363–371, 1992.
126. Cytosar-U [prescribing information]. Kalamazoo, MI, Upjohn Company, 1999.
127. Cerubidine [prescribing information]. Bedford, OH, Ben Venue Laboratories, 1999.
128. Ochs HR, Greenblatt DJ, Eckardt B, et al: Repeated diazepam dosing in cirrhotic patients: cumulation and sedation. *Clin Pharmacol Ther* 33(4):471–476, 1983.
129. VALIUM [prescribing information]. Nutley, NJ, Roche Laboratories, Inc, 2000.
130. Taxotere® [prescribing information]. Bridgewater, NJ, Aventis Pharmaceuticals, 2004.
131. Adriamycin RDF [prescribing information]. Kalamazoo, MI, Pharmacia & Upjohn Company, 1999.
132. Twelves CJ, O'Reilly SM, Coleman RE, et al: Weekly epirubicin for breast cancer with liver metastases and abnormal liver biochemistry. *Br J Cancer* 60(6):938–941, 1989.
133. Ellence [prescribing information]. Bentley, WA, Pharmacia & Upjohn, Rev, 1999.
134. Sjovall H, Hagman I, Holmberg J, et al: Pharmacokinetics of esomeprazole in patients with liver cirrhosis (abstract 346). *Gastroenterology* 118(4):A21, 2000.
135. Nexium [prescribing information]. Wilmington, DE, AstraZeneca, 2001.
136. Donelli MG, Zucchetti M, Munzone E, et al: Pharmacokinetics of anticancer agents in patients with impaired liver function. *Eur J Cancer* 34(1): 33–46, 1998.
137. Perry MC: Hepatotoxicity of chemotherapeutic agents. *Semin Oncol* 9(1):65–74, 1982.
138. ZETIA [prescribing information]. North Wales, PA, Merck/Schering-Plough Pharmaceuticals, 2005.
139. Glucotrol [prescribing information]. New York, NY, Pfizer Pharmaceuticals, 1993.
140. Diabeta [prescribing information]. Somerville, NJ, Hoechst-Roussel Pharmaceuticals, Inc., 1994.
141. Lu K, Savaraj N, Kavanagh J, et al: Clinical pharmacology of 4-demethoxydaunorubicin (DMDR). *Cancer Chemother Pharmacol* 17(2):143–148, 1986.
142. IDAMYCIN PFS [prescribing information]. Kalamazoo, MI, Pharmacia & Upjohn, 2003.
143. Ifex [prescribing information]. Princeton, NJ, Bristol-Myers Oncology Division, 1994.
144. Ramanathan RK, Egorin MJ, Takimoto CH, et al: Phase I and pharmacokinetic study of imatinib mesylate in patients with advanced malignancies and varying degrees of liver dysfunction: a study by the National Cancer Institute Organ Dysfunction Working Group. *J Clin Oncol* 26(4):563–569, 2008.
145. Gleevec [prescribing information]. East Hannover, NJ, Novartis Pharmaceuticals Corporation, 2003.
146. LAMICTAL [prescribing information]. Research Triangle Park, NC, GlaxoSmithKline, 2009.
147. COZAAR [prescribing information]. Whitehouse Station, NJ, Merck & Co., Inc, 2004.
148. Methadone Hydrochloride [prescribing information]. Columbus, OH, Roxane Laboratories, INC., 2000.
149. Naltrexone Hydrochloride [prescribing information]. St. Louis, MO, Mallinckrodt Inc, 2003.
150. Cardene [prescribing information]. Nutley, NJ, Roche Laboratories, Inc, 1999.
151. Gengo FM, Fagan SC, Krol G, et al: Nimodipine disposition and haemodynamic effects in patients with cirrhosis and age-matched controls. *Br J Clin Pharmacol* 23(1):47–53, 1987.
152. Taxol [prescribing information]. Princeton, NJ, Bristol-Myers Squibb Company, 1999.
153. Dalhoff K, Almdal TP, Bjerrum K, et al: Pharmacokinetics of paroxetine in patients with cirrhosis. *Eur J Clin Pharmacol* 41(4):351–354, 1991.
154. PAXIL [prescribing information]. Research Triangle Park, NC, GlaxoSmithKline, 2005.
155. PEXEVA [prescribing information]. Miami, FL, Noven Therapeutics LLC, 2009.
156. PAXIL CR [prescribing information]. Research Triangle Park, NC, GlaxoSmithKline, 2005.
157. Procanbid [prescribing information]. Division of Warner-Lambert, Morris Plains, NJ, Parke-Davis, 1995.
158. Green B: Focus on quetiapine. *Curr Med Res Opin* 15(3):145–151, 1999.
159. Seroquel [prescribing information]. Wilmington, DE, Zeneca Pharmaceuticals, 1997.
160. Risperdal [prescribing information]. Titusville, NJ, Janssen Pharmaceutica, 1999.
161. Bumgardner GL, Roberts JP: New immunosuppressive agents. *Gastroenterol Clin North Am* 22(2):421–449, 1993.
162. Rapamune [prescribing information]. Philadelphia, PA, Wyeth Laboratories, 1999.
163. TYGACIL [prescribing information]. Philadelphia, PA, Wyeth Pharmaceuticals, Inc, 2008.
164. Ultram [prescribing information]. Raritan, NJ, Ortho-McNeil Pharmaceutical, 1998.
165. ULTRAM [prescribing information]. Raritan, NJ, Ortho-McNeil Pharmaceutical, Inc, 2004.
166. HALCION [prescribing information]. New York, NY, Pharmacia & Upjohn Company, 2008.
167. Velban [prescribing information]. Indianapolis, IN, Eli Lilly and Co, 2000.
168. Navelbine [prescribing information]. Research Triangle, NC, Glaxo Wellcome, Inc., 2000.
169. Langtry HD, Benfield P: Zolpidem. A review of its pharmacodynamic and pharmacokinetic properties and therapeutic potential. *Drugs* 40(2):291–313, 1990.
170. Bendayan R: Renal drug transport: a review. *Pharmacotherapy* 16(6):971–985, 1996.
171. Reed WE, Sabatini S: The use of drugs in renal failure. *Semin Nephrol* 6(3):259–295, 1986.
172. Manninen V, Apajalahti A, Melin J, et al: Altered absorption of digoxin in patients given propantheline and metoclopramide. *Lancet* 1(7800):398–400, 1973.
173. Plaisance KI, Drusano GL, Forrest A, et al: Effect of renal function on the bioavailability of ciprofloxacin. *Antimicrob Agents Chemother* 34(6):1031–1034, 1990.
174. Matzke GR, Millikin SP: Influence of renal function and dialysis on drug disposition, in Evans WE, Schentag JJ, Jusko WJ (eds): *Applied Pharmacokinetics: Principles of Therapeutic Drug Monitoring*. 3rd ed. Vancouver, BC, Canada, Applied Therapeutics, Inc., 1992, p 91.
175. Doucet J, Fresel J, Hue G, et al: Protein binding of digitoxin, valproate and phenytoin in sera from diabetics. *Eur J Clin Pharmacol* 45(6):577–579, 1993.
176. MacKichan JJ: Influence of protein binding and the use of unbound (free) drug concentrations, in Evans WE, Schentag JJ, Jusko WJ (eds): *Applied Pharmacokinetics: Principles of Therapeutic Drug Monitoring*. 3rd ed. Vancouver, BC, Canada, Applied Therapeutics, Inc, 1992, p 192.
177. Swan S, Bennett WM: Drug dosing guidelines in patients with renal failure. *West J Med* 156 (6):633–638, 1992.
178. Pichette V, Leblond FA: Drug metabolism in chronic renal failure. *Curr Drug Metab* 4(2):91–103, 2003.
179. Dreisbach AW: The influence of chronic renal failure on drug metabolism and transport. *Clin Pharmacol Ther* 86(5):553–556, 2009.
180. Touchette MA, Slaughter RL: The effect of renal failure on hepatic drug clearance. *DICP* 25(11):1214–1224, 1991.
181. National Kidney Foundation: K/DOQI clinical practice guidelines for chronic kidney disease: evaluation, classification, and stratification. *Am J Kidney Dis* 39:S1–S266, 2002.
182. Stevens LA, Nolin TD, Richardson MM, et al: Comparison of drug dosing recommendations based on measured GFR and kidney function estimating equations. *Am J Kidney Dis* 54(1):33–42, 2009.
183. Golik MV, Lawrence KR: Comparison of dosing recommendations for antimicrobial drugs based on two methods for assessing kidney function: Cockcroft-Gault and modification of diet in renal disease. *Pharmacotherapy* 28(9):1125–1132, 2008.
184. Hermsen ED, Maiefski M, Florescu MC, et al: Comparison of the modification of diet in renal disease and Cockcroft-Gault equations for dosing antimicrobials. *Pharmacotherapy* 29(6):649–655, 2008.
185. Matzke GR, Frye RF: Drug therapy individualization for patients with renal insufficiency, in DiPiro JT, Talbert RL, Yee GC, et al (eds): *Pharmacotherapy: A Pathophysiologic Approach*. 7th ed. New York, McGraw-Hill, 2008.

186. Pea F, Viale P, Pavan F, et al: Pharmacokinetic considerations for antimicrobial therapy in patients receiving renal replacement therapy. *Clin Pharmacokinet* 46(12):997–1038, 2007.
187. Hasselstrom J, Eriksson S, Peterson A, et al: The metabolism and bioavailability of morphine in patients with severe liver cirrhosis. *Br J Clin Pharmacol* 29(3):289–297, 1990.
188. Pentikainen PJ, Valisalmi L, Himberg JJ, et al: Pharmacokinetics of midazolam following intravenous and oral administration in patients with chronic liver disease and in healthy subjects. *J Clin Pharmacol* 29(3):272–277, 1989.
189. Homeida M, Jackson L, Roberts CJ: Decreased first-pass metabolism of labetalol in chronic liver disease. *Br Med J* 2(6144):1048–1050, 1978.
190. Paintaud G, Bechtel Y, Brientini MP, et al: Effects of liver diseases on drug metabolism. *Therapie* 51(4):384–389, 1996.
191. Murray M: P450 enzymes. Inhibition mechanisms, genetic regulation and effects of liver disease. *Clin Pharmacokinet* 23(2):132–146, 1992.
192. Greenblatt DJ: Clinical pharmacokinetics of oxazepam and lorazepam. *Clin Pharmacokinet* 6(2):89–105, 1981.
193. McKindley DS, Boucher BA, Hess MM, et al: Effects of the acute phase response on phenytoin metabolism in neurotrauma patients. *J Clin Pharmacol* 37(2):129–139, 1997.
194. Rodighiero V: Effects of liver disease on pharmacokinetics: an update. *Clin Pharmacokinet* 37(5):399–431, 1999.
195. Tegeder I, Lotsch J, Geisslinger G: Pharmacokinetics of opioids in liver diseases. *Clin Pharmacokinet* 37(1):17–40, 1999.

CHAPTER 75 ■ RENAL REPLACEMENT THERAPY IN THE INTENSIVE CARE UNIT

GLENN KERSHAW, MATTHEW J. TRAINOR AND PANG-YEN FAN

INTRODUCTION

Rapid deterioration of kidney function in acutely ill patients is common and potentially catastrophic. Acute kidney injury (AKI) occurs in up to 70% of patients admitted to the intensive care unit (ICU) and is associated with a twofold increase in the already high mortality rate for this population. Medical therapy is often inadequate for management of the metabolic disturbances and fluid overload that complicate AKI. In this setting, renal replacement therapy (RRT) is essential to the survival of the patient. In addition, patients with end-stage renal disease (ESRD) have high rates of hospitalization, particularly for cardiovascular disease and infection. These patients often require ICU care including RRT.

We are now entering the fifth decade of providing dialysis support to ICU patients with AKI. Despite many technical advances, mortality remains alarmingly high (40% to 60%). The high death rate is largely due to the severity and the array of nonrenal organ system dysfunction, as mortality for patients with AKI is now primarily due to multiorgan system failure (MOSF). Accumulating evidence suggests that the acutely injured kidney may in turn injure distant organs and that some forms of RRT may prevent MOSF [1].

The objectives of modern day RRT now extend beyond correction of metabolic disturbances and volume overload to include facilitation of nutritional support and drug therapy, optimization of volume status, and even promotion of nonrenal organ system recovery. Treatment strategies have shifted from reactive to proactive approaches, leading to a trend toward earlier initiation of dialysis. For example, with growing recognition that fluid overload increases mortality and that volume control can improve outcomes [2–4], RRT is applied more aggressively to prevent volume overload. An important principle of renal support strategies is that of "capacity (supply) and demand mismatch." Critically ill patients have increased "demand" for renal function. Such patients often generate increased solute from their hypercatabolic metabolism and intensive nutritional support. In addition, they receive enormous amounts of fluid because of medications, blood products, enteral and parenteral nutrition, and volume resuscitation. The stress of high solute and fluid loads may overwhelm the capacity of even a minimally injured kidney. Furthermore, the limited "supply" of renal function from kidneys already compromised by AKI is further reduced by tenuous hemodynamics and endogenous/exogenous renal pressor activity. RRT expands the limited capacity of the injured kidney to match the high fluid and solute demand, thereby restoring balance [5].

PRINCIPLES OF SOLUTE CLEARANCE AND FLUID REMOVAL BY DIALYTIC TECHNIQUES

Dialysis therapies involve the movement of solute and plasma water across a semipermeable membrane separating a blood compartment and a dialysate compartment. For intermittent hemodialysis (IHD) and continuous renal replacement therapies (CRRT), this process occurs within a cartridge called a hemofilter or hemodialyzer as shown in Figure 75.1. For peritoneal dialysis (PD), the peritoneum serves as the semipermeable membrane separating blood in the mesenteric vasculature from the dialysate in the peritoneal cavity. Characteristics such as membrane thickness and pore dimensions determine the size and transfer rate of molecules that move between the blood and dialysate.

Removal of solute and water in RRT may occur by diffusion or convection. Diffusion involves movement of solute down a concentration gradient, that is, from areas of high concentration to low concentration. Conversely, water will move from an area of low osmolality to an area of high osmolality. Solute molecules have kinetic energy and move in solution. They collide with one another and with water molecules resulting in an even dispersion throughout the solution. Dialysis is diffusion across a semipermeable membrane. When solute in

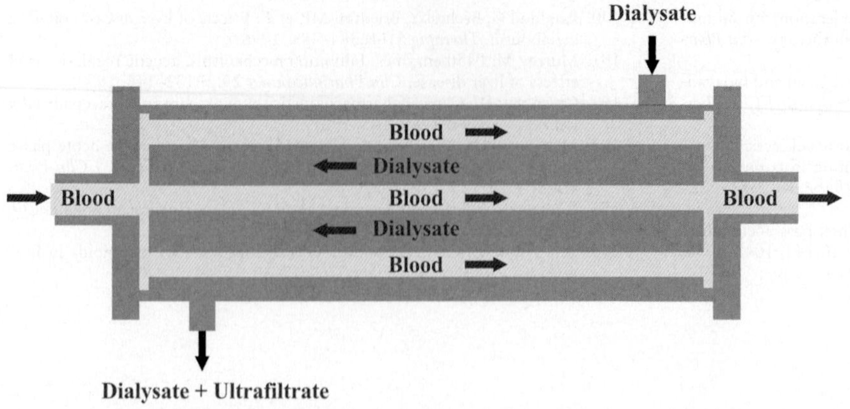

FIGURE 75.1. Schematic diagram of a hollow fiber dialyzer. Blood enters the hemofilter, passes through hollow fibers, and exits at the opposite end. Dialysate enters through the side port, flows around the blood-filled fibers in the opposite direction as the blood, combines with ultrafiltrate, and exits via the side port near the blood entry port.

motion encounters a membrane pore of sufficient dimensions, it moves through the membrane into the adjacent compartment. Small molecules with greater molecular velocity are more readily cleared than are larger molecules even if both fit through the membrane pore. A high concentration of solute in a given compartment favors a high frequency of membrane collisions and passage through the pore. Water will also pass easily through the membrane to the compartment with higher osmolality. Large shifts of water may pull some solute through the membrane, a phenomenon known as solvent drag. In a static system, net transfer (dialysis) ceases when solute concentrations equilibrate in the compartments. For RRT, blood and dialysate are continuously replenished to maintain the high concentration gradients favoring maximum transfer of solute and water.

Convection involves the transfer of solute across a semipermeable membrane driven by a hydrostatic pressure gradient. Those solutes small enough to pass through pores are swept along with water by solvent drag. The membrane acts as a sieve, retaining molecules that exceed the pore size. All filtered solutes below the membrane pore size are removed at rates proportionate to their concentration. The convective removal of fluid in this manner is termed *hemofiltration* or sometimes *ultrafiltration*. This technique does not change the plasma concentration of small solutes (blood urea nitrogen [BUN], creatinine, electrolytes, glucose), since water is removed in proportion to solute. In contrast, the concentration of larger molecules (albumin) and formed elements (hematocrit) increase as they are sieved off by the smaller membrane pores. Thus, the chemical composition of the filtrate (often referred to as ultrafiltrate) is almost identical to that of the plasma except for the absence of large molecules such as albumin. Some thought leaders opt for convection-based RRT because of greater clearance of medium-sized and large molecules than with diffusion-based techniques.

OVERVIEW OF DIALYSIS MODALITIES

The general features of different dialysis modalities are summarized in Table 75.1.

TABLE 75.1

DIALYSIS MODALITIES

Technique	Dialyzer	Physical principle
Hemodialysis		
IHD	Hemodialyzer	Concurrent diffusion (solute clearance) and convection (fluid removal)
UF	Hemodialyzer	Convection (fluid removal, limited solute clearance)
CRRT		
SCUF	Hemofilter	Convection (fluid removal, limited solute clearance)
CAVH	Hemofilter	Convection (solute clearance and fluid removal)
CAVHD	Hemofilter	Principally diffusion with some convection
CAVHDF	Hemofilter	Concurrent diffusion and convection
CVVH	Hemofilter	Convection (solute clearance and fluid removal)
CVVHD	Hemofilter	Principally diffusion with some convection
CVVHDF	Hemofilter	Concurrent diffusion and convection
Peritoneal dialysis		
CAPD	None	Principally diffusion with some convection
CCPD	None	Principally diffusion with some convection

CAPD, continuous ambulatory peritoneal dialysis; CAVH, continuous arteriovenous hemofiltration; CAVHD, continuous arteriovenous hemodialysis; CAVHDF, continuous arteriovenous hemodiafiltration; CCPD, continuous cycling peritoneal dialysis; CRRT, continuous renal replacement therapies; CVVH, continuous venovenous hemofiltration; CVVHD, continuous venovenous hemodialysis; CVVHDF, continuous venovenous hemodiafiltration; IHD, intermittent hemodialysis; SCUF, slow continuous ultrafiltration; UF, ultrafiltration.

Intermittent Hemodialysis

Intermittent hemodialysis is the standard form of RRT for the majority of stable ESRD patients in the United States. In IHD, blood is circulated through a dialysis machine and hemodialysis cartridge and then returned to the patient. Utilizing diffusion (principally for solute clearance) and convection (principally for ultrafiltration), this highly efficient modality provides rapid solute and volume removal but requires both specialized equipment and trained staff. Both blood and dialysate are pumped through the hemofilter at high flow rates. The dialysate flow is countercurrent to blood flow to maximize concentration gradients throughout the course of the filter (Fig. 75.1). Diffusion of solute across the filter is bidirectional. Urea, creatinine, and potassium move from plasma to dialysate, whereas bicarbonate and usually calcium diffuse in an opposite path (Fig. 75.2).

Standard dialysis machines can also perform isolated ultrafiltration which results in fluid removal but does not significantly alter the chemical composition of plasma. During ultrafiltration, the dialysis machine pumps only blood, but not dialysate through the hemofilter. This process generates a hydrostatic pressure gradient across the hemofilter membrane, resulting in convective fluid removal. However, no dialysate is used, so there is no diffusive solute clearance. Isolated ultrafiltration is typically used when volume overload is the sole concern.

Solute clearance can be adjusted changing the dialyzer size and membrane, blood and dialysate flow, and dialysis time as detailed later in this chapter. Fluid removal can be adjusted by changing the hydrostatic pressure gradient between the blood and dialysate compartments within the hemofilter, an automated process performed by the dialysis machine. Although this technique is commonly used in the ICU setting, the rapid shifts in solute and fluid can precipitate hemodynamic instability and may therefore be less suitable for critically ill patients. IHD treatments are typically performed for several hours three to four times per week. However, since the technique is labor and resource intensive, more frequent treatments may be limited by staffing and cost.

Peritoneal Dialysis

Peritoneal dialysis is the main form of RRT for approximately 5% to 10% of ESRD patients in the United States. In PD, dialysate is instilled into the peritoneal cavity. Through diffusion, solute and volume enter the dialysate, which is periodically drained and replaced with fresh dialysate. Solute clearance is adjusted by altering the volume of dialysate or varying the duration of each "dwell" (the interval between dialysate exchanges). More frequent exchanges will enhance solute removal, provided there is sufficient time between dialysate instillation and drainage to permit diffusion across the peritoneum. Volume is removed by maintaining a high dialysate osmolality through a high concentration of dextrose. This osmolar gradient results in the movement of water into the peritoneal cavity and also contributes to solute clearance through solvent drag. Fluid removal is adjusted by altering the dialysate dextrose content.

PD can be performed as a series of manual dialysate exchanges done during the day (chronic ambulatory peritoneal dialysis or CAPD) or through automated exchanges utilizing a PD machine (cycler) typically done at night (continuous cycled peritoneal dialysis or CCPD). For CAPD, dialysate is changed every 4 to 6 hours with a longer overnight "dwell." For CCPD, the exchanges are typically done every 2 to 3 hours through the night, and the abdomen is often left empty or with only a small volume of dialysate (sometimes called a "cushion") during the day. PD is much less efficient than IHD but is better tolerated hemodynamically, since solute and fluid shifts occur gradually. In the ICU setting, PD is generally reserved for ESRD patients who are already maintained on this modality. PD is generally not used for AKI because of technical difficulty in establishing dialysis access (discussed later in this chapter) as well as the

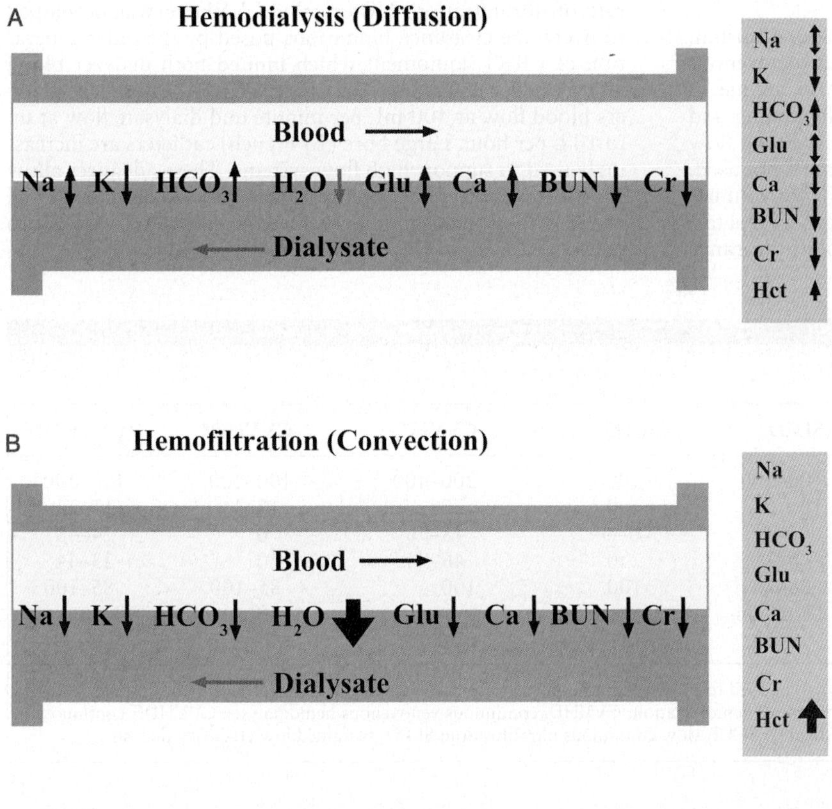

FIGURE 75.2. Solute and water movement across the dialyzer membrane in hemodialysis and hemofiltration. Net effect on serum chemistries and hematocrit shown in box at right. **A:** Significant flux in solute with relatively small shift in water in hemodialysis. Postdialyzer chemistries significantly altered with small increase in hematocrit. **B:** Significant removal of water with concomitant removal of solute in hemofiltration. Posthemofilter chemistries unchanged, since solute is removed in proportion to plasma concentration; however, hematocrit is significantly increased due to high filtration fraction. See text for more detail.

low efficiency of solute clearance. Furthermore, instillation of 1 to 2 L of dialysate into the peritoneal cavity can impair ventilation in patients with compromised oxygenation, particularly in the setting of abdominal distention or ileus.

Continuous Renal Replacement Therapies

The continuous renal replacement therapies encompass a family of dialytic modalities that vary in their mode of solute removal and duration of treatment, but share the characteristic of slow solute and volume removal maintained over an extended period of time rather than high clearances over 3 to 4 hours as with IHD. Although less efficient than IHD, CRRT provides much higher clearances than PD. Like PD, these techniques are better tolerated hemodynamically than IHD, since solute and volume are removed gradually. These modalities require intensive monitoring and necessitate ICU admission. They are widely used in the critical care setting. CRRT can be performed by a number of methods detailed later in the chapter. The operating parameters of different CRRT systems are summarized in Table 75.2. A schematic of the circuitry of the different techniques is presented in Figure 75.3.

Continuous Arteriovenous Hemofiltration, Hemodialysis, and Hemodiafiltration

Arteriovenous (AV) systems were used at the dawn of CRRT. AV systems relied on the pressure gradient between the arterial and venous circulation to drive ultrafiltration across the hemofilter membrane. However, variations in arterial pressure led to inconsistent rates of ultrafiltration and solute clearance. AV systems also required the placement and long-term maintenance of large bore arterial catheters at the femoral site. With the development of reliable double-lumen venous catheters and advanced pump-driven venovenous systems, these modalities have largely fallen out of favor.

Continuous Venovenous Hemofiltration, Hemodialysis, and Hemodiafiltration

In CRRT, solute removal is achieved by convection, diffusion, or a combination of these methods. Continuous venovenous hemofiltration (CVVH) is a purely convective technique in which a pump system drives blood through the hemofilter and generates ultrafiltration rates of 1 to 4 L per hour. Blood flow rate is generally lower than with IHD and dialysate is not used. Solute clearance is achieved by replacing these large volumes of ultrafiltrate with fluid that does not contain the solutes targeted for removal (e.g., urea and potassium). Solute clearance and volume removal are adjusted by altering the ultrafiltration rate and the rate of infusion of replacement fluid (RF). The administration of RF maintains fluid balance and lowers the plasma concentration of solute by dilution. RF can be infused before or after the filter along the course of the dialyzer circuit (Fig. 75.3).

In diffusion-based techniques such as continuous venovenous hemodialysis (CVVHD), a dual pump system drives both blood and dialysate through the hemofilter. Dialysate flow and blood flow rates are typically much lower than with IHD. The technique creates less ultrafiltrate (2 to 5 L per day) than CVVH, since the infusion of dialysate lowers the pressure gradient across the hemofilter membrane. As with IHD, diffusion of solute across the filter is bidirectional (Fig. 75.2). No RF is administered. In CVVHD, the flow of dialysate through the filter is countercurrent to the flow of blood, but the dialysate flow rate is significantly slower (1 to 2 L per hour = 17 to 34 mL per minute) than the blood flow rate (100 to 200 mL per minute). This disparity permits full equilibration of plasma urea across the membrane and complete saturation of dialysate.

For all forms of CRRT, the effluent volume (Qef) relates directly to solute clearance and is a therapeutic target to assure dosing adequacy. The effluent volume is the product of the filtration process. It comprises the ultrafiltrate in CVVH, the "spent" (equilibrated) dialysate in CVVHD, and the combination of ultrafiltrate and spent dialysate in continuous venovenous hemodiafiltration (CVVHDF). Since urea is freely filtered in CVVH, its concentration in the ultrafiltrate is identical to that of plasma. Thus, 48 L of ultrafiltrate (effluent) represents 48 L of plasma fully cleared of urea. Similarly, in CVVHD, the effluent (spent dialysate) is fully saturated with urea. Each liter of spent dialysate reflects a liter of plasma fully cleared of urea. In diffusive systems, blood flow has little impact on clearance at low dialysate flow (1 to 2 L per hour) but increasing impact as dialysate flow increases.

CVVHDF combines diffusion and convection into a single procedure. Dialysate is infused at 1 to 2 L per hour to boost the convective clearance generated by high (1 to 2 L per hour) ultrafiltration rates. RF is needed to offset the high rate of ultrafiltration. Historically, CVVHDF was developed to overcome clearance limitations posed by the older generation of CRRT equipment which limited both dialyzer blood and dialysate flow. However, current CRRT equipment delivers blood flow at 400 mL per minute and dialysate flow at up to 10 L per hour. Large bore (13 French) catheters are increasingly used to support high flow systems. These advances allow high volume ultrafiltrate generation with less complex CVVH or CVVHD systems and have called the role of CVVHDF into question.

TABLE 75.2

COMPARISON OF RRT MODALITIES

	IHD	SLED	SCUF	CVVH[a]	CVVHD[a]	CVVHDF[a]
Blood flow *(mL/min)*	250–400	100–200	<100	200–400	100–200	100–200
Dialysate flow *(mL/min)*	500–800	100	0	0	17–34	17–34
Filtrate *(L/d)*	0–4	0–4	0–4	48–96	0	24–48
Replacement fluid *(L/d)*	0	0	0	46–94	0	23–44
Effluent saturation *(%)*	15–40	60–70	100	100	85–100	85–100
Solute clearance	Diffusion	Diffusion	Convection	Convection	Diffusion	Both
Duration *(h)*	3–5	8–12	Variable	>24	>24	>24

[a]In the absence of a blood pump, arteriovenous circuits can be used to provide continuous therapy (CAVH, CAVHD, CAVHDF).
IHD, intermittent hemodialysis; CVVH, continuous venovenous hemofiltration; CVVHD, continuous venovenous hemodialysis; CVVHDF, continuous venovenous hemodiafiltration; RRT, renal replacement therapy; SCUF, slow continuous ultrafiltration; SLED, sustained low efficiency dialysis.

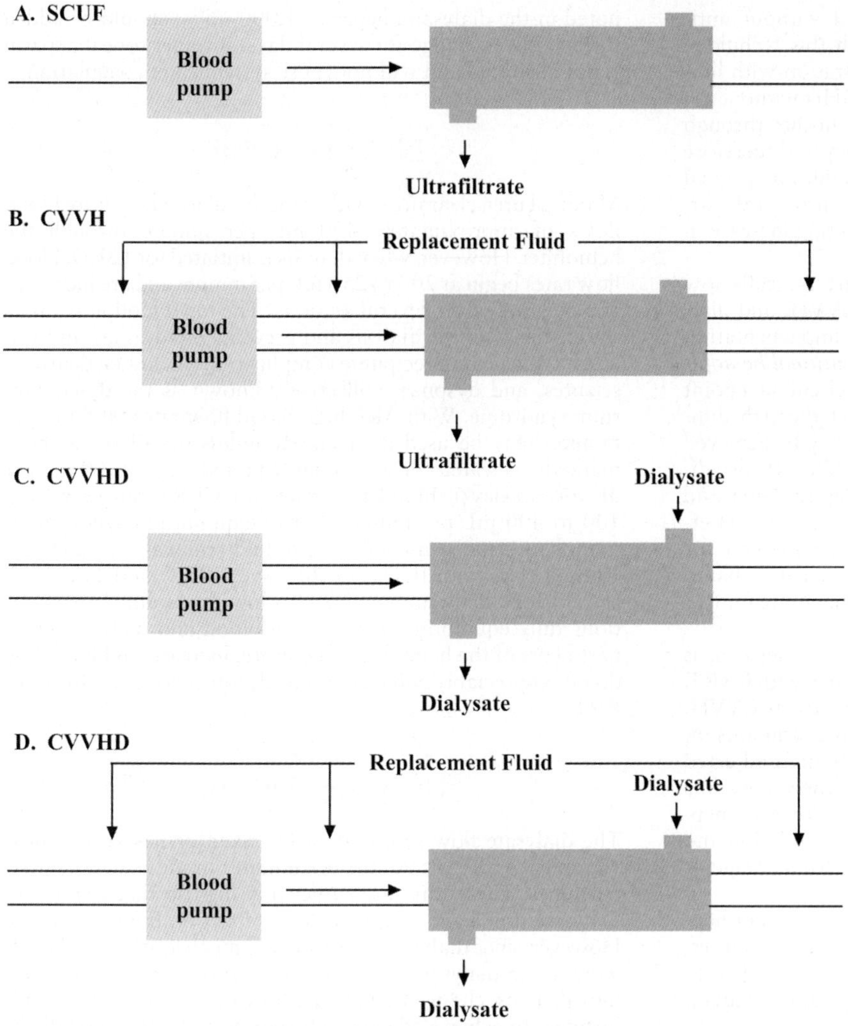

FIGURE 75.3. Schematic diagram of various CRRT configurations. A: SCUF (slow continuous ultrafiltration). Ultrafiltrate is generated by the transmembrane pressure gradient produced by the blood pump. B: CVVH (continuous venovenous hemofiltration). Large volume ultrafiltrate is generated and replacement fluid is infused preblood pump, prehemofilter, or posthemofilter. C: CVVHD (continuous venovenous hemofiltration). Dialysate is pumped through the filter to generate diffusive solute clearance. D: CVVHD (continuous venovenous hemodiafiltration). The system utilizes high ultrafiltration with replacement fluid as well as dialysate.

Slow Continuous Ultrafiltration

In slow continuous ultrafiltration (SCUF), a pump system maintains low blood flow (usually no more than 100 mL per minute) through a hemofilter and generates low rates of ultrafiltration (typically 100 to 300 mL per hour). This modality provides volume removal but does not alter the chemistry of plasma, since water is removed in proportion to solute. Compared with other CRRT modalities, SCUF is a low intensity nursing procedure. The procedure is often used in settings of severe volume overload with acceptable chemistries. At our institution, SCUF is often employed as an adjunct to IHD in the hemodynamically stable, volume overloaded patient.

Sustained Low Efficiency Dialysis

Hybrid therapies apply the CRRT principle of low solute clearance over an extended, but not continuous, period of time. Sustained low efficiency dialysis (SLED) is better tolerated hemodynamically than IHD and can be performed with either standard hemodialysis machines or with CRRT equipment. Lower blood flow (100 to 200 mL per minute) and dialysate flow (100 mL per minute) rates achieve adequate diffusive solute clearance and convective volume removal over a typical 8- to 12-hour session. SLED done with standard hemodialysis machines expands the clinical utility of these devices, but generally requires the presence of a trained dialysis nurse. However, this modality can be done with a CRRT machine by an ICU nurse. There are no data comparing SLED outcomes with either IHD or CRRT.

TECHNICAL CONSIDERATIONS FOR RENAL REPLACEMENT THERAPY

Anticoagulation

Hemofilter fibers are prone to thrombosis, as removal of fluid through ultrafiltration leads to hemoconcentration at the distal end of the dialyzer. As the filtration fraction (FF), that is, the proportion of plasma flow that is filtered, increases, the risk of filter thrombosis also rises. The FF can be calculated as follows:

$$\begin{aligned} FF &= \text{ultrafiltration rate plasma flow rate} \\ &= \text{ultrafiltration rate}/[\text{blood flow rate} \times (100\text{-Hct})] \end{aligned}$$

Thus, higher rates of ultrafiltration, especially if coupled with low blood flows, predispose to hemofilter thrombosis. Poor filter performance and filter clotting increases sharply at FF greater than 20%. Higher blood flow rates permit greater rates of fluid removal, since hemoconcentration within the filter is limited by the short transit time of blood through the dialysis cartridge.

Hemodialysis can generally be performed without anticoagulation. The high blood flows used with this technique permit adequate solute clearance and ultrafiltration with limited risk of dialyzer thrombosis [6]. However, IHD without anticoagulation also necessitates frequent saline flushes through the hemodialyzer to help maintain fiber patency and therefore is more labor intensive than standard IHD. In addition, packed red blood cell transfusions cannot be infused through the arterial line of the dialyzer circuit, since the resulting increase in hematocrit will lead to hemofilter clotting.

However, with CCRT, blood flow rates are typically low and ultrafiltration rates high, especially for CVVH, and filter thrombosis is a significant barrier to effective implementation of these therapies. One approach called *predilutional hemofiltration* involves infusion of RF into the CRRT circuit at a point before the filter, thus lowering the hematocrit through dilution. As a result, a higher ultrafiltration rate may be achieved without compromising filter life. However, prefilter RF also dilutes the solute concentration of blood entering the filter and reduces effective clearance. With this approach, the target effluent volume should be increased by 25% to compensate for the dilutional effect. Other CRRT parameters such as blood and ultrafiltration rate must be adjusted to compensate for this inefficiency.

Anticoagulation, typically with unfractionated heparin, is generally necessary to maintain hemofilter patency with CRRT, especially for principally convective modalities such as CVVH. After an initial bolus of 1,000 to 2,000 units, a continuous infusion of approximately 10 units per kg per hour is adjusted to maintain the partial thromboplastin time in the venous line of the blood circuit at 1.5 to 2 times control. However, heparin infusions do result in some systemic anticoagulation and may be contraindicated in patients with active hemorrhage or heparin-induced thrombocytopenia (HIT).

Despite theoretical advantages, low-molecular-weight heparins do not appear to offer any significant advantages in efficacy or safety over unfractionated heparin for RRT [7]. In addition, these agents are more costly and their anticoagulant effects more difficult to monitor.

For patients with active hemorrhage, regional anticoagulation limited to the CRRT blood circuit is preferred. Citrate regional anticoagulation is widely used and has become the primary mode of anticoagulation in many centers. Citrate infused in the arterial limb of the CRRT circuit prevents hemofilter thrombosis by chelating calcium, a critical component of the clotting cascade. Calcium chloride infused into the venous line of the system restores normal systemic calcium levels. This approach appears to reduce the risk of hemorrhage and extend hemofilter patency [8]. In addition, citrate can be used for patient with HIT.

Serum and ionized calcium levels must be carefully monitored, especially in patients with significant liver dysfunction, and the calcium infusion appropriately adjusted. Citrate is hepatically metabolized into bicarbonate and can cause metabolic alkalosis. In the setting of hepatic failure, citrate accumulation results in elevated serum but low ionized calcium levels, reflecting increased circulating calcium bound to citrate. Trisodium citrate solution, typically used in this form of anticoagulation, may also cause hypernatremia.

Other methods of regional anticoagulation such as prostacyclin infusion or heparin reversal with protamine have been less successful. Prostacyclin, an arachidonic acid metabolite, has a half-life of only 3 to 5 minutes and inhibits platelet aggregation. However, it induces vasodilatation and is associated with hypotension and it is costly. Protamine binds and neutralizes heparin, but infusions are technically complex and may be associated with rebound bleeding.

Anticoagulation is unnecessary for PD. However, intraperitoneal fibrin can occlude the dialysis catheter. If fibrin clots are noted in the dialysate, heparin (1,000 units) should be added to each PD exchange for several days. Intraperitoneal heparin is not absorbed and will not cause systemic anticoagulation.

Blood Flow Rate

Maximal urea clearances with standard dialyzers require blood flows of approximately 400 mL per minute through the hemofilter. However, when dialysis is initiated for ESRD, blood flow rates begin at 200 to 250 mL per minute and are increased incrementally over several sessions. The low blood flow limits the efficiency of the dialysis and prevents rapid solute and water shifts that can precipitate complications including delirium, seizures, and dyspnea, collectively known as the dysequilibrium syndrome. With AKI, high blood flow rates (400 mL per minute) may be used immediately unless the BUN has been markedly elevated for a prolonged period (e.g., >100 mg per dL for >3 days). Blood flow rates for CRRT can vary from 100 to 400 mL per minute, but dysequilibrium syndrome is not a concern because solute and fluid removal are much less efficient than with IHD. For diffusive CRRT modalities such as CVVHD, dialysate flows are so low that solute concentrations fully equilibrate between the blood and dialysate compartments of the hemofilter. Therefore, increases in blood flow do not appreciably enhance solute clearance for these forms of RRT.

Dialysate Flow Rate

The dialysate flow rate is typically fixed or has very limited variability (500 to 800 mL per minute) in most hemodialysis machines. These rates are sufficiently high so that changes in dialysate flow have relatively little impact on IHD clearances. However, since dialysate flow rates are much lower with CRRT, increases in dialysate flow can significantly enhance solute removal. Thus, change in dialysate flow rate is an important adjustment to achieve adequate clearances with these modalities. With PD, clearances can also be increased by increasing total dialysate volumes, either by instilling more dialysate with each exchange or by increasing the frequency of exchanges. The maximal of volume per exchange is limited by abdominal discomfort and/or respiratory compromise, and high exchange volumes can predispose to leakage of dialysate from the catheter tunnel. Exchanges done more often than every 2 hours provide little additional solute clearance, as shorter dwell time limits diffusion across the peritoneum.

Dialyzer Membrane

Most hemodialyzers and hemofilters are constructed as cylinders containing hollow fibers composed of a semipermeable membrane (Fig. 75.1). The surface area of the membrane depends on the number and length of these fibers. Membrane surface area affects solute clearance and ultrafiltration. Membrane size or surface area varies with the specific model of hemodialyzer or hemofilter. Bigger dialysis cartridges are used for large patients or those needing high solute clearances. Children usually require specially downsized hemofilters.

The hemofilter membrane may consist of nonorganic, synthetic compounds (e.g., polysulfone, polyacryl nitrate) or cellulose-derived materials (cellulosic membranes). In vitro exposure of blood to cellulosic membranes leads to complement activation and leukocyte adherence and these membranes are categorized as bioincompatible. Synthetic membranes are inert and are termed *biocompatible*. A seminal randomized trial reported better survival and higher rates of recovery from AKI among patients dialyzed on biocompatible membranes [9]. This outcome advantage was challenged in subsequent trials and meta-analyses [10]. Modern day cellulosic membranes claim biocompatibility, since the offending, complement-activating moiety (hydroxyl group) is now buried deep within the membrane. Regardless, we recommend exclusive use of synthetic (biocompatible) dialyzers in patients with AKI. The cost differential between synthetic and cellulosic membranes is minimal.

Pore dimensions determine the size selectivity of molecular flux across the membrane. Low flux (small pore) membranes clear small molecules (urea, potassium, and creatinine) but do not clear the larger "middle molecules" which may act as toxins. High flux membranes (large pore) clear middle molecules, such as β_2 microglobulin and perhaps inflammatory cytokines generated by AKI and MOSF. This theoretic advantage of high flux membranes may be compromised in settings of low water quality. Large pore size would permit backflow (dialysate to blood) into the patient of endotoxin fragments and other harmful water-borne molecules, such as heavy metals. In settings with high-quality water systems (generally available in the United States), we recommend the use of high flux, large surface area, biocompatible membranes.

Dialysate Composition

Dialysate solutions are composed of specific concentrations of sodium, potassium, bicarbonate, calcium, chloride, glucose, and magnesium. The range and standard concentrations of contents of dialysates for both IHD and PD are summarized in Table 75.3. For IHD, chloride, glucose, and magnesium concentrations are generally fixed. The usual dialysate sodium concentration is 140 mEq per L, but higher concentrations (148 to 150 mEq per L) are often used early in an IHD session to prevent hypotension. Dialysis against a high sodium concentration (148 to 150 mEq per L) results in diffusion of sodium into plasma. This maintains plasma osmolality at a time when urea and other small solutes are being rapidly cleared across the membrane, thus preventing acute intracellular shifts of water that can precipitously lower plasma volume. Later in the dialysis procedure, when urea mobilization is proceeding at a slower pace, dialysate (serum) sodium concentration is returned to normal (140 mEq per L) to prevent hypernatremia. This process of sodium profiling (or sodium modeling) is one of the major strategies employed to prevent hypotension in the AKI patient managed with IHD. Modern dialysis machines offer a variety of sodium modeling profiles. This technique is not needed for CRRT, since solute and volume removal occurs slowly.

TABLE 75.3

DIALYSATE FORMULATION FOR HEMODIALYSIS AND PERITONEAL DIALYSIS

Solute	Range (usual concentration)
Intermittent hemodialysis	
Na^+	138–145 mEq/L (140)
K^+	0–4 mEq/L (2)
Cl^-	100–110 mEq/L (106)
HCO_3^-	35–45 mEq/L (35)
Ca^+	1.0–3.5 mEq/L (2.5)
Mg^+	1.5 mEq/L (1.5)
Glucose	0–200 mg/dL (200)
Peritoneal dialysis	
Na^+	132 mEq/L
K^+	0
Cl^-	96 mEq/L
Lactate	35 mEq/L
Ca^+	2.5 or 3.5 mEq/L
Mg^+	0.5 or 1.5 mEq/L
Glucose	1.5%, 2.5%, or 4.25% g/dL

The dialysate potassium concentration generally ranges from 2.0 to 4.0 mEq per L. It is adjusted to normalize the serum potassium after the postdialysis equilibration period and for the next 24 hours. A rapid rate of rise of serum potassium is best treated with daily IHD or CRRT rather than alternate day IHD using low potassium (1.0 mEq per L) dialysate because of the risk of arrhythmias precipitated by intradialytic hypokalemia. Low potassium dialysate is reserved for patients with life-threatening hyperkalemia. In this setting, intradialytic potassium levels should be monitored hourly and the dialysate potassium increased as soon as the potassium is lowered to below the life-threatening range (<6 to 6.5 mEq per L). The dialysate potassium concentration is adjusted based on the predialysis serum potassium:

serum K^+ <4.0	dialysate K^+ 4.0
serum K^+ 4.0–5.5	dialysate K^+ 3.0–3.5
serum K^+ 5.6–7.5	dialysate K^+ 2.0
serum K^+ >7.5	dialysate K^+ 1.0

The buffer used in dialysate is now uniformly bicarbonate. The concentration of bicarbonate in dialysate usually varies from 33 to 35 mEq per L. Higher bicarbonate concentrations (40 mEq per L) are used in severe acidosis or to offset elevations of carbon dioxide resulting from the permissive hypercapnia that attends low tidal volume ventilation.

Dialysate calcium concentration in maintenance hemodialysis is 2.5 mEq per L of diffusible calcium. Since 50% of total calcium is protein bound, this value approximates the diffusible or ionized calcium in plasma at a total serum calcium concentration of 10 mg per dL (10 mg per dL total calcium = 5 mg per dL ionized calcium = 2.5 mEq per L ionized calcium). Since hypocalcemia is common in AKI and correction of acidosis may further depress ionized calcium, some experts advocate higher dialysate calcium concentration (3.0 to 3.5 mEq per L) in patients with AKI. High calcium dialysate may be used to correct hypocalcemia but should be used with caution. Calcium loading in animal models of sepsis increases mortality [11].

For CRRT, a wide variety of dialysate and RFs may be used. These may be custom compounded by hospital pharmacies, by regional pharmacies or may be purchased as commercially prepared solutions. The composition of dialysate employed in CVVHD may be identical to that of RF employed in CVVH. Potassium and calcium concentrations are selected to meet patient needs. Base composition may be bicarbonate, lactate, or citrate. The latter two buffers are metabolized to bicarbonate and effectively address acidosis in most patients with adequate hepatic function.

A decade ago, commercially prepared lactate buffered solutions were widely used because of their stability and extended shelf life. Bicarbonate-based solutions were unstable and available only if compounded on site. Now a number of commercially prepared bicarbonate-based solutions are available. Prolonged shelf life is achieved by a partition in the infusion bag that separates bicarbonate from the remaining solution. Breaking the partition just before use mixes the two compartments. Bicarbonate provides better hemodynamic stability than does lactate and is the buffer of choice in hepatic failure. Citrate-based RF has also been used successfully in CVVH systems.

In contrast to IHD, the composition of peritoneal dialysate is relatively constant. These commercially produced solutions are available in 2- and 5-L bags and vary only in dextrose content (1.5%, 2.5%, and 4.25% concentrations). Icodextrin, a glucose polymer which is absorbed more slowly than dextrose, has been used for selected patients with poor ultrafiltration [12]. If necessary, potassium, insulin, or even certain antibiotics can be added to the dialysate.

Dialysis Access

Establishing and maintaining adequate access is paramount to the delivery of all types of RRT. Access is best considered in two distinct settings: the ESRD patient with permanent access and the AKI patient requiring temporary access.

Arteriovenous Fistula and Graft

For the ESRD patient maintained with IHD, permanent dialysis access options include an arteriovenous fistula (AVF), arteriovenous graft (AVG), or, rarely, a tunneled central venous catheter (discussed later in the chapter). Created by connecting an artery directly to a vein, typically in the upper extremity, an AVF must "mature," a process during which high blood flow causes gradual dilatation and thickening or "arterialization" of the veins proximal to the AV anastomosis. Once mature, the AVF can be repetitively cannulated with large bore needles several times a week for IHD. Consider the optimal access for hemodialysis, AVF provides high blood flow (>500 mL per minute), durable long-term vascular access, relatively low thrombosis rates, and low infection rates. However, AVFs require long maturation time (typically several months), making them unsuitable for patients with AKI. In addition, AVFs cannot withstand prolonged cannulation, precluding their use for CRRT.

For an AVG, a synthetic graft, usually composed of material such as polytetrafluoroethylene, is used to connect the artery and vein. AVGs are used when the native veins are deemed of insufficient size or quality and unlikely to mature into a functional AVF. Although maturation time is only a few weeks, AVGs cannot be used for AKI. AVGs are not as durable as AVFs because the graft material deteriorates with multiple cannulations. In addition, AVGs have much higher rates of thrombosis and infection and they also cannot be used for CRRT.

To preserve the patency of AVFs and AVGs, measurement of blood pressure, venipuncture, and constricting dressings or tourniquets should be avoided in the access extremity. Acute thrombosis may also occur in the setting of hypotension or severe volume depletion, two conditions commonly seen in critically ill patients.

Peritoneal Dialysis Catheters

Unlike IHD and CRRT, patients on PD do not require vascular access. Instead, PD catheters allow for infusion and drainage of dialysate from the peritoneal cavity. There are several different catheters used for ESRD, but none have established superiority over the others. Most are made of silicone and have two synthetic cuffs, one placed beneath the skin and one beneath the abdominal fascia, which prevent displacement and infection of the catheter. The connectors between these catheters and dialysate fluid bags vary with each manufacturer, necessitating the use of adapters to join equipment or dialysate solutions from different companies. These catheters are typically not used for 1 or 2 weeks after placement to permit healing of the insertion site and catheter tunnel. Premature use increases the risk of dialysate leak and infection. In urgent situations, early use of permanent catheters can be attempted with low volume exchanges and the patient supine.

Although very rarely used, when access is required for AKI, a noncuffed catheter can be placed at the bedside and used immediately. This procedure should be reserved for unique situations and be performed by a skilled operator because of the risks of bowel perforation or organ puncture. Acute catheters can only be used for 3 days before the risk of peritonitis rises dramatically. At that point, the catheter must be removed and a new catheter placed at a different insertion site.

Catheters

For most patients with AKI, dialysis access is achieved by placement of a temporary central venous catheter. These devices fall into two different categories, acute noncuffed, nontunneled lines or long-term cuffed, tunneled catheters, but all are large diameter (12 to 15 French) and of dual lumen design. The acute catheters are typically constructed of materials such as polyurethane and are relatively stiff at room temperature, but become pliable at body temperature. For patients with urgent or emergent need of dialysis, acute catheters provide rapid access for IHD and CRRT and are typically inserted at the bedside into the internal jugular or femoral veins. The subclavian site is generally avoided due to the risk of developing venous stenosis after placement of relatively stiff acute dialysis catheters. Subclavian vein stenosis can preclude future placement of an AVF or AVG graft in the ipsilateral arm by restricting venous flow. Other complications of these catheters include infection, thrombosis, and vascular perforation and are discussed below.

Cuffed, tunneled catheters are placed when the expected duration of dialytic support exceeds 2 weeks. Composed of soft material such as silicone, they are usually inserted under fluoroscopic guidance into the internal jugular, external jugular, subclavian, or femoral vein and exit through a subcutaneous tunnel. These devices are available in different configurations and may have a single or dual lumen. For appropriate function, the catheters are placed so that the tips extend into the right atrium, thus permitting higher blood flows. Unlike the stiffer acute noncuffed dialysis lines, the softer cuffed catheters do not pose a significant risk for perforation. The subcutaneous cuff and insertion tunnel serve to anchor the catheter and also inhibit infection such that these lines may remain in place for several months or longer. Given the duration of use, these devices should not be placed in patients with bacteremia. Complications are similar to those with uncuffed catheters and will also be discussed below.

INDICATIONS FOR AND TIMING OF INITIATION OF RENAL REPLACEMENT THERAPY

Remarkably, there is no consensus on the absolute indications for initiation of RRT in AKI. The absence of rigorous or quantitatively defined clinical or biochemical findings that warrant dialytic support have resulted in wide variation in clinical practice. Even the limits of medical therapy and diuretic therapy are poorly defined. Conventional indications are as follows:

- Volume overload refractory to or inadequately controlled with diuretic therapy
- Hyperkalemia or metabolic acidosis refractory to medical management
- Concomitant intoxication with a dialyzable drug or toxin
- Overt uremic signs or symptoms
  - encephalopathy
  - pericarditis
  - uremic bleeding diathesis
- Progressive and advanced asymptomatic azotemia

Reserving RRT for patients who meet one of these criteria may have little impact on the high mortality of AKI, particularly in the setting of MOSF. A management strategy that merely prevents uremic complications follows the old paradigm for AKI: these patients die *with*, but not *of*, their renal dysfunction. The modern paradigm recognizes that AKI is an independent risk factor for death [13–15] and that the aggressive management of RRT may affect outcomes and reduce mortality [16–18]. However, no consensus guideline exists which defines the optimal time to initiate RRT. No threshold of azotemia or duration of oliguria has been identified beyond which dialysis support is indicated.

Early Versus Late Initiation of RRT

The evidence for early initiation of RRT in AKI is summarized in Table 75.4. Prior to 1999, all studies employed IHD. Results were often conflicting and difficult to interpret, since both timing of RRT initiation and intensity of RRT varied. Three retrospective studies from the 1960s and 1970s reported a survival advantage with early dialysis [19–21]. It is noteworthy that BUN values that defined "early dialysis" (<93 to 150 vs. >160 to 200 mg per dL) are rather high by today's standards. A small prospective trial conducted on a US Navy Hospital Ship during the Viet Nam War reported better survival with early initiation [22]. The early dialysis group also received more intensive dialysis. Ten years later, the same investigator prospectively studied early and intensive dialysis in a population with nontraumatic AKI [23]. The target BUN in the early/intensive group was 60 mg per dL, whereas the target BUN in the late/less intensive group was 100 mg per dL. No survival advantage was observed in the early/intensive group. This small underpowered study led to the general view that in the absence of life-threatening complications or uremic symptoms, HD need not be initiated until the BUN exceeded 100 mg per dL.

Studies on early initiation over the last 10 years involve primarily CRRT. A retrospective review of 100 trauma patients with AKI [24] reported a distinct survival advantage (39% vs. 20%) of "early starters" (BUN <60) over "late starters" (BUN >60). The early group started CRRT on hospital day 10 with a mean BUN of 43 and late starters on hospital day 19 with a mean BUN of 93. Late starters had more MOSF. One interpretation of this observation is that early CRRT improves survival by preventing MOSF.

A single modern-day, prospective, randomized trial has been published on early initiation of RRT [25]. Dutch investigators randomized 106 oliguric patients to early high volume CVVHD, early low volume CVVHD, and late low volume CVVHD. The criterion for early starters was oliguria more than 6 hours after optimizing hemodynamics or creatinine clearance less than 20 mL per minute on a 3-hour collection. Late starters initiated CVVHD at a BUN more than 112, K more than 6.5 or for pulmonary edema. Survival at 28 days was no different in the three groups. We suggest caution when interpreting this negative study. It is likely underpowered for the primary outcome (death). The overall mortality (27%) was much lower than the typical patient with AKI requiring CRRT support (>60%).

A survival advantage to early CRRT is reported in two retrospective studies of AKI following cardiac surgery [26,27]. Both studies report better survival when the indication for CRRT was set as diuretic resistant oliguria (urine output <100 mL per 8 hours) rather than traditional laboratory parameters. CRRT was initiated less than 24 hours postoperatively in early starters and 2.5 days postoperatively in the late starter group.

A recent large ($n = 243$) multicenter, observational study reported a survival advantage with early initiation [28]. Early and late starts were defined by an initiation BUN less than 76 mg per dL (low azotemia) and greater than 76 mg per dL (high azotemia), respectively. After adjusting for comorbid variables and for propensity for initiation of RRT, the relative risk of death at 60 days in the high azotemia group was nearly twofold.

A recent meta-analysis on the timing of initiation of RRT analyzed 18 (retrospective) cohort studies involving more than 2,000 patients [29]. A 28% risk reduction in mortality was observed with early dialysis. Publication bias, variations in technology over the 50-year span of cited studies, and heterogeneity of the definitions of early and late therapy preclude definitive conclusions.

A major methodological limitation of all observational studies is the omission of patients who never receive RRT from the analysis. Less than 15% of patients who meet RIFLE criteria (threefold increase in creatinine) receive RRT during their hospitalization. Some patients with AKI recover renal function and survive while others may expire before initiating RRT. Yet, neither outcome is integrated into a retrospective analysis. Among AKI patients managed with RRT, patients destined to recover and survive may enrich early start groups, whereas patients destined to die of MOSF after an extended ICU course may be overrepresented in late start groups. Future studies on early RRT versus late RRT, whether prospective or observational, must integrate a "No RRT" arm into the study design [30].

The best attempt to provide quantitative sample guidelines for RRT was formulated by the Acute Kidney Injury Network (AKIN) in 2008 [31]. This expert panel of critical care nephrologists references key outcome studies in justifying specific parameters to trigger RRT and are summarized in Table 75.5.

Several points are emphasized as follows:

Indications for and timing of RRT are viewed within the context of the patient's entire clinical condition. A specific indication may be absolute or relative. An absolute indication represents a stand-alone condition that makes RRT mandatory. A relative indication requires a concomitant condition without which RRT is not mandatory but could be recommended. The presence of an indication in a relatively stable patient with oliguric AKI as single organ system failure would be viewed differently from the same parameter existing in a critically ill patient with MOSF.

Trends and trajectories of illness may be more important than absolute parameters. The strength of an indication for RRT depends on whether the patient's clinical condition is improving, deteriorating, or static.

Comorbid severity scores were discussed but never formulated into the guideline.

The AKIN panel underscores a growing body of evidence that volume overload in AKI carries high morbidity and mortality [2]. Early and meticulous control of volume with CRRT can improve outcomes especially in the pediatric population with AKI and following cardiac surgery [3,4].

The panel makes no particular comment on sepsis-related AKI. The intriguing concept of cytokine clearance by convective CRRT systems in septic shock remains unproven [32–34]. Metabolic or oliguric thresholds for initiating CRRT often exist early in the course of sepsis. We advocate early CRRT in the oliguric, hypotensive septic patient even when specific metabolic indications have not been met.

Dialysis Dose

There is no benchmark for the dose or intensity of RRT used to treat AKI. Many experts suggest that IHD in this setting should at least achieve the urea clearance recommended for patients with ESRD, although there are no data validating this approach. Urea clearance can be quantitated through the *Kt*/*V* or urea reduction ratio (URR). The *Kt*/*V* is a dimensionless

TABLE 75.4

SUMMARY OF STUDIES EVALUATING TIMING OF INITIATION OF RENAL REPLACEMENT THERAPY

Study	RRT modality	Study design	Patients	Criteria for early RRT	Criteria for late RRT	Survival (%), early RRT	Survival (%), late RRT	Comment
Parsons et al. [19]	IHD	Retrospective	33	BUN 120–150	BUN >200	75	12	Historical control
Fischer et al. [20]	IHD	Retrospective	162	BUN ~150	BUN >200	43	26	Historical control
Kleinknecht et al. [21]	IHD	Retrospective	500	BUN <93	BUN >163	73	58	Historical control
Conger [22]	IHD	RCT	18	BUN <70 or Creat <5	BUN ~150 Creat ~10	64	20	Posttrauma, Navy ship Tests intensity + timing
Gillum et al. [23]	IHD	RCT	34	Creat 8 Treatment goal: BUN <60, Creat <5	BUN ~100 or Creat ~9	41	53	Intensity + timing study Survival difference NS
Gettings et al. [24]	CRRT	Retrospective	100	BUN <60	BUN >60	39	20	More MOSF/sepsis in late group
Bouman et al. [25]	CRRT	RCT	106	<12 h after AKI criteria met: UOP <30 mL/h Ccreat <20 mL/min	Standard criteria: BUN >112, K >6.5 Pulmonary edema	LV: 69 HV: 74	LV: 75	Low mortality (27%) Underpowered No CRRT in 6/36 late starts
Demirkiliç et al. [26]	CRRT	Retrospective	61	UOP <100 mL/8 h despite furosemide	Creat >5 or K >6.5	77	45	Postcardiac surgery TTI (days) 0.9 vs. 2.6
Elahi et al. [27]	CRRT	Retrospective	64	UOP <100 mL/8 h despite furosemide	BUN >84, K >6.0	78	57	Postcardiac surgery TTI (days) 0.8 vs. 2.6
Liu et al. [28]	CRRT	Retrospective	80	<12 h after ICU admission	Conventional indications	55	28	Sepsis + oliguria Historical controls Early hemofiltration
Seabra et al. [29]	IHD and CRRT	Observational	243	BUN <76	BUN >76	65	59	Adjusted RR (death) 1.85 for high BUN
Palevsky [30]	IHD and CRRT	Meta-analysis RCT, cohort	2,378	Variable	Variable			Early start risk reduction Cohort: 28% RR RCTs: 36% RR

BUN, blood urea nitrogen; Ccreat, creatinine clearance; CRRT, continuous renal replacement therapy; HV, high-volume hemofiltration; IHD, intermittent hemodialysis; LV, low-volume hemofiltration; MOSF, multiorgan system failure; RCT, randomized controlled trial; TTI, time to initiation; UOP, urine output.

TABLE 75.5

INDICATIONS FOR RENAL REPLACEMENT THERAPY IN PATIENTS WITH ACUTE KIDNEY INJURY

Indication	Characteristics	Absolute/Relative
Metabolic abnormality	BUN >76 mg/dL	Relative
	BUN >100 mg/dL	Absolute
	Hyperkalemia >6 mEq/L	Relative
	Hyperkalemia >6 mEq/L with ECG changes	Absolute
	Dysnatremia	Relative
Acidosis	pH >7.15	Relative
	PH <7.15	Absolute
	Lactic acidosis related to metformin use	Absolute
Anuria/oliguria	<0.5 mL/kg/h × 6 h	Relative
	<0.5 mL/kg/ h × 12 h	Relative
	<0.3 mL/kg/h × 24 h or anuria × 12 h	Relative
Fluid overload	Diuretic sensitive	Relative
	Diuretic resistant	Absolute

index of dialysis dose for which K is the urea clearance of the dialyzer, t is the duration of dialysis, and V is the volume of distribution of urea; the Kt/V is thought to be a measure of time-averaged urea clearance and is determined by applying predialysis and postdialysis urea and volume data to a published formula. The Kt/V for each IHD should exceed 1.2, assuming single pool urea kinetics. Alternatively, some programs target a URR of more than 65% or 70%. The URR is calculated from the following formula:

URR = (predialysis BUN − postdialysis BUN)/predialysis BUN

Finally, RRT can be used simply to maintain the BUN below a target level such as less than 80 to 100 mg per dL.

Methods of increasing urea clearance include maintaining high dialysis blood flows, often necessitating the use of large bore catheters and high gauge needles, using larger dialyzers, and extending dialysis time or frequency. It is important to note that adequate urea clearance does not ensure that ultrafiltration needs are met and additional RRT may be required to address volume overload.

There is little data regarding the dosage or intensity of PD for patients with AKI. Guidelines for stable ESRD patients on this form of RRT remain incompletely validated, even for commonly used techniques such as CCPD. When employed in the ICU setting, the patient's maintenance outpatient regimen is typically continued. However, adjustments such as increased exchange frequency, altered dialysate dextrose concentration, and, rarely, increased dialysate volume can be used to enhance solute and volume removal as clinically indicated.

Guidelines for the intensity of renal support in critically ill patients with AKI, particularly those on CRRT, are based primarily on the Acute Renal Failure Trial Network (ATN Trial) published in 2008 [35]. Prior to this, several single-center studies suggested that more dialysis leads to better outcomes. One study compared daily to alternate day IHD and reported lower mortality (28% vs. 46%) and shorter duration of AKI (9 vs. 16 days) in the daily IHD group [36]. Of note, the dose of dialysis delivered to the alternate day IHD group was very low (Kt/V_{urea}, 0.94). In addition, this study has been criticized for several methodologic irregularities. A seminal study by Ronco et al. reported improved survival with high-volume CVVH [37]. Four hundred and twenty-five patients were randomized to CVVH at variable ultrafiltration rates: 20, 35, and 45 mL per kg per hour. Survival was 41%, 57%, and 58%, respectively. This study set a standard minimum ultrafiltration rate of 35 mL per kg per hour for patients with AKI undergoing CRRT. This standard of care was reinforced by a latter prospective trial that compared CVVH at 25 mL per kg per hour to an augmented dose delivered by CVVHDF [38]. In the later group, the addition of dialysate at 18 mL per kg per hour to an ultrafiltration rate of 24 mL per kg per hour improved 28-day survival from 39% to 59%.

A large multicenter US trial, the ATN trial, tested the hypothesis that more intensive RRT in critically ill patients would decrease mortality and promote recovery of renal function [35]. A total of 1,124 patients at 27 centers were randomized to intensive therapy (IT) and less intensive therapy (LIT). An integrated treatment strategy was used. Hemodynamically stable patients were managed by IHD, whereas unstable patients were managed with CVVHD or SLED. Patients were permitted to move from one modality to another as their hemodynamic status changed. In the IT group, IHD and SLED were performed six times per week and CVVHDF provided an effluent flow rate of 35 mL per kg per hour. In the LIT group, IHD and SLED was performed three times per week and CVVHDF provided an effluent flow of 20 mL per kg per hour. The 60-day mortality was no different (53.6% in IT and 51.5% in LIT). There was no difference between the two groups in duration of RRT, rate of recovery of renal function, or recovery from nonrenal organ failure. Another multicenter, randomized trial conducted in Australia and New Zealand compared the effect of CRRT at two levels of intensity [39]. Higher intensity therapy did not reduce mortality at 90 days.

The results of the ATN trial do not imply that the dose of RRT is unimportant in managing AKI. Patients in the LIT group were better dialyzed than patients receiving usual care in typical clinical practice. Dialysis treatment (IHD, SLED) in the LIT group delivered a mean single pool Kt/V_{urea} of 1.30 that generated a mean predialysis BUN of 70. Among patients managed CVVHDF, the median time of treatment was 21 hours per day, substantially longer than times achieved in clinical practice. We support the dosing recommendation of the ATN investigators:

- IHD or SLED
  - Provide hemodialysis three times per week (alternate days).
  - Monitor the delivered dose to ensure delivery of a single pool Kt/V of 1.20 or more.

- CRRT
  - Employ large caliber catheters and systems of anticoagulation to maximize filter life.
  - Ensure effluent flow rate (hemofiltration rate + dialysate flow rate) of 20 mL or more per kg per hour.
  - In convective systems which employ RF, add 25% to the prescribed effluent flow rate (RF rate) to adjust for dilutional effects if prefilter RF is used.

MODALITY SELECTION

In the United States, the hemodynamically stable patient with AKI is generally managed with IHD. The technique provides rapid solute clearance and volume removal, but it is of limited utility in the setting of hypotension. Unstable patients are more often managed by one of the CRRTs. Patients may move from one modality to another with changes in hemodynamic status. Dialysis sessions are delivered at a minimum of three times per week. More frequent sessions are often required to achieve specific volume and metabolic targets. The average ICU patient with AKI receives 3.5 L of fluid daily. It is challenging if not impossible to mobilize this volume (24 L per week) over three IHD sessions alone. IHD may be supplemented with additional ultrafiltration sessions to meet volume needs.

The principal RRT options are IHD and CRRTs. PD management of AKI has declined markedly over the past 30 years, though it remains an important ICU modality in developing countries. SLED is used in a minority of programs, often in response to resource considerations.

IHD Versus CRRT

Modality selection in AKI is highly variable and appears to be changing in favor of CRRT. Ten years ago, most patients in the United States were treated with IHD. However, a recent survey of VA and US Academic Medical Centers reports a mix of IHD and CRRT modalities [40]. In the United Kingdom and Australia, CRRT is used as initial support in the vast majority of patients with AKI [41]. The shift toward CRRT is driven by a number of important practical as well some theoretical advantages for CRRT over IHD:

- CRRT induces less hypotension and is better tolerated by the patient with unstable hemodynamics.
- CRRT permits removal of large fluid volumes without inducing or exacerbating hypotension.
- Since CRRT induces less hypotension, it may promote renal recovery from AKI
- CRRT provides greater solute clearance than alternate day IHD.
- Since CRRT minimizes/limits hypotension and disequilibrium, it may better preserve cerebral perfusion in acute brain injury and in hepatic failure.
- The convective clearance of CRRT, particularly CVVH, may remove harmful immunomodulatory substances in sepsis.

The major trials comparing IHD with CRRT are summarized in Table 75.6. Retrospective studies from the 1990s show no survival advantage of modality selection in AKI [49,50]. Most report higher unadjusted mortality among the CRRT treated patients, but this difference is lost after adjusting for severity of illness. A modern day multicenter, observational series reported *increased* mortality with CRRT even after adjusting for study site, age, hepatic failure, and sepsis [48]. Incomplete adjustment for severity of illness may have confounded these findings. Nevertheless, the authors raise the possibility that aspects of care associated with CRRT (anticoagulation, medical errors, and removal of nutrients or drugs) may induce harm.

However, several prospective randomized trials have compared the effect of modality selection on outcomes in AKI (Table 75.6). In a small (n = 30) study of septic patients with AKI [51], CVVH preserved systemic hemodynamics better than

TABLE 75.6

MAJOR TRIALS COMPARING IHD AND CRRT

Study	Design	N	Mortality (IHD)	Mortality (CRRT)	Odds of death in IHD (95% CI)	RR,[a] CRRT vs. IHD	Comments
Mehta et al. [42]	RCT	166	48	66	0.63 (0.30–1.10)	35% vs. 33%	More liver failure, more MOSF in CRRT group
Augustine et al. [43]	RCT	80	70	68	1.12 (0.40–3.20)	No difference	More fluid removal, less hypotension in CRRT
Uehlinger et al. [44]	RCT	125	51	47	1.16 (0.50–2.50)	50% vs. 42%	
Vinsonneau et al. [45]	RCT	359	68	67	1.05 (0.60–1.7)	90% vs. 93%	5–6 h IHD 4× per wk Rigorous IHD protocol
Uchino et al. [46]	Observational Study	1,218	48	64		85% vs. 66%	CRRT predicted independence from dialysis
Bell et al. [47]	Observational Study	2,202	46	51		92% vs. 83%	32 ICUs in Sweden Dialysis dependence at 90 d: 8% vs. 16%
Cho et al. [48]	Multicenter, observational study	398	42	55	RR of death for CRRT, 1.82 (1.26–2.62)	Not reported	Mortality risk of CRRT persists after adjustment for sepsis/liver failure

[a]Independence from dialysis.
CI, confidence interval; CRRT, continuous renal replacement therapy; ICU, intensive care unit; IHD, intermittent hemodialysis; RCT, randomized controlled trial; RR, renal recovery.

did IHD over the first 24 hours, but long-term ICU mortality was 70% in both groups. In a larger single-center study of 80 patients [46], CVVHD induced less hypotension and better-controlled volume, but these factors did not improve survival, preservation of urine flow, or recovery of renal function. A potential benefit of CVVHD may have been lost in an attempt to control dialysis dose among modalities. Average dialysis times in IHD patients were 5 to 6 hours. In CVVHD patients, dialysate flow rates were often reduced to less than 1 L per hour. A US multicenter trial reported higher mortality among patients randomized to CRRT, but the randomization process was flawed [42]. Patients assigned to CRRT had more liver failure, higher APACHE scores, and a greater number of failed organ systems than did their IHD counterparts. After covariate adjustment, there was no mortality difference attributable to modality of RRT.

The French conducted the largest and most rigorous prospective multicenter trial to date [45]. In the Hemodiafe study, 359 patients from 21 medical centers were randomized to IHD or CVVHDF. Severity of illness was similar among groups. Pressor support was common at randomization (86% and 89%, IHD and CVVHD) as was sepsis (69% and 56%). Crossover from the IHD group to CVVHDF was low (3.3%) and both groups used the same dialyzer membranes. Sixty-day survival and recovery of renal function were identical between the groups. Unlike other prospective studies, Hemodiafe reported similar rates of hypotension. Hemodynamic stability among IHD patients was meticulously promoted by routine use of cool dialysate (35°C), very high dialysate sodium concentration (150 mmol), isovolemic connections, progressive ultrafiltration, and extended dialysis time (>5 hours). This study stands as evidence that all patients could be managed with IHD irrespective of hemodynamics.

Three recent meta-analysis and systematic reviews also conclude that no specific modality of renal support provides a survival advantage in AKI [52–54]. Similarly, none of the meta-analyses reported an advantage of CRRT in preserving renal function. However, two observational studies excluded from these analyses suggest some differences between IHD and CRRT. In one analysis of 1,281 patients with AKI, independence from dialysis at discharge was more common in patients treated with CRRT (85% vs. 66%), but CRRT patients had lower survival (36% vs. 52%) [46]. Multivariate adjustment identified CRRT as predictive of dialysis independence but not predictive of survival. A second analysis of 2,200 patients, managed in 32 ICUs throughout Sweden, reported twofold higher rates of dialysis dependency (16% vs. 8%) among 90-day AKI survivors managed with IHD [47]. However, mortality was higher (50.6% vs. 45.7%) among the CRRT group.

In summary, no evidence exists to support a survival advantage of specific modality support in AKI. Some prospective trials suggest improved hemodynamic stability with CRRT, and some retrospective analyses suggest enhanced recovery of renal function. In many circumstances, modality selection is guided by medical and nursing expertise and by availability of equipment or nursing support. When both modalities are available, selection should be individualized according to clinical status. Most US tertiary care centers opt for CRRT in settings of hemodynamic instability. The French experience suggests IHD can be used successfully in hemodynamically unstable patients, provided ultrafiltration rates are reduced by increasing the frequency and duration of treatment. Acute hemodialysis programs may be insufficiently staffed to perform high frequency (five to six times per week) and/or extended (>5 hours) dialysis. The same staffing limitations have lead many US programs to extend the indications for CRRT to the patient with stable hemodynamics but with severe volume overload and large obligate fluid intake.

Recommendations

We support the practice of most US centers and recommend CRRT over IHD for the management of AKI in the following clinical settings:

- Hypotension requiring pressor support
- Massive volume overload with high obligate fluid intake
- Highly catabolic patients who have failed to reduce BUN less than 80 mg per dL over three IHD sessions
- AKI in the setting of severe liver failure

Technical recommendations:

- We favor pump-driven venovenous systems over arteriovenous systems.
- We practice CVVH because of its simplicity and theoretic advantage of clearing middle molecules and harmful immunomodulatory cytokines. There is no evidence that CVVH is associated with better outcomes than CVVHD or CVVHDF.
- Regardless of the CRRT modality, the prescribed effluent volume should be 20 to 25 mL per kg per hour.
- When RF is administered in the predilution (prefilter) mode, increase target effluent volume by 25%.

Discontinuation of Therapy

Recovery of renal function is traditionally defined by the reversal of oliguria and progressive decline in serum creatinine. Increased urine volume may not be apparent in the nonoliguric patient. If the CRRT patient is intensively treated, the serum creatinine may be normal, making it impossible to detect a spontaneous decline. We define recovery of renal function according to the criteria used in the ATN study [35]:

- Urine volume exceeding 30 mL per hour (720 mL per day)
- 6-hour timed urine collection to compute creatinine clearance:

$$C_{creat} = U_{creat} \times \text{volume}/P_{creat} \div 360$$

<12 mL per minute	continue CRRT
12–20 mL per minute	individualize ongoing CRRT
20 mL per minute	discontinue CRRT

COMPLICATIONS OF RRT

A comprehensive discussion of RRT complications is beyond the scope of this chapter. For example, complications of central venous catheter placement are discussed in Chapter 2. However, we will review selected complications of dialytic support that are common in the ICU setting.

Infection

Infection is a common complication of all RRT modalities. For IHD and CRRT, infection is usually associated with hemodialysis catheter use and may result in interruption of RRT and increased mortality. Early studies showed higher infection rates with femoral versus subclavian and internal jugular vein cannulation [55,56]. However, the largest prospective randomized study comparing internal jugular and femoral catheters showed no difference in the risk of infection after 5 days [57]. This trial randomly assigned 750 patients to receive either jugular or femoral vein catheterization. The rate of catheter-related sepsis was the same for both groups (1.5 vs. 2.3 per 1,000 catheter days for femoral and jugular venous catheterization, respectively). Hematomas were significantly more common for jugular compared with femoral cannulation (3.6 vs. 1.1%).

Peritonitis is a common infectious complication of PD and is the leading cause of catheter removal and modality conversion. It typically results from bacterial contamination during the exchange procedure or migration along the catheter tunnel. Symptoms and signs include fever, abdominal pain and tenderness, and cloudy dialysate effluent. The peritoneal fluid white blood cell count of greater than 100 cells per mL with at least 50% neutrophils indicates bacterial infection; however, a lymphocyte-predominate cell count may accompany fungal or mycobacterium infections. When peritonitis is suspected, cultures should be done prior to antibiotic therapy. *Staphylococcus aureus* and *Staphylococcus epidermidis* account for less than 50% of cases; however, polymicrobial and fungal infections should receive special consideration in the ICU. Patients with suspected peritonitis should receive empiric antibiotics to cover both Gram-positive and Gram-negative organism, pending culture results.

Electrolyte and Acid–Base Disorders

All forms of RRT can cause a variety of electrolyte and acid–base disturbances. These are most common with CVVH, as convective losses of large volumes of plasma can easily lead to hypocalcemia, hypomagnesemia, hypophosphatemia, hypokalemia, and metabolic acidosis if RF and solute supplementation are not carefully adjusted. Measurements of serum electrolytes are needed at least daily and may be required more frequently in many clinical situations. With IHD and CVVHD, metabolic disturbances are less frequent, since the dialysate composition is adjusted to avoid excessive potassium removal and usually maintains calcium and magnesium levels while supplementing bicarbonate. Hypophosphatemia is uncommon with intermittent and continuous dialysis modalities because phosphorus clearance is much lower for diffusion-based RRT when compared with convective RRT.

Access Thrombosis

Thrombosis of vascular access is a frequent complication of RRT. For patients with dialysis catheters, thrombus can form around the catheter. Clinically, patients will often present with dramatic edema of the ipsilateral extremity. In some cases, the only sign is impaired blood flow through the catheter. The diagnosis can be established with venous duplex studies or venography, though the latter approach necessitates radiocontrast exposure. If the catheter remains functional, the patient can usually be anticoagulated and the line left in place and safely used for dialysis.

Dialysis catheters may also develop impaired blood flow due to the formation of a thin layer of thrombus, also known as a fibrin sheath, along the outer surface of the line. In such cases, radiologic evaluation and procedures such as removal of the thrombus with a wire (catheter stripping) or localized infusion of thrombolytics may be needed to restore function. In severe cases, the catheter must be replaced.

For patients with ESRD, thrombosis of the AVF or AVG often occurs in the setting of hypotension or severe volume depletion, particularly if there is stenosis of the venous system proximal to the access. AVGs are much more prone to thrombosis than AVFs. The diagnosis is usually obvious, as the access will no longer have a palpable thrill or audible bruit. In cases of incomplete or impending thrombosis, cannulation of the access may reveal the presence of clots. Rarely, duplex of the access is needed to confirm thrombosis. If possible, the access patency should be reestablished by either surgical thrombectomy or mechanical or chemical thrombolysis. The decision to repair or revise the AVF or AVG, as well as the approach used, will depend on the patient's clinical status and the expertise and equipment available.

Hypotension

Hypotension often complicates volume removal by IHD. Severe reductions in blood pressure during dialysis limit ultrafiltration, perpetuate renal injury, and compromise perfusion to other vital organs. The pathophysiology of intradialytic hypotension involves left ventricular (LV) underfilling and inadequate reactive (pressor) response to decreasing volume. The rate of ultrafiltration, the magnitude of fluid shifts between the extracellular and intracellular compartments, and the plasma refill rate (as fluid moves from the interstitium to plasma) determine LV filling pressure. The risk of hypotension during IHD can be reduced by several methods:

- Reduce ultrafiltration rate by extending the duration of treatment
- Reduce ultrafiltration rate by increasing frequency of treatment
- Minimize intracellular fluid shifts by employing sodium modeling
- Potentiate vasoconstrictor tone by cooling the dialysate to 35°C

Effective strategies employed less frequently are as follows:

- Enhance plasma refill rate by infusions of albumin
- Promote vasoconstrictor tone with high concentration of calcium in dialysate
- Promote vasoconstrictor tone with oral midodrine prior to dialysis
- Promote vasoconstrictor tone with infusion of norepinephrine or vasopressin

Noninvasive monitoring tools are available to titrate volume removal to specific targets. Techniques involve bioimpedance analysis, pulse contour analysis, and echocardiography. The utility of these technologies in preventing intradialytic hypotension is still unproven.

References

1. Scheel PJ, Liu M, Rabb H: Uremic lung: new insights into a forgotten condition. *Kidney Int* 74:849–851, 2008.
2. Foland JA, Fortenberry JD, Warshaw BL, et al: Fluid overload before continuous hemofiltration and survival in critically ill children: a retrospective analysis. *Crit Care Med* 32:1771–1776, 2004.
3. Goldstein SL, Currier H, Graf Cd, et al: Outcome in children receiving continuous venovenous hemofiltration. *Pediatrics* 107:1309–1312, 2001.
4. Bent P, Tan HK, Bellomo R, et al: Early and intensive continuous hemofiltration for severe renal failure after cardiac surgery. *Ann Thorac Surg* 71:832–837, 2001.
5. Mehta RL: Indications for dialysis in the ICU: renal replacement vs. renal support. *Blood Purif* 19:227–232, 2001.
6. Schwab SJ, Onorato JJ, Sharar LR, et al: Hemodialysis without anticoagulation. One-year prospective trial in hospitalized patients at risk for bleeding. *Am J Med* 83:405–410, 1987.
7. Lim W, Cook DJ, Crowther MA: Safety and efficacy of low molecular weight heparins for hemodialysis in patients with end-stage renal failure: a meta-analysis of randomized trials. *J Am Soc Nephrol* 15:3192–3206, 2004.
8. Kutsogiannis DJ, Gibney RT, Stollery D, et al: Regional citrate versus

systemic heparin anticoagulation for continuous renal replacement in critically ill patients. *Kidney Int* 67:2361–2367, 2005.
9. Hakim RM, Wingard RL, Parker RA: Effect of the dialysis membrane in the treatment of patients with acute renal failure. *N Engl J Med* 331(20):1338–1342, 1994.
10. Jorres A, Gahl GM, Dobis C, et al: Haemodialysis-membrane biocompatibility and mortality of patients with dialysis-dependent acute renal failure: a prospective randomised multicentre trial. International Multicentre Study Group. *Lancet* 354(9187):1337–1341, 1999.
11. Malcolm DS, Zaloga GP, Holaday JW: Calcium administration increases the mortality of endotoxic shock in rats. *Crit Care Med.* 17(9):900–903, 1989.
12. Moberly JB, Mujais S, Gehr T, et al: Review of clinical trial experience with icodextrin. *Kidney Int* 62[Suppl 81]:S46, 2002.
13. Levy EM, Viscoli CM, Horwitz RI: The effect of acute renal failure on mortality. A cohort analysis. *JAMA* 275:1489–1494, 1996.
14. Chertow GM, Levy EM, Hammermeister KE, et al: Independent association between acute renal failure and mortality following cardiac surgery. *Am J Med* 104:343–348, 1998.
15. Metnitz PG, Krenn CG, Steltzer H, et al: Effect of acute renal failure requiring renal replacement therapy on outcome in critically ill patients. *Crit Care Med* 30:2051–2058, 2002.
16. Liano F, Junco E, Pascual J, et al: The spectrum of acute renal failure in the intensive care unit compared with that seen in other settings. The Madrid Acute Renal Failure Study Group. *Kidney Int* 66 [Suppl]:S16–S24, 1998.
17. Liano F, Pascual J: Epidemiology of acute renal failure: a prospective, multicenter, community-based study. Madrid Acute Renal Failure Study Group. *Kidney Int* 50:811–818, 1996.
18. Uchino S, Kellum JA, Bellomo R, et al: Acute renal failure in critically ill patients: a multinational, multicenter study. *JAMA* 294:813–818, 2005.
19. Parsons FM, Hobson SM, Blagg CR, et al: Optimum time for dialysis in acute reversible renal failure. Description and value of an improved dialyser with large surface area. *Lancet* 1:129–134, 1961.
20. Fischer RP, Griffen WO Jr, Reiser M, et al: Early dialysis in the treatment of acute renal failure. *Surg Gynecol Obstet* 123:1019–1023, 1966.
21. Kleinknecht D, Jungers P, Chanard J, et al: Uremic and non-uremic complications in acute renal failure: evaluation of early and frequent dialysis on prognosis. *Kidney Int* 1:190–196, 1972.
22. Conger JD: A controlled evaluation of prophylactic dialysis in post-traumatic acute renal failure. *J Trauma* 15:1056–1063, 1975.
23. Gillum DM, Dixon BS, Yanover MJ, et al: The role of intensive dialysis in acute renal failure. *Clin Nephrol* 25:249–255, 1986.
24. Gettings LG, Reynolds HN, Scalea T: Outcome in post-traumatic acute renal failure when continuous renal replacement therapy is applied early vs. late. *Intensive Care Med* 25:805–813, 1999.
25. Bouman CS, Oudemans-Van Straaten HM, Tijssen JG, et al: Effects of early high-volume continuous venovenous hemofiltration on survival and recovery of renal function in intensive care patients with acute renal failure: a prospective, randomized trial. *Crit Care Med* 30:2205–2211, 2002.
26. Demirkiliç U, Kuralay E, Yenicesu M, et al: Timing of replacement therapy for acute renal failure after cardiac surgery. *J Card Surg* 19:17–20, 2004.
27. Elahi MM, Lim MY, Joseph RN, et al: Early hemofiltration improves survival in postcardiotomy patients with acute renal failure. *Eur J Cardiothorac Surg* 26:1027–1031, 2004.
28. Liu KD, Himmelfarb J, Paganini E, et al: Timing of initiation of dialysis in critically ill patients with acute kidney injury. *Clin J Am Soc Nephrol* 1:915–919, 2006.
29. Seabra VF, Balk EM, Liangos O, et al: Timing of renal replacement therapy initiation in acute renal failure: a meta-analysis. *Am J Kidney Dis* 52:272–284, 2008.
30. Palevsky PM: Indications and timing of renal replacement therapy in acute kidney injury. *Crit Care Med* 36[Suppl 4]:S224–S228, 2008.
31. Gibney N, Hoste E, Burdmann EA, et al: Timing of initiation and discontinuation of renal replacement therapy in AKI: unanswered key questions. *Clin J Am Soc Nephrol* 3:876–880, 2008.
32. Piccinni P, Dan M, Barbacini S, et al: Early isovolemic haemofiltration in oliguric patients with septic shock. *Intensive Care Med* 32:80–86, 2006.
33. Schetz M: Evidence-based analysis of the role of hemofiltration in sepsis and multiorgan dysfunction syndrome. *Curr Opin Crit Care* 3:434–441, 1997.
34. Cole L, Bellomo R, Hart G, et al: A phase II randomized, controlled trial of continuous hemofiltration in sepsis. *Crit Care Med* 30:100–106, 2002.
35. Palevsky PM, Zhang JH, O'Connor TZ, et al: Intensity of renal support in critically ill patients with acute kidney injury. *N Engl J Med* 359:7–20, 2008.
36. Schiffl H, Lang SM, Fischer R: Daily hemodialysis and the outcome of acute renal failure. *N Engl J Med* 346:305–310, 2002.
37. Ronco C, Bellomo R, Homel P, et al: Effects of different doses in continuous veno-venous haemofiltration on outcomes of acute renal failure: a prospective randomised trial. *Lancet* 356:26–30, 2000.
38. Saudan P, Niederberger M, De Seigneux S, et al: Adding a dialysis dose to continuous hemofiltration increases survival in patients with acute renal failure. *Kidney Int* 70:1312–1317, 2006.
39. Bellomo R, Cass A, Cole L, et al: Intensity of continuous renal-replacement therapy in critically ill patients. *N Engl J Med* 361:1627–1638, 2009.
40. Overberger P, Pesacreta M, Palevsky PM: Management of renal replacement therapy in acute kidney injury: a survey of practitioner prescribing practices. *Clin J Am Soc Nephrol* 2:623–630, 2007.
41. Gatward JJ, Gibbons GJ, Wrathall G, et al: Renal replacement therapy for acute renal failure: a survey of practice in adult ICUs in the United Kingdom. *Anaesthesia* 63:959–966, 2008.
42. Mehta RL, McDonald B, Gabbai FB, et al: A randomized clinical trial of continuous versus intermittent dialysis for acute renal failure. *Kidney Int* 60:1154–1163, 2001.
43. Augustine JJ, Sandy D, Seifert TH, et al: A randomized controlled trial comparing intermittent with continuous dialysis in patients with ARF. *Am J Kidney Dis* 44:1000–1007, 2004.
44. Uehlinger DE, Jakob SM, Ferrari P, et al: Comparison of continuous and intermittent renal replacement therapy for acute renal failure. *Nephrol Dial Transplant* 20:1630–1637, 2005.
45. Vinsonneau C, Camus C, Combes A, et al: Continuous venovenous haemodiafiltration versus intermittent haemodialysis for acute renal failure in patients with multiple-organ dysfunction syndrome: a multicentre randomized trial. *Lancet* 368:379–385, 2006.
46. Uchino S, Bellomo R, Kellum JA, et al: Patient and kidney survival by dialysis modality in critically ill patients with acute kidney injury. *Int J Artif Organs* 30:281–292, 2007.
47. Bell M, Granath F, Schon S, et al: Continuous renal replacement therapy is associated with less chronic renal failure than intermittent haemodialysis after acute renal failure. *Intensive Care Med* 33:773–780, 2007.
48. Cho KC, Himmelfarb J, Paganini E, et al: Survival by dialysis modality in critically ill patients with acute kidney injury. *J Am Soc Nephrol* 17:3132–3138, 2006.
49. Swartz RD, Messana JM, Orzol S, et al: Comparing continuous hemofiltration with hemodialysis in patients with severe acute renal failure. *Am J Kidney Dis* 34:424, 1999.
50. Guerin C, Girard R, Selli JM, et al: Intermittent versus continuous renal replacement therapy for acute renal failure in intensive care units: results from a multicenter epidemiological survey. *Intensive Care Med* 28:1411, 2002.
51. John S, Griesbach D, Baumgartel M, et al: Effects of continuous haemofiltration vs intermittent haemodialysis on systemic haemodynamics and splanchnic regional perfusion in septic shock patients: a prospective, randomized clinical trial. *Nephrol Dial Transplant* 16:320–327, 2001.
52. Rabindranath K, Adams J, Macleod AM, et al: Intermittent versus continuous renal replacement therapy for acute renal failure in adults. *Cochrane Database Syst Rev* (3):CD003773, 2007.
53. Pannu N, Klarenbach S, Wiebe N, et al: Renal replacement therapy in patients with acute renal failure: a systematic review. *JAMA* 299:793–805, 2008.
54. Bagshaw SM, Berthiaume LR, Delaney A, et al: Continuous versus intermittent renal replacement therapy for critically ill patients with acute kidney injury: a meta-analysis. *Crit Care Med* 36:610–617, 2008.
55. Kairaitis LK, Gottlieb T: Outcome and complications of temporary haemodialysis catheters. *Nephrol Dial Transplant* 14(7):1710–1714, 1999.
56. Oliver MJ, Callery SM, Thorpe KE, et al: Risk of bacteremia from temporary hemodialysis catheters by site of insertion and duration of use: a prospective study. *Kidney Int* 58(6):2543–2545, 2000.
57. Parienti JJ, Thirion M, Megarbane B, et al: Femoral vs. jugular venous catheterization and risk of nosocomial events in adults requiring acute renal replacement therapy: a randomized controlled trial. *JAMA* 299(20):2413–2422, 2008.

SECTION VI ■ INFECTIOUS DISEASE PROBLEMS IN THE INTENSIVE CARE UNIT

RICHARD T. ELLISON, III

CHAPTER 76 ■ APPROACH TO FEVER IN THE ICU PATIENT

RAUL E. DAVARO AND RICHARD H. GLEW

Humanity has but three great enemies: fever, famine and war; of these by far the greatest, by far the most terrible, is fever [1].

Sir William Osler

APPROACH TO THE FEBRILE PATIENT

Fever is identified as the body's host defense mechanism and although it is commonly associated with infections, the relationship between infection and elevation of body's temperature is poorly understood [2]. The incidence of fever in the intensive care unit (ICU) ranges from 28% to 70% [3].

Pathophysiology

The normal core body temperature of approximately 37°C is well conserved in vertebrates with minimal changes [2]. Core temperature typically exhibits diurnal rhythmicity, with a nadir of about 36.2°C in the morning and a peak of approximately 37.7°C in the afternoon [4]. Temperature elevates to 39°C to 40°C in febrile response to infection or other stress [2].

The febrile response is a complex physiologic reaction to disease involving cytokine-mediated rise in core temperature, generation of acute-phase reactants, and activation of numerous physiologic endocrinologic and immunologic systems [5]. In contrast, simple heat illness or malignant hyperthermia is an unregulated rise in body temperature caused by inability to eliminate heat adequately [4]. Physiologically, fever begins with the production of one or more proinflammatory cytokines in response to exogenous pyrogenic substances (such as microorganisms, toxic agents) or immunologic mediators. Interleukin-1 (IL-1) was the first purified protein with demonstrated pyrogenic properties; subsequently, other cytokines such as tumor necrosis factor (TNF), lymphotoxin, interferons (IFNs), and interleukin (IL–6) were documented to induce fever independently. Cytokines interact with receptors located at the organum vasculosum of the lamina terminalis causing synthesis and release of prostaglandins, chiefly prostaglandin E_2, which raise body temperature by initiating local cAMP production, which resets the thermoregulatory set point of the hypothalamus, and by coordinating other adaptive responses such as shivering and peripheral vasoconstriction [5,6]. Fever induces the production of heat shock proteins (HSPs), a class of proteins critical for cellular survival during stress. HSPs that act as molecular chaperones may have an anti-inflammatory role and indirectly decrease the level of proinflammatory cytokines [2].

Measurement

No single normal body temperature exists, and temperatures measured at different times of day and sites may vary. The Society of Critical Care Medicine and the Infectious Disease Society of America issued a consensus statement recommending that core temperature of higher than 38.3°C (101°F) be considered fever [7].

All ICU patients should be monitored with regular reliable temperature determinations. Rectal temperature is about 0.3° to 0.4°C higher than simultaneous oral temperature. Electronic thermometers operate in a predictive manner and complete a temperature reading before thermal equilibrium is reached, thereby providing rapid accurate reading. However, in a tachypneic patient, oral temperature, even obtained with an electronic thermometer, may be misleadingly low. Infrared detection tympanic thermometers appear equivalent to rectal probes when placed properly in the external auditory canal.

In general, axillary measurements and skin temperature recordings and chemical dot thermometers are unreliable and should not be used in the ICU [7]. Fever patterns are not helpful in suggesting or establishing specific diagnosis [8].

ETIOLOGY OF FEVER IN THE INTENSIVE CARE PATIENT

Approximately one third of medical inpatients will develop fever during their hospitalization and nowhere is this more common than in the ICU [9].

Noninfectious Causes of Fever

Although acute bacterial infections are among the most common and serious causes of fever in the ICU patients, fever may result from noninfectious illnesses as well (Table 76.1) [7,10]. Pseudosepsis is a clinical picture of noninfectious etiology characterized by fever, leukocytosis and hemodynamic parameters consistent with sepsis, that can occur in critically ill patients with large hematomas, acute vasculitis, subarachnoid hemorrhage, dissection of an aortic aneurysm, mesenteric ischemia, heat stroke, pancreatitis, or hyperthyroidism [11]. Fever may appear in the patient in whom the stress of surgery unmasks adrenal insufficiency or in the patient in whom malignant hyperpyrexia develops during surgery or in association with administration of nonanesthetic agents such as phenothiazines [12]. Bilateral adrenal hemorrhage, noted to occur in patients with a history of thromboembolic disease, recent surgery, and/or anticoagulant therapy, can present with fever,

TABLE 76.1

NONINFECTIOUS SOURCES OF FEVER IN THE ICU PATIENT

A. Inflammatory conditions
1. Reaction to medications
2. Reaction to blood products
3. Collagen vascular diseases
a. Systemic lupus erythematous
b. Rheumatoid arthritis
4. Vasculitis
a. Hypersensitivity vasculitis
b. Henoch–Schonlein purpura
c. Wegener's granulomatosis
d. Giant cell arteritis
5. Microcrystalline arthritis
a. Gout
b. Pseudogout
6. Postpericardiotomy syndrome
7. Pancreatitis
8. Local reaction to intramuscular injections
B. Vascular conditions
1. Deep venous thrombophlebitis
2. Pulmonary embolism
3. Dissecting aortic aneurysm
4. Mesenteric ischemia/infarction
5. Hemorrhage into
a. CNS
b. Retroperitoneum
c. Joint
d. Lung
e. Adrenals
6. Myocardial infarction
C. Metabolic conditions
1. Heat stroke
2. Malignant hyperthermia secondary to anesthesia or medications
3. Hyperthyroidism
4. Adrenal insufficiency/hemorrhage
5. Alcohol withdrawal
6. Seizures
7. Neuroleptic malignant syndrome
D. Neoplasia
1. Lymphoma
2. Renal cell carcinoma
3. Hepatocellular carcinoma
4. Malignancy metastatic to liver
5. Colon carcinoma

ICU, intensive care unit; CNS, central nervous system.

hypotension, and abdominal or flank pain [13]. Fever is a cardinal manifestation of delirium tremens in patients with acute alcohol withdrawal, although it is necessary to exclude other complications of alcohol abuse such as pneumonia or spontaneous bacterial peritonitis [14]. Likewise, fever associated with seizures must be differentiated from possible underlying causes of seizure, such as meningitis, encephalitis, brain abscess, or stroke [4].

Fever and hyperthermia can be the sole manifestation of an adverse drug reaction in 3% to 5% of cases. Drug fever can occur several days after initiation of the drug and takes few days to subside after cessation of its administration [15].

Particular diagnostic and therapeutic difficulties arise with the appearance of fever in patients with malignancy, because it is important to differentiate between neoplastic fever (especially common with lymphoma, primary and metastatic liver tumors, hypernephroma, and colon carcinoma), fever due to mechanical complications caused by the malignancy (perforation, obstruction, or hemorrhage), and fever due to infection [8].

The patient infected with the human immunodeficiency virus (HIV) who develops fever poses a formidable diagnostic challenge because opportunistic infections may occur on occasion with more than one problem at a time. In addition, HIV-infected patients have a greater incidence of adverse reactions to drugs. Intermittent fevers without discernible etiology also occur in these patients [16].

Conspicuously absent from Table 76.1 is atelectasis. Although this process is widely regarded as a cause of fever, especially in the postoperative patient where atelectasis is common, there is no clear evidence of such [17].

Accurate and timely recognition of noninfectious causes of fever can avoid unnecessary use of antibiotics, reducing the risks of untoward reactions.

Infectious Causes of Fever

Nosocomial infections are an endemic problem in the ICU, in part because of the numerous invasive devices used to monitor and support critically ill patients, and also because of the acute illnesses that predispose critically ill patients to the development of infections. Although hospital-associated infections can arise in many sites, the most common sources of bacterial infection in the ICU are bacteremia, infections associated with intravenous lines, pneumonia, intra-abdominal infection, urinary tract infection, and sinusitis (Table 76.2) [18,19].

Bacteremias

Secondary bacteremia may originate from multiple sources (e.g., lungs, genitourinary tract, abdomen, skin, and soft tissues) or can develop as a consequence of vascular invasion via intravenous and intra-arterial lines and monitors, temporary transvenous pacemakers, and intra-aortic assist devices.

Healthcare-Associated Pneumonia

Ventilator-associated pneumonia (VAP) is the most common infection acquired in the ICU. Necrotizing bacterial and fungal pneumonias occur in patients receiving antibiotics, chemotherapy, and/or corticosteroids, on ventilatory assistance, following abdominal surgery or in the setting of malignancy, neutropenia, or vascular access devices [20].

Intra-Abdominal Infections

The gastrointestinal tract can serve as the source of serious nosocomial infections. Intra-abdominal abscesses must be suspected in patients who develop postoperative fever after abdominal surgery. Acute acalculous cholecystitis complicated by biliary sepsis may occur after surgery or severe trauma [21]. Pseudomembranous colitis caused by *Clostridium difficile* in patients receiving broad-spectrum antibiotics is a common source of fever in the ICU [22].

Urinary Tract Infections

In hospital, ICUs have the highest rate of urinary tract infections, the majority of which are associated with the use of indwelling urine catheters. Partial or total obstruction or local complications (e.g., intrarenal or perinephric abscesses) must be suspected in patients with bacteremic pyelonephritis if fever and bacteremia persist [23].

TABLE 76.2

INFECTIOUS SOURCES OF FEVER IN THE ICU PATIENT

A. Urinary tract
1. Pyelonephritis
2. Prostatitis, prostatic abscess
B. Vascular devices
1. Intravenous access site
a. Phlebitis
b. Bacteremia or fungemia
c. Cellulitis
2. Intra-arterial access site
a. Bacteremia
b. Fungemia
C. Respiratory
1. Tracheobronchitis
2. Pneumonia
3. Sinusitis
4. Empyema
5. Lung abscess
D. Surgical-related wound
1. Wound infection (superficial/incisional or deep)
2. Deep-seated abscess (liver, spleen, kidney, brain, subphrenic, bowel)
E. Skin/soft tissue
1. Decubitus ulcer, with cellulitis/fasciitis/myositis
2. Cellulitis
F. Gastrointestinal
1. Antibiotic-associated colitis/*Clostridium difficile* colitis
2. Ischemic colitis (mesenteric ischemia/infarction)
3. Biliary
a. Cholecystitis, including acalculous
b. Cholangitis
4. Hepatitis (transfusion related)
a. Cytomegalovirus
b. Hepatitis C
c. Hepatitis B
5. Intra-abdominal abscess
6. Diverticulitis
G. Prosthetic device infection
1. Cardiac valve/pacemaker
2. Joint replacement prosthesis
3. Peritoneal dialysis catheter/peritonitis
4. CNS intraventricular shunt
H. Miscellaneous
1. Pyarthrosis
2. Osteomyelitis (including vertebral osteodiscitis in adults)
3. Meningitis

ICU, intensive care unit; CNS, central nervous system.

Nosocomial Sinusitis

Nosocomial sinusitis may develop in patients who require extended periods of intensive care. Nasogastric and nasotracheal tubes, facial fractures, and nasal packing are common predisposing factors. However, sinusitis alone is responsible for fever in only a minority of intubated patients [24].

DIAGNOSTIC CONSIDERATIONS

In some ICUs, the finding of fever triggers an automatic fever workup resulting in many tests that are time consuming, costly, and disruptive to the patient and staff. The American College of Critical Care Medicine and the Infectious Disease Society of America convened a task force to provide guidelines for evaluation of new fever in patients older than 18 years in the ICU setting [7].

History and Physical Examination

If able to communicate, the patient should be interviewed to identify localizing complaints. The patient and hospital chart should be reviewed thoroughly for a history of relevant antecedent problems (e.g., previous infections, cancer, allergic reactions to drugs). If the patient is unable to communicate, the medical record and medical personnel can provide insightful information concerning duration of intravascular accesses, amount and purulence of sputum or wound drainage, changes in skin condition, apparent abdominal or musculoskeletal pain or tenderness, difficulty in handling respiratory secretions and feeding, and changes in ventilator support parameters. Relatives and friends of the patient can provide epidemiologic information related to the patient's exposures and risk factors for infections.

Physical examination of the febrile ICU patient may be difficult to conduct due to limitations imposed by catheters, ventilator tubes, and monitors but nonetheless should be thorough. Skin examination may demonstrate findings suggestive of drug reaction, vasculitis, endocarditis, or soft tissue necrosis. All intravenous and intra-arterial line sites should be inspected; a tender intravenous access site, with or without purulence, can indicate septic thrombophlebitis. Spreading erythema, warmth, and tenderness that appear to indicate cellulitis of an extremity also can be the hallmarks of deep venous thrombophlebitis, pyarthrosis, or gout. After the first 24 hours postoperatively, wounds should be examined; this may require fenestrating or changing a cast to allow examination of a fractured extremity if no other source of fever is found.

Head and neck examination can provide important signs of systemic and localized infection. Funduscopic examination, preferably by an ophthalmologist, can provide clues to systemic fungal or viral infections in the immune compromised [25]. Hospital-associated sinusitis often develops in patients who required extensive period of intensive care and it may have a paucity of associated symptoms. Oral lesions of recrudescent herpetic stomatitis are common in the ICU setting and often obscured by the presence of oral endotracheal tubes or orogastric feeding tubes. These lesions may be extensive, more ulcerated and necrotic, and less vesicular in appearance in a seriously ill patient.

Examination of the lungs can be difficult in the intubated ICU patient and often is unrewardingly nonlocalizing and nonspecific. More sensitive (although nonspecific) indicators of pneumonia include the chest roentgenogram and the occurrence of unexplained deterioration in arterial oxygenation and changes in the color and amount of respiratory secretions [26]. Unfortunately, pulmonary infiltrates and arterial hypoxemia also can be seen with congestive heart failure, atelectasis, aspiration pneumonitis, pulmonary embolism, acute respiratory distress syndrome, and, less commonly, reactions to medications and pulmonary hemorrhage. Cardiac examination may demonstrate a new or changing murmur possibly due to endocarditis.

Abdominal findings can be misleadingly unremarkable in the elderly, in the patient with obtunded sensorium, and in the patient receiving sedatives. Abdominal examination can be confounding in the patient with recent abdominal or thoracic surgery. Abdominal pain and tenderness may be localized (cholecystis, intra-abdominal abscess, diverticulitis) or generalized (diffuse peritonitis, ischemic bowel, antibiotic-associated colitis). Examination of the genitalia and rectum may demonstrate unsuspected epididymitis, prostatitis, prostatic abscess, or perirectal abscess [27].

Unexplained noninfectious fever is common in patients in the neurologic ICU such as in patients with subarachnoid hemorrhage and is associated with the development of symptomatic vasospasm [28].

Diagnostic Studies

Because the information provided by positive blood cultures has important prognostic and therapeutic implications, blood cultures should be obtained in patients with new fever when clinical evaluation suggests an infectious cause. It is recommended to draw three to four blood cultures from separate sites within the first 24 hours of the onset of fever [7]. When urinary tract may be the source of fever, a urine specimen (aspirated from the catheter sampling port) should be obtained and evaluated by microscopy, and quantitative culture [7].

In patients with clinical suspicion for pneumonia, a portable chest radiograph is mandatory, and efforts should be made to obtain secretions for stains and cultures. Sputum samples should be subjected to microscopic examination to document paucity of squamous cells and to assess the approximate number of polymorphonuclear leukocytes and numbers and types of bacteria as a guide for empiric antibiotic decision making and ultimate interpretation of the results of sputum culture. Techniques aimed at obtaining samples of secretions and tissue from the distal respiratory tract include protected and nonprotected bronchoalveolar lavage (BAL), transbronchial biopsy, protected specimen brush, telescoping plugged catheter, video-assisted lung biopsy, and open lung biopsy; respiratory secretions from these sampling methods may use quantitative culture thresholds to improve the diagnostic accuracy. BAL is the preferred diagnostic approach, with a low rate of complications (2%) and a diagnostic yield between 30% and 90% depending on the type of population studied, prior antibiotic treatment, and the definition of pneumonia used [26]. The triggering receptor expressed on myeloid cells (TREM-1) is upregulated by exposure to bacteria and fungi. Measurement soluble TREM-1 in BAL has been proposed in establishing or excluding the diagnosis of bacterial of fungal pneumonia [29].

In general, abnormal fluid collections (pleural effusion, joint effusion, ascites) should be sampled for microscopic, hematologic, and chemical analysis, as well as microbiologic culture. Microbiologic yield from ascites culture has been shown to be greater when ascitic fluid is placed into blood culture or fungal isolator media [30]. Infection, crystal-induced disease, trauma, and a variety of systemic diseases can create a painful, swollen peripheral joint; arthrocentesis is indicated to establish the nature of the effusion [31]. Meningitis is an uncommon nosocomial infection, except in cases of head trauma, CSF leakage, neurosurgery, or high-grade bacteremia with virulent invasive pathogens such as *Staphylococcus aureus* or Gram-negative bacilli. Thus, sampling of cerebrospinal fluid usually should not be considered in the initial workup for nosocomial fever. However, lumbar puncture should be considered in the febrile ICU patient with sudden, unexplained change in mental status and in the febrile patient who has undergone recent neurosurgery or head trauma and whose mental status is difficult to evaluate [32].

Symptomatic complaints or physical findings referable to the abdomen dictate the need for determination of liver chemistries and serum amylase, as well as CT abdominal diagnostic imaging [21].

Examination of fluid from an inflamed, effused joint necessarily includes analysis for crystals (as well as hematological analysis) smears, and cultures. Exacerbations of gout and pseudogout mimic the symptoms, physical examination, and leukocytosis of the septic joint, and coexistence of gout and joint infection, although uncommon, can occur [31,33].

Many patients in the ICU experience diarrhea, and by far the most common enteric cause of fever in the ICU is *C. difficile*, which should be suspected in any patient with fever or leukocytosis who received an antibacterial agent or *chemotherapy* within 60 days before the onset of diarrhea [7].

Serum procalcitonin levels can be employed as an adjunctive diagnostic tool for discriminating infection as the cause of fever [7].

TREATMENT CONSIDERATIONS

Initial Antibiotic Therapy

Compelling evidence suggests that in infected critically ill patients, source control of the pathogen and early and appropriate antibiotic therapy remain the most important intervention that the clinician can implement for such patients [34]. Antimicrobial therapy should be evaluated daily to optimize efficacy, prevent resistance, and avoid toxicity [35]. Positive cultures may permit narrowing of the spectrum of antibiotic coverage or may dictate that additional organisms need to be covered by added antimicrobial therapy. Negative cultures in a patient who is unimproved yet stable on broad therapy indicate that antibiotics should be discontinued and the patient reevaluated. Negative cultures in a febrile patient who is unimproved or worsened may be a clue to disseminated fungal infection, and empiric antifungal therapy should be considered.

Once efforts have been made to determine the most likely site or sites of infection, one can make a reasonable estimate of infecting pathogens. In an ICU patient, one should assume that in addition to the usual expected pathogens at a given site, infection is likely to involve more opportunistic hospital-associated pathogens such as *S. aureus* (including methicillin-resistant *S. aureus* or MRSA), coagulase-negative staphylococci, and multidrug-resistant enteric Gram-negative bacilli and lactose nonfermenting Gram-negative bacilli (e.g., *Pseudomonas aeruginosa*, *Acinetobacter* species) and yeast (*Candida* sp). In light of possible impairment of mechanical and immunologic defenses and the presence of intravascular lines, the febrile ICU patient should be considered to be bacteremic until proven otherwise. Patients with intravascular lines and bacteremia should have their lines removed, if possible [36].

Once the spectrum of potential infecting organisms has been narrowed to one or a few likely candidates, empiric antibiotic therapy should be changed according to generally accepted principles as outlined later in the chapter (Table 76.3). However, such guidelines must be interpreted in light of the types of organisms and patterns of drug resistance prevalent in the specific institution and ICU. Definitive antibiotic therapy is determined by review of the final microbiologic data, with identification of the isolated infecting microorganism and its antibiotic susceptibilities [38].

Dosage and Route of Administration

Critically ill patients with severe sepsis and septic shock possess unique characteristics that affect the choice of antimicrobial therapy [38]. As a rule, the intravenous route is preferred because of possible unreliable absorption from muscle and the gastrointestinal tract due to impaired hemodynamics and/or gastrointestinal function.

Antibiotics such as the penicillins, cephalosporins, macrolides, and fluoroquinolones, which exhibit a high therapeutic/toxic ratio, usually are administered to adults according to a standardized dosage regimen (g per day) independent of the patient's weight. For antibiotics such as the aminoglycosides,

TABLE 76.3

PRESUMPTIVE ANTIBIOTIC THERAPY IN THE ICU OR CCU PATIENT

Site/diagnosis	Potential causes	Initial therapy	Alternative therapy
Vascular/line-associated bacteremia [36]	*Staphylococcus aureus*, GNR, coagulase-negative *staphylococci*	Vancomycin **plus** a third-generation cephalosporin[a]; suspect MRSA.	Linezolid **plus** a fluoroquinolone
Vascular/acute endocarditis [37]	*S. aureus*, *Enterococcus* spp	Vancomycin (modify according to susceptibilities MRSA, MSSA, VRE)	Linezolid or daptomycin; consider adding an aminoglycoside in *Enterococcus* spp is the pathogen
Vascular/bacteremia [36]	GNR	Third-generation cephalosporin[b] or imipenem or piperacillin–tazobactam	Linezolid **plus** fluoroquinolone
Pulmonary/pneumonia [3,21,26–55]	GNR, *Haemophilus influenzae*, *Streptococcus pneumoniae*	Piperacillin–tazobactam or third-generation cephalosporin[b] **plus** metronidazole if anaerobes suspected	Imipenem or meropenem or ertapenem
Pulmonary/pneumonia [3,21,26–55]	*S. aureus*	Vancomycin or linezolid until MRSA excluded	Cefazolin or oxacillin or nafcillin if MSSA
Pulmonary/pneumonia [3,21,26–55]	*Legionella pneumophila*	Azithromycin or fluoroquinolone	Doxycycline or clarithromycin
Urinary tract/pyelonephritis [56]	GNR, *Enterococcus* spp	Third-generation cephalosporin[b] or fluoroquinolone	Aztreonam or ampicillin or piperacillin–tazobactam (if *Enterococcus* spp suspected)
Abdomen/peritonitis, abscess, pelvic infection [21]	GNR, anaerobes, *Enterococcus* spp	Piperacillin–tazobactam or fluoroquinolone **plus** metronidazole	Vancomycin **plus** metronidazole **plus** aztreonam or imipenem or tigecycline
Abdominal/biliary tract [21]	GNR, enterococcus, anaerobes (less often)	Piperacillin–tazobactam or fluoroquinolone **plus** metronidazole	Vancomycin **plus** metronidazole **plus** aztreonam or imipenem
CNS/meningitis (community acquired) [54]	*Streptococcus pneumoniae*, *Neisseria meningitidis*	Ceftriaxone or cefotaxime **plus** vancomycin	Vancomycin **plus** aztreonam
CNS/meningitis (elderly) [54]	*S. pneumoniae*, *Listeria monocytogenes*, GNR	Ampicillin **plus** third-generation cephalosporin[b] possibly **plus** vancomycin	Vancomycin **plus** third-generation cephalosporin[b] or aztreonam **plus** trimethoprim–sulfamethoxazole if *Listeria* suspected
CNS/meningitis (nosocomial) [32]	GNR, *S. aureus*, coagulase-negative *staphylococci*, *S. pneumoniae*	Vancomycin **plus** ceftazidime	Oxacillin[c] or nafcillin[c] **plus** ceftazidime or aztreonam
CNS/abscess [57]	*S. aureus*, GNR, anaerobes, microaerophilic *Streptococcus* spp	Third-generation cephalosporin[b] **plus** metronidazole **plus** vancomycin if MRSA suspected	Vancomycin **plus** metronidazole **plus** fluoroquinolone[b]
Sepsis syndrome [35]	GNR, *S. aureus*	Piperacillin–tazobactam or ceftazidime **plus** vancomycin	Fluoroquinolone **plus** linezolid

[a]Gentamicin, tobramycin, or amikacin.
[b]Cefotaxime, ceftriaxone, or ceftazidime.
[c]Vancomycin if methicillin-resistant *S. aureus* common.
GNR, Gram-negative rod; MRSA, methicillin-resistant *S. aureus*; MSSA, methicillin-sensitive *S. aureus*; VRE, vancomycin-resistant enterococci.

which exhibit a narrow toxic–therapeutic ratio and with which likelihood of toxicity is proportional to serum and tissue levels, dosing should be based on the patient's estimated lean body weight and renal function. The creatinine clearance can be calculated readily using the modification of diet in renal disease equation (MDRD); see Chapter 73.

Serum creatinine concentrations should be checked frequently, and serum antibiotic concentrations (especially trough) monitored periodically and more often if renal function or hemodynamics are unstable.

Dosing intervals for most antibiotics are selected so that the drugs are administered every three to four serum half-lives ($t_{1/2}$). Because most of the older parenterally administered β-lactam antibiotics have a $t_{1/2}$ of about 1 hour, intravenous penicillins and cephalosporins traditionally were given every 4 hours. However, the $t_{1/2}$ for cefazolin, cefotaxime, ceftazidime is 1.5 to 2.5 hours, and these agents can be administered less frequently, perhaps ever 6 to 8 hours, even for serious infections; for ceftriaxone, the $t_{1/2}$ is 8 hours and the administration frequency is every 12 to 24 hours. Levofloxacin and the macrolide azithromycin are administered once a day.

Antimicrobial Therapy

Antimicrobial administration within the first hour of documented hypotension is associated with increased survival in adult patients with septic shock [39]. Antimicrobial therapy should be initiated at maximal recommended doses in all patients with suspected life-threatening infections without delay.

Initial Therapy of Life-Threatening Infection

Antimicrobial therapy for both Gram-negative and Gram-positive bacteria is the mainstay in the treatment of critically ill patients with severe sepsis. For example, suspected acute overwhelming infection of unknown or uncertain source in an ICU patient warrants therapy with vancomycin to cover *S. aureus*, including MRSA, plus a third-generation cephalosporin or a fluoroquinolone to treat Gram negative bacilli. If hospital-acquired, ventilator-associated, or healthcare-associated pneumonia is likely, a fluoroquinolone such as levofloxacin or gatifloxacin along with piperacillin–tazobactam and vancomycin provides optimal coverage for Gram-negative enteric bacilli; atypical bacterial pathogens, such as *Legionella*, *Chlamydia trachomatis*, and *Mycoplasma*; and MRSA [26]. In patients with febrile neutropenia, an antipseudomonal penicillin (piperacillin/tazobactam) or cephalosporin (ceftazidime) or carbapenem (imipenem) is recommended [40]: vancomycin is added for clinical or bacteriological evidence of MRSA, such as severe mucositis, catheter-related sepsis, and hypotension [40,41]. It is important when choosing empiric regimens to consider recent antibiotic therapy that might have resulted in selection of resistant pathogens. Empiric treatment must be streamlined once the cultures confirm a pathogen to avoid selection of resistant flora.

The use of recombinant human activated protein C, aggressive volume resuscitation, daily hemodialysis in patients with acute renal failure, and early noninvasive ventilation recently have been added to the armamentarium in treating patients with septic shock [42].

Therapy of Mixed Bacterial Infections

Combination therapy is necessary to provide broad effective coverage in specific infections expected to involve diverse microorganisms. For example, intra-abdominal and intrapelvic infections frequently involve complex infecting flora, including aerobic and anaerobic pathogens. Definitive treatment of such infections often includes an extended spectrum β-lactam (ESBL) or a fluoroquinolone for members of the *Enterobacteriaceae* family; clindamycin or metronidazole for *Bacteroides fragilis* and other anaerobes; and penicillin G, ampicillin, or piperacillin for enterococci. An alternative regimen particularly in the patient with known or suspected (long-term residence in the ICU or recent receipt of broad-spectrum antibiotic therapy) multiresistant Gram-negative bacteria is imipenem, meropenem, or piperacillin/tazobactam.

Synergism of Antibiotic Regimens

Although there are numerous examples of in vitro synergy, in vivo synergy has proved effective in a limited number of clinical scenarios. The best documented application of this principle is in patients with infective endocarditis due to *Enterococcus* sp, where treatment with penicillin G or ampicillin plus an aminoglycoside achieves cure levels unmatched by single therapy [43,44]. Although bacteremic infections with *P. aeruginosa* have been treated traditionally with an antipseudomonas penicillin or cephalosporin plus an aminoglycoside, there is no difference in terms of mortality, clinical efficacy, or prevention of resistance when compared with monotherapy [45].

Fungal Infections

The incidence of fungal sepsis increased threefold between 1979 and 2000 and mycosis-related deaths are on the rise. Fungi account for about 5% of all cases of sepsis, and most cases are caused by *Candida* spp [46]. Trauma, burns, abdominal surgery, parenteral nutrition, broad-spectrum antibiotics, malignancy, cancer chemotherapy, and immunosuppressive therapy following major organ transplantation are factors that increase the risk of invasive fungal infections [25].

Early recognition and aggressive medical therapy is key to the successful treatment of this complication [47]. Recently issued guidelines for treatment of candidiasis recommend fluconazole, caspofungin (an echinocandin with fungicidal activity), or an Amphotericin B preparation [47].

Emerging fungal pathogens include *Aspergillus* spp, *Fusarium* spp, *Trichosporon* spp, *Zygomycetes*, *Pseudallescheria boydii*, and dematiaceous fungi, particularly in neutropenic patients and in recipients of solid organ transplantation. *Cryptococcus neoformans* is a major cause of meningitis (less often pneumonia and fungemia) in patients with AIDS and in patients receiving cytotoxic drugs, anti-TNF, or corticosteroids [48].

Multidrug-Resistant Organisms

Over the past decade, hospitalizations with resistant infections (coagulase-negative staphylococci, MRSA, *C. difficile*–associated disease, vancomycin-resistant enterococcus, *P. aeruginosa*, *Acinetobacter baumannii*, *Klebsiella oxytoca*, and *Candida* infection) nearly doubled [49,50]. Gram-negative bacilli resistance is a persistent problem in the ICU. ESBLs have been identified in the *Enterobacteriaceae*, particularly *Klebsiella* sp, *Escherichia coli*, and *Proteus mirabilis* for several decades, and strains producing carbapenemases have been more recently identified.Strains that produce ESBLs demonstrate resistance to third-generation cephalosporins (cefotaxime, ceftriaxone, and ceftazidime), and the strains producing carbapenemase are in general resistant to all classes of β-lactam agents. These organisms also typically carry other resistance genes and are frequently resistant to trimethoprim-sulfamethoxazole, fluoroquinolones, and aminoglycosides. In addition, *P. aeruginosa* and *A. baumannii* display resistance to β-lactams, including monobactams and carbapenems, as well as fluoroquinolones and aminoglycosides; these bacteria can be pan resistant, defined as resistant to all available antibiotics [51].

Vancomycin-resistant *Enterococcus* spp emerged in the past decade as a major nosocomial pathogen. Enterococcal infections occur in patients as complications of prolonged hospitalization, particularly in patients with intravenous lines, intra-abdominal surgery, on mechanical ventilation, or who received broad-spectrum antibiotics that are devoid of activity against enterococci. Newer antibiotics such as linezolid, daptomycin, and tigecycline are treatment options for the treatment of serious nosocomial infections due to vancomycin-resistant enterococci [52].

The recent discovery of strains of MRSA with reduced susceptibility to glycopeptides (VISA) and with resistance to vancomycin (VRSA) emphasizes the importance of using antibiotics in a rationale manner to minimize the impact of resistance [52,53].

Treatment of Fever

Several factors must be considered when determining whether to treat fever symptomatically using antipyretics. Antipyretic therapy may relieve discomfort and decrease the metabolic rate associated with fever [12]. Despite these premises, neither the detrimental consequences of fever nor the beneficial effects of antipyretic therapy have been confirmed experimentally or clinically, and we recommend that antipyretic therapy be withheld unless the temperature exceeds 41°C.

Physical methods of external cooling are the treatment of choice in hyperthermia, but the use of these methods in the treatment of fever remains controversial because it can lead to adverse effects such as shivering, discomfort, and worsening hemodynamic instability [54].

References

1. Beam LJ (ed): *Selected Aphorism*. Birmingham, AL, The Classics of Medicine Library, 1985.
2. Hua-Gang Z, Mehta K, Cohen P, et al: Hyperthermia on immune regulation. *Cancer Lett* 271(2):191–204, 2008.
3. Kiekkas P, Brokakali H, Theodorakopoulou G, et al: Physical antipyresis in critically ill adults. *Am J Nurs* 108(7):40–49, 2008.
4. Axelrod YK, Diringer MN: Temperature management in acute neurologic disorders. *Crit Care Clin* 22(4):767–785, 2007.
5. Plaisance KL, Mackowiack PA: Antipyretic therapy; physiologic rationale, diagnostic implications and clinical consequences. *Arch Intern Med* 160(4):449–456, 2000.
6. Mackowiak PA, Barlett JG, Bordon EC, et al: Concepts of fever: recent advances and lingering dogma. *Clin Infect Dis* 25(1):119–138, 1997.
7. O'Grady NP, Barie PS, Barlett JG, et al: Guidelines for evaluation of new fever in critically ill adult patients: 2008 update from the American College of Critical Care Medicine and the Infectious Disease Society of America. *Crit Care Med* 36(4):1330–1349, 2008.
8. Cunha B: Fever of unknown origins: clinical overview of classic and current concepts. *Infect Dis Clin North Am* 21(4):867–915, 2007.
9. Ryan M, Levy MM: Clinical review: fever in intensive care unit patients. *Crit Care Med* 7(3):221–225, 2003.
10. Peres Bota D, Lopes Ferreira F, Melot C, et al: Body temperature alterations in the critically ill. *Intensive Care Med* 30(5):811–816, 2004.
11. Hamid NS, Spadafora PF, Khalife ME, et al: Pseudosepsis: rectus hematoma mimicking septic shock. *Heart Lung* 35(6):434–437, 2006.
12. Henker R, Carlson KK: Fever: applying research to bedside practice. *AACN Adv Crit Care* 18(1):76–87, 2007.
13. Cooper MS, Stewart PM: Corticosteroid insufficiency in acutely ill patients. *N Engl J Med* 248(8):727–734, 2003.
14. Kosten TR, O'Connor PG: Management of drug and alcohol withdrawal. *N Engl J Med* 348(18):1786–1795, 2003.
15. Eyer F, Ziker T: Bench to bedside review: mechanisms and management of hyperthermia due to toxicity. *Crit Care* 11(6):236–243, 2007.
16. Davaro RE, Thirumalai A: Life threatening complications of HIV infection. *J Intensive Care Med* 22(2):73–81, 2007.
17. Peroni DG, Boner AL: Atelectasis: mechanisms, diagnosis and management. *Paediatr Respir Rev* 1(3):274–278, 2000.
18. Calandra T, Cohen J: The international sepsis forum consensus conference on definitions of infections in the intensive care unit. *Crit Care Med* 33(7):1538–1548, 2005.
19. Vincent JL: Nosocomial infections in the intensive care units. *Lancet* 361(9604):2068–2077, 2003.
20. Poch DS, Ost DE: What are the important risk factors for health care associated pneumonia? *Semin Respir Crit Care Med* 30(1); 26–35, 2009.
21. Marshall JC, Innes M: Intensive care unit management of intra-abdominal infection. *Crit Care Med* 31(4):2228–2237, 2003.
22. Clark T, Wiselka M: *Clostridium difficile* infection. *Clin Med* 8(5); 544–547, 2008.
23. Clech C, Schwebel C, Français A, et al: Does catheter associated urinary tract infection increase mortality in critically ill patients? *Infect Control Hosp Epidemiol* 28(12):1367–1373, 2007.
24. Brook I: Acute and chronic bacterial sinusitis. *Infect Dis Clin North Am* 21(2):427–448, 2007.
25. Ostrosky-Zeichner L, Rex JH, Bennet J, et al: Deeply invasive candidiasis. *Infect Dis Clin North Am* 16(4):821–835, 2002.
26. American Thoracic Society; Infectious Diseases Society of America: Guidelines for the management of adults with hospital acquired, ventilator associated, and health care associated pneumonia. *Am J Respir Crit Care Med* 171(4):388–416, 2004.
27. Avecillas JF, Mazzone P, Arroliga AC: A rational approach to the evaluation and treatment of the infected patient in the intensive care unit. *Clin Chest Med* 24(4):645–669, 2003.
28. Rabinstein A, Sandhu K: Non-infectious fever in the neurological intensive care unit: incidence, causes and predictors. *J Neurol Neurosurg Psychiatry* 78(11):1278–1280, 2007.
29. Mizgerd JP. Acute lower respiratory tract infections. *N Engl J Med* 357:716–727, 2008.
30. Wong CL, Holroyd-Leduc J, Thorpe KE, et al: Does this patient have bacterial peritonitis or portal hypertension? How do I perform a paracentesis and analyze the results? *JAMA* 299(10):1166–1178, 2008.
31. Margaretten ME, Kohlwes J, Moore D, et al: Does this adult patient have septic arthritis? *JAMA* 297(13):1478–1488, 2007.
32. Weisfelt M, van de Beek D, Spanjaard L, et al: Nosocomial bacterial meningitis in adults: a prospective series of 50 cases. *J Hosp Infect* 66(1):71–78, 2007.
33. Yu KH, Liou LB, Wu YJ, et al: Concomitant septic and gouty arthritis—an analysis of 30 cases. *Rheumatology* 42(10):1062–1066, 2003.
34. Roberts JA, Lipmann J: Pharmacokinetic issues for antibiotics in the critically ill patient. *Crit Care Med* 37(3):840–851, 2009.
35. Sharma A, Kumar A: Antimicrobial management of sepsis and septic shock. *Clin Chest Med* 29(4):677–687, 2008.
36. Mermet LA, Allon M, Bouza E, et al: Clinical practice guidelines for the diagnosis and management of intravascular catheter-related infections: 2009 Update by the Infectious Disease Society of America. *Clin Infect Dis* 49(5):491–545, 2009.
37. Badour LM, Wilson WR, Bayer AS, et al: Infective endocarditis. *Circulation* 111:e394–e433, 2005.
38. Bochud PY, Bonten M, Marchetti O, et al: Antimicrobial therapy for patients with severe sepsis and septic shock: an evidence-based review. *Crit Care Med* 32(11, Suppl):S495–S512, 2004.
39. Kumar A, Roberts D, Wood KE, et al: Duration of hypotension before initiation of effective antimicrobial therapy is the critical determinant of survival in human septic shock. *Crit Care Med* 34(6):1589–1596, 2006.
40. Ellis M: Febrile neutropenia: evolving strategies. *Ann N Y Acad Sci* 1138:329–350, 2008.
41. Sipsas NV, Bodey GP, Kontoyiannis DP: Perspectives for the management of febrile neutropenic patients with cancer in the 21st century. *Cancer* 103(6):1103–1113, 2005.
42. Martin JB, Wheeler AP: Approach to the patient with sepsis. *Clin Chest Med* 30(1):1–16, 2009.
43. Patterson JE, Sweeney AH, Simms M, et al: An analysis of 110 serious enterococcal infections. *Medicine* 74(4):191–200, 1995.
44. Moellering RC Jr, Wennersten C, Weinberg AN: Studies on antibiotic synergism against enterococci. I. Bacteriologic studies. *J Lab Clin Med* 77:821–828, 1971.
45. Giamarellou H, Kanellakopoulou K: Current therapies for *Pseudomonas aeruginosa*. *Crit Care Clin* 24(2):261–278, 2008.
46. Chowdhry R, Marshall WL: Antifungal therapy in the intensive care unit. *J Intensive Care Med* 23(3):151–158, 2008.
47. Pappas PG, Kauffman CA, Andes D, et al: Clinical practice guidelines for the management of Candidiasis: 2009 update of the Infectious Diseases Society of America. *Clin Infect Dis* 48(5):503–535, 2009.
48. Nucci M, Marr K: Emerging fungal diseases. *Clin Infect Dis* 41(4):521–526, 2005.
49. Zilberberg MD, Shorr AF, Kollef MH: Growth and geographic variation in hospitalizations with resistant infections, United States, 2000–2005. *Emerg Infect Dis* 14(11):1756–1758, 2008.
50. Hidron AI, Edwards JR, Patel J, et al: Antimicrobial resistant pathogens associated with health care associated infections: annual summary of data reported to the national health care safety network at the Centers for Disease Control and Prevention, 2006–2007. *Infect Control Hosp Epidemiol* 29(11):996–1011, 2008.
51. Nicasio AM, Kuti JL, Nicolau DP: The current status of multi drug resistant gram negative bacilli in North America. *Pharmacotherapy* 28(2):235–249, 2008.
52. Arias CA, Murray BE: Emergence and management of drug resistant enterococcal infections. *Expert Rev Anti Infect Ther* 6(5):637–655, 2008.
53. Courvalin P: Vancomycin resistant in gram positive cocci. *Clin Infect Dis* 42[Suppl 1]:S25–S34, 2006.
54. Tunkel AR, Hartman BJ, Kaplan SL, et al: Practice guidelines for the management of bacterial meningitis. *Clin Infect Dis* 39(9):1267–1284, 2004.
55. Mandell AL, Wunderink RG, Anzueto A, et al: Infectious Disease Society of America/American Thoracic Society Consensus Guidelines on the management of community acquired pneumonia. *Clin Infect Dis* 44:S27–S72, 2007.
56. Ksycki MF, Namias N: Nosocomial urinary tract infections. *Surg Clin North Am* 89(1):475–481, 2009.
57. Greenberg BM: Central nervous system infections in the intensive care unit. *Semin Neurol* 28(5):682–689, 2008.

CHAPTER 77 ■ USE OF ANTIMICROBIALS IN THE TREATMENT OF INFECTION IN THE CRITICALLY ILL PATIENT

IVA ZIVNA, RICHARD H. GLEW AND JENNIFER S. DALY

This chapter reviews antimicrobial agents used in the treatment of bacterial, viral, fungal, and protozoan infections in the intensive care unit (ICU).

PENICILLINS

The classes of penicillins include penicillin G, ampicillin, the antistaphylococcal (semisynthetic) penicillins, and the expanded spectrum (antipseudomonal) penicillins alone and in combination with a β-lactamase inhibitor [1,2]. The serum half-life ($t_{1/2}$) of most penicillins is short, and rapid clearance occurs via the kidneys. Some semisynthetic penicillins, particularly nafcillin and oxacillin, are metabolized to a large extent by the liver; therefore, adjustment in dosage is not required in patients with renal insufficiency; for piperacillin, dosing adjustment is necessary only in severe renal insufficiency. For most other penicillins, moderate adjustments should be made in dosage in patients with severe renal insufficiency (Table 77.1). Penicillins are relatively nontoxic at usual doses, and side effects most commonly involve hypersensitivity reactions. Bone marrow and hepatic toxicity caused by semisynthetic penicillins have been described, with neutropenia more commonly seen with nafcillin and hepatitis more likely to occur with oxacillin.

Penicillin G

In the ICU, aqueous penicillin G is appropriate in the therapy of severe, overwhelming infections caused by susceptible organisms, including pneumococcal pneumonia and bacteremia caused by penicillin-susceptible strains [1], necrotizing fasciitis due to group A *Streptococcus* (in combination with clindamycin), and for streptococcal bacteremia. Because of the prevalence of penicillin-resistant pneumococci, life-threatening infections (especially meningitis) due to these organisms should be treated initially with ceftriaxone, cefotaxime, or vancomycin [3]. Although aspiration pneumonia commonly involves mouth anaerobes that are susceptible to penicillin G, penicillin-resistant anaerobes can be found in putrid, cavitary pneumonia, and empyema, and clindamycin with or without a third-generation cephalosporin (or an extended-spectrum β-lactam plus metronidazole) is the preferred regimen [4–6]. Therapy for penicillin-susceptible *Enterococcus* spp causing endocarditis is penicillin G or ampicillin plus an aminoglycoside, generally gentamicin [7]. The activity of penicillin G and ampicillin against most Gram-negative bacilli is poor [2]. *Staphylococcus aureus* should be presumed to be resistant to penicillin, ampicillin, and piperacillin, as most strains produce a penicillinase.

Penicillinase-Resistant Semisynthetic Penicillins

Because most strains of *S. aureus* are resistant to penicillin G by virtue of β-lactamase production, treatment of severe infections caused by these organisms involves one of the β-lactamase–resistant penicillins (see Table 77.1). Nafcillin and oxacillin are interchangeable: Both exhibit excellent in vitro activity against most susceptible isolates of *S. aureus*, but are slightly less active (although generally effective) than penicillin G against streptococci, and are sufficiently metabolized by the hepatic route so that no adjustment in dose is necessary in patients with renal insufficiency. Because of high prevalence of community-acquired methicillin-resistant *S. aureus* (MRSA), vancomycin should be used for empiric therapy of suspected staphylococcal infections [8]. In patients with overwhelming or disseminated infection caused by β-lactam–susceptible *S. aureus*, therapy should be instituted with 9 to 12 g per day of intravenous (IV) oxacillin or nafcillin, in divided doses every 4 hours (see Table 77.1).

Anti–Gram-Negative Penicillins

The expanded-spectrum penicillin (piperacillin) and the combination agent piperacillin/tazobactam exhibit activity against many *Enterobacteriaceae* that are resistant to ampicillin [9].

In the ICU patient with suspected bacteremia or overwhelming infection due to Gram-negative bacilli, therapy should be chosen with knowledge of local ICU resistance patterns and include agents that the patient has not recently received. Pharyngeal colonization with Gram-negative bacilli rapidly develops in patients in the ICU, and initial therapy of nosocomial aspiration pneumonia requires the addition of an antipseudomonal penicillin, carbapenem, or cephalosporin, usually in combination with an aminoglycoside or fluoroquinolone [10]. In patients with *Pseudomonas aeruginosa* infections, the intensivist should consider using higher dosages or continuous infusions of piperacillin or piperacillin/tazobactam with or without an aminoglycoside [11]. The addition of the aminoglycoside to extended-spectrum penicillins is controversial [12] but has been shown to provide broader Gram negative coverage and synergistic killing against *P. aeruginosa*.

β-Lactamase–Inhibitor Combinations

Clavulanic acid, sulbactam, and tazobactam are β-lactamase inhibitors that bind irreversibly to β-lactamases derived from *S. aureus* and anaerobes, as well as some β-lactamases from Gram-negative bacilli. Thus, the combination of one of these

TABLE 77.1

EXAMPLES OF PARENTERAL PENICILLINS

		Dose based on creatinine clearance			
Penicillin	Indication	>80 mL/min (normal)	50–80 mL/min	10–50 mL/min	<10 mL/min
Penicillin G	Meningitis	2 million U q2h	4 million U q4h	4 million U q4h	2 million U q6h
	Endocarditis	3–4 million U q4h	3–4 million U q4h	3 million U q4h	2 million U q6h
Ampicillin	Meningitis	2–3 g q4h	2–3 g q6h	2–3 g q8 h	2–3 g q12h
	Endocarditis	2 g q4h	2 g q6h	2 g q8 h	2 g q12h
Nafcillin or oxacillin	*Staphylococcus aureus* bacteremia, meningitis	2 g q4h	2 g q4h	2 g q4h	2 g q4h
	Skin, soft tissue infections	1–2 g q4–6h	1–2 g q4–6h	1–2 g q4–6h	1–2 g q4–6h
Piperacillin (use with an aminoglycoside for *Pseudomonas*)	*Pseudomonas aeruginosa*	3 g q4h or 4 g q6h	3 g q4h or 4 g q6h	3–4 g q8h	3–4 g q12h
	Enterobacteriaceae	3–4 g q6h	4 g q6h	3–4 g q8h	3–4 g q12h
Piperacillin plus tazobactam (use with an aminoglycoside for *Pseudomonas*)	*Enterobacteriaceae*	3.375 g q4–6h	3.375 g q6h	2.25 g q6h	2.25 g q8h
Ampicillin plus sulbactam	*Enterobacteriaceae*	3 g q6h	3 g q8h	3 g q12h	3 g q24h

β-lactamase inhibitors with ampicillin or piperacillin results in a drug combination that is active against β-lactamase–producing strains of *S. aureus*, *Bacteroides* sp, *Haemophilus influenzae*, *Neisseria gonorrhoeae*, and enteric Gram-negative bacilli such as *Escherichia coli* and *Klebsiella* and *Proteus* spp. However, chromosomally mediated β-lactamases of other Gram-negative bacilli are unaffected by these β-lactamase inhibitors, and therefore these combinations are ineffective against many isolates of *P. aeruginosa*, *Enterobacter cloacae*, *Citrobacter freundii*, and *Serratia marcescens*.

Formulations of β-lactamase combinations available parenterally include ampicillin–sulbactam and piperacillin–tazobactam. Piperacillin–tazobactam can be effective in the treatment of mixed infections, such as nosocomial pneumonia, intra-abdominal infections, and synergistic skin soft tissue infections. However, depending on local resistance patterns, the lack of efficacy against multiple-resistant Gram-negative bacilli commonly found in the ICU warrants monitoring of local resistance patterns and using a carbapenem, or adding an aminoglycoside as part of a combination regimen to ensure broad efficacy against nosocomial Gram-negative bacilli [10,13].

The usual suggested dosages of the available combinations are given in Table 77.1. For treatment of *P. aeruginosa* infections, the dosage of piperacillin–tazobactam should be increased to 3.375 g IV every 4 hours or 4.5 g IV every 6 hours for pneumonia. The pharmacology of the β-lactamase inhibitors is similar to that for other β-lactams: Clearance is by renal mechanisms, and dosage adjustments must be made with these combinations in the setting of renal impairment. Continuous infusion of piperacillin/tazobactam after a bolus has a pharmacodynamic advantage for organisms with relatively high minimum inhibitory concentrations (MICs) to piperacillin and in patients on continuous venovenous hemofiltration (CVVH) [11].

CEPHALOSPORINS

Cephalosporin antibiotics exhibit relative safety and an antibacterial spectrum that includes activity against Gram-positive and Gram-negative bacteria. Examples of parenteral cephalosporins that are currently available are listed in Table 77.2. Cephalosporins are not active against MRSA, *Enterococcus* spp, or *Stenotrophomonas maltophilia*. Many strains of *Enterobacter* possess an inducible chromosomal β-lactamase and may become resistant during therapy [14].

First-Generation Cephalosporins

First-generation cephalosporins exhibit a virtually identical spectrum of antibacterial activity, and they differ only in their pharmacokinetic properties. These agents are active against staphylococci (β-lactam–susceptible staphylococci) but are not effective against enterococci, *Listeria monocytogenes*, MRSA, or the majority of coagulase-negative staphylococci. Community-acquired strains of *E. coli*, *Proteus mirabilis*, and *Klebsiella pneumoniae* often are susceptible to the first-generation cephalosporins, but in general, third-generation agents are far more potent against Gram-negative bacilli and are preferred in the treatment of such infections in ICU patients. Nosocomial isolates of *Enterobacteriaceae* usually are resistant to first-generation cephalosporins, as are *Pseudomonas* and *Acinetobacter* spp.

Second-Generation Cephalosporins

Second-generation cephalosporins (e.g., cefuroxime) have only limited activity against hospital-acquired Gram-negative bacilli and therefore are not recommended for treatment of Gram negatives in the ICU setting.

Third-Generation Cephalosporins

Third-generation cephalosporins exhibit an expanded spectrum and increased potency against Gram-negative organisms, especially *Enterobacteriaceae* [15]. A number of these agents, particularly ceftazidime, are less active than first-generation cephalosporins against Gram-positive cocci. However, ceftriaxone has significant activity against *Streptococcus*

TABLE 77.2

EXAMPLES OF PARENTERAL CEPHALOSPORINS AND RELATED β-LACTAMS

	Dosage based on creatinine clearance			
Antibiotic	>80 mL/min (normal)	50–80 mL/min	<10–50 mL/min	10 mL/min
First-generation cephalosporins				
Cefazolin	1–2 g q8h	1–2 g q8h	1 g q8–12h	1–2 g q24h
Second-generation cephalosporins				
Cefuroxime	0.75–1.50 g q8h	0.75–1.50 g q8h	0.75–1.50 g q12h	0.75–1.50 g q24h
Third-generation cephalosporins				
Cefotaxime	1–2 g q6–8h	1–2 g q6–8h	1 g q8–12h	1–2 g q24h
Ceftriaxone	1–2 g q12–24h	1–2 g q24h	1–2 g q24h	1–2 g q24h
Ceftizoxime	1–2 g q8–12h	1–2 g q8–12h	1–2 g q12h	1 g q24h
Ceftazidime	1–2 g q8h	1–2 g q8h	1–2 g q12–24h	1 g q48h
Newest-generation cephalosporins				
Cefepime	1–2 g q8–12h	1–2 g q8–12h	1 g q12–24h	0.5–1.0 g q24h
Monobactams				
Aztreonam	1–2 g q8h	1–2 g q8h	1 g q8–12h	1–2 g q24h
Carbapenems				
Imipenem/cilastatin	0.5–1.0 g q6h	0.5–1.0 g q6–8h	0.5–1.0 g q8–12h	0.25–1.0 g q12h
Ertapenem	1 g q24h	1 g q24h	0.5 g q24h	0.5 g q24h
Meropenem	1 g q8h	1 g q8–12h	1 g q12h	1 g q24h
Doripenem	0.5 g q8h	0.5 g q8h	0.25 g q8–12h	Unknown

pneumoniae and other oral streptococci, and has been recommended for use in severely ill patients with community-acquired pneumonia (CAP), bacterial meningitis, and bacterial endocarditis [16–18].

The activity of most third-generation cephalosporins against *P. aeruginosa* is variable and unpredictable; only ceftazidime and cefepime, a fourth-generation cephalosporin, are considered active against this organism and should be used in combination with an aminoglycoside when infection with *P. aeruginosa* is likely [19]. If a third-generation cephalosporin is used as a single agent, gaps in coverage may occur, including (a) enterococcal superinfection; (b) *P. aeruginosa* infections in neutropenic patients; (c) emergence of broad-spectrum resistance by means of chromosomally mediated inducible β-lactamases during cephalosporin monotherapy of deep-seated infections by species of *Enterobacter*, *Providencia*, *Serratia*, *Pseudomonas*, and *Acinetobacter*; (d) intra-abdominal or intrapelvic infections likely to involve *Bacteroides fragilis*; and (e) *S. aureus* bacteremia, endocarditis, or meningitis. Thus, in ICU patients, third-generation cephalosporins generally should be used empirically as part of combination therapy or as specific single-agent treatment of Gram-negative bacillary infections involving organisms documented to be susceptible to the agent in vitro.

Newer Cephalosporins

Cefepime, a fourth-generation cephalosporin [20], has activity against Gram-positive organisms similar to that of cefotaxime and ceftriaxone and activity against *Pseudomonas* similar to that of ceftazidime. Compared with third-generation cephalosporins, cefepime has a lower affinity for β-lactamases and is not an inducer of chromosomal β-lactamases. The pharmacokinetics of cefepime are similar to those of ceftazidime: $t_{1/2}$ is 2.1 hours, and 80% to 90% of the dose is recovered in the urine. For treatment of infections due to *P. aeruginosa*, cefepime (often in conjunction with an aminoglycoside) should be dosed every 8 hours, but for moderate infections due to more susceptible species, it can be dosed every 12 hours (see Table 77.2).

Adverse Reactions

Cephalosporins are relatively nontoxic agents. The most commonly noted adverse effects are hypersensitivity reactions, including rashes, fever, interstitial nephritis, and anaphylaxis. In patients with documented penicillin allergy, the risk of cross-reactive allergic reactions to the cephalosporins is cited as 5% to 10%, and generally it is felt that cephalosporins should be avoided in patients with a history of documented anaphylaxis or immediate hypersensitivity (urticaria) reaction to the penicillins, but can be given to patients with a history of other types of reactions to penicillins, including morbilliform rash and fever. Enterococcal superinfections occur with any of the extended-spectrum cephalosporins because none of these agents has significant activity against enterococci [15,20].

Dosage

When used in the treatment of severe infections in ICU patients, all cephalosporins should be used, at least initially, at maximal doses and short dosing intervals (Table 77.2). In patients with severe impairment of renal function, dosages of all cephalosporins except ceftriaxone must be adjusted to avoid accumulation [20].

CARBAPENEMS

Four carbapenem antibiotics—imipenem, meropenem, ertapenem, and doripenem—are approved for clinical use [21–23]. Imipenem is a carbapenem and is administered in combination with cilastatin, a specific enzymatic inhibitor of a renal dehydropeptidase, which inhibits metabolism of imipenem by the kidney, increasing the $t_{1/2}$ and decreasing the nephrotoxicity of imipenem. Imipenem exhibits activity against Gram-negative bacilli at least equal to that of the third-generation cephalosporins (including anti-*Pseudomonas* potency equal to that of ceftazidime); against Gram-positive cocci similar to that of oxacillin, nafcillin, and cefazolin; and against anaerobic bacteria equal to metronidazole or clindamycin. MRSA are resistant to imipenem. *Enterococcus faecalis* appears susceptible in vitro, but *Enterococcus faecium* usually is resistant and imipenem should not be regarded as effective therapy for serious infections caused by enterococci. Among nonfermentative Gram-negative bacilli associated with nosocomial infections, *S. maltophilia*, *Burkholderia cepacia*, and *Flavobacterium* spp usually are resistant to imipenem. Resistance to imipenem arises infrequently (most commonly with *P. aeruginosa*) during therapy, usually via alteration in porin channels in the bacterial cell outer membrane, resulting in diminished intracellular concentrations of the drug, and the organism usually remains susceptible to other β-lactams if the organism is susceptible initially.

The usual dosage of imipenem/cilastatin is 2 g per day in four divided doses, with up to 4 g per day in life-threatening infections by less susceptible organisms (e.g., *P. aeruginosa*). Dosage adjustment (see Table 77.2) is necessary for patients with renal dysfunction because serum concentration-related myoclonus and seizures can occur. Treatment of highly resistant Gram-negative bacilli (e.g., *P. aeruginosa*, *E. cloacae*, and *Acinetobacter* sp) with imipenem may involve initial coadministration of a second agent, such as an aminoglycoside.

Adverse reactions to imipenem include rash and fever. The frequency of cross-reactivity with other classes of β-lactams is estimated to be approximately that observed with penicillins and cephalosporins. Risk of seizures can be minimized by adjustment of dosing in the elderly and in patients with reduced renal function; usage should be avoided when possible in patients with a history of seizures or central nervous system (CNS) lesions.

Meropenem and ertapenem are broad-spectrum carbapenem antibiotics similar to imipenem [21,22]. Meropenem is more active against Gram-negative rods, including *Pseudomonas* spp, and slightly less active against Gram-positive cocci, including *S. aureus*. Ertapenem is not active against *Pseudomonas* sp or *Enterococcus* spp but has activity against extended-spectrum β-lactamase (ESBL) producing *Klebsiella*. The standard dosing for ertapenem is 1 g IV every 24 hours and for meropenem 1 g IV every 8 hours (see Table 77.2). Meropenem and ertapenem are excreted via the kidney, but, in contrast to imipenem, their renal metabolism is negligible and cilastatin is not coadministered [22]. Meropenem and ertapenem seem less likely than imipenem to cause seizures.

Doripenem is a novel carbapenem with a broad spectrum of activity against Gram-positive pathogens, anaerobes, and Gram-negative bacteria, including *P. aeruginosa* [23]. Doripenem exhibits rapid bactericidal activity with two- to fourfold lower MIC values for Gram-negative bacteria, compared with other carbapenems. It has significant in vitro activity against *Enterobacteriaceae* (including ESBL strains), *P. aeruginosa*, *Acinetobacter* spp, and *B. fragilis*.

Doripenem is dosed at 500 mg IV every 8 hours, and dose and/or interval needs to be adjusted based on creatinine clearance (see Table 77.2). A low risk of seizures has been demonstrated in clinical studies [23].

AZTREONAM

Aztreonam is a monobactam, differing from penicillins and cephalosporins in that it has a monocyclic rather than a bicyclic nucleus, granting aztreonam little cross-allergenicity with other β-lactams. Although skin rashes occur occasionally with this drug, aztreonam has been given safely to patients with immediate hypersensitivity-type reactions (anaphylaxis, urticaria) to penicillins or cephalosporins [24].

Aztreonam has no activity against Gram-positive or anaerobic bacteria. Against most facultative aerobic Gram-negative bacilli, aztreonam exhibits a spectrum and potency much like that of third-generation cephalosporins including activity against some strains of *Pseudomonas* spp. The usual dosage of aztreonam is 1 to 2 g IV every 6 to 8 hours. Aztreonam is cleared by the kidneys, and dosage must be reduced in patients with renal insufficiency.

AMINOGLYCOSIDES

Aminoglycoside antibiotics are bactericidal agents of value in the treatment of Gram-negative infections in ICU patients [25]. Aminoglycosides in common clinical use in the critically ill patient include gentamicin, tobramycin, and amikacin. Streptomycin occasionally is used for enterococcal or mycobacterial infections.

Pharmacology

All available aminoglycosides exhibit similar pharmacologic properties: (a) absorption from the gastrointestinal (GI) tract is negligible, and adequate serum levels are obtained only by the IV or intramuscular routes; (b) volume of distribution is similar to that of total volume of extracellular fluid and therefore can be somewhat unpredictable under conditions of abnormal extracellular fluid such as dehydration, third-space losses, congestive heart failure, or ascites; (c) protein binding is minimal; (d) penetration into the cerebrospinal fluid (CSF) is poor even in the presence of meningeal inflammation; (e) drug levels in bronchial secretions are only two thirds of those in serum and are poor in vitreous fluid, prostate, and bile; (f) excretion is predominantly by glomerular filtration, and $t_{1/2}$ of the aminoglycosides in the presence of normal renal function is approximately 2 to 3 hours (longest for amikacin) and is prolonged in patients with renal impairment, approaching 24 hours in those with end-stage renal failure; (g) all aminoglycosides are dialyzable, and greater efficacy of removal occurs with hemodialysis (approximately 60% to 75% cleared in 6 hours) than with peritoneal dialysis; and (h) aminoglycoside activity is reduced under conditions of reduced pH and oxygen tension, such as in purulent, particularly anaerobic, fluids, and tissues [25].

Spectrum of Action and Indications for Therapy

The primary clinical indication for aminoglycoside therapy is serious infection caused by Gram-negative bacilli. Aminoglycosides are also used in combination with a cell wall agent for therapy of enterococcal endocarditis. Another indication is treatment of mycobacterial disease. Although more toxic than penicillins and cephalosporins, aminoglycosides provide the broadest range of potent, bactericidal antibiotic activity against Gram-negative bacilli, particularly when multiple-resistant enteric Gram-negative bacilli (e.g., *Enterobacter* sp) or nonfermentative Gram-negative organisms such as *Pseudomonas* and *Acinetobacter* spp are considered possible pathogens.

Resistance to aminoglycosides generally emerges slowly and infrequently. However, resistance to aminoglycosides has increased dramatically among *Enterococcus* spp, and currently in many hospitals, up to one fourth of isolates are gentamicin resistant [26]. Some high-level gentamicin-resistant isolates remain susceptible to high levels of streptomycin [27].

Gentamicin and Tobramycin

In many ICUs, gentamicin (or tobramycin) resistance is prevalent among local isolates of Gram-negative bacilli, and amikacin may be preferred in the initial management of Gram-negative bacillary infections, pending results of microbiologic studies and susceptibility testing. In addition, gentamicin in combination with ampicillin, penicillin, or vancomycin is indicated for treatment of endocarditis due to enterococci or viridans group streptococci and can be used with vancomycin and rifampin for treatment of prosthetic valve endocarditis caused by coagulase-negative staphylococci.

Tobramycin is more potent than gentamicin against *P. aeruginosa* in vitro and, along with amikacin, may be effective against gentamicin-resistant strains of this organism. However, the frequency of cross-resistance is unpredictable and may be alarmingly common [28]. In addition, tobramycin is less active than gentamicin against some organisms, such as *Serratia* and *Acinetobacter* spp.

Amikacin

Amikacin is the semisynthetic aminoglycoside most resistant to aminoglycoside-inactivating enzymes. For most gentamicin-resistant Gram-negative bacilli such as multiresistant ESBL-producing *Klebsiella*, amikacin is the most active aminoglycoside and should be the empiric aminoglycoside of choice in hospitals or ICUs in which gentamicin and tobramycin resistance is prevalent.

Adverse Reactions

Unlike β-lactam antibiotics, aminoglycosides are characterized by a narrow therapeutic–toxic ratio, and therapy with these agents can be associated with considerable toxicity. Hypersensitivity reactions such as fever and rash are uncommon but have been reported in up to 3% of patients who receive these drugs. Anaphylaxis has been observed on rare occasions. Neuromuscular blockade has been described uncommonly and appears to be of concern only in patients with myasthenia gravis or severe hypocalcemia or those who are receiving neuromuscular blocking agents. Ototoxicity appears to occur with equal frequency (up to 10% of patients) among the modern aminoglycosides [25]. Vestibular damage has been described more commonly with gentamicin and tobramycin, whereas impairment of auditory acuity seems more common with amikacin [25]. Ototoxicity occurs unpredictably (either early or late in therapy), is related only partially to elevated serum levels, most closely correlates with duration of therapy and total dosage administered, and often is irreversible. Patients expected to receive aminoglycoside therapy for extended duration and who are conscious and communicative should be questioned periodically about symptoms of eighth cranial nerve dysfunction, such as tinnitus, diminished auditory acuity, lightheadedness, and dizziness.

Nephrotoxicity has been reported to occur in 2% to 10% of all patients receiving aminoglycoside therapy and in up to 10% to 25% of critically ill patients. However, renal damage usually is mild and reversible promptly with cessation of therapy. Aminoglycoside-induced nephrotoxicity appears to be related to dose and duration of therapy as well as to serum concentrations, especially elevated trough levels. It is seen more commonly in elderly patients, those with preexisting renal disease, those with diminished tissue perfusion caused by cardiogenic or peripheral vascular factors, and patients receiving other nephrotoxic agents. The most useful laboratory tests that are available to reduce and detect aminoglycoside nephrotoxicity are the serum creatinine levels and determinations of trough serum aminoglycoside concentrations.

Therapy and Determination of Serum Levels

Recommended dosage schedules and desired serum concentrations for the aminoglycosides are shown in Table 77.3. The use of the once-daily dosing method for aminoglycosides (see Table 77.3) may reduce nephrotoxicity and enhance efficacy against Gram-negative bacilli [30,31]. These agents induce a postantibiotic effect, and, hence, are suited for less frequent dosing. Postantibiotic effect is uncertain for Gram-positive bacteria, and the desired peak and trough levels are lower when you are using aminoglycosides for synergistic activity against Gram-positive pathogens.

In patients with impaired renal function, serum concentrations (and serum creatinine and blood urea nitrogen values) should be monitored to ensure safe and effective concentrations. Trough concentrations should be monitored frequently (and dosage/frequency adjusted accordingly) in patients with fluctuating cardiovascular function/fluid volumes or renal function and in those who are anticipated to receive prolonged therapy [25]. Trough serum concentrations should be less than 1 μg per mL (or undetectable) when large doses are given at intervals of 24 hours or greater.

In patients undergoing hemodialysis, it can be estimated that approximately two thirds to three fourths of a dose (i.e., 1 mg per kg gentamicin or tobramycin or 5 mg per kg amikacin) is required at the end of each hemodialysis session, and serum concentrations (trough before dialysis, peak after supplemental dose given) should be monitored. In patients undergoing peritoneal dialysis, instillation of the aminoglycoside into the dialysate at a therapeutic concentration (i.e., 4 μg per mL = 4 mg per L for gentamicin and tobramycin; and 20 μg per mL = 20 mg per L for amikacin) eliminates a serum-dialysis concentration gradient and minimizes loss of drug through dialysis.

FLUOROQUINOLONES

Fluoroquinolones are broad-spectrum agents that exert their antimicrobial activity by inhibiting deoxyribonucleic acid (DNA) synthesis by binding to two enzymes, bacterial DNA gyrase and topoisomerase IV, enzymes that introduce superhelical twists into double-stranded bacterial DNA. Fluoroquinolones broadly in use include ciprofloxacin, levofloxacin, and moxifloxacin.

These agents are active and generally bactericidal against susceptible enteric Gram-negative bacilli (including enteric pathogens such as *Salmonella* and *Shigella* spp), *H. influenzae*. Resistance to these agents among Gram-negative bacteria such as *P. aeruginosa*, *Acinetobacter* spp, and *Aeromonas hydrophila* is increasing and non–lactose-fermenting Gram-negative bacilli such as *B. cepacia*, *Pseudomonas fluorescens*, and *S. maltophilia* are often resistant to the quinolones. Of the quinolones, ciprofloxacin has greatest potency against *P. aeruginosa*. Activity of quinolones against aerobic Gram-positive cocci is variable, and activity against methicillin-susceptible *S. aureus* and coagulase-negative staphylococci has diminished; MRSA commonly are resistant [32]. Although, in general, streptococci (particularly *S. pneumoniae*, *Streptococcus pyogenes* [group A streptococcus], and enterococci) exhibit poor susceptibility to older quinolones, moxifloxacin and levofloxacin are considered efficacious in treatment of pneumococcal pneumonia. Moxifloxacin has in vitro activity against *B. fragilis*, but there is little clinical experience with

TABLE 77.3

RECOMMENDED DOSAGE REGIMENS AND SERUM CONCENTRATIONS OF AMINOGLYCOSIDES IN INTENSIVE CARE UNIT PATIENTS BASED ON CALCULATED CREATININE CLEARANCE[a]

Drug/renal function	Route	Loading dose (mg/kg)	Regimen (mg/kg)	Target serum concentration (μg/mL)[b]		
				Peak[c]	Trough[c]	8 h after dose
Traditional regimen						
Gentamicin, tobramycin						
>80 mL/min	IV, IM	2.0–2.5	1.3–1.7 q8h	4–8	1.0–1.5	
60–79 mL/min		2.0–2.5	1.3–1.7 q12h	4–8	1.0–1.5	
40–59 mL/min		2.0–2.5	3 q24h	4–8	1.0–1.5	
30–39 mL/min		2.0–2.5	2 q24h	4–8	1.0–1.5	
10–29 mL/min		2.0–2.5	2–3 q48h	4–8	1.0–1.5	
<10 mL/min		2.0–2.5	1–2 q48h	4–8	1.0–1.5	
Amikacin	IV, IM					
>80 mL/min		7.5–10.0	7.5 q12h	20–25	5–10	
60–79 mL/min		7.5–10.0	5.0 q12h	20–25	5–10	
40–59 mL/min		7.5–10.0	7.5 q24h	20–25	5–10	
30–39 mL/min		7.5–10.0	5.0 q24h	20–25	5–10	
10–29 mL/min		7.5–10.0	7.5 q48h	20–25	5–10	
<10 mL/min		7.5–10.0	5.0 q48h	20–25	5–10	
Once-daily dosing[d]						
Gentamicin, tobramycin						
80 mL/min	IV	Not needed	5–7 q24h	NA[e]	Undetectable (<0.3)	2–6
60–79 mL/min	IV	Not needed	5–7 q36–48h (based on serum concentration at 6–14 h after dose)	NA[e] [29]	Undetectable (<0.3)	6–11
Amikacin	IV	Not needed	15–20 q24h	NA[e]	Undetectable (<0.3)	6–18

[a]Creatinine clearance; for women, multiply the result by 0.85.
[b]Lower concentrations are desired when using aminoglycosides for treatment of gram-positive infections
[c]Serum for peak levels should be drawn 30 minutes after a 30-minute infusion, and trough levels should be obtained within the 30 minutes before the next dose.
[d]Patient exclusions—age <12 y, pregnancy, burns >20% body surface area, ascites, dialysis, endocarditis, creatinine clearance <60 mL/min.
[e]NA—with once-daily dosing, peak concentrations are high transiently and measurement of peaks is not applicable.

its use against this pathogen. Quinolones have activity mycobacteria, including *Mycobacterium tuberculosis*, *Mycobacterium kansasii*, and *Mycobacterium fortuitum*, but susceptibility results should be used to guide therapy. Levofloxacin and moxifloxacin are more active than ciprofloxacin against *Mycoplasma* sp, *Chlamydophilia trachomatis*, and *Ureaplasma urealyticum*. All demonstrate activity against *Legionella pneumophila*.

The $t_{1/2}$ of the fluoroquinolones is relatively long (3 to 4 hours for ciprofloxacin and levofloxacin, and 9 to 10 hours for moxifloxacin). Levofloxacin is cleared primarily by the kidneys and require dosage adjustment for patients with renal insufficiency. Moxifloxacin is cleared by the liver, and dosage adjustments in renal failure are unnecessary. Some component of hepatic excretion occurs with ciprofloxacin, and major dosage adjustment (50% of dose, 12-hour interval) is required only at creatinine clearance rates of less than 20 mL per minute [33]. The fluoroquinolones are not eliminated by hemodialysis or peritoneal dialysis.

Although available oral fluoroquinolone formulations can achieve adequate serum and tissue concentrations to treat infections outside the urinary tract, parenteral therapy is preferred in the acute management of serious infections in the ICU, as oral absorption may not occur due to problems with intestinal motility or perfusion. Ciprofloxacin, moxifloxacin, and levofloxacin are available in IV preparations. GI tract absorption of fluoroquinolones can be impaired by concomitant administration of antacids, sucralfate, and multivitamins containing zinc or iron.

Adverse Reactions

In general, the fluoroquinolones are safe and well tolerated. The most common adverse reactions include GI tract symptoms (nausea, vomiting, dyspepsia, abdominal pain, and diarrhea), CNS symptoms (insomnia, restlessness, headache, dizziness, confusion, and, rarely, seizures), tendon rupture, and occasional hypersensitivity reactions (rash, pruritus, and drug fever). Ciprofloxacin increases serum concentrations and potentiates the effects of theophylline, warfarin, and cyclosporine.

Indications

The fluoroquinolones are indicated in the treatment of (a) complicated urinary tract infections involving susceptible Gram-negative bacilli; (b) prostatitis; (c) bacterial pneumonia, especially due to Gram-negative bacilli, *H. influenzae*, *Legionella* sp, or high-level penicillin-resistant *S. pneumoniae*; (d) bacterial diarrhea of diverse causes, including traveler's diarrhea and enteritis due to *Shigella*, *Salmonella*, and *Campylobacter* spp; (e) invasive (malignant) external otitis; (f) intra-abdominal and intrapelvic infections (in combination with anaerobic coverage); (g) outpatient treatment of CAP; and (h) septic shock due to urinary tract infections in combination with a β-lactam agent. In treating nosocomial pneumonia, it must be remembered that the older fluoroquinolones (e.g., ciprofloxacin) have limited activity against streptococci and no activity against anaerobes, and addition of an agent active against these organisms should be considered. In addition, resistance to fluoroquinolones is becoming increasingly common in *S. aureus* and among Gram-negative bacilli, especially *P. aeruginosa*.

VANCOMYCIN

Vancomycin is bactericidal at low concentrations against most Gram-positive cocci and bacilli, including *S. aureus* (including MRSA), coagulase-negative staphylococci, *S. pneumoniae* (including drug-resistant strains), viridans group *Streptococcus* spp, *Streptococcus bovis*, *Clostridium* sp, and *Diphtheroid* spp [34]. Although most enterococci are inhibited by low concentrations of vancomycin, bactericidal killing of these organisms requires the addition of an aminoglycoside such as gentamicin or streptomycin [7,35]. Resistance to vancomycin is an emerging problem, particularly in strains of *E. faecium*. The first strain of *S. aureus* with reduced susceptibility to vancomycin was reported in 1997 from Japan [36].

Because of poor absorption from the GI tract and severe pain with intramuscular injection, vancomycin is given IV for the treatment of systemic infections. Oral vancomycin is used only in patients with antibiotic-associated colitis caused by *Clostridium difficile*. Oral metronidazole is preferred for this process in non-ICU patients due to emerging problems with vancomycin-resistant organisms. In severely ill patients with *C. difficile* infection, oral vancomycin or a combination of oral vancomycin and IV metronidazole is recommended [29].

Vancomycin is excreted primarily by the kidneys. In patients with normal renal function, serum $t_{1/2}$ of IV-administered vancomycin varies from 2.7 to 13.3 hours, and peak and trough serum concentrations are unpredictable. The usual recommended dose for adults with normal renal function is 2 to 3 g per day in divided doses every 8 to 12 hours. The dose should be administered IV over 60 minutes. For complicated infections in seriously ill patients, a loading dose of 25 to 30 mg per kg (based on actual body weight) may be used to achieve target concentration rapidly, followed with 15 to 20 mg per kg per dose every 8 to 12 hours. Nomograms are available to guide vancomycin dosing in patients with varying degrees of renal insufficiency [37]. Serum trough concentrations should be monitored in patients with reduced renal function or unstable hemodynamics; monitoring of peak concentrations usually is not helpful. For pneumonia due to MRSA and meningitis, dosing to achieve higher troughs of 15 to 20 μg per mL should be used. For endocarditis dosing to achieve troughs of 10 to 15 μg per mL are recommended [38].

Adverse Reactions

Because there is no cross-reaction, vancomycin is the drug of choice in the therapy of serious Gram-positive infections in patients who are allergic to penicillins and cephalosporins. Vancomycin is associated with hypersensitivity reactions such as rash and fever in approximately 3% to 5% of patients. Rapid IV administration of vancomycin can produce a histamine-associated reaction characterized by flushing, tingling, pruritus, tachycardia, hypotension, and an erythematous rash over the upper trunk and face. This red-person syndrome is a histamine-release phenomenon, not a manifestation of hypersensitivity, and can be avoided by slow IV administration of the drug (i.e., at a rate no faster than 15 mg per minute or 0.5 g over 60 minutes and 1 g over 60 to 90 minutes) or by pretreatment with antihistamines [39]. Neutropenia occurs occasionally [40]. Ototoxicity appears to occur uncommonly in patients who receive vancomycin, usually in association with elevated serum levels (at least 50 μg per mL), and generally is reversible with discontinuation of therapy. Nephrotoxicity occurs rarely in patients who receive vancomycin alone, is usually associated with elevated serum vancomycin levels, and is more common in patients with recent concomitant aminoglycoside administration.

TELAVANCIN

A glycopeptide analog of vancomycin, telavancin, shows promise as alternative treatment for patients with serious infections caused by Gram-positive pathogens [41]. Telavancin exhibits low potential for resistance development and is active against resistant pathogens, including MRSA. Telavancin is currently approved only for treatment of complicated skin and skin structure infections (cSSSIs). Similar to vancomycin, it demonstrates activity in vitro against a variety of Gram-positive pathogens, including but not limited to MRSA and penicillin-resistant *S. pneumoniae*. Modifications to vancomycin's structure expanded telavancin's spectrum of activity in vitro to include organisms such as glycopeptide-intermediate *S. aureus* (GISA), vancomycin-resistant *S. aureus* (VRSA), and vancomycin-resistant enterococci (VRE). Dose of 10 mg per kg per day is recommended for patients with normal renal function. Since telavancin is cleared extensively by the kidneys, dosage adjustments will be required in patients with moderate-to-severe renal impairment. Renal toxicity was reported more frequently with telavancin than with vancomycin in two phase III clinical trials (3% vs. 1%). Potential teratogenicity of this agent must be considered in women who are pregnant or may become pregnant.

THERAPY OF ANAEROBIC INFECTIONS

As reviewed previously, excellent efficacy against anaerobes is provided by carbapenems as well as β-lactam/β-lactamase combination agents. Additional agents with anaerobic activity include metronidazole and clindamycin.

Metronidazole

Metronidazole is highly active against obligate anaerobes. Although orally administered metronidazole is absorbed nearly completely, critically ill patients with infections other than *C. difficile*–associated diarrhea should receive therapy by the IV route. Metronidazole is administered at 500 mg (7.5 mg per kg) IV every 8 hours [42]. Metronidazole is metabolized by the liver; no dose adjustment is required in patients with renal insufficiency, but dosages must be reduced in individuals with severe hepatic insufficiency. Penetration into CSF and brain is excellent. Reported serious adverse events include neutropenia, pancreatitis, peripheral neuropathy, and hepatitis. Metallic taste occurs commonly, and up to 12% of patients have minor GI tract side effects. A disulfiram-like reaction can occur with concomitant alcohol intake.

Metronidazole is active in vitro against anaerobic Gram-negative bacilli and is probably the most potent agent for treatment of infections caused by *B. fragilis* [5]. Metronidazole must be used in conjunction with an agent active against aerobic organisms in the treatment of intra-abdominal, intrapelvic, and pulmonary infections where aerobic organisms can be expected to be concurrent pathogens. It has become the drug of first choice for treatment of *C. difficile*–associated diarrhea because of limitations on the use of oral vancomycin in an attempt to decrease selective pressure for the emergence of VRE, although oral vancomycin, often with IV metronidazole, is preferred in critically ill patients [43].

Clindamycin

Clindamycin is active in vitro against a wide variety of anaerobic bacteria. It has been used with great success in the treatment of anaerobic infections of the head, neck, and lungs/pleural space. The use of clindamycin in addition to penicillin is recommended in the treatment of necrotizing fasciitis due to β-hemolytic *Streptococcus* spp because of its apparent activity against organisms that are present in very high inoculum [44]. Clindamycin-resistant strains of *B. fragilis* group are becoming more prevalent, with 29% of isolates resistant in 2001 versus 10% in 1988 [45].

Usual parenteral therapy with clindamycin for severe infections consists of 600 to 900 mg IV every 8 hours (25 to 40 mg per kg per day) [46]. Because clindamycin is metabolized by the liver and excreted in inactive form in bile, no adjustment in dosage is required in patients with renal insufficiency.

The most important side effects of clindamycin are gastrointestinal. The incidence of diarrhea during therapy with clindamycin has been reported to range from 3% to 30%. Pseudomembranous colitis due to *C. difficile* has been reported to occur in up to 10% of patients who receive clindamycin [29,47].

MACROLIDES

The macrolides are bacteriostatic antibiotics that act on the 50 S ribosome subunit. The most common use of macrolides is to treat primary atypical pneumonia due to *Mycoplasma pneumoniae*, *Chlamydophilia pneumoniae*, or *Legionella* spp; pharyngitis due to *S. pyogenes*; *Bordetella pertussis* infections; enteritis due to *Campylobacter* spp; and eradication of the diphtheria carrier state.

Erythromycin is the oldest agent in current use in this class, and now used less frequently than azithromycin or clarithromycin. Erythromycin is used occasionally in the ICU setting to enhance gut motility [48].

Azithromycin is available in oral and IV preparations and clarithromycin in an oral form [49]. In addition to sharing the microbiologic spectrum of activity of erythromycin, azithromycin is more active against *C. trachomatis* but is less active than erythromycin or clarithromycin against staphylococci and streptococci. Clarithromycin shares the antimicrobial spectrum of erythromycin but is more active against Gram-positive cocci. Both agents have activity against *Mycobacterium avium-intracellulare* and *Mycobacterium chelonae* and are used prophylactically and therapeutically for disseminated *M. avium* complex infection in patients with advanced human immunodeficiency virus (HIV) disease. These agents are bacteriostatic and not usually used as first-line agents for treatment of Gram-positive infections in the ICU.

Oxazolidinones

Linezolid, the first available oxazolidinone antimicrobial, exerts its action by inhibiting the initiation of protein synthesis by stopping assembly of bacterial ribosomes [50,51]. Linezolid has bacteriostatic activity against MRSA, VRSA, and VRE and is bactericidal against penicillin-resistant *S. pneumoniae*. It is approved for treatment of nosocomial pneumonia and cSSSIs caused by *S. aureus* (including MRSA). It is available for IV or oral use at a dosage of 600 mg every 12 hours and has excellent oral bioavailability. Dosage adjustments are not necessary for patients with renal insufficiency [52]. The oxazolidinones have the potential for interaction with monoamine oxidase inhibitors, selective serotonin receptor uptake inhibitors (SSRIs), adrenergic agents used to support blood pressure in the ICU, and foods that contain a high tyramine content, with potential to trigger the serotonin syndrome, which can involve cognitive, autonomic, and somatic manifestations, and present variously as confusion, agitation, coma, autonomic instability, flushing, low-grade fever, nausea, diarrhea, diaphoresis, myoclonus, rigidity, and rarely myoclonus and death [53]. Reversible thrombocytopenia may occur if treatment is given longer than 14 days. Resistance may develop in enterococci with long-term use and has been described in *S. aureus* [54,55].

Quinupristin/Dalfopristin

Quinupristin/dalfopristin is a combination of two streptogramin antibiotics used in combination to treat vancomycin-resistant *E. faecium* infection and other Gram-positive bacteria including *S. aureus* [56]. This agent is given by the IV route, and, due to a high incidence of phlebitis, has to be administered through a central vascular catheter. It has bacteriostatic activity against *E. faecium*. The dose is 7.5 mg per kg every 8 hours for serious infections and 7.5 mg per kg every 12 hours for skin and skin structure infections. This drug is reserved for patients with difficult-to-treat infections. Quinupristin/dalfopristin has been used in a few patients with meningitis, and CSF concentrations appear to be higher than the MIC for susceptible organisms. Myalgias and arthralgias occur in up to 10% of patients and may limit its use [57].

Daptomycin

Daptomycin, a cyclic lipopeptide antimicrobial agent with rapid, concentration-dependent bactericidal activity against aerobic and facultative Gram-positive microorganisms, is active against a range of Gram-positive bacteria, including many multidrug-resistant isolates. Daptomycin is approved for treatment of cSSSIs caused by susceptible strains of *S. aureus* (including MRSA), *S. pyogenes*, and other streptococcal and *Enterococcus species* [58]. The dosage of daptomycin for soft tissue infections is 4 mg per kg every 24 hours by IV infusion given over 30 minutes for patients with a creatinine clearance greater than 30 mL per minute. A dose of 6 mg per kg every 24 hours is recommended for bacteremia and right-sided endocarditis caused by susceptible strains of *S. aureus* (including MRSA). In the lung, daptomycin is bound to surfactant, and it is not clinically effective for pneumonia [59]. The drug is excreted primarily via the kidney with low potential for interference with hepatically metabolized drugs. If the creatinine clearance is less than 30 mL per minute, the dosage interval should be extended to 48 hours. Reported adverse effects include diarrhea, vomiting, sickle-cell crisis, hypersensitivity reactions, dermatitis, myalgias, and creatinine kinase elevations [60,61].

Tigecycline

Tigecycline is the first antibiotic in the glycylcycline class and is a minocycline derivative [62]. Tigecycline is one of the few new antimicrobials with activity against Gram-negative bacteria including multiresistant *Acinetobacter* spp and organisms that produce ESBL. In addition, it is active against Gram positives such as MRSA and enterococci including VRE. Tigecycline is approved treatment of cSSSIs and complicated intra-abdominal infections. Tigecycline is available only for IV administration, given as a 100-mg initial dose, then 50 mg every 12 hours. The most common treatment adverse effects are nausea and vomiting which occur generally during the first 2 days of therapy.

THERAPY OF FUNGAL INFECTIONS

Invasive and disseminated fungal infections are increasingly common in ICU patients, especially those who receive immunosuppressive therapy or broad-spectrum antibiotics; in patients with lymphoreticular malignancies or transplants; and in individuals with advanced HIV disease. Newer antifungals of the triazole class (fluconazole, itraconazole, voriconazole, and posaconazole) and echinocandin class (caspofungin, micafungin, and anidulafungin) have become available for the treatment of systemic mycoses. However, amphotericin B remains important for empiric initial therapy for life-threatening fungal infections when the infecting organism is not yet identified or is resistant to triazoles.

Amphotericin B

Amphotericin B is a polyene antibiotic, insoluble in water, and solubilized by the addition of sodium deoxycholate, forming a colloidal dispersion. Its mechanism of action is due to its binding to ergosterol, a sterol present in the cell membrane of susceptible fungi, resulting in altered membrane permeability and causing leakage of cell components and resultant cell death. Amphotericin B is effective against most species of fungi that are pathogenic in humans [63]. Either amphotericin B deoxycholate or one of the liposomal preparations is the initial drug of choice for empiric therapy of life-threatening, invasive, or systemic fungal infections including mucormycosis, cryptococcosis, histoplasmosis, and coccidioidomycosis and is effective for blastomycosis and extracutaneous sporotrichosis. Although *Candida albicans* generally is susceptible to amphotericin B, non-*albicans* species of *Candida* often are less susceptible, and fluconazole or an echinocandin is the drug of choice once the infecting species is identified and susceptibility is known. Amphotericin B preparations have variable activity that is evident against *Aspergillus* spp, *Zygomycetes* spp, *Scedosporium boydii*, *Fusarium* spp, and dematiaceous fungi. The combination of amphotericin B plus flucytosine is synergistic against *Candida* sp and *Cryptococcus neoformans* and is used to treat meningitis due to these fungi.

Amphotericin B for IV administration should be prepared in 5% dextrose because saline solutions result in drug precipitation. The drug is highly protein bound and is distributed into many tissues (liver, spleen, lung, muscle, kidney, skin, and adrenals); because penetration into CSF is poor, intrathecal/intracisternal administration or the use of triazoles may be necessary for some CNS mycoses. The metabolism of amphotericin B is obscure, but renal and hepatic insufficiency has little effect on serum levels of the drug and hemodialysis does not affect serum levels.

Amphotericin B usually is given by IV infusion once a day over 2 to 6 hours, at a concentration of 0.1 mg per mL. Daily and total doses are adjusted according to the fungal species, sites, and extent of infection and the individual tolerance of the patient. A test dose of 1 mg (in 25 to 100 mL 5% dextrose) is infused over 30 minutes. For patients who are critically ill with apparently rapidly progressive fungal disease, the full daily dose of 0.5 to 1.0 mg per kg can be given immediately following the test dose. For patients who exhibit poor tolerance with the test dose or subsequent increased doses, amphotericin B dosing can be increased in a gradual fashion, with increase in the dosage by 5 to 10 mg per day until the final daily dose is reached. The usual duration of amphotericin B therapy for systemic mycoses is 4 to 12 weeks, to a total dose of 1 to 2 g. For infections caused by less susceptible fungi (e.g., *Aspergillus* spp, *Zygomycetes* spp [*Mucor*], and *Coccidioides immitis*), treatment warrants daily doses of up to 1.0 to 1.5 mg per kg and a total dose of 2 g. Cryptococcosis can be treated successfully with reduced (0.3 mg per kg per day) dosages of amphotericin B plus flucytosine (150 mg per kg per day orally) for 6 weeks.

Adverse Reactions

Adverse effects of amphotericin B most frequently include infusion-associated constitutional symptoms such as fever, chills, hypotension, and tachypnea, most common and most severe with the first few doses of the drug and during escalation of dosage and can be minimized by increasing daily dosage slowly (if the clinical situation permits) or by pretreatment with acetaminophen, hydrocortisone (25 to 50 mg IV), or meperidine (25 mg IV). Dantrolene (10 mg IV) has been used successfully as an alternative or adjunctive agent in patients with severe rigors [64]. Nephrotoxicity occurs frequently with amphotericin B deoxycholate therapy, and thus patients with renal insufficiency or administration of other nephrotoxic agents should be given one of the liposomal preparations. Potassium levels should be monitored closely and supplementation with potassium begun as soon as serum potassium decreases toward the low end of normal range. Mild anemia occurs commonly during amphotericin B therapy, but thrombocytopenia, leukopenia, and severe hepatitis are rare.

Alternative lipid preparations of amphotericin B have become available in an attempt to decrease renal toxicity [65]. The lipid formulations are notably more expensive than amphotericin B deoxycholate but are advantageous in patients with, or at risk of, renal insufficiency, those on other nephrotoxic medications, or those whose renal function worsens during treatment with amphotericin B. The ability to deliver a higher dose with the lipid complex than with amphotericin B alone has resulted in reports of patients responding to the lipid formulation at high dose (5 to 10 mg per kg) when traditional therapy with amphotericin B had been ineffective [65].

Flucytosine

Flucytosine is an orally administered pyrimidine analog with a narrow spectrum of action, generally used in combination with an amphotericin preparation for therapy of *C. neoformans* and *Candida* meningitis. Most strains of *C. neoformans* and *Candida* sp are susceptible initially, whereas most other fungi that are pathogenic for humans are resistant. The use of combination therapy with flucytosine allows a reduction in dosage and duration (0.3 mg per kg per day for 6 weeks) of amphotericin B in the treatment of cryptococcal meningitis and improves efficacy in the treatment of *Candida* meningitis because of its excellent penetration into this site. The drug is cleared by the kidneys, with a serum $t_{1/2}$ of 3 hours in patients with normal renal function and 85 hours in anuric patients. The usual recommended dosage in patients with normal renal function is 150 mg per kg daily in four divided doses; the interval between doses should be doubled (every 12 hours) when the creatinine clearance rate is 20 to 40 mL per minute and quadrupled (every 24 hours) when the creatinine clearance rate is 10 to 20 mL per minute. The serum level of flucytosine should be monitored, particularly in patients with renal impairment, and the dose should be adjusted to maintain a level of 50 to 100 μg per mL. Leukopenia is the most serious complication of flucytosine therapy and occurs most commonly in patients with renal insufficiency and when serum levels exceed 100 μg per mL. GI tract intolerance (nausea, vomiting, anorexia, or diarrhea), hepatitis, and rash occur occasionally.

TRIAZOLES

Fluconazole

Fluconazole is a water-soluble triazole available for IV and oral use and exhibits good activity in vitro against *Candida* spp and *C. neoformans* [66]. As with all the triazoles, its mode of action is mediated through inhibition of ergosterol synthesis. Oral absorption is excellent, resulting in serum levels nearly as high as with IV administration and is independent of gastric acidity. Fluconazole penetrates well into bodily fluids, including CSF (50% to 90% of serum concentrations) and the eye. Fluconazole has a long (30 hours) $t_{1/2}$; because of its renal clearance, adjustments must be made in dosing in patients with renal impairment. For patients with oropharyngeal or esophageal candidiasis, the usual dosage (oral or IV) of fluconazole is 200 mg on the first day of therapy, followed by 100 mg once a day; therapy is continued until clinical findings resolve and for a total of 2 to 3 weeks. Fluconazole (800 mg loading dose, then 400 mg once daily) is effective in the treatment of systemic or hepatic candidiasis due to susceptible strains of *C. albicans* [67]. Non-albicans species of *Candida* may be less susceptible. For severe systemic mycoses (i.e., coccidioidomycosis, cryptococcosis) or candidemia, the usual daily dosage is 800 mg then 400 mg IV daily. Side effects of fluconazole are relatively minor and uncommon, with GI tract symptoms (nausea) most frequent. Mild, transient elevation of serum transaminase levels occurs occasionally. Fluconazole inhibits the metabolism and potentiates the effects of warfarin, phenytoin, cyclosporine, tacrolimus, and oral hypoglycemic agents.

Itraconazole

Itraconazole, a broad-spectrum triazole antifungal with notable activity against *Aspergillus* sp, *H. capsulatum*, *C. immitis*, and *Sporothrix schenckii*, is available for IV or oral use [68]. Itraconazole is widely distributed in most tissues but with poor levels in CSF. Clinical experience indicates that itraconazole has a role in the treatment of sporotrichosis, blastomycosis, histoplasmosis, paracoccidioidomycosis, and chromomycosis and may be of use in treating patients with coccidioidomycosis, cryptococcosis, or aspergillosis who have failed prior therapy with amphotericin B or other azoles. Daily dosage is 200 to 800 mg orally, with the higher doses indicated in patients with CNS infection. Clearance is by hepatic metabolism, and no adjustment of dosage is required in patients with renal failure. Like voriconazole, the IV form of itraconazole includes cyclodextrin to improve solubility, and as cyclodextrin is cleared by the kidney, the IV formulation should not be used if the creatinine clearance is less than 30 mL per minute. Itraconazole is well tolerated, with occasional GI tract symptoms (abdominal discomfort, nausea, and diarrhea) or minor elevation of liver chemistry values noted. Itraconazole requires an acidic environment for optimal GI tract absorption. Absorption of the elixir form of the drug is greater than with the capsules, and absorption is better with multiple daily dosing. Itraconazole has only a minimal effect on the synthesis of androgens or cortisol but appears to be able to produce a picture of mineralocorticoid excess with hypokalemia, edema, and hypertension.

Voriconazole

Voriconazole is a second-generation, broad-spectrum triazole that is a synthetic derivative of fluconazole. Voriconazole is active against strains of *Candida krusei* and *Candida glabrata* that are inherently fluconazole resistant and against strains of *C. albicans* that have acquired resistance to fluconazole. Voriconazole has a broad activity against many species of *Aspergillus* spp, including *Aspergillus terreus*, which often is resistant to amphotericin B [69]. It is a drug of choice for invasive aspergillosis and refractory infections with *Pseudoallescheria/Scedosporium* and *Fusarium* spp.

Voriconazole is available in oral and IV formulations. The standard loading dose is 6 mg per kg repeated in 12 hours. Patients who weigh more than 40 kg should receive 200 mg every 12 hours for maintenance therapy and the dosage should be adjusted in patients with mild-to-moderate liver disease. Because the azoles are metabolized by the hepatic cytochrome P450 systems, a variety of drug interactions can occur; however, voriconazole generally is well tolerated. Reported toxicities include elevations in liver enzymes, rash, and, in a third of patients, transient ocular toxicity [70]. The IV form contains cyclodextrin and should be used for short periods (<2 weeks) in patients with renal insufficiency due to accumulation of the metabolites.

Posaconazole

Posaconazole is a second-generation triazole approved for the treatment of oropharyngeal candidiasis, including infections refractory to itraconazole and/or fluconazole [71]. It is approved also as prophylaxis for invasive *Aspergillus* and *Candida* infections in patients older than 13 years who are at high risk of developing fungal infections, such as hematopoietic stem cell transplant recipients with graft-versus-host disease and neutropenic patients with hematologic malignancies [72,73]. Limited clinical experience suggests efficacy for the treatment of infections due to Zygomycetes and as salvage therapy for patients with invasive aspergillosis and coccidioidomycosis. Posaconazole currently is available only as an oral tablet or suspension and requires administration with food or a nutritional supplement to assure adequate bioavailability. Dose adjustment is not required in the presence of renal or hepatic insufficiency. Although not a substrate of hepatic CYP450 3A4, posaconazole inhibits this enzyme and thus has the potential for significant pharmacokinetic interactions with drugs metabolized by this isoform. Its use in combination with CYP450 substrates that prolong the QTc interval is contraindicated, as is its use with ergot alkaloids. The recommended dosage for posaconazole antifungal prophylaxis is 200 mg (5 mL) three times daily. Recommended therapy of oropharyngeal candidiasis is a loading dose of 200 mg (100 mg twice daily), followed by 100 mg daily for 13 days. Refractory oropharyngeal candidiasis may be treated with 400 mg twice daily with the duration based on clinical response and the patient's underlying disease. Experimental treatment of invasive fungal infections with posaconazole at doses 200 mg orally four times daily and maintenance therapy at 400 mg orally twice daily is based on pharmacokinetic data; however, package labeling does not include this indication [74]. The most common adverse effects associated with the use of posaconazole include headache, fever, nausea, vomiting, and diarrhea.

ECHINOCANDINS

Caspofungin/Micafungin/Anidulafungin

Caspofungin, micafungin, and anidulafungin are echinocandins, a class of antifungal agents that act on the fungal cell wall by inhibiting glucan synthesis. Echinocandins are available only for IV administration and are active against most species of Candida.

Caspofungin can be used for refractory cases of invasive aspergillosis for patients intolerant of voriconazole and amphotericin B. All of these agents may be used to treat candidemia with similar success but with fewer side effects than amphotericin B [58]. These agents are highly protein bound and distribute into all major organ sites including the brain; however, concentration in uninfected CSF is low. For caspofungin, the recommended dosage for adults is 70 mg as a loading dose, then 50 mg per day. Dose alteration is recommended in the presence of moderate hepatic insufficiency. Caspofungin is metabolized by the liver, and dose adjustment is required when it is given with other drugs that alter cytochrome P450 activity. In general, caspofungin is well tolerated with the most frequently reported adverse effects being increased serum transaminases, GI upset, and headaches. Caspofungin is classified as pregnancy category C and should be used during pregnancy only if the potential benefit outweighs the potential fetal risk.

These three agents exhibit a fungicidal effect against most *Candida* sp and have become the drugs of choice for empiric therapy of candidemia in the ICU. However, they are not active against *C. neoformans* and it is important to consider the possibility of cryptococcal disease when using them empirically. They have a fungistatic effect against *Aspergillus* spp. Micafungin appears comparable to fluconazole as antifungal prophylaxis in patients undergoing hematopoietic stem-cell transplantation [75,76] and anidulafungin has been used in neutropenic children. Absence of antagonism in combination with other antifungal agents suggests that combination antifungal therapy is an area that needs further study, particularly for severe aspergillosis and candidiasis [77].

Trimethoprim–Sulfamethoxazole

Trimethoprim–sulfamethoxazole (cotrimoxazole) works through sequential, two-stage inhibition of folate synthesis. It has activity against Gram-positive and Gram-negative bacteria, *Nocardia* spp, and *Pneumocystis jiroveci* (previously known as *P. carinii*). Trimethoprim–sulfamethoxazole can be used in the therapy of Gram-negative infections, including those caused by *Enterobacter* spp in the ICU patient. Sometimes this agent is effective against β-lactam–resistant nosocomial bacteria including MRSA. The dose for serious bacterial infections is 8 to 10 mg per kg per day (of the trimethoprim component), divided every 6 to 12 hours.

Trimethoprim–sulfamethoxazole is the drug of choice for *Pneumocystis* pneumonia [78,79]. In moderately to severely ill patients, it is administered IV or orally at a dosage of 15 to 20 mg per kg per day of the trimethoprim component in three to four divided doses for a total course of 14 days in non-AIDS patients and at a dosage of 15 mg per kg of the trimethoprim component daily (or 75 mg per kg of the sulfa component daily) for 21 days in patients with AIDS. Failure to obtain satisfactory response in 5 days (7 days in individuals with HIV infection) warrants change to an alternative regimen (see HIV chapter 85 for *Pneumocystis* pneumonia therapy). Adverse reactions to trimethoprim–sulfamethoxazole occur in approximately 10% to 15% of patients who are uninfected with HIV-1 and in up to two thirds of patients with AIDS. The most common problems are neutropenia or thrombocytopenia, or both (particularly in patients with advanced HIV-1–induced immunodeficiency or receiving zidovudine); rash or fever; nausea or vomiting; and abnormalities of hepatic enzymes.

Pyrimethamine–Sulfadiazine

For the treatment of systemic and invasive (including encephalitis) toxoplasmosis in the compromised host, the alternate double-antifolate combination of pyrimethamine–sulfadiazine usually is used. Pyrimethamine is administered orally with a loading dose of 200 mg, then at 75 mg daily (with folinic acid 5 mg daily) together with sulfadiazine orally at 6 g daily in four divided doses. Adverse reactions occur in similar frequency and type as with cotrimoxazole. Alternative therapy for CNS toxoplasmosis is clindamycin (900 mg IV every 6 hours) plus pyrimethamine [80].

THERAPY OF VIRAL INFECTIONS

As viral infections have become more common and more severe in an era of expanding populations of immunocompromised hosts, several antiviral agents have become available (Table 77.4). Nevertheless, antiviral therapy remains problematic and limited in scope as compared with antibacterial treatments. Antiretroviral therapy is discussed in Chapter 85.

Acyclovir and Related Compounds

Acyclovir is a nucleoside analog of guanosine with antiviral activity against herpes viruses, particularly herpes simplex virus (HSV) types 1 and 2 and varicella-zoster virus (VZV) [81]. Administered as a prodrug, acyclovir requires phosphorylation to a monophosphate form by a virus-generated thymidine kinase and then to a triphosphate form by host cellular enzymes. Because cytomegalovirus (CMV) lacks a thymidine kinase, acyclovir has limited activity against this virus.

Acyclovir is available in topical, oral, and IV preparations, with the last route preferred for serious infections in critically ill patients and for milder illnesses in those unable to take medications by mouth. Dosage varies according to the condition under treatment. After oral administration, absorption is slow and incomplete, with oral bioavailability of only 15% to 30%. Serum $t_{1/2}$ is 2 to 3 hours in patients with normal renal function. Because 85% of clearance is renal, dosage must be reduced in patients with impaired renal function. Acyclovir is well tolerated. Reversible renal impairment, due to crystalluria, occurs occasionally, usually in patients who are receiving high doses by rapid IV infusion or those who are elderly, dehydrated, or have antecedent renal insufficiency. At high doses, especially IV, neurologic reactions (confusion, delirium, hallucinations, seizures, and tremors) have occurred in approximately 1% of patients. Occasionally, patients have nausea, vomiting, or rash.

Intravenous acyclovir at 10 to 12 mg per kg every 8 hours is the drug of choice for HSV encephalitis (for a course of 14 to 21 days), for congenital HSV infection (10 to 14 days), and for VZV infections (chickenpox or shingles) in immunocompromised patients (7 to 10 days). Acyclovir at 5 mg per kg IV every 8 hours is effective against mucocutaneous HSV in immunocompromised patients.

Valacyclovir, a prodrug for acyclovir, is more completely absorbed than acyclovir and is hydrolyzed rapidly to acyclovir in the intestinal wall and the liver [82]. In general, it is well tolerated, but thrombocytopenia and hemolytic-uremic syndrome

TABLE 77.4

ANTIVIRAL THERAPY

Antiviral agent	Indication	Dose	Route	Duration of treatment	Adjust for renal failure
Acyclovir	Herpes simplex virus				
	Encephalitis	10–12 mg/kg q8h	IV	10–14 d	Yes
	Neonatal infection	10 mg/kg q8h	IV	10–14 d	Yes
	Mucocutaneous disease	5 mg/kg q8h	IV	7–10 d	Yes
	Herpes varicella-zoster	10 mg/kg q8h	IV	7–10 d	Yes
Ganciclovir	Cytomegalovirus				
	Induction	5 mg/kg q12h	IV	14–21 d	Yes
	Maintenance	5 mg/kg qd or	IV	Indefinite	
		6 mg/kg 5 d/wk	IV	Indefinite	
		3,000 mg qd	PO	Indefinite	
Foscarnet	Cytomegalovirus				
	Induction	60 mg/kg q8h or	IV	14–21 d	Yes
		90 mg/kg q12h	IV		
	Maintenance	90 mg/kg qd	IV	Indefinite	
Cidofovir (+ probenecid premedication)	Cytomegalovirus Induction Maintenance	5 mg/kg q wk IV 5 mg/kg q 2 wk	IV	14 d Indefinite	Contraindicated in patients with baseline creatinine >1.5 mg/dL or increase to >2.0 mg/dL

have been reported in immunocompromised patients. Other side effects are similar to those of acyclovir and include encephalopathy, fevers, seizures, and rash. Acyclovir, or valacyclovir, is used prophylactically in patients who are undergoing bone marrow or solid organ transplantation.

Famciclovir, a prodrug for penciclovir, is active against VZV and HSV. Side effects are similar to those of acyclovir. Both of the newer oral agents, famciclovir and valacyclovir, are dosed three times a day orally rather than the five times a day that is needed with acyclovir for VZV infections.

Ganciclovir

Ganciclovir is highly active against CMV, in part because of the high concentration of the triphosphorylated form of the drug in infected cells. The most problematic adverse effect is myelosuppression, particularly neutropenia. Other side effects include nausea and vomiting and CNS abnormalities. Ganciclovir is effective in the treatment of disseminated CMV and CMV retinitis, GI tract infection (colitis, esophagitis, and gastritis), and pneumonitis. In bone marrow transplant patients, the drug sometimes is used in combination with IV CMV hyperimmune globulin for the treatment of CMV pneumonitis [83]. Valganciclovir is a prodrug for ganciclovir [84]. It is more completely absorbed from the GI tract, achieving higher serum levels than possible with oral therapy with the parent drug.

Treatment with ganciclovir in AIDS patients with CMV retinitis usually involves induction therapy with 5 mg per kg IV twice a day for 14 to 21 days, followed by maintenance therapy with oral valganciclovir. It is given for 3 weeks or until serum CMV molecular assays are negative in immunocompromised patient with disseminated CMV infection. Ganciclovir and valganciclovir are cleared by the kidney and dosage adjustments must be made in patients with renal impairment, especially in light of the relationship between drug serum levels and myelosuppression. Valganciclovir is used as prophylaxis or preemptive therapy for CMV in transplant patients.

Cidofovir

Cidofovir is a nucleotide analog that is active against herpes viruses, including CMV, HSV, and VZV. It is a prodrug that is converted to cidofovir diphosphate by host cellular enzymes. In contrast to ganciclovir and acyclovir, activation by viral-encoded enzymes is not required, so it may be used to treat CMV infections when the virus is resistant to ganciclovir because of the UL97 mutation.

Foscarnet

Foscarnet (trisodium phosphonoformate) is an inorganic pyrophosphate analog that acts by inhibiting viral DNA polymerases of most human herpes viruses (particularly CMV) and reverse transcriptases of human retroviruses (particularly HIV-1) [83]. Foscarnet has been demonstrated to be effective in the therapy of CMV retinitis in patients with AIDS and has been used alone and in combination with ganciclovir to treat ganciclovir-resistant CMV in immunocompromised patients (especially transplant recipients) [85]. Foscarnet is associated with a significant (25%) incidence of nephrotoxicity. Therapy involves IV administration at a dosage of 60 mg per kg three times a day for induction and at 90 to 120 mg per kg once a day for maintenance therapy. Clearance is by renal excretion, and dosage adjustment is required in patients with renal impairment. Nonrenal adverse effects include nausea, vomiting, anemia, seizures, and metabolic abnormalities (hyperphosphatemia and hypophosphatemia, hypercalcemia and hypocalcemia, hypokalemia, and hypomagnesemia).

Anti-influenza Agents

Amantadine and rimantadine are oral antiviral compounds that inhibit influenza A, and zanamivir and oseltamivir are neuraminidase inhibitors that inhibit both influenza A and B viruses. If initiated within 48 hours of the start of symptoms, all four agents may reduce the intensity of influenza infection in patients infected with susceptible viruses [86]. For patients who are immunocompromised or who have ongoing viral replication and progressive symptoms, therapy after 48 hours may also be beneficial, although supporting data are not available. Zanamivir is given by the inhaled route and oseltamivir by the oral route. The dose of oseltamivir is 100 mg per day and for zanamivir 20 mg by inhalation daily. Resistance to the antiviral agents has occurred in influenza viruses, and clinicians need to be aware of the susceptibility of prevailing influenza strains in the community to appropriately choose an agent for use in the ICU.

References

1. Tleyjeh IM, Tlaygeh HM, Hejal R, et al: The impact of penicillin resistance on short-term mortality in hospitalized adults with pneumococcal pneumonia: a systematic review and meta-analysis. *Clin Infect Dis* 42:788–797, 2006.
2. Wright AJ, Wilkowske CJ: The penicillins. *Mayo Clin Proc* 66:1047–1063, 1991.
3. van de Beek D, de Gans J, Tunkel AR, et al: Community-acquired bacterial meningitis in adults. *N Engl J Med* 354:44–53, 2006.
4. Levison ME, Mangura CT, Lorber B, et al: Clindamycin compared with penicillin for the treatment of anaerobic lung abscess. *Ann Intern Med* 98:466–471, 1983.
5. Erwin ME, Fix AM, Jones RN: Three independent yearly analyses of the spectrum and potency of metronidazole: a multicenter study of 1,108 contemporary anaerobic clinical isolates. *Diagn Microbiol Infect Dis* 39:129–132, 2001.
6. Allewelt M, Schüler P, Bölcskei PL, et al: Ampicillin + sulbactam vs clindamycin +/− cephalosporin for the treatment of aspiration pneumonia and primary lung abscess. *Clin Microbiol Infect* 10:163–170, 2004.
7. Moellering RC Jr: Emergence of Enterococcus as a significant pathogen. *Clin Infect Dis* 14:1173–1176, 1992.
8. Francis JS, Doherty MC, Lopatin U, et al: Severe community-onset pneumonia in healthy adults caused by methicillin-resistant *Staphylococcus aureus* carrying the Panton-Valentine leukocidin genes [see comment]. *Clin Infect Dis* 40:100–107, 2005.
9. Perry CM, Markham A: Piperacillin/tazobactam: an updated review of its use in the treatment of bacterial infections. *Drugs* 57:805–843, 1999.
10. American Thoracic Society, Infectious Diseases Society of America: Guidelines for the management of adults with hospital-acquired, ventilator-associated, and healthcare-associated pneumonia [see comment]. *Am J Respir Crit Care Med* 171:388–416, 2005.
11. Roberts JA, Roberts MS, Robertson TA, et al: Piperacillin penetration into tissue of critically ill patients with sepsis—bolus versus continuous administration? *Crit Care Med* 37:926–933, 2009.
12. Paul M, Silbiger I, Grozinsky S, et al: Beta lactam antibiotic monotherapy versus beta lactam-aminoglycoside antibiotic combination therapy for sepsis. *Cochrane Database Syst Rev* (1):CD003344, 2006.
13. Jacoby GA, Munoz-Price LS: The new beta-lactamases. *N Engl J Med* 352:380–391, 2005.
14. Talon D, Bailly P, Bertrand X, et al: Clinical and molecular epidemiology of chromosome-mediated resistance to third-generation cephalosporins in Enterobacter isolates in eastern France. *Clin Microbiol Infect* 6:376–384, 2000.
15. Gustaferro CA, Steckelberg JM: Cephalosporin antimicrobial agents and related compounds. *Mayo Clin Proc* 66:1064–1073, 1991.
16. Tunkel AR, Hartman BJ, Kaplan SL, et al: Practice guidelines for the management of bacterial meningitis [see comment]. *Clin Infect Dis* 39:1267–1284, 2004.
17. Niederman MS, Mandell LA, Anzueto A, et al: Guidelines for the management of adults with community-acquired pneumonia. Diagnosis, assessment of severity, antimicrobial therapy, and prevention. *Am J Respir Crit Care Med* 163:1730–1754, 2001.
18. Baddour LM, Wilson WR, Bayer AS, et al: Infective endocarditis: diagnosis, antimicrobial therapy, and management of complications: a statement for healthcare professionals from the Committee on Rheumatic Fever, Endocarditis, and Kawasaki Disease, Council on Cardiovascular Disease in the Young, and the Councils on Clinical Cardiology, Stroke, and Cardiovascular Surgery and Anesthesia, American Heart Association: endorsed by the Infectious Diseases Society of America [erratum appears in *Circulation* 2005;112(15):2373]. *Circulation* 111:e394–434, 2005.
19. Safdar N, Handelsman J, Maki DG: Does combination antimicrobial therapy reduce mortality in Gram-negative bacteraemia? A meta-analysis. *Lancet Infect Dis* 4:519–527, 2004.
20. Marshall WF, Blair JE: The cephalosporins. *Mayo Clin Proc* 74:187–195, 1999.
21. Hellinger WC, Brewer NS: Carbapenems and monobactams: imipenem, meropenem, and aztreonam. *Mayo Clin Proc* 74:420–434, 1999.
22. Keating GM, Perry CM: Ertapenem: a review of its use in the treatment of bacterial infections. *Drugs* 65:2151–2178, 2005.
23. Paterson DL, Depestel DD: Doripenem. *Clin Infect Dis* 49:291–298, 2009.
24. Saxon A, Hassner A, Swabb EA, et al: Lack of cross-reactivity between aztreonam, a monobactam antibiotic, and penicillin in penicillin-allergic subjects. *J Infect Dis* 149:16–22, 1984.
25. Edson RS, Terrell CL: The aminoglycosides. *Mayo Clin Proc* 74:519–528, 1999.
26. Chow JW: Aminoglycoside resistance in enterococci. *Clin Infect Dis* 31:586–589, 2000.
27. Dodge RA, Daly JS, Davaro R, et al: High-dose ampicillin plus streptomycin for treatment of a patient with severe infection due to multiresistant enterococci. *Clin Infect Dis* 25:1269–1270, 1997.
28. John JF Jr, Rubens CE, Farrar WE Jr: Characteristics of gentamicin resistance in nosocomial infections. *Am J Med Sci* 279:25–30, 1980.
29. Riddle DJ, Dubberke ER: *Clostridium difficile* infection in the intensive care unit. *Infect Dis Clin North Am* 23:727–743, 2009.
30. Demczar DJ, Nafziger AN, Bertino JS Jr: Pharmacokinetics of gentamicin at traditional versus high doses: implications for once-daily aminoglycoside dosing. *Antimicrob Agents Chemother* 41:1115–1119, 1997.
31. Barclay ML, Kirkpatrick CM, Begg EJ: Once daily aminoglycoside therapy. Is it less toxic than multiple daily doses and how should it be monitored? *Clin Pharmacokinet* 36:89–98, 1999.
32. Van Bambeke F, Michot JM, Van Eldere J, et al: Quinolones in 2005: an update [erratum appears in *Clin Microbiol Infect* 2005;11(6):513]. *Clin Microbiol Infect* 11:256–280, 2005.
33. Drusano GL, Weir M, Forrest A, et al: Pharmacokinetics of intravenously administered ciprofloxacin in patients with various degrees of renal function. *Antimicrob Agents Chemother* 31:860–864, 1987.
34. Wilhelm MP, Estes L: Symposium on antimicrobial agents—Part XII. Vancomycin. *Mayo Clin Proc* 74:928–935, 1999.
35. Megran DW: Enterococcal endocarditis [see comment]. *Clin Infect Dis* 15:63–71, 1992.
36. Centers for Disease Control and Prevention (CDC): Reduced susceptibility of *Staphylococcus aureus* to vancomycin—Japan, 1996. *MMWR Morb Mortal Wkly Rep* 46:624–626, 1997.
37. Rybak MJ: The pharmacokinetic and pharmacodynamic properties of vancomycin. *Clin Infect Dis* 42[Suppl 1]:S35–39, 2006.
38. Rybak M, Lomaestro B, Rotschafer JC, et al: Therapeutic monitoring of vancomycin in adult patients: a consensus review of the American Society of Health-System Pharmacists, the Infectious Diseases Society of America, and the Society of Infectious Diseases Pharmacists. *Am J Health Syst Pharm* 66:82–98, 2009.
39. Renz CL, Thurn JD, Finn HA, et al: Antihistamine prophylaxis permits rapid vancomycin infusion [see comment]. *Crit Care Med* 27:1732–1737, 1999.
40. Segarra-Newnham M, Tagoff SS: Probable vancomycin-induced neutropenia. *Ann Pharmacother* 38:1855–1859, 2004.
41. Smith WJ, Drew RH: Telavancin: a new lipoglycopeptide for gram-positive infections. *Drugs Today (Barc)* 45:159–173, 2009.
42. Freeman CD, Klutman NE, Lamp KC: Metronidazole. A therapeutic review and update. *Drugs* 54:679–708, 1997.
43. Zar FA, Bakkanagari SR, Moorthi KM, et al: A comparison of vancomycin and metronidazole for the treatment of *Clostridium difficile*-associated diarrhea, stratified by disease severity. *Clin Infect Dis* 45:302–307, 2007.
44. Bisno AL, Stevens DL: Streptococcal infections of skin and soft tissues. *N Engl J Med* 334:240–245, 1996.
45. Aldridge KE, Ashcraft D, Cambre K, et al: Multicenter survey of the changing in vitro antimicrobial susceptibilities of clinical isolates of *Bacteroides fragilis* group, *Prevotella*, *Fusobacterium*, *Porphyromonas*, and *Peptostreptococcus* species. *Antimicrob Agents Chemother* 45:1238–1243, 2001.
46. Guay D: Update on clindamycin in the management of bacterial, fungal and protozoal infections. *Expert Opin Pharmacother* 8:2401–2444, 2007.
47. Gerding DN: Clindamycin, cephalosporins, fluoroquinolones, and *Clostridium difficile*-associated diarrhea: this is an antimicrobial resistance problem. *Clin Infect Dis* 38:646–648, 2004.
48. Ray WA, Murray KT, Meredith S, et al: Oral erythromycin and the risk of sudden death from cardiac causes [see comment]. *N Engl J Med* 351:1089–1096, 2004.
49. Clarithromycin and azithromycin. *Medical Letter on Drugs & Therapeutics* 34:45–47, 1992.
50. Perry CM, Jarvis B: Linezolid: a review of its use in the management of serious gram-positive infections [erratum appears in *Drugs* 2003;63(19):2126]. *Drugs* 61:525–551, 2001.
51. Moellering RC Jr: A novel antimicrobial agent joins the battle against resistant bacteria. *Ann Intern Med* 130:155–157, 1999.
52. Diekema DJ, Jones RN: Oxazolidinones: a review. *Drugs* 59:7–16, 2000.

53. Bergeron L, Boule M, Perreault S: Serotonin toxicity associated with concomitant use of linezolid. *Ann Pharmacother* 39:956–961, 2005.
54. Schulte B, Heininger A, Autenrieth IB, et al: Emergence of increasing linezolid-resistance in enterococci in a post-outbreak situation with vancomycin-resistant Enterococcus faecium. *Epidemiol Infect* 136:1131–1133, 2008.
55. Miller K, O'Neill AJ, Wilcox MH, et al: Delayed development of linezolid resistance in *Staphylococcus aureus* following exposure to low levels of antimicrobial agents. *Antimicrob Agents Chemother* 52:1940–1944, 2008.
56. Lamb HM, Figgitt DP, Faulds D: Quinupristin/dalfopristin: a review of its use in the management of serious gram-positive infections. *Drugs* 58:1061–1097, 1999.
57. Olsen KM, Rebuck JA, Rupp ME: Arthralgias and myalgias related to quinupristin-dalfopristin administration. *Clin Infect Dis* 32:e83–86, 2001.
58. Morrison VA: Caspofungin: an overview. *Expert Rev Anti Infect Ther* 3:697–705, 2005.
59. Silverman JA, Mortin LI, Vanpraagh AD, et al: Inhibition of daptomycin by pulmonary surfactant: in vitro modeling and clinical impact. *J Infect Dis* 191:2149–2152, 2005.
60. Levine DP: Clinical experience with daptomycin: bacteraemia and endocarditis. *J Antimicrob Chemother* 62[Suppl 3]:iii35–iii39, 2008.
61. Arbeit RD, Maki D, Tally FP, et al: The safety and efficacy of daptomycin for the treatment of complicated skin and skin-structure infections. *Clin Infect Dis* 38:1673–1681, 2004.
62. Livermore DM: Tigecycline: what is it, and where should it be used? *J Antimicrob Chemother* 56:611–614, 2005.
63. Barrett JP, Vardulaki KA, Conlon C, et al: A systematic review of the antifungal effectiveness and tolerability of amphotericin B formulations. *Clin Ther* 25:1295–1320, 2003.
64. Gross MH, Fulkerson WJ, Moore JO: Prevention of amphotericin B-induced rigors by dantrolene [erratum appears in *Arch Intern Med* 1986;146(12):2328]. *Arch Intern Med* 146:1587–1588, 1986.
65. Wong-Beringer A, Jacobs RA, Guglielmo BJ: Lipid formulations of amphotericin B: clinical efficacy and toxicities. *Clin Infect Dis* 27:603–618, 1998.
66. Charlier C, Hart E, Lefort A, et al: Fluconazole for the management of invasive candidiasis: where do we stand after 15 years? *J Antimicrob Chemother* 57:384–410, 2006.
67. Eggimann P, Garbino J, Pittet D: Management of Candida species infections in critically ill patients. *Lancet Infect Dis* 3:772–785, 2003.
68. Sharkey PK, Rinaldi MG, Dunn JF, et al: High-dose itraconazole in the treatment of severe mycoses. *Antimicrob Agents Chemother* 35:707–713, 1991.
69. Denning DW, Ribaud P, Milpied N, et al: Efficacy and safety of voriconazole in the treatment of acute invasive aspergillosis [see comment]. *Clin Infect Dis* 34:563–571, 2002.
70. Lazarus HM, Blumer JL, Yanovich S, et al: Safety and pharmacokinetics of oral voriconazole in patients at risk of fungal infection: a dose escalation study. *J Clin Pharmacol* 42:395–402, 2002.
71. Nagappan V, Deresinski S: Reviews of anti-infective agents: posaconazole: a broad-spectrum triazole antifungal agent [see comment]. *Clin Infect Dis* 45:1610–1617, 2007.
72. Cornely OA, Maertens J, Winston DJ, et al: Posaconazole vs. fluconazole or itraconazole prophylaxis in patients with neutropenia. *N Engl J Med* 356:348–359, 2007.
73. Ullmann AJ, Lipton JH, Vesole DH, et al: Posaconazole or fluconazole for prophylaxis in severe graft-versus-host disease [Erratum appears in *N Engl J Med* 2007;357(4):428]. *N Engl J Med* 356:335–347, 2007.
74. Morris MI: Posaconazole: a new oral antifungal agent with an expanded spectrum of activity. *Am J Health Syst Pharm* 66:225–236, 2009.
75. Hiramatsu Y, Maeda Y, Fujii N, et al: Use of micafungin versus fluconazole for antifungal prophylaxis in neutropenic patients receiving hematopoietic stem cell transplantation. *Int J Hematol* 88:588–595, 2008.
76. van Burik J-AH, Ratanatharathorn V, Stepan DE, et al: Micafungin versus fluconazole for prophylaxis against invasive fungal infections during neutropenia in patients undergoing hematopoietic stem cell transplantation. *Clin Infect Dis* 39:1407–1416, 2004.
77. Chandrasekar PH, Sobel JD: Micafungin: a new echinocandin. *Clin Infect Dis* 42:1171–1178, 2006.
78. Davey RT Jr, Masur H: Recent advances in the diagnosis, treatment, and prevention of *Pneumocystis carinii* pneumonia. *Antimicrob Agents Chemother* 34:499–504, 1990.
79. Masters PA, O'Bryan TA, Zurlo J, et al: Trimethoprim-sulfamethoxazole revisited [see comment]. *Arch Intern Med* 163:402–410, 2003.
80. Katlama C, De Wit S, O'Doherty E, et al: Pyrimethamine-clindamycin vs. pyrimethamine-sulfadiazine as acute and long-term therapy for toxoplasmic encephalitis in patients with AIDS. *Clin Infect Dis* 22:268–275, 1996.
81. Whitley RJ, Gnann JW Jr: Acyclovir: a decade later [erratum appears in *N Engl J Med* 1993;328(9):671]. *N Engl J Med* 327:782–789, 1992.
82. Valacyclovir. *Med Lett Drugs Ther* 38:3–4, 1996.
83. Balfour HH Jr: Management of cytomegalovirus disease with antiviral drugs. *Rev Infect Dis* 12[Suppl 7]:S849–860, 1990.
84. Pescovitz MD, Rabkin J, Merion RM, et al: Valganciclovir results in improved oral absorption of ganciclovir in liver transplant recipients. *Antimicrob Agents Chemother* 44:2811–2815, 2000.
85. Manion DJ, Vibhagool A, Chou TC, et al: Susceptibility of human cytomegalovirus to two-drug combinations in vitro. *Antiviral Therapy* 1:237–245, 1996.
86. Antiviral drugs for prophylaxis and treatment of influenza. *Med Lett Drugs Ther* 48:87–88, 2006.

CHAPTER 78 ■ PREVENTION AND CONTROL OF HEALTHCARE-ACQUIRED INFECTIONS IN THE INTENSIVE CARE UNIT

MIREYA WESSOLOSSKY AND RICHARD T. ELLISON, III

INTRODUCTION

Preventing healthcare-acquired infections in intensive care units (ICUs) is a daily concern of physicians providing care for critically ill patients. Patients in ICUs are at increased risk for infection for multiple reasons, including their underlying illness, the use of medical devices for organ system support and hemodynamic monitoring, impaired nutritional status that contributes immune function compromise, and ongoing exposure to hospital antibiotic-resistant bacterial flora. The focus of this chapter is to review the general epidemiology of these infections, the factors contributing to their development, preventative strategies, and important characteristics of key healthcare-acquired pathogens.

EPIDEMIOLOGY OF HEALTHCARE-ACQUIRED ICU INFECTIONS

Studies performed over the last two decades have found that infections in ICU patients are both common and significant. Work by Craven and colleagues in the early 1980s at Boston City Hospital in adult medical and surgical ICUs found that overall 28% of the patients developed at least one nosocomial infection, and once infected patients had threefold increases in mortality [1]. Similarly, in 1995, European investigators assessed the prevalence of nosocomial infections in a multinational survey of 1,417 ICUs in 17 nations on one single day (the EPIC Study), and found an overall prevalence of ICU-acquired infection of 21% [2]. A more recent study in a single US medical ICU performed over 20 months in 2000 to 2001 found that 42% of patients requiring at least 48 hours of ICU care had a microbiologically confirmed infection, and patients with infection had a 1.9-fold increased risk of in-hospital mortality ($p < 0.001$) [3].

The types of infection seen in ICU patients have varied slightly over time and between types of ICU units, but several types of infections have predominated. In the Boston City Hospital study, the incidence of infections was higher in surgical ICU than in medical ICU patients; and pneumonia, surgical wound infections, urinary tract infections (UTIs), and bloodstream infections (BSIs) were the most frequent infections [1]. In the European Prevalence of Infection in Intensive Care (EPIC) study, the principal infections identified were ventilator-associated pneumonia (47% of infections), tracheobronchitis (18%), UTI (18%), and bacteremias (12%) [2]. Klevens and others, using a multistep approach, estimated 394,288 hospital-associated infections among adults and children in ICU in 2002 from US hospitals. The infection rate per 1,000 patient-days was 13.0: among all, UTI was the highest (3.38) followed by pneumonia (3.33) and BSI (2.71) [4]. The use of medical devices is a predominant cause of infection with the majority of episodes of nosocomial pneumonia associated with mechanical ventilation, healthcare-acquired infection (HAI) UTIs associated with urinary catheterization, and primary BSIs linked to central venous catheters.

Additional data through the National Nosocomial Infection Surveillance (NNIS) system of the Centers for Disease Control and Prevention (CDC) has assessed nosocomial infections in differing types of ICUs, and found that trauma/surgical and neurosurgical ICUs tend to have more nosocomial pneumonia than medical or coronary care ICUs; and that pediatric, trauma, and burn ICUs have more BSIs than medical ICUs [5,6]. The differences in infection rates noted are likely related to the size of the unit (small vs. large), the type of more predominant device use (urinary catheters, endotracheal tubes, and vascular catheters), the age group of the patients (pediatric vs. adults), and the most predominant illness of the patients (coronary, surgical, burn, medical, and pediatric).

Pediatric intensive care units differ from adult ICUs in many ways. First, they are typically combined units (medical and surgical). Second, their beds are not commonly physically separated as adults ICU beds. Third, pediatric patients usually have less comorbidity than adults. Data from the CDC NNIS system during the years 1992 through 1997 found a mean overall patient infection rate of 6.1%, with the principal infections being venous catheter–associated BSIs, followed by pneumonia and UTIs [6].

MICROBIOLOGY OF ICU INFECTIONS

The predominant causes of ICU infections are a limited number of bacterial and fungal pathogens. In general, the pathogens that are seen can be characterized as those that survive well in a moist environment (e.g., Gram-negative bacteria including *Enterobacter* strains, *Pseudomonas aeruginosa*, and *Acinetobacter* species), those that colonize the skin and produce biofilm to allow adherence to catheters and other devices (e.g., *Staphylococcus aureus* and coagulase-negative staphylococci), and those which are resistant to commonly used antibiotics (e.g., methicillin-resistant *S. aureus* [MRSA], vancomycin-resistant enterococci [VRE], multidrug-resistant Gram-negative bacteria, and *Candida* species). In the EPIC study, the predominant pathogens were *Enterobacteriaceae* (34.4%), *S. aureus* (30.1%), and *P. aeruginosa* (28.7%) [2]. It was notable that 60% of the *S. aureus* isolates were MRSA, and that coagulase-negative staphylococci (19.1%) and fungi (17.1%) were common [2]. During the last 12 years, there has been an increasing trend toward highly antibiotic-resistant pathogens in the ICU setting. Data from the NNIS system on US ICUs comparing data from 1998 through 2003 has shown a progressive rise in the prevalence of MRSA to 60%, as well as dramatic increases in the prevalence of *Klebsiella* strains resistant to third-generation cephalosporins and *P. aeruginosa* resistant to cephalosporins and imipenem (Fig. 78.1) [5].

In the NNIS pediatric ICU study noted previously, for primary BSIs, coagulase-negative staphylococci were the most common pathogens (38%) followed by Gram-negative bacilli (25%) [6]. For nosocomial pneumonia, *P. aeruginosa* (22%) was the most frequent pathogen followed by *S. aureus* (17%), and for UTI, Gram-negative aerobic bacilli were the most frequent pathogens (57%) followed by fungi, most frequently *Candida albicans* (14%).

In addition to these predominant pathogens, there are several situations where other pathogens are a concern in the ICU. A number of institutions have noted the emergence of extended-spectrum β-lactamases (ESBL) producing *Klebsiella* and *Escherichia coli* strains [7,8]. In addition, in a few institutions that have used carbapenems extensively (often to try to treat ESBL-positive Gram-negative bacilli), the carbapenem-resistant Gram-negative pathogens *Stenotrophomonas maltophilia*, *Klebsiella pneumoniae*, *Acinetobacter baumannii*, and *Burkholderia cepacia* have emerged [9–13]. Finally, the fungal pathogens *Candida parapsilosis* and *Malassezia furfur* have been seen in patients receiving total parenteral nutrition, the latter being seen only with lipid supplementation [14,15].

RISK FACTORS

The length of ICU stay is the predominant risk factor for nosocomial infection followed by the use of medical devices [2,3,6]. In the NNIS surveillance studies and subsequent studies by the CDC's current National Healthcare Safety Network (NHSN), nosocomial infection rates for nosocomial pneumonia, BSIs, and UTIs have correlated strongly with device use [4,16]. Other risk factors include the patient's underlying illness, selected medications, and the type of healthcare facility. In the EPIC study, seven risk factors were determined for ICU-acquired infection: increased length of stay (>48 hours), mechanical ventilation, diagnosis of trauma, central venous, pulmonary artery, urinary catheterization, and stress ulcer prophylaxis [2]. Teaching hospitals with higher rates of device utilization have had higher device-associated infection rates [4,16]. As in adult ICUs, the most important risk factors for nosocomial infection in pediatric ICUs appears to be the length of ICU stay and rate of device utilization [2,6].

A potential risk factor undergoing intense study at this time is hyperglycemia. Hyperglycemia is common in the ICU setting due to underlying disease, physiologic stress, and parenteral nutritional support. In vitro investigations suggest that hyperglycemia can impair polymorphonuclear leukocyte and monocyte phagocytic and bactericidal activities [17]. A large randomized trial performed in a single surgical ICU found that tight control of blood glucose during the ICU stay (maintaining blood glucose 80 to 110 mg per dL) reduced overall mortality, the incidence of bacteremias, and the number of patients who required more than 10 days of antibiotic therapy [18].

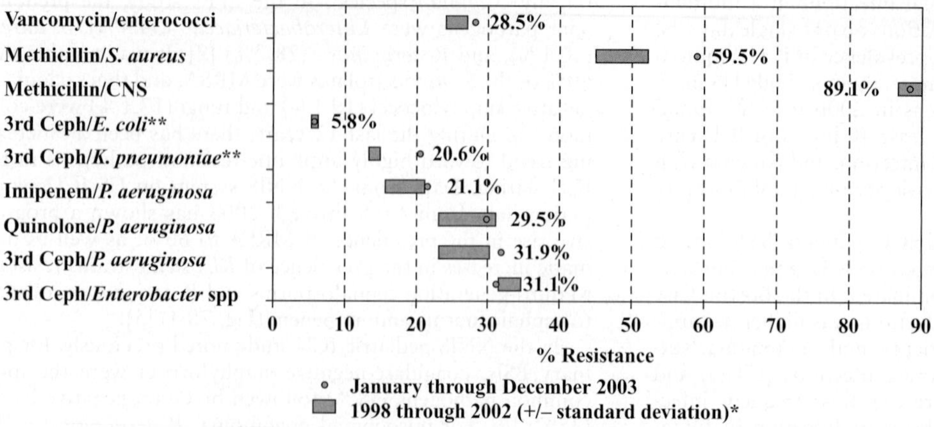

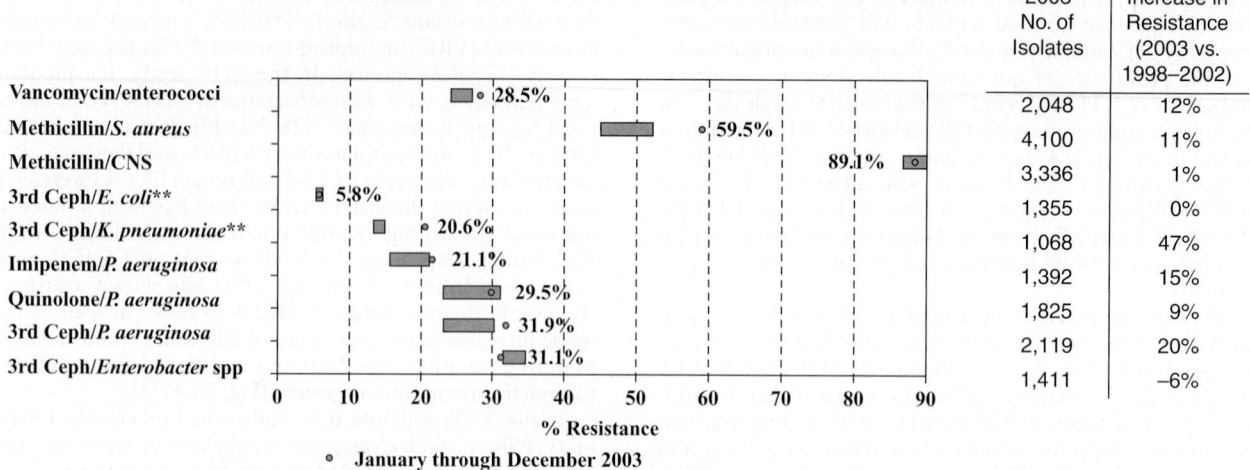

2003 No. of Isolates	Increase in Resistance (2003 vs. 1998–2002)
2,048	12%
4,100	11%
3,336	1%
1,355	0%
1,068	47%
1,392	15%
1,825	9%
2,119	20%
1,411	–6%

FIGURE 78.1. Selected antimicrobial-resistant pathogens associated with nosocomial infections in ICU patients, comparison of resistance rates from January through December 2003 with 1998 through 2002, NNIS System. CNS, coagulase-negative staphylococci; 3rd Ceph, resistance to 3rd-generation cephalosporins (ceftriaxone, cefotaxime, or ceftazidime); Quinolone, resistance to either ciprofloxacin or ofloxacin. *Percent (%) increase in resistance rate of current year (January–December 2003) compared with mean rate of resistance over previous 5 years (1998–2002): [(2003 rate – previous 5-year mean rate)/previous 5-year mean rate] × 100. **"Resistance" for *Escherichia coli* or *Klebsiella pneumoniae* is the rate of nonsusceptibility of these organisms to either 3rd group or aztreonam. [From the American Journal of Infection Control 2004; 32: 470–485. A report from the NNIS System. This report is public domain and can be copied freely.]

However, a subsequent study of the impact of tight glycemic control on outcomes in a medical ICU did not find the same benefit, and further investigation of both the risk of infection with hyperglycemia and optimal treatment is needed [19].

PREVENTIVE AND CONTROL MEASURES

A number of approaches have been found to help prevent ICU-associated infections. The comprehensive use of standard infection control practices as well as enhanced infection control precautions for selected pathogens, limiting the use of medical devices, and careful attention to architectural design are key components of strategies to prevent ICU infections. In addition, the implementation of targeted quality improvement programs for central vascular catheter infections and ventilator-associated pneumonia have been shown to be highly effective approaches to decreasing infection rates.

Infection Control Precautions

The CDC and the Hospital Infection Control Practices Advisory Committee have prepared guidelines on isolation precautions to prevent the transmission of microorganisms from colonized or infected patients to other patients, visitors, and healthcare workers [20]. The current guidelines were last updated in 2007 and recommend a two-tiered approach to patient care. Standard precautions are used for the care for all patients. Additional, more stringent transmission-based precautions are used for the care of patients who are suspected or known to be colonized or infected with specific pathogens that are readily transmitted through direct contact, through large respiratory droplets, or through smaller airborne particles. The current guidelines are summarized in Table 78.1.

A key component of these guidelines is the need for healthcare workers to practice good hand hygiene [20,21]. Approaches that have been shown to improve compliance with this practice have included the provision of water free alcohol-based hand rubs throughout institutions as well as intensified educational and monitoring programs on hand hygiene. Alcohols have excellent in vitro germicidal activity against Gram-positive and Gram-negative pathogens, fungi, and many viruses including human immunodeficiency virus, influenza virus, and respiratory syncytial virus.

There have been several additional approaches recently developed to further control of healthcare-acquired infection that should be considered in the ICU setting, particularly in the setting of high infection rates. The performance of daily bathing of patients with chlorhexidine gluconated using either impregnated clothes or dilute bathing solutions has been associated with reductions in rates of MRSA and VRE acquisition and central line–associated BSIs, potentially by decreasing the bioburden of microbial pathogens on the body surface [22–24]. Although not associated with alterations in infection rates, the institution of programs to monitor the actual performance of housekeeping staff has been found to improve the disinfection of the hospital environment in ICUs, including disinfection of computer stations [25]. Finally, equipment has been developed that allows for the use of total room disinfection with a hydrogen peroxide mist which can eradicate vegetative bacteria, fungi, spores, viruses, and prions. While its use as part of routine care remains unclear, it may be of value in controlling outbreaks due to *Clostridium difficile* or multidrug-resistant Gram-negative bacteria [26,27].

Architectural Design and Hospital Construction

Modern ICU design includes the use of single-patient rooms, adequate physical space for equipment and personnel, individual patient sinks, adequate hand hygiene stations, and adequate room ventilation with filtered air and at least six air changes per hour [28]. In addition, there are defined guidelines

TABLE 78.1

ISOLATION PRECAUTIONS

		Transmission based		
	Standard	**Airborne**	**Droplet**	**Contact**
Definition	Reduce risk of transmission of blood-borne pathogens and pathogens from moist body substances, and applies to all patients	Prevent transmission of disease by airborne droplet nuclei ($\leq$5 μm size)	Reduce risk of transmission of microorganism by droplets ($\geq$5 μm size) generated by the patient sneezing, coughing, talking, or performance of procedure	Reduce transmission of epidemiologic important organism from an infected or colonized patient through direct or indirect contact
Room		Private-negative pressure room with air exhausted to outdoors or through high-efficient filtration; door kept closed	Private room; door may remain open	Private room or cohorted with a patient with similar organism. Patient care items should be dedicated to a single patient
Mask	Mask, goggles, and face shields provide barrier protection to reduce the transmission of pathogens when splashes or spray of blood, body fluids, secretions, or excretions are likely	N95 mask or comparable respirator. Surgical mask should be worn by the patient during transportation outside the negative pressure room	Mask if entering the room	
Gown	Provide barrier protection, prevents contamination of clothing, and protects the skin of personnel from blood and body fluid exposures			
Gloves	Anticipated blood, body fluid, secretions/excretions, nonintact skin, contaminated items, and mucous membranes			
Hand hygiene	Before and after patient contact; immediately after glove removal; after contact with blood, body fluids, secretions/excretions, or mucous membranes			
Suspected or confirmed pathogens	Used for all patients independent of the presence of known pathogens	Tuberculosis Varicella (including disseminated zoster) SARS Measles Disseminated zoster Viral hemorrhagic fevers Smallpox Monkeypox Varicella Avian influenza	Meningitis due to *Neisseria meningitides* or *Haemophilus influenzae* Diphtheria (pharyngeal) Pertussis Mumps *Mycoplasma pneumoniae* Pneumonic plague Streptococcal (Group A) pharyngitis, pneumonia Influenza Rubella Parvovirus B19	MDR bacterial (MRSA, VRE, GISA, VRSA, Gram-negative bacilli) *Clostridium difficile* Viral hemorrhagic fevers Scabies Lice HSV (neonatal; disseminated) Disseminated zoster

GISA, glycopeptide-intermediate *Staphylococcus aureus*; MDR, multidrug resistant; MRSA, methicillin-resistant; *Staphylococcus aureus* SARS, severe acute respiratory syndrome; VRE, vancomycin-resistant enterococci; VRSA, vancomycin-resistant *Staphylococcus aureus*.

for the design of airborne isolation infection rooms for patients requiring management of tuberculosis or other infections readily transmitted by the airborne route.

Ongoing construction and renovation activities in healthcare facilities have also been recognized as significant risk factors for infections with environmental pathogens. There can be concerns with environmental Gram-negative organisms, particularly *Legionella* species. More frequently is a concern with disease due to environmental molds, in particular *Aspergillus* species [28,29]. United States healthcare institutions are now required to have procedures in place to ascertain that construction and renovation activities are performed in a manner that protects patients from being exposed to environmental pathogens [28].

Infection Control Surveillance Programs

In 1970, the CDC initiated the NNIS system as an approach to identifying secular trends in these infections. The program initially included 10 to 20 hospitals and expanded to nearly 300 hospitals. A subsequent study that analyzed healthcare-acquired infection rates at differing institutions before and after the distribution of infection rate data found that institutional infection rates diminished after institutions were made aware of their infection rates [30]. In addition, an analysis of ICU-associated, device-related infection rates during the 1990s for all the participating hospitals in the NNIS system showed a decreasing incidence of these infections, as institutions were able to compare their infection rates with national standards [31]. These results have been mirrored in data on central line–associated BSIs reported through the NHSN system [16]. Disseminating data in a simple and routine manner, to those who need to know, enables clinicians to make decisions on the basis of scientific data and to alter practice (Table 78.2).

Quality Improvement Initiatives

A major advance in medical care in the last decade has been the adoption of quality improvement strategies used in other industries such as air transportation. The development of standardize approaches to the provision of care has been particularly effective in the prevention of device-related infections in the ICU stetting. Several institutions have documented a significant reduction in BSIs linked to central venous catheters after the implementation of quality improvement programs targeted against these infections [32,33]. Principal components of these programs have included, providing education on appropriate infection control practices to staff involved in central catheter placement and care, standardizing the location of catheter placement to preferentially use the subclavian location and avoid femoral lines when possible, centralizing the location of all equipment required for catheter placement, the use of maximal sterile-barrier precautions (i.e., use of cap, surgical masks, sterile gown, sterile gloves, and large sterile drape) during catheter insertion, and trying to remove these catheters as quickly as possible [33–38].

A similar approach has been taken to the prevention of ventilator-associated pneumonia in the ICU with the use of targeted education programs [39–41]. These quality improvement education programs have in general followed CDC guidelines on measures to prevent healthcare-acquired pneumonia and have been directed at medical staff, ICU nursing staff, and respiratory therapists [42]. Key elements of the program include a focus on hand hygiene, maintaining the patient in a semirecumbent position with the head of the bed elevated to 30 degrees, standardizing the approach to changing ventilator circuitry, avoiding nasal intubations, avoiding gastric distension, removing nasogastric tubes, and weaning patients as rapidly as possible [39].

SELECTED HEALTHCARE-ACQUIRED PATHOGENS

Clostridium difficile–Associated Colitis

C. difficile is the most frequent etiology for healthcare-acquired diarrhea [43]. The organism may asymptomatically colonize the gut or cause illness extending from watery diarrhea through pseudomembranous colitis, toxic megacolon, perforation, and even death [43,44]. Transmission in the healthcare setting appears to occur through transient hand carriage of healthcare workers, close contact to other colonized or infected patients, or exposure to spores present on contaminated environmental surfaces [44,45]. Exposure to antibiotics increases the risk for developing disease. Practically all antibiotics have been implicated in the development of Clostridium difficile Associated-Diarrhea (CDAD), but disease is especially common with clindamycin, penicillins, and cephalosporins. Current strains of *C. difficile* are more resistant to the fluoroquinolones than previous historical strains [46], and the widespread use of fluoroquinolones for the treatment of a variety of infections (e.g., UTI, community-acquired pneumonia) may in part be contributing to an increasing incidence of CDAD. In addition, there is also evidence that current *C. difficile* strains are both less responsive to treatment with metronidazole and associated with increased virulence [43,46,47].

Approaches to the prevention of CDAD are directed toward preventing horizontal transmission of the pathogen, as well as reducing the individual patient's risks of disease if they acquire the organism through the judicious use of antibiotic therapy. Barrier methods such as private rooms or cohorting patients remain fundamental to prevent the spread of CDAD. Alcohol hand hygiene preparations are not active against bacterial spores including those of *C. difficile*, and in a study where the introduction of alcohol hand hygiene reduced the incidence of other nosocomial pathogens, the incidence of *C. difficile* was unchanged [48]. The use of soap and water for enhanced mechanical clearance during hand hygiene should be considered in the setting of increased transmission of *C. difficile* [20,21].

In addition, healthcare workers should wear gloves when caring for patients with CDAD, and the use of gowns is also recommended when soiling of the patient's cloth is likely [21,49].

Methicillin-Resistant *Staphylococcus aureus*

The prevalence of MRSA in ICUs in the United States has risen markedly in the last 10 years, from an incidence of 30% to 40% in the middle of the 1990s to more than 60% in 2004 [5,46]. This increasing prevalence of MRSA in hospitals has also augmented the use of vancomycin therapy, leading to problems with both VRE and the rare (to date) emergence of vancomycin-intermediate *S. aureus* (VISA) and vancomycin-resistant *S. aureus* (VRSA) [5,50–54]. Risk factors associated with acquisition of healthcare-acquired strains of MRSA include recent hospitalization, recent surgery, and residence in a long-term facility or injection drug use [55]. In addition, in the last 7 years, community-associated MRSA (CA-MRSA) strains have appeared in patients lacking these previous risk factors [55]. The CA-MRSA strains are distinct from traditional MRSA in several ways. First, they carry a unique gene cassette leading to methicillin resistance, type IV *mecA*. Second, they are significantly more likely to carry a gene for the Panton–Valentine leukocidin (PVL) toxin which has been associated with the development of necrotizing pneumonia and necrotic abscesses [31,55]. During the last 7 years, the prevalence of CA-MRSA has increased dramatically throughout the United States [56,57].

Current CDC guidelines recommend the use of "contact precautions" for patients known or suspected to be colonized with either healthcare-acquired MRSA or the CA-MRSA strains [20]. In the settings of outbreaks of MRSA, institutions may also consider instituting patient/staff cohorting, attempting to decolonize patients with topical nasal mupirocin and total body chlorhexidine baths/showers, and rarely screening healthcare workers for MRSA colonization [58,59]. Enhanced infection control policies with stringent contact precautions have been recommended for patients with VRSA [60].

Vancomycin-Resistant Enterococci

VRE was first recognized in Europe in 1988 and in the United States soon thereafter. By 1993, there had 20-fold increase in VRE prevalence in ICUs in the United States [61], and by 2003, VRE represented approximately 28% of enterococcal isolates in ICUs participating in the NNIS system [5]. Although not as virulent a pathogen as MRSA, VRE can cause infections in the debilitated ICU patient. Also, as the gene inducing vancomycin resistance in VRE, *vanA*, can be transferred to *S. aureus*, the presence of VRE in ICU patients increases the potential for the emergence of VRSA strains.

Infection control policies for contact precautions have been recommended for patients colonized or infected with VRE, and as with MRSA, the use of screening policies for patients at high risk for VRE can be considered. If treatment of VRE infection is necessary, the best therapeutic options at this time appear to be linezolid, daptomycin, and quinupristin/dalfopristin [62–64].

Multidrug-Resistant Gram-Negative Bacilli

The CDC NNIS database reported that in 2003, 20% of *P. aeruginosa* isolates recovered from ICU patients were resistant to carbapenems and approximately 30% were resistant to third-generation cephalosporins and fluoroquinolones [5]. *K. pneumoniae* isolates from ICU that were nonsusceptible to third-generation cephalosporin had increased to almost 50%, with many of these strains expressing ESBLs [5]. The emergence of *K. pneumoniae* species producing a carbapenemase enzyme (KPC) has appeared globally, and is a major threat due to limited options for treatment, and the KPC enzyme has now been seen in other related *Enterobacteriaceae* species [65–67]. The emergence of these strains appears related to independent risk factors including (i) severe illness, (ii) prior fluoroquinolones use, and (iii) prior extended-spectrum cephalosporin use [67]. Detection of KPC-producing strains based on routine antimicrobial susceptibility assays may be unreliable; therefore, methods are still being formalized the identification of these organisms to promptly treat and implement efficient infection control measures to contain the spread of these bacteria. Tigecycline and colistin appears among the remaining therapeutic options with the caveat of unknown clinical efficacious and toxicities.

A. baumannii has also emerged as a major ICU pathogen [65]. Overall, it is the fifth most common Gram-negative pathogen seen in NHSN ICUs [13]. Among them, 29% were resistant to carbapenems and only susceptible to colistin, an old and toxic agent. Unfortunately, this organism survives well in the environment and has been associated with significant ICU outbreaks. Infections due to this organism are associated with poor outcome, including higher rate of morbidity, mortality, and medical expenses. Control measures involve both the use of "contact precautions" and enhanced environmental cleaning efforts [20,68].

Given this rapidly increasing incidence of resistant Gram-negative strains, it is important for institutions to track rates of antibiotic resistance in their ICUs independent of overall institutional antibiotic resistance rates. Empiric antibiotic coverage for Gram-negative pathogens in given ICUs should be targeted at the known Gram-negative pathogens present in the environment. Enhanced infection control contact precautions should be used for patients who are colonized or infected with ESBL- or KPC-positive Gram-negative pathogens or multidrug-resistant *P. aeruginosa* or *A. baumannii*. Infection control measures effective in the ICU setting that are supported by well-designed clinical trials are summarized in Table 78.2

TABLE 78.2

EVIDENCE-BASED MEDICINE SUPPORTING INFECTION CONTROL MEASURES TO DECREASE HEALTHCARE-ACQUIRED INFECTIONS IN THE ICU

1. Use of a central venous catheter bundle intervention produced a large and sustained reduction in central venous catheter-related bloodstream infections in the ICU setting [32].
2. Daily patient bathing with chlorhexidine containing solution reduced the incidence of MRSA and VRE acquisition and the incidence of VRE bacteremia in the ICU setting [24].

ICU, intensive care unit; VRE, vancomycin-resistant enterococci.

References

1. Craven DE, Kunches LM, Lichtenberg DA, et al: Nosocomial infection and fatality in medical and surgical intensive care unit patients. *Arch Intern Med* 148(5):1161–1168, 1988.
2. Vincent JL, Bihari DJ, Suter PM, et al: The prevalence of nosocomial infection in intensive care units in Europe. Results of the European Prevalence of Infection in Intensive Care (EPIC) Study. EPIC International Advisory Committee. *JAMA* 274(8):639–644, 1995.
3. Osmon S, Warren D, Seiler SM, et al: The influence of infection on hospital mortality for patients requiring >48 h of intensive care. *Chest* 124(3):1021–1029, 2003.
4. Klevens RM, Edwards JR, Richards CL Jr, et al: Estimating health care-associated infections and deaths in U. S. hospitals, 2002. *Public Health Rep* 122(2):160–166, 2007.
5. National Nosocomial Infections Surveillance System: National Nosocomial Infections Surveillance (NNIS) System Report, data summary from January 1992 through June 2004, issued October 2004. *Am J Infect Control* 32(8):470–485, 2004.
6. Richards MJ, Edwards JR, Culver DH, et al: Nosocomial infections in medical intensive care units in the United States. National Nosocomial Infections Surveillance System. *Crit Care Med* 27(5):887–892, 1999.
7. Quale JM, Landman D, Bradford PA, et al: Molecular epidemiology of a city-wide outbreak of extended-spectrum beta-lactamase-producing *Klebsiella pneumoniae* infection. *Clin Infect Dis* 35(7):834–841, 2002.
8. D'Agata EM: Rapidly rising prevalence of nosocomial multidrug-resistant, Gram-negative bacilli: a 9-year surveillance study. *Infect Control Hosp Epidemiol* 25(10):842–846, 2004.
9. Gales AC, Jones RN, Forward KR, et al: Emerging importance of multidrug-resistant *Acinetobacter* species and *Stenotrophomonas maltophilia* as pathogens in seriously ill patients: geographic patterns, epidemiological features, and trends in the SENTRY Antimicrobial Surveillance Program (1997–1999). *Clin Infect Dis* 32[Suppl 2]:S104–S113, 2001.
10. Kuti JL, Moss KM, Nicolau DP, et al: Empiric treatment of multidrug-resistant *Burkholderia cepacia* lung exacerbation in a patient with cystic fibrosis: application of pharmacodynamic concepts to meropenem therapy. *Pharmacotherapy* 24(11):1641–1645, 2004.
11. Modakkas EM, Sanyal SC: Imipenem resistance in aerobic gram-negative bacteria. *J Chemother* 10(2):97–101, 1998.
12. Woodford N, Tierno PM Jr, Young K, et al: Outbreak of *Klebsiella pneumoniae* producing a new carbapenem-hydrolyzing class A beta-lactamase, KPC-3, in a New York Medical Center. *Antimicrob Agents Chemother* 48(12):4793–4799, 2004.
13. Hidron AI, Edwards JR, Patel J, et al: NHSN annual update: antimicrobial-resistant pathogens associated with healthcare-associated infections: annual summary of data reported to the National Healthcare Safety Network at the Centers for Disease Control and Prevention, 2006–2007. *Infect Control Hosp Epidemiol* 29(11):996–1011, 2008.
14. Clark TA, Slavinski SA, Morgan J, et al: Epidemiologic and molecular characterization of an outbreak of *Candida parapsilosis* bloodstream infections in a community hospital. *J Clin Microbiol* 42(10):4468–4472, 2004.
15. Sizun J, Karangwa A, Giroux JD, et al: *Malassezia furfur*-related colonization and infection of central venous catheters. A prospective study in a pediatric intensive care unit. *Intensive Care Med* 20(7):496–499, 1994.
16. Edwards JR, Peterson KD, Mu Y, et al: National Healthcare Safety Network (NHSN) report: data summary for 2006 through 2008, issued December 2009. *Am J Infect Control* 37(10):783–805, 2009.
17. Van den Berghe G: How does blood glucose control with insulin save lives in intensive care? *J Clin Invest* 114(9):1187–1195, 2004.
18. van den Berghe G, Wouters P, Weekers F, et al: Intensive insulin therapy in the critically ill patients. *N Engl J Med* 345(19):1359–1367, 2001.
19. Van den Berghe G, Wilmer A, Hermans G, et al: Intensive insulin therapy in the medical ICU. *N Engl J Med* 354(5):449–461, 2006.
20. Siegel JD, Rhinehart E, Jackson M, et al: 2007 Guideline for isolation precautions: preventing transmission of infectious agents in health care settings. *Am J Infect Control* 35[10, Suppl 2]:S65–S164, 2007.
21. Boyce JM, Pittet D: Guideline for hand hygiene in health-care settings: recommendations of the Healthcare Infection Control Practices Advisory Committee and the HICPAC/SHEA/APIC/IDSA Hand Hygiene Task Force. *Infect Control Hosp Epidemiol* 23[12, Suppl]:S3–S40, 2002.
22. Bleasdale SC, Trick WE, Gonzalez IM, et al: Effectiveness of chlorhexidine bathing to reduce catheter-associated bloodstream infections in

medical intensive care unit patients. *Arch Intern Med* 167(19):2073–2079, 2007.
23. Vernon MO, Hayden MK, Trick WE, et al: Chlorhexidine gluconate to cleanse patients in a medical intensive care unit: the effectiveness of source control to reduce the bioburden of vancomycin-resistant enterococci. *Arch Intern Med* 166(3):306–312, 2006.
24. Climo MW, Sepkowitz KA, Zuccotti G, et al: The effect of daily bathing with chlorhexidine on the acquisition of methicillin-resistant *Staphylococcus aureus*, vancomycin-resistant Enterococcus, and healthcare-associated bloodstream infections: results of a quasi-experimental multicenter trial. *Crit Care Med* 37(6):1858–1865, 2009.
25. Carling PC, Parry MF, Bruno-Murtha LA, et al: Improving environmental hygiene in 27 intensive care units to decrease multidrug-resistant bacterial transmission. *Crit Care Med* 38(4):1054–1059, 2010.
26. Shapey S, Machin K, Levi K, et al: Activity of a dry mist hydrogen peroxide system against environmental *Clostridium difficile* contamination in elderly care wards. *J Hosp Infect* 70(2):136–141, 2008.
27. Otter JA, Puchowicz M, Ryan D, et al: Feasibility of routinely using hydrogen peroxide vapor to decontaminate rooms in a busy United States hospital. *Infect Control Hosp Epidemiol* 30(6):574–577, 2009.
28. Sehulster L, Chinn RY: Guidelines for environmental infection control in health-care facilities. Recommendations of CDC and the Healthcare Infection Control Practices Advisory Committee (HICPAC). *MMWR Recomm Rep* 52(RR-10):1–42, 2003.
29. Panackal AA, Dahlman A, Keil KT, et al: Outbreak of invasive aspergillosis among renal transplant recipients. *Transplantation* 75(7):1050–1053, 2003.
30. Gaynes RP: Surveillance of nosocomial infections: a fundamental ingredient for quality. *Infect Control Hosp Epidemiol* 18(7):475–478, 1997.
31. Centers for Disease Control and Prevention (CDC): Monitoring hospital-acquired infections to promote patient safety—United States, 1990–1999. *MMWR Morb Mortal Wkly Rep* 49(8):149–153, 2000.
32. Pronovost P, Needham D, Berenholtz S, et al: An intervention to decrease catheter-related bloodstream infections in the ICU. *N Engl J Med* 355(26): 2725–2732, 2006.
33. Berenholtz SM, Pronovost PJ, Lipsett PA, et al: Eliminating catheter-related bloodstream infections in the intensive care unit. *Crit Care Med* 32(10): 2014–2020, 2004.
34. Raad II, Hohn DC, Gilbreath BJ, et al: Prevention of central venous catheter-related infections by using maximal sterile barrier precautions during insertion. *Infect Control Hosp Epidemiol* 15(4, Pt 1):231–238, 1994.
35. Warren DK, Yokoe DS, Climo MW, et al: Preventing catheter-associated bloodstream infections: a survey of policies for insertion and care of central venous catheters from hospitals in the prevention epicenter program. *Infect Control Hosp Epidemiol* 27(1):8–13, 2006.
36. Merrer J, De Jonghe B, Golliot F, et al: Complications of femoral and subclavian venous catheterization in critically ill patients: a randomized controlled trial. *JAMA* 286(6):700–707, 2001.
37. Sherertz RJ, Ely EW, Westbrook DM, et al: Education of physicians-in-training can decrease the risk for vascular catheter infection. *Ann Intern Med* 132(8):641–648, 2000.
38. Warren DK, Zack JE, Mayfield JL, et al: The effect of an education program on the incidence of central venous catheter-associated bloodstream infection in a medical ICU. *Chest* 126(5):1612–1618, 2004.
39. Babcock HM, Zack JE, Garrison T, et al: An educational intervention to reduce ventilator-associated pneumonia in an integrated health system: a comparison of effects. *Chest* 125(6):2224–2231, 2004.
40. Baxter AD, Allan J, Bedard J, et al: Adherence to simple and effective measures reduces the incidence of ventilator-associated pneumonia. *Can J Anaesth* 52(5):535–541, 2005.
41. Salahuddin N, Zafar A, Sukhyani L, et al: Reducing ventilator-associated pneumonia rates through a staff education programme. *J Hosp Infect* 57(3): 223–227, 2004.
42. From the Centers for Disease Control and Prevention: Four pediatric deaths from community-acquired methicillin-resistant *Staphylococcus aureus*—Minnesota and North Dakota, 1997–1999. *JAMA* 282(12):1123–1125, 1999.
43. Dallal RM, Harbrecht BG, Boujoukas AJ, et al: Fulminant *Clostridium difficile*: an underappreciated and increasing cause of death and complications. *Ann Surg* 235(3):363–372, 2002.
44. Gerding DN, Johnson S, Peterson LR, et al: *Clostridium difficile*-associated diarrhea and colitis. *Infect Control Hosp Epidemiol* 16(8):459–477, 1995.
45. Brooks SE, Veal RO, Kramer M, et al: Reduction in the incidence of *Clostridium difficile*-associated diarrhea in an acute care hospital and a skilled nursing facility following replacement of electronic thermometers with single-use disposables. *Infect Control Hosp Epidemiol* 13(2):98–103, 1992.
46. Boyce JM, Havill NL, Otter JA, et al: Impact of hydrogen peroxide vapor room decontamination on *Clostridium difficile* environmental contamination and transmission in a healthcare setting. *Infect Control Hosp Epidemiol* 29(8):723–729, 2008.
47. Warny M, Pepin J, Fang A, et al: Toxin production by an emerging strain of *Clostridium difficile* associated with outbreaks of severe disease in North America and Europe. *Lancet* 366(9491):1079–1084, 2005.
48. Gordin FM, Schultz ME, Huber RA, et al: Reduction in nosocomial transmission of drug-resistant bacteria after introduction of an alcohol-based handrub. *Infect Control Hosp Epidemiol* 26(7):650–653, 2005.
49. Johnson S, Gerding DN, Olson MM, et al: Prospective, controlled study of vinyl glove use to interrupt *Clostridium difficile* nosocomial transmission. *Am J Med* 88(2):137–140, 1990.
50. Chang S, Sievert DM, Hageman JC, et al: Infection with vancomycin-resistant *Staphylococcus aureus* containing the vanA resistance gene. *N Engl J Med* 348(14):1342–1347, 2003.
51. Sakoulas G, Moellering RC Jr, Eliopoulos GM: Adaptation of methicillin-resistant *Staphylococcus aureus* in the face of vancomycin therapy. *Clin Infect Dis* 42[Suppl 1]:S40–S50, 2006.
52. Tenover FC, Pearson ML: Methicillin-resistant *Staphylococcus aureus*. *Emerg Infect Dis* 10(11):2052–2053, 2004.
53. Whitener CJ, Park SY, Browne FA, et al: Vancomycin-resistant *Staphylococcus aureus* in the absence of vancomycin exposure. *Clin Infect Dis* 38(8):1049–1055, 2004.
54. Centers for Disease Control and Prevention (CDC): Vancomycin-resistant *Staphylococcus aureus*—New York, 2004. *MMWR Morb Mortal Wkly Rep* 53(15):322–323, 2004.
55. Herold BC, Immergluck LC, Maranan MC, et al: Community-acquired methicillin-resistant *Staphylococcus aureus* in children with no identified predisposing risk. *JAMA* 279(8):593–598, 1998.
56. Fridkin SK, Hageman JC, Morrison M, et al: Methicillin-resistant *Staphylococcus aureus* disease in three communities. *N Engl J Med* 352(14):1436–1444, 2005.
57. Seybold U, Kourbatova EV, Johnson JG, et al: Emergence of community-associated methicillin-resistant *Staphylococcus aureus* USA300 genotype as a major cause of health care-associated blood stream infections. *Clin Infect Dis* 42(5):647–656, 2006.
58. Boyce JM: MRSA patients: proven methods to treat colonization and infection. *J Hosp Infect* 48[Suppl A]:S9–S14, 2001.
59. Sandri AM, Dalarosa MG, Ruschel de Alcantara L, et al: Reduction in incidence of nosocomial methicillin-resistant *Staphylococcus aureus* (MRSA) infection in an intensive care unit: role of treatment with mupirocin ointment and chlorhexidine baths for nasal carriers of MRSA. *Infect Control Hosp Epidemiol* 27(2):185–187, 2006.
60. Edmond MB, Wenzel RP, Pasculle AW: Vancomycin-resistant *Staphylococcus aureus*: perspectives on measures needed for control. *Ann Intern Med* 124(3):329–334, 1996.
61. Centers for Disease Control and Prevention (CDC): Nosocomial enterococci resistant to vancomycin—United States, 1989–1993. *MMWR Morb Mortal Wkly Rep* 42(30):597–599, 1993.
62. Perry CM, Jarvis B: Linezolid: a review of its use in the management of serious gram-positive infections. *Drugs* 61(4):525–551, 2001.
63. Hsueh PR, Chen WH, Teng LJ, et al: Nosocomial infections due to methicillin-resistant *Staphylococcus aureus* and vancomycin-resistant enterococci at a university hospital in Taiwan from 1991 to 2003: resistance trends, antibiotic usage and in vitro activities of newer antimicrobial agents. *Int J Antimicrob Agents* 26(1):43–49, 2005.
64. Raad I, Hachem R, Hanna H, et al: Treatment of vancomycin-resistant enterococcal infections in the immunocompromised host: quinupristin-dalfopristin in combination with minocycline. *Antimicrob Agents Chemother* 45(11):3202–3204, 2001.
65. Souli M, Galani I, Giamarellou H: Emergence of extensively drug-resistant and pandrug-resistant Gram-negative bacilli in Europe. *Euro Surveill* 13(47), 2008.
66. Souli M, Galani I, Antoniadou A, et al: An outbreak of infection due to beta-lactamase *Klebsiella pneumoniae* Carbapenemase 2-producing *K. pneumoniae* in a Greek University Hospital: molecular characterization, epidemiology, and outcomes. *Clin Infect Dis* 50(3):364–373, 2010.
67. Nordmann P, Cuzon G, Naas T: The real threat of *Klebsiella pneumoniae* carbapenemase-producing bacteria. *Lancet Infect Dis* 9(4):228–236, 2009.
68. Karageorgopoulos DE, Falagas ME: Current control and treatment of multidrug-resistant *Acinetobacter baumannii* infections. *Lancet Infect Dis* 8(12):751–762, 2008.

CHAPTER 79 ■ CENTRAL NERVOUS SYSTEM INFECTIONS

HEIDI L. SMITH AND ALAN L. ROTHMAN

The central nervous system (CNS) infections of major interest in the intensive care unit (ICU) are bacterial meningitis, encephalitis, brain abscess, and other parameningeal foci of infection. The clinical presentations of these diseases may overlap. *Meningitis* means inflammation of the leptomeninges; its hallmark is stiff neck. *Encephalitis* is a syndrome consisting of disturbance of cerebral function and cerebrospinal fluid (CSF) pleocytosis. Many cases of bacterial meningitis also fit this definition of encephalitis due to the occurrence of mental status changes, seizures, or coma. Focal infections, such as brain abscesses, may present more as space-occupying lesions than with classical infectious signs or symptoms.

CSF examination is the major tool used in diagnosis of CNS infections. The terms *purulent* and *aseptic* describe contrasting CSF formulas, though overlap exists. The typical purulent CSF has a white blood cell count of more than 1,000 cells per mm^3 (most of which are neutrophils), a depressed glucose concentration (<40 mg per dL), and an elevated protein level (>100 mg per dL); it is most commonly seen in bacterial meningitis. In contrast, an "aseptic" formula has a lower total leukocyte count with a predominance of mononuclear cells, a glucose concentration greater than 40% to 50% of the blood level, and less marked elevation of protein; this picture characterizes most other CNS infections. An intermediate CSF formula, in which a moderate lymphocytic pleocytosis is accompanied by depressed glucose and elevated protein, suggests granulomatous disease.

GENERAL CLINICAL APPROACH

Initial evaluation of the patient with suspected CNS infection should focus on defining the nature of the symptoms (meningitic vs. encephalitic) and the presence and pattern of neurologic involvement (focal vs. diffuse).

If bacterial meningitis is suspected, expeditious analysis of CSF is critical. This must be balanced with the need to administer antibiotics promptly, because delays as short as 3 hours have been shown to lead to unfavorable outcomes [1,2]. If lumbar puncture (LP) is delayed for any reason, antibiotics (and dexamethasone; see later) should be started as soon as blood cultures have been obtained while efforts to obtain CSF proceed [3].

LP is not without risk. In patients with bleeding disorders, it should be delayed until the defect(s) can be corrected [4]. LP may be hazardous in the settings of intracranial mass lesion with edema and lumbar spinal epidural abscess. Concern for cerebral herniation as a consequence of the procedure has led to the common practice of routinely performing computed tomography (CT) scanning prior to LP. This practice is not well founded, however [5,6]. A prospective study has confirmed that CT scans rarely discover abnormalities that would represent a contraindication to LP except in patients who have a prior history of CNS disease, an immunosuppressive disorder, seizures, moderate-to-severe impairment of consciousness, papilledema, or focal neurological findings [7].

BACTERIAL MENINGITIS

Bacterial meningitis is perhaps the most clear-cut emergency in the field of infectious diseases. Delayed or inadequate treatment increases the risk of death or significant neurologic impairment [1].

Etiology

The predominant organisms vary based on the age and underlying condition of the host. Historically, bacterial meningitis in the United States has been primarily caused by five organisms: *Streptococcus pneumoniae*, *Neisseria meningitidis*, *Listeria monocytogenes*, *Haemophilus influenzae*, and group B streptococcus. However, immunization of young children against *H. influenzae* and *S. pneumoniae* has had a marked impact on meningitis in the United States, raising the average age of meningitis due to these five pathogens from 15 months old to 25 years old [8].

S. pneumoniae accounts for almost half of the cases of community-acquired bacterial meningitis in the United States in all age groups beyond the neonatal period [8]. It is associated with a sixfold higher risk of unfavorable outcome (death, neurologic sequelae) than other pathogens [9]. Pneumococcal meningitis is more common in the setting of a CSF leak, hypogammaglobulinemia, asplenia, alcoholism, head trauma, or cochlear implant [10,11]. Routine infant immunization against *S. pneumoniae* has also reduced the incidence of pneumococcal meningitis in older children and adults due to a reduction in *S. pneumoniae* carriage in the younger population [12,13].

N. meningitidis accounts for approximately one fourth of cases of meningitis in the United States [8]. Nasal carriage of *N. meningitidis* gradually increases from infancy and peaks in the teenage years [14]; it is the most common cause of meningitis in older children and young adults. It is the one form of bacterial meningitis associated with epidemic spread. A polysaccharide-protein conjugate vaccine is available in the United States but does not provide protection against serogroup B strains. The vaccine is currently recommended for preadolescents, freshman entering college, and military recruits [15].

L. monocytogenes is a common cause of meningitis in the neonatal period or in the setting of malignancy, immunosuppression, or alcoholism. Approximately 30% of patients have no apparent immunocompromising condition; most of these individuals are older than 50 years [8,16,17].

H. influenzae type B was formerly the most common cause of bacterial meningitis in young children. Vaccination of children has reduced the incidence of invasive *H. influenzae* type B disease by more than 80% [8,18]. Sporadic cases have recently been reported in unimmunized and partially immunized children, however [19]. *H. influenzae* in adults is uncommon and is usually associated with predisposing factors, such as anatomic defects (head trauma, CSF leaks) or defects in humoral immunity [20].

Gram-negative bacillary meningitis occurs in the neonatal period or after neurosurgery or trauma [21]. Community-acquired Gram-negative bacillary meningitis is rare in adults [21]. When it occurs, it is usually a complication of bacteremia from a distant site, often the urinary tract.

Staphylococcus aureus meningitis is associated with neurosurgery or trauma. Community-acquired cases occur in the presence of a focus of infection outside the CNS, such as endocarditis or soft tissue infections, and have a worse prognosis [22]. Meningitis in patients with CSF shunts is most commonly caused by skin flora (*S. aureus*, *Staphylococcus epidermidis*, *Propionibacterium acnes*) and Gram-negative bacilli [23]. These infections can have an indolent presentation and milder CSF abnormalities [3,23]. Use of shunt catheters impregnated with antibiotics has shown some promise in reducing the incidence of infection [24].

Several additional species of streptococci can cause meningitis. Group B streptococcus, *Streptococcus agalactiae*, is the most common cause of neonatal meningitis [8]. Rates of group B streptococcal invasive disease in adults are increasing, particularly in diabetic patients, but only a small proportion present as meningitis [25]. *Streptococcus suis* is an increasingly common cause of meningitis in Asia and should be considered in travelers, particularly those who may have ingested raw pork or had contact with pigs [26,27]. LP associated with the use of catheters for anesthesia and imaging procedures has been associated with the introduction of α-hemolytic streptococci in rare cases [28]. Anaerobic bacteria and other streptococci are otherwise uncommon causes of meningitis that are usually related to spread from brain abscess or parameningeal foci [29].

Pathogenesis

Bacterial seeding of the meninges usually arises from hematogenous spread. Spread from contiguous foci of infection is more often a cause of intracranial abscess. Bacteremia can arise from simple colonization of the nasopharynx, though colonization alone is obviously not sufficient, since 10% of the population is colonized with *N. meningitidis* at any given time [30]. The bacterial species most commonly associated with meningitis bind the laminin receptor on microvascular endothelial cells, potentially facilitating entry to the CNS [31]. Most meningitis pathogens also secrete immunoglobulin A proteases, facilitating immune evasion at mucosal sites [14]. Inadequate levels of antibody specific for the invading organism (such as occurs at the extremes of age or in acquired immunodeficiencies) and opsonophagocytic deficiencies (such as in asplenia, diabetes, or alcoholism) are the most commonly recognized risk factors for meningitis [32]. Individuals with terminal complement component deficiencies may experience recurrent episodes of meningococcal meningitis, though with lower mortality rates [33].

Once bacteria reach the CSF, both bacterial and host factors contribute to disease. Recognition of bacterial components, including cell wall molecules and bacterial DNA, leads to elaboration of inflammatory mediators such as tumor necrosis factor-α (TNF-α), interleukin-1, and interleukin-6 by leukocytes and endothelial cells. One of the major consequences is the disruption of the tight junctions of the blood–brain barrier. Additional inflammation, caused in part by increased migration and activation of neutrophils, triggers release of tissue factor (which aids thrombus formation and disrupts cerebral perfusion), nitric oxide (which disrupts autoregulation of blood flow and can have direct toxic effects on neurons), and matrix metalloproteinases (which can also disrupt endothelial junctions and impair neuronal function). Neuronal damage is further worsened by resulting increases in intracranial pressure [34,35].

Antibiotics that rapidly lyse bacteria generate a transient increase in inflammation as a response to the release of bacterial cell wall components [36]. Adjunctive steroid therapy acts to decrease inflammation associated with bacterial lysis [37]. The body also deploys endogenous immunomodulators such as TNF-related apoptosis-inducing ligand (TRAIL), which has been shown to reduce neuronal damage in animal models [38].

The clinical consequence of these pathologic processes is a generalized disturbance of cerebral function. An early phase of agitation or mania may be noted. Lethargy progresses to obtundation and sometimes coma. Seizures occur early in 20% to 30% of adults with meningitis [21]. Hyponatremia, caused by the syndrome of inappropriate antidiuretic hormone (SIADH) secretion, may contribute to obtundation and seizures. Focal neurologic deficits may be observed; sensorineural deafness is particularly common. Neurologic impairment persists in approximately 30% of survivors of meningitis in adulthood [6].

Diagnosis

History

Patients with meningitis may be unable to give a coherent history. Patients found unresponsive should be evaluated with a high level of suspicion for meningitis. Patients with fever and derangement of cerebral function, even if there is another cause for the latter, must have meningitis excluded. Persons with coexistent alcoholism, general debility, head trauma, or neurosurgery are at higher risk for meningitis.

Classic meningeal symptoms are headache (often with photophobia), neck pain, fever, and mental status changes; in a recent case series, 95% of patients with bacterial meningitis had at least two of these four symptoms [9]. Symptoms of other foci of infection, such as pneumonia, otitis, or sinusitis, may also be present [39]. Any history of head trauma (including remote events) or recent clear nasal or ear discharges should be obtained. Recent antibiotics, which could interfere with culture results, should be noted. A history of exposure to a patient with known meningococcal disease is usually forthcoming if present. In children, immunization history and history of school or daycare exposures should be elicited. Travel history may aid the identification of regionally endemic pathogens.

Physical Examination

Nuchal rigidity suggests meningitis when present. Limitation of motion caused by degenerative cervical arthritis may be a confounding variable in the elderly. Kernig's and Brudzinski's signs have low sensitivity but high specificity [40]. The initial neurologic examination should evaluate the mental status and the presence of focal deficits. Papilledema is rarely observed in meningitis [21,41] but alters the approach to LP when present. Serial examinations document any functional progression or improvement.

The systemic examination may give clues to the cause of meningitis. A thorough ear, nose, and throat examination can reveal possible foci leading to contiguous extension to the meninges. Petechiae or purpuric lesions strongly suggest meningococcal disease, though they may also be seen in *S. pneumoniae* and *H. influenzae* meningitis [39]. Petechiae may also be seen in aseptic meningitis caused by enteroviruses or Rocky Mountain spotted fever. Needle aspiration or punch biopsy of skin lesions should be used to obtain material for Gram stain and culture. In one series of patients with *N. meningitidis* infection, bacteria were detected on either culture or stain in more than 60% of skin specimens. In addition, the Gram stain was positive in samples obtained as late as 45 hours after initiation of antibiotics [42].

Laboratory Tests

Evaluation of the CSF is essential for the diagnosis of meningitis. The typical features of purulent CSF have been noted earlier. Neutrophils constitute more than 50% of the cells in nearly all bacterial meningitis cases and more than 80% in the majority [21]. In rare cases, the CSF shows many organisms on Gram stain but few cells, implying rapidly progressive disease [9]. Elevated protein is also almost always present [21]. Severe depression of the CSF glucose (<20 mg per dL) is strong evidence for a pyogenic process, but CSF glucose is normal in up to 50% of patients with bacterial meningitis [21]. Patients with *L. monocytogenes* meningitis may have milder CSF abnormalities with relatively modest changes in glucose and protein and white blood cell counts of less than 2,000 cells per mm^3 [16,17]. Treatment with antibiotics prior to LP may alter CSF chemistries, resulting in higher glucose levels and lower protein levels, though cell counts are usually unaffected [43].

Cultures remain the mainstays of diagnosis. Blood cultures can be useful in identifying the causative agent of meningitis in cases where CSF cultures are unrevealing [44,45]. Ultimately, 60% to 90% of patients with community-acquired meningitis and purulent CSF have an organism isolated in culture [21,39]. Antibiotic administration is more likely to render cultures negative [43,46]. Bacterial antigen detection tests offer little additional information [47]. Newer techniques such as polymerase chain reaction (PCR) detection of bacterial DNA may provide more rapid and sensitive diagnosis, particularly in the setting of antibiotic pretreatment; however, these assays are not yet widely available [48].

Imaging studies are of secondary importance in the diagnosis of meningitis. Imaging of the chest and paranasal sinuses may identify other foci of infection. CT and magnetic resonance imaging (MRI) of the brain are most useful for evaluating complications of meningitis. Rapid deterioration should lead to consideration of subdural empyema, a collection between the dura and the arachnoid membrane, best visualized on MRI [6,49]. A new focal neurologic abnormality, decreased level of consciousness, or cerebrovascular accident with a nonarterial distribution should prompt imaging for venous thrombophlebitis, also best seen on MRI [6,49].

Differential Diagnosis

Several pathogens other than pyogenic bacteria can cause clinical presentations and/or spinal fluid formulas that overlap with bacterial meningitis.

Viral meningitis can have initial clinical presentations similar to bacterial meningitis. It can be caused by a wide range of pathogens including enteroviruses, arboviruses such as West Nile virus (WNV) [50], herpes viruses such as herpes simplex virus (HSV) [51], and acute HIV infection [52]. Mumps and lymphocytic choriomeningitis are the viruses most often associated with low CSF glucose levels. Very high CSF white blood cell counts and a high proportion of neutrophils occur in a few cases of enteroviral meningitis and eastern equine encephalitis. PCR assays for detection of enteroviruses can provide timely clarification [53]. Recurrent culture-negative meningitis, sometimes referred to as Mollaret's meningitis, can have an early neutrophil predominance; most cases have a positive HSV PCR in the CSF [51]. Other types of viral meningitis may also display an early neutrophil predominance, with a shift to lymphocytes taking place with time [3].

Tuberculous meningitis most commonly presents with a mononuclear predominance in the CSF along with low glucose and high protein. However, some cases have a total leukocyte count in the range of purulent meningitis with a polymorphonuclear predominance [54]. A history of tuberculosis, risk factors for exposure, or the presence of an immunocompromising condition should raise suspicion. If an initial diagnosis of bacterial meningitis is not confirmed by culture and the patient's condition does not improve, repeat LP with studies for acid-fast bacilli should be performed. A switch to lymphocytic predominance, additional decrease in CSF glucose and increase in protein, positive chest radiograph, or well-founded clinical suspicion mandates institution of antituberculous therapy [54,55]. The reported yield of acid-fast stains of CSF ranges from 15% to 60% but improves with repeat sampling [56,57]. Nucleic acid amplification tests may facilitate earlier diagnosis, but there is a wide variability in their availability and sensitivity [58]. MRI is more likely than CT to visualize tuberculomas [59].

Parasitic infections can cause purulent meningitis. Primary amebic meningitis with *Naegleria fowleri* is acquired through freshwater swimming and presents similarly to acute bacterial meningitis. Diagnosis is made on wet mount of CSF [60]. The nematode *Strongyloides stercoralis* is capable of establishing a cycle of autoinfection in immunosuppressed hosts, including those on oral corticosteroids. Migration of larvae from the gut can result in the deposition of enteric bacteria in the CNS, causing Gram-negative or polymicrobial meningitis [61].

Fungal meningitis may present with hypoglycorrhachia. An indolent course and lymphocytic CSF pleocytosis usually distinguish these from pyogenic infections, but *Coccidioides immitis*, an endemic fungus of the southwest United States, can have neutrophil predominance [62]. *Cryptococcus neoformans* is a major cause of meningitis in patients with immunosuppressive conditions, though it can occur in normal hosts. Cryptococcal antigen assay of the CSF provides a sensitive means of diagnosis [63].

Parameningeal foci of infection, including epidural abscess, can present a purulent picture, usually with elevated protein and a normal glucose concentration [64]. Brain abscess that has ruptured into the ventricles may duplicate the clinical picture of bacterial meningitis. Localizing neurologic findings or isolation of an anaerobe or multiple organisms from the CSF should suggest one of these diagnoses.

Noninfectious conditions can cause meningeal signs and CSF findings that overlap with those of bacterial meningitis. Hypoglycorrhachia may be seen in carcinomatous meningitis. Drug-induced meningitis may have a CSF formula indistinguishable from pyogenic infection; the most commonly implicated agents are nonsteroidal anti-inflammatories, antibiotics, and intravenous immunoglobulin [65]. Postneurosurgical chemical meningitis, believed to be an inflammatory reaction to surgical manipulation, blood, or bone dust, can present with a CSF profile similar to bacterial meningitis. Although symptoms, CSF leukocytosis, and hypoglycorrhachia are usually less severe, no single parameter has been proven to distinguish between the two conditions. Given the risk of postsurgical bacterial meningitis in this population, antibiotics are often administered until CSF culture results are finalized [66–68].

Therapy

The appropriate management of patients with bacterial meningitis involves prompt initiation of antimicrobial and anti-inflammatory therapy, aggressive control of the potential complications, and prevention of spread of disease [3]. Overall mortality from bacterial meningitis is in the range of 20% to 30% [9,21,69]. However, mortality rates are significantly influenced by both the pathogen, with *S. pneumoniae* among the most deadly, and the host, with elderly patients among the most susceptible [9,21]. Consequently, most patients should be treated in an intensive care setting.

Antimicrobial Therapy

The principal consideration in choosing an antibiotic regimen for bacterial meningitis is that the agent(s) reach the CSF in concentrations that are bactericidal for the likely pathogens. Table 79.1 lists recommendations for therapy of bacterial meningitis in a variety of clinical settings. Initial therapy is usually selected empirically based on the age and underlying condition of the patient. Once the result of Gram stain of CSF is available, antimicrobial therapy can be targeted appropriately.

The third-generation cephalosporins (ceftriaxone or cefotaxime) are the mainstays of therapy for community-acquired meningitis. These agents are active against most strains of *S. pneumoniae* and provide excellent coverage against *N. meningitidis* and Gram-negative bacilli (except *Pseudomonas aeruginosa*). *S. pneumoniae* with reduced susceptibility to the cephalosporins has increased in frequency; this organism remains universally susceptible to vancomycin [70]. If the CSF Gram stain suggests pneumococci or is unrevealing, vancomycin should be given in addition to the cephalosporin until culture and sensitivity results are available [3]. Meropenem also demonstrates activity against many, but not all, cephalosporin-resistant strains of *S. pneumoniae* and has demonstrated clinical effectiveness for treatment of meningitis [70,71].

Ampicillin (or penicillin) should be included in the regimen for empiric therapy in neonates (<1 month old), individuals older than 50 years, patients with alcoholism, or those who are debilitated or immunosuppressed, for coverage of *L. monocytogenes* [16,72]. Initial therapy for postneurosurgical bacterial meningitis should include vancomycin plus either ceftazidime or cefepime to provide adequate coverage for methicillin-resistant staphylococci and *P. aeruginosa*. Resistance to antimicrobials, either at the outset or developing during treatment, can complicate therapy for Gram-negative organisms [73]. An increasing number of cases due to multidrug-resistant hospital-acquired organisms such as *Acinetobacter* sp have been reported [74].

Few good treatment regimens exist for the cephalosporin-intolerant patient. Consequently, a trial of the third-generation cephalosporins (or meropenem) should be strongly considered unless there is a documented, serious intolerance. Vancomycin is the preferred alternative for treatment of pneumococcal meningitis. The fluoroquinolone moxifloxacin has activity against pneumococci, meningococci, and *H. influenzae* and has shown promise in animal models of meningitis, but clinical experience is limited [3]. Trimethoprim–sulfamethoxazole is effective for the treatment of meningitis caused by *L. monocytogenes* and many Gram-negative bacilli other than *P. aeruginosa* [75].

If *S. pneumoniae* is isolated, adjustment of therapy should be based on the results of drug susceptibility testing. Fully susceptible organisms can be treated with third-generation cephalosporin alone. For resistant organisms, vancomycin and cephalosporin should be continued and the addition of rifampin considered [76]. Repeated examination of the CSF after 24 to 36 hours of therapy is warranted to monitor sterilization of the CSF in these cases [77]. Regardless of the causative organism, continued clinical instability after 48 hours of appropriate antibiotic therapy is also an indication for repeat LP [3]. Repeat CSF samples should have a negative Gram stain and culture after at least 24 hours of effective antibiotic therapy [6].

The recommended duration of antimicrobial therapy for meningitis depends on the etiology and the clinical response. For infection with *H. influenzae* or meningococci, 7 to 10 days of therapy is adequate. *S. pneumoniae* is usually treated for 10 to 14 days, but longer durations may be needed for drug-resistant organisms. Gram-negative bacillary meningitis is typically treated for 3 weeks and staphylococcal disease, when accompanied by bacteremia, for 4 to 6 weeks [3].

TABLE 79.1

ANTIMICROBIAL AGENTS RECOMMENDED FOR THERAPY OF BACTERIAL MENINGITIS

Clinical situation	Recommended therapy[a]
Initial cerebrospinal fluid (CSF) Gram stain negative or delayed	
Age <3 mo	Ampicillin plus ceftriaxone[b]
Age 3 mo to 50 y	Ceftriaxone[b] plus vancomycin[c]
Age >50 y	Ampicillin plus ceftriaxone[b] plus vancomycin[c]
After neurosurgery or penetrating cranial trauma	Vancomycin[c] plus ceftazidime[d]
Immunosuppression, alcoholism, debilitation	Ampicillin plus ceftriaxone[b] plus vancomycin[c]
Initial CSF Gram stain positive (community-acquired bacterial meningitis)	
Gram-positive cocci	Vancomycin[c] plus ceftriaxone[b]
Gram-negative cocci	Ceftriaxone[b]
Gram-positive bacilli	Ampicillin ± gentamicin[e]
Gram-negative bacilli	Ceftazidime[d] ± aminoglycoside[f]
Organism known, susceptibility not yet known	
Streptococcus pneumoniae	Vancomycin[c] plus ceftriaxone[b]
Streptococcus, group A or B	Penicillin G ± gentamicin[e]
Enterococcus	Penicillin G ± gentamicin[e]
Staphylococcus aureus	Vancomycin[c] (and/or nafcillin[g])
Listeria monocytogenes	Ampicillin ± gentamicin[e]
Neisseria meningitidis	Penicillin G
Haemophilus influenzae	Ceftriaxone[b]
Pseudomonas aeruginosa	Ceftazidime[d] plus tobramycin[f]
Other Gram-negative bacilli (e.g., *Escherichia coli, Klebsiella, Proteus*)	Ceftriaxone[b] plus gentamicin[f]

[a]Usual daily doses (schedules) for adults are as follows: ampicillin, 12 g/d (q4h); ceftriaxone, 4 g/d (q12h); ceftazidime, 6 g/d (q8h); nafcillin, 12 g/d (q4h); penicillin G, 24 million U/d (q2–4h).
[b]Cefotaxime, 8 to 12 g/d, given q4–6h, is equally effective.
[c]Usual daily dose of vancomycin for adults is 2–3g/d, given q8–12h, with body weight guiding dose and creatinine clearance guiding frequency of dosing. Troughs should be monitored with a goal of 15–20 mg/dL.
[d]Cefepime, 6 g/d given q8h, may be used as an alternative.
[e]Although CSF penetration of aminoglycosides is poor, some specialists recommend their use in these settings.
[f]Consideration should be given to initial intrathecal administration in addition to intravenous administration.
[g]In most areas, where methicillin resistance is common among isolates of *S. aureus*, vancomycin should be used and addition of nafcillin can be considered. In areas where methicillin resistance among *S. aureus* is still rare, nafcillin is the preferred agent.

TABLE 79.2

CHEMOPROPHYLAXIS FOR *NEISSERIA MENINGITIDIS* AND *HAEMOPHILUS INFLUENZAE*

Pathogen	Antibiotic	Dose and duration
N. meningitidis	Ceftriaxone[a]	125 mg for children or 250 mg for adults as a single intramuscular injection
	Ciprofloxacin[b]	500 mg as a single dose in adults
	Rifampin	10 mg per kg (maximum dose, 600 mg) by mouth twice a day for 2 d
H. influenzae	Rifampin	20 mg per kg (maximum dose, 600 mg) by mouth once a day for 4 d

[a]Preferred agent in pregnant women.
[b]In geographic areas where ciprofloxacin-resistant *N. meningitidis* has been reported, azithromycin 10 mg per kg for children or 500 mg for adults as a single dose can be used as an alternative.

Anti-inflammatory Therapy

The role of endogenous mediators of inflammation in the pathogenesis of meningitis has provided a rationale for the use of anti-inflammatory agents. Dexamethasone, 0.15 mg per kg every 6 hours for 4 days, has been shown to be of benefit in both childhood and adult meningitis [69,78]. Dexamethasone accelerated the normalization of CSF glucose, improved cerebral perfusion pressure, and reduced the incidence of hearing loss and other neurologic abnormalities in children, particularly those with *H. influenzae* meningitis [78], though there is renewed debate about the routine use of steroids in children given the decline in incidence of *H. influenzae* [79]. In adults, dexamethasone has been shown to reduce both mortality and neurologic sequelae [37,69]. The greatest benefits have been obtained when dexamethasone therapy was initiated before or simultaneously with the first antimicrobial dose [69]; the time period beyond the first antibiotic dose where steroids are effective is probably short but has not been well defined [37]. The recommended duration of steroid therapy is 4 days, but some studies in children suggest that 2 days may be adequate [37,80].

Adjunctive steroid therapy is not indicated in immunosuppressed individuals or postneurosurgical meningitis, as few of these patients were included in the clinical trials of dexamethasone and they are often infected with organisms not sufficiently evaluated in steroid trials [81]. In experimental animals infected with penicillin-resistant pneumococci, dexamethasone therapy reduced the penetration of vancomycin into the CSF, resulting in delayed sterilization of CSF [82]. However, given the demonstrated benefit of steroids and the lack of evidence for a similar effect in humans, steroids are still recommended in pneumococcal meningitis [3].

The benefits of steroid therapy seen in studies performed in industrialized countries have not been observed in the developing world [83,84]; therefore, adjunctive dexamethasone is not routinely recommended in these settings. Oral glycerol therapy is being explored as an alternative therapy to decrease cerebral pressure without immunosuppression, but is still in investigational stages [85,86].

Supportive Therapy

Treatment of meningitis also requires management of seizures and increased intracranial pressure. Seizures should be controlled by anticonvulsants as necessary (see Chapter 172), and aspiration and hypoxia must be prevented. Severe cerebral edema with evidence of uncal or cerebellar herniation can be managed with mannitol and steroids; several small case series have suggested that wider application of strategies for aggressive management of intracranial pressure is appropriate [87]. Fluid management should be directed at maintenance of euvolemia [88].

Bacterial meningitis in the setting of CSF shunts presents additional considerations. The highest rates of cure (88%) are obtained with initiation of antibiotics, removal of the entire shunt, temporary external drainage, and replacement of the shunt if follow-up cultures are negative upon repeat sampling of CSF. One stage removal with immediate replacement of the device followed by antibiotics is associated with a 64% rate of cure. Antibiotics alone, usually only considered for less virulent organisms such as *P. acnes* and non-aureus staphylococci, are successful 34% of the time [3,89].

Infection Control

Patients with *N. meningitidis* or *H. influenzae* type B meningitis should be managed with droplet precautions until 24 hours after initiation of antibiotics. Chemoprophylaxis is recommended in the situations described below. Dosing and duration are detailed in Table 79.2.

For *N. meningitidis*, household and day care contacts as well as hospital personnel who have performed unprotected cardiopulmonary resuscitation, intubation, or suctioning should receive chemoprophylaxis. Rifampin, ciprofloxacin, or ceftriaxone are the recommended agents. A small number of ciprofloxacin-resistant *N. meningitidis* isolates have been recently reported in North Dakota and Minnesota [90]. Primary rifampin resistance is similarly rare but may develop secondarily in individuals who receive rifampin for prophylaxis [91]. Quadrivalent (serogroups A, C, Y, and W-135) meningococcal vaccine can be used as an adjunct to chemoprophylaxis to prevent late secondary cases in contacts or to control outbreaks of disease [15,92].

For *H. influenzae* type B disease, chemoprophylaxis is recommended for household contacts only if there is at least one child younger than 4 years who is not fully vaccinated or if there is an immunocompromised child in the household [93]. In addition, if two or more cases have occurred in the same day care group within 60 days, chemoprophylaxis is recommended. Rifampin is the recommended agent.

ENCEPHALITIS

Encephalitis is a more rare infection than meningitis and a far less uniform one. Although a specific diagnosis provides important prognostic and epidemiologic information, there are only a handful of treatable causes of encephalitis.

Efforts should focus on identifying and addressing these causes. Infections of the brain that do not present as acute encephalitis but rather as subacute to chronic processes are not discussed further in this chapter.

Etiology

The causes of encephalitis endemic to the United States are predominantly viruses, although many other pathogens, including

TABLE 79.3

PROGNOSTIC CATEGORIZATION OF ENCEPHALITIDES INDIGENOUS TO THE UNITED STATES

Agent	Comments
Group 1: Causes of encephalitis that tend to resolve spontaneously and rarely leave neurologic residua	
Epstein-Barr virus	
Human herpes virus type 6	
Enteroviruses	
Mumps	
Lymphocytic choriomeningitis virus	
California encephalitis	Arbovirus
St. Louis encephalitis	Arbovirus
Colorado tick fever	Arbovirus
Herpes zoster	
Bartonellosis (cat scratch disease)	Especially acute cerebellar ataxia
Mycoplasma pneumonia	Especially acute cerebellar ataxia
Rocky Mountain spotted fever	Contingent on recovery from the systemic illness
Leptospirosis	Contingent on recovery from the systemic illness
Group 2: Causes of encephalitis that carry a small but definite risk of death and a sizable risk of sequelae	
Measles	
Powassan virus	Arbovirus
Western equine encephalitis	Arbovirus
West Nile virus	Arbovirus
Venezuelan equine encephalitis	Arbovirus
Smallpox vaccine	Vaccine is no longer in routine use
Group 3: Causes of encephalitis with a large risk of death; most survivors have significant residua	
Herpes simplex	
Cytomegalovirus	Immunosuppressed hosts
Eastern equine encephalitis	Arbovirus
Rabies	Six reported survivors

rickettsiae, *Mycoplasma pneumoniae*, *Bartonella* sp, *Treponema pallidum*, *Borrelia burgdorferi*, amoebae, *L. monocytogenes*, and *Toxoplasma gondii*, have all been associated with the syndrome [94,95]. *T. gondii* and cytomegalovirus (CMV) cause encephalitis only in patients with immunodeficiencies (see Chapters 84 and 85). In contrast, most of the acute viral encephalitides exhibit no particular predilection for the immunosuppressed host. In recent years, pressure to diagnose herpes simplex because of the potential for therapy has led to its documentation more frequently than any other form [95,96]. However, most cases of encephalitis elude diagnosis. Table 79.3 lists the causes of encephalitis that are indigenous to the United States in general prognostic categories. Despite the favorable prognosis, encephalitis caused by organisms listed in group 1 may be extremely severe, with prolonged unresponsiveness followed by gradual clearing.

Pathogenesis

Although HSV is the most common organism identified in encephalitis cases, the pathogenesis of herpes simplex encephalitis (HSE) is not entirely clear. The characteristic feature of HSE is its focal nature. It is an acute hemorrhagic necrotizing process with a predilection for the temporal lobe [97]. The virus is known to persist in the trigeminal ganglia and is thought to travel up to the trigeminal or olfactory nerves at the time of reactivation [97]. Recent studies of children with HSE have revealed defects in innate immunity [98,99].

Arboviruses are transmitted by the bite of their insect vector [100]. Blood transfusions and organ transplantation have also been a mechanism for transmission of WNV [101,102]. The mosquito-borne infections have seasonal prevalence in late summer and early fall. Prevalence in a given year can depend on weather trends affecting vectors. With the exception of the California group viruses, birds are a reservoir. Surveillance of bird populations is used to track the localities at risk for human disease [103,104]. The various arboviruses differ in their likelihood of producing overt disease, nonspecific febrile illness, or encephalitis, but they all affect young children and the elderly more severely. Eastern equine encephalitis is the most virulent, causing death or severe neurologic sequelae in more than 60% of cases [105,106]. The insect vector inoculates the arboviruses, producing viremia as an early event. The organisms replicate in reticuloendothelial tissues, where a secondary viremia arises and infects the CNS. By the time encephalitic symptoms develop, the virus has usually been cleared from the circulation and specific antibody is present, facilitating diagnosis [100].

Rabies virus reaches the brain by spreading up neural pathways from its site of inoculation, a process that may take weeks to years. Saliva contains the virus, which is usually introduced by a bite or salivary contamination of an open wound [107]. In the past 30 years, the majority of cases in North America have been caused by bat rabies [108]. Human-to-human transmission has occurred through organ transplantation from donors with undiagnosed rabies [109]. Although it has never been documented, human-to-human transmission through saliva is theoretically possible; therefore, patients should be placed in strict isolation. Prophylaxis for rabies exposure consists of a combination of passive immunization with rabies immunoglobulin plus active immunization with rabies vaccine [110].

There are numerous noninfectious processes that can produce a clinical picture overlapping with infection-related encephalitis. Anti-N-methyl-D-aspartate (anti-NMDA) receptor antibodies cause a severe form of encephalitis, sometimes associated with undiagnosed ovarian teratomas in young women [111]. Other autoantibodies, such as anti-Yo and anti-Hu, are associated with paraneoplastic syndromes, but their role in pathogenesis is less clear [112]. CNS vasculitis or sarcoidosis may manifest as acute or subacute encephalitis. Although the underlying etiologies are diverse, they share the common feature of vessel wall inflammation leading to ischemia and infarction [113].

Diagnosis

The diagnostic process is directed principally at identifying treatable causes of encephalitis, especially HSE or nonviral pathogens [96,97,114].

History

The epidemiologic features reviewed earlier (see Pathogenesis) are major contributors to diagnosis. In some cases of rabies, no apparent source can be determined. A history of foreign travel may widen the differential diagnosis beyond the considerations reviewed here. Establishing the host's immune status, and potential for occult HIV infection, will also help guide the diagnostic workup [115].

Fever is nearly universal in encephalitis. Headache is also common. A neurologic presentation may occur, with seizures, mania, personality change, or another neuropsychiatric disorder as the principal signs [115]. Focal neurologic findings, including aphasia, suggest a diagnosis of HSE [114]. Aversion to water, refusal to swallow, and delirious behavior are classic features of "furious" rabies but are absent in about 20% of cases which present with flaccid paralysis, known as "dumb" rabies [107]. Flaccid paralysis mimicking poliomyelitis has also been observed in WNV encephalitis and with certain enteroviruses [50,116].

Physical Examination

The critical component of the physical examination is to determine whether an anatomic focus of abnormality is present, increasing the likelihood of HSE. Typical skin findings may suggest alternative diagnoses, such as Rocky Mountain spotted fever, measles, or herpes zoster.

Laboratory Tests

Analysis of CSF is the most important diagnostic procedure. The CSF in encephalitis usually fits the aseptic picture described earlier. It may be normal at the outset in 10% to 20% of patients subsequently proven to have HSE [114]. The presence of red blood cells suggests a hemorrhagic type of encephalitis, such as HSE, but is not diagnostic [97]. Eosinophils suggest infection with helminths, treponemes, rickettsiae, coccidiomycosis, toxoplasmosis, or *M. pneumoniae* [96].

Given its prevalence and the availability of specific therapy, PCR for HSV should be performed on CSF in all cases [96]. PCR can be positive even after several days of antiviral therapy. False-negative results can occur early in the disease, particularly in children [117]. A repeat HSV PCR in 3 to 7 days is recommended if the clinical scenario remains consistent with HSV and no alternative diagnosis has emerged [96,115].

Advancements have been made in molecular diagnostics for other forms of encephalitis. Reliable CSF PCR assays are available for VZV, CMV, and enteroviruses. PCR of serum can aid the diagnosis of ehrlichiosis, whereas PCR of lymph node tissue can detect *B. henselae* [96].

Diagnosis of most other causes of encephalitis relies on serologic testing. In arboviral infection, antibody is usually present at the onset of neurologic signs and is sufficiently rare in the general population to permit presumptive diagnosis [96]. The presence of antibody to *T. pallidum*, *B. burgdorferi*, rickettsia, or ehrlichia may reflect prior infection but is sufficient evidence to warrant treatment. Detection of pathogen-specific antibody in the CSF can provide more convincing evidence of the etiology of encephalitis, with a serum to CSF antibody ratio of less than 20 suggesting intrathecal production of antibody. Testing CSF for antibody to *T. pallidum* or *B. burgdorferi* is warranted when encephalitis secondary to syphilis or Lyme disease is suspected [96,115,118]. For most other causes of encephalitis listed in Table 79.3, the demonstration of a significant increase in antibody titer is required for diagnosis. The preferred approach is the comparison of a stored sample from the acute phase of infection to a sample obtained 2 to 4 weeks later [96].

Premortem noninvasive diagnosis of rabies is difficult. The reference standard is detection of viral nucleocapsid by fluorescent antibody staining of brain tissue, but this is often only obtained postmortem. Premortem diagnostic techniques exploit the fact that rabies virus nucleocapsids are concentrated in the nerve endings surrounding the base of hair follicles; nuchal skin biopsy followed by fluorescent staining or RT-PCR for virus has the highest sensitivity [119].

Although they share no distinct profile, patients with encephalitis due to noninfectious causes generally have lower CSF white blood cell counts and protein levels [120]. Recurrent encephalitis, patients with cerebellar dysfunction, and presentations with psychotic features are somewhat more likely to be secondary to noninfectious etiologies [120]. These characteristics would prompt additional imaging of the cerebral vasculature, assay of CSF for known paraneoplastic antibodies, or serum studies for markers of autoimmune disease.

CT and MRI are recommended for the evaluation of all patients with suspected encephalitis [96]. The findings in viral encephalitis are most often nonspecific, but the identification of mass lesions or infarcts will redirect the diagnostic workup toward brain abscess, vasculitis, or endocarditis. The finding of focal encephalitis, particularly involving the temporal lobes, is suggestive of HSE. MRI is more sensitive than CT in demonstrating temporal lobe involvement [49]. Characteristic abnormalities may not be seen initially, however [117]. If the clinical suspicion is high, imaging studies should also be repeated after several days.

Electroencephalography (EEG) may provide early clues to a diagnosis before CT changes are apparent, but the abnormalities seen are less specific. In patients with HSE, 80% have a temporal focus, although serial studies are often required to detect these changes [115].

With the advent of new molecular approaches and improved serologic diagnostics, brain biopsy is less commonly performed. However, it should be considered in select situations, such as when a patient continues to deteriorate on acyclovir. In the largest series reported, 9% of all patients with suspected HSE had another treatable disorder [121]. Neuroimaging should be used to guide sampling of abnormal tissue. Yield is likely to be higher earlier in disease. Specimens should be sent directly for culture, PCR, and immunofluorescence as well as fixed for routine histology with staining for pathogen detection [96].

Therapy

Empiric therapy with acyclovir (10 mg per kg every 8 hours in adults) should be initiated in all patients with encephalitis pending results of the diagnostic workup for HSE [96]. Subsequent management depends on the clinical response and the results of PCR testing. Total duration of therapy in confirmed HSE is at least 14 to 21 days. Repeat HSV PCR is recommended prior to stopping therapy in HSE patients who continue to exhibit encephalitic features, with continuation of acyclovir if the repeat PCR is positive [96].

Empiric doxycycline therapy (100 mg twice a day) should be considered for patients presenting with clinical suspicion of rickettsial or ehrlichial diseases in the summer months [96]. Early institution of tetracyclines reduces mortality in Rocky Mountain spotted fever. Therapy should be given in confirmed cases until the patient has been afebrile for 2 to 3 days [122].

Specific therapy is available for most nonviral microbial causes of encephalitis. Neurosyphilis should be treated with 10 to 14 days of high-dose penicillin G [123]. Meningoencephalitis caused by the Lyme disease spirochete is treated with ceftriaxone (2 g IV once daily) for 14 days [124]. Treatment for toxoplasmic encephalitis consists of pyrimethamine plus either sulfadiazine or clindamycin [125].

Antiviral therapy may be efficacious in some non-HSE forms of viral encephalitis. Although herpes zoster–associated encephalitis is usually self-limited, acyclovir therapy is recommended based on limited evidence of improved outcomes in small case series. CMV encephalitis can be treated with a combination of ganciclovir and foscarnet. Ribavirin can be considered in cases of encephalitis secondary to rabies or measles viruses, but there is little published experience. In influenza-related encephalitis with a susceptible strain, oseltamivir is recommended [96].

Treatment for most cases of encephalitis is supportive, with particular attention to the management of cerebral edema,

SIADH, and seizures. Status epilepticus (see Chapter 172) may produce additional neurologic damage. Intubation may frequently be necessary to prevent aspiration and to provide ventilatory assistance. The risks of nosocomial infection, particularly pneumonia, are very high for patients with prolonged periods of unconsciousness.

BRAIN ABSCESS

Etiology and Pathogenesis

Brain abscesses most commonly arise from chronic infections of the paranasal sinuses, middle ear, or mastoid [29,126]. Streptococci and anaerobes are the major organisms; *S. aureus* is involved less frequently. Enteric Gram-negative bacilli are commonly found in otogenic brain abscesses. Following penetrating trauma or surgery, staphylococci and Gram-negative bacilli are important pathogens [29]. Most brain abscesses are likely polymicrobial. Recent 16S ribosomal RNA gene sequencing of brain abscess aspirates has revealed a more diverse array of organisms than had previously been isolated in culture [127].

Hematogenous seeding of brain abscesses occurs in patients with cyanotic congenital heart disease and anaerobic pleuropulmonary infections as well as some normal hosts. Microaerophilic streptococci and anaerobes are the most common organisms. *S. aureus* endocarditis can also cause hematogenous brain abscess [29]. Brain abscesses caused by fungi, mycobacteria, or atypical organisms can be seen in immunosuppressed patients. In patients infected with HIV, mass lesions are most often caused by *T. gondii* [128]. Nocardia brain abscesses are commonly associated with defects in cell-mediated immunity, but at least half of cases occur in immunocompetent patients. They may occur as isolated lesions or in conjunction with pulmonary or cutaneous disease [29].

In the development of brain abscesses, initial infection of brain tissue leads to a focus of inflammation known as early cerebritis. This area appears hypodense on CT scan and will enhance with contrast administration. The area of cerebritis expands and develops a central area of necrosis in the late cerebritis stage. A ring-enhancing wall of well-vascularized tissue then separates the necrotic, infected area from healthy surrounding tissue in the capsule stage [29,49].

Diagnosis

Brain abscess usually presents more as a focal mass lesion—with headache, seizures, or neurological deficit—than as an infectious disease [126]. Low-grade fever is present in approximately half of patients. Blood cultures are helpful to assess for a hematogenous source. Cranial CT or MRI aids localization of abscesses, staging the disease, and evaluation of the underlying cause [49].

Therapy

Brain abscess is best treated with a combination of antibiotics and surgery. Initial antimicrobial therapy should be based on the pathogens predicted by the probable underlying source. Ceftriaxone plus metronidazole has been a successful approach and provides appropriate coverage for aerobic Gram-positive cocci, anaerobes, and aerobic Gram-negative bacilli [129]. Antistaphylococcal therapy may also be required. Duration of therapy is not well defined. Most cases require a prolonged 6- to 8-week course of intravenous antibiotics with serial cranial imaging to assess response to therapy. Some clinicians add an additional 2 to 3 months of oral antibiotic therapy and follow the collection to full resolution [29].

Prolonged antimicrobial therapy alone is curative in some patients, especially when the lesions are small (<2.5 cm) and do not have a well-defined capsule by CT criteria. However, in the absence of a contraindication, most specialists recommend prompt aspiration of the abscess contents using CT-guided stereotactic techniques. This provides confirmation of the diagnosis, material for culture, and possible adequate drainage of the focus of infection. In patients with multiple abscesses, the largest lesions are usually aspirated. The hospital stay and need for second surgical procedures are reduced by excision, but deep or multiple abscesses, abscesses in the early cerebritis stage, or abscesses in vital regions are poor candidates for this approach [130].

PARAMENINGEAL FOCI

Subdural Empyema

Subdural empyema usually arises from the same foci as brain abscess or as a complication of meningitis [6,131]. The infection spreads through venous drainage into intracranial vessels, which course through the subdural space. The clinical features of subdural empyema relate to local inflammation and cerebral edema, leading to increased intracranial pressure and herniation. Patients demonstrate depression of consciousness, hemiplegia, focal seizures, papilledema, and meningitic signs [131]. MRI is the most sensitive diagnostic modality [49]. Surgical decompression and drainage are urgent adjuncts to antibiotic therapy [131].

Dural Sinus Thrombophlebitis

Major dural sinus thrombophlebitis may occur in pyogenic meningitis but more often arises from contiguous spread of sinusitis, mastoiditis, otitis, or cranial skin and soft tissue infection. The microbiology reflects that of acute infection at these sites: *S. aureus*, *S. pneumoniae* or other streptococci, and anaerobes. Clinical signs and symptoms vary with the thrombus location. For instance, sagittal sinus thrombophlebitis may cause seizures and hemiplegia, whereas cavernous sinus thrombophlebitis presents with proptosis, marked chemosis, and ophthalmoplegia. Sigmoid sinus thrombophlebitis may give no neurologic signs but produce persistent fever in a case of chronic otitis media and mastoiditis. CT and MRI often can demonstrate thrombosis in the dural sinuses. Antibiotics and drainage or excision of the focus from which the problem originates are the mainstays of therapy. The merits of anticoagulation are controversial due to the propensity of venous infarcts to become hemorrhagic [132].

Spinal Epidural Abscess

Spinal epidural abscess is an infection that may be seeded during bacteremia or occur as a complication of vertebral osteomyelitis or surgery. More than half of cases are caused by *S. aureus*. *Pseudomonas* spp are also a common pathogen in injection drug users [64,133].

The classic triad of symptoms is back pain, fever, and neurologic deficit, though many patients do not demonstrate all three [64]. Percussion tenderness over the vertebral spinous processes should raise the suspicion of spinal epidural abscess. Meningismus may develop in some patients before neurologic deficits [133]. Most patients have elevated C-reactive protein

TABLE 79.4

SUMMARY RECOMMENDATIONS FOR MANAGEMENT OF CENTRAL NERVOUS SYSTEM INFECTIONS BASED ON RANDOMIZED CONTROLLED CLINICAL TRIALS

- Dexamethasone treatment begun just prior to the institution of antibiotic therapy reduces the incidence of hearing loss in children with acute bacterial meningitis [78].
- Outcome of 2 vs. 4 days of therapy with dexamethasone was equivalent in childhood bacterial meningitis [80].
- Dexamethasone treatment begun just prior to the institution of antibiotic therapy reduces mortality and the incidence of neurologic sequelae in adults with acute bacterial meningitis [69].
- Acyclovir treatment reduces the mortality and the incidence of neurologic sequelae in herpes simplex virus encephalitis [135].

or erythrocyte sedimentation rate, two thirds have leukocytosis, and approximately 60% have positive blood cultures [64]. Early recognition of epidural abscess is critical because neurologic progression may be rapid and irreversible. MRI should be performed quickly to distinguish the extent of spinal involvement and to evaluate adjacent structures; contrast enhancement aids sensitivity [133].

Immediate neurosurgical consultation is mandatory. The goals of prompt surgical intervention are to prevent or relieve paraplegia and to obtain material for microbiological diagnosis. A nonoperative approach has been used with increasing frequency, particularly in patients with poor medical condition or if the neurologic condition is stable and a microbial etiology is identified quickly from cultures of blood or aspirated material [134]. However, the neurologic condition may deteriorate rapidly even after several weeks of antimicrobial therapy. MRI scanning and neurosurgical consultation should be available on an urgent basis for patients who are managed nonoperatively.

Blood cultures and image-guided abscess aspirate cultures should be obtained prior to initiation of antibiotic therapy in the neurologically stable patient [133]. Antistaphylococcal antibiotics should be started after cultures are obtained; Gram-negative coverage should be considered in intravenous drug abusers or patients with a documented Gram-negative focus elsewhere, such as the urinary tract. Therapy is adjusted based on the results of Gram stains and cultures. There are no controlled studies to support a specific duration of antibiotic therapy. Six to 8 weeks of therapy with close clinical monitoring, serial measurement of inflammatory markers, and repeat imaging is the most common approach [133,134].

Advances in CNS infections, based on randomized, controlled trials or meta-analyses of such trials, are summarized in Table 79.4.

References

1. Auburtin M, Wolff M, Charpentier J, et al: Detrimental role of delayed antibiotic administration and penicillin-nonsusceptible strains in adult intensive care unit patients with pneumococcal meningitis: the PNEUMOREA prospective multicenter study. *Crit Care Med* 34(11):2758–2765, 2006.
2. Lepur D, Barsic B: Community-acquired bacterial meningitis in adults: antibiotic timing in disease course and outcome. *Infection* 35(4):225–231, 2007.
3. Tunkel AR, Hartman BJ, Kaplan SL, et al: Practice guidelines for the management of bacterial meningitis. *Clin Infect Dis* 39(9):1267–1284, 2004.
4. Straus SE, Thorpe KE, Holroyd-Leduc J: How do I perform a lumbar puncture and analyze the results to diagnose bacterial meningitis? *JAMA* 296(16):2012–2022, 2006.
5. Oliver WJ, Shope TC, Kuhns LR: Fatal lumbar puncture: fact versus fiction—an approach to a clinical dilemma. *Pediatrics* 112(3, Pt 1):e174–e176, 2003.
6. van de Beek D, de Gans J, Tunkel AR, et al: Community-acquired bacterial meningitis in adults. *N Engl J Med* 354(1):44–53, 2006.
7. Hasbun R, Abrahams J, Jekel J, et al: Computed tomography of the head before lumbar puncture in adults with suspected meningitis. *N Engl J Med* 345(24):1727–1733, 2001.
8. Schuchat A, Robinson K, Wenger JD, et al: Bacterial meningitis in the United States in 1995. *N Engl J Med* 337(14):970–976, 1997.
9. van de Beek D, de Gans J, Spanjaard L, et al: Clinical features and prognostic factors in adults with bacterial meningitis. *N Engl J Med* 351(18):1849–1859, 2004.
10. Reefhuis J, Honein MA, Whitney CG, et al: Risk of bacterial meningitis in children with cochlear implants. *N Engl J Med* 349(5):435–445, 2003.
11. Wei BP, Robins-Browne RM, Shepherd RK, et al: Can we prevent cochlear implant recipients from developing pneumococcal meningitis? *Clin Infect Dis* 46(1):e1–e7, 2008.
12. Hsu HE, Shutt KA, Moore MR, et al: Effect of pneumococcal conjugate vaccine on pneumococcal meningitis. *N Engl J Med* 360(3):244–256, 2009.
13. Tsai CJ, Griffin MR, Nuorti JP, et al: Changing epidemiology of pneumococcal meningitis after the introduction of pneumococcal conjugate vaccine in the United States. *Clin Infect Dis* 46(11):1664–1672, 2008.
14. Virji M: Pathogenic neisseriae: surface modulation, pathogenesis and infection control. *Nat Rev Microbiol* 7(4):274–286, 2009.
15. American Academy of Pediatrics: Meningococcal infections, in Pickering L, Baker C, Kimberlin D, et al (eds): *Red Book: 2009 Report of the Committee on Infectious Diseases*. 28th ed. Elk Grove Village, IL, American Academy of Pediatrics, 2009, pp 455–463.
16. Brouwer MC, van de Beek D, Heckenberg SG, et al: Community-acquired *Listeria monocytogenes* meningitis in adults. *Clin Infect Dis* 43(10):1233–1238, 2006.
17. Mylonakis E, Hohmann EL, Calderwood SB: Central nervous system infection with *Listeria monocytogenes*. 33 years' experience at a general hospital and review of 776 episodes from the literature. *Medicine (Baltimore)* 77(5):313–336, 1998.
18. Swingler G, Fransman D, Hussey G: Conjugate vaccines for preventing *Haemophilus influenzae* type B infections. *Cochrane Database Syst Rev* (2):CD001729, 2007.
19. Center for Disease Control and Prevention (CDC): Invasive *Haemophilus influenzae* Type B disease in five young children—Minnesota, 2008. *MMWR Morb Mortal Wkly Rep* 58(3):58–60, 2009.
20. Spagnuolo PJ, Ellner JJ, Lerner PI, et al: *Haemophilus influenzae* meningitis: the spectrum of disease in adults. *Medicine* 61(2):74–85, 1982.
21. Durand ML, Calderwood SB, Weber DJ, et al: Acute bacterial meningitis in adults. A review of 493 episodes. *N Engl J Med* 328(1):21–28, 1993.
22. Pedersen M, Benfield TL, Skinhoej P, et al: Haematogenous *Staphylococcus aureus* meningitis. A 10-year nationwide study of 96 consecutive cases. *BMC Infect Dis* 6:49, 2006.
23. Conen A, Walti LN, Merlo A, et al: Characteristics and treatment outcome of cerebrospinal fluid shunt-associated infections in adults: a retrospective analysis over an 11-year period. *Clin Infect Dis* 47(1):73–82, 2008.
24. Parker SL, Attenello FJ, Sciubba DM, et al: Comparison of shunt infection incidence in high-risk subgroups receiving antibiotic-impregnated versus standard shunts. *Childs Nerv Syst* 25(1):77–83; discussion 85, 2009.
25. Skoff TH, Farley MM, Petit S, et al: Increasing burden of invasive group B streptococcal disease in nonpregnant adults, 1990–2007. *Clin Infect Dis* 49(1):85–92, 2009.
26. Lee GT, Chiu CY, Haller BL, et al: *Streptococcus suis* meningitis, United States. *Emerg Infect Dis* 14(1):183–185, 2008.
27. Lun ZR, Wang QP, Chen XG, et al: *Streptococcus suis*: an emerging zoonotic pathogen. *Lancet Infect Dis* 7(3):201–209, 2007.
28. Baer ET: Post-dural puncture bacterial meningitis. *Anesthesiology* 105(2):381–393, 2006.
29. Mathisen GE, Johnson JP: Brain abscess. *Clin Infect Dis* 25(4):763–779, 1997.
30. van Deuren M, Brandtzaeg P, van der Meer JW: Update on meningococcal disease with emphasis on pathogenesis and clinical management. *Clin Microbiol Rev* 13(1):144–166, 2000.
31. Orihuela CJ, Mahdavi J, Thornton J, et al: Laminin receptor initiates bacterial contact with the blood brain barrier in experimental meningitis models. *J Clin Invest* 119(6):1638–1646, 2009.
32. Overturf GD: Indications for the immunological evaluation of patients with meningitis. *Clin Infect Dis* 36(2):189–194, 2003.
33. Tebruegge M, Curtis N: Epidemiology, etiology, pathogenesis, and diagnosis of recurrent bacterial meningitis. *Clin Microbiol Rev* 21(3):519–537, 2008.
34. Scheld WM, Koedel U, Nathan B, et al: Pathophysiology of bacterial meningitis: mechanism(s) of neuronal injury. *J Infect Dis* 186[Suppl 2]:S225–S233, 2002.

35. van der Flier M, Geelen SP, Kimpen JL, et al: Reprogramming the host response in bacterial meningitis: how best to improve outcome? *Clin Microbiol Rev* 16(3):415–429, 2003.
36. Arditi M, Ables L, Yogev R: Cerebrospinal fluid endotoxin levels in children with *H. influenzae* meningitis before and after administration of intravenous ceftriaxone. *J Infect Dis* 160(6):1005–1011, 1989.
37. van de Beek D, de Gans J, McIntyre P, et al: Corticosteroids for acute bacterial meningitis. *Cochrane Database Syst Rev* (1):CD004405, 2007.
38. Hoffmann O, Priller J, Prozorovski T, et al: TRAIL limits excessive host immune responses in bacterial meningitis. *J Clin Invest* 117(7):2004–2013, 2007.
39. Geiseler PJ, Nelson KE, Levin S, et al: Community-acquired purulent meningitis: a review of 1,316 cases during the antibiotic era, 1954-1976. *Rev Infect Dis* 2(5):725–745, 1980.
40. Attia J, Hatala R, Cook DJ, et al: The rational clinical examination. Does this adult patient have acute meningitis? *JAMA* 282(2):175–181, 1999.
41. Hussein AS, Shafran SD: Acute bacterial meningitis in adults. A 12-year review. *Medicine (Baltimore)* 79(6):360–368, 2000.
42. van Deuren M, van Dijke BJ, Koopman RJ, et al: Rapid diagnosis of acute meningococcal infections by needle aspiration or biopsy of skin lesions. *BMJ* 306(6887):1229–1232, 1993.
43. Nigrovic LE, Malley R, Macias CG, et al: Effect of antibiotic pretreatment on cerebrospinal fluid profiles of children with bacterial meningitis. *Pediatrics* 122(4):726–730, 2008.
44. Ragunathan L, Ramsay M, Borrow R, et al: Clinical features, laboratory findings and management of meningococcal meningitis in England and Wales: report of a 1997 survey. Meningococcal meningitis: 1997 survey report. *J Infect* 40(1):74–79, 2000.
45. Fuglsang-Damgaard D, Pedersen G, Schonheyder HC: Positive blood cultures and diagnosis of bacterial meningitis in cases with negative culture of cerebrospinal fluid. *Scand J Infect Dis* 40(3):229–233, 2008.
46. Kanegaye JT, Soliemanzadeh P, Bradley JS: Lumbar puncture in pediatric bacterial meningitis: defining the time interval for recovery of cerebrospinal fluid pathogens after parenteral antibiotic pretreatment. *Pediatrics* 108(5):1169–1174, 2001.
47. Tarafdar K, Rao S, Recco RA, et al: Lack of sensitivity of the latex agglutination test to detect bacterial antigen in the cerebrospinal fluid of patients with culture-negative meningitis. *Clin Infect Dis* 33(3):406–408, 2001.
48. Chiba N, Murayama SY, Morozumi M, et al: Rapid detection of eight causative pathogens for the diagnosis of bacterial meningitis by real-time PCR. *J Infect Chemother* 15(2):92–98, 2009.
49. Foerster BR, Thurnher MM, Malani PN, et al: Intracranial infections: clinical and imaging characteristics. *Acta Radiol* 48(8):875–893, 2007.
50. Nash D, Mostashari F, Fine A, et al: The outbreak of West Nile virus infection in the New York City area in 1999. *N Engl J Med* 344(24):1807–1814, 2001.
51. Shalabi M, Whitley RJ: Recurrent benign lymphocytic meningitis. *Clin Infect Dis* 43(9):1194–1197, 2006.
52. Hanson KE, Reckleff J, Hicks L, et al: Unsuspected HIV infection in patients presenting with acute meningitis. *Clin Infect Dis* 47(3):433–434, 2008.
53. Archimbaud C, Chambon M, Bailly JL, et al: Impact of rapid enterovirus molecular diagnosis on the management of infants, children, and adults with aseptic meningitis. *J Med Virol* 81(1):42–48, 2009.
54. Christie LJ, Loeffler AM, Honarmand S, et al: Diagnostic challenges of central nervous system tuberculosis. *Emerg Infect Dis* 14(9):1473–1475, 2008.
55. Thwaites GE, Chau TT, Stepniewska K, et al: Diagnosis of adult tuberculous meningitis by use of clinical and laboratory features. *Lancet* 360(9342):1287–1292, 2002.
56. Paganini H, Gonzalez F, Santander C, et al: Tuberculous meningitis in children: clinical features and outcome in 40 cases. *Scand J Infect Dis* 32(1):41–45, 2000.
57. Thwaites GE, Caws M, Chau TT, et al: Comparison of conventional bacteriology with nucleic acid amplification (amplified mycobacterium direct test) for diagnosis of tuberculous meningitis before and after inception of antituberculosis chemotherapy. *J Clin Microbiol* 42(3):996–1002, 2004.
58. Pai M, Ramsay A, O'Brien R: Evidence-based tuberculosis diagnosis. *PLoS Med* 5(7):e156, 2008.
59. Abdelmalek R, Kanoun F, Kilani B, et al: Tuberculous meningitis in adults: MRI contribution to the diagnosis in 29 patients. *Int J Infect Dis* 10(5):372–377, 2006.
60. Barnett ND, Kaplan AM, Hopkin RJ, et al: Primary amoebic meningoencephalitis with *Naegleria fowleri*: clinical review. *Pediatr Neurol* 15(3):230–234, 1996.
61. Keiser PB, Nutman TB: *Strongyloides stercoralis* in the immunocompromised population. *Clin Microbiol Rev* 17(1):208–217, 2004.
62. Johnson RH, Einstein HE: Coccidioidal meningitis. *Clin Infect Dis* 42(1):103–107, 2006.
63. Bicanic T, Harrison TS: Cryptococcal meningitis. *Br Med Bull* 72:99–118, 2004.
64. Darouiche RO: Spinal epidural abscess. *N Engl J Med* 355(19):2012–2020, 2006.
65. Moris G, Garcia-Monco JC: The challenge of drug-induced aseptic meningitis. *Arch Intern Med* 159(11):1185–1194, 1999.
66. Brown EM, de Louvois J, Bayston R, et al: Distinguishing between chemical and bacterial meningitis in patients who have undergone neurosurgery. *Clin Infect Dis* 34(4):556–558, 2002.
67. Forgacs P, Geyer CA, Freidberg SR: Characterization of chemical meningitis after neurological surgery. *Clin Infect Dis* 32(2):179–185, 2001.
68. Sanchez GB, Kaylie DM, O'Malley MR, et al: Chemical meningitis following cerebellopontine angle tumor surgery. *Otolaryngol Head Neck Surg* 138(3):368–373, 2008.
69. de Gans J, van de Beek D, European Dexamethasone in Adulthood Bacterial Meningitis Study Investigators: Dexamethasone in adults with bacterial meningitis. *N Engl J Med* 347(20):1549–1556, 2002.
70. Jones ME, Draghi DC, Karlowsky JA, et al: Prevalence of antimicrobial resistance in bacteria isolated from central nervous system specimens as reported by U.S. hospital laboratories from 2000 to 2002. *Ann Clin Microbiol Antimicrob* 3:3, 2004.
71. Odio CM, Puig JR, Feris JM, et al: Prospective, randomized, investigator-blinded study of the efficacy and safety of meropenem vs. cefotaxime therapy in bacterial meningitis in children. Meropenem Meningitis Study Group. *Pediatr Infect Dis J* 18(7):581–590, 1999.
72. Safdar A, Armstrong D: Antimicrobial activities against 84 *Listeria monocytogenes* isolates from patients with systemic listeriosis at a comprehensive cancer center (1955–1997). *J Clin Microbiol* 41(1):483–485, 2003.
73. Briggs S, Ellis-Pegler R, Raymond N, et al: Gram-negative bacillary meningitis after cranial surgery or trauma in adults. *Scand J Infect Dis* 36(3):165–173, 2004.
74. Kim BN, Peleg AY, Lodise TP, et al: Management of meningitis due to antibiotic-resistant *Acinetobacter* species. *Lancet Infect Dis* 9(4):245–255, 2009.
75. Levitz RE, Quintiliani R: Trimethoprim-sulfamethoxazole for bacterial meningitis. *Ann Intern Med* 100(6):881–890, 1984.
76. Paris MM, Ramilo O, McCracken GH Jr: Management of meningitis caused by penicillin-resistant *Streptococcus pneumoniae. Antimicrob Agents Chemother* 39(10):2171–2175, 1995.
77. Kaplan SL, Mason EO Jr: Management of infections due to antibiotic-resistant *Streptococcus pneumoniae. Clin Microbiol Rev* 11(4):628–644, 1998.
78. Schaad UB, Lips U, Gnehm HE, et al: Dexamethasone therapy for bacterial meningitis in children. *Lancet* 342:457–461, 1993.
79. Mongelluzzo J, Mohamad Z, Ten Have TR, et al: Corticosteroids and mortality in children with bacterial meningitis. *JAMA* 299(17):2048–2055, 2008.
80. Syrogiannopoulos GA, Lourida AN, Theodoridou MC, et al: Dexamethasone therapy for bacterial meningitis in children: 2- versus 4-day regimen. *J Infect Dis* 169(4):853–858, 1994.
81. van de Beek D, de Gans J, McIntyre P, et al: Steroids in adults with acute bacterial meningitis: a systematic review. *Lancet Infect Dis* 4(3):139–143, 2004.
82. Paris MM, Hickey SM, Uscher MI, et al: Effect of dexamethasone on therapy of experimental penicillin- and cephalosporin-resistant pneumococcal meningitis. *Antimicrob Agents Chemother* 38(6):1320–1324, 1994.
83. Nguyen TH, Tran TH, Thwaites G, et al: Dexamethasone in Vietnamese adolescents and adults with bacterial meningitis. *N Engl J Med* 357(24):2431–2440, 2007.
84. Scarborough M, Gordon SB, Whitty CJ, et al: Corticosteroids for bacterial meningitis in adults in sub-Saharan Africa. *N Engl J Med* 357(24):2441–2450, 2007.
85. Peltola H, Roine I, Fernandez J, et al: Adjuvant glycerol and/or dexamethasone to improve the outcomes of childhood bacterial meningitis: a prospective, randomized, double-blind, placebo-controlled trial. *Clin Infect Dis* 45(10):1277–1286, 2007.
86. Saez-Llorens X, McCracken GH Jr: Glycerol and bacterial meningitis. *Clin Infect Dis* 45(10):1287–1289, 2007.
87. Lindvall P, Ahlm C, Ericsson M, et al: Reducing intracranial pressure may increase survival among patients with bacterial meningitis. *Clin Infect Dis* 38(3):384–390, 2004.
88. Singhi SC, Singhi PD, Srinivas B, et al: Fluid restriction does not improve the outcome of acute meningitis. *Pediatr Infect Dis J* 14(6):495–503, 1995.
89. Schreffler RT, Schreffler AJ, Wittler RR: Treatment of cerebrospinal fluid shunt infections: a decision analysis. *Pediatr Infect Dis J* 21(7):632–636, 2002.
90. Wu HM, Harcourt BH, Hatcher CP, et al: Emergence of ciprofloxacin-resistant *Neisseria meningitidis* in North America. *N Engl J Med* 360(9):886–892, 2009.
91. Rainbow J, Cebelinski E, Bartkus J, et al: Rifampin-resistant meningococcal disease. *Emerg Infect Dis* 11(6):977–979, 2005.
92. Weiss D, Stern EJ, Zimmerman C, et al: Epidemiologic investigation and targeted vaccination initiative in response to an outbreak of meningococcal disease among illicit drug users in Brooklyn, New York. *Clin Infect Dis* 48(7):894–901, 2009.
93. American Academy of Pediatrics: *Haemophilus influenzae* infections, in Pickering L, Baker C, Kimberlin D, et al (eds): *Red Book: 2009 Report of the Committee on Infectious Diseases*. 28th ed. Elk Grove Village, IL, American Academy of Pediatrics, 2009, pp 316–319.
94. Khetsuriani N, Holman RC, Anderson LJ: Burden of encephalitis-associated hospitalizations in the United States, 1988–1997. *Clin Infect Dis* 35(2):175–182, 2002.
95. Glaser CA, Gilliam S, Schnurr D, et al: In search of encephalitis etiologies: diagnostic challenges in the California Encephalitis Project, 1998-2000. *Clin Infect Dis* 36(6):731–742, 2003.

96. Tunkel AR, Glaser CA, Bloch KC, et al: The management of encephalitis: clinical practice guidelines by the Infectious Diseases Society of America. *Clin Infect Dis* 47(3):303–327, 2008.
97. Whitley RJ: Herpes simplex encephalitis: adolescents and adults. *Antiviral Res* 71(2-3):141–148, 2006.
98. Casrouge A, Zhang SY, Eidenschenk C, et al: Herpes simplex virus encephalitis in human UNC-93B deficiency. *Science* 314(5797):308–312, 2006.
99. Zhang SY, Jouanguy E, Ugolini S, et al: TLR3 deficiency in patients with herpes simplex encephalitis. *Science* 317(5844):1522–1527, 2007.
100. Davis LE, Beckham JD, Tyler KL: North American encephalitic arboviruses. *Neurol Clin* 26(3):727–757, ix, 2008.
101. Iwamoto M, Jernigan DB, Guasch A, et al: Transmission of West Nile virus from an organ donor to four transplant recipients. *N Engl J Med* 348(22):2196–2203, 2003.
102. Pealer LN, Marfin AA, Petersen LR, et al: Transmission of West Nile virus through blood transfusion in the United States in 2002. *N Engl J Med* 349(13):1236–1245, 2003.
103. Center for Disease Control and Prevention (CDC). Arboviral infections of the central nervous system–United States, 1996–1997. *MMWR Morb Mortal Wkly Rep* 47(25):517–522, 1998.
104. Center for Disease Control and Prevention. West Nile virus activity—United States, 2007. *MMWR Morb Mortal Wkly Rep* 57(26):720–723, 2008.
105. Deresiewicz RL, Thaler SJ, Hsu L, et al: Clinical and neuroradiographic manifestations of eastern equine encephalitis. *N Engl J Med* 336(26):1867–1874, 1997.
106. Center for Disease Control and Prevention (CDC). Eastern equine encephalitis—New Hampshire and Massachusetts, August-September 2005. *MMWR Morb Mortal Wkly Rep* 55(25):697–700, 2006.
107. Jackson AC: Rabies. *Neurol Clin* 26(3):717–726, ix, 2008.
108. De Serres G, Dallaire F, Cote M, et al: Bat rabies in the United States and Canada from 1950 through 2007: human cases with and without bat contact. *Clin Infect Dis* 46(9):1329–1337, 2008.
109. Srinivasan A, Burton EC, Kuehnert MJ, et al: Transmission of rabies virus from an organ donor to four transplant recipients. *N Engl J Med* 352(11):1103–1111, 2005.
110. Rupprecht CE, Briggs D, Brown CM, et al: Use of a reduced (4-dose) vaccine schedule for postexposure prophylaxis to prevent human rabies: recommendations of the advisory committee on immunization practices. *MMWR Recomm Rep* 59(RR-2):1–9, 2010.
111. Dalmau J, Gleichman AJ, Hughes EG, et al: Anti-NMDA-receptor encephalitis: case series and analysis of the effects of antibodies. *Lancet Neurol* 7(12):1091–1098, 2008.
112. Graus F, Saiz A, Dalmau J: Antibodies and neuronal autoimmune disorders of the CNS. *J Neurol* 257(4):509–517, 2009.
113. Scolding NJ: Central nervous system vasculitis. *Semin Immunopathol* 31(4):527–536, 2009.
114. Whitley RJ, Soong SJ, Linneman C Jr, et al: Herpes simplex encephalitis. Clinical assessment. *JAMA* 247(3):317–320, 1982.
115. Steiner I, Budka H, Chaudhuri A, et al: Viral encephalitis: a review of diagnostic methods and guidelines for management. *Eur J Neurol* 12(5):331–343, 2005.
116. Modlin JF: Enterovirus deja vu. *N Engl J Med* 356(12):1204–1205, 2007.
117. De Tiege X, Heron B, Lebon P, et al: Limits of early diagnosis of herpes simplex encephalitis in children: a retrospective study of 38 cases. *Clin Infect Dis* 36(10):1335–1339, 2003.
118. Debiasi RL, Tyler KL: Molecular methods for diagnosis of viral encephalitis. *Clin Microbiol Rev* 17(4):903–925, table of contents, 2004.
119. Dacheux L, Reynes JM, Buchy P, et al: A reliable diagnosis of human rabies based on analysis of skin biopsy specimens. *Clin Infect Dis* 47(11):1410–1417, 2008.
120. Glaser CA, Honarmand S, Anderson LJ, et al: Beyond viruses: clinical profiles and etiologies associated with encephalitis. *Clin Infect Dis* 43(12):1565–1577, 2006.
121. Whitley RJ, Cobbs CG, Alford CA Jr, et al: Diseases that mimic herpes simplex encephalitis. Diagnosis, presentation, and outcome. NIAD Collaborative Antiviral Study Group. *JAMA* 262(2):234–239, 1989.
122. Dantas-Torres F: Rocky Mountain spotted fever. *Lancet Infect Dis* 7(11):724–732, 2007.
123. Centers for Disease Control and Prevention, Workowski KA, Berman SM: Sexually transmitted diseases treatment guidelines, 2006. *MMWR Recomm Rep* 55(RR-11):1–94, 2006.
124. Wormser GP, Dattwyler RJ, Shapiro ED, et al: The clinical assessment, treatment, and prevention of lyme disease, human granulocytic anaplasmosis, and babesiosis: clinical practice guidelines by the Infectious Diseases Society of America. *Clin Infect Dis* 43(9):1089–1134, 2006.
125. Kaplan JEBC, Holmes KH, Brooks JT, et al: Guidelines for prevention and treatment of opportunistic infections in HIV-infected adults and adolescents: recommendations from CDC, the National Institutes of Health, and the HIV Medicine Association of the Infectious Diseases Society of America. *MMWR Recomm Rep* 58(RR-4):1–207, 2009.
126. Kao PT, Tseng HK, Liu CP, et al: Brain abscess: clinical analysis of 53 cases. *J Microbiol Immunol Infect* 36(2):129–136, 2003.
127. Al Masalma M, Armougom F, Scheld WM, et al: The expansion of the microbiological spectrum of brain abscesses with use of multiple 16S ribosomal DNA sequencing. *Clin Infect Dis* 48(9):1169–1178, 2009.
128. Ammassari A, Cingolani A, Pezzotti P, et al: AIDS-related focal brain lesions in the era of highly active antiretroviral therapy. *Neurology* 55(8):1194–1200, 2000.
129. Jansson AK, Enblad P, Sjolin J: Efficacy and safety of cefotaxime in combination with metronidazole for empirical treatment of brain abscess in clinical practice: a retrospective study of 66 consecutive cases. *Eur J Clin Microbiol Infect Dis* 23(1):7–14, 2004.
130. Mampalam TJ, Rosenblum ML: Trends in the management of bacterial brain abscesses: a review of 102 cases over 17 years. *Neurosurgery* 23(4):451–458, 1988.
131. Greenlee JE: Subdural empyema. *Curr Treat Options Neurol* 5(1):13–22, 2003.
132. Stam J: Thrombosis of the cerebral veins and sinuses. *N Engl J Med* 352(17):1791–1798, 2005.
133. Pradilla G, Ardila GP, Hsu W, et al: Epidural abscesses of the CNS. *Lancet Neurol* 8(3):292–300, 2009.
134. Siddiq F, Chowfin A, Tight R, et al: Medical vs surgical management of spinal epidural abscess. *Arch Intern Med* 164(22):2409–2412, 2004.
135. Whitley RJ, Alford CA, Hirsch MS, et al: Vidarabine versus acyclovir therapy in herpes simplex encephalitis. *N Engl J Med* 314(3):144–149, 1986.

CHAPTER 80 ■ INFECTIVE ENDOCARDITIS AND INFECTIONS OF INTRACARDIAC PROSTHETIC DEVICES

KAREN C. CARROLL, SARAH H. CHEESEMAN AND SARA E. COSGROVE

Infective endocarditis (IE) is an infection of the endothelial lining of the heart, characterized on pathologic study by vegetations. The infected site is usually a valve, but endocarditis may be situated on mural thrombi (rare) or the endothelial surface on which the jet stream from a stenotic lesion (patent ductus, ventricular septal defect, or stenotic valve) impinges. The term encompasses infection of the endothelial surface of any blood vessel, which most frequently occurs on hemodynamically or structurally abnormal ones such as abdominal aortic aneurysms, arteriovenous fistulas, and prosthetic grafts. The peculiarities of these infections are beyond the scope of this chapter, and the general principles of diagnosis and treatment are the same.

Significant changes in the epidemiology and character of IE have been noted over the past three decades [1–9]. Shifting demographics, an expanding pool of elderly, chronically ill and immunocompromised patients, and rising rates of nosocomial bacteremia have been observed [1–9]. Unanticipated increases in societal behaviors that predispose to bacteremia, such as injection drug use, body art (including piercing and tattooing [10]), and acupuncture [11], have also contributed to the steady incidence of IE. All of the above have contributed to changes in the microbiology of IE [1–9]. Simultaneously, advances in diagnostic criteria and methods and improvements in cardiothoracic surgery have occurred. Taken together, there has not been a noticeable decline in either the incidence or mortality of IE [1–9].

Since 1990, among published series of more than 100 patients, reported mortality ranged from 10% to 37% [1–4,9], with the lowest mortality rates attributed to earlier and higher rates of surgery, short delay before treatment, and high doses of bactericidal drugs. Decline in mortality has occurred predominantly among young patients. Mortality remains high in the elderly [2,3,12], diabetics [13], patients with other predisposing diseases such as chronic renal failure requiring hemodialysis and immunosuppression [1,2,9,14–17], patients with discernible valvular vegetations [15], patients with healthcare-associated infections [16], and those infected with staphylococci, particularly methicillin-resistant *Staphylococcus aureus* (MRSA) [2,8,15,18].

Traditionally two clinical forms of endocarditis have been delineated: acute and subacute. Subacute disease denotes insidious onset, with slow development of the characteristic lesions and absence of marked toxicity for a long period. A high proportion of these cases occur on previously damaged valves and many are caused by organisms of relatively low virulence, such as α-hemolytic streptococci (viridans streptococci). In contrast, acute bacterial endocarditis presents as a fulminant infection, with abrupt onset, high fever, more frequent leukocytosis, and rapid downhill course with respect to both valve destruction and systemic toxicity. This is most frequently secondary to *S. aureus* and may occur on previously normal valves. Among patients who require intensive care, the acute form of infection will be the more frequent problem.

A classification that more accurately characterizes current trends in IE has been proposed [6]. Dividing IE into four major categories as follows may provide better delineation of clinical conditions and microbial pathogens [6]. These categories are (a) native valve endocarditis; (b) prosthetic valve endocarditis (PVE)—early (<12 months following surgery) and late (>12 months following surgery); (c) IE in the injection drug user; and (d) nosocomial IE.

All observers of IE have noted a decrease in the frequency of rheumatic heart disease as a predisposing lesion and an increase in degenerative disease [3,6,7,9] and other previously unrecognized conditions such as mitral valve prolapse and idiopathic hypertrophic subaortic stenosis [14,15]. Taking these trends together, the universal observation of an increasing proportion of cases in older age groups is not surprising. Incidence of IE is higher among men compared with women in patients younger than 65 years and has remained relatively stable over the last several decades. In contrast, the incidence among women has significantly increased since 2000 especially among the elderly (>65 years) [8,9,12].

Populations particularly at risk for endocarditis are injection drug users and patients with prosthetic valves. Since the 1990s, other populations at risk have increased: transplant recipients [19,20], burn patients [21], patients with medical devices that put them at risk for bacteremia [9,16,22,23], and, most notably, persons on chronic hemodialysis [16,17,24,25].

Problems in endocarditis particularly relevant to patients in cardiac or intensive care units include the following:

1. Acute bacterial endocarditis,
2. Prosthetic valve endocarditis,
3. Endocarditis in patients with intravascular foreign bodies, such as pacemakers and indwelling vascular catheters,
4. Indications for surgery in endocarditis.

ETIOLOGY

The term *infective endocarditis* properly includes the whole world of microorganisms that can cause the disease. Fungi, rickettsiae (*Coxiella burnetii*, which causes Q fever), *Chlamydia* sp, and perhaps even viruses have been implicated in endocarditis, although bacteria are still the predominant cause. Substantial advances in the isolation of microorganisms and improvements in serologic testing and molecular detection have widened the spectrum of causative organisms. Uncommon species of streptococci, emerging pathogens such as *Bartonella* sp and *Tropheryma whipplei*, the increase in fungal pathogens among nosocomial cases and immunocompromised patients, and increasing resistance among "typical" endocarditis pathogens such as enterococci present unique diagnostic or therapeutic challenges [5,6,16,19–22,25].

Table 80.1 summarizes the most common pathogens from large series of endocarditis cases occurring since 1985 [1–4, 6–9,14,26–29]. Those series with a large number of injection drug users [1,6,14,18,27], patients on chronic hemodialysis [1,2,17,22], transplant recipients [19,20], and those series reporting healthcare-associated IE [1,6,7,16,22,23,25] tend to report more cases caused by *S. aureus*. Viridans streptococci occur more frequently but no longer predominate among non-injection drug user populations and the elderly [9]. Identification to species level among the viridans streptococci may have important therapeutic and prognostic implications. The *Streptococcus anginosus* (*milleri*) groups (*S. anginosus*, *S. constellatus*, and *S. intermedius*) are frequently associated with abscess formation and tend to cause severe disease but cause endocarditis less often than other viridans streptococci [30,31].

TABLE 80.1

ETIOLOGY OF ENDOCARDITIS FROM REPORTED LARGE SERIES SINCE 1985

Etiologic agents	Attributable range[a,b] (%)
Staphylococcus aureus	18–57
Viridans streptococci	11–53
Coagulase-negative staphylococci	1–15
Enterococci	4–10
Streptococcus bovis	1–13
β-Hemolytic streptococci	3–9
Streptococcus pneumoniae	1–3
Other streptococci	3–7
HACEK[c]	1–6
Enterobacteriaceae	1–4
Yeast	1–2
Molds	<1
Polymicrobial	1–6
Other bacteria[d]	2–11
Culture negative	2–39

[a] All figures are the percentage ranges of episodes reported.
[b] Rounded to nearest whole percentage.
[c] *HACEK, Haemophilus sp, Aggregatibacter actinomycetemcomitans, Cardiobacterium hominis, Eikenella corrodens, Kingella kingae.*
[d] Includes a variety of single isolates of species not represented by above genera, including *Neisseria sp, Pseudomonas, Legionella, Lactobacilli.*
Compiled from references [1–4,8,9,14,26–30].

S. anginosus is the least likely among the three species to cause abscesses and the most likely to be associated with endocarditis [31,32]. The nutritionally deficient streptococci include the following genus and species: *Abiotrophia defectiva*, *Granulicatella adiacens*, *Granulicatella para-adiacens*, *Granulicatella balaenopterae*, and *Granulicatella elegans* [33,34]. Together these organisms constitute 3% to 5% of cases of endocarditis caused by viridans streptococci [34]. These organisms require pyridoxal, the active form of vitamin B_6, for growth. Unlike other species of viridans streptococci, these organisms are tolerant to penicillin, and at least one series [33] has found decreased susceptibility to penicillin, extended spectrum cephalosporins, and macrolide antibiotics. High relapse rates are described especially when patients are treated with penicillin alone [34]. Most cases of viridans streptococcal endocarditis (80%) are caused by *Streptococcus sanguis*, *Streptococcus mitis*, or *Streptococcus mutans* [14,18,29,30]. There do not appear to be any statistically significant differences in the symptoms, demographics, or complications among patients with infections caused by this group of organisms. Newer species of viridans streptococci continue to be described.

Enterococci rank third in frequency of isolation in most series, including healthcare-associated cases and those among patients on hemodialysis. Among the non–viridans streptococci, pneumococci are still relatively uncommon causes of endocarditis (1% to 3% of all cases). The proportion of cases caused by β-hemolytic streptococci has not increased since 1980; infections with group B and group G are seen most frequently [32,35,36]. Patients with these infections usually have underlying valvular disease, numerous predisposing factors, most notably diabetes mellitus, and acute onset of their infection [32,35,36]. *Streptococcus bovis* deserves mention for several reasons. First, this organism group has undergone extensive reclassification based upon DNA–DNA reassociation studies, a description of which is beyond the scope of this chapter [37]. Second, some of the newly described species and subspecies (*S. gallolyticus* spp *gallolyticus*) are more frequently associated with endocarditis and with benign and malignant disorders of the gastrointestinal tract, while others are more frequently associated with meningitis (*S. gallolyticus* spp *pasteurianus*). In some series, this organism group has been increasing in frequency in Europe and South America [9], particularly among the elderly and among patients with chronic liver disease [4,37–39]. When this organism is isolated, the patient should be carefully evaluated for gastrointestinal tract malignancy, although it may occur months to years after the bacteremic episode [38]. Since these species and subspecies are difficult to differentiate using traditional microbiological methods, most clinical laboratories will likely continue to call them *S. bovis* or nonenterococcal Group D streptococci.

S. aureus has increased in frequency and accounts for more than 50% of cases in more recent series [1,2,6,9,16,17,19,25,27]. In several recent prospective studies, including data from the International Collaboration on Endocarditis-Prospective Cohort Study (ICE-PCS), patients with *S. aureus* endocarditis were more likely than patients with IE due to other pathogens to have a shorter duration of symptoms before diagnosis, to be hemodialysis dependent, and to have other serious comorbidities such as diabetes mellitus or other chronic illnesses [9,40–43]. Patients with *S. aureus* IE were also more likely to have severe sepsis with persistent bacteremia, major neurologic events, systemic embolization, and death than patients with IE caused by other bacteria [41–43]. In these studies, patients with *S. aureus* IE frequently had healthcare-associated or nosocomial acquisition and were more likely to have MRSA infection than patients with community-acquired *S. aureus*. In the ICE-PCS series [38], a multivariate model identified the following patient characteristics associated with MRSA IE: persistent bacteremia, chronic immunosuppressive therapy, intravascular devices as sources, and diabetes mellitus. Overall, MRSA now accounts for 25% to 50% of the cases attributable to *S. aureus* [2,25,40–43]. Persistent bacteremia correlated with infection caused by MRSA, and risk of embolic phenomena was negatively associated with oxacillin resistance [40–43].

Coagulase-negative staphylococci (CoNS) are recognized pathogens on prosthetic valves and close to 8% of cases on native valves are now caused by these organisms [44]. The majority of the CoNS species recovered are *Staphylococcus epidermidis* [44]. *Staphylococcus lugdunensis* has emerged as a particularly aggressive pathogen that causes a destructive native valve endocarditis, frequently following vasectomy or other procedures involving breaks in the skin in the perineal area [45]. In spite of universal susceptibility to β-lactams and other agents, mortality attributable to this pathogen is high, possibly related to the large vegetations frequently seen with this organism, leading to valvular dehiscence, abscess formation, and systemic embolization [45].

Before 1980, endocarditis caused by Gram-negative organisms comprised less than 3% of cases. Recent series report that Gram-negative organisms now account for 4% to 10% of all native valve endocarditis [3,6,15,46], but these rates vary by geographic location, whether the infection is community or healthcare associated and the type of Gram-negative pathogen involved. Within this subset is the HACEK group (*Haemophilus* sp, *Aggregatibacter* [previously *Actinobacillus*] *actinomycetemcomitans*, *Cardiobacterium hominis*, *Eikenella corrodens*, *Kingella kingae*), which accounts for 2% to 5% of cases [8,9,26,46]. *A. actinomycetemcomitans* is the HACEK species most frequently involved in IE [46]. HACEK organisms are fastidious, nonmotile, slow-growing coccobacilli that require a mean of 3.3 days of incubation in automated blood culture systems for growth [46]. The HACEK organisms rarely cause endocarditis in patients without preexisting valvular disease or in the absence of predisposing factors [46]. Non-HACEK Gram-negative endocarditis (*Enterobacteriaceae* and others) remains relatively rare and is seen primarily among debilitated patients with healthcare-associated infections related to medical devices or surgery [21,47,48].

Among the emerging pathogens of the 1990s are *Bartonella* sp. This genus continues to expand [49,50]. Seven species and subspecies, namely *B. quintana*, *B. henselae* (the agent of cat scratch disease), *B. elizabethae*, *B. vinsonii* spp *berkhoffii*, *B. vinsonii* spp *arupensis*, *B. koehlerae*, and *B. alsatica* have been implicated in cases of endocarditis [49,50]. *B. quintana*, the agent of trench fever, has been reported to infect middle aged, homeless male alcoholics without known underlying valvular disease. Contact with animals is a frequent association, and ectoparasites such as scabies, lice, and fleas are proposed as possible vectors of disease [49–51]. The majority of patients with *B. henselae* endocarditis have a previous history of underlying valvular disease and report contact with cats [49–51]. Characteristically, patients with *Bartonella* endocarditis present with a subacute course and large vegetations [49–51]. Because of the fastidious nature of the organism and serologic cross-reactivity between antibodies to *B. quintana* and *Chlamydia* sp, it is likely that cases of *Bartonella* endocarditis constitute a proportion of cases previously diagnosed as culture negative or due to *Chlamydia* sp [49–51]. Currently, approximately 3% of cases of endocarditis are secondary to *Bartonella* sp [51].

In spite of improvements in blood culture and serological techniques, negative blood cultures can occur in up to 31% of cases [1,2,3,7,52]. There are several reasons cited for negative blood cultures in IE: (a) prior antibiotic administration; (b) infection with fastidious, slow-growing organisms (e.g., *Bartonella* sp, fungi, *Chlamydia* and *Coxiella* spp); (c) infection with nonbacterial organisms such as fungi; and (d) endocarditis in patients with an indwelling cardiac device such as a pacemaker [52,53]. Two recent surveys [52,53] of culture-negative cases in France over two decades used serological studies and molecular methods to augment blood cultures in determining the etiology for more than 348 [52] and 740 [53] patients, respectively. In the initial study of definite cases of IE, in the 79% of patients in whom an etiologic agent was determined, *C. burnetii* and *Bartonella* sp predominated, accounting for 76% of the total [52]. Other rare bacteria included *T. whipplei*, *Mycoplasma hominis*, various streptococci, and *Legionella pneumophila* [52]. Twenty-one percent did not have an etiology determined of whom 79% had received prior administration of antibiotics [52]. In the more recent prospective series, both definitive and possible cases were included and an etiologic diagnosis was determined in 64.6%. The same group of organisms predominated [53].

IE among injection drug-users has increased in the new millennium and *S. aureus* is by far the most common cause [54,55]. Enterococci, enteric Gram-negative bacilli, *Pseudomonas*, *Candida*, and other yeasts are also important [6,9,54]. Polymicrobial endocarditis is more common among injection drug users than in noninjection drug users [6,9,18].

The common causes of early-onset PVE are CoNS (mostly *S. epidermidis*), *S. aureus*, enterococci, diphtheroids, Gram-negative bacilli, and fungi. Among the fungi, *Candida* sp are most common and have emerged as causes of both early- and late-onset disease especially among patients with healthcare-associated infection [56]. However, late-onset disease is still caused mainly by organisms such as CoNS and streptococci, although *S. aureus* accounts for about 11% of cases [9,18,57,58]. This difference is thought to be explained by intraoperative or early postoperative contamination of the prosthesis with resistant hospital flora in early PVE. Late cases represent either smoldering infection with relatively avirulent organisms seeded at the original surgery or subsequent transient bacteremias, such as those that induce endocarditis on native valves [58].

PATHOPHYSIOLOGY

The laboratory model of endocarditis is a rabbit in which a catheter passed through a valve produces mild trauma with the elaboration of a fibrin–platelet thrombus. Subsequent injection of bacteria either through the catheter or at a distant vascular site leads to infection of the traumatized valve [59]. It appears that the fibrin–platelet thrombus allows for avid binding of the bacteria [6]. Adherent bacteria induce blood monocytes to produce cytokines that contribute to further enlargement of the vegetation [60]. As the vegetation matures, the bacteria become fully enveloped, which allows for persistence by avoiding host defenses.

This model conforms to the propensity of damaged human valves toward endocarditis. Transient bacteremia with mouth flora, predominantly viridans streptococci, during chewing, tooth brushing, and the like explains the pattern observed in subacute bacterial endocarditis [6]. More virulent organisms such as *S. aureus* seem to be able to invade even normal hearts. There are several factors expressed by this pathogen that make it more virulent. In addition to surface fibronectin-binding proteins that facilitate adherence, *S. aureus* produces exoenzymes and exotoxins that are controlled by global regulators, such as accessory gene regulator (*agr*) and staphylococcal accessory regulator (*sar*), the expression of which permit tissue invasion and destruction [6]. Intravenous drug users combine the injection of contaminated materials with particulate and often irritant matter, probably accounting for the frequency of endocarditis in this setting and the propensity for right-heart involvement [54,61,62]. The use of intravascular central lines reaching near the tricuspid valve or even crossing tricuspid and pulmonic valves reproduces the rabbit model of endocarditis in humans. The introduction of bacteria through these lines causes the specter of iatrogenic endocarditis.

Once the fibrin–platelet thrombus has become infected, the pathologic process is the enlargement of this mass into a vegetation and invasion of tissue by the infection with eventual disruption. In addition to the mass of the vegetation, there are perforations or total erosions of valve cusps, rupture of chordae tendineae, fistulas from the sinus of Valsalva to atrium or pericardium, and burrowing myocardial abscesses.

Depending on the valve involved, the physiologic consequences may be predicted. Rarely, a vegetation will be so large as to function as an occlusive or stenotic lesion [62]. More often, the tissue destruction process predominates and valvular incompetence results. New regurgitant murmurs of mitral, tricuspid, or aortic origin may acutely stress the heart with resultant congestive failure. Aortic valve disease carries the worst prognosis [62] for several reasons: (a) the heart tolerates acute aortic insufficiency least well; (b) pericardial tamponade or massive left-to-right shunt may develop if a sinus of Valsalva aneurysm erodes into the pericardium or right atrium, respectively; (c) heart block may occur if a myocardial abscess invades the conducting system; and (d) aortic valve ring vegetations are most likely to be flipped into the coronary arteries, infarcting already overworked muscle. These catastrophes are all even more likely in the presence of a prosthetic aortic valve, in which case the infection has its seat at the annulus. Tricuspid valve endocarditis is the most benign. Even total tricuspid insufficiency can be tolerated for a time, and acute right-side heart failure is not as life threatening as is the pulmonary edema of left-sided failure.

The vegetations themselves may break off in whole or part as emboli to the brain, viscera (spleen and kidney are particularly common targets), coronary arteries, and notably in fungal endocarditis, large arteries of the extremities. Septic emboli to the lungs can result in pulmonary infiltrates, often nodular and sometimes cavitating. Emboli to other organs produce infarction, which is usually bland, although splenic abscess, brain abscess, and even purulent meningitis may occur in staphylococcal endocarditis. The most common cerebral lesion, however, is embolic infarct with the clinical appearance of a stroke [62,63]. The smaller vascular lesions of endocarditis may be of an immunologic, vasculitic nature or truly embolic and suppurative in character. Emboli to the vasa vasorum or vasculitis of the arteries lead to mycotic aneurysms of both cerebral and peripheral vessels. The cerebral aneurysms are generally asymptomatic until they rupture and present as subarachnoid or intracerebral hemorrhage. Peripheral mycotic aneurysms may come to attention because of their obvious enlargement and frequent overlying inflammation. Other phenomena that fall into this category are the cutaneous stigmata of endocarditis—Osler's nodes, Janeway lesions, splinter hemorrhages, and petechiae—as well as the frequent renal involvement. Kidney pathology may take several forms: localized renal infarcts, vasculitic glomerulonephritis, acute diffuse glomerulonephritis thought to represent immune complex disease, renal cortical necrosis, and interstitial nephritis likely related to antibiotic administration [62].

DIAGNOSIS

Endocarditis is diagnosed on the basis of signs and symptoms that reflect the pathology: fever, embolic phenomena, and evidence of valvular dysfunction. A continuous bacteremia is characteristic and, indeed, highly suggestive of endovascular infection, although the entity of culture-negative endocarditis also exists. The frequency of various findings in IE is shown in Table 80.2 [1,3,4,9,14,18,27].

TABLE 80.2

CLINICAL FEATURES OF ENDOCARDITIS

Feature	Frequency range (%)
History	
Fever	81–98
Malaise/weakness	49–96
Weight loss	6–30
Musculoskeletal complaints	9–25
Mental status change/neurologic event	11–32
Previous heart disease	25–55
Physical examination	
Fever	54–95
Murmur	76–95
Change in murmur	10–67
Splenomegaly	1–29
Petechiae	12–16
Osler's nodes	3–16
Janeway lesions	3–5
Splinters	3–35
Fundoscopic abnormalities	0–3
Clubbing	6–20
Lab tests	
Hematuria	26–53
↑ ESR	22–89
Rheumatoid factor	5–51
Anemia	66–68
Echocardiographic vegetations[a]	60–86

[a] Combined transthoracic and transesophageal results.
↑ ESR, elevated erythrocyte sedimentation rate.
Data compiled from references [1,3,4,14,18,27].

Criteria

Proof of the diagnosis, in terms of histopathologic confirmation of vegetation with infecting organisms on the affected valve, may be obtained only in cases requiring cardiac surgery or, in the event of death, with autopsy. Clinical criteria for the diagnosis sufficiently stringent to allow for analysis of case characteristics, epidemiology, and the outcome of therapy have been devised and revised over the years with the latest version known as the Duke criteria [26]. The Duke criteria incorporate echocardiographic findings in addition to giving heavy weight to clinical circumstances such as the type of organisms recovered from blood and injection drug use as a predisposing factor. Major and minor criteria analogous to the Jones criteria for diagnosis of rheumatic fever are summarized in Table 80.3. A definite diagnosis requires the presence of two major criteria, one major and three minor criteria, or five minor criteria. The diagnosis is rejected if a firm alternate diagnosis adequately explains the clinical findings, they resolve with less than 4 days of antibiotic therapy, or histopathologic evidence is lacking at autopsy or surgery performed after no more than 4 days of antibiotic therapy. All other clinically suspect cases meriting more than 4 days of antibiotic treatment are classified as possible [26].

Several studies have demonstrated very good sensitivity and excellent specificity (92% to 99%) for the Duke criteria [64–66]. Moreover, these criteria have been evaluated for the diagnosis of IE in children [67] and the elderly [68], as well as in patients with PVE [69]. Several criticisms and proposed modifications have followed these rigorous studies. The inability of the Duke criteria to reject cases that receive more than 4 days of

TABLE 80.3

DUKE CRITERIA AND PROPOSED MODIFIED DUKE CRITERIA FOR DEFINITIVE CLINICAL DIAGNOSIS OF ENDOCARDITIS

Major criteria

1. Positive blood culture for infective endocarditis
   - Typical microorganisms for infective endocarditis from two separate blood cultures
   - Viridans streptococci, *Streptococcus bovis*, HACEK group, or *Staphylococcus aureus* or community-acquired enterococci in the absence of a primary focus, or
   - Persistently positive blood culture, defined as recovery of a microorganism consistent with infective endocarditis from
     - A. Blood cultures drawn more than 12 hours apart, or
     - B. All of three or a majority of four or more separate blood cultures, with first and last drawn at least 1 hour apart
     - C. Single positive blood culture for *Coxiella burnetii* or antiphase IgG antibody titer >1:800
2. Evidence of endocardial involvement
   - Positive echocardiogram for IE (TEE recommended in patients with prosthetic valves, rated at least "possible IE" by clinical criteria, or complicated IE [paravalvular abscess]; TTE as first test in other patients), defined as:
     - A. Oscillating intracardiac mass on valve or supporting structures, or in the path of regurgitant jets, or on implanted material, in the absence of an alternative anatomic explanation, or
     - B. Abscess, or
     - C. New partial dehiscence of prosthetic valve, or new valvular regurgitation (increase or change in preexisting murmur not sufficient)

Minor criteria

1. Predisposition: predisposing heart condition or intravenous drug use
2. Fever: $\geq$38.0°C (100.4°F)
3. Vascular phenomena: major arterial emboli, septic pulmonary infarcts, mycotic aneurysm, intracranial hemorrhage, conjunctival hemorrhages, Janeway lesions
4. Immunologic phenomena: glomerulonephritis, Osler's nodes, Roth spots, rheumatoid factor
5. Microbiologic evidence; positive blood culture but not meeting major criterion as noted previously or serologic evidence of active infection with organism[a] consistent with infective endocarditis
6. Echocardiogram: consistent with infective endocarditis but not meeting major criterion as noted previously. Echocardiographic minor criteria eliminated (Proposed modifications, [72])

[a] Excluding single positive blood cultures for coagulase-negative staphylococci and organisms that do not cause endocarditis.
HACEK, *Haemophilus* sp, *Aggregatibacter actinomycetemcomitans*, *Cardiobacterium hominis*, *Eikenella corrodens*, *Kingella kingae*; IE, infective endocarditis; TEE, transesophageal echocardiography.
Modified from Durack DT, Lukes AS, Bright DK, et al: New criteria for the diagnosis of infective endocarditis: utilization of specific echocardiographic findings. *Am J Med* 96:200–209, 1994; and Li JS, Sexton DJ, Mick N, et al: Proposed modifications to the Duke criteria for the diagnosis of infective endocarditis. *Clin Infect Dis* 30:633–638, 2000, with permission.
Note: A definite diagnosis requires the presence of two major criteria, one major and three minor criteria, or five minor criteria.

antibiotic therapy may lead to occasional overdiagnosis of endocarditis [70]. Sensitivity may possibly be enhanced in those patients with suspected late PVE by the addition of heart failure and atrioventricular conduction disturbances to the minor criteria [69]. Likewise, others have suggested inclusion of positive serologic studies for Q fever as a major criterion, especially in endemic regions [71,72], and other physical findings, such as splenomegaly, and laboratory results, such as a high C-reactive protein, to the minor criteria [73]. Proposed modifications to the definitions have not been evaluated in large prospective studies [72]. Modifications to the major and minor criteria are listed in Table 80.3.

History

The most frequent symptoms reported by patients with endocarditis are fever and malaise, but some present with acute musculoskeletal symptoms, most frequently lower back pain or polyarthralgia [74], and others, because of an embolus, without complaining of or even noticing fever [71]. A common feature of endocarditis is loss of appetite, and its return may be the first clinical sign of response to treatment. Any febrile illness in a patient with known valvular heart disease must bring to mind the question of endocarditis. Similarly, a history of recent dental cleaning or extraction or genitourinary manipulation may indicate an opportunity for bacteremia and seeding of the valve and should be sought, as should suggestions of injection drug abuse. The history of appropriate antibiotic prophylaxis for these procedures is not sufficient to exclude the possibility of endocarditis because failures occasionally occur with currently recommended regimens.

It is important to establish the duration and tempo of the illness by history. Abrupt onset of symptoms, shaking chills, and body temperature greater than 38.9°C (102°F) strongly suggest acute endocarditis. Subacute bacterial endocarditis, in contrast, is characterized by a vague illness occurring over a period of several weeks or months.

Physical Examination

In contrast to the vagueness of the symptoms of endocarditis, many findings on physical examination are characteristic. Most pertinent to the diagnosis are cardiac murmurs and mucocutaneous embolic phenomena. Any heart murmur is compatible with a diagnosis of endocarditis because it is evidence of the turbulent flow that provides the proper nidus for infection. The fact that a murmur has been documented for a long time in no way excludes the possibility of active endocarditis. Changing murmurs, particularly new regurgitant murmurs, are much less commonly observed but are highly significant with respect to both certainty of the diagnosis and functional consequences. Thus, patients must be examined both supine and sitting up leaning forward so that an aortic regurgitant murmur is not missed. Careful listening on both sides of the sternum during inspiration is important to detect tricuspid insufficiency. Signs of congestive heart failure are not early findings in endocarditis but must be watched for because the onset of failure signals a need to consider cardiac surgical intervention.

The most commonly observed mucocutaneous lesions of endocarditis are petechiae. They most often appear on the plantar surface of the toes and fingertips, as well as the conjunctival and buccal mucosa (see Fig. 80.1B). They may be larger and more irregular in outline than conventional petechiae and sometimes have a white or even pustular center. Conjunctival petechiae commonly occur in patients on cardiopulmonary bypass [75], so it is necessary to record their presence or absence on first encounter with a patient after cardiac surgery and to interpret only those that develop under observation. The same necessity applies to subungual splinter hemorrhages, which are so commonly a result of trauma that many patients will have one or two on admission; only those which appear subsequently, while the patient is at rest in the hospital, have diagnostic usefulness [76].

Osler's nodes and Janeway lesions favor the plantar and palmar surfaces but are uncommon in recent series of endocarditis. Osler's node is a painful, tender, bluish-purple nodular lesion located on the pads of the fingers or toes. The Janeway lesion is a painless, pink, nontender macular lesion that is located commonly on the palms or soles [76,77].

Fundoscopic examination may also show evidence of endocarditis. Showering of emboli often occurs, as in the patient whose findings are illustrated in Figure 80.1. The fingertip, subungual, conjunctival, and retinal lesions all developed the day after admission for acute staphylococcal endocarditis. Splenomegaly is found in nearly half of patients with subacute bacterial endocarditis and in very few of those with acute disease.

Laboratory Tests

The key to the diagnosis of endocarditis is blood cultures. Two or three separate blood cultures within a 24-hour interval are recommended based on early studies that showed that 99.3% of all septic episodes will be detected by the first two blood cultures [78]. Strict aseptic technique and optimal skin preparation should be used when collecting blood cultures and the blood cultures should be obtained prior to administration of antibiotics [78]. In adults, 20 to 30 mL of blood per culture is optimal [78]. In cases that appear to be culture negative [52,53,78], the advice of a clinical microbiologist should be sought regarding the need for special media, such as those adequate for the propagation of *Brucella* sp, *Bartonella* organisms, or other nonculture-based tests such as serology and molecular methods (see later). Prolonging the incubation of standard blood culture bottles beyond 7 days has not been demonstrated to be necessary for successful recovery of HACEK organisms, nor does it significantly improve diagnostic yield of other fastidious pathogens [78–80].

Diphtheroids and CoNS should not be disregarded as skin contaminants if isolated repeatedly; they are well reported as causes of endocarditis. A particularly troublesome problem is the recovery of CoNS of different colony types or susceptibility patterns from different blood cultures. This is not necessarily evidence for multiple contaminated cultures because the pattern can be observed in true coagulase-negative staphylococcal endocarditis.

Fungal endocarditis has increased in frequency. Fungi most commonly isolated include *Candida albicans*, non-albicans species of *Candida*, *Aspergillus* sp, and *Histoplasma* sp [56,81]. In a recent review, emerging fungi accounted for 25% of cases [81]. In patients with fungal endocarditis, the overall frequency of positive blood cultures is 54% [81]. In cases of endocarditis caused by *Candida* sp, the percentage of positive blood cultures may be as high as 83% to 95% if appropriate methods are used [78].

Current commercially available routine manual and automated blood culture systems are usually able to recover yeasts within 5 to 7 days of incubation. The best chances for recovery of filamentous fungi such as *Aspergillus* or *Histoplasma* require the use of the lysis centrifugation method (Isolator, Wampole Laboratories, Cranbury, NJ) [78]. Premortem microbiologic diagnosis may often be made by culture and special histologic stains of large arterial emboli or cardiac vegetations [53,81].

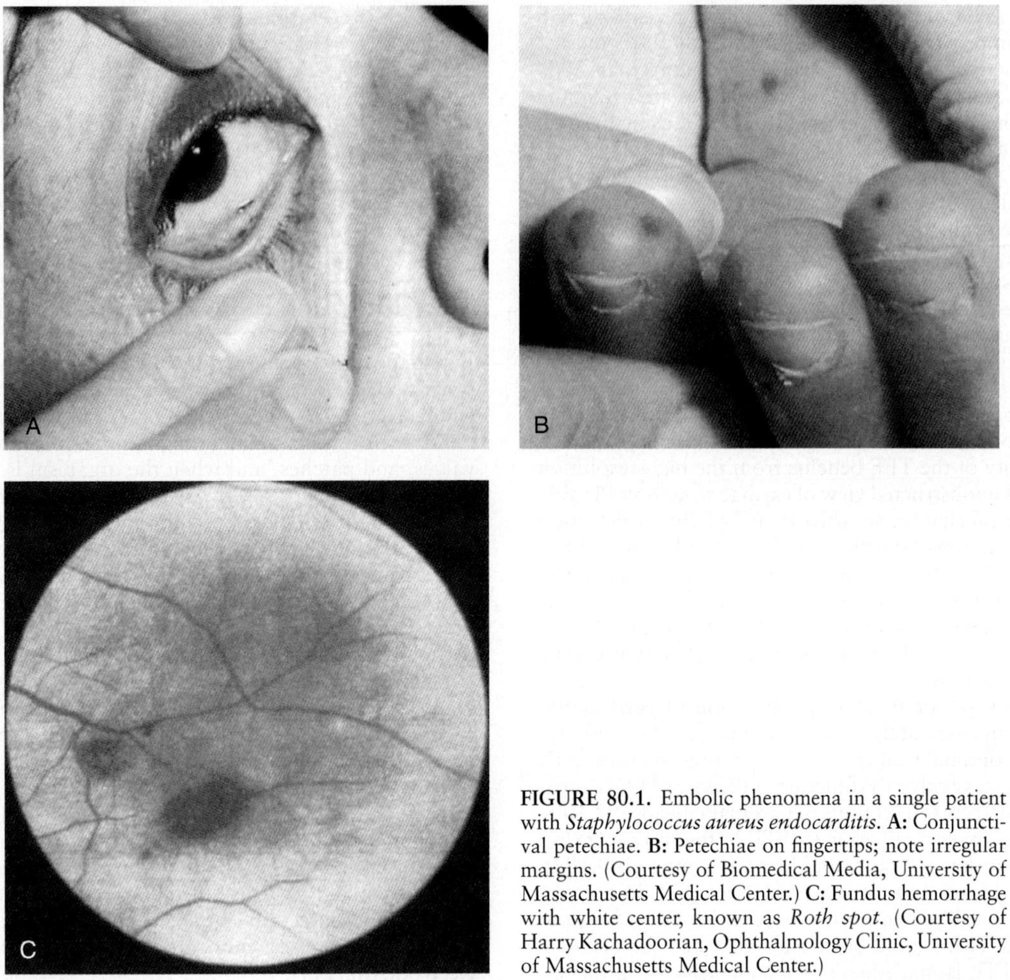

FIGURE 80.1. Embolic phenomena in a single patient with *Staphylococcus aureus endocarditis*. **A:** Conjunctival petechiae. **B:** Petechiae on fingertips; note irregular margins. (Courtesy of Biomedical Media, University of Massachusetts Medical Center.) **C:** Fundus hemorrhage with white center, known as *Roth spot*. (Courtesy of Harry Kachadoorian, Ophthalmology Clinic, University of Massachusetts Medical Center.)

Noncultivatable or difficult to cultivate organisms may be detected by serologic or molecular studies. Such organisms include *C. burnetii*, the agent of Q-fever endocarditis, *Chlamydia* sp, *Bartonella* sp, and some fungi [49–53,81,82]. Timely inclusion of serologic studies, particularly in environments where Q fever, *Brucella*, and *Bartonella* sp are prevalent, can enhance the definitive diagnosis of cases of endocarditis as demonstrated in the studies by Raoult et al. [53,83].

Molecular techniques such as polymerase chain reaction and sequence analysis of the amplified DNA have been applied both to blood cultures and to valvular tissue removed at the time of surgery [53,84,85]. Several studies have demonstrated the utility of these methods in assessing patients with high pretest probability of endocarditis but who have negative blood cultures by standard methods. Many of these studies are well summarized in the review by Syed et al. [84]. Advantages include high sensitivity, rapid results, and accurate identification. Limitations include potential for contamination and lack of an organism to test for antimicrobial susceptibility [53,84,85].

Other Diagnostic Tests

The electrocardiogram (ECG) is the simplest test for evaluation of perivalvular extension of infection in endocarditis [86]. Persistent (2 to 3 days) prolongation of the PR interval in the absence of digitalis toxicity, new persistent bundle-branch block, or complete heart block is quite specific for predicting extension into myocardial or aortic root tissue and the subsequent need for surgery [86]. However, the absence of PR prolongation does not rule out perivalvular extension.

Echocardiography plays an essential role in the diagnosis and management of IE and should be performed in all cases of suspected endocarditis [87]. Current roles for echocardiography include (a) diagnosis of IE by demonstration of vegetations, (b) characterization of underlying valvular disease, (c) clarification of the destructive nature of endocarditis, (d) assessment of the persistently febrile patient for evidence of perivalvular extension of infection, and (e) assessment of valvular function in PVE.

Studies performed in the period between 1988 and 1998 demonstrated that transthoracic two-dimensional (2D) echocardiography (TTE) has an overall sensitivity of vegetation detection of 50%, with a range of 14% to 78% in published series [88–90]. Sensitivity is affected by vegetation size, with 25% of vegetations less than 5 mm and 70% between 6 and 10 mm detected [91]. Obesity, chronic lung disease, and thoracic deformity may preclude obtaining the high-quality images needed to detect vegetations in as many as 30% of patients [91,92]. Equivocal results due to thickening or myxomatous degeneration of native valves and artifact from prosthetic valves are problems with TTE [89,92]. Diagnostic yield is also influenced by experience and skill of the person performing the procedure and the pretest probability of endocarditis. TTE has very limited ability to detect valve perforations and abscess extension, especially on prosthetic heart valves. Recent technological advances such as harmonic imaging and digital processing and storage have improved TTE image quality [84,93]. At least one report describes improved sensitivity to more than 80% using contemporary TTE [93]. Likewise studies are beginning to emerge on the improved performance of TTE using live/real time three-dimensional (3D) probes and ultrasound systems, but these have yet to be evaluated in large series [84,94].

Transesophageal echocardiography (TEE) is a significant advance in the evaluation of the patient with IE [84,89,95]. Unlike TTE, TEE has a high negative predictive value in patients with suspect native valve endocarditis (86% to 97%) [84,89,95]. Despite the somewhat invasive nature of TEE, the procedure is quite safe when performed by a skilled physician, with interruption of the procedure or complications occurring less than 1% of the time [96]. Relative contraindications include esophageal diseases, severe atlantoaxial joint disease, prior irradiation to the chest, and perforated viscus [97].

Image quality of the TEE benefits from the high-resolution transducer and unobstructed view of cardiac structures [86,89–92]. The TEE is much more sensitive than TTE for the detection of valvular vegetations; sensitivity with current biplane TEE is 90%, with vegetations as small as 1 mm being seen [96,98–100]. Early studies on 3D TEE demonstrate the potential of this technology to enhance localization of vegetations [101]. Like the situation with 3D TTE, however, large series demonstrating superiority are lacking.

TEE is also superior to TTE for detection of perivalvular abscess, with approximately 87% sensitivity [88,98]. TEE appears to be the optimal tool to detect vegetations on prosthetic valves and to assess valve dysfunction. Likewise, TEE is superior to TTE in detecting infections of pacemaker leads [92,100–103]. TEE also appears superior to TTE in the intraoperative assessment of cardiac structure and hemodynamics [100,102]. The American Heart Association Guidelines [87] do not recommend TEE for all patients with suspected endocarditis, but do suggest that TEE should be considered when the diagnostic quality of TTE is inadequate or inconclusive or in the situations described earlier where TEE is clearly superior [87]. Other applications of TEE are summarized in several recent reviews [87,103,104–106].

The European Society of Cardiology practice guidelines recommend the use of echocardiography in the evaluation of patients suspected on clinical grounds as follows [107]. Patients with native valves should be screened initially by TTE. If the study images are deemed of good quality and clinical suspicion is low, then in the presence of a negative TTE, other diagnoses should be considered. If the suspicion is high, TEE should be performed when TTE is negative.

In suspected PVE and when the TTE is positive and/or when complications are suspected (e.g., the patient has a highly virulent organism in blood cultures), TEE should be performed. If TEE is negative and suspicion remains, the TEE should be repeated in 7 days. Repeatedly negative studies exclude the diagnosis of IE [107]. Some investigators advocate that if the pretest probability is high (ranging from 4% to 60%), it is more cost-effective to proceed directly to TEE as the first and only study [108].

Some investigators have attempted to determine cost-effective uses of echocardiography for patients with suspected endocarditis [108,109]. In determination of duration of therapy for catheter-associated *S. aureus* bacteremia (SAB), TEE is probably most cost-effective when used to stratify patients to short (2 weeks) or long (4 weeks) course therapy, when long-course therapy would have otherwise been chosen for an at-risk, native valve population without immunocompromise [109].

The prognostic implications of vegetations identified by echocardiographic studies remain controversial. Some recent studies have indicated an increased risk of embolization in patients with vegetations greater than or equal to 10 mm in size, particularly in patients with mitral valve disease [105,106]. Still others have found that the predictive value of size for embolization depended on the organism and the mobility of the vegetation [105,106,110]. Most investigators agree that the presence of a vegetation alone is not an independent indication for valve replacement [105,106]. However, echocardiography may be useful for stratifying patients to high-risk subgroups where early surgery should be considered [105,106,110].

DIFFERENTIAL DIAGNOSIS

By far, the most common difficulty confronting the present-day practitioner is deciding which episodes of bacteremia represent endocarditis. The question becomes particularly acute in patients with intravascular foreign bodies, such as pacemakers, valves, and patches, and when the organism is *S. aureus*. The approach to this problem must take into account the propensity for the foreign body to become infected, the propensity of the organism to cause endocarditis, and the duration of bacteremia. Because sustained bacteremia characterizes infection of endovascular sites, the longer the bacteremia lasts, the greater the concern for an endothelial origin. In addition, even if the origin is distant and known, the longer the organisms circulate, the greater is the risk that they have settled out and seeded the intravascular foreign body secondarily.

Prosthetic valves, both mechanical and of biologic origin, have a very high risk of becoming infected, whereas permanent pacemakers (PPMs), once endothelialized, appear to carry a relatively low risk. Infection usually occurs at the skin-catheter junction and thus is most likely to invade the circulation when the vessel is in close proximity to the skin wound. However, in patients with a PPM, sustained bacteremia without an obvious focus implies infection of the pacemaker electrode, the tricuspid valve, or fibrotic endocardial regions in contact with the electrode tip [111].

Enteric Gram-negative bacilli are among the most common blood culture isolates at most hospitals but are less common as a cause of endocarditis (see Table 80.1). Notable exceptions to this characterization of enteric Gram-negative bacilli are salmonellae, particularly *S. typhimurium* and *S. choleraesuis*, which seem to have an affinity for damaged vascular endothelium and have infected aortic aneurysms as well as cardiac devices [112]. AIDS patients older than 50 years who develop salmonella bacteremia in the setting of predisposing valvular disease appear to be at particular risk for endocarditis [48,113].

Nosocomial bacteremia with Gram-negative bacilli has been shown to constitute a risk for development of PVE. Fang et al. [114] found that 26% of new cases of PVE occurred in patients who developed nosocomial Gram-negative bacteremia, in most cases from an identifiable portal of entry. Thus, patients with Gram-negative bacteremia in the setting of a prosthetic valve should receive antibiotic therapy adequate for possible endocarditis.

SAB always raises the question of whether treatment as endocarditis is warranted. A classic study reported that 64% of all bacteremias with *S. aureus* from 1940 to 1954 represented endocarditis, proved by autopsy in 38% of cases [115]. A subsequent report from the same center defined 16% of 134 patients with SAB from 1975 to 1977 as having definite or probable endocarditis [116]. These and other studies have amply demonstrated the ability of *S. aureus* to produce endocarditis on a valve previously presumed normal and have shown that established endocarditis may be found at postmortem examination in patients in whom no murmur was ever heard during their lifetime [43,115]. The changing demographics of staphylococcal endocarditis have been discussed in detail in the "Etiology" section of this chapter.

The absence of a primary focus appears to be a powerful predictor of endocarditis in community-acquired staphylococcal bacteremia [43,117]. Injection drug users are also at high risk for endocarditis and metastatic abscesses, and SAB should be treated in a fashion appropriate to endocarditis whenever it occurs in this group.

TEE has been valuable in identifying which patients have endocarditis in the setting of staphylococcal bacteremia [40,109,118]. IE has been shown to be clinically occult in a high proportion of patients with staphylococcal bacteremia [119]. Several studies support the use of a 2-week course of antibiotic therapy for catheter-associated SAB in patients at low risk for endocarditis. This would include patients without valvular heart disease (or prosthetic valves) and in whom the catheter has been removed promptly, subsequent blood cultures are negative, defervescence occurred within 72 hours, and TEE is normal [109,118,120]. Failures may still occur in patients assessed as low risk using these criteria in up to 16% of cases [120], with a range of 5% to 24% of patients with catheter-associated bacteremia presenting with recurrences, usually within 10 weeks of discontinuing therapy [121,122]. Clearly, patients who have prolonged fever or bacteremia after catheter removal should receive the longer course of antibiotic therapy because of the high mortality with catheter-associated *S. aureus* endocarditis [41,121,122]. All patients with SAB whether treated with short or longer courses of therapy should be followed closely for at least 3 months following treatment, preferably by an infectious diseases specialist [123].

The overall mortality rate for staphylococcal endocarditis in one multicenter study ranged from 16.7% to 23.7% [41]. Overall mortality rates of 36% to 48% have been reported in the last decade [124]. In contrast, human immunodeficiency virus (HIV)–seronegative parenteral drug users with this disease have a 2% to 4% mortality rate, although considerable morbidity, including congestive heart failure, occurs in 23% [124]. The more favorable outcome of addicts is generally attributed to their younger age and absence of underlying systemic illness, as well as the location of their valve involvement (right-sided valvular disease). In the HIV-seropositive injection drug user, mortality is related to the degree of immunosuppression [125]. In one study, in patients with CD4 counts of 200 or more, there was no difference in mortality between HIV-positive and HIV-negative individuals and mortality was directly related to the valve involved [124].

The epidemiology of enterococcal bacteremia has also changed [126]. Enterococci have emerged as major causes of healthcare-associated infections and in so doing have become increasingly resistant to antimicrobial agents, most importantly the penicillins, aminoglycosides, and glycopeptides [16,126–128]. Frequently, the enterococcus occurs in polymicrobial bacteremic infections along with enteric Gram-negative bacilli [128]. Mortality attributed to bacteremia is high, ranging from 13% to 42%, and seems to correlate directly with the severity of underlying illness as well as with antimicrobial resistance [128,129]. Higher mortality rates are seen among patients infected with strains that have high-level aminoglycoside resistance and resistance to vancomycin [128–130].

Two case series of patients with enterococcal bacteremia examined the risk factors for development of endocarditis [126,127]. These studies refute previous reports that nosocomial bacteremia and polymicrobial infections with enterococci are rarely associated with endocarditis. In both studies, *E. faecalis* was the predominant enterococcal species. Approximately 60% of the patients had nosocomial infections and polymicrobial bacteremia varied from 17% to 37%. Factors that were significantly associated with endocarditis included three or more positive blood cultures, the presence of a prosthetic valve, underlying valvular disease, and infection with *E. faecalis* [126,127].

INFECTIONS OF CARDIOVASCULAR IMPLANTABLE ELECTRONIC DEVICES: PACEMAKERS, AUTOMATIC IMPLANTABLE CARDIOVERTER DEFIBRILLATORS, AND VENTRICULAR-ASSIST DEVICES

Cardiovascular implantable electronic devices (CIEDs) are essential in the management of cardiac disease, and their use has increased significantly in the United States [131]. A recent population-based survey on the use of CIEDs reported that 70% of device recipients are elderly and many of these patients have multiple coexisting illnesses placing them at risk for CIED infections [132]. Despite improvements in the technology and greater ease of implantation, CIED infections appear to be increasing with the probability of infection being higher among patients with implantable cardioverter defibrillators (ICDs) than with PPMs [131,133].

Several recent studies have identified risk factors for PPM infection including long-term corticosteroid use, the presence of more than 2 pacing leads versus 2 leads, fever within 24 hours of implantation, early reinterventions, and the use of temporary pacing before the implantation [134,135]. Other patients at risk include those individuals with diabetes mellitus, renal dysfunction, heart failure, and oral anticoagulant use [131]. All of the above studies show a lowered risk of infection when patients are given perioperative antimicrobial prophylaxis [131,134,135].

Infections of pacemakers can be divided into the following distinct syndromes:

1. Generator pocket infections, which tend to occur within 2 months of surgery and are usually caused by *S. aureus*.
2. Infections associated with the lead wire and electrode, which generally present months later and more typically are caused by CoNS.
3. Endocarditis, which usually follows contiguous spread of infection along the pacer system.

Local erythema, erosion over the generator site, or drainage characterizes pocket infections, whereas electrode infections and endocarditis present more typically with sepsis and sustained bacteremia. In cases of pacemaker endocarditis, TEE is a useful diagnostic tool for defining the pacemaker as the source of bacteremia by visualizing vegetations on the leads or the tricuspid valve [103,136].

Infections that involve pacemaker wires and electrodes are almost never cured with antibiotics alone, and the entire system should be removed [131,136]. This usually can be accomplished in a one-stage procedure in which the old system is removed and the new system placed at a site remote from the infection (usually the contralateral side), followed by a course of antibiotics [131]. However, new lead placement should probably be delayed until blood cultures have been negative for 72 hours in cases of bacteremia [131]. The optimal duration of antimicrobial therapy depends upon the extent of infection and whether bacteremia is present. Short-course therapy following extraction is possible with infections confined to the pacer pocket and in the absence of bacteremia, whereas much longer duration of treatment is essential in patients with bacteremia. Patients with SAB and no obvious source should have all hardware removed. Guidelines for management are discussed in detail in reference [131].

Removal of the old system may not always be easy to accomplish. Sometimes defective or infected electrodes become firmly enclosed by fibrous tissue and are adherent to the vessel endothelium, precluding easy extraction through the venous system. Removal of a retained wire using traction devices has been successful in some instances, but serious complications such as avulsion of the tricuspid valve and creation of atrioventricular fistulae have been reported [136].

Specialized tools have been developed to remove leads from fibrotic tissue. The newest technologies are laser sheath devices. These consist of a hollow core that slides over the lead. An optical device at the proximal end of the core inserted into a laser generates pulses of ultraviolet light at various calibrated intensities. An outer sheath is loaded onto the laser sheath core prior to the procedure [137]. A multicenter study reviewed the experience with laser sheath extraction in the United States where 1,684 patients (2,561 leads) were treated with a laser sheath [137]. Complete success, defined as removal of all lead material from the vasculature, was seen in 90% of the patients. There was complete failure of lead extraction in 7% of the procedures attempted. Major complications such as tamponade and hemothorax were seen in 1.9% of patients with death occurring in 10 cases, and 1.4% of patients experienced a "minor" complication such as perforation or myocardial avulsion. The most predictive factor in failure to remove a lead by this procedure was lead implant duration of more than 10 years. Cardiopulmonary bypass surgery with dissection of the electrode is recommended for patients who can tolerate surgery when the measures discussed earlier are not successful [136].

Infection is one of the most serious complications of automatic implantable cardioverter defibrillators (AICDs). Infection rates of older AICDs, in which one of the electrodes is a surgically implanted epicardial patch, range from 1% to 7% [138]. Early infections typically involve the generator pocket and are caused by *S. aureus* [138]. Late infections tend to involve the patch with resultant purulent pericarditis, usually caused by CoNS and corynebacteria [139]. There is now agreement that these infections, whether early or late, require removal of the entire system [131,139]. Radical debridement of the pericardium is necessary if infection extends beyond the electrode patch capsule [139]. Prolonged antibiotic therapy (i.e., 6 weeks) follows these procedures. Reimplantation of the generator following disinfection and appropriate gas sterilization using new electrodes and wires after the patient has been on antibiotic therapy for 2 weeks has been successful [138] but is not recommended [131].

More recent AICDs use intracardiac defibrillating electrodes placed transvenously; management of infections involving these systems is similar to that of PPMs [131].

Ventricular-assist devices have revolutionized the management of patients with end-stage cardiac pump failure. They may be used temporarily in patients who are expected to have recovery of natural heart function, as a "bridge" in the group who are awaiting cardiac transplantation and more recently for destination therapy in patients ineligible for transplantation [140]. A ventricular-assist device consists of an encased pumping chamber usually placed in a preperitoneal or intra-abdominal position, a driveline tunneled to an exit point in the lower quadrant, and inflow and outflow conduits with unidirectional valves attached with a Dacron graft to the left ventricular apex and the ascending aorta, respectively [140].

Incidence of infection following left ventricular assist device (LVAD) implantation ranges from 18% to 59% and most infections occur between 2 weeks and 2 months of implantation [140]. Infections range in severity from local driveline exit site infection to pocket infection and bacteremia. The most serious of these infections is LVAD endocarditis, defined as infection of the LVAD surface or valves associated with persistent bacteremia or fungemia [140]. Clinical features include persistent fever, cachexia, septic cerebral embolization, and device failure [140,141]. Pathogens are typical nosocomial organisms such as *S. epidermidis*, *S. aureus*, enterococci, *Candida* sp, *Pseudomonas aeruginosa*, and other Gram-negative bacilli [140]. Mortality with LVAD endocarditis is high, approaching 50% in one series [141]. Treatment requires explantation of the device, prolonged antibiotics, and, often, emergent transplantation. Data indicate that patients with LVAD-related infections may be successfully transplanted, but reports are conflicting regarding posttransplantation survival [140]. Operative cultures and pathological examination of the LVAD at the time of transplantation can be used to guide therapy postoperatively [140].

TREATMENT

Treatment of IE encompasses antimicrobial therapy, close clinical monitoring, and the decision as to whether and when surgical intervention should be undertaken. In a consecutive series of patients admitted to medical intensive care units at a single hospital in France between 1993 and 2000, the in-hospital mortality rate was 45% (102 of 228) [142]. In an international collaborative study on native valve endocarditis managed between 2000 and 2005 at 61 centers in 28 countries, the in-hospital mortality was 143 of 1,065 (13%) in patients with community-associated disease and 138 of 557 (25%) in patients with healthcare-associated infection [16]. Mortality in prosthetic-valve endocarditis is higher and ranges from 13% to 45% [143]. In the years since 2000, antimicrobial resistance has increased among the usual causative organisms, particularly staphylococci and enterococci, increasing the challenge of treating these infections.

Antimicrobial Therapy

Antimicrobials used to treat IE must provide bactericidal activity in the bloodstream, bathing the infected vegetation and heart valve, since neither possesses an intrinsic vascular supply, and bacteria within the vegetation may be shielded by the surrounding fibrin–platelet thrombus. Certain organisms also produce a slime around indwelling devices that provides a further barrier to antimicrobial penetration and alters killing conditions. In vitro and animal model systems can suggest potential approaches to therapy, but clinical outcomes are the final arbiter of whether a particular drug or combination of drugs works in endocarditis. There have been very few controlled clinical trials [144–147]. Rather, regimens have been evaluated by comparing cure rates to those expected. In the clearest case, "Bacteriologic cure rates $\geq$98% may be anticipated in patients who complete 4 weeks of therapy with parenteral penicillin or ceftriaxone for endocarditis caused by highly penicillin-susceptible viridans group streptococci or *S. bovis* group" [87]. For other etiologies of IE, the expectation of success in therapy is less uniform. Extensive reviews of published data and the clinical wisdom of experts in the field provide the basis for therapeutic recommendations in various guidelines ([87], United States; [107], Europe; [148], United Kingdom).

In the following discussion, we review the major US recommendations [87], but urge that the reader consult the most up-to-date version of them at the time of need and take care to note the specifics of the organism, valve type, and dosing recommendations (see reference [87] for Web site address). As an example, for the highly penicillin-susceptible viridans group streptococci or *S. bovis* mentioned above (penicillin MIC $\leq$0.12 μg per mL), the dose of aqueous crystalline penicillin G is 12 to 18 million units IV divided into four to six daily doses, or ceftriaxone 2 g IV may be given as a single daily dose. A randomized controlled trial has shown that the addition of gentamicin, 3 mg per kg IV once daily, given in close temporal proximity to the dose of the cell-wall active agent (penicillin or ceftriaxone), can reduce the duration of treatment to 2 weeks in patients without cardiac complications or extracardiac sites of infection [144]. For prosthetic valve infection, 6-week therapy with the cell-wall active agent is recommended, and gentamicin is optional. For strains with MIC greater than 0.12 but less than or equal to 0.5 μg per mL, the penicillin dose is higher (18 to 24 million units per day), short-course therapy is not an option, and gentamicin is recommended for the first 2 weeks in native valve endocarditis and for the entire 6-week course in prosthetic valve disease. Ampicillin, 2 g IV every 4 hours, may be used in place of penicillin in all of the above. Vancomycin is recommended for patients with endocarditis due to these organisms only if they are unable to tolerate penicillin or ceftriaxone, in which case gentamicin is not given. The vancomycin dose is 15 mg per kg IV every 12 hours, adjusted to yield peak levels of 30 to 45 μg per mL and trough levels of 10 to 15 μg per mL (and is the same for all other organisms causing endocarditis). Desensitization to a β-lactam antibiotic, rather than use of vancomycin, should be strongly considered in patients with anaphylactic β-lactam allergies.

Most centers must now use vancomycin as the initial therapy for suspected *S. aureus* infection, despite slower killing and inferior clinical response, due to the frequency of oxacillin resistance both in healthcare-associated and community-acquired strains. Empiric vancomycin should be changed to nafcillin or oxacillin, 2 g IV every 4 hours (or cefazolin, 2 g IV every 8 hours, for patients with nonanaphylactoid type of β-lactam hypersensitivity) when *S. aureus* is determined to be susceptible to oxacillin; desensitization to oxacillin or nafcillin should be strongly considered in patients with anaphylactic β-lactam allergies. Controlled trials have shown that the addition of gentamicin does not improve outcome in native valve *S. aureus* endocarditis [145–147]. Recent data also suggest that even short courses of low doses of gentamicin are associated with nephrotoxicity in patients with SAB and endocarditis, particularly in patients with any degree of baseline renal dysfunction, advanced age, or diabetes [149]. If gentamicin is used at all, it should be given only for the first 3 to 5 days, in two or three equally divided doses totaling 3 mg per kg per 24 hours [87]. However, gentamicin is recommended for the first 2 weeks of therapy of PVE caused by gentamicin-susceptible staphylococci. If the organism is gentamicin resistant but susceptible to a fluoroquinolone, then a fluoroquinolone should be used for PVE. Rifampin has a special role in PVE because of its ability to sterilize devices (probably due to activity within the slime) and 300 mg by mouth (preferred) or IV every 8 hours should be given for the entirety of the course, if the isolate is susceptible. The usual duration of therapy for *S. aureus* endocarditis is 4 weeks for uncomplicated cases, 6 weeks for complicated cases, and 6 or more weeks for PVE, although a 2-week course of nafcillin or oxacillin can be used in selected cases of native valve *S. aureus* endocarditis limited to the right side of the heart [87].

For MRSA endocarditis, vancomycin is still the current first-line recommendation. Daptomycin is an alternative therapy based on a recent trial that found that daptomycin was not inferior to standard therapy (as described earlier) for SAB and right-sided endocarditis [150]. The dose studied was 6 mg per kg daily, although some experts recommend consideration of high doses of 8 to 12 mg per kg daily for endocarditis because of the finding that 5% of patients in the daptomycin arm had emergence of reduced susceptibility to daptomycin during treatment [150,151,151A]. However, it is unknown whether higher doses of daptomycin prevent emergence of resistance or improve outcomes. The addition of synergistic gentamicin is not thought to be more useful in this situation than for oxacillin-susceptible disease, and coadministration with vancomycin may increase toxicity. Addition of rifampin to vancomycin therapy is not recommended due to a lack of benefit on either survival or duration of bacteremia [152]. Although the optimal approach is unknown, for patients who do not respond to standard therapies, a variety of salvage approaches have been attempted including addition of or switches to agents such as trimethoprim/sulfamethoxazole, linezolid, and quinupristin/dalfopristin. CoNS, best known for causing prosthetic valve and other device infections, should be assumed to be oxacillin resistant until proven otherwise by rigorous testing (not available in all laboratories). The same antimicrobial regimens are recommended as for MRSA, although there are occasional reports of successful therapy with linezolid [153,154].

Enterococcal endocarditis is one instance where combination of penicillin, ampicillin, or vancomycin with either streptomycin or gentamicin is required for clinical efficacy [155]. With the exception of piperacillin, other cell-wall active agents (oxacillin, nafcillin, ticarcillin, aztreonam, cephalosporins, cephamycins, and meropenem) cannot be used for this purpose, nor can the other aminoglycosides. The penicillin dose is 18 to 30 million units per day administered either as a continuous infusion or as 3 to 5 million units IV every 4 hours. The ampicillin dose is 2 g IV every 4 hours. Either of these agents should be used in preference to vancomycin unless the organism is resistant or the patient cannot tolerate the β-lactam. Gentamicin is administered in three equally divided doses at 1 mg per kg or as required to achieve peak serum concentrations of 3 to 4 μg per mL and trough concentration of less than 1 μg per mL. For enterococci with high-level resistance (MIC $\geq$500 μg per mL) to gentamicin but not to streptomycin, streptomycin is given at a dose of 15 mg per kg IV or intramuscular every 12 hours. When combination therapy with a β-lactam and gentamicin or streptomycin is used for native valve endocarditis of less than 3 months' duration, the recommended duration for both components of therapy is 4 weeks. For disease of longer duration, prosthetic-valve involvement, or vancomycin-based therapy, treatment is prolonged to 6 weeks with both drugs. A report from Sweden describes success with aminoglycoside therapy given for a median of 15 days [156]; although the guidelines do not yet recommend that approach, they do point out that the information may help in deciding whether to continue an aminoglycoside in the face of nephro- or ototoxicity [87].

Enterococci with high-level resistance to streptomycin and gentamicin, as well as strains resistant to penicillin and/or vancomycin, pose additional challenges for treatment. Resistance to ampicillin and penicillin mediated by β-lactamases may be overcome by the use of ampicillin–sulbactam, 3 g IV every 6 hours for 6 weeks. Testing at high inocula may be necessary to detect inducible β-lactamases; these organisms are frequently high-level resistant to streptomycin and gentamicin as well, in which case the duration of ampicillin–sulbactam therapy should be extended beyond 6 weeks. Double β-lactam combinations (ampicillin plus either ceftriaxone or imipenem) may provide synergistic activity in some cases of high-level aminoglycoside resistance but should be supported by in vitro studies using the patient's isolate [87,157]. Enterococci with intrinsic penicillin resistance are treated with vancomycin plus gentamicin for 6 weeks.

Endocarditis due to vancomycin-resistant enterococci (VRE) warrants infectious disease consultation and may require specialized laboratory investigation [87,107,148]. A recent review identified 19 reported cases, 14 of whom survived [158]. Three patients had organisms susceptible to ampicillin and with high-level susceptibility to gentamicin; all of these responded to combination therapy with those two drugs (one patient also had valve replacement). The others received a variety of regimens directed by the susceptibility of their organisms; four had surgery. The surprisingly high survival in this series may reflect a bias toward reporting successful outcomes, but there was also considerable use of newer agents. Daptomycin has in vitro activity against VRE, and time–kill curves demonstrated synergy with gentamicin and rifampin in a case where that combination was used [158]. Quinupristin–dalfopristin is active only against *E. faecium*, and in this series was never the sole component of successful therapy [158]. The guidelines note that quinupristin–dalfopristin was effective in 4 out of 9 patients with endocarditis [87], but the compassionate-plea program reported clinical and bacteriologic response in only 2 out of 10 (0 of 1 evaluable) patients [159]. Linezolid 600 mg IV or orally every 12 hours proved successful in 10 (77%) of 13 evaluable cases of VRE endocarditis (9 courses of therapy were not evaluable) [160].

First-choice therapy for HACEK endocarditis is ceftriaxone 2 g IV every 24 hours (or other third- or fourth-generation cephalosporin) for 4 weeks in native valve disease and 6 weeks with prosthetic valves. Ampicillin–sulbactam may be used, but the combination of ampicillin and gentamicin is no longer recommended. Therapeutic failures with this combination in *A. actinomycetemcomitans* endocarditis include a nearly 30% mortality in one series [161,162]. Ciprofloxacin at 500 mg orally every 12 hours or 400 mg IV every 8 hours is the suggested alternative for patients who cannot tolerate ceftriaxone or ampicillin–sulbactam.

The choice of empiric therapy while awaiting results of blood cultures should reflect the clinical presentation and epidemiologic risks of the patient. Patients who present with acute native valve endocarditis should receive treatment appropriate for *S. aureus* and possibly enterococcus, whereas those with subacute presentation should be treated for viridans group streptococci and HACEK organisms, as well as the possibility of *S. aureus*. The European guidelines provide the clearest guidance for this situation and specify vancomycin plus gentamicin for native valve endocarditis requiring urgent therapy, or when cultures remain negative, and vancomycin, rifampin, and gentamicin for PVE [107]. However, as previously mentioned, the use of gentamicin must be weighed against the potential for increased nephrotoxicity [149]. The U.S. guidelines recommend addition of cefepime (2 g every 8 hours IV) in culture-negative PVE with onset within 2 months of surgery, directed at nosocomially acquired Gram-negative bacilli [87], and that possibility should also be considered in the choice of empiric therapy. For late-onset disease on prosthetic valves, many would concur with a recommendation for therapy appropriate for MRSA (vancomycin, rifampin, and gentamicin) with the possible addition of ceftriaxone [87].

When culture-negative endocarditis more likely represents infection with a fastidious or noncultivable organism than antibiotic interference with blood cultures, treatment directed against *Bartonella* (gentamicin plus doxycycline) should be added to ceftriaxone (for native valve disease) [87]. In the United Kingdom and Europe, Q fever (*C. burnetii*) causes a larger proportion of cases of endocarditis than in the United States, usually culture negative but proved by serology. Therapy for this pathogen is doxycycline plus ciprofloxacin or rifampin [107]. Duration of treatment is at least 3 years [148], perhaps lifelong after valve replacement [107]. *Candida* endocarditis has generally been regarded as an indication for valve replacement surgery, but often the patients who get this infection have been too ill for surgery. Factors associated with survival of some of these high-risk patients in the absence of cardiac surgery include receiving initial combination antifungal therapy (most often amphotericin B plus 5-flucytosine) followed by long-term suppressive therapy with fluconazole [163,164]. There are also case reports of good outcome in patients treated with caspofungin, including four who did not have valve replacement [165–167].

Supportive Care and Monitoring

Careful clinical monitoring of the patient on therapy for endocarditis includes surveillance for fever, evidence of congestive heart failure or other cardiac complication, metastatic infection, adverse effects of antimicrobial drugs (and levels, when appropriate), change in renal function, and superinfection. Repeat blood cultures should be obtained every 48 hours until they are repeatedly sterile. The duration of antimicrobial therapy is counted from the first day of sustained blood culture negativity [87]. In aortic and mitral valve endocarditis, serial ECGs should be obtained to look for prolongation of the PR interval or other conduction abnormality that would signal invasion of the interventricular septum by the infection. Echocardiographic imaging, should be repeated at 7 to 10 days into therapy, to look for enlarging vegetations or other complications and to better define disease in patients whose initial echocardiography was unrevealing. This study should also be repeated at the end of therapy as the patient's new baseline [87,107].

Recrudescence of fever after initial resolution most often indicates a new problem outside the heart, such as catheter-associated sepsis, drug fever, or antibiotic-associated *Clostridium difficile* colitis, but superinfection of the endocarditic valve may occur. Unless there is another immediately obvious cause, persistent or recurrent fever should prompt repeat echocardiography.

The possible need for cardiac surgery mandates discontinuation of warfarin and substitution of heparin when the diagnosis of endocarditis is made in patients on anticoagulant therapy for prosthetic valves or other indications [87,107]. Anticoagulation in endocarditis carries the risk of converting bland emboli (infarcts) to hemorrhagic ones, and thus should be carefully monitored and continued with caution. When emboli with hemorrhage occur, anticoagulant therapy should be withheld for a period of time. The risk of central nervous system (CNS) hemorrhage in *S. aureus* PVE is so high that some recommend discontinuation of all anticoagulation during the acute phase of this illness [168].

Role of Cardiac Surgery

At times, failure of antibiotics to sterilize the blood necessitates surgical debridement and removal of the infected focus—the valve. Even if bacteriologic cure is achieved, some patients have sufficient valvular damage that they will die of hemodynamic compromise unless a valve is replaced. The surprisingly favorable outcomes of a number of patients operated on in these desperate circumstances have led to consideration of cardiac surgery much earlier in the course of endocarditis [169–172]. The two indications for surgery already mentioned—microbiologic failure and congestive heart failure—are now well accepted. The challenge is to identify patients who would eventually meet these criteria before their clinical condition deteriorates.

Harbingers of microbiologic failure include difficult-to-treat and aggressive organisms, such as *S. lugdunensis*, *S. aureus*, *P. aeruginosa* or other Gram-negative bacilli involving the aortic or mitral valve, and fungi, particularly molds. *C. burnetii*, *Bartonella*, *Brucella*, and other unusual organisms associated with true culture-negative endocarditis are also difficult to eradicate with antimicrobial therapy alone. The risk of microbiologic failure or relapse is elevated in the presence of prosthetic material, resulting in the recommendation for valve replacement in most cases of early PVE and the necessity of removing infected intracardiac devices such as pacemakers and other CIEDs. Conventional blood cultures should become sterile within 7 days after the institution of appropriate antibiotic therapy [78,87,167,172]. The median time for clearance of *S. aureus* varies in different studies but may be as long as 9 days [146], placing this organism among those for which cardiac surgery should be considered. Patients should defervesce within 9 to 10 days. Persistent fever may indicate continued active infection, myocardial abscess, or embolic complication.

Many patients with endocarditis have preexisting congestive failure as a result of their underlying valvular disease, but new-onset or worsening heart failure carries an ominous prognosis—a mortality of 56% in one series [171]. Urgent surgery is indicated for these patients, and a number of authors have noted that medical stabilization may be impossible once severe progressive failure begins [171]. Acute aortic and mitral regurgitation, due to perforation, valve rupture, or paravalvular leak (in the case of PVE), are frequent mechanisms of congestive failure [172]. Valvular obstruction is less common but does occur on prosthetic valves and is an equally urgent indication for surgery. Rupture of sinus of Valsalva aneurysm into the right heart or pericardium also mandates surgery [173]. It cannot be overemphasized that once surgery is clearly indicated it should not be delayed, because of the unpredictability of the clinical course and the increasing risk of the operation as failure progresses [171,172,174].

Echocardiography may be very helpful in defining the presence of complications that do require surgery, including destruction of the valve or extension of infection beyond the valve ring as a myocardial abscess. Myocardial abscess may be the reason for prolonged fever [172,175], lead to conduction defects [86,172], or cavitate into the pericardium with resultant purulent pericarditis [172]. Myocardial abscess is generally an indication for surgery to extirpate all infected tissue as well as correct the accompanying hemodynamic abnormalities [87,107,172,173]. Occasionally, abscesses that are less than 1 cm, that do not progress on therapy, and that are not complicated by disruption of other structures may be followed with serial TEE and do not require surgery [87,172].

The risk of embolization is often viewed as an indication for surgery, but this risk diminishes greatly over the first 2 weeks of antimicrobial therapy [87,107,172,173]. In one recent large study, 56% of embolic events in 629 patients with IE occurred before hospital admission or on the day antibiotic treatment started [176], and in another, only 7.3% of 384 patients had new embolic events after the initiation of therapy [177]. The difficulty is in defining when there is sufficient risk of clinically significant systemic or cerebral embolization to justify cardiac surgery not required for any other reason but before serious target organ damage has already occurred. There have been many attempts to establish echocardiographic predictors of embolization; vegetation length more than 10 mm by TEE was associated with a ninefold increase in risk of systemic or cerebral embolization on therapy and "severe mobility," defined as "prolapsing vegetation that crosses the coaptation plane of the leaflets during the cardiac cycle," with a 2.4-fold increase [177]. The U.S. guidelines deem one or more embolic events during the first 2 weeks of therapy a class I indication for surgery (condition for which there is evidence, general agreement, or both that a given procedure or treatment is useful and effective) [87]. Anterior mitral valve leaflet vegetations, especially those greater than 10 mm, and the presence of persistent vegetations after systemic embolization are class IIa indications (the weight of evidence/opinion is in favor of usefulness/efficacy), but increase in size of vegetation despite therapy is less well established as an indication for surgery [87]. European guidelines advise consideration of surgery for recurrent emboli despite adequate antibiotic therapy or mobile vegetation greater than 10 mm before or during the first week of antibiotic therapy [107]. U.S. experts recommend delaying valve surgery for a minimum of 2 weeks after a CNS embolic event [87,172] and at least a month after CNS hemorrhage [172], but European guidelines suggest that surgery can be performed within the first 72 hours of CNS embolism if a computed tomographic scan of the brain performed immediately preoperatively shows no hemorrhage [107].

Right-sided endocarditis requires surgical intervention much less frequently than left-sided disease. Persistent fever for longer than 3 weeks is an indication for surgery, but pulmonary emboli are not [107,172]. In patients with isolated right-sided lesions, most often addicts, tricuspid vegetectomy, valve repair, or valvulectomy may permit cure of endocarditis due to resistant organisms without the risk of subsequent PVE. In the absence of pulmonary hypertension, tricuspid regurgitation may be tolerated without valve replacement [107,172].

The surgical approach for endocarditis is changing, with increasing interest in vegetectomy and valve repair rather than replacement. Repair is most often performed on the mitral valve and offers improved outcome over replacement [178,179]. Complete debridement of all infected tissue is mandatory. The European guidelines advocate consideration of early surgery for "kissing mitral vegetation," defined as secondary infection of the mitral valve by contact with a large aortic vegetation prolapsing during diastole, to preserve the structure and function of the native mitral valve, implying that the surgical procedure would be vegetectomy or valve repair, not replacement [107]. The reconstructive techniques developed for valve repair may also facilitate the surgical approach in cases with extensive perivalvular infection, where homografts and pericardial patches may be used to construct an annulus to which to attach a prosthetic valve when large amounts of normal tissue have been lost. The current view is that the risk of recurrent endocarditis on bioprosthetic and mechanical valve replacements is

TABLE 80.4

INDICATIONS FOR CONSIDERATION OF SURGERY IN PATIENTS WITH INFECTIVE ENDOCARDITIS

Indications	Evidence Grade
Congestive heart failure	I B
Fungal or highly resistant organisms	I B
Echocardiographic evidence of valve dehiscence, perforation, rupture, fistula, or large perivalvular abscess	I B
Mobile vegetation >10 mm (particularly on the anterior leaflet of the MV) or persistent vegetation after systemic embolization	IIa B
Increase in vegetation size on appropriate therapy	IIb C

I, evidence or general agreement that cardiac surgery is useful and effective; IIa, inconclusive or conflicting evidence or a divergence of opinion about the usefulness/efficacy of cardiac surgery, but weight of evidence/opinion of the majority is in favor; IIb, inconclusive or conflicting evidence or a divergence of opinion; lack of clear consensus on the basis of evidence/opinion of the majority; Level of evidence B, data derived from a single randomized trial or nonrandomized studies; Level of evidence C, consensus of opinion of experts; MV, mitral valve. Adapted from reference 87.

TABLE 80.5

SUMMARY RECOMMENDATIONS FOR MANAGEMENT OF ENDOCARDITIS BASED ON RANDOMIZED CLINICAL TRIALS

- Native valve endocarditis caused by highly penicillin-susceptible viridans streptococci or *Streptococcus bovis* is effectively treated with a 2-week regimen of ceftriaxone 2 g every 24 h IV with gentamicin 3 mg/kg/24 h IV given in a single dose [144]
- Addition of 2 weeks of gentamicin to 4 weeks of oxacillin or nafcillin therapy for methicillin-susceptible *Staphylococcus aureus* endocarditis does not improve outcome [145,146]
- Uncomplicated tricuspid valve endocarditis caused by methicillin-susceptible *Staphylococcus aureus* is effectively treated with a 2-week regimen of either nafcillin or oxacillin 12 g/24 h IV in 4 to 6 equally divided doses ([87], based on a trial comparing cloxacillin 2 g IV q4h with and without gentamicin 1 mg/kg IV q8h in injection drug users [147])

comparable, about 2% to 3% [87,107]. If valve cultures from surgery are negative, the duration of the antibiotic course originally planned should be completed, as long as it extends at least 7 to 15 days postoperatively. If intraoperative cultures are positive, the full recommended duration of antibiotics for the infecting organism should be administered counting from the day of surgery [87].

There is little difference in the clinical indications for surgery in native and PVE, but the proportion of patients requiring surgery is higher among those with prosthetic valves, approximately 50% [143,172,178,180–184]. Staphylococcal etiology and CNS embolization are uniformly identified as poor prognostic features. Early surgical intervention reduces the overall mortality of PVE [172,182,184]. More recent studies have identified patients with PVE in whom medical therapy has equivalent outcomes to surgery as those with late-onset streptococcal disease who have no significant heart failure, no new valvular regurgitation or other intracardiac complication, and no CNS or systemic embolization [144,180,181]. Most important is that cardiac surgical treatment reduces the mortality rate among patients with poor prognostic factors to the level experienced by the patients with more favorable disease characteristics [143].

Table 80.4 lists indications for surgery in patients with endocarditis by the strength of evidence supporting each indication [172,173,184]. Individual patient situations may modify the readiness to resort to surgery. For instance, in a patient with another condition that makes the risk of general anesthesia prohibitive, such as severe restrictive lung disease, one might elect to operate only in the event of congestive heart failure. The guidelines for surgical intervention are not absolute predictors of failure of medical management but overall can predict a low success rate.

Overall, therapy for endocarditis requires skillful manipulation of antibiotics and careful day-to-day judgment of the relative risks of expectant versus surgical management. It should be stressed that in cases with any adverse prognostic features, including all patients with staphylococcal or PVE, it is wise to make provisions for possible urgent surgery early in the course. This includes discussions of surgery with the patient and family and consultation with the cardiac surgical team. Table 80.5 provides a summary of recommendations for management of endocarditis supported by randomized controlled clinical trials.

References

1. Bouza E, Menasalvas A, Munoz P, et al: Infective endocarditis—a prospective study at the end of the twentieth century. New predisposing conditions, new etiologic agents, and still a high mortality. *Medicine (Baltimore)* 80:298, 2001.
2. Cabell CH, Jollis JG, Peterson GE, et al: Changing patient characteristics and the effect of mortality in endocarditis. *Arch Intern Med* 162:90, 2002.
3. Fefer P, Raveh D, Rudensky B, et al: Changing epidemiology of infective endocarditis: a retrospective survey of 108 cases, 1990–1999. *Eur J Clin Microbiol Infect Dis* 21:432, 2002.
4. Hoen B, Alla F, Selton-Suty C, et al: Changing profile of infective endocarditis: results of a 1-year survey in France. *JAMA* 288:75, 2002.
5. Millar BC, Moore JE: Emerging issues in infective endocarditis. *Emerg Infect Dis* 10:1110, 2004.
6. Moreillon P, Que YA: Infective endocarditis. *Lancet* 363:139, 2004.
7. Mouly S, Ruimy R, Launay O, et al: The changing clinical aspects of infective endocarditis: descriptive review of 90 episodes in a French teaching hospital and risk factors for death. *J Infect* 45:246, 2002.
8. de Sa DD, Tleyjeh IM, Anavekar NS, et al: Epidemiological trends of infection endocarditis: a population-based study in Olmsted County, Minnesota. *Mayo Clin Proc* 85:422, 2010.
9. Murdoch DR, Corey GR, Hoen B, et al: Clinical presentation, etiology and outcome of infective endocarditis in the 21st century: the International Collaboration on Endocarditis-Prospective Cohort Study. *Arch Intern Med* 169:463, 2009.
10. Armstrong ML, DeBoer S, Cetta F: Infective endocarditis after body art: a review of the literature and concerns. *J Adolesc Health* 43:217, 2008.
11. Cheng TO: Infective endocarditis, cardiac tamponade, and AIDS as serious complications of acupuncture [letter]. *Arch Intern Med* 164:1464, 2004.
12. Durante-Mangoni E, Bradley S, Selton-Suty C, et al: Current features of infective endocarditis in elderly patients: results of the International Collaboration on Endocarditis Prospective Cohort Study. *Arch Intern Med* 168:2095, 2008.
13. Kourany WM, Miro JM, Moreno A, et al: Influence of diabetes mellitus on the clinical manifestations and prognosis of infective endocarditis: a report from the International Collaboration on Endocarditis-Merged Database. *Scand J Infect Dis* 38:613, 2006.
14. Hogevik H, Olaison L, Andersson R, et al: Epidemiologic aspects of infective endocarditis in an urban population. A 5-year prospective study. *Medicine* 74:324, 1995.
15. Weng MC, Chang FY, Young TG, et al: Analysis of 109 cases of infective endocarditis in a tertiary care hospital. *Chin Med J* 58:18, 1996.
16. Benito N, Miro JM, de Lazzari E, et al: Health care-associated native valve endocarditis: importance of non nosocomial acquisition. *Ann Intern Med* 150:586, 2009.
17. Kamalakannan D, Pai RM, Johnson LB, et al: Epidemiology and clinical outcomes of infective endocarditis in hemodialysis patients. *Ann Thorac Surg* 83:2081, 2007.
18. Sandre RM, Shafran SD: Infective endocarditis: review of 135 cases over 9 years. *Clin Infect Dis* 22:276, 1996.
19. Ruttmann E, Bonatti H, Legit C, et al: Severe endocarditis in transplant recipients—an epidemiologic study. *Transpl Int* 18:690, 2005.
20. Sherman-Weber S, Axelrod P, Suh B, et al: Infective endocarditis following orthotopic heart transplantation: 10 cases and a review of the literature. *Transpl Infect Dis* 6:165, 2004.
21. Regules JA, Glasser JS, Wolfe SE, et al: Endocarditis in burn patients: clinical and diagnostic considerations. *Burns* 34:610, 2008.
22. Ben-Ami R, Giladi M, Carmeli Y, et al: Hospital-acquired infective endocarditis: should the definition be broadened? *Clin Infect Dis* 38:843, 2004.
23. Martin-Davila P, Fortun J, Navas E, et al: Nosocomial endocarditis in a tertiary hospital: an increasing trend in native valve cases. *Chest* 128:772, 2005.
24. Chang CF, Kuo BI, Chen TL, et al: Infective endocarditis in maintenance hemodialysis patients: fifteen years' experience in one medical center. *J Nephrol* 17:228, 2004.
25. Nucifora G, Badano LP, Viale P, et al: Infective endocarditis in chronic haemodialysis patients: an increasing clinical challenge. *Eur Heart J* 28:2307, 2007.
26. Durack DT, Lukes AS, Bright DK, et al: New criteria for the diagnosis of infective endocarditis: utilization of specific echocardiographic findings. Duke Endocarditis Service. *Am J Med* 96:200–209, 1994.
27. Siddiq S, Missri J, Silverman DI: Endocarditis in an urban hospital in the 1990s. *Arch Intern Med* 156:2454, 1996.

28. Olaison L, Hogevik H: Comparison of the von Reyn and Duke criteria for the diagnosis of infective endocarditis: a critical analysis of 161 episodes. *Scand J Infect Dis* 28:399, 1996.
29. Kjerulf A, Tvede M, Aldershvile J, et al: Bacterial endocarditis at a tertiary hospital—how do we improve diagnosis and delay of treatment? A retrospective study of 140 patients. *Cardiology* 89:79, 1998.
30. Kurland S, Enghoff E, Landelius J, et al: A 10-year retrospective study of infective endocarditis at a university hospital with special regard to the timing of surgical evaluation in *S. viridans* endocarditis. *Scand J Infect Dis* 31:87, 1999.
31. Woo PC, Tse H, Chan KM, et al: "*Streptococcus milleri*" endocarditis caused by *Streptococcus anginosus*. *Diagn Microbiol Infect Dis* 48:81, 2004.
32. Lefort A, Lortholary O, Casassus P, et al: Comparison between adult endocarditis due to beta-hemolytic streptococci (serogroups A, B, C, and G) and *Streptococcus milleri*: a multicenter study in France. *Arch Intern Med* 162:2450, 2002.
33. Liao CH, Teng LJ, Hsueh PR, et al: Nutritionally variant streptococcal infections at a University Hospital in Taiwan: disease emergence and high prevalence of *beta*-lactam and macrolide resistance. *Clin Infect Dis* 38:452, 2004.
34. Lin CH, Hsu RB: Infective endocarditis caused by nutritionally variant streptococci. *Am J Med Sci* 334:235, 2007.
35. Gallagher P, Watanakunakorn C: Group B streptococcal endocarditis: report of seven cases and review of the literature, 1962–1985. *Rev Infect Dis* 8:175, 1986.
36. Baddour LM: Infective endocarditis caused by β-hemolytic streptococci. Infectious Diseases society of America's Emerging Infections Network. *Clin Infect Dis* 26:66, 1998.
37. Beck M, Frodl R, Funke G: Comprehensive study of strains previously designated *Streptococcus bovis* consecutively isolated from human blood cultures and emended description of *Streptococcus gallolyticus* and *Streptococcus infantarius* subsp. *coli*. *J Clin Microbiol* 46:2966, 2008.
38. Hoen B, Chirouze C, Cabell CH, et al: Emergence of endocarditis due to group D streptococci: findings derived from the merged database of the International Collaboration on Endocarditis. *Eur J Clin Microbiol Infect Dis* 24:12, 2005.
39. Tripodi MF, Adinolfi LE, Ragone E, et al: *Streptococcus bovis* endocarditis and its association with chronic liver disease: an underestimated risk factor. *Clin Infect Dis* 38:1394, 2004.
40. Fowler VG, Sanders LL, Kong LK, et al: Infective endocarditis due to *Staphylococcus aureus*: 59 prospectively identified cases with follow-up. *Clin Infect Dis* 28:106, 1999.
41. Fowler VG, Miro JM, Hoen B, et al: *Staphylococcus aureus* endocarditis: a consequence of medical progress. *JAMA* 293:3012, 2005.
42. Nadji G, Remadi JP, Coviaux F, et al: Comparison of clinical and morphological characteristics of *Staphylococcus aureus* endocarditis with endocarditis caused by other pathogens. *Heart* 91:932, 2005.
43. Chang FY, MacDonald BB, Peacock JE, et al: A prospective multicenter study of *Staphylococcus aureus* bacteremia. Incidence of endocarditis, risk factors for mortality, and clinical impact of methicillin resistance. *Medicine (Baltimore)* 82:322, 2003.
44. Chu VH, Woods CW, Miro JM, et al: Emergence of coagulase-negative staphylococci as a cause of native valve endocarditis. *Clin Infect Dis* 46:232, 2008.
45. Frank KL, Del Pozo JL, Patel R: From clinical microbiology to infection pathogenesis: how daring to be different works for *Staphylococcus lugdunensis*. *Clin Microbiol Rev* 21:111, 2008.
46. Paturel L, Casalta JP, Habib G, et al: *Actinobacillus actinomycetemcomitans* endocarditis. *Clin Microbiol Infect* 10:98, 2004.
47. Morpeth S, Murdoch D, Cabell CH, et al: Non-HACEK gram-negative bacillus endocarditis. *Ann Intern Med* 147:829, 2007.
48. Aubron C, Charpentier J, Trouillet JL, et al: Native-valve infective endocarditis caused by *Enterobacteriaceae*: report of 9 cases and literature review. *Scand J Infect Dis* 38:873, 2006.
49. Avidor B, Graidy M, Efrat G, et al: *Bartonella koehlerae*, a new cat-associated agent of culture-negative human endocarditis. *J Clin Microbiol* 42:3462, 2004.
50. Dreier J, Vollmer T, Freytag CC, et al: Culture-negative infectious endocarditis caused by *Bartonella* spp.: 2 case reports and a review of the literature. *Diagn Microbiol Infect Dis* 61:476, 2008.
51. Raoult D, Fournier PE, Drancourt M, et al: Diagnosis of 22 new cases of *Bartonella* endocarditis. *Ann Intern Med* 125:646, 1996.
52. Houpikian P, Raoult D: Blood-culture-negative endocarditis in a reference center: etiologic diagnosis of 348 cases. *Medicine (Baltimore)* 84:162, 2005.
53. Fournier PE, Thuny F, Richet H, et al: Comprehensive diagnostic strategy for blood culture-negative endocarditis: a prospective study of 819 new cases. *Clin Infect Dis* 51:131, 2010.
54. Wilson LE, Thomas DL, Astemborski J, et al: Prospective study of infective endocarditis among injection drug users. *J Infect Dis* 185:1761, 2002.
55. Cooper HL, Brady JE, Ciccarone D, et al: Nationwide increase in the number of hospitalizations for illicit injection drug use-related infective endocarditis. *Clin Infect Dis* 45:1200, 2007.
56. Baddley JW, Benjamin DK, Patel M, et al: *Candida* infective endocarditis. *Eur J Clin Microbiol Infect Dis* 27:519, 2008.
57. Castillo JC, Anguita MP, Torres F, et al: Long-term prognosis of early and late prosthetic valve endocarditis. *Am J Cardiol* 93:1185, 2004.
58. Alonso-Valle H, Farinas-Alvarez C, Garcia-Palomo JD, et al: Clinical course and predictors of death in prosthetic valve endocarditis over a 20-year period. *J Thorac Cardiovasc Surg* 139:887, 2010.
59. Wright AJ, Wilson WR: Experimental animal endocarditis: *Mayo Clin Proc* 57:10, 1982.
60. Veltrop MH, Bancsi MJ, Bertina RM, et al: Role of monocytes in experimental *Staphylococcus aureus* endocarditis. *Infect Immun* 68:4818, 2000.
61. Frontera JA, Gradon JD: Right-side endocarditis in injection drug users: review of proposed mechanisms of pathogenesis. *Clin Infect Dis* 30:374, 2000.
62. Bashore TM, Cabell C, Fowler V Jr: Update on infective endocarditis. *Curr Probl Cardiol* 31: 274, 2006.
63. Snygg-Martin U, Gustaffson L, Rosengren L, et al: Cerebrovascular complications in patients with left-sided infective endocarditis are common: a prospective study using magnetic resonance imaging and neurochemical brain damage markers. *Clin Infect Dis* 47:23, 2008.
64. Bayer AS, Ward JI, Ginzton LE, et al: Evaluation of new clinical criteria for the diagnosis of infective endocarditis. *Am J Med* 96:211, 1994.
65. Hoen B, Béguinot I, Rabaud C, et al: The Duke criteria for diagnosing infective endocarditis are specific: analysis of 100 patients with acute fever or fever of unknown origin. *Clin Infect Dis* 23:298, 1996.
66. Dodds GA, Sexton DJ, Durack DT, et al: Negative predictive value of the Duke criteria for infective endocarditis. *Am J Cardiol* 77:403, 1996.
67. Stockheim JA, Chadwick EG, Kessler S, et al: Are the Duke criteria superior to the Beth Israel criteria for the diagnosis of infective endocarditis in children? *Clin Infect Dis* 27:1451, 1998.
68. Gagliardi JP, Nettles RE, McCarty DE, et al: Native valve infective endocarditis in elderly and younger adult patients: comparison of clinical features and outcomes with use of the Duke criteria and the Duke endocarditis database. *Clin Infect Dis* 26:1165, 1998.
69. Perez-Vasquez A, Farinas MC, Garcia-Palomo JD, et al: Evaluation of the Duke criteria in 93 episodes of prosthetic valve endocarditis. *Arch Intern Med* 160:1185, 2000.
70. Sekeres MA, Abrutyn E, Berlin JA, et al: An assessment of the usefulness of the Duke criteria for diagnosing active infective endocarditis. *Clin Infect Dis* 24:1185, 1997.
71. Habib G, Derumeaux G, Avierinos JF, et al: Value and limitations of the Duke criteria for the diagnosis of infective endocarditis. *J Am Coll Cardiol* 33:2023, 1999.
72. Li JS, Sexton DJ, Mick N, et al: Proposed modifications to the Duke criteria for the diagnosis of infective endocarditis. *Clin Infect Dis* 30:633–638, 2000.
73. Lamas CC, Eykyn SJ: Suggested modifications to the Duke criteria for the clinical diagnosis of native valve and prosthetic valve endocarditis: analysis of 118 pathologically proven cases. *Clin Infect Dis* 25:713, 1997.
74. Llinas L, Harrington T: Musculoskeletal manifestations as the initial presentation of infective endocarditis [letter]. *South Med J* 98:127, 2005.
75. Willerson JT, Moellering RC Jr, Buckley MJ, et al: Conjunctival petechiae after open-heart surgery. *N Engl J Med* 284:539, 1971.
76. Silverman ME, Upshaw CB Jr: Extracardiac manifestations of infective endocarditis and their historical descriptions. *Am J Cardiol* 100:1801, 2007.
77. Marrie TJ: Osler's nodes and Janeway lesions. *Am J Med* 121:105, 2008.
78. CLSI: Principles and Procedures for Blood Cultures; Approved Guideline. CLSI document M47-A. Wayne, PA: Clinical and Laboratory Standards Institute, 2007.
79. Petti CA, Bhally HS, Weinstein MP, et al: Utility of extended blood culture incubation for isolation of *Haemophilus, Actinobacillus, Cardiobacterium, Eikenella*, and *Kingella* organisms: a retrospective multicenter evaluation. *J Clin Microbiol* 44:257, 2006.
80. Baron EJ, Scott JD, Tompkins LS: Prolonged incubation and extensive subculturing do not increase recovery of clinically significant microorganisms from standard automated blood cultures. *Clin Infect Dis* 41:1677, 2005.
81. Ellis ME, Al-Abdely H, Sandridge A, et al: Fungal endocarditis in the world literature, 1965–1995. *Clin Infect Dis* 32:50, 2001.
82. Houpikian P, Raoult D: Diagnostic methods. Current best practices and guidelines for identification of difficult-to-culture pathogens in infective endocarditis. *Infect Dis Clin North America* 16:377, 2002.
83. Raoult D, Casalta JP, Richet H, et al: Contribution of systemic serological testing in diagnosis of infective endocarditis. *J Clin Microbiol* 43:5238, 2005.
84. Syed FF, Millar BC, Prendergast BD: Molecular technology in context: a current review of diagnosis and management of infective endocarditis. *Prog Cardiovasc Dis* 50:181, 2007.
85. Millar BC, Moore JE: Current trends in the molecular diagnosis of infective endocarditis. *Eur J Clin Microbiol Infect Dis* 23:353, 2004.
86. Carpenter JL: Perivalvular extension of infection in patients with infectious endocarditis. *Rev Infect Dis* 13:127, 1991.
87. Baddour LM, Wilson WR, Bayer AS, et al: Infective endocarditis: diagnosis, antimicrobial therapy, and management of complications: a statement for healthcare professionals from the Committee on Rheumatic Fever, Endocarditis, and Kawasaki disease, Council on Cardiovascular Disease in the Young, and the Councils on Clinical Cardiology, Stroke, and

Cardiovascular Surgery and Anesthesia, American Heart Association: endorsed by the Infectious Disease Society of America. *Circulation* 111:e394–e434, 2005.
88. Daniel WG, Mugge A, Martin RP, et al: Improvement in the diagnosis of abscesses associated with endocarditis by transesophageal echocardiography. *N Engl J Med* 324:795, 1991.
89. Kemp WE Jr, Citrin B, Byrd BF III: Echocardiography in infective endocarditis. *South Med J* 92:744, 1999.
90. Bayer AS, Bolger AF, Taubert KA, et al: Diagnosis and management of infective endocarditis and its complications. *Circulation* 98:2936, 1998.
91. Erbel R, Rohmann S, Drexler M, et al: Improved diagnostic value of echocardiography in patients with infective endocarditis by transesophageal approach: a prospective study. *Eur Heart J* 9:43, 1988.
92. Birmingham GD, Rahko PS, Ballantyne F: Improved detection of infective endocarditis with transesophageal echocardiography. *Am Heart J* 123:774, 1992.
93. Casella F, Rana B, Casazza G, et al: The potential impact of contemporary transthoracic echocardiography on the management of patients with native valve endocarditis: a comparison with transesophageal echocardiography. *Echocardiography* 26:900, 2009.
94. Singh P, Inamdar V, Hage FG, et al: Usefulness of live/real time three-dimensional transthoracic echocardiography in evaluation of prosthetic valve function. *Echocardiography* 26:1236, 2009.
95. Daniel WG, Mugge A, Grote J, et al: Evaluation of endocarditis and its complications by biplane and multiplane transesophageal echocardiography. *Am J Cardiac Imaging* 9:100, 1995.
96. Daniel WG, Erbel R, Kasper W, et al: Safety of transesophageal echocardiography. A multicenter survey of 10,419 examinations. *Circulation* 83:817, 1991.
97. Spier BJ, Larue SJ, Teelin TC, et al: Review of complications in a series of patients with known gastro-esophageal varices undergoing transesophageal echocardiography. *J Am Soc Echocardiogr* 22:396, 2009.
98. Shapiro SM, Young E, De Guzman S, et al: Transesophageal echocardiography in diagnosis of infective endocarditis. *Chest* 105:377, 1994.
99. Pedersen WR, Walker M, Olson JD, et al: Value of transesophageal echocardiography as an adjunct to transthoracic echocardiography in evaluation of native and prosthetic valve endocarditis. *Chest* 100:251, 1991.
100. Shively BK, Gurule FT, Roldan CA: Diagnostic value of transesophageal compared with transthoracic echocardiography in infective endocarditis. *J Am Coll Cardiol* 18:391, 1991.
101. Hansalia S, Biswas M, Dutta R, et al: The value of live/real time three-dimensional transesophageal echocardiography in the assessment of valvular vegetations. *Echocardiography* 26:1264, 2009.
102. Daniel WG, Mugge A, Grote J, et al: Comparison of transthoracic and transesophageal echocardiography for detection of abnormalities of prosthetic and bioprosthetic valves in the mitral and aortic positions. *Am J Cardiol* 71:210, 1993.
103. Evangelista A, Gonzalez-Alujas MT: Echocardiography in infective endocarditis. *Heart* 90:614, 2004.
104. Kuhl HP, Hanrath P: The impact of transesophageal echocardiography on daily practice. *Eur J Echocardiography* 5:455, 2004.
105. Sachdev M, Peterson GE, Jollis JG: Imaging techniques for diagnosis of infective endocarditis. *Cardiol Clin* 21:185, 2003.
106. Jacob S, Tong AT: Role of echocardiography in the diagnosis and management of endocarditis. *Curr Opin Cardiol* 17:478, 2002.
107. Habib G, Hoen B, Tornos P, et al: Guidelines on the prevention, diagnosis, and treatment of infective endocarditis (new version 2009): the Task Force on the Prevention, Diagnosis, and Treatment of Infective Endocarditis of the European Society of Cardiology (ESC). Endorsed by the European Society of Clinical Microbiology and Infectious Diseases (ESCMID) and the International Society of Chemotherapy (ISC) for Infection and Cancer. *Eur Heart J* 30:2369, 2009.
108. Heidenrich PA, Masoudi FA, Maini B, et al: Echocardiography in patients with suspected endocarditis: a cost-effectiveness analysis. *Am J Med* 107:198, 1999.
109. Rosen AB, Fowler VG, Corey GR, et al: Cost effectiveness of transesophageal echocardiography to determine the duration of therapy for intravascular catheter-associated *Staphylococcus aureus* bacteremia. *Ann Intern Med* 130:810, 1999.
110. Hill EE, Herijgers P, Claus P, et al: Clinical and echocardiographic risk factors for embolism and mortality in infective endocarditis. *Eur J Clin Microbiol Infect Dis* 27:1159, 2008.
111. Arber N, Pras E, Copperman Y, et al: Pacemaker endocarditis: report of 44 cases and review of the literature. *Medicine (Baltimore)* 73:299, 1994.
112. Fernandez Guerrero ML, Aguado JM, Arribas A, et al: The spectrum of cardiovascular infections due to *Salmonella enterica*: a review of clinical features and factors determining outcome. *Medicine (Baltimore)* 83:123, 2004.
113. Guerrero MLF, Perea RT, Rodrigo JG, et al: Infectious endocarditis due to non-*typhi Salmonella* in patients infected with human immunodeficiency virus: report of two cases and review. *Clin Infect Dis* 22:853, 1996.
114. Fang G, Keys TF, Gentry LO, et al: Prosthetic valve endocarditis resulting from nosocomial bacteremia: a prospective, multicenter study. *Ann Intern Med* 119:560, 1993.
115. Wilson R, Hamburger M: Fifteen years' experience with *Staphylococcus* septicemia in a large city hospital: analysis of fifty-five cases in the Cincinnati General Hospital, 1940–1954. *Am J Med Sci* 22:437, 1957.
116. Shah M, Watanakunakorn C: Changing patterns of *Staphylococcus aureus* bacteremia. *Am J Med Sci* 278:115, 1979.
117. del Rio A, Cervera C, Moreno A, et al: Patients at risk of complications of *Staphylococcus aureus* bloodstream infection. *Clin Infect Dis* 48:S246, 2009.
118. Fowler VG, Li J, Corey GR, et al: Role of echocardiography in evaluation of patients with *Staphylococcus aureus* bacteremia: experience in 103 patients. *J Am Coll Cardiol* 30:1072, 1997.
119. Abraham J, Mansour C, Veledar E, et al: *Staphylococcus aureus* bacteremia and endocarditis: the Grady Memorial Hospital experience with methicillin-sensitive *S aureus* and methicillin-resistant *S aureus* bacteremia. *Am Heart J* 147:536, 2004.
120. Fowler VG Jr, Olsen MK, Corey GR, et al: Clinical identifiers of complicated *Staphylococcus aureus* bacteremia. *Arch Intern Med* 163:2066, 2003.
121. Jernigan JA, Farr BM: Short-course therapy of catheter-related *Staphylococcus aureus* bacteremia: a meta-analysis. *Ann Intern Med* 119:304, 1993.
122. Raad II, Sabbagh MF: Optimal duration of therapy for catheter-related *Staphylococcus aureus* bacteremia: a study of 55 cases and review. *Clin Infect Dis* 14:75, 1992.
123. Mitchell DH, Howden BP: Diagnosis and management of *Staphylococcus aureus* bacteraemia. *Intern Med J* 35:S17, 2005.
124. Fernandez Guerrero ML, Gonzalez Lopez JJ, Goyenechea A, et al: Endocarditis caused by *Staphylococcus aureus*: a reappraisal of the epidemiologic, clinical, and pathologic manifestations with analysis of factors determining outcome. *Medicine (Baltimore)* 88:1, 2009.
125. Gebo KA, Burkey MD, Lucas GM, et al: Incidence of, risk factors for, clinical presentation, and 1-year outcomes of infective endocarditis in an urban HIV cohort. *J Acquir Immune Defic Syndr* 43:426, 2006.
126. Fernandez-Guerrero ML, Herrero L, Bellver M, et al: Nosocomial enterococcal endocarditis: a serious hazard for hospitalized patients with enterococcal bacteremia. *J Intern Med* 252:510, 2002.
127. Anderson DJ, Murdoch DR, Sexton DJ, et al: Risk factors for infective endocarditis in patients with enterococcal bacteremia: a case-control study. *Infection* 32:72, 2004.
128. McBride SJ, Upton A, Roberts SA: Clinical characteristics of patients with vancomycin-susceptible *Enterococcus faecalis* and *Enterococcus faecium* bacteraemia—a five-year retrospective review. *Eur J Clin Microbiol Infect Dis* 29:107, 2010.
129. Shaked H, Carmeli Y, Schwartz D, et al: Enterococcal bacteraemia: epidemiological, microbiological, clinical and prognostic characteristics, and the impact of high level gentamicin resistance. *Scand J Infect Dis* 38:995, 2006.
130. Chou YY, Lin TY, Lin JC, et al: Vancomycin-resistant enterococcal bacteremia: comparison of clinical features and outcome between *Enterococcus faecium* and *Enterococcus faecalis*. *J Microbiol Immunol Infect* 41:124, 2008.
131. Baddour LM, Epstein AE, Erickson CC, et al: Update on cardiovascular implantable electronic device infections and their management: a scientific statement from the American Heart Association. *Circulation* 121:458, 2010.
132. Zhan C, Baine WB, Sedrakyan A, et al: Cardiac device implantation in the United States from 1997 through 2004: a population-based analysis. *J Gen Intern Med* 23[Suppl 1]:13, 2007.
133. Uslan DZ, Sohail MR, St Sauver JL, et al: Permanent pacemaker and implantable cardioverter defibrillator infection: a population-based study. *Arch Intern Med* 167:669, 2007.
134. Sohail MR, Uslan DZ, Khan AH, et al: Risk factor analysis of permanent pacemaker infection. *Clin Infect Dis* 45:166, 2007.
135. Klug D, Balde M, Pavin D, et al: Risk factors related to infections of implanted pacemakers and cardioverter-defibrillators: results of a large prospective study. *Circulation* 116:1349, 2007.
136. del Rio A, Anguera I, Miro JM, et al: Surgical treatment of pacemaker and defibrillator lead endocarditis. The impact of electrode lead extraction on outcome. *Chest* 124:1451, 2003.
137. Byrd CL, Wilkoff BL, Love CJ, et al: Clinical study of the laser sheath for lead extraction: the total experience in the United States. *J Pacing Clin Electrophysiol* 25:804, 2002.
138. Wunderly D, Maloney J, Edel T, et al: Infections in implantable cardioverter defibrillator patients. *Pacing Clin Electrophysiol* 13:1360, 1990.
139. Alamassi GH, Oinger GN, Troup PJ, et al: Delayed infection of the automatic implantable cardioverter-defibrillator. Current recognition and management. *J Thorac Cardiovasc Surg* 95:908, 1988.
140. Gordon RJ, Quagliarello B, Lowy FD: Ventricular assist device-related infections. *Lancet Infect Dis* 6:426, 2006.
141. Oz MC, Argenziano M, Catanese KA, et al: Bridge experience with long-term implantable left ventricular assist devices. Are they an alternative to transplantation? *Circulation* 95:1844, 1997.
142. Mourvillier B, Trouillet J-L, Timsit J-F, et al: Infective endocarditis in the intensive care unit: clinical spectrum and prognostic factors in 228 consecutive patients. *Intensive Care Med* 30:2046, 2004.

143. Wang A, Pappas P, Anstrom KJ, et al: The use and effect of surgical therapy for prosthetic valve infective endocarditis: a propensity analysis of a multicenter, international cohort. *Am Heart J* 150:1086, 2005.
144. Sexton DJ, Tenenbaum MJ, Wilson WR, et al: Ceftriaxone once daily for four weeks compared with ceftriaxone plus gentamicin once daily for two weeks for treatment of endocarditis due to penicillin-susceptible streptococci. *Clin Infect Dis* 27:1470–1474, 1998.
145. Korzeniowski O, Sande MA, National Collaborative Endocarditis Study Group: Combination antimicrobial therapy for *Staphylococcus aureus* endocarditis in patients addicted to parenteral drugs and in nonaddicts. *Ann Intern Med* 97:496–503, 1982.
146. Abrams B, Sklaver A, Hoffman T, et al: Single or combination therapy of staphylococcal endocarditis in intravenous drug abusers. *Ann Intern Med* 90:789–791, 1979.
147. Ribera E, Gomez-Jimenez MJ, Cortes E, et al: Effectiveness of cloxacillin with and without gentamicin in short-term therapy for right-sided *Staphylococcus aureus* endocarditis. A randomized, controlled trial. *Ann Intern Med* 125:969–974, 1996.
148. Elliott TSJ, Foweraker J, Gould FK, et al: Guidelines for the antibiotic treatment of endocarditis in adults: report of the Working Party of the British Society for Antimicrobial Chemotherapy. *J Antimicrob Chemother* 54:971, 2004.
149. Cosgrove SE, Vigliani GA, Campion M, et al: Initial low-dose gentamicin for *Staphylococcus aureus* bacteremia and endocarditis is nephrotoxic. *Clin Infect Dis* 48:713, 2009.
150. Fowler VG, Boucher HW, Corey GR, et al: Daptomycin versus standard therapy for bacteremia and endocarditis caused by *Staphylococcus aureus*. *N Engl J Med* 355:653, 2006.
151. Cosgrove SE, Fowler VG Jr, et al: Management of methicillin-resistant *Staphylococcus aureus* bacteremia. *Clin Infect Dis* 46:S386, 2008.
151A. Liu C, Bayer A, Cosgrove SE, et al: Clinical practice guidelines by the Infectious Diseases Society of America for treatment of methicillin-resistant *Staphylococcus aureus* infections in adults and children. *Clin Infect Dis* 52:e18–55, Epub 2011.
152. Levine DP, Fromm BS, Reddy BR: Slow response to vancomycin or vancomycin plus rifampin in methicillin-resistant *Staphylococcus aureus* endocarditis. *Ann Intern Med* 115:674, 1991.
153. de Feiter PW, Jacobs JA, Jacobs MJ, et al: Successful treatment of *Staphylococcus epidermidis* prosthetic valve endocarditis with linezolid after failure of treatment with oxacillin, gentamicin, rifampicin, vancomycin, and fusidic acid regimens. *Scand J Infect Dis* 37:173, 2005.
154. Wareham DW, Abbas H, Karcher AM, et al: Treatment of prosthetic valve infective endocarditis due to multi-resistant Gram-positive bacteria with linezolid. *J Infect* 52:300, 2006.
155. Sande MA, Scheld WM: Combination antibiotic therapy of bacterial endocarditis. *Ann Intern Med* 92:390, 1980.
156. Olaison L, Schadewitz K, Swedish Society of Infectious Diseases Quality Assurance Study Group for Endocarditis: Enterococcal endocarditis in Sweden, 1995–1999: can shorter therapy with aminoglycosides be used? *Clin Infect Dis* 34:159, 2002.
157. Tascini C, Doria R, Leonildi A, et al: Efficacy of the combination ampicillin plus ceftriaxone in the treatment of a case of enterococcal endocarditis due to *Enterococcus faecalis* highly resistant to gentamicin: efficacy of the "ex vivo" synergism method. *J Chemother* 16:400, 2004.
158. Stevens MP, Edmond MB: Endocarditis due to vancomycin-resistant enterococci: case report and review of the literature. *Clin Infect Dis* 41:1134, 2005.
159. Linden PK, Moellering RC Jr, Wood CA, et al: Treatment of vancomycin-resistant *Enterococcus faecium* infections with quinupristin/dalfopristin. *Clin Infect Dis* 33:1816, 2001.
160. Birmingham MC, Rayner CR, Meagher AK, et al: Linezolid for the treatment of multidrug-resistant, gram-positive infections: experience from a compassionate-use program. *Clin Infect Dis* 36:159, 2003.
161. Kaplan AH, Weber DJ, Oddone EZ, et al: Infection due to *Actinobacillus actinomycetemcomitans*: 15 cases and review. *Rev Infect Dis* 11:46, 1989.
162. Schack SH, Smith PW, Penn RG, et al: Endocarditis caused by *Actinobacillus actinomycetemcomitans*. *J Clin Microbiol* 20:579, 1986.
163. Steinbach WJ, Perfect JR, Cabell CH, et al: A meta-analysis of medical versus surgical therapy for *Candida* endocarditis. *J Infect* 51:230, 2005.
164. Pappas PG, Kauffman CA, Andes D, et al: Clinical practice guidelines for the management of candidiasis: 2009 update by the Infectious Diseases Society of America. *Clin Infect Dis* 48:503, 2009.
165. Rajendram R, Alp NJ, Mitchell AR, et al: *Candida* prosthetic valve endocarditis cured by caspofungin therapy without valve replacement. *Clin Infect Dis* 40:e72, 2005.
166. Lye DCB, Hughes A, O'Brien D, et al: *Candida glabrata* prosthetic valve endocarditis treated successfully with fluconazole plus caspofungin without surgery: a case report and literature review. *Eur J Clin Microbiol Infect Dis* 24:753, 2005.
167. Bacak V, Biocina B, Starcevic B, et al: *Candida albicans* endocarditis treatment with caspofungin in an HIV-infected patient—case report and review of literature. *J Infect* 53:e11–14, 2006.
168. Tornos P, Almirante B, Mirabet S, et al: Infective endocarditis due to *Staphylococcus aureus*: deleterious effect of anticoagulant therapy. *Arch Intern Med* 159:473–475, 1999.
169. Olaison L, Hogevik H, Myken P, et al: Early surgery in infective endocarditis. *Q J Med* 89:267, 1996.
170. Mullany CJ, Chua YL, Schaff HV, et al: Early and late survival after surgical treatment of culture-positive endocarditis. *Mayo Clin Proc* 70:517, 1995.
171. Middlemost S, Wisenbaugh T, Meyerowitz C, et al: A case for early surgery in native left-sided endocarditis complicated by heart failure: results in 203 patients. *J Am Coll Cardiol* 18:663, 1991.
172. Prendergast BD, Tornos P: Surgery for infective endocarditis: who and when? *Circulation* 121:1141, 2010.
173. Olaison L, Pettersson G: Current best practices and guidelines: indications for surgical intervention in infective endocarditis. *Infect Dis Clin North Am* 16:453, 2002.
174. Larbalestier RI, Kinchla NM, Aranki SF, et al: Acute bacterial endocarditis: optimizing surgical results. *Circulation* 86 [Suppl II]:68, 1992.
175. Blumberg EA, Robbins N, Adimora A, et al: Persistent fever in association with infective endocarditis. *Clin Infect Dis* 15:983, 1992.
176. Fabri J Jr, Issa VS, Pomertantzeff PM, et al: Time-related distribution, risk factors and prognostic influence of embolism in patients with left-sided infective endocarditis. *Int J Cardiol* 110:334, 2006.
177. Thuny F, Di Salvo G, Belliard O, et al: Risk of embolism and death in infective endocarditis: prognostic value of echocardiography: a prospective multicenter study. *Circulation* 112:69, 2005.
178. Gammie JS, O'Brien SM, Griffith BP, et al: Surgical treatment of mitral valve endocarditis in North America. *Ann Thorac Surg* 80:2199, 2005.
179. Ruttman E, Legit C, Poelzl G, et al: Mitral valve repair provides improved outcome over replacement in active infective endocarditis. *J Thorac Cardiovasc Surg* 130:765, 2005.
180. Truninger K, Attenhofer Jost CH, Seifer B, et al: Long term follow up of prosthetic valve endocarditis: what characteristics identify patients who were treated successfully with antibiotics alone? *Heart* 82:714, 1999.
181. Habib G, Tribouilloy C, Thuny F, et al: Prosthetic valve endocarditis: who needs surgery? A multicentre study of 104 cases. *Heart* 91:954, 2005.
182. Wolff M, Witchitz S, Chastang C, et al: Prosthetic valve endocarditis in the ICU. Prognostic factors of overall survival in a series of 122 cases and consequences for treatment decision. *Chest* 108:688, 1995.
183. John MDV, Hibberd PL, Karchmer AW, et al: *Staphylococcus aureus* prosthetic valve endocarditis: optimal management and risk factors for death. *Clin Infect Dis* 26:1302, 1998.
184. ACC/AHA 2006 guidelines for the management of patients with valvular heart disease: a report of the American College of Cardiology/American Heart Association Task Force on Practice Guidelines (writing committee to revise the 1998 Guidelines for the Management of Patients with Valvular Heart Disease): developed in collaboration with the Society of Cardiovascular Anesthesiologists: endorsed by the Society for Cardiovascular Angiography and Interventions and the Society of Thoracic Surgeons. *Circulation* 114(5):e84–231, 2006.

CHAPTER 81 ■ INFECTIONS ASSOCIATED WITH VASCULAR CATHETERS

SUZANNE F. BRADLEY AND CAROL A. KAUFFMAN

Medical technology has led to the creation of a variety of indwelling vascular catheters that have greatly improved our ability to deliver care to critically ill patients, but also have led to increased risks of infection. It is estimated that more than 200 million intravascular devices will be inserted every year in the United States [1]. Approximately 250,000 to 500,000 episodes of healthcare-associated bloodstream infections occur per year in the United States, and are commonly associated with the use of central venous catheters. It is estimated that 12% to 25% of these device-related infections will result in death [1,2]. As a consequence of catheter-associated bloodstream infections, hospital length of stay is prolonged by 10 to 40 days, and mean attributable costs are increased by $18,432 ($3,592 to $34,410) per episode [1–3].

Guidelines for the prevention and treatment of catheter-associated infections have been published in the past few years [4–6]. Recommendations in this chapter are based on these published guidelines. The reader is referred to these publications for a more in-depth review of the topics of prevention and treatment of catheter-associated infections.

PATHOGENESIS

Foreign bodies that penetrate the cutaneous barriers of the host induce a chronic inflammatory response and are coated with host proteins, including fibronectin, fibrin, laminin, and others [7]. The coated catheter can then provide a niche for microorganisms that adhere by fimbriae and adhesins, which bind to surface receptors present on some of the coating proteins, or by electromagnetic interactions leading to the formation of biofilms within days of insertion [7,8].

Microorganisms gain entry to the catheter primarily at the insertion site. Particularly in catheters used for short term, there is a correlation between organisms isolated from the catheter and those obtained from the insertion site. Contamination of the catheter hub and ultimately the internal lumen of the catheter plays a larger role in the development of infections in catheters remaining in place for more than 1 month [7,8]. Less common are catheter-associated infections occurring as a result of hematogenous seeding from a distant focus of infection or from contaminated infusates [8].

DIAGNOSIS

Diagnostic Methods

The diagnosis of catheter-associated infection still relies primarily on the recognition of clinical signs and symptoms in a patient who has an intravascular device in place, absence of an alternative cause for those clinical findings, and microbiological evidence for infection [2]. The clinical signs noted in some, but not all, patients with a catheter-associated infection are development of warmth, erythema, and pain at the site of current or recent venous or arterial catheter placement. Patients with catheter-associated bloodstream infection generally have fever, with or without hypotension, and other signs of sepsis. Finding microorganisms on culture of a catheter in an asymptomatic patient is not indicative of infection, and conversely, impressive local findings may reflect only phlebitis or reaction to the infusate. Thus, differentiating catheter-associated infection from colonization of the catheter can be difficult, and no perfect diagnostic method has been established.

Blood Culture with Catheter Retention

Positive blood cultures in a patient who has an indwelling vascular catheter and who has no other source of infection raise the possibility of catheter-associated infection. A variety of approaches have been devised to help differentiate whether a positive blood culture represents catheter-associated infection or has arisen from another source. Quantitative cultures of blood taken simultaneously from the catheter and from peripheral blood that demonstrate a difference of more than threefold microorganisms from the catheter are probably the most accurate method to determine if catheter-associated infection is present without removing the catheter [1,2]. However, few, if any, clinical laboratories routinely perform quantitative blood cultures.

Differential time to positivity of blood cultures taken from a central line compared with those taken from a peripheral vein is another diagnostic method. Blood cultures obtained from an infected central catheter may turn positive a least 2 hours sooner than blood drawn simultaneously from a peripheral vein [2].

Another method that does not require the removal of the catheter involves culture of peripheral blood as well as the insertion site and hub. Growth of more than 15 colonies of the same organism from all three sites suggests short-term catheter-related infection [4,9].

It is important to minimize the possibility of contamination when obtaining blood for culture by having specifically trained personnel obtain the samples. Disinfection of the skin and hub using alcohol, tincture of iodine, or alcoholic chlorhexidine, but not povidone-iodine, is recommended. Blood samples taken from a peripheral vein are preferred as they are less likely to be contaminated than blood samples obtained from catheter hubs. However, all of the techniques listed above require sampling from the catheter as well as from a peripheral vein.

Catheter Culture Following Catheter Removal

Although very helpful in the diagnosis of catheter-associated infection, culture of the catheter necessitates removal of the catheter before the diagnosis can be made. For optimum culture, the catheter tip, or the introducer tip for pulmonary artery catheters, should be cultured. Quantitative cultures obtained by vortexing or sonicating the catheter tip most accurately determine the numbers of microorganisms present on both the internal and external surfaces of the catheter. However, this method is not practical in the clinical setting [2].

Rolling the distal segment of the catheter on an agar plate yields semiquantitative results that compare favorably with quantitative methods and has gained the greatest acceptance. The presence of ≥15 bacterial colonies on an agar plate correlates significantly with the presence of local inflammation and signs and symptoms of bloodstream infection. No similar cutoff has been established when yeasts are grown from the catheter tip. Some patients with catheter-associated infection will have fewer colonies, and catheter tips from asymptomatic patients will sometimes yield ≥15 colonies. A drawback of this technique is that only the external portion of the catheter is cultured, not the lumen, which may be the primary site of infection in long-term catheters. The roll-plate technique is the recommended method for diagnosis of presumed infection in short-term catheters after they have been removed [2,4].

Definitions

Adherence to standardized definitions of catheter-related infection is critical to make informed comparisons among the myriad studies that have been performed in this area. Although definitions may vary slightly from investigator to investigator, consensus has been reached in recent years [2,4,5].

Catheter colonization: The patient has no signs and symptoms of infection but a quantitative or semiquantitative culture of the catheter tip or catheter hub yields significant growth of a microorganism.

Catheter-associated bloodstream infection: Bacteremia/fungemia in a patient who has an intravascular catheter in place and who has at least one positive blood culture taken from a peripheral vein, clinical manifestations of infection (fever, chills, and/or hypotension), and no apparent source except the catheter. Additionally, there should be evidence linking the catheter to the infection using one of the semiquantitative or quantitative techniques described earlier.

Exit site infection: These infections manifest erythema, induration, and/or tenderness within 2 cm of the catheter exit site, and exudate at the exit site yields a microorganism. There may or may not be concomitant bloodstream infection.

Tunnel infection: Tenderness, erythema, and/or induration are present more than 2 cm from the exit site along the subcutaneous tract of a tunneled catheter with or without concomitant bloodstream infection.

PREVENTION OF CATHETER-RELATED INFECTIONS

Catheter Insertion

Local Skin Flora

Regardless of the type of catheter inserted, the major risk factor for the development of catheter-associated infection is the breach of a major host defense against infection—the skin. Catheter-associated infections are usually due to normal skin flora, particularly Gram-positive cocci, such as coagulase-negative staphylococci and *Staphylococcus aureus*. However, the distribution of microorganisms on the skin varies. For example, Gram-negative bacilli, *Candida* species, and anaerobes are increased in the groin area and on the lower extremities [10].

The ecology of normal human flora is further altered by illness, hospitalization, and the presence of foreign bodies. The use of antimicrobial agents inhibits the growth of normal flora and contributes to the emergence of resistant Gram-negative bacilli, *S. aureus*, vancomycin-resistant enterococci, and yeasts. Patients who have a productive cough or a tracheostomy can easily contaminate their skin with organisms from their respiratory tract. The hands of healthcare personnel may facilitate the transfer of potential pathogens from patient to patient [6].

Choice of Insertion Site

The site of catheter insertion influences the risk of infection. Central venous catheters inserted in the internal jugular vein become infected more often than those in the subclavian vein, perhaps because of difficulties in dressing the area and contamination with respiratory secretions [5,11]. Catheter insertion in the lower extremities should be avoided in adults because of increased risk of phlebitis and infection in this area of poor blood flow [5,6]. Placement of femoral lines should be a last resort in emergent situations or when no other vascular access is available, and these lines should be removed as soon as possible [5].

Insertion Techniques

Catheter-associated phlebitis and infection are more likely to occur when catheters are inserted by inexperienced personnel rather than personnel who are trained in these techniques. Prospective, randomized trials have shown that strict adherence to sterile technique (i.e., mask, cap, and large sterile drape, gloves, and gown) is beneficial in preventing central venous catheter infections, and also highly cost effective [5,6]. The importance of sterile techniques using maximal barrier precautions for short-term central catheters cannot be overemphasized and should become a part of house staff training [5,6]. Use of a catheter checklist to ensure and document adherence to infection prevention practices at the time of insertion is recommended [6,12].

Ultrasound guidance for the insertion of central vascular catheters, especially internal jugular catheters, has been shown in a meta-analysis to decrease the risk of mechanical complications associated with placement [5]. A biodegradable collagen cuff impregnated with silver ions is commercially available to attach to short-term central venous catheters before insertion. Two initial randomized controlled trials showed protection against catheter-associated colonization and bacteremia, but subsequent trials have failed to show a decrease in infection rates [5,8]. Currently, it is recommended that these cuffs not be used [5].

Cutaneous Antisepsis

Several different antiseptics, 70% alcohol, chlorhexidine, and iodine-based solutions, have been found to reduce microbial contamination at the insertion site of the catheter [4,5]. Several studies and a meta-analysis have found that chlorhexidine-based aqueous or alcoholic solutions are superior to povidone-iodine solutions in reducing colonization at the catheter insertion site and catheter-associated bacteremia [5,13,14]. Current recommendations are to use 2% chlorhexidine gluconate for antisepsis of the insertion site, allowing it to dry before catheter insertion [5,6]. Chlorhexidine products have not been approved for children less than 2 months of age.

Antimicrobial ointments have been shown to increase the risk of infection with *Candida* and antibiotic-resistant bacteria and may affect the integrity of some catheters. With the exception of povidone-iodine ointment for some hemodialysis catheters, routine use of ointments at the catheter insertion site is discouraged [5,6,15].

A chlorhexidine-impregnated patch (BIOPATCH, Ethicon, Somerville, NJ) has proved efficacious in reducing colonization at the catheter site, and in reducing bloodstream infections [8,16,17]. There currently are no firm recommendations as to whether this device should be routinely used with short-term central venous catheters [5]. However, a recent guideline suggests considering use of this patch when the rates of catheter-associated infection remain above target rates despite consistent use of evidence-based prevention bundles [6]. Use of these patches also should be considered in patients who have limited access and a history of recurrent catheter-associated infections and in those who have a heightened risk of severe sequelae if infection should occur, such as patients with recently implanted intravascular devices [6]. The use of systemic antibiotics as prophylaxis before the placement of central venous devices is strongly discouraged because selection for antibiotic-resistant microorganisms is highly likely [5,6].

Type of Catheter

Nontunneled Central Venous Catheters

These catheters are inserted into the subclavian vein, the internal jugular vein, and rarely the femoral vein. They can be single or multilumen, depending on the specific needs of each patient. Some studies, but not all, have shown that multilumen catheters are associated with a higher rate of colonization and infection than single-lumen catheters, particularly when used for an extended period of time [18–22].

Increased risk for infection, especially with multilumen catheters, occurs with the frequent manipulations that are required in the care of critically ill patients. In one study, only one of three lumens was used in most of the multilumen catheters that were inserted [21]. Therefore, it is recommended that a central venous catheter be chosen with the minimum number of ports or lumens required for the care of the patient [5]. It is recommended that the care of these multilumen lines be limited to a few well-trained personnel and that the catheter be changed to a single-lumen catheter if all the ports are no longer needed [5]. These catheters should be used predominantly in patients in the intensive care setting.

Antimicrobial Impregnated or Coated Central Venous Catheters

Numerous antimicrobial agents (tetracyclines, rifamycins, glycopeptides, β-lactams, micafungin), antiseptics (benzalkonium chloride, chlorhexidine, tridodecylmethylammonium chloride, iodine, gentian violet, and silver molecules), and antithrombotic agents (heparin, ethylenediaminetetraacetate [EDTA]) alone or in various combinations have been bound to polymer material or used to coat the surfaces of catheters in the hope of reducing colonization, thrombosis, and subsequent infection [2,8,23,24]. Heparin-coated catheters should not be used because of concerns for developing heparin-induced thrombocytopenia.

Minocycline/rifampin-coated catheters (Cook Medical, Bloomington, IN), chlorhexidine/silver sulfadiazine-coated catheters (Arrow International, Reading, PA), and a silver-platinum-carbon–impregnated catheter (Vantex CVC with Oligon, Edwards Life Sciences, Irvine, CA) are currently available. All of these catheters have been shown to reduce catheter-associated colonization [2,5,8,23,25]. In some controlled trials, the rates of catheter-associated bacteremia were sufficient to demonstrate significant reductions in infection rates when antimicrobial catheters were compared with standard catheters [2,5,8,26]. One study showed that a minocycline/rifampin-containing device was more effective at reducing both catheter colonization and catheter-associated bloodstream infections than a chlorhexidine/silver sulfadiazine-coated catheter [27]. However, that study was performed using the first-generation chlorhexidine/silver sulfadiazine catheter (ArrowGard) that was coated only on the external surface. Subsequent studies assessing the second-generation catheter that is coated on both external and internal surfaces (ArrowGard Plus) against the minocycline/rifampin catheter have not been performed.

Several meta-analyses have noted both reduced infection rates and costs when coated catheters are used for 5 to 14 days [2,23]. The recommendations are to strongly consider the use of antimicrobial-coated catheters for those adult patients who will likely require a central catheter for 5 to 14 days if the rates of catheter-associated bloodstream infections are unacceptably high in spite of adherence to other measures, such as maximal sterile barriers and use of chlorhexidine antisepsis [5]. Use of these catheters also should be considered for patients who have limited venous access and a history of catheter-associated bloodstream infection and for those with heightened risk for severe sequelae if they develop systemic infections, such as patients with recently implanted devices [6]. Each hospital must decide, based on their rates of catheter-associated bloodstream infection, whether the higher costs of purchasing antimicrobial-coated catheters are justified.

Peripherally Inserted Central Venous Catheters

Peripherally inserted central venous catheters (PICC) have become increasingly popular and appear to have lower rates of infectious complications when compared with other central venous catheters [2,4,5,8]. Initial insertion costs are lower than those for tunneled central venous catheters, but rates of mechanical complications and phlebitis are higher. These catheters must be inserted by specially trained healthcare workers or interventional radiologists. A PICC can be left in place for weeks to months as long as there is no malfunction, evidence of phlebitis, or infection.

Semipermanent Tunneled Catheters (Long-Term Central Venous Catheter)

In the 1970s, Broviac introduced a cuffed, silicone rubber central venous catheter for the purpose of hyperalimentation, and Hickman devised a similar catheter of larger gauge that allowed the administration and withdrawal of blood. The double-lumen catheter resulted when both Hickman and Broviac catheters were combined for the purpose of infusing parenteral nutrition solutions as well as other drugs. The risk of infection with semipermanent tunneled catheters appears to be low [2,4,28]. They are especially useful for administration of chemotherapy and other agents in cancer patients and in those requiring long-term parenteral nutrition. Routine use in the intensive care setting is not practical.

Pulmonary Artery Catheters

The risk of infection of percutaneously inserted heparin-bonded benzalkonium-impregnated pulmonary artery catheters appears to be low in those patients in whom the catheter requires little manipulation and is left in place for less than 7 days. The use of plastic sleeves to cover the pulmonary artery catheter is recommended to reduce the risk of contamination and prevent bloodstream infection [5]. Autopsy evidence of right-sided endocardial damage has been noted in most patients with pulmonary artery catheters, but endocarditis is relatively rare [29].

Peripheral Arterial Catheters

Indwelling arterial catheters appear to have rates of complications similar to those for venous catheters [5,8]. It has been estimated that thrombosis complicates as many as 19% to 38% of arterial catheterizations, and infection may occur in as many as 4% to 23% of patients with arterial catheters in place [30]. Signs and symptoms of infection in arterial catheters are similar to those for venous catheters; however, the absence of local signs of inflammation does not preclude infection. Distal embolic lesions and hemorrhage are highly predictive of arterial catheter-associated bloodstream infection. Late complications such as pseudoaneurysm formation and rupture of the artery may occur [31]. The rate of bloodstream infection increases the longer the catheter remains in place, with one study noting increasing risk of infection after day 4 of catheterization [30].

Midline Catheters

Midline catheters are midsized (3 to 8 in.) peripheral catheters that are inserted into the antecubital fossa or upper arm veins and extend no further than the distal portion of the subclavian vein. They can remain in place for 4 weeks, are convenient to insert, are associated with fewer infections than central venous catheters, and cause less phlebitis than peripheral catheters [4,5].

Care of the Catheter and Insertion Site

Insertion Site Dressings

Either traditional gauze and tape bandages or transparent semipermeable dressings can be used for peripheral and central catheters. Transparent dressings are changed every 5 to 7 days and gauze dressings every 2 days or more frequently if the dressing is soiled, loose, or damp [6]. Site care should be performed with a chlorhexidine-based antiseptic with each dressing change [6]. In some centers, chlorhexidine patches are placed on catheters during routine dressing changes.

Catheter Hub Disinfection

Local disinfection of the hubs of central venous catheters must be performed using either a chlorhexidine-based preparation or 70% alcohol before attempting access [5,6]. With either preparation, it is very important to allow the antiseptic to dry to ensure antimicrobial activity before accessing the catheter.

Catheter Replacement

Peripheral Catheters

Phlebitis of a peripheral vein is a well-recognized harbinger of infection and may be quite uncomfortable for the patient. A catheter causing phlebitis should be removed promptly and the tip cultured. Complications of peripheral venous catheter insertion, including phlebitis and catheter-associated infection, increase after 72 hours of insertion. Recommendations to remove and change these catheters to another site every 72 hours are aimed at decreasing the risk for infection and the discomfort associated with phlebitis [5]. The longer midline catheters and PICC lines should not be removed and changed routinely unless phlebitis or signs of infection develop [5].

Central Catheters

The risk of infection increases during the time that a central catheter is in place, but several studies have shown that routine replacement of these catheters does not reduce rates of catheter-associated bloodstream infections [5]. Routine rotation of a central catheter to a different site is associated with increased risk for pneumothorax, laceration of a vessel with hemothorax, and arrhythmias and, thus, is not recommended [5].

The use of routine catheter change over a guidewire has also been tried as a means to decrease catheter-related infections. However, a meta-analysis of studies employing this technique failed to show an effect on decreasing infections, and routine catheter changes over a guidewire are not recommended [5,32].

Thrombosis requires removal of an indwelling catheter [33]. An exception is made for the patient who has poor access and is dependent on a surgically implanted semipermanent central catheter. Under these circumstances, an attempt to salvage the catheter is reasonable [4].

Infusion-Related Issues

Local Effects

Intravenous solutions and drugs that are acidic, hypertonic, or directly irritating to vascular endothelium (KCl, certain antibiotics, chemotherapeutic agents) may lead to a local inflammatory response, thrombosis, and phlebitis, with an increased risk of infection, particularly in small-caliber peripheral veins. When such infusions are necessary, a central catheter should be used.

Infusion Tubing

Most infusion tubing should be used no longer than 96 hours [6]. However, tubing used to administer blood products or lipid emulsions should be changed every 24 hours [5].

In-Line Devices and Filters

In-line devices can be a significant source of catheter-associated infection. Pressure transducers have been implicated in outbreaks of catheter-associated bloodstream infection, particularly those due to water-associated Gram-negative bacilli, including *Pseudomonas, Serratia, Enterobacter, Citrobacter*, and *Acinetobacter* spp [34]. Stopcocks are easily contaminated through manipulation by personnel or by injection with contaminated syringes and may be an important source of infection; use of a closed system rather than stopcocks has been shown to lead to less contamination of the line [5,6]. Some studies suggest that needleless mechanical valve devices may pose a greater risk of infection than split septum devices [35,36]. Disposable transducer domes, stopcocks, needleless components, and other in-line devices should be changed with the rest of the infusion set. In-line filters do not decrease the rate of infection, and their use is not recommended [5]. All catheter hubs, needleless connectors, and injection ports should be disinfected with a chlorhexidine preparation before accessing the device [6].

Contamination of Infusates

Although contamination with microorganisms during manufacture now occurs rarely, breaks in sterile technique by hospital personnel continue to be important in causing sporadic outbreaks of infusion-related bloodstream infection. Several Gram-negative bacilli, including *Enterobacter, Klebsiella, Serratia, Citrobacter*, and *Erwinia* spp, are particularly adept at proliferating in the acidic environment of intravenous fluids containing minimal nutrients [37]. Other organisms, such as *Candida* species, have a propensity to grow in total parenteral nutrition (TPN) solutions [38,39]. The addition of albumin directly to TPN solutions increases the growth of bacteria and fungi, and the addition of fat emulsions has been associated

TABLE 81.1

SUMMARY OF RECOMMENDATIONS FOR PREVENTION OF CENTRAL VENOUS CATHETER-ASSOCIATED INFECTIONS BASED ON RANDOMIZED CONTROLLED CLINICAL TRIALS [4–6]

- Use maximal sterile barriers (sterile full-sized drape, sterile gown, sterile gloves, face mask, head cap) during insertion.
- Perform insertion site antisepsis with chlorhexidine.
- Consider the use of a chlorhexidine-impregnated patch at the insertion site.
- Cover the insertion site with either a transparent or gauze dressing.
- Do not routinely change central intravascular catheters.
- Consider use of central intravascular catheters coated with antimicrobial agents (minocycline-rifampin) or chlorhexidine-silver sulfadiazine when infection rates are high.

with the growth of corynebacteria and the yeast *Malassezia furfur* [38,40].

Multifaceted Approach to Infection Prevention

An optimum approach to prevent catheter-associated infection likely involves the use of several infection control strategies. In Michigan, 108 intensive care units assessed the impact of five-evidence–based procedures recommended by the Centers for Disease Control and Prevention to prevent catheter-associated bloodstream infection [12]. This bundle, consisting of full-barrier precautions for catheter insertion, hand washing, insertion site cleansing with chlorhexidine, avoidance of femoral insertion site, and removal of unnecessary catheters, was implemented in conjunction with clinician education, use of a designated central-line cart, a checklist to ensure adherence, and empowerment of the assistant to stop the procedure if the practices in the bundle were not being followed. This intervention led to a sustained 66% reduction in catheter-associated bloodstream infections over 18 months. This "bundle" approach has become standard of care and has been incorporated into practice recommendations endorsed by the infection control community, the Joint Commission, and the American Hospital Association to prevent catheter-associated infections [6].

Advances in prevention of infections associated with vascular catheters, based on randomized controlled trials or meta-analyses of such trials, are summarized in Table 81.1.

CATHETER-ASSOCIATED INFECTIONS

Microbiology

Coagulase-negative staphylococci (*S. epidermidis* and other species) are most commonly implicated in catheter-associated infections, followed by *S. aureus,* a variety of Gram-negative bacilli, other Gram-positive cocci and bacilli, and *Candida* and other yeasts [4,41–44]. The most common pathogens, coagulase-negative staphylococci, are associated with less severe disease than most other organisms. *S. aureus* bloodstream infection is most likely to cause complications, and *Candida* species have a propensity to seed to other structures, especially the eye [4,45,46].

Complications

Major complications of catheter-associated infection include septic shock, suppurative phlebitis, metastatic infection, endocarditis, and arteritis [4]. Complicated catheter-associated infection often requires aggressive management combining appropriate antimicrobial therapy as well as surgical intervention. Complications of bloodstream infection should be suspected, especially if the catheter has been removed, when a patient has persistence or relapse of the same organism in blood cultures after 72 hours of appropriate medical therapy and no alternative explanation is found.

Suppurative Phlebitis

Suppurative phlebitis associated with vascular catheters is manifested by fever and positive blood cultures; signs of phlebitis may or may not be obvious. For peripheral catheters, old healed insertion sites may require exploration by needle aspiration or incision; purulent material may occasionally be expressed if the vein is "milked." Suppurative phlebitis of central veins, particularly of the subclavian veins and superior vena cava, should be confirmed by detection of a thrombus by computerized tomography, magnetic resonance imaging, venography, or ultrasound [47,48]. Surgical or interventional radiological procedures to remove the thrombus are technically difficult. Most patients will respond to 3 to 4 weeks of treatment with systemic antimicrobial therapy. Surgical resection should be considered if bloodstream infection persists despite conservative management or if purulence extends beyond the vessel wall [4].

Endocarditis

Endocarditis can occur after the use of peripheral or central catheters [4,49]. The aortic and mitral valves are involved most often; presumed normal valves as well as those damaged from congenital, rheumatic, and degenerative diseases may be infected. Right atrial catheters that cross the tricuspid valve can cause endothelial damage and turbulence, predisposing the patient to the development of right-sided endocarditis if transient bacteremia or fungemia occurs. Persistent or intermittent bacteremia or fungemia despite catheter removal, or evidence of pulmonary, cutaneous, central nervous system, or other emboli by physical or laboratory examination, suggests the diagnosis of endocarditis [4]. Transesophageal echocardiography (TEE) is extremely useful in determining the presence and size of vegetations, the valves involved and their function, and the presence of myocardial abscesses [4,50]. Even if endocarditis is not present, metastatic foci to bone and visceral organs often occur as a consequence of catheter-associated *S. aureus* bacteremia [45].

Initial Treatment

In the febrile patient in whom catheter-associated bloodstream infection is suspected, empiric treatment should include antimicrobial agents that cover both Gram-positive cocci and Gram-negative bacilli [4]. Vancomycin is chosen most frequently because it is consistently active against methicillin-resistant strains of *S. aureus* (MRSA) and coagulase-negative staphylococci. An alternative agent, such as daptomycin, should be considered in settings in which MRSA isolates commonly have vancomycin minimum inhibitory concentrations (MIC) ≥ 2 μg/mL. For Gram-negative bacilli, the choice of a β-lactam/β-lactamase inhibitor combination, an antipseudomonal cephalosporin, or a carbapenem, with or without an aminoglycoside, should be based on local antimicrobial susceptibility data. Use of an antifungal agent should be considered

TABLE 81.2

SYSTEMIC TREATMENT OF INTRAVASCULAR CATHETER-ASSOCIATED BLOODSTREAM INFECTION

Pathogen	First-line agent	Alternative agents	Comments
Coagulase (−) staphylococci			
Methicillin-susceptible	Nafcillin, oxacillin	Cefazolin, vancomycin	
Methicillin-resistant	Vancomycin	Daptomycin, linezolid	
Staphylococcus aureus			
Methicillin-susceptible	Nafcillin, oxacillin	Cephazolin, vancomycin	
Methicillin-resistant	Vancomycin	Daptomycin, linezolid	Use an alternative agent if the vancomycin MIC ≥2 mg/mL
Gram-negative bacilli			
Enterobacteriaceae			
ESBL (−)	Ceftriaxone, ceftazidime Ampicillin + sulbactam Piperacillin + tazobactam	Ciprofloxacin, aztreonam, cefepime	
ESBL (+)	Carbapenem	Ciprofloxacin, cefepime	
Pseudomonas	Cefepime, carbapenem Penicillin + tazobactam	Ciprofloxacin, aztreonam	Consider addition of an aminoglycoside
Candida species	Echinocandin fluconazole	Lipid amphotericin formulations	Use an echinocandin for severely ill patients when *Candida glabrata* is likely and fluconazole in patients without prior exposure

ESBL, extended spectrum beta-lactamase; MIC, minimum inhibitory concentration.

in a patient who is clinically septic and who has a femoral catheter, parenteral nutrition, broad-spectrum antibiotic therapy, a hematological malignancy, prior transplant, and with a history of colonization with *Candida* species at multiple sites [4]. Once the organism has been identified, then appropriate systemic antibiotic therapy can be chosen based on antimicrobial susceptibilities and expert recommendations (Table 81.2).

Should the Catheter Be Removed?

It is recommended that peripheral catheters with pain, erythema, induration, or exudate be removed. Also catheters associated with a tunnel infection should be removed. For exit site infections without gross purulence, systemic signs of infection, or associated positive blood cultures, treatment with topical agents as well as systemic agents can be tried based on culture data from a sample taken at the exit site. If treatment fails, then the catheter should be removed.

In the febrile patient who is clinically stable and without localizing signs of infection along the catheter insertion site, short-term central catheters need not be removed until a microbiological assessment that includes samples of blood with or without culture of insertion sites and hubs is performed. Cultures that are positive from a single blood sample for organisms that are part of the normal skin flora, such as coagulase negative staphylococci, diphtheroids, or propionibacteria, should be repeated to establish whether a true bloodstream infection is present [2,4]. Once true bacteremia has been established and in the absence of an alternative source, short-term catheters should be removed because they serve as a persistent nidus of infection [4]. If a catheter has been changed over a guidewire, and there is significant growth of organisms from the tip of the removed catheter, the newly placed catheter is almost certainly infected and should be removed [5].

Catheter Salvage

In the case of long-term, tunneled, semipermanent catheters or ports that cannot be easily removed or in patients who have limited vascular access, treatment of catheter-associated infection with antibiotics without catheter removal has been accomplished. Catheter salvage is not recommended in patients with complications of catheter infection, such as suppurative phlebitis, endocarditis, tunnel infection, or in patients who have severe sepsis or have an implanted intravascular device, such as a prosthetic cardiac valve [4].

If salvage is a consideration, most success has occurred with coagulase-negative staphylococcal infections; in one series 80% of infections were cured without removal of the central catheter [2]. Candidates for salvage therapy should have resolution of fever and bloodstream infection within 72 hours of initiation of appropriate treatment. For bloodstream infections due to *S. aureus* and *Candida* species, catheter salvage should be reserved for extenuating circumstances, that is, when there is no alternative access. These infections and those due to Gram-negative bacilli almost always require catheter removal [4]. Thrombolytics are not recommended as an adjunct to the treatment of catheter-associated bloodstream infection [33].

Antibiotic lock therapy, as an adjunct to systemic antimicrobial therapy, has been suggested for salvage of long-term catheters [4]. In general, lock therapy involves the instillation of 2 to 5 mL of an antibiotic, often with an anticoagulant, into the catheter, allowing it to dwell until the catheter is reaccessed. Ethanol and ethylenediaminetetraacetic acid (EDTA) have also been used for lock therapy. Short-term catheters are less likely to have an intraluminal source of infection and are less likely to benefit from antibiotic lock therapy. The lock therapy antimicrobial agents and systemic antibiotics should be used concomitantly; the duration of both treatments varies widely depending on the organism and the investigator [2,4]. In general, the duration of lock and systemic therapy ranges from 7 to 14 days (Table 81.3). If antibiotic lock therapy cannot be given, then systemic treatment should be administered directly through the infected catheter. If patients with no alternative access do not respond to antibiotic treatment, exchange over a guidewire can be attempted; in this situation, exchange with an antimicrobial-impregnated catheter has been suggested [4,51].

For treatment of infections due to common Gram-positive cocci, an antibiotic lock solution containing a combination of

TABLE 81.3

APPROACH TO THE PATIENT WITH A CENTRAL VASCULAR CATHETER-ASSOCIATED BLOODSTREAM INFECTION

Initial decision	CNS	*Staphylococcus aureus*	Gram-negative bacilli	Candida species
Short-term (nontunneled) catheters				
Removed	SysRx 5–7 d[a]	SysRx >14 d[a] if no metastatic infection, & echo (−)	SysRx 7–14 d[a]	SysRx 14 d[a] after 1st (−) culture
Retained	SysRx 10–14 d[a] LT 10–14 d	Not recommended	Not recommended	Not recommended
Long-term (tunneled/implanted) catheters				
Removed	SysRx 5–7 d[a]	SysRx 4–6 wk echo (+), septic phlebitis (+), or deep infection (+); otherwise ≥ 14 d	SysRx 10–14 d[a]	IV 14 d after 1st (−) culture
Retained	SysRx 7–14 d[a] LT 10–14 d[a]	SysRx ≥14 d[a] LT ≥14 d[a] echo (−)	SysRx 14 d[a] LT 14 d[a] No other access Not recommended	Not recommended

[a]Recommended duration assumes that the bloodstream infection is uncomplicated, fever has resolved in <72 h, and the patient has no implanted intravascular devices or evidence of endocarditis or suppurative phlebitis. For *S. aureus*, no immunosuppression or active malignancy should be present.
CNS, coagulase-negative *Staphylococcus*; LT, antibiotic lock therapy; SysRx, systemic antibiotics.
Adapted from references [2] and [4].

vancomycin plus heparin or saline is used most often; the vancomycin instilled should be 1,000-fold higher than the MIC for the bacteria involved [2]. Anecdotal use of lock therapy using gentamicin, amikacin, ciprofloxacin, ampicillin, cefazolin, ceftazidime, and also minocycline/EDTA has been reported [4,52]. Compatibility issues are important; some antibiotics precipitate in heparin at higher concentrations, and some solutions may influence the integrity of the catheter structure [4]. There are insufficient data to recommend the use of ethanol alone as a lock solution at this time [4].

Staphylococcus aureus Infections

It is very difficult for physicians to distinguish uncomplicated from complicated infection due to catheter-associated *S. aureus* bloodstream infection; this has resulted in considerable debate concerning the appropriate length of therapy for these infections. Several studies suggest that physicians cannot predict which patients have endocarditis or other complications by clinical history and physical examination alone [45,50,53]. Echocardiography should be done if the results will change duration of antibiotics or the need for surgery. If transthoracic echocardiography (TTE) is equivocal, then TEE should be performed for *S. aureus* bloodstream infection without a known source [54]. If the catheter is promptly removed and a TEE examination is negative for vegetations, *S. aureus* bacteremia can be treated with a minimum of 2 weeks of a penicillinase-resistant β-lactam antibiotic or a first-generation cephalosporin. Vancomycin should be used if the patient is allergic to β-lactam antibiotics or if the organism is methicillin resistant [4]. However, even those patients who appear to be appropriate candidates for short-course therapy may later present with metastatic foci or endocarditis, so it is essential to reassess "uncomplicated" cases if the patient develops relapse of fever, bacteremia, or embolic phenomena [4,55].

Candida Species Infections

Current recommendations are to treat all patients with catheter-associated fungemia with antifungal therapy [46]. The possibility that the organism has seeded to distant sites, especially the eye, is high, and the consequences of infection may be catastrophic. All candidemic patients should have a dilated retinal examination, preferably by an ophthalmologist [46]. Most studies show that outcome is improved if the catheter is promptly removed [46], but the point has been argued that many patients with neutropenia have the gut as the source, and the catheter does not have to be removed. In the nonneutropenic patient, the recommendations remain to remove all central catheters in patients with candidemia. Treatment with an echinocandin (anidulafungin, caspofungin, micafungin) or fluconazole is recommended [46]. Treatment should continue for 2 weeks after the first negative blood culture is obtained; however, if a metastatic focus of infection is noted, prolonged therapy will be required.

References

1. Safdar N, Fine JP, Maki DG: Meta-analysis: methods for diagnosing intravascular device-related bloodstream infection. *Ann Intern Med* 142:451, 2005.
2. Raad I, Hanna H, Maki D: Intravascular catheter-related infections: advances in diagnosis, prevention, and management. *Lancet Infect Dis* 7:645, 2007.
3. Perencevich EN, Stone PW, Wright SB, et al: Raising standards while watching the bottom line: making a business case for infection control interventions. *Infect Control Hosp Epidemiol* 28:1121, 2007.
4. Mermel LA, Allon M, Bouza E, et al: Clinical practice guidelines for the diagnosis and management of intravascular catheter-related infection: 2009 Update by the Infectious Diseases Society of America. *Clin Infect Dis* 49:1, 2009.
5. O'Grady NP, Alexander M, Dellinger EP, et al: Guidelines for the prevention of intravascular catheter-related infections. *Clin Infect Dis* 35:1281, 2002.
6. Marschall J, Mermel LA, Classen D, et al: Strategies to prevent central line-associated bloodstream infections in acute care hospitals. *Infect Control Hosp Epidemiol* 29:S22, 2008.
7. Donlan RM, Costerton JW: Biofilms: Survival mechanisms of clinically relevant microorganisms. *Clin Microbiol Rev* 15:167, 2002.
8. Crnich CJ, Maki DG: The promise of novel technology for the prevention of intravascular device-related bloodstream infection. I. Pathogenesis and short-term devices. *Clin Infect Dis* 34:1232, 2002.
9. Bouza E, Alvarado N, Alcala L, et al: A randomized and prospective study of 3 procedures for the diagnosis of catheter-related bloodstream infection without catheter withdrawal. *Clin Infect Dis* 44:820, 2007.
10. Parienti J-J, Thirion M, Megarbane B, et al: Femoral vs jugular venous catheterization and risk of nosocomial events in adults requiring acute renal replacement therapy: a randomized controlled trial. *JAMA* 299:2413, 2008.

11. Merrer J, De Jonghe B, Golliot F, et al: Complications of femoral and subclavian venous catheterization in critically ill patients: a randomized controlled trial. *JAMA* 286:700, 2001.
12. Pronovost P, Needham D, Berenholtz S, et al: An intervention to decrease catheter-related bloodstream infections in the ICU. *N Engl J Med* 355:2725, 2006.
13. Chaiyakunapruk N, Veenstra DL, Lipsky BA, et al: Vascular catheter site care: the clinical and economic benefits of chlorhexidine gluconate compared with povidone iodine. *Clin Infect Dis* 37:764, 2003.
14. Milstone AM, Passaretti CL, Perl TM: Chlorhexidine: expanding the armamentarium for infection control and prevention. *Clin Infect Dis* 46:274, 2008.
15. James MT, Conley J, Tonelli M, et al: Meta-analysis: antibiotics for prophylaxis against hemodialysis catheter-related infections. *Ann Intern Med* 148:596, 2008.
16. Timsit J-F, Schwebel C, Bouadma L, et al: Clorhexidine-impregnated sponges and less frequent dressing changes for prevention of catheter-related infections in critically ill adults: a randomized controlled trial. *JAMA* 301:1231, 2009.
17. Crawford AG, Fuhr JP, Rao B: Cost-benefit analysis of chlorhexidine gluconate dressing in the prevention of catheter-related bloodstream infections. *Infect Control Hosp Epidemiol* 25:668, 2004.
18. Miller JJ, Venus B, Mathru M: Comparison of the sterility of long-term central venous catheterization using single lumen, triple lumen, and pulmonary artery catheters. *Crit Care Med* 12:634, 1984.
19. Yeung C, May J, Hughes R: Infection rate for single lumen vs. triple lumen subclavian catheters. *Infect Control Hosp Epidemiol* 9:154, 1988.
20. Hilton E, Haslett TM, Borenstein MT, et al: Central catheter infections: single- versus triple-lumen catheters: influence of guide wires on infection rates when used for replacement of catheters. *Am J Med* 84:667, 1988.
21. Gil RT, Kruse JA, Thill-Baharozian MC, et al: Triple- vs single-lumen central venous catheters: a prospective study in a critically ill population. *Arch Intern Med* 149:1139, 1989.
22. Ma TY, Yoshinaka R, Banaag A, et al: Total parenteral nutrition via multilumen catheters does not increase the risk of catheter-related sepsis: a randomized, prospective study. *Clin Infect Dis* 27:500, 1998.
23. Casey AL, Mermel LA, Nightingale P, et al: Antimicrobial central venous catheters in adults: a systematic review and meta-analysis. *Lancet Infect Dis* 8:763, 2007.
24. Hanna H, Bahna P, Reitzel R, et al: Comparative in vitro efficacies and antimicrobial durabilities of novel antimicrobial central venous catheters. *Antimicrob Agents Chemother* 50:3283, 2006.
25. Lorente L, Lecuona M, Ramos MJ, et al: The use of rifampicin-miconazole-impregnated catheters reduces the incidence of femoral and jugular catheter-related bacteremia. *Clin Infect Dis* 47:1171, 2008.
26. Rupp ME, Lisco SJ, Lipsett PA, et al: Effect of a second-generation venous catheter impregnated with chlorhexidine and silver sulfadiazine on central catheter-related infections: a randomized controlled trial. *Ann Intern Med* 143:570, 2005.
27. Darouiche RO, Raad II, Heard SO, et al: A comparison of two antimicrobial central venous catheters. *N Engl J Med* 340:1, 1999.
28. Crnich CJ, Maki DG: The promise of novel technology for the prevention of intravascular device-related bloodstream infection. II. Long-term devices. *Clin Infect Dis* 34:1362, 2002.
29. Rowley KM, Clubb KS, Walker Smith GJ, et al: Right-sided infective endocarditis as a consequence of flow-directed pulmonary-artery catheterization: a clinicopathological study of 55 autopsied patients. *N Engl J Med* 311:1152, 1984.
30. Band JD, Maki DG: Infections caused by arterial catheters used for hemodynamic monitoring. *Am J Med* 67:735, 1979.
31. Arnow PM, Costas CO: Delayed rupture of the radial artery caused by catheter-related sepsis. *Rev Infect Dis* 10:1035, 1988.
32. Cook D, Randolph A, Kernerman P, et al: Central venous catheter replacement strategies: a systematic review of the literature. *Crit Care Med* 25:1417, 1997.
33. Baskin JL, Pui C-H, Reiss U, et al: Management of occlusion and thrombosis associated with long-term indwelling central venous catheters. *Lancet* 374:159, 2009.
34. Rudnick JR, Beck-Sague CM, Anderson RL, et al: Gram-negative bacteremia in open-heart-surgery patients traced to probable tap-water contamination of pressure-monitoring equipment. *Infect Control Hosp Epidemiol* 17:281, 1996.
35. Field K, McFarlane C, Cheng AC, et al: Incidence of catheter-related bloodstream infection among patients with a needleless, mechanical valve-based intravenous connector in an Australian hematology-oncology unit. *Infect Control Hosp Epidemiol* 28:610, 2007.
36. Salgado CD, Chinnes L, Paczesny TH, et al: Increased rate of catheter-related bloodstream infection associated with use of a needleless mechanical valve device at a long-term acute care hospital. *Infect Control Hosp Epidemiol* 28:684, 2007.
37. Centers for Disease Control and Prevention: Epidemiologic notes and reports. Nosocomial bacteremias associated with intravenous fluid therapy—USA. *MMWR Morb Mortal Wkly Rep* 46:1227, 1997.
38. Mirtallo JM, Caryer K, Schneider PJ, et al: Growth of bacteria and fungi in parenteral nutrition solutions containing albumin. *Am J Hosp Pharm* 38:1907, 1981.
39. Solomon SL, Khabbaz RF, Parker RH, et al: An outbreak of *Candida parapsilosis* bloodstream infections in patients receiving parenteral nutrition. *J Infect Dis* 149:98, 1984.
40. Dankner WM, Spector SA, Fierer J, et al: *Malassezia* fungemia in neonates and adults: complication of hyperalimentation. *Rev Infect Dis* 4:743, 1987.
41. Arnow PM, Quimosing EM, Beach M: Consequences of intravascular catheter sepsis. *Clin Infect Dis* 16:778, 1993.
42. Gill MV, Klein NS, Cunha BA: Unusual organisms causing intravenous line infections in compromised hosts: I. Bacterial and algal infections. *Infect Dis Clin Pract* 5:244, 1996.
43. Engelhard D, Elishoov H, Strauss N, et al: Nosocomial coagulase negative staphylococcal infections in bone marrow transplantation recipients with central vein catheter. *Transplantation* 61:430, 1996.
44. Elting LS, Bodey GP: Septicemia due to *Xanthomonas* species and non-*aeruginosa Pseudomonas* species: increasing incidence of catheter-related infections. *Medicine (Baltimore)* 69:196, 1990.
45. Fowler VG, Justice A, Moore C, et al: Risk factors for hematogenous complications of intravenous catheter-associated *Staphylococcus aureus*. *Clin Infect Dis* 40:695, 2005.
46. Pappas PG, Kauffman CA, Andes D, et al: Clinical practice guidelines for the management of candidiasis: 2009 Update by the Infectious Diseases Society of America. *Clin Infect Dis* 48:503, 2009.
47. Andes DR, Urban AW, Acher CW, et al: Septic thrombosis of the basilic, axillary, and subclavian veins caused by a peripherally inserted central venous catheter. *Am J Med* 105:446, 1998.
48. Timsit J-F, Farkas J-C, Boyer J-M, et al: Central vein catheter-related thrombosis in intensive care patients. Incidence, risk factors, and relationship with catheter-related sepsis. *Chest* 114:207, 1998.
49. Murdoch DR, Corey GR, Hoen R, et al: Clinical presentation, etiology, and outcome of infective endocarditis in the 21st century: the International Collaboration on Endocarditis—Prospective Cohort Study. *Arch Intern Med* 169:463, 2009.
50. Fowler VG, Li J, Corey GR, et al: Role of echocardiography in evaluation of patients with *Staphylococcus aureus* bacteremia: experience in 103 patients. *J Am Coll Cardiol* 30:1072, 1997.
51. Martinez E, Mensa J, Rovira M, et al: Central venous catheter exchange by guidewire for treatment of catheter-related bacteraemia inpatients undergoing BMT or intensive chemotherapy. *Bone Marrow Transplant* 23:41, 1999.
52. Raad I, Hanna H, Dvorak T, et al: Optimal antimicrobial lock solution, using different combinations of minocycline, EDTA, and 25-percent ethanol, rapidly eradicates organisms embedded in biofilm. *Antimicrob Agents Chemother* 51:78, 2007.
53. Fowler VG, Olsen MK, Corey GR, et al: Clinical identifiers of complicated *Staphylococcus aureus* bacteremia. *Arch Intern Med* 163:2066, 2003.
54. Cheitlin MD, Armstrong WF, Aurigemma GP, et al: ACC/AHA/ASE 2003 Guideline Update for the Clinical Application of Echocardiography: summary Article: a Report of the American College of Cardiology/American Heart Association Task Force on Practice Guidelines (ACC/AHA/ASE Committee to Update the 1997 Guidelines for the Clinical Application of Echocardiography). *Circulation* 108:1146, 2003.
55. Raad II, Sabbagh MF: Optimal duration of therapy for catheter-related *Staphylococcus aureus* bacteremia: a study of 55 cases and review. *Clin Infect Dis* 14:75, 1992.

CHAPTER 82 ■ URINARY TRACT INFECTIONS

STEVEN M. OPAL

Urinary tract infection (UTI) remains a common nosocomially acquired infection, accounting for approximately 25% to 40% of all infectious complications in hospitalized patients [1–5]. In a nation-wide surveillance study of nearly one-half million intensive care unit (ICU) patients in the United States, UTI accounted for 23% of all infections and was associated with urinary catheters in 97% of patients [2]. Similar findings have recently been reported from surveys from Spain [3], Germany [4], and Brazil [5] with an overall incidence of urinary catheter-associated UTI of about 1 to 10 episodes per 1,000 catheter days. Furthermore, the urinary tract is the most frequently recognized source of Gram-negative bacteremia, which constitutes a major cause of infectious morbidity and mortality in the critically ill patient [1,6–8]. Approximately 100,000 annual admissions to acute care hospitals in the United States have been attributed to severe infections of the urinary tract [9]. Complicated UTI, progressive antimicrobial resistance, and the prevention of UTI with the widespread use of indwelling urinary catheters remain major challenges in critical care practice.

THE PATHOPHYSIOLOGY OF URINARY TRACT INFECTIONS

UTIs are primarily caused by Gram-negative bacilli (71%), with Gram-positive pathogens and fungi accounting for the remainder of microorganisms [6]. *Escherichia coli* is by far the most common cause of community-acquired and nosocomially acquired UTI. Most UTIs arise from ascending infection by enteric organisms that colonize the perineum and distal urethra. Specific clones of *E. coli* have evolved that readily colonize the uroepithelium and cause UTI. These clones possess the requisite set of virulence genes needed to successfully attach, survive, and invade the urinary tract in nonimmunocompromised patients with anatomically normal genitourinary (GU) tracts [10].

An essential characteristic of uropathogenic *E. coli* is its ability to adhere to uroepithelial membranes. Urinary isolates of *E. coli* possess an array of adhesions including type I (common pili), S pili, FIC pili, and P pili. These bacterial surface structures facilitate attachment to epithelial surfaces. Type I pili bind to mannose-containing polysaccharides on the cell surface of epithelial membranes. This allows the organism to attach and persist within the urinary tract and avoid elimination during micturition [11].

Another important adhesin of uropathogenic *E. coli* is the expression of P pili on the bacteria's outer membrane [12]. P pili bind to α-D-galactose 1 $\rightarrow$ 4 β-D-galactose (Gal-Gal) containing disaccharides of the globoseries of glycolipids. These glycolipids are found primarily on the epithelial surfaces of the upper urinary tract, enterocytes, and erythrocytes. The ability of *E. coli* to express P pili is particularly important in the establishment of upper UTIs where Gal-Gal disaccharide-containing glycolipids are found in large concentration. Recent genetic analysis reveals that bacterial pathogens cluster their virulence factors in discreet loci along the chromosome known as pathogenicity-associated islands (PAIs). These genetic elements contain a large number of genes associated with virulence and distinguish uropathogenic strains from nonpathogenic colonizing strains [13].

Other genera of the Enterobacteriaceae, including *Citrobacter, Klebsiella, Enterobacter, Serratia, Proteus, Morganella,* and *Providencia* spp, become more common causes of UTI when patients receive antibiotics or have anatomic or functional abnormalities in urine flow [14]. The microbiology of UTI after short-term urinary catheterization is similar to that observed in the noncatheterized patient. However, long-term (>30 days) catheterization generates an environment that supports a complex and often polymicrobial microflora. An extensive extracellular array of microbial-derived polysaccharides surrounds bacterial microcolonies within the lumen of the long-term urinary catheter. This biofilm structure protects bacterial populations for immune, phagocytic, or antibacterial clearance [15]. Bacteria found in the urine in chronically catheterized patients differ from noncatheterized patients. *Proteus, Providencia, Morganella,* and *Pseudomonas* species become more common, whereas *E. coli* and *Klebsiella* species become less common (Fig. 82.1). *Proteus* species, some other Gram-negative enteric organisms, and *Staphylococcus saprophyticus* synthesize the enzyme urease, a known bacterial virulence factor in the urinary tract. The generation of ammonia from the breakdown of urea increases regional pH, favoring the generation of the "triple-phosphate crystals" struvite and apatite in urine. Struvite crystals can block urinary catheter flow and promote the formation of urinary calculi [16].

Gram-positive bacteria occasionally cause UTIs in critically ill patients. The isolation of *S. aureus* in the urine is significant as it often accompanies staphylococcal bacteremia. *S. aureus* isolation in urine cultures, particularly in noncatheterized patients, should prompt a search for extrarenal sources of staphylococcal infection. *S. aureus* may also colonize chronically catheterized patients. This is particularly true for methicillin-resistant *S. aureus* strains, which may thrive in hospital settings with many elderly, catheterized patients [8].

Enterococci are prevalent in the GU tract of elderly populations and in patients with long-term urinary catheters. The remarkable ability of this organism to resist antimicrobial agents, including β-lactam antibiotics, aminoglycosides, quinolones, and recently vancomycin, makes this organism a frequent urinary pathogen in hospitalized patients [6–8]. *Candida* species and other fungal organisms may colonize or infect the GU tract. Candiduria may be associated with hematogenous dissemination ("descending UTI") or ascending UTIs from perineal surfaces. The unique problems associated with the isolation of *Candida* species of the urinary tract are considered in the final section of this chapter.

HOST DEFENSE MECHANISMS AGAINST URINARY TRACT INFECTION

The human GU tract is remarkably resistant to UTI by mechanical, mucosal, and immunologic mechanisms. The flushing action of urinary flow itself is an important defense against UTI.

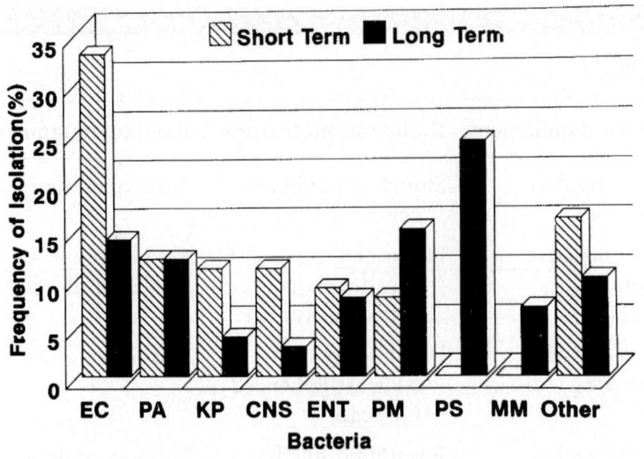

FIGURE 82.1. Distribution of bacterial isolation associated with catheter-related UTI. CNS, coagulase-negative staphylococci; EC, *Escherichia coli*; ENT, Enterococci; KP, *Klebsiella pneumoniae*; MM, *Morganella morganii*; PA, *Pseudomonas aeruginosa*; PM, *Proteus mirabilis*; PS, *Providencia stuartii.*

The frequent occurrence of UTI after obstruction or incomplete bladder emptying attests to the importance of micturition in clearing potential pathogens. Patients with neurogenic bladder or vesicoureteral reflux are highly susceptible to UTI and renal scarring. While urinary pathogens must possess a full complement of virulence factors to cause infection in the anatomically normal urinary tract, UTI in the obstructed urinary tract occurs with bacterial species devoid of special urinary virulence factors [10].

Urinary osmolarity, urea concentration, pH, and oxygen concentration limit the growth potential of many bacterial pathogens in the urinary tract. Continuous sloughing of uroepithelial cells, urinary mucosal glycocalyx (slime), and secretion of the Tamm–Horsfall protein assist in the mechanical removal of adherent bacteria that have entered the urinary tract [17].

The ability of bacteria to adhere to the mucosal surface of uroepitheilial cells is dependent on the mucopolysaccharide content of this surface and its chemical composition. Patients with high concentrations of Gal-Gal disaccharides on the cell surfaces in the urinary tract are predisposed to UTI from P-piliated *E. coli* [10]. Patients who are nonsecretors of blood group antigens have an increased risk of UTI [18]. Blood group antigens coat uroepithelial cells when secreted onto the mucosal surface. These antigens prevent attachment of bacteria to adhesin-receptor oligosaccharides on the surface of epithelial cells. Individuals who fail to secrete blood group antigens are rendered infection prone to UTI.

Although secretory immunoglobulin, neutrophils, and cell-mediated immunity contribute to the host defense against UTI, their roles are secondary to mechanical and physical barriers to infection. Uroepithelial cells produce the chemokine interleukin-8 (IL-8) in response to *E. coli* infection. IL-8 promotes neutrophil migration to the urinary tract which reduces the risk of disseminated infection. Patients differ in their level of expression of the IL-8 receptor CXCR1. Decreased CXCR1 expression in the urinary tract might contribute to increased susceptibility to pyelonephritis in some patients [19].

Adult women are much more likely to develop UTI than men. Women are more likely to develop pyelonephritis if they are sexually active, use spermicidal agents, experience urinary incontinence, have diabetes mellitus, or a family history of UTI [16]. The increased anatomic distance from the urethral orifice to the urinary bladder, the infrequent presence of Gram-negative bacteria around the male urethra, and the production of inhibitory prostatic secretions protect men from UTI until they become elderly [20]. Bladder neck obstruction from age-related benign prostatic hypertrophy causes urinary obstruction and UTI in elderly men.

SEVERE URINARY TRACT INFECTION

Acute Pyelonephritis

Acute pyelonephritis can precipitate in severe sepsis/septic shock when complicated by urinary obstruction, papillary necrosis, or other local suppurative complications. Failure of the patient to respond clinically within 72 hours to seemingly appropriate antimicrobial therapy should prompt a search for complications of UTI. Functional or mechanical obstruction to urinary flow is the principal underlying cause of treatment failure in UTI. Obstruction may arise from extrarenal causes such as retroperitoneal or pelvic masses or abnormalities intrinsic to the GU tract such as renal calculi or ureteral obstruction. Alleviation of obstruction facilitates antimicrobial treatment and is often essential to successfully eradicate infections in the upper urinary tract system [21].

Suppurative Complications of Urinary Tract Infection

Abscess formation within the GU tract may take several forms and pose a diagnostic and therapeutic challenge. It is important to distinguish between these entities because the clinical implications and medical-surgical management of each process differ substantially (see Table 82.1). Radiographic findings in a typical case of emphysematous pyelonephritis (usually caused by enteric bacteria, not *Clostridium* spp or other anaerobes) are seen in Figure 82.2A, B. Suppurative complications of UTI necessitate urgent urologic intervention with percutaneous or surgical drainage [21].

Diagnostic Methods in Urinary Tract Infection

The clinical diagnosis of acute UTI of the upper urinary tract in the noncatheterized patient is usually straightforward, with a history of urinary frequency and dysuria accompanied with costovertebral angle (CVA) tenderness and signs of systemic toxicity. The urinalysis often shows positive "dipstick" results for leukocyte esterase and nitrite, markers for leukocytes, and enteric bacteria. The presence of excess numbers of urinary leukocytes and bacteria in the urinary sediment, in the absence of contamination by epithelial cells, is indicative of a UTI in symptomatic patients. Pyuria alone without bacteriuria is indicative of GU inflammation (e.g., allergic interstitial nephritis, prostatitis, urethritis) or infection by difficult-to-culture pathogens (*Mycobacterium, Chlamydia, Mycoplasma* spp, etc.) and warrants further investigation to determine its etiology.

The urinary Gram stain of unspun urine is helpful in determining the most likely agent causing the UTI. Gram-negative rods in the urine are readily identifiable and this confirms the presence of significant bacteriuria. The finding of more than one organism per high-powered field in unspun urine equates with $>10^5$ colony-forming units (CFU) per mL [22,23]. Urinary Gram stain can also detect Gram-positive microorganisms, such as enterococci and staphylococci, and fungal elements. Polymicrobial bacteriuria is often apparent by urinary Gram stain and may be seen in UTI from long-standing urinary catheterization, enterovesical fistula, or complicated UTI associated with obstruction or foreign bodies.

Patients with severe UTIs requiring critical care management should have quantitative urinary culture performed,

TABLE 82.1

SUPPURATIVE COMPLICATIONS OF URINARY TRACT INFECTION

Disease process	Pathogenesis	Predisposing factors	Common pathogens	Radiographic features	Standard treatment
Papillary necrosis	Ischemia, necrosis, infection	Analgesics, diabetes, obstruction	Gram-negative enterics	Sloughed papilla in calyx	Antibiotics alone
Pyonephritis	Infection with hydronephrosis	Ureteral obstruction, calculi	Gram-negative enterics	Hydronephrosis with gas, debris in collecting system	Nephrostomy tube, antibiotics
Focal bacterial nephritis	Ascending UTI with focal renal inflammation	UTI with upper tract involvement	Gram-negative enterics	Focal defect on contrast-enhanced CT scan	Antibiotics alone
Corticomedullary abscess	Ascending UTI with focal renal liquefaction	UTI with obstruction, diabetes	Gram-negative enterics	Focal fluid-filled defect on CT or ultrasound	Antibiotics alone or percutaneous drainage
Xanthogranulomatous pyelonephritis	Enlarging granulomatous process with cholesterol-laden macrophages	Chronic obstruction with infection	*Proteus* spp, *Klebsiella* spp	Large heterogenous mass	Partial or complete nephrectomy
Emphysematous pyelonephritis	Ischemic necrosis with infection from gas-forming organisms	Elderly diabetic	Gram-negative enterics, rarely anaerobes	Gas on plain film, CT	Closed or open drainage or nephrectomy, antibiotics
Cortical abscess (renal carbuncle)	Hematogenous seeding of kidney	Extrarenal infection with *Staphylococcus aureus*	*S. aureus*	Semisolid intrarenal mass with caliceal distortion	Antibiotics alone or with percutaneous drainage
Perinephritic abscess	Rupture of intrarenal abscess	Obstruction, diabetes, renal transplants	*Escherichia coli*, *Proteus* spp, *S. aureus*, others	Displaced renal tissue, perinephric mass	Closed or open surgical drainage, antibiotics

CT, computed tomography; UTI, urinary tract infection.

preferably before the initiation of antimicrobial therapy. The urine culture confirms the diagnosis and defines the most appropriate antimicrobial agent for treatment. The progressive increase in antimicrobial resistance makes it imperative to carefully select antimicrobial agents based on susceptibility patterns of the infecting microorganism. Greater than 10^5 CFU per mL in clean catch, midstream urine is generally diagnostic. The quantitative level of bacteriuria diagnostic for acute UTI varies depending on the clinical situation.

In clinical surveys of symptomatic women with UTI, repeated isolation of as few as $>10^2$ pathogenic microorganisms per mL is diagnostic [21]. Catheterized patients may also have UTI with $<10^5$ CFU per mL. The presence of an indwelling urinary catheter may not allow ongoing replication of microorganisms in the urinary tract to achieve levels greater than 10^5 CFU per mL. Moreover, urinary cultures from noninstrumented men are significant with as little as 10^3 CFU per mL [24].

The absence of pyuria and significant bacteriuria does not exclude the possibility of a potentially serious UTI. Patients with severe neutropenia may not have significant levels of pyuria. Urine cultures may be negative in more than 40% of patients with perinephric abscess, and most patients with renal cortical abscesses have urinalyses without significant bacteriuria [25]. Complete unilateral urinary obstruction associated with pyonephrosis can fail to show the primary pathogen within voided urine. Urinary stent placement increases the risk of UTI. In a recent survey, voided urine specimens taken at the time of stent removal were negative in the presence of microbial colonization in 40% of the patients [26].

Blood cultures should be obtained on all patients who are septic as a result of a UTI. Urine cultures should also be performed from nephrostomy tube drainage in patients with prior urinary diversion procedures. It is generally unnecessary to change a urinary catheter before the acquisition of urine cultures in patients with acute UTI.

RADIOGRAPHIC PROCEDURES FOR THE DIAGNOSIS OF URINARY TRACT INFECTION

Complicated UTIs often require radiologic methods to establish the correct diagnosis. Routine abdominal radiographs may assist in the diagnosis of complicated forms of UTI. The presence of radiopaque renal calculi can be readily detected on abdominal radiography. Emphysematous pyelonephritis appears as an abnormal collection of gas within the renal parenchyma. Gas is detectable in the urinary collecting system in many patients with pyonephrosis. Abnormal renal shadows and loss of psoas margins may suggest the presence of a perinephric abscess. Renal ultrasonography and computed tomography (CT) have replaced the intravenous pyelogram (or excretory urogram) as the principal radiographic technique in the detection of complicated UTI. The anatomic definition of the kidney and

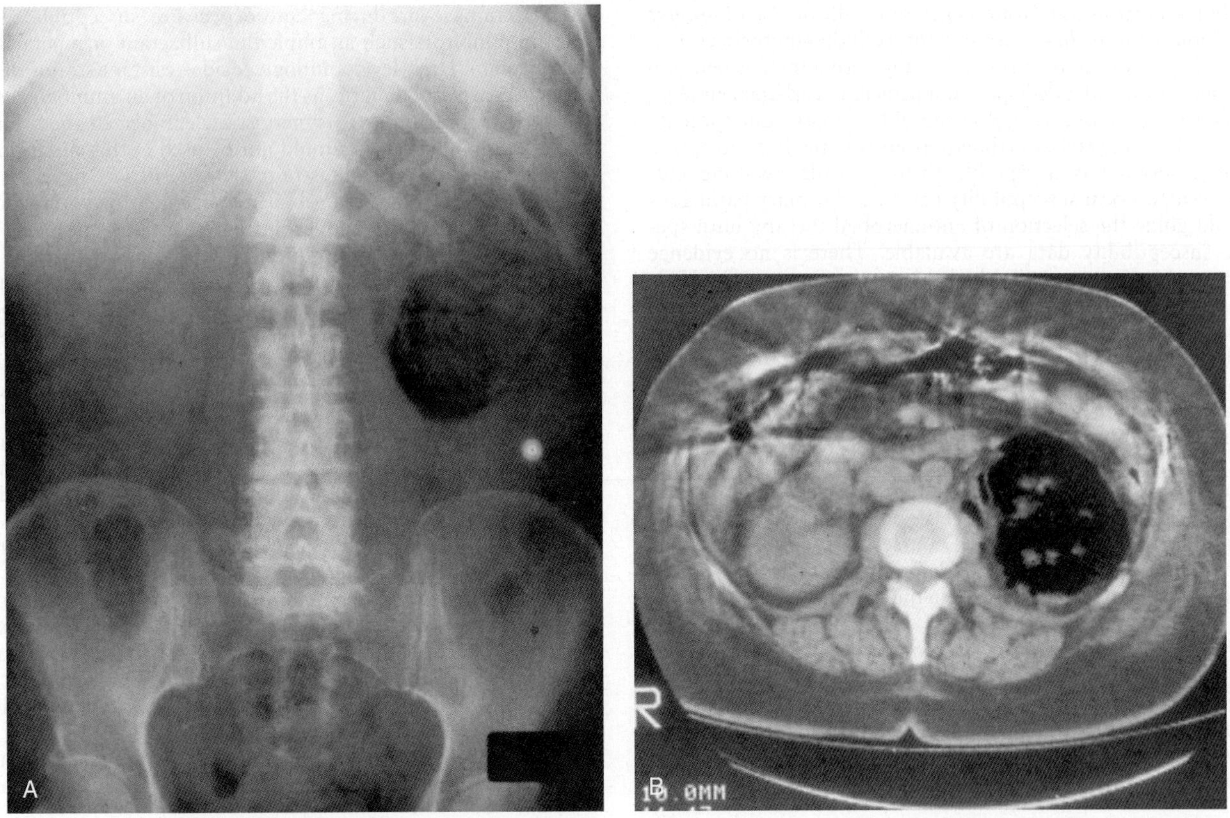

FIGURE 82.2. Radiographic findings in a diabetic woman with emphysematous pyelonephritis caused by *Escherichia coli*. **A:** Plain abdominal radiograph with evidence for gas in the left renal fossa. **B:** Computed tomography scan confirming gas in the left kidney. This patient recovered following emergency nephrectomy and antimicrobial therapy.

perirenal tissues is superior with a contrast-enhanced abdominal CT scan and is generally the preferred imaging method for complicated UTI (see Table 82.1). Renal ultrasound provides another rapid method of detecting hydronephrosis and anatomic detail of the renal parenchyma. Ultrasonography can also determine the solid or cystic nature of a renal mass detected on abdominal CT. Ultrasound can study the kidney on any plane and may be performed urgently in the absence of intravenous contrast media. The CT scan or renal ultrasound is indispensable in the localization of inflammatory processes during diagnostic aspiration or percutaneous drainage procedures. Magnetic resonance imaging (MRI) provides detailed information about the renal structures and retroperitoneal space, but the CT has sufficient resolving power in most forms of renal inflammatory disease.

The gallium-67–scan or indium-111–labeled leukocyte studies can occasionally be useful in the diagnosis of complicated UTI. These nuclear medicine studies assist in the differentiation between a renal neoplasm and a focal inflammatory process of the kidney. These studies are useful in the evaluation of patients with fever of unknown origin secondary to perinephric abscess or renal cortical abscess [27].

Intravenous pyelography (IVP) provides refined details of the calyces and ureters and remains an excellent diagnostic method for the diagnosis of papillary necrosis or small, radiolucent urinary calculi. The need for intravenous contrast media carries attendant risks of hypersensitivity reactions and radiocontrast-induced renal failure. The potential toxicity and limited resolution outside the urinary collecting system has relegated the IVP to an infrequently performed procedure in the workup of UTI in ICU patients [28].

MEDICAL MANAGEMENT OF URINARY TRACT INFECTION

Patients admitted to the ICU for management of UTI usually suffer from severe infections complicated by a systemic inflammatory response (sepsis) or suppurative complications of the GU tract. Medical management initially consists of stabilization of the patient's hemodynamic parameters and supportive measures in the management of septic shock. After the completion of appropriate diagnostic studies, empiric antimicrobial therapy should be directed toward the most likely infecting urinary pathogen(s). A urinary Gram stain usually provides evidence of either a Gram-negative or Gram-positive bacterial pathogen. If this is unavailable or nondiagnostic, then broad-spectrum, empiric antimicrobial therapy is indicated.

In the septic patient with UTI, the initial use of a β-lactam antibiotic (assuming there is no history of allergic reactions to β-lactams) in combination with an aminoglycoside has been the traditional therapeutic regimen in hospitalized patients. The β-lactam/aminoglycoside combination supplies optimal therapy for systemic infections with enteric Gram-negative bacilli, enterococci, and nonfermentative, multiresistant, Gram-negative bacterial pathogens. Severely ill septic patients who are immunocompromised also warrant combination antimicrobial therapy [21]. Increasingly, the therapeutic trend in empiric therapy is away from aminoglycosides to monotherapy with β-lactams alone, β-lactam/β-lactamase inhibitors, and/or fluoroquinolones [29].

Community-acquired UTIs in nonimmunocompromised patients who have not received antimicrobial agents infrequently harbor multiresistant Gram-negative bacilli or *Pseudomonas* sp. Should the urinary Gram stain exclude enterococci as a potential pathogen, then single therapy with a third-generation cephalosporin, extended-spectrum penicillin, carbapenem (e.g., imipenem or meropenem), β-lactam/β-lactamase inhibitor (e.g., piperacillin-tazobactam) trimethoprim-sulfamethoxazole, or a fluoroquinolone is acceptable therapy while awaiting culture results. Local susceptibility patterns of urinary pathogens should guide the selection of antimicrobial therapy until specific susceptibility data are available. There is no evidence that combination antimicrobial therapy is necessary for UTIs caused by Gram-negative bacilli unless *Pseudomonas aeruginosa* infection with neutropenia is present. A single antimicrobial agent known to be active against the infecting uropathogen should be employed once the causative organism is known. Parenteral therapy is generally administered until the patient has been rendered nontoxic and afebrile for 24 to 48 hours. Therapy may then be administered orally and should be given for a total of approximately 2 weeks [21,24]. Patients with obstructive lesions and complicated UTIs not amenable to corrective surgery may require prolonged courses of antimicrobial therapy, as indicated by their underlying urologic disorder. Common antimicrobial agents useful in the treatment of severe UTIs are listed in Table 82.2.

Standard therapy for severe enterococcal UTIs has been ampicillin and an aminoglycoside. Although this regimen remains active against most enterococcal isolates, progressive antimicrobial resistance to aminoglycosides, ampicillin, and other β-lactams and vancomycin has complicated the antimicrobial therapy for enterococcal infections [30]. Rare strains of β-lactamase–producing enterococci are susceptible to β-lactam inhibitors such as ampicillin/sulbactam or piperacillin/tazobactam. High-level aminoglycoside-resistant strains of enterococci are problematic, as the addition of an aminoglycoside no longer contributes to synergistic clearance of these infections. Aminoglycosides should not be used in this situation.

Glycopeptide-resistant strains of enterococci pose a serious threat to the antimicrobial management of enterococcal infections. Some of these isolates remain susceptible to β-lactam agents. Newer fluoroquinolones occasionally have activity against enterococci and may be useful in the treatment of glycopeptide- and β-lactam–resistant strains of enterococci. Tetracyclines and nitrofurantoin are useful alternatives for uncomplicated, enterococcal UTI if susceptibility testing indicates activity. Quinupristin/dalfopristin is a streptogramin antibiotic useful in the treatment of vancomycin-resistant *Enterococcus faecium* (but not *Enterococcus faecalis*) infections [30]. Linezolid, an oxazolidinone that inhibits the initiation of translation at the 30S ribosome of bacteria, has activity against vancomycin-resistant enterococci [31]. Multidrug-resistant enterococci are an infection control hazard in the ICU and contact precautions are recommended.

Antistaphylococcal penicillins such as nafcillin or oxacillin are indicated in the empiric therapy of renal cortical abscesses (renal carbuncle). Vancomycin should be instituted if there is a suspicion of the presence of methicillin-resistant staphylococcal isolates in a patient with a cortical abscess or perinephric abscess.

Urgent percutaneous nephrotomy tube placement for urinary drainage and abscess management is indicated in severely

TABLE 82.2

COMMON ANTIMICROBIAL AGENTS FOR SEVERE URINARY TRACT INFECTION

Agent	Dose and frequency[a]	Principal indications	Comments
Ampicillin–sulbactam	3.0 g IV q6–8 h	Gram-negative enterics	Other β-lactam/inhibitor combinations also effective
Aztreonam	1 g IV q8 h[b]	Gram-negative enterics *Pseudomonas* spp	Useful in penicillin-allergic patients
Cefazolin	1.0 g IV q8 h		
Cefotaxime	1–2 g IV q8 h	Gram-negative enterics	Other second- and third-generation cephalosporins also effective
Ciprofloxacin	400 mg IV q12 h	Gram-negative enterics *Pseudomonas* spp	Other fluoroquinolones may not be effective; moxifloxacin and gemifloxacin do not achieve high levels in urine
Fluconazole	200 mg loading 100 mg q24 h	*Candida* spp UTI	If non-*albicans Candida* spp, check susceptibility or use Amphotericin B
Gentamicin[c]	1.5 mg/kg IV q12 h or 5 mg/kg/d	Gram-negative enterics *Pseudomonas* spp enterococci	Dosing interval dependent on renal function
Piperacillin/tazobactam	3.375 g IV q8 h[d]	Gram-negative enterics *Pseudomonas* spp	Other extended-spectrum penicillins also effective
Trimethoprim/sulfamethoxazole	160/800 mg IV q12 h	Gram-negative enterics	Watch for sulfa allergies
Vancomycin	500 mg IV q12 h	MRSA	Watch renal function carefully
Linezolid	600 mg IV or PO q12 h	MRSA, VRE	Monitor complete blood counts

[a] Adult dosing in patients with normal renal function; follow susceptibility test results and treat parenterally until systemic toxicity resolves.
[b] Aztreonam dose can be increased to 2 g q8 h for *P. aeruginosa* infection.
[c] Gentamicin or other aminoglycosides often given with a β-lactam agent in Gram-negative septic shock or severe enterococcal infections.
[d] Piperacillin/tazobactam dose can be increased to 4.5 g q8 h for *P. aeruginosa* infection.
MRSA, methicillin-resistant *S. aureus*; UTI, urinary tract infection; VRE, vancomycin-resistant enterococci.

septic patients with obstructed urinary collecting systems. Percutaneous catheter drainage of perinephric abscesses, renal carbuncles, and infected urinary cysts is often necessary in combination with antimicrobial therapy to manage these complicated UTIs. Open surgical drainage is reserved for patients who fail to respond to attempted percutaneous drainage.

PREVENTIVE MEASURES AGAINST URINARY TRACT INFECTION IN THE INTENSIVE CARE UNIT SETTING

The most efficacious method of preventing UTIs in critically ill patients is not using urinary catheters at all or limiting their duration of use as much as possible [32]. Asymptomatic bacteriuria should generally not be treated whether an indwelling urinary catheter is present or not. Asymptomatic bacteriuria in pregnant women and immunocompromised patients should be treated with specific antimicrobial agents as the risk of ascending UTI is considerable and may be avoided by early medical intervention [21,33].

The Management of Catheter-Related Urinary Tract Infection

The ubiquitous presence of the indwelling urinary catheter in hospitalized patients provides microbial pathogens ready access to the urinary tract with subsequent development of UTI. It is estimated that 10% of all hospitalized patients in the United States will have a urinary catheter inserted during their hospitalization, resulting in over 1 million UTIs per year [6,21,22,24]. The overall incidence of catheter-acquired UTI in patients within critical care units varies from 0.5 to 10 UTI per 1,000 catheter days [3–5,22]. The risk factors for acquisition of catheter-related UTI include duration of catheter placement, increasing patient age, female gender, severity of underlying illness, and perhaps obesity [22,23]. The estimated risk of bacteriuria after urinary tract catheterization is approximately 5% for each day of catheterization. Chronically catheterized (more than 30 days) patients almost invariably have bacteriuria, and their admission to the ICU poses a threat of cross-contamination of urinary pathogens to other ICU patients. Despite continued infection control efforts to decrease the frequency of contamination, UTI remains the major complication of urinary catheters. The average, calculated, incremental cost associated with the hospital care of a patient with a catheter-related UTI is $589.00 [32,34].

Pathogenesis

The catheter itself interferes with physiologic host defense mechanisms against UTI. Trauma produced by an indwelling catheter may damage the bladder mucosa and the mucous layer that coats uroepithelial cells [35]. This exposes the cell surface of epithelial cells to bacterial adhesions and increases the risk of UTI. Indwelling catheters prevent complete bladder emptying. Residual urine serves as a culture medium for bacteria in an inadequately drained urinary bladder. Additionally, temporary obstruction of urine flow caused by kinking or clamping of the urinary catheter can lead to bladder distension, vesicoureteral reflux, and infection.

Bacteria gain access to the urinary tract in catheterized patients by one of three mechanisms: (a) during insertion, (b) along the external surface after insertion, or (c) via the inner lumen of the urinary catheter. Implantation of bacteria into the bladder during catheter placement occurs at a frequency of approximately 0.5% to 8% [35]. This risk varies with the experience of the healthcare worker placing the catheter and with the level of periurethral colonization by potential uropathogens. Ascending infection from within the lumen accounts for approximately 20% of catheter-related UTIs [21]. The use of sterile, closed urinary collecting devices with a sterile vent to avoid a standing column of urine from the bladder to the collecting bag has decreased the frequency of UTI. Optimal catheter design includes a sterile sampling port that obviates the need to open the system to collect urine samples. The collecting bag should have a large reservoir with a device to measure urine output with minimal manipulation of the catheter system.

Most catheter-related UTIs are derived from microorganisms that enter the urinary bladder along the external surface of the catheter [35,36]. The periurethral space becomes colonized with enteric organisms, which then migrate along the periurethral mucous sheath that surrounds the surface of the catheter. Continued movement of the catheter in and out of the urinary bladder occurs upon repositioning of the patient or catheter manipulations. This process provides ample opportunity for organisms coating the catheter surface to gain access to the urinary bladder and cause infection.

Numerous enteric organisms avidly adhere to the mucosal surface of the urinary bladder. Some organisms, such as *Providencia stuartii* and *P. aeruginosa*, also possess surface adhesins that bind directly to the urinary catheter itself. The urinary catheter becomes an ecologic niche for these organisms, resulting in prolonged infections that may persist for months in the catheterized patient [37]. More than 90% of *P. stuartii* bacteremias occur as the result of urinary catheter-induced UTIs [38]. The urease produced by *Proteus* species affects the local pH surrounding the catheter, which facilitates the deposition of struvite microcrystals on the surface of the catheter. These encrustations serve as a nidus for persistent colonization with urinary pathogens. Adherent bacteria establish microcolonies coated with extracellular polysaccharides. The continued buildup of this biofilm within the lumen of the urinary catheter eventually leads to obstruction of urinary flow [15,39]. The presence of a foreign body within the urinary bladder interferes with the penetration and antimicrobial action of antibiotics. Bactericidal agents inhibit, but often fail to kill, microorganisms that adhere to catheter materials. Furthermore, the catheter serves as a foreign body inducing early degranulation and loss of bactericidal activity of neutrophils. These factors contribute to the difficulties eradicating urinary pathogens in the catheterized patient.

Diagnosis

The presence of bacteriuria in the catheterized patient documents colonization of the urinary tract but does not necessarily confirm the presence of an actual UTI. A UTI develops when a host response occurs to the presence of microbial pathogens in the urine. As many as 70% of patients who develop catheter-related bacteriuria remain symptom free and resolve spontaneously with the catheter removal [40]. It is generally acknowledged that the treatment of asymptomatic bacteriuria in the catheterized patient is not warranted, except in some specific circumstances [41]. The severely neutropenic patient with asymptomatic bacteriuria should be treated because of the risk of systemic infection in this patient population. In addition, treating asymptomatic bacteriuria in catheterized patients might be warranted in an outbreak setting of nosocomially acquired infection to prevent further spread of specific urinary pathogens [42].

It is often difficult to recognize that a symptomatic UTI is present in the catheterized patient. Altered levels of consciousness may interfere with the patient's awareness of the UTI. Furthermore, the presence of a urinary catheter removes the symptoms of urinary frequency and the perception of dysuria. Hematuria and pyuria may be found in the catheterized patient in the absence of urinary colonization with bacteria. Isolated pyuria in patients with asymptomatic bacteriuria is not an indication for antimicrobial treatment [41]. This is presumably related to sterile inflammation and trauma induced by the catheter itself. High-grade pyuria (>50 white blood cells per high power field) with fever supports the diagnosis of a UTI in the catheterized patient [43].

The presence of lower numbers of bacteria than the traditional $>10^5$ CFU per mL can indicate infection in catheterized patients [44]. Quantitative counts as low as 10^2 CFU per mL may be significant in the catheterized patient. Low colony counts in catheterized urine can progress to high-grade bacteriuria in catheterized patients. Clinical laboratories should isolate and characterize urinary isolates from catheterized patients with low-grade bacteriuria. A recent consensus review recommended the cutoff of $>10^3$ CFU per mL for significant bacteriuria in catheterized patients [43]. The high flow rate of catheterized urine, presence of inhibitors to bacterial growth, and significance of slow-growing organisms such as enterococci and *Candida* make it incumbent on the laboratory to characterize even low numbers of uropathogens in these patients. Moreover, polymicrobial bacteriuria occurs in more than 15% of patients with catheter-related UTI [44]. Multiple organisms must be isolated, characterized, and subjected to susceptibility testing to ensure adequate treatment of catheter-related UTIs.

Most patients with catheter-associated UTIs have lower urinary tract involvement. Upper tract involvement occurs in up to one-third of catheter-related UTIs and may have serious consequences [45]. The clinical and laboratory recognition of upper urinary tract involvement in persons with UTI (with or without a catheter) remains imprecise and unsatisfactory. ICU patients with UTIs may have altered levels of consciousness and may not be able to relate the symptoms of upper tract involvement. Antibody-coated bacteria have not proved to be sufficiently reproducible to distinguish upper from lower UTI [21]. Bladder washout techniques are effective [46] but are cumbersome and infrequently used in the ICU setting. Upper tract involvement can be detected in ICU patients by ultrasound or CT imaging demonstrating kidney enlargement and focal nephritis. Evidence of systemic toxicity from a UTI is highly indicative of upper tract disease and should be treated accordingly. Bacteria confined to the urinary bladder, in contrast, readily clear with removal of the catheter and a short course of antimicrobial therapy, if necessary.

Treatment

The most important therapeutic modality in catheter-related UTIs is the removal of the urinary catheter itself. Up to two thirds of patients with bacteriuria associated with urinary catheterization spontaneously resolve within 1 week after catheter removal [37]. If persistent bacteriuria is present after short course therapy, upper tract involvement should be assumed and the patient treated with a 14-day course of an active antimicrobial agent. If patients have persistent bacteriuria after short-course therapy, upper tract infection is assumed to be present and a 14-day course of an active antimicrobial agent is indicated [41,43].

If a patient becomes systemically ill from a UTI, treatment is warranted even if the catheter must remain in place. It is possible to successfully treat UTIs in patients with indwelling catheters, although treatment failures and reinfection occur at a greater frequency than in noncatheterized patients [21]. Antimicrobial agents useful in the treatment of catheter-related UTI are described in Table 82.2.

Routine replacement of indwelling urinary catheters complicated by UTI is generally unnecessary. Nonetheless, some organisms such as *Proteus, Providencia, Morganella,* and *Pseudomonas* species and enterococci may colonize the urinary catheter in greater quantities than the bladder itself. Despite the fact that the microbiology of urine samples from indwelling catheters and replacement catheters does not differ markedly in the presence of a UTI [47], catheters should be replaced if they malfunction, leak, or have been in place for prolonged periods (longer than 2 weeks). Leaking urinary catheters generally indicate luminal obstruction and require replacement.

Long-term urinary catheterization may be associated with other local suppurative complications, particularly in adult men. These include prostatitis, prostatic abscess, epididymitis, scrotal abscess, and other urethral complications [48]. These local complications require urologic management and necessitate the removal of the urethral catheter.

Prevention

Alternatives to Urethral Catheterization

The high frequency of catheter-related UTIs has led to concerted efforts to find alternative methods to manage the incontinent patient and patients with urinary outflow obstruction. Bladder training, meticulous nursing care, special linens, and adult diapers may assist some incontinent patients and avoid long-term catheterization.

Condom catheterization has been used for men with urinary incontinence and consists of the application of an external collector about the penis with a collection tube and drainage bag. Condom catheterization may be a reasonable alternative in highly motivated, cooperative, selected patients. However, leakage of the catheter, kinking and disruption of the collecting system, and maceration and ulceration of the epithelium of the penis are frequent complications of condom drainage. The overall incidence of UTIs with condom drainage does not differ significantly from indwelling catheter drainage [49].

Catheter Design, Maintenance, and Care

Because most catheter-related infections are derived from endogenous perineal organisms adherent to the exterior surface of the catheter itself, daily application of antimicrobial materials at the urethral orifice would seem to be a logical preventive measure. However, randomized controlled clinical trials with meatal care and application of povidone-iodine solution or topical poly-antimicrobial applications have failed to convincingly demonstrate a reduction in catheter-related infections [36]. This procedure cannot be recommended as a means of prevention of catheter-associated UTI.

Considerable effort is under way to develop a urinary catheter that prevents binding with bacteria, inhibits biofilm formation, or possesses antibacterial properties. The value of siliconized catheters [50], antibacterial-coated catheters, and other catheter innovations designed to decrease the risk of UTI is an active research priority [51,52]. A recent evidence-based systematic review of the existing literature indicates that antibiotic-coated catheters reduce the incidence of bacteriuria following short-term catheterization; however, there is no clear evidence of reduced symptomatic UTI or major complications such as bacteremia [53]. Such catheters may be considered in selected patients at great risk of complications for UTI such

TABLE 82.3

EVIDENCE-BASED RECOMMENDATIONS FOR URINARY TRACT INFECTION

Summary of recommendations for the prevention and management of bacteriuria and urinary tract infections in catheterized patients

- Screening for asymptomatic bacteriuria in a patient with an indwelling urinary catheter is not recommended [41].
- Treatment of asymptomatic bacteriuria is not recommended in the chronically catheterized patient [41,43].
- The use of antimicrobial-coated urinary catheters to prevent catheter-associated urinary tract infections is effective in preventing bacteriuria in patients with short-term urinary catheterizations; however, the cost implications and impact of these catheters on other urinary catheter-associated infectious complications such as bacteremia is unclear [50–53].
- There are insufficient data to support the use of chemical disinfection of the urinary drainage systems as a means of preventing catheter-associated urinary tract infections [54,55].
- Daily meatal care to prevent contamination of the external surface of the urinary catheter is not recommended as a means of preventing catheter-associated urinary tract infections [36].
- Persistent bacteriuria >48 h after removal of a urinary catheter should be treated with antimicrobial agents [41].

Summary of recommendations in the management of candiduria in the ICU patient

- Quantitative cultures with $>10^3$ CFU/mL of *Candida* spp in a catheterized patient or $>10^4$ CFU/mL of *Candida* spp in a noncatheterized patient is considered clinically significant [43,60,61,63].
- The finding of a fungus ball within the urinary collecting system, papillary necrosis, fungal casts in the urine, or renal abscess in the presence of candiduria is considered clinically significant [43,64,66].
- In medically stable patients without major immunocompromised states, simple removal of an indwelling urinary catheter without specific antifungal therapy may be an acceptable treatment option [43,57,66].
- Because of high levels of urinary excretion, fluconazole is preferred over caspofungin, other β-glucan inhibitors, and other triazoles (such as voriconazole, itraconazole, or posaconazole) in the treatment of genitourinary candidiasis [43,66].
- Bladder irrigation with a short course of amphotericin B (2 d) remains a viable treatment option in catheterized patients with candiduria in the absence of evidence of disseminated candidiasis [70].
- A short course of fluconazole (5–7 d) is usually sufficient to treat urinary tract infections due to *Candida* spp [73].

as a patient with severe neutropenia, but such patients are uncommon in most critical care units.

Exogenous contamination of urine within the collection bag remains a potential problem associated with indwelling urethral catheters. The instillation of antiseptic agents within the drainage bag as a means of prevention of catheter-related UTIs has met with conflicting results [54,55]. The procedure may decrease the risk of colonization but increase the acquisition of multiple drug-resistant Gram-negative bacilli. Urinary irrigation with antimicrobial agents or the instillation of antiseptic in the urinary drainage bag to prevent UTI is not recommended based upon current clinical evidence. The urinary collection bag should not be allowed to be elevated above the urinary bladder. This results in reflux of voided urine back into the bladder with its attendant risk of inducing UTI. Collecting bags with antireflux valves should be used to avoid this complication of urinary catheterization.

Short-term systemic antimicrobial prophylaxis against catheter-related UTI might be useful in special circumstances such as renal transplantation or foreign body implant surgery. A summary of evidence to support prevention and treatment recommendations for urinary catheter-associated UTI is listed in Table 82.3.

THE PROBLEM OF CANDIDURIA

The clinical interpretation of the isolation of *Candida* species from the urine is problematic in that candiduria may occur in a spectrum of illnesses ranging from simple urinary contamination to life-threatening systemic candidiasis. *Candida* species are normal inhabitants of the vaginal tract of women and may contaminate inadequately collected urine specimens. This is particularly true in older women, diabetics, and patients receiving antibacterial therapy. Additionally, *Candida* species frequently colonize the urinary tract in catheterized patients. These organisms are of marginal clinical significance and frequently disappear on removal of the urinary catheter without any specific antifungal therapy [56]. In a recent survey of 861 patients with funguria by the national mycoses study group, no treatment was given in 155 patients and funguria resolved spontaneously in 76% of these patients [57].

However, tissue invasive infection of the urinary bladder has been documented cystoscopically in patients with GU candidiasis. *Candida cystitis* may produce a friable white pseudomembrane on the bladder mucosa similar to the findings of oral thrush. Furthermore, ascending urinary infection of the kidney and renal pelvis may follow GU candidiasis. Papillary necrosis, fungus ball formation, urinary obstruction, bladder rupture, and perinephric abscess have all been described from ascending infection with *Candida* species [58,59]. *Candida* infection of the upper urinary tract may arise from hematogenous dissemination of *Candida* organisms from extrarenal sites. Microabscesses of the renal parenchyma with subsequent candiduria are a frequent finding in disseminated candidiasis. A positive urine culture for *Candida* species may be the first indication of disseminated candidiasis in the critically ill patient. Therefore, the clinical significance of *Candida* in the urine remains a diagnostic dilemma.

Quantitative culture of the urine has been used in an attempt to determine the clinical ramifications of candiduria. Unfortunately, the quantitative colony counts of *Candida* species in the urine do not have the same diagnostic and prognostic implications as quantitative bacteriology of the urine [43,60]. Large studies and review of this topic [43,60,61] indicate that quantitative values for candiduria of clinical significance are seen at more than 10^3 CFU per mL (catheterized patients) or more than 10^4 CFU per mL (noncatheterized patients). The finding of urinary casts made up of *Candida* elements is of diagnostic significance and indicates invasive upper tract candidiasis. Candiduria associated with a fungus ball in the urinary collecting system dictates the need for antifungal therapy, as does papillary necrosis or abscess formation within the renal parenchyma. Recurrent isolation of *Candida* species in urine cultures in immunocompromised patients, or patients with unexplained fever and pyuria, suggests UTI with *Candida* species. Evidence of concomitant infection with *Candida* organisms in other organ systems increases the likelihood of the significance of *Candida* isolates in the urine. Disseminated candidiasis should be considered in patients with repeated and unexplained *Candida* isolates in the urinary tract [62–64].

THE TREATMENT OF GENITOURINARY CANDIDIASIS

There are several management options available for candiduria, depending on the clinical circumstances in each patient. The discontinuation of antibacterial agents, removal of immunosuppression, or removal of urinary catheters may be sufficient to spontaneously clear candiduria in medically stable patients [65].

Published treatment guidelines for GU candidiasis recommend fluconazole in place of amphotericin B as the preferred treatment in the ICU setting [66]. This triazole compound is water soluble, available as oral or intravenous formulations, and is excreted as the active compound in the urine. Posaconazole, itraconazole, caspofungin, and voriconazole are not as useful in GU candidiasis as they are hepatically excreted and do not uniformly achieve fungicidal levels in the urine. Fluconazole also provides systemic antifungal activity if unrecognized disseminated candidiasis is present.

It is now recommended that antifungal susceptibility testing be performed for serious *Candida* infections for fluconazole, itraconazole, and flucytosine [67]. Resistance among *Candida albicans* isolates is increasingly recognized and these findings emphasize the necessity of antifungal susceptibility testing [68]. *Candida krusei* is intrinsically resistant to fluconazole; *Candida lusitaniae* is resistant to amphotericin B; and *Candida glabrata* is variably sensitive to antifungal agents. *Candida parapsilosis* appears to be less susceptible to the echinocandins [66]. Amphotericin B in vitro susceptibility testing is technically difficult and the methodology has not yet been standardized for routine clinical laboratory testing [67]. High doses of amphotericin B instilled into the bladder may be potentially toxic to uroepithelial cells [69]. However, a 2-day infusion of 50 mg of amphotericin B in 1,000 cc of sterile water per day is effective [70]; a single systemic dose of amphotericin B can also clear candiduria [71]. Systemic fluconazole or amphotericin B is indicated in candiduria patients with suspected systemic candidiasis, renal abscess formation, and fungus balls within the urinary collecting system [72]. *Candida* UTI may be readily treated with oral or intravenous fluconazole. A short course of fluconazole at 200 mg orally followed by 100 mg daily for 5 to 7 days is generally sufficient for the treatment of *Candida* [73] cystitis while upper urinary tract disease is generally treated with 200 to 400 mg fluconazole for 2 weeks [66]. Clinical evidence in support of the current management strategies for GU candidiasis is provided in Table 82.3.

References

1. Haley RW, Colver DH, White JW, et al: The nationwide nosocomial infection rate: a need for vital statistics. *Am J Epidemiol* 121:159–167, 1985.
2. Richards MJ, Edwards JR, Culver DH, et al: Nosocomial infections in combined medical-surgical intensive care units in the United States. *Infect Control Hosp Epidemiol* 21:510–515, 2000.
3. Lizan-Garcia M, Peyro R, Cortina M, et al: Nosocomial surveillance in a surgical intensive care unit in Spain, 1996–2000: a time-trend analysis. *Infect Control Hosp Epidemiol* 27(1):54–59, 2006.
4. Wagenlehner FM, Loibl E, Vogel H, et al: Incidence of nosocomial urinary tract infections on a surgical intensive care unit and implications for management. *Int J Antimicrob Agents* 28[Suppl 1]:S86–S90, 2006.
5. Salomao R, Rosenthal VD, Grimberg G, et al: Device-associated infection rates in intensive care units of Brazilian hospitals: findings of the International Nosocomial Infection Control Consortium. *Rev Panam Salud Publica* 24(3):195–202, 2008.
6. Gaynes R, Edwards JR: Overview of nosocomial infections caused by gram-negative bacilli. *Clin Infect Dis* 41(6):848–854, 2005.
7. Rosenthal VD: Device-associated nosocomial infections in limited-resources countries: findings of the International Nosocomial Infection Control Consortium (INICC). *Am J Infect Control* 36(10):7–12, 2008.
8. Weber DJ, Sickbert-Bennett EE, Brown V, et al: Comparison of hospital wide surveillance and targeted intensive care unit surveillance of healthcare-associated infections. *Infect Control Hosp Epidemiol* 28(12):1361–1366, 2007.
9. Richards MJ, Edwards JR, Culver DH, et al: Nosocomial infections in medical intensive care units in the United States: national nosocomial infections surveillance system. *Crit Care Med* 27:887–892, 1999.
10. Johnson JR, Kuskowski MA, Gajewske A, et al: Virulence characteristics and phylogenetic background of multidrug-resistant and antimicrobial-susceptible clinical isolates of Escherichia coli from across the United States, 2000–2001. *J Infect Dis* 190:1739–1744, 2004.
11. De Man P, Jodal U, Lincoln K, et al: Bacterial attachment and inflammation in the urinary tract. *J Infect Dis* 158:29–35, 1988.
12. Dominque GJ, Roberts JA, Laucirica R, et al: Pathogenic significance of P fimbriated Escherichia coli in urinary tract infections. *J Urol* 133:983–989, 1985.
13. Hall RM, Collins CM, Kim MJ, et al: Mobile gene cassettes and integrons in evaluation. *Ann NY Acad Sci* 870:68–80, 1999.
14. Warren JW, Tenney JH, Woopes JM, et al: A prospective microbiologic study of bacteriuria in patients with chronic indwelling urethral catheters. *J Infect Dis* 146:719–723, 1982.
15. Casterton JW, Stewart PS, Greenberg ED: Bacterial biofilms: a common cause of persistent infections. *Science* 284:1318–1322, 1999.
16. Scholes D, Hooton TM, Roberts PL, et al: Risk factors associated with acute pyelonephritis in healthy women. *Ann Intern Med* 142:20–27, 2005.
17. Sobel JD, Kaye D: Reduced uromucoid excretion in the elderly. *J Infect Dis* 152:653, 1985.
18. Sheinfeld J, Schaeffer AJ, Cordon-Cardo C, et al: Association of Lewis blood group phenotype with recurrent urinary tract infections in women. *N Engl J Med* 320:773–777, 1989.
19. Svanborg C, Frendeus B, Godaly L, et al: Toll-like receptor signaling and chemokine receptor expression influence the severity of urinary tract infection. *J Infect Dis* 183(1):S61, 2001.
20. Stamey TA, Fair WR, Timothy MM: Antibacterial nature of prostatic fluid. *Nature* 218:444–447, 1968.
21. Stamm WE, Hooten TM: Management of urinary tract infections in adults. *N Engl J Med* 329:1328–1334, 1993.
22. Laupland KB, Zygun DA, Davies HD, et al: Incidence and risk factors for acquiring nosocomial urinary tract infection in the critically ill. *J Crit Care* 17(1):50–57, 2002.
23. Bochicchio GV, Joshi M, Bochicchio SD, et al: Reclassification of urinary tract infections in critically ill trauma patients: a time-dependent analysis. *Surg Infect* 4(4):379–385, 2003.
24. Lipsky BA: Urinary tract infection in men: epidemiology, pathophysiology, diagnosis and treatment. *Ann Intern Med* 110:138–150, 1989.
25. Meng MV, Mario LA, McAninch JW: Current treatment and outcomes of perinephric abscesses. *J Urol* 168(4 Pt 1):1337–1340, 2002.
26. Kehinda EO, Rotimi VO, Al Hunayan A, et al: Bacteriology of urinary tract infection associated with indwelling J ureteral stents. *J Endourol* 18(9):891, 2004.
27. Piccirillo M, Rigsby C, Rosenfield AT: Contemporary imaging of renal inflammatory disease. *Infect Dis Clin North Am* 1:927–964, 1987.
28. Kanel KT, Kroboth FJ, Schwentker FN, et al: The intravenous pyelogram in acute pyelonephritis. *Arch Intern Med* 148:2144–2148, 1988.
29. Czaja CA, Scholes D, Hooton TM, et al: Population-based epidemiologic analysis of acute pyelonephritis. *Clin Infect Dis* 45:273–280, 2007.
30. Linden PK: Clinical implications of nosocomial Gram-positive bacteremia and superimposed antimicrobial resistance. *Am J Med* 104:24S–33S, 1998.
31. Noskin G, Siddique F, Stosor V, et al: Successful treatment of persistent vancomycin-resistant Enterococcus faecium bacteremia with linezolid and gentamicin. *Clin Infect Dis* 28:689–690, 1999.
32. Wald HL, Kramer AM: Nonpayment for harms resulting from medical care. *JAMA* 298(23):2782–2784, 2007.
33. Millar LK, Cox SM: Urinary tract infections complicating pregnancy. *Infect Dis Clin North Am* 11:13–26, 1997.

34. Tambyah PA, Knasinski V, Maki DG: The direct costs of nosocomial catheter-associated urinary tract infection in the era of managed care. *Infect Control Hosp Epidemiol* 23(1):27–31, 2002.
35. Kunin CM: Care of the urinary catheter, in Kunin CM (ed): *Detection, Prevention, and Management of Urinary Tract Infections*. Philadelphia, Lea and Febiger, 1987, p 245.
36. Garibaldi RA, Burke JP, Britt MR, et al: Meatal colonization and catheter-associated bacteriuria. *N Engl J Med* 303:316–318, 1980.
37. Mobley HL, Chippendale GR, Tenney JH, et al: MR/K hemagglutination of Providencia stuartii correlates with adherence to catheters and with persistence in catheter-associated bacteriuria. *J Infect Dis* 157:264–271, 1988.
38. Woods TD, Watanakunakorn C: Bacteremia due to Providencia stuartii: a review of 49 episodes. *South Med J* 89:221–224, 1996.
39. Mobley HL, Warren JW: Urease-positive bacteriuria and obstruction of long-term urinary catheters. *J Clin Micro* 25(11):2216–2217, 1987.
40. Harding GKM, Nicolle LE, Ronald AR, et al: How long should catheter-acquired urinary tract infection in women be treated. *Ann Intern Med* 114:713–719, 1991.
41. Nicolle LE, Bradley S, Colgan R, et al: Infectious Diseases Society of America guidelines for the diagnosis and treatment of asymptomatic bacteriuria. *Clin Infect Dis* 40:643–654, 2005.
42. Okuda T, Endo N, Osada Y, et al: Outbreak of nosocomial urinary tract infections caused by *Serratia marcescens*. *J Clin Microbiol* 20:691–695, 1984.
43. Calandra T, Cohen J: The international sepsis forum definition of infection in the ICU consensus conference. *Crit Care Med* 33(7):1538–1548, 2005.
44. Stark RP, Maki D: Bacteriuria in the catheterized patient: what quantitative level of bacteriuria is relevant? *N Engl J Med* 311:560–564, 1984.
45. Warren JW, Damron D, Tenney JH, et al: Fever, bacteremia, and death as complications of bacteriuria in women with long-term urethral catheters. *J Infect Dis* 155:1151–1158, 1987.
46. Fairley KF, Bond AG, Brown RB, et al: Simple test to determine the site of urinary tract infection. *Lancet* 2:427–428, 1967.
47. Grahn D, Norman DC, White ML, et al: Validity of urinary catheter specimens for the diagnosis of urinary tract infection in the elderly. *Arch Intern Med* 145:1858–1860, 1985.
48. Weinberger M, Cytron S, Servadio C, et al: Prostatic abscess in the antibiotic era. *Rev Infect Dis* 10:239–249, 1988.
49. Warren JW: Urethral catheters, condom catheters, and nosocomial urinary tract infections. *Infect Control Hosp Epidemiol* 17:212–214, 1996.
50. López-López G, Pascual A, Martínez-Martínez L, et al: Effect of a siliconized latex urinary catheter on bacterial adherence in human neutrophil activity. *Diagn Microbiol Infect Dis* 14:1–6, 1991.
51. Stensballe J, Tvede M, Looms D, et al: Infection risk with nitrofurazone-impregnated urinary catheters in trauma patients. *Ann Intern Med* 147:285–293, 2007.
52. Johnson JR, Roberts PL, Olsen RJ, et al: Prevention of catheter-associated urinary tract infection with a silver oxide-coated urinary catheter: clinical and microbiologic correlates. *J Infect Dis* 162:1145–1150, 1990.
53. Johnson JR, Kushowski MA, Wilt TJ: Systemic review: antimicrobial urinary catheters to prevent catheter-associated urinary tract infection in hospitalized patients. *Ann Intern Med* 144:116–126, 2006.
54. Thompson RL, Haley CE, Searcey MA, et al: Catheter-associated bacteriuria: failure to reduce attack rates using periodic instillations of a disinfectant into urinary drainage systems. *JAMA* 251:747–751, 1984.
55. Holliman RC, Seal DV, Archer H, et al: Controlled trial of chemical disinfection of urinary drainage bags: reduction in hospital-acquired, catheter-associated infection. *Br J Urol* 60(5):419–422, 1987.
56. Jacobs LG: Fungal urinary tract infections in the elderly: treatment guidelines. *Drugs Aging* 8(2):89–96, 1996.
57. Kauffman CA, Vazquez JA, Sobel JD, et al: Prospective multicenter surveillance study of funguria in hospitalized patients. The National Institute of Allergy (NIAID) mycoses study group. *Clin Infect Dis* 30:14–18, 2000.
58. Paul N, Mathai E, Abraham OC, et al: Factors associated with candiduria and related mortality. *J Infect* 55(5):450–455, 2007.
59. Carvalho J, Guimarães CM, Mayer JR, et al: Hospital-associated funguria: analysis of risk factors, clinical presentation and outcome. *Braz J Infect Dis* 5(6):313–318, 2001.
60. Kaufman CA: Candiduria. *Clin Infect Dis* 41[Suppl 6]:S371–S376, 2005.
61. Tambyah PA, Maki DG: The relationship between pyuria and infection in patients with indwelling urinary catheters: a prospective study of 761 patients. *Arch Intern Med* 160:673–677, 2000.
62. Magill SS, Swoboda SM, Johnson EA, et al: The association between anatomic site of Candida colonization, invasive candidiasis, and mortality in critically ill surgical patients. *Diagn Microbiol Infect Dis* 55(4):293–301, 2006.
63. Lundstrom T, Sobel J: Nosocomial candiduria: a review. *Clin Infect Dis* 32:1602–1607, 2001.
64. Martino P, Girmenia C, Venditti M, et al: Candida colonization and systemic infection in neutropenic patients. *Cancer* 64:2030–2034, 1989.
65. Apisarnthanarak A, Rutjanawech S, Wichansawakun S, et al: Initial inappropriate urinary catheters use in a tertiary-care center: incidence, risk factors, and outcomes. *Am J Infect Control* 35(9):594–599, 2007.
66. Pappas PG, Kaufman CA, Andes D, et al: Clinical practice guidelines for the management of candidiasis: 2009 update by the Infectious Disease Society of America. *Clin Infect Dis* 48:503–535, 2009.
67. Rex JH, Pfaller MA, Gulgiani JN, et al: Development of interpretive breakpoints for antifungal susceptibility testing: conceptual framework and analysis of in vitro–in vivo correlation data for fluconazole, itraconazole, and *Candida* infections. *Clin Infect Dis* 24:235–247, 1997.
68. Malani AN, Kauffman CA: Candida urinary tract infections: treatment options. *Expert Rev Anti Infect Ther* 5(2):277–284, 2007.
69. Sanford JP: The enigma of Candiduria: evolution of bladder irrigation with amphotericin B for management: from anecdote to dogma with a lesson from Machiavelli. *Clin Infect Dis* 16:145–147, 1993.
70. Hsu CCS, Chang R: Two-day continuous bladder irrigation with amphotericin B. *Clin Infect Dis* 20:1570–1571, 1995.
71. Fisher JF, Woeltje K, Espinel-Ingroff A, et al: Efficacy of a single intravenous dose of amphotericin B for Candida urinary tract infections: further favorable experience. *Clin Microbiol Infect* 9(10):1024–1027, 2003.
72. Rex JH, Bennett JE, Sugar AM, et al: A randomized trial comparing fluconazole with amphotericin B for the treatment of candidemia in patients without neutropenia. *N Engl J Med* 331:1325–1330, 1994.
73. Boodeker KS, Kilzoi WJ: Fluconazole dose recommendation in urinary tract infection. *Ann Pharmacother* 35(3):369–372, 2001.

CHAPTER 83 ■ LIFE-THREATENING COMMUNITY-ACQUIRED INFECTIONS: TOXIC SHOCK SYNDROME, OVERWHELMING POSTSPLENECTOMY INFECTION, MENINGOCOCCEMIA, MALARIA, ROCKY MOUNTAIN SPOTTED FEVER, AND OTHERS

MARY T. BESSESEN

This chapter covers several infections of low incidence and high mortality, a combination of factors that challenges the physician to recognize a life-threatening disease he or she may never have seen before and institute appropriate therapy promptly. To assist in this challenge, as these diseases are discussed, key historical points and clinical clues will be emphasized.

The critically ill febrile patient should undergo a thorough history and physical examination. Family members may need to be interviewed if the patient is too ill to participate fully in the history. Key points of the exposure history include travel, employment, hobbies, and exposure to pets, wildlife, and livestock. This portion of the interview will yield better results if it is carried out in a slow-paced conversational fashion, allowing the patient or family member to chat a bit. It is less focused than a standard social history and review of symptoms due to the heterogeneous nature of the exposures being sought. A complete physical examination should be performed. In assessing vital signs, one must evaluate hypothermia (temperature less than 36°C) in the same light as fever (temperature higher than 38°C). Laboratory studies should include a complete blood count with platelet and differential counts; prothrombin and partial thromboplastin times; electrolytes, including calcium and magnesium; blood glucose; renal and liver functions; two sets of blood cultures, urine for culture and urinalysis; and a chest radiograph. If a serious infection is under diagnostic consideration, the hematology laboratory should supplement the automated differential leukocyte count with a manual differential count by microscopic examination of the peripheral blood film. This may require a specific request from the physician, especially if the total leukocyte count falls within the normal range.

TOXIC SHOCK SYNDROMES

There are two toxic shock syndromes commonly recognized, one caused by *Staphylococcus aureus* (*S. aureus*), and the other caused by *Streptococcus pyogenes* (*S. pyogenes*) (group A streptococcus). To further complicate this picture, it has recently been reported that group C and group G streptococci may occasionally cause toxic shock syndrome [1]. In addition, *Clostridium sordellii* has been reported to cause a similar, but clinically distinct, toxic shock syndrome in obstetric patients, injection drug users, and recipients of musculoskeletal tissue allografts. Each of these three syndromes is discussed in the following sections.

Staphylococcal Toxic Shock Syndrome

Staphylococcal toxic shock syndrome (TSS) was first described in 1978 [2], and gained notoriety in the early 1980s when menstrual-associated cases struck large numbers of young women [3]. It is a multisystem disease characterized by acute onset of high fever, hypotension, diffuse macular rash, severe myalgia, vomiting, diarrhea, headache, and nonfocal neurologic abnormalities. The primary focus of staphylococcal infection may be mucosal, typically vaginal, associated with tampon or diaphragm use, or a wound. Currently there are four well-recognized forms of staphylococcal TSS: menstrual [3], postsurgical [4], influenza associated [5], and recalcitrant erythematous desquamating syndrome in acquired immunodeficiency syndrome (AIDS) [6].

Etiology

Staphylococcal toxic shock syndrome is a toxin-mediated illness caused by *S. aureus* strains that produce superantigens (SAgs). Menstrual-associated TSS is almost always caused by a strain that carries the SAg TSS toxin-1 (TSST-1), which is able to cross-intact mucous membranes. Nonmenstrual TSS may be caused by any of 15 described SAgs, but is most commonly associated with TSST-1, staphylococcal enterotoxin B (SEB), or staphylococcal enterotoxin C (SEC) [7]. Staphylococcal enterotoxins B and C are not absorbed across mucous membranes, but can cause TSS in cases of staphylococcal infection of wounds. There are rare case reports of staphylococcal TSS associated with nosocomial strains of methicillin-resistant *S. aureus* (MRSA) [8]. TSS has not been a feature of the epidemic of the community-associated MRSA strain, USA300, nor was TSS identified in a large collection of USA300 isolates [9].

Pathogenesis

In TSS, bacterial toxins function as superantigens. Conventional antigens presented in the context of major histocompatibility molecules on antigen-presenting cells (APC) must be processed by the APC and recognized by multiple elements of the T-cell receptor (TCR). In contrast, superantigens do not require processing by an antigen-presenting cell but instead bind directly to the TCR to activate T-cells. Expansion of T-cell populations expressing particular TCR Vβ chains results in massive release of proinflammatory cytokines such as gamma-interferon (IF-γ), tumor necrosis factor-α (TNF-α), interleukin 1-β (IL-1β), and interleukin-2 (IL-2), leading to a capillary leak syndrome [7]. The absence of preexisting antibody to the pertinent bacterial toxin is a critical host factor in TSS. Among cases of menstruation-associated TSS, 90% do not have preexisting antibody to TSST-1. In contrast, more than 90% of healthy persons over the age of 25 years have antibody to TSST-1.

Diagnosis

Clinical Features. The classic case profile is a young (15 to 25 years old), menstruating female. However, any staphylococcal infection can predispose to TSS, including surgical wound infections, furuncles, and abscesses. Postpartum cases can occur after vaginal or cesarean delivery. Nasal reconstructive surgery carries an especially high risk of TSS. Cases may also occur after nasal packing for epistaxis.

The typical presentation is one of high fever, rash, and confusion. There may be a prodromal period of 2 to 3 days, consisting of malaise, myalgia, and chills. Patients are listless, but focal neurologic findings are not seen. Examination of patients with menstruation-associated TSS reveals vaginal hyperemia and exudate that yields *S. aureus* on culture. In nonmenstrual cases, a careful examination usually reveals a focus of staphylococcal infection. It is important to note that this focus may be subtle, with only serous drainage [4]. This is a toxin-mediated disease, and the local appearance is not one of intense purulence. Drainage of local infections is essential to a favorable outcome.

Laboratory Findings. Leukocytosis with marked left shift, thrombocytopenia, azotemia, sterile pyuria, and elevated transaminases are common, although nonspecific findings. Cultures of blood and cerebrospinal fluid (CSF) are usually sterile. Cultures of the local site of infection are usually, but not invariably, positive for *S. aureus*.

Differential Diagnosis. Streptococcal scarlet fever, measles, leptospirosis, Rocky Mountain spotted fever, Stevens–Johnson syndrome, and Kawasaki's disease can mimic TSS. Multiorgan involvement is usually absent in streptococcal scarlet fever, and the primary focus yields *S. pyogenes*. Exclusion of measles, leptospirosis, ehrlichiosis, and Rocky Mountain spotted fever requires a careful history for potential exposures and serologic testing. Stevens–Johnson syndrome is characterized by target lesions and is commonly associated with exposure to medications. Kawasaki's disease is characterized by fever and rash without multisystem involvement, is most commonly seen in children under the age of 6 years, and is associated with thrombocytosis rather than thrombocytopenia.

Treatment

The primary intervention consists of fluid resuscitation and supportive care. Any focus of staphylococcal infection must be drained. In women, a vaginal examination must be performed as soon as the patient is stabilized, and any foreign bodies (such as tampon or diaphragm) removed. After cultures of the local site and the blood are obtained, antistaphylococcal therapy should be administered intravenously.

Empiric antibacterial therapy for the critically ill patient should include an agent which is active against 100% of suspected pathogens, if feasible. At this time, the antibiotic that is most likely to cover all *S. aureus* isolates is vancomycin. There is in vitro evidence that clindamycin [10] and linezolid [11] inhibit staphylococcal toxin production, whereas β-lactam agents increase TSST-1 in culture supernatants, probably due to cell lysis releasing toxin [12]. The initial treatment of choice for menstrual TSS is nafcillin or oxacillin combined with clindamycin. After 48 hours, clindamycin can be discontinued. First-generation cephalosporins (cefazolin) may be substituted for an antistaphylococcal penicillin in patients with a history of non–life-threatening allergy to penicillins. If a healthcare-associated source of *S. aureus* infection is suspected, vancomycin should be used in place of the β-lactam agent until susceptibility tests are completed.

Intravenous immune globulin (IVIG) may be a useful adjunctive therapy. Higher doses of IVIG may be required for staphylococcal TSS than for streptococcal TSS [13].

Outcomes

The mortality of menstrual staphylococcal TSS is 3%, and 2 to 3 times higher in nonmenstrual-associated cases. Poor outcomes are associated with prolonged and refractory hypovolemic shock, acute respiratory distress syndrome, acute renal failure, electrolyte and acid-base imbalances, cardiac dysrhythmia, and disseminated intravascular coagulation (DIC) with thrombocytopenia.

Staphylococcal TSS may recur in patients with menstrual or nonmenstrual disease [14,15]. Recurrence is associated with continued use of tampons and absence of antistaphylococcal therapy for the initial episode.

Streptococcal Toxic Shock Syndrome

The clinical presentation and pathophysiology of streptococcal TSS are similar to staphylococcal TSS with a few notable differences: bacteremia is commonly seen, rash is less common, and mortality is markedly higher (30% to 70%) [7].

Like staphylococcal TSS, streptococcal TSS is a toxin-mediated disease. Streptococcal toxins that function as superantigens are streptococcal pyrogenic exotoxins A (SPE A) and B (SPE B). In addition, M-protein, a classic streptococcal virulence factor, may be released from the cell surface, bind to fibrinogen, and form large aggregates that activate intravascular polymorphonuclear leukocytes, leading to a vascular leak syndrome [16]. Blood cultures are usually positive in streptococcal TSS. Underlying infections are varied and include cellulitis, necrotizing fasciitis, postpartum myometritis, surgical wound infection, and occasionally pharyngitis [17]. Diagnosis is made by Gram stain and culture of blood and other bodily fluids.

Treatment is similar to that for staphylococcal TSS in that supportive care, including fluids, vasopressors, and ventilatory assistance, should be administered as needed, and surgical drainage of pyogenic sites is imperative. For confirmed streptococcal TSS, the antibiotic of choice is intravenous penicillin. For those who are intolerant to penicillin, other suitable agents are cephalosporins and vancomycin. Until the bacteriologic diagnosis is confirmed by culture, staphylococcal coverage should be included in the antibiotic regimen. Clindamycin is also very active against *S. pyogenes*. In an animal model of streptococcal myositis, clindamycin was more effective than penicillin [18]. This may be due to greater activity against high burdens of organisms (inoculum effect). An alternative explanation is that inhibition of protein synthesis blocks toxin production by the pathogen and reduces TNF production by the host [19]. A case control study has shown improved outcomes among children with invasive *S. pyogenes* infections whose therapy included clindamycin or erythromycin in the first 24 hours [20]. The usual adult dose of clindamycin in this setting is 600 mg per kg every 8 hours. Adjunctive therapy of streptococcal TSS with IVIG is recommended by many experts, based on retrospective studies employing doses ranging from 400 mg per kg to

2 g per kg for variable durations [21,22]. A randomized controlled trial was attempted but halted prior to completion, and it showed a trend toward improved survival in the treatment group [23]. In that trial, the dose of IVIG was 1 g per kg on day 1 and 0.5 g per kg on days 2 and 3.

Clostridium Sordellii Toxic Shock Syndrome

Clostridium sordellii is an anaerobic, Gram-positive spore-forming bacillus that has been an occasional cause of obstetric infections for many years [24]. Recently there have been reports of a TSS due to this pathogen in association with surgical and medical abortion [24,25], subcutaneous injection of black-tar heroin [26], and musculoskeletal tissue allografts [27]. The distinctive features of this syndrome are hypothermia and profound hemoconcentration. Management consists of supportive care including aggressive volume resuscitation, drainage of purulent foci, and broad-spectrum antibacterial therapy to include anaerobic organisms. Antitoxin therapy is of theoretical interest but clinically unproven.

OVERWHELMING POSTSPLENECTOMY INFECTION

Overwhelming postsplenectomy sepsis is a catastrophic illness with high morbidity and mortality in patients who have undergone splenectomy or who have severe splenic dysfunction. The spleen provides three major functions in protection from infection. It acts as a mechanical filter for infected or senescent erythrocytes; it participates in the production of soluble immune factors, including immunoglobulins and tuftsin; and it provides a site for components of the cellular immune system to act in proximity to one another [28].

Splenic function may be lost due to surgical removal, irradiation, several disease processes, and therapies [29], including sickle cell anemia, systemic lupus erythematosus, celiac disease, liver disease, acute alcoholism, high-dose corticosteroid therapy, splenic irradiation [30], and bone marrow transplantation. Normal aging has also been associated with a decrease in splenic function [31].

Splenectomy was the accepted procedure for splenic trauma for centuries, due to the belief that it served no important physiologic function, repair of trauma was difficult due to the friable nature of the organ, and expected high mortality of attempted conservative management. This prevailing wisdom was challenged in the 1970s, and currently splenic salvage is reported in 90% of cases of splenic rupture [32]. Splenic salvage in the trauma setting is associated with marked reductions in the risk of infection during the acute hospitalization, including surgical site infections and pneumonia [33]. Implantation of splenic fragments into the peritoneum has been performed in an attempt to maintain splenic function. Immune protection by these splenic fragments is incomplete at best, due to the loss of the normal splenic circulation. The presence of Howell–Jolly bodies on the peripheral blood smear indicates decreased splenic function, placing the patient at risk for overwhelming postsplenectomy infection (OPSI) [34]. Although Howell–Jolly bodies may be detected by autoanalyzers, a manual blood film should be reviewed if there is a clinical question of hyposplenism.

Epidemiology

The incidence of OPSI is impacted by many factors, including underlying disease, patient age, age at the time of splenectomy, time elapsed since splenectomy, pneumococcal vaccination, and antibiotic prophylaxis. Reported incidence rates are highest among patients with underlying thalassemia; intermediate in patients with sickle cell anemia, malignancy, or hematologic disorders; and lowest among patients who undergo splenectomy for trauma.

Encapsulated bacteria are the most common organisms causing OPSI. *Streptococcus pneumoniae, Neisseria meningitidis,* and *Haemophilus influenzae* are the organisms of greatest concern. *S. pneumoniae* is the most frequently isolated pathogen, representing over 50% of cases of OPSI. Other bacterial pathogens include *Salmonella* spp [28], *Capnocytophaga canimorsus* [35], which is associated with dog bites, and *Campylobacter* spp [36].

Asplenic individuals are also at risk for severe infection with the intraerythrocytic pathogens *Babesia microti* and *Babesia bovis*. Both organisms are transmitted by tick bites; *B. microti* is endemic on islands off the northeastern coast of the United States (Long Island, Nantucket Island, Martha's Vineyard), whereas *B. bovis* is found in Europe. The acute phase of malaria may be more severe in splenectomized individuals, but splenectomy may be protective in the chronic phase. Atypically severe cases of *Plasmodium vivax* and *Plasmodium ovale* have been reported in splenectomized individuals, and relapse of malaria following splenectomy has occurred [28].

Diagnosis

Clinical Presentation

OPSI should be considered in any febrile patient with a history or abdominal scar consistent with splenectomy or disease process associated with hyposplenism. The initial symptoms of OPSI are fever, headache abdominal pain, vomiting, and diarrhea. There may be a nonspecific prodrome characterized by low-grade fever and myalgias. If untreated, the disease evolves into fulminant septic shock and death over 2 to 5 days [37]. In advanced cases, acute tubular necrosis, adrenal cortical necrosis, and disseminated intravascular coagulation may occur. A petechial or purpuric rash may be seen. Meningitis or pneumonia occurs in approximately one-half of cases; in the remaining cases septicemia occurs, which is presumed to arise from colonization of the pharynx.

Laboratory Features

Blood cultures yield the causative organism in most cases of OPSI. Infections of lesser severity also occur and may not be associated with detectable bacteremia. Hematologic findings of DIC (thrombocytopenia, elevated prothrombin time, D-dimer, and fibrin split products), elevated serum creatinine, and blood urea nitrogen are frequently seen. Howell–Jolly bodies are found on a peripheral blood film. In the immediate post-splenectomy period, mild elevation in the platelet and leukocyte numbers are physiologic, but a leukocyte count higher than 15,000 cells per μL after the fourth postoperative day suggests infection is likely the cause [38].

Differential Diagnosis

OPSI may be mistaken for uncomplicated sepsis if the history of asplenia or hyposplenism is not appreciated. Thrombotic thrombocytopenic purpura may also have a similar presentation, with fever, thrombocytopenia, and acute renal failure.

Management

In addition to supportive care, antimicrobial therapy should be initiated promptly. Third-generation cephalosporins are active against *S. pneumoniae, N. meningitidis,* and *H. influenzae* in most locales. Cefotaxime 2 g intravenously every 8 hours or ceftriaxone 1 to 2 g intravenously once daily [39] may be used for uncomplicated cases. If meningitis is suspected, the dose of cefotaxime should be increased to 2 g every 4 to 6 hours; ceftriaxone should be given in a dose of 2 g twice daily. If pneumococci with high-grade resistance to penicillin and cephalosporins are prevalent in the region, vancomycin should be added until culture and susceptibility data become available. Patients with a severe allergy to penicillins and cephalosporins may be treated with vancomycin given with chloramphenicol or a fluoroquinolone [29]. Expert consultation should be sought in such cases.

Prevention

Guidelines for management of the postsplenectomy patient were published [40] prior to the advent of the quadrivalent conjugate meningococcal vaccine. Recommendations include timely vaccination with the 23-valent pneumococcal vaccine, preferably 2 weeks or longer prior to splenectomy. If that is impractical, it is recommended that patients be immunized as soon as possible postoperatively. Recent observations that antibody levels are improved if vaccination is delayed until 14 days postoperatively [41] must be weighed against the risk that vaccination may be overlooked if it is not carried out prior to hospital discharge. A reasonable compromise may be to immunize the patient at hospital discharge. Pneumococcal vaccine boosters should be administered every 5 years. Meningococcal conjugate vaccine (MCV4) should be administered to patients who are asplenic or who have splenic dysfunction. Due to the ongoing risk for meningococcal disease in asplenic persons, MCV4 vaccination should be repeated at 3- to 5-year intervals [42,43]. The conjugate *H. influenzae* vaccine should be administered to asplenic patients according to the standard schedule for all children [40].

Lifelong antibiotic prophylaxis is recommended by some authors [40], whereas others question this approach [28]. The data supporting prophylaxis are stronger in the pediatric population than in adults [29]. In the first 2 years following splenectomy in a child, or a patient with thalassemia or immune deficiency, antibiotic prophylaxis is recommended by most experts. Penicillin remains the drug of choice despite the emergence of resistance among some isolates. Ideally it should be dosed twice daily, but if adherence is an issue, it may be given once daily. Erythromycin may be substituted for patients who are allergic to penicillin. "Standby" antibiotics, to be taken early in the course of a febrile illness, is a strategy favored by all [28,40]. Amoxicillin-clavulanate is a good choice for this indication. Patients must be counseled to seek medical care if they are ill, and not rely on standby antibiotics alone.

MENINGOCOCCEMIA

The Centers for Disease Control (CDC) estimates that each year 1,400 to 2,800 cases of invasive meningococcal disease occur in the United States [42,44]. This section will cover *Neisseria meningitidis* bacteremia. Meningitis is covered in Chapter 79. Although infants are at highest risk for meningococcal disease, case rates also rise in the early teenage years, and 32% of cases occur among persons aged 30 years or older [44]. There are five serogroups, A, B, C, Y, and W-135. In the United States, serogroups B, C, and Y cause 93% of cases, with each representing about one third of cases. Serogroup B disease is more common among infants. Disease rates vary seasonally, with the lowest rates in the summer and early autumn months [42].

Pathophysiology

Neisseria meningitidis colonizes the nasopharynx in normal individuals by adherence to epithelial cells via pili and other adhesion factors. In the majority of individuals, it never causes disease. Invasive disease has been associated with a variety of factors, including antecedent viral infection, exposure to passive smoking, and inhalation of dry, dusty air [45]. Specific antibody and the complement system are key protective components of the host immune system. Deficiency of components of the complement system due to genetic defects or underlying disease predisposes to invasive meningococcal disease [46]. When bacteria invade the bloodstream, endotoxin activates the host immune system and proinflammatory cytokines cause a vascular leak syndrome. The endothelial thrombomodulin-endothelial protein C receptor pathway is downregulated, leading to thrombosis and purpura fulminans [47]. Profound vasoconstriction leads to peripheral ischemia and gangrene [45], and depression of myocardial contractility by cytokines contributes to shock.

Diagnosis

Clinical Manifestations

Few disease states are as impressive as full-blown meningococcal sepsis. The challenge is early recognition and intervention before irreversible damage occurs. Early in the course of meningococcal sepsis, nonspecific symptoms and signs are the only manifestations. Fever, malaise, myalgias, vomiting, tachypnea, and tachycardia are typical. The rash begins as an erythema, progressing to the characteristic petechiae and purpura only later in the course of disease. As the disease progresses it evolves to septic shock, with hypotension, poor peripheral perfusion, impaired mentation, and anuria or oliguria. Other manifestations include hemorrhage, cardiac failure, acute renal failure, and thrombocytopenia with or without DIC [48]. Other, less common complications of meningococcal sepsis include adrenal hemorrhage and failure (Waterhouse–Friedrichson syndrome), chronic renal failure necessitating hemodialysis, cutaneous necrosis with sloughing requiring skin grafting, extremity gangrene requiring subsequent amputation, and often several surgical revisions, septic arthritis, endophthalmitis, and pericarditis. Mortality remains high, despite antibiotics and intensive care; 20% to 50% of children who develop shock from meningococcal sepsis die. Transfer to a specialist unit is associated with a marked reduction in mortality [49].

Laboratory Findings

Leukocytosis or leukopenia, with a shift to immature forms, and thrombocytopenia are typical. There may be laboratory evidence of DIC. Chemistries may demonstrate acidemia, hypoglycemia, decreased cortisol levels, and elevated blood urea nitrogen and creatinine. Diagnosis is confirmed by isolation of *N. meningitidis* from cultures of blood or other normally sterile body fluids. If the diagnosis of meningococcal sepsis is clinically apparent, some experts caution against performing a lumbar puncture for cerebrospinal fluid culture due to concerns for brain herniation or clinical deterioration related to positioning the patient for the procedure. Latex agglutination and polymerase chain reaction assays provide increased sensitivity [50].

Differential Diagnosis

Purpura fulminans is characteristic of meningococcemia, but may also be caused by *S. pneumoniae* or *H. influenzae* type B.

Other infections that may mimic meningococcemia are fulminant *S. aureus* sepsis, *S. pyogenes* bacteremia, Gram-negative sepsis, Rocky Mountain spotted fever, vasculitis, thrombotic thrombocytopenic purpura, Henoch–Schonlein purpura, and any febrile illness in a patient with thrombocytopenia.

Therapy

Third-generation cephalosporins are the treatment of choice for meningococcemia due to reports of penicillin resistance [51]. Ceftriaxone, 4 g intravenously daily in one or two divided doses or cefotaxime 8 to 12 g intravenously daily in four to six divided doses should be administered to adults with suspected meningococcal disease. There is limited clinical experience with alternative antibacterial agents for patients with a history of cephalosporin allergy. Based on in vitro susceptibility data, options include meropenem and chloramphenicol [51,52]. Fluoroquinolones may be useful in postpubertal persons, but rare cases of fluoroquinolone resistance have been reported [53].

Patients should be admitted to an intensive care unit and placed in respiratory isolation until 24 hours of appropriate antibiotic therapy has been administered. Supportive care is critical to a favorable outcome. Surgical intervention may be indicated for necrotic skin lesions and gangrenous limbs. Early fasciotomy appears to limit the extent of amputation that is ultimately required [54]. Adrenal insufficiency may occur; in hypotensive patients corticosteroids should be administered pending return of results of cosyntropin stimulation test. Use of plasmapheresis has been reported in uncontrolled series [55,56].

Drotrecogin-α has been approved for severe sepsis syndrome in adults, based on randomized controlled trials that included patients with meningococcal sepsis [57], and the pathophysiology of purpura fulminans suggests that activated protein C may be beneficial. However, the most significant toxicity of drotrecogin-α is spontaneous bleeding events, and risk of bleeding would be predicted to increase in patients with meningococcal sepsis due to the thrombocytopenia and hypoprothrombinemia that are commonly observed. Retrospective analysis of patients with purpura fulminans, meningitis, or meningococcal disease treated with drotrecogin in several trials showed no overall increased risk of bleeding as compared to patients with sepsis of other etiologies, but the risk of intracranial hemorrhage was increased [58]. Most of the intracranial hemorrhages that were observed were in patients with meningitis. Systemic arterial hypertension, thrombocytopenia, and age greater than 65 years were also commonly observed in patients with intracranial hemorrhage. Drotrecogin-α, given as an intravenous infusion of 24 μg per kg per hour for 96 hours, may be used for adult patients with meningococcemia who otherwise meet criteria for APC therapy. Caution is advisable in patients with concomitant meningitis, thrombocytopenia, or a history of hypertension.

Prophylaxis

The CDC recommends chemoprophylaxis after exposure to people with *N. meningitidis* infection for household, day care, and other close contacts; for people in close contact with infected respiratory secretions, such as those performing mouth-to-mouth resuscitation; and for travelers in contact with respiratory secretions of, or seated next to, an index case for 8 hours or more [42]. The agents recommended for chemoprophylaxis are rifampin (600 mg orally for adults, 10 mg per kg orally for children) given every 12 hours for four doses; or ceftriaxone, 125 mg intramuscularly in children younger than 15 years or 250 mg intramuscularly in people aged 15 years or older [42]. Resistance to ciprofloxacin, which has been widely used for prophylaxis, has recently been reported in several cases of meningococcal infection in North Dakota and Minnesota, leading to a recommendation to use alternative agents for prophylaxis in those areas [59]. Routine chemoprophylaxis is recommended for medical staff only if they have had prolonged close contact before the institution of antibiotic therapy.

Immunization with the tetravalent (serogroups A, C, W135, and Y) MCV4 is indicated for the following populations: children at their 11- to 12-year-old preadolescent healthcare visit, college freshmen living in dormitories, travelers to areas where *N. meningitidis* is epidemic or hyperendemic, microbiologists with frequent exposure to *N. meningitidis,* military recruits, those at risk during an outbreak (such as school or dormitory mates), and those with increased susceptibility (e.g., persons with complement deficiencies or asplenia) [42].

MALARIA

In developed countries malaria is primarily seen in travelers, immigrants, and military personnel, but in the developing world it is a major cause of morbidity and mortality. Worldwide there are between 300 and 660 million cases that occur annually, resulting in 700,000 to 2.7 million deaths each year [60]. Imported cases have increased throughout the world; in the United States, approximately 1,300 cases have been reported annually to the National Malaria Surveillance System, a passive reporting system administered by the CDC, over the past decade [61]. In 2003, *Plasmodium falciparum* was identified as the causative species in 53% of cases; 70% of the cases were acquired in Africa. Virtually all of the fatal cases of malaria in the United States are caused by *P. falciparum.* Although the great majority of cases occurred among persons who did not follow a CDC-recommended prophylaxis regimen, it must be noted that approximately 20% of patients with malaria reported taking appropriate chemoprophylaxis. Failure to take a recommended regimen resulted in fatal malaria in seven reported cases since 1992 [62]. There have been small clusters of mosquito-borne malaria transmission within the United States as well as occasional congenital cases and transmission via blood transfusion [63]. This discussion will focus on severe malaria and its management in critical care settings.

Etiology

Plasmodium is an intracellular parasite that sequentially infects hepatocytes and then erythrocytes, resulting in clinical malaria. Four species cause disease in humans: *P. falciparum, P. malariae, P. ovale,* and *P. vivax*. *Plasmodium* is transmitted to human hosts by its vector, the female *Anopheles* mosquito.

Pathophysiology

Severe malaria is almost always due to *P. falciparum*, which, because of its ability to infect erythrocytes of all ages, can produce very high levels of parasitemia. Cerebral malaria is the most common clinical presentation of severe malaria. Many factors can contribute to diminished brain function in severe malaria, including obstruction of microvascular flow, elevated intracranial pressure, cerebral edema, disruption of the blood–brain barrier, hypoglycemia, hypovolemia, and seizure activity.

Obstruction of microvascular flow is caused by sequestration of erythrocytes in brain capillaries, autoagglutination, and decreased erythrocyte deformability due to intracellular parasites. Cytoadherence, a process in which *P. falciparum* derived proteins on infected erythrocytes attach to the CD36 receptor on vascular endothelial cells, appears to mediate sequestration [64].

In endemic areas, malaria is largely a disease of children. By the time they reach adulthood, residents of endemic areas develop partial immunity to *Plasmodium* infections, limiting the severity of disease. Travelers, conversely, are generally not immune; nonimmune adults who become infected are almost always symptomatic, and severe disease may develop.

Diagnosis

Clinical Features

Although imported malaria may occur at any time after leaving an endemic area, there are epidemiologic clues to help guide the evaluation. Among returning travelers presenting with fever, the most common specific diagnosis is malaria, occurring in 9% of cases [65]. Among cases diagnosed in New York, 80% of patients had symptom onset within 1 month of leaving the endemic area. Most of the cases presenting later than 1 month post-departure had *P. vivax*, which rarely causes life-threatening disease.

Patients with malaria present with a history of fever and chills, but fever may not be present at the time of the initial examination. The classic descriptions of tertian and quartan fever are rarely seen; their absence is not evidence against the diagnosis of malaria. Chills, headache, fatigue, and myalgias are common complaints. Signs include hypotension, jaundice, and hepatosplenomegaly, but these are seen in a minority of patients [66]. If hypotension is present, Gram-negative bacteremia must be excluded and treated empirically until cultures return. Cough, dyspnea, and tachypnea may dominate the clinical picture in children, causing confusion with pneumonia in areas of the developing world where chest radiography is not readily available [67].

Malaria in pregnancy presents with similar, although more severe, manifestations. Hypoglycemia and lactic acidosis are more frequently seen in maternal malaria, and the mortality of cerebral malaria is increased [68]. The partial immunity of residents of endemic areas is blunted in pregnancy [69]. Other complications include preterm delivery, intrauterine growth retardation, anemia, postpartum hemorrhage, and eclampsia [68]. Human immunodeficiency virus (HIV)–infected gravida are both at increased risk of infection with *Plasmodium* species, and have a more severe course of malaria. Additionally, malaria is associated with an increased maternal HIV viral load, and may increase HIV transmission to the fetus [70]. Placental malaria may be present even if peripheral blood films are negative for parasites [71].

Complications

The most common complications of malaria are cerebral malaria, severe anemia, metabolic acidosis, and noncardiogenic pulmonary edema. Gram-negative sepsis and metabolic acidosis are less common, but potentially grave complications of severe malaria.

Variability in host susceptibility and in the definition of cerebral malaria may account for the wide range of reported incidence. The World Health Organization defines cerebral malaria as coma that cannot be explained by hypoglycemia, postictal state, or other nonmalarial causes, such as sedative drugs, in a patient with parasitemia. Common findings are decerebrate or decorticate posturing, flaccid tone, seizures, and retinal hemorrhages. A recent study on imported severe *falciparum* malaria reported cerebral malaria in 37% of cases [61]. Overall mortality of severe malaria in that series of cases treated in a highly experienced intensive care unit setting was 11%. Cerebral malaria was present in 90% of nonsurvivors.

Laboratory Features

Common laboratory findings are anemia, thrombocytopenia, and hyperbilirubinemia. Hypoglycemia, elevated creatinine, and hypothrombinemia may also be present [61].

Microscopic examination for parasites on thick and thin films of peripheral blood remains the standard for diagnosis of malaria. Sensitivity is increased when blood for malaria smears is obtained from a capillary-rich area, such as the fingertip or earlobe, rather than by venipuncture. A thick smear examined by an experienced microscopist can detect 50 parasites per μL of blood, which is equivalent to 0.001% of erythrocytes infected [71]. Sensitivity is approximately 10-fold lower in routine clinical laboratories. In addition, patients with *falciparum* malaria may have parasites sequestered in deep capillaries in the spleen, liver, bone marrow, or placenta, with a false negative peripheral smear. Because the sensitivity of the smear is imperfect, empiric therapy for malaria should be administered when clinical suspicion is high. The thin blood film is used to identify the species and to quantitatively follow the parasitemia on serial samples. Real-time polymerase chain reaction (PCR) is more sensitive than microscopy, especially at low levels of parasitemia, and although it is not FDA-approved, the assay is readily available from reference laboratories.

Differential Diagnosis

Cerebral malaria may mimic meningoencephalitis due to viral, bacterial, fungal, or other parasitic causes. Dengue, typhoid, rickettsial infection, or mononucleosis may present with an undifferentiated fever in a returned traveler. The differential diagnosis of jaundice in this population includes leptospirosis, yellow fever, viral hepatitis, sepsis, and relapsing fevers [67]. Bacterial sepsis must also be considered as a separate or a complicating diagnosis.

Treatment

Management in an intensive care unit is indicated for patients with severe malaria. Careful management of fluids and electrolytes is critical, as well as monitoring for hypoglycemia. Renal, cardiac, and neurologic function should also be carefully monitored.

Intravenous quinidine has been used in the United States for treatment of severe malaria since 1991, when the CDC stopped providing intravenous quinine [72]. At that time, quinidine was readily available on most hospital formularies, and therapy could be initiated rapidly. The declining use of intravenous quinidine for cardiac dysrhythmias has reduced the ready availability of quinidine, but a replacement strategy has not yet been developed [73] and it remains the drug of choice. It should be initiated for severe malaria, defined as a positive blood smear with any one of the following criteria: impaired consciousness/coma, severe normocytic anemia, renal failure, pulmonary edema, acute respiratory distress syndrome, circulatory shock, disseminated intravascular coagulation, spontaneous bleeding, acidosis, hemoglobinuria, jaundice, repeated generalized convulsions, or parasitemia greater than 5%.

Hypoglycemia, QT interval prolongation, cardiac dysrhythmias, and hypotension may complicate quinidine infusion. Intensive care unit monitoring and consultation with an infectious disease specialist and a cardiologist are recommended. Cardiac complications may require slowing or stopping the infusion. When dosage is calculated, it is important to distinguish the salt from the base to ensure accuracy. The usual dose is 6.25 mg base per kg (10 mg salt per kg) loading dose intravenously over 1 to 2 hours, then 0.0125 mg base per kg per minute (0.02 mg salt per kg per minute) continuous infusion for at least 24 hours. If the patient has received mefloquine or more than 40 mg per kg of quinine in the 12 hours prior to beginning quinidine infusion, the loading dose should be omitted. Dosage adjustment for renal failure is not necessary in the first 48 hours of therapy [74]. Thin smears to assess the degree of parasitemia should be performed every 12 to 24 hours. Oral quinine 542 mg base (650 mg salt) three times daily for 3 to 7 days should be substituted when the patient is able to swallow, parasitemia is less than 1%, and mental status is normal. For infections acquired in Southeast Asia, the CDC recommends that therapy continue for 7 days; for disease acquired in Africa therapy should be stopped after 3 days.

Patients with malaria normally show improvement in 1 to 3 days [75]. If the course is more prolonged, drug resistance or inadequate serum drug levels should be suspected. In addition to quinine, the patient should be treated with one of the following: doxycycline 100 mg orally twice daily for 7 days, tetracycline 250 mg four times daily for 7 days, or clindamycin 20 mg base per kg per day orally in three divided doses for 7 days.

Artesunate, a new agent that was developed in China, has been shown in a randomized controlled trial to be superior to quinine for therapy of severe malaria [76]. Although it is not FDA approved for use in the United States, it may be available by making a treatment investigational new drug (IND) request from the CDC for cases of severe malaria. Physicians who encounter a case of *falciparum* malaria should contact the CDC malaria hotline 770-488-7788 for updated information on treatment recommendations, including changes in the availability of artesunate.

Treatment of a pregnant woman with malaria requires additional considerations [68]. High doses of quinine are reported to be abortifacient. Nevertheless, treatment with quinine has not been associated with an increased risk of congenital abnormalities, low birth weight, or stillbirth, and it is considered to be safe in the first trimester [77]. Chloroquine is safe for use in pregnant women for the treatment of non-*falciparum* or chloroquine-sensitive *falciparum* malaria. As discussed earlier, quinidine is substituted for quinine in the United States. Quinidine is listed as category C and is considered safe for breastfeeding women. Clindamycin may be used as a second agent, after completion of quinidine or oral quinine treatment. Artesunate-atovaquone-proguanil has been shown to be superior to quinine during the second and third trimesters, with no differences in birth weight, duration of gestation, or congenital abnormality rates in newborns [78]. As discussed later, exchange transfusion has also been used for severe *falciparum* malaria during pregnancy [79]. If fetal distress is observed on monitoring, emergency cesarean delivery may be necessary [67,79].

Exchange transfusion is controversial due to the lack of randomized trial data, but its use is recommended by the World Health Organization for patients with parasitemia greater than 30%, and for patients with parasitemia greater than 10% and severe disease, failure to respond to chemotherapy within 12 to 24 hours, or baseline poor prognostic factors such as advanced age or schizonts on peripheral blood film [67].

A randomized controlled trial has shown that corticosteroids were of no benefit and potentially harmful in the treatment of cerebral malaria [80]. Other adjunctive therapies that should not be used include heparin, sodium bicarbonate, mannitol, immunoglobulins, and iron chelators [67,80].

Advances in cerebral malaria, based on randomized controlled trials or meta-analyses of such trials, are summarized in Table 83.1.

TABLE 83.1

SUMMARY RECOMMENDATIONS FOR MANAGEMENT OF CEREBRAL MALARIA BASED ON RANDOMIZED CONTROLLED CLINICAL TRIALS

- Corticosteroids are harmful and should not be used.[a]
- Artesunate is the antimalarial of choice for cerebral malaria. When it becomes available in the United States, it should replace quinidine for this indication. Physicians who encounter a case of cerebral malaria should contact the CDC for an update on availability of artesunate.[b]

[a]Warrell DA, Looareesuwan S, Warrell MJ, et al: Dexamethasone proves deleterious in cerebral malaria. A double-blind trial in 100 comatose patients. *N Engl J Med* 306(6):313–319, 1982.
[b]Dondorp A, Nosten F, Stepniewska K, et al: Artesunate versus quinine for treatment of severe *falciparum* malaria: a randomised trial. *Lancet* 366(9487):717–725, 2005.

ROCKY MOUNTAIN SPOTTED FEVER

Rocky Mountain spotted fever (RMSF) is a potentially fatal zoonosis caused by the agent *Rickettsia rickettsii*, which is transmitted by ticks. Although the classic constellation of findings is fever, rash, and tick bite occurring in the summer months, it is important to consider the disease even when some of these features are lacking. A history of tick bite is reported in only 60% of documented cases [81], and rash may be absent in 20%. Recognition of RMSF is critical, as outcome is much improved with timely, appropriate therapy [82].

RMSF is transmitted by the hard ticks *Dermacentor andersoni, Dermacentor variabilis, Amblyomma cajennense,* and *Rhipicephalus sanguineus*. The latter tick, previously a recognized vector for RMSF in Mexico, was implicated in a recent outbreak of RMSF in Arizona, an area that had previously been spared this disease [83]. The incidence of reported RMSF has increased threefold in the 2002–2006 period compared to 1996–2001 [84]. Although the peak incidence is in the summer months, cases occur throughout the year. Classically it has been taught that children and males are at highest risk, but recent CDC data show that females and adults have only a slightly lower incidence. Native Americans have a higher incidence than other ethnic groups. RMSF was first described in Montana, thus its name, but is more frequently seen in the southeastern United States, especially the Carolinas, Oklahoma, Arkansas, and Missouri.

Pathophysiology

Rickettsia rickettsii parasitize endothelial cells of many organs and vascular smooth muscle. The organisms cause a direct cytopathic effect, leading to vascular injury, clotting activation, and a vascular leak syndrome. In severe cases, this manifests as multiorgan failure. Renal failure, respiratory failure, and coma may ensue.

Diagnosis

The presentation of RMSF is protean due to the multisystem nature of the disease. Symptoms include fever, malaise, headache, rash, myalgia, nausea, vomiting, abdominal pain, and diarrhea. Two thirds of cases have a temperature above 102°F at presentation; 90% have temperature above 102°F within 48 hours of presentation. Rash generally appears by the second or third day of illness and classically starts at the wrists and ankles, but is frequently generalized. It may involve the palms and soles; the face is spared. Rash may be missed in persons with dark skin. Gastrointestinal symptoms may be prominent, despite the systemic nature of the disease. Headache is typically present and is often severe. The key to the diagnosis is to consider it in any febrile patient who has been spending time outdoors in an endemic area.

Laboratory findings include a white blood cell count that is typically in the normal range, although a manual differential count reveals a shift to immature neutrophils. Platelets are usually decreased. Other nonspecific findings reflect the multisystem nature of the process and include hyponatremia, elevated creatine phosphokinase, hepatic transaminases, and creatinine and clotting indices (prothrombin time, partial thromboplastin time, and fibrin degradation products). CSF examination commonly demonstrates a mononuclear pleocytosis and occasionally an elevated CSF protein and low CSF glucose levels [82]. Diagnosis may be confirmed by biopsy of skin involved with rash and processed with immunofluorescence or immunoperoxidase staining, or by serologic testing.

Differential Diagnosis

RMSF is frequently misdiagnosed as pharyngitis or scarlet fever, despite the low incidence of sore throat [85]. Gastroenteritis is also a common initial diagnosis due to prominent gastrointestinal symptoms. RMSF must also be distinguished from rheumatic fever, encephalitis, meningitis, pneumonia, measles, meningococcemia, leptospirosis, acute abdominal illness, idiopathic thrombocytopenic purpura, thrombotic thrombocytopenic purpura, drug reaction, ehrlichiosis, and vasculitis [82,85,86].

Therapy

Specific therapy should not be delayed while awaiting confirmation of the diagnosis. Most broad-spectrum antibacterial agents such as cephalosporins, penicillins, and sulfa drugs are inactive against *R. rickettsii.* The treatment of choice for nonpregnant adults and children weighing more than 45 kg is doxycycline [87], 100 mg twice daily for 7 to 10 days. Children who weigh less than 45 kg should be given 2.2 mg per kg twice daily [81,88]. The risk of dental staining by tetracyclines in children is small for short courses of therapy; this consideration should not delay treatment [89]. Therapy of pregnant women is problematic because tetracyclines are associated with maternal hepatotoxicity and fluorescent yellow discoloration of fetal deciduous teeth. Calcification of permanent teeth does not begin until after birth; discoloration of permanent teeth would not be expected. The U.S. Food and Drug Administration and the Australian Drug Evaluation Committee have assigned pregnancy category D to doxycycline. Chloramphenicol is considered pregnancy category A by the Australian Drug Evaluation Committee [90]. Although teratogenicity has not been proven with chloramphenicol, maternal aplastic anemia or reversible bone marrow suppression may occur. Gray baby syndrome has occurred in neonates treated with chloramphenicol, and may occur in infants born to women treated with chloramphenicol near term. Doxycycline may be used for women presenting with RMSF near term [91]. Most authorities recommend therapy of pregnant women in the first or second trimester with chloramphenicol, 50 to 75 mg per kg per day in divided doses. Corticosteroid therapy has not been studied in a controlled fashion, although older literature has recommended it for patients with widespread vasculitis and encephalitis [92].

Prognosis

Outcome is directly related to timely, appropriate therapy. Mortality rates are as high as 20% for untreated cases, and 5% with proper therapy [93,94]. Risk factors for mortality include central nervous system involvement, renal dysfunction at presentation, a delay in the institution of therapy, therapy with an agent other than a tetracycline [87], and increased age.

MISCELLANEOUS INFECTIOUS DISEASES

There are many unusual infectious diseases that occasionally lead to intensive care unit admission. Several of these diseases are discussed briefly below and others such as serious epidemic viral pneumonias (Chapter 90) and biologic agents of mass destruction (Chapter 213).

Ehrlichiosis and *anaplasmosis* are tick-borne rickettsial diseases that present as a fever with few localizing symptoms or signs. Headache, myalgias, malaise, and rigors are seen in nearly all cases; gastrointestinal or respiratory symptoms may occur in a minority of cases [95]. Human monocytic ehrlichiosis (HME), caused by *Ehrlichia chaffeensis,* is most commonly seen in the southeastern United States. HME may present with meningoencephalitis, acute respiratory distress syndrome (ARDS), and a toxic shock–like illness [96]. Human granulocytic anaplasmosis (HGA), caused by *Anaplasma phagocytophilum,* is most commonly seen in the upper midwestern states and the northeastern United States [86]. HGA is typically a less severe disease than HME. It is found in the same geographic areas as babesiosis and Lyme disease and transmitted by *Ixodes scapularis* and by *Ixodes pacificus,* the same ticks that transmit *Borrelia burgdorferi* and *Babesia* species. Coinfection with *A. phagocytophilum, Babesia* spp, and *B. burgdorferi* has been reported [86,97]. *Ehrlichia ewingii* infection has been reported to cause a granulocytic ehrlichiosis in the southeastern United States, primarily in immunocompromised hosts [86]. In contrast to most tick-borne illnesses, ehrlichiosis and anaplasmosis are more frequently seen in middle-aged and older individuals [96,97]. Cases most often present in spring and summer, but have been reported in every month of the year [96]. HME may follow a fulminant course in HIV-infected individuals [98]. Leukocyte counts are generally low or normal with a shift to immature forms, elevated transaminases, and thrombocytopenia typically found if patients are followed carefully [95,97]. The diagnosis may be confirmed by the observation of clumps of organisms within leukocytes, termed morulae, but the sensitivity of microscopy in the first week of illness is only 60%, even in very experienced hands [97]. Sensitivity is even lower later in the course. The diagnosis may be confirmed serologically or by a polymerase chain reaction assay at a reference laboratory [86], but therapy may need to be initiated while awaiting results if suspicion is high. The treatment of choice is doxycycline; rifampin has been used if doxycycline is contraindicated [97]. Due to the overlap in clinical syndromes and the uncertainty of diagnosis early in the course, it is important to be certain that RMSF has been ruled out if an alternative agent to doxycycline is selected.

Capnocytophaga spp are fastidious Gram-negative rods that cause soft tissue infections, fever of unknown origin, bacteremia, and meningitis [99,100]. *C. canimorsus* is normal oral flora in dogs, and infection is often associated with a dog bite. Cases have been reported in association with cat bites and with nontraumatic exposure to the oral secretions of dogs. Several other species of the *Capnocytophaga* genus are normal oral flora of humans, and may cause bacteremia in the setting of cancer chemotherapy [101,102]. Compromised hosts may follow a severe course of illness, especially if bacteremia is complicated by disseminated intravascular coagulation. *Capnocytophaga* spp are resistant to many antibacterial agents that are commonly used to treat skin and soft tissue infections, including oxacillin and cefazolin. Ampicillin-sulbactam is a good empiric choice for serious soft tissue infection when there is a history of a dog bite. Clindamycin can be used for culture-proven cases of monomicrobial infection with *Capnocytophaga* in the case of penicillin allergy [101], but it is not active against *Pasteurella multocida,* which is a common pathogen in cases of dog or cat bites. Imipenem-cilastin is another alternative active against *Capnocytophaga* and *P. multocida* as well as other common pathogens of skin and soft tissue except MRSA.

References

1. Hashikawa S, Iinuma Y, Furushita M, et al: Characterization of group C and G streptococcal strains that cause streptococcal toxic shock syndrome. *J Clin Microbiol* 42:186–192, 2004.
2. Todd J, Fishaut M, Kapral F, et al: Toxic-shock syndrome associated with phage-group-I Staphylococci. *Lancet* 2:1116–1118, 1978.
3. Chesney PJ, Davis JP, Purdy WK, et al: Clinical manifestations of toxic shock syndrome. *JAMA* 246:741–748, 1981.
4. Bartlett P, Reingold AL, Graham DR, et al: Toxic shock syndrome associated with surgical wound infections. *JAMA* 247:1448–1550, 1982.
5. Todd JK: Toxic shock syndrome, *Staphylococcus aureus*, and influenza. *JAMA* 257:3070–3071, 1987.
6. Cone LA, Woodard DR, Byrd RG, et al: A recalcitrant, erythematous, desquamating disorder associated with toxin-producing staphylococci in patients with AIDS. *J Infect Dis* 165:638–643, 1992.
7. McCormick JK, Yarwood JM, Schlievert PM: Toxic shock syndrome and bacterial superantigens: an update. *Ann Rev Microbiol* 55:77–104, 2001.
8. Jamart S, Denis O, Deplano A, et al: Methicillin-resistant *Staphylococcus aureus* toxic shock syndrome. *Emerg Infect Dis* 11:636–637, 2005.
9. Limbago B, Fosheim GE, Schoonover V, et al: Characterization of methicillin-resistant *Staphylococcus aureus* isolates collected in 2005 and 2006 from patients with invasive disease: a population-based analysis. *J Clin Microbiol* 47(5):1344–1351, 2009.
10. Dickgiesser N, Wallach U: Toxic shock syndrome toxin-1 (TSST-1): influence of its production by subinhibitory antibiotic concentrations. *Infection* 15:351–353, 1987.
11. Stevens DL, Wallace RJ, Hamilton SM, et al: Successful treatment of staphylococcal toxic shock syndrome with linezolid: a case report and in vitro evaluation of the production of toxic shock syndrome toxin type 1 in the presence of antibiotics. *Clin Infect Dis* 42:729–730, 2006.
12. Stevens DL: The toxic shock syndromes. *Infect Dis Clin North Am* 10:727–746, 1996.
13. Darenberg J, Soderquist B, Normark BH, et al: Differences in potency of intravenous polyspecific immunoglobulin G against streptococcal and staphylococcal superantigens: implications for therapy of toxic shock syndrome. *Clin Infect Dis* 38:836–842, 2004.
14. Andrews MM, Parent EM, Barry M, et al: Recurrent nonmenstrual toxic shock syndrome: clinical manifestations, diagnosis, and treatment. *Clin Infect Dis* 32:1470–1479, 2001.
15. Kass EH: Toxic shock syndrome: a reprise. *Ann Intern Med* 97:608–611, 1982.
16. Brown EJ: The molecular basis of streptococcal toxic shock syndrome. *N Engl J Med* 350:2093–2094, 2004.
17. Chiang MC, Jaing TH, Wu CT, et al: Streptococcal toxic shock syndrome in children without skin and soft tissue infection: report of four cases. *Acta Paediatr* 94:763–765, 2005.
18. Stevens DL, Gibbons AE, Bergstrom R, et al: The Eagle effect revisited: efficacy of clindamycin, erythromycin, and penicillin in the treatment of streptococcal myositis. *J Infect Dis* 158:23–28, 1988.
19. Stevens DL, Bryant AE, Hackett SP: Antibiotic effects on bacterial viability, toxin production, and host response. *Clin Infect Dis* 20:S154–S157, 1995.
20. Zimbelman J, Palmer A, Todd J: Improved outcome of clindamycin compared with beta-lactam antibiotic treatment for invasive *Streptococcus pyogenes* infection. *Pediatr Infect Dis J* 18:1096–1100, 1999.
21. Kaul R, McGeer A, Norrby-Teglund A, et al: Intravenous immunoglobulin therapy for streptococcal toxic shock syndrome—a comparative observational study. The Canadian Streptococcal Study Group. *Clin Infect Dis* 28:800–807, 1999.
22. Cawley MJ, Briggs M, Haith LR Jr, et al: Intravenous immunoglobulin as adjunctive treatment for streptococcal toxic shock syndrome associated with necrotizing fasciitis: case report and review. *Pharmacotherapy* 19:1094–1098, 1999.
23. Darenberg J, Ihendyane N, Sjolin J, et al: Intravenous immunoglobulin G therapy in streptococcal toxic shock syndrome: a European randomized, double-blind, placebo-controlled trial. *Clin Infect Dis* 37:333–340, 2003.
24. Sinave C, Le Templier G, Blouin D, et al: Toxic shock syndrome due to Clostridium sordellii: a dramatic postpartum and postabortion disease. *Clin Infect Dis* 35:1441–1443, 2002.
25. Fischer M, Bhatnagar J, Guarner J, et al: Fatal toxic shock syndrome associated with *Clostridium sordellii* after medical abortion. *N Engl J Med* 353:2352–2360, 2005.
26. Kimura AC, Higa JI, Levin RM, et al: Outbreak of necrotizing fasciitis due to *Clostridium sordellii* among black-tar heroin users. *Clin Infect Dis* 38:e87–e91, 2004.
27. Kainer MA, Linden JV, Whaley DN, et al: Clostridium infections associated with musculoskeletal-tissue allografts. *N Engl J Med* 350:2564–2571, 2004.
28. Styrt B: Infection associated with asplenia: risks, mechanisms, and prevention. *Am J Med* 88:33–42, 1990.
29. Brigden ML, Pattullo AL: Prevention and management of overwhelming postsplenectomy infection—an update. *Crit Care Med* 27:836–842, 1999.
30. Coleman CN, McDougall IR, Dailey MO, et al: Functional hyposplenia after splenic irradiation for Hodgkin's disease. *Ann Intern Med* 96:44–47, 1982.
31. Markus HS, Toghill PJ: Impaired splenic function in elderly people. *Age Ageing* 20:287–290, 1991.
32. Upadhyaya P: Conservative management of splenic trauma: history and current trends. *Pediatr Surg Int* 19:617–627, 2003.
33. Gauer JM, Gerber-Paulet S, Seiler C, et al: Twenty years of splenic preservation in trauma: lower early infection rate than in splenectomy. *World J Surg* 32:2730–2735, 2008.
34. Corazza GR, Ginaldi L, Zoli G, et al: Howell-Jolly body counting as a measure of splenic function. A reassessment. *Clin Lab Haematol* 12:269–275, 1990.
35. Sawmiller CJ, Dudrick SJ, Hamzi M: Postsplenectomy *Capnocytophaga canimorsus* sepsis presenting as an acute abdomen. *Arch Surg* 133:1362–1365, 1998.
36. Sakran W, Raz R, Levi Y, et al: Campylobacter bacteremia and pneumonia in two splenectomized patients. *Eur J Clin Microbiol Infect Dis* 18:496–498, 1999.
37. Hansen K, Singer DB: Asplenic-hyposplenic overwhelming sepsis: postsplenectomy sepsis revisited. *Pediatr Dev Pathol* 4:105–121, 2001.
38. Toutouzas KG, Velmahos GC, Kaminski A, et al: Leukocytosis after posttraumatic splenectomy: a physiologic event or sign of sepsis? *Arch Surg* 137:924–929, 2002.
39. Working Party of the British Committee for Standards in Haematology Clinical Haematology Task Force: Guidelines for the prevention and treatment of infection in patients with an absent or dysfunctional spleen. *BMJ* 312:430–434, 1996.
40. Davies JM, Barnes R, Milligan D, et al: Update of guidelines for the prevention and treatment of infection in patients with an absent or dysfunctional spleen. *Clin Med* 2:440–443, 2002.
41. Shatz DV, Schinsky MF, Pais LB, et al: Immune responses of splenectomized trauma patients to the 23-valent pneumococcal polysaccharide vaccine at 1 versus 7 versus 14 days after splenectomy. *J Trauma* 44:760–766, 1998.
42. Bilukha OO, Rosenstein N: Prevention and control of meningococcal disease. Recommendations of the Advisory Committee on Immunization Practices (ACIP). *MMWR Recomm Rep* 54:1–21, 2005.
43. Centers for Disease Control and Prevention: Updated recommendation from the Advisory Committee on Immunization Practices for revaccination of persons at prolonged increased risk for meningococcal disease. *MMWR Morb Mortal Wkly Rep* 58:1042–1043, 2009.
44. Rosenstein NE, Perkins BA, Stephens DS, et al: The changing epidemiology of meningococcal disease in the United States, 1992–1996. *J Infect Dis* 180:1894–1901, 1999.
45. Pathan N, Faust SN, Levin M: Pathophysiology of meningococcal meningitis and septicaemiae. *Arch Dis Child* 88:601–607, 2003.
46. Ellison RT III, Kohler PF, Curd JG, et al: Prevalence of congenital or acquired complement deficiency in patients with sporadic meningococcal disease. *N Engl J Med* 308:913–916, 1983.
47. Faust SN, Levin M, Harrison OB, et al: Dysfunction of endothelial protein C activation in severe meningococcal sepsis. *N Engl J Med* 345:408–416, 2001.
48. Havens PL, Garland JS, Brook MM, et al: Trends in mortality in children hospitalized with meningococcal infections, 1957 to 1987. *Pediatr Infect Dis J* 8:8–11, 1989.
49. Booy R, Habibi P, Nadel S, et al: Reduction in case fatality rate from meningococcal disease associated with improved healthcare delivery. *Arch Dis Child* 85(5):386–390, 2001.
50. Hazelzet JA: Diagnosing meningococcemia as a cause of sepsis. *Pediatr Crit Care Med* 6:S50–S54, 2005.
51. Jorgensen JH, Crawford SA, Fiebelkorn KR: Susceptibility of *Neisseria meningitidis* to 16 antimicrobial agents and characterization of

resistance mechanisms affecting some agents. *J Clin Microbiol* 43:3162–3171, 2005.
52. Brigham KS, Sandora TJ: *Neisseria meningitidis*: epidemiology, treatment and prevention in adolescents. *Curr Opin Pediatr* 21:437–443, 2009.
53. Centers for Disease Control and Prevention (CDC): Emergence of fluoroquinolone-resistant *Neisseria meningitidis*–Minnesota and North Dakota, 2007–2008. *MMWR Morb Mortal Wkly Rep* 57:173–175, 2008.
54. Warner PM, Kagan RJ, Yakuboff KP, et al: Current management of purpura fulminans: a multicenter study. *J Burn Care Rehabil* 24:119–126, 2003.
55. Churchwell KB, McManus ML, Kent P, et al: Intensive blood and plasma exchange for treatment of coagulopathy in meningococcemia. *J Clin Apheresis* 10:171–177, 1995.
56. Valbonesi M, Pallavicini FB, Cannella G, et al: MOF induced by meningococcal sepsis: successful outcome after intensive multidisciplinary approaches. *Transfus Apher Sci* 33:75–77, 2005.
57. Bernard GR, Vincent JL, Laterre PF, et al: Efficacy and safety of recombinant human activated protein C for severe sepsis. *N Engl J Med* 344:699–709, 2001.
58. Vincent JL, Nadel S, Kutsogiannis DJ, et al: Drotrecogin alfa (activated) in patients with severe sepsis presenting with purpura fulminans, meningitis, or meningococcal disease: a retrospective analysis of patients enrolled in recent clinical studies. *Crit Care (London, England)* 9:R331–R343, 2005.
59. Wu HM, Harcourt BH, Hatcher CP, et al: Emergence of ciprofloxacin-resistant *Neisseria meningitidis* in North America. *N Engl J Med* 360:886–892, 2009.
60. Snow RW, Guerra CA, Noor AM, et al: The global distribution of clinical episodes of *Plasmodium falciparum* malaria. *Nature* 434:214–217, 2005.
61. Bruneel F, Hocqueloux L, Alberti C, et al: The clinical spectrum of severe imported falciparum malaria in the intensive care unit: report of 188 cases in adults. *Am J Respir Crit Care Med* 167:684–689, 2003.
62. Centers for Disease Control and Prevention: Malaria deaths following inappropriate malaria chemoprophylaxis—United States, 2001. *MMWR Morb Mortal Wkly Rep* 50:597–599, 2001.
63. Zucker JR: Changing patterns of autochthonous malaria transmission in the United States: a review of recent outbreaks. *Emerg Infect Dis* 21:37–43, 1996.
64. Ho M, White NJ: Molecular mechanisms of cytoadherence in malaria. *Am J Physiol* 276:C1231–C1242, 1999.
65. Freedman DO, Weld LH, Kozarsky PE, et al: Spectrum of disease and relation to place of exposure among ill returned travelers. *N Engl J Med* 354:119–130, 2006.
66. Winters RA, Murray HW: Malaria—the mime revisited: fifteen more years of experience at a New York City teaching hospital. *Am J Med* 93:243–246, 1992.
67. Severe falciparum malaria. World Health Organization, Communicable Diseases Cluster. *Trans R Soc Trop Med Hyg* 94:S1–S90, 2000.
68. Alvarez JR, Al Khan A, Apuzzio JJ: Malaria in pregnancy. *Infect Dis Obstet Gynecol* 13:229–236, 2005.
69. Whitty CJ, Edmonds S, Mutabingwa TK: Malaria in pregnancy. *BJOG* 112:1189–1195, 2005.
70. Brentlinger PE, Behrens CB, Micek MA: Challenges in the concurrent management of malaria and HIV in pregnancy in sub-Saharan Africa. *Lancet Infect Dis* 6:100–111, 2006.
71. Rogerson SJ, Mkundika P, Kanjala MK: Diagnosis of Plasmodium falciparum malaria at delivery: comparison of blood film preparation methods and of blood films with histology. *J Clin Microbiol* 41:1370–1374, 2003.
72. Centers for Disease Control and Prevention: Availability and use of parenteral quinidine gluconate for severe or complicated malaria. *MMWR Morb Mortal Wkly Rep* 49:1138–1140, 2000.
73. Magill A, Panosian C: Making antimalarial agents available in the United States. *N Engl J Med* 353:335–337, 2005.
74. Griffith KS, Lewis LS, Mali S, et al: Treatment of malaria in the United States: a systematic review. *JAMA* 297:2264–2277, 2007.
75. Miller KD, Greenberg AE, Campbell CC: Treatment of severe malaria in the United States with a continuous infusion of quinidine gluconate and exchange transfusion. *N Engl J Med* 321:65–70, 1989.
76. Dondorp A, Nosten F, Stepniewska K, et al: Artesunate versus quinine for treatment of severe falciparum malaria: a randomised trial. *Lancet* 366:717–725, 2005.
77. McGready R, Thwai KL, Cho T, et al: The effects of quinine and chloroquine antimalarial treatments in the first trimester of pregnancy. *Trans R Soc Trop Med Hyg* 96:180–184, 2002.
78. McGready R, Ashley EA, Moo E, et al: A randomized comparison of artesunate-atovaquone-proguanil versus quinine in treatment for uncomplicated falciparum malaria during pregnancy. *J Infect Dis* 192:846–853, 2005.
79. Wong RD, Murthy AR, Mathisen GE, et al: Treatment of severe falciparum malaria during pregnancy with quinidine and exchange transfusion. *Am J Med* 92:561–562, 1992.
80. Warrell DA, Looareesuwan S, Warrell MJ, et al: Dexamethasone proves deleterious in cerebral malaria. A double-blind trial in 100 comatose patients. *N Engl J Med* 306:313–319, 1982.
81. Masters EJ, Olson GS, Weiner SJ, et al: Rocky Mountain spotted fever: a clinician's dilemma. *Arch Intern Med* 163:769–774, 2003.
82. Kirk JL, Fine DP, Sexton DJ, et al: Rocky Mountain spotted fever. A clinical review based on 48 confirmed cases, 1943–1986. *Medicine* 69:35–45, 1990.
83. Demma LJ, Traeger MS, Nicholson WL, et al: Rocky Mountain spotted fever from an unexpected tick vector in Arizona. *N Engl J Med* 353:587–594, 2005.
84. McNabb SJ, Jajosky RA, Hall-Baker PA, et al: Summary of notifiable diseases—United States, 2006. *MMWR Morb Mortal Wkly Rep* 55:1–92, 2008.
85. Helmick CG, Bernard KW, D'Angelo LJ: Rocky Mountain spotted fever: clinical, laboratory, and epidemiological features of 262 cases. *J Infect Dis* 150:480–488, 1984.
86. Chapman AS, Bakken JS, Folk SM, et al: Diagnosis and management of tickborne rickettsial diseases: Rocky Mountain spotted fever, ehrlichioses, and anaplasmosis—United States: a practical guide for physicians and other health-care and public health professionals. *MMWR Recomm Rep* 55:1–27, 2006.
87. Holman RC, Paddock CD, Curns AT, et al: Analysis of risk factors for fatal Rocky Mountain spotted fever: evidence for superiority of tetracyclines for therapy. *J Infect Dis* 184:1437–1444, 2001.
88. Centers for Disease Control and Prevention: Fatal cases of Rocky Mountain spotted fever in family clusters—three states, 2003. *MMWR Morb Mortal Wkly Rep* 53:407–410, 2004.
89. Lochary ME, Lockhart PB, Williams WT Jr: Doxycycline and staining of permanent teeth. *Pediatr Infect Dis J* 17:429–431, 1998.
90. Anonymous. Micromedex. 2010.
91. Stallings SP: Rocky Mountain spotted fever and pregnancy: a case report and review of the literature. *Obstet Gynecol Surv* 56:37–42, 2001.
92. Woodward TE: Rocky Mountain spotted fever: epidemiological and early clinical signs are keys to treatment and reduced mortality. *J Infect Dis* 150:465–468, 1984.
93. Kirkland KB, Wilkinson WE, Sexton DJ: Therapeutic delay and mortality in cases of Rocky Mountain spotted fever. *Clin Infect Dis* 20:1118–1121, 1995.
94. Dalton MJ, Clarke MJ, Holman RC, et al: National surveillance for Rocky Mountain spotted fever, 1981–1992: epidemiologic summary and evaluation of risk factors for fatal outcome. *Am J Trop Med Hyg* 52:405–413, 1995.
95. Bakken JS, Krueth J, Wilson-Nordskog C, et al: Clinical and laboratory characteristics of human granulocytic ehrlichiosis. *JAMA* 275:199–205, 1996.
96. Demma LJ, Holman RC, McQuiston JH, et al: Epidemiology of human ehrlichiosis and anaplasmosis in the United States, 2001–2002. *Am J Trop Med Hyg* 73:400–409, 2005.
97. Bakken JS, Dumler JS: Human granulocytic ehrlichiosis. *Clin Infect Dis* 31:554–560, 2000.
98. Paddock CD, Suchard DP, Grumbach KL, et al: Brief report: fatal seronegative ehrlichiosis in a patient with HIV infection. *N Engl J Med* 329:1164–1167, 1993.
99. Brenner DJ, Hollis DG, Fanning GR, et al: *Capnocytophaga canimorsus sp. nov.* (formerly CDC group DF-2), a cause of septicemia following dog bite, and *C. cynodegmi sp. nov.*, a cause of localized wound infection following dog bite. *J Clin Microbiol* 27:231–235, 1989.
100. Janda JM, Graves MH, Lindquist D, et al: Diagnosing *Capnocytophaga canimorsus* infections. *Emerg Infect Dis* 12:340–342, 2006.
101. Bonatti H, Rossboth DW, Nachbaur D, et al: A series of infections due to *Capnocytophaga* spp in immunosuppressed and immunocompetent patients. *Clin Microbiol Infect* 9:380–387, 2003.
102. Martino R, Ramila E, Capdevila JA, et al: Bacteremia caused by *Capnocytophaga species* in patients with neutropenia and cancer: results of a multicenter study. *Clin Infect Dis* 33:e20–e22, 2001.

CHAPTER 84 ■ ACUTE INFECTION IN THE IMMUNOCOMPROMISED HOST

JENNIFER S. DALY AND ROBERT W. FINBERG

Advances in the management of neoplastic diseases, transplant immunology, and the therapy of autoimmune diseases have resulted in marked improvements in life expectancy and the quality of patients' lives. However, patients with autoimmune diseases, neoplasia, or transplants become highly susceptible to infection by virtue of their associated therapies or by the nature of their underlying illness. Infection has been and remains a leading cause of death in patients with leukemia and lymphoma and a major cause of morbidity and mortality in patients with solid tumors or transplants [1–4]. Rapid progression of fungal, bacterial, and mycobacterial infections occurs in patients given monoclonal antibodies to treat Crohn's disease and autoimmune diseases such as rheumatoid arthritis [5–8]. The epidemic of human immunodeficiency virus (HIV)-1 infection has added to the numbers of immunocompromised hosts by virtue of the central event of the virus's pathogenesis—a progressive, irreversible weakening of cell-mediated immunity unless the patient responds to antiretroviral agents. See Chapter 85.

Traditionally, infection has accounted for up to 75% of deaths in patients with acute leukemia or Hodgkin's disease [1,9] or in transplant recipients [4,10], but with advances in prophylaxis and management, deaths due to infections have decreased to about 50% while deaths due to graft versus host disease, relapse of malignancy, and multiorgan failure have increased [3,11–13]. Once patients require the care of an intensive care unit (ICU), the mortality increases, and the 1-year survival of cancer patients that require mechanical ventilation in the ICU is below 11% in some centers [14] with acute mortality between 44% and 74% [15–17]. While intensive efforts are clearly beneficial in stem cell transplant patients requiring ICU care in the pre-engraftment period, patients with graft versus host disease following engraftment have the worst prognosis [14]. Early ICU admission has been advocated based on one small study demonstrating that among patients initially thought to be too sick to benefit from ICU care, many were subsequently admitted to the ICU, and did well [18].

Although a great variety of microorganisms have been noted to cause severe, life-threatening infections in immunocompromised hosts, the clinician can formulate a diagnostic plan and decide on empiric therapy by giving careful consideration to the nature, duration, and severity of the immunosuppression that is causing the patient's predisposition to infection. Infection can arise as a consequence of derangements in host defenses that result from the primary disease, the medical and surgical treatment of the condition, or a combination of these factors. Additionally, immunocompromised patients are likely to manifest their infections in ways that are characteristically different from those of patients with intact immune responses.

IMMUNE DEFECTS AND ASSOCIATED ORGANISMS AND INFECTIONS

Underlying disease or treatments affect different aspects of the immune system and, depending on the type of defect, are associated with predisposition to infection with specific classes of organisms or disease syndromes. A level of suspicion of infection with certain organisms depends on the specific immune defect, the duration of immunosuppression, surgical and medical interventions, colonization with nosocomial pathogens, and previous latent or asymptomatic infections that may reactivate after immunosuppression. In general, the most common sites of serious, definable infection in the immunocompromised host are the bloodstream [including infection related to intravenous (IV) access devices], lung, and mucocutaneous surfaces (including oral, gastrointestinal, skin, and perirectal areas). The diverse organisms frequently or uniquely associated with infections in the compromised host are listed in Table 84.1. As a general rule, patients whose underlying disease or treatment leads to a lack of T cells or any abnormality in T cell-macrophage activation will be subject to infections with organisms that live intracellularly such as viruses, fungi, and intracellular bacteria (e.g., *Listeria*, *Legionella*, mycobacteria). Patients with profound neutropenia will be subject to infection with aerobic Gram-positive and Gram-negative bacteria that live on the skin and within the gut. Patients lacking antibodies or a spleen will be unusually susceptible to infection with encapsulated bacteria (*Streptococcus pneumoniae, Haemophilus influenzae,* and *Neisseria meningitidis*). As for any patient in the ICU, the immunocompromised patient is susceptible to infection with bacteria that are found in ventilators or spread in the ICU. The most common organisms found in patients with bloodstream infections vary by center and whether or not patients are on prophylactic antimicrobials [19]. *Escherichia coli* and *Staphylococcus aureus*, including methicillin-resistant *S. aureus* (MRSA), continue to be common, followed by coagulase-negative staphylococci, enterococci including vancomycin-resistant enterococci, *Pseudomonas aeruginosa*, *Klebsiella* spp, *Enterobacter* spp, and various streptococci [20–23]. In patients with neutropenia and documented bacteremia, Gram-positive organisms predominate over Gram-negative bacilli in patients in most centers, and the presence of an intravascular device is associated with having a positive blood culture [24]. Fungal infections increase in frequency with increasing duration of the immunocompromised state and therapy with broad-spectrum antibiotics.

Anatomic Barriers

The skin and mucosal surfaces serve a primary role in the defense of the host against invasion by endogenous and exogenous microorganisms. Mucous membrane ulceration in the mouth and gastrointestinal tract can occur spontaneously in patients with acute leukemia, although this complication more commonly arises after chemotherapy. In patients with solid tumors, disruption of mucocutaneous barriers can result from invasion, obstruction, or perforation by the malignancy. Iatrogenic disruption of the normal skin and mucosal barriers results from medical and surgical support interventions common to the ICU, including intravascular and urinary catheters [25]

TABLE 84.1

ORGANISMS COMMONLY OR UNIQUELY ASSOCIATED WITH ACUTE INFECTION IN THE IMMUNOCOMPROMISED HOST

Organism	Type of immune deficiency most likely to predispose to this organism
Bacteria	
Enteric Gram-negative bacilli (*Escherichia coli, Klebsiella, Enterobacter*, or *Proteus* spp	All immunocompromised patients, especially those with neutropenia and those on mechanical ventilation or medications that suppress gastric acid
Staphylococcus aureus	All immunocompromised patients, especially those with skin infections or intravascular catheters
Pseudomonas aeruginosa	Especially common in neutropenic patients and those on mechanical ventilation
Listeria monocytogenes	Patients with T cell or macrophage deficiencies, HIV/AIDS patients
Legionella pneumophila and related organisms	Patients with T cell or macrophage deficiencies and anyone exposed to water sources contaminated with Legionella
Skin/mucous membrane saprophytes	All immunocompromised patients
Corynebacterium jeikeium	Neutropenic patients, especially those with indwelling catheters; splenectomized patients
Capnocytophaga spp	Splenectomized patients
Coagulase-negative staphylococci	Patients with indwelling vascular catheters or prosthetic material
Nocardia spp	Patients with T cell or macrophage abnormalities
Streptococcus pneumoniae	Patients with immunoglobulin deficiencies or hyposplenism
Haemophilus influenzae	Patients with immunoglobulin deficiencies or hyposplenism
Neisseria meningitidis	Patients with immunoglobulin deficiencies or hyposplenism
Mycobacteria	Patients with a history of high risk exposure for tuberculosis (lived in an endemic area or history of a positive tuberculin skin test) or long-standing immune defects and/or chronic lung disease
Fungi	
Candida albicans and other *Candida* spp	Patients with vascular catheters after abdominal surgery, including liver transplantation; patients with prolonged neutropenia; and those receiving intravenous hyperalimentation
Torulopsis glabrata	Same as Candidiasis, increased in patients with diabetes and urinary tract colonization
Aspergillus spp	Patients with prolonged neutropenia, after transplantation, or on medications such as steroids and cytotoxic agents
Zygomycetes spp	Patients with neutropenia, after transplantation, with diabetes, or on medications such as steroids and cytotoxic agents
Trichosporon spp	Patients with neutropenia, after transplantation, or on medications such as steroids and cytotoxic agents, with vascular catheters and those receiving intravenous hyperalimentation
Fusarium spp	Patients with neutropenia, after transplantation, or on medications such as steroids and cytotoxic agents, with vascular catheters and those receiving intravenous hyperalimentation
Pneumocystis jiroveci	Patients with T cell or macrophage deficiencies, especially those receiving steroids, antirejection agents, or with lymphocytic leukemia or HIV/AIDS
Endemic fungi and yeasts	
Cryptococcus neoformans	Patients with HIV/AIDS, after transplantation, or receiving steroids
Histoplasma capsulatum	Patients from an endemic area
Coccidioides immitis	Patients from an endemic area
Protozoa	
Toxoplasma gondii	Patients with HIV/AIDS, after transplantation, or on medications such as steroids and cytotoxic agents
Parasites	
Strongyloides stercoralis	Patients from an endemic area and after transplantation, or on medications such as steroids and cytotoxic agents
Viruses	
Cytomegalovirus	Patients after bone marrow or solid organ transplantation
Varicella-zoster virus	Patients with T cell or macrophage abnormalities, especially those not receiving antiviral prophylaxis with cancer, or after bone marrow or solid organ transplantation
Herpes simplex virus	Patients with T cell or macrophage abnormalities and ICU patients, especially those not receiving antiviral prophylaxis with cancer, or after bone marrow or solid organ transplantation

(see Chapter 81 on catheter infections). Organisms that most frequently cause infection of intravascular catheters include coagulase-negative staphylococci, *S. aureus*, enterococci, *Corynebacterium* spp (including *C. jeikeium*), and *Candida* spp [1,25,26]. Percutaneously inserted central catheters (PICC) are associated with an increased risk of both infection and thrombosis [27]. The risk of these infections can be reduced, although not eliminated, through the use of permanent, subcutaneously tunneled catheters (e.g., Hickman, Broviac, Groshong, or Portacath systems) [28]. Genitourinary tract infections are associated with disruption of the urinary tract integrity, as occurs with urinary catheter drainage, pelvic tumors, or radiation with resultant ureteral obstruction, or after renal transplant.

The gastrointestinal tract is a source of occult bacteremia or fungemia, as chemotherapy and neutropenia cause breakdown in normal mucosal defenses of the gut, facilitating entry of bacteria or yeast into the bloodstream. Clinically apparent intestinal problems seen in neutropenic patients include typhlitis, anorectal cellulitis/fasciitis/abscess, necrotizing colitis, and *Clostridium difficile*-associated colitis caused by chemotherapy or antibiotics [29]. Typhlitis, an inflammatory disease of the cecum, may lead to toxic megacolon and perforation and requires a high index of suspicion and prompt diagnosis. Unusually severe and prolonged viral gastroenteritis caused by cytomegalovirus (CMV), adenovirus, rotavirus, and Coxsackie virus has been observed in marrow transplant recipients [30–32]. Herpes simplex virus (HSV) should be suspected as a possible cause for any lesion of mucous membranes in an immunocompromised host, and may also cause fatal hepatitis [33]. Adenovirus may cause hepatitis, pneumonitis, or hemorrhagic cystitis [32], and BK and JC viruses may cause persistent fever and renal insufficiency [34,35]. Necrotizing gingivostomatitis caused by oral anaerobes as well as severe periodontal infection may also complicate neutropenia.

Defective Phagocytosis

Neutrophils and macrophages provide defense against infection by bacteria and many fungi. Patients with leukemia, particularly an acute type of leukemia, commonly have a reduction in their absolute number of circulating neutrophils; qualitative defects of neutrophil function have also been described in these patients. Aplastic anemia, as well as extensive bone marrow involvement caused by lymphoma or metastatic solid tumors, may result in neutropenia. By far the most common cause of neutropenia, however, is cytotoxic chemotherapy. Patients whose neutrophils are reduced in number by malignancy or chemotherapy are at risk for development of spontaneous bacteremia. The risk becomes significant at absolute neutrophil counts that are persistently below 500 per mm^3 (or below 1,000 per mm^3 and falling) and increases dramatically at counts below 100 per mm^3 [32,36].

Invasive and disseminated fungal infections also may be a consequence of neutropenia and become more common after the neutropenic patient has received broad-spectrum antibiotic therapy [32,37]. *Candida* and *Aspergillus* spp are the most common fungal pathogens observed in neutropenic hosts, but unusual genera such as *Fusarium, Trichosporon, Scedosporium (Pseudallescheria),* and *Cunninghamella* have been described with increasing frequency [38,39]

Altered Humoral Immunity

B-cell lymphocytic function and antibody production may be impaired in untreated patients with chronic lymphocytic leukemia, multiple myeloma, and lymphoma. Acquired deficits in antibody production may also be encountered in otherwise healthy patients (e.g., immunoglobulin A deficiency, common variable immunodeficiency). Hypogammaglobulinemia or impaired antibody response predisposes patients to infections attributable to encapsulated bacteria such as *S. pneumoniae, H. influenzae,* and *N. meningitidis*; moreover, these infections are likely to be sudden, severe, and associated with fulminant bacteremia [32]. Infections caused by enteric Gram-negative bacilli and *P. aeruginosa* also may be seen in previously untreated patients with defective humoral immunity secondary to B-cell malignancies.

Impaired Cell-Mediated Immunity

T cell-mediated immunity includes cytotoxic (killer) T cells, activated macrophages, and antibody-dependent cellular cytotoxicity. These critical components of immunity are impaired in patients with Hodgkin's disease [40] and other lymphomas and in those taking antirejection drugs (e.g., cyclosporine, mycophenolate mofetil, tacrolimus, sirolimus, and antilymphocyte antibodies), antibodies against tumor necrosis factor-α, or corticosteroids [4,6,8,41]. Patients infected with HIV-1 experience a progressive and devastating loss of T cell-mediated immunity. This virus selectively infects and lyses CD4$^+$ lymphocytes that play a central role in governing humeral and cellular immune responses. Defects in cell-mediated immunity are commonly associated with primary or reactivation of infection by herpes viruses (varicella-zoster virus, CMV, HSV), protozoa (*Toxoplasma gondii* and *Cryptosporidium* spp), fungi (*Pneumocystis jiroveci, Cryptococcus neoformans, Histoplasma capsulatum, Coccidioides immitis,* and *Candida* spp), helminths (*Strongyloides stercoralis*), mycobacteria (*M. tuberculosis, M. avium-intracellulare, M. kansasii, M. chelonae*), and other intracellular bacteria (*Listeria monocytogenes, Salmonella,* and *Legionella* spp) [4,40,42].

Immunosuppressive Medications

Cytotoxic chemotherapy, corticosteroids, anticytokine antibodies, and other immunosuppressive therapeutic regimens can alter host defenses in several ways. Immunosuppressive effects depend on the class of drug, dose and duration of therapy, and timing relative to other therapeutic modalities (e.g., radiation, which may contribute to neutropenia). Several new inhibitors of cytokines and cytokine activation (including anti-TNF and anti-IL-1 antibodies) used to treat autoimmune disorders have resulted in the reactivation of latent tuberculosis and histoplasmosis as well as invasive aspergillosis [6,43,44]. Physicians need to be aware of the fact that patients on such agents have a risk of reactivation of intracellular organisms.

Antimicrobial Therapy

Antibiotic therapy is highly effective in the management of documented infections and febrile episodes in the compromised host. These agents are double-edged swords, however, and promote a shift toward increasing frequency of infections caused by progressively more resistant organisms, including *P. aeruginosa, Enterobacter* spp, expanded spectrum β-lactamase producing *Klebsiella* spp, multiply resistant enterococci, methicillin-resistant *S. aureus*, and fluconazole-resistant *Candida* spp. Unusual, intrinsically resistant bacteria (e.g., *Capnocytophaga* and *Corynebacterium* spp) and fungi (e.g., *Scedosporium* and *Fusarium* spp) are being seen with increasing frequency in oncology centers.

Splenectomy

Splenectomy, which results in the loss of the reticuloendothelial capacity to clear organisms from the bloodstream, predisposes patients to fulminant, overwhelming bacteremia caused by encapsulated bacteria (*S. pneumoniae, H. influenzae,* and *N. meningitidis*) as well as *S. aureus*. Although the syndrome of overwhelming postsplenectomy infection is most common in patients whose splenectomy was for malignancy or reticuloendothelial disease, overwhelming postsplenectomy infection can occur in any splenectomized patient regardless of underlying disease or interval since surgery (see Chapter 3). Accordingly, fever higher than 38°C in the splenectomized patient warrants immediate investigation and empiric therapy for possible bacteremia or focal bacterial infection. Consideration of ICU admission and presumptive antibiotic therapy is appropriate if the patient appears systemically toxic. A third-generation cephalosporin (e.g., ceftriaxone or cefotaxime) is reasonable empiric therapy, although if skin or skin structure infection is present, vancomycin should be added because of the increasing likelihood of community-acquired methicillin-resistant *S. aureus*.

DIAGNOSTIC APPROACH TO FEVER

In the evaluation of acutely ill, immunocompromised patients with fever in the ICU, a meticulous and thorough history and physical examination must be performed initially and repeated daily. Particular attention should be directed to sites of high risk, such as the oropharynx, anorectal region, lungs, skin, optic fundi, and vascular catheter sites [32,45]. Patients with focal abnormalities such as solid tumors, organ transplants, or recent surgery need to have these specific sites investigated with special care. Patients with neutropenia and infection exhibit fewer and less striking physical findings of infection (e.g., local warmth, swelling, adenopathy, exudate, or fluctuance) than are ordinarily encountered in immunocompetent individuals (see Chapter 76).

Initial laboratory studies that should be performed in the evaluation of the acutely ill, febrile, compromised host include (a) cultures of blood; (b) cultures of urine if symptoms or abnormal urinalysis; (c) routine sputum culture if the patient has symptoms or signs of pulmonary disease; (d) swab, aspiration, or biopsy of suspect skin, mucous membrane, or other lesions for smears, cultures, and pathologic examination; (e) semiquantitative culture of IV catheters in place when fever develops, if possible (if the cannula is a critical lifeline or a subcutaneously tunneled device that shows no local signs of infection, removal can be deferred pending results of routine blood cultures); (f) chest radiography; and (g) serum chemistries (i.e., electrolytes, liver chemistries, creatinine), in part to detect possible visceral involvement or multiorgan failure caused by disseminated infection and also to serve as baselines for monitoring possible adverse reactions to subsequent antimicrobial therapy.

Patients with defects in cell-mediated immunity (e.g., HIV-1 infection, lymphoma, transplant recipients) often harbor organisms that are best diagnosed by histological examination (e.g., *Pneumocystis jiroveci, T. gondii*) or special culture techniques (e.g., mycobacteria, viruses). In instances in which such organisms are high in the differential diagnosis, initial evaluation often entails immediate biopsy of the pathologic process. Localizing symptoms and signs may indicate the need for other studies, such as computed tomography (CT), magnetic resonance imaging (MRI), or nuclear medicine scans [e.g., gallium-67 scan to detect *P. jiroveci* pneumonia (PCP)]. Tachypnea warrants arterial blood gas studies because progressive hypoxemia in the absence of radiographic findings can be an early indicator of pulmonary infection, especially PCP, and may indicate a need for bronchoscopy. Depending on the nature of the abnormality and the state of immunosuppression, consider lung biopsy and/or quantitative culture of washings or protected brushings obtained through the bronchoscope if patient presents with pulmonary symptoms and a new finding on chest X-ray [46,47].

APPROACH TO SPECIFIC INFECTIOUS DISEASE PRESENTATIONS

Acute Fever without Obvious Source: Neutropenia

In patients with fever and neutropenia, shock may be an early complication of bacteremia. Consequently, even though the wide use of antibiotic prophylaxis during episodes of neutropenia has decreased the incidence of documented infection in febrile neutropenic patients to only 20% to 30% [48,49], multiple randomized trials and consensus guidelines support the initiation of empiric broad-spectrum antibiotic therapy for all patients with fever greater than 38°C and absolute neutrophil counts less than 500 per μL (or less than 1,000 per μL and falling) [36,37,45,50]. The immediate institution of such therapy in these patients (even in the absence of documentation of bacterial infection) dramatically reduces morbidity and mortality. The most rapidly fatal infectious agents that are documented to cause acute fever in the critically ill neutropenic cancer patient are enteric Gram-negative bacilli (e.g., *E. coli, Klebsiella* spp, *Proteus* spp), *P. aeruginosa*, and *S. aureus* [36,37]. In the patient without an obvious site of infection, initial empiric antibiotic therapy should be directed against these pathogens (Table 84.2). Such therapy should take into consideration idiosyncrasies of the antimicrobial susceptibility patterns of organisms in the institutions where the patient has resided in the months before infection and recent antibiotic use in a particular patient.

Despite the testing of hundreds of antibacterial regimens for use in patients with fever and neutropenia, there is no consensus on one best regimen. For patients who have not received prior antibiotic prophylaxis or therapy, a single antipseudomonal third-generation cephalosporin (e.g., ceftazidime or cefepime), piperacillin/tazobactam, or a carbapenem (imipenem or meropenem) constitutes an appropriate regimen [51,52]. Although the use of cefepime or piperacillin/tazobactam alone is somewhat controversial, none of the β-lactam agents discussed earlier are clearly preferred, except as dictated by local resistance patterns or cost [45,51,52]. Current data indicate that the empiric use of aminoglycosides with broad-spectrum β-lactam agents is not needed [53].

In a patient in septic shock who is admitted to the ICU or in institutions with endemic-resistant Gram-negative bacteria, a multidrug regimen may be indicated. For patients with immediate hypersensitivity reactions to cephalosporins and penicillins, aztreonam has activity against Gram-negative bacilli and can be used with an antimicrobial agent with activity against a broad spectrum of Gram-positive organisms (e.g., vancomycin typically is added to this regimen because aztreonam has no Gram-positive activity). Because of the increased prevalence of methicillin-resistant staphylococci, recent guidelines have recommended routine initial inclusion of vancomycin in empiric regimens for patients in shock, particularly in patients on antimicrobial prophylaxis and those with evidence for skin or

TABLE 84.2

EMPIRIC REGIMENS FOR INITIAL THERAPY OF CRITICALLY ILL, FEBRILE, ADULT ICU PATIENTS WITH NEUTROPENIA AND CANCER (DOSAGES PROVIDED FOR PATIENTS WITH NORMAL RENAL FUNCTION)

Choice of β-lactam or monobactam[a]	Plus or minus additional antimicrobial to treat skin/soft tissue infections if present (must use for patients given aztreonam) or patient suspected of having staphylococcal infection[a]
Piperacillin/tazobactam 3.375 g IV q 4 or 4.5 g IV q6h OR Ceftazidime 2 g IV q8h OR Imipenem/cilastatin 500–750 mg IV q6h OR meropenem 1 g IV q8h For penicillin and cephalosporin allergic patients: aztreonam, 2 g IV q6–8h, plus vancomycin, 2 g/d divided q6–12h	Vancomycin 1–1.5 g IV q12 (weight based—15 mg/kg q12h) (alternatives for allergic patients include linezolid, daptomycin, quinupristin/dalfopristin, or clindamycin)

[a]The choice of regimen should be based on local resistance patterns and the individual patient's most recent prior antimicrobial therapy.

skin structure infections or with inflammation at the site of or dysfunction of indwelling plastic venous access catheters [45]. Randomized controlled trials have demonstrated no benefit to continuing vancomycin after 72 hours unless patients demonstrated a Gram-positive infection [45,54].

Most standard regimens are designed for patients who have not previously received antibiotics. The development of fever with systemic symptoms such as shock or respiratory distress in a patient on antibiotic therapy requires a change in therapy to include organisms that are known to be resistant to classes of antibacterials the patient has received. For example, in a patient who recently has received cephalosporins, the choice of piperacillin, piperacillin/tazobactam, or imipenem may be preferable to ceftazidime especially if expanded spectrum β-lactamase–producing organisms are established flora in the local ICU.

After initial evaluation of the patient and initiation of empiric antibiotic therapy, subsequent management is based on (a) identification of a focus of infection, (b) isolation of an etiologic agent, (c) defervescence versus continued fever, and (d) duration of neutropenia. In the patient for whom an infection has been documented clinically or by culture, antibiotics should be continued as appropriate for the site of infection, susceptibility profile of pathogens, and the patient's clinical response. Even when a specific pathogen is identified by culture, in patients who are neutropenic a broad-spectrum regimen usually is maintained for the duration of neutropenia [37,45,55]. In patients likely to have permanent or extremely prolonged granulocytopenia, attempts to stop therapy are reasonable but should be made with continuing close clinical observation [45,56].

If fever has not been eliminated or the patient continues to have evidence of ongoing sepsis, the search should continue for potential sites of focal infection (skin, optic fundi, oropharynx, chest, abdomen, and perirectal area). The serial, empiric addition of one antibiotic after another without culture data is not efficacious in most settings and may lead to confusion in the event that an adverse reaction occurs [45]. Cephalosporins and vancomycin can cause bone marrow suppression and lead to colonization with resistant organisms. The addition or sequential substitution of multiple cephalosporins may induce β-lactamase production by some organisms.

Persistent or Recurrent Fever without Obvious Source: Neutropenia

Should fevers persist for 4 to 7 days of neutropenia, randomized controlled trials have found that empiric antifungal therapy with an amphotericin B preparation, voriconazole, or caspofungin [57–59] is appropriate. The rationale for such therapy is that it is difficult to culture fungi before they cause disseminated disease, and that the mortality from disseminated fungal disease in neutropenic hosts is high. *Candida* and *Aspergillus* spp are common pathogens, and *Fusarium, Trichosporon*, and *Bipolaris* spp are seen occasionally but are becoming more common [60–63]. The use of the serum assay for galactomannan as a marker for *Aspergillus* infection is controversial as sensitivity is low, and there may be false-positive results in patients receiving piperacillin [64,65]. Another serum assay that tests for 1,3-β-D-glucan antigenemia shows promise but serial monitoring is needed and predictive value for invasive fungal infections varies in different centers [66,67]. More research is needed on both these assays.

Patients at particularly high risk of disseminated fungal disease include those with (a) prolonged granulocytopenia, (b) parenteral nutrition, (c) *Candida* colonization in oropharynx or urine, (d) corticosteroid therapy, and (e) advancing multiple organ dysfunction (renal, hepatic, pulmonary). Moreover, multiorgan failure often is a reflection of disseminated candidiasis [68]. The use of antifungal prophylaxis with the imidazoles (fluconazole) has caused a shift in the species of *Candida* causing infection from *C. albicans* and *C. tropicalis* to the more imidazole-resistant *C. krusei* and *C. glabrata* [69], and with the use of posaconazole or voriconazole a shift has started to occur to more infections due to *Zygomycetes* [70]. Hepatosplenic (also called *chronic disseminated*) candidiasis presents with fevers and elevation of serum alkaline phosphatase that continue through the return of neutrophils to greater than 1,000 cells per mm^3 [71]. Multiple embolic lesions are present in liver and spleen, and prolonged therapy with amphotericin B, itraconazole, fluconazole, or caspofungin, depending on the sensitivity of the organism, is beneficial [72].

Based on the findings from a randomized clinical trial of primary therapy and randomized studies of salvage therapy, voriconazole is the drug of choice for infections caused by *Aspergillus* [73,74]. However, an amphotericin preparation continues to be the drug of choice when a fungal infection is suspected in patients already receiving an azole antifungal [70]. Amphotericin has activity against *Aspergillus*, the *Zygomycetes*, and many other filamentous fungi. According to data from randomized clinical trials, the newer preparations of amphotericin B appear to decrease renal toxicity while maintaining efficacy; therefore, amphotericin B complexed with cholesteryl sulfate, with liposomal vesicles, or with a bilayered lipid membrane have become standard for use in patients on other nephrotoxic drugs or those with impaired renal function, despite their higher cost [75] (see Chapter 77). Prognosis remains poor, however, for patients treated for documented invasive fungal infection in the setting of persistent neutropenia [60,76]. Most ICU patients who remain febrile and neutropenic after 4 to 7 days of broad-spectrum antibacterials should be treated with either voriconazole, an amphotericin B preparation, or echinocandin, although in selected low-risk patients (where the risk of *Aspergillus* or *Zygomycetes* is low), itraconazole or fluconazole is equally efficacious, as shown in open randomized clinical trails and endorsed in expert reviews of these studies [59,77–80].

Pneumonia in the Compromised Host

The lung is one of the most common identifiable sites of infection in immunocompromised patients [2,46,81]. Pulmonary disease can be caused by a wide variety of agents, including bacteria, protozoa, helminths, viruses, fungi, and mycobacteria (Table 84.3) (see Chapter 68). The differential diagnosis is made even more difficult by the various noninfectious pulmonary complications that can present abruptly with acute respiratory symptoms and fever. These include underlying malignancy or vasculitis, drug toxicity, interstitial fibrosis, diffuse alveolar hemorrhage, radiation pneumonitis, cardiogenic pulmonary edema, bronchiolitis obliterans organizing pneumonia (BOOP), diffuse alveolar damage syndrome, acute fibrinous organizing pneumonia (AFOP), pulmonary alveolar proteinosis, and pulmonary embolism [46,81].

Pneumonia in the immunocompromised patient often presents without the symptoms and signs seen in normal hosts. Regardless of cause, fever and progressive shortness of breath (and concomitant tachypnea and arterial hypoxemia) tend to be common symptoms; in the neutropenic patient, cough, sputum production, and physical examination (as well as radiographic) findings are likely to be unimpressive or absent. Chest radiographs should be obtained promptly in the compromised patient with fever or dyspnea. High-resolution CT or MRIs will often reveal infiltrates or masses that cannot be appreciated on conventional X-rays and thus are recommended in cases in which there is question about the diagnosis [82].

Differential Diagnosis

Developing an appropriate differential diagnosis for the causative agents of pneumonia in the immunocompromised host rests first on an appreciation of the nature, severity, and duration of the immune suppression. In addition to being susceptible to conventional respiratory tract pathogens (*S. pneumoniae*, *H. influenzae*), hospitalized immunocompromised hosts are prone to Gram-negative bacillary pneumonia; those with prolonged (greater than 7 days) or profound (less than 100 neutrophils per mm^3) neutropenia may become infected with *Aspergillus* or *Zygomycetes* spp [2]. T cell-deficient hosts (e.g., patients with HIV infection, transplant, or lymphoma) are more likely to acquire PCP [83] or infection with CMV, HSV [84–86], endemic fungi (*Cryptococcus, Histoplasma*) [44,87,88], *Nocardia* spp, or intracellular bacteria (mycobacteria, *Legionella* spp) [89–91]. Patients who have resided in tropical countries may reactivate latent infection by *Strongyloides stercoralis* in the setting of altered cell-mediated immunity. Pulmonary infiltrates, polymicrobial bacteremia, and bacterial meningitis are the hallmarks of this syndrome [92]. Patients with deficient neutrophil and T cell function (e.g., bone marrow transplant recipients) may be at risk for all of these pathogens.

Chest radiographs may provide useful clues; focal or multifocal infiltrates tend to suggest infections by bacteria or fungi, but are unlikely to provide a definitive diagnosis. Computerized tomographic scanning often provides more information, including the detection of lesions not seen on routine chest radiograph [46]. Diffuse disease is more characteristic of viral causes (HSV, CMV), PCP, or noninfectious processes (drug toxicity, lymphangitic carcinomatosis, and radiation pneumonitis). Cavitary disease can be seen with certain of the necrotizing Gram-negative bacilli such as *P. aeruginosa* as well as *S. aureus* and anaerobes (e.g., postaspiration or postobstructive). Cavities also can be a late finding with pneumonia due to *Aspergillus, Zygomycetes*, and *Nocardia* spp. It is impossible, however, to make firm rules with regard to radiographic patterns. Gram-negative bacilli or *Legionella* may progress to diffuse disease or incite the acute respiratory distress syndrome. Patients with severe defects in cell-mediated immunity may manifest a miliary pattern caused by disseminated tuberculosis or histoplasmosis. Conversely, radiation pneumonitis may present as focal, sharply demarcated infiltrates confined to the irradiated portion of the lung.

TABLE 84.3

COMMON CAUSES OF ACUTE PULMONARY DISEASE IN IMMUNOCOMPROMISED PATIENTS

Infectious causes

Bacteria
- *Streptococcus pneumoniae*
- *Haemophilus influenzae*
- *Pseudomonas aeruginosa*
- Enteric Gram-negative bacilli
- *Staphylococcus aureus*
- *Legionella* spp
- *Nocardia* spp
- Mycobacteria

Fungi
- *Aspergillus* spp
- *Pneumocystis jiroveci*
- *Candida* spp
- *Zygomycetes* spp
- *Cryptococcus neoformans*

Viruses
- Cytomegalovirus
- Herpes simplex virus

Protozoa
- *Toxoplasma gondii*

Parasite
- *Strongyloides stercoralis*

Noninfectious causes

Primary disease (malignancy, autoimmune, or other illnesses that led to immunocompromising condition)

Malignancy
- Primary
- Metastatic

Vasculitis

Alveolar damage, fibrosis, and organizing pneumonia
- Bronchiolitis obliterans and organizing pneumonia (BOOP)
- Acute fibrinous organizing pneumonia (AFOP)
- Diffuse alveolar damage syndrome

Drug toxicity
- Bleomycin
- Busulfan
- Cyclophosphamide

Hemorrhage
Congestive heart failure
Radiation

Diagnostic Approach and Empiric Therapy

The diagnostic approach to pulmonary disease in the immunocompromised host also depends on the nature of the immune deficit. As a general rule, all accessible sites (blood, urine, and sputum) should be cultured, although sputum of high quality is obtained rarely in these circumstances. In neutropenic hosts, empiric antibacterial therapy is begun at the outset regardless of radiographic pattern, using one of the regimens discussed previously for fever and neutropenia [36,37]. In the case of ventilated inpatients, treatment of pneumonia must include antibiotic(s) that are effective against organisms that are likely to be present in the ICU (some of these organisms are typically resistant to antibiotics typically used in treating febrile, neutropenic patients). These regimens typically contain more than one antibiotic and they should be adjusted based on the cumulative susceptibility report of the hospital or unit. While logical, the use of "protected specimen brushes" has not been shown to be of clear clinical value and should not be a reason to perform an invasive procedure in an immunocompromised patient [93].

If a clinical response occurs in a neutropenic patient, therapy is continued until neutropenia resolves. In the setting of persistent neutropenia, a clinical picture of progressive pulmonary disease despite antibiotic therapy suggests invasive disease caused by fungi found in the environment (a variety of "saprophytic" fungi are a major concern, especially *Aspergillus,* but also *Rhizopus, Fusarium,* and *Trichosporon* spp) [38,62,63]. Expectorated sputum, bronchial brush specimen cultures, or bronchial lavage fluid may provide presumptive evidence of these pathogens, but prompt definitive diagnosis often requires open or thoracoscopically guided lung biopsy. Transbronchial biopsy is often nondiagnostic. Typically, pneumonia caused by *Aspergillus* or *Zygomycetes* spp causes areas of lung infarction that may be missed by transbronchial biopsy [94,95]. Computed tomographic scans may show the classic "crescent" sign in patients with aspergillosis but this is a sign of late disease, and although it may be helpful diagnostically in patients who are recovering, early diagnosis is important to prevent mortality in persistently neutropenic patients. Unlike bacteria, which are usually easy to culture, fungi are often not isolated in cases where histopathology eventually demonstrates their presence. While PCR (polymerase chain reaction)-based techniques have yet to be of demonstrated clinical usefulness in these clinical situations, measurements of polysaccharide antigen in serum or other body fluids has been of demonstrated utility in the diagnosis of both *Cryptococcus*- and *Histoplasma*-associated pneumonia.

The standard approach to therapy of confirmed pulmonary disease caused by *Aspergillus* is to treat with voriconazole as this agent has been shown to be superior to treatment with amphotericin B preparations [74,96]. While the use of combinations of antifungal agents (including echinocandins and azoles as well as echinocandins and amphotericin) has rationale, support from animal data, and anecdotal human experience, large trials have yet to be performed, making it difficult to recommend this approach at this time unless single agents have failed. There is no established therapy for some emerging fungal pathogens such as *Trichosporon* or *Fusarium* spp, although encouraging results have been reported in a few cases using posaconazole and voriconazole [96].

In patients with compromised T cell immunity, the list of diagnostic possibilities is longer and more diverse, making a single formula for empiric therapy a virtual impossibility. Clinicians caring for these patients should be guided both by the type of the underlying immunodeficiency as well as the patent's previous experiences with both pathogens and antimicrobial agents. Expectorated or induced sputum may demonstrate the organism by special stains in a minority of cases (*P. jiroveci, M. tuberculosis, Nocardia asteroides*), but flexible bronchoscopy with lavage or transbronchial biopsy and open or thoracoscopically assisted lung biopsy may be required in order to make a diagnosis for these patients [46,97,98] (see Chapters 9 and 69). Bronchoscopy is particularly helpful for diffuse or interstitial disease, in which it not only provides lavage fluid with reasonable diagnostic accuracy for infectious agents such as *P. jiroveci* and bacteria but also pathologic specimens that may allow diagnosis of CMV infection, drug pneumonitis, hemorrhage, or lymphangitic carcinomatosis. In patients with focal or nodular disease, thoracoscopically assisted biopsy is likely to yield the best results.

In the immunocompromised host (non-HIV infected), the diagnosis of PCP often requires bronchoscopy with bronchoalveolar lavage with or without biopsy. A variety of other infections also require biopsy for diagnosis. It is reasonable to treat (empirically) with trimethoprim-sulfamethoxazole (15 per kg of the trimethoprim component IV daily divided every 6 or 8 hours) while arrangements are made for diagnostic procedures, as the organisms persist for the first few days of treatment. It is usually an error to postpone performing bronchoscopy (with biopsy) or thoracoscopically guided lung biopsy in severely ill immunocompromised patients with pulmonary infiltrates in the hope that they will improve, because clinical deterioration may make the procedure (and the diagnosis) impossible. If PCP is confirmed and the patient has severe renal insufficiency, serum drug concentration monitoring, if available, should be used to adjust therapy to obtain a peak serum sulfamethoxazole level of 100 μg per mL or trimethoprim levels of 5 to 8 mg per μL [99]. An alternative diagnosis, established by histologic or microbiologic diagnosis, allows

TABLE 84.4

ADVANCES IN MANAGEMENT BASED UPON RANDOMIZED CONTROLLED CLINICAL TRIALS AND META-ANALYSES OF THESE TRIALS

Acute fever without obvious source: neutropenia

- Broad-spectrum antibiotic therapy should be started for all immunocompromised patients with fever greater than 38°C and absolute neutrophil counts less than 500/mm^3 (or less than 1,000/mm^3 and falling) [36,37,50–52].
- There is no benefit to continuing vancomycin after 72 h unless a Gram-positive infection is documented [51,54].
- There is no benefit to adding an aminoglycoside to a β-lactam agent in patients with fever and neutropenia [52,53].

Persistent fever or recurrent fever with obvious source: neutropenia

- Empiric antifungal with an amphotericin B preparation, voriconazole, or an echinocandin should be started for the immunocompromised patient with neutropenia and fever of 4–7 d duration [57–59,77,78].

Treatment of aspergillosis

- Voriconazole is the drug of choice for documented infections due to *Aspergillus* [73].

Prophylaxis of fungal infections

- In patients undergoing chemotherapy for acute myelogenous leukemia or the myelodysplastic syndrome, posaconazole prevented invasive fungal infections more effectively than did either fluconazole or itraconazole and improved overall survival. There were more serious adverse events possibly or probably related to treatment in the posaconazole group [103,104].
- Both fluconazole and itraconazole have shown benefit for prophylaxis in patients after allogeneic stem cell transplant [108].

institution of specific therapy, such as acyclovir for HSV pneumonia, ganciclovir for CMV pneumonia, trimethoprim-sulfamethoxazole for nocardiosis, or corticosteroids for radiation pneumonitis, BOOP, AFOP, or drug-induced disease [46,97,100,101].

PREVENTION OF INFECTION

Increasing emphasis is being placed on the prevention of opportunistic infections in immunocompromised hosts. These strategies have taken many different forms. Early efforts were directed at modifications of the environment of neutropenic patients through laminar airflow, nonabsorbable antibiotics, and elaborate efforts at disinfecting the inanimate environment. These approaches have proven expensive and laborious and since they did not affect either disease remission or mortality, they have been abandoned by most centers.

Oral fluoroquinolone (and trimethoprim-sulfamethoxazole) administration has been studied in patients with prolonged neutropenia. These agents reduce levels of aerobic Gram-negative bacilli in the gut lumen, the major reservoir for dissemination of infection in the neutropenic host, and studies document the efficacy of levofloxacin in preventing infections and hospitalizations in patients with chemotherapy-induced neutropenia [102].

Antifungal prophylaxis with oral fluconazole (400 mg orally daily or 200 mg IV every 12 hours) has proved effective in reducing infection by *Candida* spp in bone marrow transplant recipients [81]. See Chapter 188. Recent studies suggest that posaconazole, which has a much broader spectrum than fluconazole (including *Aspergillus*), is efficacious in preventing fungal infections in severely neutropenic patients, hematopoietic stem cell transplant patients, and those with graft versus host disease [103,104].

Antiviral prophylaxis with acyclovir has been shown to reduce mucositis and mucocutaneous infections by HSV in transplant recipients and in patients with leukemia [105,106]. Although prophylactic administration of ganciclovir has been demonstrated to decrease CMV disease in solid organ transplant recipients, the administration of this agent to bone marrow transplant patients results in neutropenia. Consequently, most centers are now using "preemptive" treatment with ganciclovir (beginning treatment only when DNA levels are increased in the serum of patients at risk). See Chapter 188.

Administration of granulocyte-colony–stimulating factors hasten bone marrow recovery and shorten the duration of neutropenia in some patients receiving chemotherapy. Consensus guidelines suggest that they should be used to support dose-intense chemotherapy and have little impact on mortality in patients with existing neutropenia and fever and should not be used as a routine adjunct to antimicrobials [107].

Advances in infection in the immunocompromised host, based on randomized controlled trials or meta-analyses of such trials, are summarized in Table 84.4.

References

1. Bodey GP, Bolivar R, Fainstein V: Infectious complications in leukemic patients. *Semin Hematol* 19:193, 1982.
2. Winston DJ, Emmanouilides C, Busuttil RW: Infections in liver transplant recipients. *Clin Infect Dis* 21:1077, 1995.
3. Jurado M, Deeg HJ, Storer B, et al: Hematopoietic stem cell transplantation for advanced myelodysplastic syndrome after conditioning with busulfan and fractionated total body irradiation is associated with low relapse rate but considerable nonrelapse mortality. *Biol Blood Marrow Transplant* 8:161, 2002.
4. Fishman JA: Infection in solid-organ transplant recipients. *N Engl J Med* 357:2601, 2007.
5. Warris A, Bjorneklett A, Gaustad P: Invasive pulmonary aspergillosis associated with infliximab therapy. *N Engl J Med* 344:1099, 2001.
6. Keane J, Gershon S, Wise RP, et al: Tuberculosis associated with infliximab, a tumor necrosis factor alpha-neutralizing agent. *N Engl J Med* 345:1098, 2001.
7. Keane J: TNF-blocking agents and tuberculosis: new drugs illuminate an old topic. *Rheumatology (Oxford)* 44:714, 2005.
8. Crum NF, Lederman ER, Wallace MR: Infections associated with tumor necrosis factor-alpha antagonists. *Medicine (Baltimore)* 84:291, 2005.
9. Notter DT, Grossman PL, Rosenberg SA, et al: Infections in patients with Hodgkin's disease: a clinical study of 300 consecutive adult patients. *Rev Infect Dis* 2:761, 1980.
10. Zander DS, Baz MA, Visner GA, et al: Analysis of early deaths after isolated lung transplantation. *Chest* 120:225, 2001.
11. Kobayashi K, Kami M, Murashige N, et al: Outcomes of patients with acute leukaemia who relapsed after reduced-intensity stem cell transplantation from HLA-identical or one antigen-mismatched related donors. *Br J Haematol* 129:795, 2005.
12. Yoo JH, Choi SM, Lee DG, et al: Prognostic factors influencing infection-related mortality in patients with acute leukemia in Korea. *J Korean Med Sci* 20:31, 2005.
13. Gratwohl A, Brand R, Frassoni F, et al: Cause of death after allogeneic haematopoietic stem cell transplantation (HSCT) in early leukaemias: an EBMT analysis of lethal infectious complications and changes over calendar time. *Bone Marrow Transplant* 36:757, 2005.
14. Pene F, Aubron C, Azoulay E, et al: Outcome of critically ill allogeneic hematopoietic stem-cell transplantation recipients: a reappraisal of indications for organ failure supports. *J Clin Oncol* 24:643, 2006.
15. Azoulay E, Thiery G, Chevret S, et al: The prognosis of acute respiratory failure in critically ill cancer patients. *Medicine (Baltimore)* 83:360, 2004.
16. Huynh TN, Weigt SS, Belperio JA, et al: Outcome and prognostic indicators of patients with hematopoietic stem cell transplants admitted to the intensive care unit. *J Transplant* 2009:917294, 2009.
17. Nishida K, Palalay MP: Prognostic factors and utility of scoring systems in patients with hematological malignancies admitted to the intensive care unit and required a mechanical ventilator. *Hawaii Med J* 67:264, 2008.
18. Thiery G, Azoulay E, Darmon M, et al: Outcome of cancer patients considered for intensive care unit admission: a hospital-wide prospective study. *J Clin Oncol* 23:4406, 2005.
19. Reuter S, Kern WV, Sigge A, et al: Impact of fluoroquinolone prophylaxis on reduced infection-related mortality among patients with neutropenia and hematologic malignancies. *Clin Infect Dis* 40:1087, 2005.
20. Paul M, Gafter-Gvili A, Leibovici L, et al: The epidemiology of bacteremia with febrile neutropenia: experience from a single center, 1988–2004. *Isr Med Assoc J* 9:424, 2007.
21. Ramphal R: Changes in the etiology of bacteremia in febrile neutropenic patients and the susceptibilities of the currently isolated pathogens. *Clin Infect Dis* 39[Suppl 1]:S25, 2004.
22. Wisplinghoff H, Seifert H, Wenzel RP, et al: Current trends in the epidemiology of nosocomial bloodstream infections in patients with hematological malignancies and solid neoplasms in hospitals in the United States. *Clin Infect Dis* 36:1103, 2003.
23. Avery R, Kalaycio M, Pohlman B, et al: Early vancomycin-resistant enterococcus (VRE) bacteremia after allogeneic bone marrow transplantation is associated with a rapidly deteriorating clinical course. *Bone Marrow Transplant* 35:497, 2005.
24. Zinner SH: Fluoroquinolone prophylaxis in patients with neutropenia. *Clin Infect Dis* 40:1094, 2005.
25. Fatkenheuer G, Buchheidt D, Cornely OA, et al: Central venous catheter (CVC)-related infections in neutropenic patients—guidelines of the Infectious Diseases Working Party (AGIHO) of the German Society of Hematology and Oncology (DGHO). *Ann Hematol* 82[Suppl 2]:S149, 2003.
26. Sepkowitz KA: Treatment of patients with hematologic neoplasm, fever, and neutropenia. *Clin Infect Dis* 40[Suppl 4]:S253, 2005.
27. Cheong K, Perry D, Karapetis C, et al: High rate of complications associated with peripherally inserted central venous catheters in patients with solid tumours. *Intern Med J* 34:234, 2004.
28. Mermel LA, Allon M, Bouza E, et al: Clinical practice guidelines for the diagnosis and management of intravascular catheter-related infection: 2009 update by the Infectious Diseases Society of America. *Clin Infect Dis* 49:1, 2009.
29. Maschmeyer G, Haas A: The epidemiology and treatment of infections in cancer patients. *Int J Antimicrob Agents* 31:193, 2008.
30. Sandherr M, Einsele H, Hebart H, et al: Antiviral prophylaxis in patients with haematological malignancies and solid tumours: guidelines of the Infectious Diseases Working Party (AGIHO) of the German Society for Hematology and Oncology (DGHO). *Ann Oncol* 17(7):1051–1059, 2006.

31. Yolken RH, Bishop CA, Townsend TR, et al: Infectious gastroenteritis in bone-marrow-transplant recipients. *N Engl J Med* 306:1010, 1982.
32. Pizzo PA: Fever in immunocompromised patients. *N Engl J Med* 341:893, 1999.
33. Herget GW, Riede UN, Schmitt-Graff A, et al: Generalized herpes simplex virus infection in an immunocompromised patient—report of a case and review of the literature. *Pathol Res Pract* 201:123, 2005.
34. Hirsch HH, Randhawa P: BK virus in solid organ transplant recipients. *Am J Transplant* 9[Suppl 4]:S136, 2009.
35. Drachenberg CB, Hirsch HH, Papadimitriou JC, et al: Polyomavirus BK versus JC replication and nephropathy in renal transplant recipients: a prospective evaluation. *Transplantation* 84:323, 2007.
36. Pizzo PA: Management of fever in patients with cancer and treatment-induced neutropenia. *N Engl J Med* 328:1323, 1993.
37. Hughes WT, Armstrong D, Bodey GP, et al: 2002 guidelines for the use of antimicrobial agents in neutropenic patients with cancer. *Clin Infect Dis* 34:730, 2002.
38. Husain S, Munoz P, Forrest G, et al: Infections due to Scedosporium apiospermum and Scedosporium prolificans in transplant recipients: clinical characteristics and impact of antifungal agent therapy on outcome. *Clin Infect Dis* 40:89, 2005.
39. Walsh TJ, Groll A, Hiemenz J, et al: Infections due to emerging and uncommon medically important fungal pathogens. *Clin Microbiol Infect* 10[Suppl 1]:48, 2004.
40. Fisher RI, DeVita VT Jr, Bostick F, et al: Persistent immunologic abnormalities in long-term survivors of advanced Hodgkin's disease. *Ann Intern Med* 92:595, 1980.
41. Hellmann DB, Petri M, Whiting-O'Keefe Q: Fatal infections in systemic lupus erythematosus: the role of opportunistic organisms. *Medicine (Baltimore)* 66:341, 1987.
42. Patel R, Roberts GD, Keating MR, et al: Infections due to nontuberculous mycobacteria in kidney, heart, and liver transplant recipients. *Clin Infect Dis* 19:263, 1994.
43. Giles JT, Bathon JM: Serious infections associated with anticytokine therapies in the rheumatic diseases. *J Intensive Care Med* 19:320, 2004.
44. Wood KL, Hage CA, Knox KS, et al: Histoplasmosis after treatment with anti-tumor necrosis factor-alpha therapy. *Am J Respir Crit Care Med* 167:1279, 2003.
45. *NCCN Clinical Practice Guidelines in Oncology: Prevention and Treatment of Cancer-Related Infections V2.2009*. 2009 [cited April 23, 2010]; Available from: http://www.nccn.org/professionals/physician_gls/PDF/infections.pdf.
46. Shorr AF, Susla GM, O'Grady NP: Pulmonary infiltrates in the non-HIV-infected immunocompromised patient: etiologies, diagnostic strategies, and outcomes. *Chest* 125:260, 2004.
47. Fagon JY, Chastre J, Wolff M, et al: Invasive and noninvasive strategies for management of suspected ventilator-associated pneumonia. A randomized trial. *Ann Intern Med* 132:621, 2000.
48. Klastersky J, Ameye L, Maertens J, et al: Bacteraemia in febrile neutropenic cancer patients. *Int J Antimicrob Agents* 30[Suppl 1]:S51, 2007.
49. Zinner SH: New pathogens in neutropenic patients with cancer: an update for the new millennium. *Int J Antimicrob Agents* 16:97, 2000.
50. Pizzo PA, Hathorn JW, Hiemenz J, et al: A randomized trial comparing ceftazidime alone with combination antibiotic therapy in cancer patients with fever and neutropenia. *N Engl J Med* 315:552, 1986.
51. Paul M, Yahav D, Fraser A, et al: Empirical antibiotic monotherapy for febrile neutropenia: systematic review and meta-analysis of randomized controlled trials. *J Antimicrob Chemother* 57:176, 2006.
52. Pereira CA, Petrilli AS, Carlesse FA, et al: Cefepime monotherapy is as effective as ceftriaxone plus amikacin in pediatric patients with cancer and high-risk febrile neutropenia in a randomized comparison. *J Microbiol Immunol Infect* 42:141, 2009.
53. Paul M, Schelsinger A, Grozinsky-Glasberg S, et al: Beta-lactam versus beta-lactam-aminoglycoside combination therapy in cancer patients with neutropenia. *Cochrane Database Syst Rev* (2):CD003038, 2002.
54. Wade JC, Glasmacher A: Vancomycin does not benefit persistently febrile neutropenic people with cancer. *Cancer Treat Rev* 30:119, 2004.
55. Pizzo PA, Robichaud KJ, Gill FA, et al: Duration of empiric antibiotic therapy in granulocytopenic patients with cancer. *Am J Med* 67:194, 1979.
56. DiNubile MJ: Stopping antibiotic therapy in neutropenic patients. *Ann Intern Med* 108:289, 1988.
57. Pizzo PA, Robichaud KJ, Gill FA, et al: Empiric antibiotic and antifungal therapy for cancer patients with prolonged fever and granulocytopenia. *Am J Med* 72:101, 1982.
58. Walsh TJ, Pappas P, Winston DJ, et al: Voriconazole compared with liposomal amphotericin B for empirical antifungal therapy in patients with neutropenia and persistent fever. *N Engl J Med* 346:225, 2002.
59. Martino R, Viscoli C: Empirical antifungal therapy in patients with neutropenia and persistent or recurrent fever of unknown origin. *Br J Haematol* 132:138, 2006.
60. Shaukat A, Bakri F, Young P, et al: Invasive filamentous fungal infections in allogeneic hematopoietic stem cell transplant recipients after recovery from neutropenia: clinical, radiologic, and pathologic characteristics. *Mycopathologia* 159:181, 2005.
61. Pagano L, Offidani M, Fianchi L, et al: Mucormycosis in hematologic patients. *Haematologica* 89:207, 2004.
62. Husain S, Alexander BD, Munoz P, et al: Opportunistic mycelial fungal infections in organ transplant recipients: emerging importance of non-Aspergillus mycelial fungi. *Clin Infect Dis* 37:221, 2003.
63. Singh N: Trends in the epidemiology of opportunistic fungal infections: predisposing factors and the impact of antimicrobial use practices. *Clin Infect Dis* 33:1692, 2001.
64. Weisser M, Rausch C, Droll A, et al: Galactomannan does not precede major signs on a pulmonary computerized tomographic scan suggestive of invasive aspergillosis in patients with hematological malignancies. *Clin Infect Dis* 41:1143, 2005.
65. Marr KA, Laverdiere M, Gugel A, et al: Antifungal therapy decreases sensitivity of the Aspergillus galactomannan enzyme immunoassay. *Clin Infect Dis* 40:1762, 2005.
66. Ellis M, Al-Ramadi B, Finkelman M, et al: Assessment of the clinical utility of serial beta-D-glucan concentrations in patients with persistent neutropenic fever. *J Med Microbiol* 57:287, 2008.
67. Senn L, Robinson JO, Schmidt S, et al: 1,3-Beta-D-glucan antigenemia for early diagnosis of invasive fungal infections in neutropenic patients with acute leukemia. *Clin Infect Dis* 46:878, 2008.
68. Maksymiuk AW, Thongprasert S, Hopfer R, et al: Systemic candidiasis in cancer patients. *Am J Med* 77:20, 1984.
69. Rex JH, Pappas PG, Karchmer AW, et al: A randomized and blinded multicenter trial of high-dose fluconazole plus placebo versus fluconazole plus amphotericin B as therapy for candidemia and its consequences in nonneutropenic subjects. *Clin Infect Dis* 36:1221, 2003.
70. Chamilos G, Marom EM, Lewis RE, et al: Predictors of pulmonary zygomycosis versus invasive pulmonary aspergillosis in patients with cancer. *Clin Infect Dis* 41:60, 2005.
71. Thaler M, Pastakia B, Shawker TH, et al: Hepatic candidiasis in cancer patients: the evolving picture of the syndrome. *Ann Intern Med* 108:88, 1988.
72. Pappas PG, Kauffman CA, Andes D, et al: Clinical practice guidelines for the management of candidiasis: 2009 update by the Infectious Diseases Society of America. *Clin Infect Dis* 48:503, 2009.
73. Herbrecht R, Denning DW, Patterson TF, et al: Voriconazole versus amphotericin B for primary therapy of invasive aspergillosis. *N Engl J Med* 347:408, 2002.
74. Walsh TJ, Anaissie EJ, Denning DW, et al: Treatment of aspergillosis: clinical practice guidelines of the Infectious Diseases Society of America. *Clin Infect Dis* 46:327, 2008.
75. Herbrecht R, Natarajan-Ame S, Nivoix Y, et al: The lipid formulations of amphotericin B. *Expert Opin Pharmacother* 4:1277, 2003.
76. Cordonnier C, Ribaud P, Herbrecht R, et al: Prognostic factors for death due to invasive aspergillosis after hematopoietic stem cell transplantation: a 1-year retrospective study of consecutive patients at French transplantation centers. *Clin Infect Dis* 42:955, 2006.
77. Winston DJ, Hathorn JW, Schuster MG, et al: A multicenter, randomized trial of fluconazole versus amphotericin B for empiric antifungal therapy of febrile neutropenic patients with cancer. *Am J Med* 108:282, 2000.
78. Boogaerts M, Winston DJ, Bow EJ, et al: Intravenous and oral itraconazole versus intravenous amphotericin B deoxycholate as empirical antifungal therapy for persistent fever in neutropenic patients with cancer who are receiving broad-spectrum antibacterial therapy. A randomized, controlled trial. *Ann Intern Med* 135:412, 2001.
79. Bennett JE, Powers J, Walsh T, et al: Forum report: issues in clinical trials of empirical antifungal therapy in treating febrile neutropenic patients. *Clin Infect Dis* 36:S117, 2003.
80. Perfect JR: Management of invasive mycoses in hematology patients: current approaches. *Oncology (Williston Park)* 18:5, 2004.
81. Sharma S, Nadrous HF, Peters SG, et al: Pulmonary complications in adult blood and marrow transplant recipients: autopsy findings. *Chest* 128:1385, 2005.
82. Franquet T: High-resolution computed tomography (HRCT) of lung infections in non-AIDS immunocompromised patients. *Eur Radiol* 16:707, 2006.
83. Sepkowitz KA, Brown AE, Telzak EE, et al: Pneumocystis carinii pneumonia among patients without AIDS at a cancer hospital. *JAMA* 267:832, 1992.
84. Sia IG, Patel R: New strategies for prevention and therapy of cytomegalovirus infection and disease in solid-organ transplant recipients. *Clin Microbiol Rev* 13:83, 2000.
85. Graham BS, Snell JD Jr: Herpes simplex virus infection of the adult lower respiratory tract. *Medicine (Baltimore)* 62:384, 1983.
86. Ramsey PG, Rubin RH, Tolkoff-Rubin NE, et al: The renal transplant patient with fever and pulmonary infiltrates: etiology, clinical manifestations, and management. *Medicine (Baltimore)* 59:206, 1980.
87. Wheat LJ: Diagnosis and management of histoplasmosis. *Eur J Clin Microbiol Infect Dis* 8:480, 1989.
88. Chang WC, Tzao C, Hsu HH, et al: Pulmonary cryptococcosis: comparison of clinical and radiographic characteristics in immunocompetent and immunocompromised patients. *Chest* 129:333, 2006.
89. Wiesmayr S, Stelzmueller I, Tabarelli W, et al: Nocardiosis following solid organ transplantation: a single-centre experience. *Transpl Int* 18:1048, 2005.
90. Alp E, Yildiz O, Aygen B, et al: Disseminated nocardiosis due to unusual species: two case reports. *Scand J Infect Dis* 38:545, 2006.

91. O'Reilly KM, Urban MA, Barriero T, et al: Persistent culture-positive Legionella infection in an immunocompromised host. *Clin Infect Dis* 40:e87, 2005.
92. Nucci M, Portugal R, Pulcheri W, et al: Strongyloidiasis in patients with hematologic malignancies. *Clin Infect Dis* 21:675, 1995.
93. Fujitani S, Yu VL: Diagnosis of ventilator-associated pneumonia: focus on nonbronchoscopic techniques (nonbronchoscopic bronchoalveolar lavage, including mini-BAL, blinded protected specimen brush, and blinded bronchial sampling) and endotracheal aspirates. *J Intensive Care Med* 21:17, 2006.
94. Shelhamer JH, Toews GB, Masur H, et al: NIH conference. Respiratory disease in the immunosuppressed patient. *Ann Intern Med* 117:415, 1992.
95. Rosenow EC III, Wilson WR, Cockerill FR III: Pulmonary disease in the immunocompromised host. 1. *Mayo Clin Proc* 60:473, 1985.
96. Pfaller MA, Messer SA, Hollis RJ, et al: Antifungal activities of posaconazole, ravuconazole, and voriconazole compared to those of itraconazole and amphotericin B against 239 clinical isolates of Aspergillus spp. and other filamentous fungi: report from SENTRY Antimicrobial Surveillance Program, 2000. *Antimicrob Agents Chemother* 46:1032, 2002.
97. Maschmeyer G, Beinert T, Buchheidt D, et al: Diagnosis and antimicrobial therapy of pulmonary infiltrates in febrile neutropenic patients—guidelines of the Infectious Diseases Working Party (AGIHO) of the German Society of Hematology and Oncology (DGHO). *Ann Hematol* 82[Suppl 2]:S118, 2003.
98. Patel NR, Lee PS, Kim JH, et al: The influence of diagnostic bronchoscopy on clinical outcomes comparing adult autologous and allogeneic bone marrow transplant patients. *Chest* 127:1388, 2005.
99. Sattler FR, Cowan R, Nielsen DM, et al: Trimethoprim-sulfamethoxazole compared with pentamidine for treatment of Pneumocystis carinii pneumonia in the acquired immunodeficiency syndrome: a prospective, noncrossover study. *Ann Intern Med* 109:280, 1988.
100. Bhatti S, Hakeem A, Torrealba J, et al: Severe acute fibrinous and organizing pneumonia (AFOP) causing ventilatory failure: successful treatment with mycophenolate mofetil and corticosteroids. *Respir Med* 103:1764, 2009.
101. Peikert T, Rana S, Edell ES: Safety, diagnostic yield, and therapeutic implications of flexible bronchoscopy in patients with febrile neutropenia and pulmonary infiltrates. *Mayo Clin Proc* 80:1414, 2005.
102. Bucaneve G, Micozzi A, Menichetti F, et al: Levofloxacin to prevent bacterial infection in patients with cancer and neutropenia. *N Engl J Med* 353:977, 2005.
103. Ullmann AJ, Lipton JH, Vesole DH, et al: Posaconazole or fluconazole for prophylaxis in severe graft-versus-host disease. *N Engl J Med* 356:335, 2007.
104. Cornely OA, Maertens J, Winston DJ, et al: Posaconazole vs. fluconazole or itraconazole prophylaxis in patients with neutropenia. *N Engl J Med* 356:348, 2007.
105. Seale L, Jones CJ, Kathpalia S, et al: Prevention of herpesvirus infections in renal allograft recipients by low-dose oral acyclovir. *JAMA* 254:3435, 1985.
106. Wade JC, Newton B, Flournoy N, et al: Oral acyclovir for prevention of herpes simplex virus reactivation after marrow transplantation. *Ann Intern Med* 100:823, 1984.
107. Aapro MS, Cameron DA, Pettengell R, et al: EORTC guidelines for the use of granulocyte-colony stimulating factor to reduce the incidence of chemotherapy-induced febrile neutropenia in adult patients with lymphomas and solid tumours. *Eur J Cancer* 42:2433, 2006.
108. Glasmacher A, Prentice AG: Evidence-based review of antifungal prophylaxis in neutropenic patients with haematological malignancies. *J Antimicrob Chemother* 56[Suppl 1]:i23, 2005.

CHAPTER 85 ■ INTENSIVE CARE OF PATIENTS WITH HIV INFECTION

SARAH H. CHEESEMAN AND MARK J. ROSEN

At the start of the pandemic in the 1980s, AIDS was considered to be rapidly fatal in almost all cases, and the benefits of aggressive interventions, including treatment in the intensive care unit (ICU), were questioned for patients with advanced disease. Respiratory failure due to *Pneumocystis jiroveci* pneumonia (PCP) was by far the most common disorder that prompted ICU admission, outcomes were uniformly dismal, and intensive care admission was often discouraged by clinicians and declined by patients. HIV-infected persons who now have access to effective combination antiretroviral therapy (ART) for HIV infection enjoy much better outcomes. Since the use of these drugs became the standard of care in 1996, U.S. mortality rates due to AIDS declined from an annual high of around 45,000 per year to the current plateau of around 14,000 by 2007 [1]. Until recently, the hopeful prognosis in the United States and developed nations stood in sharp contrast to the global epidemic, where an estimated 2.7 million people acquired HIV infection in 2008 and 2 million died [2], but dramatically scaled-up access to combination ART is now reducing HIV-related mortality in sub-Saharan Africa [1].

With the use of ART, the spectrum of critical illness in HIV infection is changing along with the short- and long-term prognosis following these illnesses. In addition, the use of antiretrovirals entails risk of drug interactions and toxicity, requiring vigilance in the multidrug complexity of ICU care.

REASONS FOR INTENSIVE CARE UNIT ADMISSION

The literature on the frequency and reasons for ICU admission in patients with HIV infection must be interpreted with the understanding that with rare exception, each study reviews the experience of a single center and reflects local ICU admission criteria and practice patterns. Care of patients with HIV infection and with critical illness in general may vary widely, so the conclusions of these reports cannot be generalized [3]. The decision on whether to admit HIV-infected patients to the ICU or withhold such treatment varies by hospital characteristics (county/state, Veterans Affairs Medical Centers, church affiliated, voluntary, and for profit) and geographic location, and these differences are maintained after controlling for severity of illness and patient demographic and socioeconomic characteristics. Thus, data on diseases and outcomes from one center cannot be applied reliably to others. Endemic fungi and other pathogens influence ICU admission rates for different diseases; this may be important in the United States, where the epidemic has shifted from the east and west coasts to the southern states [1].

There is emerging evidence that the reasons for ICU admission have changed over the last three decades of the AIDS epidemic, largely due to reduced incidence of opportunistic infections owing to ART. In the era before ART, an estimated 5% to 10% of hospitalizations of patients with HIV infection involved an ICU admission; most patients were admitted for respiratory failure, and PCP was the most common diagnosis [4–6]. Although PCP has always been the most common cause of respiratory failure in patients with HIV infection, it appears that ICU admissions for PCP, and for respiratory failure in general, continue to decline [7,8]. The few studies of intensive care in the era of ART suggest that overall ICU utilization by HIV-infected persons has not declined; respiratory failure is still the most common reason for admission, but its relative frequency is declining as other organ failures are increasing [8]. Patients are also less likely to be admitted for PCP and other HIV-associated opportunistic infections, and are now more likely to have life-threatening bacterial pneumonia, sepsis, neurologic disorders, and complications of end-stage liver disease [7–11]. Patients may also become critically ill from the toxic effects of antiretroviral medications and from an accelerated inflammatory response related to immune reconstitution resulting from the use of ART.

PULMONARY DISORDERS

Pneumocystis Pneumonia

Pneumonia caused by *Pneumocystis jiroveci* (formerly classified as *Pneumocystis carinii*) has always been a major cause of illness and death in patients with HIV infection. Once thought to be a parasite, genomic analysis revealed that *P. jiroveci* is in fact a fungus that infects only humans, while *P. carinii* is pathogenic only in immunodeficient rats [12]. Although the taxonomy of this pathogen changed, the term PCP is still acceptable shorthand for *Pneumocystis* pneumonia.

Despite immune restoration from ART and effective specific chemoprophylaxis for PCP, this infection still occurs for several reasons: many patients do not know that they have HIV infection until they develop an opportunistic infection; others know that they have HIV but are not receiving medical care; and some are in care but are either not prescribed or choose not to take prophylaxis or ART [13]. Adherence to complex regimens with difficult-to-tolerate side effects is often problematic, and suboptimal adherence leads to selection of HIV mutations that confer drug resistance. Some patients take prophylaxis for PCP, but are still so profoundly immunocompromised that it is ineffective [14]. Nevertheless, the incidence of PCP has declined in the era of ART.

PCP should be suspected in a patient with known or suspected HIV infection, fever, and progressive cough and dyspnea. Radiographically, the diagnosis is strongly suggested by perihilar or diffuse ground glass opacities, but this pattern is not specific for PCP. Other presentations include pneumatoceles, pneumothorax, nodules, lobar consolidation, and normal images [15]. The diagnosis can be confirmed only by identifying the organism in specimens obtained from the respiratory tract, either in sputum induced by inhalation of hypertonic saline or by bronchoscopy. Although establishing a diagnosis is not difficult, many clinicians treat patients with suspected PCP empirically, reserving bronchoscopy for patients who do not respond to treatment. A decision-analysis model and a retrospective study comparing these two strategies suggest that the outcomes are similar, but no clinical trial has ever evaluated whether initial empiric therapy or a more aggressive diagnostic strategy that includes bronchoscopy is preferable [16,17]. In intubated patients, the diagnosis may be established easily with bronchoalveolar lavage.

The treatment of PCP is outlined in Table 85.1 [18]. Trimethoprim-sulfamethoxazole (TMP-SMX) is the preferred treatment for PCP in patients who have not had an adverse reaction to this drug [18]. Many physicians are willing to use TMP-SMX despite a history of a prior adverse reaction in patients receiving adjunctive corticosteroid therapy and ICU support, because it is not clear whether any of the alternatives is as effective for moderate-to-severe disease. Patients with severe PCP who do not respond or who are intolerant of this medication are usually given pentamidine, but this drug is associated with adverse reactions that are more serious than those associated with TMP-SMX. Clindamycin with primaquine is effective for moderate-to-severe PCP, but primaquine cannot be administered parenterally, potentially limiting its use.

When treatment of PCP is delayed or ineffective, patients may develop hypoxemic respiratory failure. The clinical and radiographic features of severe PCP resemble the acute respiratory distress syndrome (ARDS), with hypoxemia, intrapulmonary shunting, reduced pulmonary compliance, and diffuse radiographic opacities [19]. As the disease progresses and pulmonary compliance diminishes, pneumothorax is common and is associated with a particularly poor prognosis [20,21]

TABLE 85.1

TREATMENT OF MODERATE-TO-SEVERE *PNEUMOCYSTIS* PNEUMONIA

Drug	Dose	Comments
Trimethoprim-sulfamethoxazole	15–20 mg/kg/d TMP plus 75–100 mg/kg/d SMX *IV* or *PO* in 3 or 4 divided doses	Drug of choice, but toxicity (rash, fever, nausea, leukopenia) is frequent
Pentamidine isethionate	3–4 mg/kg IV daily	Toxicity: dysglycemia, renal failure, QT interval prolongation, arrhythmias, pancreatitis, hypotension; 50% dextrose must be available
Clindamycin plus primaquine	Clindamycin 600–900 mg q6–8 h *IV* or *PO* plus 30 mg primaquine base *qd* (15 mg primaquine base = 26.3 mg primaquine phosphate)	Screen for glucose-6-phosphate dehydrogenase deficiency
Prednisone	40 mg PO *bid* days 1–5, 20 mg PO *bid* or 40 mg PO daily, days 6–10 20 mg PO daily, days 11–21	Recommended as adjunctive therapy for severe disease [$PaO_2 \leq 70$ mm Hg, or $P(A\text{-}a)O_2 > 35$ mm Hg breathing room air] within 72 h of PCP therapy

IV, intravenous; PO, by mouth; SMX, sulfamethoxazole; TMP, trimethoprim.

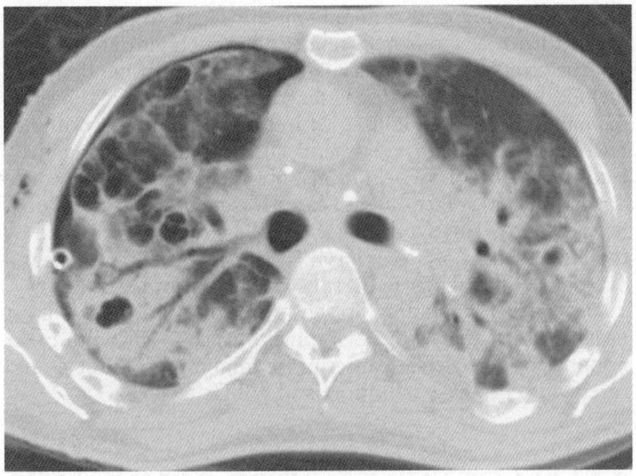

FIGURE 85.1. Selected computerized tomographic image of a patient with severe *Pneumocystis* pneumonia. This patient has significant cystic changes, as well as areas of dense pulmonary consolidation. Note the pneumothorax and chest tube in the right lung.

(Fig. 85.1). Just as severe PCP resembles ARDS clinically, the supportive treatment is similar, including intubation, mechanical ventilation, application of positive end-expiratory pressure, and lung-protective ventilation strategies [22].

Animal models of PCP indicate that the clinical severity of infection correlates more closely with markers of inflammation than with the organism burden, suggesting that the immune response and its attendant inflammation account for the clinical manifestations of pneumonia [23]. Respiratory compromise is believed to be mediated by activated CD8+ cells and neutrophils in the lung in response to killed organisms, and patients with PCP typically have deterioration of gas exchange during the first few days of treatment with anti-*Pneumocystis* agents alone [24]. When corticosteroids are administered to patients with moderate-to-severe PCP (defined as a PaO_2 less than 70 mm Hg while breathing room air or an arterial-alveolar oxygen difference greater than 35 mm Hg) at the start of anti-*Pneumocystis* treatment, there is a reduced likelihood of respiratory failure, deterioration of oxygenation, and death [25,26]. Corticosteroids may attenuate lung injury caused by the inflammatory response to killed organisms, allowing the patient to survive to receive more antimicrobial therapy. Corticosteroids offer no benefit in patients with less severe abnormalities in gas exchange at the start of therapy, or in whom they are administered more than 72 hours after anti-*Pneumocystis* treatment has begun.

Other Pulmonary Disorders

A wide variety of infectious and noninfectious HIV-associated pulmonary disorders may lead to respiratory failure. Bacterial pneumonias, most commonly caused by *Streptococcus pneumoniae,* have probably surpassed PCP as the cause of respiratory failure in the era of ART [27]. In patients with severe immune compromise, pulmonary infection or disseminated disease with *Pseudomonas aeruginosa*, *Mycobacterium tuberculosis*, cytomegalovirus, endemic fungi, and *Aspergillus* spp may also lead to respiratory failure [28].

COINFECTION WITH HIV AND HEPATITIS VIRUSES

With improved treatment of HIV with antiretroviral agents, complications of hepatitis B (HBV) and C viruses (HCV) have emerged as a major cause of mortality in HIV-infected persons [29–31]. An estimated 15% to 30% of patients with HIV are coinfected with HCV, an eightfold increase in HCV infection compared with the general population [32]. Patients coinfected with HCV and HIV are more likely to develop cirrhosis than those with HCV alone. Thus, many patients with HIV infection are admitted to ICUs with end-stage liver disease and associated encephalopathy and gastrointestinal hemorrhage. Although a number of antiretroviral agents are also active against HBV, permitting construction of regimens effective against both pathogens for HIV-HBV coinfected patients, management of coinfection with HIV and HCV entails separate combination drug regimens with interactions and overlapping toxicities, administered for at least 6 months and often more than 12 months. Such therapy requires close supervision by experienced personnel and may exacerbate liver dysfunction in cases of decompensated cirrhosis.

IMMUNE RECONSTITUTION DISORDERS

Initiation of antiretroviral therapy may be followed by paradoxic worsening of known opportunistic infections after an initial response to therapy, characterized by an unusual degree of inflammatory reaction. Alternatively, patients with an infection not yet manifested clinically may develop an inflammatory reaction at the infected site (so-called unmasking). These reactions are not typical of the usual clinical presentation of the infectious agent, and are now termed "immune reconstitution inflammatory syndrome" (IRIS) or "immune restoration disease" (IRD) [33,34]. For instance, *Mycobacterium avium* complex, which usually produces disseminated disease with no histologic evidence of host response in persons with advanced HIV infection and CD4+ lymphocyte counts <50 per μL, may present with fever and pain due to focal necrotizing lymphadenitis. A meta-analysis of 64 reports comprising 13,103 persons initiating antiretroviral therapy found that 13% developed IRIS; some series report much higher rates, particularly in patients with cytomegalovirus retinitis [35]. The time to onset of IRIS is reported to vary from 3 to 658 days after starting ART with a median of 29 to 49 days [34,36,37]. The risk is higher for patients with lower CD4+ counts before initiation of ART, but the occurrence of IRIS seems to correlate better with rapid decline in viral load than with increase in CD4+ lymphocyte count [36,37], and the meta-analysis found a case-fatality rate of 6.7% [35]. IRIS-related respiratory compromise is reported in association with mycobacterial infection and PCP [38,39]. Corticosteroids may be used to suppress the aberrant inflammatory reaction, but there are no guidelines as to when to use them or the optimal dose and duration. Corticosteroids are usually reserved for patients with severe inflammatory disease.

OTHER CRITICAL ILLNESSES

HIV-infected persons are not spared any of the diseases that can bring non-HIV-infected persons with otherwise similar characteristics to the ICU, including severe bacterial infections, gastrointestinal hemorrhage, trauma, drug overdose, violence, and cardiovascular disease. Injection drug users are obviously at increased risk of developing infective endocarditis.

Patients with HIV infection have accelerated atherosclerosis and increased risk of coronary artery disease; this was previously attributed to therapy, particularly protease inhibitors which are known to increase plasma lipid levels [40,41]. However, the risk of major cardiovascular disease outcomes increased in patients randomized to interrupt ART when CD4+ lymphocyte count rose above 400 compared to those who continued therapy and who had more drug exposure [42]. Subsequent analyses have correlated cardiovascular disease risk to higher levels of viremia [43] and abnormalities of endothelial function that improve with ART [44].

Laboratory abnormalities, including pancytopenia, eosinophilia, and transaminase elevations, may either represent the patient's baseline or indicate significant disease or drug toxicity. Among laboratory abnormalities that may safely be ignored are macrocytosis as a normal accompaniment of zidovudine, stavudine, or tenofovir therapy (provided there are no hypersegmented polymorphonuclear leukocytes), mild indirect hyperbilirubinemia in patients on atazanavir or indinavir, and hyperuricemia in patients taking didanosine. Elevations of creatine phosphokinase in patients taking zidovudine or tenofovir may also be asymptomatic and benign, but some reflect clinical myositis caused by these drugs. Hyponatremia seems to be relatively common and well tolerated in advanced HIV infection, but frank adrenal insufficiency or isolated hypoaldosteronism may require specific diagnosis and management.

TOXIC EFFECTS OF ANTIRETROVIRAL THERAPY

The drugs used in antiretroviral therapy are associated with several life-threatening toxicities that prompt admission to the ICU. Nucleoside analog reverse transcriptase inhibitors (NRTIs), especially didanosine and stavudine (and zalcitabine, which is no longer available in the United States), can cause pancreatitis, which may be severe. In a retrospective study of 73 HIV-infected patients with pancreatitis, 46% of cases were attributed to drug toxicity, with didanosine and pentamidine (used to treat PCP) the most common offending agents [45]. Didanosine may cause portal hypertension without cirrhosis [46]. Patients who received this drug even many years before may present with life-threatening hemorrhage from esophageal varices.

Nucleoside reverse transcriptase inhibitors can cause lactic acidosis by inhibiting DNA polymerase-γ, disrupting mitochondrial DNA. This may also cause hepatic steatosis or mitochondrial myopathy [47]. Lactic acidosis is the consequence of increased anaerobic glycolysis by damaged mitochondria, coupled with decreased lactate clearance by the fatty liver. Mild hyperlactatemia occurs commonly in patients receiving NRTIs and is not clinically important, but severe lactic acidosis occurs at a rate of 1.3 to 3.2 cases per 1,000 person-years of nucleoside exposure and may be life threatening [48,49]. The appearance of nausea, vomiting, abdominal pain, dyspnea, or weakness in persons on long-term therapy with these agents may herald the onset of this life-threatening illness and should prompt measurement of serum lactate. This entity should be considered in the differential diagnosis of apparent sepsis, hepatic failure, and pancreatitis requiring ICU admission of patients on antiretroviral therapy. Since patients may also develop severe lactic acidosis due to sepsis, empiric antibiotics should be administered pending the results of microbiologic evaluation. If severe hyperlactatemia or lactic acidosis is found, all antiretroviral therapy must be stopped immediately since continuation of a partial regimen may lead to viral resistance. In addition to standard care, case reports suggest that this disorder may improve with use of riboflavin, thiamine, L-carnitine, and coenzyme Q [50–52]. The same drugs and mechanism underlie a syndrome of severe neuromuscular weakness and respiratory failure that may mimic Guillain–Barré syndrome or botulism, and the same therapies have been proposed [53]. The newer NRTIs (tenofovir, emtricitabine, lamivudine, and abacavir) produce less inhibition of DNA polymerase-γ and largely replace the agents most commonly implicated (stavudine, didanosine, and zidovudine); this seems to have reduced the incidence of syndromes related to mitochondrial toxicity.

Abacavir hypersensitivity is a protean syndrome that may include fever, chills, nausea, diarrhea, rash, myalgia, aseptic meningitis, hepatitis, cough, or influenza-like illness within a few weeks of starting treatment. Discontinuation of the drug leads to resolution of symptoms, but rechallenge can produce an anaphylactic reaction with cardiovascular collapse and high fever [54,55]. This syndrome should be virtually eliminated by the introduction of screening for the HLA-B*5701 allele and avoidance of abacavir in persons who carry it [56,57].

Severe rash, including Stevens–Johnson syndrome, is most notably associated with nevirapine, but can occur with other nonnucleoside reverse transcriptase inhibitors (NNRTIs) and rarely with protease inhibitors and NRTIs.

MANAGEMENT OF PROPHYLAXIS AND ANTIRETROVIRAL AGENTS

Even when critically ill, patients who received prophylaxis against opportunistic infections like PCP before the ICU admission should generally continue to receive it, and initiation of appropriate measures should be considered in those who have not. However, even a single dose of glucocorticoids can reduce the CD4+ lymphocyte count dramatically, so decisions should be based on recent values before receiving corticosteroids if they are available. In patients who stopped taking ART for more than a month, it is usually best to assume that the risk of a patient developing opportunistic infections corresponds to that before starting ART.

The use of ART in critically ill patients requires expertise in selection of drugs and consideration of their doses, toxicity, and interactions with other treatments. The critical care clinician is well-advised to manage these patients in close collaboration with an expert in antiretroviral treatment. Patients receiving ART should continue to receive these drugs whenever possible, as discontinuing therapy is associated with viral replication, emergence of resistance, and clinical progression of HIV infection. In patients coinfected with HBV, discontinuation of lamivudine (and presumably emtricitabine and tenofovir, the other antivirals active against HBV) may result in exacerbations of hepatitis B that may be fatal [58,59].

The feasibility of continuing antiretroviral therapy depends on that of enteral administration. When the gastrointestinal tract is significantly dysfunctional, all of the drugs in a patient's regimen will inevitably be stopped at the same time, and no harm is likely if they can be resumed in a few days. Still, the NNRTIs (efavirenz, nevirapine, and etravirine) are eliminated very slowly, and stopping all agents at the same time may lead to a prolonged period of inadvertent NNRTI monotherapy and the selection of drug-resistance mutations. When ART therapy must be interrupted for more than a few days, consultation with an expert is in order.

Continuing antiretroviral therapy entails potentially complex interactions with other drugs prescribed, including effects on absorption and metabolism that result in either suboptimal or toxic levels of both the antiretrovirals and other drugs. For example, administration of proton-pump inhibitors causes significant reductions in the protease inhibitor atazanavir; an H_2 blocker can be given safely 12 hours before or after atazanavir. Protease inhibitors significantly reduce the metabolism and increase the activity of midazolam. Lorazepam and temazepam may be safer alternatives for sedation, but dose titration with close monitoring of effect in the ICU setting may suffice to overcome the potential risks of midazolam administration. Given the frequency of cardiovascular disease as a cause of ICU admission among HIV-infected persons, HMG-CoA reductase inhibitors may be prescribed, but protease inhibitors have significant and varying interactions with most of these drugs; simvastatin and lovastatin are contraindicated with all of the protease inhibitors because of massive increases in their plasma levels.

The presence of acute kidney injury necessitates dose adjustments of all the nucleoside analogs except abacavir, and the components of fixed-dose combinations require individual adjustments. If renal function varies or is impaired for several days, the best way to assure consistently adequate and nontoxic levels of antiretrovirals is to change the regimen to drugs that do not require adjustment for renal insufficiency, when possible.

In considering whether to start antiretroviral therapy in a critically ill patient who did not receive it before, a few questions may guide the decision. First, is the enteral route expected to remain available to permit consistent and continuous drug administration? If not, antiretroviral therapy must wait. Second, does the patient have an infection for which there is no effective therapy other than the potential offered by improved immunologic status (e.g. cryptosporidiosis or progressive multifocal leukoencephalopathy)? In this situation, all other care is futile unless antiretroviral therapy is begun, and it should be. Third, did the patient not receive ART because the diagnosis of HIV infection was never established, by choosing not to take ART because of personal reasons, or because of repeatedly opting to stop ART? The latter two do not lend themselves to easy answers, and it may be well to wait at least until the patient is no longer critically ill and able to make an informed choice. Patients with advanced neurocognitive disease may have marked improvement on antiretroviral therapy and may regain functional independence; for them, treatment is as imperative as for those with otherwise untreatable infections. When therapy is started in patients who are deemed to be at high risk of abandoning it, the regimen should have minimal adverse consequences if discontinued abruptly (e.g., NNRTIs should be avoided).

The risk of IRIS has been a deterrent to starting antiretroviral therapy early in patients with opportunistic infection, but more recent studies have clarified this issue considerably. A randomized trial of early versus deferred ART in patients with acute opportunistic infections excluding tuberculosis found that fewer patients who received early therapy had progression of AIDS or death, with no difference in the rate of IRIS [60]. Other studies support a survival advantage for patients who started on ART in the ICU [61,62]. In patients with tuberculosis, IRIS occurred in 12.4% of patients randomized to early ART (started at a mean of 70 days after the initiation of antituberculous therapy) and only 3.8% of those whose ART was delayed until completion of treatment for tuberculosis (mean of 260 days), but mortality was significantly higher in the delayed-ART group (12.1% versus 5.4%), and no deaths were attributed to IRIS [63]. However, in patients with cryptococcal meningitis treated with a suboptimal fluconazole regimen that is the only one commonly available in Africa, early initiation of ART (within 72 hours of diagnosis) resulted in nearly threefold increased mortality compared to initiation after 10 weeks, with median survivals of 28 and 637 days, respectively [64]. Although firm conclusions are not yet available about the timing of ART in patients with serious opportunistic infections, it seems that the opportunistic infection should be under good control before initiating ART and that the clinician must anticipate the potential emergence of serious effects from IRIS [65].

PREDICTORS OF OUTCOME

Overall, it seems that critically ill patients with HIV infection have similar short-term outcomes as other patients with a comparable severity of illness, and survival rates seem to be improving [7,8,10,66,67]. Most studies in patients with HIV infection are limited by selection bias, as they are usually retrospective analyses where the admitting physician's knowledge of the patient's serostatus may have affected the decision to admit to ICU or vigor of care. In a study conducted in a South African surgical ICU, HIV testing was performed but results not divulged and there were no differences in ICU or hospital mortality or duration of stay when outcome was adjusted for age, despite a higher incidence of sepsis and organ failure in the HIV-infected patients [68]. Thus, evidence from a variety of settings supports the concept that HIV-infected and uninfected persons have similar outcomes of intensive care, and that decisions regarding the appropriateness of ICU interventions should not use HIV status alone as a criterion.

Studies examining the value of laboratory tests and scoring systems in predicting ICU outcomes for HIV-infected patients, including lactate dehydrogenase (LDH), serum albumin, CD4+ lymphocyte count, APACHE II score, and multisystem organ failure scores yield conflicting data on their reliability. It now seems clear that patients with HIV/AIDS have similar short-term outcomes to those of other patients with a similar severity of illness. Long-term survival is related to the severity of the HIV disease, other comorbid illness, and whether the patient has been treated with ART. In addition to the patient's illness, the experience of the hospital and healthcare providers in treating HIV infection and its complications also influences mortality. In one large study, adjusted mortality for patients with AIDS was 30% lower among hospitals with the most experience treating these patients [69].

Since the outcome of intensive care does not depend directly on the patient's HIV status, determination of whether or not a patient has HIV infection or determination of CD4+ lymphocyte counts should not be overriding considerations in deciding whether to offer or withhold intensive care. Rather, these decisions should be made using the same criteria as for all patients, namely, the likelihood of benefit and the patient's wishes.

RISK TO HEALTHCARE WORKERS AND POSTEXPOSURE PROPHYLAXIS

The risk of acquiring HIV-1 infection by mucous membrane exposure is approximately 0.09% (just under 1 in 10,000) and by percutaneous (e.g., needlestick) exposure, approximately 0.3%, or 1 in 300 instances [70,71]. Virtually all documented infections have involved accidents with hollow-bore needles. The risk is higher when inflicted by a device that came directly from the HIV-infected patient's artery or vein, had visible blood on it, produced deep injury, or came from a source patient with terminal illness (defined as death due to AIDS within 60 days of the healthcare worker's exposure). Each of these features increases the risk of infection independently. In a case-control study where healthcare workers infected by needlestick exposures were compared with healthcare workers who sustained exposures from HIV-infected patients but did not become infected, the only factor that was shown to reduce the risk of infection was postexposure use of zidovudine by the healthcare worker [72]. Zidovudine prophylaxis appeared to reduce the risk of infection by 81%. This study led to much stronger recommendations for antiretroviral therapy in healthcare workers with percutaneous or mucous membrane exposure to HIV-1.

Current recommendations reflect the failure rate of single-agent postexposure prophylaxis, the prevalence of zidovudine-resistant virus, the proven antiviral efficacy of three-drug regimens in infected individuals, and the importance of tolerability of the regimen to ensure completion of a full 4-week course [73]. Most percutaneous exposures from a known HIV-positive source warrant three or more drugs, with the exception of superficial injury from a solid needle used for a patient with asymptomatic HIV infection or known low viral load of less than 1,500 HIV RNA copies per mL, for which two-drug therapy is recommended. Three or more drugs are also recommended for large-volume splashes to mucous membranes or nonintact skin from patients with symptomatic HIV infection, AIDS, acute seroconversion, or known high viral load. Two-drug regimens are recommended for small-volume exposures to mucous membranes or nonintact skin. The National Institutes of Health AIDS Information Web site provides the most current drug recommendations [73]; expert consultation is advised, especially for cases involving drug-resistant virus and pregnant or breastfeeding personnel. Recommendations for postexposure prophylaxis emphasize initiating treatment within an hour or two of exposure, and data from infants of HIV-positive mothers not treated during pregnancy and delivery suggest little benefit to therapy delayed beyond 48 to 72 hours [74]. However, the time after which therapy will not be successful has not been defined.

The list of potential side effects of antiretroviral drugs is daunting, and most healthcare workers will experience some of them, along with justifiable anxiety. They should be reassured that most HIV-infected people tolerate these regimens with the help of adequate psychosocial support and proper medical follow-up.

TABLE 85.2

SUMMARY RECOMMENDATION FOR MANAGEMENT OF PULMONARY COMPLICATIONS OF HUMAN IMMUNODEFICIENCY VIRUS INFECTION

- Early adjunctive treatment with corticosteroids reduces the risks of respiratory failure and death in patients with acquired immunodeficiency syndrome (AIDS) and moderate-to-severe *Pneumocystis* pneumonia [18,25,26].
- Early versus deferred ART in patients with acute opportunistic infections excluding tuberculosis decreases progression to AIDS or death, with no difference in the rate of IRIS [60].
- Early versus deferred ART in patients with tuberculosis decreases mortality, but increases risk of IRIS [63].

ART, antiretroviral therapy; IRIS, immune reconstitution inflammatory syndrome.

SUMMARY

In summary, the evolution of the AIDS epidemic and the introduction of effective antiretroviral therapy have changed the spectrum of critical illnesses in patients with HIV infection. The use of ART led to reduced risk of AIDS-associated illness and improved survival, but raises new and complex questions about how best to use these treatments in patients with critical illness. Clearly, large-scale multidisciplinary studies of critical care of patients with HIV infection would yield valuable insights, but until the important clinical questions are answered, critical care clinicians must work closely not only with the ICU multidisciplinary team, but also with colleagues with backgrounds in infectious diseases, pharmacology, and palliative care. Advances in HIV infection, based on randomized controlled trials or meta-analyses of such trials, are summarized in [18] and Table 85.2.

References

1. Centers for Disease Control and Prevention. HIV/AIDS Surveillance Report, 2007. Vol. 19. Atlanta: U.S. Department of Health and Human Services, Centers for Disease Control and Prevention; 2009:1–63. Available at: http://www.cdc.gov/hiv/topics/surveillance/resources/reports/
2. UNAIDS. AIDS Epidemic Update: November 2009. Available at: http://data.unaids.org/pub/Report/2009/JC1700_Epi_Update_2009_en.pdf
3. Curtis JR, Bennett CL, Horner RE, et al: Variations in intensive care unit utilization for patients with human immunodeficiency virus-related Pneumocystis carinii pneumonia: importance of hospital characteristics and geographic location. *Crit Care Med* 26:668–675, 1998.
4. Rosen M, De Palo VD: Outcome of intensive care for patients with AIDS. *Crit Care Clin* 19:107–114, 1993.
5. Rosen M, Clayton K, Schneider R, et al: Intensive care of patients with HIV infection: utilization, critical illnesses and outcomes. *Am J Respir Crit Care Med* 155:67–71, 1997.
6. Afessa B, Green B: Clinical course, prognostic factors and outcome prediction for HIV patients in the ICU. *Chest* 118:138–145, 2000.
7. Narasimhan M, Posner A, DePalo V, et al: Intensive care in patients with HIV infection in the era of highly active antiretroviral therapy. *Chest* 125:1800–1804, 2004.
8. Powell K, Davis L, Morris AM, et al: Survival for patients with HIV admitted to the ICU continues to improve in the current era of combination antiretroviral therapy. *Chest* 135:11–17, 2009.
9. Rosenberg A, Seneff M, Atiyeh L, et al: The importance of bacterial sepsis in intensive care unit patients with acquired immunodeficiency syndrome: implications for future care in the age of increasing antiretroviral resistance. *Crit Care Med* 29:548–556, 2001.
10. Huang L, Quartin A, Jones D, et al: Intensive care of patients with HIV infection. *N Engl J Med* 355:173–181, 2006.
11. Valdez H, Chowdhry T, Asaad R, et al: Changing spectrum of mortality due to human immunodeficiency virus: analysis of 260 deaths during 1995–1999. *Clin Infect Dis* 32:1487–1503, 2001.
12. Stringer J, Beard C, Miller R, et al: A new name (*Pneumocystis jiroveci*) for Pneumocystis from humans. *Emerg Infect Dis* 8:891–896, 2002.
13. Kaplan J, Hanson D, Dworkin M, et al: Epidemiology of human immunodeficiency virus-associated opportunistic infections in the United States in the era of highly active antiretroviral therapy. *Clin Infect Dis* 30:S5–S14, 2000.
14. Saah A, Hoover D, Peng Y, et al: Predictors of failure of Pneumocystis carinii pneumonia prophylaxis. Multicenter AIDS Cohort Study. *JAMA* 273:1197–1202, 1995.
15. Thomas CF Jr, Limper AH: Pneumocystis pneumonia. *N Engl J Med* 350: 2487–2498, 2004.
16. Tu J, Biem H, Detsky A: Bronchoscopy versus empirical therapy in HIV-infected patients with presumptive Pneumocystis carinii pneumonia. *Am Rev Respir Dis* 148:370–377, 1993.
17. Parada JP, Deloria-Knoll M, Chmiel JS, et al: Relationship between health insurance and medical care for patients hospitalized with human immunodeficiency virus-related Pneumocystis carinii pneumonia, 1995–1997: Medicaid, bronchoscopy, and survival. *Clin Infect Dis* 37:1549–1555, 2003.
18. Centers for Disease Control and Prevention: Guidelines for prevention and treatment of opportunistic infections among HIV-infected adults and adolescents. Recommendations from CDC, the National Institutes of Health, and the HIV Medicine Association/Infectious Diseases Society of America. *MMWR* 58(RR-04):1–198, 2009. Available at: http://www.cdc.gov/hiv/resources/guidelines/.
19. Maxfield RA, Sorkin B, Fazzini EP, et al: Respiratory failure in patients with acquired immunodeficiency syndrome and Pneumocystis carinii pneumonia. *Crit Care Med* 14:443–449, 1986.
20. Afessa B: Pleural effusion and pneumothorax in hospitalized patients with HIV infection. *Chest* 117:1031–1037, 2000.
21. Wachter R, Luce J, Safrin S, et al: Cost and outcome of intensive care for patients with AIDS, Pneumocystis carinii pneumonia and severe respiratory failure. *JAMA* 273:230–235, 1995.
22. Davis JL, Morris A, Kallet RH, et al: Low tidal volume ventilation is associated with reduced mortality in HIV-infected patients with acute lung injury. *Thorax* 63:988–993, 2008.
23. Beck J, Rosen M, Peavy H: Pulmonary complications of HIV infection. Report of the Fourth NHLBI Workshop. *Am J Respir Crit Care Med* 164:2120–2126, 2001.
24. Montaner J, Russell J, Lawson L, et al: Acute respiratory failure secondary to Pneumocystis carinii pneumonia in the acquired immunodeficiency syndrome: a potential role for systemic corticosteroids. *Chest* 95:881–884, 1989.
25. Bozzette SA, Sattler FR, Chiu J, et al: A controlled trial of early adjunctive treatment with corticosteroids for Pneumocystis carinii pneumonia in the

acquired immunodeficiency syndrome. California Collaborative Treatment Group. *N Engl J Med* 323:1451–1457, 1990.
26. Gagnon S, Boota AM, Fischl MA, et al: Corticosteroids as adjunctive therapy for severe Pneumocystis carinii pneumonia in the acquired immunodeficiency syndrome. A double-blind, placebo-controlled trial. *N Engl J Med* 323:1444–1450, 1990.
27. Barbier F, Coquet I, Legriel S, et al: Etiologies and outcome of acute respiratory failure in HIV-infected patients. *Intensive Care Med* 35:1678–1686, 2009.
28. Masur H: Management of patients with HIV in the intensive care unit. *Proc Am Thorac Soc* 3:96–102, 2006.
29. Bica I, McGovern B, Dhar R, et al: Increasing mortality due to end-stage liver disease in patients with human immunodeficiency virus infection. *Clin Infect Dis* 32:492–497, 2001.
30. Monga H, Rodriguez-Barrada M, Breaux K, et al: Hepatitis-C infection-related morbidity and mortality among patients with human immunodeficiency virus infection. *Clin Infect Dis* 33:240–247, 2001.
31. Sulkowski M, Thomas D: Hepatitis C in HIV-infected persons. *Ann Intern Med* 138:197–207, 2003.
32. Sherman K, Rouster S, Chung R, et al: Hepatitis C virus prevalence among patients coinfected with human immunodeficiency virus: a cross-sectional analysis of the U.S. Adult AIDS Clinical Trials Group. *Clin Infect Dis* 34:831–837, 2002.
33. Shelburne SA, Hamill RJ, Rodriguez-Barradas, et al: Immune reconstitution inflammatory syndrome: Emergence of a unique syndrome during highly active antiretroviral therapy. *Medicine* 81:213–227, 2002.
34. Shelburne SA, Visnegarwala F, Darcourt J, et al: Incidence and risk factors for immune reconstitution inflammatory syndrome during highly active antiretroviral therapy. *AIDS* 19:399–406, 2005.
35. Muller M, Wandel S, Colebunders R, et al: Immune reconstitution inflammatory syndrome in patients starting antiretroviral therapy for HIV infection: a systematic review and meta-analysis. *Lancet Infect Dis* 10:251–261, 2010.
36. Manabe YC, Campbell JD, Sydnor E, et al: Immune reconstitution inflammatory syndrome: risk factors and treatment implications. *J Acquir Immune Defic Syndr* 46:456–462, 2007.
37. Murdoch DM, Venter WDF, Feldman C, et al: Incidence and risk factors for the immune reconstitution inflammatory syndrome in HIV patients in South Africa: a prospective study. *AIDS* 22:601–610, 2008.
38. Narita M, Ashkin D, Hollender E, et al: Paradoxical worsening of tuberculosis following antiretroviral therapy in patients with AIDS. *Am J Respir Crit Care Med* 158:157–161, 1998.
39. Wislez M, Bergot E, Antoine M, et al: Acute respiratory failure following HAART introduction in patients treated for Pneumocystis carinii pneumonia. *Am J Respir Crit Care Med* 164:847–851, 2001.
40. Friis-Moller N, Sabvin CA, Weber R, et al: Combination antiretroviral therapy and the risk of myocardial infarction. *N Engl J Med* 349:1993–2003, 2003.
41. Barbaro G, DiLorenzo G, Cirelli A, et al: An open-label, prospective, observational study of the incidence of coronary artery disease in patients with HIV infection receiving highly active antiretroviral therapy. *Clin Ther* 25:2405–2418, 2003.
42. The Strategies for Management of Antiretroviral Therapy (SMART) Study Group: CD4+ count-guided interruption of antiretroviral treatment. *N Engl J Med* 355:2283–2296, 2005.
43. Marin B, Thiébaut R, Bucher HC, et al: Non-AIDS-defining deaths and immunodeficiency in the era of combination antiretroviral therapy. *AIDS* 23:1743–1753, 2009.
44. Torriani FJ, Komarow L, Parker RA, et al: Endothelial function in human immunodeficiency virus-infected antiretroviral-naïve subjects before and after starting potent antiretroviral therapy: the ACTG (AIDS Clinical Trials Group) Study 5152s. *J Am Coll Cardiol* 52:569–576, 2008.
45. Gan I, May G, Raboud J, et al: Pancreatitis in HIV infection: predictors of severity. *Am J Gastroenterol* 98:1278–1283, 2003.
46. Kovari H, Ledergerber B, Peter U, et al: Association of non-cirrhotic portal hypertension in HIV-infected persons and antiretroviral therapy with didanosine: a nested case-control study. *Clin Infect Dis* 49: 626–635, 2009.
47. Miller K, Cameron M, Wood L, et al: Lactic acidosis and hepatic steatosis associated with use of stavudine: report of four cases. *Ann Intern Med* 133:192–196, 2000.
48. Sundar K, Suarez M, Banogon P, et al: Zidovudine-induced fatal lactic acidosis and hepatic failure in patients with acquired immunodeficiency syndrome: report of two patients and review of the literature. *Crit Care Med* 25:1425–1430, 1997.
49. Moyle GJ, Datta D, Mandalia S, et al: Hyperlactataemia and lactic acidosis during antiretroviral therapy: relevance, reproducibility and possible risk factors. *AIDS* 16:1341–1349, 2002.
50. Brinkman K, ter Hofstede H, Burgur D, et al: Adverse effects of reverse transcriptase inhibitors: mitochondrial toxicity as a common pathway. *AIDS* 12:1735–1744, 1998.
51. Fouty B, Frerman F, Reves R: Riboflavin to treat nucleoside analogue-induced lactic acidosis. *Lancet* 352:291–292, 1998.
52. Schramm C, Wanitschke R, Galle P: Thiamine for the treatment of nucleoside analogue-induced severe lactic acidosis. *Eur J Anaesthesiol* 16:733–735, 1999.
53. Simpson D, Estanislao L, Evans S, et al: HIV-associated neuromuscular weakness syndrome. *AIDS* 18:1403–1412, 2004.
54. Walensky R, Goldberg J, Daily J: Anaphylaxis after rechallenge with abacavir. *AIDS* 13:999–1000, 1999.
55. Escaut L, Liotier J, Albengres E, et al: Abacavir rechallenge has to be avoided in cases of hypersensitivity reaction. *AIDS* 13:1419–1420, 1999.
56. Mallal S, Phillips E, Carosi G, et al: HLA-B*5701 screening for hypersensitivity to abacavir. *N Engl J Med* 358:568–579, 2008.
57. Saag M, Balu R, Phillips E, et al: High sensitivity of human leukocyte antigen-b*5701 as a marker for immunologically confirmed abacavir hypersensitivity in white and black patients. *Clin Infect Dis* 46:1111–1118, 2008.
58. Bessesen M, Ives D, Condreay L, et al: Chronic active hepatitis B exacerbations in human immunodeficiency virus-infected patients following development of resistance to or withdrawal of lamivudine. *Clin Infect Dis* 28:1032–1035, 1999.
59. Sellier P, Clevenbergh P, Mazeron M-C, et al: Fatal interruption of a 3TC-containing regimen in a HIV-infected patient due to re-activation of chronic hepatitis B virus infection. *Scand J Infect Dis* 36:533–535, 2004.
60. Zolopa AR, Andersen J, Komarow L, et al: Early antiretroviral therapy reduces AIDS progression/death in individuals with acute opportunistic infections: a multicenter randomized strategy trial. *PLoS One* 4:1–10, 2009.
61. Morris A, Wachter RM, Luce J, et al: Improved survival with highly active antiretroviral therapy in HIV-infected patients with severe Pneumocystis carinii pneumonia. *AIDS* 17:73–80, 2003.
62. Croda J, Croda MG, Neves A, et al: Benefit of antiretroviral therapy on survival of human immunodeficiency virus-infected patients admitted to an intensive care unit. *Crit Care Med* 37:1605–1611, 2009.
63. Abdool Karim SS, Naidoo K, Grobler A, et al: Timing of initiation of antiretroviral drugs during tuberculosis therapy. *N Engl J Med* 362:697–706, 2010.
64. Makadzange AT, Ndhlovu CE, Takarinda K, et al: Early versus delayed initiation of antiretroviral therapy for concurrent HIV infection and cryptococcal meningitis in sub-Saharan Africa. *Clin Infect Dis* 50:1532–1538, 2010.
65. Bicanic T, Meintjes G, Rebe K, et al: Immune reconstitution inflammatory syndrome in HIV-associated cryptococcal meningitis: a prospective study. *J Acquir Immune Defic Syndr* 51:130–134, 2009.
66. Casalino E, Mendoza-Sassi G, Wolff M, et al: Predictors of short- and long-term survival in HIV-infected patients admitted to the ICU. *Chest* 13:421–429, 1998.
67. Dickson SJ, Batson S, Copas AJ, et al: Survival of HIV-infected patients in the intensive care unit in the era of highly active antiretroviral therapy. *Thorax* 62:964–968, 2007.
68. Bhagwanjee S, Muckart D, Jeena P, et al: Does HIV status influence the outcome of patients admitted to a surgical intensive care unit? A prospective double-blind study. *BMJ* 314:1077–1084, 1997.
69. Cunningham W, Tisnado D, Lui H, et al: The effect of hospital experience on mortality among patients hospitalized with acquired immune deficiency syndrome in California. *Am J Med* 107:137–143, 1999.
70. Bell D: Occupational risk of human immunodeficiency virus infection in healthcare workers: an overview. *Am J Med* 102[Suppl 5B]:9–15, 1997.
71. Ippolito G, Puro V, DeCarli G, et al: The risk of occupational human immunodeficiency virus in health care workers. *Arch Intern Med* 153:1451–1458, 1993.
72. Cardo D, Culver D, Ciesielski C, et al: A case-control study of HIV seroconversion in health care workers after percutaneous exposure. *N Engl J Med* 337:1485–1490, 1997.
73. Centers for Disease Control and Prevention: Updated U.S. Public Health Service guidelines for the management of occupational exposures to HIV and recommendations for postexposure prophylaxis. *MMWR* 2005;54(No. RR-9):1–17. (Access most recent version at http://www.aidsinfo.nih.gov/)
74. Wade N, Birkhead G, Warren B, et al: Abbreviated regimens of zidovudine prophylaxis and perinatal transmission of the human immunodeficiency virus. *N Engl J Med* 339:1409–1414, 1998.

CHAPTER 86 ■ INFECTIOUS COMPLICATIONS OF DRUG ABUSE

AFROZA LITON AND WILLIAM L. MARSHALL

Drug abuse, the deliberate taking of an unprescribed drug dose or illicit substance, is a pervasive problem in our society [1]. A variety of drugs are abused, including opiates, depressants, stimulants, and hallucinogens. This chapter will focus on infections that occur as a consequence of drugs that are either explicitly illegal or those which are legal but are used by the patient for purposes other than for which they were prescribed. Abused drugs can be administered by a variety of means, including "snorting" through the nasal mucosa, via inhalation through smoking, and orally by parenteral routes, including injection into the soft tissues, called "skin popping," or directly into the vascular system.

Drug abuse is attended by an increased risk in a number of infections, some of which may lead patients to be admitted to the intensive care unit (ICU) [2]. Infections associated with parenteral drug abuse include skin and soft tissue infection, endocarditis, bone and joint infections, pneumonia, ophthalmologic infections, and hepatitis [2–4]. Illicit drugs are often "cut" or mixed with adulterants, which may be contaminated with bacteria or may suppress the immune response—as is the case with agranulocytosis caused by levamisole-containing cocaine leading to bacterial or fungal infection [5]. Illicit drug injection occurs under unsanitary conditions, using drugs that are not sterile and injection equipment that has often been used more than once. Such practices provide a mechanism for passage of a variety of infectious agents. Although in some instances, particularly for the hepatitis viruses and human immunodeficiency virus (HIV), the infectious agent is passed directly from blood-contaminated drug paraphernalia to the patient, the mode of spread is less clear for other agents. Prevention of infectious complications of drug use is directed at treating addiction, or failing that, mitigating infectious complications via needle exchange programs [6]. Finally, many patients with substance abuse problems are homeless, have poor nutrition, and live under crowded conditions, placing them at increased risk for tuberculosis.

FEVER

Fever is one of the most common complaints of parenteral drug users presenting to the hospital. Self-limited illnesses are the most common causes of fever in this population. More significant etiologies include pneumonia, cellulitis, and soft tissue abscesses. Endocarditis accounts for fewer than 15% of all cases of fever [7].

All febrile parenteral drug users should undergo a thorough history, physical examination, and have routine blood laboratories and chest radiographs taken. Particular attention should be paid to abnormalities of the skin and soft tissues, cardiac valvular abnormalities, bony tenderness, and pulmonary abnormalities. However, clinical evaluation alone often does not differentiate major disease from trivial illness in these patients. Parenteral drug users who are febrile should be admitted to the hospital for further observation.

Weisse et al. have developed an algorithm for febrile parenteral drug abusers with no apparent source of infection [7]. In this approach, blood cultures are obtained on all patients and empiric antibiotic therapy is started. If blood cultures are positive or if the patient has clinical stigmata indicative of endocarditis, an echocardiogram is performed. If valvular vegetations are seen, the diagnosis of endocarditis is considered established. On the other hand, if blood cultures are negative and the patient is clinically well, antibiotic therapy may be stopped. However, parenteral drug users commonly self-administer antibiotics and this practice may substantially reduce the likelihood of positive blood cultures, as can prophylactic antibiotics in HIV+ patients [8,9]. Hence, careful clinical evaluation is advised when making antibiotic decisions in these patients.

BACTEREMIA

Bacteremia is a frequent occurrence in the febrile parenteral drug user [10,11]. Approximately 60% of bacteremias in parenteral drug abusers are due to causes other than endocarditis [12]. Of these, the majority are due to either skin or soft tissue infections or to mycotic aneurysms of peripheral arteries. A smaller number of bacteremias are due to miscellaneous causes, such as septic arthritis, septic thrombophlebitis, or pneumonia. In about 3% of cases, the source of the bacteremia is undiscovered.

Although the organisms associated with bacteremias in the parenteral drug user may vary based on geographic location and the type of drug abused, some generalizations can be made [12,13]. Drug users have an increased incidence of staphylococcal carriage of the skin, nose, and throat [14]. Bacterial infection derives principally from the user's own flora, so that *Staphylococcus aureus* constitutes the majority of bacteremias in these patients. In this regard, methicillin-resistant *S. aureus* (MRSA) infections are now being encountered with increasing frequency in parenteral drug users and in the community [14,15].

Streptococci and Gram-negative aerobic bacilli are the next most frequently isolated organisms. Polymicrobial bacteremias occur in about 10% of cases, and in about two-thirds of these cases at least one of the organisms isolated is a *Staphylococcus* spp [12]. Bacteremia and other infections due to the facultative anaerobe *Eikenella corrodens* are particularly associated with injecting drug users who contaminate the injection needle or the injection site with saliva [16].

The approach toward the bacteremic parenteral drug user should be to search for an underlying etiology and to begin empiric antibiotic treatment. The isolation of a group A β-hemolytic streptococci from the blood should prompt a search for a cutaneous or soft tissue focus of infection [17]. Empiric antibiotic therapy may be based on local experience but should generally include agents directed against staphylococci and streptococci as well as aerobic Gram-negative bacilli. If

MRSA infections have previously occurred in parenteral drug users in the community, vancomycin should be considered.

SOFT TISSUE INFECTIONS

Skin and soft tissue infections occur commonly in the parenteral drug user and are increasing in frequency [18,19]. Such infections are often polymicrobial and appear to derive from either the skin or oral cavity [18,20,21]. The most common pathogens are *S. aureus,* streptococci, oral anaerobes, and aerobic Gram-negative bacilli [16–21]. Cutaneous infection in the intravenous drug user generally occurs in the antecubital fossa, forearm, and hand since these are the sites of the most accessible veins. However, intravenous drug users may also avail themselves of other, less available sites with infection occurring in the feet, legs, anterior neck, groin, and axilla [22,23].

The most common skin infections in the injecting drug user (IDU) are simple cellulitis and localized skin abscess. These occur more frequently among those who "skin pop" compared to those who inject intravenously [24]. Simple cellulitis usually requires only antibiotic therapy directed against staphylococci and streptococci. Since the incidence of MRSA infections is rising, and the IDU is particularly at risk for MRSA infections of the skin and soft tissues [14], patients requiring intravenous therapy should receive vancomycin. Localized soft tissue abscesses that do not penetrate into the deep subcutaneous tissue should be drained. Given the risk of occult bacteremia in this population, antibiotic therapy should be given as directed by Gram stain of the drained material. In all patients with a history of injection drug use, blood cultures should be obtained in the workup of skin and soft tissue infections.

The presence of vesicles or bullae, an area of central necrosis within a larger area of erythema, and the presence of subcutaneous crepitation in a patient with systemic toxicity is suggestive of necrotizing fasciitis [25]. Gas seen in the soft tissues on radiographs is also indicative of deep infection [26]. However, extensive necrosis may be present even in the absence of these signs, and surgical exploration should be considered in any case that manifests local erythema, fluctuance, and induration [27]. Suspicion for needles or other foreign bodies should similarly prompt surgical exploration. Any abnormal material from this exploration should be immediately examined using Gram stain to provide the basis for empiric antimicrobial therapy. Examination of a sample of tissue using frozen-section biopsy may also be useful [28]. Magnetic resonance imaging (MRI) typically reveals increased T2 signal along fascial planes and gadolinium enhancement, whereas contrast-enhanced computed tomography (CT) scanning is a less sensitive diagnostic tool for necrotizing fasciitis [26].

Necrotizing fasciitis, pyomyositis, or gangrene requires immediate, aggressive debridement in the operating room in association with parenteral antibiotics [27]. Gram stain and culture are imperative to guide antimicrobial therapy. Empiric therapy should be directed against staphylococci, streptococci, anaerobes, and aerobic Gram-negative bacilli. Surgical debridement may be required on multiple occasions before infection is controlled [29]. There have been multiple outbreaks of soft tissue infection with or without systemic symptoms associated with *Clostridium* spp discussed later in this chapter.

PERIPHERAL VASCULAR INFECTIONS

Because parenteral drug use often involves vascular injection of material under non-sterile conditions, it is not surprising that a wide range of vascular complications may result from these practices [30]. The most frequent manifestations of such infections are fever associated with pain, redness, and swelling over the involved area. When the injecting site is into the deep tissues of the groin or neck, it may be difficult to distinguish involvement of vascular structures from simple cellulitis, soft tissue abscess, or fasciitis. If there is any question, angiography should be performed to determine if vascular tissue is involved. Septic thrombophlebitis usually presents as fever, bacteremia, and swelling over the involved vein. This can often be treated with antibiotics alone, although incision, drainage, and removal of the vein are sometimes necessary. Anticoagulation is generally not required [12].

Mycotic aneurysms result when the user injects directly into the artery [12,30]. Aneurysms most frequently occur in the femoral arteries. Carotid aneurysms and brachial artery aneurysms occasionally occur [30]. The classic presentation of this syndrome is a febrile patient with a tender, pulsatile mass, usually in the groin or the neck. Sometimes, there is a small amount of bleeding at the site. If there is any question of an aneurysm, a vascular surgical consultation should be obtained prior to any exploration of the lesion. Angiography will confirm the site and extent of the aneurysm. The most frequent microbiological agents isolated are *S. aureus* and streptococci, with aerobic Gram-negative bacilli occasionally being identified [12]. Empiric antibiotic therapy should be directed against these organisms. Ligation and excision of the involved arterial segment is usually successful [31].

ENDOCARDITIS

Endocarditis in the parenteral drug abuser differs in several respects from endocarditis in the nonaddict. It is more likely to occur in persons without underlying valvular heart disease, to involve the tricuspid valve, to be due to *S. aureus*, and to have a more benign outcome [3,32]. Certain types of intravenous drug abuse may predispose to the development of endocarditis. Heroin use has long been associated with this complication [33].

Tricuspid-valve endocarditis is the prototypical presentation of endocarditis in the parenteral drug user [33]. The patient complains of fever, usually for less than 1 week. There may be a history of chills and pleuritic chest pain and occasionally hemoptysis. On physical examination, fever is a nearly universal finding. A systolic murmur may or may not be present on admission, but often develops during the course of therapy. Signs of peripheral embolization, such as petechiae, splinter hemorrhages, Janeway lesions, or Roth spots, are uncommon. Osler's nodes are frequently absent. On chest radiograph, multiple patchy infiltrates indicative of pulmonary emboli are strongly suggestive of the diagnosis of tricuspid endocarditis. Blood cultures are usually positive and in the majority of instances, *S. aureus* is isolated. When blood cultures are negative in the face of the appropriate clinical syndrome, one should suspect that the patient has recently taken antibiotics.

Endocarditis involving the valves of the left side of the heart may also occur in the parenteral drug user. Compared to patients with tricuspid-valve endocarditis alone, there is more likely to be a history of underlying heart disease [12]. On examination, a heart murmur is usually evident on presentation, and peripheral emboli are frequent. Streptococci are more likely to be isolated from the blood, but *S. aureus* is still frequently isolated [3,12,33].

In addition to staphylococci and streptococci, a variety of other organisms have been associated with endocarditis in the parenteral drug user, including aerobic Gram-negative bacilli, particularly *P. aeruginosa*, and fungi, notably *Candida* spp [3]. Moreover, polymicrobial bacteremia is a well-recognized complication of endocarditis in this population and is usually indistinguishable on clinical grounds from that due to a single organism [34].

Bacteremia and pulmonary emboli on chest radiograph are highly predictive of tricuspid-valve endocarditis in the parenteral drug user [3,12]. However, all individuals with clinically suspected endocarditis should have echocardiography performed. Transesophageal echocardiography is more sensitive than transthoracic echocardiography in identifying valvular vegetations [35]. When echocardiographic findings are combined with clinical manifestations, the diagnosis of endocarditis can usually be established with high sensitivity and specificity using the Duke criteria or modifications of the Duke criteria [36], even in IDUs with HIV infection [37].

Empiric therapy for endocarditis in the parenteral drug user should be directed against staphylococci, streptococci, and aerobic Gram-negative bacilli. Nafcillin, oxacillin, and cefazolin are reasonable choices only if methicillin resistance among staphylococci has not been encountered. Vancomycin is the current alternative for the treatment of MRSA infections and for the β-lactam-allergic patient. Until cultures return, a broad-spectrum antibiotic, such as ceftazidime, should also be added for initial empiric therapy of aerobic Gram-negative bacilli because of the frequency of this type of endocarditis in addicts [38].

The prognosis for tricuspid-valve staphylococcal endocarditis in the parenteral drug user is good, with a mortality of less than 10% employing a choice of several therapies [3,12,37]. There was no difference in outcome between treatments with a β-lactam antibiotic alone and in combination with an aminoglycoside for 4 weeks [39]. Although a combination of a penicillinase-resistant penicillin with an aminoglycoside has been advocated for 2-week therapy for right-sided endocarditis [40], one study found that results for combination therapy were no different from those when a penicillinase-resistant penicillin was used alone [41].

Nonstaphylococcal endocarditis, particularly that involving the aortic and mitral valves, has a significantly worse prognosis. Left-sided endocarditis secondary to *P. aeruginosa* has a particularly poor outcome, with a mortality rate of nearly 70% [12]. To achieve cure, a 6-week course of intravenous therapy with an antipseudomonal β-lactam antibiotic plus an aminoglycoside, both at high doses, combined with early surgical removal of the involved valve is usually required [38]. *Candida* endocarditis also has an extremely high mortality rate even with prompt valve replacement and systemic antifungal therapy [42].

The role of surgery in endocarditis in the parenteral drug user is no different from endocarditis in the general population. Hemodynamic decompensation, persistently positive blood cultures in the face of appropriate antimicrobial therapy, multiple embolic episodes after therapy is initiated, fungal endocarditis, and evidence of extravalvular extension of infection constitute major criteria for valve replacement [43]. Tricuspid valvulotomy is successful in the majority of patients with isolated tricuspid-valve involvement and intractable infection. Only about 10% of patients require a subsequent prosthetic valve to control congestive right-heart failure [44].

SKELETAL INFECTIONS

Infections of the bones and joints represent a distinct clinical syndrome in the drug abuser. Most cases have been reported among intravenous heroin users, and many cases occur in association with endocarditis [45]. Bacterial osteomyelitis of the vertebral column is the most frequent skeletal infection reported. The lumbar, cervical, and thoracic spine are involved, in that order. Patients generally present with weeks to months of pain in the involved area. High fevers are unusual, and many patients are afebrile. There is usually tenderness over the involved vertebral bodies and radiographic evidence of osteomyelitis. Laboratory values are generally normal, although the peripheral white blood cell count may be modestly elevated. The erythrocyte sedimentation rate and/or C-reactive protein are almost always elevated and may serve as useful markers of a response to therapy [46]. Because of the chronicity of symptoms and the general lack of toxicity of these patients, it is not unusual for the diagnosis to be missed for weeks or even months. The complaint of low back or neck pain in an intravenous drug user should always suggest the diagnosis of vertebral osteomyelitis. Septic arthritis often involves the sacroiliac and sternoarticular joints and the symphysis pubis. There is usually weeks to months of pain at the site and tenderness to palpation at the site of involvement. Radiographs are usually normal at presentation. MRI is preferable to contrast-enhanced CT of the spine to make the diagnosis of vertebral osteomyelitis [47].

The bacteriology of skeletal infections among drug users is quite different from that seen in other patients. Gram-positive cocci, such as staphylococci and streptococci, as well as aerobic Gram-negative bacilli, particularly *P. aeruginosa*, are frequently isolated [45]. Skeletal infections due to *Candida* spp may also occur, either alone or as part of a dissemination syndrome [48]. Because of this, it is imperative that a bacteriologic diagnosis be established in such patients. In most cases, this can be achieved by needle aspirate of the involved bone or joint. For sternoarticular infections, open surgical exploration is often required. Therapy involves long-term antibiotic therapy and in some cases surgical debridement [49].

SYSTEMIC SYNDROMES WITH SPORE-FORMING BACTERIA

Anaerobic spore-forming bacilli of the genus *Clostridium* are ubiquitous in the environment; exospores can remain viable indefinitely. If illicit substances become contaminated with these spores, subsequent injection of the substances may result in severe illness or death. The first reports of infections in people addicted to morphine injection were of tetanus in 1876. By the 1950s in New York, drug addiction accounted for the majority of cases of tetanus. Wound botulism caused by *Clostridium botulinum* was first observed in IDUs in the United States in 1982. Cases increased during the 1990s with the use of black-tar heroin, and a similar outbreak was seen in Germany in 2005. These patients presented with abscesses associated with symmetrical descending paralysis, some requiring mechanical ventilation. Treatment included antitoxin, antimicrobials, and surgical drainage of abscesses [50]. In the last decade, there have been outbreaks of serious illness and death among IDUs in the United Kingdom due to *Clostridium novyi* and *Clostridium histolyticum* [51]. Skin poppers using subcutaneous and intramuscular injection appear to be particularly at risk [52].

Similar to infections with *Clostridium* spp, since 2009 there have been cases of anthrax confirmed in heroin users in Scotland [53]. All injection routes have been implicated, but smoking or snorting may also pose a significant risk. Most had severe soft tissue infections with significant soft-tissue edema but differed from classic necrotizing fasciitis or classic cutaneous anthrax. Patients had vague prodromal symptoms, appeared very ill, but their symptoms had nonspecific systemic features. Some developed septic shock leading to multiorgan failure.

HUMAN IMMUNODEFICIENCY VIRUS INFECTION

Injecting drug use represents the third most common risk behavior for infection with HIV in the United States and is associated with 75% of HIV cases among heterosexual men. Black and Hispanic ethnic groups are disproportionately represented among IDUs with HIV infection [54]. In some metropolitan regions, notably Atlanta, Detroit, and San Francisco, the rate of HIV infection among IDUs is approximately 10%. There is great geographic variability in the prevalence of HIV infection among IDUs. The highest rates are in the northeastern United States and Puerto Rico.

Certain practices increase the risk for a drug user to acquire HIV infection. These include frequent intravenous drug injections, injection in "shooting galleries," places where users rent the injecting paraphernalia and return it after use, injection with used needles, or sharing needles. Additional factors associated with an increased risk include use of cocaine or other drugs that prompts HIV risk behaviors and having sex partners who use intravenous drugs. The latter is significantly associated with HIV infection in women [55]. Finally, the use of methamphetamine, "crystal meth," has been linked to an increase in the sexual transmission of HIV, including highly antiretroviral-resistant strains [56]. In vitro studies show that opiates, methamphetamine, and cocaine can potentiate HIV replication and can enhance neurotoxicity [57].

HIV-positive IDUs are more likely to develop infections that are not AIDS-defining illnesses. Disease patterns in this group may differ from the other HIV-infected groups [58]. In particular, they have a high risk of developing bacterial pneumonia and bacterial sepsis, especially due to encapsulated organisms such as *Streptococcus pneumoniae* or *Haemophilus influenzae*. This observation highlights the importance of pneumococcal and *H. influenzae* type B vaccines in this group [58]. Progressive decline of CD4 lymphocyte counts to less than 200 per μL, and smoking illicit drugs significantly increase the risk of bacterial pneumonia [59]. In one study, *Pneumocystis* pneumonia, community-acquired bacterial pneumonia, and tuberculosis were the three most frequent pulmonary diseases seen among a group of illicit drug users in Washington, DC [60].

Any intravenous drug user should be considered at risk for HIV infection, and such patients should be offered testing for infection [54]. In areas of high prevalence, the clinician should be aware that HIV-related immunodeficiency might be complicating the clinical course in an IDU. In the United States, IDUs are also the highest risk group for human T-cell lymphotropic virus type I or II (HTLV-I or HTLV-II) infection [4]. The impact of this on HIV-related mortality is unclear, but coinfection with HIV and HTLV-I has been associated with myelopathy [61].

VIRAL HEPATITIS

Acute and chronic hepatitis have long been recognized as common reasons for hospital admission among drug users [4]. Of the infectious causes, hepatitis B virus (HBV) remains a principal pathogen. It is estimated that from 60% to 80% of parenteral drug users in the United States are infected with hepatitis B, and that nearly 10% are chronic carriers [62]. Moreover, coinfection with the hepatitis delta virus, a hepatotropic agent that requires hepatitis B for replication, has been reported in 8% to 40% of IDUs infected with hepatitis B and is associated with a more fulminant course [63]. Hepatitis A has also been documented as a cause of acute hepatitis among intravenous drug users [64].

After HIV infection, infection with hepatitis C virus (HCV) is the next emerging infectious disease epidemic in the United States. The vast majority of cases of HCV infection are associated with injecting drug use. Acute infection, which occurs relatively soon after injection drug practices begin, is rarely symptomatic, but chronic infection occurs in 85% of all cases. Patients may develop chronic liver disease and cirrhosis. In one survey, HCV infection was identified in 80% of intravenous drug users [65], but more recent studies report a decrease in HCV seroprevalence among IDUs from 65% to 35% [66]. Psychiatric comorbidities in drug users complicate the treatment of HCV with interferon.

Parenteral drug abusers may suffer multiple attacks of acute hepatitis and are also likely to have significant structural and functional abnormalities of their liver, even if they are asymptomatic. Noninfectious factors, particularly the use of alcohol and other drugs, may act synergistically with the hepatitis viruses to lead to a poorer outcome [62].

In addition, coinfection with HIV, although decreasing [6] may also cause increased activity of these viruses, particularly HCV, promotes liver damage and lower response to the treatment [67]. Finally, concomitant HCV and either HBV or hepatitis A virus (HAV) can lead to severe hepatitis or death, underlining the importance of vaccinating eligible parenteral drug users for HAV and HBV [68]. Special attention is required to choose therapies in patients with HIV and HBV coinfection. Antiretroviral medications like lamivudine or tenofovir are only partially active as monotherapy against both viruses, requiring thoughtful combination therapy to be effective against both viruses. There is an increase in the incidence of hepatocellular carcinoma and hepatotoxic effects associated with antiretroviral drugs in patients with HIV and HCV/HBV coinfection [69].

Sexually Transmitted Diseases

Sexually transmitted infections such as Chlamydia and gonorrhea are closely associated with substance abuse, both due to frequent exchange of sex for money or drugs and because of the sexual disinhibition that result from the use of psychoactive substances, especially alcohol and cocaine. Crack use has also been linked to an increased risk of syphilis and other ulcerative genital infections [70]. The high false-positive rate of nontreponemal tests for syphilis (rapid plasma reagin test and the Venereal Disease Research Laboratory test) in IDUs requires use of specific treponemal tests (e.g., the fluorescent treponemal antibody absorption test). Standard therapy for syphilis appears to be effective in both HIV-seropositive and HIV-seronegative IDUs. HIV-infected women have higher risk of cervical dysplasia and cancer associated with concurrent human papillomavirus infection that warrants at least yearly Papanicolaou smears in this group [58].

PULMONARY DISEASE AND TUBERCULOSIS

As noted earlier, community-acquired pneumonia, tuberculosis (TB), HIV-associated *Pneumocystis* pneumonia, and septic pulmonary emboli due to right-sided endocarditis are the major pulmonary complications of illicit drug use [12,60]. In addition, pulmonary edema may acutely attend drug injection. This is not associated with infection and usually clears in 1 to 2 days.

A unilateral infiltrate on chest radiograph in a drug abuser should suggest a bacterial pneumonia. Antibiotic therapy should be directed against community-acquired pathogens, such as *S. pneumoniae*, *S. aureus*, and nonpseudomonal Gram-negative bacilli, such as *H. influenzae* and *Klebsiella pneumoniae*. If there is a recent history of unconsciousness suggesting aspiration of oropharyngeal contents, antimicrobial therapy directed against anaerobes should be considered.

Nearly 1 out of 3 U.S.-born persons older than 15 years of age who has TB is substance abuser. In addition to poor socioeconomic condition, substance abuse often takes place in enclosed spaces with poor ventilation and high volumes of human traffic, and increases the likelihood of TB transmission

[71]. The risk of developing active tuberculosis among IDUs is significant, particularly if they are coinfected with HIV. Many drug users with HIV infection and TB may not demonstrate cutaneous tuberculin reactivity probably because of anergy. These patients have a high risk for developing active TB that is more likely to be extrapulmonary [72]. Data indicate the effectiveness of preventive isoniazid therapy for all drug users who are HIV infected and live in areas of high prevalence of TB [73]. Some experts advocate treatment of latent TB regardless of tuberculin skin test reaction but the spread of multidrug-resistant TB in HIV+, drug-using populations suggests that this approach may not always be successful [74].

The clinician should maintain a high index of suspicion of TB in any drug user with pulmonary disease, particularly if the patient is infected with HIV. If there is any possibility of pulmonary TB, patients should be placed in respiratory isolation. Acid-fast smears should be performed on at least three respiratory specimens before active pulmonary TB is ruled out. If smears are positive, antituberculous therapy should be initiated [75] (see Chapter 87). Clinicians must address barrier to treatment adherence to reduce the risk of treatment failure that will lead to developing drug resistance [58].

DISSEMINATED CANDIDIASIS

A distinctive form of disseminated candidiasis has been described in injecting drug abusers who use brown heroin. *Candida albicans* has been specifically implicated in these cases. The source of infection is unclear but appears to be derived from the drug user's own flora [76]. The syndrome is characterized by fever within hours after injection, followed days to weeks later by skin, eye, and osteoarticular lesions. The skin lesions consist of deep subcutaneous nodules confined to the scalp or other hairy areas, and painful pustules on an erythematous base found in all areas of the body. Direct examination of expressed material from these pustules will demonstrate budding yeast. Costochondral tumors are a unique part of the syndrome, presenting as pain and swelling over the involved ribs. Biopsy of such lesions is often diagnostic, demonstrating both pseudohyphae and yeast. Optimal therapy is not established. Azole antifungals have been used successfully in many cases of skin involvement alone, but amphotericin B and surgery have been required with ocular or osteoarticular involvement [76].

OCULAR INFECTIONS

IDUs have an increased risk of eye infections, usually secondary to hematogenous spread from another site. Most cases are secondary to *Candida* spp, either as part of the disseminated candidiasis syndrome described earlier or with eye involvement alone. *Aspergillus* and *Fusarium* spp have also been associated with endophthalmitis in the parenteral drug user. Usually only one eye is involved, and there are no other sites of infection [77]. Treatment generally requires vitrectomy combined with systemic antifungal therapy such as voriconazole or amphotericin B.

Endophthalmitis due to bacteria is far less common than that due to fungi. Unlike fungal endophthalmitis, which often presents indolently, the onset of bacterial endophthalmitis is usually explosive with acute pain, redness, and decreased visual acuity. It may be mistaken initially for conjunctivitis. Progressive destruction of the eye may occur rapidly and immediate ophthalmologic consultation is requisite. Unusual organisms have been frequently isolated in this disease, such as *Bacillus* spp and *Staphylococcus epidermidis* [77].

CENTRAL NERVOUS SYSTEM INFECTIONS

Epidural abscess is the most frequent central nervous system infection in the IDUs [2,78]. A common presentation is indolent radicular pain associated with an underlying vertebral osteomyelitis. Imaging studies, such as myelography, CT scan, or MRI, are useful in defining the extent of the infectious process. Needle aspiration under radiographic visualization can establish the microbiologic etiology. Staphylococci are the most frequent cause, although other pathogens, including *P. aeruginosa* and *M. tuberculosis*, have also been recognized. Neurosurgical consultation should be obtained at the time the diagnosis is first suspected [2,78].

Brain abscesses may occur, usually as a result of embolization from either endocarditis or a mycotic aneurysm. They are usually multiple and generally due to *S. aureus*. Antibiotic therapy alone has led to cure in some cases [79]. Cerebral mucormycosis is another complication of intravenous drug use and is suggested by the finding of lesions in the basal ganglia [80].

References

1. Schulden JD, Thomas YF, Compton WM: Substance abuse in the United States: findings from recent epidemiologic studies. *Curr Psychiatry Rep* 11(5):353–359, 2009.
2. Calder KK, Severyn FA: Surgical emergencies in the intravenous drug user. *Emerg Med Clin North Am* 21(4):1089–1116, 2003.
3. Brown PD, Levine DP: Infective endocarditis in the injection drug user. *Infect Dis Clin North Am* 16(3):645–665, viii–ix, 2002.
4. Contoreggi C, Rexroad VE, Lange WR: Current management of infectious complications in the injecting drug user. *J Subst Abuse Treat* 15(2):95–106, 1998.
5. Knowles L, Buxton JA, Skuridina N, et al: Levamisole tainted cocaine causing severe neutropenia in Alberta and British Columbia. *Harm Reduct J* 6:30, 2009.
6. Des Jarlais DC, Perlis T, Arasteh K, et al: Reductions in hepatitis C virus and HIV infections among injecting drug users in New York City, 1990–2001. *AIDS* 19[Suppl 3]:S20–S25, 2005.
7. Weisse AB, Heller DR, Schimenti RJ, et al: The febrile parenteral drug user: a prospective study in 121 patients. *Am J Med* 94(3):274–280, 1993.
8. Novick DM, Ness GL: Abuse of antibiotics by abusers of parenteral heroin or cocaine. *South Med J* 77(3):302–303, 1984.
9. Styrt BA, Chaisson RE, Moore RD: Prior antimicrobials and staphylococcal bacteremia in HIV-infected patients. *AIDS* 11(10):1243–1248, 1997.
10. Trilla A, Miro JM: Identifying high risk patients for Staphylococcus aureus infections: skin and soft tissue infections. *J Chemother* 7[Suppl 3]:37–43, 1995.
11. Manfredi R, Costigliola P, Ricchi E, et al: Sepsis-bacteraemia and other infections due to non-opportunistic bacterial pathogens in a consecutive series of 788 patients hospitalized for HIV infection. *Clin Ter* 143(4):279–290, 1993.
12. Levine DP, Crane LR, Zervos MJ: Bacteremia in narcotic addicts at the Detroit Medical Center. II. Infectious endocarditis: a prospective comparative study. *Rev Infect Dis* 8(3):374–396, 1986.
13. Mouly S, Ruimy R, Launay O, et al: The changing clinical aspects of infective endocarditis: descriptive review of 90 episodes in a French teaching hospital and risk factors for death. *J Infect* 45(4):246–256, 2002.
14. El-Sharif A, Ashour HM: Community-acquired methicillin-resistant Staphylococcus aureus (CA-MRSA) colonization and infection in intravenous and inhalational opiate drug abusers. *Exp Biol Med (Maywood)* 233(7):874–880, 2008.
15. Frazee BW, Lynn J, Charlebois ED, et al: High prevalence of methicillin-resistant Staphylococcus aureus in emergency department skin and soft tissue infections. *Ann Emerg Med* 45(3):311–320, 2005.
16. Armstrong O, Fisher M: The treatment of Eikenella corrodens soft tissue infection in an injection drug user. *W V Med J* 92(3):138–139, 1996.
17. Bernaldo de Quiros JC, Moreno S, Cercenado E, et al: Group A streptococcal bacteremia. A 10-year prospective study. *Medicine (Baltimore)* 76(4):238–248, 1997.
18. Irish C, Maxwell R, Dancox M, et al: Skin and soft tissue infections and vascular disease among drug users, England. *Emerg Infect Dis* 13(10):1510–1511, 2007.
19. Centers for Disease Control and Prevention (CDC): Soft tissue infections among injection drug users—San Francisco, California, 1996–2000. *MMWR Morb Mortal Wkly Rep* 50(19):381–384, 2001.
20. Ebright JR, Pieper B: Skin and soft tissue infections in injection drug users. *Infect Dis Clin North Am* 16(3):697–712, 2002.

21. Harris HW, Young DM: Care of injection drug users with soft tissue infections in San Francisco, California. *Arch Surg* 137(11):1217–1222, 2002.
22. Espiritu MB, Medina JE: Complications of heroin injections of the neck. *Laryngoscope* 90(7, Pt 1):1111–1119, 1980.
23. Somers WJ, Lowe FC: Localized gangrene of the scrotum and penis: a complication of heroin injection into the femoral vessels. *J Urol* 136(1):111–113, 1986.
24. Thomas WO III, Almand JD, Stark GB, et al: Hand injuries secondary to subcutaneous illicit drug injections. *Ann Plast Surg* 34(1):27–31, 1995.
25. Smolyakov R, Riesenberg K, Schlaeffer F, et al: Streptococcal septic arthritis and necrotizing fasciitis in an intravenous drug user couple sharing needles. *Isr Med Assoc J* 4(4):302–303, 2002.
26. Johnston C, Keogan MT: Imaging features of soft-tissue infections and other complications in drug users after direct subcutaneous injection ("skin popping"). *AJR Am J Roentgenol* 182(5):1195–1202, 2004.
27. Callahan TE, Schecter WP, Horn JK: Necrotizing soft tissue infection masquerading as cutaneous abscess following illicit drug injection. *Arch Surg* 133(8):812–817; discussion 817–819, 1998.
28. Majeski J, Majeski E: Necrotizing fasciitis: improved survival with early recognition by tissue biopsy and aggressive surgical treatment. *South Med J* 90(11):1065–1068, 1997.
29. Chen JL, Fullerton KE, Flynn NM: Necrotizing fasciitis associated with injection drug use. *Clin Infect Dis* 33(1):6–15, 2001.
30. al Zahrani HA: Vascular complications following intravascular self-injection of addictive drugs. *J R Coll Surg Edinb* 42(1):50–53, 1997.
31. Tsao JW, Marder SR, Goldstone J, et al: Presentation, diagnosis, and management of arterial mycotic pseudoaneurysms in injection drug users. *Ann Vasc Surg* 16(5):652–662, 2002.
32. Martin-Davila P, Navas E, Fortun J, et al: Analysis of mortality and risk factors associated with native valve endocarditis in drug users: the importance of vegetation size. *Am Heart J* 150(5):1099–1106, 2005.
33. Jain V, Yang MH, Kovacicova-Lezcano G, et al: Infective endocarditis in an urban medical center: association of individual drugs with valvular involvement. *J Infect* 57(2):132–138, 2008.
34. Baddour LM, Meyer J, Henry B: Polymicrobial infective endocarditis in the 1980s. *Rev Infect Dis* 13(5):963–970, 1991.
35. Maisch B, Drude L: Value and limitations of transesophageal echocardiography in infective endocarditis. *Herz* 18(6):341–360, 1993.
36. Li JS, Sexton DJ, Mick N, et al: Proposed modifications to the Duke criteria for the diagnosis of infective endocarditis. *Clin Infect Dis* 30(4):633–638, 2000.
37. Cecchi E, Imazio M, Tidu M, et al: Infective endocarditis in drug addicts: role of HIV infection and the diagnostic accuracy of Duke criteria. *J Cardiovasc Med (Hagerstown)* 8(3):169–175, 2007.
38. Levitsky S, Mammana RB, Silverman NA, et al: Acute endocarditis in drug addicts: surgical treatment for gram-negative sepsis. *Circulation* 66(2 Pt 2):I135–I138, 1982.
39. Abrams B, Sklaver A, Hoffman T, et al: Single or combination therapy of staphylococcal endocarditis in intravenous drug abusers. *Ann Intern Med* 90(5):789–791, 1979.
40. DiNubile MJ: Short-course antibiotic therapy for right-sided endocarditis caused by Staphylococcus aureus in injection drug users. *Ann Intern Med* 121(11):873–876, 1994.
41. Ribera E, Gomez-Jimenez J, Cortes E, et al: Effectiveness of cloxacillin with and without gentamicin in short-term therapy for right-sided Staphylococcus aureus endocarditis. A randomized, controlled trial. *Ann Intern Med* 125(12):969–974, 1996.
42. Popescu GA, Prazuck T, Poisson D, et al: A "true" polymicrobial endocarditis: Candida tropicalis and Staphylococcus aureus–to a drug user. Case presentation and literature review. *Rom J Intern Med* 43(1–2):157–161, 2005.
43. Baddour LM, Wilson WR, Bayer AS, et al: Infective endocarditis: diagnosis, antimicrobial therapy, and management of complications: a statement for healthcare professionals from the Committee on Rheumatic Fever, Endocarditis, and Kawasaki Disease, Council on Cardiovascular Disease in the Young, and the Councils on Clinical Cardiology, Stroke, and Cardiovascular Surgery and Anesthesia, American Heart Association: endorsed by the Infectious Diseases Society of America. *Circulation* 111(23):e394–e434, 2005.
44. Arbulu A, Holmes RJ, Asfaw I: Surgical treatment of intractable right-sided infective endocarditis in drug addicts: 25 years experience. *J Heart Valve Dis* 2(2):129–137; discussion 138–139, 1993.
45. Sapico FL, Liquete JA, Sarma RJ: Bone and joint infections in patients with infective endocarditis: review of a 4-year experience. *Clin Infect Dis* 22(5):783–787, 1996.
46. Beronius M, Bergman B, Andersson R: Vertebral osteomyelitis in Goteborg, Sweden: a retrospective study of patients during 1990–95. *Scand J Infect Dis* 33(7):527–532, 2001.
47. Gotway MB, Marder SR, Hanks DK, et al: Thoracic complications of illicit drug use: an organ system approach. *Radiographics* 22 Spec No:S119–S135, 2002.
48. Lafont A, Olive A, Gelman M, et al: Candida albicans spondylodiscitis and vertebral osteomyelitis in patients with intravenous heroin drug addiction. Report of 3 new cases. *J Rheumatol* 21(5):953–956, 1994.
49. Brancos MA, Peris P, Miro JM, et al: Septic arthritis in heroin addicts. *Semin Arthritis Rheum* 21(2):81–87, 1991.
50. Cooper JG, Spilke CE, Denton M, et al: Clostridium botulinum: an increasing complication of heroin misuse. *Eur J Emerg Med* 12(5):251–252, 2005.
51. Brazier JS, Gal M, Hall V, et al: Outbreak of clostridium histolyticum infections in injecting drug users in England and Scotland. *Euro Surveill* 9(9):15–16, 2004.
52. Brazier JS, Duerden BI, Hall V, et al: Isolation and identification of Clostridium spp. from infections associated with the injection of drugs: experiences of a microbiological investigation team. *J Med Microbiol* 51(11):985–989, 2002.
53. Booth MG, Hood J, Brooks TJ, et al: Anthrax infection in drug users. *Lancet* 375(9723):1345–1346, 2010.
54. Centers for Disease Control and Prevention (CDC): Trends in HIV/AIDS diagnoses—33 states, 2001–2004. *MMWR Morb Mortal Wkly Rep* 54(45):1149–1153, 2005.
55. Schoenbaum EE, Hartel D, Selwyn PA, et al: Risk factors for human immunodeficiency virus infection in intravenous drug users. *N Engl J Med* 321(13):874–879, 1989.
56. Nakamura N, Mausbach BT, Ulibarri MD, et al: Methamphetamine use, attitudes about condoms, and sexual risk behavior among HIV-positive men who have sex with men [published online ahead of print October 24, 2009]. *Arch Sex Behav*, 2009.
57. Nath A: Human immunodeficiency virus-associated neurocognitive disorder: pathophysiology in relation to drug addiction. *Ann N Y Acad Sci* 1187:122–128, 2010.
58. O'Connor PG, Selwyn PA, Schottenfeld RS: Medical care for injection-drug users with human immunodeficiency virus infection. *N Engl J Med* 331(7):450–459, 1994.
59. Caiaffa WT, Vlahov D, Graham NM, et al: Drug smoking, Pneumocystis carinii pneumonia, and immunosuppression increase risk of bacterial pneumonia in human immunodeficiency virus-seropositive injection drug users. *Am J Respir Crit Care Med* 150(6 Pt 1):1493–1498, 1994.
60. O'Donnell AE, Selig J, Aravamuthan M, et al: Pulmonary complications associated with illicit drug use. An update. *Chest* 108(2):460–463, 1995.
61. Beilke MA, Theall KP, O'Brien M, et al: Clinical outcomes and disease progression among patients coinfected with HIV and human T lymphotropic virus types 1 and 2. *Clin Infect Dis* 39(2):256–263, 2004.
62. Haverkos HW, Lange WR: From the alcohol, drug abuse, and mental health administration. Serious infections other than human immunodeficiency virus among intravenous drug abusers. *J Infect Dis* 161(5):894–902, 1990.
63. Kreek MJ, Des Jarlais DC, Trepo CL, et al: Contrasting prevalence of delta hepatitis markers in parenteral drug abusers with and without AIDS. *J Infect Dis* 162(2):538–541, 1990.
64. Centers for disease control (CDC). Hepatitis A among drug abusers. *MMWR Morb Mortal Wkly Rep* 37(19):297–300, 305, 1988.
65. Hagan H, Des Jarlais DC: HIV and HCV infection among injecting drug users. *Mt Sinai J Med* 67(5–6):423–428, 2000.
66. Amon JJ, Garfein RS, Ahdieh-Grant L, et al: Prevalence of hepatitis C virus infection among injection drug users in the United States, 1994–2004. *Clin Infect Dis* 46(12):1852–1858, 2008.
67. Smit C, van den Berg C, Geskus R, et al: Risk of hepatitis-related mortality increased among hepatitis C virus/HIV-coinfected drug users compared with drug users infected only with hepatitis C virus: a 20-year prospective study. *J Acquir Immune Defic Syndr* 47(2):221–225, 2008.
68. Soriano V, Vispo E, Labarga P, et al: Viral hepatitis and HIV co-infection. *Antiviral Res* 85(1):303–315, 2010.
69. Koziel MJ, Peters MG: Viral hepatitis in HIV infection. *N Engl J Med* 356(14):1445–1454, 2007.
70. Siegal HA, Falck RS, Wang J, et al: History of sexually transmitted diseases infection, drug-sex behaviors, and the use of condoms among midwestern users of injection drugs and crack cocaine. *Sex Transm Dis* 23(4):277–282, 1996.
71. Pevzner ES, Robison S, Donovan J, et al: Tuberculosis transmission and use of methamphetamines and other drugs in Snohomish County, WA, 1991–2006. *Am J Public Health*, 100(12):2481–2486, 2010.
72. Selwyn PA, Sckell BM, Alcabes P, et al: High risk of active tuberculosis in HIV-infected drug users with cutaneous anergy. *JAMA* 268(4):504–509, 1992.
73. Scholten JN, Driver CR, Munsiff SS, et al: Effectiveness of isoniazid treatment for latent tuberculosis infection among human immunodeficiency virus (HIV)-infected and HIV-uninfected injection drug users in methadone programs. *Clin Infect Dis* 37(12):1686–1692, 2003.
74. Hannan MM, Peres H, Maltez F, et al: Investigation and control of a large outbreak of multi-drug resistant tuberculosis at a central Lisbon hospital. *J Hosp Infect* 47(2):91–97, 2001.
75. Aaron L, Saadoun D, Calatroni I, et al: Tuberculosis in HIV-infected patients: a comprehensive review. *Clin Microbiol Infect* 10(5):388–398, 2004.
76. Bisbe J, Miro JM, Latorre X, et al: Disseminated candidiasis in addicts who use brown heroin: report of 83 cases and review. *Clin Infect Dis* 15(6):910–923, 1992.
77. Kim RW, Juzych MS, Eliott D: Ocular manifestations of injection drug use. *Infect Dis Clin North Am* 16(3):607–622, 2002.
78. Chuo CY, Fu YC, Lu YM, et al: Spinal infection in intravenous drug abusers. *J Spinal Disord Tech* 20(4):324–328, 2007.
79. Tunkel AR, Pradhan SK: Central nervous system infections in injection drug users. *Infect Dis Clin North Am* 16(3):589–605, 2002.
80. Hopkins RJ, Rothman M, Fiore A, et al: Cerebral mucormycosis associated with intravenous drug use: three case reports and review. *Clin Infect Dis* 19(6):1133–1137, 1994.

CHAPTER 87 ■ TUBERCULOSIS

ROBERT W. BELKNAP AND RANDALL R. REVES

EPIDEMIOLOGY

Tuberculosis (TB) continues to cause significant morbidity and mortality worldwide. In 2007, there were an estimated 9.27 million new cases, 13.7 million prevalent cases, and 1.75 million deaths due to TB [1]. Globally, the total number of TB cases is increasing but because of population growth, the overall incidence rate per 100,000 persons has declined minimally. In the United States, incident TB cases have been declining since 1992 and reached a historic low in 2009 at 11,545 [2]. The challenge for TB controllers is continuing to progress toward the goal of TB elimination. Concurrent with the decline, TB in the United States has increasingly become a disease of foreign-born, minority, and other underserved populations.

A threat to TB control efforts worldwide has been the rise of multidrug-resistant (MDR) and extensively drug-resistant (XDR) forms of TB. Both forms have been present in relatively low numbers for decades but an outbreak of XDR TB in rural South Africa associated with a high and rapid mortality brought this issue to international attention [3]. The World Health Organization's 4th report on drug-resistant TB estimated that 0.5 million MDR-TB cases occur annually and approximately 7% of these are XDR TB [4]. The accuracy of these estimates is limited by the absence of culture and susceptibility testing in many high-burden countries. Nevertheless, the overall trend appears to be increasing and may have important implications for choosing empiric treatment in hospitalized patients and for infection control.

The proportion of newly diagnosed TB patients who require hospitalization each year is poorly characterized. One large urban hospital reported that TB accounted for 1% of medical intensive care unit (ICU) admissions over a 15-year period [5]. Epidemiological studies show that between 3% and 24% of hospitalized TB patients require treatment in an ICU and between 2% and 13% require mechanical ventilation [5,6]. While overall mortality from TB in the United States has been around 5% for the past decade [2], mortality remains particularly high (50% to 60%) among patients with TB-associated respiratory failure requiring mechanical ventilation [6–8]. Factors associated with mortality include multiorgan failure, malnutrition, renal failure, immunosuppression, and delayed diagnosis [6–10].

PATHOGENESIS

The pathogenesis of TB is a two-stage process, which can be divided into TB infection and progression to disease [11,12]. These stages are reflective of the risk factors that should be considered when determining the likelihood that a patient has TB (Table 87.1). TB infection, with rare exceptions, results from the airborne transmission of tubercle bacilli. In a susceptible host upon reaching the alveoli, the tubercle bacilli multiply to produce a localized pneumonia, spread to involve the hilar lymph nodes, then enter the bloodstream through the thoracic duct, and disseminate throughout the body. This primary infection is usually clinically unapparent. Most patients develop cell-mediated immunity to *Mycobacterium tuberculosis*, which brings the infection under control over a period of weeks. Despite initial immunologic control of TB infection, viable tubercle bacilli remain in scattered foci as latent TB infection that if untreated may persist for life [13].

The second stage is the development of active TB, which occurs at a variable rate dependent on the person's age at infection and other medical conditions [12]. Progression from latent to active TB, termed reactivation, is much more frequent in people with certain conditions, particularly HIV infection (Table 87.1) [12,14]. Patients with advanced HIV have a 10

TABLE 87.1

FACTORS THAT SHOULD PROMPT CONSIDERATION OF TUBERCULOSIS IN THE DIFFERENTIAL DIAGNOSIS

Risks for tuberculosis infection

1. History of active tuberculosis, particularly if never or inadequately treated
2. History of a positive tuberculin skin test
3. Other risk factors for infection (tuberculin status unknown)
   - Contact with known or suspected tuberculosis
   - Presence of fibrotic lung lesions compatible with inactive tuberculosis
   - Immigration from countries with high risk for tuberculosis
   - Advanced age
   - Medically underserved populations
   - Alcohol or other drug use
   - Institutional exposure
   - Homeless shelters
   - Correctional facilities
   - Nursing homes
   - Some hospitals and mental institutions

Risks for progression to active tuberculosis (tuberculin status positive or unknown)

1. Known or suspected HIV infection
2. Other immunosuppressive conditions
   - Lymphatic and reticuloendothelial disorders
   - High-dose corticosteroids, tumor necrosis factor-α inhibitors, and other immunosuppressive therapy
3. Recent tuberculosis infection
4. Presence of upper lobe scars compatible with inactive tuberculosis
5. Certain medical conditions
   - Silicosis
   - Chronic renal failure
   - Diabetes mellitus
   - Intravenous drug use
   - Gastrectomy or other conditions associated with weight loss

times greater risk while those on effective antiretroviral therapy (ART) still have twice the risk of an uninfected person [12]. In most cases, reactivation of TB causes pulmonary disease, but reactivation can occur at any site where a latent focus was established during the initial infection [11]. Disseminated disease may also occur and is believed to result from the erosion of a tuberculous focus directly into a blood vessel [15]. In a critically ill patient, the presence of any risk factor for infection or progression should prompt consideration of TB in the differential diagnosis.

CLINICAL MANIFESTATIONS AND DIAGNOSIS

Physicians in intensive care settings face the challenge of maintaining an appropriate index of suspicion for TB when it is a relatively rare cause of critical illness. Prompt recognition of TB and early institution of effective multiple-drug therapy are required to achieve the dual goals of successfully treating patients and preventing nosocomial TB transmission. Delays in diagnosis are unfortunately common and have been noted in more than half of patients admitted to community hospitals [16]. Concomitant nontuberculous infections occur in up to a third of patients and can lead to delays in diagnosis [8]. Fluoroquinolones are quite active against *M. tuberculosis,* and patients with unrecognized pulmonary TB are increasingly being treated initially with these agents for presumed community-acquired pneumonia. An initial clinical response to fluoroquinolones has been documented as a cause for delays in diagnosing TB [17].

TB may present as the primary cause of a life-threatening illness, but it may also be a coincidental illness in patients being treated for another condition [8] (Fig. 87.1). The symptoms and signs of TB are variable and depend on the site and extent of disease [6–8]. The history of a chronic, progressive illness with fever, night sweats, and weight loss, with or without a chronic cough, is most suggestive of TB. However, obtaining an accurate history can be difficult and TB patients often report the acute onset of symptoms [7,18,19]. A variety of laboratory abnormalities have been associated with TB, including anemia, hypoalbuminemia, elevated alkaline phosphatase, and hyponatremia, but are nonspecific [11,20].

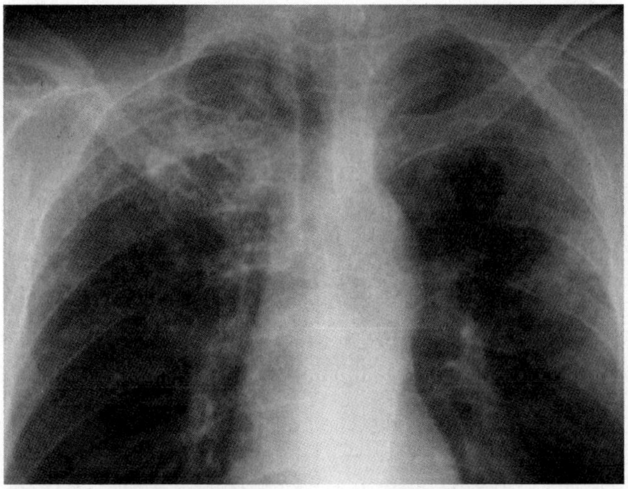

FIGURE 87.1. Chest radiograph of a 41-year-old homeless patient who was hospitalized with multiple fractures, including the right clavicle, after being hit by a car. The patient denied all respiratory symptoms despite having extensive bilateral upper lobe fibronodular and cavitary disease. Sputum samples were smear positive and grew *Mycobacterium tuberculosis.*

Pulmonary Tuberculosis

Pulmonary TB is the most common form of disease accounting for 80% of cases in the United States [2]. Extrapulmonary TB is more common among patients who are female, born outside the United States, and with HIV infection [21]. Acute respiratory failure, which occurs in 2% to 13% of hospitalized TB cases, is the most common reason for admission to an ICU [5,6,10,19]. While chronic cough and fevers are usually present, other symptoms suggestive of pulmonary TB include weight loss, dyspnea, and hemoptysis [11]. Of note, dyspnea may be minimal despite fairly extensive lung destruction. Hemoptysis occurs in about 20% of patients and occasionally can be massive [22]. Pulmonary TB may also be asymptomatic, occurring in patients with primarily extrapulmonary disease, or may be a coincidental finding (Fig. 87.1).

Definitively diagnosing pulmonary TB relies on the collection of respiratory samples for smear and culture. Sputum samples should be considered in symptomatic patients at risk for TB even when the chest radiograph appears normal. Positive sputum cultures in the absence of radiographic abnormalities were relatively rare in the pre-AIDS era [23] but appear more commonly among TB cases associated with AIDS [24]. The proportion of hospitalized TB patients who have a positive sputum smear ranges between 35% and 65% [7,9]. A minimum of three sputa or other lower respiratory tract specimens should be collected when pulmonary, pleural, or disseminated TB is suspected. The samples should be collected 8 to 24 hours apart preferably with at least one early morning specimen [25].

Patients who are unable to spontaneously produce sputum should have samples induced using nebulized hypertonic saline [11]. Bronchoscopic specimens are not more sensitive, and should not be considered a replacement for three expectorated or induced sputa [26]. Bronchoscopy is generally helpful if alternative diagnoses are being sought or if a tissue biopsy is needed. For select patients, including young children, who either cannot tolerate the nebulizer or who still do not produce an adequate sputum sample, gastric aspirates should be obtained. When acid-fast bacilli (AFB) smears of respiratory secretions are negative, other specimens that may yield a diagnosis include pleural fluid, pleural biopsy, or transbronchial biopsy [11,27]. More invasive procedures such as transthoracic needle biopsy of the lung or mediastinal lymph nodes or open lung biopsy may be necessary in certain circumstances.

Pleural Tuberculosis

Pleural TB presents in two forms, commonly as tuberculous pleuritis and rarely as tuberculous empyema [11,28]. Tuberculous pleuritis occurs in 6% of HIV-negative and 11% of HIV-positive patients [29], and the incidence increases with declining CD4 cell counts [30]. It results from the rupture of a granuloma into the pleural space and may occur alone or in conjunction with pulmonary disease [28]. Often patients are asymptomatic but some present with acute symptoms of fever and chest pain, suggesting a viral or bacterial cause. The pathogenesis is primarily an immunologic reaction with very few tubercle bacilli actually present in the pleural space. Radiographically, a unilateral effusion covering less than half the hemithorax is typical. Untreated, tuberculous pleuritis often resolves but these patients are at high risk for recurrent pulmonary disease. Tuberculous empyema is much less common and results from the entry of large numbers of bacilli into the pleural space due to the rupture of an adjacent cavity or development of a bronchopleural fistula [31].

Pleural fluid and tissue biopsy are typically needed to definitively diagnose tuberculous pleuritis. Sputum specimens should also be collected to evaluate for concurrent pulmonary disease. The pleural fluid most often shows a serous exudate with elevated protein and lactate dehydrogenase levels, low-to-normal glucose levels, and a pH range between 7.05 and 7.45 [29,32]. Early in the process, the fluid has a predominance of polymorphonuclear leukocytes that are replaced by lymphocytes within days. Adenosine deaminase (ADA) and other biochemical markers have been studied extensively, alone and in combination, as markers for diagnosing tuberculous pleuritis. Recent studies have supported measuring ADA levels, especially isoenzyme 2, showing additive diagnostic sensitivity and specificity when combined with other tests [33]. Interferon-gamma release assays (IGRA) are also undergoing investigation as diagnostic tools for pleural TB [34]. Both ADA and IGRA tests may be useful in settings that lack the capacity to do cultures, but should not replace a pleural biopsy which provides tissue for culture and pathology review.

AFB smears of pleural fluid and pleural biopsies are rarely positive (10% to 20%). The earliest presumptive diagnosis is provided by pathologic findings of granulomas with or without caseation, which are seen histologically in 60% of specimens [28]. Pleural fluid cultures are positive in only 20% to 30%. The yield increases slightly with multiple samples but usually delays the initiation of TB treatment [35]. Pleural biopsies are culture positive in 55% to 85% of specimens and should be sought whenever TB is considered a likely diagnosis.

Disseminated Tuberculosis

Disseminated TB refers to multiorgan involvement and may occur during progressive primary infection or as a complication of chronic TB [27,36]. The term *miliary tuberculosis*, which refers to the histologic appearance of diffuse nodular lesions resembling millet seeds, has historically been used interchangeably with disseminated disease. Now the term miliary is generally reserved to describe a diffuse micronodular infiltrate on the chest radiograph (Fig. 87.2). Young children and immunocompromised patients are at greatest risk for disseminated TB. However, a chronic, cryptic form of disease, termed *late generalized tuberculosis*, can occur in the elderly or those with other underlying illnesses [15]. In this cryptic form of disseminated TB, miliary infiltrates are rare and a diagnosis is often made postmortem.

Clinical evidence of dissemination is seen in up to 10% of HIV-associated and 33% of solid-organ-transplant–associated TB cases [37,38]. The presentations range from generalized lymphadenopathy to fulminant respiratory failure [39]. The duration of symptoms before diagnosis may vary from 1 week to over a year. Fever and other constitutional symptoms are seen in over 90%, respiratory symptoms in 75%, abdominal symptoms in 25%, and central nervous system (CNS) symptoms in 20%. In some reports, the presentation of disseminated TB has been similar to that of Gram-negative sepsis [40]. Acute respiratory failure is uncommon but a well-characterized complication of disseminated or miliary TB [19,41]. Laboratory abnormalities in disseminated disease are nonspecific. Anemia is common, but leukocyte and platelet counts range from markedly elevated to severely depressed [36]. Alkaline phosphatase levels are frequently elevated, likely related to granulomatous hepatitis. Chest radiographic findings are variable and may demonstrate miliary nodules of 1 to 3 mm in diameter or larger nodules of 5 to 7 mm. In about 10% of disseminated cases, radiographs will be normal, particularly early in the illness.

Virtually any body fluid, tissue, or organ may yield a diagnosis, particularly with clinical or laboratory abnormalities that suggest an extrapulmonary site of disease. Because extrapulmonary TB usually involves a lower burden of organisms compared with pulmonary disease, histologic examination and culture of biopsy specimens often provides the greatest diagnostic yield. Sputum smears should be examined for AFB but are positive in less than a third of patients with miliary TB. Histology and cultures of transbronchial, thoracoscopic, or traditional open lung biopsy will usually confirm the diagnosis. However, a careful search for chronic skin lesions, scrotal involvement, or lymphadenopathy may disclose other more accessible sites for a diagnostic biopsy [42]. Urine and stool cultures are easily obtainable and also may provide the diagnosis. Lumbar puncture should be considered in patients with headache or other CNS symptoms since meningitis is found in nearly 20% of patients with disseminated TB. A mycobacterial blood culture is

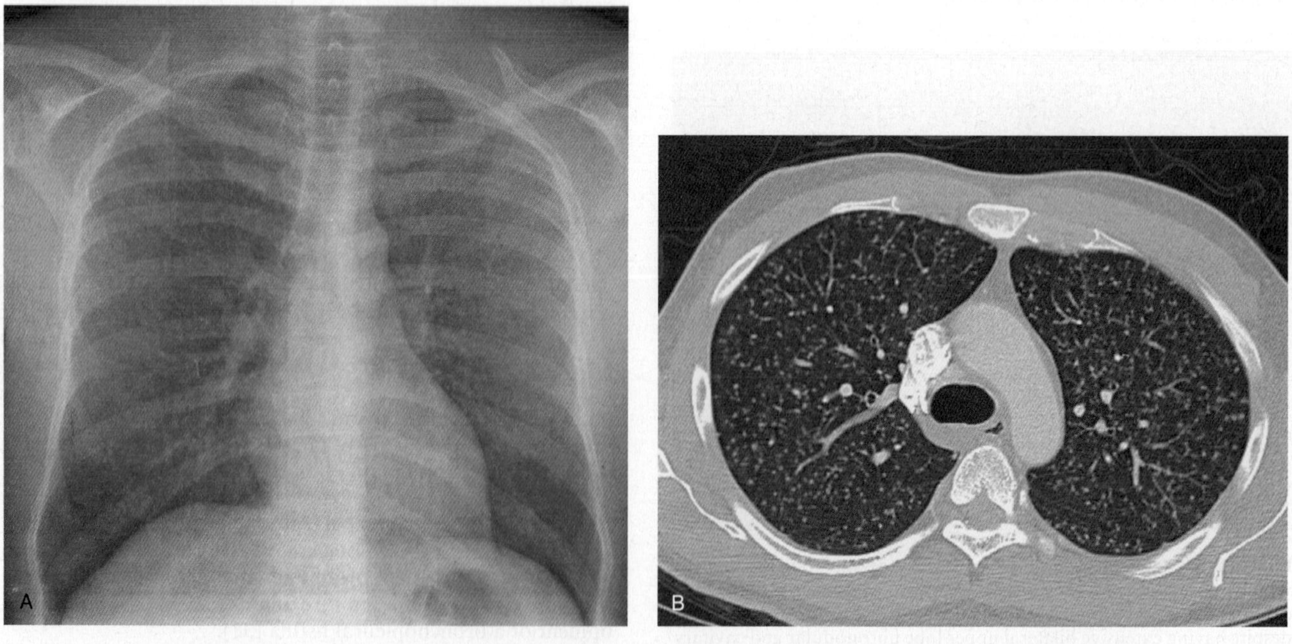

FIGURE 87.2. Chest radiograph (A) and CT scan (B) showing miliary disease in a 36-year-old patient who presented with several months of fever, weight loss, and abdominal pain.

positive in about 26% to 42% of HIV-infected individuals, and is the only culture-positive specimen in some [43]. Other potentially useful diagnostic tests include culture of gastric aspirates and biopsy specimens of liver or bone marrow. In disseminated TB, granulomas are seen in about 90% of liver biopsies; the yield is lower from bone marrow biopsy unless pancytopenia is present [44].

Central Nervous System Tuberculosis

TB involving the CNS may present as meningitis, as one or more parenchymal tuberculomas, or as a combination of both [45,46]. The clinical presentation varies from an indolent illness with headache and subtle changes in mental status to more acute presentations. Focal neurologic symptoms and signs may result from a tuberculoma causing a localized mass effect or from basilar meningitis affecting the cranial nerves directly or causing infarction of intracranial arteries [45]. Evidence of active or inactive TB at another site is noted in about three-fourths of cases, most often miliary infiltrates on chest radiographs. Tuberculomas of the CNS are readily detected by computed tomography (Fig. 87.3), but magnetic resonance imaging is often needed to detect basilar meningitis [46]. Tuberculous meningitis and tuberculomas are more common among HIV-infected individuals and present with signs, symptoms, and laboratory findings that are similar to those found in individuals who are HIV-negative [47].

Rapid diagnosis and treatment is critical to patient survival and neurological outcomes in tuberculous meningitis. A definitive diagnosis can be difficult though and antituberculous treatment should be initiated immediately in suspect cases since delays in therapy are correlated with outcomes. Evaluation of cerebral spinal fluid (CSF), although often nonspecific, is important for diagnosing CNS TB. The CSF findings classically described are a lymphocytic pleocytosis, low glucose, and an elevated protein. However, the absence of these findings does not exclude the diagnosis since the white cell count may range widely, a polymorphonuclear predominance occurs in up to 30%, and the protein and glucose may be normal [45,46]. AFB smears of CSF are positive in only 10% to 20% of cases and cultures are positive in <50%. Because disseminated disease is common with tuberculous meningitis, AFB cultures sent from other sources, including sputum, urine, and stool, may provide a diagnostic smear or culture. CNS tuberculomas may be diagnosed by a typical radiographic appearance and response to treatment, but definitive diagnosis usually requires biopsy or surgical excision.

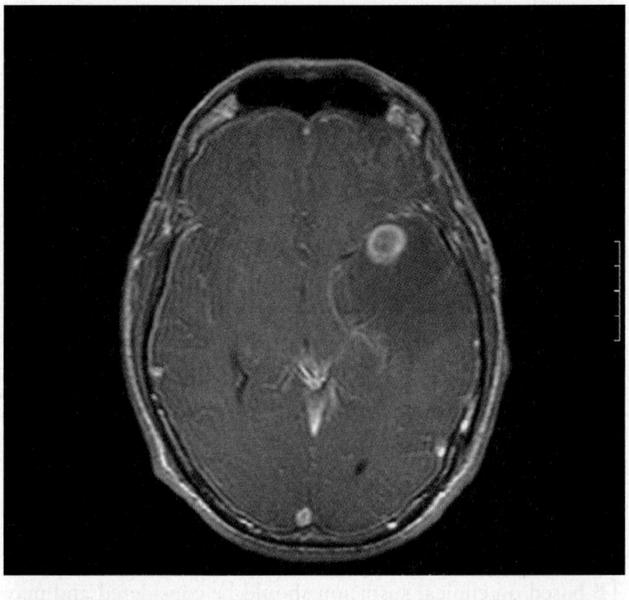

FIGURE 87.3. Computed tomographic scan of a 45-year-old patient with AIDS, known to be TST (+) but never completed latent treatment, who presented with a headache, expressive aphasia, and neologisms. The scan shows a tuberculoma with marked surrounding edema. Cerebral spinal fluid (CSF) showed a white blood cell count of 675 (100% lymphocytes), glucose 42 mg/dL, and protein 246 mg/dL. CSF cultures were negative but the diagnosis of isoniazid-resistant tuberculosis was confirmed by excisional biopsy.

Other Forms of Extrapulmonary Tuberculosis

Other forms of TB, such as lymphatic, pericardial, gastrointestinal, cutaneous, skeletal, and genitourinary, may be either coincidental findings or may provide clues to the diagnosis of disseminated disease in critically ill patients [11].

TB patients on therapy also may present to the ICU after developing an immune reconstitution syndrome or paradoxical reaction. This syndrome is characterized by a worsening of symptoms and/or radiographic studies despite effective chemotherapy with microbiologic improvement [48]. Typical manifestations are the recurrence or development of fever and other systemic manifestations, enlargement and suppuration of lymphatic tissue, worsening of pulmonary infiltrates, and life-threatening complications such as respiratory failure or enlargement of intracranial lesions. These reactions can occur in any TB patient but are most common in patients with TB and advanced AIDS who are started on antiretroviral therapy (ART) within the first few months of TB treatment [49].

Chest Radiography

Routine chest radiography is an invaluable screening and diagnostic tool for patients at risk for TB. Radiographs are able to detect most active pulmonary TB cases, particularly the most infectious cases with extensive parenchymal disease and cavitation. Radiographs can demonstrate fibrosis from previously active TB that identifies patients at higher risk for reactivation, and can provide clues to the diagnosis in patients with extrapulmonary disease. The classic radiographic appearance of active TB is a fibrotic, cavitary upper lobe opacity (Fig. 87.1), but pulmonary TB can present with a variety of findings on chest radiograph, including a normal film. The radiographic appearance of TB depends primarily on the duration of illness and the host's immune function. For example, primary TB typically presents as a lower lobe infiltrate often with ipsilateral hilar adenopathy. Primary TB occurs most often in young children but can be seen at any age including the elderly, as described among recently infected nursing home residents [50]. Other radiographic appearances, which can be seen alone or in combination, are alveolar opacities, mixed alveolar-interstitial infiltrates, miliary disease, and intrathoracic adenopathy (Figs. 87.2 and 87.4) [8]. These "atypical" presentations of pulmonary TB have been reported in up to 34% to 45% of HIV-negative individuals in some series [51,52]. In the presence of advanced immunodeficiency, there is greater variation in the radiographic patterns of TB with more frequently lower lobe involvement, diffuse infiltrates, hilar or mediastinal adenopathy, and pleural effusions [37,53].

Tuberculin Skin Testing and Interferon-Gamma Release Assays

The tuberculin skin test (TST) had been the only licensed test for detecting TB infection, but newer blood tests, IGRAs, are now commercially available [11,54]. IGRAs measure the

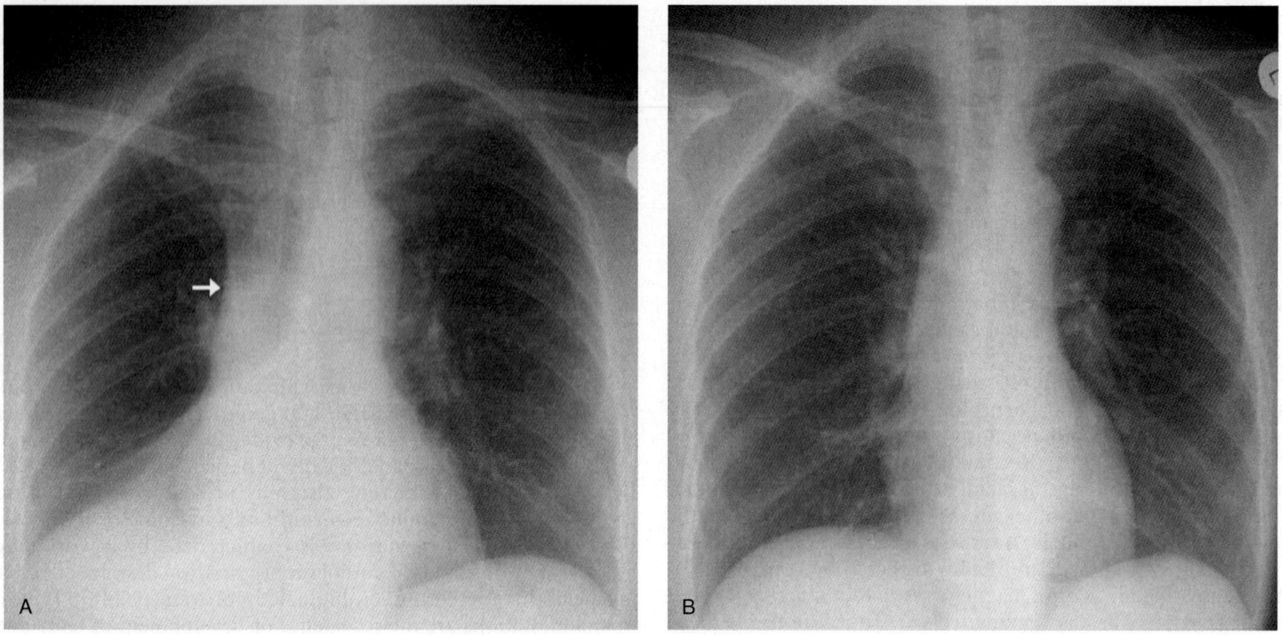

FIGURE 87.4. Chest radiographs of a 49-year-old patient who had undergone a liver transplant 6 months prior for hepatitis-B–associated liver disease. The initial radiograph (**A**) showed right paratracheal adenopathy (*arrow*) with partial right lung collapse that resolved by the end of treatment (**B**). The patient received standard tuberculosis therapy with the substitution of rifabutin for rifampin to minimize the drug interaction with tacrolimus.

interferon gamma produced by peripheral blood lymphocytes after stimulation with mycobacterial antigens. Both the TST and IGRAs are useful adjunctive tests but must be interpreted with caution. A positive result indicates the patient has been infected and may increase your clinical suspicion for active disease but is nondiagnostic. Similarly, a negative test does not rule out active TB since between 10% and 25% of patients with culture-confirmed disease will have a negative TST or IGRA [55,56]. Anergy testing is of no diagnostic value and is no longer recommended for any patient population [11].

Nucleic Acid Amplification Tests

Culture remains the gold standard for diagnosing all forms of TB but is not always rapid or highly sensitive. One approach to overcome these limitations has been the development of nucleic acid amplification (NAA) tests [57]. These tests offer several advantages including a rapid result, high specificity, and broad application to tissue samples, and in some cases even formalin fixed tissue [58]. The unfortunate limitation to NAA tests has been the somewhat disappointingly low sensitivity, particularly in paucibacillary disease. The approximate sensitivity of these tests in diagnosing smear negative pulmonary, pleural, and meningeal TB is 50%, and therefore should be interpreted in the context of clinical suspicion [46,59].

Culture and Drug Susceptibility Testing

The importance of using rapid diagnostic techniques in clinical mycobacteriology has been tragically illustrated in outbreaks of drug-resistant TB among immunocompromised hosts whose median survival with standard, ineffective therapy was 16 days [3]. Liquid culture systems containing radiometric or colorimetric material permit detection of mycobacterial growth in 2 to 6 days. The traditional use of biochemical testing for identification of isolates as *M. tuberculosis* has been largely replaced by the more accurate and rapid methods using commercial nucleic acid probes or high-performance liquid chromatography. Drug susceptibility testing can also be done more rapidly with the commercial liquid cultures systems. Rapid susceptibility testing is most important for identifying *M. tuberculosis* isolates with resistance to at least isoniazid and rifampin. These isolates are referred to as multidrug resistant because TB due to these strains can be expected to fail standard therapy [60]. Many hospital laboratories now lack the expertise and the number of specimens to conduct the full range of testing on a daily basis [11]. More timely results may be achieved by sending specimens, particularly those that are AFB smear positive to a full-service mycobacteriology laboratory. Molecular methods for rapidly detecting drug resistance have been developed and are proving highly sensitive and specific, particularly for isoniazid and rifampin [61]. Where available, these tests provide the earliest evidence for MDR TB.

TREATMENT

Principles of Therapy for Tuberculosis

Two characteristics of *M. tuberculosis* dictate the requirements for successful therapy—a high frequency of spontaneous mutations and a slow, intermittent growth cycle. Overcoming these characteristics requires multiple drugs to prevent the selection of drug-resistant mutants and an extended duration of therapy to kill the dormant mycobacteria [60]. Culture confirmation should always be pursued aggressively, but empiric therapy for TB based on clinical suspicion should be considered and may be important for the survival of critically ill patients.

Recommendations for Initial Therapy

The choice of initial TB therapy in the ICU should be made after considering the risk for MDR disease. The potential for drug-resistant TB can be estimated by knowing the patient's country of birth and whether they have a history of prior TB treatment. In 2008, the percentage of patients with MDR TB among U.S.-born and foreign-born persons with no prior TB treatment was low, 0.6% and 1.2%, respectively. Among those with a history of prior treatment, these rates increased to 1.3% in U.S.-born and 6.0% in foreign-born persons [2]. Drug resistance should also be suspected in patients who fail while on treatment or who relapse after treatment has ended, particularly patients who did not get directly observed therapy [62,63].

For most patients, the four-drug, oral regimen of isoniazid, rifampin, pyrazinamide, and ethambutol will be appropriate [60]. The choice of therapy, when drug resistance is suspected, should be made in consultation with a physician experienced in treating MDR TB, and generally should include two or more agents likely to have activity. The agents usually chosen include an aminoglycoside (amikacin, kanamycin, or capreomycin), a quinolone (typically levofloxacin, moxifloxacin, or gatifloxacin), and one or two of the "second-line" agents such as ethionamide, cycloserine, or *p*-aminosalicylic acid (PAS) [60,64]. Of note, ethambutol, pyrazinamide, ethionamide, cycloserine, and PAS can only be given orally or enterally via a feeding tube [60,64]. Due to the relatively poor anti-TB activity of second-line drugs, some experts have recommended measuring serum drug levels to allow dose increases in order to achieve concentrations above the in vitro minimum inhibitory concentration [65]. Although not examined in a comparative trial, surgical resection may be a useful adjunct in the therapy of MDR TB after weeks or months of medical therapy [64].

More detailed information regarding TB treatment is available on the CDC Web site, http://www.cdc.gov/tb/publications/guidelines/Treatment.htm. Other complicating factors that may need consideration when starting TB therapy in a critically ill patient are shown in Table 87.2.

TABLE 87.2

SELECT THERAPEUTIC CHALLENGES IN TREATING CRITICALLY ILL TUBERCULOSIS PATIENTS (WHEN DRUG SUSCEPTIBLE DISEASE IS KNOWN OR EXPECTED)

1. Documented or anticipated malabsorption—medications which can be given parenterally:
   a. Rifampin
   b. Quinolone—levofloxacin, moxifloxacin, or gatifloxacin (ofloxacin or ciprofloxacin may be used if the others are not available)
   c. Aminoglycoside—amikacin (streptomycin can be used if drug susceptibility is known); second-line agents are kanamycin and capreomycin
   d. Isoniazid—when available but it may be difficult to obtain
2. Hepatic failure—acute or severe
   a. Empiric therapy: aminoglycoside, quinolone (levofloxacin may be preferred since moxifloxacin is hepatically cleared), ethambutol (consider including rifampin if not fulminant hepatic failure)
   b. Avoid: isoniazid and pyrazinamide
3. Renal failure
   a. Dose adjust: ethambutol, pyrazinamide, aminoglycosides, and levofloxacin
   b. No change in dosing: isoniazid, rifampin, and moxifloxacin
4. Pregnancy
   a. Empiric therapy: isoniazid, rifampin, ethambutol
   b. Avoid: pyrazinamide (may be safe but data lacking), aminoglycosides, and quinolones (both could be considered for critically ill patients when malabsorption is likely or drug resistance is a concern)

Adjunctive Corticosteroids

In certain circumstances, corticosteroids may be useful in TB treatment by reducing the intensity of the inflammatory response [60]. In a randomized, placebo-controlled trial, corticosteroids were shown to lower the mortality and morbidity of patients with tuberculous meningitis [66]. Corticosteroids also reduce the need for pericardiocentesis in patients being treated for tuberculous pericarditis [67], but there does not appear to be a long-term benefit in reducing the late complication of constrictive pericarditis. Corticosteroids also appear beneficial for treating severe pulmonary TB with more rapid defervescence, weight gain, and radiographic improvement [68]. The initial corticosteroid dose in most studies has been the equivalent of 40 to 80 mg of daily prednisone, tapering off over 1 to 3 months.

Management of Adverse Drug Effects

During the treatment of TB, serious mistakes can result from the failure to appropriately recognize and manage adverse drug effects [69]. Most mistakes fall into three categories: (a) failing to discontinue therapy in the face of a serious adverse effect; (b) abandoning important first-line drugs because of minor adverse effects; and (c) failing to recognize serious drug-drug interactions. Drug-induced hepatitis is probably the greatest concern for clinicians treating TB, particularly when patients have underlying liver disease. Fortunately, the risk of fulminant hepatitis is low and generally occurs when TB medications are continued despite evidence of toxicity.

While clinically significant or fulminant hepatitis is rare, increased transaminase levels are common with the combination of isoniazid, rifampin, and pyrazinamide. Clinicians should also remember that patients with severe or disseminated TB might have elevated liver function tests, particularly alkaline phosphatase, as a result of their disease. Patients with abnormal liver function tests and no known cause should have TB treatment held if transaminases are three times the upper limit of normal and the patient has symptoms of toxicity (i.e., nausea, vomiting, loss of appetite, or jaundice) or if transaminases are five times the upper limit in asymptomatic patients [70]. Patients with underlying liver disease and/or baseline liver function abnormalities should generally start standard TB treatment with close monitoring of symptoms and liver function tests.

The decision to stop or change therapy due to liver dysfunction must be made on a case-by-case basis. When therapy is held due to hepatotoxicity, the drugs are usually restarted cautiously, resuming one drug at a time. Pyrazinamide is the most frequent cause of liver injury in patients receiving the standard four-drug regimen, and may best be avoided if rifampin and isoniazid are reintroduced without difficulty. In critically ill patients for whom holding therapy may pose a significant risk, reasonable short-term therapy can be achieved with an aminoglycoside, fluoroquinolone, and ethambutol (Table 87.2). Patients who develop a rapid rise in transaminases to levels of 10 to 20 times normal should probably not be rechallenged with pyrazinamide or isoniazid. Other serious side effects that should result in the permanent discontinuation of the offending medication are severe rifampin-associated hypersensitivity reactions like acute renal failure, hemolysis, or thrombocytopenia.

When minor side effects occur, all attempts should be made to treat the symptoms and to determine if an alternative cause exists before discontinuing standard first-line TB medications. Minor side effects such as gastrointestinal upset can often be managed by adjusting the dosing schedule or by prescribing an antiemetic. Isolated bilirubin elevation caused by rifampin-associated cholestasis may occur but resolves despite continued therapy. Transient minor rashes or pruritus are often associated with pyrazinamide and may be managed using antihistamines without interrupting therapy.

Finally, recognizing potentially serious drug-drug interactions and adjusting therapy accordingly can avoid many drug-associated adverse events. Rifampin and to a lesser extent rifabutin are inducers of the hepatic cytochrome P450 enzyme system. Therefore, particular caution should be used when HIV-infected TB patients are taking or may be starting ART [71]. In general, few HIV-infected patients in the ICU will be able to take ART, but for those who can recent observational and randomized trials have shown a mortality benefit from early initiation of ART particularly for patients with CD4 counts below 200. Updated recommendations for the combined use of TB and HIV drugs can be found on the CDC Web site, http://www.cdc.gov/tb/publications/guidelines/TB_HIV_Drugs/default.htm. Other notable interactions with rifamycins include warfarin, most antiseizure medications, and many antirejection medications given for bone marrow and solid-organ transplants. The safest practice is to review all medications when treating someone with a rifamycin.

TABLE 87.3

SUMMARY OF RECOMMENDATIONS FOR TUBERCULOSIS TREATMENT THAT ARE SUPPORTED BY RANDOMIZED CONTROLLED TRIALS

Treatment for known or suspected drug-susceptible tuberculosis, initial phase
1. INH, RIF, PZA, EMB 7 d/wk for 56 doses (8 wk) [60]
Adjunctive corticosteroids are recommended for:
1. Tuberculous meningitis—improved survival and fewer serious adverse events [66]
2. Tuberculous pericarditis—improved survival and decreased need for repeat pericardiocentesis but no decreased risk of constrictive pericarditis [67]
Early initiation of antiretroviral therapy is recommended for patients co-infected with TB and HIV
1. Start ART in the first 2 weeks of TB treatment for HIV-infected patients with a CD4 < 200 [71]

INFECTION CONTROL AND RESPIRATORY ISOLATION

Preventing Nosocomial Transmission

Early suspicion for TB is the most important step in preventing transmission because it allows the appropriate use of effective respiratory isolation, prompt diagnostic evaluation, and initiation of effective treatment. Screening for active TB is generally achieved through the collection of three successive morning sputa for AFB smear. However, nearly half of patients with pulmonary TB are smear negative, and smear-negative patients are able to transmit infection [72]. Therefore, hospitalized patients with negative sputum smears but a high risk for TB should be kept in respiratory isolation until an alternative diagnosis is made or empiric TB treatment has been initiated for several days. The infectiousness of TB begins to decrease within days after initiating effective therapy, probably by decreasing the cough as well as by reducing the number of tubercle bacilli. Decisions about discontinuing isolation once treatment is instituted should be carefully individualized, avoiding a decision based only on the number of days on therapy. The safest approach in a patient receiving treatment in the hospital is to continue isolation until three sputum smears are negative, particularly when drug susceptibilities are unknown. Other measures that may be of benefit in intubated patient include the use of a closed suctioning system to avoid generating infectious aerosols and the use of submicron filters for air exhausted from ventilators [25].

All healthcare workers who will be exposed to potentially infectious TB patients should use personal protective devices. Properly fitted masks capable of filtering at least 95% of particles 1 μm in size are recommended with fit-testing to ensure a face-seal leakage of less than 10%. Powered air-purifying respirators with a helmet or hood are a more effective and more expensive option. These could be considered in certain high-risk situations such as an unavoidable bronchoscopy of an infectious case of TB. Periodic tuberculin testing of hospital personnel should be continued as a means of monitoring the effectiveness of other measures and of evaluating tuberculin converters and providing treatment when appropriate [25].

Public Health Aspects

Presumptive and confirmed cases of TB should be promptly reported to the local public health department as required by law in every state. The function of this reporting is to provide the opportunity to conduct timely contact investigations, which may be critical to prevent life-threatening complications of TB among small children or immunocompromised household members. In addition, many health departments can assist in ensuring completion of outpatient therapy and thus prevent a hospital readmission for treatment failure or relapse with drug-resistant TB.

Treatment recommendations for TB, based on randomized controlled trials, are summarized in Table 87.3.

References

1. World Health Organization: *Global Tuberculosis Control*. Geneva, Switzerland, 2009.
2. CDC. Reported Tuberculosis in the United States, 2009. Atlanta, GA: U.S. Department of Health and Human Services, CDC, October 2010.
3. Gandhi NR, Moll A, Sturm AW, et al: Extensively drug-resistant tuberculosis as a cause of death in patients co-infected with tuberculosis and HIV in a rural area of South Africa. *Lancet* 368(9547):1575–1580, 2006.
4. World Health Organization: *Anti-Tuberculosis Drug Resistance in the World, Fourth Global Report*. Geneva, Switzerland, 2008.
5. Frame RN, Johnson MC, Eichenhorn MS, et al: Active tuberculosis in the medical intensive care unit: a 15-year retrospective analysis. *Crit Care Med* 15(11):1012–1014, 1987.
6. Rao VK, Iademarco EP, Fraser VJ, et al: The impact of comorbidity on mortality following in-hospital diagnosis of tuberculosis. *Chest* 114(5):1244–1252, 1998.
7. Lee PL, Jerng JS, Chang YL, et al: Patient mortality of active pulmonary tuberculosis requiring mechanical ventilation. *Eur Respir J* 22(1):141–147, 2003.
8. Zahar JR, Azoulay E, Klement E, et al: Delayed treatment contributes to mortality in ICU patients with severe active pulmonary tuberculosis and acute respiratory failure. *Intensive Care Med* 27(3):513–520, 2001.
9. Sacks LV, Pendle S: Factors related to in-hospital deaths in patients with tuberculosis. *Arch Intern Med* 158(17):1916–1922, 1998.

10. Erbes R, Oettel K, Raffenberg M, et al: Characteristics and outcome of patients with active pulmonary tuberculosis requiring intensive care. *Eur Respir J* 27(6):1223–1228, 2006.
11. American Thoracic Society/Centers for Disease Control and Prevention. Diagnostic standards and classification of tuberculosis in adults and children. *Am J Respir Crit Care Med* 161(4 Pt 1):1376–1395, 2000.
12. Horsburgh CR Jr: Priorities for the treatment of latent tuberculosis infection in the United States. *N Engl J Med* 350(20):2060–2067, 2004.
13. Lillebaek T, Dirksen A, Baess I, et al: Molecular evidence of endogenous reactivation of *Mycobacterium tuberculosis* after 33 years of latent infection. *J Infect Dis* 185(3):401–404, 2002.
14. Centers for Disease Control and Prevention. Targeted tuberculin testing and treatment of latent tuberculosis infection. *MMWR Morb Mortal Wkly Rep* 49(RR-6), 2000.
15. Slavin RE, Walsh TJ, Pollack AD: Late generalized tuberculosis: a clinical pathologic analysis and comparison of 100 cases in the preantibiotic and antibiotic eras. *Medicine* 59:352–366, 1980.
16. Greenaway C, Menzies D, Fanning A, et al: Delay in diagnosis among hospitalized patients with active tuberculosis—predictors and outcomes. *Am J Respir Crit Care Med* 165(7):927–933, 2002.
17. Dooley KE, Golub J, Goes FS, et al: Empiric treatment of community-acquired pneumonia with fluoroquinolones, and delays in the treatment of tuberculosis. *Clin Infect Dis* 34(12):1607–1612, 2002.
18. Penner C, Roberts D, Kunimoto D, et al: Tuberculosis as a primary cause of respiratory failure requiring mechanical ventilation. *Am J Respir Crit Care Med* 151(3 Pt 1):867–872, 1995.
19. Levy H, Kallenbach JM, Feldman C, et al: Acute respiratory failure in active tuberculosis. *Crit Care Med* 15(3):221–225, 1987.
20. Braidy J, Pothel C, Amra S: Miliary tuberculosis presenting as adrenal failure. *Can Med Assoc J* 124(6):748–749, 1981.
21. Peto HM, Pratt RH, Harrington TA, et al: Epidemiology of extrapulmonary tuberculosis in the United States, 1993–2006. *Clin Infect Dis* 49(9):1350–1357, 2009.
22. Sanyika C, Corr P, Royston D, et al: Pulmonary angiography and embolization for severe hemoptysis due to cavitary pulmonary tuberculosis. *Cardiovasc Intervent Radiol* 22(6):457–460, 1999.
23. Husen L, Fulkerson LL, Del Vecchio E, et al: Pulmonary tuberculosis with negative findings on chest x-ray films: a study of 40 cases. *Chest* 60(6):540–542, 1971.
24. Pedro-Botet J, Gutierrez J, Miralles R, et al: Pulmonary tuberculosis in HIV-infected patients with normal chest radiographs. *AIDS* 6(1):91–93, 1992.
25. Centers for Disease Control and Prevention. Guidelines for preventing the transmission of *Mycobacterium tuberculosis* in health-care settings. *MMWR Morb Mortal Wkly Rep* 54(RR-17), 2005.
26. Brown M, Varia H, Bassett P, et al: Prospective study of sputum induction, gastric washing, and bronchoalveolar lavage for the diagnosis of pulmonary tuberculosis in patients who are unable to expectorate. *Clin Infect Dis* 44(11):1415–1420, 2007.
27. Sharma SK, Mohan A, Sharma A, et al: Miliary tuberculosis: new insights into an old disease. *Lancet Infect Dis* 5(7):415–430, 2005.
28. Ferrer J: Tuberculous pleural effusion and tuberculous empyema. *Semin Respir Crit Care Med* 22(6):637–646, 2001.
29. Frye MD, Pozsik CJ, Sahn SA: Tuberculous pleurisy is more common in AIDS than in non-AIDS patients with tuberculosis. *Chest* 112(2):393–397, 1997.
30. Keiper MD, Beumont M, Elshami A, et al: CD4 T lymphocyte count and the radiographic presentation of pulmonary tuberculosis. A study of the relationship between these factors in patients with human immunodeficiency virus infection. *Chest* 107(1):74–80, 1995.
31. Johnson TM, McCann W, Davey WN: Tuberculous bronchopleural fistula. *Am Rev Respir Dis* 107(1):30–41, 1973.
32. Epstein DM, Kline LR, Albelda SM, et al: Tuberculous pleural effusions. *Chest* 91(1):106–109, 1987.
33. Zemlin AE, Burgess LJ, Carstens ME: The diagnostic utility of adenosine deaminase isoenzymes in tuberculous pleural effusions. *Int J Tuberc Lung Dis* 13(2):214–220, 2009.
34. Dheda K, van Zyl-Smit RN, Sechi LA, et al: Utility of quantitative T-cell responses versus unstimulated interferon-{gamma} for the diagnosis of pleural tuberculosis. *Eur Respir J* 34(5):1118–1126, 2009.
35. Kirsch CM, Kroe DM, Azzi RL, et al: The optimal number of pleural biopsy specimens for a diagnosis of tuberculous pleurisy. *Chest* 112(3):702–706, 1997.
36. Maartens G, Willcox PA, Benatar SR: Miliary tuberculosis: rapid diagnosis, hematologic abnormalities, and outcome in 109 treated adults. *Am J Med* 89(3):291–296, 1990.
37. Singh N, Paterson DL: *Mycobacterium tuberculosis* infection in solid-organ transplant recipients: impact and implications for management. *Clin Infect Dis* 27(5):1266–1277, 1998.
38. Hill AR, Premkumar S, Brustein S, et al: Disseminated tuberculosis in the acquired immunodeficiency syndrome era. *Am Rev Respir Dis* 144(5):1164–1170, 1991.
39. Gachot B, Wolff M, Clair B, et al: Severe tuberculosis in patients with human immunodeficiency virus infection. *Intensive Care Med* 16(8):491–493, 1990.
40. Ahuja SS, Ahuja SK, Phelps KR, et al: Hemodynamic confirmation of septic shock in disseminated tuberculosis. *Crit Care Med* 20(6):901–903, 1992.
41. Kim JY, Park YB, Kim YS, et al: Miliary tuberculosis and acute respiratory distress syndrome. *Int J Tuberc Lung Dis* 7(4):359–364, 2003.
42. Kennedy C, Knowles GK: Miliary tuberculosis presenting with skin lesions. *Br Med J* 3:356, 1975.
43. Bouza E, Diaz-Lopez MD, Moreno S, et al: *Mycobacterium tuberculosis* bacteremia in patients with and without human immunodeficiency virus infection. *Arch Intern Med* 153(4):496–500, 1993.
44. Cucin RL, Coleman M, Eckardt JJ, et al: The diagnosis of miliary tuberculosis: utility of peripheral blood abnormalities, bone marrow and liver needle biopsy. *J Chronic Dis* 26(6):355–361, 1973.
45. Rock RB, Olin M, Baker CA, et al: Central nervous system tuberculosis: pathogenesis and clinical aspects. *Clin Microbiol Rev* 21(2):243–261, table of contents, 2008.
46. Thwaites G, Fisher M, Hemingway C, et al: British Infection Society guidelines for the diagnosis and treatment of tuberculosis of the central nervous system in adults and children. *J Infect* 59(3):167–187, 2009.
47. Dube MP, Holtom PD, Larsen RA: Tuberculous meningitis in patients with and without human immunodeficiency virus infection. *Am J Med* 93(5):520–524, 1992.
48. Breen RA, Smith CJ, Bettinson H, et al: Paradoxical reactions during tuberculosis treatment in patients with and without HIV co-infection. *Thorax* 59(8):704–707, 2004.
49. Lawn SD, Bekker LG, Miller RF: Immune reconstitution disease associated with mycobacterial infections in HIV-infected individuals receiving antiretrovirals. *Lancet Infect Dis* 5(6):361–373, 2005.
50. Stead WW: Tuberculosis among elderly persons: an outbreak in a nursing home. *Ann Intern Med* 94(5):606–610, 1981.
51. Khan MA, Kovnat DM, Bachus B, et al: Clinical and roentgenographic spectrum of pulmonary tuberculosis in the adult. *Am J Med* 62(1):31–38, 1977.
52. Miller WT, MacGregor RR: Tuberculosis: frequency of unusual radiographic findings. *Am J Roentgenol* 130(5):867–875, 1978.
53. Burman WJ, Jones BE: Clinical and radiographic features of HIV-related tuberculosis. *Semin Respir Infect* 18(4):263–271, 2003.
54. Centers for Disease Control and Prevention. Guidelines for using the QuantiFERON-TB Gold test for detecting *Mycobacterium tuberculosis* infection, United States. *MMWR Morb Mortal Wkly Rep* 54(RR-15):49–55, 2005.
55. Holden M, Dubin MR, Diamond PH: Frequency of negative intermediate-strength tuberculin sensitivity in patients with active tuberculosis. *N Engl J Med* 285(27):1506–1509, 1971.
56. Pai M, Zwerling A, Menzies D: Systematic review: T-cell-based assays for the diagnosis of latent tuberculosis infection: an update. *Ann Intern Med* 149(3):177–184, 2008.
57. Piersimoni C, Scarparo C: Relevance of commercial amplification methods for direct detection of *Mycobacterium tuberculosis* complex in clinical samples. *J Clin Microbiol* 41(12):5355–5365, 2003.
58. Ruiz-Manzano J, Manterola JM, Gamboa F, et al: Detection of mycobacterium tuberculosis in paraffin-embedded pleural biopsy specimens by commercial ribosomal RNA and DNA amplification kits. *Chest* 118(3):648–655, 2000.
59. Pai M, Flores LL, Pai N, et al: Diagnostic accuracy of nucleic acid amplification tests for tuberculous meningitis: a systematic review and meta-analysis. *Lancet Infect Dis* 3(10):633–643, 2003.
60. American Thoracic Society, CDC, Infectious Disease Society of America: Treatment of tuberculosis. *MMWR Recomm Rep* 52(RR-11), 2003
61. Bwanga F, Hoffner S, Haile M, et al: Direct susceptibility testing for multi drug resistant tuberculosis: a meta-analysis. *BMC Infect Dis* 9:67, 2009.
62. Centers for Disease Control and Prevention: Reported tuberculosis in the United States, 2004. Atlanta, GA, U.S. Department of Health and Human Services, CDC, 2005.
63. Weis SE, Slocum PC, Blais FX, et al: The effect of directly observed therapy on the rates of drug resistance and relapse in tuberculosis. *N Engl J Med* 330:1179–1184, 1994.
64. Iseman MD: Treatment of multidrug-resistant tuberculosis. *N Engl J Med* 329:784–791, 1993.
65. Peloquin CA: Using therapeutic drug monitoring to dose the antimycobacterial drugs. *Clin Chest Med* 18:79–87, 1997.
66. Thwaites GE, Nguyen DB, Nguyen HD, et al: Dexamethasone for the treatment of tuberculous meningitis in adolescents and adults. *N Engl J Med* 351(17):1741–1751, 2004.
67. Strang JI, Kakaza HH, Gibson DG, et al: Controlled clinical trial of complete open surgical drainage and of prednisolone in treatment of tuberculous pericardial effusion in Transkei. *Lancet* 2:759–764, 1988.
68. Smego RA, Ahmed N: A systematic review of the adjunctive use of systemic corticosteroids for pulmonary tuberculosis. *Int J Tuberc Lung Dis* 7(3):208–213, 2003.
69. Davidson PT, Le HQ: Drug treatment of tuberculosis—1992. *Drugs* 43(5):651–673, 1992.
70. Saukkonen JJ, Cohn DL, Jasmer RM, et al: An official ATS statement: hepatotoxicity of antituberculosis therapy. *Am J Respir Crit Care Med* 174(8):935–952, 2006.
71. Piggott DA, Karakousis PC: Timing of antiretroviral therapy for HIV in the setting of TB treatment. *Clin Dev Immunol* 2011. Article ID 103917, 10 pages.
72. Behr MA, Warren SA, Salamon H, et al: Transmission of *Mycobacterium tuberculosis* from patients smear-negative for acid-fast bacilli. *Lancet* 353(9151):444–449, 1999.

CHAPTER 88 ■ BOTULISM

MARY DAWN T. CO AND RICHARD T. ELLISON, III

The name botulism is derived from the Latin term *botulus* for sausage. Justinus Kerner (1786–1862) first recognized the association between the mysterious "sausage poison" and paralytic illnesses in 1820. *Clostridium botulinum*, the etiologic agent of botulism, is an anaerobic, spore-forming organism that elaborates a neurotoxin that prevents the release of acetylcholine. Illness develops after toxin exposure, and patients present with a symmetric descending paralysis that characteristically begins with dysarthria, diplopia, dysphonia, or dysphagia. The most common botulism syndromes include food-borne, wound, and infant botulism. Botulism toxin is also now used therapeutically in neuromuscular and ophthalmologic disorders as well as a cosmetic enhancement tool, and cases of iatrogenic botulism have occurred. Although the majority of cases are due to infant botulism, food-borne botulism is considered a public health emergency as there is always a potential that a large number of individuals may have been exposed. Additionally, botulinum is a category A biological agent, and any case must initially be considered as potentially linked to a bioterrorist event (see Chapter 213).

PATHOGENESIS

C. botulinum is an anaerobic Gram-positive bacillus that produces heat-resistant spores that can survive boiling. Under conditions of an anaerobic environment, low acidity (pH greater than 4.6), and low temperature, the organism can germinate, grow, and produce a neurotoxin that itself is readily inactivated by heat (greater than 85°C for 5 minutes) [1].

Seven distinct antigenic neurotoxins (A through G) may be produced by *C. botulinum* but only four types—A, B, E, and F—are associated with human disease. Food-borne botulism occurs after the ingestion of preformed toxin in foods contaminated by spores. Wound botulism occurs when spores infect traumatized or contaminated skin. Infant botulism occurs in infants 3 to 26 weeks old after intestinal colonization by *C. botulinum* [2]. Botulism of undetermined etiology occurs in adults whose intestinal flora has been altered or whose gastric barrier has been compromised because of intestinal surgery, gastric achlorhydria, or antibiotic therapy [2,3].

All botulinum toxins have the same mechanism of action [2]. The toxin is carried via the bloodstream to the neuromuscular junction where it binds irreversibly and thereby produces paralysis. However, it does not affect the central nervous system or the adrenergic nervous system [1]. The toxin is a zinc-containing endopeptidase that cleaves to specific sites on three proteins (VAMP, SNAP25, syntaxin), interfering with the release of acetylcholine [4].

EPIDEMIOLOGY

There have been approximately 20 cases of food-borne botulism yearly in the United States, with the majority of cases caused by toxin type A (50%), followed by toxin type E (37%), and then toxin type B (10%) [5]. Food-borne botulism has traditionally been associated with home-processed foods. However, an increasing number of cases have been associated with commercially prepared foods that have inadvertently been processed in a manner that allowed the production of the toxin.

Wound botulism has primarily been seen in intravenous drug users who present with cranial nerve palsies in the setting of abscesses from heroin use [6]. California has accounted for over 75% of U.S. cases, with an epidemic noted in individuals injecting black tar heroin [7].

Iatrogenic botulism has rarely developed after botulinum toxin (Botox) has been injected for cosmetic or neurologic purposes [8,9]. Although the normal concentration of botulinum toxin A in the therapeutic preparation allows for a large margin of safety with minimal treatment side effects, therapeutic doses have been reported to cause generalized muscle weakness with widespread electromyogram (EMG) abnormalities typical of botulism [10]. In addition, four individuals have contracted botulism after receiving unlicensed preparations of botulinum toxin for cosmetic purposes [11].

Botulism toxin is the most poisonous substance known to man with 1 g of toxin able to potentially kill 1 million people [9]. Given its ease of production and transport, it is a major bioterrorism threat and is classified as a category A biological agent. Botulism toxin was used as a bioweapon in the 1930s by the Japanese military who fed cultures of *C. botulinum* to prisoners during that country's occupation of Manchuria [12]. Aerosols derived from botulism toxin were also dispersed in Japan on at least three different occasions by a Japanese cult, although for unclear reasons these terrorist attempts failed [12] (see Chapter 213).

CLINICAL MANIFESTATIONS

Clinical manifestations of all forms of botulism are similar. Cardinal features include (a) cranial nerve palsies, (b) descending paralysis, (c) symmetry in symptoms, (d) absence of fever, (e) clear sensorium, and (f) lack of sensory findings [1]. Food-borne botulism may be preceded by gastrointestinal symptoms such as cramps, nausea, vomiting, and diarrhea [2,12]. Infant botulism is usually characterized by a history of constipation and feeding difficulties [2,12].

Patients may complain of dry mouth secondary to parasympathetic blockade as well as neurologic symptoms such as dysphagia, dysphonia, diplopia, and dysarthria related to palsies of the bulbar musculature. Symptoms then progress to involve lower extremity weakness and loss of the protective gag reflex requiring respiratory support. Physical examination is significant for a lack of fever except in cases of wound botulism with secondarily infected wounds. Sensory findings are absent except for periorbital paresthesias secondary to hyperventilation. Deep tendon reflexes, although present initially, usually disappear. Ocular findings are common and include dilated, poorly reactive, or fixed pupils, ptosis, nystagmus, and sixth cranial nerve dysfunction. A clear sensorium is usually present because the toxin does not usually penetrate the central nervous system [2,12].

The incubation period of food-borne botulism is usually 12 to 36 hours after toxin ingestion but may be as short as 2 hours [2,12]. Severity of disease depends on the amount of toxin that is absorbed into the system. Mortality has improved with the advances in critical care, and eventual recovery is seen in 95% of cases in the United States [8]. The recovery period may be protracted and is dependent on the reinnervation of paralyzed muscle fibers [13,14].

DIAGNOSIS

Successful diagnosis of botulism requires a high index of suspicion for the disease, given that the symptoms and laboratory values are often nonspecific. If there is a suspected case of botulism, the local state health department should be notified [15]. The Centers for Disease Control (CDC) can also be contacted through its 24-hour botulism consultation service for additional information [8]. Prior to the administration of antitoxin, a serum sample (10 to 15 mL) should be collected and refrigerated. Anaerobic cultures and toxin assays of stool, serum, and gastric aspirates, suspected foodstuff, or wounds should be collected. Early cases are more likely to be diagnosed by toxin detection, while later cases are confirmed by culture [16]. The only acceptable method for the detection of the botulism neurotoxin is the mouse bioassay in which a patient's serum or supernatant from a culture of the patient specimens suspected to contain toxin is administered to pairs of mice with and without toxin, serving to confirm the diagnosis and define the circulating toxin. However, a recent study on clinical wound botulism revealed the sensitivity of the assay to be only 68% [17].

DIFFERENTIAL DIAGNOSIS

Diseases mistaken for botulism include brainstem infarction, polyradiculopathies such as the Guillain–Barre syndrome or its Miller Fisher variant, myasthenia gravis (MG), brainstem infarction, tick paralysis, polio, meningitis or encephalitis, and poisonings such as carbon monoxide, shellfish, or organophosphate poisoning [1,7]. An improvement of strength after the edrophonium test is suggestive of MG but has also been reported in botulism [18]. The Guillain–Barre syndrome is characterized by an ascending paralysis and usually, but not always, an elevated cerebrospinal fluid protein level initially. Electrophysiologic studies may be helpful in distinguishing between causes of flaccid paralysis such as MG, the Guillain–Barre syndrome, and the Lambert–Eaton syndrome. Normal nerve conduction velocity, absence of sensory deficits, and a small increment of motor response seen on repetitive nerve stimulation at 20 Hz (as compared to the 4 Hz in MG) are characteristic of botulism. Tick paralysis is diagnosed by the presence of an embedded *Dermacentor* tick. Altered mental status is usually seen in encephalitis, organophosphate, and carbon monoxide poisonings rather than botulism. Shellfish poisoning presents with tremors and paresthesias that are usually absent in botulism [1].

TREATMENT

The mortality rate from botulism has decreased dramatically since the first decades of the 20th century to its current rate of 3% to 5% with the advent of intensive care units [19], and all patients suspected of botulism should initially be monitored in an intensive care setting.

Therapy consists of toxin removal, supportive care, including nutritional support and treatment of secondary infections, and passive immunization with equine antitoxin [2]. Patients should be assessed and monitored for the adequacy of cough, the control of oropharyngeal secretions, and ventilation. Readers can refer to the Chapter 50 on extrapulmonary causes of respiratory failure for guidelines on how to monitor for the adequacy of ventilation and when to consider endotracheal intubation (Chapters 1 and 58), and to the Chapter 59 on invasive mechanical ventilation for guidelines on how to ventilate patients with respiratory failure due to neuromuscular diseases. Studies in infants have suggested that a reverse Trendelenburg position (20 to 25 degrees) may be helpful in nonintubated patients by reducing the entry of oral secretions and also by improved respiratory mechanics [4].

For adults and older children, passive immunization with equine antitoxin should be administered as soon as botulism is diagnosed. Antitoxin will only neutralize toxin molecules that have not bound to nerve endings. Timely administration minimizes subsequent nerve damage and severity of disease but will not reverse existing paralytic damage [20]. There are several antitoxins available including an FDA (U.S. Food and Drug Administration)-approved bivalent antitoxin containing antibodies to toxins A and B, and a non–FDA approved BAT-E (Botulism antitoxin E); both of these are available through the CDC [12]. Additionally, there is a heptavalent (A–G) despeciated antitoxin available through the U.S. Army. Clinicians should contact their local state health departments or the CDC (770-488-7100) or U.S. Army Medical Research Institute of Infectious Diseases (USAMRIID) (888-872-7443) to obtain these antitoxins. Patients should be skin tested prior to antitoxin administration and desensitized using the protocol enclosed with the antitoxin if there is any evidence of a wheal and flare reaction.

Equine antitoxin is not recommended for treatment of infants suspected of botulism because of the potential serious side effects of serum sickness and anaphylaxis. However, a recent study found that the administration of human botulism immune globulin intravenous within 72 hours of hospitalization for suspected infant botulism decreased illness severity, shortened hospital stays, and reduced costs [21]. This preparation, human botulism immune globulin (Baby-BIG), is now FDA agent approved and available through the California Department of Public Health.

Patients with wound botulism also require aggressive wound debridement regardless of how well the wound appears as toxin is produced until the infection is eliminated. Antitoxin should be administered prior to surgery to neutralize toxin released by the procedure. Penicillin therapy, 10 to 20 million units per day, is appropriate [4,7]. Aminoglycosides and clindamycin should be avoided because of the potential for neuromuscular blockade [22,23].

Because botulinum toxin is not absorbed through intact skin, standard precautions should be undertaken when caring for patients suspected of botulism. There have been no cases of human-to-human transmission described [8].

Advances in botulism, based on randomized controlled trials, are summarized in Table 88.1.

TABLE 88.1

RECOMMENDATIONS FOR THE TREATMENT OF BOTULISM BASED ON RANDOMIZED CLINICAL TRIALS

- Treatment with the drug, human botulism immune globuliln, intravenously given within 3 d of hospital admission for infant botulism shortens length and cost of the hospital stay and the length of illness.[a]

[a] Arnon SS, Schechter R, Maslanka SE, et al: Human botulism immune globulin for the treatment of infant botulism. *N Engl J Med* 354(5): 462–471, 2006.

References

1. Gantz N: Botulism, in Rippe JM, Fink MP, Cerra FB (eds): *Intensive Care Medicine*, 3rd ed. Boston, MA, Little, Brown and Company, 1996, pp 1224–1227.
2. Centers for Disease Control: *Botulism in the United States 1899–1996: Handbook for Epidemiologists, Clinicians and Laboratory Workers*. Atlanta, GA, CDC, 1998.
3. Bartlett JC: Infant botulism in adults. *N Engl J Med* 1315:254–255, 1986.
4. Arnon SS, Schechter R, Inglesby TV, et al: Botulinum toxin as a biological weapon: medical and public health management. *JAMA* 285:1059–1070, 2001.
5. Sobel J, Tucker N, Sulka A, et al: Foodborne botulism in the United States, 1990–2000. *Emerg Infect Dis* 10:1606–1611, 2004.
6. MacDonald KL, Rutherford GW, Friedman SM, et al: Botulism and botulism-like illness in chronic drug abusers. *Ann Intern Med* 102:616–618, 1985.
7. Werner SB, Passaro D, McGee J, et al: Wound botulism in California 1951–1998: recent epidemic in heroin injectors. *Clin Infect Dis* 31:1018–1024, 2000.
8. Sobel J: Botulism. *Clin Infect Dis* 41:1167–1173, 2005.
9. Ting PT, Freiman A: The story of Clostridium botulinum: from food poisoning to Botox. *Clin Med* 4:258–261, 2004.
10. Bakheit AM, Ward CD, McLellan DL: Generalised botulism-like syndrome after intramuscular injections of botulinum toxin type A: a report of two cases. *J Neurol Neurosurg Psychiatry* 62:198, 1997.
11. Chertow DS, Tan ET, Maslanka SE, et al: Botulism in 4 adults following cosmetic injections with an unlicensed, highly concentrated botulinum preparation. *JAMA* 296:2476–2479, 2006.
12. Dembek ZF, Smith LA, Rusnak JM: Botulism: cause, effects, diagnosis, clinical and laboratory identification, and treatment modalities. *Disaster Med Public Health Prep* 1:122–134, 2007.
13. Duchen LW: Motor nerve growth induced by botulinum toxin as a regenerative phenomenon. *Proc R Soc Med* 65:196–197, 1972.
14. Mann JM, Martin S, Hoffman R, et al: Patient recovery from type A botulism: morbidity assessment following a large outbreak. *Am J Public Health* 71:266–269, 1981.
15. Shapiro RL, Hatheway C, Becher J, et al: Botulism surveillance and emergency response. A public health strategy for a global challenge. *JAMA* 278:433–435, 1997.
16. Woodruff BA, Griffin PM, McCroskey LM, et al: Clinical and laboratory comparison of botulism from toxin types A, B, and E in the United States, 1975–1988. *J Infect Dis* 166:1281–1286, 1992.
17. Wheeler C, Inami G, Mohle-Boetani J, et al: Sensitivity of mouse bioassay in clinical wound botulism. *Clin Infect Dis* 48:1669–1673, 2009.
18. Cherington M: Electrophysiologic methods as an aid in diagnosis of botulism: a review. *Muscle Nerve* 5:S28–S29, 1982.
19. Gangarosa EJ, Donadio JA, Armstrong RW, et al: Botulism in the United States, 1899–1969. *Am J Epidemiol* 93:93–101, 1971.
20. Tacket CO, Shandera WX, Mann JM, et al: Equine antitoxin use and other factors that predict outcome in type A foodborne botulism. *Am J Med* 76:794–798, 1984.
21. Arnon SS, Schechter R, Maslanka SE, et al: Human botulism immune globulin for the treatment of infant botulism. *N Engl J Med* 354:462–471, 2006.
22. Santos JI, Swensen P, Glasgow LA: Potentiation of Clostridium botulinum toxin aminoglycoside antibiotics: clinical and laboratory observations. *Pediatrics* 68:50–54, 1981.
23. Schulze J, Toepfer M, Schroff KC, et al: Clindamycin and nicotinic neuromuscular transmission. *Lancet* 354:1792–1793, 1999.

CHAPTER 89 ■ TETANUS

MARY DAWN T. CO AND RICHARD T. ELLISON, III

Tetanus, caused by the neurotoxin tetanospasmin, is produced by the anaerobic spore forming Gram-positive bacterium *Clostridium tetani*. Clinically, tetanus presents with skeletal muscle rigidity and spasms that classically involve the muscles of the face (lockjaw). It is a relatively rare clinical entity in developed countries because of the broad use of tetanus toxoid immunization. However, tetanus still occurs frequently in the Third World, and in individuals who have never been or have been inadequately vaccinated in the setting of a wound infection or another portal of entry. Diagnosis is based on clinical suspicion and the exclusion of other entities because of a lack of timely confirmatory testing. Treatment relies mainly on respiratory support and symptomatic management of the muscular rigidity and spasms and the autonomic manifestations of the disease.

PATHOGENESIS

Clostridium tetani is an obligate anaerobic spore-forming bacillus. Mature organisms develop spores that are widely distributed in soil and dust as well as in the intestines and feces of animals. While the bacteria are sensitive to heat and aerobic conditions, the spores are resistant to ethanol, phenol, and formalin. However, they do not survive treatment with iodine, glutaraldehyde, hydrogen peroxide, or autoclaving at 121°C and 103 kPa (15 psi) for 15 minutes [1].

The vegetative form of *C. tetani* produces two types of zinc metalloproteinase toxins, tetanospasmin and tetanolysin, with tetanospasmin playing more of a prominent role in pathogenesis. Unlike the toxin produced by *Clostridium botulinum*, the *C. tetani* neurotoxin is of a single antigenic type and specifically targets the central nervous system (CNS), including the peripheral motor end plates, spinal cord, brain, and the sympathetic nervous system [1,2]. Although this toxin can exert an excitatory effect, it acts primarily by blocking the release of neurotransmitters such as glycine and γ-aminobutyric acid (GABA), which normally acts to inhibit the transmission of motor nerve impulses. Specifically, the toxin degrades synaptobrevin, a protein required for contact of inhibitory neurotransmitter vesicles with their release site on the presynaptic membrane [3].

Antitoxin is of therapeutic value only in protecting neurons that have not already bound the toxin. As the effect of the toxin on a synapse does not appear reversible, recovery from tetanus depends on the generation of new nerve terminals and new synapse formation.

EPIDEMIOLOGY

Tetanus is endemic in the developing world with neonatal tetanus accounting for the majority (>50%) of deaths due to tetanus [4]. Tetanus is a rare disease in the developed world with morbidity and mortality in the United States declining steadily, due to the availability of tetanus vaccines, improved wound management, and the use of tetanus immunoglobulin for postexposure prophylaxis [5]. According to the 1998 to 2000 surveillance data, an average of 43 tetanus cases occurred yearly in the United States with the majority of cases related to acute injuries such as puncture wounds, lacerations, and abrasions [6]. The highest incidences were reported in individuals ≥60 years old, persons of Hispanic origin, older adults with diabetes, and intravenous drug users. No deaths were reported in those individuals who received adequate immunization.

CLINICAL MANIFESTATIONS

Tetanus usually occurs in the setting of necrotic or infected tissue in which anaerobic bacterial growth is facilitated. However, in up to 30% of cases, no acute injury is reported [6]. The incubation period for tetanus varies from 3 to 21 days, with the length of the incubation period dependent on how far the injury site is from the CNS [7]. The first nerves affected are the shortest, accounting for the early symptoms of facial distortion and neck stiffness. It has been found that the shorter the incubation period, the worse the prognosis [8].

Clinical tetanus can present in three forms—local, cephalic, and generalized—with 80% of cases being generalized. Local tetanus presents as a focal region of muscle contraction at a site of spore inoculation [1]. Symptoms may persist but usually resolve spontaneously. *Cephalic tetanus* develops after a traumatic head injury, but has been reported after otitis media when *C. tetanus* was present in the middle ear [9]. Typically, there is involvement of the cranial nerves, especially cranial nerve VII in the facial area.

Generalized tetanus typically presents with involvement of facial musculature, starting with masseter rigidity (lockjaw or trismus) and risus sardonicus (orbicularis oris), and then progresses in a descending fashion with difficulty swallowing and abdominal rigidity [1]. Spasms, which are often triggered by sensory stimuli, are common and may resemble seizures with flexion of the arms and the extension of legs (opisthotonus). The patient does not lose consciousness and severe pain usually accompanies the spasms. Laryngospasm and respiratory compromise may result from vocal cord or diaphragmatic spasms and upper airway obstruction. In addition, fractures of the spine or the long bones, dislocations, and rhabdomyolysis may occur as a result of spasms. The course of this illness occurs over 2 weeks, reflecting the time it takes for intraaxonal toxin to travel to the CNS. Spasms occur within the first 2 weeks of illness followed by autonomic disturbances such as extremes in blood pressure and cardiac arrhythmias including sinus tachycardia and cardiac arrest [10,11]. Individuals with tetanus are at high risk for nosocomial pneumonia with an incidence of approximately 35%. Autonomic dysfunction is an independent risk factor for pneumonia in patients with tetanus [12].

Neonatal tetanus, more often seen in developing countries, is a form of generalized tetanus that commonly arises when an unhealed umbilical stump becomes infected after an incision with an unsterile instrument and if the mother has not been adequately immunized [1,7].

DIAGNOSIS

No laboratory test is available that provides a definitive diagnosis of tetanus. Diagnosis is clinical and primarily based on the presence of trismus, dysphagia, muscular rigidity, and spasm, and confirmed by the detection of toxin in bodily fluids using mouse bioassays, microbiologic isolation from infected wounds, or by the use of real-time polymerase chain reaction (PCR) assays that detect a fragment of the neurotoxin gene of *C. tetani* [2]. The organism is isolated only 30% of the time in wound tetanus [7]. In addition, the presence of the bacteria does not necessarily indicate tetanus, since not all strains of *C. tetani* carry the toxin producing plasmid [2,13]. Antitetanus antibodies can be measured, although a minimally protective level of antibody concentration has not been established [14]. In individuals with tetanus, with the "spatula" test (sensitivity of 94% and specificity of 100%), insertion of a spatula into the patient's mouth induces a reflex spasm of the masseter instead of a gag reflex, leading to the patient biting the spatula [15].

Few other conditions present with muscular rigidity and sympathetic hyperreactivity except for strychnine poisoning. Strychnine blocks the inhibitory glycine receptor in the spinal cord and the brain. Unlike tetanus, however, the sudden contraction of all striated muscles is usually followed by complete relaxation of these muscles. Additional conditions that can mimic the spasms seen in tetanus include hypocalcemia and reactions to certain medications including neuroleptic drugs and central dopamine antagonists. Odontogenic infections can produce trismus but not the other manifestations of tetanus [1].

TREATMENT

The mortality rate in tetanus varies from 6% in mild to moderate tetanus up to 60% in the severest of cases [1,16]. Autonomic nervous system dysfunction has been shown to predict a poor outcome in mild to moderate cases of tetanus [17]. Illness is less severe among patients who have received a complete immunization series of tetanus toxoid compared with those who were never or inadequately vaccinated [18].

Individuals suspected of generalized tetanus should be observed in an intensive care setting with minimal stimuli. Initial management consists of airway stabilization and general intensive care support including mechanical ventilation, nutritional support, and deep venous thrombosis prophylaxis. Diagnostic evaluation should include blood samples for antitoxin levels, strychnine and dopamine antagonist assays, and electrolytes (including creatinine kinase), along with urine samples for toxicology and myoglobin levels [1]. Antihistamines such as benztropine or diphenhydramine should be administered to rule out a dystonic reaction to a dopamine-blocking agent.

Benzodiazepines such as midazolam, lorazepam, and diazepam have been the mainstay of treatment [1]. This class of agents acts as GABA agonists, thus indirectly opposing the effects of the toxin by competing for receptor sites [2]. Doses are initially titrated to produce sedation and limit reflex spasms. Propofol (alone or in combination with benzodiazepines) and intrathecal baclofen are alternative options that have been used [19,20]. Intravenous diazepam and lorazepam contain propylene glycol, which may increase the risk of lactic acidosis at the recommended doses of treatment [21]. If the muscle spasms cannot be controlled with these agents, a paralytic agent such as vecuronium can be added [1]. Once the symptoms have resolved, benzodiazepines should be tapered to prevent withdrawal.

If a portal of entry can be identified, the wound should be debrided and an antibiotic active against anaerobic organisms should be administered with metronidazole for 7 to 10 days now considered to be the first line of therapy. Treatment courses of 7 to 10 days using regimens of penicillin, either as a single-dose intramuscular benzathine dose or intravenous benzyl penicillin, are alternative regimens [1,22]. Passive immunization with human tetanus immunoglobulin (at a dose of

TABLE 89.1

RECOMMENDATIONS FOR THE TREATMENT OF *CLOSTRIDIUM TETANI* BASED ON RANDOMIZED CLINICAL TRIALS

- Treatment with metronidazole, benzyl penicillin, or intramuscular benzathine penicillin has a comparable impact on the need for tracheostomy; the use of neuromuscular blockade; the need for mechanical ventilation; and the incidences of dysautonomia, nosocomial pneumonia, and in hospital death [22].
- Treatment with intrathecal rather than intramuscular administration of antitetanus immunoglobulin showed better clinical progression including fewer respiratory complications and a significantly shorter duration of spasms [24].

500 units) may shorten the course and severity of tetanus by neutralizing toxin that has not reached the CNS [23]. A randomized clinical trial has found that patients treated with intrathecal rather than intramuscular administration of human antitetanus immunoglobulin showed better clinical progression including fewer respiratory complications and significantly shorter duration of spasms [24].

Autonomic dysfunction is usually related to excessive catecholamine release and can be treated by a combined alpha- and beta-blocker such as labetalol. Beta-blockade alone may result in severe hypertension due to an unopposed α effect [25].

Since the amount of toxin causing disease may be too small to induce a consistent immunological response, immunization with tetanus toxoid should be given at diagnosis, at 4 to 6 weeks and 1 year later to prevent future attacks [1,7].

Advances in tetanus, based on randomized controlled trials, are summarized in Table 89.1.

References

1. Bleck T: Clostridium tetani, in Mandell GL, Bennett JE, Dolin R (eds): *Principles and Practice of Infectious Diseases*. 6th ed. Philadelphia, Elsevier-Churchill Livingstone, 2005, pp 2817–2822.
2. Akbulut D, Grant KA, McLauchlin J: Improvement in laboratory diagnosis of wound botulism and tetanus among injecting illicit-drug users by use of real-time PCR assays for neurotoxin gene fragments. *J Clin Microbiol* 43(9):4342–4348, 2005.
3. Cornille F, Martin L, Lenoir C, et al: Cooperative exosite-dependent cleavage of synaptobrevin by tetanus toxin light chain. *J Biol Chem* 272(6):3459–3464, 1997.
4. Roper MH, Vandelaer JH, Gasse FL: Maternal and neonatal tetanus. *Lancet* 370(9603):1947–1959, 2007.
5. Kretsinger K, Srivastava P: Tetanus, in Roush SW, McIntyre L, Baldy LM (eds): *Manual for the Surveillance of Vaccine-Preventable Diseases*, Chapter 16, 4th ed. Atlanta, GA, Center for Disease Control and Prevention, 2008.
6. Pascual FB, McGinley EL, Zanardi LR, et al: Tetanus surveillance—United States, 1998–2000. *MMWR Surveill Summ* 52(3):1–8, 2003.
7. Centers for Disease Control and Prevention: in Atkinson W, Wolfe S, Hamborsky J, McIntyre L (eds): *Epidemiology and Prevention of Vaccine-Preventable Diseases*. 11th ed. Washington DC, Public Health Foundation, 2009, pp 273–282.
8. Veronesi R, Focaccia R: The Clinical Picture, in: Veronesi R (ed): *Tetanus: Important New Concepts*. Amsterdam, Excerpta Medica, 1981, pp 183–206.
9. Raghuram J, Ong YY, Wong SY: Tetanus in Singapore: report of three cases. *Ann Acad Med Singapore* 24(6):869–873, 1995.
10. Mitra RC, Gupta RD, Sack RB: Electrocardiographic changes in tetanus: a serial study. *J Indian Med Assoc* 89(6):164–167, 1991.
11. Kanarek DJ, Kaufman B, Zwi S: Severe sympathetic hyperactivity associated with tetanus. *Arch Intern Med* 132(4):602–604, 1973.
12. Cavalcante NJ, Sandeville ML, Medeiros EA: Incidence of and risk factors for nosocomial pneumonia in patients with tetanus. *Clin Infect Dis* 33(11):1842–1846, 2001.
13. Bleck T: Clinical aspects of tetanus, in Simpson L (ed): *Botulinum Neurotoxin and Tetanus Toxin*. New York, Academic Press, 1989, pp 379–398.
14. Goulon M, Girard O, Grosbuis S, et al: Antitetanus antibodies. Assay before anatoxinotherapy in 64 tetanus patients. *Nouv Presse Med* 1(45):3049–3050, 1972.
15. Apte NM, Karnad DR: Short report: the spatula test: a simple bedside test to diagnose tetanus. *Am J Trop Med Hyg* 53(4):386–387, 1995.
16. Nolla-Salas M, Garces-Bruses J: Severity of tetanus in patients older than 80 years: comparative study with younger patients. *Clin Infect Dis* 16(4):591–592, 1993.
17. Wasay M, Khealani BA, Talati N, et al: Autonomic nervous system dysfunction predicts poor prognosis in patients with mild to moderate tetanus. *BMC Neurol* 5(1):2, 2005.
18. Wassilak S, Orenstein W, Sutter R: Tetanus toxoid, in Plotkin S, Orenstein W (eds): *Vaccines*. 3rd ed. Philadelphia, WB Saunders, 1999, pp 441–474.
19. Borgeat A, Popovic V, Schwander D: Efficiency of a continuous infusion of propofol in a patient with tetanus. *Crit Care Med* 19(2):295–297, 1991.
20. Santos ML, Mota-Miranda A, Alves-Pereira A, et al: Intrathecal baclofen for the treatment of tetanus. *Clin Infect Dis* 38(3):321–328, 2004.
21. Kapoor W, Carey P, Karpf M: Induction of lactic acidosis with intravenous diazepam in a patient with tetanus. *Arch Intern Med* 141(7):944–945, 1981.
22. Ganesh Kumar AV, Kothari VM, Krishnan A, et al: Benzathine penicillin, metronidazole and benzyl penicillin in the treatment of tetanus: a randomized, controlled trial. *Ann Trop Med Parasitol* 98(1):59–63, 2004.
23. Blake PA, Feldman RA, Buchanan TM, et al: Serologic therapy of tetanus in the United States, 1965–1971. *JAMA* 235(1):42–44, 1976.
24. Miranda-Filho Dde B, Ximenes RA, Barone AA, et al: Randomised controlled trial of tetanus treatment with antitetanus immunoglobulin by the intrathecal or intramuscular route. *BMJ* 328(7440):615, 2004.
25. Domenighetti GM, Savary G, Stricker H: Hyperadrenergic syndrome in severe tetanus: extreme rise in catecholamines responsive to labetalol. *Br Med J (Clin Res Ed)* 288(6429):1483–1484, 1984.

CHAPTER 90 ■ SERIOUS EPIDEMIC VIRAL PNEUMONIAS

DANIEL H. LIBRATY

There are a number of established, emerging, and reemerging viruses that can lead to severe respiratory illness in immunocompetent individuals. The etiologic agents of serious viral pneumonias can generally be divided into three groups:

1. *Human-adapted respiratory viruses*. The primary site of entry, replication, and disease for these viruses is the human respiratory tract. They are spread efficiently by person-to-person transmission. The most significant members of this group are the human influenza A and B viruses; others are respiratory syncytial virus (RSV) and adenovirus.
2. *Human-adapted viruses—respiratory disease after a viremic phase*. Viral entry and person-to-person spread of these viruses is via the respiratory tract. However, these viruses cause respiratory illness after a phase of systemic viral replication and dissemination. Members of this group include varicella zoster virus (chickenpox) and rubeola virus (measles).
3. *Zoonotic viruses*. Viruses in this group include the severe acute respiratory syndrome (SARS) coronavirus, New World hantaviruses producing the hantavirus cardiopulmonary syndrome (HCPS), and the H5N1 avian influenza A virus.

PATHOGENESIS

A virus must first gain access to the lower respiratory tract in order to produce severe pneumonia. The most common mode of entry is via droplet transmission. Airborne virus-containing droplets 5 to 10 μm in diameter are filtered and deposited in the upper respiratory tract. Virus reaches the lower respiratory tract after efficient replication and spread within squamous epithelial cells, often in the setting of impaired mucociliary clearance (due to extremes of age, antecedent or concurrent infections, and drugs). This is the usual mode of entry for many human-adapted respiratory viruses, such as influenza, RSV, adenovirus, and coronavirus. Person-to-person spread via droplets is limited to a distance of approximately 1 m. Other viruses such as varicella and rubeola are transmitted via aerosols (particles 1 to 5 μm in diameter) that can deposit directly in the lower respiratory tract. As such, they are highly infectious and can be transmitted over greater distances and time than agents transmitted by droplets. Although deposited directly in alveoli, viral dissemination in the lung typically occurs hematogenously after a viremic phase [1,2].

Once in the lower respiratory tract, there are a limited number of ways that the lung can respond to a viral infection and produce respiratory illness. Viral invasion and replication can directly produce a necrotizing bronchopneumonia with highly inflammatory, purulent, and exudative reactions. This is not common, but can be seen with influenza and adenovirus infections. Respiratory viral infections can impair host lung defenses in a way that leads to secondary bacterial pneumonias, particularly with *Streptococcus pneumoniae* or *Staphylococcus aureus*. The classic examples are postinfluenza or measles pneumonias. Finally, viral infection of the lower respiratory tract may produce severe disease by triggering a common tissue response to acute lung injuries termed *diffuse alveolar damage* or *acute respiratory distress syndrome*. The acute lung injury may progress from an early exudative phase, often with profound noncardiogenic pulmonary edema (especially in HCPS), to a proliferative or organizing phase that produces interstitial inflammation, and a late resolving phase [3].

CLINICAL MANIFESTATIONS

The limited host response patterns to virus-induced lung injury means that there is significant overlap in the clinical manifestations of viral pneumonias. The clues to a specific viral etiology are often found in assessing host risk factors and epidemiology on presentation. A summary of the common clinical manifestations for specific viral pneumonias is presented in Table 90.1. Many of the viral infections discussed in this chapter are characterized by a “flu-like illness” prodrome. Symptoms begin with the acute onset of headache, chills, and myalgias. Within a few days, a cough and sore throat develop along with upper respiratory tract infection. The presence or absence of upper respiratory symptoms at this stage may provide one clue to the specific viral etiology. The human-adapted respiratory viruses (human influenza, RSV, adenovirus, non-SARS coronavirus) generally all produce upper respiratory symptoms. Measles is characterized by coryza and conjunctivitis in the prodrome. The absence of upper respiratory symptoms has been reported to be characteristic of infections with several of the zoonotic viruses: SARS coronavirus, hantavirus, and the H5N1 avian influenza virus [4–6]. The lower respiratory tract signs and symptoms in viral pneumonias are generally nonspecific and progress to dyspnea, tachypnea, and inspiratory crackles. Sputum production is variable. If the clinical course is biphasic (dyspnea and productive cough after improvement of a flu-like illness), then a secondary bacterial pneumonia should be suspected.

Routine laboratory tests are generally of little help in distinguishing among the viruses that can produce severe respiratory illness. Total leukocyte counts are typically within the normal range or slightly elevated. One exception is measles virus infection, which can produce a marked leukopenia [7]. The most common hematologic finding in the viral pneumonias is a relative lymphopenia. The complete blood count may be useful for diagnosing HCPS. In HCPS caused by Sin Nombre virus (a New World hantavirus), the triad of thrombocytopenia (platelet count less than 150 K per mm^3), absolute neutrophilia, and the presence of immunoblasts was a sensitive and specific predictor of HCPS in one study [5]. Electrolyte abnormalities and hepatic transaminase elevation can occur among any of the severe viral pneumonias.

TABLE 90.1

PRESENTATION AND MANIFESTATIONS OF SPECIFIC VIRAL PNEUMONIAS

Virus	Transmission	Epidemiology/settings	Pulmonary manifestations	Extrapulmonary manifestations	Laboratory findings	Radiographic findings
Human influenza A and B viruses	Airborne droplet transmission ($\geq$10 μm) Small aerosol (rare) Fomite contact	Yearly and seasonal (peak season November–April in temperate climates) Attack rates highest at extremes of age Predisposing risk factors for pulmonary complications: chronic heart, lung, renal disease; pregnancy Nosocomial transmission in hospitals and institutional settings	Flu-like illness prodrome (see text) with upper respiratory signs/symptoms Bronchitis Croup Unilateral and bilateral primary viral pneumonia Secondary bacterial pneumonias (*Streptococcus pneumoniae* and *Staphylococcus aureus*)	Secondary bacterial otitis media Myositis (early convalescence) Myocarditis/pericarditis Reye's syndrome (children)	(Nonspecific) Relative lymphopenia in adults Leukocytosis in children	(Nonspecific) Segmental and bilateral alveolar and/or interstitial infiltrates Consolidation suggests superimposed bacterial process Diffuse hemorrhagic alveolitis seen in primary influenza pneumonia
Respiratory syncytial virus	Airborne droplet transmission ($\geq$10 μm)	Yearly and seasonal (overlaps with human influenza) Severe illness at extremes of age: <2 and >65 years old High-risk individuals: children with underlying cardiopulmonary disorders; adults with congestive heart failure or chronic pulmonary disease Outbreaks in long-term care facilities	Prodrome with upper respiratory signs/symptoms as with human influenza Bronchiolitis (common in infants) Pneumonia, unilateral and bilateral	Otitis media	(Nonspecific) Same as influenza	(Nonspecific) Segmental and multiple areas of interstitial and/or alveolar infiltrates In children, hyperaeration is reported as common finding
Adenovirus	Airborne droplet transmission ($\geq$10 μm)	Endemic: mild respiratory disease year round Epidemic: outbreaks in military barracks, hospitals, and institutional settings	Flu-like illness prodrome with upper respiratory signs/symptoms Progression to severe pneumonia, can be necrotizing	The adenovirus serotypes that produce severe pneumonia are generally not the ones that produce extrapulmonary disease such as diarrhea, epidemic keratoconjunctivitis, or hemorrhagic cystitis	(Nonspecific) Relative lymphopenia	(Nonspecific) Segmental and multiple areas of interstitial and/or alveolar infiltrates Focal infiltrates reported as a common presentation
Varicella virus	Airborne: aerosol transmission	Year-round transmission with peaks in late winter and early spring in temperate climates Intimate contact with index case of primary varicella infection (chickenpox) Incubation period is 10–20 d after infection Risk factors for developing pneumonia: nonimmune adults; smoking; chronic obstructive pulmonary disease; >100 skin lesions; pregnancy, third trimester	Pneumonia presents 1–6 d after onset of typical rash (chickenpox) Fever, dyspnea, tachypnea in absence of upper respiratory symptoms	Cutaneous lesions (chickenpox) CNS involvement (uncommon): acute cerebellar ataxia, encephalitis, CNS vasculitis	(Nonspecific)	Nodular or interstitial pneumonitis common

Rubeola virus	Fomite and direct contact with respiratory droplets Airborne: aerosol transmission	Epidemic transmission, localized outbreaks in household and community settings Outbreaks in doctor's offices and emergency departments Infectivity greatest in the 3 d before onset of rash in index case (incubation period 10–14 d) Risk factors for severe illness: nonimmune adults and children <5 years old; crowding; pregnancy; HIV infection; malnourished children, developing countries; vitamin A deficiency	Prodrome: cough, coryza, conjunctivitis Unilateral and bilateral primary viral pneumonia Secondary bacterial pneumonias (*S. pneumoniae*, *S. aureus*, and others)	Typical morbilliform rash (see text) CNS involvement: acute or chronic encephalitis (typically after respiratory disease)	Leukopenia	(Nonspecific)
SARS coronavirus	Airborne droplet transmission ($\geq 10\ \mu m$) Fomites	Epidemic/outbreak settings Originated in Asia Person-to-person transmission after contact with symptomatic, SARS CoV-infected person No transmission seen since 2003	Fever, myalgias, cough Upper respiratory signs/symptoms are uncommon Dyspnea, tachypnea, respiratory decompensation develop around second week of illness	Watery diarrhea in 25% of patients around second week of illness	Absolute lymphopenia common	Ground-glass opacifications Unilateral and bilateral focal infiltrates Pneumomediastinum without preceding intubation or positive pressure ventilation reported as characteristic sign
New World hantaviruses	Small-particle aerosols generated from rodent excreta	Sporadic, clustered cases in Americas Exposure to rodents, their droppings and urine, especially in closed spaces In general, no person-to-person transmission (except possibly with Andes virus)	Febrile/flu-like prodrome usually without any upper respiratory signs/symptoms Rapid progression to noncardiogenic pulmonary edema/ARDS with hypotension	Renal dysfunction with proteinuria and microscopic hematuria	Thrombocytopenia (early and nearly all cases) Absolute neutrophilia Relative lymphopenia with immunoblasts on peripheral smear Elevated hepatic transaminases (nearly all cases)	Bilateral noncardiogenic pulmonary edema/ARDS
Avian influenza A virus H5N1	Presumed droplet transmission and/or direct contact from bird to human	Sporadic cases in countries with animal influenza A H5N1 Close contact/exposure to live or dead domestic fowl or wild birds or domestic ducks Few reports of limited person-to-person transmission by intimate contact only	Flu-like prodrome often without upper respiratory signs/symptoms Early development of primary viral pneumonia	Watery diarrhea Multiorgan failure	(Nonspecific) Lymphopenia Mild-to-moderate thrombocytopenia Elevated hepatic transaminases	(Nonspecific) Unilateral and bilateral infiltrates Multifocal consolidations ARDS

ARDS, acute respiratory distress syndrome; CNS, central nervous system; HIV, human immunodeficiency virus; SARS, severe acute respiratory syndrome.

The radiographic findings in viral pneumonias are also broad and nonspecific. Radiographic infiltrates can have interstitial, alveolar, or combined patterns. The presence of only a diffuse alveolar pattern might suggest a primary influenza pneumonia with hemorrhagic alveolitis [8] or the capillary leak syndrome of acute respiratory distress syndrome, especially due to HCPS. Peribronchial nodular infiltrates is a pattern often reported with varicella pneumonia [9]. Computed tomography (CT) scans are better at detecting the presence, extent, and complications of respiratory infections than chest radiographs. However, they are no better at defining particular radiographic patterns of specific viral or bacterial causes [9].

DIAGNOSIS

The diagnostic modalities available for viral pneumonias rely on detection of a viral component (nucleic acid or protein), growth of the virus in vitro, or development of a virus-specific antibody response. Definitive serologic evidence of a viral infection requires a rise in virus-specific antibody titers between paired acute illness and convalescent sera. With a few exceptions, serologic assays are therefore not generally helpful for the clinician in the acute setting of a viral pneumonia. This section will focus on diagnostic tests that may assist the clinician faced with a critically ill patient and suspected viral pneumonia.

Human Influenza A and B

Rapid, direct, antigen-detection assays are commercially available for diagnosing human influenza A and B virus infections. These assays rely on detection of the influenza virus nucleoprotein in respiratory secretions, and results can be obtained within 1 hour. Because they are based on the viral nucleoprotein, none of the rapid antigen tests provide information about influenza A hemagglutinin subtypes (e.g., H1, H3). Details regarding the available rapid antigen tests for influenza are provided by the Centers for Disease Control (CDC) (http://www.cdc.gov/flu/professionals/diagnosis/rapidclin.htm). The test specificities for diagnosing an influenza virus infection are generally high (more than 90%), but reported sensitivities are lower (33% to 80%) and may vary for different human influenza A virus subtypes [10–12]. In clinical practice, the timing and method of sample collection can greatly affect test sensitivity. Influenza A virus shedding from the upper respiratory tract typically peaks 2 to 3 days after symptom onset [13,14]. The window available to reliably detect viral antigen from upper respiratory tract secretions may extend only 5 to 6 days after symptom onset. Influenza virus nucleoprotein is most abundant in the columnar respiratory epithelium. Posterior nasopharyngeal swabs or aspirates that collect columnar epithelial cells are usually the preferred samples for rapid antigen detection assays [10,15,16], even for mechanically ventilated patients in the intensive care unit (ICU).

Reverse transcriptase polymerase chain reaction (RT-PCR) assays and viral culture are the next most commonly used diagnostic tests for human influenza virus infections. Posterior nasopharyngeal swabs or washes, and samples of lower respiratory tract secretions such as endotracheal aspirates or bronchoalveolar lavages, are acceptable samples. Virus typing and influenza A subtyping can be accomplished with either method. Due to its high sensitivity, specificity, and throughput, RT-PCR assays have generally supplanted virus culture in many clinical microbiology laboratories. Unlike viral culture, the detection of influenza viral RNA by RT-PCR cannot assess the presence of live virus in respiratory secretions.

Respiratory Syncytial Virus

Rapid antigen-detection assays and direct immunofluorescent staining for RSV from respiratory secretions have been the primary diagnostic tests used in children. These tests have >80% sensitivity and >90% specificity [17]. RT-PCR assays and respiratory viral culture are the other common diagnostic approaches in pediatric populations. In adults, the RSV rapid antigen assays and viral culture are generally insensitive due to low virus shedding and preexisting anti-RSV antibody in respiratory secretions [18,19]. Direct fluorescent antibody staining in nasopharyngeal specimens was reported to be the only rapid assay at least equivalent to viral culture in adults [17]. A RT-PCR assay on respiratory secretions is the preferred acute illness diagnostic method for RSV infection in adults [20,21].

Adenovirus

PCR of adenovirus DNA or respiratory viral culture from a nasopharyngeal swab or aspirate, sputum, or lower respiratory tract secretions is the diagnostic test of choice for adenoviral pneumonia. Direct adenovirus antigen assays that cover most serotypes, such as immunofluorescent antibody staining, are not as sensitive as PCR assays or viral culture.

Varicella

Varicella pneumonia typically develops within 1 to 6 days after the characteristic rash of chickenpox has appeared [22]. If desired, a specific microbiological diagnosis can be obtained by PCR assay or viral culture from a swab or scraping at the base of an unroofed vesicle. Viral detection in respiratory secretions is generally not required.

Rubeola (Measles)

Pulmonary involvement with measles is generally diagnosed on the basis of history and physical findings. In outbreak settings, pneumonia should be suspected in patients who develop respiratory distress and persistent or recurrent fevers during the course of typical measles. Measles is characterized by malaise and fever, followed rapidly by coryza, conjunctivitis, and cough [23]. Early in illness, the presence of Koplik spots on the buccal mucosa is pathognomonic of measles. The classic morbilliform rash begins 3 to 4 days after onset of illness and starts to fade after another 3 days. Worsening respiratory symptoms as the rash is fading is suspicious for rubeola pneumonia. Laboratory confirmation may be useful, particularly in suspected sporadic cases within a highly immunized population. Viral isolation or rapid detection of measles antigen in nasopharyngeal secretions is difficult and not readily available. A presumptive serologic diagnosis can be made by detection of serum antimeasles virus immunoglobulin M (IgM) or immunoglobulin G (IgG) in unimmunized individuals. Serum antibodies appear 1 to 3 days after onset of the rash [24]. Definitive serologic diagnosis requires paired acute and convalescent sera. In immunocompromised patients with overwhelming pneumonia, the antibody response may be minimal. Viral antigen staining of cells or RT-PCR assays on nasal exudates or urinary sediment may be useful in this setting [23].

Severe Acute Respiratory Syndrome Coronavirus

The most practical diagnostic approach for SARS coronavirus is a RT-PCR assay on nasopharyngeal specimens within

2 weeks after symptom onset [25]. The other primary site where SARS coronavirus RNA can be detected is stool (week 2 onward). Lower respiratory tract secretions harbor a greater viral load than upper respiratory tract secretions early in illness. However, lower respiratory tract aspiration, lavage, or intubation pose serious nosocomial transmission risks and should not be pursued solely for diagnostic purposes. IgM seroconversion does not occur until after the first week of illness and therefore is also of limited diagnostic utility [4]. With resolution of SARS viral transmission in 2003, and the apparent subsequent mutation of the virus [26], any initial positive test for SARS coronavirus must be viewed as a potential false-positive finding.

Hantavirus

There are nearly a dozen New World hantaviruses that have been associated with HCPS. Sin Nombre virus (in the southwestern United States) and Andes virus (in South America) are the two best known HCPS-associated hantaviruses. The diagnosis of HCPS can be made by detection of antihantavirus IgM antibodies in acute illness serum. Nearly all patients with HCPS have detectable IgM in their sera at the onset of pulmonary edema. The currently available IgM capture enzyme-linked immunosorbent assay using a recombinant Sin Nombre virus antigen can be used to diagnose all New World hantavirus infections [27]. RT-PCR assay on blood or lung tissue is a research assay of limited utility and not widely available. Because of low yield and biosafety issues, attempted culture of hantaviruses in clinical microbiology laboratories is not recommended.

Avian Influenza Virus (H5N1)

If H5N1 influenza A virus infection is suspected on epidemiologic grounds, then all avenues for making a definitive diagnosis should be pursued. The diagnostic approach to H5N1 influenza is to collect nasopharyngeal and lower respiratory tract specimens for rapid antigen detection, RT-PCR assay, and viral culture. Aerosol-generating procedures for specimen collection should be performed with appropriate infection control precautions. Detection of viral RNA in respiratory specimens by RT-PCR is the most sensitive and rapid method for detecting influenza A/H5N1. A hallmark of H5N1 influenza has been a higher frequency of virus detection and viral loads in pharyngeal and lower respiratory tract samples than in nasal samples between 2 and 16 days after the onset of illness [6,28]. Viral RNA has also been detected in fecal samples. The CDC has provided guidance for the laboratory testing of suspected H5N1 cases (http://www.cdc.gov/flu/avian/professional/guidance-labtesting.htm). The clinical microbiology laboratory should be notified if H5N1 influenza A virus infection is suspected and specimens are collected for viral culture. This is to ensure that the specimens will be handled and processed with the appropriate biosafety containment level.

TREATMENT AND MANAGEMENT

Caring for a patient with a severe viral pneumonia can be complex; however, the approach to such a patient is often identical to that of other acute severe pneumonias. First, a clinical assessment of disease severity is made so that an appropriate level of care can be established. This process can be assisted by standardized scoring algorithms established for critically ill patients or community-acquired pneumonias [29,30]. Supportive care with maintenance of ventilation, oxygenation, and hemodynamic parameters is based on general principles previously outlined in Chapter 68. Next, diagnostic procedures to try to establish the cause of the severe pneumonia can be pursued. Finally, one needs to evaluate the role of specific antiviral and/or immunomodulatory therapies in the care of the patient. As with most infectious pneumonias, the decision to treat with these therapies is often made empirically or with limited diagnostic information. A summary of potential therapeutic options, dosages, and adverse effects is presented in Table 90.2.

Human Influenza A and B

There are two classes of antiviral drugs currently available for the treatment of human influenza virus infections: adamantanes (amantadine and rimantadine) and neuraminidase inhibitors (oseltamivir, zanamivir, peramivir). The adamantanes are older, established compounds, but they are not active against influenza B. In placebo-controlled trials, when amantadine or rimantadine therapy was initiated within 48 hours of symptom onset in influenza A virus infections, there was a 1 to 2 day reduction in duration of fever and overall illness symptom scores [31]. However, there are no controlled data on the utility of adamantanes in the treatment of severe influenza A lower respiratory tract infections, and several factors make them less than ideal for patients in the ICU. In several studies, rimantadine treatment produced small initial decreases in viral titers, but later in therapy, similar or higher frequencies of viral shedding compared to placebo [32]. The incidence of adamantane resistance among influenza A viruses worldwide has increased in recent years [33]. Resistance emerges at a high frequency during treatment with adamantanes, and resistant virus can be transmitted to the close contacts of patients in community and nosocomial settings [32,34].

The neuraminidase inhibitors have activity against influenza A and B. As with the adamantanes, oseltamivir and zanamivir decrease the duration and severity of generalized symptoms by approximately 1 day when started within 48 hours after onset of illness [35]. Some lines of evidence make the neuraminidase inhibitors attractive for treatment of patients with severe influenza virus pneumonias. They markedly reduce viral load during the first 48 hours of treatment, can decrease viral shedding, and may lower the incidence of influenza-related lower respiratory tract complications [36–38]. However, the latter benefit has been questioned by a recent meta-analysis [39]. Development of resistance to oseltamivir or zanamivir has been uncommon in immunocompetent adults, but appears to be higher in children and immunocompromised individuals [40,41]. Importantly, person-to-person transmission of resistant virus has not been documented. Zanamivir may be active against some oseltamivir-resistant strains.

Despite the lack of randomized controlled trials in the ICU setting, most practitioners would initiate treatment with a neuraminidase inhibitor in patients with suspected or confirmed severe influenza pneumonia. Some clinicians advocate the use of oseltamivir at twice the recommended dose for patients with severe influenza pneumonia or a combination of oseltamivir and rimantadine. There are no randomized clinical trial data to support these approaches at the present time, but they are being actively investigated. Zanamivir should not be nebulized for patients on mechanical ventilation due to possible obstruction of the ventilation circuit (http://www.fda.gov/safety/medwatch/safetyinformation/safetyalertsforhumanmedicalproducts/ucm186081.htm). Peramivir is an intravenous neuraminidase inhibitor that received emergency use authorization by the U.S. Food and Drug Administration in the setting of the 2009 novel H1N1 influenza A pandemic. Pregnant women,

TABLE 90.2

SUMMARY OF ANTIVIRAL AGENTS AND THERAPEUTIC OPTIONS FOR SPECIFIC VIRAL PNEUMONIAS

Virus	Drug	Adult dosage (duration)	Dosage adjustments[a]	Potential adverse effects	Comments
Human influenza viruses	Oseltamivir	75 mg PO b.i.d (5 d)	Decrease to 75 mg PO qd in patients with CrCl between 10 and 30 mL/min	Nausea, vomiting, headache	Neuraminidase inhibitors effective against human influenza A and B viruses Some consider increase to 150 mg PO b.i.d × 7–10 d—no randomized trial
	Zanamivir	2 × 5 mg oral inhalations bid (5 d)	None	Cough, nasal and throat discomfort, bronchospasm, decreased lung function	Use with caution in patients with asthma or COPD
	Amantadine	100 mg PO b.i.d or 200 mg PO qd (3–5 d)	Decrease to 100 mg/d for patients >65 y old or CrCl <50 mL/min	Anticholinergic effects: CNS effects can include insomnia, delirium, hallucinations, and seizures	Adamantanes not effective against human influenza B viruses
	Rimantadine	100 mg PO b.i.d or 200 mg PO qd (3–5 d)	Decrease to 100 mg/d for patients >65 y old, CrCl <10 mL/min, or with severe hepatic dysfunction	Same as amantadine, except CNS adverse effects less common	
Adenovirus	Cidofovir	5 mg/kg IV × 1	Contraindicated in patients with CrCl ≤55 mL/min	Renal toxicity: acute renal failure, proteinuria Neutropenia Metabolic acidosis Uveitis	Cidofovir given with probenecid (2 g PO 3 h before cidofovir infusion, and 1 g PO 2 and 8 h after the infusion) Also, prehydrate with 1 L IV NS
Varicella	Acyclovir	10 mg/kg IV q8 h × 7–10 d	Decrease to 10 mg/kg IV q12 h for CrCl 10–50 mL/min 10 mg/kg IV q24 h for CrCl <10 mL/min	Occasional mild nausea, vomiting, diarrhea Crystal formation and renal tubular obstruction Dizziness, delirium, obtundation (rare)	IV hydration to avoid renal toxicity CNS toxicity seen with high drug levels
Rubeola (measles)	Vitamin A	200,000 IU PO qd × 1–2 d (100,000 IU PO qd if ≤1 y old)	None		
	Ribavirin?	20–35 mg/kg/d IV × 7 d	None	Dose-related hemolytic anemia (common) Cough, dyspnea, nausea, headache, fatigue Hypocalcemia with IV ribavirin	Data from small case series; no randomized trial
New World hantaviruses	Ribavirin?	33 mg/kg IV load, then 16 mg/kg IV q6 h × 4 d, 8 mg/kg IV q8 h × 3 d	None	Same as previously noted	No suggestion of benefit if ribavirin started in cardiopulmonary phase of HCPS; unknown if there would be benefit if initiated earlier during prodromal phase
Avian influenza A H5N1 virus	Oseltamivir	75 mg PO b.i.d × 5 d or consider increase to 150 mg PO b.i.d × 7–10 d	Same as previously noted	Same as previously noted	Most experience to date in treating H5N1 infections has been with oseltamivir, but no randomized trials
	Zanamivir	2 × 5 mg oral inhalations b.i.d (5 d)	None	Same as previously noted	Same cautions as previously noted

[a]Consult appropriate references for potential drug–drug interactions.
Note: Zanamavir may be useful for oseltamivir-resistant H5N1 strains, but no experience as either single agent or in combination with other antivirals.
b.i.d, twice daily; CrCl, creatinine clearance; COPD, chronic obstructive pulmonary disease; CNS, central nervous system; HCPS, hantavirus cardiopulmonary syndrome; IV, intravenous; PO, orally; NS, normal saline.

infants and children younger than 2 years, individuals with chronic cardiopulmonary or renal disease, and those immunosuppressed were at higher risk of developing severe illness during the 2009 H1N1 influenza pandemic (same as in all human influenza outbreaks). The 2009 novel H1N1 virus has now become the dominant circulating influenza A H1N1 strain worldwide. There are no data to support the use of corticosteroids in the treatment of influenza pneumonia, and inhaled ribavirin is not beneficial [42]. An important addition to the treatment of influenza pneumonia is antibacterial therapy. There is a high incidence of secondary bacterial infections complicating influenza pneumonia, particularly with *S. pneumoniae* or *S. aureus* [43]. In this setting, antibiotic therapy directed against *S. aureus* should be added to the antibiotic regimen used for community-acquired pneumonia bacterial pathogens. In areas where there is a high prevalence of community-acquired methicillin-resistant *S. aureus*, vancomycin should be used as the initial antistaphylococcal antibiotic.

Respiratory Syncytial Virus

Because RSV is a frequent cause of serious lower respiratory tract infections in infants and young children, data on potential therapies come from pediatric studies. There have been no trials of anti-RSV therapies in adults to date. Current treatment strategies for RSV lower respiratory tract infections are essentially supportive. Aerosolized ribavirin therapy of infants with RSV lower respiratory tract infections had no significant effects on clinical outcome in two randomized trials [44,45]. Palivizumab, a humanized anti-RSV neutralizing monoclonal antibody, has been successful in reducing hospitalizations of high-risk children for RSV lower respiratory tract infections when given prophylactically [46]. However, the utility of palivizumab or anti-RSV immune globulin as a potential treatment of serious RSV infections is unknown. Clinical observations and a mouse model of RSV infection have demonstrated airway hyperresponsiveness and other asthmatic changes in RSV-infected lungs [47], and prompted trials of anti-inflammatory therapies. Unfortunately, two randomized trials failed to demonstrate any overall beneficial effect of intravenous dexamethasone in RSV lower respiratory tract infections [48,49]. On subgroup analysis in one study, dexamethasone treatment was beneficial in mechanically ventilated patients with bronchiolitis and mild gas exchange abnormalities (PaO_2/FIO_2 more than 200 mm Hg or mean airway pressure $\leq$10 cm H_2O) [48]. These findings have yet to be confirmed in a prospective fashion.

Adenovirus

Adenoviral pneumonia occurs in isolated outbreaks among immunocompetent adults or sporadically in immunocompromised individuals. As such, there are no prospective randomized trials of antiviral medications. Cidofovir is an antiviral drug with potent in vitro activity against adenovirus. Cidofovir has been reported to be successful in treating adenoviral pneumonia in small case series [50–52], and is currently considered the antiviral agent of choice. Because severe adenovirus disease is associated with defects in cellular or humoral immunity, donor lymphocyte infusions and intravenous immunoglobulin have been used as adjunctive therapy [50]. Their efficacy in the treatment of adenoviral pneumonia is unknown.

Varicella

Intravenous acyclovir is considered standard therapy for the treatment of varicella pneumonia. There have been no randomized controlled trials of acyclovir for varicella pneumonia. Its efficacy in reducing the severity of pox lesions [53,54] and apparent benefit in numerous case series of varicella pneumonia support its use. A compilation of 46 case reports and 227 patients with varicella pneumonia suggested that mortality was 3.6-fold higher in untreated compared to acyclovir-treated patients [22]. In a small uncontrolled retrospective study, patients who received adjunctive corticosteroids had shorter ICU and hospital stays than those who did not receive corticosteroids [55]. There are no prospective controlled studies supporting the use of adjunctive corticosteroid therapy in varicella pneumonia.

Rubeola (Measles)

Pneumonia is the most common severe complication of measles and accounts for most measles-associated deaths [56]. There is no specific antiviral therapy for measles. In developing countries, treatment with vitamin A has been associated with a 50% reduction in the mortality of severe measles. Hospitalized children with measles in the United States often have a measurable deficiency in Vitamin A, and they are more likely to have pneumonia or diarrhea. The World Health Organization recommends vitamin A therapy for all children with measles, and the American Academy of Pediatrics recommends vitamin A therapy for hospitalized children older than 2 years with measles in the United States [56]. Data in older children and adults are lacking, but vitamin A treatment should probably be extended to all individuals with severe measles [57,58]. Intravenous ribavirin was reported to have beneficial effects in a small case series of measles pneumonia in adults [59], but there are no data from prospective randomized studies. Another important point in the treatment of measles pneumonia is antibacterial therapy. Secondary bacterial pneumonia and laryngotracheobronchitis are frequent complications of measles. As with influenza, *S. aureus* and *S. pneumoniae* are the most commonly isolated bacterial pathogens. Less frequent bacterial causes of pneumonia following measles include *Neisseria meningitidis, Klebsiella pneumoniae, Escherichia coli, Haemophilus influenzae*, and *Pseudomonas* spp [56]. Broad-spectrum antibiotic therapy, including coverage for *S. aureus* and *S. pneumoniae*, should be instituted.

Severe Acute Respiratory Syndrome Coronavirus

The SARS epidemic of 2003 was marked by the empiric use of several antiviral and immunomodulatory strategies because controlled trials were not possible. Ribavirin was the most commonly used antiviral agent, but its poor in vitro activity against the SARS coronavirus and its apparent limited ability to reduce early viral shedding in patients makes its usefulness questionable [60]. Corticosteroids were used extensively during the SARS outbreak of 2003 at varying doses and durations. Retrospective analyses on the effects of corticosteroids in SARS suggest that they did not provide any significant benefits and may have been associated with some adverse outcomes [60,61].

Hantavirus

There has been one placebo-controlled, double-blind trial of intravenous ribavirin for treatment of HCPS due to Sin Nombre virus [62]. The accrual of study subjects was low and inadequate to clearly assess the efficacy of ribavirin. There were no trends to support the use of ribavirin in patients presenting in the cardiopulmonary phase of HCPS. Whether ribavirin may have a beneficial effect if initiated during the prodromal phase is unknown. Intravenous ribavirin was beneficial when given early to patients with another hantavirus disease, hemorrhagic fever with renal syndrome caused by Hantaan virus [63]. There is no evidence that pharmacologic doses of corticosteroids provide any benefit in HCPS.

At the present time, clinical management of HCPS involves supportive care with several caveats. Excessive fluid resuscitation will exacerbate the pulmonary edema of HCPS without commensurate improvement in cardiac output. Recommendations are to fluid resuscitate with 1 to 2 L of isotonic crystalloid and then maintain as low a wedge pressure (8 to 12 mm Hg) as is compatible with satisfactory cardiac output (cardiac index more than 2.2 L per minute per m^2). The use of loop diuretics is discouraged. Inotropic agents (e.g., dobutamine, dopamine, norepinephrine) should be initiated earlier in resuscitation than in other conditions, instead of continued fluid boluses [5].

Avian Influenza Virus (H5N1)

The H5N1 influenza A viruses are susceptible in vitro to the neuraminidase inhibitors, and neuraminidase inhibitors have been protective in animal models of influenza A H5N1 infection [64–66]. Although prospective clinical trials have not been performed, the current recommendation is that patients with suspected influenza A H5N1 infection promptly receive a neuraminidase inhibitor, preferably within 48 hours of infection [6,67]. Doubling the standard doses of oseltamivir and increasing the duration of treatment for 7 to 10 days are considerations for severe H5N1 infections [6]. Emergence of resistance to oseltamivir has been documented in a few patients with H5N1 infections treated with oseltamivir [68]. These strains remain susceptible to zanamivir. Whether combination therapy with zanamivir or other antivirals is beneficial and would reduce the emergence of oseltamivir resistance is unknown. The influenza A H5N1 isolates from Asia are highly resistant to the adamantanes, and therefore these drugs do not play a therapeutic role [6]. Corticosteroids have been used in the treatment of sporadic influenza A H5N1 infections, but their routine use cannot be recommended. In a randomized trial in Vietnam, all four patients given dexamethasone died [69].

INFECTION CONTROL ISSUES FOR THE INTENSIVE CARE UNIT

Most of the viruses presented in this chapter can be transmitted in the nosocomial setting via direct contact with an infected patient and through inhalation of droplets or aerosols. Efforts to reduce transmission to healthcare workers and other patients are often guided by the transmission efficiency of the specific viral agents. Human influenza, RSV, adenovirus, varicella, and measles are efficiently transmitted person to person. SARS coronavirus and avian influenza A H5N1 virus are transmitted less efficiently, but nosocomial transmission may be promoted by aerosol-generating procedures. The New World hantaviruses are generally not transmitted person to person, except possibly the Andes virus.

Strategies to prevent nosocomial transmission include iso-·on precautions for patients, chemoprophylaxis and immu-ı of healthcare workers if possible, and surveillance and ·ification of healthcare workers' exposures. In gen- ·with suspected epidemic viral pneumonias should · combination of standard, contact, droplet, ·on precautions. When feasible, limit the number of healthcare workers with direct access to the patient and limit their contact with other patients. Restrict visitors to a minimum and provide them appropriate personal protective equipment. High-efficiency N-95 masks or powered air-purifying respirators are preferred for healthcare workers. If high-efficiency masks are limited or unavailable, surgical masks may be considered if the primary mode of agent transmission is via droplets and no aerosol-generating procedures are performed. Detailed guidelines can be found on the CDC Web site (http://www.cdc.gov/ncidod/dhqp/guidelines.html).

Advances in antiviral or immunomodulatory therapy of viral pneumonias based on randomized controlled trials or meta-analyses of such trials is summarized in Table 90.3.

TABLE 90.3

SUMMARY RECOMMENDATIONS FOR ANTIVIRAL OR IMMUNOMODULATORY THERAPY OF VIRAL PNEUMONIAS BASED ON RANDOMIZED CONTROLLED CLINICAL TRIALS

Human influenza

- Neuraminidase inhibitors given within 48 h of flu symptom onset decrease the duration of symptoms, viral load, and viral shedding; controversy as to whether they lower the incidence of influenza-related lower respiratory tract complications [35,39]; no randomized controlled trials for treatment of severe pneumonia.
- Aerosolized ribavirin does not provide any clinical benefit [42].

Respiratory syncytial virus (RSV)

- Aerosolized ribavirin has no significant effect on outcome in infants with RSV lower respiratory tract infections [44,45].
- Intravenous dexamethasone does not provide any overall beneficial effect in RSV lower respiratory tract infections [48,49].
- On post hoc analysis, dexamethasone (0.6 mg/kg IV q6 h × 48 h) may be beneficial in mechanically ventilated patients with bronchiolitis and mild gas exchange abnormalities (PaO_2/FIO_2 >200 mm Hg or mean airway pressure ≤10 cm H_2O) [48].

Adenovirus

- No randomized controlled trials of cidofovir for adenovirus pneumonia.

Varicella

- No randomized controlled trials of IV acyclovir for varicella pneumonia. A meta-analysis of published case series suggests that IV acyclovir decreases mortality [22].

Rubeola (measles)

- Oral vitamin A therapy decreases mortality and improves recovery from pneumonia in children [56,57].

SARS coronavirus

- No randomized controlled trials for antivirals or corticosteroids.

Hantavirus cardiopulmonary syndrome (HCPS)

- No trends to support the use of ribavirin in patients presenting in the cardiopulmonary phase of HCPS [62].

Avian influenza A virus (H5N1)

- Neuraminidase inhibitors have been protective in animal models of influenza A H5N1 infection. There are no patient-based randomized controlled trials.
- No trends to support the use of dexamethasone from a small, unpublished, randomized trial [69].

IV, intravenous; SARS, severe acute respiratory syndrome.

References

1. Bryant RE: Viral pneumonia, in Braude AI, Davis CE, Fierer J (eds): *Infectious Diseases and Medical Microbiology*. Philadelphia, WB Saunders, 1986, p 815.
2. Dermody TS, Tyler KL: Introduction to viruses and viral diseases, in Mandell GL, Bennett JE, Dolin R (eds): *Principles and Practice of Infectious Diseases*. Philadelphia, Churchill Livingstone, 2000, p 1536.
3. Barrios R: Diffuse alveolar damage, in Cagle PT (ed): *Color Atlas and Text of Pulmonary Pathology*. Philadelphia, Lippincott Williams & Wilkins, 2005, p 361.
4. Peiris JS, Yuen KY, Osterhaus AD, et al: The severe acute respiratory syndrome. *N Engl J Med* 349:2431, 2003.
5. Hantavirus in the Americas. *Wkly Epidemiol Rec* 74(22):173, 1999.
6. Beigel JH, Farrar J, Han AM, et al: Avian influenza A (H5N1) infection in humans. *N Engl J Med* 353:1374, 2005.
7. Bernstein DL, Reuman PD, Schiff GM: Rubeola (measles) and subacute sclerosing panencephalitis virus, in Gorbach SL, Bartlett JG, Blacklow NR (eds): *Infectious Diseases*. Philadelphia, WB Saunders, 1992, p 1754.
8. Lindsay MI Jr, Morrow GW Jr: Primary influenzal pneumonia. *Postgrad Med* 49:173, 1971.
9. Donowitz GR, Mandell GL: Acute pneumonia, in Mandell GL, Bennett JE, Dolin R (eds): *Principles and Practice of Infectious Diseases*. Philadelphia, Churchill Livingstone, 2000, p 717.
10. Fiore AE, Shay DK, Broder K, et al: Prevention and control of seasonal influenza with vaccines: recommendations of the Advisory Committee on Immunization Practices (ACIP), 2009. *MMWR Recomm Rep* 58(RR-8):1–52, 2009.
11. Kok J, Blyth CC, Foo H, et al: Comparison of a rapid antigen test with nucleic acid testing during cocirculation of pandemic influenza A/H1N1 2009 and seasonal influenza A/H3N2. *J Clin Microbiol* 48(1):290–291, 2010.
12. Faix DJ, Sherman SS, Waterman SH: Rapid-test sensitivity for novel swine-origin influenza A (H1N1) virus in humans. *N Engl J Med* 361(7):728–729, 2009.
13. Dolin R: Influenza: current concepts. *Am Fam Physician* 14:72, 1976.
14. Douglas RGJ: Influenza in man, in Kilbourne ED (ed): *The Influenza Viruses and Influenza*. New York, Academic Press, 1975, p 395.
15. Hers JF: Disturbances of the ciliated epithelium due to influenza virus. *Am Rev Respir Dis* 93[Suppl]:162, 1996.
16. Schmid ML, Kudesia G, Wake S, et al: Prospective comparative study of culture specimens and methods in diagnosing influenza in adults. *BMJ* 316:275, 1998.
17. Ohm-Smith MJ, Nassos PS, Haller BL: Evaluation of the Binax NOW, BD Directigen, and BD Directigen EZ assays for detection of respiratory syncytial virus. *J Clin Microbiol* 42:2996, 2004.
18. Casiano-Colon AE, Hulbert BB, Mayer TK, et al: Lack of sensitivity of rapid antigen tests for the diagnosis of respiratory syncytial virus infection in adults. *J Clin Virol* 28:169, 2003.
19. Falsey AR, Formica MA, Treanor JJ, et al: Comparison of quantitative reverse transcription-PCR to viral culture for assessment of respiratory syncytial virus shedding. *J Clin Microbiol* 41:4160, 2003.
20. Falsey AR, Formica MA, Walsh EE: Diagnosis of respiratory syncytial virus infection: comparison of reverse transcription-PCR to viral culture and serology in adults with respiratory illness. *J Clin Microbiol* 40:817, 2002.
21. Falsey AR, Hennessey PA, Formica MA, et al: Respiratory syncytial virus infection in elderly and high-risk adults. *N Engl J Med* 352:1749, 2005.
22. Mohsen AH, McKendrick M: Varicella pneumonia in adults. *Eur Respir J* 21:886, 2003.
23. Gershon AA: Measles virus (rubeola), in Mandell GL, Bennett JE, Dolin R (eds): *Principles and Practice of Infectious Diseases*. Philadelphia, Churchill Livingstone, 2000, p 1801.
24. Bernstein DI, Schiff GM: Measles, in Gorbach SL, Bartlett JG, Blacklow NR (eds): *Infectious Diseases*. Philadelphia, WB Saunders, 1992, p 1088.
25. Lau SK, Che XY, Woo PC, et al: SARS coronavirus detection methods. *Emerg Infect Dis* 11:1108, 2005.
26. Li F, Li W, Farzan M, et al: Structure of SARS coronavirus spike receptor-binding domain complexed with receptor. *Science* 309:1864, 2005.
27. Organization PAHO: *Hantavirus in the Americas: Guidelines for Diagnosis, Treatment, Prevention, and Control*. Washington, DC, PAHO, 1999.
28. Peiris JS, Yu WC, Leung CW, et al: Re-emergence of fatal human influenza A subtype H5N1 disease. *Lancet* 363:617, 2004.
29. Knaus WA, Draper EA, Wagner DP, et al: APACHE II: a severity of disease classification system. *Crit Care Med* 13:818, 1985.
30. Buising KL, Thursky KA, Black JF, et al: A prospective comparison of severity scores for identifying patients with severe community acquired pneumonia: reconsidering what is meant by severe pneumonia. *Thorax* 61:419, 2006.
31. Jefferson T, Deeks JJ, Demicheli V, et al: Amantadine and rimantadine for preventing and treating influenza A in adults. *Cochrane Database Syst Rev* 3:CD001169, 2004.
32. Hayden FG, Sperber SJ, Belshe RB, et al: Recovery of drug-resistant influenza A virus during therapeutic use of rimantadine. *Antimicrob Agents Chemother* 35:1741, 1991.
33. Bright RA, Medina MJ, Xu X, et al: Incidence of adamantane resistance among influenza A (H3N2) viruses isolated worldwide from 1994 to 2005: a cause for concern. *Lancet* 366:1175, 2005.
34. Shiraishi K, Mitamura K, Sakai-Tagawa Y, et al: High frequency of resistant viruses harboring different mutations in amantadine-treated children with influenza. *J Infect Dis* 188:57, 2003.
35. Cooper NJ, Sutton AJ, Abrams KR, et al: Effectiveness of neuraminidase inhibitors in treatment and prevention of influenza A and B: systematic review and meta-analyses of randomised controlled trials. *BMJ* 326(7401):1235, 2003.
36. Puhakka T, Lehti H, Vainionpaa R, et al: Zanamivir: a significant reduction in viral load during treatment in military conscripts with influenza. *Scand J Infect Dis* 35:52, 2003.
37. Nicholson KG, Aoki FY, Osterhaus AD, et al: Efficacy and safety of oseltamivir in treatment of acute influenza: a randomised controlled trial. Neuraminidase Inhibitor Flu Treatment Investigator Group. *Lancet* 355:1845, 2000.
38. Kaiser L, Wat C, Mills T, et al: Impact of oseltamivir treatment on influenza-related lower respiratory tract complications and hospitalizations. *Arch Intern Med* 163:1667, 2003.
39. Jefferson T, Jones M, Doshi P, et al: Neuraminidase inhibitors for preventing and treating influenza in healthy adults: systematic review and meta-analysis. *BMJ* 339:b5106, 2009.
40. Kiso M, Mitamura K, Sakai-Tagawa Y, et al: Resistant influenza A viruses in children treated with oseltamivir: descriptive study. *Lancet* 364:759, 2004.
41. Ison MG, Gubareva LV, Atmar RL, et al: Recovery of drug-resistant influenza virus from immunocompromised patients: a case series. *J Infect Dis* 193:760, 2006.
42. Rodriguez WJ, Hall CB, Welliver R, et al: Efficacy and safety of aerosolized ribavirin in young children hospitalized with influenza: a double-blind, multicenter, placebo-controlled trial. *J Pediatr* 125:129, 1994.
43. Oliveira EC, Lee B, Colice GL: Influenza in the intensive care unit. *J Intensive Care Med* 18:80, 2003.
44. Guerguerian AM, Gauthier M, Lebel MH, et al: Ribavirin in ventilated respiratory syncytial virus bronchiolitis. A randomized, placebo-controlled trial. *Am J Respir Crit Care Med* 160:829, 1999.
45. Rodriguez WJ, Kim HW, Brandt CD, et al: Aerosolized ribavirin in the treatment of patients with respiratory syncytial virus disease. *Pediatr Infect Dis J* 6:159, 1987.
46. Feltes TF, Cabalka AK, Meissner HC, et al: Palivizumab prophylaxis reduces hospitalization due to respiratory syncytial virus in young children with hemodynamically significant congenital heart disease. *J Pediatr* 143:532, 2003.
47. Mejias A, Chavez-Bueno S, Jafri HS, et al: Respiratory syncytial virus infections: old challenges and new opportunities. *Pediatr Infect Dis J* 24[Suppl 11]:S189, 2005.
48. van Woensel JB, van Aalderen WM, de Weerd W, et al: Dexamethasone for treatment of patients mechanically ventilated for lower respiratory tract infection caused by respiratory syncytial virus. *Thorax* 58:383, 2003.
49. Buckingham SC, Jafri HS, Bush AJ, et al: A randomized, double-blind, placebo-controlled trial of dexamethasone in severe respiratory syncytial virus (RSV) infection: effects on RSV quantity and clinical outcome. *J Infect Dis* 185:1222, 2002.
50. Bordigoni P, Carret AS, Venard V, et al: Treatment of adenovirus infections in patients undergoing allogeneic hematopoietic stem cell transplantation. *Clin Infect Dis* 32:1290, 2001.
51. Ribaud P, Scieux C, Freymuth F, et al: Successful treatment of adenovirus disease with intravenous cidofovir in an unrelated stem-cell transplant recipient. *Clin Infect Dis* 28:690, 1999.
52. Barker JH, Luby JP, Sean Dalley A, et al: Fatal type 3 adenoviral pneumonia in immunocompetent adult identical twins. *Clin Infect Dis* 37:e142, 2003.
53. Dunkle LM, Arvin AM, Whitley RJ, et al: A controlled trial of acyclovir for chickenpox in normal children. *N Engl J Med* 325:1539, 1991.
54. Wallace MR, Bowler WA, Murray NB, et al: Treatment of adult varicella with oral acyclovir. A randomized, placebo-controlled trial. *Ann Intern Med* 117:358, 1992.
55. Mer M, Richards GA: Corticosteroids in life-threatening varicella pneumonia. *Chest* 114:426, 1998.
56. Perry RT, Halsey NA: The clinical significance of measles: a review. *J Infect Dis* 189[Suppl 1]:S4, 2004.
57. Rupp ME, Schwartz ML, Bechard DE: Measles pneumonia. Treatment of a near-fatal case with corticosteroids and vitamin A. *Chest* 103:1625, 1993.
58. Tatsukawa M, Sawayama Y, Nabeshima S, et al: A case of severe adult measles pneumonia—efficacy of combination of steroid pulse therapy, high-dose vitamin A and gamma globulins. *Kansenshogaku Zasshi* 75:989, 2001.
59. Forni AL, Schluger NW, Roberts RB: Severe measles pneumonitis in adults: evaluation of clinical characteristics and therapy with intravenous ribavirin. *Clin Infect Dis* 19:454, 1994.
60. Yu WC, Hui DS, Chan-Yeung M: Antiviral agents and corticosteroids in the treatment of severe acute respiratory syndrome (SARS). *Thorax* 59:643, 2004.

61. Auyeung TW, Lee JS, Lai WK, et al: The use of corticosteroid as treatment in SARS was associated with adverse outcomes: a retrospective cohort study. *J Infect* 51:98, 2005.
62. Mertz GJ, Miedzinski L, Goade D, et al: Placebo-controlled, double-blind trial of intravenous ribavirin for the treatment of hantavirus cardiopulmonary syndrome in North America. *Clin Infect Dis* 39:1307, 2004.
63. Huggins JW, Hsiang CM, Cosgriff TM, et al: Prospective, double-blind, concurrent, placebo-controlled clinical trial of intravenous ribavirin therapy of hemorrhagic fever with renal syndrome. *J Infect Dis* 164:1119, 1991.
64. Govorkova EA, Leneva IA, Goloubeva OG, et al: Comparison of efficacies of RWJ-270201, zanamivir, and oseltamivir against H5N1, H9N2, and other avian influenza viruses. *Antimicrob Agents Chemother* 45:2723, 2001.
65. Gubareva LV, McCullers JA, Bethell RC, et al: Characterization of influenza A/HongKong/156/97 (H5N1) virus in a mouse model and protective effect of zanamivir on H5N1 infection in mice. *J Infect Dis* 178:1592, 1998.
66. Leneva IA, Goloubeva O, Fenton RJ, et al: Efficacy of zanamivir against avian influenza A viruses that possess genes encoding H5N1 internal proteins and are pathogenic in mammals. *Antimicrob Agents Chemother* 45:1216, 2001.
67. Chotpitayasunondh T, Ungchusak K, Hanshaoworakul W, et al: Human disease from influenza A (H5N1), Thailand, 2004. *Emerg Infect Dis* 11:201, 2005.
68. de Jong MD, Tran TT, Truong HK, et al: Oseltamivir resistance during treatment of influenza A (H5N1) infection. *N Engl J Med* 353:2667, 2005.
69. Tran TH, Nguyen TL, Nguyen TD, et al: Avian influenza A (H5N1) in 10 patients in Vietnam. *N Engl J Med* 350:1179, 2004.

SECTION VII ■ GASTROINTESTINAL DISEASE PROBLEMS IN THE INTENSIVE CARE UNIT

DOMINIC J. NOMPLEGGI

CHAPTER 91 ■ UPPER AND LOWER GASTROINTESTINAL BLEEDING

RYAN F. PORTER, GARY R. ZUCKERMAN AND CHANDRA PRAKASH GYAWALI

Acute gastrointestinal (GI) bleeding is a common emergency that often necessitates admission to the intensive care unit (ICU). There are compelling differences in incidence, clinical presentation, severity, and mortality between lower and upper GI hemorrhage. The annual incidence rate of lower intestinal bleeding is estimated at 20.5 to 33 cases per 100,000 adult populations [1,2], while that of upper GI bleeding is estimated between 60 and 125 cases per 100,000 [3,4]. The incidence of upper GI bleeding has declined in those younger than age 70 years to as low as 47 per 100,000 over the past decade [2,5]. *Helicobacter pylori* eradication efforts and widespread use of proton pump inhibitor (PPI) therapy may account for this decline. The incidence in older populations, however, remains stable possibly from more frequent use of aspirin and nonsteroidal anti-inflammatory drugs (NSAIDs) [4,6]. The majority of upper GI bleeds are nonvariceal (80% to 90%), of which 28% to 59% are attributable to peptic ulcer bleeding [3,4]. Patients with lower GI bleeding are half as likely to present with hemodynamic compromise or require blood transfusion, and have significantly higher hemoglobin concentrations at presentation compared to upper GI bleeding [7]. The mortality rate from upper GI bleeding has remained stable at 5% to 12%, while mortality rates for lower intestinal bleeding remain below 5% [4,7]. Newer surgical, endoscopic, and medical therapies, as well as improved ICU care, will hopefully improve survival rates for both upper and lower GI bleeding in the coming years.

INITIAL EVALUATION AND RESUSCITATION

Resuscitating the actively bleeding patient takes priority over localizing the bleeding source. The immediate goals are to replete intravascular volume and prevent irreversible shock. However, even in situations of exsanguinating hemorrhage, limited attempts to localize bleeding while resuscitation continues may be required to help direct a surgical or angiographic approach.

An initial brief history and physical examination that includes serial measurement of vital signs and evaluation of the volume and character of bleeding helps determine the urgency and degree of resuscitation necessary. Tachycardia (pulse >100 beat per minute), hypotension (systolic blood pressure <100 mm Hg), or orthostatic hypotension (an increase in the pulse of ≥20 beats per minute or a drop in systolic blood pressure of ≥20 mm Hg on standing) indicates significant intravascular volume depletion [4]. Insight into volume status can also be gained from evaluation of mucous membranes and neck veins, and measurement of urine output [4]. Bleeding patients will need large bore intravenous-access catheters (e.g., peripheral catheters 16 or 18 guage or central venous access), supplemental oxygen, correction of coagulopathies and prompt packed red blood cell transfusion for tachycardia, hypotension or hemoglobin less than 10 g/dL [4]. Clinical parameters and evidence of gross bleeding will dictate the approach, but preparedness should be for the potential of massive bleeding.

Older patients with hemodynamic compromise or shock have a poor outcome (Table 91.1) and need urgent resuscitation and close monitoring. In situations of massive hematemesis, endotracheal intubation provides airway protection and facilitates endoscopic evaluation and therapy. Chest pain may imply a superimposed myocardial infarction or dissecting aneurysm, whereas a history of abdominal vascular surgery adds aortoenteric fistula to the differential diagnoses. GI bleeding is generally not associated with significant abdominal pain, and its presence could signify hematobilia, intestinal infarction, or intestinal perforation.

FURTHER EVALUATION AND MANAGEMENT

Resuscitation may need to continue even after the initial volume deficit has been corrected if there is evidence of ongoing or renewed bleeding. Because of the laxative properties of fresh blood in the GI tract, repeated passage of liquid blood per rectum implies ongoing or recurrent bleeding. As bleeding stops, the stool becomes formed and converts from red or maroon blood to darker stool and eventually to brown stool that contains occult blood, which may persist for as long as 2 weeks after GI bleeding has ceased.

TABLE 91.1

CLINICAL RISK FACTORS FOR MORTALITY IN ACUTE UPPER GASTROINTESTINAL BLEEDING

Clinical feature	Mortality (%)
Age ≥60 y	11
Age <60 y	1
Shock on admission	23
No shock	4
Rebleeding in 72 h	30
No rebleeding	3
Failure to clear red nasogastric aspirate	50
Red-to-clear nasogastric return	8

Data derived from Branicki FJ, Boey J, Fok PJ, et al: Bleeding duodenal ulcer: a prospective evaluation of risk factors for rebleeding and death. *Ann Surg* 211:411, 1989; Hunt PS: Bleeding gastroduodenal ulcers: selection of patients for surgery. *World J Surg* 11:289, 1987; and MacLeod IA, Mills PR: Factors predicting the probability of further hemorrhage after upper gastrointestinal hemorrhage. *Br J Surg* 69:256, 1982, with permission.

TABLE 91.2

COMPLETE ROCKALL SCORE FOR RISK STRATIFICATION OF ACUTE UPPER GASTROINTESTINAL BLEEDING

Variable	Points
Clinical Rockall score	
Age	
<60 y	0
60–79 y	1
≥80 y	2
Shock	
Heart rate >100 beats/min	1
Systolic blood pressure <100 mm Hg	2
Coexisting illness	
Coronary artery disease, congestive heart failure, other major illness	2
Renal failure, hepatic failure, metastatic cancer	3
Endoscopic diagnosis	
No finding, Mallory–Weiss tear	0
Peptic ulcer, erosive disease, esophagitis	1
Cancer of the upper GI tract	2
Endoscopic stigmata of recent bleeding	
Clean based ulcer, flat pigmented spot	0
Blood in upper GI tract, active bleeding visible vessel, clot	2

Note: Patients with a clinical Rockall score of 0 or a complete Rockall score of <2 are considered to be at low risk for rebleeding or mortality. Higher scores indicate higher risks.
Adapted from Gralnek IM, Barkum AN, Bardou M: Management of acute bleeding from a peptic ulcer. *N Engl J Med* 359:928–937, 2008.

In patients without hematemesis, a nasogastric (NG) tube aspirate of red blood may be a poor prognostic sign [3,4], but the lack of red blood or coffee ground material does not exclude an upper GI bleeding source [4]. Clinical variables at presentation in combination with endoscopic findings have been used to triage and risk-stratify patients, assess risk of poor outcomes, and aid in guiding management [3,4]. The Glasgow-Blatchford Score is a validated tool based solely on clinical variables scored from 0 to 23, with higher values predictive of higher risk. Scores of 0 are at low risk of rebleeding and mortality and can be considered for outpatient management [4,8]. The Rockall Score can be calculated prior to and after endoscopy (Table 91.2), with higher scores predictive of higher risk of a poor outcome [4,9]. While their exact role in clinical management continues to be evaluated, these scores will likely continue to have an increasing role in patient care.

DIAGNOSTIC EVALUATION

Bedside Diagnosis

While hematemesis is clearly a symptom of upper GI bleeding, black tarry melenic stool predicts an upper GI bleeding source, and brighter colors of red in the stool are more often associated with a distal colonic bleeding source. However, color of bloody stool may not always be helpful in predicting the level of GI bleeding and is subject to interpretation variability of both patients and physicians. A pocket-sized color card is helpful in confirming the stool color, as described by the patient, and suggesting the level of bleeding in the GI tract [10]. When bright blood in the stool (implying a lower GI bleed) is associated with hemodynamic compromise, as many as 11% of patients may have an upper GI bleeding source, even if the NG aspirate is negative [3,4]. In this setting, an upper endoscopy may be the first endoscopic evaluation even though the presenting symptom is hematochezia.

Upper Endoscopy

When bleeding is suspected to originate proximal to the jejunum, esophagogastroduodenoscopy (upper endoscopy) is the diagnostic procedure of choice. This identifies the bleeding source in 80% to 90% of cases with a high degree of accuracy, provides therapeutic options, and carries low morbidity [3,4]. Endoscopy has the added advantage of detecting prognostic signs (Table 91.2) and classifies bleeding stigmata as high or low risk for rebleeding based on the Forrest grade (Table 91.3) [11].

Even when an exact diagnosis cannot be made, localizing the bleeding to a specific region within the upper GI tract can be helpful to the surgeon (if resection is indicated) or interventional radiologist (if embolization of the bleeding vessel is recommended). Erythromycin or metoclopramide can be administered intravenously to induce gastric emptying and clear the stomach of blood and clots prior to endoscopy [12,13]; repeated lavage with saline through a wide-bore orogastric tube also may be used for this purpose. However, routine gastric lavage may not be necessary and is not endorsed by the authors. Complications related to endoscopy are higher when the procedure is performed on an emergency basis.

The timing of endoscopy in upper GI bleeding continues to be evaluated. Endoscopy within 12 hours of presentation increased the use of endoscopic therapy but did not reduce rebleeding rates or improve survival rates [14]. However, endoscopy within 24 hours did demonstrate a reduction in the length of hospital stay and need for surgical intervention [15,16]. Patients with bloody NG aspirate did benefit from

TABLE 91.3

RISK FACTORS FOR CONTINUED BLEEDING OR REBLEEDING FROM PEPTIC ULCER

Endoscopic finding	Forrest grade	Proportion that continues to bleed or rebleed (%)
Arterial bleeding	IA	90
Nonbleeding visible vessel	IIA	40–50
Adherent clot	IIB	10–25
Oozing	IB	<20
Flat pigmented spot	IIC	<10
Clean ulcer base	III	<5
Ulcer of posterior-inferior duodenal bulb (gastroduodenal artery)		[a]
Ulcer of lesser-curve gastric body (left gastric artery)		[a]

[a] Percent unknown but frequent finding at surgery for ongoing bleeding.
Note: Forrest grades IIC and III are considered low risk for rebleeding.
Data from NIH Consensus Conference: Therapeutic endoscopy and bleeding ulcers. *JAMA* 262:1369, 1989; Swain CP: Pathology of bleeding lesions, in Sugawa C, Schuman B, Lucas C (eds): *Gastrointestinal Bleeding*. New York, Igaku-Shoin, 1992, p 26; Lane L: Rolling review: upper gastrointestinal bleeding. *Aliment Pharmacol Ther* 7:207, 1993; Forrest JA, Finlayson ND, Shearman DJ: Endoscopy in gastrointestinal bleeding. *Lancet* 2:394–397, 1974.

endoscopy within 12 hours to reduce the blood transfusion requirements and length of hospital stay [14]. Therefore, endoscopy offered within 24 hours of upper GI bleeding presentation appears appropriate, with consideration for early endoscopy within 12 hours for patients with bloody NG aspirate or clinical suspicion for high-risk lesions [17]. The benefit of a repeat "second-look" endoscopy is an area of investigation, especially in the presence of factors associated with an increased risk of rebleeding (history of peptic ulcer disease, previous ulcer bleeding, presence of shock at presentation, ulcers >2 cm, large underlying bleeding vessel ≥2 mm diameter, and ulcers located in lesser curve of stomach or posterior/superior duodenal bulb) [18,19]. A meta-analysis in 2003 concluded that second-look endoscopy was associated with a decreased risk of recurrent bleeding but did not alter subsequent surgery rates or mortality [20]. Scheduled repeat endoscopy therefore is not routinely recommended, but can be considered on an individual case basis if clinical signs of recurrent bleeding are present or if there are questions about adequate hemostasis [21,22].

Enteroscopy

If a small bowel lesion is suspected after a negative upper endoscopy, a longer endoscope can be used to evaluate the proximal small bowel (push enteroscopy), which allows visual inspection and endoscopic hemostasis of bleeding lesions as far distal as the proximal jejunum [23]. Further evaluation of small bowel bleeding lesions can be provided by capsule endoscopy. Disadvantages of capsule endoscopy in acute bleeding include the lack of accurate localization of visualized lesions, and the fact that the test is not performed in real time [23]. Bleeding lesions beyond the reach of a push enteroscope can potentially be approached using single- and double-balloon enteroscopy, techniques that allow for visualization of most of the small bowel. Balloons at the endoscope tip and an overtube can be consecutively inflated and deflated while inserting and pulling out the endoscope to allow bowel to pleat over the overtube, thus allowing deep endoscope insertion into the small bowel, either through the mouth or the anus [23].

Sigmoidoscopy/Colonoscopy

When a distal lower GI bleeding source is suspected, early sigmoidoscopy may be helpful if the bleeding is not of a magnitude that would prevent adequate visualization. For most situations, however, colonoscopy replaces sigmoidoscopy in the diagnostic approach. Early colonoscopy provides a higher yield of the bleeding source compared to radiologic studies, especially when performed within 24 hours of presentation [24,25]. In patients with severe hematochezia and diverticulosis, urgent colonoscopy (within 6 to 12 hours of hospitalization or diagnosis of hematochezia) after rapid bowel purge can provide endoscopic treatment of diverticular hemorrhage and may prevent recurrent bleeding and decrease the need for surgery [26]. Only 20% of patients with lower GI bleeding, however, have a lesion amenable to endoscopic intervention [27]. Even when the exact cause of bleeding cannot be determined, colonoscopy may localize fresh blood to a segment of colon and direct further therapies such as angiotherapy or surgery. Patients with subacute bleeding or hemorrhage that has ceased can undergo adequate bowel preparation followed by semiurgent colonoscopy [28].

Radionuclide Bleeding Scan

The technetium-99m–labeled red blood cell scan performed at the bedside offers a noninvasive diagnostic approach to patients suspected of having GI bleeding originating beyond the reach of an endoscope, especially in unstable patients where bowel preparation or endoscopy cannot be safely performed. Although bleeding rates as low as 0.1 mL per minute can be detected by this method, the patient should have evidence of ongoing bleeding during the study [7]. If the test localizes bleeding, angiography or endoscopy (push enteroscopy, colonoscopy, double-balloon enteroscopy, capsule endoscopy) is needed to confirm the site, to further define the cause, and to offer therapy for ongoing bleeding [7]. If the test is negative, colonoscopy followed by capsule endoscopy is usually performed to evaluate potential colonic and small bowel bleeding sources [23].

Mesenteric Arteriography

Because a more rapid bleeding rate is necessary for a positive arteriogram (0.5 mL per minute), this procedure typically is performed after active bleeding is documented on a radionuclide bleeding scan [7]. However, because of the intermittent nature of bleeding and the variable timing of mesenteric arteriography, a positive red blood cell scan does not always result in a diagnostic arteriogram [7]. Arteriography is also useful for upper GI bleeding sources not visualized on upper endoscopy because of rapid bleeding or a blood-filled stomach.

THERAPEUTIC PROCEDURES FOR HEMOSTASIS

Evidence-based recommendations for the therapy of GI bleeding are summarized in Table 91.4.

Endoscopic Therapy (Endotherapy)

Endotherapy offers a convenient and expedient method for treatment of GI bleeding. Although endotherapy was primarily used for the treatment of upper GI and peptic ulcer bleeding, these modalities can also be applied to patients with lower GI bleeding [4,29–31]. Endotherapy is indicated for all patients with high-risk lesions because of the significant risk of persistent or recurrent bleeding (22% to 55%) and even death

TABLE 91.4

SUMMARY OF EVIDENCE-BASED FINDINGS FOR THERAPY OF GASTROINTESTINAL (GI) BLEEDING

- Octreotide infusion is an effective adjunct to endoscopic therapy for variceal bleeding [51,57,58].
- Endoscopic variceal band ligation is the therapy of choice for esophageal variceal bleeding [71].
- Identification of patients at high risk for rebleeding and mortality, and early diagnostic endoscopy with hemostatic therapy in patients with high-risk stigmata of rebleeding improve outcome in acute nonvariceal upper GI bleeding [8,9,11,101].
- Intravenous proton pump inhibitors, especially when administered as an infusion after a bolus dose, are superior to intravenous histamine-2 receptor antagonists in the reduction of rebleeding after successful endoscopic therapy in acute nonvariceal upper GI bleeding [105,106,108].
- Early colonoscopy for acute lower GI bleeding may identify a bleeding source more often compared to radiologic studies, but the choice of diagnostic test may not affect patient outcome [25].

if left untreated [3,4,32]. Randomized trials demonstrate that endotherapy for upper GI bleeding decreases further bleeding, shortens hospital stay, decreases transfusions, decreases emergency surgery, decreases mortality, and lowers costs [17]. Optimal therapy for adherent clots remains controversial; a recent meta-analysis demonstrated reduced rebleeding rates (RR 0.35, 95% CI 0.14–0.82) with endoscopic removal of clot and treating of the uncovered lesion, but no change in length of hospitalization, need for surgery, transfusion requirements, and mortality compared to only medical therapy [33–35].

The most common modalities used are thermal therapy (heater probe, bipolar probe, argon laser coagulation), injection therapy (epinephrine, hypertonic saline, sclerosing solutions), and mechanical therapy (hemoclips, endoloops, and band ligation). The treatment modalities are generally comparable with respect to efficacy and safety even when used in combination [3,36]. In a Cochrane database systemic review, addition of an alternative modality of endotherapy to epinephrine injection alone reduced further bleeding from 18.8% to 10.4% (OR 0.51), need for emergency surgery from 10.8% to 7.1% (OR 0.63), and mortality from 5% to 2.5% (OR 0.50) in high-risk ulcers [37]. These findings are similar to prior meta-analysis and mirrors published guidelines [38]. However, despite successful endotherapy, rebleeding can occur in up to 30% of patients (Table 91.3). The Baylor bleeding score, using patient age, number of illnesses, illness severity, site of bleeding, and stigmata of bleeding, has been proposed to predict the likelihood of rebleeding [39].

Angiotherapy

Intra-arterial vasopressin and/or embolization are used for angiographic control of various bleeding lesions [7]. A recent randomized study comparing urgent colonoscopy to radionuclide scanning followed by angiography demonstrated no differences in hospital stay and transfusion requirements, despite the fact that colonoscopy identified a definitive bleeding source more often. However, this study used only vasopressin infusion and did not use embolization as a mode of angiotherapy [24]. Vasopressin has potential to cause cardiovascular complications. Gelfoam and metal coil used for embolic therapy after superselective cannulation of the bleeding artery are effective because they can be delivered close to the terminal bleeding vessel and result in localized thrombosis with vessel occlusion. Embolization successfully controls bleeding in 52% to 94% of patients, with approximately 10% of these patients requiring repeat embolization for recurrent bleeding [40]. Angiotherapy may be a first-line treatment for uncontrolled lower GI bleeding from lesions such as diverticula and angiodysplasia, but its use in the upper gut is reserved for peptic ulcer bleeding that is not localized or controlled by endotherapy in the presence of a prohibitive surgical risk. Angiotherapy can be comparable to surgical intervention when endoscopic therapy fails for bleeding peptic ulcers. A retrospective analysis demonstrated no difference between embolization and surgery in recurrent bleeding (29.0% and 23.1%), additional surgery required (16.1% and 30.8%), and mortality (25.8% and 20.5%) despite an older population and higher prevalence of heart disease within embolization group [41]. The timing for the use of angiography and angiotherapy must be individualized and usually is a consensus decision by the involved physicians.

Surgical Therapy

The appropriate timing of when a surgeon should be involved in the care of a bleeding patient is physician and institution dependent, and ranges from an early team approach at presentation to involvement once the risk of significant morbidity and mortality are established after a poor response to medical and endoscopic therapy. Surgical intervention is an effective and safe alternative for patients with uncontrollable bleeding or those unable to tolerate additional bleeding [42]. Prior to surgical intervention, a repeat endoscopy for a patient with persistent or recurrent bleeding can be considered due to lower risks of side effects from endoscopy compared to surgery [43,44]. A possible exception may be ulcers >2 cm in hypotensive patients where the risk of rebleeding is extremely high with repeat endoscopic therapy [44,45].

Patients with massive hemorrhage that overwhelms the resuscitation effort may need to proceed directly to the surgical suite during ongoing resuscitation. If these patients are high-risk surgical candidates, angiotherapy for variceal bleeding or a percutaneously or surgically placed portal-hepatic shunt for variceal bleeding may be alternatives.

SPECIFIC BLEEDING LESIONS

Variceal Upper Gastrointestinal Bleeding

Portal hypertension, most frequently a consequence of cirrhosis, leads to portosystemic collateral circulations at the squamocolumnar junctions in the gut (i.e., gastroesophageal, anal, and peristomal), which progressively enlarge to form varices. Bleeding from gastroesophageal varices characteristically is brisk and typically presents as hematemesis, melena, or hematochezia in association with hemodynamic instability. The presentation may be less dramatic, as acute blood loss can be self-limited in 50% to 60% of cases [46]. One-half to two-thirds of patients with cirrhosis and acute upper GI bleeding have nonvariceal sources of hemorrhage documented by endoscopy [47,48]. Upper GI variceal bleeding occurs in at least 20% of all patients with cirrhosis who develop varices, with bleeding episodes carrying a mortality rate of at least 20% at 6 weeks [49,50]. Once active bleeding stops, the likelihood of recurrent variceal hemorrhage is 40% within 72 hours and 60% within 10 days if no definitive treatment is pursued [33]. Risk factors associated with variceal rupture include a portal pressure gradient greater than 12 mm Hg, large variceal size (greater than 5 mm), and progressive hepatic dysfunction [51]. Endoscopic findings that implicate esophageal or gastric varices as the bleeding source include the red sign, where one varix is brighter red than the others from microtelangiectasia (red-sign variants include red-wale marks, cherry-red spots, hematocystic spots, and diffuse redness of varix), and the white-nipple sign, in which a fresh fibrin clot may be seen protruding from a varix [51–53]. Endotracheal intubation protects the airway from aspiration of blood in obtunded patients, especially in the setting of massive bleeding [54]. Additional complications that must be addressed include alcohol withdrawal, aspiration, infection, and electrolyte imbalances.

Octreotide is a somatostatin analog that decreases splanchnic blood flow and portal pressure, controlling variceal bleeding in as many as 85% of patients [55–57] with an efficacy approaching that of endoscopic therapy (Table 91.4) and providing improved visibility during subsequent endoscopy [57–61]. Octreotide typically is administered intravenously as a bolus dose of 50 to 100 μg followed by continuous infusion of 25 to 50 μg per hour continued 3 to 5 days after diagnosis, but tachyphylaxis may limit efficacy of repeated bolus administrations [51,58–60,62–64]. Aside from transient nausea and abdominal pain with bolus doses, significant adverse effects from octreotide are rare [65]. Vasopressin, once widely used in this setting, has a significant cardiovascular side-effect profile and for this reason has been replaced by octreotide.

Infection (specifically spontaneous bacterial peritonitis) occurs in patients with cirrhosis and GI bleeding of any type in 25% to 50% of cases, leading to increased bleeding and mortality [66–68]. Antibiotic prophylaxis with a fluoroquinolone (norfloxacin or ciprofloxacin) in all cirrhotics with GI hemorrhage reduces the rate of bacterial infections and improves survival [69,70]. Intravenous ceftriaxone is an alternative for patients with advanced cirrhosis or when quinolone-resistant organisms are suspected [51].

Endoscopic band ligation has gained acceptance as the preferred endoscopic treatment for patients with bleeding esophageal varices, with rapid obliteration of varices, and low rates of complications and rebleeding (Table 91.4) [51,71]. Endoscopic variceal sclerotherapy (injecting a sclerosing solution into the variceal lumen or into the adjacent submucosa), although successful in controlling variceal bleeding, is associated with a 20% to 40% incidence of complications, and has largely been relegated to a second-line therapeutic modality [51,72]. Complications of band ligation include recurrent bleeding from treatment-induced esophageal ulcers, stricture formation, esophageal perforation, and acceleration of portal hypertensive gastropathy [72,73]. Repeat variceal band ligation is performed at 2- to 3-month intervals until varices are obliterated, as this approach reduces the incidence of rebleeding [51].

Gastric varices are detected in approximately 20% of patients with portal hypertension, but can also occur from splenic vein thrombosis. Gastric varices bleed less often, but blood loss can be more substantial compared to esophageal varices [74]. When available, endoscopic injection of a tissue adhesive such as butyl cyanoacrylate is effective, with hemostasis rates approaching that of TIPS with fewer recurrences [51,75,76]. Complications include a propensity for embolic phenomenon posttreatment, including massive pulmonary embolism [77]. Gastric variceal hemorrhage dictates earlier consideration of nonendoscopic therapeutic approaches such as transjugular intrahepatic portosystemic shunt (TIPS) placement. Embolization of the short gastric veins and varices is a potential management option for isolated gastric varices. In the setting of splenic vein thrombosis, splenectomy may be an appropriate therapy.

A TIPS (an iatrogenic fistula between the hepatic vein and portal vein) decreases portal pressure gradient to less than the 10 mm Hg necessary for the formation of esophagogastric varices [78,79]. TIPS commonly is recommended if esophageal variceal bleeding recurs after two or more endoscopic attempts at therapy [80], if active bleeding is not responsive to variceal ligation or sclerotherapy, or as first-line treatment for gastric variceal bleeding [51]. Complications include transient deterioration of liver function, new or worsened hepatic encephalopathy (25%), and shunt insufficiency from thrombosis or stenosis [79]. When placed in an emergency setting to control active bleeding, a 10% in-hospital mortality and 40% 30-day mortality have been reported [79,81–83].

Surgically created shunts reliably control acute bleeding (>90%) and prevent rebleeding (<10%) [84–87] but are limited by high operative mortality and postprocedure encephalopathy. Therefore, surgical shunts are only considered in well-compensated cirrhotic patients with good long-term prognoses [87].

Esophageal or gastric balloon devices may be used for direct tamponade of the bleeding source when definitive therapy is not immediately available. There are two basic types of balloon tubes: those with gastric and esophageal balloons (Sengstaken–Blakemore and Minnesota tubes), and those with a large gastric balloon alone (Linton–Nachlas). The incidence of rebleeding is expectedly high. Other complications (aspiration, balloon migration, airway occlusion, perforation, pressure necrosis) occur in 15% to 30% of patients, including death in 6% [88,89]. Instructions for correctly placing and maintaining a specific balloon device are included as a product insert and should be reviewed before balloon use.

Peptic Ulcer Bleeding

The most important etiologic factors for peptic ulcer disease are *H. pylori* infection and NSAID use. Although the role of *H. pylori* infection in ulcer formation is established, its exact role in precipitating ulcer bleeding is controversial [90–92]. With long-term NSAID use, there is a greater risk of gastric ulceration compared to duodenal ulceration. Bleeding risk varies depending on NSAID dose and agent used. Other cofactors, including older age, a history of past peptic ulcers (especially with ulcer bleeding), and a history of coronary disease, may be independent risk factors for ulcer bleeding [93,94]. Population-based studies have suggested that ulcer formation and bleeding occur even with COX-2 inhibitors, albeit at a lower rate [95]. Both COX-2 inhibitors and their nonselective analogs are associated with increased risk of ulcer bleeding when taken in conjunction with anticoagulants such as warfarin [96]. This risk with nonselective NSAIDs and anticoagulation taken together may be as high as 13 times that of patients taking neither NSAIDs nor anticoagulants [97]. Less than 1% of peptic ulcers result from hypersecretory states such as Zollinger–Ellison syndrome. In a proportion of patients, the disorder remains idiopathic, either because of inability to demonstrate *H. pylori* or lack of a history of obvious NSAID use.

Although 80% or more patients with acute GI bleeding eventually stop bleeding [98], it is important to recognize factors associated with higher risk for morbidity and mortality, including older age, large ulcer size (more than 2 cm), large-volume bleeding, and onset of bleeding while hospitalized (Table 91.1). Other prognostic information can be obtained from endoscopy findings, which should detail whether stigmata of recent bleeding (active bleeding, nonbleeding visible vessel, adherent clot, flat pigment spots) or no stigmata (clean ulcer base) were found in association with the ulcer (Table 91.3). These criteria can be used to predict rebleeding and the need for therapeutic intervention [32,98–100]. Patient age, hemodynamic parameters, comorbidities, and endoscopic findings have been compiled into scoring system by Rockall et al. [101] and Blatchford [4]. The Rockall score (Table 91.2) has been validated as a predictor of short-term mortality, but not recurrent bleeding [9].

In vitro data suggest that gastric acid plays an important role in impairing platelet aggregation, clot lysis, and increased fibrinolytic activity that is reversible at pH values above 6 to 6.5 [102–104]. Proton pump inhibitors (PPIs) can effectively raise gastric pH >4.0 but their ability to elevate pH to >6.0 is unclear [102]. However, these differences in gastric pH may not translate into clinical benefit. In contrast to histamine-2 receptor antagonists, PPIs have been established as beneficial in acute nonvariceal upper GI bleeding (Table 90.4), with a rapid increase in gastric pH, especially with IV PPI, when a mean pH of 6 is reached approximately 1 hour sooner than oral PPI [105]. A recent Cochrane meta-analysis reaffirmed the established understanding that IV PPI therapy in the setting of peptic ulcer disease decreased rebleeding rates (OR 0.40, 95% CI 0.24–0.67), need for urgent surgery (OR 0.50, 95% CI 0.33–0.76), and risk of death (OR 0.53, 95% CI 0.31–0.91) [106]. Intravenous PPI therapy upon presentation (when compared to IV PPI therapy initiated after endoscopic therapy) decreases the need for endoscopic therapy but not rebleeding rates, blood transfusion requirements, or mortality, a result supported by meta-analysis [107,108]. This approach has been demonstrated to be cost effective, reducing need for endoscopic therapy by 7.4% [109].

Therefore, the current clinical practice is to administer intravenous PPI therapy at presentation of acute upper GI bleeding. Intravenous PPI dosing regimens continue to be debated. A pooled randomized controlled trial suggested that IV bolus followed by continuous infusion decreased rebleeding rates and need for surgery compared to bolus dosing alone [110], leading recent reviews in the topic to suggest a regimen of IV PPI (80 mg bolus dose plus continuous infusion at 8 mg per hour) for 72 hours after endoscopic therapy of nonvariceal upper GI bleeding for any patient with a high-risk Forrest grade bleeding lesion [4]. Oral administration can be substituted after the initial intravenous period once oral intake is resumed.

Mallory–Weiss Tear

A Mallory–Weiss tear represents bleeding from a mucosal disruption at the area of the esophagogastric junction and is found in approximately 5% to 15% of cases of upper GI bleeding. The classic history is a patient with vomiting of nonbloody gastric contents followed by hematemesis, although this presentation is variable (29% to 86%) [111]. Blood with the initial emesis does not exclude the diagnosis. The great majority of patients (80% to 90%) bleeding from a Mallory–Weiss tear stop bleeding without therapeutic intervention, and rebleeding rates are low (less than 5%). Endoscopy offers diagnosis and the option for endotherapy; rarely nonendoscopic measures such as angiography and embolic therapy are required.

Angiodysplasia

Angiodysplasia lesions are small (3 to 15 mm) vascular mucosal abnormalities that can cause GI bleeding from the stomach, small bowel, or colon. Bleeding upper GI lesions frequently occur in patients with chronic renal failure [112,113], whereas vascular heart disease is associated with colonic lesions [114]. The character of the bleeding usually is subacute and recurrent rather than massive. Angiodysplasia typically is diagnosed at endoscopy; bleeding colonic angiodysplasia lesions can also be detected with angiography. Angiodysplasia lesions are the most frequent finding in the small bowel on wireless capsule endoscopy performed for evaluation of obscure GI bleeding. Endoscopic thermal therapy typically is successful in obliterating the lesions [115]. When large lesions are encountered, the periphery is cauterized first to obliterate the feeder vessels, and the center of the lesion is treated last [116]. Angiotherapy and surgery can be used to treat bleeding vascular lesions.

Dieulafoy's Lesion

Dieulafoy's lesion, an unusual cause of massive bleeding, represents a mucosal defect, not an ulcer, that exposes an end artery of the same caliber as its feeding submucosal artery [117]. The lesions are typically located in the gastric cardia/proximal stomach but are rarely found in the duodenum and other parts of the GI tract including the colon and rectum [118]. Bleeding often is massive and recurrent yet difficult to diagnose. The site is minute, innocent-looking, and frequently not appreciated at endoscopy once bleeding has stopped. Upper endoscopy can offer diagnosis and treat a lesion that was previously considered amenable only to surgical resection [119]. Endoscopic band ligation is one method that has been successful for hemostasis [120].

Colonic Diverticular Bleeding

Bleeding colonic diverticula are the most frequent cause of lower GI bleeding, but a definitive diagnosis (e.g., finding stigmata of recent bleeding) is established in only 20% of patients with hematochezia and colonic diverticula [121]. Diverticular bleeding demonstrated by angiography usually is localized to the right colon, whereas the left colon is the more common location when colonoscopy is performed as the diagnostic study (descending colon, 21%; rectosigmoid, 35%) [122,123]. The character of diverticular bleeding invariably is bright red or maroon blood per rectum, sometimes associated with orthostasis or hypotension. The majority of patients stop bleeding spontaneously, but approximately 20% to 30% rebleed.

Urgent colonoscopy after a rapid colonic purge (more than 4 to 6 hours) is recommended as an option in patients with ongoing bleeding, once the patient is resuscitated and hemodynamically stable [29,31]. However, a recent randomized controlled study failed to demonstrate an outcome benefit between urgent colonoscopy and radiologic studies for localization of bleeding, despite a higher likelihood of finding the bleeding source in the urgent colonoscopy group (Table 90.3) [24]. When a bleeding diverticulum is identified by the finding of a visible vessel or a pigmented protuberance [123], epinephrine injection, thermal contact therapy, or hemoclip application can be considered [30,31,124]. One study demonstrated that visualized diverticular bleeding treated with endoscopic therapy had no recurrent bleeding during a 30-month follow-up compared to 53% of patients with medical therapy alone [31]. Surgical intervention, either segmental or subtotal colectomy, is required in 18% to 25% of patients requiring blood transfusion [125]. Angiotherapy with vasopressin infusion or embolization after superselective cannulation of the bleeding vessel is an alternative approach in patients unstable for surgery.

There is limited evidence that endoscopic therapy may prevent recurrent bleeding and the need for surgery [31]. Alternatively, in patients who have stopped bleeding, elective colonoscopy can be performed during the same hospital stay, after adequate bowel preparation.

Aortoenteric Fistula

The key to recognizing an aortoenteric fistula is inclusion within the differential diagnosis of every patient with bleeding and a history of aortic graft surgery. Although fistulas can occur rarely between a native aortic aneurysm and the intestinal lumen, they more commonly occur in patients who have undergone abdominal aortic graft surgery (0.5% to 2.4%) [126]. This communication with resultant bleeding presents, on average, 4 years after the surgery. The point of intestinal breach can be anywhere from the esophagus to the colon, but occurs most often in the third duodenum (75%). A massive bleeding episode may be preceded by a small "herald bleed" that stops spontaneously. The interval between the first event and the exsanguinating hemorrhage can be hours, weeks, or months (average, 1 to 3 weeks). Making the diagnosis is difficult, but upper endoscopy is useful in excluding the diagnosis by identifying another lesion that is actively bleeding or has stigmata of recent bleeding. Endoscopic visualization of the graft eroding through the intestinal wall is diagnostic but uncommon. In some cases, computed tomography of the abdomen can identify graft abnormalities such as air–fluid levels that may indicate an enteric communication [127]. Angiography has not usually been helpful in the diagnosis unless bleeding is ongoing. If available, a vascular surgeon and an interventional radiologist should be part of the evaluating team. Graft repair surgery or an endovascular approach may be required for a confirmed diagnosis, and exploratory surgery likely is necessary for a presumed diagnosis of a fistulized or infected graft site.

References

1. Longstreth GF: Epidemiology and outcome of patients hospitalized with acute lower gastrointestinal hemorrhage: a population-based study. *Am J Gastroenterol* 92:419, 1997.
2. Lanas A, García-Rodríquz LA, Polo-Tomás M, et al: Time trends and impact of upper and lower gastrointestinal bleeding and perforation in clinical practice. *Am J Gastroenterol* 104:1633–1641, 2009.
3. Shajan P, Wilcox CM: Modern endoscopic therapy of peptic ulcer bleeding. *Dig Dis* 26:291, 2008.
4. Gralnek IM, Barkum AN, Bardou M: Management of acute bleeding from a peptic ulcer. *N Engl J Med* 359:928, 2008.
5. Loperfido S, Baldo V, Piovesana E, et al: Changing trends in acute upper-GI bleeding: a population-based study. *Gastrointest Endosc* 70:212, 2009.
6. Higham J, Kang JY, Majeed A: Recent trends in admissions and mortality due to peptic ulcer in England: increasing frequency of haemorrhage among older subjects. *Gut* 50:460, 2002.
7. Zuckerman GR, Prakash C: Acute lower intestinal bleeding, Part I. clinical presentation and diagnosis. *Gastrointest Endosc* 48:606, 1998.
8. Stanley AJ, Ashley D, Dalton HR, et al: Outpatient management of patients with low-risk upper-gastrointestinal haemorrhage: multicentre validation and prospective evaluation. *Lancet* 373:42–47, 2009.
9. Church NI, Dallal HJ, Masson J, et al: Validity of the Rockall scoring system after endoscopic therapy for bleeding peptic ulcer: a prospective cohort study. *Gastrointest Endosc* 63:606, 2006.
10. Zuckerman GR, Trellis DR, Sherman TM, et al: An objective measure of stool color for differentiating upper from lower gastrointestinal bleeding. *Dig Dis Sci* 40:1614, 1995.
11. Forrest JA, Finlayson ND, Shearman DJ: Endoscopy in gastrointestinal bleeding. *Lancet* 2:394–397, 1974.
12. Carbonell N, Pauwels A, Serfaty L, et al: Erythromycin infusion prior to endoscopy for acute upper gastrointestinal bleeding: a randomized controlled, double blind trial. *Am J Gastroenterol* 101:1211, 2006.
13. Coffin B, Pocard M, Panis Y, et al: Erythromycin improves the quality of EGD in patients with acute upper GI bleeding: a randomized controlled study. *Gastrointest Endosc* 56:174, 2002.
14. Lin HJ, Wang K, Perng CL, et al: Early or delayed endoscopy for patients with peptic ulcer bleeding: a prospective randomized study. *J Clin Gastroenterol* 22:267–271, 1996.
15. Cooper GS, Chak A, Conners AF Jr, et al: The effectiveness of early endoscopy for upper gastrointestinal hemorrhage: a community-based analysis. *Med Care* 36:462–474, 1998.
16. Copper GS, Chak A, Way LE, et al: Early endoscopy in upper gastrointestinal hemorrhage: associations with recurrent bleeding, surgery, and length of hospital stay. *Gastrointest Endosc* 49:145–152, 1999.
17. Tsoi KK, Ma TK, Sung JJ: Endoscopy for upper gastrointestinal bleeding: how urgent is it? *Nat Rev Gastroenterol Hepatol* 6(8):463–469, 2009.
18. Chung IK, Kim EJ, Lee MS, et al: Endoscopic factors predisposing to rebleeding following endoscopic hemostasis in bleeding peptic ulcers. *Endoscopy* 33:969–975, 2001.
19. Thompoulos KC, Theochrais GJ, Vagenas KA, et al: Predictors of hemostatic failure after adrenaline injection in patients with peptic ulcers with non-bleeding visible vessel. *Scand J Gastroenterol* 39:600–604, 2004.
20. Marmo R, Rotondano G, Bianco MA, et al: Outcome of endoscopic treatment for peptic ulcer bleeding: Is a second look necessary? A meta-analysis. *Gastrointest Endosc* 57:62–67, 2003.
21. Barkun A, Bardou M, Marshall JK: Consensus recommendation for managing patients with nonvariceal upper gastrointestinal bleeding. *Ann Intern Med* 139:843–857, 2003.
22. Das A, Wong RC: Prediction of outcome of acute GI hemorrhage: a review of risk scores and predicative models. *Gastrointest Endosc* 60:85–93, 2004.
23. Raju GS, Gerson L, Das A, et al: American gastroenterological association (AGA) institute medical position statement on obscure gastrointestinal bleeding. *Gastroenterology* 133:1694–1696, 2007.
24. Jensen DM: Management of patients with severe hematochezia—with all current evidence available. *Am J Gastroenterol* 100:2403–2406, 2005.
25. Green BT, Rockey DC, Portwood G, et al: Urgent colonoscopy for evaluation and management of acute lower gastrointestinal bleeding: a randomized controlled trial. *AJG* 100:2395–2402, 2005.
26. Jensen DM, Machicado GA: Diagnosis and treatment of severe hematochezia: the role of urgent colonoscopy after purge. *Gastroenterology* 95:1567, 1998.
27. Zuckerman GR, Prakash C: Acute lower intestinal bleeding. Part II: etiology, therapy, and outcomes. *Gastrointest Endosc* 49:228, 1999.
28. Rossini FP, Ferrari A, Spandre M, et al: Emergency colonoscopy. *World J Surg* 13:190–192, 1989.
29. NIH Consensus Conference: Therapeutic endoscopy and bleeding ulcers. *JAMA* 262:1369, 1989.
30. Prakash C, Chokshi H, Walden D, et al: Endoscopic management of acute diverticular bleeding. *Endoscopy* 31:460, 1999.
31. Jensen DM, Machicado GA, Jutabha RJ, et al: Urgent colonoscopy for the diagnosis and treatment of severe diverticular hemorrhage. *N Engl J Med* 342:78, 2000.
32. Lin HJ, Lo WC, Lee FY, et al: A prospective randomized comparative trial showing that omeprazole prevents rebleeding in patients with bleeding peptic ulcer after successful endoscopic therapy. *Arch Intern Med* 158:54, 1998.
33. Kahi CJ, Jensen DM, Sung JJ, et al: Endoscopic therapy versus medical therapy for bleeding peptic ulcer with adherent clot: a meta-analysis. *Gastroenterology* 129:855–862, 2005.
34. Laine L: Systemic review of endoscopic therapy for ulcers with clots: can a meta-analysis be misleading? *Gastroenterology* 129:2127–2128, 2005.
35. Sung JJ, Chan FK, Lau JY, et al. The effect of endoscopic therapy in patients receiving omeprazole for bleeding ulcers with non-bleeding ulcers with non-bleeding visible vessels or adherent clots: a randomized comparison. *Ann Intern Med* 139:237–243, 2003.
36. Marmo R, Rotondano G, Piscopo R, et al: Dual therapy versus monotherapy in the endoscopic treatment of high-risk bleeding ulcers: a meta-analysis of controlled trials. *Am J Gastroenterol* 102:279–289, 2007.
37. Vergara M, Calvet X, Gisbert JP: Epinephrine injection versus epinephrine injection and a second endoscopic method in high risk bleeding ulcers. *Cochrane Database Syst Rev* 2:CD005584, 2007.
38. Calvet X, Vergara M, Brullet E, et al: Addition of second endoscopic treatment following epinephrine injection improves outcome in high-risk bleeding ulcers. *Gastroenterology* 126:441–450, 2004.
39. Saeed ZA, Ramirez FC, Hepps KS, et al: Prospective validation of the Baylor bleeding score for predicting the likelihood of rebleeding after endoscopic hemostasis of peptic ulcers. *Gastrointest Endosc* 41:561–565, 1995.
40. Ljungdahl M, Eriksson LG, Nyman R, et al: Arterial embolisation in management of massive bleeding from gastric and duodenal ulcers. *Eur J Surg* 168:384–390, 2002.
41. Ripoll C, Bañares R, Beceiro I, et al: Comparison of transcatheter arterial embolization and surgery for treatment of bleeding peptic ulcer after endoscopic treatment failure. *J Vasc Interv Radiol* 15:447–450, 2004.
42. Imhof M, Ohmann C, Röher HD, et al: Endoscopic versus operative treatment in high-risk ulcer bleeding patients—results of a randomized study. *Langenbecks Arch Surg* 387:327–336, 2003.
43. Barkun A, Sabbah S, Enns R, et al: The Canadian Registry on Nonvariceal Upper Gastrointestinal Bleeding and Endoscopy (RUGBE): endoscopic hemostasis and proton pump inhibition are associated with improved outcomes in real-life setting. *Am J Gastroenterol* 99:1238–1246, 2004.
44. Lau JYW, Sung JJY, Lam Y, et al: Endoscopic retreatment compared with surgery in patients with recurrent bleeding after initial endoscopic control of bleeding ulcers. *N Engl J Med* 340:751–756, 1999.
45. Adler DG, Leighton JA, Davila RE, et al: ASGE guideline: the role of endoscopy in acute non-variceal upper-GI hemorrhage. *Gastrointest Endosc* 60:497–504, 2004. [Erratum, *Gastrointest Endosc* 61:356, 2005.]
46. Sanyal AJ, Preston PP, Luketic VA, et al: Bleeding gastroesophageal varices. *Semin Liver Dis* 13:328, 1993.
47. Dagradi AE, Mehler R, Tan DTD, et al: Sources of upper gastrointestinal bleeding in patients with liver cirrhosis and large esophagogastric varices. *Am J Gastroenterol* 54:458, 1970.
48. Peifer KJ, Zuckerman GR, Lisker-Melman M, et al: Frequency of variceal upper gastrointestinal bleeding in patients with established varices. *Gastrointest Endosc* 59:AB163, 2004.
49. El-Serag HB, Everhart JE: Improved survival after variceal hemorrhage over an 11-year period in the Department of Veterans Affairs. *Am J Gastroenterol* 95:3566–3573, 2000.
50. D'Amico G, de Franchis R: Upper digestive bleeding in cirrhosis. Post-therapeutic outcome and prognostic indicators. *Hepatology* 38:599–612, 2003.
51. Garcia-Tsao G, Sanyal AJ, Grace ND, et al: Prevention and management of gastroesophageal varices and variceal hemorrhage in cirrhosis. *Hepatology* 46:922–938, 2007.
52. Hirata M, Ishihama S, Sanjo K, et al: Study of new prognostic factors of esophageal variceal rupture by use of image processing with a video endoscope. *Surgery* 116:8, 1994.
53. Kleber G, Sauerbruch T, Ansari H, et al: Prediction of variceal hemorrhage in cirrhosis: a prospective follow-up study. *Gastroenterology* 100:1332, 1991.
54. Bornman PC, Krige JEJ, Terblanche J: Management of oesophageal varices. *Lancet* 343:1079, 1994.
55. Avgerinos A, Armonis A, Raptis S: Somatostatin and octreotide in the management of acute variceal hemorrhage. *Hepatogastroenterology* 42:145, 1995.
56. McKee R: A study of octreotide in oesophageal varices. *Digestion* 45[Suppl 1]:60, 1990.
57. Bildozola M, Kravetz D, Argonz J, et al: Efficacy of octreotide and sclerotherapy in the treatment of acute variceal bleeding in cirrhotic patients. A prospective, multicentric and randomized clinical trial. *Scand J Gastroenterol* 35:419, 2000.
58. Imperiale TF, Teran JC, McCullough AJ: A meta-analysis of somatostatin versus vasopressin in the management of acute esophageal variceal hemorrhage. *Gastroenterology* 109:1289, 1995.
59. Sung JJY, Chung SCS, Lai CW, et al: Octreotide infusion or emergency sclerotherapy for variceal hemorrhage. *Lancet* 342:637, 1993.
60. Hwang SJ, Lin HC, Chang CF, et al: A randomized controlled trial comparing octreotide and vasopressin in the control of acute esophageal variceal bleeding. *J Hepatol* 16:320, 1992.
61. Katkov WN: Hold that needle: octreotide for acute variceal hemorrhage. *Hepatology* 19:1051, 1994.

62. Sung JJY, Chung SCS, Yung MY, et al: Prospective randomised study of effect of octreotide on rebleeding from oesophageal varices after endoscopic ligation. *Lancet* 346:1666, 1995.
63. Besson I, Ingrand P, Person B, et al: Sclerotherapy with or without octreotide for acute variceal bleeding. *N Engl J Med* 333:555, 1995.
64. Escorsell A, Bandi JC, Andreu V, et al: Desensitization to the effects of intravenous octreotide in cirrhotic patients with portal hypertension. *Gastroenterology* 120:161, 2001.
65. Burroughs AK: Octreotide in variceal bleeding. *Gut* 35[Suppl 3]:S23, 1994.
66. Bleichner G, Boulanger R, Squara P, et al: Frequency of infections in cirrhotic patients presenting with acute gastrointestinal haemorrhage. *Br J Surg* 73:724, 1986.
67. Bernard B, Grange JD, Khac EN, et al: Antibiotic prophylaxis for the prevention of bacterial infections in cirrhotic patients with gastrointestinal bleeding: a meta-analysis. *Hepatology* 29:1655, 1999.
68. Goulis J, Armonis A, Patch D, et al: Bacterial infection is independently associated with failure to control bleeding in patients with gastrointestinal hemorrhage. *Hepatology* 27:1207, 1998.
69. Bernard B, Grange JD, Khac EN, et al: Antibiotic prophylaxis for the prevention of bacterial infections in cirrhotic patients with gastrointestinal bleeding: a meta-analysis. *Hepatology* 29:1655–1661, 1999.
70. Soares-Weiser K, Brezis M, Tur-Kaspa R, et al: Antibiotic prophylaxis for cirrhotic patients with gastrointestinal bleeding. *Cochrane Database Syst Rev* 2:CD002907, 2002.
71. Masci E, Stigliano R, Mariani A, et al: Prospective multicenter randomized trial comparing banding ligation with sclerotherapy of esophageal varices. *Hepatogastroenterology* 46:1769, 1999.
72. Schuman BM, Beckman JW, Tedesco FJ, et al: Complications of endoscopic injection sclerotherapy: a review. *Am J Gastroenterol* 82:823, 1987.
73. Lo GH, Lai KH, Cheng JS, et al: The effects of endoscopic variceal ligation and propranolol on portal hypertensive gastropathy: a prospective, controlled trial. *Gastrointest Endosc* 53:579, 2001.
74. Sarin SK, Lahoti D, Saxena SP, et al: Prevalence, classification and natural history of gastric varices: a long-term follow-up study in 568 portal hypertension patients. *Hepatology* 16:1343, 1992.
75. Tan P, Hou M, Lin H, et al: A randomized trail of endoscopic treatment of acute gastric variceal hemorrhage: *N*-butyl-2-cyanoacrylate injection versus band ligation. *Hepatology* 43:690, 2006.
76. Noh du Y, Park SY, Joo Sy, et al: Therapeutic effect of the endoscopic *N*-butyl-2-cyanoacrylate injection for acute esophagogastric variceal bleeding: comparison with transjugular intrahepatic portosystemic shunt. *Korean J Gastroenterol* 43:186, 2004.
77. Hwang SS, Kim HH, Park SH, et al: *N*-butyl-2-cyanoacrylate pulmonary embolism after endoscopic injection sclerotherapy for gastric variceal bleeding. *J Comput Assist Tomogr* 25:16, 2001.
78. Dib N, Oberti F, Cales P: Current management of the complications of portal hypertension: variceal bleeding and ascites. *CMAJ* 174:1433, 2006.
79. Jalan R, Redhead DN, Hayes PC: Transjugular intrahepatic portasystemic stent-shunt in the treatment of variceal hemorrhage. *Br J Surg* 82:1158, 1995.
80. Paquet KJ, Feussner H: Endoscopic sclerosis and esophageal balloon tamponade in acute hemorrhage from esophagogastric varices: a prospective controlled randomized trial. *Hepatology* 5:580, 1985.
81. O'Connor JFB, Gacad R, Newman JS, et al: What role for TIPS in managing variceal bleeding? A practical approach to choosing the best therapy for your patient. *J Critical Illness* 12:103, 1997.
82. Sanyal AJ, Freedman AM, Luketic VA, et al: Transjugular intrahepatic portosystemic shunts for patients with active variceal hemorrhage unresponsive to sclerotherapy. *Gastroenterology* 111:138, 1996.
83. McCormick PA, Dick R, Panagou EB, et al: Emergency transjugular intrahepatic portasystemic stent shunting as salvage treatment for uncontrolled variceal bleeding. *Br J Surg* 81:1324, 1994.
84. Cavallari A, DeRaffele E, Bellusci R: Bleeding esophageal varices: today's role of portosystemic shunts. *Dig Dis* 10[Suppl 1]:74, 1992.
85. Spina G, Santambrogio R: The role of portosystemic shunting in the management of portal hypertension. *Baillieres Clin Gastroenterol* 6:497, 1992.
86. Orozco H, Mercado MA, Chan C, et al: A comparative study of the elective treatment of variceal hemorrhage with beta-blockers, transendoscopic sclerotherapy, and surgery: a prospective, controlled, and randomized trial during 10 years. *Ann Surg* 232:216, 2000.
87. Henderson JM, Nagle A, Curtas S, et al: Surgical shunts and TIPS for variceal decompression in the 1990s. *Surgery* 128:540, 2000.
88. Panes J, Teres J, Bosch J, et al: Efficacy of balloon tamponade in treatment of bleeding gastric and esophageal varices: results in 151 consecutive episodes. *Dig Dis Sci* 33:454, 1988.
89. Haddock G, Garden OJ, McKee RF, et al: Esophageal tamponade in the management of acute variceal hemorrhage. *Dig Dis Sci* 34:913, 1989.
90. Boonpongmanee S, Fleischer DE, Pezzullo JC, et al: The frequency of peptic ulcer as a cause of upper-GI bleeding is exaggerated. *Gastrointest Endosc* 59:788, 2004.
91. Hosking SW, Yung MY, Chung CS, et al: Different prevalence of Helicobacter in bleeding and non-bleeding ulcers. *Gastroenterology* 102:85, 1992.
92. Hawkey CJ: Risk of ulcer bleeding in patients infected with Helicobacter pylori taking non-steroidal anti-inflammatory drugs. *Gut* 46:310, 2000.
93. Soll AH, Weinstein WM, Kurata J, et al: Non-steroidal anti-inflammatory drugs and peptic ulcer disease. *Ann Intern Med* 114:307, 1991.
94. Silverstein FE, Graham DY, Senior JR, et al: Misoprostol reduces serious gastrointestinal complications in patients with rheumatoid arthritis receiving non-steroidal anti-inflammatory drugs: a randomized double-blind, placebo-controlled trial. *Ann Intern Med* 123:241, 1995.
95. Mamdani M, Juurlink DN, Kopp A, et al: Gastrointestinal bleeding after the introduction of COX-2 inhibitors: ecological study. *BMJ* 328:1415, 2004.
96. Battisella M, Mamdami MM, Juurlink DN, et al: Risk of upper gastrointestinal hemorrhage in warfarin users treated with non-selective NSAIDs or COX-2 inhibitors. *Arch Intern Med* 165:189, 2005.
97. Shorr RI, Ray WA, Daugherty JR, et al: Concurrent non-steroidal anti-inflammatory drugs and oral anticoagulants places elderly persons at high risk for hemorrhagic peptic ulcer disease. *Arch Intern Med* 153:1665, 1993.
98. Schaffalitzky de Muckadell OB, Havelund T, Harling H, et al: Effect of omeprazole on the outcome of endoscopically treated bleeding peptic ulcers. Randomized double-blind placebo-controlled multicenter study. *Scand J Gastroenterol* 32:320, 1997.
99. Lau JYW, Sung JJY, Lee KKC, et al: Effect of intravenous omeprazole on recurrent bleeding after endoscopic treatment of bleeding peptic ulcers. *N Engl J Med* 343:310, 2000.
100. Zuckerman GR, Welch R, Douglas A, et al: Controlled trial of medical therapy for active upper gastrointestinal bleeding and prevention of rebleeding. *Am J Med* 76:361, 1984.
101. Rockall TA, Logan RFA, Devlin HB, et al: Risk assessment after acute upper gastrointestinal haemorrhage. *Gut* 38:316, 1996.
102. Metz DC, Amer F, Hunt B, et al: Lansoprazole regimens that sustain intragastric pH >6.0 an evaluation of intermittent oral and continuous intravenous infusion dosages. *Aliment Pharmacol Ther* 23:985–995, 2006.
103. Ponsky J, Hoffman M, Swaynigim D: Saline irrigation in gastric hemorrhage: the effect of temperature. *J Surg Res* 28:204, 1980.
104. Patchett SE, Enright H, Afdhal N, et al: Clot lysis by gastric juice: an in vitro study. *Gut* 30:1704, 1989.
105. Laine L, Shah A, Bemanian S: Intragastric pH with oral vs. intravenous bolus plus infusion proton-pump inhibitor therapy in patients with bleeding ulcers. *Gastroenterology* 134:1838–1841, 2008.
106. Leontiadis GI, Sharma VK, Howden CW: Proton pump inhibitor treatment for acute peptic ulcer bleeding. *Cochrane Database Syst Rev* 1:CD002094, 2006.
107. Lau JY, Leung WK, Wu JC, et al: Omeprazole before endoscopy in patients with gastrointestinal bleeding. *N Engl J Med* 356:1631–1640, 2007.
108. Dorward S, Sreedharan A, Leontiadis GI, et al: Proton pump inhibitor treatment initiated prior to endoscopic diagnosis in upper gastrointestinal bleeding. *Cochrane Database Syst Rev* 4:CD005415, 2006.
109. Tsoi KK, Lau JY, Sung JJ: Cost-effectiveness analysis of high-dose omeprazole infusion before endoscopy for patients with upper gastrointestinal bleeding. *Gastrointest Endosc* 67:1056–1063, 2008.
110. Morgan D: Intravenous proton pump inhibitors in critical care setting. *Crit Care Med* 30[6, Suppl]:S369–S372, 2002.
111. Graham DY, Schwartz JT: The spectrum of the Mallory-Weiss tear. *Medicine* 57:302, 1997.
112. Zuckerman GR, Cornette GL, Clouse RE, et al: Upper gastrointestinal bleeding in patients with chronic renal failure. *Ann Intern Med* 102:588, 1985.
113. Clouse RE, Costigan DJ, Mills BA, et al: Angiodysplasia as a cause of upper gastrointestinal bleeding. *Arch Intern Med* 145:458, 1985.
114. Boley SJ, Sammartano R, Adams A, et al: On the nature and etiology of vascular ectasias of the colon. *Gastroenterology* 72:650, 1977.
115. Santos JC, Aprilli F, Guimaraes AS, et al: Angiodysplasia of the colon: endoscopic diagnosis and treatment. *Br J Surg* 75:256, 1988.
116. Krevsky B: Detection and treatment of angiodysplasia. *Gastrointest Endosc Clin North Am* 7:509, 1997.
117. Eidus LB, Rasuli P, Manion D, et al: Caliber-persistent artery of the stomach (Dieulafoy's vascular malformation). *Gastroenterology* 99:1507, 1990.
118. McClave SA, Goldschmid S, Cunningham JT, et al: Dieulafoy's cirsoid aneurysm of the duodenum. *Dig Dis Sci* 33:801, 1988.
119. Lin HJ, Lee FY, Tsai YT, et al: Therapeutic endoscopy for Dieulafoy's disease. *J Clin Gastroenterol* 11:507, 1989.
120. Nikolaidis N, Zezos P, Giouleme O, et al: Endoscopic band ligation of Dieulafoy-like lesions in the upper gastrointestinal tract. *Endoscopy* 33:754, 2001.
121. Casarella WJ, Kanter IE, Seaman WB: Right-sided colonic diverticula as a cause of acute rectal hemorrhage. *N Engl J Med* 286:450, 1972.
122. Hurwich DB, Gostout CJ, Balm RK: Acute lower GI bleeding from diverticulosis: prevalence, clinical features and outcome [Abstract]. *Gastrointest Endosc* 39:297, 1993.
123. Foutch PG, Zimmerman K: Diverticular bleeding and the pigmented protuberance (sentinel clot): clinical implications, histopathological correlation, and results of endoscopic intervention. *Am J Gastroenterol* 91:2589, 1996.
124. Binmoeller KF, Thonke F, Soehendra N: Endoscopic hemo-clip treatment for gastrointestinal bleeding. *Endoscopy* 25:167, 1993.
125. Bounds BC, Fiedman LS: Lower gastrointestinal bleeding. *Gastroenterol Clin N Am* 32:1107, 2003.
126. Champion MC, Sullivan S, Coles JC, et al: Aortoenteric fistula: incidence, presentation, recognition, and management. *Ann Surg* 195:314, 1982.
127. Low RN, Wall SD, Jeffrey RB Jr, et al: Aortoenteric fistula and perigraft infection: evaluation with CT. *Radiology* 175:157, 1990.

CHAPTER 92 ■ STRESS ULCER SYNDROME

SONAL KUMAR, CHANDRA PRAKASH GYAWALI AND GARY R. ZUCKERMAN

Stress ulcer syndrome refers to the acute onset of upper gastrointestinal (GI) bleeding, usually from proximally located gastric ulcers and erosions, in patients admitted to an intensive care unit (ICU) for other illnesses. Gastric mucosal erosions have been found at protocol endoscopy within hours of ICU admission [1–4], typically without clinical bleeding at this early stage, and sometimes are referred to as *stress-related mucosal disease*. Descriptions of acute ulcerations of the intestines in the setting of acute burns date back more than 150 years [5]. The "stress" tag dates back to 1950 [6] and refers to extreme physiologic stress during critical illness that necessitates an ICU admission. Stress ulcer syndrome has been related temporally to a number of acute disorders including burns [3,7], cerebral lesions, stroke [4,8], various surgical procedures [1,9,10], and other acute medical illnesses found in an ICU [2]. The goal of management is prophylaxis, preventing the formation of the early acute gastric precursor lesions and/or preventing progression to clinically significant GI bleeding.

CLINICAL CHARACTERISTICS AND PRESENTATION

Stress ulcers frequently are asymptomatic and come to clinical attention only when they manifest bleeding. Progression to stress ulcer syndrome (SUS) (i.e., clinical bleeding or intestinal perforation) is uncommon. When it occurs, GI bleeding typically presents within 14 days of the onset of physiologic stress or ICU admission [11]. Hematemesis, gross blood from the nasogastric tube, and melena are the usual presentations of SUS [1–4,12,13]. The true incidence of overt GI bleeding resulting from stress ulceration is difficult to ascertain and varies depending on the definition of bleeding and the category of ICU patients. The finding at preemptive endoscopy of a small amount of blood adjacent to an ulcer without clinically evident overt bleeding has been noted in 22% to 36% of ICU admissions [2,3]. Significant stress ulcer bleeding occurs in 2% to 7% of critically ill patients [14,15]. Patients with thermal injury from burns or with acute intracranial disease including head trauma and coma appear to be at increased risk of developing stress ulcer–related bleeding [3,12]. Evidence is surfacing that the incidence of stress ulcer bleeding is decreasing, from as high as 22% in the 1970s to 1.6% to 6.0% of patients admitted to ICUs in more recent studies [3,16–19]. Our recent experience suggests that SUS now occurs in less than 1% of ICU admissions [20]. This may be related to the common use of prophylactic agents and improved care of critically ill patients in the present-day ICU setting.

Stress ulceration with clinically significant bleeding is associated with a mortality rate as high as 50% to 80% [16–19,21], although death often is a result of the underlying disease and not directly linked to GI bleeding [16]. Thus, stress ulcer bleeding may serve more as a marker for the severely ill patient having a cascade of complications rather than represent a unique clinical entity.

RISK FACTORS FOR STRESS ULCER SYNDROME

Clinical risk factors commonly associated with SUS include mechanical ventilation, coagulopathy, major surgery, hemorrhagic shock, hypotension, trauma, and sepsis [11]. A statistically significant predisposition to stress ulceration has been demonstrated in ICU patients with coagulopathy or a requirement for prolonged mechanical ventilation (over 48 hours) [16,17]. Hypotension and shock also are more frequent among patients with bleeding attributed to stress ulceration but do not reach statistical significance as independent risk factors [16]. Patients with thermal injury from burns (>35% body surface area) and patients with acute intracranial disease including head trauma and coma also are at increased risk of having stress ulcers (Curling's and Cushing's ulcers, respectively) [22,23]. Conditions that present a low risk for SUS include myocardial infarction, congestive heart failure, arrhythmias, chronic renal failure on dialysis, chronic obstructive pulmonary disease, and malignancy [11]. Recent studies emphasize that although the incidence of GI bleeding increases with up to two risk factors, additional risk factors do not further increase bleeding potential [24].

PATHOPHYSIOLOGY

Stress ulcer is a misnomer in that many of the lesions appear as shallow mucosal erosions without the depth of an ulcer (Table 92.1). The earliest mucosal changes have been described in the most proximal parts of the stomach [25], but the process can eventually involve the distal stomach and duodenum [17,20]. Early mucosal changes include pallor, mottling, and submucosal petechiae which coalesce to form superficial linear erosions and ulcers. This can progress to diffuse mucosal damage with bleeding and in rare cases, perforation. On endoscopy, mucosal erosions have been found as early as 5 hours after ICU admission, and most are evident within 72 hours. Within 24 hours of ICU admission, they have the appearance of small (1 to 2 mm), round, shallow erosions, and by 48 hours, the lesions can be larger (2 to 25 mm), deeper, and associated with a clot. When patients bleed, 10 or more gastric mucosal erosions usually are observed at endoscopy [25,26]. The result is a diffuse area of involvement that can result in a spectrum of manifestations ranging from oozing of blood to massive hemorrhage or perforation [11,16].

Although the precise etiology of stress ulceration is not known, a number of factors have been implicated and studied in animal models. Animal studies using endoscopic and pathologic analyses have demonstrated progressive gastric mucosal injury from the physiologic stress of induced shock [27], a process that has been observed in humans under similar stress [1,27,28]. Gastric acid, but not hypersecretion, appears to be an essential prerequisite for the development of stress ulceration [29,30]. The classic lesion has been associated with a

TABLE 92.1

CHARACTERISTICS OF STRESS ULCER SYNDROME

Endoscopic evidence of gastric erosions within 72 h of intensive care unit admission
Multiple ulcers located in the proximal stomach, in contrast to peptic ulcers, which typically are found in the distal stomach
Duodenal ulcers uncommon; when present, usually associated with proximal gastric ulcers
Onset of hemorrhage within 14 d of intensive care unit admission
Abdominal pain unusual except in the infrequent setting of gastroduodenal perforation

TABLE 92.2

RECOMMENDED AND PUTATIVE CATEGORIES OF ICU PATIENTS WHO COULD BENEFIT FROM STRESS ULCER PROPHYLAXIS

ICU patients with
Coagulopathy
Requirement for mechanical ventilation for >48 h
Head injury (with Glasgow Coma Score of ≤10)
Burns involving >35% of body surface area
Multiple trauma, including spinal cord injuries
Partial hepatectomy
Peri- or postoperative status, especially after hepatic or renal transplantation
Acute hepatic failure
Acute renal failure
History of gastric ulceration or bleeding during year before admission

ICU, intensive care unit.

normal or even decreased intraluminal gastric acid secretion [31–33], suggesting that a breakdown in the mucosal defense mechanism must also be present for stress ulceration to occur. Mucosal ischemia is thought to be the inciting event in the pathogenesis [31,32]. In experimental models, stress causes a decrease in gastric mucosal blood flow, resulting in decreased delivery of oxygen and nutrients and leading to a deficit in aerobic metabolism and high-energy phosphate compounds [30,34,35]. Diminished intramucosal blood flow decreases the availability of systemic bicarbonate to buffer back-diffused hydrogen ions, thereby allowing a fall in the intramural gastric pH [30,31,36]. Mucosal ischemia and subsequent reperfusion result in the formation of toxic oxygen-derived free radicals and superoxides [33,37,38] while decreasing the synthesis of cytoprotective prostaglandins [38], thereby creating a favorable scenario for mucosal damage.

Factors such as elevated gastrin and pepsin levels, increased intraluminal bile and urea concentrations, and decreased gastric motility from enhanced vagal stimulation appear to be contributory to the development of a stress ulcer but are inadequate by themselves to induce the lesion [31,39]. The impact, if any, of *Helicobacter pylori* on the risk and development of stress ulcer is unknown. *H. pylori* seropositivity has been found to be lower in patients with stress ulcer bleeding when compared with controls [40]. In fact, it is possible that some of the *H. pylori*–positive cases diagnosed as stress ulcer actually represent *H. pylori*–associated peptic ulcer disease.

PROPHYLAXIS

The logic of prophylaxis lies in the assumption that the formation of stress ulcers can be prevented, or that, once formed, the progression from ulcer to bleeding or perforation can be halted. Several studies have suggested that the risk of bleeding from stress ulcer and the overall prognosis are related primarily to the severity of the underlying disease [2,12,41,42], and aggressive management of the underlying disease while attempting to maintain visceral perfusion should always take precedence. If those patients at risk can be identified sufficiently early in their ICU stays, the administration of any standard prophylactic agent shortly after ICU admission decreases the rate of stress ulcer bleeding. The international guidelines of early goal-directed therapy also include stress ulcer prophylaxis with histamine-2 receptor antagonists (H2RAs) or proton pump inhibitors (PPIs) as part of initial management in patients with severe sepsis or septic shock [43]. Decreasing or neutralizing gastric acid is the most common prophylactic approach, and antacids and H2RA initially fulfilled this role effectively. The ideal pH threshold and the duration of pH elevation required to prevent bleeding are not known. In fact, stress ulcer bleeding is not always pH dependent, as bleeding has been noted in patients with a mean gastric pH greater than 4.0 [44].

More recently, PPIs have been shown to be comparable with H2RA [45], and an orally administered PPI has been approved by the Food and Drug Administration (FDA) for prophylaxis [14]. The difficulties of evaluating and comparing studies involving prophylaxis of stress ulcers include the variability in patient populations, severity of disease, definition of bleeding, and the type and method of drug delivery.

A national survey of clinicians demonstrated a lack of consensus in the use of stress ulcer prophylaxis, with many patients receiving prophylaxis for an extended period without clear-cut indications or documented benefit [46]. Development and implementation of institution-specific guidelines (taking into account drug cost and availability), with prophylaxis reserved for patients at highest risk for stress ulcer bleeding (Table 92.2), has been demonstrated to increase appropriateness of prophylaxis and decrease cost of care without increasing the incidence of stress ulcers or frequency of clinically significant GI bleeding [47–49].

Regimens for Prophylaxis

Histamine-2 Receptor Antagonists

H2RAs are commonly used agents for the prophylaxis of stress ulcers [46]. They have been found to be comparable or superior to antacids in preventing bleeding, and antacids and H2RAs are superior to no treatment or placebo [50–52]. Intravenous (IV) H2RA prophylaxis confers a significantly lower bleeding rate from stress ulceration in critically ill ventilated patients [53]. H2RAs are administered intravenously as a standard intermittent bolus or by continuous infusion, though continuous infusion more effectively maintains the desired gastric pH [54]. Nevertheless, studies using intermittent bolus IV doses of H2RA achieved the goal of prevention of bleeding as well as studies using continuous titrated dosing [21]. This would suggest that 24-hour pH control is not necessary for the prophylactic effect. Of note, patients with a creatinine clearance of less than 30 mL per minute should receive half the recommended dose, and caution should be exercised in patients with thrombocytopenia [54].

Proton Pump Inhibitors

PPIs block the final pathway for acid secretion by irreversibly inhibiting H+/K+-ATPase in gastric parietal cells. They can be administered enterally or intravenously at once-daily dosing, provide predictable and sustained pH control, and have been demonstrated to be safe and effective in stress ulcer prophylaxis [50–52,55]. Omeprazole administered orally as a suspension at a dose of 40 mg daily was effective in preventing clinically significant GI bleeding in trauma patients requiring mechanical ventilation and with at least one other risk factor for stress ulcer development [50]. IV PPIs may also be effective for stress ulcer prophylaxis, although studies of patients at risk for stress ulcer bleeding are lacking. A randomized, double-blind study utilizing immediate-release omeprazole suspension (40-mg dose followed in 6 to 8 hours with a second 40-mg loading dose and 40 mg daily thereafter via nasogastric or orogastric tube), compared with IV cimetidine (50-mg bolus and 50 mg per hour thereafter), showed that the immediate-release omeprazole suspension was as effective as cimetidine in preventing upper GI bleeding (a "noninferiority" analysis utilizing cimetidine as the benchmark). The omeprazole suspension was also more effective than IV cimetidine in maintaining gastric pH greater than 4 in these critically ill patients [14]. Another recent randomized, "noninferiority" study compared multiple doses of IV pantoprazole to continuous infusion cimetidine, finding effective control of gastric pH and no episodes of clinically significant upper GI bleeding, and demonstrated similar outcomes with either prophylactic approach [52]. Trends in recent years have been toward the use of some form of prophylaxis in patients at risk, more often PPIs than H2RAs [20,56].

Antacids

Antacids can be administered through a nasogastric tube every 1 to 2 hours to control gastric pH. Studies evaluating the efficacy of antacids in the prophylaxis of stress ulcer have emphasized maintaining gastric intraluminal pH above 3.5 to 4.0 to prevent bleeding [41,57]. This involves the time-consuming process of frequent monitoring of gastric pH by gastric fluid aspiration or using indwelling probes and titrating antacids to pH findings. In fact, the optimal gastric pH level is unknown, the practice of titrating gastric pH is not of proven necessity for adequate prophylaxis, and the need for continuous 24-hour pH control does not appear to be critical. Antacids may cause diarrhea, may be contraindicated in renal failure, and may affect bioavailability of oral medications. In spite of these disadvantages, antacids have demonstrated efficacy in the prevention of stress ulcer bleeding [41,57]. Various antacids have had previous FDA approval for stress ulcer prophylaxis, and the doses varied with the preparation.

Sucralfate

Sucralfate is the aluminum salt of sulfated sucrose and does not affect gastric acidity. Some studies report efficacy similar to H2RA in the prevention of stress ulcer bleeding [58,59]. The primary mechanism of action likely is related to its intestinal mucosal cytoprotection and the ability to preserve microvascular integrity while coating early mucosal erosions and protecting them from further acid and pepsin damage. Its use may be associated with a lower risk of nosocomial pneumonia at a lower cost to the patient [60–65], although more recent data suggest no increase in the incidence of pneumonia with H2RA [66]. Sucralfate usually is administered in the form of slurry through a nasogastric tube at a dose of 4 to 6 g per day. Sucralfate can be incorporated into liquid slurry by dissolving a 1-g tablet in 5 to 15 mL of water. Sucralfate suspension (Hoechst Marion Roussel, Kansas City, MO) currently is available at the strength of 1 g in 10 mL; however, equivalence of the suspension to similar doses of sucralfate tablets has not been demonstrated. Although generally safe for short-term use in critically ill patients [67], toxic plasma aluminum levels may result in patients with impaired renal function [68], and therefore sucralfate is not generally recommended for "first-line" prophylaxis.

TABLE 92.3

SUMMARY OF EVIDENCE-BASED FINDINGS FOR PREVENTION OF STRESS ULCER SYNDROME

- Intravenous histamine-2 receptor antagonists (cimetidine, ranitidine) significantly reduce the incidence of clinically important gastrointestinal bleeding in mechanically ventilated patients, without increasing the risk for ventilator-associated pneumonia [53]. Although cimetidine has been shown to be an effective prophylactic agent, its safety profile (various drug–drug interactions, thrombocytopenia) has decreased its clinical usage.
- Sucralfate administered by nasogastric tube also reduces the bleeding risk, but intravenous ranitidine may be superior [53,69].
- Omeprazole administered orally or through a nasogastric tube (particularly immediate-release formulation) may be as effective as intravenous cimetidine infusion in preventing stress ulcer bleeding [14,51].
- Pantoprazole IV effectively controls gastric pH and may prevent stress ulcer bleeding [49].
- The results of "noninferiority" studies of a few PPIs have been extrapolated to the usage of all PPIs in many ICUs.

ICU, intensive care unit; PPIs, proton pump inhibitors.

Other Measures

There is evidence that stress-related upper GI bleeding may be reduced by enteral feeding [51,53,69]. Prostaglandins; free-radical scavengers, such as dimethylsulfoxide and allopurinol; and the bioflavonoid meciadanol also have been used in stress ulcer prophylaxis with varying results [70–72]. The use of these novel therapies over conventional prophylactic agents currently is not recommended, although some show promise for stress ulcer prophylaxis in limited studies [47].

A summary of evidence-based findings for management of SUS is provided in Table 92.3.

Complications of Prophylaxis

Although therapeutic agents are superior to no prophylaxis in preventing stress ulcer bleeding, there is a growing concern about potential complications of prophylaxis, particularly nosocomial pneumonia. The incidence of nosocomial pneumonia is approximately 20-fold higher in mechanically ventilated patients, in whom the mortality rate from the pneumonia can be as high as 60% [73,74]. Gastric alkalinization and colonization with Gram-negative bacilli is thought to play a causal role [74,75], rendering pH-altering drugs potentially disadvantageous. Although a persistently alkaline gastric environment increases the likelihood of bacterial colonization, it is unclear if this is influenced by the pharmacologic agent used for stress ulcer prophylaxis, as several meta-analyses have provided conflicting results [76–78]. Studies show a higher incidence of nosocomial pneumonia in patients treated with antacids when compared with sucralfate, a drug that does not alter the gastric pH and appears to have bactericidal properties [79,80]. Other studies and one meta-analysis have shown no statistically significant difference in the rate of pneumonia in sucralfate- and H2RA-treated, mechanically ventilated patients [58,59,65, 81–83]. Thus, the relationship of stress ulcer prophylaxis and nosocomial pneumonia needs further clarification before one prophylactic agent can be recommended over another.

Additional issues with stress ulcer prophylaxis include patients being inappropriately continued on acid-suppressive therapy after transfer out of the ICU. A recent study demonstrated that as many as 86% of patients remained on either PPI or H2RA after transfer from the surgical ICU, and 24% of patients were discharged from the hospital with continuation of the medications in the absence of risk factors for SUS-related GI bleeding [84]. There has been no evidence to suggest that noncritically ill patients are also at risk for developing stress ulcers, and continuation of prophylaxis is likely inappropriate [56,85]. In addition to potential side effects of taking medications, there is also a significant economic impact of overutilization of stress ulcer prophylaxis, both in the noncritically ill patient population and in patients on discharge from the hospital [86]. Therefore, it is essential to identify patients at risk for developing stress ulcers and utilize prophylaxis in only that setting.

THERAPY FOR ESTABLISHED BLEEDING

Once clinically significant bleeding commences, upper GI endoscopy should be performed as soon as possible to establish the diagnosis and to determine the need for endoscopic hemostasis. Although multiple stress ulcers or erosions have the potential to bleed at the same time, it is not unusual for only one or two ulcers to be actively bleeding and to respond to endoscopic therapy (authors' personal experience, Gary R. Zuckerman, C. Prakash Gyawali). If endoscopic measures fail, it may be necessary to resort to angiography with intra-arterial vasopressin or embolization, as used in peptic ulcer bleeding. Surgical therapy should be reserved for patients with continuing life-threatening hemorrhage that is unresponsive to endoscopic therapy. Surgical procedures that leave significant amounts of gastric mucosa intact are associated with a recurrent bleeding rate that approaches 50%, mainly because of the proximal gastric locations and multiplicity of the bleeding lesions [87]. The mortality associated with total gastrectomy in these critically ill patients approaches 100%, however. The addition of vagotomy may decrease the high rebleeding rate and has prompted the use of subtotal gastrectomy with vagotomy and oversewing of any ulcers in the residual stomach [88].

OUTCOME

The mortality rate for critically ill patients with or without stress ulcer bleeding varies in large part with the type and severity of the underlying disease [16]. Although mortality in ICU patients with stress ulcer bleeding can be as high as 80% [3,9,12,34], the relationship of stress ulcer bleeding and mortality is unclear. An earlier natural history study from a medical ICU that did not use prophylaxis found that the overall mortality rate for patients who bled was 90%, whereas it was only 13% for nonbleeders [16]. Meta-analyses of studies performed to evaluate stress ulcer prophylaxis have shown no effect on mortality with the use of antacids or H2RA [76,77]. One analysis found a reduced mortality rate with the use of sucralfate relative to antacids and a trend toward reduced mortality compared with H2RA [65], whereas another meta-analysis did not find any overall mortality advantage for sucralfate-treated patients [76].

The advantage, if any, of a specific prophylactic agent over any other or of a non–pH-altering drug over one that does affect gastric pH has not been clarified at this time. The choice of a prophylactic agent is influenced not only by one's interpretation of the scientific literature but also by the willingness of the ICU staff to adhere to a particular protocol for stress ulcer prophylaxis.

References

1. Lucas CE, Sugawa C, Riddle J, et al: Natural history and surgical dilemma of stress gastric bleeding. *Arch Surg* 102:266, 1971.
2. Peura DA, Johnson LF: Cimetidine for prevention and treatment of gastroduodenal mucosal lesions in patients in an intensive care unit. *Ann Intern Med* 103:173, 1985.
3. Czaja AJ, McAlhany JC, Pruitt BA: Acute gastroduodenal disease after thermal injury: an endoscopic evaluation of incidence and natural history. *N Engl J Med* 291:925, 1974.
4. Kitamura T, Ito K: Acute gastric changes in patients with acute stroke. *Stroke* 7:460, 1976.
5. Curling TB: On acute ulceration of the duodenum in cases of burns. *Med Chir Trans* 25:260, 1842.
6. Selye H: Gastrointestinal system, in *The Physiology and Pathology of Exposure to Stress: A Treatise Based on the Concepts of the General Adaptation Syndrome and the Diseases of Adaptations*. Montreal, QC, Canada, ACTA, 1950, p 688.
7. Czaja AJ, McAlhany JC Jr, Andes WA, et al: Acute gastric disease after cutaneous thermal injury. *Arch Surg* 110:600–605, 1975.
8. Cushing H: Peptic ulcers and the interbrain. *Surg Gynecol Obstet* 55:1, 1932.
9. Beil AR Jr, Mannix H Jr, Beal JM: Massive upper gastrointestinal hemorrhage after operation. *Am J Surg* 108:324, 1964.
10. Goodman AA, Frey CF: Massive upper gastrointestinal hemorrhage following surgical operations. *Ann Surg* 167:180, 1968.
11. Zuckerman GR, Cort D, Shuman RB: Stress ulcer syndrome. *J Intensive Care Med* 3:21, 1988.
12. Kamada T, Fusamoto H, Kawano S, et al: Gastrointestinal bleeding following head injury: a clinical study of 433 cases. *J Trauma* 17:44, 1977.
13. LeGall JR, Mignon FC, Rapin M, et al: Acute gastroduodenal lesions related to severe sepsis. *Surg Gynecol Obstet* 142:377, 1976.
14. Conrad SA, Gabrielli A, Margolis B, et al: Randomized, double-blind comparison of immediate-release omeprazole oral suspension versus intravenous cimetidine for the prevention of upper gastrointestinal bleeding in critically ill patients. *Crit Care Med* 33:760–765, 2005.
15. Kantorova I, Svoboda P, Scheer P, et al: Stress ulcer prophylaxis in critically ill patients: a randomized controlled trial. *Hepatogastroenterology* 51:757–761, 2004.
16. Schuster DP, Rowley H, Feinstein S, et al: Prospective evaluation of the risk of upper gastrointestinal bleeding after admission to a medical intensive care unit. *Am J Med* 76:623, 1984.
17. Cook DJ, Fuller HD, Guyatt GH, et al: Risk factors for gastrointestinal bleeding in critically ill patients. *N Engl J Med* 330:377, 1994.
18. Cook DJ, Pearl RG, Cook RJ, et al: Incidence of clinically important bleeding in mechanically ventilated patients. *J Intensive Care Med* 6:167, 1991.
19. Skillman JJ, Bushnell LS, Goldman H, et al: Respiratory failure, hypotension, sepsis and jaundice: a clinical syndrome associated with lethal hemorrhage from acute stress ulceration of the stomach. *Am J Surg* 147:451, 1984.
20. Kumar S, Zuckerman GR, Micek ST, et al: Stress ulcer syndrome: a reappraisal. *Gastroenterology* 130:A464, 2006.
21. Zuckerman GR, Shuman R: Therapeutic goals and treatment options for prevention of stress ulcer syndrome. *Am J Med* 83[Suppl 6A]:29, 1987.
22. Haglund U: Stress ulcers. *Scand J Gastroenterol* 25[Suppl 175]:27, 1990.
23. Fitts C, Cathcart R, Artz C, et al: Acute gastrointestinal tract ulceration: Cushing's ulcer, steroid ulcer, Curling's ulcer, and stress ulcer. *Am J Surg* 37:218, 1971.
24. Metz CA, Livingston DH, Smith S, et al: Impact of multiple risk factors and ranitidine prophylaxis on the development of stress-related upper gastrointestinal bleeding: a prospective, multicenter, double-blind, randomized trial. *Crit Care Med* 21:1844, 1993.
25. Brown TH, Davidson PF, Larson GM: Acute gastritis occurring within 24 hours of severe head injury. *Gastrointest Endosc* 35:37, 1989.
26. Martin LF, Booth FV, Reines D, et al: Stress ulcers and organ failure in intubated patients in surgical intensive care units. *Ann Surg* 215:332, 1991.
27. Goodman AA, Osborne MP: An experimental model and clinical definition of stress ulceration. *Surg Gynecol Obstet* 134:563, 1972.
28. Skillman JJ, Bushnell LS, Goldman H, et al: Respiratory failure, hypotension, sepsis, and jaundice. *Am J Surg* 117:523, 1969.

29. Harjola PT, Sivula A: Gastric ulceration following experimentally induced hypoxia and hemorrhagic shock: in vivo study of pathogenesis in rabbits. *Ann Surg* 163:21, 1966.
30. Skillman JJ, Gould SA, Chung RSK, et al: The gastric mucosal barrier: clinical and experimental studies in critically ill and normal man, and in the rabbit. *Ann Surg* 172:564, 1970.
31. Marrone GC, Silen W: Pathogenesis, diagnosis and treatment of acute gastric mucosal lesions. *Clin Gastroenterol* 3:635, 1984.
32. Hase T, Moss BJ: Microvascular changes of gastric mucosa in the development of stress ulcer in rats. *Gastroenterology* 65:224, 1973.
33. Yabana T, Yachi A: Stress-induced vascular damage and ulcer. *Dig Dis Sci* 33:751, 1988.
34. Menguy R: Role of gastric mucosal energy metabolism in the etiology of stress ulceration. *World J Surg* 5:175, 1981.
35. Chamberlain CE: Acute hemorrhagic gastritis. *Gastroenterol Clin North Am* 22:843, 1993.
36. Cheung LY: Gastric mucosal blood flow: its measurement and importance in mucosal defense mechanisms. *J Surg Res* 36:282, 1984.
37. Mantor PC, Tuggle DW, Perkins TA, et al: Stress-induced gastric ulcers. *Curr Surg* 46:388, 1989.
38. Das D, Banerjee RK: Effect of stress on the antioxidant enzymes and gastric ulceration. *Mol Cell Biochem* 125:115, 1993.
39. Bresalier RS: The clinical significance and pathophysiology of stress related gastric mucosal hemorrhage. *J Clin Gastroenterol* 13[Suppl 2]:S35, 1991.
40. Schilling D, Haisch G, Sloot N, et al: Low seroprevalence of *Helicobacter pylori* infection in patients with stress ulcer bleeding—a prospective evaluation of patients on a cardiosurgical intensive care unit. *Intensive Care Med* 26:1832, 2000.
41. Hastings PR, Skillman JJ, Bushnell LS, et al: Antacid titration in the prevention of acute gastrointestinal bleeding. A controlled, randomized trial in 100 critically ill patients. *N Engl J Med* 298:1041, 1978.
42. Zinner MJ, Zuidema GD, Smith PL, et al: The prevention of upper gastrointestinal tract bleeding in patients in an intensive care unit. *Surg Gynecol Obstet* 153:214, 1981.
43. Dellinger RP, Levy MM, Carlet JM, et al: Surviving sepsis campaign: international guidelines for management of severe sepsis and septic shock. *Crit Care Med* 36:296–327, 2008.
44. Martin L, Booth F, Karlstadt R, et al: Continuous intravenous cimetidine decreased stress-related upper gastrointestinal hemorrhage without promoting pneumonia. *Crit Care Med* 17:862, 1989.
45. Powell H, Morgan M, Li SK, et al: Inhibition of gastric acid secretion in the intensive care unit after coronary artery bypass graft. A pilot study of intravenous omeprazole by bolus and infusion, ranitidine and placebo. *Theor Surg* 8:125, 1993.
46. Lam NP, Le PD, Crawford SY, et al: National survey of stress ulcer prophylaxis. *Crit Care Med* 27:16, 1999.
47. Anonymous: ASHP therapeutic guidelines on stress ulcer prophylaxis. Developed through the ASHP commission on therapeutics. *Am J Health Syst Pharm* 56:347, 1999.
48. Pitimana-aree S, Forrest D, Brown G, et al: Implementation of a clinical practice guideline for stress ulcer prophylaxis increases appropriateness and decreases cost of care. *Intensive Care Med* 24:217, 1998.
49. Devlin JW, Ben-Menachem T, Ulep SK, et al: Stress ulcer prophylaxis in medical ICU patients: annual utilization in relation to the incidence of endoscopically proven stress ulceration. *Ann Pharmacother* 32:869, 1998.
50. Lasky MR, Metzler MH, Phillips JO: A prospective study of omeprazole suspension to prevent clinically significant gastrointestinal bleeding from stress ulcers in mechanically ventilated trauma patients. *J Trauma* 44:527, 1998.
51. Levy MJ, Seelig CB, Robinson NJ, et al: Comparison of omeprazole and ranitidine for stress ulcer prophylaxis. *Dig Dis Sci* 42:1255, 1997.
52. Somberg L, Morris J Jr, Fantus R, et al: Intermittent intravenous pantoprazole and continuous cimetidine infusion: effect on gastric pH control in critically ill patients at risk of developing stress-related mucosal disease. *J Trauma* 64:1202–1210, 2008.
53. Cook D, Guyatt G, Marshall J, et al: A comparison of sucralfate and ranitidine for the prevention of upper gastrointestinal bleeding in patients requiring mechanical ventilation. Canadian Critical Care Trials Group. *N Engl J Med* 338:791, 1998.
54. Ostro MJ, Russel JA, Soldin SJ, et al: Control of gastric pH with cimetidine: boluses versus primed infusions. *Gastroenterology* 89:532, 1985.
55. Merki HS, Wilder-Smith CH: Do continuous infusions of omeprazole and ranitidine retain their effect with prolonged dosing? *Gastroenterology* 106:60, 1994.
56. Hwang KO, Kolarov S, Cheng L, et al: Stress ulcer prophylaxis for non-critically ill patients on a teaching service. *J Eval Clin Pract* 13:716–721, 2007.
57. McAlhany JC, Czaja AJ, Pruitt BA: Antacid control of complications from acute gastroduodenal disease after burns. *J Trauma* 16:645, 1976.
58. Fabian TC, Boucher BA, Croce MA, et al: Pneumonia and stress ulceration in severely injured patients. A prospective evaluation of the effects of stress ulcer prophylaxis. *Ann Surg* 128:185, 1993.
59. Ryan P, Dawson J, Teres D, et al: Nosocomial pneumonia during stress ulcer prophylaxis with cimetidine and sucralfate. *Arch Surg* 128:1353, 1993.
60. Schuster DP: Stress ulcer prophylaxis: in whom? With what? *Crit Care Med* 21:4, 1993.
61. Prodihom G, Leuenberger P, Koerfer J, et al: Nosocomial pneumonia in mechanically ventilated patients receiving antacid, ranitidine, or sucralfate as prophylaxis for stress ulcer. A randomized controlled trial. *Ann Intern Med* 120:653, 1994.
62. Maier RV, Mitchell D, Gentilello L: Optimal therapy for stress gastritis. *Ann Surg* 220:353, 1994.
63. Cook DJ, Reeve BK, Scholes LC: Histamine-2-receptor antagonists and antacids in the critically ill population: stress ulceration versus nosocomial pneumonia. *Infect Control Hosp Epidemiol* 15:437, 1994.
64. Cook DJ: Stress ulcer prophylaxis: gastrointestinal bleeding and nosocomial pneumonia. Best evidence synthesis. *Scand J Gastroenterol Suppl* 210:48, 1995.
65. Cook DJ, Reeve BK, Guyatt GH, et al: Stress ulcer prophylaxis in critically ill patients. Resolving discordant meta-analysis. *JAMA* 275:308, 1996.
66. Hanisch EW, Encke A, Naujoks F, et al: A randomized, double-blind trial for stress ulcer prophylaxis shows no evidence of increased pneumonia. *Am J Surg* 176:453, 1998.
67. Tryba M, Kurz-Muller K, Donner B: Plasma aluminum concentrations in long-term mechanically ventilated patients receiving stress ulcer prophylaxis with sucralfate. *Crit Care Med* 22:1769, 1994.
68. Mulla H, Peek G, Upton D, et al: Plasma aluminum levels during sucralfate prophylaxis for stress ulceration in critically ill patients on continuous venovenous hemofiltration: a randomized controlled trial. *Crit Care Med* 29:267, 2001.
69. Pingleton SK, Hadzima SK: Enteral alimentation and gastrointestinal bleeding in mechanically ventilated patients. *Crit Care Med* 11:13, 1983.
70. Zinner MJ, Rypins EB, Martin LR, et al: Misoprostol versus antacid titration for preventing stress ulcers in postoperative surgical ICU patients. *Ann Surg* 210:590, 1989.
71. Salim AS: Protection against stress-induced acute gastric mucosal injury by free radical scavengers. *Intensive Care Med* 17:455, 1991.
72. Kitler ME, Hays A, Enterline JP, et al: Preventing postoperative acute bleeding of the upper part of the gastrointestinal tract. *Surg Gynecol Obstet* 171:366, 1990.
73. Fisher RL, Pipkin GA, Wood JR: Stress-related mucosal disease. Pathophysiology, prevention and treatment. *Crit Care Clin* 11:323, 1995.
74. Tryba M, Cook DJ: Gastric alkalinization, pneumonia, and systemic infections: the controversy. *Scand J Gastroenterol Suppl* 210:53, 1995.
75. Heyland D, Mandell LA: Gastric colonization by gram-negative bacilli and nosocomial pneumonia in the intensive care unit patient. Evidence for causation. *Chest* 101:187, 1992.
76. Cook DJ, Witt LG, Cook RJ, et al: Stress ulcer prophylaxis in the critically ill: a meta-analysis. *Am J Med* 91:519, 1991.
77. Tryba M: Prophylaxis of stress ulcer bleeding: a meta-analysis. *J Clin Gastroenterol* 13[Suppl 2]:S44, 1991.
78. Ortiz JE, Sottile FD, Sigel P, et al: Gastric colonization as a consequence of stress ulcer prophylaxis: a prospective randomized trial. *Pharmacotherapy* 18:486, 1998.
79. Driks MR, Craven DE, Celli BR, et al: Nosocomial pneumonia in intubated patients given sucralfate as compared with antacids or histamine type 2 blockers. *N Engl J Med* 317:1376, 1987.
80. Tryba M: Risk of acute stress bleeding and nosocomial pneumonia in ventilated intensive care unit patients: sucralfate versus antacids. *Am J Med* 83[Suppl 3B]:117, 1987.
81. Pickworth KK, Falcone RE, Hoogeboom JE, et al: Occurrence of nosocomial pneumonia in mechanically ventilated trauma patients: a comparison of sucralfate and ranitidine. *Crit Care Med* 21:1856, 1993.
82. Laggner AN, Lenz K, Base W, et al: Prevention of upper gastrointestinal bleeding in long term ventilated patients. Sucralfate versus ranitidine. *Am J Med* 86[Suppl 6A]:81, 1989.
83. Simms HH, DeMaria E, McDonald L, et al: Role of gastric colonization in the development of pneumonia in critically ill trauma patients: results of a prospective randomized trial. *J Trauma* 31:531, 1991.
84. Murphy CE, Stevens AM, Ferrentino N, et al: Frequency of inappropriate continuation of acid suppressive therapy after discharge in patients who began therapy in the surgical intensive care unit. *Pharmacotherapy* 28:968–976, 2008.
85. Qadeer MA, Richter JE, Brotman DJ: Hospital-acquired gastrointestinal bleeding outside the critical care unit: risk factors, role of acid suppression, and endoscopy findings. *J Hosp Med* 1:13–20, 2006.
86. Heidelbaugh JJ, Inadomi JM: Magnitude and economic impact of inappropriate use of stress ulcer prophylaxis in non-ICU hospitalized patients. *Am J Gastroenterol* 101:2200–2205, 2006.
87. Hubert JP, Kiernan PD, Welch JS, et al: The surgical management of bleeding stress ulcers. *Ann Surg* 191:672, 1980.
88. Ritchie WP: Stress ulceration, in Nyhus LM, Wastell C (eds): *Surgery of the Stomach and Duodenum*. 4th ed. Boston, MA, Little, Brown and Company, 1986, p 663.

CHAPTER 93 ■ GASTROINTESTINAL MOTILITY IN THE CRITICALLY ILL PATIENT

FILIPPO CREMONINI, ANTHONY J. LEMBO, BRENNAN M.R. SPIEGEL AND INDER M. SINGH

The gastrointestinal tract is a series of coordinated organs that propels its contents through the precise regulation of neural, chemical, and endocrine signals. Although a detailed review of the physiology of motility is beyond the scope of this chapter, it is important for the critical care provider to understand that the closely coordinated movements of the gastrointestinal tract, from mouth to rectum, can frequently be disrupted and deranged in the setting of severe illness.

Unfortunately, the bowels are not a teleologic priority when systematic illness strikes. Rather, during severe illnesses, physiologic reserve shifts away from the gastrointestinal tract to critical organs such as the lungs, brain, and cardiovascular system, resulting in significant dysfunction of the gastrointestinal tract. This presents most often as delayed transit, or even bowel paralysis, which may occur at any level of the gastrointestinal tract causing gastroparesis or bowel ileus. These conditions can lead to a range of clinically significant consequences, including aspiration, erosive esophagitis, decreased oral intake, nosocomial pneumonia, abdominal pain and distention, obstipation, and even life-threatening bowel perforation.

Because alterations in bowel motility are extremely prevalent in the critically ill population, providers must be prepared to identify and treat these common, morbid, and sometimes fatal disorders. Although there has been surprisingly little research dedicated to understanding the pathophysiologic basis of motility abnormalities in the critically ill patient [1], there have nonetheless been several advances in the treatment of these disorders. This chapter will focus on the clinical presentations of the most common motility disorders in the critically ill patients, including gastroesophageal reflux disease (GERD), gastroparesis, ileus, and colonic pseudoobstruction and will review the current evidence supporting diagnostic and therapeutic approaches for these conditions.

GASTROESOPHAGEAL REFLUX DISEASE

Critically ill patients are especially prone to developing gastroesophageal reflux and related complications, particularly erosive esophagitis, which is one of the leading causes of inpatient upper gastrointestinal tract hemorrhage in mechanically ventilated patients, after stress-related mucosal disease [2,3]. GERD is particularly prevalent in the critically ill patient for several important reasons (Fig. 93.1). First, critically ill patients are often in the recumbent position, which promotes acid reflux [4–6] and reduces acid clearance from the esophagus. Second, many critically ill patients are intubated, sedated, or too ill to report symptoms of acid reflux. Significant reflux can thus go unrecognized until significant complications occur. This prolonged acid exposure is exacerbated in patients who are *nihil per os (nothing by mouth)*, in whom decreased swallowing leads to poor clearance of esophageal contents. Third, critically ill patients are more likely to have increased transient relaxation of the lower esophageal sphincter (LES), due to use of drugs (e.g., morphine, atropine, theophylline, barbiturates) and to the frequent use of indwelling nasogastric tubes [7–9]. Fourth, mechanically ventilated patients are prone to acid reflux and microaspiration, at least in part due to mechanical deformities of the upper esophageal sphincter created by the pressure of the endotracheal tube cuff [4]. Fifth, critically ill patients often develop concomitant gastroparesis (see following discussion) from a host of factors, which, in turn, favors retrograde flow of gastric contents toward the distal esophagus. Taken together, these multiple mechanisms concur to clinically significant acid reflux and to its related complications.

Several steps can be taken in the critical care setting to minimize complications of acid reflux in the critically ill patient. First, patients should be kept in the semirecumbent or upright position as often as possible. This maneuver can minimize acid stasis in the distal esophagus and improve emptying of stomach contents, thereby reducing complications of acid reflux [4,5]. The effectiveness of this maneuver in patients who are mechanically ventilated remains controversial [5,6]. Nevertheless, as positional changes are generally a low risk and easy to enact measure, it seems prudent to position patients in a semirecumbent or upright position when feasible and be wary when patients remain in the supine position for prolonged periods.

Another step is to minimize the use of nasogastric tubes. Data indicate that indwelling nasogastric tubes promote GERD and subsequent microaspiration of bacterially contaminated contents into the lower airways [7–9]. Thus, gastroesophageal reflux also can lead to nosocomial pneumonia [10,11]. Results from a small ($n = 17$) randomized trial suggests that the nasogastric tube size (i.e., 2.85 mm vs. 6.0 mm) does not appear to reduce GERD [9], although clearly this study was not powered to demonstrate statistically significant differences in clinically relevant outcomes (such as bleeding or pneumonia). Placement of a gastrostomy tube in mechanically ventilated patients may reduce GERD and potentially its complications, although such intervention is not without its own risks and side effects [12].

A final step is to minimize the use of medications known to relax the LES. Many of these agents (Table 93.1) are commonly used in the intensive care setting. It should be noted that while these agents are known to decrease LES resting pressure, the clinical significance on the development of complication of GERD including erosive esophagitis or upper gastrointestinal hemorrhage is unknown. Thus, the agents listed in Table 93.1 should not be avoided on the basis of theoretical concerns alone, assuming their use is otherwise medically justified.

Pharmacological therapy is often necessary especially in the intensive care unit (ICU) to reduce the potential complications of GERD. Treatment relies primarily on acid suppression. Traditionally, intravenous (IV) histamine-2 receptor antagonists (H2RAs) have served as the mainstay antisecretory therapy in the critical care setting. H2RAs are particularly useful for prophylaxis against stress-related mucosal disease [13] and are therefore primarily used for stress ulcer prophylaxis (as opposed to GERD prophylaxis) (see Chapter 92). However, IV

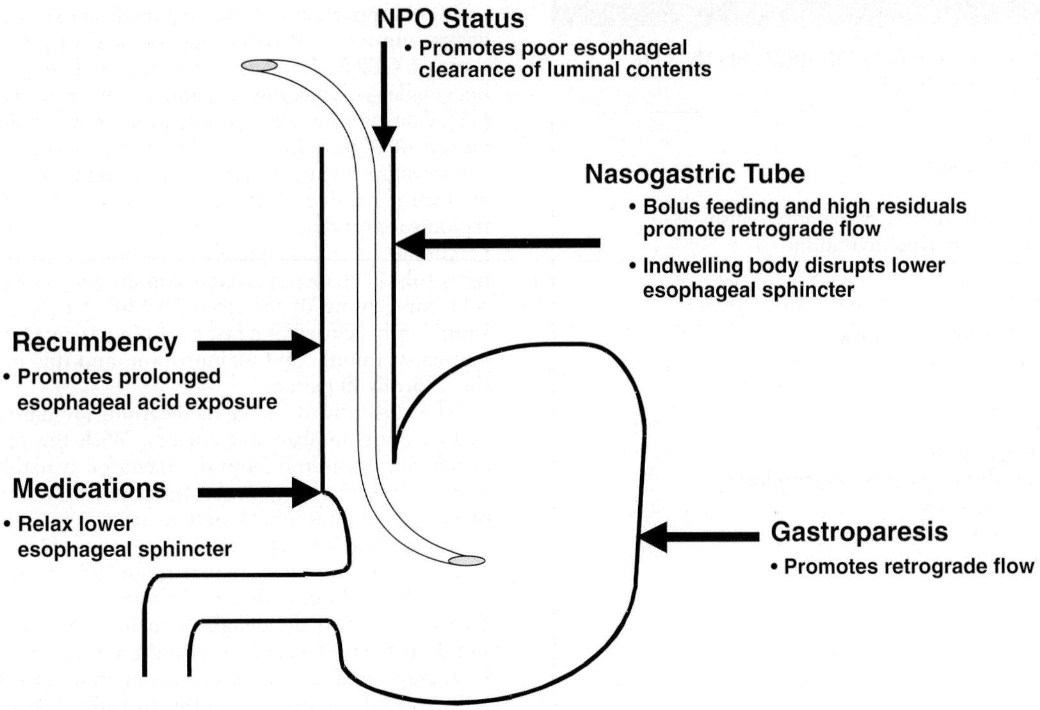

FIGURE 93.1. The combination of factors contributing to gastroesophageal reflux disease (GERD) in the critically ill patient. Patients in the intensive care unit setting are highly susceptible to each of these factors making GERD a prevalent problem. NPO, nothing by mouth.

proton pump inhibitors (PPIs) (pantoprazole, esomeprazole) have since replaced H2RAs as the antisecretory of choice in the hospital setting. IV PPIs have excellent effectiveness in reducing recurrent hemorrhage following endoscopic hemostasis for bleeding peptic ulcer [14]. Although there are limited data regarding their use for erosive esophagitis, experimental data have shown that IV PPIs produce potent and longer-lasting acid inhibition [15], making them the preferred antisecretory medication in patients at risk for GERD-related complications [16].

GASTROPARESIS

Gastroparesis, or delayed gastric emptying in the absence of mechanical obstruction, may lead to several complications in critically ill patients, including malnutrition, erosive esophagitis (as previously noted), and aspiration of gastric contents with resulting nosocomial pneumonia.

As with GERD, gastroparesis arises from a confluence of several common factors (Table 93.2) in the critically ill patient, including medications (especially narcotics and anticholinergic agents), autonomic dysfunction, postsurgical states, and endocrine abnormalities, among others.

Patients with gastroparesis typically present with nausea, vomiting, abdominal pain, early satiety, and postprandial bloating. In patients receiving tube feeding, high gastric residuals are a common early sign of delayed gastric emptying. Because the symptoms of gastroparesis are often nonspecific, the clinician should maintain a low threshold for considering the diagnosis. A combination of physical examination findings and imaging studies confirm gastroparesis and exclude competing diagnoses, including mechanical obstruction and mucosal diseases. On examination, patients with gastroparesis may demonstrate epigastric distention with tenderness but typically lack abdominal rigidity or guarding, signs of a potentially more ominous and acute diagnosis. The examiner should evaluate for a succussion splash by placing the stethoscope over the left upper quadrant while gently shaking the abdomen laterally by holding either side of the pelvis. A positive test occurs when a splash is heard over the stomach and favors the diagnosis of mechanical gastric outlet obstruction over gastroparesis. Of note, the maneuver is only valid if the patient has not ingested solids or liquids within the previous 3 hours.

Laboratory testing may help determine the underlying cause of the decreased motility. Serum electrolyte levels, serum glucose level, serum cortisol level, thyroid-stimulating hormone level, amylase, and white blood cell count (screen for infection) should be measured. A host of other tests can be used in the outpatient setting to investigate chronic gastroparesis (e.g., erythrocyte sedimentation rate [scleroderma, myopathies, lupus], urinary protein [amyloidosis], chest radiography [lung cancer with gastroparesis as a paraneoplastic syndrome], and antineuronal or anti-Hu antibodies [paraneoplastic gastroparesis]), but these are rarely useful in the critically ill patient.

Plain films of the abdomen should be obtained to evaluate for evidence of gastric distention and to screen for overt evidence of gastric obstruction. Upper endoscopy should be considered if there is suggestion of gastric outlet obstruction,

TABLE 93.1

CLASSES OF MEDICATIONS COMMONLY USED IN THE INTENSIVE CARE UNIT SETTING THAT RELAX THE LOWER ESOPHAGEAL SPHINCTER

Anticholinergic agents
Aminophylline
Benzodiazepines
β-Adrenergic agonists
Nitrates

TABLE 93.2

COMMON CAUSES OF GASTROPARESIS IN THE CRITICALLY ILL PATIENT[a]

Endocrinopathies
Adrenal insufficiency
Diabetes
Hypoparathyroidism or hyperparathyroidism
Hypothyroidism or hyperthyroidism
Infections
Pneumonia
Abdominal or pelvic infections
Urinary tract infections
Sepsis
Medications
Anticholinergic agents
Aluminum-hydroxide–containing products
β-Adrenergic agonists
Calcium channel blockers
Diphenhydramine
Levodopa
Narcotics
Octreotide
Tricyclics
Neurologic disorders
Multiple sclerosis
Parkinson's disease
Stroke
Postsurgical settings
Esophagectomy with gastric pull-through
Fundoplication
Gastroplasty
Gastric bypass surgery
Roux-en-Y gastrojejunostomy
Vagotomy
Whipple procedure
Vascular disorders
Mesenteric ischemia
Superior mesenteric artery syndrome
Median arcuate ligament syndrome

[a]This list is not comprehensive but is specifically relevant to the critically ill patient.

because significant amounts of retained food, feedings, and secretions can be found in the stomach even in the absence of an obstruction to the pyloric outlet. Additional imaging tests for the investigation of gastroparesis in the ICU setting are infrequently indicated. If the problem is suspected by the presentation, becomes a primary issue, and is not easily linked to other disorders in the ICU patient, then confirming the diagnosis by other methods may be merited once the patient leaves the ICU. The most accepted diagnostic test, usually performed in the outpatient setting, is a scintigraphic emptying study. Most centers use a 4-hour gastric emptying test, with a ^{99}Tc-labeled-egg meal. In health, gastric retention of more than 10% at 4 hours suggests delayed gastric emptying [17]. Alternative diagnostic tests include stable isotope-labeled breath tests, magnetic resonance imaging, catheter-based manometry, and newly developed wireless capsule-based manometry. Still, the simple finding of persistent high gastric tube residuals should be sufficient to formulate a presumptive diagnosis in the critically ill patient.

Once diagnosed, gastroparesis is treated by reversing known underlying causes of decreased motility, providing adequate nutritional support, and employing medical therapies to promote gastric motility and reduce gastric acid to prevent complications of GERD. Principles of nutritional support include using smaller volume, low-fat, and low-fiber meals or tube feeds [18]. Consultation with the nutrition or metabolic support services is often warranted to help select between available liquid caloric supplements. In general, parenteral nutrition should be avoided if possible. Rather, patients who need long-term nutrition support due to gastroparesis should be considered for a percutaneous endoscopically or radiologically placed jejunostomy tube [19], often placed in conjunction with a gastrostomy tube for venting of the stomach [20]. Surgical interventions should only be used as a last resort in patients with intractable nausea, vomiting, and malnutrition, and this has no place in the critically ill patient.

The currently available medications are unfortunately limited in both number and efficacy. With the removal of cisapride and tegaserod from the menu of available promotility agents, clinicians have limited options. Most authorities recommend metoclopramide, despite its neurologic side effects (e.g., akathisia) that impact up to 30% of users [21]. Reducing the rate of IV infusion may reduce frequency of neurological side effects. Metoclopramide has multiple actions, including coordination of antral, duodenal, and pyloric muscle function while simultaneously serving as a centrally acting antiemetic [22,23]. Metoclopramide can be administered orally, intravenously, rectally, and subcutaneously. In the critically ill patient, metoclopramide typically is dosed at 10 to 20 mg IV every 6 hours. The major disadvantage of IV bolus dosing is that plasma levels are often erratic, largely because levels peak rapidly and the half-life is short. Subcutaneous dosing (two to four times per day in 2-mL aliquots) has been promoted as an alternative route, as it is associated with more stable plasma levels [24]. Although the tardive dyskinesia side effects have been known for decades, the Food and Drug Administration (FDA) recently issued a "black box" warning in reference to metoclopramide, which indirectly has put some pressure on clinicians toward less use of this medication.

Erythromycin, an antibiotic with motilin-receptor agonist properties, also has promotility effects. Oral tablets generally have poor efficacy in gastroparesis [25], the preferred route of oral administration being liquid suspension at low doses of 125 to 250 mg twice daily. Erythromycin may be used in combination with metoclopramide for patients with an incomplete response to either agent alone. IV dosing of erythromycin (100 to 200 mg every 6 hours) improves gastric contractility by invoking high-amplitude gastric contractions [26]. It is particularly effective in diabetic patients and has also shown benefits in reducing high tube feed residuals [27]. Unfortunately, long-term use of erythromycin leads to tachyphylaxis from down-regulation of motilin receptors [25] and also is associated with antimicrobial resistance.

Nonpharmacologic therapies include gastric pacing and pyloric botulin toxin injection [28]. These options are currently available at limited centers but rarely used in critically ill patients.

ILEUS

Any disease state affecting neurohormonal mediators, vascular perfusion, electrolyte balance, and muscular contraction has the potential to affect the coordinated propulsive small and large intestinal motility, resulting in ileus. Virtually all causes of ileus can present in the critically ill patient. The postoperative state, inflammation, metabolic derangement, neurogenic impairment, and drug-induced aperistalsis are all common occurrences in the ICU. As a result of decreased impaired propulsive activity, patients develop obstipation and, eventually,

TABLE 93.3

DIFFERENTIATION OF ILEUS AND SMALL BOWEL OBSTRUCTION

Clinical feature	Ileus	Small bowel obstruction
Bowel sounds	Generally absent	High-pitched and active
Peritoneal signs	Less common	More common, although inconsistent
Involved bowel on radiograph	Small and large bowel dilated	Small bowel dilated
Rectal gas	Present	Absent
Air fluid levels	Absent	Present, although inconsistent
Luminal "cut point"	Absent	Present, although inconsistent

inability to tolerate enteral intake. Patients typically present with abdominal distention, nausea, vomiting, abdominal pain, and high tube feed residuals.

Distinguishing ileus from small bowel obstruction is critical, as prolonged mechanical obstruction can lead to bowel ischemia and peritonitis. Table 93.3 compares classical physical examination and radiographic findings of adynamic ileus and small bowel obstruction. These conditions share many clinical manifestations, including abdominal distention, obstipation, pain, vomiting, and decreased ability to tolerate oral intake. Peritoneal signs and auscultation of high-pitched bowel sounds favor the diagnosis of small bowel obstruction, whereas a silent bowel suggests ileus. Although the skilled clinician often can reliably distinguish small bowel obstruction from ileus on the basis of history and physical examination alone, plain abdominal radiographs may serve to confirm the clinical impression. Ileus typically is characterized by the presence of both small and large bowel dilatation, the presence of gas throughout the bowel and into the rectum, lack of a luminal "cut point" or caliber transition, and an elevated diaphragm. In contrast, small bowel obstruction typically presents with small bowel distention in the absence of colonic gas, a paucity of gas in the rectum, air fluid levels on upright positioning, and evidence of a luminal cut point. Despite the stereotypical features of small bowel obstruction and ileus, plain film imaging does not always provide a definitive diagnosis, as long-standing ileus or partial small bowel obstruction may appear similar on abdominal imaging. In addition, late-stage mechanical obstruction may lead to exhaustion of intestinal propulsive activity, resembling adynamic ileus without high-pitched bowel sounds and a similar air distribution pattern on plain abdominal X-rays. In cases in which the plain films are inadequate, contrast-enhanced computed tomography (CT) should be considered [29]. A CT scan may provide additional information to complement the clinical picture, such as the presence or absence of intra-abdominal inflammation (e.g., pancreatitis, abdominal abscess) or retroperitoneal pathology.

Once ileus has been diagnosed and small bowel obstruction excluded, the next step is to identify and treat reversible causes of hypomotility. Bearing in mind that common causes of ileus in the critically ill patient include electrolyte abnormalities, sepsis, inflammation, postoperative hypomotility, and medications (Table 93.4), initial laboratory studies should include serum potassium, magnesium, calcium, bicarbonate, lipase, blood urea nitrogen, creatinine, and white blood cell count. Electrolyte abnormalities can often be easily reversed, leading to improvement in small bowel motility. Medications should be carefully reviewed, and potentially causative agents discontinued or limited if otherwise warranted. There are no specific rules about how and when to discontinue medications in the setting of ileus, especially when necessary pain medications (e.g., narcotics) are implicated. Ultimately, the decision rests on a careful balance of clinical factors and meticulous attention to the progress and clinical sequelae of the ileus. In particular, if there is concomitant evidence of significant cecal or large bowel distention to suggest colonic pseudoobstruction and impending perforation, then all the medications contributing to aperistalsis must be discontinued.

In contrast, if there are no clinical signs of deterioration and no worsening on serial abdominal X-rays, the ileus is nonprogressive and stable, and a supportive, conservative treatment is preferred, the treatment plan should include adequate IV hydration, electrolytes replacement, and treatment of the underlying condition, with close clinical and radiological follow-up. There is little evidence [30–40] to support insertion of a nasogastric tube for decompression of prolonged ileus and worsening abdominal distention; however, when vomiting is present, this is routinely performed. One caveat to this widespread approach is the trend in favor of more atelectasis and pneumonia in patients receiving nasogastric decompression in randomized controlled trials [30–40]. Overall, individual trials' data and meta-analyses on tube decompression, mostly in postoperative ileus patients, do not support the need for this intervention [33,41].

Active treatments for ileus remain limited, and the usual promotility agents are generally ineffective.

Opioid-induced bowel dysfunction can occur after the initial dose of opioids and not resolve for some time after therapy is discontinued. The constipating effect of narcotics is not characterized by tolerance [42]. While stool softeners, stimulant, and osmotic laxative are traditionally used, a subset of critically ill patients will not respond to traditional measures and will go on to develop inability to tolerate enteral feedings and laxatives [43]. Opioid reversing agents, with limited systemic bioavailability, have been traditionally used, such as Naloxone, naltrexone, and nalmefene. However, early transit across the blood–brain barrier by these agents caused concomitant analgesia reversal and the onset of opioid withdrawal, without consistent restoration of peristalsis [44]. The newer naltrexone derivative methylnaltrexone is less lipid-soluble than

TABLE 93.4

COMMON CAUSES OF ILEUS IN INTENSIVE CARE UNIT PATIENTS

Electrolyte disorders
Medications
Peritoneal inflammation
Postsurgical setting
Mesenteric ischemia
Sepsis
Retroperitoneal disease
Myocardial infarction

the previous agents and does not cross the blood–brain barrier. Methylnaltrexone is efficacious in treating opioid-induce bowel dysfunction both orally and intravenously, and in most patients, it is effective within 4 hours of the first dose [45].

Postoperative ileus, the interruption of colonic motor activity after surgery, has a multifactorial pathophysiology, with surgical stress hormones, activation of the endogenous opioid system, exogenous opioids given for pain, and inflammation compounding imbalances in fluid and electrolytes.

Traditional prokinetics have been used for reversal of postoperative ileus. Although metoclopramide has proven efficacy in the foregut, it provides little or no benefit for postoperative ileus [46–50]. There have been few studies of metoclopramide in postoperative ileus, so it is difficult to conclude whether its ineffectiveness in postoperative ileus extends to other forms of ileus. Similarly, randomized controlled trials of erythromycin in postoperative ileus demonstrated minimal, if any, benefit [51]. The somatostatin analog, octreotide, has been used empirically, although no good randomized controlled data exist for its use in humans with postoperative ileus, and there are potential detrimental effects on gastric emptying with octreotide that need to be considered before administering in severe whole gut dysmotility.

One trial of 65 postcolectomy patients demonstrated efficacy of methylnaltrexone (see earlier) 0.3 mg given intravenously every 6 hours to achieve a first bowel movement and to hasten discharge from the hospital [52]. These observations support a role for opioid reversal even in the absence of a previous effect of exogenous opioids on gut motor function. Larger trials on methylnaltrexone are needed.

Another opioid antagonist, the selective μ-opioid receptor antagonist, alvimopan, is approved by the FDA for the treatment of postoperative ileus [53,54]. Oral alvimopan is administered preoperatively and postoperatively. In one randomized, controlled, blinded clinical trial of postoperative ileus, alvimopan, 6 mg twice daily, led to a faster passage of flatus (by 21 hours), earlier initiation of bowel movements (by 41 hours), and faster time to discharge (by 23 hours) than placebo [53]. A subsequent larger trial in 510 patients demonstrated similar results [54]. These dramatic effects in postoperative ileus set the stage for the use of alvimopan in other forms of ileus. In a study of 522 patients with noncancer pain requiring an equivalent dose of narcotics more than 30 mg of oral morphine daily, alvimopan was superior to placebo in increasing bowel movement frequency and other endpoints correlated to severe opioid-induced constipation. Although this study was not in a critical care population, the data suggest that alvimopan could be administered after the bowel dysfunction ensues and could prove efficacious for opioids-induced ileus in the critically ill patient [55].

ACUTE COLONIC PSEUDOOBSTRUCTION (OGILVIE'S SYNDROME)

Acute colonic pseudoobstruction, or Ogilvie's syndrome, is characterized by marked dilatation of the cecum and ascending colon in the absence of mechanical obstruction (Fig. 93.2). Similar to ileus, colonic pseudoobstruction generally occurs in critically ill patients with sepsis, recent surgery, electrolyte abnormalities, and trauma, among other conditions. The diagnosis rests on radiographic evaluation of the cecum, where a diameter of more than 9 cm suggests evidence of pseudoobstruction in the absence of a mechanical obstruction. This threshold is somewhat arbitrary and is based on an early series from 1956 that linked this diameter with clinically significant sequelae, namely colonic perforation [56]. More recent case series suggest that a cecal diameter exceeding 12 cm correlates most highly with bowel perforation and should serve as a critical threshold to track in patients with suspected pseudoobstruction [57,58].

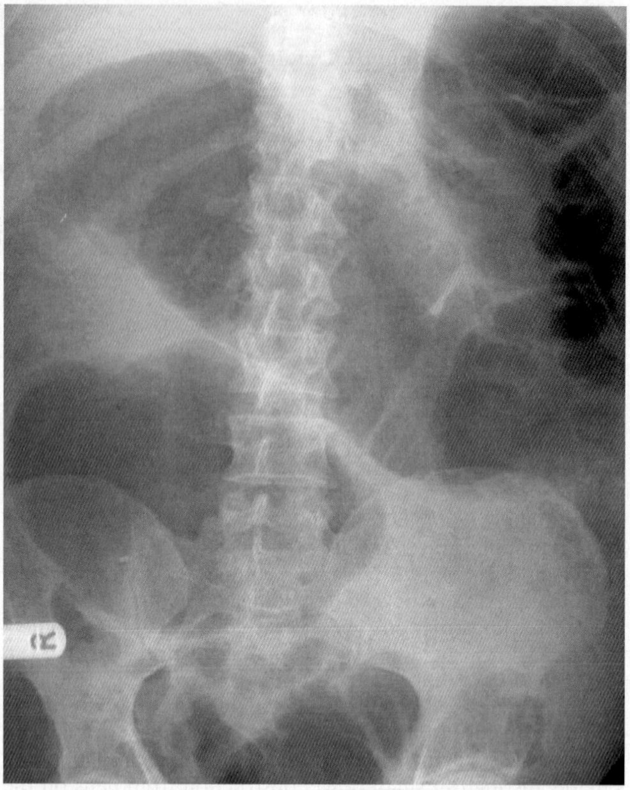

FIGURE 93.2. Marked dilatation of the cecum and other colonic regions in colonic pseudoobstruction. When the cecal diameter exceeds 12 cm, the risk for perforation rises substantially. [From the Scottish Radiological Society (SRS-X: www.radiology.com.uk/srs-x), with permission.]

The exact mechanism by which cecal dilatation occurs remains unclear. There are two competing theories [59]. The first theory, originally postulated by Ogilvie himself in 1948 [60], suggests that sympathetic drive to the enteric nervous system is interrupted, thereby promoting unopposed parasympathetic stimulation. This, in turn, could promote unabated distal colonic luminal contractions and a potential source of obstruction. The second theory, espoused by Hutchinson and Griffiths [61], contends that colonic pseudoobstruction arises from a combination of sympathetic overdrive and parasympathetic suppression, both described in the setting of physiologic stress, thereby leading to colonic hypomotility and eventual paralysis. The proven effectiveness of neostigmine in colonic pseudoobstruction (see following discussion) supports the validity of the latter theory. In contrast, there are few physiologic data to support Ogilvie's original concept of sympathetic interruption. It must be noted that the autonomic nervous system is not the sole player in colonic motility, as the regulators of the enteric nervous system are potentially innumerable, including, among the many, neurohormonal factors and gut peptides.

The clinical presentation of acute colonic pseudoobstruction is typical of obstructive colonic processes, with the patient demonstrating marked abdominal distention, nausea, vomiting, and abdominal pain. If left untreated, colonic pseudoobstruction can lead to ischemia, perforation (in approximately 3% of cases overall), peritonitis, and death [62–65]. Thus, the clinician must keep a high index of suspicion for colonic pseudoobstruction in patients with risk factors, as the consequences of late diagnosis can be grave.

Fortunately, conservative measures are sufficient in most cases, and the cecal dilatation resolves spontaneously. Conservative measures consist of ceasing oral intake, frequent repositioning of the patient, and treating potential underlying causes of dysmotility (as with ileus). Although nasogastric tubes are often employed in cases of colonic pseudoobstruction, there are no data from randomized controlled studies to support its effectiveness in reducing clinically significant endpoints. Because nasogastric decompression has limited, if any, role in ileus [40–49], there is little a priori reason to believe that the maneuver would be of benefit in colonic pseudoobstruction, a condition that is even more distal to the tip of a nasogastric tube than ileus. In contrast, case series do support the effectiveness of colonoscopic decompression, which reduces the cecal diameter in nearly 70% of patients [62,65]. Unfortunately, colonoscopic decompression alone is often short lived, and recurrent distention occurs in approximately half of patients [59,62]. Thus, colonoscopic decompression usually is accompanied by placement of a rectal tube or stent with its proximal tip in the ascending colon. Although colonoscopic decompression and tube placement is conceptually attractive, the procedure is challenging and often unsuccessful and it must be conducted in an unprepared bowel without the benefit of full air insufflation.

In patients failing to respond to conservative measures after 24 to 48 hours, including correction of electrolyte abnormalities, IV hydration, correction of underlying medical causes, and minimization of culprit medications, pharmacologic therapy is generally warranted. Moreover, if at any time the cecal diameter exceeds 12 cm, or if there is evidence of worsening clinical status, then aggressive treatment should be pursued immediately, because these findings constitute a gastroenterological emergency, which mandates early consultative involvement of a surgeon. In patients with markedly dilated large bowel, some specialists would defer even an initial attempt at colonoscopic decompression to a trial of medical therapy. The acetylcholinesterase inhibitor neostigmine increases the postsynaptic concentration of acetylcholine, thereby favoring a boost in the deranged colonic motor function. Neostigmine is effective in colonic pseudoobstruction, and its IV administration has been accepted as initial therapy. This recommendation is largely based on a pivotal controlled trial in which 10 of 11 patients randomized to receive neostigmine had prompt evacuation of their colonic contents and normalization of their cecal diameter, whereas none of 10 patients randomized to placebo had these outcomes [63]. Moreover, all of the patients in the placebo arm achieved a response when crossed over to neostigmine in an open-label fashion. The dosage used was 2 mg IV in one infusion followed by an additional 2 mg infusion 3 hours later if there was no initial response or adverse event. Being an anticholinesterase inhibitor, neostigmine has an array of well-defined cholinergic side effects, including bronchoconstriction, abdominal cramping, hypersalivation, diaphoresis, and bradycardia. Hemodynamically relevant side effects, including cardiac arrest and cardiovascular collapse, can occur, requiring neostigmine to be administered in a monitored setting. It is contraindicated in patients with bradycardia, active bronchospasm, and mechanical bowel obstruction. Existing electrolyte imbalances and use of antimotility agents were predictors of poor response to neostigmine. Patients with postoperative colonic ileus had the best response rate [64]. The combined administration of 2 mg neostigmine with glycopyrrolate, an anticholinergic agent that has limited activity on the muscarinic receptors of the colon and has the potential of reducing the incidence of cholinergic side effects of neostigmine, has been evaluated in a randomized, controlled study of 13 patients with neurogenic bowel using videofluorographic assessment of evacuation [65]. The neostigmine–glycopyrrolate combination resulted in bowel evacuation with significantly less bradycardia and increase in airways resistance than with neostigmine alone, suggesting that the coadministration would make treatment with neostigmine safer in clinical settings where cardiorespiratory function is compromised.

When severe colonic pseudoobstruction fails to respond to conservative measures, neostigmine, and colonic decompression, surgery must be considered. In these settings, surgery has a high morbidity and may lead to poor outcomes in patients who are already critically ill. Indeed, case series indicate that one quarter of patients with colonic pseudoobstruction die in the perioperative period, even in the absence of bowel perforation [60], although the presence of underlying critical illness is arguably the strongest predictor of such a guarded prognosis. Alternatively, endoscopic cecostomy with placement of a percutaneous tube using a modified Seldinger technique similar to percutaneous gastrostomy has been described [66].

SUMMARY

Gastrointestinal motility requires coordinated neural, chemical, and endocrine signals. Faced with serious systemic illness, the gastrointestinal tract often becomes dysfunctional, leading to syndromes such as GERD, gastroparesis, ileus, and colonic pseudoobstruction. Although there are no randomized trials to support IV PPI therapy versus IV H2RA therapy in the critically ill patient, there is a biological rationale to consider using IV PPI therapy.

In general, the critical care provider should aim to maintain the appropriate physiologic environment (e.g., normalize electrolytes imbalances, maximize blood flow) and limit known causes of dysmotility (e.g., narcotics, anticholinergics) to ensure at least some level of gastrointestinal motor function. When these measures fail, providers should employ therapies that are supported by the highest level of evidence, namely randomized controlled trials, when available (Table 93.5). Among the therapies described in this chapter, there is high level of

TABLE 93.5

SUMMARY OF EVIDENCE-BASED MANAGEMENT RECOMMENDATIONS

- Treatment and prevention of complications from gastroesophageal reflux should include encouraging the semirecumbent or upright position, avoidance of nasogastric tubes, and use of potent antisecretory therapy, such as intravenous proton pump inhibitors.
- Medical therapy for gastroparesis often is ineffective, although modest benefits are seen with metoclopramide (especially subcutaneous administration) and erythromycin.
- Evidence for placement of a nasogastric tube for decompression in postoperative ileus is weak, as indicated by meta-analyses.
- Data indicate that there is little or no benefit of metoclopramide or erythromycin in the setting of ileus.
- Methylnaltrexone is an opioid reversal agent that does not cross the blood–brain barrier and achieves sustained laxation in opioid-induced bowel dysfunction.
- Alvimopan, a highly selective opioid receptor antagonist, has demonstrated excellent results in postoperative ileus in randomized controlled trials.
- Neostigmine was shown in effective medical therapy for the treatment of acute colonic pseudoobstruction in the presence of colonic diameter >12 cm as determined by direct abdominal X-ray. Endoscopic bowel decompression with insertion of a decompression tube is an effective alternative management option.

evidence to support neostigmine in colonic pseudoobstruction, alvimopan in postoperative ileus, methylnaltrexone in opioid-induced bowel dysfunction, and good evidence supporting the use of metoclopramide in gastroparesis. Future research on critical care patients should study the effects of novel medications under development on endpoints of motor function, morbidity, and mortality, with fewer systemic side effects and an excellent risk profile.

References

1. Quigley EM: Critical care dysmotility: abnormal foregut motor function in the ICU/ITU patient. *Gut* 54:1351–1352; discussion 1384–1390, 2005.
2. Mutlu GM, Mutlu EA, Factor P: Prevention and treatment of gastrointestinal complications in patients on mechanical ventilation. *Am J Respir Med* 2:395–411, 2003.
3. Newton M, Burnham WR, Kamm MA: Morbidity, mortality, and risk factors for esophagitis in hospital inpatients. *J Clin Gastroenterol* 30:264–269, 2000.
4. Torres A, Serra-Batlles J, Ros E, et al: Pulmonary aspiration of gastric contents in patients receiving mechanical ventilation: the effect of body position. *Ann Intern Med* 116:540–543, 1992.
5. Ibanez J, Penafiel A, Raurich JM, et al: Gastroesophageal reflux in intubated patients receiving enteral nutrition: effect of supine and semirecumbent positions. *JPEN J Parenter Enteral Nutr* 16:419–422, 1992.
6. Orozco-Levi M, Torres A, Ferrer M, et al: Semirecumbent position protects from pulmonary aspiration but not completely from gastroesophageal reflux in mechanically ventilated patients. *Am J Respir Crit Care Med* 152:1387–1390, 1995.
7. Nagler R, Spiro HM: Persistent gastroesophageal reflux induced during prolonged gastric intubation. *N Engl J Med* 269:495–500, 1963.
8. Ibanez J, Penafiel A, Marse P, et al: Incidence of gastroesophageal reflux and aspiration in mechanically ventilated patients using small-bore nasogastric tubes. *JPEN J Parenter Enteral Nutr* 24:103–106, 2000.
9. Ferrer M, Bauer TT, Torres A, et al: Effect of nasogastric tube size on gastroesophageal reflux and microaspiration in intubated patients. *Ann Intern Med* 130:991–994, 1999.
10. DeVault KR: Gastroesophageal reflux disease: extraesophageal manifestations and therapy. *Semin Gastrointest Dis* 12:46–51, 2001.
11. Torres A, El-Ebiary M, Soler N, et al: Stomach as a source of colonization of the respiratory tract during mechanical ventilation: association with ventilator-associated pneumonia. *Eur Respir J* 9:1729–1735, 1996.
12. Douzinas EE, Tsapalos A, Dimitrakopoulos A, et al: Effect of percutaneous endoscopic gastrostomy on gastro-esophageal reflux in mechanically-ventilated patients. *World J Gastroenterol* 12:114–118, 2006.
13. Cook D, Guyatt G, Marshall J, et al: A comparison of sucralfate and ranitidine for the prevention of upper gastrointestinal bleeding in patients requiring mechanical ventilation. Canadian Critical Care Trials Group. *N Engl J Med* 338:791–797, 1998.
14. Lau JY, Sung JJ, Lee KK, et al: Effect of intravenous omeprazole on recurrent bleeding after endoscopic treatment of bleeding peptic ulcers. *N Engl J Med* 343:310–316, 2000.
15. Pisegna JR: Pharmacology of acid suppression in the hospital setting: focus on proton pump inhibition. *Crit Care Med* 30:S356–S361, 2002.
16. Fennerty MB: Pathophysiology of the upper gastrointestinal tract in the critically ill patient: rationale for the therapeutic benefits of acid suppression. *Crit Care Med* 30:S351–S355, 2002.
17. Abell TL, Camilleri M, Donohoe K, et al: Consensus recommendations for gastric emptying scintigraphy: a joint report of the American Neurogastroenterology and Motility Society and the Society of Nuclear Medicine. *Am J Gastroenterol* 103:753–763, 2008.
18. McCallum RW, George SJ: Gastric dysmotility and gastroparesis. *Curr Treat Options Gastroenterol* 4:179–191, 2001.
19. Koretz RL, Lipman TO, Klein S: AGA technical review on parenteral nutrition. *Gastroenterology* 121:970–1001, 2001.
20. Devendra D, Millward BA, Travis SP: Diabetic gastroparesis improved by percutaneous endoscopic jejunostomy. *Diabetes Care* 23:426–427, 2000.
21. Ganzini L, Casey DE, Hoffman WF, et al: The prevalence of metoclopramide-induced tardive dyskinesia and acute extrapyramidal movement disorders. *Arch Intern Med* 153:1469–1475, 1993.
22. Chen JD, Pan J, McCallum RW: Clinical significance of gastric myoelectrical dysrhythmias. *Dig Dis* 13:275–290, 1995.
23. Ricci DA, Saltzman MB, Meyer C, et al: Effect of metoclopramide in diabetic gastroparesis. *J Clin Gastroenterol* 7:25–32, 1985.
24. McCallum RW, Valenzuela G, Polepalle S, et al: Subcutaneous metoclopramide in the treatment of symptomatic gastroparesis: clinical efficacy and pharmacokinetics. *J Pharmacol Exp Ther* 258:136–142, 1991.
25. Richards RD, Davenport K, McCallum RW: The treatment of idiopathic and diabetic gastroparesis with acute intravenous and chronic oral erythromycin. *Am J Gastroenterol* 88:203–207, 1993.
26. Kendall BJ, Chakravarti A, Kendall E, et al: The effect of intravenous erythromycin on solid meal gastric emptying in patients with chronic symptomatic post-vagotomy-antrectomy gastroparesis. *Aliment Pharmacol Ther* 11:381–385, 1997.
27. Keshavarzian A, Isaac RM: Erythromycin accelerates gastric emptying of indigestible solids and transpyloric migration of the tip of an enteral feeding tube in fasting and fed states. *Am J Gastroenterol* 88:193–197, 1993.
28. Rayner CK, Horowitz M: New management approaches for gastroparesis. *Nat Clin Pract Gastroenterol Hepatol* 2:454–462; quiz 493, 2005.
29. Peck JJ, Milleson T, Phelan J: The role of computed tomography with contrast and small bowel follow-through in management of small bowel obstruction. *Am J Surg* 177:375–378, 1999.
30. Bauer JJ, Gelernt IM, Salky BA, et al: Is routine postoperative nasogastric decompression really necessary? *Ann Surg* 201:233–236, 1985.
31. Cheadle WG, Vitale GC, Mackie CR, et al: Prophylactic postoperative nasogastric decompression. A prospective study of its requirement and the influence of cimetidine in 200 patients. *Ann Surg* 202:361–366, 1985.
32. Cunningham J, Temple WJ, Langevin JM, et al: A prospective randomized trial of routine postoperative nasogastric decompression in patients with bowel anastomosis. *Can J Surg* 35:629–632, 1992.
33. Cheatham ML, Chapman WC, Key SP, et al: A meta-analysis of selective versus routine nasogastric decompression after elective laparotomy. *Ann Surg* 221:469–476; discussion 476–478, 1995.
34. Wolff BG, Pembeton JH, van Heerden JA, et al: Elective colon and rectal surgery without nasogastric decompression. A prospective, randomized trial. *Ann Surg* 209:670–673; discussion 673–675, 1989.
35. Petrelli NJ, Stulc JP, Rodriguez-Bigas M, et al: Nasogastric decompression following elective colorectal surgery: a prospective randomized study. *Am Surg* 59:632–635, 1993.
36. Otchy DP, Wolff BG, van Heerden JA, et al: Does the avoidance of nasogastric decompression following elective abdominal colorectal surgery affect the incidence of incisional hernia? Results of a prospective, randomized trial. *Dis Colon Rectum* 38:604–608, 1995.
37. Pearl ML, Valea FA, Fischer M, et al: A randomized controlled trial of postoperative nasogastric tube decompression in gynecologic oncology patients undergoing intra-abdominal surgery. *Obstet Gynecol* 88:399–402, 1996.
38. Huerta S, Arteaga JR, Sawicki MP, et al: Assessment of routine elimination of postoperative nasogastric decompression after Roux-en-Y gastric bypass. *Surgery* 132:844–848, 2002.
39. Akbaba S, Kayaalp C, Savkilioglu M: Nasogastric decompression after total gastrectomy. *Hepatogastroenterology* 51:1881–1885, 2004.
40. Yoo CH, Son BH, Han WK, et al: Nasogastric decompression is not necessary in operations for gastric cancer: prospective randomised trial. *Eur J Surg* 168:379–383, 2002.
41. Nelson R, Edwards S, Tse B: Prophylactic nasogastric decompression after abdominal surgery. *Cochrane Database Syst Rev* CD004929, 2005.
42. McNicol E, Horowicz-Mehler N, Fisk RA, et al: Management of opioid side effects in cancer-related and chronic noncancer pain: a systematic review. *J Pain* 4:231–256, 2003.
43. De Schepper HU, Cremonini F, Park MI, et al: Opioids and the gut: pharmacology and current clinical experience. *Neurogastroenterol Motil* 16:383–394, 2004.
44. Becker G, Galandi D, Blum HE: Peripherally acting opioid antagonists in the treatment of opiate-related constipation: a systematic review. *J Pain Symptom Manage* 34:547–565, 2007.
45. Thomas J, Karver S, Cooney GA, et al: Methylnaltrexone for opioid-induced constipation in advanced illness. *N Engl J Med* 358:2332–2343, 2008.
46. Davidson ED, Hersh T, Brinner RA, et al: The effects of metoclopramide on postoperative ileus. A randomized double-blind study. *Ann Surg* 190:27–30, 1979.
47. Jepsen S, Klaerke A, Nielsen PH, et al: Negative effect of Metoclopramide in postoperative adynamic ileus. A prospective, randomized, double blind study. *Br J Surg* 73:290–291, 1986.
48. Tollesson PO, Cassuto J, Faxen A, et al: Lack of effect of metoclopramide on colonic motility after cholecystectomy. *Eur J Surg* 157:355–358, 1991.
49. Seta ML, Kale-Pradhan PB: Efficacy of metoclopramide in postoperative ileus after exploratory laparotomy. *Pharmacotherapy* 21:1181–1186, 2001.
50. Cheape JD, Wexner SD, James K, et al: Does metoclopramide reduce the length of ileus after colorectal surgery? A prospective randomized trial. *Dis Colon Rectum* 34:437–441, 1991.
51. Smith AJ, Nissan A, Lanouette NM, et al: Prokinetic effect of erythromycin after colorectal surgery: randomized, placebo-controlled, double-blind study. *Dis Colon Rectum* 43:333–337, 2000.
52. Viscusi E, Rathmell J, Fichera A, et al: A double-blind, randomized, placebo-controlled trial of methylnaltrexone (MNTX) for post-operative bowel dysfunction in segmental colectomy. *Proc Am Soc Anesth* 103:A893, 2005.
53. Taguchi A, Sharma N, Saleem RM, et al: Selective postoperative inhibition of gastrointestinal opioid receptors. *N Engl J Med* 345:935–940, 2001.
54. Wolff BG, Michelassi F, Gerkin TM, et al: Alvimopan, a novel, peripherally acting mu opioid antagonist: results of a multicenter, randomized, double-blind, placebo-controlled, phase III trial of major abdominal surgery and postoperative ileus. *Ann Surg* 240:728–734; discussion 734–735, 2004.

55. Webster L, Jansen JP, Peppin J, et al: Alvimopan, a peripherally acting mu-opioid receptor (PAM-OR) antagonist for the treatment of opioid-induced bowel dysfunction: results from a randomized, double-blind, placebo-controlled, dose-finding study in subjects taking opioids for chronic non-cancer pain. *Pain* 137:428–440, 2008.
56. Davis L, Lowman RM: An evaluation of cecal size in impending perforation of the cecum. *Surg Gynecol Obstet* 103:711–718, 1956.
57. Vanek VW, Al-Salti M: Acute pseudo-obstruction of the colon (Ogilvie's syndrome). An analysis of 400 cases. *Dis Colon Rectum* 29:203–210, 1986.
58. Gierson ED, Storm FK, Shaw W, et al: Caecal rupture due to colonic ileus. *Br J Surg* 62:383–386, 1975.
59. Laine L: Management of acute colonic pseudo-obstruction. *N Engl J Med* 341:192–193, 1999.
60. Ogilvie H: Large-intestine colic due to sympathetic deprivation: a new clinical syndrome. *Br Med J* 2:671–673, 1948.
61. Hutchinson R, Griffiths C: Acute colonic pseudo-obstruction: a pharmacological approach. *Ann R Coll Surg Engl* 74:364–367, 1992.
62. Rex DK: Colonoscopy and acute colonic pseudo-obstruction. *Gastrointest Endosc Clin N Am* 7:499–508, 1997.
63. Ponec RJ, Saunders MD, Kimmey MB: Neostigmine for the treatment of acute colonic pseudo-obstruction. *N Engl J Med* 341:137–141, 1999.
64. Mehta R, John A, Nair P, et al: Factors predicting successful outcome following neostigmine therapy in acute colonic pseudo-obstruction: a prospective study. *J Gastroenterol Hepatol* 21:459–461, 2006.
65. Korsten MA, Rosman AS, Ng A, et al: Infusion of neostigmine-glycopyrrolate for bowel evacuation in persons with spinal cord injury. *Am J Gastroenterol* 100:1560–1565, 2005.
66. Ramage JI Jr, Baron TH: Percutaneous endoscopic cecostomy: a case series. *Gastrointest Endosc* 57:752–755, 2003.

CHAPTER 94 ■ FULMINANT COLITIS AND TOXIC MEGACOLON

STEPHEN B. HANAUER

Ulcerative colitis is characterized by a diffuse, continuous inflammatory process usually limited to the superficial mucosa of the colon. *Fulminant colitis* implies progression of mucosal inflammation into deeper (muscular) layers of the colon wall. It generally is associated with severe bloody diarrhea, fever, tachycardia, and abdominal tenderness. Systemic manifestations result from transmural colitis, which may also produce circular muscle paralysis precipitating dilatation. *Toxic megacolon* refers to acute dilatation of the colon, generally as a complication of ulcerative colitis, but it may occur with any severe inflammatory colitis. Toxic megacolon has been described with idiopathic and infectious colitis, including ulcerative colitis, Crohn's disease, amebic colitis, pseudomembranous colitis, and other infections [1]. Toxic megacolon has been reported to complicate from 1% to 13% of all ulcerative colitis cases [2] and from 2% to 3% of Crohn's colitis cases [1]. Although mortality in early series was as high as 25% (reaching 50% if colonic perforation occurred), early recognition and management of toxic megacolon has substantially lowered mortality to below 15% [3] and usually below 2% in experienced centers [4]. Factors associated with increased mortality include age older than 40 years, the presence of colonic perforation, and delay of surgery [3,4]. Colonic perforation, whether free or localized, is the greatest risk factor leading to increased morbidity or death.

PREDISPOSING FACTORS

The severity of disease activity is the most important predictor of toxic megacolon, which is more common in extensive colitis than in proctitis or proctosigmoiditis [5]. Limited right- or left-sided segmental colitis also has been associated with toxic megacolon. Concomitant *Clostridium difficile* infection often occurs in hospitalized patients with inflammatory bowel disease and can be associated with refractory disease [6,7]. Similarly, cytomegalovirus (CMV) infections frequently complicate colitis in the setting of immune suppression with corticosteroids or cyclosporine [8,9]. Treatment of CMV with ganciclovir usually is not necessary unless there are systemic manifestations such as fever or associated hepatitis.

Toxic megacolon typically occurs early in the course of ulcerative colitis, usually within the first 5 years of disease, and 25% to 40% of cases present with the initial attack [1]. The onset of toxic megacolon has been linked to patients who have recently undergone diagnostic examinations, such as barium enemas or colonoscopy, suggesting that manipulation of the inflamed bowel or vigorous laxative preparation may exacerbate the process, possibly through electrolyte imbalance (Table 94.1) [3,10].

Certain drug therapies have been implicated in the development of toxic megacolon. Diphenoxylate hydrochloride/atropine sulfate (Lomotil), loperamide, and other inhibitors of colonic motility such as opiates and narcotics may contribute to the development of toxic megacolon by inhibiting colon muscle function in severe transmural disease [11].

Electrolyte and pH disturbances are risk factors for toxic megacolon. Severe potassium depletion, secondary to severe diarrhea or corticosteroid therapy, or both, is known to inhibit colonic motility. Potassium requirements of patients with colitis

TABLE 94.1

POTENTIAL PRECIPITANTS OF TOXIC MEGACOLON

Concurrent pathogens (*Clostridium difficile*, CMV)
Narcotics
Anticholinergics
Antidiarrheal agents (diphenoxylate with atropine, loperamide, opiates)
Barium enema
Colonoscopy

CMV, cytomegalovirus.

may be massive, and restoration of serum potassium alone may not be adequate to replenish body stores [1,11].

Despite early speculations on the role of corticosteroids in inducing toxic megacolon, most experienced clinicians do not accept the implication that corticosteroids or adrenocorticotropic hormone are precipitating factors [1,11–13]. Concern remains, however, that corticosteroids may suppress signs of perforation, thereby delaying surgical therapy.

CLINICAL FEATURES

Toxic megacolon usually occurs on the background of chronic inflammatory bowel disease [1,3]. The presentation typically evolves with progressive diarrhea, bloody stool, and cramping abdominal pain. Occasionally, in patients treated for inflammatory bowel disease over long periods of time, a paradoxic decrease in stool frequency with passage of only bloody discharge or bloody membranes may be an ominous sign (Table 94.2). Thereafter, clinical signs of toxemia, including pyrexia (temperature >101.5°F), tachycardia, and leukocytosis (total white blood cell count >10,500 cells per μL), develop as abdominal pain and distention become progressive and bowel sounds diminish or cease. Signs of peritoneal irritation, including rebound tenderness and abdominal guarding, represent transmural inflammation to the serosa, even in the absence of free perforation. Conversely, peritoneal signs may be minimal or absent in elderly patients or those receiving high-dose or prolonged corticosteroid therapy. In such patients, loss of hepatic dullness may be the first clinical indication of colonic perforation. Mental status changes, including confusion, agitation, and apathy, occasionally are noted. Leukocytosis with a left shift generally is present. Anemia, hypokalemia, and hypoalbuminemia are common. The presence of anemia, requirement for transfusion hypoalbuminemia, and malnutrition are poor prognostic factors [14,15].

Plain films of the abdomen usually are sufficient radiographic studies, revealing loss of haustration with segmental or total colonic dilatation. Clinical studies have demonstrated a strong correlation between colonic dilatation and deep ulceration involving the muscle layers [16]. The magnitude of dilatation may not be severe, averaging 8 to 9 cm (normal is <5 to 6 cm), although colonic diameter may reach 15 cm before rupture. Maximal dilatation can occur in any part of the colon. Accompanying mucosal thumbprinting or pneumatosis cystoides coli reflect severe transmural disease. Free peritoneal air should serve as an immediate indication for surgery [3]. Infrequently, retroperitoneal tracking of air from a colonic perforation may produce subcutaneous emphysema and pneumomediastinum without pneumoperitoneum. In patients with severe colitis, small bowel ileus may herald toxic megacolon and is a bad prognostic sign for medical success. Discrepancies may exist between physical and radiographic findings. Abdominal distention by physical examination can be minimal despite massive colonic dilatation. Conversely, physical findings may dominate the presentation, and peritoneal signs in the absence of free air or dilatation should not be ignored.

A limited proctoscopic or flexible sigmoid examination generally shows extensive ulceration with friable, bleeding mucosa. In rare instances, however, such as with rectal enema therapy or Crohn's disease, the rectum may be normal [17]. An abdominal radiograph after cautious proctoscopic examination can assist in determining the extent and severity of colitis. Computed tomography scans can demonstrate thinning of the colonic wall or evidence of perforation or abscess [1]. More extensive endoscopic examinations, although controversial, generally are contraindicated. If performed, the presence of severe colitis (deep penetrating ulcers) in conjunction with clinical features of severe disease is a poor prognostic sign [16]. Similarly, the presence of extensive and deep ulcerations is a poor prognostic marker in Crohn's disease [17].

TABLE 94.2

CLINICAL FEATURES OF TOXIC MEGACOLON

Symptoms and signs
Increased diarrhea and bleeding
Fever >101.5°F
Abdominal distention
Decreased or absent bowel sounds
Peritoneal signs (potentially masked by corticosteroids)
Hemodynamic instability
Mental status changes
Radiographic findings
Progressive segmental or pancolonic dilatation (may not correlate with physical findings)
Pneumocystoides intestinalis
Laboratory test findings
White blood cell count >10,000/μL, with pronounced left shift
Anemia (may not be reflected in initial measurement if dehydrated)
Hypernatremia (if dehydrated)
Hypokalemia
Metabolic alkalosis (diarrhea)/acidosis (sepsis)
Hypomagnesemia
Hypophosphatemia
Hypoalbuminemia

MANAGEMENT

Few medical emergencies require as close cooperation between medical and surgical personnel as fulminant colitis and toxic megacolon [3,13,18]. A team approach with early management and continuous assessment is vital not only to determine whether surgery is indicated but also to support the critically ill patient preoperatively and postoperatively. Early recognition and institution of therapy by an experienced team can alter the outcome of this life-threatening illness (Table 94.3).

TABLE 94.3

MANAGEMENT OF TOXIC MEGACOLON

Team approach toward management, including medical and surgical personnel
Resuscitation and stabilization—electrolyte and fluid repletion, central venous pressure measurements, blood transfusions to maintain hematocrit greater than 30%, nasogastric suctioning, broad-spectrum antibiotics, administration of intravenous corticosteroids (e.g., methylprednisolone, 40 mg/d, and hydrocortisone, 400 mg/d)
Evaluate status—abdominal examination every 6 h, radiographs of abdomen every 12–24 h
Surgical intervention required for clinical deterioration at any time, failure of medical management to improve status within 48 h, evidence of perforation, shock, persistent hemorrhage
Consider cyclosporine A or infliximab for nontoxic patients without response to intravenous corticosteroids after 3–5 d

Medical Treatment

Despite the fact that "bowel rest" is ineffective as primary therapy for severe colitis, oral intake of fluids should be discontinued in fulminant colitis or once colonic dilatation is recognized [11,13,18]. A nasogastric tube is indicated for patients with associated small bowel ileus. Rolling the less toxic patient from front to back may redistribute colonic air and assist in decompression. Rarely, patients who have been made "nothing by mouth" with colonic dilatation *in the absence of toxic signs or symptoms* may benefit from resumption of oral feeding. Anticholinergic and narcotic agents should be discontinued [11]. Resuscitative measures, including vigorous fluid, electrolyte, and blood replacement, are paramount. Extracellular fluid loss may be severe and, when combined with a low oncotic pressure from hypoalbuminemia, the hemodynamic state often is unstable. The goal of fluid replacement should be to restore previous losses and continue replenishing ongoing losses from diarrhea, fever, and third spacing of fluids. Transfusion of packed red blood cells should be instituted to maintain the serum hematocrit above 30%. Although severe hypokalemia may not be present, total body potassium depletion is common, and resuscitative measures should include adequate potassium replacement. Phosphate, calcium, and magnesium depletion should be corrected parenterally.

Aminosalicylates, a mainstay of maintenance therapy and the treatment of mild-to-moderate disease, have no role in the treatment of fulminant colitis or toxic megacolon. Their activity, limited to superficial inflammation, is insufficient to abort or control the transmural disease, while the potential adverse effects (e.g., nausea, vomiting, or worsening colitis) may confuse the clinical picture [13]. They should be withheld until the patient has recovered and resumed a normal diet. Broad-spectrum antibiotics, with adequate Gram-negative and anaerobic coverage, are considered standard therapy and should be administered without delay once transmural inflammation or toxic megacolon is suspected [13,18]. Antibiotics should be continued until the patient stabilizes over several days to a week, or through the initial postoperative period. Unfortunately, the evidence base is weak regarding the role of antibiotics in fulminant colitis or toxic megacolon and, hence, the ultimate benefits (or risks) have not been adequately determined.

Corticosteroids have long been used in the management of ulcerative colitis as well as in Crohn's colitis [12]. In general, parenteral corticosteroids are essential to patients with toxic megacolon, and most patients are likely to be receiving the drugs before toxic megacolon develops [11]. Augmented doses of corticosteroids should be administered in view of the additional stress of the toxic state. There is no general agreement regarding which corticosteroid preparation or dose should be given. Prednisone, 20 mg intravenously every 6 hours, and prednisolone sodium phosphate have been used successfully. Hydrocortisone, 100 mg every 6 hours, and methylprednisolone, 6 to 15 mg every 6 hours, also are available for intravenous (IV) administration. A continuous infusion of corticosteroids may be beneficial to maintain steady plasma levels [11]. Patients who fail to respond with a reduction in bowel movements, cessation of transfusion requirements, and normalization of C-reactive protein within 5 to 7 days are unlikely to respond [11,18,19].

Cyclosporin A, 2 to 4 mg per kg per 24 hours administered as an IV continuous infusion, in severe ulcerative colitis has been effective for patients failing to improve after 7 to 10 days of intensive IV hydrocortisone therapy [11,13]. Most recently, cyclosporin A, without steroids, was also effective in a small pilot trial in patients with severe ulcerative colitis (not toxic) [20]. Most recently, a trial comparing 2 mg per kg with 4 mg per kg of cyclosporin A in conjunction with corticosteroids in severe colitis demonstrated that the lower dose was equally efficacious with less adverse effects [21]. In contrast, the role of cyclosporin A in toxic megacolon is controversial [22,23]. There are scant data regarding the long-term outlook after cyclosporin A therapy for fulminant or severe colitis, although patients who respond and are maintained on azathioprine have improved, long-term outcomes [11].

TABLE 94.4

EVIDENCE-BASED THERAPY OF FULMINANT COLITIS AND TOXIC MEGACOLON

Cyclosporin A at 4 mg/kg is effective either alone or with corticosteroids to treat severe fulminant ulcerative colitis (toxic megacolon excluded from trials) [11].

Cyclosporin A at 2 mg/kg is equally effective as 4 mg/kg in conjunction with corticosteroids in severe ulcerative colitis (toxic megacolon excluded) [21].

Infliximab is effective in moderate-to-severe, refractory ulcerative colitis in the outpatient setting [24]; the role in severe-to-fulminant colitis is less established [11].

Most recently, the biologic chimeric anti–tumor necrosis factor monoclonal antibody, infliximab, has been used to treat ulcerative colitis [11]. Formal studies have not been performed in the setting of fulminant colitis or toxic megacolon, although, in the setting of *severe* colitis in hospitalized patients, infliximab may have acute benefits [11]. Nevertheless, the long-term outcome has not been assessed for this group of patients. A summary of the evidence-based medical management approaches for fulminant colitis and toxic megacolon is provided in Table 94.4 and a recently proposed algorithm by Hart and Ng is presented in Figure 94.1 [11].

Resuscitative measures for fulminant infectious colitis resulting in toxic megacolon should be initiated in the same manner as for idiopathic ulcerative colitis. Broad-spectrum antibiotic coverage should be followed by pathogen-specific therapy after the causative organism has been identified. Vancomycin may be preferred over metronidazole in the setting of severe or fulminant colitis if *C. difficile* is considered likely because of prior antibiotic exposure or the presence of pseudomembranes [7]. The same criteria for surgical treatment should be used [3].

Surgical Intervention

When no improvement or deterioration occurs, despite 12 to 24 hours of intensive medical management, surgical intervention is required for toxic megacolon [3,11]. Failure to substantially improve within 5 to 7 days of intensive corticosteroid or cyclosporin A therapy is an indication for surgery [3,11,18,19]. Some physicians actually view early surgical management of toxic megacolon as the conservative approach, noting that delay of operative therapy may promote higher mortality [25,26].

Evidence of colonic perforation is an unequivocal indication for emergent surgery. If physical signs of perforation are absent, 12- to 24-hour radiographic surveillance is necessary. Perforation is associated with severe complications, including peritonitis, extreme fluid and electrolyte imbalance, and hemodynamic instability. Early recognition of perforation should lessen morbidity or mortality [3]. Other indications for emergent surgery precluding protracted medical management include signs of septic shock and imminent transverse colon rupture (diameter >12 cm). Hypoalbuminemia, persistently elevated C-reactive protein or erythrocyte sedimentation rate, small bowel ileus,

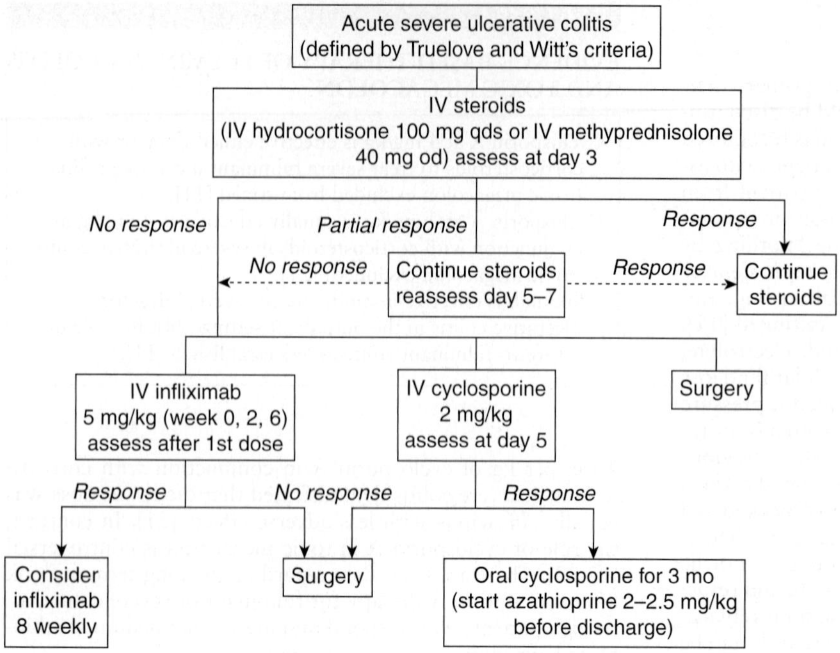

FIGURE 94.1. Proposed algorithm for the treatment of hospitalized patients with severe ulcerative colitis. [From Hart AL, Ng SC. Review article: the optimal medical management of acute severe ulcerative colitis. *Aliment Pharmacol Ther* 32(5):615–627, 2010.]

and deep colonic ulcers are poor prognostic factors for successful medical therapy [11].

Although the medical management of fulminant colitis is similar to that of toxic megacolon, the absence of acute colonic dilatation may permit delay of surgical intervention. The timing of surgical intervention in these less urgent cases requires experienced clinical judgment, however. Early intervention to reduce mortality must be balanced against the potential for intensive medical management to control the inflammatory process and complications; these efforts aimed at preventing the psychosocial and medical stigmata of a colectomy. In general, in the absence of colonic dilatation, medical management may be continued for 5 to 7 days in a further attempt to reverse transmural inflammation, as long as the patient is stable and improving. The option between cyclosporine and infliximab for patients with severe, nontoxic ulcerative colitis is controversial and has yet to be addressed in controlled, comparative effectiveness trials [11]. Patients who do not begin to respond to the intensive IV steroid regimen should be referred to centers experienced in biologic (infliximab) or cyclosporin therapy in severe colitis, or undergo colectomy [11,13,18].

The type of operation performed for treatment of fulminant colitis or toxic megacolon depends on the clinical status of the patient and the experience of the surgeon [3,4,14]. A one-stage procedure that cures ulcerative colitis without the need for a second operation is appropriate for older patients or those not desiring restorative ileal pouch-anal anastomosis. Most surgeons prefer a limited abdominal colectomy with ileostomy, leaving the rectosigmoid as a mucous fistula or the rectum alone, using a Hartmann procedure [3,11]. This approach has the advantages of limiting the lengthy pelvic dissection in acutely ill patients while allowing for the option of a subsequent restorative, sphincter-saving procedure (ileoanal anastomosis). In patients with indeterminate colitis or Crohn's disease, preservation of the rectum may provide the opportunity for an eventual ileorectal or ileoanal anastomosis to preserve anal continence after temporary diversion and pathologic review of the colectomy specimen.

The surgical management of toxic megacolon must be individualized for each patient. The type of operation selected depends on the clinical condition of the patient and the experience of the surgeon [3,27,28].

References

1. Gan SI, Beck PL: A new look at toxic megacolon: an update and review of incidence, etiology, pathogenesis, and management. *Am J Gastroenterol* 98:2363–2371, 2003.
2. Daperno M, Sostegni R, Rocca R, et al: Review article: medical treatment of severe ulcerative colitis. *Aliment Pharmacol Ther* 16[Suppl 4]:7–12, 2002.
3. Ausch C, Madoff RD, Gnant M, et al: Aetiology and surgical management of toxic megacolon. *Colorectal Dis* 8:195–201, 2006.
4. Jakobovits SL, Travis SP: Management of acute severe colitis. *Br Med Bull* 75–76:131–44, 2005.
5. Farmer RG, Easley KA, Rankin GB: Clinical patterns, natural history, and progression of ulcerative colitis. A long-term follow-up of 1116 patients. *Dig Dis Sci* 38:1137–1146, 1993.
6. Jodorkovsky D, Young Y, Abreu MT: Clinical outcomes of patients with ulcerative colitis and co-existing *Clostridium difficile* infection. *Dig Dis Sci* 55:415–420, 2010.
7. Ananthakrishnan AN, Issa M, Binion DG: *Clostridium difficile* and inflammatory bowel disease. *Med Clin North Am* 94:135–153, 2010.
8. Lawlor G, Moss AC: Cytomegalovirus in inflammatory bowel disease: pathogen or innocent bystander? *Inflamm Bowel Dis* 16(9):1620–1627, 2010.
9. Kim JJ, Simpson N, Klipfel N, et al: Cytomegalovirus infection in patients with active inflammatory bowel disease. *Dig Dis Sci* 55:1059–1065, 2010.
10. Kumar S, Ghoshal UC, Aggarwal R, et al: Severe ulcerative colitis: prospective study of parameters determining outcome. *J Gastroenterol Hepatol* 19:1247–1252, 2004.
11. Hart AL, Ng SC. Review article: the optimal medical management of acute severe ulcerative colitis. *Aliment Pharmacol Ther* 32(5):615–627, 2010.
12. Lichtenstein GR, Abreu MT, Cohen R, et al: American Gastroenterological Association Institute technical review on corticosteroids, immunomodulators, and infliximab in inflammatory bowel disease. *Gastroenterology* 130:940–987, 2006.
13. Kornbluth A, Sachar DB: Ulcerative colitis practice guidelines in adults: American College of Gastroenterology, Practice Parameters Committee. *Am J Gastroenterol* 105:501–523; quiz 24, 2010.
14. Ho GT, Mowat C, Goddard CJ, et al: Predicting the outcome of severe ulcerative colitis: development of a novel risk score to aid early selection of patients for second-line medical therapy or surgery. *Aliment Pharmacol Ther* 19:1079–1087, 2004.
15. Ananthakrishnan AN, McGinley EL, Binion DG, et al: Simple score to

identify colectomy risk in ulcerative colitis hospitalizations. *Inflamm Bowel Dis* 16:1532–1540, 2010.
16. Carbonnel F, Lavergne A, Lemann M, et al: Colonoscopy of acute colitis. A safe and reliable tool for assessment of severity. *Dig Dis Sci* 39:1550–1557, 1994.
17. Allez M, Lemann M, Bonnet J, et al: Long term outcome of patients with active Crohn's disease exhibiting extensive and deep ulcerations at colonoscopy. *Am J Gastroenterol* 97:947–953, 2002.
18. Travis SP: Review article: the management of mild to severe acute ulcerative colitis. *Aliment Pharmacol Ther* 20[Suppl 4]:88–92, 2004.
19. Travis SP, Farrant JM, Ricketts C, et al: Predicting outcome in severe ulcerative colitis. *Gut* 38:905–910, 1996.
20. D'Haens G, Lemmens L, Geboes K, et al: Intravenous cyclosporine versus intravenous corticosteroids as single therapy for severe attacks of ulcerative colitis. *Gastroenterology* 120:1323–1329, 2001.
21. Van Assche G, D'Haens G, Noman M, et al: Randomized, double-blind comparison of 4 mg/kg versus 2 mg/kg intravenous cyclosporine in severe ulcerative colitis. *Gastroenterology* 125:1025–1031, 2003.
22. Garcia-Lopez S, Gomollon-Garcia F, Perez-Gisbert J: Cyclosporine in the treatment of severe attack of ulcerative colitis: a systematic review. *Gastroenterol Hepatol* 28:607–614, 2005.
23. Pham CQ, Efros CB, Berardi RR: Cyclosporine for severe ulcerative colitis. *Ann Pharmacother* 40:96–101, 2006.
24. Rutgeerts P, Sandborn WJ, Feagan BG, et al: Infliximab for induction and maintenance therapy for ulcerative colitis. *N Engl J Med* 353:2462–2476, 2005.
25. D'Amico C, Vitale A, Angriman I, et al: Early surgery for the treatment of toxic megacolon. *Digestion* 72:146–149, 2005.
26. Randall J, Singh B, Warren BF, et al: Delayed surgery for acute severe colitis is associated with increased risk of postoperative complications. *Br J Surg* 97(3):404–409, 2010.
27. Berg DF, Bahadursingh AM, Kaminski DL, et al: Acute surgical emergencies in inflammatory bowel disease. *Am J Surg* 184:45–51, 2002.
28. Randall J, Singh B, Warren BF, et al: Delayed surgery for acute severe colitis is associated with increased risk of postoperative complications. *Br J Surg* 97:404–409, 2010.

CHAPTER 95 ■ EVALUATION AND MANAGEMENT OF LIVER FAILURE

GOWRI KULARATNA AND MAURICIO LISKER-MELMAN

INTRODUCTION

Liver failure results from progressive deterioration of hepatic function in the setting of either acute or chronic liver disease. *Acute* or *fulminant hepatic failure* (FHF) is a devastating condition in which the liver fails within a short period of time, encompassing a range of clinical syndromes. FHF is an uncommon entity, estimated to affect approximately 2,000 patients annually in the United States. Prompt evaluation and aggressive management, including liver transplantation, play an integral part in successfully treating patients with FHF in the intensive care unit (ICU). In contrast, *chronic liver failure* is a more frequent medical condition that may evolve into end-stage liver disease, independent of its cause (e.g., viral, autoimmune, metabolic, toxic). It usually develops after years of hepatocyte insult. The definition, etiology, clinical features, complications, and management of fulminant and chronic liver failure are reviewed in this chapter. The role of liver transplantation and future therapies for fulminant and chronic liver disease are discussed briefly.

FULMINANT HEPATIC FAILURE

Definition

Fulminant hepatic failure (FHF) is a rare condition which includes evidence of coagulation abnormalities (international normalized ratio [INR] >1.5) and any degree of mental alteration (encephalopathy) in a patient without preexisting cirrhosis and with an illness of no more than 24-week duration. This definition can be further classified by length of illness: *hyperacute liver failure* (7 days), *acute liver failure* (8 to 28 days), *subacute liver failure* (29 to 60 days), *late-onset hepatic failure* (8 to 24 weeks), and *subfulminant hepatic failure* (jaundice to encephalopathy in 2 to 12 weeks). These terms, however, are not helpful, as they do not provide prognostic or practical information separate from etiology. Terms such as *late-onset hepatic failure* (8 to 24 weeks from the beginning of symptoms) and *subfulminant hepatic failure* (jaundice and encephalopathy in 2 to 12 weeks) are not commonly used. Patients with acute liver failure superimposed on a chronic liver disease do not fit the classic definition of FHF. There are classifications [1,2], however, that allow for the inclusion of these patients with previously asymptomatic chronic conditions as having FHF.

Etiology

Numerous causes of FHF are recognized, and their relative importance differs around the world. Some authors classify them into four major categories: infectious (e.g., viral hepatitis), drugs/chemicals/toxins (e.g., acetaminophen, isoniazid, *Amanita phalloides*), vascular (e.g., Budd–Chiari syndrome, ischemic hepatitis, tamponade), and metabolic (e.g., Wilson's disease, Reye's syndrome, acute fatty liver of pregnancy). In the United States, acetaminophen accounts for nearly 50% of cases followed by idiosyncratic drug reactions (12%). Acute viral hepatitis (hepatitis A and hepatitis B) is the etiologic factor in 12% of cases and has become an infrequent cause of FHF over the last few decades due to effective immunization programs. In contrast, in the developing world, viral hepatitis is the dominant etiology of fulminant hepatitis. Hepatitis C is a rare source of FHF [3].

The identification of the cause of FHF is important because it can provide important prognostic information as well as dictate treatments and antidotes. In the case of viral hepatitis, patient contacts must be identified and informed of the potential need for prophylaxis as indicated. Approximately 20% of adult cases with acute liver failure have indeterminate causes, with women affected more often than men [4,5]. Initial laboratory

TABLE 95.1

INITIAL LABORATORY TESTING FOR FHF

Initial laboratory testing for FHF	
■ Complete blood count ■ Basic metabolic panel ■ INR ■ Liver chemistry panel ■ Lactate ■ Blood gas ■ HIV (rapid antibody test) ■ Pregnancy testing ■ Blood and urine cultures ■ Imaging and other testing – CXR/ECG – RUQ US with Dopplers	■ Viral markers – Hepatitis A IgM antibody – Hepatitis B markers – Hepatitis C antibody ■ Autoimmune markers – Antinuclear antibody – Anti–smooth muscle antibody ■ Toxicology screen and drug panel – Urine and serum drug screen including acetaminophen, cocaine, alcohol

CXR, chest x-ray; ECG, electrocardiogram; INR, international normalized ratio; HIV, human immunodeficiency virus; RUQ US, right upper quadrant ultrasound.
Liver chemistry panel: aspartate aminotransferase, alanine aminotransferase, alkaline phosphatase, total and direct bilirubin, albumin, total protein.
Hepatitis B markers: hepatitis B surface antigen, hepatitis B surface antibody, hepatitis B core antibodies (IgG, IgM).

testing to delineate etiology and assess degree of injury is obligatory (Table 95.1).

Acetaminophen is the most common cause of FHF in the United States and the United Kingdom. This drug is a constituent in numerous over-the-counter preparations and is also commonly combined with prescription analgesics. Although the recommended doses of acetaminophen (up to 4 g per day) are safe in healthy individuals, dose-dependent hepatotoxicity can occur. Hepatotoxicity can occur through intentional (e.g., suicide attempt) or unintentional (e.g., combined with alcohol, barbiturates, or other inducers of the cytochrome P450 system) overdose. Approximately one third of cases can occur in association with efforts at pain relief; these "therapeutic misadventures" occur with lower cumulative doses of ingested acetaminophen [6]. These patients may seek late medical attention resulting in delayed physician recognition.

Acetaminophen is 95% eliminated by hepatic conjugation. Approximately 5% of acetaminophen is converted to *N*-acetyl-p-benzoquinone-imine (NAPQI), which is inactivated after reaction with cellular glutathione and excreted rapidly. If glutathione stores are depleted, NAPQI becomes highly toxic and produces massive liver necrosis. NAPQI accumulates at a higher rate in the setting of increased cytochrome P450–2E1 activity, as seen with chronic alcohol ingestion, and with medications that induce the P450 system. As a result, patients with chronic moderate alcohol intake can develop toxicity with ingestion of less than 10 g of acetaminophen. For more detail on this topic, please refer to chapter 120.

Patients with acetaminophen toxicity present in three phases. The first phase involves acute gastrointestinal (GI) symptoms of nausea, vomiting, and abdominal pain within the first few hours after ingestion. During the second phase (12 to 48 hours), asymptomatic liver test abnormalities occur, with marked elevation of liver enzymes and a high aspartate aminotransferase (AST)/alanine aminotransferase (ALT) ratio. The third phase presents with manifestations of hepatic failure, including jaundice and encephalopathy. The mortality of acetaminophen toxicity is higher when associated with severe acidosis, coagulopathy, renal failure, mental status changes, and cerebral edema (CE) [6] (Table 95.2).

The effective antidote, *N*-acetylcysteine (NAC), is potentially lifesaving when administered early, especially within 24 hours of acute ingestion. Thus, suspicion and early identification of acetaminophen toxicity are of vital importance in treating patients presenting with FHF. NAC replenishes glutathione stores, preventing depletion and subsequent tissue hypoxia and ischemic damage. Both, the oral and intravenous forms can be used with similar efficacy [7]. Oral NAC is given over 72 hours with a loading dose of 140 mg per kg and subsequent doses of 70 mg per kg every 4 hours for a total of 17 doses. Because of its sulfur moiety, NAC has a strong odor and taste, and it needs to be diluted (usually in cola) to be tolerated. It is not uncommon for oral NAC to induce nausea and vomiting. A nasogastric or nasoduodenal feeding tube

TABLE 95.2

INDICATORS OF POOR PROGNOSIS IN ACUTE LIVER FAILURE

Etiology	Parameter
Acetaminophen-induced liver failure	Arterial pH $<7.30^a$ PT >100 s INR >6.5 Creatinine >300 μmol/L (2.3 mg/dL) Encephalopathy grade 3–4
Nonacetaminophen liver failure	PT >100 s[b] INR >6.7[b] Age <10 or >40 Serum bilirubin >300 μmol/L (2.3 mg/dL) Seronegative hepatitis or drug reaction

[a]Highest sensitivity (49%), specificity (99%), and positive predictive value (81%).
[b]Highest specificity (100%) but lower sensitivity (34%) and positive predictive value (46%).
INR, international normalized ratio; PT, prothrombin time; s, seconds.
Modified from the Kings College Criteria indicating a poor prognosis in acute liver failure.

may be placed in this situation to reliably deliver the medication. If the patient develops significant nausea or vomiting, has a polysubstance overdose requiring gastric decontamination, GI bleeding, or intestinal obstruction, IV NAC is the preferable administration route. IV NAC is given as a 150 mg per kg loading dose, then 50 mg per kg over 4 hours, followed by 100 mg per kg over 16 hours. It has been our experience that dosing of both, oral and IV NAC, can be administered beyond the recommended doses until improvement in liver chemistry parameters is noted. Anaphylactoid reactions are seen in 5% to 14% of patients, typically occurring with the IV loading dose [8,9]. Because this reaction may be rate dependent, the loading dose has to be administered over 15 to 60 minutes.

The decision to administer NAC is dependent on serum levels of acetaminophen and time after ingestion (consult nomogram in acetaminophen chapter 120). Although the therapeutic benefit of NAC is best when given within 10 hours, its effects can still be of value within 36 hours of ingestion. When administered early, NAC leads to greater than 95% survival. The administration of NAC to patients with nonacetaminophen FHF has shown possible benefit [10]. However, combined analyses of these data do not demonstrate a mortality benefit in nonacetaminophen hepatotoxicity cases [11]. Larger controlled trials are needed to better assess the use of NAC in these patients.

Clinical Manifestations and Management

Despite timely intervention, multisystem organ failure can develop in patients with FHF. Hepatic encephalopathy (HE) and CE affect patients with FHF in varying degrees. Coagulopathy and jaundice are often present before severe encephalopathy occurs. Cardiorespiratory failure, renal failure, and infectious complications can develop and further complicate the management of these patients. Unfortunately, multisystem organ failure is a cause of ineligibility for transplantation in 20% of patients with FHF [12].

Hepatic Encephalopathy

HE is a syndrome of disordered consciousness and altered neuromuscular activity. HE is present in all patients with FHF, with symptoms ranging from subclinical confusion (grade 0) to coma (grade 4) (Table 95.3). The mechanism of HE is complex with interplay of many hypothesized factors including CE; toxins such as ammonia, glutamate, and endogenous benzodiazepines; and cytokine-like mediators such as interleukin (IL-1), IL-6, and tumor necrosis factor [13–15]. Alterations in cerebral blood flow due to loss of intracranial autoregulation may be a minor contributor to HE [16]. The diagnosis of mild HE is made through interviewing the patient for signs of impaired cognition. This may manifest itself through mild agitation, inability to concentrate, or more subtly, as an inability to perform counting tasks. HE may progress rapidly to grade 3 or 4, and frequent monitoring is essential. Arterial ammonia level more than 200 μg per dL is associated with cerebral herniation, although levels do not correlate with the degree of HE [17]. Mechanical intubation is indicated in the setting of significant acidosis or grade 4 HE, to protect patient's airway and decrease metabolic stress. Treatment is directed at the correction of precipitating factors such as sepsis, GI bleeding, medications, and fluid and electrolyte imbalance [18]. Standard therapy for HE in chronic liver disease, such as lactulose, neomycin, or rifaximin, have no proven benefits in FHF and can induce significant side effects such as bloating, abdominal pain, nausea, and electrolyte disturbances from diarrheal losses [19]. Flumazenil, a benzodiazepine antagonist, had limited success in one trial treating HE in children with FHF, and no definitive data are available for its use in adults [20].

TABLE 95.3

STAGES OF HEPATIC ENCEPHALOPATHY

- *Grade I*: sleep reversal pattern, mild confusion, irritability, tremor
- *Grade II*: lethargy, disorientation, inappropriate behavior, asterixis
- *Grade III*: somnolence, severe confusion, aggressive behavior, asterixis
- *Grade IV*: Coma

Cerebral Edema

CE is a devastating complication of FHF that accounts for about 25% of deaths. It is seen in up to 80% of patients with FHF and advanced encephalopathy [21]. The pathogenesis of CE is thought to be the result of progressive accumulation of water in the brain. Two main mechanisms have been proposed to explain CE. The first is water influx down an osmotic gradient into the gray matter, astrocytes in particular [22]. Osmotic and metabolic alterations in the astrocytes lead to cellular swelling and accumulation of glutamine. The second mechanism is reduced cerebral flow and loss of autoregulation, resulting in increased intracranial pressure (ICP) [23].

The early clinical manifestations of CE often overlap with advanced encephalopathy (grades 3 and 4) and include agitation, headache, nausea, or vomiting. The most feared complications are brain herniation and death. Frequent evaluation of mental status (avoiding sedation and neuromuscular blockade if possible), assessment for hyperreflexia, pupillary changes, and sudden systemic hypertension play an important role in monitoring these patients. The neurologic examination and computed tomography (CT) of the brain are often unreliable methods to follow CE or ICP [24]. However, head CT can be helpful if there is clinical suspicion for structural lesions or hemorrhage. Severe CE, cerebral herniation, or a large intracranial bleed from an underlying coagulopathy eliminate the possibility of transplantation.

ICP measurements obtained by placement of intraparenchymal, subdural or epidural pressure transducers, accurately determine ICP and help direct therapy. Monitoring of ICP has always provoked controversy. Some suggest that these patients can be monitored without the need of invasive placement of intracranial bolts, while others suggest that ICP monitors facilitate the care of patients with CE [25,26]. ICP monitoring should be considered in patients with progressive mental status impairment (HE grades 3 and 4) and under consideration for liver transplantation. Placement of ICP monitors may be complicated by intracranial bleeding (<5%) in the setting of severe coagulopathy [27,28] and volume overload from the use of blood products in an effort to correct coagulation abnormalities. Activated recombinant factor VII (see "Coagulopathy" section in the chapter) may help ameliorate these complications. Infections from monitor placement are also potential life-threatening complications. As a result, the efficacy and indication for ICP monitoring in patients with encephalopathy has been questioned [29]. Once the decision to place an ICP monitor is made, epidural pressure transducers are preferred because of a lower rate of bleeding complications (approximately 5%) compared with the intraparenchymal and subdural types (approximately 20%). Measurement of ICP with these monitors requires experience and familiarity with the equipment [30]. Monitoring mean arterial pressures (MAPs) and maintaining cerebral perfusion pressures (CPPs) (MAP minus ICP) are important. Ideally, ICP should be maintained around 15 mm Hg, with CPP greater than 40 to 50 mm Hg. Recovery of neurologic function is optimized by maintaining CPPs at greater than 40 mm Hg.

Simple recognized strategies to stabilize or decrease the ICP include elevation of the head of the bed to 30 degrees to improve venous drainage and minimization of endotracheal suction and external stimuli [31], control of fever, correction of hyponatremia and hypoosmolality, and short-term hyperventilation to a Pco_2 of 30 to 35 mm Hg [32]. Intravenous administration of mannitol (100 mL of 20% solution given intravenously at 0.5 to 1.0 mg per kg) and intravenous hypertonic saline boluses (20 mL 30% saline) to obtain sodium levels of 145 to 155 mEq per L are considered first-line treatment strategy for CE. Mannitol draws water osmotically from brain tissue reducing the ICP and may be helpful to "bridge" patients to liver transplantation. It should be avoided in patients with renal failure. Hypertonic saline infusions have been used to decrease the incidence and severity of increased ICP in FHF [33]. Hyponatremia increases ammonia-induced CE and has been recognized as a cause of this complication in postoperative patients treated with excessive 5% glucose solutions [23].

No established role exists for the use of regular diuretics. Administration of corticosteroids such as dexamethasone has failed to show any benefit in treating elevated ICP [34]. Hypothermia (32°C to 34°C) reduces the production of inflammatory mediators, decreases arterial and cerebrospinal spinal fluid ammonia levels, and attenuates ICP pressure; however, no control studies are available, and its use as a therapeutic option remains uncertain [35–38]. Barbiturates have been investigated as a treatment option for CE in FHF; however, with the exception of patients with seizures and CE, barbiturates are not useful. Experimental use of NAC and prostaglandin I_2 infusions increases cerebral microcirculation and blood flow. The role of these agents remains to be determined in human studies.

Definitive treatment of CE in FHF is liver transplantation. Prolonged low CPPs and increased ICP are contraindications to liver transplantation given the high risk of brain death and significant neurologic sequelae. Despite the most appropriate care and stringent inclusion criteria, residual neurologic deficits may persist after transplantation [39].

Coagulopathy

Because of the loss of hepatocyte function in FHF, there is reduced synthesis of coagulation and anticoagulation factors that results in marked elevation of the INR, prolongation of the prothrombin, and activated partial thromboplastin times. These parameters should be followed to monitor hepatic function recovery (in the absence of fresh frozen plasma). Factor V has the shortest half-life and is a sensitive marker of defective synthesis of coagulation factors, but it is rarely measured. Along with clotting factor deficiencies and consumption, there may be platelet dysfunction, thrombocytopenia, and fibrinolysis resulting in a clinical picture similar to disseminated intravascular coagulation [40].

In the setting of coagulopathy due to clotting factor synthesis deficiency, overt bleeding does not frequently occur. However, when severe coagulopathy develops along with platelet dysfunction, GI and oropharyngeal bleeding can result. Protection of the gastric mucosa with proton pump inhibitors, H2 blockers, or sucralfate is important. The skin, lungs, and urogenital tract are also potential sites of significant blood loss. Fresh frozen plasma and platelets are indicated in patients with active bleeding or before invasive procedures. Packed cell replacement is required for significant blood loss. However, due to risk of worsening CE and fluid overload, blood products use must be judicious.

Factor VII is a central figure in the clotting cascade. Its activation is in response to tissue factor release after endothelial injury [41]. Recombinant activated factor VII (rFVIIa) has emerged as a potential treatment and prophylaxis option for bleeding in patients with liver disease. Prophylactic use of rFVIIa is not standard of care. In a group of children with FHF, prophylactic rFVIIa allowed for decreased transfusion requirements and better maintenance of fluid balance [42]. Data also supports rFVIIa use in patients who are undergoing placement of ICP monitors. In seven patients receiving rFVIIa, complete normalization of the prothrombin time (PT) allowed ICP monitor placement in comparison with three out of eight historical controls managed by conventional means. The patients receiving rFVIIa also had a significant decrease in mortality and anasarca due to fluid overload. The high cost of rFVIIa limits its more frequent use (approximately $2,000 for a 60 kg patient). However, the cost savings from decreased transfusion requirements and hemofiltration for fluid overload may offset the additional costs of rFVIIa [43].

Cardiac Complications

Elevated cardiac output (hyperdynamic circulation), decreased peripheral oxygen extraction (tissue hypoxia), and low systemic vascular resistance are present in patients with FHF [44]. These hemodynamic parameters, possibly due to the release of vasoactive mediators from dying hepatocytes, are similar to sepsis. Splanchnic and peripheral vasodilatation leading to systemic hypotension should be treated with volume replacement. Pulmonary artery catheter, central venous pressure, or esophageal Doppler monitoring can be crucial in assessing and correcting fluid status in these patients. MAP should be maintained above 50 mm Hg. Norepinephrine is generally used as the primary vasopressor due to its consistent effects on CPP. Conflicting data exist regarding vasopressin and terlipressin and their effects on ICP and systemic hemodynamics. A progressive rise in systolic blood pressure, within minutes or hours, can be indicative of ICP elevation and should be treated as discussed earlier.

Respiratory Complications

Respiratory complications occur frequently in patients with FHF. Hypoxemia can result from acute lung injury, cardiogenic or noncardiogenic pulmonary edema, pneumonia, intraalveolar hemorrhage, or intrapulmonary vascular shunting (hepatopulmonary syndrome). These patients should be treated with supplemental oxygen or intubation as clinically indicated. Intubation, however, is used more frequently for airway protection rather than for respiratory failure. Positive pressure ventilation should be used to optimize compliance with caution, as the resulting decreased vascular return can lead to increased ICP and cardiac output. The combination of rising ICP and metabolic acidosis in patients with FHF leads to a compensatory hyperventilation and hypocapnia.

Monitoring the development of CE becomes difficult in patients who are intubated, sedated, and paralyzed. As a result, intubation should be performed in those who are unresponsive in a grade 3 or 4 HE and require airway protection with ventilatory assistance.

Renal Failure

The development of renal failure in FHF is a poor prognostic indicator and is the result of a variety of factors. Up to 75% of patients with acetaminophen toxicity develop acute renal failure from direct renal toxicity of NAPQI. Renal failure also occurs in approximately 30% of patient with FHF from other causes [8]. The most frequent causes of renal failure are intravascular volume depletion (relative hypovolemia caused by vasodilatation), acute tubular necrosis, and hepatorenal syndrome (HRS). Type I HRS predominates in FHF. It is rapidly progressive and carries a dismal prognosis.

Oliguric renal failure in FHF is defined as urine output less than 300 mL per 24 hours [45] or serum creatinine 3.4 mg per dL (>300 mmol per L). Renal failure leads to a variety of metabolic disorders including hyperkalemia, hypercalcemia, hyperphosphatemia, hypophosphatemia, and hypermagnesemia that can further complicate patient management.

Diagnosis requires close monitoring of urine output, volume status (see "Cardiac Complications" section in the chapter), and measurement of urinary sodium and creatinine. Urinary sodium and creatinine can help identify the presence of acute tubular necrosis (high or normal urine sodium) but cannot differentiate between prerenal azotemia and HRS (low urine sodium). Nephrotoxic agents and mannitol should be avoided in renal failure, and careful renal dosing is vital. Some patients will require hemodialysis or hemofiltration to control the volume status, especially in the setting of CE, correct acidosis, improve electrolyte imbalance, and azotemia. Patients with tenuous hemodynamics who require hemodialysis or hemofiltration are best served with continuous modes of renal replacement [46].

Metabolic Disorders

Lactic acidosis is a severe metabolic complication of FHF. Serum lactate accumulates as a result of tissue hypoxia from hypotension as well as impaired hepatic uptake and metabolism of lactate. Renal dysfunction and other metabolic abnormalities can easily contribute to increase the underlying acidosis. Severe, refractory lactic acidosis requires intravenous bicarbonate infusion or dialysis.

Hypoglycemia also frequently complicates FHF given the primary metabolic role of the liver in glycogen storage and gluconeogenesis. Massive hepatic damage is required before serum glucose drops to levels that impair neurologic and cellular function. Nonetheless, frequent glucose monitoring and infusion of concentrated dextrose solutions may be required [47].

Sepsis

Patients with FHF are at high risk for septic complications. Abnormal neutrophil and Kupffer cell function, decreased bacterial opsonization, bacterial gut translocation, and altered cytokines contribute to immunologic impairment [48]. Up to 80% of patients with FHF will develop a bacterial infection. The urinary tract and pulmonary system are the most frequent sources of infection. Skin wounds, indwelling vascular access catheters, and ICP monitors are also potential sources of infection. The most common organisms identified are *Staphylococcus*, *Streptococcus*, Gram-negative organisms, and *Candida* species. Fungal infections occur late in the course of illness and are associated with high mortality.

Because the hemodynamic, metabolic, and hematologic parameters of FHF are often indistinguishable, hospital staff must maintain a high level of suspicion for infectious complications. In fact, one third of septic patients maintain a normal white cell count and remained afebrile. Since sepsis may be easily overlooked, early surveillance cultures should be obtained with a low threshold to start broad-spectrum antibiotics. If possible, aminoglycosides should be avoided owing to their nephrotoxicity. The use of prophylactic antibiotics is controversial. The addition of enteral decontamination regimens has not been shown to decrease the incidence of infection [49]. Sepsis can be catastrophic, since it compromises the opportunity to proceed with transplantation and contribute to multisystem organ failure.

The systemic inflammatory response syndrome (SIRS) presents clinically with manifestations compatible with sepsis: fever or hypothermia, tachycardia, leucocytosis or leucopenia, and tachypnea or hyperventilation, and it can be triggered by a variety of infectious and noninfectious conditions [50]. In FHF, SIRS can be associated with infection or by the release of inflammatory cytokines from the necrotic hepatocytes; as such, high level of suspicion and early identification of infectious sources are needed for adequate treatment and ICU support.

Prognosis

Prognostic factors in patients with FHF have been investigated to determine patient survival and identify those who would be best treated by transplantation. The Kings College criteria [51] produced the first prognosis model and have been used most often worldwide (Table 95.2) for this purpose. These criteria have a high positive predictive value and remain useful today [52]. Recent papers suggest that elevated lactate levels on admission improves the sensitivity of the model to predict mortality in acetaminophen-induced FHF [53]. On admission to the ICU, the Acute Physiology and Chronic Health Evaluation (APACHE) II system has been found comparable with the Kings College criteria in those with acetaminophen-induced liver failure [54]. However, more recent studies have shown that the absence of these criteria may not be as reliable in predicting survival [55].

Age does not appear to play an important prognostic role in the situation of transplantation for FHF. Although the grade of encephalopathy may influence posttransplant outcome, its reliability has been debated. The role of serial Doppler ultrasounds has been investigated in predicting outcome by measuring the mean hepatic artery resistive index. Results have indicated that as the mean hepatic arterial resistive index increases, there is an associated poorer prognosis in those patients who meet transplant criteria [56]. Assessing patients with CT has also been investigated. A prior study indicates that patients with liver volumes of less than 1,000 mL have a poorer prognosis [57].

Measurements of serum alpha-fetoprotein (AFP) and serum protein Gc-globulin (an actin-binding protein released during massive tissue injury) have been investigated with promising results [58]. Of these potential markers, AFP has been investigated the most. Early AFP elevation in FHF is suggestive of regeneration and thus has garnered interest as a marker of survival. In a recent study, a threshold level of AFP of 3.9 μg per L or above was highly sensitive in predicting survival. In this study, AFP was measured 1 day after ALT levels peaked [59]. Despite these results, no marker or clinical finding has proven to be reliably predictive of outcome.

CHRONIC LIVER DISEASE

Chronic liver disease is a result of continuous, long-term hepatic injury. Chronic viral hepatitis is arbitrarily defined as the presence of persistent liver inflammation, liver chemistry abnormalities, and positive serologic and molecular markers for more than 6 months. The persistent nature of the hepatic insult leads to a sequence of damage and repair processes that may ultimately progress to the development of fibrosis, cirrhosis, and hepatocellular carcinoma (HCC). Damage to the hepatic parenchyma, with or without fibrosis, is a common outcome in chronic liver disease. Regardless of whether the insult to the hepatocytes, the biliary ducts, or the hepatic vasculature is toxic, viral, metabolic, autoimmune, or ischemic, the reparative process often leads to similar results.

Cirrhosis is a chronic diffuse condition characterized by replacement of liver cells by fibrotic tissue, which creates a nodular-appearing distortion of the normal liver architecture. Chronic liver disease and cirrhosis affects nearly 5.5 million Americans. Cirrhosis is the 10th leading cause of death in the United States.

Etiology

Chronic hepatitis C and B infection, chronic alcohol use, and nonalcoholic fatty liver disease (NAFLD) are the most common causes of chronic liver disease in the United States.

Hepatitis C virus (HCV) is a global health problem with approximately 200 million carriers worldwide. The incidence of HCV has declined in the last 30 years. The prevalence in the U.S. population is 1.8%, making HCV infection the most common chronic blood-borne infection. In the United States, 4 million people have been infected with this virus and 2.7 million have chronic infection. HCV is the leading cause of death from chronic liver disease [60–62].

Two billion people worldwide have serological evidence of past or present infection with the hepatitis B virus; approximately 400 million people are chronic carriers. HBV is unevenly distributed throughout the world. In endemic areas (Asia and sub-Saharan Africa), infection is usually acquired in childhood. In contrast, in Western countries where HBV is relatively rare, the infection is acquired in adulthood [63]. HBV causes 60% to 80% of HCC worldwide. It is estimated that between 500,000 and 1,000,000 deaths per year occur worldwide due to this disease.

Alcoholic liver disease also is a significant medical and socioeconomic problem worldwide. Although alcohol exerts a direct toxic effect on the liver, significant liver damage develops in only 10% to 20% of those patients with chronic alcohol abuse. The spectrum of alcoholic liver disease is broad, and a single patient may be affected by more than one of the following conditions: fatty liver (90% of alcoholics), alcoholic hepatitis, or alcoholic cirrhosis (common cause of end-stage liver disease and HCC).

NALFD is a clinicopathologic syndrome that encompasses several clinical entities that range from simple steatosis, steatohepatitis, fibrosis, and end-stage liver disease in the absence of significant alcohol consumption [64]. NAFLD is a worldwide phenomenon with an estimated prevalence of about 30% in the general population. The prevalence of NASH ranges from 3% to 9% with substantial variation among ethnic groups. It affects both children and adults, and the incidence increases with age. NAFLD is associated with an increasing prevalence of type II diabetes and obesity in the U.S. population. The metabolic syndrome including abdominal obesity, dyslipidemia, hypertension, and insulin resistance is also associated with NAFLD. NALFD-induced cirrhosis may progress to HCC (13% of all cases of HCC) [65].

Other causes of chronic liver disease include autoimmune liver disease, primary sclerosing cholangitis, primary biliary cirrhosis, hemochromatosis, Wilson's disease, α_1-antitrypsin deficiency, and Budd–Chiari syndrome.

Clinical Manifestations and Diagnosis

Clinical manifestations of chronic liver disease vary according to the functional and histologic stage of the liver disease. Patients may be asymptomatic or have one or several manifestations of liver dysfunction. Physical findings described in patients with cirrhosis include temporal wasting, jaundice, telangiectasia, gynecomastia, ascites, splenomegaly, caput medusae, palmar erythema, and testicular atrophy. Some laboratory abnormalities are suggestive of cirrhosis. Serum albumin and prothrombin time/INR, which are good indicators of hepatic synthetic function, are frequently abnormal. These markers reflect degree and progression of chronic liver disease and play an important role in determining patient prognosis. Bilirubin levels rise with disease progression, resulting in jaundice and pruritus. Hypoglycemia, frequently seen in FHF, rarely occurs in the setting of chronic liver disease.

The severity of chronic liver disease is often scored by the Child-Turcotte-Pugh (CTP) classification, which considers variables such as serum albumin, serum bilirubin, prothrombin time, and the degree of ascites and encephalopathy (Table 95.4). The model for end-stage liver disease (MELD), calculated from the INR, total bilirubin, and creatinine, predicts survival in patients with chronic liver disease awaiting transplant. Initially envisioned as a tool to evaluate patients undergoing transjugular intrahepatic portosystemic shunt (TIPS), it is now primarily used to prioritize liver allocation for liver transplantation in patients with end-stage liver disease.

Noninvasive imaging techniques including ultrasonography, CT, and magnetic resonance imaging (MRI) can identify hepatic steatosis, cirrhosis, and HCC. Liver biopsy remains the gold standard to establish the severity of liver inflammation and fibrosis.

Complications and Management

Portal hypertension is the most frequent complication in patients with cirrhosis. Clinical manifestations of portal hypertension include esophageal and gastric varices, portal hypertensive

TABLE 95.4

CHILD-TURCOTTE-PUGH SCORING SYSTEM

	Points scored for increasing abnormality		
Clinical and biochemical measurements	**1**	**2**	**3**
Albumin (g/dL)	>3.5	2.8–3.5	<2.8
Bilirubin (mg/dL)	1–2	2–3	>3
For cholestatic disease: bilirubin (mg/dL)	<4	4–10	>10
PT	1–4	4–6	>6
or			
INR	<1.7	1.7–2.3	>2.3
Ascites	Absent	Slight	Moderate
Encephalopathy (grade)	None	1 and 2	3 and 4

Child A, 5–6 points; Child B, 7–9 points; Child C, 10–15 points.
Prothrombin time (PT) or international normalized ratio (INR) may be used for scoring.
From Pugh RNH, Murray-Lyon IM, Dawson JL, et al: Transection of the esophagus for bleeding esophageal varices. *Br J Surg* 60:646–649, 1983, with permission.

gastropathy, colopathy, splenomegaly, hypersplenism, ascites, spontaneous bacterial peritonitis (SBP), and HRS. HE that ranges from subtle cerebral dysfunction to deep coma is also a frequent complication of end-stage liver disease. Complications of chronic liver disease may result in frequent admissions to the ICU.

Portal Hypertensive Bleeding

Portal hypertension is characterized by increased resistance to portal flow and increased portal venous inflow. Portal hypertension is defined by measuring the pressure difference between the hepatic vein and the portal vein (normal pressure gradient 3 mm Hg) through transjugular approach. Varices do not form at hepatic venous pressure gradient less than 12 mm Hg [66,67].

Portal hypertension induces hemodynamic changes in the hepatic and splanchnic blood flow, with development of portosystemic collateral circulation (esophagus, stomach, rectum, umbilicus, retroperitoneum) and splenomegaly. Bleeding from gastric and esophageal varices is a common indication for ICU admission in patients with cirrhosis. Variceal bleeding presents with hematemesis, melena, or hematochezia. The bleeding event is often dramatic and associated with severe hemodynamic instability and frequently followed by HE. Patients with portal hypertensive gastropathy or colopathy usually present with less severe bleeding and often with chronic anemia. Given advances in medical and endoscopic therapy, acute variceal bleeding mortality has decreased significantly [68,69]. Recent studies show an associated in-hospital, 6-week, and overall mortality rates of 14.2%, 17.5%, and 33.5%, respectively [70]. Rebleeding episodes remain frequent (29%). Comprehensive management of patients with GI bleeding related to portal hypertension must include the following considerations: primary prophylaxis (banding of esophageal varices or use of nonselective beta-blockers), treatment of the active hemorrhage (blood/volume resuscitation, banding of esophageal varices, octreotide infusion, antibiotic prophylaxis), and prevention of rebleeding (secondary prophylaxis with nonselective beta-blockers). The management of variceal hemorrhage is discussed in Chapter 92. In esophageal bleeding refractory to endoscopic treatment, consideration has to be given to salvage therapy with TIPS [71].

Thrombocytopenia is common in patients with splenomegaly secondary to cirrhosis and it is one of the features of hypersplenism. The importance of thrombocytopenia in bleeding from portal hypertension is unclear. In our experience, transfusion of platelets should be limited to those patients who are actively bleeding or undergoing an invasive procedure.

Ascites

Mechanisms responsible for the formation of ascites are complicated, multifactorial, and result in sodium and water retention. Circulatory dysfunction characterized by arterial vasodilation with hypotension, high cardiac output, and hypervolemia is frequently seen in patients with portal hypertension and ascites. Levels of nitric oxide, a potent vasodilator, are elevated in the splanchnic circulation of patients with ascites. The ensuing arterial vasodilation triggers activation of baroreceptor-mediated systems, the renin–angiotensin–aldosterone system, and the sympathetic nervous system, inducing sodium retention. Regulation of water balance is also disrupted in patients with cirrhosis. As a result of the reduced effective intravascular volume, arginine vasopressin levels are elevated. The major clinical consequence of this elevation is dilutional hyponatremia, which occurs despite a sodium avid state [72].

Patients with large volume ascites generally present with abdominal distension with a fluid wave or shifting dullness on examination. Respiratory compromise from associated pleural effusion (hepatic hydrothorax) or increase intra-abdominal pressure may result. Large volume ascites may also induce the development of ventral and umbilical hernias, with increase risk of intestinal strangulation or rupture. At times, ascites may only be a radiologic finding (e.g., ultrasound, CT, or MRI).

Analysis of the ascitic fluid is essential for the appropriate management of patients with decompensated liver disease. Small volume (60 mL) diagnostic paracentesis should be performed in patients hospitalized with ascites. Even in the presence of severe coagulopathy, it is safe to remove fluid [73]. Infection and bleeding are rare complications (<1%) [74]. The ascitic fluid should be sent for cell count and differential, culture, albumin, triglycerides (chylous ascites), amylase (pancreatic ascites), adenosine deaminase (peritoneal tuberculosis), and cytology (malignant ascites), as clinically indicated. A serum-to-ascites albumin gradient (SAAG) more than 1.1 g per dL indicates portal hypertension with 97% specificity. A SAAG less than 1.1 g per dL is found in nephrotic syndrome, peritoneal carcinomatosis, serositis, tuberculosis, and biliary and pancreatic ascites.

Restriction of sodium intake to 2,000 mg per day and minimizing IV sodium load (fluids, antibiotics, total parenteral nutrition, blood transfusions) play an important therapeutic role. Fluid restriction to 1,000 to 1,200 mL a day is helpful in patients with severe hyponatremia (serum sodium <125 mEq per L). In cirrhotics, hyponatremia develops in the setting of ascites in an environment of avid renal sodium retention and increased extracellular fluid volume (hypervolemic hyponatremia) or due to excessive losses of sodium and extracellular fluid (hypovolemic hyponatremia). New V2-receptor antagonists that block the action of arginine vasopressin in the distal tubule of the kidneys are promising pharmacologic agents to treat patients with cirrhosis, dilutional hyponatremia, and ascites [75].

Potassium-sparing diuretics acting at the distal tubule (spironolactone, amiloride, triamterene) and loop diuretics (furosemide, bumetanide) are frequently used in combination in patients with cirrhosis. Spironolactone inhibits sodium reabsorption in the distal tubule and collecting ducts by antagonizing aldosterone. Spironolactone is very effective in managing cirrhotic ascites, but its use is associated with hyperkalemia and painful gynecomastia. Loop diuretics also have a natriuretic effect and can be used in combination with distal tubule diuretics to achieve a more rapid extravascular fluid loss. Furosemide is not as effective as spironolactone as a single agent in the long-term management of ascites because of its lack of inhibition of distal sodium reabsorption. Intravenous furosemide should be avoided as it can result in intravascular volume depletion and precipitate renal failure. Renal function should be closely monitored to avoid prerenal azotemia. The use of aspirin and nonsteroidal anti-inflammatory agents should be avoided because the inhibition of prostaglandin affects renal hemodynamics and natriuresis [76].

Large-volume paracentesis (LVP) can safely remove 8 to 10 L as a therapeutic measure in patients with significant abdominal discomfort or respiratory compromise. The administration of albumin (6 to 8 g per L of ascites removed) during LVP has been associated with a lower incidence of hemodynamic disturbances without affecting survival [77,78]. Refractory ascites is a condition that develops in patients who do not respond adequately to maximum doses of diuretics [79]. Progressive intravascular volume depletion, renal failure, and electrolyte abnormalities may limit the use of high-dose diuretics. A reasonable alternative in patients with refractory ascites requiring frequent LVPs with preserved liver function is a TIPS [80]. Complications associated with TIPS include HE, cardiopulmonary compromise, transient pulmonary hypertension, infection, bleeding, ischemic hepatitis, and shunt occlusion.

Spontaneous Bacterial Peritonitis

Spontaneous bacterial peritonitis (SBP) is an infectious complication resulting from bacterial translocation that occurs through altered gut permeability and bacterial overgrowth. It is the most common infection in patients with cirrhosis and primarily seen in hospitalized patients. SBP develops in the setting of reticuloendothelial system depression and leukocyte dysfunction along with decreased opsonic activity in the ascitic fluid [81,82]. Almost 30% of patients with ascites admitted to the hospital for any reason have SBP [82,83]. Patients may present with abdominal pain, fevers, or mental status change; however, the diagnosis is often overlooked because clinical manifestations may be subtle or nonspecific. SBP is associated with high in-hospital mortality (10% to 30%). Advanced age and ICU stay are associated with increased mortality [84,85]. Recurrent SBP is common, with a 43% chance of recurrence at 6 months and 69% at 1 year [82,86]. Renal insufficiency occurs in up to one third of patients with SBP [87]. The median long-term survival of patients who develop SBP is 9 months [86].

A polymorphonuclear count of more than 250 per mm^3, a leukocyte count of more than 500 per mm^3, or the presence of a positive bacterial culture in the ascitic fluid establishes the diagnosis of SBP [88]. Ascitic fluid or blood cultures will be positive in at least one half of patients with SBP [88]. Identification of more than one organism raises the possibility of secondary bacterial peritonitis usually related to another intra-abdominal process. The most common organisms responsible for SBP are the Gram-negative enteric bacteria, *Escherichia coli*, and *Klebsiella*, accounting for 46% and 10% of cases, respectively [89]. *Streptococcus* sp (19%), *Staphylococcus* (1%), and anaerobic bacteria (6%) are less frequently implicated. Since identification of organisms is not immediately available, treatment should be targeted at the most likely culprits. The ideal antibiotic should have both Gram-negative and enteric organism coverage without nephrotoxicity. A third- or fourth-generation cephalosporin (cefotaxime, ceftriaxone), ampicillin/sulbactam, or ciprofloxacin at a renal adjusted dose are preferred therapies. Repeat paracentesis should be performed in patients who are not responding to therapy after 48 hours. If a 50% decrease in polymorphonuclear leukocyte count is not seen after 72 hours of antibiotic use, coverage should be broadened.

Two studies have demonstrated that administration of intravenous albumin in addition to antibiotics in the setting of SBP results in a lower incidence of renal impairment, improving short-term survival [90,91]. Due to the high recurrence rate of infection (70%), prophylactic, oral long-term antibiotic therapy is recommended after recovery. Secondary prophylaxis can be achieved with norfloxacin 400 mg daily. Primary antibiotic prophylaxis for SBP is indicated in the setting of acute GI bleeding [92].

Hepatic Encephalopathy

HE is a syndrome of disordered consciousness and altered neuromuscular activity, found in up to one third of patients with chronic liver failure [75]. Pathogenesis of this disorder is complex and incompletely understood. Inflammatory cytokines, benzodiazepine-like compounds, defective clearance of ammonia, and increased neuronal inhibition through the γ-aminobutyric acid (GABA) receptor supramolecular complex play a role in the pathogenesis of HE [93].

Clinical features range in severity from subclinical encephalopathy, manifested by disturbances in psychometric testing, to coma [94]. Symptoms may wax and wane over the clinical course of decompensated liver disease. Grade 1 encephalopathy involves personality changes and alterations in sleep patterns. Loss of orientation and lethargy develop as the grade of encephalopathy progresses. Asterixis and abnormal reflexes are seen on physical examination and are important clinical indicators of encephalopathy. The development of coma with decerebrate posturing indicates grade 4 encephalopathy. Although electroencephalograms are rarely used for the diagnosis, triphasic waves are present in grades 1 to 3 encephalopathy. Delta waves are frequently encountered in patients with coma (grade 4). CE and elevated ICP seen in acute liver failure is not present in patients with HE and end-stage liver disease. Serum ammonia is a popular marker for encephalopathy in chronic liver disease. However, there is poor correlation between ammonia levels and clinical disease [95] and in many cases results are of uncertain [96]. No single test is available to accurately assess for the presence or degree of encephalopathy.

Encephalopathy is usually precipitated by an acute event such as increased nitrogen load (GI bleeding, excess dietary protein intake, azotemia, constipation), the use of certain medications (sedatives, narcotics, diuretics), infection (SBP, pneumonia, urinary tract infection), electrolyte abnormalities (hypokalemia, hyponatremia), TIPS, surgical shunting, or superimposed acute liver disease. Noncompliance with medication used in the treatment of encephalopathy also may trigger this entity. Progression of underlying liver disease can also account for worsening encephalopathy.

Evaluation of patients with encephalopathy should start with identification of the precipitating event. Metabolic abnormalities such as abnormal serum sodium, potassium, and glucose as well as hypoxemia should be corrected. Hyponatremia should be treated with special caution, as rapid correction can lead to central pontine myelinolysis and neurologic damage [97]. Hypovolemia can be corrected with fluid resuscitation. A source of infection or sepsis should be investigated, even in the absence of fever, with cultures obtained from urine, blood, sputum, and ascites. Given the coagulopathy associated with chronic liver disease, a lumbar puncture should be pursued only if clinically imperative and after correction of blood clotting abnormalities. The presence of GI bleeding should be investigated. Prior history of medications or toxic ingestions should be reviewed.

Medications that decrease endogenous nitrogen production and nitrogen delivery to the liver play an important role in treating encephalopathy. Lactulose is a nonabsorbable disaccharide that reduces the intestinal production and absorption of ammonia [98]. The dose of lactulose should be titrated to achieve three to five soft stools a day, starting at 30 mL every 2 to 4 hours orally or via nasogastric tube. Lactulose can also be given as an enema in patients with an ileus or in those at increased risk of aspiration (300 mL lactulose in 700 mL distilled water). Rifaximin is a nonabsorbable rifamycin antibiotic, with broad-spectrum activity against Gram-positive and Gram-negative aerobes and anaerobes [99] with minimal side effects and no reported drug interactions. A dose of 1,200 mg per day (400 mg tid) is used as monotherapy or in combination with lactulose in the treatment of acute or chronic HE [100–103]. It is a safe drug in patients with renal impairment. Neomycin is a minimally absorbed antibiotic (1% to 3%) that efficaciously controls HE. It is given orally (500 to 1,000 mg every 6 hours) or as a retention enema (1% solution in 100 to 200 mL isotonic saline), as monotherapy or in combination with lactulose. It alters the colonic bacterial flora by acting against urease-producing bacteria. Neomycin is nephrotoxic and should be avoided in patients with renal insufficiency. Ototoxicity can also be associated with long-term use of neomycin. Metronidazole (250 mg orally every 8 hours) is also used to treat encephalopathy; side effects include metallic taste and peripheral neuropathy [104].

Dietary intake of protein should be reduced but not to the degree of inducing or exacerbating the catabolic effects of chronic liver disease. Patients with prolonged ICU admissions should receive 40 to 60 g per day of protein. Tube feeds with high-branched chain amino acid concentrations are expensive and have no clinical benefits over formulas [105].

Hepatorenal Syndrome

Hepatorenal syndrome (HRS), a feared consequence of end-stage liver disease, occurs in up to 10% of patients hospitalized with cirrhosis and ascites [106]. It is characterized by functional renal failure in the absence of obvious abnormalities in kidney structure. The primary mechanism in the generation of HRS involves intense renal vasoconstriction in response to activation of neurohumoral factors including the renin–angiotensin–aldosterone system and the sympathetic nervous system [107] leading to low renal perfusion and glomerular filtration rate.

HRS is divided into two clinically distinct types. Type I HRS progresses rapidly and has a close temporal association with a precipitating event that results in either a doubling of the initial serum creatinine to greater than 2.5 mg per dL or a 50% reduction in the initial 24-hour creatinine clearance to less than 20 mL per minute in less than 2 weeks [107]. Type II HRS progresses in a slower but relentless fashion as a form of expression of circulatory dysfunction, and clinically manifests as diuretic-resistant ascites. In contrast to patients with type II HRS that present with better-preserved liver function, patients with type I HRS have a very poor prognosis. They are usually severely ill with marked edema, ascites, sodium retention, hyponatremia, and hypotension. Precipitants of HRS include SBP, LVP without plasma expansion, and GI bleeding [107,108].

Although diagnostic criteria for HRS and oliguric renal failure have been established (Table 95.5), the distinction between type I HRS and prerenal azotemia may be extremely difficult. Patients with type I HRS can be supported by hemodialysis or hemofiltration, but prognosis is poor, with a median survival of approximately 2 weeks [109]. Ultimately, the treatment of choice is liver transplantation [110]. In the absence of prior renal disease, patients with HRS may show recovery of renal function after transplantation [111]. Patients with type II HRS show manifestations of liver failure with severe ascites that is refractory to treatment with sodium restriction. Median survival in type II HRS is 6 months.

Pharmacologic therapy with splanchnic vasoconstrictor drugs and volume expansion has shown promise as a bridge to transplantation. The rationale behind the use of splanchnic vasoconstrictors is the reduction in portal blood flow and pressure [112]. Splanchnic vasoconstrictors used in the treatment of HRS include vasopressin, ornipressin, terlipressin, and norepinephrine or in combination with the α-agonist midodrine [110]. The most promising results have been shown with terlipressin in combination with albumin. Terlipressin administered at progressive dosage (0.5 to 1 mg intravenously at 4- to 6-hour intervals) is associated with improvement in renal function and hemodynamic status [110]. Reported side effects have been minimal and reversible with dose reduction or discontinuation. Albumin should be given concomitantly at a loading dose of 1 g per kg followed by 20 to 40 g per day [113]. Patients with type I HRS treated with terlipressin and albumin pretransplant have similar posttransplant outcome as patients without HRS [106]. A combination of octreotide, midodrine, and albumin also has been beneficial in the treatment of HRS in smaller studies [110,112].

HRS may occasionally be prevented by timely administration of albumin and antibiotics in the treatment of SBP [90,106,112]. Preliminary reports of TIPS as a treatment of types I and II HRS have shown success, although more data are needed before promoting its widespread use for these entities [114–116].

TABLE 95.5

DIAGNOSTIC CRITERIA OF HEPATORENAL SYNDROME

Major criteria

- Low glomerular filtration rate, as indicated by serum creatinine >1.5 mg/dL or 24-h creatinine clearance <40 mL/min
- Absence of shock, ongoing bacterial infection, fluid losses, and current treatment with nephrotoxic drugs
- No sustained improvement in renal function (decrease in serum creatinine to 1.5 mg/dL or increase in creatinine clearance to 40 mL/min) after diuretic withdrawal and expansion of plasma volume with 1.5 L of a plasma expander
- Proteinuria <500 mg/d and no ultrasonographic evidence of obstructive uropathy or parenchymal renal disease

Additional criteria

- Urine volume <500 mL/d
- Urine sodium <10 mEq/L
- Urine osmolality greater than plasma osmolality
- Urine RBCs <50/high-power field
- Serum sodium concentration <130 mEq/L

Note: All major criteria must be present for the diagnosis of hepatorenal syndrome. Additional criteria are not necessary for the diagnosis but provide supportive evidence.

From Arroyo V, Gines P, Gerbes AL, et al: Definition and diagnostic criteria of refractory ascites and hepatorenal syndrome in cirrhosis. International Ascites Club. *Hepatology* 23:164, 1996, with permission.

LIVER TRANSPLANTATION

Fulminant Hepatic Failure

For many patients with FHF, liver transplantation provides the only realistic opportunity to stay alive. Of all liver transplants, approximately 5% are for patients with FHF. It has been estimated that 40% of patients with FHF admitted to transplant centers ultimately undergo transplantation. With supportive ICU care alone, only 25% will survive, while the remaining 35% perish despite the best intensive care available [55] and highest priority (status 1) assigned to these patients for liver transplantation by the United Network for Organ Sharing. The rapidly progressive nature of FHF and difficulty in obtaining organs prevents many potential recipients from receiving a transplant in a timely fashion. Patients listed as status 1 have an unacceptably high mortality rate while on the waiting list.

There is a favorable 3-year survival (75%) in those patients who undergo liver transplantation for FHF [55], and the outcome and prognosis of these patients is dependent on the specific etiology that induced the acute failure. Patients with FHF from acute hepatitis A, hepatitis B, and acetaminophen toxicity have better survival rates. Conversely, patients with FHF from idiosyncratic drug reactions, halothane exposure, and acute Wilson's disease tend to fare worse [55]. Regardless of the cause, early referral and evaluation for liver transplantation is imperative. Although most living donor transplantations are performed in patients with chronic liver disease, its role has been investigated in FHF. Survival up to 90% at 5 years has been reported in pediatric patients undergoing living donor transplants [117].

TABLE 95.6

SUMMARY OF EVIDENCE-BASED MANAGEMENT APPROACHES IN THE MANAGEMENT OF FULMINANT HEPATIC FAILURE AND CHRONIC LIVER DISEASE

Fulminant hepatic failure	
Hepatic encephalopathy	
Cerebral edema	■ There is no proven effective therapy. ■ There are no controlled trials to prove efficacy of ICP monitoring, and experience is variable across centers. ■ Mannitol has been shown in a controlled trial to decrease ICP and to improve survival. ■ Uncontrolled investigations show a benefit of hypothermia, but there are no controlled trials. ■ A randomized controlled trial has demonstrated that hypertonic saline and maintenance of hypernatremia (145–155 mmol/L) resulted in decreased incidence and severity of intracranial hypertension.
Acetaminophen toxicity	■ Based on controlled trials, *N*-acetylcysteine administration in oral or intravenous form can be recommended in suspected acetaminophen overdose.
Chronic liver disease	
Bleeding from portal hypertension	■ See Chapter 92
Ascites	■ Randomized controlled trials have demonstrated that the combination of sodium restriction to <2 g/d and oral diuretics is effective in reduction of ascites (AASLD guidelines). ■ Controlled trials have demonstrated that serial therapeutic paracentesis are equally as effective in controlling ascites as the combination of sodium restriction and oral diuretics; concomitant administration of albumin has been shown in uncontrolled trials to have a significant effect on electrolyte and creatinine levels without effect on clinical morbidity and mortality. It use remains controversial (AASLD guidelines). ■ Randomized controlled trials have demonstrated that TIPS is effective for controlling refractory ascites (AASLD guidelines).
Spontaneous bacterial peritonitis	■ Patients with SBP should receive antibiotics. ■ One randomized controlled trial demonstrated that administration of albumin (1.5 g/kg initially, then 1 g/kg on day 3) with antibiotics in SBP resulted in decreased mortality.
Hepatic encephalopathy	■ Lactulose and neomycin are the most frequently used agents in the treatment of hepatic encephalopathy; rifaximin has been shown in controlled trials to be an effective alternative or adjuvant to lactulose and neomycin.
Hepatorenal syndrome	■ Several uncontrolled studies and one small randomized study have demonstrated the use of terlipressin in combination with albumin improves renal function in type I HRS. ■ Small uncontrolled studies have demonstrated an improvement in renal function with the use of octreotide, midodrine, and albumin.

AASLD, American Association for the Study of Liver Diseases; HRS, hepatorenal syndrome; ICP, intracranial pressure; SBP, spontaneous bacterial peritonitis; TIPS, transjugular intrahepatic portosystemic shunt.

End-Stage Liver Disease

Liver transplantation is frequently indicated in patients with end-stage liver disease. The timing of liver transplantation in these patients is a complex issue. Transplant evaluation should be initiated when there is a decline in hepatic synthetic function, ascites, HE, or other complications such as ascending cholangitis, SBP, HRS, and HCC. Liver allocation in the United States is currently based on the MELD score. MELD is an accurate predictor of short-term survival (3 months) in patients with cirrhosis awaiting liver transplantation [118–121]. Contraindications for liver transplantation include sepsis, advanced cardiac or pulmonary disease, extrahepatic malignancy, multiorgan failure, and unresolved alcoholism, drug addiction, as well as psychosocial and compliance issues.

The 1-year survival for liver transplantation in the setting of chronic liver disease is currently 85% to 90% [122,123]. With increasing numbers of patients listed for transplantation and the relatively static number of cadaveric organs available, death is not uncommon while awaiting organ donation [124]. Because of the worldwide shortage of cadaveric liver donors, interest has developed in the role of living donors [125]. Living donors may provide a valuable option for some patients. Despite promising results, a number of donor deaths have occurred, raising questions regarding the suitability of this mode of transplantation [126].

Alternative Therapies

The severe and rapidly progressive consequences of FHF have led to investigate and develop other supportive modalities that could allow time for liver recovery or serve as a "bridge" to liver transplantation.

Prostaglandin E_1 (PGE_1) has been investigated as a possible therapy for patients with FHF. Benefits of intravenous PGE_1, especially if administered 10 days after the onset of symptoms, have not been verified [97,127]. Hepatic arterial infusions of

PGE_1 seem to be superior to IV administration in postsurgical acute liver failure based on very limited data [97].

Substitution of hepatocyte function with liver assist devices has been studied extensively [128–130]. These devices can be divided into biological (using whole animal livers), hybrid bioartificial (using cultured immortalized hepatocytes with both excretory and synthetic function), combination of both and nonbiological extracorporeal liver assist devices. Promise has been shown by the bioartificial hybrid systems which implement both mechanical toxin removal and biologic function provided by sliced or granulated livers or hepatocytes from low-grade tumor cells or pigs housed within a "bioreactor" [131]. In extracorporeal devices, albumin is the molecular absorbent used to remove toxins such as ammonia, bilirubin, aromatic amino acids, which accumulate as a result of liver failure and lead to the development of HE and renal failure. The most well studied of these dialysis systems is the molecular adsorbent recirculation system (MARS). It improves biochemical markers in both FHF and acute-on-chronic liver failure [132,133]. However, conclusive mortality benefits have not been shown and further trials are needed.

Human hepatocyte transplantation has also been investigated as an emergent alternative. There have been more than 80 cases of human hepatocyte transplantations, mostly in patients with inborn errors of metabolism (Crigler Najjar syndrome, Glycogen storage disease 1a and 1b, etc.) with short-term benefits [134,135]. In FHF and chronic liver failure, there is a reduction in bilirubin and ammonia with improvement in HE. Again, larger randomized clinical trials are needed to evaluate their efficacy. There are many barriers to overcome before this method can have widespread clinical use [136,137].

Evidence-Based Therapies

FHF and chronic liver disease are managed depending on the presentation and the presence and type of complications, as described in the earlier sections. In many instances, clinicians are guided by management strategies that have proved successful in the clinical setting. Some of the evidence-based approaches used in the treatment of these forms of liver disease are outlined in Table 95.6.

References

1. Bernuau J, Rueff B, Benhamou JP: Fulminant and subfulminant liver failure: definitions and causes. *Semin Liver Dis* 6:97, 1986.
2. Lee W: Etiologies of acute liver failure. *Semin Liver Dis* 28:142–152, 2008.
3. Bowen DG, Shackel NA, Mccaughan GW: East meets West: acute liver failure in the global village. *J Gastroenterol Hepatol* 15:467, 2000.
4. Ostapowicz G, Fontana RJ, Schidt FV, et al: Results of a prospective study of acute liver failure at 17 tertiary care centers in the United States. *Ann Intern Med* 137:947, 2005.
5. Larson AM: Acetaminophen hepatotoxicity. *Clin Liver Dis* 11(3):525–48, vi, 2007.
6. Chun LJ, Tong MJ, Busuttil RW, et al: Acetaminophen hepatotoxicity and acute liver failure. *J Clin Gastroenterol* 43(4):342–349, 2009.
7. Kanter MZ: Comparison of oral and i.v. acetylcysteine in the treatment of acetaminophen poisoning. *Am J Health Syst Pharm* 63(19):1821–1827, 2006.
8. Ben-Ari Z, Vaknin H, Tur-Kaspa R: *N*-acetylcysteine in acute liver failure (non-paracetamol induced). *Hepatogastroenterology* 47:786, 2000.
9. Montanini S, Sinardi D, Pratico C, et al: Use of acetylcysteine as the life-saving antidote in *Amanita phalloides* (death cap) poisoning. Case report on 11 patients. *Arzneimittelforschung* 49(12):1044, 1999.
10. Sklar GE, Subramaniam M: Acetylcysteine treatment for nonacetaminophen-induced acute liver failure. *Ann Pharmacother* 38:498, 2004.
11. Bihari DJ, Gimson AES, Williams R: Cardiovascular, pulmonary, and renal complications of fulminant hepatic failure. *Semin Liver Dis* 6:119, 1986.
12. Blei AT: Medical therapy of brain edema in fulminant hepatic failure. *Hepatology* 32:666, 2000.
13. Odeh M: Pathogenesis of hepatic encephalopathy: the tumour necrosis factor-alpha theory. *Eur J Clin Invest* 37(4):291–304, 2007.
14. Ahboucha S, Butterworth RF: The neurosteroid system: implication in the pathophysiology of hepatic encephalopathy. *Neurochem Int* 52(4–5):575–587, 2008.
15. Llansola M, Rodrigo R, Monfort P, et al: NMDA receptors in hyperammonemia and hepatic encephalopathy. *Metab Brain Dis* 22(3–4):321–335, 2007.
16. Strauss G, Hansen BA, Kirkkegard P, et al: Liver function, cerebral blood flow autoregulation, and hepatic encephalopathy in fulminant hepatic failure. *Hepatology* 25:837, 1997.
17. Elgouhari H, O'Shea R: What is the utility of measuring the serum ammonia level in patients with altered mental status ? *Cleve Clin J Med* 76:252–254, 2009.
18. Eroglu Y, Byrne WJ: Hepatic encephalopathy. *Emerg Med Clin North Am* 27(3):401–414, 2009.
19. Festi D, Vestito A, Mazzella G, et al: Management of hepatic encephalopathy: focus on antibiotic therapy. *Digestion* 73:94–101, 2006.
20. Devictor D, Tahiri C, Lanchier C, et al: Flumazenil in the treatment of hepatic encephalopathy in children with fulminant liver failure. *Intensive Care Med* 21(3):253, 1995.
21. Ware AJ, D'Agostino AN, Combes B: Cerebral edema is a major complication of massive hepatic necrosis. *Gastroenterology* 61:877, 1971.
22. Blei AT: The pathophysiology of brain edema in acute liver failure. *Neurochem Int* 47:71, 2005.
23. Wendon J, Lee W: Encephalopathy and cerebral edema in the setting of acute liver failure: pathogenesis and management. *Neurocrit Care* 9(1):97–102, 2008.
24. Lidofsky SD, Bass NM, Prager MC, et al: Intracranial pressure monitoring and liver transplantation for fulminant hepatic failure. *Hepatology* 16:1, 1992.
25. Bernuau J, Durand F: Intracranial pressure monitoring in patients with acute liver failure: a questionable invasive surveillance. *Hepatology* 44:502–504, 2006.
26. Wendon J, Larsen F: Intracranial pressure monitoring in acute liver failure. A procedure with clear indications. *Hepatology* 44:504–506, 2006.
27. Vaquero J, Fontana RJ, Larson AM, et al: Complications and use of intracranial pressure monitoring in patients with acute liver failure and severe encephalopathy. *Liver Transpl* 11:1581–1589, 2005.
28. Keays RT, Alexander GJ, Williams RJ: The safety and value of extradural intracranial pressure monitors in fulminant hepatic failure. *Hepatology* 18(2):205–209, 1993.
29. Blei AT, Olafsson S, Webster S, et al: Complications of intracranial pressure monitoring in acute liver failure. *Lancet* 341:157, 1993.
30. Cordoba J, Blei AT: Cerebral edema and intracranial pressure monitoring. *Liver Transpl Surg* 1(3):187, 1995.
31. Nora LM, Bleck TP: Increased intracranial pressure complicating hepatic failure. *J Crit Illness* 4:87, 1989.
32. Lidofsky SD: Liver transplantation for fulminant hepatic failure. *Gastroenterol Clin North Am* 22:257, 1993.
33. Murphy N, Auzinger G, Bernel W, et al: The effect of hypertonic sodium chloride on intracranial pressure in patients with acute liver failure. *Hepatology* 39(2):464, 2004.
34. Canalese J, Gimson AES, Davies C, et al: Controlled trial of dexamethasone and mannitol for cerebral edema in fulminant hepatic failure. *Gut* 23:625, 1982.
35. Nemoto EM, Klementavicius R, Melick JA, et al: Suppression of cerebral metabolic rate for oxygen ($CMRO_2$) by mild hypothermia compared with thiopental. *J Neurosurg Anesthesiol* 8:52, 1996.
36. Vaquero J, Rose C, Butterworth RF: Keeping cool in liver failure: rationale for the use of mild hypothermia. *J Hepatol* 43(6):1067, 2005.
37. Stravitz RT, Larsen FS: Therapeutic hypothermia for acute liver failure. *Crit Care Med* 37[7, Suppl]:S258–S264, 2009.
38. Jalan R, Olde Damink SW, Deutz NE, et al: Moderate hypothermia prevents cerebral hyperemia and increase in intracranial pressure in patients undergoing liver transplantation for acute liver failure. *Transplantation* 75(12):2034–2039, 2003.
39. O'Brien CJ, Wise RJ, O'Grady JG, et al: Neurologic sequelae in patients recovered from fulminant hepatic failure. *Gut* 28:93, 1987.
40. Munoz SJ, Stravitz RT, Gabriel DA: Coagulopathy of acute liver failure. *Clin Liver Dis* 13(1):95–107, 2009.
41. Caldwell SH, Chang C, Macik BG: Recombinant activated factor VII (rFVIIa) as a hemostatic agent in liver disease: a break from convention in need of controlled trials. *Hepatology* 39:592, 2004.
42. Brown JB, Emerick KM, Brown DL, et al: Recombinant factor VIIa improves coagulopathy caused by liver failure. *Liver Transpl* 9(2):138, 2003.
43. Shami VM, Caldwell SH, Hespenheide EE, et al: Recombinant activated factor VII for coagulopathy in fulminant hepatic failure compared with conventional therapy. *Liver Transpl* 9:138, 2003.
44. Williams R, Gimson AES: Intensive care and management of acute hepatic liver failure. *Dig Dis Sci* 36:820, 1991.

45. Garcia-Tsao G, Parikh CR, Viola A: Acute kidney injury in cirrhosis. *Hepatology* 48(6):2064–2077, 2008.
46. Davenport A, Will EJ, Davidson AM: Improved cardiovascular stability during continuous modes of renal replacement therapy in critically ill patients with acute hepatic and renal failure. *Crit Care Med* 21(3):328, 1993.
47. Shakil AO, Kramer D, Mazariegos GV, et al: Acute liver failure: clinical features, outcome analysis, and applicability of prognostic criteria. *Liver Transpl* 6:163, 2000.
48. Bernal W, Auzinger G, Sizer E, et al: Intensive care management of acute liver failure. *Semin Liver Dis* 28:188–200, 2008.
49. Rolando N, Wade J, Stangou A, et al: Prospective study comparing the efficacy of prophylactic parenteral antimicrobials, with or without enteral decontamination, in patients with acute liver failure. *Liver Transpl Surg* 2:8, 1996.
50. Robertson CM, Coopersmith CM: The systemic inflammatory response syndrome. *Microbes Infect* 8(5):1382–1389, 2006.
51. O'Grady JG, Alexander GJ, Hayallar KM: Early indicators of prognosis in fulminant hepatic failure. *Gastroenterology* 97:439, 1989.
52. Anand A, Nightingale P, Neuberger J: Early indicators of prognosis in fulminant hepatic failure: an assessment of the King's criteria. *J Hepatol* 26:62, 1997.
53. Benal W, Donaldson N, Wyncoll D, et al: Blood lactate as an early predictor of outcome in paracetamol-induced acute liver failure: a cohort study. *Lancet* 359:558, 2002.
54. Mitchell I, Bihari D, Chang R, et al: Earlier identification of patients at risk for acetaminophen induced acute liver failure. *Crit Care Med* 26:279, 1998.
55. Schiodt FV, Atillasoy E, Shakil AO, et al: Etiology and outcome for 295 patients with acute liver failure in the United States. *Liver Transpl Surg* 5:86, 1999.
56. Deasy NP, Wendon J, Meine HB, et al: The role of serial Doppler examination as a predictor of clinical outcome and the need for transplantation in fulminant and severe acute liver failure. *Br J Radiol* 72:134, 1999.
57. Shakil OA, Jones BC, Lee RG, et al: Prognostic value of abdominal CT scanning and hepatic histopathology in patients with acute liver failure. *Dig Dis Sci* 45:334, 2000.
58. Lee WM, Galbraith RM, Watt GH, et al: Predicting survival in fulminant hepatic failure using serum Gc protein concentrations. *Hepatology* 21:101, 1995.
59. Schmidt LE, Dalhoff K: Alpha-fetoprotein is a predictor of outcome in acetaminophen-induced liver injury. *Hepatology* 41(1):26, 2005.
60. Alter M, Kruson-Moran D, Nainan OV, et al: The prevalence of hepatitis C virus infection in the United States, 1988 through 1994. *NEJM*. 341:556–562, 1999.
61. Ray K: The burden of hepatitis C in the United States. *Hepatology* 36:S30–S40, 2002.
62. Centers for Disease Control and Prevention: Recommendations for prevention and control of hepatitis C virus (HCV) infection and HCV-related chronic disease. *MMWR Morb Mortal Wkly Rep* 40(RR-19):1, 1998.
63. Lok AS, McMahon BJ: Chronic hepatitis B: *Hepatology* 45(2):507–539, 2007.
64. Sanyal A: AGA technical review on nonalcoholic fatty liver disease. *Gastroenterology* 123:1705–1725, 2002.
65. Clark JM: The epidemiology of nonalcoholic fatty liver disease in adults. *J Clin Gastroenterol* 40[Suppl 1]:S5, 2006.
66. Garcia-Tsao G: Portal hypertension. *Curr Opin Gastroenterol* 21:313–322, 2005.
67. Sass DA, Chopra KB: Portal hypertension and variceal hemorrhage. *Med Clin North Am* 93(4):837–853, vii–viii, 2009.
68. Van Dam J, Brugge WR: Endoscopy of the upper gastrointestinal tract. *N Engl J Med* 341:1738, 1999.
69. Graham DY, Smith JL: The course of patients after variceal hemorrhage. *Gastroenterology* 80:800, 1981.
70. Nietsch HH: Management of portal hypertension. *J Clin Gastroenterol* 39(3):232, 2005.
71. Owen AR, Stanley AJ, Vijayananthan A, et al: The transjugular intrahepatic portosystemic shunt (TIPS). *Clin Radiol* 64:664–674, 2009.
72. Cardenas A, Arroyo V: Mechanisms of water and sodium retention in cirrhosis and the pathogenesis of ascites. *Best Pract Res Clin Endocrinol Metab* 17(4):607, 2003.
73. Runyon BA: Paracentesis of ascitic fluid: a safe procedure. *Arch Intern Med* 146:2259, 1986.
74. Hoefs JC: Diagnostic paracentesis: a potent clinical tool. *Gastroenterology* 98:230, 1990.
75. Gines P, Cardenas A: The management of ascites and hyponatremia in cirrhosis. *Semin Liver Dis* 28:43–58, 2008.
76. Mirouze D, Zipser RD, Reynolds TB: Effects of inhibitors of prostaglandin synthesis on induced diuresis in cirrhosis. *Hepatology* 3:50, 1983.
77. Tito L, Gines P, Arroyo V, et al: Randomized comparative study of therapeutic paracentesis with and without intravenous albumin in cirrhosis. *Gastroenterology* 94:1493, 1988.
78. Gines A, Fernandez-Esparrach G, Monescillo A, et al: Randomized trial comparing albumin, dextran-70 and polygeline in cirrhotic patients with ascites treated by paracentesis. *Gastroenterology* 111:1002, 1996.
79. Bahaa E, Dragonov P: Evaluation and management of patients with refractory ascites. *World J Gastroenterol* 15(1):67–80, 2009.
80. Cardenas A, Arroyo V: Refractory ascites. *Dig Dis* 23(1):30, 2005.
81. Runyon BA: Low-protein-concentration ascitic fluid is predisposed to spontaneous bacterial peritonitis. *Gastroenterology* 91:1343, 1986.
82. Parsi MA, Atreja A, Zein NN: Spontaneous bacterial peritonitis: recent data on incidence and treatment. *Cleve Clin J Med* 71(7):569, 2004.
83. Amadal TP, Skinhoj P: Spontaneous bacterial peritonitis in cirrhosis. Incidence, diagnosis, and prognosis. *Scand J Gastroenterol* 22:295, 1987.
84. Runyon BA, Umland ET, Merlin T: Inoculation of blood culture bottles with ascitic fluid. Improved detection of spontaneous bacterial peritonitis. *Arch Intern Med* 147:73, 1987.
85. Thuluvath PJ, Morss S, Thompson R: Spontaneous bacterial peritonitis—in-hospital mortality, predictors of survival, and health care costs from 1988 to 1998. *Am J Gastroenterol* 96(4):1232, 2001.
86. Tito L, Rimola A, Gines P, et al: Recurrence of spontaneous bacterial peritonitis in cirrhosis: frequency and predictive factors. *Hepatology* 8:27, 1988.
87. Follo A, Llovet JM, Navasa M, et al: Renal impairment following spontaneous bacterial peritonitis in cirrhosis: incidence, clinical course, predictive factors and prognosis. *Hepatology* 20:1495, 1994.
88. Runyon BA: Spontaneous bacterial peritonitis: an explosion of information. *Hepatology* 8:171, 1988.
89. Garcia-Tsao G: Spontaneous bacterial peritonitis. *Gastroenterol Clin North Am* 21:257, 1992.
90. Sort P, Navasa M, Arroyo V, et al: Effect of intravenous albumin on renal impairment and mortality in patients with cirrhosis and spontaneous bacterial peritonitis. *N Engl J Med* 341:403, 1999.
91. Fernández J, Monteagudo J, Bargallo X, et al: A randomized unblinded pilot study comparing albumin versus hydroxyethyl starch in spontaneous bacterial peritonitis. *Hepatology* 42(3):627–634, 2005.
92. Hsieh WJ, Lin HC, Hwang SJ, et al: The effect of ciprofloxacin in the prevention of bacterial infection in patients with cirrhosis after upper gastrointestinal bleeding. *Am J Gastroenterol* 93:962, 1998.
93. Sundaram V, Obaid OS: Hepatic encephalopathy: pathophysiology and emerging therapies. *Med Clin North Am* 43:819–836, 2009.
94. Lizardi-Cervera J, Almeda P, Guevara L, et al: Hepatic encephalopathy: a review. *Ann Hepatol* 2(3):122, 2003.
95. Phear EA, Sherlock S, Summerstill WHJ: Blood ammonia levels in liver disease and hepatic coma. *Lancet* 1:836, 1955.
96. Ong JP, Aggarwal A, Krieger D, et al: Correlation between ammonia levels and the severity of hepatic encephalopathy. *Am J Med* 114:188–193, 2003.
97. Stearns RH: Severe symptomatic hyponatremia: treatment and outcome. *Ann Intern Med* 107:656, 1987.
98. Van Leeuwen PA, van Berlo CL, Soeters PB: New mode of action for lactulose. *Lancet* 1(8575–8576):55–56, 1988.
99. Festi D, Vestito A, Mazzella G, et al: Experimental and clinical pharmacology of rifaximin, a gastrointestinal selective antibiotic. *Digestion* 73[Suppl 1]:13, 2006.
100. Mas A, Rodes J, Sunyer L, et al: Spanish Association for the Study of the Liver Hepatic Encephalopathy Cooperative Group. Comparison of rifaximin and lactitol in the treatment of acute hepatic encephalopathy: results of a randomized, double-blind, double-dummy, controlled clinical trial. *J Hepatol* 38(1):51, 2003.
101. Williams R, James OF, Warnes TW, et al: Evaluation of the efficacy and safety of rifaximin in the treatment of hepatic encephalopathy: a double-blind, randomized, dose-finding multi-centre study. *Eur J Gastroenterol Hepatol* 12(2):203, 2000.
102. Miglio F, Valpiani D, Rossellini SR, et al: Rifaximin, a non-absorbable rifamycin, for the treatment of hepatic encephalopathy. A double-blind, randomised trial. *Curr Med Res Opin* 13(10):593, 1997.
103. Puxeddu A, Quartini M, Massimetti A, et al: Rifaximin in the treatment of chronic hepatic encephalopathy. *Curr Med Res Opin* 13(5):274, 1995.
104. Hobson-Webb L, Metronidazole: Newly recognized cause of autonomic neuropathy. *J Child Neurol* 21(5):429–431, 2006.
105. Marchesini G, Bianchi G, Rossi B, et al: Nutritional treatment with branched-chain amino acids in advanced liver cirrhosis. *J Gastroenterol* 35[Suppl]:7, 2000.
106. Cardenas A: Hepatorenal syndrome: a dreaded complication of end-stage liver disease. *Am J Gastroenterol* 100(2):460, 2005.
107. Arroyo V, Gines P, Gerbes AL, et al: Definition and diagnostic criteria of refractory ascites and hepatorenal syndrome in cirrhosis. *Hepatology* 23:164, 1996.
108. Arroyo V, Fernandez J, Gines P: Pathogenesis and treatment of hepatorenal syndrome. *Semin Liver Dis* 28:81–95, 2008.
109. Gines A, Escorsell A, Gines P, et al: Incidence, predictive factors and prognosis of the hepatorenal syndrome in cirrhosis with ascites. *Gastroenterology* 105:229, 1993.
110. Sandhu BS, Sanyal AJ: Hepatorenal syndrome. *Curr Treat Options Gastroenterol* 8(6):443, 2005.
111. Gonwa TA, Klintmalm GB, Levy M, et al: Impact of pretransplant renal function on survival after liver transplantation. *Transplantation* 59:361, 1995.
112. Pham PT, Pham PC, Rastogi A, et al: Review article: current management of renal dysfunction in the cirrhotic patient. *Aliment Pharmacol Ther* 21(8):949, 2005.
113. Fernandez J, Navasa J, Garcia-Pagan JC, et al: Effect of intravenous albumin on systemic and hepatic hemodynamics and vasoactive neurohormonal

systems in patients with cirrhosis and spontaneous bacterial peritonitis. *J Hepatol* 41:384–390, 2004.
114. Guevara M, Gines P, Bandi JC, et al: Transjugular intrahepatic portosystemic shunts in hepatorenal syndrome: effects on renal function and vasoactive substances. *Hepatology* 28:416, 1999.
115. Wong F: Midodrine, octreotide, albumin, and TIPS in selected patients with cirrhosis and type 1 hepatorenal syndrome. *Hepatology*. 40(1):55–64, 2004.
116. Brensing KA, Textor J, Perz J, et al: Long term outcome after transjugular intrahepatic portosystemic stent-shunt in non-transplant cirrhotics with hepatorenal syndrome: a phase II study. *Gut* 47:288–295, 2000.
117. Miwa S, Hashikura Y, Mita A, et al: Living-related liver transplantation for patients with fulminant and subfulminant hepatic failure. *Hepatology* 30:521, 1999.
118. Meerman L, Zijlstra JG, Schweizer JJ, et al: Acute liver failure: spontaneous recovery or transplantation. *Scand J Gastroenterol* 223[Suppl]:55, 1997.
119. Wang VS, Saab S: Liver transplantation in the era of model for end-stage liver disease. *Liver Int* 24(1):1, 2004.
120. Botta F, Giannini E, Romagnoli P, et al: MELD scoring system is useful for predicting prognosis in patients with liver cirrhosis and is correlated with residual liver function: a European study. *Gut* 52(1):134, 2003.
121. Kamath PS, Weisner RH, Malinchoc M, et al: A model to predict survival in patients with end stage liver disease. *Hepatology* 33:464, 2001.
122. Keeffe EB: Liver transplantation: current status and novel approaches to liver replacement. *Gastroenterology* 120:749, 2001.
123. Busuttil RW, Farmer DG, Yersiz H, et al: Analysis of long-term outcomes of 3,200 liver transplantations over two decades: a single-center experience. *Ann Surg* 241(6):905, 2005.
124. Keeffe EB: Summary guidelines on organ allocation and patient listing for liver transplantation. *Liver Transpl Surg* 4:S108, 1998.
125. Marcos A: Right lobe liver donor liver transplantation: a review. *Liver Transpl* 6:3, 2000.
126. Neuberger JM, Lucey MR: Living related liver donation: the inevitable donor deaths highlight the need for greater transparency. *Transplantation* 77(4):489, 2004.
127. Sterling RK, Luketic VA, Sanyal AJ, et al: Treatment of fulminant hepatic failure with intravenous prostaglandin E_1. *Liver Transpl Surg* 4:424, 1998.
128. Watanabe FD, Multon CJ, Hewitt WR, et al: Clinical experience with bioartificial liver in the treatment of severe liver failure. A phase I clinical trial. *Ann Surg* 225:484, 1997.
129. Cao S, Esquivel CO, Keeffe EB: New approaches to supporting the failing liver. *Ann Rev Med* 49:85, 1998.
130. Pless G, Sauer IM: Bioartificial liver: current status. *Transplant Proc* 37(9):3893, 2005.
131. Tsiaoussis J, Newsome PN, Nelson LJ, et al: Which hepatocyte will it be? Hepatocyte choice for bioartificial liver support systems. *Liver Transpl* 7:2, 2001.
132. Tan HK: Molecular Adsorbent Recirculating System (MARS). *Ann Acad Med* 33:329–335, 2004.
133. Karvellas CJ, Gibney N, Kutsogiannis D, et al: Bench to bedside review: Current evidence for extracorporeal albumin dialysis systems in liver failure. *Crit Care* 11:215–223, 2007.
134. Chowdhury JR: Forward prospects of liver cell transplantation and liver-directed gene therapy. *Semin Liver Dis* 19:1, 1999.
135. Fox I, Chowdhury J, Kaufman S, et al: Treatment of the Crigler-Najjar syndrome type I with hepatocyte transplantation. *N Engl J Med* 338:1422, 1998.
136. Fitzpatrick E, Mitry R, Dhawan A. Human hepatocyte transplantation: state of art. *J Intern Med* 266:339–357, 2009.
137. Najimi M, Sokal E: Liver cell transplantation. *Minerva Pediatr* 57(5):243, 2005.

CHAPTER 96 ■ DIARRHEA

COLIN T. SWALES, LAURA HARRELL, EUGENE CHANG AND JOHN K. ZAWACKI

Diarrhea frequently complicates the course of the critically ill patient, occurring in 40% to 50% of patients in the intensive care unit (ICU). Diarrhea is the most common nonhemorrhagic gastrointestinal (GI) complication in this patient population [1–3]. Despite its high prevalence in the ICU patient population, diarrhea is frequently overlooked by physicians and the ICU team, especially when more emergent cardiovascular, respiratory, and infectious issues are present. Inattention to excessive stool output, however, can often result in serious perturbations of fluid and electrolyte balance, promote skin breakdown and infection, and create difficulty in the administration of proper nutritional support. In these instances, proper and immediate evaluation and management are essential to prevent further complications in a critically ill patient. The evaluation of diarrhea is often limited by the patient's status and practical limitations in performing diagnostic studies in the ICU setting.

The term diarrhea often carries a different meaning for patients and healthcare providers. Increases in stool frequency or fluidity do not necessarily indicate the presence of diarrhea. In a general patient population, an increase in daily stool weight or volume (exceeding 200 g per day) has been used as an objective-defining criterion [4]. In the critically ill patient, however, accurate measurement of stool output may be difficult, if not impossible. Physicians, therefore, must use their best judgment to decide whether diarrhea is present and to determine whether it represents a clinical problem requiring attention. This chapter provides helpful insights for making these decisions, presents guidelines for rapid and directed evaluation, and suggests effective approaches for the management of diarrhea in this setting.

ETIOLOGY

The causative factors of diarrhea in the ICU patient differ considerably from those of diarrhea in the general population. Numerous causes of diarrhea in the ICU setting exist and can be broadly divided into three categories: (i) diarrhea secondary to iatrogenic causes, (ii) diarrhea secondary to underlying diseases, and (iii) diarrhea resulting as a primary manifestation of specific diseases. Careful review of clinical information will allow physicians to narrow the diagnostic possibilities and avoid overlooking simple and common causes of diarrhea (Table 96.1). In some patients, diarrhea is the result of a combination of factors. Thus, it is incumbent on the physician to carefully review available data to identify the cause or causes of diarrhea.

Iatrogenic Causes

Iatrogenic factors are the most common and the most frequently overlooked cause of diarrhea in the critically ill patient. Furthermore, rapid and successful treatment of iatrogenic diarrhea can often be achieved by eliminating the offending agent or process.

Medications

Medications are a frequent cause of iatrogenic diarrhea in the ICU setting. Many of the drugs commonly used in the ICU can cause diarrhea (Table 96.2). Therefore, any medication

TABLE 96.1

DIFFERENTIAL DIAGNOSIS OF DIARRHEA IN THE INTENSIVE CARE UNIT SETTING

Iatrogenic causes
Medications
Enteral feeding
Pseudomembranous colitis
Diarrhea secondarily related to underlying disease
Infections in immunosuppressed patients
Neoplastic disease in immunosuppressed patients
Gastrointestinal bleeding
Neutropenic enteropathy
Ischemic bowel disease
Postsurgical diarrhea (postcholecystectomy, following gastric surgery)
Surgically induced short bowel syndrome or pancreatic insufficiency
Fecal impaction
Opiate withdrawal
Diarrhea as a primary manifestation of disease
Diabetic diarrhea
Renal failure
Sepsis
Adrenal insufficiency
Graft-versus-host disease
Vasculitis
Diarrhea-causing pathogens
Inflammatory bowel disease
Celiac sprue

TABLE 96.2

MEDICATIONS ASSOCIATED WITH DIARRHEA[a]

Antibiotics (especially erythromycin, ampicillin, clindamycin, azithromycin, cephalosporins)
Antacids (magnesium containing)
Magnesium and phosphorus supplements
Proton pump inhibitors
Lactulose
Colchicine
Digitalis
Quinidine
Theophylline
Levothyroxine
Aspirin
Nonsteroidal anti-inflammatory agents
Cimetidine
Misoprostol
Diuretics
Beta-blocking agents
Chemotherapeutic agents
Immunosuppressants (tacrolimus, sirolimus, mycophenolate mofetil, cyclosporine, azathioprine)
HIV medications (especially protease inhibitors, e.g., nelfinavir)
Oral hypoglycemics, e.g., metformin

[a]Additives in the physical formulation of medications (e.g., sorbitol, lactose) may produce diarrhea independently of the primary medication.

or combination of medications should be suspected, and uncertainty on the part of the physician warrants consultation with a pharmaceutical reference. Antibiotic-associated diarrhea occurs in 3% to 29% of hospitalized patients [5]. The frequency of diarrhea varies considerably depending on the antibiotic administered. The rate of diarrhea associated with parenterally administered antibiotics is comparable to orally administered antibiotics, especially antibiotics excreted into the enterohepatic circulation. Antibiotics most commonly associated with diarrhea include ampicillin, tetracycline, clindamycin, azithromycin, clarithromycin, fluoroquinolones, and many of the cephalosporins [6]. Antibiotic agents often cause a nonspecific, noninflammatory diarrhea associated with nausea, abdominal cramping, and bloating. In these instances, diagnostic studies generally are negative. Fluid and electrolyte losses are minimal and symptoms often abate after withdrawal or change of the medication. Alterations in intestinal flora, breakdown of dietary carbohydrate products, and prokinetic effects (e.g., from erythromycin) are all postulated mechanisms of diarrhea [7].

Clostridium difficile infection (CDI) is the most common cause of infectious diarrhea in the ICU [8]. In fact, residence in the ICU has been identified as a risk factor for developing CDI [9], and some authors believe that *C. difficile* toxins are responsible for 50% of the cases of diarrhea in the ICU setting. CDI in the ICU is increasing in not only in incidence but also in severity [10]. It can present as a serious and sometimes life-threatening complication. CDI must always be considered in ICU patients with diarrhea who are commonly exposed to various mediations, particularly antibiotics that predispose to the development of CDI. Classically, clindamycin, penicillin, and broad-spectrum cephalosporins have been implicated. However, CDI may be caused by any antibiotic, including metronidazole and vancomycin, the agents typically used to treat CDI. The risk factors associated with CDI, besides antibiotic exposure and environmental factors, include age greater than 60, severe underlying disease, gastric acid suppression, and immunologic susceptibility [7].

C. difficile produces multiple toxins, two of which have been well characterized. Toxin-induced changes in colonocyte function, cytokine release, and alterations in intestinal motility result in the signs and symptoms characteristic of CDI [11]. One strain of *C. difficile*, NAP1 (North American pulsed-field electrophoresis type 1), has been associated with both an increased morbidity and mortality [12]. Prompt recognition and treatment of CDI are essential because severe cases of CDI can progress to fulminant colitis and toxic megacolon requiring urgent surgical intervention.

Agents that increase the osmotic load in the gut lumen are also frequent causes of diarrhea in the ICU patient. Magnesium-containing antacids (e.g., Maalox and Mylanta) are common examples of such agents. The gut lumen osmotic load can also be increased as a result of aggressive enteral repletion of nutrients such as magnesium and phosphorus. Lactulose, a useful agent in the treatment of hepatic encephalopathy, provides an osmotic gradient resulting in increased fluid secretion and stool output. Many medications contain inert additives, sorbitol or lactose, which may also cause an osmotic diarrhea. In one study including 29 tube-fed patients with diarrhea, 48% of the cases were attributed to sorbitol-containing elixirs [13].

Proton pump inhibitors (PPIs), another commonly used class of medication in the ICU setting, frequently cause diarrhea, particularly when administered in higher doses. In fact, in a large study of more than 40,000 patients treated with omeprazole, lansoprazole, or pantoprazole, the most common adverse event was diarrhea [14].

Immunosuppressants used in transplantation (e.g., tacrolimus, sirolimus, mycophenolate mofetil, cyclosporine, and azathioprine) are associated with diarrhea. However, these agents may not be causative. As an example, an alternative explanation was found in 50% of kidney transplant patients who developed diarrhea while receiving mycophenolate [15]. In patients with HIV who are treated with highly active antiretroviral therapy (HAART), drug-induced diarrhea occurs in up to 75% of patients, and the protease inhibitors as well as integrase inhibitors are the most common drug-related cause of diarrhea in this population [16]. Symptoms are lessened by dose reduction or eliminated by discontinuation of therapy.

Withdrawal from medications (e.g., long-term sedatives, analgesics) may also be associated with diarrhea [17].

Other medications associated with diarrhea include colchicine, quinidine, digitalis, metoclopramide, theophylline, levothyroxine, aspirin, nonsteroidal anti-inflammatory drugs, misoprostol, cimetidine, diuretics, cholinergic agents (e.g., bethanechol), and beta-blockers.

Enteral Feedings

Enteral feedings are the most common cause of diarrhea in the ICU setting, occurring in up to 63% of ICU patients [1,18]. Numerous studies have investigated the role of enteral feedings in causing diarrhea in the critically ill patient. Certain aspects, such as concurrent administration of antibiotics, osmolality of solution, type of solution, and serum albumin, have been assessed to determine their contributing roles in the occurrence and severity of diarrhea in these patients [19]. In most instances, diarrhea in enterally fed patients is associated with concurrent antibiotic administration [18,20]. However, enteral feeds also cause changes in gut function that can result in diarrhea. The osmolarity of the enteral solution may play a role when elemental-type diets are used, and especially when feedings are rapidly administered directly into the small intestine. Bolus feeding may be more physiologic, especially with regard to glucose homeostasis; however, feedings administered in this manner distal to the pylorus introduce high-osmolar contents rapidly into the small bowel, resulting in a higher incidence of diarrhea [21]. The impact of enteral nutrition-related complications, including diarrhea, was illustrated in a prospective, multicenter cohort study of 400 patients [22]. In this study, 62.8% (251 of 400) patients suffered GI complication with 14.7% of the studied patients experiencing enteral nutrition-related diarrhea. These authors found that patients with GI complications had a reduction in their tube feed volumes, longer length of stay in the ICU, and higher mortality.

Enteral formulas high in lactose or fat content may also be a factor in susceptible patients. Starved or chronically parenterally fed patients who have developed small bowel villus atrophy and a decrease in mucosal disaccharidase enzyme activity may experience diarrhea when enteral feedings are initiated.

The relationship between hypoalbuminemia and diarrhea is controversial. Hwang et al. [2] compared ICU patients with and without diarrhea and found that the albumin level was statistically different between groups (1.90 g per dL vs. 3.40 g per dL in the groups with or without diarrhea, respectively). Hypoalbuminemia with resulting lowered oncotic pressure may cause diarrhea by inducing changes in the Starling forces sufficient to inhibit intestinal fluid absorption. Some authors claim that concurrent nutritional intake and correction of the albumin deficit with intravenous salt-poor albumin may result in normalization and maintenance of albumin levels with an improved tolerance to enteral feedings and resolution of diarrhea [23]. Conversely, patients with severe hypoalbuminemia secondary to cirrhosis or nephrotic syndrome do not uniformly have diarrhea. Until further studies show efficacy, routine use of intravenous albumin repletion cannot be recommended.

Studies investigating the role of the intestinal response to tube feedings have revealed that intraduodenal infusion resulted in a normal postprandial pattern of small intestinal motility and an increase in the volume of fluid entering the colon, but did not result in diarrhea [24]. Intragastric infusion, on the contrary, resulted in small intestinal motility and colonic flow similar to fasting, and the majority of subjects developed diarrhea [25]. This has led to the conclusion that enteral feeding–related diarrhea may be secondary to a disorder in colonic function. Further supporting this hypothesis are studies that have shown that the ascending colon, normally the site of maximal absorption of water and electrolytes, actually secretes water, sodium, and chloride during intragastric and intraduodenal infusion [26]. Up to 3.2 L per day was secreted by the ascending colon in these studies. Although this is well within the estimated 5.7 L per day maximal absorptive capacity of the colon, diarrhea still occurred, suggesting that this reversal of normal colonic physiology seriously impairs the absorptive capacity of the colon [27].

Diarrhea Secondarily Related to Underlying Disease

Diarrhea may result from various processes or pathogens associated with disease states commonly seen in the critically ill patient. Diarrhea may occur more frequently in patients who are immunosuppressed, have alterations in cardiac output and blood flow, or have various primary GI diseases.

In immunosuppressed patients, multiple infectious agents may be responsible for the development of diarrhea. Cytomegalovirus (CMV), herpes simplex virus, *Giardia*, *Salmonella*, *Shigella*, *Cryptosporidium*, *Isospora*, *Campylobacter*, and *Mycobacteria* are among the most common identifiable pathogens. Postchemotherapy patients can also experience diarrhea as a result of direct injury to the bowel, ranging from bowel edema to frank infarction. The cause of these changes is unclear; however, infections, direct toxic effects of chemotherapeutic agents, neutropenia, and primary intestinal injury have been postulated as initiating factors [28]. Strongyloides stercoralis should be remembered as a cause of diarrhea in patients who lived or traveled to endemic areas. Untreated immunosuppressed patients may develop hyperinfection with pulmonary infiltrates and infection of the CSF and blood with enteric Gram-negative bacilli [29].

In patients with acquired immunodeficiency syndrome (AIDS), diarrhea is perhaps the most commonly experienced symptom. Aside from iatrogenic causes, these patients can develop diarrhea from a single or multiple pathogens. CMV, *Mycobacterium* spp, *Cryptosporidium*, and *Microsporidium* are the most common agents. *Cryptosporidium* typically results in a severe large-volume secretory diarrhea (often in excess of 1 L per day) [30]. Other pathogens such as *Entamoeba histolytica*, *Isospora belli*, *Giardia lamblia*, *Microsporidium*, adenoviruses, and other species described above are capable of causing diarrhea in patients with AIDS [31]. Bacillary dysentery may become chronic and relapsing, posing challenges with treatment. The herpes simplex virus may cause perianal ulceration, urgency, and frequent mucopurulent discharge, which may be interpreted as diarrhea [32]. The CD4 count (cluster of differentiation 4 count) indicates the degree of immunocompromise in these patients, and a lower count broadens the differential diagnosis of the etiology of diarrhea. *Cryptosporidium parvum*, *Enterocytozoon bieneusi*, *Encephalitozoon intestinalis*, *Mycobacterium avium* complex (MAC), and enteroaggregative *Escherichia coli* cause self-limited disease in normal and mildly immunosuppressed individuals, but may cause persistent, severe diarrhea in patients with CD4 counts less than 200 cells per mm [3,33–37]. CMV rarely causes diarrhea in patients with CD4 counts greater than 50 cells per mm [3,38]. Patients with AIDS also may develop high-grade intestinal lymphomas predominantly of B-cell origin, which may present as diarrhea. Kaposi's sarcoma may cause GI bleeding but rarely causes diarrhea [39].

Intestinal ischemia, especially involving the colon, may result in abdominal pain and diarrhea in the ICU patient. Postsurgical patients, especially those who have undergone repair of an abdominal aortic aneurysm, may have as high as a 6% incidence of colonoscopically documented ischemia [40]. Patients who have undergone an abdominoperineal resection or therapeutic angiography are also at risk. Compromise of the inferior mesenteric artery with left-sided colonic involvement is the primary etiologic factor. Symptoms may occur within hours to a few days following the procedure and may even be delayed for weeks. Patients in shock with depressed cardiac output may be more likely to present with right-sided colonic involvement, which is associated with a worse prognosis [41]. Severity can range from mild, transient ischemic changes to mucosal ulceration or bowel necrosis. Sympathomimetic drugs, vasopressin, ergot preparations, migraine therapies, alosetron, bevacizumab, and digoxin may further place susceptible patients at risk [42]. Likewise, small intestinal ischemia, especially venous ischemia, may present with bloody or nonbloody diarrhea. Bleeding of either the upper or lower GI tract is a frequent cause of bloody diarrhea in the ICU setting. Blood acts as both an irritant and osmotic agent resulting in diarrhea. Common causes of upper GI bleeding include esophagitis, gastric and duodenal ulcer disease, and hemorrhagic gastropathy, whereas infectious colitis, diverticulosis, and ischemia may result in lower GI bleeding.

Fecal impaction in both medical and surgical patients may cause diarrhea and should be considered in the ICU patient with diarrhea. Drugs such as analgesics, sedatives, aluminum-containing antacids, and sucralfate may decrease intestinal motility and fecal fluidity, resulting in formation of a partially obstructing fecal mass and diarrhea. Diverticulitis also may present with an accompanying diarrhea.

Diarrhea as a Primary Manifestation of Disease

Several common diseases are occasionally characterized by diarrhea during their courses. For instance, patients with diabetes can experience severe bouts of diarrhea. Diabetic diarrhea is thought to result from an autonomic neuropathy and its subsequent effect on intestinal fluid absorption [43]. These patients invariably have other signs of autonomic neuropathy including orthostatic hypotension, gastroparesis, anhidrosis, abnormalities in RR wave variation on electrocardiogram, and neurogenic bladder [44]. Abnormalities in motility with intestinal stasis and bacterial overgrowth may also play a role in the development of diarrhea in diabetic patients.

Other endocrine disorders such as adrenal insufficiency and hyperthyroidism should also be considered in the critically ill patient with diarrhea. Adrenal insufficiency, either primary adrenal failure as a result of result of bilateral adrenal hemorrhage or infarction, or relative deficiency induced by stress in patients chronically exposed to corticosteroids, may present with secretory diarrhea. The symptoms and signs of an adrenal crisis include shock, nausea, vomiting, diarrhea, abdominal pain, fever, fatigue, and sometimes confusion or coma. Patients with hyperthyroidism have increased fecal output largely due to increased intestinal motility [45].

Graft-versus-host disease (GVHD) may complicate both the short- and long-term course of patients who have undergone transplant (most commonly following allogeneic hematopoietic stem cell transplantation) [46,47]. Acute GVHD, occurring less than 100 days after transplant, typically is characterized by dermatitis, hepatitis, and gastroenteritis usually manifesting with nausea, abdominal pain, and diarrhea. Chronic GVHD (occurring more than 100 days after transplantation) may mimic autoimmune diseases, such as systemic lupus erythematosus, systemic sclerosis, or Sjogren's syndrome [48] and often is characterized by a less severe form of diarrhea.

Vasculitic diseases such as systemic lupus erythematosus, dermatomyositis, polyarteritis, and Wegener's granulomatosis can involve medium- and small-sized vessels supplying the GI tract. Abdominal pain, fever, bleeding, and diarrhea are common resulting symptoms.

Finally, one must always consider causes of diarrheal disease that are not unique to the critically ill patient. Infectious causes of diarrhea in immunocompetent hospitalized patients are possible, but are unusual in clinical practice unless the onset of the diarrhea is within the first few days of hospitalization or a nosocomial outbreak of infection is present [49]. Infectious causes that should be considered include *Salmonella*, *Shigella*, *Campylobacter*, *Giardia*, or *E. histolytica*, although other pathogens have also been implicated [50]. Nonenteric infectious causes of diarrhea include toxic shock syndrome and Legionnaires' disease. Other causes to be considered include lactose intolerance, inflammatory bowel disease, and celiac sprue.

DIAGNOSIS

History and Physical Examination

The history is important in establishing the diagnosis and etiology of diarrhea in the ICU patient; however, depressed neurological function as the result of the disease state or iatrogenic sedation and intubation may make obtaining a history impossible. Attention to onset, duration, character, relation to enteral intake, and associated symptoms of diarrhea may be helpful etiologic clues. Information on prior episodes of diarrhea, the patient's underlying medical conditions (which may be associated with diarrhea), or prior use of antibiotics is also important to elucidate. Next, a careful review of the patient's current medications and their administration relative to the onset of diarrhea should be performed. Any suspected agent should be discontinued if at all possible or changed to an alternative medication. Every effort should be made at decreasing the number of medications and continuing only those that are absolutely necessary. The physician should also determine whether the initiation of enteral feedings has correlated with the onset of symptoms.

A history of abdominal pain may suggest ischemia, infection, or various inflammatory conditions such as vasculitis or GVHD. Bloody diarrhea may suggest primary GI bleeding, ischemia, or occasionally pseudomembranous colitis secondary to CDI. Passage of frequent small-volume stools with urgency and tenesmus suggests distal, left-sided colonic involvement, whereas passage of less frequent, large-volume stools suggests more proximal involvement (small intestine or right colon). These historical clues, however, are not mutually exclusive, and in disease states with extensive bowel involvement, the distinction may not be appreciable.

Physical examination may provide further clues to the etiology of diarrhea, but findings are usually nonspecific. More important, the physical examination is essential in assessing the clinical severity of diarrhea. Orthostasis suggests severe volume loss, adrenal insufficiency, or autonomic neuropathy (e.g., from diabetes). Fever may occur in individuals with infection, vasculitis, adrenal insufficiency, or hyperthyroidism. Abdominal tenderness may suggest infectious, ischemic, or vasculitic causes. Skin rashes or mucosal ulcerations in appropriate patients may suggest inflammatory bowel disease, vasculitis, or GVHD. Clinical manifestations of AIDS may be apparent. Abdominal distention, palpable bowel loops, or abnormal rectal examination may suggest a partially obstructing fecal impaction.

Laboratory Studies

Serum electrolytes especially sodium, potassium, magnesium, and phosphorus should be obtained and carefully monitored in patients with diarrhea. Severe diarrhea may result in a hyperchloremic metabolic acidosis and prerenal azotemia. The serum sodium may be normal, elevated, or depressed depending on the severity of diarrhea, oral/parenteral water intake, type of intravenous fluid administered, and other disease states (e.g., hepatic or renal dysfunction). The serum potassium, magnesium, and phosphorus may be normal or depressed, whereas elevations (e.g., in potassium) may suggest adrenal insufficiency or uremia. Leukocytosis may suggest infection or ischemia, whereas neutropenia may suggest an immunosuppressed state or sepsis. Low serum protein levels may be a clue to the presence of a protein-losing gastroenteropathy.

Examination of the stool may be the single most important and most overlooked laboratory investigation in the ICU patient with diarrhea. The presence of fecal leukocytes should be determined, and when present may suggest infection, ischemia, or mucosal inflammation. Newer assays for fecal calprotectin and lactoferrin have been validated for use in dysentery and inflammatory bowel disease, but its usefulness in the ICU setting requires study [51]. An assay for *C. difficile* should always be obtained; most toxin assays are enzyme immunoassays and are typically very specific, although 100 to 1,000 pg of toxin A or B must be present to obtain a positive result. Because testing two or three samples for the toxins improves the diagnostic yield by only 5% to 10% [14], consideration should be given for obtaining polymerase chain reaction (PCR) testing rather than ordering serial toxin assays if the clinical suspicion remains high. Cytopathic effect on cultured fibroblasts is more sensitive than the toxin assay but is not offered in many laboratories.

Fresh stool specimens for culture and ova and parasite examination should be requested in patients where there is a clinical suspicion, for example, in dysenteric presentations or when either fecal leukocytes or an elevated fecal calprotectin is found. Indiscriminate ordering of stool culture and O&P is not warranted. Immunosuppressed patients, however, require more extensive examination of the stool. Often, opportunistic pathogens are not detected readily through stool studies, and endoscopic examination with biopsies is required. Some pathogens such as CMV or MAC isolated from stool do not necessarily represent infection and require evidence of tissue invasion on biopsy for diagnosis.

Qualitative examination of the stool for fat using a Sudan III stain is the best screening test if a malabsorptive state is suspected. Determination of the stool osmolar gap, which is $290 - [(\text{stool } [Na^+] + \text{stool } [K^+]) \times 2]$, helps to distinguish osmotic and secretory causes of watery diarrhea. A gap grater than 125 mOsm per L is conventional for an osmotic diarrhea. High-volume stool output that persists with fasting suggests a secretory etiology, whereas an elevated stool osmolar gap suggests osmotic causes. A low stool pH may suggest bacterial overgrowth or carbohydrate malabsorption [4].

Special Diagnostic Investigations

Plain abdominal radiographs are sometimes helpful and may show signs of ischemia, obstruction, perforation, or a megacolon associated with colitis. Contrast studies better define GI pathology that may result in diarrhea but often cannot be performed in a critically ill patient. Both the above study types have been in practice supplanted by computed tomography (CT); newer imaging modalities, such as CT enterography and magnetic resonance enterography, are quickly replacing the more cumbersome enteroclysis and may be useful in selected cases.

Flexible sigmoidoscopy, colonoscopy, and upper endoscopy can be extremely useful in diagnosing various causes of diarrhea. Colitides, including infectious, ischemic/vasculitic, and pseudomembranous colitis, will often have a characteristic endoscopic appearance. The classic findings in *C. difficile* colitis include distinct, adherent, raised plaques (pseudomembranes) 2 to 5 mm in size that may be confluent. More commonly, the mucosa is normal; a normal appearance should not exclude the diagnosis of CDI, as mucosal biopsies may reveal pseudomembranes histologically. CMV or herpes colitis are best diagnosed endoscopically. CMV colitis may manifest as discrete ulcerations or widespread mucosal edema, erythema, and erosion. The characteristic vesicles of herpes may or may not be present and can be replaced by extensive ulceration. MAC (aforementioned) usually is diagnosed histologically; small bowel or colonic biopsies reveal abundant acid-fast bacilli. *Cryptosporidium* and *Giardia* can be made by histologic evaluation of small bowel biopsies, whereas identification of *Microsporidium* is more difficult and requires the use of electron microscopy. GVHD is confirmed most commonly by histopathological findings seen in biopsies obtained during flexible sigmoidoscopy.

Video capsule endoscopy, where a 12 mm capsule is either swallowed or placed in the small bowel endoscopically, captures via telemetry images of the entire small bowel. The mucosal detail provided is excellent, and so small bowel ulcerations, villus abnormalities, strictures, and other mucosal lesions are now more readily detected. Small bowel ulcerations, villus abnormalities, strictures, and other mucosal lesions are now more readily detected. For example, capsule endoscopy allows for a more precise gauge of the extent of Crohn's disease and celiac disease, and eosinophilic gastroenteritis has a characteristic capsule endoscopic appearance [52]. Although this technology permits detection of occult small bowel pathology not previously appreciated, its possible role and value in the diagnosis of persisting diarrhea in the ICU patient is unknown.

MANAGEMENT

Initial Management

The first and most important step in management of patients with diarrhea regardless of the etiology is correction of fluid and electrolyte imbalances (Fig. 96.1). Careful monitoring of the patient's physical and laboratory parameters will help guide replacement therapy. Most often, free water, sodium, potassium, phosphorus, or magnesium repletion will be required. If fluid losses are particularly severe or the patient's circulatory status is tenuous or compromised, central venous access and monitoring are essential. Physicians and nursing staff should ensure that proper patient hygiene and skin care are maintained. Suspected infectious causes of diarrhea warrant patient isolation and enteric precautions until a diagnosis is made and proper treatment instituted.

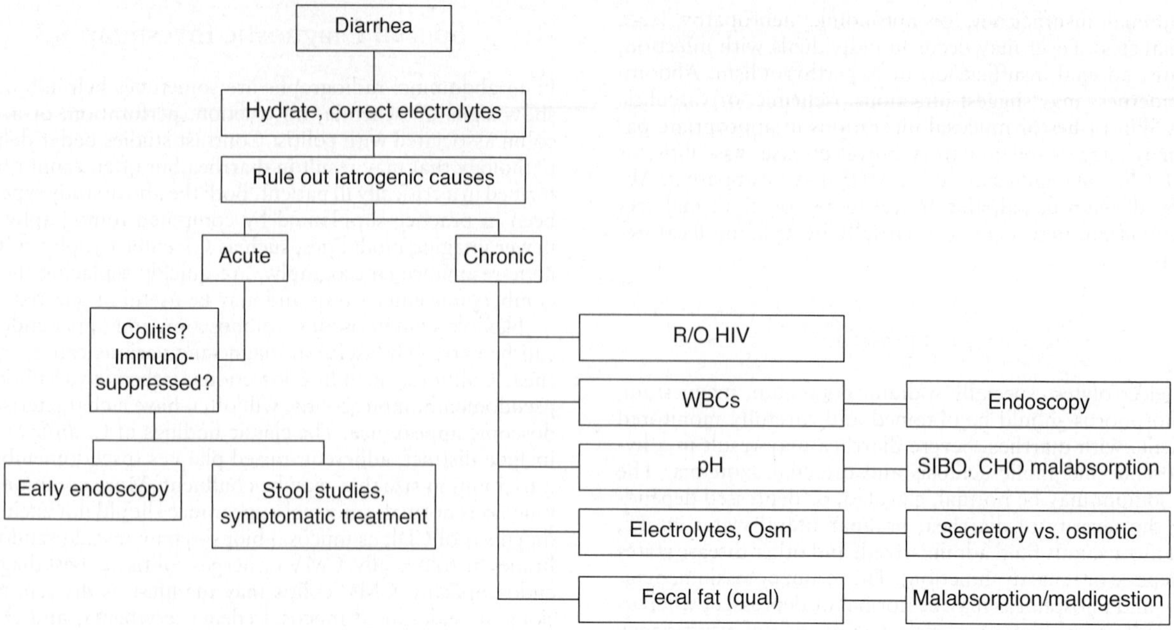

FIGURE 96.1. Algorithm for management of diarrhea in the intensive care unit.

Therapy of Iatrogenic Causes

Iatrogenic causes of diarrhea are among the most readily diagnosed and easily treated etiologies. Suspect medications, especially antibiotics, should be withdrawn or changed to those less likely to cause diarrhea.

If a diagnosis of *C. difficile* colitis is suspected or made, the offending antibiotic should be discontinued, or if necessary, replaced by agents less likely to cause CDI (Table 96.3). Vancomycin administered by the enteral route (0.5 to 2 g per day) has been a time-honored and highly efficacious therapy, resulting in improvement in more than 95% of patients [53]. Expense and concern over the selection of vancomycin-resistant bacteria, however, are major drawbacks. Several trials and a recent Cochrane meta-analysis show equal efficacy between metronidazole and vancomycin [54–56]. Thus, vancomycin should be reserved for those patients who cannot tolerate, do not respond to metronidazole, or suffer repeated relapses of infection. Metronidazole can be given 250 mg four times daily or 500 mg three times daily for 10 to 14 days. Patients will generally respond within 24 to 48 hours with improvement in diarrhea, pain, fever, and leukocytosis. Although there are limited data, two small studies have suggested that intravenous metronidazole is also useful for the treatment of CDI [55]. Intravenous vancomycin should not be used to treat CDI, as it is not excreted in the stool [57,58]. In severe cases of *C. difficile* colitis, high doses of oral vancomycin (500 mg four times daily) are preferred. If the patient has an ileus or toxic megacolon, intravenous metronidazole should be administered. One small series demonstrated benefit with the administration of vancomycin enemas in patients with severe pseudomembranous colitis [59]. Relapse rates may be high, occurring in as many as 24% of patients [60]. Case reports of successful salvage of toxic pseudomembranous colitis using intravenous immune globulin were not supported by a single-center, retrospective cohort [61]. Bile salt–binding resins such as cholestyramine or colestipol may be useful as adjunctive therapy in mild cases or in relapses but should not be used exclusively, especially in moderate to severe diarrhea. These agents can bind vancomycin, making this combination less desirable.

Small trials have suggested a benefit using probiotics for both primary and secondary prevention of antibiotic-associated diarrhea. A recent meta-analysis of these trials concluded that they may reduce the incidence of antibiotic-associated diarrhea (AAD) by about half, although there was significant heterogeneity in the trials [62]. Treatment studies for CDI have not demonstrated a significant benefit [63], and there have been several case reports of *Saccharomyces cerevisiae* fungemia in critically ill and immunocompromised patients who had been given probiotics containing *Saccharomyces boulardii*, which has identical DNA fingerprinting to *S. cerevisiae*. Given these case reports, probiotics cannot be recommended for the treatment of antibiotic-associated diarrhea in the critically ill patient [64].

Data are now emerging that exposure to PPIs is associated with increased odds of CDI in hospitalized patients. The postulate that acid suppression causes enteric infections seems reasonable but remains controversial. These data are observational and thus may be subject to uncontrolled confounding.

TABLE 96.3

TREATMENT OF *CLOSTRIDIUM DIFFICILE* COLITIS

General
Discontinue offending antibiotic if possible
Avoid antimotility agents
Isolation with enteric precautions
Antimicrobial
Metronidazole 250 mg PO q.i.d. or 500 mg t.i.d. for 10–14 d[a]
Vancomycin 125–500 mg PO q.i.d. for 7–14 d
Anion exchange resins (in combination with metronidazole in mild cases)
Cholestyramine 4 g PO t.i.d.
Colestipol 5 g PO t.i.d.

[a]If the patient has an ileus or toxic megacolon, metronidazole should be administered intravenously.

TABLE 96.4

A SUMMARY OF THE EVIDENCE-BASED MANAGEMENT APPROACHES FOR *CLOSTRIDIUM DIFFICILE*–RELATED DIARRHEA

- Vancomycin and metronidazole are equally effective in treating diarrhea from *C. difficile* colitis[a,b]
- Rates of recurrent *C. difficile*–associated disease following treatment with vancomycin or metronidazole are not significantly different[b]
- Tapered or pulsed dosing regimens of vancomycin are more effective than a 10- to 14-day course of vancomycin for the treatment of recurrent *C. difficile*–associated disease[c]

[a]Teasley DG, Gerding DN, Olson M, et al: Prospective randomised trial of metronidazole versus vancomycin for *Clostridium difficile*–associated diarrhea and colitis. *Lancet* 2:1043, 1983.
[b]Wenisch C, Parschalk B, Hasenhündl M, et al: Comparison of vancomycin, teicoplanin, metronidazole, and fusidic acid for the treatment of *Clostridium difficile*–associated diarrhea. *Clin Infect Dis* 22:813, 1996.
[c]McFarland LV, Elmer GW, Surawicz CM, et al: Breaking the cycle: treatment strategies for 163 cases of recurrent *Clostridium difficile* disease. *Am J Gastroenterol* 97:1769, 2002.

Nonetheless, it is prudent to review the indication for PPI prescription in all patients and restrict use of these drugs appropriately [65].

Antimotility agents should not be used in colitis, because they may lengthen the course of illness and may precipitate toxic megacolon [66]. If the patient with *C. difficile* colitis develops peritoneal signs, bacteremia unresponsive to antibiotics, progressive fever, rigors, or radiologic evidence of significant pericolonic inflammation with increasing bowel wall edema, surgical intervention is indicated [67]. The recommended procedure is subtotal colectomy with ileostomy, with possible ileorectal anastomosis after the inflammation has subsided. A summary of the evidence-based treatment approaches for *C. difficile*–related diarrhea is provided in Table 96.4.

There are several controlled trials now available which demonstrate the effectiveness of octreotide in chemotherapy and radiation-associated acute diarrhea. Doses range in these studies from 100 to 500 μg given subcutaneously twice or three times daily. Budesonide is not helpful in these settings [68].

Enteral feedings suspected of causing diarrhea should be reduced in volume, given by continuous infusion, or temporarily discontinued. Lactose-free feeds should be used, as the high incidence of stress-induced GI mucosal injury in the ICU population affects loss of disaccharidase activity. Fiber-containing formulas or fiber added to standard formulas may benefit ICU patients with tube feeding-associated diarrhea [69,70]. Elemental diet supplements may also be considered in patients with short bowel syndrome, pancreatic insufficiency, radiation enteritis, fistula, and inflammatory bowel disease. Their major disadvantages are high cost and increased osmolarity [71].

Treatment of Diarrhea Related to Disease

Efforts should always be made to treat the underlying disease causing diarrhea in the critically ill patient, although such efforts may or may not improve the diarrhea. Diarrhea secondary to sepsis will typically resolve, as the source of sepsis is treated, whereas diarrhea secondary to diabetes or uremia may not improve despite treatment of the primary disease.

Diarrhea-causing pathogens should, in general, be treated. The detection of *Blastocystis hominis* in parasite exams may indicate coinfection with other pathogens, and empiric nitazoxanide or metronidazole may be beneficial [72]. Infections in patients with AIDS and other immunocompromised settings are treatable with currently available therapy [73,74].

Patients with ischemic colitis without transmural necrosis may be managed with supportive care. Drugs that exacerbate ischemia should be discontinued if possible. Aggressive efforts at maintaining circulatory blood volume and maximizing oxygen delivery should be emphasized. Signs of infarction or perforation warrant operative management.

Fistulas should be managed by bowel rest or surgery depending on the clinical circumstances. Postcholecystectomy diarrhea may respond to bile acid sequestrants such as cholestyramine. Surgically induced cases of short bowel syndrome or malabsorption may be aided by enteral nutrition in the form of elemental diets or, if unsuccessful, parenteral nutrition. Fecal impactions should be removed by manual disimpaction followed by cleansing enemas consisting of tap water, sodium phosphate, or diatrizoate (water-soluble contrast) enemas. More proximal and firm impactions can be broken up using a sigmoidoscope and an irrigating device by directing a water jet into the fecal mass under direct vision. Prevention following treatment with appropriate laxatives or enemas is paramount.

Treatment of Diarrhea as a Primary Manifestation of Disease

Every effort should be made to treat the disease responsible for the diarrheal syndrome. General supportive measures previously discussed should also be employed in all patients. Diseases such as vasculitis should be managed with corticosteroid or immunosuppressive therapy. Adrenal insufficiency will respond promptly to the administration of corticosteroids. Hyperthyroid patients should receive appropriate therapies. GVHD should be managed with corticosteroids and immunosuppressive agents. The chronic form of the disease may be

TABLE 96.5

ANTIDIARRHEAL AGENTS AND DOSAGES

Loperamide (Imodium)
- Available forms: capsules (2 mg) and liquid (5 mL [1 tsp] = 1 mg)
- Dosage: 4 mg initially, followed by 2 mg after each diarrheal stool
- Maximum daily recommended dose: 16 mg per day

Diphenoxylate with atropine (Lomotil)
- Available forms: 1 tablet or 5 mL liquid = 2.5 mg diphenoxylate and 0.025 atropine
- Dosage: 2 tablets or 10 mL 4 times a day (20 mg of diphenoxylate) initially, then decrease and titrate to symptoms
- Maximum daily recommended dose: 20 mg/d (based on diphenoxylate)

Deodorized opium tincture
- Available form: 10 mg morphine per mL
- Dosage: 0.6 mL 4 times a day (range: 0.3–1 mL 4–6 times a day)
- Maximum daily recommended dose: 6 mL/d

Camphorated opium tincture (paregoric)
- Available form: 0.4 mg morphine per mL
- Dosage: 5–10 mL 1–4 times a day
- Maximum daily recommended dose: 40 mL/d

more effectively treated, whereas the acute variety may be less responsive, with a substantial mortality rate. Treatment of the inflammatory bowel diseases is address in another chapter, but generally includes aminosalicylates, corticosteroids, immunomodulating agents, biologics, and surgery. Celiac sprue will respond to supportive measures and a gluten-free diet.

Palliative Measures

The aforementioned diagnostic and therapeutic approaches will result in proper diagnosis and directed treatment in a majority of patients with diarrhea in the critical care setting. In a modest number of patients, however, a cause for diarrhea will not be found or a specific treatment will not be readily available. For this category of patients, palliative therapies are available with the goal to lessen fluid losses, patient discomfort, and morbidity (Table 96.5). Antimotility agents such as loperamide, diphenoxylate with atropine, and deodorized tincture of opium (DTO) may decrease frequency and severity of diarrhea in patients with diarrhea of unclear etiology or diarrhea due to enteral feeding or other noninfectious causes. Advantages of loperamide include the absence of central nervous system activity and resultant side effects, whereas DTO is administered in drop form, enhancing dosing flexibility. Octreotide can be used for palliation of diarrhea in patients with AIDS, GVHD, hormone-producing tumors, radiation- and chemotherapy-induced diarrhea, and other causes of secretory diarrhea [75].

CONCLUSION

Diarrhea is a frequently occurring complication in the ICU setting. It is a symptom that tends to be overshadowed by other processes in the ICU, but in and of itself may result in significant morbidity. In most instances, it can be managed following institution of proper diagnostic, therapeutic, or palliative measures.

References

1. Kelly T, Patrick M, Hillman K, et al: Study of diarrhea in critically ill patients. *Crit Care Med* 11:7, 1983.
2. Hwang TL, Lue MC, Nee YJ, et al: The incidence of diarrhea in patients with hypoalbuminemia due to acute or chronic malnutrition during enteral feeding. *Am J Gastroenterol* 89:376; 1994.
3. Dark D, Pingleton S: Nonhemorrhagic gastrointestinal complications in acute respiratory failure. *Crit Care Med* 17:755, 1989.
4. Fine KD, Schiller L: AGA technical review on the evaluation and management of chronic diarrhea. *Gastroenterology* 116:1464, 1999.
5. McFarland LV: Diarrhea acquired in the hospital. *Gastroenterol Clin North Am* 22:563, 1993.
6. Gilbert DN: Aspects of the safety profile of oral antimicrobial agents. *Infect Dis Clin Pract* 4[Suppl 2]:S103, 1995.
7. Dublerke ER, Reshe KA, Yan Y, et al: *Clostridium difficile* associated disease in a setting of endemicity: identification of novel risk factors. *Clin Infect Disease* 45:1543–1549, 2007.
8. Lialios A, Oropello JM, Benjamin E: Gastrointestinal complications in the intensive care unit. *Clin Chest Med* 20:329–345, 1999.
9. Brown E, Talbot G, Axelrod P, et al: Risk factors for *Clostridium difficile* toxin-associated diarrhea. *Infect Control Hosp Epidemiol* 11:283, 1990.
10. Zilberberg MD: *Clostridium difficile*–related hospitalization among US adults, 2006. *Emerg Infect Dis* 15:122–124, 2009.
11. Voth DE, Ballard JD: *Clostridium difficile* toxins: mechanism of action and role in disease. *Clin Microbiol Rev* 18:247–263, 2005.
12. Loo VG, Poirier L, Miller MA, et al: A pre-dominantly clonal multi-institutional outbreak of *C. difficile* associated diarrhea with high morbidity and mortality. *N Engl J Med* 353:2442–2449, 2005.
13. Edes T, Walk B, Austin J: Diarrhea in tube fed patients: feeding formula not necessarily the cause. *Am J Med* 88:91, 1990.
14. Martin R, Dunn N, Freemantle S, et al: The rates of common adverse events reported during treatment with proton pump inhibitors used in general practice in England. *Br J Clin Pharmacol* 50:366, 2000.
15. Maes B, Hadaya K, de Moor B, et al: Severe diarrhea in renal transplant patients: results of the DIDACT study. *Am J Transplant* 6:1466, 2006.
16. Reijers M, Weigel H, Hart A, et al: Toxicity and drug exposure in a quadruple drug regimen in HIV-1 infected patients participating in the ADAM study. *AIDS* 14:59, 2000.
17. Isto E, VanDyke M, Gimble C, et al: Withdrawal symptoms in critically ill children after long-term administration of sedatives and/or analgesics: a first evaluation. *Crit Care Med* 36:2427–2432, 2008.
18. Keohane P, Attrill H, Love M, et al: Relation between osmolality of diet and gastrointestinal side effects in enteral nutrition. *Br Med J* 288:678, 1984.
19. Cataldi-Betcher E, Seltzer M, Slocum B, et al: Complications occurring during enteral nutritional support: a prospective study. *JPEN J Parenter Enteral Nutr* 7:546, 1983.
20. Keohane P, Attrill H, Jones B, et al: Roles of lactose and *Clostridium difficile* in the pathogenesis of enteral feeding associated diarrhoea. *Clin Nutr* 1:259, 1983.
21. McHugh P, Moran T: Calories and gastric emptying: a regulatory capacity with implications for feeding. *Am J Physiol* 236:254, 1979.
22. Montejo J: Enteral nutrition-relation gastrointestinal complications in critically ill patients: a multicenter study. *Crit Care Med* 27:1447, 1999.
23. Ford E, Jennings L, Andrassy RJ: Serum albumin (oncotic pressure) correlates with enteral feeding tolerance in the pediatric surgical patient. *J Pediatr Surg* 22:7, 1987.
24. Raimundo A, Rogers J, Grimble G, et al: Colonic inflow and small bowel motility during intraduodenal enteral nutrition. *Gut* 29:A1469, 1988.
25. Raimundo A, Rogers J, Silk D: Is enteral feeding related to diarrhoea initiated by an abnormal colonic response to intragastric diet infusion? [abstract] *Gut* 31:A1195, 1990.
26. Bowling T, Raimundo A, Grimble G, et al: Colonic secretory effect in response to enteral feeding in man. *Gut* 35:1734, 1994.
27. Bowling T, Silk D: Colonic responses to enteral tube feeding. *Gut* 42:147, 1998.
28. Starnes H, Moore F, Mentzer S, et al: Abdominal pain in neutropenic cancer patients. *Cancer* 57:616, 1986.
29. Longworth DL, Weller PF: Hyperinfection syndrome with strongyloidiasis. *Curr Clin Top Infect Dis* 7:1–26, 1986.
30. Rodgers V, Kagnoff M: Gastrointestinal manifestations of the acquired immunodeficiency syndrome. *West J Med* 146:57, 1987.
31. Santangelo W, Krejs G: Southwestern Internal Medicine Conference. The gastrointestinal manifestations of the acquired immunodeficiency syndrome. *Am J Med Sci* 292:328, 1986.
32. Baker R, Peppercorn M: Gastrointestinal ailments of homosexual men. *Medicine (Baltimore)* 61:390, 1982.
33. Flanigan T, Whalen C, Turner J, et al: Cryptosporidium infection and CD4 counts. *Ann Intern Med* 116:840, 1992.
34. Asmuth D, DeGirolami P, Federman M, et al: Clinical features of microsporidiosis in patients with AIDS. *Clin Infect Dis* 18:819, 1994.
35. Horsburgh CJ: *Mycobacterium avium* complex infection in the acquired immunodeficiency syndrome. *N Engl J Med* 324:1332, 1991.
36. Durrer P, Zbinden R, Fleisch F, et al: Intestinal infection due to enteroaggregative *Escherichia coli* among human immunodeficiency virus-infected persons. *J Infect Dis* 182:1540, 2000.
37. Wanke C, Mayer H, Weber R, et al: Enteroaggregative *Escherichia coli* as a potential cause of diarrheal disease in adults infected with human immunodeficiency virus. *J Infect Dis* 178:185, 1998.
38. Gallant J, Moore R, Richman D, et al: Incidence and natural history of cytomegalovirus disease in patients with advanced human immunodeficiency virus disease treated with zidovudine. *J Infect Dis* 166:1223, 1992.
39. Weber J, Carmichael D, Boylston A, et al: Kaposi's sarcoma of the bowel presenting as apparent ulcerative colitis. *Gut* 26:295, 1985.
40. Ernst C, Hagihara P, Daugherty M, et al: Ischemic colitis incidence following aortic reconstruction: a prospective study. *Surgery* 80:417, 1976.
41. Sotiriadis J, Brandt LJ: Ischemic colitis has a worse prognosis when isolated to the right side of the colon. *Am J Gastroenterol* 102:2247, 2007.
42. Mueller P, Benowitz N: Toxicologic causes of acute abdominal disorders. *Emerg Med Clin North Am* 7:667, 1989.
43. Chang E, Bergenstal R, Field M: Diarrhea in streptozocin treated rats. *J Clin Invest* 75:1666, 1985.
44. Whalen G, Soergel K, Geenen J: Diabetic diarrhea. *Gastroenterology* 56:1021, 1969.
45. Ryan J, Sleisenger M: Effects of systemic and extraintestinal disease on the gut, in Slesenger M, Fordtran J (eds): *Gastrointestinal Disease*. Philadelphia, WB Saunders, 1993, p 193.
46. McDonald G, Shulman H, Sullivan K, et al: Intestinal and hepatic complications of human bone marrow transplantation. Part I. *Gastroenterology* 90:460, 1986.
47. McDonald G, Shulman H, Sullivan K, et al: Intestinal and hepatic complications of human bone marrow transplantation. Part II. *Gastroenterology* 90:770, 1986.
48. Flowers ME, Kansu E, Sullivan KM: Pathophysiology and treatment of graft-versus-host disease. *Hematol Oncol Clin North Am* 13:1091, 1999.

49. Siegel D, Edelstein P, Nachamkin I: Inappropriate testing of diarrheal diseases in the hospital. *JAMA* 263:979, 1990.
50. Fine K, Krejs G, Fordtran J: Infectious diarrhea, in Sleisenger M, Fordtran J (eds): *Gastrointestinal Disease*. Philadelphia, WB Saunders, 1993, p 1128.
51. Shastri YM, Bergis D, Povse N, et al: Prospective multicenter study evaluating fecal calprotectin in adult acute bacterial diarrhea. *Am J Med* 121:1099, 2008.
52. May A, Manner H, Schneider M, et al: Prospective multicenter trial of capsule endoscopy in patients with chronic abdominal pain, diarrhea and other signs and symptoms (CEDAP-Plus Study). *Endoscopy* 39:606, 2007.
53. Bartlett J: Treatment of *Clostridium difficile* colitis. *Gastroenterology* 89:1192, 1985.
54. Teasley D, Gerding D, Olson M, et al: Prospective randomized trial of metronidazole versus vancomycin for *Clostridium difficile* associated diarrhea and colitis. *Lancet* 2:1043, 1983.
55. Zar FA, Bakkanagari SR, Moorthi KM, et al: A comparison of vancomycin and metronidazole for the treatment of *Clostridium difficile*-associated diarrhea, stratified by disease severity. *Clin Infect Dis* 45:302, 2007.
56. Nelson, RL: Antibiotic treatment for *Clostridium difficile*-associated diarrhea in adults. *Cochrane Database Syst Rev* 18:CD004610, 2007.
57. Bolton R, Culshaw M: Faecal metronidazole concentrations during oral and intravenous therapy for antibiotic associated colitis due to *Clostridium difficile*. *Gut* 27:1169, 1986.
58. Friedenberg F, Fernandez A, Kaul V, et al: Intravenous metronidazole for the treatment of *Clostridium difficile* colitis. *Dis Colon Rectum* 44:1176, 2001.
59. Apisarnthanarak A, Razari B, Mundy LM, et al: Adjunctive intracolonic vancomycin for severe *Clostridium difficile* colitis. *Dis Colon Rectum* 44:1176, 2001.
60. Bartlett J, Tedesco F, Schull S, et al: Relapse following oral vancomycin therapy of antibiotic-associated pseudomembranous colitis. *Gastroenterology* 78:431, 1979.
61. Juang P, Skledar SJ, Zgheib NK, et al: Clinical outcomes of intravenous immune globulin in severe *Clostridium difficile*-associated diarrhea. *Am J Infect Control* 35:131, 2007.
62. McFarland LV: Meta-analysis of probiotics for the prevention of antibiotic associated diarrhea and the treatment of *Clostridium difficile* disease. *Am J Gastroenterol* 101:812, 2006.
63. Dendukuri N, Costa V, McGregor M, et al: Probiotic therapy for the prevention and treatment of *Clostridium difficile*-associated diarrhea: a systematic review. *CMAJ* 173(2):167, 2005.
64. Munoz P, Bouza E, Cuenca-Estrella M, et al: *Saccharomyces cerevisiae* fungemia: an emerging infectious disease. *Clin Infect Dis* 40(11):1625, 2005.
65. Dial MS: Proton pump inhibitor use and enteric infections. *Am J Gastroenterol* 104:S10, 2007.
66. Rubin M, Bodenstein L, Kent C: Severe *Clostridium difficile* colitis. *Dis Colon Rectum* 38:350, 1995.
67. Lipsett P, Samantaray D, Tam M, et al: Pseudomembranous colitis: a surgical disease. *Surgery* 116:491, 1994.
68. Karthaus M, Ballo H, Abenhardt W, et al: Prospective, double-blind, placebo-controlled, multicenter, randomized phase III study with orally administered budesonide for prevention of irinotecan (CPT-11)-induced diarrhea in patients with advanced colorectal cancer. *Oncology* 68:326, 2005.
69. Shimoni Z, Averbuch Y: The addition of fiber and the use of continuous infusion decrease the incidence of diarrhea in elderly tube-fed patients in medical wards of a general regional hospital: a controlled clinical trial. *J Clin Gastroenterol* 41:901, 2007.
70. Rushdi TA, Pichard C, Khater YH: Control of diarrhea by fiber-enriched diet in ICU patients on enteral nutrition: a prospective randomized controlled trial. *Clin Nutr* 23:1344, 2004.
71. Randall H: Enteral nutrition: tube feeding in acute and chronic illness. *J Parenter Enteral Nutr* 8:113, 1984.
72. Rossignol JF, Kabil SM, Said M, et al: Effect of nitazoxanide in persistent diarrhea and enteritis associated with *Blastocystis hominis*. *Clin Gastroenterol Hepatol* 3:987, 2005.
73. Gilbert DN, Moellering RC, Eliopoulos G, et al: *The Sanford Guide to Antimicrobial Therapy 2009*. Sperryville, VA, Antimicrobial Therapy, 2009.
74. Bartlett J: *The Johns Hopkins Hospital 2004 Guide to Medical Care of Patients with HIV Infection*. Philapelphia, PA: Williams & Wilkins, 2004.
75. Gorden P, Comi R, Maton P, et al: Somatostatin and somatostatin analogue (SMS201995) in treatment of hormone-secreting tumors of the pituitary and gastrointestinal tract and non-neoplastic diseases of the gut. *Ann Intern Med* 110:35, 1989.

CHAPTER 97 ■ SEVERE AND COMPLICATED BILIARY TRACT DISEASE

JOHN M. ISKANDER, SREENIVASA S. JONNALAGADDA AND RIAD AZAR

A wide spectrum of biliary tract diseases may be seen in the intensive care unit (ICU). Presentations vary from mildly abnormal blood chemistries to life-threatening septic shock. Unrecognized biliary disease can lead to significant morbidity. Awareness of the different biliary disorders commonly encountered in the ICU, in conjunction with a logical approach to noninvasive and invasive patient evaluation, allows the clinician to diagnose and treat these conditions appropriately.

The anatomy of the biliary tract is depicted in Figure 97.1. Approximately 500 mL of bile is secreted at the level of the canaliculus each day. Bile flows through progressively larger ductules until reaching the main bile ducts. The bile duct courses through or immediately adjacent to the head of the pancreas in more than 90% of patients. Hence, any pathology in the head of the pancreas can result in biliary obstruction. Bile flow into the duodenum is regulated by the sphincter of Oddi, which consists of muscle fibers that surround the distal bile duct in the wall of the duodenum at the major ampulla. Tonic contraction of the sphincter increases pressure in the common bile duct and allows the gallbladder to fill in a retrograde fashion through the cystic duct. A gallstone passing from the gallbladder to the duodenum typically would encounter resistance to passage in the region of the cystic duct and at the sphincter of Oddi. Biliary tree pathology can be diagnosed by transabdominal ultrasonography, computed tomography (CT), magnetic resonance cholangiopancreatography, endoscopic retrograde cholangiopancreatography (ERCP), or endoscopic ultrasonography (EUS). Access to the biliary tree for therapeutic purposes may be obtained via ERCP, percutaneously, or at open surgery.

DIAGNOSTIC EVALUATION

Physical Examination

Physical signs in patients with biliary tract disease may encompass a spectrum from the acute abdomen with localized right upper quadrant pain to nonspecific findings including ileus, fever, or sepsis with hemodynamic instability. When biliary tract disease is suspected, careful inspection and examination for findings of icterus, hepatomegaly, ascites, and focal tenderness over the liver or gallbladder should be undertaken.

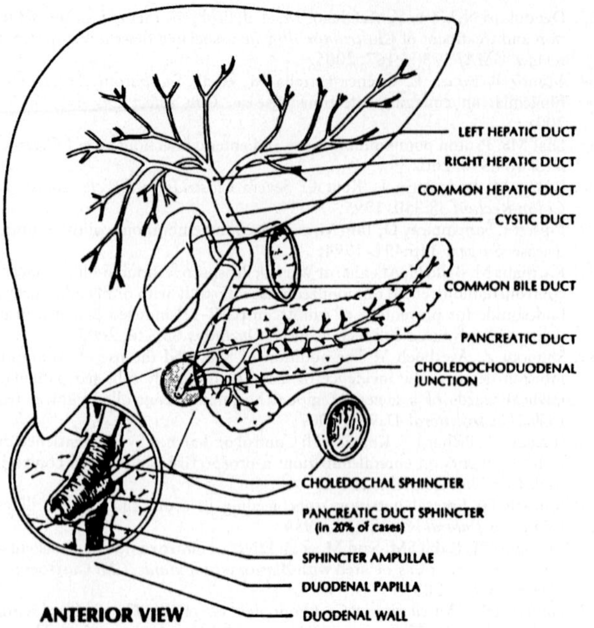

FIGURE 97.1. Normal anatomy of the biliary tract. [From Turner MA, Cho S-R, Messmer JM: Pitfalls in cholangiographic interpretation. *Radiographics* 7:1067, 1987, with permission.]

Laboratory Evaluation

In the obtunded or otherwise compromised ICU patient, abnormal laboratory values often are the first clue to biliary tract disease. All ICU patients should have appropriate laboratory testing on admission, including serum bilirubin, alkaline phosphatase, and transaminases (aspartate aminotransferase or alanine aminotransferase). Although elevations in bilirubin should result in an evaluation for an obstructive process, other processes such as sepsis, drug effects, hemolysis, or other nonbiliary etiologies should be considered in an acutely ill patient (see Chapters 99 and 150). Alkaline phosphatase elevation is often seen in patients with biliary tract disease, but it is not specific. The hepatobiliary origin of an elevated serum level of this enzyme can be confirmed by detection of concomitantly elevated 5′-nucleotidase or γ-glutamyltransferase. Serum transaminase elevations are the hallmark of hepatocellular injury. However, an elevation in transaminases can also be seen in patients with bile duct obstruction, and may precede elevation of bilirubin and alkaline phosphatase in the acute setting. Occasionally, a patient with significant biliary disease may present with a normal laboratory evaluation, as in cholecystitis without involvement of the common bile duct and without substantial pericholecystitic hepatitis.

Noninvasive Imaging Studies

Noninvasive radiologic imaging is essential in the evaluation of patients with suspected biliary tract disease.

Plain Abdominal Radiograph

The plain radiographic features of biliary tract disease usually are nonspecific [1]. The most common bowel gas finding seen in patients with acute biliary disease is a generalized ileus. Gallstones rarely are detected on plain radiographs, because only 20% of stones have a sufficient calcium concentration to make them radiopaque. Air in the biliary tree may result from a biliary-enteric fistula, prior sphincterotomy, or a biliary-enteric surgical anastomosis. Infections with gas-producing organisms rarely present with gas in the biliary tree or gallbladder wall.

Ultrasonography

Ultrasonography of the biliary tree is an extremely useful diagnostic test in the ICU setting and can be performed at bedside with good results [2]. It is a sensitive test for determining biliary ductal dilatation, and the accuracy of ultrasonography in detecting cholelithiasis exceeds 95%. However, its accuracy in detecting choledocholithiasis may be limited, as gas in the duodenum can obscure visualization of the distal bile duct. In the presence of cholelithiasis or gallbladder sludge, the findings of ductal dilatation, elevated liver enzymes, abdominal pain, and fever are strongly suggestive of cholangitis. Findings on ultrasonography that may indicate acute gallbladder disease include focal tenderness over the gallbladder, thickening of the gallbladder wall, and pericholecystitic fluid collections, but none is specific for cholecystitis. The technique also may detect other abnormalities, including liver lesions, pancreatic masses, abscesses, and ascites.

Hepatobiliary Scanning

Scanning the abdomen after an intravenous injection of technetium-99m iminodiacetic acid yields physiologic and structural information regarding the biliary tract. Filling the gallbladder with radionuclide confirms the patency of the cystic duct and virtually excludes the diagnosis of acute cholecystitis. False-positive examinations can be seen in patients with chronic cholecystitis, on long-term parenteral hyperalimentation, or after prolonged fasting. Delayed views and routine pretreatment with cholecystokinin increase the accuracy of technetium-99m iminodiacetic acid scanning for acute cholecystitis to greater than 93% [3]. Hepatobiliary scanning is also useful in identifying structural abnormalities of the biliary tree such as significant bile duct leaks, which can be identified in almost all patients with this problem. Scanning has a limited role in patients with poor hepatocellular function, complete biliary obstruction, and cholangitis because these defects often prevent adequate uptake or excretion of the radiopharmaceutical into the biliary tree.

Computed Tomography

CT is highly accurate for the detection of biliary tract disease [4]. The sensitivity for detecting choledocholithiasis is as high as 88% using helical CT. Unlike ultrasonography or radionuclide scanning, however, CT cannot be used portably in the ICU. Findings on CT for gallbladder disease include thickening of the gallbladder wall, pericholecystitic fluid, and adjacent abscesses. In addition, CT is highly accurate for the detection of biliary tract obstruction (i.e., the level and the cause). It also allows detailed visualization of the pancreas, vessels, and surrounding organs and can be used to assess the severity of pancreatitis including complications such as necrotizing pancreatitis or the formation of pseudocysts.

Magnetic Resonance Imaging

Advances in magnetic resonance imaging (MRI) technology have greatly improved the resolution of biliary imaging [5]. The use of magnetic resonance cholangiogram images can be manipulated to display highly accurate representations of the biliary tree. The sensitivity of this technique rivals that of direct cholangiography. In one study, the overall sensitivity and specificity of magnetic resonance cholangiograms for diagnosis of bile duct stones were 100% and 95.6%, respectively, with corresponding positive and negative predictive values of 92.6% and 100% [6]. This technique also permits visualization of any mass contiguous to a bile duct stricture. In the intensive care setting, its use may be limited as patients must be transported to the scanner, and problems with magnetic compatibility of support equipment must be overcome. The noninvasive images of the biliary tree obtained, however, can be highly diagnostic and preclude other more invasive studies.

Summary

When evaluating the ICU patient with suspected biliary tract disease, ultrasonography should be the initial procedure of choice, followed by hepatobiliary scanning if cystic duct obstruction or bile leakage is suspected. Both are portable and noninvasive. Ultrasonography is highly accurate for the detection of gallstones and structural pathology. Hepatobiliary scanning, on the contrary, provides physiologic information, primarily regarding patency of the cystic duct. Such physiologic data are especially important for patients with suspected calculous or acalculous cholecystitis. CT or MRI should be reserved for those patients in whom sonographic or radionuclide findings are equivocal, if other intra-abdominal pathology needs to be excluded, or if ductal dilatation is seen on ultrasonography without a clearly defined etiology.

Invasive Diagnostic Tests

Endoscopic Retrograde Cholangiopancreatography

The technique of ERCP is used for both diagnostic and therapeutic purposes as described in Chapter 13. In brief, a side-viewing endoscope is passed through the mouth into the second duodenum, where the major ampulla is identified and cannulated. The biliary tree is then opacified with contrast injected through a catheter, allowing a retrograde cholangiogram to be obtained. Fluoroscopy and standard radiographs are used to examine the biliary tree and define such abnormalities as stones, strictures, leaks, and obstruction. Endoscopic therapy, including stone removal, biliary drainage, or stricture dilatation, can be accomplished in the same setting. ERCP can be used in the evaluation and therapy of the ICU patient, especially if the patient can be stabilized for endoscopy and transported to a fluoroscopy room. Rarely is it necessary to perform emergent biliary decompression at the bedside using portable fluoroscopy. Coagulopathies should be corrected before the procedure, especially if an endoscopic sphincterotomy (electrocautery incision of the sphincter of Oddi in the duodenal wall for stone removal or drainage) is anticipated. If coagulopathies cannot be satisfactorily corrected, a stent can be placed into the bile duct to ensure drainage without performing a sphincterotomy. Major morbidity from the diagnostic procedure includes pancreatitis, cholangitis, perforation, and hemorrhage. The complication rates of ERCP in a recent review noted reduced rates, compared with prior reporting, of pancreatitis at 3.5%, infection at 1.4%, and perforation at 0.6% under standard conditions [7]. The value of ERCP is largely operator dependent and can be highly successful in the delineation and treatment of biliary disease in the ICU patient [8].

Endoscopic Ultrasonography

EUS involves the transoral passage of an endoscope with an ultrasonic transducer at the tip. The limitations of transabdominal ultrasonography are overcome with this modality because all areas of the biliary tree, including the intrapancreatic portion of the bile duct as well as the pancreas, can be imaged without interference from gas in the intestines. EUS can reliably identify cholelithiasis and is more sensitive than transabdominal ultrasonography in detecting choledocholithiasis in patients with biliary pancreatitis. Although EUS is typically an elective procedure and uncommonly used in the ICU, the test may be useful in identifying those patients who would benefit from endoscopic stone extraction by ERCP [9].

Percutaneous Transhepatic Cholangiography

Percutaneous transhepatic cholangiography (PTC) also may be used in evaluating the ICU patient. The technique requires fluoroscopy to guide passage of a needle into the intrahepatic bile ducts. The biliary tree is then filled with contrast and images are taken. The use of PTC for the diagnosis of biliary tract pathology has been supplanted by ERCP and noninvasive examinations, such as ultrasonography, CT, and MRI. Currently, PTC is used primarily as an initial step in percutaneous transhepatic biliary drainage. Decompression of the biliary tree via a percutaneous catheter is a highly effective method for rapid nonoperative and nonendoscopic biliary decompression. This procedure is indicated when a patient requires emergent biliary drainage but is not stable enough to undergo ERCP under conscious sedation, if the major papilla cannot be reached endoscopically because of postsurgical anatomy or a technical failure in cannulating the bile duct. The technique involves an initial PTC to delineate the biliary anatomy, followed by selective cannulation of an appropriate intrahepatic bile duct with an 18-gauge needle. A guidewire is then passed into the biliary tree, the tract is dilated, and a drainage catheter placed. Successful drainage can be established in almost all patients. Percutaneous biliary drainage is an invasive procedure, and acute complications, including hemorrhage, sepsis, and bile leakage, occur in 1% to 5% of patients [10].

Percutaneous Liver Biopsy

Liver biopsy is an important technique in the evaluation of selected patients with hepatobiliary abnormalities who do not have obvious biliary ductal dilatation. Liver biopsy may lead to a rapid pathologic diagnosis in patients with intrinsic liver disease. In cases of infection, tissue can also be cultured. In patients with a coagulopathy, a liver biopsy may be obtained by way of the hepatic vein using a transjugular approach or percutaneously using a sheath, embolizing the tract after completion of the biopsy [11].

BILIARY TRACT DISORDERS ENCOUNTERED IN THE INTENSIVE CARE UNIT

Cholangitis

Acute cholangitis is a life-threatening illness. The presentation of patients with cholangitis may range from intermittent low-grade fevers to fulminant septic shock. This diagnosis must be considered and excluded in all patients who present to the ICU with shock and sepsis of unknown origin because of the high mortality if urgent biliary decompression is not accomplished. As partial or complete biliary obstruction is a prerequisite to the pathophysiology of cholangitis, it typically occurs in patients with biliary stasis secondary to stones, strictures, or recent manipulations of the biliary tree [12]. Bacteremia occurs when bacterial infection of the biliary tree is associated with an elevated intraductal pressure that allows reflux of bacteria into the portal venous circulation and bloodstream.

The clinical manifestations of cholangitis include fever or chills, abdominal pain, and jaundice. The classic triad of fever, right upper quadrant pain, and jaundice was described by Charcot [13] in 1877 and is seen in a small percentage of patients presenting with cholangitis [12]. Laboratory abnormalities are present in the overwhelming majority of patients, with more than 90% having elevation of bilirubin, alkaline phosphatase, or transaminases. Blood cultures are positive in more than a third of patients [13,14], and solitary isolates of *Escherichia coli*, *Klebsiella pneumoniae*, or enterococcus are found most commonly. Polymicrobial infections, including anaerobes, are identified frequently if bile is cultured at operation [15,16]. Often it is difficult to prospectively diagnose cholangitis in the ICU population, and this entity should be considered in the differential diagnosis of all patients who present with sepsis.

Since most patients with cholangitis will demonstrate gallstones or a dilated biliary tree, an abdominal ultrasound is the best initial evaluation. This, in association with elevated liver enzymes, fever, or sepsis, is strongly indicative of this diagnosis and should prompt early consultation for therapeutics.

Treatment

Once cholangitis is suspected, the patient should be treated empirically with broad-spectrum antibiotics. Recent trials demonstrated the use of the extended-spectrum penicillins, cephalosporins, and ciprofloxacin in this setting [16,17]. Although most patients respond to antibiotic therapy alone, those with biliary obstruction may progress to a more fulminant state despite general resuscitative measures and broad-spectrum antibiotics. These patients must be identified rapidly and treated with emergent biliary decompression. This can be accomplished by endoscopic, percutaneous, or surgical means. Selection of a particular approach should be tailored to the patient's condition, local expertise, and the rapid availability of the procedure. Initial efforts in decompensated patients should concentrate on decompression of the biliary tree via ERCP or percutaneous drainage. Definitive therapy may be accomplished at a later time, even if this requires a second procedure. It must be recognized that even with modern support, biliary decompressive techniques, and broad-spectrum antibiotics, the mortality from acute fulminant cholangitis ranges from 10% to 50% [12,14].

Biliary Obstruction

Biliary obstruction may present in the ICU patient without cholangitis. The multiple causes of biliary obstruction are listed in Table 97.1, the most common being stone disease, benign stricture, and malignancy. The patient with physical findings and laboratory studies suggesting obstruction should initially be evaluated with noninvasive imaging to define the level of obstruction and determine the etiology. In the noninfected patient, an elective direct cholangiogram by ERCP or PTC should be obtained when the patient's condition allows. This provides anatomic details of the biliary tree and allows for definitive therapy planning. Care must be taken to ensure that the entire biliary tree is visualized at cholangiography and that adequate prophylactic antibiotics are administered. In addition, adequate biliary decompression after the procedure is essential to prevent the development of cholangitis.

Biliary obstruction without cholangitis is seen more often with malignancy than with stone disease or inflammatory strictures. The diagnosis can usually be made before laparotomy with ERCP or PTC. Definitive therapy for stone disease and benign strictures as well as palliative therapy for malignant strictures may also be accomplished during either procedure. Reviews of endoscopic or transhepatic stenting of malignancies demonstrate the use of these approaches when compared with surgical decompression for unresectable disease [18,19]. Surgical approaches are preferred in those patients who are good operative candidates and who may have resectable malignancy. Bile duct stenting often serves as a bridge to surgery in such patients.

TABLE 97.1

CAUSES OF BILIARY OBSTRUCTION

Intrinsic lesions
Stones
Cholangiocarcinoma
Benign stricture
Sclerosing cholangitis
Periarteritis nodosa
Ampullary stenosis
Parasites
Extrinsic lesions
Pancreatic carcinoma
Metastatic carcinoma
Pancreatitis
Pancreatic pseudocyst
Visceral artery aneurysm
Lymphadenopathy
Choledochal cyst
Hepatic cyst(s)
Duodenal diverticulum
Iatrogenic lesions
Postoperative stricture
Hepatic artery infusion chemotherapy

Bile Leaks

A bile leak may be seen after open or laparoscopic cholecystectomy, hepatic resection, liver transplantation, or trauma to the liver from penetrating abdominal injuries. In a postcholecystectomy setting, such a leak may occur from the cystic duct stump or branches of the right intrahepatic ductal system via the gallbladder fossa. The extravasated bile may accumulate focally to form a biloma or freely flow within the peritoneal cavity. The resultant bile peritonitis usually is associated with abdominal pain, ascites, leukocytosis, and fever. Occasionally, collections of bile become infected, resulting in an abscess if untreated. Seldom, patients may present solely with new-onset ascites and an elevated serum bilirubin level. Diagnosis of a biliary leak can usually be made with hepatobiliary scanning. Ultrasonography and CT may reveal a biloma or free fluid in the abdominal cavity. This can be followed by ERCP to determine the exact location of the leak and provide definitive therapy.

Patients with suspected bile leaks should be placed on broad-spectrum antibiotics, and the presence of a bile leak should be confirmed with hepatobiliary scanning followed by direct cholangiography. ERCP with therapeutic intent should be performed as soon as possible after diagnosis to limit the degree of bile leakage and patient symptoms. Postoperative leaks or premature removal of a T-tube often can be managed definitively with endoscopic decompression at the same setting as ERCP. This is accomplished by placing a biliary stent across the major papilla with or without concomitant biliary sphincterotomy. Rarely, if endoscopic therapy is unsuccessful in healing a bile leak, surgical repair may be required.

Acute Cholecystitis

Acute cholecystitis is a frequent and important event that occurs in the ICU. The signs and symptoms of acute cholecystitis often are not readily apparent in the compromised ICU patient. A high degree of suspicion and prompt use of noninvasive testing, including ultrasonography and hepatobiliary scanning, are essential to arrive at a timely and correct diagnosis of this entity. Acalculous cholecystitis deserves special mention because it can result in significant morbidity and mortality in the ICU patient [20]. Although the signs and symptoms may be similar to those seen with calculous cholecystitis, the presentation in the postoperative or acutely ill ICU patient may be masked by the complicated underlying situation. In this setting, an aggressive diagnostic and therapeutic approach is essential because significant morbidity and even mortality continues to occur from complicated acalculous cholecystitis.

Supportive measures should be undertaken while the patient is being evaluated with noninvasive testing. Antibiotic therapy with broad-spectrum coverage should be initiated in patients with clinical evidence of sepsis, leukocytosis, or fever. Percutaneous cholecystostomy has become the therapy of choice for patients with acute calculous or acalculous cholecystitis who do not respond to conservative therapy and are too unstable for operative cholecystectomy. Percutaneous cholecystostomy is performed at the bedside using ultrasound guidance. A 22-gauge needle is inserted transhepatically into the gallbladder, and bile is aspirated. A guidewire is passed through this needle and the tract is dilated, allowing placement of a drainage catheter, with success rates exceeding 95%. Complications are few and include local wound infection, bleeding, and, rarely, bile peritonitis. The primary advantage of percutaneous cholecystostomy is that it can be done at the bedside without general anesthesia. Percutaneous cholecystostomy often is helpful in patients with suspected gallbladder disease, even if cholecystitis is not found, by excluding the diagnosis. Therefore, percutaneous cholecystostomy should be performed early if gallbladder disease is suspected. The cholecystostomy drainage catheter is left in place until acute symptoms resolve, at which time an elective surgical cholecystectomy or, in the setting of a patent cystic duct and functioning gallbladder, simple tube removal may be performed. In patients with acute calculous cholecystitis and severe underlying medical problems, the gallstones can be removed through the percutaneous tract using various techniques [21]. Such percutaneous gallstone removal is an effective alternate therapy to cholecystectomy for patients with other significant medical conditions.

Gallstone Pancreatitis

Acute pancreatitis often results from biliary stone disease. Although most cases are self-limited and respond to conservative management, fulminant pancreatitis may occur with mortality in excess of 10%. There are several theories regarding the pathogenesis of gallstone pancreatitis, the most accepted being that stone passage or impaction in the ampulla is responsible for this entity. Gallstone pancreatitis should be considered and excluded in the evaluation of all patients with acute pancreatitis because it is a recurrent and treatable cause of this presentation. Standard abdominal ultrasound in combination with laboratory screening for biliary obstruction can be used to exclude gallstones as the cause for the pancreatitis in most patients [22]. Patients with acute pancreatitis should be classified into risk groups based on one of the accepted prognostic scales [23]. These scales include the Ranson criteria, the Glasgow criteria, the Acute Physiology and Chronic Health Evaluation III scoring system, and CT criteria for grading severity of pancreatitis. Grading by CT is based on the degree of inflammation, the presence of fluid collections, and the area of pancreatic necrosis seen during bolus infusion of intravenous contrast while scanning. These prognostic scales allow physicians to identify patients who are at risk for developing severe pancreatitis and a complicated hospital course. Three or more of the following criteria defined by Ranson [23] at any time during the first 48 hours of hospitalization predict severe pancreatitis.

At admission or diagnosis:

1. Age older than 55 years
2. White blood cell count greater than 16,000 cells per mm^3
3. Blood glucose greater than 200 mg per dL
4. Serum lactate dehydrogenase greater than 350 IU per L
5. Serum aspartate aminotransferase greater than 250 Sigma-Frankel units per dL

During the initial 48 hours:

1. Hematocrit fall greater than 10%
2. Blood urea nitrogen rise greater than 5 mg per dL
3. Serum calcium level less than 8.0 mg per dL
4. Arterial oxygen partial pressure less than 60 mm Hg
5. Base deficit greater than 4 mEq per L
6. Estimated fluid sequestration greater than 6,000 mL

Patients with acute pancreatitis from biliary stone disease should be managed initially as detailed in Chapter 99. Although most patients improve with conservative therapy alone, patients with severe gallstone pancreatitis (three or more prognostic criteria) and high likelihood of having choledocholithiasis, cholangitis, or persisting biliary colic may benefit from early intervention with ERCP. Early ERCP [24,25] allows the removal of impacted or retained common bile duct stones, limiting further pancreatic inflammation and preventing cholangitis. Consultation with a skilled biliary endoscopist should be obtained early in the course of all patients with severe gallstone pancreatitis. It is generally accepted that patients with gallstone pancreatitis require definitive therapy to prevent recurrent bouts. This may be accomplished by cholecystectomy or endoscopic sphincterotomy with stone extraction in nonoperative candidates. Although debate continues regarding the timing of surgery, it is generally accepted that all patients who are operative candidates should undergo cholecystectomy during the initial hospital admission after the pancreatitis has subsided [26]. Early operative intervention in patients with active severe gallstone pancreatitis has been associated with unacceptably high morbidity [26].

Summary

The management of biliary tract disorders encountered in the ICU varies with the specific disorder. Several of the evidence-based treatment approaches are listed in Table 97.2.

TABLE 97.2

EVIDENCE-BASED MANAGEMENT APPROACHES FOR BILIARY TRACT DISORDERS ENCOUNTERED IN THE INTENSIVE CARE UNIT

- Early ERCP is beneficial in the management of biliary pancreatitis [25].
- ERCP is highly effective in the management of postoperative bile leaks [27].
- In patients with cholangitis, empiric antibiotic therapy should be directed against Gram-negative bacteria [28].
- Percutaneous cholecystostomy offers an important therapeutic alternative for critically ill patients with acute cholecystitis [29].

ERCP, endoscopic retrograde cholangiopancreatography.

References

1. Roszler MH: Plain film radiologic examination of the abdomen. *Crit Care Clin* 10:277, 1994.
2. Romano WM, Platt JF: Ultrasound of the abdomen. *Crit Care Clin* 10:297, 1994.
3. Davis LP, Fink-Bennett D: Nuclear medicine in the acutely ill patient. I. *Crit Care Clin* 10:365, 1994.
4. Zingas AP: Computed tomography of the abdomen in the critically ill. *Crit Care Clin* 10:321, 1994.
5. Reinhold C, Bret PM: Current status of MR cholangiopancreatography. *AJR Am J Roentgenol* 166:1285, 1996.
6. Demartines N, Eisner L, Schnabel K, et al: Evaluation of magnetic resonance cholangiography in the management of bile duct stones. *Arch Surg* 135:148, 2000.
7. Andriulli A, Loperfido S, Napolitano G, et al: Incidence rates of post-ERCP complications: a systematic survey of prospective studies. *Am J Gastroenterol* 102(8):1781–8, 2007.
8. Cohen SA, Siegel JH: Biliary tract emergencies endoscopic and medical management. *Crit Care Clin* 11:273, 1995.
9. Chak A, Hawes RH, Cooper GS, et al: Prospective assessment of the utility of EUS in the evaluation of gallstone pancreatitis. *Gastrointest Endosc* 49:599, 1999.
10. Zparchez Z: Percutaneous biliary drainage. Indications, performances, and complications. *J Gastrointestin Liver Dis* 13(2):139–146, 2004.
11. Sawyer AM, McCormick PA, Tennyson GS, et al: A comparison of transjugular and plugged-percutaneous liver biopsy in patients with impaired coagulation. *J Hepatol* 17:81, 1993.
12. Lai EC, Chu K, Ngan H: Acute cholangitis, in Pitt HA, Carr-Locke DL, Ferrucci JT (eds): *Hepatobiliary and Pancreatic Disease, The Team Approach to Management*. Boston, MA, Little, Brown and Company, 1995, p 229.
13. Charcot JM: *Lecons sur les maladies du foie des voiesbiliaires et des viens*. Paris, Faculte de Medecine de Paris. Recueilles et publiees par Bourneville et Sevestre, 1877.
14. Sinanan MN: Acute cholangitis. *Infect Dis Clin North Am* 6:571, 1992.
15. Pitt HA, Postier RG, Cameron JL: Consequences of preoperative cholangitis and its treatment on the outcome of surgery for choledocholithiasis. *Surgery* 94:447, 1983.
16. Leung JWL, Ling TKW, Chan RCY, et al: Antibiotics, biliary sepsis, and bile duct stones. *Gastrointest Endosc* 40:716, 1994.
17. Sung JJ, Lyon DJ, Suen R, et al: Intravenous ciprofloxacin as treatment for patients with acute suppurative cholangitis: a randomized, controlled clinical trial. *J Antimicrob Chemother* 35:855, 1995.
18. Brandabur JJ, Kozarek RA, Ball TJ, et al: Non-operative versus operative treatment of obstructive jaundice in pancreatic cancer: cost and survival analysis. *Am J Gastroenterol* 83:1132, 1988.
19. Shepherd HA, Royle G, Ross APR, et al: Endoscopic biliary endoprosthesis in the palliation of malignant obstruction of the distal common bile duct: a randomized trial. *Br J Surg* 75:1166, 1988.
20. Barie PS, Fischer E: Acute acalculous cholecystitis. *J Am Coll Surg* 180:232, 1995.
21. Picus D, Hicks ME, Darcy MD, et al: Percutaneous cholecystolithotomy: analysis of results and complications in 58 consecutive patients. *Radiology* 183:799, 1992.
22. Wang SS, Lin XZ, Tsai YT, et al: Clinical significance of ultrasonography, computed tomography, and biochemical tests in the rapid diagnosis of gallstone-related pancreatitis: a prospective study. *Pancreas* 3:153, 1988.
23. Ranson JH: The current management of acute pancreatitis. *Adv Surg* 28:93, 1995.
24. Carr-Locke DL: Role of endoscopy in gallstone pancreatitis. *Am J Surg* 165:519, 1993.
25. Fan ST, Edward CS, Lai EC, et al: Early treatment of acute biliary pancreatitis by endoscopic papillotomy. *N Engl J Med* 328:228, 1993.
26. Kelly TR, Wagner DS: Gallstone pancreatitis: a prospective randomized trial of the timing of surgery. *Surgery* 104:600, 1988.
27. Barkun AN, Rezieg M, Mehta SN, et al: Postcholecystectomy biliary leaks in the laparoscopic era: risk factors, presentation, and management. McGill Gallstone Treatment Group. *Gastrointest Endoscopy* 45:277, 1997.
28. Rerknimitr R, Fogel EL, Kalayci C, et al: Microbiology of bile in patients with cholangitis or cholestasis with and without plastic biliary endoprosthesis. *Gastrointest Endoscopy* 56:885, 2002.
29. Melin MM, Sarr MG, Bender CE, et al: Percutaneous cholecystostomy: a valuable technique in high-risk patients with presumed acute cholecystitis. *Br J Surg* 82:1274, 1995.

CHAPTER 98 ■ HEPATIC DYSFUNCTION

MAURICIO LISKER-MELMAN AND GOWRI KULARATNA

Liver function abnormalities are detected in about 50% of intensive care unit (ICU) patients, often leading to hepatology consultation [1]. The presentation of hepatic dysfunction range from simple abnormalities in biochemical tests with little impact on a patient's clinical course to complex manifestations of liver failure that require prompt intervention and have high morbidity and mortality. Etiologies of hepatic dysfunction are many and variable in this setting. Sometimes, a detailed clinical history is sufficient to establish the cause of the derangement; however, a combination of clinical experience and judicious use of supplemental testing is required to establish a specific diagnosis and suggest a therapeutic course of action. Understanding the anatomic interactions between the liver and other organs and the physiologic principles that determine hepatic function is essential for establishing a rational therapeutic approach for each disorder. In this chapter, we outline aspects of liver physiology that are altered in critically ill patients and review common disorders of hepatic dysfunction seen in this setting.

PHYSIOLOGIC CONSIDERATIONS

Blood Flow

In resting conditions, the liver receives 25% of the cardiac output and 10% to 15% of the total body blood volume. About 25% of the liver volume consists of blood (capacitance function). The human liver has dual blood supply. Approximately one third of the hepatic blood flow is supplied by the hepatic artery (low-flow, high-pressure system, well-oxygenated blood) and two thirds by the portal vein (high-flow, low-pressure system, poorly oxygenated blood). The hepatic artery supplies the capsule of the liver and bile ducts. The portal vein is formed by the splenic vein, superior mesenteric vein, and inferior mesenteric vein (it drains into the splenic vein). The left gastric vein branches from the portal vein and plays a fundamental role in the formation of esophageal varices in patients with portal hypertension. The portal vein provides venous drainage for several abdominal organs: pancreas, stomach, intestine, and spleen. Once within the liver, arterial and venous bloods mix in the hepatic sinusoids [2]. The sinusoids are involved in the exchange between the blood, space of Disse, and the hepatocytes. The blood flowing through the sinusoids is collected in the central veins and then into the hepatic veins and inferior vena cava.

The sinusoids are composed of fenestrated endothelial cells, Kupffer cells, stellate cells, and natural killer (NK) cells. Endothelial cells represent 50% of the sinusoidal cells. They contain numerous fenestrae (not uniform in size or distribution) with dynamic structure and function. Endothelial cells have several functions including endocytosis, secretion (interleukins, interferon, eicosanoids, endothelin, and nitric oxide), and expression of adhesion molecules. Kupffer cells are phagocytic and remove infective, toxic, and foreign substances from the portal blood. They also release substances involved in the immune response by the liver. Stellate cells, also known as lipocytes, fat storing cells, or Ito cells, store fat vacuoles (major storage sites of retinoids). They have contractile activity regulating the blood flow through the sinusoids. The NK cells, also known as Pit cells are liver-associated lymphocytes with azurophilic granules with lysosomal activity [3,4].

Blood flow through the liver varies considerably under different physiologic conditions. In the normal state, the liver extracts less than half of its supplied oxygen (4.6 mg per minute per 100 g liver). Thus, in most conditions of increased oxygen demand, the liver can increase oxygen extraction without an alteration in blood flow [5]. Regulation of total hepatic blood flow occurs primarily at the level of the hepatic artery. If portal venous inflow decreases, compensation is accomplished through vasodilatation of the hepatic artery. However, reductions in mean arterial pressure below 50 mm Hg exceed the capacity of the autoregulatory mechanisms to maintain adequate liver perfusion [6].

Bilirubin Metabolism

The majority of bilirubin (80%) is generated from the breakdown of heme released by senescent red blood cells. Unconjugated bilirubin (indirect bilirubin) circulates bound to albumin before entering the hepatocyte through an active process mediated by transporter proteins. Once inside the hepatocyte, unconjugated bilirubin is transferred to the smooth endoplasmic reticulum, where it is conjugated with glucuronic acid (conjugated or direct bilirubin) and, in turn, secreted into the biliary canaliculi by a pump called multidrug resistance protein 2. Once in the gastrointestinal tract, bilirubin is deconjugated by gut bacteria enzymes and oxidized to stercobilin and eliminated in the stool. Stercobilin is also reabsorbed in the small intestine, passes the liver, and is reexcreted through the kidney (urobilirubin) in the so-called enterohepatic circulation [7].

Unconjugated hyperbilirubinemia results from increased bilirubin production (e.g., ineffective erythropoiesis, hemolytic disorders), impaired uptake (e.g., Gilbert's syndrome, use of certain drugs such as rifampin), or defective conjugation (e.g., Gilbert's syndrome, Crigler–Najjar syndrome types I and II). In the physiological jaundice of the newborn, the bilirubin metabolism is affected at various levels (increased disruption of hepatocytes, reduced hepatocyte uptake, intracellular transport and conjugation, and increased enterohepatic circulation) resulting in unconjugated hyperbilirubinemia. Breast milk jaundice is another form of unconjugated hyperbilirubinemia attributed to the ingestion of breast milk components that affect the enzyme that conjugates bilirubin [8]. Conjugated hyperbilirubinemia results from a wide spectrum of familial (Dubin Johnson syndrome and Rotor syndrome), hepatocyte, and biliary disorders that are associated with a benign course, acute or chronic liver cell damage, cholestatic injury, or biliary tree obstruction (intra- or extrahepatic) [9].

Drug Metabolism

The liver is positioned strategically between the digestive tract and the systemic circulation. Only those substances absorbed by the oral mucosa and the rectum bypass the liver, reaching the systemic circulation directly. Several diverse pathways participate in the metabolism of drugs and toxins by the liver. Three main enzymatic pathways participate in drug metabolism: oxidation, hydrolysis, and reduction, catalyzed by oxidoreductases, hydrolases, and transferases. The oxidoreductases and hydrolases catalyze phase I reactions that increase polarity (or water solubility) of substances and potentially generate toxic metabolites. The transferases catalyze phase II reactions through conjugation and produce less toxic and biologically less active products when compared with the parent compound. The most important drug-oxidation system is the P450 system (the electron-transport chain associated with the microsomal system). The central protein in this system is cytochrome P450, a hemoprotein [10]. The primary reactions, biochemical or physiologic changes, and toxic consequences to the liver of drug and toxin exposure may be variable and in part dependent on the interaction with the host [11,12].

Drug-induced liver injury (DILI) has a difficult to calculate incidence, ranging from asymptomatic liver chemistry abnormalities with a small potential impact to life or function to fulminant liver failure with high morbidity and mortality. A thorough medication history obtained from the patient, relatives, friends, caregivers, and pharmacy records is essential to identify and substantiate this challenging clinical problem. Factors to be considered when assessing patients with suspected DILI include clinical presentation and timeline of symptoms, timeline of drug ingestion, concurrent liver disease and other potential etiologies of liver injury, concomitant medications, herbal and substance abuse, biochemical pattern of liver injury, histologic findings, and response to rechallenge [13].

Hemostatic Function

The liver is the primary site of synthesis of most of the coagulation factors and the major inhibitors of the activated coagulation cascade. The synthesis of procoagulant factors II, VII, IX, and X and anticoagulant factor proteins C and S depends on the presence of vitamin K. The adequacy of hepatic synthetic function can be estimated by the prothrombin time or international normalized ratio (INR) [14]. In the presence of liver disease, there is reduced synthesis of clotting factors and inhibitors of coagulation. The synthesis of abnormal clotting proteins with anticoagulant activity leads to disseminated intravascular coagulation (DIC) and enhanced fibrinolytic activity [15,16]. In addition, thrombocytopenia, associated with portal hypertension and hypersplenism, and thrombocytopathy are usually identified in patients with end-stage liver disease. Consequently, most patients with liver disease have some measurable defect in hemostasis involving the coagulation system, fibrinolytic system, platelets, and reticuloendothelial system (Kupffer cells). The resultant clinical impact of this bleeding diathesis, however, is of variable importance. When and how the physician institutes therapeutic or prophylactic hemostatic interventions is debated and must be individually assessed for each patient.

CLINICAL DISORDERS

Ischemic Hepatitis

Liver ischemia is the consequence of hypoxic liver insult and presents in the setting of reduced liver blood flow, persistent hypotension, or severe hypoxemia. Common synonyms for ischemic hepatitis include acute hepatic infarction, shock liver, and hypoxic hepatitis [17,18]. The hepatic insult is diffuse, noninflammatory in nature, and results in variable degrees of central vein (zone 3) necrosis and collapse. The syndrome typically is recognized through detailed clinical history and biochemical evaluation, as the precipitating factor may not be apparent. Dehydration, heat stroke, hemorrhage, cardiogenic shock, acute decline in cardiac output in the absence of hypotension, traumatic shock, respiratory failure, aortic dissection, pulmonary embolus, and extensive burns have been associated with ischemic hepatitis [19–22]. In patients with congestive heart failure (left ventricular failure) and chronic passive liver congestion (right ventricular failure), even minor, additional insults may precipitate liver ischemia [23]. It is difficult to estimate the prevalence of ischemic hepatitis, but approximately 1% of patients in the ICU develop severe hypotension, cardiac failure, or respiratory failure and are susceptible to developing this condition [24].

The clinical presentation is highly variable. Biochemically, there is a characteristic rapid rise in serum aminotransferases, reaching 10 to 40 times the upper limits of normal. The lactate dehydrogenase also increases dramatically, whereas abnormalities in serum bilirubin, alkaline phosphatase, and prothrombin time are less striking. Peak elevations occur in the first 72 hours. In situations in which the triggering factor resolves, normalization of laboratory tests may occur over 7 to 10 days. Other chemistry abnormalities include renal failure with increased blood urea nitrogen and serum creatinine. Patients may present with hepatic encephalopathy, mild jaundice, weakness, or general malaise. More typically, the dominant clinical features are those of the disorder that triggered the ischemic insult [25]. The differential diagnosis includes other disorders associated with significant, rapid increases in liver enzymes, such as acute viral hepatitis, alcoholic hepatitis, and drug-induced hepatotoxicity. In only rare instances is a liver biopsy necessary for diagnosis [24].

Treatment of ischemic hepatitis is directed at correction of the underlying disease or factor that initiated the liver damage. The aim of treatment is to improve cardiac output, optimize liver and peripheral organ perfusion, and improve tissue oxygenation. The specific intervention depends on the precipitating factor and varies from case to case [26,27]. Ischemic hepatitis frequently is self-limiting, and recovery is associated with normalization of the hepatic architecture. From the liver standpoint, the prognosis depends on the presence of a normal or previously damaged liver and on the etiology of the underlying disorder [24,25,28].

Congestive Hepatopathy

Congestive hepatopathy and passive hepatic congestion are interchangeable terms used to refer to the outcome of increased hepatic vein pressure from a variety of causes. The increased pressure is transmitted through the hepatic veins and venules to the hepatocytes resulting in initial damage to cells in zone 3 [29]. Additional liver damage is thought to occur from decreased hepatic flow and decreased arterial oxygen saturation [30]. The most common causes are ischemic cardiomyopathy, heart failure, valvular heart disease, restrictive lung disease, and pericardial disease. Right-sided heart failure of any etiology (constrictive pericarditis, tricuspid regurgitation, mitral valve stenosis, or cardiomyopathy) increases the pressure of the inferior vena cava and the hepatic veins and ultimately produces liver congestion [31–33]. Although the clinical presentation of hepatic vein thrombosis (Budd–Chiari syndrome), primary thrombosis limited to hepatic venules, sinusoidal obstructive syndrome (formerly known as venoocclusive disease), and inferior vena cava thrombosis at its hepatic portion (obliterative hepatocavopathy) may be similar to congestive hepatopathy, accurate differential diagnosis is imperative. The workup of these conditions includes various imaging modalities, such as ultrasound with Doppler flow, fluoroscopic cavography, and magnetic resonance venography; at times, liver biopsy is needed for a definitive diagnosis. These medical conditions have different etiologic factors and treatment approaches [34–37].

The patient with liver congestion may present with signs and symptoms of right-sided heart failure and only subtle abnormalities in liver chemistries. The aminotransferases may be mildly elevated, reflecting limited degree of liver cell necrosis. Mild elevations of the alkaline phosphatase and total bilirubin are also common. In more severe presentations, the patient may be deeply jaundiced, suggesting extrahepatic biliary obstruction. Congestive hepatopathy can eventually lead to development of hepatocellular necrosis, broad fibrous septa deposition, regenerative nodule formation, architectural derangement, and frank cirrhosis, previously termed *cardiac cirrhosis*. Congestion produces tender hepatomegaly, and a pulsatile liver can occur with tricuspid regurgitation. Hepatojugular reflux may be elicited, and ascites is a frequent finding. In these patients, the ascitic fluid albumin is high (>2 g per dL); in contrast, in noncardiac cirrhosis, the ascitic fluid albumin is typically lower (<2 g per dL) [33,38]. The serum albumin to ascites albumin gradient (SAAG) is more than 1.1 g per dL in both conditions. Diagnosis rests on a combination of a high index of suspicion and studies that confirm the presence of cardiopulmonary disease. Pressure measurements through cardiac catheterization, transjugular hepatic venous pressure gradients, and cardiac imaging studies are diagnostic.

A transjugular liver biopsy, ideally obtained at the time of pressure measurements, can be helpful in difficult cases. Classic biopsy findings include centrilobular parenchymal atrophy, sinusoidal and terminal hepatic venular distention, and red blood cell congestion and extravasation into the space of Disse. In addition, perisinusoidal collagen deposition is seen in chronic congestion. Treatment is focused on management of the underlying pulmonary, cardiac, or pericardial disease. Ascites is managed with diuretics, low-salt diet, or large-volume paracentesis. Transjugular intrahepatic portosystemic shunts (TIPSs) are contraindicated in this condition, as the resulting marked increase in the right heart and pulmonary arterial pressures may precipitate severe heart failure [25].

Total Parenteral Nutrition

Total parenteral nutrition (TPN) remains a vital medical intervention, and its use has become routine to provide nutrition to those who are unable to eat or tolerate enteral nutrition (short gut syndrome, Crohn's disease, radiation enteritis, severe pancreatitis, post-op periods, etc.). Hepatobiliary dysfunction is recognized as a major adverse effect of short-term and long-term TPN use [39,40]. Variable degrees of liver dysfunction, ranging from subtle laboratory abnormalities to clinically apparent liver disease, develop in 40% to 60% of infants and 15% to 40% of adults who require long-term TPN [41–43]. The wide prevalence ranges reflect the difficulty in ascribing liver dysfunction to TPN, particularly in the ICU where the etiology of liver abnormalities may be multifactorial. The spectrum of hepatobiliary complications attributable to TPN includes hepatic steatosis, intrahepatic cholestasis, biliary sludge, and cholelithiasis [44]. TPN-related complications are more commonly seen after prolonged periods of parenteral nutrition. Cholestasis predominates in infants (occurring in 40% to 60%), hepatic steatosis and steatohepatitis predominate in adults (occurring in up to 40% to 55%), while biliary sludge and cholelithiasis affect both groups [43]. Progression to cirrhosis and portal hypertension is rare and occurs more frequently in infants and neonates than in adults [43].

Most patients with hepatic steatosis are asymptomatic. Mild elevations of aminotransferases, alkaline phosphatase, and total bilirubin may be identified in up to 70% of patients [45]. Enzyme levels usually peak within 1 to 4 weeks of TPN initiation. The elevation is often transient and complete resolution may occur spontaneously despite continued use of TPN. Hepatic steatosis is most likely a direct consequence of a high carbohydrate load and defective secretion of triglycerides by the liver. Glucose or dextrose overfeeding (>50 kcal per kg per day) should be avoided [46]. With the development of currently accepted protocols for caloric intake (25 to 40 kcal per kg per day), including lipids as an alternative calorie source, the prevalence of liver steatosis has declined significantly [47,48]. In a prospective study, a 53% versus 17% reduction in hepatic steatosis was reported in patients who received only dextrose infusion when compared with mixed dextrose and lipid emulsion [49]. The use of fish oil–based lipid emulsions (instead of safflower or soybean oil) appears to be "hepatoprotective" in children receiving TPN, but this strategy has not been studied in adults [50].

Essential fatty acid and choline deficiency are less common causes of hepatic steatosis. Essential fatty acid deficiency may manifest with skin rash, neuropathy, hepatosplenomegaly, and thrombocytopenia. It can be avoided as long as patients receive 2% to 4% of their calories as linoleic acid [51,52]. Intravenous (IV) lipid emulsion preparations typically contain 50% linoleic acid [46]. Low plasma choline has also been observed in patients on TPN. Choline is necessary for the synthesis of very low-density lipoproteins (VLDL). Deficiency of VLDL promotes the accumulation of triglycerides (defective triglyceride transport) in the liver and steatosis. Restoration of normal plasma choline concentrations, in the form of lecithin, decreases hepatic steatosis [43,49,51,53,54].

Cholestasis is uncommon in adults on short-term TPN (<3 weeks) [45]. In contrast, in adults on long-term TPN, cholestasis has been reported in up to 65% [55]. In the same series of 90 patients, 41.5% developed serious liver disease–related complications including portal hypertension, ascites, gastrointestinal bleeding, coagulopathy, encephalopathy, and extensive fibrosis or cirrhosis [55]. The degree of laboratory abnormality does not necessarily correlate with the degree of injury [45]. Large doses of lipid emulsion (>1 g per kg per day), short bowel syndrome (small bowel remnant <50 cm), bacterial translocation, hypoxia, and sepsis have been associated with the development of chronic cholestasis [43,45,56]. Micronutrients found in TPN such as manganese, aluminum, and copper may play a toxic role. Administration of these additives is discontinued in patients who demonstrate signs of cholestasis [46,49,57,58]. Low levels of antioxidants such as vitamin A, vitamin E, and selenium are found in TPN solutions; however, supplementation does not always improve cholestasis [57,58]. In patients with transplanted allografts, the combination of cyclosporine and TPN may also induce cholestasis.

The major concern with cholestasis in those receiving long-term TPN is the risk of progression to chronic liver disease and liver failure [59]. In this setting, TPN may need to be discontinued. TPN-dependent individuals with intestinal failure, who have persistent liver enzyme abnormalities or evidence of impending liver failure, should be considered for isolated intestine transplantation. In the presence of end-stage liver disease, however, combined intestine and liver transplantation may become necessary [46]. Survival post-isolated intestine or combined intestine–liver transplantation is 50% at 5 years, making this a viable therapeutic option [46]. Ursodeoxycholic acid (10 to 30 mg per kg per day) has shown variable success in preterm infants and adults with TPN-induced cholestasis by improving bile flow and reducing gallbladder stasis [46,60].

Biliary sludge develops in 50% to 100% of individuals after more than 6 weeks on TPN [61]. Again, clinical manifestations vary significantly. Some patients may be asymptomatic, whereas others develop striking gallbladder distention, acalculous cholecystitis, or gallstone cholecystitis. Decreased release of cholecystokinin (biliary stasis), use of narcotics (increase in bile duct pressure), and increased bile lithogenicity are contributing factors. Early introduction of oral feeding decreases the incidence of biliary complications. Trials with cholecystokinin injections have mostly been conducted in the pediatric population. Overall, they have shown inconsistent results and its long-term effects in preventing sludge formation and cholelithiasis remain unknown [62–64]. Changes in the rate or composition of the TPN infusion to stimulate gallbladder contraction are impractical and not universally successful [65,66]. Acute acalculous cholecystitis is a serious condition that requires the use of broad-spectrum antibiotics, a percutaneous drainage procedure, or a surgical intervention (i.e., cholecystectomy).

Sepsis and Multiorgan System Failure

The liver often sustains injury and develops dysfunction in sepsis and in systemic inflammatory response syndrome. The injury that occurs in the first hours is most often a consequence of liver hypoperfusion, usually in the setting of shock. This can lead to alterations in liver function including DIC and bleeding complications. Progressive liver injury then accompanies systemic effects with release of bacterial and inflammatory mediators [67]. The liver also contributes to the host immune response through a variety of mechanisms. The portal circulation, which arises from the splanchnic vasculature, is susceptible to vasoconstriction and bacterial translocation during sepsis [68]. The liver is composed of several types of cells, including hepatocytes, Kupffer, endothelial sinusoidal, Stellate, NK cells, and others. All these cells contribute to the hepatic response in sepsis through a series of intercellular interactions as well as through circulating or secreted factors. Kupffer cells are responsible for production and clearance of inflammatory mediators, bacterial scavenging, and toxin inactivation [69]. The hepatocytes respond by altering their basic metabolic pathways toward gluconeogenesis and increased production of cytokines and coagulants. Lactate clearance and protein synthesis are reduced. Endothelial cells are responsible for production of cytokines in response to endotoxins. They further contribute to antimicrobial activity and host defense through production of nitric oxide. Activated neutrophils also are recruited to the liver and respond by release of oxygen-free radicals and destructive enzymes such as protease and elastase.

The acute-phase reactants produced in this setting promote a procoagulant state and induce activation of other cells involved in the immune response. However, the liver can be damaged by cytokines released by Kupffer cells as well as by factors released from activated neutrophils. The subsequent fibrin deposition and hepatocyte damage can adversely affect the microcirculation of the liver, thereby leading to progressive liver damage and systemic toxicity [70]. The role that the liver plays in the immune and metabolic responses to infection can lead to significant clinical sequelae. The majority of patients with bacteremia from either Gram-positive or Gram-negative bacteria have abnormal liver tests. Aminotransferase elevation is characteristic in this setting and is reflective of cellular and mitochondrial injury. Abnormal liver enzymes and jaundice can occur in 2 to 3 days after the onset of bacteremia. It is not uncommon to see liver enzyme elevations reaching two to three times the upper limit of normal. The serum bilirubin level also may reach 5 to 10 times normal in the setting of sepsis [71].

Prompt treatment of sepsis with supportive care and antibiotic therapy can result in normalization of enzymes and reversal of the associated hepatic dysfunction. There is no evidence that antibodies directed toward endotoxins or cytokines play an important role in management [72]. The use of a stress dose of steroids has been found to favorably affect host defenses and reduce bacterial colonization of the liver during endotoxemia. Activated protein C (APC) in multicenter placebo-controlled trials has reduced mortality by 6% in severe clinical sepsis cases. Through its interactions with epithelial cells and macrophages, APC is thought to modulate inflammatory responses and increase microvascular perfusion. Effect of APC on hepatic microvasculature, however, has not been documented [73].

Multisystem organ failure is an ominous sign of progressive critical illness. Hepatic dysfunction in this setting is a poor prognostic indicator [74]. Sepsis, hemorrhage, severe trauma, or tissue injury such as pancreatitis can precipitate this clinical picture. Hepatic hypermetabolism leads to relative systemic hypoperfusion, and multiple organ injury develops as tissue perfusion is continually compromised. In these conditions, the liver reduces protein synthesis, increases protein catabolism, and decreases detoxification potential. Disproportionately high bilirubin levels compared with aminotransferase levels develop in patients with hepatic dysfunction. Patients with elevations in serum bilirubin greater than 8 mg per dL, without the presence of hemolysis or biliary obstruction, have a mortality rate greater than 90% [74]. Prompt reversal of hypotension can greatly reduce hepatic necrosis, bacterial translocation, and impaired Kupffer cell activity seen in patients with shock.

Drug-Induced Liver Injury

While DILI is suspected to be a common clinical problem in both out- and inpatients, its true incidence is unknown. Detection of DILI requires an elevated index of suspicion and probably its presence is frequently missed. In many instances, it is discovered unexpectedly and associated with only transient and asymptomatic abnormalities in liver chemistry. In contrast, patients with drug-induced cholestasis manifested with jaundice have an 11% probability of progressing to death or liver transplantation [75]. The incidence in DILI increases with age and is higher after the age of 40 [76]. As a result of an increasing number of available pharmacologic agents, the incidence of hepatotoxicity is rising [10]. A DILI network has been established as the first broad registry in the United States to understand and assess this problem [13]. According to the DILI network (apart from acetaminophen), antimicrobials and central nervous system drugs (45.5% and 15%, respectively) are the most common drug classes causing liver damage. The most common antibiotics found related with DILI were amoxicillin–clavulanate, trimethoprim–sulfamethoxazole, isoniazid, and nitrofurantoin.

DILI is a consequence of either a biochemical or an immune-mediated injury mechanism [77]. Biochemical injury develops from the direct effect of the drugs or their metabolites during hepatic detoxification process. Toxic by-products produced by the cytochrome P450 system or through conjugation can alter plasma cell membranes, cellular enzyme activity, or mitochondria. Drugs and their metabolites can also induce a host immune defense response with inflammatory cytokines, complement system activation, and nitric oxide, playing integral roles in the development of hepatocyte damage.

Mild or subclinical hepatic dysfunction occurs more frequently than overt dysfunction, and medications are responsible for up to 25% of cases of fulminant hepatic failure [78]. Drug hepatotoxicity can be intrinsic or idiosyncratic. Intrinsic hepatotoxicity is dose dependent, and, as seen with acetaminophen, the damage is predictable and uniform in presentation. Because the offending agent is directly toxic, close monitoring of drug levels may be preventative. In the case of idiosyncratic reactions, such as with isoniazid and phenytoin, the damage is dose independent and unpredictable. The drug or metabolite may either be directly hepatotoxic or induce a specific host immune response. Chronic liver disease can develop in the case of continuous or repeated exposure to an offending medication, inducing either type of reaction (such as amiodarone or methotrexate) [79].

Elevations in the serum aminotransferase levels from drug hepatotoxicity are typically mild and present in asymptomatic patients with mild dysfunction [80]. These elevations are observed within a few days to weeks after starting the offending agent and resolve without residual effect after its discontinuation. In more unusual cases, severe elevations of serum aminotransferases and submassive hepatic necrosis can develop and lead to fulminant hepatic failure. Histologic findings of autoimmune liver disease can be seen with some drugs that cause chronic active hepatitis [80].

Isolated serum enzyme abnormalities can be simply related to induction of cytochrome P450 enzymes and are not necessarily indicative of hepatotoxicity. Medications such as phenytoin and rifampicin induce the microsomal oxidase systems and can cause elevated gamma glutamyl transpeptidase (GGT) levels. These elevations are usually present in asymptomatic patients and do not represent cholestasis. Drug-induced cholestasis manifests as elevations in serum alkaline phosphatase, total bilirubin, and GGT. Cholestasis can occur with hepatocellular inflammation and necrosis, with associated systemic symptoms such as fever, myalgias, arthropathy, and rash. Toxicity from erythromycin, chlorpromazine, or oral hypoglycemic agents can present with this clinical picture. Cholestasis with minimal or no systemic symptoms can also occur and is the presentation typically associated with anabolic steroid or estrogen use [80]. Because the presentation of drug-induced cholestasis can resemble biliary obstruction, hepatobiliary imaging is often necessary to exclude biliary ductal dilation or a hepatic or pancreatic mass. Complete recovery after cessation of the offending agent may take several months.

The identification of specific markers of DILI to predict hepatotoxicity, pharmacogenomics, and pharmacovigilance, and the DILI network holds the promise of increasing our understanding of this challenging problem in this era of polypharmacy [81].

Sinusoidal Obstruction Syndrome

Sinusoidal obstruction syndrome (SOS), previously referred as hepatic venoocclusive disease, is a well-recognized complication of high-dose chemotherapy and total body irradiation in stem cell transplantation recipients [82]. SOS has also been reported in patients who ingested food contaminated with pyrrolizidine alkaloids (bush tea), following liver transplantation, after long-term use of azathioprine and other chemotherapeutic agents [83,84]. Although the incidence of SOS varies considerably, there is a perception of a declining occurrence due to newer nonmyeloablative conditioning regimens, avoidance of cyclophosphamide, and better patient selection.

Initially, the syndrome was thought to occur primarily as a result of injury directed toward the hepatic venules, with progressive venular obliteration, hepatocyte necrosis, and fibrosis. More recent studies indicate that venular involvement is not essential to pathogenesis, and that sinusoidal obstruction is the primary mechanism behind disease development [82,85]. In SOS, damage to hepatocytes and sinusoidal endothelial cells is a central pathogenic event.

Classically, 3 to 4 weeks after the triggering event, the affected patient develops weight gain (fluid retention and ascites), right upper quadrant pain (tender hepatomegaly), and jaundice. Laboratory abnormalities begin with isolated hyperbilirubinemia (mostly conjugated or direct), followed by elevations in alkaline phosphatase and aminotransferases [36,86]. A high index of clinical suspicion must be maintained for a successful diagnosis, as several other conditions have similar presentations [82]. Clinical presentation may be similar to Budd–Chiari syndrome, congestive hepatopathy (i.e., right-sided heart failure, constrictive pericarditis, tricuspid regurgitation, pulmonary hypertension), graft-versus-host disease, or disseminated fungal infections [87,88].

The initial diagnosis of SOS is often made on clinical grounds, but the gold standard for diagnosis is liver histology. The major histological features are sinusoidal congestion and fibrosis, necrosis of pericentral hepatocytes, narrowing and eventually fibrosis, and obliteration of sublobular and central venules [89]. In early stages, the histological changes may be patchy and that may lead to erroneous interpretation. A transjugular approach to measure the hepatic venous pressure gradient (>10 mm Hg) may have differential diagnosis and prognostic implications, and in addition, it is useful to obtain a liver biopsy. Numerous biochemical markers including plasminogen activator inhibitor-1 (PAI-1) have been investigated as diagnostic markers in SOS. One study of 350 stem cell recipient patients showed that PAI-1 was elevated in all patients with SOS. Plasma levels not exceeding 120 ng per mL had a strong negative predictive value for SOS (100% sensitivity and 30.6% specificity) [90,91]. Imaging modalities such as ultrasonography, magnetic resonance imaging, and computed tomography are more useful in excluding other causes of liver dysfunction, such as biliary obstruction or malignancy, than in establishing the diagnosis of SOS [92].

Prognosis depends on the extent of hepatic injury and is classified into three stages: mild, moderate, and severe. The degree and rate of bilirubin elevation appear to be the best biochemical markers of prognosis [82]. Mild to moderate disease is characterized by eventual resolution of liver dysfunction, whereas severe disease is associated with multiorgan failure and a mortality rate approaching 100%. Death usually is a consequence of renal, pulmonary, or cardiac failure other than liver failure [82,92,93].

A variety of pharmacologic and preventive strategies for this form of circulatory obstruction are under investigation. Anticoagulants and thrombolytics have used in patients with SOS with variable success. Anticoagulants such as antithrombin III, and low dose and low-molecular-weight heparins, are awaiting randomized studies to confirm positive preliminary results. Potent thrombolytics such as tissue plasminogen activator (tPA) has been used with variable success for SOS. In a study of 16 patients with SOS diagnosed post–stem cell transplant treated with tPA, with and without heparin, 29% showed a response (defined as downward trend or stabilization in serum bilirubin). However, the probability of bleeding complications was high and the survival only 33% at day 100 [92,94].

Defibrotide, a single-stranded oligonucleotide with antithrombotic, thrombolytic, and anti-ischemic effects, is a promising agent for SOS. In several uncontrolled trials of patients with moderate to severe SOS, the IV administration of defibrotide was associated with resolution of symptoms (36% to 64% of patients) and with improve survival without noticing significant side effects [85,95]. The initial enthusiasm generated with defibrotide as a treatment agent for SOS has generated studies that explore its use as a prophylactic agent [95]; while results are optimistic, trials are small and retrospective.

Other therapeutic options for SOS such as TIPS, ursodeoxycholic acid, and pentoxifylline are under investigation [96]. Spontaneous resolution has been reported in 70% to 85% of patients in mild cases. Supportive care is paramount and includes minimizing sodium load, administration of diuretics, and therapeutic paracentesis [82,86,97].

CONCLUSION

Timely identification of contributors to hepatic dysfunction is the foundation of adequate management in critically ill patients. A history of alcohol use or risk factors for viral hepatitis may suggest the presence of acute or chronic liver disease, factors that may further complicate management of patients with liver chemistry abnormalities in the ICU. A complete medical history seeking explanations for liver dysfunction is at times difficult to obtain in ICU patients, and relevant medications may be overlooked by patients, family, or caregivers. No singular therapy is available for the patient in whom hepatic dysfunction develops in the ICU. Identification of the etiology and correction of the initial insult through applying a counteracting drug, volume resuscitation, cardiopulmonary support, treatment of infection, or withdrawal of an offending medication have an important management role. The few evidence-based management points related to this topic are summarized in Table 98.1. In patients with previously normal livers who survive, residual effects on hepatic function are infrequent.

TABLE 98.1

EVIDENCE FOR MANAGEMENT APPROACHES THAT ARE RELEVANT TO HEPATIC DYSFUNCTION IN THE ICU PATIENT

Clinical disorder	Management evidence
■ TPN-associated hepatic steatosis	■ Controlled trials have demonstrated that choline is a required nutrient in TPN preparation.
■ TPN-associated cholestasis	■ Uncontrolled trials indicate that ursodeoxycholic acid has variable success in preventing this complication of TPN; controlled studies are lacking.
■ Drug hepatotoxicity	■ Discontinue offending agent (see Acetaminophen toxicity chapter 120); specific controlled data are lacking.
■ Sinusoidal obstruction syndrome	■ Defibrotide has been shown to improve symptoms in uncontrolled investigations; controlled studies are in progress.

TPN, total parenteral nutrition.

References

1. Strassburg CP: Shock liver. *Best Pract Res Clin Gastroenterol* 17(3):369, 2003.
2. Bioulac-Sage P, Saric J, Balabaud C: Microscopic anatomy of the intrahepatic circulatory system, in Okuda K, Benhamou J-P (eds): *Portal Hypertension. Clinical and Physiologic Aspects*. Tokyo, Springer-Verlag, 1991, p 13.
3. McCuskey Robert S: The hepatic microvascular system in health and its response to toxicants. *Anat Rec (Hoboken)* 291:661–671, 2008.
4. Soon RK Jr, Yee HF Jr: Stellate cell contraction: role, regulation, and potential therapeutic target. *Clin Liver Dis* 12(4):791–803, 2008.
5. Greenway CV, Stark RD: Hepatic vascular bed. *Physiol Rev* 51:23, 1971.
6. Lautt WW: Hepatic vasculature: a conceptual review. *Gastroenterology* 73:1163, 1977.
7. Fabris L, Cadamuro M, Okolicsanyi L: The patient presenting with isolated hyperbilirubinemia. *Dig Liver Dis* 41(6):375–381, 2009.
8. Maruo Y, Nishizawa K, Sato H, et al: Prolonged unconjugated hyperbilirubinemia associated with breast milk and mutations of the bilirubin uridine diphosphate- glucuronosyltransferase gene. *Pediatrics* 106(5):E59, 2000.
9. Gollan JL: Pathobiology of bilirubin and jaundice. *Semin Liver Dis* 8:1, 1988.
10. Lewis JH: Drug-induced liver disease. *Med Clin North Am* 84:1275, 2000.
11. Porter TD, Coon MJ: Cytochrome P450. Multiplicity of isoforms, substrates and catalytic and regulatory mechanisms. *J Biol Chem* 266:134, 1991.
12. Assis D, Navarro V: Human drug hepatotoxicity: a contemporary clinical perspective. *Expert Opin Drug Metab Toxicol* 5(5):463–473, 2009.
13. Chalasani N, Fontana RJ, Bonkovsky HL, et al: Causes, clinical features, and outcomes from a prospective study of drug-induced liver injury in the United States. *Gastroenterology* 135:1924–1934, 2008.
14. Amitrano L, Guardascione MA, Brancaccio V, et al: Coagulation disorders of the liver. *Semin Liver Dis* 22:83, 2002.
15. Pereira SP, Langley PG, Williams R: The management of abnormalities of hemostasis in acute liver failure. *Semin Liver Dis* 16:403, 1996.
16. Paramo JA, Rocha E: Hemostasis in advanced liver disease. *Semin Thromb Hemost* 19:184, 1993.
17. Fuchs S, Bogomolski-Yahalom V, Patel O, et al: Ischemic hepatitis: clinical and laboratory observations in 34 patients. *J Clin Gastroenterol* 26:183, 1998.
18. Gitlin N, Serio KM: Ischemic hepatitis: widening horizons. *Am J Gastroenterol* 87:831, 1992.
19. Ischaemic hepatitis (editorial). *Lancet* 1:1019, 1985.
20. Bynum TE, Boitnott JK, Maddrey WC: Ischemic hepatitis. *Dig Dis Sci* 24:129, 1979.
21. Kew M, Bersohn I, Seftel H, et al: Liver damage in heatstroke. *Am J Med* 49:192, 1970.
22. Alcorn JM, Miyai K: Aortic dissection and hepatic ischemia. *J Clin Gastroenterol* 14(2):180–182, 1992.
23. Nouel O, Henrion J, Bernuau J, et al: Fulminant hepatic failure due to transient circulatory failure in patients with chronic heart disease. *Dig Dis Sci* 25:49, 1980.
24. Birrer R, Takuda Y, Takara T: Hypoxic hepatopathy: pathophysiology and prognosis. *Intern Med* 46(14):1063–1070, 2007.
25. Giallourakis CC, Rosenberg PM, Friedman LS: The liver in heart failure. *Clin Liver Dis* 6(4):947–967, 2002.
26. Naschitz JE, Yeshurun D: Compensated cardiogenic shock: a subset with damage limited to liver and kidney. The possible salutary effect of low-dose dopamine. *Cardiology* 74:212, 1986.
27. Hawker F: Liver dysfunction in critical illness. *Anaesth Intensive Care* 19:165, 1991.
28. Hickmann PE, Potter JM: Mortality associated with ischemic hepatitis. *Aust N Z J Med* 20:32, 1990.
29. Safran AP, Schaffner F: Chronic passive congestion of the liver in man: electron microscopic study of cell atrophy and intralobular fibrosis. *Am J Pathol* 50:447, 1967.
30. Giallourakis CC, Rosenberg PM, Friedman LS: The liver in heart failure. *Clin Liver Dis* 6(4):947, 2002.
31. Valla D: Cirrhosis of vascular origin. *Rev Prat* 41:1170, 1991.
32. Runyon BA: Cardiac ascites: a characterization. *J Clin Gastroenterol* 10:410, 1988.
33. Sheth AA, Lim JK: Liver disease from asymptomatic constrictive pericarditis. *J Clin Gastroenterol* 42(8):956–958, 2008.
34. Valla D: Hepatic vein thrombosis (Budd-Chiari syndrome). *Semin Liver Dis* 22:5, 2002.
35. Okuda K: Inferior vena cava thrombosis at its hepatic portion (obliterative hepatocavopathy). *Semin Liver Dis* 22:15, 2002.
36. DeLeve LD, Shulman HM, McDonald GB: Toxic injury to hepatic sinusoids: sinusoidal obstruction syndrome (veno-occlusive disease). *Semin Liver Dis* 22:27, 2002.
37. Sarin SK, Agarwal SR: Extrahepatic portal vein obstruction. *Semin Liver Dis* 22:43, 2002.
38. Runyon BA, Montano AA, Akriviadis EA, et al: The serum-ascites albumin gradient is superior to the exudate-transudate concept in the differential diagnosis of ascites. *Ann Intern Med* 117:215, 1992.
39. Buchman AL: Complications of long-term home total parenteral nutrition: their identification, prevention and treatment. *Dig Dis Sci* 46:1, 2001.
40. Delaney HM: The interrelationship of the liver and gut. *Nutrition* 12:54, 1996.
41. Kelly DA: Liver complications of pediatric parenteral nutrition—epidemiology. *Nutrition* 14:153, 1998.
42. Archer SB, Burnett RJ, Fischer JE: Current uses and abuses of total parenteral nutrition. *Adv Surg* 29:165, 1996.
43. Kelly DA: Intestinal failure-associated liver disease: what do we know today? *Gastroenterology* 130:S70–S77, 2006.
44. Raman M, Allard JP: Parenteral nutrition related hepato-biliary disease in adults. *Appl Physiol Nutr Metab* 32(4):646–654, 2007.
45. Kwan V, George J: Liver disease due to parenteral and enteral nutrition. *Clin Liver Dis* 8(4):893–913, 2004.
46. Buchman AL, Iyer K, Fryer J: Parenteral nutrition-associated liver disease and the role for isolated intestine and intestine/liver transplantation. *Hepatology* 43(1):9–19, 2006.
47. Lowry SF, Brennan MF: Abnormal liver function during parenteral nutrition: relation to infusion excess. *J Surg Res* 26:300, 1979.
48. Meguid MM, Akahoshi MP, Jeffers S, et al: Amelioration of metabolic complications of conventional total parenteral nutrition. *Arch Surg* 119:1294, 1984.
49. Ukleja A, Romano MM: Complications of parenteral nutrition. *Gastroenterol Clin North Am* 36(1):23–46, 2007.
50. De Meijer VE, Gura KM, Le HD, et al: Fish oil-based lipid emulsions prevent and reverse parenteral nutrition-associated liver disease: the Boston experience. *J Parenter Enteral Nutr* 33(5):541–547, 2009.
51. Langer B, McHattie JD, Zohrab WJ, et al: Prolonged survival after complete bowel resection using intravenous alimentation at home. *J Surg Res* 15:226, 1973.
52. Reif S, Tano M, Oliverio R, et al: Total parenteral nutrition–induced steatosis: reversal by parenteral lipid infusion. *J Parenter Enteral Nutr* 15:102, 1991.
53. Buchman AL, Dubin MD, Moukarzel AA, et al: Choline deficiency: a cause of hepatic steatosis during parenteral nutrition that can be reversed with intravenous choline supplementation. *Hepatology* 22:1399, 1995.
54. Lombardi B, Ugazio G, Raick AN: Choline-deficiency-fatty liver: relation of plasma phospholipids to liver triglycerides. *Am J Physiol* 210:31, 1968.
55. Cavicchi M, Beau P: Prevalence of liver disease and contributing factors in patients receiving home parenteral nutrition for permanent intestinal failure. *Ann Int Med* 132(7):525–532, 2000.
56. Chambier C, Lemann M, Vahedi K, et al: Chronic cholestasis in patients supported by prolonged parenteral nutrition. *J Parenter Enteral Nutr* 22(S):16, 1998.
57. Guglielmi FW, Boggio-Bertinet D, Federico A, et al: Total parenteral nutrition-related gastroenterological complications. *Dig Liver Dis* 38(9): 623–642, 2006.
58. Guglielmi FW, Regano N, Mazzuoli S, et al: Cholestasis induced by total parenteral nutrition. *Clin Liver Dis* 12(1):97–110, 2008.
59. Stanko RT, Nathan G, Mendelow H, et al: Development of hepatic cholestasis and fibrosis in patients with massive loss of intestine supported by prolonged parenteral nutrition. *Gastroenterology* 92:197, 1987.
60. Kowdley KV: Ursodeoxycholic acid therapy in hepatobiliary disease. *Am J Med* 108:481, 2000.
61. Messing B, Bories C, Kunstlinger F, et al: Does total parenteral nutrition induce gallbladder sludge formation and lithiasis? *Gastroenterology* 84:1012, 1983.
62. Doty JE, Pitt HA, Porter-Fink V, et al: Cholecystokinin prophylaxis of parenteral nutrition–induced gallbladder disease. *Ann Surg* 201:76, 1985.
63. Sitzman JV, Pitt HA, Steinborn PA, et al: Cholecystokinin prevents parenteral nutrition induced biliary sludge in humans. *Surg Gynecol Obstet* 170:25, 1991.
64. Prescott W, Btaiche IF: Sincalide in patients with parenteral nutrition-associated gallbladder disease. *Ann Pharmacother* 38:1942–1945, 2004.
65. Doty JE, Pitt HA, Porter-Fink V, et al: The effect of intravenous fat and total parenteral nutrition on biliary physiology. *J Parenter Enteral Nutr* 8:263, 1984.
66. Priori P, Lezzilli R, Panuccio D, et al: Stimulation of gallbladder emptying by intravenous lipids. *J Parenter Enteral Nutr* 21:350, 1997.
67. Cerra FB, Siegel JH, Border JR, et al: The hepatic failure of sepsis: cellular versus substrate. *Surgery* 86:409, 1979.
68. Szabo G: Liver in sepsis and systemic inflammatory response syndrome. *Clin Liver Dis* 6(4):1045–1066, 2002.
69. Spapen H: Liver perfusion in sepsis, septic shock, and multiorgan failure. *Anat Rec (Hoboken)* 291:714–720, 2008.
70. Dhainaut JF, Marin N, Mignon A, et al: Hepatic response to sepsis: interaction between coagulation and inflammatory processes. *Crit Care Med* 29(S):42, 2001.
71. Sikuler E, Guetta V, Kenyan A, et al: Abnormalities in bilirubin and liver enzyme levels in adult patients with bacteremia: a prospective study. *Arch Intern Med* 149:2246, 1989.

72. Fink MP: Adoptive immunotherapy of gram-negative sepsis: use of monoclonal antibodies to lipopolysaccharide. *Crit Care Med* 21(S):32, 1993.
73. Lee S, Clemens M, Lee S: Role of Kupffer cells in vascular stress genes during trauma and sepsis. *J Surg Res* 158(1):104–111, 2010.
74. Barton R, Cerra FB: The hypermetabolism: multiple organ failure syndrome. *Chest* 96:1153, 1989.
75. Andrade RJ, Lucena MI, Fernández MC, et al: Drug-induced liver injury: an analysis of 461 incidences submitted to the Spanish registry over a 10-year period. *Gastroenterology* 129(2):512–521, 2005.
76. Marti L, del Olmo JA, Tosca J, et al: Clinical evaluation of drug induced hepatitis. *Rev Esp Enferm Dig* 97(4):258–265, 2005.
77. Losser MR, Payen D: Mechanisms of liver damage. *Semin Liver Dis* 16:357, 1996.
78. Bass NM, Ockner RK: Drug-induced liver disease, in Zakim D, Boyer TD (eds): *Hepatology: A Textbook of Liver Disease*. Philadelphia, WB Saunders, 1996, pp 962–1017.
79. Lee MG, Hanchard B, Williams NP: Drug-induced acute liver disease. *Postgrad Med J* 65:367, 1989.
80. Zimmerman HJ: Drug-induced liver disease, in Schiff ER, Sorrell MF, Maddrey WC (eds): *Schiff's Diseases of the Liver*. Philadelphia, Lippincott–Raven Publishers, 1999, p 973.
81. Tarantino G, Di Minno MN, Capone D: Drug-induced liver injury: is it somehow foreseeable? *World J Gastroenterol* 15(23):2817–2833, 2009.
82. Kumar S, DeLeve LD, Kamath PS, et al: Hepatic veno-occlusive disease (sinusoidal obstruction syndrome) after hematopoietic stem cell transplantation. *Mayo Clin Proc* 78(5):589–598, 2003.
83. Sebagh M, Debette M, Samuel D, et al: "Silent" presentation of veno-occlusive disease after liver transplantation as part of the process of cellular rejection with endothelial predilection. *Hepatology* 30:1144–1150, 1999.
84. Chojkier M: Hepatic sinusoidal-obstruction syndrome: toxicity of pyrrolizidine alkaloids. *J Hepatol* 39(3):437–446, 2003.
85. Poreddy V: Hepatic circulatory diseases associated with chronic myeloid disorders. *Clin Liver Dis* 6(4):909–931, 2002.
86. Wadleigh M, Ho V, Momtaz P, et al: Hepatic veno-occlusive disease: pathogenesis, diagnosis, and treatment. *Curr Opin Hematol* 10:451–462, 2003.
87. Carreras E, Granena A, Navasa M, et al: On the reliability of clinical criteria for the diagnosis of hepatic veno-occlusive disease. *Ann Hematol* 66:77–80, 1993.
88. Bayraktar UD, Seren S, Bayraktar Y: Hepatic venous outflow obstruction: three similar syndromes. *World J Gastroenterol.* 13(13):1912–1927, 2007.
89. Khan AZ, Morris-Stiff G, Makuuchi M: Patterns of chemotherapy-induced hepatic injury and their implications for patients undergoing liver resection for colorectal liver metastases. *J Hepatobiliary Pancreat Surg* 16(2):137–144, 2009.
90. Salat C, Holler E, Kolb HJ, et al: Plasminogen activator inhibitor-1 confirms the diagnosis of hepatic veno-occlusive disease in patients with hyperbilirubinemia after bone marrow transplantation. *Blood* 89:2184–2188, 1997.
91. Pihusch M, Wegner H: Diagnosis of hepatic veno-occlusive disease by plasminogen activator inhibitor-1 plasma antigen levels: a prospective analysis in 350 allogeneic hematopoietic stem cell recipients. *Transplantation* 80(10):1376–1382, 2005.
92. Helmy A: Review article: updates in the pathogenesis and therapy of hepatic sinusoidal obstruction syndrome. *Aliment Pharmacol Ther* 23(1):11–25, 2006.
93. McDonald GB, Sharma P, Matthews DE, et al: Venoocclusive disease of the liver after bone marrow transplantation: diagnosis, incidence, and predisposing factors. *Hepatology* 4(1):116–122, 1984.
94. Kularni S, Rodrigueq M: Recombinant tissue plasminogen activator (rtPA) for the treatment of hepatic veno-occlusive disease. *Bone Marrow Transplant* 23(8):803–807, 1999.
95. Ho VT, Revta C, Richardson PG: Hepatic veno-occlusive disease after hematopoietic stem cell transplantation: update on defibrotide and other current investigational therapies. *Bone Marrow Transplant* 41:229–237, 2008.
96. Boyer TD, Haskal ZJ: The role of transjugular intrahepatic portosystemic shunt in the management of portal hypertension. *Hepatology* 41:386–400, 2005.
97. Wingard JR, Nichols WG, McDonald GB: Supportive care. *Hematology Am Soc Hematol Educ Program* 372–389, 2004.

CHAPTER 99 ■ ACUTE PANCREATITIS

MICHAEL L. STEER

DEFINITION, CLASSIFICATION, AND PATHOLOGY

Pancreatitis, an inflammatory disease of the pancreas, can be classified as *acute* or *chronic* on the basis of clinical, morphologic, or functional criteria. The classification of any particular patient's disease depends on the criteria being used. Clinically, acute pancreatitis is defined as a process that is of rapid onset and usually associated with pain and alterations in exocrine function. With successful treatment, complete resolution can be expected. Chronic pancreatitis, on the contrary, is usually associated with repeated episodes of pain or diminished exocrine function, or both, that recur even after successful treatment of an attack. The morphologic or functional classification of pancreatitis, which has been the subject of several international symposia [1–4], also distinguishes between an acute and a chronic form of the disease, but that distinction is based on the reversibility of morphologic or functional changes, or both, in the pancreas. According to this scheme, *acute pancreatitis* is defined as an inflammatory process that occurs in a gland that was morphologically and functionally normal before the attack and can return to that state after resolution of the attack. In contrast, *chronic pancreatitis* is defined as an inflammatory disease involving a pancreas that was morphologically or functionally abnormal, or both, before the onset of symptoms or that will remain abnormal even after the attack has resolved. For the most part, the term *acute pancreatitis* is used in this chapter in its clinical rather than its morphologic or functional context. For reasons of completeness, however, the pathologic, etiologic, and therapeutic issues that are of particular relevance to morphologically or functionally defined chronic pancreatitis also are discussed.

The pathologic changes associated with acute pancreatitis vary to a great extent with the severity of an attack [5]. Mild acute pancreatitis is associated with interstitial edema, a mild infiltration of inflammatory cells, and evidence of intrapancreatic or peripancreatic fat necrosis, or both. In contrast, severe attacks of acute pancreatitis usually are associated with acinar cell necrosis that may be either focal or diffusely distributed throughout the gland. In addition, thrombosis of intrapancreatic vessels, vascular disruption with intraparenchymal hemorrhage, and abscess formation may be noted. Because chronic pancreatitis involves inflammation in a previously diseased gland, areas of scarring with fibrosis along with atrophy of acinar tissue can be seen even in tissue taken during the early stages of an attack. Varying degrees of acute inflammation are usually observed to be superimposed on these more chronic changes.

ETIOLOGY

Pancreatitis is associated with a number of other disease states or conditions that collectively are referred to as the *etiologies* of pancreatitis [6–8]. In developed countries, 70% to 80% of patients with pancreatitis have the disorder in association with either ethanol abuse or biliary tract stone disease. Another 10% to 20% of patients have no identifiable cause for pancreatitis and are considered to have idiopathic pancreatitis. In the remaining 5% to 10% of patients, pancreatitis develops in association with one of the various etiologies listed in Table 99.1. In the less well-developed countries, particularly those in Africa and Asia, disease develops as a result of malnutrition or ingestion of potentially toxic agents, or both, in a significant fraction of patients with acute pancreatitis [9–12]. Their pancreatitis has been termed *nutritional* or *tropical* pancreatitis. This entity is particularly common in the Indian subcontinent, but its cause is unknown [12].

Biliary Tract Stone Disease

Biliary tract stones are the most frequent cause of morphologic and functionally defined acute pancreatitis and, along with ethanol abuse, account for 60% to 80% of patients with clinically acute pancreatitis in developed countries. The frequency of either biliary tract stones or ethanol abuse among any group of patients being evaluated with acute pancreatitis depends on the socioeconomic composition of that group; that is, in affluent suburban groups, biliary tract stones account for more attacks, whereas ethanol abuse is more commonly found to be associated with pancreatitis when inner-city and poorer patients are studied [6]. Biliary tract stone disease is a frequent cause of acute pancreatitis among American Indians of the desert Southwest, who are prone to development of stones, and among many Asian groups, who have a high incidence of stone formation as a consequence of chronic bactibilia.

Reports by Acosta and Ledesma [13] and Acosta et al. [14] indicated that the onset of pancreatitis associated with biliary tract stones is related to the passage of those stones through the terminal biliopancreatic duct and into the duodenum. The mechanism by which stone passage triggers this so-called gallstone pancreatitis has been the subject of considerable speculation and experimental investigation. Three theories have been proposed. The first was the "common channel" theory proposed by Opie [15] in 1901 after he noted gallstones impacted in the ampulla of Vater when patients dying of gallstone pancreatitis underwent autopsy examination. He suggested that such stones might create a common biliopancreatic channel proximal to the stone-induced obstruction and that, as a consequence, bile could reflux into the pancreatic ductal system. He reasoned that bile reflux would be injurious to the pancreas and trigger pancreatitis. Subsequent investigations by many groups, however, have challenged the validity of this theory pointing out that pancreatic duct pressure normally exceeds biliary duct pressure, and therefore pancreatic juice reflux into the biliary tract rather than bile reflux into the pancreas would be expected if an obstruction were to create a common channel [16]. Furthermore, many patients develop pancreatitis but lack a common channel that could permit reflux [17], and bile perfused into the pancreatic duct at normal pressure does not induce pancreatitis [18].

The second theory proposed to explain gallstone-induced pancreatitis suggested that the stone passing through the sphincter of Oddi could render that sphincter incompetent and, as a result, permit reflux of duodenal juice containing activated digestive enzymes into the pancreas [19]. This "duodenal reflux" would seem an unlikely explanation for the development of pancreatitis because it is now clear that neither endoscopic nor surgical procedures that make the sphincter of Oddi incompetent lead to subsequent attacks of acute pancreatitis.

The third theory suggests that either the stone or edema and inflammation resulting from stone passage cause pancreatic duct obstruction and that pancreatic duct obstruction is the event that triggers acute pancreatitis. Studies using a model of acute necrotizing biliary pancreatitis induced in opossums support this theory [20], but in virtually all other species (dog, cat, mouse, rat, rabbit, etc.), pancreatic duct obstruction leads to atrophy of the pancreas with little or no evidence of pancreatitis. This observation has cast considerable doubt on the duct obstruction theory.

Most students of acute pancreatitis favor the "common channel-bile reflux theory" but, clearly, uncertainty regarding mechanisms responsible for gallstone-induced pancreatitis persists. It is generally believed that acute pancreatitis results from an autodigestive injury to the pancreas by enzymes that it normally synthesizes and secretes. Normally, those digestive enzymes are synthesized, intracellularly transported, and secreted from acinar cells as inactive zymogens. Activation normally occurs within the duodenum where the brush border enzyme enterokinase activates trypsinogen and trypsin activates the other zymogens. During pancreatitis, however, zymogen activation appears to occur inside acinar cells, perhaps as a result of pathological changes in cytoplasmic calcium levels and co-localization of digestive zymogens with lysosomal hydrolases such as cathepsin B, and, subsequently, zymogen activation leads to the acinar cell injury/death which is the hallmark of severe pancreatitis [21–25].

Recent studies in our laboratory have revealed that the bile acid receptor Gpbar1 is expressed at the apical (luminal) pole of pancreatic acinar cells and that activation of Gpbar1 in acinar cells can cause pathological rises in cytoplasmic calcium levels, zymogen activation, and cell injury. These very recent findings

TABLE 99.1

MISCELLANEOUS ETIOLOGIES OF ACUTE PANCREATITIS

Trauma
Postoperative setting
Common duct exploration
Sphincteroplasty
Distal gastrectomy
Cardiopulmonary bypass
Cardiac or renal transplantation
Endoscopic retrograde cholangiopancreatography
Translumbar aortography
Metabolic disorders
Hyperparathyroidism
Hyperlipoproteinemias types I, IV, and V
Penetrating ulcer
Connective tissue disorders
Scorpion bite
Renal failure
Hereditary pancreatitis
Pancreatic duct obstruction from duodenal diverticulum, ampullary tumor, sphincter of Oddi dysfunction, duodenal Crohn's disease, pancreatic tumor
Drugs
Bacterial, viral, fungal infections, parasites
Pancreatic trauma
Ischemia or acidosis
Autoimmune

[24] suggest that indeed, biliary pancreatitis may be triggered by bile reflux into the pancreatic duct through a common biliopancreatic duct and that bile acids contained within that bile may trigger pancreatitis via events that are set in motion following activation of Gpbar1.

Ethanol Abuse

In most patients with ethanol-associated pancreatitis, their first clinical attack of pancreatitis develops after many years of ethanol abuse. The incidence of pancreatitis is related to the logarithm of alcohol consumption, but there is no threshold below which alcohol ingestion is not associated with an increased incidence of pancreatitis. The mean consumption of ethanol among patients with ethanol-associated pancreatitis is 150 to 175 g per day. The mean duration of consumption before the first attack is 18 ± 11 years for men and 11 ± 8 years for women [26]. Ethanol-associated pancreatitis, like ethanol abuse itself, is more common among men than among women. Epidemiologic studies suggested that ethanol-associated pancreatitis is most common among those ingesting a high-protein diet with either high or low fat content [26]. The mechanism by which chronic ethanol abuse leads to chronic pancreatic injury is not clear, although some studies suggest that injury may result from secretion of a juice that is high in proteolytic enzyme content, low in proteolytic enzyme inhibitors, and contains lysosomal hydrolases capable of activating trypsin either within acinar cells or in the pancreatic ductal space [26–28].

In some patients with ethanol-induced pancreatitis, the disease develops after only one or several exposures to ethanol. This observation, along with the finding that a substantial number of patients dying of ethanol-associated disease do not have pancreatic fibrosis at autopsy [29], suggested that ethanol might be a cause of morphologic and/or functional and clinical acute pancreatitis.

The mechanism by which ethanol might cause acute injury to the pancreas is not clear. Some suggested possibilities include a direct toxic drug-like effect on acinar cells or, alternatively, induction of ductal hypertension as a result of stimulating exocrine secretion and sphincteric contraction [30,31]. Recent reports have suggested that direct cellular injury may be mediated by ethanol metabolites [30–35], and that circulating levels of bacterial endotoxin, perhaps released by the intestinal effects of ethanol, may be important contributing events [34]. It is possible that the chronic pancreatitis associated with prolonged ethanol abuse represents the cumulative effect of repeated subclinical attacks of acute pancreatitis. Thus, mild episodes associated with minimal necrosis may progress to fibrosis (i.e., the necrosis–fibrosis concept) [36]. It is also possible that chronic exposure to ethanol interferes with the resolution of inflammation and fibrosis, which normally follow episodes of injury, and that, in this way, ethanol favors the persistence of pancreatic fibrosis/inflammation even after relatively mild episodes of injury [37].

Drugs

Exposure to certain drugs represents perhaps the third most common cause of acute pancreatitis [38–41] (Table 99.2). The relationship between drug exposure and the development of pancreatitis can be categorized as definite, probable, or equivocal on the strength of the data that indicate that the drug actually causes pancreatitis. The former category includes those drugs whose use is associated with an increased incidence of pancreatitis and that, on specific rechallenge, have been found to induce the disease. On the contrary, drugs in the equivocal category include those that are anecdotally associated with the disease but never demonstrated in prospective studies to be capable of inducing pancreatitis. Historically, diuretic agents such as the thiazides, ethacrynic acid, and furosemide were considered the most likely drugs to cause pancreatitis. More recently, however, drug-related pancreatitis has been reported to be the most common among individuals with acquired immunodeficiency syndrome or acquired immunodeficiency syndrome–related complex receiving dideoxyinosine [42], pentamidine, or related compounds and among transplant patients receiving immunosuppressant agents such as azathioprine. Although previously considered to cause pancreatitis, histamine-2 (H_2)–blockers and steroids are not currently believed to be capable of causing acute pancreatitis.

TABLE 99.2

DRUGS ASSOCIATED WITH ACUTE PANCREATITIS

Definite	
Thiazide diuretics	Valproic acid
Ethacrynic acid	Estrogens
Furosemide	Tetracycline
Azathioprine	Sulfonamides
Asparaginase	Mercaptopurine
Mesalamine	Pentamidine
Dideoxyinosine	
Probable	
Methyldopa	Iatrogenic hypercalcemia
Enalapril	Procainamide
Octreotide	Erythromycin
Chlorthalidone	Phenformin
Equivocal	
Isoniazid	Rifampin
Acetaminophen	Steroids
Histamine-2–blockers	Propoxyphene

Pancreatic Duct Obstruction

Obstruction of the pancreatic duct is considered by most investigators to be the mechanism by which biliary tract stones trigger acute pancreatitis. Other events or processes that cause pancreatic duct obstruction also can result in pancreatitis. Thus, pancreatitis may be caused by duodenal, ampullary, biliary duct, or pancreatic tumors that obstruct the duct or by inflammatory lesions (e.g., peptic ulcer, duodenal Crohn's disease, periampullary diverticulitis) that interfere with pancreatic duct drainage [6]. Pancreatic cysts and pseudocysts and periampullary diverticula filled with food and debris can interfere with duct drainage and as a consequence precipitate pancreatitis. Ductal strictures, frequently the result of traumatic duct injury or previous pancreatitis, can be a cause for obstructive pancreatitis. Finally, certain parasites, such as *Ascaris* and *Clonorchis*, can trigger pancreatitis by physically obstructing the pancreatic duct [6,43]. An association between pancreas divisum and pancreatitis has been claimed, presumably reflecting relative obstruction to pancreatic juice flow at the lesser papilla [44], but this is quite controversial [45,46].

Other Miscellaneous Causes of Acute Pancreatitis

Many of the remaining miscellaneous causes of pancreatitis are listed in Table 99.1. Traumatic pancreatitis usually follows blunt abdominal trauma, during which the body of the pancreas is compressed against the vertebral column. As a result, the gland is "cracked," and the duct is either partially or completely transected [47]. Lesser degrees of blunt trauma may be associated with pancreatic contusion, whereas penetrating injury can affect any portion of the pancreas. Traumatic injury to the pancreas also can be associated with surgical procedures performed on or near the pancreas [48–50]. Postoperative pancreatitis is also frequently associated with procedures performed on or near the sphincter of Oddi (duct exploration, sphincteroplasty, distal gastrectomy), procedures associated with hypoperfusion or atheroembolism of the pancreatic circulation (cardiopulmonary bypass, cardiac transplantation, renal transplantation, translumbar aortography) [51,52], or procedures involving pancreatic duct injection (endoscopic retrograde cholangiopancreatography [ERCP]) [53].

Chronic pancreatitis can also be a familial disease transmitted by a mutation on chromosome 7 that is transmitted as an autosomal dominant with incomplete penetrance [54]. Reports indicate that the mutation results in synthesis of a cationic trypsinogen that is resistant to autoinactivation after activation has occurred [55]. Patients with classic cystic fibrosis mutations can present with pancreatitis even in the absence of pulmonary disease. Studies indicate that a substantial number of patients with so-called idiopathic pancreatitis may have nonclassic cystic fibrosis mutations or polymorphisms [56].

Pancreatitis can also develop on an autoimmune basis in association with other autoimmune processes such as primary sclerosing cholangitis, Sjogren's syndrome, and primary biliary cirrhosis. A number of recent reports, particularly from Japan, have drawn attention to a form of autoimmune pancreatitis characterized by extensive lymphoplasmacytic infiltration into the pancreas and sclerosis of the pancreatic and bile ducts. Patients with this form of pancreatitis frequently present with both bile and pancreatic duct obstruction and a mass in the head of the pancreas. They can easily be thought to have neoplastic disease of the pancreas but, if placed on steroid treatment, the changes of autoimmune pancreatitis rapidly resolve. Many, but not all, of these patients have elevated circulating levels of IgG4 and this may permit their identification [57].

Idiopathic Pancreatitis

Approximately 5% to 10% of patients with acute pancreatitis have the disease in the absence of biliary tract stones, ethanol abuse, or any other identifiable etiology. Reports suggest that many of these patients have biliary sludge, that their attacks can be prevented by cholecystectomy, and that they actually have biliary rather than idiopathic pancreatitis [58,59]. Approximately 40% of individuals with chronic pancreatitis neither abuse ethanol nor have malnutrition. As a result, they are considered to have idiopathic chronic pancreatitis [60]. Studies in Europe and the United States suggest that these individuals can be divided into a juvenile group, with an onset of disease at a median age of 18, and a senile group, whose disease begins at a mean age of 60. Disease in the former group is characterized by pain, whereas that in the senile group is most often painless and associated with calcifications, diabetes mellitus, or both [61].

CLINICAL PRESENTATION

Symptoms

The symptoms of acute pancreatitis include abdominal pain, nausea, and vomiting [6,7,43,62,63] (Table 99.3). The pain typically is localized to the epigastrium but frequently involves one or both upper quadrants. On occasion, it may be felt in the lower abdomen, one or both shoulders, or the lower chest. The pain is usually described as being of rapid onset, slowly increasing to a maximal severity, and then remaining constant. It usually lacks the waxing and waning character of intestinal or ureteral colic, but it may be diminished by assuming an upright position, leaning forward, or lying on the side with the knees drawn upward. The pain may have a pleuritic component and may be associated with rapid but shallow respirations. Frequently, the pain is described as being a boring or knifelike sensation that passes straight through to the midcentral back from the epigastrium.

TABLE 99.3

SIGNS AND SYMPTOMS OF ACUTE PANCREATITIS

Observation	Incidence (%)
Pain	95
Nausea/vomiting	80
Distention	75
Guarding	50
Pain radiating to back	50
Jaundice	20
Abdominal mass	15
Melena	4
Hematemesis	3

Nausea and vomiting commonly are noted in patients with acute pancreatitis. The vomiting typically persists even after the stomach has been emptied and may result in gastroesophageal tears with bleeding (i.e., Mallory–Weiss syndrome). The vomiting and retching may be relieved by passage of a nasogastric tube, but neither the vomiting nor gastric decompression results in reduction of the abdominal pain.

Physical Examination

Patients with acute pancreatitis typically appear anxious and ill. They may be diaphoretic and hyperthermic. Tachycardia, tachypnea, and hypotension are common. Patients often roll or move around in search of a more comfortable position. In this respect, they are quite unlike those with peritonitis caused by a perforated viscus, which remain motionless because movement exacerbates their pain. Most patients with acute pancreatitis have a clear sensorium, but some have mild or even severe alterations in their mental status as a result of drug or ethanol exposure, hypoxemia, hypotension, or release of circulating toxic agents from the inflamed pancreas. Jaundice is common, even in patients with nonbiliary pancreatitis, among whom the hyperbilirubinemia may reflect nonobstructive cholestasis.

The abdominal examination of patients with acute pancreatitis usually reveals abdominal tenderness and voluntary and involuntary guarding. These findings may be limited to the epigastrium or diffusely present throughout the abdomen. A mass, located in the epigastrium or left upper quadrant of the abdomen, or both, may be felt. Direct, percussion, and rebound tenderness usually can be elicited. Abdominal distention also can be seen. Hypovolemia and dehydration are commonly present and can be detected by the presence of hypotension, tachycardia, collapsed neck veins, dry skin, dry mucous membranes, and decreased subcutaneous elasticity. Bowel sounds are often diminished or absent. Flank ecchymoses (Grey Turner's sign) or other evidence of retroperitoneal bleeding (Cullen's sign) may be noted. Examination of the chest may reveal evidence of pleural effusion that may be on either or both sides but is most commonly present on the left. Because of pleuritic and abdominal pain, deep breathing is difficult, and atelectasis, particularly at the bases, is common. Examination of the skin may reveal areas of tender subcutaneous induration and erythema that resemble erythema nodosum. These lesions are believed to result from fat digestion by circulating pancreatic lipases.

LABORATORY TESTS AND RADIOLOGIC EXAMINATIONS

Routine Blood Tests

Acute pancreatitis is associated with significant losses of intravascular fluid. A substantial amount of fluid is lost as a result of the anorexia, nausea, and vomiting that accompanies the disease. In addition to these fluid losses, large volumes of fluid can be sequestered in the retroperitoneum as a result of the pancreatic inflammatory process. In addition, a systemic "capillary leak" process may result in additional fluid sequestration. Taken together, these losses of fluid from the intravascular compartment can cause the hematocrit, hemoglobin, blood urea nitrogen, and serum creatinine to rise. Hypoalbuminemia is common, but the serum electrolytes may remain normal unless vomiting has been significant. Because of the pancreatic inflammatory process, the white blood cell count usually is elevated and the differential may show a shift to the left. Hyperglycemia, which commonly is noted, may result from the combined effects of elevated circulating catecholamines, decreased insulin release, and hyperglucagonemia [64,65]. A mild rise in serum bilirubin from nonobstructive cholestasis frequently is seen even in nonbiliary acute pancreatitis. When the disease is induced by the passage of gallstones, the hyperbilirubinemia is even more marked, and superimposed cholangitis with bacteremia and positive blood cultures can occur [66]. Markedly elevated circulating triglyceride levels always are seen in individuals whose pancreatitis is caused by hyperlipoproteinemia [67], but hypertriglyceridemia with lactescent serum also can be seen in alcohol-induced acute pancreatitis [68].

Hypocalcemia is relatively common among individuals with acute pancreatitis [69]. For the most part, the hypocalcemia is caused by hypoalbuminemia, and as a result, the ionized calcium level is actually normal. In some patients, however, hypocalcemia can develop that is out of proportion to the degree of hypoalbuminemia and that reflects a true decrease in circulating ionized calcium levels. Tetany and carpopedal spasm and other complications of their hypocalcemia may develop in some patients. Marked hypocalcemia has been considered to be a sign of a poor prognosis. In patients with severe pancreatitis, disseminated intravascular coagulation may develop [70], and as a result, they may have thrombocytopenia, elevated levels of fibrin degradation products, decreased fibrinogen levels, and prolongations of the partial thromboplastin and prothrombin times.

Amylase

The serum amylase concentration is usually, but not always, elevated during an attack of pancreatitis [7]. The magnitude of that rise does not depend on the severity of pancreatitis, and some reports indicate that as many as 10% of patients with normal or near-normal serum amylase levels may have lethal pancreatitis [71]. To a great extent, this may reflect the fact that amylase elevations during pancreatitis typically are transient, with an increase to 2 to 12 hours after the onset of an attack and a decline in serum amylase values to near-normal levels 3 to 6 days after the attack has begun. Thus, patients presenting long after the onset of an attack may have normal or only slightly increased serum amylase levels.

TABLE 99.4

CAUSES OF HYPERAMYLASEMIA

Pancreatic causes
Pancreatitis, pseudocyst, ascites
Pancreatic cancer
Pancreatic duct obstruction
Pancreatic trauma
Endoscopic retrograde cholangiopancreatography
Nonpancreatic intra-abdominal causes
Perforated hollow viscus
Bowel obstruction
Cholangitis, cholecystitis
Mesenteric infarction
Ovarian cyst
Renal failure
Ruptured ectopic pregnancy
Extra-abdominal causes
Salivary gland tumors, trauma, infection, obstruction
Lung tumors
Burns
Diabetic acidosis
Pneumonia

Serum amylase activity also may be increased in a number of diseases other than pancreatitis [7,63,72]. Amylase may be synthesized at extrapancreatic sites (e.g., salivary glands, fallopian tube, lung) or produced by nonpancreatic tumors (e.g., lung, prostate, ovary), and release of the nonpancreatic amylase into the circulation may result in hyperamylasemia (Table 99.4). Patients with these nonpancreatic extra-abdominal causes for hyperamylasemia rarely are confused with those who have pancreatitis, because the clinical features of pancreatitis usually are absent in the former group. On the contrary, some patients with disorders that might be clinically confused with acute pancreatitis also may have hyperamylasemia. This is particularly true for patients with acute cholecystitis, perforated gastric or duodenal ulcers, small bowel obstruction, intestinal ischemia, and intestinal infarction. It may also be true for some patients passing common bile duct stones into the duodenum who do not have pancreatitis.

The overall sensitivity and specificity of amylase determination in the diagnosis of pancreatitis depends on the value chosen as the cutoff level [73] and the presence or absence of clinical features of pancreatitis. Patients with hyperamylasemia but not pancreatitis usually have mild elevations of the circulating amylase level (approximately 200 IU per L) or lack clinical features of pancreatitis, or both, whereas those with pancreatitis usually manifest profound hyperamylasemia (>1,000 IU per L) in association with clinical features of the disease.

Approximately 0.5% of individuals have a condition referred to as *macroamylasemia* in which amylase is bound to an abnormal circulating protein and, as a result, the amylase is not cleared by the kidney [63,74,75]. Some of these individuals may develop abdominal pain and may be incorrectly suspected of having pancreatitis. In this setting, measurement of urinary amylase activity may be particularly helpful because, in macroamylasemia, urinary amylase levels usually are very low. Renal clearance of amylase also may be reduced as a result of renal failure, and this reduced clearance can lead to mild hyperamylasemia. On the contrary, enhanced renal clearance of amylase can occur in pancreatitis, and this phenomenon can result in an increase in the clearance ratio for amylase compared with creatinine [75,76]. However, measurement of the so-called amylase to creatinine clearance ratio has not been helpful in the diagnosis of pancreatitis. Alterations of this ratio appear to represent a nonspecific response to an acute illness. Thus, the clearance ratio may be elevated in many patients who lack pancreatitis but may be normal in many who have pancreatitis [74–80].

Other Enzyme Assays and Blood Tests

The urine amylase level may remain elevated long after serum amylase levels have returned to normal [7,81]. As a result, measurement of urinary amylase activity may be particularly helpful in patients who are first seen several days after an attack of pancreatitis and who are found to have normal or near-normal serum amylase activity [63]. Hyperlipasemia also may persist after serum amylase levels have returned to normal, and in such patients, measurement of serum lipase activity may be useful [63,71]. Circulating levels of other pancreatic enzymes (trypsinogen, chymotrypsinogen, phospholipase, elastase) or urinary levels of the activation peptide released when trypsinogen is activated (i.e., trypsinogen activation peptide) can also be measured, but there is little or no evidence to suggest that these determinations are more helpful in the diagnosis of pancreatitis than the simpler measurement of serum amylase activity [71,82,83]. Acute pancreatitis also can be associated with methemalbuminemia [84] and with increased circulating levels of several cytokines (e.g., interleukin-1 [IL-1], IL-6, tumor necrosis factor-α) [85] and acute-phase reactants (e.g., C-reactive protein) [86,87]. The magnitude and duration of these changes may have some prognostic value in pancreatitis, but these changes are not specific to pancreatitis and are therefore of little diagnostic value.

Routine Radiography

Routine chest radiographs may reveal basal atelectasis as a result of splinted respiration, elevated diaphragms, or both. A pleural effusion, more common on the left than on the right, also can be seen. Abdominal films may reveal pancreatic calcifications in patients with chronic pancreatitis. These calcifications result from calcium precipitation in the proteinaceous intraductal plugs that develop in chronic pancreatitis. In general, plain abdominal films reveal evidence of a paralytic ileus, whereas contrast gastrointestinal studies may reveal displacement of peripancreatic organs by pancreatic masses. Retroperitoneal air may be seen when pancreatic abscess is caused by a gas-forming organism. In general, however, the value of routine radiographs when pancreatitis is suspected lies in the failure of those films to reveal evidence of nonpancreatic diseases that might mimic acute pancreatitis (e.g., pneumonia, perforated hollow viscus, and mechanical bowel obstruction).

Ultrasonography

Ultrasonography in patients with acute pancreatitis usually is limited by the presence of intestinal gas in the upper abdomen during the early stages of the disease. Even in this setting, ultrasonography may be helpful in detecting gallbladder stones, bile duct dilatation, or both. Later during the course of pancreatitis, ultrasonography may be very useful in detecting and monitoring pancreatic inflammatory masses and pseudocysts [88].

Computed Tomography

In acute pancreatitis, particularly during the early stages of the disease, computed tomography (CT) is the most useful imaging modality because it can define the gross features of the pancreas and peripancreatic organs without being limited by the presence of distended gas-filled loops of bowel in the upper abdomen [89]. The pancreas may be normal or slightly swollen in appearance on CT in mild cases of pancreatitis. Evidence of peripancreatic inflammation, including streaking in the retroperitoneal and transverse mesocolic fat, may also be seen. With more severe attacks, peripancreatic and intrapancreatic fluid collections can be detected. Dynamic CT, performed by rapidly imaging the pancreas during bolus injection of contrast material, can define areas of pancreatic necrosis because those areas do not enhance as a result of contrast administration [90–92]. Detection of these changes may be of prognostic value in acute pancreatitis [93] (see "Prognosis" section in the chapter), but their major value in the early stages of the disease lies in the fact that their presence confirms the diagnosis of acute pancreatitis. Conversely, the finding of a normal pancreas without signs of peripancreatic inflammation on the CT of a patient suspected of having severe pancreatitis, particularly if that patient's condition is deteriorating, should suggest that the patient does not have pancreatitis.

Magnetic resonance imaging (MRI) can also be of great value in the diagnosis of acute pancreatitis. It can reveal the presence of an inciting stone in the distal bile duct. In addition, MRI may be more accurate than CT in defining the extent of pancreatitis-associated necrosis [94].

DIFFERENTIAL DIAGNOSIS

The differential diagnosis of acute pancreatitis includes other processes that may cause upper abdominal pain, nausea, vomiting, and abdominal tenderness. The serum amylase or lipase, or both, is usually elevated in acute pancreatitis and normal or near normal in many other processes that may cause similar symptoms. On the contrary, serum levels of pancreatic enzymes may be elevated in some states that can mimic acute pancreatitis (Table 99.5). For the most part, these states are associated with only one- to twofold elevations in circulating enzyme levels and with a normal appearance of the pancreas and peripancreatic tissues on CT examination. On occasion, however, the diagnosis may be uncertain, and operative intervention may be indicated to establish the diagnosis, particularly in patients whose conditions are deteriorating despite aggressive nonoperative therapy.

PROGNOSIS

Most patients with acute pancreatitis have a relatively mild self-limited attack that resolves with only supportive treatment. On the other hand, roughly 5% to 10% of patients in most series have a severe attack that is associated with considerable

TABLE 99.5

DIFFERENTIAL DIAGNOSIS OF ACUTE PANCREATITIS

Perforated hollow viscus
Cholecystitis/cholangitis
Bowel obstruction
Mesenteric ischemia/infarction

TABLE 99.6

RANSON'S PROGNOSTIC SIGNS

On admission	
	Age >55 y
	White blood cell count >16,000/μL
	Blood glucose >200 mg/dL
	Lactate dehydrogenase >350 IU/L
	Glutamic oxaloacetic transaminase >250 Sigma–Frankel units/dL
During initial 48 h	
	Hematocrit decrease >10%
	Blood urea nitrogen rise >5 mg/dL
	Serum Ca^{2+} <8 mg/dL
	Partial pressure of oxygen <60 mm Hg
	Base deficit >4 mEq/L
	Fluid sequestration >6 L

morbidity and a mortality that can approach 40%. Certain clinical features have been identified that are associated with a poor prognosis. These include age older than 60 years, a "first attack" of pancreatitis, obesity, postoperative pancreatitis, hypocalcemia, methemalbuminemia, and the presence of either Grey Turner's or Cullen's sign [95]. Investigators in New York and Glasgow evaluated large groups of patients with pancreatitis and identified clinical and laboratory features that are available during the initial 48 hours of diagnosis that can be used to define the prognosis of an attack. These criteria, frequently referred to as the *Ranson* [96] and *Imrie* [97] *criteria*, are listed in Tables 99.6 and 99.7, respectively. The presence of fewer than three of the Ranson criteria is associated with mild pancreatitis, little morbidity, and a mortality of less than 1%. In contrast, many patients with three or more of these prognostic signs have severe pancreatitis, with a 34% incidence of septic complications and a mortality that, with seven to eight prognostic signs, may reach 90%. Using the Imrie criteria, severe pancreatitis has been found when three or more of the criteria are present, whereas mild pancreatitis is associated with fewer of the prognostic signs.

Although the criteria developed by the New York and Glasgow groups have proved to be of considerable value in allowing prospective trials in the evaluation of new therapies and interventions for acute pancreatitis, these prognostic criteria are not particularly helpful in the management of an individual patient and should never be used as criteria for the diagnosis of pancreatitis. It has been suggested that the Acute Physiology and Chronic Health Evaluation-2 (APACHE-2) system [98] might be a useful method for evaluating the severity of an attack, predicting its risk of morbidity and mortality, and comparing groups of patients with acute pancreatitis. It is likely that reports using this system will appear in the future, and that the APACHE-2 system will replace the Ranson and the Imrie systems for evaluating the prognosis of acute pancreatitis, because this system allows ongoing modifications in the grading of severity as the disease progresses.

TABLE 99.7

IMRIE'S PROGNOSTIC SIGNS

Age >55 y
White blood cell count >15,000/μL
Blood glucose >10 mmol/L
Serum urea >16 mmol/L
Partial pressure of oxygen <60 mm Hg
Serum Ca^{2+} <2.0 mmol/L
Lactic dehydrogenase >600 μg/L
Aspartate aminotransferase/alanine aminotransferase >100 μg/L
Serum albumin <32 g/L

The morbidity of an individual attack of pancreatitis is closely related to the presence of peripancreatic fluid collections demonstrable by CT. Ranson et al. [99], in a prospective study involving 83 patients with acute pancreatitis, noted that those with two or more peripancreatic fluid collections seen on CT had a 61% incidence of late pancreatic abscess, those with only one fluid collection or inflammation confined to the pancreas and peripancreatic fat had a 12% to 17% incidence of pancreatic abscess, and those with either no CT changes of pancreatitis or with only pancreatic enlargement on CT had a zero incidence of pancreatic abscess. The morbidity, incidence of abscess formation, and mortality of an attack of pancreatitis also have been shown to be related to the amount of pancreatic tissue that is not enhanced on CT after bolus administration of contrast material during dynamic CT. Beger et al. [91] suggested that patients might benefit from surgical intervention and necrosectomy of the pancreas when dynamic CT indicates that considerable portions of the pancreas are poorly perfused or nonperfused (i.e., necrotic).

In addition to these scoring systems, other factors characterizing acute pancreatitis may be helpful in predicting the severity and, thus, the outcome of an attack. Most notable in this regard are the presence or onset, shortly after presentation, of evidence suggesting organ failure and/or evidence of extravascular extravasation of normally intravascular fluid [7,100,101]. This fluid loss can result in renal failure, respiratory failure, or both as well as hemoconcentration, and each of these changes is predictive of a poor outcome. In contrast, the absence of hemoconcentration on admission usually suggests that pancreatic necrosis is unlikely [102,103]. Elevated circulating levels of other factors (e.g., C-reactive protein, certain cytokines, phospholipase A2, trypsinogen activation peptide, and trypsinogen-2) are also suggestive of a severe attack and predictive of a poor outcome [7].

TREATMENT OF ACUTE PANCREATITIS

Initial Management

During the early stages of an acute attack of pancreatitis, efforts should be made to confirm the diagnosis, control pain, and support fluid and electrolyte needs [104]. Establishing the diagnosis of acute pancreatitis may be difficult and, at times, impossible without exploratory laparotomy. Usually, the clinical picture combined with hyperamylasemia, a convincing CT, and favorable response to aggressive nonoperative therapy are sufficient, but when doubt persists, exploration may be warranted if the dire consequences of an overlooked bowel perforation, infarction, or obstruction are to be avoided [105]. On the contrary, reports have suggested that laparotomy may increase the incidence of septic complications in pancreatitis [106]; therefore, exploration should be avoided if possible.

Treatment of Pain

The pain of pancreatitis is often severe and difficult to control. Most patients require narcotic medications. Meperidine rather than morphine would appear to be the narcotic drug of choice for gallstone pancreatitis because it relaxes the sphincter of Oddi, whereas morphine causes sphincteric contraction [107].

Fluid and Electrolyte Replacement

The early stage of severe acute pancreatitis is characterized by major fluid and electrolyte losses. External losses, caused by repeated episodes of vomiting and exacerbated by nausea and diminished fluid intake, can lead to hypochloremic alkalosis. Internal losses caused by leakage of intravascular fluid into the inflamed retroperitoneum, pulmonary parenchyma, and soft tissues elsewhere in the body contribute to hypovolemia. The most sensitive indicator of the magnitude of fluid loss during this stage of pancreatitis is the hematocrit; serum electrolytes may remain normal, because electrolyte composition of the lost fluid is similar to that in plasma. On the contrary, the blood pH may fall as hypovolemia and poor tissue perfusion lead to metabolic acidosis. Hypoalbuminemia and hypomagnesemia, caused by preexisting malnutrition in chronic alcoholics, losses during the early stages of pancreatitis, or both, may warrant replacement therapy. Tetany, carpopedal spasm, or other manifestations of hypocalcemia are rare but when they occur should prompt aggressive calcium replacement.

The hemodynamic parameters during severe pancreatitis may resemble those of septic shock [108]. Thus, heart rate, cardiac output, and cardiac index rise and total peripheral resistance falls. The arterial-venous oxygen difference and intrapulmonary shunt rise, and marked hypoxemia may result. The basis for these changes is, most likely, multifactorial and includes hypovolemia, atelectasis, and the release of vasoactive agents and cytokines, including IL-1, IL-6, and tumor necrosis factor-α [85,109].

Treatment requires meticulous management of fluid and electrolyte needs. A fluid balance flow sheet may prove extremely useful in this regard. Endotracheal intubation and mechanical ventilatory support may be needed. For the most part, patients with severe pancreatitis should be in an ICU where facilities for close monitoring are available. Volume status can best be followed using a Swan-Ganz catheter to track filling pressures and an indwelling urethral catheter to monitor urine output. Arterial oxygenation can be followed using an indwelling arterial catheter and frequent blood gas determinations.

Aggressive and adequate fluid resuscitation, instituted during the early stages of acute pancreatitis, is essential. A growing body of evidence indicates that inadequate fluid resuscitation may promote progression of otherwise mild pancreatitis into severe pancreatitis, with its associated major morbidity and high mortality.

Other Treatments

The role of prophylactic antibiotics in the management of acute pancreatitis is not clear. Early randomized studies, performed primarily in patients with mild alcohol-induced pancreatitis, suggested that prophylactic antibiotics did not alter the incidence of septic complications or the mortality of pancreatitis [110,111]. More recently, however, studies evaluating this issue have focused on patients with severe gallstone-induced pancreatitis. Some have indicated that prophylactic treatment with broad-spectrum agents, such as imipenem, or a third-generation cephalosporin may be of benefit to these patients [112,113], whereas others have suggested that prophylactic antibiotics may be of little or no value in the management of patients with severe pancreatitis [114]. In some cases, the prophylactic use of broad-spectrum antibiotics may promote the emergence of resistant bacteria or fungi, or both. The latter problem may be reduced, to some extent, by the concomitant administration of an antifungal agent such as fluconazole [115].

The peritoneal exudate that develops during acute pancreatitis contains a number of potentially harmful vasoactive agents and enzymes. It is believed that these substances are absorbed from the peritoneal cavity into the circulation and contribute to the morbidity of pancreatitis by causing complications such as vasomotor collapse, myocardial depression, acute respiratory distress syndrome, and renal failure [116–119]. Peritoneal lavage has been used in an attempt to remove these substances, and early anecdotal reports suggested that peritoneal lavage was beneficial [106,120–123]. However, a large multi-institutional prospectively randomized and controlled trial in the United Kingdom indicated that short-term peritoneal lavage did not alter the morbidity or mortality of pancreatitis [124]. On the contrary, Ranson and Berman [125] reported the results of a study in which peritoneal lavage was performed for a prolonged period in a small group of severely ill patients with pancreatitis. They concluded that prolonged peritoneal lavage might indeed be of value in the management of such patients. Thus, at present, the actual value and the ideal method of performing peritoneal lavage in this setting remain unclear.

TABLE 99.8

TREATMENTS OF LIMITED OR UNPROVEN VALUE

Nasogastric suction
Histamine-2 receptor antagonists
Antacids
Atropine
Glucagon
Calcitonin
Somatostatin
Indomethacin
Steroids
Hypothermia
Thoracic duct drainage
Plasmapheresis
Prostaglandins
Procainamide
Gabexate mesilate
Aprotinin
Isoproterenol
Heparin
Dextran
Vasopressin
Propylthiouracil
Epsilon-aminocaproic acid
Peritoneal lavage

Many other methods of treating pancreatitis have been examined, but to date, no controlled trials have been reported that demonstrate a beneficial effect of these forms of therapy in pancreatitis (Table 99.8). Nasogastric suction has not been shown to alter the morbidity or mortality of pancreatitis, but many clinicians, including myself, believe that it improves patient comfort. Histamine-2 receptor antagonists, antacids, or both may diminish the risk of stress ulcers, but these drugs do not alter the severity or course of pancreatitis. Agents that reduce pancreatic function (atropine, glucagon, calcitonin, somatostatin), inhibit inflammation or cytotoxic responses (indomethacin, steroids, prostaglandins), inhibit digestive enzymes (procainamide, gabexate, aprotinin), or improve flow in the pancreatic microcirculation (isoproterenol, heparin, dextrans) have not been found to alter the course of pancreatitis in humans, although many of these approaches have been found to be of benefit if begun early in the course of experimental pancreatitis in laboratory animals [126,127]. A multicenter, prospective, controlled, randomized trial was reported, suggesting that the platelet-activating factor antagonist lexipafant might favorably affect the course of acute pancreatitis [128]. Administration of lexipafant was found to reduce the mortality and incidence of organ failure in patients treated within 72 hours of the onset of acute severe pancreatitis. However, a more recent trial specifically focusing on the use of lexipafant during the initial 48 to 72 hours of pancreatitis found that it did not alter outcome [129]. Thus, at present, there is no evidence to support the use of this agent in pancreatitis.

By convention, most patients with severe pancreatitis are treated by a combination of bowel rest and either parenteral or enteral nutrition. The mortality rate for patients treated with enteral or parenteral nutrition has been found to remain unaltered, but those treatments have been reported to reduce the incidence of infections, complication, and the need for surgical intervention [130,131]. Furthermore, recent reports suggest that enteral nutrition can be successfully administered by either the nasogastric or the nasojejunal route and that the benefits of using either route are comparable [132,133].

Role of Surgery and Endoscopy in Gallstone Pancreatitis

Most patients with biliary tract stone–induced pancreatitis recover quickly and uneventfully, as the offending stone is either passed into the duodenum or disimpacts itself from the ampulla of Vater by moving proximally in the duct. The role of early interventions designed to remove obstructing stones in this disease has been extremely controversial. Acosta et al. [134] and Stone et al. [135] concluded that early surgical intervention could reduce the severity of pancreatitis and shorten the duration of hospitalization. In contrast, Kelly and Wagner [136] found that early surgical intervention was associated with greater morbidity and mortality than was delayed surgery. Three prospectively randomized controlled trials and a recent observational, prospective, multicenter trial have evaluated the benefit of early endoscopic sphincterotomy and stone extraction in the management of patients with gallstone pancreatitis [66,137–139]. Each study concluded that early intervention did not alter the course of mild pancreatitis, but three studies [66,137,139] suggested that the morbidity of severe pancreatitis, particularly if it was associated with cholestasis, was reduced by early stone removal. It appears that early stone removal by endoscopic sphincterotomy benefits these patients by reducing the incidence of associated cholangitis. On the basis of currently available data, it seems most appropriate that patients with mild pancreatitis do not undergo either early surgical or endoscopic intervention. On the contrary, early intervention seems warranted for patients with severe gallstone pancreatitis and intervention could either be surgical or endoscopic, depending on the local availability of expertise in these areas. It is possible that the benefit of early surgical or endoscopic intervention could also be achieved by the use of prophylactic antibiotics that are designed to prevent cholangitis, but a trial evaluating this approach has not been reported.

Recurrent attacks of gallstone pancreatitis may develop if stones either in the gallbladder or biliary ducts remain after resolution of the index attack. For that reason, most clinicians recommend that some form of treatment designed to prevent recurrent attacks should be administered before discharge of the patient from the hospital [130]. That might be accomplished by laparoscopic or open cholecystectomy combined with surgical or endoscopic duct clearance if choledocholithiasis is discovered by preoperative magnetic resonance cholangiopancreatography (MRCP). Alternatively, in patients whose only symptoms are those of duct disease and who lack symptoms of cholecystolithiasis, endoscopic sphincterotomy and duct clearance may be sufficient, particularly if those patients are poor surgical risks.

TABLE 99.9

COMPLICATIONS OF ACUTE PANCREATITIS

Systemic complications
■ Cardiovascular collapse
■ Respiratory failure
■ Renal failure
■ Metabolic encephalopathy
■ Disseminated intravascular coagulation
■ Gastrointestinal bleeding
Local complications
■ Acute fluid collection
■ Pancreatic necrosis ± infection
■ Pancreatic pseudocyst
■ Pancreatic abscess
■ Pancreatic ascites
■ Pancreatic-pleural fistula
■ Duodenal obstruction
■ Bile duct obstruction
■ Splenic vein thrombosis
■ Pseudoaneurysm + hemorrhage

Treatment of Systemic Complications

Systemic complications of acute pancreatitis include cardiovascular collapse, respiratory failure, renal failure, metabolic encephalopathy, disseminated intravascular coagulation, and gastrointestinal bleeding (Table 99.9). For the most part, the pathogenesis and management of these manifestations of acute pancreatitis are identical to those involved when these processes are superimposed on other diseases that result in severe peritonitis and hypovolemic shock. In other words, there may be nothing specific about these systemic complications of pancreatitis, although they may be worsened by circulating vasoactive agents, activated digestive enzymes, and protein breakdown fragments absorbed from the inflamed pancreas.

Treatment of the cardiovascular collapse of acute pancreatitis requires aggressive and meticulous fluid and electrolyte administration. Measurement of venous filling pressures, hematocrit, cardiac output, and urinary output may be extremely helpful in gauging fluid needs. The growing consensus is that aggressive fluid and electrolyte therapy may be the most effective method of preventing the appearance of pulmonary and renal failure in these patients. Theoretically, peritoneal dialysis, by removing the yet unabsorbed but potentially harmful agents released by the inflamed pancreas, and plasmapheresis, which could permit removal of circulating harmful agents, could also prevent or reduce the severity of these systemic complications of pancreatitis. Their value, however, has not been shown by definitive clinical studies.

Treatment of the atelectasis and acute respiratory distress syndrome associated with acute pancreatitis is similar to the treatment of these problems when they are associated with other causes of peritonitis. Thus, good pulmonary toilet combined with close monitoring of pulmonary function by measurement of mechanics and blood gases are indicated. With deterioration in function, intubation and respiratory support may be needed. Similarly, the management of the renal failure of pancreatitis is not different from that of acute renal failure caused by other diseases. The renal failure of pancreatitis is prerenal and, when it occurs, is associated with a poor prognosis.

Dialysis, usually in the form of hemodialysis, may be needed in the most severely affected.

Disseminated intravascular coagulation, manifested by decreased platelet counts and fibrinogen levels, prolonged prothrombin and partial thromboplastin times, and increased circulating levels of fibrin-split products, occurs in some patients with severe acute pancreatitis. Bleeding caused by disseminated intravascular coagulation, however, is rare. Thus, prophylactic anticoagulation with heparin in patients with biochemical evidence of disseminated intravascular coagulation is not indicated and may be associated with significant problems, including retroperitoneal hemorrhage.

The gastrointestinal bleeding that sometimes is seen in patients with pancreatitis usually results from stress-induced gastroduodenal lesions. Thus, prophylaxis with antacids, H_2-blockers, or proton pump inhibitors may be useful in preventing this problem. Rarely, massive bleeding may result from injury to gastrointestinal structures by the inflammatory process in the peripancreatic retroperitoneum. Thus, thrombosis of gastrointestinal vessels may lead to ischemic injury and bleeding from the stomach, intestine, or colon. In extreme cases, infarction and perforation of the viscus may occur. The inflammatory process may lead to erosion into retroperitoneal vessels near the pancreas. In these situations, treatment is dictated by the lesions present but usually involves resection of nonviable tissues.

LOCAL COMPLICATIONS OF PANCREATITIS

Definitions

Considerable confusion has surrounded the terminology used to describe the local complications of an acute attack of pancreatitis. At a symposium in Atlanta, an international group of clinicians and scientists attempted to resolve this confusion by proposing the use of the following definitions [140]:

1. *Acute pancreatic and peripancreatic fluid collections*: Fluid collections in or near the pancreas that occur early in the course of acute pancreatitis and that lack a wall of granulation or fibrous tissue.
2. *Pancreatic necrosis*: An area of nonviable pancreatic tissue that may be diffuse or focal and that typically is associated with peripancreatic fat necrosis. Pancreatic necrosis may be either *sterile* or *infected*.
3. *Pancreatic pseudocyst*: A collection of pancreatic juice that usually is rich in digestive enzymes and that is enclosed by a nonepithelialized wall of fibrous or granulation tissue (Figs. 99.1 and 99.2). It usually is round or ovoid in shape and not present until 4 to 6 weeks have elapsed from the onset of acute pancreatitis. Before this time, the fluid collection usually lacks a defined wall and may be either an *acute fluid collection* or a localized area of *pancreatic necrosis*. Bacteria may be present in a pseudocyst as a result of contamination, but in this setting, clinical signs of infection usually are absent. When pus is present, however, the lesion should be referred to as a *pancreatic abscess*. Leakage of pseudocysts into the peritoneal cavity or chest leads to the development of *pancreatic ascites* or *pancreatic-pleural fistula*, respectively.
4. *Pancreatic abscess*: A circumscribed intra-abdominal collection of pus, usually in proximity to the pancreas, which contains little or no pancreatic necrosis that arises as a consequence of either acute pancreatitis or pancreatic trauma (Fig. 99.3). The relative absence of necrosis distinguishes *pancreatic abscess* from *infected pancreatic necrosis*.

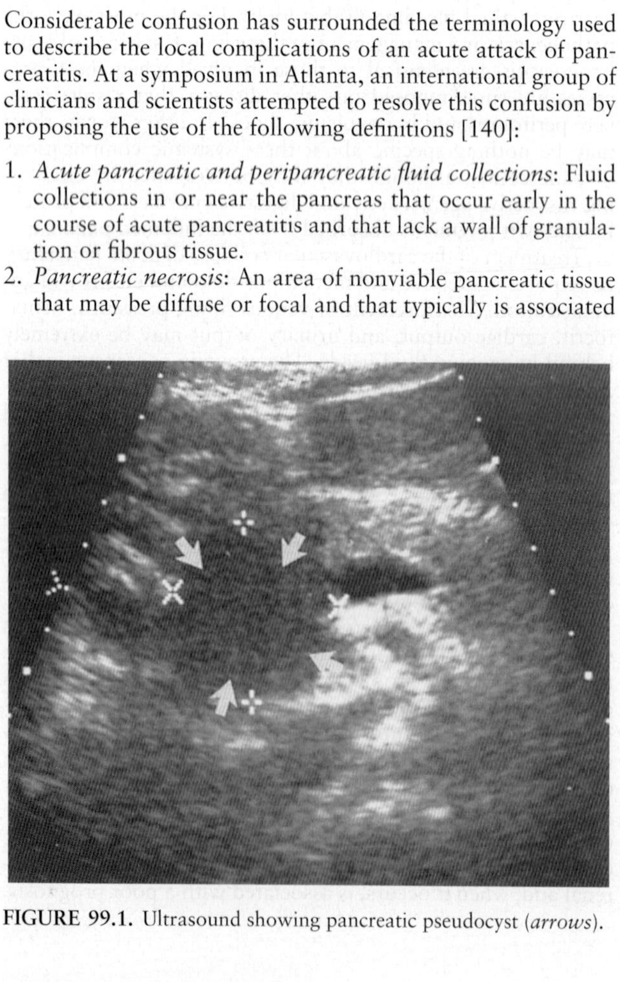

FIGURE 99.1. Ultrasound showing pancreatic pseudocyst (*arrows*).

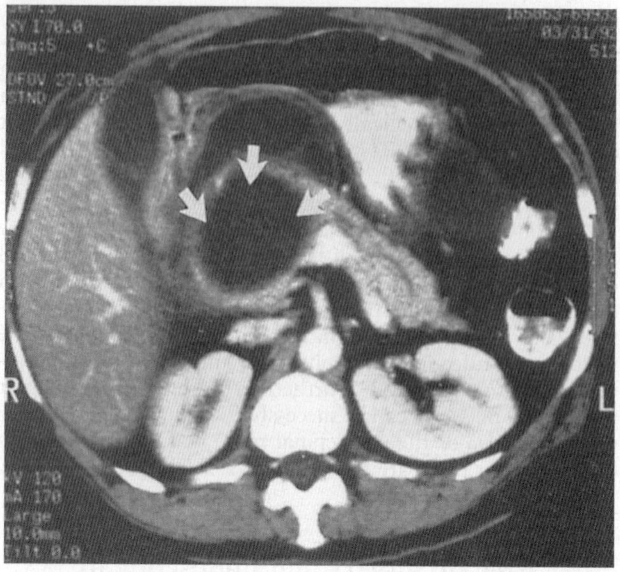

FIGURE 99.2. Computed tomography showing pseudocyst (*arrows*) in the head of the pancreas.

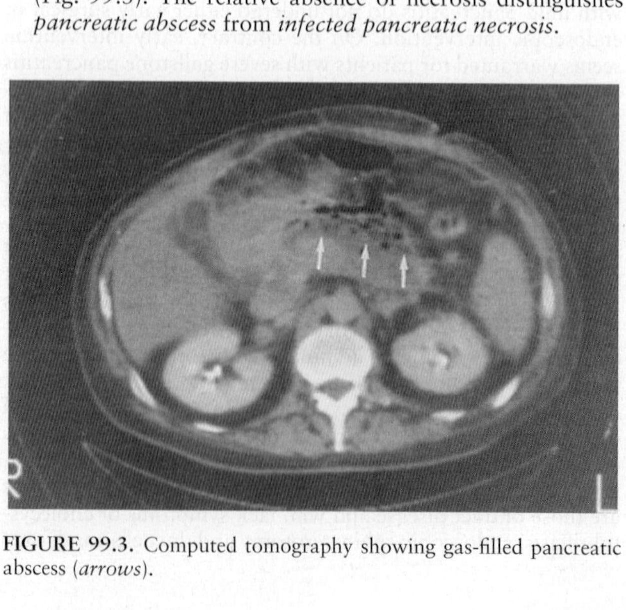

FIGURE 99.3. Computed tomography showing gas-filled pancreatic abscess (*arrows*).

Diagnosis

Patients with uncomplicated pancreatitis usually are judged by the various prognostication schemes to have mild pancreatitis at the time of diagnosis, and they generally recover uneventfully within the subsequent 1 to 2 weeks. In contrast, patients with severe pancreatitis, who remain ill for longer periods, frequently have one or more of the local complications of pancreatitis. In the past, these lesions were identified on the basis of physical examination, contrast radiography, and blood chemistry studies. For the most part, these relatively crude and inaccurate methods have been replaced by the techniques of ultrasonography (both transcutaneous and endoscopic), CT, and MRI. Ultrasonography and either CT or MRI can be used to diagnose and define the extent of acute fluid collections and pseudocysts accurately. These techniques can be used to follow the progression of these lesions and determine whether or not a wall, which distinguishes a pseudocyst from an acute fluid collection, is present.

Dynamic contrast-enhanced CT and MRI are the most accurate means of identifying and quantitating areas of pancreatic necrosis, whereas ERCP may be useful in determining whether or not fluid collections communicate with the main pancreatic duct. In addition, ERCP can be used to localize the point of duct rupture in patients with either pancreatic ascites or pancreatic-pleural fistulas. The presence of extraintestinal gas on either ultrasonography or CT is diagnostic of either infected necrosis or abscess, but this finding is only occasionally noted. More often, patients with either infected necrosis or abscess are found to have poorly enhanced areas on dynamic CT or fluid collections on ultrasonography, or both, in a clinical setting of suspected sepsis. When doubt about the presence or absence of infection persists, fine-needle aspiration of these areas, under either ultrasonographic or CT guidance, may yield material that, on Gram's stain, reveals the presence of bacteria [141,142].

Management

Acute Fluid Collections

Acute fluid collections generally require no specific treatment. They usually resolve spontaneously within several weeks of an attack. Attempts to drain these collections either by percutaneously placed catheters or by early surgical intervention should be discouraged.

Sterile Necrosis

In the past, sterile necrosis was treated during the early stages of pancreatitis by surgical necrosectomy combined with postoperative lavage of the peripancreatic area [143], particularly when large portions of the pancreas were devitalized. There has been considerable controversy, however, regarding this practice and, at present, the consensus view is that patients with sterile necrosis, even if extensive, should be managed nonoperatively during the initial few weeks of their illness [144]. Surgical intervention in such patients may be associated with considerable morbidity and may even result in secondary infection of the inflamed, but previously sterile, pancreas.

Although the consensus view is that patients with sterile necrosis do not need intervention during the early phases of their disease, the potential value of intervention at later times is not entirely clear. Some of these patients experience a very prolonged illness and full recovery may only be possible after the devitalized pancreatic and peripancreatic tissue has been removed. This can be accomplished surgically by exposing the involved area and removing the necrotic tissue—a procedure that may require repeated operations and can lead to considerable morbidity. Recently, alternatives to this approach have been proposed. They involve transpapillary or transcutaneous placement of irrigating catheters into the involved area followed by debridement achieved by continuous lavage [145–147]. In another approach, debridement is achieved using a percutaneously placed operating nephroscope or laparoscope [148,149]. The experience with these minimally invasive methods of debriding the inflamed pancreas is, to date, mostly anecdotal but suggests that debridement with little additional morbidity can be achieved.

Infected Necrosis

Infected necrosis usually is an indication for surgical intervention, whether it is detected by the presence of extraintestinal gas on CT examination or by fine-needle aspiration of an area of pancreatic necrosis. Organisms recovered in areas of infected pancreatic necrosis usually are those that are present in the gastrointestinal tract (*Klebsiella* spp, *Pseudomonas* spp, *Escherichia coli*, *Enterococcus*, *Proteus* spp) [150]. In addition, yeast such as *Candida albicans* may be encountered. It is believed that most of these organisms reach the inflamed pancreas via transmigration from adjacent segments of the intestine. Antibiotic therapy, although indicated, by itself usually represents an inadequate approach to the management of infected pancreatic necrosis. Similarly, because of the presence of large amounts of necrotic puttylike material, percutaneous drainage of these areas using indwelling catheters may prove unsuccessful and, for the most part, patients with infected necrosis require urgent, aggressive, and repeated surgical debridement and drainage. This is especially true for the unstable or septic patient who is doing poorly with nonoperative management. On the other hand, recent reports have suggested that stable patients with infected necrosis can be managed more electively and conservatively. For those stable patients, delay in performing surgical debridement may actually be beneficial, since it appears to improve survival, decrease surgical complications, and decrease the need for repeated operations when compared with early operation in this group [151]. Furthermore, although most of these patients will eventually need debridement, recent anecdotal reports have indicated that some may be definitively treated with either antibiotics alone or with antibiotics combined with percutaneous drainage [152].

Pseudocyst

Pseudocysts may cause symptoms either because they are themselves tender or because they result in obstruction of adjacent organs such as the stomach, duodenum, and bile duct. On occasion, pancreatic pseudocysts contribute to the progression of pancreatitis by causing pancreatic duct obstruction. On the other hand, many pseudocysts do not cause symptoms. Until relatively recently, the general consensus was that pseudocysts should be treated regardless of their size or whether they caused symptoms [153]. Several more recent reports, however, indicated that chronic pseudocysts, even those greater than 6 cm in diameter, can be safely observed and that treatment is only needed for those that become symptomatic [154,155].

Several methods of treating pseudocysts have been proposed, including either open or laparoscopic internal surgical drainage (cystogastrostomy, cystoduodenostomy, Roux-en-Y cystojejunostomy), endoscopic drainage (cystogastrostomy, cystoduodenostomy), and percutaneous drainage (aspiration, aspiration followed by administration of somatostatin, and catheter drainage, with or without administration of somatostatin) [156]. My experience with percutaneous drainage has, to a great extent, been disappointing because of a considerable incidence of either recurrence after aspiration or infection after catheter drainage. On the other hand, endoscopic drainage, via endoscopic cystoduodenostomy or cystgastrostomy, is a highly effective way of managing cysts located in the pancreatic head or body, particularly if they are pressing inward on the duodenum or stomach and there is little in the way of tissue or blood vessels interposed between the cyst and the duodenal or gastric lumen [157]. Surgical internal drainage (i.e., cystojejunostomy, cystogastrostomy) would seem most appropriate for management of cysts in the pancreatic tail or the head/body cysts that cannot be safely accessed endoscopically.

Pancreatic Ascites, Fistulas, and Abscesses

Patients with pancreatic ascites or pancreatic-pleural fistulas may respond to nonoperative therapy with bowel rest, parenteral nutrition, and administration of somatostatin or other agents designed to inhibit pancreatic secretion [158–165]. Most, however, fail this method of treatment, and some form of intervention is needed. An ERCP should be performed to identify the site of duct disruption [166–168] that, if in the pancreatic tail, can be treated easily by distal pancreatectomy. Alternatively, anastomosis of a Roux-en-Y loop of jejunum to the site of rupture, particularly if it is in the head or neck of the gland, may be preferable. Endoscopically placed stents also can be used to prevent leakage of juice from the duct, and this nonoperative approach can be useful in the management of these complications [169].

Pancreatic abscess, like infected pancreatic necrosis, always requires some form of intervention, but, because pancreatic abscesses contain liquid pus rather than the paste-like material in pancreatic necrosis, percutaneous drainage of pancreatic abscesses might be considered. Alternatively, surgical or endoscopic intervention and placement of drainage catheters in the abscess may be appropriate. I have, for the most part, treated such patients with surgical drainage, but recent advances in endoscopy and in the field of invasive radiology may permit successful nonoperative management of such individuals.

TABLE 99.10

SUMMARY OF ADVANCES IN THE MANAGEMENT OF ACUTE PANCREATITIS

- Early, aggressive fluid resuscitation is beneficial in cases of severe acute pancreatitis associated with shock [170].
- In contrast to morphine, meperidine relaxes the sphincter of Oddi and is thus a favored analgesic in cases of pancreatitis [107,171].
- Use of enteral nutrition has shown benefit over parenteral nutrition in terms of duration of hospital stay, infectious morbidity, and need for surgery in meta-analysis [172–174]. Enteral nutrition, because it is associated with fewer complications, may be the better of these two treatment modalities.
- Antibiotic use remains controversial; meta-analyses have shown utility in preventing infection of pancreatic necrosis [175,176], although a large, randomized, controlled trial failed to demonstrate benefit [114].
- In cases of severe necrotizing pancreatitis, conservative management in an intensive care setting trends toward a survival benefit when compared with early surgical intervention [177].
- Early endoscopic sphincterotomy and stone extraction are beneficial in preventing sepsis in cases of severe gallstone pancreatitis in patients with jaundice [66,137,178].

Most aspects of the management of acute pancreatitis and its complications are based on information derived from clinical experience, case series, and retrospective comparisons. A summary of recent advances in the management of acute pancreatitis is provided in Table 99.10.

References

1. Sarles H: Introduction and proposal adopted unanimously by the participants of the symposium, in Sarles H (ed): *Pancreatitis-Symposium*. Basel, Switzerland, Verlag S. Karger, 1965, p VI.
2. Sarner M, Cotton PB: Classification of pancreatitis. *Gut* 25:756, 1984.
3. Singer MV, Gyr K: Revised classification of pancreatitis—Marseilles 1984. *Gastroenterology* 89:683, 1985.
4. Dervenis C, Johnson CD, Bassi C, et al: Diagnosis, objective assessment of severity, and management of acute pancreatitis. Santorini consensus conference. *Int J Pancreatol* 25:195, 1999.
5. Kloppel G, Maillet B: Histopathology of acute pancreatitis, in Beger HG, Warshaw AL, Buchler MW, et al (eds). *The Pancreas*. Oxford, Blackwell, 1998, pp 404–409.
6. Steer ML: Acute pancreatitis, in Wolfe MM, Davis G, Farraye FA, et al (eds). *Therapy of Digestive Disorders*. 2nd ed. New York, Elsevier, 2006, pp 417–426.
7. Frossard JL, Steer ML, Pastor CM: Acute pancreatitis. *Lancet* 371:143–152, 2008.
8. Turi S, Kraft M, Lerch MM: Acute pancreatitis associated with metabolic, infectious, and drug-related diseases, in Beger H, Warshaw A, Buchler M, et al (eds). *The Pancreas*. 2nd ed. Oxford. Blackwell, 2008, pp 172–183.
9. Pitchumoni CS: Special problems of tropical pancreatitis. *Clin Gastroenterol* 13:541, 1984.
10. Narendranathan M: Chronic calcific pancreatitis of the tropics. *Trop Gastroenterol* 2:40, 1981.
11. Pitchumoni CS, Jain NK, Lowenfels AF, et al: Chronic cyanide poisoning. Unifying concept for alcoholic and tropical pancreatitis. *Pancreas* 3:220, 1988.
12. Sidu SS, Nundy S, Tandon RK: The effect of the modified Puestow procedure on diabetes in patients with tropical chronic pancreatitis—a prospective study. *Am J Gastroenterol* 96:107, 2001.
13. Acosta JL, Ledesma CL: Gallstone migration as a cause for acute pancreatitis. *N Engl J Med* 290:484, 1974.
14. Acosta JL, Ross R, Ledesma CL: The usefulness of stool screening for diagnosing cholelithiasis in acute pancreatitis: a description of the technique. *Am J Dig Dis* 22:168, 1977.
15. Opie EL: The relationship of cholelithiasis to disease of the pancreas and fat necrosis. *Am J Med Surg* 12:27, 1901.
16. Menguy RB, Hallenbeck GA, Bollman JL, et al: Intraductal pressures and sphincteric resistance in canine pancreatic and biliary ducts after various stimuli. *Surg Gynecol Obstet* 106:306, 1958.
17. Mann FC, Giordano AS: The bile factor in pancreatitis. *Arch Surg* 6:1, 1923.
18. Robinson TM, Dunphy JE: Continuous perfusion of bile protease activators through the pancreas. *JAMA* 183:530, 1963.
19. McCutheon AD: Reflux of duodenal contents in the pathogenesis of pancreatitis. *Gut* 5:260, 1964.
20. Lerch MM, Saluja AK, Runzi M, et al: Pancreatic duct obstruction triggers acute necrotizing pancreatitis in the opossum. *Gastroenterology* 104:853, 1993.
21. Steer ML, Meldolesi J, Figarella C: Pancreatitis: the role of lysosomes. *Dig Dis Sci* 29:934, 1984.
22. Steer ML: The early intraacinar cell events which occur during acute pancreatitis. The Frank Brooks Memorial Lecture. *Pancreas* 17:31, 1998.
23. Steer ML, Sharma A, Tao XH, et al: Where and how does pancreatitis begin? in Amman RW, Buchler MW, Adler G, et al (eds): *Pancreatitis: Advances in Pathobiology, Diagnosis, and Treatment. Falk Symposium 143*. New York, NY, Springer, 2005, pp 3–12.
24. Perides G, Laukkarinen JM, Vassileva G, et al: Biliary acute pancreatitis in mice is mediated by the G protein-coupled cell surface bile acid receptor Gpbar1. *Gastroenterology* 138(2):715–725, 2010.
25. Saluja AK, Donovan EA, Yamaguchi Y, et al: Caerulein-induced in vitro activation of trypsinogen in rat pancreatic acini is mediated by cathepsin B. *Gastroenterology* 113:304, 1997.
26. Sarles H: Chronic pancreatitis: etiology and pathophysiology, in Go VLW, Gardner JD, Brooks EP, et al. (eds): *The Exocrine Pancreas: Biology, Pathobiology, and Diseases*. New York, Raven Press, 1986, p 37.
27. Steer ML, Glazer G, Manabe T: Direct effects of ethanol on exocrine secretion from the in-vitro rabbit pancreas. *Dig Dis Sci* 24:769, 1979.
28. Rinderknecht H, Renner IG, Koyama HH: Lysosomal enzymes in pure pancreatic juice from normal healthy volunteers and chronic alcoholics. *Dig Dis Sci* 24:180, 1979.

29. Apte MV, Pirola RC, Wilson JS: Molecular mechanisms of alcoholic pancreatitis. *Dig Dis* 23:232, 2005.
30. Pandol SJ, Raraty M: Pathobiology of alcoholic pancreatitis. *Pancreatology* 7:105, 2007.
31. Vonlaufen A, Wilson JS, Apte MV: Molecular mechanisms of pancreatitis: current opinion, *J Gastroenterol Hepatol* 23:1339, 2008.
32. Criddle DN, Murphy J, Fistetto G, et al: Fatty acid ethyl esters cause pancreatic calcium toxicity via inositol trisphosphate receptors and loss of ATP synthesis, *Gastroenterology* 130:781, 2006.
33. Criddle DN, Raraty MG, Neoptolemos JP, et al: Ethanol toxicity in pancreatic acinar cells: mediation by nonoxidative fatty acid metabolites. *Proc Natl Acad Sci USA* 101:10738, 2004.
34. Vonlaufen A, Xu Z, Kumar DB, et al: Bacterial endotoxin: a trigger factor for alcoholic pancreatitis? Evidence from a novel, physiologically relevant animal model. *Gastroenterology* 134:640, 2008.
35. Renner IG, Savage WE III, Pantoja H, et al: Death due to acute pancreatitis. A retrospective analysis of 405 autopsy cases. *Dig Dis Sci* 30:1005, 1985.
36. Kloppel G: Progression from acute to chronic pancreatitis. A pathologist's view. *Surg Clin North Am* 79:801, 1999.
37. Perides G, Tao X, West N, et al: A mouse model of ethanol-dependent chronic pancreatitis. *Gut* 54:1461, 2005.
38. Thomas FB: Drug-induced pancreatitis: facts vs fiction. *Drug Ther Hosp* 7:60, 1982.
39. Greenberger NJ, Toskes P, Isselbacher KJ: Diseases of the pancreas, in Braunwald E, et al. (eds): *Harrison's Principles of Internal Medicine*. New York, McGraw-Hill, 1988, p 1372.
40. McArthur K: Drug induced pancreatitis. *Aliment Pharmacol Ther* 10:238, 1996.
41. Trivedi CD, Pitchumoni CS: Drug-induced pancreatitis: an update. *J Clin Gastroenterol* 39:709, 2005.
42. Lambert JS, Seidlin M, Reichman RC, et al: 2′, 3′-Dideoxyinosine (ddI) in patients with the acquired immunodeficiency syndrome of AIDS-related complex. A phase I trial. *N Engl J Med* 322:1333, 1990.
43. Durr GH: Acute pancreatitis, in Howatt HT, Sarles H (eds): *The Exocrine Pancreas*. London, WB Saunders, 1979, p 352.
44. Warshaw AL, Simeone JF, Schapiro RH, et al: Evaluation and treatment of the dominant dorsal duct syndrome (pancreas divisum redefined). *Am J Surg* 159:59, 1990.
45. Delhaye M, Cremer M: Clinical significance of pancreas divisum. *Acta Gastroenterol Belg* 55:306, 1992.
46. Fogel EL, Toth TG, Lehman GA, et al: Does endoscopic therapy favorably affect the outcome of patients who have recurrent acute pancreatitis and pancreas divisum? *Pancreas* 34:21, 2007.
47. Wilson RH, Moorehead RJ: Current management of trauma to the pancreas. *Br J Surg* 78:1196, 1991.
48. Bardenheier JA, Kaminski DL, William VL: Pancreatitis after biliary tract surgery. *Am J Surg* 16:773, 1968.
49. Peterson LM, Collins JJ, Wilson RE: Acute pancreatitis occurring after operation. *Surg Gynecol Obstet* 127:23, 1968.
50. White TT, Morgan A, Hopton D: Postoperative pancreatitis: a study of seventy cases. *Am J Surg* 120:132, 1970.
51. Adiseshia M: Acute pancreatitis after cardiac transplantation. *World J Surg* 7:519, 1983.
52. Feiner H: Pancreatitis after cardiac surgery. *Am J Surg* 131:684, 1976.
53. Sherman S, Lehman GA: Endoscopic retrograde cholangiopancreatography- and endoscopic sphincterotomy-induced pancreatitis, in Beger HG, Warshaw AL, Buchler MW, et al (eds), *The Pancreas*. Oxford, Blackwell, 1998, pp 291–310.
54. Whitcomb DC, Preston RA, Aston CE, et al: A gene for hereditary pancreatitis maps to chromosome 7g35. *Gastroenterology* 110:1975, 1996.
55. Whitcomb DC, Gorry MC, Preston RA, et al: Hereditary pancreatitis is caused by a mutation in the cationic trypsinogen gene. *Nat Genet* 14:141, 1996.
56. Cohn JA, Friedman KJ, Noone PG, et al: Relation between mutations of the cystic fibrosis gene and idiopathic pancreatitis. *N Engl J Med* 339:653, 1998.
57. Hamano H, Kawa S, Horiuchi A, et al: High serum IgG4 concentrations in patients with sclerosing pancreatitis. *N Engl J Med* 344:732, 2001.
58. Ros E, Navarro S, Bru C, et al: Occult microlithiasis in "idiopathic" acute pancreatitis: prevention of relapses by cholecystectomy or ursodeoxycholic acid therapy. *Gastroenterology* 101:1701, 1991.
59. Lee SP, Nicholls JF, Park HZ: Biliary sludge as a cause of acute pancreatitis. *N Engl J Med* 326:589, 1992.
60. Owyang C, Levitt M: Chronic pancreatitis, in Yamada T, Owyang C, Powell DW, et al (eds): *Textbook of Gastroenterology*. Philadelphia, PA, JB Lippincott Co, 1991, p 1874.
61. Layer P, Kalthoff L, Clain JE, et al: Nonalcoholic chronic pancreatitis—two diseases? *Dig Dis Sci* 30:980, 1985.
62. Silen W: *Cope's Early Diagnosis of the Acute Abdomen*. 15th ed. New York, NY, Oxford University Press, 1979.
63. Leavitt MD, Edkfeldt JH: Diagnosis of acute pancreatitis, in Go VLW, Gardner JD, Brooks EP, et al. (eds): *The Exocrine Pancreas: Biology, Pathobiology, and Diseases*. New York, Raven Press, 1986, p 481.
64. Solomon SS, Duckworth WC, Jallepalli P, et al: The glucose intolerance of acute pancreatitis. *Diabetes* 29:22, 1980.
65. Drew SI, Joffe B, Vinik A, et al: The first 24 hours of acute pancreatitis. *Am J Med* 64:795, 1978.
66. Fan ST, Lai ECS, Mok FPT, et al: Early treatment of acute biliary pancreatitis by endoscopic papillotomy. *N Engl J Med* 328:228, 1993.
67. Toskes P: Hyperlipidemic pancreatitis. *Gastroenterol Clin North Am* 19:783, 1990.
68. Cameron JL, Crisler C, Margolis S, et al: Acute pancreatitis with hyperlipemia. *Surgery* 70:53, 1971.
69. Imrie CW, Beastall GH, Allam BF, et al: Parathyroid hormone and calcium homeostasis in acute pancreatitis. *Br J Surg* 65:717, 1978.
70. Ranson JHC, Lackner H: Coagulopathies, in Bradley EL (ed): *Complications of Pancreatitis*. Philadelphia, PA, WB Saunders, 1982, p 154.
71. Steer ML: Acute pancreatitis, in Yamada T, Owyang C, Powell DW, et al (eds): *Textbook of Gastroenterology*. Philadelphia, PA, JB Lippincott Co, 1991, p 1859.
72. Salt WB, Schenker S: Amylase—its clinical significance: a review of the literature. *Medicine* 55:269, 1976.
73. Steinberg WM, Goldstein SS, Davis ND, et al: Diagnostic assays in acute pancreatitis. A study of sensitivity and specificity. *Ann Intern Med* 102:576, 1985.
74. Berk JE, Kizu H, Wilding P: A newly recognized cause for elevated serum amylase activity. *N Engl J Med* 277:941, 1967.
75. Levitt MD, Rapoport M, Cooperband SR: The renal clearance of amylase in renal insufficiency, acute pancreatitis, and macroamylasemia. *Ann Intern Med* 71:919, 1969.
76. Warshaw AL, Fuller AF: Specificity of increased renal clearance of amylase in diagnosis of acute pancreatitis. *N Engl J Med* 292:325, 1975.
77. McMahon MJ, Playforth MJ, Rashid SA, et al: The amylase-to-creatinine clearance—a nonspecific response to acute illness? *Br J Surg* 69:29, 1982.
78. Levitt MD, Gross JB Jr: Postoperative elevation of amylase/creatinine clearance ratio in patients without pancreatitis. *Gastroenterology* 77:497, 1979.
79. Levin RJ, Galuser FL, Berk JE: Enhancement of the amylase-creatinine clearance ratio in disorders other than acute pancreatitis. *N Engl J Med* 292:329, 1975.
80. Morton WJ, Tedesco FJ, Harter H, et al: Serum amylase determinations and amylase to creatinine clearance ratios in patients with chronic renal insufficiency. *Gastroenterology* 71:594, 1976.
81. Matuli WR, Pereira SP, O'Donohue JW: Biochemical markers of acute pancreatitis. *J Clin Pathol* 59:340, 2006.
82. Banks PA: Acute pancreatitis: clinical presentation, in Go VLW, Gardner JD, Brooks EP, et al (eds): *The Exocrine Pancreas: Biology, Pathobiology, and Diseases*. New York, NY, Raven Press, 1986, p 475.
83. Tenner S, Fernandez-del Castillo C, Warshaw A, et al: Urinary trypsinogen activation peptide (TAP) predicts severity in patients with acute pancreatitis. *Int J Pancreatol* 21:105, 1997.
84. Bank S, Barbezat GO, Marks IN, et al: Methemalbuminaemia in acute abdominal emergencies. *BMJ* 2:86, 1968.
85. Kusske AM, Rungione AJ, Reber HA: Cytokines and acute pancreatitis. *Gastroenterology* 110:639, 1996.
86. Buchler M, Malfertheiner P, Beger HG: Correlation of imaging procedures, biochemical parameters and clinical stage in acute pancreatitis, in Malfertheiner P, Ditschuneit H (eds): *Diagnostic Procedures in Pancreatic Disease*. Berlin, Springer-Verlag, 1986, p 123.
87. Mayer AD, McMahon MJ, Bowen M, et al: C-reactive protein: an aid to assessment and monitoring of acute pancreatitis. *J Clin Pathol* 37:207, 1984.
88. Lees WR: Pancreatic ultrasonography. *Clin Gastroenterol* 13:763, 1984.
89. Freeny PC: Radiology of acute pancreatitis: diagnosis, detection of complications, and interventional therapy, in Glazer G, Ranson JHC (eds): *Acute Pancreatitis*. London, Bailliere Tindall, 1988, p 275.
90. Kivisarri L, Somer K, Standertskjold-Nordenstam C-G, et al: A new method for the diagnosis of acute hemorrhagic-necrotizing pancreatitis using contrast-enhanced CT. *Gastrointest Radiol* 9:27, 1984.
91. Beger HG, Krautzberger W, Bittner R, et al: Results of surgical treatment of necrotizing pancreatitis. *World J Surg* 9:972, 1985.
92. Runzi M, Raptopoulos V, Saluja AK, et al: Evaluation of necrotizing pancreatitis in the opossum by dynamic contrast-enhanced computed tomography: correlation between radiographic and morphologic changes. *J Am Coll Surg* 180:673, 1995.
93. Balthazar EJ: Acute pancreatitis: assessment of severity with clinical and CT evaluation. *Radiology* 223:603, 2002.
94. Matos C, Bali MA, Delhaye M, et al: Magnetic resonance imaging in the detection of pancreatitis and pancreatic neoplasms. *Best Pract Res Clin Gastroenterol* 20:157, 2006.
95. Ranson JHC: Prognostication in acute pancreatitis, in Glazer G, Ranson JHC (eds): *Acute Pancreatitis*. London, Bailliere Tindall, 1988, p 303.
96. Ranson JHC, Rifkind KM, Roses DF, et al: Prognostic signs and the role of operative management in acute pancreatitis. *Surg Gynecol Obstet* 139:69, 1974.
97. Imrie CW, Benjamin IS, Ferguson JC, et al: A single-centre double-blind trial of Trasylol therapy in primary acute pancreatitis. *Br J Surg* 65:337, 1978.
98. Larvin M, McMahon MJ: APACHE-2 score for assessment and monitoring of acute pancreatitis. *Lancet* 2:201, 1989.
99. Ranson JHC, Balthazar E, Caccavale R, et al: Computed tomography and the prediction of pancreatic abscess in acute pancreatitis. *Ann Surg* 201:656, 1985.

100. Halonen KJ, Pettila V, Leppaniemi AK, et al: Multiple organ dysfunction associated with severe acute pancreatitis. *Crit Care Med* 30:1274, 2002.
101. Vincent JL, de Mendoca A, Cantraine F, et al: Use of the SOFA score to assess the incidence of organ dysfunction/failure in intensive care units: results of a multicenter, prospective study. *Crit Care Med* 26:1793, 1998.
102. Brown A, Orav J, Banks PA: Hemoconcentration is an early marker for organ failure and necrotizing pancreatitis. *Pancreas* 20:367, 2000.
103. Lankisch PG, Mahike R, Blum T, et al: Hemoconcentration: an early marker of severe and/or necrotizing pancreatitis? A critical appraisal. *Am J Gastroenterol* 96:2081, 2001.
104. UK Working Party on Acute Pancreatitis: UK guidelines for the management of acute pancreatitis. *Gut* 54:1, 2001.
105. Uhl W, Warshaw AL, Imrie CW, et al: IAP guidelines for the surgical management of acute pancreatitis. *Pancreatology* 2:565, 2002.
106. Ranson JHC, Spencer FC: The role of peritoneal lavage in severe acute pancreatitis. *Ann Surg* 187:565, 1978.
107. Thune A, Baker RA, Saccone GT, et al: Differing effects of pethidine and morphine on human sphincter of Oddi motility. *Br J Surg* 77:992, 1990.
108. Beger HG, Bittner R, Buchler M, et al: Hemodynamic data pattern in patients with acute pancreatitis. *Gastroenterology* 90:70, 1986.
109. Yamanaka K, Saluja AK, Brown GE, et al: Protective effects of prostaglandin E_1 on the acute lung injury of caerulein-induced acute pancreatitis in rats. *Am J Physiol* 272:G23, 1997.
110. Finch WT, Sawyers JL, Schenker S: A prospective study to determine the efficacy of antibiotics in acute pancreatitis. *Ann Surg* 183:667, 1976.
111. Howes R, Zuidema GD, Cameron J: Evaluation of prophylactic antibiotics in acute pancreatitis. *J Surg Res* 18:197, 1975.
112. Bassi C, Vesentini S, Abbas H, et al: Result of the Italian Multicenter Trial with imipenem (I) in necrotizing pancreatitis (NP). *Pancreas* 7:732, 1992.
113. Sainio V, Kemppainen E, Puolakkainen P, et al: Early antibiotic treatment in acute necrotizing pancreatitis. *Lancet* 346:663, 1995.
114. Isenmann R, Runzi M, Kron M, et al: Prophylactic antibiotic treatment in patients with predicted severe acute pancreatitis: a placebo-controlled double-blind trial. *Gastroenterology* 126:997, 2004.
115. Gotzinger P, Wamser P, Barlan M, et al: *Candida* infection of local necrosis in severe acute pancreatitis is associated with increased mortality. *Shock* 14:320, 2000.
116. McMahon MJ, Lankisch PG: Peritoneal lavage and dialysis for the treatment of acute pancreatitis, in Beger HG, Buchler M (eds): *Acute Pancreatitis*. Berlin, Springer-Verlag, 1987, p 278.
117. Frey CF, Wong HN, Hickman D, et al: Toxicity of hemorrhagic ascitic fluid associated with hemorrhagic pancreatitis. *Arch Surg* 117:401, 1982.
118. Traverso LW, Pullos TG, Frey CF: Haemodynamic characterisation of porcine haemorrhagic pancreatitis ascites fluid. *J Surg Res* 34:254, 1983.
119. Ellison EC, Pappas TN, Johnson JA, et al: Demonstration and characterisation of the hemoconcentrating effect of ascitic fluid that accumulates during haemorrhagic pancreatitis. *J Surg Res* 30:241, 1981.
120. Geokas MC, Olsen H, Barbour B, et al: Peritoneal lavage in the treatment of acute hemorrhagic pancreatitis. *Gastroenterology* 58:950, 1970.
121. Wall AJ: Peritoneal dialysis in the treatment of severe acute pancreatitis. *Med J Australia* 2:281, 1965.
122. Bolooki H, Gliedman ML: Peritoneal dialysis in the treatment of acute pancreatitis. *Surgery* 64:466, 1978.
123. Lasson A, Balldin G, Genell S, et al: Peritoneal lavage in severe acute pancreatitis. *Acta Chir Scand* 150:479, 1984.
124. Mayer AD, McMahon MJ, Corfield AP, et al: Controlled clinical trial of peritoneal lavage for the treatment of severe acute pancreatitis. *N Engl J Med* 312:399, 1985.
125. Ranson JH, Berman RS: Long peritoneal lavage decreases pancreatic sepsis in acute pancreatitis. *Ann Surg* 211:708, 1990.
126. Goebell H, Singer MV: Acute pancreatitis: standards of conservative treatment, in Beger HG, Buchler M (eds): *Acute Pancreatitis*. Berlin, Springer-Verlag, 1987, p 259.
127. Steinberg WM, Schlesselman SN: Treatment of pancreatitis. Comparison of animal and human studies. *Gastroenterology* 93:1420, 1987.
128. Kingsnorth AW, Galloway SW, Formeka LLJ: Randomized, double-blind phase II trial of lexipafant, a platelet-activating factor antagonist, in human acute pancreatitis. *Br J Surg* 82:1414, 1995.
129. Johnson CD, Kingsnorth AN, Imrie CW, et al: Double blind, randomised, placebo controlled study of a platelet activating factor antagonist, lexipafant, in the treatment and prevention of organ failure in predicted severe acute pancreatitis. *Gut* 48:62, 2001.
130. Heinrich S, Schafer M, Rousson V, et al: Evidence-based treatment of acute pancreatitis: a look at established paradigms, *Ann Surg* 243:154, 2006.
131. Marik PE, Zaloga GP: Meta-analysis of parenteral nutrition versus enteral nutrition in patients with acute pancreatitis. *BMJ* 328:1407, 2004.
132. Whitcomb DG: Acute pancreatitis. *N Engl J Med* 354:2142, 2006.
133. Estock FC, Chong P, Menezes N, et al: A randomized study of early nasogastric versus nasojejunal feeding in severe acute pancreatitis. *Am J Gastroenterol* 100: 432, 2005.
134. Acosta JM, Rossi R, Galli OMR, et al: Early surgery for acute gallstone pancreatitis: evaluation of a systemic approach. *Surgery* 83:367, 1978.
135. Stone HH, Fabian TC, Dunlop WE: Gallstone pancreatitis. Biliary tract pathology in relation to time of operation. *Ann Surg* 194:305, 1981.
136. Kelly TR, Wagner DS: Gallstone pancreatitis: a prospective randomized trial of the timing of surgery. *Surgery* 104:600, 1988.
137. Neoptolemos JP, Carr-Locke DL, London NJ, et al: Controlled trial of urgent endoscopic retrograde cholangiopancreatography and endoscopic sphincterotomy versus conservative treatment for acute pancreatitis due to gallstones. *Lancet* 2:979, 1988.
138. Folsch OR, Nitsche R, Ludtke R, et al: Early ERCP and papillotomy compared with conservative treatment for acute biliary pancreatitis. The German Study Group on Acute Biliary Pancreatitis. *N Engl J Med* 336:237, 1997.
139. Van Santvoort HC, Besselink MG, de Vries AC, et al: Early endoscopic retrograde cholangiopancreatography in predicted severe acute biliary pancreatitis: a prospective multicenter study. *Ann Surg* 250:68, 2009.
140. Bradley EL: A clinically based classification system for acute pancreatitis. Summary of the International Symposium on Acute Pancreatitis, Atlanta, GA, September 11 through 13, 1992. *Arch Surg* 128:586, 1993.
141. Gerzoff SG, Banks PA, Robbins AH, et al: Early diagnosis of pancreatic infection by computed tomography-guided aspiration. *Gastroenterology* 93:1315, 1987.
142. Banks PA, Gerzoff SG: Indications and results of fine needle aspiration of pancreatic exudate, in Beger HG, Buchler M (eds): *Acute Pancreatitis*. Berlin, Springer-Verlag, 1987, p 171.
143. Beger HG, Buchler M, Bittner R, et al: Necrosectomy and postoperative local lavage in necrotizing pancreatitis. *Br J Surg* 75:207, 1988.
144. Bradley EL, Allen K: A prospective longitudinal study of observation versus surgical intervention in the management of necrotizing pancreatitis. *Am J Surg* 161:19, 1991.
145. Baron TH, Morgan DE: Endoscopic transgastric irrigation tube placement via PEG for debridement of organized pancreatic necrosis. *Gastrointest Endosc* 50:574, 1999.
146. Freeney PC, Hauptmann E, Althaus AJ, et al: Percutaneous CT-guided catheter drainage of infected acute necrotizing pancreatitis: techniques and results. *Am J Roentgenol* 170:969, 1998.
147. Kozarek RA, Ball TJ, Patterson DJ, et al: Endoscopic transpapillary therapy for disrupted pancreatic duct and peripancreatic fluid collections. *Gastroenterology* 100:1362, 1991.
148. Carter CR, McKay CJ, Imrie CW: Percutaneous necrosectomy and sinus tract endoscopy in the management of infected pancreatic necrosis: an initial experience. *Ann Surg* 232:175, 2000.
149. Horvath KD, Kao LS, Wherry KL, et al: A technique for laparoscopic-assisted percutaneous drainage of infected pancreatic necrosis and pancreatic abscess. *Surg Endosc* 15:1221, 2001.
150. Pemberton JH, Nagorney DM, Dozois RR: Pancreatic abscess, in Go VLW, Gardner JD, Brooks EP, et al. (eds): *The Exocrine Pancreas: Biology, Pathobiology, and Diseases*. New York, Raven Press, 1986, p 513.
151. Hartwig W, Maksan SM, Foitzik T, et al: Reduction in mortality with delayed surgical therapy of severe pancreatitis. *J Gastrointest Surg* 30:195, 2002.
152. Runzi M, Niebel W, Goebell H, et al: Severe acute pancreatitis: nonsurgical treatment of infected necroses. *Pancreas* 30:195, 2005.
153. Bradley EL, Clements JL, Gonzales AC: The natural history of pancreatic pseudocysts: a unified concept of management. *Am J Surg* 137:135, 1979.
154. Yeo CJ, Bastidas JA, Lynch-Nyhan A, et al: The natural history of pancreatic pseudocysts documented by computed tomography. *Surg Gynecol Obstet* 170:411, 1990.
155. Vitas GJ, Sarr MG: Selected management of pancreatic pseudocysts: operative versus expectant management. *Surgery* 111:123, 1992.
156. Morali GA, Braverman DZ, Shemesh D, et al: Successful treatment of pancreatic pseudocysts with a somatostatin analogue and catheter drainage. *Am J Gastroenterol* 86:515, 1991.
157. Beckingham IJ, Crige EJ, Bornman PC, et al: Long-term outcome of endoscopic drainage of pancreatic pseudocysts. *Am J Gastroenterol* 94:71, 1999.
158. Sankaran S, Walt AJ: Pancreatic ascites: recognition and management. *Arch Surg* 111:430, 1976.
159. Cameron JL, Kieffer RS, Anderson WJ, et al: Internal pancreatic fistulas: pancreatic ascites and pleural effusions. *Ann Surg* 184:587, 1976.
160. Kavin H, Sobel JD, Dembo AJ: Pancreatic ascites treated by irradiation of pancreas. *BMJ* 2:503, 1971.
161. DeWale B, Van der Spek P, Devis G: Peritoneovenous shunt for pancreatic ascites. *Dig Dis Sci* 32:550, 1987.
162. Variyam EP: Central vein hyperalimentation in pancreatic ascites. *Am J Gastroenterol* 78:178, 1983.
163. Ward PA, Raju S, Suzuki H: Preoperative demonstration of pancreatic fistula by endoscopic pancreatography in a patient with pancreatic ascites. *Ann Surg* 185:232, 1977.
164. Cameron JL, Brawley RK, Bender HW, et al: The treatment of pancreatic ascites. *Ann Surg* 170:668, 1969.
165. Gislason H, Growbech JE, Soreide O: Pancreatic ascites: treatment by continuous somatostatin infusion. *Am J Gastroenterol* 86:519, 1991.
166. Sankaran S, Sugawa C, Walt AJ: Value of endoscopic retrograde pancreatography in pancreatic ascites. *Surg Gynecol Obstet* 148:185, 1979.
167. Rawlings W, Bynum TE, Pasternak G: Pancreatic ascites: diagnosis of leakage site by endoscopic pancreatography. *Surgery* 81:363, 1977.
168. Levine JB, Warshaw AL, Falchuk KR, et al: The value of endoscopic retrograde pancreatography in the management of pancreatic ascites. *Surgery* 81:360, 1977.

169. Kozarek RA, Ball TJ, Paterson DJ, et al: Endoscopic transpapillary therapy for disrupted pancreatic duct and peripancreatic fluid collections. *Gastroenterology* 100:1362, 1991.
170. Rivers E, Nguyen B, Havstad S, et al: Early goal-directed therapy in the treatment of severe sepsis and septic shock. *N Engl J Med* 345:1368, 2001.
171. Helm JF, Venu RP, Geenen JE, et al: Effects of morphine on the human sphincter of Oddi. *Gut* 29:1402, 1988.
172. McClave SA, Chang WK, Dhaliwal R, et al: Nutrition support in acute pancreatitis: a systematic review of the literature. *JPEN J Parenter Enteral Nutr* 30:143, 2006.
173. Marik PE, Zaloga GP: Meta-analysis of parenteral nutrition versus enteral nutrition in patients with acute pancreatitis. *BMJ* 328:1407, 2004.
174. Al-Omran M, Groof A, Wilke D: Enteral versus parenteral nutrition for acute pancreatitis. *Cochrane Database Syst Rev* CD002837, 2003.
175. Bassi C, Larvin M, Villatoro E: Antibiotic therapy for prophylaxis against infection of pancreatic necrosis in acute pancreatitis. *Cochrane Database Syst Rev* CD002941, 2003.
176. Golub R, Siddiqi F, Pohl D: Role of antibiotics in acute pancreatitis: a meta-analysis. *J Gastrointest Surg* 2:496, 1998.
177. Mier J, Leon EL, Castillo A, et al: Early versus late necrosectomy in severe necrotizing pancreatitis. *Am J Surg* 173:71, 1997.
178. Folsch UR, Nitsche R, Ludtke R, et al: Early ERCP and papillotomy compared with conservative treatment for acute biliary pancreatitis. The German Study Group on Acute Biliary Pancreatitis. *N Engl J Med* 336:237, 1997.

SECTION VIII ■ ENDOCRINE PROBLEMS IN THE INTENSIVE CARE UNIT

NEIL ARONIN • DAVID M. HARLAN

CHAPTER 100 ■ MANAGEMENT OF HYPERGLYCEMIA IN CRITICALLY ILL PATIENTS

MICHAEL J. THOMPSON, DAVID M. HARLAN, SAMIR MALKANI AND JOHN P. MORDES

INTRODUCTION

Hyperglycemia is a common problem that complicates the delivery of intensive care. About 7.8% of the U.S. population was reportedly diabetic in 2007 [1]. National Health Interview Survey and census projections suggest that between 2000 and 2050, the number of persons with diabetes will rise from 12 million to 48.3 million persons of all ages and that the prevalence will increase to 12% [2]. Perhaps, as many as one in three people born in the United States in 2000 will develop diabetes at some time [3]. In addition, the growing worldwide prevalence of obesity is increasing the prevalence of diabetes in many nations [4]. The world prevalence of diabetes among adults is predicted to be 7.7%, or 439 million adults, by 2030 [5].

Epidemiology alone would make diabetes a common problem in the intensive care unit (ICU), but poorly controlled diabetes also predisposes to cardiovascular [6,7], renal [8–10], and infectious [11–16] complications that often require intensive surgical and medical care. In addition, hyperglycemia frequently occurs in severely ill ICU patients who have no prior history of diabetes [17].

Whatever the primary problem, hyperglycemia amplifies the challenges of intensive care. Often, pre-existing diabetes itself is the primary problem, as in ketoacidosis and hyperosmolar coma. These conditions are discussed in Chapter 101.

ETIOLOGY AND PATHOPHYSIOLOGY

Metabolic Homeostasis

Individuals with normal glucose tolerance maintain their blood glucose concentration between 60 and 120 mg per dL. Maintenance of glucose within this narrow range is controlled by the degree of tissue insulinization (Fig. 100.1) [18]. This is a function of the amount of insulin available and the responsiveness of target tissues. After eating, blood glucose concentration rises but remains within the normal range as a result of increased insulin secretion. Insulin first promotes the transport of glucose into cells and the repletion of glycogen and protein stores. It then mediates the storage of excess glucose as triglyceride. When absorption of nutrients is complete, the concentrations of all metabolites and hormones return to basal levels.

In the fasting state, two mechanisms keep blood glucose concentration in the normal range, glycogenolysis and gluconeogenesis. Initially, hepatic glycogen is mobilized. If fasting persists longer than 12 to 18 hours, peripheral tissues begin to use free fatty acids for fuel, thereby sparing glucose. A low level of circulating insulin is permissive to the lipolytic release of these fatty acids. At the same time, gluconeogenesis supplies glucose for obligate glycolytic tissues, most notably the central nervous system.

If starvation continues for more than 72 hours, the brain begins to use ketone bodies as an alternative fuel, further sparing glucose utilization [18]. At this stage, a progressive decrease in hepatic gluconeogenesis occurs as a consequence of decreased amino acid release in the periphery. As starvation continues, lactate, pyruvate, and glycerol become the main gluconeogenic precursors in place of amino acids. At all times, a low level of circulating insulin regulates the rate of lipolysis, glucose transport, and gluconeogenesis. Healthy humans are always insulinized to an appropriate degree.

Metabolic Stress

Major surgery and critical illness are physiologically stressful events that provoke complex metabolic responses. Tissue hypoxia and hypoxemia adversely affect normal oxidative phosphorylation, and counterregulatory hormones are secreted. These hormones include epinephrine, norepinephrine, cortisol, growth hormone, glucagon, and various cytokines (e.g., tumor necrosis factor-α). They raise blood glucose concentration, mobilize alternative fuels, and increase peripheral resistance to the effects of insulin. In the ICU, their effects may be further amplified by the concurrent administration of exogenous vasopressors, glucocorticoids, and other drugs that can affect intermediary metabolism.

Stress and the Diabetic State

Stress-induced changes in metabolism normally lead to increased insulin release. This in turn enhances peripheral glucose utilization and inhibits alternative fuel mobilization. In this way, the body resists stress without losing control of the biochemical machinery. In patients with decreased insulin reserves (i.e., diabetes mellitus), failure of this feedback loop produces hyperglycemia and related metabolic complications. To preclude these complications, careful management of insulin, fluid, and electrolytes is necessary.

Classification of Diabetes

Diabetes is not one disease but rather a family of syndromes that have in common hyperglycemia resulting from inadequate insulinization. These syndromes vary with respect to

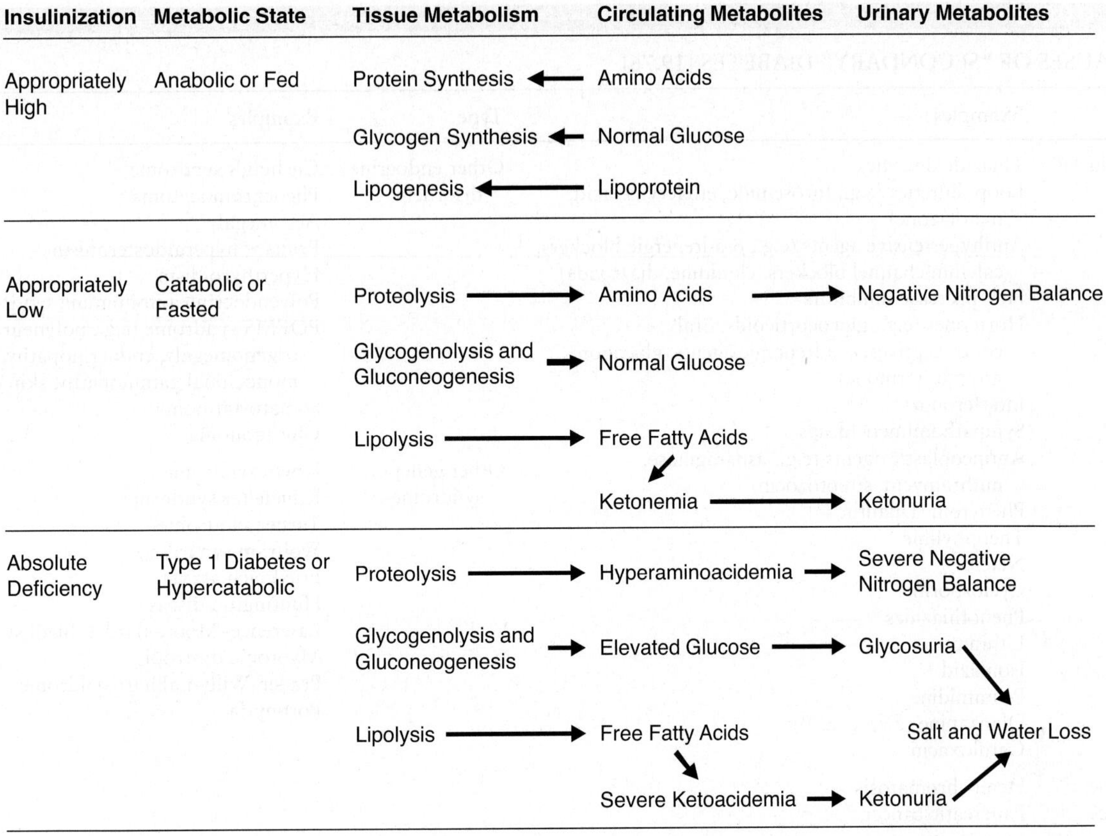

FIGURE 100.1. Metabolic effects of insulin in normal and diabetic states. *Upper* entries illustrate the anabolic, storage-promoting effects of insulin that occur with eating. *Middle* entries illustrate the controlled catabolic effects that occur during fasting. *Bottom* entries illustrate the *uncontrolled catabolism that ensues from absolute deficiency of insulin in type 1 diabetes.*

genetics, pathophysiology, and appropriate treatment modalities [19]. Table 100.1 outlines the American Diabetes Association's (ADA's) classification system.

Type 1 Diabetes

In type 1 diabetes, the insulin-producing β cells in the pancreatic islets are destroyed, resulting in near total deficiency of insulin [18,20]. Hyperglycemia develops rapidly, most commonly during childhood and adolescence. Most cases of type 1 diabetes are autoimmune in origin [20]. About 10% of persons with diabetes have this form of the disorder.

Patients with type 1 diabetes require exogenous insulin for survival (Fig. 100.1). The insulin can be given either as a continuous insulin infusion or as conventional subcutaneous injections. The key ICU issue is continuity of treatment. Inappropriate discontinuation of insulin treatment, even for relatively brief intervals, can lead to serious metabolic complications.

Patients with type 1 diabetes who are not given insulin can neither store nor use glucose, and unregulated gluconeogenesis and lipolysis occur (Fig. 100.1). In this hypercatabolic state, accelerating amino acid and fat mobilization produce hyperglycemia, hyperlipidemia, and ketosis. The excess glucose produced by uncontrolled gluconeogenesis remains in the circulation because there is no insulin to stimulate transport into cells. The osmotic diuresis of glucose and the buffering of ketoacids produce secondary fluid and electrolyte shifts. Ultimately, diabetic ketoacidosis occurs. This disorder is discussed in Chapter 101.

TABLE 100.1

CLASSIFICATION OF DIABETIC SYNDROMES [19]

Type 1 diabetes (β-cell destruction) autoimmune (Type 1 A) and idiopathic (Type 1B)
Type 2 diabetes (insulin resistance with variable insulin secretory defect)
Other specific types
Genetic defects of β-cell function (e.g., MODY, mitochondrial DNA)
Genetic defects in insulin action (e.g., lipoatrophic diabetes)
Diseases of the exocrine pancreas (see Table 100.2)
Endocrinopathies (see Table 100.2)
Drug or chemical induced (see Table 100.2)
Infections (e.g., congenital rubella)
Uncommon forms of immune-mediated diabetes (e.g., stiff-man syndrome)
Other genetic syndromes associated with diabetes
Gestational diabetes mellitus

MODY, maturity-onset diabetes of the young.

Type 2 Diabetes

Type 2 diabetes is characterized by relative, rather than absolute, deficiency of insulin. It involves defects in both insulin action and insulin secretion. Impaired response to insulin in peripheral tissues is often the dominant feature [21–23]. It develops insidiously, most commonly in obese individuals older than 40 years. It may go undetected for years, only to be discovered serendipitously or during the stress of surgery or other illness. Patients with type 2 diabetes account for more than 80% of the diabetic population.

TABLE 100.2

SOME CAUSES OF "SECONDARY" DIABETES [19,76]

Type	Examples	Type	Examples
Drug induced	Thiazide diuretics	Other endocrine disorders	Cushing's syndrome
	Loop diuretics (e.g., furosemide, ethacrynic acid, metolazone)		Pheochromocytoma
	Antihypertensive agents (e.g., β-adrenergic blockers, calcium channel blockers, clonidine, diazoxide)		Acromegaly
	HIV protease inhibitors		Primary hyperaldosteronism
	Hormones (e.g., glucocorticoids, oral contraceptives, α-adrenergic agents, glucagon, growth hormone)		Hyperthyroidism
	Interferon-α		Polyendocrine autoimmune syndromes
	Sympathomimetic drugs		POEMS syndrome (e.g., polyneuropathy, organomegaly, endocrinopathy, monoclonal gammopathy, skin changes)
	Antineoplastic agents (e.g., asparaginase, mithramycin, streptozocin)		Somatostatinoma
	Phenytoin (Dilantin™)		Glucagonoma
	Theophylline	Other genetic syndromes	Down syndrome
	Niacin		Klinefelter syndrome
	Cyclosporin		Turner syndrome
	Phenothiazines		Wolfram syndrome
	Lithium		Friedreich ataxia
	Isoniazid		Huntington disease
	Pentamidine		Lawrence–Moon–Bardet–Biedl syndrome
	Olanzapine (Zyprexa™)		Myotonic dystrophy
	Gatifloxacin		Prader–Willi–Labhart syndrome
Pancreatic diseases	Hemochromatosis		Porphyria
	Pancreatic cancer		
	Pancreatitis		
	Cystic fibrosis		
	Fibrocalculous pancreatopathy		
	Abdominal trauma		

Many patients with type 2 diabetes can be treated with diet, exercise, and oral hypoglycemic agents. Some patients, especially those who are not obese, need insulin to control their hyperglycemia. This is done to prevent symptoms (e.g., polyuria) and long-term complications. Even when type 2 diabetes is untreated, there is usually enough insulin present to control lipid mobilization and prevent ketoacidosis when the patient is otherwise well.

In the ICU, patients with type 2 diabetes whose diabetes is uncontrolled should be treated with insulin. Keys to management include attention to both blood glucose concentration and acid–base balance. Infection, metabolic stress, and many medications commonly used in the ICU can exacerbate type 2 diabetes and lead to ketoacidosis [24], hyperosmolar coma, or lactic acidosis. These disorders are discussed in Chapter 101.

Other Types of Diabetes

Additional forms of diabetes involve specific genetic defects or are secondary to intercurrent diseases, infections, medications, or a combination of these [19]. The broad categories into which these other specific types of diabetes fall are given in Table 100.1. A partial listing of the other types of diabetes and precipitants of secondary diabetes is given in Table 100.2.

ICU patients with any form of uncontrolled hyperglycemia require insulin to control hyperglycemia and prevent short-rm metabolic complications. Patients who have undergone pancreatectomy have absolute insulin deficiency, are ke-ne, and are insulin dependent. Patients with other dis-xocrine pancreas (e.g., pancreatitis) can develop variable degrees of insulin deficiency and, in the ICU, should be considered potentially at risk for ketoacidosis. Gestational diabetes in an ICU setting should also be treated with insulin.

DIAGNOSIS OF HYPERGLYCEMIA IN THE INTENSIVE CARE UNIT

Diagnostic Criteria

All acutely ill patients should have their blood glucose level measured at entry into the ICU and at regular intervals throughout their stay. In the outpatient setting, diabetes is diagnosed by a fasting blood glucose level greater than 126 mg per dL or a glucose level greater than or equal to 200 mg per dL measured 2 hours after a 75-g oral-glucose tolerance test. It is required that this be a persistent condition confirmed by repeating the test on another day. A formal diagnosis of new onset diabetes should be made tentatively during the stress of an ICU admission as hyperglycemia may subsequently resolve. Hyperglycemic ICU patients with no prior history of diabetes should be evaluated for persistence of impaired glucose tolerance after recovery.

The majority of seriously ill patients with hyperglycemia do not have a preexisting diagnosis of diabetes. In one study of 1,200 subjects treated in a medical ICU, 70% of individuals at some time experienced a plasma glucose concentration of more than 215 mg per dL, and only about 17% of these patients had a prior history of diabetes [25].

Assessment of Severity

Whenever the glucose concentration in any patient is greater than about 250 mg per dL, actual or impending ketoacidosis and hyperosmolality must be excluded. Ketoacidosis can be diagnosed on the basis of history, physical findings, and the presence of an anion gap acidosis and ketonemia. Osmolarity can be measured by the laboratory or calculated from the serum concentrations of glucose, blood urea nitrogen, sodium, and potassium (Table 100.1; Chapter 101). Hyperosmolar states in the setting of diabetes are usually associated with severe dehydration, obtundation, and extreme hyperglycemia. Diabetic ketoacidosis and hyperosmolar coma require urgent treatment (see Chapter 101). In this chapter, we describe the goals, methods, and pitfalls of treating intercurrent diabetes mellitus in the ICU when neither ketoacidosis nor hyperosmolar coma is the primary disease process.

TREATMENT OF CRITICALLY ILL PATIENTS WITH PREEXISTING DIABETES

Initial Evaluation

Physicians caring for patients with diabetes in an ICU should attempt to determine the type of diabetes, its duration, the presence of diabetic complications, and the degree of previous glycemic control. Patients with type 1 diabetes require insulin treatment at all times; those with type 2 diabetes may or may not require insulin. Patients with diabetes that is secondary to some other disorder (Table 100.2) require diagnosis and treatment of the precipitating factors.

Long-standing diabetes is associated with complications that tend to be worse in patients with either type 1 [26] or type 2 [27] disease that is poorly controlled. These sequelae of diabetes complicate the management of critical illness. Diabetes is a leading cause of cardiovascular and peripheral vascular disease. Assessments of both cardiac function and peripheral circulation are advisable for all patients with diabetes. Diabetic neuropathy can affect the autonomic nervous system, with implications for management of blood pressure, heart rate, and voiding. Autonomic neuropathy should be suspected in patients with an abnormal pupillary response to light or absence of heart rate response (R-R interval change in the electrocardiogram) during Valsalva maneuver. Assessment of kidney function should include a urinalysis for protein; albuminuria precedes abnormalities in blood urea nitrogen and creatinine levels. Diabetic eye disease is not a contraindication to anticoagulation, but its severity should be documented before instituting therapy.

A history of poor control should alert the clinician to other potential problems. Poorly controlled diabetes may imply poor nutrition. This has important implications for resistance to infection and wound healing; nutritional assessment and vitamin repletion may be required. Thiamine in particular is a critical cofactor in carbohydrate metabolism, and patients with uncontrolled diabetes may be thiamine deficient. Occult infections to which individuals with diabetes are particularly susceptible include osteomyelitis, cellulitis, tuberculosis, cholecystitis, gingivitis, sinusitis, cystitis, and pyelonephritis [11,12,28,29]. Patients with type 2 diabetes are frequently hyperlipidemic and may develop pancreatitis when poorly controlled [30].

Systems are now available for accurately measuring a patient's blood glucose levels at the point of care and with near-immediate results using hospital-grade bedside machines, and should be on hand in all emergency departments, ICUs, operating suites, and recovery rooms [31,32]. It should be noted that glucose meter measurements can be influenced by hematocrit, creatinine concentration, plasma protein concentration, and PO_2, all of which can be very abnormal in ICU patients [33–35]. Test strips based on glucose dehydrogenase-pyrroloquinoline quinone (GDH-PQQ) methodology can falsely elevate blood glucose readings in patients receiving maltose or icodextrin by more than 100 mg per dL [36]. Maltose is used in a number of biological preparations and peritoneal dialysis solutions may contain icodextrin. Extremely elevated blood glucose concentrations may be outside the range accurately measured by the bedside monitor and should be verified with a serum sample sent to the laboratory [37]. In general, however, therapy should not be delayed by waiting for confirmatory results of laboratory glucose concentration.

Why Control Hyperglycemia in the Intensive Care Unit?

Hyperglycemia in the Intensive Care Unit Predicts Adverse Outcome

It is intuitively plausible to assume that glucose concentration should always be in the normal range, and studies show that hyperglycemia in the ICU is associated with adverse outcome. Even minimal hyperglycemia, plasma glucose concentration more than 110 mg per dL, has been shown to predict increased in-hospital mortality and the risk of congestive heart failure in patients with acute myocardial infarction [38]. Hyperglycemic patients also have an increased risk of wound infection as well as overall mortality following cardiac surgery [39,40]. Hyperglycemia is also associated with poor outcome in patients with stroke [41]. Patients in whom diabetes is diagnosed for the first time during an ICU admission reportedly have an 18-fold increase in their risk of in-hospital mortality [42].

How Does Hyperglycemia Adversely Affect Outcome?

Hyperglycemia predisposes to disturbances in sodium, potassium, and phosphate concentrations. Because uncontrolled hyperglycemia also provokes an osmotic diuresis, symptomatic hyponatremia can result. Hypokalemia predisposes to arrhythmia, and hypophosphatemia may interfere with platelet function and white cell motility. Control of glycemia prevents these problems and the need for compensatory correction. The susceptibility of patients with diabetes to infection is well recognized [11,12,28]. Uncontrolled glycemia appears to impair innate immunity (cytokine responses), granulocyte function (chemotaxis, phagocytosis, and killing), and, possibly, lymphocyte function and antibody formation [43–46]. Some microorganisms become more virulent in a high-glucose environment [43]. Endothelial function may also be impaired by hyperglycemia [47]. In general, better regulation of blood glucose leads to improvement in these parameters.

What is the Evidence that Control of Blood Glucose Concentration Alters Clinical Outcome in Intensive Care Unit Patients?

Recognizing that hyperglycemia is bad is not the same as saying that control of hyperglycemia in the ICU is beneficial. Attempting to normalize blood glucose concentration in the ICU is not without risk. The available evidence does not yet establish that intensive management of hyperglycemia within the normal is unequivocally beneficial [48].

The best evidence for benefit attributable to intensive management derives from studies performed in a surgical ICU setting. Intensive insulin treatment reportedly improves myocardial performance and results in faster recovery after coronary artery bypass grafting [49]. Continuous intravenous insulin infusion also reduces the risk of sternal wound infection in diabetic patients after cardiac surgical procedures [39]. The studies reporting benefit, however, did not seek to reduce plasma glucose concentration all the way to the "normal" range. In 2001, an influential study of surgical ICU patients by Van den Berghe et al. [50] reported that intensive insulin therapy with a target plasma glucose concentration less than 110 mg per dL reduced in-hospital mortality by 34%, septicemia by 46%, acute renal failure by 41%, and critical-illness polyneuropathy by 44%. This study, together with the results of retrospective studies [40,51,52], generated widespread acceptance of the concept that intensive glycemic control is important in critically ill patients. This then led to implementation of intensive glycemic control protocols in a majority of academic ICU programs.

A question raised after the release of the results of the 2001 study by Van den Berghe et al. was whether intensive management would show similar benefit in the medical ICU. To some extent, this was a reflection of several atypical features in the original study, which involved only a single center and was not blinded [50]. In addition, the mortality among the cardiac surgery patients in the control group (5.1%) was several times higher than expected. Finally, all study subjects received 200 to 300 g of glucose daily, that is, 2 to 3 L of 10% dextrose and early enteral or parenteral feeding. These characteristics are not the norm for cardiothoracic surgery patients worldwide. A subsequent report from the Van den Berghe group [25] reported that intensive insulin therapy of patients in a medical ICU, while improving several indices of morbidity, did not reduce in-hospital mortality. Disturbingly, hypoglycemia (<40 mg per dL) occurred in 18% of subjects in the intensively treated group versus 3% of those in the conventionally treated group, and hypoglycemia was identified as an independent risk factor for death. The data concerning hypoglycemia were surprising, as this problem had not been encountered in several other studies designed to evaluate the safety and practicality of implementing intensive insulin protocols in ICU settings [52–54].

The lack of a consistent, evidence-based dataset led to several multicenter randomized controlled trials of blood glucose management in heterogeneous ICU populations. The GLUControl trial randomized 3,000 medical and surgical ICU patients in several centers in Europe to two regimens of insulin therapy targeted to achieve a plasma glucose concentration of either 80 to 110 mg per dL or 140 to 180 mg per dL [55]. The trial was stopped early due to an increased frequency of hypoglycemia together with lack of clinical benefit in the intensive insulin therapy cohort.

The NICE-SUGAR (Normoglycemia in Intensive Care Evaluation and Survival Using Glucose Algorithm Regulation) trial randomized 5,000 medical and surgical ICU patients at multiple centers in Australia, New Zealand, and Canada to intensive (81 to 108 mg per dL) or conventional (≤180 mg per dL) management [56]. The investigators reported that intensive glucose control increased mortality and the rate of hypoglycemia compared with the conventional target cohort. It should be noted, however, that two features of this study are atypical. First, the protocol required measurement of glucose in the ICU only every 4 hours. Second, a substantial fraction of mortality occurred late, after discharge from the ICU, for reasons that are not clear.

A possible adverse effect of increased incidence of hypoglycemia resulting from intensive glycemic control efforts was …o suggested by the results of the COIITSS (Corticosteroid …ment and Intensive Insulin Therapy for Septic Shock in …ial [57]. In this trial, critically ill patients with sepsis who were treated both with intensive insulin therapy and with glucocorticoids. The investigators reported a higher frequency of hypoglycemia (16.4%) in the intensive insulin cohort than in the conventional treatment group (7.8%) with no reduction in mortality.

Finally, the VISEP (Volume Substitution and Insulin Therapy in Severe Sepsis) planned to randomize 600 patients to receive either intensive insulin therapy to maintain euglycemia or conventional insulin therapy and either 10% pentastarch or modified Ringer's lactate for fluid resuscitation [58]. The trial was stopped early because at 28 days, there was no significant difference between the two groups in mortality, but the rate of severe hypoglycemia and other serious adverse events was higher in the intensive therapy group.

In critically ill patients, an association exists between even mild or moderate hypoglycemia and mortality [59,60]. Tight glycemic control has also been specifically associated with a high incidence of hypoglycemia and an increased risk of death in patients not receiving parenteral nutrition [61].

Recommended Glycemic Targets

The American Association of Clinical Endocrinologists (AACE) and the ADA have jointly recommended a glycemic target of 140 to 180 mg per dL in the ICU setting, noting that greater benefit may be realized at the lower end of this range [48]. Most experts have abandoned the target of less than 110 mg per dL suggested by the original Van den Berge study [50]. Glucose concentrations less than 80 mg per dL should be stringently avoided because they pose the hazard of hypoglycemia and might contribute to mortality [50,59,60]. An intensive insulin treatment program to achieve the AACE/ADA targets requires a strong institutional commitment. It is a team effort requiring participation of physicians, nursing, and pharmacy staff.

Treatment of Hyperglycemia in the Critically Ill

The majority of ICU patients will require treatment for hyperglycemia and we recommend that they be treated with a continuous intravenous infusion of regular insulin. This applies to all patients, irrespective of prior history of diabetes or previous treatment modalities. Patients known to have type 1 diabetes are absolutely insulin dependent, and they must be treated with exogenous insulin at all times. Oral hypoglycemic agents (see Chapter 106) should not be used in the ICU for many reasons. Their absorption, metabolism, and excretion cannot be predicted in the critically ill patient. Sulfonylureas can cause severe hypoglycemia [62] (see Chapter 106). Metformin should be discontinued because it can cause lactic acidosis in the setting of renal failure [63].

Our recommendations for the management of patients with ketoacidosis or hyperosmolar syndrome are given elsewhere (see Chapter 106). For patients whose primary ICU diagnosis is not diabetic ketoacidosis or hyperosmolar hyperglycemic syndrome, we recommend the treatment program advocated by the AACE and ADA [48].

Insulin Therapy

Although optimal glycemic targets are now agreed to, insulin infusion algorithms to achieve those targets necessarily will vary from ICU to ICU and need to be individualized by a multidisciplinary team. Every protocol will require development of guidelines for adjustment of the insulin infusion rate in response to *both* the absolute value *and* the rate of change of the glucose concentration. Glucose concentration should be checked hourly until it is in the target range of 140 to 180 mg per dL, and every 2 hours thereafter. During the initial period, adjustments to the insulin infusion rate will depend on the patient's sensitivity to insulin (see later) and the observed response to therapy, which cannot be exactly predicted. Concurrent glucose infusions or parenteral or enteral feeding will also affect the dose required.

Diluted insulin solutions prepared for continuous insulin infusions have a limited storage life, since insulin adheres to the plastic infusion bag. There is no advantage to the use of rapid-acting semisynthetic insulin for this purpose, but it can be used when regular insulin is unavailable. It should be stressed that it is entirely appropriate to infuse insulin at low rates (e.g., 0.5 U per hour). A low rate of insulin infusion is often all that is needed to prevent ketoacidosis in a patient with type 1 diabetes.

Adjustment of the Insulin Infusion Rate

The amount of insulin required by a given ICU patient will depend in large part on the degree of insulin resistance induced by the primary illness, the agents used in its treatment, and the patient's body mass index. It will also depend on the type and amount of nutritional support being given. An escalating insulin infusion requirement is a sensitive indicator of increasing insulin resistance and requires careful reevaluation of the patient's overall metabolic status. Stressors that increase insulin resistance include sepsis, occult infections, heart disease, tissue ischemia, hypoxemia, and various medications. The most common offending medications are glucocorticoids and pressors.

In otherwise stable patients, instituting or increasing enteral or parenteral nutrition typically increases insulin requirements. Insulin-mediated glucose disposal is impaired in stressed patients with hyperglycemia, and even extremely high insulin infusion rates cannot prevent hyperglycemia due to unmanageable carbohydrate loads. To control hyperglycemia in the ICU, a choice must sometimes be made between increasing insulin infusion rates and reducing carbohydrate feeding. We recommend that insulin infusion rates should not be increased beyond 20 units per hour (480 units per day) without first decreasing any exogenous carbohydrate loads, especially in patients who are obese. This suggestion is based on the fact that maximal insulin effects are achieved when only some of the available insulin receptors are occupied [64,65]. High concentrations of insulin, such as those achieved during continuous intravenous infusions at high rates, desensitize target tissues at both the receptor and postreceptor levels, paradoxically enhancing insulin resistance [66].

Factors that increase insulin sensitivity in the ICU include improvement in intercurrent illnesses, changes in medication, and reductions in enteral or parenteral feeding. Occasionally, hepatic failure, renal failure, or adrenal insufficiency leads to a decreased insulin requirement.

When plasma glucose concentrations are lower than 140 mg per dL, a common response is to discontinue insulin completely. For patients with type 1 diabetes, this is always inappropriate because it can precipitate hyperglycemia and ketosis within hours. The proper response is to reduce the insulin infusion rate to 1 or even 0.5 units per hour and, if necessary, to give glucose in the form of 5% dextrose in water. We recommend the same strategy for most other hyperglycemic ICU patients as well. Unless their primary disease state has improved dramatically, they frequently experience recurrent hyperglycemia. Patients with hyperglycemia in the ICU should receive continuous intravenous insulin until they demonstrate clear improvement in overall clinical status and stability of glycemic control that extends over several blood glucose determinations.

Transition to Other Forms of Therapy

When the condition of an ICU patient with hyperglycemia has improved to such an extent that continuous insulin infusion is no longer needed, subsequent therapy will depend on the cause of the hyperglycemia. Patients with "secondary diabetes" (e.g., catecholamine or steroid induced) may need no further treatment for glucose control after the offending drug is stopped. In contrast, all patients with type 1 and most with type 2 diabetes will continue to require insulin. This should include intermediate or long-acting insulin, for example, neutral protamine hagedorn (NPH), glargine, or detemir (see Table 106.1 in hypoglycemia chapter for details).

It is not uncommon for glycemic control to deteriorate during the transition from intravenous insulin therapy to subcutaneous insulin therapy. It is essential that the intravenous infusion of regular insulin be continued for 2 to 3 hours after the first subcutaneous injection of insulin is given. The initial dose of subcutaneous insulin should be estimated from a review of the preceding intravenous insulin requirements. Presumably, the individual ready to transition to subcutaneous therapy will have had reasonably stable insulin requirements. We recommend basing this dose on the average hourly insulin requirement during the 6 hours prior to discontinuation of the insulin drip using the following procedure:

Calculating the starting intermediate (NPH) or long-acting (Glargine or Detemir) insulin dose

1. The average hourly insulin drip rate for the last 6 hours is ___ units per hour.
2. Multiply by 24 to give a daily usage rate: ___ units per day.
3. Multiply by 70% to estimate the first day's total insulin dose: ___ units.
4. All can be administered in divided doses twice daily; glargine can be given once daily. Dose adjustment may be necessary after first dose given. Review daily thereafter.

When patients are able to eat, a rapid-acting insulin (e.g., lispro, aspart, or glulisine) should be given before each meal. Some stable patients with type 2 diabetes can be managed with oral hypoglycemic agents (Chapter 106; Table 106.2) or diet alone, but that therapeutic decision is best made after discharge from the ICU on a regimen of subcutaneous insulin.

SURGERY IN THE CRITICALLY ILL PATIENT WITH DIABETES

Critically ill patients frequently require invasive procedures, surgery, and intensive postoperative care. In such situations, the treatment of intercurrent diabetes is obviously of importance. The possibility of diabetes must be considered in all surgical emergencies, and both glucose and electrolytes must be measured immediately. A critically ill patient with diabetes, even if previously undiagnosed, can rapidly develop metabolic derangements.

It is generally accepted that good perioperative control of glucose is desirable, but the target levels of glucose and the ideal method of insulin delivery during surgery need to be individualized [67]. Perioperative control of blood pressure and vascular responses may be as important as glucose control for prevention of adverse perioperative events.

Abdominal pain accompanied by guarding and rebound tenderness is a common symptom of diabetic ketoacidosis. The diagnosis of diabetic ketoacidosis has on occasion been made at laparotomy, and this disorder must be excluded in every patient being evaluated for an abdominal surgery. The patient with trauma being prepared for surgery should also be evaluated for diabetes, regardless of mental status. The stress of major trauma and shock is less likely to be survived if ketoacidosis or hyperosmolarity is present or allowed to develop. Severe trauma causes the release of counterregulatory hormones, cytokines, and other unidentified factors that can rapidly induce a state of severe insulin resistance.

Transfers from the Intensive Care Unit to the Operating Room

The ICU patient with diabetes who requires surgery should be sent to the operating room or procedure suite with infusions of both insulin and 5% dextrose in half-normal saline.

Management During Emergency Surgery

Treatment of hyperglycemia in diabetic patients being prepared for urgent major surgery is also best achieved with an intravenous insulin infusion. Frequent monitoring of blood glucose is essential. Proper fluid and electrolyte balance must accompany the proper degree of insulinization; the amount and the type of fluid administered must be assessed on an individual basis.

In general, premedication in patients with diabetes should be kept to a minimum. With respect to the type and the route of anesthesia, the regional and local are preferred if possible. Inhalant and parenteral anesthetics affect carbohydrate metabolism either directly through impairment of insulin secretion or indirectly through interference with the peripheral action of insulin on glucose utilization [67,68]. Halothane can inhibit insulin release, and nitrous oxide, trichloroethylene, and cyclopropane promote sympathetic stimulation and catecholamine release. Barbiturates share some of these effects and also block the removal of glucose and perhaps free fatty acids from the circulation. Some anesthetic agents, including halothane, have also been associated with hypoglycemia (see Chapter 106; Table 106.3).

Management After Emergency Procedures

Patients managed with an insulin infusion must either be maintained on the infusion or switched to subcutaneous intermediate-acting insulin. Those kept on the infusion must have frequent blood glucose testing. Patients no longer critically ill who are able to resume oral feedings can generally resume their usual insulin regimen. The most important point is that insulin should not be abruptly discontinued because severe hyperglycemia and ketosis may ensue. Patients who remain critically ill should remain on a continuous intravenous insulin infusion.

Postoperative recovery in the ICU may be accompanied by reduced levels of counterregulatory hormones and cytokines and may require reduced insulin doses. An increase in insulin requirements in the postoperative period may signify increasing insulin resistance and should prompt the search for infection or another complication.

TABLE 100.3

DIABETES TREATMENT GOALS IN CRITICALLY ILL AND SURGICAL PATIENTS[a]

Zone	Target Blood Glucose (mg/dL)
Too low for safety	<120
Goal	140–180
Hyperglycemia	181–300
Severe hyperglycemia	>300
Surgical range	140–200

[a]At our institutions, we recommend that all intensive care unit patients with blood glucose concentrations >140 mg/dL be treated with a continuous intravenous infusion of regular insulin with a target as close as possible to 140 [48]. A less stringent target range may be referred during the perioperative period and whenever staffing or ...ing constraints prevent the implementation of more intensive ... Patients with type 1 diabetes must be treated with insulin at

Hyperalimentation and Diabetes

If blood glucose rises above 140 mg per dL in a severely ill patient on hyperalimentation, an insulin infusion should be administered. The hyperalimentation should be continuous. The admixture of insulin with parenteral nutrition formulations, although a common practice, can be problematic. There is too much variability among severely ill patients to rely on a fixed ratio of insulin to carbohydrate. If insulin is added to parenteral nutrition formulations, the dose should be limited to less than 50% of the individuals total insulin requirement, with the residual administered by intravenous insulin infusion or subcutaneous injection. This allows rapid adjustment of the insulin dose for changing metabolic needs. If an obese patient receiving hyperalimentation develops severe hyperglycemia and a large insulin requirement, consideration should be given to reducing the amount of carbohydrate administered [69,70]. ICU physicians should be aware that infusions of fructose, sorbitol, and other total parenteral nutrition formulations have occasionally led to lactic acidosis [71].

PITFALLS IN THE CARE OF THE CRITICALLY ILL PATIENT WITH HYPERGLYCEMIA

Sliding Scales

We cannot overstate the need to obtain frequent blood glucose specimens for evaluating glucose control. In an ICU, these should be used to guide adjustments of the rate of insulin infusion. There is no role for intermittent insulin boluses that are given only after hyperglycemia has occurred [72]; the use of "sliding scales" should be actively discouraged [73]. Patients with type I diabetes whose insulin is withheld until hyperglycemia occurs can quickly become ketoacidotic.

A patient who has begun taking insulin should continue to receive it daily until the need has unequivocally disappeared. A previously normoglycemic patient who develops hyperglycemia in the course of a severe illness should be treated continuously with insulin until the stress of the illness has been reduced to the point at which an independent assessment of the need for insulin can be made.

Sporadic Insulin Administration

Unfortunately, some patients are treated with regular insulin injections on an intermittent schedule, whenever a very high blood glucose concentration is noticed. This disorganized approach to the management of hyperglycemia leads to erratic glycemic control and potentially serious shifts in fluids and electrolytes. The best way to avoid these problems is to maintain

ICU patients with hyperglycemia on a continuous infusion of regular insulin.

Hypoglycemia Due to Sensitivity to Short-Acting Insulin

Unusual sensitivity to insulin can be observed in two situations. The first is in some patients presenting with hyperosmolar hyperglycemic syndrome. When treated with short-acting insulin, their glucose concentration may decline very rapidly. This problem is discussed in Chapter 106. The second situation occurs in patients with long-standing type 1 diabetes. They sometimes develop extreme sensitivity to the glucose-lowering effects of short-acting insulin. The reason is unclear, but this sensitivity frequently contributes to increased risk of hypoglycemia. This is principally a problem in outpatient management and should rarely complicate insulin infusion therapy. However, in the insulin-dependent patient with long-standing diabetes, the initial use of short-acting insulin should be approached with some caution. Hypoglycemia can result from the use of as little as 5 to 10 units given either subcutaneously or intravenously. When short-acting insulin is needed for patients who are suspected to be sensitive, the initial doses should be small (2 to 4 units) and the response monitored by bedside blood glucose determinations.

The Diabetic Kidney and Radiographic Contrast Agents

Acute hyperglycemia appears to be an independent risk factor for the development of contrast-induced nephropathy (CIN). The risk of CIN is even greater for the diabetic patient with preexisting renal insufficiency, hypotension, congestive heart failure, or anemia. Mehran et al. [74] have developed a scoring system that can be used to quantify the risk of CIN. The evidence that any pharmaceutical intervention (e.g., acetylcysteine) can prevent CIN is limited [75]. Current evidence supports the use of an infusion of sodium bicarbonate (154 mEq per L) at a rate of 3 mL per kg per hour for 1 hour before contrast exposure, followed by an infusion of 1 mL per kg per hour for 6 hours after the procedure.

CONCLUSIONS

The key to successful care of the very ill patient with diabetes is careful monitoring of glycemia and fastidious treatment with a continuous infusion of insulin. These patients have a defect in normal metabolic regulation, and only attentive treatment can compensate for the diabetes during the metabolic stress of critical illness or surgery. Careful monitoring of blood glucose followed by adjustment of insulin infusion rates minimizes swings to either hyperglycemia or hypoglycemia. Point of care glucose determinations make this intensive metabolic care possible not only in the ICU but also in the operating room, recovery room, emergency department, and procedure suite. Evidence-based glycemic targets have now been developed. Advances in therapy, based on randomized, controlled trials or meta-analyses of such trials, are summarized in Table 100.4. Although achieving recommended targets demands time and attention, achieving them will minimize the special risks faced by patients with hyperglycemia complicating the stress of severe illness or surgery.

TABLE 100.4

ADVANCES IN MANAGEMENT OF DIABETES IN CRITICALLY ILL PATIENTS

Recommendation	Comments
Anticipate hyperglycemia at any time during an ICU admission.	New onset of hyperglycemia due to stress is very common [25,77]. We recommend treating diabetes in all patients whose plasma glucose concentration is >140 mg/dL [48]. ICU patients with newly recognized hyperglycemia should be evaluated for persistence of impaired glucose tolerance after recovery.
Avoid hyperglycemia in the ICU because it is associated with poor outcome.	Observational studies have documented an adverse association of hyperglycemia with wound infection, congestive heart failure, recovery from stroke, and overall mortality [38,39,41,42].
Avoid hypoglycemia in the ICU because it is associated with increased mortality	Two recent clinical studies document increased mortality in critically ill patients who experience hypoglycemia during hospitalization [59,60].
With current technology it is not safe to seek to lower glucose concentration to <110 mg/dL in ICU patients	Five large randomized clinical trials have demonstrated either no reduction [25,55,57,58] or an increase in ICU mortality [56] associated with intensive insulin treatment. All showed increased risk of hypoglycemia. Only one of these showed reduced morbidity [25].
Be alert to the presence of type 1 diabetes.	Patients with type 1 diabetes are absolutely insulin dependent, and they must be treated with insulin at all times.
Treatment of diabetes using only "sliding scale" boluses of insulin, whether intravenous or subcutaneous, should be avoided.	Sliding scale prescriptions given only after hyperglycemia has occurred amplify the risk of hypoglycemia, recurrent hyperglycemia, and even ketoacidosis. There is no role for them in the ICU [72] and their use is actively discouraged [73]. Continuous insulin infusion is the treatment of choice for diabetes in the ICU.
Oral hypoglycemic agents should not be used in the ICU.	Insulin is the only acceptable agent for control of diabetes in the ICU. The absorption, metabolism, distribution, and excretion of oral agents cannot be predicted in the critically ill patient. As a result, for example, sulfonylureas can cause persistent hypoglycemia [62] and metformin can cause lactic acidosis in the setting of renal failure [63].

References

1. Centers for Disease Control, National Institutes of Health, National Diabetes Fact Sheet, 2007. 2010 http://www.cdc.gov/diabetes/pubs/pdf/ndfs_2007.pdf.
2. Narayan KM, Boyle JP, Geiss LS, et al: Impact of recent increase in incidence on future diabetes burden: U.S., 2005–2050. *Diabetes Care* 29:2114, 2006.
3. Narayan KMV, Boyle JP, Thompson TJ, et al: Lifetime risk for diabetes mellitus in the United States. *JAMA* 290:1884, 2003.
4. Hossain P, Kawar B, El Nahas M: Obesity and diabetes in the developing world—a growing challenge. *N Engl J Med* 356:213, 2007.
5. Shaw JE, Sicree RA, Zimmet PZ: Global estimates of the prevalence of diabetes for 2010 and 2030. *Diabetes Res Clin Pract* 87:4, 2010.
6. Nesto RW: Correlation between cardiovascular disease and diabetes mellitus: Current concepts. *Am J Med* 116:11, 2004.
7. Sobel BE, Schneider DJ: Cardiovascular complications in diabetes mellitus. *Curr Opin Pharmacol* 5:143, 2005.
8. Gruden G, Gnudi L, Viberti G: Pathogenesis of diabetic nephropathy, in LeRoith D, Taylor SI, Olefsky JM (eds): *Diabetes Mellitus. A Fundamental and Clinical Text.* 3rd ed. Philadelphia, PA, Lippincott Williams & Wilkins, 2004, p. 1315–1330.
9. Molitch ME, DeFronzo RA, Franz MJ, et al: Diabetic nephrology. *Diabetes Care* 23:S69–S72, 2000.
10. Balakumar P, Arora MK, Ganti SS, et al: Recent advances in pharmacotherapy for diabetic nephropathy: current perspectives and future directions. *Pharmacol Res* 60:24, 2009.
11. Shah BR, Hux JE: Quantifying the risk of infectious diseases for people with diabetes. *Diabetes Care* 26:510, 2003.
12. Joshi N, Caputo GM, Weitekamp MR, et al: Infections in patients with diabetes mellitus. *N Engl J Med* 341:1906, 1999.
13. Shilling AM, Raphael J: Diabetes, hyperglycemia, and infections 1. *Best Pract Res Clin Anaesthesiol* 22:519, 2008.
14. Jeffcoate WJ, Lipsky BA, Berendt AR, et al: Unresolved issues in the management of ulcers of the foot in diabetes. *Diabet Med* 25:1380, 2008.
15. Samaras K: Prevalence and pathogenesis of diabetes mellitus in HIV-1 infection treated with combined antiretroviral therapy. *J Acquir Immune Defic Syndr* 50:499, 2009.
16. Dooley KE, Chaisson RE: Tuberculosis and diabetes mellitus: convergence of two epidemics. *Lancet Infect Dis* 9:737, 2009.
17. Cely CM, Arora P, Quartin AA, et al: Relationship of baseline glucose homeostasis to hyperglycemia during medical critical illness. *Chest* 126:879, 2004.
18. Flakoll PJ, Jensen MD, Cherrington AD: Physiologic action of insulin, in LeRoith D, Taylor SI, Olefsky JM (eds): *Diabetes mellitus. A fundamental and clinical text.* 3rd ed. Philadelphia, PA, Lippincott Williams & Wilkins, 2004, pp. 165–181.
19. American Diabetes Association: Diagnosis and classification of diabetes mellitus. *Diabetes Care* 33[Suppl 1]:S62–S69, 2010.
20. Barker JM, Eisenbarth GS: The natural history of autoimmunity in type 1 A diabetes mellitus, in LeRoith D, Taylor SI, Olefsky JM (eds): *Diabetes mellitus. A fundamental and clinical text.* 3rd ed. Philadelphia, PA, Lippincott Williams & Wilkins, 2004, pp. 471–482.
21. LeRoith D: Beta-cell dysfunction and insulin resistance in type 2 diabetes: role of metabolic and genetic abnormalities. *Am J Med* 113:3S, 2002.
22. Petersen KF, Shulman GI: Etiology of insulin resistance. *Am J Med* 119:S10–S16, 2006.
23. Reaven GM: Insulin resistance and its consequences: type 2 diabetes mellitus and the insulin resistance syndrome, in LeRoith D, Taylor SI, Olefsky JM (eds): *Diabetes Mellitus. A Fundamental and Clinical text.* 3rd ed. Philadelphia, PA, Lippincott Williams & Wilkins, 2004, pp. 899–916.
24. Westphal SA: Occurrence of diabetic ketoacidosis in non-insulin-dependent diabetes and newly diagnosed diabetic adults. *Am J Med* 101:19, 1996.
25. Van den Berghe G, Wilmer A, Hermans G, et al: Intensive insulin therapy in the medical ICU. *N Engl J Med* 354:449, 2006.
26. Diabetes Control and Complications Trial Research Group: The effect of intensive treatment of diabetes on the development and progression of long-term complications in insulin-dependent diabetes mellitus. *N Engl J Med* 329:977, 1993.
27. Genuth S, Eastman R, Kahn R, et al: Implications of the United Kingdom prospective diabetes study. *Diabetes Care* 22:S27–S31, 1999.
28. Boyko EJ, Lipsky BA: Infection and diabetes, in National Diabetes Data Group (Ed): *Diabetes in America.* 2nd ed. Bethesda, National Institutes of Health, 1995, pp. 485–499.
29. Nicolle LE: Urinary tract infection in diabetes. *Curr Opin Infect Dis* 18:49, 2005.
30. Goldberg IJ: Clinical review 124—diabetic dyslipidemia: causes and consequences. *J Clin Endocrinol Metab* 86:965, 2001.
31. Lacara T, Domagtoy C, Lickliter D, et al: Comparison of point-of-care and laboratory glucose analysis in critically ill patients. *Am J Crit Care* 16:336, 2007.

ldstein DE, Little RR, Lorenz RA, et al: Tests of glycemia in diabetes. *tes Care* 27:1761, 2004.

K, Maruta H, Usuda Y, et al: Influence of blood sample oxygen od glucose concentration measured using an enzyme-electrode *Care Med* 25:231, 1997.

34. Desachy A, Vuagnat AC, Ghazali AD, et al: Accuracy of bedside glucometry in critically ill patients: influence of clinical characteristics and perfusion index. *Mayo Clin Proc* 83:400, 2008.
35. Eastham JH, Mason D, Barnes DL, et al: Prevalence of interfering substances with point-of-care glucose testing in a community hospital. *Am J Health Syst Pharm* 66:167, 2009.
36. Kirrane BM, Duthie EA, Nelson LS: Unrecognized hypoglycemia due to maltodextrin interference with bedside glucometry. *J Med Toxicol* 5:20, 2009.
37. Kanji S, Buffie J, Hutton B, et al: Reliability of point-of-care testing for glucose measurement in critically ill adults. *Crit Care Med* 33:2778, 2005.
38. Capes SE, Hunt D, Malmberg K, et al: Stress hyperglycaemia and increased risk of death after myocardial infarction in patients with and without diabetes: a systematic overview. *Lancet* 355:773, 2000.
39. Furnary AP, Zerr KJ, Grunkemeier GL, et al: Continuous intravenous insulin infusion reduces the incidence of deep sternal wound infection in diabetic patients after cardiac surgical procedures. *Ann Thorac Surg* 67:352, 1999.
40. Furnary AP, Gao G, Grunkemeier GL, et al: Continuous insulin infusion reduces mortality in patients with diabetes undergoing coronary artery bypass grafting. *J Thorac Cardiovasc Surg* 125:1007, 2003.
41. Capes SE, Hunt D, Malmberg K, et al: Stress hyperglycemia and prognosis of stroke in nondiabetic and diabetic patients: a systematic overview. *Stroke* 32:2426, 2001.
42. Umpierrez GE, Isaacs SD, Bazargan N, et al: Hyperglycemia: an independent marker of in-hospital mortality in patients with undiagnosed diabetes. *J Clin Endocrinol Metab* 87:978, 2002.
43. Geerlings SE, Hoepelman AIM: Immune dysfunction in patients with diabetes mellitus (DM). *FEMS Immunol Med Microbiol* 26:259, 1999.
44. Alexiewicz JM, Kumar D, Smogorzewski M, et al: Polymorphonuclear leukocytes in non-insulin-dependent diabetes mellitus: abnormalities in metabolism and function. *Ann Intern Med* 123:919, 1995.
45. McMahon MM, Bistrian BR: Host defenses and susceptibility to infection in patients with diabetes mellitus. *Infect Dis Clin North Am* 9:1, 1995.
46. Abrass CK: Fc receptor-mediated phagocytosis: abnormalities associated with diabetes mellitus. *Clin Immunol Immunopathol* 58:1, 1991.
47. Langouche L, Vanhorebeek I, Vlasselaers D, et al: Intensive insulin therapy protects the endothelium of critically ill patients. *J Clin Invest* 115:2277, 2005.
48. Moghissi ES, Korytkowski MT, DiNardo M, et al: American Association of Clinical Endocrinologists and American Diabetes Association consensus statement on inpatient glycemic control. *Diabetes Care* 32:1119, 2009.
49. Lazar HL, Chipkin S, Philippides G, et al: Glucose-insulin-potassium solutions improve outcomes in diabetics who have coronary artery operations. *Ann Thorac Surg* 70:145, 2000.
50. Van den Berghe G, Wouters P, Weekers F, et al: Intensive insulin therapy in critically ill patients. *N Engl J Med* 345:1359, 2001.
51. Krinsley JS: Effect of an intensive glucose management protocol on the mortality of critically ill adult patients. *Mayo Clin Proc* 79:992, 2004.
52. Kanji S, Singh A, Tierney M, et al: Standardization of intravenous insulin therapy improves the efficiency and safety of blood glucose control in critically ill adults. *Intensive Care Med* 30:804, 2004.
53. Goldberg PA, Siegel MD, Sherwin RS, et al: Implementation of a safe and effective insulin infusion protocol in a medical intensive care unit. *Diabetes Care* 27:461, 2004.
54. Taylor BE, Schallom ME, Sona CS, et al: Efficacy and safety of an insulin infusion protocol in a surgical ICU. *J Am Coll Surg* 202:1, 2006.
55. Preiser JC, Devos P, Ruiz-Santana S, et al: A prospective randomised multi-centre controlled trial on tight glucose control by intensive insulin therapy in adult intensive care units: the Glucontrol study. *Intensive Care Med* 35:1738, 2009.
56. Finfer S, Chittock DR, Su SY, et al: Intensive versus conventional glucose control in critically ill patients. *N Engl J Med* 360:1283, 2009.
57. Annane D, Cariou A, Maxime V, et al: Corticosteroid treatment and intensive insulin therapy for septic shock in adults: a randomized controlled trial. *JAMA* 303:341, 2010.
58. Brunkhorst FM, Engel C, Bloos F, et al: Intensive insulin therapy and pentastarch resuscitation in severe sepsis. *N Engl J Med* 358:125, 2008.
59. Egi M, Bellomo R, Stachowski E, et al: Hypoglycemia and outcome in critically ill patients. *Mayo Clin Proc* 85:217, 2010.
60. Hermanides J, Bosman RJ, Vriesendorp TM, et al: Hypoglycemia is associated with intensive care unit mortality. *Crit Care Med* 38:1430, 2010.
61. Marik PE, Preiser JC: Toward understanding tight glycemic control in the ICU: a systematic review and metaanalysis. *Chest* 137:544, 2010.
62. Kagansky N, Levy S, Rimon E, et al: Hypoglycemia as a predictor of mortality in hospitalized elderly patients. *Arch Intern Med* 163:1825, 2003.
63. Luft FC: Lactic acidosis update for critical care clinicians. *J Am Soc Nephrol* 12:S15–S19, 2001.
64. Shulman GI: Cellular mechanisms of insulin resistance. *J Clin Invest* 106:171, 2000.
65. Shepherd PR, Kahn BB: Mechanisms of disease—glucose transporters and insulin action: implications for insulin resistance and diabetes mellitus. *N Engl J Med* 341:248, 1999.

66. Olefsky JM, Nolan JJ: Insulin resistance and non-insulin-dependent diabetes mellitus: cellular and molecular mechanisms. *Am J Clin Nutr* 61[Suppl]: 980S, 1995.
67. Dierdorf SF: Anesthesia for patients with diabetes mellitus. *Curr Opin Anaesthesiol* 15:351, 2002.
68. Tuttnauer A, Levin PD: Diabetes mellitus and anesthesia. *Anesthesiol Clin* 24:579, 2006.
69. Choban PS, Burge JC, Scales D, et al: Hypoenergetic nutrition support in hospitalized obese patients: a simplified method for clinical application. *Am J Clin Nutr* 66:546, 1997.
70. Shikora SA, Jensen GL: Hypoenergetic nutrition support in hospitalized obese patients. *Am J Clin Nutr* 66:679, 1997.
71. Cohen RD, Woods HF: Lactic acidosis revisited. *Diabetes* 32:181, 1983.
72. Queale WS, Seidler AJ, Brancati FL: Glycemic control and sliding scale insulin use in medical inpatients with diabetes mellitus. *Arch Intern Med* 157:545, 1997.
73. Baldwin D, Villanueva G, McNutt R, et al: Eliminating inpatient sliding-scale insulin: a reeducation project with medical house staff. *Diabetes Care* 28:1008, 2005.
74. Mehran R, Aymong ED, Nikolsky E, et al: A simple risk score for prediction of contrast-induced nephropathy after percutaneous coronary intervention: development and initial validation. *J Am Coll Cardiol* 44:1393, 2004.
75. Tepel M, Aspelin P, Lameire N: Contrast-induced nephropathy: a clinical and evidence-based approach. *Circulation* 113:1799, 2006.
76. Ganda OP: Prevalence and incidence of secondary and other types of diabetes, in National Diabetes Data Group (Ed): *Diabetes in America*. 2nd ed. Bethesda, National Institutes of Health, 1995, pp. 69–84.
77. Conner TM, Flesner-Gurley KR, Barner JC: Hyperglycemia in the hospital setting: the case for improved control among non-diabetics. *Ann Pharmacother* 39:492, 2005.

CHAPTER 101 ■ HYPERGLYCEMIC DIABETIC COMA

SAMIR MALKANI, ALDO A. ROSSINI, DAVID M. HARLAN, MICHAEL J. THOMPSON AND JOHN P. MORDES

INTRODUCTION

The Acute Metabolic Complications of Diabetes: The Overlap Concept

The most urgent metabolic complications of diabetes are the four diabetic comas: hypoglycemia, diabetic ketoacidosis (DKA), hyperglycemic hyperosmolar syndrome (HHS), and alcoholic ketoacidosis (ethanol-induced hypoglycemia). These diagnostic possibilities must be considered in any lethargic or comatose patient. In addition to being life-threatening conditions, they account for thousands of hospitalizations and substantial costs [1]. Recognition of these diabetic comas is particularly important because these conditions are reversible with appropriate treatment. We use diabetic coma as a generic term that encompasses both frank coma and the milder metabolic abnormalities that precede loss of consciousness. This chapter considers the hyperglycemic crises; hypoglycemia and alcoholic ketoacidosis are discussed in Chapter 106.

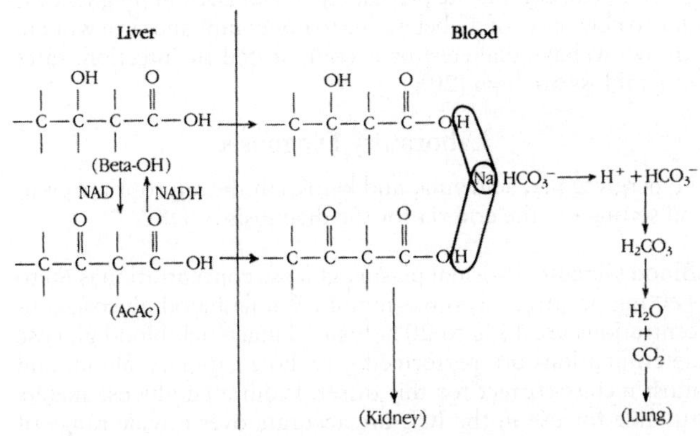

FIGURE 101.1. Neutralization of ketoacids. Hydrogen ion from ketoacids is neutralized by bicarbonate, producing carbonic acid that then decomposes to H_2O and CO_2. The latter is expelled by the lungs. The neutralized salts of ketone bodies are excreted in the urine. NAD, nicotinamide adenine dinucleotide; NADH, reduced form of NAD; AcAc, acetoacetate; Beta-OH, β-hydroxybutyrate.

Although DKA and HHS are discussed separately, it is important to recognize that metabolic decompensation related to hyperglycemia can take many forms depending on the severity of insulin deficiency, underlying genetic predispositions, and intercurrent illnesses. There is frequent overlap in clinical phenotypes, and clinicians should be aware of this concept [1,2]. DKA can occur in a patient with type 2 diabetes; up to a third of patients with HHS have no prior history of diabetes [1]; both DKA and HHS can be complicated by lactic, uremic, or other form of metabolic acidosis, and ketoacidosis itself can occur in the setting of profound hypoglycemia [3]. These metabolic disturbances can overlap to yield both classical DKA and nonclassical presentations of HHS and other ketotic and acidotic states.

In a comatose patient if the blood glucose concentration is less than 50 mg per dL or if for any reason the blood glucose cannot be measured rapidly, the first diagnostic and therapeutic step should be the infusion of 50 mL of a 50% dextrose solution. The hypoglycemic patient who awakens is resuscitated; coma of any other origin is not adversely affected.

DIABETIC KETOACIDOSIS

DKA comprises the triad of hyperglycemia, metabolic acidosis, and ketonemia. Any person with diabetes can develop DKA [4], but it most often occurs in those with type 1 diabetes. Before the discovery of insulin, most patients with type 1 diabetes died of DKA. With the advent of insulin and intensive care, mortality from DKA has fallen to less than 5% [5]. Deaths are associated with intercurrent heart disease or infection in older patients, cerebral edema in younger patients, and, occasionally, therapeutic errors.

Pathophysiology and Etiology

Normal Glucose Homeostasis

After a meal, pancreatic islet β cells release insulin into the circulation, enabling fuels to enter cells and activating enzymes for their storage or metabolism. Glucose enters most tissues only in the presence of insulin; erythrocytes, heart, and brain are exceptions. Glucose is stored in liver and muscle as glycogen. Some glucose is metabolized; some is converted into triglyceride.

In adipose tissue, insulin activates lipoprotein lipase, clears lipoproteins from the circulation, and stores them intracellularly. Insulin also inhibits the breakdown and release of previously stored fat. Insulin has similar effects on skeletal muscle, permitting both amino acids and glucose to enter cells for oxidation or storage [6,7].

During starvation, insulin concentrations decrease, catabolic pathways are activated, and stored fuels (glucose, amino acids, and fats) are mobilized to meet energy needs. Liver glycogen provides glucose for only several hours. Muscle glycogen is not directly available due to lack of glucose-6-phosphatase in muscle. To support plasma glucose, muscle glycogen undergoes anaerobic glycolysis, generating lactate that is converted into glucose in the liver. After glycogen stores are exhausted, the liver synthesizes glucose from muscle-derived amino acids through the process of gluconeogenesis [8]. To conserve muscle mass during starvation, glucose consumption is reduced and fatty acids released from adipose tissue become the principal fuel source. Some fatty acids are transformed by the liver into ketoacids [9].

The rate of catabolism is regulated by insulin. As circulating glucose concentration decreases, insulin concentration also decreases—but never to zero. Low insulin levels permit lipolysis and proteolysis while stimulating gluconeogenesis, and maintaining normal glucose concentration. Increased glucose concentration stimulates insulin secretion, which in turn reduces or halts catabolism. Precise regulation of insulin secretion, even in the absence of food intake, achieves continuous control of carbohydrate metabolism.

Abnormal Glucose Homeostasis

DKA can be viewed as a "super-fasted" state that occurs when there is insufficient insulin available to regulate carbohydrate metabolism [7]. Without insulin, glucose no longer enters most cells and is neither stored nor metabolized. Glucagon secretion is increased and hepatic glucose production increases without restraint. When the renal threshold for glucose is exceeded (180 to 200 mg per dL), an osmotic diuresis ensues and water and electrolytes are lost. If insulin deficiency persists, the stress-response hormones cortisol, epinephrine, norepinephrine, glucagon, and growth hormone are released and accelerate catabolism. Glucagon excess is responsible for oxidation of fatty acids to ketone bodies in the liver. Once this happens, DKA ensues with the life-threatening combination of hyperglycemia, acidemia, ketonemia, loss of free water, and depletion of electrolytes.

The cause of ketoacidosis is insulin deficiency. New onset type 1 diabetes commonly presents as ketoacidosis, but most ᵉs occur in individuals known to have diabetes. Dietary in- ᵗion in a person with known treated diabetes may pro- ic hyperglycemia, polydipsia, and polyuria but never ᵑuria in any hyperglycemic diabetic patient should sence of DKA. Such patients must be carefully evaluated for the presence of acidemia. Ketoacidosis occurs most often in patients who have omitted their insulin or who have an intercurrent infection.

Infection and other stressors produce a state of insulin resistance, in part because of the presence of high levels of tumor necrosis factor α; infection may be the most common trigger of DKA in the ICU setting [10]. Severe stress occasionally causes ketosis in patients with type 2 diabetes [4]. African Americans with type 2 diabetes may be particularly susceptible to the development of ketosis [11,12]. Other factors that can precipitate ketosis include acute myocardial infarction, emotional stress, cancer, drugs that interfere with insulin release or action, pregnancy, menstruation, and various endocrinopathies. Occasionally, no precipitating factor can be identified.

Clinical Manifestations

Most patients with DKA are lethargic; about 10% are comatose [13]. They have lost large quantities of fluid; their skin, lips, and tongue are dry; and their eyes are soft to palpation. Postural hypotension is common, but shock is rare [14].

Patients with DKA have rapid deep (Kussmaul) respiration, and their breath has a sweet fruity odor. Some patients with new-onset DKA have been misdiagnosed as having psychological hyperventilation [15]. If a patient with DKA is not tachypneic, the physician should suspect that severe acidosis (pH <7.1) is depressing the respiratory drive [16].

It is important to measure the temperature accurately. Because the patient is hyperventilating, rectal or tympanic temperature should be measured. Patients with DKA do not have fever unless an intercurrent process, usually infection, is present. Similarly, the rare cases of hypothermia in DKA are associated with sepsis [17].

Abdominal pain is common and may be accompanied by a tender guarded abdomen with diminished or absent bowel sounds. DKA should always be excluded when evaluating abdominal pain [18]. What may appear to be a surgical condition will resolve with correction of the acidosis.

Patients with DKA may be nauseous and vomit guaiac-positive coffee grounds–like material. This is probably due to gastric atony, distention, and rupture of mucosal blood vessels. Pleuritic chest pain may also be present. The cause is unknown, but it resolves with treatment of the DKA.

The nose and sinuses of all patients with DKA should be examined. Acute sinusitis and a black intranasal eschar should suggest mucormycosis, an opportunistic fungal infection that disseminates rapidly in acidotic patients. Mucormycosis is often fatal; survival requires prompt diagnosis [19].

DKA can complicate pregnancy. When DKA in pregnancy is due to new onset of diabetes, due to noncompliance in a woman known to have diabetes, or is complicated by infection, rates of fetal loss are high [20].

Laboratory Diagnosis

Hyperglycemia, acidemia, and ketosis in the appropriate clinical setting are the criteria for the diagnosis of DKA.

Blood Glucose. Normal plasma glucose concentration is 60 to 120 mg per dL (3.3 to 6.7 mmol). Whole blood glucose concentrations are 15% to 20% lower. Fingerstick blood glucose determinations are performed on whole capillary blood, and most meters correct for this offset. Calibrated glucose meters suitable for use in the ICU are accurate over a wide range of concentrations, but very high and low concentrations are less consistently accurate and should be confirmed by a clinical laboratory. Meters intended for home use may give less reproducibly accurate results [21].

In DKA, blood glucose concentration of 400 to 800 mg per dL is typical, but as many as 15% of cases of DKA may present with blood glucose concentrations less than 300 mg per dL—so called euglycemic DKA [22]. Typically, these are younger patients with a high glomerular filtration rate (GFR). In one series, approximately 1% of patients with DKA presented with a blood glucose concentration less than 180 mg per dL and a bicarbonate concentration less than 10 mEq per L [23]. More often, the solute diuresis causes dehydration, decreases the GFR, and further increases circulating blood glucose concentration.

Electrolytes

Sodium. Serum sodium concentration is quite variable in DKA and must be interpreted in the context of serum glucose and lipid concentrations. If extremely abnormal, it may need special attention during management. Large amounts of sodium are lost during the osmotic diuresis of DKA, and the serum concentration does not necessarily reflect this loss. Because sodium resides principally in the extracellular fluid space, elevated sodium concentration may simply reflect the degree of dehydration and free water loss.

Abnormally low sodium concentrations may be due to the osmotic effect of large amounts of extracellular glucose. The osmotic activity of glucose, drawing free water from the intracellular to the extracellular space, produces a fall of 1.6 mEq per L of sodium for every increase of 100 mg per dL in blood glucose concentration more than 100 mg per dL [24]. The "corrected" serum sodium in a patient with a measured concentration of 135 mEq per L and a glucose concentration of 600 mg per dL is $[1.6 \times (6 - 1) + 135]$, or 143 mEq per L. The patient presenting with an elevated serum sodium concentration despite hyperglycemia has a severe total body free water deficit.

It is also important to be certain that abnormally low serum sodium concentrations in DKA are not factitious. Sodium resides only in the aqueous phase of plasma and when the nonaqueous constituents such as triglycerides increase substantially, the reported concentration of sodium will be spuriously low unless "ion-specific" technology is used for the measurement [4].

Chloride. Chloride concentrations are usually not helpful in the diagnosis of DKA, although they may provide useful information. Hyperchloremia may sometimes represent a more chronic ketoacidotic state [25] and may be associated with slower recovery [26]. Extremely low levels of chloride may result from vomiting [27]. Hyperchloremic acidosis can also occur during recovery from DKA as a consequence of the loss of neutralized ketone body salts [28].

Potassium. Potassium is the electrolyte that must be watched most carefully and often during therapy. All patients with DKA are at risk for life-threatening hypokalemia during treatment, despite the fact that the serum potassium concentration is usually elevated at presentation [26,29]. This elevation is due to catabolism of tissue, dehydration, and shifts of potassium from the intracellular to the extracellular space as hydrogen ions are buffered. An initially elevated serum potassium concentration should never obscure the fact that total body potassium loss (in the range of 200 to 700 mEq) occurs in ketoacidosis. The greatest potassium loss accompanies the osmotic diuresis of glucose. Additional losses are due to the excretion of ketone bodies as potassium salts, dehydration-induced secondary hyperaldosteronism, and vomiting. Potassium replacement early in the course of therapy for DKA is always necessary. It should be started as soon as the potassium concentration is at the upper end of the normal range because continued insulin therapy will invariably cause the potassium concentration to fall further. Normal or low concentrations of potassium early in ketoacidosis reflect a very severe potassium deficit.

TABLE 101.1

CALCULATIONS

Anion gap	$(Na^+ + K^+) - (Cl^- + HCO_3^-) + 17 = 0$
or	
	$Na^+ - (Cl^- + HCO_3^-) + 12 = 0$
Osmolality[a]	$2(Na^+ + K^+) + \text{Glucose}/18 + \text{BUN}/2.8$

[a]Normal osmolality: 285–295 mOsm/kg.
BUN, blood urea nitrogen.

Magnesium. Like potassium, serum magnesium concentrations in patients with untreated DKA tend to be elevated initially, but they fall with subsequent hydration.

Bicarbonate. Serum bicarbonate concentration is low in ketoacidosis [16] because of neutralization of ketone bodies, which are acids. Bicarbonate buffer in the extracellular compartment represents the first line of defense in acid–base homeostasis. The process is summarized in Figure 101.1. Hydrogen ion (H^+) from ketoacids is neutralized by bicarbonate, producing carbonic acid, water, and CO_2. As CO_2 is expelled through the lungs, the neutralized salts of the ketone bodies are excreted in the urine. In patients with established DKA, the serum bicarbonate concentration is less than 15 mEq per L.

Phosphorous. Elevated serum phosphate concentrations are common in untreated DKA; the mechanism is not clear. After therapy, there is a precipitous decline to subnormal levels [30]. It has been estimated that as much as 1 mM per kg of phosphate is lost during DKA. Hypophosphatemia of less than 0.5 mM per L has been described in both DKA and HHS [30].

Acidosis. Arterial blood gas and pH measurements are essential in the management of all but the mildest cases of DKA. The arterial pH in DKA is almost always less than 7.3. If arterial samples cannot be obtained, venous or capillary samples may be used, although they provide less information [31]. DKA classically presents as an anion gap acidosis. The anion gap should be calculated for all acidemic patients (Table 101.1). In addition to confirming the diagnosis of DKA, the anion gap can be used together with plasma ketone measurements to obtain important additional insight into the nature and severity of a given case [32]. More chronic ketoacidotic states may be associated with hyperchloremic rather than anion gap acidosis [25], probably as a consequence of the loss of neutralized ketone body salts [28]. Rare cases of DKA are complicated by intercurrent metabolic alkalosis, most often from severe vomiting [27,33].

Plasma Ketones and β-Hydroxybutyrate

Plasma ketones should be measured in all comatose patients with diabetes at the time of presentation. When the nitroprusside test is used, the results are usually expressed as the highest dilution of serum that gives a positive reaction. This test is always positive (>1:2 dilution) in DKA, but its result may not reflect the full extent of ketogenesis. This is because the test measures only acetoacetate (AcAc) and acetone. It does not measure beta-hydroxybutyrate (BOHB), which, although a "ketone body," is a hydroxyacid and not a ketone (Fig. 101.2). Normally, the BOHB-to-AcAc ratio is 3:1, but acidosis increases the ratio to 6:1 or even 12:1 as pH decreases. The BOHB-to-AcAc ratio at pH 7.1 is at least 6:1.

BOHB can be measured directly, and the test is available in many hospital laboratories. Measurement of BOHB concentration, if the result is available rapidly, can also be used to establish the diagnosis of DKA. The advantage of BOHB measurement derives from the fact that it is the major ketone

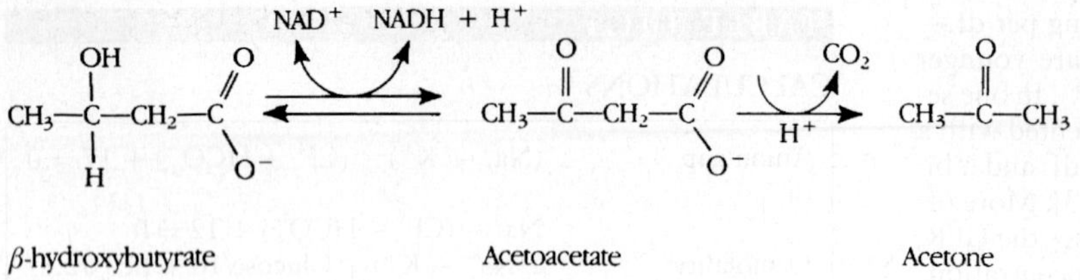

FIGURE 101.2. Biochemical interrelationships of the ketone bodies. Acetoacetate and acetone are ketones, whereas β-hydroxybutyrate, although a "ketone body," is β-hydroxy carboxylic acid and not a ketone. NAD^+, nicotine adenine dinucleotide; NADH, reduced form of NAD.

body and its concentration is a better indicator of the severity of ketoacidosis.

The results of plasma ketone, BOHB, anion gap, and arterial pH measurements can be used to determine whether a pure or mixed anion gap acidosis is present. The highest positive ketone dilution is multiplied by 0.1 mM per L to obtain an estimate of AcAc concentration; the BOHB can be measured directly. If a patient's anion gap as calculated in Table 101.1 is greater than the estimated contribution of ketone bodies (AcAc plus BOHB), the presence of an additional unmeasured anion should be considered (e.g., lactate, salicylate, uremic compounds, methanol, or ethylene glycol; see Chapter 119).

Ketone body measurements are also useful for monitoring the resolution of DKA. In cases of severe acidosis, ketones initially rise rather than fall as the acidosis improves. This is due to conversion of BOHB back to AcAc. Clearance of ketone bodies occurs slowly; measurement of ketones and BOHB more often than every 12 hours is generally unnecessary.

It is worth noting that certain newer home blood monitors have the capacity to measure not only glucose but also "ketones." These meters measure BOHB rather than AcAc using strips distinct from those used to measure glucose. They can warn patients of impending or established ketoacidosis prior to hospital presentation.

Blood Urea Nitrogen and Creatinine. The blood urea nitrogen (BUN) of patients with DKA is typically elevated to values between 25 and 50 mg per dL due not only to prerenal azotemia from volume depletion but also to increased ureagenesis. Patients with DKA are in a state of uncontrolled gluconeogenesis; the large quantities of amino acids released from muscle for conversion to glucose produce hyperaminoacidemia. These amino acids increase substrate availability for ureagenesis. Although the serum creatinine concentration usually reflects the degree of dehydration and prerenal azotemia in DKA accurately [34], spurious elevations occasionally occur because AcAc interferes with some older creatinine assays [35].

Complete Blood Count. Hematocrit and hemoglobin in DKA are usually high and in proportion to the degree of dehydration. Low values suggest preexisting anemia or acute blood loss. A characteristic hematologic finding in DKA is leukocytosis. White blood cell counts in the range of 15,000 to 90,000 per μL with a significant left shift often occur in the absence of intercurrent illness [13,36]. Leukocytosis and a left shift in DKA do not necessarily imply concurrent infection. The absence of leukocytosis suggests possible folic acid or vitamin B_{12} deficiency.

Triglycerides. Insulin deficiency impairs clearance of lipid from the circulation and accelerates hepatic production of very low-density lipoprotein (VLDL) [6]. In DKA, there is marked elevation of serum triglyceride concentrations that may be clin-[illegible]ly obvious in the form of lactescent serum. With insulin ther-[illegible]s biochemical derangement reverses. If a patient can eat [illegible] onset of DKA, hyperchylomicronemia may also be

Urine. Urinary glucose and acetone should be measured. If pyuria is present, a urine specimen should be sent for culture and sensitivity. To avoid iatrogenic infection, catheterization should be avoided unless the patient is comatose or anuric. A pregnancy test should be performed in women of childbearing age, as pregnancy can precipitate DKA.

Serum Amylase and Lipase. Serum amylase and lipase concentrations are sometimes elevated in acute ketoacidosis, but they do not necessarily imply exocrine pancreatic disease [37,38]. In some cases, the amylase may be of salivary gland origin.

Other Laboratory Findings. Uric acid concentrations may be elevated during acute DKA [39] as a result of impaired renal function or competition from ketone bodies at sites of tubular secretion. Hepatic enlargement with fatty infiltration of parenchymal cells may occur during acute DKA. Increased levels of C-reactive protein and interleukin-6 may be indicative of underlying infection in DKA [40].

Treatment

Patients with severe DKA should be hospitalized in an intensive care unit (ICU). Delaying intensive care greatly increases morbidity, and detaining patients in the emergency room long after the diagnosis is established should be avoided. Treatment should be directed at three main problems—fluid, electrolytes, and insulin—in that order [41].

Recording of Data

The comprehensive flow sheet of vital signs, laboratory data, and treatment that is part of the modern electronic ICU greatly enhances management. For ICUs that do not have advanced capabilities, a comprehensive paper flow sheet is essential to follow the response to therapy.

Fluid Replacement

Fluid and electrolyte therapy always takes precedence over insulin administration in the treatment of DKA. As described later in "Complications" section of this chapter, insulin administration before volume and potassium repletion can cause shock and arrhythmias [42].

The free water deficit in adults with DKA generally ranges between 5 and 11 L, typically about 100 mL per kg, and is due primarily to the osmotic diuresis of glucose [41,43]. Vomiting and hyperventilation may also contribute to water loss. Initial fluid resuscitation should be an infusion of 0.9% saline. Approximately 2 L should be given during the first hour to restore blood volume, stabilize blood pressure, and establish urine flow. Another liter of 0.9% saline can typically be given during the next 2 hours. The subsequent rate of fluid replacement depends on individual clinical circumstances. During the first 24 hours, 75% of the estimated total water deficit should be replaced. Urine flow should be maintained at approximately

30 to 60 mL per hour. Fluid replacement after the first 2 L may be changed to hypotonic 0.45% saline if hypernatremia is present [44].

Electrolytes

Sodium, Chloride, and Potassium. Sodium and chloride are replaced together with free water as just described. Potassium must be added to the saline. Because serum potassium concentration does not accurately reflect total body potassium, replacement should be initiated early in treatment. Until the serum potassium concentration is known, replacement should be carried out cautiously. The recommended initial repletion rate is 20 mEq per hour as KCl or K_3PO_4. When the serum value is known, the rate of potassium administration can be adjusted. If a nasogastric tube is in place, electrolyte losses due to gastric suctioning must also be considered. Typical potassium deficits in DKA are 3 to 5 mEq per kg, but if hypokalemia or normokalemia is present at the time of admission, the deficit may be much higher, up to 10 mEq per kg.

Potassium concentration often falls precipitously after starting therapy. K^+ shifts from the extracellular to the intracellular space in the presence of glucose and insulin. As acidemia resolves, buffered intracellular H^+ is exchanged for extracellular K^+, further lowering the serum potassium concentration. The electrocardiogram can be helpful in monitoring potassium treatment but cannot substitute for serum potassium determinations. A sudden reduction in serum potassium concentration can cause flaccid paralysis, respiratory failure, and life-threatening cardiac arrhythmias. If a patient in mild DKA is alert and able to tolerate liquids, potassium should be given orally.

Phosphate. Depletion of phosphate occurs in DKA. Initially, the concentration of phosphate is elevated, but levels may decrease to less than 1 mM per L within 4 to 6 hours of starting insulin treatment. Persistent severe hypophosphatemia can cause neurological disturbances, arthralgias, muscle weakness with respiratory impairment, rhabdomyolysis, and liver dysfunction [45].

Except when hypophosphatemia is severe ($\leq$1.0 mg per dL), however, the need for phosphate replacement in DKA may be more theoretical than real. No studies have demonstrated that replacement of phosphate affects the course or outcome of ketoacidosis [46–48].

For treating severe hypophosphatemia, potassium phosphate (20 mEq K^+; 16 mM PO_4^{3-}) can be added to replacement fluids in place of KCl. Because phosphate deficits in DKA average only 1.0 mM per kg, it is rarely necessary to administer more than one 5-mL ampule of potassium phosphate. Thereafter, potassium should be replaced as KCl. The hazards of parenteral phosphate administration include hypomagnesemia, hypocalcemia, and metastatic calcification [49]. If a patient with DKA can tolerate oral medication, phosphate-containing antacids (e.g., Neutra-Phos®) can be given.

Bicarbonate. Despite the presence of a low serum bicarbonate concentration and severe acidemia, most authorities now concur that there is no need for the routine use of bicarbonate therapy in DKA [50–55]. Neutralization is intuitively appealing, but fluid and electrolyte replacement alone will ameliorate acidosis, and bicarbonate therapy may produce adverse effects. These include severe acute hypokalemia [56], late alkalosis due to paradoxical cerebrospinal fluid acidosis [57], a shift of the oxygen dissociation curve to the left that results in tissue hypoxia and lactic acidosis [58], and increased hepatic ketogenesis [52]. In children, bicarbonate therapy may increase the risk of cerebral edema [59]. Bicarbonate replacement in DKA should be used only when hypotensive shock is unresponsive to rapid fluid replacement [60], buffering capability is completely exhausted, respiratory responses are maximal, and acidemia is worsening [41]. Even in these circumstances, bicarbonate can only "buy time" until metabolic treatment reverses the acidosis. On those rare occasions when it may possibly be beneficial, two ampules of sodium bicarbonate (100 mEq each) should be given over 1 hour.

Magnesium. Hypermagnesemia may occur early in the course of DKA [61], but serum Mg^{2+} concentrations generally return to normal without specific treatment. In some patients, Mg^{2+} stores may be depleted, and hypomagnesemia may rarely lead to cardiac arrest [62]. Dysrhythmia should alert the physician to the possible need for magnesium supplementation.

Insulin

Insulin therapy in DKA is essential but should be instituted only after fluid and electrolyte resuscitation is underway [41]. Continuous low-dose infusion after an intravenous loading dose is the preferred method [63]. For adults, we recommend a bolus of 10 U of short-acting insulin followed by a continuous intravenous infusion starting at 5 to 10 U per hour. In children, the recommended initial bolus is 0.1 U per kg of body weight and the infusion rate is 0.1 U per kg per hour [64–66]. If for some reason continuous infusion cannot be given, the older bolus method can still be used. For adults, initially give 10 to 25 U of short-acting insulin intravenously plus 10 to 25 U subcutaneously. Regular (crystalline) insulin is typically used in intravenous infusions; semisynthetic rapid acting insulins approved for intravenous administration offer no advantage by this route. The onset of action of intravenous regular insulin occurs within minutes; bolus doses peak within 30 minutes, and the duration of action is 2 to 3 hours.

If DKA is treated with frequent subcutaneous insulin injections, very short-acting analogues may be advantageous because of their rapid onset of action. Their shorter duration of action may, however, require more frequent monitoring of blood glucose concentration. The safety and efficacy of repeated subcutaneous injections of rapid acting insulin analogues every 1 to 2 hours for the treatment of uncomplicated DKA is well documented [67].

Insulin for infusion should be added to 0.45% saline (at a concentration of 0.5 U per mL), and the container swirled before use. Blood glucose concentration should be measured every 1 to 2 hours after starting the infusion. If the glucose concentration has not decreased by 100 mg per dL, the insulin infusion rate should be doubled. When the glucose concentration has fallen by more than 150 mg per dL, the infusion rate should be decreased by 50%, but it should never be stopped.

The minimum blood glucose concentration during the first 24 hours of treatment should be $\approx$200 mg per dL. If it falls to below 200 mg per dL, glucose infusion (D5 W) should be started, and the insulin infusion rate should be adjusted to $\approx$1.0 U per hour to maintain insulinization and inhibit ketogenesis. Never stop insulin entirely during the treatment of DKA, even if the infusion rate is reduced to only 0.5 U per hour or less. This is particularly important in children with DKA because their high GFR and high rate of urinary glucose excretion can lead to a low blood glucose concentration before ketone production has been reversed by insulin.

As noted above, resolving DKA is often accompanied by an increase in plasma ketones (principally AcAc) as BOHB is reoxidized. Total ketone bodies (AcAc plus BOHB) slowly fall throughout treatment, and the increase in measured ketones is transient. An increase in conventionally measured "plasma ketones" during the early hours of DKA treatment does not necessarily mean that treatment is inadequate and that more insulin is needed. The entire clinical picture must be assessed, and if the acidosis and hyperglycemia are resolving, the rise in ketones should be interpreted as a sign of improvement.

Complications

The morbidity and mortality associated with DKA are proportional to the severity of coma and acidemia at the time of presentation. Many complications can occur despite appropriate therapy.

Hypotension and Shock

Hypotension is an important complication of DKA. It is usually caused by volume depletion, and normally fluid replacement alone will reverse it [68]. Persistent hypotension should prompt consideration of fluid shifts, bleeding, severe acidosis, hypokalemia, arrhythmia, myocardial infarction, sepsis, and adrenal insufficiency.

When insulin is administered to a patient with DKA, both glucose and water move to the intracellular space. Blood pressure may then fall as extracellular and intravascular volumes decrease. Increasing the rate of fluid replacement can usually reverse this.

If shock persists despite fluid replacement, occult blood loss should be considered. Patients with gastric ulcer, colitis, or hemorrhagic pancreatitis can bleed into the gut lumen or peritoneum. Physical examination and an inappropriately low hematocrit in the face of dehydration are clues to this complication.

A shift in K^+ from the extracellular to the intracellular fluid space after insulin administration can lower serum potassium concentration and cause cardiac arrhythmias which may compromise blood pressure.

Patients with hypotension and increased central venous pressure should be investigated for heart disease. Myocardial infarction is the most common finding, but other conditions such as cardiac tamponade can occur. Myocardial infarction is a common complication in long-standing diabetes, and its classic symptoms may be less obvious in the diabetic population. Patients in DKA who have had a myocardial infarction have a poorer prognosis [69].

Gram-negative sepsis is another cause of shock in ketoacidosis [60]. Pyelonephritis and pneumonia are common in such cases and must be treated appropriately when encountered. Ketoacidosis per se does not cause fever.

It is not uncommon for patients with type 1 diabetes to have other autoimmune diseases, and adrenal insufficiency should be considered in cases of ketoacidosis with refractory shock. The stress of DKA may uncover a state of partial adrenal insufficiency requiring glucocorticoid replacement.

The initial approach to the patient in shock is additional fluid replacement. (See Chapters 157 and 158 for a detailed discussion of the subsequent management of this problem.) Thereafter, further diagnostic procedures are necessary. Cardiovascular monitoring systems should be used as needed.

Thrombosis

The dehydration and intravascular volume contraction common in DKA may activate coagulation factors [70]. Thrombosis of cerebral vessels and stroke are recognized complications of DKA. Some authorities suggest the routine use of low-dose heparin in the management of DKA, but there are no controlled studies to document its efficacy [71].

Cerebral Edema

Subclinical brain edema may be common in DKA [72], but clinically important cerebral edema is a rare complication in adults. It occurs more commonly in children [65], with a reported frequency of 0.3% to 0.5% in pediatric cases of DKA [64,73]. Cerebral edema has been associated with very high mortality (24%) [73]. It usually occurs a few hours after the initiation of therapy. Children who develop cerebral edema during treatment for DKA may initially have a relatively normal serum osmolality and then experience a progressive decline in serum sodium concentration [74]. Treatment with bicarbonate increases the risk of cerebral edema in children with DKA who present with azotemia and a low PCO_2 [59]. Greater baseline acidosis, higher potassium and urea concentrations, and large volumes of administered fluid are also risk factors for cerebral edema [75].

The exact mechanism of cerebral edema is unknown, but it may involve a combination of fluid shifts, thrombosis of intracerebral vessels, and effects on ion exchange mechanisms [76]. The most effective treatment for cerebral edema is probably mannitol [77]. Hypertonic saline has also been used [78]. Steroids are not recommended [79,80]. Unfortunately, even when diagnosed early, cerebral edema may cause permanent neurologic damage or death.

Renal Failure

Hyperglycemic patients given intravenous fluids should have brisk urine flow. Patients in DKA who do not void within a few hours of therapy should be considered oliguric. A common cause of oliguria is postrenal obstruction. A dilated atonic bladder is common in comatose patients and even more common in diabetic patients with severe neuropathy and DKA. Occasionally, patients with DKA precipitated by pyelonephritis develop acute tubular necrosis. Acute renal failure in the absence of infection is an uncommon complication of DKA [81].

Recurrent Diabetic Ketoacidosis

If ketoacidosis reappears in a patient who has received adequate amounts of insulin, infection or a severe contra-insulin state (e.g., Cushing's syndrome) should be suspected. More commonly, the problem is iatrogenic. The physician treating DKA notes that the blood glucose concentration has fallen, mistakenly assumes the condition has been cured, and discontinues insulin treatment. Because the duration of action of intravenous insulin is brief and these patients make no insulin, ketone production resumes and ketosis soon recurs [2]. Insulin infusions should be continued, if only at 0.5 to 1 U per hour, until the patient is well enough to be switched to subcutaneous injections of longer-acting insulin. The intravenous infusion of insulin can be discontinued 2 to 3 hours after the first subcutaneous injection of intermediate-acting insulin is given. Cases of insulin-resistant DKA with recurrent hyperglycemia that respond to treatment with insulin-like growth factor I have been described [82], but these are extremely uncommon.

Low Blood Glucose Concentration

The blood glucose concentration in DKA usually decreases rapidly as a result of renal excretion as soon as fluid is administered and urine flow is established [68]. After insulin is given, glucose is metabolized as well as excreted, and blood glucose concentrations may fall rapidly. The physician must be alert to the possibility of precipitous reductions in glycemia. To avoid cerebral edema, the goal of the first 24 hours of DKA treatment is a blood glucose concentration not less than 200 mg per dL.

When the blood glucose concentration falls to 200 mg per dL, D5 W should be administered together with insulin. Use of D10 W is unnecessary [83]. Dual therapy inhibits ketone production while precluding hypoglycemia. For the first 24 hours of treatment, continuous intravenous infusion of insulin is recommended.

Follow-up Care of Diabetic Ketoacidosis

After a patient has recovered from DKA, the physician's goal should be the prevention of further episodes [84]. This requires the identification of any precipitating factors. Lack of education regarding diabetes should be remedied.

HYPERGLYCEMIC HYPEROSMOLAR SYNDROME

Severe hyperglycemia, dehydration, and coma have long been known to occur in the absence of significant acidosis or ketonemia in older patients with diabetes [85]. This syndrome is designated as HHS. Mortality in HHS has historically been high, on the order of approximately 50%, but increasing recognition and improved ICU-based treatment have substantially improved this figure; mortality more recently is on the order of 15% [69,86]. With optimal care, HHS managed in an ICU setting can carry a relatively favorable prognosis. Of note is the fact that, with the increasing prevalence of obesity and type 2 diabetes in children, a similar disorder is being reported in the pediatric population [87–89]. The syndrome can be the initial presentation of type 2 diabetes and, in the United States, may occur with disproportionate frequency in African American youth.

Pathophysiology and Etiology

The pathophysiology that gives rise to HHS requires that three interrelated elements be present: insulin deficiency, renal impairment, and cognitive impairment.

Insulin Deficiency

Relative lack of insulin is the fundamental defect in HHS. Patients have sufficient insulin to inhibit ketone body formation but not enough to prevent hyperglucagonemia, glycogenolysis, and gluconeogenesis [90]. The resulting hyperglycemia induces an osmotic diuresis, with resultant fluid and electrolyte losses.

Paradoxically, venous insulin concentration levels in patients with HHS are comparable with those sometimes observed in DKA [91]. Animals with experimentally induced HHS have portal insulin concentrations higher than those of animals with experimental ketoacidosis [92]. The data suggest that partial insulinization of the liver in HHS enables affected patients to metabolize free fatty acids and thereby avoid ketogenesis in the face of severe hyperglycemia. Additional data indicate, however, that hepatic insulinization alone cannot account for the absence of ketosis in HHS. Ketone bodies can be induced when medium-chain triglycerides (precursors of fatty acids) are administered to animals with an experimental HHS syndrome [93]. The result suggests that patients with HHS would produce ketones despite hepatic insulinization if enough substrate in the form of free fatty acids were present. Their resistance to ketosis must therefore depend on limited availability of circulating free fatty acids [94].

The low concentrations of free fatty acids in HHS may be due to relatively low concentrations of lipolytic hormones [95] including growth hormone and cortisol. Concentrations of these hormones are lower in HHS than in DKA [96]. Another explanation is that hyperosmolality itself inhibits the release of free fatty acids [97]. Additional unidentified factors may play a role.

Renal Impairment

Some degree of renal impairment accompanies all cases of HHS. Younger patients with diabetes have a normal GFR and, even in the event of DKA, filter enough glucose into the urine to prevent extreme hyperglycemia. In contrast, typical patients with HHS are older. Their renal blood flow and GFR are reduced, and they cannot readily excrete a glucose load. When they become hyperglycemic, the glucose is neither metabolized nor excreted. It remains in the extracellular fluid space. The resulting increase in osmolality, together with the decreased GFR, causes still less glucose to be excreted (Fig. 101.3).

The underlying renal abnormality in HHS may be prerenal, renal, or postrenal. The common result is that affected patients are unable to compensate for the hyperglycemia with an osmotic diuresis. The result is an extremely high glucose

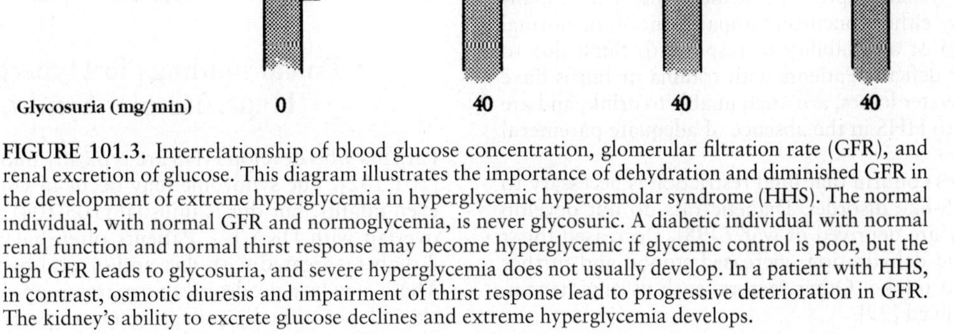

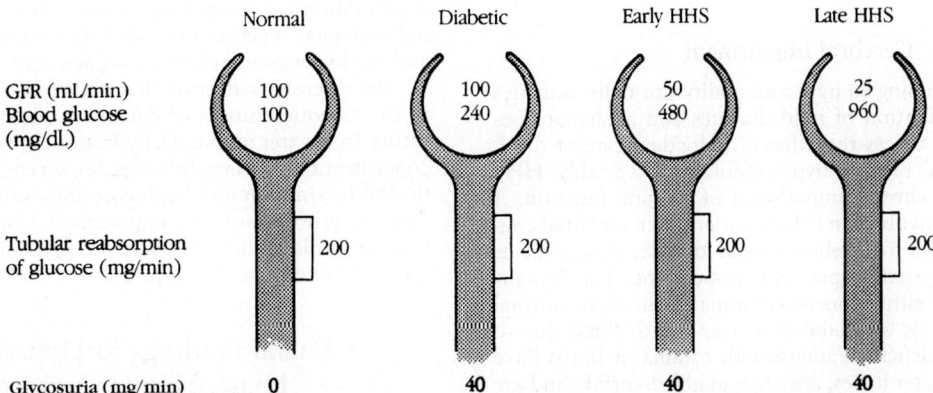

FIGURE 101.3. Interrelationship of blood glucose concentration, glomerular filtration rate (GFR), and renal excretion of glucose. This diagram illustrates the importance of dehydration and diminished GFR in the development of extreme hyperglycemia in hyperglycemic hyperosmolar syndrome (HHS). The normal individual, with normal GFR and normoglycemia, is never glycosuric. A diabetic individual with normal renal function and normal thirst response may become hyperglycemic if glycemic control is poor, but the high GFR leads to glycosuria, and severe hyperglycemia does not usually develop. In a patient with HHS, in contrast, osmotic diuresis and impairment of thirst response lead to progressive deterioration in GFR. The kidney's ability to excrete glucose declines and extreme hyperglycemia develops.

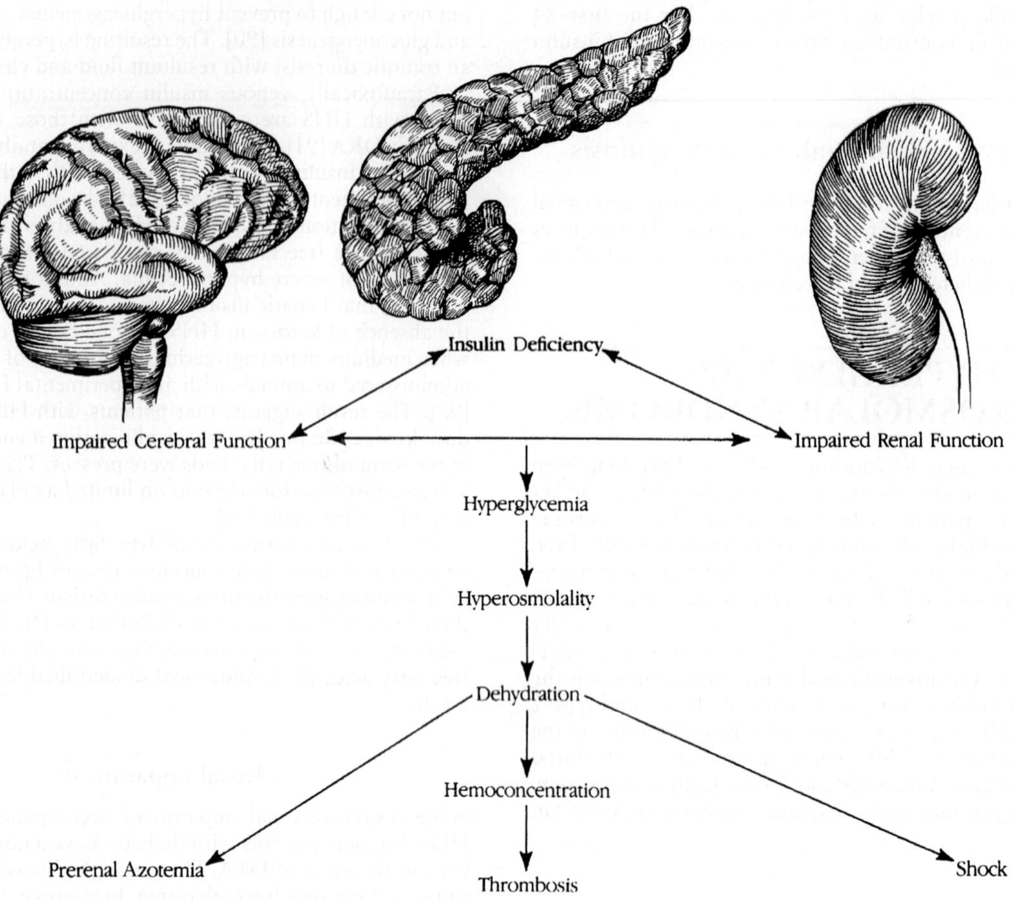

FIGURE 101.4. Pathogenesis of hyperglycemic hyperosmolar syndrome (HHS). Three interrelated factors give rise to HHS: insufficient insulin leads to hyperglycemia and glycosuria, impaired renal function exaggerates the hyperglycemia and hyperosmolality, and impaired cognition leads to decreased free water intake. Together, these factors lead to dehydration and the hyperosmolar hyperglycemic state.

concentration. Severe hyperglycemia itself can cause prerenal azotemia because glycosuria causes a hypotonic osmotic diuresis resulting in urinary loss of free water. If not replaced orally, this loss causes a reduction in intravascular volume and renal perfusion.

Cerebral Impairment

Hyperglycemia leading to hyperosmolality normally activates thirst. The combination of mild diabetes and azotemia does not lead to HHS unless the affected individual cannot drink sufficient water to prevent hyperosmolality. Invariably, HHS involves acute or chronic impairment of cerebral function. A common history involves an elderly patient with impaired cognitive function due to cerebrovascular disease, dementia, or central nervous system–depressant medications. This impairment may involve either concurrent impairment of the normal thirst mechanism or an inability to respond to thirst due to speech or motor deficits. Patients with trauma or burns have large insensible water losses, are often unable to drink, and are also susceptible to HHS in the absence of adequate parenteral fluids.

Animal studies confirm that fluid restriction is necessary to produce an HHS-like disorder. Diabetic rats do not develop HHS unless they are deprived of water [98]. Decreased thirst leads to increased dehydration, increased stupor, and further decreases in fluid intake. Other factors, such as angiotensin, may also be involved [99].

Interrelationships

To summarize, three interrelated factors are required for HHS. Insulin deficiency leads to hyperglycemia and glycosuria. Impaired renal function exaggerates the hyperglycemia and leads to hyperosmolality. Decreased free water intake precludes dilutional compensation and further exacerbates prerenal azotemia. Together, these three factors produce dehydration and the hyperosmolar hyperglycemic state (Fig. 101.4).

The severe dehydration that occurs in this syndrome is due to the osmotic diuresis of glucose in the absence of compensatory free water intake. Dehydration, in turn, leads to hemoconcentration, setting the stage for severe prerenal azotemia, thrombosis, and shock. As glucose and osmolality rise, cerebral function is progressively compromised. Coma ensues when the serum osmolality is 350 mOsm per kg [100]. Severe HHS may take several days to develop.

Clinical Findings in Hyperglycemic Hyperosmolar Syndrome

Patients who develop HHS are typically middle aged or elderly [101,102]. The syndrome may occur in younger patients and even infants, but this is unusual [103,104] and may represent overlap with DKA [2]. Patients often have a history of type 2 diabetes treated with diet and/or oral hypoglycemic agents. There may be a prodrome of progressive polyuria and polydipsia and, occasionally, polyphagia lasting days to several weeks.

Most patients have underlying diseases. Renal and cardiovascular disorders are most common. Other intercurrent problems include infection, myocardial infarction, stroke, hemorrhage, and trauma [102]. Additional predisposing factors include dialysis [105], hyperalimentation [106], and medications. Diazoxide [107], phenytoin [108], propranolol [109], immunosuppressive agents [110], cimetidine [111], and the antipsychotic drugs clozapine and olanzapine [112,113] all impair insulin secretion or action and have been implicated as causes of HHS. The disorder has also been associated with treatment of HIV with nucleoside analogue didanosine [114] and lithium-induced diabetes insipidus [115,116].

Fever is a common finding in HHS even in the absence of infection, but infection must be rigorously excluded in all cases. Patients may have hypotension and tachycardia due to dehydration, and they frequently hyperventilate. Neurological manifestations include tremors and fasciculations. Mental status ranges from mild disorientation to obtundation and coma depending on the degree of abnormalities in osmolality and perfusion [117]. Up to a third of patients with HHS may seize [118], and many in this group are misdiagnosed as having primary intracerebral disease. Once treatment has been instituted, neurologic symptoms may clear rapidly. The hyperventilation may reflect lactic acidosis, a common complication of severe dehydration and hypotension. Rapid respiration in a hyperglycemic patient does not always imply ketoacidosis.

Diagnosis

The key to the diagnosis of HHS is the demonstration of hyperglycemia and hyperosmolality without significant ketosis in the appropriate clinical setting.

Blood Glucose Concentration

Blood glucose concentrations in HHS are generally higher than in DKA, usually greater than 600 mg per dL. Values as high as 2,000 mg per dL occur.

Acetone

Most patients in HHS are not ketonemic. Serum acetone levels are usually normal or only slightly elevated, seldom exceeding 1:2. Occasional patients in HHS develop a severe intercurrent metabolic acidosis. In these very ill patients, a severe hyperosmolar state may overlap with ketoacidosis. Such cases are uncommon.

Osmolality

Serum osmolality in comatose patients is usually more than 350 mOsm per kg. It can be measured directly in the laboratory but is easily and quickly approximated from BUN, sodium, potassium, and glucose concentrations as shown in Table 101.1.

Acid–Base Balance

Most patients in HHS are only mildly acidotic. Serum bicarbonate concentration and arterial pH are usually close to normal. The average pH is about 7.25 before treatment, and HCO_3 is typically $\geq$15 mEq per L. The acidemia most often represents either mild lactic acidosis or uremic acidosis. If there is a significant anion gap (see Table 101.1), other causes of acidosis should be considered. These include salicylate, methanol, and ethylene glycol ingestions.

Renal Function

As outlined above, renal function is always impaired in patients with HHS. In addition to any preexisting renal disease, dehydration induces prerenal azotemia, and the ratio of BUN to creatinine is usually greater than 30:1. BUN and creatinine should be repeated after treatment to determine the degree of intrinsic renal impairment.

Electrolytes

The serum sodium concentration in early HHS is highly variable, ranging between 100 and 180 mEq per L. Hyponatremia may result from the dilutional effect of osmotically active glucose in patients with high free water intake in the face of impaired renal function. As mentioned previously, for each 100 mg per dL increase in blood glucose in excess of 100 mg

TABLE 101.2

EVIDENTIARY BASIS OF MANAGEMENT

Recommendation	Comments
Begin fluid resuscitation of DKA and HHS before insulin therapy.	Studies have shown that hydration lowers plasma glucose by improvement in glomerular filtration and increase in net urinary glucose loss. There is partial correction of pH and plasma bicarbonate with hydration [41].
Low dose (0.1 unit/kg/h) infusion of rapid-acting insulin is recommended.	Randomized controlled trials (RCTs) have shown lower rates of insulin infusion to be as effective as higher rates. Lower insulin rates confer reduced risk of hypokalemia and hypoglycemia [63].
Potassium replacement should begin early.	Studies have shown that insulin administration before volume and potassium repletion can cause shock and arrhythmias [26,29].
Bicarbonate replacement is not recommended in managing DKA.	Trials have shown no benefit of bicarbonate use in patients with pH >6.9 with respect to resolution of ketonemia, acidosis, or hyperglycemia [50–55]. No trials of bicarbonate use in patients with pH <6.9 have been reported.
Phosphate replacement has not been shown to be of benefit in DKA.	Randomized trials have not demonstrated clinical benefit from the routine use of phosphate replacement in DKA [46–48].
Intravenous insulin infusion is preferred for moderate to severe DKA, whereas repeated doses of subcutaneous insulin may be used instead in mild DKA.	Trials comparing intravenous insulin infusion to subcutaneous insulin injections showed similar eventual outcomes, but quicker resolution of ketosis and hyperglycemia with intravenous insulin. In patients with mild DKA, trials show subcutaneous injections of fast-acting insulin every 1–2 hours to be as effective as intravenous infusion of regular insulin [67].

Note: Treatment of the diabetic comas has evolved incrementally over many decades. This table summarizes the validation of key components of therapy.

per dL, serum sodium concentration falls approximately 1.6 mEq per L. When severe hypotonic fluid losses occur in the later stages of HHS, patients may become hypernatremic. Because sodium remains in the extracellular fluid compartment, this electrolyte should be followed to assess the state of hydration.

Serum potassium concentration in HHS syndrome is also variable. It may range from 2.2 to 7.8 mEq per L [85]. Hypokalemia requires immediate potassium replacement. As mentioned later, serum potassium concentrations decrease after treatment with insulin is begun. Hyperkalemia often responds to fluid replacement and improvement in urinary output. Patients with HHS, like those with DKA, lose substantial quantities of electrolytes.

Treatment

Overview

The best treatment for HHS is prevention. The condition can be avoided by periodic attention to blood glucose control and mental status. Susceptible individuals are those with mildly impaired glucose metabolism. They are often the elderly living alone. They may be hospitalized inpatients who have experienced trauma, undergone extensive surgery, or been placed on hyperalimentation regimens. They may also be residents of nursing homes, although improvements in care appear to have reduced this risk [102]. Individuals in all of these settings can be at risk for hyperglycemia and hyperosmolality. When HHS does occur, continuous vigilance in monitoring the details of the patient's clinical progress at the bedside is the key to achieving a successful outcome.

Fluid Replacement

Patients with HHS are, without exception, profoundly dehydrated. Within the first 2 hours, 1 to 2 L of 0.9% saline should be given. Normal saline is recommended, even if hypernatremia is present, to expand the extracellular fluid compartment rapidly. After initial volume expansion and restoration of normotension, subsequent treatment for dehydration in this syndrome emphasizes free water replacement. The osmotic diuresis of glucose produces free water loss in excess of solute loss. The initial infusion of normal saline must never be overlooked, however, because it rapidly expands the extracellular compartment and helps reestablish adequate perfusion pressure. The corrected serum sodium can be used to help decide when the switch from 0.9% saline to 0.45% saline should be made.

The typical HHS patient requires 6 to 8 L of fluids (100 to 200 mL per kg) during the first 12 hours of treatment. The rate of fluid administration must be adjusted as appropriate to the patient's clinical status. Elderly patients with cardiovascular impairment may require less aggressive replacement.

Electrolytes

As soon as adequate urine flow has been established and the degree of hypokalemia estimated, potassium supplementation should be added to the intravenous fluids. During the initial phases of therapy, serum potassium concentration should be checked frequently and the electrocardiogram monitored for changes in morphology and rhythm. A sudden fall in serum potassium concentration frequently accompanies the initiation of insulin therapy [94]. Cardiac arrhythmias induced by hypokalemia may be irreversible, particularly in the elderly. The potassium deficit in HHS can be ≥5 mEq per kg [85], but generally, the magnitude of the loss is not as great as that encountered in DKA [119].

Insulin

Most patients with HHS are more sensitive to insulin than are patients with DKA [94]. In addition, blood glucose concentration in HHS can fall rapidly when urine output is reestablished after volume expansion with saline. The combination of insulin sensitivity and glucose diuresis puts patients in HHS at risk of sudden unexpected hypoglycemia. Treatment with insulin is essential but should be instituted with careful monitoring and only after fluid and electrolyte resuscitation is underway.

Only short-acting insulin should be used. Continuous infusion is now standard but must be used with great caution. We do not recommend an initial intravenous insulin bolus. For the infusion, we recommend a starting dose of 1 to 5 U per hour, depending on individual circumstances. This dose is sufficient to insulinize the patient and is usually not high enough to cause severe hypoglycemia. If continuous insulin infusion therapy is not possible, treatment should be with boluses of intravenous regular insulin. The initial dose should not exceed 10 to 30 U. Boluses should be given every 2 to 4 hours, with dose adjusted on the basis of blood glucose determinations.

As emphasized repeatedly, normalization of glucose is not the primary goal of treatment; fluid and electrolyte resuscitation take precedence and often improve glycemia substantially before any insulin is given. An attempt should be made to maintain blood glucose concentration near 250 mg per dL for the first 24 hours. Rapid fall in blood glucose concentration correlates with the development of cerebral edema [100,120].

Complications

Hypotension

When insulin is administered to patients with HHS syndrome, glucose shifts from the extracellular to the intracellular compartment. Because glucose is osmotically active, the movement of glucose intracellularly draws free water from the extracellular compartment. The rapid intracellular movement of free water compromises intravascular volume and may precipitate hypotension and shock [121]. The use of normal (0.9%) saline for initial volume replacement helps prevent hypotension. The higher osmolality of normal (308 mOsm per L) compared with half-normal (154 mOsm per L) saline reduces the osmotic effect of the glucose shifts that follow insulin administration [122].

The magnitude of the fluid shifts that can be induced by insulin was illustrated in a dramatic case report. A patient with congestive heart failure and preexisting renal disease was found to have severe hyperglycemia. Because fluid replacement was contraindicated, the patient was treated with insulin alone. The insulin treatment resulted in a shift of fluid from the extracellular to the intracellular compartment sufficient to ameliorate the congestive heart failure [123].

Cerebral Edema

Blood glucose concentrations should never be reduced precipitously. Rapid reduction is a major contributor to the development of cerebral edema and a fatal outcome in HHS. The exact cause of cerebral edema in HHS is unknown, but animal studies suggest that neuronal intracellular osmolality increases in HHS. The osmotically active solute has not been identified. The term idiogenic osmoles is used to describe these uncharacterized, osmotically active, nondiffusible substances [124]. They draw water into neurons when the extracellular osmolality drops as a result of the intracellular movement of glucose. This is followed by severe edema, increased intracranial pressure, and disturbed hypothalamic function.

Thrombosis

Large vessel thromboembolic events are an important cause of mortality in HHS. Severe dehydration and hyperosmolality lead to reduced cardiac output and hyperviscosity, predisposing

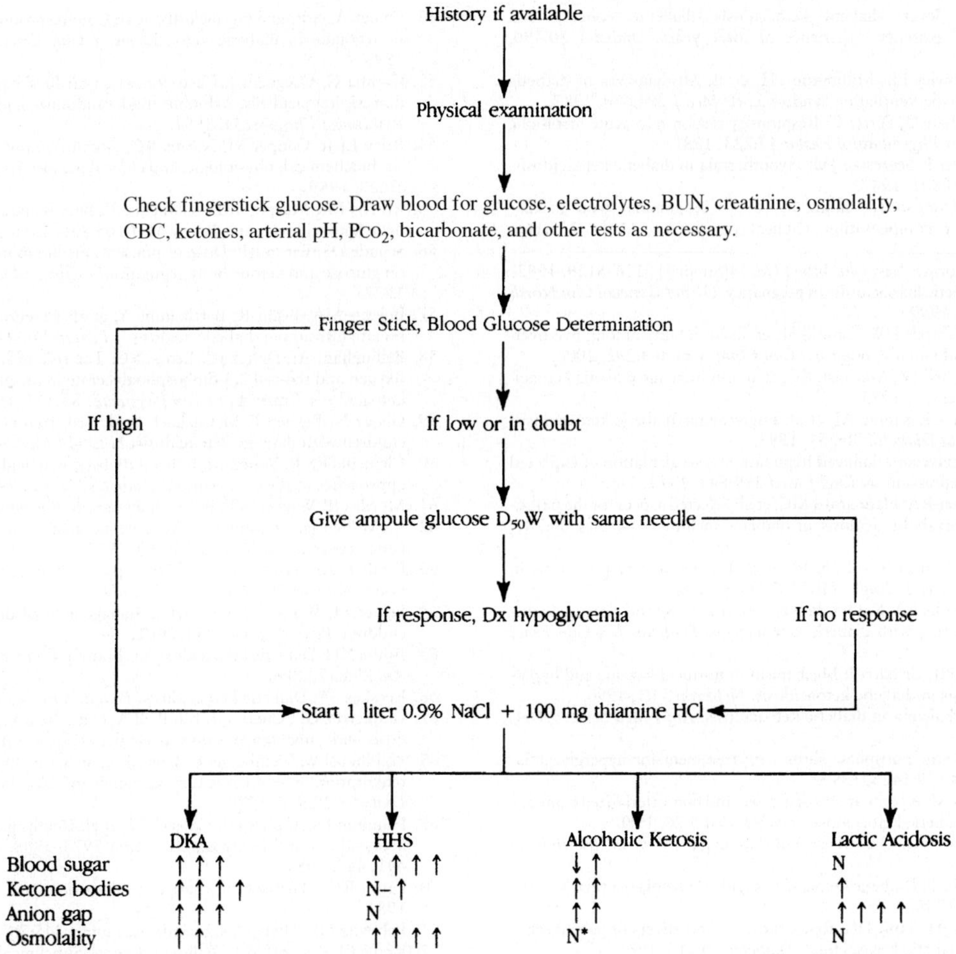

FIGURE 101.5. Algorithm for the diagnosis of diabetic coma. Measured osmolality is greater than predicted; result in freezing point depression test is increased by 1 mOsm/5 mg% EtOH. CBC, complete blood count; N, normal; ↑, mildly elevated; ↓, mildly depressed; ↑↑, moderately elevated; ↑↑↑, severely elevated; ↑↑↑↑, extremely elevated. BUN, blood urea nitrogen. [Adapted from Lindsey CA, Faloon GR, Unger RH: Plasma glucagon in hyperosmolar coma. *JAMA* 229:1771, 1974, with permission. Illustration by Albert Miller.]

to venous and arterial thrombosis. Use of low-dose heparin prophylaxis is recommended in high-risk patients [125].

CONCLUSIONS

The diabetic comas are often described as discrete entities, but they frequently present as overlapping disorders [2]. Patients in DKA often have concurrent mild lactic acidosis and may also develop hyperosmolality. Initial treatment of all diabetic comas must always emphasize fluid and electrolytes. DKA and HHS also require careful management of insulin therapy. Physicians must obtain the relevant history, perform a thorough physical examination, classify the disorder, and treat appropriately. The approach to treatment is summarized in Fig. 101.5. With care, nearly all patients with DKA and most with HHS can survive.

References

1. Kitabchi AE, Nyenwe EA: Hyperglycemic crises in diabetes mellitus: diabetic ketoacidosis and hyperglycemic hyperosmolar state. *Endocrinol Metab Clin North Am* 35:725, viii, 2006.
2. Hare JW, Rossini AA: Diabetic comas: the overlap concept. *Hosp Pract* 14:95:1028, 1979.
3. McGuire LC, Cruickshank AM, Munro PT: Alcoholic ketoacidosis. *Emerg Med J* 23:417, 2006.
4. Kitabchi AE, Umpierrez GE, Murphy MB, et al: Management of hyperglycemic crises in patients with diabetes. *Diabetes Care* 24:131, 2001.
5. American Diabetes Association: Hyperglycemic crises in patients with diabetes mellitus. *Diabetes Care* 24:154, 2001.
6. Flakoll PJ, Carlson MG, Cherrington AD: Physiologic action of insulin, in LeRoith D, Taylor SI, Olefsky JM (eds): *Diabetes Mellitus. A Fundamental and Clinical Text.* 2nd ed. Philadelphia, PA, Lippincott Williams & Wilkins, 2000, pp. 148–161.
7. Cahill GF Jr: The Banting Memorial Lecture 1971. Physiology of insulin in man. *Diabetes* 20:785, 1971.
8. Cherrington AD: Banting Lecture 1997. Control of glucose uptake and release by the liver in vivo. *Diabetes* 48:1198, 1999.
9. Beylot M: Regulation of in vivo ketogenesis: role of free fatty acids and control by epinephrine, thyroid hormones, insulin and glucagon. *Diabetes Metab* 22:299, 1996.
10. Azoulay E, Chevret S, Didier J, et al: Infection as a trigger of diabetic ketoacidosis in intensive care-unit patients. *Clin Infect Dis* 32:30, 2001.
11. Umpierrez GE, Kelly JP, Navarrete JE, et al: Hyperglycemic crises in urban blacks. *Arch Int Med* 157:669, 1997.
12. Banerji MA, Chaiken RL, Huey H, et al: GAD antibody negative NIDDM in adult black subjects with diabetic ketoacidosis and increased frequency of human leukocyte antigen DR3 and DR4: flatbush diabetes. *Diabetes* 43:741, 1994.
13. Snorgaard O, Eskildsen PC, Vadstrup S, et al: Diabetic ketoacidosis in Denmark: epidemiology, incidence rates, precipitating factors and mortality rates. *J Intern Med* 226:223, 1989.

14. Beigelman PM: Severe diabetic ketoacidosis (diabetic "coma"). 482 episodes in 257 patients: experience of three years. *Diabetes* 20:490, 1971.
15. Treasure RA, Fowler PB, Millington HT, et al: Misdiagnosis of diabetic ketoacidosis as hyperventilation syndrome. *Br Med J* 294:630, 1987.
16. Verdon F, van Melle G, Perret C: Respiratory response to acute metabolic acidosis. *Bull Eur Physiopathol Respir* 17:223, 1981.
17. Guerin JM, Meyer P, Segrestaa JM: Hypothermia in diabetic ketoacidosis. *Diabetes Care* 10:801, 1987.
18. Campbell IW, Duncan LJ, Innes JA, et al: Abdominal pain in diabetic metabolic decompensation. Clinical significance. *JAMA* 233:166, 1975.
19. Sugar AM: Mucormycosis. *Clin Infect Dis* 14[Suppl 1]:S126–S129, 1992.
20. Ramin KD: Diabetic ketoacidosis in pregnancy. *Obstet Gynecol Clin North Am* 26:481, viii, 1999.
21. Kimberly MM, Vesper HW, Caudill SP, et al: Variability among five over-the-counter blood glucose monitors. *Clin Chim Acta* 364:292, 2006.
22. Munro JF, Campbell IW, McCuish AC, et al: Euglycaemic diabetic ketoacidosis. *Br Med J* 2:578, 1973.
23. Jenkins D, Close CF, Krentz AJ, et al: Euglycaemic diabetic ketoacidosis: does it exist? *Acta Diabetol* 30:251, 1993.
24. Katz MA: Hyperglycemia-induced hyponatremia—calculation of expected serum sodium depression. *N Engl J Med* 289:843, 1973.
25. Halperin ML, Bear RA, Hannaford MC, et al: Selected aspects of the pathophysiology of metabolic acidosis in diabetes mellitus. *Diabetes* 30:781, 1981.
26. Adrogué HJ, Wilson H, Boyd AE III, et al: Plasma acid-base patterns in diabetic ketoacidosis. *N Engl J Med* 307:1603, 1982.
27. Elisaf MS, Tsatsoulis AA, Katopodis KP, et al: Acid-base and electrolyte disturbances in patients with diabetic ketoacidosis. *Diabetes Res Clin Pract* 34:23, 1996.
28. Oh MS, Carroll HJ, Uribarri J: Mechanism of normochloremic and hyperchloremic acidosis in diabetic ketoacidosis. *Nephron* 54:1, 1990.
29. Fulop M: Hyperkalemia in diabetic ketoacidosis. *Am J Med Sci* 299:164, 1990.
30. Bohannon NJ: Large phosphate shifts with treatment for hyperglycemia. *Arch Intern Med* 149:1423, 1989.
31. Hale PJ, Nattrass M: A comparison of arterial and non-arterialized capillary blood gases in diabetic ketoacidosis. *Diabet Med* 5:76, 1988.
32. Emmett M, Narins RG: Clinical use of the anion gap. *Medicine (Baltimore)* 56:38, 1977.
33. Zonszein J, Baylor P: Diabetic ketoacidosis with alkalemia—a review. *West J Med* 149:217, 1988.
34. Owen OE, Licht JH, Sapir DG: Renal function and effects of partial rehydration during diabetic ketoacidosis. *Diabetes* 30:510, 1981.
35. Molitch ME, Rodman E, Hirsch CA, et al: Spurious serum creatinine elevations in ketoacidosis. *Ann Intern Med* 93:280, 1980.
36. Slovis CM, Mork VG, Slovis RJ, et al: Diabetic ketoacidosis and infection: leukocyte count and differential as early predictors of serious infection. *Am J Emerg Med* 5:1, 1987.
37. Vinicor F, Lehrner LM, Karn RC, et al: Hyperamylasemia in diabetic ketoacidosis: sources and significance. *Ann Intern Med* 91:200, 1979.
38. Nsien EE, Steinberg WM, Borum M, et al: Marked hyperlipasemia in diabetic ketoacidosis. A report of three cases. *J Clin Gastroenterol* 15:117, 1992.
39. Goldberg LH: Hyperuricemia, diabetes mellitus, and diabetic ketoacidosis. *Pa Med* 79:40, 1976.
40. Gogos CA, Giali S, Paliogianni F, et al: Interleukin-6 and C-reactive protein as early markers of sepsis in patients with diabetic ketoacidosis or hyperosmosis. *Diabetologia* 44:1011, 2001.
41. DeFronzo RA, Matsuda M, Barrett EJ: Diabetic ketoacidosis: a combined metabolic-nephrologic approach to therapy. *Diab Rev* 2:209, 1994.
42. Soler NG, Bennet MA, Dixon K, et al: Potassium balance during treatment of diabetic ketoacidosis with special reference to the use of bicarbonate. *Lancet* ii:665, 1972.
43. Lang F: Osmotic diuresis. *Ren Physiol* 10:160, 1987.
44. Foster DW, McGarry JD: The metabolic derangements and treatment of diabetic ketoacidosis. *N Engl J Med* 309:159, 1983.
45. Subramanian R, Khardori R: Severe hypophosphatemia. Pathophysiologic implications, clinical presentations, and treatment. *Medicine (Baltimore)* 79:1, 2000.
46. Fisher JN, Kitabchi AE: A randomized study of phosphate therapy in the treatment of diabetic ketoacidosis. *J Clin Endocrinol Metab* 57:177, 1983.
47. Wilson HK, Keuer SP, Lea AS, et al: Phosphate therapy in diabetic ketoacidosis. *Arch Intern Med* 142:517, 1982.
48. Becker DJ, Brown DR, Steranka BH, et al: Phosphate replacement during treatment of diabetic ketosis. Effects on calcium and phosphorus homeostasis. *Am J Dis Child* 137:241, 1983.
49. Zipf WB, Bacon GE, Spencer ML, et al: Hypocalcemia, hypomagnesemia, and transient hypoparathyroidism during therapy with potassium phosphate in diabetic ketoacidosis. *Diabetes Care* 2:265, 1979.
50. Viallon A, Zeni F, Lafond P, et al: Does bicarbonate therapy improve the management of severe diabetic ketoacidosis? *Crit Care Med* 27:2690, 1999.
51. Green SM, Rothrock SG, Ho JD, et al: Failure of adjunctive bicarbonate to improve outcome in severe pediatric diabetic ketoacidosis. *Ann Emerg Med* 31:41, 1998.
52. Okuda Y, Adrogue HJ, Field JB, et al: Counterproductive effects of sodium bicarbonate in diabetic ketoacidosis. *J Clin Endocrinol Metab* 81:314, 1996.
53. Gamba G, Oseguera J, Castrejon M, et al: Bicarbonate therapy in severe diabetic ketoacidosis. A double blind, randomized, placebo controlled trial. *Rev Invest Clin* 43:234, 1991.
54. Riley LJ Jr, Cooper M, Narins RG: Alkali therapy of diabetic ketoacidosis: biochemical, physiologic, and clinical perspectives. *Diabetes Metab Rev* 5:627, 1989.
55. Morris LR, Murphy MB, Kitabchi AE: Bicarbonate therapy in severe diabetic ketoacidosis. *Ann Intern Med* 105:836, 1986.
56. Schade DS, Eaton RP: Dose response to insulin in man: differential effects on glucose and ketone body regulation. *J Clin Endocrinol Metab* 44:1038, 1977.
57. Bureau MA, Begin R, Berthiaume Y, et al: Cerebral hypoxia from bicarbonate infusion in diabetic acidosis. *J Pediatr* 96:968, 1980.
58. Bellingham AJ, Detter JC, Lenfant C: The role of hemoglobin affinity for oxygen and red-cell 2,3-diphosphoglycerate in the management of diabetic ketoacidosis. *Trans Assoc Am Physicians* 83:113, 1970.
59. Glaser N, Barnett P, McCaslin I, et al: Risk factors for cerebral edema in children with diabetic ketoacidosis. *N Engl J Med* 344:264, 2001.
60. Clements RS Jr, Vourganti B: Fatal diabetic ketoacidosis: major causes and approaches to their prevention. *Diabetes Care* 1:314, 1978.
61. Mordes JP, Wacker WE: Excess magnesium. *Pharmacol Rev* 29:273, 1977.
62. McMullen JK: Asystole and hypomagnesaemia during recovery from diabetic ketoacidosis. *Br Med J* 1:690, 1977.
63. Kitabchi AE: Low-dose insulin therapy in diabetic ketoacidosis: fact or fiction? *Diabetes Metab Rev* 5:337, 1989.
64. Felner EI, White PC: Improving management of diabetic ketoacidosis in children. *Pediatrics* 108:735, 2001.
65. White NH: Diabetic ketoacidosis in children. *Endocrinol Metab Clin North Am* 29:657, 2000.
66. Kecskes SA: Diabetic ketoacidosis. *Pediatr Clin North Am* 40:355, 1993.
67. Umpierrez GE, Cuervo R, Karabell A, et al: Treatment of diabetic ketoacidosis with subcutaneous insulin aspart. *Diabetes Care* 27:1873, 2004.
68. Waldhausl W, Kleinberger G, Korn A, et al: Severe hyperglycemia: effects of rehydration on endocrine derangements and blood glucose concentration. *Diabetes* 28:577, 1979.
69. Hamblin PS, Topliss DJ, Chosich N, et al: Deaths associated with diabetic ketoacidosis and hyperosmolar coma 1973–1988. *Med J Aust* 151:439, 441, 444, 1989.
70. Paton RC: Haemostatic changes in diabetic coma. *Diabetologia* 21:172, 1981.
71. Lebovitz HE: Diabetic ketoacidosis. *Lancet* 345:767, 1995.
72. Krane EJ, Rockoff MA, Wallman JK, et al: Subclinical brain swelling in children during treatment of diabetic ketoacidosis. *N Engl J Med* 312:1147, 1985.
73. Edge JA, Hawkins MM, Winter DL, et al: The risk and outcome of cerebral oedema developing during diabetic ketoacidosis. *Arch Dis Child* 85:16, 2001.
74. Hale PM, Rezvani I, Braunstein AW, et al: Factors predicting cerebral edema in young children with diabetic ketoacidosis and new onset type I diabetes. *Acta Paediatr* 86:626, 1997.
75. Edge JA, Jakes RW, Roy Y, et al: The UK case-control study of cerebral oedema complicating diabetic ketoacidosis in children. *Diabetologia* 49:2002, 2006.
76. Silver SM, Clark EC, Schroeder BM, et al: Pathogenesis of cerebral edema after treatment of diabetic ketoacidosis. *Kidney Int* 51:1237, 1997.
77. Rosenbloom AL, Hanas R: Diabetic ketoacidosis (DKA): treatment guidelines. *Clin Pediatr (Phila)* 35:261, 1996.
78. Dunger DB, Sperling MA, Acerini CL, et al: ESPE/LWPES consensus statement on diabetic ketoacidosis in children and adolescents. *Arch Dis Child* 89:188, 2004.
79. Strachan MW, Nimmo GR, Noyes K, et al: Management of cerebral oedema in diabetes. *Diabetes Metab Res Rev* 19:241, 2003.
80. Levin DL: Cerebral edema in diabetic ketoacidosis. *Pediatr Crit Care Med* 9:320, 2008.
81. Murdoch IA, Pryor D, Haycock GB, et al: Acute renal failure complicating diabetic ketoacidosis. *Acta Paediatr* 82:498, 1993.
82. Usala A-L, Madigan T, Burguera B, et al: Brief report: treatment of insulin-resistant diabetic ketoacidosis with insulin-like growth factor I in an adolescent with insulin-dependent diabetes. *N Engl J Med* 327:853, 1992.
83. Krentz AJ, Hale PJ, Singh BM, et al: The effect of glucose and insulin infusion on the fall of ketone bodies during treatment of diabetic ketoacidosis. *Diabet Med* 6:31, 1989.
84. Flexner CW, Weiner JP, Saudek CD, et al: Repeated hospitalization for diabetic ketoacidosis. *Am J Med* 76:691, 1984.
85. Ennis ED, Stahl EJVB, Kreisberg RA: The hyperosmolar hyperglycemic syndrome. *Diab Rev* 2:115, 1994.
86. Pinies JA, Cairo G, Gaztambide S, et al: Course and prognosis of 132 patients with diabetic non ketotic hyperosmolar state. *Diabete Metab* 20:43, 1994.
87. Bhowmick SK, Levens KL, Rettig KR: Hyperosmolar hyperglycemic crisis: an acute life-threatening event in children and adolescents with type 2 diabetes mellitus. *Endocr Pract* 11:23, 2005.

88. Morales AE, Rosenbloom AL: Death caused by hyperglycemic hyperosmolar state at the onset of type 2 diabetes. *J Pediatr* 144:270, 2004.
89. Kershaw MJ, Newton T, Barrett TG, et al: Childhood diabetes presenting with hyperosmolar dehydration but without ketoacidosis: a report of three cases. *Diabet Med* 22:645, 2005.
90. Lindsey CA, Faloona GR, Unger RH: Plasma glucagon in nonketotic hyperosmolar coma. *JAMA* 229:1771, 1974.
91. Henry DP II, Bressler R: Serum insulin levels in non-ketotic hyperosmotic diabetes mellitus. *Am J Med Sci* 256:150, 1968.
92. Joffe BI, Seftel HC, Goldberg R, et al: Factors in the pathogenesis of experimental nonketotic and ketoacidotic diabetic stupor. *Diabetes* 22:653, 1973.
93. Wilson HK, Keuer SP, Lea AS, et al: Experimental hyperosmolar diabetic syndrome. Ketogenic response to medium-chain triglycerides. *Diabetes* 24:301, 1975.
94. Gerich JE, Martin MM, Recant L: Clinical and metabolic characteristics of hyperosmolar nonketotic coma. *Diabetes* 20:228, 1971.
95. Turpin BP, Duckworth WC, Solomon SS: Simulated hyperglycemic hyperosmolar syndrome. Impaired insulin and epinephrine effects upon lipolysis in the isolated rat fat cell. *J Clin Invest* 63:403, 1979.
96. Van der Meulen JA, Klip A, Grinstein S: Possible mechanism for cerebral oedema in diabetic ketoacidosis. *Lancet* 2:306, 1987.
97. Gerich J, Penhos JC, Gutman RA, et al: Effect of dehydration and hyperosmolarity on glucose, free fatty acid and ketone body metabolism in the rat. *Diabetes* 22:264, 1973.
98. Bavli S, Gordon EE: Experimental diabetic hyperosmolar syndrome in rats. *Diabetes* 20:92, 1971.
99. Malvin RL, Mouw D, Vander AJ: Angiotensin: physiological role in water-deprivation-induced thirst of rats. *Science* 197:171, 1977.
100. Arieff AI, Carroll HJ: Cerebral edema and depression of sensorium in nonketotic hyperosmolar coma. *Diabetes* 23:525, 1974.
101. Cahill GF Jr: Hyperglycemic hyperosmolar coma: a syndrome almost unique to the elderly. *J Am Geriatr Soc* 31:103, 1983.
102. Wachtel TJ, Silliman RA, Lamberton P: Predisposing factors for the diabetic hyperosmolar state. *Arch Intern Med* 147:499, 1987.
103. Foster DW: Insulin deficiency and hyperosmolar coma. *Adv Intern Med* 19:159, 1974.
104. Ginsberg-Fellner F, Primack WA: Recurrent hyperosmolar nonketotic episodes in a young diabetic. *Am J Dis Child* 129:240, 1975.
105. Emder PJ, Howard NJ, Rosenberg AR: Non-ketotic hyperosmolar diabetic pre-coma due to pancreatitis in a boy on continuous ambulatory peritoneal dialysis. *Nephron* 44:355, 1986.
106. Sypniewski E Jr, Mirtallo JM, Schneider PJ: Hyperosmolar, hyperglycemic, nonketotic coma in a patient receiving home total parenteral nutrient therapy. *Clin Pharm* 6:69, 1987.
107. Balsam MJ, Baker L, Kaye R: Hyperosmolar nonketotic coma associated with diazoxide therapy for hypoglycemia. *J Pediatr* 78:523, 1971.
108. Gharib H, Munoz JM: Endocrine manifestations of diphenylhydantoin therapy. *Metabolism* 23:515, 1974.
109. Podolsky S, Pattavina CG: Hyperosmolar nonketotic diabetic coma: a complication of propranolol therapy. *Metabolism* 22:685, 1973.
110. Woods JE, Zincke H, Palumbo PJ, et al: Hyperosmolar nonketotic syndrome and steroid diabetes. Occurrence after renal transplantation. *JAMA* 231:1261, 1975.
111. Pomare EW: Hyperosmolar non-ketotic diabetes and cimetidine [letter]. *Lancet* 1:1202, 1978.
112. Nugent BW: Hyperosmolar hyperglycemic state. *Emerg Med Clin North Am* 23:629, 2005.
113. Newcomer JW: Second-generation (atypical) antipsychotics and metabolic effects: a comprehensive literature review. *CNS Drugs* 19[Suppl 1]:1, 2005.
114. Munshi MN, Martin RE, Fonseca VA: Hyperosmolar nonketotic diabetic syndrome following treatment of human immunodeficiency virus infection with didanosine. *Diabetes Care* 17:316, 1994.
115. MacGregor D, Baker AM, Appel RG, et al: Hyperosmolar coma due to lithium-induced diabetes insipidus. *Lancet* 346:413, 1995.
116. Azam H, Newton RW, Morris AD, et al: Hyperosmolar nonketotic coma precipitated by lithium-induced nephrogenic diabetes insipidus. *Postgrad Med J* 74:39, 1998.
117. Maccario M: Neurological dysfunction associated with nonketotic hyperglycemia. *Arch Neurol* 19:525, 1968.
118. Daniels JC, Chokroverty S, Barron KD: Anacidotic hyperglycemia and focal seizures. *Arch Intern Med* 124:701, 1969.
119. Walsh CH, Soler NG, James H, et al: Studies on whole-body potassium in non-ketoacidotic diabetics before and after treatment. *Br Med J* 4:738, 1974.
120. Maccario M, Messis CP: Cerebral oedema complicating treated non-ketotic hyperglycaemia. *Lancet* 2:352, 1969.
121. Brown RH, Rossini AA, Callaway CW, et al: Caveat on fluid replacement in hyperglycemic, hyperosmolar, nonketotic coma. *Diabetes Care* 1:305, 1978.
122. Feig PU, McCurdy DK: The hypertonic state. *N Engl J Med* 297:1444, 1977.
123. Axelrod L: Response of congestive heart failure to correction of hyperglycemia in the presence of diabetic nephropathy. *N Engl J Med* 293:1243, 1975.
124. Arieff AI, Kleeman CR: Cerebral edema in diabetic comas. II. Effects of hyperosmolality, hyperglycemia and insulin in diabetic rabbits. *J Clin Endocrinol Metab* 38:1057, 1974.
125. Kian K, Eiger G: Anticoagulant therapy in hyperosmolar non-ketotic diabetic coma. *Diabet Med* 20:603, 2003.

CHAPTER 102 ■ SEVERE HYPERTHYROIDISM

MARJORIE S. SAFRAN

Patients with thyrotoxicosis rarely need hospitalization. However, some patients with severe thyrotoxicosis develop a decompensated clinical presentation called *thyroid storm.* It is characterized by hyperpyrexia, tachycardia, and delirium [1] and generally occurs in a patient with severe thyrotoxicosis who then experiences a stressful event. The cause of this rapid decompensation is unknown, but it may be partly due to a sudden inhibition in thyroid hormone binding to plasma proteins, resulting in a rise in the already elevated free hormone pool [2]. Thyroid storm accounts for no more than 2% of hospital admissions for all forms and complications of thyrotoxicosis, and the diagnosis is often difficult to make because there is a fine line between severe thyrotoxicosis and thyroid storm. Even when properly treated, thyroid storm has a mortality rate of 7% to 30% [3].

ETIOLOGY

Before the preoperative use of iodides and the antithyroid drugs propylthiouracil (PTU) and methimazole (MMI; Tapazole), thyroid storm was most frequently seen during and after subtotal thyroidectomy. Because these agents are used to restore euthyroidism before surgery, thyroid storm is rarely seen in this context. Thyroid storm now occurs most commonly in patients with severe underlying thyrotoxicosis, frequently undiagnosed, who become ill for other reasons, such as infections, trauma, labor, diabetic ketoacidosis, or pulmonary and cardiovascular disorders. It can occur during or after nonthyroid surgery, and has been reported after external beam radiation to the neck [4], ingestion of sympathomimetic drugs (such as pseudoephedrine) in a thyrotoxic patient [5], and rarely with intentional or accidental overdoses [6,7]. Thyroid storm may rarely occur approximately 10 to 14 days after the administration of large doses of iodine 131 in patients with large goiters who have not been adequately pretreated with PTU or MMI to deplete the gland of stored thyroxine (T_4) and triiodothyronine (T_3) [8]. Beta-blockers are used to decrease symptoms of excess thyroid hormone release, but *may not* prevent thyroid storm.

CLINICAL MANIFESTATIONS

There is no absolute level of circulating thyroid hormones indicative of thyroid storm, and the diagnosis is made on a clinical basis [3]. Patients with thyroid storm are almost always febrile (temperature usually higher than 100°F) and have rapid sinus tachycardia and tachyarrhythmias (especially atrial fibrillation in elderly patients) out of proportion to the degree of fever that can frequently result in congestive heart failure. Patients are often agitated, delirious, and tremulous, with hot, flushed skin due to vasodilation. The skin may be moist or dry, depending on the state of hydration. Diarrhea occurs frequently and contributes to dehydration and hypovolemia. Vascular collapse and shock, which are poor prognostic signs, may occur in these patients. Hepatomegaly with abnormal liver enzymes and splenomegaly can be present; jaundice portends a poor prognosis.

Most patients display the classic signs of thyrotoxic Graves' disease, including ophthalmopathy, or toxic uninodular or multinodular goiter. However, in elderly patients, apathy, severe myopathy, profound weight loss, and congestive heart failure may be the predominant findings. As thyroid storm progresses, coma, hypotension, vascular collapse, and death may ensue unless active therapy is instituted.

DIAGNOSIS AND DIFFERENTIAL DIAGNOSIS

The diagnosis of thyroid storm is made on clinical grounds. Thyroid function tests do not differentiate between severe thyrotoxicosis and thyroid storm. Serum T_4 concentrations are usually similar, although it has been suggested that the serum-free T_4 concentration is significantly higher in patients with thyroid storm [2], which might partially explain their more severe symptoms. On the other hand, the serum T_3 concentrations are not higher and in fact may be less elevated or even normal in these patients when the precipitating cause is an intercurrent illness or surgery because peripheral T_3 production from T_4 is markedly impaired in a wide variety of acute and chronic systemic illnesses. Liver function tests are frequently abnormal, especially in elderly patients with congestive heart failure. Elevations in total and free serum calcium concentrations may occur.

The differential diagnosis for a patient presenting with hyperpyrexia, delirium, and tachycardia includes severe infection, malignant hyperthermia [9], neuroleptic malignant syndrome, and acute mania with lethal catatonia. Thyroid storm can be distinguished from these disorders clinically by a history of thyroid disease, thyroid hormone, or iodine ingestion and the presence on physical examination of a goiter or the stigmata of Graves' disease, including ophthalmopathy, onycholysis, and pretibial myxedema. However, any of the disorders mentioned in the differential diagnosis can coexist with thyroid storm since they may precipitate decompensation in a patient with preexisting hyperthyroidism.

TREATMENT

Treatment of thyroid storm is directed toward therapy of the underlying illness, supportive care, blocking peripheral effects of thyroid hormone, and inhibition of thyroid hormone synthesis and release (Table 102.1).

Underlying Illness

Nonthyroidal illness and surgery in previously undiagnosed or only partially treated patients with hyperthyroidism are the most common causes of thyroid storm. Thus, the precipitating disease should be vigorously treated. Cardiac arrhythmias and congestive heart failure require approximately twice the dose of digoxin needed in euthyroid patients, and refractory arrhythmias should alert the physician to the presence of thyrotoxicosis. Patients may also be refractory to heparin and insulin, with higher doses required. It is evident that these patients must receive adequate antibiotic therapy; careful fluid, electrolyte, and vitamin supplementation; vigorous pulmonary therapy; and careful pre- and postoperative care. If emergency surgery is required in a thyrotoxic patient, propranolol, PTU or MMI, iodides, and perhaps corticosteroids should be given before, during, and after surgery.

Supportive Care

A cooling blanket can be used if the temperature rises above 101°F, but the shivering response should be decreased by using drugs that block the central thermoregulatory centers, such as chlorpromazine or meperidine, 25 to 50 mg every 4 to 6 hours. Antipyretics other than salicylates may also be given because salicylates displace thyroid hormones from serum-binding proteins and can increase the free hormone concentrations [10]. Dehydration is frequently present and should be treated while monitoring for congestive heart failure.

Blockade of Peripheral Effects of Thyroid Hormone

Many of the clinical manifestations of hyperthyroidism can be alleviated by the administration of drugs that deplete or block the peripheral action of the catecholamines. Beta-adrenergic blocking agents are currently the drugs of choice in alleviating the catecholamine-dependent signs and symptoms of thyrotoxicosis and thyroid storm. The widest experience has been achieved with propranolol, which also has the advantage of decreasing T_4 to T_3 conversion (see later). Tachycardia and tremors can be improved within minutes of intravenous administration. Oral doses in the range of 60 to 120 mg every 6 hours may be required [11].

Because propranolol may be contraindicated in patients with congestive heart failure, it is frequently debated whether to use beta-blockers in patients with severe thyrotoxicosis or thyroid storm. However, tachycardia and tachyarrhythmias are major contributing factors to the congestive failure in many of these patients, so beta-blockers may be used cautiously along with digoxin and other cardiotropic drugs and diuretics. Rarely, hypotension and cardiac arrest occur after intravenous administration of beta-blockers in patients with severe congestive failure and severe thyrotoxicosis [12]. In patients with asthma, the more selective beta$_1$-blocking drugs, such as metoprolol and atenolol, may be used with less risk. A short-acting beta$_1$-blocker, esmolol [13], and diltiazem can also be used to control the tachyarrhythmias associated with thyrotoxicosis [14].

TABLE 102.1

TREATMENT OF THYROID STORM

Therapy of underlying intercurrent illness	
Digoxin, diuretics, antibiotics, IV fluid supplemented with B-complex vitamins, and insulin for diabetic ketoacidosis	
Supportive care	
Cooling blanket, antipyretics (*not* aspirin), or both for hyperpyrexia	
Block peripheral effects of thyroid hormone	
β-Adrenergic blocking drugs	
Propranolol ($beta_1$- and $beta_2$-blocker)	1 mg IV/min for a total of 2–10 mg 40–120 mg PO q4–6h
Metoprolol ($beta_1$-blocker)	100–400 mg PO q12h
Atenolol ($beta_1$-blocker)	50–100 mg PO daily
Esmolol ($beta_1$-blocker)	500 μg/kg over 1 min, then 50–100 μg/kg/min
Deplete catecholamines	
Reserpine	Test dose of 0.25 mg IM, then initial dose of 1–5 mg 1.0–2.5 mg IM q4–6h
Guanethidine	1–2 mg/kg PO q4–6h
Inhibition of synthesis of thyroid hormones	
Propylthiouracil (PTU)	~ 800mg PO stat and 200–300 mg q8h 600 mg in 90 mL of water by rectum as a retention enema, followed by 250 mg q4h
Methimazole (MMI)	~ 80mg PO stat and 40 mg PO q12h 40 mg dissolved in aqueous solution by rectum q6h
Block release of thyroid hormone from thyroid gland	
Saturated solution of potassium iodide	5 drops PO q8h
Lugol's solution	10 drops PO q8h
Lithium	300 mg q6h, adjust to serum lithium level ~1 mEq/L
Inhibition of peripheral 5′-monodeiodination of thyroxine (T_4) to triiodothyronine (T_3)	
Corticosteroids	Equivalent to 300–400 mg hydrocortisone daily, especially dexamethasone, 2 mg q6h
Propranolol, metoprolol, atenolol, and possibly esmolol	
Propylthiouracil	
Remove thyroid hormones from the circulation	
Plasmapheresis	
Charcoal hemoperfusion	
Cholestyramine	4 g PO q6h

IM, intramuscularly; IV, intravenous; PO, oral.

Inhibition of Thyroid Hormone Synthesis

The antithyroid drugs, PTU and MMI, are potent inhibitors of the synthesis of both T_4 and T_3. Although the onset of action is rapid, PTU and MMI only partially block thyroid hormone synthesis. Weeks are required to deplete the thyroid of stored hormone and observe clinical effects of these drugs. Intravenous MMI is available in Europe, but in the United States, administration by either nasogastric tube or by rectum may be used [15]. PTU has the added advantage of partially blocking the peripheral conversion of T_4 to T_3 and therefore may be the drug of choice. These drugs are not effective if thyroid storm is due to excess ingestion of thyroid hormone (see the section Thyrotoxicosis Factitia) or painful or silent thyroiditis because they affect the synthesis of thyroid hormone and do not affect its release or peripheral activity.

Blockade of Thyroid Hormone Release

Iodide administration plays a major role in the treatment of thyroid storm because of its rapid inhibition of thyroid hormone release from the gland [16]. This effect occurs almost immediately after oral or intravenous administration. Some inhibition of hormone synthesis may also occur in the hyperfunctioning gland. As with PTU and MMI, iodide therapy is not useful in thyroid storm caused by ingestion of excess amounts of thyroid hormone (thyrotoxicosis factitia) because it affects the synthesis and release of endogenously synthesized thyroid hormone.

Lugol's solution or saturated solution of potassium iodide can be given orally or as a potassium iodide enema, 1 g in 60 mL of water, followed by 500 mg of potassium iodide in 20 mL of water every 6 hours, given rectally in a patient who is unable to receive oral medication. Iodide therapy results in dramatic improvement and should be maintained until the serum T_4 and T_3 concentrations are normal or near-normal. However, iodides can exacerbate hyperthyroidism if the patient is not pretreated with PTU or MMI and also delay the option of radioactive iodine for subsequent, definitive treatment. Escape from the iodide effect often occurs when PTU or MMI is not concomitantly used [17]. In patients allergic to iodine, lithium has been used to inhibit thyroid hormone release and partially inhibit thyroid hormone synthesis [18].

Inhibition of Peripheral Generation of Triiodothyronine

It is generally believed that the major bioactive hormone is T_3, that the major source of circulating T_3 is derived from T_4, and that most, if not all, of the metabolic effects of T_4 result from the intracellular generation of T_3 from T_4. A variety of drugs impair the outer-ring monodeiodination of T_4 to T_3, thus decreasing the peripheral generation of T_3. Propranolol, some selective beta$_1$-blocking drugs [19], and PTU are relatively weak inhibitors of T_4 to T_3 conversion. The corticosteroids, especially dexamethasone, are potent inhibitors when administered in high doses and also have an inhibitory effect on thyroid hormone hypersecretion. Their importance in treating thyroid storm has been well documented; the survival rate in thyroid storm was improved when corticosteroids were added to the treatment regimen. Because relative adrenal insufficiency may be present in patients with thyroid storm, glucocorticoid therapy would also correct this possibility. Indeed, combination therapy of severe hyperthyroidism with PTU, iodides, and dexamethasone has resulted in a marked reduction of serum T_3 concentration within 24 hours.

The gallbladder dyes, iopanoic acid (Telepaque) and ipodate (Oragrafin), are potent inhibitors of T_4 to T_3 conversion, but are no longer available in the United States. Similarly, amiodarone also decreases T_3 levels. In addition, it is rich in iodine, and may also block entrance of T_4 into the cell. Although this drug has been used in the short-term (2 weeks) treatment of thyrotoxicosis, it should not be used in the treatment of thyroid storm because its long half-life and high iodide content can cause persistent, severe hyperthyroidism [20].

Removal of Thyroid Hormone from the Circulation

Direct removal of thyroid hormone from the circulation is occasionally required in patients who do not respond to conventional medical treatment. There are case reports of successful use of plasmapheresis [21] and charcoal plasma perfusion [22]. Cholestyramine, which binds T_3 and T_4 in the gut and decreases serum T_3 and T_4 concentrations by increasing the fecal excretion of these hormones [23], may also be useful, particularly if used early in a patient with an overdose.

Thyrotoxicosis Factitia

The inadvertent ingestion of excess amounts of thyroid hormone most commonly occurs in children, although adults may also ingest excess hormone for weight reduction or as a suicide attempt [6,7,24]. Gastric lavage or emesis induction should be performed as soon as possible after ingestion. Occasionally, oral charcoal administration can be useful. As previously mentioned, this form of thyrotoxicosis is not due to endogenous production of thyroid hormone; therefore, drugs that inhibit the synthesis of T_4 and T_3 or those that block thyroid hormone release are not helpful. Therapy should focus on preventing the peripheral effects of excessive thyroid hormone with β-adrenergic blocking drugs and possibly high-dose corticosteroids Cholestyramine may also be useful to decrease serum thyroid hormone levels, as above.

CONCLUSIONS

It is evident that each patient must be treated individually and that a set protocol cannot be advised for all patients. Specific therapy should be directed toward inhibiting the synthesis and release of T_4 and T_3 from the thyroid, blocking the peripheral conversion of T_4 to T_3, relieving the catecholamine-mediated effects by β-adrenergic blockade, and treating the possibility of decreased adrenal reserve with corticosteroids. Associated and precipitating diseases should, of course, be vigorously treated. Iodine often works quickly to improve thyroid hormone levels, but will delay the use of radioactive iodine treatment of hyperthyroidism and thus should be saved for patients with thyroid storm, not just severe thyrotoxicosis.

References

1. Abend SL, Braverman LE: Acute thyroid disorders, in May HL (ed): *Emergency Medicine*. 2nd ed. Boston, Little, Brown and Company, 1992, p 1274.
2. Brooks MH, Waldstein SS: Free thyroxine concentration in thyroid storm. *Ann Intern Med* 93:694, 1980.
3. Burch HB, Wartofsky L: Life-threatening thyrotoxicosis. Thyroid storm. *Endocrinol Metab Clin North Am* 22:263, 1993.
4. Diaz R, Blakey MD, Murphy PB, et al: Thyroid storm after intensity-modulated radiation therapy: a case report and discussion. *Oncologist* 14:233, 2009.
5. Wilson BE, Hobbs WN: Case report: pseudoephedrine-associated thyroid storm: thyroid hormone-catecholamine interactions. *Am Med Sci* 306:317, 1993.
6. Bhasin S, Wallace W, Lawrence JB, et al: Sudden death associated with thyroid hormone abuse. *Am J Med* 71:887, 1981.
7. Hartung B, Schott M, Daldrup T, et al: Lethal thyroid storm after uncontrolled intake of liothyronine in order to lose weight. *Int J Legal Med* 124(6):637–640, 2010.
8. Kadmon PM, Noto RB, Boney CM, et al: Thyroid storm in a child following radioactive iodine (RAI) therapy: a consequence of RAI versus withdrawal of antithyroid medication. *J Clin Endocrinol Metab* 86:1865, 2001.
9. Nishiyama K, Kitahara A, Natsume H, et al: Malignant hyperthermia in a patient with Graves' disease during subtotal thyroidectomy. *Endocr J* 48:227, 2001.
10. Larsen PR: Salicylate-induced increases in free triiodothyronine in human serum. *J Clin Invest* 51:1125, 1972.
11. Ringel MD: Management of hypothyroidism and hyperthyroidism in the intensive care unit. *Crit Care Clin* 17:59, 2001.
12. Dalan R, Leow MK: Cardiovascular collapse associated with beta blockade in thyroid storm. *Exp Clin Endocrinol Diabetes* 115(6):392–396, 2007.
13. Vijayakumar HR, Thomas WO, Ferrara JJ: Peri-operative management of severe thyrotoxicosis with esmolol. *Anaesthesia* 44:406, 1989.
14. Roti E, Montermini M, Roti S, et al: The effect of diltiazem, a calcium channel-blocking drug, on cardiac rate and rhythm in hyperthyroid patients. *Arch Intern Med* 148:1919, 1988.
15. Jongjaroenprasert W, Akarawut W, Chantasart D, et al: Rectal administration of propylthiouracil in hyperthyroid patients: comparison of suspension enema and suppository form. *Thyroid* 12:627, 2002.
16. Wartofsky L, Ransil BJ, Ingbar SH: Inhibition by iodine of the release of thyroxine from the thyroid glands of patients with thyrotoxicosis. *J Clin Invest* 49:78, 1970.
17. Emerson CH, Anderson AJ, Howard WJ, et al: Serum thyroxine and triiodothyronine concentrations during iodide treatment of hyperthyroidism. *J Clin Endocrinol Metab* 40:33, 1975.
18. Nayak B, Burman K: Thyrotoxicosis and thyroid storm. *Endocrinol Metab Clin North Am* 35:663, 2006.
19. Perrild H, Hansen JM, Skovsted L, et al: Different effects of propranolol, alprenolol, sotalol, atenolol and metoprolol on serum T_3 and serum rT_3 in hyperthyroidism. *Clin Endocrinol* 18:139, 1983.
20. Bogazzi F, Bartalena L, Martino E: Approach to the patient with amiodarone-induced thyrotoxicosis. *J Clin Endocrinol Metab* 95:2529, 2010.
21. Vyas A, Vyas P, Vijayakrishnan R, et al: Successful treatment of thyroid storm with plasmapheresis in methimazole-induced agranulocytosis. *Endocr Pract* 16:673, 2010.
22. Kreisner E, Lutzky M, Gross JL. Charcoal hemoperfusion in the treatment of levothyroxine intoxication. *Thyroid* 20:209, 2010.
23. Solomon B, Wartofsky L, Burman KD: Adjunctive cholestyramine therapy for thyrotoxicosis. *Clin Endocrinol (Oxf)* 38:39, 1993.
24. Cohen JH III, Ingbar SH, Braverman LE: Thyrotoxicosis due to ingestion of excess thyroid hormone. *Endocr Rev* 10:113, 1989.

CHAPTER 103 ■ MYXEDEMA COMA

MIRA SOFIA TORRES AND CHARLES H. EMERSON

Myxedema coma is a syndrome that occurs in advanced untreated hypothyroidism [1–5]. It is defined by a group of characteristic clinical features and not by laboratory evidence of severe hypothyroidism (Table 103.1). Myxedema coma is generally preceded by increasingly severe signs and symptoms of thyroid insufficiency. Fortunately, it is quite rare. Hypothyroid patients who are neglectful or whose contact with family and friends is limited are most vulnerable. Despite early and intensive treatment, mortality from myxedema coma is still as high as 30% to 50% [2,4,6–8].

ETIOLOGY AND PATHOPHYSIOLOGY

By definition, myxedema coma does not occur in the absence of hypothyroidism. If hypothyroidism is due to hypothalamic or pituitary insufficiency, the condition is even more serious because it is also accompanied by adrenal failure. Pituitary tumors are the major cause of central hypothyroidism in the United States. In countries with poor access to health care, postpartum pituitary necrosis is quite prevalent and is therefore another important cause of secondary hypothyroidism.

More than 95% of patients with hypothyroidism have primary thyroid disease. Most patients with primary hypothyroidism have either autoimmune thyroid failure or hypothyroidism secondary to ablative procedures on the thyroid. These include radioactive iodine and surgery for hyperthyroidism, thyroid resection for thyroid cancer, and external thyroid irradiation for head and neck tumors. Certain drugs, such as lithium carbonate and amiodarone, can cause hypothyroidism but are only rarely associated with myxedema coma.

Myxedema coma is distinguished from uncomplicated hypothyroidism by a variety of features that relate to central nervous system (CNS) dysfunction. The pathophysiology of myxedema coma will become clearer when there is a better understanding of the effects of thyroid hormone on the brain. Narcotics and hypnotics should be used with caution in hypothyroid patients because these patients are very sensitive to their sedative effects. These agents, alone or in combination with other factors, may precipitate myxedema coma in hypothyroid patients. Other precipitating factors are trauma, surgery, and severe infection [1–9]. The most important factor in temperate climates, however, is cold stress. In one series, 9 of 11 patients with myxedema coma were admitted in the late fall or winter [2].

TABLE 103.1

CLINICAL FEATURES OF MYXEDEMA COMA

Mental obtundation
Course, dry skin
Myxedema facies
Hypothermia
Hypoglycemia
Bradycardia and hypotension
Electrocardiographic changes
Atonic gastrointestinal tract
Atonic bladder
Pleural, pericardial, and peritoneal effusions

CLINICAL MANIFESTATIONS

Patients are partially or completely obtunded. Therefore, the history must often be obtained from other sources. Friends, relatives, and acquaintances might have noted increasing lethargy, complaints of cold intolerance, and changes in the voice. An outdated container of L-thyroxine discovered with the patient's belongings suggests that he or she has been remiss in taking medication. The medical record may also indicate that the patient was taking thyroid hormone or may refer to previous treatment with radioactive iodine. A thyroidectomy scar suggests the possibility of hypothyroidism. Other than coma itself, the cardinal manifestations are hypothermia and hypotension. Hypotonia of the gastrointestinal tract is common and often so severe as to suggest an obstructive lesion. Urinary retention due to a hypotonic bladder is related but less frequent. Most patients have the physical features of severe hypothyroidism, including bradycardia and slow relaxation of the deep tendon reflexes. A myxedematous facies (Fig. 103.1) results from the dry puffy skin, pallor, hypercarotenemia, periorbital edema, and patchy hair loss.

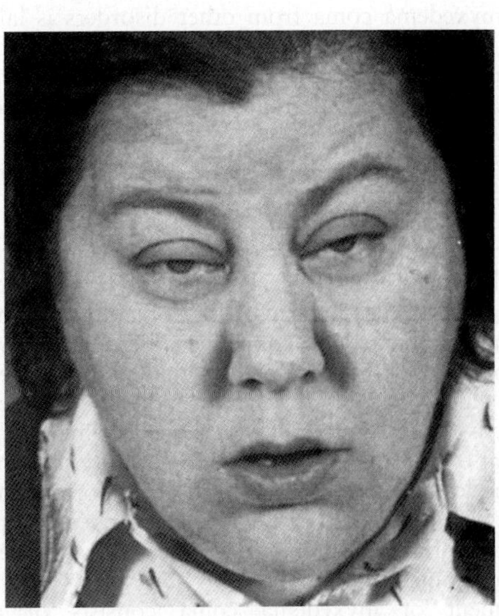

FIGURE 103.1. Characteristic facies of severe hypothyroidism. Note the facial and periorbital puffiness and the dull, lethargic expression.

DIAGNOSIS AND DIFFERENTIAL DIAGNOSIS

The diagnosis of myxedema coma is based on the presence of the characteristic clinical syndrome in a patient with hypothyroidism. The laboratory's role is to confirm that the patient is hypothyroid and determine whether there are treatable complications of myxedema coma, such as hypoventilation, hypoglycemia, and hyponatremia. Because of the gravity of hypothyroidism, treatment must be instituted before laboratory tests confirm the diagnosis.

The diagnostic laboratory features of primary hypothyroidism are a subnormal serum-free thyroxine index or serum-free thyroxine (T_4) concentration and an elevated serum thyroid-stimulating hormone (TSH) concentration. The serum-free thyroxine index is also low in severely ill patients with a wide variety of conditions. This is the so-called "sick euthyroid syndrome" or nonthyroidal illness. Unlike patients with myxedema coma, however, serum TSH concentrations are not elevated in patients with the sick euthyroid syndrome, except in a small percentage, and only as they are clearly recovering from their severe illness. Distinction between hypothyroidism secondary to pituitary or hypothalamic disease (i.e., central hypothyroidism) and the sick euthyroid syndrome is difficult because serum TSH concentrations are low or, when TSH bioactivity is reduced as in secondary hypothyroidism, only mildly elevated in patients with central hypothyroidism. It is important to measure TSH as well as the serum-free thyroxine or free thyroxine index in patients presenting with myxedema coma. In central hypothyroidism, the typical clinical presentation of the myxedematous patient would help establish the diagnosis. The sick euthyroid syndrome is discussed in Chapter 107. The measurement of the total serum triiodothyronine (T_3) concentration is of no value in the diagnosis of hypothyroidism or myxedema coma. It lacks sensitivity in the diagnosis of hypothyroidism and is depressed not only by illness but also by fasting.

Alone, few of the signs and symptoms described in this chapter are unique to myxedema coma. For example, the differential diagnosis of hypothermia (see Chapter 65) includes numerous conditions, such as protein-calorie malnutrition, sepsis, hypoglycemia, and exposure to certain drugs and toxins [10]. Hypotension and hypoventilation, other cardinal features of myxedema coma, occur in other disease states. What distinguishes myxedema coma from other disorders is laboratory evidence of hypothyroidism, characteristic myxedema facies with periorbital puffiness, skin changes, obtundation, and, frequently, a constellation of other physical signs characteristic of severe hypothyroidism.

TREATMENT

As noted earlier, in most patients with myxedema coma, hypothyroidism is due to primary thyroid disease. The initial management of myxedema coma due either to primary thyroid disease or central (pituitary or hypothalamic) disease is similar, since glucocorticoids are recommended in all patients. The only proviso is that in patients with central hypothyroidism, additional evaluation of the CNS for the presence of space-occupying lesions may be warranted. Therefore, the management team must be alert for evidence of space-occupying lesions within or in the region of the pituitary in all patients with myxedema coma.

Treatment of myxedema coma consists of management of hypoglycemia, respiratory depression, hyponatremia, hypothermia, hypotension, and administration of thyroid hormone (Table 103.2). All patients require continuous monitoring of the electrocardiogram and an intravenous line to administer fluids and drugs. Baseline thyroid function tests, serum cortisol, complete blood count, blood urea nitrogen, creatinine, plasma glucose, and electrolytes are mandatory. Pneumonia commonly develops or may be the precipitating factor and must be treated promptly (see Chapter 68). Hypothyroidism and myxedema coma are also associated with hemostatic abnormalities, particularly capillary bleeding and cerebral hemorrhage. Although bleeding should be anticipated in many patients, few strategies have evolved to counter this disorder.

TABLE 103.2

TREATMENT OF MYXEDEMA COMA

Assisted ventilation for hypoventilation
Intravenous glucose for hypoglycemia
Water restriction or hypertonic saline for severe hyponatremia
Passive rewarming for hypothermia
Administration of T_4 or T_3 IV[a]
Administration of hydrocortisone[a]
Treatment of underlying infection and other illnesses, if present
Avoidance of all sedatives, hypnotics, and narcotics

IV, intravenously; T_3, triiodothyronine; T_4, thyroxine.
[a]Dosage must be individualized (see text).

Hypoglycemia

Because hypoglycemia is not unusual in myxedema coma, 50 mL of 50% glucose should immediately be administered intravenously to avoid any delay in confirming the presence of this complication. Chapter 106 details the management of hypoglycemia.

Hypoventilation

Respiratory center depression is common in severe hypothyroidism and myxedema coma. Arterial blood gases should be routinely obtained, therefore, to rule out hypoventilation. If respiratory center depression is clinically obvious, assisted ventilation with oxygen supplementation must be started without delay, taking care not to correct chronic hypercapnia too rapidly (see Chapter 62).

Hyponatremia

Hyponatremia, which results from impaired free water clearance, is most deleterious to CNS function when it develops rapidly. Although hyponatremia is present in some patients, it is usually not the cause of coma because its onset is likely to be gradual. A limiting factor is that water intake decreases as myxedema coma develops, offsetting the tendency toward hyponatremia. Treatment consists of restriction of free water. If the serum sodium concentration is less than 110 mEq per L, hypertonic saline and, in some cases, furosemide should be administered (see Chapter 72).

Hypothermia

Hypothermia is one of the hallmarks of myxedema coma. It can be overlooked or its severity underestimated, however, if an out-of-date or poorly calibrated thermometer is used. Regardless of the cause, hypothermia is associated with a decrease in the basal metabolic rate, myocardial irritability, and blood pressure alterations. Blood pressure initially rises and then gradually falls. Changes in the cardiovascular status are accompanied by electrocardiographic changes. First, there is sinus bradycardia, then T wave inversion, and finally the development of a J wave [10]. At core temperatures below 28°C, ventricular fibrillation is a major threat to life. For an in-depth discussion of this complication, see Chapter 65.

Despite its gravity, the management of the hypothermia of myxedema coma differs from the treatment of exposure-induced hypothermia in euthyroid subjects. In myxedema coma, the patient should be kept in a warm room and covered with blankets. Active heating should be avoided because it increases oxygen consumption and promotes peripheral vasodilation and circulatory collapse. Active heating is recommended only for situations of severe hypothermia in which ventricular fibrillation is an immediate threat. In these cases, the rate of rewarming should not exceed 0.5°C per hour and core temperature should be raised to approximately 31°C.

Hypotension

Hypotension is another ominous feature of myxedema coma. Hypothermia and thyroid hormone deficiency per se are the two most important causes of hypotension, but bleeding and, perhaps in some cases, decreased adrenal reserve may also play a role. Because hypothermia itself produces hypotension, some improvement in blood pressure can be expected if passive measures to restore body temperature are successful. Intravenous fluids should be administered carefully as patients undergo rewarming. Anemia is common in hypothyroidism and has a multifactorial basis. In patients in whom anemia is severe or there appears to be active bleeding, a case can be made for transfusion. If this course is chosen, it must be done with great caution because patients with myxedema coma are extremely prone to circulatory collapse. Sympathomimetic vasoconstrictors or drugs intended to increase myocardial contractility, such as isoproterenol or digitalis, have very limited use in myxedema coma. The response to these drugs is poor, and myxedematous patients are very sensitive to their toxic effects.

Glucocorticoid Therapy

Although there is little evidence that hypotension in myxedema coma results from adrenal insufficiency, there are at least theoretic reasons for considering that these patients have decreased adrenal reserve. Furthermore, it is sometimes unclear whether the myxedema coma is due to primary or pituitary-hypothalamic hypothyroidism. Therefore, one of the immediate measures in treating myxedema coma is to administer 300 mg hydrocortisone intravenously in three divided doses during the first 24 hours. Gradually decreasing doses of hydrocortisone should be administered over the next few days, depending on the patient's response. This protocol is recommended even in the absence of hypotension.

Sepsis

Infections, especially pneumonia and urosepsis, are precipitants or comorbidities in up to 80% of patients with myxedema coma, and sepsis is an important cause of death in these patients [2,4,6–8]. Some signs of sepsis such as tachycardia and fever may be absent in the initial presentation of patients with myxedema. A careful evaluation for underlying infections should be conducted in each patient. When suspected, such infections should be treated aggressively. The management of sepsis is discussed in detail in Chapter 159.

Thyroid Hormone

Administration of thyroid hormone is the definitive treatment of myxedema coma and is essential for reversing hypotension, hypothermia, and depressed consciousness. The sensorium may be improved in a few patients when glucose is given or hypoventilation corrected, but deterioration recurs if thyroid hormone is not given. The gastrointestinal absorption of thyroid hormone is often markedly reduced in myxedema coma. Therefore, thyroid hormone must be given by the intravenous route. To ensure proper dosing, synthetic preparations should be used.

There are no large controlled studies of the optimum form of thyroid hormone for myxedema coma or, for that matter, any aspect of the treatment of myxedema coma. Both T_4 and T_3 have been used with varying degrees of success, and each has its theoretic advantages. T_4 is advantageous because most thyroid hormone is secreted in the form of T_4. For this and other reasons, plasma and intracellular T_4 and T_3 profiles are more stable and representative of the normal condition if T_4 rather than T_3 is administered. Conversely, T_3 is advantageous because it has a more rapid onset of action than T_4.

The best doses for treating myxedema coma have not been studied in a rigorous fashion. As is the case when deciding between T_4 and T_3, the choice is not straightforward. In patients with long-standing untreated hypothyroidism, thyroid hormone treatment is usually initiated at low doses. These patients frequently have underlying arteriosclerotic cardiovascular disease, and initial therapy with full replacement doses of thyroid hormone can precipitate angina or myocardial infarction. On the other hand, in near-terminal patients with myxedema coma, the need for thyroid hormone is urgent. In this setting, the blood pressure and body temperature can increase within hours after thyroid hormone is started.

We prefer to use T_4 in all but the most severe cases of myxedema coma. Except in elderly patients, the initial intravenous dose of T_4 should be between 0.2 and 0.5 mg, with the larger doses in this range used for more comatose patients, those with more severe hypotension or hypothermia, and those with large body mass. In the elderly patient or those with a history of heart disease, the initial T_4 dose should probably not exceed 0.4 mg. If there is no improvement in the state of consciousness, blood pressure, or core temperature at first 6 to 12 hours after the initial dose, T_4 should again be administered to bring the total dose during the first 24 hours to 0.5 mg. Thyroid hormone should then be given again 24 hours later and every 24 hours thereafter. After the first 24 hours, the subsequent doses should range from 0.05 to 0.2 mg daily, depending on the clinical response. If the treatment is not maintained, coma may recur. A recent prospective study randomly assigned 11 patients to two groups: one received a loading dose of 0.5 mg of T_4 intravenously followed by a daily maintenance dose of 0.1 mg intravenously ("high-dose" group); the other group received only the maintenance dose of 0.1 mg daily ("low-dose" group). Four of eleven patients died, but only one of them was in the high-dose group. The mortality rate was lower in the high-dose group, but did not reach statistical significance [7]. However, the sample size was small. Based on this information, it was suggested that patients who receive a loading dose fared better than those on less vigorous regimens. A smaller dose in comatose patients is probably indicated in very elderly patients [6], or in patients who are normotensive and euthermic and have another explanation for their comatose state, such as CNS trauma or recent sedative ingestion. Another situation that calls for lower doses is the patient who has had an acute myocardial infarction and whose hypotension appears to be secondary to the myocardial infarction, which is a major contributor to the patient's depressed sensorium. In these cases, ventilatory support should be given and intravenous doses of as little as 0.05 to 0.1 mg of T_4 administered in the first 24 hours. Care must be taken in making the diagnosis of myocardial infarction, however, since creatine kinase-MB activity is increased in the absence of myocardial infarction in a few patients with myxedema coma [11,12].

In the most severe cases of myxedema coma, intravenous T_3 may be a better choice as the initial therapy. If T_3 is used, however, greater caution must be exercised to avoid overstimulation of the cardiovascular system [2] and too rapid an increase in oxygen consumption. It is clear that T_3 has been lifesaving in some patients, but an inverse correlation between survival and calculated plasma T_3 concentrations has actually been reported in myxedema coma [2]. Although doses as high as 0.2 mg of T_3 in the first 24 hours have been used, as little as 0.0025 mg has been reported to increase cardiac output, heart rate, ventricular stroke work, oxygen consumption, and oxygen delivery in myxedema coma [13]. Based on these and other considerations, a reasonable starting dose of T_3 is 0.0125 mg (12.5 μg) given intravenously [1]. This dose should be repeated every 6 hours for the first 48 hours. If there is no apparent response after 15 to 21 hours, as shown by heart rate, blood pressure, and body temperature, the next two doses could be increased to 0.025 mg (25 μg). If, on the other hand, signs of myocardial ischemia develop, the dose should be reduced. Particularly worrisome would be a decrease in blood pressure in the face of an increase in body temperature, suggesting that cardiovascular decompensation is occurring in the face of increased oxygen demands. If there is gradual improvement of metabolic parameters, the T_3 should be tapered and T_4 treatment introduced, starting with doses of 0.05 mg given intravenously every 24 hours. When the patient stabilizes and is fully conscious, T_4 can be given by the oral instead of the intravenous route. T_4 therapy must be closely monitored, however, as T_4 malabsorption can be a serious problem in a variety of clinical settings. If the clinical response to oral T_4 is not maintained or serum T_4 concentrations fall, the patient should be switched back to intravenous T_4 therapy.

Although myxedema coma is associated with a high mortality, many patients survive by using judicious therapy aimed at correcting the secondary metabolic disturbances and reversing the hypothyroid state. This must be done in a sustained but gradual fashion, however, because an effort to correct hypothyroidism too rapidly may completely negate the beneficial effects of the initial treatment.

Pertinent clinical studies of myxedema coma are listed in Table 103.3.

TABLE 103.3

PERTINENT CLINICAL STUDIES OF MYXEDEMA COMA

- Myxedema coma has a high mortality rate and is often the first manifestation of thyroid disease [2,5–8].
- Old age is associated with increased mortality in myxedema coma [2,6].
- Sepsis and infection are important contributors to mortality [2,4,6–8].
- High-dose thyroid hormone treatment has been associated with a worse outcome in myxedema coma. It is not known if this association is due to patients with more severe forms of myxedema coma being treated with higher doses of thyroid hormone [2,6].

References

1. Pereira VG, Haron ES, Lima-Neto N, et al: Management of myxedema coma: report on three successfully treated cases with nasogastric or intravenous administration of triiodothyronine. *J Endocrinol Invest* 5(5):331–334, 1982.
2. Hylander B, Rosenqvist U: Treatment of myxoedema coma—factors associated with fatal outcome. *Acta Endocrinol (Copenh)* 108(1):65–71, 1985.
3. Nicoloff JT, LoPresti JS: Myxedema coma. A form of decompensated hypothyroidism. *Endocrinol Metab Clin North Am* 22(2):279–290, 1993.
4. Jordan RM: Myxedema coma. Pathophysiology, therapy, and factors affecting prognosis. *Med Clin North Am* 79(1):185–194, 1995.
5. Reinhardt W, Mann K: Incidence, clinical picture and treatment of hypothyroid coma. Results of a survey. *Med Klin (Munich)* 92(9):521–524, 1997.
6. Yamamoto T, Fukuyama J, Fujiyoshi A: Factors associated with mortality of myxedema coma: report of eight cases and literature survey. *Thyroid* 9(12):1167–1174, 1999.
7. Rodriguez I, Fluiters E, Perez-Mendez LF, et al: Factors associated with mortality of patients with myxoedema coma: prospective study in 11 cases treated in a single institution. *J Endocrinol* 180(2):347–350, 2004.
8. Dutta P, Bhansali A, Masoodi SR, et al: Predictors of outcome in myxoedema coma: a study from a tertiary care centre. *Crit Care* 12(1):R1, 2008.
9. Ragaller M, Quintel M, Bender HJ, et al: Myxedema coma as a rare postoperative complication. *Anaesthesist* 42(3):179–183, 1993.
10. Reuler JB: Hypothermia: pathophysiology, clinical settings, and management. *Ann Intern Med* 89(4):519–527, 1978.
11. Hickman PE, Silvester W, Musk AA, et al: Cardiac enzyme changes in myxedema coma. *Clin Chem* 33(4):622–624, 1987.
12. Nee PA, Scane AC, Lavelle PH, et al: Hypothermic myxedema coma erroneously diagnosed as myocardial infarction because of increased creatine kinase MB. *Clin Chem* 33(6):1083–1084, 1987.
13. McCulloch W, Price P, Hinds CJ, et al: Effects of low dose oral triiodothyronine in myxoedema coma. *Intensive Care Med* 11(5):259–262, 1985.

CHAPTER 104 ■ HYPOADRENAL CRISIS AND THE STRESS MANAGEMENT OF THE PATIENT ON CHRONIC STEROID THERAPY

NEIL ARONIN

The adrenal glands secrete five types of hormone, but two are critical in the intensive care unit (ICU) setting. Mineralocorticoids (primarily aldosterone) regulate electrolyte balance. Glucocorticoids (primarily cortisol) promote gluconeogenesis and have many other actions. Aldosterone and cortisol are life sustaining; deficiency of either can result in hypoadrenal crisis. The other three types of adrenal hormones (dehydroepiandrosterone and its sulfate, estrone, and catecholamines) do not play a major role in acute care settings.

Hypoadrenal crisis can occur as an acute event in individuals lacking a prior history of adrenal disorders. A high index of suspicion arises in patients who have inadequate responses to initial therapies. Patients treated with glucocorticoids have a heightened risk for inadequate cortisol response to stress. Diagnosis of cortisol deficiency can be elusive; conditions that contribute to ICU admission (e.g., sepsis, acute respiratory failure) might interfere with traditional tests of adrenal function.

The sometime uncertainty in biochemical diagnosis of adrenal hypofunction invokes the use of clinical judgment in starting therapy. Recent studies indicate that varied disease in ICU patients do not allow a unified algorithm of treatment. Because excess cortisol is beset with side effects and exacerbation of illness, it is prudent to have mastery of the normal regulation and actions of aldosterone and cortisol; the strengths and foibles of diagnostic tests of adrenal insufficiency; and the evidence for appropriate, effective, and safe use of glucocorticoids in ICU patients.

ETIOLOGY

The most common cause of primary adrenal failure is Addison's disease, an autoimmune disease that is frequently known before the ICU admission. Addison's disease often coexists with additional autoimmune endocrinopathies, especially Hashimoto's thyroiditis. Other causes of adrenal failure present a difficult diagnosis in the ICU: overwhelming sepsis, hemorrhage secondary to trauma, circulating anticoagulants or anticoagulant therapy, tuberculosis, fungal disease, amyloidosis, acquired immune deficiency syndrome, antiphospholipid syndrome, infarction, irradiation, metastatic disease, and drugs [1–5]. Critical illness can cause or unmask adrenal insufficiency.

The most common cause of secondary adrenal insufficiency is suppression of corticotrophin (adrenocorticotrophic hormone [ACTH]) release by prior glucocorticoid therapy. ACTH regulates the maintenance of cells in the zona fasciculata and the synthesis and release of cortisol from these cells. Glucocorticoid therapy suppresses ACTH, thereby causing involution of the cortisol-producing cells. The anterior pituitary regains its ability to respond to stress before normal adrenal function is restored. There are no cutoffs on duration of glucocorticoid therapy, its route of administration, and its dosage that can cause adrenal cortical atrophy (zona fasciculata) and inadequate cortisol reserve. Adrenal suppression may occur in patients without obvious clinical signs of Cushing's syndrome. Symptoms of withdrawal mimic those of Addison's disease, such as weakness, lethargy, abdominal discomfort, arthralgias, myalgias, and weight loss. After short-term glucocorticoid treatment, symptoms may arise despite an intact hypothalamic-pituitary-adrenal axis by standard tests of adrenal reserve. These findings underscore the widespread and differential action of glucocorticoids in selected patients.

Pituitary dysfunction can also result in cortisol insufficiency, but not aldosterone lack. Noteworthy causes of impaired pituitary function are tumors in the region of the sella turcica and irradiation of the pituitary or hypothalamus.

Actions of Aldosterone and Cortisol

The adrenal cortex secretes aldosterone from the zona glomerulosa and cortisol from the zona fasciculata. Aldosterone promotes the reabsorption of sodium and the secretion of potassium and hydrogen in the renal tubule [6]. This mineralocorticoid is controlled mainly by the renin-angiotensin system; regulation of blood pressure is coordinated in the short term (angiotensin action on a membrane-bound receptor) and in the longer term (aldosterone, nuclear action on gene expression). Glucocorticoid suppression of ACTH, or primary ACTH loss, does not suppress aldosterone in the zona glomerulosa. Glucocorticoids promote gluconeogenesis and protein wasting and increase the secretion of free water by the kidney [7,8]. In large doses, cortisol binds to aldosterone receptors in the kidney, thereby increasing sodium reabsorption and potassium and hydrogen ion excretion. Glucocorticoids act on numerous tissues, including the central nervous system, and affect the sense of well-being, appetite, and mood. They inhibit ACTH release through hypothalamic and pituitary actions. Glucocorticoids have direct effects on the cardiovascular system and maintain blood pressure, although mechanisms are not established. Critical illness and glucocorticoid deficiency affect physiological systems in common.

Excess glucocorticoid therapy causes lymphopenia, leukocytosis, and eosinopenia [9], can lead to osteoporosis and reduction of hypercalcemia [10], and can impair host defenses to infectious diseases. These properties should be considered in the decision to treat ICU patients with glucocorticoids; the decision is not risk free.

Aldosterone deficiency results in sodium wasting, with concomitant loss of water and an increase in renal reabsorption of potassium. A decrease in plasma volume and dehydration occurs, with subsequent increases in blood urea nitrogen and plasma renin activity.

Reduction in circulating levels of cortisol causes a marked increase in circulating levels of ACTH and a corresponding increase in β-lipotropin, from which melanocyte-stimulating hormone activity increases; in longstanding adrenal insufficiency, the skin (especially creases and scars) develops hyperpigmentation [11]. Orthostatic hypotension can progress to frank shock in a crisis. Hypoglycemia and an increase in sensitivity to insulin are commonplace. Hyponatremia is a hallmark of aldosterone deficiency, but may also be found in cortisol deficiency. The mechanism for the latter may invoke increased sensitivity to vasopressin [12–14]; serum potassium levels would be normal.

DIAGNOSIS

Clinical manifestations that suggest adrenal insufficiency include a nonspecific history of progressive weakness, lassitude, fatigue, anorexia, vomiting, and constipation. Patients in adrenal crisis are volume depleted and hypotensive or in frank shock [15–18]. They often have fever and stupor or coma. As a precipitous event (adrenal hemorrhage, overwhelming infection, anticoagulant therapy, trauma, surgery), adrenal crisis lacks hyperpigmentation. Flank pain may be present in adrenal hemorrhage or infection. Severely ill patients are suspected of developing adrenal hypofunction, but actual incidence is not established, a conundrum in making the diagnosis of adrenal crisis. To further complicate recognition of adrenal dysfunction, glucocorticoid resistance has been postulated in critical illness.

In critical illness, the diagnosis of adrenal hypofunction is less apparent than it is in ambulatory medicine. Severe illness can interfere with the adrenal response to ACTH, making difficult interpretation of cortisol reserve and adrenal function. Lack of ACTH shares symptoms of primary glucocorticoid deficiency, in particular hypoglycemia. ACTH deficiency in pituitary disease generally occurs after deficiency in other pituitary hormones; deficits in overall pituitary secretion can lead to signs of other endocrine gland dysfunctions.

In primary adrenal insufficiency, plasma concentrations of cortisol are usually low or in the low normal range. Response to ACTH stimulation is inadequate and is the definitive test for a diagnosis of adrenal hypofunction. After administering 250 μg of cosyntropin (Cortrosyn; synthetic ACTH 1–24) intravenously to the patient, an adequate adrenal response shows a 10 μg increase of cortisol over baseline at 30 or 60 minutes, or a stimulated cortisol level >20 μg per dL.

The altered adrenal response to ACTH in critical illness limits interpretation of standard stimulation tests. Recognition of the complexity of adrenal hypofunction has led to reconsideration of its diagnosis in the ICU. Serum-free cortisol measurement is shown to be more accurate than total serum cortisol in determining cortisol adequacy [19]. ICU patients often have hypoproteinemia. Most circulating cortisol is bound to protein. Changes in protein abundance or dynamics therefore affect interpretation of total cortisol measurements. A serum-free cortisol of <9 μg per dL is sufficient to initiate glucocorticoid replacement [20]. However, measurement of free cortisol is unavailable in most hospitals. A random total cortisol of <10 μg per dL is useful as a threshold for glucocorticoid therapy. It is a practical guideline, but not supported by extensive clinical study. The American College of Critical Care considers this recommendation to be weak with moderate quality of evidence [18]. The concept of situational adrenal insufficiency is an idea inchoate, but a threshold concentration of total cortisol provides a mark for intervention. The term *critical illness-related corticosteroid insufficiency* is preferred in assessing adrenal function in severe illness, because of the uncertainties in diagnosis.

Other diagnostic clues are useful in the diagnosis of adrenal crisis in ICU patients. Computed tomography scan can reveal adrenal hemorrhage or infiltration. Electrolytes vary, but hyponatremia is found in primary adrenal failure with hyperkalemia (sometimes not to a major degree) and in secondary adrenal failure without hyperkalemia. Hypoglycemia, elevated blood urea nitrogen, hypercalcemia, eosinophilia, lymphocytosis, and a normocytic, normochromic anemia are noted.

TREATMENT

The management of the hypoadrenalism has been vetted by a committee of international experts and the American College of Critical Care Medicine [18]. Recommendations have been provided as guidelines for the usefulness of glucocorticoid therapy in hypoadrenal function and critical illness (Fig. 104.1). There is agreement that hypoadrenalism needs to be treated. In critical illness in which primary adrenal function is suspected (e.g., evidence of hemorrhage), a bolus of 100 mg of hydrocortisone should be administered intravenously and then 100 mg over the next 24 hours. The patient ought to receive saline to maintain volume. After the initial therapy and stabilization of the patient, hydrocortisone can be decreased by 50% each day. Maintenance is 20 to 30 mg per day. Fludrocortisone 0.1 mg per day is started at the time of the maintenance glucocorticoid dose.

Dexamethasone can be used in place of initial hydrocortisone therapy if adrenal reserve of cortisol needs to be studied. Saline infusion is necessary with glucocorticoid administration. Fludrocortisone (because its main activity is regulation of gene transcription) does not act quickly; the saline will maintain circulating volume. Hydrocortisone has mineralocorticoid properties; dexamethasone does not.

In patients with functional adrenals, use of glucocorticoids in septic shock or early severe adult respiratory distress syndrome has not been established. A recommendation should be based on strong evidence of at least moderate quality. Few studies have sufficiently large subject groups for proper analysis. Intravenous hydrocortisone (50 mg q6 h) has been indicated in patients with septic shock [21]. A caveat is that the placebo-treated group had an unusually high mortality, which might have skewed the results to favor the treatment group. The study also promoted the use of fludrocortisones, a recommendation that was not explained.

The Corticosteroid Therapy of Septic Shock (CORTICUS) trial showed no effect of glucocorticoid treatment on outcome in shock [22]. Like Annane et al. 2002 [21], in CORTICUS subjects received either hydrocortisone 50 mg q6 h for 5 days or placebo. An important distinction in CORTICUS is that the placebo treatment group yielded a 32% mortality rate whereas glucocorticoid-treated subjects had a 35% mortality rate.

There is no ready explanation for the difference in placebo deaths, 73% in Annane et al. [21] compared with 32% in

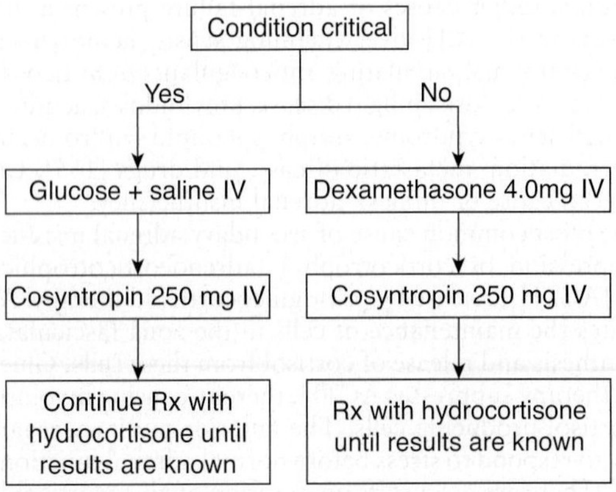

FIGURE 104.1. Management of suspected hypoadrenal crisis. IV, intravenously; Rx, treatment.

CORTICUS, except possibly the severity of shock in test subjects. Both trials were randomized and had seemingly sufficient subjects. Annane et al. [21] enrolled subjects in more severe shock than did the CORTICUS trial and started the glucocorticoid therapy sooner (8 hours vs. 72 hours, respectively). The difference in severity of shock might have accounted for the disparity in placebo mortality. Therefore, the trials do not have comparable study groups. Based on these studies that lack compelling, high-quality data, glucocorticoid therapy would not be expected to be effective in reducing mortality in subjects with less severe shock. In patients with severe shock, the evidence indicates (with caveats) that glucocorticoid therapy is useful if given early in the course of the shock. Rationale for fludrocortisone treatment is unclear and not established.

Studies on the use of mineralocorticoids (fludrocortisone), the rate of tapering of glucocorticoids in treated ICU patients, and duration of the use of glucocorticoids in septic shock and respiratory failure have weak evidence of moderate or low quality. High-dose methylprednisolone (continuous infusion; 1 mg per kg per day) might be useful in acute respiratory distress syndrome, but additional confirmation is needed. Offering definitive recommendations could be misleading in these settings. The compelling evidence, to date, is the use of glucocorticoids early in severe shock, data leading to a weak recommendation based on moderate-quality study.

GLUCOCORTICOID USE IN STRESSED PATIENTS ON GLUCOCORTICOID TREATMENT

General Principles

In healthy subjects, the secretion rate of cortisol increases from 10 mg per day to 50 to 150 mg per day during surgical procedures, but rarely exceeds 200 mg per day [17]. The degree of response depends, in part, on the extent and duration of surgery.

Historically, the withdrawal of chronic glucocorticoid therapy (and adrenal suppression) has been linked to the development of shock. Although in theory glucocorticoid withdrawal could lead to hypotension, documentation is sparse. Shock in the acutely ill or surgical patient on steroid therapy (or within 1 year of withdrawal) should not be attributed solely to decreased adrenal responsiveness. Adrenal glucocorticoids should be administered, but other causes of hypotension should be sought. Suppression of the hypothalamic-pituitary-adrenal axis can occur after only 5 days of glucocorticoid treatment and, after their long-term administration, the adrenal axis may respond inadequately to appropriate stimulation up to 1 year after glucocorticoid withdrawal. To emphasize, adrenal suppression cannot be predicted based on glucocorticoid dosage and duration, or the measurement of normal serum, basal cortisol [23].

Diagnosis and Treatment

Patients with high risk for adrenal suppression took pharmacologic or replacement doses of glucocorticoids for at least 4 weeks or stopped this treatment within the prior year. The cosyntropin test provides an assessment of adrenal cortisol reserve and estimates the adequacy of a stress response. A subnormal response (see earlier) predicts the need for supplemental glucocorticoids. For minor surgical procedures, the patient's usual dose of glucocorticoid is often sufficient, but a single dose of 25 mg hydrocortisone or its equivalent can be given. The glucocorticoid dose should be increased from 50 to 75 mg per day hydrocortisone (or equivalent) for 2 days in surgery of moderate severity and duration and to 150 mg hydrocortisone (or equivalent) for up to 3 days in the most severe surgery. Excessive glucocorticoid dosing can have untoward effects [24]; more is not necessarily better.

Hydrocortisone can be rapidly tapered and the patient returned to the usual dose of glucocorticoid, if needed.

TABLE: SUMMARY OF ADVANCES IN MANAGING HYPOADRENAL CRISIS

- Primary adrenal hypofunction in crisis (glucocorticoid and aldosterone insufficiency) presents with hypotension, fever, volume depletion, and often stupor and coma [13,25].
- The most common cause of secondary adrenal failure is glucocorticoid suppression, which can occur in as few as 5 days after prednisone treatment and last up to 1 year after chronic glucocorticoid withdrawal [26–28].
- Because cortisol is bound to corticosteroid-binding globulin and albumin, which is often reduced in critical care patients, interpretation of the cosyntropin stimulation test should consider the serum albumin concentration [19].
- Supplementation with glucocorticoid and mineralocorticoid improves survival in a subset of critically ill patients (renal failure, hypotension with poor response to pressor agents, lactic acidosis) who have documented inadequate cortisol response to cosyntropin [29].
- In patients with functional adrenals, use of glucocorticoids has not been established with high-quality data. Use of glucocorticoids early in severe shock might be useful [18,21].

References

1. Rusnak RA: Adrenal and pituitary emergencies. *Emerg Med Clin North Am* 7:903–925, 1989.
2. Szalados JE, Vukmir RB: Acute adrenal insufficiency resulting from adrenal hemorrhage as indicated by post-operative hypotension. *Intensive Care Med* 20:216–218, 1994.
3. Vella A, Nippoldt TB, Morris JC III: Adrenal hemorrhage: a 25-year experience at the Mayo Clinic. *Mayo Clin Proc* 76:161–168, 2001.
4. Hofbauer LC, Heufelder AE: Endocrine implications of human immunodeficiency virus infection. *Medicine (Baltimore)* 75:262–278, 1996.
5. Xarli VP, Steele AA, Davis PJ, et al: Adrenal hemorrhage in the adult. *Medicine (Baltimore)* 57:211–221, 1978.
6. Loffing J, Zecevic M, Feraille E, et al: Aldosterone induces rapid apical translocation of ENaC in early portion of renal collecting system: possible role of SGK. *Am J Physiol Renal Physiol* 280:F675–F682, 2001.
7. White PC: Corticosteroid action, in Becker KL (ed): *Principles and Practice of Endocrinology and Metabolism*. Philadelphia, Lippincott Williams & Wilkins, 2001, p 714.
8. Boykin J, DeTorrente A, Erickson A, et al: Role of plasma vasopressin in impaired water excretion of glucocorticoid deficiency. *J Clin Invest* 62:738–744, 1978.
9. Ilfeld DN, Krakauer RS, Blaese RM: Suppression of the human autologous mixed lymphocyte reaction by physiologic concentrations of hydrocortisone. *J Immunol* 119:428–434, 1977.
10. Lukert BP, Raisz LG: Glucocorticoid-induced osteoporosis: pathogenesis and management. *Ann Intern Med* 112:352–364, 1990.
11. Krieger DT, Liotta AS, Brownstein MJ, et al: ACTH, beta-lipotropin, and related peptides in brain, pituitary, and blood. *Recent Prog Horm Res* 36:277–344, 1980.
12. Oelkers W: Hyponatremia and inappropriate secretion of vasopressin (antidiuretic hormone) in patients with hypopituitarism. *N Engl J Med* 321:492–496, 1989.
13. Oelkers W: Adrenal insufficiency. *N Engl J Med* 335:1206–1212, 1996.
14. Papanek PE, Raff H: Chronic physiological increases in cortisol inhibit the vasopressin response to hypertonicity in conscious dogs. *Am J Physiol* 267:R1342–R1349, 1994.

15. Annane D, Bellissant E, Bollaert PE, et al: Corticosteroids in the treatment of severe sepsis and septic shock in adults: a systematic review. *JAMA* 301:2362–2375, 2009.
16. Kehlet H, Binder C: Value of an ACTH test in assessing hypothalamic-pituitary-adrenocortical function in glucocorticoid-treated patients. *Br Med J* 2:147–149, 1973.
17. Lamberts SW, Bruining HA, de Jong FH: Corticosteroid therapy in severe illness. *N Engl J Med* 337:1285–1292, 1997.
18. Marik PE, Pastores SM, Annane D, et al: Recommendations for the diagnosis and management of corticosteroid insufficiency in critically ill adult patients: consensus statements from an international task force by the American College of Critical Care Medicine. *Crit Care Med* 36:1937–1949, 2008.
19. Hamrahian AH, Oseni TS, Arafah BM: Measurements of serum free cortisol in critically ill patients. *N Engl J Med* 350:1629–1638, 2004.
20. Siraux V, De Backer D, Yalavatti G, et al: Relative adrenal insufficiency in patients with septic shock: comparison of low-dose and conventional corticotropin tests. *Crit Care Med* 33:2479–2486, 2005.
21. Annane D, Sebille V, Charpentier C, et al: Effect of treatment with low doses of hydrocortisone and fludrocortisone on mortality in patients with septic shock. *JAMA* 288:862–871, 2002.
22. Sprung CL, Annane D, Keh D, et al: Hydrocortisone therapy for patients with septic shock. *N England J Med* 358:111–124, 2008.
23. Henzen C, Suter A, Lerch E, et al: Suppression and recovery of adrenal response after short-term, high-dose glucocorticoid treatment. *Lancet* 355:542–545, 2000.
24. Udelsman R, Ramp J, Gallucci WT, et al: Adaptation during surgical stress. A reevaluation of the role of glucocorticoids. *J Clin Invest* 77:1377–1381, 1986.
25. Malchoff CD, Carey RM: Adrenal insufficiency. *Curr Ther Endocrinol Metab* 6:142–147, 1997.
26. Streck WF, Lockwood DH: Pituitary adrenal recovery following short-term suppression with corticosteroids. *Am J Med* 66:910–914, 1979.
27. Graber AL, Ney RL, Nicholson WE, et al: Natural history of pituitary-adrenal recovery following long-term suppression with corticosteroids. *J Clin Endocrinol Metab* 25:11–16, 1965.
28. Schlaghecke R, Kornely E, Santen RT, et al: The effect of long-term glucocorticoid therapy on pituitary-adrenal responses to exogenous corticotropin-releasing hormone. *N Engl J Med* 326:226–230, 1992.
29. Loriaux L: Glucocorticoid therapy in the intensive care unit. *N Engl J Med* 350:1601–1602, 2004.

CHAPTER 105 ■ DISORDERS OF MINERAL METABOLISM

SETH M. ARUM AND DANIEL T. BARAN

Disorders of mineral metabolism, although common, are rarely the primary cause of admission to an intensive care unit (ICU). However, these disorders frequently exacerbate life-threatening medical situations. Calcium, magnesium, and phosphorus are the main, clinically relevant minerals that can have an important impact on general health and on the course of a critical care admission. Calcium ions regulate membrane potentials, the coagulation cascade, neurotransmitter release, hormone-receptor interactions, and intercellular communication through channels and ion exchange. Magnesium is necessary for parathyroid hormone (PTH) secretion and maintenance of serum calcium, neuromuscular function, and membrane sodium-potassium adenosine triphosphatase (ATPase) activity. Phosphate, the major intracellular anion, is also instrumental for normal cellular function. It is a component of nucleic acids, phospholipids, and high-energy nucleotides and is necessary to facilitate oxygen delivery to cells. Phosphorus can also bind calcium in the body, and thus phosphorus metabolism is related to calcium and magnesium homeostasis. Therefore, symptoms of abnormal phosphorus metabolism often reflect the abnormalities in circulating calcium and magnesium. Calcium, magnesium, and phosphate balance are controlled through the interactions of PTH, 1α, 25-dihydroxyvitamin D (1,25 D), and calcitonin (CT).

CALCIUM DISORDERS

Calcium Physiology

Ninety-nine percent of total body calcium is stored in bone, whereas less than 1% is located in extracellular fluids. The calcium found in the extracellular fluids is either free (40%) or bound to albumin or other anions (60%) [1]. It is the free ionized calcium that is biologically active. Acid-base balance affects the binding of calcium to albumin. Hyperventilation, and the resultant respiratory alkalosis, enhances the binding of calcium to albumin, thereby acutely decreasing the ionized calcium and causing symptoms of hypocalcemia despite unchanged levels of total calcium. Similarly, changes in serum protein levels affect total serum calcium. The measured total calcium level in the serum can be corrected to account for changes in serum proteins by using the following formula:

$$\text{Corrected total calcium (mg/dL)} = \text{measured total calcium (mg/dL)} + (0.8 \times [4 - \text{measured albumin (g/dL)}])$$

Although the formula takes into account changes in serum proteins, it does not consider the impact of alterations in pH which frequently occur during acute illness. Measuring the ionized calcium directly is another option which should not be affected by either the serum proteins or the pH.

Calcium homeostasis is a function of absorption from the intestine (primarily the small intestine by active transport and facilitated diffusion), bone resorption/formation, and urinary excretion. The average diet contains 500 to 1,500 mg of calcium per day. In young individuals, the efficiency of intestinal absorption varies inversely with the amount of calcium ingested. Approximately 300 mg of calcium is exchanged daily between plasma and bone. Serum calcium is in equilibrium with intracellular calcium and calcium in bone and is filtered through the kidney. Urinary calcium excretion (normally 100 to 300 mg of calcium per day) depends on the glomerular filtration rate and the tubular sodium resorption. Loop diuretics enhance urinary calcium excretion in conjunction with their effect on sodium excretion. It is this property that serves as a useful adjunct to lower elevated serum calcium levels in the hydrated patient.

Hormonal Regulation of Calcium

Calcium absorption, excretion, and bone resorption/formation are in large part regulated by three hormones: PTH, 1,25 D, and CT.

Parathyroid Hormone

PTH is an 84-amino acid polypeptide produced and secreted by the chief cells of the parathyroid gland [1]. Secretion of PTH is stimulated by low levels of calcium in the cytoplasm of the parathyroid chief cells. The rapid release of PTH in response to hypocalcemia is essential for calcium homeostasis. The target organs for PTH are bone and kidneys. Chronic PTH secretion stimulates osteoclasts. This results in bone resorption and dissolution of hydroxyapatite crystals, resulting in the release of calcium and phosphate. This effect is augmented in the presence of 1,25 D. The renal effects of PTH include decreased proximal tubular reabsorption of phosphate (phosphate wasting), enhanced distal tubular calcium reabsorption (calcium retention), and increased renal mitochondrial 1α-hydroxylase activity (enhanced 1,25 D production). It is through the increased production of 1,25 D that PTH indirectly increases intestinal absorption of calcium.

Magnesium is mandatory for PTH secretion and end-organ response. Studies have shown that hypomagnesemia impairs PTH secretion and the renal response to PTH administration. Much of this seems reversible with magnesium repletion [2]. Clinically, correction of the hypocalcemia can often only be achieved after correcting the hypomagnesemia.

PTH can have both anabolic and catabolic effects on bone. Anabolic effects occur with intermittent administration of low-dose PTH [3]. In fact, daily subcutaneous injections of PTH derivatives have been shown to increase bone density and decrease fracture risk in various populations [4,5]. The catabolic, bone-resorptive effects of chronic PTH secretion are likely mediated through its effects on osteoprotegerin (OPG) and receptor activator of nuclear factor kappa ligand (RANK-ligand), resulting in increased osteoclast maturation and activity. Intermittent administration of PTH does not impact the OPG/RANK-ligand system as it does with constant administration, likely explaining the differing effects on bone mass [6].

Vitamin D

Vitamin D is a steroid hormone that is essential for calcium balance and is also likely important in numerous other cellular functions [7]. Activation of vitamin D requires 25-hydroxylation in the liver and 1-hydroxylation in the kidney to form the active hormone 1,25 D. Negative feedback is exerted by 1,25 D on its own production by suppressing 1-hydroxylase activity and stimulating the enzyme 24-hydroxylase to produce the biologically inactive steroids 24,25$(OH)_2$D and 1,24,25 $(OH)_3$D [8].

The effects of 1,25 D are exerted through interactions with nuclear receptors located in a variety of cells, including enterocytes, parathyroid chief cells, osteoblasts, and renal tubular cells. 1,25 D increases intestinal absorption of calcium and phosphate. It has also been shown to suppress PTH gene expression as a negative feedback mechanism [8].

Calcitonin

CT is a 32-amino acid polypeptide produced by the C-cells of the thyroid [9]. It is secreted in response to elevations in serum calcium. It can also be stimulated by certain gastrointestinal (GI) tract hormones (e.g., gastrin). The primary physiologic function of CT in humans remains unclear. Medullary carcinoma of the thyroid is a malignant neoplasm of the C-cells and is characterized by elevated CT levels. However, calcium, phosphate, and PTH levels remain normal. Also, patients can have undetectable levels of CT after a thyroidectomy with no clear detrimental systemic effects.

Despite the lack of clinical consequences from endogenous CT excess or deficiency, exogenous CT is a potent inhibitor of bone resorption. It also acts on the kidneys to enhance excretion of calcium, phosphate, magnesium, and sodium [9]. Both of these mechanisms make CT useful in the treatment of hypercalcemia. The effect of CT on bone resorption is lost over time due to tachyphylaxis [9]. This phenomenon, possibly due to downregulation of CT receptors, is of clinical importance when treating patients with hypercalcemia. The excellent short-term effects of CT to lower serum calcium (within 12 to 48 hours) allow the institution of therapies that require several days to attain maximal effectiveness (e.g., bisphosphonates).

CT can also be used in the treatment of osteoporosis. The administration of a salmon CT nasal spray has been shown to decrease markers of bone turnover, increase bone mineral density at the spine, and decrease the risk of vertebral fractures in postmenopausal women with osteoporosis [10].

Hypercalcemia

Hypercalcemia is an abnormality of the balance between different body compartments and can result from increased bone resorption, decreased renal excretion, increased GI absorption, or any combination of these mechanisms.

The signs and symptoms of hypercalcemia are protean and can be divided into four groups: (a) mental, (b) neurologic and musculoskeletal, (c) GI and urologic, and (d) cardiovascular. The mental manifestations of hypercalcemia include stupor, obtundation, apathy, lethargy, confusion, disorientation, and coma. In general, for a given level of hypercalcemia, older patients exhibit more of the mental signs than younger patients. The neurologic and musculoskeletal effects of hypercalcemia are reduced muscle tone and strength, myalgias, and decreased deep tendon reflexes. The GI and urologic signs are vomiting, constipation, polyuria, and polydipsia. The major cardiovascular effect of hypercalcemia, which the intensive care physician must address, is shortening of the QT interval. In the presence of ventricular ectopic beats, the calcium-induced shortening of the QT interval increases the potential for fatal arrhythmias or asystole.

Differential Diagnosis

Elevated serum calcium measurements have been reported in approximately 1% of the general population [11]. The causes of hypercalcemia can be differentiated into two broad groups defined by whether or not the process is driven by abnormal parathyroid tissue. Hence, the groups are termed: (a) PTH-independent hypercalcemia; and (b) PTH-dependent hypercalcemia. In PTH-independent hypercalcemia, the hypercalcemia is not mediated by abnormal parathyroid tissue, and the PTH level should be appropriately suppressed. In PTH-dependent hypercalcemia, the process is driven by abnormal parathyroid tissue, and the PTH level should be elevated, or inappropriately normal.

PTH-independent hypercalcemia is more common in hospitalized patients. Hypercalcemia of malignancy is the most common cause of PTH-independent hypercalcemia. The malignancies most often associated with hypercalcemia include lung (35%), breast (25%), hematologic (myeloma and lymphoma [14%]), head and neck (6%), and renal (3%) [12]. The hypercalcemia can be mediated by secretion of parathyroid hormone–related peptide (PTH-RP), most commonly seen in squamous cell carcinomas (often lung or head and neck tumors); autonomous activation of 1,25 D (occasionally seen with lymphomas); or by lytic bone lesions/metastases [13]. See Chapter 116 for a complete discussion of the hypercalcemia of malignancy.

Other possible causes of PTH-independent hypercalcemia include granulomatous diseases, immobilization, milk-alkali syndrome, thyrotoxicosis, vitamin D or A intoxication, or Addison's disease.

Granulomatous diseases, such as sarcoidosis and tuberculosis, can cause hypercalcemia due to autonomous 1,25 D production by the granulomas (similar to certain lymphomas). These patients have increased intestinal calcium absorption and sensitivity to vitamin D intake. Hypercalcemia occurs in 10% of patients, though hypercalciuria has been documented in as many as 20% [14].

Immobilization causes hypercalcemia as a result of decreased bone formation and persistent bone resorption. Hypercalcemia in the immobilized individual occurs most commonly in patients with high bone turnover (e.g., adolescents during the growth spurt or individuals with Paget's disease or thyrotoxicosis).

PTH-dependent hypercalcemia is much more common in the outpatient setting, though these patients can be hospitalized due to other issues. PTH-dependent hypercalcemia can be caused by primary or tertiary hyperparathyroidism. Another possible cause is familial hypocalciuric hypercalcemia (FHH). The routine measurement of serum calcium has altered the clinical presentation of hyperparathyroidism with most patients presenting with asymptomatic hypercalcemia.

Primary or tertiary hyperparathyroidism results from autonomous secretion of PTH despite elevated serum calcium levels. The latter occurs typically after chronic secondary hyperparathyroidism in the setting of end-stage renal failure. Hypercalcemia develops due to increased bone resorption, increased intestinal calcium absorption from stimulation of 1,25 D production, and increased renal tubular calcium reabsorption. The patient can be hypophosphatemic due to the phosphaturic effect of PTH. The hormone also induces renal bicarbonate wasting, resulting in a mild hyperchloremic acidosis. In primary hyperparathyroidism, a single adenoma is present in 80% to 85% of cases, whereas four-gland hyperplasia occurs in 15% to 20% of cases [15]. Parathyroid cancer is present in less than 1% of these patients and typically presents with much higher serum calcium levels [16].

Parathyroid hyperplasia or adenomas can also occur as part of the multiple endocrine neoplasia (MEN) syndromes. Type I MEN involves tumors of the pituitary, pancreas, and parathyroid (usually hyperplasia), whereas type II is associated with pheochromocytoma, medullary cancer of the thyroid, and primary hyperparathyroidism (hyperplasia or adenoma).

FHH is an autosomal dominant disorder characterized by hypercalcemia with inappropriately normal or elevated PTH levels. It is usually caused by a mutation in the calcium-sensing receptor gene [17]. In contrast to primary hyperparathyroidism, patients with FHH have relative hypocalciuria (fractional excretion of calcium <0.01), do not develop nephrolithiasis or bone disease, and cannot be cured surgically, unless rendered hypocalcemic by removal of all parathyroid tissue [18].

Several medications can induce hypercalcemia as well. Hypercalcemia associated with the use of thiazide diuretics is often an indicator of underlying primary hyperparathyroidism. Vitamins D and A intoxication can also cause hypercalcemia. Lithium may also affect parathyroid function and is associated with hypercalcemia and either elevated or inappropriately normal PTH levels [19].

Laboratory Evaluation

Hypercalcemia should always be considered in the patient with altered mental status. A total serum calcium level alone usually makes the diagnosis. However, altered binding of calcium to proteins, as can occur with hypoalbuminemia or with abnormal proteins (e.g., myeloma), or an acid–base imbalance may affect the free calcium level. Ionized calcium levels should not be affected by these issues. Because of the interrelationships of calcium, magnesium, and phosphorus, the latter two minerals should be measured in all cases involving altered calcium metabolism. An electrocardiogram to determine the QT interval is very important to assess the severity and urgency of the patient's hypercalcemia.

The differential diagnosis of the hypercalcemia can be narrowed down with a serum intact PTH measurement. If PTH levels are physiologically suppressed by the hypercalcemia, then PTH-independent sources should be sought, with malignancy being the most common. If malignancy is suspected, obtaining PTH-RP and 1,25 D levels can provide useful clues. In the absence of PTH, elevated 1,25 D levels imply autonomous production, most commonly associated with lymphomas and granulomatous diseases [13,14]. A bone scan may identify a metastatic process. Because myeloma is characterized by bone resorption with little bone formation, the bone scan is usually negative, but a skeletal survey may find lytic lesions. The diagnosis would then be confirmed by urine immunoelectrophoresis, serum protein electrophoresis, and bone marrow examination.

The diagnosis of milk-alkali syndrome is made by the patient's history, often revealing large quantities of calcium carbonate ingestion. In this instance, the patient should also be alkalotic with an elevated bicarbonate level. Thyrotoxicosis and Addison's disease can be ruled out with thyroid function tests and a Cortrosyn stimulation test, respectively (see Chapter 104 for a discussion about evaluating adrenal function in the critically ill). Vitamin D intoxication is quite rare, but the possibility can be eliminated by measuring 25-hydroxyvitamin D levels. Vitamin A levels can be measured if the diagnosis remains unclear.

If PTH-dependent hypercalcemia is confirmed with elevated or inappropriately normal PTH levels, a 24-hour urine for a fractional excretion of calcium can be done to differentiate primary or tertiary hyperparathyroidism from FHH, though this test may be altered by renal failure or the use of various diuretics.

Management

The aim of treatment of hypercalcemia is to minimize its effects on central nervous system (CNS), renal, and cardiovascular function. Appropriate treatment of hypercalcemia depends, in part, on the cause. General concepts in the management involve attempts to (a) increase renal calcium clearance, (b) decrease bone resorption, and (c) decrease intestinal calcium absorption. To this end, it is critical that the pathophysiology of the disease process be understood. If, for example, the hypercalcemia in a patient with myeloma is due to a combination of increased bone resorption plus decreased renal calcium clearance, successful management of the hypercalcemia requires that both processes be treated. Specific measures directed toward the pathophysiology of the hypercalcemia are discussed next.

Hydration and Diuresis. Saline hydration creates a diuresis that increases renal calcium excretion by decreasing calcium reabsorption in the proximal tubule. Hydration plays a critical role in the initial management of hypercalcemia because the onset of the therapeutic response is rapid. The aim of therapy is to achieve a urine output of 3 to 5 L per 24 hours. This often requires the administration of 200 to 500 mL per hour of normal saline [13]. Because a potential complication of administration of this amount of saline is congestive heart failure, extreme care must be taken in treating the patient with underlying cardiac disease or renal insufficiency. The concomitant administration of a loop diuretic helps prevent fluid overload and further increases renal calcium excretion by inhibiting distal tubular calcium reabsorption. Furosemide 20 to 40 mg can be administered by intravenous (IV) route once rehydration has been achieved. Measurement of serum electrolytes, phosphorus, and magnesium is mandatory during saline hydration to replace adequately the quantities lost in the urine. If renal or cardiac failure precludes the use of saline hydration, dialysis with a calcium-free dialysate is an effective alternative.

Calcitonin. CT reduces the resorption of calcium from bone by inhibiting osteoclasts. It also exerts transient effects to increase the renal excretion of calcium, along with sodium, potassium, magnesium, and phosphate. The benefits of CT in the treatment of hypercalcemia include (a) rapid onset within 2 hours, (b) maximal effect within 24 to 48 hours, and (c) low toxicity [9]. It can be used safely in patients with renal failure, and its side effects are limited to transient nausea, facial flushing, and occasional hypersensitivity at the injection site. The dose is 4 to 8 IU per kg body weight subcutaneously or intramuscularly every 12 hours [13]. Usually CT is effective for only 4 to 7 days [9], but it is still used for the rapid response, as bisphosphonates often require several days to attain maximal effectiveness.

Bisphosphonates. Bisphosphonates are organic compounds that are potent inhibitors of bone resorption through inhibition of osteoclastic activity and survival. Because of the delay in reduction of serum calcium with bisphosphonates, these agents are often used in conjunction with other therapies. Pamidronate can be infused intravenously as 60 or 90 mg over 2 hours with hydration. Zoledronate, at a dose of 4 mg intravenously over not less than 15 minutes, has been shown to be more effective at normalizing serum calcium in patients with hypercalcemia of malignancy [20]. Renal function must be monitored, and the doses of either medication may be repeated after a minimum of 7 days to allow a full response to the initial dose.

Denosumab. Denosumab is a monoclonal antibody directed against RANK-ligand, preventing the binding of RANK-ligand to osteoclasts, thereby inhibiting their development/activity and decreasing bone resorption [21]. This agent has recently been approved for the treatment of postmenopausal women with osteoporosis and has been shown to reduce the incidence of vertebral, non-vertebral, and hip fractures [21]. It has also been approved for the prevention of skeletal related events in patients with bone metastases from solid tumors [22]. It is also being studied in hypercalcemia of malignancy [23]. Therefore, this class of agents may prove to offer another treatment option for hypercalcemia of malignancy in the near future.

Hypocalcemia

Hypocalcemia is frequently encountered in critically ill patients. Although low serum albumin concentrations may explain some hypocalcemia, up to 18% of hospitalized patients and 85% of patients in ICUs were found to have hypocalcemia [24]. The symptoms of hypocalcemia can range from paresthesias and tetany to seizures or fatal laryngospasm. A positive Chvostek's sign (muscle spasm in response to tapping the facial nerve) is suggestive, but not diagnostic, of hypocalcemia. Trousseau's sign (carpal spasm precipitated by inflation of a blood pressure cuff above the systolic blood pressure) is more sensitive and specific. In contrast to the QT interval shortening in hypercalcemia, hypocalcemia is attended by an increase in the QT interval on the electrocardiogram, predisposing patients to cardiac arrhythmias. Chronic hypocalcemia is associated with basal ganglia calcification, cataract formation, and behavioral abnormalities [25].

Differential Diagnosis

Risk factors for the development of hypocalcemia in hospitalized patients include alkalosis, renal failure, and multiple transfusions. Although pancreatitis is associated with hypocalcemia, the mechanism is unclear. Hyperphosphatemia is the suspected cause of hypocalcemia attending tumor lysis and rhabdomyolysis.

Inadequate, or absent, PTH secretion is a cause of hypocalcemia. Hypoparathyroidism can occur after surgery, neck irradiation, as a result of iron deposition in hemochromatosis or thalassemia, or in severe magnesium deficiency [25]. Idiopathic hypoparathyroidism can be familial or sporadic. An autoimmune phenomenon may explain the idiopathic variety and may be found together with other autoimmune endocrine dysfunction. Target tissue unresponsiveness due to a defect in the cell membrane G protein is characterized by hypocalcemia and hyperphosphatemia in the presence of elevated PTH levels. This is commonly known as pseudohypoparathyroidism, and can be associated with somatic abnormalities (short, stocky habitus; round facies; and short metacarpals, metatarsals, or both).

Hypocalcemia can also signify vitamin D deficiency. Although nutritional rickets is rare in the United States, vitamin D deficiency is not [8]. Vitamin D deficiency may be the result of liver or renal failure with impaired hydroxylation of the parent compound, but is most often caused by inadequate sun exposure or malabsorption.

Laboratory Evaluation

A low corrected serum calcium or ionized calcium level confirms the diagnosis. Studies to discern the cause may include creatinine, phosphate, amylase, and magnesium levels; liver function tests; and 25-hydroxyvitamin D and PTH levels. In hypoparathyroidism due to the absence of PTH or target tissue unresponsiveness, serum phosphate levels tend to be high as a result of the absent phosphaturic effect of PTH.

Management

Treatment of hypocalcemia depends on its severity and chronicity. Symptomatic patients should be treated with IV calcium. A 10-mL vial of 10% calcium gluconate provides 93 mg of elemental calcium. One or two 10-mL vials should be administered in 100 mL 5% dextrose in water over 10 minutes. Calcium to be administered intravenously should always be diluted because concentrated solutions are very irritating to veins. Electrocardiographic monitoring during calcium supplementation is recommended as arrhythmias can occur from overcorrection. Often, the initial bolus needs to be followed by a continuous infusion which can be started with 10 vials of calcium gluconate in 1 L of 5% dextrose in water running at 50 mL per hour. This can then be adjusted to maintain the serum calcium levels in the lower portion of the normal range [24]. Hypocalcemia may mask digitalis toxicity. In these situations, a slower rate of calcium administration is recommended to prevent cardiac arrhythmias.

Oral supplementation should be instituted concurrently to provide 500 to 1,000 mg of elemental calcium three times daily. If calcium supplementation alone cannot maintain serum calcium levels, vitamin D preparations may be administered. Ergocalciferol (vitamin D_2) has a wide safety margin and relatively low cost. The usual dose is 25,000 to 100,000 IU daily. This preparation has a slow onset of action because it must be 25-hydroxylated in the liver and 1α-hydroxylated in the kidney. The preparation has a long half-life because it is stored in fat. Activated vitamin D preparations that act more rapidly are also available. Calcitriol is 1,25 D_3 and can be given as 0.25 to 1.0 μg, once or twice daily. This has a shorter half-life than vitamin D but is more potent. It can be used for long-term management but has a narrower therapeutic window [25].

The goal of treating hypocalcemia is to prevent symptoms attributable to low calcium and to avoid hypercalciuria and hypercalcemia. In a hypoparathyroid patient, total serum calcium should be maintained between 8.0 and 8.5 mg per dL. In the absence of PTH, circulating calcium levels greater than 9.0 mg per dL are often attended by hypercalciuria and an increased risk of nephrolithiasis or nephrocalcinosis. If hypercalciuria occurs despite lower serum calcium concentrations, thiazide diuretics can be used to try and enhance tubular reabsorption of calcium [25].

MAGNESIUM DISORDERS

Magnesium Physiology

Magnesium is the major intracellular divalent cation. Two-thirds of the total body content of magnesium is found in bone and only 2% is found in the extracellular space. Muscle and liver are the soft tissues that contain the greatest amount of magnesium. Thirty percent of extracellular magnesium circulates bound to protein [1]. Therefore, as with circulating calcium levels, albumin concentration must be known to interpret total magnesium levels. Magnesium absorption occurs throughout the small intestine. Absorption is enhanced by 1,25 D. Like calcium, magnesium is reabsorbed in the kidney tubules.

Magnesium is necessary for normal sodium- and potassium-activated ATPase, PTH secretion, and neuromuscular function. Decreased sodium- and potassium-activated ATPase due to hypomagnesemia can result in intracellular potassium depletion [26]. Magnesium-induced decreases in PTH secretion result in hypocalcemia that can only be corrected by magnesium replacement. Magnesium inhibits the release of acetylcholine by presynaptic fibers and decreases the sensitivity of the motor end plate to the neurotransmitter. Therefore, hypomagnesemia is often attended by CNS hyperexcitability, whereas hypermagnesemia results in CNS depression.

Hypermagnesemia

Hypermagnesemia is often attended by a loss of deep tendon reflexes and CNS depression. Flaccid paralysis, hypotension, confusion, and coma may result from magnesium levels greater than 6 mg per dL [26]. The most common cause of hypermagnesemia in the hospitalized patient is renal failure. The hypermagnesemia may be aggravated by the administration of magnesium-containing antacids. Diabetic ketoacidosis is usually attended by hypermagnesemia, but this typically reflects dehydration, which masks the total body magnesium depletion resulting from the glucose-induced osmotic diuresis.

Management

The actions of magnesium on neuromuscular function are antagonized by calcium. Emergency treatment of the magnesium-induced CNS depression includes IV administration of one to two 10-mL vials of calcium gluconate diluted in 100 mL 5% dextrose in water over 5 to 10 minutes to prevent venous irritation [26]. The dose may be repeated as necessary. Total serum calcium must be monitored and not allowed to exceed 11 mg per dL.

Definitive treatment of the hypermagnesemia requires increasing renal magnesium excretion. In the presence of normal renal function, increased magnesium excretion can be achieved by IV administration of furosemide, 20 to 40 mg IV, every 1 to 2 hours, along with fluid hydration, though there is little literature to support its use [26]. Serum electrolytes, particularly potassium, must be closely monitored. Dialysis is the treatment of choice when kidney function is impaired and the patient is symptomatic from the hypermagnesemia.

Hypomagnesemia

Hypomagnesemia is much more common than hypermagnesemia in the hospitalized patient [1]. The increased CNS excitability in the patient with hypomagnesemia is partly due to the accompanying hypocalcemia, which results from impaired PTH secretion and decreased peripheral tissue responsiveness to PTH. The intracellular potassium depletion seen with hypomagnesemia can also exacerbate digitalis toxicity.

Hypomagnesemia may result from decreased intestinal absorption (e.g., steatorrhea), or more commonly from increased renal excretion due to an osmotic diuresis (e.g., hyperglycemia), or drugs (e.g., ethanol, aminoglycosides, or cisplatin). Dietary deficiency alone is rarely the explanation for hypomagnesemia. The exceptions are starvation or prolonged parenteral feeding [26].

The drugs that most commonly increase renal magnesium excretion are alcohol and diuretics. Hypomagnesemia in the alcohol abuser may also be partly attributable to dietary deficiency. Hypomagnesemia is encountered in 30% of alcoholics [26].

Management

Magnesium may be administered orally or parenterally. If serum magnesium levels are below 1 mg per dL, or if the patient is symptomatic, parenteral treatment is indicated. The patient with symptoms usually has a total body magnesium deficit of 1 to 3 mEq per kg body weight. Because approximately half of the administered magnesium is lost due to renal excretion, replacement of the deficit requires administration of 2 to 6 mEq per kg body weight. It is recommended to give 8 to 12 g of magnesium sulfate over the first 24 hours followed by 4 to 6 g per day for 3 to 4 days to replete body stores [26]. Serum magnesium and calcium levels should be monitored. The dose should be reduced by 75% in patients with renal failure.

In the patient with mild magnesium deficiency, oral therapy is usually satisfactory. Magnesium oxide 400 mg (241 mg of elemental magnesium) can be given as 1 to 2 tablets daily. Diarrhea is the most common side effect. As with all magnesium supplementation, levels must be monitored closely in the patient with renal insufficiency.

PHOSPHORUS DISORDERS

Phosphorus Physiology

Eighty-five percent of total body phosphorus is found in bone [1]. Extracellular phosphate accounts for only 1% of total body phosphorus. Because of shifts in phosphate between intracellular and extracellular compartments, serum phosphate levels do not accurately reflect total body stores. For example, because acidosis causes a shift in phosphate from within cells to the extracellular compartment, serum phosphate levels may be normal in the acidotic patient despite depletion of total body stores [27]. As the acidosis is corrected, serum phosphate levels may fall.

Phosphorus is a component of nucleic acids and phospholipids and is a cofactor for a number of enzymes. Low phosphate levels increase renal 1α-hydroxylase activity and 1,25 D production, whereas high phosphate levels suppress its production [1]. Thus, phosphorus metabolism is closely related to calcium and magnesium metabolism.

Hyperphosphatemia

Increased phosphate levels are most often encountered in patients with renal failure or hypoparathyroidism. Both of these conditions result in impaired phosphate excretion. Hyperphosphatemia can also be seen from cellular leaks as in hemolysis, rhabdomyolysis, or the tumor lysis syndrome. The hyperphosphatemia, along with diminished renal 1,25 D production, results in hypocalcemia. The symptoms are usually attributable to the accompanying hypocalcemia, and not the hyperphosphatemia per se [27]. Therefore, in the symptomatic patient, therapy should be directed at correction of the hypocalcemia.

Chronic management of hyperphosphatemia can be accomplished with limiting phosphate intake as well as using phosphate binders, such as calcium acetate 667 mg, 2 tablets with meals or sevelamer 800 mg, 1 to 2 tablets with meals [27].

Hypophosphatemia

Hypophosphatemia can be seen in up to 3% of hospitalized patients or 34% of patients in the ICU [28]. It can result from impaired intestinal phosphate absorption or increased renal phosphate excretion. The cause of hypophosphatemia in alcoholics is often multifactorial but most likely reflects malnutrition and the accompanying vomiting. When taken in excess, phosphate-binding antacids impair phosphate absorption. The resulting hypophosphatemia can stimulate 1,25 D production and cause hypercalcemia, which has been confused with hyperparathyroidism.

Renal phosphate excretion is increased in hyperparathyroidism, vitamin D deficiency, and with osmotic diuresis. There are also rare genetic and paraneoplastic conditions that cause excess phosphate excretion due to excess "phosphatonins" such as fibroblast growth factor 23 [1]. PTH inhibits renal tubular phosphate reabsorption, resulting in hypophosphatemia when secreted in excess. Serum phosphate levels are reduced in vitamin D deficiency due to impaired intestinal phosphate absorption and increased renal phosphate excretion (the result of secondary hyperparathyroidism in response to the associated hypocalcemia). The patient in diabetic ketoacidosis has a total body phosphorus deficit, despite normal serum phosphorus levels. In the early stages of the illness, the rising serum glucose levels cause an osmotic diuresis with increased renal phosphate loss. However, the developing acidosis causes a shift in phosphorus from the intracellular to the extracellular compartment. This shift, along with the accompanying volume depletion, tends to normalize the serum phosphorus levels. Rehydration and insulin treatment with resolution of the acidosis may cause a rapid fall in serum phosphorus levels.

The potential consequences of severe hypophosphatemia are impaired oxygen delivery to the tissues due to decreased 2,3-diphosphoglycerate levels, muscle weakness, and rhabdomyolysis. The latter is most likely to occur when severe hypophosphatemia occurs after prolonged mild hypophosphatemia (e.g., in the hospitalized alcoholic in whom phosphate level falls precipitously during carbohydrate administration).

Management

Severe hypophosphatemia (<1.5 mg per dL) requires parenteral therapy [27]. Potassium phosphate or sodium phosphate can be used depending on the patient's potassium level. Fifteen mmol may be added to 5% dextrose in water and given intravenously over 2 hours [28]. Further treatment depends on the serum phosphate levels and clinical condition. The dose may be repeated up to three times in the first 24 hours until phosphate levels normalize.

Parenteral therapy should be limited in the patient with renal failure or hypocalcemia. In the patient with renal failure, IV therapy can cause hyperphosphatemia, worsen hypocalcemia, and cause metastatic calcification, primarily in the kidney. The latter can occur if the patient is hypercalcemic or if the phosphate is administered too rapidly. Initial doses should be 50% lower if the patient is under renal failure or hypercalcemic [27].

Oral preparations of potassium phosphate (K-Phos Neutral) can be used for milder hypophosphatemia or for chronic management. The usual oral dose is 1 to 4 g per day in divided doses. The most common side effect is diarrhea.

References

1. Moe SM: Disorders involving calcium, phosphorus, and magnesium. *Prim Care* 35(2):215–237, v–vi, 2008.
2. Rude RK, Oldham SB, Singer FR: Functional hypoparathyroidism and parathyroid hormone end-organ resistance in human magnesium deficiency. *Clin Endocrinol* 5:209, 1976.
3. Canalis E, Giustina A, Bilezikian JP: Mechanisms of anabolic therapies for osteoporosis. *N Engl J Med* 357:905, 2007.
4. Neer RM, Arnaud CD, Zanchetta JR, et al: Effect of parathyroid hormone (1–34) on fractures and bone mineral density in postmenopausal women with osteoporosis. *N Engl J Med* 344:1434, 2001.
5. Saag KG, Shane E, Boonen S, et al: Teriparatide or alendronate in glucocorticoid-induced osteoporosis. *N Engl J Med* 357:2028, 2007.
6. Khosla S: The OPG/RANKL/RANK System. *Endocrinology* 142:5050, 2001.
7. Nagpal S, Na S, Rathnachalam R: Noncalcemic actions of vitamin D receptor ligands. *Endocr Rev* 26:662, 2005.
8. Holick MF: Vitamin D deficiency. *N Engl J Med* 357:256, 2007.
9. Wisneski LA: Salmon calcitonin in the acute management of hypercalcemia. *Calcif Tissue Int* 46:S26, 1990.
10. Chesnut CH III, Silverman S, Andriano K, et al: A randomized trial of nasal spray salmon calcitonin in postmenopausal women with established osteoporosis: the Prevent Recurrence of Osteoporotic Fractures Study. *Am J Med* 109:267, 2000.
11. Palmer M, Jakobsson S, Akerstrom G, et al: Prevalence of hypercalcaemia in a health survey: a 14-year follow-up study of serum calcium values. *Eur J Clin Invest* 18:39, 1988.
12. Mundy GR, Martin TJ: The hypercalcemia of malignancy: pathogenesis and management. *Metabolism* 31:1247, 1982.
13. Stewart AF: Hypercalcemia associated with cancer. *N Engl J Med* 352:373, 2005.
14. Horwitz MJ, Hodak SP, Stewart AF: Non-parathyroid hypercalcemia, in Rosen CJ (ed): *Primer of the Metabolic Bone Diseases and Disorders of Mineral Metabolism*. Washington, DC, ASBMR, 2008, p 307.
15. Bilekizian JL, Silverberg SJ: Asymptomatic primary hyperparathyroidism. *N Engl J Med* 350:1746, 2004.
16. Rodgers SE, Perrier ND: Parathyroid carcinoma. *Curr Opin Oncol* 18:16, 2006.
17. Pollak MR, Brown EM, Chou YHW, et al: Mutations in the human Ca^{2+}-sensing receptor gene cause familial hypocalciuric hypercalcemia and neonatal severe hyperparathyroidism. *Cell* 75:1297, 1993.
18. Marx SJ, Spiegel AM, Brown EM, et al: Divalent cation metabolism: familial hypocalciuric hypercalcemia versus typical primary hyperparathyroidism. *Am J Med* 65:235, 1978.
19. Saunders BD, Saunders EFH, Gauger PG: Lithium therapy and hyperparathyroidism: an evidence-based assessment. *World J Surg* 33:2314, 2009.
20. Major P, Lortholary A, Hon J, et al: Zoledronic acid is superior to pamidronate in the treatment of hypercalcemia of malignancy: a pooled analysis of two randomized, controlled, clinical trials. *J Clin Oncol* 19:558, 2001.
21. Cummings SR, San Martin J, McClung MR, et al: Denosumab for prevention of fractures in postmenopausal women with osteoporosis. *N Engl J Med* 361:756, 2009.
22. Body JJ, Lipton A, Gralow J, et al: Effects of denosumab in patients with bone metastases with and without previous bisphosphonate exposure. *J Bone Miner Res* 25:440, 2010.
23. http://clinicaltrials.gov/ct2/show/NCT00896454.
24. Cooper MS, Gittoes NJL: Diagnosis and management of hypocalcemia. *BMJ* 336:1298, 2008.
25. Shoback D: Hypoparathyroidism. *N Engl J Med* 359:391, 2008.
26. Topf JM, Murray PT: Hypomagnesemia and hypermagnesemia. *Rev Endocr Metab Disord* 4:195, 2003.
27. Kraft MD, Btaiche IF, Sacks GS, et al: Treatment of electrolyte disorders in adult patients in the intensive care unit. *Am J Health-Syst Pharm* 62:1663, 2005.
28. Brunelli SM, Goldfarb S: Hypophosphatemia: clinical consequences and management. *J Am Soc Nephrol* 18:1999, 2007.

CHAPTER 106 ■ HYPOGLYCEMIA

JOHN P. MORDES, MICHAEL J. THOMPSON, DAVID M. HARLAN AND SAMIR MALKANI

Hypoglycemia occurs often in the intensive care unit (ICU) as both an admission diagnosis and a consequence of therapy. In a 2001 study of intensive insulin therapy in a surgical ICU population, hypoglycemia occurred in up to 5.1% of patients [1]. Another study of more than 2,200 ICU patients reported that nearly 7% experienced at least one episode of hypoglycemia [2]. Estimates of prevalence range as high as 25% [3]. Hypoglycemia is a marker of poor outcome in hospitalized patients in general [4–6], and among the critically ill in particular [7,8]. Severe, prolonged hypoglycemia can cause permanent neurological and cardiovascular damage.

DEFINITION OF HYPOGLYCEMIA

No specific blood glucose concentration defines hypoglycemia. Whipple proposed a symptom-based definition of hypoglycemia in the 1930s that remains valid [9]. "Whipple's triad" defines hypoglycemia as (a) documentation of a low blood glucose concentration, (b) concurrent symptoms of hypoglycemia, and (c) resolution of symptoms after administration of glucose. Typically, this concentration in serum is less than 50 mg per dL (2.8 mM). The physiologic definition is a blood glucose concentration low enough to cause the release of counterregulatory hormones (e.g., catecholamines) and impair the function of the central nervous system (CNS).

SYMPTOMS AND SIGNS OF HYPOGLYCEMIA

Counterregulatory hormones released in response to low glucose concentrations cause sympathoadrenal symptoms and signs. Prominent symptoms include hunger, tingling, shakiness, weakness, palpitations, and anxiety [10]. Corresponding signs include diaphoresis, tachycardia, peripheral vasoconstriction, and widening of the pulse pressure. These findings may be absent in patients receiving sympatholytic drugs (e.g., beta-blockers) and in patients with diabetes who have autonomic neuropathy.

Early symptoms and signs of neuroglycopenia include difficulty thinking and sensations of warmth, weakness, and fatigue. These may be followed by confusion, slurred speech, and other nonspecific behavioral changes [10]. Severe neuroglycopenia can cause disturbances of integrative function, obtundation, seizures, coma, and, rarely, a permanent vegetative state.

Hypoglycemia can be associated with acute pulmonary edema [11], supraventricular and ventricular tachycardias, atrial fibrillation, and junctional dysrhythmias [12–14]. Electrocardiographic abnormalities associated with hypoglycemia include T wave flattening, increased Q-T interval, ST segment depression, and repolarization abnormalities [15–17]. Bradycardias have also been attributed to hypoglycemia, but only rarely [18]. Prolonged hypoglycemia can be associated with hypothermia [19–21], respiratory failure [22], and hypokalemia and hypophosphatemia [23].

NORMAL GLUCOSE REGULATORY PHYSIOLOGY

Glucose Utilization

Plasma glucose concentration is maintained in a narrow range (~60 to ~120 mg per dL; ~3.3 to ~6.7 mmol). The organ most dependent on glucose is the brain, which consumes ~150 g per day. Unlike fat or muscle, the CNS does not require insulin for glucose transport. During starvation, the brain uses ketone bodies as a substitute fuel (see Chapter 100), but acquisition of the capability to use this alternate substrate requires hours to days. Even during prolonged starvation, the brain still needs ~44 g per day of glucose. Other tissues with obligate glucose needs include erythrocytes (~36 g per day) and renal medulla (~25 g per day).

Sources of Plasma Glucose

There are two sources of blood glucose: endogenous and ingested carbohydrate. In the postprandial state, the concentration of circulating insulin rises in response to the increase in glucose concentration. The insulin promotes (a) transport of glucose into skeletal muscle for immediate use or storage as muscle glycogen and (b) hepatic storage of glucose in the form of liver glycogen. When all other metabolic demands for glucose are being met, some excess glucose is used for synthesis of triglyceride.

During brief starvation, such as when asleep, the principal source of glucose is hepatic glycogen. During prolonged starvation, glucose is derived principally from conversion of muscle-derived amino acids. Smaller contributions to gluconeogenesis are made by (a) glycerol derived from fat and (b) lactate produced by anaerobic glycolysis. When euglycemia is maintained by glycogenolysis or gluconeogenesis, insulin levels are low but never zero.

The liver stores only 60 to 80 g of glycogen, a supply that is exhausted by an overnight fast. Muscle glycogen stores are ~120 g, but this glycogen is not directly available for the maintenance of systemic glucose concentrations due to the lack of glucose-6-phosphatase in muscle. Muscle glycogen contributes to plasma glucose only via anaerobic glycolysis, leading to the production of lactate, which is transported to the liver and converted into glucose. The shuttling of glucose to muscle and lactate to the liver comprises the Cori cycle. Muscle can also amidate pyruvate to form alanine, which is then exported to the liver and converted to glucose. Gluconeogenesis occurs principally in the liver using amino acids, glycerol, and lactate as substrates. The enzymes and pathways required for gluconeogenesis are shown in Figure 106.1.

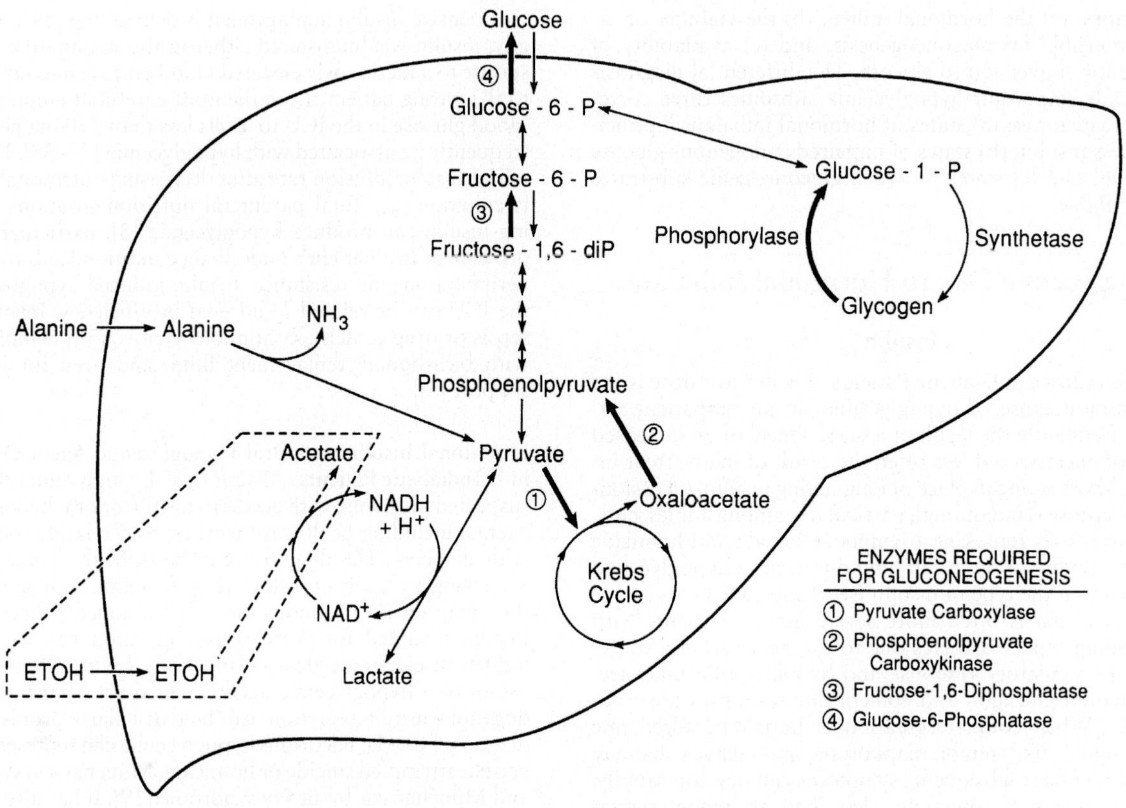

FIGURE 106.1. Metabolic pathways important in the response to hypoglycemia. The thick, annotated arrows indicate the key steps in glycogen breakdown and gluconeogenesis. In the presence of low circulating insulin concentrations, phosphorylase activity is increased, leading to the release of glucose-1-phosphate, which is then converted to glucose-6-phosphate and finally to glucose through the action of glucose-6-phosphatase. Glucose is also generated from three carbon precursors by gluconeogenesis. This process essentially reverses glycolysis and is controlled by four enzymes: (1) pyruvate carboxylase, (2) phosphoenolpyruvate carboxykinase, (3) fructose-1,6-diphosphatase, and (4) glucose-6-phosphatase. Within the box delimited by dotted lines, the metabolic effects of ethanol ingestion are indicated. Ethanol is converted to acetaldehyde and then to acetate, producing reduced nicotinamide adenine dinucleotide (NADH). The high concentration of NADH favors the generation of lactate from pyruvate, decreasing the concentration of the latter. As the availability of pyruvate as a gluconeogenic precursor declines, glucose production via gluconeogenesis also declines, and hypoglycemia can ensue.

Hormonal Regulation of Plasma Glucose Concentration

Insulin is the most important regulator of glycemia, promoting glucose uptake and storage in the fed state, and regulating glycogenolysis, gluconeogenesis, and lipolysis in the fasted state. Glucagon, glucocorticoids, catecholamines, growth hormone, and, to a lesser degree, thyroxine promote the formation of glucose in the fasted state and in general counteract the actions of insulin. Foremost among these "counterregulatory" hormones is glucagon, which is secreted in response to low glucose. It promotes both glycogenolysis (an immediate effect) and gluconeogenesis (a delayed but more enduring effect). Glucocorticoids antagonize the action of insulin, stimulating gluconeogenesis and inhibiting extrahepatic glucose utilization. Catecholamines also promote glycogenolysis and gluconeogenesis. The mechanism by which growth hormone promotes blood glucose elevation is not fully understood. The influence of thyroxine on blood glucose concentration is probably indirect. Fasting glucose tends to be elevated and decreased in hyperthyroid and hypothyroid patients, respectively. Absence of liver glycogen has been observed in hyperthyroid animals [24].

CLASSIFICATION OF HYPOGLYCEMIA

Hypoglycemia can be classified as fasting (or postabsorptive) or postprandial (or "reactive"). The former always represents a major health problem that requires further evaluation. Hypoglycemia that occurs only after eating can be more difficult to assess. It is usually minimally symptomatic and is attributed variously to exaggerated insulin response, renal glycosuria, defects in glucagon responses, and high insulin sensitivity [25,26]. Some cases of postprandial hypoglycemia, however, are severe and associated with health issues including mutations in the insulin receptor [27], autoantibodies against insulin [28], gastric "dumping" after bypass surgery, and nesidioblastosis, all of which are described later. Postprandial hypoglycemia generally does not require intensive care.

DIFFERENTIAL DIAGNOSIS OF HYPOGLYCEMIA

Hypoglycemia that fulfills Whipple's triad always implies a major disturbance in glucose homeostasis, which is dependent on three factors: (a) the hormonal milieu, (b) the viability of organs responsible for gluconeogenesis, and (c) availability of substrate for conversion to glucose. The differential diagnosis of medically important hypoglycemia subsumes three corresponding categories: (a) states of hormonal imbalance, principally excess insulin, (b) states of impaired endogenous glucose production, and (c) states in which gluconeogenic substrates are unavailable.

Hypoglycemia Due to Hormonal Imbalance

Insulin

Insulin Overdoses in Diabetic Patients. Insulin overdose is the most common cause of hypoglycemia. In an outpatient setting, it is frequently the result of a missed meal or an increased amount of exercise and less often the result of inadvertent injection of short acting in place of long-acting insulin. Occasionally, an overdose is intentional, particularly among adolescents. Rarely, overdoses represent attempts at suicide and homicide [29]. The rapidity of onset [30] and duration of hypoglycemia [31] depend on the type of insulin (see Table 106.1).

Hypoglycemia is often more severe among patients with long-standing type 1 diabetes due to the presence of a defective counterregulatory response and hypoglycemia unawareness. Impaired glucagon and epinephrine responses are common [32]. When counterregulation is impaired, adrenergic warning signals like tremor, diaphoresis, and tachycardia may not occur and neuroglycopenic symptoms can develop rapidly. The phenomenon is sometimes described as hypoglycemia-associated autonomic failure [33]. Inadequate counterregulatory responses can also delay recovery from hypoglycemia.

Hypoglycemia in ICU patients can result from rapid changes in clinical status, medications that impair counterregulation (e.g., high-dose β-adrenergic blockers), and the presence of intercurrent disease processes. Although insulin-induced hypoglycemia is easily diagnosed in the ICU, it is crucial to determine exactly why it occurred.

Intensive insulin management is demanding [34]; occasionally, insulin is administered either in the wrong dose or in response to a factitiously elevated blood glucose measurement or to the wrong patient. Even the most careful attempts to lower blood glucose in the ICU to levels less than 110 mg per dL can frequently be associated with hypoglycemia [35–39]. Failure to adjust insulin infusion rate after decreasing nutritional support is common [2]. Total parenteral nutrition solutions containing insulin can produce hypoglycemia [3], particularly if improvement in a patient's underlying condition leads to reduced peripheral insulin resistance. Insulin-induced hypoglycemia in the ICU can be related to adrenal insufficiency, renal failure, sepsis or drug toxicity, continuous venovenous hemofiltration with bicarbonate replacement fluid, and need for inotropic support [3].

Intentional Insulin and Oral Hypoglycemic Agent Overdoses in Nondiabetic Patients. "Factitious" hypoglycemia should be suspected in anyone with access to insulin or oral hypoglycemic agents, including healthcare workers and relatives of persons with diabetes. The diagnosis can be difficult. These patients are trying to frustrate rather than facilitate a diagnosis, and they may devise ingenious methods to conceal their actions. Insulin intended for surreptitious injection has been found hidden in electronic devices and body cavities. Surreptitious use of oral hypoglycemic agents, which act by increasing endogenous insulin secretion, can be particularly problematic to diagnose [40,41]. Factitious hypoglycemia can represent malingering, attempted suicide or homicide, Münchausen syndrome, and Münchausen-by-proxy syndrome [29]. It has also been reported to result from adulteration of herbal and counterfeit prescription drugs with oral agents [42,43].

Insulinoma. Insulinomas are insulin-secreting pancreatic islet tumors. They are uncommon but do represent the most common form of pancreatic islet neoplasm. Most (>90%) are nonmalignant. They are typically small and difficult to visualize radiographically. To evaluate a patient with suspected

TABLE 106.1

INSULIN PREPARATIONS

Class	Preparation	Onset of action	Peak	Duration
Short-acting				
	Aspart (NovoLog™)[a]	15 min	45–90 min	3–5 h
	Glulisine (Apidra™)[a]	15 min	50–60 min	~ 4 h
	Lispro (Humalog™)[a]	15–30 min	30 min–2.5 h	3–6 h
	Regular (Humulin R™, Novolin R™)	30–60 min	1–5 h	5–10 h
Intermediate-acting				
	NPH (Humulin N™, Novolin N™)	1–2 h	4–14 h	16–24 h
Long-acting				
	Glargine (Lantus™)[a]	1.5–5 h	No peak	18 to >24 h[b]
	Detemir (Levemir™)[a]	1 h	No peak	Up to 24 h
Combinations				
	70% NPH, 30% Regular (Humulin 70/30™, Novolin 70/30™)	30 min	4–8 h	24 h
	75% Protamine lispro, 25% lispro[a]	15 min	1.5 h	10–16 h
	70% Protamine aspart, 30% aspart[a]	15 min	1.5 h	10–16 h
	50% Protamine lispro, 50% lispro[a]	15 min	1.5 h	10–16 h

Notes: Data are for recombinant human insulin or semisynthetic insulin administered subcutaneously. Protamine lispro and protamine aspart insulins are available only in fixed-ratio combinations.
[a]Semisynthetic insulin.
[b]Study ended at 24 h. Trade names are given in parentheses. Additional semisynthetic insulins are under development.

insulinoma, fasting immunoreactive insulin (IRI; measured in microunits [μU] per milliliter) and glucose (milligrams per deciliter) should be obtained. Insulinoma is usually associated with an IRI/glucose ratio >0.3. Elevated levels of C-peptide and proinsulin help confirm the diagnosis by documenting that the source of insulin is endogenous. Proinsulin is typically elevated up to 25% of the insulin concentration in cases of insulinoma [44].

It can be difficult to differentiate among insulinoma, factitious hypoglycemia due to self-administration of insulin, and abuse of oral hypoglycemic agents. When intentional insulin overdose is suspected, insulin measurements are of limited value. Patients with factitious hypoglycemia may have circulating anti-insulin antibodies that interfere with the radioimmunoassay for insulin. This is true even if human insulin is injected. These patients may appear to have elevated levels of insulin, just as would patients with an insulinoma. In this circumstance, simultaneous glucose, insulin, and C-peptide concentrations are helpful. Insulin and C-peptide are normally cosecreted by the pancreas in equimolar quantities, but the latter is not present in insulin for injection. Absence of C-peptide in a patient with unexplained fasting hypoglycemia strengthens the possibility of surreptitious use of insulin. If oral hypoglycemic agent abuse is suspected, both serum and urine should be screened.

Nonislet Tumors that Secrete Insulin. Rarely, complex endocrine tumors may secrete insulin [45]. Hypoglycemia due to ectopic secretion of insulin by nonendocrine tumors is very rare [46–49].

Nesidioblastosis or Persistent Hyperinsulinemic Hypoglycemia (PHH). Nesidioblastosis (nonmalignant islet cell hyperplasia) is a rare form of nonmalignant islet cell adenomatosis that leads to insulin-mediated hypoglycemia. In infants, nesidioblastosis is typically characterized by islet hyperplasia, β-cell hypertrophy, and increased β-cell mass. It can be either diffuse or focal and is sometimes termed persistent hyperinsulinemic hypoglycemia of infancy (PHHI) [50–53]. Rapid diagnosis of the childhood form is crucial to avoid hypoglycemic damage to the maturing CNS. Several different genetic mutations have been associated with the disorder cases [51,52,54–57]. Special cases of hyperinsulinemic hypoglycemia in infancy include Costello syndrome [58] and the Beckwith–Wiedemann syndrome, which is due to defects in pancreatic β-cell potassium channels [59].

A small number of cases of adult nesidioblastosis have been reported [51,60,61]. The pathological findings are reportedly less consistent than in infants [62], and the cause is unknown. Additional cases of PHH have been diagnosed in adults who had previously undergone Roux-en-Y gastric bypass surgery for weight reduction [63]. Whether these cases represent nesidioblastosis [63,64], "dumping syndrome," or a reactive process leading to or unmasking a defect in β-cell function [65] is unclear, perhaps in part because the pathological diagnosis of nesidioblastosis is difficult [62]. Treatment options include diazoxide, streptozocin, calcium channel blockade [66], octreotide (discussed later), percutaneous gastrostomy into the remnant stomach [67], as well as partial pancreatectomy [64].

Antibody-Mediated ("Autoimmune") Hypoglycemia. Autoimmune hypoglycemia can result from autoantibodies directed against insulin itself or autoantibodies directed against the insulin receptor [68]. Both can occur in either insulin-treated [69] or nondiabetic individuals, and both types of autoantibodies can be found in the same patient [70]. About 90% of cases have been reported from Japan [71]. Serum insulin concentrations typically are extremely high, usually higher than those produced by insulinomas. It is assumed that in these cases, glucose administration causes excessive insulin response because the antibodies buffer most of the insulin secreted [72].

Endogenous antibodies that bind to and activate the insulin receptor can also cause hypoglycemia [73]. Some, but not all cases, are associated with other autoimmune disorders [74–76], and a few have occurred in patients with myeloma [77]. Previous exposure to exogenous insulin is not necessary, but some patients may have an abnormal insulin molecule [78]. Metformin may be helpful in the management of some cases [79]. Some cases respond to immunosuppressive therapy [73]. The natural history of this syndrome is that the antireceptor antibodies disappear and the syndrome resolves over a time course of months to years [28].

Pancreas and Islet Transplantation. Hypoglycemia can occur after pancreas and islet transplantation [80], but it is generally not a significant clinical problem [81,82]. Islet transplantation has been reported to resolve hypoglycemia unawareness [83]. There is a report of nesidioblastosis-like transformation of a successful pancreas allograft [84].

Nonislet Tumors with Insulin-Like Activity. Certain tumors not of pancreatic islet origin are associated with fasting hypoglycemia clinically indistinguishable from that caused by islet cell neoplasms. Whereas insulinomas are typically quite small, nonpancreatic neoplasms associated with hypoglycemia tend to be large mesenchymal tumors. The large size initially suggested that excessive glucose utilization by the tumor was the cause of the hypoglycemia, but subsequent studies suggest that most cases result from secretion of high-molecular-weight insulin-like growth factor II (pro-IGF-II or "big IGF-II") [85,86]. Pro-IGF-II levels decrease significantly and hypoglycemia resolves after successful tumor resection [87–92]. Abnormal processing of the IGF-II molecule may play a role in some cases [88,90,93]. Nonislet cell neoplasms associated with hypoglycemia include gastrointestinal stromal cell tumors [94], hemangiopericytoma [95–97], hepatoma [98,99], uterine tumors [100], renal tumors [101], mesenteric sarcomas [102], colorectal cancer [103], gastric cancer [104], adrenocortical carcinoma, lymphoma, poorly differentiated thyroid cancer [105], somatostatinoma [106], phylloides tumor [107], and leukemia [108]. Multiple myeloma may also cause hypoglycemia via an antibody-mediated mechanism described later [76].

The diagnosis of hypoglycemia due to production of pro-IGF-II by nonislet cell tumors requires the exclusion of insulinoma. As noted earlier, this can be done by obtaining simultaneous insulin and glucose measurements during hypoglycemia. The observation of increased blood glucose concentration after intravenous administration of glucagon, an index of adequate glycogen stores, may also help discriminate between insulin and IGF-secreting tumors [109]. Methods have been developed for measuring serum pro-insulin-like growth factor-II directly [86]. Hypoglycemia associated with high levels of IGF-I has rarely been reported [110].

Hypoglycemia Due to Noninsulin Hypoglycemic Agents

Pharmaceuticals other than insulin that are used to treat type 2 diabetes fall into two classes. "Hypoglycemic agents" enhance insulin secretion and can cause hyperinsulinemic hypoglycemia. The sulfonylureas and meglitinides belong to this class; all are taken orally. "Antidiabetic agents" promote normoglycemia through mechanisms other than enhancement of insulin secretion; they include both oral and injectable agents. When given as monotherapy they do not cause hypoglycemia, but they can amplify the glucose-lowering activity of insulin

TABLE 106.2

ORAL HYPOGLYCEMIC AGENTS

	Usual total daily dose (mg)	Half-life (h)	Duration of action (h)
First-generation sulfonylureas			
Acetohexamide (Dymelor™)	500–750	0.8–2.4	12–24
Chlorpropamide (Diabinese™)	250–375	25–60	24–72
Tolazamide (Tolinase™)	250–500	5–11	14–16
Tolbutamide (Orinase™)	1,000–2,000	4–25	6–12
Second- and third-generation sulfonylureas			
Glimepiride (Amaryl™)	1–4	2–8	12–24
Glipizide (Glucotrol™)	10–20	1.1–3.7	12–24
Glyburide (DiaBeta™, Glynase™, Micronase™)	3–20	0.7–3.0	12–24
Other insulin secretagogues			
Nateglinide (Starlix™)	180–360	1.5	<4
Repaglinide (Prandin™)	1.5–16	1	4

Notes: Oral hypoglycemic agents available in the United States. Glipizide is also known as glibenclamide. Gliclazide and gliquidone are second-generation sulfonylureas available outside the United States. Overdoses with any of these drugs can cause hypoglycemia. Some trade names are given in parentheses.

and oral hypoglycemic agents. The thiazolidinediones (TZDs), biguanides, α-glucosidase inhibitors, glistens, and bromocriptine mesylate (Cycloset™) are oral antidiabetic agents. Exenatide, liraglutide, and pramlintide are injectable antidiabetic agents. As discussed later, many drugs not used in the treatment of diabetes can also amplify the glucose-lowering activity of oral hypoglycemic agents, and a complete medication history can be critical in the diagnosis of hypoglycemia.

Sulfonylureas. After insulin, these are the most common cause of hypoglycemia [111] (Tables 106.2 and 106.3). Sulfonylureas reduce serum glucose by increasing insulin secretion, inhibiting glycogenolysis and gluconeogenesis, and enhancing the response of target tissues to the effects of insulin [112]. Severe hypoglycemia is not common with appropriate administration of these drugs [113], but it can be observed in several contexts [114]. In all age groups, the condition is most often observed in the context of decreased carbohydrate intake. Maternal treatment of diabetes with glyburide can lead to postpartum hypoglycemia in neonates [115]. In patients between the ages of 11 and 30 years, perhaps two-thirds of hypoglycemic comas are due to sulfonylurea agents [41]. Half of these cases are suicide attempts [111]. In patients with type 2 diabetes older than 60 years, sulfonylurea-induced hypoglycemia is a frequent complication [114,116].

Liver disease decreases the clearance of tolbutamide, acetohexamide, tolazamide, glipizide, glyburide, and glimepiride (Table 106.2). Metabolites of sulfonylureas are excreted in urine with one exception; 50% of glyburide metabolites are excreted in bile. Accordingly, sulfonylurea-induced hypoglycemia is often observed in older individuals in the setting of acute or chronic starvation superimposed on mild to moderate liver or renal failure.

The half-life of some sulfonylureas is >24 hours and the duration of action is often even longer (Table 106.1). Hepatic and renal insufficiency can extend their half-lives. Patients with sulfonylurea-induced hypoglycemia should therefore be hospitalized after initial resuscitation with glucose. They require continued treatment with oral and intravenous glucose for a minimum of 18 to 24 hours.

When oral agent overdosage is suspected, serum and urine should be screened for sulfonylurea compounds. Sulfonylurea drugs circulate bound to proteins, and drugs of several classes can displace sulfonylureas and enhance their hypoglycemic effect (Table 106.3). The constellation of insulin concentration ≥3.9 μU per mL, C-peptide ≥1.4 ng per mL, and glucose <49 mg per dL may be helpful in diagnosing sulfonylurea-induced hypoglycemia [40].

Repaglinide and Nateglinide. Repaglinide (Prandin™) and nateglinide (Starlix™) belong to a different class of oral hypoglycemic agents (Table 106.1). Like the sulfonylureas, they increase endogenous insulin secretion but do so by a different mechanism. They appear to be associated with fewer episodes of hypoglycemia than are sulfonylureas. Both are rapidly eliminated. Surreptitious use of repaglinide has been reported [117].

Antidiabetic Agents. Biguanides, when given as monotherapy, induce hypoglycemia much less often than do sulfonylureas [118,119], probably by inhibiting gluconeogenesis. Metformin is the only biguanide currently available in the United States. It is also available in combination with the oral hypoglycemic agents glyburide (Glucovance™), glipizide (Metaglip™), and repaglinide (PrandiMet™); overdosage with these combination drugs can cause severe hypoglycemia. Thiazolidinediones and gliptins are also available in fixed ratio combinations with metformin; some of these have been associated with hypoglycemia.

Drugs of the thiazolidinedione class, including pioglitazone (Actos™) and rosiglitazone (Avandia™) in the United States, do not cause hypoglycemia when used as monotherapy but can potentiate hypoglycemia caused by insulin or sulfonylureas. They act by increasing insulin sensitivity.

Acarbose (Precose™) and miglitol (Glyset™) are α-glucosidase inhibitors that inhibit the digestion of complex carbohydrates; they have not been reported to cause hypoglycemia when used as monotherapy. Patients treated with insulin or sulfonylureas in addition to acarbose who experience hypoglycemia may not respond to the oral administration of complex sugars, but should respond to monomeric glucose.

TABLE 106.3

DRUGS AND TOXINS ASSOCIATED WITH HYPOGLYCEMIA

Agents that increase circulating insulin	Agents that impair gluconeogenesis	Uncertain or other mechanisms of action	
Direct stimulants of insulin secretion	*Hepatotoxins*	ACE inhibitors	Haloperidol [223]
Oral hypoglycemic agents (Table 106.2)	Acetaminophen (Tylenol™, Tempra™)	Acetazolamide (Diamox™)	Halothane
β_2-Adrenergic agonists (e.g., Albuterol™ [225])	Propoxyphene (Darvon™)	Aspirin	Herbal extracts
Calcium	Amanitotoxin	Aluminum hydroxide (Dialume™)	Imatinib (Gleevec™) [224]
Chloroquine (Aralen™)	*Inhibition of gluconeogenesis*	Anabolic steroids	Indomethacin
Cibenzoline	Akee fruit	Azapropazone	Interferon-α
Disopyramide (Norpace™)	Ethanol	Chlorpromazine (Thorazine™)	Isoxsuprine
Quinidine	Metformin	Cimetidine	Lidocaine
Quinine	Metoprolol (Lopressor™)	Ciprofloxacin, gatifloxacin, clinafloxacin	Lithium
Ritodrine (Yutopar™)	Nadolol (Corgard™)	Clofibrate	Mefloquine
Terbutaline	Phenformin	Dandelions [217]	Nefazodone
Trimethoprim/sulfamethoxazole (Bactrim™) [141,142]	Pindolol (Visken™)	Dexmedetomidine [218]	NSAIDs
Destruction of β cells with insulin release	Propranolol (Inderal™)	Diphenhydramine	Orphenadrine
Pentamidine (Pentam™)		Doxepin (Sinequan™, Adapin™)	Oxytetracycline
Streptozotocin		"Ecstasy" (MDMA) [219]	Para-aminobenzoic acid
Agents that enhance the action of oral agents		Enflurane Formestane	Para-aminosalicylic acid
Clarithromycin [226]		Ethylenediaminetetraacetic acid (Versene™)	Perhexiline
Imipramine (Tofranil™)		Etanercept [220,221]	Phenytoin (Dilantin™)
NSAIDs		Etomidate [222]	Ranitidine (Zantac™)
Phenylbutazone (Butazolidin™)		Fenoterol	Salicylates
Salicylates		Fluoxetine	Selegiline
Sulfonamides			Sulfadiazine
Warfarin (Coumadin™)			Sulfisoxazole (Gantrisin™)
			Valproate

Notes: A sampling of common trade names is shown in parentheses; the enumeration of trade names is not exhaustive. Data for some listed agents is very limited or anecdotal or involved treatment with more than one drug. Drugs for which better documentation is available are indicated in bold italic.
ACE, angiotensin-converting enzyme; MDMA, methylenedioxymethamphetamine; NSAIDs, nonsteroid anti-inflammatory drugs.
Adapted from Seltzer [111], Marks and Teale [29], and Murad et al. [124].

Exenatide (Byetta™) and liraglutide (Victoza™) are injectable mimetics of gut incretins [120,121]. They augment glucose-dependent insulin secretion and reduce postprandial glucagon secretion. When given with a sulfonylurea, they can cause hypoglycemia. Gliptins are inhibitors of the enzyme dipeptidyl peptidase-4. They inhibit the degradation of endogenous gut incretins and have glucose lowering effects similar to those of exenatide. Drugs in this class include sitagliptin (Januvia™) and saxagliptin (Onglyza™). Pramlintide (Symlin™) is a mimetic of the islet hormone amylin [121]. It suppresses postmeal glucagon secretion and delays gastric emptying. It is targeted at controlling postmeal hyperglycemia in diabetic patients who are also taking insulin. Like exenatide, it has been associated with hypoglycemia.

Bromocriptine is an oral dopamine agonist that is used in the treatment of pituitary tumors and Parkinson's disease. A micronized formulation (Cycloset™) is approved for treating type 2 diabetes [122]. Its mechanism of action is unclear. It has not been reported to cause hypoglycemia, but experience with the drug is limited.

Medication Errors. Severe hypoglycemia can result from inadvertent substitution of an oral hypoglycemic agent for a different medication. Medication errors due to phonetic similarity in name are exemplified by cases in which acetazolamide (Diamox™) has been prescribed but acetohexamide (Dymelor™) inadvertently dispensed [111,123]. Examples of such substitution errors are listed in Table 106.4.

Other Drugs and Poisons That Cause Hypoglycemia

Hundreds of drugs and toxins have been reported to cause or predispose to hypoglycemia (Table 106.3). For some, like ethanol, the association is well documented and the mechanism well understood. For most, however, the evidence supporting an association is poor and the mechanism of action is unknown. Some are based only on a single case report. In some instances, drug–drug interactions may be amplifying the hypoglycemic

TABLE 106.4

MEDICATION ERRORS THAT CAN RESULT IN HYPOGLYCEMIA

Prescribed medication	Dispensed medication
Acetazolamide (Diamox)	Acetohexamide (Dymelor)
Chlorpromazine	Chlorpropamide
Chloroquine	Chlorpropamide
Dyazide	Dymelor
Dialume	Diabinese
Tolectin	Tolinase
Diamox	Diabinese

effect of concurrently administered oral hypoglycemic agents. In other instances, the data are contaminated by intercurrent sepsis or other disease. Few rechallenge data to support the association are available. An analysis of the quality of the evidence implicating many drugs as the cause of hypoglycemia is available [124]. Some drugs with stronger supporting evidence are indicated in Table 106.3.

Ethanol-Induced Hypoglycemia (Alcoholic Ketoacidosis)

Ethanol-induced hypoglycemia is most often observed in children and chronic alcohol abusers. The most common history is binge drinking in the setting of poor intake of other dietary carbohydrates. Patients usually present in a stuporous or comatose state; nausea, vomiting, and abdominal pain are common. Ethanol concentration is typically low, and alcoholic hypoglycemia can occur up to 30 hours after the ingestion of alcoholic beverages. Blood glucose as low as 5 mg per dL has been recorded. Ketonuria and ketonemia are frequently present and reflect the appropriately low circulating insulin concentration [125].

Ethanol causes hypoglycemia by suppressing hepatic gluconeogenesis. Glycogenolysis is not affected. When ethanol is oxidized to acetaldehyde and acetate, NAD^+ is reduced to NADH. The reduced NAD^+:NADH ratio produces an unfavorable intracellular environment for the oxidation of substrates of gluconeogenesis such as lactate and glutamate to pyruvate and α-ketoglutarate, respectively (Fig. 106.1). As a result, intracellular levels of pyruvate are below the Michaelis constant (Km) of pyruvate carboxylase, one of the rate-limiting steps in gluconeogenesis. Ethanol also inhibits hepatic uptake of the gluconeogenic precursors glycerol, alanine, and lactate and inhibits the release of alanine from muscle [126].

Management consists of rehydration with intravenous fluids and glucose to correct hypoglycemia. Parenteral thiamine (100 mg) should be given to prevent Wernicke's encephalopathy. Treatment with glucose and fluids rapidly reverses the condition and sodium bicarbonate is generally unnecessary.

β-Adrenergic Receptor Antagonists

The nonselective beta-blockers propranolol, pindolol, and nadolol reportedly predispose to hypoglycemia in diverse clinical settings. Both diabetic and nondiabetic patients undergoing hemodialysis are susceptible. Neonates may also have hypoglycemia during their first 24 hours of life as a result of propranolol treatment of the mother for cardiac arrhythmias, hypertension, or thyrotoxicosis. Hypoglycemia in infants treated with propranolol for cyanotic heart disease or neonatal thyrotoxicosis has also been reported. These drugs increase the risk of hypoglycemia in patients who are undernourished or who have liver disease [126] and occasionally when administered prior to cardiac surgery [111,127].

Antiarrhythmic Agents

Quinidine can enhance insulin secretion and produce hypoglycemia in ill, fasting patients [128]. Hypoglycemia has been reported in patients treated with disopyramide, an antiarrhythmic agent with pharmacologic properties similar to those of quinidine [129,130]. In neither case is supporting evidence strong. The investigational antiarrhythmic cibenzoline is more convincingly associated with hypoglycemia [131].

Antibiotics

There is evidence [124] that pentamidine, used to treat *Pneumocystis carinii* infection, can be toxic to pancreatic β cells, causing transient hypoglycemia due to the release of stored insulin. It eventually results in diabetes in some patients [111]. Similarly, quinine, chemically related to quinidine, is known to elevate insulin concentrations in patients being treated for malaria [132,133]. Those with cerebral malaria are most prone to hypoglycemia, possibly due to the high intake of glucose by malarial parasites, coupled with the increased insulin release. Quinine may rarely cause hypoglycemia in normal individuals [134].

Gatifloxacin (Tequin™) [135–138], levofloxacin (Levaquin™) [135], ciprofloxacin (Cipro™) [139,140], and other fluoroquinolones reportedly cause hypoglycemia, particularly when administered to patients who are also receiving sulfonylureas. Gatifloxacin may carry the highest risk of hypoglycemia, yet paradoxically some patients treated with this drug also experience new onset of hyperglycemia [135]. Trimethoprim/sulfamethoxazole has also been reported to cause hyperinsulinemic hypoglycemia in the setting of malnutrition and infection, renal failure [141], and oral hypoglycemic therapy [142].

Salicylates

Salicylate intoxication reportedly causes hypoglycemia occasionally in children but only very rarely in adults [111,143]. In children, it may be a component of aspirin-associated Reye's syndrome [144]. The frequency of salicylate-induced hypoglycemia is difficult to ascertain due to intercurrent acidosis and renal or hepatic impairment in many cases of intoxication.

Angiotensin-Converting Enzyme Inhibitors

Cases of hypoglycemia associated with angiotensin-converting enzyme inhibitors have been reported in persons with both types 1 and 2 diabetes [145–148], but the quality of the evidence is low [124]. No mechanism for the effect has been identified, and a retrospective analysis of nearly 14,000 persons with diabetes failed to identify an increased risk of hypoglycemia associated with this class of drugs [149].

Poisons

Several plant substances can cause hypoglycemia. Hypoglycin A toxin is found in akee fruit, a staple of the Jamaican diet. The ripe fruit is edible, but immature fruit causes vomiting a few days after ingestion. Affected patients have severe hypoglycemia due to inhibition of hepatic gluconeogenesis by hypoglycin [150]. Amanita toxins produced by the mushroom *Amanita phalloides* are inhibitors of RNA polymerase and cause hepatocellular necrosis. Fatal hypoglycemia can result from the ensuing complete depletion of hepatic glycogen and decreased capacity for gluconeogenesis [126].

Hypoglycemia Associated with Deficiencies in Counterregulatory Hormones

Glucocorticoid insufficiency can cause hypoglycemia in children by decreasing glycogenolysis and gluconeogenesis. In adults, it causes hypoglycemia uncommonly [151]. Malnutrition may contribute to the development of hypoglycemia in these cases. Patients with panhypopituitarism are prone to hypoglycemia and have increased sensitivity to insulin [151]. Although catecholamines play a significant role in preventing and reversing hypoglycemia, their absence does not commonly predispose to hypoglycemia. Adrenalectomized patients with sympathetic denervation due to spinal cord transection maintain euglycemia. Glucagon deficiency may very rarely cause hypoglycemia.

Fasting Hypoglycemia Due to Inadequate Production of Endogenous Glucose

Liver Damage

About 90% of gluconeogenesis occurs in the liver. Hepatic injury can cause hypoglycemia but only when the insult is very severe; only about 20% of normal liver biosynthetic capability is needed to maintain normal glucose homeostasis [152]. Hypoglycemia seldom occurs in the setting of isolated, limited hepatic failure and is not the cause of hepatic coma [126]. Hypoglycemia due to toxic or infectious hepatitis is rare but does occur when the disorder is fulminant. Hepatotoxins that can impair gluconeogenesis and cause hypoglycemia include carbon tetrachloride, the *A. phalloides* mushroom toxin, and urethane. Drugs that cause hypoglycemia by inducing hepatocellular necrosis include acetaminophen, isoniazid, sodium valproate, methyldopa, tetracycline, and halothane [126]. Neither tests of hepatocellular integrity (e.g., transaminases) nor tests of hepatic function (e.g., bilirubin concentration) nor the presence of structural damage (e.g., cirrhosis, chronic active hepatitis, and metastatic liver disease) correlate well with the capability of the liver to maintain normoglycemia.

Congestive heart failure (CHF) from any cause can lead to hepatic congestion and hypoglycemia in adults and children. Patients with this syndrome usually have severe failure with cardiac cachexia, malnutrition, and muscle wasting. The mechanism by which CHF leads to hypoglycemia is not completely understood. Changes in hepatic blood flow may alter the delivery of gluconeogenic precursors or changes in intracellular redox state may decrease the gluconeogenic capacity of the hepatocyte. Hypoglycemia in this setting resolves with successful treatment of the CHF [126].

Renal Damage

Some patients with diabetes develop improved glucose tolerance with the onset of renal failure. A decrease in insulin requirements and more frequent episodes of hypoglycemia may also occur [153]. There is no correlation between degree of renal failure and severity of hypoglycemia in these patients, and the underlying mechanisms are not completely understood. Investigators variously implicate delayed insulin clearance, deficiencies in the delivery of gluconeogenic substrate [151], and hepatic insufficiency secondary to uremia [154].

Symptomatic hypoglycemia occurs in many diabetic patients receiving either hemodialysis or ambulatory peritoneal dialysis [155,156]. Any dialysis patient who experiences a change in mental status should be evaluated for hypoglycemia. The symptoms and signs of neuroglycopenia resemble those of the dialysis disequilibrium syndrome commonly induced by fluid shifts. These include fatigue, confusion, lethargy, and even coma. Postdialysis hypoglycemia in diabetic patients, if prolonged, can be fatal [157].

Spontaneous fasting hypoglycemia has also been reported to occur in nondiabetic patients with end-stage renal disease [158–160]. It is not clear, however, whether these rare cases represent a distinct clinical entity [161] or instances of renal failure enhancing intercurrent disorders that predispose to hypoglycemia [162]. These might include drug ingestion, liver disease, and adrenal or pituitary insufficiency.

Fasting Hypoglycemia Due to the Unavailability of Gluconeogenic Substrate

Substrate deficiency leads to hypoglycemia in ketotic hypoglycemia of childhood [163]. Patients with this condition, a variant of the normal response to starvation, are usually diagnosed between 18 months and 5 years of age. The hallmark of the condition is a low basal concentration of the gluconeogenic precursor alanine, and the hypoglycemia can be corrected with either glucose or alanine.

Other Causes of Hypoglycemia

Sepsis

Sepsis has occasionally been implicated as a cause of hypoglycemia [164–167]. Shock and liver failure were intercurrent problems in some cases [165]. Under conditions of decreased hepatic reserve, the combination of circulatory failure and impairment of gluconeogenesis by endotoxin may lead to hypoglycemia. Septic hypoglycemic patients are often acidotic, and the fatality rate is high [164,165]. In one report, only 1 of 15 such patients survived 1 month after the onset of hypoglycemia and hypotension [165].

Congenital Disorders

The commonest cause of neonatal hypoglycemia is maternal diabetes [168]. Congenital enzyme deficiencies and other abnormalities in the function of specific enzymes typically produce hypoglycemia in the context of glycogen storage disease, impaired hepatic gluconeogenesis, or respiratory chain defects [169]. Mutations of the sulfonylurea receptor can also cause this disorder [55]. These uncommon conditions usually present as hypoglycemia in infancy, but they can rarely present as unexplained persistent hypoglycemia in a critically ill adult [70,170]. The pediatric disorders are reviewed elsewhere [52,53].

Exercise-Induced Hypoglycemia

Exercise-induced hyperinsulinemic hypoglycemia is an autosomal-dominant hyperinsulinemia syndrome [171]. The cause appears to be failure of β-cell–specific transcriptional silencing of a gene, monocarboxylate transporter 1, important in pyruvate stimulated insulin release [172].

LABORATORY DIAGNOSIS OF HYPOGLYCEMIA

Normal Blood Glucose Concentration

Normal plasma glucose is 60 to 120 mg per dL (3.3 to 6.7 mmol). Whole blood glucose concentrations are 15% to 20% lower. Fingerstick blood glucose determinations are performed on whole capillary blood, and most meters reflect this offset. Symptoms of hypoglycemia generally occur when plasma glucose is <50 mg per dL (2.8 mmol) or the whole blood glucose concentration is <40 mg per dL (2.2 mmol). Calibrated hospital-quality glucose meter technology is accurate over a wide range of concentrations; values between 40 and 350 mg per dL generally agree well with values obtained using standard laboratory methods. Glucose meters for home use can be less accurate [173]. Because fingerstick blood glucose determinations can be less accurate at the lower end of their scale, they may require confirmation by a clinical laboratory. Interpretation of fingerstick glucose should take into account the clinical context, symptoms, and response to glucose administration. They can be misleading in patients who are hypoperfused [174,175], in shock [176], or undergoing cardiopulmonary resuscitation [177]. Certain meter technologies are inaccurate in the presence of various interfering substances [178,179].

There are several physiologic exceptions to guideline values for diagnosing hypoglycemia in very ill patients. After about 48 hours of starvation, many individuals, particularly women, have a plasma glucose concentration <50 mg per dL (2.8 mmol). After 72 hours of fasting, the plasma glucose may approach 40 mg per dL (2.2 mmol). Starved individuals are nonetheless asymptomatic, do not fulfill Whipple's triad, and are not physiologically or clinically hypoglycemic. The absence of symptoms is due to the shift to ketones for CNS metabolism. Comparably low plasma glucose, 60 mg per dL (3.3 mmol) or less, is also encountered in pregnancy. Again, there are no symptoms of hypoglycemia per se in these cases. Finally, rare individuals may have an anomalously low "set point" for blood glucose concentration, and such individuals appear asymptomatic in the face of persistent glycemia in the range of 35 to 45 mg per dL [180].

Spurious Hypoglycemia

This term applies to glucose concentrations that are reported to be low but come from a normoglycemic patient. This most commonly occurs as a result of storing blood samples at room temperature for long periods before laboratory analysis. As a result of anaerobic glycolysis by blood elements, the actual glucose concentration in the test tube may decline. The effect is enhanced if large numbers of white blood cells are present in the sample as a result of severe leukocytosis or leukemia [181].

Spurious Hyperglycemia Leading to Insulin Overdose

Falsely elevated glucose readings can lead to inappropriate insulin administration and hypoglycemia. The commonest cause of spurious hyperglycemia in the ICU is measurement of glucose in blood obtained from an extremity into which glucose is being infused. An uncommon cause of hypoglycemia in the ICU results from a "drug–device interaction" affecting patients receiving parenteral nutrition products containing maltose or galactose. These products cause certain monitoring systems to give falsely elevated glucose readings leading to inappropriate insulin treatment [178].

Testing for Ketonuria

Urinary ketone testing can facilitate the differential diagnosis of hypoglycemia. Normally, fasting is associated with low circulating insulin that promotes gluconeogenesis and lipolysis. Hypoglycemia in association with ketonuria enhances the likelihood that the cause is not excess insulin.

Other Studies

In addition to glucose and urinary ketones, additional tests should be ordered as appropriate to the patient's underlying medical condition. In general, these should always include studies of hepatic and renal function. Additional serum and plasma samples from any comatose, hypoglycemic patient, when they are first seen, should be obtained. This permits assays for medications, IRI/glucose ratios, proinsulin, and C-peptide to be performed later, if indicated. Testing for oral hypoglycemic agents requires sophisticated laboratory methods, and it is recommended that laboratory personnel be consulted to ensure that appropriate specimens (urine, blood, or both) are ordered. A cosyntropin (Cortrosyn^{TM}) test should be performed if adrenal insufficiency is suspected.

MANAGEMENT OF HYPOGLYCEMIA

Initial Management with Glucose

When symptomatic hypoglycemia is suspected, remember Whipple's triad. After fingerstick glucose determination, the treatment is glucose administration, and the diagnostic outcome is resolution of symptoms. It is important to document the presence of hypoglycemia before giving glucose. Most patients with depressed mental status are not hypoglycemic [182] (Table 106.5).

The practice of giving intravenous glucose empirically assumes that it could be useful and is always harmless [183]. This belief has been called into question. In cases of stroke, in particular ischemic stroke, hyperglycemia may be predictive of poor outcome [184,185], and empiric use of hypertonic dextrose has been discouraged by many authors [177,182,186,187]. In addition, even in those cases in which empiric glucose appears to be resuscitative, there is no way to back-calculate what might have been the antecedent glucose concentration [188]. In the hospital, treatment of hypoglycemia is with intravenous D-glucose (dextrose) if a patient is unresponsive or might aspirate, but if a patient is alert and cooperative, oral carbohydrate (e.g., sucrose in orange juice or glucose tablets or gel) is preferable.

In general, all comatose patients, including trauma patients, should undergo fingerstick glucose determination, and the threshold for administration of intravenous glucose in addition to standard life-support measures should be low. Treatment with glucose is lifesaving in the presence of hypoglycemic coma. Early responders recognize that altered mental status due to hypoglycemia is sometimes the root cause of an accident [189].

The initial treatment of hypoglycemia in the patient with stupor or coma has traditionally consisted of the intravenous injection of 50 mL of 50% dextrose in water ($D_{50}W$) over 3 to 5 minutes. Care must be taken to avoid subcutaneous extravasation; the solution is hypertonic and can cause local tissue damage and severe pain. Alternatively, 10% dextrose delivered in 5 g (50 mL) aliquots can be equally efficacious and results in lower posttreatment blood glucose levels [190]. If hypoglycemia is present, treatment with glucose usually leads to improved mental status within minutes. It is difficult, however, to predict the magnitude of the glucose response to a bolus of intravenous glucose [187], and elderly patients and patients with very prolonged hypoglycemia may have a delayed response.

Subsequent Management

Glucose

The prompt improvement that usually occurs in hypoglycemic patients treated with intravenous glucose can be misleading. When hypoglycemia occurs in a diabetic patient taking insulin, no additional treatment may be needed, but there are many other causes of hypoglycemia. The initial bolus of glucose treats the symptoms of hypoglycemia but *not their cause*. The most common error in the management of hypoglycemia is inadequate treatment leading to recurrence of symptoms.

After the first bolus of $D_{50}W$, an infusion of D_5W or $D_{10}W$ glucose should be started in any patient whose hypoglycemic episode is not clearly due simply to excess short- or intermediate-acting insulin. The choice of D_5W or $D_{10}W$ glucose depends on the severity of the initial hypoglycemia. This infusion allows the critical care physician to evaluate the cause

TABLE 106.5

HYPOGLYCEMIA: DIAGNOSIS, MANAGEMENT, EVIDENCE

Recommendation	Comments
Suspect hypoglycemia in all cases of altered mental status	Hypoglycemia is a very common reversible cause of altered mental status.
Be aware that intensive therapy with insulin infusions carries a risk of hypoglycemia	Attempting to lower blood glucose in the ICU to levels <110 mg/dL is frequently associated with hypoglycemia [35–39]. (See Chapter 100 on Diabetes Management.)
Always determine blood glucose concentration before administering glucose	Most patients with altered mental status are not hypoglycemic [182] and empiric glucose administration should not be assumed to be completely risk free [177,182,184–186].
Consider 10% dextrose rather than 50% dextrose	D_{10} W can be as efficacious as D_{50} W while lessening the risk of subsequent hyperglycemia [190].
Fingerstick glucose concentrations can at times be misleading	Measurements from an extremity in which glucose is being infused or in the setting of shock [176], CPR [177], and parenteral nutrition products containing maltose or galactose [227] may be inaccurate.
Suspect overdose of an antidiabetic medication when unexplained hypoglycemia is encountered in the ICU	Medication errors are common in hospitals [228]. Hypoglycemia is commonly caused by overdosage with exogenous insulin and overdosage with oral hypoglycemic agents that enhance endogenous insulin secretion.
If hypoglycemia is thought to be due to a drug not used to treat diabetes, evaluate the case thoughtfully	Many medications reportedly cause hypoglycemia (Table 106.3), but evidence supporting the association is often poor [124]. Hypoglycemia may be due to a drug–drug interaction, and discontinuation of a suspect medication may not always be appropriate.
When treating refractory hypoglycemia always exclude adrenal insufficiency	Cortisol is an important glucose-counterregulatory hormone and renal insufficiency predisposes to hypoglycemia in persons being treated for diabetes.
The role of continuous glucose monitoring in the ICU is promising but still investigational	Continuous monitoring of glucose concentration holds out the promise of enhanced detection and reduced frequency of hypoglycemia in the ICU setting. How this technology will affect glycemic control [215] or the management of neonatal hypoglycemia [214] remains to be determined, and studies to validate its use in the setting of intercurrent illness are at an early stage [216].

Key elements in the diagnosis and management of hypoglycemia in the intensive care unit (ICU). CPR, cardiopulmonary resuscitation.

of the hypoglycemic episode while protecting the patient from recurrence. An appropriate target glucose concentration is 100 mg per dL (5.6 mM). It is advisable not to overtreat with glucose, especially in the case of oral hypoglycemic agent poisoning. Extremely high serum glucose may stimulate endogenous insulin secretion, causing rebound hyperinsulinemia and recurrent hypoglycemia [191].

Hypoglycemia Due to Long-Acting Insulin

If long-acting insulin (Table 106.1) might have caused the hypoglycemic episode, continuation of the glucose infusion, fingerstick blood glucose testing, and periodic adjustment of the infusion rate may be required. The duration of therapy depends on the particular insulin preparation and the dose taken. Massive insulin overdose (2,500 units of NPH) has been associated with persistent hypoglycemia for up to 6 days [189].

Hypoglycemia Due to Sulfonylureas

When the cause of hypoglycemia is sulfonylurea ingestion (Table 106.2), the patient should usually be admitted to hospital because of the prolonged duration of action of most members of this class of drugs. Efforts to prevent drug absorption and increase elimination should be considered. Activated charcoal adsorbs sulfonylureas, and urinary alkalinization may enhance excretion [192,193]. Charcoal hemoperfusion is probably not indicated, except in the setting of renal failure and massive overdose [194]. Continuous intravenous glucose is mandatory. Oral carbohydrate should be provided if the patient can eat. It is particularly important that the glucose infusion be continued while the patient recovering from a sulfonylurea overdose is asleep. Cases of persistent sulfonylurea-induced hypoglycemia requiring up to 27 days of intravenous glucose have been reported [195]. The typical patient with this condition requires 2 to 3 days of intravenous glucose therapy [111,196]. As discussed later, octreotide and diazoxide may be helpful adjuvant therapies in some cases.

Refractory Hypoglycemia

If the history and physical examination do not immediately establish the underlying cause of hypoglycemia, continuation of the infusion and glycemia monitoring are required. Persistent severe hypoglycemia requires intensive monitoring. Blood glucose should be measured every 1 to 3 hours and the serum glucose concentration maintained at a target level of 100 mg per dL (5.6 mmol per L). Diagnostic studies can be obtained as appropriate during continuous glucose infusion.

Intravenous glucose should continue until normoglycemia is achieved. To determine whether parenteral glucose is no longer needed, the infusion should be discontinued and blood glucose concentration measured every 15 minutes. If blood glucose falls to <50 mg per dL or if the patient becomes symptomatic, glucose infusion is resumed. Depending on the etiology of the hypoglycemia, parenteral glucose infusion may be required for many days and the use of additional drugs should be considered (see below). When hypoglycemia is due to impaired gluconeogenesis in the setting of liver disease, renal disease, or CHF, only treatment of the underlying condition will prevent recurrence. When a tumor is the course of hypoglycemia, surgery is the definitive therapy.

Drugs Other Than Glucose in the Management of Hypoglycemia

Most cases of hypoglycemia in the ICU can be treated with glucose alone. When recurrent severe hypoglycemia and volume management are problems, intensivists may consider the addition of adjunctive therapies. Particularly when hypoglycemia is due to an insulinoma, nesidioblastosis, or other tumor, it may be necessary to supplement the glucose infusion with drugs that inhibit insulin secretion.

Glucocorticoids

Parenteral adrenocortical steroids can increase gluconeogenic substrates and inhibit insulin action in the periphery. Hydrocortisone sodium succinate can be given at a dose of 100 mg per L of glucose infused. This therapy is beneficial in patients whose hypoglycemia is in the context of adrenocortical insufficiency; one case report describes utility in hemangiopericytoma-associated hypoglycemia [96]. It is not helpful in sulfonylurea poisoning [197].

Octreotide (Sandostatin™)

Somatostatin is produced in pancreatic islet delta cells and inhibits insulin secretion. The long-acting analog octreotide can inhibit sulfonylurea-induced insulin secretion, and it has been used as supplemental therapy for insulinomas [198], oral agent-induced hypoglycemia [199–205], and quinine-induced hypoglycemia in malaria [133]. The dose is 1 to 2 units per kg every 8 hours [202].

Diazoxide (Hyperstat™)

Diazoxide is a benzothiadiazine nondiuretic antihypertensive agent that blocks the secretion of insulin from both normal and neoplastic β cells. To treat hypoglycemia, diazoxide is infused at a dose of 300 mg (1 to 3 mg per kg in children) in D_5W over 30 minutes every 4 hours, or as a constant infusion of 1 mg per kg per hour. It has been reported to be effective in reversing severe, refractory hypoglycemia due to sulfonylurea poisoning [197] and neonatal hyperinsulinemic hypoglycemia due to certain gene mutations [206].

Glucagon

The primary action of exogenous glucagon in the treatment of hypoglycemia is the promotion of glycogenolysis. It is most effective in patients with ample liver glycogen stores. Glucagon is a useful drug for out-of-hospital treatment of hypoglycemia due to excess insulin in known diabetic patients. It is good practice to teach family members of diabetic patients to administer parenteral glucagon. In the intensive care setting, however, there is seldom a need to administer glucagon unless vascular access cannot be maintained. In addition, glucagon can stimulate insulin secretion and promote recurrent hypoglycemia [207]. It has also been associated with hypoglycemia when used as premedication for endoscopy [208].

Rapamycin

In a single case report, rapamycin was effective in controlling intractable hypoglycemia in a patient with metastatic insulinoma [209]. The drug was thought to act both by reducing the malignant β-cell proliferation and by inhibiting insulin production.

PREVENTION OF HYPOGLYCEMIA IN THE ICU

With reported prevalence rates of 5% and higher [1–3], prevention of hypoglycemia is central to the metabolic management of the ICU patient. In general, oral antidiabetic agents like sulfonylureas should be discontinued in seriously ill patients [210]. Insulin infusions require meticulous management. Several studies have demonstrated that hypoglycemia can be avoided while achieving glycemic control by using structured insulin orders and management algorithms [211,212]. Such protocols are discussed in detail in Chapter 100. Up to a third of patients admitted to an emergency department with severe hypoglycemia may experience recurrent hypoglycemia in the hospital [213]. Strategies for preventing recurrent hypoglycemia have been outlined earlier.

Finally, it is becoming clear that promising new technology for continuous monitoring of glucose concentration has the potential to prevent hypoglycemia in ICU. Initial reports suggest that this technology enhances the detection of hypoglycemia in neonates [214] and reduces the frequency of hypoglycemic events in the adult ICU [215,216]. How this technology will affect glycemic control [215] or the management of neonatal hypoglycemia [214] or ICU outcomes remains to be determined but is potentially transformative.

CONCLUSION

Hypoglycemia is a serious problem in all hospitalized patients and a predictor of mortality in the critically ill [7,8]. It must be considered in all cases of stupor and coma. Diagnosis is based on Whipple's triad, and evaluation should take no more than a few minutes. After initial therapy with glucose, remember that only the symptoms and not the cause have been treated. The most common cause of hypoglycemia is insulin overdosage in individuals with diabetes; in the ICU, this is often a complication of strict glucose control protocols. Hypoglycemia due to intercurrent medical conditions requires correction of the underlying disorder. Patients with sulfonylurea- or insulinoma-induced hypoglycemia may require aggressive treatment of hypoglycemia with parenteral glucose for many days.

References

1. Van den Berghe G, Wouters P, Weekers F, et al: Intensive insulin therapy in critically ill patients. *N Engl J Med* 345:1359, 2001.
2. Vriesendorp TM, van Santen S, DeVries JH, et al: Predisposing factors for hypoglycemia in the intensive care unit. *Crit Care Med* 34:96, 2006.
3. Mechanick JI, Handelsman Y, Bloomgarden ZT: Hypoglycemia in the intensive care unit. *Curr Opin Clin Nutr Metab Care* 10:193, 2007.
4. Mendoza A, Kim YN, Chernoff A: Hypoglycemia in hospitalized adult patients without diabetes. *Endocr Pract* 11:91, 2005.
5. Kagansky N, Levy S, Rimon E, et al: Hypoglycemia as a predictor of mortality in hospitalized elderly patients. *Arch Intern Med* 163:1825, 2003.
6. Mortensen EM, Garcia S, Leykum L, et al: Association of hypoglycemia with mortality for subjects hospitalized with pneumonia. *Am J Med Sci* 339:239, 2010.
7. Egi M, Bellomo R, Stachowski E, et al: Hypoglycemia and outcome in critically ill patients. *Mayo Clin Proc* 85:217, 2010.
8. Hermanides J, Bosman RJ, Vriesendorp TM, et al: Hypoglycemia is associated with intensive care unit mortality. *Crit Care Med* 38:1430, 2010.
9. Whipple AO: The surgical therapy of hyperinsulinism. *J Int Chirurgie* 3:237, 1938.

10. Cryer PE: Symptoms of hypoglycemia, thresholds for their occurrence, and hypoglycemia unawareness. *Endocrinol Metab Clin North Am* 28:495, 1999.
11. Margulescu AD, Sisu RC, Cinteza M, et al: Noncardiogenic acute pulmonary edema due to severe hypoglycemia—an old but ignored cause. *Am J Emerg Med* 26:839, 2008.
12. Navarro-Gutierrez S, Gonzalez-Martinez F, Fernandez-Perez MT, et al: Bradycardia related to hypoglycaemia. *Eur J Emerg Med* 10:331, 2003.
13. Chelliah YR: Ventricular arrhythmias associated with hypoglycaemia. *Anaesth Intensive Care* 28:698, 2000.
14. Odeh M, Oliven A, Bassan H: Transient atrial fibrillation precipitated by hypoglycemia. *Ann Emerg Med* 19:565, 1990.
15. Shimada R, Nakashima T, Nunoi K, et al: Arrhythmia during insulin-induced hypoglycemia in a diabetic patient. *Arch Intern Med* 144:1068, 1984.
16. Lindstrom T, Jorfeldt L, Tegler L, et al: Hypoglycaemia and cardiac arrhythmias in patients with type 2 diabetes mellitus. *Diabet Med* 9:536, 1992.
17. Marques JL, George E, Peacey SR, et al: Altered ventricular repolarization during hypoglycaemia in patients with diabetes. *Diabet Med* 14:648, 1997.
18. Pollock G, Brady WJ Jr, Hargarten S, et al: Hypoglycemia manifested by sinus bradycardia: a report of three cases. *Acad Emerg Med* 3:700, 1996.
19. Hillson RM: Hypoglycemia and hypothermia. *Diabetes Care* 6:211, 1983.
20. Kedes LH, Field JB: Hypothermia: a clue to the diagnosis of hypoglycemia. *N Engl J Med* 271:785, 1964.
21. Passias TC, Meneilly GS, Mekjavic IB: Effect of hypoglycemia on thermoregulatory responses. *J Appl Physiol* 80:1021, 1996.
22. Arem R, Zoghbi W: Insulin overdose in eight patients: insulin pharmacokinetics and review of the literature. *Medicine (Baltimore)* 64:323, 1985.
23. Matsumura M, Nakashima A, Tofuku Y: Electrolyte disorders following massive insulin overdose in a patient with type 2 diabetes. *Intern Med* 39:55, 2000.
24. Butler PC, Rizza RA: Regulation of carbohydrate metabolism and response to hypoglycemia. *Endocrinol Metab Clin North Am* 18:1, 1989.
25. Brun JF, Fedou C, Mercier J: Postprandial reactive hypoglycemia. *Diabetes Metab* 26:337, 2000.
26. Hofeldt FD: Reactive hypoglycemia. *Endocrinol Metab Clin North Am* 18:185, 1989.
27. Hojlund K, Hansen T, Lajer M, et al: A novel syndrome of autosomal-dominant hyperinsulinemic hypoglycemia linked to a mutation in the human insulin receptor gene. *Diabetes* 53:1592, 2004.
28. Taylor SI, Barbetti F, Accili D, et al: Syndromes of autoimmunity and hypoglycemia. Autoantibodies directed against insulin and its receptor. *Endocrinol Metab Clin North Am* 18:123, 1989.
29. Marks V, Teale JD: Drug-induced hypoglycemia. *Endocrinol Metab Clin North Am* 28:555, 1999.
30. Stapczynski JS, Haskell RJ: Duration of hypoglycemia and need for intravenous glucose following intentional overdoses of insulin. *Ann Emerg Med* 13:505, 1984.
31. Samuels MH, Eckel RH: Massive insulin overdose: detailed studies of free insulin levels and glucose requirements. *J Toxicol Clin Toxicol* 27:157, 1989.
32. Cryer PE: Hypoglycemia: still the limiting factor in the glycemic management of diabetes. *Endocr Pract* 14:750, 2008.
33. Cryer PE: Mechanisms of hypoglycemia-associated autonomic failure and its component syndromes in diabetes. *Diabetes* 54:3592, 2005.
34. Sauer P, Van Horn ER: Impact of intravenous insulin protocols on hypoglycemia, patient safety, and nursing workload. *DCCN—Dimensions of Critical Care Nursing* 28:95, 2009.
35. Finfer S, Chittock DR, Su SY, et al: Intensive versus conventional glucose control in critically ill patients. *N Engl J Med* 360:1283, 2009.
36. Annane D, Cariou A, Maxime V, et al: Corticosteroid treatment and intensive insulin therapy for septic shock in adults: a randomized controlled trial. *JAMA* 303:341, 2010.
37. Van den Berghe G, Wilmer A, Hermans G, et al: Intensive insulin therapy in the medical ICU. *N Engl J Med* 354:449, 2006.
38. Preiser JC, Devos P, Ruiz-Santana S, et al: A prospective randomised multicentre controlled trial on tight glucose control by intensive insulin therapy in adult intensive care units: the Glucontrol study. *Intensive Care Med* 35:1738, 2009.
39. Brunkhorst FM, Engel C, Bloos F, et al: Intensive insulin therapy and pentastarch resuscitation in severe sepsis. *N Engl J Med* 358:125, 2008.
40. DeWitt CR, Heard K, Waksman JC: Insulin and C-peptide levels in sulfonylurea-induced hypoglycemia: a systematic review. *J Med Toxicol* 3:107, 2007.
41. Klonoff DC, Barrett BJ, Nolte MS, et al: Hypoglycemia following inadvertent and factitious sulfonylurea overdosages. *Diab Care* 18:563, 1995.
42. Kao SL, Chan CL, Tan B, et al: An unusual outbreak of hypoglycemia. *N Engl J Med* 360:734, 2009.
43. Dalan R, Leow MK, George J, et al: Neuroglycopenia and adrenergic responses to hypoglycaemia: insights from a local epidemic of serendipitous massive overdose of glibenclamide. *Diabet Med* 26:105, 2009.
44. Mathur A, Gorden P, Libutti SK: Insulinoma. *Surg Clin North Am* 89:1105, 2009.
45. Furrer J, Hättenschwiler A, Komminoth P, et al: Carcinoid syndrome, acromegaly, and hypoglycemia due to an insulin-secreting neuroendocrine tumor of the liver. *J Clin Endocrinol Metab* 86:2227, 2001.
46. Seckl MJ, Mulholland PJ, Bishop AE, et al: Hypoglycemia due to an insulin-secreting small-cell carcinoma of the cervix. *N Engl J Med* 341:733, 1999.
47. Morgello S, Schwartz E, Horwith M, et al: Ectopic insulin production by a primary ovarian carcinoid. *Cancer* 61:800, 1988.
48. Shetty MR, Boghossian HM, Duffell D, et al: Tumor-induced hypoglycemia: a result of ectopic insulin production. *Cancer* 49:1920, 1982.
49. Uysal M, Temiz S, Gul N, et al: Hypoglycemia due to ectopic release of insulin from a paraganglioma. *Horm Res* 67:292, 2007.
50. Raffel A, Krausch MM, Anlauf M, et al: Diffuse nesidioblastosis as a cause of hyperinsulinemic hypoglycemia in adults: a diagnostic and therapeutic challenge. *Surgery* 141:179, 2007.
51. Kaczirek K, Niederle B: Nesidioblastosis: an old term and a new understanding. *World J Surg* 28:1227, 2004.
52. Sperling MA, Menon RK: Differential diagnosis and management of neonatal hypoglycemia. *Pediatr Clin North Am* 51:703, 2004.
53. Straussman S, Levitsky LL: Neonatal hypoglycemia. *Curr Opin Endocrinol Diabetes Obes* 17:20, 2010.
54. Thompson GB, Service FJ, Andrews JC, et al: Noninsulinoma pancreatogenous hypoglycemia syndrome: an update in 10 surgically treated patients. *Surgery* 128:937, 2000.
55. Magge SN, Shyng SL, MacMullen C, et al: Familial leucine-sensitive hypoglycemia of infancy due to a dominant mutation of the β-cell sulfonylurea receptor. *J Clin Endocrinol Metab* 89:4450, 2004.
56. Sperling MA, Menon RK: Hyperinsulinemic hypoglycemia of infancy—recent insights into ATP-sensitive potassium channels, sulfonylurea receptors, molecular mechanisms, and treatment. *Endocrinol Metab Clin North Am* 28:695, 1999.
57. Otonkoski T, Ämmälä C, Huopio H, et al: A point mutation inactivating the sulfonylurea receptor causes the severe form of persistent hyperinsulinemic hypoglycemia of infancy in Finland. *Diabetes* 48:408, 1999.
58. Alexander S, Ramadan D, Alkhayyat H, et al: Costello syndrome and hyperinsulinemic hypoglycemia. *Am J Med Genet A* 139:227, 2005.
59. Hussain K, Cosgrove KE, Shepherd RM, et al: Hyperinsulinemic hypoglycemia in Beckwith-Wiedemann syndrome due to defects in the function of pancreatic beta-cell adenosine triphosphate-sensitive potassium channels. *J Clin Endocrinol Metab* 90:4376, 2005.
60. Rinker RD, Friday K, Aydin F, et al: Adult nesidioblastosis—a case report and review of the literature. *Dig Dis Sci* 43:1784, 1998.
61. Anlauf M, Wieben D, Perren A, et al: Persistent hyperinsulinemic hypoglycemia in 15 adults with diffuse nesidioblastosis—diagnostic criteria, incidence, and characterization of β-cell changes. *Am J Surg Pathol* 29:524, 2005.
62. Klöppel G, Anlauf M, Raffel A, et al: Adult diffuse nesidioblastosis: genetically or environmentally induced? *Hum Pathol* 39:3, 2008.
63. Service GJ, Thompson GB, Service FJ, et al: Hyperinsulinemic hypoglycemia with nesidioblastosis after gastric-bypass surgery. *N Engl J Med* 353:249, 2005.
64. Patti ME, McMahon G, Mun EC, et al: Severe hypoglycaemia post-gastric bypass requiring partial pancreatectomy: evidence for inappropriate insulin secretion and pancreatic islet hyperplasia. *Diabetologia* 48:2236, 2005.
65. Meier JJ, Butler AE, Galasso R, et al: Hyperinsulinemic hypoglycemia after gastric bypass surgery is not accompanied by islet hyperplasia or increased beta-cell turnover. *Diab Care* 29:1554, 2006.
66. Guseva N, Phillips D, Mordes JP: Successful treatment of persistent hyperinsulinemic hypoglycemia with nifedipine in an adult patient. *Endocr Pract* 16:107, 2010.
67. McLaughlin T, Peck M, Holst J, et al: Reversible hyperinsulinemic hypoglycemia after gastric bypass: a consequence of altered nutrient delivery. *J Clin Endocrinol Metab* 95:1851, 2010.
68. Lupsa BC, Chong AY, Cochran EK, et al: Autoimmune forms of hypoglycemia. *Medicine (Baltimore)* 88:141, 2009.
69. Koyama R, Nakanishi K, Kato M, et al: Hypoglycemia and hyperglycemia due to insulin antibodies against therapeutic human insulin: treatment with double filtration plasmapheresis and prednisolone. *Am J Med Sci* 329:259, 2005.
70. Kim CH, Park JH, Park TS, et al: Autoimmune hypoglycemia in a type 2 diabetic patient with anti-insulin and insulin receptor antibodies. *Diab Care* 27:288, 2004.
71. Burch HB, Clement S, Sokol MS, et al: Reactive hypoglycemic coma due to insulin autoimmune syndrome: case report and literature review. *Am J Med* 92:681, 1992.
72. Vogeser M, Parhofer KG, Furst H, et al: Autoimmune hypoglycemia presenting as seizure one week after surgery. *Clin Chem* 47:795, 2001.
73. Redmon JB, Nuttall FQ: Autoimmune hypoglycemia. *Endocrinol Metab Clin North Am* 28:603, 1999.
74. Varga J, Lopatin M, Boden G: Hypoglycemia due to antiinsulin receptor antibodies in systemic lupus erythematosus. *J Rheumatol* 17:1226, 1990.
75. Uchigata Y, Takayama-Hasumi S, Kawanishi K, et al: Inducement of antibody that mimics insulin action on insulin receptor by insulin autoantibody directed at determinant at asparagine site on human insulin B chain. *Diabetes* 40:966, 1991.

76. Selinger S, Tsai J, Pulini M, et al: Autoimmune thrombocytopenia and primary biliary cirrhosis with hypoglycemia and insulin receptor autoantibodies. A case report. *Ann Intern Med* 107:686, 1987.
77. Redmon B, Pyzdrowski KL, Elson MK, et al: Hypoglycemia due to a monoclonal insulin-binding antibody in multiple myeloma. *N Engl J Med* 326:994, 1992.
78. Seino S, Fu ZZ, Marks W, et al: Characterization of circulating insulin in insulin autoimmune syndrome. *J Clin Endocrinol Metab* 62:64, 1986.
79. Miranda-Garduno LM, Gomez-Perez FJ, Rull JA: Improvement of autoimmune hypoglycemia by decreasing circulating free insulin concentrations with metformin. *Endocr Pract* 14:511, 2008.
80. Shen J, Gaglia J: Hypoglycemia following pancreas transplantation. *Curr Diab Rep* 8:317, 2008.
81. Redmon JB, Teuscher AU, Robertson RP: Hypoglycemia after pancreas transplantation. *Diab Care* 21:1944, 1998.
82. Stagner JI, Mokshagundam SP, Samols E: Induction of mild hypoglycemia by islet transplantation to the pancreas. *Transplant Proc* 30:635, 1998.
83. Leitao CB, Tharavanij T, Cure P, et al: Restoration of hypoglycemia awareness after islet transplantation. *Diab Care* 31:2113, 2008.
84. Semakula C, Pambuccian S, Gruessner R, et al: Clinical case seminar: hypoglycemia after pancreas transplantation: association with allograft nesidiodysplasia and expression of islet neogenesis-associated peptide. *J Clin Endocrinol Metab* 87:3548, 2002.
85. Christofilis MA, Remacle-Bonnet M, Atlan-Gepner C, et al: Study of serum big-insulin-like growth factor (IGF)-II and IGF binding proteins in two patients with extrapancreatic tumor hypoglycemia, using a combination of Western blotting methods. *Eur J Endocrinol* 139:317, 1998.
86. Miraki-Moud F, Grossman AB, Besser M, et al: A rapid method for analyzing serum pro-insulin-like growth factor-II in patients with non-islet cell tumor hypoglycemia. *J Clin Endocrinol Metab* 90:3819, 2005.
87. Daughaday WH, Trivedi B: Measurement of derivatives of proinsulin-like growth factor-II in serum by a radioimmunoassay directed against the E-domain in normal subjects and patients with nonislet cell tumor hypoglycemia. *J Clin Endocrinol Metab* 75:110, 1992.
88. Daughaday WH, Trivedi B, Baxter RC: Serum "big insulin-like growth factor II" from patients with tumor hypoglycemia lacks normal E-domain O-linked glycosylation, a possible determinant of normal propeptide processing. *Proc Natl Acad Sci USA* 90:5823, 1993.
89. Daughaday WH, Emanuele MA, Brooks MH, et al: Synthesis and secretion of insulin-like growth factor II by a leiomyosarcoma with associated hypoglycemia. *N Engl J Med* 319:1434, 1988.
90. Daughaday WH, Wu JC, Lee SD, et al: Abnormal processing of pro-IGF-II in patients with hepatoma and in some hepatitis B virus antibody-positive asymptomatic individuals. *J Lab Clin Med* 116:555, 1990.
91. Cotterill AM, Holly JM, Davies SC, et al: The insulin-like growth factors and their binding proteins in a case of non-islet-cell tumour-associated hypoglycaemia. *J Endocrinol* 131:303, 1991.
92. Trivedi N, Mithal A, Sharma AK, et al: Non-islet cell tumour induced hypoglycaemia with acromegaloid facial and acral swelling. *Clin Endocrinol (Oxf)* 42:433, 1995.
93. Baxter RC, Daughaday WH: Impaired formation of the ternary insulin-like growth factor-binding protein complex in patients with hypoglycemia due to nonislet cell tumors. *J Clin Endocrinol Metab* 73:696, 1991.
94. Escobar GA, Robinson WA, Nydam TL, et al: Severe paraneoplastic hypoglycemia in a patient with a gastrointestinal stromal tumor with an exon 9 mutation: a case report. *BMC Cancer* 7:13, 2007.
95. Lawson EA, Zhang X, Crocker JT, et al: Hypoglycemia from IGF2 overexpression associated with activation of fetal promoters and loss of imprinting in a metastatic hemangiopericytoma. *J Clin Endocrinol Metab* 94:2226, 2009.
96. Anaforoglu I, Simsek A, Turan T, et al: Hemangiopericytoma-associated hypoglycemia improved by glucocorticoid therapy: a case report. *Endocrine* 36:151, 2009.
97. Adams J, Lodge JPA, Parker D: Liver transplantation for metastatic hemangiopericytoma associated with hypoglycemia. *Transplantation* 67:488, 1999.
98. Saigal S, Nandeesh HP, Malhotra V, et al: A case of hepatocellular carcinoma associated with troublesome hypoglycemia: management by cytoreduction using percutaneous ethanol injection. *Am J Gastroenterol* 93:1380, 1998.
99. Atiq M, Safa M: Recurrent hypoglycemia associated with poorly differentiated carcinoma of the liver. *Am J Clin Oncol* 30:213, 2007.
100. Wakami K, Tateyama H, Kawashima H, et al: Solitary fibrous tumor of the uterus producing high-molecular-weight insulin-like growth factor II and associated with hypoglycemia. *Int J Gynecol Pathol* 24:79, 2005.
101. Korn E, Van Hoff J, Buckley P, et al: Secretion of a large molecular-weight form of insulin-like growth factor by a primary renal tumor. *Med Pediatr Oncol* 24:392, 1995.
102. Sato R, Tsujino M, Nishida K, et al: High molecular weight form insulin-like growth factor II-producing mesenteric sarcoma causing hypoglycemia. *Intern Med* 43:967, 2004.
103. Ko AH, Bergsland EK, Lee GA: Tumor-associated hypoglycemia from metastatic colorectal adenocarcinoma: case report and review of the literature. *Dig Dis Sci* 48:192, 2003.
104. Kato A, Bando E, Shinozaki S, et al: Severe hypoglycemia and hypokalemia in association with liver metastases of gastric cancer. *Intern Med* 43:824, 2004.
105. Rosario PW, Furtado MS, Castro AF, et al: Non-islet cell tumor hypoglycemia in a patient with poorly differentiated thyroid cancer. *Thyroid* 17:84, 2007.
106. He X, Wang J, Wu X, et al: Pancreatic somatostatinoma manifested as severe hypoglycemia. *J Gastrointestin Liver Dis* 18:221, 2009.
107. Hino N, Nakagawa Y, Ikushima Y, et al: A case of a giant phyllodes tumor of the breast with hypoglycemia caused by high-molecular-weight insulin-like growth factor II. *Breast Cancer* 17:142, 2010.
108. Daughaday WH: Hypoglycemia in patients with non-islet cell tumors. *Endocrinol Metab Clin North Am* 18:91, 1989.
109. Hoff AO, Vassilopoulou-Sellin R: The role of glucagon administration in the diagnosis and treatment of patients with tumor hypoglycemia. *Cancer* 82:1585, 1998.
110. Ogiwara Y, Mori S, Iwama M, et al: Hypoglycemia due to ectopic secretion of insulin-like growth factor-I in a patient with an isolated sarcoidosis of the spleen. *Endocr J* 57:325, 2010.
111. Seltzer HS: Drug-induced hypoglycemia. A review of 1418 cases. *Endocrinol Metab Clin North Am* 18:163, 1989.
112. Gerich JE: Oral hypoglycemic agents. *N Engl J Med* 321:1231, 1989.
113. Aldhahi W, Armstrong J, Bouche C, et al: β-cell insulin secretory response to oral hypoglycemic agents is blunted in humans *in vivo* during moderate hypoglycemia. *J Clin Endocrinol Metab* 89:4553, 2004.
114. Shorr RI, Ray WA, Daugherty JR, et al: Individual sulfonylureas and serious hypoglycemia in older people. *J Am Geriatr Soc* 44:751, 1996.
115. Langer O, Conway DL, Berkus MD, et al: A comparison of glyburide and insulin in women with gestational diabetes mellitus. *N Engl J Med* 343:1134, 2000.
116. Ben-Ami H, Nagachandran P, Mendelson A, et al: Drug-induced hypoglycemic coma in 102 diabetic patients. *Arch Intern Med* 159:281, 1999.
117. Hirshberg B, Skarulis MC, Pucino F, et al: Repaglinide-induced factitious hypoglycemia. *J Clin Endocrinol Metab* 86:475, 2001.
118. Bodmer M, Meier C, Krahenbuhl S, et al: Metformin, sulfonylureas, or other antidiabetes drugs and the risk of lactic acidosis or hypoglycemia: a nested case-control analysis. *Diab Care* 31:2086, 2008.
119. Bailey CJ, Turner RC: Metformin. *N Engl J Med* 334:574, 1996.
120. DeFronzo RA, Ratner RE, Han J, et al: Effects of exenatide (exendin-4) on glycemic control and weight over 30 weeks in metformin-treated patients with type 2 diabetes. *Diab Care* 28:1092, 2005.
121. Kendall DM, Riddle MC, Rosenstock J, et al: Effects of exenatide (exendin-4) on glycemic control over 30 weeks in patients with type 2 diabetes treated with metformin and a sulfonylurea. *Diab Care* 28:1083, 2005.
122. Pijl H, Ohashi S, Matsuda M, et al: Bromocriptine—a novel approach to the treatment of type 2 diabetes. *Diab Care* 23:1154, 2000.
123. Hargett NA, Ritch R, Mardirossian J, et al: Inadvertent substitution of acetohexamide for acetazolamide. *Am J Ophthalmol* 84:580, 1977.
124. Murad MH, Coto-Yglesias F, Wang AT, et al: Clinical review: drug-induced hypoglycemia: a systematic review. *J Clin Endocrinol Metab* 94:741, 2009.
125. McGuire LC, Cruickshank AM, Munro PT: Alcoholic ketoacidosis. *Emerg Med J* 23:417, 2006.
126. Arky RA: Hypoglycemia associated with liver disease and ethanol. *Endocrinol Metab Clin North Am* 18:75, 1989.
127. Brown DR, Brown MJ: Hypoglycemia associated with preoperative metoprolol administration. *Anesth Analg* 99:1427, 2004.
128. Phillips RE, Looareesuwan S, White NJ, et al: Hypoglycaemia and antimalarial drugs: quinidine and release of insulin. *Br Med J* 292:1319, 1986.
129. Goldberg IJ, Brown LK, Rayfield EJ: Disopyramide (Norpace)-induced hypoglycemia. *Am J Med* 69:463, 1980.
130. Nappi JM, Dhanani S, Lovejoy JR, et al: Severe hypoglycemia associated with disopyramide. *West J Med* 138:95, 1983.
131. Takada M, Fujita S, Katayama Y, et al: The relationship between risk of hypoglycemia and use of cibenzoline and disopyramide. *Eur J Clin Pharmacol* 56:335, 2000.
132. White NJ, Warrell DA, Chanthavanich P, et al: Severe hypoglycemia and hyperinsulinemia in falciparum malaria. *N Engl J Med* 309:61, 1983.
133. Phillips RE, Looareesuwan S, Molyneux ME, et al: Hypoglycaemia and counterregulatory hormone responses in severe falciparum malaria: treatment with Sandostatin. *Q J Med* 86:233, 1993.
134. Limburg PJ, Katz H, Grant CS, et al: Quinine-induced hypoglycemia. *Ann Intern Med* 119:218, 1993.
135. Park-Wyllie LY, Juurlink DN, Kopp A, et al: Outpatient gatifloxacin therapy and dysglycemia in older adults. *N Engl J Med* 354:1352, 2006.
136. Khovidhunkit W, Sunthornyothin S: Hypoglycemia, hyperglycemia, and gatifloxacin. *Ann Intern Med* 141:969, 2004.
137. Brogan SE, Cahalan MK: Gatifloxacin as a possible cause of serious postoperative hypoglycemia. *Anesth Analg* 101:635, table, 2005.
138. Menzies DJ, Dorsainvil PA, Cunha BA, et al: Severe and persistent hypoglycemia due to gatifloxacin interaction with oral hypoglycemic agents. *Am J Med* 113:232, 2002.
139. Lin G, Hays DP, Spillane L: Refractory hypoglycemia from ciprofloxacin and glyburide interaction. *J Toxicol Clin Toxicol* 42:295, 2004.
140. Kelesidis T, Canseco E: Quinolone-induced hypoglycemia: a life-threatening but potentially reversible side effect. *Am J Med* 123:e5-e6, 2010.

141. Strevel EL, Kuper A, Gold WL: Severe and protracted hypoglycaemia associated with co-trimoxazole use. *Lancet Infect Dis* 6:178, 2006.
142. Roustit M, Blondel E, Villier C, et al: Symptomatic hypoglycemia associated with trimethoprim/sulfamethoxazole and repaglinide in a diabetic patient. *Ann Pharmacother* 44:764, 2010.
143. Raschke R, Arnold-Capell PA, Richeson R, et al: Refractory hypoglycemia secondary to topical salicylate intoxication. *Arch Intern Med* 151:591, 1991.
144. Maheady DC: Reye's syndrome: review and update. *J Pediatr Health Care* 3:246, 1989.
145. Arauz-Pacheco C, Ramirez LC, Rios JM, et al: Hypoglycemia induced by angiotensin-converting enzyme inhibitors in patients with non-insulin-dependent diabetes receiving sulfonylurea therapy. *Am J Med* 89:811, 1990.
146. Buller GK, Perazella M: ACE inhibitor-induced hypoglycemia. *Am J Med* 91:104, 1991.
147. Herings RMC, De Boer A, Stricker BHC, et al: Hypoglycaemia associated with use of inhibitors of angiotensin converting enzyme. *Lancet* 345:1195, 1995.
148. Morris AD, Boyle DIR, McMahon AD, et al: ACE inhibitor use is associated with hospitalization for severe hypoglycemia in patients with diabetes. *Diab Care* 20:1363, 1997.
149. Shorr RI, Ray WA, Daugherty JR, et al: Antihypertensives and the risk of serious hypoglycemia in older persons using insulin or sulfonylureas. *JAMA* 278:40, 1997.
150. Billington D, Osmundsen H, Sherratt HS: The biochemical basis of Jamaican akee poisoning. *N Engl J Med* 296:1482, 1976.
151. Arky RA: Hypoglycemia, in DeGroot LJ, Cahill GF Jr, Martini L, Nelson DH, Odell WD, Potts JT Jr, Steinberger E, Winegrad AI (eds): *Endocrinology*. New York, NY, Grune and Stratton, 1979, pp 1099–1123.
152. Marks V: Hepatogenous and nephrogenic hypoglycemia, in Marks V, Rose FC, (eds): *Hypoglycemia*. 2nd ed. Oxford, Blackwell Scientific, 1981, pp 216–226.
153. Muhlhauser I, Toth G, Sawicki PT, et al: Severe hypoglycemia in type I diabetic patients with impaired kidney function. *Diab Care* 14:344, 1991.
154. Garber AJ, Bier DM, Cryer PE, et al: Hypoglycemia in compensated chronic renal insufficiency. Substrate limitation of gluconeogenesis. *Diabetes* 23:982, 1974.
155. Comty CM, Leonard A, Shapiro FL: Nutritional and metabolic problems in the dialyzed patient with diabetes mellitus. *Kidney Int* 1[Suppl]:51, 1974.
156. Tzamaloukas AH, Murata GH, Eisenberg B, et al: Hypoglycemia in diabetics on dialysis with poor glycemic control: hemodialysis versus continuous ambulatory peritoneal dialysis. *Int J Artif Organs* 15:390, 1992.
157. Greenblatt DJ: Insulin sensitivity in renal failure. Fatal hypoglycemia following dialysis. *N Y State J Med* 74:1040, 1974.
158. Rutsky EA, McDaniel HG, Tharpe DL, et al: Spontaneous hypoglycemia in chronic renal failure. *Arch Intern Med* 138:1364, 1978.
159. Avram MM, Wolf RE, Gan A, et al: Uremic hypoglycemia. A preventable life-threatening complication. *N Y State J Med* 84:593, 1984.
160. Bansal VK, Brooks MH, York JC, et al: Intractable hypoglycemia in a patient with renal failure. *Arch Intern Med* 139:101, 1979.
161. Pun KK: Hypoglycaemia and insulin resistance in uraemia associated with insulin fragments. *Med Hypotheses* 17:243, 1985.
162. Toth EL, Lee DW: "Spontaneous"/uremic hypoglycemia is not a distinct entity: substantiation from a literature review. *Nephron* 58:325, 1991.
163. Pagliara AS, Kari IE, De Vivo DC, et al: Hypoalaninemia: a concomitant of ketotic hypoglycemia. *J Clin Invest* 51:1440, 1972.
164. Miller SI, Wallace RJ Jr, Musher DM, et al: Hypoglycemia as a manifestation of sepsis. *Am J Med* 68:649, 1980.
165. Nouel O, Bernuau J, Rueff B, et al: Hypoglycemia. A common complication of septicemia in cirrhosis. *Arch Intern Med* 141:1477, 1981.
166. Scheetz A: Hypoglycemia and sepsis in two elderly diabetics. *J Am Geriatr Soc* 38:492, 1990.
167. Romijn JA, Godfried MH, Wortel C, et al: Hypoglycemia, hormones and cytokines in fatal meningococcal septicemia. *J Endocrinol Invest* 13:743, 1990.
168. Maayan-Metzger A, Lubin D, Kuint J: Hypoglycemia rates in the first days of life among term infants born to diabetic mothers. *Neonatology* 96:80, 2009.
169. Mochel F, Slama A, Touati G, et al: Respiratory chain defects may present only with hypoglycemia. *J Clin Endocrinol Metab* 90:3780, 2005.
170. Kluge S, Kühnelt P, Block A, et al: A young woman with persistent hypoglycemia, rhabdomyolysis, and coma: recognizing fatty acid oxidation defects in adults. *Crit Care Med* 31:1273, 2003.
171. Otonkoski T, Kaminen N, Ustinov J, et al: Physical exercise-induced hyperinsulinemic hypoglycemia is an autosomal-dominant trait characterized by abnormal pyruvate-induced insulin release. *Diabetes* 52:199, 2003.
172. Otonkoski T, Jiao H, Kaminen-Ahola N, et al: Physical exercise-induced hypoglycemia caused by failed silencing of monocarboxylate transporter 1 in pancreatic beta cells. *Am J Hum Genet* 81:467, 2007.
173. Kimberly MM, Vesper HW, Caudill SP, et al: Variability among five over-the-counter blood glucose monitors. *Clin Chim Acta* 364:292, 2006.
174. Kulkarni A, Saxena M, Price G, et al: Analysis of blood glucose measurements using capillary and arterial blood samples in intensive care patients. *Intensive Care Med* 31:142, 2005.
175. Desachy A, Vuagnat AC, Ghazali AD, et al: Accuracy of bedside glucometry in critically ill patients: influence of clinical characteristics and perfusion index. *Mayo Clin Proc* 83:400, 2008.
176. Atkin SH, Dasmahapatra A, Jaker MA, et al: Fingerstick glucose determination in shock. *Ann Intern Med* 114:1020, 1991.
177. Thomas SH, Gough JE, Benson N, et al: Accuracy of fingerstick glucose determination in patients receiving CPR. *South Med J* 87:1072, 1994.
178. Kirrane BM, Duthie EA, Nelson LS: Unrecognized hypoglycemia due to maltodextrin interference with bedside glucometry. *J Med Toxicol* 5:20, 2009.
179. Eastham JH, Mason D, Barnes DL, et al: Prevalence of interfering substances with point of care glucose testing in a community hospital. *Am J Health Syst Pharm* 66:167, 2009.
180. Sood V, Costello BA, Burge MR: How low can you go? Chronic hypoglycemia versus normal glucose homeostasis. *J Invest Med* 49:205, 2001.
181. Astles JR, Petros WP, Peters WP, et al: Artifactual hypoglycemia associated with hematopoietic cytokines. *Arch Pathol Lab Med* 119:713, 1995.
182. Hoffman JR, Schriger DL, Votey SR, et al: The empiric use of hypertonic dextrose in patients with altered mental status: a reappraisal. *Ann Emerg Med* 21:20, 1992.
183. Plum F, Posner JB: *The diagnosis of stupor and coma*. Philadelphia, PA, FA Davis Co., 1982, pp 1–352.
184. Candelise L, Landi G, Orazio EN, et al: Prognostic significance of hyperglycemia in acute stroke. *Arch Neurol* 42:661, 1985.
185. Pulsinelli WA, Levy DE, Sigsbee B, et al: Increased damage after ischemic stroke in patients with hyperglycemia with or without established diabetes mellitus. *Am J Med* 74:540, 1983.
186. Browning RG, Olson DW, Stueven HA, et al: 50% dextrose: antidote or toxin? *Ann Emerg Med* 19:683, 1990.
187. MacLeod DB, Montoya DR, Fick GH, et al: The effect of 25 grams i.v. glucose on serum inorganic phosphate levels. *Ann Emerg Med* 23:524, 1994.
188. Balentine JR, Gaeta TJ, Kessler D, et al: Effect of 50 milliliters of 50% dextrose in water administration on the blood sugar of euglycemic volunteers. *Acad Emerg Med* 5:691, 1998.
189. Luber SD, Brady WJ, Brand A, et al: Acute hypoglycemia masquerading as head trauma: a report of four cases. *Am J Emerg Med* 14:543, 1996.
190. Moore C, Woollard M: Dextrose 10% or 50% in the treatment of hypoglycaemia out of hospital? A randomised controlled trial. *Emerg Med J* 22:512, 2005.
191. Losek JD: Hypoglycemia and the ABC'S (sugar) of pediatric resuscitation. *Ann Emerg Med* 35:43, 2000.
192. Neuvonen PJ, Karkkainen S: Effects of charcoal, sodium bicarbonate, and ammonium chloride on chlorpropamide kinetics. *Clin Pharmacol Ther* 33:386, 1983.
193. Kannisto H, Neuvonen PJ: Adsorption of sulfonylureas onto activated charcoal in vitro. *J Pharm Sci* 73:253, 1984.
194. Ludwig SM, McKenzie J, Faiman C: Chlorpropamide overdose in renal failure: management with charcoal hemoperfusion. *Am J Kidney Dis* 10:457, 1987.
195. Ciechanowski K, Borowiak KS, Potocka BA, et al: Chlorpropamide toxicity with survival despite 27-day hypoglycemia. *J Toxicol Clin Toxicol* 37:869, 1999.
196. Sills MN, Ogu CC, Maxa J: Prolonged hypoglycemic crisis associated with glyburide. *Pharmacotherapy* 17:1338, 1997.
197. Palatnick W, Meatherall RC, Tenenbein M: Clinical spectrum of sulfonylurea overdose and experience with diazoxide therapy. *Arch Intern Med* 151:1859, 1991.
198. Viola KV, Sosa JA: Current advances in the diagnosis and treatment of pancreatic endocrine tumors. *Curr Opin Oncol* 17:24, 2005.
199. Boyle PJ, Justice K, Krentz AJ, et al: Octreotide reverses hyperinsulinemia and prevents hypoglycemia induced by sulfonylurea overdoses. *J Clin Endocrinol Metab* 76:752, 1993.
200. Green RS, Palatnick W: Effectiveness of octreotide in a case of refractory sulfonylurea-induced hypoglycemia. *J Emerg Med* 25:283, 2003.
201. Crawford BA, Perera C: Octreotide treatment for sulfonylurea-induced hypoglycaemia. *Med J Aust* 180:540, 2004.
202. McLaughlin SA, Crandall CS, McKinney PE: Octreotide: an antidote for sulfonylurea-induced hypoglycemia. *Ann Emerg Med* 36:133, 2000.
203. Gonzalez RR, Zweig S, Rao J, et al: Octreotide therapy for recurrent refractory hypoglycemia due to sulfonylurea in diabetes-related kidney failure. *Endocr Pract* 13:417, 2007.
204. Sherk DK, Bryant SM: Octreotide therapy for nateglinide-induced hypoglycemia. *Ann Emerg Med* 50:745, 2007.
205. Vallurupalli S: Safety of subcutaneous octreotide in patients with sulfonylurea-induced hypoglycemia and congestive heart failure. *Ann Pharmacother* 44:387, 2010.
206. Flanagan SE, Kapoor RR, Mali G, et al: Diazoxide-responsive hyperinsulinemic hypoglycemia caused by HNF4 A gene mutations. *Eur J Endocrinol* 162:987, 2010.
207. Thoma ME, Glauser J, Genuth S: Persistent hypoglycemia and hyperinsulinemia: caution in using glucagon. *Am J Emerg Med* 14:99, 1996.
208. Hashimoto T, Adachi K, Ishimura N, et al: Safety and efficacy of glucagon as a premedication for upper gastrointestinal endoscopy—a comparative study with butyl scopolamine bromide. *Aliment Pharmacol Ther* 16:111, 2002.

209. Bourcier ME, Sherrod A, DiGuardo M, et al: Successful control of intractable hypoglycemia using rapamycin in an 86-year-old man with a pancreatic insulin-secreting islet cell tumor and metastases. *J Clin Endocrinol Metab* 94:3157, 2009.
210. Varghese P, Gleason V, Sorokin R, et al: Hypoglycemia in hospitalized patients treated with antihyperglycemic agents. *J Hosp Med* 2:234, 2007.
211. Maynard G, Lee J, Phillips G, et al: Improved inpatient use of basal insulin, reduced hypoglycemia, and improved glycemic control: effect of structured subcutaneous insulin orders and an insulin management algorithm. *J Hosp Med* 4:3, 2009.
212. Kaukonen KM, Rantala M, Pettila V, et al: Severe hypoglycemia during intensive insulin therapy. *Acta Anaesthesiol Scand* 53:61, 2009.
213. Lin YY, Hsu CW, Sheu WH, et al: Risk factors for recurrent hypoglycemia in hospitalized diabetic patients admitted for severe hypoglycemia. *Yonsei Med J* 51:367, 2010.
214. Harris DL, Battin MR, Weston PJ, et al: Continuous glucose monitoring in newborn babies at risk of hypoglycemia. *J Pediatr* 157:198, 2010.
215. Holzinger U, Warszawska J, Kitzberger R, et al: Real-time continuous glucose monitoring in critically ill patients: a prospective randomized trial. *Diab Care* 33:467, 2010.
216. Holzinger U, Warszawska J, Kitzberger R, et al: Impact of shock requiring norepinephrine on the accuracy and reliability of subcutaneous continuous glucose monitoring. *Intensive Care Med* 35:1383, 2009.
217. Goksu E, Eken C, Karadeniz O, et al: First report of hypoglycemia secondary to dandelion (Taraxacum officinale) ingestion. *Am J Emerg Med* 28:111, 2010.
218. Bernard PA, Makin CE, Werner HA: Hypoglycemia associated with dexmedetomidine overdose in a child? *J Clin Anesth* 21:50, 2009.
219. Montgomery H, Myerson S: 3,4-methylenedioxymethamphetamine (MDMA, or "ecstasy") and associated hypoglycemia. *Am J Emerg Med* 15:218, 1997.
220. Wambier CG, Foss-Freitas MC, Paschoal RS, et al: Severe hypoglycemia after initiation of anti-tumor necrosis factor therapy with etanercept in a patient with generalized pustular psoriasis and type 2 diabetes mellitus. *J Am Acad Dermatol* 60:883, 2009.
221. Cheung D, Bryer-Ash M: Persistent hypoglycemia in a patient with diabetes taking etanercept for the treatment of psoriasis. *J Am Acad Dermatol* 60:1032, 2009.
222. Banerjee A, Rhoden WE: Etomidate-induced hypoglycaemia. *Postgrad Med J* 72:510, 1996.
223. Walter RB, Hoofnagle AN, Lanum SA, et al: Acute, life-threatening hypoglycemia associated with haloperidol in a hematopoietic stem cell transplant recipient. *Bone Marrow Transplant* 37:109, 2006.
224. Haap M, Gallwitz B, Thamer C, et al: Symptomatic hypoglycemia during imatinib mesylate in a non-diabetic female patient with gastrointestinal stromal tumor. *J Endocrinol Invest* 30:688, 2007.
225. Ozdemir D, Yilmaz E, Duman M, et al: Hypoglycemia after albuterol overdose in a pediatric patient. *Pediatr Emerg Care* 20:464, 2004.
226. Khamaisi M, Leitersdorf E: Severe hypoglycemia from clarithromycin-repaglinide drug interaction. *Pharmacotherapy* 28:682, 2008.
227. U.S. Food and Drug Administration: Important safety information on interference with blood glucose measurement following use of parenteral maltose/parenteral galactose/oral xylose-containing products. Available at: www.fda.gov/cber/safety/maltose110405.htm. Accessed 11-10-2005.
228. Dean-Franklin B, Vincent C, Schachter M, et al: The incidence of prescribing errors in hospital inpatients: an overview of the research methods. *Drug Saf* 28:891, 2005.

CHAPTER 107 ■ NONTHYROIDAL ILLNESS SYNDROME (SICK EUTHYROID SYNDROME) IN THE INTENSIVE CARE UNIT

SHIRIN HADDADY AND ALAN P. FARWELL

INTRODUCTION

Critical illness causes multiple alterations in thyroid hormone concentrations in patients who have no previously diagnosed intrinsic thyroid disease [1–6]. These effects are nonspecific and relate to the severity of the illness. Despite abnormalities in serum thyroid hormone parameters, there is little evidence that these patients have clinically significant thyroid dysfunction. Because a wide variety of illnesses tend to result in the same changes in serum thyroid hormones, such alterations in thyroid hormone indexes have been termed the *sick euthyroid syndrome* or, more recently, the *nonthyroidal illness syndrome*. These changes are rarely isolated and often are associated with alterations in other endocrine systems, such as reductions in serum gonadotropin and sex hormone concentrations [7] and increases in serum corticotropin and cortisol levels [8]. Similar changes in endocrine function have been shown experimentally by the administration of cytokines from the interleukin (IL) and interferon families as well as tumor necrosis factor-α (TNF-α) [9]. Thus, the sick euthyroid syndrome should not be viewed as an isolated pathologic event but as part of a coordinated systemic reaction to illness that involves both the immune and endocrine systems.

The differentiation between patients with the sick euthyroid syndrome and those with intrinsic thyroid disease is a frequent diagnostic problem in the intensive care unit (ICU). This chapter will first review normal thyroid physiology and discuss the changes in thyroid hormone metabolism seen with critical illness. Management of these patients and the identification of those with intrinsic thyroid disease will then be discussed. Finally, the use of thyroid hormone replacement in the sick euthyroid syndrome will be reviewed.

NORMAL THYROID HORMONE ECONOMY

Regulation

The synthesis and secretion of thyroid hormone is under the control of the anterior pituitary hormone, thyrotropin (TSH). In a classic negative feedback system, TSH secretion increases when serum thyroid hormone levels fall and decreases when they rise (Fig. 107.1). TSH secretion is also under the regulation of the hypothalamic hormone, thyrotropin-releasing hormone (TRH). The negative feedback of thyroid hormone is targeted mainly at the pituitary level but likely affects TRH release from the hypothalamus as well. In addition, input from higher cortical centers can affect hypothalamic TRH secretion.

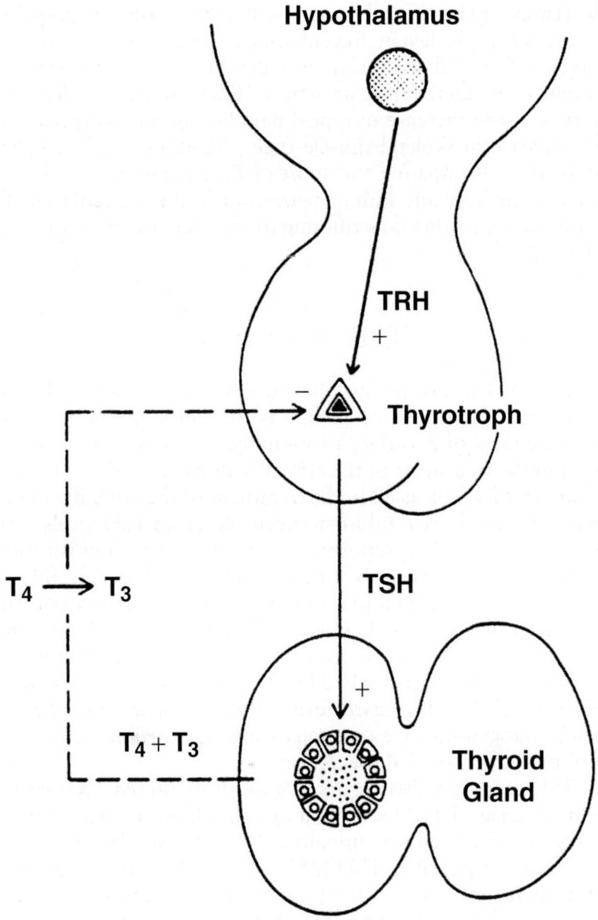

FIGURE 107.1. Diagram of the hypothalamic-pituitary-thyroid axis. The inhibitory effect of T_4 and T_3 on thyrotropin (TSH) secretion is shown by the dashed line and minus sign, and the stimulatory effects of thyrotropin-releasing hormone (TRH) on TSH secretion and TSH on thyroid secretion are shown by the solid lines and plus signs. T_4 and T_3 may also have an inhibitory effect on TRH secretion. [From Toft AD: Thyrotropin: assay, secretory physiology, and testing of regulation, in Braverman LE, Utiger RD (eds): *The Thyroid: A Fundamental and Clinical Text*. Philadelphia, JB Lippincott, 1991, with permission.]

Under the influence of TSH, the thyroid gland synthesizes and releases thyroid hormone. Thyroxine (T_4, 65% iodine by weight) is the principal secretory product of the thyroid gland, comprising ~90% of secreted thyroid hormone under normal conditions [10]. While T_4 may have direct actions in some tissues, T_4 primarily functions as a hormone precursor that is metabolized in peripheral tissues to the transcriptionally active 3,5,3′-triiodothyronine (T_3, 59% iodine by weight).

Metabolic Pathways

The major pathway of metabolism of T_4 is by sequential monodeiodination [11] (Fig. 107.2). At least three deiodinases, each with its unique expression in different organs, catalyze the deiodination reactions involved in the metabolism of T_4. Removal of the 5′-, or outer ring, iodine by type 1 iodothyronine 5′deiodinase (type 1 deiodinase, D1) is the "activating" metabolic pathway, leading to the formation of T_3. Removal of the inner ring, or 5-, iodine by type 3 iodothyronine deiodinase (type 3 deiodinase, D3) is the "inactivating" pathway, producing the metabolically inactive hormone, 3,3′,5′-triiodothyronine (reverse T_3, rT_3). Type 1 deiodinase (D1) is found most abundantly in the liver, kidneys, and thyroid. It is upregulated in hyperthyroidism and downregulated in hypothyroidism. Type 3 deiodinase is expressed primarily in the brain, in skin, and in placental and chorionic membranes. The actions of D3 also include the inactivation of T_3 to form T_2, another inactive metabolite. Under normal conditions, ~41% of T_4 is converted to T_3, ~38% is converted to rT_3, and ~21% is metabolized via other pathways, such as conjugation in the liver and excretion in the bile [4,5].

T_3 is the metabolically active thyroid hormone and exerts its actions via binding to chromatin-bound nuclear receptors and regulating gene transcription in responsive tissues [12]. Important in the understanding of the alterations in circulating thyroid hormone levels seen in critical illness is the fact that only ~10% of circulating T_3 is secreted directly by the thyroid gland while >80% of T_3 is derived from conversion of T_4 in peripheral tissues [10,11]. Thus, factors that affect peripheral T_4 to T_3 conversion will have significant effects on circulating T_3 levels. Serum levels of T_3 are approximately 100-fold less than those of T_4, and, like T_4, T_3 is metabolized by deiodination to form diiodothyronine (T_2) and by conjugation in the liver. The half-lives of circulating T_4 and T_3 are 5 to 8 days and 1.3 to 3 days, respectively [13].

Serum-Binding Proteins

Both T_4 and T_3 circulate in the serum as bound hormones to several proteins synthesized by the liver [14]. thyroxine-binding globulin (TBG) is the predominant transport protein and binds

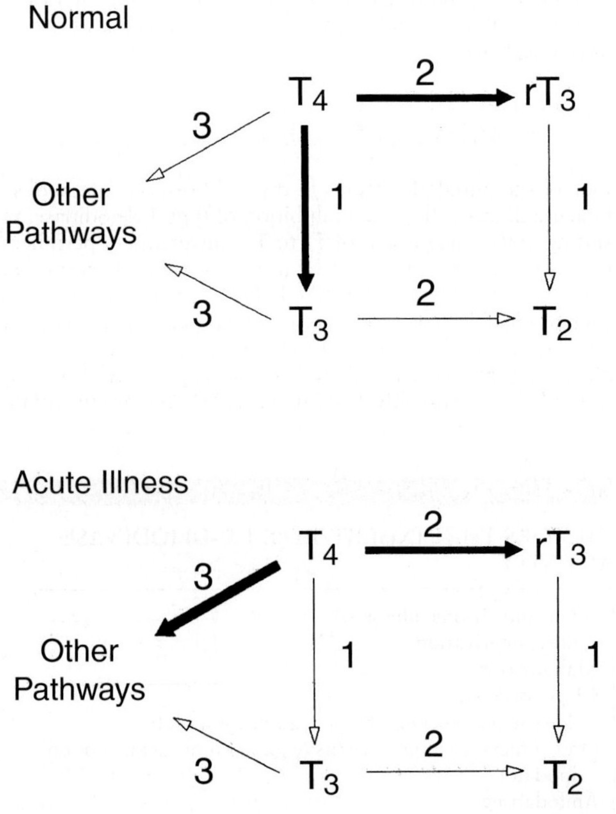

FIGURE 107.2. Pathways of thyroid hormone metabolism. Thyroid hormones are metabolized by outer ring deiodination (*1*, type 1 and type 2 5′-deiodinase), inner ring deiodination (2, type 3 5-deiodinase) or by nondeiodinative pathways (*3*). Deiodination is the major route of T_4 metabolism in healthy individuals, and nondeiodinative pathways of metabolism assume a greater role in critically ill patients.

~80% of the circulating serum thyroid hormones. The affinity of T_4 for TBG is approximately 10-fold greater than that of T_3 and is part of the reason that circulating T_4 levels are higher than T_3 levels. Other serum-binding proteins include transthyretin [15], which binds ~15% of T_4 but little, if any T_3, and albumin, which has a low affinity but a very large binding capacity for T_4 and T_3. Overall, 99.97% of circulating T_4 and 99.7% of circulating T_3 is bound to plasma proteins.

Free Hormone Concept

Essential to the understanding of the regulation of thyroid function and the alterations of circulating thyroid hormones seen in critical illness is the "free hormone" concept, which is that only the unbound hormone has any metabolic activity. Under the regulation by the pituitary, overall thyroid function is affected when there are any changes in free hormone concentrations. Changes in either the concentrations of binding proteins or the binding affinity of thyroid hormone to the serum-binding proteins have significant effects on the total serum hormone levels due to the high degree of binding of T_4 and T_3 to these proteins. Despite these changes, this does not necessarily translate into thyroid dysfunction.

THYROID HORMONE ECONOMY IN CRITICAL ILLNESS

The widespread changes in thyroid hormone economy in the critically ill patient occur as a result of: (a) alterations in the peripheral metabolism of the thyroid hormones, (b) alterations in TSH regulation, and (c) alterations in the binding of thyroid hormone to TBG.

Peripheral Metabolic Pathways

One of the initial alterations in thyroid hormone metabolism in acute illness is the acute inhibition of type 1 deiodinase, resulting in the impairment of T_4 to T_3 conversion in peripheral tissues [16]. D1 is inhibited by a wide variety of factors, including acute illness (Table 107.1) [11], resulting in the acute decrease in T_3 production in critically ill patients. In contrast, inner ring deiodination by D3 may be increased by acute illness, resulting in increased levels of rT_3 [17,18]. Additionally, since rT_3 is subsequently deiodinated by D1, degradation of rT_3 decreases and levels of this inactive hormone rise in proportion to the fall in T_3 levels. Recent studies on postmortem tissues have confirmed that alterations in deiodinase enzymes occur in patients who died during an acute critical illness, with decrease in type 1 and increase in type 3 deiodinases and, surprisingly, an increase in skeletal muscle type 2 deiodinase [18,19]. Finally, there is impaired transport of T_4 into peripheral tissues, such as the liver and kidney where much of the circulating T_3 is produced, further contributing to the decrease in production of T_3 [20].

TABLE 107.1

FACTORS THAT INHIBIT TYPE 1 5′-DEIODINASE ACTIVITY

Acute and chronic illness
Caloric deprivation
Malnutrition
Glucocorticoids
β-Adrenergic blocking drugs (e.g., propranolol)
Oral cholecystographic agents (e.g., iopanoic acid, sodium ipodate)
Amiodarone
Propylthiouracil
Fatty acids
Fetal/neonatal period
Selenium deficiency
Cytokines (interleukin 1 and 6)

TSH Regulation

Serum TSH levels are usually normal early in acute illness. However, TSH levels often fall as the illness progresses due to the effects of a variety of inhibitory factors that are common in the treatment of the critically ill patient (Table 107.2). Many medications used in the treatment of the critically ill patient may also have inhibitory effects on serum TSH levels. Van den Berghe et al. [21] reported that intravenous administration of dopamine for as short a time as 15 to 21 hours is able to acutely decrease TSH levels and its withdrawal results in a tenfold increase in serum TSH levels. In one study, children who received dopamine infusions during a pediatric ICU admission for meningococcal sepsis had lower TSH levels than those who did not [22,23]. Increased levels of glucocorticoids, whether from endogenous or exogenous sources, also have direct inhibitory effects on TSH secretion.

TSH secretion also occurs as a result of altered TRH secretion. Decreased TRH secretion due to inhibitory signals from higher cortical centers, impaired TRH metabolism [24], the alteration of pulsatile TSH [25], and the decrease or absence of a nocturnal TSH surge [25,26] may all decrease TSH levels. Serum levels of Leptin, the ob gene product that has been shown to vary directly with thyroid hormone levels [27], also fall as illness progresses [28] and hypothalamic TRH secretion falls, which in turn leads to lowered TSH levels [29]. The decrease of hypothalamic TRH gene expression in animal models is, however, not associated with increased serum T_4 and T_3

TABLE 107.2

FACTORS THAT ALTER TSH SECRETION

Increase	Decrease
Chlorpromazine	Acute and chronic illness
Cimetidine	Adrenergic agonists
Domperidone	Caloric restriction
Dopamine antagonists	Carbamazepine
Haloperidol	Clofibrate
Iodide	Cyproheptadine
Lithium	Dopamine and dopamine agonists
Metoclopramide	Endogenous depression
Sulfapyridine	Glucocorticoids
Radiographic contrast agents	Insulin-like growth factor-1
	Metergoline
	Methysergide
	Opiates
	Phenytoin
	Phentolamine
	Pimozide
	Somatostatin
	Serotonin
	Surgical stress
	Thyroid hormone metabolites

TABLE 107.3

FACTORS THAT ALTER BINDING OF T_4 TO TBG

Increase binding	Decrease binding
	Drugs
Estrogens	Glucocorticoids
Methadone	Androgens
Clofibrate	L-Asparaginase
5-Fluorouracil	Salicylates
Heroin	Mefenamic acid
Tamoxifen	Antiseizure medications (phenytoin, Tegretol)
Raloxifene	
Liver disease	Furosemide
Porphyria	Heparin
HIV infection	Systemic factors
Inherited	Inherited
	Acute illness
	Nonesterified free fatty acids

HIV, human immunodeficiency virus.

levels [30]. Finally, certain thyroid hormone metabolites that are increased during acute nonthyroidal illness may play a role in the inhibition of TSH and TRH secretion [1].

Serum-Binding Proteins

The affinity of thyroid hormones binding to transport proteins and the concentrations of serum-binding proteins are altered with acute illness (Table 107.3). Serum levels of transthyretin and albumin decrease, especially during prolonged illness, malnutrition, and in high catabolic states. TBG levels may be increased, as seen with liver dysfunction and HIV infection, or decreased, as seen with severe or prolonged illness [14]. TBG may also be rapidly degraded by protease cleavage during cardiac bypass, thereby partially explaining the rapid fall of serum T_3 levels in patients undergoing cardiac surgery [31].

An acquired binding defect of T_4 to TBG is commonly seen in patients with critical illness. This is believed to result from the release of some as yet unidentified factor from injured tissues that has the characteristics of unsaturated nonesterified fatty acids (NEFA) [32], which also inhibit T_4 to T_3 conversion [33]. In systemically ill patients, NEFA levels rise in parallel with the severity of the illness [34], and drugs such as heparin stimulate the generation of NEFA [35]. Many drugs, including high-dose furosemide, antiseizure medications, and salicylates also alter binding of T_4 to TBG. The alterations in serum-binding proteins in critical illness make the estimation of the free hormone concentrations difficult (see later).

Role of Cytokines in the Pathogenesis of the Sick Euthyroid Syndrome

Cytokines are medium-sized polypeptide hormones secreted by mononuclear cells of the lymphoid system in response to a variety of stimuli, including infection by foreign organisms, invasion by foreign cells, metabolic derangements, and organ system dysfunction [36]. Cytokines have an array of systemic and local actions characteristic of illness, such as fever, prostration, inflammation, and the initiation of wound repair. Cytokine production by lymphoid cells is essential for the development and maintenance of immunity. The actions of cytokines include both autocrine and paracrine effects on cell proliferation and differentiation and on induction of other cytokines. Classes of cytokines include the interleukins (1 to 12), interferons (α, β, and γ), tumor necrosis factors (α and β), and other assorted growth factors. Of these cytokines, TNF-α and several interleukins (IL-1, 6, and 10) have been extensively studied for their role in the pathogenesis of the sick euthyroid syndrome [9,37].

TNF-α, IL-1, and IL-6 concentrations are increased in systemic illness and are implicated as mediators of endotoxemia-induced shock, fever, and metabolic acidosis. TNF-α and IL-1 both induce the production of IL-6 and TNF-α also induces IL-1 production [38] and activates nuclear factor-kappa B (NF-κB), which has been shown to inhibit hepatic type 1 5′-deiodinase activity [39]. Serum concentrations of these cytokines have shown to be inversely proportional to serum T_3 concentrations in children (IL-6 and TNF-α [40]); postoperative patients (IL-6 [41]); hospitalized patients, including those with acute myocardial infarction (IL-6 [42–44]) and after bone marrow transplant (IL-6 and TNF-α [45]); and nursing home patients (TNF-α [46]). However, there have been reports of a lack of correlation between IL-6 and TNF-α after abdominal surgery [47] and in rheumatoid arthritis [48].

The administration of cytokines to animals produces an acute fall in serum T_3 concentrations in rats (TNF-α [49], IL-1 [50,51], IL-6 [52]) and mice (IL-1 [53,54], IL-6 [55]) and shows a direct inhibitory effect on thyroid cells in culture (TNF-α [49,56,57] and IL-1 [57–59]). Variable effects on deiodinase enzymes have been reported, including an inhibition of type 1 5′-deiodinase (IL-1β [60], NF-κB [39]) and inhibition (TNF-α, IL-1, and IL-6 [61]) and induction of type 2 5′-deiodinase (response to lipopolysaccharide [62]).

The administration of TNF-α [63] or IL-6 [64] to healthy human volunteers as well as isolated limb perfusion of cancer patients with TNF-α [65] also produced an acute decrease in both serum T_3 and TSH concentrations and a rise in serum rT_3 concentrations, while the administration of an IL-1α receptor antagonist failed to alter the decrease in serum thyroid hormone concentrations observed after infusion of endotoxin in healthy males [66]. In addition, recovery from these changes in thyroid hormone parameters was associated with a rise in TSH [65], similar to the recovery phase of the sick euthyroid syndrome (see later).

Other cytokines have been variably investigated as to their role in the pathogenesis of the sick euthyroid syndrome. Interferon α causes a decrease in serum T_3 and TSH and a rise in serum rT_3 concentrations in both humans [67] and mice [58] and has been shown to directly inhibit thyroidal type 1 5′-deiodinase activity [56,57] while interferon γ appears to have no effect on thyroid hormone parameters [68]. An increase in TSH has been observed in patients treated with IL-2 [69]. Soluble cytokine receptors may play a regulatory role in the cytokine cascade by functioning either as carrier proteins or cytokine inhibitors [36,38], and serum T_3 levels were found to be inversely proportional to soluble receptors for TNF-α, IL-1, and IL-2 in hospitalized patients [58].

From the data discussed earlier, it is likely that cytokines play a role in the alterations in thyroid hormone metabolism that occurs with systemic illness. While all cytokines examined to date can produce the sick euthyroid syndrome in either man or rodents when administered in pharmacologic doses, no one cytokine can be singled out as the primary mediator of the syndrome. This is not unexpected, given the diverse interrelationships and cascade nature of the cytokine network. Whether the sick euthyroid syndrome results from activation of the cytokine network or simply represents an endocrine response to systemic illness resulting from the same mediators that trigger the cytokine cascade remains to be determined.

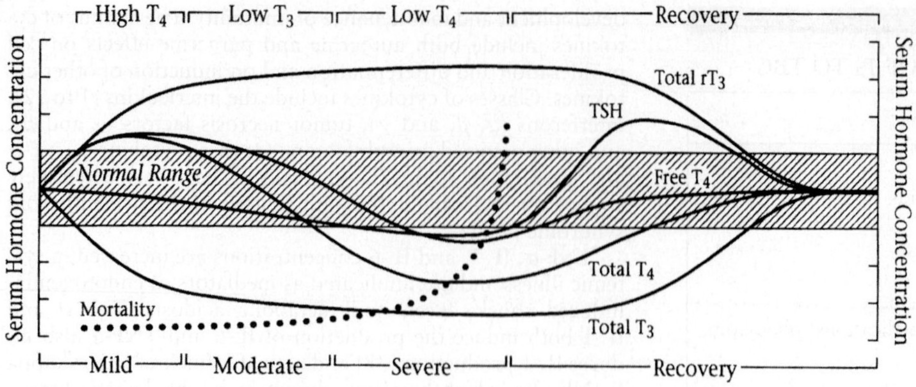

FIGURE 107.3. Alterations in thyroid hormone concentrations with critical illness. Schematic representation of the continuum of changes in serum thyroid hormone levels in patients with nonthyroidal illness. These alterations become more pronounced with increasing severity of the illness and return to the normal range as the illness subsides and the patient recovers. A rapidly rising mortality accompanies the fall in total and free T_4 levels.

Stages of the Sick Euthyroid Syndrome

As discussed earlier, critical illness causes multiple nonspecific alterations in thyroid hormone concentrations in patients without intrinsic thyroid dysfunction that relate to the severity of the illness [3,70,71]. One author has postulated that sick euthyroid syndrome may be a compensatory mechanism in response to the oxidative stress of acute illness [72]. Whatever the underlying cause, these alterations in thyroid hormone parameters represent a continuum of changes that depends on the severity of the illness and that can be categorized into several distinct stages (Fig. 107.3) [1]. The wide spectrum of changes observed often results from the differing points in the course of the illness that the thyroid function tests were obtained. Importantly, these changes are rarely isolated and often associated with alterations of other endocrine systems, such as decreases in serum gonadotropin and sex hormone concentrations [73] and increases in serum adrenocorticotropic hormone and cortisol levels [74]. Thus, the sick euthyroid syndrome should not be viewed as an isolated pathologic event but as part of a coordinated systemic reaction to illness involving both the immune and endocrine systems.

Low T_3 State

Common to all of the abnormalities in thyroid hormone concentrations seen in critically ill patients is a substantial depression of serum T_3 levels, which can occur as early as 24 hours after the onset of illness. Over half of the patients admitted to the medical service will demonstrate depressed serum T_3 concentrations [75,76]. The development of the low T_3 state arises from the impairment of peripheral T_4 to T_3 conversion through the inhibition of type 1 deiodinase (discussed earlier). This results in the marked reduction of T_3 production and rT_3 degradation [77], thereby leading to the reciprocal changes in serum T_3 and serum rT_3 concentrations. Low T_3 levels are also found in the peripheral tissues [18]. Previously, it was thought that the inhibition of type 1 deiodinase was the sole cause of the low T_3 syndrome by decreasing T_3 production. Recent studies suggest that increased type 3 deiodinase in critical illness increases T_3 disposal, adding to the decrease in serum T_3 levels [17,18]. Thyroid hormone receptor expression is also decreased in acute nonthyroidal illness [78], possibly in response to the decrease in tissue T_3 levels.

High T_4 State

Serum T_4 levels may be elevated early in acute illness due to either the acute inhibition of type 1 deiodinase or increased TBG levels. This is seen most often in the elderly and in patients with psychiatric disorders. As the duration of illness increases, nondeiodinative pathways of T_4 degradation increase serum T_4 levels to the normal range [75].

Low T_4 State

As the severity and the duration of the illness increases, serum total T_4 levels decrease into the subnormal range. Contributors to this decrease in serum T_4 levels are (a) a decrease in the binding of T_4 to serum carrier proteins, (b) a decrease in serum TSH levels leading to decreased thyroidal production of T_4, and (c) an increase in nondeiodinative pathways of T_4 metabolism. The decline in serum T_4 levels correlates with prognosis in the ICU, with mortality increasing as serum T_4 levels drop below 4 μg per dL and approaching 80% in patients with serum T_4 levels below 2 μg per dL [79–81]. Despite marked decreases in serum total T_4 and T_3 levels in the critically ill patient, the free hormone levels have been reported to be normal or even elevated [82,83], providing a possible explanation for why most patients appear euthyroid despite thyroid hormone levels in the hypothyroid range. Thus, the low T_4 state is unlikely to be a result of a hormone-deficient state and is probably more of a marker of multisystem failure in these critically ill patients.

Recovery State

As acute illness resolves, so do the alterations in thyroid hormone concentrations. This stage may be prolonged and is characterized by modest increases in serum TSH levels [84]. Full recovery, with restoration of thyroid hormone levels to the normal range, may require several weeks [85] or months after hospital discharge [76]. One study reported that 35 of 40 patients with nonthyroidal illness after coronary artery bypass grafting were able to regain normal thyroid function within 6 months after surgery [86].

ALTERATIONS IN THYROID FUNCTION IN SPECIFIC CRITICAL ILLNESSES

Caloric Deprivation

Most, if not all, nonthyroidal illness is associated with decreased caloric intake, catabolism, and/or malnutrition. Caloric deprivation is the most common inhibitory factor of type 1 5′-deiodinase [11,87,88]. Serum T_3 levels decrease and rT_3 levels increase within 24 hours of the onset of a fast. The decrease in serum T_3 levels may possibly be an adaptive response in order to preserve the total body protein stores. Indeed, restoring the serum T_3 to normal during starvation results in a marked increase in urinary nitrogen excretion [89]. Thus, the inhibition of T_4 to T_3 conversion in starvation can be viewed as a condition of adaptive hypothyroidism. Further support for the role of caloric deprivation in the development of the sick euthyroid syndrome is the demonstration that serum thyroid hormone levels in critically ill patients receiving nutritional support return to normal levels [90].

HIV Infection

A unique pattern of changes in circulating thyroid hormone levels is seen in patients with HIV infection and in those with AIDS [91]. A progressive increase in TBG levels is commonly observed and T_4 levels rarely decrease below the normal range. Serum rT_3 levels fail to rise with advancing infections and are only modestly increased in preterminal AIDS patients. Most striking is the observation that serum T_3 levels remain in the normal range despite progression of the HIV infection and are only mildly decreased in the critically ill AIDS patient, suggesting that these "inappropriately normal" T_3 levels play a role in the wasting and weight loss seen in the terminal phases of this disease. In contrast to T_4 levels in the sick euthyroid syndrome, it is the decreased serum T_3 levels in AIDS patients admitted to the ICU with *Pneumocystis carinii* infections that correlate with increased mortality [92].

Liver Disease

In contrast to the decrease in thyroid hormone levels seen in critically ill patients, individuals suffering from acute and chronic hepatocellular dysfunction often have marked elevations in total T_4 levels similar to those seen in patients with thyrotoxicosis [93]. T_3 levels are also higher than expected with illness and tend to fall late in the course of terminal liver disease. The etiology of these increased thyroid hormone concentrations is the increased discharge of TBG following destruction of hepatocytes. Free hormone measurements remain in the normal range. As with other illnesses, the low T_4 syndrome can be seen in patients with cirrhosis and is associated with increased mortality [94].

Cardiac Disease

Thyroid hormones have profound effects on the cardiovascular system [95]. Cardiac contractility, systolic time intervals, and heart rate are all increased in thyrotoxicosis and decreased in hypothyroidism. Multiple cardiac genes are either positively or negatively altered by thyroid hormone [96,97]. Serum T_4 and T_3 levels fall acutely following myocardial infarction [98], cardiac arrest [99–101], and cardiopulmonary bypass [86,102–105]. A significant inverse relationship between free T_3 and global oxygen consumption has been demonstrated after coronary artery bypass grafting with and without cardiopulmonary bypass [105]. Nonthyroidal illness syndrome has also been found with prevalence of 62.2% in patients with stress cardiomyopathy [106]. In contrast to other medical illnesses where serum T_4 levels are correlated with prognosis, serum T_3 concentrations are a negative prognostic factor in patients with congestive heart failure [107,108] and with coronary artery disease [109], raising a question as to what, if any, role thyroid hormones play in acute cardiac injury.

MANAGEMENT OF THE CRITICALLY ILL PATIENT WITH ABNORMAL THYROID FUNCTION TESTS

Evaluation

The identification of the critically ill patient with intrinsic thyroid disease is often difficult and always a diagnostic challenge. The routine screening of an ICU population for the presence of thyroid dysfunction is not recommended due to the high prevalence of abnormal thyroid function tests and low prevalence of true thyroid dysfunction. Whenever possible, it is best to defer evaluation of the thyroid-pituitary axis until the patient has recovered from his or her acute illness. In principal, when thyroid function tests are ordered in a hospitalized patient, it should be with a high clinical index of suspicion for the presence of thyroid dysfunction. For example, thyroid function should be evaluated in the patient admitted to the ICU with tachyarrhythmias when that patient also has a goiter, proptosis, and a tremor. Similarly, the patient with a large pericardial effusion, hypothermia, a goiter, and "hung-up" deep tendon reflexes should suggest the diagnosis of hypothyroidism. In practice, however, thyroid function tests are ordered in the patient with less-specific clinical findings and often present a diagnostic dilemma. Because every test of thyroid hormone function can be altered in the critically ill patient, no single test can definitively rule in or rule out the presence of intrinsic thyroid dysfunction.

Primary Tests

Sensitive Thyrotropin Assays

The development of the sensitive TSH assay has both helped and hindered the evaluation of thyroid function in the critically ill. These new assays have greatly expanded the lower range of the TSH assay, so the typical sensitive TSH assay has a lower limit of detection of 0.01 to 0.03 mU per L, which is 20- to 30-fold lower than the lower limit of the normal range. With this improved sensitivity has come the recognition of an increased frequency of subnormal TSH values in hospitalized patients, indicating that transient abnormalities in TSH secretion are commonplace in acute illness. To what degree this TSH dysregulation represents clinically significant alterations in thyroid function is uncertain.

Abnormal thyroid function tests have been reported in 20% to 40% of acutely ill patients, of which >80% have no intrinsic thyroid dysfunction after the resolution of the illness [75,76,110]. In a study of 1,580 hospitalized patients, only 24% of patients with suppressed TSH values (TSH < assay limit of detection) and 50% of patients with TSH values >20 mU per L were found to have thyroid disease [75,76]. More importantly, none of the patients with subnormal but detectable TSH values and only 14% of patients with elevated TSH values <20 mU per L were subsequently diagnosed with intrinsic thyroid dysfunction. The development of sensitive third-generation TSH assays has led to small improvements in discerning between overt hyperthyroidism and nonthyroidal illness [76]. Overall, however, while a normal TSH level has a high predictive value of normal thyroid function, an abnormal TSH value alone is not helpful in the evaluation of thyroid function in the critically ill patient.

Serum T_4 Assays

Measurement of free thyroid hormone concentrations in the patient with nonthyroidal illness is fraught with difficulty [83]. The gold standard of the determination of free hormone levels is by equilibrium dialysis. However, this technique is labor intensive and time consuming and, thus, is rarely used. The most commonly available laboratory tests of thyroid hormone concentrations, the free T_4 index, free T_4, and free T_3, are measured by analog methods, which represent estimates of the free hormone concentration and are therefore subject to inaccuracies [82].

The free T_4 index is determined by multiplying the total T_4 concentration by the T_3- or T_4-resin uptake, which is an inverse estimate of serum TBG concentrations [111]. Recent developments have allowed the measurement of free T_4 levels by the analog method, a less-expensive alternative to the free T_4 index [112], but the two tests are likely comparably accurate [113]. In a healthy population, there is a close correlation between the free T_4 index and free T_4 levels. In the critically ill patient, this association is no longer seen, mainly due to difficulties in estimating TBG binding with resin uptake tests. In spite of this, the sensitivity of the free T_4 index in a large study of hospitalized patients was 92.3%, as compared to 90.7% for the sensitive TSH test [76].

Secondary Tests

Serum T_3 and rT_3 Assays

As previously discussed, serum T_3 concentrations are affected to the greatest degree by the alterations in thyroid hormone economy resulting from acute illness. Therefore, there is no indication for the routine measurement of serum T_3 levels in the initial evaluation of thyroid function in the critically ill patient. This test should only be obtained if thyrotoxicosis is clinically suspected in the presence of a suppressed sensitive TSH value and an elevated or high normal free T_4 index or free T_4 determination. Thus, in patients with an elevated free T_4 index or free T_4 and a suppressed TSH, the finding of an elevated serum T_3 concentration will differentiate between thyrotoxicosis and the high T_4 state of the sick euthyroid syndrome. The total T_3 assay is preferable to the free T_3 (analog) assay, due to the variability between laboratories with the latter test [111].

Although some investigators have reported that serum rT_3 levels are a significant prognostic indicator of mortality in the ICU [114], rT_3 levels are generally unreliable and should not be used to distinguish between intrinsic thyroid dysfunction and nonthyroidal illness [115].

Serum Thyroid Autoantibodies

Autoantibodies to thyroglobulin and thyroid peroxidase (TPO), two intrinsic thyroid proteins, are commonly ordered tests [111]. While significant titers of either or both of these antibodies indicate the presence of autoimmune thyroid disease, the presence of thyroid autoantibodies alone does not necessarily indicate thyroid dysfunction, as they are present in approximately 12% to 26% of the general population [116]. Thyroid autoantibodies do, however, add to the sensitivity of abnormal TSH and free thyroxine index values in diagnosing known intrinsic thyroid disease [75,76].

Imaging Studies

Imaging studies are rarely essential to the diagnosis of thyroid disorders in the critically ill patient. Occasionally, functional analysis of the thyroid gland using the radioisotope ^{123}I may be useful in the patient with suspected thyrotoxicosis and equivocal laboratory tests. However, these studies are labor intensive and the management of the underlying acute illness often overshadows the benefits of obtaining these studies. While anatomical studies such as ultrasound, isotopic imaging, CT, and MRI are useful in the evaluation of thyroid nodules and goiter, these conditions rarely are the cause of acute illness; as such, these studies are not usually helpful in the critically ill patient.

Diagnosis

As indicated, the diagnostic significance of a single abnormal thyroid function test is low. The best single test to screen for thyroid dysfunction is either the free T_4 index or the free T_4, realizing that subtle changes in thyroid function will be missed. However, a reasonable approach to the initial evaluation of the thyroid function in the critically ill patient is to obtain either free T_4 index or free T_4 and TSH measurements in patients with a high clinical suspicion for intrinsic thyroid dysfunction. Assessment of these values in the context of the duration, severity, and stage of illness of the patient will allow the correct diagnosis in most patients. For example, a mildly elevated TSH coupled with a low free T_4 index or free T_4 is more likely to indicate primary hypothyroidism early in an acute illness as opposed to the same values obtained during the recovery phase of the illness. Similarly, the combination of an elevated TSH and low normal free T_4 index or free T_4 is more likely to indicate thyroid dysfunction in the hypothermic, bradycardic patient than the tachycardic, normothermic individual. If both the free T_4 index or free T_4 and TSH are normal, thyroid dysfunction is effectively eliminated as a significant contributing factor to the clinical picture. If the diagnosis is still unclear, measurement of thyroid antibodies is helpful as a marker of intrinsic thyroid disease and increases the sensitivity of both the free T_4 index or free T_4 and the TSH. Only in the case of a suppressed TSH and a mid-to-high normal free T_4 index or free T_4 is measurement of serum T_3 levels indicated.

Prognosis

Both serum T_4 and serum T_3 concentrations have been associated as negative indicators of prognosis when they are low. As mentioned previously, a direct relationship exists between low serum T_4 levels and poor outcomes in critically ill patient [110]. In acutely ill older patients with nonthyroidal illness syndrome, mortality rate was significantly higher, with an inverse relationship between free T_3 values and death rate [117]. The same relationship was found in burn patients, with free T_3 and TSH levels lower in nonsurvivors compared to survivors [118]. In patients on mechanical ventilation, patients with low free T_3 had higher mortality rate and longer duration of mechanical ventilation and ICU length of stay [119]. In different types of cardiac disease the prognostic value of low T_3 has been shown, including coronary artery disease and chronic heart failure [107–109]. Whether this is a causal association or simply reflecting multiorgan failure is unclear.

TREATMENT OF THE SICK EUTHYROID SYNDROME WITH THYROID HORMONE

Thyroid Hormone Therapy of General ICU Patients

There are only a few studies examining the use of supplemental thyroid hormone therapy in the critically ill general medical patient. The initial study in medical ICU patients by Brent and

Hershman examined the effect of thyroid hormone therapy in patients with serum T_4 levels <5 μg per dL but with no evidence of intrinsic thyroid dysfunction [120]. Either T_4 or placebo was given intravenously on a daily basis, with subsequent normalization of serum T_4 levels by day 5 in the T_4-treated group. There was no difference in mortality between the two groups and the elevation of TSH and serum T_3 concentrations seen in the recovery phase of acute illness was delayed in the T_4-treated group, suggesting that T_4 replacement was detrimental to the restoration of normal pituitary-thyroid regulation. A double-blind study with T_4 in patients with acute renal failure [121] showed that the mortality in the non-T_4-treated control group was significantly less than in the T_4-treated group; however, the mortality in the T_4-treated group was similar to that institution's experience and in historical controls, so a specific deleterious effect of T_4 could not be proved. A follow-up double-blind study with T_4 in patients after renal transplant by the same group [122] also failed to show any benefit.

One could argue that L-T_4 therapy in the sick euthyroid syndrome would be unlikely to have any effect due to the marked inhibition of T_4 to T_3 conversion in the patients, preventing significant increases in serum T_3 concentrations. Addressing this issue, Becker et al. [123] examined the effect of treatment with T_3 in 36 patients with acute burn injuries. Treatment with L-T_3 200 μg daily in four divided doses orally normalized serum T_3 concentrations but resulted in no change in either mortality or basal metabolic rate. Thus, despite the poor prognosis of the general ICU patients with the sick euthyroid syndrome [110], it does not appear that treatment with either L-T_4 or L-T_3 provides any benefit to these patients.

Thyroid Hormone Therapy in Premature Infants

Fetal thyroid function begins between 8 and 10 weeks' gestation and continues to mature throughout pregnancy [124,125]. Serum T_4 concentrations remain low throughout most of the second trimester and then steadily increase, with a twofold rise occurring between 24 and 34 weeks, at which time serum T_4 levels plateau [126]. There has been a remarkable increase in the number of surviving premature infants, especially in those <30 weeks' gestation. All premature infants have some degree of transient hypothyroxinemia, with serum T_4 concentrations varying directly with the gestational age [127]. Approximately 50% of infants born <30 weeks' gestation have serum T_4 concentrations <6.5 μg per dL [126,128,129]. Superimposed on this physiological hypothyroxinemia often are concurrent illnesses such as respiratory distress syndrome, infections, and malnutrition that contribute to the development of the sick euthyroid syndrome. Severe hypothyroxinemia with concentrations <4 μg per dL were seen in 21% of preterm babies, ranging from 40% at 23 weeks' gestation to 10.2% at 29 weeks [127]. Unlike adults, in whom most abnormalities resulting from clinical hypothyroxinemia are reversible, untreated congenital hypothyroxinemia can potentially have a devastating effect on brain development in the neonate [130–132].

Reuss et al. [133] showed that severe hypothyroxinemia in premature infants of <33 weeks' gestation correlated with a fourfold increase in a diagnosis cerebral palsy. In the study with the longest follow-up, hypothyroxinemia in premature infants of <32 weeks' gestation was associated with a 30% increase in school failure, poor school performance, and need for special education by 9 years of age [134].

The initial double-blind study of T_4 treatment in 23 premature infants of gestational age 26 to 28 weeks with hypothyroxinemia showed no differences between the groups in developmental indices at 1 year of age [135]. In the largest study to date, 200 infants born at 25 to 30 weeks' gestation received either thyroxine or placebo for 6 weeks and neurological development was assessed periodically up to 24 months [136]. While there appeared to be a beneficial effect for thyroxine in the very young (25 to 26 weeks' gestation), there also appeared to be a deleterious effect on the infants of 27 to 30 weeks' gestation. This study group was reevaluated 3 years later at early school age and reported a trend toward a benefit of T_4 supplementation on IQ and behavioral issues at 24/25 weeks' gestation but a significant deleterious effect on IQ and no effect on behavioral issues in those treated at 29 weeks' gestation [137]. Three other studies, two using T_4 [138,139] and one using T_3 [140], failed to show any significant effects of thyroid hormone treatment. Finally, an extensive meta-analysis and review of the literature concluded that thyroid hormone treatment failed to reduce neonatal mortality, improve neurodevelopmental outcome, or reduce the severity of the respiratory distress syndrome [141]. Thus, there is no indication currently for the use of thyroid hormone treatment in premature infants.

Thyroid Hormone Therapy in Cardiac Surgery

Within 15 to 30 minutes after placing the patient on bypass, serum T_4 and T_3 levels fall and serum rT_3 levels increase [142]. These alterations may persist for several days postoperatively [86,102]. These changes also have been observed in off-pump cardiopulmonary bypass [104]. Alterations in thyroid hormone parameters during and after cardiopulmonary bypass have been confirmed in multiple human and animal studies [86,102,103,143–146]. The etiology of these rapid changes in thyroid hormone concentrations remains unclear; one proposal suggests that these alterations may result from enhanced degradation of TBG [31]. Experimental studies in animals have shown that T_3 replacement after cardiopulmonary bypass significantly improves cardiac contractility and left ventricular function and decreases systemic vascular resistance [147–150]. Initial studies on the use of T_3 in humans undergoing cardiac surgery suggested that hormone-treated patients may require less ionotropic support [151] and have improved hemodynamic parameters [152]. However, the clearly demonstrable benefit of T_3 repletion in animals has not been translated into similar benefit in humans undergoing coronary artery bypass in controlled clinical trials.

A large placebo-controlled trial [153] found no effect of T_3 on any postoperative hemodynamic parameters, although a follow-up report of this same patient group suggested a lower incidence in atrial fibrillation in the T_3-treated group after the first postoperative day [154]. However, a lack of effect for T_3 was shown conclusively in a double-blind, placebo controlled trial [155], as there was no significant difference in the incidence of arrhythmia or the need for ionotropic support or vasodilator drugs in the 24 hours following surgery or in perioperative mortality or morbidity between the T_3 and the placebo groups. Somewhat more promising results have been reported in children undergoing cardiac surgery with improved hemodynamic parameters and a suggestion that the need for intensive postoperative care is decreased with intravenous L-T_3 [156,157]. Further studies may be indicated in this population. However, despite the promise in animal studies, there is no indication for the routine use of T_3 in adult patients undergoing cardiac surgery.

T_3 in Brain-Dead Potential Heart Donors

After brain death occurs, there is a progressive reduction in cardiac contractility, depletion of high-energy phosphates, and accumulation of tissue lactate [158,159]. These changes coincide with a rapid decline in serum T_3 concentrations and an increase in serum rT_3 concentrations within minutes to hours. An initial study in human heart donors [159] showed that T_3 treatment in human heart donors results in hemodynamic stability, a decrease in ionotropic support required, and preservation of cardiac function prior to transplantation. At least four other groups have subsequent beneficial effects of T_3 therapy in conjunction with other hormones in organ donors, especially those that are unstable [160]. Two other groups found no significant clinical effects of T_3 over placebo on human donor cardiac function [158,161], provided there was no antecedent cardiac dysfunction in the donor. Another study examined the use of T_3 to resuscitate impaired donor hearts with lower ejection fractions, higher filling pressures, and increased ionotropic support prior to transplantation [158,162]. Subsequently, several consensus conferences held in the United States and Canada have recommended the use of hormonal resuscitation consisting of T_3 (4 μg bolus followed by a 3 μg per hour infusion), vasopressin, methylprednisolone, and insulin in donors whose cardiac ejection fraction is less than 45% in an effort to increase the suitability of hearts for transplantation [160,163]. Thus, T_3 may be beneficial to stabilize or improve cardiac function in donors prior to cardiac transplantation.

Thyroid Hormone Therapy in Congestive Heart Failure

When T_3 and thyroid hormone analogs were initially studied as adjuncts to the treatment of heart failure [164,165], the rationale for the use of these hormones had been as pharmacological agents for their potential ionotropic properties and interactions with the adrenergic system rather than as hormonal replacement therapy to correct abnormal serum thyroid hormone concentrations. Recently, more attention has been paid to the interactions between the heart and the thyroid hormones in cardiac disease states. In both cardiac failure and in hypothyroidism, cardiac output and cardiac contractility is decreased. Decreased serum T_3 concentrations typical of the sick euthyroid syndrome are often observed in patients with congestive heart failure, while serum T_4 concentrations remain normal [166–168]. Importantly, the T_3 found in cardiac myocytes appears to come from the circulating T_3 pool rather than from local deiodination of T_4, indicating that the heart may be more responsive to changes in circulating serum T_3 concentrations [96,97]. Consistent with this observation, similar decreases in cardiac genes, including α-myosin heavy chain, SR calcium ATPase, and β1 adrenergic receptors, have been observed in both hypothyroidism and in heart failure [96,97]. Finally, low T_3 levels have been determined to be a strong predictor of mortality in patients with congestive heart failure [107,108]. These observations have led several investigators to examine the role of thyroid hormone treatment in patients with congestive heart failure.

An initial uncontrolled study examined the effect of oral T_4 therapy on 20 patients with dilated cardiomyopathy [169]. Cardiac output and functional capacity was increased and systemic vascular resistance decreased. Hamilton et al. [170] examined the effect of a supraphysiologic intravenous infusion of T_3 on cardiac function in patients with New York Heart Association (NYHA) Class III or IV heart failure. Cardiac output increased and systemic vascular resistance decreased without any untoward effects. More recently, Pingitore et al. [171] randomized 20 patients with NYHA Class III or less heart failure to a 3-day intravenous infusion of T_3 or placebo. During the first day of the T_3 infusion, serum T_3 levels were supraphysiologic and then declined to the high normal range on day 2 and 3. The T_3 infusion produced a significant improvement in the neurohumoral profile, with a decrease in serum noradrenaline, N-terminal pro-B-type natriuretic peptide, and aldosterone concentrations, and an increase in the left ventricular end diastolic volume. Since above-normal serum T_3 concentrations were achieved during all or part of these two studies, there is a question of whether the beneficial effects of T_3 are a pharmacologic effect rather than a physiologic one. There are currently no studies on the long-term use of T_3 in the treatment of congestive heart failure. However, as with children undergoing cardiac surgery, more studies may be indicated in this patient population.

Thyroid Hormone Therapy in the Hypothyroid Patient in the Intensive Care Unit

This chapter has discussed the evaluation and management of patients without intrinsic thyroid dysfunction who present with abnormal thyroid hormone parameters as a result of nonthyroidal illness. However, thyroid hormone therapy is needed when the hypothyroid patient presents to the ICU. By definition, the nonthyroidal illness syndrome excludes patients with intrinsic thyroid dysfunction; however, all of the changes in TSH secretion, thyroid hormone metabolism, and thyroid-binding proteins discussed earlier also occur in the hypothyroid patient. As such, the same caveats toward measuring thyroid hormone parameters exist. Most importantly, an admission to the ICU is not the time to determine the adequacy of thyroid hormone replacement in a hypothyroid patient on a previously stable outpatient regimen.

Hypothyroid patients should be continued on their outpatient L-T_4 dose. Oral L-T_4 is the preferred method for replacing thyroid hormone in a hypothyroid patient. Because of the long half-life of about 7 days of L-T_4, the L-T_4 dose can be held for 1 to 2 days if the oral route is unavailable. If oral therapy cannot be resumed within 3 days, intravenous L-T_4 should be administered. Because 50% to 70% of an oral dose of L-T_4 is absorbed, the intravenous L-T_4 dose should be 30% to 50% less than the oral dose. Neither oral nor intravenous L-T_3 is indicated in the hypothyroid patient in the absence of myxedema coma.

If hypothyroidism is diagnosed in the ICU setting and initiation of thyroid hormone replacement is required, special consideration should be given to the patients with coronary artery disease. In patients with significant preexisting coronary artery disease, starting thyroid hormone may aggravate the angina. It is recommended that the initial dose of L-T_4 should not exceed 25 μg for those with known ischemic hearth disease and 50 μg for patients aged 65 years or older without such a preexisting diagnosis.

The oral dose of L-T_4 may differ in the ICU setting, due to pharmacological agents or gastrointestinal conditions that may decrease the absorption of L-T_4. Patients with jejunoileal bypass surgery, bowel resection, malabsorptive disorders (like celiac disease), and conditions that impair gastric acidity may need adjustment in the dose of L-T_4. L-T_4 should not be administered within 2 to 3 hours of calcium carbonate, bile acid sequestrants, ferrous sulfate, phosphate binders, sucralfate, and aluminium-containing antacids since they may interfere with the absorption of L-T_4. Also by their effect on decreasing the gastric acidity, proton pump inhibitors, if given for a long period, may decrease the absorption of L-T_4.

SUMMARY

In summary, the spectrum of alterations in thyroid hormone concentrations and regulation seen in the critically ill patient are the result of a coordinated systemic reaction to illness. The

TABLE 107.4

SUMMARY OF CLINICAL TRIALS ON THE EFFECTS OF TREATMENT OF THE SICK EUTHYROID SYNDROME WITH THYROID HORMONE [70]

General ICU patients
- No benefit of L-T_4 on general medical patients [120], patients with acute renal failure [121], or renal transplant [122].
- No benefit of L-T_3 on burn patients [123].

Premature infants
- No benefit of L-T_4 on developmental indices of premature infants at 26–28 weeks' gestation [135].
- Possible beneficial effect of L-T_4 on infants of at 25–26 weeks' gestation but possible deleterious effects on infants of 27–30 weeks' gestation [136].
- No benefit of L-T_3 [140].
- Meta-analysis shows no significant effects of thyroid hormone treatment of premature infants [141].

Cardiac surgery patients
- Small studies suggest improved hemodynamic parameters with L-T_3 [151,152].
- Large trials show no benefit of L-T_3 noted in patients undergoing cardiac bypass [153,155,176].
- Possible improvement in hemodynamic parameters and hospital stay with L-T_3 in children undergoing cardiac surgery [156,157].

Cardiac donors
- Variable results (helpful [159,160], no benefit [158,161]) on the effects of L-T_3 in preserving function of normal hearts in brain-dead cardiac donors prior to transplantation.
- Possible benefits of L-T_3 in improving function of impaired hearts prior to transplant, potentially increasing the pool of organs available for transplantation [158,162].
- Consensus conferences recommend the use of L-T_3 as part of the hormonal resuscitation in donors whose cardiac ejection fraction is <45% [160].

Congestive heart failure
- Small uncontrolled study suggested short term L-T_4 therapy increased cardiac output and functional capacity and decreased systemic vascular resistance [169].
- Improved hemodynamic parameters and neurohumoral profiles with short-term intravenous L-T_3 infusion, possibly requiring supraphysiologic concentrations [170,171].

question of whether the sick euthyroid syndrome in critically ill patients represents pathologic alterations in thyroid function that negatively impacts these patients or simply reflects the multisystem failure (i.e., respiratory, cardiac, renal, hepatic failure) that occurs in critically ill patients is still debatable [172–175]. The interpretation of thyroid function tests in the ICU patient and the identification of those patients with intrinsic thyroid dysfunction is often difficult and must take into consideration both the clinical assessment of the patient and the duration and severity of the illness. Whenever possible, it is best to defer the evaluation of thyroid function until the patient has recovered from the critical illness. Thyroid hormone replacement therapy has not been shown to be of benefit in the vast majority of these patients in the published studies to date (Table 107.4 [70]). At the present time, in the absence of any clinical evidence of hypothyroidism, there does not appear to be any compelling evidence for the use of thyroid hormone therapy in any patient with decreased thyroid hormone parameters due to the sick euthyroid syndrome.

References

1. Farwell AP: Sick euthyroid syndrome in the intensive care unit, in Irwin RS, Rippe JM (eds): *Intensive Care Medicine.* Philadelphia, Lippincott Williams & Wilkins, 2008, pp 1309–1322.
2. Mebis L, Debaveye Y, Visser TJ, et al: Changes within the thyroid axis during the course of critical illness. *Endocrinol Metab Clin North Am* 35(4):807–821, x, 2006.
3. Burman KD, Wartofsky L: Thyroid function in the intensive care unit setting. *Crit Care Clin* 17(1):43–57, 2001.
4. DeGroot LJ: "Non-thyroidal illness syndrome" is functional central hypothyroidism, and if severe, hormone replacement is appropriate in light of present knowledge. *J Endocrinol Invest* 26(12):1163–1170, 2003.
5. Farwell AP: Sick euthyroid syndrome. *J Intensive Care Med* 12:249–260, 1997.
6. Langton JE, Brent GA: Nonthyroidal illness syndrome: evaluation of thyroid function in sick patients. *Endocrinol Metab Clin North Am* 31(1):159–172, 2002.
7. Brierre S, Kumari R, Deboisblanc B: The endocrine system during sepsis. *Am J Med Sci* 328(4):238–247, 2004.
8. Hamrahian AH, Oseni TS, Arafah BM: Measurements of serum free cortisol in critically ill patients. *N Engl J Med* 350(16):1629–1638, 2004.
9. Papanicolaou DA: Euthyroid sick syndrome and the role of cytokines. *Rev Endocr Metab Disord* 1(1–2):43–48, 2000.
10. Larsen PR, Silva JE, Kaplan MM: Relationships between circulating and intracellular thyroid hormones: physiological and clinical implications. *Endocr Rev* 2(1):87–102, 1981.
11. Bianco AC, Larsen PR: Intracellular pathways of iodothyronine metabolism, in Braverman LE, Utiger RD (eds): *Werner and Ingbar's The Thyroid.* Philadelphia, Lippincott Williams and Wilkins, 2005, pp 109–134.
12. Yen PM: Physiological and molecular basis of thyroid hormone action. *Physiol Rev* 81(3):1097–1142, 2001.
13. Zimmermann MB: Iodine deficiency. *Endocr Rev* 30(4):376–408, 2009.
14. Benvenga S: Thyroid hormone transport proteins and the physiology of hormone binding, in Braverman LE, Utiger RD (eds): *Werner and Ingbar's The Thyroid.* Philadelphia, Lippincott Williams & Wilkins, 2005, pp 97–108.
15. Palha JA: Transthyretin as a thyroid hormone carrier: function revisited. *Clin Chem Lab Med* 40(12):1292–1300, 2002.
16. Koenig RJ: Regulation of type 1 iodothyronine deiodinase in health and disease. *Thyroid* 15(8):835–840, 2005.
17. Huang SA, Bianco AC: Reawakened interest in type III iodothyronine deiodinase in critical illness and injury. *Nat Clin Pract Endocrinol Metab* 4(3):148–155, 2008.
18. Peeters RP, van der Geyten S, Wouters PJ, et al: Tissue thyroid hormone levels in critical illness. *J Clin Endocrinol Metab* 90(12):6498–6507, 2005.
19. Mebis L, Langouche L, Visser TJ, et al: The type II iodothyronine deiodinase is up-regulated in skeletal muscle during prolonged critical illness. *J Clin Endocrinol Metab* 92(8):3330–3333, 2007.
20. Hennemann G, Krenning EP: The kinetics of thyroid hormone transporters and their role in non-thyroidal illness and starvation. *Best Pract Res Clin Endocrinol Metab* 21(2):323–338, 2007.

21. Van den Berghe G, de Zegher F, Lauwers P, et al: Dopamine and the sick euthyroid syndrome in critical illness. *Clin Endocrinol* 41:731–737, 1994.
22. den Brinker M, Dumas B, Visser TJ, et al: Thyroid function and outcome in children who survived meningococcal septic shock. *Intensive Care Med* 31(7):970–976, 2005.
23. den Brinker M, Joosten KF, Visser TJ, et al: Euthyroid sick syndrome in meningococcal sepsis: the impact of peripheral thyroid hormone metabolism and binding proteins. *J Clin Endocrinol Metab* 90(10):5613–5620, 2005.
24. Duntas LH, Nguyen TT, Keck FS, et al: Changes in metabolism of TRH in euthyroid sick syndrome. *Eur J Endocrinol* 141(4):337–341, 1999.
25. Adriaanse R, Romijn JA, Brabant G, et al: Pulsatile thyrotropin secretion in nonthyroidal illness. *J Clin Endocrinol Metab* 77:1313–1317, 1993.
26. Romijn JA, Wiersinga WM: Decreased nocturnal surge of thyrotropin in nonthyroidal illness. *J Clin Endocrinol Metab* 70:35–42, 1990.
27. Hsieh CJ, Wang PW, Wang ST, et al: Serum leptin concentrations of patients with sequential thyroid function changes. *Clin Endocrinol (Oxf)* 57(1):29–34, 2002.
28. Corsonello A, Buemi M, Artemisia A, et al: Plasma leptin concentrations in relation to sick euthyroid syndrome in elderly patients with nonthyroidal illnesses. *Gerontology* 46(2):64–70, 2000.
29. Warner MH, Beckett GJ: Mechanisms behind the non-thyroidal illness syndrome: an update. *J Endocrinol* 205(1):1–13, 2010.
30. Mebis L, Debaveye Y, Ellger B, et al: Changes in the central component of the hypothalamus-pituitary-thyroid axis in a rabbit model of prolonged critical illness. *Crit Care* 13(5):R147, 2009.
31. Afandi B, Schussler GC, Arafeh AH, et al: Selective consumption of thyroxine-binding globulin during cardiac bypass surgery. *Metabolism* 49(2):270–274, 2000.
32. Lim CF, Munro SL, Wynne KN, et al: Influence of non-esterified fatty acids and lysolecithins on thyroxine binding to thyroxine-binding globulin and transthyretin. *Thyroid* 4:319–324, 1995.
33. Chopra IJ, Huang TS, Solomon DS, et al: The role of T_4-binding serum proteins in oleic acid-induced increase in free T_4 in nonthyroidal illnesses. *J Clin Endocrinol Metab* 63:776–779, 1986.
34. Lim CF, Docter R, Visser TJ, et al: Inhibition of thyroxine transport into cultured rat hepatocytes by serum of nonuremic critically ill patients: effects of bilirubin and non-esterified fatty acids. *J Clin Endocrinol Metab* 76:1165–1172, 1993.
35. Stockigt JR, Lim CF: Medications that distort in vitro tests of thyroid function, with particular reference to estimates of serum free thyroxine. *Best Pract Res Clin Endocrinol Metab* 23(6):753–767, 2009.
36. Charo IF, Ransohoff RM: The many roles of chemokines and chemokine receptors in inflammation. *N Engl J Med* 354(6):610–621, 2006.
37. Nylen ES, Seam N, Khosla R, et al: Endocrine markers of severity and prognosis in critical illness. *Crit Care Clin* 22(1):161–179, viii, 2006.
38. Rees RC: Cytokines as biological response modifiers. *Clin Pathol* 45:93–98, 1992.
39. Nagaya T, Fujieda M, Otsuka G, et al: A potential role of activated NF-kappa B in the pathogenesis of euthyroid sick syndrome. *J Clin Invest* 106(3):393–402, 2000.
40. Hashimoto H, Igarashi N, Yachie A, et al: The relationship between serum levels of interleukin-6 and thyroid hormone in children with acute respiratory infection. *J Clin Endocrinol Metab* 78:288–291, 1994.
41. Murai H, Murakami S, Ishida K, et al: Elevated serum interleukin-6 and decreased thyroid hormone levels in postoperative patients and effects of Il-6 on thyroid cell function in vitro. *Thyroid* 6:601–606, 1996.
42. Boelen A, Platvoet-Ter SMC, Wiersinga WM: Association between serum interleukin-6 and serum 3,5,3'-triiodothyronine in non-thyroidal illness. *J Clin Endocrinol Metab* 77:1695–1699, 1993.
43. Kimura T, Kanda T, Kotajima N, et al: Involvement of circulating interleukin-6 and its receptor in the development of euthyroid sick syndrome in patients with acute myocardial infarction. *Eur J Endocrinol* 143(2):179–184, 2000.
44. Kimur T, Kotajima N, Kanda T, et al: Correlation of circulating interleukin-10 with thyroid hormone in acute myocardial infarction. *Res Commun Mol Pathol Pharmacol* 110(1–2):53–58, 2001.
45. Lee WY, Kang MI, Oh KW, et al: Relationship between circulating cytokine levels and thyroid function following bone marrow transplantation. *Bone Marrow Transplant* 33(1):93–98, 2004.
46. Mooradian AD, Reed RL, Osterweil D, et al: Decreased serum triiodothyronine is associated with increased concentrations of tumor necrosis factor. *J Clin Endocrinol Metab* 71:1239–1242, 1990.
47. Michalaki M, Vagenakis AG, Makri M, et al: Dissociation of the early decline in serum T_3 concentration and serum IL-6 rise and TNFalpha in nonthyroidal illness syndrome induced by abdominal surgery. *J Clin Endocrinol Metab* 86(9):4198–4205, 2001.
48. Wellby ML, Kennedy JA, Pile K, et al: Serum interleukin-6 and thyroid hormones in rheumatoid arthritis. *Metabolism* 50(4):463–467, 2001.
49. Pang X-P, Hershman JM, Mirell CJ, et al: Impairment of hypothalamic-thyroid function in rats treated with human recombinant tumor necrosis factor a. *Endocrinology* 125:76–84, 1989.
50. Dubuis JM, Dayer JM, Siegrist-Kaiser CA, et al: Human recombinant interleukin-1b decreases plasma thyroid hormone and thyroid stimulating hormone levels in rats. *Endocrinology* 123:2175–2181, 1988.
51. Hermus ARMM, Sweep CGJ, van der Meet MJM, et al: Continuous infusion of interleukin-1b induces an nonthyroidal illness syndrome in the rat. *Endocrinology* 131:2139–2146, 1992.
52. Bartalena L, Grasso L, Brogioni S, et al: Interleukin 6 effects on the pituitary-thyroid axis in the rat. *Eur J Endocrinol* 131:302–306, 1994.
53. Enomoto T, Sugawa H, Kosugi S, et al: Prolonged effects of recombinant human interleukin-1 a on mouse thyroid function. *Endocrinology* 127:2322–2327, 1990.
54. Fujii T, Sato K, Ozawa M, et al: Effect of Interleukin-1 (Il-1) on thyroid hormone metabolism in mice: Stimulation by Il-1 of iodothyronine 5'-deiodinating activity (type I) in the liver. *Endocrinology* 124:167–174, 1989.
55. Boelen A, Platvoet MC, Wiersinga WM: Systemic and local illness in interleukin-6 knock-out mice: the role of Il-6 in the sick euthyroid syndrome. *J Endocrinol Invest* 19:S79, 1996.
56. Tang K-T, Braverman LE, De Vito WJ: Tumor necrosis factor-a and interferon-g modulate gene expression of type I 5′-deiodinase, thyroid peroxidase and thyroglobulin in FRTL-5 rat thyroid cells. *Endocrinology* 136:881–888, 1995.
57. Pekary AE, Berg L, Santini F, et al: Cytokines modulate type I iodothyronine deiodinase mRNA levels and enzyme activity in FRTL-5 rat thyroid cells. *Mol Cell Endocrinol* 101:R31–R35, 1994.
58. Boelen A, Platvoet-ter Schiphorst MC, Bakker O, et al: The role of cytokines in the lipopolysaccharide-induced sick euthyroid syndrome in mice. *J Endocrinol* 146:475–483, 1995.
59. Rasmussen AK, Bendtzen K, Feldt-Rasmussen U: Thyrocyte-interleukin-1 interactions. *Exp Clin Endocrinol Diabetes* 108(2):67–71, 2000.
60. Jakobs TC, Mentrup B, Schmutzler C, et al: Proinflammatory cytokines inhibit the expression and function of human type I 5′-deiodinase in HepG2 hepatocarcinoma cells. *Eur J Endocrinol* 146(4):559–566, 2002.
61. Molnar I, Czirjak L: Euthyroid sick syndrome and inhibitory effect of sera on the activity of thyroid 5'-deiodinase in systemic sclerosis. *Clin Exp Rheumatol* 18(6):719–724, 2000.
62. Fekete C, Gereben B, Doleschall M, et al: Lipopolysaccharide induces type 2 iodothyronine deiodinase in the mediobasal hypothalamus: implications for the nonthyroidal illness syndrome. *Endocrinology* 145(4):1649–1655, 2004.
63. van der Poll F, Romijn JA, Endert E, et al: Tumor necrosis factor: a putative mediator of the sick euthyroid syndrome in man. *J Clin Endocrinol Metab* 71:1567–1572, 1990.
64. Stouthard JML, van der Poll T, Endert E, et al: Effects of acute and chronic interleukin-6 administration on thyroid hormone metabolism in humans. *J Clin Endocrinol Metab* 79:1342–1346, 1994.
65. Feelders RA, Swaak AJ, Romijn JA, et al: Characteristics of recovery from the euthyroid sick syndrome induced by tumor necrosis factor alpha in cancer patients. *Metab Clin Exp* 48(3):324–329, 1999.
66. van der Poll T, Van Zee KJ, Endert E, et al: Interleukin-1 receptor blockade does not affect endotoxin-induced changes in plasma thyroid hormone and thyrotropin concentrations in man. *J Clin Endocrinol Metab* 80:1341–1346, 1995.
67. Corssmit EPM, Heyligenberg R, Endert E, et al: Acute effects of interferon-a administration on thyroid hormone metabolism in healthy men. *J Clin Endocrinol Metab* 80:3140–3144, 1995.
68. de Metz J, Romijn JA, Endert E, et al: Administration of interferon-gamma in healthy subjects does not modulate thyroid hormone metabolism. *Thyroid* 10(1):87–91, 2000.
69. Witzke O, Winterhagen T, Saller B, et al: Transient stimulatory effects on pituitary-thyroid axis in patients treated with interleukin-2. *Thyroid* 11(7):665–670, 2001.
70. Farwell A: Thyroid hormone therapy is not indicated in the majority of patients with the sick euthyroid syndrome. *Endocr Pract* 14:1180–1187, 2008.
71. DeGroot LJ: Dangerous dogmas in medicine: the nonthyroidal illness syndrome. *J Clin Endocrinol Metab* 84(1):151–164, 1999.
72. Selvaraj N, Bobby Z, Sridhar MG: Is euthyroid sick syndrome a defensive mechanism against oxidative stress? *Med Hypotheses* 71(3):404–405, 2008.
73. Woolf PD, Hamill RW, McDonald JV, et al: Transient hypogonadism caused by critical illness. *J Clin Endocrinol Metab* 60(3):444–450, 1985.
74. Parker LN, Levin ER, Lifrak ET: Evidence for adrenocortical adaptation to severe illness. *J Clin Endocrinol Metab* 60(5):947–952, 1985.
75. Spencer CA: Clinical utility and cost-effectiveness of sensitive thyrotropin assays in ambulatory and hospitalized patients. *Mayo Clin Proc* 63(12):1214–1222, 1988.
76. Spencer C, Elgen A, Shen D, et al: Specificity of sensitive assays of thyrotropin (TSH) used to screen for thyroid disease in hospitalized patients. *Clin Chem* 33(8):1391–1396, 1987.
77. Rodriguez-Perez A, Palos-Paz F, Kaptein E, et al: Identification of molecular mechanisms related to nonthyroidal illness syndrome in skeletal muscle and adipose tissue from patients with septic shock. *Clin Endocrinol (Oxf)* 68(5):821–827, 2008.
78. Beigneux AP, Moser AH, Shigenaga JK, et al: Sick euthyroid syndrome is associated with decreased TR expression and DNA binding in mouse liver. *Am J Physiol Endocrinol Metab* 284(1):E228–E236, 2003.

79. Kaptein EM, Weiner JM, Robinson WJ, et al: Relationship of altered thyroid hormone indices to survival in nonthyroidal illness. *Clin Endocrinol (Oxf)* 16:565–574, 1982.
80. Slag MF, Morley JE, Elson MK, et al: Hypothyroxinemia in critically ill patients as a predictor of high mortality. *JAMA* 245:43–45, 1981.
81. Maldonado LS, Murata GH, Hershman JM, et al: Do thyroid function tests independently predict survival in the critically ill? *Thyroid* 2(2):119–123, 1992.
82. Nelson JC, Weiss RM: The effect of serum dilution on free thyroxine concentration in the low T_4 syndrome of nonthyroidal illness. *J Clin Endocrinol Metab* 61:239–246, 1985.
83. Chopra IJ: Simultaneous measurement of free thyroxine and free 3,5,3'-triiodothyronine in undiluted serum by direct equilibrium dialysis/radioimmunoassay: evidence that free triiodothyronine and free thyroxine are normal in many patients with the low triiodothyronine syndrome. *Thyroid* 8(3):249–257, 1998.
84. Hamblin S, Dyer SA, Mohr VS, et al: Relationship between thyrotropin and thyroxine changes during recovery from severe hypothyroxinemia of critical illness. *J Clin Endocrinol Metab* 62:717–722, 1986.
85. Iglesias P, Munoz A, Prado F, et al: Alterations in thyroid function tests in aged hospitalized patients: prevalence, aetiology and clinical outcome. *Clin Endocrinol (Oxf)* 70(6):961–967, 2009.
86. Cerillo AG, Storti S, Mariani M, et al: The non-thyroidal illness syndrome after coronary artery bypass grafting: a 6-month follow-up study. *Clin Chem Lab Med* 43(3):289–293, 2005.
87. Douyon L, Schteingart DE: Effect of obesity and starvation on thyroid hormone, growth hormone, and cortisol secretion. *Endocrinol Metab Clin North Am* 31(1):173–189, 2002.
88. Visser TJ, Lamberts SWJ, Wilson JHP, et al: Serum thyroid hormone concentrations during prolonged reduction of dietary intake. *Metabolism* 27(4):405–409, 1978.
89. Gardner DF, Kaplan MM, Stanley CA, et al: Effect of tri-iodothyronine replacement on the metabolic and pituitary responses to starvation. *New Engl J Med* 300(11):579–584, 1979.
90. Richmond DA, Molitch ME, O'Donnell TF: Altered thyroid hormone levels in bacterial sepsis: the role of nutritional adequacy. *Metabolism* 29:936–942, 1980.
91. Koutkia P, Mylonakis E, Lewis RM: Human immunodeficiency virus infection and the thyroid. *Thyroid* 12(7):577–582, 2002.
92. Fried JC, LoPresti JS, Micon M, et al: Serum triiodothyronine values: prognostic indicators of acute mortality due to *Pneumocystis carinii* pneumonia associated with the acquired immunodeficiency syndrome. *Arch Intern Med* 150:406–409, 1990.
93. Yamanaka T, Ido K, Kimura K, et al: Serum levels of thyroid hormones in liver diseases. *Clinica Chimica Acta* 101:45–55, 1980.
94. Caregaro L, Alberino F, Amodio P, et al: Nutritional and prognostic significance of serum hypothyroxinemia in hospitalized patients with liver cirrhosis. *J Hepatology* 28(1):115–121, 1998.
95. Klein I, Danzi S: Thyroid disease and the heart. *Circulation* 116(15):1725–1735, 2007.
96. Danzi S, Klein I: Thyroid hormone-regulated cardiac gene expression and cardiovascular disease. *Thyroid* 12(6):467–472, 2002.
97. Klein I, Ojamaa K: Thyroid hormone and the cardiovascular system. *N Engl J Med* 344(7):501–509, 2001.
98. Wiersinga WM, Lie KI, Touber JL: Thyroid hormones in acute myocardial infarction. *Clin Endocrinol (Oxf)* 14:367–374, 1984.
99. Worstman J, Premachandra BN, Chopra IJ, et al: Hypothyroxinemia in cardiac arrest. *Arch Intern Med* 147:245–248, 1987.
100. Longstreth WT Jr, Manowitz NR, DeGroot LJ, et al: Plasma thyroid hormone profiles immediately following out-of-hospital cardiac arrest. *Thyroid* 6:649–653, 1996.
101. Iltumur K, Olmez G, Ariturk Z, et al: Clinical investigation: thyroid function test abnormalities in cardiac arrest associated with acute coronary syndrome. *Crit Care* 9(4):R416–R424, 2005.
102. Reinhardt W, Mocker V, Jockenhovel F, et al: Influence of coronary artery bypass surgery on thyroid hormone parameters. *Horm Res* 47:1–8, 1997.
103. Holland FW, Brown PS, Weintraub BD, et al: Cardiopulmonary bypass and thyroid function: a euthyroid sick syndrome. *Ann Thorac Surg* 52:46–50, 1991.
104. Cerillo AG, Sabatino L, Bevilacqua S, et al: Nonthyroidal illness syndrome in off-pump coronary artery bypass grafting. *Ann Thorac Surg* 75(1):82–87, 2003.
105. Velissaris T, Tang AT, Wood PJ, et al: Thyroid function during coronary surgery with and without cardiopulmonary bypass. *Eur J Cardiothorac Surg* 36(1):148–154, 2009.
106. Lee SJ, Kang JG, Ryu OH, et al: The relationship of thyroid hormone status with myocardial function in stress cardiomyopathy. *Eur J Endocrinol* 160(5):799–806, 2009.
107. Iervasi G, Pingitore A, Landi P, et al: Low-T_3 syndrome: a strong prognostic predictor of death in patients with heart disease. *Circulation* 107(5):708–713, 2003.
108. Pingitore A, Landi P, Taddei MC, et al: Triiodothyronine levels for risk stratification of patients with chronic heart failure. *Am J Med* 118(2):132–136, 2005.
109. Coceani M, Iervasi G, et al: Thyroid hormone and coronary artery disease: from clinical correlations to prognostic implications. *Clin Cardiol* 32(7):380–385, 2009.
110. Plikat K, Langgartner J, Buettner R, et al: Frequency and outcome of patients with nonthyroidal illness syndrome in a medical intensive care unit. *Metabolism* 56(2):239–244, 2007.
111. Baloch Z, Carayon P, Conte-Devolx B, et al: Laboratory medicine practice guidelines. Laboratory support for the diagnosis and monitoring of thyroid disease. *Thyroid* 13(1):3–126, 2003.
112. Midgley JE: Direct and indirect free thyroxine assay methods: theory and practice. *Clin Chem* 47(8):1353–1363, 2001.
113. Liewendahl K, Mahonen H, Tikanoja S, et al: Performance of direct equilibrium dialysis and analogue-type free thyroid hormone assays, and an immunoradiometric TSH method in patients with thyroid dysfunction. *Scand J Clin Lab Invest* 47(5):421–428, 1987.
114. Peeters RP, Wouters PJ, van Toor H, et al: Serum 3,3',5'-triiodothyronine (rT_3) and 3,5,3'-triiodothyronine/rT_3 are prognostic markers in critically ill patients and are associated with postmortem tissue deiodinase activities. *J Clin Endocrinol Metab* 90(8):4559–4565, 2005.
115. Burmeister LA: Reverse T_3 does not reliably differentiate hypothyroid sick syndrome from euthyroid sick syndrome. *Thyroid* 5(6):435–441, 1995.
116. Prummel MF, Wiersinga WM: Thyroid peroxidase autoantibodies in euthyroid subjects. *Best Pract Res Clin Endocrinol Metab* 19(1):1–15, 2005.
117. Tognini S, Marchini F, Dardano A, et al: Non-thyroidal illness syndrome and short-term survival in a hospitalised older population. *Age Ageing* 39(1):46–50, 2010.
118. Gangemi EN, Garino F, Berchialla P, et al: Low triiodothyronine serum levels as a predictor of poor prognosis in burn patients. *Burns* 34(6):817–824, 2008.
119. Bello G, Pennisi MA, Montini L, et al: Nonthyroidal illness syndrome and prolonged mechanical ventilation in patients admitted to the ICU. *Chest* 135(6):1448–1454, 2009.
120. Brent GA, Hershman JM: Thyroxine therapy in patients with severe nonthyroidal illnesses and low thyroxine concentration. *J Clin Endocrinol Metab* 63(1):1–8, 1986.
121. Acker CG, Singh AR, Flick RP, et al: A trial of thyroxine in acute renal failure. *Kid Int* 57(1):293–298, 2000.
122. Acker CG, Flick R, Shapiro R, et al: Thyroid hormone in the treatment of post-transplant acute tubular necrosis (ATN). *Am J Transplant* 2(1):57–61, 2002.
123. Becker RA, Vaughan GM, Ziegler MG, et al: Hypermetabolic low triiodothyronine syndrome of burn injury. *Crit Care Med* 10(12):870–875, 1982.
124. Obregon MJ, Calvo RM, Del Rey FE, et al: Ontogenesis of thyroid function and interactions with maternal function. *Endocr Dev* 10:86–98, 2007.
125. Burrow GN, Fisher DA, Larsen PR: Maternal and fetal thyroid function. *N Engl J Med* 331:1072–1078, 1994.
126. Fisher DA: Euthyroid low thyroxine and triiodothyronine states in prematures and sick neonates. *Ped Clin N Amer* 37:1297–1312, 1990.
127. Reuss ML, Leviton A, Paneth N, et al: Thyroxine values from newborn screening of 919 infants born before 29 weeks' gestation. *Am J Public Health* 87(10):1693–1697, 1997.
128. Uhrmann S, Marks KH, Maisels MJ, et al: Frequency of transient hypothyroxinemia in low birthweight infants. *Arch Dis Child* 56:214–217, 1981.
129. Frank JE, Faix JE, Hermos RJ, et al: Thyroid function in very low birth weight infants: effects on neonatal hypothyroidism screening. *J Peds* 128:548–554, 1996.
130. Bernal J: Thyroid hormones and brain development. *Vitam Horm* 71:95–122, 2005.
131. Rovet J, Daneman D: Congenital hypothyroidism: a review of current diagnostic and treatment practices in relation to neuropsychologic outcome. *Paediatr Drugs* 5(3):141–149, 2003.
132. Anderson GW: Thyroid hormones and the brain. *Front Neuroendocrinol* 22(1):1–17, 2001.
133. Reuss ML, Paneth N, Pinto-Martin JA, et al: The relationship of transient hypothyroxinemia in preterm infants to neurologic development at two years of age. *New Engl J Med* 334:821–827, 1996.
134. Den Ouden AL, Kok JH, Verkerk PH, et al: The relation between neonatal thyroxine levels and neurodevelopmental outcome at age 5 and 9 years in a national cohort of very preterm and/or very low birth weight infants. *Pediatr Res* 39:142–145, 1996.
135. Chowdhry P, Scanlon JW, Auerbach R, et al: Results of controlled double-blind study of thyroid replacement in very-low-birth-weight premature infants with hypothyroxinemia. *Pediatrics* 73:301–305, 1984.
136. van Wassenaer AG, Kok JH, de Vijlder JJM, et al: Effects of thyroxine supplementation on neurologic development in infants born at less than 30 weeks' gestation. *N Engl J Med* 336(1):21–26, 1997.
137. Briet JM, van Wassenaer AG, Dekkar FW, et al: Neonatal thyroxine supplementation in very preterm children: developmental outcome evaluated at early school age. *Pediatrics* 107(4):712–718, 2001.
138. Smith LM, Leake RD, Berman N, et al: Postnatal thyroxine supplementation in infants less than 32 weeks' gestation: effects on pulmonary morbidity. *J Perinatol* 20(7):427–431, 2000.
139. Vanhole C, Aerssens P, Naulaers G, et al: L-thyroxine treatment of preterm newborns: clinical and endocrine effects. *Pediatr Res* 42(1):87–92, 1997.

140. Amato M, Guggisberg C, Schneider H: Postnatal triiodothyronine replacement and respiratory distress syndrome of the preterm infant. *Horm Res* 32(5–6):213–217, 1989.
141. Osborn DA: Thyroid hormones for preventing neurodevelopmental impairment in preterm infants. *Cochrane Database Syst Rev* (4):CD001070, 2001.
142. Bremner WF, Taylor KM, Baird S, et al: Hypothalamo-pituitary-thyroid axis during cardiopulmonary bypass. *J Thorac Cardiovasc Surg* 75:392–399, 1978.
143. Chu SH, Huang TS, Hsu RB, et al: Thyroid hormone changes after cardiovascular surgery and clinical implications. *Ann Thorac Surg* 52:791–796, 1991.
144. Robuschi G, Medici D, Fesani F, et al: Cardiopulmonary bypass: "a low T_4 and T_3 syndrome" with blunted thyrotropin response to thyrotropin-releasing hormone. *Horm Res* 23:151–158, 1986.
145. Clark RE: Cardiopulmonary bypass and thyroid hormone metabolism. *Ann Thorac Surg* 56:S35–S42, 1993.
146. Broderick TJ, Wechsler AS: Triiodothyronine in cardiac surgery. *Thyroid* 7:133–137, 1997.
147. Novitzky D, Human PA, Cooper DK, et al: Ionotropic effect of triiodothyronine following myocardial ischemia and cardiopulmonary bypass: an experimental study in pigs. *Ann Thorac Surg* 45:50–55, 1988.
148. Novitzky D, Human PA, Cooper DK, et al: Effect of triiodothyronine on myocardial high energy phosphates and lactate after ischemia and cardiopulmonary bypass. *J Thorac Cardiovasc Surg* 96:600–607, 1988.
149. Novitzky D, Matthews N, Shawley D, et al: Triiodothyronine replacement on the recovery of stunned myocardium in dogs. *Ann Thorac Surg* 51:10–17, 1991.
150. Kazmierczak P, Polak A, Mussur M: Influence of preischemic short-term triiodothyronine administration on hemodynamic function and metabolism of reperfused isolated rat heart. *Med Sci Monit* 10(10):BR381–BR387, 2004.
151. Novitzky D, Cooper DKC, Swanepoel A, et al: Inotropic effect of triiodothyronine following myocardial ischemia and cardiopulmonary bypass: an initial experience in patients undergoing open-heart surgery. *Eur J Cardiothor Surg* 3:140–145, 1989.
152. Novitzky D, Cooper DKC, Barton CI, et al: Triiodothyronine as an ionotropic agent after open-heart surgery. *J Thorac Cardiovasc Surg* 98:972–978, 1989.
153. Klemperer JD, Klein I, Gomez M, et al: Thyroid hormone treatment after coronary-artery bypass surgery. *N Engl J Med* 333(23):1522–1527, 1995.
154. Klemperer JD, Klein IL, Ojamaa K, et al: Triiodothyronine therapy lowers the incidence of atrial fibrillation after cardiac operations. *Ann Thorac Surg* 61(5):1323–1327; discussion 1328–1329, 1996.
155. Bennett-Guerrero E, Jimenez JL, White WD, et al: Cardiovascular effects of intravenous triiodothyronine in patients undergoing coronary artery bypass surgery. A randomized, double-blind, placebo-controlled trial. *JAMA* 275:687–692, 1996.
156. Bettendorf M, Schmidt KG, Grulich-Henn J, et al: Tri-iodothyronine treatment in children after cardiac surgery: a double-blind, randomised, placebo-controlled study. *Lancet* 356(9229):529–534, 2000.
157. Chowdhury D, Ojamaa K, Parnell VA, et al: A prospective randomized clinical study of thyroid hormone treatment after operations for complex congenital heart disease. *J Thorac Cardiovasc Surg* 122(5):1023–1025, 2001.
158. Jeevanandam V: Triiodothyronine: spectrum of use in heart transplantation. *Thyroid* 7:139–145, 1997.
159. Novitzky D: Novel actions of thyroid hormone: the role of triiodothyronine in cardiac transplantation. *Thyroid* 6:531–536, 1996.
160. Novitzky D, Cooper DK, Barton CI, et al: Hormonal therapy of the brain-dead organ donor: experimental and clinical studies. *Transplantation* 82(11):1396–1401, 2006.
161. Goarin J-P, Cohen S, Riou B, et al: The effects of triiodothyronine on hemodynamic status and cardiac function in potential heart donors. *Anesth Anal* 83:41–47, 1996.
162. Jeevanandam V, Todd B, Regillo T, et al: Reversal of donor myocardial dysfunction by triiodothyronine replacement therapy. *J Heart Lung Trans* 13:681–687, 1994.
163. Zaroff JG, Rosengard BR, Armstrong WF, et al: Consensus conference report: maximizing use of organs recovered from the cadaver donor: cardiac recommendations, March 28–29, 2001, Crystal City, Va. *Circulation* 106(7):836–841, 2002.
164. Morkin E, Pennock GD, Raya TE, et al: Studies on the use of thyroid hormone and a thyroid hormone analogue in the treatment of congestive heart failure. *Ann Thorac Surg* 56:S54–S60, 1993.
165. Tielens ET, Forder JR, Chatham JC, et al: Acute L-triiodothyronine administration potentiates ionotropic responses to beta-adrenergic stimulation in the isolated perfused rat heart. *Cardiovasc Res* 32:306–310, 1996.
166. Hamilton MA: Prevalence and clinical implications of abnormal thyroid hormone metabolism in advanced heart failure. *Ann Thorac* 56:S48–S53, 1993.
167. Gomberg-Maitland M, Frishman WH: Thyroid hormone and cardiovascular disease. *Am Heart J* 135(2, Pt 1):187–196, 1998.
168. Shanoudy H, Soliman A, Moe S, et al: Early manifestations of "sick euthyroid" syndrome in patients with compensated chronic heart failure. *J Card Fail* 7(2):146–152, 2001.
169. Moruzzi P, Doria E, Agostoni PG: Medium-term effectiveness of L-thyroxine treatment in idiopathic dilated cardiomyopathy. *Am J Med* 101(5):461–467, 1996.
170. Hamilton MA, Stevenson LW, Fonarow GC, et al: Safety and hemodynamic effects of intravenous triiodothyronine in advanced congestive heart failure. *Am J Cardiol* 81(4):443–447, 1998.
171. Pingitore A, Galli E, Barison A, et al: Acute effects of triiodothyronine (t3) replacement therapy in patients with chronic heart failure and low-t3 syndrome: a randomized, placebo-controlled study. *J Clin Endocrinol Metab* 93(4):1351–1358, 2008.
172. Bello G, Paliani G, Annetta MG, et al: Treating nonthyroidal illness syndrome in the critically ill patient: still a matter of controversy. *Curr Drug Targets* 10(8):778–787, 2009.
173. Lechan RM: The dilemma of the nonthyroidal illness syndrome. *Acta Biomed* 79(3):165–171, 2008.
174. De Groot LJ: Non-thyroidal illness syndrome is a manifestation of hypothalamic-pituitary dysfunction, and in view of current evidence, should be treated with appropriate replacement therapies. *Crit Care Clin* 22(1):57–86, vi, 2006.
175. Farwell AP: Thyroid hormone therapy is not indicated in the majority of patients with the sick euthyroid syndrome. *Endocr Pract* 14(9):1180–1187, 2008.
176. Teiger E, Menasche P, Mansier P, et al: Triiodothyronine therapy in open-heart surgery: from hope to disappointment. *Eur Heart J* 14:629–633, 1993.

SECTION IX ■ HEMATOLOGIC AND ONCOLOGIC PROBLEMS IN THE INTENSIVE CARE UNIT

PATRICK F. FOGARTY

CHAPTER 108 ■ DISORDERS OF HEMOSTASIS IN CRITICALLY ILL PATIENTS

JEREMIAH BOLES AND ALICE D. MA

Disorders of hemostasis are common in critically ill patients. This chapter will review hemostasis, pathophysiology of commonly encountered congenital and acquired bleeding disorders along with their associated symptoms, laboratory findings, and management.

REVIEW OF NORMAL HEMOSTASIS

Hemostasis can be broken into a series of steps occurring in overlapping sequence. Primary hemostasis refers to the interactions between the platelet and the injured vessel wall, culminating in the formation of a platelet plug. The humoral phase of clotting, or secondary hemostasis, encompasses a series of enzymatic reactions, resulting in a hemostatic fibrin plug. Finally, fibrinolysis and wound repair occur. Each of these steps is carefully regulated, and perturbations can predispose to either hemorrhage or thrombosis. Depending on the nature of the defect, the hemorrhagic or thrombotic tendency can be either profound or subtle.

Primary hemostasis begins at the site of vascular injury, with platelets adhering to the subendothelium, utilizing interactions between molecules such as collagen and von Willebrand factor (vWF) in the vessel wall with glycoprotein (GP) receptors on the platelet surface. Upon exposure to agonists present at a wounded vessel, signal transduction leads to platelet activation. Via a process known as inside-out signaling, the platelet membrane integrin $\alpha_{2b}\beta_3$ (also known as GP IIbIIIa) undergoes a conformational change to be able to bind fibrinogen, which cross-links adjacent platelets, leading to platelet aggregation. Secretion of granular contents is also triggered by outside signals, potentiating further platelet activation (Fig. 108.1). Lastly, the surface of the platelet changes to serve as an adequate scaffold for the series of biochemical reactions resulting in thrombin generation.

Following platelet activation, a series of enzymatic reactions take place on phospholipid surfaces, culminating in the formation of a stable fibrin clot. Several models have attempted to make sense of these reactions. The cascade model was developed by two groups nearly simultaneously [1,2] and explained the extrinsic, intrinsic, and common pathways leading to fibrin formation (Fig. 108.2). While the cascade model accounts for the physiologic reactions underlying the prothrombin time (PT) and the activated partial thromboplastin time (aPTT), it fails to explain completely the bleeding diathesis seen in individuals deficient in factors XI, IX, and VIII, as well as the lack of bleeding in those deficient only in contact factors. A cell-based model of hemostasis has been developed to address these deficiencies. In this model, upon vascular injury, the membrane of a tissue factor (TF)-bearing cell such as an activated monocyte or fibroblast serves as a platform for generation of a small amount of thrombin and FIXa, which then serves to activate platelets and cleave FVIII from vWF. Newly formed FVIIIa participates in the tenase complex on the surface of activated platelets to form FXa that interacts with the FVa generated on the platelet surface to form the prothrombinase complex. This complex generates a large burst of thrombin which is sufficient to cleave fibrinogen, activate FXIII, and activate the thrombin activatable fibrinolysis inhibitor (TAFI), thus allowing for formation of a stable fibrin clot (Fig. 108.2).

Fibrinolysis leads to clot dissolution once wound healing has occurred, in order to restore normal blood flow. Plasminogen is activated to plasmin by the action of either tissue plasminogen activator (t-PA) or urokinase plasminogen activator (u-PA). Plasmin degrades fibrin and fibrinogen and can thus dissolve both formed clot as well as its soluble precursor. Plasmin is inhibited by a number of inhibitors, of which α_2-plasmin inhibitor is the most significant. Plasminogen activation is also inhibited by a number of molecules; chief among them is plasminogen activator inhibitor-1 (PAI-1). Lastly, cellular receptors act to localize and potentiate or clear plasmin and plasminogen activators (see Chapter 111 for further discussion).

APPROACH TO THE BLEEDING PATIENT

Physicians in the intensive care unit (ICU) often encounter bleeding patients and it can be difficult to identify which of these patients require further evaluation. Patients who experience bleeding that is excessive, spontaneous, or delayed following surgery or tissue injury require further investigation, which must begin with a thorough clinical history. A bleeding history should assess a patient's exposure and response to all hemostatic challenges in the past such as trauma, surgery, and childbirth. Characterization of menses in females also may be revealing. Several bleeding assessment tools have been developed and are useful in the evaluation for an underlying coagulopathy, particularly von Willebrand disease (vWD) [3]. This history should also identify coexisting medical conditions such as liver, kidney, or thyroid disorders. A careful medication history is also important, including use of all over-the-counter medications which may contain aspirin, as well as any herbal preparations. Also of cardinal importance is an evaluation for a family history of abnormal bleeding. An inherited or congenital bleeding disorder is suggested by abnormal bleeding with onset shortly after birth and persistence throughout life. It is further supported by a family history with a consistent genetic pattern. However, it is important to note that a negative family history does not exclude a congenital bleeding disorder. For instance, approximately one third of all cases of hemophilia A arise from spontaneous mutations. Many of the rare coagulation disorders, including deficiency of factors II, V, VII, X,

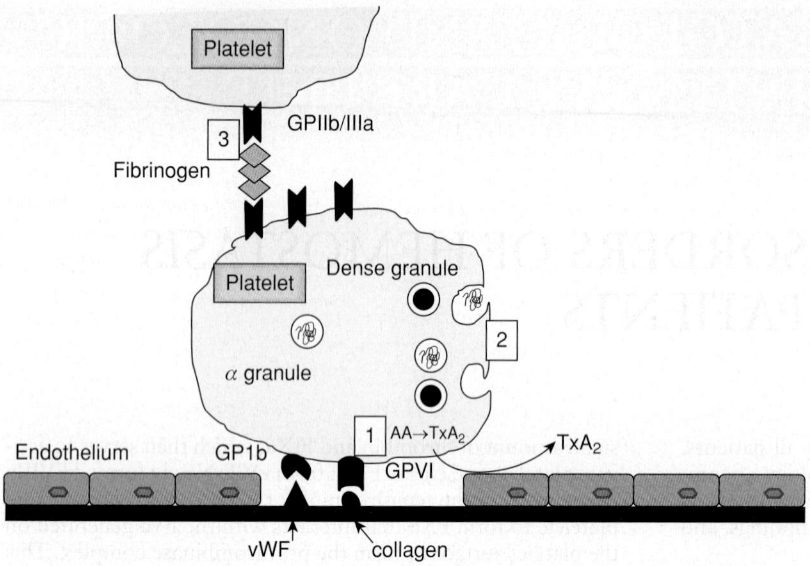

FIGURE 108.1. Primary hemostasis. (1) Exposure of subendothelium at sites of vascular disruption results in platelet adhesion via GPIb and GP VI with exposed von Willebrand factor (vWF) and collagen, respectively. Following platelet adhesion TxA_2 is produced and released which promotes vasoconstriction and platelet aggregation. (2) Platelet adhesion also results in fusion of cytoplasmic granules to the plasma membrane. Release of alpha and dense granules activates nearby platelets. (3) Platelet activation results in exposure of GPIIb/IIIa on the platelet surface allowing fibrinogen to cross bridge platelets resulting in a platelet plug.

as well as vWD type 2 N, among others, are inherited in an autosomal recessive fashion, and the parents of the patient may be entirely asymptomatic.

A bleeding history should also ascertain past sites/mechanisms of bleeding. Surgical bleeding in patients with an underlying hemorrhagic condition is typically described as "diffuse oozing," without the readily identifiable bleeding source seen with a surgical mishap such as a severed vessel. Patients with platelet disorders typically manifest mucocutaneous bleeding such as gingival bleeding and epistaxis as well as menorrhagia, petechiae, and ecchymoses. Platelet defects impact primary hemostasis and therefore the bleeding in these disorders is often immediate following surgery or trauma, whereas delayed bleeding is more classically associated with coagulation disorders. Patients with coagulation defects typically present with hemorrhages into soft tissues such as muscles and joints.

A physical examination should pay particular attention to the skin, joints, mucosal surfaces, and liver and spleen size.

LABORATORY ASSAYS OF PRIMARY AND SECONDARY HEMOSTASIS

While the history and physical examination can increase suspicion for the presence of a bleeding disorder, laboratory confirmation is required for precise diagnosis and treatment.

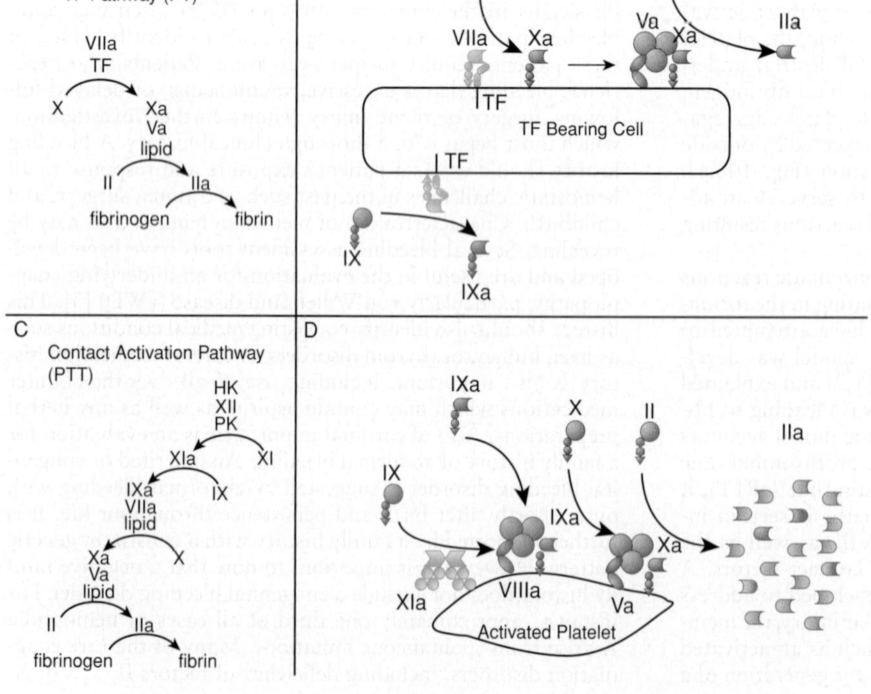

FIGURE 108.2. Secondary hemostasis. **A:** Tissue factor (TF) pathway cascade model of coagulation—basis for prothrombin time (PT) laboratory assay. **B:** Circulating FVIIa binds TF on a TF-bearing cell. TF/FVIIa along with calcium (Ca) and phospholipid (lipid) form the "extrinsic tenase" complex and converts FX to FXa. FXa combines with FVa, calcium, and phospholipid, "prothrombinase" complex, to activate FII to FIIa which in turn converts fibrinogen into fibrin. **C:** Contact activation pathway model of coagulation—basis for partial thromboplastin time (PTT) laboratory assay. **D:** On an activated platelet surface, FXIa activates FIXa. FIXa is also formed on the surface of a TF-bearing cell (B). FIXa, along with FVIIIa, Ca, and lipid, constitute the "intrinsic tenase" complex. This complex converts FX to FXa with subsequent FIIIa generation through the prothrombinase complex. (Courtesy of Dougald Monroe.)

Laboratory evaluation is particularly crucial in individuals who are suspected of having a bleeding disorder but in whom prior bleeding is absent, such as those with mild congenital bleeding disorders who never previously underwent a sufficient hemostatic challenge, or those with acquired hemorrhagic disorders.

Initial Evaluation of Primary Hemostasis—Platelet Function

An assessment of a patient's platelet count is fundamental in evaluating primary hemostasis. This is typically part of a complete blood count (CBC). Reduced platelet counts, or thrombocytopenia, may be seen in a large number of acquired and congenital conditions. Evaluation and management of thrombocytopenia is further discussed in Chapter 109.

An evaluation of the peripheral smear is also cardinal in any evaluation of a bleeding patient. It allows one to assess platelet size and morphology, presence of platelet clumping (pseudothrombocytopenia), leukocyte inclusions, and red cell fragments, among other aberrancies, which may further direct workup and treatment.

Traditionally, platelet function was evaluated by bleeding time (BT). However, many institutions have discontinued using this test given the difficulty in standardization. Furthermore, the BT has been shown to be an inadequate predictor of bleeding, particularly in preoperative risk assessment [4]. More recently, automated tests have been developed to assess platelet function. The most widely used is the platelet function analyzer (PFA-100®). This assay measures the time required (closure time) for flowing whole, citrated blood to occlude an aperture in a membrane impregnated with a combination of either collagen and epinephrine or collagen and adenosine diphosphate (ADP). Closure time is affected by platelet count, hematocrit, platelet function, and vWF [5]. The PFA-100® appears to assess platelet function with greater sensitivity and reproducibility than the BT; however, a recent position statement from the Platelet Physiology Subcommittee of the Scientific and Standardization Committee of the International Society of Thrombosis and Hemostasis noted that although the PFA-100® is abnormal in some platelet disorders, it was not felt to have sufficient sensitivity or specificity to be used as a screening tool for platelet disorders [6].

Evaluation of Secondary Hemostasis—Coagulation

The PT and the aPTT are assays performed on citrated plasma, which require enzymatic generation of thrombin on a phospholipid surface. Prolongation of the PT and the aPTT can be seen in individuals with either deficiencies of, or inhibitors to, humoral clotting factors, though not all patients with prolongations of these assays will have bleeding diatheses (Table 108.1).

The PT measures the time needed for formation of an insoluble fibrin clot once citrated plasma has been recalcified and thromboplastin has been added, indicating activity of factors VII, V, X, and II and fibrinogen. It commonly is used to monitor anticoagulation with vitamin K antagonists such as warfarin. Since thromboplastin from various sources and different lots can affect the rates of clotting reactions, the International Normalized Ratio (INR) measurement was developed

TABLE 108.1

LABORATORY TEST ABNORMALITIES IN COMMON ACQUIRED AND CONGENITAL BLEEDING DISORDERS

	Acquired bleeding disorders	Congenital bleeding disorders
PT elevated, aPTT wnl	Liver disease DIC Vitamin K deficiency Vitamin K antagonists (e.g., warfarin)	FVII deficiency
PT wnl, aPTT elevated	Heparin Lupus inhibitor Acquired FVIII inhibitor	Hemophilia A and B FXI deficiency Severe vWD
Both PT and aPTT elevated	Heparin overdose Warfarin overdose FVI inhibitors FX inhibitors Severe DIC Severe vitamin K deficiency Severe liver disease Direct thrombin inhibitors	Afibrinogenemia Hypo- or dysfibrino-genemia Prothrombin deficiency FV deficiency Combined deficiency of FV and FVIII
Both PT and aPTT wnl	LMWH therapy Fondaparinux therapy Antiplatelet agents Acquired vWD Scurvy Acquired thrombocytopenia	vWD FXIII deficiency Congenital platelet dysfunction Congenital thrombocytopenia Collagen disorders (e.g., Ehlers–Danlos syndrome)

wnl, within normal limits; DIC, disseminated intravascular coagulation; LMWH, low-molecular-weight heparin; PT, prothrombin time; PTT; partial thromboplastin time; vWD, von Willebrand disease.

to avoid some of this variability in PT measurement. Each batch of thromboplastin reagent has assigned to it a numerical International Sensitivity Index (ISI) value, which is used in the formula:

$$\mathrm{INR} = (\mathrm{PT}_{\mathrm{patient}}/\mathrm{PT}_{\mathrm{normal\ mean}})^{\mathrm{ISI}}$$

The INR is less predictive of bleeding in patients with liver disease, and can be inaccurate in patients with lupus anticoagulants that are strong enough to affect the PT.

The aPTT tests the activity of factors XII, XI, IX, VIII, X, V, and II, and fibrinogen, high-molecular-weight kininogen (HMWK), and plasma prekallikrein (PK) [7]. Citrated plasma is recalcified, and phospholipids (to provide a scaffold for the clotting reactions) and an activator of the intrinsic system such as kaolin, celite, or silica are added. The reagents used show variable sensitivities to inhibitors such as lupus anticoagulants and heparin, and to deficiencies (if any) in involved clotting factors, and normal ranges will vary from laboratory to laboratory. aPTT values that are vastly different from one laboratory to another should prompt suspicion of a lupus anticoagulant.

The Thrombin Clotting Time and Reptilase Time

The thrombin clotting time (TCT) or thrombin time (TT) measures the time needed for clot formation once thrombin is added to citrated plasma. Thrombin enzymatically cleaves fibrinopeptides A and B from the α- and β-chains of fibrinogen, allowing for polymerization into fibrin. The TT is prolonged in the presence of any thrombin inhibitor such as heparin, lepirudin, or argatroban; by low levels of fibrinogen or structurally abnormal fibrinogen (dysfibrinogens); and by elevated levels of fibrinogen or fibrin degradation products, which can serve as nonspecific inhibitors of the reaction. Patients with paraproteins can have a prolonged TT because of the inhibitory effect of the paraprotein on fibrin polymerization.

Reptilase is snake venom from *Bothrops atrox* which also enzymatically cleaves fibrinogen. Reptilase cleaves only fibrinopeptide A from the α-chain of fibrinogen, but fibrin polymerization still occurs. Reptilase time (RT) is not affected by heparin but may be more sensitive than the TT to the presence of a dysfibrinogenemia.

Mixing Studies

Mixing studies are used to evaluate prolongations of the aPTT (less commonly the PT or the TT) and are useful in making the distinction between an inhibitor and a clotting factor deficiency. The patient's plasma is mixed 1:1 with normal control plasma, and the assay is repeated (with or without prolonged incubation at 37°C). Correction of the clotting test signifies factor deficiency, since the normal plasma will supply the deficient factor. Incomplete correction of the clotting test after mixing suggests the presence of an inhibitor, since an inhibitor will prolong clotting in normal plasma. Incomplete correction can sometimes be seen with nonspecific inhibitors such as lupus anticoagulants, elevated fibrin split products, or a paraprotein. Less commonly, deficiencies of multiple clotting factors can lead to incomplete correction of the mixing study, since the mixing study was designed to correct deficiency of a single factor.

Tests of specific factor activity levels as well as evaluation for vWD will be discussed in the following sections.

CONGENITAL DISORDERS OF HEMOSTASIS

Due to a requirement for specialized management, all cases of suspected or proven congenital hemostatic defects require consultation with a hematologist upon admission to the critical care setting.

Von Willebrand Disease

It has been estimated that lower-than-reference levels of vWF occur in 1% of the population worldwide and therefore vWD is the most common congenital bleeding disorder [8]. However, only a fraction of the aforementioned individuals are symptomatic (approximately 5% of those with low levels) [9]. vWD is inherited in an autosomal manner with the more common type I disease being autosomal dominant.

vWD constitutes a quantitative or qualitative deficiency in vWF, and is divided into three subtypes according to the pathophysiology. Types 1 and 3 are the result of a partial (type 1) or virtually a complete (type 3) quantitative deficiency of vWF, while type 2 is a qualitative defect in vWF. Type 1 vWD represents the most common subtype accounting for approximately 70% of patients, while type 2 accounts for 15% to 20% and type 3 for only 2% to 5% of vWD patients [10].

Because bleeding symptoms in persons with vWD may be absent or overlooked until a major hemorrhage due to surgery or trauma has occurred, the diagnosis should be considered in an ICU patient with otherwise unexplained excessive bleeding, particularly if there is a significant family history including an autosomal pattern of inheritance. The most common historical bleeding symptoms include epistaxis, increased bleeding after dental extractions, and menorrhagia. A validated bleeding assessment tool has been developed to screen outpatients who may benefit from formal vWD laboratory testing [3], but its usefulness in the critical care setting has not been established.

A formal diagnosis of vWD should be based on three components: (a) a history of excessive bleeding, either spontaneous mucocutaneous and/or postsurgical, (b) a positive family history for excessive bleeding, and (c) confirmatory laboratory testing. Diagnostic tests for vWD, reviewed elsewhere [11], should be performed in a specialized laboratory and are summarized in Table 108.2.

The goals of treatment in vWD are to correct the quantitative or qualitative deficiencies in vWF, platelets, and FVIII. Treatment options include desmopressin (DDAVP), vWF-containing concentrates, and/or antifibrinolytics. See Tables 108.3 and 108.4 for general treatment guidelines.

In normal volunteers, DDAVP increases plasma levels of FVIII, vWF, and tissue plasminogen activator [12]. It may be given IV or SQ [13]. When given intravenously, the FVIII and vWF levels are usually increased three- to fivefold above basal levels within 30 minutes. vWD patients should undergo a DDAVP trial to gauge their individual response since there is considerable interindividual variability. Dosing of DDAVP for vWD is generally recommended at 0.3 μg per kg (IV or SQ), or 300 μg intranasally, which can be repeated at intervals of 12 to 24 hours. Tachyphylaxis (due to depletion of FVIII/vWF from repeated endothelial exocytosis into plasma) following repeated dosing is expected; DDAVP given as a second dose is 30% less effective than the first dose [14]. For this reason, and due to the risk of hyponatremia (which can lead to seizures), serial dosing should be limited to two to three doses in a 72-hour period with concurrent free water restriction and monitoring of serum sodium levels. DDAVP is most effective in type 1 vWD. It is relatively contraindicated in type 2B vWD because of the transient induction of thrombocytopenia [15]. Patients

TABLE 108.2

EXPECTED LABORATORY VALUES IN vWD FROM THE NHLBI

	Normal	Type 1	Type 2A	Type 2B	Type 2M	Type 2N	Type 3	PLT-vWD[a]
vWF:Ag	N	L, ↓ or ↓↓	↓ or L	↓ or L	↓ or L	N or L	Absent	↓ or L
vWF:RCo	N	L, ↓ or ↓↓	↓↓ or ↓↓↓	↓↓	↓↓	N or L	Absent	↓↓
FVIII	N	N or ↓	N or ↓	N or ↓	N or ↓	↓↓	1-9 IU/dL	N or L
RIPA	N	Often N	↓	Often N	↓	N	Absent	Often N
LD-RIPA	Absent	Absent	Absent	↑↑↑	Absent	Absent	Absent	↑↑↑
PFA-100® CT	N	N or ↑	↑	↑	↑	N	↑↑↑	↑
BT	N	N or ↑	↑	↑	↑	N	↑↑↑	↑
Platelet count	N	N	N	↓ or N	N	N	N	↓
vWF	N	N	Abnormal	Abnormal	N	N	Absent	Abnormal
multimer pattern	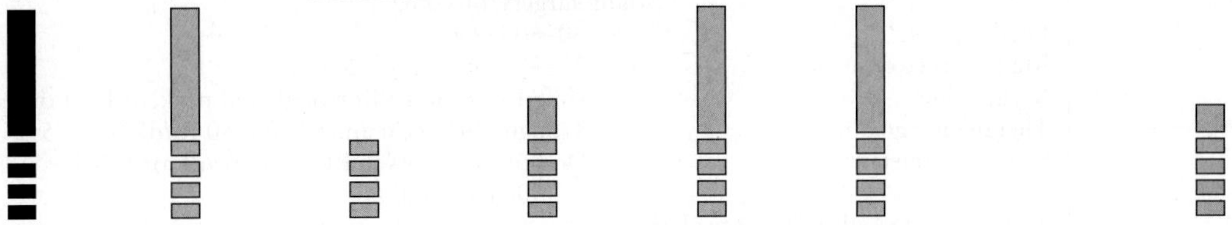							

[a]The symbols and values represent prototypical cases. In practice, laboratory studies in certain patients may deviate slightly from these expectations.
L, 30–50 IU/dL; ↓, ↓↓, ↓↓↓, relative decrease; ↑, ↑↑, ↑↑↑, relative increase; BT, bleeding time; FVIII, factor VIII activity; LD RIPA, low-dose ristocetin-induced platelet aggregation (concentration of ristocetin ≤0.6 mg/mL); N, normal; PFA-100® CT, platelet function analyzer closure time; RIPA, ristocetin-induced platelet aggregation; vWF, von Willebrand factor; vWF:Ag, vWF antigen; vWF:RCo, vWF ristocetin cofactor activity.
Reprinted from The National Heart, Lung, and Blood Institute. The Diagnosis, Evaluation, and Management of von Willebrand Disease. Bethesda, MD: National Institutes of Health Publication 08-5832, 2008.

with type 3 vWD are usually unresponsive to DDAVP. Certain hemophilia treatment centers caution against use of DDAVP in patients with coronary artery disease, since this agent may also activate platelets.

Antifibrinolytic agents (epsilon aminocaproic acid and tranexamic acid) can be used alone or as adjunctive treatment in vWD patients with mucosal bleeding. These drugs inhibit fibrinolysis by inhibiting plasminogen activation, thereby promoting clot stability. They are contraindicated in the setting of gross hematuria as resultant ureteral obstruction by insoluble clot has been described. Given a concern for thrombosis, antifibrinolytics should be avoided in patients with

TABLE 108.3

DOSING GUIDELINES FOR VON WILLEBRAND DISEASE (vWD) TREATMENT

Medication	Dose	Comments
DDAVP	Nasal spray: 300 μg (1 spray in each nostril) If weight <50 kg 150 μg (1 spray in 1 nostril) IV: 0.3 μg/kg (not to exceed 20–25 μg)	Most useful in type 1 vWD, ineffective in type 3. Requires challenge to document efficacy. Relatively contraindicated in type 2B as may exacerbate thrombocytopenia May repeat dose in 12 h and/or 24 h. Tachyphylaxis occurs with repeat dosing. Due to risk of hyponatremia, if dosing serially, limit doses to no more than 2–3 in a 72-h period, fluid restrict, and follow serum sodium levels. Avoid in patients with coronary disease.
Antifibrinolytic agents: epsilon-aminocaproic acid (EACA)	50 mg/kg PO up to q 6h (lower doses may be effective) or 1 g/h IV continuous infusion Do not exceed 24 g/24 h	Especially useful for mucocutaneous bleeding, especially for dental procedures May be used as adjunctive treatment (DDAVP, factor concentrates)
Tranexamic acid	25 mg/kg q 8 h (not yet available in the United States)	Avoid in upper urinary tract bleeding
vWF-containing FVIII concentrates (e.g., Humate-P, Alphanate)	60–80 RCoF U/kg as an initial dose, then 40–60 u/kg IV every 12 h (see Table 108.4)	FVIII activity levels are often used in the monitoring of response to vWF-containing products as real-time vWF activity measures are not always available Dosed in RCoF units. Individual product is labeled with ratio of RCoF units:FVIII

DDAVP, desmopressin; vWD, von Willebrand disease; vWF, von Willebrand factor; RCoF, ristocetin cofactor.

TABLE 108.4

SUGGESTED INITIAL DOSING OF vWF CONCENTRATES FOR PREVENTION OR MANAGEMENT OF BLEEDING

Major surgery/bleeding	
Loading dose[a]	60–80 RCoF U/kg
Maintenance dose	40–60 RCoF U/kg, typically every 12 h initially
Monitoring	vWF:RCo and FVIII trough and peak, at least daily
Therapeutic goal	Trough vWF:RCo and FVIII >50 IU/dL for 7–14 d
Safety parameter	Do not exceed vWF:RCo 200 IU/dL or FVIII 250–300 IU/dL
May alternate with DDAVP for latter part of treatment	
Minor surgery/bleeding	
Loading dose[a]	30–60 U/kg
Maintenance dose	20–40 U/kg every 12–48 h
Monitoring	vWF:RCo and FVIII trough and peak, at least once
Therapeutic goal	Trough vWF:RCo and FVIII >50 IU/dL for 3–5 d
Safety parameter	Do not exceed vWF:RCo 200 IU/dL or FVIII 250–300 IU/dL
May alternate with DDAVP for latter part of treatment	

[a]Loading dose is in vWF:RCo IU/dL.
Adapted from The National Heart, Lung, and Blood Institute. The Diagnosis, Evaluation, and Management of von Willebrand Disease. Bethesda, MD: National Institutes of Health Publication 08-5832, 2008.

prothrombotic conditions, disseminated intravascular coagulation (DIC), or when receiving prothrombin complex concentrates (PCCs).

vWF factor-containing FVIII concentrates are appropriate for patients with severe vWD or in situations when other therapies (including DDAVP) are ineffective and are preferred to cryoprecipitate, which contains vWF, but has not undergone viral inactivation. When used in the treatment of vWD, they are dosed in ristocetin cofactor (RCoF) units, as opposed to FVIII units (Table 108.4). Limited data suggest a role for rFVIIa in patients with type 3 vWD who have developed alloantibodies to vWF [16].

The National Heart Lung and Blood Institute has recently published guidelines for the diagnosis, evaluation, and management of vWD [17].

Hemophilia

The hemophilias are congenital bleeding disorders characterized by X-linked inheritance and result in a deficiency of FVIII (hemophilia A) or FIX (hemophilia B). In the United States, they have a combined incidence of 1 in 5,000 male births. Hemophilia A is more common than hemophilia B and accounts for approximately 80% of cases. Since hemophilia is an X-linked disorder, all daughters of affected males are obligate carriers and all sons are healthy. Females may rarely manifest bleeding symptoms if they (a) are the homozygous offspring from a carrier mother and affected father, (b) have a high degree of lyonization, or (c) are a carrier with concomitant Turner's syndrome (XO).

The clinical phenotype of hemophilia patients depends on the residual level of circulating procoagulant protein (FVIII or FIX). It is possible to differentiate three degrees of clinical severity: (a) mild hemophilia (5% to 50% factor activity) in which bleeding is prolonged but typically only occurs following trauma or surgery, (b) moderate hemophilia (1% to 5% factor activity) in which prolonged bleeding follows minor trauma, and (c) severe hemophilia (<1% factor activity) where patients experience spontaneous hemorrhage into joints (hemarthrosis) and muscles.

In severe and moderate hemophilia, the PT is normal and the aPTT is prolonged. However, the PTT may be normal in patients with mild hemophilia whose residual factor activity is >20%. If the aPTT is prolonged, it should correct with a mixing study, since hemophilia is a factor deficiency syndrome. Specific factor assays should be performed to confirm a diagnosis of hemophilia A or B.

The management of most cases of hemophilia, thanks to the availability of replacement clotting factor concentrates, occurs in the outpatient setting, but individuals who previously have escaped diagnosis (mild or moderate hemophilia) or who have sustained major trauma or complications from a bleeding episode (compartment syndrome) may present to critical care. If not previously diagnosed, hemophilia should be suspected in male patients who have a personal history of bleeding into joints or muscles, a history of excessive bleeding upon surgical challenge, and/or a positive sex-linked family history of bleeding.

Hemarthrosis, a hallmark of hemophilia, accounts for approximately 85% of all bleeding events in severe hemophilia and most commonly involves the ankles, knees, and elbows [18]. Intramuscular hematomas in persons with hemophilia may expand to the point where blood flow is compromised to surrounding neurovascular structures resulting in tissue gangrene and compartment syndrome; the condition requires surgery and aggressive clotting factor replacement therapy [19] (Table 108.5). Gastrointestinal bleeding is uncommon in hemophilia. However, patients with an underlying structural lesion may present with hematemesis, hematochezia, or melena. Hemophilia patients who present with evidence for gastrointestinal bleeding should have a complete endoscopic evaluation to assess for and treat any underlying lesion. Approximately 90% of persons with severe hemophilia will develop hematuria during their life, although the condition is typically painless, benign, and unassociated with a structural lesion. As discussed earlier, antifibrinolytic agents are contraindicated in patients with genitourinary bleeding.

TABLE 108.5

RECOMMENDED HEMOSTATIC LEVELS IN HEMOPHILIA[a]

Clinical situation	Hemophilia target factor activity (%)[a]
Mild hemorrhage (joint, muscle)	30–40
Mucosal hemorrhage (oral, dental)	30–40 with EACA
Major hemorrhage	>50
Life-threatening hemorrhage or perioperative management (major and orthopedic procedures)	100

[a]Minimum recommended goal factor activity levels.
EACA, epsilon-aminocaproic acid.

Hemorrhage into head and neck structures is a medical emergency in persons with hemophilia. Retropharyngeal hematoma, which may occur spontaneously or following dental or surgical procedures, may present with inability to control saliva, neck swelling, and pain. If untreated, it may result in airway compromise and in some cases may require tracheostomy. Hemorrhage into the central nervous system is a severe and potentially fatal (albeit rare) complication of hemophilia. Intracranial hemorrhage (ICH) may occur spontaneously in severe hemophilia or as the result of trauma. Prompt recognition of ICH is paramount and factor replacement therapy should be given immediately while the diagnostic workup is underway (Table 108.5).

The approach to treating major bleeding episodes in hemophilia A and B is similar. The clinical scenario dictates the target factor activity level (Table 108.5). For example, an ICH requires a target activity level of 100% initially, while levels of 30% to 40% may be sufficient for minor bleeds such as uncomplicated hemarthrosis. Prior to completion of the diagnostic (radiologic or otherwise) workup, clotting factor concentrate should be administered immediately to a person with hemophilia and a suspected life- or limb threatening bleed. Plasma-derived and recombinant factor concentrates [20] contain much higher concentrations of the desired factor compared to fresh frozen plasma (FFP) or cryoprecipitate. If possible, avoidance of FFP or cryoprecipitate is advised to avoid volume overload, transfusion-related lung injury (TRALI), and potential viral transmission (see Chapter 114).

DDAVP may be used instead of factor concentrate in selected patients with mild hemophilia A who have minor bleeding or a requirement for an enhanced FVIII activity level prior to a short-lived bleeding challenge. Any mild hemophilia A patient should undergo a DDAVP trial to gauge his or her individual response in lieu of assuming efficacy of the agent. FVIII levels in plasma increase two- to six-fold following administration. For mild hemophilia A, the recommended dose is 0.3 μg per kg (IV or SQ) or 300 μg intranasally; as previously discussed, tachyphylaxis and hyponatremia may develop after serial dosing.

Antifibrinolytic agents are a useful adjunctive treatment in hemophilia patients with mucosal bleeding. However, hemophilic patients with hematuria, DIC, receiving a PCC, or other prothrombotic conditions should not be treated with antifibrinolytics.

One of the most significant complications of hemophilia treatment is the development of an inhibitor. Inhibitors are alloantibodies against exogenously administered clotting factor that neutralize the factor. The development of a new inhibitor is more common in hemophilia A than in hemophilia B [21], in severe hemophilia, and among previously untreated patients (as opposed to adults who typically have been extensively exposed to clotting factor concentrate).

Inhibitors, if present at high titer, neutralize exogenous factor rendering factor concentrates ineffective. Therefore, an inhibitor should be suspected when administration of factor concentrate at a dose previously sufficient to achieve hemostasis, or improve bleeding, fails to do so. Once suspected, a Bethesda assay should be performed to document the titer of the inhibitor (reported in Bethesda units, BU). Of the two goals of treatment in patients with inhibitors, namely, to achieve adequate hemostasis and to eradicate the inhibitor, only the former is typically relevant to the critical care setting. Bleeding should be treated with bypassing agents, typically an activated prothrombin complex concentrate (aPCC) or rFVIIa [22]. If the titer is <5 BU, high doses of FVIII or FIX may be given as initial treatment in cases of life- or limb-threatening bleeding episodes. In patients with a long-standing inhibitor, however, the anamnestic response negates factor activity after 5 to 7 days, at which point bypassing agents become necessary.

RARE CONGENITAL COAGULATION DISORDERS

Less Common Coagulation Factor Deficiencies

The hemophilias and vWD represent approximately 85% of congenital bleeding disorders. The remaining disorders will be briefly discussed next.

Disorders of Fibrinogen

Congenital fibrinogen disorders result from a quantitative (afibrinogenemia) or qualitative (dysfibrinogenemia) defect in fibrinogen synthesis. Congenital afibrinogenemia has a variable bleeding phenotype with the majority of patients experiencing moderate bleeding [23]. Afflicted individuals present typically in the neonatal period with umbilical stump bleeding or bleeding following circumcision [23]. Patients may also experience hemarthrosis, intramuscular hemorrhage, spontaneous abortion, mucosal surface bleeds, ICH, or spontaneous splenic rupture [24]. Heterozygotes are typically asymptomatic. The clinical phenotype in patients with congenital dysfibrinogenemia is variable and includes (a) asymptomatic (55%), (b) hemorrhagic (25%), (c) thrombotic (10% to 20%), or (d) a combination of both hemorrhagic and thrombotic complications (1% to 2%) [25]. Treatment of congenital fibrinogen disorders should be individualized given the clinical variability. In general, replacement therapy in the form of fibrinogen concentrates, cryoprecipitate, or (not recommended) FFP should be given to patients with a hemorrhagic presentation to achieve a goal fibrinogen level of 50 to 100 mg per dL [26].

Prothrombin (FII) Deficiency

Congenital prothrombin deficiency is characterized by a concordant decrease in prothrombin antigen and activity [27]. Aprothrombinemia has not been reported. Patients with hypoprothrombinemia present with severe hemorrhage including ICH, mucocutaneous bleeding, hemarthrosis, spontaneous abortions, and significant postoperative bleeding. Heterozygotes are usually asymptomatic; however, they may experience increased postoperative bleeding [28]. Prothrombin deficiency is treated with factor replacement in the form of FFP or PCC to a goal prothrombin level of 30% [29].

Factor V Deficiency

FV deficiency is associated with mucocutaneous bleeding and rarely with ICH [30]. There are mild, moderate, and severe deficiency states. Patients with severe deficiency usually present with umbilical stump and mucocutaneous bleeding. Older individuals may present with postoperative bleeding or menorrhagia. FV deficiency is treated with FFP to a goal activity level of 20% to 30%. Alpha granules in platelets contain FV and platelet transfusions have been used in the treatment of FV deficiency when patients have developed neutralizing inhibitors to FV with varying success [31]. Combined deficiency of FV and FVIII should always be considered in the differential diagnosis of patients who present with FV deficiency. This is discussed next [32].

Combined Factor V and VIII Deficiency

Combined FV and FVIII deficiency (F5F8D) is a rare disorder where patients have detectable, but low antigen and activity levels of both factors, typically in the 5% to 15% range. Patients present with increased bleeding following trauma or surgery. Patients are treated with a combination of FFP and FVIII concentrates.

Factor VII Deficiency

Patients with less than 1% FVII activity manifest a severe bleeding disorder, predominantly involving the mucous membranes, muscles, joints, and following surgery or trauma, while those with more than 5% have relatively mild symptoms. Factor VII activity correlates poorly with bleeding severity, but in general, only modest amounts of circulating FVII are required for adequate hemostasis, and bleeding is uncommon, even with surgery, in individuals with FVII activity levels >15% to 20% [33,34]. In the United States, rFVIIa is used to treat FVII deficiency. Plasma-derived FVII concentrates are available in Europe to treat this disorder [35,36]. When rFVIIa and/or FVII concentrates are unavailable, PCC (depending on factor formulation) or FFP may be used.

Factor X Deficiency

In congenital FX deficiency, severity of bleeding appears to correlate with residual FX activity and may be quite severe. In a case series of Iranian patients with congenital FX deficiency, the most common symptoms were epistaxis, menorrhagia, and hemarthrosis [37]. FX deficiency is treated with PCCs.

Factor XI Deficiency

FXI deficiency, previously known as hemophilia C, is common amongst Ashkenazi Jews where the gene frequency is 8% to 9% [38]. The inheritance is autosomal rather than X linked as with hemophilia A and B. Severe FXI deficiency (<15% to 20% FXI activity) occurs in homozygotes or compound heterozygotes. Heterozygous individuals have a partial FXI deficiency (20% to 70% FXI activity) [39]. Bleeding is unpredictable as some severe FXI deficiency patients are asymptomatic, while an analysis of 50 kindreds demonstrated that 30% to 50% of heterozygotes experienced significant bleeding [40].

Treatment for FXI deficiency includes FFP, antifibrinolytic agents [41], FXI concentrates (available in the United Kingdom and France) [42], and rFVIIa (not FDA approved for this purpose) [43]. There is concern of a prothrombotic potential associated with FXI concentrates as DIC and arterial thrombosis have been described in up to 10% of patients. Heparin has been added to these concentrates to reduce this thrombotic potential, but there is a general recommendation to maintain FXI levels at no greater than 70 IU per dL [44].

Factor XIII Deficiency

The most common presentation for FXIII-deficient patients is umbilical stump bleeding [45]. FXIII-deficient patients may also experience ICH, hemarthrosis, menorrhagia, and increased bleeding following surgery or trauma [46]. FXIII has a half-life of 8 to 12 days and levels required to maintain hemostasis are only in the range of 2% to 5%. Treatment includes FXIII concentrates, FFP, or cryoprecipitate. Given FXIII's long half-life, factor concentrates may be given once every several weeks as prophylactic therapy [47].

Vitamin K-Dependent Factor Deficiencies

Patients with combined deficiency of the vitamin K-dependent factors (FII, FVII, FIX, FX, proteins C and S) may present with umbilical stump bleeding or ICH [48]. Factor activity levels are variable and generally range from 1% to 30%. High doses of supplemental vitamin K may significantly improve or completely correct deficient factor activities. In acute bleeding episodes, patients may be treated with FFP or PCCs.

Congenital Qualitative Platelet Disorders

Defects in Platelet Adhesion

Bernard–Soulier syndrome (BSS) is a rare, autosomal recessive, severe bleeding disorder characterized by thrombocytopenia, giant platelets, and severe mucocutaneous bleeding [49]. Deficient platelet binding to subendothelial vWF is due to abnormalities (either qualitative or quantitative) in the GP Ib/IX/V complex. The mainstay of treatment in BSS is platelet transfusion during clinically significant hemorrhagic episodes. However, alloimmunization to transfused platelets is often encountered when patients develop neutralizing antibodies to GP Ib/IX/V on transfused platelets which renders those platelets useless. rFVIIa has been used to treat patients with these inhibitors and has proven successful in many cases [50].

Defects in Platelet Aggregation

Glanzmann thrombasthenia is a rare, autosomal recessive disorder characterized by absent platelet aggregation secondary to defective GP IIb/IIIa on the platelet surface. Affected patients present with severe to life-threatening mucocutaneous bleeding. Treatment includes platelet transfusion. However, many patients may become refractory as alloantibodies to transfused platelets form. rFVIIa has been used to treat bleeding in this disorder [51].

Disorders of Platelet Secretion: The Storage Pool Diseases

Platelets contain two types of intracellular granules, alpha and delta (or dense), which are required for an optimal secondary wave of platelet aggregation. The gray platelet syndrome is the most common alpha granule storage pool disease (SPD) and may predispose to early onset myelofibrosis, a probable consequence of the impaired storage of growth factors such as PDGF [52]. Hermansky–Pudlak syndrome and Chediak–Higashi syndrome are SPDs affecting dense granules. The Hermansky–Pudlak syndrome is associated with oculocutaneous albinism and increased accumulation of an abnormal fat-protein compound, ceroid, in the reticuloendothelial system [53]. The Chediak–Higashi syndrome is characterized by oculocutaneous albinism, neurologic abnormalities, immune deficiency with a tendency to infections, and giant inclusions in the cytoplasm of platelets and leukocytes [54]. The primary treatment for clinically significant bleeding in patients with SPDs is platelet transfusion.

ACQUIRED COAGULATION DISORDERS

Anticoagulant Drugs

Use of anticoagulants in the critical care setting is ubiquitous. The pharmacology, monitoring, and appropriate reversal of anticoagulant drugs are reviewed in detail in Chapter 110.

Generally, patients on anticoagulants who develop clinically insignificant bleeding may be closely monitored while the drug is continued; appropriate therapeutic monitoring (e.g., INR, aPTT, anti-Xa) should also be obtained and followed closely. Major bleeding, except in rare instances, typically should prompt discontinuation of anticoagulant drugs. Consideration should also be given to holding subsequent doses or reducing doses based on laboratory or clinical evolution.

Heparins, Low-Molecular-Weight Heparins, and Fondaparinux

These agents, and management of associated bleeding complications, are discussed in Chapter 110.

Warfarin (Coumadin)

Given its widespread use, warfarin is a common cause of iatrogenic, serious bleeding that frequently requires critical care. Warfarin is an oral vitamin K antagonist that exerts its anticoagulant effects through inhibition of vitamin K-dependent γ carboxylation of the vitamin K-dependent factors (FII, FVII, FIX, and FX). γ carboxylation is required for these coagulation factors to become biologically active. Warfarin also inhibits γ carboxylation of the vitamin K-dependent regulatory proteins C and S. Treatment with warfarin reduces the biologically active levels of all these vitamin K-dependent factors, both pro- and anti-coagulant. However, the net effect at steady state is anticoagulation. Given the half-life of the independent factors affected by warfarin, patients may become relatively prothrombotic in the first several days after warfarin initiation as proteins C and S are the first to become significantly reduced. This is the rationale for "bridging" with unfractionated heparin (UFH) or low-molecular-weight heparin (LMWH) for the first several days of warfarin administration to abrogate extension of existing thrombosis or development of new ones [55].

Warfarin is monitored via the PT and INR with a typical therapeutic range of 2.0 to 3.0 but this is patient and indication specific [55]. At supratherapeutic doses, the aPTT may also become prolonged.

When asymptomatic, supratherapeutic anticoagulation with warfarin does not generally require treatment beyond reducing the dose or holding warfarin for a period of time to allow for correction in the INR. Consideration may also be given to administering a small dose of vitamin K (1 to 5 mg) which will significantly lower the INR within 24 hours, depending on the INR and clinical scenario. If the patient is experiencing significant or life-threatening bleeding, reversal of anticoagulation is indicated and accomplished by replenishing the vitamin K-dependent factors. This can be achieved using either FFP or PCCs (Table 108.6).

TABLE 108.6

REVERSAL OF WARFARIN-INDUCED ANTICOAGULATION MANAGEMENT OF SUPRATHERAPEUTIC INR

Clinical situation	INR	Actions
No significant bleeding	<5.0	■ Lower dose, or ■ Hold dose and restart at a lower dose once INR in desired range, or ■ Check INR in 24 h if INR only mildly prolonged
	5.0–9.0	■ Hold warfarin, repeat INR in 24 h ■ Give vitamin K_1 1–2.5 mg PO × 1 if at increased risk of bleeding ■ Check INR in 24 h—when INR in desired range, restart warfarin at adjusted dose
	≥9.0	■ Hold warfarin and give vitamin K_1 2.5–5 mg PO × 1 (may repeat in 24 h if INR not improved) ■ When INR in desired range, restart warfarin at adjusted dose
Serious or life-threatening bleeding	Any prolongation in INR due to warfarin administration	■ Hold warfarin ■ Give vitamin K_1 10 mg slow IV push (over 30 min); may repeat in 12–24 h ■ Give FFP, prothrombin complex concentrate (PCC), or rFVIIa for acute reversal ■ Monitor INR and repeat intervention as necessary

Adapted from Ansell J, Hirsh J, Hylek E, et al: Pharmacology and management of the vitamin K antagonists: American College of Chest Physicians Evidence-Based Clinical Practice Guidelines (8th Edition). *Chest* [6, Suppl]:175s, 2008.

PCCs are plasma-derived products enriched in vitamin K-dependent factors. The typical dose is 25 to 50 U per kg depending on the degree of anticoagulation. There are two types of PCCs available, activated PCC (aPCC) and nonactivated (simply referred to as PCC). The activated form contains activated coagulation proteases that are used in the treatment of hemophilia with inhibitors. The nonactivated formulations were originally licensed for the treatment of hemophilia B, given their high FIX content. Furthermore, there are two types of nonactivated PCCs: 4-factor (FII, FVII, FIX, FX)–containing products and a 3-factor (FII, FIX, FX) product. While the 3-factor product does contain some FVII, it is at a low concentration (less than one-third that of FIX) and therefore is considered a 3-factor concentrate. If a 3-factor concentrate is used for warfarin reversal, rFVIIa may be required as adjunctive treatment to replenish FVII [55]. Notably, only 3-factor PCCs are currently available in the United States; however, a phase III clinical trial is currently enrolling to evaluate the efficacy and safety of a 4-factor PCC in reversal of oral vitamin K antagonist-induced bleeding. Both activated and nonactivated PCCs contain heparin and are therefore contraindicated in patients with heparin-induced thrombocytopenia [56]. As the effects of FFP, PCC, and rFVIIa are transient, 10 mg of parenteral vitamin K (IV over 30 minutes) should also be given to reverse the INR more durably [55]. When available, PCCs are preferred over FFP because they are concentrated into much smaller volumes, can be virally inactivated, and have a lower risk of TRALI (see Chapter 114). The pharmacodynamics of warfarin is discussed further in Chapter 110.

Superwarfarins

The superwarfarins are a group of pharmacologic compounds that are long-acting rat poisons. They have considerably longer half-lives than warfarin (weeks to months versus 1 to 2 days) and are considerably more potent. Superwarfarin poisoning has been associated with homicide and suicide attempts, accidental ingestion, and occupational exposure. Patients typically present with bleeding symptoms and laboratory findings similar to those of warfarin overdose; however, the PT/INR does not appropriately normalize with standard doses of vitamin K. An assay for each of the superwarfarins is necessary to confirm the diagnosis. Patients require high doses of vitamin K for prolonged periods to control bleeding risk. FFP or rFVIIa may be required in episodes of life-threatening bleeding [57].

Direct Thrombin Inhibitors (Argatroban, Lepirudin, Bivalirudin)

Reversal of anticoagulation due to direct thrombin inhibitors (DTIs) in cases of clinically significant bleeding is typically achieved through cessation of drug given a short half-life (<1 hour). No specific antidote is available and supportive care is the standard. The pharmacodynamics of DTIs are discussed in greater detail in Chapter 110.

Vitamin K Deficiency

Vitamin K deficiency is a frequently encountered problem in hospitalized medical patients. It is particularly common in those with chronic malabsorption syndromes (e.g., cystic fibrosis), malnutrition, and those on broad-spectrum antibiotics [58]. Patients on warfarin and with vitamin K deficiency present with similar laboratory and physical findings, namely prolongation primarily of the PT as well as easy bruising or soft tissue bleeding. Vitamin K deficiency is managed by supplementation of vitamin K. If a patient has a malabsorptive syndrome, parenteral vitamin K is typically recommended.

Since vitamin K-dependent coagulation factors are synthesized in the liver, it can be difficult to distinguish between vitamin K deficiency and a coagulopathy of liver disease (decreased hepatic synthesis of coagulation factors). In clinical scenarios where underlying liver disease is present, it may be beneficial to evaluate coagulation factor levels, both vitamin K-dependent and independent (e.g., FII and FV, respectively). In this example, if both FII and FV levels are decreased, then the patient likely has hepatic synthetic dysfunction. If FV is normal and FII is decreased, then the patient likely has vitamin K deficiency.

Coagulopathy of Liver Disease

An unfortunate hallmark of liver disease is coagulopathy. It stands to reason that since all of the coagulation factors (except FVIII, which is also synthesized in extrahepatic endothelial cells) are made in the liver, end-stage liver disease (ESLD) is marked by multiple coagulation factor deficiencies [59,60]. However, increased extravascular redistribution and increased factor consumption also contribute. The degree of coagulation factor reduction as well as the number of factors reduced typically parallel the severity of liver disease [61]. Factors V and VII appear to be sensitive markers of hepatic synthetic dysfunction with FVII levels typically the most notably affected secondary to its short half-life [62]. A prolongation in the PT is therefore an early marker of liver disease. As hepatic dysfunction progresses and other coagulation factors in the common and contact activation pathway are decreased, the aPTT prolongs. In contrast, FVIII levels are typically elevated in compensated cirrhosis. This may be secondary to an increase in vWF that is seen in cirrhotics [60]. In addition, proteins required for FVIII clearance such as low-density lipoprotein receptor-related protein (LRP) are present in decreased amounts, thus raising FVIII levels. Patients with liver disease may have normal fibrinogen levels, given its long half-life, but they may develop an acquired dysfibrinogenemia associated with abnormal fibrinogen glycosylation that disrupts fibrin polymerization [63,64]. This may be reflected by a normal fibrinogen quantitative assay but an abnormal functional assay such as the TT or RT.

In addition to coagulation factor deficiency, a number of other variables associated with advanced liver disease may contribute to coagulopathy in this population. These include (a) vitamin K deficiency secondary to malnutrition, malabsorption/maldigestion from bile salt insufficiency, and altered intestinal motility [63]; (b) portal hypertension with resultant hypersplenism and secondary thrombocytopenia [65]; (c) decreased thrombopoietin (the principle regulator of platelet production) synthesis by hepatocytes with resultant thrombocytopenia [66]; (d) impaired platelet function as demonstrated by abnormal platelet function, as assessed by PFA-100® [66]; and (e) hyperfibrinolysis secondary to impaired synthesis of plasminogen activator inhibitors and decreased clearance of plasminogen activators (reviewed in reference [67]). Chronic, low-grade DIC may also contribute to coagulopathy (discussed later).

Despite evidence for a significant coagulopathy based on laboratory tests as well as evident petechiae, ecchymosis, purpura, and bleeding after invasive procedures, patients with ESLD rarely bleed spontaneously. It is much more common for them to present with hemorrhage as a result of an underlying anatomic lesion such as from an esophageal varix. There remains active debate as to the actual net degree of coagulopathy in these patients. For instance, Mannucci has argued that defects in platelet number and function may be balanced by increased levels of vWF. Furthermore, decreased levels of coagulation factors and inhibitors of fibrinolysis are balanced by decreased levels of inhibitors of coagulation and profibrinolytic factors [68]. The end result is a potential rebalancing of hemostasis. The fact that the degree of PT and aPTT prolongation correlates poorly with bleeding after liver biopsy and other potentially hemorrhagic procedures supports this rebalancing notion [69,70]. Ultimately, a more comprehensive assessment of hemostasis is needed as PT and aPTT only assess thrombin generation in a closed system devoid of anticoagulant factors and do not address fibrinolysis at all.

Given that we lack a comprehensive hemostatic assessment tool, many physicians prefer to prophylactically give FFP or other hemostatic agents to patients with ESLD who are to undergo procedures or who have significantly abnormal coagulation laboratory values. Unfortunately, we have little data to support these measures. The current guidelines recommend FFP transfusions only when hemostasis is needed for bleeding or invasive procedures and the PT or aPTT is >1.5 times normal (reviewed in reference [71]). FFP is generally given at a dose of 10 to 15 mL per kg repeated every 8 hours. Notably, despite repeated infusions of FFP, the PT may not completely correct and therefore clinical response should be monitored rather than relying on the PT as a measure of efficacy [72]. As discussed earlier, patients with ESLD may also develop hypofibrinogenemia or a dysfibrinogenemia. This should be suspected in a patient with a prolonged TT or RT or in a patient who continues to bleed despite FFP infusion. Cryoprecipitate may be required to treat hypo/dysfibrinogenemia as FFP typically does not sufficiently replace fibrinogen. Cryoprecipitate is typically given in doses of 10 pooled units. Patients should be transfused to a goal fibrinogen level of >100 mg per dL. There are a number of human fibrinogen concentrates available in Europe, and in 2009 the Food and Drug Administration approved the first human fibrinogen concentrate in the United States. It is currently indicated for the treatment of patients with congenital afibrinogenemia and hypofibrinogenemia. Some authors have reported beneficial outcomes in patients given rFVIIa and PCCs in ESLD. However, there are currently no guidelines or randomized trials that address dosing or efficacy [63]. However, given the hypervolemia typical of patients with ESLD, multiple infusions of FFP may not be possible and treatment with PCCs may be considered to reduce volume overload as well as decrease the risk of TRALI. If a 3-factor PCC is used, adjunctive rFVIIa may be indicated [73].

Many have argued for controlled trials to evaluate the role of prophylactic hemostatic agents in this patient population as current practice typically involves using expert opinion and case series data [74].

Disseminated Intravascular Coagulation

DIC is a well-recognized syndrome characterized by both thrombotic and hemorrhagic complications in the setting of a number of defined disorders that are typically associated with systemic inflammation (Table 108.7) [75]. The pathogenesis of DIC is complex and is characterized by widespread activation of the TF coagulation pathway with a marked imbalance between procoagulant and anticoagulant processes resulting in unopposed thrombin generation and diffuse fibrin clot formation with subsequent microvascular occlusion and tissue hypoxia [76]. When severe, these changes may culminate in multiple organ dysfunction syndrome (MODS). The pathogenesis is further reviewed elsewhere [75,77].

The clinical presentation of DIC is variable and the majority of patients do not demonstrate a significant hemorrhagic phenotype [78]. A clinical suspicion for DIC is paramount in establishing its diagnosis. In addition to a compatible underlying condition (e.g., sepsis), abnormal laboratory studies consistent with increased thrombin generation and fibrinolysis (consumptive coagulopathy) are also required. A DIC screening panel is typically composed of PT, aPTT, platelet count, fibrinogen, and D-dimer. DIC is suggested when the laboratories demonstrate increased activation of coagulation (elevated PT/aPTT, decreased fibrinogen) as well as evidence of fibrinolysis (elevated D-dimer or fibrin degradation products). An elevation in PT is a very sensitive measure for DIC but has lower specificity since it may be normal, especially in chronic DIC [79]. Since fibrinogen is an acute phase reactant, it may be normal or even elevated in chronic DIC, thereby limiting its specificity in low-grade DIC. Elevation of D-dimer is a sensitive marker for DIC, in the range of 90% to 100% in one report; however, its specificity limits its utility as a single screening test [80].

The International Society on Thrombosis and Hemostasis established a subcommittee on DIC to develop and validate a scoring system to aid in the diagnosis of DIC. This system is based on platelet count, fibrin degradation products, PT, and fibrinogen level [81]. A prospective validation study demonstrated this scoring system to be 91% sensitive and 97% specific for the diagnosis of DIC, with higher scores correlated with higher 28-day mortality (Table 108.8) [82].

Identification and treatment of the underlying disorder remains the hallmark of treatment for DIC [78]. Treatment of DIC should be based on both the clinical presentation as well as the laboratory results [75]. Recommendations for the management of DIC are based on expert opinion given a lack of published, randomized data. In general, patients who experience

TABLE 108.7

DISORDERS ASSOCIATED WITH DISSEMINATED INTRAVASCULAR COAGULATION

Infection
Gram-negative or Gram-positive septicemia
Rickettsiae—especially Rocky Mountain spotted fever
Spirochetes
Fungi
Viruses—especially herpes
Protozoa—especially malaria
Tissue damage
Trauma
Crush injury
Burn
Heat stroke
Hemolytic transfusion reaction
Neoplasia
Metastatic carcinoma
Leukemia—especially acute promyelocytic leukemia
Chemotherapy
Obstetric disasters
Abruptio placentae
Retained dead fetus
Preeclampsia/eclampsia
Amniotic fluid embolism
Placenta previa, accreta, and percreta
Miscellaneous
Fat embolism
Shock
Cardiac arrest
Giant hemangioma (Kasabach–Merritt syndrome)
Vasculitis
Toxins (snake venom, brown recluse spider bite)
Near drowning—especially fresh water

TABLE 108.8

DIAGNOSTIC SCORE FOR DISSEMINATED INTRAVASCULAR COAGULATION

1. Underlying disorder associated with DIC—if yes → proceed, if no → do not proceed, search for alternative process
2. Obtain global coagulation tests: platelet count, PT, fibrinogen, D-dimer
3. Assign score based on laboratory tests
   a. Platelet count
      i. >100 = 0, <100 = 1, <50 = 2
   b. D-dimer or fibrin degradation products
      i. No increase = 0, moderate increase = 2, strong increase = 3
   c. Prolonged PT
      i. <3 s = 0, >3 s but <6 s = 1, >6 s = 2
   d. Fibrinogen level
      i. >1.0 g/L = 0, <1.0 g/L = 1
4. Calculate score
   a. If ≥5, compatible for DIC
   b. If <5, suggestive, but not confirmed DIC, repeat in 1–2 d

Adapted from Bakhtiara K, Meijers JC, de Jonge E, et al: Prospective validation of the International Society of Thrombosis and Haemostasis scoring system for disseminated intravascular coagulation. *Crit Care Med* 32(12):2416–2421, 2004.

significant bleeding or who require invasive procedures should be treated with FFP to replace coagulation factors. PCCs may also be considered when hypervolemia complicates FFP administration, but they may lack certain depleted factors such as FV. Furthermore, the literature discusses increased risk for thrombosis given trace amounts of activated factors contained in the preparations [83]. It is unclear if this risk is still present in today's products. Cryoprecipitate should be used to replace fibrinogen if the plasma level is <100 g per dL. While there is no established threshold at which to transfuse platelets in DIC, in the setting of active bleeding or in anticipation of invasive procedures, platelet transfusions may be indicated.

In contrast to replacing coagulation factors, fibrinogen, and platelets, some investigators have evaluated the role of anticoagulants, namely UFH, in the treatment of DIC. This putative measure is based on the pathologic activation of coagulation-associated with DIC as well as the depletion of endogenous anticoagulants. Initial animal studies evaluating anticoagulants in DIC suggested a benefit [84]; however, subsequent human trials have yielded conflicting results [78,85,86]. To date there are no data from randomized, controlled trials to support the use of UFH in the management of DIC.

More recently, trials of recombinant anticoagulant proteins have been conducted in patients with sepsis-related DIC. Similar to UFH, early trials evaluating tissue factor pathway inhibitor (TFPI) were promising; however, a subsequent phase III trial did not demonstrate survival benefit [87,88]. Large trials evaluating the use of antithrombin concentrates to restore the anticoagulant pathway have also been disappointing [89]. Most recently, considerable attention has been directed toward activated protein C (APC) and sepsis/DIC. Animal models suggest a link between downregulation of the protein C/thrombomodulin system and endotoxin-induced DIC (reviewed in reference [90]). Recombinant human APC (drotrecogin alfa) has been demonstrated to improve mortality and organ function in septic patients. Furthermore, it appears that patients with the most severe sepsis (APACHE score >25) received the largest benefit [91]. Drotrecogin alfa is not used in DIC unassociated with severe sepsis.

DIC is discussed in further detail in Chapter 109.

Trauma-Induced Coagulopathy

Trauma-induced coagulopathy includes the coagulopathy associated with the stresses of trauma as well as unintended consequences of its treatment. Historically it was felt that the coagulopathy associated with trauma was largely secondary to dilution of the coagulation system with volume and blood replacement. However, it is becoming increasingly apparent that this process is much more dynamic and complicated. Traumatic events requiring massive transfusion of blood lead to significant coagulopathy through a number of mechanisms that include (a) dilution of coagulation proteins and platelets from volume resuscitation, (b) consumptive coagulopathy and thrombocytopenia (through DIC associated with trauma), (c) acidemia which impairs function of the coagulation cascade, (d) hypothermia which impairs function of platelets and coagulation factors, and (e) electrolyte perturbations, particularly hypocalcemia which impairs the calcium-dependent coagulation processes [92]. Prompt attention is required to mitigate the coagulopathy associated with trauma and to rapidly correct it. Clinically, patients have a compatible history of massive trauma requiring aggressive resuscitation and typically have a prolongation of PT and aPTT that corrects on mixing study, as well as thrombocytopenia and often hypofibrinogenemia. Treatment is targeted at correcting or preventing the occurrence of the above listed mechanisms that have been associated with the development of trauma induced coagulopathy. Most guidelines recommend transfusion of red blood cells to a target hemoglobin of 7 to 10 g per dL to maintain rheology, FFP administration to a goal PT/aPTT of <1.5 × upper limit of normal, platelet transfusion to keep platelets $>50 \times 10^9$/L (or $>100 \times 10^9$ in patients with brain injury), and fibrinogen >100 mg per dL [93,94]. Notably, recent large animal models of dilutional coagulopathy suggest that treatment with PCC was as effective as FFP in correcting coagulopathy and warranted further investigation [95]. Some studies also suggest that rFVIIa may be beneficial (reviewed in reference [96]).

Acquired Hemophilia A

The most common antibodies that affect clotting factor activity with a resultant hemorrhagic phenotype are directed against FVIII. Acquired hemophilia A, or acquired FVIII deficiency, is a rare disorder with an estimated incidence of 1.0 per million that is caused by autoantibodies directed against a patient's endogenous FVIII, resulting in low FVIII activity levels [97]. Acquired hemophilia A is most commonly an idiopathic condition that occurs in the elderly but can also be associated with malignancy, drugs, autoimmune disorders, and the postpartum state.

Acquired hemophilia should be suspected in patients without a prior bleeding history who present later in life with significant, large ecchymoses, hematomas, mucosal, gastrointestinal bleeding, or who experience significant bleeding following surgery or trauma. Hemarthroses that are a hallmark of congenital hemophilia are not typical of acquired hemophilia.

Patients with acquired hemophilia present with bleeding symptoms and a prolonged aPTT in contrast to patients with a lupus anticoagulant who typically present with a prolonged aPTT and thrombotic complications [97]. Once acquired hemophilia is suspected based on clinical presentation and a prolonged aPTT, an incubated aPTT mixing study should be performed. Since FVIII inhibitors are commonly time and temperature dependent, the mixing study should be performed at 37°C for 1 to 2 hours. In the case of an acquired FVIII inhibitor, the incubated aPTT will not completely correct into the normal range which indicates the presence of an inhibitor. A FVIII activity level may also be helpful to identify the inhibitor as FVIII specific. The strength of the inhibitor may be quantified in a Bethesda assay. The strength of the inhibitor has treatment implications.

Treatment goals of these patients are twofold: (a) control of bleeding and (b) eradication of the inhibitor. Bleeding in patients with low-titer inhibitors (<5 BU) can often be treated with high doses of FVIII concentrates [98]. Bleeding in patients with high-titer inhibitors is treated with a FVIII inhibitor bypassing agent, such as an aPCC or rFVIIa [99]. Porcine FVIII was also an option for patients with a low-titer inhibitor since the inhibitor titer to porcine FVIII is only 5% to 10% of the titer against human FVIII [100]. Unfortunately, this product was removed from production in 2004 given concerns for porcine parvovirus contamination. Clinical trials are currently underway evaluating recombinant porcine FVIII. Inhibitor eradication typically involves immunosuppression, though spontaneous resolution of the inhibitor can occur [98]. There is an unfortunate relapse rate of approximately 20%; however, 70% of these patients can be brought back into a second remission [101].

ACQUIRED PLATELET DISORDERS/DYSFUNCTION

Medications

The antiplatelet effect of medications is the most common cause for acquired platelet dysfunction. Aspirin and nonsteroidal anti-inflammatory drugs (NSAIDs) are the most commonly used medications that affect platelet function (Table 108.9) [102]. Their predominant antiplatelet effect is achieved through the inhibition of platelet cyclooxygenase (COX-1) which in turn ultimately inhibits vasoconstriction and platelet aggregation [103]. Inhibition of COX-1 by aspirin is irreversible for the life of the platelet and is dose-dependent. There is an increased risk of bleeding in patients taking aspirin, and two recent meta-analyses have described an approximate 1% increase in absolute risk of bleeding in patients taking aspirin compared to placebo [104,105]. Notably, this bleeding risk does not appear to be dose dependent when the total daily dose is ≤325 mg per day but does increase with concomitant administration of other anticoagulants or antiplatelet agents [106,107]. The primary site of bleeding associated with aspirin is gastrointestinal. NSAIDs, on the other hand, reversibly inhibit COX-1 for the length of time that the medication remains metabolically active. Platelet function is not affected by the newer COX-2 specific inhibitors or acetaminophen.

TABLE 108.9

DRUGS THAT COMMONLY AFFECT PLATELET FUNCTION

Analgesics
Aspirin
NSAIDs
Cardiovascular medications
Dipyridamole
P2Y12 receptor blockers—thienopyridines
Ticlid (ticlopidine)
Plavix (clopidogrel)
Effient (prasugrel)
GP IIb/IIIa inhibitors
ReoPro (abciximab)
Aggrastat (tirofiban)
Integrilin (eptifibatide)
Antibiotics
β-Lactam antibiotics—e.g., PCN, cephalosporins
Psychotropic
Antidepressants (fluoxetine)
Phenothiazines
Herbal supplements
Fish oil
Cumin
Garlic
Ginkgo biloba
Turmeric

Dipyridamole is a less frequently used antiplatelet drug with an unclear mechanism of action. It has historically been used for stroke prophylaxis. There does not appear to be a significant increase in bleeding risk for patients taking dipyridamole versus placebo in several randomized trials evaluating the efficacy of dipyridamole in stroke prevention [108].

Clopidogrel (Plavix) belongs to a class of antiplatelet agents known as the thienopyridines and is being used with increasing frequency in the treatment of cardio- and cerebrovascular disease. Thienopyridines are irreversible antagonists to the platelet P2Y12 receptor which inhibits ADP-mediated platelet aggregation. The thienopyridines, particularly ticlopidine (Ticlid), have been implicated in the development of thrombotic thrombocytopenic purpura (TTP) [109].

The GP IIb/IIIa antagonists are a group of antiplatelet agents that are primarily used during coronary procedures. These drugs impair aggregation by inhibiting the cross bridging of platelets by fibrinogen. This class is associated with an increased risk of bleeding, particularly at the puncture site for percutaneous coronary intervention. There does not appear to be an increased risk for intracerebral hemorrhage for patients receiving GP IIb/IIIa inhibitors versus heparin [110]. These agents are also associated with thrombocytopenia, often profound, that may result in significant bleeding complications [111].

Many other medications including large doses of penicillins, psychotropic drugs such as fluoxetine, dietary supplements such as fish oil, gingko, garlic, and cumin may impair platelet function, although not typically to a significant degree [102].

Laboratory testing to confirm an acquired platelet defect secondary to medication is rarely necessary as clinical history and medication record usually suffice. However, if needed for confirmation, platelet function testing may be useful. Treatment for drug-induced platelet dysfunction depends on the severity of bleeding as well as the medication involved. In most cases, minor bleeding may be addressed by withholding the medication. In more severe cases, platelet transfusion may be indicated depending on timing of the last dose as well as its specific platelet effect. In general, platelets have a life span on average of 7 to 10 days. As a result, the bone marrow replaces approximately 10% of the body's platelets each day. Therefore, if a medication irreversibly inhibits platelet function, platelet transfusion may be needed to reverse the antiplatelet effect until the bone marrow has sufficiently replenished the affected platelets. For most situations, a single platelet transfusion is sufficient to correct bleeding association with disordered platelets.

Acquired platelet dysfunction due to antiplatelet agents is discussed in further detail in Chapter 109.

Uremia

The multisystem organ dysfunction encountered in critically ill patients often includes acute kidney injury and subsequent uremia. Bleeding associated with uremia has long been recognized and has historically been associated with a prolonged bleeding time. However, the degree of BT prolongation neither correlates with the degree of azotemia nor the severity of bleeding symptoms. The clinical manifestations of uremic bleeding are predominantly mucocutaneous though patients may present with epistaxis, gastrointestinal bleeding, hematuria, or increased bleeding following surgery or procedures [112].

Despite this long-recognized association between uremia and a bleeding diathesis, the exact pathophysiology remains poorly defined though impairment in platelet function appears integral [113]. There are data to suggest that this is a multifactorial process and includes an acquired platelet defect as well as impairment in platelet–endothelium interaction. Additional factors include vWF abnormalities, anemia which affects rheology, thrombocytopenia, uremic toxins, and increased nitrous oxide (NO) production [114]. The presence of a uremic toxin is supported by the improvement in platelet function in patients following dialysis. Notably, urea is unlikely to be the primary toxin as there is no positive correlation between blood urea nitrogen and bleeding risk [115]. NO is produced by endothelial cells and platelets and inhibits platelet aggregation. Plasma from uremic patients has increased NO and the addition of an NO synthesis inhibitor to uremic rats improved BT [116,117].

Treatment for uremic bleeding often includes aggressive dialysis which may correct the bleeding and has been suggested to prevent uremic bleeding. DDAVP has been recommended as the first-line therapy for uremic bleeding (2 to 4 μg per kg intranasally or 0.3 μg per kg by slow intravenous infusion); it improves platelet function in uremia, most likely due to release of FVIII and vWF [118]. If no improvement is noted after the first dose, further doses should not be given. If DDAVP is ineffective or contraindicated, cryoprecipitate may be given (10 units every 12 to 14 hours). Improvement in bleeding in response to cryoprecipitate is likely related to FVIII and vWF [119]. Correction of anemia to a goal hematocrit of 30% corrects the BT in many patients through improved rheology. This may be accomplished via red cell transfusions in the acute period or erythropoietin over prolonged periods. Erythropoietin may also have beneficial effects on platelet function [120]. Conjugated estrogens may improve uremic bleeding and appears to do so in a dose-dependent manner presumably by reducing NO production [121,122] (reviewed in reference [123]).

Hematologic Disorders

Abnormal platelet function is frequently noted in patients with a number of primary hematologic disorders, including myelodysplastic syndromes and myeloproliferative disorders. The bleeding diathesis occurs out of proportion to what would be expected in patients with similar quantitative platelet defects. In general, the mechanisms underlying the platelet dysfunction seen in these disorders are poorly understood but probably reflect the genetic and developmental abnormalities in stem cells that underlie these disorders. The severity of the predisposition to bleeding cannot be reliably predicted from the results of the bleeding time, platelet count, or in vitro platelet function tests.

The bleeding complications of the myeloproliferative disorders have been estimated in the literature to range from 1.7% to 37%, depending on the disorder and population screened [124]. The bleeding manifestations in both polycythemia vera (PV) and essential thrombocythemia (ET) involve the skin and mucous membranes and include menorrhagia, epistaxis, ecchymosis, and gastrointestinal bleeding. This pattern of bleeding suggests an underlying platelet or vWD defect. It has long been assumed that dysfunctional platelets derived from abnormal stem cells were responsible for increased bleeding with these disorders. Recently, however, there are increasing data to suggest that extreme thrombocytosis may paradoxically result in an acquired type 2 vWD which contributes to the bleeding diathesis [125]. Other conditions associated with acquired vWD include Heyde's syndrome, which is the association of tight aortic stenosis with gastrointestinal arteriovenous malformations. In this condition, the shear stress associated with the stenotic aortic valve consumes the high-molecular-weight multimers of vWF [126].

Treatment of the underlying disorder remains the mainstay though platelet transfusions may be needed for clinically significant bleeding. If acquired vWD is suspected, it should be confirmed through appropriate testing (to be discussed later) prior to initiating directed treatment. Treatment depends largely on the degree of defect and could include intravenous immune globulin, DDAVP, or vWF replacement [125].

OTHER ACQUIRED BLEEDING DISORDERS

Acquired vWD

Acquired vWD is a heterogenous disorder that is associated with a number of different disease states. Several distinct pathophysiological mechanisms are involved which include increased vWF clearance or proteolysis, vWF adsorption to cells with subsequent increased clearance, decreased synthesis, and antibody formation against vWF [127]. Lymphoproliferative and autoimmune disorders are most commonly associated with acquired vWD.

In general, mechanisms underlying acquired vWD are divided into immune- and nonimmune-mediated categories. Immune-mediated acquired vWD is suggested by mixing studies which show an inhibition of vWF in a functional assay. Proposed nonimmune mechanisms include (a) vWF being adsorbed onto cells (e.g., Wilm's tumor, platelets in myeloproliferative disorders, plasma cells in multiple myeloma, and Waldenström's macroglobulinemia), (b) increased proteolysis of HMW multimers at sites of high blood shear flow rates in patients with aortic stenosis, angiodysplasia, and congenital heart disease, (c) decreased synthesis in hypothyroidism, and (d) proteolysis by plasmin during increased periods of fibrinolysis such as with thrombolytic therapy and DIC. A diagnosis should be expected if a patient has a bleeding phenotype similar to a patient with vWD, a compatible underlying disorder, an absence of lifelong bleeding symptoms, and a negative family history [128]. Treatment for acquired vWD is aimed at correcting the underlying disorder if possible and while promoting hemostasis as one would in patients with congenital vWD (e.g., DDAVP, factor concentrates, antifibrinolytics).

Acquired FII (Prothrombin) Inhibitors

Clinically, patients with antiphospholipid antibodies most commonly have a thrombotic phenotype; however, rarely these patients may also have an antibody directed against prothrombin. This antibody binds to prothrombin and increases its clearance, which results in low FII activity levels and clinically significant bleeding. This disorder should be considered in a bleeding patient with evidence for prolongation in PT and PTT. The PT should correct with mixing, the PTT will not. Tests for the lupus inhibitor will be positive, and measurements of FII activity as well as FII antigen will be low. Treatment for acute hemorrhage involves FFP, typically at a dose of 15 to 20 mL per kg with a goal FII activity of >30% [129]. PCCs may also be used.

Acquired FV Inhibitors

Acquired FV inhibitors are noted to occasionally occur following cardiac surgery after exposure to topical thrombin or fibrin-glue preparations. These preparations may be contaminated with bovine FV and antibodies may form which cross-react with human FV. A recent retrospective analysis of acquired FV patients noted that 68% of patients presented with bleeding events that most commonly manifested as mucocutaneous events [130]. Patients typically present with a significant prolongation in both the PT and PTT. This prolongation fails to correct in a mixing study. Inhibitor specificity to FV is demonstrated with a low FV activity. FFP is not recommended as a treatment since FV is present in such a low concentration that it is quickly neutralized by the inhibitor. PCCs are likewise felt to be unhelpful given their low FV content. Plasma exchange and platelet transfusions have been used successfully to control bleeding. It is thought that FV contained in the alpha granules of circulating platelets is protected from inhibition until the platelet becomes activated at the site of vessel damage. More recently, rFVIIa has been reported to successfully promote hemostasis in a small case series [131].

Acquired FX Deficiency

Acquired FX deficiency is associated with amyloidosis. It is thought that amyloid fibrils bind to FX and thereby remove it from circulation. Treatment of the underlying amyloidosis and/or splenectomy has been shown to improve the circulating FX level [132]. PCCs are the preferred treatment for acute bleeding episodes.

ACKNOWLEDGMENT

This work was supported in part by a grant from the National Hemophilia Foundation-Baxter Fellowship (JB).

References

1. Davie EW, Ratnoff OD: Waterfall Sequence for Intrinsic blood clotting. *Science* 145:1310–1312, 1964.
2. Macfarlane RG: An enzyme cascade in the blood clotting mechanism, and its function as a biochemical amplifier. *Nature* 202:498–499, 1964.
3. Rodeghiero F, Castaman G, Tosetto A, et al: The discriminant power of bleeding history for the diagnosis of type 1 von Willebrand disease: an international, multicenter study. *J Thromb Haemost* 3:2619–2626, 2005.
4. De Caterina R, Lanza M, Manca G, et al: Bleeding time and bleeding: an analysis of the relationship of the bleeding time test with parameters of surgical bleeding. *Blood* 84:3363–3370, 1994.
5. Franchini M: The platelet-function analyzer (PFA-100) for evaluating primary hemostasis. *Hematology* 10:177–181, 2005.
6. Hayward CP, Harrison P, Cattaneo M, et al: Platelet function analyzer (PFA)-100 closure time in the evaluation of platelet disorders and platelet function. *J Thromb Haemost* 4:312–319, 2006.
7. Langdell RD, Wagner RH, Brinkhous KM: Effect of antihemophilic factor on one-stage clotting tests; a presumptive test for hemophilia and a simple one-stage antihemophilic factor assay procedure. *J Lab Clin Med* 41:637–647, 1953.
8. Rodeghiero F, Castaman G, Dini E: Epidemiological investigation of the prevalence of von Willebrand's disease. *Blood* 69:454–459, 1987.
9. Sadler JE, Mannucci PM, Berntorp E, et al: Impact, diagnosis and treatment of von Willebrand disease. *Thromb Haemost* 84:160–174, 2000.
10. Sadler JE, Budde U, Eikenboom JC, et al: Update on the pathophysiology and classification of von Willebrand disease: a report of the Subcommittee on von Willebrand Factor. *J Thromb Haemost* 4:2103–2114, 2006.
11. Favaloro EJ, Smith J, Petinos P, et al: Laboratory testing for von Willebrand's disease: an assessment of current diagnostic practice and efficacy by means of a multi-laboratory survey. RCPA Quality Assurance Program (QAP) in Haematology Haemostasis Scientific Advisory Panel. *Thromb Haemost* 82:1276–1282, 1999.
12. Mannucci PM, Ruggeri ZM, Pareti FI, et al: 1-Deamino-8-d-arginine vasopressin: a new pharmacological approach to the management of haemophilia and von Willebrands' diseases. *Lancet* 1:869–872, 1977.
13. Rodeghiero F, Castaman G, Mannucci PM: Prospective multicenter study on subcutaneous concentrated desmopressin for home treatment of patients with von Willebrand disease and mild or moderate hemophilia A. *Thromb Haemost* 76:692–696, 1996.
14. Mannucci PM, Bettega D, Cattaneo M: Patterns of development of tachyphylaxis in patients with haemophilia and von Willebrand disease after repeated doses of desmopressin (DDAVP). *Br J Haematol* 82:87–93, 1992.
15. Holmberg L, Nilsson IM, Borge L, et al: Platelet aggregation induced by 1-desamino-8-D-arginine vasopressin (DDAVP) in type IIB von Willebrand's disease. *N Engl J Med* 309:816–821, 1983.
16. Grossmann RE, Geisen U, Schwender S, et al: Continuous infusion of recombinant factor VIIa (NovoSeven) in the treatment of a patient with type III von Willebrand's disease and alloantibodies against von Willebrand factor. *Thromb Haemost* 83:633–634, 2000.
17. The National Heart, Lung, and Blood Institute: The Evaluation and Management of Von Willebrand Disease, National Heart, Lung, and Blood Institute, National Institutes of Health, Bethesda, 2007. Available at: www.nhlbi.nih.gov/guidelines/vwd.
18. Roosendaal G, Lafeber FP: Blood-induced joint damage in hemophilia. *Semin Thromb Hemost* 29:37–42, 2003.
19. Balkan C, Kavakli K, Karapinar D: Iliopsoas haemorrhage in patients with haemophilia: results from one centre. *Haemophilia* 11:463–467, 2005.
20. Key NS, Negrier C: Coagulation factor concentrates: past, present, and future. *Lancet* 370:439–448, 2007.
21. Lusher JM, Arkin S, Abildgaard CF, et al: Recombinant factor VIII for the treatment of previously untreated patients with hemophilia A. Safety, efficacy, and development of inhibitors. Kogenate Previously Untreated Patient Study Group. *N Engl J Med* 328:453–459, 1993.
22. Kempton CL, White GC II: How we treat a hemophilia A patient with a factor VIII inhibitor. *Blood* 113:11–17, 2009.
23. al-Mondhiry H, Ehmann WC: Congenital afibrinogenemia. *Am J Hematol* 46:343–347, 1994.
24. Shima M, Tanaka I, Sawamoto Y, et al: Successful treatment of two brothers with congenital afibrinogenemia for splenic rupture using heat- and solvent detergent-treated fibrinogen concentrates. *J Pediatr Hematol Oncol* 19: 462–465, 1997.
25. Haverkate F, Samama M: Familial dysfibrinogenemia and thrombophilia. Report on a study of the SSC Subcommittee on Fibrinogen. *Thromb Haemost* 73:151–161, 1995.
26. Mannucci PM, Duga S, Peyvandi F: Recessively inherited coagulation disorders. *Blood* 104:1243–1252, 2004.
27. Akhavan S, Mannucci PM, Lak M, et al: Identification and three-dimensional structural analysis of nine novel mutations in patients with prothrombin deficiency. *Thromb Haemost* 84:989–997, 2000.
28. Girolami A, Scarano L, Saggiorato G, et al: Congenital deficiencies and abnormalities of prothrombin. *Blood Coagul Fibrinolysis* 9:557–569, 1998.
29. Bolton-Maggs PH, Perry DJ, Chalmers EA, et al: The rare coagulation disorders—review with guidelines for management from the United Kingdom Haemophilia Centre Doctors' Organisation. *Haemophilia* 10: 593–628, 2004.
30. Salooja N, Martin P, Khair K, et al: Severe factor V deficiency and neonatal intracranial haemorrhage: a case report. *Haemophilia* 6:44–46, 2000.
31. Chediak J, Ashenhurst JB, Garlick I, et al: Successful management of bleeding in a patient with factor V inhibitor by platelet transfusions. *Blood* 56:835–841, 1980.
32. Peyvandi F, Tuddenham EG, Akhtari AM, et al: Bleeding symptoms in 27 Iranian patients with the combined deficiency of factor V and factor VIII. *Br J Haematol* 100:773–776, 1998.
33. Barnett JM, Demel KC, Mega AE, et al: Lack of bleeding in patients with severe factor VII deficiency. *Am J Hematol* 78:134–137, 2005.
34. Giansily-Blaizot M, Verdier R, Biron-Adreani C, et al: Analysis of biological phenotypes from 42 patients with inherited factor VII deficiency: can biological tests predict the bleeding risk? *Haematologica* 89:704–709, 2004.
35. Scharrer I: Recombinant factor VIIa for patients with inhibitors to factor VIII or IX or factor VII deficiency. *Haemophilia* 5:253–259, 1999.
36. Mariani G, Testa MG, Di Paolantonio T, et al: Use of recombinant, activated factor VII in the treatment of congenital factor VII deficiencies. *Vox Sang* 77:131–136, 1999.
37. Peyvandi F, Mannucci PM, Lak M, et al: Congenital factor X deficiency: spectrum of bleeding symptoms in 32 Iranian patients. *Br J Haematol* 102:626–628, 1998.
38. Seligsohn U: Factor XI deficiency. *Thromb Haemost* 70:68–71, 1993.
39. Bolton-Maggs PH, Young Wan-Yin B, McCraw AH, et al: Inheritance and bleeding in factor XI deficiency. *Br J Haematol* 69:521–528, 1988.
40. Bolton-Maggs PH, Patterson DA, Wensley RT, et al: Definition of the bleeding tendency in factor XI-deficient kindreds—a clinical and laboratory study. *Thromb Haemost* 73:194–202, 1995.

41. Berliner S, Horowitz I, Martinowitz U, et al: Dental surgery in patients with severe factor XI deficiency without plasma replacement. *Blood Coagul Fibrinolysis* 3:465–468, 1992.
42. Mannucci PM, Bauer KA, Santagostino E, et al: Activation of the coagulation cascade after infusion of a factor XI concentrate in congenitally deficient patients. *Blood* 84:1314–1319, 1994.
43. O'Connell NM: Factor XI deficiency. *Semin Hematol* 41:76–81, 2004.
44. Bolton-Maggs PH, Colvin BT, Satchi BT, et al: Thrombogenic potential of factor XI concentrate. *Lancet* 344:748–749, 1994.
45. Kitchens CS, Newcomb TF: Factor XIII. *Medicine (Baltimore)* 58:413–429, 1979.
46. Abbondanzo SL, Gootenberg JE, Lofts RS, et al: Intracranial hemorrhage in congenital deficiency of factor XIII. *Am J Pediatr Hematol Oncol* 10:65–68, 1988.
47. Brackmann HH, Egbring R, Ferster A, et al: Pharmacokinetics and tolerability of factor XIII concentrates prepared from human placenta or plasma: a crossover randomised study. *Thromb Haemost* 74:622–625, 1995.
48. Brenner B, Tavori S, Zivelin A, et al: Hereditary deficiency of all vitamin K-dependent procoagulants and anticoagulants. *Br J Haematol* 75:537–542, 1990.
49. Nurden P, Nurden AT: Congenital disorders associated with platelet dysfunctions. *Thromb Haemost* 99:253–263, 2008.
50. Tefre KL, Ingerslev J, Sorensen B: Clinical benefit of recombinant factor VIIa in management of bleeds and surgery in two brothers suffering from the Bernard–Soulier syndrome. *Haemophilia* 15:281–284, 2009.
51. Di Minno G, Coppola A, Di Minno MN, et al: Glanzmann's thrombasthenia (defective platelet integrin alphaIIb-beta3): proposals for management between evidence and open issues. *Thromb Haemost* 102:1157–1164, 2009.
52. Nurden AT, Nurden P: The gray platelet syndrome: clinical spectrum of the disease. *Blood Rev* 21:21–36, 2007.
53. Walker M, Payne J, Wagner B, et al: Hermansky–Pudlak syndrome. *Br J Haematol* 138:671, 2007.
54. Kaplan J, De Domenico I, Ward DM: Chediak-Higashi syndrome. *Curr Opin Hematol* 15:22–29, 2008.
55. Ansell J, Hirsh J, Hylek E, et al: Pharmacology and management of the vitamin K antagonists: American College of Chest Physicians Evidence-Based Clinical Practice Guidelines (8th Edition). *Chest* 133:160S–198S, 2008.
56. Leissinger CA, Blatt PM, Hoots WK, et al: Role of prothrombin complex concentrates in reversing warfarin anticoagulation: a review of the literature. *Am J Hematol* 83:137–143, 2008.
57. Spahr JE, Maul JS, Rodgers GM: Superwarfarin poisoning: a report of two cases and review of the literature. *Am J Hematol* 82:656–660, 2007.
58. Vermeer C, Hamulyak K: Pathophysiology of vitamin K-deficiency and oral anticoagulants. *Thromb Haemost* 66:153–159, 1991.
59. Trotter JF: Coagulation abnormalities in patients who have liver disease. *Clin Liver Dis* 10:665–678, x–xi, 2006.
60. Hollestelle MJ, Thinnes T, Crain K, et al: Tissue distribution of factor VIII gene expression in vivo—a closer look. *Thromb Haemost* 86:855–861, 2001.
61. Rodriguez-Inigo E, Bartolome J, Quiroga JA, et al: Expression of factor VII in the liver of patients with liver disease: correlations with the disease severity and impairment in the hemostasis. *Blood Coagul Fibrinolysis* 12:193–199, 2001.
62. Green G, Poller L, Thomson JM, et al: Factor VII as a marker of hepatocellular synthetic function in liver disease. *J Clin Pathol* 29:971–973, 1976.
63. Kujovich JL: Hemostatic defects in end stage liver disease. *Crit Care Clin* 21:563–587, 2005.
64. Roberts HR, Stinchcombe TE, Gabriel DA: The dysfibrinogenaemias. *Br J Haematol* 114:249–257, 2001.
65. Bashour FN, Teran JC, Mullen KD: Prevalence of peripheral blood cytopenias (hypersplenism) in patients with nonalcoholic chronic liver disease. *Am J Gastroenterol* 95:2936–2939, 2000.
66. Peck-Radosavljevic M, Wichlas M, Zacherl J, et al: Thrombopoietin induces rapid resolution of thrombocytopenia after orthotopic liver transplantation through increased platelet production. *Blood* 95:795–801, 2000.
67. Ferro D, Celestini A, Violi F: Hyperfibrinolysis in liver disease. *Clin Liver Dis* 13:21–31, 2009.
68. Mannucci PM: Abnormal hemostasis tests and bleeding in chronic liver disease: are they related? No. *J Thromb Haemost* 4:721–723, 2006.
69. Ewe K: Bleeding after liver biopsy does not correlate with indices of peripheral coagulation. *Dig Dis Sci* 26:388–393, 1981.
70. Boks AL, Brommer EJ, Schalm SW, et al: Hemostasis and fibrinolysis in severe liver failure and their relation to hemorrhage. *Hepatology* 6:79–86, 1986.
71. Ramsey G: Treating coagulopathy in liver disease with plasma transfusions or recombinant factor VIIa: an evidence-based review. *Best Pract Res Clin Haematol* 19:113–126, 2006.
72. Youssef WI, Salazar F, Dasarathy S, et al: Role of fresh frozen plasma infusion in correction of coagulopathy of chronic liver disease: a dual phase study. *Am J Gastroenterol* 98:1391–1394, 2003.
73. Lorenz R, Kienast J, Otto U, et al: Efficacy and safety of a prothrombin complex concentrate with two virus-inactivation steps in patients with severe liver damage. *Eur J Gastroenterol Hepatol* 15:15–20, 2003.
74. Tripodi A, Mannucci PM: Abnormalities of hemostasis in chronic liver disease: reappraisal of their clinical significance and need for clinical and laboratory research. *J Hepatol* 46:727–733, 2007.
75. Levi M: Disseminated intravascular coagulation. *Crit Care Med* 35:2191–2195, 2007.
76. Levi M: Current understanding of disseminated intravascular coagulation. *Br J Haematol* 124:567–576, 2004.
77. Gando S: Microvascular thrombosis and multiple organ dysfunction syndrome. *Crit Care Med* 38:S35–S42, 2010.
78. Levi M: Disseminated intravascular coagulation: What's new? *Crit Care Clin* 21:449–467, 2005.
79. Toh CH: Laboratory testing in disseminated intravascular coagulation. *Semin Thromb Hemost* 27:653–656, 2001.
80. Carr JM, McKinney M, McDonagh J: Diagnosis of disseminated intravascular coagulation. Role of D-dimer. *Am J Clin Pathol* 91:280–287, 1989.
81. Taylor FB Jr, Toh CH, Hoots WK, et al: Towards definition, clinical and laboratory criteria, and a scoring system for disseminated intravascular coagulation. *Thromb Haemost* 86:1327–1330, 2001.
82. Bakhtiari K, Meijers JC, de Jonge E, et al: Prospective validation of the International Society of Thrombosis and Haemostasis scoring system for disseminated intravascular coagulation. *Crit Care Med* 32:2416–2421, 2004.
83. Hellstern P, Halbmayer WM, Kohler M, et al: Prothrombin complex concentrates: indications, contraindications, and risks: a task force summary. *Thromb Res* 95:S3–S6, 1999.
84. Slofstra SH, van't Veer C, Buurman WA, et al: Low molecular weight heparin attenuates multiple organ failure in a murine model of disseminated intravascular coagulation. *Crit Care Med* 33:1365–1370, 2005.
85. Corrigan JJ Jr: Heparin therapy in bacterial septicemia. *J Pediatr* 91:695–700, 1977.
86. Feinstein DI: Diagnosis and management of disseminated intravascular coagulation: the role of heparin therapy. *Blood* 60:284–287, 1982.
87. Abraham E, Reinhart K, Svoboda P, et al: Assessment of the safety of recombinant tissue factor pathway inhibitor in patients with severe sepsis: a multicenter, randomized, placebo-controlled, single-blind, dose escalation study. *Crit Care Med* 29:2081–2089, 2001.
88. Abraham E, Reinhart K, Opal S, et al: Efficacy and safety of tifacogin (recombinant tissue factor pathway inhibitor) in severe sepsis: a randomized controlled trial. *JAMA* 290:238–247, 2003.
89. Warren BL, Eid A, Singer P, et al: Caring for the critically ill patient. High-dose antithrombin III in severe sepsis: a randomized controlled trial. *JAMA* 286:1869–1878, 2001.
90. Levi M, van der Poll T: Recombinant human activated protein C: current insights into its mechanism of action. *Crit Care* 11[Suppl 5]:S3, 2007.
91. Dhainaut JF, Yan SB, Claessens YE: Protein C/activated protein C pathway: overview of clinical trial results in severe sepsis. *Crit Care Med* 32:S194–S201, 2004.
92. Sihler KC, Napolitano LM: Complications of massive transfusion. *Chest* 137:209–220, 2010.
93. Armand R, Hess JR: Treating coagulopathy in trauma patients. *Transfus Med Rev* 17:223–231, 2003.
94. Fries D, Innerhofer P, Reif C, et al: The effect of fibrinogen substitution on reversal of dilutional coagulopathy: an in vitro model. *Anesth Analg* 102:347–351, 2006.
95. Dickneite G, Pragst I: Prothrombin complex concentrate vs fresh frozen plasma for reversal of dilutional coagulopathy in a porcine trauma model. *Br J Anaesth* 102:345–354, 2009.
96. Monroe DM: Modeling the action of factor VIIa in dilutional coagulopathy. *Thromb Res* 122[Suppl 1]:S7–S10, 2008.
97. Franchini M, Gandini G, Di Paolantonio T, et al: Acquired hemophilia A: a concise review. *Am J Hematol* 80:55–63, 2005.
98. Franchini M, Lippi G: Acquired factor VIII inhibitors. *Blood* 112:250–255, 2008.
99. Kessler CM: New perspectives in hemophilia treatment. *Hematology Am Soc Hematol Educ Program* 1:429–435, 2005.
100. Morrison AE, Ludlam CA, Kessler C: Use of porcine factor VIII in the treatment of patients with acquired hemophilia. *Blood* 81:1513–1520, 1993.
101. Collins PW, Hirsch S, Baglin TP, et al: Acquired hemophilia A in the United Kingdom: a 2-year national surveillance study by the United Kingdom Haemophilia Centre Doctors' Organisation. *Blood* 109:1870–1877, 2007.
102. Shen YM, Frenkel EP: Acquired platelet dysfunction. *Hematol Oncol Clin North Am* 21:647–661, vi, 2007.
103. Roth GJ, Majerus PW: The mechanism of the effect of aspirin on human platelets. I. Acetylation of a particulate fraction protein. *J Clin Invest* 56:624–632, 1975.
104. Derry S, Loke YK: Risk of gastrointestinal haemorrhage with long term use of aspirin: meta-analysis. *BMJ* 321:1183–1187, 2000.
105. Weisman SM, Graham DY: Evaluation of the benefits and risks of low-dose aspirin in the secondary prevention of cardiovascular and cerebrovascular events. *Arch Intern Med* 162:2197–2202, 2002.
106. Delaney JA, Opatrny L, Brophy JM, et al: Drug drug interactions between antithrombotic medications and the risk of gastrointestinal bleeding. *CMAJ* 177:347–351, 2007.
107. McQuaid KR, Laine L: Systematic review and meta-analysis of adverse events of low-dose aspirin and clopidogrel in randomized controlled trials. *Am J Med* 119:624–638, 2006.

108. Leonardi-Bee J, Bath PM, Bousser MG, et al: Dipyridamole for preventing recurrent ischemic stroke and other vascular events: a meta-analysis of individual patient data from randomized controlled trials. *Stroke* 36:162–168, 2005.
109. Bennett CL, Kim B, Zakarija A, et al: Two mechanistic pathways for thienopyridine-associated thrombotic thrombocytopenic purpura: a report from the SERF-TTP Research Group and the RADAR Project. *J Am Coll Cardiol* 50:1138–1143, 2007.
110. Memon MA, Blankenship JC, Wood GC, et al: Incidence of intracranial hemorrhage complicating treatment with glycoprotein IIb/IIIa receptor inhibitors: a pooled analysis of major clinical trials. *Am J Med* 109:213–217, 2000.
111. Merlini PA, Rossi M, Menozzi A, et al: Thrombocytopenia caused by abciximab or tirofiban and its association with clinical outcome in patients undergoing coronary stenting. *Circulation* 109:2203–2206, 2004.
112. Molino D, De Lucia D, Gaspare De Santo N: Coagulation disorders in uremia. *Semin Nephrol* 26:46–51, 2006.
113. Weigert AL, Schafer AI: Uremic bleeding: pathogenesis and therapy. *Am J Med Sci* 316:94–104, 1998.
114. Sohal AS, Gangji AS, Crowther MA, et al: Uremic bleeding: pathophysiology and clinical risk factors. *Thromb Res* 118:417–422, 2006.
115. Steiner RW, Coggins C, Carvalho AC: Bleeding time in uremia: a useful test to assess clinical bleeding. *Am J Hematol* 7:107–117, 1979.
116. Remuzzi G, Perico N, Zoja C, et al: Role of endothelium-derived nitric oxide in the bleeding tendency of uremia. *J Clin Invest* 86:1768–1771, 1990.
117. Noris M, Benigni A, Boccardo P, et al: Enhanced nitric oxide synthesis in uremia: implications for platelet dysfunction and dialysis hypotension. *Kidney Int* 44:445–450, 1993.
118. Zeigler ZR, Megaludis A, Fraley DS: Desmopressin (d-DAVP) effects on platelet rheology and von Willebrand factor activities in uremia. *Am J Hematol* 39:90–95, 1992.
119. Janson PA, Jubelirer SJ, Weinstein MJ, et al: Treatment of the bleeding tendency in uremia with cryoprecipitate. *N Engl J Med* 303:1318–1322, 1980.
120. Zhou XJ, Vaziri ND: Defective calcium signalling in uraemic platelets and its amelioration with long-term erythropoietin therapy. *Nephrol Dial Transplant* 17:992–997, 2002.
121. Zoja C, Noris M, Corna D, et al: L-arginine, the precursor of nitric oxide, abolishes the effect of estrogens on bleeding time in experimental uremia. *Lab Invest* 65:479–483, 1991.
122. Vigano G, Gaspari F, Locatelli M, et al: Dose-effect and pharmacokinetics of estrogens given to correct bleeding time in uremia. *Kidney Int* 34:853–858, 1988.
123. Hedges SJ, Dehoney SB, Hooper JS, et al: Evidence-based treatment recommendations for uremic bleeding. *Nat Clin Pract Nephrol* 3:138–153, 2007.
124. Elliott MA, Tefferi A: Thrombosis and haemorrhage in polycythaemia vera and essential thrombocythaemia. *Br J Haematol* 128:275–290, 2005.
125. Federici AB, Rand JH, Bucciarelli P, et al: Acquired von Willebrand syndrome: data from an international registry. *Thromb Haemost* 84:345–349, 2000.
126. Vincentelli A, Susen S, Le Tourneau T, et al: Acquired von Willebrand syndrome in aortic stenosis. *N Engl J Med* 349:343–349, 2003.
127. Franchini M, Lippi G: Acquired von Willebrand syndrome: an update. *Am J Hematol* 82:368–375, 2007.
128. Tiede A, Priesack J, Werwitzke S, et al: Diagnostic workup of patients with acquired von Willebrand syndrome: a retrospective single-centre cohort study. *J Thromb Haemost* 6:569–576, 2008.
129. Erkan D, Bateman H, Lockshin MD: Lupus anticoagulant-hypoprothrombinemia syndrome associated with systemic lupus erythematosus: report of 2 cases and review of literature. *Lupus* 8:560–564, 1999.
130. Ang AL, Kuperan P, Ng CH, et al: Acquired factor V inhibitor. A problem-based systematic review. *Thromb Haemost* 101:852–859, 2009.
131. William BM: Adjunctive role for recombinant activated factor VII in the treatment of bleeding secondary to a factor V inhibitor. *Blood Coagul Fibrinolysis* 19:327–328, 2008.
132. Furie B, Voo L, McAdam KP, et al: Mechanism of factor X deficiency in systemic amyloidosis. *N Engl J Med* 304:827–830, 1981.

CHAPTER 109 ■ THROMBOCYTOPENIA

THOMAS G. DELOUGHERY

Thrombocytopenia is common in the intensive care unit (ICU). Platelet counts below 100,000 per μL occur in 25% to 38% of ICU patients and counts fewer than 10,000 per μL occur in 2% to 3% [1–4]. A variety of disease processes can lead to thrombocytopenia, ranging from an epiphenomenon of the illnesses that lead to the ICU admission to a devastating complication of therapy (Table 109.1).

The immediate priorities in thrombocytopenic patients are to establish the validity and severity of the thrombocytopenia, evaluate for life-threatening processes such as heparin-induced thrombocytopenia or thrombotic thrombocytopenic purpura, and initiate therapy. In the critical care setting, therapeutic decisions often have to be made before a definitive cause of the thrombocytopenia is established.

INITIAL EVALUATION

The initial assessment should be rapid, focusing on whether the patient is bleeding or experiencing thrombosis; the underlying disorder(s) leading to ICU admission; current medications; and (if available) past medical history.

In the assessment of bleeding, one should detect whether the patient is suffering from "structural" aberrancies (e.g., bleeding from a gastric ulcer) or generalized bleeding, which may suggest a hemostatic defect such as may occur due to thrombocytopenia. One should inspect sites of instrumentation, such as IV sites or chest tube drainage, and the mucosa for bleeding. The fingertips and toes should be examined for evidence of emboli or ischemia.

TABLE 109.1

DIFFERENTIAL DIAGNOSIS OF THROMBOCYTOPENIA

Disseminated intravascular coagulation
Drug-induced thrombocytopenia
HELLP syndrome
Hemophagocytic syndrome
Heparin-induced thrombocytopenia
Liver disease
Posttransfusion purpura
Pseudothrombocytopenia
Thrombotic thrombocytopenia purpura

HELLP, hemolysis, elevated liver tests, and low platelets.

TABLE 109.2

LABORATORY TESTS IN EVALUATION OF THROMBOCYTOPENIA

Prothrombin time/INR
Activated partial thromboplastin time
D-dimer
LDH
Creatinine
Bun
Peripheral smear

LDH, lactate dehydrogenase level.

Exposure to medicines is a common cause of thrombocytopenia [5,6]. One should carefully review the record of current and recently administered medications and ask the patient (if possible) and family about medications (prescribed, over the counter, and herbal) [7,8] that the patient has recently taken.

Laboratory Testing

In the patient with thrombocytopenia, examination of the blood smear can quickly reveal whether pseudothrombocytopenia (artifactual platelet clumping) [9] is present and verify the degree of thrombocytopenia (Table 109.2). Although exceptions do exist, the magnitude of thrombocytopenia can be an aid in the differential diagnosis of low platelet counts (Table 109.3). Heparin-induced thrombocytopenia and thrombotic microangiopathy (including thrombotic thrombocytopenic purpura, TTP) often present with modest thrombocytopenia (50 to 100 × 10^9 per L). The smear should be carefully reviewed for presence of fragmented red cells (schistocytes). Laboratory assessment of liver function and renal function also should be assessed. A markedly elevated level of lactate dehydrogenase level (LDH) out of proportion to other liver function abnormalities characteristically occurs in TTP and hantavirus infection [10,11]. If there is any suspicion of HIT, all heparin should be stopped and alternative antithrombotic agents should be started [12,13]. Assessment of platelet function can be difficult and must be based largely on clinical judgment. The bleeding time or the platelet function assay (PFA) is rarely useful in the evaluation of a thrombocytopenic patient, because the low platelet count leads to prolongations in the test endpoint [14].

TABLE 109.3

TYPICAL PLATELET COUNTS IN VARIOUS DISEASE STATES

Moderate thrombocytopenia (50–100,000 per μL)
Thrombotic thrombocytopenic purpura
Heparin-induced thrombocytopenia
Disseminated intravascular coagulation
Hemophagocytic syndrome
Severe thrombocytopenia (<20,000 per μL)
Drug-induced thrombocytopenia
Posttransfusion purpura
Immune thrombocytopenia

Diagnostic Clues

The reason for the ICU admission is a very important indicator in evaluation of thrombocytopenia (Table 109.4) [15]. For example, thrombocytopenia in patients who present with sudden-onset multiorgan system failure may indicate TTP or sepsis. In long-term critical care patients, new-onset thrombocytopenia may be a manifestation of HIT, drug-induced thrombocytopenia, occult or established sepsis, or bacteremia [16].

IMMEDIATE THERAPY—PLATELET TRANSFUSION

Although platelet thresholds below which critically ill patients are at risk for severe bleeding are likely to vary among patients, clinical practice generally dictates that a platelet count above 10,000 per μL does not require platelet transfusion, as long as the patient is stable without signs of bleeding, is not receiving platelet inhibitors, has preserved renal function, does not require an invasive procedure, and does not have aggressive DIC [17]. If any of these is present, especially major or life-threatening hemorrhage (such as intracranial), then a threshold of greater than 50,000 per μL is reasonable [18,19]. An exception is thrombocytopenia due to thrombotic microangiopathy (TTP), wherein platelet transfusion is contraindicated unless perhaps the platelets are transfused slowly and plasma exchange already is underway. Platelet transfusions should comprise six to eight platelet concentrates or one single-donor plateletpheresis unit. Additional discussion regarding transfusion of blood products in critically ill patients is found in Chapter 114.

THROMBOCYTOPENIA

Heparin-Induced Thrombocytopenia

HIT occurs due to the formation of antibodies directed against the complex of heparin and platelet factor 4 [12,20]. This complex in a minority of cases binds to the FcγRIIA receptor, activating platelets and macrophages. The frequency of HIT is 1% to 5% when unfractionated heparin is used but less than 1% with low-molecular-weight heparin [21]. HIT is more common in women and more common in surgery patients than medical patients [22].

HIT should be suspected when there is a sudden onset of thrombocytopenia with either at least a 50% drop in the platelet count from baseline or the platelet count falling to less than 100 × 10^9/L in a patient receiving heparin in *any* form. HIT usually occurs at least 4 days after starting heparin but may occur suddenly in patients with recent (less than 3 months) exposure [23]. An often overlooked feature of HIT is recurrent thrombosis in a patient receiving heparin despite a normal platelet count [24]. Recently, a scoring system—the four Ts—has been validated in several critical care studies as a means of assessing the pretest probability of HIT [25,26] (Table 109.5).

Patients with very low scores are very unlikely to have HIT and can forgo PF4-heparin antibody testing and empiric therapy. A biphasic pattern of thrombocytopenia following cardiac surgery—namely, recovery from the postsurgical thrombocytopenia followed by recurrent thrombocytopenia—is strongly predictive for HIT [27].

The diagnosis of HIT can be challenging in the critical care patient who has multiple reasons for being thrombocytopenic.

TABLE 109.4

DIAGNOSTIC CLUES TO THROMBOCYTOPENIA

Clinical setting	Differential diagnosis
Cardiac surgery	Cardiopulmonary bypass, HIT, dilutional thrombocytopenia, TTP
Interventional cardiac procedure	Abciximab or other IIb/IIIa blockers, HIT
Sepsis syndrome	DIC, ehrlichiosis, sepsis hemophagocytic syndrome, drug-induced, misdiagnosed TTP, mechanical ventilation, pulmonary artery catheters
Pulmonary failure	DIC, H1N1, infection hantavirus pulmonary syndrome, mechanical ventilation, pulmonary artery catheters
Mental status changes/ seizures	TTP, ehrlichiosis
Renal failure	TTP, dengue, HIT, DIC
Cardiac failure	HIT, drug-induced, pulmonary artery catheter
Postsurgery	Dilutional, drug-induced, HIT, TTP
Pregnancy	HELLP syndrome, fatty liver of pregnancy, TTP/HUS
Acute liver failure	Splenic sequestration, HIT, drug-induced, DIC

DIC, disseminated intravascular coagulation; HELLP, hemolysis, elevated liver function tests, and low platelets; HIT, heparin-induced thrombocytopenia; TTP, thrombotic thrombocytopenic purpura.

In this situation, the laboratory assay for HIT may be helpful. Two levels of HIT testing exist. Increasingly, an ELISA assay that detects the presumed pathogenic antiheparin-platelet factor 4 antibodies is evaluated initially [13]. This test is very sensitive but in some populations not specific. For example, 25% to 50% of cardiac surgery patients will show positive results (presumably due to platelet activation in the bypass circuit) [28,29]. A negative test rules out HIT in all but the highest-risk patients.

A second type of test, a (functional) platelet aggregation assay, such as the serotonin release assay, comprises patient plasma, donor platelets, and heparin. If added heparin induces platelet aggregation, the test is considered to be positive. The test is technically demanding, but if performed carefully can be sensitive and specific [12,13,30]. One caveat is that early in the HIT disease process, the test can be negative but then turns positive 24 hours later as the antibody titer increases. Due to substantial frequency of false positivity of PF4-heparin ELISA among cardiovascular, dialysis, and vascular surgery patients, a diagnosis of HIT should be confirmed by a serotonin release assay, even if treatment for HIT already has been initiated.

The first step in therapy of HIT consists of stopping *all* heparin. Low-molecular-weight heparins cross-react with the HIT antibodies and therefore these agents are also contraindicated. Institution of warfarin therapy alone following a diagnosis of HIT has been associated with an increased risk of thromboses and is also contraindicated. Due to the high risk of thrombosis (53% in one study) [21] among HIT patients, antithrombotic therapy should be administered to all patients [12]. For immediate therapy of HIT patients, several antithrombotic agents are available [12,20,31] (Table 109.6).

Argatroban is a synthetic thrombin inhibitor with a short half-life of 40 to 50 minutes [12,32]. Dosing is 2 μg per kg per minute with the infusion adjusted to keep the aPTT 1.5 to 3 times normal. One advantage of argatroban is that it is not renally excreted and no dose adjustment is necessary in renal disease [33]. These characteristics make it the most useful agent for patients in the critical care unit. However, argatroban

TABLE 109.5

PREDICTION RULE FOR HEPARIN-INDUCED THROMBOCYTOPENIA

Points	2	1	0
Thrombocytopenia	>50% fall from baseline and nadir 20–100 × 10^9/L	30%–50% fall or nadir 10–19 × 10^9/L	Fall <30% or nadir <10 × 10^9/L
Timing of platelet fall	Onset day 5–10 of heparin or <1 d if patient recently exposed to heparin	Consistent but not clear records or count falls after day 10	Platelets fall <5 d and no recent (100 d) heparin
Thrombosis	New thrombosis or skin necrosis or systemic reaction with heparin	Progressive or recurrent thrombosis or suspected but not proven thrombosis	None
Other cause for thrombocytopenia	None	Possible	Definite

Notes: Patients with a low probability score are very unlikely to have HIT and can forgo PF4-heparin antibody testing and empiric therapy. Patients with intermediate and high scores should receive empiric therapy until definitive testing can be obtained.
Total score: 6–8, high probability; 4–5, intermediate probability; 0–3, low probability.
Adapted from Lo et al. [25] and Crowther et al. [26].

TABLE 109.6

TREATMENT OF HEPARIN-INDUCED THROMBOCYTOPENIA

Argatroban
Therapy: initial dose of 2 μg/kg/min adjusted to an aPTT of 1.5–3.0 times normal
Reversal: no antidote but $T_{1/2} \sim 40$ min
In severe liver disease (jaundice) dose at 0.5 μg/kg/min adjusted to an aPTT 1.5–3.0 times normal
For patients with multiorgan system failure: 1 μg/kg/min adjusted to aPTT 1.5–3.0 times normal
Post-CABG—0.5–1 μg/kg/min adjusted to aPTT 1.5–3.0 times normal
Indication: prevention and treatment of thrombosis in HIT

Bivalirudin
Bolus: 1 mg/kg
Infusion: 2.5 mg/kg/h for 4 h and then 0.2 mg/kg/h for 14–20 h
Renal adjustment:
- For creatinine clearance of 30–59 mL/min, decrease dose by 20%
- For creatinine clearance of 10–29 mL/min, decrease dose by 60%
- For creatinine clearances less than 10 mg/min, decrease dose by 90%

Note: Antilepirudin antibodies may cross-react with bivalirudin
Indication: Percutaneous coronary intervention, in patients with or without HIT

Lepirudin
Therapy: VERY sensitive to renal function—half-life can go from less than an hour to over 100 h in renal failure. Not recommended in renal insufficiency. May be used in hepatic failure.
- Initial IV bolus 0.4 mg/kg IV push (may be omitted or reduced to 0.2 mg/kg, unless there is life- or limb-threatening thrombosis):
- Continuous infusion: initial rate determined by renal function:
  - GFR >60 mL/min: 0.10 mg/kg/h
  - GFR 45–60 mL/min: 0.075 mg/kg/h
  - GFR <45 mL/min: lepirudin not recommended (consider argatroban)
- Perform aPTT at 4-h intervals until steady state within the therapeutic range (1.5–2.0 times patient baseline aPTT) is achieved

Notes: Antilepirudin antibodies form in 60%–80% of patients on lepirudin and can prolong lepirudin effect. Rare patients may have fatal anaphylaxis.
Indication: Prevention and treatment of thrombosis in HIT

Fondaparinux[a]
Therapy: 7.5 mg every 24 h (consider 5.0 mg in patients under 50 kg and 10 mg in patients over 100 kg)
Reversal: protamine ineffective; see Chapter 110: Antithrombotic Therapy.

[a]Fondaparinux is not approved for treatment of HIT. Its use, however, may be considered after initial anticoagulation with a direct thrombin inhibitor has been administered and the platelet count has recovered, while awaiting a therapeutic INR from therapy with warfarin.
Adapted from Laposata et al. [31], Kondo et al. [32], Hyers et al. [212], Hirsh et al. [213], Hirsh et al. [214].

must be used with caution in patients with severe liver disease by using an initial dose of 0.5 μg per kg per minute [32]. Also metabolism appears to be decreased in patients with multiorgan system failure and these patients should receive a dose of 1 μg per kg [34]. Argatroban (like all thrombin inhibitors) prolongs the prothrombin time/INR (PT/INR) making initiation of warfarin therapy difficult. If available, the chromogenic Xa assay can be used to adjust warfarin therapy [35]. Also, if the patient is on a drip of 2 μg per kg per minute or less, one can simply aim for a PT/INR of more than 4.0 as therapeutic. Unfortunately, there is no agent that can reverse argatroban.

Lepirudin, another direct inhibitor of thrombin, is also monitored using the aPTT. The half-life of lepirudin is short, but the drug accumulates in renal insufficiency with the half-life increasing to more than 50 to 100 hours. Recent data indicate that a lower dosing regimen that is recommended on the package insert may result in lower bleeding rates [12]. There is no antidote for lepirudin. Patients with even slight renal insufficiency (creatinine greater than 1.5) must have their lepirudin doses adjusted to avoid overanticoagulation [36]. Up to 80% of patients receiving long-term lepirudin therapy will develop antibodies that reduce the metabolism of hirudin and *increase* the therapeutic effect of lepirudin [37,38]. Patients on long-term (>6 days) lepirudin therapy should still continue to have monitoring to avoid overanticoagulation.

Bivalirudin is a semisynthetic direct thrombin inhibitor. Its indication involves patients undergoing percutaneous coronary intervention, but other patients may receive it as a treatment for HIT.

The indirect anti-Xa inhibitor fondaparinux does not cross-react with HIT antibodies [12,39], suggesting a potential role in therapy of HIT [40]. However, it has not been studied as extensively in HIT as have the DTIs. Additionally, exposure to fondaparinux has been rarely associated with a syndrome similar to delayed-onset HIT [41]. In the future, newer agents such as dabigatran and rivaroxaban may be suitable for management of patients with HIT.

The issue of platelet transfusion remains controversial [42]. Patients with HIT rarely bleed, which reduces clinical concern over the potential for platelet transfusions, but a prudent approach would be to reserve transfusion of platelets for the rare patient with severe thrombocytopenia who also has life-threatening bleeding.

As mentioned earlier, initiation of warfarin as the sole antithrombotic agent in the initial treatment of HIT has been associated with limb gangrene. In patients receiving a direct thrombin inhibitor, warfarin can be started in small doses (2 to 5 mg daily) once the platelet count has recovered. These often malnourished patients tend to have a dramatic response to warfarin therapy and excessive anticoagulation can easily occur. One should overlap warfarin and parental therapy by 2 to 3 days as there is evidence that patients may do worse if therapy with a DTI is truncated [32].

Patients with HIT should be carefully screened for any thrombosis, at least by performing lower extremity Doppler ultrasound. If thrombosis is present, at least 3 months of therapeutic anticoagulation are required, whereas HIT without thrombosis usually is treated with 30 days of therapeutic anticoagulation.

Thrombotic Thrombocytopenic Purpura

TTP should be suspected when any patient presents with thrombocytopenia and microangiopathic hemolytic anemia (as evidenced by schistocytes on the blood smear and biochemical evidence of hemolysis); end-organ damage, mostly manifesting as renal insufficiency or neurologic phenomena, and fever also may occur, although the minority of patients with TTP present with all of the aforementioned features [43–45]. Critical care patients with TTP most often present with intractable seizures, strokes, or sequela of renal insufficiency. Postsurgical TTP may occur 1 to 2 weeks after major surgery, and is heralded by decreasing platelet counts and renal insufficiency [46]. Many patients who present to the critical care unit with TTP have been misdiagnosed as having sepsis, "lupus flare," or vasculitis.

Evidence is strong that many patients with the classic form of TTP have an inhibitor against an enzyme that is responsible for cleaving newly synthesized von Willebrand factor (vWF) [45,47,48]. vWF is synthesized as an ultra large multimer that can spontaneously aggregate platelets. The enzyme, ADAMTS13, cleaves vWF into a smaller form that can circulate [48,49]. Presumably when ADAMTS13 is inhibited in TTP, the ultra large multimers can spontaneously aggregate platelets leading to the clinical syndrome of TTP. However, many patients with classic TTP have normal activity of ADAMTS13 and reduced levels are found in other diseases implying other factors are important in pathogenesis of TTP [50–52].

There is currently not a single diagnostic test for TTP but rather the diagnosis is based on the clinical presentation [43,45]. Patients uniformly will have a microangiopathic hemolytic anemia with the presence of schistocytes on the peripheral smear. Renal insufficiency and not frank renal failure is the most common renal manifestation. Thrombocytopenia may range from a mild decrease in platelet number to platelets being undetectable. The findings of thrombocytopenia with a relative normal prothrombin time help eliminate DIC from the differential [53]. The LDH is often extremely elevated and is a prognostic factor in TTP [54]. Finding very low levels of ADAMTS13 due to an inhibitor may also be a negative prognostic factor [55]. However, lack of standardization and slow turnaround time still make this assay difficult to use clinically.

Untreated TTP is rapidly fatal. Mortality in the preplasma exchange era ranged from 95% to 100%. Today plasma exchange therapy is the cornerstone of TTP treatment and has reduced mortality to less than 20% [11,43,56–58].

Glucocorticoid therapy, either 1 to 2 mg per kg of methylprednisolone until remission or 1 g of methylprednisolone initially, may be given to patents presumed to have TTP, although this intervention is not practiced in all centers [45]. The glucocorticoid may be continued until the patient has fully recovered and perhaps longer, given the presumed autoimmune nature of the disease and the high relapse rates. Plasma infusion is beneficial but [47] plasma exchange has been shown to be superior to simple plasma infusion in therapy of TTP [56]. This may be due to the ability of plasma exchange to give very large volumes of fresh frozen plasma and removal of inhibitory antibodies. In patients who cannot be immediately exchanged, plasma infusions should be started at a dose of one unit every 4 hours. Patients with all but the mildest cases of TTP should receive 1 to 1.5 plasma volume exchange each day for at least 5 days [43]. Daily plasma exchange should be continued daily until the LDH has normalized, at which point the frequency of exchange may be taped, starting with every-other-day exchange. If the platelet count falls or LDH level rises, daily exchange should be reinstated [59]. Since the platelet count can be affected by a variety of external influences, the LDH level tends to be the most reliable marker of disease activity [60]. There is increasing evidence that the use of the anti-CD20 therapy may reduce the incidence of relapses and shorten the duration of therapy in refractory disease [48].

Renal insufficiency should be managed in the typical fashion. About 50% of patients require renal replacement therapy.

Hemolytic Uremic Syndrome

Classically, hemolytic uremic syndrome (HUS) comprises the triad of renal failure, microangiopathic anemia, and thrombocytopenia [61,62]. Two major forms are recognized: a "typical" form, which occurs in young children with an antecedent diarrheal illness, and an "atypical" form.

Typical HUS

Typical HUS (also referred to as HUS D+) occurs typically in children under the age of 4, although cases in adolescents and adults may occur. Children often have a prodrome of diarrhea, usually bloody [63,64]. Children come to medical attention due to symptoms of renal failure. In HUS, thrombocytopenia can be mild in the 50,000 per μL range. Extrarenal involvement is common in typical HUS. Neurologic involvement can be seen in 40% of patients with seizure being the predominant feature. Elevated liver function tests are seen in 40% of patients and 10% of patients will have pancreatitis. Patients with classic HUS will respond to conservative therapy and renal replacement therapy, but severe cases or those with prominent extrarenal manifestations may require response to plasma exchange [65]. Unfortunately, although most patients recover some renal function, many patients will have long-term renal damage.

Atypical HUS

Atypical HUS is best described as HUS without preceding *Escherichia coli* infection [66,67]. This description obviously lacks diagnostic precision, but in general, this term has been applied to HUS which has prominent extrarenal symptomatology, and the prognosis is thought to be worse for atypical HUS [65]. HUS in older patients and HUS without preceding diarrhea may also better be described as having atypical HUS. Therapy for atypical HUS is plasma exchange but the effectiveness of this intervention is debatable [68]. Patients with atypical HUS, especially older patients, may require months of plasma exchange several times each week to control the disease. Chronic renal insufficiency or failure often ensues. Some patients are found to have defects in the regulatory proteins of complement such as factor H [69].

Therapy-Related TTP/HUS

TTP/HUS syndromes can complicate a variety of therapies [70,71]. TTP/HUS can be associated with medications such as cyclosporine, tacrolimus, gemcitabine, and clopidogrel. Cyclosporine/tacrolimus-associated TTP/HUS occurs within days after the agent is started manifesting as a falling platelet count, falling hematocrit, and rising serum LDH level [71,72]. Some cases have been fatal but often the TTP/HUS resolves with decreasing the dose of the calcineurin inhibitor or changing to another agent.

In the past TTP/HUS was most commonly seen with the antineoplastic agent mitomycin C, with a frequency of 10% when a dose of more than 60 mg was used [73]. Anecdotal reports indicated that treatment with staphylococcal A columns was useful for this condition [74]. Now, the most common antineoplastic drug causing TTP/HUS is gemcitabine [75–78]. Like with mitomycin, the appearance of the TTP/HUS syndrome associated with gemcitabine can be delayed, and the condition often is fatal. Severe hypertension often precedes the clinical appearance of the TTP/HUS [79]. The use of plasma exchange is controversial [80], since advanced cancer itself can be associated with a TTP-like syndrome that is typically poorly responsive to plasma exchange. The increasing use of vascular endothelial growth factor (VEGF) inhibitors such as bevacizumab and sunitinib has been associated with observation of related TTP/HUS syndromes as well [81–83].

TTP/HUS has been reported with other drugs including the thienopyridines, ticlopidine, and clopidogrel [84]. The frequency of ticlopidine-associated TTP may be as high as 1:1,600, and since this drug was often prescribed for patient with vascular disease, these patients may have been initially misdiagnosed as having recurrent strokes or angina [75,78]. The frequency of TTP using clopidogrel is much less—0.0001%—but since it is widely prescribed, it is the second most common cause of drug-induced TTP [84]. Almost all cases of clopidogrel-induced TTP occur within 2 weeks of starting the drug. All patients with thienopyridine-associated TTP should receive plasma exchange.

TTP/HUS can complicate both autologous and allogeneic hematopoietic stem cell transplants [85–89]. The frequency ranges widely, depending on the criteria used to diagnose TTP/HUS, but it is in the range of 15% for allogeneic and 5% for autologous hematopoietic stem cell transplantation procedures [86,87]. One type, characterized by fulminant multiorgan failure occurs early after transplantation (e.g., within 20 to 60 days), has multiorgan system involvement, is often fatal, and has been associated with severe cytomegalovirus (CMV) infection. Another type of TTP/HUS is similar to cyclosporine/tacrolimus-associated HUS. TTP/HUS that is associated with the conditioning regimen used in the transplantation protocol occurs 6 months or more after total body irradiation, and is associated with primary renal involvement. Finally, patients with systemic CMV infections may present with a TTP/HUS syndrome related to vascular infection with CMV. The etiology of hematopoietic stem cell transplantation-related TTP appears to be different from that of "classic" TTP since alterations of ADAMTS13 have not been found in bone marrow transplant-related TTP implicated in therapy-related vascular damage [90]. The best management of hematopoietic stem cell transplantation-related TTP/HUS is uncertain. Patients should have doses of cyclosporine or tacrolimus decreased, if taking calcineurin inhibitors. Although plasma exchange is often tried, patients with fulminant or conditioning-related TTP/HUS or those with TTP/HUS and concomitant acute graft versus host disease typically do not respond [91–93].

Pregnancy-Related Thrombocytopenic Syndromes

One should consider three syndromes in the critically ill pregnant woman who presents with thrombocytopenia. These are the HELLP syndrome, fatty liver of pregnancy, and TTP (Table 109.7) [94,95].

The acronym HELLP syndrome (Hemolysis, Elevated Liver tests, Low Platelets) describes a variant of pre-eclampsia [96,97]. Classically, HELLP syndrome occurs after 28 weeks of gestation in a patient suffering from pre-eclampsia but can occur as early as 22 weeks in patients with the antiphospholipid antibody syndrome [98]. The pre-eclampsia need not be severe. The first sign of HELLP is a decrease in the platelet count followed by abnormal liver function tests. Signs of hemolysis are present with abundant schistocytes on the smear and a high LDH. HELLP can progress to liver failure and deaths are also reported due to hepatic rupture. Unlike TTP, fetal involvement is present in the HELLP syndrome with fetal thrombocytopenia reported in 30% of cases. In severe cases, elevated D-dimers consistent with DIC are also found. Delivery of the child will most often result in cessation of the HELLP syndrome but refractory cases will require dexamethasone and plasma

TABLE 109.7

PREGNANCY-RELATED DISEASES—TTP/HUS, HELLP SYNDROME, AND ACUTE FATTY LIVER OF PREGNANCY (AFLP)

	HELLP	TTP/HUS	AFLP
Hypertension	Always present	Sometimes present	Sometimes present
Proteinuria	Always present	Sometimes present	Sometimes present
Thrombocytopenia	Always	Always	Always
LDH elevation	Present	Marked	Present
Fibrinogen	Normal to low	Normal	Normal to very low
Schistocytes	Present	Present	Absent
Liver tests	Elevated	Normal	Elevated
Ammonia	Normal	Normal	Elevated
Glucose	Normal	Normal	Low

HELLP, hemolysis, elevated liver tests, and low platelets; TTP/HUS, thrombotic thrombocytopenic purpura/hemolytic uremia syndrome.
Adapted from Sibai [94], Steingrub [95], Egerman and Sibai [104], Esplin and Branch [105].

exchange [99]. About a quarter of women who suffer from HELLP will have a recurrence with a later pregnancy [100].

Fatty liver of pregnancy also occurs late in pregnancy and is only associated with pre-eclampsia in 50% of cases [101–103]. Patients first present with nonspecific symptoms of nausea and vomiting but can progress to fulminant liver failure. Patients develop thrombocytopenia early in the course but in the later stages can develop DIC and very low fibrinogen levels. Mortality rates without therapy can be as high as 90%. Low glucose and high ammonia levels can help distinguish fatty liver from other pregnancy complications [104]. Treatment consists of prompt delivery of the child and aggressive blood product support.

TTP can occur anytime during pregnancy often leading to diagnostic confusion due to the overlap symptoms between TTP and HELLP syndrome [100,104]. There does appear to be a unique presentation of TTP that occurs in the second trimester at 20 to 22 weeks [105]. The fetus is uninvolved with no evidence of infarction or thrombocytopenia if the mother survives. The pregnancy appears to promote the TTP since the TTP will resolve with termination of the pregnancy and can recur with the next pregnancy [106]. Therapy includes terminations of the pregnancy or attempting to support the patient with plasma exchange until delivery. Many patients will have relapses with future pregnancies so this information must be weighed in planning future pregnancies. An unusual complication of pregnancy is a HUS-type syndrome seen up to 28 weeks' postpartum. This form of HUS is severe, and permanent renal failure often results despite aggressive therapy. When evaluated, many of these patients will be found to have defects in regulatory proteins of complement such as factor H deficiency, perhaps explaining the virulence of their renal failure [107].

Disseminated Intravascular Coagulation

At the most basic level, DIC is the clinical manifestation of inappropriate thrombin activation [108–111]. Inappropriate thrombin activation can be due to causes such as sepsis, obstetric disasters, etc. The activation of thrombin leads to (a) conversion of fibrinogen to fibrin, (b) activation of platelets (and their consumption), (c) activation of factors V and VIII, (d) activation of protein C (and degradation of factors Va and VIIIa), (e) activation of endothelial cells, and (f) activation of fibrinolysis.

The clinical manifestations of DIC in a given patient depend on the balance of thrombin activations and secondary fibrinolysis plus the patient's ability to compensate for the DIC. Patients with DIC can present in one of four patterns [108,110]:

1. Asymptomatic. Patients can present with laboratory evidence of DIC but no bleeding or thrombosis. This is often seen in patients with sepsis or cancer. However, with further progression of the underlying disease, these patients can rapidly become symptomatic.
2. Bleeding. The bleeding is due to a combination of factor depletion, platelet dysfunction, thrombocytopenia, and excessive fibrinolysis [108]. These patients may present with diffuse bleeding from multiple sites—IV sites, areas of instrumentation, etc.
3. Thrombosis. Despite the general activation of the coagulation process, thrombosis is unusual in most patients with acute DIC. The exceptions include cancer patients, trauma patients, and certain obstetrical patients. Most often the thrombosis is venous, but arterial thrombosis and nonbacterial thrombotic endocarditis have been reported [112].
4. Purpura fulminans. This severe form of DIC is described in more detail later.

TABLE 109.8

MANAGEMENT OF DISSEMINATED INTRAVASCULAR COAGULATION (DIC): TRANSFUSION

The five basic tests of hemostasis[a]
Hematocrit
Platelet count
Prothrombin time (PT)
Activated partial thromboplastin time (aPTT)
Fibrinogen level
Guidelines for transfusion in patients at high risk of bleeding[b]
A. Platelets <50,000 per μL: give platelet concentrates or 1 unit of single-donor platelets.
B. Fibrinogen <80–100 mg/dL: give 10 units of cryoprecipitate[c]
C. Hematocrit below 30%: give red cells
D. Protime >twofold the upper limit of normal *and* aPTT abnormal: give 2–4 units of FFP[d]

[a]These laboratory tests should be repeated after administering blood products serially. A record of the test and the blood products administered should be maintained.
[b]Patients with DIC who are not actively bleeding generally do not require replacement of platelets or coagulation factors, unless an invasive procedure is planned or other circumstances are present; see text.
[c]For a fibrinogen level less then 100 mg/dL, transfusion of 10 units of cryoprecipitate is expected to increase the plasma fibrinogen level by 100 mg/dL.
[d]In patients with DIC and a markedly prolonged PT and aPTT, one can give 2–4 units of fresh frozen plasma (FFP) initially.

The best way to treat DIC is to treat the underlying cause that is driving the thrombin generation [108,109,111, 113,114]. In the past, there was concern about replacement of depleted blood cells and coagulation proteins in DIC due to fears of "feeding the fire." However, such hesitation has not been well validated, and one must provide replacement if depletion occurs and bleeding ensues [115]. Measurement of laboratory tests that will reflect the basic parameters essential for both blood volume and hemostasis may be helpful [18,116]. Replacement therapy is based on the results of these laboratories and the clinical situation of the patient (Table 109.8). Additional discussion regarding transfusion of blood products in critically ill patients is found in Chapter 114. DIC complicating acute promyelocytic leukemia is discussed in detail in Chapter 115.

Heparin therapy is reserved for the patient who has thrombosis as a component of their DIC [109,117,118]. Given the coagulopathy that is often present, one should use specific heparin levels instead of the aPTT to monitor anticoagulation [119,120].

Purpura Fulminans

DIC in association with necrosis of the skin may occur in two situations [121,122]. One, primary purpura fulminans, is most often seen after a viral infection [123]. In these patients, the purpura fulminans starts with a painful red area on an extremity that rapidly progresses to a black ischemic lesion. In many patients, acquired deficiency of protein S is found [121, 124,125].

Secondary purpura fulminans is most often associated with meningococcemia infections, but it can occur in any patient with overwhelming infection [126–128]. Postsplenectomy sepsis syndrome patients and those with functional hyposplenism due to chronic liver diseases are also at risk [129]. Patients present with signs of sepsis, and the skin lesions often involve the extremities that may lead to amputation. As opposed to primary purpura fulminans, those with secondary purpura fulminans will have symmetrical ischemic at the distal parts of the body (toes and fingers) that ascend as the process progresses. Rarely, adrenal infarction (Waterhouse–Friderichsen syndrome) can occur which leads to severe hypotension [130].

Therapy for purpura fulminans is controversial. Primary purpura fulminans, especially cases with postvaricella autoimmune protein S deficiency, may respond to plasma infusion titrated to keep the protein S level more than 25% [121]. Intravenous immune globulin has also been reported to help decrease the antiprotein S antibodies. Heparin has been reported to control the DIC and extent of necrosis [131]. The starting dose in these patients is 5 to 8 units per kg per hour [109].

Sick patients with secondary purpura fulminans have been treated with plasma drips, plasmapheresis, and continuous plasma ultrafiltration [131–134]. Heparin therapy alone has not been shown to improve survival [135]. Much attention has been given to replacement of natural anticoagulants such as protein C and antithrombin as therapy for purpura fulminans but unfortunately randomized trials using antithrombin have shown mostly negative results [121,125,136–138]. Trials using either zymogen protein C concentrates or rAPC have shown more promise in controlling the coagulopathy of purpura fulminans and improving outcomes in sepsis [132,139–143]. Although bleeding is a concern with use of protein C, most complications occur in patients with platelet counts under 30×10^9/L or in those who have meningitis [144]. If recombinant activated protein C is used, one should also very carefully monitor other parameters of coagulation. Unfortunately, many patients will need debridement and amputation; in one review approximately 66% of patients required amputation [122].

Drug-Induced Hemolytic-DIC Syndromes

A severe variant of the drug-induced immune complex hemolysis associated with DIC has been recognized. Rare patients who receive certain second- and third-generation cephalosporins (especially cefotetan and ceftriaxone) [145] have developed this syndrome [146–151]. The clinical syndrome starts 7 to 10 days after receiving the drug, and often the patient has only received the antibiotic for surgical prophylaxis. Severe Coombs'-positive hemolysis with hypotension and DIC develops. The patients are often believed to have sepsis and often re-exposed to the cephalosporin, resulting in worsening of the clinical status. The outcome is often fatal due to massive hemolysis and thrombosis [148,152–154].

Quinine is associated with a unique syndrome of drug-induced DIC [155–158]. Approximately 24 to 96 hours after quinine exposure, the patient becomes acutely ill with nausea and vomiting. The patient then develops a microangiopathic hemolytic anemia, DIC, and renal failure. Some patients, besides having antiplatelet antibodies, also have antibodies that bind to red cells and neutrophils that may lead to the more severe syndrome. Despite therapy, patients with quinine-induced TTP frequently manifest chronic renal failure.

Treatment of the drug-induced hemolytic-DIC syndrome is based on anecdotal reports. Patients have responded to aggressive therapy including plasma exchange, dialysis, and prednisone. Early recognition of the hemolytic anemia (and the suspicion that it is drug-related) is important for early diagnosis so that the incriminating drug can be discontinued. DIC associated with acute promyelocytic leukemia is discussed in detail in Chapter 115.

Drug-Induced Thrombocytopenia

Patients with drug-induced thrombocytopenia typically present with very low platelet counts 1 to 3 weeks after starting a new medication [159,160]. One of the agents most commonly associated with drug-induced thrombocytopenia in the critical care setting is vancomycin. The thrombocytopenia is acute and severe (below $<10 \times 10^9$/L), is durably refractory to platelet transfusions, and resolves within days of stopping the drug [161]. In patients with a possible drug-induced thrombocytopenia, the primary therapy is to stop the suspect drug, although patients with severe thrombocytopenia generally should receive platelet transfusions due to the risk of fatal bleeding [159,162]. However, with vancomycin-induced thrombocytopenia, the patient may be refractory to platelet transfusion [161,163]. If there are multiple new medications, the best approach is to stop any drug that is strongly associated with thrombocytopenia [164] (Table 109.9). Immune globulin, corticosteroids, and intravenous anti-D have been suggested as useful in drug-related thrombocytopenia. However, since most of these thrombocytopenic patients recover when the agent is cleared from the body, this therapy is probably not necessary and avoids exposing the patient to additional drug-associated adverse events.

TABLE 109.9

CRITICAL CARE DRUGS COMMONLY IMPLICATED IN THROMBOCYTOPENIA

Antiarrhythmics
Procainamide
Quinidine
Anti-GP IIb/IIIa agents
Abciximab
Eptifibatide
Tirofiban
Antimicrobial
Amphotericin B
Fluoroquinolones
Rifampin
Trimethoprim-sulfamethoxazole
Vancomycin
H_2-blockers
Cimetidine
Ranitidine
Acetaminophen
Bevacizumab
Carbamazepine
Danazol
Efalizumab
Gold
Heparin
Hydrochlorothiazide
Interferon
Methyldopa
Nonsteroidal anti-inflammatory agents
Trastuzumab
Quinine

Adapted from DeLoughery [5], George et al. [6], George and Aster [160], Warkentin and Kwon [215], Leal and Robins [216], Cheah et al. [217], Jara et al. [218].

Sepsis

Thrombocytopenia associated with sepsis syndromes classically has been attributed to DIC or destruction by autoimmune mechanisms [165–167]. Increasing evidence, however, points to cytokine-driven hemophagocytosis of platelets [168–171]. Patients with hemophagocytosis appear to have higher rates of multiple organ system failure and higher mortality rates. Inflammatory cytokines, especially monocyte-colony stimulating factor (M-CSF), are thought responsible for inducing the hemophagocytosis [166,172].

Thrombocytopenia may be a diagnostic clue to infection with unusual organisms [173]. Three members of the Ehrlichia family have been reported to cause infections in humans [174,175]. They are transmitted by ticks and the diseases that they produce are similar. Most patients have a febrile illness with high fevers, headaches, and myalgias [174,176]. Patients may have central nervous system signs and marked elevation of the serum levels of liver enzymes. Rarely patients may present with a toxic shock-like syndrome [177]. Although many cases are mild, severe disease is common and the case fatality rate is 2% to 5% [176]. The typical hematologic picture is leukopenia (1.3 to 4 × 10^9 per L) and mild thrombocytopenia (30 to 60 × 10^9 per L). In many patients, the buffy coat reveals the organisms bundled in a 2 to 5 μm morula in the cytoplasm of the granulocytes or monocytes. Consideration of ehrlichiosis is important because highly specific therapy is doxycycline, which is a drug not routinely used for therapy of sepsis syndrome.

The classical hematological presentation of Hantavirus pulmonary syndrome (HPS) can be helpful in the diagnosis of this severe illness. Patients suffer a flu-like prodrome and then rapidly develop a noncardiac pulmonary edema resulting in profound respiratory failure [10,178]. Ventilatory support is required in 75% of cases and the mortality is approximately 50%. A powerful indicator to the presence of Hantavirus is found on the peripheral smear [10,179]. The triad of thrombocytopenia, increased and left-shifted white cell count, and more than 10% circulating immunoblasts can identify all cases of HPS and was seen in only 2.6% non-HPS controls in a recent study [10]. Marked hemoconcentration is also present due to capillary leak syndrome with the hematocrit reaching in some patients as high as 68%.

Viral Hemorrhagic Fevers

Viral hemorrhagic fevers (VHFs) are a diverse group of viral infections that can result in massive bleeding [180–182]. VHFs are an important problem in certain parts of the world but travelers may carry the disease anywhere. In the Southern United States, dengue is becoming an increasing problem and fatal cases of arenavirus have been reported in California [183]. As described in Table 109.10, there are four groups of viruses which can lead to VHFs [184,185].

The typical pattern is a febrile illness that proceeds over a few days to shock and diffuse bleeding with the patient developing signs of thrombocytopenia and in some cases DIC. A key sign is that patients will experience profuse bleedıng from the gastrointestinal track and mucosal bleeding often out of proportion to the observed coagulation defects. This finding should serve as a diagnostic clue. Most VHFs are also associated with leukopenia and hemoconcentration. Therapy is aggressive supportive care of the patients and replacement of coagulation factors. As noted in Table 109.10, ribavirin can treat certain VHFs. Given the propensity of many of these infections to spread to healthcare workers, precautions should be taken to prevent nosocomial spread [186].

TABLE 109.10

VIRAL HEMORRHAGIC FEVER-ASSOCIATED THROMBOCYTOPENIA

Arenaviridae
- Diseases: Lassa fever, New World arenaviruses
- Distribution: West Africa (Lassa), South America [rare California] (New World)
- Vector: rodents
- Incubation: 5–16 d
- Therapy: ribavirin
- Unique clinical features: pharyngitis, late deafness (Lassa); neurological involvement–seizures (New World)

Bunyaviridae
- Diseases: Crimean–Congo hemorrhagic virus (CCHF), Rift Valley fever, hemorrhagic fever with renal syndrome (HFRS)
- Distribution: Africa, central Asia, eastern Europe, Middle East (CCHF), Africa, Middle East (Rift), Asia, Balkans, Europe (HFRS)
- Vector: ticks (CCHF), mosquitoes (Rift Valley), rodents (HFRS)
- Incubation: 1–6 d (CHHF), 2 wk to 2 mo (HFRS)
- Therapy: ribavirin
- Unique clinical features: retinitis, hepatitis (Rift Valley), prominent bleeding with DIC, jaundice (CCHF); renal disease (CCHF)

Filoviridae
- Diseases: Ebola, Marburg viruses
- Distribution: Africa
- Vector: ?
- Incubation: 2–21 d
- Unique clinical features: maculopapular rash, high mortality

Flaviviridae
- Diseases: dengue, yellow fever
- Distribution: widespread (dengue), Africa, tropical Americans (yellow)
- Vector: mosquitoes
- Incubation: 3–15 d
- Unique clinical feature: liver involvement (yellow)

Adapted from DeLoughery [185], Nimmannitya [219], Taylor and Strickland [220].

Bleeding in the Platelet-Refractory Patient

Bleeding in patients who are refractory to platelet transfusion presents a difficult clinical problem (Table 109.11) [187,188]. If patients are demonstrated to have HLA antibodies, one can transfuse HLA-matched platelets [189]. Unfortunately, matched platelet transfusions do not work in 20% to 70% of these patients. Also, since some loci are difficult to match, effective products may be unavailable. As many as 25% of patients have antiplatelet antibodies in which HLA-matched products will be ineffective. One can perform platelet cross-matching to find compatible units for these patients but this may not always be successful. In the patient who is totally refractory to platelet transfusion, consider drugs as an etiology of antiplatelet antibodies (especially vancomycin) [163]. Use of antifibrinolytic agents such as epsilon aminocaproic acid or tranexamic acid may decrease the incidence of minor bleeding but are ineffective for major bleeding [190]. "Platelet drips" consisting of infusing either a platelet concentrate per hour or one plateletpheresis unit every 6 hours may be given as a continuous infusion [191,192]. For life-threatening bleeding

TABLE 109.11

EVALUATION AND MANAGEMENT OF PLATELET ALLOIMMUNIZATION

1. Check platelet count 15 min after platelet transfusion.
2. If rise in platelet count is less than 5,000 per μL, check for HLA antibodies.
3. Administer HLA-matched platelets and evaluate for response.
4. If three sequential HLA-matched platelet transfusions are ineffective, discontinue HLA-matched platelets.
5. In completely refractory patients:
   A. Evaluate for other causes of thrombocytopenia (HIT, drugs).
   B. Consider institution of antifibrinolytic therapy
   1. Epsilon aminocaproic acid 1 g/h IV, or
   2. Tranexamic acid 10 mg/kg IV every 8 h
   C. Platelet "drip"—continuous infusion of platelets at the rate of 1 unit over 6 h
   D. Recombinant activated VII for life-threatening bleeding

rVIIa may be of use [193]. For platelet refractory patients with arterial bleeding, the use of angiographic delivery of platelets has been reported to be successful in stopping bleeding [194].

Catastrophic Antiphospholipid Antibody Syndrome

Rarely patients with antiphospholipid antibody syndrome can present with fulminant multiorgan system failure [195–199]. Catastrophic antiphospholipid antibody syndrome is caused by widespread microthrombi in multiple vascular fields. These patients will develop renal failure, encephalopathy, adult respiratory distress syndrome (often with pulmonary hemorrhage), cardiac failure, dramatic livedo reticularis, and worsening thrombocytopenia. Many of these patients have preexisting autoimmune disorders and high titer-anticardiolipin antibodies. It appears that the best therapy for these patients is aggressive immunosuppression, plasmapheresis, and anticoagulation, then (perhaps) IV cyclophosphamide monthly [198]. Early recognition of this syndrome can lead to quick therapy and resolution of the multiorgan system failure.

Posttransfusion Purpura

Patients with this disorder develop severe thrombocytopenia ($<10 \times 10^9$ per L), and often severe bleeding, 1 to 2 weeks after receiving blood products [200]. Affected patients usually lack the platelet antigen PLA1. For unknown reasons, exposure to the antigens from the transfusion leads to rapid destruction of the patient's own platelets. The diagnostic clue is thrombocytopenia in a patient, typically female, who has received a red cell or platelet blood product in the past 7 to 10 days. Treatment consists of intravenous immunoglobulin [201] and plasmapheresis to remove the offending antibody. If patients with a history of posttransfusion purpura require further transfusions, only PLA1-negative platelets should be given.

Liver Disease

Patients with severe liver disease have multiple hemostatic defects [202–206] (see Chapter 108, Disorders of Hemostasis). Splenomegaly (due to cirrhosis) and infections (e.g., HCV) may be contributory. Additionally, the liver is the source of thrombopoietin and lack of this platelet growth factor may worsen thrombocytopenia [207–209]. Patients may have platelet dysfunction due to the increase in fibrinogen degradation products and circulating plasmin [210]. Platelet transfusion should be given only to patients with platelet counts that are reliably less than 10×10^9 per L who are actively bleeding, or who require a higher platelet count due to an invasive procedure. The thrombopoietin receptor agonist eltrombopag has been used in patients with HCV-associated thrombocytopenia enabling administration of eradication therapy for HCV [211], but the delayed onset of action may make use in the critical care unit, where a need for immediate correction in the platelet count is more likely to be encountered, less feasible.

References

1. Hanes SD, Quarles DA, Boucher BA: Incidence and risk factors of thrombocytopenia in critically ill trauma patients. *Ann Pharmacother* 31(3):285–289, 1997.
2. Bonfiglio MF, Traeger SM, Kier KL, et al: Thrombocytopenia in intensive care patients: a comprehensive analysis of risk factors in 314 patients. *Ann Pharmacother* 29(9):835–842, 1995.
3. Chakraverty R, Davidson S, Peggs K, et al: The incidence and cause of coagulopathies in an intensive care population. *Br J Haematol* 93(2):460–463, 1996.
4. Stéphan F, Hollande J, Richard O, et al: Thrombocytopenia in a surgical ICU. *Chest* 115(5):1363–1370, 1999.
5. DeLoughery T: Drug induced immune hematological disease. *Immunol Allergy Clin* 18(4):829–841, 1998.
6. George JN, Raskob GE, Shah SR, et al: Drug-induced thrombocytopenia: a systematic review of published case reports. *Ann Intern Med* 129:886–890, 1998.
7. Heck AM, DeWitt BA, Lukes AL: Potential interactions between alternative therapies and warfarin. *Am J Health-Syst Pharm* 57:1221–1230, 2000.
8. Royer DJ, George JN, Terrell DR: Thrombocytopenia as an adverse effect of complementary and alternative medicines, herbal remedies, nutritional supplements, foods, and beverages. *Eur J Haematol* 84(5):421–429, 2010.
9. Bizzaro N: EDTA-dependent pseudothrombocytopenia: a clinical and epidemiological study of 112 cases, with 10-year follow-up. *Am J Hematol* 50(2):103–109, 1995.
10. Mertz GJ, Hjelle BL, Bryan RT: Hantavirus infection. *Dis Mon* 44:89–138, 1998.
11. Bell WR, Braine HG, Ness PM, et al: Improved survival in thrombotic thrombocytopenic purpura-hemolytic uremic syndrome—clinical experience in 108 patients. *N Engl J Med* 325:398–403, 1991.
12. Warkentin TE, Greinacher A, Koster A, et al: Treatment and prevention of heparin-induced thrombocytopenia: American College of Chest Physicians Evidence-Based Clinical Practice Guidelines (8th Edition). *Chest* 133[Suppl 6]:340S–380S, 2008.
13. Arepally GM, Ortel TL: Heparin-induced thrombocytopenia. *Annu Rev Med* 61:77–90, 2010.
14. Kundu S, Sio R, Mitu A, et al: Evaluation of platelet function by PFA-100. *Clin Chem* 40:1827–1828, 1994.
15. Alving BM, Spivak JL, DeLoughery TG: Consultative hematology: hemostasis and transfusion issues in surgery and critical care medicine. *Hematology* 1998:320–341, 1998.
16. Oguzulgen IK, Ozis T, Gursel G: Is the fall in platelet count associated with intensive care unit acquired pneumonia? *Swiss Med Wkly* 134(29–30):430–434, 2004.
17. Rebulla P, Finazzi G, Marangoni F, et al: The threshold for prophylactic platelet transfusions in adults with acute myeloid leukemia. *N Engl J Med* 337:1870–1875, 1997.
18. Counts RB, Haisch C, Simon TL, et al: Hemostasis in massively transfused trauma patients. *Ann Surg* 190(1):91–99, 1979.
19. Miller RD, Robbins TO, Tong MJ, et al: Coagulation defects associated with massive blood transfusions. *Ann Surg* 174(5):794–801, 1971.
20. Shantsila E, Lip GY, Chong BH: Heparin-induced thrombocytopenia. A contemporary clinical approach to diagnosis and management. *Chest* 135(6):1651–1664, 2009.

21. Warkentin TE, Levine MN, Hirsh J, et al: Heparin-induced thrombocytopenia in patients treated with low-molecular-weight heparin or unfractionated heparin. *N Engl J Med* 332:1330–1335, 1995.
22. Warkentin TE, Sheppard JA, Sigouin CS, et al: Gender imbalance and risk factor interactions in heparin-induced thrombocytopenia. *Blood* 108(9): 2937–2941, 2006.
23. Warkentin TE, Kelton JG: Temporal aspects of heparin-induced thrombocytopenia. *N Engl J Med* 344(17):1286–1292, 2001.
24. Hach-Wunderle V, Kainer K, Krug B, et al: Heparin-associated thrombosis despite normal platelet counts. *Lancet* 344:469–470, 1994.
25. Lo GK, Juhl D, Warkentin TE, et al: Evaluation of pretest clinical score (4 T's) for the diagnosis of heparin-induced thrombocytopenia in two clinical settings. *J Thromb Haemost* 4(4):759–765, 2006.
26. Crowther MA, Cook DJ, Albert M, et al: The 4Ts scoring system for heparin-induced thrombocytopenia in medical-surgical intensive care unit patients. *J Crit Care* 25:287–293, 2010.
27. Pouplard C, May MA, Regina S, et al: Changes in platelet count after cardiac surgery can effectively predict the development of pathogenic heparin-dependent antibodies. *Br J Haematol* 128(6):837–841, 2005.
28. Trossaert M, Gaillard A, Commin PL, et al: High incidence of anti-heparin/platelet factor 4 antibodies after cardiopulmonary bypass surgery. *Br J Haematol* 101(4):653–655, 1998.
29. Visentin GP, Malik M, Cyganiak KA, et al: Patients treated with unfractionated heparin during open heart surgery are at high risk to form antibodies reactive with heparin:platelet factor 4 complexes. *J Lab Clin Med* 128:376–383, 1996.
30. Warkentin TE, Greinacher A: Laboratory testing for heparin-induced thrombocytopenia, in Warkentin TE, Greinacher A (eds): *Heparin-Induced Thrombocytopenia*. New York, Marcel Dekker, 2000, pp 211–244.
31. Laposata M, Green D, Van Cott EM, et al: College of American Pathologists Conference XXXI on Laboratory Monitoring of Anticoagulant Therapy—The clinical use and laboratory monitoring of low-molecular-weight heparin, danaparoid, hirudin and related compounds, and argatroban. *Arch Pathol Lab Med* 122:799–807, 1998.
32. Kondo LM, Wittkowsky AK, Wiggins BS: Argatroban for prevention and treatment of thromboembolism in heparin-induced thrombocytopenia. *Ann Pharmacother* 35(4):440–451, 2001.
33. Swan SK, Hursting MJ: The pharmacokinetics and pharmacodynamics of argatroban: effects of age, gender, and hepatic or renal dysfunction. *Pharmacotherapy* 20(3):318–329, 2000.
34. Baghdasarin SB, Singh I, Militello MA, et al: Argatroban dosage in critically ill patients with HIT. *Blood* 104(11):1779, 2004.
35. Moll S, Ortel TL: Monitoring warfarin therapy in patients with lupus anticoagulants [see comments]. *Ann Intern Med* 127(3):177–185, 1997.
36. Greinacher A, Janssens U, Berg G, et al: Lepirudin (recombinant hirudin) for parenteral anticoagulation in patients with heparin-induced thrombocytopenia. Heparin-Associated Thrombocytopenia Study (HAT) investigators. *Circulation* 100(6):587–593, 1999.
37. Song X, Huhle G, Wang L, et al: Generation of anti-hirudin antibodies in heparin-induced thrombocytopenic patients treated with r-hirudin. *Circulation* 100(14):1528–1532, 1999.
38. Huhle G, Hoffmann U, Song X, et al: Immunologic response to recombinant hirudin in HIT type II patients during long-term treatment. *Brit J Haem* 106(1):195–201, 1999.
39. Bauer KA: Fondaparinux sodium: a selective inhibitor of factor Xa. *Am J Health Syst Pharm* 58[Suppl 7], 2001.
40. Lobo B, Finch C, Howard A, et al: Fondaparinux for the treatment of patients with acute heparin-induced thrombocytopenia. *Thromb Haemost* 99(1):208–214, 2008.
41. Warkentin TE, Maurer BT, Aster RH: Heparin-induced thrombocytopenia associated with fondaparinux. *N Engl J Med* 356(25):2653–2655, 2007.
42. Hopkins CK, Goldfinger D: Platelet transfusions in heparin-induced thrombocytopenia: a report of four cases and review of the literature. *Transfusion* 48(10):2128–2132, 2008.
43. George JN: How I treat patients with thrombotic thrombocytopenic purpura-hemolytic uremic syndrome. *Blood* 96:1223–1229, 2000.
44. Murrin RJ, Murray JA: Thrombotic thrombocytopenic purpura: aetiology, pathophysiology and treatment. *Blood Rev* 20(1):51–60, 2006.
45. George JN: Clinical practice. Thrombotic thrombocytopenic purpura. *N Engl J Med* 354(18):1927–1935, 2006.
46. Saltzman DJ, Chang JC, Jimenez JC, et al: Postoperative thrombotic thrombocytopenic purpura after open heart operations. *Ann Thorac Surg* 89(1):119–123, 2010.
47. Furlan M, Robles R, Galbusera M, et al: Von Willebrand factor-cleaving protease in thrombotic thrombocytopenic purpura and the hemolytic-uremic syndrome. *N Engl J Med* 339:1578–1584, 1998.
48. Sadler JE: Von Willebrand factor, ADAMTS13, and thrombotic thrombocytopenic purpura. *Blood* 112(1):11–18, 2008.
49. Levy GG, Nichols WC, Lian EC, et al: Mutations in a member of the ADAMTS gene family cause thrombotic thrombocytopenic purpura. *Nature* 413(6855):488–494, 2001.
50. Veyradier A, Obert B, Houllier A, et al: Specific von Willebrand factor-cleaving protease in thrombotic microangiopathies: a study of 111 cases. *Blood* 98(6):1765–1772, 2001.
51. Peyvandi F, Ferrari S, Lavoretano S, et al: von Willebrand factor cleaving protease (ADAMTS-13) and ADAMTS-13 neutralizing autoantibodies in 100 patients with thrombotic thrombocytopenic purpura. *Br J Haematol* 127(4):433–439, 2004.
52. Vesely SK, George JN, Lammle B, et al: ADAMTS13 activity in thrombotic thrombocytopenic purpura-hemolytic uremic syndrome: relation to presenting features and clinical outcomes in a prospective cohort of 142 patients. *Blood* 102(1):60–68, 2003.
53. Park YA, Waldrum MR, Marques MB: Platelet count and prothrombin time help distinguish thrombotic thrombocytopenic purpura-hemolytic uremic syndrome from disseminated intravascular coagulation in adults. *Am J Clin Pathol* 133(3):460–465, 2010.
54. Patton JF, Manning KR, Case D, et al: Serum lactate dehydrogenase and platelet count predict survival in thrombotic thrombocytopenic purpura. *Am J Hematol* 47:94–99, 1994.
55. Coppo P, Wolf M, Veyradier A, et al: Prognostic value of inhibitory anti-ADAMTS13 antibodies in adult-acquired thrombotic thrombocytopenic purpura. *Br J Haematol* 132(1):66–74, 2006.
56. Rock GA, Shumak KH, Buskard NA, et al: Comparison of plasma exchange with plasma infusion in the treatment of thrombotic thrombocytopenic purpura. *N Engl J Med* 325:393–397, 1991.
57. Kaplan BS, Trachtman H: Improve survival with plasma exchange thrombotic thrombopenic purpura-hemolytic uremic syndrome. *Am J Med* 110(2):156–157, 2001.
58. Viswanathan S, Rovin BH, Shidham GB, et al: Long-term, sub-clinical cardiac and renal complications in patients with multiple relapses of thrombotic thrombocytopenic purpura. *Br J Haematol* 149(4):623–625, 2010.
59. George JN: Thrombotic Thrombocytopenic purpura—hemolytic uremic syndrome. *Hematology* 1998;379–383, 1998.
60. van Genderen PJ, Michiels JJ: Acquired von Willebrand disease. [Review] [54 refs]. *Bail Clin Haem* 11(2):319–330, 1998.
61. Copelovitch L, Kaplan BS. The thrombotic microangiopathies. *Pediatr Nephrol* 23(10):1761–1767, 2008.
62. Razzaq S. Hemolytic uremic syndrome: an emerging health risk. *Am Fam Physician* 74(6):991–996, 2006.
63. Karch H, Friedrich AW, Gerber A, et al: New aspects in the pathogenesis of enteropathic hemolytic uremic syndrome. *Semin Thromb Hemost* 32(2):105–112, 2006.
64. Kavanagh D, Goodship TH, Richards A: Atypical haemolytic uraemic syndrome. *Br Med Bull* 77–78:5–22, 2006.
65. Dundas S, Murphy J, Soutar RL, et al: Effectiveness of therapeutic plasma exchange in the 1996 Lanarkshire *Escherichia coli* O157:H7 outbreak. *Lancet* 354(9187):1327–1330, 1999.
66. Noris M, Remuzzi G: Atypical hemolytic-uremic syndrome. *N Engl J Med* 361(17):1676–1687, 2009.
67. Taylor CM, Machin S, Wigmore SJ, et al: Clinical practice guidelines for the management of atypical haemolytic uraemic syndrome in the United Kingdom. *Br J Haematol* 148(1):37–47, 2010.
68. Michael M, Elliott EJ, Craig JC, et al: Interventions for hemolytic uremic syndrome and thrombotic thrombocytopenic purpura: a systematic review of randomized controlled trials. *Am J Kidney Dis* 53(2):259–272, 2009.
69. Caprioli J, Noris M, Brioschi S, et al: Genetics of HUS: the impact of MCP, CFH, and IF mutations on clinical presentation, response to treatment, and outcome. *Blood* 108(4):1267–1279, 2006.
70. Moake JL, Byrnes JJ: Thrombotic microangiopathies associated with drugs and bone marrow transplantation. [Review] [66 refs]. *Hematol Oncol Clin North Am* 10(2):485–497, 1996.
71. Zakarija A, Bennett C: Drug-induced thrombotic microangiopathy. *Semin Thromb Hemost* 31(6):681–690, 2005.
72. Gharpure VS, Devine SM, Holland HK, et al: Thrombotic thrombocytopenic purpura associated with FK506 following bone marrow transplantation. *Bone Marrow Transplant* 16(5):715–716, 1995.
73. Wu DC, Liu JM, Chen YM, et al: Mitomycin-C induced hemolytic uremic syndrome: a case report and literature review. [Review] [27 refs]. *Jpn J Clin Oncol* 27(2):115–118, 1997.
74. Borghardt EJ, Kirchertz EJ, Marten I, et al: Protein A-immunoadsorption in chemotherapy associated hemolytic-uremic syndrome. *Transfus Sci* 19[Suppl 7], 1998.
75. Saif MW, McGee PJ: Hemolytic-uremic syndrome associated with gemcitabine: a case report and review of literature. *JOP* 6(4):369–374, 2005.
76. Brodowicz T, Breiteneder S, Wiltschke C, et al: Gemcitabine-induced hemolytic uremic syndrome: a case report. *J Natl Cancer Inst* 89:1895–1896, 1997.
77. Fung MC, Storniolo AM, Nguyen B, et al: A review of hemolytic uremic syndrome in patients treated with gemcitabine therapy. *Cancer* 85(9):2023–2032, 1999.
78. Izzedine H, Isnard-Bagnis C, Launay-Vacher V, et al: Gemcitabine-induced thrombotic microangiopathy: a systematic review. *Nephrol Dial Transplant* 21(11):3038–3045, 2006.
79. Walter RB, Joerger M, Pestalozzi BC: Gemcitabine-associated hemolytic-uremic syndrome. *Am J Kidney Dis* 40(4):E16, 2002.
80. Gore EM, Jones BS, Marques MB: Is therapeutic plasma exchange indicated for patients with gemcitabine-induced hemolytic uremic syndrome? *J Clin Apher* 24(5):209–214, 2009.
81. Eremina V, Jefferson JA, Kowalewska J, et al: VEGF inhibition and renal thrombotic microangiopathy. *N Engl J Med* 358(11):1129–1136, 2008.

82. Bollee G, Patey N, Cazajous G, et al: Thrombotic microangiopathy secondary to VEGF pathway inhibition by sunitinib. *Nephrol Dial Transplant* 24(2):682–685, 2009.
83. Benz K, Amann K: Thrombotic microangiopathy: new insights. *Curr Opin Nephrol Hypertens* 19(3):242–247, 2010.
84. Zakarija A, Kwaan HC, Moake JL, et al: Ticlopidine- and clopidogrel-associated thrombotic thrombocytopenic purpura (TTP): review of clinical, laboratory, epidemiological, and pharmacovigilance findings (1989–2008). *Kidney Int Suppl* 112:S20–S24, 2009.
85. Schriber JR, Herzig GP: Transplantation-associated thrombotic thrombocytopenic purpura and hemolytic uremic syndrome. [Review] [76 refs]. *Semin Hematol* 34(2):126–133, 1997.
86. Clark RE: Thrombotic microangiopathy following bone marrow transplantation [see comments]. [Review] [97 refs]. *Bone Marrow Transplant* 14(4):495–504, 1994.
87. Fuge R, Bird JM, Fraser A, et al: The clinical features, risk factors and outcome of thrombotic thrombocytopenic purpura occurring after bone marrow transplantation. *Br J Haematol* 113(1):58–64, 2001.
88. Daly AS, Xenocostas A, Lipton JH: Transplantation-associated thrombotic microangiopathy: twenty-two years later. *Bone Marrow Transplant* 30(11):709–715, 2002.
89. Choi CM, Schmaier AH, Snell MR, et al: Thrombotic microangiopathy in haematopoietic stem cell transplantation: diagnosis and treatment. *Drugs* 69(2):183–198, 2009.
90. Van der Plas RM, Schiphorst ME, Huizinga EG, et al: von Willebrand factor proteolysis is deficient in classic, but not in bone marrow transplantation-associated, thrombotic thrombocytopenic purpura. *Blood* 93(11):3798–3802, 1999.
91. Sarode R, McFarland JG, Flomenberg N, et al: Therapeutic plasma exchange does not appear to be effective in the management of thrombotic thrombocytopenic purpura/hemolytic uremic syndrome following bone marrow transplantation. *Bone Marrow Transplant* 16(2):271–275, 1995.
92. Magann EF, Martin JN Jr: Twelve steps to optimal management of HELLP syndrome. [Review] [20 refs]. *Clin Obstet Gynecol* 42(3):532–550, 1999.
93. Kennedy GA, Kearney N, Bleakley S, et al: Transplantation-associated thrombotic microangiopathy: effect of concomitant GVHD on efficacy of therapeutic plasma exchange. *Bone Marrow Transplant* 45(4):699–704, 2010.
94. Sibai BM: Imitators of severe pre-eclampsia/eclampsia. *Clin Perinatol* 31(4):835–852, vii–viii, 2004.
95. Steingrub JS: Pregnancy-associated severe liver dysfunction. *Crit Care Clin* 20(4):763–776, xi, 2004.
96. Baxter JK, Weinstein L: HELLP syndrome: the state of the art. *Obstet Gynecol Surv* 59(12):838–845, 2004.
97. Leeman L, Fontaine P: Hypertensive disorders of pregnancy. *Am Fam Physician* 78(1):93–100, 2008.
98. Le Thi TD, Tieulie N, Costedoat N, et al: The HELLP syndrome in the antiphospholipid syndrome: retrospective study of 16 cases in 15 women. *Ann Rheum Dis* 64(2):273–278, 2005.
99. Martin JN Jr, Perry KG Jr, Blake PG, et al: Better maternal outcomes are achieved with dexamethasone therapy for postpartum HELLP (hemolysis, elevated liver enzymes, and thrombocytopenia) syndrome. *Am J Obstet Gynecol* 177(5):1011–1017, 1997.
100. Habli M, Eftekhari N, Wiebracht E, et al: Long-term maternal and subsequent pregnancy outcomes 5 years after hemolysis, elevated liver enzymes, and low platelets (HELLP) syndrome. *Am J Obstet Gynecol* 201(4):385, 2009.
101. Jwayyed SM, Blanda M, Kubina M: Acute fatty liver of pregnancy. *J Emerg Med* 17(4):673–677, 1999.
102. Bacq Y: Acute fatty liver of pregnancy. [Review] [56 refs]. *Semin Perinatol* 22(2):134–140, 1998.
103. Sibai BM: Imitators of severe preeclampsia. *Obstet Gynecol* 109(4):956–966, 2007.
104. Egerman RS, Sibai BM: Imitators of preeclampsia and eclampsia. [Review] [65 refs]. *Clin Obstet Gynecol* 42(3):551–562, 1999.
105. Esplin MS, Branch DW: Diagnosis and management of thrombotic microangiopathies during pregnancy. [Review] [32 refs]. *Clin Obstet Gynecol* 42(2):360–367, 1999.
106. Dashe JS, Ramin SM, Cunningham FG: The long-term consequences of thrombotic microangiopathy (thrombotic thrombocytopenic purpura and hemolytic uremic syndrome) in pregnancy. *Obstet Gynecol* 91(5, Pt 1):t-8, 1998.
107. Fakhouri F, Roumenina L, Provot F, et al: Pregnancy-associated hemolytic uremic syndrome revisited in the era of complement gene mutations. *J Am Soc Nephrol* 21(5):859–867, 2010.
108. Carey MJ, Rodgers GM: Disseminated intravascular coagulation: clinical and laboratory aspects. *Am J Hematol* 59:65–73, 1998.
109. De Jonge E, Levi M, Stoutenbeek CP, et al: Current drug treatment strategies for disseminated intravascular coagulation. *Drugs* 55:767–777, 1998.
110. Baker WF Jr: Clinical aspects of disseminated intravascular coagulation: a clinician's point of view. [Review] [635 refs]. *Semin Thromb Hemost* 15(1):1–57, 1989.
111. Levi M, ten Cate H: Disseminated intravascular coagulation. [Review] [52 refs]. *New Engl J Med* 341(8):586–592, 1999.
112. Sharma S, Mayberry JC, DeLoughery TG, et al: Fatal cerebroembolism from nonbacterial thrombotic endocarditis in a trauma patient: case report and review. *Mil Med* 165(1):83–85, 2000.
113. Hoffman JN, Faist E: Coagulation inhibitor replacement during sepsis: useless? [Review] [44 refs]. *Crit Care Med* 28[9, Suppl]:S74–S76, 2000.
114. Wada H, Asakura H, Okamoto K, et al: Expert consensus for the treatment of disseminated intravascular coagulation in Japan. *Thromb Res* 125(1):6–11, 2010.
115. Feinstein DI: Diagnosis and management of disseminated intravascular coagulation: the role of heparin therapy. *Blood* 60:284, 1982.
116. Stainsby D, MacLennan S, Hamilton PJ: Management of massive blood loss: a template guideline. *Br J Anaesth* 85(3):487–491, 2000.
117. Feinstein DI: Diagnosis and management of disseminated intravascular coagulation: the role of heparin therapy. [Review] [34 refs]. *Blood* 60(2):284–287, 1982.
118. Callander N, Rapaport SI: Trousseau's syndrome. *West J Med* 158(4):364–371, 1993.
119. Brill-Edwards P, Ginsberg JS, Johnston M, et al: Establishing a therapeutic range for heparin therapy [see comments]. *Ann Int Med* 119(2):104–109, 1993.
120. Olson JD, Arkin CF, Brandt JT, et al: College of American Pathologists Conference XXXI on laboratory monitoring of anticoagulant therapy: laboratory monitoring of unfractionated heparin therapy. [Review] [182 refs]. *Arch Pathol Lab Med* 122(9):782–798, 1998.
121. Darmstadt GL: Acute infectious purpura fulminans: pathogenesis and medical management. [Review] [149 refs]. *Pediatr Dermatol* 15(3):169–183, 1998.
122. Davis MD, Dy KM, Nelson S: Presentation and outcome of purpura fulminans associated with peripheral gangrene in 12 patients at Mayo Clinic. *J Am Acad Dermatol* 57(6):944–956, 2007.
123. Spicer TE, Rau JM: Purpura fulminans. [Review] [44 refs]. *Am J Med* 61(4):566–571, 1976.
124. Josephson C, Nuss R, Jacobson L, et al: The varicella-autoantibody syndrome. *Pediatr Res* 50(3):345–352, 2001.
125. Smith OP, White B: Infectious purpura fulminans: diagnosis and treatment. [Review] [50 refs]. *Brit J Haem* 104(2):202–207, 1999.
126. Gamper G, Oschatz E, Herkner H, et al: Sepsis-associated purpura fulminans in adults. *Wien Klin Wochenschr* 113(3–4):107–112, 2001.
127. Ward KM, Celebi JT, Gmyrek R, et al: Acute infectious purpura fulminans associated with asplenism or hyposplenism. *J Am Acad Dermatol* 47(4):493–496, 2002.
128. Childers BJ, Cobanov B: Acute infectious purpura fulminans: a 15-year retrospective review of 28 consecutive cases. *Am Surg* 69(1):86–90, 2003.
129. Carpenter CT, Kaiser AB: Purpura fulminans in pneumococcal sepsis: case report and review. [Review] [41 refs]. *Scand J Infect Dis* 29(5):479–483, 1997.
130. Yoshikawa T, Tanaka KR, Guze LB: Infection and disseminated intravascular coagulation. *Medicine (Baltimore)* 50(4):237–258, 1971.
131. Duncan A: New therapies for severe meningococcal disease but better outcomes? [comment] [see comments]. *Lancet* 350(9091):1565–1566, 1997.
132. Smith OP, White B, Vaughan D, et al: Use of protein-C concentrate, heparin, and haemodiafiltration in meningococcus-induced purpura fulminans [see comments]. *Lancet* 350(9091):1590–1593, 1997.
133. Branson HE, Katz J: A structured approach to the management of purpura fulminans. *J Natl Med Assoc* 75(8):821–825, 1983.
134. Nolan J, Sinclair R: Review of management of purpura fulminans and two case reports. *Br J Anaesth* 86(4):581–586, 2001.
135. Manios SG, Kanakoudi F, Maniati E: Fulminant meningococcemia. Heparin therapy and survival rate. *Scand J Infect Dis* 3(2):127–133, 1971.
136. Giudici D, Baudo F, Palareti G, et al: Antithrombin replacement in patients with sepsis and septic shock. [Review] [54 refs]. *Haematologica* 84(5):452–460, 1999.
137. Fourrier F, Jourdain M, Tournoys A: Clinical trial results with antithrombin III in sepsis. [Review] [27 refs]. *Crit Care Med* 28[9, Suppl]:S38–S43, 2000.
138. Levi M, De Jonge E, van der PT, et al: Novel approaches to the management of disseminated intravascular coagulation. [Review] [37 refs]. *Crit Care Med* 28[9, Suppl]:S20–S24, 2000.
139. Rivard GE, David M, Farrell C, et al: Treatment of purpura fulminans in meningococcemia with protein C concentrate. *J Pediatr* 126:646–652, 1995.
140. White B, Livingstone W, Murphy C, et al: An open-label study of the role of adjuvant hemostatic support with protein C replacement therapy in purpura fulminans-associated meningococcemia. *Blood* 96(12):3719–3724, 2000.
141. Aoki N, Matsuda T, Saito H, et al: A comparative double-blind randomized trial of activated protein C and unfractionated heparin in the treatment of disseminated intravascular coagulation. *Int J Hematol* 75(5):540–547, 2002.
142. Schellongowski P, Bauer E, Holzinger U, et al: Treatment of adult patients with sepsis-induced coagulopathy and purpura fulminans using a plasma-derived protein C concentrate (Ceprotin). *Vox Sang* 90(4):294–301, 2006.
143. Toussaint S, Gerlach H: Activated protein C for sepsis. *N Engl J Med* 361(27):2646–2652, 2009.
144. Taylor FB, Kinasewitz G: Activated protein C in sepsis. *J Thromb Haemost* 2(5):708–717, 2004.

145. Garratty G: Drug-induced immune hemolytic anemia. *Hematology Am Soc Hematol Educ Program* 73–79, 2009.
146. Garratty G: Immune cytopenia associated with antibiotics. [Review] [108 refs]. *Transfus Med Rev* 7(4):255–267, 1993.
147. Chenoweth CE, Judd WJ, Steiner EA, et al: Cefotetan-induced immune hemolytic anemia. *Clin Infect Dis* 15(5):863–865, 1992.
148. Garratty G, Nance S, Lloyd M, et al: Fatal immune hemolytic anemia due to cefotetan [see comments]. *Transfusion* 32(3):269–271, 1992.
149. Endoh T, Yagihashi A, Sasaki M, et al: Ceftizoxime-induced hemolysis due to immune complexes: case report and determination of the epitope responsible for immune complex-mediated hemolysis. *Transfusion* 39(3):306–309, 1999.
150. Arndt PA, Leger RM, Garratty G: Serology of antibodies to second- and third-generation cephalosporins associated with immune hemolytic anemia and/or positive direct antiglobulin tests. *Transfusion* 39(11–12):1239–1246, 1999.
151. Martin ME, Laber DA: Cefotetan-induced hemolytic anemia after perioperative prophylaxis. *Am J Hematol* 81(3):186–188, 2006.
152. Bernini JC, Mustafa MM, Sutor LJ, et al: Fatal hemolysis induced by ceftriaxone in a child with sickle cell anemia [see comments]. *J Pediatr* 126(5 Pt 1):813–815, 1995.
153. Borgna-Pignatti C, Bezzi TM, Reverberi R: Fatal ceftriaxone-induced hemolysis in a child with acquired immunodeficiency syndrome. *Pediatr Infect Dis J* 14(12):1116–1117, 1995.
154. Lascari AD, Amyot K: Fatal hemolysis caused by ceftriaxone [see comments]. *J Pediatr* 126(5 Pt 1):816–817, 1995.
155. Gottschall JL, Elliot W, Lianos E, et al: Quinine-induced immune thrombocytopenia associated with hemolytic uremic syndrome: a new clinical entity. *Blood* 77(2):306–310, 1991.
156. Gottschall JL, Neahring B, McFarland JG, et al: Quinine-induced immune thrombocytopenia with hemolytic uremic syndrome: clinical and serological findings in nine patients and review of literature. [Review] [15 refs]. *Am J Hematol* 47(4):283–289, 1994.
157. Crum NF, Gable P: Quinine-induced hemolytic-uremic syndrome. *South Med J* 93(7):726–728, 2000.
158. Kojouri K, Vesely SK, George JN: Quinine-associated thrombotic thrombocytopenic purpura-hemolytic uremic syndrome: frequency, clinical features, and long-term outcomes. *Ann Intern Med* 135(12):1047–1051, 2001.
159. Aster RH, Bougie DW: Drug-induced immune thrombocytopenia. *N Engl J Med* 357(6):580–587, 2007.
160. George JN, Aster RH: Drug-induced thrombocytopenia: pathogenesis, evaluation, and management. *Hematology Am Soc Hematol Educ Program* 153–158, 2009.
161. Von DA, Curtis BR, Bougie DW, et al: Vancomycin-induced immune thrombocytopenia. *N Engl J Med* 356(9):904–910, 2007.
162. Zondor SD, George JN, Medina PJ: Treatment of drug-induced thrombocytopenia. *Expert Opin Drug Saf* 1(2):173–180, 2002.
163. Christie DJ, van Buren N, Lennon SS, et al: Vancomycin-dependent antibodies associated with thrombocytopenia and refractoriness to platelet transfusion in patients with leukemia. *Blood* 75(2):518–523, 1990.
164. Pedersen-Bjergaard U, Andersen M, Hansen PB: Drug-induced thrombocytopenia: clinical data on 309 cases and the effect of corticosteroid therapy. *Eur J Clin Pharmacol* 52(3):183–189, 1997.
165. Harris RL, Musher DM, Bloom K, et al: Manifestations of sepsis. [Review] [234 refs]. *Arch Intern Med* 147(11):1895–1906, 1987.
166. van Gorp EC, Suharti C, ten Cate H, et al: Review: infectious diseases and coagulation disorders. [Review] [176 refs]. *J Infect Dis* 180(1):176–186, 1999.
167. Tiab M, Mechinaud F, Harousseau JL: Haemophagocytic syndrome associated with infections. *Baillieres Clin Haematol* 13, 163–178, 2000.
168. Francois B, Trimoreau F, Vignon P, et al: Thrombocytopenia in the sepsis syndrome: role of hemophagocytosis and macrophage colony-stimulating factor. *Am J Med* 103(2):114–120, 1997.
169. Risdall RJ, Brunning RD, Hernandez JI, et al: Bacteria-associated hemophagocytic syndrome. *Cancer* 54(12):2968–2972, 1984.
170. Stephan F, Thioliere B, Verdy E, et al: Role of hemophagocytic histiocytosis in the etiology of thrombocytopenia in patients with sepsis syndrome or septic shock. *Clin Infect Dis* 25(5):1159–1164, 1997.
171. Dhote R, Simon J, Papo T, et al: Reactive hemophagocytic syndrome in adult systemic disease: report of twenty-six cases and literature review. *Arthritis Rheum* 49(5):633–639, 2003.
172. Baker GR, Levin J: Transient thrombocytopenia produced by administration of macrophage colony-stimulating factor: investigations of the mechanism. *Blood* 91:89–99, 1998.
173. Amsden JR, Warmack S, Gubbins PO: Tick-borne bacterial, rickettsial, spirochetal, and protozoal infectious diseases in the United States: a comprehensive review. *Pharmacotherapy* 25(2):191–210, 2005.
174. Dumler JS, Bakken JS: Human ehrlichiosis: newly recognized infections transmitted by ticks. *Annu Rev Med* 49:201–213, 1998.
175. McQuiston JH, McCall CL, Nicholson WL: Ehrlichiosis and related infections. *J Am Vet Med Assoc* 223(12):1750–1756, 2003.
176. Bakken JS, Krueth J, Wilson-Nordskog C, et al: Clinical and laboratory characteristics of human granulocytic ehrlichiosis. *JAMA* 275(3):199–205, 1996.
177. Fichtenbaum CJ, Peterson LR, Weil GJ: Ehrlichiosis presenting as a life-threatening illness with features of the toxic shock syndrome [see comments]. *Am J Med* 95(4):351–357, 1993.
178. Butler JC, Peters CJ: Hantaviruses and hantavirus pulmonary syndrome. [Review] [21 refs]. *Clin Infect Dis* 19(3):387–394, 1994.
179. Nolte KB, Feddersen RM, Foucar K, et al: Hantavirus pulmonary syndrome in the United States: a pathological description of a disease caused by a new agent. *Hum Pathol* 26(1):110–120, 1995.
180. Barry M: Viral hemorrhagic fevers. *Hematology* 414–423, 2000.
181. Schnittler HJ, Feldmann H: Viral hemorrhagic fever—a vascular disease? [Review] [25 refs]. *Thromb Haemost* 89(6):967–972, 2003.
182. Geisbert TW: Emerging viruses: advances and challenges. *Curr Mol Med* 5(8):733–734, 2005.
183. Fatal illnesses associated with a new world arenavirus—California, 1999–2000. *MMWR Morb Mortal Wkly Rep* 49(31):709–711, 2000.
184. Lupi O, Tyring SK: Tropical dermatology: viral tropical diseases. [Review] [179 refs]. *J Am Acad Dermatol* 49(6):979–1000, 2003.
185. DeLoughery TG: Critical care clotting catastrophes. *Crit Care Clin* 21(3):531–562, 2005.
186. Casillas AM, Nyamathi AM, Sosa A, et al: A current review of Ebola virus: pathogenesis, clinical presentation, and diagnostic assessment. [Review] [29 refs]. *Biol Res Nurs* 4(4):268–275, 2003.
187. Dan ME, Schiffer CA: Strategies for managing refractoriness to platelet transfusions. *Curr Hematol Rep* 2(2):158–164, 2003.
188. Brand A: Alloimmune platelet refractoriness: incidence declines, unsolved problems persist. *Transfusion* 41(6):724–726, 2001.
189. Schiffer CA: Diagnosis and management of refractoriness to platelet transfusion. *Blood Rev* 15(4):175–180, 2001.
190. Fricke W, Alling D, Kimball J, et al: Lack of efficacy of tranexamic acid in thrombocytopenic bleeding. *Transfusion* 31:345–348, 1991.
191. Hod E, Schwartz J: Platelet transfusion refractoriness. *Br J Haematol* 142(3):348–360, 2008.
192. Narvios A, Reddy V, Martinez F, et al: Slow infusion of platelets: a possible alternative in the management of refractory thrombocytopenic patients. *Am J Hematol* 79(1):80, 2005.
193. Kirkpatrick BD, Alston WK: Current immunizations for travel. *Curr Opin Infect Dis* 16(5):369–374, 2003.
194. Madoff DC, Wallace MJ, Lichtiger B, et al: Intraarterial platelet infusion for patients with intractable gastrointestinal hemorrhage and severe refractory thrombocytopenia. *J Vasc Interv Radiol* 15(4):393–397, 2004.
195. Asherson RA: The catastrophic antiphospholipid syndrome [editorial]. *J Rheumatol* 19(4):508–512, 1992.
196. Asherson RA, Piette JC: The catastrophic antiphospholipid syndrome 1996: acute. *Lupus* 5(5):414–417, 1996.
197. Asherson RA, Cervera R: Catastrophic antiphospholipid syndrome. *Curr Opin Hematol* 5:325–329, 2000.
198. Merrill JT, Asherson RA: Catastrophic antiphospholipid syndrome. *Nat Clin Pract Rhuem* 2:81–89, 2006.
199. Cervera R, Bucciarelli S, Plasin MA, et al: Catastrophic antiphospholipid syndrome (CAPS): descriptive analysis of a series of 280 patients from the "CAPS Registry." *J Autoimmun* 32(3–4):240–245, 2009.
200. Mueller-Eckhardt C: Post-transfusion purpura. *Brit J Haematol* 64(3):419–424, 1986.
201. Mueller-Eckhardt C, Kiefel V: High-dose IgG for post-transfusion purpura-revisited. [Review] [19 refs]. *Blut* 57(4):163–167, 1988.
202. DeLoughery TG: Management of bleeding with uremia and liver disease. [Review] [32 refs]. *Curr Opin Hematol* 6(5):329–333, 1999.
203. Carr JM: Hemostatic disorders in liver disease, in Schiff L, Schiff ER (eds): *Disease of the Liver*. 7th ed. Philadelphia, PA, J.B. Lippincott, 1993, pp 1061–1076.
204. Kelly DA, O'Brien FJ, Hutton RA, et al: The effect of liver disease on factors V, VIII and protein C. *Brit J Haematol* 61(3):541–548, 1985.
205. Spector I, Corn M: Laboratory tests of hemostasis. The relation to hemorrhage in liver disease. *Arch Intern Med* 119(6):577–582, 1967.
206. Roberts LN, Patel RK, Arya R: Haemostasis and thrombosis in liver disease. *Br J Haematol* 2009.
207. Martin TG 3rd, Somberg KA, Meng YG, et al: Thrombopoietin levels in patients with cirrhosis before and after orthotopic liver transplantation. *Ann Intern Med* 127(4):285–288, 1997.
208. Peck-Radosavljevic M, Zacherl J, Meng YG, et al: Is inadequate thrombopoietin production a major cause of thrombocytopenia in cirrhosis of the liver? *J Hepatol* 27(1):127–131, 1997.
209. Hugenholtz GG, Porte RJ, Lisman T: The platelet and platelet function testing in liver disease. *Clin Liver Dis* 13(1):11–20, 2009.
210. Thorsen LI, Brosstad F, Gogstad G, et al: Competitions between fibrinogen with its degradation products for interactions with the platelet-fibrinogen receptor. *Thromb Res* 44(5):611–623, 1986.
211. McHutchison JG, Dusheiko G, Shiffman ML, et al: Eltrombopag for thrombocytopenia in patients with cirrhosis associated with hepatitis C. *N Engl J Med* 357(22):2227–2236, 2007.
212. Hyers TM, Agnelli G, Hull RD, et al: Antithrombotic therapy for venous thromboembolic disease. *Chest* 114[Suppl]:561S–578S, 1998.
213. Hirsh J, Warkentin TE, Raschke R, et al: Heparin and low-molecular-weight heparin: mechanisms of action, pharmacokinetics, dosing considerations, monitoring, efficacy, and safety. [Review] [246 refs]. *Chest* 114[5, Suppl]:489S–510S, 1998.

214. Hirsh J, Warkentin TE, Shaughnessy SG, et al: Heparin and low molecular weight heparin. *Chest* 119:64S–94S, 2001.
215. Warkentin TE, Kwon P: Immune thrombocytopenia associated with efalizumab therapy for psoriasis. *Ann Intern Med* 143(10):761–763, 2005.
216. Leal T, Robins HI: Bevacizumab induced reversible thrombocytopenia in a patient with recurrent high-grade glioma: a case report. *Cancer Chemother Pharmacol* 65(2):399–401, 2010.
217. Cheah CY, De KB, Leahy MF: Fluoroquinolone-induced immune thrombocytopenia: a report and review. *Intern Med J* 39(9):619–623, 2009.
218. Jara SC, Olier GC, Garcia-Donas JJ, et al: Drug-induced thrombocytopenia induced by trastuzumab: a special challenge in a curable disease. *Ann Oncol* 20(9):1607–1608, 2009.
219. Nimmannitya S: Dengue and dengue hemorrhagic fever, in Cook GC, Zumla A (eds): *Manson's Tropical Diseases*. 21st ed. Philadelphia, PA, W.B. Saunders, 2004.
220. Taylor TE, Strickland GT: Malaria, in Hunter GW, Strickland TG, Magill AJ, et al. (eds): *Hunter's Tropical Medicine and Emerging Infectious Diseases*. 8th ed. Philadelphia, PA, W.B. Saunders, 2004, pp 614–643.

CHAPTER 110 ■ ANTITHROMBOTIC PHARMACOTHERAPY

CHRISTOPHER D. ADAMS, KEVIN E. ANGER, BONNIE C. GREENWOOD AND JOHN FANIKOS

INTRODUCTION

Thromboembolic disease is commonly encountered among critically ill patients [1]. While these patients are at high risk for developing arterial and venous thrombosis due to underlying comorbidities, central venous catheter placement, and immobility, they are also at high risk for hemorrhagic complications resulting from gastrointestinal stress ulcerations, invasive procedures, liver dysfunction, uremia, or coagulopathy [2]. These divergent features often complicate antithrombotic treatments for prevention or management of thrombosis. Limitations in administration routes, hemodynamic instability, alterations in renal and hepatic function, and drug interactions further complicate the administration of these high-risk medications [3].

This chapter focuses on the mechanism of action, pharmacokinetics, pharmacodynamics, clinical indications, complications of therapy, and reversal options for antithrombotic pharmacotherapy in critically ill patients.

ANTIPLATELET PHARMACOTHERAPY

Overview of Antiplatelet Pharmacotherapy

Antiplatelet agents target mechanisms in platelet activation, adhesion, and aggregation. Pharmacological inhibitors of platelet function fall into four general categories: thromboxane (TXA) inhibitors, antagonists of adenosine diphosphate (ADP)-mediated platelet activation, glycoprotein (GP) IIb/IIIa inhibitors, and phosphodiesterase inhibitors (Fig. 110.1).

Antiplatelet "resistance" and "nonresponse" are terms applied to clinical outcomes characterized by failure to prevent a thrombotic event due to inadequate platelet inhibition [4]. Resistance is conferred by underlying clinical, cellular, and genetic mechanisms. It is best confirmed by platelet function testing [5]. While several methods are available for measuring overall and drug-specific platelet aggregation, standard testing protocols have yet to be established [6].

Aspirin and Aspirin Derivatives

Pharmacology, Pharmacodynamics, and Monitoring

Aspirin, or acetylsalicylic acid, is a prodrug of salicylic acid that blocks platelet activation. Aspirin irreversibly inhibits both cyclooxygenase enzymes (COX-1, COX-2), reducing prostaglandin and TXA byproducts generated from arachidonic acid. Thromboxane A_2 stimulates platelet activation, aggregation, and recruitment. COX-1 enzymes are present in most tissues, but larger amounts are found in the stomach, kidneys, and platelets. The prostaglandin products of COX enzyme activity provide protection from gastrointestinal mucosal injury. COX-2 is found in both nucleated and nonnucleated cells and is responsive to inflammatory stimuli. Inhibition of COX-1 appears to be the primary mechanism by which aspirin inhibits hemostasis. The acetylation of platelet COX-1 enzymes by aspirin causes inhibition of platelet TXA_2 production. The irreversible antiplatelet effect lasts for the life of platelet (7 to 10 days). Saturation of the mechanism occurs at doses as low as 30 mg. Large doses of aspirin (>3,000 mg daily) are required to inhibit COX-2 and produce systemic anti-inflammatory effects. Consequently, there is a 50- to 100-fold variation between the daily doses required to suppress inflammation and inhibit platelet function [7,8].

Enteric-coated and delayed release formulations have diminished bioavailability, take 3 to 4 hours to reach peak plasma levels, and have delayed onset. Rectally administered aspirin has variable absorption with a bioavailability of 20% to 60% over a 2- to 5-hour retention time [9]. For acute thrombosis, immediate-release aspirin is preferred [10].

The optimal aspirin dose that maximizes efficacy and minimizes toxicity is controversial. Evidence-based recommendations vary from 75 to 325 mg daily. There is currently no data suggesting inferiority of lower (75 to 100 mg) to higher (>100 mg) maintenance dosing in preventing thromboembolic events [11].

Recurrent vascular thrombotic episodes despite aspirin therapy occur at rates between 2% and 6% of patients per year [4]. Aspirin resistance occurs in 5.5% to 45% of aspirin-treated patients. Possible mechanisms of aspirin resistance

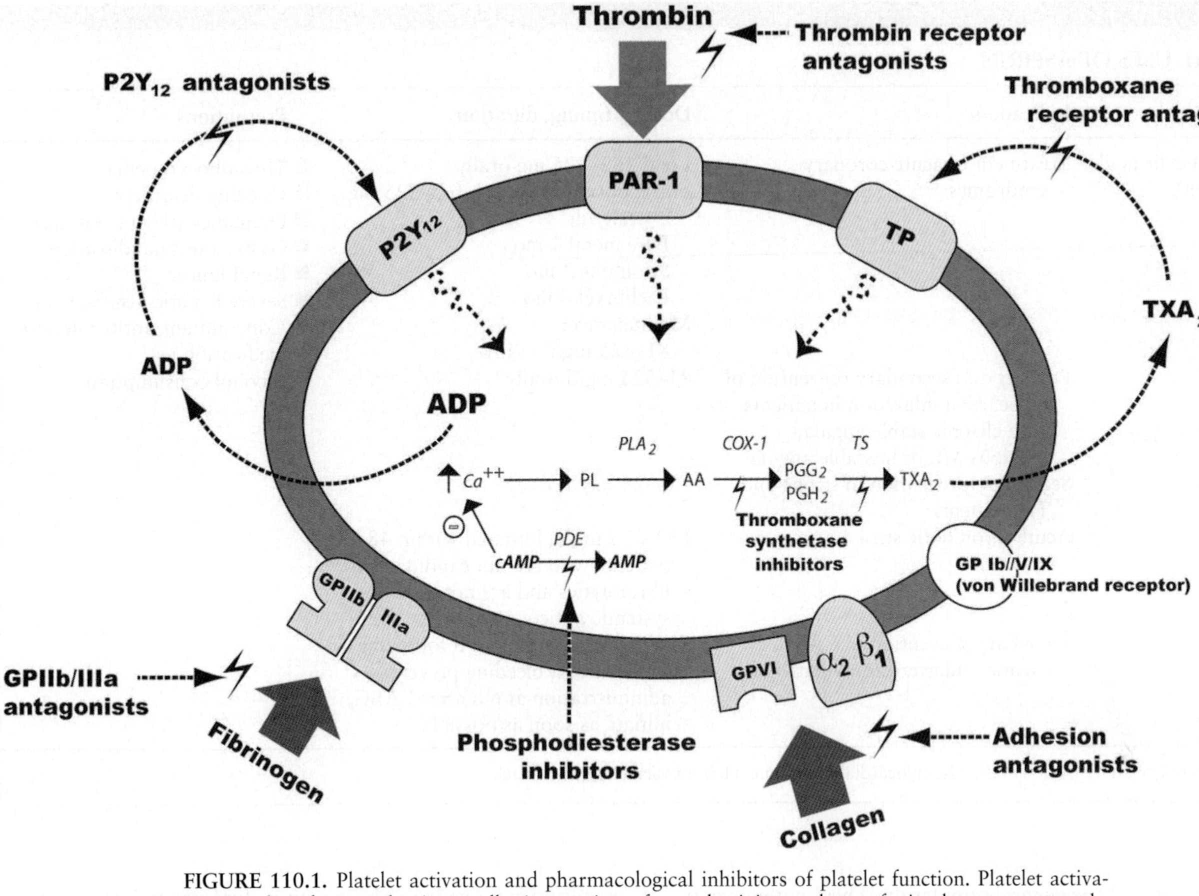

FIGURE 110.1. Platelet activation and pharmacological inhibitors of platelet function. Platelet activation involves four mechanisms: adhesion to sites of vascular injury, release of stimulatory compounds, aggregation, and priming of coagulation. Pharmacological inhibitors of platelet function target adhesion, release, and aggregation mechanisms. Platelet adhesion is a four-step process involving tethering of von Willebrand factor (VWF) to glycoprotein (GP) Ib platelet receptors, a potential target of investigational agents. The rolling phase of adhesion involves interaction between vascular collagen with GP VI and GP Ia/IIa receptors, another potential target of investigational agents. The activation phase of adhesion involves release of thromboxane A_2 (TXA_2) and adenosine diphosphate (ADP) which can be blocked with use of aspirin and $P2Y_{12}$ inhibitors, respectively. The stable adhesion phase involves the interaction of GP IIb/IIIa receptors with fibrinogen and VWF, which can be blocked with the use of GP IIb/IIIa inhibitors.

include extrinsic factors (compliance, absorption, dosage formulation, and smoking) and intrinsic factors (pharmacodynamic alterations, receptor polymorphisms, upregulation of nontargeted platelet activation pathways). In clinical trials, aspirin resistance has been associated with an increased risk of death, acute coronary syndromes (ACS), and stroke [5,12,13].

Clinical Indications

Aspirin is indicated for the primary and secondary prevention of arterial and venous thrombosis (Table 110.1). Aspirin is effective in reducing atherothrombotic disease morbidity and mortality in ACS, stable angina, coronary bypass surgery, peripheral arterial disease (PAD), transient ischemic attack, acute ischemic stroke, and polycythemia vera. A meta-analysis of 145 randomized studies in patients with coronary artery and cerebrovascular disease demonstrated that aspirin 75 to 300 mg per day reduced the risk of nonfatal myocardial infarction (MI) by 35% and the risk of vascular events by 18% [14]. Aspirin provides effective thromboprophylaxis in patients on warfarin with prosthetic heart valves and in patients with nonvalvular atrial fibrillation [15].

Complications and Reversal of Effect

Aspirin increases the incidence of major, gastrointestinal, and intracranial bleeding [15]. The recommended interval for discontinuation of aspirin prior to elective surgery or procedures is 7 to 10 days. Therapy can be resumed approximately 24 hours or the next morning after surgery when there is adequate hemostasis [16]. For patients exhibiting clinically significant bleeding or requiring emergent surgery, platelet transfusion may be warranted. Intravenous desmopressin antagonizes aspirin's effect, suggesting a role in emergent situations as well [17].

Aspirin produces gastrointestinal ulcerations and hemorrhage through direct irritation of the gastric mucosa and via inhibition of prostaglandin synthesis. Aspirin, in recommended doses, increases the risk of gastrointestinal bleeding 1.5- to 3-fold [14,18]. Enteric-coated and buffered aspirin doses $\leq$325 mg do not reduce the incidence of gastrointestinal bleeding [19]. Aspirin-induced gastric toxicity can be prevented with concurrent use of acid-suppressive therapy [20].

Underlying aspirin allergy can exacerbate respiratory tract disease, angioedema, urticaria, or anaphylaxis and is estimated

TABLE 110.1

CLINICAL USES OF ASPIRIN

Drug	Indications	Dosing, timing, duration	Precautions
Acetylsalicylic acid (aspirin)	Treatment of acute coronary syndromes	Load 162–325 mg orally Initial dosing for stents 162–325 mg orally/d: Bare metal 1 mo Sirolimus 3 mo Paclitaxel 6 mo Maintenance: 81–325 mg/d orally	■ Thrombocytopenia ■ Bleeding disorders ■ Pregnancy (third trimester) ■ Gastrointestinal disorders ■ Renal failure ■ Severe hepatic insufficiency ■ Concomitant antithrombotic medication use ■ Alcohol consumption
	Primary and secondary prevention of myocardial infarction in patients with chronic stable angina, previous MI, or unstable angina	81–325 mg/d orally	
	Secondary prevention in stroke and TIA patients	75–325 mg/d orally	
	Acute thrombotic stroke	160–325 mg/d, initiated within 48 h (in patients who are not candidates for fibrinolytics and are not receiving systemic anticoagulation)	
	Secondary prevention in CABG, carotid endarterectomy patients	75–325 mg/d starting 6 h following procedure; if bleeding prevents administration at 6 h after CABG, initiate as soon as possible	

CABG, coronary artery bypass graft; MI, myocardial infarction; TIA, transient ischemic attack.

to occur in 10% of the general population. These patients may be converted to alternative antiplatelet therapies. Leukotriene-modifying agents may reduce aspirin-provoked respiratory reactions but do not eliminate the risk. For patients with a compelling indication for therapy, aspirin desensitization may be considered [21].

$P2Y_{12}$ Inhibitors

Pharmacology, Pharmacodynamics, and Monitoring

$P2Y_{12}$ inhibitors prevent platelet activation by blocking ADP binding to $P2Y_{12}$ receptors. This action prevents activation of the GP IIb/IIIa receptor complex on the platelet surface [10].

Thienopyridine derivatives, clopidogrel, prasugrel, and ticlopidine, are prodrugs requiring hepatic activation via the cytochrome P450 (CYP450) isoenzyme system (Table 110.2). Metabolism by CYP450 plays a key role in the onset of action, potency, and drug interaction profile of these agents [22,23]. A loading dose provides a rapid increase in plasma concentration and a faster onset of action. Both clopidogrel and ticlopidine require a two-step activation process via CYP450. Prasugrel undergoes one-step oxidation by multiple CYP450 isoenzyme pathways which are believed to be responsible for its more predictable action.

While thienopyridine metabolites have a short plasma elimination half-life (1 to 8 hours), their irreversible activity at $P2Y_{12}$ receptors spans the life of the platelet (7 to 10 days). The onset of action, duration of antiplatelet effect, and unpredictable levels of platelet inhibition have led to the development of newer agents [24–26]. Three investigational nonthienopyridine derivatives are currently under investigation for the management of ACS. These agents do not require hepatic activation resulting in immediate, short-acting, dose-dependent inhibition of platelet aggregation [26].

Resistance to clopidogrel occurs in 4% to 34% of patients and depends on the agent, type, and timing of platelet function test, as well as underlying comorbidities such as diabetes and obesity [23]. Possible mechanisms of $P2Y_{12}$ inhibitor resistance include extrinsic factors and intrinsic factors. Recent literature highlighted the importance of genetic and drug-induced alterations of CYP3A4 enzymes, the pathway responsible for thienopyridine activation [27]. Clopidogrel resistance has been associated with an increased risk of death, MI, and stroke. For patients with presumed or confirmed clopidogrel resistance, maintenance dosing up to 150 mg daily or use of more potent agents may be necessary, particularly in patients with in-stent thrombosis [27].

Monitoring the antiplatelet effect of $P2Y_{12}$ inhibitors using platelet function testing is an evolving area of research [27]. The high incidence of varied responses to thienopyridines due to CYP450 polymorphisms and potential drug interactions have suggested a strategy for improving response by using point-of-care platelet function testing.

Clinical Indications

$P2Y_{12}$ inhibitors are indicated for primary and secondary thrombosis prevention in a variety of disease states (Table 110.3). Ticlopidine reduces thrombotic events in patients with stroke, but is associated with neutropenia, thrombocytopenia, and thrombotic thrombocytopenic purpura [28]. Clopidogrel is indicated alone or in combination with aspirin for primary and secondary prevention of ischemic events in ACS, PAD, stroke, and coronary artery disease. Prasugrel is indicated alone or in combination with aspirin for the prevention of thrombotic cardiovascular events, including in-stent

TABLE 110.2

PHARMACOKINETIC AND PHARMACODYNAMIC PROPERTIES OF $P2Y_{12}$ INHIBITORS

	Ticlopidine	Clopidogrel	Prasugrel	Ticagrelor[a]	Cangrelor[a]	Elinogrel[a]
Route	Oral	Oral	Oral	Oral	IV	Oral/IV
Receptor binding	Irreversible	Irreversible	Irreversible	Reversible	Reversible	Reversible
Prodrug	Yes	Yes	Yes	No	No	No
Metabolism	CYP3A4	CYP3A4, 2B6	CYP3A4, 2B6, 2C9, 2C19	CYP3A4	Plasma esterase	Not reported
Clearance	Renal 60% Fecal 23%	Renal 50% Fecal 46%	Renal 68% Fecal 27%	Renal 1%	—	Renal 52% Fecal 48%
Time to peak platelet inhibition	2–5 d	300 mg LD: 6 h 600 mg LD: 2 h	1–2 h	2 h	30 min	20 min (IV)
Duration of antiplatelet effect	7–10 d	7–10 d	7–10 d	1 d	20–60 min	1 d
Genetic polymorphisms	Yes	Yes	No	No	Not reported	Not reported

[a]Investigational agent.
IV, intravenous; CYP, cytochrome P; LD, loading dose.

thrombosis, in ACS patients who are managed with percutaneous coronary intervention (PCI) [23].

Complications and Reversal of Effect

The incidence of major bleeding with $P2Y_{12}$ inhibitors varies between agents, dosing, patient populations, and concomitant antithrombotic therapies. Gastrointestinal hemorrhage is a common complication of $P2Y_{12}$ inhibitor therapy [20]. Endoscopic evaluations at 1 week demonstrated less gastrointestinal damage with clopidogrel 75 mg daily than with aspirin 325 mg daily [29]. For patients exhibiting clinically significant bleeding, platelet transfusion may be warranted.

$P2Y_{12}$ inhibitors should be avoided in patients undergoing neuraxial analgesia due to the risk of subdural hematoma [30]. Therapy should be discontinued 7 to 10 days prior to elective surgery or invasive procedure and resumed approximately 24 hours or the next morning after surgery.

TABLE 110.3

CLINICAL USES OF $P2Y_{12}$ INHIBITORS

Drug	Indications	Dosing, timing, duration	Precautions
Clopidogrel (Plavix™)	Treatment of acute coronary syndromes +/− percutaneous intervention	Load 300 mg ×1 PCI load: 300–600 mg × 1 Maintenance 75 mg/d orally Drug-eluting stents: duration of clopidogrel ideally 12 mo following drug-eluting stent	■ Age >75 y (prasugrel) ■ Interruption of clopidogrel may cause in-stent thrombosis with subsequent fatal and nonfatal myocardial infarction
	Primary and Secondary prevention of myocardial infarction in patients with chronic stable angina, previous MI, or unstable angina	75 mg orally once daily	■ Indwelling epidural catheter ■ Combination of aspirin and clopidogrel in patients with recent TIA or stroke
	Cerebrovascular accident Arteriosclerotic vascular disease		■ Liver disease ■ Thrombotic thrombocytopenic purpura may occur (rare)
	Peripheral arterial occlusive disease		■ Recent trauma, surgery/biopsy ■ Hematologic disorders
Ticlopidine (Ticlid™)	Placement of stent in coronary artery Secondary prevention in thromboembolic stroke	250 mg orally twice a day	■ Discontinue if ANC less than 1,200/μL or platelet count less than 80,000/μL (ticlopidine)
Prasugrel (Effient™)	Treatment of acute coronary syndromes +/− percutaneous intervention	Load 60 mg × 1 Maintenance: 10 mg/d orally Weight <60 kg, consider using a lower maintenance dose of 5 mg/d	■ Elevated triglycerides (ticlopidine)

ANC, absolute neutrophil count; MI, myocardial infarction; PCI, percutaneous coronary intervention; TIA, transient ischemic attack.

TABLE 110.4

PHARMACOKINETIC AND PHARMACODYNAMIC PROPERTIES OF GLYCOPROTEIN IIB/IIIA INHIBITORS

	Abciximab	Eptifibatide	Tirofiban
Agent type	Fab fragment of human–mouse chimeric monoclonal antibody	Cyclic heptapeptide	Nonpeptide
Antigenicity	Yes	No	No
Receptor binding effect	Reversible	Reversible	Reversible
Receptor affinity	High	Moderate	Moderate
Excretion	Renal and reticuloendothelial system	50% renal	39%–69% renal
Dosage reduction in renal failure	No	Yes, decrease infusion dose by 50% if CrCl <50 mL/min	Yes, decrease infusion dose by 50% if CrCl <30 mL/min
Removable by dialysis	No	Yes	Yes
Duration of antiplatelet effect	24–48 h	4–8 h	4–8 h

CrCl; creatinine clearance using Cockcroft–Gault equation.

Glycoprotein IIb/IIIa Inhibitors

Pharmacology, Pharmacodynamics, and Monitoring

GP IIb/IIIa receptors are expressed on the platelet surface, with approximately 50,000 to 80,000 copies per platelet. Blocking GP IIb/IIIa receptors prevents platelet activation, aggregation, and fibrinogen-mediated platelet to platelet bridging.

Intravenous GP IIb/IIIa inhibitors (abciximab, eptifibatide, and tirofiban) vary in their structure and pharmacokinetic properties (Table 110.4) [10,31]. Although the exact threshold required for efficacy with these agents has not been established, >80% platelet inhibition is thought to be a target associated with adequate antiplatelet activity in patients with ACS and in those undergoing PCI [32].

Abciximab is a human–murine chimeric monoclonal antibody that demonstrates a dose-dependent inhibition of GP IIb/IIIa receptors. After an initial intravenous bolus and infusion, the onset of platelet inhibition is rapid (5 minutes) and 80% to 90% of ADP-induced platelet aggregation is suppressed [31]. Abciximab has a strong affinity for the receptor, resulting in occupancy that persists for weeks. Once discontinued, platelet function recovers gradually, with bleeding time normalizing at 12 hours and ADP-induced aggregation returning at 24 to 48 hours [31,32].

Both eptifibatide, a synthetic peptide, and tirofiban, a synthetic small molecule, demonstrate high selectivity, but reduced affinity for the GP IIb/IIIa receptor when compared to abciximab. Both exhibit platelet inhibition that is linear and dose dependent. An intravenous eptifibatide or tirofiban bolus dose followed by an infusion provides >80% inhibition of ADP-induced platelet aggregation. For patients undergoing PCI, a second eptifibatide bolus 10 minutes after the initial dose further enhances platelet inhibition at 1 hour. Since both agents dissociate from the GP IIb/IIIa receptor rapidly, normal platelet aggregation is restored within 4 to 8 hours after drug discontinuation [33–35].

Platelet counts should be monitored within the first 24 hours while taking GP IIb/IIIa inhibitors. For abciximab, platelet counts should be evaluated within 2 to 4 hours of initiation due to a higher risk of thrombocytopenia.

Clinical Indication

GP IIb/IIIa inhibitors are included in evidence-based guidelines as adjunctive therapy for patients with ACS and those undergoing PCI (Table 110.5).

Optimal use of GP IIb/IIIa inhibitors involves appropriate patient risk stratification, use with other antithrombotic agents, appropriate dose, and duration of therapy [36].

Complications and Reversal of Effect

The frequency of major bleeding with GP IIb/IIIa therapy ranges from 1% to 14% of patients and depends on the agent, concomitant therapies, and settings of ACS or PCI [32–34]. Failure to adjust dosing in renal dysfunction further increases the risk of bleeding [37]. Factors associated with bleeding risk include age, female gender, body weight, diabetes, congestive heart failure, renal function, concomitant fibrinolytic use, prolonged femoral sheath placement, and heparin dosing [38,39].

The duration of the antiplatelet effect is agent specific and is influenced by platelet binding (abciximab binds to platelets for up to 10 days) and renal function (tirofiban and eptifibatide have half-lives of 1.5 to 3 hours with normal renal function). An intravenous desmopressin dose of 0.3 μg per kg may be beneficial in reducing bleeding time [17].

Nonhemorrhagic side effects of GP IIb/IIIa inhibitors include severe thrombocytopenia. The incidence of thrombocytopenia with eptifibatide and tirofiban is similar to placebo, with rates ranging from 0.2% to 0.3% of treated patients. With abciximab, the incidence is reported as 5%; however, up to 4% of cases can be due to pseudothrombocytopenia as a result of platelet clumping. The onset of thrombocytopenia usually occurs within the first 24 hours of infusion, but delayed onset has been reported [40,41].

Platelet or red blood cell transfusions may be warranted for patients with persistent thrombocytopenia or clinically significant bleeding and must take into account drug concentrations in the plasma or drug bound to platelets [31]. Abciximab has been associated with antibody formation in 6% of patients. The risk of thrombocytopenia and immune-mediated reactions may limit repeat use [8,10,32]. GP IIb/IIIa inhibitor administration should be avoided in patients requiring neuraxial analgesia due to risk of subdural hematoma [30].

Dipyridamole

Pharmacology, Pharmacodynamics, and Monitoring

Dipyridamole inhibits adenosine binding to platelets and endothelial cells. The increase in adenosine leads to a rise in cyclic adenosine monophosphate (cAMP), which in turn decreases platelet responsiveness to various stimuli. Dipyridamole is

TABLE 110.5

CLINICAL USES OF GLYCOPROTEIN IIB/IIIA INHIBITORS

Drug	Indications	Dosing, timing, duration	Precautions
Eptifibatide (Integrilin™)	Treatment of acute coronary syndromes +/− percutaneous coronary intervention	IV bolus 180 μg/kg ABW (maximum 22.6 mg) as soon as possible, followed by 2 μg/kg ABW/min (maximum 15 mg/h) infusion until discharge or CABG surgery, up to 72 h If undergoing PCI, administer a second 180 μg/kg IV bolus 10 min after the first and continue the infusion up to discharge, or for up to 18–24 h after procedure, whichever comes first, allowing for up to 96 h of therapy Renal adjustment CrCl <50 mL/min, 180 μg/kg actual body weight (maximum 22.6 mg) IV bolus as soon as possible, followed by 1 μg/kg/min (maximum 7.5 mg/h) infusion	■ Concomitant use of fibrinolytics, anticoagulants, antiplatelet agents, and nonsteroidal anti-inflammatory agents ■ Indwelling epidural catheter ■ Do not remove arterial sheath unless aPTT is less than 45 s or ACT less than 150 s and heparin discontinued for 3–4 h ■ Platelet count below 150,000/μL ■ Renal insufficiency (eptifibatide) ■ Severe renal insufficiency, chronic hemodialysis (tirofiban) ■ Readministration of abciximab may result in hypersensitivity, thrombocytopenia, or diminished benefit due to antibody formation ■ Hemorrhagic retinopathy
Abciximab (Reopro™)	Treatment of acute coronary syndromes +/− percutaneous coronary intervention	Initial, 0.25 mg/kg IV bolus (over 5 min), followed by 0.125 μg/kg/min (maximum 10 μg/min) IV infusion for 12 h in combination with fibrinolytic treatment or after PCI, unless complications No adjustment required for renal dysfunction	
Tirofiban (Aggrastat™)	Treatment of acute coronary syndromes	0.4 μg/kg/min IV for 30 min, then 0.1 μg/kg/min for 12–24 h after PCI Severe renal impairment (CrCl less than 30 mL/min): give half the usual dose–0.2 μg/kg/min IV for 30 min, then 0.05 μg/kg/min	

ABW, actual body weight; ACT, activated clotting time; aPTT, activated thromboplastin time; CABG, coronary artery bypass graft; CrCl; creatinine clearance using Cockcroft–Gault equation; IV, intravenous; PCI, percutaneous coronary intervention.

metabolized hepatically and has a half-life of approximately 10 hours [10].

Clinical Indications

Dipyridamole is indicated as adjunctive therapy for the prevention of thromboembolism in patients with cardiac valve replacement. Combined with aspirin, dipyridamole is indicated for secondary prevention of cerebrovascular accidents and TIA. The combination of aspirin and extended-release dipyridamole was associated with reductions in major vascular events in patients with stroke or TIA (Table 110.6) [10,42].

Complications and Reversal of Effect

While headache is the most common adverse effect associated with dipyridamole therapy, hemorrhage may also occur. For patients exhibiting clinically significant bleeding, platelet transfusion may be warranted.

Cilostazol

Pharmacology, Pharmacodynamics, and Monitoring

Cilostazol blocks platelet activation via phosphodiesterase 3 (PDE3) inhibition. PDE3 inhibition increases cAMP concentrations resulting in inhibition of platelet aggregation and an increase in vasodilation [43].

Cilostazol is extensively metabolized by CYP 450-3A4 subclass. Avoidance of therapy or reduced dosing may be required for patients taking potent CYP3A4 inhibitors [44].

Clinical Indication

Cilostazol is indicated for treatment of intermittent claudication symptoms and has shown benefit in reducing symptoms and improving walking distance [44].

Complications and Reversal of Effect

Nonhemorrhagic complications of cilostazol therapy include headache, peripheral edema, and tachycardia [44].

Overview of Anticoagulant Pharmacotherapy

Blood coagulation has been summarized previously in Chapter 108. Anticoagulant agents inhibit thrombosis and propagation by inhibiting thrombin directly or indirectly by attenuating thrombin generation (Fig. 110.2). Unfractionated heparin (UFH) and low-molecular-weight heparin (LMWH) are effective in acute thrombosis due to their rapid onset. Since heparins are dependent on the presence of antithrombin (AT) for clotting factor inhibition, they are considered indirect anticoagulants. Heparins contain a pentasaccharide sequence that binds to AT, producing a conformational change that accelerates AT inactivation of coagulation factors XIIa, IXa, XIa, Xa, and IIa (thrombin). Of these, thrombin and Xa play the most critical role in the coagulation cascade. The active pentasaccharide sequence responsible for catalyzing AT is found on one-third and one-fifth of the chains of heparin and LMWH, respectively. Fondaparinux is a synthetic analog of this naturally occurring pentasaccharide [45–47].

TABLE 110.6

CLINICAL USES OF PHOSPHODIESTERASE INHIBITORS

Drug	Indications	Dosing, timing, duration	Precautions
Dipyridamole (Persantine™)	Radionuclide myocardial perfusion study VTE prophylaxis after heart valve replacement	0.142 mg/kg/min IV for 4 min (0.57 mg/kg total) prior to thallium; maximum 60 mg With concomitant warfarin therapy: 75–100 mg orally four times daily	■ Aminophylline injection should be readily available for relieving adverse effects such as chest pain and bronchospasm ■ Hypotension ■ Severe coronary artery disease, abnormal cardiac rhythm ■ Avoid in patients with severe hepatic insufficiency ■ Avoid in patients with severe renal failure (CrCl less than 10 mL/min)
Dipyridamole extended-release/aspirin (Aggrenox™)	Secondary prevention in stroke and TIA patients	200 mg dipyridamole, 25 mg aspirin (1 capsule) orally twice daily Patients with intolerable headache 200 mg dipyridamole, 25 mg aspirin orally daily at bedtime, with 81 mg of aspirin in the morning Return to usual dose as soon as tolerance to headache develops (usually within a week)	■ Severe coronary artery disease ■ Coagulation abnormalities ■ Severe renal impairment
Cilostazol (Pletal™)	Intermittent claudication	100 mg orally twice a day	

CrCl, creatinine clearance using Cockcroft–Gault equation; IV, intravenous; TIA, transient ischemic attack; VTE, venous thromboembolism.

Unfractionated Heparin

Pharmacology, Pharmacodynamics, and Monitoring

UFH is composed of a heterogeneous mixture of highly sulfated polysaccharide chains that vary in molecular weight, anticoagulant activity, and pharmacokinetic properties. A minimum of 18 saccharide units are required for UFH to form a ternary complex with AT and inhibit thrombin. Once bound to AT molecules, UFH can readily dissociate and bind to other AT molecules. Alternatively, the only requirement for factor Xa inhibition is for the heparin-AT complex to be formed. Heparin has equal inhibitory activity against factor Xa and thrombin, binding in a 1:1 ratio.

Since UFH is poorly absorbed orally, intravenous or subcutaneous injections are the preferred administration routes [47]. When given as subcutaneous injection with therapeutic intent, UFH doses need to be large enough (>30,000 units per day) to overcome erratic bioavailability. UFH readily binds to plasma proteins after parenteral administration which contributes to variable anticoagulant response. Despite these limitations, intravenous administration rapidly achieves therapeutic plasma concentrations that can be monitored and adjusted based on infusion rates [45].

UFH clearance from systemic circulation is dose related and occurs through two independent mechanisms [46,48]. The initial phase is rapid and saturable binding to endothelial cells, macrophages, and local proteins where UFH is depolymerized. The second phase is a slower, nonsaturable, renal-mediated clearance. At therapeutic doses, UFH is cleared primarily in the initial phase with higher-molecular-weight chains being cleared more rapidly than lower-weight counterparts. As elimination becomes dependent on renal clearance, increased or prolonged UFH dosing provides a disproportionate increase in both the intensity and duration of anticoagulant effect. With therapeutic intravenous doses of heparin, the half-life of UFH is approximately 60 minutes [46,48].

The anticoagulant response to UFH is monitored using activated partial thromboplastin time (aPTT), a measurement sensitive to the inhibitory effects of thrombin. The aPTT should be measured every 6 hours, and doses adjusted accordingly, until the patient sustains therapeutic levels. Once steady state is reached, the frequency of monitoring can be extended.

Weight-based dosing nomograms are recommended for treatment of thromboembolic disease. Such nomograms have been associated with a shorter time to reach a therapeutic level without an increase in bleeding events. Heparin dosing nomograms differ between hospitals due to differences in thromboplastin agents and interlaboratory standards in aPTT measurements [49].

Clinical Indications

Clinical indications for UFH include treatment of ACS, treatment or prevention of venous thromboembolism (VTE), bridge therapy for atrial fibrillation, and cardioversion (Table 110.7) [36,48,50]. Due to UFH's short half-life and reversibility, it remains the best option in patients with bleeding risk or organ dysfunction. Patients with fluctuating renal function or a calculated creatinine clearance less than 30 mL per minute are not candidates for LMWH or fondaparinux due to the risk of accumulation and increased bleeding risk, and should be given UFH [51]. When used for thromboprophylaxis in medical patients, three times daily heparin dosing provides better efficacy in reducing VTE events compared to twice daily dosing, but generates more major, but not minor, bleeding episodes [52].

Complications and Reversal of Effect

The major complications of UFH therapy include bleeding (major bleeding, 0% to 7%; fatal bleeding, 0% to 3%), heparin-induced thrombocytopenia (1% to 5%), and osteoporosis (2% to 3% risk of vertebral fracture with less than 1 month of treatment) [53]. Hemorrhagic episodes are associated with anticoagulation intensity, route of administration (continuous infusions are associated with lower rates), and concomitant use of

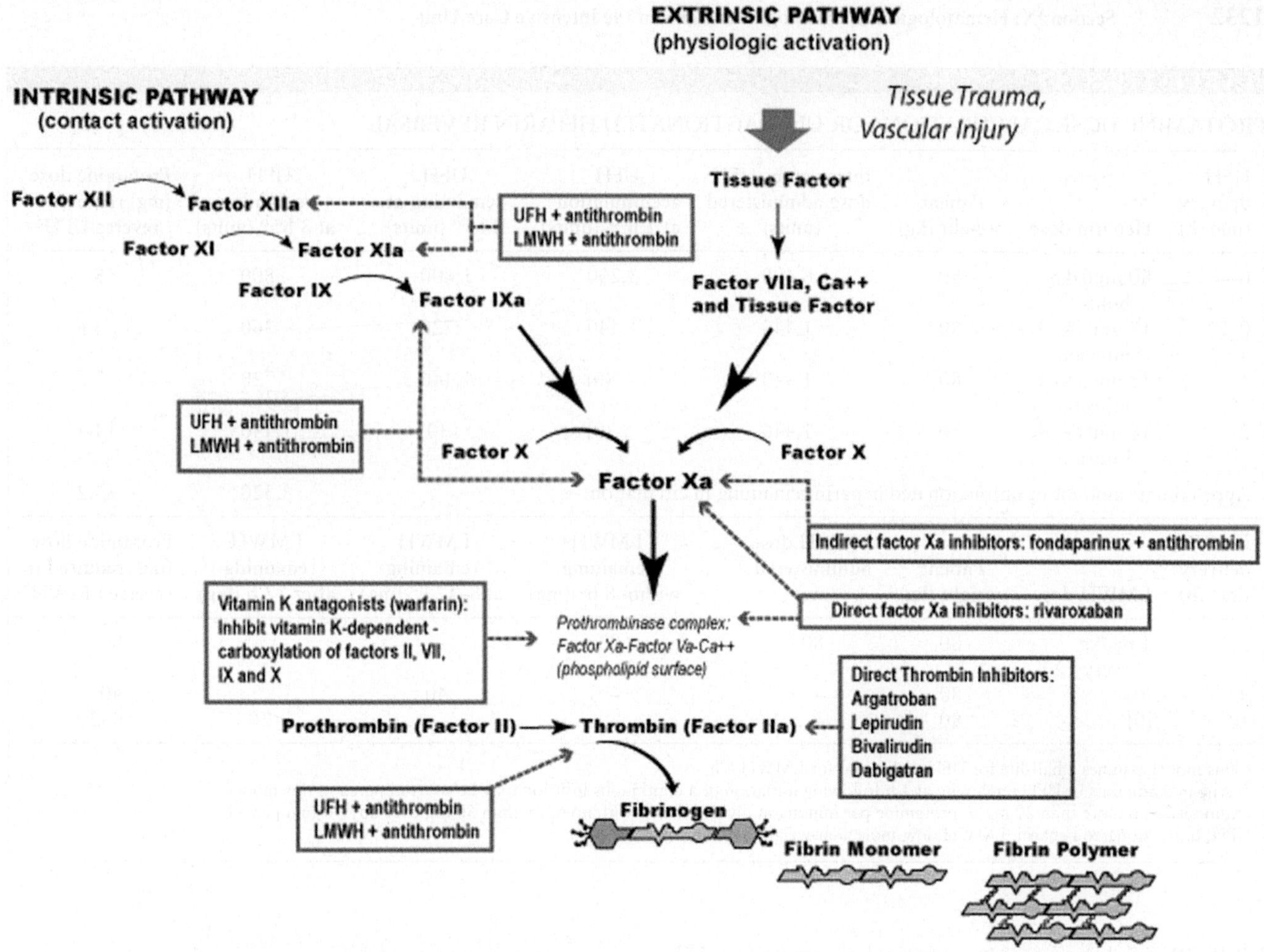

FIGURE 110.2. The coagulation cascade comprises the intrinsic (contact activation) pathway and the extrinsic (tissue factor) pathway. Each pathway generates a series of reactions in which inactive circulating enzymes and their cofactors are activated. These activated factors then catalyze the next reaction in the cascade. Thrombin plays a pivotal role by triggering the conversion of soluble fibrinogen in insoluble fibrin monomers, which serve as the foundation for thrombus formation. Thrombin also activates factors VIII, V, and XIII. Factor XIII generates the covalent bonds that link fibrin strands, ensuring structural integrity. Anticoagulants, either through their interaction with antithrombin, or through a direct inhibition of thrombin, interrupt these enzymatic reactions.

TABLE 110.7

CLINICAL USES OF UNFRACTIONATED HEPARIN

Drug	Indications	Dosing, timing, duration	Precautions
Unfractionated heparin	Treatment of VTE	80 units/kg bolus, then 18 units/kg/h infusion adjusted per local heparin nomogram	■ Allergic or hypersensitivity-type reactions ■ Congenital or acquired bleeding disorders ■ Indwelling epidural catheter ■ Gastrointestinal ulceration and ongoing tube drainage of the small intestine or stomach ■ Hepatic disease with impaired hemostasis ■ Hereditary antithrombin III deficiency and concurrent use of antithrombin ■ Menstruation ■ Neonates and infants weighing <10 kg ■ Premature infants weighing less than 1 kg
	Treatment of ACS	IV bolus: 60 units/kg (max 4,000 units) 12 units/kg/h (max 1,000 units) +/− fibrinolysis, adjusted to maintain aPTT 1.5–2 times control or per local heparin nomogram	
	Bridge therapy for atrial fibrillation, cardioversion	IV infusion: 60–80 units/kg bolus Target aPTT, 60 s, range, 50–70 s	
	Prophylaxis of VTE in the medically ill or surgical population	5,000 units SC every 8–12 h	
	Prophylaxis of VTE in pregnancy (with prior VTE)	7,500–15,000 units SC every 12 h	

ACS, acute coronary syndrome; aPTT, activated partial thromboplastin time; IV, intravenous; SC, subcutaneous; VTE, venous thromboembolism.

TABLE 110.8

PROTAMINE DOSE CALCULATION FOR UNFRACTIONATED HEPARIN REVERSAL

UFH delivery time (h)	Heparin dose	Patient weight (kg)	Intravenous UFH dose administered (units)	UFH accumulation at 1 h[a,b] (units)	UFH remaining at 2 h[a,b] (units)	UFH remaining at 3 h[a,b] (units)	Protamine dose (mg) required to reverse UFH[c]
0	80 units/kg bolus	80	6,400	3,200	1,600	800	8
0	18 units/kg/h infusion	80	1,440	1,440	720	360	3.6
1	18 units/kg/h infusion	80	1,440	(0)	1,440	720	7.2
2	18 units/kg/h infusion	80	1,440	(0)	(0)	1,440	14.4
Approximate amount of unfractionated heparin remaining in circulation →						3,320	33.2
LMWH delivery time (h)	**LMWH dose**	**Patient weight (kg)**	**LMWH dose administered (mg)**	**LMWH remaining within 8 h[a] (mg)**	**LMWH remaining at 8–12 h[a] (mg)**	**LMWH remaining after 12 h (mg)**	**Protamine dose (mg) required to reverse LMWH[c]**
0	1 mg/kg every 12 h	80	80	80	–	–	80
8	(0)	80	–	–	40	–	40
12	(0)	80	–	–	–	≤20	0–20

[a]This model assumes a half-life for UFH of 1 h and for LMWH 8 h.
[b]Estimated amounts of UFH remaining at 1 h following initiation of a continuous infusion may be overestimated in this model.
[c]Administer no more than 20 mg of protamine per minute, in divided doses, with no more than 50 mg over any 10-min period.
UFH, unfractionated heparin, LMWH, low-molecular-weight heparin.

GP IIb/IIIa inhibitors, aspirin or fibrinolytic agents [53–55]. Patient-specific risk factors for bleeding include age, gender, renal failure, low body weight, and excessive alcohol consumption [53].

Perioperative anticoagulation must be individualized based on the surgery or procedure and the patient's risks for thrombosis and bleeding. Discontinuing therapeutic doses of heparin 4 hours before surgery and measuring an aPTT is usually sufficient since normal hemostasis is restored in this time frame [16,56,57]. Therapeutic-dose heparin therapy can be restarted 12 hours after major surgery, but should be delayed if evidence of bleeding is present. There is no contraindication to neuraxial techniques in patients receiving twice daily, low-dose UFH subcutaneously, as the risk for developing spinal hematoma appears to be minimal [16,30].

Treatment of UFH-related bleeding includes protamine sulfate, transfusion, and supportive care. Protamine sulfate binds to UFH to form a stable salt, which renders heparin inactive. Protamine dosing is dependent on timing of the last heparin dose. For immediate reversal (<30 minutes since last heparin dose), 1 mg of protamine is administered for every 100 units of heparin and a followup aPTT can evaluate the reversal response. When UFH is given as a continuous IV infusion, only UFH delivered during the preceding 2 to 2.5 hours should be included in the calculation to determine the protamine dose (Table 110.8) [58]. If the dose of heparin is unknown, the maximal tolerated protamine dose of 50 mg can be slowly administered followed by serial measurements of aPTT. Adverse reactions, such as hypotension and bradycardia, are common. However, reaction severity can be reduced by slowly administering protamine over 1 to 3 minutes. Allergic responses to protamine are more common in patients who have been previously exposed to the drug, but patients can be pretreated with corticosteroids and antihistamines [53,59,60].

Low-Molecular-Weight Heparins

Pharmacology, Pharmacodynamics, and Monitoring

LMWHs are derived from UFH by chemical or enzymatic depolymerization, yielding fragments approximately one-third the molecular weight of UFH. All LMWH molecules contain the active pentasaccharides that catalyze AT inhibition of factor Xa. Because of their smaller size, LMWHs have decreased affinity for plasma proteins and cellular binding sites, resulting in a superior pharmacokinetic profile compared to UFH. LMWHs also have increased bioavailability after subcutaneous injection, renal clearance that is dose-independent, and a longer half-life (17 to 21 hours). LMWHs are administered in fixed doses for thromboprophylaxis or in total body weight-adjusted doses for therapeutic anticoagulation (Table 110.9) [45,61].

With their predictable dose response (peak anti-Xa activity occurs 3 to 5 hours after injection), laboratory monitoring is usually not necessary. Anti-Xa monitoring is optional in high-risk patient populations, specifically renal insufficiency, obesity, and pregnancy. In these cases, anti-Xa plasma levels are drawn 4 hours after administration, and subsequent doses are adjusted to a target range of 0.5 to 1.1 IU per mL [62].

Clinical Indications

LMWHs are suitable replacements for UFH for many indications [63]. LMWHs require fewer injections and produce fewer adverse events. In hospitalized medical patients receiving thromboprophylaxis, LMWH was associated with a lower risk of DVT, fewer injection site hematomas, and no difference in bleeding when compared with UFH [64]. LMWHs have largely replaced intravenous UFH in patients with acute VTE who are able to receive unmonitored anticoagulation in the ambulatory setting. UFH remains the preferred option for ACS patients,

TABLE 110.9

CLINICAL USES OF LOW-MOLECULAR-WEIGHT HEPARINS

Drug	Indications	Dosing, timing, duration	Precautions
Enoxaparin (Lovenox™)	Treatment of VTE	1 mg/kg SC every 12 h OR 1.5 mg/kg SCevery 24 h CrCl <30 mL/min: 1 mg/kg SC every 24 h	■ Indwelling epidural catheter ■ Recent spinal or ophthalmologic surgery ■ History of recent major bleed (gastrointestinal, intracranial, etc.) ■ Congenital or acquired bleeding disorders ■ History of heparin-induced thrombocytopenia ■ Liver disease ■ Renal impairment (CrCl <30 mL/min), consider unfractionated heparin ■ Concomitant use of antithrombotic drugs ■ Diabetic retinopathy ■ Uncontrolled hypertension
	Treatment of ACS	30 mg bolus IV followed by 1 mg/kg SC every 12 h WITH tenecteplase CrCl <30 mL/min: not recommended	
	Prophylaxis/bridge therapy for atrial fibrillation/ cardioversion	1 mg/kg SC every 12 h OR 1.5 mg/kg SC every 24 h CrCl <30 mL/min: 1 mg/kg SC every 24 h	
	Prophylaxis of VTE in the medically ill or surgical population	40 mg SC every 24 h CrCl <30 mL/min: 1 mg/kg SC daily	
	Prophylaxis of VTE in the trauma patients	30 mg SC every 12 h OR 40 mg SC every 24 h	
Dalteparin (Fragmin™)	Treatment of VTE	<56 kg: 10,000 IU daily 57–68 kg: 12,500 IU daily 69–82kg: 15,000 IU daily 83–98 kg: 18,000 IU daily >99 kg: 18,000 IU daily	
	Treatment of ACS	120 IU/kg SC every 12 h (MAX 10,000 IU/dose)	
	Prophylaxis of VTE after hip or other major surgery (first month)	Initial dose: 2500 IU once Maintenance: 2,500–5,000 IU SC every 24 h	
	Prophylaxis of VTE in the medically ill or surgical population	5,000 IU SC every 24 h	
Tinzaparin (Innohep™)	Treatment of DVT	175 international units anti-Xa/kg SC daily	

ACS, acute coronary syndrome; CrCl, creatinine clearance using Cockcroft–Gault equation; IU, international units; IV, intravenous; SC, subcutaneous; VTE, venous thromboembolism.

those who may require an urgent surgical intervention, those with compromised renal function, or those requiring intensive monitoring for other reasons [48].

Complications and Reversal of Effect

Hemorrhage is the major complication of LMWH therapy, with data suggesting lower rates when compared to UFH. Major bleeding is reported to occur in 0% to 3% of patients [53]. Preprocedural thromboembolic risk assessment, bleeding risk assessment, and physician preference will play a role in determining whether LMWH prophylaxis is continued or withheld in the surgical setting. For patients receiving therapeutic LMWH, therapy should be discontinued 12 to 24 hours prior to the procedure, or earlier in patients with renal dysfunction. Therapeutic doses of LMWH should not be restarted for 24 hours after a major procedure or with neuraxial anesthesia [16,30].

In the setting of overdose or hemorrhage, protamine completely reverses the antithrombin activity of LMWH, but only reverses 60% of the antifactor Xa activity. If immediate reversal is warranted within 8 hours of LMWH administration, a protamine dose of 1 mg neutralizes 100 anti-Xa units or 1 mg of LMWH (Table 110.8). Should bleeding continue, a second dose of 0.5 mg of protamine per 100 anti-Xa units may be administered. Smaller protamine doses are required if the LMWH administration interval is beyond 8 hours [65,66].

Heparin-induced thrombocytopenia (HIT) is an immune-mediated, hypercoagulable disorder that results from antibodies formed against the heparin-platelet factor 4 complex. The incidence in critically ill patients ranges from 1% to 5% and is associated with thrombocytopenia and life-threatening thrombosis in approximately 30% to 50% of antibody-positive patients [67]. HIT typically occurs in patients who have been exposed to UFH or LMWH for 5 to 7 days, or even sooner in patients with prior exposure. A 50% decrease in platelet count occurring 4 to 10 days after the initiation of UFH or LMWH therapy or formation of a new thrombus during therapy may be indicative of HIT. Platelet counts should be measured prior to the initiation of UFH or LMWH and monitored every other day for the first 4 to 10 days of therapy. Since heparin alternatives must be used in patients with HIT, direct thrombin inhibitors are the treatment of choice [68,69].

Patients receiving heparin for a period of greater than 1 month are at risk for developing osteoporosis and vertebral

TABLE 110.10

CLINICAL USES OF FONDAPARINUX

Drug	Indications	Dosing, timing, duration	Precautions
Fondaparinux (Arixtra™)	Treatment of VTE Treatment is for 5–9 d; continue treatment until a therapeutic oral anticoagulant effect is established	<50 kg: 5.0 mg SC daily 50–100 kg: 7.5 mg SC daily >100 kg: 10 mg SC daily Renal impairment CrCL 50–80 mL/min—25% reduction in total clearance; consider empiric dosage reduction CrCL 30–50 mL/min—40% reduction in total clearance; consider empiric dosage reduction CrCL less than 30 mL/min—contraindicated	■ Indwelling epidural catheter ■ Recent spinal or ophthalmologic surgery ■ History of recent major bleed (gastrointestinal, intracranial, etc.) ■ Congenital or acquired bleeding disorders
	Treatment of STEMI and NSTEMI[a]	2.5 mg SC daily	
	Prophylaxis of VTE in major surgery and acute medically ill[a]	2.5 mg SC daily	

[a]Indicates off-label use of medication.
CrCl, creatinine clearance using Cockcroft–Gault equation; NSTEMI, non ST-elevation myocardial infarction; SC, subcutaneous; STEMI, ST-elevation myocardial infarction; VTE, venous thromboembolism.

fractures. Osteoporosis reportedly occurs less frequently in patients treated with LMWHs as compared to UFH [48].

Fondaparinux

Fondaparinux is a synthetic analog of the naturally occurring pentasaccharide found in heparins. Fondaparinux selectively and irreversibly binds to AT. This results in neutralization of factor Xa, which ultimately inhibits thrombin formation and thrombus development [48].

Pharmacology, Pharmacodynamics, and Monitoring

After subcutaneous administration, fondaparinux has a half-life of 17 to 21 hours in patients with normal renal function. Fondaparinux is excreted in the urine with clearance reduced in patients with renal impairment. As with LMWHs, monitoring of anti-Xa levels is not required during fondaparinux administration (Table 110.10) [48].

Clinical Indications

Fondaparinux is as safe and effective as the heparins for treatment of deep venous thrombosis (DVT) and pulmonary embolism (PE) and for thromboprophylaxis in surgical and medically ill patients [70–73]. Fondaparinux showed superior efficacy in reducing VTE in patients undergoing knee arthroplasty, hip arthroplasty, and hip fracture surgery [74–76]. In a combined analysis, the overall incidence of major bleeding was statistically higher with fondaparinux (2.7%) compared with LMWH (1.7%) [77]. However, the incidence of clinically relevant bleeding, defined as bleeding leading to death, reoperation, or occurring in a critical organ, did not differ between the agents. Differences in efficacy and safety outcomes could be related to the timing of perioperative drug administration. Fondaparinux given less than 6 hours after surgery has been associated with an increased frequency of major bleeding [77]. Fondaparinux may be an option for thromboprophylaxis in the setting of HIT but conclusive data are not available [78].

Complications and Reversal of Effect

Fondaparinux is contraindicated in patients with severe renal impairment (calculated creatinine clearance <30 mL per minute) and should not be used for VTE prophylaxis in patients weighing less than 50 kg. No antidote exists for fondaparinux-related hemorrhage and reversal is further complicated by its prolonged half-life [79]. Recombinant factor VIIa (rVIIa) reverses the coagulation defect induced by fondaparinux, but the clinical utility is unknown [80,81]. With a short half-life (2 to 3 hours), rVIIa may require repeat dosing. The use of fondaparinux and neuraxial anesthesia or analgesia should follow the conditions used in clinical trials as closely as possible [30].

Direct Thrombin Inhibitors

The direct thrombin inhibitors (DTIs) are lepirudin, bivalirudin, and argatroban. They exert their antithrombotic effect by binding to the active site of thrombin and inhibiting thrombin-catalyzed reactions. This prevents fibrin formation, activation of coagulant factors V, VIII, XIII, protein C, and platelet aggregation [82].

Pharmacology, Pharmacodynamics, and Monitoring

Lepirudin (*r*-hirudin) is a recombinant derivative of hirudin, produced from leech salivary glands. Bivalirudin is the synthetic analog of r-hirudin. Argatroban, derived from the amino acid arginine, is a small synthetic molecule. The DTIs differ in their pharmacokinetic parameters (Table 110.11) [82]. Lepirudin is eliminated through renal clearance, argatroban by hepatic metabolism, and bivalirudin by proteolytic cleavage in the plasma. Bivalirudin has the shortest half-life, making it a particularly useful agent in the procedural or periprocedural period. DTI selection is predicated on patient-specific characteristics such as hemodynamic stability, hepatic function, and renal function. Critically ill patients typically require lower doses than recommended by the manufacturer [82,83]. DTIs are monitored using aPTT (Table 110.12). The aPTT level should be measured every 6 hours until the patient has sustainable therapeutic levels, then the monitoring frequency can be extended [69].

Clinical Indications

Lepirudin and argatroban significantly reduce the rates of thromboembolic complications in patients with HIT [84,85].

TABLE 110.11

PHARMACOKINETIC AND PHARMACODYNAMIC PROPERTIES OF DIRECT THROMBIN INHIBITORS

Feature	Lepirudin	Argatroban	Bivalirudin
Molecular weight (Da)	6,979	526	2,180
FDA-approved indication	Management of HIT	Management of HIT, or use in patients with HIT who are undergoing PCI	Use in patients with or at risk for HIT or HITTS who are undergoing PCI
Primary elimination route	Renal	Hepatic	Enzymatic
Elimination half-life	1.3 h	39–51 min	10–24 min
Fraction eliminated unchanged by kidney (%)	35	16	20
Laboratory test to monitor	aPTT, ECT	aPTT, ECT	aPTT, ACT, ECT
Target range	aPTT: 1.5–2.5 × control	aPTT: 1.5–3 × control	aPTT: 1.5–2.5 × control
Effects on INR	Minimal	Moderate to clinically significant	Minimal to moderate

ACT, activated clotting time; aPTT, activated partial thromboplastin time; Da, dalton; ECT, ecarin clotting time; FDA, Food and Drug Administration; HIT, heparin-induced thrombocytopenia; HITTS, HIT with thrombosis syndrome; INR, international normalized ratio; PCI, percutaneous coronary intervention.

Bivalirudin has been safely used in critically ill HIT patients [86]. Argatroban and bivalirudin are indicated for prophylaxis of thrombosis in patients with, or at risk for, HIT undergoing PCI. Bivalirudin is also indicated in the treatment of patients undergoing PCI as well as those with unstable angina/non-ST segment elevation myocardial infarction undergoing PCI (see Table 110.12) [87].

Complications and Reversal of Effect

No specific reversal agent is available for DTI-induced hemorrhage.

For lepirudin, hemofiltration may be an alternative in the setting of life-threatening hemorrhage. Anecdotally, rVIIa has been reported to be useful as well [88]. DTIs can produce elevation in the international normalized ratio (INR), an effect that is most pronounced with argatroban, and magnified when coadministered with warfarin. This laboratory interaction has misled clinicians to discontinue argatroban therapy prematurely, predisposing patients to venous limb gangrene [78]. With concurrent administration, the argatroban infusion should be stopped and the INR measured 4 to 6 hours. If the INR is within therapeutic range on warfarin alone, warfarin monotherapy can be continued, otherwise argatroban therapy should be resumed.

Oral Anticoagulants—Vitamin K Antagonists

Warfarin, a vitamin K antagonist (VKA), inhibits the enzyme vitamin K epoxide reductase complex (VKORC), which converts vitamin K to an active form. The absence of vitamin K reduces the hepatic production of functional coagulation factors II (thrombin), VII, IX, and X and the regulatory anticoagulant proteins C, S, and Z. Since thrombin has a longer half-life (60 to 72 hours) compared to the other factors (6 to 24 hours), at least 6 days of warfarin treatment is required for an antithrombotic effect [89].

Warfarin is extensively metabolized by the CYP450 isoenzyme system including CYP2C9, CYP1A1, CYP1A2, and CYP3A4. Several genetic polymorphisms have been identified with CYP2C9 and VKORC that may influence warfarin clearance and dose sensitivity [90,91].

In critically ill patients, alterations in coagulation factors, caused by reduced dietary vitamin K intake, hypoalbuminemia, antibiotic administration, acute hepatic injury, or hypermetabolic states, will impact the effects of warfarin [90,91]. Furthermore, drug interactions alter warfarin absorption, clearance, and plasma protein binding. The interactions could have either synergistic or antagonistic effects [89].

Warfarin's anticoagulant effect is measured using the INR [92]. The INR uses the international sensitivity index of the local thromboplastin reagent to standardize the laboratory result. The INR target range will vary based on indication and the patient's risk for thromboembolic and bleeding complications (see Table 110.13). Nomogram-based warfarin dosing is considered safer and more effective for reaching target INR goals. To prevent excessive anticoagulation, loading doses are avoided and low doses are employed for the elderly [93]. Frequent INR monitoring is necessary during initiation of therapy until steady state is reached.

Clinical Indications

Warfarin is effective for primary and secondary prevention of venous thromboembolism, for prevention of systemic embolism in patients with prosthetic heart valves or atrial fibrillation, and for prevention of stroke, recurrent infarction, or death in patients with acute myocardial infarction [89,94–96].

Complications and Reversal of Effect

Treatment with warfarin increases the risk of major bleeding by 0.3% to 0.5% per year and the risk of intracerebral hemorrhage by approximately 0.2% per year compared to controls [53]. Important risk factors for hemorrhage include anticoagulant intensity, time within therapeutic range, and patient age. Higher goal INR (INR >3) has been directly associated with increased hemorrhage rates. Elevated INR can be managed by withholding or decreasing warfarin doses. In patients experiencing or at risk of bleeding, vitamin K administration will reverse the anticoagulant effects of warfarin. Vitamin K is given orally or parenterally. Oral vitamin K normalizes supratherapeutic INRs more rapidly than subcutaneous vitamin K [97]. Intravenous vitamin K corrects excessive warfarin anticoagulation quicker and more completely than subcutaneous administration [98].

For patients with an INR >5.0 but <9.0 and no significant bleeding, the next two doses of warfarin should be held, and low dose (1 to 2.5 mg) oral vitamin K administered. For patients with an INR >9.0, the vitamin K dose can be increased to 2.5 to 5 mg [89].

In the setting of serious or life-threatening hemorrhage, warfarin should be held and vitamin K 10 mg administered by slow IV infusion. The supplementation of coagulation factors with

TABLE 110.12

CLINICAL USES OF DIRECT THROMBIN INHIBITORS

Drug	Indications	Dosing, timing, duration	Precautions
Bivalirudin (Angiomax™)	PCI (with glycoprotein IIB/IIIA inhibitor)	0.75 mg/kg IV bolus dose, followed by an infusion of 1.75 mg/kg/h for the duration of the procedure CrCl less than 30 mL/min, a reduction of initial infusion rate to 1 mg/kg/h should be considered; no bolus dose reduction is necessary	■ Indwelling epidural catheter ■ Recent major, spinal or ophthalmologic surgery, or cerebrovascular accident ■ History of recent major bleed (gastrointestinal, intracranial, etc.) ■ Congenital or acquired bleeding disorders ■ Repeat lepirudin courses may require more frequent monitoring due to antibody formation ■ Hepatic impairment (argatroban) ■ Renal dysfunction (bivalirudin and lepirudin)
	Treatment of ACS[a]	Initial IV bolus dose of 0.1 mg/kg, followed by 0.25 mg/kg/h. Titration to aPTT 1.5–2 times control	
	Treatment and prophylaxis of HITT[a]	0.1–0.2 mg/kg/h, titration to aPTT 1.5–2 times control	
Argatroban	Treatment and prophylaxis of HITT	0.5–1.2 μg/kg/min continuous IV infusion to start titration to goal aPTT between 50 and 85 s. Begin VKA therapy, measure INR daily. Stop argatroban when INR >4. Repeat INR in 4–6 h, if INR is below desired range then resume argatroban infusion	
	Treatment of ACS	Bolus: 100 μg/kg Initial infusion: 1–3 μg/kg/min for 6–72 h; maintain aPTT between 50 and 85 s	
Lepirudin (Refludan™)	Treatment and prophylaxis of HITT ■ aPTT ratio target: between 1.5 and 2.5; begin monitoring aPTT 4 h after initiation of infusion and daily thereafter; recheck aPTT 4 h after any dosage changes ■ aPTT greater than 2.5: discontinue infusion for 2 h, decrease infusion rate by 50% when reinstated ■ aPTT less than 1.5: increase infusion rate in 20% increments until target aPTT is achieved	Bolus: 0.4 mg/kg IV (up to 44 mg) Initial infusion: 0.05–0.15 mg/kg/h (up to 16.5 mg/h) for 2–10 d, adjust infusion rate according to aPTT ratio Renal impairment CrCl <60 mL/min): Bolus: 0.2 mg/kg IV Initial infusion: 0.001–0.01 mg/kg/h (up to 16.5 mg/h) for 2–10 d, adjust infusion rate according to aPTT ratio	

[a]Indicates off-label use of medication.
ACS, acute coronary syndrome; ACT, activated clotting time; aPTT, activated partial thromboplastin time; CBC, complete blood count; CrCl, creatinine clearance using Cockcroft–Gault equation; HITT, heparin-induced thrombocytopenia and thrombosis; INR, international normalized ratio; IV, intravenous; PCI, percutaneous coronary intervention; PT, prothrombin time; VKA, vitamin K antagonist.

fresh frozen plasma (FFP) or prothrombin complex concentrate may be more effective in cases where immediate reversal of the INR is necessary [98]. Recombinant factor VIIa may be beneficial in patients with refractory bleeding in the setting of elevated INRs, or those requiring an invasive procedure [89,99–101].

Nonhemorrhagic adverse events of warfarin include acute skin necrosis and limb gangrene. These complications are typically observed on the third to eighth day of therapy [89].

In patients scheduled for surgery, warfarin may be continued, interrupted for approximately 5 days, or replaced with short-term parenteral or bridge therapy depending on the patient's risk for venous or arterial thromboembolism. Warfarin is resumed after surgery. Most bridging regimens have been developed from observational studies since there is not a standardized definition of bridging [101,102].

For warfarin-treated patients receiving neuraxial anesthesia with an indwelling catheter, the catheter should be removed when the INR is less than 1.5. Patients with a low risk of bleeding may undergo surgery with an INR of 1.3 to 1.5 [30,101].

TABLE 110.13

CLINICAL USES OF WARFARIN

Drug	Indications	Dosing, timing, duration	Precautions
Warfarin (Coumadin™)	Treatment of VTE	Initial dosing: 2.5–10 mg every 24 h (see precautions) titrated to range INR: 2.0–3.0; target of 2.5	■ Lower initial dosing (<5 mg may be warranted in patients who are debilitated, or are taking medications known to increase sensitivity to warfarin ■ Cerebrovascular disease ■ Coronary disease ■ CYP2C9 and VKORC1 genetic variation ■ Moderate to severe hypertension ■ Malignancy ■ Renal impairment ■ Recent trauma ■ Malignancy ■ Collagen vascular disease ■ Conditions that increase risk of hemorrhage, necrosis, and/or gangrene, pre-existing ■ Congestive heart failure ■ Excessive dietary vitamin K ■ Vitamin K deficiency ■ Elderly or debilitated patients (lower dosing may be required) ■ Hepatic impairment ■ Hyperthyroidism/hypothyroidism ■ Epidural catheters ■ Infectious diseases or disturbances of intestinal flora, such as sprue or antibiotic therapy ■ Poor nutritional state ■ Protein C deficiency ■ Heparin-induced thrombocytopenia
	Atrial fibrillation	Initial dosing: 2.5–10 mg every 24 h (see precautions) titrated to range INR: 2.0–3.0; target of 2.5	
	Post MI	Initial dosing: 2.5–10 mg every 24 h (see precautions) titrated to range INR 2.0–3.0; target of 2.5	
	Mechanical valve in the atrial position	Initial dosing: 2.5–5 mg every 24 h (see precautions) titrated to range INR 2.0–3.0; target of 2.5	
	Mechanical valve in the mitral position	Initial dosing: 2.5–5 mg every 24 h (see precautions) titrated to range INR 2.5–3.5; target of 3.0	
	Mechanical valve in both the atrial and mitral position	Initial dosing: 2.5–5 mg every 24 h (see precautions) titrated to target INR 2.5–3.5; target of 3.0	
	Bioprosthetic valve in the mitral position	Initial dosing: 2.5–5 mg every 24 h (see precautions) titrated to target INR 2.0–3.0; target of 2.5 for 3 months	

[a]Indicates off label use of medication.
INR, international normalized ratio; MI, myocardial infarction; VTE, venous thromboembolism.

FIBRINOLYTIC THERAPY

Overview of Fibrinolytic Pharmacotherapy

Fibrinolytic agents have been used clinically since the 1950s when streptokinase was shown to be effective in dissolving occlusive thrombi.

Pharmacology, Pharmacodynamics, and Monitoring

Fibrinolytic agents promote the conversion of plasminogen to plasmin, which subsequently causes the degradation of fibrin clots [103]. Streptokinase and urokinase are naturally occurring first-generation fibrinolytic agents [104]. Recombinant tissue plasminogen activator (rt-PA) is a second-generation fibrinolytic that causes less overall systemic depletion of fibrinogen

TABLE 110.14

PHARMACOKINETIC AND PHARMACODYNAMIC PROPERTIES OF FIBRINOLYTICS

	Streptokinase	Urokinase	Alteplase	Reteplase	Tenecteplase
	First-generation		Second-generation	Third-generation	
Source	Group C β-hemolytic strep	Synthesized from urine or kidney cell tissue	Recombinant DNA technology	Recombinant DNA technology	Recombinant DNA technology
Molecular weight (Da)	47,000	Variable	70,000	39,000	70,000
Administration	Continuous infusion	Continuous infusion	Rapid continuous infusion	Sequential bolus	Single bolus
Half-life	20–80 min	15–20 min	5 min	15–18 min	20 min

Da, dalton; DNA, deoxyribonucleic acid;

TABLE 110.15

CLINICAL USES OF FIBRINOLYTICS

Drug	Indications	Dosing, timing, duration	Precautions
Alteplase (Activase™ and Cathflo Activase™)	Acute myocardial infarction (accelerated infusion)	>67 kg 15 mg IV bolus, followed by 50 mg infusion over 30 min, then 35 mg infusion over 60 min (total = 100 mg) ≤67 kg 15 mg IV bolus, followed by 0.75 mg/kg infusion over 30 min (max 50 mg), then 0.5 mg/kg over 60 min (max 35 mg)	■ Recent major or minor surgery (within 10 d) ■ Cerebrovascular diseases ■ Recent gastrointestinal or genitourinary bleeding ■ Recent trauma ■ Hypertension: systolic BP greater than or equal to 175–180 mmHg and/or diastolic BP greater than or equal to 110 mmHg
	Pulmonary embolism	Routine administration for PE (noncardiac arrest): 100 mg IV administered over 120 min During cardiopulmonary resuscitation: 50 mg IV single dose administered over 5 min	■ Left heart thrombus ■ Acute pericarditis ■ Subacute bacterial endocarditis
	Acute ischemic stroke (within 3 h of symptom onset)	0.9 mg/kg IV (not to exceed 90 mg total dose) infused over 60 min with 10% of the total dose administered as an initial intravenous bolus over 1 min	■ Hemostatic defects ■ Severe hepatic or renal dysfunction ■ Pregnancy
	Arterial thrombosis	Catheter-directed administration: 1.5 mg/h by transcatheter intra-arterial infusion until lysis of thrombus	■ Diabetic hemorrhagic retinopathy or other hemorrhagic ophthalmic conditions
	Central venous catheter occlusion	Weight >30 kg 2 mg/2 mL Weight >10 kg but <30 kg 110% of the internal lumen volume, not to exceed 2 mg/2 mL	■ Septic thrombophlebitis or occluded arteriovenous cannula at a seriously infected site ■ Advanced age
Reteplase (Retavase™)	Acute myocardial infarction	10 unit IV bolus, two doses given 30 min apart	■ Patients receiving oral anticoagulants
	Central venous catheter occlusion[a]	0.4 units/2 mL	■ Known or suspected infection in the catheter during use for catheter clearance
Tenecteplase (TNKase™)	Acute myocardial infarction	<60 kg: 30 mg dose ≥60 to <70 kg: 35 mg ≥70 to <80 kg: 40 mg ≥80 to <90 kg: 45 mg ≥90 kg: 50 mg Single IV bolus over 5 s	■ Severe neurological deficit (NIHSS >22) (ischemic stroke) ■ Patients with major early infarct signs on computerized cranial tomography (ischemic stoke) ■ History of streptococcal infection within 5 d–12 mo (streptokinase)
Streptokinase (Streptase™)	Acute myocardial infarction	1.5 million IU over 60 min	■ Previous streptokinase administration (within 5 d–12 mo)
	Pulmonary embolism	250,000 IU IV over 30 min, then 100,000 IU/h for 24 h	
	Deep venous thrombosis	250,000 IU IV over 30 min, then 100,000 IU/h for 72 h	
	Arterial thrombosis	250,000 IU IV over 30 min, then 100,000 IU/h for 24 h	
Urokinase (Abbokinase™ or Kinlytic™)	Pulmonary embolism	Loading dose: 4,400 IU/kg IV over 10 min, then 4,400 IU/kg/h IV for 12 h	
	Central venous catheter occlusion[a]	5,000 IU, fill volume of catheter for 1–4 h. May repeat with 10,000 IU in catheter if first dose fails.	

[a] Indicates off-label use of medication.
BP, blood pressure; IU, international units; IV, intravenous; MI, myocardial infarction; NIHSS, National Institute of Health Stroke Scale.

and plasminogen compared with streptokinase and urokinase. The half-life of rt-PA is less than 5 minutes when administered as a bolus followed by rapid continuous infusion. Third-generation fibrinolytic agents are synthetic agents with increased fibrin specificity compared to first-generation fibrinolytics and extended half-lives compared to rt-PA [104]. Reteplase is administered in sequential intravenous bolus doses while tenecteplase is administered as a single bolus (Table 110.14). The beneficial properties of the newer agents continue to be evaluated in clinical trials.

Clinical Indications

Fibrinolytic therapy is administered to patients with acute ischemic stroke, venous thromboembolism, acute myocardial

TABLE 110.16

SELECTED EVIDENCE-BASED CLINICAL TRIALS OR META-ANALYSES RELEVANT TO THE CARE OF INTENSIVE CARE UNIT PATIENTS

Indication	Comparison	Result	Reference
Antiplatelet therapies	Meta-analysis of 2,930 patients with cardiovascular disease treated with aspirin regimens ranging from 75 to 325 mg daily	Overall, 28% of patients were classified as aspirin resistant. A cardiovascular-related event occurred in 41% of patients, an acute coronary syndrome in 40%, and death in 6%. Aspirin-resistant patients are at a greater risk of clinically important cardiovascular morbidity.	[14]
	Double-blind trial comparing ticagrelor (180-mg loading dose, 90 mg twice daily) versus clopidogrel (300–600-mg loading dose, 75 mg daily thereafter) for the prevention of cardiovascular events in 18,624 patients admitted to the hospital with an acute coronary syndrome.	Over 12 mo the composite of death from vascular causes, myocardial infarction, or stroke occurred in 9.8% ticagrelor patients vs 11.7% of those receiving clopidogrel. There were no significant differences in the rates of major bleeding (11.6% vs 11.2%).	[25]
Antithrombotic therapies Thromboprophylaxis in medically ill patients	Meta-analysis comparing the incidence of DVT and PE in hospitalized medically ill patients receiving thromboprophylaxis with UFH twice daily, to UFH tree times daily and to LMWH.	UFH dosage of 5,000 units three times daily was more effective in preventing DVT than UFH 5,000 units twice daily. LMWH was associated with a lower risk of DVT and injection site hematoma but no difference was seen in the risk of bleeding or thrombocytopenia.	[64]
Treatment of acute pulmonary embolism (MATISSE PE)	Open-label trial comparing fondaparinux to aPTT-monitored intravenous UFH for the initial treatment of hemodynamically stable patients with PE.	The 3-mo incidence of the composite end point of symptomatic, recurrent PE (nonfatal or fatal) and new or recurrent deep-vein thrombosis was similar in fondaparinux-treated patients (3.8%) and those assigned to UFH (5.0%). Major bleeding occurred in 1.3% of patients treated with fondaparinux and 1.1% of those treated with unfractionated heparin.	[71]
Reversal of warfarin anticoagulant effect with vitamin K	Open-label trial comparing vitamin K subcutaneous vs intravenous administration in patients with an INR >6.0 without active bleeding.	Intravenous vitamin K corrects excessive warfarin anticoagulation quicker and more completely than subcutaneous administration.	[98]
Thrombolytic therapies Treatment of acute ischemic stroke	Double-blind trial comparing the safety and efficacy of alteplase administered between 3 and 4.5 h after the onset of a stroke. The primary end point was disability.	More patients had a favorable outcome at 90 d with alteplase (52%) than with placebo (45%) when measured using the modified Rankin scale. The incidence of intracranial hemorrhage was higher with alteplase than with placebo. Mortality did not differ significantly between the groups.	[108]
Treatment of submassive pulmonary embolism	Meta-analysis of randomized trials comparing thrombolytic therapy with UFH in patients with acute pulmonary embolism.	Thrombolytic therapy was associated with a nonsignificant reduction in recurrent pulmonary embolism, death, and a nonsignificant increase in major bleeding when compared to UFH. When thrombolytic therapy was compared with UFH in patients with major (hemodynamically unstable) PE, thrombolysis was associated with a significant reduction in recurrent PE or death.	[111]
Treatment of acute myocardial infarction	Open-label trial comparing the efficacy and safety of tenecteplase plus enoxaparin or abciximab with that of tenecteplase plus weight-adjusted unfractionated heparin in patients with acute MI.	There were significantly fewer efficacy (composites of 30-d mortality, in-hospital reinfarction, or in-hospital refractory ischemia) and efficacy plus safety end points (in-hospital intracranial hemorrhage or in-hospital major bleeding complications) in the enoxaparin and abciximab groups than in the UFH group.	[113]

MATISSE PE, Mondial Assessment of Thromboembolism Treatment Initiated by Synthetic Pentasaccharide with Symptomatic Endpoints—Pulmonary Embolism; UFH, unfractionated heparin; DVT, deep venous thrombosis; LMWH, low-molecular-weight heparin; aPPT, activated partial prothrombin time; MI, myocardial infarction; PE, pulmonary embolism.

infarction, peripheral arterial occlusion, and in those patients requiring venous catheter maintenance (Table 110.15).

The goal of fibrinolytic therapy in acute ischemic stroke is to recanalize vessels and rapidly restore oxygenation to ischemic but salvageable brain tissue. rt-PA has been shown to improve long-term neurological recovery [105,106]. Pooled analysis of six trials comparing rt-PA to placebo showed that treatment benefit increased as time to start of therapy decreased [107]. While recent guidelines recommend intravenous rt-PA treatment within 3 hours of symptom onset, emerging evidence suggests additional benefit without increased bleeding risk in patients treated between 3 and 4.5 hours [108]. The intra-arterial route is recommended for patients with angiographically demonstrated middle cerebral artery occlusion and without major early infarct signs on CT or MRI scan, who can be treated within 6 hours of symptom onset in a center with the appropriate expertise [109]. Streptokinase is not recommended for acute ischemic stroke due to increased mortality and symptomatic intracranial hemorrhage [109]. Anticoagulants and antiplatelet agents should be held for 24 hours, or until coagulation parameters have returned to normal, after treatment with intravenous rt-PA therapy.

Fibrinolytic therapy is indicated for treatment of acute massive PE to accelerate lysis, provide hemodynamic improvement, and reverse cardiogenic shock. Fibrinolytic use is controversial in patients with submassive PE. Treatment is based on risk stratification of PE severity, bleeding risk, and prognosis [110]. A meta-analysis comparing fibrinolytic therapy with heparin alone for initial treatment, however, showed no benefit of fibrinolytic therapy in decreasing recurrent PE or death [111] (Table 110.16).

In centers with expertise, catheter-direct fibrinolytic therapy is a management option for treatment of acute DVT and may reduce long-term complications of postthrombotic syndrome [112].

The goal of therapy for patients presenting with ST-elevation myocardial infarction is rapid reperfusion. For patients presenting to centers without PCI capabilities, or timely transfer to those facilities, fibrinolytic therapy is recommended within 30 minutes of arrival of medical contact or within 30 minutes of hospital arrival if the emergency medical service does not have fibrinolytic capabilities. Fibrinolytic agents have been combined with various anticoagulants and antiplatelet agents to improve outcomes and reduce bleeding [113–115].

A clear role for fibrinolytic therapy, compared with surgical revascularization, for acute limb ischemia has yet to be defined. There is wide variation in fibrinolytic agents employed, doses studied, patient populations, and endpoints of therapy. The greatest benefit has been shown for patients presenting with acute ischemia <14 days who are at low risk for irreversible ischemia [116].

A common use for fibrinolytic agents is to clear thrombotic occlusions within central venous and dialysis catheters. This therapy is both effective and safe since little to no active drug reaches the systemic circulation [117].

Complications and Reversal of Effect

Because of its derivation from *Streptococcus*, patients may have preformed antibodies to streptokinase from prior streptococcal infections. Adverse drug events include allergic reactions, anaphylaxis, and fever.

Bleeding is the most common and severe complication of fibrinolytic therapy. The most common areas of bleeding are the gastrointestinal and genitourinary tracts as well as sites of interrupted vascular integrity, including catheter access sites, gingiva, and skin [118]. Symptomatic intracerebral hemorrhage rates range between 0.5% and 11% of patients treated with fibrinolytic therapy [119]. A review of six randomized controlled trials of rt-PA for patients with ischemic stroke found an intracerebral hemorrhage rate of 5.9% compared with 1.1% in the placebo groups [107]. Various risk factors for hemorrhage have been identified, but application to clinical practice is limited [120].

Patients receiving fibrinolytic therapy should be closely monitored for intracerebral hemorrhage. Intracerebral hemorrhage should be suspected in patients with sudden focal neurological deterioration (over minutes to hours), decreased level of consciousness, new-onset headache, nausea, vomiting, or acute increases in blood pressure during and within 24 hours of fibrinolytic treatment. Prompt treatment should ensue with replacement of coagulation factors, platelets, FFP, red blood cells, and aminocaproic acid.

References

1. Martinelli I, Bucciarelli P, Mannucci PM: Thrombotic risk factors: basic pathophysiology. *Crit Care Med* 38[2, Suppl]:S3, 2010.
2. Steinberg KP: Stress-related mucosal disease in the critically ill patient: risk factors and strategies to prevent stress-related bleeding in the intensive care unit. *Crit Care Med* 30[6, Suppl]:S362, 2002.
3. Power BM, Forbes AM, van Heerden PV, et al: Pharmacokinetics of drugs used in critically ill adults. *Clin Pharmacokinet* 34:25, 1998.
4. Sanderson S, Emery J, Baglin T, et al: Narrative review: aspirin resistance and its clinical implications. *Ann Intern Med* 142:370, 2005.
5. Pamukcu B: A review of aspirin resistance; definition, possible mechanisms, detection with platelet function tests, and its clinical outcomes. *J Thromb Thrombolysis* 23:213, 2007.
6. Williams CD, Cherala G, Serebruany V: Application of platelet function testing to the bedside. *Thromb Haemost* 103:29, 2010.
7. Patrono C, Rocca B: Aspirin, 110 years later. *J Thromb Haemost* 7[Suppl 1]:258, 2009.
8. Billett HH: Antiplatelet agents and arterial thrombosis. *Cardiol Clin* 26: 189, 2008.
9. Nowak MM, Brundhofer B, Gibaldi M: Rectal absorption from aspirin suppositories in children and adults. *Pediatrics* 54:23, 1976.
10. Patrono C, Baigent C, Hirsh J, et al: Antiplatelet drugs: American College of Chest Physicians Evidence-Based Clinical Practice Guidelines (8th Edition). *Chest* 133[Suppl 6]:199S, 2008.
11. Spinler SA: Safety and tolerability of antiplatelet therapies for the secondary prevention of atherothrombotic disease. *Pharmacotherapy* 29:812, 2009.
12. Krasopoulos G, Brister SJ, Beattie WS, et al: Aspirin "resistance" and risk of cardiovascular morbidity: systematic review and meta-analysis. *BMJ* 336:195, 2008.
13. Christie DJ, Kottke-Marchant K, Gorman RT: Hypersensitivity of platelets to adenosine diphosphate in patients with stable cardiovascular disease predicts major adverse events despite antiplatelet therapy. *Platelets* 19:104, 2008.
14. McQuaid KR, Laine L: Systematic review and meta-analysis of adverse events of low-dose aspirin and clopidogrel in randomized controlled trials. *Am J Med* 119:624, 2006.
15. The ACTIVE Investigators: Effect of clopidogrel added to aspirin in patients with arterial fibrillation. *N Engl J Med* 360:2066, 2009.
16. Douketis JD, Berger PB, Dunn AS, et al: The perioperative management of antithrombotic therapy: American College of Chest Physicians Evidence-Based Clinical Practice Guidelines (8th Edition). *Chest* 133[6, Suppl]:299S, 2008.
17. Reiter RA, Mayr F, Blazicek H: Desmopressin antagonizes the in-vitro platelet dysfunction induced by GP IIb-IIIa inhibitors and aspirin. *Blood* 102:4594, 2003.
18. Derry S, Loke YK: Risk of gastrointestinal haemorrhage with long-term use of aspirin: meta-analysis. *BMJ* 321:1183, 2000.
19. Kelly J, Kaufman D, Jurgelon J, et al: Risk of aspirin-associated major upper-gastrointestinal bleeding with enteric-coated or buffered product. *Lancet* 348:1413, 1996.
20. Cryer B: Management of patients with high gastrointestinal risk on antiplatelet therapy. *Gastroenterol Clin North Am* 38:289, 2009.
21. Gollapudi RR, Teirstein PS, Stevenson DD, et al: Aspirin sensitivity: implications for patients with coronary artery disease. *JAMA* 292:3017, 2004.
22. Cattaneo M: New P2Y(12) inhibitors. *Circulation* 121:171, 2010.
23. Reinhart KM, White CM, Baker WL: Prasugrel: a critical comparison with clopidogrel. *Pharmacotherapy* 29:1441, 2009.

24. Bhatt DL, Lincoff AM, Gibson CM, et al: Intravenous platelet blockade with cangrelor during PCI. *N Engl J Med* 361:2330, 2009.
25. Wallentin L, Becker RC, Budaj A, et al: Ticagrelor versus clopidogrel in patients with acute coronary syndromes. *N Engl J Med* 361:1045, 2009.
26. Siller-Matula JM, Krumphuber J, Jilma B: Pharmacokinetic, pharmacodynamic and clinical profile of novel antiplatelet drugs targeting vascular diseases. *Br J Pharmacol* 159:502, 2010.
27. Braunwald E, Angiolillo D, Bates E, et al: Antiplatelet therapy and platelet function testing. *Clin Cardiol* 31:I36, 2008.
28. Gent M, Blakely JA, Easton JD, et al: The Canadian American Ticlopidine Study (CATS) in thromboembolic stroke. *Lancet* 1:1215, 1989.
29. Fort FT, Lafolie P, Tóth E, et al: Gastroduodenal tolerance of 75 mg clopidogrel versus 325 mg aspirin in healthy volunteers: a gastroscopic study. *Scand J Gastroenterol* 35:464, 2000.
30. Horlocker TT, Wedel D, Rowlingson JC, et al: Regional anesthesia in the patient receiving antithrombotic or thrombolytic therapy: American Society of Regional Anesthesia and Pain Medicine Evidenced-Based Guidelines (Third Edition) anticoagulation. *Reg Anesth Pain Med* 35:64, 2010.
31. Crouch MA, Nappi JM, Cheang KI: Glycoprotein IIb/IIIa receptor inhibitors in percutaneous coronary intervention and acute coronary syndrome. *Ann Pharmacother* 37:860, 2003.
32. EPIC Investigators: Use of a monoclonal antibody directed against the platelet glycoprotein IIb/IIIa receptor in high risk coronary angioplasty. *N Engl J Med* 330:956, 1994.
33. The ESPRIT Investigators: Novel dosing regimen of eptifibatide in planned coronary stent implantation (ESPRIT): a randomised, placebo-controlled trial. *Lancet* 356:2037, 2000.
34. The IMPACT-II Investigators: Randomised placebo-controlled trial of effect of eptifibatide on complications of percutaneous coronary intervention: IMPACT-II. Integrilin to Minimize Platelet Aggregation and Coronary Thrombosis-II. *Lancet* 349:1422, 1997.
35. Topol EJ, Moliterno DJ, Herrmann HC, et al: Comparison of two platelet glycoprotein IIb/IIIa inhibitors, tirofiban and abciximab, for the prevention of ischemic events with percutaneous coronary revascularization. *N Engl J Med* 344:1888, 2001.
36. Braunwald E, Antman EM, Beasley JW, et al: ACC/AHA 2002 Guideline Update for the Management of Patients with Unstable Angina and Non–ST-Segment Elevation Myocardial Infarction—Summary Article. *JACC* 40:1366, 2002.
37. Alexander KP, Chen AY, Roe MT, et al: Excess dosing of antiplatelet and antithrombin agents in the treatment of non-ST-segment elevation acute coronary syndromes. *JAMA* 294:3108, 2005.
38. Kirtane AJ, Piazza G, Murphy SA, et al: Correlates of bleeding events among moderate- to high-risk patients undergoing percutaneous coronary intervention and treated with eptifibatide: observations from the PROTECT-TIMI-30 trial. *J Am Coll Cardiol* 47:2374, 2006.
39. Hernandez AV, Westerhout CM, Steyerberg EW, et al: Effects of platelet glycoprotein IIb/IIIa receptor blockers in non-ST segment elevation acute coronary syndromes: benefit and harm in different age subgroups. *Heart* 93:450, 2007.
40. Sane DC, Damaraju LV, Topol E, et al: Occurrence and clinical significance of pseudothrombocytopenia during abciximab therapy. *J Am Coll Cardiol* 36:75, 2001.
41. Curtis BR, Divgi A, Garritty M, et al: Delayed thrombocytopenia after treatment with abciximab: a distinct clinical entity associated with the immune response to the drug. *J Thromb Haemost* 2:985, 2004.
42. Sacco RL, Diener HC, Yusuf S, et al: Aspirin and extended-release dipyridamole versus clopidogrel for recurrent stroke. *N Engl J Med* 359:1238, 2008.
43. Dawson DL, Cutler BS, Meissner MH, et al: Cilostazol has beneficial effects in treatment of intermittent claudication: results from a multicenter, randomized, prospective, double blind trial. *Circulation* 98:678, 1998.
44. Jacoby D, Mohler ER: Drug treatment of intermittent claudication. *Drugs* 64:1657, 2004.
45. Weitz DS, Weitz JI: Update on Heparin: what do we need to know? *J Thromb Thrombolysis* 29:199, 2010.
46. Bussey H, Francis J, the Heparin Consensus Group: Heparin overview and issues. *Pharmacotherapy* 24:103S, 2004.
47. Hull RD, Raskob GE, Hirsh J, et al: Continuous intravenous heparin compared with intermittent subcutaneous heparin in the initial treatment of proximal-vein thrombosis. *N Engl J Med* 315:1109, 1986.
48. Hirsh J, Bauer KA, Donati MB, et al: Parenteral anticoagulants: American College of Chest Physicians Evidenced-Based Practice Guidelines (8th Edition). Chest 133:141S–159S.
49. Raschke RA, Reilly BM, Guidry JR, et al: The weight-based heparin dosing nomogram compared with a "standard care" nomogram: a randomized controlled trial. *Ann Intern Med* 119:874, 1993.
50. Turpie AGG, Robinson JG, Doyle DJ, et al: Comparison of high-dose with low-dose subcutaneous heparin to prevent left ventricular mural thrombosis in patients with acute transmural anterior myocardial infarction. *N Engl J Med* 320:352, 1989.
51. Lim W, Dentali F, Eikelboom JW, et al: Meta analysis: low-molecular-weight heparin and bleeding in patients with severe renal insufficiency. *Ann Intern Med* 144:673, 2006.
52. King CS, Holley AB, Jackson JL, et al: Twice vs three times daily heparin dosing for thromboprophylaxis in the general medical population. A meta-analysis. *Chest* 131:507–516, 2007.
53. Schulman S, Beth RJ, Kearon C, et al: Hemorrhagic complications of anticoagulant and thrombolytic treatment: American College of Chest Physicians Evidence-Based Clinical Practice Guidelines (8th Edition). *Chest* 133:257, 2008.
54. Saour JN, Sieck JO, Mamo LAR, et al: Trial of different intensities of anticoagulation in patients with prosthetic heart valves. *N Engl J Med* 322:428, 1990.
55. The Stroke Prevention in Atrial Fibrillation Investigators: bleeding during antithrombotic therapy in patients with atrial fibrillation. *Arch Intern Med* 156:409, 1996.
56. Kearon C, Hirsh J: Management of anticoagulation before and after elective surgery. *New Engl J Med* 336:1506, 1997.
57. Smith MS, Muir H, Hall R: Perioperative management of drug therapy, clinical considerations. *Drugs* 51:238, 1996.
58. Cuker A, Sood SL: Hematologic problems in the intensive care unit, in Irwin RS, Rippe JM (eds): *Manual of Intensive Care Medicine*. Philadelphia, Lippincott Williams & Wilkins, 2010, p 563.
59. Carr JA, Silverman N: The heparin-protamine interaction: a review. *J Cardiovasc Surg (Torino)* 40:659, 1999.
60. McEvoy GK, Litvak K, Welsh OH, et al: *Protamine Sulfate Antiheparin Agents in AHFS Drug Information*. Bethesda, American Society of Health-System Pharmacists, 1999, p 1265.
61. Barrowcliffe TW: Low-molecular-weight heparins. *Br J Haematol* 90:1, 1995.
62. Nutescu EA, Spinler SA, Wittkowsky A, et al: Low-molecular-weight heparin in renal impairment and obesity: available evidence and clinical practice recommendations across medical and surgical settings. *Ann Pharmacother* 43:1064–1083, 2009.
63. Weitz JI: Drug therapy: low-molecular-weight heparins. *N Engl J Med* 337:688, 1997.
64. Wein L, Wein S, Haas SJ, et al: Pharmacologic venous thromboembolism prophylaxis in hospitalized medical patients: a meta-analysis of randomized controlled trials. *Arch Intern Med* 167:1476, 2007.
65. Host J, Lindblad B, Bergqvist D, et al: Protamine neutralization of intravenous and subcutaneous low-molecular-weight heparin (tinzaparin, logiparin): an experimental investigation in healthy volunteers. *Blood Coagul Fibrinolysis* 5:795, 1994.
66. Van Ryn-McKenna J, Cai L, Ofosu FA, et al: Neutralization of enoxaparin-induced bleeding by protamine sulfate. *Thromb Haemost* 63:271, 1990.
67. Selleng K, Warkentin TE, Greinacher A: Heparin-induced thrombocytopenia in intensive care patients. *Crit Care Med* 35:1, 2007.
68. Warkentin TE, Kelton JG: Temporal aspects of heparin-induced thrombocytopenia. *N Engl J Med* 344:1286, 2001.
69. Warkentin TE, Greinacher A, Koster A, et al: Treatment and prevention of heparin-induced thrombocytopenia: American College of Chest Physicians Evidence-Based Clinical Practice Guidelines (8th Edition). *Chest* 133:340, 2008.
70. Buller HR, Davidson BL, Decousus H, et al: Fondaparinux or enoxaparin for the initial treatment of symptomatic deep venous thrombosis: a randomized trial. *Ann Intern Med* 140:867, 2004.
71. The Matisse Investigators: Subcutaneous fondaparinux versus intravenous unfractionated heparin in the initial treatment of pulmonary embolism. *N Engl J Med* 349:1695, 2003.
72. Cohen AT, Davidson BL, Gallus AS, et al: For the ARTEMIS Investigators. Efficacy and safety of fondaparinux for the prevention of venous thromboembolism in older acute medical patients: randomized placebo controlled trial. *BMJ* 332:325, 2006.
73. Agnelli G, Bergqvist D, Cohen AT, et al: Randomized clinical trial of postoperative fondaparinux versus perioperative dalteparin for prevention of venous thromboembolism in high-risk abdominal surgery. *Br J Surg* 92:1212, 2005.
74. Bauer KA, Eriksson BI, Lassen MR, et al: For the Steering Committee of the Pentasaccharide in Major Knee Surgery Study. *N Engl J Med* 345:1305, 2001.
75. Lassen MR, Bauer KA, Eriksson BI, et al: Postoperative fondaparinux versus preoperative enoxaparin for prevention of venous thromboembolism in elective hip-replacement surgery: a randomised double-blind comparison. *Lancet* 359:1715, 2002.
76. Eriksson BI, Bauer KA, Lassen MR, et al: Fondaparinux compared with enoxaparin for the prevention of venous thromboembolism after hip-fracture surgery. *N Engl J Med* 345:1298, 2001.
77. Turpie AGG, Bauer KA, Eriksson BI, et al: Fondaparinux vs enoxaparin for the prevention of venous thromboembolism in major orthopedic surgery. *Arch Intern Med* 162:1833, 2002.
78. Dager WE, Dougherty JA, Nguyen PH, et al: Heparin-induced thrombocytopenia: treatment options and special considerations. *Pharmacotherapy* 27:564, 2007.
79. Smythe MA, Dager WE, Patel NM: Managing complications of anticoagulant therapy. *J Pharm Pract* 17:327, 2004.
80. Bijsterveld NR, Moons AH, Boekholdt SM, et al: Ability of recombinant factor VIIa to reverse the anticoagulant effect of the pentasaccharide fondaparinux in healthy volunteers. *Circulation* 106:2550, 2002.

81. Gerotziafas GT, Depasse F, Chakroun T, et al: Recombinant factor VIIa partially reverses the inhibitory effect of fondaparinux on thrombin generation after tissue factor activation in platelet rich plasma and whole blood. *Thromb Haemost* 91:53, 2004.
82. Di Nisio M, Middeldorp A, Buller HR: Direct thrombin inhibitors. *N Engl J Med* 353:1028, 2005.
83. Hursting MJ, Soffer J: Reducing harm associated with argatroban; practical considerations of argatroban therapy in heparin-induced thrombocytopenia. *Drug Safety* 32:203, 2009.
84. Greinacher A, Eichler P, Lubenow N, et al: Heparin-induced thrombocytopenia with thromboembolic complications: meta-analysis of 2 prospective trials to assess the value of parenteral treatment with lepirudin and its therapeutic aPTT range. *Blood* 96:846, 2000.
85. Lewis BE, Wallis DE, Hursting MJ, et al: Effects of argatroban therapy, demographic variables, and platelet count on thrombotic risks in heparin-induced thrombocytopenia. *Chest* 129:1407, 2006.
86. Kiser TH, Fish DN: Evaluation of bivalirudin treatment for heparin-induced thrombocytopenia in critically Ill patients with hepatic and/or renal dysfunction. *Pharmacotherapy* 26:452, 2006.
87. Stone GW, White HD, Ohman EM, et al: For the acute catheterization and urgent intervention triage strategy (ACUITY) trial investigators. Bivalirudin in patients with acute coronary syndromes undergoing percutaneous coronary intervention: a subgroup analysis from the Acute Catheterization and Urgent Intervention Triage strategy (ACUITY) trial. *Lancet* 369:907, 2007.
88. Elg M, Carlsson S, Gustafsson D: Effect of activated prothrombin complex concentrate or recombinant factor VIIa on the bleeding time and thrombus formation during anticoagulation with a direct thrombin inhibitor. *Thromb Res* 101:145, 2001.
89. Ansell J, Hirsh J, Hylek E, et al: The pharmacology and management of the vitamin K antagonists: American College of Chest Physicians Evidence-Based Clinical Practice Guidelines (8th Edition). *Chest* 133:160, 2008.
90. Rieder MJ, Reiner AP, Gage BF, et al: Effect of VKORC1 haplotypes on transcriptional regulation and warfarin dose. *N Engl J Med* 352:2285, 2005.
91. Higashi M, Veenstra DL, Wittkowsky AK, et al: Influence of CYP2C9 genetic variants on the risk of over anticoagulation and of bleeding events during warfarin therapy. *JAMA* 287:1690, 2002.
92. Johnston M, Harrison L, Moffat K, et al: Reliability of the international normalized ratio for monitoring the induction phase of warfarin: comparison with the prothrombin time ratio. *J Lab Clin Med* 128:214, 1996.
93. Crowther MA, Ginsberg JB, Kearon C, et al: A randomized trial comparing 5 mg and 10 mg warfarin loading doses. *Arch Intern Med* 159:46, 1999.
94. Kearon C, Ginsberg J, Kovacs MJ, et al: Comparison of low-intensity warfarin therapy with conventional-intensity warfarin therapy for long-term prevention of recurrent thromboembolism. *N Engl J Med* 349:631, 2003.
95. Hylek EM, Skates SJ, Sheehan MA, et al: An analysis of the lowest intensity of prophylactic anticoagulation for patients with nonrheumatic atrial fibrillation. *N Engl J Med* 335:540, 1996.
96. Hering D, Piper C, Bergemann R, et al: Thromboembolic and bleeding complications following St. Jude medical valve replacement: results of the German Experience with Low-Intensity Anticoagulation Study. *Chest* 127:53, 2005.
97. Crowther MA, Douketis JD, Schnurr T, et al: Oral vitamin K lowers the international normalized ratio more rapidly than subcutaneous vitamin K in the treatment of warfarin-associated coagulopathy: a randomized, controlled trial. *Ann Intern Med* 137:251, 2002.
98. Raj G, Kumar R, McKinney P: Time course of reversal of anticoagulant effect of warfarin by intravenous and subcutaneous Phytonadione. *Arch Intern Med* 159:2721, 1999.
99. Makris M, van Veen JJ, Maclean R: Warfarin anticoagulation reversal: management of the asymptomatic and bleeding patient. *J Thromb Thrombolysis* 29(2):171–181, 2010.
100. Deveras REA, Kessler CM: Reversal of warfarin-induced excessive anticoagulation with recombinant human factor VIIa concentrate. *Ann Intern Med* 137:884, 2002.
101. O'Donnell M, Kearon C: Perioperative management of oral anticoagulation. *Cardiol Clin* 26:200, 2008.
102. Douketis JD, Berger PB, Dunn AS, et al: Perioperative management of antithrombotic therapy. American College of Chest Physicians Evidence-Based Clinical Practice Guidelines (8th Edition). *Chest* 133[Suppl 6]:299S, 2008.
103. Haire WD: Pharmacology of fibrinolysis. *Chest* 101:91S, 1992.
104. Verstraete M: Third-generation thrombolytic drugs. *Am J Med* 109:52, 2000.
105. National Institute of Neurological Disorders and Stroke rt-PA Stroke Study Group: Tissue plasminogen activator for acute ischemic stroke. *N Engl J Med* 333:1581, 1995.
106. Clarke WM, Wissman S, Albers GW, et al: Recombinant tissue-type plasminogen activator (Alteplase) for ischemic stroke 3 to 5 hours after symptom onset: the ATLANTIS Study; a randomized controlled trial. Alteplase Thrombolysis for Acute Noninterventional Therapy in Ischemic Stroke. *JAMA* 282:2019, 1999.
107. Hacke W, Donnan G, Fieschi C, et al: Association of outcome with early stroke treatment: pooled analysis of ATLANTIS, ECASS, and NINDS rt-PA stroke trials. *Lancet* 363:768, 2004.
108. Hacke W, Kaste M, Bluhmki E, et al: Thrombolysis with alteplase 3 to 4.5 hours after acute ischemic stroke. *N Engl J Med* 359:1317, 2008.
109. Albers GW, Amarenco P, Easton JD, et al: Antithrombotic and thrombolytic therapy for ischemic stroke: American College of Chest Physicians Evidence-Based Clinical Practice Guidelines (8th Edition). *Chest* 133:630S, 2008.
110. Konstantinides S, Geibel A, Heusel G, et al: For the Management Strategies and Prognosis of Pulmonary Embolism-3 Trial Investigators. *N Engl J Med* 347:1143, 2002.
111. Wan S, Quinlan DJ, Agnelli G, et al: Thrombolysis compared with heparin for the initial treatment of pulmonary embolism: a meta-analysis of the randomized controlled trials. *Circulation* 110:744, 2004.
112. Mewissen MW, Seabrook GR, Meissner MH, et al: Catheter-directed thrombolysis for lower extremity deep vein thrombosis: report of a national multi center registry. *Radiology* 211:39–49, 1999.
113. The Assessment of the Safety and Efficacy of a New Thrombolytic Regimen (ASSENT)-3 Investigators: Efficacy and safety of tenecteplase in combination with enoxaparin, abciximab, or unfractionated heparin: the ASSENT-3 randomised trial in acute myocardial infarction. *Lancet* 358:605, 2001.
114. Sabatine MS, Cannon CP, Gibson CM, et al: Addition of clopidogrel to aspirin and fibrinolytic therapy for myocardial infarction with ST-segment elevation. *N Engl J Med* 352:1179, 2005.
115. Antman EM, Morrow DA, McCabe CH, et al: Enoxaparin versus unfractionated heparin with fibrinolysis for ST-elevation myocardial infarction. *N Engl J Med* 354:1477, 2006.
116. Ouriel K, Kandarpa K: Safety of thrombolytic therapy with urokinase or recombinant tissue plasminogen activator for peripheral arterial occlusion: a comprehensive compilation of published work. *J Endovasc Ther* 11:436, 2004.
117. Baskin JL, Pui CH, Reiss U, et al: Management of occlusion and thrombosis associated with long-term indwelling central venous catheters. *Lancet* 374:159, 2009.
118. Conway Donovan B: How to give thrombolytic therapy safely. *Chest* 95:290S, 1989.
119. Broderick J, Connolly S, Feldmann E, et al: Guidelines for the management of spontaneous intracerebral hemorrhage in adults: 2007 update: a guideline from the American Heart Association/American Stroke Association Stroke Council, High Blood Pressure Research Council, and the Quality of Care and Outcomes in Research Interdisciplinary Working Group. *Stroke* 38:2001, 2007.
120. Fiumara K, Kucher N, Fanikos J: Predictors of major hemorrhage following fibrinolysis for acute pulmonary embolism. *Am J Cardiol* 97:127–129, 2006.

CHAPTER 111 ■ DIAGNOSIS AND MANAGEMENT OF PROTHROMBOTIC DISORDERS IN THE INTENSIVE CARE UNIT

ASHKAN EMADI AND MICHAEL B. STREIFF

INTRODUCTION

Arterial and venous thromboembolism are among the most common causes of hospitalization in the United States [1,2]. Given the severity of illness of patients in the intensive care unit (ICU), critical care physicians are likely to manage patients with prothrombotic conditions. In this chapter, we will review the regulation of normal hemostasis (which is required to prevent excessive activity of platelets and/or coagulation factors) and the biology, diagnosis and management of selected prothrombotic disorders in the critical care setting.

Prophylaxis and the general approach to treatment of venous thromboembolism (VTE) are discussed in Chapter 52, "Venous Thromboembolism: Pulmonary Embolism and Deep Venous Thrombosis."

REGULATION OF NORMAL HEMOSTASIS

Hemostasis maintains the integrity of the closed circulatory system after vascular injury. A tenuous balance of prothrombotic (i.e., platelets, coagulation proteins) and endogenous antithrombotic (i.e., antithrombin, nitric oxide) mechanisms ensures hemostasis without pathologic thrombosis. Disruptions of this balance are common in critically ill patients and can lead to clinically significant bleeding or thrombosis. Additional information regarding the normal control of bleeding is present in Chapter 108, "Disorders of Hemostasis in Critically Ill Patients."

The potentially prothrombotic activity of coagulation factors and platelets, however, is opposed by negative regulators of hemostasis. Platelet activation is inhibited by endothelial-derived nitric oxide, prostacyclin, and the ectonucleotidase CD39, which together antagonize platelet activation. The tissue factor pathway is inhibited by tissue factor pathway inhibitor (TFPI). TFPI is synthesized by the endothelium and binds to factor Xa and inhibits its function as well as the activation of factor X by the tissue factor/factor VIIa complex. Since its concentrations increase dramatically with heparin administration, TFPI probably contributes to the antithrombotic efficacy of unfractionated and low-molecular-weight heparin (LMWH) [3,4].

Antithrombin (AT) (formerly antithrombin III) is a liver-derived serine protease inhibitor that inhibits factors XIIa, XIa, IXa, and, in particular, Xa and thrombin by binding to their active sites. Heparin accelerates this reaction to several thousand-fold, thus explaining its potent anticoagulant activity. Protein C (PC) is a liver-derived, vitamin K–dependent protease that is activated on the surface of intact endothelium by thrombin bound to thrombomodulin. This activation event is enhanced by the presence of endothelial PC receptor. Activated protein C (APC) when complexed with its cofactor, protein S (PS), on phospholipid-rich surfaces catalyzes the inactivation of activated forms of factors V and VIII (also known as factor Va and factor VIIIa). PS is a liver-derived, vitamin K–dependent protein that binds to the APC and accelerates its inactivation of factors Va and VIIIa. It exists in the plasma in an active free form that can complex with PC and an inactive form bound to C4b-binding protein [5].

Further regulation of the coagulation cascade is provided by the fibrinolytic system, whose components include plasminogen, tissue plasminogen activator (TPA), plasminogen activator inhibitor I and II, α_2-antiplasmin, and thrombin activatable fibrinolysis inhibitor (TAFI). Plasminogen is a liver-synthesized plasma protein that is converted to plasmin on activation by TPA. Plasmin cleaves fibrin and is principally responsible for clot dissolution and remodeling in the intravascular compartment. Activation of plasminogen is opposed by plasminogen activator inhibitors I and II which inhibit TPA from activating plasminogen. α_2-Antiplasmin is synthesized in the liver and binds to plasmin and prevents it from digesting fibrin clot. TAFI is a carboxypeptidase that is activated by the thrombin–thrombomodulin complex. It removes C-terminal lysine residues from partially digested fibrin clot, thereby downregulating the binding of additional plasminogen to the fibrin clot and thus slowing fibrinolysis [6].

THROMBOPHILIC DISORDERS

Thrombophilic disorders are inherited or acquired conditions that variably increase the risk of venous or arterial thromboembolism depending on the particular alteration and the severity of its impact on the hemostatic mechanism. From a practical diagnostic standpoint, it is most useful to divide these disorders into conditions that are associated with venous or arterial thromboembolism (Table 111.1). A more detailed description of each thrombophilic state follows below along with the appropriate approach to diagnosis.

Factor V Leiden

Factor V Leiden (FVL) is the most common inherited thrombophilic condition affecting approximately 5% of Caucasian European Americans, 2% of Hispanic Americans, 1% of African Americans and Native Americans, and 0.5% of Asian Americans [7]. FVL refers to a single base change (Arg506Gln) in the factor V gene (G1691A) that eliminates the first and most important of three APC cleavage sites. The mutation slows down the inactivation of factor Va by APC leading to more thrombin generation. FVL heterozygosity is associated

TABLE 111.1

INHERITED AND ACQUIRED PROTHROMBOTIC CONDITIONS

Venous thromboembolism	Arterial thromboembolism
Inherited	Inherited
Factor V Leiden	Hyperhomocysteinemia
Prothrombin gene mutation	Dysfibrinogenemia
Antithrombin (III) deficiency	
Protein C deficiency	
Protein S deficiency	
Elevated factor VIII activity	
Elevated factor IX level	
Elevated factor XI level	
Hyperhomocysteinemia	
Dysfibrinogenemia	
Acquired	Acquired
Antiphospholipid syndrome	Antiphospholipid syndrome
Heparin-induced thrombocytopenia	Heparin-induced thrombocytopenia
Cancer	Cancer
Surgery	Surgery
Trauma	Trauma
Pregnancy/postpartum	Inflammation
Central venous catheters	
Vena cava filters	
Immobilization	
Infection/inflammation	
Cardiopulmonary failure	
Exogenous estrogens	

with a 5-fold increased risk of VTE, whereas homozygosity increases this risk by at least 10-fold [8]. FVL does not appear to be associated with an increased risk of arterial thromboembolism [9]. FVL heterozygosity and homozygosity increase the risk of recurrent VTE modestly by 1.56-fold (95% confidence interval [CI], 1.14 to 2.12) and 2.65-fold (95% CI, 1.18 to 5.97), respectively [10]. Diagnosis of FVL relies on a functional screening assay, the APC resistance assay, and confirmatory DNA-based testing.

The Prothrombin G20210A Mutation

The prothrombin gene mutation G20210A (PGM) is present in 1.1% of non-Hispanic Whites and Mexican Americans and in 0.3% of African Americans [11]. It is associated with a 30% increase in prothrombin levels in heterozygotes resulting in a 2.8-fold increased risk of VTE [12]. Homozygosity for the FII mutation is rare, so reliable risk estimates are not available. The PGM does not appear to increase the risk of arterial thromboembolism or recurrent VTE [10,13]. Diagnosis of the PGM is based on DNA testing of peripheral blood.

Compound Heterozygotes for the FVL and FII Mutations

Given the relatively high frequency of FVL and the PGM in the population, double heterozygotes for these mutations are occasionally identified. Compound heterozygosity for both FVL and the PGM is associated with a 20-fold increased risk for first-ever VTE and a 4.8-fold risk for recurrent VTE (95% CI, 0.50 to 46.3) [8,10].

Protein C Deficiency

PC is an important endogenous anticoagulant protein that inactivates factors Va and VIIIa. Heterozygous PC deficiency affects 0.2% of the general population and 3.2% of unselected patients with their first episode of VTE [14]. It is associated with a sevenfold increased risk of VTE [15,16]. Homozygous PC deficiency is a rare thrombophilic syndrome that produces life-threatening thrombotic complications shortly after birth, a condition called *neonatal purpura fulminans*. PC deficiency may result from mutations that produce quantitative (type I deficiency) or qualitative (type II) defects. Therefore, accurate diagnostic testing should include both PC activity and antigen levels. Acquired causes of PC deficiency include disseminated intravascular coagulation/acute thrombosis, vitamin K deficiency, vitamin K antagonist (VKA) therapy (i.e., warfarin), and liver disease. Therefore, diagnostic testing should be performed in the absence of these conditions to ensure that laboratory results are interpretable [17].

Protein S Deficiency

PS is the nonenzymatic cofactor for activated PC. PS circulates in two forms: approximately 60% is bound to C4b binding protein, while the remaining 40% is free. Only free PS has cofactor activity. The incidence of PS deficiency is estimated to be 0.03% to 0.13%. PS deficiency affects 7.3% of unselected patients with venous thrombosis [14,18]. PS deficiency is associated with an eightfold increased risk of VTE [15] and may be a risk factor for arterial thromboembolism [19,20].

Deficiency of PS may by quantitative (type I deficiency) or qualitative (type II). An additional type of deficiency (type III) can be acquired during pregnancy, inflammatory states, and estrogen therapy, which increase C4b binding protein levels leading to reduced free PS. Other acquired causes of PS deficiency include vitamin K deficiency, VKA therapy (i.e., warfarin), acute thrombosis, and liver disease. For accurate diagnosis of PS deficiency, all three tests including PS activity, total PS antigen and free PS antigen should be checked in the absence of conditions associated with acquired PS deficiency [18].

Antithrombin (III) Deficiency

AT inhibits serine protease coagulation factors by binding to the active site of the target protease and forming an inactive complex. Heterozygous type I AT deficiency is rare, affecting 1 in 2,000 in the population. It is associated with an 8- to 10-fold increased risk of thrombosis and is present in 1% to 2% of patients with thrombosis [21]. AT deficiency does not increase the risk of arterial thromboembolism [19,20].

Deficiency of AT may by quantitative (type I deficiency) or qualitative (type II). Complete AT deficiency is incompatible with life. The diagnosis of AT deficiency is made by measuring AT activity and antigen levels. Acquired AT deficiency may occur in acute thrombosis, disseminated intravascular coagulation, and during heparin therapy. Artifactual increases in AT can be seen during therapy with VKAs (e.g., warfarin) [21].

Dysfibrinogenemia

Dysfibrinogenemia is a rare inherited thrombophilic state caused by mutations in the Aα, Bβ, or γ fibrinogen genes and affects fewer than 1% of patients with venous thrombosis. Acquired dysfibrinogenemia is associated with chronic liver disease and cirrhosis as well as liver cancers and renal cell carcinoma. Approximately one third of cases of dysfibrinogenemia are complicated by thrombosis (venous more commonly than arterial), possibly because of reduced thrombin binding or inhibition of fibrinolysis. Diagnosis of dysfibrinogenemia is made by measuring fibrinogen function (e.g., Clauss fibrinogen assay) as well as fibrinogen antigen. Typically, the fibrinogen activity level is much lower than the fibrinogen antigen level [22,23].

Hyperhomocysteinemia

Homocysteine is a thiol-containing amino acid that is converted to methionine by methionine synthase with vitamin B_{12} and 5-methyltetrahydrofolate as cofactors. Homocysteine is also converted to cysteine by cystathionine β-synthase, which requires pyridoxine (vitamin B_6) as a cofactor. Congenital causes of hyperhomocysteinemia include homocystinuria (deficiency of cystathionine β-synthase) and inheritance of the thermolabile mutation in the methylene tetrahydrofolate reductase (MTHFR) gene. Homocystinuria is associated with markedly increased levels of homocysteine (>100 μmol per L) and developmental delay, arterial and venous thromboembolism, eye abnormalities, and premature coronary artery disease. Thermolabile mutations in MTHFR produce much more modest elevations in homocysteine (15 to 30 μmol per L) in only a minority of cases, and generally in association with folate deficiency. Acquired causes of hyperhomocysteinemia include deficiency of vitamin B_{12}, folate and pyridoxine, and renal insufficiency [24].

Hyperhomocysteinemia has been associated with a 20% increase in cardiovascular disease for each 5 μmol per L increase in fasting homocysteine levels [25]. Homozygosity for the MTHFR mutation is associated with a 1.16-fold increased risk of coronary artery disease [26]. This risk appeared to be significantly modified by folate status. Hyperhomocysteinemia is also associated with a two- to threefold higher risk of initial and recurrent VTE [27,28]. However, randomized studies of vitamin supplementation in patients with venous and arterial thrombotic disease did not demonstrate improved clinical outcomes [29–31]. Therefore, the utility of homocysteine lowering therapy is in question. The diagnosis of hyperhomocysteinemia is based on demonstrating elevated levels of homocysteine in a fasting blood sample. Methionine loading prior to sampling can increase the sensitivity of testing.

Elevated Coagulation Factor Levels

Elevated factor VIII (>95 percentile) has been associated with an increased risk of initial and recurrent VTE [32,33]. Elevated factor VIII levels appear to be inherited, but the responsible genetic alterations have yet to be completely characterized. Factor VIII activity levels are the diagnostic test of choice. This test should be done at least 6 months after an episode of VTE and in the absence of inflammation to avoid spurious elevations. Elevated factor IX and XI antigen levels have been associated with a 2.5- and 2.2-fold increased risk of initial VTE, respectively [34,35].

ACQUIRED PROTHROMBOTIC DISORDERS

Although inherited thrombophilic conditions may lead to thrombosis, the attention paid to their potential presence by physicians and patients alike is often disproportionate, because acquired prothrombotic disorders are much more common and, in many cases, more potent causes of thromboembolism. A list of inherited and acquired prothrombotic disorders is displayed in Table 111.1. In this section, we will review several important acquired thrombotic disorders of relevance to the intensive care.

Cancer

Patients with cancer are at four- to sevenfold increased risk of thromboembolism (venous and arterial) compared with patients without cancer [36,37]. The risks of thromboembolism are influenced by the primary site of cancer, its histology, and stage as well as our treatments for cancer including surgery, chemotherapy, and growth factors such as erythropoietic stimulatory agents. High-risk organ sites include pancreas, brain, and stomach, while lung cancer and colon cancer are associated with intermediate risk and breast cancer and prostate cancer are associated with a lower risk. Adenocarcinoma is associated with a higher risk of thromboembolism than squamous cell carcinoma, and metastatic disease is associated with a higher risk than localized disease. Myeloproliferative disorders, in particular polycythemia vera (PV), are associated with an increased risk of thromboembolism that is mediated at least in part by an increased red cell volume. Therefore, it is essential to control erythrocytosis in patients with PV with phlebotomy (see "Hematologic Conditions" section in the chapter and Chapter 113, "Therapeutic Apheresis: Technical Considerations and Indications in Critical Care"). Surgery increases the risk of thromboembolism by 10-fold, whereas chemotherapy further increases the relative risk of thromboembolism by 50% in cancer patients. Erythropoietic stimulatory agents have been noted to be associated with an increased risk of thrombosis when hemoglobin values exceed 12 g per dL [38].

Unlike congenital thrombophilic states, cancer is associated with both arterial and venous thromboembolism. Thromboembolism can be the first clue to the presence of an occult malignancy. Idiopathic events are 4.8-fold more commonly associated with the presence of occult malignancy than triggered episodes of thromboembolism. The risk of occult malignancy in patients with thromboembolism declines to the background rate in the population over 6 months [39]. Although an randomized clinical trial (RCT) was unable to identify a survival benefit with extensive cancer screening in patients with idiopathic VTE [40], we think it is worthwhile to ensure that patients are up-to-date with preventive healthcare cancer screening (colonoscopy, etc.) and consider computed tomographic scanning to identify occult primaries in patients aged 50 or older presenting with idiopathic VTE.

Cancer patients are also two- to threefold more likely to suffer recurrent VTE and bleeding during therapy [41]. LMWH has been shown to reduce the incidence of recurrent VTE by 50% in patients with cancer, and therefore LMWH rather than oral VKAs should be considered the agent of choice for long-term management of VTE in cancer patients [42].

Heparin-Induced Thrombocytopenia

Thrombocytopenia affects 20% of patients in the ICU [43]. While the true prevalence of heparin-induced thrombocytopenia (HIT) in the ICU is debatable [44], accurate diagnosis and treatment are essential due to the potential thrombotic and hemorrhagic risks associated with the condition.

HIT is an immune-mediated, prothrombotic disorder caused by heparin-dependent, platelet-activating IgG antibodies directed against platelet factor 4 (PF4) that trigger activation of platelets, endothelial cells, and monocytes resulting in consumptive thrombocytopenia and, in 50% of untreated cases, venous and/or arterial thromboses. Digital/extremity gangrene is a classic finding. Less commonly, skin reactions/necrosis at heparin injection sites or acute systemic reactions (fever, hypotension) occur after heparin administration. Surgical patients (particularly, orthopedic and cardiothoracic) are at high risk for HIT, while medical patients are at intermediate risk and obstetric and pediatric patients are at low risk [45,46]. The clinical probability of HIT can be assessed using the "4 T score," a validated, clinical prediction rule (see Chapter 109 for the elements of the 4 T score) [47]. Management of any patient in whom HIT is being seriously considered requires elimination of exposure to all forms of heparin, and prompt initiation of anticoagulation with a direct thrombin inhibitor (see Chapter 109, "Thrombocytopenia and Platelet Dysfunction"). The clinical diagnosis of HIT should be confirmed with objective laboratory testing, such as the widely available enzyme-linked immunosorbent assay (ELISA assay) for heparin-PF4 antibodies. Patients who develop HIT without thrombosis are typically treated with anticoagulation for 1 to 3 months, whereas patients with thrombosis should be at least 3 to 6 months or longer with warfarin as dictated by the thrombotic event. Without treatment, the mortality of HIT is as high as 20% to 25% with a similar percentage of patients surviving with major complications (e.g., stroke or limb loss). Early diagnosis and treatment has improved mortality and morbidity to 5% to 10% [45,46]. Additional information regarding the pathophysiology and management of HIT is discussed in Chapter 109, "Thrombocytopenia and Platelet Dysfunction."

Major Trauma

Major trauma is an important cause of VTE in the ICU. Fifty-eight percent of trauma patients develop venographic VTE in the absence of thromboprophylaxis [48]. Trauma is a potent stimulus for clot formation because it impacts all three elements of Virchow's triad. Patients are immobilized (stasis) and have extensive vascular and tissue injury (vessel wall damage) leading to tissue factor and collage exposure resulting in activated coagulation (hypercoagulability). Risk factors for VTE in the major trauma patient are listed in Table 111.2 [49,50]. Thromboprophylaxis with enoxaparin (30 mg subcutaneously twice daily), which is much more effective than unfractionated heparin (5,000 units twice daily), can reduce the incidence of VTE by 50% [51]. Mechanical prophylaxis with sequential compression devices and/or graduated compression stocking are a useful adjunctive measure if feasible based on the patient's injuries. Given the high incidence of VTE, intensivists should maintain a high index of suspicion and confirm any clinical findings indicative of thrombosis with objective radiologic testing. Although some have advocated routine radiologic surveillance and prophylactic vena cava filter placement as strategies to reduce VTE in trauma patients, the value of these strategies remains unproven [52,53]. Acute VTE should be managed with conventional anticoagulation. If contraindications to anticoagulation exist, an optional vena cava filter can be placed until the patient is safe for anticoagulation. Once anticoagulation is tolerated, the filter can be removed. As with other patients' triggered episodes of VTE, trauma patients should be treated with warfarin for at least 3 to 6 months, as dictated by their thrombotic event. Catheter-directed or systemic thrombolysis should be reserved for patients with life- or limb-threatening thrombotic events. Catheter or surgical embolectomy is also an option for life-threatening thromboembolism.

TABLE 111.2

RISK FACTORS FOR VENOUS THROMBOEMBOLISM IN TRAUMA PATIENTS

Age >40
Pelvic and or lower extremity fractures with AIS ≥3
Head injury with AIS ≥3
Mechanical ventilation >3 d
Major venous injuries
Injuries requiring major surgery
Spinal cord injury
Prolonged immobility
Delayed institution of thromboprophylaxis
Blood transfusions
Femoral venous catheters

AIS, Abbreviated Injury Scale.

Antiphospholipid Antibody Syndrome

The antiphospholipid antibody syndrome (APS) is an acquired, autoimmune hypercoagulable disorder that is associated with venous and/or arterial thromboembolism, recurrent pregnancy losses, thrombocytopenia, renal insufficiency, vasculitis, and cardiac valvular abnormalities. APS may be primary (not due to any immediately apparent underlying disorder) or secondary, most commonly in association with rheumatologic diseases such as systemic lupus erythematosus (SLE). The diagnostic criteria for APS require the occurrence of one or more objectively documented episodes of thromboembolism or recurrent pregnancy losses in association with positive laboratory testing for a lupus anticoagulant or moderate or high-titer IgG or IgM anticardiolipin antibodies or β_2-glycoprotein I antibodies, performed on at least two occasions 12 or more weeks apart, and at least 12 weeks after the thrombotic insult [54].

The prevalence of elevated anticardiolipin antibodies or lupus anticoagulants in the general population varies from 1% to 5%. In patients with SLE, 15% to 30% have an Lupus Anticoagulants (LA) and 20% to 40% have anticardiolipin antibodies. The mean age of onset of symptoms of APS is 31 years and onset after age 50 years is uncommon [54]. In a mixed population of patients with and without SLE, the incidence of thromboembolism was 2.8% per year [55]. In a cohort of lupus patients, 50% of patients suffered a thromboembolic event over 20 years (2.5% per year) [56]. Patients with a positive lupus anticoagulant or β_2-glycoprotein I antibodies appear to be at higher risk for thromboembolism than patients with anticardiolipin antibodies [57]. In addition, IgG β_2-glycoprotein I antibodies appear to confer a greater risk of thrombosis than IgM antibodies [55,58]. Triple positive patients (i.e., patients positive for lupus anticoagulants, β_2-glycoprotein I antibodies and anticardiolipin antibodies) appear to be very high risk for thromboembolism (recurrent thromboembolism 44% over 10 years) [59].

The most common manifestation of APS that would bring patients to the ICU is venous or arterial thromboembolism. A retrospective review of APS patients noted that 59% had VTE, 28% had arterial thromboembolism, and 13% had both venous and arterial thromboembolism [60]. The diagnosis of APS is made by objectively confirming clinical manifestations (thromboembolism, pregnancy morbidity) and documenting laboratory evidence of antiphospholipid antibodies.

Treatment of VTE of patients with APS is similar to patients with other thrombophilic disorders with several important caveats. APS patients who have an LA often have baseline prolongation of their activated thromboplastin time (aPTT). If the standard therapeutic range is used, these patients' unfractionated heparin may be underdosed. Therefore, patients with a prolonged aPTT at baseline should be treated with an LMWH or have their unfractionated heparin therapy monitored with an anti-Xa heparin activity assay. For chronic antithrombotic therapy of APS, conventional intensity anticoagulation with a VKA targeting an international normalized ratio (INR) of 2 to 3 is appropriate [57,61,62]. Occasional APS patients will suffer recurrent thromboembolic events despite conventional intensity anticoagulation. In these patients, higher INR targets (INR 3 to 4) or use of alternative anticoagulants (e.g., LMWH, fondaparinux) is appropriate. If a VKA is considered for long-term therapy, it is important to confirm that the patient's antiphospholipid antibody does not prolong the baseline prothrombin time. In occasional APS patients, the INR is not an accurate reflection of anticoagulation and specialized tests such as a chromogenic factor X activity assay must be use for VKA management [63]. Since APS patients are at increased risk for recurrent VTE in the absence of anticoagulation, indefinite anticoagulation is appropriate [64].

For patients with APS and arterial thromboembolism, we also prefer anticoagulation rather than aspirin or antiplatelet agents. Although one study suggested that aspirin and warfarin were equally effective for arterial thromboembolism, participants in this study did not fulfill diagnostic criteria for APS; therefore, we prefer conventional intensity anticoagulation (INR 2 to 3) to aspirin [65].

Catastrophic Antiphospholipid Syndrome

A devastating and life-threatening form of APS that occasionally brings a patient to the ICU is the catastrophic antiphospholipid syndrome (CAPS). CAPS is a rare (<1% of APS patients present with CAPS) life-threatening manifestation of APS characterized by multiorgan (kidneys, brain, skin, liver, etc.) failure resulting from diffuse microvascular thrombosis. CAPS is often triggered by infections, major surgery, discontinuation of immunosuppression, or anticoagulation. Almost all patients with CAPS require ICU level of care. The mortality associated with CAPS approaches 50%. Common manifestations of CAPS-associated organ involvement are displayed in Table 111.3 [66].

CAPS is thought to result from widespread activation of the endothelium, monocytes, and platelets with tissue factor expression and diffuse activation of the coagulation cascade resulting in widespread microvascular thrombosis and tissue infarction. The diagnostic criteria for CAPS are displayed in Table 111.4. *The differential diagnosis* in patients suspected to have CAPS usually includes severe sepsis, thrombotic thrombocytopenic purpura (TTP), hemolytic-uremic syndrome (HUS), disseminated intravascular coagulation (DIC), infectious purpura fulminans, and heparin induced thrombocytopenia thrombosis (HIT/T).

Multimodality therapy is necessary for effective treatment of CAPS. The mainstay of therapy includes anticoagulation (e.g., weight-based unfractionated heparin (UFH) titrated to a therapeutic aPTT) and immunosuppression with corticosteroids (e.g., IV pulse methylprednisolone 1,000 mg per day for 3 to 5 days followed by 1 to 2 mg per kg per day is the most commonly administered dosage). Second-line therapies that are frequently employed in addition to anticoagulation and corticosteroids include intravenous immunoglobulins (IVIG) (total dose of IVIG is 2 g per kg [400 mg per kg for 5 days or 1,000 mg per kg for 2 days]), plasmapheresis, and rituximab (375 mg per m^2 weekly for 4 weeks). Fibrinolytic agents are often used to treat life- or limb-threatening venous or arterial thrombosis. Third-line therapies include cyclophosphamide, prostacyclin (5 ng per kg per minute for 7 days [per case reports]), and defibrotide (100 to 275 mg per kg per day for a minimum of 3 weeks).

TABLE 111.3

CLINICAL MANIFESTATIONS OF CATASTROPHIC ANTIPHOSPHOLIPID SYNDROME

Organ system	Manifestations
Blood	Coombs positive hemolytic anemia, autoimmune thrombocytopenia, disseminated intravascular coagulation, bone marrow infarct
Brain	Infarcts, encephalopathy, seizure, transient ischemic attack
Heart	Valvular lesions (Libman-Sacks endocarditis), myocardial infarction, heart failure
Kidney	A 50% increase in serum creatinine, severe systemic hypertension (>180/100 mm Hg), and/or proteinuria (>500 mg/24 h)
Lung	Acute respiratory distress syndrome: most common, pulmonary hypertension with normal cardiac output and pulmonary capillary wedge pressure, pulmonary hemorrhage
Skin	Livedo reticularis, skin ulcers, digital ischemia, purpura, skin necrosis
Vasculature	Venous and/or arterial thromboembolism: most common include deep venous thrombosis, pulmonary embolism, extremity artery thromboembolism, portal vein and inferior vena cava thrombosis, retinal artery, and vein thrombosis

TABLE 111.4

DIAGNOSTIC CRITERIA OF CATASTROPHIC ANTIPHOSPHOLIPID SYNDROME

Diagnostic criteria
1. Evidence of involvement (vascular occlusions) affecting three or more organs, systems, and/or tissues[a]
2. Development of manifestations simultaneously or within 1 week or less
3. Confirmation by histopathology of small vessel occlusion in one organ or tissue[b]
4. Laboratory confirmation of the presence of antiphospholipid antibodies (lupus anticoagulant or anticardiolipin antibodies)[c]
Definite catastrophic antiphospholipid syndrome
All four criteria are met
Probable catastrophic antiphospholipid syndrome
All four criteria are present but only two organs, systems, or tissues are involved
All four criteria are present but confirmation of laboratory tests 6 wk apart not performed
Criteria 1, 2, and 4 are present
Criteria 1, 3, and 4 are present

[a]Objective evidence of vessel occlusions. A 50% rise in serum creatinine, severe systemic hypertension (>180/100 mm Hg), and/or significant proteinuria (>500 mg/24 h) are alternative manifestations of renal involvement.
[b]Thrombosis must be present on histopathology. Vasculitis may be present but is not diagnostic in isolation.
[c]If the patient has not had previous laboratory testing for APS, then laboratory confirmation requires that the presence of antiphospholipid antibodies must be detected on two or more occasions at least 12 wk apart (not necessarily at the time of the event).

Treatment of potential precipitating factors is also extremely important. Such measures include broad-spectrum antibiotics for infections, aggressive hemodynamic resuscitation in case of shock, debridement or amputation for necrotic tissues, mechanical ventilation, renal replacement therapy, tight glycemic control, stomach acid suppression, and control of malignant hypertension in case of renal artery/vein thrombosis. Intravascular instrumentation, especially arterial, should be minimized because of the potential for new clot formation [67].

CAPS mortality rate remains as high as 48% despite all therapies. The clinical manifestations related to poor prognosis and mortality include renal involvement, splenic involvement, pulmonary involvement, adrenal involvement, and SLE diagnosis. CAPS recurrence is unusual. Patients usually have a stable course with continued anticoagulation. One fourth of the survivors will develop further APS-related events, but it is rare to develop recurrent CAPS [67].

Drugs

Certain medications have been associated with an increased risk of thrombosis (Table 111.5). Detection of acute thrombosis in a patient receiving one of these medications typically is a sufficient criterion for discontinuation, and use of such agents in patients with a prior history of thromboembolism must be considered very carefully, weighing the potential benefit against the potential for recurrent thrombosis.

TABLE 111.5

MEDICATIONS COMMONLY ASSOCIATED WITH THROMBOEMBOLISM

Medication	Risk of thromboembolism	Risk factors for thromboembolism	Prevention
Chemotherapy	Two- to sixfold increase	Cancer site—(highest risk—pancreatic, gastric; high risk—lymphoma, gynecologic, bladder, testicular)[a] Prechemotherapy platelet count $\geq$350,000/μL[a] Hemoglobin >10 g/dL or use of ESA[a] Prechemotherapy WBC >11,000/μL[a] BMI >35 kg/m^2[a]	LMWH? In high-risk patients
Estrogen receptor modulators (tamoxifen, raloxifene)	Two- to threefold increase (healthy women breast cancer prophylaxis) 1.5–7 fold increase (adjuvant therapy early breast cancer)	Postmenopausal threefold more likely than premenopausal	N/A
Hormone replacement therapy	Two- to threefold increase	Older age, obesity, thrombophilia, oral > transdermal	N/A
Erythropoietin	1.5-fold	Hemoglobin >12 g/dL	N/A
Thalidomide, lenalidomide	Alone (1%–3%) With high-dose dexamethasone, combination chemotherapy (10%–20%)	Individual VTE risk factors—obesity, previous VTE, cardiac or renal disease, diabetes, infection immobility, surgery, trauma, erythropoietin use, thrombophilia, recent diagnosis, hyperviscosity[b] Treatment risk factors—high-dose dexamethasone, doxorubicin, or combination chemotherapy[b]	Low risk—(0–1 VTE risk factors, no treatment risk factors)—aspirin[b] High risk—2 or more VTE risk factors or a treatment risk factor)—prophylactic dose LMWH or warfarin (INR 2–3)[b]
Hormonal contraceptives	Three- to fourfold increased risk	Age >35 y, smoking, obesity, thrombophilia, third > second generation, oral > transdermal, progestin mini-pill < estrogens or combined estrogen/progestins	N/A
Antipsychotics	Twofold	Low potency antipsychotics (e.g., chlorpromazine) > high-potency antipsychotics (e.g., haloperidol); initial 3 mo of therapy, two or more antipsychotics, supratherapeutic serum levels	N/A

[a]Khorana AA, Kuderer NM, Culakova E, et al: Development and validation of a predictive model for chemotherapy-associated thrombosis. *Blood* 111:4902–4907, 2008.
[b]Agnelli G, Gussoni G, Bianchini C, et al; PROTECHT Investigators: Nadroparin for the prevention of thromboembolic events in ambulatory patients with metastatic or locally advanced solid cancer receiving chemotherapy: a randomised, placebo-controlled, double-blind study. *Lancet Oncol* 10:943–949, 2009.
BMI, body mass index; ESA, erythropoietin stimulating agent; LMWH, low-molecular-weight heparin; INR, international normalized ratio; VIE, venous thromboembolism; WBC, white blood cell.

Hematologic Conditions

Myeloproliferative disorders such as PV and essential thrombocythemia (ET) are associated with an increased risk of thrombotic (arterial and venous) and bleeding complications due to increased blood viscosity associated with erythrocytosis as well as functional abnormalities in leukocytes and platelets and acquired form of von Willebrand disease associated with thrombocytosis. Risk factors for thrombohemorrhagic events include age older than 60 (PV, ET), a previous history of thromboembolism (PV, ET), poorly controlled erythrocytosis (PV), leukocytosis (PV, ET), thrombocytosis (PV, ET), thrombophilia (PV, ET), JAK2 mutation status (PV, ET), and traditional cardiovascular risk factors (hyperlipidemia, smoking, diabetes, and hypertension) (PV, ET). In PV patients, adequate phlebotomy to control erythrocytosis is essential to prevent thrombohemorrhagic complications. Aspirin is useful in PV and ET patients 60 years or older to prevent arterial thromboembolism [68]. In patients who have thrombohemorrhagic events despite these measures, cytoreductive therapy with hydroxyurea, anagrelide, or α-interferon should be prescribed. Anticoagulation is appropriate for patients who suffer VTE [68,69].

Paroxysmal nocturnal hemoglobinuria (PNH) is a rare clonal hematopoietic stem cell disorder that results in the loss of expression of complement regulatory proteins (CD55, CD59) on blood cell membranes. This acquired genetic alteration results in chronic intravascular hemolysis, pancytopenia, and a strong predisposition to venous (more common) and arterial (less common) thrombosis [70,71]. Unusual locations for thrombosis (e.g., hepatic vein thrombosis/Budd–Chiari syndrome, cerebral venous sinus thrombosis, dermal vessel thrombosis) are not uncommon in PNH patients. The diagnosis of PNH can be easily made using flow cytometry to detect the presence/absence of CD55 and CD59 (using antibodies) or glycosylphosphatidylinositol-anchored proteins (GPI-AP) (using fluorescein-labeled aerolysin, a bacterial toxin that binds to all GPI-AP, more sensitive than first technique) on the surface of blood cell membranes. Symptomatic patients with significant hemolysis, fatigue, or end-organ damage or thromboembolism should be treated with eculizumab, a humanized monoclonal antibody against complement protein C5a [71]. For patients with thromboembolism, conventional anticoagulation is appropriate although not always effective in preventing recurrent events. Preliminary data suggest that eculizumab may control the disease process to such an extent that patients with thromboembolism may be able to discontinue anticoagulation [72,73].

DIAGNOSIS APPROACH TO THROMBOPHILIA

Since thrombophilia testing is expensive and has yet to be demonstrated to significantly influence the outcome of patients with thromboembolism [74,75], there should be a strong clinical rationale for considering a thrombophilia evaluation and testing should be focused on patients likely to benefit from the results (Table 111.6). In selected patients, thrombophilia testing may influence the duration of anticoagulation (i.e., in patients with high-risk thrombophilia—AT, PC, or PS deficiency; homozygous FVL; antiphospholipid syndrome; compound heterozygosity for FVL; and the PGM), the management of future pregnancies, provide additional insight into the etiology of a thrombotic event, or improve the adequacy of subsequent VTE prophylaxis efforts during risk periods. These benefits, however, must be weighed against the risks that include increased healthcare insurance costs and unnecessary testing of unaffected family members. Clearly testing should only be performed if it will influence the care of the patient. Therefore, testing should not be performed in patients with idiopathic or recurrent VTE whom you plan to treat indefinitely regardless of the results. Conversely, if the patient has continuing risk factors for bleeding, perhaps the presence of a high-risk thrombophilic state would be sufficient reason to continue anticoagulation despite the presence of these risk factors. In sum, thrombophilia testing should only be done after consideration of its costs and the risks and benefits to the patient [76].

If thrombophilia testing is planned, it should be performed at a time when accurate results can be obtained. Acute thrombosis can result in reductions in AT, PC, and PS activity. Therefore, abnormal results should be interpreted with caution and repeated if possible when the patient is not on anticoagulation. However, if normal results are obtained prior to the initiation of therapy, the patient does not have AT, PC, or PS deficiency. Testing for FVL and PGM may be performed during the acute thrombotic event, as the APC resistance assay and the DNA-based tests are not affected by therapeutic doses of anticoagulation. Fibrinogen assays are generally also insensitive to therapeutic anticoagulation as are antigen assays for factors IX and XI and homocysteine levels. Factor VIII activity should not be measured during an acute episode of thrombosis [76]. Testing for anticardiolipin and β_2-glycoprotein I antibodies can be done during anticoagulation, but lupus anticoagulant testing can be affected by anticoagulation therapy [54]. The timing and recommended tests for prothrombotic conditions are listed in Table 111.7.

It is also important to tailor hypercoagulable testing to the patient's thrombotic process (Table 111.8). FVL and PGM have not been associated with arterial thromboembolism. Therefore, in patients with arterial thrombosis, these tests are not worthwhile ordering, and in patients who are known carriers of FVL or the PGM who suffer an arterial thrombotic event, it is worthwhile looking for another reason for hypercoagulability or for a right-left shunt such as a patent foramen ovale. The link between AT, PC, and, to a somewhat lesser extent, PS and arterial thromboembolism is tenuous and so similar limitations should be considered when testing for these entities. In contrast, cancer, HIT/T, APS, and hyperhomocysteinemia have all been associated with arterial and venous thromboembolism.

TABLE 111.6

CANDIDATE SELECTION FOR LABORATORY TESTING FOR PROTHROMBOTIC CONDITIONS

High yield	Low yield
Young patients (age ≤50)	Older patients (age >50)
Patients with positive family history (first degree relatives)	Patients in situations when artifactual test results may occur (pregnancy, warfarin therapy, etc.)
Patients with idiopathic TE	Patients with cancer
Patients with TE in unusual sites	Patients with strong transient risk factors (major trauma, surgery, etc.)
Patients with recurrent TE	Patients in whom testing will not influence therapy
Patients with warfarin skin necrosis	Patients with arterial TE should not be tested for venous thrombophilic states
Patients planning future pregnancies	

TE, thromboembolism.

TABLE 111.7

LABORATORY TESTING FOR PROTHROMBOTIC CONDITIONS

Condition	Test	Timing	Potential causes of erroneous results
Factor V Leiden	Activated protein C resistance assay	Anytime	Heparin (anti-Xa) level >1.0 units/mL
	Factor V Leiden DNA-based testing	Anytime	DNA contamination
Prothrombin (factor II) gene mutation	Factor II DNA-based testing	Anytime	DNA contamination
Protein C deficiency	Protein C activity (if abnormal then protein C antigen)	Prior to anticoagulation or after discontinuation	Acute thrombosis, DIC, warfarin, vitamin K deficiency, heparin (anti-Xa) level >1.0 units/mL, lupus anticoagulant, elevated factor VIII concentrations, liver disease
Protein S deficiency	Protein S activity (if abnormal then total and free protein S antigen)	Prior to anticoagulation or after discontinuation	Acute thrombosis, DIC, warfarin, vitamin K deficiency, estrogen therapy, pregnancy/postpartum, heparin (anti-Xa) level >1.0 units/mL, lupus anticoagulant, elevated factor VIII concentrations, liver disease
Antithrombin (III) deficiency	Antithrombin activity (if abnormal, antithrombin antigen)	Prior to anticoagulation or after discontinuation	Acute thrombosis, DIC, warfarin, vitamin K deficiency, heparin (anti-Xa) level >1.0 units/mL, lupus anticoagulant, elevated factor VIII concentrations, liver disease, nephrotic syndrome
Dysfibrinogenemia	Fibrinogen activity (i.e., standard Clauss fibrinogen assay), thrombin time, fibrinogen antigen, reptilase time	Prior to anticoagulation with heparin or direct thrombin inhibitors	Heparin (thrombin time is very sensitive to heparin, fibrinogen less sensitive, reptilase time and fibrinogen antigen insensitive), direct thrombin inhibitors affect thrombin time and fibrinogen activity, myeloma proteins, liver disease
Hyperhomocysteinemia	Homocysteine level	Fasting, with or without methionine loading at anytime	Renal insufficiency, vitamin B_{12} deficiency, folate deficiency
Elevated factor VIII levels	Factor VIII activity	At least 6 mo after thrombotic event in the absence of inflammation	Acute phase response (e.g., infection, inflammation, postsurgery), heparin, direct thrombin inhibitors, DIC
Elevated factor IX levels	Factor IX antigen	At least 6 mo after thrombotic event after discontinuation of warfarin	Acute thrombosis, DIC, warfarin, vitamin K deficiency, liver disease
Elevated factor XI levels	Factor XI antigen	At least 6 mo after thrombotic event	Acute thrombosis, DIC, severe liver disease
Heparin-induced thrombocytopenia	Platelet factor 4 antibody ELISA assay	Anytime	Elevated immune complexes/ immunoglobulin level
	Serotonin release assay	Anytime	
Antiphospholipid syndrome	Activated partial thromboplastin time (low phospholipid reagent) + mixing studies with normal plasma	At diagnosis of thrombotic event and at least 12 wk later	Heparin, direct thrombin inhibitors
	Dilute Russell Viper venom time with confirm procedure	At diagnosis of thrombotic event and at least 12 wk later	Heparin (anti-Xa) level >1.0 units/mL, direct thrombin inhibitor, fondaparinux, warfarin (?), factor X, V, and II inhibitors
	Platelet neutralization procedure	At diagnosis of thrombotic event and at least 12 wk later	Heparin, factor V deficiency/inhibitors
	Anticardiolipin antibody ELISA	At diagnosis of thrombotic event and at least 12 wk later	Rheumatoid factor, Syphilis and HIV can result in positive test and must be ruled out
	β_2-Glycoprotein I antibody ELISA	At diagnosis of thrombotic event and at least 12 wk later	Rheumatoid factor can produce false-positive results

DIC, disseminated intravascular coagulation; HIV, human immunodeficiency virus; ELISA, enzyme-linked immunosorbent assay.

TABLE 111.8

SELECTED META-ANALYSES AND PROSPECTIVE STUDIES IN THROMBOPHILIC DISORDERS

Thrombophilic disorder	Characteristic	Study methodology	Reference
Factor V Leiden (FVL)	FVL heterozygosity and homozygosity are associated with a 5- and 10-fold increased risk of VTE	Meta-analysis of eight case–control studies including 2,310 cases and 3,204 controls	Emmerich J et al. [8]
	FVL is not a risk factor for myocardial infarction (OR, 1.24 [95% CI, 0.91–1.69] and RR, 0.83 [0.58–1.20]) or stroke (OR, 0.92 [95% CI, 0.56–1.53] and RR, 0.68 (0.45–1.04)	Meta-analysis of three case-control studies and three prospective observational studies	Juul K et al. [9]
	FVL heterozygosity and homozygosity increase the risk of recurrent thrombosis by 1.56-fold (95% CI, 1.14–2.12) and 2.65-fold (95% CI, 1.18–5.97), respectively; FVL is not	Meta-analysis of 46 studies	Segal J et al. [10]
Prothrombin gene mutation	Heterozygous factor II mutation associated with a 3.8-fold increased risk of VTE	Meta-analysis of 8 case–control studies including 2,310 cases and 3,204 controls	Emmerich J et al. [8]
	Prothrombin gene mutation is not associated with myocardial infarction (RR, 0.8 [0.4–1.6]) or stroke (RR, 1.1 [0.5–2.4])	Prospective cohort study of 14,916 U.S. men	Ridker P et al. [13]
	The prothrombin gene mutation is not associated with recurrent VTE (OR, 1.45; 95% CI, 0.96–2.2).	Meta-analysis of 46 studies	Segal J et al. [10]
Compound heterozygotes for FVL and the prothrombin gene mutation	Compound heterozygotes for FVL and the factor II mutation are at 20-fold (95% CI, 11.1–36.1) increased risk for VTE	Meta-analysis of eight case–control studies including 2,310 cases and 3,204 controls	Emmerich J et al. [8]
	The OR for recurrent VTE in compound heterozygotes for FVL and the factor II mutation is 4.81 (95% CI, 0.50–46.3)	Meta-analysis of 46 studies	Segal J et al. [10]
Hyperhomocysteinemia	Homocysteine lowering vitamin supplementation does not reduce the incidence of recurrent VTE	Two prospective, randomized, controlled trials	Ray JG et al. [29] and den Heijer M et al. [30]
	Homocysteine lowering vitamin supplementation does not reduce the incidence of cardiovascular disease in post-MI patients	Prospective, randomized, controlled trial of 5,522 patients	Lonn E et al. [31]
Antiphospholipid syndrome	High intensity vitamin K antagonist therapy (INR, 3–4) is not superior to conventional intensity therapy (INR, 2–3) for treatment of APS patients with previous VTE9	Two prospective, randomized, controlled trials	Crowther M et al. [61] and Finazzi G et al. [62]

CI, confidence interval; INR, international normalized ratio; MI, myocardial infarction; OR, odds ratio; RR, relative risk; VTE, venous thromboembolism.

References

1. Heit JA: The epidemiology of venous thromboembolism in the community. *Arterioscler Thromb Vasc Biol* 28(3):370–372, 2008.
2. Lloyd-Jones D, Adams RJ, Brown TM, et al: Executive summary: heart disease and stroke statistics—2010 update: a report from the American Heart Association. *Circulation* 121(7):948–954, 2010.
3. Furie B, Furie BC: Mechanisms of thrombus formation. *N Engl J Med* 359(9):938–949, 2008.
4. Mann KG, Brummel-Ziedins K, Orfeo T, et al: Models of blood coagulation. *Blood Cells Mol Dis* 36(2):108–117, 2006.
5. Dahlback B: Advances in understanding pathogenic mechanisms of thrombophilic disorders. *Blood* 112(1):19–27, 2008.
6. Rijken DC, Lijnen HR: New insights into the molecular mechanisms of the fibrinolytic system. *J Thromb Haemost* 7(1):4–13, 2009.
7. Ridker PM, Miletich JP, Hennekens CH, et al: Ethnic distribution of factor V Leiden in 4047 men and women. Implications for venous thromboembolism screening. *JAMA* 277(16):1305–1307, 1997.
8. Emmerich J, Rosendaal FR, Cattaneo M, et al: Combined effect of factor V Leiden and prothrombin 20210A on the risk of venous thromboembolism–pooled analysis of 8 case-control studies including 2310 cases and 3204 controls. Study Group for Pooled-Analysis in Venous Thromboembolism. *Thromb Haemost* 86(3):809–816, 2001.
9. Juul K, Tybjaerg-Hansen A, Steffensen R, et al: Factor V Leiden: the Copenhagen City Heart Study and 2 meta-analyses. *Blood* 100(1):3–10, 2002.
10. Segal JB, Brotman DJ, Necochea AJ, et al: Predictive value of factor V Leiden and prothrombin G20210A in adults with venous thromboembolism and in family members of those with a mutation: a systematic review. *JAMA* 301(23):2472–2485, 2009.
11. Chang MH, Lindegren ML, Butler MA, et al: Prevalence in the United States of selected candidate gene variants: third National Health and Nutrition Examination Survey, 1991–1994. *Am J Epidemiol* 169(1):54–66, 2009.
12. Poort SR, Rosendaal FR, Reitsma PH, et al: A common genetic variation in the 3′-untranslated region of the prothrombin gene is associated with elevated plasma prothrombin levels and an increase in venous thrombosis. *Blood* 88(10):3698–3703, 1996.
13. Ridker PM, Hennekens CH, Miletich JP: G20210A mutation in prothrombin gene and risk of myocardial infarction, stroke, and venous thrombosis in a large cohort of US men. *Circulation* 99(8):999–1004, 1999.
14. Mateo J, Oliver A, Borrell M, et al: Laboratory evaluation and clinical characteristics of 2,132 consecutive unselected patients with venous thromboembolism–results of the Spanish Multicentric Study on Thrombophilia (EMET-Study). *Thromb Haemost* 77(3):444–451, 1997.
15. Martinelli I, Mannucci PM, De Stefano V, et al: Different risks of thrombosis in four coagulation defects associated with inherited thrombophilia: a study of 150 families. *Blood* 92(7):2353–2358, 1998.
16. Koster T, Rosendaal FR, Briet E, et al: Protein C deficiency in a controlled series of unselected outpatients: an infrequent but clear risk factor for venous thrombosis (Leiden Thrombophilia Study). *Blood* 85(10):2756–2761, 1995.
17. Khor B, Van Cott EM: Laboratory tests for protein C deficiency. *Am J Hematol* 85(6):440–442, 2010.
18. Castoldi E, Hackeng TM: Regulation of coagulation by protein S. *Curr Opin Hematol* 15(5):529–536, 2008.
19. Douay X, Lucas C, Caron C, et al: Antithrombin, protein C and protein S levels in 127 consecutive young adults with ischemic stroke. *Acta Neurol Scand* 98(2):124–127, 1998.
20. Mahmoodi BK, Brouwer JL, Veeger NJ, et al: Hereditary deficiency of protein C or protein S confers increased risk of arterial thromboembolic events at a young age: results from a large family cohort study. *Circulation* 118(16):1659–1667, 2008.
21. Patnaik MM, Moll S: Inherited antithrombin deficiency: a review. *Haemophilia* 14(6):1229–1239, 2008.
22. de Moerloose P, Neerman-Arbez M: Congenital fibrinogen disorders. *Semin Thromb Hemost* 35(4):356–366, 2009.
23. Cunningham MT, Brandt JT, Laposata M, et al: Laboratory diagnosis of dysfibrinogenemia. *Arch Pathol Lab Med* 126(4):499–505, 2002.
24. Ray JG: Hyperhomocysteinemia: no longer a consideration in the management of venous thromboembolism. *Curr Opin Pulm Med* 14(5):369–373, 2008.
25. Humphrey LL, Fu R, Rogers K, et al: Homocysteine level and coronary heart disease incidence: a systematic review and meta-analysis. *Mayo Clin Proc* 83(11):1203–1212, 2008.
26. Klerk M, Verhoef P, Clarke R, et al: MTHFR 677 C→T polymorphism and risk of coronary heart disease: a meta-analysis. *JAMA* 288(16):2023–2031, 2002.
27. Eichinger S, Stumpflen A, Hirschl M, et al: Hyperhomocysteinemia is a risk factor of recurrent venous thromboembolism. *Thromb Haemost* 80(4):566–569, 1998.
28. Ray JG: Meta-analysis of hyperhomocysteinemia as a risk factor for venous thromboembolic disease. *Arch Intern Med* 158(19):2101–2106, 1998.
29. Ray JG, Kearon C, Yi Q, et al; Heart Outcomes Prevention Evaluation 2 (HOPE-2) Investigators: Homocysteine-lowering therapy and risk for venous thromboembolism: a randomized trial. *Ann Intern Med* 146(11):761–767, 2007.
30. den Heijer M, Willems HP, Blom HJ, et al: Homocysteine lowering by B vitamins and the secondary prevention of deep vein thrombosis and pulmonary embolism: a randomized, placebo-controlled, double-blind trial. *Blood* 109(1):139–144, 2007.
31. Lonn E, Yusuf S, Arnold MJ, et al: Homocysteine lowering with folic acid and B vitamins in vascular disease. *N Engl J Med* 354(15):1567–1577, 2006.
32. Koster T, Blann AD, Briet E, et al: Role of clotting factor VIII in effect of von Willebrand factor on occurrence of deep-vein thrombosis. *Lancet* 345(8943):152–155, 1995.
33. Kyrle PA, Minar E, Hirschl M, et al: High plasma levels of factor VIII and the risk of recurrent venous thromboembolism. *N Engl J Med* 343(7):457–462, 2000.
34. van Hylckama Vlieg A, van der Linden IK, Bertina RM, et al: High levels of factor IX increase the risk of venous thrombosis. *Blood* 95(12):3678–3682, 2000.
35. Meijers JC, Tekelenburg WL, Bouma BN, et al: High levels of coagulation factor XI as a risk factor for venous thrombosis. *N Engl J Med* 342(10):696–701, 2000.
36. Heit JA, Silverstein MD, Mohr DN, et al: Risk factors for deep vein thrombosis and pulmonary embolism: a population-based case-control study. *Arch Intern Med* 160(6):809–815, 2000.
37. Blom JW, Doggen CJ, Osanto S, et al: Malignancies, prothrombotic mutations, and the risk of venous thrombosis. *JAMA* 293(6):715–722, 2005.
38. Khorana AA, Connolly GC: Assessing risk of venous thromboembolism in the patient with cancer. *J Clin Oncol* 27(29):4839–4847, 2009.
39. Lee AY, Levine MN: Venous thromboembolism and cancer: risks and outcomes. *Circulation* 107[23, Suppl 1]:I17–I21, 2003.
40. Carrier M, Le Gal G, Wells PS, et al: Systematic review: the Trousseau syndrome revisited: should we screen extensively for cancer in patients with venous thromboembolism? *Ann Intern Med* 149(5):323–333, 2008.
41. Prandoni P, Lensing AW, Piccioli A, et al: Recurrent venous thromboembolism and bleeding complications during anticoagulant treatment in patients with cancer and venous thrombosis. *Blood* 100(10):3484–3488, 2002.
42. Lee AY, Levine MN, Baker RI, et al: Low-molecular-weight heparin versus a coumarin for the prevention of recurrent venous thromboembolism in patients with cancer. *N Engl J Med* 349(2):146–153, 2003.
43. Crowther MA, Cook DJ, Meade MO, et al: Thrombocytopenia in medical-surgical critically ill patients: prevalence, incidence, and risk factors. *J Crit Care* 20(4):348–353, 2005.
44. Crowther MA, Cook DJ, Albert M, et al: The 4Ts scoring system for heparin-induced thrombocytopenia in medical-surgical intensive care unit patients. *J Crit Care* 25(2):287–293, 2010.
45. Warkentin TE, Greinacher A, Koster A, et al; American College of Chest Physicians: Treatment and prevention of heparin-induced thrombocytopenia: American College of Chest Physicians Evidence-Based Clinical Practice Guidelines (8th Edition). *Chest* 133[6, Suppl]:340S–380S, 2008.
46. Arepally GM, Ortel TL: Heparin-induced thrombocytopenia. *Annu Rev Med* 61:77–90, 2010.
47. Lo GK, Juhl D, Warkentin TE, et al: Evaluation of pretest clinical score (4 T's) for the diagnosis of heparin-induced thrombocytopenia in two clinical settings. *J Thromb Haemost* 4(4):759–765, 2006.
48. Geerts WH, Code KI, Jay RM, et al: A prospective study of venous thromboembolism after major trauma. *N Engl J Med* 331(24):1601–1606, 1994.
49. Knudson MM, Ikossi DG, Khaw L, et al: Thromboembolism after trauma: an analysis of 1602 episodes from the American College of Surgeons National Trauma Data Bank. *Ann Surg* 240(3):490–496; discussion 496–498, 2004.
50. Geerts WH, Bergqvist D, Pineo GF, et al: Prevention of venous thromboembolism: American College of Chest Physicians Evidence-Based Clinical Practice Guidelines (8th Edition). *Chest* 133[6, Suppl]:381S–453S, 2008.
51. Geerts WH, Jay RM, Code KI, et al: A comparison of low-dose heparin with low-molecular-weight heparin as prophylaxis against venous thromboembolism after major trauma. *N Engl J Med* 335(10):701–707, 1996.
52. Adams RC, Hamrick M, Berenguer C, et al: Four years of an aggressive prophylaxis and screening protocol for venous thromboembolism in a large trauma population. *J Trauma* 65(2):300–306; discussion 306–308, 2008.
53. Greenfield LJ, Proctor MC, Rodriguez JL, et al: Posttrauma thromboembolism prophylaxis. *J Trauma* 42(1):100–103, 1997.
54. Giannakopoulos B, Passam F, Ioannou Y, et al: How we diagnose the antiphospholipid syndrome. *Blood* 113(5):985–994, 2009.
55. Forastiero R, Martinuzzo M, Pombo G, et al: A prospective study of antibodies to beta2-glycoprotein I and prothrombin, and risk of thrombosis. *J Thromb Haemost* 3(6):1231–1238, 2005.
56. Somers E, Magder LS, Petri M: Antiphospholipid antibodies and incidence of venous thrombosis in a cohort of patients with systemic lupus erythematosus. *J Rheumatol* 29(12):2531–2536, 2002.
57. Giannakopoulos B, Krilis SA: How I treat the antiphospholipid syndrome. *Blood* 114(10):2020–2030, 2009.
58. Galli M, Luciani D, Bertolini G, et al: Anti-beta 2-glycoprotein I, antiprothrombin antibodies, and the risk of thrombosis in the antiphospholipid syndrome. *Blood* 102(8):2717–2723, 2003.

59. Pengo V, Ruffatti A, Legnani C, et al: Clinical course of high-risk patients diagnosed with antiphospholipid syndrome. *J Thromb Haemost* 8(2):237–242, 2010.
60. Provenzale JM, Ortel TL, Allen NB: Systemic thrombosis in patients with antiphospholipid antibodies: lesion distribution and imaging findings. *AJR Am J Roentgenol* 170(2):285–290, 1998.
61. Crowther MA, Ginsberg JS, Julian J, et al: A comparison of two intensities of warfarin for the prevention of recurrent thrombosis in patients with the antiphospholipid antibody syndrome. *N Engl J Med* 349(12):1133–1138, 2003.
62. Finazzi G, Marchioli R, Brancaccio V, et al: A randomized clinical trial of high-intensity warfarin vs. conventional antithrombotic therapy for the prevention of recurrent thrombosis in patients with the antiphospholipid syndrome (WAPS). *J Thromb Haemost* 3(5):848–853, 2005.
63. Moll S, Ortel TL: Monitoring warfarin therapy in patients with lupus anticoagulants. *Ann Intern Med* 127(3):177–185, 1997.
64. Lim W, Crowther MA, Eikelboom JW: Management of antiphospholipid antibody syndrome: a systematic review. *JAMA* 295(9):1050–1057, 2006.
65. Levine SR, Brey RL, Tilley BC, et al: Antiphospholipid antibodies and subsequent thrombo-occlusive events in patients with ischemic stroke. *JAMA* 291(5):576–584, 2004.
66. Bucciarelli S, Espinosa G, Cervera R: The CAPS Registry: morbidity and mortality of the catastrophic antiphospholipid syndrome. *Lupus* 18(10):905–912, 2009.
67. Cervera R: Update on the diagnosis, treatment, and prognosis of the catastrophic antiphospholipid syndrome. *Curr Rheumatol Rep* 12(1):70–76, 2010.
68. Tefferi A, Elliott M: Thrombosis in myeloproliferative disorders: prevalence, prognostic factors, and the role of leukocytes and JAK2V617 F. *Semin Thromb Hemost* 33(4):313–320, 2007.
69. Spivak JL: Polycythemia vera: myths, mechanisms, and management. *Blood* 100(13):4272–4290, 2002.
70. Hillmen P, Lewis SM, Bessler M, et al: Natural history of paroxysmal nocturnal hemoglobinuria. *N Engl J Med* 333(19):1253–1258, 1995.
71. Brodsky RA: How I treat paroxysmal nocturnal hemoglobinuria. *Blood* 113(26):6522–6527, 2009.
72. Hillmen P, Muus P, Duhrsen U, et al: Effect of the complement inhibitor eculizumab on thromboembolism in patients with paroxysmal nocturnal hemoglobinuria. *Blood* 110(12):4123–4128, 2007.
73. Emadi A, Brodsky RA: Successful discontinuation of anticoagulation following eculizumab administration in paroxysmal nocturnal hemoglobinuria. *Am J Hematol* 84(10):699–701, 2009.
74. Cohn D, Vansenne F, de Borgie C, et al: Thrombophilia testing for prevention of recurrent venous thromboembolism. *Cochrane Database Syst Rev* (1):CD007069, 2009.
75. Christiansen SC, Cannegieter SC, Koster T, et al: Thrombophilia, clinical factors, and recurrent venous thrombotic events. *JAMA* 293(19):2352–2361, 2005.
76. Khor B, Van Cott EM: Laboratory evaluation of hypercoagulability. *Clin Lab Med* 29(2):339–366, 2009.

CHAPTER 112 ■ ANEMIA IN THE CRITICAL CARE SETTING

MARC S. ZUMBERG, MARC J. KAHN AND ALICE D. MA

GENERAL PRINCIPLES

Anemia is common in the critical care setting. Recent studies have shown that 29% to 62% of patients have anemia at the time of admission to critical care units and 20% to 30% have moderate or severe anemia (hemoglobin <9 g per dL) [1–5]. Anemia will develop in nearly all patients at some point during the course of a prolonged intensive care unit (ICU) stay, and as a result, the majority of patients admitted more than 7 days receive a red blood cell (RBC) transfusion [1–5].

Certain anemias may be encountered more frequently in patients who are admitted to critical care units than in other settings, including anemias arising from iatrogenic sources (e.g., mechanical hemolysis caused by ventricular assist devices or intra-aortic balloon pumps); those producing hemodynamic or systemic compromise that leads to a requirement for critical care (e.g., massive blood loss due to trauma, gastrointestinal lesions, or surgical invasion; thrombotic microangiopathies); and those arising in the context of prolonged critical illness (e.g., anemia of chronic disease/inflammation [ACD]). Losses from an enhanced frequency of phlebotomy for diagnostic testing in the critical care unit may contribute to the development or maintenance of anemia and have been estimated to account for 1 to 2 units lost during a typical hospital stay [5,6].

This chapter provides an overview of the evaluation and laboratory workup of anemia, with a focus on diagnoses that provoke the most clinical concern, are important to recognize quickly, and are the most likely to be encountered in the critical care setting. Accordingly, the hemolytic anemias, including the microangiopathic hemolytic anemias, autoimmune hemolytic anemia (AIHA), and sickle cell syndromes, will be covered in the most detail (Table 112.1). The ACD often develops in patients in the ICU and will also be a focus of this chapter. Anemia due to massive blood loss including trauma and gastrointestinal bleeding is essential to recognize, obtain proper consultation for, and treat appropriately, but the diagnosis is usually self-evident.

Initial Evaluation

The etiologies of anemia in the critical care setting are diverse, but the evaluation of anemia in a critical care patient initially should be approached in a manner similar to the noncritical care setting.

The patient's volume status should be considered first, as an increase in the plasma volume may lead to a decrease in the measured hemoglobin or hematocrit that does not represent a decrease in the red cell mass or oxygen carrying capacity. This situation is known as dilutional or spurious anemia and is particularly common in ICU patients requiring fluid resuscitation [5]. Dilutional anemia does not require treatment.

To better come up with a differential diagnosis of the anemia, it should be determined whether the anemia predated the patient's critical illness, developed in conjunction with the critical illness, or developed during the ICU stay (Table 112.2).

TABLE 112.1

CLASSIFICATION OF THE HEMOLYTIC ANEMIAS: CONGENITAL VERSUS ACQUIRED

Congenital hemolytic anemias

Defects in the erythrocyte membrane
- e.g., hereditary spherocytosis

Deficiencies in erythrocyte metabolic enzymes
- ex. pyruvate kinase deficiency
- ex. glucose-6-phosphate dehydrogenase deficiency

Defects in globin structure and synthesis
- ex. sickle cell disease
- ex. thalassemia

Acquired hemolytic anemias

Autoimmune hemolytic anemias
- ex. warm autoimmune hemolytic anemia
- ex. cold agglutinin disease
- ex. paroxysmal cold hemoglobinuria
- ex. drug-induced hemolytic anemia

Microangiopathic hemolytic anemia
- ex. thrombotic thrombocytopenic purpura
- ex. hemolytic uremic syndrome
- ex. disseminated intravascular coagulation

Hemolytic transfusion reaction

Paroxysmal nocturnal hemoglobinuria

Infectious agents
- ex. malaria

Chemicals, drugs, and physical agents
- ex. arsenic

Advanced liver disease

Laboratory Studies

Anemias can be classified by the size of the RBCs as reflected by the mean corpuscular volume (MCV): microcytic (MCV, <80 fL), normocytic (80 to 100 fL), and macrocytic (>100 fL). A finite number of diagnoses constitute each of these categories, allowing the practitioner to narrow the differential diagnosis (Table 112.3). One should take caution to review the MCV prior to the transfusion of RBCs, as donor RBCs may increase or decrease the MCV depending on the pretransfusion value.

TABLE 112.2

SAMPLE DIFFERENTIAL DIAGNOSIS OF ANEMIA BASED ON THE TIME COURSE OF ANEMIA IN RELATION TO THE CRITICAL ILLNESS

Anemia predating the critical illness
- Primary bone marrow disorders
- Vitamin deficiencies
- Hemoglobinopathies
- Congenital anemias

Anemia developing in conjunction with the critical illness
- Anemia of chronic disease/inflammation
- Hemolytic anemias
- Thrombotic thrombocytopenic purpura

Anemia developing during the course of the intensive care unit stay
- Gastrointestinal bleeding
- Frequent phlebotomies
- Drug-induced hemolytic anemia
- Anemia of chronic disease/inflammation

TABLE 112.3

DIFFERENTIAL DIAGNOSIS OF SELECTED ANEMIAS BASED ON RED CELL MEAN CORPUSCULAR VOLUME (MCV)

Microcytic (MCV ≤80 fl)
- Fe deficiency
- α-Thalassemia
- β-Thalassemia
- Anemia of chronic disease/inflammation
- Lead poisoning
- Sideroblastic anemia

Normocytic (MCV 80–100 fl)
- Acute blood loss
- Primary bone marrow disorders
- Anemia of chronic disease/inflammation
- Splenomegaly
- Hemolytic anemia with low or normal reticulocyte count
- Endocrine disorders

Macrocytic (MCV >100 fl)
- Megaloblastic anemia
  - B_{12} deficiency
  - Folic acid deficiency
  - Drug induced
- Hypothyroidism
- Liver disease
- Hemolytic anemia with reticulocytosis
- Myelodysplastic syndrome

Several additional tests may be helpful in the evaluation of anemia. The reticulocyte count, which is a measure of the bone marrow's ability to produce new RBCs, should be the initial test performed. The reticulocyte count is typically elevated in hemolytic anemias, gastrointestinal bleeding, or after supplementation of a missing nutrient such as iron or vitamin B_{12}. The reticulocyte count is typically low in primary bone marrow failure disorders, nutritional deficiencies, the anemia of chronic disease/inflammation, and any condition leading to the underproduction of or resistance to erythropoietin (e.g., renal disease). If a hemolytic anemia is suspected (i.e., due to consistently hemolyzed blood specimens, characteristic findings on physical examination [see later], or refractoriness to erythrocyte transfusion), measurement of total and unfractionated bilirubin (elevated), lactate dehydrogenase (LDH) (elevated), and haptoglobin (decreased) may be useful, although the results are not specific to hemolysis and may be similar in patients with advanced liver disease.

The blood smear itself may help to narrow the diagnosis and quickly identify anemias due to causes that require expeditious, specialized management (e.g., thrombotic microangiopathies). Examples of erythrocyte abnormalities include schistocytes (Fig. 112.1), sickle cells (Fig. 112.2), bite cells (Fig. 112.3), or spherocytes (Fig. 112.4) and identification of these aberrant forms is critical in making the correct diagnosis (Table 112.4).

Further laboratory testing should be guided by the results of the MCV, reticulocyte count, review of the blood smear, and any clinical suspicion of likely diagnoses (Table 112.5).

Therapeutic Red Cell Transfusion

Clinicians caring for patients in critical care settings are often confronted with the decision to transfuse RBCs even before results of laboratory testing or other evaluation has elucidated

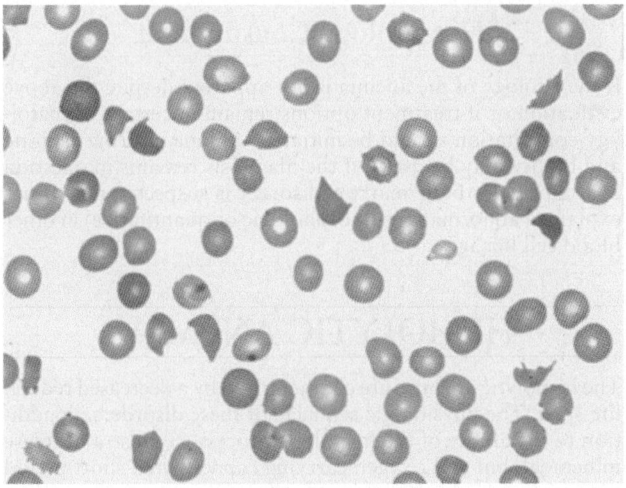

FIGURE 112.1. Peripheral smear from a patient with disseminated intravascular coagulation shows characteristic "helmet: cells. [Reused with permission from Maslak P. ASH Image Bank 2008;2008:8-00102.]

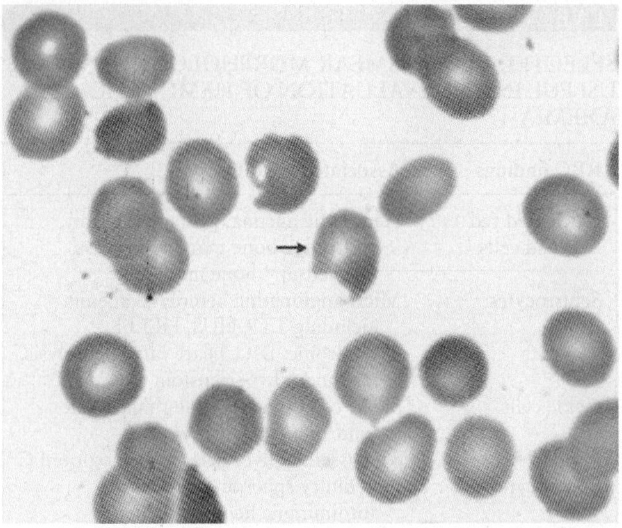

FIGURE 112.3. The RBC deformity (*arrow*) shown in this image is referred to as a "bite" cell. [Reused with permission from Lazarchick J. ASH Image Bank 2008;2008:8-00151.]

the cause of the anemia. Erythrocyte transfusion in this setting may be guided by hemodynamic considerations, rather than a finite transfusion trigger [7]. Because of the (albeit low) risk of transmission of infectious pathogens and the potential for transfusion reactions and immunomodulation, and in light of increasing evidence from randomized trials that anemia is well tolerated in individuals without cardiopulmonary compromise, more restrictive transfusion policies are becoming more common [8–12]. Principles of transfusion are discussed in greater detail in Chapter 114.

Use of Erythropoiesis-Stimulating Agents

In multiple randomized clinical studies, use of erythropoiesis-stimulating agents (ESAs) in critically ill patients as compared with placebo or no intervention had no statistically significant effect on overall mortality, length of hospital stay, ICU stay, or duration of mechanical ventilation [13,14]. A recent meta-analysis, however, has shown that use of ESAs reduced the odds of a patient receiving at least one transfusion and modestly decreased the mean number of units of blood transfused by 0.41 units [13]. The optimal dosing and schedule of erythropoietin remains to be determined [13,15–17], and the need for concomitant supplemental intravenous iron, which may be considered when the serum ferritin drops below 100 to 200 ng per mL or iron saturation drops below 20% [2,15], still is debated. In a recent U.S. multicenter, retrospective, observational study of ESA utilization in anemic critically ill patients admitted to the ICU, practice patterns were highly variable [18]. Thus, at the present time, there remains insufficient evidence to recommend the routine use of ESAs in critically ill anemic patients [13].

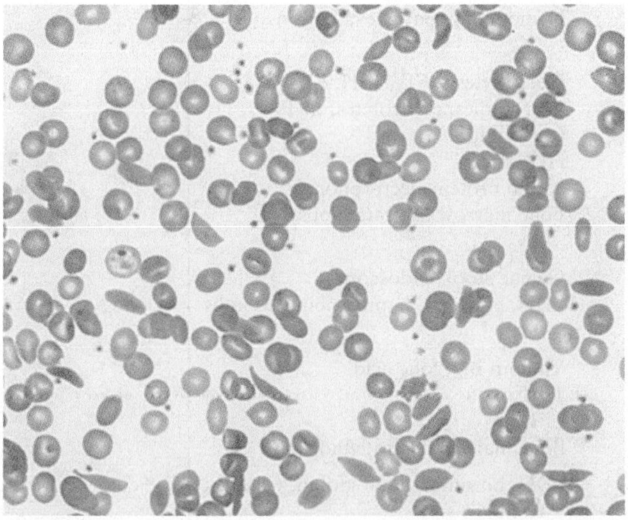

FIGURE 112.2. Peripheral smear from a patient with sickle cell disease illustrates the spectrum of RBC findings in this disorder including sickle cells, polychromatophilic RBCs, target cells, and Howell-Jolly bodies. [Reused with permission from Lazarchick J. ASH Image Bank 2009;2009:9-00044.]

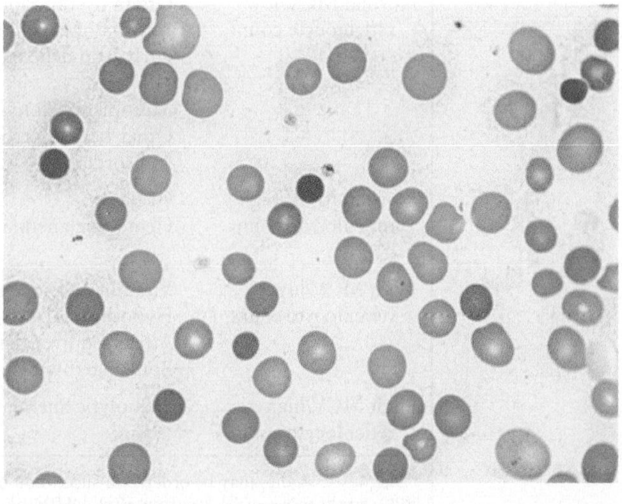

FIGURE 112.4. Spherocytes lack central pallor and may appear smaller than typical red cells. [Reused with permission from Maslak P. ASH Image Bank 2008;2008:8-00103.]

TABLE 112.4

SELECTED BLOOD SMEAR MORPHOLOGIC FINDINGS USEFUL IN THE EVALUATION OF HEMOLYTIC ANEMIA

RBC findings	Associated conditions
Nucleated red blood cells	Hemolytic anemia, postsplenectomy, infiltrative bone marrow process, "revved-up" bone marrow
Schistocytes	Microangiopathic hemolytic anemia including TTP, HUS, HELLP syndrome, DIC, heart valve hemolysis, malignant hypertension
Sickle cells	Sickle cell disease, sickle-thalassemic syndromes
Target cells	Thalassemia, liver disease, hemoglobin C
Spherocytes	Hereditary spherocytosis, warm autoimmune hemolytic anemia
Bite cells	G6PD deficiency
Tear drop cells	Myelofibrosis, infiltrative bone marrow process
RBC agglutination	Cold agglutinin disease
Rouleaux formation	Multiple myeloma, Waldenstrom's macroglobulinemia

DIC, disseminated intravascular coagulation; G6PD, glucose 6 phosphate dehydrogenase; HELLP syndrome, hemolysis, elevated liver enzymes, low platelets; HUS, hemolytic uremic syndrome; RBC, red blood cell; TTP, thrombotic thrombocytopenic purpura.

Hematology Consultation

If the etiology of the anemia is not apparent despite the above evaluation or if treatment options remain uncertain, hematology consultation should be initiated. A bone marrow aspirate and biopsy may be useful if the diagnosis remains in question or if a primary bone marrow disorder is suspected due to unexplained abnormalities (morphologic or quantitative) in other blood cell lineages.

HEMOLYTIC ANEMIAS

The hemolytic anemias are characterized by a decreased red cell life span. The physiologic sequelae of these disorders, in addition to the ability of the hemolytic process to cause a decrease in hemoglobin and oxygen carrying capacity in a short period of time, may lead to a requirement for critical care. The patient with hemolysis may be very or only minimally symptomatic, depending on the rate of red cell destruction and the degree of compensation by the bone marrow, which produces young red cells (reticulocytes) in response to the decreased hemoglobin.

Overview of Laboratory Features

Pathologic features of hemolysis differ greatly depending on whether the red cell destruction is primarily intravascular or extravascular. Biochemical evidence for intravascular hemolysis includes elevated levels of LDH and unconjugated bilirubin and decreased levels of haptoglobin, which is cleared from the

TABLE 112.5

SUGGESTED INITIAL SAMPLE LABORATORY EVALUATION BASED ON THE MCV AND RETICULOCYTE COUNT

Laboratory finding	Suspected diagnoses	Diagnostic studies[a]
Decreased MCV/low reticulocyte count	Iron deficiency Thalassemia trait Sideroblastic anemia	Iron studies Hemoglobinopathy evaluation Bone marrow aspirate/biopsy
Decreased MCV/high reticulocyte count	Thalassemia	Hemoglobinopathy evaluation
Normal MCV/low reticulocyte count	Organ dysfunction Anemia of chronic disease Early iron deficiency HIV Multiple myeloma Other bone marrow disorders	Electrolytes, LFTs, TSH, EPO Iron studies, electrolytes, LFTs Iron studies HIV studies Serum protein electrophoresis Bone marrow aspirate/biopsy
Normal MCV/high reticulocyte count	GI bleed Hemolytic anemia	Guaiac stool, endoscopy LDH, bilirubin, haptoglobin, Coombs test
High MCV/low reticulocyte count	Vitamin deficiencies Hypothyroidism Advanced liver disease Bone marrow disorders	Vitamin B_{12}, folic acid TSH LFTs Bone marrow aspirate/biopsy
High MCV/high reticulocyte count	Hemolytic anemia	LDH, bilirubin, haptoglobin, Coombs test

[a]Diagnostic studies may be ordered in succession until diagnostic result is reached.
EPO, erythropoietin; GI, gastrointestinal; HIV, human immunodeficiency virus; LDH, lactate dehydrogenase; LFTs, liver function tests; MCV, mean corpuscular volume; TSH, thyroid stimulating hormone.

circulation after binding free hemoglobin. Hemoglobinuria results when free hemoglobin is filtered through the glomerulus and is released into the urine, imparting a reddish color. Some hemoglobin in the urine is taken up by tubular cells and is converted to hemosiderin. This can be detected by checking for intracellular iron in the urine by staining the urine with Prussian blue stain. Extravascular hemolysis may be evidenced by only a declining hemoglobin level, although cases of brisk destruction of red cells may show elevations in LDH and unconjugated bilirubin.

Increased red cell production is evidenced by an increase in the number of circulating reticulocytes, which are young red cells whose large size typically results in an elevated red cell MCV and red cell distribution width. Circulating nucleated red blood cells (NRBCs) may be seen in cases of brisk hemolysis. Morphologic evidence of red cell destruction may be evident on the blood smear (see following sections and Figs. 112.1 to 112.4).

Immune-Mediated Hemolysis

The pathophysiology of immune-mediated hemolysis involves antibodies binding to red cells, with or without the activation of complement, leading to red cell destruction. If the antibody on the red cell surface is immunoglobulin G (IgG), then red cell destruction is mediated via Fc receptors on macrophages within the reticuloendothelial (RE) system. Complete or partial phagocytosis occurs causing the red cells to take a spherocytic shape as opposed to the normal, more pliable, biconcave disc shape.

Antibodies which lead to hemolysis can be divided into two categories: warm and cold, referring to the temperature at which the antibody optimally reacts with the red cell. Warm antibodies react with red cells best at temperatures 37°C and typically do not agglutinate red cells [19]. Cold antibodies typically react best at temperatures less than 32°C, with maximal reactivity at 4°C and lead to red cell agglutination [20]. The hallmark of AIHA is a positive direct Coombs test, which will detect the presence of either IgG or C3 bound to red cells (Table 112.6).

Warm Autoimmune Hemolytic Anemia

In warm autoimmune hemolytic anemia (WAIHA), IgG antibodies are directed against red cell surface membrane antigens [19]. Most commonly, these antibodies are directed against members of the Rh blood group, but the specificity of the pathogenic IgG antibodies is not always identified. The IgG antibodies coat the red cells and may or may not fix complement (C3). IgG-coated red cell membrane fragments are engulfed by macrophages in the RE system (usually the spleen) [19,21]. As the red cell loses surface area, it loses the ability to retain its biconcave disc shape. Since the shape with the smallest surface area-to-volume ratio is a sphere, the red cell becomes progressively more spherocytic with each pass through the splenic circulation [19].

WAIHA can manifest as a primary disorder, or alternatively, it can be secondary to an underlying disorder, such as collagen vascular disease (e.g., lupus) or a lymphoproliferative disorder (e.g., lymphoma). Approximately 30% of patients with chronic lymphocytic leukemia have a positive Coombs test, although a much lower proportion develops hemolysis [22]. AIHA may be associated with immune thrombocytopenia, a condition called Evans syndrome. AIHA can also be provoked by infection or can be induced by various drugs. Causes of WAIHA are listed in Table 112.7.

TABLE 112.6

INTERPRETATION OF THE COOMBS TEST AND DIFFERENTIAL DIAGNOSIS

	IgG positive	IgG negative
C3 positive	WAIHA	Drug-induced hemolysis
	Drug-induced hemolysis	Cold agglutinin disease
		PCH
C3 negative	WAIHA	WAIHA (rare)

Notes: In performing this test, red cells from the patient are washed to remove nonspecific proteins and antibodies. Next, antibodies to human IgG, human C3, or both are added to the cells. If the patient's red cells have either IgG or C3 attached to them, the red cells will agglutinate, indicating a positive test. The specificity of the antibody can be tested by testing the patient's serum against panels of red cells that express different subsets of red cell antigens.
IgG, immunoglobulin G; PCH, paroxysmal cold hemoglobinuria; WAIHA, warm autoimmune hemolytic anemia.

TABLE 112.7

CAUSES OF IMMUNE HEMOLYTIC ANEMIAS

Warm autoimmune hemolytic Anemia
- Idiopathic
- Lymphoproliferative disease
- Autoimmune disease
- Drugs
- Infections
- Solid tumors

Cold agglutinin disease
- Idiopathic
- Lymphoproliferative disease
- Infections

Clinical Features. Almost all patients present with worsening and often debilitating fatigue. Older patients, and those with rapid hemolysis and ensuing severe anemia, may present with evidence of organ compromise such as dyspnea, angina, or syncope and can suffer myocardial ischemia, hypotension, and/or renal failure. Physical findings can include pallor, jaundice, and splenomegaly. Laboratory findings include an increased reticulocyte count, increased bilirubin (total and indirect), and increased LDH. The direct Coombs test should be positive (Table 112.6), and typically spherocytes, microspherocytes, NRBCs, and/or anisocytosis are seen on the blood smear.

Transfusion in Patients with Warm Autoimmune Hemolytic Anemia. If the patient has heart failure, angina, shock, or evidence of hypoperfusion to vital organs, or if compensatory erythrocytosis is absent or inadequate due to an underlying illness that suppresses the bone marrow, such as leukemia, prior chemotherapy, or renal failure, then red cell transfusion should be performed [19]. The anti-erythrocyte autoantibody itself also occasionally can be directed against red cell precursors in the marrow, leading to an inappropriately low reticulocyte count [19,23]. Any transfusion in patients with WAIHA needs to be coordinated closely with the blood bank or transfusion service. The offending antibody will frequently interfere with performing a crossmatch to identify compatible blood for transfusion. It is critical to obtain a thorough transfusion and pregnancy history to determine the likelihood of an underlying alloantibody which may be masked by the autoantibody; testing a red cell eluate may be helpful in this regard. Crossmatching can be done using low ionic strength solution (LISS) which will minimize nonspecific interactions, allowing the stronger alloantibody interactions to appear. If time allows, phenotyping can be performed to identify any antigens on the patient's red cells that may be likely to engender an immune reaction when exposed to transfused blood; such a maneuver may help to minimize the risk of a delayed hemolytic transfusion reaction (DHTR). If crossmatched units are not available, phenotypically matched red cells are preferred. If not available, due to time constraints or the patient's condition, then ABO and Rh type-specific, noncrossmatched, or "least incompatible" units should be used. Each unit should be transfused slowly, while the patient's clinical status is closely assessed for evidence of worsening hemolysis. The blood bank may require that samples of the patient's blood be drawn soon after the transfusion begins to record any evidence of hemolysis. This is termed an in vivo crossmatch.

Treatment. After hemostatic instability has been addressed through transfusion of RBCs, the initial treatment of WAIHA consists of immunosuppression which, if successful, may attenuate antibody production and allow the patient's RBCs to survive normally in the circulation. First-line therapy consists of glucocorticosteroids, either intravenously such as methylprednisolone or oral prednisone, typically at 1 to 2 mg per kg daily [19]. Intravenous immunoglobulin (IVIG) has also been used but is less effective than in immune thrombocytopenic purpura (ITP) [19,24]. If steroids are ineffective, or if relapse occurs, then alternative immunosuppression should be considered. Agents which have been reported to be useful in WAIHA include rituximab, cyclophosphamide, mycophenolate mofetil, and azathioprine [19,25–27]. Splenectomy should also be considered as a reasonable second-line treatment option in eligible patients [19]. As with all hemolytic anemias, the administration of folic acid 1 to 5 mg per day, at least as long as hemolysis is ongoing, is recommended. The reticulocyte count and complete blood cell count (CBC) should be followed closely to monitor the effectiveness of therapy. The amount of blood drawn may be minimized by using pediatric tubes or "bullet" tubes, if available.

Cold Agglutinin Disease

In cold agglutinin disease (CAD), immunoglobulin M (IgM) antibodies target red cell surface antigens, typically with specificity to either "I" or "i." These IgM antibodies optimally bind to red cells at "cold" temperatures (typically <32°C and most strongly at 4°C) [20], and, given their ability to bind more than one RBC simultaneously, lead to the agglutination and clumping of RBCs in the distal microvasculature. IgM anti-erythrocyte antibodies fix complement to the red cell, leading to either intravascular or extravascular hemolysis. CAD may be primary or secondary due to disorders such as lymphoproliferation or infection [28,29].

Clinical Features. In most patients, CAD is a chronic condition characterized by mild to moderate hemolysis and episodic cyanosis and ischemia of the ears, tip of the nose, and digits [29]. When episodic, cold-induced hemolytic episodes occur, intravascular hemolysis may be associated with shock, rigors, back pain, and renal failure.

Laboratory Evaluation. Cold-agglutinin titers can be measured. On Coombs testing, complement (C3) is typically positive while IgG is negative, reflecting the underlying IgM autoantibody which more efficiently fixes complement (Table 112.6). The thermal amplitude of the autoantibody, not the antibody titer, however, best determines the severity of clinical symptoms. If binding occurs only at 4°C to 30°C, it is less clinically important than if significant binding occurs at temperatures more than 34°C, approximating more physiologic conditions. In fact, many normal individuals will have cold agglutinins detected at 4°C but have no clinical symptoms.

Treatment. In patients with chronic, mild CAD, the mainstay of treatment is avoidance of cold temperatures. Corticosteroids and splenectomy are typically ineffective in CAD as compared with WAIHA. Other agents, such as chlorambucil, cyclophosphamide, and rituximab, have been used successfully [20,30]. In patients who present with impending or actual end-organ damage such as myocardial ischemia or stroke, plasmapheresis may be effective because IgM remains primarily intravascular and can be efficiently removed. Plasmapheresis may need to be performed preoperatively in surgeries requiring cardiopulmonary bypass or cardioplegia [20,31]. In all patients, care must be taken to keep the extracorporeal tubing warm and to warm intravenous fluids and blood products, or hemolysis may worsen. Folic acid repletion is recommended in all patients.

Paroxysmal Cold Hemoglobinuria

IgG is the pathogenic antibody in this rare condition. Similar to IgM antibodies in CAD, the IgG antibody in paroxysmal cold hemoglobinuria (PCH) binds to red cells only at cold temperatures where it fixes complement. Unlike the antibody in CAD, however, it is activated at warmer temperatures and does not agglutinate red cells. This antibody is called the Donath-Landsteiner antibody and is directed against the "P" red cell antigen [20]. Red cell destruction occurs primarily via activation of the complement cascade and leads to subsequent intravascular hemolysis. In the past, PCH was primarily a disease associated with tertiary syphilis and, therefore, has become much less common in the penicillin era. Currently, PCH is primarily a pediatric disorder (often following a viral infection), only rarely affecting adults. Patients suffer episodic, cold-induced hemolysis. There is no cold-induced digital ischemia.

The diagnosis is made by detection of the Donath-Landsteiner antibody. The Coombs test is typically negative for IgG and positive for C3 (Table 112.6). The blood bank should be alerted to the possibility of this diagnosis, as special considerations are required for detection. Serum is collected from the patient and kept at 37°C. Patient serum and normal red cells are next chilled to 4°C then warmed to 37°C. The presence of lysis is revealed by detection of free hemoglobin in the sample. Controls must be performed where red cells and serum are incubated at 37°C and in a separate test tube at 4°C. In both of these scenarios, there should be no lysis detected [32], as a positive test requires the extremes of temperature.

Drug-Induced Hemolytic Anemias

More than 130 drugs have been reported to cause immune-mediated hemolytic anemia [33]. Drugs can induce hemolytic anemia by three general mechanisms: the innocent bystander mechanism, hapten mechanism, and a true autoimmune mechanism [34,35]. These are described in Table 112.8. It should be noted that many drugs may lead to a positive direct Coombs test in the absence of overt hemolysis. Thus, a positive direct Coombs test should not be inferred to represent hemolysis unless there is worsening anemia in conjunction with consistent laboratory evaluation.

Other drugs may cause hemolysis by alternative mechanisms. Oxidant agents such as dapsone and other sulfa drugs may cause hemolysis in a dose-dependent fashion, especially in individuals with glucose 6-phosphate dehydrogenase (G6PD) deficiency who are impaired in their ability to detoxify the oxidant damage to hemoglobin (see "Glucose 6-Phosphate Dehydrogenase Deficiency" section later in the chapter). Ribavirin,

TABLE 112.8

MECHANISMS OF DRUG-INDUCED HEMOLYSIS

Mechanism	Pathophysiology	Examples
Innocent bystander mechanism	Antibodies develop against the drug. The drug and antibody bind together to form immune complexes, which deposit on the surface of the red cell, where they are recognized by the RE system. The drug must be present in order for hemolysis to occur	Quinine Quinidine Isoniazid
Hapten mechanism	Drug binds to the red cell surface, and antibodies form which are directed against the complex of RBC/drug	Penicillins Cephalosporins, especially Cefotetan
True autoimmune mechanism	Certain drugs appear to induce formation of antibodies directed against red cell surface components, independent of any binding to the RBC surface. Once the process has been initiated, antibody production can continue, even in the absence of drug	Alpha methyldopa Levodopa Procainamide Fludarabine

RBC, red blood cell; RE, reticuloendothelial.

used to treat hepatitis C, causes hemolysis in a dose-dependent fashion. Its mechanism of red cell damage is unclear, but it may relate to nucleotide depletion. Other agents such as cyclosporine and tacrolimus may cause a microangiopathic hemolytic anemia due to endothelial damage (see section "Microangiopathic Hemolytic Anemia").

MICROANGIOPATHIC HEMOLYTIC ANEMIA

The microangiopathic hemolytic anemias are defined as disorders in which narrowing or obstruction of small blood vessels results in distortion and fragmentation of erythrocytes leading to hemolysis and subsequent anemia [36]. The hallmark finding on the blood smear is the schistocyte, a fragmented RBC (Fig. 112.1). It is essential that the intensivist recognize the differential diagnosis of microangiopathic hemolytic anemia as many of the diagnoses, some of which may be apparent given the patient's current or recent medical history, require prompt recognition and treatment (Table 112.9) [36,37]. If the underlying etiology of microangiopathic hemolytic anemia is in question, immediate hematology consultation is strongly recommended to evaluate for life threatening diagnosis such as thrombotic TTP.

TTP, once almost uniformly fatal, can now be treated effectively in the majority of patients with prompt recognition and initiation of therapeutic plasma exchange (TPE) [36–38]. The diagnosis should be suspected in any patient who presents with unexplained microangiopathic hemolytic anemia and thrombocytopenia [36–38]. The "classic pentad" of microangiopathic hemolytic anemia, thrombocytopenia, mental status changes, renal failure, and fever is present in fewer than 25% of patients at presentation. Only unexplained microangiopathic hemolytic anemia and thrombocytopenia are required to suspect the diagnosis; the clinical sequela are likely late manifestations of the disease [39].

Moake and others first noted unusually large von Willebrand factor (vWF) multimers in the plasma of affected patients and proposed them to be central in the pathophysiology of the disorder [40]. In the late 1990s, two groups reported that a vWF-cleaving protease (later termed ADAMTS-13, as a member of a disintegrin and metalloproteinase with thrombospondin components family of proteins) was found to be absent in familial TTP and inhibited by an antibody in the majority of cases of acquired TTP [41,42]. The absence of ADAMTS-13 was subsequently shown to prevent the breakdown and lead to the accumulation of ultra large molecular weight vWF multimers [40,43,44]. These ultra large vWF multimers efficiently bind to glycoprotein receptors on platelet surfaces leading to adhesion of platelets to the blood vessel endothelium and subsequently to small vessel occlusion affecting a variety of organs [38,40]. Hemolytic anemia occurs due to the mechanical shearing of RBCs as they transverse the turbulent and occluded microvasculature, thus leading to the classic findings of schistocytes seen on the peripheral blood smear (Fig. 112.1) [36,45].

TABLE 112.9

DIFFERENTIAL DIAGNOSIS OF MICROANGIOPATHIC HEMOLYTIC ANEMIA

Thrombotic thrombocytopenic purpura
Hemolytic uremic syndrome
Disseminated intravascular coagulation
HELLP syndrome (Hemolysis, Elevated Liver enzymes, Low Platelets)
Preeclampsia
Malignant hypertension
Malfunctioning prosthetic heart valve with turbulent flow
Severe vasculitis
Scleroderma renal crisis
Catastrophic antiphospholipid antibody syndrome
Malignancy
Intravascular foreign bodies
- Left ventricular assist device
- Intra-aortic balloon pump

Drugs
- Cyclosporine
- Tacrolimus
- Ticlopidine
- Clopidogrel
- Chemotherapeutic agents such as mitomycin C and gemcitabine

Clinical Manifestations

As discussed earlier, the clinical manifestations of TTP can be quite varied. Neurologic symptoms may range from subtle confusion to frank seizures or coma. Renal dysfunction may range from mild proteinuria or azotemia to acute renal failure. Occlusion in the blood vessels of the cardiac conduction system may lead to arrhythmias and sudden cardiac death. Pancreatitis has been described and should be considered in patients with abdominal pain. Fever is often noted. Any organ maybe affected leading to a wide range of symptoms.

Laboratory Features

Laboratory evaluation usually reveals a hemolytic anemia with at least (and often more than) 2 schistocytes or greater than 1% of RBCs per 100× field on microscopic exam (Table 112.4 and Fig. 112.1) [37,38]. Coagulation studies such as the activated partial thromboplastin time and the prothrombin time are typically normal, whereas they are usually prolonged in disseminated intravascular coagulation (DIC). The Coombs test is negative. Most cases of classic acquired TTP are associated with a severe deficiency of ADAMTS-13 (<5%), and an inhibitory antibody can be demonstrated [41–43,45]. ADAMTS-13 results are often not available in real time, are not required to make the diagnosis, and should not routinely be used to make therapeutic decisions regarding the initiation of plasma exchange. ADAMTS-13 levels have prognostic value regarding the risk of relapse but are less useful in determining the likelihood of initial response to plasma exchange. Moderate decreases in ADAMTS-13 are not specific and may be seen in a variety of disorders including sepsis [43].

Schistocytes may be seen in conditions other than TTP (Table 112.9). These conditions usually have in common damage to the blood vessel endothelium, leading to the release of ultra large vWF multimers. The presentation of these syndromes may mimic TTP, although the hemolytic uremic syndrome (HUS) often presents with a primary component of renal failure [36]. Conditions other than TTP are not typically associated with a severe (<5%) deficiency of ADAMTS-13 and TPE may not be effective, although it is often initiated if HUS is suspected [36,41].

The distinction between TTP and HUS may be difficult to make. Classic childhood HUS is usually preceded by hemorrhagic diarrhea caused by *Escherichia coli* 0157:H7. Atypical HUS as seen in adults may be difficult to differentiate from TTP. Typically, renal failure is more severe and extra renal manifestations are less or absent in HUS [36,38]. Thrombocytopenia and the presence of schistocytes may be more marked. ADAMTS-13 is not usually severely depressed in HUS, suggesting a different pathophysiology between these two related conditions [41]. Atypical HUS has been linked to uncontrolled activation of the complement system due to either congenital or acquired mutations or antibodies against various factors in the complement pathway [46]. As the ability to differentiate between TTP and atypical HUS is often unclear, prompt TPE is often initiated in atypical HUS, even though efficacy may be less as compared to TTP [36,38].

Treatment

TPE with fresh frozen plasma at a 1.0 to 1.5× plasma volume should be initiated as soon as idiopathic TTP is suspected [36,38,44,45]. A dual-lumen, large bore, dialysis-type catheter is often needed for the procedure and should be promptly placed despite the coexisting thrombocytopenia. With prompt TPE, 80% to 90% of patients with classic TTP survive this once uniformly fatal disease [36–38]. The effectiveness of TPE is thought to be due to both the removal of an anti-ADAMTS-13 antibody and the replacement of ADAMTS-13 in donor fresh frozen plasma. If TPE is not readily available, FFP should be infused at a rate of 30 mL per kg per day while arrangements for TPE are made [44]. Randomized trials have supported the efficacy of TPE over simple plasma infusion which could become problematic given the large volume of FFP needed [45,47].

TPE should be continued until the platelet count and LDH have normalized for 2 days [39]. Plasma exchange is often tapered down to every other day upon remission, but this practice has not been critically studied and its efficacy in preventing relapse is uncertain. In refractory or relapsing patients, cryosupernatant plasma, devoid of vWF, should be considered [45,48]. Catheter-related infections should also be investigated and have been documented to lead to relapse. Immunosuppressants such as glucocorticoids and cyclosporine as adjuncts to plasma exchange have been used, but efficacy remains uncertain [36,38]. Aspirin has also been used for its antiplatelet effects but is often avoided until the platelet counts begin to rise [39]. Platelet transfusion is generally avoided, as it was thought to exacerbate the disease although recent data calls this into question [49].

In small case reports and case series, rituximab has been found to be effective in relapsing and refractory cases and should be considered [50,51]. Recombinant ADAMTS-13 is under development and may prove to be effective in the future.

Disseminated Intravascular Coagulation

Although microangiopathic hemolytic anemia may be present in patients with DIC, typically the thrombotic or bleeding manifestations of DIC are more clinically significant. DIC, which is often due to an underlying serious or catastrophic event such as septicemia or an obstetric emergency, will be covered in greater detail in Chapters 108 and 109.

Other Causes of Microangiopathic Hemolytic Anemia

The differential diagnosis of microangiopathic hemolytic anemia includes the other diagnoses listed in Table 112.9. Appropriate consultation and treatment should be pursued dependent on the most likely diagnosis.

HEMOGLOBINOPATHIES

Sickle Cell Anemia

Sickle cell anemia results from the presence of a point mutation leading to an amino acid substitution (valine for glutamic acid) in the sixth position of the beta chain of hemoglobin. An unstable form of hemoglobin (hemoglobin S) is produced which polymerizes in the setting of dehydration or hypoxia, a term referred to as sickling. The sickling of red cells is responsible for a variety of clinical conditions including extremely painful episodes in the back and extremities. Patients may be symptomatic if they are homozygous for hemoglobin S; if they are compound heterozygotes for hemoglobin S, hemoglobin C, hemoglobin D, and hemoglobin E; or if they also have concomitant beta thalassemia. The most common complications of sickling disorders leading to ICU admission are listed in Table 112.10.

Transfusion. Although patients with sickling disorders are nearly always anemic, transfusions are not indicated for hemodynamically stable anemia, routine vasoocclusive crisis, routine

TABLE 112.10

CRITICAL CARE COMPLICATIONS OF SICKLE CELL DISEASE

Acute chest syndrome
Acute stroke
Acute cholecystitis
Congestive heart failure
Hyperhemolysis
Pulmonary hypertension
Sepsis
Severe aplastic crisis
Delayed transfusion reaction

pregnancies, or simple surgical procedures that do not require general anesthesia. In general, hematology consultation is indicated if transfusion is considered, as the need for transfusion usually suggests a more complicated clinical scenario. Transfusion therapy can be simple, chronic, or performed via RBC exchange. Simple transfusion involves infusion of a sufficient volume of red cells to improve tissue oxygenation. Chronic simple transfusions are primarily used to prevent stroke recurrence. RBC exchange, performed (where available) via erythrocytapheresis using a noncollapsible, large bore, dialysis-type catheter, involves the removal of the patient's hemoglobin S red cells, followed by replacement of RBCs from a non–hemoglobin S donor targeting a final hemoglobin no higher than 8 to 10 g per dL with hemoglobin S less than 30%. RBC exchange is often used in the management of acute stroke or severe acute chest syndrome (ACS) as a more rapid and efficient way to remove hemoglobin S and improve oxygen delivery. Alternatively, manual exchange transfusion involves removing 500 cc of blood, followed by infusion of 300 cc normal saline, followed by another 500 cc removal of blood, and subsequent transfusion of 4 to 5 units of packed red cells [52]. Care should be taken to keep the end hemoglobin value no higher than 10 g per dL to minimize the risk for hyperviscosity.

Alloimmunization, typically to the Rh (E, C), Kell (K), Duffy (Fya, Fyb), and Kidd (Jk) antigens, occurs in up to 30% of patients [53]. Alloimmunization can be minimized by transfusing red cells that have been phenotypically matched for these red cell antigens. If phenotypically matched units are not available, crossmatched red cell units that are negative for C, E, and Kell are recommended.

Acute Chest Syndrome

Pulmonary complications frequently cause significant morbidity and mortality in patients with sickling disorders and are a common reason for ICU admission. Among the pulmonary complications, the ACS is among the most frequently observed in the ICU setting.

Clinical Features. ACS can be defined by a constellation of fever, hypoxemia, chest pain, leukocytosis, and new pulmonary infiltrate in a patient with a sickling disorder [54]. Although most common in patients homozygous for hemoglobin S, ACS can also be seen in decreasing frequency in patients with hemoglobin SC disease and $S/\beta+$ thalassemia. Importantly, the clinical definition of ACS does not indicate a specific etiology. ACS can be caused by infection, thrombosis, fat embolism, or any combination of these conditions. A large multicenter study showed that a specific cause of ACS could be identified in more than 50% of patients studied [55]. The most common etiologies observed were fat embolism and infection. Specific

TABLE 112.11

CAUSES OF THE ACUTE CHEST SYNDROME IN A 30-CENTER STUDY

Cause	Percentage
Fat embolism, with or without infection	8.8
Chlamydia	7.2
Mycoplasma	6.6
Virus	6.4
Bacteria	4.5
Mixed infections	3.7
Legionella	0.6
Miscellaneous infections	0.4
Infarction	16.1
Unknown	45.7

Adapted from Vichinsky EP, Neumayr LD, Earles AN, et al: Causes and outcomes of the acute chest syndrome in sickle cell disease. *N Engl J Med* 342:1855–1865, 2000.

etiologies of ACS from this study of 671 episodes are listed in Table 112.11.

Physiologic Markers. Secretory phospholipase A2, a potent inflammatory mediator, has been implicated as a cause of lung damage in patients with ACS [56], and serum levels may be predictive of impending ACS [57]. In addition, circulating activated endothelial progenitor cells have been proposed as a potential etiology of ACS [58].

Treatment. Treatment of ACS depends in part on the clinical presentation. If the sputum Gram stain suggests infection with a particular organism, targeted antibiotic therapy should be initiated without delay. Interestingly, although pneumococcus is a frequent cause of infection in children with ACS, it is much less common in adults, in whom mycoplasma is more frequently implicated [54]. However, when an infectious etiology of ACS is suspected, empiric coverage for pneumococcus remains appropriate. In addition, because of the high mortality associated with ACS, empiric antibiotic coverage for mycoplasma and chlamydia should also be strongly considered. Maintaining hydration and oxygenation during episodes of ACS are imperative to prevent further sickling. However, fluids must be administered carefully to avoid fluid overload. There is no data to support the routine use of anticoagulants in ACS, and in the absence of data, this practice should be avoided.

Patients with ACS and hypoxia (PO_2 <75 mm Hg) should be transfused red cells by either simple or exchange transfusion [59]. One small single-institution study found no difference between the two transfusion modalities [60]. Clinically, decisions between these two strategies are usually based on the degree of hypoxia, the pace of respiratory failure, as well as other comorbidities. Red cell exchange transfusion may be favored in the more severe or rapidly progressive cases and in critically ill patients with hemoglobin SC disease because such patients typically have baseline hemoglobin levels in the 10 to 11 g per dL range. In addition to providing a source of oxygen delivery, exchange transfusion also decreases levels of inflammatory mediators such as soluble vascular cell adhesion molecule-1 [61].

Acute Stroke

Stroke is one of the most morbid complications of sickle cell disease, with a prevalence of more than 20% in some series [62]. In addition to overt stroke, more than 60% of patients with sickle cell disease have evidence of brain damage from occult infarction that is incidentally found on magnetic resonance imaging [63]. The pathophysiology of stroke in sickle cell patients is complicated. Stroke is related to nitric oxide depletion, hypercoagulability, and abnormalities of the major cerebral arteries. Unfortunately, stroke recurrence is common with more than 50% of cases occurring within 36 months following the initial event [64]. The presence of constricted cerebral arteries with collateralization (moyamoya syndrome) is associated with recurrent stroke and may be alleviated by surgical vascular bypass [65]. Although transcranial Doppler measurement of blood velocity has predictive value for stroke in pediatric patients with sickle cell disease, the measurement of cranial blood flow velocity is less able to stratify the risk of stroke for adults [66].

Treatment. Although there have been no specific trials addressing the issue, antiplatelet agents can be used in the treatment of acute stroke in adults with sickle cell disease, similar to patients without sickle cell disease [67]. Although there are no randomized trials, retrospective studies suggest that the use of red cell exchange transfusion to increase oxygen carrying capacity to the brain in the setting of acute stroke may be of some benefit [59]. For acute stroke in patients with sickle cell disease, emergent red cell exchange transfusion to reduce hemoglobin S to less than 30% has been recommended by some experts [68]. Similarly, consensus opinion suggests that conventional angiography can be used in sickle cell patients suspected of having an aneurysmal subarachnoid hemorrhage [59]. Because of the osmotic dye load which might increase intracerebral sickling, experts also suggest exchange transfusion prior to angiography [59]. Acute retinal artery occlusion can be considered as an ophthalmic stroke. The exact pathophysiology of retinal artery occlusion in sickle cell disease and risk factors for the condition are not known [69]. Similarly, there is scant data on the treatment of retinal artery occlusion in sickle cell anemia. At this time, it is reasonable for sickle cell patients presenting with acute thrombotic stroke or acute retinal artery occlusion to undergo red cell exchange transfusion. In addition, antiplatelet agent administration appears reasonable.

Acute Cholecystitis

Patients with hemolytic disorders, including sickle cell disease, form gallstones composed of the insoluble salt, calcium bilirubinate. For sickle cell patients presenting with acute cholecystitis, laparoscopic cholecystectomy appears safe and effective [70]. A prospective trial supports the idea that most sickle cell patients undergoing cholecystectomy should receive transfusion support [71]. A randomized trial has suggested that simple preoperative transfusion to a hemoglobin level of 10 g per dL is not associated with more complications than preoperative red cell exchange transfusion to a target hemoglobin S less than 30% [72]. In addition, simple transfusion is associated with a lower rate of alloantibody formation, as fewer units of RBCs are transfused. The use of postoperative incentive spirometry is strongly encouraged due to a decreased incidence of ACS [73].

Pulmonary Hypertension

Pulmonary hypertension is a recently recognized cause of morbidity and mortality in sickle cell disease occurring in more than 30% of patients and conferring an increased death rate ratio of 10.1 [74]. Pulmonary hypertension may be secondary to nitric oxide scavenging by free hemoglobin released during hemolysis. Such scavenging can lead to synthesis of vasoconstrictors such as vascular-cell adhesion molecule 1 and E-selectin. Hemolysis also leads to the release of arginase from hemolyzed red cells, reducing nitric oxide synthesis. The formation of reactive oxygen and nitrogen species catalyzed by free hemoglobin may also lead to pulmonary vasoconstriction. Pulmonary hypertension, in conjunction with high cardiac output, is a major cause of congestive heart failure in patients with sickle cell disease.

The management of patients with sickle cell disease and pulmonary hypertension remains controversial. Some authors have noted a decreased incidence of pulmonary hypertension in retrospective studies of patients treated with hydroxyurea [75], but this finding is not universal. A small study found that therapy with sildenafil improved exercise capacity in patients with sickle cell disease and pulmonary hypertension [76]. However, a recent trial using sildenafil in children with sickle cell disease and pulmonary hypertension was prematurely suspended due to an increase incidence of adverse events including painful crisis. Speculation exists that endothelin antagonists, such as bosentan, may also be effective in reducing pulmonary pressures, although prospective trials are lacking. Such is also the case for epoprostenol and oral arginine [77].

Currently, there is insufficient evidence in the medical literature to suggest specific treatment strategies for patients with sickle cell disease and pulmonary hypertension. At a minimum, conservative management including oxygen therapy to treat hypoxia and aggressive treatment of right heart failure are recommended.

Hyperhemolysis

Patients with hyperhemolysis, characterized by a lower post-transfusion hemoglobin compared with the pretransfusion value, present with profound anemia and hemolysis despite red cell transfusion support [78]. The pathophysiology of hyperhemolysis in sickle cell disease remains unclear but may be related to a combination of bystander hemolysis, suppression of erythropoiesis, and destruction of RBCs due to contact lysis via activated macrophages [79]. There are case reports supporting the use of IVIG and corticosteroids in addition to transfusion to maintain enough RBCs to support the circulation [80]. Erythropoietin administration may also be of benefit in cases where the reticulocyte count is inadequate. Although hyperhemolysis can recur, typically it occurs as an isolated event. Prompt recognition is important to avoid life-threatening anemia in the setting of continued erythrocyte transfusion.

Aplastic Crisis

Aplastic crisis in sickle cell disease is usually secondary to either folic acid deficiency or infection with parvovirus B19. Aplasia secondary to folic acid deficiency is more common in late pregnancy when folic acid requirements are increased. Infection with parvovirus can be accompanied by marked marrow necrosis [81]. Treatment of parvovirus infection–induced aplasia in immunocompetent individuals is supportive and resolves upon clearance of the virus.

Sepsis

Because patients with sickling disorders are functionally asplenic, infection remains a common reason for hospitalization. Pneumonia is the most common infection and may be due to pneumococcal species, especially if the patient did not receive appropriate immunizations. Treatment of patient with sickle cell disease and sepsis parallels the treatment of similar patients without a coexistent hemoglobinopathy. Broad-spectrum antibiotics which can later be tailored to the most likely organism should be administered immediately. Adequate hydration must be maintained during an infectious episode to prevent further sickling of erythrocytes. Organisms responsible for sepsis in the sickle cell population can be found in Table 112.12. Consideration of immunization status is important when considering the most likely organism.

TABLE 112.12

ORGANISMS RESPONSIBLE FOR BLOOD-BORNE INFECTIONS IN PATIENTS WITH SICKLING DISORDERS

Gram-positive cocci
Staphylococcus aureus
Coagulase-negative staphylococci
Streptococcus pneumoniae
Viridans Streptococci
Enterococci
Streptococcus bovis
Gram-negative bacilli
Acinetobacter baumannii
Escherichia coli
Klebsiella spp
Anaerobes
Bacteroides spp
Fusobacterium sp
Fungi

Adapted from Chulamokha L, Scholand SJ, Riggio JM, et al: Bloodstream infections in hospitalized adults with sickle cell disease: a retrospective analysis. *Am J Hematol* 81:723–728, 2006.

Thalassemia

Patients with thalassemia can develop high output heart failure that can lead to ICU admissions. Treatment of heart failure in thalassemic patients is similar to the management of heart failure in other patient populations including the use of diuretics, angiotensin-converting enzyme inhibitors, and beta-blockers. Chelation therapy with deferasirox is recommended in patients with thalassemia major and iron overload especially if iron overload has caused cardiac toxicity. Transfusion support is required in symptomatic anemia. Unless a coexistent hemoglobinopathy is present, stroke, ACS, and other common complications of sickle cell disease are not typically seen.

Hemolytic Transfusion Reactions

Patients may experience hemolytic transfusion reactions that are either immediate (acute) or delayed. Acute hemolytic transfusion reactions (AHTRs) typically manifest with a feeling of impending doom. Subsequently, back pain, hypotension, red urine, and shock develop. Renal failure due to the massive hemoglobin load may occur, and DIC often ensues. Between the years 1990 and 1992, the majority of the 150 preventable transfusion-related fatalities reported to the Food and Drug Administration (FDA) were due to ABO-incompatible RBC transfusions leading to an AHTR [82–84]. Indeed, AHTR is typically the result of human error, in specimen collection, labeling, or transfusion [83]. Errors within the laboratory are much less common. Although this dramatic presentation is classic, it is important to note that a rise in temperature of 1°C above baseline may be the sole initial presentation of a hemolytic transfusion reaction and necessitates the cessation of transfusion of that unit of red cells and initiation of workup for transfusion reaction. In the case of an immediate hemolytic transfusion reaction, hemoglobinuria and hemoglobinemia may be seen, and reaction between the remnant of the transfused unit and the patient's pretransfusion serum can be identified. Treatment consists of stopping the transfusion as soon as the reaction is suspected, hydration, forced diuresis, and maintenance of blood pressure.

Delayed hemolytic transfusion reactions (DHTRs) typically present 1 to 4 weeks after transfusion of a unit of red cells. The patient may present with fatigue, jaundice, pallor, or red- or tea-colored urine. Patients with sickling disorders may come to medical attention due to a new or worsening pain crisis. The hemoglobin will be lower than that seen posttransfusion. The LDH and bilirubin will be increased, the reticulocyte count will likely be elevated, and the antibody screen will be positive, and a new alloantibody often identified. The DHTR is typically due to mismatches of non-ABO red cell antigens. Patients should be issued a card stating the antigen to which they have made a new alloantibody and told to present this card prior to all future transfusions. This is especially important in cases of antibodies to the Kidd antigen, as these alloantibodies are typically transient and may not be detectable on future antibody screens.

Glucose 6-Phosphate Dehydrogenase Deficiency

G6PD deficiency, a sex-linked trait primarily affecting men most commonly of African American or Mediterranean descent, is the most common erythrocyte enzyme defect in the world [85]. G6PD is necessary to maintain glutathione in its reduced state in the erythrocyte. Patients deficient in this enzyme are subject to oxidative hemolysis when exposed to certain drugs and toxins, or during episodes of infection. A sample list of drugs to be avoided in G6PD-deficient patients is provided in Table 112.13. Because acute infection makes oxidative hemolysis more likely, there has been confusion about the safety of certain drugs in G6PD-deficient patients. A list of drugs that can be safely administered to G6PD-deficient patients is shown in Table 112.14. A more exhaustive drug list can be found at many Web sites dedicated to G6PD deficiency (ex. www.g6pd.org). G6PD deficiency is seldom a major issue in critically ill patients because the anemia is typically not severe, and the patients are closely monitored. However, in solid organ transplant recipients who are exposed to oxidant drugs such as trimethoprim–sulfamethoxazole or dapsone, the diagnosis should be strongly considered in the setting of a new hemolytic or unexplained acute anemia [86].

In the more common African American variant of G6PD, enzyme levels are elevated in young reticulocytes, and therefore measurement of this enzyme should not be attempted in the

TABLE 112.13

DRUGS TO BE AVOIDED IN G6PD-DEFICIENT PATIENTS

Dapsone
Methylene blue
Nalidixic acid
Nitrofurantoin
Phenazopyridine
Primaquine
Sulfacetamide
Sulfanilamide
Sulfapyridine
Toluidine blue
Urate oxidase

Note: List is not intended to be all inclusive.
Adapted from Lichtman MA, Beutler E, Kipps TJ, et al: Williams hematology, 7th ed. New York: McGraw-Hill Medical, 2006.

TABLE 112.14

DRUGS THAT ARE SAFE IN G6PD-DEFICIENT PATIENTS

Acetaminophen
Acetylsalicylic acid
Ascorbic acid
Chloramphenicol
Chloroquine
Colchicine
Diphenhydramine
Isoniazid
Phenytoin
Procainamide
Pyrimethamine
Quinine
Streptomycin
Sulfadiazine
Sulfamethoxazole
Trimethoprim
Vitamin K

Note: List is not intended to be all inclusive.
Adapted from Lichtman MA, Beutler E, Kipps TJ, et al: Williams hematology. 7th ed. New York: McGraw-Hill Medical, 2006.

setting of an acute hemolytic episode, where the majority of circulating red cells are young.

Paroxysmal Nocturnal Hemoglobinuria

Paroxysmal nocturnal hemoglobinuria (PNH) is an acquired disease in which an abnormal stem cell clone gives rise to red cells, white cells, and platelets that lack proteins which are normally attached to the cell surface by a glycerophosphatidylinositol (GPI) anchor. Among these proteins are CD55 and CD59, which are responsible for inactivating complement on the surface of red cells. PNH cells are therefore more susceptible to complement-mediated lysis [87]. Patients with PNH may come to the attention of the intensivist with complications such as hemolysis, pancytopenia, arterial, or venous thrombosis (including the Budd–Chiari syndrome/hepatic vein thrombosis). Patients may also develop pancytopenia due to marrow hypoplasia, as there is an association with primary bone marrow disorders such as aplastic anemia, myelodysplastic syndrome (MDS), and acute myelogenous leukemia [88,89].

Flow cytometry showing the absence of GPI-linked surface molecules CD55 and CD59 on erythrocytes and granulocytes has supplanted older testing (such as the Ham's test) for the diagnosis of PNH [88]. Eculizumab has been FDA approved for the treatment of hemolysis due to PNH. Patients treated with eculizumab show markedly lower rates of hemolysis and also thrombosis [90–94] but are at increased risk for infection with meningococcus, requiring immunization prior to use [88].

Hereditary Spherocytosis

Hereditary spherocytosis (HS) is an autosomal dominant disorder, of red cell membrane skeletal proteins leading to a lack of anchoring of the red cell lipid bilayer to its skeletal backbone [95–97], leading to a characteristic spherocytic shape. Patients have lifelong hemolysis which is often well compensated. However, with even mild infections, the hemolysis can accelerate, and the patient can become more anemic. Splenomegaly is present in many patients and splenic rupture may occur after trauma. Patients with HS may present with an aplastic crisis manifested by severe reticulocytopenia and anemia often due to parvovirus B-19 infection which transiently suppresses the bone marrow's ability to produce red cells and compensate for the accelerated hemolysis [97,98]. The Coombs test will be negative and should be used to differentiate HS from warm autoimmune hemolytic anemia, which can present similarly. RBC transfusion may be administered to patients with aplastic crisis.

Hemolysis from Infectious Agents

Certain infectious pathogens cause hemolysis that can be severe or life threatening. Malaria is prototypic; infection with falciparum malaria is known as blackwater fever, due to the massive hemolysis caused by this agent. *Babesia microti* is another intracellular parasite that can lead to hemolysis. It is carried by the same tick as Lyme disease and can look like malarial forms on peripheral smear. *Bartonella bacilliformis*, the agent responsible for Oroya fever, and *Verruca peruvianis*, an extracellular parasite, can lyse red cells leading to dramatic hemolysis. In endemic regions of the world, these organisms are leading causes of hemolysis in critically ill patients. The toxin of *Clostridium welchii*, an agent of gas gangrene, may cause severe hemolysis. The bacterium produces a lysolecithinase, which attacks the red cell membrane bilayer. *Clostridium perfringens*, another agent causing gas gangrene, also leads to hemolysis via the action of phospholipases produced in its exotoxin [99]. In certain cases, the hemolysis can be severe enough to produce a disparity between the hemoglobin and the hematocrit. This infectious complication typically follows bowel or gynecologic surgery.

Hemolysis Associated with Chemical and Physical Agents

Arsenic, especially arsine gas, can lead to hemolysis, as it can elevate levels of copper in the blood. Wilson's disease, which is a disorder of copper metabolism, may present with hemolysis as part of its clinical picture [100]. Some dialysis centers have had difficulty with copper contamination of their water supply, leading to severe hemolysis [101]. Insect and spider bites, especially the bite of the brown recluse spider (*Loxosceles reclusa*), can lead to hemolysis, as can certain snakebites [102]. Severe burns can lead to hemolysis, since the red cell membrane is sensitive to temperatures more than 55°C.

Other Causes of Anemia in the Critical Care Setting

Iron deficiency leads to a hypoproliferative anemia due to the inability to synthesize hemoglobin. Iron deficiency may be caused by chronic blood loss, decreased iron intake (either from dietary reasons or from iron malabsorption as occurs in celiac sprue or following gastrointestinal bypass), or both. In the ICU, red cell transfusion is the most immediate way to correct the anemia, but in patients with a low hemoglobin but no hemodynamic compromise, oral or intravenous iron is preferred. Parenteral iron may be preferred in iron-deficient patients who have undergone gastrointestinal bypass, cancer patients, those who suffer from functional iron deficiency, patients undergoing treatment with erythropoietin, or patients with chronic kidney disease [103–106]. Iron dextran, iron sucrose, iron gluconate, and ferumoxytol are all available for intravenous use. The newer formulations of iron dextran have a lower rate of severe allergic reactions compared with older dextran preparations, but the incidence continues to remain higher than with the newer nondextran iron preparations [107–114].

TABLE 112.15

MECHANISMS OF THE ANEMIA OF CHRONIC DISEASE/CRITICAL ILLNESS

Blood loss
Phlebotomy
Active bleeding
Decreased red cell production
Decreased production of erythropoietin
Blunted response to erythropoietin
Sequestration of iron through up regulation of hepcidin
Renal dysfunction
Increased red cell destruction
Reduced red blood cell deformability

The iron deficit is calculated by the following formula: (desired hemoglobin − actual hemoglobin) × (weight in pounds) + storage iron. Storage iron is estimated at 1,000 g for men and 600 mg for women.

Megaloblastic Anemia

Megaloblastic anemia is a rare cause of anemia in the ICU but should be suspected in the individuals presenting with a macrocytic, hypoproliferative anemia (high MCV, low reticulocyte count) (Table 112.5). Vitamin B_{12} and folic acid levels should be measured, but accuracy may be affected in the acute setting. The measurement of homocysteine and methylmalonic acid (MMA) is a more sensitive way to asses for these nutritional deficiencies but can also be altered in the critically ill patient [115]. Typically, both homocysteine and MMA are elevated in B_{12} deficiency, while homocysteine alone is elevated in folic acid deficiency. Elevation of homocysteine and MMA may be the first laboratory signs of subclinical B_{12} deficiency. The peripheral smear may show oval macrocytes and hypersegmented neutrophils. Other anemias which are hypoproliferative and macrocytic include the MDS, aplastic anemia, the anemia of hypothyroidism, and liver disease (Table 112.5).

Anemia of Chronic Disease (ACD)/Inflammation

The anemia of chronic disease/inflammation is common in the ICU and its etiology is multifactorial (Table 112.15) [1]. Once thought to occur over weeks to months, the ACD has been shown to occur in less than a week and is thus thought to be a major contributor to anemia in critically ill patients [1,116]. Several studies have shown elevated levels of cytokines such as tumor necrosis factor-alpha; interleukin-6; C-reactive protein; and interferons alpha, beta, and gamma in ACD [1,117,118]. This cytokine response has been shown to inhibit erythropoietin production, blunt the erythropoietic response, and play a central role in iron metabolism, leading to the sequestration of iron. Iron metabolism is primarily mediated by the antimicrobial peptide hepcidin, which impairs the ability to export iron from gut epithelial cells and hepatocytes into the bloodstream [119]. Hepcidin is upregulated in the ACD, leading to the sequestration of iron. In the ACD, the serum iron (Fe), total iron-binding capacity (TIBC), and percentage iron saturation (iron/TIBC) are typically low. Ferritin, an acute phase reactant, is often normal or elevated, as opposed to iron deficiency where it is low. Renal failure is common in the ICU and also may contribute to the ACD, especially when progressive [1,120]. Increased red cell destruction has also been noted in the ACD due to decreased RBC deformability [1].

CONCLUSION

As demonstrated in this chapter, anemia is exceedingly common in the critical care setting, but its etiology remains very diverse. A rational approach to the evaluation of anemia includes review of the white blood count, platelet count, MCV, reticulocyte count, peripheral blood smear, and any prior CBCs that may be available. If hemolysis is suspected, LDH, bilirubin, and haptoglobin will provide additional information to support or refute this diagnosis. A Coombs test is often sent if the etiology of hemolysis remains in question. As highlighted in the chapter, certain causes of anemia such as blood loss, microangiopathic hemolytic anemia, complications of sickle cell disease, hemolysis from drugs as well as foreign devices, and ACD are seen with increased frequency in critically ill patients and should be considered in the ICU patient population. Specific treatment recommendations are based on the underlying diagnosis. Minimization of the volume and frequency of blood draws is essential. Conservative transfusion thresholds are increasingly being used in the absence of hemodynamic compromise or acute blood loss. The role of ESAs has been investigated but remains uncertain. If the etiology of the anemia remains obscure, or the management of an underlying diagnosis remains uncertain, hematology consultation is recommended.

References

1. Asare K: Anemia of critical illness. *Pharmacotherapy* 28:1267–1282, 2008.
2. Corwin HL, Gettinger A, Pearl RG, et al: The CRIT Study: anemia and blood transfusion in the critically ill—current clinical practice in the United States. *Crit Care Med* 32:39–52, 2004.
3. Corwin H, Rodriguez R, Pearl R, et al: Erythropoietin response in critically ill patients [abstract]. *Crit Care Med* 25:A82, 2010.
4. Vincent JL, Baron JF, Reinhart K, et al: Anemia and blood transfusion in critically ill patients. *JAMA* 288:1499–1507, 2002.
5. Walsh TS, Saleh EE: Anaemia during critical illness. *Br J Anaesth* 97:278–291, 2006.
6. Smoller BR, Kruskall MS, Horowitz GL: Reducing adult phlebotomy blood loss with the use of pediatric-sized blood collection tubes. *Am J Clin Pathol* 91:701–703, 1989.
7. Practice strategies for elective red blood cell transfusion. American College of Physicians. *Ann Intern Med* 116:403–406, 1992.
8. Carson JL, Duff A, Poses RM, et al: Effect of anaemia and cardiovascular disease on surgical mortality and morbidity. *Lancet* 348:1055–1060, 1996.
9. Hebert PC, Wells G, Blajchman MA, et al: A multicenter, randomized, controlled clinical trial of transfusion requirements in critical care. Transfusion Requirements in Critical Care Investigators, Canadian Critical Care Trials Group. *N Engl J Med* 340:409–417, 1999.
10. McIntyre L, Hebert PC, Wells G, et al: Is a restrictive transfusion strategy safe for resuscitated and critically ill trauma patients? *J Trauma* 57:563–568, 2004.
11. Welch HG, Meehan KR, Goodnough LT: Prudent strategies for elective red blood cell transfusion. *Ann Intern Med* 116:393–402, 1992.
12. Lacroix J, Hebert PC, Hutchison JS, et al: Transfusion strategies for patients in pediatric intensive care units. *N Engl J Med* 356:1609–1619, 2007.
13. Zarychanski R, Turgeon AF, McIntyre L, et al: Erythropoietin-receptor agonists in critically ill patients: a meta-analysis of randomized controlled trials. *CMAJ* 177:725–734, 2007.
14. Corwin HL, Gettinger A, Fabian TC, et al: Efficacy and safety of epoetin alfa in critically ill patients. *N Engl J Med* 357:965–976, 2007.
15. Napolitano LM: Current status of blood component therapy in surgical critical care. *Curr Opin Crit Care* 10:311–317, 2004.
16. Arroliga AC, Guntupalli KK, Beaver JS, et al: Pharmacokinetics and pharmacodynamics of six epoetin alfa dosing regimens in anemic critically ill patients without acute blood loss. *Crit Care Med* 37:1299–1307, 2009.
17. Cook D, Crowther M: Targeting anemia with erythropoietin during critical illness. *N Engl J Med* 357:1037–1039, 2007.
18. Brophy GM, Sheehan V, Shapiro MJ, et al: A US multicenter, retrospective, observational study of erythropoiesis-stimulating agent utilization in anemic, critically ill patients admitted to the intensive care unit. *Clin Ther* 30:2324–2334, 2008.
19. Packman CH: Hemolytic anemia due to warm autoantibodies. *Blood Rev* 22:17–31, 2008.
20. Petz LD: Cold antibody autoimmune hemolytic anemias. *Blood Rev* 22: 1–15, 2008.

21. Mollison PL: Measurement of survival and destruction of red cells in haemolytic syndromes. *Br Med Bull* 15:59–67, 1959.
22. Gribben JG: How I treat CLL up front. *Blood* 115:187–197, 2010.
23. Conley CL, Lippman SM, Ness P: Autoimmune hemolytic anemia with reticulocytopenia. A medical emergency. *JAMA* 244:1688–1690, 1980.
24. Flores G, Cunningham-Rundles C, Newland AC, et al: Efficacy of intravenous immunoglobulin in the treatment of autoimmune hemolytic anemia: results in 73 patients. *Am J Hematol* 44:237–242, 1993.
25. Valent P, Lechner K: Diagnosis and treatment of autoimmune haemolytic anaemias in adults: a clinical review. *Wien Klin Wochenschr* 120:136–151, 2008.
26. Hoffman PC: Immune hemolytic anemia—selected topics. *Hematology Am Soc Hematol Educ Program* 80–86, 2009.
27. Bussone G, Ribeiro E, Dechartres A, et al: Efficacy and safety of rituximab in adults' warm antibody autoimmune haemolytic anemia: retrospective analysis of 27 cases. *Am J Hematol* 84:153–157, 2009.
28. Berentsen S, Bo K, Shammas FV, et al: Chronic cold agglutinin disease of the "idiopathic" type is a premalignant or low-grade malignant lymphoproliferative disease. *APMIS* 105:354–362, 1997.
29. Berentsen S, Beiske K, Tjonnfjord GE: Primary chronic cold agglutinin disease: an update on pathogenesis, clinical features and therapy. *Hematology* 12:361–370, 2007.
30. Berentsen S, Ulvestad E, Gjertsen BT, et al: Rituximab for primary chronic cold agglutinin disease: a prospective study of 37 courses of therapy in 27 patients. *Blood* 103:2925–2928, 2004.
31. Gertz MA: Management of cold haemolytic syndrome. *Br J Haematol* 138: 422–429, 2007.
32. Eder AF: Review: acute Donath-Landsteiner hemolytic anemia. *Immunohematology* 21:56–62, 2005.
33. Salama A: Drug-induced immune hemolytic anemia. *Expert Opin Drug Saf* 8:73–79, 2009.
34. Johnson ST, Fueger JT, Gottschall JL: One center's experience: the serology and drugs associated with drug-induced immune hemolytic anemia—a new paradigm. *Transfusion* 47:697–702, 2007.
35. Garratty G: Drug-induced immune hemolytic anemia. *Hematology Am Soc Hematol Educ Program* 73–79, 2009.
36. George JN: Evaluation and management of patients with thrombotic thrombocytopenic purpura. *J Intensive Care Med* 22:82–91, 2007.
37. Burns ER, Lou Y, Pathak A: Morphologic diagnosis of thrombotic thrombocytopenic purpura. *Am J Hematol* 75:18–21, 2004.
38. George JN: Clinical practice. Thrombotic thrombocytopenic purpura. *N Engl J Med* 354:1927–1935, 2006.
39. Allford SL, Hunt BJ, Rose P, et al: Guidelines on the diagnosis and management of the thrombotic microangiopathic haemolytic anaemias. *Br J Haematol* 120:556–573, 2003.
40. Moake JL, Rudy CK, Troll JH, et al: Unusually large plasma factor VIII: von Willebrand factor multimers in chronic relapsing thrombotic thrombocytopenic purpura. *N Engl J Med* 307:1432–1435, 1982.
41. Furlan M, Robles R, Galbusera M, et al: von Willebrand factor-cleaving protease in thrombotic thrombocytopenic purpura and the hemolytic-uremic syndrome. *N Engl J Med* 339:1578–1584, 1998.
42. Tsai HM, Lian EC: Antibodies to von Willebrand factor-cleaving protease in acute thrombotic thrombocytopenic purpura. *N Engl J Med* 339:1585–1594, 1998.
43. Lammle B, Kremer Hovinga JA, George JN: Acquired thrombotic thrombocytopenic purpura: ADAMTS13 activity, anti-ADAMTS13 autoantibodies and risk of recurrent disease. *Haematologica* 93:172–177, 2008.
44. Sadler JE: Von Willebrand factor, ADAMTS13, and thrombotic thrombocytopenic purpura. *Blood* 112:11–18, 2008.
45. Boulmay B, Kitchens C: Evidence-based approach to the diagnosis and management of thrombotic thrombocytopenic purpura, in Crowther M, Ginsberg J, Schünemann H, et al (eds): *Evidence-Based Hematology*, Oxford, UK: Blackwell Publishing, 131–135, 2008.
46. Noris M, Remuzzi G: Atypical hemolytic-uremic syndrome. *N Engl J Med* 361:1676–1687, 2009.
47. Rock GA, Shumak KH, Buskard NA, et al: Comparison of plasma exchange with plasma infusion in the treatment of thrombotic thrombocytopenic purpura. Canadian Apheresis Study Group. *N Engl J Med* 325:393–397, 1991.
48. Obrador GT, Zeigler ZR, Shadduck RK, et al: Effectiveness of cryosupernatant therapy in refractory and chronic relapsing thrombotic thrombocytopenic purpura. *Am J Hematol* 42:217–220, 1993.
49. Swisher KK, Terrell DR, Vesely SK, et al: Clinical outcomes after platelet transfusions in patients with thrombotic thrombocytopenic purpura. *Transfusion* 49:873–887, 2009.
50. Elliott MA, Heit JA, Pruthi RK, et al: Rituximab for refractory and or relapsing thrombotic thrombocytopenic purpura related to immune-mediated severe ADAMTS13-deficiency: a report of four cases and a systematic review of the literature. *Eur J Haematol* 83:365–372, 2009.
51. Ling HT, Field JJ, Blinder MA: Sustained response with rituximab in patients with thrombotic thrombocytopenic purpura: a report of 13 cases and review of the literature. *Am J Hematol* 84:418–421, 2009.
52. Charache S: Treatment of sickle cell anemia. *Annu Rev Med* 32:195–206, 1981.
53. Roseff SD: Sickle cell disease: a review. *Immunohematology* 25:67–74, 2009.
54. Charache S, Scott JC, Charache P: "Acute chest syndrome" in adults with sickle cell anemia. Microbiology, treatment, and prevention. *Arch Intern Med* 139:67–69, 1979.
55. Vichinsky EP, Neumayr LD, Earles AN, et al: Causes and outcomes of the acute chest syndrome in sickle cell disease. National Acute Chest Syndrome Study Group. *N Engl J Med* 342:1855–1865, 2000.
56. Kuypers FA, Styles LA: The role of secretory phospholipase A2 in acute chest syndrome. *Cell Mol Biol (Noisy-le-grand)* 50:87–94, 2004.
57. Styles LA, Aarsman AJ, Vichinsky EP, et al: Secretory phospholipase A(2) predicts impending acute chest syndrome in sickle cell disease. *Blood* 96: 3276–3278, 2000.
58. van Beem RT, Nur E, Zwaginga JJ, et al: Elevated endothelial progenitor cells during painful sickle cell crisis. *Exp Hematol* 37:1054–1059, 2009.
59. Danielson CF: The role of red blood cell exchange transfusion in the treatment and prevention of complications of sickle cell disease. *Ther Apher* 6:24–31, 2002.
60. Turner JM, Kaplan JB, Cohen HW, et al: Exchange versus simple transfusion for acute chest syndrome in sickle cell anemia adults. *Transfusion* 49: 863–868, 2009.
61. Liem RI, O'Gorman MR, Brown DL: Effect of red cell exchange transfusion on plasma levels of inflammatory mediators in sickle cell patients with acute chest syndrome. *Am J Hematol* 76:19–25, 2004.
62. Verduzco LA, Nathan DG: Sickle cell disease and stroke. *Blood* 114:5117–5125, 2009.
63. Steen RG, Emudianughe T, Hankins GM, et al: Brain imaging findings in pediatric patients with sickle cell disease. *Radiology* 228:216–225, 2003.
64. Kirkham FJ: Therapy insight: stroke risk and its management in patients with sickle cell disease. *Nat Clin Pract Neurol* 3:264–278, 2007.
65. Fryer RH, Anderson RC, Chiriboga CA, et al: Sickle cell anemia with moyamoya disease: outcomes after EDAS procedure. *Pediatr Neurol* 29: 124–130, 2003.
66. Valadi N, Silva GS, Bowman LS, et al: Transcranial Doppler ultrasonography in adults with sickle cell disease. *Neurology* 67:572–574, 2006.
67. Sacco RL, Adams R, Albers G, et al: Guidelines for prevention of stroke in patients with ischemic stroke or transient ischemic attack: a statement for healthcare professionals from the American Heart Association/American Stroke Association Council on Stroke: co-sponsored by the Council on Cardiovascular Radiology and Intervention: the American Academy of Neurology affirms the value of this guideline. *Stroke* 37:577–617, 2006.
68. Lottenberg R, Hassell KL: An evidence-based approach to the treatment of adults with sickle cell disease. *Hematology Am Soc Hematol Educ Program* 58–65, 2005.
69. Liem RI, Calamaras DM, Chhabra MS, et al: Sudden-onset blindness in sickle cell disease due to retinal artery occlusion. *Pediatr Blood Cancer* 50:624–627, 2008.
70. Al-Mulhim AS, Al-Mulhim AA: Laparoscopic cholecystectomy in 427 adults with sickle cell disease: a single-center experience. *Surg Endosc* 23: 1599–1602, 2009.
71. Haberkern CM, Neumayr LD, Orringer EP, et al: Cholecystectomy in sickle cell anemia patients: perioperative outcome of 364 cases from the National Preoperative Transfusion Study. Preoperative Transfusion in Sickle Cell Disease Study Group. *Blood* 89:1533–1542, 1997.
72. Vichinsky EP, Haberkern CM, Neumayr L, et al: A comparison of conservative and aggressive transfusion regimens in the perioperative management of sickle cell disease. The Preoperative Transfusion in Sickle Cell Disease Study Group. *N Engl J Med* 333:206–213, 1995.
73. Bellet PS, Kalinyak KA, Shukla R, et al: Incentive spirometry to prevent acute pulmonary complications in sickle cell diseases. *N Engl J Med* 333: 699–703, 1995.
74. Gladwin MT, Sachdev V, Jison ML, et al: Pulmonary hypertension as a risk factor for death in patients with sickle cell disease. *N Engl J Med* 350: 886–895, 2004.
75. Ataga KI, Moore CG, Jones S, et al: Pulmonary hypertension in patients with sickle cell disease: a longitudinal study. *Br J Haematol* 134:109–115, 2006.
76. Machado RF, Martyr S, Kato GJ, et al: Sildenafil therapy in patients with sickle cell disease and pulmonary hypertension. *Br J Haematol* 130: 445–453, 2005.
77. Benza RL: Pulmonary hypertension associated with sickle cell disease: pathophysiology and rationale for treatment. *Lung* 186:247–254, 2008.
78. Petz LD, Calhoun L, Shulman IA, et al: The sickle cell hemolytic transfusion reaction syndrome. *Transfusion* 37:382–392, 1997.
79. Win N, New H, Lee E, et al: Hyperhemolysis syndrome in sickle cell disease: case report (recurrent episode) and literature review. *Transfusion* 48: 1231–1238, 2008.
80. Win N, Yeghen T, Needs M, et al: Use of intravenous immunoglobulin and intravenous methylprednisolone in hyperhaemolysis syndrome in sickle cell disease. *Hematology* 9:433–436, 2004.
81. Godeau B, Galacteros F, Schaeffer A, et al: Aplastic crisis due to extensive bone marrow necrosis and human parvovirus infection in sickle cell disease. *Am J Med* 91:557–558, 1991.
82. Goodnough LT, Brecher ME, Kanter MH, et al: Transfusion medicine. First of two parts—blood transfusion. *N Engl J Med* 340:438–447, 1999.
83. Linden JV: Errors in transfusion medicine. Scope of the problem. *Arch Pathol Lab Med* 123:563–565, 1999.

84. Mummert TB, Tourault MA: Transfusion-related fatality reports—a summary. *Nurs Manage* 25:80I, 80L, 80O, 1994.
85. Nkhoma ET, Poole C, Vannappagari V, et al: The global prevalence of glucose-6-phosphate dehydrogenase deficiency: a systematic review and meta-analysis. *Blood Cells Mol Dis* 42:267–278, 2009.
86. Cappellini MD, Fiorelli G: Glucose-6-phosphate dehydrogenase deficiency. *Lancet* 371:64–74, 2008.
87. Brodsky RA: Advances in the diagnosis and therapy of paroxysmal nocturnal hemoglobinuria. *Blood Rev* 22:65–74, 2008.
88. Hill A: Eculizumab in the treatment of paroxysmal nocturnal hemoglobinuria. *Clin Med Insights Ther* 2009:1467, 2009.
89. Hillmen P, Lewis SM, Bessler M, et al: Natural history of paroxysmal nocturnal hemoglobinuria. *N Engl J Med* 333:1253–1258, 1995.
90. Brodsky RA, Young NS, Antonioli E, et al: Multicenter phase 3 study of the complement inhibitor eculizumab for the treatment of patients with paroxysmal nocturnal hemoglobinuria. *Blood* 111:1840–1847, 2008.
91. Hill A, Hillmen P, Richards SJ, et al: Sustained response and long-term safety of eculizumab in paroxysmal nocturnal hemoglobinuria. *Blood* 106: 2559–2565, 2005.
92. Hillmen P, Hall C, Marsh JC, et al: Effect of eculizumab on hemolysis and transfusion requirements in patients with paroxysmal nocturnal hemoglobinuria. *N Engl J Med* 350:552–559, 2004.
93. Hillmen P, Young NS, Schubert J, et al: The complement inhibitor eculizumab in paroxysmal nocturnal hemoglobinuria. *N Engl J Med* 355: 1233–1243, 2006.
94. Young NS, Antonioli E, Rotoli B, et al: Safety and efficacy of the terminal complement inhibitor Eculizumab in patients with paroxysmal nocturnal hemoglobinuria: Interim Shepherd Phase III Clinical Study. ASH Annual Meeting Abstracts 108:971, 2006.
95. Gallagher PG, Ferriera JD: Molecular basis of erythrocyte membrane disorders. *Curr Opin Hematol* 4:128–135, 1997.
96. Mohandas N, Gallagher PG: Red cell membrane: past, present, and future. *Blood* 112:3939–3948, 2008.
97. Perrotta S, Gallagher PG, Mohandas N: Hereditary spherocytosis. *Lancet* 372:1411–1426, 2008.
98. Summerfield GP, Wyatt GP: Human parvovirus infection revealing hereditary spherocytosis. *Lancet* 2:1070, 1985.
99. Boyd SD, Mobley BC, Regula DP, et al: Features of hemolysis due to *Clostridium perfringens* infection. *Int J Lab Hematol* 31:364–367, 2009.
100. Balkema S, Hamaker ME, Visser HP, et al: Haemolytic anaemia as a first sign of Wilson's disease. *Neth J Med* 66:344–347, 2008.
101. Ivanovich P, Manzler A, Drake R: Acute hemolysis following hemodialysis. *Trans Am Soc Artif Intern Organs* 15:316–320, 1969.
102. McDade J, Aygun B, Ware RE: Brown recluse spider (*Loxosceles reclusa*) envenomation leading to acute hemolytic anemia in six adolescents. *J Pediatr* 156:155–157, 2010.
103. Aggarwal HK, Nand N, Singh S, et al: Comparison of oral versus intravenous iron therapy in predialysis patients of chronic renal failure receiving recombinant human erythropoietin. *J Assoc Physicians India* 51:170–174, 2003.
104. Auerbach M, Ballard H, Trout JR, et al: Intravenous iron optimizes the response to recombinant human erythropoietin in cancer patients with chemotherapy-related anemia: a multicenter, open-label, randomized trial. *J Clin Oncol* 22:1301–1307, 2004.
105. Henry DH, Dahl NV, Auerbach M, et al: Intravenous ferric gluconate significantly improves response to epoetin alfa versus oral iron or no iron in anemic patients with cancer receiving chemotherapy. *Oncologist* 12:231–242, 2007.
106. Van Wyck DB, Roppolo M, Martinez CO, et al: A randomized, controlled trial comparing IV iron sucrose to oral iron in anemic patients with nondialysis-dependent CKD. *Kidney Int* 68:2846–2856, 2005.
107. Chertow GM, Mason PD, Vaage-Nilsen O, et al: Update on adverse drug events associated with parenteral iron. *Nephrol Dial Transplant* 21: 378–382, 2006.
108. Faich G, Strobos J: Sodium ferric gluconate complex in sucrose: safer intravenous iron therapy than iron dextrans. *Am J Kidney Dis* 33:464–470, 1999.
109. Kosch M, Bahner U, Bettger H, et al: A randomized, controlled parallel-group trial on efficacy and safety of iron sucrose (Venofer) vs iron gluconate (Ferrlecit) in haemodialysis patients treated with rHuEpo. *Nephrol Dial Transplant* 16:1239–1244, 2001.
110. Laman CA, Silverstein SB, Rodgers GM: Parenteral iron therapy: a single institution's experience over a 5-year period. *J Natl Compr Canc Netw* 3: 791–795, 2005.
111. Michael B, Coyne DW, Fishbane S, et al: Sodium ferric gluconate complex in hemodialysis patients: adverse reactions compared to placebo and iron dextran. *Kidney Int* 61:1830–1839, 2002.
112. Michael B, Coyne DW, Folkert VW, et al: Sodium ferric gluconate complex in haemodialysis patients: a prospective evaluation of long-term safety. *Nephrol Dial Transplant* 19:1576–1580, 2004.
113. Silverstein SB, Rodgers GM: Parenteral iron therapy options. *Am J Hematol* 76:74–78, 2004.
114. Zumberg M, Kahn M: Acquired anemias: iron deficiency, cobalamin deficiency, and autoimmune hemolytic anemia, in Crowther M, Ginsberg J, Holger J, et al (eds): *Evidence Based Hematology*. Oxford, UK: Wiley-Blackwell, 197–205, 2008.
115. Wickramasinghe SN: Diagnosis of megaloblastic anaemias. *Blood Rev* 20: 299–318, 2006.
116. Patteril MV, vey-Quinn AP, Gedney JA, et al: Functional iron deficiency, infection and systemic inflammatory response syndrome in critical illness. *Anaesth Intensive Care* 29:473–478, 2001.
117. Jelkman W: Proinflammatory cytokines lowering erythropoietin production. *Interferon Cytokine Res* 18:555–559, 1998.
118. von AN, Muller C, Serke S, et al: Important role of nondiagnostic blood loss and blunted erythropoietic response in the anemia of medical intensive care patients. *Crit Care Med* 27:2630–2639, 1999.
119. Ganz T: Molecular pathogenesis of anemia of chronic disease. *Pediatr Blood Cancer* 46:554–557, 2006.
120. Radtke HW, Claussner A, Erbes PM, et al: Serum erythropoietin concentration in chronic renal failure: relationship to degree of anemia and excretory renal function. *Blood* 54:877–884, 1979.

CHAPTER 113 ■ THERAPEUTIC APHERESIS: TECHNICAL CONSIDERATIONS AND INDICATIONS IN CRITICAL CARE

THERESA A. NESTER AND MICHAEL LINENBERGER

TECHNICAL RATIONALE AND INSTRUMENTS

Apheresis means *to remove*. Apheresis instruments are designed to separate whole blood into its component parts to selectively remove one component and return the remaining components to the patient. By processing one or more blood volumes, a significant amount of pathologic solutes or cells may be removed while the intravascular compartment remains relatively euvolemic. In an exchange procedure, replacement fluid or blood is given back to the patient to allow plasma or red cells to be removed. With any apheresis procedure, some type of anticoagulant is added to the circuit to ensure that blood flows freely.

Centrifugation apheresis instruments use either a continuous or a discontinuous flow method to deliver blood to the separation device where blood cells and plasma are differentially sedimented according to their specific gravity. Continuous flow methods draw blood into the extracorporeal circuit, separate blood into components in the centrifugation chamber,

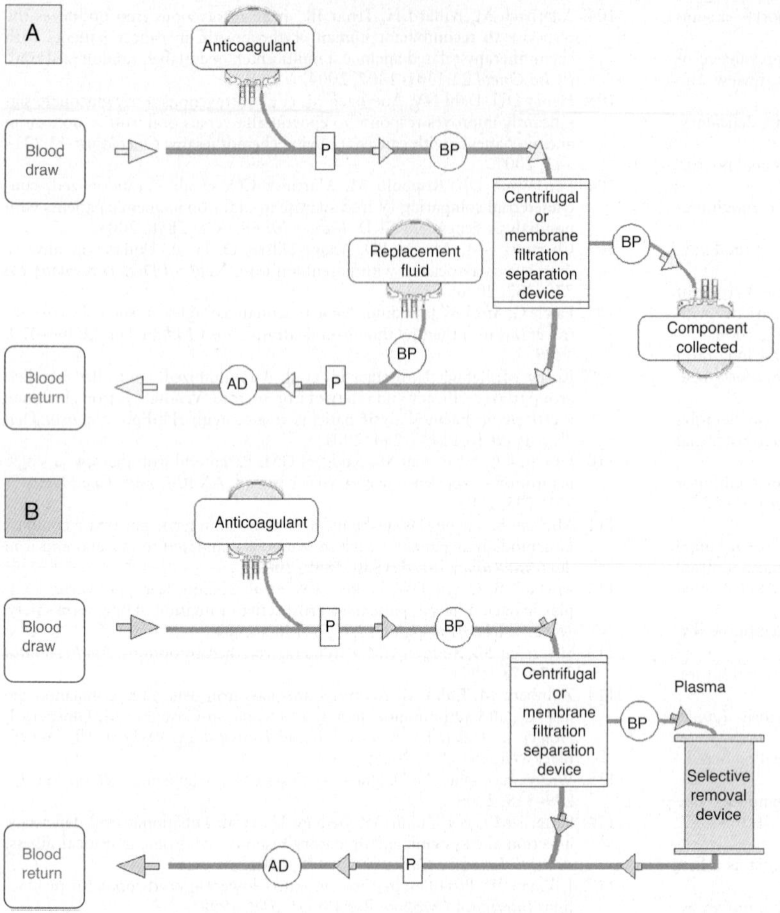

FIGURE 113.1. **A:** Basic circuitry and instrumentation of component removal in a therapeutic apheresis procedure. Anticoagulant is added to the patient's blood as it is drawn and pumped to the separation device. The component to be collected is pumped from the device to a collection bag, and the remainder of the blood is returned, along with appropriate replacement fluid, to the patient. **B:** Circuitry and instrumentation for selective removal of pathogenic substance from the patient's plasma. The patient's anticoagulated blood is pumped to the separation device, and separated plasma is then delivered to the selective removal device. The purified plasma is then combined with the cellular portion of the patient's blood and returned to the patient. AD, air detector; BP, blood pump; P, pressure monitor. [From Linenberger ML, Price TH: Use of cellular and plasma apheresis in the critically ill patient: part 1: technical and physiological considerations. *J Intensive Care Med* 20:18–27, 2005, with permission.]

divert the unwanted component into a collection bag, and return nonpathologic components to the patient without interruption (Fig. 113.1). Dual venous/catheter access is required for these procedures. Discontinuous, or intermittent, flow methods accomplish the same steps but draw, process, and return a discrete amount of blood extracorporeally before another discrete volume of blood is removed. Discontinuous procedures take a longer time than continuous procedures but require only single vein/catheter access [1].

Some apheresis instruments, predominantly used in Asia and Europe, use a membrane filtration technique to isolate plasma. The extracorporeal membrane consists of either a flat plate or a hollow fiber with a pore size that excludes cellular components from the filtrate. The plasma that is separated in the instrument is diverted for disposal or treatment, while the other blood components are returned to the patient [2].

Specialized columns and instruments have been developed over the years to treat separated plasma, with the goal of selectively removing pathogenic proteins or other solutes [3–8]. One example is hypercholesterolemia therapy. Two different columns are approved for patients with familial hypercholesterolemia who have failed combination drug therapy. The heparin-induced extracorporeal low-density lipoprotein (LDL) precipitation (HELP) system and Liposorber LA-15 system target the removal of LDLs from separated plasma [4]. Additional columns and systems have been tested and used outside the United States [5]. These include a dextran-sulfate column to remove anti-DNA and anticardiolipin antibodies and immobilized polymyxin B or other adsorbers to remove inflammatory cytokines and mediators of sepsis [6–8]. One specialized methodology, called extracorporeal photopheresis (ECP), involves isolating peripheral white blood cells by leukapheresis, treating the cells with a psoralen drug, and exposing them to ultraviolet A light before returning the photoactivated cells to the patient [9]. A dedicated instrument approved by the Food and Drug Administration (FDA) is used to perform ECP, which is beneficial for some patients with cutaneous T cell lymphoma, graft-versus-host disease after hematopoietic stem cell transplantation, systemic sclerosis, and solid organ transplant allorejection. Although ECP is usually an elective procedure, a critically ill patient may undergo treatment as part of a multimodality therapeutic approach.

PHYSIOLOGIC PRINCIPLES

The effectiveness of an apheresis procedure in reducing a plasma molecule or cellular component depends on two factors: (a) the distribution of that component between the intravascular and extravascular space and (b) the rate of regeneration of the component [10]. For solutes that move freely between intravascular and extravascular compartments, complete reequilibration between the compartments occurs at approximately 48 hours after a plasma exchange. Circulating blood cells also traffic between sites of vascular margination and/or splenic sequestration and this, in turn, can affect the efficiency of a therapeutic cytapheresis procedure.

The rate of intravascular regeneration of a pathologic solute or blood cell population after apheresis also depends on the rates of synthesis or production and decay or cell death. Plasma exchange typically removes large molecules at a rate that greatly exceeds their natural synthetic rate; thus, a simple one-compartment mathematical model is used to predict the depletion of soluble plasma substances. Assumptions of

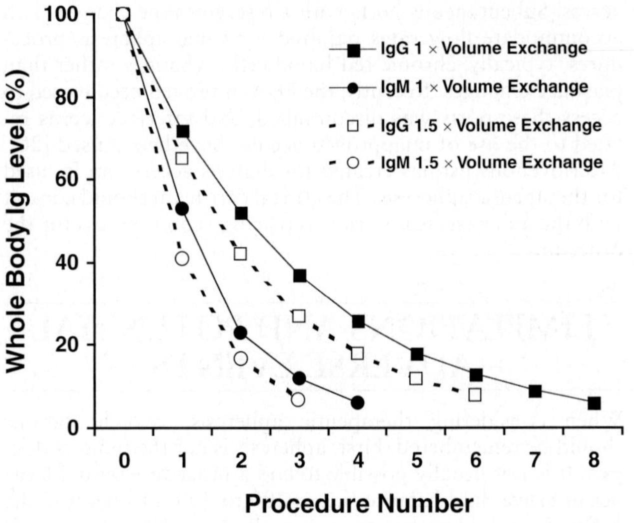

FIGURE 113.2. Hypothetical depletion of whole body immunoglobulin (Ig) levels by therapeutic plasma exchange. The 1-compartment model predicts that approximately 60% of the soluble substance will be removed from the plasma with a 1× plasma volume therapeutic exchange, and approximately 80% will be removed with a 1.5× volume exchange. Because roughly 50% of IgG distributes to the extravascular space, reequilibration between the intravascular and extravascular compartments occurs between sequential procedures, and 6 or 7 1× volume exchanges are needed to deplete whole body IgG to less than 10% of the pretreatment level. By comparison, IgM is predominantly intravascular, and, therefore, only 3 or 4 1× volume exchanges are needed to deplete whole body IgM to less than 10%. By increasing the processing to 1.5× plasma volumes, the same therapeutic goal would require three procedures to deplete IgM and five procedures to deplete IgG. [From Linenberger ML, Price TH: Use of cellular and plasma apheresis in the critically ill patient: part 1: technical and physiological considerations. *J Intensive Care Med* 20:18–27, 2005, with permission.]

the model are that the plasma removed is replaced with a fluid devoid of the target substance, and that complete mixing of the replacement fluid with the remaining intravascular plasma volume occurs [10]. Figure 113.2 depicts the kinetics of removal and regeneration of plasma immunoglobulin G (IgG) and IgM after therapeutic plasma exchange (TPE). The reliability of the one-compartment model to predict removal of soluble substances may be limited by conditions that cause an expanded plasma volume, such as paraproteinemia, molecules with rapid synthetic rates, and situations where rebound IgG production occurs, such as in the setting of humoral solid organ rejection due to a preformed antibody [11].

The efficiency of cell depletion by cytapheresis is less predictable than soluble substance removal by plasma exchange. Factors that may hinder the prediction include a rapid rate of cell production, such as occurs with untreated acute leukemia; the propensity of the spleen to sequester abnormal circulating cells or platelets; and miscalculation of the plasma volume of the patient. In general, a cytapheresis procedure in which 1.5 to 2.0 blood volumes are processed can be expected to remove approximately 35% to 85% of the target cells [12].

ANTICOAGULATION AND FLUID REPLACEMENT

Citrate is the most commonly used anticoagulant for plasma exchange and cytapheresis procedures. Heparin is often used with ECP, specialized column extraction systems, and plasma membrane filtration. Current apheresis instruments limit both the anticoagulant (citrate or heparin) dose and rate of blood return based on the patient's total blood volume. The operator can also adjust the ratio of anticoagulant to whole blood being processed.

The acid-citrate-dextrose (ACD) solution effectively chelates free or ionized plasma calcium, thereby preventing coagulation of blood and plasma in the apheresis circuit. The precise decrease in ionized calcium in vivo during an apheresis procedure is difficult to predict, as this depends on dilution, metabolism, redistribution, and excretion of infused citrate [13]. Fluid replacement with fresh frozen plasma (FFP) or albumin may decrease the ionized calcium further because of citrate in the FFP or calcium binding by albumin. Ionized calcium may typically decrease by 23% to 33%, as measured during donor apheresis procedures [14].

Citrate does not produce an anticoagulant effect in vivo. The half-life in patients with normal renal and hepatic function is approximately 30 minutes. In a patient with severe liver disease, where citrate will not be as quickly metabolized, the operator should reduce the amount and/or rate of ACD used during an exchange. In critically ill patients needing plasma exchange, it is advised that ionized calcium be monitored and intravenous calcium replacement be provided as needed. Some apheresis services use protocols for the infusion of intravenous calcium gluconate or calcium chloride during all TPEs [15].

Continuous reinfusion of extracorporeal heparin during an apheresis procedure will affect the patient's hemostatic parameters. The effect is measurable until the drug is metabolized, usually within 60 to 120 minutes of finishing the procedure. For patients already therapeutically anticoagulated with heparin, the anticoagulation normally used with apheresis may be reduced or eliminated. The primary providers of critically ill patients must communicate with the apheresis team all information regarding systemic anticoagulation, coagulopathy, and contraindications to anticoagulation, especially when heparin is planned for a therapeutic procedure. It is particularly important to document if the patient has known or suspected heparin-induced thrombocytopenia.

Replacement fluid used in plasma exchange may consist of FFP, albumin, or saline. The type of fluid depends on (a) the patient's baseline hemostatic parameters, particularly fibrinogen; (b) the anticipated number and frequency of procedures; and (c) the condition being treated. For a patient with a neurologic illness, such as acute Guillain–Barré syndrome, 1 to 1.5 plasma volume exchanges are typically performed every other day with 5% albumin as replacement fluid. This regimen and schedule allows the fibrinogen level to recover between procedures. Alternatively, if a condition requires that plasma exchange be performed daily, some FFP replacement will likely be needed to maintain the patient's fibrinogen at a hemostatic level. For conditions where a plasma component is felt to be an important part of the therapy, such as with thrombotic thrombocytopenic purpura, FFP should comprise at least half of the replacement fluid [16]. In such cases, fibrinogen and other coagulation factors will not be depleted.

An apheresis instrument that uses a centrifugation technique must deliver a specific volume of packed red cells to the separation chamber to maintain the cell/plasma density gradient necessary for efficient selective extraction. The extracorporeal blood volume (ECV) necessary for this purpose varies according to the specifications of the instrument and disposable tubing kit and the hematocrit of the patient. The AABB (formerly American Association of Blood Banks) recommends that the ECV for a general procedure should not exceed 15% of a patient's total blood volume [17]. The implications for a therapeutic apheresis procedure can be illustrated by the following example. A 60-kg adult with a hematocrit of 40% has a total blood volume of: 60 kg × 70 mL per kg (the standard conversion factor for an adult male) = 4,200 mL; and a red cell volume of 4,200 mL × 40/100 = 1,680 mL. If the instrument requires 200 mL of extracorporeal red cell volume, then the ECV required to deliver that 200 mL will be 200/1,680 = 0.12, or 12% of the total blood volume. If, however, the same patient has a hematocrit of 20%, the red cell volume will be 4,200 mL × 20/100 = 840 mL; and the required ECV will be 200/840 = 0.24 or 24% of the total blood volume, which exceeds the AABB safety limit. Allogeneic red cells are required when the ECV exceeds 15%. These are either given to the patient as a transfusion prior to the procedure (to increase their pretreatment red cell volume), or used to "prime" the apheresis circuit at the beginning of the procedure (and returned to the patient as part of the return fluid).

VASCULAR ACCESS

The type of vascular access required for therapeutic apheresis depends on the status of the patient's peripheral veins, the condition being treated, and the anticipated treatment schedule. The vein or catheter must be able to withstand negative pressures associated with inlet rates ranging from 30 to 150 mL per minute for the draw line and up to 150 mL per minute for blood being returned to the patient. For a patient needing only one exchange, it may be possible to use antecubital or forearm veins. A 16- to 18-gauge Teflon or silicone-coated steel, back-eye apheresis, or dialysis-type needle is required for the draw line. The patient ideally will be able to help by squeezing a ball during the exchange.

A large bore central venous catheter is often required for critically ill patients, especially those requiring daily procedures [18,19]. Temporary or long-term tunneled catheters for adults weighing more than 40 kg should be at least 10-French size (Table 113.1). Smaller diameter short-term catheters are acceptable for smaller adults and pediatric patients. Plastic central venous catheters such as those used for cardiac pressure monitoring are not adequate for the draw line because they collapse under the negative pressure generated from the high inlet flow rate. These catheters or a peripheral vein may be useful as return access under certain circumstances.

Peripherally inserted central venous catheter (PICC) lines and standard port-a-catheters are also not options for venous access. Subcutaneous ports with a reservoir-type chamber can accommodate flow rates required for some apheresis procedures, typically, chronic red blood cell exchanges rather than plasma exchanges. Recently, the FDA-approved needle used to access these ports was discontinued, and safety concerns related to the use of unapproved needles have been raised [20]. Arteriovenous fistulas created for dialysis access can be used for therapeutic apheresis. The critical care team should consult with the apheresis team prior to placing venous access for the procedure.

LIMITATIONS AND POTENTIAL ADVERSE EVENTS

When considering therapeutic apheresis, two limitations should be remembered. First, apheresis is not the same as dialysis. It is not usually possible to end a procedure with a large net negative fluid balance (i.e., >200 to 400 mL) because the deficit is colloid rather than crystalloid, and hypotension is likely to occur. A safe end fluid balance is plus or minus 10% to 15% of the total blood volume. In addition, it is not recommended that red cells be transfused during the apheresis procedure (other than at the start as a blood "prime") because the cell separation gradient and cell/plasma interface in the separation chamber may be disturbed. The second limitation is that the procedure is almost always an adjunctive, rather than definitive, therapy for the condition being treated. Thus, while apheresis can be performed on very ill patients, one must carefully consider the risks that are associated with hemodynamic instability, hematologic abnormalities, the need for vascular access, and the priorities for more urgent primary treatments.

Possible adverse complications related to therapeutic apheresis are shown in Table 113.2. Central line complications include procedure-related events, infection, and bleeding (Chapter 2). Citrate toxicity occurs in approximately 0.8% to 1.2% of therapeutic procedures [21]. Higher risk is associated with larger process volumes, longer procedure duration, nonphysiological bleeding, severe anemia, unstable vital signs, liver failure, alkalosis due to hyperventilation, and use of replacement fluid consisting of blood components that contain citrate as the anticoagulant [17,22]. Signs and symptoms of hypocalcemia can include a metallic taste in the mouth, muscle

TABLE 113.1

CATHETER RECOMMENDATIONS BASED ON PATIENT WEIGHT

Patient weight	Catheter name	Manufacturer	Size/Gauge
Percutaneous (nontunneled) catheters for short-term apheresis			
35–70 kg	Quinton Mahurkar	Kendall	10–11.5 Fr 12 Fr (triple lumen)
	Duo-Flow XTP	Medcomp	9 Fr
>70 kg	Quinton Mahurkar	Kendall	10–11.5 Fr 12 Fr (triple lumen)
	Hemo-Cath	Medcomp	11.5 Fr
Tunneled catheters for long-term apheresis			
35–70 kg	Quinton Permcath	Kendall	10 Fr
>70 kg	Hickman TriFusion	BARD	12 Fr (triple lumen)
	VasCath	BARD	
	Ash Split Cath	Medcomp	13 Fr
	Mahurkar Cuffed	Kendall	14 Fr
	TAL PALINDROME	Kendall	13.5 Fr 14.5 Fr

Fr, French.

TABLE 113.2

POSSIBLE ADVERSE EFFECTS OF THERAPEUTIC APHERESIS

Central venous catheter-associated complications
Signs and symptoms of hypocalcemia and/or hypomagnesemia
Hypotension related to vasovagal reactions or fluid shifts
Transfusion reactions
Altered hemostatic parameters
Bradykinin reaction in patients on ACE inhibitors undergoing plasma exchange or plasma treatment
Removal of highly protein-bound drugs or immunoglobulins (with frequent plasma exchanges)

ACE, angiotensin-converting enzyme.

or gastrointestinal cramps, perioral numbness, distal paresthesias, and chest tightness. In sedated or unconscious patients, severe citrate toxicity may manifest as tetany, muscle spasm including laryngospasm, a prolonged QTc interval and decreased myocardial contractility [23]. Hypomagnesemia and hypokalemia may also occur, as the kidneys increase cation excretion into the urine to facilitate excretion of the citrate load. Although rare, fatal arrhythmias have occurred during therapeutic apheresis. To avoid these complications, ionized calcium should be monitored and intravenous calcium infused, as indicated, either through the return line or as an additive with the albumin replacement fluid.

Hypotension or vasovagal reactions occur in roughly 0.5% to 2.9% of therapeutic apheresis procedures [23,24]. Patients with preexisting hemodynamic instability or diminished vascular tone, as seen in certain neurologic disorders, may be at particular risk. In such patients, a net negative end fluid balance must be avoided. Transfusion reactions may occur if blood components are part of the replacement fluid. Allergic reactions have also been reported in some patients receiving albumin as the replacement fluid.

Hemostatic alterations and bleeding may occur in severely ill patients with baseline coagulopathy and/or severe thrombocytopenia. A typical 1.3-volume plasma exchange using albumin depletes most coagulation factors to approximately 25% to 45% of their preprocedure values [25]. Repletion time of these coagulation factors depends on their respective rates of synthesis, with most factors returning to baseline values by 24 hours. The exception is fibrinogen, which takes about 3 days to return to baseline values. Because fibrinogen levels are the most severely affected during the course of a series of plasma exchanges, preprocedure fibrinogen levels should be monitored, especially if the replacement fluid does not include at least 50% plasma. Therapeutic leukapheresis removes a portion of circulating platelets, and this decrement could be clinically significant in a patient with preprocedure severe thrombocytopenia. The postprocedure platelet count and coagulation status should be monitored in a critically ill patient, particularly if an invasive procedure is needed shortly after apheresis.

In some patients undergoing plasma exchange with albumin as the replacement fluid, a severe reaction consisting of flushing, hypotension, bradycardia, and dyspnea has been linked to concomitant use of angiotensin-converting enzyme (ACE) inhibitors [26]. This reaction is mediated by bradykinin, which is thought to be generated by prekallikrein-activating factor in the albumin preparation. These reports have led to the recommendation that ACE inhibitors be withheld for 24 to 48 hours (depending on the half-life of the specific drug) before plasma exchange using albumin [26]. If an emergency exchange is required in a patient on an ACE inhibitor, FFP should be used as the replacement fluid to avoid this reaction. Similar reactions involving ACE inhibitors have been seen in patients undergoing plasma treatment with specialized columns; thus, similar precautions must be followed [27].

An additional potential adverse effect of repeated plasma exchange is the removal of highly protein-bound therapeutic drugs and plasma immunoglobulins. The exact effects of exchange on individual drug levels have not been delineated. To avoid this complication, medications should be administered following a plasma exchange procedure whenever possible. Immunoglobulin levels should also be measured periodically in immunosuppressed patients undergoing a series of plasma exchanges, as these proteins will be nonselectively depleted from the circulation, and severe hypogammaglobulinemia could further predispose the patient to infections [28].

INDICATIONS IN CRITICAL CARE

Evidence-based guidelines for clinical applications are published by the American Society for Apheresis (ASFA) every few years [29]. Medical conditions are placed into categories from I to IV, with I indicating that therapeutic apheresis is known to be an effective primary or adjunct therapy based on randomized controlled clinical trials or broad noncontroversial experience, and category IV indicating no demonstrated efficacy, and possibly even a negative impact of therapeutic apheresis for the condition. Examples of evidence-based indications for therapeutic apheresis are shown in Table 113.3.

Therapeutic Plasma Exchange

In the intensive care unit, TPE is likely to be the most frequent apheresis procedure used. Antibody-mediated conditions known to respond to plasma exchange include idiopathic thrombotic thrombocytopenic purpura [16,30,31]; demyelinating diseases including acute inflammatory demyelinating polyneuropathy/Guillain–Barré syndrome [32–34]; severe, acute idiopathic inflammatory demyelinating diseases (Table 113.4); myasthenic crisis [43,44]; demyelinating polyneuropathy with IgG and IgA [45,46]; antiglomerular basement membrane (Goodpasture's) disease; and pulmonary hemorrhage associated with other forms of rapidly progressive glomerulonephritis (RPGN) [47,48]. Among patients with RPGN, the evidence supporting a potential benefit of plasma exchange derives from retrospective and case-control studies among more severely affected patients [49,50], whereas randomized controlled trials have yielded supportive results in some studies [38] but not others [39,40] (see Table 113.4). For patients with renal vasculitis due to causes other than anti-GBM disease, a review of randomized controlled clinical trials demonstrated a significant reduction in end-stage renal disease with use of TPE [41].

With the muscle-specific receptor tyrosine kinase antibody (MuSK-Ab) form of myasthenia gravis, TPE appears to be a more effective therapy than intravenous immunoglobulin (IVIg) infusion [51]. By comparison, with the acetyl cholinesterase receptor (AChR-Ab) form of myasthenia gravis, and with Guillain–Barré syndrome, plasma exchange is effective but not superior to or as tolerable as IVIg infusion [33,34,41] (see Table 113.4). For patients with acute attacks of demyelination, plasma exchange may be useful. Although there is only one randomized controlled trial [37], observations from this study and retrospective data indicate that at least 50% of patients with neuromyelitis optica (NMO), characterized by spinal and visual involvement, achieve increased function with plasma exchange, and that patients with steroid-refractory optic neuritis may also achieve some benefit [52]. A potential

TABLE 113.3

EVIDENCE-BASED INDICATION CATEGORIES FOR THERAPEUTIC APHERESIS FOR DISORDERS POTENTIALLY AFFECTING CRITICALLY ILL PATIENTS

Disease	Apheresis procedure	Indication Category	Recommendation Grade
Renal			
Antiglomerular basement membrane antibody disease	Plasma exchange	I	1A
ANCA-associated rapidly progressive glomerulonephritis (dialysis dependence or diffuse alveolar hemorrhage [DAH])	Plasma exchange	I	1A 1C for DAH
Immune complex rapidly progressive glomerulonephritis	Plasma exchange	III	2B
Myeloma cast nephropathy	Plasma exchange	II	2B
Hemolytic uremic syndrome (typical, diarrhea associated)	Plasma exchange	IV	1C
Allograft rejection (antibody mediated)	Plasma exchange	I	IB
Autoimmune and rheumatologic			
Cryoglobulinemia (severe/symptomatic)	Plasma exchange	I	IB
Idiopathic thrombocytopenic purpura	Plasma exchange	IV	1C
Systemic lupus erythematosus cerebritis or DAH	Plasma exchange	II	2C
Systemic lupus erythematosus nephritis	Plasma exchange	IV	1B
Catastrophic antiphospholipid syndrome	Plasma exchange	II	2C
Hematologic			
Thrombotic thrombocytopenic purpura	Plasma exchange	I	1A
Hyperleukocytosis with leukostasis	Leukapheresis	I	1B
Sickle cell disease with acute stroke	Red cell exchange	I	1C
Sickle cell disease with acute chest syndrome	Red cell exchange	II	1C
Thrombocytosis (symptomatic, myeloproliferative origin)	Plateletpheresis	II	2C
Posttransfusion purpura	Plasma exchange	III	2C
Polycythemia vera or erythrocytosis	Erythrocytapheresis	III	2C
Hyperviscosity (monoclonal IgM, IgA, IgG)	Plasma exchange	I	1B
Coagulation factor inhibitors	Plasma exchange	IV	2C
Babesiosis (severe)	Red cell exchange	I	1B
Malaria (severe)	Red cell exchange	II	2B
Neurologic			
Acute inflammatory demyelinating polyradiculopathy (Guillain–Barré syndrome)	Plasma exchange	I	1A
Acute disseminated encephalomyelitis	Plasma exchange	II	2C
Chronic inflammatory demyelinating polyradiculopathy	Plasma exchange	I	1B
Myasthenia crisis	Plasma exchange	I	1A
Demyelinating polyneuropathy with IgG and IgA	Plasma exchange	I	1B
Demyelinating polyneuropathy with IgM	Plasma exchange	I	1C
Lambert-Eaton myasthenia syndrome	Plasma exchange	II	2C
Multiple sclerosis (acute, fulminant)	Plasma exchange	II	1B
Neuromyelitis optica	Plasma exchange	II	1C
Other disorders			
Drug overdose and poisoning	Plasma exchange	III	2C
Acute hepatic failure	Plasma exchange	III	2B
Toxic epidermal necrolysis	Plasma exchange	N/A	N/A
Severe sepsis and multiple-organ dysfunction syndrome	Plasma exchange	III	2B
Burn shock resuscitation	Plasma exchange	IV	2B

IgA, immunoglobulin A; IgG, immunoglobulin G; IgM, immunoglobulin M.
Category I: Disorders for which apheresis is accepted as first-line therapy, either as a primary standalone treatment or in conjunction with other modes of treatment. *Category II*: Disorders for which apheresis is accepted as second-line therapy, either as a standalone treatment or in conjunction with other modes of treatment. *Category III*: Disorders for which the optimum role of apheresis therapy is not established. Decision making should be individualized. *Category IV*: Disorders in which published evidence demonstrates or suggests apheresis to be ineffective or harmful. IRB approval is desirable if apheresis treatment is undertaken in these circumstances. N/A indicates that the disorder is not ranked by the ASFA criteria.
Note: The Grade system has also been assigned in an effort to parallel an approach more commonly used to evaluate therapeutic recommendations. Adapted from Guyatt G, Gutterman D, Baumann MH, et al: Grading strength of recommendations and quality of evidence in clinical guidelines: report from an American college of chest physicians task force. *Chest* 129:174–181, 2006; also Adapted from evidence-based indications categorizations generated by the American Society for Apheresis (ASFA) Apheresis Applications Committee. Zbigniew M, Szczepiorkowski (eds): Clinical applications of therapeutic apheresis: an evidence based approach. 5th edition. *J Clin Apher* 25(3), 2010.

TABLE 113.4

RANDOMIZED CONTROLLED TRIALS AND SYSTEMATIC REVIEWS OF RANDOMIZED CONTROLLED TRIALS THAT UTILIZED THERAPEUTIC APHERESIS FOR DISORDERS IN CRITICAL CARE PATIENTS

Disease category [Ref.]	n	Intervention	Outcome
Severe sepsis and septic shock [35]	106	Plasma exchange (PE) vs. standard therapy	**28-d mortality** 18/54 (33%) PE 28/52 (54%) Control ($p = 0.05$)
Sepsis syndrome [36]	30	Plasma filtration (PF) vs. standard therapy	**14-d mortality** 8/14 (57%) PF 8/16 (50%) Control ($p = 0.73$)
Acute inflammatory demyelinating polyradiculopathy/Guillain–Barré syndrome (systematic review of six trials) [33]	649	PE vs. supportive care	**Mechanical ventilation at 4 wk** 85/315 (27%) Control 44/308 (14%) PE (RR 0.53; 95% CI 0.39–0.74, $p = 0.0001$) **Severe sequelae at 1 y** 55/328 (17%) Control 35/321 (11%) PE (RR 0.65; 95% CI 0.44–0.96, $p = 0.03$) **1-y mortality** 18/328 (5.5%) Control 15/321 (4.7%) PE (RR 0.85; 95% CI 0.42–1.45, $p = 0.70$)
Acute inflammatory demyelinating polyradiculopathy/Guillain–Barré syndrome (systematic review of five trials) [34]	582	PE vs. intravenous immunoglobulin (IVIg)	**Median time to discontinuation of mechanical ventilation (two studies)** 34 d ($n = 34$) PE vs. 27 d ($n = 29$) IVIg (p = NS) 29 d ($n = 40$) PE vs. 26 d ($n = 44$) IVIg (p = NS) **Mortality during follow-up** 9/286 (3.1%) PE 7/296 (2.4%) IVIg (RR 0.78; 95% CI 0.31–1.95, p = NS)
Severe, acute idiopathic inflammatory demyelinating diseases of the central nervous system, including multiple sclerosis [37]	22	Active PE vs. sham PE (crossover allowed)	**≥Moderate acute improvement** 8/19 (42%) Active PE therapy 1/17 (6%) Sham PE therapy
Rapidly progressive glomerulonephritis (RPGN), including antiglomerular basement membrane (anti-GBM) disease and antineutrophil cytoplasmic antibody (ANCA) associated disease [38]	44	PE vs. immunoadsorption (IA)	**6-mo median creatinine clearance** 49 mL/min PE 49 mL/min IA **6-mo mortality** 1/23 (4.3%) PE 2/21 (9.5%) IA (p = NS)
RPGN, including anti-GBM disease and ANCA-associated disease [39]	33	PE vs. standard therapy with immunosuppression	**Dialysis-free survival among patients with type III RPGN** 42% PE ($n = 18$) 49% Control ($n = 15$; p = NS)
RPGN, including anti-GBM disease and ANCA-associated disease [40]	32	PE vs. standard therapy with immunosuppression	**Patients on dialysis at study end** 3/16 (19%) PE 5/16 (31%) Control (p = NS)
Renal vasculitis (adult) other than anti-GBM (systematic review of six trials) [41]		Use of PE	**3-mo response rate** Significant reduction in risk of end-stage renal disease ($p = 0.01$) **12-mo response rate** Significant reduction in risk of end-stage renal disease ($p = 0.002$)
Thrombotic thrombocytopenic purpura [16]	102	PE vs. plasma infusion (PI)	**6-mo response rate** 40/51 (78%) PE 25/51 (49%) PI ($p = 0.002$) **6-mo mortality** 11/51 (22%) PE 19/51 (37%) PI ($p = 0.036$)
Myasthenia gravis [42]	87	PE vs. intravenous immunoglobulin (IVIg)	**Day 15 variation of myasthenic muscular score** +18 PE ($n = 41$) +15.5 IVIg ($n = 46$; $p = 0.65$)

CI, confidence interval; n, number; NS, not significant; RR, relative risk; vs., versus.

mechanism of action of TPE with NMO is modulation of the serum autoantibody NMO-IgG, which has been implicated in disease pathophysiology [53].

The optimum role of TPE in the setting of severe sepsis and multiorgan dysfunction is not established. Two randomized controlled trials in adults using either continuous plasma filtration versus supportive care [36] or plasma exchange versus standard care [35] have been published. No differences were observed in the 14-day mortality rates of 14 patients with sepsis syndrome receiving 34 hours of continuous plasma filtration and 16 untreated control patients (57% vs. 50%) [36] (see Table 113.4). By comparison, the 28-day mortality rate was 33.3% among 54 patients with sepsis and septic shock treated with one or two TPE treatments compared with 53.8% among 52 nontreated control patients ($p = 0.05$) [35] (see Table 113.4). When differences between the control and experimental groups were considered using multiple logistic regression, the significance of the treatment variable on mortality was $p = 0.07$.

A nonrandomized observational cohort study evaluated hemodynamic and mortality outcomes in critically ill surgical patients with sepsis treated with TPE and continuous venovenous hemofiltration [54]. No overall difference in mortality was observed between treated patients and an untreated historical control group (42% vs. 46%); however, patients with organ failure limited to one or two systems appeared to benefit, with mortality rates of 10% among 10 treated patients versus 38% among 16 untreated control patients [54]. Although encouraging, these data must be supported by results from additional well-designed randomized controlled trials before plasma exchange can be recommended as a noninvestigational therapy for this indication [55].

Use of red blood cell exchange may be warranted for selected patients with sickle cell disease who are experiencing stroke, acute chest syndrome (ACS), priapism, or multiple organ failure as a complication of their disease [56]. Because automated red cell exchange (also called erythrocytapheresis) can more rapidly reduce the level of hemoglobin S-positive cells (to the goal of <30%) while maintaining euvolemia and minimizing hyperviscosity complications, this modality has been utilized in preference to simple transfusion by many centers. Although this makes intuitive sense, the data needed to show a clear advantage of automated red cell exchange over simple transfusion are lacking. An observational, retrospective cohort analysis found no differences in postprocedure and total lengths of stay for patients with ACS treated with automated red cell exchange ($n = 20$) compared with those who received simple transfusion support ($n = 20$) [57]. Moreover, the apheresis group required, on average, four times as many units of donor red cells.

Manual exchange transfusion, in which phlebotomized blood is replaced by simple transfusions of allogeneic red cells and FFP, has the added theoretical advantage of reducing the levels of plasma inflammatory mediators, which might augment vaso-occlusive tissue injury in patients with ACS [58]. One nonrandomized trial used a combination of TPE and automated red cell exchange for 7 patients with severe ACS and multiorgan failure, and observed an 86% 1-year survival [59]. Despite these observations, the optimal approach for critically ill patients with ACS and other severe complications remains undefined, in part because crossmatch-compatible blood may be very difficult to locate for heavily transfused sickle cell patients with multiple alloantibodies. Adequately powered randomized clinical trials are sorely needed to clarify the indications for automated or manual red cell exchange versus simple transfusion support and the potential role of TPE.

Red cell exchange may also be useful in patients with severe clinical manifestations of falciparum malaria or babesiosis [60,61]. Although a meta-analysis performed in 2002 showed no survival benefit of red cell exchange compared with antimalarials and aggressive supportive care alone [62], many case reports and series suggest a benefit in clinical status with rapid reduction of hyperparasitemia using adjunctive manual or automated red cell exchange [61,63,64]. The Centers for Disease Control and Prevention (CDC) also recommends consideration of red cell exchange as adjunctive therapy if *Plasmodium falciparum* parasitemia is greater than 10%, or if the patient has severe malaria manifested by nonvolume overload pulmonary edema, renal complications, or cerebral malaria [65]. Quinidine administration should not be delayed and may be given concurrently with the exchange. As in fulminant malaria, several case reports demonstrate that patients with overwhelming parasitemia from Babesia also quickly respond to red cell exchange [61].

Automated red cell exchange may be considered as an alternative to large volume phlebotomy in selected patients with uncontrolled erythrocytosis and polycythemia vera with acute thromboembolism, severe microvascular complications, or bleeding [66]. This method can quickly and more safely normalize the hematocrit in patients who are hemodynamically unstable.

Leukapheresis

Leukapheresis (i.e., selective removal of white blood cells) is commonly used in patients with acute myeloid leukemia (AML) experiencing symptoms of intravascular leukostasis. Signs and symptoms typically manifest as neurologic alterations (confusion, mental status changes, altered level of consciousness) or pulmonary compromise (hypoxemia, diffuse lung infiltrates). Leukapheresis is indicated in patients with AML and a circulating blast count greater than 50,000 per μL who are clearly demonstrating signs of intravascular leukostasis (i.e., symptoms not attributable to infection, bleeding, or metabolic derangements) [67,68]. Leukapheresis may be warranted sooner in monocytic subtypes of AML, as signs of intravascular leukostasis may be seen at blast counts less than 50,000 per μL or after the start of chemotherapy. Prophylactic leukapheresis should be considered in AML patients with circulating blast counts greater than 100,000 per μL, particularly if the count is rapidly rising and definitive therapy with induction chemotherapy is delayed [refer to ASFA Guideline Ref]. In comparison with AML, leukostasis complications are rare in patients with acute lymphoblastic leukemia (ALL) and circulating blast counts less than 400,000 per μL. Studies have shown that prophylactic leukapheresis for asymptomatic patients with ALL and hyperleukocytosis does not offer additional benefit above aggressive supportive care and chemotherapy [69].

Plateletpheresis

Plateletpheresis should be considered as an urgent intervention in patients experiencing thrombosis or hemorrhage in the setting of uncontrolled thrombocytosis associated with a stem cell disorder [70]. Such stem cell disorders include essential thrombocythemia, polycythemia vera, idiopathic myelofibrosis, or unclassified myeloproliferative neoplasm. The goal of the plateletpheresis is to decrease the count below 1 million per μL, with a target closer to 500,000 per μL [70]. Plateletpheresis may also be indicated for the management of perioperative thrombohemorrhagic complications in patients with myeloproliferative neoplasms undergoing splenectomy [71].

For any apheresis procedure, consultation with the apheresis team can be useful in assessing experience and available data for a given condition. The apheresis physician and team should be viewed as partners in determining the treatment plan. Initial discussion with the apheresis physician will include whether the indication is urgent or routine, the impact of apheresis on other treatment modalities, volume management, fluid replacement, and vascular access. Ongoing discussions should continue through the patient's course so that appropriate adjustments can be made to optimize the therapy.

References

1. Burgstaler EA: Current instrumentation for apheresis, in McLeod BC, Price TH, Weinstein R (eds): *Apheresis: Principles and Practice*. 2nd ed. Bethesda, MD, AABB, 2003, pp 95–130.
2. Siami GA, Siami FS: Membrane plasmapheresis in the United States: a review over the last 20 years. *Ther Apher* 5:315–332, 2001.
3. Levi J, Degani N: Correcting immune imbalance: the use of Prosorba column treatment for immune disorders. *Ther Apher Dial* 7:197–205, 2003.
4. Mabuchi H, Koizumi J, Shimzu M, et al: Long-term efficacy of low-density lipoprotein apheresis on coronary heart disease in familial hypercholesterolemia. *Am J Cardiol* 82:1489–1495, 1998.
5. Siami GA, Siami FS: The current status of therapeutic apheresis devices in the United States. *Int J Artif Organs* 25:499–502, 2002.
6. Schneider M, Gaubitz M, Perniok A: Immunoadsorption in systemic connective tissue diseases and primary vasculitis. *Ther Apher* 2:117–120, 1997.
7. Kutsuki H, Takata S, Yamamoto K, et al: Therapeutic selective adsorption of anti-DNA antibody using dextran sulfate cellulose column (Selesorb) for the treatment of systemic lupus erythematosus. *Ther Apher* 2:18–24, 1998.
8. Kodama M, Tani T, Hanasawa H, et al: Treatment of sepsis by plasma endotoxin removal: hemoperfusion using a polymyxin-B immobilized column. *J Endotoxin Res* 4:293–297, 1997.
9. Knobler R, Barr LM, Couriel DR, et al: Extracorporeal photopheresis: past, present, and future. *J Am Acad Dermatol* 61:652–665, 2009.
10. Brecher ME: Plasma exchange: why we do what we do. *J Clin Apher* 17: 207–211, 2002.
11. Tobian AA, Shirey RS, Montogomery RA, et al: The critical role of plasmapheresis in ABO-incompatible renal transplantation. *Transfusion* 48: 2453–2460, 2008.
12. Hester J: Therapeutic cell depletion, in McLeod BC, Price TH, Weinstein R (eds): *Apheresis: Principles and Practice*. 2nd ed. Bethesda, MD, AABB, 2003, pp 283–294.
13. Crookston KP, Simon TL: Physiology of apheresis, in McLeod BC, Price TH, Weinstein R (eds): *Apheresis: Principles and Practice*. 2nd ed. Bethesda, MD, AABB, 2003, pp 71–79.
14. Bolan CD, Greer SE, Cecco SA, et al: Comprehensive analysis of citrate effects during plateletpheresis in normal donors. *Transfusion* 41:1165–1171, 2001.
15. Weinstein R: Prevention of citrate reactions during therapeutic plasma exchange by constant infusion of calcium gluconate with the return fluid. *J Clin Apher* 11:204–210, 1996.
16. Rock GA, Shumak KH, Buskard NA, et al: Comparison of plasma exchange with plasma infusion in the treatment of thrombotic thrombocytopenic purpura. The Canadian Apheresis Study Group. *N Engl J Med* 325:393–397, 1991.
17. Jones HG, Bandarenko N: Management of the therapeutic apheresis patient, in McLead BC, Price TH, Weinstein R (eds): *Apheresis: Principles and Practice*. 2nd ed. Bethesda, MD, AABB, 2003, pp 253–282.
18. Schonermarck U, Bosch T: Vascular access for apheresis in intensive care patients. *Ther Apher Dial* 7:215–220, 2003.
19. Feller-Kopman D: Ultrasound-guided internal jugular access: a proposed standardized approach and implications for training and practice. *Chest* 132:302–309, 2007.
20. Powers ML, Lublin D, Eby D, et al: Safety concerns related to use of unapproved needles for accessing implantable venous access devices. *Transfusion* 49:2008–2009, 2009.
21. McLeod BC, Sniecinski I, Ciavarella D, et al: Frequency of immediate adverse effects associated with therapeutic apheresis. *Transfusion* 39:282–288, 1999.
22. Lu Q, Nedelcu E, Ziman A, et al: Standardized protocol to identify high-risk patients undergoing therapeutic apheresis procedures. *J Clin Apher* 23: 111–115, 2008.
23. Korach JM, Berger P, Giraud C, et al: Role of replacement fluids in the immediate complications of plasma exchange. French Registry Cooperative Group. *Intensive Care Med* 24:452–458, 1998.
24. Bramiage CP, Schroder K, Bramlage P, et al: Predictors of complication in therapeutic plasma exchange. *J Clin Apher* 24:225–231, 2009.
25. Chirnside A, Urbaniak SJ, Prowse CV, et al: Coagulation abnormalities following intensive plasma exchange on the cell separator, II: effects on factors I, II, V, VII, VIII, IX, X, and antithrombin III. *Br J Haematol* 48:627–634, 1981.
26. Owen HG, Brecher ME: Atypical reactions associated with use of angiotensin-converting enzyme inhibitors and apheresis. *Transfusion* 34: 891–894, 1994.
27. Olbricht CJ, Schaumann D, Fischer D: Anaphylactoid reactions, LDL apheresis with dextran sulfate, and ACE inhibitors [letter]. *Lancet* 340:908–909, 1992.
28. Wing EJ, Bruns FJ, Fraley DS, et al: Infectious complications with plasmapheresis in rapidly progressive glomerulonephritis. *JAMA* 244:2423–2426, 1980.
29. Zbigniew M, Szczepiorkowski (eds): Clinical applications of therapeutic apheresis: an evidence based approach. 5th edition. *J Clin Apher* 25(3), 2010.
30. Michael M, Elilott EJ, Ridley GF, et al: Interventions for haemolytic uremic syndrome and thrombotic thrombocytopenic purpura. *Cochrane Database Syst Rev* (1):CD003595, 2009.
31. Loirat C, Girma J, Desconclois C, et al: Thrombotic thrombocytopenic purpura related to severe ADAMTS13 deficiency in children. *Pediatr Nephrol* 24:19–29, 2009.
32. Van der Meche FG, Schmitz PI: A randomized trial comparing intravenous immune globulin and plasma exchange in Guillain-Barré syndrome. Dutch Guillain-Barré Study Group. *N Engl J Med* 326:1123–1129, 1992.
33. Raphael JC, Chevret S, Hughes RAC, et al: Plasma exchange for Guillain-Barré syndrome. *Cochrane Database Syst Rev* (2):CD001798, 2002.
34. Hughes RA, Raphael JC, Swan AV, et al: Intravenous immunoglobulin for Guillain-Barré syndrome. *Cochrane Database Syst Rev* (1):CD002063, 2006.
35. Busund R, Koukline V, Utrobin U, et al: Plasmapheresis in severe sepsis and septic shock: a prospective, randomized, controlled trial. *Intensive Care Med* 28:1434–1439, 2002.
36. Reeves JH, Butt WW, Sham F, et al: Continuous plasmafiltration in sepsis syndrome. Plasmafiltration in Sepsis Study Group. *Crit Care Med* 27: 2096–2104, 1999.
37. Weinshenker BG, O'Brien PC, Petterson TM, et al: A randomized trial of plasma exchange in acute central nervous system inflammatory demyelinating disease. *Ann Neurol* 46:878–886, 1999.
38. Stegmayr BG, Almroth G, Berlin G, et al: Plasma exchange or immunoadsorption in patients with rapidly progressive crescentic glomerulonephritis. A Swedish multicenter study. *Int J Artif Organs* 22:81–87, 1999.
39. Zauner I, Bach D, Braun N, et al: Predictive value of initial histology and effect of plasmapheresis on long-term prognosis of rapidly progressive glomerulonephritis. *Am J Kidney Dis* 39:28–35, 2002.
40. Cole E, Cattran D, Magil A, et al: A prospective randomized trial of plasma exchange as additive therapy in idiopathic crescentic glomerulonephritis. The Canadian Apheresis Study Group. *Am J Kidney Dis* 20:261–269, 1992.
41. Walters G, Willis NS, Graig JC: Interventions for renal vasculitis in adults. *Cochrane Database System Rev* (3):CD003232, 2008.
42. Gajdos P, Chevret S, Clair B, et al: Clinical trial of plasma exchange and high-dose intravenous immunoglobulin in myasthenia gravis. Myasthenia Gravis Clinical Study Group. *Ann Neurol* 41:789–796, 1997.
43. Chaudhuri A, Behan PO: Myasthenic Crisis. *Q J Med* 102:97–107, 2009.
44. Batocchi AP, Evoli A, Di Schino C, et al: Therapeutic apheresis in myasthenia gravis. *Ther Apher* 4:275–279, 2000.
45. Weinstein R: Therapeutic apheresis in neurological disorders. *J Clin Apher* 15:74–128, 2000.
46. Kiprov DD, Hofmann JC: Plasmapheresis in immunologically mediated polyneuropathies. *Ther Apher Dial* 7:189–196, 2003.
47. Madore F: Plasmapheresis. Technical aspects and indications. *Crit Care Clin* 18:375–392, 2002.
48. Szczepiorkowski ZM: TPE in renal, rheumatic, and miscellaneous disorders, in McLeod BC, Price TH, Weinstein R (eds): *Apheresis: Principles and Practice*. 2nd ed. Bethesda, MD, AABB, 2003, pp 375–409.
49. Frasca GM, Soverini ML, Falaschini A, et al: Plasma exchange treatment improves prognosis of antineutrophil cytoplasmic antibody-associated crescentic glomerulonephritis: a case-control study in 26 patients from a single center. *Ther Apher Dial* 7:540–546, 2003.
50. Klemmer PJ, Chalermskulrat W, Reif MS, et al: Plasmapheresis therapy for diffuse alveolar hemorrhage in patients with small-vessel vasculitis. *Am J Kidney Dis* 42:1149–1153, 2003.
51. Oh SJ: Muscle-specific receptor tyrosine kinase antibody positive myasthenia gravis current status. *J Clin Neurol* 5:53–64, 2009.
52. Ruprecht K, Klinker E, Dintelmann T, et al: Plasma exchange for severe optic neuritis. *Neurology* 63:1081–1083, 2004.
53. Watanabe S, Nakashima I, Misu T, et al: Therapeutic efficacy of plasma exchange in NMO-IgG-positive patients with neuromyelitis optica. *Mult Scler* 13:128–132, 2007.
54. Schmidt J, Mann S, Mohr VD, et al: Plasmapheresis combined with continuous venovenous hemofiltration in surgical patients with sepsis. *Intensive Care Med* 26:532–537, 2000.
55. Stegmayer B: Apheresis in patients with severe sepsis and multi organ dysfunction syndrome. *Transfus Apher Sci* 38:203–208, 2008.
56. Swerdlow PS: Red cell exchange in sickle cell disease. *Hematology Am Soc Hematol Educ Program* 48–53, 2006.

57. Turner JM, Kaplan JB, Cohen HW, et al: Exchange versus simple transfusion for acute chest syndrome in sickle cell anemia adults. *Transfusion* 49:863–868, 2009.
58. Liem RI, O'Gorman MR, Brown DL: Effect of red cell exchange transfusion on plasma levels of inflammatory mediators in sickle cell patients with acute chest syndrome. *Am J Hematol* 76:19–25, 2004.
59. Boga C, Kozanoglu I, Ozdogu H, et al: Plasma exchange in critically ill patients with sickle cell disease. *Transfus Apher Sci* 37:17–22, 2007.
60. Shelat SG, Lott JP, Braga MS, et al: Considerations on the use of adjunct red blood cell exchange transfusion in the treatment of severe *plasmodium falciparum* malaria. *Transfusion* 50(4):875–880, 2009.
61. Spaete J, Patrozou E, Rich JD, et al: Red cell exchange transfusion for babesiosis in Rhode Island. *J Clin Apher* 24:97–105, 2009.
62. Riddle MS, Jackson JL, Sanders JW, et al: Exchange transfusion as an adjunct therapy in severe *Plasmodium falciparum* malaria: a meta-analysis. *Clin Infect Dis* 34:1192–1198, 2002.
63. Nieuwenhuis JA, Meertens JHJM, Zijlstra JG, et al: Automated erythrocytapheresis in severe falciparum malaria: a critical appraisal. *Acta Trop* 98:201–206, 2006.
64. van Genderen PJJ, Hesselink DA, Bezemer JM, et al: Efficacy and safety of exchange transfusion as an adjunct therapy for severe *Plasmodium falciparum* malaria in non immune travelers: a 10-year single-center experience with a standardized treatment protocol. *Transfusion* 50(4):787–794, 2009.
65. Centers for Disease Control and Prevention: Available at: http://www.cdc.gov/malaria/facts.htm.
66. Vecchio S, Leonardo P, Musuraca V, et al: A comparison of the results obtained with traditional phlebotomy and with therapeutic erythrocytapheresis in patients with erythrocytosis. *Blood Transfus* 5:20–23, 2007.
67. Bug G, Anargyrou K, Tonn T, et al: Impact of leukapheresis on early death rate in adult acute myeloid leukemia presenting with hyperleukocytosis. *Transfusion* 47:1843–1850, 2007.
68. Inaba H, Fan Y, Pounds S, et al: Clinical and biologic features and treatment outcome of children with newly diagnosed acute myeloid leukemia and hyperleukocytosis. *Cancer* 113:522–529, 2008.
69. Lowe EJ, Pui CH, Hancock ML, et al: Early complications in children with acute lymphoblastic leukemia presenting with hyperleukocytosis. *Pediatr Blood Cancer* 45:10–15, 2005.
70. Zarkovic M, Kwaan HC: Correction of hyperviscosity by apheresis. *Semin Thromb Hemost* 29:535–542, 2003.
71. Mesa R, Nagorney DS, Schwager S, et al: Palliative goals, patient selection, and perioperative platelet management. Outcomes and lessons from 3 decades of splenectomy for myelofibrosis with myeloid metaplasia at the Mayo Clinic. *Cancer* 107:361–370, 2006.

CHAPTER 114 ■ TRANSFUSION THERAPY: BLOOD COMPONENTS AND TRANSFUSION COMPLICATIONS

TERRY GERNSHEIMER

Transfusion support can be a key element in decreasing morbidity and mortality of the critically ill patient by the support of oxygen delivery and correction of hemostatic abnormalities. An understanding of the benefits, limitations, and risks of blood component therapy is of fundamental importance in the intensive care setting. This chapter will outline blood components available for transfusion, their appropriate dosages, and therapeutic effects. Complications of transfusion therapy, including infectious risks, transfusion reactions, effects of storage, and immunomodulatory effects, as well as methods to minimize these complications, will be discussed.

BLOOD COMPONENT THERAPY

Cellular Blood Components

Red Blood Cells

One unit of "packed" red blood cells (pRBC) is processed by the removal of platelet rich plasma from a donated unit of whole blood and contains approximately 200 mL red blood cells, usually less than 50 mL plasma, and an additive that brings the component to 300 to 350 mL in total volume. Depending upon the additive, the storage life at 4°C will be from 35 to 42 days. Red blood cell storage has multiple theoretic and measurable effects. Any platelets still present in the component are rendered inactive by the cold storage. As red blood cells are stored, intracellular potassium leaks into the plasma space. 2,3-Diphosphoglyceric acid (2,3-DPG) may also be depleted from the red blood cells, which theoretically could cause increased oxygen affinity and decreased release of oxygen at the tissues [1]. This effect reverses after several hours in vivo but may be clinically significant in the patient undergoing massive transfusion. Stored pRBC also have elevated plasma ammonia levels, elevated PCO_2, lowered pH, and increased amounts of microaggregates. These all have theoretic effects on oxygen delivery when given rapidly in large amounts. Massive transfusion can also theoretically result in hypocalcemia and hyperkalemia.

In 1993, Marik and Sibald [2] reported the incidental finding of increased gastric pH in 23 patients with septic shock transfused with 3 units of pRBC, but Walsh failed to find a similar effect in a small randomized control trial in 22 patients with septic shock transfused with pRBC stored for less than 5 or more than 20 days [3]. Hébert found a higher incidence of mortality and life-threatening complications who received blood stored less than 8 days when compared with standard therapy in a randomized study of 66 patients undergoing cardiac surgery [4]. Although van der Watering did find longer ICU stays and decreased survival in a retrospective study of 2,732 patients undergoing coronary artery bypass graft (CABG) who received blood that had undergone a median age of $\geq$18 days or more versus less than 18 days of storage, this difference was not apparent in a multivariate analysis [5]. A retrospective report of a large number of patients (5,902) by Koch et al. [6] showed a significant increase in mortality and complications at 1 year in patients undergoing CABG who received blood >14 days of age versus <15 days of age, but differences in characteristics of the two patient groups complicated the analysis. The effect of storage age remains controversial [7] and will require careful prospective randomized clinical trials in adequate numbers of patients before the true clinical significance of storage age and the nature of the effect becomes clear [8].

Other than factors V and VIII, the activity of most coagulation factors are quite stable during storage, even after 2 weeks, and therefore whole blood (without the plasma removed), when available, may be used in selected patients with coagulopathy and bleeding, and can reduce donor exposure by limiting administration of multiple products (e.g., red cells and plasma) [9]. Factor V levels in stored whole blood are well above 50% and therefore adequate for hemostasis. Factor VIII is produced by endothelial cells as well as by the liver, and levels increase in the setting of inflammation, so a decrease with storage may be less clinically relevant. Whole blood may also be the preferred form of red cell transfusion in patients who require intravascular volume expansion as well as increased oxygen carrying capacity.

The primary function of hemoglobin in RBCs is to transport oxygen efficiently from the lungs to the various tissues of the body. Oxygen transport is a complex process regulated by several different mechanisms of control, involving the heart and vascular system. The most important functional feature of the hemoglobin molecule is its ability to combine loosely and reversibly with oxygen. Decreased hemoglobin oxygen affinity and increased tissue oxygen delivery occur with increased temperature and decreased pH, when there are increased tissue requirements. Oxygen is also less tightly bound with increased 2,3-DPG levels, which increases in the chronically ill patient [10]. In the seriously ill patient with severe acidosis and septic shock, however, 2,3-DPG levels may decrease resulting in decreased tissue oxygen delivery.

In a normovolemic, otherwise healthy individual, the effect of a decreased hematocrit is decreased blood viscosity and a compensatory augmentation of cardiac output and blood flow to most organs [11]. Human and animal studies reveal remarkable tolerance for hematocrit levels as low as 15% [12,13], but an optimum value has not been well defined and is very dependent on the patient's physiologic state. A decrease in the hematocrit also involves a redistribution of blood flow away from the endocardium and may have adverse effects on ischemic cardiac tissue. A retrospective analysis of patients older than 65 years hospitalized with acute myocardial infarction found that in patients with a hematocrit less than 30.0% (and perhaps <33.0%) on admission, transfusion was associated with a lower 30-day mortality rate [14]. However, in patients who had undergone elective CABG, postoperative transfusion for hemoglobin levels greater than 8 did not improve morbidity, mortality, or complication rates [15]. Postoperative patients with known vascular disease and hematocrits less than 28% have been shown to have a significant increase in myocardial ischemia and morbid cardiac events [16], and in one study that retrospectively evaluated patients refusing transfusion on religious grounds, low preoperative hemoglobin was associated with increased morbidity and mortality in patients with cardiovascular disease undergoing surgery [17]. In a large multicenter, randomized trial, there was no difference in adverse outcomes when patients with cardiac disease were transfused at a hemoglobin threshold of 7.0 g versus 10 g [18]. In this study of more than 800 patients, less acutely ill, younger patients (<55 years of age) without cardiac disease who were randomized to the more liberal (higher) transfusion trigger had an overall higher mortality rate. A restrictive RBC transfusion strategy also did not adversely affect outcomes related to mechanical ventilation [19]. In postoperative patients without cardiovascular disease, few data support interference with wound healing or increased anesthesia risk at hemoglobin levels of less than 10 g per dL [20], and hemoglobin values as low as 7 g per dL appear to be safe in otherwise healthy individuals [21].

Advocates of restrictive transfusion strategies point out that transfusing to normal hemoglobin concentrations does not improve organ failure and mortality in the critically ill patient [22] and to data that transfusion may actually be associated with increased infection rates, morbidity and mortality [23]. Proponents of more liberal transfusion strategies point out the possible detrimental effects that may be associated with oxygen debt [24]. A thoughtful transfusion policy is dependent on the time the anemia developed over and can be expected to continue; additional medical problems that may make a patient more susceptible to anemia, such as tissue ischemia and pulmonary disease; and whether there is rapid, ongoing blood loss.

Blunted erythropoietin responses have been noted in critically ill pediatric [25] and adult patients [26]. Long-term intensive care patients may not only fail to increase their erythropoietin level in response to anemia but may have correctable nutritional deficiencies and iron profiles consistent with anemia of chronic disease. Although erythropoietin therapy increases red blood cell production and appears to decrease transfusion needs [27–29], the effect can take weeks and may reduce blood cell transfusion only minimally. It is an expensive alternative to more restrictive transfusion strategies to reduce transfusion exposure in appropriately chosen patients.

Studies in animal models [30] and in humans [31,32] reveal that platelet function and interaction with subendothelium decline at lower hematocrits. In the thrombocytopenic and thrombocytopathic (e.g., uremic) patient, transfusion to higher hematocrit values is appropriate in the patient at risk of bleeding.

Therapeutic Effect. The response to red cell transfusion will depend on intravascular volume, but it can be estimated that one unit of pRBC will increase the hematocrit by approximately 3%. It may take up to 24 hours while intravascular volume equilibrates for full effect. Rapid ongoing red cell destruction or splenic sequestration may also affect the hematocrit increment as well as the red cell survival.

Emergency Blood Usage. Uncrossmatched type O RBCs can be used for a bleeding patient in dire emergency. Type O, Rh-negative RBCs can be transfused to people of any blood type with only a slight risk of hemolysis. This risk increases in patients who have previously been transfused or pregnant and may have formed antibodies [33]. Type O, Rh-positive RBCs are sometimes used for women who are beyond childbearing age and in adult males. When Rh-positive RBCs are used in an Rh-negative patient, there is a chance of a D immunization, and if the patient requires emergency transfusion in the future, they may have preformed antibodies. Anti-D antibodies do not generally cause immediately intravascular hemolysis but rather a slow extravascular hemolysis, so the risk is small overall. Anti–Rh-D (Rhogam®) may be given within 48 hours of giving transfusion of Rh-positive blood to an Rh-negative woman of childbearing age, but the amounts required limit its use in prevention of immunization.

Platelets

Platelets are essential for the initial phase of hemostasis. Following exposure of subendothelial substances, platelets adhere to the subendothelial tissues by von Willebrand factor and other adhesive proteins. This initial adhesion activates platelets, causing release of platelet alpha and dense granules. Some of these granule contents, including factor V, fibrinogen, von Willebrand factor, and calcium, move to the extracellular space via the open canalicular system, increasing their concentrations in the immediate "neighborhood" of the platelet. With platelet activation, anionic phospholipids move to the platelet surface, forming binding sites collectively known as platelet factor 3, upon which coagulation factors can interact with calcium to form IXa, Xa, and thrombin. Platelet glycoprotein IIb-IIIa is exposed and binds fibrinogen. Thrombin generation causes further platelet activation and converts fibrinogen to fibrin, resulting in a platelet-fibrin mass that can effectively cease bleeding from a break in the endothelium. Fifteen percent of the platelet's protein is actin and myosin, which, upon coupling in the presence of increased concentrations of adenosine diphosphate (ADP) and calcium, leads to cytoskeletal movement and clot retraction.

The threshold of thrombocytopenia at which bleeding may occur will vary depending on the patient's clinical condition. In general, spontaneous bleeding does not occur until the platelet count falls below 5,000 to 10,000/μL [34–37]. The recommended "trigger" for prophylactic platelet transfusions in patients undergoing chemotherapy or hematopoietic stem cell transplantation (HSCT) without bleeding or other comorbid conditions is less than 10,000/μL. For the majority of invasive procedures, a platelet count of 30 to 50,000/μL will be adequate. For high-risk procedures, such as neurologic or ophthalmologic surgeries, a platelet count of 100,000/μL is recommended by the American Society of Anesthesiology [38] and the College of American Pathologists [39]. Technique and experience appear to be as least as important predictors of bleeding following placement of catheters as clotting abnormalities, even in patients with isolated platelet counts less than 20,000/μL [40]. The risk of bleeding with thrombocytopenia increases when complicated by other hemostatic abnormalities.

Platelet counts less than 50,000/μL are associated with increased risk of microvascular bleeding in the massively transfused patient [41]. For this reason, platelet transfusion has been advocated with replacement of every blood volume to avoid the effect of dilutional thrombocytopenia [42]; however, some investigators have found that patients receiving prophylactic platelet transfusion were no less likely to develop microvascular bleeding [43]. In patients with brisk ongoing blood loss, rapid turnaround of platelet counts can direct diagnosis and are important in managing transfusion therapy.

Higher transfusion triggers may be indicated with abnormal platelet function [44]. Platelet function abnormalities may be congenital or acquired. Medications, sepsis, malignancy, tissue trauma, obstetrical complications, and extra corporeal circulation may all adversely affect platelet function. Liver and kidney disease may be associated with severe thrombocytopathy. Hypothermia prolongs bleeding time in trauma patients [45] and arterial hemorrhage in animals [46]. Glycoprotein IIb-IIIa inhibitors may affect platelet number as well as function. If platelet dysfunction is present, the patient with a disrupted vascular system (e.g., trauma or surgery) will require a higher platelet count to achieve hemostasis. Higher counts may be necessary to prevent spontaneous bleeding as well. The transfused platelets may quickly become dysfunctional in the patient, and other therapy may be necessary, such as dialysis and dialysis and desmopressin acetate (DDAVP) for bleeding in renal failure, rewarming of the hypothermic patient, or correction of acidosis.

In several situations, platelet transfusions may not be indicated unless there is significant bleeding. In autoimmune thrombocytopenias (e.g., immune thrombocytopenia (ITP) and posttransfusion purpura), transfusion increments are usually poor and platelet survival is short. Administration of intravenous immune globulin in high doses may improve transfusion response and survival as well as treat the underlying disease [47]. There have been reports of rapid exacerbation of the thrombotic process in the cerebrovascular circulation in patients with thrombotic thrombocytopenic purpura (TTP) following platelet transfusion [48]. These reports are anecdotal and may represent disease progression, but in general, platelet transfusions are felt to be relatively contraindicated in TTP unless there is clinically significant bleeding.

TABLE 114.1

EXPECTED PLATELET INCREMENT WITH TRANSFUSION[a]

	1 unit[b]	4 units	6 units
	0.8×10^{11}	3.2×10^{11}	4.8×10^{11}
50 lb/23 kg	17,600/μL	70,400/μL	105,600/μL
100 lb/45 kg	8,800	35,200	52,800
150 lb/68 kg	5,900	23,500	35,200
200 lb/91 kg	4,400	17,600	26,400

[a]In a patient with a normal sized spleen and without platelet antibodies.
[b]Whole blood platelets. An apheresis platelet component contains the equivalent of 4–8 units of whole blood platelets.

Pooled random donor platelet concentrates are prepared from platelets that have been harvested by centrifuging units of donated whole blood. Up to 8 units of platelets, each from a separate donor, can be pooled into a single bag for transfusion. All units are from the same ABO type. If ABO compatible platelets are unavailable, in most cases, pooled ABO incompatible platelets can be substituted with very little risk. The usual adult dose is 1 unit per 15 kg of body weight. Four to six units of pooled random donor platelets are frequently used in patients receiving prophylactic transfusions; however, a study of more than 1,200 hospitalized patients with thrombocytopenia due to chemotherapy or HSCT for hematologic malignancy showed no difference in bleeding incidence and decreased platelet exposure overall when transfused with low ($1.1 \times 10^{11}/m^2$), medium ($2.2 \times 10^{11}/m^2$), or high ($4.4 \times 10^{11}/m^2$) doses of platelets prophylactically for platelet counts of less than 10,000/μL [49], suggesting that a dose of only 3 or 4 units of pooled random donor platelets is adequate. Patients who received smaller doses did require more frequent transfusions, making this strategy less appropriate for outpatient transfusion.

In a 70-kg patient with a normal sized spleen, each unit is expected to increase the platelet count by approximately 7,000/μL (Table 114.1) when checked 10 minutes to 1 hour after transfusion [50]. The survival of transfused platelets averages 3 to 5 days but will decrease if a consumptive process is present. Platelet concentrates also contain about 60 mL of plasma per unit and small numbers of red blood cells and leukocytes. Platelet units must be maintained at room temperature, as platelets lose shape and release their granular contents when refrigerated. Apheresis platelets, collected from a single donor, are prepared in components equivalent to 4 to 6 pooled units. An apheresis platelet concentrate contains 200 to 400 mL of plasma and, if the plasma is of an incompatible type, may be reduced in volume by centrifugation, although this results in an approximate 10% to 15% loss of platelets and probably some loss of function. Apheresis platelets may be collected for a specific recipient from a family member or other human leukocyte antigen (HLA) compatible donor for patients that have become refractory to random donor platelet transfusions due to alloimmunization. Leukocyte reduction of transfused cellular blood components has been clearly shown to reduce the rate of alloimmunization in patients undergoing chemotherapy for acute myelocytic leukemia [51].

Granulocytes

The degree of granulocytopenia is directly related to the risk of infection [52]. Although antibiotics have improved morbidity and mortality in patients affected by prolonged periods of neutropenia, most antimicrobials are less effective in the presence of granulocytopenia. Bacterial and, more particularly fungal, infections remain a major cause of death in HSCT patients despite shortening of the period of neutropenia with hematopoietic growth factors [53]. Granulocytes collected by continuous flow centrifugation and filtration leukapheresis function normally in vitro in the quantitative nitroblue tetrazolium, oxygen consumption, and chemotaxis assays [54]. Bacterial killing by filtration leukapheresis granulocytes, which circulate for several hours posttransfusion, is only slightly decreased compared with granulocytes collected by continuous flow centrifugation. Transfused granulocytes rapidly migrate to sites of infection [55].

Early studies showed promise for the use of granulocyte transfusion for treatment of documented infections in neutropenic patients [56–58]; however, their usefulness in the prevention of infection has been more controversial [59], due to limitations in the inability to collect cells in sufficient amounts to provide an effective transfusion dose, poor response to granulocytes in heavily transfused, alloimmunized patients [60], and the early development of alloimmunization in patients transfused with granulocytes [61]. To this end, HLA-compatible donors have been administered corticosteroids prior to granulocyte collection with some limited success.

The administration of granulocyte colony-stimulating factor has been shown to be safe when given to normal donors [62] and has been administered to donors prior to collection to increase collection and posttransfusion increments [63,64]. Whether this will increase the efficacy of granulocyte transfusion in treatment of infection will require further study.

Plasma Components

Fresh Frozen Plasma

One unit of fresh frozen plasma (FFP) is the plasma taken from a unit of whole blood. It is frozen within 8 hours of collection and contains all coagulation factors in normal concentrations. It is free of red blood cells, leukocytes, and platelets. Plasma may also be provided as "frozen plasma" or "thawed plasma." These components are prepared by methods similar to plasma, and their factor concentrations differ only slightly. All will be considered here collectively as "FFP." One unit contains approximately 200 to 250 mL and must be ABO compatible (type AB is the universal donor type). Rh factor need not be considered. Since there are no viable leukocytes, FFP carries minimal risk of cytomegalovirus (CMV) transmission or graft versus host disease (GVHD).

FFP transfusion is indicated in patients with documented coagulation factor deficiencies and active bleeding. FFP should not be used to correct isolated deficiencies in clotting factors when a concentrated replacement source, such as factor VIII or IX, is available, as these concentrates are either recombinant or have undergone processing to inactivate viruses and can correct the deficiency using a much smaller infused volume. Factor deficiencies may be congenital or acquired secondary to liver disease, warfarin anticoagulation, disseminated intravascular coagulation (DIC), or massive replacement with red blood cells and crystalloid/colloid solutions. Usually, there is an increase of at least 1.6 times the normal prothrombin time (PT) or activated partial thromboplastin time (aPTT) before clinically important factor deficiency exists. This corresponds to levels of most factors less than 20% of normal. Above these levels, most routine non–major invasive procedures such as line placement [27], liver biopsy [65], and thoracentesis [66] are not associated with an increased risk of bleeding complications; however, the acceptable upper limits of PT and PTT prior to invasive procedures have not been evaluated in a large prospective randomized study to date [67–69].

TABLE 114.2

FRESH FROZEN PLASMA (FFP)—DOSAGE FOR TRANSFUSION

Volume of 1 unit FFP: 200–250 mL
1 mL plasma contains 1 unit coagulation factors
1 Unit FFP contains 220 units coagulation factors
Factor recovery with transfusion = 40%
1 Unit FFP provides ~80 units coagulation factors
70 kg × 0.05 = plasma volume of 35 dL (3.5 L)
$\frac{80\text{ unit}}{35\text{ dL}}$ = 2.3 unit/dL = 2.3% (of normal 100 unit/dL)
In a 70-kg patient:
1 Unit FFP increases most factors ~2.5%
4 Units FFP increase most factors ~10%

In the massively transfused patient, consumption and dilution of coagulation factors may cause rapid development of coagulopathy. Patients with a PT or aPTT ratio (reference midrange normal value divided by actual) 1.8 or more had an 80% to 85% chance of exhibiting microvascular bleeding, and either of these tests should be closely monitored during resuscitation of the bleeding patient [33]. FFP transfusion is indicated when the ratio exceeds 1.5 times the midrange normal value in these patients [30]. Usually an increase in factor levels of at least 10% will be needed for any significant change in coagulation status, so the usual dose is 3 to 4 units (approximately 10 to 15 mL per kg), but the amount will vary depending on the patient's size and clotting factor levels (Table 114.2). Reversal of warfarin anticoagulation is indicated only if significant bleeding or risk of bleeding is present. FFP may be used for this purpose, but often, recurrent transfusion is required to maintain normal factor levels.

FFP is indicated in the treatment of TTP, most commonly in conjunction with plasmapheresis. Many other disorders are treated by plasmapheresis, but usually FFP replacement is not used. FFP should *not* be used for volume expansion unless the patient also has a significant coagulopathy and is bleeding.

Cryoprecipitate

Cryoprecipitate is prepared from plasma and contains fibrinogen, von Willebrand factor, factor VIII, factor XIII, and fibronectin. Cryoprecipitate is supplied in bags (each made from one whole blood unit) from multiple donors that have been resuspended in saline or plasma and pooled prior to transfusion. It must be kept at room temperature. The concentration of fibrinogen in cryoprecipitate units is up to 10 times that in FFP and therefore blood levels can be increased rapidly with much smaller volumes.

Fibrinogen levels can drop rapidly in DIC and is usually associated with other coagulation abnormalities that may in combination be treated with FFP. Isolated hypofibrinogenemia is infrequently associated with bleeding in adults, and correction should be reserved for patients with clinical bleeding or patients who are a risk of bleeding due to imminent invasive procedures or trauma [26] with significant hypofibrinogenemia (<100 mg per dL).

Cryoprecipitate should not be used for patients with von Willebrand disease or hemophilia A (factor VIII deficiency) unless they do not (or are not known to) respond to DDAVP, and recombinant and/or virally inactivated preparations are not available. It is usually given for factor XIII deficiency, when virus-inactivated concentrates of this protein are not available.

Cryoprecipitate is sometimes useful if platelet dysfunction associated with renal failure does not respond to dialysis or DDAVP and in other platelet function defects [70].

The amount of fibrinogen per bag of cryoprecipitate can vary widely between blood centers depending on the donor's fibrinogen concentration. The approximate fibrinogen increment with each bag of cryoprecipitate transfused can be calculated by the formula: 25 mg/plasma volume (in liters). Six bags will increase the fibrinogen level of a 70-kg patient approximately 45 mg per dL. To replace factor VIII or von Willebrand factor when specific factor concentrates are unavailable, the usual dose is 1 bag per 10 kg of body weight. Approximately 150 units of factor VIII and von Willebrand factor are provided per bag. Although single units of cryoprecipitate can be used in the preparation of locally applied fibrin glue for surgery, commercially available, virally inactivated concentrates have a higher fibrinogen concentration and are preferred for this purpose. A patient may donate autologous plasma for processing into cryoprecipitate prior to a planned surgical procedure.

Human fibrinogen concentrate (RiaSTAP®) is a heat-treated, lyophilized fibrinogen (coagulation factor I) powder made from pooled human plasma. It is indicated for bleeding or procedure prophylaxis in patients with congenital hypofibrinogenemia or dysfibrinogenemia.

COMPLICATIONS OF TRANSFUSION

Transfusion-Related Risks

Infectious Complications

Since the recognition that human immunodeficiency virus (HIV) could be transmitted by blood transfusion in the mid-1980s, exclusion of donors with high risk has done more to decrease transfusion transmitted infection than any testing that has been implemented since that time [71]. Enzyme-linked immunosorbent assay (ELISA) testing for anti-HIV antibody was instituted in 1985 dropping the risk of HIV transmitted infection to 1 in 667,000 units [72]. The addition of P24 antigen decreased the window period between infection and detection to approximately 16 days [73].

Blood centers began clinical trials in April 1999 to screen blood with a polymerase chain reaction (PCR) test for hepatitis C virus (HCV) and HIV RNA. Although confirmed data are not available, the current estimated risks/unit are as low as 1:2,000,000 for HIV and HCV [74]. Risks for other viral transmissions are estimated to be 1:500,000–750,000 for hepatitis B and 1:3,000,000 for human T-lymphotropic virus I and II [75,76].

CMV is a DNA virus acquired as a primary infection with body secretions, blood products, or organ allografts. Infection in a normal host usually is asymptomatic but remains latent for life and can cause recurrent infection when it reactivates. CMV infection and seropositivity are extremely common, being 40% in highly industrialized areas, and is close to 100% in warmer climates, densely populated areas, and developing countries [77]. Transfusion-associated CMV infection in the immunocompetent patient with a normal immune system is usually asymptomatic, occurring 4 to 12 weeks after blood component exposure in 0.9% to 17% of patients [78]. In CMV-negative, immunosuppressed neonates and transplant and HIV-positive patients, the risk of CMV infection leading to severe end-organ disease and organ allograft rejection is high [79]. Leukocyte depletion of blood is equivalent to CMV seronegative blood in preventing CMV infection through transfusion [80] but may be more expensive and indicated only if CMV-negative blood is not available or leukocyte-depleted blood components are being provided for another reason. Although CMV seronegative blood is transfused to organ transplant recipients in some centers to prevent infection with secondary strains, the clinical relevance of this practice has not been demonstrated.

Bacterial contamination of red blood cell and platelet units may occur during collection. Red blood cell units may be contaminated with cold-loving organisms such as Yersinia. Platelets are stored at room temperature and multiple organisms can grow in those conditions. Although staphylococcus and streptococcus are most frequently implicated, Gram-negative organisms have also been identified [81]. The incidence of bacterial contamination of platelets has been estimated to be as high as 0.1% [82]. The institution of bacterial testing of platelets in 2004 in the United States is expected to decrease this risk [83]. Symptoms of hypotension, fever, and chills almost always occur within 3 hours of the transfusion and may be complicated by severe shock and DIC [84]. Both the patient and the blood component bag should be cultured if bacterial contamination is suspected.

Other organisms that can be transmitted by blood transfusion include other hepatitis viruses, malaria, and, rarely, syphilis. Trypanosoma cruzi, the parasite responsible for Chagas disease is becoming a commonly transfusion transmitted disease in Central and South America and has been reported in some Southern Border states. Fear of transfusion transmission of new variant Creutzfeldt-Jakob disease has led to stringent criteria on blood donor eligibility and institution of universal leukoreduction in some European countries, but the risk of infection by transfusion is low [85] and testing is not universal.

Transfusion Reactions

A transfusion should be stopped immediately whenever a transfusion reaction is suspected.

An **acute hemolytic transfusion reaction** (AHTR) occurs following transfusion of an incompatible blood component. Most are due to naturally occurring antibodies in the ABO antigen system, but AHTR may occur with incompatibility of Rh, Kell, Kidd, Lewis, and other red blood cell antigen systems. The vast majority of cases are due to failure of appropriate systems to identify the correct transfusion recipient [86]. Signs and symptoms include fever, hypotension, tachycardia, dyspnea, chest or back pain, flushing, and severe anxiety. Release of cytokines, such as tumor necrosis factor, interleukin 8, and monocyte chemoattractant protein-1 [87], is followed by fever, capillary leak, and activation of the hemostatic mechanism. If the reaction is severe, it may go on to cause a consumptive coagulopathy (DIC) and renal failure due to shock and deposition of thrombi in arterioles. Hemoglobinuria may be the first sign of hemolysis in the sedated patient. Centrifuging a tube of blood and examining the plasma for a reddish discoloration can quickly make the diagnosis. Treatment should first of all be immediate discontinuation of the transfusion as soon as AHTR is suspected and maintenance of venous access and fluid resuscitation if necessary. Pressor support may be necessary along with central venous pressure or Swann Ganz monitoring. AHTR is rare, estimated at 1:77,000 units [88].

Delayed hemolytic transfusion reactions (DHTRs) usually occur in patients who have been previously sensitized to an antigen through transfusion or pregnancy. A fall in titer over time may make incompatibility undetectable. A subsequent transfusion causes recall of the antibody followed by a falling hematocrit 5 to 10 days later. The hematocrit will continue to fall until all of the incompatible transfused cells have been destroyed. DHTR can result in symptomatic or asymptomatic hemolysis but has only rarely been reported to cause severe morbidity or mortality [89]. Once recognized, the patient is usually easily supported by transfusion of compatible red blood cells.

Febrile nonhemolytic transfusion reaction (FNHTR) is a 1°C rise in temperature or greater that cannot be explained by the patient's clinical condition. FNHTR usually occurs within 1 hour of completion of the transfusion. Reactions are more common with platelet transfusions and in patients who have been heavily transfused and can be quite severe. FNHTR is often due to sensitization to antigens on donor leukocytes [90]. Cytokines, released from the white cells during storage of cellular blood components, also appear to play a role [91]. Prestorage leukocyte depletion of red blood cells and platelets by filtration may be helpful in patients for whom this is a problem. Leukocyte-reduced single-donor apheresis platelets are a possible alternative to leukocyte depletion by filtration of pooled random donor platelets. Occasionally, patients with persistent febrile reactions will require removal of most of the plasma (volume reduction) from platelet preparations. FNHTR should be differentiated from bacterial contamination, which is usually associated with higher fevers and other symptoms of sepsis. Antipyretics can be used to prevent or treat FNHTR. Meperidine may be useful in the treatment of rigors.

Transfusion-related acute lung injury (TRALI) can be indistinguishable from adult respiratory distress syndrome [92,93], involving severe bilateral pulmonary edema and hypoxemia. Symptoms of dyspnea, hypotension, and fever typically begin 30 minutes to 6 hours after transfusion and the chest x-ray shows diffuse nonspecific infiltrates. Ventilatory support may be required for several days before resolution but approximately 80% of patients improve within 48 to 96 hours. TRALI occurs when donor plasma contains an antibody, usually against the patient's HLA or leukocyte specific antigens. Lipids generated during prior storage of the transfused product and preexisting lung damage also appear to play parts in the pathogenesis of TRALI. Less often, the patient may have antibodies against donor leukocytes in the component. The blood center should be notified promptly so that components from the donor can be quarantined and the donor tested for antibodies against the patient.

Transfusion-associated cardiovascular overload (TACO) may occur in patients sensitive to increased amounts of intravascular volume with transfusion and may initially present a clinical picture similar to TRALI. Unlike TRALI, diuresis is usually effective in its treatment.

Allergic and anaphylactic reactions are common and are usually due to preformed immunoglobulin E antibodies to specific proteins in the donor's plasma. Mild urticaria complicates up to 3% of plasma infusions [94] and can be avoided with future transfusions by pretreatment with antihistamines, and in severe cases with corticosteroids. Only in cases of severe reactions (anaphylaxis), is washing of RBCs and platelets to remove all plasma indicated. Slowing of the rate of transfusion and centrifugation to remove some of the plasma in a platelet component will sometimes be effective in preventing future reactions in patients for whom this is a recurrent problem.

Transfusion-related graft versus host disease (TRGVHD) is due to infusion of donor lymphocytes that engraft and then proliferate in response to stimulation by foreign (host) antigens. TRGVHD typically begins 2 to 50 days after transfusion with rash, diarrhea, signs of hepatic inflammation, and pancytopenia [95]. TRGVHD occurs in patients with severe defects of cellular immunity, most notably HSCT patients, neonates, and patients with lymphoproliferative disorders. Transfusion from relatives and HLA compatible donors are at risk of causing GVHD. It can be prevented by gamma irradiation of cellular blood components.

Immune Modulation

Transfusions have been known to induce immune tolerance following the observation made more than 20 years ago that multiply transfused kidney transplant recipients had an increased graft survival rate [96]. Transfusion-induced immunosuppression has been implicated in postoperative infection, increased cancer recurrence rates, and development of non-Hodgkin lymphoma [97,98]. There is also evidence from animal studies

TABLE 114.3

RANDOMIZED CLINICAL TRIALS IN TRANSFUSION MEDICINE THAT HAVE RESULTED IN CHANGES IN CLINICAL PRACTICE

Appropriate hemoglobin threshold for RBC transfusion	Hebert et al. [18] Hebert et al. [19] (The TRICC Trial)	A hemoglobin threshold of 7.0 g/dL vs. 9.0 g/dL is not associated with increased morbidity, mortality, or prolonged ventilatory support.
Appropriate platelet count threshold for prophylactic platelet transfusion	Gmur et al. [35] Wandt et al. [36] Rebulla et al. [37]	Platelet transfusion "triggers" of $<10{,}000/\mu L$ are safe for the prevention of bleeding in chemotherapy-induced thrombocytopenia in patients without comorbid conditions.
Prevention of transfusion transmitted CMV infection	Bowden et al. [80]	Leukocyte reduction of cellular blood components is as effective in reducing the risk of CMV transmission as the use of CMV seronegative blood components.
Prevention of platelet alloimmunization	TRAP Study Group [51]	Leukoreduction of cellular blood components prevents HLA alloimmunization in patients with acute leukemia undergoing induction chemotherapy.
Use of leukoreduction to decrease postoperative infection	van de Watering et al. [99]	Leukoreduction of cellular blood components decreases postoperative infection in patients undergoing cardiac surgery.
Appropriate platelet transfusion dose for prophylactic transfusion of thrombocytopenia	Slichter et al. [49]	Low-dose platelet transfusion results in an overall decrease in the number of total platelets transfused and no increase in bleeding. Platelet transfusion frequency is increased.

that transfusion increases the risk of metastatic disease, although data in humans are inconclusive. Removal of donor leukocytes has been shown to decrease the immunomodulatory effects of blood transfusions. The clinical usefulness is clear only in prevention of alloimmunization in patients undergoing chemotherapy for acute myelocytic leukemia [50]. A prospective randomized study in patients undergoing cardiac surgery showed a decrease in infection rates when leukocyte-reduced blood components were used [99]. This has led some centers to adopt policies of universal leukoreduction, but this remains controversial.

Table 114.3 summarizes some of the most important recent advances in transfusion medicine based on randomized, controlled trials or meta-analyses of such trials.

References

1. Valeri CR, Hirsch NM: Restoration in vivo of erythrocyte adenosine triphosphate, 2,3-diphosphoglycerate, potassium ion, and sodium ion concentrations following the transfusion of acid-citrate-dextrose stored human blood cells. *J Lab Clin Med* 73:722–33, 1969.
2. Marik PE, Sibbald WJ: Effect of stored-blood transfusion on oxygen delivery in patients with sepsis. *JAMA* 269:3024–3029, 1993.
3. Walsh TS, McArdle F, McLellan SA, et al: Does the storage time of transfused red blood cells influence regional or global indexes of tissue oxygenation in anemic critically ill patients? *Crit Care Med* 32:364–371, 2004.
4. Hébert PC, Chin-Yee I, Fergusson D, et al: A pilot trial evaluating the clinical effects of prolonged storage of red cells. *Anesth Analg* 100:1433–1438, 2005.
5. van de Watering L, Lorinser J, Versteegh M, et al: Effects of storage time of red blood cell transfusions on the prognosis of coronary artery bypass graft patients. *Transfusion* 46:1712–1718, 2006.
6. Koch CG, Li L, Sessler DI: Duration of red-cell storage and complications after cardiac Surgery. *N Engl J Med* 358:1229–1239, 2008.
7. Gauvin F, Spinella PC, Lacroix J, et al: Association between length of storage of transfused red blood cells and multiple organ dysfunction syndrome in pediatric intensive care patients. *Transfusion* 50(9):1902–1913, 2010.
8. Lee JS, Gladwin MT: The risks of red cell storage. *Nat Med* 16:381–382, 2010.
9. Counts RB, Haisch C, Simon TL, et al: Hemostasis in massively transfused trauma patients. *Ann Surg* 190:91–99, 1979.
10. Allen JB, Allen FB: The minimum acceptable level of hemoglobin. *Int Anesthesiol Clin* 20:1–22, 1982.
11. Messmer KFW: Acceptable hematocrit levels in surgical patients. *World J Surg* 11:41–46, 1987.
12. Jan KM, Chien S: Effect of hematocrit variations on coronary hemodynamics and oxygen utilization. *Am J Physiol* 233:H106–H113, 1977.
13. Brazier J, Cooper N, Maloney JV Jr, et al: The adequacy of myocardial oxygen delivery in acute normovolemic anemia. *Surgery* 75:508–516, 1974.
14. Wu WC, Rathore SS, Wang Y, et al: Blood transfusion in elderly patients with acute myocardial infarction. *N Engl J Med* 345:1230–1236, 2001.
15. Bracey AW, Radovancevic R, Riggs SA, et al: Lowering the hemoglobin threshold for transfusion in coronary artery bypass procedures: effect on patient outcome. *Transfusion* 39:1070–1077, 1999.
16. Nelson AH, Fleisher LA, Rosenbaum SH. Relationship between postoperative anemia and cardiac morbidity in high-risk vascular patients in the intensive care unit: *Crit Care Med* 21:860–866, 1993.
17. Carson JL, Duff A, Poses RM, et al: Effect of anaemia and cardiovascular disease on surgical mortality and morbidity. *Lancet* 348:1055–1060, 1996.
18. Hebert PC, Wells G, Blajchman MA, et al: A multicenter, randomized, controlled clinical trial of transfusion requirements in critical care. *N Engl J Med* 340:409–417, 1999.
19. Hebert PC, Blajchman MA, Cook DJ, et al: Do blood transfusions improve outcomes related to mechanical ventilation? *Chest* 119:1850–1857, 2001.
20. Perioperative Red Cell Transfusion: National Institute of Health Consensus Development Statement 4:1–6, 1988.
21. Carson JL, Hill S, Carless P, et al: Transfusion triggers: a systematic review of the literature. *Transfus Med Rev* 16:187–199, 2002.
22. Alvarez G, Hebert PC: Debate: transfusing to normal hemoglobin levels will not improve outcome. *Crit Care* 5:56–63, 2001.
23. Vincent JL, Baron JF, Reinhart K, et al: Anemia and blood transfusion in critically ill patients. *JAMA* 288:1499–1507, 2002.
24. Haupt MT: Debate: transfusing to normal hemoglobin levels improves outcome: *Crit Care* 5:64–66, 2001.
25. Krafte-Jacobs B, Levetown ML, Bray GL, et al: Erythropoietin response to critical illness. *Crit Care Med* 22:821–826, 1994.
26. Rogiers P, Zhang H, Leeman M, et al: Erythropoietin response is blunted in critically ill patients. *Intensive Care Med* 23:159–162, 1997.
27. Gabriel A, Chiari K, Grabner FR, et al: High dose recombinant human erythropoietin stimulates reticulocyte production in patients with multiple organ dysfunction syndrome. *J Trauma* 44:361–367, 1998.
28. van Iperen CE, Gaillard CA, Kraaijenhagen RJ, et al: Response of erythropoiesis and iron metabolism to recombinant human erythropoietin in intensive care unit patients. *Critical Care Med* 28:2773–2778, 2000.
29. Corwin HL, Gettinger A, Rodriguez RM, et al: Efficacy of recombinant human erythropoietin in the critically ill patient: a randomized, double blind, placebo-controlled trial. *Crit Care Med* 27:2346–2350, 1999.
30. Blajchman MA, Bordin JO, Bardossy L, et al: The contribution of the haematocrit to thrombocytopenic bleeding in experimental animals. *Br J Haematol* 86:347–350, 1994.
31. Anand A, Feffer SE: Hematocrit and bleeding time: an update. *South Med J* 87:299–301, 1994.
32. Valeri CR, Cassidy G, Pivicek LE, et al: Anemia-induced increase in the bleeding time: implications for treatment of nonsurgical blood loss. *Transfusion* 41:977–983, 2001.
33. Oberman HA, Barnes BA, Friedman BA: The risk of abbreviating the major crossmatch in urgent or massive transfusion. *Transfusion* 18:137–141, 1978.
34. Slichter SJ, Harker LA: Thrombocytopenia: mechanisms and management of defects in platelet function. *Clin Haematol* 7:523–529, 1978.
35. Gmur J, Burger J, Schanz U, et al: Safety of stringent prophylactic platelet transfusion policy for patients with acute leukaemia. *Lancet* 338:1223–1236, 1991.
36. Wandt H, Frank M, Ehninger, et al: Safety and cost effectiveness of a 10 × 10^9/L trigger for prophylactic platelet transfusions compared to the traditional 20 × 10^9/L: a prospective comparative trial in 105 patients with acute myeloid leukemia. *Blood* 91:3601–3606, 1998.
37. Rebulla P, Finazzi G, Marangoni F, et al: The threshold for prophylactic platelet transfusions in adults with acute myeloid leukemia. *New Engl J Med* 337:1870–1875, 1997.
38. ASA Task Force on Blood Transfusion and Adjuvant Therapies: Practice guidelines for perioperative blood transfusion and adjuvant therapies. *Anesthesiology* 105:198–208, 2006.
39. Development Task Force of the College of American Pathologists: Practice parameter for the use of fresh-frozen plasma, cryoprecipitate, and platelets. *JAMA* 271:777–781, 1994.
40. DeLoughery TG, Liebler JM, Simonds V, et al: Invasive line placement in critically ill patients: do hemostatic defects matter? *Transfusion* 36:827–831, 1996.
41. Ciavarella D, Reed RL, Counts RB, et al: Clotting factor levels and the risk of diffuse microvascular bleeding in the massively transfused patient. *Br J Haematol* 67:365–368, 1987.
42. Leslie SD, Toy PT: Laboratory hemostatic abnormalities in massively transfused patients given red blood cells and crystalloid. *Am J Clin Pathol* 96:770–773, 1991.
43. Reed RL II, Heimbach DM, Counts RB: Prophylactic platelet administration during massive transfusion. *Ann Surg* 203:41–48, 1986.
44. Contreras M: The appropriate use of platelets: an update from the Edinburgh consensus conference. *Br J Haematol* 101[Suppl 1]:10–12, 1998.
45. Leben J, Tryba M, Bading B, et al: Clinical consequences of hypothermia in trauma patients. *Acta Anaesthesiol Scand Suppl* 109:39–41, 1996.
46. Oung CM, Li MS, Shum-Tim D, et al: In vivo study of bleeding time and arterial hemorrhage in hypothermic versus normothermic animals. *J Trauma* 32:251–254, 1993.
47. Spahr JE, Rodgers GM: Treatment of immune-mediated thrombocytopenia purpura with concurrent intravenous immunoglobulin and platelet transfusion: a retrospective review of 40 patients. *Am J Hematol* 83(2):122–125, 2008.
48. Gordon LI, Kwaan HC, Rossi EC: Deleterious effects of platelet transfusions and recovery thrombocytosis in patients with thrombotic microangiopathy. *Semin Hematol* 24:194–201, 1987.
49. Slichter SJ, Kaufman RM, Assman SF, et al: Dose of prophylactic platelet transfusions and prevention of hemorrhage. *N Engl J Med* 362:600–613, 2010.
50. Slichter SJ: Principles of platelet transfusion therapy, in Hoffman R, Benz EJ, Shattil SJ, et al (eds): *Hematology Basic Principles and Practice*. New York, NY, Churchill-Livingstone, 1991, pp 1610–1622.
51. The Trial to Reduce Alloimmunization to Platelets Study Group: Leukocyte reduction and ultraviolet B irradiation of platelets to prevent alloimmunization and refractoriness to platelet transfusions. *N Engl J Med* 337:1861–1869, 1997.
52. Pizzo PA: Management of fever in patients with cancer and treatment-induced neutropenia. *N Engl J Med* 328:1323–1332, 1993.
53. Engels EA, Ellis CA, Supran SE, et al: Early infection in bone marrow transplantation: quantitative study of clinical factors that affect risk. *Clin Infect Dis* 28:256–266, 1999.

54. McCullough J, Weiblen B, Deinard AR, et al: In vitro function and post-transfusion survival of granulocytes collected by continuous-flow centrifugation and by filtration leukapheresis. *Blood* 2:315–326, 1976.
55. Dutcher J, Schiffer C, Johnston G: Rapid migration of 111indium-labeled granulocytes to sites of infection. *N Engl J Med* 304:586–589, 1981.
56. Lowenthal RM, Grossman L, Goldman JM, et al: Granulocyte transfusions in treatment of infections in patients with acute leukemia and aplastic anemia. *Lancet* i:353–358, 1975.
57. Alavi J, Root R, Djerassi I, et al: A randomized clinical trial of granulocyte transfusions for infection in acute leukemia. *N Engl J Med* 13:706–711, 1977.
58. Vogler W, Winton E: A controlled study of the efficacy of granulocyte transfusions in patients with neutropenia. *Am J Med* 4:548–555, 1977.
59. Clift RA, Sanders JE, Thomas ED, et al: Granulocyte transfusions for the prevention of infection in patients receiving bone marrow transplants. *N Engl J Med* 298:1052–1057, 1978.
60. Adkins D, Goodnough L, Shenoy S, et al: Effect of leukocyte compatibility on neutrophil increment after transfusion of granulocyte colony-stimulating factor-mobilized prophylactic granulocyte transfusions and on clinical outcomes after stem cell transplantation. *Blood* 11:3605–3612, 2000.
61. Schiffer C, Aisner J, Daly PA, et al: Alloimmunization following prophylactic granulocyte transfusion. *Blood* 54:766–774, 1979.
62. Bensinger WI, Price TH, Dale DC: The effects of daily recombinant human granulocyte colony-stimulating factor administration on normal granulocyte donors undergoing leukapheresis. *Blood* 81:1883–1888, 1993.
63. Caspar CB, Seger RA, Burger J, et al: Effective stimulation of donors for granulocyte transfusions with recombinant methionyl granulocyte colony-stimulating factor. *Blood* 81:2866–2871, 1993.
64. Price TH, Bowden RA, Boeckh M, et al: Phase I/II trial of neutrophil transfusions from donors stimulated with G-CSF and Dexamethasone for treatment of patients with infections in hematopoietic stem cell transplantation. *Blood* 95:3302–3309, 2000.
65. McVay PA, Toy PT: Lack of increased bleeding after liver biopsy in patients with mild hemostatic abnormalities. *Am J Clin Pathol* 94:747–753, 1990.
66. McVay PA, Toy PT: Lack of increased bleeding after paracentesis and thoracentesis in patients with mild coagulation abnormalities. *Transfusion* 31: 164–71, 1991.
67. Wallis J, Dzik W: Is FFP over-transfused in the USA? *Transfusion* 44:1674–1675, 2004.
68. http://consensus.nih.gov/cons/045/045_statement.htm.
69. Contreras M, Ala FA, Greaves M, et al: Guidelines for the use of fresh frozen plasma. British Committee for Standards in Haematology, Working Party of the Blood Transfusion Task Force. *Transfus Med* 2:57–63, 1992.
70. Weigert AL, Schafer AL: Uremic bleeding: pathogenesis and therapy. *Am J Med Sci* 316:94–104. 1998.
71. Busch MP, Young MJ, Samson SM, et al: Risk of human immunodeficiency virus (HIV) transmission by blood transfusions before the implementation of HIV-1 antibody screening. The Transfusion Safety Study Group. *Transfusion* 31(1):4–11, 1991.
72. Schreiber GB, Busch MP, Kleinman SH, et al: The risk of transfusion-transmitted viral infections. *N Engl J Med* 337(26):1685–1690, 1996.
73. Benjamin RJ: Nucleic acid testing: update and applications. *Semin Hematol* 38:11–16, 2001.
74. Busch MP, Glynn SA, Stramer SL, et al: NHLBI-REDS NAT Study Group. A new strategy for estimating risks of transfusion-transmitted viral infections based on rates of detection of recently infected donors. *Transfusion* 45:254–264, 2005.
75. Dodd RY: Current safety of the blood supply in the United States. *Int J Hematol* 80:301–305,2004.
76. Pomper GJ, Wu Y, Snyder EL: Risks of transfusion-transmitted infections: 2003. *Curr Opin Hematol* 10:412–418,2003.
77. Clair P, Embil J, Fahey J: A seroepidemiologic study of cytomegalovirus infection in a Canadian recruit population. *Mil Med* 155(10):489–492, 1990.
78. Tegtmeier GE: Post transfusion cytomegalovirus infections. *Arch Pathol Lab Med* 113:236–245, 1989.
79. Bowden RA: Transfusion-transmitted cytomegalovirus infection. *Hematol Oncol Clin North Am* 9:155–166, 1995.
80. Bowden RA, Slichter SJ, Sayers MH, et al: A comparison of filtered leukocyte-reduced and cytomegalovirus (CMV) seronegative blood products for the prevention of transfusion-associated CMV infection after marrow transplant. *Blood* 86:3598–3603, 1995.
81. Perez P, Salmi LR, Follea G, et al: BACTHEM Group; French Haemovigilance Network: Determinants of transfusion-associated bacterial contamination: results of the French BACTHEM Case-Control Study. *Transfusion* 41:862–872, 2001.
82. Blajchman MA: Bacterial contamination of blood products and the value of pre-transfusion testing. *Immunol Invest* 24:163–170, 1995.
83. Centers for Disease Control and Prevention: Fatal bacterial infections associated with platelet transfusions—United States, 2004. *MMWR Morb Mortal Wkly Rep* 54:168–170, 2005.
84. Goldman M, Sher G, Blajchman M: Bacterial contamination of cellular blood products: the Canadian perspective. *Transfus Sci* 23:17–19, 2000.
85. Krailadsiri P, Seghatchian J, MacGregor I, et al: The effects of leukodepletion on the generation and removal of microvesicles and prion protein in blood components. *Transfusion* 46:407–417, 2006.
86. Lumadue JA, Manabe YC, Moore RD, et al: Adherence to a strict specimen-labeling policy decreases the incidence of erroneous blood grouping of blood bank specimens. *Transfusion* 37:1169–1172, 1997.
87. Capon SM, Goldfinger D: Acute hemolytic transfusion reaction, a paradigm of the systemic inflammatory response: new insights into pathophysiology and treatment. *Transfusion* 35:513–520, 1995.
88. Linden JV, Wagner K, Voytovich AE, et al: Transfusion errors in New York State: an analysis of 10 years' experience. *Transfusion* 40:1207–1213, 2000.
89. Sazama K: Reports of 355 transfusion-associated deaths: 1976 through 1985. *Transfusion* 30:583–590, 1990.
90. Brubaker DB: Clinical significance of white cell antibodies in febrile nonhemolytic transfusion reactions. *Transfusion* 30:733–737, 1990.
91. Heddle NM, Kelton JG: Febrile nonhemolytic transfusion reactions, in Popovsky MA (ed): *Transfusion Reactions*. 2nd ed. Bethesda, MD, AABB Press, 2001, pp 55–62.
92. Kleinman S, Caulfield T, Chan P, et al: Toward an understanding of transfusion-related acute lung injury: Statement of a consensus panel. *Transfusion* 44:1774–1789, 2004.
93. Moore SB: Transfusion-related acute lung injury (TRALI): Clinical presentation, treatment, and prognosis. *Crit Care Med* 34[5, Suppl]:S114–S117.2006.
94. Stephen CR, Martin RC, Bourgeois-Cavardin M: Antihistaminic drugs in the treatment of nonhemolytic transfusion reactions. *JAMA* 158:525–529, 1955.
95. Gorlin JB, Mintz PD: Transfusion-associated graft-vs-host-disease, in Mintz PD (ed). *Transfusion Therapy: Clinical Principles and Practice*. Bethesda, MD, AABB Press, 1999, pp 341–357.
96. Opelz G, Sengar DP, Michkey MR, et al: Effect of blood transfusions on subsequent kidney transplants. *Transplant Proc* 5:253–259, 1973.
97. Vamvakas EC, Blajchman MA: Deleterious clinical effects of transfusion-associated Immunomodulation: fact or fiction? *Blood* 97:1180–1195, 2001.
98. Vamvakas EC: Allogeneic blood transfusion as a risk factor for the subsequent development of non-Hodgkin's lymphoma. *Transfus Med Rev* 14:258–268, 2000.
99. van de Watering LM, Hermans J, Houbiers JG, et al: Beneficial effects of leukocyte depletion of transfused blood on postoperative complications in patients undergoing cardiac surgery: a randomized clinical trial. *Circulation* 97:562–568, 1998.

CHAPTER 115 ■ CRITICAL CARE OF PATIENTS WITH HEMATOLOGIC MALIGNANCIES

MATTHEW J. WIEDUWILT AND LLOYD E. DAMON

INTRODUCTION

Although the incidence of aggressive hematologic malignancies like acute myeloid leukemia (AML), acute lymphoblastic leukemia (ALL), and intermediate- and high-grade non-Hodgkin lymphomas is low, these potentially curable diseases frequently require intensive care unit (ICU) management at presentation to prevent early mortality and achieve disease remission. Patients with hematologic malignancies account for approximately 2% of all ICU admissions [1,2]. Approximately 7% of patients with hematologic malignancies admitted to the hospital will become critically ill [3]. The most frequently reported indications for ICU admission in patients with hematologic malignancies are respiratory failure (26% to 91%), severe sepsis (8% to 64%), neurologic impairment (14% to 23%), and acute renal failure (14% to 23%). For all critically ill patients with hematologic malignancies, ICU mortality, in hospital mortality and 6-month mortality rates are 23% to 62%, 54% to 82%, and 66% to 83%, respectively [1–11]. Risk factors for death in the ICU include high disease severity score (APACHE II, SAPS II, SOFA), vasopressor use, leukopenia, increasing number of organ failures, and acute renal failure (see Table 115.1). Notably, mechanical ventilation has not been consistently associated with increased risk of death in this patient population, and some studies suggest improved outcomes with early endotracheal intubation [2,12]. In addition, survival in patients with hematologic malignancies admitted to the ICU after chemotherapy alone versus hematopoietic stem cell transplant (HSCT) are not different, suggesting that critically ill HSCT patients should be treated aggressively on ICU admission [13,14]. In fact, when matched for severity of acute illness upon ICU admission, survival of patients with hematologic malignancies and nononcologic patients appears to be similar [1].

OVERVIEW OF HEMATOLOGIC MALIGNANCIES

Acute Myeloid Leukemia

AML accounts for 22% to 54% of hematologic malignancy admissions to the ICU [1,2,4,6–11]. Patients with AML may require ICU admission for disease- or treatment-related complications including sepsis (frequently complicated by neutropenia), bleeding due to thrombocytopenia and occasionally acute disseminated intravascular coagulation and multiple organ failure.

The incidence of AML in the United States is 3.5 cases per 100,000 persons per year with approximately 12,000 new cases diagnosed annually [15]. More than half of newly diagnosed AML patients are over 65 years of age and a third are older than 75 years. Five-year survival rates are approximately 50% in adults under the age of 45 years but drop to less than 10% in patients over the age of 65 [16]. The risk factors for the development of AML, including genetic and environmental factors, have been well defined [17–27].

AML arises from the acquisition of genetic mutations in myeloid precursors or stem cells leading to various degrees of maturation arrest, unregulated proliferation, and resistance to apoptosis. By the World Health Organization 2008 classification system, the diagnosis of AML requires myeloid blasts to comprise 20% or more of nucleated cells in the peripheral blood or bone marrow except in cases of AML with the recurrent cytogenetic abnormalities t(15;17), t(8;21), inv(16)/t(16;16), myeloid sarcoma (a tumor of myeloblasts), and some cases of erythroleukemia [28]. The recurrent cytogenetic abnormalities t(15;17), t(8;21), inv(16)/t(16;16) and normal cytogenetics accompanied by gene mutations in NPM1 or CEBP-alpha confer a better prognosis in terms of risk of relapse, and the majority of patients obtain durable complete remissions with chemotherapy alone [28,29]. Conversely, patients with poor-risk cytogenetics and those with normal cytogenetics accompanied by mutations in the FLT3 protooncogene have a low likelihood of durable remission with chemotherapy alone and typically undergo allogeneic HSCT [29].

Standard induction chemotherapy for AML using 3 days of intravenous (IV) anthracycline (daunorubicin, idarubicin) or anthracenedione (mitoxantrone) and 7 days of cytarabine by continuous IV infusion, ideally initiated within 5 days of diagnosis, leads to complete remission rates of 60% to 80% in young adults under 60 years of age and 50% in patients over 60 years of age. Postremission therapy is tailored to pretreatment risk status, performance status and age and may consist of three to four cycles of high-dose cytarabine, autologous HSCT or, for younger patients at high risk of relapse, allogeneic HSCT [30].

Acute Promyelocytic Leukemia

APL accounts for 5% to 6% of all acute myeloid leukemia with approximately 600 to 800 new diagnoses made each year in the Unites States [31,32]. APL frequently presents with acute disseminated intravascular coagulation (DIC) that can be rapidly fatal due to intracerebral, pulmonary, or gastrointestinal hemorrhage, in all accounting for 50% to 60% of early deaths [33]. Early suspicion and treatment of APL, even prior to definitive genetic diagnosis, is important to reduce the risk of life-threatening hemorrhage [34]. Paradoxically, patients are also at risk for thrombotic events that complicate about 10% to 12% of cases, frequently in those with expression of CD2, CD15, and FLT3-ITD mutation [35,36].

APL occurs due to arrest of myeloid differentiation at the promyelocyte stage leading to accumulation of leukemic promyelocytes in the bone marrow, blood, and tissues. Morphologically, leukemic promyelocytes typically have variable

TABLE 115.1

OUTCOMES OF PATIENTS WITH HEMATOLOGIC MALIGNANCIES ADMITTED TO THE ICU

Number of patients	ICU mortality (%)	In-hospital mortality (%)	Risk factors for death	Reference
7,689	43	59	HSCT, Hodgkin lymphoma, severe sepsis, age, length of hospital stay prior to ICU admission, respiratory failure, neurologic failure, renal failure, anemia	[2]
22	55	82	APACHE II score, number of failing organs, mechanical ventilation	[4]
60	—	78	APACHE II score >30, number of failing organs, resistant disease, leukopenia	[5]
92	—	77	Progression of underlying malignancy	[6]
78	26	—	Number of failing organs, liver failure	[7]
104	44	—	SAPS II score, mechanical ventilation	[8]
124	42	54	Leukopenia, vasopressors, renal failure	[9]
58	62	—	SAPS II score, SOFA score	[10]
24	—	75	SAPS II score >66, liver failure, neurologic failure, number of failing organs	[3]
92	50	55	SAPS II, SOFA, ODIN, and LODS scores, allogeneic HSCT, neutropenia, severe sepsis, vasopressor use, invasive mechanical ventilation	[11]
101	23	—	SAPS II score, SOFA score, mechanical ventilation, renal replacement therapy	[1]

HSCT, hematopoietic stem cell transplant; SAPS II, Simplified Acute Physiology Score II; APACHE II, Acute Physiology and Chronic Health Evaluation II; SOFA, Sequential Organ Failure Assessment; ODIN, Organ Dysfunction and/or Infection Score; LODS, Logistic Organ Dysfunction Score.

nuclear morphology with bilobed or reniform nuclei, prominent cytoplasmic granules, and numerous large Auer rods, frequently in bundles [37]. Approximately 5% of APL presents as a microgranular variant characterized by few or absent granules [38]. Patients with this microgranular variant tend to have higher presenting white blood cell counts, placing them at higher risk for complications and relapse. Except in rare instances, APL is characterized by the presence of the recurrent cytogenetic abnormality t(15;17)(q22;q12) leading to a PML-RAR-alpha fusion gene that can be demonstrated by cytogenetic analysis, FISH and quantitative RT-PCR [37]. The chimeric PML-RAR-alpha protein is the target of therapy with all-*trans*-retinoic acid (ATRA) and arsenic trioxide (ATO), agents that cause degradation of the PML-RAR-alpha oncoprotein thereby promoting terminal differentiation of leukemic promyelocytes [39,40].

The diagnosis of APL should be considered in any patient with a new diagnosis of leukemia especially if accompanied by clinical and laboratory evidence of acute DIC. Early institution of treatment with the differentiating agent ATRA is indicated upon suspicion of APL [32,34]. Careful review of the peripheral blood smear from new leukemia patients in consultation with hematologists and hematopathologists should be performed to look for characteristic hypergranular leukemic promyelocytes. Expedited performance of flow cytometry, specifically evaluating for coexpression of CD34, CD15, and CD13 on the surface of leukemic cells can aide in diagnosing the microgranular variant of APL [41].

Greater than 70% of APL patients attain prolonged remissions with current treatment strategies. Induction chemotherapy regimens generally combine ATRA with an anthracycline, typically idarubicin or daunorubicin [32]. ATO is highly active against APL and in combination with ATRA produces CR rates over 90% [42–44]. ATRA or ATO, however, may cause a fatal differentiation syndrome characterized by fever, dyspnea, pulmonary infiltrates, pleuropericardial effusions, weight gain, peripheral edema, renal failure, and hypotension.

Acute Lymphoblastic Leukemia

ALL results from the acquisition of genetic mutations in lymphoid progenitor or stem cells resulting in the arrest of cells at an early stage of differentiation [45]. In 2009, about 5,760 people were diagnosed with ALL in the United States with a median age of 13 years [15]. ALL patients comprise 9% to 27% of ICU admissions for hematologic malignancies [1,2,4,6–11]. The 10-year survival among adults with ALL is less than 30% [45–47]. Favorable disease characteristics in ALL include ages 1 to 15 years, presenting WBC <50,000 per μL and rapid achievement of complete remission, whereas age >35 years is unfavorable. Cases with the t(9;22)/BCR-ABL (Philadelphia chromosome, Ph), representing 15% to 20% of adult cases of ALL, and the t(4;11)/MLL-AF4 translocations typically fare poorly, with survival rates of less than 10% with chemotherapy alone and long term survival after allogeneic HSCT ranging 20% to 45% [48–53].

Clinical trial regimens in the last decade have improved complete remission rates to 74% to 93% with 5-year survival rates as high as 48% [54]. Therapy for ALL typically spans 2 to 3 years and includes induction therapy, postremission therapy, central nervous system (CNS) prophylaxis and maintenance chemotherapy in patients who do not undergo HSCT. Induction therapy for ALL typically combines vincristine, an anthracycline (e.g. daunorubicin), and a corticosteroid (prednisone or dexamethasone) with L-asparginase and/or cyclophosphamide. Prophylaxis against CNS relapse includes intrathecal chemotherapy with methotrexate with or without cytarabine and frequently high-dose IV systemic methotrexate. Postremission therapy typically includes the same agents used in induction as well as cytarabine and 6-mercaptopurine. Maintenance therapy consists of oral methotrexate and 6-mercaptopurine often with pulses of vincristine and corticosteroids. Imatinib (Gleevec®) and dasatinib (Sprycel®) inhibit the chimeric BCR-ABL tyrosine kinase produced by the Philadelphia chromosome and improve complete remission and survival rates in Ph+ ALL [55–63]. Ideally, allogeneic HSCT is performed in patients with poor-risk disease.

Aggressive Non-Hodgkin Lymphomas

Diffuse large B-cell lymphoma (DLBCL) is an aggressive non-Hodgkin lymphoma of intermediate grade that typically presents with rapidly enlarging lymph nodes or extranodal masses frequently with symptoms of organ compromise from lymphomatous involvement of extranodal sites. Diagnosis is typically made by excisional biopsy of a lymph node or mass showing large lymphoid cells that completely efface lymph node architecture. Malignant B-cells express CD19, CD20, and CD22 with variable expression of surface immunoglobulin, CD5 and CD10 [64]. Common genetic abnormalities in DLBCL include constitutive expression of the transcriptional repressor Bcl-6, the antiapoptotic protein Bcl-2, and/or the transcription factor c-myc [65]. The International Prognostic Index for aggressive lymphomas uses five unfavorable variables to establish risk status: age greater than 60 years, poor performance status, advanced stage (Ann Arbor Stage III or IV disease), extranodal involvement at more than one site and elevated serum lactate dehydrogenase [66]. First-line combination chemotherapy with cyclophosphamide, doxorubicin, vincristine, and prednisone (CHOP) in combination with the humanized monoclonal anti-CD20 antibody rituximab results in 2-year overall survival rates of 70% to 90% [65].

Burkitt lymphoma (BL), which has the fastest growth rate of any human malignancy, is an aggressive non-Hodgkin lymphoma with endemic, sporadic, and immunodeficiency-associated clinical variants. BL typically presents with rapidly progressive nodal and extranodal disease, commonly in the abdomen and gastrointestinal tract leading to nausea, vomiting, anorexia, bowel obstruction, and gastrointestinal bleeding. Advanced stage is common at diagnosis with bone marrow involvement in 30% to 38% and CNS involvement in 13 to 17% of adults [67]. Morphologically, lymphoma cells are medium-sized with deeply basophilic cytoplasm containing cytoplasmic lipid vacuoles and a high proliferative index of greater than 90%. A leukemic variant exists and can be distinguished from ALL by surface expression of immunoglobulin, CD20 and CD10, without coexpression of TdT or CD34. BL is genetically characterized by chromosomal translocations that lead to constitutive expression of c-myc, typically t(8;14) and rarely t(2;8) or t(8;22)[68]. High-intensity, brief-duration chemotherapy, typically with cyclophosphamide, doxorubicin, vincristine, and antimetabolite-containing regimens, with intensive CNS prophylaxis, have led to 1-year remission rates as high as 86% [67]. The bulky disease and high cell proliferation rates seen in both DLBCL and Burkitt lymphoma place patients at high risk for tumor lysis syndrome and prophylactic treatment with allopurinol to prevent hyperuricemia is typically given prior to chemotherapy.

Other Malignancies

Other notable hematologic malignancies frequently requiring ICU level care are multiple myeloma, Waldenstrom macroglobulinemia and myeloproliferative neoplasms such as chronic myeloid leukemia, essential thrombocythemia, polycythemia vera, and chronic idiopathic myelofibrosis. In multiple myeloma, spinal cord compression may occur due to encroachment of the spinal canal by epidural plasmacytomas and from pathologic fracture of spinal vertebrae. Emergent imaging of the entire spine with MRI is required for diagnosis (see Chapter 116). In Waldenstrom macroglobulinemia, high concentrations of monoclonal IgM paraprotein in the serum can lead to the hyperviscosity syndrome manifest as mucosal bleeding, confusion, seizures, coma, visual disturbance, and/or headache as well as cryoglobulinemia, cold agglutinin hemolytic anemia, and plasma volume expansion leading to congestive heart failure [69]. Myeloproliferative neoplasms may lead to life-threatening hemorrhage or thrombosis, requiring critical care (see Chapter 111).

DISEASE AND TREATMENT RELATED COMPLICATIONS

Hyperleukocytosis and Leukostasis

In AML, hyperleukocytosis, generally defined as a circulating blast count greater than 50,000 to 100,000 per μL, occurs in 5% to 18% of patients at initial presentation [70,71]. Early mortality during initial treatment of patients with hyperleukocytic AML ranges from 5% to 30% with advanced age, poor performance status, coagulopathy, respiratory compromise, and organ failure associated with early death [70–75]. Hyperleukocytosis in AML is frequently associated with leukostasis manifesting as respiratory failure, visual disturbance, intracranial hemorrhage, and renal failure.

Leukostasis, although typically associated with hyperleukocytosis, can occur at white blood cell counts less than 50,000 per μL (likely due to interpatient variability in leukemia cell biology and individual susceptibility). Myeloid leukemic blasts are less deformable than mature white blood cells possibly predisposing to formation of aggregates of cells in the small blood vessels, tissue ischemia, endothelial damage and tissue infiltration [76–78]. In addition, expression of specific cell surface adhesion molecules on leukemia cells and endothelial cell activation by cytokines secreted by leukemic blasts may play important roles in promoting leukostasis. The expression of CD56/NCAM on the surface of leukemia cells in myelomonocytic AML correlates with the development of leukostasis [79]. In vitro, myeloid blasts promote their own adhesion to the vascular endothelium by upregulating expression of ICAM-1, VCAM-1, and E-selectin on endothelial cells [80]. In ALL, hyperleukocytosis is rarely associated with symptomatic leukostasis except with extreme hyperleukocytosis (WBC >400,000 per μL) possibly due to the smaller size, easier deformability, and decreased vascular endothelium adherence of lymphoblasts [81]. Notably, lymphoblasts in the rare ALL patients with symptomatic leukostasis are less deformable than lymphoblasts from ALL patients without leukostasis [82]. In AML with hyperleukocytosis, most studies have not shown a demonstrable difference in complete response rates, disease free survival or overall survival after treatment [83]. However, the presence of pulmonary leukostasis, hepatomegaly, hyperbilirubinemia, and hypofibrinogenemia are predictors of poor outcome in patients with hyperleukocytosis [74,75,84].

Hydroxyurea at doses of 20 to 30 mg per kg per day or more can reduce peripheral leukocyte counts, and generally requires 1 to 2 days to take effect. Red blood cell transfusions should be avoided until the leukocyte count is less than 50,000 per μL to avoid ischemic events such as stroke or acute coronary syndrome. Although invasive, leukapheresis is a relatively safe procedure and is frequently used in combination with hydroxyurea to rapidly lower circulating blast counts and theoretically decrease the risk of tumor lysis syndrome and progressive leukostasis. Two blood volumes (140 mL per kg) are processed in the typical leukapheresis procedure. Studies have failed to show a consistent clinical benefit with the use of leukapheresis in hyperleukocytic leukemias [85–88], although some uncontrolled retrospective single institution studies show reduction of early mortality in patients undergoing leukapheresis without an overall survival benefit [87,88]. Despite the poor prognosis of APL presenting with hyperleukocytosis and organ failure, leukapheresis is contraindicated in this group of patients due to risk of exacerbating acute DIC, initiating vasomotor instability, and increasing induction death [89].

Hyperviscosity Syndrome

The hyperviscosity syndrome occurs in 30% of patients with Waldenstrom macroglobulinemia (also called lymphoplasmacytic lymphoma with IgM monoclonal gammopathy) at presentation and is defined by the presence of increased serum viscosity with neurologic symptoms related to impaired blood flow including headache, vertigo, dizziness, visual impairment, hearing impairment, tinnitus, nystagmus, stupor, stroke, dementia, and coma [90–95]. In addition, mucosal bleeding, including GI hemorrhage, renal failure, and congestive heart failure due to plasma volume expansion and concomitant anemia may occur. Elevated serum IgM, with its large pentameric structure, is most commonly associated with hyperviscosity, although the syndrome has been reported with IgA, IgG, and kappa light chain multiple myeloma [96–101]. Normal serum viscosity measures 1.4 to 1.8 centipoises [102,103] and symptomatic hyperviscosity typically occurs at greater than 4 centipoises [69].

Emergent plasmapheresis is indicated for symptomatic hyperviscosity. One to two plasma volumes are typically exchanged and replaced with 5% albumin in patients with low bleeding risk or fresh frozen plasma (FFP) in patients at high risk for bleeding. Symptoms typically resolve quickly but neurologic deficits can remain. Red blood cell transfusions should be avoided if possible until serum viscosity is lowered. Definitive treatment for the underlying malignancy should be instituted quickly to control paraprotein production. Procedural risks include depletion of clotting factors when 5% albumin is used as the exchange fluid, hypocalcemia from citrate anticoagulant use, dialysis catheter-related infection, pneumothorax or thrombosis, and complications from FFP administration including anaphylaxis, blood-borne infections, and transfusion-related acute lung injury.

Bleeding

Bleeding in hematologic malignancies is a common cause of morbidity and mortality. DIC and thrombocytopenia are common etiologies, but acquired clotting factor deficiencies can also predispose to life-threatening hemorrhage.

Disseminated Intravascular Coagulation

Acute DIC is a common cause of morbidity and mortality during the treatment of many hematologic malignancies and is especially characteristic of acute promyelocytic leukemia and to a lesser degree other forms of acute leukemia. Sepsis, especially gram-negative sepsis occurring in the setting of disease or treatment related neutropenia, is a common cause of DIC as well. Complicating the diagnosis of DIC is the frequent presence of hepatic failure due to malignant infiltration of the liver or treatment-related hepatotoxicity. Clinically, patients are at high risk for death from bleeding and can develop oozing from IV lines and surgical sites, purpura, pulmonary hemorrhage, intracranial hemorrhage, gastrointestinal bleeding, and multiple organ failure.

Acute DIC results from pathologic coagulation within small blood vessels, typically from the release of tissue factor or endotoxin exposure, leading to unmitigated activation of coagulation and consumption of coagulation factors and platelets. Depletion of clotting factors and platelets, activation of plasmin, and the production of anticoagulant fibrin split products can lead to severe bleeding. Laboratory hallmarks of acute DIC include thrombocytopenia, prolongation of clotting times, hypofibrinogenemia, elevated fibrin split products, and sometimes schistocytes on the peripheral blood smear.

The coagulopathy observed in APL resembles acute DIC but with some subtle differences [104]. In APL, leukemic cells produce tissue factor and high levels of a cysteine protease called cancer procoagulant, both of which are downregulated by ATRA treatment in primary and cultured leukemic APL blasts [105–109]. Tissue factor in conjunction with activated Factor VII activates Factor X, whereas cancer procoagulant can directly activate Factor X leading to pathologic coagulation [104,110]. In addition, rapid death of malignant cells leads to increased thrombin generation [111]. Unlike acute DIC, antithrombin and protein C levels are maintained in the coagulopathy of APL [112]. Increased fibrinolysis also complicates APL and can lead to bleeding. APL cells express both cell surface u-PA (urokinase-plasminogen activator) and t-PA (tissue-plasminogen activator). u-PA is transiently upregulated upon differentiation of leukemic cells with ATRA [113,114]. Dexamethasone administered with ATRA suppresses the upregulation of u-PA. Annexin II is highly expressed on leukemic promyelocytes and interacts with plasminogen and t-PA to increase plasmin production [115]. In addition, annexin II is highly expressed on cerebral endothelial cells potentially explaining the high rates of intracerebral hemorrhage in APL [116,117]. Notably, treatment with ATRA downregulates the expression of annexin II on leukemic promyelocytes [115,118].

Reversal of acute DIC requires effective treatment of the underlying cause. Supportive care includes early management of sepsis including the administration of broad-spectrum antibiotic coverage with anti-Pseudomonal activity in neutropenic patients and reversal of organ dysfunction when possible. In the setting of APL, early institution of ATRA combined with cytotoxic chemotherapy in high-risk patients with WBC >10,000 per μL is indicated to reduce the burden of leukemic promyelocytes. DIC typically resolves within 48 hours of initiation of ATRA in this setting.

With acute DIC, frequent monitoring of complete blood count, prothrombin time (PT), partial thromboplastin time (PTT), and fibrinogen three to four times a day is prudent to monitor the consumptive process and guide replacement of platelets and coagulation factors. In patients with APL-associated DIC who are bleeding or who are at high risk of bleeding, maintenance of platelet count above 30,000 to 50,000 per μL and fibrinogen above 100 to 150 mg per dL with platelet and cryoprecipitate transfusions has been recommended [32]. Fresh frozen plasma also may be given to reduce the prolonged PT and PTT. By inhibiting thrombin and Factor Xa, low-dose heparin (4 to 5 U per kg per hour) could theoretically improve severe bleeding in acute DIC by limiting fibrinogen and platelet consumption, plasminogen activation, and fibrin split product production. Results of clinical studies, however, have been equivocal, and routine use of heparin to prevent or treat acute DIC-related bleeding is not universally standard [104,119–121]. Conversely, thrombosis may occur in acute DIC, and in this setting, the administration of low-dose heparin may beneficial [122,123].

Thrombocytopenia

Thrombocytopenia in patients with hematologic malignancies can be caused by bone marrow infiltration by malignant cells, myelosuppression from chemotherapy and other medications, bacterial sepsis, acute DIC, immune thrombocytopenia and/or hypersplenism from splenomegaly. The risk of major hemorrhage dramatically increases at platelet counts less than 5,000 per μL and the use of prophylactic platelet transfusions, starting in the 1970s, typically with a transfusion threshold of 20,000 per μL, reduced the frequency of fatal bleeding in this population to less than 1%. However, this strategy led to an increased demand for platelet concentrates [124,125].

The issue of the optimal platelet count to trigger a prophylactic platelet transfusion has been addressed. A 2004 Cochrane Database systematic review included three prospective randomized studies comparing prophylactic platelet transfusions at platelet counts of 10,000 per μL versus 20,000 per μL. None of these studies showed significant differences in severe bleeding events or mortality but the studies were small and possibly underpowered to show noninferiority of the lower transfusion threshold [125]. Current studies suggest that the risk of spontaneous hemorrhage in patients without concomitant coagulopathy or acute DIC, platelet dysfunction, fever, mucositis or uncontrolled hypertension is acceptable until platelets are below 10,000 per μL. Safely minimizing the platelet dose per prophylactic transfusion has recently been studied. A 2010 study randomized 1,272 patients undergoing chemotherapy or HSCT for hematologic and nonhematologic malignancies to receive 1.1×10^{11}, 2.2×10^{11}, or 4.4×10^{11} platelets per square meter of body surface area to be given prophylactically for platelet counts less than 10,000 per μL. The lowest dose group required fewer platelets overall but required more transfusions (five versus three per patient per treatment course). Bleeding rates of all grades were similar between the groups with no deaths from hemorrhage in the low- and medium-dose groups supporting the use of low-dose platelet transfusions [126]. Avoiding drugs that cause platelet dysfunction (especially aspirin, nonsteroidal anti-inflammatory agents [NSAIDs], Cox-2 inhibitors, and clopidogrel), treating underlying coagulopathy and reversing renal dysfunction are important adjuncts to preventing bleeding in thrombocytopenic patients as well.

Acquired von Willebrand Syndrome

The acquired von Willebrand syndrome (aVWS) results from a reduction in the level of von Willebrand factor (VWF) and may rarely occur in monoclonal gammopathy of undetermined significance (MGUS), Waldenstrom macroglobulinemia, multiple myeloma, non-Hodgkin lymphomas, and myeloproliferative neoplasms, especially essential thrombocythemia [127–130]. Treatment of the underlying malignancy to decrease tumor burden or reduce elevated platelet counts is generally effective in resolving acquired von Willebrand disease. Management may include platelet apheresis in the setting of extreme thrombocytosis and active bleeding [131]. High-dose IVIG (dose, 1 g per kg per day for 2 days) may be considered in patients with lymphoid neoplasms who have inhibitory antibodies to VWF [99,100,132,133]. For treatment of acute bleeding, desmopressin (dose, 0.03 μg per kg IV) or purified plasma-derived vWF/FVIII concentrates may be considered [132]. Aspirin and NSAIDs should be avoided until the aVWS has resolved.

Pulmonary Complications

Mechanical ventilation is associated with poor outcomes in patients with hematologic malignancies. Mortality ranges from 39% to 82%, although most studies of respiratory failure in patients with hematologic malignancies are retrospective and have failed to match mechanically ventilated and nonventilated patients for degree of respiratory compromise. Hampshire et al. retrospectively studied 7,689 cases of hematologic malignancies requiring ICU admission in England, Wales, and Northern Ireland. When matched for PaO_2:FiO_2 ratios, mechanically ventilated hematologic malignancy patients had reduced mortality compared with nonventilated hematologic malignancy patients (mortality 67% vs. 85% for PaO_2:FiO_2 <100 mm Hg, 50% vs. 69% for PaO_2:FiO_2 100 to 199 mm Hg)[2]. In a smaller study, invasive mechanical ventilation within 24 hours after ICU admission was associated with lower mortality rates compared with patients receiving noninvasive positive pressure ventilation [12]. After HSCT, however, patients who require mechanical ventilation appear to fare less well. Short-term mortality is 82% to 96% and worsens to 98% to 100% in the setting of combined renal and hepatic failure [101]. Only 9% to 14% of mechanically ventilated HSCT patients are alive 6 months after ICU admission [93,101].

Diagnostic approaches to identify the etiology of respiratory failure include blood cultures, blood and urine infectious serologies, diagnostic imaging, bronchoscopy, and surgical lung biopsy. Flexible bronchoscopy with bronchoalveolar lavage (BAL) detects pulmonary infections in approximately 50% of patients with hematologic malignancies presenting with respiratory deterioration leading to a change in antimicrobial therapy in 38% of patients [94,95]. In one study there was no survival advantage to BAL and respiratory deterioration requiring mechanical ventilation occurred in 36% of patients as a short-term consequence of BAL highlighting the need for careful patient selection and the broad use of noninvasive diagnostic tests prior to pursuing BAL [95]. In two retrospective studies of surgical lung biopsy among hematologic malignancy patients with unexplained pulmonary infiltrates, a specific diagnosis was made in 62% to 67% of patients and led to change in therapy 40% to 57% of the time. A specific diagnosis was significantly associated with decreased mortality in both studies (absolute reduction in mortality, 29% to 33%) [103,134].

Infection is the most common identifiable cause of respiratory distress in hematologic malignancies. Pulmonary hemorrhage, diffuse alveolar damage, pulmonary embolism, and congestive heart failure are the most common identifiable noninfectious causes. Pulmonary infections are typically due to *Pseudomonas aeruginosa*, *Staphylococcus aureus*, and streptococcal species with *Legionella pneumophila* and mycobacterial infections being less common pathogens. Prolonged neutropenia from underlying disease or myelotoxic chemotherapy places patients at risk for mycelial fungal pneumonia with *Aspergillus* spp being the most common offenders. Patients with lymphoid malignancies and those treated with allogeneic HSCT are also at risk for *Pneumocystis jiroveci* pneumonia and viral pneumonias including cytomegalovirus infection. Effective antimicrobial treatment can be difficult in this group of patients as mixed infections and antimicrobial resistance are common [135,136]. Ganciclovir and related antiviral agents in combination with IV immunoglobulin have reduced the mortality of CMV pneumonia in HSCT patients [137].

Noninfectious etiologies of respiratory failure in patients with hematologic malignancies, including those undergoing HSCT, include cardiogenic pulmonary edema, diffuse alveolar hemorrhage, engraftment syndrome, idiopathic pneumonia syndrome, bronchiolitis obliterans syndrome (BOS), cryptogenic organizing pneumonia, granulomatous inflammation and malignant infiltration of the lungs. Chemotherapeutic agents such as carmustine (BCNU), busulfan, and bleomycin are known to cause lung injury. ICU patients with hematologic malignancies are also at high risk for pulmonary embolism given immobility, active malignancy, and frequently DIC.

Diffuse alveolar hemorrhage (DAH) accounts for 20% to 30% of pulmonary complications after allogeneic HSCT [138] and is a cause of early death in 1.5% of patients with APL [33]. DAH occurs with hematopoietic engraftment in allogeneic HSCT patients and presents with cough, hemoptysis, declining hemoglobin, and hypoxemia with diffuse alveolar filling on lung imaging. Serial lavage during BAL shows increasingly bloody fluid return. Treatment for DAH includes replacement of platelets and coagulation factors to maintain hemostasis, supportive mechanical ventilation as needed, and corticosteroids. Small retrospective studies support the use of high-dose corticosteroids (methylprednisolone 30 to 1,500 mg per day) for treatment of DAH after allogeneic HSCT [139–141]. Administration of parenteral recombinant activated factor VII has been associated with resolution of DAH occurring after HSCT in several case reports [142–147].

In addition to DAH, early onset noninfectious pulmonary complications after allogeneic HSCT include pulmonary engraftment syndrome and idiopathic pneumonia syndrome. Pulmonary engraftment syndrome mimics DAH and is characterized by fever, pulmonary infiltrates, hypoxia, and a skin rash developing early after HSCT, coinciding with recovery of circulating neutrophils (ANC > 500 per μL). It is typically a self-limited process lasting 1 to 2 weeks that is treated with supportive care and a short course of standard-dose corticosteroids [118]. Idiopathic pneumonia syndrome (IPS), which occurs in about 10% of HSCT patients, presents with fever, cough, shortness of breath, hypoxemia, and diffuse bilateral pulmonary infiltrates without an identifiable infection by BAL. IPS occurs after hematopoietic engraftment with a median onset of 21 to 52 days after HSCT and carries a 60% to 90% mortality [117,148,149]. Pathologically the syndrome is characterized by an interstitial infiltrate comprised primarily of lymphocytes. In a study of 15 patients with IPS, the combination of etanercept, a tissue necrosis factor-alpha (TNF-alpha) antagonist, and corticosteroids given at 2 mg per kg daily (methylprednisolone equivalent) resulted in 10 complete responses and a 28-day survival of 73% [150].

Late-onset noninfectious pulmonary complications after HSCT typically occur more than 3 months after stem cell infusion and include BOS and cryptogenic-organizing pneumonia (COP, formerly referred to as bronchiolitis obliterans with organizing pneumonia). BOS occurs in 14% of allogeneic HSCT patients with chronic graft-versus-host disease (cGVHD). BOS is a manifestation of cGVHD whereby alloreactive donor T-cells generate fibromuscular proliferation of the walls of small airways. This produces an obstructive physiology with air trapping and occasionally the need for supplemental oxygen. There is no standard treatment for BOS beyond immunosuppression for cGVHD, although investigations are ongoing combining aerosolized corticosteroids with azithromycin and montelukast (a leukotriene receptor antagonist). COP tends to occur late after allogeneic HSCT and demonstrates restrictive pulmonary physiology. COP is associated with GVHD and may be a manifestation of the disease itself. Some insult triggers inflammation of the small airways causing a proliferative bronchiolitis and deposition of cellular matrix materials into alveoli leading to hypoxemia. Unlike BOS, COP is reversible and corticosteroid responsive [151].

Common pulmonary processes complicating hematologic malignancies are summarized in Table 115.2.

Infection

Chemotherapy for high-grade hematologic malignancies commonly causes neutropenia (phagocytic immunocompromise) and cellular and/or humoral immunosuppression. For uncertain reasons, AML patients retain adequate cellular and humoral immunity even during periods of severe bone marrow suppression. Neutropenic patients are susceptible to infections by endogenous skin, genitourinary and gastrointestinal tract flora as well as hospital-acquired infections including nosocomial and ventilator-associated pneumonias, central venous line infections, *Clostridium difficile* colitis, and infections with *Pseudomonas* spp, *Stenotrophomonas* spp, *Burkholderia* spp, vancomycin-resistant enterococcus, methicillin-resistant *S. aureus*, and extended spectrum beta-lactamase-producing Gram-negative organisms. Prolonged neutropenia, especially with concomitant corticosteroid administration or diabetes mellitus, places patients at risk for invasive fungal infections, especially *Aspergillus* spp. Immunosuppressed patients, particularly those with lymphoid malignancies and those undergoing allogeneic HSCT, are at additional risk for opportunistic infections such as *P. jiroveci*, herpes simplex virus, varicella zoster virus, and cytomegalovirus. Treatment of febrile patients with neutropenia or immunosuppression involves rapid evaluation for infectious causes and initiation of empiric broad-spectrum antibiotic therapy with adequate coverage of *Pseudomonas aeruginosa* and methicillin-resistant *S. aureus*. For patients with persistent fever and prolonged neutropenia (>7 days), the addition of antifungal therapy targeting *Aspergillus* spp is indicated. Afebrile neutropenic patients with an absolute neutrophil count less than 500 per μL should receive daily prophylactic treatment with a fluoroquinolone antibiotic. A meta-analysis of 95 trials including 52 trials using fluoroquinolone prophylaxis showed that neutropenic patients receiving fluoroquinolone prophylaxis had significant decreases in all cause mortality, infection-related mortality, fever and documented infection with a nonsignificant trend toward increasing antimicrobial resistance [152]. The use of granulocyte stimulating growth factors (e.g., G-CSF) in patients receiving myelotoxic chemotherapy reduces total days of neutropenia and hospital length of stay without promoting tumor cell growth or affecting overall survival [153].

Differentiation Syndrome

Differentiation syndrome (DS), formerly referred to as retinoic acid syndrome, is a potentially fatal process of unclear mechanism (likely, detrimental cytokine storm) that occurs in 2% to 27% of APL patients treated with ATRA or arsenic trioxide [154]. Symptoms include fever, peripheral edema, weight gain more than 5 kg, pleuropericardial effusions, shortness of breath, interstitial pulmonary infiltrates, acute renal failure and hypotension after initiating APL treatment with the differentiating agents ATRA or arsenic trioxide. The diagnosis requires at least two of the above findings. Moderate DS is defined as having two to three of the above findings whereas severe DS has four or more findings [155]. Elevation of liver transaminases may also occur. Symptoms can develop at any time within the first 4 weeks of treatment with highest incidences in the first and third weeks of treatment. Risk factors for the development of severe DS include WBC >5,000 per μL and elevated serum creatinine [154].

The diagnosis of DS is difficult at times as frequent complications of APL and its treatment, such as pneumonia, pulmonary hemorrhage, heart failure, acute renal failure, and sepsis, can mimic the syndrome. Early consideration of DS is important, however, so that prompt treatment with dexamethasone can be initiated. In both moderate and severe cases, dexamethasone is given at 10 mg PO or IV twice a day. Although no controlled studies of dexamethasone treatment have been published, since the inception of this practice the mortality rate from differentiation syndrome has dropped to less than 1% in recent studies. In moderate cases, ATRA and/or arsenic trioxide can be continued safely with close monitoring for worsening symptoms. In severe cases, ATRA and/or arsenic trioxide are held until symptoms resolve at which point it is generally safe to resume treatment. Administration of chemotherapy early in ATRA treatment has been shown to reduce the incidence if differentiation syndrome [156]. Patients with high suspicion of APL and a WBC >10,000 per μL should be treated immediately with cytotoxic chemotherapy in addition to ATRA prior

TABLE 115.2

FREQUENTLY ENCOUNTERED PULMONARY COMPLICATIONS IN HEMATOLOGIC MALIGNANCIES

Complication	Context	Timing	Diagnosis	Management
Infection	Neutropenia	Variable: ≤7 days of neutropenia: bacterial, *Candida* spp >7 days of neutropenia: bacterial, fungal including *Aspergillus* spp	Blood cultures, fungal serologies, BAL, lung biopsy (transbronchial, VATS, open) CXR/CT/HRCT	Empiric antimicrobials may include coverage of MRSA, GNRs, *Pseudomonas* spp, typical and atypical bacterial pathogens, *Candida* spp, *Aspergillus* spp
	HSCT	After engraftment: viral including CMV, RSV, Herpesviridae, fungal, bacterial, mycobacterial, *Pneumocystis jiroveci*	Blood cultures, fungal serologies, respiratory virus DFA and PCR, CMV PCR (blood), BAL, lung biopsy (transbronchial, VATS, open) CMV shell culture, viral PCR, fungal, bacterial and mycobacterial cultures with BAL and lung biopsy CXR/CT/HRCT	Prophylaxis: Herpesviridae: Acyclovir/valacyclovir. PCP: TMP/SMX, dapsone, atovaquone or inhaled pentamidine Treatment: Empiric coverage of MRSA, GNRs, *Pseudomonas* spp, typical and atypical bacterial pathogens, *Candida* spp, *Aspergillus* spp pending diagnosis Targeted therapy for diagnosed infection
Diffuse alveolar hemorrhage	DIC, APL	Anytime until DIC resolves	Cough, hemoptysis, hemoglobin drop	DIC: Treat underlying cause Platelet goal >50,000/μL Fibrinogen goal >100–150 mg/dL
	HSCT	First 3–4 wk after transplant, around engraftment	CXR/CT/HRCT: Diffuse ground glass opacities, consolidations BAL: Increasingly bloody return on serial lavage	HSCT: High-dose corticosteroids, platelet goal >50,000/μL, correct coagulopathy, consider recombinant activated factor VII
Drug toxicity	HSCT (Carmustine, Busulfan) Busulfan	3 mo–2 y after exposure	CXR/CT/HRCT: Ground glass opacities, interstitial pneumonitis PFTs: Decreased DLCO	Corticosteroids, supportive care
Pulmonary engraftment syndrome	HSCT	At count recovery (ANC >500/μL)	Associated findings: fever, rash	Self-limited lasting 1–2 wk Corticosteroids
Idiopathic pneumonia syndrome	HSCT	3 wk–4 mo after HSCT	CXR/CT/HRCT: Interstitial pulmonary infiltrate	Corticosteroids Consider etanercept
Cryptogenic organizing pneumonia	HSCT	Late (>100 d after HSCT)	CXR/CT/HRCT: Bilateral patchy alveolar filling, areas of ground glass opacities and consolidation PFTSs: Restrictive physiology	Corticosteroid responsive Reversible
Bronchiolitis obliterans syndrome	HSCT, chronic GVHD	Late (>100 d after HSCT)	CT/HRCT: Air trapping, bronchiolitis PFTs: Obstructive physiology	Treat underlying GVHD Irreversible, corticosteroids may slow progression

BAL, bronchoalveolar lavage; VATS, video-assisted thoracoscopic surgery, CXR, chest X-ray; CT, computed tomography; HRCT, high-resolution computed tomography; MRSA, methicillin-resistant *Staphylococcus aureus*; GNR, Gram-negative rod; HSCT, hematopoietic stem cell transplant; CMV, cytomegalovirus; RSV, respiratory syncytial virus; DFA, direct fluorescence assay; PCR, polymerase chain reaction; PCP, *Pneumocystis jiroveci pneumonia*; TMP/SMX, trimethoprim/sulfamethoxazole; DIC, disseminated intravascular coagulation; APL, acute promyelocytic leukemia; PFTs, pulmonary function tests; DLCO, diffusing capacity; ANC, absolute neutrophil count; GVHD, graft-versus-host disease.

to molecular diagnosis as these patients are at especially high risk for severe differentiation syndrome and death during induction therapy [157]. Even with improved recognition and treatment, 26% of patients in the LPA96 and LPA99 trials developing severe DS died during induction therapy, 11% from DS alone [154].

Therapeutic Agents

Treatment of aggressive hematologic malignancies typically requires toxic, myelosuppressive chemotherapy regimens. Patients are prone to life-threatening bacterial and

TABLE 115.3

OVERVIEW OF COMMON CHEMOTHERAPEUTIC AGENTS FOR HEMATOLOGIC MALIGNANCIES

Drug	Indication	Mechanism	Major toxicities	Management
Anthracyclines, anthracenediones	AML, APL, ALL, lymphomas, myeloma	Topoisomerase II inhibition, reactive oxygen species generation	1. Vesicant 2. Cardiac toxicity, acute and dose-dependent [158–162] 3. Myelosuppression 4. t-AML, t-MDS at 1–5 years after treatment [163]	1. CVC preferred 2. Dexrazoxane for prophylaxis [164,165] 3. G-CSF support
Cytosine arabinoside (Cytarabine, AraC)	AML, ALL, high-grade lymphomas	Inhibits DNA polymerase, incorporation into DNA [166]	1. Myelosuppression 2. Acute cytarabine syndrome: fever, rash, conjunctivitis, myalgias and bone pain 6 to 12 hours after infusion. 3. High dose ($\geq$1 g/m^2): mucositis, conjunctivitis, enterocolitis, rash, neurotoxicity, cerebellar toxicity (2%–3%, >40% with CrCl <60 mL/min) [167,168]	1. G-CSF support 2. Corticosteroids [169] 3. Twice daily showers, ophthalmic corticosteroids, systemic corticosteroids
All-*trans*-retinoic acid (ATRA)	APL	Promotes degradation of PML-RARα oncoprotein	1. Differentiation syndrome: fever, peripheral edema, weight gain more than 5 kg, pleuropericardial effusions, shortness of breath, interstitial pulmonary infiltrates, acute renal failure and hypotension 2. Bone pain, arthralgias, headache, dry skin, rash, nausea, edema, mouth sores, flu-like symptoms, pseudotumor cerebri, Sweet's syndrome [170]	1. Dexamethasone 10 mg PO or IV twice daily, hold ATRA for severe symptoms
Arsenic trioxide (ATO)	APL	Promotes degradation of PML-RARα oncoprotein	1. Differentiation syndrome identical to ATRA [32] 2. QTc prolongation [171–173] 3. Hypokalemia, hypomagnesemia 4. Myelosuppression, fatigue, fever, headache, nausea, vomiting, diarrhea, abdominal pain, chest pain, myalgias, bone pain, hyperglycemia, atrial arrhythmias	1. Dexamethasone 10 mg PO or IV twice daily, hold ATO for severe symptoms 2. Frequent EKGs, correct electrolyte abnormalities, discontinue ATO
Ifosfamide, cyclophosphamide	High-grade lymphomas, myeloma, hematopoietic cell transplant conditioning	DNA alkylation causing inter- and intrastrand DNA cross-linking	1. Hemorrhagic cystitis due to acrolein metabolite 2. Myelosuppression 3. Ifosfamide: CNS toxicity 4. Cyclophosphamide: SIADH, cardiotoxicity (>200 mg/kg) [174] 5. t-MDS and t-AML 3–5 years after treatment [175]	1. MESNA 2. G-CSF support 3. Drug cessation, methylene blue
Plant alkaloids (vincristine, vinblastine)	ALL, lymphomas	Bind β-tubulin and inhibit microtubule polymerization [176]	1. Vesicant 2. Sensory-motor and autonomic neuropathy, severe constipation, ileus, small bowel obstruction, hyponatremia	1. CVC preferred 2. Aggressive bowel regimen
Methotrexate (MTX)	ALL, lymphomas	Inhibits dihydrofolate reductase [177]	1. Myelosuppression, hepatitis, acute renal failure, mucositis, seizure	1. Urine alkalinization, hydration [145], leucovorin rescue, carboxypeptidase G-2 (cleaves MTX) [146]
6-mercaptopurine	ALL, APL maintenance therapy	Inhibits de novo purine synthesis, DNA and RNA synthesis	Myelosuppression, immunosuppression, GI irritation, biliary stasis, transaminitis	Dose reduction
L-asparaginase	ALL	Deamination of plasma asparagine and glutamine	1. Venous thrombosis from decreased antithrombotic factors, cerebral venous sinus thrombosis rate 1%–3% [147,178–180] 2. Hypersensitivity reactions 3. Hepatotoxicity, pancreatitis, hypoinsulinemia	1. 3–6 mo of anticoagulation [181,182] 2. Pegylated asparaginase [183]
Rituximab	CD20+ B-cell lymphomas, CLL [65]	Binds to CD20 on the surface of malignant and benign B-cells [184]	1. Hypersensitivity reactions 2. Tumor lysis syndrome (high risk with circulating lymphoma/leukemia cells >10,000/μL)	1. Acetaminophen, antihistamine, corticosteroids, slow infusion 2. Allopurinol, hydration, rasburicase

AML, acute myeloid leukemia; APL, acute promyelocytic leukemia; ALL. acute lymphoblastic leukemia; t-AML, treatment-related AML; t-MDS, treatment-related myelodysplastic syndrome; CVC, central venous catheter; G-CSF, Granulocyte colony stimulating factor; SIADH, syndrome of inappropriate ADH; CLL, chronic lymphocytic leukemia.

TABLE 115.4

SELECTED EVIDENCE-BASED APPROACHES FOR HEMATOLOGIC MALIGNANCIES

Clinical relevance	Comparison	Results	Reference
ICU outcomes			
Patients with hematologic malignancies have similar mortality to nononcologic patients when matched for disease severity.	Retrospective study of 101 consecutive ICU admissions of patients with hematologic malignancies vs. 3,808 nononcologic admissions.	Mortality of hematologic malignancy and nononcologic patients similar when matched for SAPS II score (OR = 0.59, 95% CI = 0.32–1.08, $p = 0.09$).	[1]
Hyperleukocytosis			
Improved short-term but not long-term survival with leukapheresis in hyperleukocytic AML.	Retrospective analysis of leukapheresis in 53 vs. no leukapheresis in 28 AML patients with hyperleukocytosis (WBC >100,000/μL).	Reduced 21-day mortality in leukapheresis group vs. no leukapheresis (16% vs. 32%, $p = 0.015$). No difference in overall survival (median 6.5 vs. 7.5 months).	[88]
Prophylactic platelet transfusion			
Equivalent bleeding rates with platelet transfusion threshold 10,000/μL vs. 20,000/μL.	Meta-analysis of three prospective randomized trials.	No difference in mortality, remission rates, severe bleeding events or RBC transfusion requirements between two threshold levels. Studies potentially underpowered.	[125]
Noninvasive positive pressure ventilation			
Improved survival with addition of noninvasive positive pressure ventilation to standard care alone in patients with early hypoxemia.	Prospective, randomized trial of 52 immunosuppressed patients with fever, pulmonary infiltrates, and early hypoxemic respiratory failure treated with NIPPV vs. supplemental oxygen-based therapy alone.	NIPPV superior to supplemental oxygen based therapy alone for incidence of endotracheal intubation (2 vs. 20 patients, $p = 0.03$), serious complications (13 vs. 21, $p = 0.02$), death in the ICU (10 vs. 18, $p = 0.03$) and death in the hospital (13 vs. 21, $p = 0.02$).	[185]
Invasive ventilation			
Improved survival with early intubation of hypoxemic patients.	Retrospective analysis of 166 consecutive admits requiring mechanical ventilation with NIPPV vs. IMV.	Intubation within 24 hours of ICU admission associated with improved survival (OR = 0.29, 95% CI = 0.11–0.78). Survival equivalent between NIPPV and IMV when matched for SAPS II score.	[12]
Prophylactic antibiotics during neutropenia			
Use of prophylactic antibiotics in afebrile neutropenic patients improves survival and supports use of fluoroquinolone prophylaxis.	Meta-analysis of 100 trials (10,275 patients).	Compared to placebo, antibiotic prophylaxis associated with reduced risk of death (RR = 0.66, 95% CI = 0.54–0.81), infection related death (RR = 0.58, 95% CI = 0.45–0.74) and fever (RR = 0.52, 95% CI = 0.37–0.84). Fluoroquinolone prophylaxis with reduced all-cause mortality (RR = 0.52, 95% CI = 0.37–0.84).	[152]
Growth factors for neutropenia			
G-CSF shortens duration of neutropenia without improving overall survival.	Prospective, randomized trial of G-CSF vs. placebo following AML induction chemotherapy.	Neutrophil recovery 15% earlier in G-CSF treated patients ($p = 0.014$). No difference in complete remission rates or 6-mo survival.	[186]
Differentiation syndrome			
Early institution of chemotherapy after starting ATRA for APL reduces the incidence of differentiation syndrome.	Randomized, prospective analysis of rates of differentiation syndrome in APL patients with WBC <5,000/μL treated with ATRA until complete remission followed by chemotherapy vs. ATRA with chemotherapy starting day 3.	Incidence of differentiation syndrome 18% in ATRA with delayed chemotherapy vs. 9.2% in ATRA with early chemotherapy ($p = 0.035$).	[156]

SAPS II, simplified acute physiology score II; AUC, area under the curve; CI, confidence interval; NIPPV, noninvasive positive pressure ventilation; IMV, invasive mechanical ventilation; OR, odds ratio; RR, relative risk; G-CSF, granulocyte colony-stimulating factor; ATRA, all-trans-retinoic acid; APL, acute promyelocytic leukemia.

fungal infections as a result of prolonged neutropenia, bleeding from thrombocytopenia, and organ failure from the toxic effects of chemotherapy. Selected toxicities of agents commonly used in the treatment of hematologic malignancies and their management are supplied in Table 115.3.

Additional complications of malignant hematologic diseases or their treatment, including tumor lysis syndrome and malignant epidural cord compression, are discussed in detail in Chapter 116.

Selected evidenced-based approaches for managing patients with hematologic malignancies are presented in Table 115.4.

References

1. Merz TM, Schär P, Bühlmann M, et al: Resource use and outcome in critically ill patients with hematological malignancy: a retrospective cohort study. *Critical Care* 12:R75, 2008.
2. Hampshire PA, Welch CA, McCrossan LA, et al: Admission factors associated with hospital mortality in patients with haematological malignancy admitted to UK adult, general critical care units: a secondary analysis of the ICNARC Case Mix Programme Database. *Critical Care* 13:R137, 2009.
3. Gordon AC, Oakervee HE, Kaya B, et al: Incidence and outcome of critical illness amongst hospitalised patients with haematological malignancy: a prospective observational study of ward and intensive care unit based care. *Anaesthesia* 60:340–347, 2005.
4. Lloyd-Thomas A, Dhaliwal H, Lister T, et al: Intensive therapy for life-threatening medical complications of haematological malignancy. *Intensive Care Med* 12:317–324, 1986.
5. Lloyd-Thomas AR, Wright I, Lister TA, et al: Prognosis of patients receiving intensive care for life-threatening medical complications of haematological malignancy. *BMJ* 296:1025–1029, 1988.
6. Yau E, Rohatiner AZ, Lister TA, et al: Long term prognosis and quality of life following intensive care for life-threatening complications of haematological malignancy. *Br J Cancer* 64:938–942, 1991.
7. Evison J, Rickenbacher P, Ritz R, et al: Intensive care unit admission in patients with haematological disease: incidence, outcome and prognostic factors. *Swiss Med Wkly* 131:681–686, 2001.
8. Kroschinsky F, Weise M, Illmer T, et al: Outcome and prognostic features of intensive care unit treatment in patients with hematological malignancies. *Intensive Care Med* 28:1294–1300, 2002.
9. Benoit D, Vandewoude K, Decruyenaere J, et al: Outcome and early prognostic indicators in patients with a hematologic malignancy admitted to the ICU for a life-threatening complication. *Crit Care Med* 31:104–112, 2003.
10. Cornet AD, Issa AI, Loosdrecht AA, et al: Sequential organ failure predicts mortality of patients with a haematological malignancy needing intensive care. *Eur J Haematol* 74:511–516, 2005.
11. Lamia B, Hellot M, Girault C, et al: Changes in severity and organ failure scores as prognostic factors in onco-hematological malignancy patients admitted to the ICU. *Intensive Care Med* 32:1560–1568, 2006.
12. Depuydt PO, Benoit DD, Vandewoude KH, et al: Outcome in noninvasively and invasively ventilated hematologic patients with acute respiratory failure. *Chest* 126:1299–1306, 2004.
13. Lim Z, Pagliuca A, Simpson S, et al: Outcomes of patients with haematological malignancies admitted to intensive care unit. A comparative review of allogeneic haematopoietic stem cell transplantation data. *Br J Haematol* 136:448–450, 2007.
14. Bruennler T, Mandraka F, Zierhut S, et al: Outcome of hemato-oncologic patients with and without stem cell transplantation in a medical ICU. *Eur J Med Res* 12(8):323–30, 2007.
15. Horner MJ, Ries LAG, Krapcho M, et al (eds): SEER Cancer Statistics Review, 1975–2006, National Cancer Institute. Bethesda, MD, http://seer.cancer.gov/csr/1975_2006/.
16. Pulte D, Gondos A, Brenner H: Expected long-term survival of patients diagnosed with acute myeloblastic leukemia during 2006–2010. *Ann Oncol* 21(2):335–341, 2010.
17. Peterson-Bjergaard J, Larsen SO: Incidence of acute nonlymphocytic leukemia, preleukemia and acute myeloproliferative syndrome up to 10 year after treatment of Hodgkin's disease. *N Engl J Med* 307:965–971, 1982.
18. Blayney DW, Longo DL, Young RC, et al: Decreasing risk of leukemia with prolonged follow up after chemotherapy for Hodgkin's disease. *N Engl J Med* 316:710–714, 1987.
19. Travis LB, Holoway EJ, Bergfeldt, et al: Risk of leukemia after platinum-based chemotherapy for ovarian cancer. *N Engl J Med* 340:351–357, 1999.
20. Boyce JD Jr, Green MH, Killen JY Jr, et al: Leukemia and preleukemia after adjuvant treatment of gastrointestinal cancer with semustine (methyl-CCNU). *N Engl J Med* 309:1079–1084, 1983.
21. Stone RM, Neuberg D, Soiffer R, et al: Myelodysplastic syndrome as a late complication following autologous bone marrow transplantation for non-Hodgkin's lymphoma. *J Clin Oncol* 12:2535–2542, 1994.
22. Pui CH, Ribeiro RC, Hancock ML, et al: Acute myeloid leukemia in children treated with epipodophyllotoxins for acute lymphoblastic leukemia. *N Engl J Med* 323:1682–1987, 1991.
23. Watson MS, Carroll Aj, Shuster JJ, et al: Trisomy 21 in childhood acute lymphoblastic leukemia: a Pediatric Oncology Group Study (8602). *Blood* 82:3098–3102, 1993.
24. Sedlacek SM, Curtis JL, Weintraub J, et al: Essential thrombocythemia and leukemic transformation. *Medicine (Baltimore)* 65:353–364, 1986.
25. Landaw SA: Acute leukemia in polycythemia vera. *Semin Hematol* 23:156–165, 1986.
26. Sterkers Y, Preudhomme C, Lai JL, et al: Acute myeloid leukemia and myelodysplastic syndromes following essential thrombocythemia treated with hydroxyurea: high proportion of cases with 17p deletion. *Blood* 91:616–622, 1998.
27. Greenberg P, Cox C, LeBeau MM, et al: International scoring system for evaluating prognosis in myelodysplastic syndromes. *Blood* 89:2079–2088, 1997.
28. Vardiman JW, Brunning RD, Arber DA, et al: Introduction and overview of the classification of myeloid neoplasms, in: Swerdlow SH, Campo E, Harris LE, et al (eds): *WHO Classification of Tumours of Haematopoietic and Lymphoid Tissues*. Lyon, France, IARC Press, 2008, pp 233–237.
29. Schlenk RF, Dohner K, Krauter J, et al: Mutations and treatment outcome in cytogenetically normal acute myeloid leukemia. *N Engl J Med* 358:1909–1918, 2008.
30. Dohner H, Estey EH, Amadori S, et al: Diagnosis and management of acute myeloid leukemia in adults: recommendations from an international expert panel, on behalf of the European LeukemiaNet. *Blood* 115(3):453–474, 2010.
31. Stanley M, McKenna RW, Ellinger G, et al: Classification of 358 cases of acute myeloid leukemia by FAB criteria: analysis of clinical and morphologic features, in Bloomfield CD (ed): *Chronic and Acute Leukemias in Adults*. Boston, MA, Martinus Nijhoff Publishers, 1985, pp 147–174.
32. Sanz MA, Grimwade D, Tallman MS, et al: Management of acute promyelocytic leukemia: recommendations from an expert panel on behalf of the European LeukemiaNet. *Blood* 113(9):1875–1890, 2009.
33. De la Serna J, Montesinos P, Vellenga E: Causes and prognostic factors of remission induction failure in patients with acute promyelocytic leukemia treated with all-trans retinoic acid and idarubicin. *Blood* 111:3395–3402, 2008.
34. Tallman MS, Altman J: How I treat acute promyelocytic leukemia. *Blood* 114(25):5126–5135, 2009.
35. Breccia M, Avvisati G, Latagliata R, et al: Occurrence of thrombotic events in acute promyelocytic leukemia correlates with consistent immunophenotype and molecular features. *Leukemia* 21:79–83, 2007.
36. Stein E, McMahon B, Kwaan H, et al: The coagulopathy of acute promyelocytic leukaemia revisited. *Best Pract Res Clin Haematol* 22(1):153–163, 2009.
37. Arber DA, Brunning RD, LeBeau MM, et al: Acute myeloid leukemia with recurrent cytogenetic abnormalities, in: Swerdlow SH, Campo E, Harris LE, et al (eds): *WHO Classification of Tumours of Haematopoietic and Lymphoid Tissues*. Lyon, France, IARC Press, 2008, pp 110–123.
38. Golomb HM, Rowley JD, Vardiman JW, et al: "Microgranular" acute promyelocytic leukemia: a distinct clinical, ultrastructural, and cytogenetic entity. *Blood* 55:253–259, 1980.
39. Raelson JV, Nervi C, Rosenauer A, et al: The PML/RAR alpha oncoprotein is a direct molecular target of retinoic acid in acute promyelocytic leukemia cells. *Blood* 88:2826–2832, 1996.
40. Lallemand-Breitenbach V, Jeanne M, Benhenda S, et al: Arsenic degrades PML or PML-RARalpha through a SUMO-triggered RNF4/ubiquitin-mediated pathway. *Nat Cell Biol* 10:547–555, 2008.
41. Orfoa A, Chillon MC, Bortoluci AM, et al: The flow cytometric pattern of CD34, CD15 and CD13 expression in acute myeloblastic leukemia is highly characteristic of the presence of PML/RARalpha gene rearrangements. *Haematologica* 84:405–412, 1999.
42. Hu J, Liu YF, Wu CF, et al: Long-term efficacy and safety of all-trans retinoic acid/arsenic trioxide- based therapy in newly diagnosed acute promyelocytic leukemia. *Proc Natl Acad Sci U S A* 106(9):3342–3347, 2009.
43. Ravandi F, Estey E, Jones D, et al: Effective treatment of acute promyelocytic leukemia with all-trans-retinoic acid, arsenic trioxide, and gemtuzumab ozogamicin. *J Clin Oncol* 27(4):504–510, 2009.
44. Dai CW, Zhang GS, Shen JK, et al: Use of all-trans retinoic acid in combination with arsenic trioxide for remission induction in patients with newly

diagnosed acute promyelocytic leukemia and for consolidation/maintenance in CR patients. *Acta Haematol* 121(1):1–8, 2009.
45. Pui CH, Robison LL, Look AT: Acute lymphoblastic leukaemia. *The Lancet* 371:1030–1043, 2008.
46. Annino L, Vegna ML, Camera A, et al: Treatment of adult acute lymphoblastic leukemia (ALL): long-term follow-up of the GIMEMA ALL 0288 randomized study. *Blood* 99:863–871, 2002.
47. Thiebaut A, Vernant JP, Degos L, et al: Adult acute lymphocytic leukemia study testing chemotherapy and autologous and allogeneic transplantation. A follow-up report of the French protocol LALA 87. *Hematol Oncol Clin North Am* 14:1353–1366, 2000.
48. Barrett AJ, Horowitz MM, Ash RC, et al: Bone marrow transplantation for Philadelphia chromosome-positive acute lymphoblastic leukemia. *Blood* 79:3067–3070, 1992.
49. Chao NJ, Blume KG, Forman SJ, et al: Long-term follow-up of allogeneic bone marrow recipients for Philadelphia chromosome-positive acute lymphoblastic leukemia. *Blood* 85:3353–3354, 1995.
50. Dombret H, Gabert J, Boiron JM, et al: Outcome of treatment in adults with Philadelphia chromosome-positive acute lymphoblastic leukemia—results of the prospective multicenter LALA-94 trial. *Blood* 100:2357–2366, 2002.
51. Thomas X, Boiron JM, Huguet F, et al: Outcome of treatment in adults with acute lymphoblastic leukemia: analysis of the LALA-94 trial. *J Clin Oncol* 22:4075–4086, 2004.
52. Yanada M, Matsuo K, Suzuki T, et al: Allogeneic hematopoietic stem cell transplantation as part of postremission therapy improves survival for adult patients with high-risk acute lymphoblastic leukemia: a metaanalysis. *Cancer* 106:2657–2663, 2006.
53. Laport GG, Alvarnas JC, Palmer JM, et al: Long-term remission of Philadelphia chromosome-positive acute lymphoblastic leukemia after allogeneic hematopoietic cell transplantation from matched sibling donors: a 20-year experience with the fractionated total body irradiation-etoposide regimen. *Blood* 112, 903–909, 2008.
54. Rowe JM: Optimal management of adults with ALL. *Br J Haematol* 144:468–483, 2009.
55. Thomas DA, Faderl S, Cortes J, et al: Treatment of Philadelphia chromosome-positive acute lymphocytic leukemia with hyper-CVAD and imatinib mesylate. *Blood* 103:4396–4407, 2004.
56. Lee KH, Lee JH, Choi SJ, et al: Clinical effect of imatinib added to intensive combination chemotherapy for newly diagnosed Philadelphia chromosome-positive acute lymphoblastic leukemia. *Leukemia* 19:1509–1516, 2005.
57. Lee S, Kim YJ, Min CK, et al: The effect of first-line imatinib interim therapy on the outcome of allogeneic stem cell transplantation in adults with newly diagnosed Philadelphia chromosome-positive acute lymphoblastic leukemia. *Blood* 105:3449–3457, 2005.
58. Yanada M, Takeuchi J, Sugiura I, et al: High complete remission rate and promising outcome by combination of imatinib and chemotherapy for newly diagnosed BCR-ABL-positive acute lymphoblastic leukemia: a phase II study by the Japan Adult Leukemia Study Group. *J Clin Oncol* 24:460–466, 2006.
59. de Labarthe A, Rousselot P, Huguet-Rigal F, et al: Imatinib combined with induction or consolidation chemotherapy in patients with de novo Philadelphia chromosome-positive acute lymphoblastic leukemia: results of the GRAAPH-2003 study. *Blood* 109:1408–1413, 2007.
60. Ottmann OG, Wassmann B, Pfeifer H, et al: Imatinib compared with chemotherapy as front- line treatment of elderly patients with Philadelphia chromosome-positive acute lymphoblastic leukemia (Ph+ALL). *Cancer* 109:2068–2076, 2007.
61. Vignetti M, Fazi P, Cimino G, et al: Imatinib plus steroids induces complete remissions and prolonged survival in elderly Philadelphia chromosome-positive patients with acute lymphoblastic leukemia without additional chemotherapy: results of the Gruppo Italiano Malattie Ematologiche dell'Adulto (GIMEMA) LAL0201-B protocol. *Blood* 109:3676–3678, 2007.
62. Talpaz M, Shah NP, Kantarjian H, et al: Dasatinib in imatinib-resistant Philadelphia chromosome-positive leukemias. *N Engl J Med* 354(24):2531–2541, 2006.
63. Ottmann O, Dombret H, Martinelli G, et al: Dasatinib induces rapid hematologic and cytogenetic responses in adult patients with Philadelphia chromosome positive acute lymphoblastic leukemia with resistance or intolerance to imatinib: interim results of a phase 2 study. *Blood* 110(7):2309–2315, 2007.
64. Stein H, Warnke RA, Chan WC, et al: Diffuse large B-cell lymphoma, not otherwise specified, in Swerdlow SH, Campo E, Harris LE, et al (eds): *World Health Organization Classification of Tumours of Haematopoietic and Lymphoid Tissues.* Lyon, France, IARC Press, 2008, pp 233–237.
65. Abramson JS, Shipp MA: Advances in the biology and therapy of diffuse large B-cell lymphoma: moving toward a molecularly targeted approach. *Blood* 106:1164–1174, 2005.
66. Armitage JO, Weisenburger DD: New approach to classifying non-Hodgkin's lymphomas: clinical features of the major histologic subtypes. Non- Hodgkin's Lymphoma Classification Project. *J Clin Oncol* 16:2780–2795, 1998.
67. Blum KA, Lozanski G, Byrd JC: Adult Burkitt leukemia and lymphoma. *Blood* 104:3009–3020, 2004.
68. Leoncini L, Raphael M, Stein H, et al: Burkitt lymphoma, in Swerdlow SH, Campo E, Harris LE, et al (eds): *World Health Organization Classification of Tumours of Haematopoietic and Lymphoid Tissues.* Lyon, France, IARC Press, 2008, pp 233–237.
69. Treon SP: How I treat Waldenstrom macroglobulinemia. *Blood* 114(12):2375–2385, 2009.
70. Hug V, Keating M, McCredie K, et al: Clinical course and response to treatment of patients with acute myelogenous leukemia presenting with high leukocyte count. *Cancer* 52:773–779, 1983.
71. Dutcher JP, Schiffer CA, Wiernik PH: Hyperleukocytosis in adult acute nonlymphocytic leukemia: impact on remission rate and duration, and survival. *J Clin Oncol* 5(9):1364–1372, 1987.
72. Berg J, Vincent PC, Gunz FW: Extreme leucocytosis and prognosis of newly diagnosed patients with acute non-lymphocytic leukaemia. *Med J Aust* 1(11):480–482, 1979.
73. Vaughan WP, Kimball AW, Karp JE, et al: Factors affecting survival of patients with acute myelocytic leukemia presenting with high WBC counts. *Cancer Treat Rep* 65(11–12):1007–1013, 1981.
74. Lester TJ, Johnson JW, Cuttner J. Pulmonary leukostasis as the single worst prognostic factor in patients with acute myelocytic leukemia and hyperleukocytosis. *Am J Med* 79(1):43–48, 1985.
75. Ventura GJ, Hester JP, Smith TL, et al: Acute myeloblastic leukemia with hyperleukocytosis: risk factors for early mortality in induction. *Am J Hematol* 27(1):34–37, 1988.
76. Lichtman MA: Rheology of leukocytes, leukocyte suspensions, and blood in leukemia. Possible relationship to clinical manifestations. *J Clin Invest* 52:350–358, 1973.
77. Sharma K. Cellular deformability studies in leukemia. *Physiol Chem Phys Med NMR* 25:293–297, 1993.
78. Rosenbluth MJ, Lam WA, Fletcher DA: Force microscopy of nonadherent cells: a comparison of leukemia cell deformability. *Biophys J* 90:2994–3003, 2006.
79. Novotny JR, Nuckel H, Duhrsen U: Correlation between expression of CD56/NCAM and severe leukostasis in hyperleukocytic acute myelomonocytic leukaemia. *Eur J Haematol* 76:299–308, 2006.
80. Stucki A, Rivier AS, Gikic M, et al: Endothelial cell activation by myeloblasts: molecular mechanisms of leukostasis and leukemic cell dissemination. *Blood* 97:2121–2129, 2001.
81. Lowe EJ, Pui CH, Hancock ML, et al: Early complications in children with acute lymphoblastic leukemia presenting with hyperleukocytosis. *Pediatr Blood Cancer* 45:10–15, 2005.
82. Lam WA, Rosenbluth MJ, Fletcher DA: Increased leukaemia cell stiffness is associated with symptoms of leucostasis in paediatric acute lymphoblastic leukaemia. *Brit J Haematol* 142:497–501, 2008.
83. Marbello L, Ricci F, Nosari AM, et al: Outcome of hyperleukocytic adult acute myeloid leukaemia: a single-center retrospective study and review of literature. *Leuk Res* 32(8):1221–1227, 2008.
84. Greenwood MJ, Seftel MD, Richardson C, et al: Leukocyte count as a predictor of death during remission induction in acute myeloid leukaemia. *Leuk Lymphoma* 47:1245–1252, 2006.
85. Porcu P, Danielson CF, Orazi A, et al: Therapeutic leukapheresis in hyperleukocytic leukemias: lack of correlation between degree of cytoreduction and early mortality rate. *Br J Haematol* 98:433–436, 1997.
86. Cuttner J, Holland JF, Norton L, et al: Therapeutic leukapheresis for hyperleukocytosis in acute myelocytic leukemia. *Med Pediatr Oncol* 11:76–78, 1983.
87. Giles FJ, Shen Y, Kantarjian HM, et al: Leukapheresis reduces early mortality in patients with acute myeloid leukaemia with high white cell counts but does not improve long-term survival. *Leuk Lymphoma* 42:67–73, 2001.
88. Bug G, Anargyrou K, Tonn T, et al: Impact of leukapheresis on early death rate in adult acute myeloid leukemia presenting with hyperleukocytosis. *Transfusion* 47(10):1843–1850, 2007.
89. Vahdat L, Maslak P, Miller WH Jr, et al: Early mortality and the retinoic acid syndrome in acute promyelocytic leukemia: impact of leukocytosis, low-dose chemotherapy, PML/RARalpha isoform, and CD13 expression in patients treated with all-trans retinoic acid. *Blood* 84:3843–3849, 1994.
90. Pavy MD, Murphy PL, Virella G: Paraprotein-induced hyperviscosity. A reversible cause of stroke. *Postgrad Med* 68(3):109–112, 1980.
91. Mueller J, Hotson JR, Langston JW: Hyperviscosity-induced dementia. *Neurology* 33(1):101–103, 1983.
92. Garcia-Sanz R, Montoto S, Torrequebrada A, et al: Waldenstrom macroglobulinaemia: presenting features and outcome in a series with 217 cases. *Br J Haematol* 115(3):575–582, 2001.
93. Pene F, Aubron C, Azoulay E, et al: Outcome of critically ill allogeneic hematopoietic stem-cell transplantation recipients: a reappraisal of indications for organ failure supports. *J Clin Oncol* 24(4):643–649, 2006.
94. Hummel M, Rudert S, Hof H, et al: Diagnostic yield of bronchoscopy with bronchoalveolar lavage in febrile patients with hematologic malignancies and pulmonary infiltrates. Ann Hematol 87:291–297, 2008.
95. Azoulay E, Mokart D, Rabbat A, et al: Diagnostic bronchoscopy in hematology and oncology patients with acute respiratory failure: prospective multicenter data. *Crit Care Med* 36:100–107, 2008.
96. Carter PW, Cohen HJ, Crawford J: Hyperviscosity syndrome in association with kappa light chain myeloma. *Am J Med* 86:591, 1989.

97. Bachrach HJ, Myers JB, Bartholomew WR: A unique case of kappa light chain disease associated with cryoglobulinemia, pyroglobulinemia and hyperviscosity syndrome. *Am J Med* 86:596, 1989.
98. Kes P, Pecanic Z, Getaldic B, et al: Treatment of hyperviscosity syndrome in the patients with plasma cell dyscrasias. *Acta Med Croatica* 50(4–5):173–177, 1996.
99. Sampson B, Anderson DR, Dugal M, et al: Acquired type 2 a von Willebrand disease: response to immunoglobulin infusion. *Haemostasis* 27(6):286–289, 1997.
100. Viallard JF, Pellegrin JL, Vergnes C, et al: Three cases of acquired von Willebrand disease associated with systemic lupus erythematosus. *Br J Haematol* 105(2):532–537, 1999.
101. Bach PB, Schrag D, Nierman DM, et al: Identification of poor prognostic features among patients requiring mechanical ventilation after hematopoietic stem cell transplantation. *Blood* 98:3234–3240, 2001.
102. Rosenson RS, McCormick A, Uretz EF: Distribution of blood viscosity values and biochemical correlates in healthy adults. *Clin Chem* 42:1189–1195, 1996.
103. Zihlif M, Khanchandani G, Ahmed HP, et al: Surgical lung biopsy in patients with hematological malignancy or hematopoietic stem cell transplantation and unexplained pulmonary infiltrates: improved outcome with specific diagnosis. *Am J Hematol* 78:94–99, 2005.
104. Stein E, McMahon B, Kwaan H, et al: The coagulopathy of acute promyelocytic leukaemia revisited. *Best Prac Res Clin Haematol* 22:153–163, 2009.
105. Falanga A, Alessio MG, Donati MB, et al: A new procoagulant in acute leukemia. *Blood* 71:870–875, 1988.
106. Falanga A, Consonni R, Marchetti M, et al: Cancer procoagulant in the human promyelocytic cell line NB4 and its modulation by retinoic acid. *Leukemia* 8:156–159, 1994.
107. Koyama T, Hirosawa S, Kawamata N, et al: All-trans retinoic acid upregulates thrombomodulin and downregulates tissue factor expression in acute promyelocytic leukemia cells: Distinct expression of thrombomodulin and tissue factor in human leukemic cells. *Blood* 84:3001–3009, 1994.
108. Falanga A, Iacoviello L, Evangelista V, et al: Loss of blast cell procoagulant activity and improvement of hemostatic variables in patients with acute promyelocytic leukemia administered all-trans retinoic acid. *Blood* 86:1072–1081, 1995.
109. De Stefano V, Teofili L, Sica S, et al: Effect of all-trans retinoic acid on procoagulant and fibrinolytic activities of cultured blast cell from patients with acute promyelocytic leukemia. *Blood* 86:3535–3541, 1995.
110. Gordon SG, Franks JJ Lewis B: Cancer procoagulant A: a factor X activating procoagulant from malignant tissue. *Thromb Res* 6:127–137, 1975.
111. Wang J, Weiss I, Svoboda K, et al: Thrombogenic role of cells undergoing apoptosis. *Br J Haematol* 115:382–391, 2001.
112. Rodeghiero F, Mannucci PM, Vigano S, et al: Liver dysfunction rather than intravascular coagulation as the main cause of low protein C and antithrombin III in acute leukemia. *Blood* 63:965–969, 1984.
113. Tapiovaara H, Alitalo R, Stephens R, et al: Abundant urokinase activity on the surface of mononuclear cells from blood and bone marrow of acute leukemia patients. *Blood* 82:914–919, 1993.
114. Tapiovaara H, Matikainen S, Hurme M, et al: Induction of differentiation of promyelocytic NB4 cells by retinoic acid is associated with rapid increase in urokinase activity subsequently downregulated by production of inhibitors. *Blood* 83:1883–1891, 1994.
115. Menell JS, Cesarman GM, Jacovina AT, et al: Annexin II and bleeding in acute promyelocytic leukemia. *N Engl J Med* 340:994–1004, 1999.
116. Kwaan HC, Wang J, Weiss I: Expression of receptors for plasminogen activators on endothelial cell surface depends on their origin. *J Thromb Haemost* 2:306–312, 2004.
117. Yen KT, Lee AS, Krowka MJ, et al: Pulmonary complications in bone marrow transplantation: a practical approach to diagnosis and treatment. *Clin Chest Med* 25:189–201, 2004.
118. Lee CK, Gingrich RD, Hohl RJ, et al: Engraftment syndrome in autologous bone marrow and peripheral stem cell transplantation. *Bone Marrow Transplant* 16(1):175–182, 1995.
119. Kantarjian HM, Keating MJ, Walters RS, et al: Acute promyelocytic leukemia. M.D. Anderson Hospital experience. *Am J Med* 80:789–797, 1986.
120. Cunningham I, Gee TS, Reich LM, et al: Acute promyelocytic leukemia: treatment results during a decade at Memorial Hospital. *Blood* 73:1116–1122, 1989.
121. Rodeghiero F, Avvisati G, Castaman G, et al: Early deaths and antihemorrhagic treatments in acute promyelocytic leukemia. A GIMEMA retrospective study in 268 consecutive patients. *Blood* 75:2112–2117, 1990.
122. Feinstein DI: Diagnosis and management of disseminated intravascular coagulation: the role of heparin therapy. *Blood* 60:284–287, 1982.
123. Sakuragawa N, Hasegawa H, Maki M, et al: Clinical evaluation of lowmolecular-weight heparin (FR-860) on disseminated intravascular coagulation (DIC)-a multicenter co-operative double-blind trial in comparison with heparin. *Thromb Res* 72:475–500, 1993.
124. Sullivan MT, McCullough J, Schreiber GB, et al: Blood collection and transfusion in the United States in 1997. *Transfusion* 42(10):1253–1260, 2002.
125. Stanworth SJ, Hyde C, Heddle N, et al: Prophylactic platelet transfusion for haemorrhage after chemotherapy and stem cell transplantation. *Cochrane Database Syst Rev* (4):CD004269, 2004.
126. Slichter SJ, Kaufman RM, Assmann SF, et al: Dose of prophylactic platelet transfusions and prevention of hemorrhage.*N Engl J Med* 362(7):600–613, 2010.
127. Richard C, Cuadrado MA, Prieto M, et al: Acquired von Willebrand disease in multiple myeloma secondary to absorption of von Willebrand factor by plasma cells. *Am J Hematol* 35:114–117, 1990.
128. Budde U, Schaefer G, Mueller N, et al: Acquired von Willebrand's disease in the myeloproliferative syndrome. *Blood* 64:981–985, 1984.
129. Fabris F, Casonato A, Del Ben MG, et al: Abnormalities of von Willebrand factor in myeloproliferative disease: a relationship with bleeding diathesis. *Br J Haematol* 63:75–83, 1986.
130. van Genderen PJ, Budde U, Michiels JJ, et al: The reduction of large von Willebrand factor multimers in plasma in essential thrombocythaemia is related to the platelet count. *Br J Haematol* 93:962–965, 1996.
131. Budde U, van Genderen: Acquired von Willebrand disease in patients with high platelets counts. *Semin Thromb Hemost* 23:425–431, 1997.
132. Federici AB, Budde U, Rand JH: Acquired von Willebrand syndrome 2004: International Registry–diagnosis and management from online to bedside. *Hamostaseologie* 24(1):50–55, 2004.
133. Mohri H, Motomura S, Kanamori H, et al: Clinical significance of inhibitors in acquired von Willebrand syndrome. *Blood* 91(10):3623–3629, 1998.
134. White DA, Wong PW, Downey R: The utility of open lung biopsy in patients with hematologic malignancies. *Am J Respir Crit Care Med* 161:723–729, 2000.
135. Dunagan DP, Baker AM, Hurd DD, et al: Bronchoscopic evaluation of pulmonary infiltrates following bone marrow transplantation. *Chest* 111(1):135–141, 1997.
136. Ewig S, Torres A, Riquelme R, et al: Pulmonary complications in patients with haematological malignancies treated at a respiratory ICU. *Eur Respir J* 12:116–122, 1998.
137. Enright H, Haake R, Weisdorf D, et al: Cytomegalovirus pneumonia after bone marrow transplantation. Risk factors and response to therapy. *Transplantation* 55(6):1339–1346, 1993.
138. Sirithanakul K, Salloum A, Klein JL, et al: Pulmonary complications following hematopoietic stem cell transplantation: diagnostic approaches. *Am J Hematol.* 80(2):137–146, 2005.
139. Chao NJ, Duncan SR, Long, GD, et al: Corticosteroid therapy for diffuse alveolar hemorrhage in autologous bone marrow transplant recipients. *Ann Intern Med* 114(2):145–146, 1991.
140. Metcalf JP, Rennard SI, Reed EC, et al: Corticosteroids as adjunctive therapy for diffuse alveolar hemorrhage associated with bone marrow transplantation. *Am J Med* 96(4):327–334, 1994.
141. Raptis A, Mavroudis D, Suffredini AF, et al: High-dose corticosteroid therapy for diffuse alveolar hemorrhage in allogeneic bone marrow stem cell transplant recipients. *Bone Marrow Transplant* 24,879–883, 1999.
142. Hicks K, Peng D, Gajewski JL: Treatment of diffuse alveolar hemorrhage after allogeneic bone marrow transplant with recombinant factor VIIa. *Bone Marrow Transplant* 30(12):975–978, 2002.
143. Pastores SM, Papadopoulos E, Voigt L, et al: Diffuse alveolar hemorrhage after allogeneic hematopoietic stem-cell transplantation: treatment with recombinant factor VIIa. *Chest* 124(6):2400–2403, 2003.
144. Shenoy A, Savani BN, Barrett AJ: Recombinant factor VIIa to treat diffuse alveolar hemorrhage following allogeneic stem cell transplantation. *Biol Blood Marrow Transplant* 13(5):622–623, 2007.
145. Stoller RG, Hande KR, Jacobs SA, et al: Use of plasma pharmacokinetics to predict and prevent methotrexate toxicity. *N Engl J Med* 297:630–634, 1977.
146. Buchen S, Ngampolo D, Melton RG, et al: Carboxypeptidase G-2 rescue in patients with methotrexate intoxication and renal failure. *Br J Cancer* 92:480–487, 2005.
147. Liebman HA, Wada K, Patch MJ, et al: Depression of functional and antigenic plasma antithrombin III (ATIII) due to therapy with L-asparaginase. *Cancer* 50:45I, 1982.
148. Clark JG, Hansen JA, Hertz MI, et al: NHLBI workshop summary: idiopathic pneumonia syndrome after bone marrow transplantation, *Am Rev Respir Dis* 147(6 Pt 1):1601–1606, 1993.
149. Kantrow SP, Hackman RC, Boeckh M, et al: Idiopathic pneumonia syndrome: changing the spectrum of lung injury after marrow transplantation. *Transplantation* 63(8):1079–1086, 1997.
150. Yanik GA, Ho VT, Levine JE, et al: The impact of soluble tumor necrosis factor receptor etanercept on the treatment of idiopathic pneumonia syndrome after allogeneic hematopoietic stem cell transplantation. *Blood* 112(8):3073–3081, 2008.
151. Palmas A, Tefferi A, Myers JL, et al: Late-onset noninfectious pulmonary complications after bone marrow transplantation. *Br J Haematol* 100(4):680–687, 1998.
152. Gafter-Gvili A, Fraser A, Paul M, et al: Meta-analysis: antibiotic prophylaxis reduces mortality in neutropenic patients. *Ann Intern Med* 142(12 Pt 1):979–995, 2005.
153. Stone RM, Berg DT, George SL, et al: Granulocyte-macrophage colony stimulating factor after initial chemotherapy for elderly patients with primary acute myelogenous leukemia. Cancer and Leukemia Group B. *N Engl J Med* 332:1671–1677, 1995.

154. Montesinos P, Bergua JM, Vellenga E, et al: Differentiation syndrome in patients with acute promyelocytic leukemia treated with all-trans retinoic acid and anthracycline chemotherapy: characteristics, outcome, and prognostic factors. *Blood* 113(4):775–783, 2009.
155. Frankel SR, Eardley A, Lauwers G, et al: The 'retinoic acid syndrome' in acute promyelocytic leukemia. *Ann Intern Med* 117:292–296, 1992.
156. de Botton S, Chevret S, Coiteux V, et al: Early onset of chemotherapy can reduce the incidence of ATRA syndrome in newly diagnosed acute promyelocytic leukemia (APL) with low white blood cell counts: results from APL 93 trial. *Leukemia* 17(2):339–342, 2003.
157. Sanz MA, Martin G, Rayon C, et al: A modified AIDA protocol with anthracycline-based consolidation results in high antileukemic efficacy and reduced toxicity in newly diagnosed PML/RAR-alpha-positive acute promyelocytic leukemia. *Blood* 94:3015–3021, 1999.
158. Bristow MR, et al: Early anthracycline cardiotoxicity. *Am J Med* 65:823–832, 1978.
159. Bosser RL, Green MD: Strategies for prevention of anthracycline cardiotoxicity, *Cancer Treat Rev* 19:57–77,1993.
160. Shan K, Lincoff AM, Young JB: Anthracycline-induced cardiotoxicity. *Ann Intern Med* 125(1):47–58, 1996.
161. Von Hoff DD, Layard MW, Basa P, et al: Risk factors for doxorubicin-induced congestive heart failure. *Ann Intern Med* 91(5):710–717, 1979.
162. Swain SM, Whaley FS, Gerber MC, et al: Cardioprotection with dexrazoxane for doxorubicin-containing therapy in advanced breast cancer. *J Clin Oncol* 15:1318–1332, 1997.
163. Smith SM, Le Beau MM, Huo D, et al: Clinical-cytogenetic associations in 306 patients with therapy-related myelodysplasia and myeloid leukemia: the University of Chicago series. *Blood* 102:43–52, 2003.
164. Wouters KA, Kremer LC, Miller TL, et al: Protecting against anthracycline-induced myocardial damage: a review of the most promising strategies. *Br J Haematol* 131:561–578, 2005.
165. van Dalen EC, Caron HN, Dickinson HO, et al: Cardioprotective interventions for cancer patients receiving anthracyclines. *Cochrane Database Syst Rev* CD003917, 2008.
166. Kufe DW, Munroe D, Herrick D, et al: Effects of 1-beta-D-arabinofuranosylcytosine incorporation on eukaryotic DNA template function. *Mol Pharmacol* 26:128, 1985.
167. Damon LE, Mass R, Linker CA: The association between high-dose cytarabine neurotoxicity and renal insufficiency. *J Clin Oncol* 7(10):1563–1568, 1989.
168. Smith GA, Damon LE, Rugo HS, et al: High-dose cytarabine dose modification reduces the incidence of neurotoxicity in patients with renal insufficiency. *J Clin Oncol* 15(2):833–839, 1997.
169. Castleberry RP, Crist WM, Holbrook T, et al: The cytosine arabinoside (Ara-C) syndrome. *Med Pediatr Oncol* 9(3):257–264, 1981.
170. Tallman MS, Altman JK: How I treat acute promyelocytic leukemia. *Blood* 10:114(25):5126–5135.
171. Beckman KJ, Bauman JL, Pimental PA, et al: Arsenic-induced torsade de pointes. *Crit Care Med* 19:290–292, 1991.
172. Barbey J, Pezzullo J, Soignet S: Effect of arsenic trioxide on QT interval in patients with advanced malignancies. *J Clin Oncol* 21:3609–3615, 2003.
173. Unnikrishnan D, Dutcher JP, Varshneya N, et al: Torsades de pointes in 3 patients with leukemia treated with arsenic trioxide. *Blood* 97:1514–1516, 2001.
174. Goldberg MA, Antin JH, Guinan EC, et al: Cyclophosphamide cardiotoxicity: an analysis of dosing as a risk factor. *Blood* 68:1114–1118, 1986.
175. Tucker MA, Coleman CN, Cox RS, et al: Risk of second cancers after treatment for Hodgkin's disease. *N Engl J Med* 318:76, 1988.
176. Jordan MA, Thrower D, Wilson L: Mechanism of inhibition of cell proliferation by Vinca alkaloids. *Cancer* 51:2212–2222, 1991.
177. Allegra CJ, Hoang K, Yeh CG, et al: Evidence for direct inhibition of de novo purine synthesis in human MCF-7 breast as a principal mode of metabolic inhibition by methotrexate. *J Biol Chem* 260:9720–9726, 1985.
178. Homans AC, Ryback ME, Baglini RL, et al: Effect of L-Asparginase administration on coagulation and platelet function in children with leukemia. *J Clin Oncol* 5:811–817, 1987.
179. Mitchell L, Hoogendoorn H, Giles AR, et al: Increased endogenous thrombin generation in children with acute lymphoblastic leukemia: risk of thrombotic complications in L'Asparaginase-induced antithrombin III deficiency. *Blood* 83:386–391, 1994.
180. Payne JH, Vora AJ: Thrombosis and acute lymphoblastic leukaemia. *Br J Haematol* 138:430–445, 2007.
181. Monagle P, Chan A, Massicotte P, et al: Antithrombotic therapy in children: the Seventh ACCP Conference on Antithrombotic and Thrombolytic Therapy. *Chest* 126:645S–687S, 2004.
182. Hirsh J, Guyatt G, Albers GW, et al: The Seventh ACCP Conference on Antithrombotic and Thrombolytic Therapy Evidence-Based Guidelines. *Chest* 126[3, Suppl]: 172S–173S, 2004.
183. Douer D, Yampolsky H, Cohen LJ, et al: Pharmacodynamics and safety of intravenous pegaspargase during remission induction in adults aged 55 years or younger with newly diagnosed acute lymphoblastic leukemia. *Blood* 109(7):2744–2750, 2007.
184. Maloney DG, Smith B, Rose A: Rituximab: mechanism of action and resistance. *Semin Oncol* 29:2–9, 2002.
185. Hilbert G, Gruson D, Vargas F, et al: Noninvasive ventilation in immunosuppressed patients with pulmonary infiltrates, fever, and acute respiratory failure. *N Engl J Med* 344:481–487, 2001.
186. Godwin JE, Kopecky KJ, Head DR, et al: A double-blind placebo-controlled trial of granulocyte-colony stimulating factor in elderly patients with previously untreated acute myeloid leukemia: a Southwest oncology group study (9031). *Blood* 91:3607–3613, 1998.

CHAPTER 116 ■ ONCOLOGIC EMERGENCIES

DAMIAN J. GREEN, JOHN A. THOMPSON AND BRUCE MONTGOMERY

The clinical presentation of oncologic emergencies has not changed dramatically over the past 50 years; however, the efficacy and variety of therapeutic interventions have improved considerably. Because a patient's prognosis has a significant impact on the choice of treatments, it is of paramount importance for the intensivist and the care team to determine the following: (a) Is the clinical scenario truly emergent? (b) Is the syndrome related to malignancy, a side effect of treatment, or a benign process? (c) What is the specific tumor type that is responsible for the syndrome? (d) What is the stage of disease? (e) What studies are necessary to establish the diagnosis? (f) What are the wishes of the patient and family? The prognostic implications and the expected impact of treatment can then be weighed and appropriate therapy instituted or modified.

SUPERIOR VENA CAVA SYNDROME

Physiology

The superior vena cava (SVC) syndrome develops as a result of impaired blood return through the SVC to the right atrium. Obstruction results in venous hypertension, with the severity of ensuing signs and symptoms dependent on the site of obstruction and the rapidity with which the block occurs. The SVC is formed by the union of the left and right brachiocephalic veins in the middle third of the mediastinum and extends inferiorly

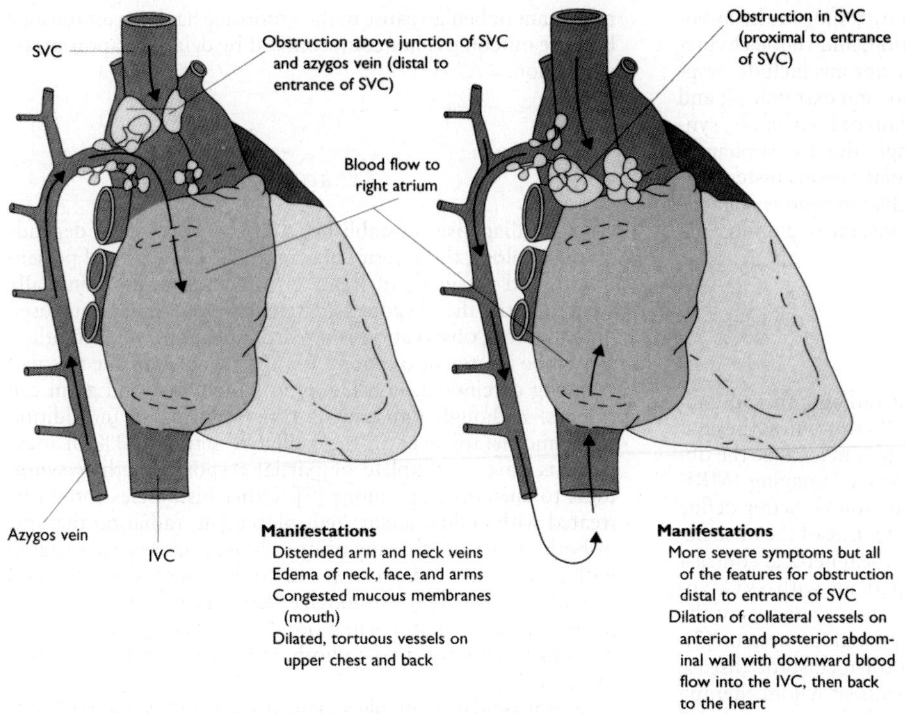
SVC
Obstruction above junction of SVC and azygos vein (distal to entrance of SVC)
Blood flow to right atrium
Azygos vein
IVC
Manifestations
Distended arm and neck veins
Edema of neck, face, and arms
Congested mucous membranes (mouth)
Dilated, tortuous vessels on upper chest and back
Obstruction in SVC (proximal to entrance of SVC)
Manifestations
More severe symptoms but all of the features for obstruction distal to entrance of SVC
Dilation of collateral vessels on anterior and posterior abdominal wall with downward blood flow into the IVC, then back to the heart

FIGURE 116.1. Anatomic locations of superior vena cava (SVC) obstruction leading to the SVC syndrome. IVC, inferior vena cava. [Reprinted from Skarin AT (ed): *Atlas of Diagnostic Oncology*. 2nd ed. St. Louis, Mosby, 1996, with permission.]

for 5 to 8 cm, terminating in the right atrium (Fig. 116.1). The SVC serves as the principal venous drainage for the head, neck, and upper extremities. The major collateral, the azygous vein, joins posteriorly just over the right mainstem bronchus and drains the posterior thorax. The SVC is thin walled and is bounded by the mediastinal parietal pleura and the right paratracheal, azygous, hilar, and subcarinal lymph nodes. As a result, it is extremely susceptible to extrinsic compression by adjacent lymph nodes or the aorta, with subsequent stasis, occlusion, or thrombosis. If obstruction occurs distal to the azygous vein, collateral flow through the azygous can adequately compensate for diminished return. However, if the obstruction is proximal to the azygous, flow must completely bypass the SVC and return via internal mammary, superficial thoracoabdominal, and vertebral venous systems to the inferior vena cava. This more circuitous route results in significantly higher venous pressures. The trachea and bronchi of children are smaller and significantly more susceptible to extrinsic compression, increasing the risk of fatal complications.

Etiology

The vast majority of patients with SVC syndrome have bronchogenic carcinoma, most commonly of the small cell histology (Table 116.1). Non-Hodgkin lymphoma, breast cancer, and other neoplasms make up the remainder of the malignant causes. Despite a high frequency of mediastinal involvement, Hodgkin lymphoma patients rarely present with SVC compression. Benign causes of SVC syndrome make up 6% to 20% of all cases and include thrombosis due to indwelling intravenous catheters or pacemakers and granulomatous disease [1,2]. Infectious causes of the SVC syndrome decreased substantially with the advent of antibiotics but must be considered in the differential diagnosis for patients from endemic areas or with potential human immunodeficiency virus infection. Blastomycosis, actinomycosis, histoplasmosis, tuberculosis, nocardia, and syphilis occasionally cause fibrosing mediastinitis and aortitis leading to SVC syndrome. An extensive list of rare causes may include idiopathic mediastinal fibrosis, goiter, thymoma, Behçet's syndrome, sarcoidosis, prior radiation with local vascular fibrosis, and unusual metastases of common malignancies.

Clinical Manifestations

The presentation of SVC syndrome depends largely on the acuity of the obstruction to flow. In patients with benign causes, extensive collateral flow often develops that minimizes symptoms

TABLE 116.1

PRIMARY DIAGNOSIS IN 125 CASES OF SVC SYNDROME

Histology	% of Cases	Total (%)
Lung carcinoma		79
Small cell	34	
Squamous cell	21	
Adenocarcinoma	14	
Large cell/other	11	
Lymphoma		14
Non-Hodgkin's lymphoma	13	
Hodgkin's lymphoma	0.8	
Other malignancy		6
Adenocarcinoma	3	
Kaposi's sarcoma	0.8	
Seminoma	0.8	
Acute myelomonocytic leukemia	0.8	
Leiomyosarcoma	0.8	

From Armstrong BA, Perez CA, Simpson JR, et al: Role of irradiation in the management of superior vena cava syndrome. *Int J Radiat Oncol Biol Phys* 13:531–539, 1987.

for months to years. Acute compression by tumor or thrombosis does not allow time for collateralization, and venous hypertension inevitably induces symptoms. Symptoms include dyspnea, edema of the face, neck, upper torso, and extremities; and cough. In rare instances, patients complain of hoarseness, syncope, headaches, chest pain, or dysphagia due to esophageal compression. Physical signs include jugular venous distention, edema of the face or upper extremities, dilated venous collaterals, plethora, and tachypnea and, in rare instances, papilledema or stridor.

Diagnosis

Initial evaluation should include a chest radiograph and contrast enhanced computed tomography (CT) to confirm the clinical diagnosis, identify a potential etiology, and localize the obstruction. Venography or magnetic resonance imaging (MRI) may be appropriate in subsequent evaluation to better define the extent of obstruction, particularly if stenting of the obstruction is considered (Fig. 116.2). Of note, focal hepatic contrast enhancement on CT has been noted in patients with SVC syndrome due to collateralization through patent remnants of the umbilical vein or of the musculophrenic venous system [3]. These abnormalities could be mistaken for metastatic disease and should be further evaluated in patients in whom therapy would be changed in the presence of isolated metastases. If a malignant cause of SVC obstruction is considered, all reasonable efforts should be made to obtain diagnostic material, as treatment depends on the underlying histology. The approach may include sputum cytology, bronchoscopy, transthoracic needle aspiration, biopsy of palpable lymph nodes, mediastinoscopy, thoracotomy, or video-assisted thoracoscopy. Despite concerns regarding surgical complications, morbidity associated with surgical procedures necessary to procure a diagnosis is not substantially different from that in patients without SVC syndrome [1,4]. The rapidity of the diagnostic workup depends on the likelihood of morbid complications at the time of presentation. Most series suggest that patients with malignant SVC syndrome have had symptoms an average of 45 days before presentation, and the vast majority of patients with malignancy do not die of SVC syndrome but of other complications of their disease [1]. The significant complications of SVC syndrome are tracheal obstruction and cerebral edema, and fatalities from cerebral edema are extremely rare. Therefore, the truly emergent situation in adults is a patient who presents with stridor or other evidence of significant airway compromise or the rare patient with cerebral edema. In essentially all other settings, treatment should be instituted only after the malignant or benign cause of the syndrome has been established because outcome is not compromised by delay for appropriate evaluation.

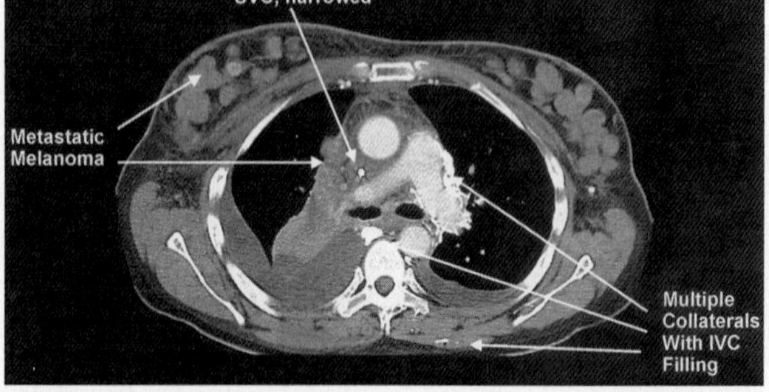

FIGURE 116.2. Upper extremity contrast injection demonstrating severe narrowing of the superior vena cava (SVC) with the development of multiple collaterals and inferior vena cava (IVC) filling.

Treatment

Once the diagnosis is established, initiation of therapy depends on the etiology, the severity of symptoms, the acuity of presentation, and the goals of treatment. If patients are minimally symptomatic, the azygous is patent, and treatment is focused on palliation, observation is a reasonable option. Chemotherapy is the treatment of choice for SVC syndrome due to small cell lung carcinoma, non-Hodgkin lymphoma, and germ cell tumors. Although radiation is often considered in addition to chemotherapy even in the palliative setting, 80% of these patients have a complete or partial response of their symptoms to chemotherapy alone [5]. Other histologies should be treated with endovascular stent placement, radiation therapy, or both. Radiation therapy prior to biopsy has been associated with a significant reduction in rates of histologic diagnosis and should be avoided [6]. Although external beam radiation effectively palliates symptoms in more than 70% of patients within 2 weeks [7], relapse after radiotherapy occurs in 15% to 30% of cases.

Endovascular stent placement, as a primary intervention, is a particularly attractive option for patients who lack a tissue diagnosis and whose symptoms on presentation require a rapid palliative intervention; including all patients, regardless of histology, who present with airway compromise or cerebral edema. In these patients, SVC stent placement provides rapid relief of symptoms (less than 48 hours) while awaiting response to systemic chemotherapy or radiation treatment. Responses to endovascular stent placement are durable (90% symptom free at time of death, versus 12% with palliative radiation) and the primary patency rates for malignant SVC syndrome are 50% to 100% [8]. Some authors have suggested a role for stent placement in first-line management of all SVC syndrome patients; however, no randomized controlled trials have been published [8].

Anticoagulation after stent placement is controversial, with some studies suggesting a high rate of thrombosis unless patients are anticoagulated, whereas other series, using no anticoagulation, report efficacy and thrombotic risk equivalent to those who use anticoagulation [9,10].

In patients with an established diagnosis, radiation therapy remains an appropriate intervention. Many fractionation protocols have been used, with the majority of patients receiving 30 Gy in 10 fractions, whereas patients treated with curative intent often receive 50 Gy in 25 fractions. Although high doses of radiation have often been given early in the treatment course to achieve rapid tumor response, there is little evidence to suggest that this is necessary [11]. In cases of SVC thrombosis with an indwelling catheter or pacemaker, thrombolytic agents may be useful as primary therapy or as an adjunct to stent placement [12]. The additional benefit of thrombolytics or anticoagulation in patients treated for malignant SVC syndrome is not well established.

Surgical resection and reconstruction of the SVC is reserved for patients with benign disease or the rare patient with tracheal obstruction in the setting of chemotherapy or radiotherapy-resistant disease.

SVC syndrome has been thought to predict for poor outcome. However, the presence of SVC syndrome is not a negative prognostic factor in small cell carcinoma and lymphoma independent of the stage and bulk of disease, and patients should be treated with curative intent if otherwise appropriate [13].

CARDIAC TAMPONADE

Physiology

Cardiac tamponade results from accumulation of fluid within the pericardium that impairs left ventricular expansion and diastolic filling. As stroke volume drops, compensatory tachycardia occurs to offset progressive hypotension. Ultimately, pressures equalize in the left atrium, pulmonary vasculature, right atrium, and SVC, and circulatory collapse ensues. As with SVC syndrome, the severity of symptoms is dependent on the speed of progression. Tamponade occurs when the pericardium cannot expand because fluid accumulation is too rapid or because the pericardium is thickened or fibrotic.

Etiology

Pericardial or cardiac involvement with malignancy occurs in 1% to 20% of patients with cancer and is often not diagnosed antemortem [14,15]. In up to 40% of unselected patients presenting with tamponade, malignancy is identified as the cause; the frequency with which tamponade develops as the initial manifestation of a patient's disease has led to standard cytologic examination of all significant effusions [16]. Tumors may involve the pericardium by direct extension from intrathoracic organs or hematogenous spread. Malignancies most often associated with pericardial effusions are lung, breast, lymphoma, and leukemia. Pericardial effusions in patients with cancer are due to pericardial or cardiac involvement in 60% of cases, with idiopathic pericarditis and radiation-induced pericarditis causing 32% and 10% of cases, respectively [17]. Other potential causes include infection, Dressler's syndrome, rheumatic disease, and hypothyroidism.

Clinical Manifestations

The common symptoms of pericardial effusion include dyspnea (85%), cough (30%), orthopnea (25%), and chest pain (20%). The common signs of pericardial effusion are jugular venous distention (100%), tachycardia (100%), pulsus paradoxus (89%), systolic blood pressure of less than 90 (52%), and pericardial rub (22%) [16]. Other signs of right- and left-sided heart failure may include hepatosplenomegaly, rales, peripheral edema, and ascites. Plain films demonstrate cardiac enlargement in at least half of all cases, and electrocardiography may reveal abnormalities suggestive of pericarditis (low-voltage, ST-segment elevation) or electrical alternans.

Diagnosis

Echocardiography is the most useful means of rapidly detecting hemodynamically significant effusions. Early signs include right atrial collapse and mitral regurgitation with later detection of left atrial or right ventricular collapse. Echocardiography also allows estimation of the volume, fluidity, and contents of the effusion, although it is difficult to distinguish tumor, thrombus, or fibrinous material from one another. The specificity of echocardiography for hemodynamic compromise has been called into question, and in many centers right heart catheterization with demonstration of equalization of pressures is required to diagnose tamponade physiology definitively. Emergent treatment of tamponade invariably involves drainage of the effusion, and cytologic evaluation of the fluid provides a very specific means of establishing a malignant etiology. The detection rate of pericardial fluid cytology ranges from 50% to 100%, and certain histologies, such as lymphoma and mesothelioma, are more difficult to demonstrate in pericardial fluid [14,18,19]. Pericardial biopsy is occasionally required to establish a diagnosis in difficult cases and can be performed under local anesthesia using a subxiphoid approach. The presence of a pericardial effusion correlates with a shortened survival among patients with cancer (median survival 15.1 weeks) and the definitive identification of neoplastic cells in the pericardial fluid by cytology portends an even worse prognosis (median survival 7.3 weeks) [20].

Treatment

Cardiac tamponade requires immediate treatment to relieve the increased end-diastolic pressure and inadequate ventricular filling. Oxygen, pressor agents, and intravenous fluids to improve cardiac output should be provided as appropriate. Inotropic agents are frequently ineffective however, because a state of intense adrenergic stimulation is already present [21]. When airway management is required, significant caution should be used because the positive intrathoracic pressure that results from initiation of mechanical ventilation places tamponade patients at particularly high risk for profound postintubation hypotension [21]. Emergent pericardiocentesis is indicated for significant hypotension, and it has been suggested that a pulse pressure of less than 20 mm Hg, a paradoxic pulse greater than 50% of the pulse pressure, or a peripheral venous pressure above 13 mm are other absolute indications for emergent intervention [22]. Fluid should be evaluated with cell counts, cultures, and cytology as noted earlier. Patients who present with malignant tamponade have recurrence after simple pericardiocentesis in 58% to 83% of cases [16,23]. Pericardial effusions without clinical tamponade may be observed if patients are asymptomatic or have minimal effusion (less than 1 cm), as progression to tamponade requiring pericardiocentesis in a single study was 20% for all patients, and progression of effusions of less than 1 cm in size to greater than 1 cm was only 4% [23]. Because of the high recurrence rate after pericardiocentesis in patients with tamponade, additional therapy is generally indicated if the patient's survival or quality of life would be otherwise compromised. Symptomatic relief with pericardiocentesis alone is 90% to 100%, with a complication rate of 3% [24]. Radiation therapy is noninvasive and allows treatment of the majority of the pericardium but carries a theoretical risk of radiation-induced pericarditis. As a single modality, radiation controls pericardial effusion in 67% of cases, with a particularly high success in hematopoietic tumors (93%). Systemic therapy is generally used only for diseases that are considered to be chemosensitive, such as breast cancer or lymphoma; in these individuals, it prevents recurrence in 73% of treated patients.

Instillation of sclerosing agents, radionuclides, and chemotherapy through indwelling catheters have been widely used with the intent to induce nonspecific inflammation with obliteration of the pericardial space or to achieve specific antineoplastic effects. Typically, a catheter is placed into the pericardial sac and drainage continued until output is less than 100 mL per day. Sclerosing agent or chemotherapy is injected into the catheter every 24 to 48 hours until fluid output is less than 25 to 50 mL per day, and the catheter is removed. A review of 20 different studies reported an overall control rate of 82% with common toxicities, including fever, pain, arrhythmias, and occasional cytopenias [24]. Tetracycline, which is no longer available, has the most extensive track record; however, doxycycline and minocycline have shown similar efficacy in malignant pericardial and pleural effusions. Chemotherapeutic agents that demonstrate response rates greater than 50%

include bleomycin, cisplatin, carboplatin, mitoxantrone, fluorouracil, and thiotepa [24–29]. In a randomized trial of 80 patients comparing intrapericardial bleomycin with observation alone following drainage, the 2-month failure free survival was 46% versus 29%; and median survival was 119 days versus 79 days for the groups, respectively. Because of the small size of this trial, these differences did not achieve statistical significance [30].

One small prospective trial ($n = 21$) comparing bleomycin with doxycycline showed bleomycin to be better tolerated, with less retrosternal pain and shorter periods of catheter drainage [28]. The use of sclerosing agents in the treatment of recurrent malignant pericardial effusions may result in an increased risk of both subsequent constrictive pericarditis and tamponade, leading some groups to favor the instillation of nonsclerosing chemotherapeutic agents [31]. In the absence of randomized studies, no single agent is accepted as the gold standard for intervention.

A surgical procedure or balloon catheter can be used to create a pericardial window to drain the fluid. This can be done by performing a subxiphoid pericardiotomy, thoracotomy or thoracoscopy with window, pleuroperitoneal window, or subcutaneous balloon pericardiotomy. These procedures control the effusion in 85% to 95% of patients [24,32–34]. An advantage of subxiphoid or balloon pericardiotomy is that both can be performed without general anesthesia, reducing operative morbidity.

Prognosis

The development of malignant pericardial effusion and tamponade usually reflects uncontrolled metastatic disease and portends a dire prognosis. Median survivals for patients treated for tamponade range from 3.3 to 4.5 months. Nonrandomized studies suggest that patients with lung and breast cancer have substantially better survival rates if systemic therapy can be instituted [35,36]. The decision to intervene in a patient with malignant cardiac tamponade depends on the patient's histology and sensitivity to treatment as well as the patient's condition. Patients for whom treatment of tamponade provides meaningful palliative benefit should be considered for the treatment that is likely to provide durable relief of symptoms with the minimum of morbidity and requirement for hospitalization.

MALIGNANT EPIDURAL CORD COMPRESSION

Few complications of malignancy are more dreaded than epidural cord compression. The associated pain, neurologic deficits, and dramatically impaired quality of life are serious problems for the patients who develop this condition and by extension for their families. Early recognition of the signs and symptoms of cord compression may prevent serious compromise in survival and functional capacity. *Epidural cord compression* is defined by compression of the dural sac and its contents by an extradural tumor mass. Minimum radiologic evidence for compression is indentation of the theca at the level of clinical features, which include pain, weakness, sensory disturbance, or evidence of sphincter dysfunction [37].

Physiology

Epidural cord compression by malignancy occurs as a result of metastasis or primary tumor involvement of the vertebral column, paravertebral space, or epidural space. Damage to the cord occurs when the tumor compromises the vertebral venous plexus or compresses neural tissue directly or when compromised bone impinges on the cord. The resulting vasogenic edema and hemorrhage induce further ischemic damage. The vertebral body is the most common source of compressive lesions, predominantly in the thoracic (70%), followed by the lumbar (20%) and cervical (10%) regions [38]. Tumor invasion through the intervertebral foramen and cord compression without bone involvement is most often seen with lymphoma, leading to normal plain films and radionuclide scans despite clinical compression. Multiple noncontiguous levels are involved in 10% to 40% of cases [39,40].

TABLE 116.2

PRIMARY DIAGNOSIS CAUSING EPIDURAL CORD COMPRESSION ($N = 896$)

Histology	% of Cases
Lung	18
Breast	13
Unknown primary	11
Lymphoma	10
Myeloma	8
Sarcoma	8
Prostate	6
Gastrointestinal tract	4
Renal	5
Other	17

Data from Weissman DE, Gilbert M, Wang H, et al: The use of computed tomography of the spine to identify patients at high risk for epidural metastases. *J Clin Oncol* 3:1541–1544, 1985; Ruff RL, Lanska DJ: Epidural metastases in prospectively evaluated veterans with cancer and back pain. *Cancer* 63:2234–2241, 1989.

Etiology

The most common causes of malignant cord compression are tumors with a propensity for bony metastases, including breast and lung, followed by hematopoietic malignancy and gastrointestinal and genitourinary primaries [41,42] (Table 116.2). Cord compression afflicts 5% of patients during their course and is found in up to 10% of patients at autopsy. Benign causes of cord compression include stenosis, epidural abscess, or hematoma.

Clinical Manifestations

The cardinal sign of malignant cord compression is pain, present in 95% of patients at diagnosis. Weakness, autonomic dysfunction, and sensory changes are present in more than 50% of cases [43]. The pain is typically worse with recumbency, coughing, straining, or exercise. Radicular pain develops later and is an important localizing sign. Weakness, sensory loss, and incontinence are also late findings. Urinary retention alone is very rarely a presentation of cord compression. Duration of symptoms before severe cord compression and paralysis is remarkably variable, ranging from years to 24 to 48 hours.

Diagnosis

The diagnosis of cord compression relies primarily on MRI, given its sensitivity, speed, and the ability to detect compression at multiple levels. The utility of radionuclide studies and radiographs for predicting cord compression is dependent entirely on the patient's disease status (known vs. initial diagnosis of malignancy), symptoms, and neurologic examination [44]. In fact, at least 20% of patients with malignancy, back pain, and cord compression have neither localizing neurologic signs nor abnormal radiographs and would be misdiagnosed without further imaging studies [44]. MRI allows evaluation of the entire neuraxis, is more sensitive for detection of paraspinal disease, and may demonstrate leptomeningeal and intramedullary disease. Because the risk of malignant cord compression at the site of plain film abnormalities in a symptomatic patient with malignancy is so high, it has been proposed to bypass MRI and to radiate the cord two segments above and below the defined lesion [41]. However, a prospective study analyzed the expected outcome with that approach compared with treatment planning on the basis of MRI and found that MRI changed the radiotherapy plan in 53% of patients [45]. These changes included 21% of patients in whom all paraspinal disease would not have been treated and 5% of those in whom additional levels of true cord compression would not have been treated. In 30% of patients, the demonstrated level of compression on MRI was more than two vertebral levels away from the level indicated by neurologic examination. If patients are unable to undergo MRI because of claustrophobia, the presence of metal implants, or access, myelography can be performed instead. CT scanning is superior to MRI for definition of vertebral body anatomy and may be useful before consideration of surgical intervention.

Treatment

Therapeutic options include corticosteroids, surgery, and radiation. In emergent situations, corticosteroids are generally given while awaiting MRI to decrease peritumoral edema and to prevent edema formation during radiation. On the basis of laboratory studies and a single randomized controlled trial that compared high-dose dexamethasone with radiation to radiation alone [46], some authors support the use of high-dose dexamethasone, defined as a 100-mg intravenous bolus followed by 96 mg per day tapered over a 2-week period. This approach is efficacious, but adverse side effects are reported in up to 30% of patients [47]. Alternatively, a more standard approach is 10 mg intravenously followed by 4 mg every 6 hours tapered over 2 weeks, especially in patients who are clinically stable. Ambulatory patients without progressive deficit may forgo steroids altogether during radiotherapy without undue risk [48]. Historically, radiation therapy and direct decompressive surgery were felt to be equally effective as initial interventions in patients with metastatic spinal cord compression. A recent randomized trial comparing direct decompressive surgery plus postoperative radiotherapy to radiotherapy alone revealed a statistically significant outcome benefit to the combined approach under certain conditions. Compared with patients who received radiotherapy alone, more patients who underwent surgery were able to walk after treatment (84% vs. 57%) and were ambulatory for a significantly longer duration (median: 122 days, versus 13 days) [49]. A secondary data analysis from this randomized trial revealed no benefit from surgical intervention for patients greater than 65 years of age [50]. First-line radiation therapy remains an important option for patients who are known to have highly radiosensitive tumors; nonsurgical candidates; patients with multiple areas of spinal cord compression; and those who experienced symptoms of total paraplegia for longer than 48 hours at presentation. Because surgical complication rates approach 20% [51], radiation therapy should generally be used as the first-line intervention in patients over age 65. Specific radiation treatment plans for cord compression vary between centers. The most common course is 30 Gy in 10 fractions over 2 weeks.

TABLE 116.3

INCIDENCE OF HYPERCALCEMIA IN ADVANCED MALIGNANCY

Histology	% Who develop hypercalcemia
Breast	19–30
Lung	10–35
Multiple myeloma	20–30
Head and neck	5–24
Renal	17

Prognosis

Early intervention is vital to preserving function. For patients who are ambulatory at the time of treatment, at least 80% remain ambulatory. The development of paraparesis decreases the ambulation rate to 50%, and patients who are paraplegic at the time of therapy recover ambulation only 10% to 19% of the time after radiation therapy alone [37,43,49,52–55]. In paraplegic patients, outcomes appeared to be better for individuals who were candidates for upfront surgical decompression (62% of patients randomized to combined surgery plus radiation regained the ability to walk compared with 19% of those who received radiation alone), the difference was statistically significant, but the sample size was small ($n = 32$) [49].

HYPERCALCEMIA

Hypercalcemia of malignancy (HCM) is the most common emergent metabolic disorder associated with cancer, affecting 10% to 20% of patients with malignancy at some time during their clinical course (Table 116.3). Diagnosis and timely interventions are life saving in the short term but also enhance patients' compliance with primary and supportive treatments and may improve quality of life.

Physiology

In healthy persons, vitamin D and parathyroid hormone (PTH) control absorption and mobilization of calcium. Calcitriol, the active form of vitamin D, enhances gastrointestinal absorption and mobilizes calcium from bone. PTH increases renal calcium resorption in the distal tubule and also mobilizes calcium from bone. In patients with HCM, increased calcium mobilization combines with renal insufficiency to cause symptomatic hypercalcemia. At least two mechanisms are proposed: direct osteolysis by tumor or increased osteoclastic resorption as a result of humoral mediators. Both mechanisms may be active in many patients. The parathyroid hormone-related protein (PTHrP) is postulated to play a role in the majority of patients with HCM, as levels are elevated in at least 80% of cases [56]. PTHrP is a 139 amino acid protein that may give rise to several peptides with differing biologic activities [57,58]. PTHrP appears to have important roles in calcium transport and developmental biology, and the N-terminal 13 amino acids share amino acid sequence and homology with intact PTH. PTHrP stimulates osteoblasts to produce receptor activator of nuclear factor-κB ligand (RANKL) which in turn activates osteoclast precursors and leads to both osteolysis and the release of bone-derived growth factors. These growth factors, including transforming growth factor-β and insulin like growth factor-1, are known to both promote tumor cell proliferation and further increase production of PTHrP, which then continues to drive renal calcium reabsorption [59]. Circulating vitamin D metabolites may be increased in some lymphomas, enhancing intestinal calcium absorption and causing or exacerbating hypercalcemia [60].

Normal kidneys are capable of filtering and excreting four to five times the normal calcium concentration in the serum to maintain serum calcium homeostasis. PTHrP increases renal tubular resorption and osteolytic calcium release, causing rapid and persistent elevation of extracellular calcium. The subsequent calciuria and osmotic diuresis result in volume depletion. Decreased glomerular filtration limits the kidney's ability to filter and excrete calcium, and proximal tubular calcium and sodium reabsorption increase, leading to further increases in serum calcium concentrations.

Symptoms of nausea and vomiting worsen the dehydration. If the concentration of calcium in the glomerular filtrate exceeds its solubility, calcium may precipitate in the renal tubules, further compromising renal function.

Etiology

HCM occurs most frequently in patients with breast cancer, multiple myeloma, and squamous cell malignancies of the lung, head and neck, and esophagus (Table 116.3). For instance, the incidence of hypercalcemia in patients with metastatic breast carcinoma is 20% to 30% [61,62]. A tumor "flare" can develop in patients with breast cancer after initiation of hormonal therapy, with associated pain and hypercalcemia, and this response may predict for better response to treatment [63]. Hypercalcemia develops in patients with metastatic lung carcinoma in 10% to 35% of cases but, almost invariably in non–small cell rather than small cell histology [64,65]. The development of hypercalcemia in patients with lung carcinoma in several series suggested that disease was unresectable and prognosis uniformly poor [66]. Some malignancies are rarely associated with hypercalcemia despite a propensity for widespread metastases, including prostate cancer and small cell lung cancer. Multiple myeloma commonly causes hypercalcemia, and up to 20% of myeloma patients may present with this complication. It represents advanced disease and, although associated with a worse prognosis, survival is substantially better than for patients with hypercalcemia resulting from solid tumors [67].

Clinical Manifestations

As with other oncologic emergencies, the rapidity with which hypercalcemia develops often determines the severity of symptoms. Patients may have significant symptoms with minimally elevated calcium and require therapy, whereas other patients are minimally symptomatic despite long-standing hypercalcemia. Many of the symptoms of hypercalcemia are relatively nonspecific, and the possibility of hypercalcemia must be kept in mind when considering patients with nausea, fatigue, lethargy, and mental status changes. Decreased intravascular volume and hypercalcemia cause malaise, fatigue, anorexia, and polyuria. Hypercalcemia decreases neuromuscular excitability and decreased muscle tone. Neuromuscular symptoms include weakness and diminished deep tendon reflexes. Neuropsychiatric manifestations may include confusion, lethargy, psychosis, or even coma. Hypercalcemia heightens cardiac contractility and irritability, and this is reflected by electrocardiographic changes, such as prolonged PR interval, widened QRS complex, and a shortened QT. With progressive hypercalcemia, bradyarrhythmias and bundle-branch block may develop, which can evolve to complete heart block and asystole.

Diagnosis

The diagnosis of hypercalcemia is documented by the presence of elevated corrected serum calcium, defined by the following formula: [4.0 − patient (Alb)] × 0.8 + [Ca], where Alb signifies albumin. Alternatively, an elevation of serum ionized calcium documents hypercalcemia and does not require the concomitant measurement of serum albumin. Other laboratory studies that should be considered include PTH, PTHrP, blood urea nitrogen and creatinine, phosphate, and magnesium. The assessment of a patient presenting with hypercalcemia should include several important aspects of disease history. Although hypercalcemia is a common complication of malignancy, other nonmalignant causes (including hyperparathyroidism, intravenous fluids, total parenteral nutrition, milk-alkali syndrome, thiazide diuretics, vitamins A and D, and lithium) are present in 10% to 15% of cancer patients who present with hypercalcemia and should be considered in the differential diagnosis.

Treatment

The decision to treat hypercalcemia should be dictated by the patient's history, current disease status, quality of life, and the wishes of the patient and family. The prognosis for most patients with HCM is poor. Severe pain, obstruction, or irreversible structural symptoms may be an indication not to pursue therapy. However, relief of the symptoms of hypercalcemia may improve quality of life and functional status for many patients during the remainder of their lifetimes. Patients who are symptomatic and who have no other potential etiology of hypercalcemia should be treated. If calcium is elevated but the patient is asymptomatic, specific hypocalcemic therapy can be held, with close observation, particularly if effective systemic therapy is to be initiated. Because most symptoms and the underlying physiology of hypercalcemia are due in part to volume depletion, intravenous hydration is the initial therapy of choice (Table 116.4). Although no randomized controlled clinical trials have been conducted to inform the approach to hydration, in general patients require repletion with 3 to 7 L intravenous saline over 24 to 36 hours to achieve euvolemia. If congestive heart failure is a concern or if the patient has severe hypercalcemia, loop diuretics can be used, but only after it is clear that adequate volume expansion has been achieved. If diuretics are used before the glomerular filtration rate has been restored, renal clearance of calcium is impaired further, and hypercalcemia may worsen despite the best intentions. Loop diuretics suppress

TABLE 116.4

ALGORITHM FOR CLINICAL MANAGEMENT OF HYPERCALCEMIA OF MALIGNANCY

Calcium Level	Symptoms	Therapy
<12 mg/dL	None	Observation, or hydration followed by observation
<12 mg/dL	Present	Hydration, bisphosphonate
12–14 mg/dL	Present	Hydration, bisphosphonate
>14	Present	Hydration, bisphosphonate
>14	Severe	Hydration, loop diuretics, calcitonin, bisphosphonate
		Alternatives: plicamycin, gallium nitrate, prednisone phosphate, dialysis

proximal absorption of sodium and calcium, augmenting calciuresis.

Bisphosphonates are the most useful hypocalcemic agents available for controlling HCM. They inhibit prenylation of small guanosine triphosphatases, which are necessary for osteoclast function and are cytotoxic to osteoclasts through a number of different mechanisms [68]. Zoledronic acid and pamidronate are the bisphosphonates currently in clinical use. Two randomized trials comparing pamidronate and zoledronic acid demonstrated improved response rates for zoledronic acid, 4- and 8-mg infusions; complete response rates by day 10 were 88.4%, 86.7%, and 69.7% for zoledronic acid, 4 mg and 8 mg, and pamidronate, 90 mg, respectively. Normalization of calcium occurred by day 4 in 50% of patients treated with zoledronic acid and 33% of those given pamidronate. Median duration of complete response favored zoledronic acid, 4 and 8 mg, over pamidronate, with response durations of 32, 43, and 18 days, respectively. Zoledronic acid is administered intravenously over 5 minutes. Optimal zoledronic acid dosage and administration schedules have not been established; the standard dose is 4 mg, with 8 mg reserved for patients with recurrent or refractory hypercalcemia. The onset of zoledronic acid's effect is apparent within 3 to 4 days, with maximal effect within 7 to 10 days, and lasts for 14 days to 2 months. Adverse effects include transient low-grade temperature elevations that typically occur within 24 to 36 hours after administration and persist for up to 2 days ($\leq$20% of patients). Other bisphosphonates (except clodronate) may also produce transient fever, and the incidence of temperature elevation, nausea, anorexia, dyspepsia, and vomiting may be increased by rapid administration. New-onset hypophosphatemia and hypomagnesemia may occur; preexisting abnormalities in the same electrolytes may be exacerbated by treatment. Serum calcium may fall below the normal range, although symptoms are rare. Renal insufficiency has occurred in ongoing clinical trials at the 8-mg dose level and must be considered in patients with existing renal insufficiency [69]. No dose reduction is recommended for patients receiving the 4-mg dose of zoledronic acid when the measured serum creatinine is less than 3.0 mg per dL [70]. Another bisphosphonate, ibandronate, has demonstrated comparable activity and a longer duration of efficacy when compared to pamidronate in a randomized study of patients with hypercalcemia. Ibandronate appears to be the least nephrotoxic bisphosphonate agent, leading some authors to advocate its use in patients with renal impairment; however ibandronate is not currently approved for the management of hypercalcemia of malignancy by the Food and Drug Administration (FDA) in the United States [71]. An association has been reported between bisphosphonate therapy and subsequent development of osteonecrosis of the jaw.

The incidence is higher with zoledronic acid than with pamidronate (10% vs. 4%) and the risk is significantly increased in individuals with underlying dental conditions or those undergoing dental procedures during treatment. Patients on chronic therapy appear to be at greatest risk [72].

Other treatments for HCM include corticosteroids, calcitonin, plicamycin, and gallium nitrate. Calcitonin rapidly inhibits bone resorption and decreases renal calcium reabsorption. Salmon calcitonin is administered at 4 IU per kg subcutaneously or intramuscularly every 12 hours, and tachyphylaxis occurs rapidly, necessitating dosing increases to 8 IU every 6 to 12 hours. Efficacy is limited to the first 24 to 48 hours after initiation of therapy, and additional treatment with bisphosphonate should be considered concurrent with calcitonin. Corticosteroids are effective in lymphoma and multiple myeloma, tumors in which steroids are often cytotoxic. The onset of action is slow, over several weeks, and the mechanism of effect is through treatment of the underlying malignancy and suppression of gastrointestinal calcium absorption. Therapies designed to interfere with RANKL binding, including the monoclonal antibody denosumab and a decoy RANLK receptor, osteoprotegerin, appear to decrease serum calcium levels in preclinical and clinical settings, however no randomized clinical trials have been performed to evaluate these agents in patients with hypercalcemia [59,73–75]. Dialysis should be considered for patients with severe renal insufficiency and associated electrolyte abnormalities, particularly in patients for whom effective therapy is available.

Hypercalcemia reflects biologically aggressive, advanced disease. For patients with solid tumors, particularly those with chemotherapy-resistant disease, the prognosis is extremely grim, with median survivals of 30 to 60 days in most studies [76]. By contrast, hypercalcemia in patients with multiple myeloma and breast cancer is associated with relatively longer survival. The argument has been made that treatment of HCM prolongs survival in patients in whom other morbid complications of their disease will develop. In fact, it is clear that hypocalcemic agents do not prolong survival but can have impressive palliative benefit in relieving symptoms from hypercalcemia, such as nausea, emesis, and constipation, and improving pain control for some patients who achieve normocalcemia [76].

LEUKOSTASIS

Physiology

Leukostasis is a potentially devastating complication of leukemia in patients who present with hyperleukocytosis, defined as a leukocyte count greater than 100,000 per μL. The syndrome of leukostasis is related to obstruction of flow in capillary beds of the central nervous system, lungs, and heart by immature, rigid blasts. Although viscosity might be expected to play a role, it is rarely elevated because the principal determinant of viscosity, red blood cells, is often low due to marrow replacement by leukemic blasts. The obstruction of capillary beds by blasts and restricted flow results in tissue hypoxia, cytokine release, and coagulation. Tissue invasion also occurs and is not affected by leukapheresis. The risk of leukostasis was evaluated by Lichtman and Rowe [77], who demonstrated that the leukocrit, which is proportional to the number and volume of circulating leukocytes and blasts, was the parameter most closely associated with the development of leukostasis. Although integrins are postulated to play a role in the syndrome, analysis of vascular endothelium in patients with leukostasis compared with controls showed no significant differences in expression of vascular cellular adhesion molecule-1, endothelial–leukocyte adhesion molecule-1, or intercellular adhesion molecule-1 [78]. In vitro studies suggest that in the presence of inflammatory cytokines, leukemic blasts can adhere to vascular endothelium and that these blasts are capable of secreting multiple mediators of endothelial damage [79]. Until clinical correlations between cytokine excretion, integrin expression, and the development of leukostasis are available, the role of integrins in development of the syndrome will remain speculative.

Etiology

Hyperleukocytosis occurs in 10% to 20% of patients with acute myelogenous leukemia (AML) at presentation and is much less common in patients with chronic myelogenous leukemia, acute lymphoblastic leukemia, or chronic lymphocytic leukemia. For equivalent degrees of leukocytosis, the risk of leukostasis is much higher with AML than with other diagnoses because of the larger size and adhesion characteristics of

TABLE 116.5

ALGORITHM FOR TREATMENT OF SYMPTOMATIC HYPONATREMIA

Acute	Mildly symptomatic	Na <125 mg/dL	Free water restriction 500–1,000 mL/d Demeclocycline Avoid in renal/hepatic dysfunction
Acute	Severe symptoms	Na <115 mg/dL	3% saline Furosemide diuresis

AML blasts. The risk of developing leukostasis depends on total white blood cell count (WBC), the percentage of blasts, and the rate at which counts are rising. The clinical presentation, diagnosis, and management of hyperleukocytosis are discussed in further detail in Chapter 115.

HYPONATREMIA

Physiology

Clinically symptomatic hyponatremia is a relatively rare complication of malignancy affecting only 1% to 2% of cancer patients. In the majority of these individuals, the syndrome of inappropriate antidiuretic hormone (SIADH) develops. Secretion of ectopic ADH occurs almost solely in patients with small cell bronchogenic carcinoma, and the majority of other patients have coincident central nervous system or pulmonary disease. As a result of excess ADH, excessive water resorption occurs in the collecting ducts, and extracellular fluid osmolality decreases inappropriately. Water is able to move freely, and the decrease in extracellular osmolality results in a shift to the intracellular compartment with associated cellular edema. When hyponatremia occurs acutely, this edema causes dramatic neuronal edema and subsequent neurologic symptoms. Plasma volume expands, and urinary sodium excretion parallels the rate of oral sodium intake. Typically, the patient with SIADH is euvolemic to slightly hypervolemic, urine sodium is greater than 20 mEq per L, and plasma urea, uric acid, creatinine, and rennin activity are normal or low.

Etiology

At presentation, hyponatremia develops in more than 50% of patients with small cell carcinoma after free water loading, but symptoms develop in fewer than 10% of patients. SIADH has also been reported in a broad variety of other malignancies but is most commonly found in the setting of central nervous system or pulmonary metastases. SIADH may also develop in patients with malignancy due to other conditions, including the use of opiates, vinca alkaloids, β agonists, chlorpropamide, and cyclophosphamide. Hypoadrenalism due to rapid tapering of therapeutic corticosteroids is also a common etiology for mild hyponatremia. Other etiologies include volume contraction due to emesis or diarrhea, renal wasting due to diuretics or intrinsic renal disease, and pseudohyponatremia from excess serum lipids or paraproteins. Hypothyroidism and pulmonary or central nervous system disease are also potential causes of SIADH.

Diagnosis

Hyponatremia is often manifested as fatigue, nausea, myalgia, headaches, and subtle neurologic symptoms. Rapid drops in serum sodium or levels less than 115 mg per dL cause altered mental status, seizures, coma, pathologic reflexes, and papilledema. The diagnostic evaluation includes a review of medications and assessment of volume status as well as serum and urine electrolytes, osmolality, and creatinine. Patients with SIADH have inappropriately elevated urine sodium, and urine osmolality is greater than plasma osmolality but never reaches maximal dilution (less than 100 μOsm). Thyroid and adrenal dysfunction cause similar electrolyte imbalances and must be ruled out if laboratory studies suggest SIADH. CT or radiographs of the chest and brain may be necessary to eliminate pulmonary or central nervous system disease as causes of excessive ADH secretion.

Treatment

Treatment of the hyponatremia is tailored to the acuity with which it developed and the extent of symptoms that the patient is experiencing. Chronic severe hyponatremia should be treated with fluid restriction alone. Treatment of the underlying malignancy may alleviate SIADH due to small cell carcinoma. Local therapy to brain or pulmonary metastases may improve serum sodium, and discontinuing offending medications should be effective. Acute symptomatic hyponatremia can be treated as indicated in Table 116.5.

Free water restriction is expected to improve hyponatremia within 7 to 10 days. Demeclocycline induces a dose-dependent, reversible nephrogenic diabetes insipidus and is expected to correct sodium within 3 to 4 days. The primary side effect of demeclocycline is renal toxicity, and the risk of toxicity is increased by renal or hepatic dysfunction. The initial dose of demeclocycline is 600 mg daily to a maximum of 1,200 mg per day in two- to three-times-a-day dosing.

Patients who are seizing, comatose, or rapidly decompensating should be treated with hypertonic saline and furosemide to induce an isotonic diuresis as originally proposed by Gross et al. [80] and Hantman et al. [81]. Once the sodium level is above 120 mg per dL, more conservative measures are appropriate. The primary risk of rapid correction of hyponatremia is central pontine myelinolysis, which typically occurs 3 to 5 days after repletion with corticobulbar spinal dysfunction, dysphasia, quadriparesis, and delirium. Although controversial, most data support the idea that the risk of pontine myelinolysis is greatest for patients with chronic, severe hyponatremia who are treated too rapidly. Generally, the sodium level should not be corrected at a rate faster than 0.5 mM per L per hour even in acute circumstances [82].

TUMOR LYSIS SYNDROME

Physiology

Tumor lysis syndrome (TLS) is a metabolic emergency that remains a significant risk for patients with hematopoietic malignancy and is being recognized with greater frequency in patients with solid tumors. TLS results from the release of intracellular purines, phosphate, and potassium from rapidly proliferating tumor cells, which may occur spontaneously or with the initiation of therapy. The massive tumor necrosis that initiates the syndrome may occur as a result of tumor hypoxia or with the use of chemotherapy, radiation, or embolization of tumor. Tumor lysis is followed by hyperuricemia, hyperkalemia, hyperphosphatemia, hypocalcemia, and renal insufficiency. The hyperuricemia, combined with metabolic acidosis, results in crystallization of uric acid in the collecting ducts of the kidneys and ureters, leading to obstructive uropathy. Hyperphosphatemia may also cause metastatic calcification in the renal tubules. The resultant renal insufficiency worsens hyperkalemia and hypocalcemia.

Etiology

Patients at highest risk include those with lymphoma, particularly high-grade Burkitt's or non-Burkitt's non-Hodgkin's lymphoma and acute leukemia. The frequency of TLS depends on the criteria used, which are not well established or accepted. In Burkitt's lymphoma the incidence may be as high as 30%, and in patients with acute leukemia with hyperleukocytosis, electrolyte disturbances develop consistent with TLS in 50% of cases [83,84]. A variety of solid tumors have been reported to cause the syndrome, but the most common appear to be small cell lung carcinoma, breast carcinoma, and neuroblastoma. Others include ovarian and vulvar carcinoma, medulloblastoma, sarcomas, seminoma, and melanoma [85,86]. The pretreatment variables that predict the occurrence of the syndrome are azotemia and elevated lactic dehydrogenase and hyperuricemia, evidence of a rapidly proliferating tumor undergoing spontaneous necrosis. Generally, these malignancies are clinically aggressive and sensitive to chemotherapy or radiation.

Diagnosis

The diagnosis of TLS is a clinical one, as there is no specific pathognomonic finding or laboratory value that is specific to the syndrome. The diagnosis of TLS is made on the basis of the presence of azotemia, hyperuricemia, hyperphosphatemia, and hypocalcemia in a patient with extensive, rapidly proliferating tumor. The incidence of hyperkalemia is somewhat more variable. Profound metabolic acidosis out of proportion to the degree of renal insufficiency is common. Many of the metabolic abnormalities of TLS may occur as a result of acute renal failure alone, and a urinary uric acid to creatinine ratio greater than 1 helps to distinguish acute uric acid nephropathy from other catabolic forms of acute renal failure in which serum urate is elevated.

Treatment

Management can be grouped into prevention/conservative therapy and hemodialysis. Allopurinol in doses of 200 to 600 mg per m^2 per day should be initiated before therapy to decrease uric acid production [87]. Intravenous allopurinol is safe and effective and is indicated for patients who are unable to take oral allopurinol because of being non per os (NPO) for surgery or having respiratory distress/intubation or abnormal gastrointestinal motility/absorption [88]. Intravenous hydration at 200 to 300 mL per hour containing 25 to 50 mEq per L $NaHCO_3$ should be given to expand volume, alkalinize the urine, and wash out the renal medulla. It is preferable to decrease urine osmolality to isotonic and to increase urinary pH to greater than 7.0. In practice this is sometimes difficult, and in our experience isotonic $NaHCO_3$ (1.4%) more effectively achieves alkaline urine, although the risk of fluid overload is somewhat greater. Increasing metastatic calcification with the development of alkalemia is also a risk; however, the incidence of this complication is far less than that of renal insufficiency related to deposition of insoluble uric acid. Hyperkalemia should be aggressively managed with potassium restriction and sodium polystyrene sulfonate as appropriate. Hemodialysis is often necessary and is indicated to control volume, reduce phosphorus and uric acid levels, and manage uremia. Some proposed criteria for initiation of hemodialysis are persistent hyperkalemia despite conventional treatment, rapidly rising phosphate, symptomatic hypocalcemia, fluid overload, severe metabolic acidosis, and hyperuricemia. Typically, daily dialysis is necessary because the catabolic rate is sharply increased in patients with TLS. Daily weights, close monitoring of fluid intake and output, and serum electrolytes, including potassium, calcium, phosphorus, and uric acid, should be performed at least twice a day in a patient at high risk and more frequently if dialysis is instituted. Allopurinol is associated with a significant number of side effects and should be discontinued within 3 days of completion of treatment if there is no evidence of tumor lysis. Rasburicase is a recombinant urate oxidase that converts uric acid to more soluble allantoin. A randomized study of rasburicase and allopurinol in pediatric patients at high risk of tumor lysis demonstrated that uric acid levels were substantially lower in patients receiving prophylactic rasburicase. The size of the trial was too small to demonstrate a significant difference in renal failure, and the incidence of tumor lysis was not reported [89]. Two compassionate-use rasburicase trials involving pediatric and adult cancer patients have documented impressive efficacy in both the prevention and treatment of hyperuricemia [90,91]. Rasburicase was approved by the U.S. FDA for the initial management of elevated plasma uric acid levels in 2009. Approval was based on findings from a postmarketing surveillance randomized multicenter trial (EFC 4978) which demonstrated a statistically significant difference in response rate (fraction of patients with a plasma uric acid levels <7.5 mg per dL) among rasburicase-treated leukemia, lymphoma, and solid tumor patients (87% response) when compared with patients treated with allopurinol (66%). Interestingly, although the serum uric acid was significantly lower in the rasburicase-treated group, there was no difference between the arms in incidence of TLS. Rasburicase was administered at a dose of 0.2 mg per kg per day for 5 days. The most common rasburicase-associated toxicities included edema (50%), vomiting (38%), hyperbilirubinemia (16%), and sepsis (12%) [92]. A subsequent randomized trial of 64 patients comparing rasburicase administered daily (0.15 mg per kg per day) for 5 days versus a single dose followed by "as needed" dosing in adult patients with hematologic malignancies at risk for developing tumor lysis syndrome. The single-dose group demonstrated a sustained response in 87% of patients demonstrating that it is reasonable to decrease the duration of administration and follow uric acid levels in selected patients [93]. When rasburicase is used, it is important to recognize that the enzyme can continue to degrade uric acid in blood samples at room temperature. Samples must be collected in prechilled heparinized tubes, transported on ice, and analyzed within 4 hours of collection. Rasburicase is contraindicated in patients with glucose-6-phosphate dehydrogenase deficiency.

Outcome with development of full-blown tumor lysis syndrome is variable. In the reported cases of solid tumor TLS, the fatality rate was very high (36%) [85]. Institution of prophylaxis in patients identified as high risk (even those with solid tumors), which includes both rasburicase and consideration

TABLE 116.6

ADVANCES IN MANAGEMENT BASED ON RANDOMIZED CONTROLLED CLINICAL TRIALS IN ONCOLOGIC EMERGENCIES

Clinical description	Comparison	Results	Significance	Reference
Spinal cord compression	Radiation +/– high dose dexamethasone	High-dose dexamethasone improved functional outcome initially and at 6 months.	Little morbidity was associated with dexamethasone with major benefit when used with radiation.	[46]
Spinal cord compression	Operable candidates: decompressive surgery followed by radiation versus radiation alone	Surgery followed by radiation therapy gave a superior functional outcome compared to radiation therapy alone.	For operable candidates whose life expectancy is more than weeks or a few months, surgery followed by radiation should be an initial consideration.	[49]
Spinal cord compression	Age stratification: decompressive surgery followed by radiation versus radiation alone	Secondary data analysis demonstrates a strong relationship between age and treatment benefit.	Age is an important variable in predicting which patients will benefit from surgical decompression in patients with epidural cord compression; no surgery benefit is seen in individuals >age 65.	[50]
Hypercalcemia	Zoledronic acid (4 vs. 8 mg) versus pamidronate (three-arm randomized study)	Zoledronic acid at 4 mg produced more rapid and sustained response compared to pamidronate with excellent side effect profile compared to pamidronate; 8 mg did not add to response effect.	Major PP, Coleman RE: Zoledronic acid in the treatment of hypercalcemia of malignancy: results of the international clinical development program. *Semin Oncol* 28[2, Suppl 6]: 17–24, 2001.	[95]
Tumor lysis syndrome	Rasburicase versus allopurinol for prophylaxis of tumor lysis in lymphoma patients (children)	Four hours after the first dose, patients randomized to rasburicase compared to allopurinol achieved an 86% versus 12% reduction ($p < 0.0001$) of initial plasma uric acid levels; sample size was small; adult trial results not available.	In patients who have evidence of pretreatment tumor lysis syndrome or patients who are allergic to allopurinol, rasburicase may be a suitable alternative to allopurinol.	[89]
Tumor lysis syndrome	Rasburicase versus rasburicase + allopurinol versus allopurinol monotherapy	Trial demonstrated a significant improvement in uric acid response rates (the proportion of patients with plasma uric acid levels less than 7.5 mg/dL from day three through day seven following initiation of antihyperuricemic treatment) among rasburicase-treated patients compared to allopurinol-treated patients.	Rasburicase was approved by the FDA for the initial management of patients with malignancy at high risk for developing tumor lysis syndrome.	[92]
Tumor lysis syndrome	Rasburicase (0.15 mg/kg) dosed daily for 5 consecutive days versus rasburicase as a single dose (0.15 mg/kg) followed by "as needed" doses (to a maximum of 5 doses)	A single dose of rasburicase resulted in a sustained response in 87% of treated adult patients.	Administration of a single dose of rasburicase can be effective in the prevention of TLS in most patients (uric acid levels can be followed thereafter for subsequent dose administration).	[93]

for early use of hemodialysis, are highly recommended. Some institutions initiate induction therapy with vincristine, oral cyclophosphamide, and corticosteroids for patients with high-grade lymphoma in an attempt to decrease tumor burden more slowly and avoid the metabolic effect of sudden lysis [94]. No reports to date quantify the effect of this intervention on the incidence of TLS.

Advances in oncologic emergencies, based on randomized, controlled trials or meta-analyses of such trials, are summarized in Table 116.6.

References

1. Yellin A, Rosen A, Reichert N, et al: Superior vena cava syndrome. The myth—the facts. *Am Rev Respir Dis* 141:1114–1118, 1990.
2. Parish JM, Marschke RF Jr, Dines DE, et al: Etiologic considerations in superior vena cava syndrome. *Mayo Clin Proc* 56:407–413, 1981.
3. Baba Y, Ohkubo K, Nakai H, et al: Focal enhanced areas of the liver on computed tomography in a patient with superior vena cava obstruction. *Cardiovasc Intervent Radiol* 22:69–70, 1999.
4. Ahmann FR. A reassessment of the clinical implications of the superior vena caval syndrome. *J Clin Oncol* 2:961–969, 1984.
5. Urban T, Lebeau B, Chastang C, et al: Superior vena cava syndrome in small-cell lung cancer. *Arch Intern Med* 153:384–387, 1993.
6. Loeffler JS, Leopold KA, Recht A, et al: Emergency prebiopsy radiation for mediastinal masses: impact on subsequent pathologic diagnosis and outcome. *J Clin Oncol* 4:716–721, 1986.
7. Armstrong BA, Perez CA, Simpson JR, et al: Role of irradiation in the management of superior vena cava syndrome. *Int J Radiat Oncol Biol Phys* 13:531–539, 1987.
8. Nicholson AA, Ettles DF, Arnold A, et al: Treatment of malignant superior vena cava obstruction: metal stents or radiation therapy. *J Vasc Interv Radiol* 8:781–788, 1997.
9. Stock KW, Jacob AL, Proske M, et al: Treatment of malignant obstruction of the superior vena cava with the self-expanding Wallstent. *Thorax* 50:1151–1156, 1995.
10. Irving JD, Dondelinger RF, Reidy JF, et al: Gianturco self-expanding stents: clinical experience in the vena cava and large veins. *Cardiovasc Intervent Radiol* 15:328–333, 1992.
11. Chan RH, Dar AR, Yu E, et al: Superior vena cava obstruction in small-cell lung cancer. *Int J Radiat Oncol Biol Phys* 38:513–520, 1997.
12. Gray BH, Olin JW, Graor RA, et al: Safety and efficacy of thrombolytic therapy for superior vena cava syndrome. *Chest* 99:54–59, 1991.
13. Wurschmidt F, Bunemann H, Heilmann HP: Small cell lung cancer with and without superior vena cava syndrome: a multivariate analysis of prognostic factors in 408 cases. *Int J Radiat Oncol Biol Phys* 33:77–82, 1995.
14. Theologides A: Neoplastic cardiac tamponade. *Semin Oncol* 5:181–192, 1978.
15. Lam KY, Dickens P, Chan AC: Tumors of the heart. A 20-year experience with a review of 12,485 consecutive autopsies. *Arch Pathol Lab Med* 117:1027–1031, 1993.
16. Markiewicz W, Borovik R, Ecker S: Cardiac tamponade in medical patients: treatment and prognosis in the echocardiographic era. *Am Heart J* 111:1138–1142, 1986.
17. Posner MR, Cohen GI, Skarin AT: Pericardial disease in patients with cancer. The differentiation of malignant from idiopathic and radiation-induced pericarditis. *Am J Med* 71:407–413, 1981.
18. Krikorian JG, Hancock EW: Pericardiocentesis. *Am J Med* 65:808–814, 1978.
19. Zipf RE Jr, Johnston WW: The role of cytology in the evaluation of pericardial effusions. *Chest* 62:593–596, 1972.
20. Gornik HL, Gerhard-Herman M, Beckman JA: Abnormal cytology predicts poor prognosis in cancer patients with pericardial effusion. *J Clin Oncol* 23:5211–5216, 2005.
21. Little WC, Freeman GL: Pericardial Disease 10.1161/CIRCULATIONAHA.105.561514. *Circulation* 113:1622–1632, 2006.
22. Spodick DH: Acute cardiac tamponade. Pathologic physiology, diagnosis and management. *Prog Cardiovasc Dis* 10:64–96, 1967.
23. Laham RJ, Cohen DJ, Kuntz RE, et al: Pericardial effusion in patients with cancer: outcome with contemporary management strategies. *Heart* 75:67–71, 1996.
24. Vaitkus PT, Herrmann HC, LeWinter MM: Treatment of malignant pericardial effusion. *JAMA* 272:59–64, 1994.
25. Moriya T, Takiguchi Y, Tabeta H, et al: Controlling malignant pericardial effusion by intrapericardial carboplatin administration in patients with primary non-small-cell lung cancer. *Br J Cancer* 83:858–862, 2000.
26. Norum J, Lunde P, Aasebo U, et al: Mitoxantrone in malignant pericardial effusion. *J Chemother* 10:399–404, 1998.
27. Colleoni M, Martinelli G, Beretta F, et al: Intracavitary chemotherapy with thiotepa in malignant pericardial effusions: an active and well-tolerated regimen. *J Clin Oncol* 16:2371–2376, 1998.
28. Liu G, Crump M, Goss PE, et al: Prospective comparison of the sclerosing agents doxycycline and bleomycin for the primary management of malignant pericardial effusion and cardiac tamponade. *J Clin Oncol* 14:3141–3147, 1996.
29. Cormican MC, Nyman CR: Intrapericardial bleomycin for the management of cardiac tamponade secondary to malignant pericardial effusion. *Br Heart J* 63:61–62, 1990.
30. Kunitoh H, Tamura T, Shibata T, et al: A randomised trial of intrapericardial bleomycin for malignant pericardial effusion with lung cancer (JCOG9811). *Br J Cancer* 100:464–469, 2009.
31. Lestuzzi C, Lafaras C, Bearz A, et al: Malignant pericardial effusion: sclerotherapy or local chemotherapy [quest]. *Br J Cancer* 101:734–735, 2009.
32. Galli M, Politi A, Pedretti F, et al: Percutaneous balloon pericardiotomy for malignant pericardial tamponade. *Chest* 108:1499–1501, 1995.
33. Ziskind AA, Pearce AC, Lemmon CC, et al: Percutaneous balloon pericardiotomy for the treatment of cardiac tamponade and large pericardial effusions: description of technique and report of the first 50 cases. *J Am Coll Cardiol* 21:1–5, 1993.
34. DeCamp MM Jr, Mentzer SJ, Swanson SJ, et al: Malignant effusive disease of the pleura and pericardium. *Chest* 112:291S–295S, 1997.
35. Swanepoel E, Apffelstaedt JP: Malignant pericardial effusion in breast cancer: terminal event or treatable complication? *J Surg Oncol* 64:308–311, 1997.
36. Wang PC, Yang KY, Chao JY, et al: Prognostic role of pericardial fluid cytology in cardiac tamponade associated with non-small cell lung cancer. *Chest* 118:744–749, 2000.
37. Loblaw DA, Laperriere NJ: Emergency treatment of malignant extradural spinal cord compression: an evidence-based guideline. *J Clin Oncol* 16:1613–1624, 1998.
38. Stark RJ, Henson RA, Evans SJ: Spinal metastases. A retrospective survey from a general hospital. *Brain* 105:189–213, 1982.
39. Weissman DE, Gilbert M, Wang H, et al: The use of computed tomography of the spine to identify patients at high risk for epidural metastases. *J Clin Oncol* 3:1541–1544, 1985.
40. Ruff RL, Lanska DJ: Epidural metastases in prospectively evaluated veterans with cancer and back pain. *Cancer* 63:2234–2241, 1989.
41. Rodichok LD, Harper GR, Ruckdeschel JC, et al: Early diagnosis of spinal epidural metastases. *Am J Med* 70:1181–1188, 1981.
42. Bruckman JE, Bloomer WD: Management of spinal cord compression. *Semin Oncol* 5:135–140, 1978.
43. Gilbert RW, Kim JH, Posner JB: Epidural spinal cord compression from metastatic tumor: diagnosis and treatment. *Ann Neurol* 3:40–51, 1978.
44. Byrne TN: Spinal cord compression from epidural metastases. *N Engl J Med* 327:614–619, 1992.
45. Husband DJ, Grant KA, Romaniuk CS: MRI in the diagnosis and treatment of suspected malignant spinal cord compression. *Br J Radiol* 74:15–23, 2001.
46. Sorensen S, Helweg-Larsen S, Mouridsen H, et al: Effect of high-dose dexamethasone in carcinomatous metastatic spinal cord compression treated with radiotherapy: a randomised trial. *Eur J Cancer* 30A:22–27, 1994.
47. Heimdal K, Hirschberg H, Slettebo H, et al: High incidence of serious side effects of high-dose dexamethasone treatment in patients with epidural spinal cord compression. *J Neurooncol* 12:141–144, 1992.
48. Maranzano E, Latini P, Beneventi S, et al: Radiotherapy without steroids in selected metastatic spinal cord compression patients. A phase II trial. *Am J Clin Oncol* 19:179–183, 1996.
49. Patchell RA, Tibbs PA, Regine WF, et al: Direct decompressive surgical resection in the treatment of spinal cord compression caused by metastatic cancer: a randomised trial. *Lancet* 366:643–648, 2005.
50. Chi JH, Gokaslan Z, McCormick P, et al: Selecting treatment for patients with malignant epidural spinal cord compression-does age matter?: results from a randomized clinical trial. *Spine (Philadelphia)*. 34:431–435, 2009.
51. Holman PJ, Suki D, McCutcheon I, et al: Surgical management of metastatic disease of the lumbar spine: experience with 139 patients. *J Neurosurg Spine* 2:550–563, 2005.
52. Landmann C, Hunig R, Gratzl O: The role of laminectomy in the combined treatment of metastatic spinal cord compression. *Int J Radiat Oncol Biol Phys* 24:627–631, 1992.
53. Maranzano E, Latini P, Checcaglini F, et al: Radiation therapy in metastatic spinal cord compression. A prospective analysis of 105 consecutive patients. *Cancer* 67:1311–1317, 1991.
54. Sundaresan N, Galicich JH, Lane JM, et al: Treatment of neoplastic epidural cord compression by vertebral body resection and stabilization. *J Neurosurg* 63:676–684, 1985.
55. Zelefsky MJ, Scher HI, Krol G, et al: Spinal epidural tumor in patients with prostate cancer. Clinical and radiographic predictors of response to radiation therapy. *Cancer* 70:2319–2325, 1992.
56. Burtis WJ, Brady TG, Orloff JJ, et al: Immunochemical characterization of circulating parathyroid hormone-related protein in patients with humoral hypercalcemia of cancer. *N Engl J Med* 322:1106–1112, 1990.
57. Broadus AE, Mangin M, Ikeda K, et al: Humoral hypercalcemia of cancer. Identification of a novel parathyroid hormone-like peptide. *N Engl J Med* 319:556–563, 1988.

58. Strewler GJ: The physiology of parathyroid hormone-related protein. *N Engl J Med* 342:177–185, 2000.
59. Lumachi F, Brunello A, Roma A, et al: Cancer-induced hypercalcemia. *Anticancer Res* 29:1551–1555, 2009.
60. Breslau NA, McGuire JL, Zerwekh JE, et al: Hypercalcemia associated with increased serum calcitriol levels in three patients with lymphoma. *Ann Intern Med* 100:1–6, 1984.
61. Scheid V, Buzdar AU, Smith TL, et al: Clinical course of breast cancer patients with osseous metastasis treated with combination chemotherapy. *Cancer* 58:2589–2593, 1986.
62. Muggia FM: Overview of cancer-related hypercalcemia: epidemiology and etiology. *Semin Oncol* 17:3–9, 1990.
63. Mortimer JE, Dehdashti F, Siegel BA, et al: Metabolic flare: indicator of hormone responsiveness in advanced breast cancer. *J Clin Oncol* 19:2797–2803, 2001.
64. Bender RA, Hansen H: Hypercalcemia in bronchogenic carcinoma. A prospective study of 200 patients. *Ann Intern Med* 80:205–208, 1974.
65. Takai E, Yano T, Iguchi H, et al: Tumor-induced hypercalcemia and parathyroid hormone-related protein in lung carcinoma. *Cancer* 78:1384–1387, 1996.
66. Coggeshall J, Merrill W, Hande K, et al: Implications of hypercalcemia with respect to diagnosis and treatment of lung cancer. *Am J Med* 80:325–328, 1986.
67. Cherng NC, Asal NR, Kuebler JP, et al: Prognostic factors in multiple myeloma. *Cancer* 67:3150–3156, 1991.
68. Rogers MJ, Gordon S, Benford HL, et al: Cellular and molecular mechanisms of action of bisphosphonates. *Cancer* 88:2961–2978, 2000.
69. Major P, Lortholary A, Hon J, et al: Zoledronic acid is superior to pamidronate in the treatment of hypercalcemia of malignancy: a pooled analysis of two randomized, controlled clinical trials. *J Clin Oncol* 19:558–567, 2001.
70. Hillner BE, Ingle JN, Chlebowski RT, et al: American Society of Clinical Oncology 2003 Update on the Role of Bisphosphonates and Bone Health Issues in Women With Breast Cancer. *J Clin Oncol* 21:4042–4057, 2003. doi: 10.1200/JCO.2003.08.017.
71. Prommer EE: Established and potential therapeutic applications of octreotide in palliative care. *Support Care Cancer* 16:1117–1123, 2008.
72. Durie BG, Harousseau JL, Miguel JS, et al: International uniform response criteria for multiple myeloma. *Leukemia* 20:1467–1473, 2006.
73. Capparelli C, Kostenuik PJ, Morony S, et al: Osteoprotegerin prevents and reverses hypercalcemia in a murine model of humoral hypercalcemia of malignancy. *Cancer Res* 60:783–787, 2000.
74. Fizazi K, Bosserman L, Gao G, et al: Denosumab treatment of prostate cancer with bone metastases and increased urine N-telopeptide levels after therapy with intravenous bisphosphonates: results of a randomized phase II trial [discussion 515–506]. *J Urol* 182:509–515, 2009.
75. Oyajobi BO, Anderson DM, Traianedes K, et al: Therapeutic efficacy of a soluble receptor activator of nuclear factor κB-IgG Fc fusion protein in suppressing bone resorption and hypercalcemia in a model of humoral hypercalcemia of malignancy. *Cancer Res* 61:2572–2578, 2001.
76. Ralston SH, Gallacher SJ, Patel U, et al: Cancer-associated hypercalcemia: morbidity and mortality. Clinical experience in 126 treated patients. *Ann Intern Med* 112:499–504, 1990.
77. Lichtman MA, Rowe JM: Hyperleukocytic leukemias: rheological, clinical, and therapeutic considerations. *Blood* 60:279–283, 1982.
78. van Buchem MA, Hogendoorn PC, Bruijn JA, et al: Endothelial activation antigens in pulmonary leukostasis in leukemia. *Acta Haematol* 90:29–33, 1993.
79. Stucki A, Rivier AS, Gikic M, et al: Endothelial cell activation by myeloblasts: molecular mechanisms of leukostasis and leukemic cell dissemination. *Blood* 97:2121–2129, 2001.
80. Gross P, Reimann D, Neidel J, et al: The treatment of severe hyponatremia. *Kidney Int Suppl* 64:S6–S11, 1998.
81. Hantman D, Rossier B, Zohlman R, et al: Rapid correction of hyponatremia in the syndrome of inappropriate secretion of antidiuretic hormone. An alternative treatment to hypertonic saline. *Ann Intern Med* 78:870–875, 1973.
82. Mulloy AL, Caruana RJ: Hyponatremic emergencies. *Med Clin North Am* 79:155–168, 1995.
83. Thiebaut A, Thomas X, Belhabri A, et al: Impact of pre-induction therapy leukapheresis on treatment outcome in adult acute myelogenous leukemia presenting with hyperleukocytosis. *Ann Hematol* 79:501–506, 2000.
84. Kemeny MM, Magrath IT, Brennan MF: The role of surgery in the management of American Burkitt's lymphoma and its treatment. *Ann Surg* 196:82–86, 1982.
85. Kalemkerian GP, Darwish B, Varterasian ML: Tumor lysis syndrome in small cell carcinoma and other solid tumors. *Am J Med* 103:363–367, 1997.
86. Lorigan PC, Woodings PL, Morgenstern GR, et al: Tumour lysis syndrome, case report and review of the literature. *Ann Oncol* 7:631–636, 1996.
87. DeConti RC, Calabresi P: Use of allopurinol for prevention and control of hyperuricemia in patients with neoplastic disease. *N Engl J Med* 274:481–486, 1966.
88. Smalley RV, Guaspari A, Haase-Statz S, et al: Allopurinol: intravenous use for prevention and treatment of hyperuricemia. *J Clin Oncol* 18:1758–1763, 2000.
89. Goldman SC, Holcenberg JS, Finklestein JZ, et al: A randomized comparison between rasburicase and allopurinol in children with lymphoma or leukemia at high risk for tumor lysis. *Blood* 97:2998–3003, 2001.
90. Bosly A, Sonet A, Pinkerton CR, et al: Rasburicase (recombinant urate oxidase) for the management of hyperuricemia in patients with cancer: report of an international compassionate use study. *Cancer* 98:1048–1054, 2003.
91. Pui CH, Jeha S, Irwin D, et al: Recombinant urate oxidase (rasburicase) in the prevention and treatment of malignancy-associated hyperuricemia in pediatric and adult patients: results of a compassionate-use trial. *Leukemia* 15:1505–1509, 2001.
92. Padzur R. Available at: http://www.cancer.gov/cancertopics/druginfo/fda-rasburicase.
93. Vadhan-Raj S, Fayad LE, Fanale M, et al: Randomized Clinical Trial of Rasburicase Administered as a Standard Fixed Five Days Dosing Vs a Single Dose Followed by as Needed Dosing in Adult Patients with Hematologic Malignancies at Risk for Developing Tumor Lysis Syndrome. In: American Society of Hematology Annual Meeting; 2009; New Orleans, LA.
94. Soussain C, Patte C, Ostronoff M, et al: Small noncleaved cell lymphoma and leukemia in adults. A retrospective study of 65 adults treated with the LMB pediatric protocols. *Blood* 85:664–674, 1995.
95. Major PP, Coleman RE: Zoledronic acid in the treatment of hypercalcemia of malignancy: results of the international clinical development program. *Semin Oncol* 28[2, Suppl 6]: 17–24, 2001.

SECTION X ■ PHARMACOLOGY, OVERDOSES, AND POISONINGS

LUKE YIP • KENNON HEARD • STEVEN B. BIRD

CHAPTER 117 ■ GENERAL CONSIDERATIONS IN THE EVALUATION AND TREATMENT OF POISONING

IAN M. BALL AND CHRISTOPHER H. LINDEN

The objective of this chapter is to provide the general intensivist with both an overview and an approach to the management of the critically ill poisoned patient. General concepts germane to the intensive care unit (ICU) will be introduced and explored. Every attempt has been made to be as evidence based as possible, within the intrinsic limitations of the medical toxicology literature.

Because overdose studies cannot ethically be performed in humans and animal data may not be available or applicable to humans, predicting the severity of poisoning must be based on toxicodynamic data from previously published reports of human poisonings. However, such data are often incomplete or altogether unavailable and are always limited by the accuracy of the overdose history.

Poisoning or *intoxication* is defined as the occurrence of harmful effects resulting from exposure to a foreign chemical or xenobiotic. Such effects may be local (i.e., limited to exposed body surfaces), subjective (i.e., symptoms only) or systemic and objective (e.g., behavioral, biochemical, cognitive, or physiologic). In the absence of signs or symptoms, external or internal body contact with a potentially harmful amount of a chemical is merely an exposure. An *overdose* is an excessive exposure to a chemical that in specified (e.g., therapeutic) amounts is normally intended for human use. Whether an exposure or overdose results in poisoning depends more on the conditions of exposure (primarily the dose) than the identity of the agent involved. Ordinarily safe chemicals, even those essential for life such as oxygen and water, in excessive amounts or by an inappropriate route can result in harmful effects. Conversely, by limiting the dose, chemicals usually thought of as poisons can be rendered harmless. Poisoning is distinguished from adverse allergic, intolerance, and idiosyncratic pharmacogenetic reactions in that effects are concentration or dose related and, hence, predictable. As such, it includes adverse drug reactions due to unwanted secondary effects and pharmacokinetic and pharmacodynamic interactions.

Poisonings, exposures, and overdoses may be characterized by the route, duration, and intent of exposure. Ingestion, dermal or ophthalmic contact, inhalation, and parenteral injection (including bites and stings) are the most common routes, but rectal, urethral, vaginal, bladder, peritoneal, intraocular, and intrathecal exposures can also occur. Events that occur once or during a short period of time are considered acute, whereas those that occur repeatedly or over a prolonged time interval are said to be chronic

EPIDEMIOLOGY

Although comprehensive data regarding the true incidence of poisoning are not available [1], it is clearly a significant medical problem. Just under two and a half million human exposures were reported to the National Poison Data System in 2007 [2]. Of these, 20% to 25% are treated at a health care facility, and approximately 6% are admitted to a hospital. Half of those admitted are treated in an ICU. In other countries, the ICU admission rate for those evaluated at a health care facility varies from 5% to 22% [3–5].

Exposures and poisonings are responsible for 1% to 5% of emergency department visits, 5% to 10% of all ambulance transports, 5% to 14% of adult ICU admissions, and 2% to 5% of pediatric hospital admissions [3–9]. In addition, 25% of routine medical admissions involve some form of drug-related adverse patient event (an adverse drug reaction or noncompliance), and up to 30% of acute psychiatric admissions are prompted by attempted self-harm via chemical exposure. Although the incidence of poisoning in children has decreased since the introduction of the Poison Prevention Packaging Act in 1970 [10], the overall incidence of poisoning is increasing, particularly that due to suicide attempts in teens, middle-aged adults, and the elderly. The volume of calls handled by United States Poison Centers increased by 7.6% in 2007 [2]. Poisoning is second only to firearms as the leading cause of suicide [5]. Poisoning is the second leading cause of injury death [2]. The yearly medical cost for the treatment of poisoning in the United States is estimated to be $26 billion [11]. Poisoning accounts for 6% of the economic costs of all injuries in the United States [11].

Most exposures reported to US poison centers are acute (90.9%), unintentional (83.2%), occur at home (92.9%), cause minor or no harmful effects (95%), result from ingestion (78.4%), and involve children 6 years of age or younger (51.2%) [2].

Poisoning accounts for 2% to 14% of all ICU admissions, with an average length of stay of about 3 days [3,5,7–9]. The mortality rate for such patients varies from 0.6% to 6.1% [3,4,6–9]. Although only 1,239 poisoning fatalities were reported by US poison centers in 2007 [2], death certificate data indicate that the true number of poisoning deaths is 20 to 50 times higher [12]. Poison center statistics vastly underestimate mortality from poisoning because they rarely capture cases in which the victim is found dead and goes directly to the medical examiner.

PHARMACOLOGIC CONCEPTS

Toxic exposures all undergo the same pharmacologic steps, as outlined in Table 117.1. Clinician familiarity with toxicokinetics is essential for predicting the effect of a particular exposure and guiding appropriate treatment and disposition. Only a

TABLE 117.1

TOXICOKINETIC STAGES

1. Absorption
2. Distribution
3. Metabolism
4. Excretion

brief overview of these concepts is presented here. The reader is referred to other sources for additional information [13–17]. Details regarding the disposition and toxic effects of specific agents can be found in subsequent chapters and other references [14–27].

Mechanism of Action

Most chemicals are absorbed and cause systemic poisoning by selectively binding to and disrupting the function of specific targets (e.g., enzymes, proteins, membrane lipids, or neurohumoral receptors). Effects may be systemic or limited to a specific organ or tissue, depending on the distribution and location of target site.

Poisoning is usually functional and reversible. Hence, if end organ function can be supported, complete patient recovery is possible upon toxin elimination. However, if normal activity of the target site is essential for cell viability, a toxic exposure may result in necrosis. Agents that can cause fatal cellular damage include acetaminophen, carbon monoxide, corrosives, toxic alcohols, heavy metals, and neurotoxic hydrocarbons.

Absorption

Absorption involves the translocation of chemicals across the membranes of cells that make up mucosal surfaces, pulmonary epithelium, and skin, all of which function as biologic barriers. Translocation occurs by filtration or passive diffusion through gaps or membrane pores by dissolving in and diffusing through the membrane itself (e.g., lipid-soluble chemicals), or by attaching to carrier molecules in the membrane, which actively or passively facilitate diffusion (e.g., water-soluble chemicals). The rate and extent of absorption depend on physical properties of the chemical and the route of exposure. In general, only chemicals that are small (i.e., <4 nm in diameter), have low molecular weight (i.e., <50 Da), and are soluble in both water and lipids at the pH of body fluids can readily cross membranes.

Absorption after intravenous injection is complete and almost instantaneous. Peak arterial and venous blood concentrations occur within 30 to 90 seconds. Most toxins cross biologic membranes by simple passive diffusion. The rate at which this occurs is governed by Fick's law of diffusion.

$$\text{Rate of Diffusion} = dQ/dt = [DAK(C1 - C2)]/d$$

where D is the diffusion constant (constant for each toxin), A is the membrane surface area, K is the partition coefficient (represents the lipid: water partitioning of the toxin), d is the membrane thickness, and C is the toxin concentration.

Pulmonary absorption is rapid but incomplete. Blood concentrations peak within seconds to minutes. The absorption of chemicals after intramuscular or subcutaneous injection is slower but relatively complete. Peak blood levels generally occur within an hour of administration. Poor water solubility (low K) is responsible for the slow absorption and long duration of action of intramuscular depot formulations (e.g., neuroleptics).

The rate and extent of absorption after ingestion are variable. Peak blood levels are typically noted within 0.5 to 2.0 hours of a therapeutic dose. The absorbed dose is proportional to, but not necessarily equal to, the administered dose. The rate and extent of absorption after contact with other mucosal surfaces (e.g., oral, nasal, ophthalmic, rectal) is similar to ingestion. Skin absorption, if it occurs at all, is usually considerably slower. Regardless of route, absorption tends to follow first-order kinetics (i.e., the amount of chemical absorbed per unit of time is directly proportional to its concentration). *Hence, threshold tissue concentrations are usually reached more quickly and effects begin sooner after an overdose than after a therapeutic dose.*

Zero-Order Kinetics: rate of reaction is not proportional to toxin concentration

First-Order Kinetics: rate of reaction is proportional to toxin concentration

The dissolution and solvation of particulate material is often a rate-limiting step in gastrointestinal (GI) drug absorption. Hence, pill, solid, and suppository formulations tend to be absorbed more slowly than liquids, powders, or suspensions. Slow dissolution and solvation also account for the delayed and prolonged absorption of enteric-coated tablets (e.g., aspirin, potassium), sustained-release preparations (e.g., cardiovascular drugs, lithium, phenytoin, theophylline), drugs that tend to form concretions (e.g., ethchlorvynol, glutethimide, heavy metals, iron, lithium, and meprobamate), and those with poor water solubility (e.g., carbamazepine and digoxin). The rate of dissolution is also inversely related to the tablet concentration. *Hence, absorption generally takes longer and peak effects occur later after an overdose than after a therapeutic one.*

Ingested chemicals are predominantly absorbed from the small intestine rather than the stomach because the small intestine has a larger surface area. Hence, decreased gastric emptying or bowel activity caused by the presence of food, disease, or the effects of ingested agents (e.g., anticholinergics, opioids, sedative–hypnotics, salicylates) can also delay or prolong absorption. Food and coingestants may decrease absorption by binding to the chemical within the gut lumen or by competitively inhibiting its dissolution and translocation. Absorption may also be decreased if intestinal motility is excessive.

Distribution

During distribution, chemicals may become bound to and inactivated by endogenous nontarget molecules such as serum proteins. The final distribution of chemical is uneven and reflects its affinity for active and inactive binding sites and the locations of such sites. It is also influenced by biologic variables such as age, sex, weight, and disease states as they relate to body composition (e.g., water, fat, muscle content) and serum protein concentrations. The extent of distribution of a chemical is reflected by its apparent volume of distribution, measured in liters per kilogram of body weight, and calculated most simply by dividing the amount of chemical in the body (i.e., the absorbed or bioavailable dose) by its plasma concentration.

$$\text{Volume of Distribution} = \text{Bioavailable Dose}/\text{Plasma Concentration}$$

Because distribution is also a translocation process, it is influenced by the same chemical characteristics as absorption and follows first-order kinetics. Distribution generally occurs much faster than absorption, as evidenced by the occurrence of peak effects within minutes of an IV drug injection. Slow distribution is partly responsible for the delayed onset of action of some agents (e.g., digitalis, heavy metals, lithium, and salicylates).

Tissue Concentration

The severity of poisoning reflects the concentration of a chemical at its site(s) of action and is proportional to the dose. Because the blood concentration of a chemical is also proportional to the dose, blood levels are sometimes used as a surrogate to assess the severity of poisoning. However, blood and target site concentrations are not always in steady-state equilibrium. When distribution occurs more slowly than absorption (e.g., after IV administration, inhalational exposure, and the ingestion of agents with inherently slow distribution), blood levels may be higher than those in tissue. Conversely, when redistribution of a chemical from tissue to blood occurs more slowly than elimination (e.g., after extracorporeal removal), blood levels may be lower than those in tissue. In both instances, blood levels do not accurately reflect those in tissue and do not correlate with the severity of poisoning.

Age, genetic influences, tolerance, underlying disease, and the presence or absence of other chemicals may have synergistic or antagonistic effects and may also influence the response to a given level of toxin exposure. The effect of metabolites must also be considered. Many chemicals have metabolites that remain pharmacologically active. Some (e.g., acetaminophen, toxic alcohols, chlorinated hydrocarbons, meperidine, paraquat, and certain organophosphate insecticides) undergo metabolic activation, resulting in the production of compounds that are more toxic than the parent one.

Metabolism/Elimination

Elimination of chemicals from the body (detoxification) is accomplished by urinary, pulmonary, GI, and glandular (e.g., bile, milk, tears, saliva, sweat) excretion or metabolic inactivation. Hepatic metabolism and renal excretion are the major routes of elimination for most agents. Pulmonary excretion also plays a major role in the elimination of gases and volatile chemicals. Elimination generally follows first-order kinetics. For some toxins, hepatic metabolism has a finite capacity (i.e., becomes "saturated") and proceeds at a constant rate (zero-order kinetics). When the primary route of elimination is a zero-order metabolism, a small increase in dose can result in a large increase in blood and tissue concentrations and potential poisoning. Chemicals exhibiting such metabolism include alcohols, phenytoin, salicylate, and theophylline.

Renal excretion is accomplished by translocation processes (e.g., glomerular filtration, tubular secretion, and reabsorption) and is therefore influenced by the same factors as absorption and distribution. Any condition that impairs hepatic or renal blood flow or function can decrease toxin elimination. Metabolic enzymes are also subject to genetic influences and to induction or inhibition resulting from past or current chemical exposures. Regardless of the kinetics and route of elimination, the time required for elimination increases as the tissue concentration of chemical increases. *Hence, the duration of the effect tends to be longer after an overdose than after a therapeutic dose.*

CLINICAL CONSIDERATIONS

The principal objectives in the diagnosis and evaluation of the poisoning are recognition of an exposure or poisoning, identification of the offending agent(s), prediction of potential toxicity, and assessment of the severity of clinical effects. Treatment objectives include resuscitation, prevention of further absorption, enhancement of elimination, and the administration of antidotal therapy (Table 117.2).

TABLE 117.2

TREATMENT OBJECTIVES—GENERAL PRINCIPLES

1. Resuscitation
2. Prevention of further exposure
3. Enhanced elimination
4. Novel/antidotal therapy

Early accurate diagnosis is a prerequisite for optimal management.

The priority of assessment and treatment objectives depends on the phase of poisoning [28]. During the preclinical phase (i.e., the time between exposure and the onset of clinical or laboratory evidence of toxicity), management priorities include chemical identification, prediction of toxicity, and prevention of absorption (i.e., decontamination). The sooner decontamination is accomplished, the greater its efficacy. Hence, the physical examination and gathering of ancillary data should initially be brief. Assessment should focus on the exposure history, whether or not poisoning is likely to ensue, and whether or not decontamination is indicated.

During the toxic phase (i.e., the time between the onset of toxicity and its peak), assessment of the severity of poisoning, resuscitation, prevention of further absorption, enhancement of elimination, and antidotal therapy are the primary objectives. If the patient is critically ill, the history, physical examination, and diagnostic testing must be conducted concurrently with resuscitation.

During the resolution phase (i.e., the time between peak toxicity and full recovery), continued supportive care, enhancement of elimination, antidotal therapy, and reassessment of severity (i.e., evaluation of the response to treatment) are the most important management considerations. Measures to prevent subsequent reexposure should also be initiated before discharge.

Recognition of Poisoning

Although poisoning can cause a wide variety of nonspecific signs and symptoms, the diagnosis can usually be established by the history, physical examination, routine and toxicologic laboratory evaluation, and the clinical course. Ideally, criteria similar to Koch's postulates for infectious disease should be met: A chemical is identified in or on the body in an amount known to cause the observed signs and symptoms within the reported time frame. In reality, the diagnosis is often made on the basis of a history of exposure, a clinical course consistent with poisoning, and exclusion of other etiologies.

Making the diagnosis is easy when an accurate history of exposure is available. However, patients may be unaware of an exposure, unwilling to admit to one, or unable to give a history at all. Patients may give a history that is vague, confusing, or intentionally disguised.

Circumstances that should arouse suspicion of occult poisoning include sudden or unexplained illness in a previously healthy individual; similar unexplained symptoms in a group of individuals; a psychiatric history, alcoholism, or drug abuse; a recent change in health, economic status, or social relationships; and the onset of illness shortly after ingesting food, drink, or medication. Poisoning should always be considered in patients with metabolic abnormalities (especially acid–base disturbances), gastroenteritis, or changes in behavior or mental status of unclear etiology. Leakage of illicit drug packets that have been ingested or concealed in body cavities should be suspected in patients with altered mental status or unusual behavior who have just arrived from abroad (especially Asia and South America) or who have recently been arrested or incarcerated for criminal activity [29,30]. Drug intoxication is a risk factor for trauma and suicide and should also be considered in all injured patients [31].

To avoid missing the diagnosis of poisoning, the physician must specifically inquire about toxin exposure. In suspicious cases, the physician should assume the role of detective to elicit historical support for the diagnosis [32]. Paramedics, police, and family, friends, employer, pharmacist, or personal physician can be questioned regarding the circumstances and events surrounding the illness, particularly the availability of chemicals and the likelihood of exposure. The patient's clothes and place of discovery should be searched for a suicide note, xenobiotics, and open or empty medication containers. Third parties should be instructed to search the house for such evidence and to bring it in for inspection.

In the absence of a history of exposure, the characteristic clinical course of poisoning may also suggest the diagnosis. Signs and symptoms of poisoning typically develop within minutes to an hour of an acute exposure, progress to a maximum within several hours, and gradually resolve over a period of hours to a few days. In such situations, toxicology screening (see later) may allow for a positive diagnosis if signs and symptoms are consistent with the known toxicity of the toxin(s) detected and other etiologies have been excluded.

Identification of the Offending Agent

History

The etiology of poisoning may or may not be disclosed by the patient history. Even when a history is available, its accuracy and reliability must be assessed. The identity of the toxin involved is incorrectly reported by up to 50% of patients with intentional ingestions [33]. The amount reportedly taken is also unreliable. Hence, in such patients, the history should be approached with caution. Layperson misidentification of acetaminophen as aspirin and vice versa is also relatively common. To avoid missing the correct diagnosis, the presence or absence of both drugs should be confirmed by laboratory analysis when an overdose of any kind is suspected.

Pill, Product, Plant, and Animal Identification

Drugs in pill form can often be identified by the imprint code, the alphabetical and numeric markings on tablets and capsules. A listing of imprint codes with the corresponding trade name and ingredient(s) can be found in the Identidex portion of *Poisindex* [27], which is available at virtually all poison centers in the United States. It also provides the identities of street drugs based on their slang names. Prescription drugs may be identified by contacting the dispensing pharmacy. Drug samples can sometimes be identified by direct chemical analysis (Toxicology Screening section). Police and government toxicology laboratories may be of assistance when illicit drug use is involved.

By US law [34], the ingredients of potentially hazardous commercial products used in and around the home must be stated on their label. This information, however, is not necessarily present or accurate, and labels may be missing or unreadable. In such cases, the ingredients may be identified by consulting *Poisindex* [27] or a regional poison center. Alternatively, the manufacturer or distributor can be called to obtain information on drugs or products that they produce or distribute. This action may be particularly helpful if the product is an outdated formulation or a recently reformulated or released one. Most large companies maintain 24-hour emergency telephone numbers for such purposes, and many employ medical consultants who can also provide management advice. Although industrial products do not have the same labeling requirements as household ones, right-to-know legislation requires that companies make information regarding the ingredients and potential toxicity of products they make, distribute, or use available to workers and health care providers [35]. Such information can be obtained by requesting a Material Data Safety Sheet (MSDS).

Information on drugs and chemical products manufactured or obtained outside the United States can be found in *Poisindex* [27] and *Martindale: The Complete Drug Reference* [21], or obtained from a domestic or foreign poison center. Information on drugs undergoing clinical trials in the United States may also be found in *Martindale*, since such drugs are often already available in other countries. Most foreign poison centers have English-speaking staff or translators available.

Plants (including fungi or mushrooms), along with their active parts and chemical constituents, can be identified by consulting *Poisindex* [27] if either their common or botanical name is known. If the name is not known but a sample is available, a representative from a local nursery, horticultural or mycologic society, or university botany department may be of assistance in identifying it. Similarly, pet stores, zoos, veterinarians, amateur or academic entomologists, herpetologists, zoologists, and field guides can be helpful in identifying potentially venomous insects, reptiles, snakes, and other animals. Poison centers usually maintain lists of local experts who are willing to help with such identifications.

Toxidromes

A toxidrome is a clinical syndrome that involves multiple physiologic systems and facilitates bedside identification of the culprit toxin [36]. The physiologic state of the patient can usually be characterized as excited (i.e., central nervous system [CNS] excitation with increased blood pressure, pulse, respirations, and temperature), depressed (i.e., decreased level of consciousness and decreased vital signs), discordant (i.e., inconsistent, mixed, or opposing CNS and vital sign abnormalities), or normal. The differential diagnosis can then be narrowed to the common or characteristic causes of these physiologic states (Table 117.3).

The *excited state* is primarily caused by sympathomimetics (agents that directly or indirectly stimulate α- and β-adrenergic receptors), anticholinergics (agents that block parasympathetic muscarinic receptors), hallucinogens, and withdrawal syndromes. The *depressed state* is primarily caused by sympatholytics (agents that block adrenergic receptors or depress cardiovascular activity), cholinergics (agents that directly or indirectly stimulate muscarinic receptors), opioids, or sedative hypnotics (which enhance the effect of the inhibitory CNS neurotransmitter gamma-aminobutyric acid [GABA] or depress neuronal membrane excitability). The *discordant state* is primarily due to asphyxiants (agents that decrease the availability, absorption, transport, or use of oxygen), membrane active agents (those that block sodium channels or otherwise alter the activity of excitable cell membranes), and agents that cause a variety of CNS syndromes due to interference with dopamine, GABA, glycine, or the synthesis, metabolism, or function of serotonin. A *normal physiologic state* may be due to a nontoxic exposure (Table 117.4), psychogenic illness, or presentation during the preclinical phase of poisoning. Agents that have a long preclinical phase (i.e., delayed onset of toxicity) are known as toxic "time bombs." Delayed onset of toxicity may result from slow absorption or distribution, metabolic activation, or a mechanism of action

TABLE 117.3

DIFFERENTIAL DIAGNOSIS OF POISONING BASED ON PHYSIOLOGIC ASSESSMENT AND UNDERLYING MECHANISMS

Excited (CNS stimulation with increased vital signs)	Depressed (CNS depression with decreased vital signs)	Discordant (mixed CNS and vital sign abnormalities)	Normal
Sympathomimetics Amphetamines Bronchodilators (β-agonists) Catecholamine analogues Cocaine Decongestants Ergot alkaloids Methylxanthines Monoamine oxidase inhibitors Thyroid hormones **Anticholinergics** Antihistamines Antispasmodics (GI-GU) Atropine and other belladonna alkaloids Cyclic antidepressants Cyclobenzaprine Mydriatics (topical) Nonprescription sleep aids Orphenadrine Parkinsonian therapeutics Phenothiazines Plants/mushrooms **Hallucinogens** LSD and tryptamine derivatives Marijuana Mescaline and amphetamine derivatives Psilocybin mushrooms Phencyclidine **Withdrawal syndromes** Baclofen β-Adrenergic blockers Clonidine Cyclic antidepressants Ethanol Opioids Sedative hypnotics	**Sympatholytics** α-Adrenergic antagonists Angiotensin-converting enzyme inhibitors β-Adrenergic blockers Calcium channel blockers Clonidine gestants Cyclic antidepressants Decongestants (imidazolines) Digitalis Neuroleptics **Cholinergics** Bethanechol Carbamate insecticides Echothiophate Myasthenia gravis therapeutics Nicotine Organophosphate insecticides Physostigmine Pilocarpine Urecholine **Opioids** Analgesics Antidiarrheal drugs Fentanyl and derivatives Heroin Opium **Sedative-hypnotics** Alcohols Anticonvulsants Barbiturates Benzodiazepines Bromide Ethchlorvynol GHB Glutethimide Methyprylon Muscle relaxants	**Asphyxiants** Carbon monoxide Cyanide Hydrogen sulfide Inert (simple) gases Irritant gases Methemoglobinemia Oxidative phosphorylation inhibitors Herbicides (nitrophenols) **AGMA inducers** Alcoholic ketoacidosis Ethylene glycol Iron Methanol (formaldehyde) Paraldehyde Metformin/phenformin (chronic) Salicylate Toluene Valproic acid **CNS syndromes** Disulfiram Extrapyramidal reactions Isoniazid (GABA lytic) Neuroleptic malignant syndrome Serotonin syndrome Solvents (hydrocarbons) Strychnine (glycinergic) **Membrane active agents** Amantadine Antiarrhythmics Beta-blockers Cyclic antidepressants Fluoride Heavy metals Lithium Local anesthetics Meperidine/propoxyphene Neuroleptics Quinine (antimalarials)	**Nontoxic exposure** **Psychogenic illness** **Toxic time bombs** Acetaminophen Agents that form concretions *Amanita phalloides* and related mushrooms Anticholinergics Cancer therapeutics Carbamazepine Chloramphenicol Chlorinated hydrocarbons Colchicine Digitalis preparations Dilantin kapseals Disulfiram Enteric-coated pills Ethylene glycol Heavy metals Fluoride Immunosuppressive agents Lithium Lomotil (atropine and diphenoxylate) Methanol Methemoglobin inducers (some) Monoamine oxidase inhibitors Paraquat Opioids Organophosphate insecticides (some) Podophyllin Salicylates Sustained-release formulations Thyroid hormone synthesis inhibitors Thyroxine valproic acid Viral antimicrobials

AGMA, anion gap metabolic acidosis; CNS, central nervous system; GABA, gamma-aminobutyric acid; GHB, gamma-hydroxybutyrate; GI–GU, gastrointestinal–genitourinary; LSD, lysergic acid diethylamide.

TABLE 117.4

CRITERIA FOR A NONTOXIC EXPOSURE

- Patient is asymptomatic by both history and physical examination
- Amount and identity of all chemicals and time of exposure are known with high degree of certainty
- Exposure dose is less than the smallest dose known or predicted to cause toxicity

that involves the disruption of metabolic or synthetic pathways. Psychogenic illness should be considered when symptoms are inconsistent with the reported exposure and cannot be substantiated by objective physical findings, laboratory abnormalities, and toxicologic testing and other etiologies have been excluded [37].

An excited or depressed state may be mischaracterized as a discordant one when the activity of a stimulant or depressant is selective for a receptor subtype or results in a compensatory or opposing autonomic response. For example, hypotension caused by an alpha-blocker, β_2-agonist, or vasodilator may be

TABLE 117.5

PHYSIOLOGIC GRADING OF THE SEVERITY OF POISONING

	Signs and symptoms	
Severity	Stimulant poisoning	Depressant poisoning
Grade 1	Agitation, anxiety, diaphoresis, hyperreflexia, mydriasis, tremors	Ataxia, confusion, lethargy, weakness, verbal, able to follow commands
Grade 2	Confusion, fever, hyperactivity, hypertension, tachycardia, tachypnea	Mild coma (nonverbal but responsive to pain); brainstem and deep tendon reflexes intact
Grade 3	Delirium, hallucinations, hyperpyrexia, tachyarrhythmias	Moderate coma (respiratory depression, unresponsive to pain); some but not all reflexes absent
Grade 4	Coma, cardiovascular collapse, seizures	Deep coma (apnea, cardiovascular depression); all reflexes absent

accompanied by tachycardia, and hypertension due to a selective α-agonist (e.g., phenylpropanolamine) may be accompanied by bradycardia. Severe stimulant or depressant poisoning can also cause what appears to be a discordant state (Table 117.5). For example, prolonged seizures and extreme hyperthermia caused by sympathomimetics can culminate in cardiovascular collapse as a consequence of anaerobic metabolism, acidosis, or depletion of neurotransmitters. Similarly, marked hypotension and hypoventilation caused by physiologic depressants can precipitate seizures and tachyarrhythmias as a result of ischemia, anoxia, and acidosis. In addition, paradoxic excitation can result from the preferential inhibition of cortical function that normally controls social activity by low doses of CNS depressants, most notably alcohol and other sedative hypnotics. In such cases, the physiologic state and its cause can often be correctly identified by the overall clinical picture and course of events.

The severity of mental status changes and the nature of associated autonomic findings can be used to narrow the differential diagnosis of physiological stimulation and depression to one of four subcategories (see Table 117.3). In the excited patient, marked vital sign abnormalities (e.g., severe hypertension with end-organ ischemia, tachyarrhythmias, hyperthermia, cardiovascular collapse) with minor mental status changes suggest an agent with peripheral sympathomimetic activity as the cause. Conversely, marked mental status abnormalities with nearly normal vital signs suggest a centrally acting hallucinogen. Anticholinergic poisoning (Table 117.6) can be differentiated from sympathomimetic (Table 117.7), hallucinogen, and withdrawal syndromes by the presence of dry, flushed, and hot skin; decreased or absent bowel sounds; and urinary retention. Other causes of excitation are usually accompanied by pallor, diaphoresis, and increased bowel or bladder activity.

In the patient with physiological depression, marked cardiovascular abnormalities (e.g., hypotension and bradycardia) with relatively clear sensorium suggest a peripherally acting sympatholytic, whereas marked CNS and respiratory depression with minimal pulse and blood pressure abnormalities suggest a centrally acting agent (opioid or sedative hypnotic). Cholinergic poisoning (Table 117.8) can be distinguished from other causes of physiologic depression by the presence of characteristic autonomic findings: *S*alivation, *l*acrimation, *u*rination, *d*efecation, *G*I cramps, and *e*mesis (SLUDGE syndrome). In addition, cholinergic poisoning causes pallor and diaphoresis, whereas the skin is usually warm and dry with opioid and sedative–hypnotic poisoning.

Other findings can sometimes help narrow the differential diagnosis further. Only the most common and diagnostically useful ones are noted here. Because of limited specificity and sensitivity, the presence or absence of a particular sign or symptom cannot be used to confirm or exclude a given etiology.

Ocular findings can sometimes help narrow the diagnostic possibilities. Although mydriasis can be caused by any agent or condition that results in physiologic excitation (see Table 117.3), it is most pronounced in anticholinergic poisoning, in which it is associated with minimal pupil response to light and accommodation. Similarly, although miosis is a nonspecific manifestation of physiologic depression, it is usually most pronounced in opioid poisoning. Notable miosis can, however, also be caused by cholinergic agents and sympatholytics with alpha-blocking effects (e.g., phenothiazines). Visual disturbances suggest anticholinergic, cholinergic, digitalis, hallucinogen, methanol, and quinine poisoning. Horizontal nystagmus and disconjugate gaze are nonspecific manifestations

TABLE 117.6

ANTICHOLINERGIC TOXIDROME

Tachycardia
Hyperthermia
Hallucination/confusion
Dry mouth/garbled speech
Mydriasis
Ileus
Urinary retention
Dry, flushed skin

TABLE 117.7

SYMPATHOMIMETIC TOXIDROME

Mydriasis
Agitation
Diaphoresis
Hypertension
Hyperthermia
Tachycardia

TABLE 117.8

CHOLINERGIC TOXIDROME

Salivation
Lacrimation
Urination
Defecation
GI cramps
Emesis

of sedative–hypnotic poisoning. Although vertical and rotary nystagmus can be seen in patients with lithium and phenytoin poisoning, they are most suggestive of phencyclidine intoxication. These etiologies should be readily distinguishable by assessing the physiologic state. Rapidly alternating lateral "ping-pong" gaze has been described in monoamine oxidase inhibitor poisoning. Except for abnormalities due to topical chemical exposure, both eyes are equally affected. Although failure to respond to topical miotics has been said to be diagnostic of drug-induced pupillary dilatation, this is only true for topical exposures. Hence, unilateral pupillary abnormalities should generally prompt evaluation for a central, structural lesion.

Dermatologic abnormalities may also be helpful. Flushed skin can be caused by anticholinergics, boric acid, a disulfiram-ethanol reaction, monosodium glutamate, niacin, scombroid (fish poisoning), and rapid infusion of vancomycin (red man syndrome). The skin is hot and dry in anticholinergic poisoning but normal or moist with other etiologies. Flushing should not be confused with the orange skin discoloration caused by rifampin. Pallor and diaphoresis may be due to cholinergics, hallucinogens, hypoglycemics, sympathomimetics, and drug withdrawal (see Table 117.3). As noted previously, manifestations of the SLUDGE syndrome distinguish cholinergic poisoning from other etiologies. Cyanosis may be due to agents that cause cardiovascular or respiratory depression, methemoglobinemia, pneumonitis, or simple asphyxia. In methemoglobinemia, it may have a chocolate-brown or slate-gray hue and is unaffected by oxygen administration. Cyanosis should not be confused with the blue discoloration of the skin caused by amiodarone or by topical exposure to blue dyes. The latter condition can be diagnosed by wiping the skin with acetone or alcohol. Hair loss, mucosal pigmentation, and nail abnormalities are suggestive of heavy metal poisoning (e.g., arsenic, lead, mercury, thallium).

Finally, the presence of neuromuscular abnormalities may suggest certain etiologies. Seizures and tremors can be caused by cholinergics, hypoglycemic agents, lithium, membrane-active agents, some narcotics (e.g., meperidine, propoxyphene), and most physiologic stimulants [38] (see Table 117.3). They can also occur in patients poisoned by agents that cause asphyxia, low lactate increased AGMA (see later), and cerebral hypoperfusion or hypoventilation (e.g., physiologic depressants; see Table 117.3). The most common causes of seizures due to poisoning are tricyclic antidepressants, sympathomimetics, antihistamines (primarily diphenhydramine), theophylline, and isoniazid. Although carbon monoxide, hypoglycemics, lithium, and theophylline can cause focal seizures, seizures due to poisoning are usually generalized. Because hypertensive and traumatic CNS hemorrhages are known complications of poisoning, the possibility of a structural lesion should be considered if focal signs and symptoms are present. Myoclonus suggests anticholinergic or sympathomimetic poisoning. Fasciculations are typical of cholinergic insecticide poisoning but can also be caused by sympathomimetics. Rigidity may be seen in phencyclidine and sympathomimetic poisoning and in those with CNS syndromes (see Table 117.3). Dystonic posturing is most often caused by antipsychotic agents. It is also a characteristic feature of strychnine poisoning.

Laboratory Findings

Acid–base status, anion gap, serum osmolality, ketone, electrolyte, glucose, and organ function abnormalities identified by routine laboratory tests can be extremely helpful in the differential diagnosis of poisoning. As with clinical manifestations, the diagnostic sensitivity and specificity of a single finding is not sufficiently high for its presence or absence to confirm or exclude a specific etiology. The use of anion and osmolar gaps and serum ketone and lactate levels in the diagnosis of poisoning of unknown etiology is summarized in Figure 117.1.

Assessing acid–base status and calculating the anion gap is particularly important because an increased AGMA may be due to advanced ethylene glycol, methanol, and salicylate poisoning. In such cases, prompt initiation of specific therapies is essential to prevent progressive, irreversible, or fatal poisoning [39,40]. The normal anion gap is 13 ± 4 mEq per L in unselected acutely hospitalized patients. In ethylene glycol and methanol poisoning, AGMA is primarily due to the accumulation of acid metabolites. In salicylate poisoning, it is caused by the accumulation of a variety of endogenous organic acids resulting from salicylate's interference with intermediary metabolism. Agents that cause hypoxemia, cellular asphyxia, seizures, shock, or extensive tissue necrosis can also cause an AGMA, but in these instances, the accumulation of lactic acid generated by anaerobic metabolism is responsible for the AGMA. When the underlying cause is unclear, measuring the serum lactate level may be helpful. The lactate concentration is usually low (<5 mEq per L) or significantly less than the anion gap in ethylene glycol, methanol, and salicylate poisoning, but high (>5 mEq per L) or nearly equal to the anion gap in conditions associated with anaerobic metabolism.

Other common toxicologic causes of a low-lactate AGMA include ethanol, which can cause ketoacidosis by disrupting intermediary metabolism in susceptible alcoholics, and toluene, which can cause renal tubular acidosis with bicarbonate wasting. Rarely, this metabolic picture occurs in poisoning by formaldehyde (which is metabolized to formic acid), paraldehyde (presumably as a result of its metabolism to acetic acid), phosphate [41], and sulfur (and possibly sulfates) [42]. It can also be seen with large overdoses of ibuprofen (and probably all nonsteroidal anti-inflammatory agents) and valproic acid (due to high levels of these acidic drugs and their metabolites) [43,44]. Metformin and nucleoside reverse transcriptase inhibitor antiretroviral agents (e.g., zidovudine or azidothymidine) can interfere with normal-lactate metabolism and cause a high-lactate AGMA at therapeutic as well as excessive doses [45,46]. A high-lactate AGMA can rarely occur soon after massive acetaminophen ingestion [47].

An abnormally low anion gap may be seen in severe bromide, calcium, iodine, lithium, magnesium, and nitrate intoxication [39,48,49]. In bromide, iodine, and lithium intoxication, the low anion gap results from spuriously elevated chloride levels, and with nitrate poisoning, it is due to falsely elevated bicarbonate levels.

Serum osmolality can help differentiate the toxic causes of a low-lactate AGMA. An increased osmole gap may be seen early in the course of ethylene glycol and methanol (when high serum levels of the parent compounds are present) but not salicylate poisoning. Although not strictly accurate from a physical chemistry perspective [50], the osmole gap is typically defined

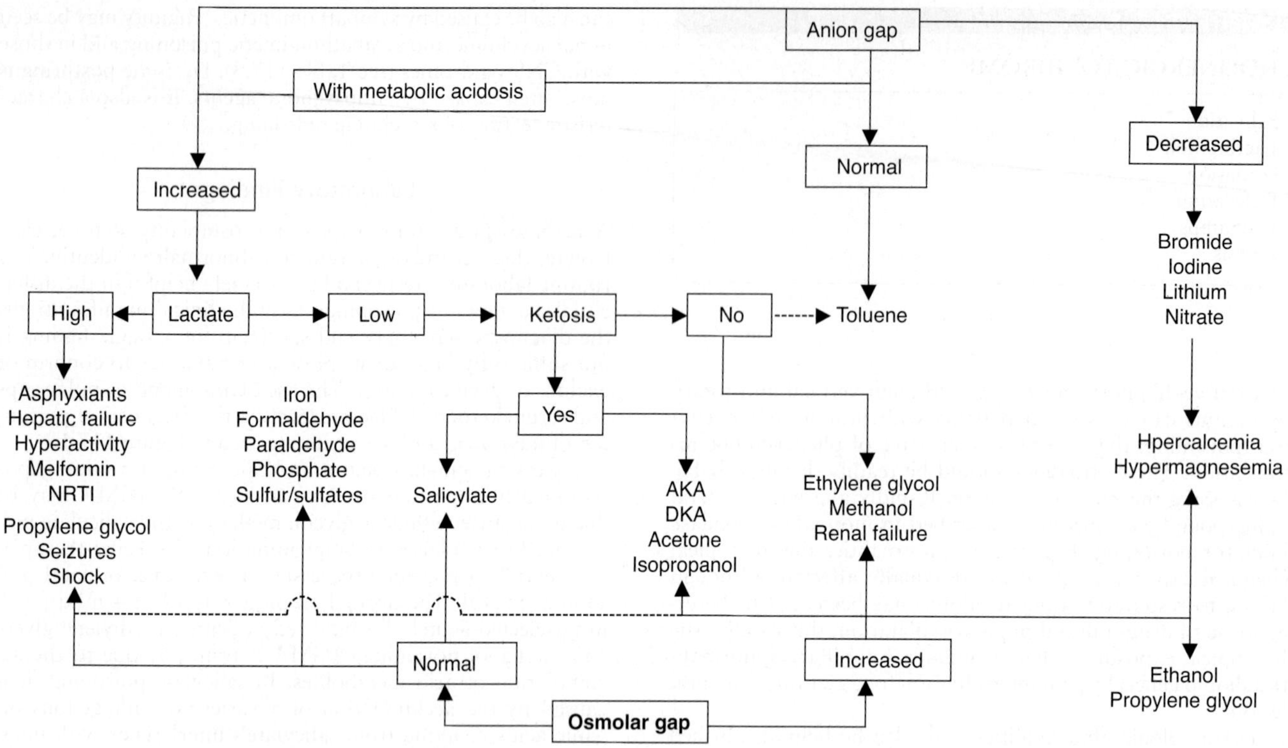

FIGURE 117.1. Use of routine laboratory findings and calculated gaps in the differential diagnosis of poisonings. AKA, alcoholic ketoacidosis; DKA, diabetic ketoacidosis; NRTI, nucleoside/nucleotide reverse transcriptase inhibitors.

as the difference between the measured serum osmolality and the calculated serum osmolality.

$$\text{Serum Osmolality } (\mu\text{mol/L}) = 2 \text{ (serum Na)} + \text{serum glucose} + \text{serum BUN}$$

where normal serum osmolality is 290 ± 10 mOsm per kg of H_2O normal osmole gap is 5 ± 7 mOsm per kg (in unselected acutely hospitalized patients [40]).

$$\text{Osmole gap} = [\text{calculated serum osmolality} - \text{measured serum osmolality}]$$

Normal osmole gap is 5 ± 7 mOsm per kg (in unselected hospitalized patients [40])

This formula assumes that all concentrations are measured in millimoles per liter. If the glucose and BUN concentrations are measured in milligrams per deciliter, dividing them by 18 and 3, respectively, gives their approximate concentrations in millimoles.

Additional causes of an increased osmolar gap include other low-molecular-weight solutes, such as acetone, ethanol, isopropyl alcohol, magnesium, mannitol, and propylene glycol [51]. The approximate concentration of these substances that will increase the serum osmolality by 1 mOsm per kg of H_2O, calculated on the basis of their molecular weights, is shown in Table 117.9. When direct measurements are not readily available, the serum concentration of these agents can be estimated by multiplying this amount by the osmolar gap. Serum osmolality must be measured by freezing point depression rather than the headspace or vapor pressure method to detect the presence of volatile agents such as acetone and toxic alcohols. An increased osmolar gap has also been reported in alcoholic ketoacidosis and conditions causing lactic acidosis [52].

Serum ketones can also help to differentiate the toxic causes of a low-lactate AGMA. Ketosis, as defined by a positive nitroprusside reaction, is relatively common in salicylate poisoning but unusual in ethylene glycol and methanol poisoning. Ketosis is also seen in alcoholic ketoacidosis and in acetone and isopropyl alcohol poisoning.

The urinalysis, serum calcium concentration, and the overall clinical picture can also be helpful in differentiating the toxic causes of a low-lactate AGMA. Crystalluria, hypocalcemia, and back pain or flank tenderness suggest ethylene glycol; visual symptoms implicate methanol; and tinnitus or impaired

TABLE 117.9

EFFECTS OF SOME SOLUTES ON SERUM OSMOLALITY

Solute	Approximate concentration required to increase serum osmolality by 1 mOsm/kg
Alcohols, glycols, and ketones	
Acetone	5.8 mg/dL
Ethanol	4.6 mg/dL
Ethylene glycol	5.2 mg/dL
Isopropanol	6.0 mg/dL
Methanol	2.6 mg/dL
Propylene glycol	7.6 mg/dL
Electrolytes	
Calcium	4.0 mg/dL (1 mEq/L)
Magnesium	2.4 mg/dL (1 mEq/L)
Sugars	
Mannitol	18 mg/dL
Sorbitol	18 mg/dL

hearing point to salicylates. Crystalluria can also be caused by acyclovir [53], felbamate [54], indinavir [55], oxalate [56], primidone [57], and sulfa drugs [58]. Hypocalcemia is also seen in fluoride and oxalate [56] intoxication.

Serum potassium and glucose abnormalities may also provide clues to the etiology of poisoning [18,59,60]. Toxicologic causes of hypokalemia include barium, β_2-adrenergic agonists, calcium channel blockers, chloroquine, diuretics, insulin, licorice, methylxanthines, and toluene. Hyperkalemia can be caused by α-adrenergic agonists, angiotensin-converting enzyme inhibitors, beta-blockers, digitalis, fluoride, potassium-sparing diuretics, and trimethoprim. Common toxicologic causes of hypoglycemia are ethanol, beta-blockers, hypoglycemics, quinine, and salicylate. Common causes of hyperglycemia include acetone, β-agonists, calcium channel blockers, iron, and methylxanthines.

Common toxicologic causes of acute liver dysfunction are acetaminophen, ethanol, halogenated hydrocarbons (e.g., carbon tetrachloride), heavy metals, and mushrooms (e.g., *Amanita phalloides* and related species) [61]. Acute renal toxicity is most often due to ethylene glycol, halogenated hydrocarbons, heavy metals, nonsteroidal anti-inflammatory drugs, toluene, envenomations, and agents that cause hemolysis or rhabdomyolysis [62]. An elevated creatinine with a normal BUN can be seen in acetone and isopropyl alcohol poisoning because acetone interferes with colorimetric assays for creatinine, resulting in falsely high results. Acute hemolysis (in the absence of glucose-6-phosphate dehydrogenase deficiency) can result from poisoning by arsine gas, naphthalene, and inducers of methemoglobinemia. Rhabdomyolysis is associated with toluene abuse, CNS syndromes (see Table 117.3), and severe physiologic dysfunction (e.g., extreme agitation, deep or prolonged coma, hyperthermia, seizures) of any etiology [63]. The most common agents involved are sympathomimetics, ethanol, heroin, and phencyclidine.

Electrocardiographic Findings

The ECG may provide clues to the cause of poisoning [18]. Ventricular tachyarrhythmias that occur in patients with normal QRS and QT intervals suggest myocardial irritation (i.e., increased automaticity) as the underlying mechanism. Sympathomimetics, digitalis, and cardiac-sensitizing agents such as chloral hydrate and aliphatic or halogenated hydrocarbons, which potentiate the action of endogenous catecholamines, are common causes [64]. In contrast, ventricular tachyarrhythmias that occur in the setting of depolarization and repolarization abnormalities, reflected by QRS and QT interval prolongation, respectively, suggest a reentrant mechanism. Causes include electrolyte abnormalities, organophosphate insecticides, and other membrane active agents (see Table 117.1) [65,66]. Torsades de pointes (polymorphous) ventricular tachycardia strongly implicates an agent that prolongs the QT interval.

Atrioventricular conduction abnormalities (atrioventricular block) and bradyarrhythmias can be caused by beta-blockers, calcium channel blockers, digitalis, membrane-active psychotherapeutic agents, organophosphate insecticides, and α-agonists such as phenylpropanolamine. With α-agonists, they are a reflex (i.e., homeostatic) response to hypertension, but with other causes, they are associated with generalized cardiovascular depression and hypotension.

Radiologic Findings

Ingested chemicals can sometimes be visualized within the GI tract by abdominal radiographic imaging, and such imaging can occasionally be helpful in suggesting the etiology or amount of an unknown ingestion. Although a large variety of chemicals can be detected by routine radiography in vitro, relatively few are visible in vivo [67]. Agents most likely to be visible on plain films are indicated by the mnemonic CHIPES (Table 117.10) [18].

TABLE 117.10

XENOBIOTICS VISIBLE ON PLAIN STOMACH RADIOGRAPHS

Chlorinated hydrocarbons
Heavy metals
Iodinated compounds
Packets of drugs
Enteric-coated drugs
Salicylates

Ingested drug packets may appear as uniform, ovoid or round, marble-sized densities scattered along the GI tract [29,30]. Ingested hydrocarbons may sometimes appear as a double gastric fluid level or "double bubble" because of the air–fluid and fluid–fluid interface lines created when less dense hydrocarbons layer on top of gastric fluids. Computed tomography may be superior to plain films in detecting ingested drug packets but the optimal test in this setting remains unclear [68,69]. Whether contrast should be used or not remains controversial. Abdominal ultrasound can detect ingested pills, particularly enteric-coated and sustained-released formulations [70]. Such imaging may be useful in confirming or refuting some recent specific (CHIPES) ingestions. Because the volume of pills can be determined, plain radiography may be used to guide GI decontamination.

Abnormal findings on chest radiography can be caused by a wide variety of chemicals [18,71]. Diffuse or patchy infiltrates (i.e., pneumonitis or acute lung injury) can be due to the inhalation of irritant gases (e.g., ammonia, chlorine, hydrogen sulfide, nitrogen oxides, phosgene, smoke, sulfur dioxide), fumes (e.g., beryllium, metal oxides, polymers), and vapors (e.g., acids, aldehydes, hydrocarbons, isocyanates, mercury). They can also be seen in patients who have ingested or injected cholinergic agents (e.g., carbamate and organophosphate insecticides), metabolic poisons (e.g., cyanide, carbon monoxide, heavy metals, hydrogen sulfide), paraquat, phencyclidine, salicylates, thiazide diuretics, and tocolytics and in patients with envenomations. Aspiration pneumonitis is quite common and can occur in patients with coma or seizures of any etiology [72]. Acute lung injury can also develop in any patient with prolonged or pronounced anoxia, hyperthermia, or hypotension (e.g., those with severe opioids or sedative–hypnotic or sympathomimetic poisoning). Chronic chemical exposure can cause pulmonary fibrosis, granulomas, or pleural plaques.

Response to Antidotes

The use of antidotes for diagnostic purposes has largely fallen from favor. The availability of point of care blood glucose measurement negates the need for empiric intravenous dextrose in altered patients. Many antidotes may be harmful if used inappropriately, including flumazenil physostigmine, glucagon, nitrites, and chelators. Naloxone remains a reasonably safe therapy in a patient with clinical signs of opiate intoxication. Clinicians should be prepared to manage acute withdrawal and its sequelae.

Toxicology Screening

Analysis of a sample of the toxin itself, or patient urine, blood, gastric contents, or hair [71,73] can sometimes be helpful in identifying the cause of poisoning. Urine is generally the best specimen to analyze because large quantities can be obtained for extraction procedures and many chemicals are normally concentrated in urine. However, toxicology testing can detect only a small fraction of all chemicals (primarily drugs) and is not always reliable [74]. Immunoassay screens are inexpensive and provide results within minutes, but they are only capable of detecting a few agents. They suffer from many false positives and false negatives. Patients may be misdiagnosed and potentially harmed by clinicians acting solely on the results of immunoassay screens [75]. Comprehensive screens are expensive and require 2 to 6 hours for completion (excluding transportation times). Although results may increase diagnostic certainty or specificity, they rarely change disposition or treatment in patients who are asymptomatic or who have signs and symptoms consistent with the reported exposure [75–80]. Noteworthy exceptions are acetaminophen and salicylate, which are widely available, commonly ingested, sometimes misidentified, require specific treatment, and cause few or nonspecific early signs and symptoms. Hence, in most overdose patients, quantitative acetaminophen and salicylate levels are the only toxicology tests likely to be clinically useful.

Critically ill poisoned patients suffering seizures, cardiovascular instability, acid–base abnormalities, multiple organ dysfunction, nonsinus cardiac rhythms, or cardiac conduction disturbance without a toxicologic diagnosis should generally have comprehensive toxicology screening.

Knowledge of the methods used for chemical detection (e.g., colorimetric spot tests; thin-layer paper or plate chromatography; gas- or high-pressure liquid chromatography; absorbance, atomic absorption, flame ionization, or fluorometric assays; enzyme-multiplied and radionuclide immunoassays; gas chromatography with mass spectrometry) is required for accurate interpretation of the results of screening tests [75,81–83]. A positive result on one assay should always be confirmed by repeat analysis using a different technique. The physician should speak directly with the laboratory technician to determine which chemicals can be detected by the screening methods used and the sensitivity and specificity of each assay. In addition, directed analysis (e.g., coma, hallucinogen, or stimulant screen), with more rapidly available results, can be performed if the technician and clinician communicate.

A negative result from a screen should never be used to exclude the diagnosis of poisoning when clinical findings suggest otherwise. It may simply mean a chemical is not detectable by the assay(s) used, its concentration is below the limit of detection of the assay(s), or its concentration is too low to be confirmed. It may also mean the time of sampling or the specimen submitted is inappropriate for testing (e.g., the chemical may be undergoing absorption and is not yet present in urine or it may already have been metabolized or eliminated). In such cases, repeating the test on a sample obtained at an earlier or later time may be revealing.

Prediction of Potential Toxicity

The prediction of toxicity requires knowledge of the dose, time, and identity of an exposure and is necessary for determining the appropriate treatment. For commercial products, the amount and concentration of every ingredient should be identified. Household products deemed hazardous by the US Consumer Product Safety Committee are required by law to bear a label describing the nature of their toxicity and first aid measures as well as a "keep out of reach of children" warning and a signal word that indicates the degree or severity of potential toxicity [34]. The signal words "caution," "warning," and "danger" identify a product or its constituent(s) as a weak irritant (i.e., may damage mucosal surfaces), strong irritant (i.e., can damage skin and mucosa), or corrosive (i.e., can cause permanent tissue damage or death) after topical exposure or moderately toxic, highly toxic, or extremely toxic (oral median lethal dose: 50 to 500 mg per kg, 1 to 50 mg per kg, or <1 mg per kg, respectively) after ingestion. Label information is frequently inaccurate or incomplete [34,84] and should generally be confirmed by consulting an independent information source.

The dose of drug in a pill or tablet can be determined using the resources cited in "Identification of the Offending Agent" section of this chapter. For liquids and powders, the dose can be estimated or measured using the container or the weights and volumes listed on the label. An exposure may also be reported in tablespoons or swallows. Standard flatware volumes can vary from 3 to 7 mL for a teaspoon and from 7 to 14 mL for a tablespoon. The volume of a swallow varies with age, height, weight, sex, the orifice size of the container, and the viscosity of the ingested liquid and ranges from 1 to 5 mL in infants to 4 to 40 mL in adults [85].

The accuracy and reliability of the history must be evaluated when assessing potential toxicity. The amount and time of ingestion are frequently erroneous when reported by patients with intentional self-poisoning. It is best always to assume a worst-case scenario: that the maximum possible dose (i.e., the entire amount available or not clearly accounted for) was ingested. The potential toxicity can then be estimated from previously reported toxicodynamic data. For drugs with CNS and cardiovascular activity, the ingestion of 5 to 10 therapeutic doses by an adult and one adult dose by a young child can result in significant toxicity. Beta-blockers, calcium channel blockers, and oral hypoglycemics can cause toxicity after only one or two therapeutic doses, particularly in those physiologically naïve to their effects. The ingestion of only one to two tablets, capsules, or teaspoonfuls of an antimalarial (e.g., chloroquine, hydroxychloroquine), antipsychotic (e.g., chlorpromazine, thioridazine), camphor, calcium channel blocker, methyl salicylate, opioid, oral hypoglycemic, theophylline, or tricyclic antidepressant (e.g., imipramine, desipramine) can be fatal to a toddler [86].

The time of exposure is important because it allows for prediction of the time of onset of toxicity and the time of peak toxicity. Only when the time elapsed since exposure clearly exceeds the longest reported or predicted interval between exposure and peak toxicity should the possibility of subsequent poisoning be excluded (see Table 117.5). Peak toxicity usually occurs within 4 to 6 hours of an oral overdose. Important exceptions to this generalization are the toxic time bombs described earlier. For some of these agents (e.g., acetaminophen, ethylene glycol, methanol, paraquat), the serum concentration measured during the preclinical phase can be used to predict subsequent toxicity. Peak toxicity may also be delayed (up to 12 to 24 hours) after exposure to irritants and corrosives. The possibility of pregnancy and potential toxicity to the fetus should also be considered.

Assessment of Severity

The severity of poisoning is primarily determined by findings on physical examination. Because poisoning is far more dynamic than most diseases and illnesses, frequent reevaluations are required. Poisoned patients can rapidly deteriorate, with few or no warning signs.

A complete physical examination should ultimately be performed in all patients. The examination should initially be directed toward assessment of cardiovascular stability, respiratory function, and neurologic status. Accurate and timely measurement of all vital signs is essential. The respiratory rate should be measured for a full minute. A core or rectal temperature should be obtained to detect severe or occult abnormalities. The sickest patients are the ones most likely to have significant temperature abnormalities. They are also the ones in whom preoccupation with cardiovascular and respiratory therapy can lead to delayed temperature measurement. In contrast, an abbreviated mental status examination is usually sufficient. The degree of physiologic dysfunction should be objectively described.

The number and type of ancillary tests required to assess metabolic or organ function is determined primarily by clinical severity and secondarily by the history. Asymptomatic but potentially poisoned patients with reliable histories and unintentional exposures should have blood and urine samples obtained on presentation. Samples can be saved and subsequently sent for (baseline) analysis in the event of deterioration. Pregnancy testing, however, is recommended in all susceptible women of childbearing age. Patients who are symptomatic or suicidal should have serum electrolytes, BUN, creatinine, and glucose measurements; urinalysis; and 12-lead ECG. Arterial blood gas, serum osmolality, and ketone and methemoglobin analyses may also be indicated. Anion, osmolal, and oxygen saturation gaps should be calculated whenever their determinants are measured. Assessment of patients with respiratory complaints or grade 2 or greater stimulant or depressant poisoning (see Table 117.5) should include a chest radiograph. A complete blood cell count, coagulation studies, serum amylase, calcium, magnesium, creatine phosphokinase, and hepatic enzyme levels should also be determined in any patient with grade 2 or greater physiologic dysfunction. Additional testing (e.g., biopsies, invasive monitoring, neurodiagnostic studies, radiologic examinations) should be individualized and based on the findings of physical examination, the history, and the results of routine ancillary studies.

The measurement of chemical concentrations in serum, whole blood, or urine can sometimes help in assessing the severity of poisoning. Agents for which quantitative measurements are necessary or desirable for optimal patient management include acetaminophen, acetone, alcohols, antiarrhythmics, antiepileptics, barbiturates, carbon monoxide, digoxin, electrolytes (including calcium and magnesium), ethylene glycol, heavy metals, lithium, salicylate, and theophylline [75,81]. Quantitative or qualitative assays for other toxins are not generally helpful because they serve only to confirm the clinical impression and do not affect treatment (which is either supportive or must be initiated long before laboratory results are available in order to be effective).

Provision of Supportive Care

Meticulous supportive care is necessary to maintain physiologic and biochemical homeostasis and to prevent secondary complications (e.g., anoxia, aspiration, bedsores, shock-induced organ injury, sepsis) until detoxification can be accomplished by normal mechanisms or therapeutic interventions. Despite advances in preventing absorption, enhancing elimination, and antidotal treatment, supportive care remains the most effective therapy for most poisoned patients. Details of supportive therapy (e.g., treatment of vital sign abnormalities and organ dysfunction) can be found in other chapters. Only considerations of special relevance to the poisoned patient are discussed here.

Monitoring

Unless toxicity is minimal and predicted with a high degree of certainty to remain so, venous access should be established and continuous cardiac monitoring initiated. Because fluid resuscitation may become necessary, normal saline is the preferred IV solution. Pulse oximetry should be performed on presentation and monitored frequently if abnormal or significant (grade 2 or greater) physiologic dysfunction (see Table 117.5) is present. Until the ultimate severity of poisoning is known, frequent or continuous visual observation is also necessary. Patients with intentional self-poisoning also need close behavioral observation until the possibility of a repeat suicide attempt has been evaluated in detail and assessed to be unlikely.

Respiratory Care

Pulmonary aspiration of gastric contents is a relatively common complication of poisoning and its treatment (e.g., GI decontamination procedures) [87,88]. Patients with CNS depression or seizures are at risk for aspiration and airway obstruction. Although spontaneously breathing patients who respond to painful stimulation can sometimes be successfully managed by aspiration-preventative positioning (e.g., left lateral decubitus and Trendelenburg position) and close observation, definitive airway management is recommended for those who cannot respond by voice. Using the gag reflex to assess the need for intubation should be abandoned [87]. Many normal individuals have an absent gag reflex, and many comatose patients will gag if sufficiently stimulated and yet be unable to protect their airway. In addition, attempting to elicit a gag reflex may itself induce vomiting and cause aspiration in a patient with an altered mental state. Prophylactic or therapeutic intubation may also be required for patients with extreme behavioral or physiologic stimulation who require aggressive pharmacologic therapy with sedative, antipsychotic, anticonvulsant, or paralyzing agents. Even in comatose patients, pretreatment with a sedative and neuromuscular blocking agent can facilitate intubation [88]. An endotracheal tube with a low-pressure high-volume cuff is recommended to reduce aspiration, but it is by no means completely effective [89]. In intubated patients who can tolerate it, elevating the head of the bed may decrease the incidence of aspiration [90]. Extracorporeal membrane oxygenation, cardiopulmonary bypass, nitric oxide, prone positioning, and oscillation should be considered in patients with reversible poisoning who cannot otherwise be adequately oxygenated or ventilated.

Cardiovascular Therapy

Because of adverse drug interactions, therapy intended to maintain or restore normal blood pressure, pulse, and sinus rhythm may worsen, rather than alleviate, cardiovascular toxicity. Hence, the severity and trend of cardiovascular abnormalities and the potential complications of treatment should be considered before instituting pharmacologic therapy. In addition, because the causes of cardiovascular toxicity are varied and multiple mechanisms may be concurrently operative, invasive hemodynamic monitoring may be necessary for accurate diagnosis and optimal treatment. Aggressive supportive measures, such as transvenous cardiac pacing and intra-aortic balloon pump or cardiopulmonary bypass should be considered in patients with reversible poisoning who are unresponsive to routine therapeutic measures [91].

In the absence of extremes of heart rate, hypotension due to poisoning is most often caused by loss of peripheral vascular tone rather than pump failure. Bedside echocardiography can also be useful to assess cardiac output. Norepinephrine is generally considered the first line vasopressor in patients who do not respond to fluid administration.

When hypertension causes end organ dysfunction, therapy is indicated. In patients with sympathomimetic poisoning, beta-blockade may result in unopposed α receptor stimulation. This leads to increased peripheral vascular resistance, increasing the demand on a beta blocked heart. Hence, treatment with a nonselective sympatholytic or with an arteriodilator followed by a beta blocker is preferred.

Sinus tachycardia can usually be managed with sympatholytics. In patients with sympathomimetic poisoning and signs or symptoms of myocardial ischemia, a beta-blocker (with or without an arteriodilator, depending on the presence or absence of coexisting hypertension) or a calcium channel blocker can be used.

Lidocaine is generally first line therapy for ventricular tachyarrhythmias. Underlying electrolyte and metabolic abnormalities should be corrected. Sodium bicarbonate or hypertonic saline may be effective in treating wide-complex tachycardias due to toxins with sodium channel blocking properties.

Normalizing electrolytes and continuous electrocardiographic monitoring is the mainstay of treatment for toxins that prolong the QT interval. The clinician must be prepared to manage Torsades des Pointes. Antibodies are available to treat serious dysrhythmias caused by cardiac glycosides. Magnesium may also be effective in digitalis poisoning. Procainamide, other class 1 A agents, beta-blockers, and physostigmine should not be used for arrhythmias caused by membrane-active agents or those associated with prolonged QRS or QT intervals because of the potential for worsening rhythm disturbances and conduction abnormalities.

Bradycardia requires treatment only if it is associated with hemodynamic instability. In most cases, atropine, dopamine, and epinephrine are the agents of choice. Calcium, glucagon, and high dose insulin can be effective in calcium channel blocker and beta-blocker poisoning.

Treatment of Neuromuscular Hyperactivity

Profound metabolic acidosis and sudden cardiac arrest can occur in patients with severe agitation who continue to struggle while being physically restrained. Prompt pharmacologic treatment of behavioral and muscular hyperactivity in such patients is critical. In general, benzodiazepines are preferred to antipsychotic agents because the latter lower the seizure threshold and prolong QTc. In phencyclidine poisoning, however, haloperidol, a central dopaminergic antagonist, may be more effective than benzodiazepines because phencyclidine has central dopaminergic activity. Similarly, chlorpromazine may be more effective than benzodiazepines in hallucinogen poisoning. The combined use of benzodiazepines and neuroleptics can be more effective than either alone; doses and side effects can often be minimized using this approach. For agitation and hallucinations due to anticholinergic poisoning, physostigmine may be considered.

Seizures can usually be effectively treated with GABA agonists such as benzodiazepines and barbiturates. Pyridoxine is usually necessary in isoniazid poisoning. Phenytoin, a Vaughn–Williams class 2 anticonvulsant, should be avoided in all cases where a toxin with sodium channel blocking properties may have been ingested. Seizures due to cyanide, hydrogen sulfide, and organophosphate insecticides usually require specific antidotes.

Severe agitation or prolonged convulsions can also cause rhabdomyolysis and hyperthermia. Because these complications can result in additional organ dysfunction, neuromuscular blocking agents should be given to patients who do not respond to sedatives and anticonvulsants. During such therapy, seizures should continue to be monitored (by electroencephalography) and treated to prevent permanent neurologic damage. Nondepolarizing agents are preferable to succinylcholine for inducing paralysis, because the latter agent may be hazardous in patients with rhabdomyolysis [23].

Prevention of Absorption

Early and effective decontamination can limit the surface exposure and systemic absorption of chemicals and reduce toxicity. Decontamination should be considered in all patients unless the exposure is clearly nontoxic (see Table 117.4), the time of predicted peak toxicity has passed, or the benefit of decontamination is minimal.

Body Cavity Exposure

The removal of chemicals from body cavities (e.g., bladder, external auditory canal, nose, rectum, vagina) can be accomplished by aspiration and irrigation using normal saline. Particulate matter (e.g., pills, suppositories, drug packages) should be manually removed, preferably under direct visualization. The removal of ingested drug packages from the GI tract is discussed in "Ingestion" section of this chapter.

Eye and Skin Exposure

Decontamination after topical exposure includes manual removal of particulate material, irrigation of exposed surfaces, and a scrub for skin exposure to noncorrosive chemicals. Because "time is damage," particularly with corrosives, tap water or any other readily available liquid that is clear and drinkable can be used in the prehospital setting. If exposure involves an unknown chemical, its pH should be measured. Searching for pH paper (e.g., pHydrion), usually available in the emergency department or the labor and delivery area, should not delay treatment. Irrigation should initially be performed for about 20 minutes. Prolonged irrigation (up to 24 hours) may be beneficial for corrosive exposures, especially those involving strong alkali.

With ocular exposures, blepharospasm secondary to pain can prevent effective irrigation unless treatment is preceded by the instillation of a topical anesthetic. Particulate material should be removed with a moist cotton-tipped swab or eye spud. Normal saline and lactated Ringer's solution are traditionally used irrigation fluids. It is unclear whether commercially available pH-balanced saline solutions and normal saline adjusted to a pH of 7.4 with sodium bicarbonate are less irritating than normal saline or lactated Ringer's solution [92,93]. Warming the solution may decrease discomfort [94], but this is not necessary if an anesthetic is used. Irrigating solutions can be administered via an IV infusion setup, directly through the tubing, or via an irrigating (Morgan) lens attachment. A low-pressure squeeze bottle also may be used. One or two liters is usually sufficient. For acid or alkali exposures, the tear pH (normally 7.3 to 7.7) should be determined after and before irrigation. Irrigation should continue until the pH is between 5 and 8.

For skin exposures, treatment should begin with the removal of contaminated clothing. Gloves should be worn to prevent contamination of caretakers. Particulate matter should be removed from the skin using a soft brush, forceps, or hand-held vacuum cleaner before irrigation. Washing the skin with soap and water or isopropyl alcohol more effectively prevents pesticide absorption than simply rinsing with water [95]. For some toxins, a triple wash (irrigation and washing with soap before and after an alcohol scrub) may provide better decontamination than irrigation alone. Because it contains 30% alcohol, tincture of green soap has been recommended as a skin detergent [27].

Inhalational Exposure

The patient should be removed from the contaminated atmosphere and supplemental oxygen administered. Under no circumstances should a rescuer enter a hazardous dust, fume, gas, or vapor environment without adequate eye, skin, and respiratory protection.

Ingestion

GI decontamination can be accomplished with activated charcoal, gastric lavage, whole-bowel irrigation, and endoscopic or surgical removal of the ingested chemical. There is little to no role for Ipecac. Cathartics, although often used in conjunction with other treatments, are not an effective method of decontamination [96,97]. Except in cases of corrosive ingestion, the same is true for diluents.

Despite extensive experimental data documenting the efficacy of GI decontamination measures in preventing chemical absorption in animals and in human volunteers, there is no conclusive evidence that these interventions improve the outcome in actual overdose patients [98–103]. Clinical efficacy is difficult to prove because the overdose history is frequently unreliable, and most overdoses do not cause severe or life-threatening toxicity. In addition, the efficacy of GI decontamination decreases as the time between ingestion and treatment increases. Experimental data showing that GI decontamination is effective in preventing chemical absorption when initiated more than 1 hour after ingestion is limited. Since the mean time between ingestion and arrival at a hospital is more than 1 hour in children and more than 3 hours in adults [104–110], most patients present for treatment at a time when the efficacy of GI decontamination remains unknown.

With the sophisticated monitoring and supportive techniques available today, it is likely that most poisoned patients will recover fully without any decontamination therapy [105,109]. However, since experimental studies show that decontamination can limit toxin absorption and shorten the duration of toxicity, and since absorption is prolonged after overdose, decontamination may be effective longer after ingestion than experimentally proven. It is therefore recommended that it be performed unless the exposure is nontoxic (see Table 117.4), or the risk of decontamination outweighs the potential benefit.

The choice of decontamination method should be based on the relative efficacy, and contraindications of the available options. Activated charcoal has equal or greater efficacy, fewer contraindications, less frequent and less serious complications than other methods of decontamination, and is the preferred treatment for most overdoses [103–114]. Emptying the stomach via lavage is rarely indicated. Overdose patients treated with gastric lavage or syrup of ipecac in the emergency department have longer emergency department stays and have a higher incidence of pulmonary aspiration (which sometimes necessitates admission of a patient who would otherwise be discharged) than those treated with activated charcoal [104,106,107].

Gastric lavage is indicated in a recent life-threatening ingestion, when the toxin is small in size or easily dissolved in the stomach, not well adsorbed by activated charcoal and not responsive to other therapies. Syrup of ipecac is virtually never the best method of GI decontamination and is no longer routinely recommended, even for the home management of ingested poisons [115]. Whole-bowel irrigation should be considered in patients who have ingested toxic amounts of agents that are slowly absorbed or not amenable to decontamination by other techniques. Endoscopy and surgery should be reserved for patients with potentially severe poisoning in whom alternative methods of decontamination are unsuccessful or contraindicated.

Activated Charcoal. Activated charcoal can prevent absorption of ingested chemicals by binding them within the gut lumen. Its clinical efficacy remains controversial [103] because it is neither absorbed nor metabolized, the toxin bound to it is normally eliminated with stool [102,105,116,117]. Activated charcoal is a fine black powder produced by the activation (i.e., pyrolysis, oxidation, and purification) of carbon-containing materials such as bone, coal, peat, petroleum, and wood. It is odorless, tasteless, and insoluble in liquids. The activation process yields particles that have an extensive internal network of minute, branching, irregular, interconnecting channels (i.e., pores) that range in size from approximately 10 to 100 nm in diameter and account for the extremely large surface area of activated charcoal. The surface area of activated charcoal in clinical use ranges from 600 to 2,000 m^2 per g.

The absorption or adherence of chemical molecules to the external and internal surfaces of activated charcoal is rapid (within minutes of contact). It is due to relatively weak van der Waals forces and can be described by the following reversible equilibrium: activated charcoal + toxin ↔ activated charcoal – toxin complex. Hence, as the amount of activated charcoal is increased, the fraction of unbound or free chemical decreases (i.e., the equilibrium shifts to the right according to the law of mass action). At an activated charcoal to chemical ratio of 10 to 1 or greater, 90% or more of most chemicals is adsorbed into charcoal in vitro. The absorptive capacity (i.e., the amount of chemical that can be absorbed by 1 g of charcoal in vitro) ranges from a few milligrams to more than 1 g depending on the molecular size, structure, and solubility of the chemical, the pore size and surface area of activated charcoal, the negative logarithm of acid ionization constant of the chemical and the pH of the solution, and the presence or absence of competing solutes. Small, highly ionized molecules of inorganic compounds, such as acids, alkali, electrolytes (e.g., potassium), and the readily dissociable salts of arsenic, bromide, cyanide, fluoride, iron, and lithium, are not well adsorbed by activated charcoal [116,117].

In animal studies and in simulated overdoses using therapeutic or slightly greater doses in human volunteers, activated charcoal prevents the GI absorption of nearly all chemicals [116]. In agreement with in vitro studies, as the ratio of activated charcoal to chemical increases, its efficacy increases; with simultaneous dosing of activated charcoal and chemical at a ratio of 10 to 1 or greater, charcoal prevents the absorption of most chemicals by more than 90%. At a constant charcoal to chemical ratio, the efficacy of activated charcoal in preventing chemical absorption increases as the amount and concentration of either agent increases [116,117], suggesting that the efficacy of activated charcoal may be relatively greater after actual overdose than it is after a simulated one. Diluting a dose of activated charcoal and administering it in aliquots by gastric lavage is less effective than administering the same dose as a single concentrated bolus [117]. Administering a dose before and after gastric lavage is more effective than giving one only after lavage.

The interval between administration of toxin and activated charcoal also has a significant effect on the in vivo efficacy of charcoal. As this interval (i.e., the time for uninhibited absorption) increases, the ability of activated charcoal to prevent chemical absorption decreases. In controlled studies using doses of activated charcoal many times greater than those of toxin, charcoal decreased chemical absorption an average of 71% (range, 10% to 100%) when it was given within 5 minutes, 52% (range, 17% to 75%) when given at 30 minutes, and 38%, 34%, 21%, 29%, and 14% when given at 1, 2, 3, 4, and 6 hours, respectively [102,105].

The ability of activated charcoal to prevent the absorption of a toxin in vivo generally correlates with its ability to adsorb that chemical in vitro [116]. However, the absorption of some toxins that are poorly adsorbed by activated charcoal (e.g., cyanide, malathion, tolbutamide) is significantly reduced. Conversely, the absorption of some toxins that are relatively well adsorbed by activated charcoal in vitro (e.g., ethanol, ipecac, *N*-acetylcysteine) is not significantly inhibited in vivo.

The presence of food in the stomach appears to enhance the efficacy of activated charcoal in preventing the absorption of ingested agents, possibly by slowing gastric emptying. Coingested antacids, cathartics, chocolate, ethanol, and excipients have variable but relatively minor or no effect on its efficacy.

Activated charcoal is administered as an aqueous suspension; a minimum of 8 mL of water should be added to each gram of powdered charcoal if a premixed formulation is not available. Premixed product containers should be thoroughly agitated to resuspend sedimented charcoal before use.

Activated charcoal can be given orally to awake patients or by gastric tube to comatose or uncooperative patients. A nipple bottle can be used for infants. Putting the suspension in an opaque container and having the patient sip it through a straw may enhance its acceptability in adults. The recommended dose is at least 10 times the weight of the ingested toxin. Because of volume constraints, the maximum single dose is generally limited to 1 to 2 g per kg of body weight.

Compared with other methods of GI decontamination, the advantages of activated charcoal are ease of administration, rapidity of action, extensively documented safety and efficacy, lack of absolute contraindications, and its ability to enhance toxin elimination (see "Multiple-Dose Activated Charcoal" section of this chapter). The main disadvantages are its color (black), gritty taste, ability to stain clothing (which can limit its acceptance by staff and patients), and low or reversible binding of some chemicals. It can also prevent the enteral absorption and enhance elimination of drugs administered for therapeutic purposes.

In controlled studies in human volunteers, activated charcoal is equal or superior to gastric lavage and emesis in preventing drug absorption [118,119]. Activated charcoal was more effective than gastric lavage and emesis in preventing the absorption of drugs from sustained-release preparations 1 hour after drug ingestion [119] but less effective than whole-bowel irrigation at 4 hours after ingestion [120]. In awake overdose patients, activated charcoal alone caused fewer adverse effects and was equal or superior to syrup of ipecac followed by charcoal in terms of clinical outcome [107–110]. It was equally or more effective than gastric lavage followed by charcoal in obtunded patients [107,108], particularly those who presented more than 1 hour after overdose [108], although this was not observed in patients treated earlier [107]. In asymptomatic overdose patients, there was no difference in clinical outcome between those who were treated with activated charcoal and those who received no decontamination [109].

Activated charcoal is nonreactive and nonabsorbable and has little or no intrinsic toxicity. Adverse effects associated with activated charcoal therapy include nausea, vomiting, abdominal cramps, diarrhea, and constipation. These effects may be related to excessive volumes or rapid administration, concomitant cathartic therapy, prior treatment with syrup of ipecac, or the ingested toxin because they are rarely observed in volunteers given activated charcoal. Aspiration of activated charcoal along with gastric contents can result in large and small airway obstruction, pneumonitis, and death [121–124]. Aspiration of an aqueous suspension of activated charcoal can also increase airway resistance, pulmonary microvascular permeability, and shunt fraction, and decrease vital capacity [125]. If activated charcoal gets into the eyes, it can cause corneal abrasions [124].

Although there are no absolute contraindications, activated charcoal is not recommended for ingestions of acids, alkali, and hydrocarbons that are poorly absorbed and have low systemic toxicity (i.e., low-viscosity petroleum distillates and turpentine) [102,103,105,112,117]. It does not adsorb these corrosives and obscures endoscopic assessment of the extent of injury. With hydrocarbons, it may promote vomiting and increase the risk of pulmonary aspiration.

Gastric Lavage. Gastric lavage can directly remove ingested chemicals from the stomach and thereby prevent their absorption [100]. As with activated charcoal, the efficacy of gastric lavage decreases as time between ingestion and treatment increases. In animal studies and in simulated overdoses using therapeutic or slightly greater doses in human volunteers, gastric lavage decreased chemical absorption an average of 42% (range, 29% to 90%) when performed within 20 minutes of chemical administration, 26% (range, 13% to 38%) when performed at 30 minutes, and 17% (range, 8% to 32%) when performed at 60 minutes [100]. Efficacy is enhanced if activated charcoal is given before and after lavage [115], but not if it is only given afterward [118].

Gastric lavage is performed by first aspirating stomach contents and then repetitively instilling and withdrawing fluid through a nasogastric or orogastric tube [125]. It appears to be most effective if the patient is placed in a left lateral decubitus Trendelenburg position. The left lateral decubitus position has also been shown to delay spontaneous drug absorption [126]. An unknown fraction of gastric contents may enter the duodenum during gastric lavage [127]. Although theoretically reasonable and commonly stated as fact, there is no direct evidence that a large-bore tube (i.e., 28 to 40 Fr) is more effective than a small-bore (i.e., 16 to 18 Fr) tube. On the contrary, no difference in the recovery of either solid (i.e., pill) or liquid formulations with respect to tube size has been found in experimental or clinical [128] studies. Most intact pills do not fit through the lumen of even the largest tube [129]. They are, however, designed to disintegrate rapidly [127]. Hence, unless lavage is accomplished very soon after ingestion, the size of the tube is probably irrelevant.

The simplest, quickest, and least expensive method to use is a funnel connected to the lavage tube, raising it 2 to 3 feet above the level of the stomach when administering fluid and lowering it 2 to 3 feet below the stomach to allow drainage [130].

Tap water is the lavage fluid of choice for patients older than 2 years. Because of the potential for inducing fluid and electrolyte disturbances, normal saline is recommended for younger patients [131]. Using warm fluids may increase pill dissolution and inhibit gastric emptying, and massaging the epigastrium may promote the mixing and suspension of gastric contents and enhance the efficacy of gastric lavage. The optimal volume of fluid for each lavage cycle is unclear. Recommended amounts range from 60 to 800 mL for adults and up to 10 mL per kg of body weight for children [100,125,127]. Larger aliquots (5 to 10 mL per kg body weight) are superior to smaller ones. The majority of chemical recovery occurs with the initial aspiration and first few lavage cycles, but estimation of recovery on the basis of visible pill fragments in the lavage effluent is unreliable [128], probably because most of what is seen consists of insoluble excipients and bears little relation to the amount of drug present. Nevertheless, it is recommended that lavage be continued until the return is relatively clear. It is rarely necessary to use more than 5 L of fluid. Injection of air into the stomach may prevent or alleviate obstructed drainage due to mucosal collapse around lavage tube orifices. When performed successfully, the amount of fluid recovered should be 90% or more of that instilled.

Endotracheal intubation is neither necessary nor sufficient to prevent aspiration during gastric lavage. On the contrary, gastric lavage can safely be performed on awake patients without endotracheal intubation [100,131,132], and the presence of an endotracheal tube does not preclude aspiration [89,100]. In both situations, however, proper positioning is essential. In awake but uncooperative patients, it is intuitively safer to use a small-bore tube rather than a large one. The practice of physically restraining a combative patient and forcibly inserting a large-bore tube invites a mechanical complication (see later) and should be abandoned. If a large-bore tube is deemed necessary (e.g., a witnessed ingestion of a highly lethal quantity of chemical), therapeutic sedation with or without paralysis, along with endotracheal intubation, is recommended. Short-acting agents should be used.

In experimental animal and human studies, gastric lavage is not as effective as activated charcoal [120]. In adult overdose patients, gastric lavage followed by activated charcoal was no more effective in preventing clinical deterioration than charcoal alone [104,108,110], except in comatose patients who presented within 1 hour of ingestion.

Gastric lavage can sometimes recover large amounts of chemicals. However, significant quantities of drugs are recovered in only a small fraction of patients. In acutely inebriated patients, gastric aspiration removed the equivalent of more than 40 mg per dL of ethanol in only 18% [133]. Gastric endoscopy after gastric lavage revealed residual solid in the stomach of 88% of overdose patients [134].

As in experimental studies, the clinical efficacy of gastric lavage decreases as the time between overdose and initiation of treatment increases. The efficacy of gastric lavage increases in cases of toxin induced gastroparesis or decreased intestinal motility.

Gastric lavage can result in significant morbidity and mortality. It is associated with an increased incidence of aspiration and ICU admission [104] and was thought to have contributed to death in 8 of 22 (36%) patients who died after this procedure [135]. Misplacement of the lavage tube in the trachea can result in pneumothorax, pneumonia, and death [136–138]. Malpositioning of the tube, primarily in the esophagus, has been reported in 50% of pediatric patients undergoing gastric lavage [139]. Basing tube insertion length on the child's height or length and radiographic imaging have been suggested as ways to improve and document tube placement. The lavage tube can also become kinked and impacted in the esophagus [140,141]. Because forceful removal can lead to esophageal perforation [141], inserting a flexible pediatric esophagoscope into the lumen of the tube under fluoroscopy and advancing the kinked area into the stomach where the tube can be straightened has been recommended as treatment for this complication. Esophageal spasm can prevent tube removal, a problem that can be reversed by administering glucagon [142]. Esophageal perforation can occur during tube insertion [143]. Laryngospasm [144], hypoxia, ECG changes and dysrhythmias [145], and cardiac arrest [128] have also been reported. Other complications include hematemesis, gastric rupture, charcoal empyema, and pneumoperitoneum [126,140,146,147]. On endoscopy, esophageal and gastric erosions are noted in almost all patients treated by gastric lavage using a large-bore tube [148].

Although there are no absolute contraindications to gastric lavage, its use in corrosive and hydrocarbon ingestions is rarely advisable [100,123,124,147–150]. With corrosives, insertion of a tube may increase the risk of esophageal perforation. Hence, it should be reserved for large ingestions of liquid acid or alkali and for agents that can cause systemic toxicity (e.g., heavy metals, hydrazine), and only done if it can be performed within 1 to 2 hours of exposure. Because lavage may increase the risk of pulmonary aspiration after hydrocarbon ingestion [150], it should be reserved for large ingestions of agents that have systemic toxicity (i.e., camphor, halogenated and aromatic derivatives, and those that contain heavy metals or pesticides).

Syrup of Ipecac. Although syrup of ipecac is simple to use, and was once widely available for home administration, it is less effective than activated charcoal in preventing chemical absorption in experimental studies and has more contraindications [99]. Vomiting exposes patients to aspiration risks and may preclude the administration of activated charcoal or other oral antidotes (e.g., *N*-acetylcysteine). There is virtually no role for Ipecac in the critically ill poisoned patient.

Whole-Bowel Irrigation. *Whole-bowel irrigation* refers to the enteral administration of large volumes of an electrolyte solution. It is commonly used to cleanse the GI tract before colonoscopy, barium enema radiography, and bowel surgery and can prevent the absorption of ingested chemicals by promoting enhancing gut motility [98,101,151–154].

In experimental studies, whole-bowel irrigation decreased chemical absorption by about 70% (range, 67% to 73%) when initiated 1 hour after simulated overdose of ampicillin, paraquat, and sustained-release formulations of aspirin and lithium and 4 hours after a supratherapeutic dose of enteric-coated aspirin [120,154–157]. Whole-bowel irrigation is also a form of dialysis. It has been used in the treatment of uremia [158] and can enhance elimination of previously absorbed chemicals [159]. Whole-bowel irrigation solutions have been found both to enhance [160,161] and to interfere [152–154,157] with the in vitro adsorptive capacity of activated charcoal.

Whole-bowel irrigation is performed by orally administering a solution of electrolytes and polyethylene glycol (e.g., CoLyte, GoLYTELY) at a rate of 0.5 L per hour in children 9 months to 6 years of age, 1 L per hour for 6- to 12-year-olds, and 2 L per hour for those older than 12 years, until the rectal effluent is clear, which typically takes 2 to 4 hours. In the ICU setting, the solution should be administered by nasogastric tube. The head of the bed should remain elevated during treatment.

In human volunteer studies, whole-bowel irrigation was more effective than gastric lavage and more or less effective than activated charcoal in preventing drug absorption [120,154,162]. The combination of charcoal followed by whole-bowel irrigation was more effective than whole-bowel irrigation alone but equally or less effective than charcoal alone [155–157]. Although no controlled studies addressing efficacy in overdose patients have been performed, it may be useful for ingestions of enteric-coated or sustained-release pharmaceuticals, foreign bodies (e.g., bezoars, button batteries, drug packets, lead paint chips), and agents that are poorly adsorbed by activated charcoal (e.g., iron and other metals), and in patients with extremely large ingestions or delayed presentation [102,151–174]. Potential complications of whole-bowel irrigation include regurgitation and aspiration of gastric contents and abdominal distension with cramping [102,151,156,175]. Fluid and electrolyte abnormalities have not been noted. Disadvantages of whole-bowel irrigation are that it is unpleasant, labor intensive, and time-consuming. Contraindications include bowel obstruction, perforation or ileus, and hemodynamic instability. It can be safely performed in intubated obtunded patients.

Endoscopy and Surgery. Gastric endoscopy, using baskets or snares to grasp or break up particulate chemicals, can be used to remove foreign bodies (e.g., button batteries that break apart or fail to pass beyond the pylorus) and gastric pill bezoars or concretions (see Absorption section) [176–178]. It should be reserved for patients with severe or potentially lethal poisoning, such as those with large amounts of heavy metal visible in the stomach on radiograph and those who continue to deteriorate and have rising drug levels despite attempts at GI decontamination by other methods. Endoscopy should never be used for the removal of drug packets, because it may cause rupture and lethal toxicity [179].

Immediate retrieval by laparotomy is indicated for patients who develop toxicity after the ingestion of packets containing cocaine [179]. Surgery should also be considered when

TABLE 117.11

CHEMICALS AND TOXIC SYNDROMES WITH SPECIFIC ANTIDOTES

Agent/condition	Antidotes
Acetaminophen	*N*-acetylcysteine
Anticholinergic poisoning	Physostigmine
Anticoagulants	Phytonadione (vitamin K), protamine
Benzodiazepines	Flumazenil
β-adrenergic antagonists	Glucagon, calcium salts
Calcium channel blockers	Calcium salts, glucagons
Carbon monoxide	Oxygen, hyperbaric oxygen
Cholinergic syndrome	Atropine, pralidoxime
Cyanide	Nitrites, thiosulfate, hydroxycobal
Digoxin (digitalis)	Fab antibody fragments, magnesium
Dystonic reactions	Benztropine, diphenhydramine
Ethylene glycol	Ethanol, 4-methylpyrazole, pyridoxine, thiamine
Envenomations (arthropod, snake)	Antivenins
Fluoride	Calcium and magnesium salts
Heavy metals (arsenic, mercury, lead)	British antilewisite (dimercaprol), dimercaptosuccinic acid, D-penicillamine, calcium disodium, ethylenediaminetetraacetic acid
Hydrogen sulfide	Oxygen, nitrites
Iron	Deferoxamine
Isoniazid (hydrazines)	Gamma-aminobutyric acid agonists, pyridoxine
Methanol	Ethanol, 4-methylpyrazole, folate
Methemoglobinemia	Methylene blue
Opioids	Naloxone, nalmefene, naltrexone
Sympathomimetics	Adrenergic blockers
Vacor (*N*-3-pyridylmethyl-*N*′-*p*-nitrophenylurea)	Nicotinamide (niacinamide)

endoscopic removal is unsuccessful or impossible because of the location of the toxin or foreign body [180,181].

Cathartics. Cathartics are osmotically active saccharides (e.g., mannitol, sorbitol) or salts (e.g., magnesium citrate, magnesium sulfate, disodium phosphate) that cause retention of fluids within the gut, thereby stimulating GI motility and the evacuation of intestinal contents [96,97,124,149,182–184]. In animal and human volunteer studies, cathartics have variable but clinically insignificant effects on chemical absorption [96,97]. Their effect on the efficacy of activated charcoal is also minimal and clinically insignificant [185–189]. There is currently no role for cathartics in the critically ill poisoned patient.

Dilution. The administration of water, milk, or other drinkable liquids is now recommended as a primary treatment only for corrosive ingestions [190]. In this setting, dilution may lower the concentration of chemical and limit its toxicity. To be effective, dilution should be accomplished as soon as possible. The volume of fluid should not exceed 5 mL per kg, because larger amounts may induce vomiting and cause further esophageal exposure. Dilution is no longer recommended to prevent toxin absorption. It may facilitate the dissolution of solid chemicals, increase the amount of chemical in solution, and stimulate gastric emptying, thereby enhancing chemical absorption.

Antidotal Therapy

Antidotes directly or indirectly counteract the effects of toxins [15,18,191–195]. They can be classified as *selective* or *nonselective*. Selective antidotes act by competing with chemicals for target sites or metabolic pathways, by binding and neutralizing them (e.g., antibodies and chelators), by promoting their metabolic detoxification, and by antagonizing their autonomic effects via activation or inhibition of opposing neuronal pathways (see Table 117.11). Nonselective antidotes act by correcting metabolic derangements or enhancing nonmetabolic toxin elimination.

Although antidotes can reduce morbidity and mortality, few are available and most are potentially harmful, and reasonable diagnostic certainty is necessary for their safe and effective use. Specific indications, contraindications, dosing, and potential complications are discussed in the chapters that deal with specific poisonings. A summary Table of antidotes can be found in the Appendix.

Enhancement of Elimination

The nonmetabolic elimination of most toxins can be accelerated by therapeutic interventions such as diuresis, urine alkalization, GI dialysis (i.e., multiple-dose activated charcoal or whole-bowel irrigation), and extracorporeal techniques. To be of potential clinical importance, a significant fraction (i.e., 25%) of the dose must be removed, or the rate of elimination, as assessed by clearance or half-life, must be significantly greater (i.e., 25%) than that accomplished by intrinsic mechanisms.

All enhanced elimination procedures are associated with potential complications, and some require specialized equipment and expertise. Reasonable diagnostic certainty is generally a prerequisite to their use. In general, invasive elimination procedures should be reserved for patients with severe poisoning who deteriorate or fail to improve despite aggressive supportive care, antidotal therapy, and noninvasive methods of toxin removal [196–199].

Diuresis and Manipulation of Urinary pH

Maintenance of a dilute urine flow enhances toxin excretion by decreasing the passive distal tubular reabsorption of toxins that have undergone glomerular filtration and proximal tubular secretion [14–18,196–200]. Increasing urinary pH (considered neutral at a pH of 6) can enhance the renal excretion of acidic toxins by the mechanism known as ion trapping. Like all membranes, those of the nephron, particularly the distal tubule, are generally more permeable to nonionized and nonpolar molecules than to ionized and polar ones. After filtration and secretion, nonionized forms of weak acids or become ionized and trapped in an alkaline urine. Diuresis and urinary alkalinization act synergistically [201].

Diuresis alone can enhance the renal excretion of alcohols, bromide, calcium, fluoride, lithium, meprobamate, potassium, and isoniazid. Except for calcium and potassium, however, clinical efficacy remains unproven.

Alkalinization of the urine can enhance the excretion of the chlorophenoxy acetic acid herbicide 2,4-D (and probably 2,4,5-T), chlorpropamide, diflunisal, fluoride, methotrexate, phenobarbital (and probably other long-acting barbiturates), sulfonamides, and salicylates. Only for phenobarbital and salicylate poisoning is urinary alkalization accepted as clinically effective [202].

The goal of diuresis is a urine flow of 3 to 8 mL per kg per hour and that of alkalinization is a urine pH of 7.5 or greater. IV administration of 0.9% saline (sodium chloride) is used for inducing diuresis. An alkaline diuresis solution can be prepared by adding three ampules (132 mEq) of sodium bicarbonate to dextrose 5% in water such that the final solution is nearly isotonic. Fluids are administered roughly at the same rate as the desired urine output. Acetazolamide should not be used to produce an alkaline urine, because it may worsen toxicity by causing a concomitant systemic acidosis, resulting in an increase in the amount of unionized drug in the blood and enhanced tissue distribution [203]. It may also compete with acidic drugs for tubular secretion and thereby inhibit their elimination.

Acid–base status, fluid balance, electrolyte parameters, and clinical response must be carefully monitored during therapy. Urine pH should be measured hourly.

Multiple-Dose Activated Charcoal

Repetitive activated charcoal administration can enhance the elimination of previously absorbed chemicals by binding them within the GI tract as they are excreted in the bile, secreted by cells of the stomach or intestine, or passively diffuse into the lumen of the gut [116,204–206]. The charcoal–chemical complex is then excreted with stool. In most cases, reverse absorption (enterocapillary exsorption) is the mechanism, with the entire surface of the gut acting as a dialysis membrane. Activated charcoal keeps the concentration of free toxin in gut fluids near zero, and chemicals merely diffuse from blood perfusing the gut into luminal fluids as a result of concentration gradients. Interruption of enterohepatic or enteroenteric recirculation appears to be the underlying mechanism of action for a minority of toxins. Theoretically, multiple-dose charcoal can enhance the elimination of any chemical whose absorption is decreased by a single dose. Efficacy is predicted to be greatest for chemicals with a high charcoal binding capacity, physical and pharmacokinetic characteristics that make them amenable to removal by extracorporeal methods (see later), and a long intrinsic elimination half-life (e.g., amiodarone, isotretinoin, organochlorine pesticides, organometallic compounds) [207].

Multiple-dose activated charcoal enhances the elimination of most chemicals regardless of whether the chemical is administered orally or parenterally [206]. As with most forms of decontamination, the clinical efficacy of this therapy remains unproven [208]. Although clinically significant reductions in half-life have been noted in patients with carbamazepine, dapsone, phenobarbital, quinine, and theophylline overdose, there are no prospective studies showing that this therapy reduces morbidity or mortality [206].

The efficacy of multiple-dose activated charcoal increases as the cumulative amount of charcoal administered increases, either by increasing the amount or frequency of charcoal dosing [209]. When the cumulative amount of charcoal remains constant, there is no difference in the efficacy of different dosing regimens (e.g., 25 g every 2 hours vs. 50 g every 4 hours) [210]. With normal bowel activity, doses of activated charcoal of 0.5 to 1.0 g per kg every 4 hours are generally well tolerated. In those with decreased GI motility, smaller doses or less frequent intervals should be used. Alternatively, charcoal can be given by a slow, continuous nasogastric infusion. This method of administration may also be better for patients who cannot retain charcoal because of vomiting. Metoclopramide and odansetron (or other serotonergic antiemetics) can also be given to control or prevent vomiting. Gastric aspiration should be performed before repeating the dose of charcoal. In the event of gastrostaxis, regurgitation, or abdominal distension, treatment should be withheld.

Complications of multiple-dose activated charcoal are similar to those for charcoal used for GI decontamination. In addition, intestinal obstruction, pseudo-obstruction, and nonocclusive intestinal infarction have been reported in patients with decreased bowel motility treated with multiple doses of activated charcoal [211–215].

Extracorporeal Methods

Peritoneal dialysis, hemodialysis, hemoperfusion, hemofiltration, plasmapheresis, and exchange transfusion are theoretically capable of removing any chemical from the blood [210,216–222]. There remains very little evidence regarding the efficacy of continuous renal replacement therapy in the management of human poisonings. Most toxins undergo significant tissue distribution, and few remain in the blood in amounts high enough to warrant extracorporeal removal. Hemodialysis is therefore most effective for toxins with volumes of distribution less than 1 L per kg. In addition, with dialysis techniques, only toxins that are small (i.e., molecular weight less than 500 to 1,500 Da), water soluble, uncharged, and not highly bound to serum proteins (90% to 95% or less) readily diffuse across dialysis membranes. (Table 117.12)

The clearance of a toxin by extracorporeal removal must be significantly greater than its intrinsic total body clearance (i.e., the sum of metabolic, renal, and other routes of clearance) to be considered effective from a pharmacokinetic perspective. As with other treatments, their clinical efficacy (i.e., ability to decrease morbidity and mortality) is based on observation, experience, and retrospective comparisons rather than on controlled prospective studies.

Hemodialysis is considered effective for the treatment of barbiturate, bromide, chloral hydrate, ethanol, ethylene glycol, isopropyl alcohol, lithium, methanol, procainamide, acetaminophen, theophylline, salicylate, and possibly heavy metal poisoning [196–198]. Because hemodialysis can remove toxins from the blood faster than they can redistribute from tissue to blood, a rebound increase in blood concentration and clinical relapse may occur within 1 or 2 hours of treatment.

Other techniques are less effective than hemodialysis. Peritoneal dialysis may be useful when these methods are not

TABLE 117.12

PROPERTIES OF A DIALYZABLE TOXIN

1. Small volume of distribution
2. Low molecular weight
3. Water soluble
4. Uncharged
5. Low protein binding

available or technically difficult (e.g., in neonates) or when anticoagulation may be hazardous [197,198]. Complications include infection, injury to intra-abdominal organs, and hypothermia. Plasma exchange may also be a useful alternative in neonates. It is effective for treating hemolysis (e.g., arsine poisoning) and methemoglobinemia. Two blood-volume exchanges are usually performed using central or peripheral arteriovenous or venovenous access. Complications include transfusion reactions and hypothermia. The roles of hemofiltration and plasmapheresis in the treatment of poisoning remain to be defined [219–222].

Safe Disposition

ICU admission is recommended for patients with coma, refractory hemodynamic instability, respiratory depression, seizures, and/or dysrhythmias [223,224]. Patients with extremes of temperature, severe agitation, or life-threatening metabolic abnormalities also benefit from intensive care. CNS depression may be the best predictor of serious complications [7]. Patients who are less ill, stable, or even asymptomatic are frequently unnecessarily admitted to the ICU because of physician uncertainty, fear of late deterioration and potential litigation, and lack of an alternative monitored setting. Some patients may require close observation and cardiac monitoring; but unless active interventions are likely to be necessary, admission to an intermediate care unit, telemetry unit, or emergency department observation unit is adequate. Length of hospital stay in patients with self-poisoning can be reduced by use of a multidisciplinary team that involves a toxicologist and psychiatrist as well as medical personnel [225].

Prevention of Recurrence

Suicidal patients require psychiatric assessment. If they are given prescriptions, the amount of drug (e.g., a 1- to 2-week supply) and number of refills should be limited. Substance abusers should be counseled regarding attendant medical risks and given the opportunity for rehabilitation through referral for behavior modification, supervised withdrawal, and abstinence or maintenance therapy.

Adults with accidental poisoning should be educated regarding the safe use of drugs and other chemicals. Assistance with the administration of medications may be required for visually impaired, elderly, developmentally delayed, or confused patients. Preventive education may be indicated for health care providers who have committed dosing errors or who are unaware of adverse drug interactions. When poisoning results from environmental or workplace exposure, the appropriate governmental agency (e.g., Environmental Protection Agency; Occupational Safety and Health Administration; National Institute of Occupational Safety and Health; or local, state, or federal health departments) should be notified. Unsafe working conditions should be brought to the attention of employers. Industrial hygiene and occupational health services should be offered if available. Finally, physicians have a duty to warn the general public (e.g., via press releases) of acute environmental hazard.

References

1. Veltri JC, McElwee NE, Schumacher MC: Interpretation and uses of data collected in poison control centres in the United States. *Med Toxicol* 2:389, 1987.
2. Bronstein AC, Spyker DA, Cantilena LR, et al: 2007 Annual Report of the American Association of Poison Control Centers' National Poison Data System: 25th Annual Report. *Clin Toxicol* 46:927–1057, 2008.
3. Strom J, Thisted B, Kranz T, et al: Self-poisoning treated in an ICU. drug pattern, acute mortality, and short-term survival. *Acta Anaesthesiol Scand* 30:148, 1986.
4. Proudfoot A: Acute poisoning: principles of management. *Med Int* 61:2499, 1989.
5. Henderson A, Wright M, Pond SM: Experience with 732 acute overdose patients admitted to an intensive care unit over six years. *Med J Aust* 158:28, 1993.
6. McCaig LF, Burt CW: Poisoning-related visits to emergency departments in the United States, 1993–1996. *Clin Toxicol* 37:817, 1999.
7. Heyman EN, LoCastro DE, Gouse LH, et al: Intentional drug overdose: predictors of clinical course in the intensive care unit. *Heart Lung* 25:246–252, 1996.
8. Zimmerman JE, Wagner DP, Draper EA, et al: Evaluation of acute physiology and chronic health evaluation: III. Predictions of hospital mortality in an independent database. *Crit Care Med* 26:1317, 1998.
9. Bosch TM, van der Werf TS, Uges DRA, et al: Antidepressants self-poisoning and ICU admissions in a university hospital in the Netherlands. *Pharm World Sci* 22:92–95, 2000.
10. Walton WW: An evaluation of the Poison Packaging Act. *Pediatrics* 69:363, 1982.
11. Centers for Disease Control and Prevention: Unintentional poisoning deaths—United States, 1999–2004. *MMWR Morb Mortal Wkly Rep* 56: 93–96, 2007.
12. Hoppe-Roberts JM, Lloyd LM, Chyka PA: Poisoning mortality in the United States: comparison of national mortality statistics and poison control center reports. *Ann Emerg Med* 35:440, 2000.
13. Kearns GL, Abdel-Rahman SM, Alander SW, et al: Developmental pharmacology—drug disposition, action, and therapy in infants and children. *N Engl J Med* 349:1157, 2003.
14. Hardman JG, Limbird LE, Goodman AG (eds): *Goodman and Gilman's The Pharmacological Basis of Therapeutics*. 10th ed. New York, McGraw-Hill, 2001.
15. Klassen CD (ed): *Casarett and Doull's Toxicology: The Basic Science of Poisons*. 6th ed. New York, McGraw-Hill, 2001.
16. Munson PL, Mueller RA, Breese GR: *Principles of Pharmacology: Basic Concepts and Clinical Applications*. New York, Chapman and Hall, 1996.
17. Niesink RJM, de Vries J, Hollinger MA: *Toxicology: Principles and Practice*. Boca Raton, FL, CRC Press, 1996.
18. Golfrank LR, Flomenbaun NE, Lewin NA, et al (eds): *Goldfrank's Toxicologic Emergencies*. 7th ed. New York, McGraw-Hill, 2002.
19. Clayton GD, Clayton FE (eds): *Patty's Industrial Hygiene and Toxicology.* 5th ed. New York, John Wiley and Sons, 2001.
20. Baselt RC: *Disposition of Toxic Drugs and Chemicals in Man*. 7th ed. Foster City, CA, Biomedical Publications, 2004.
21. Sweetman S (ed): *Martindale: The Complete Drug Reference*. 36th ed. London, Pharmaceutical Press, 2009.
22. Dart RC (ed): *Medical Toxicology*. 3rd ed. Philadelphia, Lippincott Williams & Wilkins, 2004.
23. McEvoy GK (ed): *AHFS Drug Information*. Bethesda, MD, American Society of Health-System Pharmacists, published yearly, 2011.
24. Sullivan JB, Krieger GR (eds): *Clinical Environmental Health and Toxic Exposures*. 2nd ed. Philadelphia, Lippincott Williams & Wilkins, 2001.
25. Ford MD, Delaney KA, Ling LJ, et al (eds): *Clinical Toxicology*. Philadelphia, WB Saunders, 2001.
26. Brent J, Wallace KL, Burkhart KK, et al (eds): *Critical Care Toxicology: Diagnosis and Management of the Critically Poisoned Patient*. Philadelphia, Elsevier Mosby, 2005.
27. *Poisindex System*. Greenwood Village, CO, Thomson Micromedex, updated quarterly.

28. Kulig K: Initial management of ingestions of toxic substances. *N Engl J Med* 326:1677, 1992.
29. June R, Aks SE, Keys N, et al: Medical outcome of cocaine bodystuffers. *J Emerg Med* 18:221, 2000.
30. Traub SJ, Hoffman RS, Nelson LS: Body packing—the internal concealment of illicit drugs. *N Engl J Med* 349:2519, 2003.
31. Rivara FP, Mueller BA, Fligner CL: Drug Use in Trauma Victims. *J Trauma* 29:4, 1989.
32. Fitzgerald FT, Tierney LM: The bedside Sherlock Holmes. *West J Med* 137:169, 1982.
33. Wright N: An assessment of the unreliability of the history given by self-poisoned patients. *Clin Toxicol* 16:381, 1980.
34. Federal Hazardous Substances Act, October 14, 2008 version, 15 U.S.C. 1261 et seq.
35. Greenberg MI, Cone DC, Roberts JR: Material safety data sheet: a useful resource for the emergency physician. *Ann Emerg Med* 27:347, 1996.
36. Ashton CH, Teoh R, Davies DM: Drug-induced stupor: some physical signs and their pharmacological basis. *Adverse Drug React Acute Poisoning Rev* 8:1, 1989.
37. Jones TF, Craig AS, Hoy D, et al: Mass psychogenic illness attributed to toxic exposure at a high school. *N Engl J Med* 342:96, 2000.
38. Olson KR, Kearney TE, Dyer JE, et al: Seizures associated with poisoning and drug overdose. *Am J Emerg Med* 11:565, 1993.
39. Salem MM, Mujais SK: Gaps in the anion gap. *Arch Intern Med* 152:1625, 1992.
40. Aabakken L, Johansen KS, Rydningen EB, et al: Osmolal and anion gaps in patients admitted to an emergency medical department. *Hum Exp Toxicol* 13:131, 1994.
41. Kirschbaum B: The acidosis of exogenous phosphate intoxication. *Arch Intern Med* 158:405, 1998.
42. Schwartz SM, Carroll HM, Schoschmidt LA: Sublimed (inorganic) sulfur ingestion: a cause of life-threatening metabolic high anion gap. *Arch Intern Med* 146:1437, 1986.
43. Linden CH, Townsend PL: Clinical and laboratory observations: metabolic acidosis after acute ibuprofen overdosage. *J Pediatr* 111:922, 1987.
44. Andersen GO, Ritland S: Life threatening intoxication with sodium valproate. *Clin Toxicol* 33:279, 1995.
45. Gan SC, Barr J, Arieff AI, et al: Biguanide-associated lactic acidosis: case report and review of the literature. *Arch Intern Med* 152:2333, 1992.
46. Brinkman K, Hofstede HJ, Burger DM, et al: Adverse effects of reverse transcriptase inhibitors: mitochondrial toxicity as common pathway. *AIDS* 12:1735, 1998.
47. Roth B, Woo O, Blanc P: Early metabolic acidosis and coma after acetaminophen ingestion. *Ann Emerg Med* 33:452, 1999.
48. Senecal PE, Dyer JE, Osterloh JD: Nitrate as a cause of decreased anion gap. *Vet Hum Toxicol* 33:375, 1991.
49. Sporer KA, Mayer AP: Saltpeter ingestion. *Am J Emerg Med* 9:164, 1991.
50. Koga Y, Purssell RA, Lynd LD: The irrationality of the present use of the osmole gap: applicable physical chemistry principle and recommendations to improve validity of current practices. *Toxicol Rev* 23:203, 2004.
51. Purssell RA, Lynd LD, Koga Y: The use of the osmole gap as a screening test for the presence of exogenous substances. *Toxicol Rev* 23:189, 2004.
52. Schelling JR, Howard RL, Winter SD, et al: Increased osmolal gap in alcoholic ketoacidosis and lactic acidosis. *Ann Intern Med* 113:580, 1990.
53. Blossom AP, Cleary JD, Daley WP: Acyclovir-induced crystalluria. *Ann Pharmacother* 36:526, 2002.
54. Rengstorff DS, Milstone AP, Seger DL, et al: Felbamate overdose complicated by massive crystalluria and acute renal failure. *Clin Toxicol* 38:667, 2000.
55. Tsao JW, Kogan SC: Indinavir crystalluria. *N Engl J Med* 340:1329, 1999.
56. Sanz P, Reig R: Clinical and pathological findings in fatal plant oxalosis. A review. *Am J Forensic Med Pathol* 13:342, 1992.
57. Van Heijst ANP, deJong W, Seldenrijk R, et al: Coma and crystalluria: a massive primidone intoxication treated with hemoperfusion. *Clin Toxicol* 20:307, 1983.
58. Simon DI, Brosius FC, Rothstein DM: Sulfadiazine crystalluria revisited. *Arch Intern Med* 150:2379, 1990.
59. Bradberry SM, Vale JA: Disturbances of potassium homeostasis in poisoning. *Clin Toxicol* 33:295, 1995.
60. Gennari FJ: Hypokalemia. *N Engl J Med* 339:451, 1998.
61. Lewis JH, Zimmerman HJ: Drug-induced liver disease. *Med Clin North Am* 73:775, 1989.
62. Abuelo JG: Renal failure caused by chemicals, foods, plants, animal venoms, and misuse of drugs: an overview. *Arch Intern Med* 150:505, 1990.
63. Richards JR: Rhabdomyolysis and drugs of abuse. *J Emerg Med* 19:51, 2000.
64. Boon NA: Solvent abuse and the heart. *BMJ* 294:722, 1987.
65. Stratmann HG, Kennedy HL: Torsades de pointes associated with drugs and toxins: recognition and management. *Am Heart J* 113:1470, 1987.
66. Vukimir RB: Torsades de pointes: a review. *Am J Emerg Med* 9:250, 1991.
67. Savitt DL, Hawkins HH, Roberts JR: The radiopacity of ingested medications. *Ann Emerg Med* 16:331, 1987.
68. Eng JGH, Aks SE, Waldron R, et al: False-negative abdominal CT scan in a cocaine body stuffer. *Am J Emerg Med* 17:702, 1999.
69. Hergan K, Kofler K, Oser W: Drug Smuggling by Body Packing: what radiologists should know about it. *Eur Radiol* 14, 2004.
70. Amitai Y, Silver B, Leikin JG, et al: Detection of tablets in the gastrointestinal tract by ultrasound. *Am J Emerg Med* 10:18, 1992.
71. Pragst F, Balikova MA: State of the art in hair analysis for detection of drug and alcohol use. *Clin Chim Acta* 370:1–2, 2006.
72. Reed CR, Glauser FL: Drug-induced noncardiogenic pulmonary edema. *Chest* 100:1120, 1991.
73. Klein J, Chitayat D, Koren G: Hair analysis as a marker for fetal exposure to maternal smoking. *NEJM* 328(11):67, 1993.
74. Osterloh JD: Utility and reliability of emergency toxicologic testing. *Emerg Med Clin North Am* 8:693, 1990.
75. Kozer E, Vergee Z, Koren G: Misdiagnosis of a mexiletine overdose because of a nonspecific result of urinary toxicologic screening. *N Engl J Med* 343:1971, 2000.
76. Mahoney JD, Gross PL, Stern TA, et al: Quantitative serum toxic screening in the management of suspected drug overdose. *Am J Emerg Med* 8:16, 1990.
77. Belson MG, Simon HK: Utility of comprehensive toxicologic screens in children. *Am J Emerg Med* 17:221, 1999.
78. Fabbri A, Ruggeri S, Marchesni G, et al: A combined HPLC-immunoenzymatic comprehensive screening for suspected drug poisoning in the emergency department. *Emerg Med J* 21:317, 2004.
79. Eisen JS: Screening urine for drugs of abuse in the emergency department: do test results affect physician's patient care decisions? *Can J Emerg Med* 6:104, 2004.
80. Tomaszewski C, Runge J, Gibbs M, et al: Evaluation of a rapid bedside toxicology screen in patients suspected of drug toxicity. *J Emerg* 28:389, 2005.
81. Hepler BR, Sutheimer CA, Sunshine I: Role of the toxicology laboratory in the treatment of acute poisoning. *Med Toxicol* 1:61, 1986.
82. Ashley DL, Needham U: Assessment of a scheme for prioritizing inorganic intoxicants by using signs-and-symptoms analysis. *Clin Toxicol* 24:375, 1986.
83. Nice A, Leikin JB, Maturen A: Toxidrome recognition to improve efficiency of emergency urine drug screens. *Ann Emerg Med* 17:676, 1988.
84. Alderman D, Burke M, Cohen B, et al: How adequate are warnings and first aid instructions on consumer product labels? An investigation. *Vet Hum Toxicol* 24:8, 1982.
85. Saylor JH: Volume of a swallow: role of orifice size and viscosity. *Vet Hum Toxicol* 29:79, 1987.
86. Bar-Oz B, Levichek Z, Koren G: Medications that can be fatal for a toddler with one tablet or teaspoonful: a 2004 update. *Paediatr Drugs* 6:123, 2004.
87. Mackaway-Jones K, Moulton C: Gag reflex and intubation. *Emerg Med J* 16:444, 1999.
88. Adnet F, Borron SW, Finot MA, et al: Intubation difficulty in poisoned patients: association with initial Glasgow Coma Scale score. *Acad Emerg Med* 5:123, 1998.
89. Moll J, Kerns W, Tomaszewski C, et al: Incidence of aspiration in intubated patients receiving activated charcoal. *J Emerg Med* 17:279, 1999.
90. Torres A, Serva-Battles J, Ros E, et al: Pulmonary aspiration of gastric contents in patients receiving mechanical ventilation: the effect of body position. *Ann Intern Med* 116:540, 1992.
91. Purkayastha S, Bhangoo P, Athanasiou T, et al: Treatment of poisoning induced cardiac impairment using cardiopulmonary bypass: a review. *Emerg Med J* 23:246, 2006.
92. Herr RD, White GL, Bernhisel K, et al: Clinical comparison of ocular irrigation fluids following chemical injury. *Am J Emerg Med* 9:228, 1991.
93. Jones JB, Schoenleber DB, Gillen JP: The tolerability of lactated Ringer's solution and BSS Plus for ocular irrigation with and without the Morgan therapeutic lens. *Acad Emerg Med* 5:1150, 1998.
94. Ernst AA, Thomson T, Haynes M, et al: Warmed versus room temperature saline solution of ocular irrigation: a randomized clinical trial. *Ann Emerg Med* 32:676, 1998.
95. Wester RC, Maibach HI: In vivo percutaneous absorption and decontamination of pesticides in humans. *J Toxicol Environ Health* 16:25, 1985.
96. American Academy of Clinical Toxicology and European Association of Poisons Centre and Clinical Toxicologists: Position statement: cathartics. *Clin Toxicol* 35:743, 1997.
97. American Academy of Clinical Toxicology and European Association of Poisons Centre and Clinical Toxicologists: Position paper: cathartics. *Clin Toxicol* 42:243, 2004.
98. American Academy of Clinical Toxicology and European Association of Poisons Centre and Clinical Toxicologists: Position statement: whole bowel irrigation. *Clin Toxicol* 35:753, 1997.
99. American Academy of Clinical Toxicology and European Association of Poisons Centre and Clinical Toxicologists: Position paper: ipecac syrup. *Clin Toxicol* 42:133, 2004.
100. American Academy of Clinical Toxicology and European Association of Poisons Centre and Clinical Toxicologists: Position paper: gastric lavage. *Clin Toxicol* 42:933, 2004.
101. American Academy of Clinical Toxicology and European Association of Poisons Centre and Clinical Toxicologists: Position paper: whole bowel irrigation. *Clin Toxicol* 42:843, 2004.
102. American Academy of Clinical Toxicology and European Association of Poisons Centre and Clinical Toxicologists: Position paper: single-dose activated charcoal. *Clin Toxicol* 43:61, 2005.

103. Eddleston M, Juszczak E, Buckley N, et al: Multiple-dose activated charcoal in acute self-poisoning: a randomized controlled trial. *Lancet* 371:597–607, 2008.
104. Merigian KS, Woodard M, Hedges JR, et al: Prospective evaluation of gastric emptying in the self-poisoned patient. *Am J Emerg Med* 8:479, 1990.
105. Underhill TJ, Greene MK, Dove AR: A comparison of the efficacy of gastric lavage, ipecacuanha, and activated charcoal in the emergency management of paracetamol overdose. *Arch Emerg Med* 7:148, 1990.
106. Kornberg AE, Dolgin J: Pediatric ingestions: charcoal alone versus ipecac and charcoal. *Ann Emerg Med* 20:648, 1991.
107. Bosse GM, Barefoot JA, Pfeifer MP, et al: Comparison of three methods of gut decontamination in tricyclic antidepressant overdose. *J Emerg Med* 13:203, 1995.
108. Pond SM, Lewos-Driver DJ, Williams GM, et al: Gastric emptying in acute overdose: a prospective randomised controlled trial. *Med J Aust* 163:345, 1995.
109. Cooper GM, Le Couteur DG, Richardson D, et al: A randomized clinical trial of activated charcoal for the routine management of oral drug overdose. *Clin Toxicol* 40:313, 2002.
110. Merigian KS, Blaho K: Single dose activated charcoal in the treatment of the self-poisoned patient: a prospective controlled trial. *Am J Ther* 9:301, 2002.
111. Kulig KW: Gastric lavage in acute drug overdose. *JAMA* 262:1392, 1989.
112. Olson KR: Is gut emptying all washed up? *Am J Emerg Med* 8:560, 1990.
113. Bond GR: The role of activated charcoal and gastric lavage in gastrointestinal decontamination: a state-of-the-art review. *Ann Emerg Med* 39:273, 2002.
114. American Academy of Pediatrics Committee on Injury, Violence, and Poison Prevention: Poison treatment in the home. *Pediatrics* 112:1182, 2003.
115. Manoguerra AS, Cobaugh DJ, and Members of the Guidelines for the Management of Poisonings Consensus Panel of the American Association of Poison Control Centers: Guideline on the use of ipecac syrup in the out-of-hospital management of ingested poisons. *Clin Toxicol* 1:1, 2005.
116. Palatnick W, Tenenbein M: Activated charcoal in the treatment of drug overdose: an update. *Drug Saf* 7:3, 1992.
117. Graudins A, Linden CH: The effect of charcoal and drug concentrations on the adsorption of acetaminophen to activated charcoal. *Clin Toxicol* 34:594, 1996.
118. Lapatto-Reiniluoto O, Kivisto KT, Neuvonen JP: Effect of activated charcoal alone or given after gastric lavage in reducing the absorption of diazepam, ibuprofen and citalopram. *Br J Clin Pharmacol* 48:148, 1999.
119. Minton NA, Glucksman E, Henry JA: Prevention of drug absorption in simulated theophylline overdose. *Hum Exp Toxicol* 14:170, 1995.
120. Kirschenbaum LA, Mathews SC, Sitar DS, et al: Whole-bowel irrigation versus activated charcoal in sorbitol for the ingestion of modified-release pharmaceuticals. *Clin Pharmacol Ther* 46:264, 1989.
121. Elliot CG, Colby TV, Kelly TM, et al: Charcoal lung: bronchiolitis obliterans after aspiration of activated charcoal. *Chest* 96:672, 1989.
122. Seger D: Single-dose activated charcoal—backup and re-assess. *Clin Toxicol* 42:101, 2004.
123. Arnold TC, Willis BH, Xiao F, et al: Aspiration of activated charcoal elicits an increase in lung microvascular permeability. *Clin Toxicol* 37:9, 1999.
124. McKinney P, Phillips S, Gomez HF, et al: Corneal abrasions secondary to activated charcoal. *Am J Emerg Med* 11:562, 1993.
125. Wheeler-Usher DH, Wanke LA, Bayer MJ: Gastric emptying: risk versus benefit in the treatment of acute poisoning. *Med Toxicol* 1:142, 1986.
126. Vance MV, Selden BS, Clark RF: Optimal patient position for transport and initial management of toxic ingestions. *Ann Emerg Med* 21:243, 1992.
127. Saetta JP, March S, Gaunt ME, et al: Gastric emptying procedures in the self-poisoned patient: are we forcing gastric content beyond the pylorus? *J R Soc Med* 84:274, 1991.
128. Watson WA, Leighton J, Guy J, et al: Recovery of cyclic antidepressants with gastric lavage. *J Emerg Med* 7:373, 1989.
129. Agocha A, Reyman L, Longmore W, et al: Can pills really fit through the lavage tubes? [abstract]. *Vet Hum Toxicol* 28:494, 1986.
130. Shrestha M, George J, Chiu MJ, et al: A comparison of three gastric lavage methods using the radionuclide gastric emptying study. *J Emerg Med* 14:413, 1996.
131. Rudolph JP: Automated gastric lavage and a comparison of 0.9% normal saline solution and tap water irrigant. *Ann Emerg Med* 14:1156, 1985.
132. Thomas RT, Sterling ML, Salness K, et al: Absence of pulmonary aspiration in adults after gastric lavage without endotracheal intubation [abstract]. *Vet Hum Toxicol* 23[Suppl 1]:57, 1981.
133. Gough D, Rust D: Nasogastric intubation: morbidity in an asymptomatic patient. *Am J Emerg Med* 4:511, 1986.
134. Coutselinis A, Plulos L, Boukis D, et al: A lethal complication of gastric lavage leading to malpractice suit: a case report. *Forensic Sci Int* 11:47, 1978.
135. Thomas B, Cummin D, Falcone RE: Accidental pneumothorax from a nasogastric tube. *N Engl J Med* 335:1325, 1996.
136. Scalzo AJ, Tominack RL, Thompson MW: Malposition of pediatric gastric lavage tubes demonstrated radiographically. *J Emerg Med* 13:219, 1995.
137. Calvanese JC: Midesophageal kinking and lodgment of a 34-F gastric lavage tube. *Ann Emerg Med* 14:1123, 1985.
138. Wald P, Stern J, Weiner B, et al: Esophageal tear following forceful removal of an impacted oral-gastric lavage tube. *Ann Emerg Med* 15:80, 1985.
139. Weiner BC: Management of oral-gastric lavage tube impaction of the esophagus. *Am J Gastroenterol* 81:1202, 1986.
140. Thoma ME, Glauser JM: Use of glucagon for removal of an orogastric lavage tube. *Am J Emerg Med* 13:219, 1995.
141. Askenasi R, Abramowicz M, Jeanmart J, et al: Esophageal perforation: an unusual complication of gastric lavage. *Ann Emerg Med* 13:146, 1984.
142. Thompson AM, Robins JB, Prescott LF: Changes in cardiorespiratory function during gastric lavage for drug overdose. *Hum Toxicol* 6:215, 1987.
143. Justiniani FR, Hippalgoankar R, Martinez LO: Charcoal-containing empyema complicating treatment for overdose. *Chest* 87:404, 1985.
144. Mariani PJ, Pook N: Gastrointestinal tract perforation with charcoal peritoneum complicating intubation and lavage. *Ann Emerg Med* 22:606, 1993.
145. Chaudel S, Ducluzeau R, Pacheco Y, et al: Endoscopic gastric lesions after a gastric washing-out using the Faucher tube in intoxicated comatose patients [abstract]. *Vet Hum Toxicol* 24:287, 1982.
146. Penner GE: Acid ingestion: toxicology and treatment. *Ann Emerg Med* 9:374, 1984.
147. Friedman EM, Lovejoy FH: The emergency management of caustic ingestions. *Emerg Med Clin North Am* 2:77, 1984.
148. Howel JM: Alkaline ingestions. *Ann Emerg Med* 15:820, 1986.
149. Okada Y, Iway A, Kobayashi H: Gastric lavage solution for ingestion of corrosive agents. *Jpn J Acute Med* 11:75, 1987.
150. Seger DL: The hydrocarbon controversy. *Emerg Med Surv* 1:1, 1984.
151. Tenenbein M: Whole bowel irrigation as a gastrointestinal decontamination procedure after acute poisoning. *Med Toxicol* 3:77, 1988.
152. Tennenbein M: Whole bowel irrigation for toxic ingestions. *Clin Toxicol* 23:177, 1985.
153. Tenenbein M: Whole bowel irrigation in iron poisoning. *J Pediatr* 111:142, 1987.
154. Tenenbein M, Cohen S, Sitar DS: Whole bowel irrigation as a decontamination procedure after acute drug overdose. *Arch Intern Med* 147:905, 1987.
155. Smith SW, Ling LJ, Halstenson CE: Whole-bowel irrigation as a treatment for acute lithium overdose. *Ann Emerg Med* 20:536, 1991.
156. Mizutani T, Yamashita M, Okubo N, et al: Efficacy of whole bowel irrigation using solutions with or without adsorbent in the removal of paraquat in dogs. *Hum Exp Toxicol* 11:495, 1992.
157. Kirshenbaum LA, Sitar DS, Tenenbein M: Interaction between whole-bowel irrigation solution and activated charcoal: implications for the treatment of toxic ingestions. *Ann Emerg Med* 19:1129, 1990.
158. Young TK, Lee SC, Tang CK: Diarrhea therapy of uremia. *Clin Nephrol* 11:86, 1979.
159. Porter RS, Baker EB: Drug clearance by diarrhea induction. *Am J Emerg Med* 3:182, 1985.
160. Arimori K, Furukawa E, Nakano M: Adsorption of imipramine onto activated charcoal and a cation exchange resin in macrogel-electrolyte solution. *Chem Pharm Bull* 40:3105, 1992.
161. Arimori K, Deshimaru M, Furukawa E, et al: Adsorption of mexiletine onto activated charcoal in macrogel-electrolyte solution. *Chem Pharm Bull* 41:766, 1993.
162. Rosenberg PJ, Livingstone DJ, McLellan BA: Effect of whole bowel irrigation on the antidotal efficacy of oral activated charcoal. *Ann Emerg Med* 17:681, 1988.
163. Hoffman RS, Chiang WK, Howland MA, et al: Theophylline desorption from activated charcoal caused by whole bowel irrigation solution. *Clin Toxicol* 29:191, 1991.
164. Makosiej FJ, Hoffman RS, Howland MA, et al: An in vitro evaluation of cocaine hydrochloride adsorption by activated charcoal and desorption upon addition of polyethylene glycol electrolyte lavage solution. *Clin Toxicol* 31:381, 1993.
165. Atta-Politou J, Kolioliou M, Havariotou M, et al: An in vitro evaluation of fluoxetine adsorption by activated charcoal and desorption upon addition of polyethylene glycol-electrolyte solution. *Clin Toxicol* 36:117, 1998.
166. Brown CR, Becker CE, Osterlob JD, et al: Whole gut lavage in a simulated drug overdose [abstract]. *Vet Hum Toxicol* 29:366, 1987.
167. Burkhart KK, Wuerz RC, Donovan JW: Whole bowel irrigation as an adjunctive treatment for sustained-released theophylline overdose. *Ann Emerg Med* 21:1316, 1992.
168. Minocha A, Spyker DA: Acute overdose with sustained-release drug formulations: perspectives in treatment. *Med Toxicol* 1:300, 1986.
169. Buckley N, Dawson AH, Howarth D, et al: Slow-release verapamil poisoning. Use of polyethylene glycol whole-bowel irrigation lavage and high-dose calcium. *Med J Aust* 158:202, 1993.
170. Melandri R, Re G, Morigi A, et al: Whole bowel irrigation after delayed release fenfluramine overdose. *Clin Toxicol* 33:161, 1995.
171. Hoffman RS, Smilkstein MJ, Goldfrank LR: Whole bowel irrigation and the cocaine body packer [abstract]. *Vet Hum Toxicol* 31:374, 1989.
172. Shah M, Nakanishi A: Polyethylene glycol-electrolyte solution for rectal sunflower seed bezoar. *Pediatr Emerg Care* 6:127, 1990.
173. Burkhart K, Kulig K, Rumack B: Whole bowel irrigation for zinc sulfate overdose. *Ann Emerg Med* 19:1167, 1990.
174. Roberge RJ, Martin TG: Whole bowel irrigation in an acute oral lead intoxication. *Am J Emerg Med* 10:577, 1992.
175. Palatnick W, Tenenbein M: Safety of treating poisoning patients with whole bowel irrigation. *Am J Emerg Med* 6:200, 1988.

176. Marsteller HJ, Gugler R: Endoscopic management of toxic masses in the stomach. *N Engl J Med* 296:1003, 1977.
177. Bartecchi CE: Removal of gastric drug masses. *N Engl J Med* 296:282, 1977.
178. Litovitz TL: Button battery ingestions. *JAMA* 249:2495, 1983.
179. Trent M, Kim U: Cocaine packet ingestion: surgical or medical management? *Arch Surg* 122:1179, 1987.
180. Landsman J, Bricker J, Reid BS, et al: Emergency gastrostomy: treatment of choice for iron bezoar. *J Pediatr Surg* 22:184, 1987.
181. Tenenbein M, Wiseman N, Yatscoff RW: Gastrotomy and whole bowel irrigation in iron poisoning. *Pediatr Emerg Care* 7:286, 1991.
182. Riegel JM, Becker CE: Use of cathartics in toxic ingestions. *Ann Emerg Med* 10:254, 1981.
183. Shannon M, Fish SS, Lovejoy FH: Cathartics and laxatives: do they still have a place in management of the poisoned patient? *Med Toxicol* 1:247, 1986.
184. Tenenbein M: Cathartics for drug overdose. *Ann Emerg Med* 16:832, 1987.
185. Gaudreault P, Friedman PA, Lovejoy FH: Efficacy of activated charcoal and magnesium citrate in the treatment of oral paraquat intoxication. *Ann Emerg Med* 14:123, 1985.
186. Al-Shareef AH, Buss DC, Allen EM, et al: The effects of charcoal and sorbitol (alone and in combination) on plasma theophylline concentrations after a sustained-release formulation. *Hum Exp Toxicol* 9:179, 1990.
187. Galinski RE, Levy G: Evaluation of activated charcoal-sodium sulfate combination for inhibition of acetaminophen absorption and repletion of inorganic sulfate. *Clin Toxicol* 22:21, 1984.
188. Goldberg MJ, Spector R, Park GD, et al: The effect of sorbitol and activated charcoal on serum theophylline concentrations after slow-release theophylline. *Clin Pharmacol Ther* 41:108, 1987.
189. Keller RE, Schwab RA, Krenzelok EP: Contribution of sorbitol combined with activated charcoal in prevention of salicylate absorption. *Ann Emerg Med* 19:654, 1990.
190. Dean BL, Peterson R, Garrettson LK, et al: American Association of Poison Control Centers Policy statement: gastrointestinal dilution with water as a first aid procedure in poisoning. *Clin Toxicol* 19:531, 1982.
191. Done AK: Clinical pharmacology of systemic antidotes. *Clin Pharmacol Ther* 2:750, 1961.
192. Linden CH: Antidotes in poisoning, in Callaham ML (ed): *Current Therapy in Emergency Medicine.* Philadelphia, BC Decker, 1990, p 949.
193. Goldfrank L, Cohen L, Flomenbaum N, et al: Newer antidotes and controversies in antidotal therapy, in Rund DA, Wolcott BW (eds): *Emergency Medicine Annual.* Vol. 3. Norwalk, CT, Appleton-Century-Crofts, 1984, p 223.
194. Litovitz TL: The anecdotal antidotes. *Emerg Med Clin North Am* 2:145, 1984.
195. Bolgiano EB, Barish RA: Use of new and established antidotes. *Emerg Med Clin North Am* 12:317, 1994.
196. Gelfand MC, Winchester JF: Hemoperfusion in drug overdose: a technique when conservative management is not sufficient. *Clin Toxicol* 17:583, 1980.
197. Pond SM: Diuresis, dialysis, and hemoperfusion: indications and benefits. *Emerg Med Clin North Am* 2:29, 1984.
198. Peterson RG, Peterson LN: Cleansing the blood: hemodialysis, peritoneal dialysis, exchange transfusion, charcoal hemoperfusion, forced diuresis. *Pediatr Clin North Am* 22:675, 1986.
199. Todd JW: Do measures to enhance drug removal save life? *Lancet* 1:331, 1984.
200. Barter DC: The pharmacological role of the kidney. *Drugs* 19:31, 1980.
201. Garrettson LK, Geller RJ: Acid and alkaline diuresis: when are they of value in the treatment of poisoning? *Drug Saf* 5:220, 1990.
202. Proudfoot AT, Krenzelok EP, Vale JA: Position paper on urine alkalinization. *Clin Toxicol* 42:1, 2004.
203. Sweeney K, Chapron D, Brandt L, et al: Toxic interaction between acetazolamide and salicylate: case reports and a pharmacokinetic explanation. *Clin Pharmacol Ther* 40:518, 1986.
204. Chyka PA: Multiple-dose activated charcoal and enhancement of systemic drug clearance: summary of studies in animal and human volunteers. *Clin Toxicol* 33:399, 1995.
205. Bradberry SM, Vale JA: Multiple-dose activated charcoal: a review of relevant clinical studies. *Clin Toxicol* 33:407, 1995.
206. American Academy of Clinical Toxicology and European Association of Poisons Centre and Clinical Toxicologists: Position statement and practice guidelines on the use of multi-dose activated charcoal in the treatment of acute poisoning. *Clin Toxicol* 37:731, 1999.
207. Campbell JW, Chyka PA: Physiochemical characteristics of drugs and response to repeat-dose activated charcoal. *Am J Emerg Med* 10:208, 1992.
208. Tenenbein M: Multiple doses of activated charcoal: time for reappraisal? *Ann Emerg Med* 20:529, 1991.
209. Park GD, Radomski L, Goldberg MJ, et al: Effects of size and frequency of oral doses of charcoal on theophylline clearance. *Clin Pharmacol Ther* 34:663, 1983.
210. Ilkhanipourk K, Yealy DM, Kronzelok EP: The comparative efficacy of various multiple-dose activated charcoal regimens. *Am J Emerg Med* 10:298, 1992.
211. Watson WA, Cremer KF, Chapman JA: Gastrointestinal obstruction associated with multiple-dose activated charcoal. *J Emerg Med* 4:401, 1986.
212. Ray MJ, Padin R, Condie JD, et al: Charcoal bezoar: small-bowel obstruction secondary to amitriptyline overdose therapy. *Dig Dis Sci* 33:106, 1988.
213. Olson KR, Pond SM, Verrier ED, et al: Intestinal infarction complicating phenobarbital overdose. *Arch Intern Med* 144:407, 1984.
214. Longdon P, Henderson A: Intestinal pseudo-obstruction following the use of enteral charcoal and sorbitol and mechanical ventilation with papaveretum sedation for theophylline poisoning. *Drug Saf* 7:74, 1992.
215. Goulbourne KB, Cisek JE: Small-bowel obstruction secondary to activated charcoal and adhesions. *Ann Emerg Med* 24:108, 1994.
216. Trafford A, Horn C, Sharpstone P, et al: Hemoperfusion in acute drug toxicity. *Clin Toxicol* 17:547, 1980.
217. Haapenen EJ: Hemoperfusion in acute intoxication: clinical experience with 48 cases. *Acta Med Scand* 668[Suppl]:76, 1982.
218. Papadopoulou ZL, Novello AC: The use of hemoperfusion in children: past, present, and future. *Pediatr Clin North Am* 29:1039, 1982.
219. Golper TA, Bennet WM: Drug removal by continuous arteriovenous haemofiltration: a review of the evidence in poisoned patients. *Med Toxicol* 3:341, 1988.
220. Lin JL, Jeng LB: Critical, acutely poisoned patients treated with continuous arteriovenous hemoperfusion in the emergency department. *Ann Emerg Med* 25:75, 1995.
221. Shumack KH, Rock GA: Therapeutic plasma exchange. *N Engl J Med* 310:762, 1984.
222. Jones JS, Dougherty J: Current status of plasmapheresis in toxicology. *Ann Emerg Med* 15:474, 1986.
223. Brett AS, Rothschild N, Gray R, et al: Predicting the clinical course of intentional drug overdose: implications for use of the intensive care unit. *Arch Intern Med* 147:133, 1987.
224. Kulling P, Persson H: Role of the intensive care unit in the management of the poisoned patient. *Med Toxicol* 1:375, 1986.
225. Whyte IM, Dawson AH, Buckley NA, et al: Model for the management of self-poisoning. *Med J Aust* 167:142, 1997.

CHAPTER 118 ■ ACETAMINOPHEN POISONING

STEVEN B. BIRD

PHARMACOLOGY

Acetaminophen (*N*-acetyl-para-aminophenol [APAP]) is a nonnarcotic analgesic with excellent antipyretic activity but almost no anti-inflammatory effects. It belongs to the same drug family as phenacetin and acetanilid, the coal tar or aminobenzene analgesics [1,2]. Although APAP is the active metabolite of phenacetin, unlike phenacetin it rarely, if ever, causes nephrotoxicity and does not cause methemoglobinemia and hemolytic anemia. Unlike aspirin, APAP has no barrier-breaker effect on the gastrointestinal tract and no effect on platelet function, has a high therapeutic index, and has not been implicated as a factor in Reye's syndrome. As a result, APAP is the preferred agent for the treatment of fever and mild to moderate pain when anti-inflammatory and antiplatelet action is not important.

Acetaminophen is an active ingredient in several hundred products, including pure APAP formulations, combinations with opioid analgesics, and numerous combination cough and cold preparations. It is also available in an extended-release (ER) formulation (which contains 325 mg of immediate-release and 325 mg of delayed-release acetaminophen per tablet) and as a suppository, but there is no commercial intravenous formulation.

Acetaminophen has a pK_a of 9.5 and is quickly and almost completely absorbed after ingestion of therapeutic doses of immediate-release formulations (10 to 15 mg per kg every 4 hours), yielding peak plasma concentrations between 5 and 20 μg per mL within 30 to 120 minutes. Clinical effects are noted within 30 minutes. Liquid preparations are absorbed slightly faster than solid formulations. Rectal absorption is similar to that of oral ingestion. The volume of distribution of APAP is 0.9 to 1.0 L per kg, and protein binding is negligible. Therapeutic plasma concentrations range from 10 to 20 μg per L, and elimination after therapeutic dosing follows first-order kinetics, with an average half-life of 2 to 4 hours [1]. Elimination is slower in neonates and young infants [3], the elderly [2], and in patients with hepatic dysfunction [4]. Clinical effects persist for 3 to 4 hours after therapeutic doses.

After overdose, peak acetaminophen levels are usually noted within 4 hours. The ingestion of very large doses and the concomitant ingestion of agents that delay gastric emptying (e.g., anticholinergics and opioids) may result in peak levels occurring later. Prolonged absorption with a late rise in the acetaminophen level has also been reported after an ER overdose [5].

TOXICOLOGY

The short- or long-term therapeutic use of APAP is rarely associated with adverse effects. Hypersensitivity reactions, such as urticaria, fixed drug eruption, angioedema, laryngeal edema, and anaphylaxis, are extremely rare [6]. Although high-dose APAP has been associated with chronic renal impairment [7], a cause-effect relationship has not been established.

Despite remarkable safety in appropriate doses, APAP can cause fatal hepatic necrosis after overdosage. This was first recognized in Europe more than 40 years ago and the first cases of hepatotoxicity in the United States were reported in 1975. Since that time, the incidence of APAP poisoning has increased dramatically in parallel with its increased availability and use; APAP is now the most common drug involved in exposures reported to US poison control centers, accounting for more than 140,000 calls in 2007 [8]. The incidence of occult poisoning is unknown, but based on retrospective data approximately 1 of every 70 overdose patients have a detectable acetaminophen concentration and 1 in 500 a potentially toxic APAP ingestion [9].

The metabolism of APAP explains its toxicity and the rationale for the current treatment of overdose (Fig. 118.1) (Table 118.1) [2]. After therapeutic doses, approximately 90% of APAP metabolism occurs by hepatic conjugation with sulfate or glucuronide to form inactive, nontoxic, renally eliminated metabolites. In adults, glucuronidation is the predominant route; in infants and young children, sulfation is the major pathway. Less than 5% of APAP is eliminated unchanged in the urine. The small remaining fraction (approximately 5%) undergoes oxidation by the P450 mixed-function oxidase enzyme system (CYP2E1) to yield the highly reactive, potentially toxic, electrophilic intermediate *N*-acetyl-para-benzoquinoneimine (NAPQI) [10]. NAPQI is quickly detoxified by reduced glutathione (GSH) to form nontoxic cysteine and mercapturic acid conjugates that are excreted in the urine.

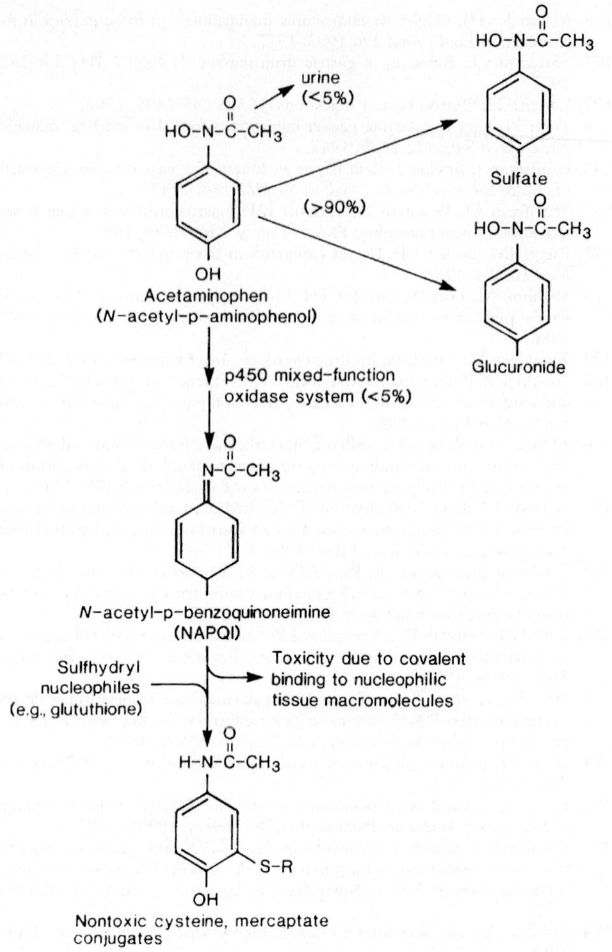

FIGURE 118.1. Postulated metabolism of acetaminophen. Toxicity occurs when the supply of sulfhydryl nucleophiles (e.g., glutathione) is inadequate to prevent the persistence of *N*-acetyl-para-benzoquinoneimine (NAPQI) and subsequent binding to hepatocyte macromolecules.

After overdose, the amount of drug metabolized by the P450 route increases, because of a greater total drug burden and saturation of alternative enzymatic pathways [11]. As a result, GSH utilization increases. If GSH regeneration is inadequate to meet demand and becomes significantly depleted, NAPQI can persist and react with hepatocyte macromolecules, resulting in the death of hepatocytes. In animal studies, such injury occurs when GSH stores reach less than 30% of normal [12]. Hepatocyte necrosis is most pronounced in areas of highest CYP2E1 activity: the centrilobular (central venule) zones of the liver. The degree of injury can range from asymptomatic

TABLE 118.1

TREATMENT OF ACETAMINOPHEN POISONING OR ASSOCIATED HEPATOTOXICITY

1. Administer activated charcoal if ingestion within 1–2 hours
2. Administer NAC either IV (preferred) or orally
3. Early consultation with hepatology and or transplant services for critically ill patients
4. Psychiatric evaluation for all intentional overdoses

elevations in aminotransferase levels to fulminant liver failure. Although far less common, the same process can occur in the kidney [13]. Very rarely, renal toxicity can occur in the absence of serious hepatotoxicity [14].

Pancreatitis, in some cases fulminant, can occur, and diffuse myocardial necrosis has been noted in fatal cases. Very rarely, with massive ingestions, early coma and metabolic acidosis may be seen [15]. Although uncommon, thrombocytopenia after acute overdose has also been described [16]. The mechanisms causing these atypical toxicities are unknown, and it is unclear to what extent these effects are directly due to APAP.

The precise dosage required to produce hepatotoxicity is unknown and almost certainly varies to some degree with individual differences in CYP2E1 activity, GSH stores, and capacity for GSH regeneration. Retrospective data suggest that significant toxicity is likely only after acute overdoses of greater than 250 mg per kg in adults [13], and prospective studies have suggested that toxicity is unlikely in unintentional pediatric ingestions of up to 200 mg per kg [17]. The possibility of toxicity at lower doses and skepticism regarding the accuracy of overdose histories have led to acceptance of a more conservative definition of risk, particularly in the United States. On the basis of APAP's volume of distribution and the well-established accuracy of APAP blood levels in predicting toxicity (see later), it is currently recommended that single ingestions of greater than 140 to 150 mg per kg be considered potentially toxic.

Elevated aminotransferase concentrations have also been reported after repeated ingestions of therapeutic or slightly greater doses of APAP [18]. Individuals who have conditions associated with increased CYP2E1 activity (e.g., chronic alcoholics) or glutathione depletion such as children younger than 10 years of age [19], those with chronic malnutrition, recent fasting (due to intercurrent illness), or recent ethanol use [20] may be at increased risk for such toxicity, but the accuracy of these reports has been challenged, and their therapeutic implications remain controversial. Such individuals are likely to have low hepatic carbohydrate and sulfate stores and, hence, decreased capacity for APAP metabolism via the glucuronidation and sulfation. There is currently no valid estimation of the amount, frequency, or duration of the dosing that defines risk. It appears that after repeated doses, accumulation of APAP to concentrations associated with toxicity after acute overdose is not required and that sustained moderate elevations are sufficient to cause GSH depletion and toxicity [21]. Such observations suggest that the APAP level at which NAPQI production exceeds GSH regeneration is near, or possibly within, the therapeutic range and that GSH stores and the capacity for its regeneration are the most important factors in the development of hepatotoxicity. They also support the concept that hepatotoxicity is more dependent on the area under the curve (time vs. concentration) of APAP than the peak drug level.

Intentional acute overdose is the most common cause of toxicity and fatalities, but accidental therapeutic overdosing and the abuse of opioids with unintentional coingestion of APAP (e.g., with codeine or propoxyphene) have also been reported. Therapeutic overdoses may result from dosing calculation errors, excessive self-treatment, the use of adult formulations or extra-strength formulations when lower dosage formulations were intended, and errors involving substitution of higher-dose rectal suppositories for similar-appearing lower dosage forms.

The importance of accurately diagnosing APAP toxicity soon after overdose extends beyond the high frequency with which it is encountered and its potential for causing morbidity and mortality. Acetaminophen is unique among common toxic exposures because effective treatment requires recognition of potential poisoning and initiation of therapy when no reliable clinical signs of overdose are present. Physicians must therefore consider occult APAP ingestion and liberally obtain APAP levels on all overdose patients to avoid missing the diagnosis.

CLINICAL MANIFESTATIONS

Acetaminophen hepatotoxicity can be divided into four clinical stages based on the time interval after ingestion: stage I (0 to 24 hours), the latent period; stage II (24 to 48 hours), the onset of hepatotoxicity; stage III (72 to 96 hours), maximal hepatic injury; and stage IV (4 days to 2 weeks), recovery [2,13].

During stage I, patients may be completely asymptomatic but often experience nausea, vomiting, and malaise, which may be accompanied by pallor and mild diaphoresis. There is no known correlation between presence or absence of early symptoms and the risk of hepatotoxicity. Although late in stage I very sensitive indicators of hepatic injury, such as γ-glutamyltransferase level, may be elevated, more widely used laboratory studies (e.g., aspartate aminotransferase [AST], alanine aminotransferase, prothrombin time, bilirubin) are completely normal. Early coma and metabolic acidosis have been reported in patients with massive ingestions [15], but these findings are so atypical that other causes should be suspected. They should be attributed to APAP only if the APAP concentration is extremely high and other etiologies have been excluded.

Symptoms during stage II are typical of hepatitis and include right upper-quadrant abdominal pain, nausea, fatigue, and malaise. Physical examination often reveals right upper-quadrant tenderness and hepatomegaly. The first elevation of aminotransferase levels usually occurs between 24 and 36 hours after APAP ingestion, but in the most severe cases, it can occur by 16 hours or earlier. Early in stage II, tests reflecting liver function, such as bilirubin and prothrombin time, are most often normal or only slightly elevated. Marked elevations of aminotransferase levels (greater than 1,000 IU per L) within 24 hours or bilirubin and prothrombin time within 36 hours should suggest that the time of ingestion was earlier than reported. Although unusual, in severe cases, marked liver function abnormalities may be evident by 36 to 48 hours. Complications during stage II are directly related to the degree of liver injury and may include coagulopathy, encephalopathy, acidosis, and hypoglycemia. With few exceptions, life-threatening problems are not seen earlier than 48 hours, and death in this period is distinctly rare. Renal dysfunction, manifested by rising creatinine and an active urinary sediment, may become evident during this stage but usually lags somewhat behind the hepatic injury. The blood urea nitrogen may also be elevated, but it can be normal in the presence of hepatic failure and resultant decreased urea formation.

Biochemical evidence of liver injury becomes most pronounced during stage III. With successful treatment, however, peak aminotransferase levels may sometimes occur earlier (Fig. 118.2). Most patients, even those with markedly elevated aminotransferase levels, go on to recover fully. Most deaths occur 3 to 7 days after ingestion and result from intractable metabolic disturbances, secondary complications such as cerebral edema or dysrhythmias, or exsanguination due to coagulopathy. Oliguric or anuric renal failure may result from acute tubular necrosis and is sometimes accompanied by flank pain. Some degree of renal dysfunction occurs in approximately 25% of patients with significant hepatotoxicity [15]. Even when severe, renal failure is almost always reversible.

During stage IV, if sufficient hepatocytes remain viable and the patient survives, the liver regenerates. Recovery is often complete by day 5 or 6 in patients with minimal toxicity, but those with more serious poisoning may not be clinically normal for 2 weeks or more. It is interesting that even patients with severe toxicity who survive regain normal liver function. There are no known cases of chronic or persistent liver abnormalities from APAP poisoning. In those who ultimately die, a slow decline in aminotransferase levels without clinical improvement may be seen. Declining enzyme levels merely

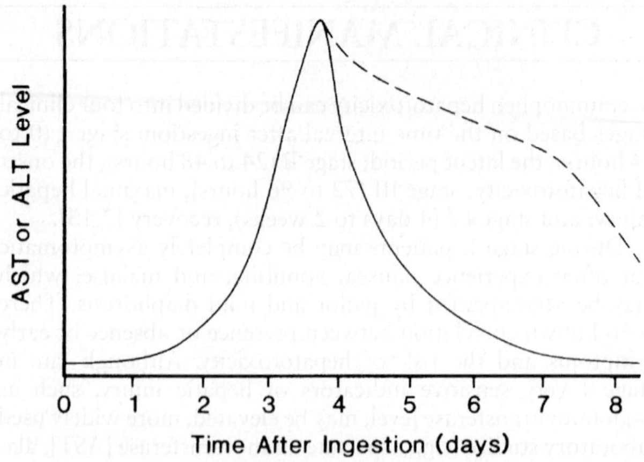

FIGURE 118.2. Expected time course of aminotransferase elevation due to acetaminophen-induced hepatotoxicity. The solid line represents typical course; the dashed line represents course of severe toxicity. ALT, alanine aminotransferase; AST, aspartate aminotransferase [Adapted from Jaeschke H, Mitchell JR: Neutrophil accumulation exacerbates acetaminophen-induced liver injury (abstract). *FASEB J* 3:A920, 1989, with permission.]

represent a washout of those released at the time of the initial insult, not a recovery of normal liver function. These patients can be identified by persistent or increasing marked elevations of bilirubin and prothrombin time. Although this pattern is occasionally seen in patients who recover, most survivors do not have significant or persistent bilirubin or prothrombin time elevation after aminotransferase levels fall.

Because of variations in dosing patterns and patient characteristics, the time course of toxicity in patients with repeated ingestions is not well defined. With chronic toxicity, dose–response patterns differ from those of acute overdose, but the clinical manifestations are the same.

DIAGNOSTIC EVALUATION

The diagnostic evaluation consists of determining the risk of toxicity and assessing for it. The serum APAP concentration is used to predict toxicity after acute overdose. If the APAP concentration between 4 and 24 hours after ingestion falls on or above the acetaminophen treatment nomogram line (Fig. 118.3), the patient should be considered at risk for hepatotoxicity, and hence, in need of antidotal therapy (see later). Conversely, if the APAP concentration is even slightly below the nomogram line, the risk of hepatotoxicity is negligible and antidotal therapy is not necessary. The original Rumack–Matthew nomogram line, which defined the risk of toxicity based on the natural course of untreated patients [22], was actually 25% higher than the line now used in the United States. Hence, the nomogram has a 25% safety margin that allows one to be fairly rigid when using the nomogram to make treatment decisions.

There are, however, some important caveats regarding use of the nomogram. First and foremost, it applies only to single acute ingestions. Second, when there is uncertainty about the exact time of ingestion, the worst-case scenario should be assumed. For example, if the ingestion was between 4 and 6 hours earlier, the 6-hour value on the nomogram should be used. And finally, when levels are obtained 20 to 24 hours after overdose, the limit of detection of the APAP assay must also be considered. Because most hospitals use immunoassays with a detection limit of 10 μg per mL, potentially toxic APAP levels during this period will be below this limit and reported as nondetectable, which does not necessarily mean nontoxic. Again,

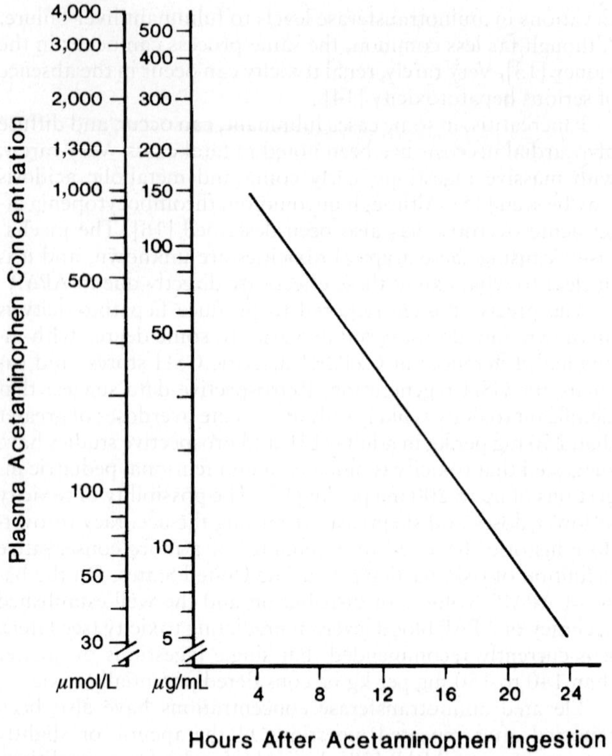

FIGURE 118.3. Acetaminophen treatment nomogram. Patients with acetaminophen concentrations on or above the line require treatment with *N*-acetylcysteine. [Adapted from Jaeschke H, Mitchell JR: Neutrophil accumulation exacerbates acetaminophen-induced liver injury (abstract). *FASEB J* 3:A920, 1989, with permission.]

a worst-case scenario should be assumed, and antidotal treatment should be given until the level is confirmed to be nontoxic by a more sensitive assay, or until it has been determined that the patient is asymptomatic and has no laboratory evidence of hepatotoxicity.

With rare exceptions (see later), a single APAP concentration within the time period specified by the nomogram is sufficient to plan appropriate therapy. Although it is true that the elimination half-life of APAP is related to the likelihood of toxicity, half-lives should not be relied on in making therapeutic decisions. The observations that half-lives greater than 4 hours were associated with toxicity and that toxicity was negligible if APAP half-life was less than 4 hours [23] were based on multiple APAP determinations in untreated patients over a 36-hour period. Because treatment must be started as early as possible [24] and treatment may alter APAP elimination [11], half-life determinations are not relevant to current standards of care.

There are three situations in which repeat measurements may be of value. The first is in the patient with a time of ingestion that is unknown but that was within 4 hours. In this situation, an increasing APAP level indicates ongoing absorption from a recent ingestion. To detect a rising level and define the peak value, repeat determinations must be frequent (every hour) until the level declines. This prevents underestimation of the peak value due to incomplete absorption at the time of the first level. It also may rule out toxicity by detecting a peak value less than 150 μg per mL.

The second situation in which repeating the APAP may be useful is after an overdose of an ER formula. Because of prolonged absorption, patients with nontoxic APAP levels soon after ingestion may have subsequent levels that are toxic by the nomogram [25]. The optimal time to repeat drug levels to detect such nomogram line-crossers is unknown. In one patient, a potentially toxic APAP level did not occur until 14 hours after ingestion [5]. The manufacturer recommends obtaining a second APAP level 4 to 6 hours after the initial one [26]. Others have recommended that to avoid missing a potentially toxic level, drug levels should be measured every 2 hours from 4 to 16 hours after overdose [27].

Finally, repeat APAP levels may be of value in the patient with very high levels and slow elimination in whom it is possible that APAP may still be present at the completion of therapy. Antidotal treatment should not be discontinued while APAP is still present. This is particularly relevant as shorter courses of antidotal therapy have become the routine.

In assessing the patient who is found to be at risk for toxicity and hence requires hospitalization and antidotal treatment, a complete blood count, electrolytes, blood urea nitrogen, creatinine, glucose, prothrombin time, aminotransferase levels, and bilirubin should be obtained at admission and repeated every 24 hours until resolution of toxicity is noted. If liver failure develops, laboratory values, particularly prothrombin time and glucose, must be obtained more frequently. Renal function, acid–base status, amylase, and electrocardiogram may also need to be evaluated or repeated. Assessment of renal, pancreatic, and myocardial toxicity should follow the same guidelines as those for other etiologies.

MANAGEMENT

Treatment includes gastrointestinal decontamination, antidotal treatment (if indicated), and support of organ function. Unless clinically significant hepatic or renal failure develops, management consists only of antidote administration and monitoring of signs, symptoms, and laboratory parameters. Although this can be accomplished outside the intensive care unit, patients often require monitoring or treatment for toxicity due to coingestions or constant observation because of suicide risk. If significant hepatic failure ensues, intensive care unit admission is required for close monitoring and treatment of complications. Invasive monitoring is infrequently required, but may be useful if multisystem failure occurs.

Gastrointestinal Decontamination

Gastrointestinal decontamination is recommended for patients who can be treated within 1–2 hours of APAP overdose. Although once considered controversial and even contraindicated, activated charcoal is now considered the method of choice. As routine treatment of APAP poisoning has moved from oral *N*-acetylcysteine (NAC) to intravenous administration, this formerly contentious point has been rendered moot.

Antidotal Treatment

The observation that hepatotoxicity occurs only when GSH is depleted led to a search for agents that might increase available sulfhydryl groups either by increasing GSH or by providing alternative sulfhydryl sources. Exogenous GSH does not readily enter cells, so various precursors and substitutes, including cysteamine, methionine, and NAC [24,28], have been tried. Although all regimens are effective when started within 8 to 10 hours of ingestion, cysteamine was abandoned because of its toxicity, and methionine has been replaced by NAC, which is more effective and probably carries less risk of worsening hepatic encephalopathy when liver failure is present.

There are several suggested mechanisms of action of NAC. In cells, NAC is converted to cysteine, a GSH precursor, and thus increases GSH stores. Second, NAC or cysteine can substitute directly for GSH because it has available sulfhydryl groups. Third, NAC augments the sulfation of APAP to nontoxic metabolite by providing sulfur substrate [11]. Fourth, NAC may promote the back conversion of NAPQI to its precursors, although this has not been demonstrated in humans. Finally, there is accumulating evidence that NAC may be beneficial, even after liver injury has occurred, through mechanisms other than its effects on APAP metabolism [29]. Suggested mechanisms for these late effects of NAC include direct antioxidant action to modify postinflammatory radical-mediated destruction, restoration of enzyme function in injured tissue, and correction of microvascular function by restoring endothelial-derived relaxing factor [29]. It is likely that the relative importance of each of the previously described effects of NAC in any given patient varies with the severity of the overdose and the delay to NAC initiation. These variations may explain apparent differences in efficacy between different NAC protocols.

Two treatment regimens are currently approved for use in the United States. The first consists of a 72-hour course of oral NAC given as a 140 mg per kg loading dose, followed by 17 doses of 70 mg per kg every 4 hours beginning 4 hours after the loading dose, for a total NAC dose of 1,330 mg per kg [30]. The second regimen, approved by the FDA in 2004, consists of an intravenous loading dose of acetylcysteine of 150 mg per kg in 200 mL dextrose 5% in water (D_5W) over 15 minutes, followed by 50 mg per kg in 500 mL D_5W over 4 hours, then 100 mg per kg in 1 L D_5W over the next 16 hours [31]. This is identical to the standard treatment regimens in Europe and Canada [28]. Because the FDA-approved dosing requires three separate intravenous formulations, some Poison Control Centers, hospitals, and medical toxicologists have simplified NAC protocols that differ from the FDA-approved dosing [32].

For oral therapy, NAC is usually supplied as a 20% solution (20 g per 100 mL), which should be diluted 3 to 1 to yield a 5% mixture with juice or a soft drink to increase its palatability and decrease gastrointestinal side effects. Antiemetics (e.g., metoclopramide, 0.1 to 1.0 mg per kg intravenous (IV), initial adult dose 10 mg; droperidol, 20 to 150 μg per kg IV, initial adult dose 1.25 mg) may be required to treat antecedent vomiting or vomiting due to NAC. Ondansetron (50 to 150 μg per kg IV, initial adult dose 4 mg) may be effective when traditional antiemetics are not. If antiemetics fail, NAC can be given by gastric or duodenal tube. Various other methods may prove helpful in decreasing emesis after dosing: chilling the solution with ice chips, using a straw and covering the container, diluting to a 10% solution, or administering the solution over 15 to 60 minutes instead of as a bolus. If vomiting occurs within 1 hour of any dose, that dose should be repeated.

The use of oral or IV NAC is dependent on the experience of the clinician, the local hospital formulary, severity of the patient, and physician preference. Most patients can be adequately treated with oral NAC if it is begun within 8 to 10 hours of ingestion. Other patients, particularly those who present after 8 to 10 hours or those with encephalopathy, should receive IV NAC therapy.

There are no well-documented serious side effects of oral NAC, although nausea and vomiting are extremely common [33]. Side effects from intravenous NAC are far less common but potentially more serious. There are several reports of serious or fatal anaphylactoid reactions (e.g., hypotension, bronchospasm, rash, death) to intravenous NAC during the 20-hour protocol, and minor dermatologic reactions are common [34,35]. It is important to recognize that adverse effects to intravenous NAC are not truly anaphylactic; they are dose and concentration dependent [34]. As a result, more dilute and slowly administered doses are better tolerated [36]. Except for an anaphylactoid reaction in one patient after an NAC overdose, there were no serious adverse reactions reported during the 48-hour intravenous protocol [36]. Transient skin rash occurred in approximately 15% of patients during the loading dose but did not necessitate discontinuing treatment. Even with more serious reactions, NAC therapy can often be continued or resumed after treatment with diphenhydramine [35].

All dosing protocols appear to be equivalent when NAC is started within 8 hours of ingestion. Efficacy decreases with longer delays in therapy, with apparent differences between the dosing regimens when NAC is started after 16 hours. With late treatment, 82% of high-risk patients treated with the 20-hour regimen developed aminotransferase values above 1,000 IU per L, an incidence not significantly different from the 89% incidence reported in untreated historical control subjects [28]. After treatment with 48 hours of intravenous NAC, only 58% of late-treated patients developed hepatotoxicity, a result that was significantly better than that with the 20-hour course or no treatment [36]. After 72 hours of oral NAC, only 41% of late-treated patients developed hepatotoxicity [24], although this was not statistically different from the 48-hour protocol [36]. These studies included only patients receiving NAC within 24 hours of ingestion.

In the first controlled study of NAC started more than 24 hours after overdose, intravenous NAC started after onset of liver failure (median 53 hours after APAP) reduced cerebral edema, need for pressors, and mortality [37]. It is interesting that this study used the same NAC dosing that had earlier been found ineffective more than 15 hours after overdose [28], but instead of discontinuing NAC after 20 hours, therapy was continued until either recovery or death occurred.

The numerous actions of NAC may explain why various NAC protocols are equivalent when started early but not when started late. When started within 8 hours of overdose, NAC probably exclusively affects APAP metabolism and GSH turnover, and its role is preventative before GSH depletion and NAPQI covalent binding. In this setting, NAC may be needed only until APAP metabolism is complete; thus, shorter courses of NAC are effective. With further treatment delay, the role of NAC may increasingly be to ameliorate the effects of NAPQI covalent binding, and by 16 hours after ingestion, this may be its sole action and would explain why longer courses of NAC, continued during the period of maximal liver injury, appear to be superior. These considerations have led to selective management, such as short-course NAC for those treated early who do not develop aminotransferase elevations or late treatment with NAC for any patient who develops liver injury (see later).

Cimetidine has been suggested as a possible antidote for APAP because of its inhibitory effect on P450 activity. Animal studies showed efficacy of high-dose cimetidine given before or soon after APAP, but there is no evidence of efficacy in humans [38]. Even if the massive dose suggested by animal studies proved to be safe and effective in humans, its theoretic effect would require early administration. In problematic cases, such as late presentation, there is no theoretic or experimental support for cimetidine use. Hence, although cimetidine is not contraindicated, it has no proven role and should never be considered an alternative to NAC.

Supportive Care

The management of hepatic failure, renal failure, or other end-organ manifestations of APAP toxicity should be treated according to usual guidelines. In view of the increased availability and success of liver transplantation, the most severely ill patients deserve this consideration. Several successful transplants have been done after APAP overdose. The greatest challenge is early identification of patients destined for irreversible hepatic failure (see "Prognosis and Outcome" section of this chapter).

SPECIAL CONSIDERATIONS

Acute Overdose in Alcoholics and Other High-Risk Patients

Certain subgroups of patients appear to be at greater or lesser risk for APAP toxicity, but this fact is of more theoretic than practical value in the management of acute overdose. Higher risk is expected in patients with increased CYP2E1 enzyme activity from chronic use of agents that induce this enzyme (e.g., ethanol, barbiturates, phenytoin, sedative–hypnotics, griseofulvin, haloperidol, tolbutamide) [39] or decreased GSH stores or low GSH turnover rates (e.g., malnourished patients or those with liver disease). Lower toxicity might be expected when CYP2E1 activity is inhibited by chronic use of agents such as cimetidine or when a patient has coingested an agent that is metabolized by this enzyme, thus competing with APAP and decreasing NAPQI formation [2].

Acute overdose studies in animals demonstrated increased toxicity after chronic ethanol use and decreased toxicity when ethanol and APAP were coingested [40]. The protective effect of ethanol coingestion appears to be due to competitive inhibition of NAPQI formation by P450 ethanol metabolism. Chronic ethanol use, particularly in an alcoholic that is currently abstinent [41] could worsen toxicity by causing P450 induction, GSH depletion, or some other unknown mechanism. For example, an alcoholic might be protected by the acute coingestion of ethanol or be nutritionally deprived and have lower P450 activity.

Despite suggestions that some of these factors may be important [42], the amount of chronic ethanol or drug use that is clinically significant is unknown and certain to be variable.

Because the treatment nomogram line is conservative, treatment decisions after acute overdose should be made in the same manner as described previously, regardless of chronic coingestants.

Acute Overdose in Pediatric Patients

Of 417 children with acute APAP overdose, 49 of whom had plasma APAP levels over the nomogram line, indicating potential toxicity, only three (6.1%) developed an AST or ALT greater than 1,000 IU per L [43]. This incidence is less than that reported in adults, leading to speculation that children are relatively protected from APAP toxicity.

Several pharmacokinetic differences between children and adults have been noted. The most consistent finding is that the ratio of APAP-sulfate to APAP-glucuronide is higher in children than in adults [44], but this difference in nontoxic routes of metabolism has not been shown to be associated with a decrease in production of NAPQI. Thus, increased sulfation has not been proven favorably to alter NAPQI formation. Decreased P450 activity, and thus decreased NAPQI formation, has also been postulated in children, but decreased P450 activity is noted only in fetal and neonatal subjects [45]. Most APAP poisonings occur outside the newborn period, when P450 activity may be even greater than in adults. Hence, this theory cannot explain a hepatoprotective effect in older children. If children are actually less susceptible to APAP toxicity, it may be because of an increased ability to regenerate GSH, but this, too, is unproven.

Perhaps the most likely explanation is that pediatric overdoses are quantitatively less severe. In adults, particularly those treated late, the outcome is worse in patients with very high APAP levels [24]. Substantial toxicity has also developed in children with very high levels, but there are too few cases to allow for any conclusions. Until larger numbers of children with very high APAP levels are studied, patients of all ages with a significant overdose must still be considered at substantial risk and managed accordingly. As with adults, the longer the time between ingestion and presentation or treatment in children with potentially toxic drug levels, the greater the incidence of hepatotoxicity and the worse the prognosis [21].

Acute Overdose in Pregnancy

Although experience with overdose in pregnancy is limited [46], certain conclusions seem valid. First, there is clear evidence that APAP overdose can result in morbidity and mortality to woman and fetus at all stages of pregnancy. Second, there currently is no evidence that NAC is harmful to a pregnant woman or her fetus. Third, NAC is hepatoprotective to the woman. Fourth, NAC crosses the human placenta [47], and this is likely to be beneficial to the fetus. On the basis of these observations, it is recommended that pregnant women be treated according to standard guidelines regardless of gestational age of the fetus and that newborns delivered during a course of maternal NAC treatment should also complete a course of NAC after delivery.

Acute Overdose of Extended-Release Acetaminophen

Because experience with ER APAP overdose is limited, the applicability of the nomogram, which was derived from clinical outcome data in patients with immediate-release APAP overdose, to those with ER APAP overdose remains to be determined [25–27]. Although it is agreed that patients who have a potentially toxic APAP level after acute acetaminophen ER overdose require NAC, the management of those with levels that are elevated but nontoxic is controversial. Some have suggested that such patients do not require NAC [48]. Given that peak drug levels after supratherapeutic but nontoxic doses of ER acetaminophen are only two-thirds of those seen after equivalent doses of an immediate-release formulation, despite nearly identical areas under the curve [49], others recommend treatment if any APAP level is two-thirds or more of the one that is indicated toxic by the nomogram [27].

Chronic Overdose

There are occasional reports of serious toxicity from chronic overdose in infants with acute febrile illness [19,21]. Chronic toxicity has also been reported after doses only slightly higher than recommended and even with therapeutic ones in adults with fasting and alcohol use [50]. Although alcoholics do appear to be at greater risk for toxicity from therapeutic doses, the validity of data on fasting has been questioned [51]. There is no evidence that this occurs in otherwise healthy individuals. Similarly, in the absence of continued ethanol abuse, there is no evidence that therapeutic dosing carries an increased risk in patients with cirrhosis or other forms of chronic liver disease [52]. On the basis of current knowledge, there is no reason to avoid APAP in any of these groups, although patients must be clearly instructed to avoid overdosing.

Evaluation of patients with chronic overdose should include a detailed history of the timing of doses, particularly the last dose; the amount ingested at each dose; possible increased risk factors (e.g., chronic alcoholism, use of other P450 inducers); symptomatology; an APAP level at least 4 hours after the last dose; and aminotransferase levels. In such cases, the nomogram has never been studied and has little or no validity. Because there are currently no reliable guidelines to assess risk, it is best then to consult with a toxicologist or regional poison center to determine the best course of action. One approach is to treat according to the guidelines discussed the next section.

Late Treatment

Treatment decisions in patients who present more than 24 hours after an overdose are problematic. Initial studies of the 20-hour intravenous NAC protocol suggested that NAC was of no value if started more than 12 to 15 hours after ingestion [28], and initial results of the 72-hour oral protocol indicated that treatment more than 16 hours after ingestion was ineffective [30]. As a result, studies of treatment initiated after 24 hours were not performed initially. More extensive data and analysis of patients treated with 72 hours of oral NAC revealed that patients first treated between 16 and 24 hours after overdose experienced less hepatotoxicity than untreated historical control subjects or historical control subjects treated late with a 20-hour course of intravenous NAC [24].

Subsequently, a series of studies showed theoretic and clinical benefit to late NAC administration [29,53,54]. In the most remarkable of these, NAC started a median of 53 hours after ingestion and after evidence of severe liver injury reduced morbidity and mortality [29]. Although the issue of which cases warrant late treatment is not well defined, the following approach to the treatment of patients who present late is offered: If the APAP level is undetectable and aminotransferase levels are normal, NAC is not indicated, because the possibility of hepatotoxicity is extremely low. If hepatotoxicity is evident, a full course of NAC is indicated. For patients who have detectable APAP levels and no hepatotoxicity, NAC therapy should be started. It can be discontinued before completing a full course of therapy when the APAP concentration falls to zero, as long as aminotransferase levels remain normal.

Short-Course ORAL Treatment

Treatment of acute APAP overdose with an abbreviated course of oral NAC is based on the observation that treatment for 20 hours with intravenous NAC [28] and for 48 hours with oral NAC [36] is just as effective as treatment with oral NAC for 72 hours [24] when treatment is started within 8 to 16 hours of ingestion (see previous section), and that patients who develop hepatotoxicity exhibit laboratory evidence of such toxicity within 24 to 36 hours of ingestion [9,55]. In short-course protocols, oral NAC is initiated in patients with toxic or potentially toxic APAP levels (by the nomogram) in the same dose as used in the standard 72-hour regimen, and APAP levels and aminotransferases are obtained at 24 and 36 hours postingestion. As with late treatment, if the APAP level becomes undetectable and aminotransferase levels are normal at either point in time, NAC is stopped, whereas if hepatotoxicity becomes evident, a full course of NAC is indicated. For patients who have detectable APAP levels and no hepatotoxicity, NAC therapy should be continued. It can be discontinued before completing a full course of therapy if the APAP concentration subsequently becomes undetectable and if aminotransferase levels remain normal. Although toxicologists have been successfully using short-course NAC therapy for years, published data are limited [56], and poison centers have been slow to adopt this approach. Hence, consultation with a toxicologist is advised when contemplating such treatment.

PROGNOSIS AND OUTCOME

Severe hepatotoxicity after APAP overdose has traditionally been defined by an ALT or AST greater than 1,000 IU per L, although most patients with such elevations have no significant short- or long-term sequelae. By using this definition, the risk of hepatotoxicity can be estimated based on the initial APAP concentration. Without NAC therapy, hepatotoxicity develops in less than 8% of all overdose patients, in 60% of probable risk cases (APAP concentration above a nomogram line intersecting 200 μg per mL at 4 hours and 50 μg per mL at 12 hours), and in 89% of high-risk cases (APAP concentration above a nomogram line intersecting 300 μg per mL at 4 hours and 75 μg per mL at 12 hours) [13].

Far less toxicity occurs in patients treated with NAC, although outcome depends on APAP concentration and the time NAC was started. Even in high-risk late-treated cases, only 41% of patients treated with oral NAC for 72 hours developed toxicity. Most important is that regardless of APAP level, NAC is extremely effective when started within 8 hours [24]. Hepatotoxicity occurred in less than 5% of patients in this subset.

Death is unusual after APAP overdose. When patients at probable risk for hepatotoxicity are considered, the reported mortality rate in untreated cases varies from 5.3% [28] to 24% [57]. A mortality rate of 1.1% has been noted in similar patients treated with the 20-hour intravenous NAC protocol [29], and it was found to be 0.68% in patients treated with the 72-hour oral NAC protocol [24]. In fact, even among high-risk cases first treated between 16 and 24 hours after overdose, the mortality rate was only 3.1% after oral NAC therapy [24].

It is not uncommon to see aminotransferase elevations greater than 10,000 IU per L during stage III, with eventual complete recovery [2]. As a result, aminotransferase levels alone are inadequate to judge prognosis. Evidence of hepatic dysfunction, such as marked elevations in prothrombin time and bilirubin, or evidence of persistent hypoglycemia, lactic acidosis, or hepatic encephalopathy, indicates true hepatic failure and a poor prognosis. Previous reports suggested that a bilirubin greater than 4 mg per dL or a prothrombin time greater than twice control indicates a poor prognosis [58]. More recently, a pH less than 7.30, prothrombin time greater than 100 seconds, serum creatinine greater than 3.4 mg per dL, and grade III or higher encephalopathy have been used to define poor prognosis [59], as has the single criterion of an increasing prothrombin time on day 4 after overdose [60] or a lactate of greater than 3.5 mmol per L shorter after admission [61]. Most recently, Schmidt and Dalhoff [62] demonstrated that an increasing alpha-fetoprotein serum concentration (particularly a concentration of more than 3.9 μg per L on the day after peak ALT) is associated with survival. As noted previously, patients meeting these criteria may benefit from NAC treatment [29,53]. Standard measures for the treatment of liver failure, including arrangements for possible liver transplantation, should also be provided.

The presence or absence of aminotransferase elevation at the time of treatment initiation appears to be the most sensitive early prognostic indicator. To date, all reported patients who died from APAP toxicity already had some degree of AST or ALT elevation at the time a 72-hour course of oral NAC was started [24]. Hence, all patients with liver enzyme values that are normal when oral NAC is started would be expected to survive.

ACKNOWLEDGMENT

Christopher H. Linden, M.D., contributed to this chapter in a previous edition.

References

1. Burke A, Smyth E, Fitzgerald GA: Analgesic-antipyretic and antiinflammatory agents; pharmacotherapy of gout, in Brunton LL, Lazo JS, Parker KL (eds): *Goodman and Gilman's The Pharmacological Basis of Therapeutics.* 11th ed. New York, McGraw Hill, 2006.
2. Linden CH, Rumack BH: Acetaminophen overdose. *Emerg Med Clin North Am* 2(1):103–119, 1984.
3. Peterson RG, Rumack BH: Pharmacokinetics of acetaminophen in children. *Pediatrics* 62(5 Pt 2 Suppl):877–879, 1978.
4. Andreasen PB, Hutters L: Paracetamol (acetaminophen) clearance in patients with cirrhosis of the liver. *Acta Med Scand Suppl* 624:99–105, 1979.
5. Bizovi KE, Aks SE, Paloucek F, et al: Late increase in acetaminophen concentration after overdose of Tylenol Extended Relief. *Ann Emerg Med* 28(5):549–551, 1996.
6. Stricker BH, Meyboom RH, Lindquist M: Acute hypersensitivity reactions to paracetamol. *Br Med J (Clin Res Ed)* 291(6500):938–939, 1985.
7. Fored CM, Ejerblad E, Lindblad P, et al: Acetaminophen, aspirin, and chronic renal failure. *N Engl J Med* 20;345(25):1801–1808, 2001.
8. Bronstein AC, Spyker DA, Cantilena LR Jr, et al: 2007 Annual Report of the American Association of Poison Control Centers' National Poison Data System (NPDS): 25th Annual Report. *Clin Toxicol (Phila)* 46(10):927–1057, 2008.
9. Ashbourne JF, Olson KR, Khayam-Bashi H: Value of rapid screening for acetaminophen in all patients with intentional drug overdose. *Ann Emerg Med* 18(10):1035–1038, 1989.
10. Corcoran GB, Mitchell JR, Vaishnav YN, et al: Evidence that acetaminophen and N-hydroxyacetaminophen form a common arylating intermediate, N-acetyl-p-benzoquinoneimine. *Mol Pharmacol* 18(3):536–542, 1980.
11. Slattery JT, Wilson JM, Kalhorn TF, et al: Dose-dependent pharmacokinetics of acetaminophen: evidence of glutathione depletion in humans. *Clin Pharmacol Ther* 41(4):413–418, 1987.
12. Mitchell JR, Thorgeirsson SS, Potter WZ, et al: Acetaminophen-induced hepatic injury: protective role of glutathione in man and rationale for therapy. *Clin Pharmacol Ther* 16(4):676–684, 1974.
13. Prescott LF: Paracetamol overdosage. Pharmacological considerations and clinical management. *Drugs* 25(3):290–314, 1983.
14. Davenport A, Finn R: Paracetamol (acetaminophen) poisoning resulting in acute renal failure without hepatic coma. *Nephron* 50(1):55–56, 1988.
15. Roth B, Woo O, Blanc P: Early metabolic acidosis and coma after acetaminophen ingestion. *Ann Emerg Med* 33(4):452–456, 1999.
16. Fischereder M, Jaffe JP: Thrombocytopenia following acute acetaminophen overdose. *Am J Hematol* 45(3):258–259, 1994.
17. Mohler CR, Nordt SP, Williams SR, et al: Prospective evaluation of mild to moderate pediatric acetaminophen exposures. *Ann Emerg Med* 35(3): 239–244, 2000.
18. Watkins PB, Kaplowitz N, Slattery JT, et al: Aminotransferase elevations in healthy adults receiving 4 grams of acetaminophen daily: a randomized controlled trial. *JAMA* 296(1):87–93, 2006.
19. Heubi JE, Barbacci MB, Zimmerman HJ: Therapeutic misadventures with acetaminophen: hepatoxicity after multiple doses in children. *J Pediatr* 132(1):22–27, 1998.
20. Whitcomb DC, Block GD: Association of acetaminophen hepatotoxicity with fasting and ethanol use. *JAMA* 272(23):1845–1850, 1994.
21. Rivera-Penera T, Gugig R, Davis J, et al: Outcome of acetaminophen overdose in pediatric patients and factors contributing to hepatotoxicity. *J Pediatr* 130(2):300–304, 1997.
22. Rumack BH, Matthew H: Acetaminophen poisoning and toxicity. *Pediatrics* 55(6):871–876, 1975.
23. Prescott LF, Roscoe P, Wright N, et al: Plasma-paracetamol half-life and hepatic necrosis in patients with paracetamol overdosage. *Lancet* 1(7698): 519–522, 1971.
24. Smilkstein MJ, Knapp GL, Kulig KW, et al: Efficacy of oral N-acetylcysteine in the treatment of acetaminophen overdose. Analysis of the national multicenter study (1976 to 1985). *N Engl J Med* 319(24):1557–1562, 1988.
25. Cetaruk EW, Dart RC, Horowitz RS, et al: Extended-release acetaminophen overdose. *JAMA* 275(9):686, 1996.
26. Temple AR, Mrazik TJ: More on extended-release acetaminophen. *N Engl J Med* 333(22):1508–1509, 1995.
27. Graudins A, Aaron CK, Linden CH: Overdose of extended-release acetaminophen. *N Engl J Med* 333(3):196, 1995.
28. Prescott LF, Illingworth RN, Critchley JA, et al: Intravenous N-acetylcysteine: the treatment of choice for paracetamol poisoning. *Br Med J* 2(6198):1097–1100, 1979.
29. Harrison PM, Wendon JA, Gimson AE, et al: Improvement by acetylcysteine of hemodynamics and oxygen transport in fulminant hepatic failure. *N Engl J Med* 324(26):1852–1857, 1991.

30. Rumack BH, Peterson RC, Koch GG, et al: Acetaminophen overdose. 662 cases with evaluation of oral acetylcysteine treatment. *Arch Intern Med* 141(3 Spec No):380–385, 1981.
31. Cumberland Pharmaceuticals Inc., Nashville, Tennessee, USA, 2004.
32. Kao LW, Kirk MA, Furbee RB, et al: What is the rate of adverse events after oral N-acetylcysteine administered by the intravenous route to patients with suspected acetaminophen poisoning? *Ann Emerg Med* 42(6):741–750, 2003.
33. Miller LF, Rumack BH: Clinical safety of high oral doses of acetylcysteine. *Semin Oncol* 10[1, Suppl 1]:76–85, 1983.
34. Dawson AH, Henry DA, McEwen J: Adverse reactions to *N*-acetylcysteine during treatment for paracetamol poisoning. *Med J Aust* 150(6):329–331, 1989.
35. Bailey B, McGuigan MA: Management of anaphylactoid reactions to intravenous *N*-acetylcysteine. *Ann Emerg Med* 31(6):710–715, 1998.
36. Smilkstein MJ, Bronstein AC, Linden C, et al: Acetaminophen overdose: a 48-hour intravenous N-acetylcysteine treatment protocol. *Ann Emerg Med* 20(10):1058–1063, 1991.
37. Keays R, Harrison PM, Wendon JA, et al: Intravenous acetylcysteine in paracetamol induced fulminant hepatic failure: a prospective controlled trial. *BMJ* 303(6809):1026–1029, 1991.
38. Burkhart KK, Janco N, Kulig KW, et al: Cimetidine as adjunctive treatment for acetaminophen overdose. *Hum Exp Toxicol* 14(3):299–304, 1995.
39. Coon MJ, Koop DR, Reeve LE, et al: Alcohol metabolism and toxicity: role of cytochrome P-450. *Fundam Appl Toxicol* 4(2 Pt 1):134–143, 1984.
40. Tredger JM, Smith HM, Read RB, et al: Effects of ethanol ingestion on the metabolism of a hepatotoxic dose of paracetamol in mice. *Xenobiotica* 16(7):661–670, 1986.
41. Ali FM, Boyer EW, Bird SB: Estimated risk of hepatotoxicity after an acute acetaminophen overdose in alcoholics. *Alcohol* 42(3):213–218, 2008.
42. Bray GP, Harrison PM, O'Grady JG, et al: Long-term anticonvulsant therapy worsens outcome in paracetamol-induced fulminant hepatic failure. *Hum Exp Toxicol* 11(4):265–270, 1992.
43. Rumack BH: Acetaminophen overdose in young children. Treatment and effects of alcohol and other additional ingestants in 417 cases. *Am J Dis Child* 138(5):428–433, 1984.
44. Miller RP, Roberts RJ, Fischer LJ: Acetaminophen elimination kinetics in neonates, children, and adults. *Clin Pharmacol Ther* 19(3):284–294, 1976.
45. Roberts I, Robinson MJ, Mughal MZ, et al: Paracetamol metabolites in the neonate following maternal overdose. *Br J Clin Pharmacol* 18(2):201–206, 1984.
46. Riggs BS, Bronstein AC, Kulig K, et al: Acute acetaminophen overdose during pregnancy. *Obstet Gynecol* 74(2):247–253, 1989.
47. Horowitz RS, Dart RC, Jarvie DR, et al: Placental transfer of N-acetylcysteine following human maternal acetaminophen toxicity. *J Toxicol Clin Toxicol* 35(5):447–451, 1997.
48. Douglas D, Smilkstein M, Sholar JB: Overdose with extended-relief acetaminophen: is a new approach necessary? *Acad Emerg Med* 2:397, 1995.
49. Stork DG, Rees S, Howland MA, et al: Pharmacokinetics of extended relief vs. regular release Tylenol in simulated human overdose. *J Toxicol* 34:157, 1996.
50. Seeff LB, Cuccherini BA, Zimmerman HJ, et al: Acetaminophen hepatotoxicity in alcoholics. A therapeutic misadventure. *Ann Intern Med* 104(3): 399–404, 1986.
51. Hall AH, Kulig KW, Rumack BH: Acetaminophen hepatotoxicity. *JAMA* 256(14):1893–1894, 1986.
52. Benson GD: Acetaminophen in chronic liver disease. *Clin Pharmacol Ther* 33(1):95–101, 1983.
53. Harrison PM, Keays R, Bray GP, et al: Improved outcome of paracetamol-induced fulminant hepatic failure by late administration of acetylcysteine. *Lancet* 335(8705):1572–1573, 1990.
54. Bruno MK, Cohen SD, Khairallah EA: Antidotal effectiveness of N-acetylcysteine in reversing acetaminophen-induced hepatotoxicity. Enhancement of the proteolysis of arylated proteins. *Biochem Pharmacol* 37(22):4319–4325, 1988.
55. Singer AJ, Carracio TR, Mofenson HC: The temporal profile of increased transaminase levels in patients with acetaminophen-induced liver dysfunction. *Ann Emerg Med* 26(1):49–53, 1995.
56. Yip L, Dart RC: A 20-hour treatment for acute acetaminophen overdose. *N Engl J Med* 348(24):2471–2472, 2003.
57. Hamlyn AN, Douglas AP, James O: The spectrum of paracetamol (acetaminophen) overdose: clinical and epidemiological studies. *Postgrad Med J* 54(632):400–404, 1978.
58. Clark R, Borirakchanyavat V, Davidson AR, et al: Hepatic damage and death from overdose of paracetamol. *Lancet* 1(7794):66–70, 1973.
59. O'Grady JG, Wendon J, Tan KC, et al: Liver transplantation after paracetamol overdose. *BMJ* 303(6796):221–223, 1991.
60. James O, Lesna M, Roberts SH, et al: Liver damage after paracetamol overdose. Comparison of liver-function tests, fasting serum bile acids, and liver histology. *Lancet* 2(7935):579–581, 1975.
61. Bernal W, Donaldson N, Wyncoll D, et al: Blood lactate as an early predictor of outcome in paracetamol-induced acute liver failure: a cohort study. *Lancet* 359(9306):558–563, 2002.
62. Schmidt LE, Dalhoff K: Alpha-fetoprotein is a predictor of outcome in acetaminophen-induced liver injury. *Hepatology* 41(1):26–31, 2005.

CHAPTER 119 ■ ALCOHOLS AND GLYCOL POISONING

JENNIFER L. ENGLUND, MARCO L.A. SIVILOTTI AND MARSHA D. FORD

The accidental or deliberate consumption of alcohols and glycols is a major cause of health problems [1,2]. Although light consumption of ethanol may be associated with health benefits in some populations [3–5], heavy consumption increases overall mortality, especially mortality due to trauma, suicide, cirrhosis, and malignancies [6]. Ethanol is estimated to contribute to 100,000 deaths annually in the United States; with economic costs in excess of $200 billion [7,8]. Ethanol is involved in at least 10% of fatalities reported to US poison centers, and other alcohols and glycols, especially methanol and ethylene glycol, are responsible for another 3% of all fatalities [9]. These so-called toxic alcohols, namely methanol and ethylene glycol, are usually involved in sporadic poisonings, often involving the accidental exposure of a young child to automotive or household products or the intentional suicidal ingestion in adults. Furthermore, multiple-victim poisonings can occur after recreational substitution for ethanol, during illicit manufacture of ethanol, or after the addition of other glycol products [10–12].

ETHANOL

Ethanol is consumed by most adults and is the most serious drug of abuse in Western society. Approximately one-third of the US population can be categorized as moderate-to-heavy drinkers, consuming four or more alcoholic drinks per week and of these, about one in five can be considered problem drinkers or alcoholics [13]. Ethanol use is a factor in about 8% of emergency department visits [14], 10% to 50% of hospital admissions [15], and its projected economic costs due to job absenteeism and poor job performance are staggering [8,13]. Chronic ethanol consumption can cause multiorgan system

TABLE 119.1

COMPARATIVE DATA ON THE TOXIC ALCOHOLS AND GLYCOLS

Substance	Formula	Molecular weight	Specific gravity	V_d (L/kg)	Elimination half-life ($t^1/_2$)	Boiling point (°C)	Onset of toxicity	Important metabolites
Ethanol	$CH_3\ CH_2OH$	46	0.79	0.6	Zero order at 15–30 mg/dL/h	78.5	30–60 min	Acetaldehyde Acetic acid
Methanol	CH_3OH	32	0.79	0.7	Zero order at 8.5 mg/dL/h without ethanol; first order: $t^1/_2$ = 46.5 h with ethanol or fomepizole and 2.5 h with hemodialysis	64.7	12–24 h[a]	Formaldehyde Formic acid
Ethylene glycol	CH_2–CH_2 | | OH OH	62	1.11	0.68	First order: $t^1/_2$ = 2.5–4.5 h without ethanol and with normal kidneys, 17 h with ethanol or fomepizole and <3 h with hemodialysis	197.6	4–12 h[a]	Glycoaldehyde Glyoxylic acid Glycolic acid Oxalic acid
Isopropanol	$CH_3\ CHCH_3$ | OH	60	0.79	0.6–0.7	First order: $t^1/_2$ = 2.5–3.5 h	82.5	30–60 min	Acetone
Propylene glycol	$CH_2\ CHCH_3$ | | OH OH	76	1.04	0.55	First order: $t^1/_2$ = 2–5 h in adults, 19.3 h in infants	188.2	Seconds with intravenous, ? with dermal	Pyruvate Lactate Acetate
Benzyl alcohol	C_6H_5–CH_2OH	108	1.04	?	?	204.7	?	Benzoic acid Hippuric acid
Diethylene glycol	$CH_2\ CH_2\ O\ CH_2\ CH_2$ | | OH OH	106	1.12	?	?	245	?	2-Hydroxyethoxyacetic acid

[a]For metabolite effects; may be longer if ethanol coingested.
V_d, volume of distribution.
Data from Refs. [74,80,81,86,91,92,94,103–105,109,127,128,130,146].

disease, nutritional disorders, and teratogenic effects. In addition to beverages (typically 4% to 50% ethanol by volume), ethanol can be found in a myriad of colognes, perfumes, mouthwashes, aftershaves, and over-the-counter medicinals. Many of these products contain 50% to 99% ethanol and can be sources for intoxication, especially for children [16].

The chemical properties and kinetics of ethanol are summarized in Table 119.1. Ethanol is a small, slightly polar aliphatic alcohol with a weak electric charge, miscible in water and lipids. It diffuses easily into all body tissues. It is postulated that ethanol influences multiple ion channels, possibly by causing subtle alterations in their tertiary structure or their dynamic interaction with cell membranes. The behavioral effects of ethanol may result from its ability to antagonize the excitatory *N*-methyl-D-aspartate–glutamate receptor and to potentiate the inhibitory γ-aminobutyric acid A receptor [17–20]. Ethanol is also known to interact with glycine, nicotinic acetylcholine, 5-HT_3, and P_{2X} purinergic receptors, as well as the L-type calcium- and potassium-channel proteins [21,22]. The major metabolite, acetate, has been shown to mimic adenosine's effects via the P_1 receptor [23]. The precise role of these and other effects in producing intoxication, dependence, and withdrawal (see Chapter 145) is uncertain.

Ethanol is readily absorbed from the gastrointestinal tract, with 57% of the absorption occurring in the small intestine. Peak ethanol levels typically occur 30 to 60 minutes after ingestion if the stomach is empty [16]. Women have higher peak ethanol concentrations after a given dose because of smaller body mass and smaller relative body water, rather than gender differences in gastric mucosal alcohol dehydrogenase (ADH) activity [24–27].

Metabolism of ethanol occurs predominantly in the liver by three enzymatic systems: the cytosolic ADH enzyme family (especially class I), the cytochrome P450 enzymes (microsomal ethanol oxidizing system, largely CYP2E1 but also 3A4 and 1A2), and peroxisomal catalase [28]. Metabolism is Michaelis–Menten with zero-order kinetics prevailing at levels over 100 mg per dL [29]. Only a small fraction of ethanol is exhaled or secreted in urine and sweat [13,30].

ADH is responsible for greater than 57% of ethanol metabolism at low doses. In the ADH metabolic pathway (Fig. 119.1), ethanol is oxidized to acetaldehyde and then to acetate in a process that reduces oxidized nicotinamide adenine dinucleotide (NAD^+) to nicotinamide adenine dinucleotide (NADH). The increased ratio of NADH to NAD^+ can inhibit NAD^+-dependent reactions, such as gluconeogenesis,

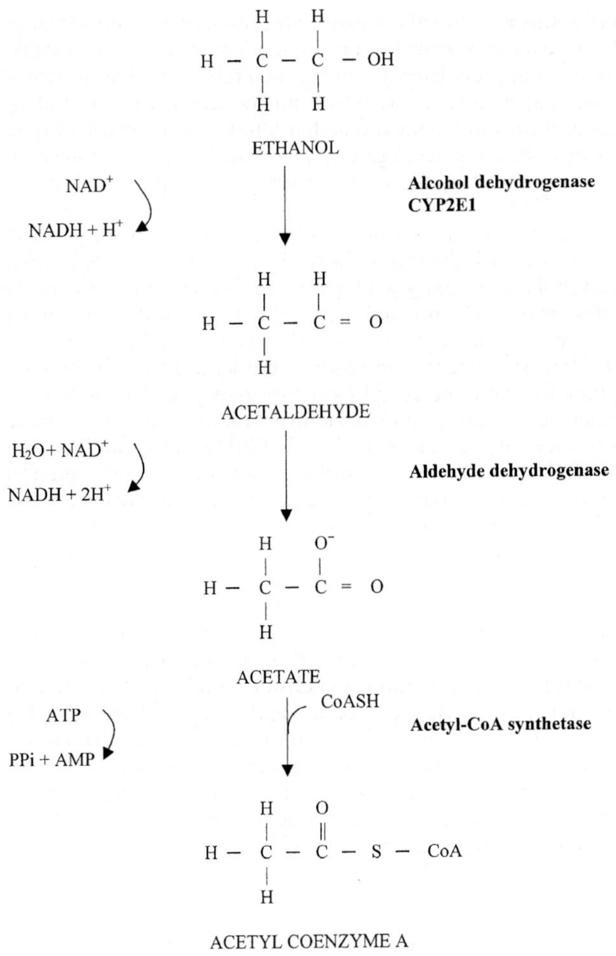

FIGURE 119.1. Ethanol metabolism. AMP, adenosine monophosphate; ATP, adenosine triphosphate; Co, coenzyme; NAD^+, oxidized form of nicotinamide adenine dinucleotide; NADH, nicotinamide adenine dinucleotide; PPi, inorganic pyrophosphate.

as well as slowing subsequent ethanol oxidation and clearance [31]. Acetate is linked to coenzyme A (acetyl-CoA), which can then participate in the citric acid cycle, fatty acid synthesis, or ketone formation [30]. Genetic variations in ADH and aldehyde dehydrogenase have been extensively characterized and may play a role in determining susceptibility to alcoholism [32–35]. Normally, the cytochrome P450 and catalase systems play minor roles in ethanol metabolism [36,37]. Chronic ethanol use can induce CYP2E1 activity 4- to 10-fold, allowing habitual users to metabolize ethanol twice as quickly as occasional drinkers [38].

Ethanol is a central nervous system (CNS) depressant. After acute ingestion, there is often an initial stage of paradoxical excitation due to release of learned social inhibitions. For nontolerant individuals, a blood ethanol concentration as low as 20 mg per dL impairs driving-related skills involving perception and attention [39]. At concentrations of 50 mg per dL, gross motor control and orientation may be affected, and intoxication may become apparent [40]. Lethargy, ataxia, and muscular incoordination may be seen at serum levels of 150 mg per dL or greater, coma at approximately 250 mg per dL, and death with levels greater than 450 mg per dL [16,41]. Tolerant drinkers can achieve higher levels before developing similar symptoms, and survival has been reported despite a serum level of 1,500 mg per dL [42]. At high doses, ethanol functions as an anesthetic, causing CNS depression, autonomic dysfunction (e.g., hypotension, hypothermia), coma, and death from respiratory depression and cardiovascular collapse. The estimated LD_{50} in adults is 5 to 8 g per kg and 3 g per kg for children [16].

Tolerance to ethanol's effects develops both acutely and after chronic consumption. With acute consumption, the physiologic effects at a given serum level of ethanol have been noted to be less when ethanol concentrations are declining rather than when levels are rising (Mellanby effect) [43]. Compared with inexperienced drinkers, chronic drinkers experience diminished effects to a given amount of ethanol. Tolerance is accompanied by changes in membrane-associated receptors [21,22].

Clinical Manifestations

Patients may present with varying degrees of altered consciousness, including agitation, stupor, and coma. The odor of ethanol or its congeners on their breath is usually present. Slurred speech, ataxia, and nystagmus are noted in patients with mild to moderate intoxication. Disconjugate gaze is frequently seen in comatose patients. Acute intoxication may be accompanied by vomiting, particularly in novice drinkers. Children younger than 10 years of age are most susceptible to alcohol-induced hypoglycemia, which can occur at relatively low serum ethanol levels (discussed later).

Diagnostic Evaluation

The physical examination should be directed toward evaluation of the airway and a search for complicating or contributing factors such as trauma, infection, and hemorrhage. In patients with moderate-to-severe poisoning, laboratory studies including complete blood cell count, serum electrolytes, blood urea nitrogen, creatinine, glucose, ethanol, magnesium, calcium, and phosphorus level, liver function tests, prothrombin time, electrocardiogram, chest radiograph, arterial or venous blood gas, and urinalysis should be obtained as clinically indicated. If the level of consciousness is inconsistent with the serum ethanol level or does not improve over a few hours, the physician should reconsider the diagnosis of ethanol intoxication (Table 119.2).

Management

Patients with stupor or coma who cannot be aroused to a verbal (but not necessarily coherent) state or who have a poor respiratory effort should be intubated to ensure airway patency and to protect against pulmonary aspiration. Intravenous (IV) naloxone (0.1 to 2 mg), dextrose (25 to 50 g) and thiamine hydrochloride (100 mg) should be administered when opioid toxicity, hypoglycemia, or Wernicke's encephalopathy are considerations.

Activated charcoal should be withheld unless potentially toxic coingestants are suspected. Hypothermia, if present, is usually mild in the absence of environmental exposure, and can be managed with warm blankets. Nutritional, electrolyte, and fluid deficiencies should be corrected. A variety of interventions trying to increase ethanol clearance or decrease its effects, including supplemental IV fluids, dextrose, and fructose, are neither clinically useful nor recommended [44,45].

ALCOHOLIC KETOACIDOSIS

Alcoholic ketoacidosis (AKA) develops as a result of hormonal, nutritional, and metabolic changes caused by ethanol (Fig. 119.2). Because ethanol retards ketogenesis, AKA usually occurs when ethanol levels are low to absent [30]. Ethanol

TABLE 119.2

DIFFERENTIAL DIAGNOSES FOR ACUTE ETHANOL INTOXICATION

Metabolic
Hypoglycemia
Hyperglycemia
Hyponatremia
Hypothermia
Hepatic encephalopathy
Disulfiram reaction
Hypercalcemia
Hypoxia
Drug intoxication
Phencyclidine
Opioids
Cyclic antidepressants
Other alcohols (methanol, isopropanol, ethylene glycol)
Other sedative-hypnotics (meprobamate, methaqualone, glutethimide, benzodiazepines, barbiturates, chloral hydrate, ethchlorvynol, methyprylon)
Anticholinergics
Carbon monoxide
Trauma
Intracranial hemorrhage (subdural, epidural, intracerebral bleed)
Infections
Central nervous system infections
Acquired immunodeficiency syndrome
Sepsis
Neurologic
Postictal
Delirium tremens
Wernicke's encephalopathy
Adapted from Adinoff B, Bone GHA, Linnoila M: Acute ethanol poisoning and the ethanol withdrawal syndrome. *Med Toxicol* 3:172, 1988.

metabolism indirectly impairs gluconeogenesis and increases fatty acid and ketone formation. Inadequate nutritional intake in alcoholics depletes glycogen, minerals, and vitamin stores. Vomiting results in decreased intravascular volume and increased catecholamine levels that blunt insulin release [46] activate lipase, and accelerate free fatty acid oxidation. Glucagon activates the carnitine acyltransferase system producing excess acetyl-CoA.

Acetyl-CoA cannot be used by mammals to form pyruvate or higher carbohydrates. Instead, it can undergo only three metabolic fates: fatty acid synthesis, oxidation to CO_2 in the citric acid cycle, and cholesterol or ketone body formation via 3-hydroxy-3-methylglutaryl-CoA. The ketogenic pathway has the largest capacity and requires the least adenosine triphosphate for handling acetyl-CoA overload [46]. Nutritional deficiencies impair acetyl-CoA conversion to triglycerides and its entrance into the citric acid cycle [30]. Finally, the increased NADH to NAD^+ redox ratio caused by ethanol oxidation favors the conversion of acetoacetate to β-hydroxybutyrate, which is largely responsible for the ketoacidosis.

Other acid–base abnormalities may occur in alcoholics. Respiratory acidosis may be caused by hypoglycemia or ethanol-induced respiratory depression. Lactic acidosis can occur secondary to seizure activity, an increase in the NADH to NAD^+ ratio that favors lactate formation from pyruvate, decreased gluconeogenesis, thiamine deficiency impairing pyruvate's entry into the citric acid cycle, and liver dysfunction [47]. Vomiting may cause volume contraction, hypokalemia, and metabolic alkalosis [46]. A mild acetic acidosis may be seen when peripheral tissues incompletely oxidize acetate. An unexplained hyperchloremic metabolic acidosis has been observed in acutely intoxicated patients [47].

Clinical Manifestations

Patients with AKA usually present with a recent history of binge alcohol drinking and poor nutritional intake followed by vomiting. The fruity odor of ketones may be detected along with Kussmaul's breathing, dry mucous membranes, tachycardia, orthostatic hypotension, and poor skin turgor [30].

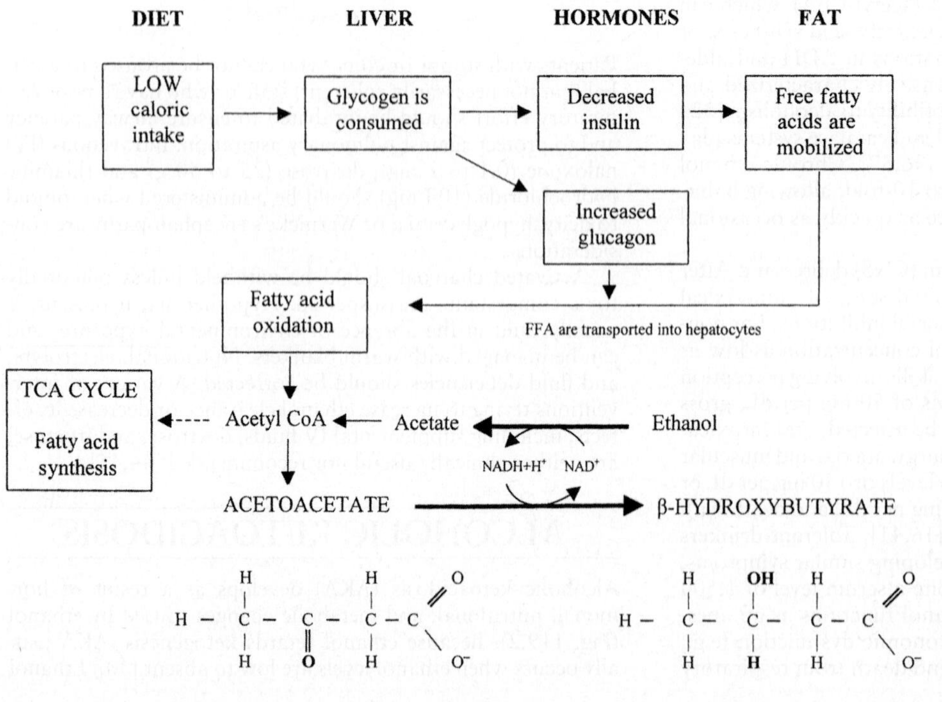

FIGURE 119.2. Mechanism of alcoholic ketoacidosis. Co, coenzyme; FFA, free fatty acids; NAD^+, oxidized form of nicotinamide adenine dinucleotide; NADH, nicotinamide adenine dinucleotide; TCA, tricarboxylic acid cycle (also known as *citric acid cycle*). [Adapted from Eckardt MJ, Harford TC, Kaelber CT, et al: Health hazards associated with alcohol consumption. *JAMA* 246:648, 1981, with permission.]

Abdominal pain is typical, with nonspecific tenderness on examination [48].

Diagnostic Evaluation

The diagnosis of AKA is a diagnosis of exclusion. Signs and symptoms of concomitant gastritis, pancreatitis, hepatitis, gastrointestinal hemorrhage, and vitamin and mineral deficiencies are often present. Laboratory studies should include those listed for acute ethanol intoxication plus serum ketones, lactate, and osmolality. Ethanol levels are often low to undetectable, and hypoglycemia may be present [49,50]. A respiratory or metabolic alkalosis may be present in addition to the anion gap metabolic acidosis. At presentation, the predominant serum ketone is usually β-hydroxybutyrate due to the altered redox state, which results in falsely low serum ketones by the semi-quantitative nitroprusside test for acetoacetate [30]. Many laboratories now measure β-hydroxybutyrate directly to mitigate this concern. Hypokalemia is uncommon, in part because acidosis shifts potassium out of the cell. The osmol gap may be elevated from glycerol, acetone, and its metabolites [51], even after correcting for the serum ethanol concentration [52].

The differential diagnosis of an anion gap metabolic acidosis includes lactic acidosis; salicylate poisoning; uremia; diabetic ketoacidosis; and intoxication from iron, ibuprofen, toluene, methanol, ethylene glycol, and diethylene glycol. Hypoxia and hypotension are the most common causes of lactic acidosis, but malignancies, leukemia, and toxicity due to cyanide, metformin, and carbon monoxide should also be considered [53]. AKA can usually be differentiated from diabetic ketoacidosis by the lack of significant hyperglycemia, minimal alteration of consciousness, a relatively mild acidosis, and rapid improvement with supportive therapy [54]. The presence of more than mild tenderness on abdominal examination should prompt investigation for other pathology such as pancreatitis, hepatitis, sepsis, or pneumonia [48].

Management

Supportive therapy is the same as that noted for acute intoxication. IV fluid resuscitation, glucose (25 to 50 g), and thiamine (100 mg) reverse the ketogenic process and are the mainstays of therapy. Maintenance fluids should consist of dextrose (5%) in normal saline [30]. Thiamine facilitates the entry of pyruvate into the citric acid cycle and protects against Wernicke's encephalopathy [55]. Once urine output is established, supplemental potassium and magnesium should be administered. Hypophosphatemia may develop with increased glycolysis and carbohydrate refeeding and should be corrected with potassium phosphate [49,54]. Hospitalization and refeeding of malnourished patients may be required.

ETHANOL-RELATED HYPOGLYCEMIA

Four types of hypoglycemia associated with or induced by ethanol have been delineated: alcohol-induced fasting hypoglycemia, reactive hypoglycemia of chronic alcoholism, alcohol potentiation of drug- or exercise-induced hypoglycemia, and alcohol-promoted reactive hypoglycemia [56]. Alcohol-induced fasting hypoglycemia is the best understood. Marginal nutritional status is the only requirement for its development, and it can occur in poorly nourished alcoholics and in young children, fasted normal subjects, patients on low-carbohydrate diets, and those with thyrotoxicosis and adrenocortical deficiency [49,56,57]. When these patients consume ethanol rather than food, their marginal glycogen stores are readily depleted by glycogenolysis and the body's metabolic needs become dependent on gluconeogenesis. Ethanol inhibits this reaction [57], however, probably by the increasing NADH to NAD^+ ratio. This effect preferentially shunts pyruvate to lactate and thus blocks pyruvate from participating in gluconeogenesis or other reactions in which it is the key intermediate (Fig. 119.3) [30].

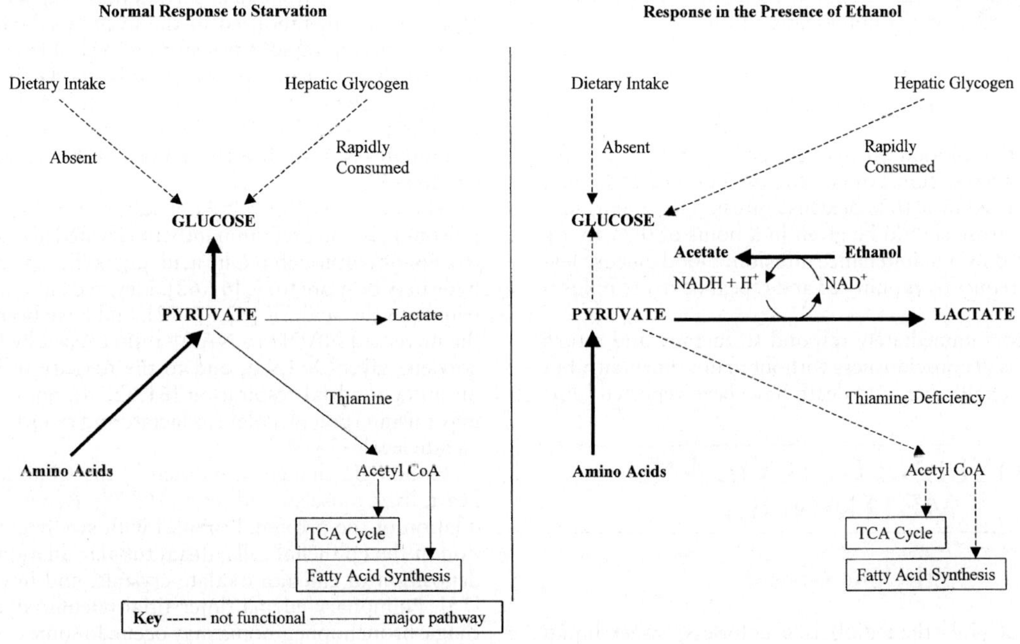

FIGURE 119.3. Ethanol-induced hypoglycemia. Co, coenzyme; NAD^+, oxidized form of nicotinamide adenine dinucleotide; NADH, nicotinamide adenine dinucleotide; TCA, tricarboxylic acid cycle (also known as *citric acid cycle*). [Adapted from Hoffman RS, Goldfrank LR: Ethanol-associated metabolic disorders. *Emerg Med Clin North Am* 7:943, 1989, with permission.]

Contributory endocrinologic abnormalities may include impaired cortisol release and decreased growth hormone secretion due to hypothalamic–pituitary dysfunction [56,57]. Lactic acidosis may result from excessive lactate production [57].

The biochemical mechanisms underlying the other types of hypoglycemia are poorly understood [56,58], but alcohol-promoted reactive hypoglycemia may be due to potentiation of insulin secretion by ethanol [56]. Liver disease is not necessary for the development of hypoglycemia [59].

Clinical Manifestations

CNS depression ranging from confusion to coma, seizures, and symptoms of increased sympathetic activity such as diaphoresis, anxiety, tremulousness, palpitations, and weakness are the hallmarks of hypoglycemia. Hypothermia occurs frequently [56].

The CNS effects of hypoglycemia and ethanol intoxication can mimic one another, whereas hypoglycemia-induced adrenergic signs and symptoms can be mistaken for ethanol withdrawal. The differential diagnoses are similar to those for acute ethanol intoxication (Table 119.2).

Diagnostic Evaluation

Laboratory evaluation is the same as for a patient with acute intoxication. If metabolic acidosis is present, the studies recommended for AKA are also indicated. Serum glucose concentrations are usually less than 40 mg per dL, ethanol levels are often low [56], and lactate levels may be elevated [57].

Caution is advised when assessing capillary blood glucose levels with point-of-care testing. Errors can be introduced by the age of the strips, and by the accuracy of machines used to read them especially outside the calibration range. The effect of varying ethanol levels on the accuracy of these strips has not been adequately studied. Given the morbidity and mortality of severe hypoglycemia, the potential errors in testing, and the benign nature of IV glucose, all symptomatic patients with an equivocal glucose reading should be treated with glucose, especially if diabetic or alcohol impaired [30].

Management

Therapy for ethanol-induced hypoglycemia parallels that for acute ethanol intoxication. An IV dextrose bolus of 25 to 50 g should be followed by a 10% dextrose infusion. In young children, 25% dextrose should be given in a bolus of 0.25 to 1 g per kg, followed by a maintenance infusion. Blood glucose levels should be frequently monitored and repeat dextrose boluses may be necessary.

Most patients immediately respond to therapy and return to normal levels of consciousness without major morbidity, but persistent encephalopathy and death have been reported [30].

ETHYLENE GLYCOL AND METHANOL

Ethylene Glycol

Ethylene glycol (1,2-ethanediol) is a colorless, sweet liquid [60,61] that imparts a warm sensation to the tongue and esophagus when swallowed. It is found primarily in automotive antifreeze solutions. Ingestions usually result from suicide attempts, intentional substitution of ethylene glycol for ethanol, or accidental exposure. Ethylene glycol itself causes little toxicity other than ethanol-like inebriation until it is metabolized in the liver into its toxic acid metabolites (Fig. 119.4). Ethylene glycol is first metabolized in the liver by ADH to glycoaldehyde, which is rapidly transformed via aldehyde dehydrogenase to glycolic acid. Glycolic acid is slowly converted to glyoxylic acid, which in turn is converted to multiple metabolites, including oxalic acid [61,62]. It is uncertain which of these metabolites is most directly responsible for renal tubular toxicity [63–65].

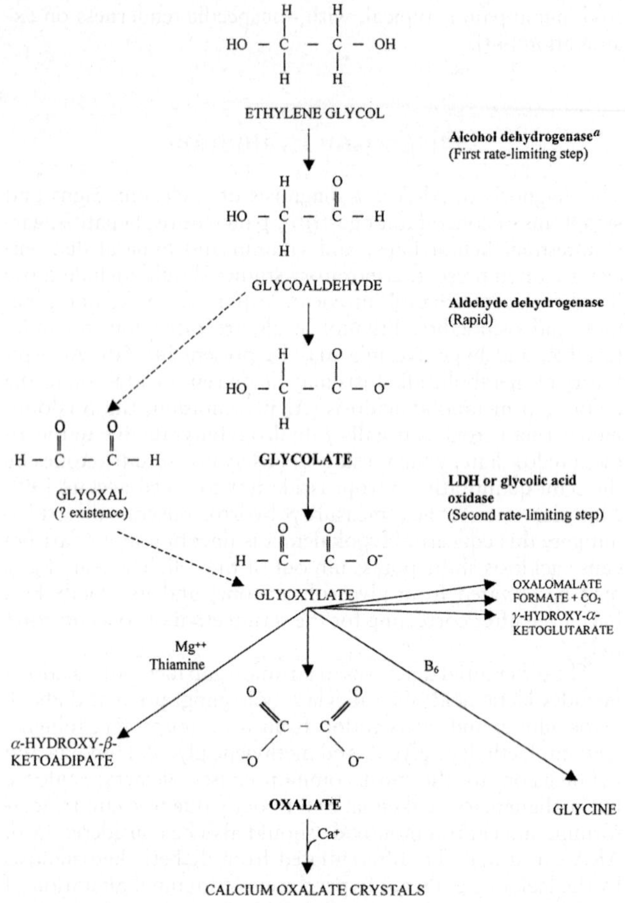

FIGURE 119.4. Ethylene glycol metabolism. [a] Blocked by ethanol and fomepizole. LDH, lactate dehydrogenase.

The anion gap metabolic acidosis seen in ethylene glycol poisoning is due predominantly to elevated glycolic acid levels, [62,66–68] although oxalic acid, glyoxylic acid and glycoaldehyde may be more toxic [61,62]. Elevated lactic acid levels contribute to the acidosis [62,67–72], and have been attributed to the increased NADH to NAD^+ ratio caused by metabolism of ethylene glycol [64,73], and to the toxicity of glyoxylic acid on mitochondrial respiration [61,62,74]. Some lactate assays may misinterpret glycolate as lactate and report falsely elevated lactate levels [75–77].

Pathologic changes are noted in the CNS, kidneys, lungs, heart, liver, muscles, and retina [16,78]. Renal findings include dilation of the proximal tubules with swelling and vacuolization of the epithelial cells, distal tubular dilation, intratubular deposition of calcium oxalate crystals, and interstitial edema [73]. Pulmonary edema, interstitial pneumonitis, and hemorrhagic bronchopneumonia may occur. In some cases, interstitial myocarditis, skeletal muscle inflammation, and centrilobular hepatic fatty infiltration may develop. CNS findings include cerebral edema, meningoencephalitis, and cerebellar changes, including focal loss of Purkinje cells [78].

The chemical properties and kinetics of ethylene glycol are summarized in Table 119.1. Oral absorption of ethylene glycol occurs rapidly. Percutaneous absorption through intact skin is negligible. Ethylene glycol has a high boiling point and toxicity from vapor inhalation does not occur. Hepatic metabolism predominates yet renal elimination of the parent compound is initially substantial. The ensuing renal failure markedly prolongs the elimination of ethylene glycol and its metabolites [67,73,79,80].

The reported minimum lethal dose is 1.6 g per kg in humans. Hence, the estimated fatal dose widely quoted for a 70-kg person is 100 mL of 100% ethylene glycol, but this value is based on limited data [81] and assumes no treatment. With early and intensive treatment, survival has been reported in patients with serum ethylene glycol concentrations as high as 1,889 mg per dL [70,82,83].

Methanol

Methanol is a colorless liquid and has an odor distinct from that of ethanol [84,85]. Dietary sources and endogenous metabolism can produce serum methanol levels of 0.15 mg per dL [86]. Exogenous sources of methanol include windshield washing fluid, de-icing fluids, carburetor cleaners, paint removers, and paint thinners.

Methanol is oxidized in the liver by ADH to formaldehyde, which is quickly converted to formic acid (formate) by hepatic aldehyde dehydrogenase (Fig. 119.5). In primates, formate accumulates due to saturation of one-carbon metabolism. High levels of formate, an inhibitor of mitochondrial cytochrome oxidase, cause histotoxic hypoxia and are responsible for the characteristic metabolic acidosis and ocular toxicity seen with methanol toxicity [73]. Formaldehyde is also very toxic, but it has a very short half-life.

Formate plays a pivotal role in methanol toxicity. Blood formate concentrations account for nearly the entire observed anion gap and base deficit [87–89]. Symptoms and prognosis also correlate better with formate than with methanol levels [90,91]. Primates infused with formic acid develop ocular toxicity, even when the acidosis is controlled with sodium bicarbonate [92]. Ocular toxicity results from the inhibition of cytochrome oxidase by formic acid in the optic nerve, leading to disruption of mitochondrial electron transport and decreased axoplasmic flow and electrical conduction [93]. Although this produces changes in the optic nerve head, direct retinal toxicity can also occur [94].

The chemical properties and kinetics of methanol are summarized in Table 119.1. Methanol is absorbed orally, dermally, and via inhalation [84,95]. Exposure can occur intentionally or accidentally, as occurred in Estonia in 2001 when 68 patients died after consuming illegal spirits contaminated with methanol [96]. A retrospective hospital record review of 16 individuals who inhaled carburetor cleaning fluid fumes identified 48 hospital presentations with serum methanol levels greater than 20 mg per dL and 19 greater than 50 mg per dL [74]. Methanol's metabolism is slower than that of ethylene glycol or ethanol [73], which may explain why methanol toxicity develops more slowly. Hepatic oxidation predominates, with only trivial amounts eliminated via the lungs and kidneys [84]. Elimination follows first-order kinetics at low doses and during hemodialysis [97–99]. At higher doses, zero-order (Michaelis–Menten) kinetics may prevail. In one untreated patient, methanol elimination occurred at a rate of 8.5 mg per dL per hour [100]. The elimination half-life of formate in one untreated patient was 3.7 hours [90], and averaged 3.4 ± 1.5 hours in eight patients treated with fomepizole (4-methylpyrazole) and leucovorin [89]. With hemodialysis, the formate elimination half-life was estimated to be between 1.1 and 2.8 hours [87,89,90].

Reported lethal doses in patients with inadequate, delayed, or no therapy vary considerably and are not well established. In one epidemic, the minimal lethal dose was 15 mL of a 40%-by-weight methanol solution. In another outbreak, one patient survived a 600-mL ingestion of pure methanol but had permanent sequelae, whereas another reportedly imbibed 500 mL without complications [10].

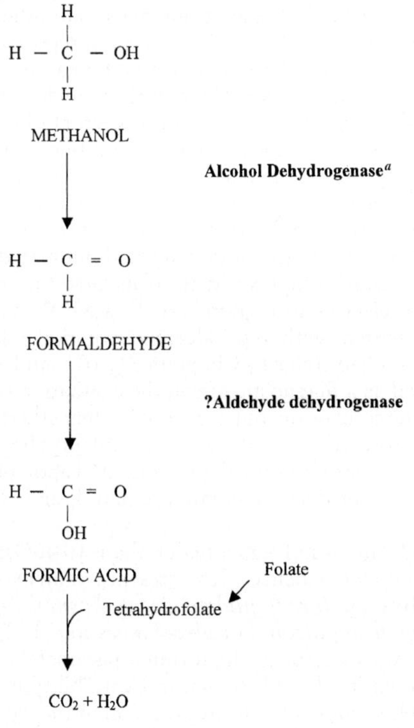

FIGURE 119.5. Methanol metabolism. [a]Blocked by ethanol and fomepizole.

Clinical Manifestations

Ethylene Glycol

Ethanol-like intoxication usually begins within an hour of ingestion. Symptoms due to toxic metabolites usually occur 4 to 12 hours after ingestion, but are delayed further if ethanol was coingested by delaying the metabolism of ethylene glycol. Patients may present alert, intoxicated, or in a coma, depending on the time since ingestion, the dose of ethylene glycol, coingestion of ethanol, and cross-tolerance [61,62,73,78,101,102]. Vital signs can be normal. Ocular exposure can produce a chemical conjunctivitis and chemosis [78], but systemic toxicity does not occur.

The classic division of ethylene glycol poisoning into three stages is primarily of historical interest. In reality, patients rarely exhibit sequential toxicity that can be readily divided into distinct stages. Shortly after ingestion and before significant metabolism of ethylene glycol has occurred, CNS effects such as ethanol-like intoxication, stupor, nausea, and vomiting predominate. As toxic metabolites begin to accumulate, a metabolic acidosis ensues with associated cardiovascular and pulmonary signs, including Kussmaul's respirations, tachycardia, cyanosis, and cardiogenic or noncardiogenic pulmonary edema [101]. As renal injury progresses, flank pain and tenderness, proteinuria, and anuria may occur. Acute renal failure occurs in nearly all untreated patients who manifest metabolic acidosis (serum bicarbonate less than 10 mmol per L). Renal dysfunction can develop within 9 hours of ingestion [103]. Patients may also develop myositis with muscle tenderness and elevated creatine kinase [61,73]. Death may result from severe metabolic derangements, cardiovascular or respiratory failure, or progressive CNS depression. Prolonged seizures, coma, and a cerebral herniation syndrome have also been reported [104]. Preterminal dysrhythmias and hypotension are rare [70]. The presence of hyperkalemia, severe acidemia, seizures, and coma at presentation demonstrate severe toxicity.

Seizures are usually generalized but do not occur in all cases. Jacksonian seizures have been reported, as have myoclonic jerks and tetanic contractions due to hypocalcemia [70,78]. Progressive CNS depression and prolonged seizures usually result from cerebral edema [73]. Transient nystagmus and cranial nerve (II, V, VI, VII, VIII, IX, and X) palsies have been reported to occur 4 to 18 days postingestion [82,104–107].

Methanol

Onset of toxicity usually occurs within 30 hours of methanol ingestion [108]. In one epidemic, a range of 40 minutes to 72 hours was reported. Factors influencing time to symptoms include the dose, ethanol coingestion, and folate stores [85,108].

Neurologic, ophthalmologic, and gastrointestinal symptoms predominate [20,21,97,98,109,110]. Methanol is a less potent CNS depressant than ethanol. Patients may be alert on admission and complain only of headache and dizziness. Amnesia, restlessness, acute mania, lethargy, confusion, coma, and convulsions may follow. Cases mimicking subarachnoid hemorrhage with severe headache, vomiting, hypertension, and bradycardia followed by loss of consciousness have been described. Dyspnea is reported by only 8% to 25% of patients [96].

Early on, many patients offer no visual complaints. Visual symptoms accompany the metabolic acidosis and usually develop when the blood pH falls below 7.2. Blurred vision, photophobia, scotomata, eye pain, partial or complete loss of vision, and visual hallucinations (e.g., bright lights, "skin over eyes," "snowstorm," dancing spots, flashes) have been reported. These disturbances can persist after formate has been completely eliminated and the acidosis has resolved.

Methanol can produce severe hemorrhagic gastritis and pancreatitis, causing upper abdominal pain, nausea, vomiting, and diarrhea. Liver function abnormalities have been documented in moderately to severely ill patients.

Vital signs may reveal tachycardia and Kussmaul's respirations, but the blood pressure is usually maintained. Untreated, patients can die from sudden respiratory arrest [84]. The skin may be cool and diaphoretic, and abdominal muscles rigid without rebound tenderness.

The most notable physical findings are those discovered on ophthalmologic examination, but these are late findings. Pupils may react sluggishly or may be fixed and dilated [10]. Funduscopic examination may show hyperemia of the optic discs followed by retinal edema, which develops initially along the retinal vessels and then spreads to the central areas of the fundus. Retinal vessel engorgement accompanies the retinal edema [110]. Papilledema may develop [20]. Ophthalmologic findings do not necessarily correlate with visual complaints.

Diagnostic Evaluation

Poisoning by ethylene glycol and methanol should be suspected in all patients with a history of ingesting ethanol substitutes or who have an unexplained anion gap metabolic acidosis.

Ethylene Glycol

Laboratory studies should include complete blood cell count; serum electrolytes; glucose; blood urea nitrogen; creatinine; arterial or venous blood gas; calcium; serum osmolality; ethanol, methanol, and ethylene glycol levels; and urinalysis. Additional laboratory studies may include electrocardiogram, chest radiograph, and head computed tomography as clinically indicated. Early after ingestion, before significant metabolism of ethylene glycol, an osmol gap may be present [111] with neither metabolic acidosis nor an anion gap (see later discussion on osmol gap). As ethylene glycol is metabolized, the osmol gap decreases and an anion gap metabolic acidosis develops. Patients who present very late may have renal failure with normal osmol and anion gaps, normal pH, and unmeasurable ethylene glycol levels.

Perhaps the greatest diagnostic challenge in managing a patient suspected to have ingested a toxic alcohol or glycol is the limited availability of methanol and ethylene glycol testing. Gas chromatography can reliably quantify the presence of ethylene glycol or methanol, but most hospitals are unable to obtain these tests in a timely fashion [112]. Moreover, some hospitals offer a "toxic alcohol screen" that detects methanol, ethanol, and isopropanol but not ethylene glycol, which is a diol. This nomenclature can mislead a clinician into interpreting a negative "toxic alcohol screen" as excluding the presence of ethylene glycol. Interference due to propionic acid, propylene glycol, glycerol, 2,3-butanediol, and β-hydroxybutyrate has been described [113–116]. Testing for glycolic acid or formic acid is even less available [76,117,118]. A rapid bedside qualitative test for ethylene glycol is available but not approved for diagnostic use in humans [119]. Breath alcohol analysis can mistake methanol for ethanol, providing indirect evidence of exposure. Therefore, diagnostic and therapeutic decisions are often based on circumstantial evidence derived from the history and available laboratory testing, pending confirmatory testing. It is essential for the physician to understand the strengths and the limitations of these indirect markers of toxicity.

Arterial pH measurements in ethylene glycol exposed patients can range from 6.7 to 7.5 [62,103]. Ethylene glycol poisoning often results in higher anion gaps than other causes of this abnormality [64]. A gap of 58 has been reported [70]. The differential diagnosis of an increased anion gap metabolic acidosis is discussed above (see Alcoholic Ketoacidosis section). In young children, child abuse and inborn errors of organic acid metabolism should be considered in the differential diagnosis [116,120]. Hyperkalemia may be seen in association with acidosis and with renal failure [61,78,101]. The creatinine and blood urea nitrogen are normal unless renal failure has supervened. Calcium levels are initially normal but may drop significantly as calcium complexes with oxalic acid to form calcium oxalate. The electrocardiogram may show ST-T wave and QTc changes consistent with hypocalcemia, hyperkalemia, or both.

The osmol gap (refer to Chapters 71, 101, and 117) is frequently used as a diagnostic test in the evaluation of these patients. Extreme caution must be used when interpreting the osmol gap, however. First, the serum osmolality should be measured by the freezing point depression, as vapor pressure osmometry will not detect methanol, ethanol, and isopropanol [121].

Although an osmol gap greater than 10 mOsm is often sought as indirect evidence of the presence of an exogenous alcohol or glycol, *failure to find an elevated osmol gap does not rule out significant alcohol or glycol ingestion* [122]. Cumulative measurement error in the formula parameters, variations in the formula itself, and the natural variability in the osmol gap at baseline contribute to imprecision in the calculated osmol gap [52,123,124]. This variability can hide a significant amount of an alcohol or glycol. Furthermore, as the parent alcohol or glycol is oxidized to the toxic charged metabolite, the osmol gap disappears. Conversely, an elevated osmol gap is not specific for alcohols or glycols, as lactic acidosis, ketoacidosis, and sepsis can also increase the osmol gap [122].

In studies of various control populations not exposed to methanol, isopropanol, or ethylene glycol, osmol gaps averaged approximately −1 to −2 mOsm per kg [125–127]. The variability was substantial, however, with standard deviations of between 5 and 8 mOsm per kg. Thus, although an arbitrary upper limit of 10 mOsm per kg has historically been used for the normal osmol gap [128], an osmol gap of 10 mOsm per kg in a patient whose usual baseline gap is 0 could represent substantial serum concentrations of ethylene glycol (62 mg per dL) or methanol (32 mg per dL) [129]. One patient with an osmol gap of only 11 mOsm per kg had an ethylene glycol level of 38 mg per dL and subsequently developed renal failure [64], whereas another patient with an osmol gap of 7.2 mOsm per kg required hemodialysis for ethylene glycol toxicity [130]. Thus, an elevated osmol gap may suggest the presence of an alcohol or glycol, but a normal gap does not rule out a small ingestion or a late presentation [122,126,131,132].

Microscopic examination of the urine for crystals is another indirect diagnostic test frequently recommended. Less than 50% of patients have crystalluria at presentation, however. Sequential urinalysis may improve sensitivity in detecting crystalluria [60,67,133]. Calcium oxalate monohydrate (needle shaped) and calcium oxalate dihydrate (envelope shaped) crystals can be seen. The monohydrate crystals are the predominant form at all concentrations and are more specific for ethylene glycol toxicity, but may be confused with uric or hippuric acid crystals [64,67]. The dihydrate crystals tend to occur at higher concentrations and convert to the monohydrate form within 24 hours [134]. They are less specific and can also be found in the urine after ingestion of oxalate-containing foods such as rhubarb. Other nonspecific urinary findings can include low specific gravity, proteinuria, hematuria, and pyuria. Some antifreeze manufacturers add fluorescein to their products to facilitate the detection of radiator leaks. Wood's lamp examination of the urine or gastric aspirate to detect fluorescence is unreliable and should not be used to make or exclude the diagnosis [135,136]. Other drugs, food products, toxins, and even endogenous compounds cause urine to fluoresce, as do many urine collection containers themselves [137,138].

Methanol

The laboratory studies listed for ethylene glycol evaluation should be obtained. Methanol can also cause an anion gap metabolic acidosis and an osmol gap [109]. The caveats noted under ethylene glycol for the evaluation and interpretation of these parameters apply equally to methanol. Elevated lactate levels, mild hypokalemia, and leukocytosis may occur. Lactic acidosis may be seen late in the course of methanol poisoning and may result from inhibition of the mitochondrial electron transport system or from poor tissue perfusion [73]. Serum lactate concentrations of 11.5 and 23 mmol per L have been reported 24 hours or more after ingestion. Amylase elevations and pancreatitis can occur in up to one half of severely poisoned patients [10,100]. Computed tomography scanning can demonstrate cerebral edema, as well as frontal lobe and basal ganglia hemorrhages and infarcts associated with poor clinical outcomes.

Management

The focus of treatment for ethylene glycol and methanol poisoning is to prevent the formation of toxic metabolites by inhibiting liver ADH and enhancing the removal of the parent compound and metabolites. Antidotal therapy, cofactor therapy, and hemodialysis may be necessary in addition to supportive care to achieve these goals.

Initial treatment includes airway management in the comatose patient, IV fluids, cardiac monitoring, and appropriate laboratory studies. Gastric aspiration via a nasogastric tube may be beneficial when performed within an hour of an intentional ingestion [83]. Oral activated charcoal is ineffective but may be considered when coingestants are suspected [81,139].

IV sodium bicarbonate should be administered to correct serum pH to at least 7.3 [100,139]. Large doses of sodium bicarbonate may be required. Sodium bicarbonate is useful in ethylene glycol and methanol poisonings for three reasons. First, unlike the metabolites in lactic acidosis and ketoacidosis, the metabolites of ethylene glycol and methanol cannot be transformed to regenerate bicarbonate [64], and the acidosis must be corrected with exogenous alkali. Second, increasing the serum pH enhances the ionization of acid metabolites, making them less diffusible, trapping them in the blood and extracellular fluid, and limiting their tissue penetration [73]. Third, urinary alkalinization may increase excretion of acid metabolites through ion trapping, provided renal function remains normal [67]. In ethylene glycol poisoning, however, the hypocalcemia that occurs as calcium complexes with oxalate may be worsened by alkali administration. Calcium chloride/gluconate should be administered to correct symptomatic hypocalcemia including seizures, but the indiscriminate use of calcium salts to correct a laboratory value should be avoided, because it may increase the precipitation of calcium oxalate crystals [140]. In methanol poisoning, increasing the serum pH may increase the concentration of ionized formate, thus diminishing formic acid access to the CNS and possibly ameliorating retinal toxicity [73].

Seizures should initially be treated with standard anticonvulsants, such as benzodiazepines and barbiturates. Hypocalcemia and hypoglycemia should be excluded. Recurrent or persistent coma or seizures should prompt evaluation for underlying cerebral edema. Cerebral edema should be managed acutely with hyperventilation, mannitol (provided renal function is intact), and potentially intracranial pressure monitoring and decompression. Cardiopulmonary complications may require inotropes and vasopressors.

Ethanol and fomepizole are antidotes for ethylene glycol and methanol poisoning. These agents inhibit liver ADH, and block the initial oxidation of ethylene glycol and methanol to their more toxic metabolites. After ADH is inhibited, ethylene glycol and methanol can be eliminated via endogenous or extracorporeal routes [85,141]. Antidotal therapy has no effect on the elimination of the acid metabolites. Indications for antidotal therapy in cases of known or possible methanol or ethylene glycol intoxication are outlined in Table 119.3 [101,103,139,142].

Recognition that ethanol is the preferred substrate for ADH [143] suggested its clinical use as a competitive inhibitor of this enzyme [144]. While most sources recommend administering sufficient ethanol to maintain serum ethanol concentrations between 100 and 150 mg per dL [97], limited data support this target concentration. Because ethanol is a competitive inhibitor of ADH, extremely high levels of ethylene glycol or methanol must by necessity be met with higher doses of ethanol. Targeting a 1:4 molar ratio [73,143] a serum ethanol concentration of 100 mg per dL should suffice for methanol concentrations as high as 257 mg per dL or ethylene glycol as high as 540 mg per dL. Dosage guidelines to achieve an ethanol concentration of 100 mg per dL are outlined in Table 119.4 [84,145].

There are disadvantages to using ethanol therapeutically [81,146,147]. Perhaps the most important limitation is the toxicity of ethanol itself, including coma, airway compromise, respiratory depression, and agitation [30,148,149]. At

TABLE 119.3

INDICATIONS FOR ALCOHOL DEHYDROGENASE INHIBITOR THERAPY

A serum methanol or ethylene glycol concentration >20 mg/dL[a]

When serum methanol or ethylene glycol levels are not readily available:
- Documented ingestion of a consequential amount of methanol or ethylene glycol, especially when it is associated with a falling serum bicarbonate level or serum osmol gap >10 mOsm/kg by freezing point depression
- History or strong clinical suspicion of methanol or ethylene glycol ingestion and one of the following:
  - A falling serum bicarbonate level or a serum bicarbonate <20 mmol
  - Arterial pH <7.3
  - Renal dysfunction or ocular toxicity

[a]Attempts should be made to obtain confirmatory methanol or ethylene glycol concentrations as soon as possible when contemplating alcohol dehydrogenase inhibitor therapy. In all cases, consultation with a medical toxicologist is strongly recommended.

recommended doses, ethanol induces inebriation in the nontolerant individual. Subsequent behavioral effects and severe mental status depression may require interventions, such as sedation and endotracheal intubation shortly after initiation of therapy. The need for these interventions as well as the continuous infusion of ethanol itself can complicate and delay interfacility transfer. Although IV ethanol administration is generally preferred over oral ethanol, this requires extemporaneous compounding from dehydrated ethanol and an infusion of a hypertonic solution (10% ethanol by volume is 1,700 mOsm per kg), usually via a central venous catheter. Maintaining an adequate ethanol level can be difficult and interindividual variation in metabolism and removal during hemodialysis necessitate frequent monitoring of serum concentrations and dosage adjustments [148]. Finally, ethanol therapy is relatively contraindicated in patients on disulfiram or similar medications, patients with hepatic disease, and patients with alcohol addiction [81]. Admission to an intensive care setting is considered mandatory for an individual receiving ethanol therapy.

TABLE 119.4

ETHANOL DOSING FOR ETHYLENE GLYCOL OR METHANOL POISONING

Loading dose of ethanol:
- 0.8 g/kg (1 mL/kg) of 100% ethanol
- Oral or via nasogastric tube: Use 20%–30% concentration (e.g., 5 mL/kg of 20% ethanol; recall "80 proof" = 40% by volume)
- Intravenous: use 5%–10% concentration, load over 1 h (e.g., 10 mL/kg of 10% ethanol in D_5 W over 1 h)

If ethanol is already present, the amount of ethanol required to achieve a serum ethanol level of 100–150 mg/dL may be calculated as follows:
- Amount ethanol (mg) = [desired concentration (mg/dL)—known concentration (mg/dL)] × V_d of ethanol (0.6 L/kg) × body weight (kg) × 10 dL/L

Maintenance doses of ethanol:
- Begin during administration of the loading dose.
- Give 80 mg/kg/h of ethanol orally or intravenously (as above). For a patient on hemodialysis, the maintenance dose should be higher: 250–350 mg/kg/h. Chronic alcoholics also require higher doses (average 150 mg/kg/h). Because of potential hypoglycemia, glucose should be given along with ethanol. Serum ethanol and glucose levels must be monitored frequently.
- D_5 W, dextrose 5% in water; V_d, volume of distribution

[a]Adapted from Ekins BR, Rollins DE, Duffy DP, et al: Standardized treatment of severe methanol poisoning with ethanol and hemodialysis. *West J Med* 142:337, 1985.

Given these limitations to ethanol therapy, fomepizole has emerged as the preferred antidote. A more potent competitive inhibitor of ADH [67,140,150–154], parenteral fomepizole is approved by the U.S. Food and Drug Administration for therapy of methanol and ethylene glycol poisoning in adults [130,142,155,156]. Fomepizole has many advantages over ethanol: wide therapeutic margin, ease of administration, fixed dosing schedule, lack of CNS or behavioral toxicity, lack of metabolic or fluid balance effects, patient and provider safety, and no need for drug concentration monitoring [81,146,147,149,154]. Currently, fomepizole is only available in a parenteral formulation, though oral administration of this same formulation has similar pharmacokinetics and efficacy [157]. Highly selected patients treated with fomepizole may also avoid hemodialysis (discussed later), intensive care unit admission, or even interfacility transfer [67,79,81,146,151,156–160]. These advantages are even more important in the setting of mass epidemics [95].

A minimum serum fomepizole concentration of 10 μM (0.8 mg per dL) [161] effectively halts ethylene glycol and methanol oxidation [79,103,142,153,162] and is much higher than the in vitro K_i of fomepizole for human ADH of 1 μM [163]. Recommended dosing (Table 119.5) achieves and maintains serum fomepizole concentrations greater than 100 μM, eliminating the need for drug concentration monitoring [164]. Adverse drug events associated with fomepizole therapy are infrequent, but include rash, eosinophilia, minimal hepatic transaminase elevations, nausea, vomiting, and abdominal pain [148,165]. Hypersensitivity to pyrazoles, such as celecoxib and zaleplon, is the only contraindication to its use. Fomepizole does not appear to affect retinol dehydrogenases

TABLE 119.5

FOMEPIZOLE INTRAVENOUS DOSING PROTOCOL

Loading dose: 15 mg/kg

Maintenance dose (beginning 12 h after loading dose):
- 10 mg/kg every 12 h; increase dose to 15 mg/kg every 12 h if more than 48 h after loading dose

Dosing during hemodialysis:
- At initiation of dialysis:
  - If <6 h since last dose, no additional dose
  - If >6 h since last dose, next scheduled dose
- During hemodialysis: next scheduled dose every 4 h
- At completion of hemodialysis:
  - If <1 h since last dose, no additional dose
  - If 1–3 h since last dose, half of next scheduled dose
  - If >3 h since last dose, next scheduled dose

Each dose diluted in 100 mL normal saline and infused over 30 min involved in vision [166,167]. Its dosing protocol is based on zero-order elimination kinetics, increased clearance during hemodialysis, and potential auto-induction of metabolism via cytochrome P450–2E1 [130,154,155,168,169] (Table 119.5).

The main disadvantage to fomepizole therapy is the higher acquisition cost of the drug compared to ethanol [170,171], although this acquisition cost must be balanced against improved patient safety and reduced intensity of monitoring and therapy [146,159,172]. Although there are no prospective clinical studies directly comparing the safety of ethanol with fomepizole, a recent hospital record review reported far fewer adverse drug events with fomepizole [184]. In this study, the *number needed to harm* with ethanol was only two, and only seven when restricted to severe harm (mostly coma, violent agitation, and hemodynamic instability) [149]. Fomepizole is the antidote of choice, when available [171], especially for a patient who has coingested other CNS depressants, for the critically ill patient with a profound anion gap metabolic acidosis of uncertain etiology, for the patient in whom hemodialysis may be technically challenging (e.g., infants), and during times of limited resources as may occur during mass poisonings [81,147,173].

Fomepizole has also been successfully used to treat combined methanol/isopropanol [174] and diethylene glycol/triethylene glycol [158] overdose in humans. Treatment with fomepizole or ethanol should be continued until the metabolic acidosis has resolved and serum methanol or ethylene glycol levels fall below 20 mg per dL.

Cofactor therapy in patients poisoned by ethylene glycol includes IV pyridoxine (100 mg) and thiamine (100 mg) once a day until ethylene glycol levels are unmeasurable and acidemia has cleared. Pyridoxine is required for the conversion of glyoxylic acid to glycine, whereas thiamine and magnesium are required for the conversion of glycolic acid to γ-hydroxy-α-ketoadipate. Administering these cofactors may shunt metabolism away from the formation of oxalic acid [60,61], although benefit has not been documented in human poisonings. Magnesium should be administered to patients with hypomagnesemia.

Patients poisoned with methanol should receive IV folinic acid (leucovorin), 1 to 2 mg per kg every 4 to 6 hours until methanol and metabolic acidosis have been cleared [90,140]. Folic acid (folate) can be substituted if leucovorin is unavailable. Hepatic formate metabolism occurs through a folate-dependent mechanism (see Fig. 119.5). The susceptibility of primates to methanol toxicity correlates with reduced hepatic 5,6,7,8-tetrahydrofolate (THF, or reduced folate) stores compared with lower mammals [140], and exogenous folinic acid (5-formyl-THF) or folate may increase their capacity to remove formate. Although human data are limited, monkeys pretreated with folic or folinic acid resulted in marked attenuation of serum formate levels and metabolic acidosis after methanol administration [175]. Folinic acid given after the onset of methanol toxicity was also beneficial.

Hemodialysis effectively removes ethylene glycol, methanol, glycolic acid, formic acid, and probably the other toxic metabolites, and should be used in nearly all cases with acidosis or end organ toxicity [66,79,89,97]. Early hemodialysis can prevent subsequent toxicity [21,134]. Addition of extra sodium bicarbonate to the dialysate can assist in correcting acidosis, and hemodialysis may assist in controlling volume status. The frequency of fomepizole dosing must be increased during hemodialysis to compensate for its removal. When using ethanol, its infusion rate should be empirically doubled at the start of hemodialysis, and serum ethanol levels should be monitored hourly.

Recommendations for hemodialysis are outlined in Table 119.6 [79,82,85,140,146,147]. Traditional criteria for hemodialysis have included a serum ethylene glycol or methanol concentration greater than 50 mg per dL, independent of symptoms, acid–base status, or other markers of end-organ toxicity [140]. Selected patients have been successfully managed with fomepizole, cofactors, and IV fluid hydration alone despite serum ethylene glycol concentrations >400 mg per dL, though consultation with a toxicologist is strongly recommended [153,159,176,177]. Such patients must be hemodynamically stabile, and have near normal acid–base status and renal function. If minimal ethylene glycol metabolism has occurred before initiation of fomepizole therapy, the endogenous ethylene glycol elimination half-life is expected to be less than 18 hours [79]. Thus, patients with a normal serum creatinine and arterial pH at the start of fomepizole therapy may forgo hemodialysis despite high serum ethylene glycol concentrations [79,81,160]. Although a similar strategy has been reported in a patient with combined methanol/isopropanol ingestion [174], the prolonged methanol elimination half-life (approximately 50 hours) after ADH inhibition [178] would favor hemodialysis when readily available and technically feasible. Acid–base status, renal function, and serum ethylene glycol or methanol levels must be closely monitored in patients in whom hemodialysis is withheld [146].

Ethylene glycol clearance rates of 156 to 226 mL per minute (fractional excretion 43% to 92%; half-life 2.3 to 3.5 hours) can be expected during hemodialysis, as compared with renal clearance rates of 27.5 ± 4.1 mL per minute (fractional excretion 26% ± 9%) in patients with normal renal function, and clearance rates of 1 to 6 mL per minute in patients with renal dysfunction [79,80]. Glycolic acid is removed by hemodialysis, with a clearance of 105 to 170 mL per minute (half-life 2.5 hours) [62,64,68]. The hemodialysis elimination rate for methanol is 142 to 286 mL per minute; for formate, it is 148 to 203 mL per minute [20,89,97,101,145].

Hemodialysis should be continued until serum ethylene glycol or methanol levels are below 20 mg per dL and acid–base derangement has been corrected [73,81]. The required duration of hemodialysis in hours can be estimated using the formula $[-V \ln (20/A)/0.06\,k]$, where V is total body water in liters, A is the initial alcohol concentration in mg per dL, and k is 57% of the dialyzer urea clearance in milliliters per minute at the observed blood flow rate [179–181]. More than one round of hemodialysis may be necessary in massive overdoses and for ethylene glycol poisoned patients with renal failure.

TABLE 119.6

INDICATIONS FOR HEMODIALYSIS IN METHANOL OR ETHYLENE GLYCOL POISONING

Renal dysfunction as evidenced by increased serum creatinine concentration[a]
Severe metabolic acidosis (pH <7.25) with evidence of end-organ toxicity (abnormal renal function for ethylene glycol, visual toxicity for methanol) independent of parent compound concentration
Serum methanol or ethylene glycol concentration >50 mg/dL

[a]Selected patients with ethylene glycol concentrations above 50 mg/dL *and* normal creatinine and arterial pH at initiation of fomepizole treatment may be eligible for conservative treatment without hemodialysis. In all cases, consultation with a medical toxicologist is strongly recommended.

Adapted from Barceloux DG, Krenzelok EP, Olson K, et al: American Academy of Clinical Toxicology practice guidelines on the treatment of ethylene glycol poisoning. *J Toxicol Clin Toxicol* 37:537, 1999.

Peritoneal dialysis is markedly inferior to hemodialysis. Continuous arteriovenous hemofiltration with dialysis has been used in a hemodynamically unstable patient, but is less efficient at toxin removal [182]. Sorbent-based hemodialysis systems were inadvertently shown to be ineffective for methanol removal due to rapid saturation of the sorbent cartridge [183] and charcoal cartridges saturate within a few hours [175].

Patients with ethylene glycol poisoning who have acute renal failure may require hemodialysis for several months. Recovery of renal function is the expected course, although renal dysfunction may be permanent [61,62,67,73,83,184]. Full neurologic recovery is possible even after prolonged coma and seizures. Transient cranial nerve palsies developing 4 to 18 days after ingestion have been reported in under- or untreated patients [80,105–107]. Bilateral basal ganglia and brainstem infarction can occur in severely ethylene glycol poisoned patients [185].

Seizures, coma, and severe acidosis in patients with methanol poisoning portend a poor prognosis [109]. Cerebral edema is a common postmortem methanol toxicity finding [160]. The development of dilated, unresponsive pupils may indicate either severe optic nerve damage or cerebral edema [110]. Other neurologic sequelae include a parkinsonian-like syndrome, spasticity, transient resting tremor, cognitive defects, and paraplegia. Computed tomography, magnetic resonance, and autopsy studies have documented frontal lobe and basal ganglia hemorrhages and infarcts, especially in the putamen [186–191]. Bilateral putaminal hemorrhage and/or insular subcortex white matter necrosis correlate with a poor clinical outcome following methanol toxicity. The etiology of these lesions remains uncertain, but they are likely due to the direct toxicity of methanol and/or its metabolites. These abnormalities usually occur in severely acidemic patients with delayed presentation or diagnosis.

Harvesting of organs for transplant is not precluded in patients who die from ethylene glycol or methanol poisoning. Several centers have reported successful experience with kidney, heart, lung, pancreatic beta cell, and liver procurement from methanol-poisoned patients [172,192–196].

ISOPROPANOL

Isopropanol (isopropyl alcohol) is a clear, colorless, volatile liquid with a disagreeable taste and characteristic odor [197]. It is commonly available over the counter in 70% solutions of "rubbing alcohol." Because of its ready availability at an inexpensive price, abusers of alcohol often ingest isopropanol as an ethanol substitute. Cases of toxicity have been reported in children who were sponge bathed with the compound [198,199].

Isopropanol produces CNS depression, coma, and death from respiratory depression. In this respect, it has twice the potency of ethanol [200,201], a phenomenon attributed to its higher molecular weight [197] and possibly the CNS depressant effects of its metabolite, acetone. Depending on individual tolerance, serum concentrations of 150 mg per dL or greater may induce coma, and levels of 200 mg per dL or greater can be fatal in untreated patients, although lower concentrations may produce severe adverse effects [202].

The chemical properties and kinetics of isopropanol are summarized in Table 119.1. Oral absorption usually occurs within 30 minutes. Eighty percent of an absorbed dose is oxidized to acetone via ADH (Fig. 119.6) [197,201]. Acetone cannot undergo further oxidation to a carboxylic acid, however. Therefore, metabolic acidosis is not a feature of isopropanol toxicity unless respiratory depression with hypoxia or

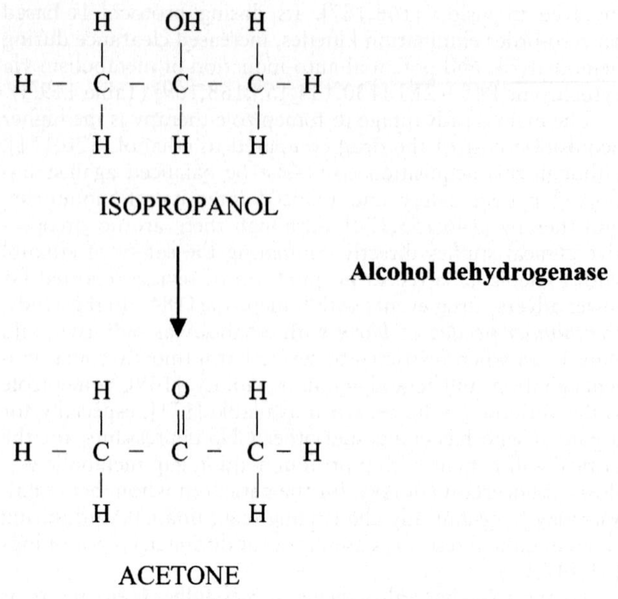

FIGURE 119.6. Isopropanol metabolism.

hypotension results in lactate production. Excretion of acetone and unchanged isopropanol (20% of an absorbed dose) is predominantly renal, with some excretion by respiratory, gastric, and salivary routes [201]. Acetone can be detected in the urine within 3 hours of ingestion [203]. The elimination half-life of isopropanol can be as long as 5.8 hours in infants [204]. Serum acetone levels frequently remain elevated after isopropanol levels are undetectable because acetone is eliminated slowly, with a half-life of 10.8 to 31.0 hours. The contribution of acetone to the prolonged duration of CNS depression remains speculative [197].

Clinical Presentation

An "intoxicated" patient without acidemia, yet with positive serum or urinary ketones and a fruity breath odor, should be suspected of isopropanol intoxication. Initial signs and symptoms usually consist of mild intoxication followed by gastritis, abdominal pain, nausea, vomiting, and possibly hematemesis [197]. Hemorrhagic tracheobronchitis may occur. As CNS depression progresses, patients become ataxic, dysarthric, confused, stuporous, and comatose. Pupils are typically miotic, but mydriasis has been reported [197,198,205,206]. Respiratory depression and hypotension may occur in severe intoxication [207]. Because of the profound and prolonged cerebral depressive effects of isopropanol, comatose patients may develop compartment syndromes and rhabdomyolysis with myoglobinuria. Delayed hypoglycemia may occur via the mechanism described for ethanol [197,198,202].

Many patients who ingest isopropanol are ethanol abusers who have a multitude of associated diseases, including chronic liver disease, pancreatitis, traumatic injuries, and chronic obstructive pulmonary disease, which may complicate the clinical picture.

Diagnostic Evaluation

Patients with known or suspected isopropanol poisoning should have quantitative isopropanol and acetone serum levels along with the laboratory studies noted for acute ethanol intoxication. The presence of high levels of acetone can interfere with older creatinine assays based on a colorimetric method, producing a falsely high creatinine value in the presence of a normal BUN [208,209]. In patients who may have also ingested other toxic alcohols, serum osmolality, ethanol, ethylene glycol, and methanol levels should also be obtained.

The differential diagnosis of isopropanol poisoning includes toxic and metabolic states in which ketonemia may develop, such as alcoholic, diabetic, and starvation ketoacidosis. Patients with these conditions have elevated acetoacetate, β-hydroxybutyrate, and acetone levels compared with the isolated acetonemia seen with isopropanol intoxication. Traces of isopropanol may be detected in patients with diabetic or AKA due to the back reduction of acetone to isopropanol [210,211]. Poisoning by salicylate, cyanide, and acetone itself (which is found in nail polish and super glue remover) and inborn errors of metabolism should also be considered in the differential diagnosis of unexplained ketosis. Some degree of metabolic acidosis is expected in most of these conditions, whereas it is absent in uncomplicated isopropanol or acetone poisoning cases.

Management

Treatment is similar to that described for acute ethanol intoxication. Airway management and evaluation for hemorrhagic gastritis are particularly important. IV fluids should contain glucose, and serum glucose levels should be periodically checked. Isopropanol and acetone are removed by hemodialysis, but such therapy is rarely indicated [205]. Occasionally, patients with serum isopropanol concentration greater than 400 mg per dL accompanied by hemodynamic instability despite IV fluids may benefit from hemodialysis [197]. Since acetone is less toxic than isopropanol, there is no indication for either fomepizole or ethanol therapy [174,212].

Most patients recover with appropriate airway management and treatment of complicating factors. CNS depression and volume depletion secondary to vomiting can cause hypotension [197]. Pulmonary edema and hemorrhage are common findings on autopsy [202] and should be anticipated in severely ill patients.

PROPYLENE GLYCOL

Propylene glycol (1,2-propanediol) is commonly used as a solvent (e.g., in laundry stain removers), as an antifreeze, and as a diluent for a number of pharmaceuticals, including IV formulations of chlordiazepoxide, lorazepam, diazepam, etomidate, phenobarbital, pentobarbital, phenytoin, procainamide, nitroglycerin, and theophylline and topical silver sulfadiazine cream. Oral and dermal absorption is usually poor, but toxic amounts may be absorbed through abraded or burned skin [213]. Approximately one-half of a dose undergoes hepatic oxidation via ADH to lactate, and then to pyruvate and acetate. The rest is excreted unchanged in the urine [214].

Although oral doses of as much as 1 g per kg are essentially nontoxic, toxicity can occur following rapid or prolonged infusion of higher doses. Rapid IV infusion, as might occur during phenytoin loading, can cause prolonged PR and QRS duration, idioventricular rhythms, and cardiorespiratory depression and arrest [215]. Infusion of smaller doses has also precipitated cardiac standstill [216]. Propylene glycol, rather than phenytoin, is responsible for such toxicity [215]. Elderly patients, especially those with severe underlying cardiac disease, are at increased risk and should be infused with medications containing propylene glycol at rates slower than those usually recommended.

Alternatively, frequent repeat IV dosing of medications using propylene glycol as a diluent, as might occur with extremely high doses of diazepam for ethanol withdrawal, massive ingestion of products containing propylene glycol, or the chronic dermal absorption of silver sulfadiazine through damaged skin, can lead to accumulation of propylene glycol and its metabolites, resulting in seizures, and decreased level of consciousness [217–219]. On laboratory testing, an osmolar gap and high serum lactate concentrations are expected. Propylene glycol can be mistaken for ethylene glycol on gas chromatography [220].

Management consists of immediately stopping IV infusion or dermal application and supportive therapy. Fomepizole has been used to block the metabolism of propylene glycol, but this therapy cannot be recommended in the absence of information on the relative toxicity of the parent compound to its metabolites [221]. Hemodialysis and continuous venovenous hemofiltration have reportedly been used to treat patients with propylene glycol toxicity [222,223].

DIETHYLENE GLYCOL

Diethylene glycol (2,2′-dihydroxydiethyl ether, ethylene diglycol, 2,2′-oxydiethanol, 3-oxapentane-1,5-diol; DEG) is a viscous and sweet tasting liquid found in resins, antifreeze, brake fluids, cosmetics, wallpaper strippers, inks, lubricants, liquid heating/cooking fuels, plasticizers, adhesives, paper, and packaging materials [12,224]. Over the years, diethylene glycol has resulted in tragic outbreaks of renal failure and death following its substitution for propylene glycol in medications [225,226]. Unlike propylene glycol, diethylene glycol can cause acute renal failure, elevated liver enzymes, encephalopathy, and delayed neurologic toxicity. Since the first reported outbreak that occurred in the United States in 1937, there have been other outbreaks worldwide, including South Africa (1969), Spain (1985), India (1986 and 1998), Nigeria (1990 and 2008), Bangladesh (1990 to 1992), Argentina (1992), Haiti (1996), Panama (2006), and China (2006). These outbreaks often involved medications, such as acetaminophen, cough syrup, or teething syrup, ingested by children. The number of identified deaths during each outbreak ranged from 5 to 236. The median toxic dose is estimated to be approximately 1 g per kg [227].

Following diethylene glycol ingestion, patients may present with gastrointestinal symptoms, inebriation, CNS depression, acidosis, and renal failure. Interestingly, additional neurologic symptoms may develop up to several weeks after the ingestion and include cranial nerve palsy, peripheral neuropathy, dysphonia, lethargy, mental status changes, quadriparesis, and seizures [225,228]. Metabolism of diethylene glycol via hepatic ADH leads to 2-hydroxyethoxyacetic acid (2-HEAA) [224]. Although 2-HEAA is believed to be the primary toxic metabolite, the parent glycol itself may also be directly toxic. Although the name suggests the potential to be metabolized to two ethylene glycol molecules, this does not occur in vivo [224]. Survivors with renal failure tend to remain dialysis dependent and the degree of renal injury may be a predictor of delayed neurologic sequelae. Treatment is similar to ethylene glycol, including ADH inhibition, extracorporeal elimination, and supportive care. Fomepizole without hemodialysis, however, is not recommended given the uncertain toxicity of the diethylene glycol itself [159,224,225].

References

1. O'Connor PG, Schottenfeld RS: Patients with alcohol problems. *N Engl J Med* 338:592, 1998.
2. McGinnis JM, Foege WH: Actual causes of death in the United States. *JAMA* 270:2207, 1993.
3. Agarwal DP: Cardioprotective effects of light-moderate consumption of alcohol: a review of putative mechanisms. *Alcohol Alcoholism* 37(5): 409–415, 2002.
4. Hines LM, Stampfer MJ, Ma J, et al: Genetic variation in alcohol dehydrogenase and the beneficial effect of moderate alcohol consumption on myocardial infarction. *N Engl J Med* 344:549, 2001.
5. Berger K, Ajani UA, Kase CS, et al: Light-to-moderate alcohol consumption and the risk of stroke among U.S. male physicians. *N Engl J Med* 341:1557, 1999.
6. Thun MJ, Peto R, Lopez AD, et al: Alcohol consumption and mortality among middle-aged and elderly U.S. adults. *N Engl J Med* 337:1705, 1997.
7. Angell M, Kassirer JP: Alcohol and other drugs—toward a more rational and consistent policy. *N Engl J Med* 331:537, 1994.
8. Wiese JG, Shlipak MG, Browner WS: The alcohol hangover. *Ann Intern Med* 132:897, 2000.
9. Bronstein AC, Spyker DA, Cantilena LR Jr, et al: 2007 Annual Report of the American Association of Poison Control Centers' National Poison Data System (NPDS): 25th Annual Report. *Clin Toxicol (Philadelphia)* 46(10):927–1057, 2008.
10. Naraqi S, Dethlefs RF, Slobodniuk RA, et al: An outbreak of acute methyl alcohol intoxication. *Aust NZ J Med* 9:65, 1979.
11. Swartz RD, Millman RP, Billi JE, et al: Epidemic methanol poisoning: clinical and biochemical analysis of a recent episode. *Medicine* 60:373, 1981.
12. Rentz ED, Lewis L, Mujica OJ, et al: Outbreak of acute renal failure in Panama in 2006: a case-control study. *Bull World Health Organ* 86(10):749–756, 2008.
13. Eckardt MJ, Harford TC, Kaelber CT, et al: Health hazards associated with alcohol consumption. *JAMA* 246:648, 1981.
14. McDonald AJ III: US emergency department visits for alcohol-related diseases and injuries between 1992 and 2000. *Arch Intern Med* 164:531, 2004.
15. Cyr MG, Wartman SA: The effectiveness of routine screening questions in the detection of alcoholism. *JAMA* 259:51, 1988.
16. Scherger DL, Wruk KM, Kulig KW, et al: Ethyl alcohol (ethanol)-containing cologne, perfume, and after-shave ingestions in children. *Am J Dis Child* 142:630, 1988.
17. Ueno S, Harris RA, Messing RO, et al: Alcohol actions on GABA(A) receptors: from protein structure to mouse behavior. *Alcohol Clin Exp Res* 25[Suppl 5]:81S, 2001.
18. Chester JA, Cunningham CL: GABA(A) receptor modulation of the rewarding and aversive effects of ethanol. *Alcohol* 26(3):131, 2002.
19. Aguayo LG, Peoples RW, Yeh HH, et al: GABA(A) receptors as molecular sites of ethanol action. Direct or indirect actions? *Curr Top Med Chem* 2(8):869, 2002.
20. Allgaier C: Ethanol sensitivity of NMDA receptors. *Neurochem Int* 41(6):377, 2002.
21. Nutt DJ, Peters TJ: Alcohol: the drug. *Br Med Bull* 50:5, 1994.
22. Crews FT, Morrow AL, Criswell H, et al: Effects of ethanol on ion channels. *Int Rev Neurobiol* 39:283, 1996.
23. Israel Y, Orrego H, Carmichael FJ: Acetate-mediated effects of ethanol. *Alcohol Clin Exp Res* 18:144, 1994.
24. Frezza M, di Padova C, Pozzato G, et al: High blood alcohol levels in women: the role of decreased gastric alcohol dehydrogenase activity and first-pass metabolism. *N Engl J Med* 322:95, 1990.
25. Lieber CS, Gentry RT, Baraona E: First pass metabolism of ethanol. *Alcohol Alcohol* 2[Suppl]:163, 1994.
26. Seitz HK, Gartner U, Egerer G, et al: Ethanol metabolism in the gastrointestinal tract and its possible consequences. *Alcohol Alcohol* 2[Suppl]:157, 1994.
27. Levitt MD, Levitt DG: Appropriate use and misuse of blood concentration measurements to quantitate first-pass metabolism. *J Lab Clin Med* 136(4):275, 2000.
28. Ramchandani VA, Bosron WF, Li TK: Research advances in ethanol metabolism. *Pathol Biol* 49(9):676, 2001.
29. Brennan DR, Betzelos S, Reed R, et al: Ethanol elimination in an ED population. *Am J Emerg Med* 13:276, 1995.
30. Hoffman RS, Goldfrank LR: Ethanol-associated metabolic disorders. *Emerg Med Clin North Am* 7:943, 1989.
31. Lands WE: A review of alcohol clearance in humans. *Alcohol* 15:147, 1998.
32. Li TK, Bosron WF: Genetic variability of enzymes of alcohol metabolism in human beings. *Ann Emerg Med* 15:997, 1986.
33. Crabb DW: Ethanol oxidizing enzymes: roles in alcohol metabolism and alcoholic liver disease. *Prog Liver Dis* 13:151, 1995.
34. Agarwal DP: Genetic polymorphisms of alcohol metabolizing enzymes. *Pathol Biol* 49(9):703, 2001.
35. Day CP, Bashir R, James OF, et al: Investigation of the role of polymorphisms at the alcohol and aldehyde dehydrogenase loci in genetic predisposition to alcohol-related end-organ damage. *Hepatology* 1991;14:798. [Erratum: *Hepatology* 1992;15:750.]
36. Teschke R, Hasumura Y, Lieber CS: Hepatic microsomal alcohol-oxidizing system: affinity for methanol, ethanol, propanol, and butanol. *J Biol Chem* 250:7397, 1975.
37. Oshino N, Jamieson D, Chance B: The properties of hydrogen peroxide production under hyperoxic and hypoxic conditions of perfused rat liver. *Biochem J* 146:53, 1975.
38. Norberg A, Jones AW, Hahn RG, et al: Role of variability in explaining ethanol pharmacokinetics: research and forensic applications. *Clin Pharmacokinet* 42(1):1, 2003.
39. Ogden EJ, Moskowitz H: Effects of alcohol and other drugs on driver performance. *Traffic Inj Prev* 5(3):185–198, 2004.
40. Crabb DW, Bosron WF, Li TK: Ethanol metabolism. *Pharmacol Ther* 34:59, 1987.
41. Charness ME, Simon RP, Greenberg DA: Ethanol and the nervous system. *N Engl J Med* 321:442, 1989.
42. Johnson RA, Noll EC, Rodney WM: Survival after a serum ethanol concentration of 1 1/2%. *Lancet* 2(8312):1394, 1982.
43. Mellanby E: *Alcohol: its absorption into and disappearance from the blood under different conditions. Special Report Series No. 31, Medical Research Committee*. London: HMSO, 1919.
44. Brown SS, Forrest JAH: A controlled trial of fructose in the treatment of acute alcoholic intoxication. *Lancet* 2:898, 1972.
45. Li J, Mills T, Erato R: Intravenous saline has no effect on blood ethanol clearance. *J Emerg Med* 17:1, 1999.
46. Halperin ML, Hammeke M, Josse RG, et al: Metabolic acidosis in the alcoholic: a pathophysiologic approach. *Metabolism* 32:308, 1983.
47. Fulop M, Bock J, Ben-Ezra J, et al: Plasma lactate and 3-hydroxybutyrate levels in patients with acute ethanol intoxication. *Am J Med* 57:191, 1986.
48. McGuire LC, Cruickshank AM, Munro PT: Alcoholic ketoacidosis. *Emerg Med J* 23:417, 2006.
49. Bluntzer ME, Blachley JD: Acid-base and electrolyte disturbances induced by alcohol. *J Crit Illness* 1:19, 1986.
50. Marinella MA: Alcoholic ketoacidosis presenting with extreme hypoglycemia. *Am J Emerg Med* 15:257, 1997.
51. Braden GL, Strayhorn CH, Germain MJ, et al: Increased osmolal gap in alcoholic acidosis. *Arch Intern Med* 153:2377, 1993.
52. Purssell RA, Pudek M, Brubacher J, et al: Derivation of a formula to calculate the contribution of ethanol to the osmolar gap. *Ann Emerg Med* 38:653, 2001.
53. Oliva PB: Lactic acidosis. *Am J Med* 48:209, 1970.
54. Wrenn KD, Slovis CM, Minion GE, et al: The syndrome of alcoholic ketoacidosis. *Am J Med* 2:119, 1991.
55. Watson AJS, Walker JF, Tomkin GH, et al: Acute Wernicke's encephalopathy precipitated by glucose loading. *Irish J Med Sci* 150:301, 1981.
56. Marks V: Alcohol and carbohydrate metabolism. *Clin Endocrinol Metab* 7:333, 1978.
57. Wilson NM, Brown PM, Juul SM, et al: Glucose turnover and metabolic and hormonal changes in ethanol-induced hypoglycaemia. *BMJ* 282:849, 1981.
58. Chalmers RJ, Bennie EH, Johnson RH, et al: The growth hormone response to insulin-induced hypoglycaemia in alcoholics. *Psychiatr Med* 7:607, 1977.
59. Haight JSJ, Keating WR: Failure of thermoregulation in the cold during hypoglycaemia induced by exercise and alcohol. *J Physiol* 229:87, 1973.
60. Haupt MC, Zull DN, Adams SL: Massive ethylene glycol poisoning without evidence of crystalluria: a case for early intervention. *J Emerg Med* 6:295, 1988.
61. Beasley VR, Buck WB: Acute ethylene glycol toxicosis: a review. *Vet Hum Toxicol* 22:255, 1957.
62. Jacobsen D, Ovrebo S, Ostborg J, et al: Glycolate causes the acidosis in ethylene glycol poisoning and is effectively removed by hemodialysis. *Acta Med Scand* 216:409, 1984.
63. Poldelski V, Johnson A, Wright S, et al: Ethylene glycol-mediated tubular injury: identification of critical metabolites and injury pathways. *Am J Kidney Dis* 38:339, 2001.
64. Gabow PA, Clay K, Sullivan JB, et al: Organic acids in ethylene glycol intoxication. *Ann Intern Med* 105:16, 1986.
65. McMartin K: Are calcium oxalate crystals involved in the mechanism of acute renal failure in ethylene glycol poisoning? *Clinical Toxicology* 47(9):859–869, 2009.
66. Clay KL, Murphy RC: On the metabolic acidosis of ethylene glycol intoxication. *Toxicol Appl Pharmacol* 39:39, 1977.
67. Jacobsen D, Hewlett TR, Webb R, et al: Ethylene glycol intoxication: evaluation of kinetics and crystalluria. *Am J Med* 84:145, 1988.
68. Moreau CL, Kerns W, Tomaszewski CA, et al: Glycolate kinetics and hemodialysis clearance. *J Toxicol Clin Toxicol* 36:659, 1998.
69. Baud FJ, Galliot M, Astier A, et al: Treatment of ethylene glycol poisoning with intravenous 4-methylpyrazole. *N Engl J Med* 319:97, 1988.
70. Scully RE, Galdabini JJ, McNeely BU: Case records of the Massachusetts General Hospital: case 38–1979. *N Engl J Med* 301:650, 1979.
71. Jacobsen D: Organic acids in ethylene glycol intoxication [letter]. *Ann Intern Med* 105:799, 1986.

72. Brown CG, Trumbull D, Klein-Schwartz W, et al: Ethylene glycol poisoning. *Ann Emerg Med* 12:501, 1983.
73. Jacobsen D, McMartin KE: Methanol and ethylene glycol poisonings: mechanism of toxicity, clinical course, diagnosis and treatment. *Med Toxicol* 1:309, 1986.
74. Wallace EA, Green AS: Methanol toxicity secondary to inhalant abuse in adult men. *Clin Toxicol* 47(3):239–242, 2009.
75. Morgan TJ, Clark C, Clague A: Artifactual elevation of measured plasma L-lactate concentration in the presence of glycolate. *Crit Care Med* 27:2177, 1999.
76. Shirey T, Sivilotti M: Reaction of lactate electrodes to glycolate. *Crit Care Med* 27:2305, 1999.
77. Manini AF, Hoffman RS, McMartin KE, et al: Relationship between serum glycolate and falsely elevated lactate in severe ethylene glycol poisoning. *J Anal Toxicol* 33(3):174–176, 2009.
78. Friedman EA, Greenberg JB, Merrill JP, et al: Consequences of ethylene glycol poisoning. *Am J Med* 32:891, 1962.
79. Sivilotti MLA, Burns MJ, McMartin KE, et al: Toxicokinetics of ethylene glycol during fomepizole therapy: implications for management. *Ann Emerg Med* 36:114, 2000.
80. Peterson CD, Collins AJ, Himes JM, et al: Ethylene glycol poisoning: pharmacokinetics during therapy with ethanol and hemodialysis. *N Engl J Med* 304:21, 1981.
81. Barceloux DG, Krenzelok EP, Olson K, et al: American Academy of Clinical Toxicology practice guidelines on the treatment of ethylene glycol poisoning. *J Toxicol Clin Toxicol* 37:537, 1999.
82. Johnson B, Meggs WJ, Bentzel CJ: Emergency department hemodialysis in a case of severe ethylene glycol poisoning. *Ann Emerg Med* 33:108, 1999.
83. Stokes JB, Aueron F: Prevention of organ damage in massive ethylene glycol ingestion. *JAMA* 243:2065, 1980.
84. Becker CE: Methanol poisoning. *J Emerg Med* 1:51, 1983.
85. Frederick LJ, Schulte PA, Apol A: Investigation and control of occupational hazards associated with the use of spirit duplicators. *Am Ind Hyg Assoc J* 45:51, 1984.
86. Eriksen SP, Kulkarni AB: Methanol in normal human breath. *Science* 141:639, 1963.
87. McMartin KE, Ambre JJ, Tephly TR: Methanol poisoning in human subjects: role for formic acid accumulation in the metabolic acidosis. *Am J Med* 68:414, 1980.
88. Sejersted OM, Jacobsen D, Ovrebo S, et al: Formate concentrations in plasma from patients poisoned with methanol. *Acta Med Scand* 213:105, 1983.
89. Kerns W II, Tomaszewski C, McMartin K, et al: Formate kinetics in methanol poisoning. *J Toxicol Clin Toxicol* 40:137, 2002.
90. Osterloh JD, Pond SM, Grady S, et al: Serum formate concentrations in methanol intoxication as a criterion for hemodialysis. *Ann Intern Med* 104:200, 1986.
91. Kostic MA, Dart RC: Rethinking the toxic methanol level. *J Toxicol Clin Toxicol* 41:793, 2003.
92. Martin-Amat G, McMartin KE, Hayreh SS, et al: Methanol poisoning: ocular toxicity produced by formate. *Toxicol Appl Pharmacol* 45:201, 1978.
93. Hayreh MS, Hayreh SS, Baumbach GL, et al: Methyl alcohol poisoning. III. Ocular toxicity. *Arch Ophthalmol* 95:1851, 1977.
94. Eells JT: Methanol-induced visual toxicity in the rat. *J Pharmacol Exp Ther* 257:56, 1991.
95. Kahn A, Blum D: Methyl alcohol poisoning in an 8-month-old boy: an unusual route of intoxication. *J Pediatr* 94:841, 1979.
96. Paasma R, Hovda KE, Tikkerberi A, Jacobsen D. Methanol mass poisoning in Estonia: outbreak in 154 patients. *Clin Toxicol* 45(2):152–157, 2007.
97. Jacobsen D, Ovrebo S, Sejersted OM: Toxicokinetics of formate during hemodialysis. *Acta Med Scand* 214:409, 1983.
98. McCoy HG, Cipolle RJ, Ehlers SM, et al: Severe methanol poisoning: application of a pharmacokinetic model for ethanol therapy and hemodialysis. *Am J Med* 67:574, 1979.
99. Jones AW: Elimination half-life of methanol during hangover. *Pharmacol Toxicol* 60:217, 1987.
100. Jacobsen D, Webb R, Collins TD, et al: Methanol and formate kinetics in late diagnosed methanol intoxication. *Med Toxicol* 3:418, 1988.
101. Catchings TT, Beamer WC, Lundy L, et al: Adult respiratory distress syndrome secondary to ethylene glycol ingestion. *Ann Emerg Med* 14:594, 1985.
102. Jacobsen D, Ostby N, Bredesen E: Studies on ethylene glycol poisoning. *Acta Med Scand* 212:11, 1982.
103. Brent J, McMartin K, Phillips S, et al: Fomepizole for the treatment of ethylene glycol poisoning. *N Engl J Med* 340:832, 1999.
104. Morgan B, Ford MD, Fullmer R: Ethylene glycol ingestion resulting in brainstem and midbrain dysfunction. *J Toxicol Clin Toxicol* 38:445, 2000.
105. Berger JR, Syyar DR: Neurological complications of ethylene glycol intoxication: report of a case. *Arch Neurol* 38:724, 1981.
106. Anderson B: Facial-auditory nerve oxalosis. *Am J Med* 88:87, 1990.
107. Spillane L, Roberts JR, Meyer AE: Multiple cranial nerve deficits after ethylene glycol poisoning. *Ann Emerg Med* 20:208, 1991.
108. Martensson E, Olofsson U, Heath A: Clinical and metabolic features of ethanol-methanol poisoning in chronic alcoholics. *Lancet* 1:327, 1988.
109. Jacobsen D, Bredesen JE, Eide I, et al: Anion and osmolal gaps in the diagnosis of methanol and ethylene glycol poisoning. *Acta Med Scand* 212:17, 1982.
110. Ingemansson SO: Clinical observations on ten cases of methanol poisoning with particular reference to ocular manifestations. *Acta Ophthalmol* 62:15, 1984.
111. Gennari FJ: Serum osmolality: uses and limitations. *N Engl J Med* 310:102, 1984.
112. Kearney J, Rees S, Chiang W: Availability of serum methanol and ethylene glycol levels: a national survey [abstract]. *J Toxicol Clin Toxicol* 35:509, 1997.
113. Blandford DE, Desjardins PR: A rapid method for measurement of ethylene glycol. *Clin Biochem* 27:25, 1994.
114. Jones AW, Nilsson L, Gladh SA, et al: 2,3-butanediol in plasma from an alcoholic mistakenly identified as ethylene glycol by gas chromatographic analysis. *Clin Chem* 37:1453, 1991.
115. Malandain H, Cano Y: Interference of glycerol, propylene glycol and other diols in enzymatic assays of ethylene glycol [abstract]. *Clin Chem* 41:S120, 1995.
116. Shoemaker JD, Lynch RE, Hoffman JW, et al: Misidentification of propionic acid as ethylene glycol in a patient with methylmalonic acidemia. *J Pediatr* 120:417, 1992.
117. Fraser AD: Importance of glycolic acid analysis in ethylene glycol poisoning. *Clin Chem* 44(8 Pt 1):1769, 1998.
118. Yao HH, Porter WH: Simultaneous determination of ethylene glycol and its major toxic metabolite, glycolic acid, in serum by gas chromatography. *Clin Chem* 42:292, 1996.
119. Long H, Nelson LS, Hoffman RS. A rapid qualitative test for suspected ethylene glycol poisoning. *Acad Emerg Med* 15(7):688–690, 2008.
120. Woolf AD, Wynshaw-Boris A, Rinalso P, et al: Intentional infantile ethylene glycol poisoning presenting as an inherited metabolic disorder. *J Pediatr* 120:421, 1992.
121. Walker JA, Schwartzbard A, Krauss EA, et al: The missing gap: a pitfall in the diagnosis of alcohol intoxication by osmometry. *Arch Intern Med* 146:1843, 1986.
122. Lynd LD, Richardson KJ, Purssell RA, et al: An evaluation of the osmole gap as a screening test for toxic alcohol poisoning. *BMC Emerg Med* 8:5, 2008.
123. Koga Y, Purssell RA, Lynd LD: The irrationality of the present use of the osmole gap. *Toxicol Rev* 23:203, 2004.
124. Krahn J, Khajuria A: Osmolality gaps: diagnostic accuracy and long-term variability. *Clin Chem* 52(4):737–739, 2006.
125. Schelling JR, Howard RL, Winter SD, et al: Increased osmolal gap in alcoholic ketoacidosis and lactic acidosis. *Ann Intern Med* 113:557, 1990.
126. Hoffman RS, Smilkstein MJ, Howland MA, et al: Osmol gaps revisited: normal values and limitations. *J Toxicol Clin Toxicol* 31:81, 1993.
127. Sivilotti MLA, Collier CP, Choi SB: Ethanol and the osmolal gap. *Ann Emerg Med* 39:656, 2002.
128. Smithline N, Gardner KD: Gaps: anionic and osmolal. *JAMA* 236:1594, 1976.
129. Purssell RA, Lynd LD, Koga Y: The use of the osmole gap as a screening test for the presence of exogenous substances. *Toxicol Rev* 23:189, 2004.
130. Jobard E, Harry P, Turcant A, et al: 4-methylpyrazole and hemodialysis in ethylene glycol poisoning. *J Toxicol Clin Toxicol* 34:379, 1996.
131. Lund ME, Banner W: Effect of alcohols and selected solvents on serum osmolality measurements. *J Toxicol Clin Toxicol* 20:115, 1983.
132. Glaser DS: Utility of the serum osmol gap in the diagnosis of methanol or ethylene glycol ingestion. *Ann Emerg Med* 27:343, 1996.
133. Jacobsen D, Akesson I, Shefter E: Urinary calcium oxalate monohydrate crystals in ethylene glycol poisoning. *Scand J Clin Lab Invest* 42:231, 1982.
134. Burns JR, Finlayson B: Changes in calcium oxalate crystal morphology as a function of concentration. *Invest Urol* 18:174, 1980.
135. Wallace KL, Suchard JR, Curry SC, et al: Diagnostic use of physicians' detection of urine fluorescence in a simulated ingestion of sodium fluorescein-containing antifreeze. *Ann Emerg Med* 38:49, 2001.
136. Casavant MJ, Shah MN, Battels R: Does fluorescent urine indicate antifreeze ingestion by children? *Pediatrics* 107:113, 2001.
137. McStay CM, Gordon PE: Images in clinical medicine. Urine fluorescence in ethylene glycol poisoning. *N Engl J Med* 356(6):611, 2007.
138. Winter ML, Snodgrass WR, Theelen T, et al: Urine fluorescence in ethylene glycol poisoning. *N Engl J Med* 356(19):2006–2007, 2007.
139. Barceloux DG, Bond GR, Krenzelok EP, et al: American Academy of Clinical Toxicology practice guidelines on the treatment of methanol poisoning. *J Toxicol Clin Toxicol* 40:415, 2002.
140. Jacobsen D, McMartin KE: Antidotes for methanol and ethylene glycol poisoning. *J Toxicol Clin Toxicol* 35:127, 1997.
141. Palatnick W, Redman LW, Sitar DS, et al: Methanol half-life during ethanol administration: implications for management of methanol poisoning. *Ann Emerg Med* 26:202, 1995.
142. Brent J, McMartin K, Phillips S, et al: Fomepizole for the treatment of methanol poisoning. *N Engl J Med* 344:424, 2001.
143. Tephly TR, McMartin KE: Methanol metabolism and toxicity, in Stegink L, File LJ (eds): *Aspartame: Physiology and Biochemistry.* New York, Marcel Dekker Inc, 1984, p 111.

144. Wacker WEC, Haynes H, Druyan R, et al: Treatment of ethylene glycol poisoning with ethyl alcohol. *JAMA* 194:173, 1965.
145. Ekins BR, Rollins DE, Duffy DP, et al: Standardized treatment of severe methanol poisoning with ethanol and hemodialysis. *West J Med* 142:337, 1985.
146. Jacobsen D: New treatment for ethylene glycol poisoning. *N Engl J Med* 340:879, 1999.
147. Tenenbein M: Recent advancements in pediatric toxicology. *Pediatr Clin North Am* 46:1179, 1999.
148. Lepik KJ, Levy AR, Sobolev BG, et al: Adverse drug events associated with the antidotes for methanol and ethylene glycol poisoning: a comparison of ethanol and fomepizole. *Ann Emerg Med* 53(4):439–450 e10, 2009.
149. Sivilotti ML: Ethanol: tastes great! Fomepizole: less filling! *Ann Emerg Med* 53(4):451–453, 2009.
150. Blomstrand R, Theorell H: Inhibitory effect on ethanol oxidation in man after administration of 4-methylpyrazole. *Life Sci* 9:631, 1970.
151. Baud FJ, Bismuth C, Garnier R, et al: 4-methylpyrazole may be an alternative to ethanol therapy for ethylene glycol intoxication in man. *J Toxicol Clin Toxicol* 24:463, 1986.
152. Connally HE, Thrall MA, Forney SD, et al: Safety and efficacy of 4-methylpyrazole for treatment of suspected or confirmed ethylene glycol poisoning in dogs: 107 cases (1983–1995). *J Am Vet Med Assoc* 209:1857, 1996.
153. Borron SW, Mégarbane B, Baud FJ: Fomepizole in treatment of uncomplicated ethylene glycol poisoning. *Lancet* 354:831, 1999.
154. Bestic M, Blackford M, Reed M: Fomepizole: a critical assessment of current dosing recommendations. *J Clin Pharmacol* 49(2):130–137, 2009.
155. Faessel H, Houze P, Baud FJ, et al: 4-methylpyrazole monitoring during hemodialysis of ethylene glycol intoxicated patients. *Eur J Clin Pharmacol* 49:211, 1995.
156. Harry P, Turcant A, Bouachour G, et al: Efficacy of 4-methylpyrazole in ethylene glycol poisoning: clinical and toxicokinetic aspects. *Hum Exp Toxicol* 13:61, 1994.
157. Megarbane B, Houze P, Baud FJ: Oral fomepizole administration to treat ethylene glycol and methanol poisonings: advantages and limitations. *Clin Toxicol* 46(10):1097, 2008.
158. Borron SW, Baud FJ, Garnier R: Intravenous 4-methylpyrazole as an antidote for diethylene glycol and triethylene glycol poisoning: a case report. *Vet Human Toxicol* 39:26, 1997.
159. Boyer EW, Mejia M, Woolf A, et al: Severe ethylene glycol ingestion treated without hemodialysis. *Pediatrics* 107:172, 2001.
160. Cheng JT, Beysolow TD, Kaul B, et al: Clearance of ethylene glycol by kidneys and hemodialysis. *J Toxicol Clin Toxicol* 25:95, 1987.
161. McMartin KE, Hedstrom KG, Tolf BR, et al: Studies on the metabolic interaction between 4-methylpyrazole and methanol using the monkey as an animal model. *Arch Biochem Biophys* 199:606, 1980.
162. Sivilotti ML, Burns MJ, McMartin KE, et al: Toxicokinetics of ethylene glycol during fomepizole therapy: implications for management. For the Methylpyrazole for Toxic Alcohols Study Group. *Ann Emerg Med* 36(2):114–125, 2000.
163. Li TK, Theorell H: Human liver alcohol dehydrogenase: inhibition by pyrazole and pyrazole analogues. *Acta Chem Scand* 23:892, 1969.
164. McMartin KE, Brent J, META Study Group: Pharmacokinetics of fomepizole (4MP) in patients. *J Toxicol Clin Toxicol* 36:450, 1998.
165. Lepik KJ, Brubacher JR, DeWitt CR, et al: Bradycardia and hypotension associated with fomepizole infusion during hemodialysis. *Clin Toxicol* 46(6):570–573, 2008.
166. Blomstrand R, Ingemansson SO: Studies on the effect of 4-methylpyrazole on methanol poisoning using the monkey as an animal model: with particular reference to the ocular toxicity. *Drug Alcohol Depend* 13:343, 1984.
167. Sivilotti MLA, Burns MJ, Aaron CK, et al: Reversal of severe methanol-induced visual impairment: no evidence of retinal toxicity due to fomepizole. *J Toxicol Clin Toxicol* 39:627, 2001.
168. Jacobsen D, Barron SK, Sebastian CS, et al: Non-linear kinetics of 4-methylpyrazole in healthy human subjects. *Eur J Clin Pharmacol* 37:599, 1989.
169. Jacobsen D, Ostensen J, Bredesen L, et al: 4-Methylpyrazole (4-MP) is effectively removed by hemodialysis in the pig model. *Hum Exp Toxicol* 15:494, 1996.
170. Sivilotti MLA, Eisen JS, Less JS, et al: Can emergency departments not afford to carry essential antidotes? *Can J Emerg Med* 4:23, 2002.
171. Dart RC, Borron SW, Caravati EM, et al. Expert consensus guidelines for stocking of antidotes in hospitals that provide emergency care. *Ann Emerg Med* 54(3):386–394 e1, 2009.
172. Caballero F, Cabrer C, Gonzalez-Segura C, et al: Short- and long-term success of organs transplanted from donors dying of acute methanol intoxication. *Transplant Proc* 31:2591, 1999.
173. Baum CR, Langman CB, Oker EE, et al: Fomepizole treatment of ethylene glycol poisoning in an infant. *Pediatrics* 106:1489, 2000.
174. Bekka R, Borron SW, Astier A, et al: Treatment of methanol and isopropanol poisoning with intravenous fomepizole. *J Toxicol Clin Toxicol* 39:59, 2001.
175. Noker PE, Eells JT, Tephly TR: Methanol toxicity: treatment with folic acid and 5-formyl tetrahydrofolic acid. *Alcohol Clin Exp Res* 4:378, 1980.
176. George M, Al Duaij N, Becker ML, et al: Re: ethylene glycol ingestion treated only with fomepizole (Journal of Medical Toxicology: volume 3, number 3, September 2007; 125–128). *J Med Toxicol* 4(1):67, 2008.
177. Velez LI, Shepherd G, Lee YC, et al: Ethylene glycol ingestion treated only with fomepizole. *J Med Toxicol* 3(3):125–128, 2007.
178. Burns MJ, Graudins A, Aaron CK, et al: Treatment of methanol poisoning with intravenous 4-methylpyrazole. *Ann Emerg Med* 30:829, 1997.
179. Youssef GM, Hirsch DJ: Validation of a method to predict required dialysis time for cases of methanol and ethylene glycol poisoning. *Am J Kidney Dis* 46:509, 2005.
180. McMurray M, Carty D, Toffelmire EB: Predicting methanol clearance during hemodialysis when direct measurement is not available. *CAANT J* 12:29, 2002.
181. Burns AB, Bailie GR, Eisele G, et al: Use of pharmacokinetics to determine the duration of dialysis in management of methanol poisoning. *Am J Emerg Med* 16:538, 1998.
182. Christiansson LK, Kaspersson KE, Kulling PE, et al: Treatment of severe ethylene glycol intoxication with continuous arteriovenous hemofiltration dialysis. *J Toxicol Clin Toxicol* 33:267, 1995.
183. Whalen JE, Richards CJ, Ambre J: Inadequate removal of methanol and formate using the sorbent based regeneration hemodialysis delivery system. *Clin Nephrol* 11:318, 1979.
184. Rasic S, Cengic M, Golemac S, et al: Acute renal insufficiency after poisoning with ethylene glycol. *Nephron* 81:119, 1999.
185. Dribben W, Furbee B, Kirk M: Brainstem infarction and quadriplegia associated with ethylene glycol ingestion. *J Toxicol Clin Toxicol* 37:657, 1999.
186. Phang PT, Passerini L, Mielke B, et al: Brain hemorrhage associated with methanol poisoning. *Crit Care Med* 16:137, 1988.
187. Anderson TJ, Shuaib A, Becker WJ: Neurologic sequelae of methanol poisoning. *Can Med Assoc J* 136:1177, 1987.
188. Ley CO, Gali FG: Parkinsonian syndrome after methanol intoxication. *Eur Neurol* 22:405, 1983.
189. Rosenberg NL: Methylmalonic acid, methanol, metabolic acidosis, and lesions of the basal ganglia [letter]. *Ann Neurol* 22:96, 1987.
190. Gaul HP, Wallace CJ, Auer RN, et al: MR findings in methanol intoxication. *AJNR Am J Neuroradiol* 16:1783, 1995.
191. Hantson P, Duprez T, Mahieu P: Neurotoxicity to the basal ganglia shown by magnetic resonance imaging (MRI) following poisoning by methanol and other substances. *J Toxicol Clin Toxicol* 35:151, 1997.
192. Chari RS, Hemming AW, Cattral M: Successful kidney pancreas transplantation from donor with methanol intoxication. *Transplantation* 66:674, 1998.
193. Hantson P, Kremer V, Lerut J, et al: Successful liver transplantation with a graft from a methanol-poisoned donor. *Transpl Int* 9:437, 1996.
194. Evrard P, Hantson P, Ferrant E, et al: Successful double lung transplantation with a graft obtained from a methanol-poisoned donor. *Chest* 115:1458, 1999.
195. Friedlaender MM, Rosenmann E, Rubinger D, et al: Successful renal transplantation from two donors with methanol intoxication. *Transplantation* 61:1549, 1996.
196. Bentley MJ, Mullen JC, Lopushinsky SR, et al: Successful cardiac transplantation with methanol or carbon monoxide-poisoned donors. *Ann Thorac Surg* 71:1194, 2001.
197. LaCouture PG, Wason S, Abrams A, et al: Acute isopropyl alcohol intoxication: diagnosis and management. *Am J Med* 75:657, 1983.
198. Lewin GA, Oppenheimer PR, Wingert WA: Coma from alcohol sponging. *J Am Coll Emerg Physicians* 6:165, 1977.
199. Vivier PM, Lewander WJ, Martin HF, et al: Isopropyl alcohol intoxication in a neonate through chronic dermal exposure: a complication of culturally based umbilical care practice. *Pediatr Emerg Care* 10:91, 1994.
200. Martinez TT, Jaeger RW, deCastro FJ, et al: A comparison of the absorption and metabolism of isopropyl alcohol by oral, dermal and inhalation routes. *Vet Hum Toxicol* 28:233, 1986.
201. Daniel DR, McAnnalley BH, Garriott JC: Isopropyl alcohol metabolism after acute intoxication in humans. *J Anal Toxicol* 5:110, 1981.
202. Alexander CB, McBay AJ, Hudson RP: Isopropanol and isopropanol deaths: ten years' experience. *J Forensic Sci* 27:541, 1982.
203. LaCouture PG, Heldreth DD, Shannon M, et al: The generation of acetonemia/acetonuria following ingestion of a subtoxic dose of isopropyl alcohol. *Am J Emerg Med* 7:38, 1989.
204. Parker KM, Lera TA: Acute isopropanol ingestion: pharmacokinetic parameters in the infant. *Am J Emerg Med* 10:542, 1992.
205. Rosansky SJ: Isopropyl alcohol poisoning treated with hemodialysis: kinetics of isopropyl alcohol and acetone removal. *J Toxicol Clin Toxicol* 19:265, 1982.
206. Kelner M, Bailey DN: Isopropanol ingestion: interpretation of blood concentrations and clinical findings. *J Toxicol Clin Toxicol* 20:497, 1983.
207. Pappas AA, Ackerman BH, Olsen KM, et al: Isopropanol ingestion: a report of six episodes with isopropanol and acetone serum concentration time data. *J Toxicol Clin Toxicol* 29:11, 1991.
208. Linden CH: Unknown alcohol. *Ann Emerg Med* 28:371, 1996.
209. Hawley PC, Falko JM: "Pseudo" renal failure after isopropyl alcohol intoxication. *South Med Assoc J* 75:630, 1982.
210. Jones AE, Summers RL: Detection of isopropyl alcohol in a patient with diabetic ketoacidosis. *J Emerg Med* 19:165, 2000.
211. Bailey DN: Detection of isopropanol in acetonemic patients not exposed to isopropanol. *J Toxicol Clin Toxicol* 28:459, 1990.
212. Su M, Hoffman RS, Nelson LS: Error in an emergency medicine textbook: isopropyl alcohol toxicity. *Acad Emerg Med* 9:175, 2002.

213. Fligner CL, Jack R, Twiggs GA, et al: Hyperosmolality induced by propylene glycol: a complication of silver sulfadiazine therapy. *JAMA* 253:1606, 1985.
214. Ruddick JA: Toxicology, metabolism, and biochemistry of 1,2-propanediol. *Toxicol Appl Pharmacol* 21:102, 1972.
215. Unger AH, Sklaroff HJ: Fatalities following intravenous use of sodium diphenylhydantoin for cardiac arrhythmias. *JAMA* 200:335, 1967.
216. York RC, Coleridge ST: Cardiopulmonary arrest following intravenous phenytoin loading. *Am J Emerg Med* 6:255, 1988.
217. Wilson KC, Reardon C, Farber HW: Propylene glycol toxicity in a patient receiving intravenous diazepam. *N Engl J Med* 343:815, 2000.
218. Arulanantham K, Genel M: Central nervous system toxicity associated with ingestion of propylene glycol. *J Pediatr* 93:515, 1978.
219. Cate JC, Hedrick R: Propylene glycol intoxication and lactic acidosis. *N Engl J Med* 303:1237, 1980.
220. Robinson CA Jr, Scott JW, Ketchum C: Propylene glycol interference with ethylene glycol procedures. *Clin Chem* 29:727, 1983.
221. Mullins ME, Barnes BJ: Hyperosmolar metabolic acidosis and intravenous lorazepam. *NEJM* 347:857–858, 2002.
222. Parker MG, Fraser GL, Watson DM, et al: Removal of propylene glycol and correction of increased osmolar gap by hemodialysis in a patient on high dose lorazepam infusion therapy. *Intensive Care Med* 28:81, 2002.
223. Al Khafaji AH, Dewhirst WE, Manning HL: Propylene glycol toxicity associated with lorazepam infusion in a patient receiving continuous venovenous hemofiltration with dialysis. *Anesth Analg* 94:1583, 2002.
224. Schep LJ, Slaughter RJ, Temple WA, et al: Diethylene glycol poisoning. *Clin Toxicol* 47(6):525–535, 2009.
225. Alfred S, Coleman P, Harris D, et al: Delayed neurologic sequelae resulting from epidemic diethylene glycol poisoning. *Clin Toxicol* 43(3):155–159, 2005.
226. Hari P, Jain Y, Kabra SK: Fatal encephalopathy and renal failure caused by diethylene glycol poisoning. *J Tropical Pediatr* 52(6):442–444, 2006.
227. O'Brien KL, Selanikio JD, Hecdivert C, et al: Epidemic of pediatric deaths from acute renal failure caused by diethylene glycol poisoning. Acute Renal Failure Investigation Team. *JAMA* 279(15):1175–1180, 1998.
228. Rollins YD, Filley CM, McNutt JT, et al: Fulminant ascending paralysis as a delayed sequela of diethylene glycol (Sterno) ingestion. *Neurology* 59(9):1460–1463, 2002.

CHAPTER 120 ■ ANTIARRHYTHMIC AGENTS

MICHAEL GANETSKY

The therapeutic use, misuse, and intentional overdose of antiarrhythmic drugs are associated with severe morbidity and mortality [1]. The recognition, management, and prevention of antiarrhythmic toxicity require an understanding of the pharmacology of these drugs as they are related to cardiac electrophysiology. A general review of the mechanisms involved as well as the principles of management of poisoning is followed by a discussion of individual agents.

PHARMACOLOGY

Antiarrhythmic drugs are most commonly classified on the basis of their predominant physiologic effect and mechanism of action as originally proposed by Vaughan Williams [2] and Campbell [3] (Tables 120.1 and 120.2; Fig. 120.1).

The major effect of class I agents is blockade of the fast inward sodium current responsible for the rapid upstroke and conduction of the action potential [4] (see Fig. 120.1). This effect is also known as *local anesthetic* or *membrane stabilizing action*. Class I drugs depress automaticity, particularly in Purkinje fibers. Class I drugs comprise a large group of antiarrhythmic agents, many of which have diverse electrophysiologic properties; consequently, this class has been subdivided into classes IA, IB, and IC (see Table 120.2) [3].

The class II antiarrhythmic drugs are β-adrenergic antagonists; they inhibit the proarrhythmic effects of catecholamines, which shorten refractory periods and facilitate reentrant circuits. The slowly conducting, calcium-channel–dependent action potentials of the normal sinoatrial (SA) and atrioventricular (AV) nodes (see Fig. 120.1) rely partially on sympathetic tone. Class II drugs depress conduction and automaticity through these specialized tissues, leading to bradycardia and AV block. Toxicity due to beta-blockers is covered further in Chapter 125.

Class III agents prolong the refractory period by increasing the cardiac action potential duration (APD), especially in phases 2 and 3 (see Fig. 120.1). This effect is produced by blockade of the major outward potassium-rectifying (repolarizing) current. Amiodarone is the prototypic class III agent, whereas ibutilide and dofetilide are newer class III agents.

Class IV drugs (calcium antagonists or calcium channel blockers) antagonize the slow inward calcium current responsible for the slow upstroke and conduction of the action potentials of SA and AV nodal cells [4] (see Fig. 120.1). Verapamil, diltiazem, and nifedipine represent the three subclasses of calcium channel antagonists. Both verapamil and diltiazem have negative inotropic and chronotropic properties and are useful for slowing the ventricular response rate in patients with atrial

TABLE 120.1

VAUGHAN WILLIAMS CLASSIFICATION OF ANTIARRHYTHMIC ACTIONS

Class	Drugs	Actions
I	Quinidine Procainamide Disopyramide Moricizine Lidocaine Tocainide Mexiletine Flecainide Propafenone	Block fast sodium current (hence slow conduction)
II	Beta-blockers	Block effects of catecholamines
III	Amiodarone Sotalol Ibutilide Bretylium	Prolong action potential and, hence, refractoriness by blocking K^+ current
IV	Verapamil Diltiazem	Block cardiac calcium channel

TABLE 120.2

SUBGROUPS OF CLASS I DRUGS

Class	Drugs	Effects on action potential	Summary of clinical effects
IA	Quinidine Procainamide Disopyramide Moricizine	Reduce rate of depolarization; prolong duration of action potential	Moderate slowing of cardiac conduction; prolongation of refractory periods
IB	Lidocaine Mexiletine Tocainide	Reduce rate of depolarization selectively in ischemic cells; shorten action potential duration	Selective depression of ischemic tissue; may shorten refractory periods
IC	Flecainide Propafenone	Marked depression of depolarization rate	Marked slowing of cardiac conduction; small increase in refractory periods

fibrillation. In therapeutic dosing, calcium channel antagonists such as nifedipine have little effect on cardiac conduction or inotropic state and are, therefore, not used for their antiarrhythmic properties. Calcium channel blocker toxicity is discussed in Chapter 126.

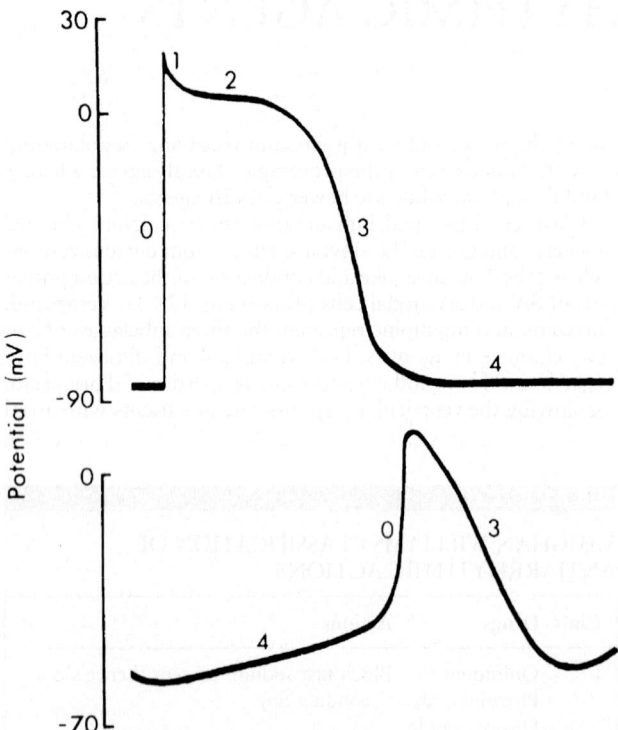

FIGURE 120.1. Typical cellular action potentials recorded from working myocardium (*upper trace*) and the atrioventricular node (*lower trace*). The nodal cell has an action potential of smaller amplitude, with a much slower rate of depolarization in phase 0. The nodal cell exhibits spontaneous diastolic (phase 4) depolarization ("pacemaker" activity). Rapid depolarization in phase 0 (atrial and ventricular cells and Purkinje fibers) is produced by a fast inward sodium current (depressed by class I drugs). A slower inward calcium current is also present but is the only inward current found in sinoatrial and atrioventricular nodal cells. This explains their slower rate of depolarization in phase 0 and their sensitivity to calcium-channel blockers. Repolarization (phase 3) is produced by a number of outward potassium currents; the rapid component of the delayed rectifier potassium current is the most important. Blockade of this current by antiarrhythmic or other drugs prolongs repolarization and action potential duration (class III action).

Adenosine and digoxin are two drugs with antiarrhythmic effects that do not fall within the Vaughan Williams classification. Adenosine is an endogenous nucleoside that produces AV nodal conduction block and vasodilation via specific adenosine-sensitive receptors. The antiarrhythmic properties and toxicity of digoxin are discussed in Chapter 127.

The cellular electropharmacology of antiarrhythmic agents involves suppression of automaticity, decreased cardiac conduction, and refractory period prolongation. Automaticity, the spontaneous depolarization of pacemaker myocytes, occurs in SA and AV nodes as well as in Purkinje fibers. In SA and AV nodal cells, the rate of firing depends on several different inward and outward currents; the combination of currents renders these cells relatively insensitive to depression by antiarrhythmic drugs [1,4,5]. In Purkinje fibers, however, automaticity occurs as an escape phenomenon that arises in the presence of AV block. Escape beats probably result from the action of a single inward sodium channel (the "pacemaker current") and are suppressed by therapeutic concentrations of most class I antiarrhythmic agents. Therefore, Purkinje fiber automaticity is more susceptible to depression by antiarrhythmic agents than is sinus node automaticity. Nonetheless, clinical suppression of the sinus node leading to asystole, particularly in the presence of the high vagal tone commonly seen in the early phases of acute myocardial infarction, is an uncommon but well-recognized complication of therapy with antiarrhythmic agents such as lidocaine.

Reentrant circuit arrhythmias depend on conduction rates around the circuit and the refractory periods of pathway components. If the conduction time falls below the refractory period of part of the circuit, the "excitable gap" disappears, the advancing wavefront meets only refractory tissue, and the arrhythmia terminates. An ideal antiarrhythmic agent would, therefore, accelerate conduction and prolong refractoriness within the substrate for reentry. Many antiarrhythmic agents prolong refractory periods in myocardium, but none accelerates conduction in therapeutic use. Almost invariably, conduction tends to slow. This combination of decreasing conduction and refractory period prolongation can be either proarrhythmic or antiarrhythmic [5]. However, clinicians cannot predict which outcome is likely for a given drug in a given patient. Some antiarrhythmic agents (in particular, class IB drugs and amiodarone [3]) show selectivity for depressing conduction in ischemic or otherwise abnormal myocardium by binding preferentially to the inactivated state of the sodium channel. A complete conduction block through an ischemic segment of a reentrant circuit may be the mechanism of arrhythmia termination; this could occur without slowing conduction in healthy myocardium. Other drugs tend to show less selectivity and depress conduction in normal myocardium at therapeutic concentrations, probably explaining the greater propensity of class IC drugs to be proarrhythmic both in therapeutic use and in overdose [3].

Although most antiarrhythmic agents prolong refractoriness, lidocaine, mexiletine, and tocainide tend to shorten it, particularly in low concentrations; this may explain some cases of drug-associated arrhythmogenesis in patients with reentrant tachycardias. Lengthening of refractoriness should be proarrhythmic, but if conduction is slowed simultaneously, the net effect on the reentrant circuit determines the outcome.

Antiarrhythmic drugs suppress most forms of automaticity known to cause tachyarrhythmias. The major exception to this rule is the form of triggered automaticity due to *early after-depolarizations* (EADs). EADs can be defined as a marked slowing of repolarization, visible on the action-potential recording and due to reduction of the normal repolarizing outward potassium current. If voltage conditions are appropriate, prolonged depolarization may trigger a series of automatic action potentials. The upstrokes of these action potentials are due to inward current flow through the normal calcium channels that had been inactivated, had recovered from inactivation, and had found the membrane potential still within their activation range. The channels then reactivate and produce a secondary upstroke. Increased intracellular calcium concentrations activate calcium-sensitive potassium channels and accelerate repolarization. This process can occur as a single event or as an oscillatory series of action potentials, depending on the prevailing conditions of voltage and calcium levels [6–8].

The induction of EADs may be the basis of arrhythmias, including torsade de pointes associated with long QT syndromes [5,6,9]. According to this theory, the slowing of repolarization leads directly to the QT wave prolongation, often with associated prominent, bizarre TU waves. Any triggered activity, should it occur, results in ventricular tachyarrhythmias.

The class IA antiarrhythmic agents quinidine, disopyramide, and procainamide are all capable of producing EADs and torsade de pointes [6]. This is also true of the class III drugs, such as amiodarone, sotalol, ibutilide, and dofetilide. The class IB agents, lidocaine, mexiletine, and tocainide, do not produce EADs and do not cause torsade de pointes. Class IC compounds infrequently cause significant slowing of repolarization and have not been shown to cause torsade de pointes. Of the class IV agents, only mibefradil has an effect on repolarization, which usually manifests as TU-wave changes. Experimental models suggest that this effect is not proarrhythmic; however, there has been a report of torsade due to QT prolongation from therapeutic dosing of mibefradil [10,11].

CLINICAL PRESENTATION

Toxicity common to therapeutic doses and overdoses of antiarrhythmic agents include depression of automaticity and cardiac conduction, which may be caused by a combination of direct electrophysiologic and secondary metabolic effects. Symptoms following acute overdose usually begin within 4 hours and can occur at any time during chronic therapy. Drug absorption may continue for many hours following the ingestion of large doses, sustained-release preparations, or agents with anticholinergic effects, resulting in delayed or progressive toxicity. Respiratory depression and hypotension produce acidosis and myocardial ischemia that further aggravate depressed conduction. Cardiac manifestations include QRS prolongation, QTc prolongation, sinus node dysfunction, bradycardia, AV block, ventricular arrhythmias, and poor ventricular function. These derangements can culminate in intractable arrhythmias, cardiogenic shock, or death. Manifestations of acute toxicity may also include dizziness, visual disturbances, psychosis, anticholinergic symptoms, hypoglycemia, hyperglycemia, and hypokalemia. Seizures may result from class I (particularly IB) toxicity. Procainamide and quinidine can cause hypotension if infused too rapidly.

Warning signs that indicate an increased risk of torsade include a QTc interval greater than 560 milliseconds, previous history of torsade, bradycardia, increased frequency and complexity of ventricular premature beats, or a ventricular premature beat falling on the T wave [12].

The electrocardiogram (ECG) may provide a clue to the agent or class involved in cases where the drug ingested is not known. Class IB drugs usually have no effect on the QT interval; whereas class IA, IC, and III agents prolong it. With class IA agents, QT prolongation is due to slowing of both depolarization and repolarization. Hence, both the QRS duration and JT interval are increased. In contrast, QT prolongation primarily results from slowed depolarization with class IC agents, resulting in an increased QRS (but not JT) duration and from prolonged repolarization with class III agents, resulting in an increased JT (but not QRS) interval.

The differential diagnosis of bradyarrhythmias includes beta-blocker, calcium channel blocker, cholinergic agent (carbamate and organophosphate insecticides), clonidine, cyclic antidepressant, and digitalis poisoning. Other agents that cause QRS and QT interval prolongation include antihistamines, antipsychotic agents, cyclic antidepressants, magnesium, and potassium. Ventricular tachyarrhythmias may occur in poisoning with sympathomimetics (see Chapter 144). Hypoglycemia, hypoxia, and metabolic disturbances should be considered in the differential diagnosis of patients with neurologic symptoms.

DIAGNOSTIC EVALUATION

Physical examination should focus on vital signs and respiratory, cardiovascular, and central nervous system (CNS) function. Frequent vital signs and continuous cardiac monitoring should be performed. Essential tests include an ECG and serum electrolytes, blood urea nitrogen, creatinine, and magnesium measurement; liver function tests and serum drug levels, if available, may also be helpful. A chest radiograph should be obtained as clinically indicated. Patients with hypotension and hypoxemia should have arterial blood gas and serum lactate measurements.

MANAGEMENT

The general features of antiarrhythmic drug overdose and their management are discussed below (Table 120.3). Care of the antiarrhythmic poisoned patient centers on general supportive and critical care principles. Unique aspects pertinent to individual drugs are discussed in later sections. All patients suspected of ingesting an overdose of antiarrhythmic agents should receive oral activated charcoal. Patients with complications of therapeutic dosing may also benefit from oral activated charcoal to reduce absorption of a recently administered drug dose. The greatest amount of absorption to charcoal will occur if given within 1 to 2 hours of ingestions. CNS and respiratory depression commonly require airway support by endotracheal intubation. Seizures are managed by benzodiazepine therapy. Phenytoin should never be used to treat seizures secondary to drug toxicity because of the risk of increased mortality.

Initial therapy for hypotension involves administration of intravenous fluids. Because poisoned patients are infrequently hypovolemic, fluid administration should be monitored closely. In general, if a response in blood pressure is not seen with 2 L of intravenous fluids, pressors such as norepinephrine should be administered. Early consideration should be given to

TABLE 120.3

MANAGEMENT OF LIFE-THREATENING ANTIARRHYTHMIC DRUG OVERDOSE

Supportive care
Activated charcoal for acute (<1 h) oral ingestions
Correct acidosis, hypoxia
Benzodiazepines for seizure control
Enhance drug elimination
Activated charcoal
Consider extracorporeal elimination if appropriate
Hypotension
Fluid administration
Alkalinization (hypertonic $NaHCO_3$) for class I drugs
Inotropes, vasopressors
Consider pulmonary artery catheter for monitoring
Circulatory assist devices
Impaired conduction
Temporary pacing for atrioventricular block or bradycardia
Alkalinization (hypertonic $NaHCO_3$) for class I drugs
Ventricular arrhythmias
Torsade de pointes
Temporary pacing
$MgSO_4$
Isoproterenol
Monomorphic ventricular tachycardia
Cardioversion, if causing hypotension
Hypertonic $NaHCO_3$ for class I drugs
Lidocaine, except for class IB drugs
Overdrive pacing
PEA cardiac arrest
Intravenous lipid emulsion for bupivacaine (may consider for other lipophilic agents or in refractory cases). Loading dose of 1.5 mL/kg administered over 1 min, repeated one to two times every 3–5 min as needed. If hemodynamic improvement is noted, the loading dose should be followed by a continuous infusion at a rate of 0.25–0.5 mL/kg/min

circulatory assist devices for patients with cardiogenic shock. Intra-aortic balloon pump counterpulsation has been used successfully to treat patients with severe quinidine or disopyramide toxicity [13,14], and partial cardiac bypass has been used to maintain circulation during massive lidocaine or flecainide toxicity [15–17].

Decreased ventricular conduction, as measured by QRS prolongation in quinidine, procainamide, flecainide, and encainide toxicity, are often treated with sodium bicarbonate infusion [18–22]. In animals, hypertonic sodium bicarbonate reverses ventricular arrhythmias caused by flecainide toxicity [23] and reverses hypotension due to tricyclic antidepressants with class IA antiarrhythmic effects [20]. Hypertonic sodium bicarbonate should be considered for the treatment of QRS widening greater than 100 milliseconds or ventricular tachyarrhythmias in the setting of class IA or IC drug toxicity. Common practice is to administer intravenous boluses of sodium bicarbonate (50 mEq of 1 mEq per mL solution) as needed to increase and maintain blood pH between 7.45 and 7.55. As an alternative, a continuous infusion of 1,000 mL of 5% dextrose in water containing 2 to 3 amps of sodium bicarbonate and potassium chloride is an option. Bicarbonate should be administered for 12 to 24 hours and then gradually withdrawn while watching for QRS lengthening to recur. At present, there is no evidence that prophylactic alkalinization before QRS widening changes outcome. In the most severely poisoned patients, however, alkalinization may be ineffective, especially if there is persistent metabolic acidosis. In a series of patients with class I antiarrhythmic drug overdose requiring cardiopulmonary resuscitation, only 2 of 29 survived despite the use of hypertonic sodium bicarbonate [24].

Sodium bicarbonate appears to act by increasing the extracellular sodium concentration and reducing the drug-induced sodium channel blockade [25]. Hypertonic sodium chloride has proven effective in animals and, anecdotally, in humans, but sodium bicarbonate is generally preferable because increasing pH is equally or more important in some models [20,25–27] (see Chapter 123 for more detail).

The treatment of recalcitrant ventricular tachycardia typically consists of repeated cardioversions, cardiopulmonary resuscitation, vasopressor support, and mechanical ventilation. Treatment with other class IA and IC antiarrhythmic drugs is contraindicated, given the potential for further arrhythmia aggravation [28]. Lidocaine may be considered because it does not depress conduction, but it is often ineffective. Suppression of ventricular tachycardia and hemodynamic improvement has been anecdotally described with sodium bicarbonate [21,22]. Overdrive pacing may also be effective.

The treatment of torsade de pointes should include 1 to 2 g of a 25% solution of intravenous magnesium sulfate. Direct-current cardioversion is often effective in terminating torsade de pointes, but it frequently recurs. Increasing the ventricular rate to greater than 90 to 110 beats per minute by an infusion of isoproterenol or ventricular pacing may also be effective [29,30]. In one study, infusion of potassium chloride at 0.5 mEq per kg for 60 to 90 minutes normalized excessive quinidine-induced QT prolongation, but simply correcting hypokalemia did not suppress torsade de pointes [31]. Lidocaine is inconsistently effective [32,33]. Treatment with class IA or III antiarrhythmic drugs is contraindicated because further prolongation of repolarization and the QT interval may exacerbate torsade de pointes. Magnesium therapy should also be considered in patients at increased risk for this arrhythmia (see earlier); it has been found to prevent occurrence of torsade in a dog model (dose of 30 to 60 mg per kg) [34].

Although most antiarrhythmic drugs are weak bases, urine acidification is contraindicated because systemic acidosis may aggravate cardiotoxicity [20]; treatment with hypertonic alkaline solution to reduce cardiotoxicity is likely to be of greater benefit. Hemodialysis is of limited benefit for antiarrhythmic toxicity because drug clearance is limited by protein binding and high lipid solubility [26,35,36]. Hemoperfusion using charcoal resin is more effective in removing drugs with high protein binding and high lipid solubility; however, this modality is rarely available. Hemoperfusion is of greatest value for disopyramide [37] or *N*-acetylprocainamide (NAPA) toxicity [38].

INDIVIDUAL AGENTS

Class IA Agents

Quinidine

Quinidine is administered orally as sulfate or gluconate. The usual dose of immediate-release quinidine sulfate is 200 to 400 mg, four times per day, with gluconate doses being approximately 30% higher. Bioavailability is approximately 70% for both forms; peak plasma levels are reached earlier for the sulfate (60 to 90 minutes) than for the gluconate. Quinidine is metabolized by CYP3A4 to 3-OH quinidine and

TABLE 120.4

DOSE AND PHARMACOKINETICS OF CLASS I AND II ANTIARRHYTHMIC AGENTS

Drug	Usual daily dose	Therapeutic or usual plasma concentration (μg/mL)	Volume of distribution (L/kg)	Elimination half-life	% Excreted unchanged in Urine	% Bound in plasma	Active metabolites	Methods of enhancing elimination
Class IA								
Quinidine	Depends on formulation (see text)	2–7	2.0–3.5	7 h	17–50[a]	80–90	3-OH quinidine	—
Procainamide	3–6 g	4–8 (NAPA, 7–15)	2 (NAPA, 1.4)	2.5–4.5 h (NAPA, 5–9 h)	40–60 (NAPA, 80)	10–20 (NAPA, 10)	NAPA	HD, HP
Disopyramide	300–600 mg	2–6	1.0–1.5	4–10 h	40–60	50–65	—	HD, HP
Moricizine	600–900 mg	0.1–3.0[b]	8–11	1.5–13.0 h	1	95	—	—
Class IB								
Lidocaine	1–3 μg/min	1.5–6.0	1.0–1.7	1.5–2.5 h[c]	<10	60–80	Monoethylglycinexylidide, glycine xylidide	?HP
Tocainide	1.2–2.4 g	3–10	1.5–3.2	11–20 h	40	10	—	HD, HP
Mexiletine	600–1,200 mg	0.5–2.0	5–7	6–17 h	8–15	50–70	—	—
Class IC								
Flecainide	100–300 mg	0.07–0.50	9	12–18 h[a,d]	70	50	—	—
Propafenone	400–800 mg	0.2–1.8	1.9–3.0	3.6 h (17 h)[e]	—	—	5-hydroxy-propafenone	—
Class III								
Amiodarone	100–400 mg	1.0–2.5[b]	70	40–49 d	<1	99	Desethylamiodarone	—
Sotalol	160–320 mg	0.6–3.2	2	12–15 h	>75	0	—	HD, HP
Bretylium	See text	?	7	4–10 h	95	1–6	—	—

[a] Shorter with lower urine pH.
[b] Correlates poorly with therapeutic effect.
[c] Longer in patients with congestive heart failure.
[d] Dose dependent.
[e] Slow metabolizers at CYP2D6 locus.
HD, hemodialysis; HP, hemoperfusion; NAPA, *N*-acetylprocainamide.

quinidine-*N*-oxide; these metabolites have less electrophysiologic activity than quinidine [39,40]. Details of pharmacokinetics are listed in Table 120.4.

Torsade de pointes is an adverse effect of therapeutic doses of quinidine (also known as *quinidine syncope*). Risk factors for this arrhythmia are recent initiation of quinidine therapy, concurrent digoxin therapy, female gender, structural heart disease, hypokalemia, and hypomagnesemia. Possible mechanisms include prolongation of the QTc interval and potentiation of EADs [40].

In therapeutic doses, sustained-release quinidine formulations produce therapeutic plasma concentrations for up to 8 hours in most patients. In overdose, however, saturation of enzymes that metabolize the drug may dramatically prolong serum concentrations. Consequently, serial serum drug monitoring is warranted (see Table 120.4), especially when potentially interactive agents, are coadministered. Agents that are CYP3A4 inhibitors, such as cimetidine, can increase quinidine serum concentration. Mild quinidine overdose presents as cinchonism (headache, tinnitus, deafness, diplopia, confusion), vertigo, visual disturbances (blurred vision, photophobia, scotomata, contracted visual fields, yellow vision), or delirium. Severe toxicity is characterized by CNS toxicity (lethargy, coma, respiratory depression, seizures), gastrointestinal tract toxicity (nausea, vomiting, diarrhea), and cardiovascular collapse [41]. Noncardiac side effects include nausea, cinchonism, thrombocytopenia, and drug-induced fever.

Initial therapy for acute quinidine overdose should include gastric decontamination with activated charcoal. Treatment of CNS toxicity is supportive, with intubation and ventilation for CNS depression and benzodiazepines for seizures. Deaths from quinidine overdose are usually secondary to arrhythmias or hypotension. When pacing is indicated for bradycardia, failure to capture is common in the face of drug-induced myocardial depression. QRS prolongation should be treated with bicarbonate infusion. Hypotension may result from vasodilation from β-adrenergic blockade, impaired contractility from sodium channel blockade, or arrhythmias. Vasodilation may be treated with fluid administration and alpha-acting vasopressors such as norepinephrine; large doses may be required.

Refractory hypotension has been successfully treated with an intra-aortic balloon pump [13] and partial circulatory bypass.

Procainamide

Procainamide is eliminated by hepatic metabolism and renal excretion [42,43]. The major metabolite is NAPA, which has potent class III and some class I antiarrhythmic activity [44]. In fast acetylators or in renal failure, as much as 40% of a dose of procainamide may be excreted as NAPA. Because the prevalence of the fast and slow acetylator phenotypes varies between ethnic groups, widely variable procainamide and NAPA concentrations may occur in specific populations [45]. Blood concentrations of NAPA may exceed those of the parent drug, given its dependence on renal elimination.

The cardiovascular side effects of procainamide are very similar to those of quinidine except that the drug has no β-adrenergic antagonist activity. Acute procainamide toxicity is manifested primarily by hypotension, but QRS widening and ventricular arrhythmias may also occur [46]. Inappropriate drug dosing in renal insufficiency or before achieving steady-state concentrations is the most common cause of procainamide toxicity. Toxic levels of NAPA (>25 μg per mL) may begin to accumulate as a result of acute or chronic renal insufficiency, potentially leading to torsade. Approximately 40% of patients receiving long-term oral therapy with procainamide develop a syndrome resembling systemic lupus erythematosus that usually resolves after drug withdrawal [47].

Signs and symptoms of acute procainamide overdose are similar to those of quinidine overdose. Patients with non–life-threatening procainamide toxicity (e.g., hypotension) and adequate renal function can be managed with supportive care. Seizure has been reported in a pediatric ingestion [48]. Hypertonic sodium bicarbonate may be useful for QRS prolongation, monomorphic ventricular tachycardia, or hypotension [18]. This therapy has minimal benefit in NAPA toxicity because this metabolite has primarily class III effects. Torsade de pointes should be treated as already discussed. Anecdotal reports have showed increased procainamide and NAPA clearance with hemodialysis or hemoperfusion; however, clinical significance is unclear [38,46].

Disopyramide

Disopyramide, unlike most other antiarrhythmic drugs, has protein binding that shows nonlinear, saturable characteristics [49,50]. This is clinically important because small increases in total plasma level within the therapeutic range (see Table 120.3) may mask larger rises in free (active) drug concentration. When administered intravenously, disopyramide produces hypotension less frequently than do quinidine or procainamide. Widening of the QRS complex, prolongation of the QT interval, and drug-induced ventricular tachyarrhythmias have all been reported as side effects [51]. There are numerous reports of QTc prolongation, torsade, or monomorphic ventricular tachycardia from the interaction of disopyramide and macrolide antibiotics. Erythromycin, clarithromycin, and azithromycin have all been implicated; a possible mechanism is inhibition of hepatic CYP3A4 [52].

Acute disopyramide overdose is similar to that of quinidine or procainamide, with QRS prolongation, severe refractory hypotension, and arrhythmias [14,53–55]. Hypoglycemia is a recognized adverse effect [55]. Data regarding management are limited, but an approach similar to that for quinidine toxicity is appropriate. Hypotension refractory to intravenous fluids and vasopressors has been treated with an intra-aortic balloon pump [14]. Because of its relatively small volume of distribution, disopyramide clearance is substantially increased by hemoperfusion [14,37,56].

Class IB Agents

Lidocaine (and Other Local Anesthetics)

Amide-type local anesthetics (e.g., articaine, bupivacaine, etidocaine, lidocaine, mepivacaine, prilocaine, and ropivacaine) are extensively metabolized by hepatic dealkylation, hydrolysis, ring hydroxylation, and conjugation. Ester-type agents are metabolized by hepatic and plasma esterases. Derivatives of para-aminobenzoic acid (e.g., benzocaine, procaine, tetracaine) are predominantly hydrolyzed by plasma pseudocholinesterase, whereas other esters (e.g., cocaine, dyclonine, proparacaine) are predominantly metabolized in the liver [57]. Allergic cross-reactivity occurs within the amide and ester groups but not between them.

Extensive first-pass metabolism prevents effective oral therapy with lidocaine and local anesthetics, but toxicity can occur after ingestion [57]. The maintenance infusion rate of lidocaine must be reduced in patients with cardiac failure or hepatic dysfunction and in the elderly [58]. Plasma concentrations should be monitored for infusions lasting longer than 24 hours. Lidocaine has two active metabolites, monoethylglycinexylidide (MEGX) and glycine xylidide (GX). Although these metabolites have short elimination half-lives of 2 hours and 1 hour, respectively, they may contribute significantly to toxicity, which can occur several hours after an infusion is started [57,58]. Most lidocaine toxicity is caused by errors in dosing and administration [59]. Life-threatening toxicity and death have occurred after inadvertent overdose, surgical procedures such as liposuction, and parenteral, mucosal, and topical anesthesia [60–62]. The safety of tumescent liposuction, in which large volumes of lidocaine solutions are infused subcutaneously, has been called into question following several reported deaths [63].

All local anesthetics have toxicity similar to lidocaine, with neurologic signs and symptoms usually preceding cardiac manifestations, except in massive acute overdose [64,65]. Neurologic symptoms, the most significant of which is seizures, include auditory disturbances, visual disturbances, paresthesias, and ataxia. Lidocaine has a bimodal concentration-dependent effect on seizures; lidocaine suppresses seizures at concentrations between 0.5 and 5 μg per mL but increases the risk at levels above 8 to 9 μg per mL. The relative contribution to epileptogenicity of the parent compound compared with the metabolites MEGX and GX is still unclear [66]. Adverse cardiac effects from lidocaine administration are unusual in the absence of severe underlying conduction-system disease, acute myocardial ischemia, or massive overdose. Persons with third-degree heart block requiring ventricular arrhythmia suppression should have a prophylactic pacemaker inserted before lidocaine administration [67]. However, lidocaine administration in asymptomatic patients with bundle-branch block or intraventricular conduction disease carries a low risk [68].

Acute massive overdose of lidocaine is characterized by seizures, coma, respiratory arrest, and cardiovascular collapse [61,64,69–71]. Hypotension is due to myocardial depression [72]. Lidocaine has little or no effect on the QT interval; however, QRS prolongation, AV block, and depressed automaticity with bradycardia or asystole can occur. Data regarding management are anecdotal. Seizures should be managed using intravenous diazepam; phenytoin should be avoided. Bradyarrhythmias may respond to isoproterenol infusion or cardiac pacing. Hypotension and shock respond to fluid administration and vasopressors such as dopamine. If QRS prolongation is present, hypertonic sodium bicarbonate may be useful. Intra-aortic balloon pump and cardiopulmonary bypass have been used successfully in patients with circulatory collapse [15,16].

Amide-type local anesthetics can also induce methemoglobinemia [57,70,73]. This effect has been described after percutaneous absorption of benzocaine-containing formulations, during use of prilocaine as an epidural anesthetic agent, and due to prilocaine found in eutectic mixture of local anesthetics (EMLA) cream. Amide agents are hydrolyzed to an amino group that exerts an oxidizing stress in susceptible individuals—such as those with G-6-PD deficiency—to produce methemoglobinemia. In some cases, patients may also exhibit red blood cell hemolysis. Methemog-lobinemia is treated with methylene blue (see Chapter 147).

Bupivacaine intoxication can lead to PEA cardiac arrest that is not responsive to standard ACLS protocols. This is a dreaded complication of regional anesthesia after inadvertent intravenous injection of bupivacaine. Intravenous lipid emulsion (Intralipid) is rapidly becoming accepted as standard treatment for bupivacaine-induced cardiac arrest. Even though no human trials exist, there is excellent animal evidence and several human case reports [74]. The mechanism is still unclear, but effects are likely from partitioning of bupivacaine away from cardiac receptors and into an intravenous lipid phase. Therefore, intralipid may be an effective therapy for other lipophilic anesthetic agents. The initial loading dose is 1.5 mL per kg (typically 100 mL in an average adult) administered over 1 minute, which can be repeated one to two times every 3 to 5 minutes. If hemodynamic improvement is noted, the loading dose should be followed by a continuous infusion at a rate of 0.25 to 0.5 mL per kg per minute [75].

Tocainide

Adverse effects are common during tocainide therapy, with up to 50% of patients requiring dosage adjustments or discontinuation [76]. The most common side effects are nausea, vomiting, and anorexia, and neurologic effects such as dizziness, paresthesias, tremor, ataxia, and confusion. Tremor suggests that the maximum tolerable dose of tocainide has been reached. Serious toxicity resulting from pulmonary fibrosis in up to 0.1% and agranulocytosis and leukopenia in 0.2% of patients has been reported [77]. Monitoring for clinical or laboratory signs of agranulocytosis has been recommended, particularly during the first 12 weeks of therapy.

Massive tocainide overdose causes effects similar to those of lidocaine overdose: loss of consciousness, seizures, high-degree AV block, asystole, and ventricular fibrillation [76,78–80]. Treatment considerations are also similar. Because 40% of tocainide elimination is renal, urine acidification theoretically increases tocainide excretion but is not recommended because of enhanced systemic toxicity.

Mexiletine

Mexiletine is structurally similar to lidocaine and undergoes extensive metabolism in the liver to largely inactive compounds [81,82]. Hepatic impairment can significantly prolong the elimination half-life to 25 hours or longer. Patients with chronic liver disease, such as hepatic cirrhosis, undergo a marked reduction in the hepatic metabolism of mexiletine [83,84]. Smoking enhances mexiletine elimination, reducing the half-life by 35% compared with nonsmokers [85]. Phenytoin, rifampin, and phenobarbital induce hepatic enzymes and lower mexiletine plasma concentrations. Antacid therapy, cimetidine, and narcotic analgesics can slow the absorption of mexiletine [86].

Mexiletine is generally well tolerated, with little effect on hemodynamics, even in patients with congestive heart failure [87]. Mexiletine shares much of the side effect profile of lidocaine, including cross-reactivity in allergic individuals. Dizziness, ataxia, and tremor are relatively common. Overdose effects resemble those of lidocaine. Heart block or asystole accompanied by hypotension occur with massive overdose [88,89]. Status epilepticus requiring diazepam and phenobarbital has been described [90]. The prolonged duration of seizures compared with lidocaine overdose may be due to mexiletine's longer elimination half-life of 5.5 to 12 hours. A urine drug immunoassay was reported as positive for amphetamines in the setting of a mexiletine overdose, likely from cross-reactivity due to structural similarity of these compounds [91].

Class IC Agents

Flecainide

Flecainide is very well absorbed orally, with negligible hepatic first-pass effect. Flecainide displays polymorphic drug metabolism because it is metabolized via CYP2D6 to active metabolites. This phenomenon effectively results in two distinct populations of patients having very different clearance rates. The average half-life is between 8 and 10 hours, with substantial individual variability. Inhibitors of the CYP2D6 pathway, such as INH, quinidine, selective serotonin-uptake inhibitors, and other agents metabolized by this pathway, may decrease or increase the clearance of flecainide when added to or deleted from therapy. Amiodarone can double the serum concentration of flecainide when the two drugs are concomitantly administered; the flecainide dose should be reduced by 50% when these drugs are coadministered. Serum concentrations can be followed but are rarely used. The proposed therapeutic range is 200 to 1,000 ng per mL.

Flecainide is approved for the management of paroxysmal atrial fibrillation or flutter associated with disabling symptoms, but there are many restrictions due to its adverse effects. Flecainide has a very narrow therapeutic index and can be toxic even at therapeutic concentrations [92]. In the Cardiac Arrhythmia Suppression Trial (CAST) [93], postinfarction patients being treated for ventricular arrhythmias demonstrated an increased mortality relative to patients treated with placebo. Furthermore, flecainide possesses considerable negative inotropic effects that limit its usefulness in the setting of congestive heart failure. Other dose-related side effects occur, including CNS toxicity such as blurred vision, dizziness, headache, nausea, and paresthesias. Flecainide also increases the ventricular pacing threshold.

Flecainide is highly toxic in overdose; in one series, the mortality rate was 10% [24]. Overdose is characterized by QRS prolongation with a normal JT interval, hypotension, coma, or seizures [24,94]. Serious cardiac effects that can occur include severe bradycardia, high-grade conduction blocks, and ventricular dysrhythmias. Cardiac arrest is not uncommon after overdose; survival after full arrest is rare [92]. Data regarding management are mostly anecdotal. In rats, hypertonic sodium bicarbonate, 3 to 6 mEq per kg, reduced flecainide-induced QRS prolongation [95], and in dogs, this treatment largely abolished ventricular tachycardia [23]. In overdose patients, both hypertonic sodium bicarbonate and sodium lactate have been reported to be effective [96,97]. Hypertonic sodium bicarbonate or sodium lactate should be considered in patients with evidence of disturbed ventricular conduction. Cardiopulmonary bypass and extracorporeal membrane oxygenation (ECMO) have been used to support perfusion until spontaneous perfusion returned [17,98]. In one report, a patient who developed refractory ventricular fibrillation due to a flecainide overdose was successfully resuscitated after a 300-mg amiodarone bolus was given [92].

Propafenone

Propafenone is used for select patients with atrial fibrillation and for refractory ventricular tachycardia and fibrillation. Like flecainide, propafenone undergoes significant first-pass hepatic metabolism via the CYP2D6 isoenzyme pathway.

Bioavailability ranges from 5% to 50%, depending on the patient's phenotype; agents that inhibit CYP2D6 lower the clearance rate. Administering propafenone with food may significantly increase bioavailability in extensive metabolizers by diminishing first-pass drug extraction [99,100].

Propafenone has other drug interactions as well. Propafenone administration may increase digoxin concentrations between 35% and 85% due to impairment of nonrenal digoxin clearance. Quinidine is a specific and potent inhibitor of CYP2D6 and can significantly increase propafenone concentration [101]. Coadministration of propafenone with warfarin may result in a 25% increase in prothrombin time from unknown mechanisms. Similar to flecainide, propafenone has a narrow therapeutic index.

Propafenone overdose is similar to that of flecainide; toxicity includes QRS prolongation, hypotension, bradycardia, coma, and seizures [24,102,103]. Seizures appear to be more common in propafenone overdose than in flecainide overdose. PR interval prolongation is a characteristic finding in propafenone toxicity [104,105]. Hypertonic sodium bicarbonate has been beneficial for QRS prolongations and aberrant ventricular conduction [106,107]. Benzodiazepines should be used for seizures; phenytoin should be avoided [108]. Management of cardiovascular toxicity is similar to that of flecainide overdose. Transvenous cardiac pacing was successful in a case with severe bradycardia due to a high-grade conduction block [104].

Class III Agents

Amiodarone

Amiodarone was first used as a vascular smooth-muscle relaxant. In addition to its class III activity (prolonging the cardiac APD), amiodarone possesses properties common to all Vaughan Williams classifications. These include calcium channel–smooth-muscle relaxant (class IV), noncompetitive antiadrenergic (class II), and some sodium-channel–blocking (class I) activity.

Amiodarone is generally considered the most effective antiarrhythmic agent for treatment and prophylaxis of most types of arrhythmia [109]. Its clinical use, however, is complicated by unusual pharmacokinetics (see Table 120.4) and prevalent side effects [110,111]. After oral administration, amiodarone widely distributes into body tissues where drug concentration generally exceeds that of the plasma. It is highly lipophilic, highly bound to plasma proteins, and has an extremely long (average, 53 days) elimination half-life [112]. Metabolism occurs in the liver and possibly in the gastrointestinal tract. The major metabolite, desethylamiodarone, accumulates in plasma and tissues and has electrophysiologic properties that are similar to the parent compound [113,114].

Many side effects are dose dependent, but therapeutic drug monitoring is of little benefit, except to determine compliance. Evidence suggests a limited correlation between drug level and antiarrhythmic effect [115] and serious noncardiac toxicity seems to be more likely at levels above 2.5 μg per mL [116,117].

Pulmonary fibrosis is an important and potentially life-threatening side effect of long-term therapy [118]. Pulmonary toxicity is somewhat dose dependant; its prevalence ranges from 5% to 15% in patients who take at least 500 mg per day, but is 0.1% to 0.5% when the dose is less than 200 mg per day [119]. Common presenting features include dyspnea, nonproductive cough, fever, and general malaise. A diffuse interstitial pattern on the chest film, similar to congestive heart failure, is the most typical radiographic finding. Symptoms usually resolve with withdrawal of amiodarone therapy. Corticosteroids may improve prognosis and prevent relapse [119].

Amiodarone generally does not produce congestive heart failure, even in patients with poor ventricular function, because its vasodilator properties may offset negative inotropic effects. Sinus bradycardia is common during therapy, and symptomatic sinus pauses or sinus arrest can occur in 2% to 4% of patients. AV block may occur in patients with underlying conduction-system disease. Torsade de pointes has been reported, but is much less likely than with other class III agents.

Amiodarone is iodinated and interferes with conversion of thyroxine to triiodothyronine, causing significant elevations of thyroxine and slight reductions in triiodothyronine concentrations [120]. Most patients are typically euthyroid, with normal thyroid stimulating hormone levels. Peripheral neuropathy, tremor, and nervousness develop initially in up to 30% of patients, but these symptoms often improve over time. Asymptomatic corneal microdeposits are present in almost all patients on long-term therapy. Dermatologic effects include increased photosensitivity and blue-gray skin discoloration.

Asymptomatic elevation of hepatic transaminase is relatively common with long-term amiodarone therapy; the reported incidence is 24% to 26%. Transaminase can reach up to 3 times normal and resolve with or without discontinuation of therapy [121]. Acute hepatitis following intravenous loading of amiodarone is much less common but not infrequently described in the literature [121,122]. Transaminitis can be severe and rarely lead to fatality. Postulated mechanisms include a polysorbate 80 additive used in the intravenous preparation, immunologic-mediated injury, or a direct hepatotoxic effect [123].

Acute amiodarone overdoses generally tend to follow a benign course. There are several reports of ingestions developing self-limited episodes of ventricular tachycardia, QT prolongation, or mild bradycardia [124,125]. No CNS depression or seizures have been reported. Cholestyramine modestly reduces the elimination half-life of amiodarone from 44 to 28 days, perhaps by interrupting enterohepatic recirculation [126]. There is likely a role for multidose activated charcoal, even up to 12 hours after the ingestion, since amiodarone has delayed an erratic enteral absorption [127].

Sotalol

Sotalol is a β-adrenergic antagonist with class III activity. It is used for the prophylaxis and treatment of AV reentrant and ventricular tachycardias. It has excellent oral bioavailability and is mostly renally excreted unchanged. Overdoses manifest both pharmacologic properties of sotalol; β-adrenergic antagonism causes bradycardia, hypotension, low cardiac output, and CNS depression, while the class III activity causes QT prolongation, ventricular ectopy, and dysrhythmias, especially torsade de pointes. Reported cases of ventricular arrhythmias due to sotalol overdose are typically associated with bradycardia [127]. Management should include treatment of the beta-blocker toxicity (see Chapter 127 for discussion) and control of QT prolongation and torsade de pointes with agents such as magnesium or isoproterenol (see earlier for further discussion). There are reports of lidocaine suppressing torsade from sotalol overdose [127,128].

Bretylium

Bretylium tosylate is the prototypic adrenergic neuron-blocking drug with antiarrhythmic activity. It was first used for the treatment of hypertension and subsequently as a prophylactic antiarrhythmic agent and for the treatment of ventricular fibrillation [129,130].

Bretylium administration produces an initial sympathomimetic effect caused by norepinephrine release from adrenergic neurons followed by adrenergic blockade. Elimination is significantly reduced in renal failure [131]. Rapid administration produces a biphasic hemodynamic response, with an initial increase followed by a subsequent decrease (within 15 to 30 minutes) in heart rate and blood pressure [132]. Patients with a fixed cardiac output from severe pump failure or aortic stenosis may be unable to compensate for the peripheral vasodilation caused by bretylium. Hypotension is postural and may be treated by placing the patient supine or in Trendelenburg's position. If this is insufficient, volume expansion or infusion of vasopressors such as dopamine or norepinephrine may be required. Patients receiving long-term bretylium infusions often demonstrate exaggerated catecholamine responsiveness [132]. After overdose, hemodynamic effects may persist for longer than 3 days.

Ibutilide and Dofetilide

Ibutilide and dofetilide, the newest class III, and first "pure" action potential–prolonging agents, are approved for termination of atrial fibrillation and flutter [133–135]. Both drugs are structurally similar to sotalol but have no beta-blockade effect. They prolong APD by a dual mode of action, initially blocking the rapid component of the delayed rectifier potassium current and enhancing the noninactivating component of the inward sodium current that flows during the plateau (phase 2) of the action potential. The net effect is to increase atrial and ventricular refractory period APD. Although very little information is available about overdose toxicity, development of torsade de pointes is the major concern. With therapeutic doses, the incidence of this arrhythmia ranged from 3.6% to 12.5% in clinical trials. Most episodes were self-limited, but some were sustained and required cardioversion. Nonsustained monomorphic ventricular tachycardia may also be provoked by ibutilide [136].

Adenosine

Adenosine is an endogenous purine nucleoside normally present in all cells in the human body. Intravenous adenosine, administered as a rapid infusion, is used for termination of supraventricular arrhythmias. An increased heart rate as compensation for peripheral vasodilation has been reported in patients with atrial fibrillation and flutter or if an atrial impulse is conducted via an accessory pathway [137–139]. Adenosine may also induce atrial fibrillation as a result of the decrease in atrial APD. It should be used with caution in patients with asthma because it can provoke bronchospasm. Short periods (longer than 6 seconds) of asystole are commonly seen after termination of supraventricular arrhythmias.

Therapeutic and toxic doses of adenosine induce intense vasodilation, flushing, and a feeling of pressure or pain in the chest that patients often describe as extremely unpleasant. The duration of these effects is extremely short (measured in seconds) with bolus therapy but can be prolonged in patients receiving continuous infusions during radionuclide studies or those patients taking dipyridamole [140].

References

1. Roden DM, George AL: The cardiac ion channels: relevance to management of arrhythmias. *Annu Rev Med* 47:135–148, 1996.
2. Vaughn Williams E: A classification of antiarrhythmic actions reassessed after a decade of new drugs. *J Clin Pharmacol* 24:129–147, 1984.
3. Campbell TJ: Subclassification of class I antiarrhythmic drugs: enhanced relevance after CAST. *Cardiovasc Drugs Ther* 65:519–528, 1992.
4. Katz AM: Cardiac ion channels. *N Engl J Med* 32817:1244–1251, 1993.
5. Campbell TJ: Proarrhythmic actions of antiarrhythmic drugs: a review. *Aust N Z J Med* 203:275–282, 1990.
6. Jackman WM, Friday KJ, Anderson JL, et al: The long QT syndromes: a critical review, new clinical observations and a unifying hypothesis. *Prog Cardiovasc Dis* 312:115–172, 1988.
7. Surawicz B: Ventricular arrhythmias: why is it so difficult to find a pharmacologic cure? *J Am Coll Cardiol* 146:1401–1416, 1989.
8. January CT, Riddle JM: Early after depolarizations: mechanism of induction and block. A role for L-type Ca2+ current. *Circ Res* 645:977–990, 1989.
9. Roden DM, Hoffman BF: Action potential prolongation and induction of abnormal automaticity by low quinidine concentrations in canine Purkinje fibers. Relationship to potassium and cycle length. *Circ Res* 566:857–867, 1985.
10. Benardeau A, Weissenburger J, Hondeghem L, et al: Effects of the T-type Ca(2+) channel blocker mibefradil on repolarization of guinea pig, rabbit, dog, monkey, and human cardiac tissue. *J Pharmacol Exp Ther* 2922:561–575, 2000.
11. Glaser S, Steinbach M, Opitz C, et al: Torsades de pointes caused by Mibefradil. *Eur J Heart Fail* 35:627–630, 2001.
12. Keren A, Tzivoni D: Torsades de pointes: prevention and therapy. *Cardiovasc Drugs Ther* 52:509–513, 1991.
13. Shub C, Gau GT, Sidell PM, et al: The management of acute quinidine intoxication. *Chest* 732:173–178, 1978.
14. Holt DW, Helliwell M, O'Keeffe B, et al: Successful management of serious disopyramide poisoning. *Postgrad Med J* 56654:256–260, 1980.
15. Freedman MD, Gal J, Freed CR: Extracorporeal pump assistance–novel treatment for acute lidocaine poisoning. *Eur J Clin Pharmacol* 222:129–135, 1982.
16. Noble J, Kennedy DJ, Latimer RD, et al: Massive lignocaine overdose during cardiopulmonary bypass. Successful treatment with cardiac pacing. *Br J Anaesth* 5612:1439–1441, 1984.
17. Yasui RK, Culclasure TF, Kaufman D, et al: Flecainide overdose: is cardiopulmonary support the treatment? *Ann Emerg Med* 295:680–682, 1997.
18. Wasserman F, Brodsky L, Dick MM, et al: Successful treatment of quinidine and procaine amide intoxication; report of three cases. *N Engl J Med* 25917:797–802, 1958.
19. Bailey DJ: Cardiotoxic effects of quinidine and their treatment. *Arch Intern Med* 105:13–22, 1960.
20. Pentel P, Benowitz N: Efficacy and mechanism of action of sodium bicarbonate in the treatment of desipramine toxicity in rats. *J Pharmacol Exp Ther* 2301:12–19, 1984.
21. Winkelmann BR, Leinberger H: Life-threatening flecainide toxicity. A pharmacodynamic approach. *Ann Intern Med* 1066:807–814, 1987.
22. Gardner ML, Brett-Smith H, Batsford WP: Treatment of encainide proarrhythmia with hypertonic saline. *Pacing Clin Electrophysiol* 1310:1232–1235, 1990.
23. Salerno DM, Murakami MM, Johnston RB, et al: Reversal of flecainide-induced ventricular arrhythmia by hypertonic sodium bicarbonate in dogs. *Am J Emerg Med* 133:285–293, 1995.
24. Koppel C, Oberdisse U, Heinemeyer G: Clinical course and outcome in class IC antiarrhythmic overdose. *J Toxicol Clin Toxicol* 284:433–444, 1990.
25. Sasyniuk BI, Jhamandas V: Mechanism of reversal of toxic effects of amitriptyline on cardiac Purkinje fibers by sodium bicarbonate. *J Pharmacol Exp Ther* 2312:387–394, 1984.
26. Nattel S, Mittleman M: Treatment of ventricular tachyarrhythmias resulting from amitriptyline toxicity in dogs. *J Pharmacol Exp Ther* 2312:430–435, 1984.
27. Woie L, Oyri A: Quinidine intoxication treated with hemodialysis. *Acta Med Scand* 1953:237–239, 1974.
28. Yang T, Roden DM: Extracellular potassium modulation of drug block of IKr. Implications for torsade de pointes and reverse use-dependence. *Circulation* 933:407–411, 1996.
29. Winkle RA, Mason JW, Griffin JC, et al: Malignant ventricular tachyarrhythmias associated with the use of encainide. *Am Heart J* 1025:857–864, 1981.
30. Kay GN, Plumb VJ, Arciniegas JG, et al: Torsade de pointes: the long-short initiating sequence and other clinical features: observations in 32 patients. *J Am Coll Cardiol* 25:806–817, 1983.
31. Choy AM, Lang CC, Chomsky DM, et al: Normalization of acquired QT prolongation in humans by intravenous potassium. *Circulation* 967:2149–2154, 1997.
32. Nguyen PT, Scheinman MM, Seger J: Polymorphous ventricular tachycardia: clinical characterization, therapy, and the QT interval. *Circulation* 742:340–349, 1986.
33. Stratmann HG, Kennedy HL: Torsades de pointes associated with drugs and toxins: recognition and management. *Am Heart J* 1136:1470–1482, 1987.
34. Yamamoto H, Bando S, Nishikado A, et al: [Efficacy of isoproterenol, magnesium sulfate and verapamil for torsade de pointes]. *Kokyu To Junkan* 393:261–265, 1991.
35. Blair AD, Burgess ED, Maxwell BM, et al: Sotalol kinetics in renal insufficiency. *Clin Pharmacol Ther* 294:457–463, 1981.
36. Singh SN, Lazin A, Cohen A, et al: Sotalol-induced torsades de pointes successfully treated with hemodialysis after failure of conventional therapy. *Am Heart J* 121(2, Pt 1):601–602, 1991.

37. Gosselin B, Mathieu D, Chopin C, et al: Acute intoxication with disopyramide: clinical and experimental study by hemoperfusion an Amberlite XAD 4 resin. *Clin Toxicol* 173:439–449, 1980.
38. Braden GL, Fitzgibbons JP, Germain MJ, et al: Hemoperfusion for treatment of N-acetylprocainamide intoxication. *Ann Intern Med* 1051:64–65, 1986.
39. Kavanagh KM, Wyse DG, Mitchell LB, et al: Contribution of quinidine metabolites to electrophysiologic responses in human subjects. *Clin Pharmacol Ther* 463:352–358, 1989.
40. Grace AA, Camm AJ: Quinidine. *N Engl J Med* 3381:35–45, 1998.
41. Kerr F, Kenoyer G, Bilitch M: Quinidine overdose. Neurological and cardiovascular toxicity in a normal person. *Br Heart J* 334:629–631, 1971.
42. Giardina EG, Dreyfuss J, Bigger JT, et al: Metabolism of procainamide in normal and cardiac subjects. *Clin Pharmacol Ther* 193:339–351, 1976.
43. Giardina EG, Fenster PE, Bigger JT Jr, et al: Efficacy, plasma concentrations and adverse effects of a new sustained release procainamide preparation. *Am J Cardiol* 465:855–862, 1980.
44. Roden DM, Reele SB, Higgins SB, et al: Antiarrhythmic efficacy, pharmacokinetics and safety of N-acetylprocainamide in human subjects: comparison with procainamide. *Am J Cardiol* 463:463–468, 1980.
45. Straka RJ, Hansen SR, Benson SR, et al: Predominance of slow acetylators of N-acetyltransferase in a Hmong population residing in the United States. *J Clin Pharmacol* 368:740–747, 1996.
46. Raja R, Kramer M, Alvis R, et al: Resin hemoperfusion for severe N-acetylprocainamide toxicity in patients with renal failure. *Trans Am Soc Artif Intern Organs* 30:18–20, 1984.
47. Hoffman BF, Rosen MR, Wit AL: Electrophysiology and pharmacology of cardiac arrhythmias. VII. Cardiac effects of quinidine and procaine amide. A. *Am Heart J* 896:804–808, 1975.
48. White SR, Dy G, Wilson JM: The case of the slandered Halloween cupcake: survival after massive pediatric procainamide overdose. *Pediatr Emerg Care* 183:185–188, 2002.
49. Hinderling PH, Garrett ER: Pharmacodynamics of the antiarrhythmic disopyramide in healthy humans: correlation of the kinetics of the drug and its effects. *J Pharmacokinet Biopharm* 43:231–242, 1976.
50. Meffin PJ, Robert EW, Winkle RA, et al: Role of concentration-dependent plasma protein binding in disopyramide disposition. *J Pharmacokinet Biopharm* 71:29–46, 1979.
51. Fechter P, Ha HR, Follath F, et al: The antiarrhythmic effects of controlled release disopyramide phosphate and long acting propranolol in patients with ventricular arrhythmias. *Eur J Clin Pharmacol* 256:729–734, 1983.
52. Granowitz EV, Tabor KJ, Kirchhoffer JB: Potentially fatal interaction between azithromycin and disopyramide. *Pacing Clin Electrophysiol* 239:1433–1435, 2000.
53. Podrid PJ, Schoeneberger A, Lown B: Congestive heart failure caused by oral disopyramide. *N Engl J Med* 30211:614–617, 1980.
54. Kotter V, Linderer T, Schroder R: Effects of disopyramide on systemic and coronary hemodynamics and myocardial metabolism in patients with coronary artery disease: comparison with lidocaine. *Am J Cardiol* 463:469–475, 1980.
55. Nappi JM, Dhanani S, Lovejoy JR, et al: Severe hypoglycemia associated with disopyramide. *West J Med* 1381:95–97, 1983.
56. Sevka MJ, Matthews SJ, Nightingale CH, et al: Disopyramide hemodialysis and kinetics in patients requiring long-term hemodialysis. *Clin Pharmacol Ther* 293:322–326, 1981.
57. Blumer J, Strong JM, Atkinson AJ Jr: The convulsant potency of lidocaine and its N-dealkylated metabolites. *J Pharmacol Exp Ther* 186(1):31–36, 1973.
58. Halkin H, Meffin P, Melmon KL, et al: Influence of congestive heart failure on blood vessels of lidocaine and its active monodeethylated metabolite. *Clin Pharmacol Ther* 176:669–676, 1975.
59. Davison R, Parker M, Atkinson AJ: Excessive serum lidocaine levels during maintenance infusions: mechanisms and prevention. *Am Heart J* 104(2 Pt 1):203–208, 1982.
60. Bryant CA, Hoffman JR, Nichter LS: Pitfalls and perils of intravenous lidocaine. *West J Med* 139(4):528–530, 1983.
61. Burlington B, Freed CR: Massive overdose and death from prophylactic lidocaine. *JAMA* 24310:1036–1037, 1980.
62. Brosh-Nissimov T, Ingbir M, Weintal I, et al: Central nervous system toxicity following topical skin application of lidocaine. *Eur J Clin Pharmacol* 60(9):683–684, 2004.
63. Rao RB, Ely SF, Hoffman RS: Deaths related to liposuction. *N Engl J Med* 34019:1471–5, 1999.
64. Denaro CP, Benowitz NL: Poisoning due to class 1B antiarrhythmic drugs. Lignocaine, mexiletine and tocainide. *Med Toxicol Adverse Drug Exp* 46: 412–428, 1989.
65. Antonelli D, Bloch L: Sinus standstill following lidocaine administration. *JAMA* 248(7):827–828, 1982.
66. DeToledo JC: Lidocaine and seizures. *Ther Drug Monit* 223:320–322, 2000.
67. Lichstein E, Chadda KD, Gupta PK: Atrioventricular block with lidocaine therapy. *Am J Cardiol* 312:277–281, 1973.
68. Gupta PK, Lichstein E, Chadda KD: Lidocaine-induced heart block in patients with bundle branch block. *Am J Cardiol* 334:487–492, 1974.
69. Hess GP, Walson PD: Seizures secondary to oral viscous lidocaine. *Ann Emerg Med* 177:725–727, 1988.
70. O'Donohue WJ Jr, Moss LM, Angelillo VA: Acute methemoglobinemia induced by topical benzocaine and lidocaine. *Arch Intern Med* 14011:1508–1509, 1980.
71. Barber K, Chen SM, Ferguson R, et al: Lidocaine removal during resin hemoperfusion for phenobarbital intoxication. *Artif Organs* 82:229–231, 1984.
72. Groban L, Deal DD, Vernon JC, et al: Cardiac resuscitation after incremental overdosage with lidocaine, bupivacaine, levobupivacaine, and ropivacaine in anesthetized dogs. *Anesth Analg* 921:37–43, 2001.
73. Haselbarth V, Doevendans JE, Wolf M: Kinetics and bioavailability of mexiletine in healthy subjects. *Clin Pharmacol Ther* 296:729–736, 1981.
74. Ludot H, Tharin JY, Belouadah M, et al: Successful resuscitation after ropivacaine and lidocaine-induced ventricular arrhythmia following posterior lumbar plexus block in a child. *Anesth Analg* 1065:1572–1574, 2008; table of contents.
75. Weinberg G: Lipid rescue resuscitation from local anaesthetic cardiac toxicity. *Toxicol Rev* 253:139–145, 2006.
76. Roden DM, Woosley RL: Drug therapy. Flecainide. *N Engl J Med* 3151:36–41, 1986.
77. Volosin KJ, Greenspon AJ: Tocainide: a new drug for ventricular arrhythmias. *Am Fam Physician* 331:233–235, 1986.
78. Nyquist O, Forssell G, Nordlander R, et al: Hemodynamic and antiarrhythmic effects of tocainide in patients with acute myocardial infarction. *Am Heart J* 100(6 Pt 2):1000–1005, 1980.
79. Wiegers U, Hanrath P, Kuck KH, et al: Pharmacokinetics of tocainide in patients with renal dysfunction and during haemodialysis. *Eur J Clin Pharmacol* 244:503–507, 1983.
80. Cohen A: Accidental overdose of tocainide successfully treated. *Angiology* 38(8):614, 1987.
81. Pringle T, Fox J, McNeill JA, et al: Dose independent pharmacokinetics of mexiletine in healthy volunteers. *Br J Clin Pharmacol* 213:319–321, 1986.
82. Upward JW, Holt DW, Jackson G: A study to compare the efficacy, plasma concentration profile and tolerability of conventional mexiletine and slow-release mexiletine. *Eur Heart J* 53:247–252, 1984.
83. Wang T, Wuellner D, Woosley RL, et al: Pharmacokinetics and nondialyzability of mexiletine in renal failure. *Clin Pharmacol Ther* 376:649–653, 1985.
84. Nitsch J, Steinbeck G, Luderitz B: Increase of mexiletine plasma levels due to delayed hepatic metabolism in patients with chronic liver disease. *Eur Heart J* 411:810–814, 1983.
85. Grech-Belanger O, Gilbert M, Turgeon J, et al: Effect of cigarette smoking on mexiletine kinetics. *Clin Pharmacol Ther* 376:638–643, 1985.
86. Stein J, Podrid P, Lown B: Effects of oral mexiletine on left and right ventricular function. *Am J Cardiol* 546:575–578, 1984.
87. Shanks RG: Hemodynamic effects of mexiletine. *Am Heart J* 107(5, Pt 2):1065–1071, 1984.
88. Hruby K, Missliwetz J: Poisoning with oral antiarrhythmic drugs. *Int J Clin Pharmacol Ther Toxicol* 235:253–257, 1985.
89. Frank SE, Snyder JT: Survival following severe overdose with mexiletene, nifedipine, and nitroglycerine. *Am J Emerg Med* 91:43–46, 1991.
90. Nelson LS, Hoffman RS: Mexiletine overdose producing status epilepticus without cardiovascular abnormalities. *J Toxicol Clin Toxicol* 326:731–736, 1994.
91. Kozer E, Verjee Z, Koren G: Misdiagnosis of a mexiletine overdose because of a nonspecific result of urinary toxicologic screening. *N Engl J Med* 343(26):1971–1972, 2000.
92. Siegers A, Board PN: Amiodarone used in successful resuscitation after near-fatal flecainide overdose. *Resuscitation* 531:105–108, 2002.
93. Echt DS, Liebson PR, Mitchell LB, et al: Mortality and morbidity in patients receiving encainide, flecainide, or placebo. The Cardiac Arrhythmia Suppression Trial. *N Engl J Med* 324(12):781–788, 1991.
94. Gotz D, Pohle S, Barckow D: Primary and secondary detoxification in severe flecainide intoxication. *Intensive Care Med* 173:181–184, 1991.
95. Keyler DE, Pentel PR: Hypertonic sodium bicarbonate partially reverses QRS prolongation due to flecainide in rats. *Life Sci* 451(7):1575–1580, 1989.
96. Hudson CJ, Whitner TE, Rinaldi MJ, et al: Brugada electrocardiographic pattern elicited by inadvertent flecainide overdose. *Pacing Clin Electrophysiol* 279:1311–1313, 2004.
97. Lovecchio F, Berlin R, Brubacher JR, et al: Hypertonic sodium bicarbonate in an acute flecainide overdose. *Am J Emerg Med* 165:534–537, 1998.
98. Auzinger GM, Scheinkestel CD: Successful extracorporeal life support in a case of severe flecainide intoxication. *Crit Care Med* 294:887–890, 2001.
99. Straka RJ, Hansen SR, Walker PF: Comparison of the prevalence of the poor metabolizer phenotype for CYP2D6 between 203 Hmong subjects and 280 white subjects residing in Minnesota. *Clin Pharmacol Ther* 581:29–34, 1995.
100. Siddoway LA, Thompson KA, McAllister CB, et al: Polymorphism of propafenone metabolism and disposition in man: clinical and pharmacokinetic consequences. *Circulation* 754:785–791, 1987.
101. Funck-Brentano C, Kroemer HK, Pavlou H, et al: Genetically-determined interaction between propafenone and low dose quinidine: role of active metabolites in modulating net drug effect. *Br J Clin Pharmacol* 274:435–444, 1989.
102. Podrid PJ, Lown B: Propafenone: a new agent for ventricular arrhythmia. *J Am Coll Cardiol* 41:117–125, 1984.

103. Buss J, Neuss H, Bilgin Y, et al: Malignant ventricular tachyarrhythmias in association with propafenone treatment. *Eur Heart J* 65:424–428, 1985.
104. Eray O, Fowler J: Severe propafenone poisoning responded to temporary internal pacemaker. *Vet Hum Toxicol* 42(5):289, 2000.
105. Rambourg-Schepens MO, Grossenbacher F, Buffet M, et al: Recurrent convulsions and cardiac conduction disturbances after propafenone overdose. *Vet Hum Toxicol* 413:153–154, 1999.
106. Molia AC, Tholon JP, Lamiable DL, et al: Unintentional pediatric overdose of propafenone. *Ann Pharmacother* 37(7–8):1147–1148, 2003.
107. Stancak B, Markovic P, Rajnic A, et al: Acute toxicity of propafenone in a case of suicidal attempt. *Bratisl Lek Listy* 105(1):14–17, 2004.
108. Ellison DW, Pentel PR: Clinical features and consequences of seizures due to cyclic antidepressant overdose. *Am J Emerg Med* 71:5–10, 1989.
109. Salerno DM, Gillingham KJ, Berry DA, et al: A comparison of antiarrhythmic drugs for the suppression of ventricular ectopic depolarizations: a meta-analysis. *Am Heart J* 120(2):340–353, 1990.
110. Myers M, Peter T, Weiss D, et al: Benefit and risks of long-term amiodarone therapy for sustained ventricular tachycardia/fibrillation: minimum of three-year follow-up in 145 patients. *Am Heart J* 119(1):8–14, 1990.
111. Bauman JL, Berk SI, Hariman RJ, et al: Amiodarone for sustained ventricular tachycardia: efficacy, safety, and factors influencing long-term outcome. *Am Heart J* 114(6):1436–1444, 1987.
112. Holt DW, Tucker GT, Jackson PR, et al: Amiodarone pharmacokinetics. *Am Heart J* 106(4 Pt 2):840–847, 1983.
113. Barbieri E, Conti F, Zampieri P, et al: Amiodarone and desethylamiodarone distribution in the atrium and adipose tissue of patients undergoing short- and long-term treatment with amiodarone. *J Am Coll Cardiol* 81:210–213, 1986.
114. Pallandi RT, Campbell TJ: Resting, and rate-dependent depression of V_{max} of guinea-pig ventricular action potentials by amiodarone and desethylamiodarone. *Br J Pharmacol* 92(1):97–103, 1987.
115. Mitchell LB, Wyse DG, Gillis AM, et al: Electropharmacology of amiodarone therapy initiation. Time courses of onset of electrophysiologic and antiarrhythmic effects. *Circulation* 801:34–42, 1989.
116. Counihan PJ, McKenna WJ: Low-dose amiodarone for the treatment of arrhythmias in hypertrophic cardiomyopathy. *J Clin Pharmacol* 295:436–438, 1989.
117. Rotmensch HH, Belhassen B, Swanson BN, et al: Steady-state serum amiodarone concentrations: relationships with antiarrhythmic efficacy and toxicity. *Ann Intern Med* 1014:462–469, 1984.
118. Magro SA, Lawrence EC, Wheeler SH, et al: Amiodarone pulmonary toxicity: prospective evaluation of serial pulmonary function tests. *J Am Coll Cardiol* 123:781–788, 1988.
119. Camus P, Bonniaud P, Fanton A, et al: Drug-induced and iatrogenic infiltrative lung disease. *Clin Chest Med* 253:479–519, 2004.
120. Nademanee K, Singh BN, Callahan B, et al: Amiodarone, thyroid hormone indexes, and altered thyroid function: long-term serial effects in patients with cardiac arrhythmias. *Am J Cardiol* 5810:981–986, 1986.
121. Ratz Bravo AE, Drewe J, Schlienger RG, et al: Hepatotoxicity during rapid intravenous loading with amiodarone: Description of three cases and review of the literature. *Crit Care Med* 331:128–134, 2005; discussion 245–246.
122. James PR, Hardman SM: Acute hepatitis complicating parenteral amiodarone does not preclude subsequent oral therapy. *Heart* 776:583–584, 1997.
123. Gregory SA, Webster JB, Chapman GD: Acute hepatitis induced by parenteral amiodarone. *Am J Med* 1133:254–255, 2002.
124. Bouffard Y, Berger Y, Delafosse B: Acute amiodarone poisoning. Clinical and pharmacokinetic study. *Arch Mal Coeur Vaiss* 7810:1589–1590, 1985.
125. Goddard CJ, Whorwell PJ: Amiodarone overdose and its management. *Br J Clin Pract* 435:184–186, 1989.
126. Nitsch J, Luderitz B: Acceleration of amiodarone elimination by cholestyramine. *Dtsch Med Wochenschr* 111(33):1241–4, 1986.
127. Leatham EW, Holt DW, McKenna WJ: Class III antiarrhythmics in overdose. Presenting features and management principles. *Drug Saf* 96:450–462, 1993.
128. Assimes TL, Malcolm I: Torsade de pointes with sotalol overdose treated successfully with lidocaine. *Can J Cardiol* 145:753–756, 1998.
129. Nowak RM, Bodnar TJ, Dronen S, et al: Bretylium tosylate as initial treatment for cardiopulmonary arrest: randomized comparison with placebo. *Ann Emerg Med* 108:404–407, 1981.
130. Anderson JL, Patterson E, Wagner JG, et al: Clinical pharmacokinetics of intravenous and oral bretylium tosylate in survivors of ventricular tachycardia or fibrillation: clinical application of a new assay for bretylium. *J Cardiovasc Pharmacol* 33:485–499, 1981.
131. Josselson J, Narang PK, Adir J, et al: Bretylium kinetics in renal insufficiency. *Clin Pharmacol Ther* 332:144–150, 1983.
132. Woosley RL, Reele SB, Roden DM, et al: Pharmacologic reversal of hypotensive effect complicating antiarrhythmic therapy with bretylium. *Clin Pharmacol Ther* 323:313–321, 1982.
133. Yang T, Snyders DJ, Roden DM: Ibutilide, a methanesulfonanilide antiarrhythmic, is a potent blocker of the rapidly activating delayed rectifier K+ current (IKr) in AT-1 cells. Concentration-, time-, voltage-, and use-dependent effects. *Circulation* 916:1799–806, 1995.
134. Ellenbogen KA, Stambler BS, Wood MA, et al: Efficacy of intravenous ibutilide for rapid termination of atrial fibrillation and atrial flutter: a dose-response study. *J Am Coll Cardiol* 281:130–136, 1996.
135. Cropp JS, Antal EG, Talbert RL: Ibutilide: a new class III antiarrhythmic agent. *Pharmacotherapy* 171:1–9, 1997.
136. Stambler BS, Wood MA, Ellenbogen KA, et al: Efficacy and safety of repeated intravenous doses of ibutilide for rapid conversion of atrial flutter or fibrillation. Ibutilide Repeat Dose Study Investigators. *Circulation* 947:1613–1621, 1996.
137. Watt AH, Bernard MS, Webster J, et al: Intravenous adenosine in the treatment of supraventricular tachycardia: a dose-ranging study and interaction with dipyridamole. *Br J Clin Pharmacol* 212:227–230, 1986.
138. Slade AK, Garratt CJ: Proarrhythmic effect of adenosine in a patient with atrial flutter. *Br Heart J* 701:91–92, 1993.
139. White RD: Acceleration of the ventricular response in paroxysmal lone atrial fibrillation following the injection of adenosine. *Am J Emerg Med* 113:245–246, 1993.
140. Klabunde RE: Dipyridamole inhibition of adenosine metabolism in human blood. *Eur J Pharmacol* 93(1–2):21–26, 1983.

CHAPTER 121 ■ ANTICHOLINERGIC POISONING†

KEITH K. BURKHART

The classic anticholinergic syndrome manifests an easily recognizable toxidrome, but patients may present with some but not all of the classic symptoms. Decreased secretions, tachycardia, mydriasis, and delirium are those most commonly seen [1]. The presence of coingestants and the multiple pharmacologic actions of many anticholinergic drugs may mask anticholinergic manifestations, although anticholinergic effects often persist longer than other pharmacologic actions [2]. The anticholinergic syndrome is more accurately an antimuscarinic syndrome. However, it is conventionally called anticholinergic and is referred to as such herein.

Anticholinergic poisoning may result in seizures, delirium, and coma, along with their associated complications. Anticholinergic-induced coma and respiratory failure may require mechanical ventilation. As with any toxicologic emergency, supportive care is of paramount importance. Physostigmine is an effective antidote with proven benefits, but also has a risk for serious adverse events.

†*The views expressed in this chapter do not necessarily represent the views of the Food and Drug Administration of the United States.*

EPIDEMIOLOGY AND SOURCES

A variety of pharmaceuticals and naturally occurring products can produce an anticholinergic syndrome (Table 121.1). Many drugs with anticholinergic effects may be classified in a manner that does not identify this activity (e.g., histamine-1 [H_1]–blockers, gastrointestinal and genitourinary tract antispasmodics, cough and cold preparations, over-the-counter sleep aids, and anticholinergic plants). For some, anticholinergic effects are desirable (e.g., atropine to treat bradycardia induces mydriasis and inhibits secretions). For others, the anticholinergic effects are an undesirable side effect (e.g., antihistamines, antipsychotics, and tricyclic antidepressants).

Pharmaceuticals and plants with anticholinergic action may be intentionally abused for mind-altering effects; especially common is the use of *Datura stramonium* (jimsonweed) [3]. Anticholinergic toxicity has occurred by a number of routes other than ingestion, including inhalation of nebulized medication [4], inhalation of pyrolysis products (e.g., the smoking of plant parts) [3], transdermal use, and ocular instillation.

PHARMACOLOGY

Anticholinergic agents antagonize the effects of the endogenous neurotransmitter acetylcholine (ACh). Receptors for ACh are widely distributed in the body, including the central nervous system and the sympathetic and parasympathetic ganglia, postganglionic parasympathetic terminals, and motor end plates of the peripheral nervous system.

ACh receptors are divided into two types, muscarinic and nicotinic, based on their ability to bind muscarine or nicotine. This division has a functional significance as well, best described in the peripheral nervous system, where muscarinic receptors predominate in the parasympathetic terminals and nicotinic receptors in autonomic ganglia and motor end plates. Most drugs have predominant effects on one of the two main ACh receptors, but at high doses, there may be some crossover effect. For example, nicotine primarily stimulates nicotinic receptors. Stimulation produces tachycardia, hypertension, muscle fasciculations, and receptor fatigue, with consequent paralysis at high doses. Nicotinic antagonists, such as the nondepolarizing muscle relaxants (e.g., pancuronium), block the action of ACh at the motor end plate and produce skeletal muscle paralysis. Excessive muscarinic receptor stimulation (e.g., organophosphate poisoning) leads to the cholinergic toxidrome (see Chapters 128 and 141). Agents that block muscarinic receptors may cause anticholinergic toxicity, the focus of this chapter.

Many drugs with anticholinergic properties undergo extensive hepatic metabolism into active and inactive metabolites. A number of these drugs may have half-lives greater than 12 to 24 hours (e.g., tricyclic antidepressants). More important may be the persistence of muscarinic receptor binding. In the intensive care unit (ICU), many patients emerge from coma into a delirious state. Reversal by physostigmine suggests persistence anticholinergic delirium rather than ICU psychosis [2].

CLINICAL PRESENTATION

Anticholinergic effects have been classically described by the mnemonic "Blind as a bat, Hot as Hades, Dry as a bone, Red as a beet, and Mad as a hatter" in reference to the consequences of ciliary muscle paralysis, hyperthermia, anhydrosis, vasodilation, and delirium, respectively. The toxidrome has been subdivided into the peripheral anticholinergic syndrome and the central anticholinergic syndrome (Table 121.2). The former

TABLE 121.1

SOME AGENTS THAT CAUSE ANTICHOLINERGIC SYNDROME[a]

Pharmaceuticals	Plants
Antihistamines (H1-blockers)	*Atropa belladonna* (deadly nightshade)
Brompheniramine	*Brugmansia arborea* (angel's trumpet)
Chlorpheniramine	*Brugmansia suaveolens* (angel's trumpet)
Clemastine	*Cestrum diurnum* (day-blooming jessamine)
Cyclizine	*Cestrum nocturnum* (night-blooming jessamine)
Cyproheptadine	*Cestrum parqui* (willow-leaved jessamine)
Dimenhydrinate	*Datura metel* (downy thorn apple)
Diphenhydramine	*Datura stramonium* (jimson weed)
Hydroxyzine	*Hyoscyamus niger* (black henbane)
Meclizine	*Lycium halimifolium* (matrimony vine)
Promethazine	Mushrooms
Pyrilamine	Myristicaceae
Tripelennamine	*Myristica fragrans* (nutmeg)
Antiparkinsonian drugs	*Amanita muscaria* (fly agaric)
Benztropine	*Amanita pantherina* (panther mushroom)
Biperiden	Physalis heterophylla (ground cherry)
Ethopropazine	Solanaceae
Procyclidine	*Solanum carolinense* (wild tomato)
Trihexyphenidyl	*Solanum dulcamara* (bittersweet)
Antipsychotics[b]	*Solanum nigrum* (black nightshade)
Acetophenazine	*Solanum pseudocapsicum* (Jerusalem cherry)
Chlorpromazine	*Solanum tuberosum* (potato)
Clozapine	Verbenaceae
Fluphenazine	*Lantana camara* (wild sage)
Haloperidol	
Iloperidone	
Loxapine	
Molindone	
Olanzapine	
Paliperidone	
Perphenazine	
Prochlorperazine	
Quetiapine	
Risperidone	
Thioridazine	
Thiothixene	
Trifluoperazine	
Ziprasidone	
Antispasmodics	
Anisotropine	
Clidinium	
Dicyclomine	
Isometheptene	
Methantheline	
Propantheline	
Stramonium	
Tridihexethyl	
Belladonna alkaloids and related synthetic congeners	
Atropine (racemic hyoscyamine)	
Glycopyrrolate	
Hyoscine	
Ipratropium	
Methscopolamine	
Scopolamine	
Cyclic antidepressants	
Amitriptyline	
Amoxapine	
Desipramine	
Doxepin	
Imipramine	
Maprotiline	
Nortriptyline	
Protriptyline	
Trimipramine	
Zimelidine	
Muscle relaxants	
Cyclobenzaprine	
Orphenadrine	
Mydriatics	
Cyclopentolate	
Homatropine	
Tropicamide	

[a]Many of these agents have other significant toxic manifestations in addition to their anticholinergic effects.
[b]Some of the antipsychotics have minimal muscarinic binding.

TABLE 121.2

MANIFESTATIONS OF THE ANTICHOLINERGIC SYNDROME

Peripheral anticholinergic signs and symptoms
Cardiovascular: hypertension and tachycardia
Skin: dry and flushed with dry mucous membranes
Eyes: mydriasis (variable)
Genitourinary: urinary retention and decreased bowel sounds (ileus)
Central anticholinergic signs and symptoms
Loss of short-term memory and confusion, disorientation, psychomotor agitation
Visual/auditory hallucinations or frank psychosis
Incoordination and ataxia
Picking or grasping movements and extrapyramidal reactions
Seizures
Coma with respiratory failure

is due to quaternary amines (e.g., glycopyrrolate), which are charged molecules that poorly penetrate the blood–brain barrier, whereas the latter is due to tertiary amines (e.g., atropine), which are uncharged and reach the central nervous system. The most serious anticholinergic manifestations include agitated delirium, hyperthermia, and seizures. Patients may present with primarily peripheral signs and symptoms, primarily central ones, or both. In addition, central symptoms may persist longer than the peripheral manifestations.

The clinical presentation may be complicated by other pharmacologic actions of the intoxicant (e.g., tricyclic antidepressants) or the actions of other potentially toxic substances (e.g., salicylates, sympathomimetics).

MANAGEMENT

Traditionally, anticholinergic-poisoned patients have been managed with conservative supportive care. Obtaining and assessing historical and physical data confirms or provides the diagnoses that guide management decisions. Historical data may be simple in terms of a single agent, such as jimsonweed, or complex, as in a polydrug overdose. An analysis of the pharmacologic properties of the known intoxicants guides management decisions.

Delirium and coma are typically the most serious anticholinergic consequences that would require ICU admission. Shortly after exposure, most patients demonstrate sinus tachycardia and hypertension. These abnormalities are usually mild, but occasionally require medical intervention. Patients' respiratory status should be continuously monitored because of potential for respiratory failure. Hyperthermia, although not often present, is occasionally severe and may require rapid cooling measures. Foley catheter insertion may be needed for urinary retention.

Laboratory studies that should be considered in patients with moderate to severe anticholinergic toxicity include serum electrolytes; blood urea nitrogen; creatinine; and creatine phosphokinase, urinalysis, and electrocardiogram. Rhabdomyolysis and dehydration may be evident. A urine toxicology screen does not detect most anticholinergic agents and typically contributes little to the diagnostic workup or patient management. Many anticholinergic agents are not detected even on comprehensive toxicology screens that take hours to return [5]. Resolution of mental status changes after physostigmine administration may be the most rapid and cost-effective way to arrive at the diagnosis and simultaneously treating the poisoning.

Gastrointestinal decontamination (see Chapter 117) should be considered, especially for plant ingestions where symptoms often persist for days. Administration of activated charcoal is recommended. Its administration, however, may be problematic for the agitated or delirious patient. Physostigmine administration has also been recommended to facilitate activated charcoal administration [6].

Hallucinations, agitation, and delirium have been traditionally treated with benzodiazepines (e.g., diazepam, lorazepam) and butyrophenones (e.g., haloperidol). Heavily sedating doses may often be required such that endotracheal intubation becomes necessary, however [2]. Furthermore, haloperidol use often worsens the anticholinergic delirium, and should not be used. Physostigmine, as an antidote, reversibly binds to acetylcholinesterase and prevents this enzyme from degrading ACh, thereby allowing the neurotransmitter to persist, accumulate, and competitively reverse muscarinic receptor inhibition at its postsynaptic sites of action. Physostigmine, as opposed to similar drugs such as neostigmine and pyridostigmine, is a tertiary rather than a quaternary amine and effectively crosses the blood–brain barrier. As a result, it is effective in reversing central as well as peripheral anticholinergic effects. A more liberal use of physostigmine has the potential to help many patients and save resources. Use as a diagnostic tool may avoid an expensive workup. It may also avoid alternative treatment with other drugs and the costs of potentially having to intubate the heavily sedated patient [7,8].

Physostigmine administration allegedly has contributed to poor outcomes, especially after cyclic antidepressant poisoning [7–9]. When administered in excessive amounts or to a patient not in an anticholinergic state, signs and symptoms of cholinergic excess may appear. Several case reports [9,10] and an animal study [11] describe asystole, seizures, and death when physostigmine was used to treat tricyclic antidepressant poisoning. A recent review of reports and studies questions the justification for an absolute contraindication to physostigmine's use in all cyclic antidepressant cases [12]. A retrospective series of 39 patients treated with physostigmine included cyclic antidepressant poisoned patients [13]. None of these patients developed dysrhythmias or needed atropine, while one patient had a self-limited seizure. Reports have also described the benefits following olanzapine poisoning [7,8]. Close observation is mandatory following reversal of anticholinergic-induced respiratory or CNS depression, especially early in the course of intoxication. The awakening and cholinergic effects theoretically could enhance gut activity and further absorption of ingested drugs such that when physostigmine is cleared the patient might have greater toxicity than at the time of first administration.

Physostigmine can be both diagnostic [13] and therapeutic (Table 121.3). Administration to the confused, febrile patient may return mental status to normal and reduce fever. A head computerized axial tomogram and lumbar puncture may be avoided if the patient awakens and provides a history that is consistent with the anticholinergic toxicity. On theoretic grounds, it has been suggested that physostigmine may be useful for seizures unresponsive to conventional treatment; severe hypertension resulting in acute symptoms or end-organ dysfunction; and supraventricular tachycardias resulting in hemodynamic instability, cardiac ischemia, or other organ dysfunction. In clinical practice, these indications rarely arise and physostigmine is almost exclusively used as a diagnostic aid and for the treatment of central nervous system excitation (psychomotor agitation) and coma.

Contraindications to the use of physostigmine include bronchospasm and mechanical obstruction of the intestine

TABLE 121.3

SUMMARY TREATMENT RECOMMENDATIONS FOR ANTICHOLINERGIC TOXICITY AND USE OF PHYSOSTIGMINE

Place patient on cardiac and pulmonary monitor
Obtain electrocardiogram—If QRS prolonged more than 100–110 msec, physostigmine should not be used
Consider a urinary catheter
Consider pretreatment with 1 mg lorazepam IV
If no QRS prolongation, administer 2 mg physostigmine IV over 4 minutes
If no resolution of delirium and no bradycardia or seizures, consider repeat dosing of 1–2 mg physostigmine IV
If appropriate response, repeat 1–2 mg physostigmine as necessary

or urogenital tract. It should be used with caution in patients with asthma, gangrene, diabetes, cardiovascular disease, or any vagotonic state, and with choline esters or depolarizing neuromuscular-blocking agents (e.g., succinylcholine). Physostigmine should also be used cautiously after cyclic antidepressant overdose and is contraindicated in patients with evidence of cardiac conduction delay (e.g., atrioventricular block and prolonged QRS interval) on electrocardiogram.

Patients receiving physostigmine should be placed on continuous cardiac monitoring and be under continuous careful observation. Recommendations for the safe use of physostigmine center on its slow intravenous infusion at a rate not to exceed 0.5 mg per minute to avoid adverse drug events such as bradydysrhythmia and seizures. Slower rates of administration can be used and simply delay the onset. The average does needed for adults is approximately 2 mg [2]. Mental status improvement is usually seen within 5 to 20 minutes of administration. If no reversal of anticholinergic effect has occurred after 10 to 20 minutes, an additional 1 to 2 mg may be administered. Administration by continuous infusion has been used following the ingestion of an anticholinergic plant, *Atropa belladonna* [14]. The recommended dose in pediatric patients is 0.02 mg per kg at 0.5 mg per minute. The half-life of physostigmine is short and its duration of action after the 2-mg dose typically is only 1 to 6 hours [15]. The action of many anticholinergic agents persists longer and, therefore, additional doses may be needed [15]. In one case series of physostigmine use for anticholinergic toxicity, two-thirds of patients required just one dose of physostigmine, and no patient required another dose more than 6.5 hours after the first dose [15]. If cholinergic toxicity emerges, atropine is not needed unless severe toxicity develops. Seizures are rare and usually self-limited; diazepam is recommended as needed. Anecdotally, some physicians have administered lorazepam, 1 mg, before the physostigmine as an additional safety measure.

References

1. Patel RJ, Saylor T, Williams SR, et al: Prevalence of autonomic signs and symptoms in antimuscarinic drug poisonings. *J Emerg Med* 26(1):89–94, 2004.
2. Burns MJ, Linden CH, Graudins A, et al: A comparison of physostigmine and benzodiazepines for the treatment of anticholinergic poisoning. *Ann Emerg Med* 35(4):374–381, 2000.
3. Gowdy J: Stramonium intoxication: review of symptomatology in 212 cases. *JAMA* 221(6):585–587, 1972.
4. Jannun DR, Mickel SF: Anisocoria and aerosolized anticholinergics. *Chest* 90(1):148–149, 1986.
5. Goldfrank L, Flomenbaum N, Lewin N, et al: Anticholinergic poisoning. *J Toxicol Clin Toxicol* 19(1):17–25, 1982.
6. Burkhart KK, Magalski AE, Donovan JW: A retrospective review of the use of activated charcoal and physostigmine in the treatment of jimson weed poisoning [abstract]. *J Toxicol Clin Toxicol* 37:389, 1999.
7. Weizberg M, Su M, Mazzola JL, et al: Altered mental status from olanzapine overdose treated with physostigmine. *Clin Toxicol (Philadelphia)* 44(3):319–325, 2006.
8. Ferraro KK, Burkhart KK, Donovan JW, et al: A retrospective review of physostigmine in olanzapine overdose. *J Toxicol Clin Toxicol* 39:474, 2001.
9. Walker WE, Levy RC, Hanenson IB: Physostigmine: its use and abuse. *J Am Coll Emerg Phys* 5(6):436–439, 1976.
10. Pentel P, Peterson CD: Asystole complicating physostigmine treatment of tricyclic antidepressant overdose. *Ann Emerg Med* 9(11):588–590, 1980.
11. Vance MA, Ross SM, Millington WR, et al: Potentiation of tricyclic antidepressant toxicity by physostigmine in mice. *Clin Toxicol* 11(4):413–421, 1977.
12. Suchard JR: Assessing physostigmine's contraindication in cyclic antidepressant ingestions. *J Emerg Med* 25(2):185–191, 2003.
13. Schneir AB, Offerman SR, Ly BT, et al: Complications of diagnostic physostigmine administration to emergency department patients. *Ann Emerg Med* 42(1):14–19, 2003.
14. Bogan R, Zimmermann T, Zilker T, et al: Plasma level of atropine after accidental ingestion of *Atropa belladonna*. *Clin Toxicol* 47(6):602–604, 2009.
15. Rosenbaum CD, Bird SB: Frequency and timing of physostigmine redosing in anticholinergic toxidrome. *Clin Toxicol* 46(7):634, 2008.

CHAPTER 122 ■ ANTICONVULSANT POISONING

STEVEN B. BIRD

Anticonvulsants can be divided into four groups based on their primary mechanism of action: those that primarily act on neuronal membranes (membrane-active agents), those that act on neurotransmitters or their receptor sites (synaptic agents), those with multiple sites of action, and those that are not yet understood. Membrane-active agents alter ion fluxes and include carbamazepine (CBZ), oxcarbazepine, ethosuximide, zonisamide, phenytoin, and lamotrigine (LTG). Synaptic agents primarily affect the activity of gamma-aminobutyric acid (GABA) and include barbiturates, benzodiazepines, gabapentin (GBP), tiagabine, and vigabatrin. Agents that have multiple sites of action include valproate, GBP, felbamate, and topiramate, and those for which mechanisms of action still are not understood are levetiracetam, stiripentol, and remacemide [1–3].

(Barbiturates and benzodiazepines are discussed in Chapter 143.) The precise action mechanisms of many of the newer anticonvulsants also remain unknown. Even within groups, the site or mechanism of action may differ. Pharmacologic differences are important from a therapeutic standpoint. In the treatment of seizures, combining agents from different groups may be effective whenever a single agent is ineffective or requires a toxic dose for efficacy. Therapeutic synergism may also occur when different agents of the same group are combined (e.g., benzodiazepines and barbiturates).

PHENYTOIN

Phenytoin (diphenylhydantoin) is the most commonly used anticonvulsant medication [4]. It is also used in the treatment of trigeminal neuralgia. Phenytoin was the antidysrhythmic of choice for digitalis toxicity before the advent of digitalis Fab fragments [5]. Iatrogenic intoxications can occur with drug interactions because distribution, protein binding, and clearance of phenytoin are affected by other medications and disease states. Toxicity may occur when the daily-administered dose exceeds endogenous metabolism and elimination [6–8]. Toxicity may also result when switching dosage forms or between generic and proprietary forms of the drug because of different release and absorption characteristics. There are idiosyncratic and hypersensitivity reactions associated with therapeutic use that are unrelated to dose, most commonly seen in patients with underlying neurologic disorders [9].

Pharmacology

Phenytoin is the prototypic membrane-active anticonvulsant. It acts on sodium pumps and channels in excitable cell membranes and is classified as a type 1B antidysrhythmic agent. By blocking the accumulation of intracellular sodium during tetanic stimulation, it limits the posttetanic potentiation of synaptic transmission and prevents seizure foci from detonating adjacent areas.

Phenytoin is a weak acid, with a pK_a of 8.5. The intravenous (IV) form has a pH of 10 to 12, contains 50 mg per mL, and is dissolved in a 40% propylene glycol and 10% ethanol vehicle. The phenytoin prodrug fosphenytoin (Cerebyx) has a pH between 8.6 and 9.0 and greater solubility. It is compatible with common IV preparations, lacks the cardiotoxic diluent propylene glycol, and may be administered intramuscularly as well as intravenously. It has a conversion half-life of 8.4 to 32.7 minutes to active phenytoin and is dosed in phenytoin equivalent (PE) units (75 mg per mL of fosphenytoin equals 50 mg per mL of phenytoin) [10]. In many institutions, fosphenytoin has replaced phenytoin.

Absorption occurs in the duodenum but depends on dosage form, gastric emptying, and bowel motility. Peak levels occur between 2.6 and 8.9 hours after oral dosing of an extended-release capsule. In overdosage, absorption may continue for up to 7 days, possibly due to decreased gastric motility and pharmacobezoar formation. The volume of distribution (V_d) of phenytoin is 0.6 L per kg, and it distributes preferentially into the brainstem and cerebellum [11]. Phenytoin is highly protein bound; decreased protein binding increases the free, pharmacologically active form of the drug and the V_d. Because usually only total phenytoin levels are measured, toxicity from increased free phenytoin may occur at lower total phenytoin levels [8].

Hepatic metabolism of phenytoin follows first-order elimination kinetics, with an average half-life of 22 hours (range: 7 to 55 hours). When plasma levels exceed 10 μg per mL, metabolism follows zero-order elimination kinetics, yielding a much longer half-life. The enzyme system may be induced or inhibited by other drugs, inherited genetic disturbances, or liver disease [12,13].

The anticonvulsant effects of phenytoin occur with plasma levels between 10 and 20 μg per mL. This can be achieved within 45 to 60 minutes by an IV-loading dose of 15 to 20 mg per kg of phenytoin or PE units of fosphenytoin. The rate of IV phenytoin administration should not exceed 50 mg per minute because of propylene glycol toxicity [14]. To avoid hypotension, fosphenytoin administration should not exceed 150 PE units per minute. Phenytoin has been successfully administered by the interosseous route in children with poor venous access. Maintenance dosing is usually 4 to 6 mg per kg per day in single or divided doses, although neonates may require higher doses (5 to 8 mg per kg per day) [15]. Death from isolated phenytoin ingestions is unusual but has been reported in young children with ingestions of 100 to 220 mg per kg [16,17]. Death results from central nervous system (CNS) depression with respiratory insufficiency and hypoxia-related complications.

Clinical Manifestations

Toxicity resulting from acute and chronic intoxication has a similar presentation. Patients with serum phenytoin concentrations between 20 and 40 μg per mL typically have nausea, vomiting, normal to dilated pupils, nystagmus in all directions, blurred vision, diplopia, slurred speech, dizziness, ataxia, tremor, and lethargy [18]. They may also be excited and agitated. As phenytoin serum concentration increases, confusion, hallucinations, and apparent psychosis may develop. Progressive CNS depression occurs, and nystagmus may improve. Pupillary response becomes sluggish, and deep tendon reflexes diminish [7]. Severe toxicity with coma and respiratory depression occurs with serum concentration exceeding 90 μg per mL [19]. Slowing of alpha wave activity is seen on electroencephalograms. As toxicity increases, brainstem evoked potentials are suppressed and may be absent. Paradoxical hyperactivity has been reported in patients with underlying neurologic deficits, with findings of dystonia, dyskinesia, choreoathetoid movements, decerebrate rigidity, and increased seizure activity [7,20]. Patients with baseline focal neurologic deficits may show contralateral abnormalities, including hemianopia, hemianesthesia, and hemiparesis. Patients recover completely if no anoxic or hypoxic complications develop during acute toxicity. Cerebellar atrophy after acute intoxication with phenytoin that was not known to be attributed to hypoxia has been reported, however [21]. Recovery may take 1 week or longer.

In rare instances, chronic toxicity has been associated with a syndrome of inappropriate antidiuretic hormone [22], encephalopathy, and cerebellar degeneration [11]. Chronic use of phenytoin causes hyperglycemia, vitamin D deficiency and osteomalacia, folate depletion, megaloblastic anemia, and peripheral neuropathy. Other adverse drug events include altered collagen metabolism that causes hirsutism, gingival hyperplasia, keratoconus, and hypertrichosis [23].

Non–dose-dependent phenytoin adverse drug events include hypersensitivity reactions such as fever, rash eosinophilia, hepatitis, lymphadenopathy, myositis, a lupuslike syndrome, rhabdomyolysis, nephritis, vasculitis, and hemolytic anemia [9]. Phenytoin administration during pregnancy has resulted in fetal hydantoin syndrome [24].

Phenytoin-induced dysrhythmias, hypotension, congestive failure, respiratory arrest, and asystole result predominately from propylene glycol toxicity during rapid IV phenytoin administration (e.g., >50 mg per minute). If the rate of infusion is slowed or temporarily halted, these effects usually resolve spontaneously but may persist for 1 to 2 hours [17,25]. Cardiovascular toxicity from phenytoin intoxication itself is rare, represents significant toxicity, and primarily occurs in patients with underlying cardiac disorders [26,27].

Diagnostic Evaluation

Essential laboratory studies should include sequential serum phenytoin levels (free and total, if available) and levels of other anticonvulsant medications, particularly when enteric-coated dosage form is involved. The interval between drug levels should be based on factors such as severity of intoxication, rate of rise of levels, and time since exposure. Intervals should be more frequent during the initial evaluation phase, while absorption is still occurring, than later, during the postabsorptive phase. In stable patients whose drug levels have peaked or started to decline, it may be appropriate to obtain levels every 12 to 24 hours until they return to the therapeutic range. Recommended laboratory studies include serum complete blood cell count, electrolytes, blood urea nitrogen, creatinine, glucose, albumin, and liver function tests. In hypoalbuminemic patients, the corrected phenytoin concentration is equal to the measured phenytoin concentration multiplied by 4.4 and divided by the serum albumin level. In all deliberate overdoses, an electrocardiogram (ECG) and acetaminophen and salicylate levels should be obtained. Arterial blood gas, chest radiograph, head computed tomography, and lumbar puncture should be obtained as clinically indicated.

The differential diagnosis of phenytoin intoxication includes sedative–hypnotic agents, other anticonvulsants, phencyclidine, neuroleptic agents, and other CNS depressant drugs. Other conditions such as diabetic ketoacidosis; hyperosmolar nonketotic coma; sepsis; CNS infection, tumor, and trauma; seizure disorders; extrapyramidal syndromes; postictal states; and cerebellar abnormalities may also mimic phenytoin intoxication.

Management

Patients should have a rapid evaluation of respiratory status followed by intubation if hypoxia or risk of aspiration is present. Vascular access should be established and the patient placed on continuous cardiac monitoring. If the mental status is abnormal, a fingerstick blood sugar should be obtained. Patients who are hyperglycemic from phenytoin intoxication can be treated with discontinuation of the drug; insulin therapy is rarely required. Flumazenil, the benzodiazepine antagonist, has no role in managing phenytoin intoxication, even if benzodiazepines are part of the polypharmacy overdose, as its use may increase the risk of status epilepticus, particularly in patients with a preexisting seizure disorder.

Hypotension occurring during phenytoin infusion is treated with discontinuation of the infusion and administration of crystalloids. Pressors are rarely necessary. Treatment of cardiac dysrhythmias is supportive, with use of the appropriate antidysrhythmics when indicated. Type IB antidysrhythmic agents should be avoided [28].

Patients with a seizure disorder should be placed on seizure precautions due to the possibility of paradoxical seizures during the acute intoxication phase or breakthrough seizures during the recovery phase when phenytoin levels may be in the subtherapeutic range. Seizures should be treated with benzodiazepines or a different anticonvulsant.

Because phenytoin has a long elimination half-life, measures to increase the rate of elimination should be considered. Gastrointestinal (GI) tract decontamination uses oral-activated charcoal administration. Phenytoin undergoes enterohepatic recirculation with active gut secretion; multiple-dose oral activated charcoal (MDAC) can increase the rate of elimination and may decrease hospital stay [29,30] (see Chapter 117). MDAC is indicated in patients with a phenytoin concentration greater than 40 μg per mL, moderate neurologic toxicity, or rising levels after GI tract decontamination. As drug levels may continue to decline for many hours after stopping MDAC, such therapy should be discontinued before drug levels reach the therapeutic range in patients who require phenytoin for therapeutic purposes. Serum levels of concurrent anticonvulsant medications may also decline when MDAC is administered, increasing the risk of breakthrough seizures. An observation period is necessary to ensure establishment of a therapeutic anticonvulsant regimen and documentation of stable therapeutic serum levels even after passage of charcoal stools. Because phenytoin has a high degree of protein binding and hepatic elimination, forced diuresis, hemodialysis, and hemoperfusion are not useful [31]. It is anticipated that hemofiltration would not be useful for similar reasons.

Disposition

Because the majority of patients with phenytoin poisoning do well with supportive therapy alone, determining the degree of toxicity is important. After adequate GI decontamination, the patient should be assessed for progression of toxicity. Patients who are not suicidal or ataxic, have no underlying cardiac dysrhythmia, can feed themselves, and are not at risk of hurting themselves can be discharged, providing serum phenytoin levels are not rising and a reliable caretaker is available. Patients who do not meet these criteria should be admitted. Severely toxic patients, those with underlying cardiac or CNS disorder, intubated patients, or patients with rapidly progressive signs of toxicity require intensive care monitoring.

VALPROIC ACID

Valproic acid (VA) 2-propylpentanoic or 2-propyl valeric acid is structurally unique among the anticonvulsants. VA is a branched-chain carboxylic acid with a pK_a of 4.8. In addition to being an anticonvulsant medication, VA is commonly used for the treatment of acute manic episodes, mood stabilization, and prophylaxis of migraine and affective disorders.

VA is marketed as a sodium salt (Depakene); in a syrup solution; in a prodrug form, divalproex sodium (Depakote); and as a sustained-release form of divalproex sodium (Depakote ER). The latter is a molecular complex that dissociates in the GI tract into two molecules of VA. There is also a parenteral form for VA.

Pharmacology

VA is thought to mediate its anticonvulsant effect by increasing cerebral and cerebellar levels of GABA [32] by blocking its metabolism through inhibition of GABA transferase and succinic aldehyde dehydrogenase. It may also prolong the recovery of inactivated sodium channels and have effects on potassium channels in neuronal cell membranes.

VA's pharmacokinetic profile is significantly altered in an overdose setting. Within its therapeutic range (50 to 100 mg per mL), VA is 80% to 95% serum protein bound [33,34]. The degree of protein binding decreases and the V_d (0.13 to 0.22 L per kg) increases as VA levels exceed 90 μg per mL [33,34]. The resultant increase in free VA levels is evident by enhanced distribution into target organ systems and better than predicted extracorporeal drug removal. This has been demonstrated by a higher cerebrospinal fluid-to-serum level and hemodialysis extraction ratio in the VA-poisoned patient [35,36]. Protein binding of VA may also be decreased in uremic patients or in the presence of other highly protein-bound agents (e.g., acetylsalicylic acid), which displace VA from its binding sites [37].

VA is highly bioavailable, with the time to peak serum levels after ingestion dependent on the dosage form and VA species. In capsule form, VA itself achieves peak serum levels after 1 to 4 hours in therapeutic dosing, whereas peak serum levels may be delayed 4 to 5 hours after ingestion of the enteric-coated divalproex sodium tablets. Peak serum levels may be delayed out to 17 hours in overdose [38]. This may be explained by the enteric-coating dissolution time and the sequential process of intestinal conversion of divalproex to the sodium salt. This is followed by the final conversion to the free acid, the only form absorbed from the GI tract. There is no evidence suggesting formation of pharmacobezoars from large numbers of VA tablets.

VA is metabolized predominantly by the liver, with 1% to 4% excreted unchanged in the urine [33]. It undergoes beta and omega oxidation to several metabolites: hydroxyvalproate, 2-propylglutarate, 2-propylpent-4-enoate, 5-hydroxyvalproate, and 4-hydroxyvalproate. At high doses of VA, the omega oxidation pathway may become saturated, leading to a decrease in total VA body clearance [35]. The metabolites undergo glucuronidation and biliary excretion, with a possible enterohepatic recirculation [35,39]. At therapeutic levels, VA elimination half-life averages 10.6 hours (range: 5 to 20 hours), but in an overdose it may extend to 30 hours.

VA disrupts amino acid and fatty acid metabolism, sequesters acetyl coenzyme A by forming valproyl coenzyme A, and interrupts the ornithine–citrulline shuttle and carnitine transport [40–42]. This may result in encephalopathy associated with hyperammonemia at therapeutic levels of VA [43,44], acutely contribute indirectly to the CNS-depressant effects, and chronically contribute to other target organ toxicity. VA metabolites have been implicated in the metabolic perturbations associated with VA poisoning [44,45], interfere with urine ketone determinations, and may be the hepatotoxic mediators of VA. There may be a link between VA- and opiate-induced CNS toxicity because of their similar influence on the GABAnergic systems [19,46]. Because VA and its metabolites are low molecular weight, branched chain carboxylic acids, they may be used as substrates for several enzymatic processes. This leads to inhibition of critical biochemical pathways, such as the urea cycle, and subsequent fatalities in some sensitive patient populations. Death has occurred after therapeutic doses of VA in patients with a congenital deficiency of ornithine carbamoyltransferase [47]. In addition, a frequently fatal Reye-like hepatitis has been observed in patients receiving therapeutic doses. Those at greatest risk appear to be very young patients (younger than 2 years of age), those being treated with multiple anticonvulsants, and those with other long-term neurologic complications. The fatality rate is 1 per 500 in this patient population [48]. This hepatotoxic reaction occurs in chronic exposure and may be mediated by metabolites formed via the cytochrome P450 pathway. These metabolites in turn depress fatty acid oxidation in the hepatocyte mitochondria [49]. This effect may parallel that seen after ingestion of ackee fruit containing hypoglycin, causing Jamaican vomiting sickness [49]. VA can produce a hyperammonemia and encephalopathy exclusive of the hepatotoxic reaction [39]. This may be associated with VA-induced carnitine deficiency [44].

Valproate as the sodium salt provides a significant sodium load (13.8 mg sodium per 100 mg VA) in overdose. VA and its metabolites are low-molecular-weight, osmotically active, free-acid, or anionic species. They may produce a slightly elevated osmolar gap and an elevated anion gap metabolic acidosis with a reduction in circulating endogenous cations, particularly calcium [35,40,49–53]. Valproate may have a dose-related toxic effect on bone marrow and platelet function, with resultant hematologic consequences such as thrombocytopenia, anemia, and leukopenia [54–56].

The morbidity and mortality from dose-related acute or acute-on-chronic VA poisoning appear to be related to hypoxic sequelae from respiratory failure, aspiration, or terminal cardiorespiratory arrest [35,50–52,57]. Although it has been speculated that VA has a direct, irreversible, neurotoxic effect, this has not been substantiated and it is indistinguishable from hypoxic injury [52].

Patients ingesting greater than 200 mg per kg are at high risk for significant CNS depression, but poor correlation exists between peak serum level and dose of VA ingested [57]. Patients who die from acute VA poisoning have had peak serum VA levels ranging from 106 to 2,728 μg per mL, whereas survival has been reported in a patient with a peak serum level of 2,120 μg per mL [40,49,56]. Although serum VA levels may not correlate with clinical effect, in general, serum levels of 180 μg per mL are usually associated with serious CNS toxicity (e.g., coma and apnea) and significant metabolic derangement (e.g., acidosis and hypocalcemia) [40,49,56,58,59]. The duration of toxicity is proportional to the peak serum VA level.

On the basis of endogenous VA clearance, it will take 3 days for the serum level to drop within the therapeutic range in a patient with a serum level greater than 1,000 μg per mL.

Clinical Manifestations

In acute intoxication, hypotension, mild tachycardia, decreased respiratory rate, and elevated or depressed temperature may be seen. Miosis may be present. The hallmarks of VA toxicity are global CNS-related depression in conjunction with unique metabolic changes. The mental status varies on a continuum from confusion and disorientation to obtundation and deep coma with respiratory failure. Tremor, hallucinations, and hyperactivity have been reported, but there is a notable lack of cerebellar–vestibular effects. Patients with an underlying seizure disorder may have breakthrough seizures. Most patients with serious acute VA poisoning manifest CNS toxicity for at least 24 hours and this may extend to several days. Laboratory abnormalities observed in patients with high serum VA levels include an anion gap metabolic acidosis, hypocalcemia, hyperosmolality, and hypernatremia. Transient rises in serum transaminase levels have been observed without evidence of functional liver toxicity. Hyperammonemia associated with vomiting, lethargy, and encephalopathy may occur at therapeutic serum levels. Although rare, complications or delayed sequelae associated with severe VA intoxication include optic nerve atrophy, cerebral edema, acute respiratory distress syndrome, and hemorrhagic pancreatitis.

Non–dose-related toxicity (e.g., hepatic failure, pancreatitis, red blood cell aplasia, neutropenia, and alopecia) has not been reported in acute overdoses with high serum levels of VA. Pancreatitis is usually considered a non–dose-related effect but has been observed [55]. Alopecia, thrombocytopenia, leukopenia, and anemia have been associated with acute and chronic VA intoxication.

The differential diagnosis should include opioid toxicity and a list of substances causing an increased anion gap metabolic acidosis. VA intoxication can be indistinguishable from opioid poisoning by signs and symptoms, and VA-poisoned patients may occasionally respond to naloxone. VA may cause a false-positive urine ketone determination, thereby misdirecting the clinician to causes of ketosis [40].

Diagnostic Evaluation

Essential laboratory studies should include sequential serum VA levels and levels of other anticonvulsant medications, particularly when the enteric-coated dosage form is involved. It should be recognized that VA metabolites are highly cross-reactive on enzyme-multiplied immunoassay technique assay for VA [35], and there may be an overestimation of serum VA levels as high as 50%. Recommended laboratory studies include complete blood cell count, reticulocyte count, serum electrolytes, blood urea nitrogen, creatinine, glucose, calcium, ammonia, and liver function tests. In addition, serum amylase and lipase levels should be obtained to rule out pancreatitis.

In all deliberate overdoses, an ECG and acetaminophen and salicylate levels should be obtained. Arterial blood gas, chest radiograph, head computed tomography, and lumbar puncture should be obtained as clinically indicated.

Management

As with any consequential CNS depressant ingestion, the patient's airway and respiratory status should be frequently assessed; early intubation and ventilation help prevent hypoxic sequelae. Vascular access and continuous cardiac monitoring should be established. Patients with altered mental status should have a fingerstick blood sugar determination or receive IV dextrose, followed by naloxone and thiamine as clinically indicated.

Naloxone (0.8 to 2.0 mg) has been reported to be effective in increasing the level of consciousness of patients with signs and symptoms of opioid toxicity and serum VA levels between 185 and 190 μg per mL [58,59]. Patients with higher VA serum levels have not responded to larger doses of naloxone [56,60]. Naloxone has been shown experimentally to antagonize GABA, the inhibitory neurotransmitter increased by VA [19,46]. It is therefore worth trying naloxone (up to 10 mg) all comatose patients with suspected VA poisoning. Flumazenil, the benzodiazepine antagonist, should be avoided in patients with a preexisting seizure disorder.

Carnitine has been used for the treatment of hyperammonemia because VA interferes with the citrulline–ornithine cycle and carnitine's availability to shuttle fatty acids across the mitochondrial membrane. There are some pediatric data suggesting that carnitine improves mental status [42,43,61–63]. The oral and parenteral carnitine doses range from 1.5 to 2.0 g, divided into 3 to 4 doses per day.

GI decontamination should be performed in patients with suspected VA, even if several hours have elapsed since ingestion [64]. Activated charcoal is preferred; gastric lavage and whole-bowel irrigation for enteric-coated preparations are additional options. Methods to enhance elimination may be effective since an increase in the free serum drug fraction, decreased protein binding, and marked prolongation in elimination half-life occur after overdose. MDAC may enhance the clearance and reduce the VA half-life by interrupting enterohepatic recirculation and GI tract dialysis [65]. Extracorporeal removal by hemodialysis or hemoperfusion is also effective. Indications for extracorporeal removal are not clearly defined, requiring a risk-benefit analysis on a case-by-case basis. It should be considered when the VA level exceeds 1,000 μg per mL and is recommended for patients with levels exceeding 2,000 μg per mL. In a patient with a level exceeding 2,000 μg per mL, prompt institution of hemodialysis led to complete resolution of toxicity within 3 days, whereas a similar patient managed with only supportive care died [40,56]. Patients not responding to conventional therapy or who have severe acid–base derangement may also benefit from hemodialysis. VA clearance during hemodialysis has been as high as 270 mL per minute, with a four- to fivefold decrease in elimination half-life [36]. Hemodialysis has the added benefit of correcting acid-base derangements secondary to VA and removal of its metabolites. Because of VA's extensive protein binding and predominate hepatic elimination, it is anticipated that forced diuresis, manipulation of urine pH, and hemofiltration would not be useful in the management of VA intoxication. Charcoal hemoperfusion used for VA intoxication has demonstrated clearance similar to that of hemodialysis [48,66]. Use of hemodialysis and hemoperfusion in series may be more advantageous due to a more consistent extraction of VA as its degree of protein binding increases coincident with declining levels and desaturation of binding sites [67].

Disposition

The disposition of the VA-poisoned patient is based on the severity of CNS toxicity, quantitative serum levels, evidence of hypoxic insult, risk of secondary complications, and the amount of VA ingested. Patients with serum VA levels exceeding 150 μg per mL are at risk for CNS and respiratory depression and should be observed until levels return to the therapeutic range. Patients with VA serum levels exceeding 1,000 μg per mL are at high risk for serious prolonged toxicity and should be admitted to an intensive care unit.

CARBAMAZEPINE

CBZ is an iminostilbene compound with a chemical structural backbone resembling that of the tricyclic antidepressants. It is stereochemically similar to phenytoin. CBZ has long been recognized as a well-tolerated and effective agent for the management of various types of seizure disorders. It is also used for the treatment of trigeminal and glossopharyngeal neuralgias, tabetic pain, and affective disorders [68]. A sustained-release formulation is available.

Pharmacology

Because CBZ is unionized and highly lipophilic, there is no parenteral dosage form, and the rate-limiting step for systemic absorption is tablet dissolution time [69]. Consequently, the pharmacokinetics and toxicokinetics of CBZ are not well defined and are subject to significant inter- and intrapatient variability. CBZ is 80% protein bound and may have twice the V_d of other anticonvulsants, such as phenytoin and phenobarbital.

In overdose, systemic absorption of CBZ may be inconsistent over time. This leads to intermittent surges of drug released into the circulation and may cause unexpected clinical deterioration of patients. This may explain the "cyclic coma" associated with CBZ poisoning [70–72]. Patients have been reported to relapse into deep coma as late as 2 days after admission to the hospital coincident with a marked increase in plasma levels of CBZ, even after the patient's condition has appeared to stabilize or improve clinically. CBZ's V_d ranges from 1.4 to 3.0 L per kg at toxic levels [4,73].

CBZ is predominantly metabolized in the liver, with 1% to 3% excreted unchanged in the urine. Endogenous clearance is 0.6 to 1.3 mL per minute per kg [4,68]. The variability in clearance may be attributed to alteration in the metabolic capabilities of hepatic enzymes, particularly the cytochrome P450 system [68]. This system is sensitive to autoinduction during chronic administration or, conversely, inhibition with concurrent administration of enzyme inhibitors such as erythromycin [74]. The elimination half-life of CBZ in naive users may exceed 24 hours, whereas in chronic users it may be less than 15 hours [4,68,69,75]. Half-life determinations of CBZ, especially in overdose, often are misleading due to erratic absorption and inability to determine the contribution of sustained absorption from the GI tract [75]. Most evidence suggests that CBZ undergoes first-order kinetics, although it is postulated that some of its metabolic pathways, such as epoxidation, may follow Michaelis–Menton kinetics and saturate at high levels [75].

Forty percent of CBZ is converted to the active metabolite CBZ-10,11-epoxide (CBZ-epoxide), further complicating the kinetic and toxicity profile of CBZ [68,72]. An inactive metabolite is also formed. CBZ-epoxide elimination half-life is 5.0 to 9.8 hours and is in turn converted to the 10,11-dihydroxide [73,75]. CBZ-epoxide is much less protein bound than CBZ (50% vs. 80%) [68]. The therapeutic CBZ concentration is 3 to 14 μg per mL. Within this range, adverse drug events including nystagmus, ataxia, dizziness, and anorexia have been noted [4,76].

CBZ may be best described as a CNS depressant with mild anticholinergic activity and a proclivity for alteration of the cerebellar–vestibular brainstem function. CBZ mediates its pharmacologic effects by mechanisms that include stabilizing the inactive sodium channel, alteration of neurotransmitter activity (norepinephrine, acetylcholine), enhancement of adenosine, stimulation of benzodiazepine receptors, and depression of evoked repetitive firings in neurons and the brainstem reticular formation [68].

CBZ has been described as similar to tricyclic antidepressants in its toxicity profile [71,77–80]. Although these agents share sedative, anticholinergic, and sodium channel blocking activity, CBZ has a higher therapeutic index, and malignant cardiac dysrhythmias and seizures do not usually occur in patients with a normal cardiac and neurologic function [81]. In overdose with extremely high CBZ levels, however, fatal dysrhythmias may develop [76,82,83].

CBZ toxicity can be defined as dose dependent or non–dose dependent. Non–dose-dependent toxicity includes idiosyncratic and immunologic-mediated reactions such as bone marrow suppression, hepatitis, tubulointerstitial renal disease, cardiomyopathy, hyponatremia, and exfoliative dermatitis. It is responsible for the majority of CBZ-related fatalities [4,80,84] and is recognized in the course of chronic therapeutic dosing. Dose-related effects in sensitive populations include those with existing neurologic deficits and myocardial disease. Dose-related toxicity has been reported in acute overdoses, with survival in adults after 80-g ingestions. Death has been reported after acute ingestion of 60 g and after a 6-g ingestion in a patient receiving long-term maintenance therapy [78,85,86].

Respiratory depression and significant neurologic toxicity and death have been reported, with peak serum CBZ levels ranging from 20 to 65 μg per mL [70,72,73,76,78,79,86–92]. Patients with serum levels in the range of 10 to 20 μg per mL usually respond to verbal stimuli unless other coexisting medical complications or additional sedative–hypnotic substances are present [76].

There is poor correlation between serum CBZ levels and clinical outcome. Prognosis appears to depend on occurrence of respiratory depression and aspiration of gastric contents [71,72,76,78,79,86–89,91,93]. All reported deaths occurred in patients with a history of seizure disorders. Surviving patients may have a protracted course (days to weeks) because of secondary complications arising from hypoxic-related sequelae from respiratory and CNS depression, prolonged GI tract absorption, and a prolonged elimination half-life.

The kinetics of CBZ toxicity are affected by the active metabolite CBZ-epoxide, which may partially account for the lack of correlation between peak CBZ levels and the severity of symptoms. The concentration of CBZ-epoxide is only 40% that of CBZ. CBZ-epoxide concentration in the free, unbound form may be equal to or greater than that of CBZ, however [94,95].

Toxicity may occur by gradual accumulation of CBZ in patients receiving therapeutic dosing because of improper dosing protocols or as a result of a drug interaction with enzyme inhibitors such as erythromycin or verapamil [74] and from generic substitution [96].

Clinical Manifestations

Patients with acute and chronic exposures have similar findings. Key findings suggestive of CBZ poisoning include the triad of coma, anticholinergic syndrome, and adventitious movements [79]. Physical findings include CNS depression with pronounced effects on the cerebellar–vestibular system (e.g., nystagmus, ataxia, ophthalmoplegia, diplopia, absent doll's eye reflex, and absent caloric reflexes), central and peripheral anticholinergic toxicity (e.g., hyperthermia, sinus tachycardia, hypertension, urinary retention, mydriasis, and ileus), and neuroleptic-type movement disorders (e.g., oculogyric crisis, dystonia, opisthotonus, choreoathetosis, and ballismus), which can occur in patients without preexisting neurologic disorders.

Other effects, which are not clearly reproducible and may be indirectly related to hypoxia or occur in patients with preexisting disease, include cardiac conduction disturbances, hypotension, hypothermia, respiratory depression, deep coma, diminished or exaggerated deep tendon reflexes, and dysarthria. Some patients may be agitated and restless, combative, or irritable, experience hallucinations, or have seizures. Because CBZ has prolonged absorption from the GI tract and prolonged elimination half-life, the clinical course may be extremely protracted and deceptive, and sudden deterioration may occur days after admission [70,72].

Seizures associated with high levels of CBZ appear to occur predominantly in patients with preexisting neurologic disorders. In many reports, it is unclear whether witnessed motor activity was a true seizure or another movement disorder and whether the seizure occurred primarily or was secondary to hypoxic insult [70,71,76,77,79,88,94].

Cardiac conduction disturbances such as prolongation of the PR, QRS, and QTC intervals and complete heart block have been reported [71,88,90,97]. Patients with an underlying abnormal cardiac conduction system may be at particular risk for the development of complete heart block [98]. In most patients, conduction defects are not seen or there is marginal prolongation of intervals without progression to malignant dysrhythmia despite extremely high CBZ levels [77–79,81,90,99].

Diagnostic Evaluation

Essential laboratory studies should include sequential serum CBZ levels and levels of other anticonvulsant medications, serum electrolytes, blood urea nitrogen, creatinine, and ECG. Recommended laboratory studies include complete blood cell count and liver function tests. In all deliberate overdoses, acetaminophen and salicylate levels should be obtained. Arterial blood gas, chest radiograph, head computed tomography, and lumbar puncture should be obtained as clinically indicated.

CBZ and CBZ-epoxide are highly cross-reactive on enzyme-multiplied immunoassay technique assays for CBZ and can result in a falsely elevated CBZ level. The clinical consequence of this is debatable, however. High-pressure liquid chromatography assay has the ability to distinguish between CBZ and CBZ-epoxide. Using the ratio of CBZ to CBZ-epoxide, an index can be generated that may reflect the rapidity of absorption of CBZ from the GI tract. A ratio greater than 2.5 is evidence of rapid or continued CBZ absorption from the GI tract. Cases in which patients appear to relapse or deteriorate may be due to an abrupt increase in absorption occurring as late as 48 hours after the initial ingestion [72,78,90,92]. In cases in which serial CBZ and CBZ-epoxide levels were monitored, the ratio greatly increased just before and coincident with the clinical deterioration [70,72,90].

Patients whose serum CBZ level continues to significantly rise, manifesting delayed symptoms, or who appear to relapse or deteriorate after appropriate GI decontamination should be suspect for harboring pharmacobezoars in their GI tract. Radiographic contrast study should be considered to confirm this diagnosis; CBZ is not radiopaque [85,99]. The differential diagnosis of CBZ toxicity includes tricyclic antidepressants, neuroleptics, sedative–hypnotics, anticholinergic agents, and other anticonvulsant poisonings.

Management

Management begins with treatment of respiratory, neurologic, and cardiovascular derangements. Early intubation and ventilation should be considered, as poor outcomes with CBZ-poisoned patients are primarily associated with pulmonary complications. Vascular access and continuous cardiac monitoring [68,70,76] should be established. Hypotension should be initially managed with crystalloid fluid challenges followed by pressor agents (e.g., dopamine) [70,78]. There is no specific antidysrhythmic regimen for CBZ-induced cardiac toxicity. IV sodium bicarbonate therapy should be considered in patients whose QRS is greater than 100 milliseconds. Patients with altered mental status should have a fingerstick blood sugar determination or receive IV dextrose, followed by naloxone and thiamine as clinically indicated. Seizures are usually self-limited but respond to IV diazepam or phenytoin [73].

GI decontamination should be initiated as soon as possible with activated charcoal. MDAC may double the elimination of systematically absorbed CBZ [100] (see Chapter 119) and should also be considered in patients with serum CBZ concentration greater than 20 μg per mL. MDAC should be discontinued before CBZ levels decline to the therapeutic range in those with an underlying seizure disorder [101]. Although MDAC therapy significantly reduces serum CBZ levels, it has not been shown to improve patient outcome [102]. In patients with rising drug levels despite initial GI tract decontamination, whole-bowel irrigation may also be useful (see Chapter 119).

Hemoperfusion has been used to enhance CBZ clearance in overdose cases but with modest results, usually no more than the increase achieved by MDAC, which is less invasive [78,87–88]. In one case, it was equivalent to an increase in CBZ excretion of 200 mg per hour [78]. If used at all, extracorporeal removal should be reserved for those with greatly elevated serum levels and concomitant deep coma. Neither urinary manipulation nor hemodialysis is useful.

Although there is one case report of a CBZ-poisoned patient (serum level: 27.8 μg per mL) who responded to a dose of flumazenil [91], this agent may precipitate seizures and is contraindicated in CBZ overdose. Physostigmine has been reported to be effective in the treatment of dystonia associated with CBZ poisoning [77]. Given that CBZ-associated dystonias are self-limited, the risks of physostigmine therapy likely outweigh its potential benefits.

Disposition

Because CBZ displays erratic absorption, the decision should be in favor of admission and a prolonged observation period in an intensive care setting for patients with a history suggestive of a large ingestion despite initial clinical presentation and CBZ serum level. CBZ-poisoned patients at greatest risk for significant sequelae should also be admitted to the intensive care unit. This would include patients whose CBZ levels exceed 20 μg per mL or are readily rising, who are obtunded or comatose, those with cardiovascular symptoms, whose ECG shows a QRS greater than 100 milliseconds, and those with seizures. The majority of patients at risk for significant sequelae require observation for a minimum of 48 hours.

NEWER ANTICONVULSANTS

Felbamate (Felbatol)

Felbamate is a phenyl dicarbamate with a structure similar to that of the sedative-hypnotic agent meprobamate. Its mechanism of action is believed to have some indirect effect on the $GABA_A$-receptor supramolecular complex [103,104], block repetitive neuronal firing, and affect the sodium channel on the neuronal membrane. Felbamate is rapidly absorbed, with a bioavailability of 90% and peak plasma concentrations occurring 1 to 4 hours after oral dosing. Its V_d is 0.75 L per kg. The drug circulates as the free drug and is only 20% to 30% protein bound. Absorption and elimination are linear and plateau at high levels. The drug undergoes partial hepatic metabolism with an inactive metabolite and renal excretion. Approximately 40% of a dose is eliminated unchanged in the urine. The elimination half-life is 20 to 23 hours. Felbamate does not induce its own metabolism [105].

Felbamate has significant drug interactions. It can inhibit and induce the P450 cytochrome system. This affects the metabolism of coadministered medications. Felbamate induces the metabolism of CBZ and inhibits the metabolism of phenytoin and VA. The effect of felbamate on metabolism takes 2 to 3 weeks to clear after discontinuation of the drug [105,106].

Although uncommon, serious adverse drug events include aplastic anemia and hepatic failure, which is associated with a 20% mortality rate. Other adverse drug events include nausea, vomiting, abdominal pains, headache, insomnia, palpitations, tachycardia, blurred vision, diplopia, tremors, and ataxia. Children are likely to demonstrate anorexia and somnolence [105].

There is limited information regarding deliberate felbamate overdose [107,108]. A 20-year-old woman developed altered mental status, massive crystalluria, and acute renal failure after an overdose of felbamate and VA. Macroscopic urinary crystals were identified by gas chromatography as containing felbamate. Crystalluria and acute renal failure resolved with hydration. A 44-year-old man who ingested an unknown amount of felbamate, haloperidol, and benztropine recovered with supportive care. Symptoms were predominately neurologic, with ataxia, nystagmus, weakness, abnormal movements, and agitation [109]. The management of felbamate overdose is supportive care. Gut decontamination with activated charcoal would appear to be reasonable. There are no data on hemodialysis, hemoperfusion, or urinary manipulation [109].

Lamotrigine (Lamictal)

LTG, or 3–5-diamino-6 (2,3-dichlorophenyl)-1,2,4-triazine, is not structurally related to other anticonvulsants. The mechanism of action of LTG is believed to involve voltage-sensitive sodium channels and stabilizes neuronal membranes. Lamotrigine has no effect on the release of GABA, acetylcholine, norepinephrine, or dopamine. In oral dosing, LTG is rapidly absorbed, with a bioavailability of 98%. Peak plasma levels are reached 1 to 4 hours after dosing. Protein binding is 55%, and the V_d ranges from 0.9 to 1.4 L per kg. LTG is metabolized in the liver and excreted as the glucuronide metabolite. LTG does not induce its own metabolism. The elimination half-life of the parent compound is 12 to 50 hours (mean: 30 hours) [103,105].

Adverse drug events include Stevens–Johnson syndrome, toxic epidermal necrolysis, drowsiness, dizziness, headache, unsteady gait, tremor, ataxia, somnolence, diplopia, blurred vision, and nausea [105].

There is limited information regarding deliberate LTG overdose [108,110–112]. One patient presented with nystagmus and ataxia 1 hour after ingestion. The initial ECG showed a normal sinus rhythm with a QRS of 112 milliseconds, which gradually resolved over 48 hours. In another case, ataxia, rotary nystagmus, and a normal ECG were noted. A 2-year-old boy developed tremor, muscle weakness, ataxia, hypertonia, and generalized tonic–clonic seizure after ingesting 800 mg of LTG.

The management of acute LTG overdose should include GI decontamination, continuous cardiac monitoring, and supportive care. It would be prudent to closely monitor a patient with serial ECGs for 24 to 48 hours if the initial ECG shows a prolonged QRS duration (greater than 100 milliseconds). IV sodium bicarbonate therapy has not been studied but should be considered. Benzodiazepines are appropriate for the treatment of seizures. There are no data on hemodialysis or hemoperfusion.

Gabapentin (Neurontin)

GBP is an engineered molecule based on GABA and altered to increase membrane permeability and entrance through the blood–brain barrier. Chemically, GBP is GABA with a cyclohexane ring (1-[aminomethyl]-cyclohexane) [105].

Gabapentin appears to bind to a specific site in the CNS but does not affect ligand binding to $GABA_A$, $GABA_B$, benzodiazepine, glutamate, glycine, and *N*-methyl-D-aspartate sites on the neuronal membrane [103,105].

GBP is 50% to 60% absorbed from the GI tract, with peak serum levels occurring 1 to 3 hours after oral administration. Its V_d is 0.8 to 1.0 L per kg. GBP is not protein bound and does not appear to be metabolized; all of a dose is excreted unchanged in the urine. The terminal elimination half-life is 5 to 7 hours. Renal elimination and half-life are proportional to renal function. The elimination rate can neither be induced, nor can the elimination half-life be altered with repetitive dosing [105,113].

Adverse drug events include CNS depression, nystagmus, blurred vision, diplopia, mood changes, headache, weight gain, seizures, fatigue, nausea, dizziness, slurred speech, and unsteady gait [106]. Lethargy, somnolence, dizziness, drowsiness, dysarthria, diplopia, sedation, ataxia, slurred speech, and GI distress have been observed after overdose [114,115]. Signs and symptoms resolved within 48 hours without specific therapy. Treatment is supportive. There are no data on binding to activated charcoal, urinary manipulation, hemodialysis, or hemoperfusion.

Oxcarbazepine (Trileptal)

Oxcarbazepine is the dihydro derivative of CBZ and can be thought of as being a prodrug, which is almost 100% biotransformed during hepatic first-pass metabolism to the active metabolite 10,11-dihydro-10-hydroxycarbamazepine. It has the same anticonvulsant effect as CBZ. The parent and the metabolite are lipophilic and pass into the CNS. Its advantages are that it has better tolerability and does not form the CBZ-epoxide. Peak serum drug levels occur 4.5 hours after an oral dose. The V_d is 49 L per kg. The elimination half-lives of oxcarbazepine and its metabolite are 1.0 to 2.5 hours and 8 to 11 hours, respectively. Adverse drug events include hyponatremia (in up to 30% of patients) headache, ataxia, dizziness, nausea, memory impairment, concentration difficulties, anorexia, and weight gain [113,116]. Evaluation and treatment considerations are the same as for CBZ. CBZ assays cannot be used to measure oxcarbazepine levels. Oxcarbazepine concentrations are not routinely available and are generally not useful in patient management [117].

Tiagabine (Gabitril)

Tiagabine is a GABA reuptake inhibitor derived from nipecotic acid to which a lipophilic moiety has been added to improve passage into the CNS. By selectively inhibiting neuronal GABA reuptake, it prolongs the action of GABA in the synapse. It is rapidly absorbed orally, with a peak level by 0.5 to 1.0 hours after ingestion. The drug is 96% protein bound and is metabolized in the liver. There is some degree of enterohepatic circulation. The elimination half-life ranges from 4 to 7 hours in patients receiving enzyme-inducing drugs [113]. Adverse drug events include CNS depression, seizures, nausea, hypertension, tachycardia, asthenia, sedation, dizziness, mild memory impairment, abdominal pain, and nausea. Treatment is supportive.

Topiramate (Topamax)

Topiramate is a sulfamate-substituted monosaccharide compound different from other anticonvulsants. Its mechanism of action may be in part due to sodium-channel blockade, enhancing the action of GABA, and diminishing kainate-induced excitatory receptor stimulation. Oral absorption is rapid, with a peak serum level at 1.8 to 4.3 hours. The plasma protein binding of topiramate is 9% to 17%, and its V_d is 0.7 L per kg. It is 70% to 97% eliminated unchanged in the urine. The elimination half-life is 18 to 24 hours.

Development of a nonanion-gap metabolic acidosis is a relative common occurrence with topiramate use, both in therapeutic dosing as well as overdose [118]. This occurs by impairing both the normal reabsorption of filtered bicarbonate by the proximal renal tubule and the excretion of hydrogen ions by the distal renal tubule. This combination of defects is termed mixed renal tubular acidosis (RTA) [119]. Treatment of the metabolic acidosis includes cessation of the topiramate and fluid resuscitation as needed. The use of parenteral sodium bicarbonate is rarely needed. Other adverse drug events include sedation, cognitive dysfunction, paresthesias, dizziness, fatigue, weight loss, diarrhea, and urolithiasis. Treatment is supportive [113].

Levetiracetam (Keppra)

Levetiracetam (Keppra) is a new anticonvulsant used to treat partial complex seizures that is also being investigated for its mood-stabilizing properties. Although its precise mechanism of action is unknown, levetiracetam does not appear to directly interact with the GABA system. There are few case reports of overdose with levetiracetam. It appears the most common adverse effects in overdose are sedation and respiratory depression [120,121]. There are no data regarding specific antidotal therapy for levetiracetam overdose. Treatment is supportive care.

Vigabatrin (Sabril)

Vigabatrin is an engineered GABA-related anticonvulsant with limited availability in the United States. Chemically, it is gamma-vinyl-GABA. It is a stereospecific GABA transaminase inhibitor, the S(+) enantiomer being biologically active. Its peak serum level occurs 0.5 to 3.0 hours after ingestion, and its V_d is 0.8 L per kg. There is virtually no plasma protein binding of the drug, and more than 80% of the drug is eliminated unchanged. The plasma half-life ranges from 4 to 8 hours. The cerebrospinal fluid level is 0% to 15% of the serum level [114]. Adverse drug events include visual field defects [122], diplopia, drowsiness, irritability, agitation, anxiety, psychomotor effects, depression, sedation, confusion, and ataxia [113]. A patient who ingested 8 to 12 g in an overdose developed a psychotic episode lasting 36 hours [123]. Supportive care is the mainstay of management.

References

1. Kwan P, Sills GJ, Brodie MJ: The mechanisms of action of commonly used antiepileptic drugs. *Pharmacol Ther* 90:21, 2001.
2. Pellock JM: Treatment of epilepsy in the new millennium. *Pharmacotherapy* 20:129, 2000.
3. Wallace SJ: Newer antiepileptic drugs: advantages and disadvantages. *Brain Dev* 23(5):277, 2001.
4. McNamara JO: Drugs effective in the therapy of the epilepsies, in Hardman JG, et al (eds): *Goodman and Gilman's The Pharmacological Basis of Therapeutic.* 10th ed. New York, McGraw-Hill, 2001, p 468.
5. Helfant RH, Seuffert GW, Patton RD, et al: The clinical use of diphenylhydantoin (dilantin) in the treatment and prevention of cardiac arrhythmias. *Am Heart J* 77(3):315, 1969.
6. Albertson TE, Fisher CJ Jr, Shragg TA, et al: A prolonged severe intoxication after ingestion of phenytoin and phenobarbital. *West J Med* 135(5):418, 1981.
7. Patel H, Crichton JU: The neurologic hazards of diphenylhydantoin in childhood. *J Pediatr* 73(5):676, 1968.
8. Reidenberg MM, Affrime M: Influence of disease on binding of drugs to plasma proteins. *Ann N Y Acad Sci* 226:115, 1973.
9. Powers NG, Carson SH: Idiosyncratic reactions to phenytoin. *Clin Pediatr (Philadelphia)* 26(3):120, 1987.
10. Boucher BA, Feler CA, Dean JC, et al: The safety, tolerability, and pharmacokinetics of fosphenytoin after intramuscular and intravenous administration in neurosurgery patients. *Pharmacotherapy* 16(4):638, 1996.
11. Kokenge R, Kutt H, McDowell FM: Neurological sequelae following dilantin overdose in a patient and in experimental animals. *Neurology* 15:823, 1965.
12. Reynolds EH: Chronic antiepileptic toxicity: a review. *Epilepsia* 16(2):319, 1975.
13. Kutt H: Interactions of antiepileptic drugs. *Epilepsia* 16(2):393, 1975.
14. Louis S, Kutt H, McDowell F: The cardiocirculatory changes caused by intravenous Dilantin and its solvent. *Am Heart J* 74(4):523, 1967.
15. Borofsky LG, Louis S, Kutt H, et al: Diphenylhydantoin: efficacy, toxicity, and dose-serum level relationships in children. *J Pediatr* 81(5):995, 1972.
16. Laubscher FA: Fatal diphenylhydantoin poisoning. A case report. *JAMA* 198(10):1120, 1966.
17. Petty CS, Muellinig RJ, Sindell HW: Accidental poisoning with diphenylhydantoin (Dilantin). *J Forensic Sci* 2:279, 1957.
18. Kutt H, Winters W, Kikenge R: Metabolism of diphenylhydantoin, blood levels and toxicity. *Arch Neurol* 11:642, 1964.
19. Dingledine R, Iversen LL, Breuker E: Naloxone as a GABA antagonist: evidence from iontophoretic, receptor binding and convulsant studies. *Eur J Pharmacol* 47(1):19, 1978.
20. Stilman N, Masdeu JC: Incidence of seizures with phenytoin toxicity. *Neurology* 35:1769, 1985.
21. Masur H, Elger CE, Ludolph AC, et al: Cerebellar atrophy following acute intoxication with phenytoin. *Neurology* 39(3):432, 1989.
22. Luscher TF, Siegenthaler-Zuber G, Kuhlmann U: Severe hypernatremic coma due to diphenylhydantoin intoxication. *Clin Nephrol* 20(5):268, 1983.
23. Wagner KJ, Zell M, Leikin JB: Metabolic effects of phenytoin toxicity. *Ann Emerg Med* 15(4):509, 1986.
24. Bodendorfer LG: Fetal effects of anticonvulsant drugs and seizure disorders. *Drug Intell Clin Pharm* 12:14, 1978.
25. Garrettson LK, Jusko WJ: Diphenylhydantoin elimination kinetics in overdosed children. *Clin Pharmacol Ther* 17(4):481, 1975.
26. Binder L, Trujillo J, Parker D, et al: Association of intravenous phenytoin toxicity with demographic, clinical, and dosing parameters. *Am J Emerg Med* 14(4):398, 1996.
27. Wyte CD, Berk WA: Severe oral phenytoin overdose does not cause cardiovascular morbidity. *Ann Emerg Med* 20(5):508, 1991.
28. Rizzon P, Di Biase M, Favale S, et al: Class 1B agents lidocaine, mexiletine, tocainide, phenytoin. *Eur Heart J* 8[Suppl A]:21, 1987.
29. Mauro LS, Mauro VF, Brown DL, et al: Enhancement of phenytoin elimination by multiple-dose activated charcoal. *Ann Emerg Med* 16(10):1132, 1987.
30. Howard CE, Roberts RS, Ely DS, et al: Use of multiple-dose activated charcoal in phenytoin toxicity. *Ann Pharmacother* 28(2):201, 1994.
31. Wilson JT, Huff JG, Kilroy AW: Prolonged toxicity following acute phenytoin overdose in a child. *J Pediatr* 95(1):135-8, 1979.
32. Faingold CL, Browning RA: Mechanisms of anticonvulsant drug action. *Eur J Pediatr* 146:8, 1987.
33. Chadwick DW: Concentration-effect relationships of valproic acid. *Clin Pharmacokinet* 10(2):155, 1985.
34. Cramer JA, Mattson RH: Valproic acid: in vitro plasma protein binding and interaction with phenytoin. *Ther Drug Monit* 1(1):105, 1979.
35. Dupuis RE, Lichtman SN, Pollack GM: Acute valproic acid overdose. Clinical course and pharmacokinetic disposition of valproic acid and metabolites. *Drug Safety* 5(1):65, 1990.
36. Brent J, Yanover M, Kulig K, et al: Valproic acid (VPA) poisoning treated by hemodialysis [abstract]. Presented at: AACT/AAPCC/ABMT/CAPCC Annual Scientific Meeting. September 1988; Baltimore, MD.
37. Goulden KJ, Dooley JM, Camfield PR, et al: Clinical valproate toxicity induced by acetylsalicylic acid. *Neurology* 37(8):1392, 1987.
38. Graudins A, Aaron CK: Delayed peak serum valproic acid in massive divalproex overdose—treatment with charcoal hemoperfusion. *J Toxicol Clin Toxicol* 34(3):335, 1996.
39. Kingsley E, Tweedale R, Gray P: The role of toxic metabolism in the hepatotoxicity of valproic acid. *Gastroenterology* 79:511, 1980.
40. Mortensen PB, Hansen HE, Pedersen B, et al: Acute valproate intoxication: biochemical investigations and hemodialysis treatment. *Int J Clin Pharmacol Ther Toxicol* 21(2):64, 1983.
41. Mortensen PB: Inhibition of fatty acid oxidation by valproate. *Lancet* 2(8199):856, 1980.
42. Cotariu D, Zaidman JL: Valproic acid and the liver. *Clin Chem* 34(5):890, 1988.
43. Coulter DL: Carnitine, valproate, and toxicity. *J Child Neurol* 6(1):7, 1991.
44. Riva R, Albani F, Gobbi G, et al: Carnitine disposition before and during valproate therapy in patients with epilepsy. *Epilepsia* 34(1):184, 1993.
45. Coulter DL, Allen RJ: Hyperammonemia with valproic acid therapy. *J Pediatr* 99(2):317, 1981.
46. Hyden H, Cupello A, Palm A: Naloxone reverses the inhibition by sodium valproate of GABA transport across the Deiters' neuronal plasma membrane. *Ann Neurol* 21(4):416, 1987.
47. Kay JD, Hilton-Jones D, Hyman N: Valproate toxicity and ornithine carbamoyltransferase deficiency. *Lancet* 2(8518):1283, 1986.
48. Dreifuss FE, Santilli N, Langer DH, et al: Valproic acid hepatic fatalities: a retrospective review. *Neurology* 37(3):379, 1987.
49. Gerber N, Dickinson RG, Harland RC, et al: Reye-like syndrome associated with valproic acid therapy. *J Pediatr* 95(1):142, 1979.
50. Schnabel R, Rambeck B, Janssen F: Fatal intoxication with sodium valproate. *Lancet* 1(8370):221, 1984.
51. Janssen F, Rambeck B, Schnabel R: Acute valproate intoxication with fatal outcome in an infant. *Neuropediatrics* 16(4):235, 1985.
52. Bigler D: Neurological sequelae after intoxication with sodium valproate. *Acta Neurol Scand* 72(3):351, 1985.
53. Eeg-Olofsson O, Lindskog U: Acute intoxication with valproate. *Lancet* 1(8284):1306, 1982.
54. Gidal B, Spencer N, Maly M, et al: Valproate-mediated disturbances of hemostasis: relationship to dose and plasma concentration. *Neurology* 44(8):1418, 1994.
55. Andersen GO, Ritland S: Life threatening intoxication with sodium valproate. *J Toxicol Clin Toxicol* 33(3):279, 1995.
56. Connacher AA, Macnab MS, Moody JP, et al: Fatality due to massive overdose of sodium valproate. *Scot Med J* 32(3):85, 1987.
57. Garnier R, Boudignat O, Fournier PE: Valproate poisoning. *Lancet* 2(8289):97, 1982.
58. Alberto G, Erickson T, Popiel R, et al: Central nervous system manifestations of a valproic acid overdose responsive to naloxone. *Ann Emerg Med* 18(8):889, 1989.
59. Steiman GS, Woerpel RW, Sherard ES Jr: Treatment of accidental sodium valproate overdose with an opiate antagonist. *Ann Neurol* 6(3):274, 1979.
60. Palatrick W, Honcharik N, Roberts D, et al: Coma, anion gap and metabolic derangements associated with a massive valproic acid poisoning. *J Anal Toxicol* 12:35, 1988.

61. Raskind JY, El-Chaar GM: The role of carnitine supplementation during valproic acid therapy. *Ann Pharmacother* 34(5):630, 2000.
62. Ohtani Y, Endo F, Matsuda I: Carnitine deficiency and hyperammonemia associated with valproic acid therapy. *J Pediatr* 101(5):782, 1982.
63. Stephens JR, Levy RH: Effects of valproate and citrulline on ammonium-induced encephalopathy. *Epilepsia* 35(1):164, 1994.
64. Lokan RJ, Dinan AC: An apparent fatal valproic acid poisoning. *J Anal Toxicol* 12(1):35, 1988.
65. Farrar HC, Herold DA, Reed MD: Acute valproic acid intoxication: enhanced drug clearance with oral-activated charcoal. *Crit Care Med* 21(2):299, 1993.
66. Van der Merwe AC, Albrecht CF, Brink MS, et al: Sodium valproate poisoning. A case report. *S Afr Med J* 67(18):735, 1985.
67. Tank JE, Palmer BF: Simultaneous "in series" hemodialysis and hemoperfusion in the management of valproic acid overdose. *Am J Kidney Dis* 22(2):341, 1993.
68. Durelli L, Massazza U, Cavallo R: Carbamazepine toxicity and poisoning. Incidence, clinical features and management. *Med Toxicol Adverse Drug Exp* 4(2):95, 1989.
69. Levy RH, Pitlick WH, Troupin AS, et al: Pharmacokinetics of carbamazepine in normal man. *Clin Pharmacol Ther* 17(6):657, 1975.
70. Sethna M, Solomon G, Cedarbaum J, et al: Successful treatment of massive carbamazepine overdose. *Epilepsia* 30(1):71, 1989.
71. Sullivan JB Jr, Rumack BH, Peterson RG: Acute carbamazepine toxicity resulting from overdose. *Neurology* 31(5):621, 1981.
72. de Zeeuw RA, Westenberg HG, van der Kleijn E, et al: An unusual case of carbamazepine poisoning with a near-fatal relapse after two days. *Clin Toxicol* 14(3):263, 1979.
73. Deng JF, Shipe JR Jr, Rogol AD, et al: Carbamazepine toxicity: comparison of measurement of drug levels by HPLC and EMIT and model of carbamazepine kinetics. *J Toxicol Clin Toxicol* 24(4):281, 1986.
74. Goulden KJ, Camfield P, Dooley JM, et al: Severe carbamazepine intoxication after coadministration of erythromycin. *J Pediatr* 109(1):135, 1986.
75. Vree TB, Janssen TJ, Hekster YA, et al: Clinical pharmacokinetics of carbamazepine and its epoxy and hydroxy metabolites in humans after an overdose. *Ther Drug Monit* 8(3):297, 1986.
76. May DC: Acute carbamazepine intoxication: clinical spectrum and management. *South Med J* 77(1):24, 1984.
77. O'Neal W Jr, Whitten KM, Baumann RJ, et al: Lack of serious toxicity following carbamazepine overdosage. *Clin Pharm* 3(5):545, 1984.
78. Nilsson C, Sterner G, Idvall J: Charcoal hemoperfusion for treatment of serious carbamazepine poisoning. *Acta Med Scand* 216(1):137, 1984.
79. Fisher RS, Cysyk B: A fatal overdose of carbamazepine: case report and review of literature. *J Toxicol Clin Toxicol* 26(7):477, 1988.
80. Hopen G, Nesthus I, Laerum OD: Fatal carbamazepine-associated hepatitis. Report of two cases. *Acta Med Scand* 210(4):333, 1981.
81. Apfelbaum JD, Caravati EM, Kerns WP Jr, et al: Cardiovascular effects of carbamazepine toxicity. *Ann Emerg Med* 25(5):631, 1995.
82. Johnson CD, Rivera H, Jimenez JE: Carbamazepine-induced sinus node dysfunction. *P R Health Sci J* 16(1):45, 1997.
83. Kenneback G, Bergfeldt L, Vallin H, et al: Electrophysiologic effects and clinical hazards of carbamazepine treatment for neurologic disorders in patients with abnormalities of the cardiac conduction system. *Am Heart J* 121(5):1421, 1991.
84. Hart RG, Easton JD: Carbamazepine and hematological monitoring. *Ann Neurol* 11(3):309, 1982.
85. Noda S, Umezaki H: Carbamazepine-induced ophthalmoplegia. *Neurology* 32(11):1320, 1982.
86. Denning DW, Matheson L, Bryson SM, et al: Death due to carbamazepine self-poisoning: remedies reviewed. *Hum Toxicol* 4(3):255, 1985.
87. Chan KM, Aguanno JJ, Jansen R, et al: Charcoal hemoperfusion for treatment of carbamazepine poisoning. *Clin Chem* 27(7):1300, 1981.
88. Gary NE, Byra WM, Eisinger RP: Carbamazepine poisoning: treatment by hemoperfusion. *Nephron* 27(4–5):202, 1981.
89. Leslie PJ, Heyworth R, Prescott LF: Cardiac complications of carbamazepine intoxication: treatment by haemoperfusion. *BMJ (Clin Res Ed)* 286(6370):1018, 1983.
90. Rockoff S, Baselt RC: Severe carbamazepine poisoning. *Clin Toxicol* 18(8):935, 1981.
91. Watson WA, Cremer KF, Chapman JA: Gastrointestinal obstruction associated with multiple-dose activated charcoal. *J Emerg Med* 4(5):401, 1986.
92. Zuber M, Elsasser S, Ritz R, et al: Flumazenil (Anexate) in severe intoxication with carbamazepine (Tegretol). *Eur Neurol* 28(3):161, 1988.
93. Kossoy AF, Weir MR: Therapeutic indications in carbamazepine overdose. *South Med J* 78(8):999, 1985.
94. Patsalos PN, Krishna S, Elyas AA, et al: Carbamazepine and carbamazepine-10,11-epoxide pharmacokinetics in an overdose patient. *Hum Toxicol* 6(3):241, 1987.
95. Schoeman JF, Elyas AA, Brett EM, et al: Correlation between plasma carbamazepine-10,11-epoxide concentration and drug side-effects in children with epilepsy. *Dev Med Child Neurol* 26(6):756, 1984.
96. Gilman JT, Alvarez LA, Duchowny M: Carbamazepine toxicity resulting from generic substitution. *Neurology* 43(12):2696, 1993.
97. Beermann B, Edhag O, Vallin H: Advanced heart block aggravated by carbamazepine. *Br Heart J* 37(6):668, 1975.
98. Durelli L, Mutani R, Sechi GP, et al: Cardiac side effects of phenytoin and carbamazepine. A dose-related phenomenon? *Arch Neurol* 42(11):1067, 1985.
99. Coutselinis A, Poulos L: An unusual case of carbamazepine poisoning with a near-fatal relapse after two days. *Clin Toxicol* 16(3):385, 1980.
100. Neuvonen PJ, Elonen E: Effect of activated charcoal on absorption and elimination of phenobarbitone, carbamazepine and phenylbutazone in man. *Eur J Clin Pharmacol* 17(1):51, 1980.
101. Patsalos PN, Stephenson TJ, Krishna S, et al: Side-effects induced by carbamazepine-10,11-epoxide. *Lancet* 2(8469–8470):1432, 1985.
102. Wason S, Baker RC, Carolan P, et al: Carbamazepine overdose—the effects of multiple dose activated charcoal. *J Toxicol Clin Toxicol* 30(1):39, 1992.
103. Macdonald RL, Kelly KM: Antiepileptic drug mechanisms of action. *Epilepsia* 34[Suppl 5]:S1, 1993.
104. White HS, Wolf HH, Swinyard EA, et al: A neuropharmacological evaluation of felbamate as a novel anticonvulsant. *Epilepsia* 33(3):564, 1992.
105. Ramsay RE: Advances in the pharmacotherapy of epilepsy. *Epilepsia* 34[Suppl 5]:S9, 1993.
106. Wagner ML, Remmel RP, Graves NM, et al: Effect of felbamate on carbamazepine and its major metabolites. *Clin Pharmacol Ther* 53(5):536, 1993.
107. Rengstorff DS, Milston AP, Seger DL, et al: Felbamate overdose complicated by crystalluria and acute renal failure. *J Toxicol Clin Toxicol* 38:667, 2000.
108. Buckley NA, Whyte IM, Dawson AH: Self-poisoning with lamotrigine. *Lancet* 342(8886–8887):1552, 1993.
109. Hwang TL, Still CN, Jones JE: Reversible downbeat nystagmus and ataxia in felbamate intoxication. *Neurology* 45(4):846, 1995.
110. Harchelroad F, Lang D, Valeriano J: Lamotrigine overdose [abstract]. *Vet Hum Toxicol* 36:372, 1994.
111. O'Donnell J, Bateman DN: Lamotrigine overdose in an adult. *J Toxicol Clin Toxicol* 38:659, 2000.
112. Briassoulis G, Kalabalikis T, Tamiolaki M, et al: Lamotrigine childhood overdose. *Pediatr Neurol* 19:239, 1998.
113. Bialer M: Comparative pharmacokinetics of the newer antiepileptic drugs. *Clin Pharmacokinet* 24:441, 1993.
114. Fischer JH, Barr AN, Rogers SL, et al: Lack of serious toxicity following gabapentin overdose. *Neurology* 44(5):982, 1994.
115. Verma A, St. Claire EW, Radtke RA: A case of sustained massive gabapentin overdose without serious side effects. *Ther Drug Monit* 21:615, 1999.
116. Dong X, Leppik IE, White J, et al: Hyponatremia from oxcarbazepine and carbamazepine. *Neurology* 65:1976, 2005.
117. Gonzalez-Esquivel DF, Ortega-Gavilan M, Alcantara-Lopez G, et al: Plasma level monitoring of oxcarbazepine in epileptic patients. *Arch Med Res* 31:202–205, 2000.
118. Garris SS, Oles KS: Impact of topiramate on serum bicarbonate concentrations in adults. *Ann Pharmacother* 39:424–426, 2005.
119. Mirza N, Marson AG, Pirmohamed M: Effect of topiramate on acid-base balance: extent, mechanism and effects. *Br J Clin Pharmacol* 68:655–661, 2009.
120. Barrueto F Jr, Williams K, Howland MA, et al: A case of levetiracetam (Keppra) poisoning with clinical and toxicokinetic data. *J Toxicol Clin Toxicol* 40:881–884, 2002.
121. Harden C: Safety profile of levetiracetam. *Epilepsia* 42[Suppl 4]:36–39, 2001.
122. Spence SJ, Sankar R: Visual defects and other ophthalmological disturbances associated with vigabatrin. *Drug Saf* 24:385, 2001.
123. Sander J, Hart YM, Sharron SD: Vigabatrin and epilepsy. *J Neurol Neurosurg Psychiatry* 55:245, 1992.

CHAPTER 123 ■ ANTIDEPRESSANT POISONING

CYNTHIA K. AARON AND ABHISHEK KATIYAR

Cyclic antidepressants constitute a major component of reported drug overdoses requiring treatment in an intensive care setting [1]. These medications are freely available to patients who are at high risk for suicide or overdose. The consequences of overdose are severe and predominantly affect the central nervous system (CNS) and cardiovascular system. Treatment of overdose is directed toward limiting drug absorption and managing complications of toxicity; there is no antidote for cyclic antidepressant toxicity.

Although iminodibenzyl was synthesized in the late nineteenth century, the pharmacology of cyclic antidepressants was not detailed until the 1940s. These compounds were designed to have antihistaminic, sedative, analgesic, and antiparkinsonian properties. Imipramine, the first of the dibenzazepines, was synthesized as a phenothiazine derivative but was found to be ineffective as a neuroleptic agent. In the late 1950s, patients taking imipramine reported that the drug had mood-elevating effects. Imipramine and later congeners have since been used in the treatment of endogenous depression. Other indications for cyclic antidepressants include therapy of enuresis in children, treatment for migraine headaches, chronic pain control, smoking cessation, panic disorders, premenstrual dysphoric syndrome, and cocaine detoxification [2,3].

Classic tricyclic antidepressants have a seven-membered central ring with a terminal nitrogen containing either three constituents (tertiary amines) or two constituents (secondary amines). Tertiary amines include amitriptyline, imipramine, doxepin, trimipramine, and chlorimipramine (clomipramine). Secondary amines include desipramine, protriptyline, and nortriptyline. Included with cyclic antidepressants are two dibenzoxazepine compounds that contain the central seven-membered ring with a heterocyclic constituent: loxapine and its demethylated metabolite amoxapine.

Maprotiline, a dibenzobicyclooctadiene, mianserin, and mirtazapine (Remeron®) are tetracyclic antidepressants [4]. Mirtazapine, a derivative of mianserin, has additional α_2-antagonist activity. Bicyclic compounds include viloxazine, venlafaxine, and zimeldine.

Trazodone and nefazodone are triazolopyridine derivatives that are structurally and pharmacologically different from the other cyclic antidepressants. Atypical antidepressants include bupropion, a unicyclic phenylaminoketone [5–10], and a large group of antidepressants called *selective serotonergic reuptake inhibitors* (SSRIs). Currently available SSRIs include fluoxetine, a straight-chain phenylpropylamine; paroxetine, a phenylpiperidine derivative; sertraline; fluvoxamine; citalopram, and escitalopram.

Venlafaxine and duloxetine are considered SSNRIs, since they have norepinephrine-reuptake inhibition effects. Although not classically considered SSRI, some antidepressant agents having serotonergic activity include mirtazapine, trazodone, nefazodone, and clomipramine. Cyclic antidepressants that are not available in the United States because of side effects include mianserin (agranulocytosis), nomifensine (hepatotoxicity and hemolytic anemia), lofepramine (hepatotoxicity and hyponatremia), and zimeldine (Guillain–Barré syndrome) [11–14].

A third class of antidepressants is the monoamine oxidase inhibitors (MAOIs; e.g., moclobemide, pargyline, phenelzine, tranylcypromine, selegiline, and isocarboxazid). They are used to treat depression, panic disorders, phobias, and obsessive-compulsive behavior. A group of MAOIs that selectively inhibit the monoamine oxidase (MAO) isoenzyme type B (MAO-B) are being used as agents to treat Parkinson's disease [15].

PHARMACOLOGY

The therapeutic effects of cyclic antidepressants are relatively similar, but their pharmacology differs considerably. The cyclic antidepressants act as neurotransmitter postsynaptic receptor blockers for histamine, dopamine, acetylcholine, serotonin, and norepinephrine (NE). They inhibit the reuptake of neurotransmitter biogenic amines and have quinidine-like membrane-stabilizing effects [3,4,11,13,14,16–19] (Tables 123.1 through 123.3). These agents may induce atrioventricular blocks [20–23] and have a direct negative cardiac inotropic effect, demonstrated by a decrease in the rate of change in left ventricular pressure and an increase in left ventricular end-diastolic pressure [17,24,25]. CNS effects may be

TABLE 123.1

CYCLIC ANTIDEPRESSANT EFFECTS ON NEUROTRANSMITTERS

Antidepressant	Effect
Receptor blockade	
Acetylcholine (antimuscarinic)	Sinus tachycardia, gastrointestinal hypomotility, warm dry skin, urinary retention, mydriasis, lethargy, hallucinations, seizures, coma
Norepinephrine	Hypotension, reflex tachycardia, orthostasis, ? seizures
Histamine	Antihistamine effects, sedation, hypotension
Serotonin	Hypotension, ejaculation disturbances
Dopamine	Endocrine disturbances (galactorrhea, impotence), dystonias
Biogenic amine reuptake blockade	
Dopamine	Hypotension, psychomotor retardation, antiparkinsonian effects
Norepinephrine	Transient hyperadrenergic state (tremor, tachycardia), adrenergic depletion (hypotension, antidepressant effects), ejaculation disturbances
Serotonin	Seizures, ejaculation disturbances, antidepressant effects

TABLE 123.2

RELATIVE POTENCIES OF CYCLIC ANTIDEPRESSANTS: RECEPTOR BLOCKADE

Compound	ACh	H_1	Alpha	5-HT	DA
Tertiary amines					
Amitriptyline	4+	3+	4+	2+	1+
Imipramine	3+	2+	4+	1+	1+
Secondary amines					
Nortriptyline	3+	3+	3+	1+	1+
Desipramine	1+	2+	2+	0	0
Dibenzoxazepines					
Amoxapine	±	2+	3+	0	2+
Tetracyclics					
Maprotiline	±	3+	3+	2+	2+
Triazolopyridines					
Trazodone	0	±	3+	0	0
SSRIs					
Fluoxetine	0	0	0	1+	0
Paroxetine	0	0	0	0	1+
Sertraline	0	0	0	0	0
Atypical					
Bupropion	0	1+	0	0	
Venlafaxine	0	0	0		

ACh, acetylcholine; DA, dopamine; H_1, histamine; 5-HT, serotonin; SSRIs, selective serotonin reuptake inhibitors.

TABLE 123.3

RELATIVE POTENCIES OF CYCLIC ANTIDEPRESSANT REUPTAKE BLOCKADE

Compound	NE	5-HT	DA	ACh
Tertiary amines				
Amitriptyline	2+	1+	1+	3+
Imipramine	2+	2+	1+	3+
Secondary amines				
Nortriptyline	3+	1+	3+	3+
Desipramine	4+	±	1+	2+
Dibenzoxazepines				
Amoxapine	3+	±	3+	2+
Tetracyclics				
Maprotiline	3+	0	1+	±
Triazolopyridines				
Trazodone	0	1+	±	0
SSRIs				
Fluoxetine	±	3+	3+	0
Paroxetine	0	4+	1+	1+
Sertraline	±	3+	0	1+
Atypical				
Bupropion	0	0	2+	1+
Venlafaxine	±	3+		

ACh, acetylcholine; DA, dopamine; 5-HT, serotonin; NE, norepinephrine; SSRIs, selective serotonin reuptake inhibitors.

related to neurotransmitter and to direct membrane effects [24,26,27]. All tricyclic antidepressants increase the density of β-adrenoreceptors.

SSRIs and SSNRIs alter serotonergic neurotransmission. The International Union of Pharmacological Societies Commission on Serotonin Nomenclature has classified at least twelve 5-hydroxytryptamine (5-HT) receptors based on operational criteria (Table 123.4). SSRIs block some serotonin receptors and inhibit the reuptake of serotonin at other receptor subtypes. Buspirone, a nonbenzodiazepine sedative-hypnotic, is a 5-HT_{1A} partial agonist and is inhibitory on serotonin neuronal firing. It has anxiolytic and antidepressant activity. Excessive stimulation can lead to hypotension. Antagonists at 5-HT_{1C}, such as ritanserin, may be anxiolytic. 5-HT_{1D} receptor subtype stimulation leads to inhibition of neurotransmitter release, and its agonist is sumatriptan, an antimigraine medication. 5-HT_2 stimulation can cause vasoconstriction. 5-HT_3 antagonists have antiemetic and antipsychotic activity (ondansetron) [28]. Classic tricyclic antidepressants affect serotonin neurotransmission by enhancing the sensitivity of postsynaptic 5-HT_{1A} postsynaptic receptors. The SSRIs alter the release of serotonin presynaptically, leading to an increase in the amount of serotonin that is available for neurotransmission without changing the sensitivity of the 5-HT_{1A} postsynaptic receptors [29]. In general, the SSRIs normalize the number and function of 5-HT_{1A} and 5-HT_2 receptors [28]. As a group, the predominant difference between SSRIs is in their effect on the hepatic cytochrome P450 system and drug–drug interactions.

Venlafaxine and duloxetine are considered selective serotonergic and NE reuptake inhibitors. Blockade of NE-α_2 receptors leads to decrease in 5-HT release. Selective serotonergic and NE reuptake inhibitors induce desensitization and downregulation of 5-HT and NE receptors, leading to disinhibition of serotonergic neurons, interruption of feedback inhibition, and increased release of synaptic 5-HT.

MAOIs inhibit the activity of MAO, a flavin-containing enzyme located in the mitochondrial membranes of most tissues [30]. MAO enzymes are divided into two families: MAO-A, which uses 5-HT as its predominant substrate, and MAO-B, whose primary substrates are 2-phenylethylamine, benzylamine, phenylethanolamine, and O-tyramine. Monoaminergic neurons contain predominantly MAO-A; serotonergic neurons have both. MAO-A metabolizes epinephrine, NE, metanephrine, and 5-HT. Both MAO-A and MAO-B metabolize tyramine, octopamine, and tryptamine [31]. MAO regulates intraneuronal catecholamine metabolism and mediates the oxidative deamination of epinephrine, NE, dopamine, and 5-HT. MAO also regulates ingested monoamine (tyramine, ethanolamine) in the gut that would normally be absorbed into the portal circulation [20,21]. The effect of MAOs is to increase the catecholamine storage pool by preventing intraneuronal degradation of catecholamines and 5-HT. These catecholamines can be released by indirectly acting sympathomimetic agents (e.g., amphetamine, tyramine, and dopamine). MAO-A is predominantly found in the intestinal mucosa, placenta, biogenic nerve terminals, liver, and brain, whereas MAO-B is found in the brain, platelets, and liver [22]. Exogenously administered catecholamines are metabolized through catechol-O-methyl transferase (COMT).

MAOIs can be divided into reversible agents (moclobemide) or irreversible (selegiline, phenylzine, isocarboxazid, and tranylcypromine). They may also be selective to MAO-A (moclobemide) or MAO-B (pargyline, selegiline). The original MAOIs (e.g., phenelzine, isocarboxazid, and tranylcypromine) are nonselective irreversible MAO-A and MAO-B inhibitors., selegiline [23]. Selegiline and tranylcypromine are metabolized to desmethylselegiline, levoamphetamine, and levomethamphetamine and will give a positive amphetamine on drugs of abuse urine screening [32].

TABLE 123.4

INTERNATIONAL UNION OF PHARMACOLOGICAL SOCIETIES COMMISSION ON SEROTONIN NOMENCLATURE[a]

Receptor	Second messenger	Location	Agonist	Effect	Antagonist	Effect
5-HT_{1A}	cAMP	CNS	Buspirone	Anxiolytic	—	—
5-HT_{1B} (rodent only)	cAMP	CNS, PNS	mCPP	—	—	—
5-HT_{1C}	cAMP	CNS	—	—	Ritanserin	Anxiolytic
5-HT_{1D}	cAMP	CNS and extracerebral vascular smooth muscle	Sumatriptan, methylsergide	Antimigraine	—	—
5-HT_{1E}	cAMP	CNS	Ergotamine	—	Methylsergide	—
5-HT_{1F}	cAMP	CNS	Ergotamine	—	Methylsergide, yohimbine	—
5-HT_{2A}	IP_3DG	Vascular smooth muscle	—	Hypertension	Ketanserin, ritanserin	Hypotension
5-HT_{2B}	IP_3DG	Stomach	Tryptamine	—	—	—
5-HT_{2C}	IP_3DG	CNS, choroid plexus	mCPP (trazodone metabolite)	—	—	—
5-HT_3	Ionic channel	CNS, PNS	—	—	Ondansetron, granisetron	Antiemetic
5-HT_4	cAMP	Cardiac (nonventricular), gastrointestinal tract, bladder	Renzapride, cisapride	Gastric motility	—	—
5-HT_5–5-HT_7	cAMP	—	—	—	—	—

[a] All 5-HT receptors are G-proteins except for 5-HT_3 receptors, which are ionic channel receptors. 5-HT_1 are negatively coupled to adenylyl cyclase; 5-HT_2 are coupled to protein kinase C via phosphoinositide breakdown; 5-HT_3 are ionic channels; 5-HT_4, 5-HT_6, and 5-HT_7 are positively coupled to adenylyl cyclase.
Data from Uhl JA: Phenytoin: the drug of choice in tricyclic antidepressant overdose? *Ann Emerg Med* 10(5):270, 1981; and Kulig K, Bar-Or, Wythe E, et al: Phenytoin as treatment for tricyclic antidepressant cardiotoxicity in a canine model. *Vet Hum Toxicol* 26:41, 1984, with permission.
cAMP, 3′,5′-cyclic adenosine monophosphate; CNS, central nervous system; 5-HT, serotonin; IP_3DG, inositol triphosphodiglyceride; mCPP, *m*-chlorophenyl piperazine; PNS, peripheral nervous system.

Cyclic antidepressants are well absorbed orally in therapeutic dosing; peak serum levels occur 2 to 6 hours after ingestion [33]. In overdose [33,34], gastrointestinal (GI) absorption may be delayed secondary to anticholinergic and antihistaminic properties of these drugs. Metabolism is predominately hepatic, with a small enterohepatic circulation [35,36]. Some cyclic antidepressants have active metabolites. The volume of distribution is large, with distribution occurring within the first several hours after ingestion [36]. Elimination half-life averages 8 to 30 hours but may be prolonged in overdose [37]. Elimination is hepatic, with minimal renal involvement. Fluoxetine has an active metabolite with an elimination half-life that extends into weeks. Cyclic antidepressants are extensively bound to serum proteins, particularly α_1-acid glycoprotein (AAG), and binding appears to be pH dependent [38]. MAO inhibitors are well absorbed orally with relatively short elimination half-lives [32]. Since the irreversible agents permanently inhibit the activity of MAO, their effects can last 4 to 6 weeks.

Toxicity from cyclic antidepressants results in CNS depression, seizures, hypotension, dysrhythmias, and cardiac conduction abnormalities [38]. Hyperthermia may occur as a result of increased muscle activity, seizures, and autonomic dysfunction [39]. These toxic effects are believed to have multiple etiologies, none of which has been fully elucidated.

Patients who ingest large amounts of cyclic antidepressants frequently present with hypotension. Several mechanisms have been suggested, including direct negative inotropic effects [17,25] and dysrhythmias, with subsequent decreases in filling time and cardiac output [39–41]. Receptor blockade produces vasodilation and autonomic dysfunction. In addition, blockade of the biogenic amine pump prevents adequate uptake and release of these neurotransmitters as active substances, thereby contributing to hypotension [11,16,40].

The CNS effects in cyclic antidepressant overdose can be quite profound. Although some of the newer cyclic antidepressants are less toxic in overdose, they can cause seizures and alteration in mental status [8,42,43]. The etiology of coma, seizures, and myoclonus is multifactorial and involves receptor blockade and direct membrane effects which all contribute to CNS derangements [42–45]. Cyclic antidepressants interact with both the $GABA_A$ and $GABA_B$-chloride ion channel in the CNS and may alter chloride flow across the receptor [46–48].

Dysrhythmias and conduction abnormalities often provide a clue to the recognition of cyclic antidepressant overdose. Action potential propagation, particularly in ventricular myocardial cells and the conduction system, is significantly affected by these drugs [49]. Cyclic antidepressants blunt phase 0 of the action potential depolarization by blocking the fast inward flux of sodium through the sodium channel [50]. This, in turn, slows the rate of rise of phase 0 (V_{max}) and slows overall action potential depolarization. As ventricular conduction slows, the QRS complex widens [50–52]. This also contributes to unidirectional blocks and reentrant dysrhythmias [52]. Because inward sodium flux is coupled to the calcium excitation in myocardial cells, the myocardial cells are unable to contract fully and become less efficient. A less toxic effect is seen on phase 4 of the action potential (spontaneous diastolic depolarization), leading to decreased automaticity [49]. Delayed repolarization occurs and may contribute to QTc interval prolongation, which has been associated with torsades de pointes [53–56]. Because cyclic antidepressants have their tightest myocardial binding during diastole, toxicity appears to be directly related to heart rate; in amitriptyline-poisoned dogs, increasing heart rate caused a decrease in V_{max} and widened the QRS complex [50–52,57,58]. Interventions that slowed the heart rate, such as beta-blockers, improved conduction but led to irreversible hypotension [53,57].

The decrease in V_{max} during phase 0 appears to be pH sensitive [51,53,58]. Alkalinization with molar sodium lactate, sodium bicarbonate, or hyperventilation, or increasing extracellular sodium concentration, produces an increase in the rate of rise of the action potential (V_{max}), narrows the QRS complex, decreases the incidence of ventricular tachycardia, and improves blood pressure [53,58–65]. These studies also show that decreasing pH worsens conduction abnormalities, produces hypotension, and increases the incidence of dysrhythmias. A combination of increased extracellular sodium and alkalosis (or hyperventilation plus sodium bicarbonate) in vitro has been shown to be equally and possibly more effective than either alone [52,58]. The use of lidocaine in animal studies decreased automaticity and ectopy and improved conduction. However, it did not have the same salutary effect on the blood pressure as alkalinization and may have worsened inotropy [58]. Although binding of cyclic antidepressants to AAG is increased at an alkalotic pH, infusion of AAG in animals to increase serum protein binding has not been shown to be beneficial [38].

SSRI toxicity results from exaggeration of its pharmacologic activity and is manifest as the serotonin syndrome. The pathophysiology is not fully understood but is believed to result from excessive 5-HT_{1A} stimulation, although dopamine and other neurotransmitters may be involved. The serotonin syndrome is associated with SSRI use alone, change in dose, overdose, or in combination with other agents [e.g., serotonin precursor or agonists, lithium, tricyclic antidepressants, 5-HT analogs, other SSRIs, meperidine, pentazocine, tramadol, cocaine, 3,4-methylenedioxy-*N*-methylamphetamine (Ecstasy), MAOIs, and herbal remedies such as St. John's Wart].

Two forms of toxicity are caused by MAOI: acute overdose and drug and food interactions. Toxicity from acute MAOI overdose results from the exaggerated pharmacologic effects of MAOI and may be associated with secondary complications [66]. The primary drug-drug interaction occurs when MAOI is taken with an indirectly acting sympathomimetic agent (e.g., ephedrine, phenylephrine, phenylpropanolamine, and amphetamine), which causes an NE surge in the peripheral sympathetic nerve terminals. MAOI and food interaction primarily involve the small amounts of tyramine or tryptophan that are normally present in certain foods (e.g., aged cheeses, smoked or pickled meats, yeast and meat extracts, red wines, Italian broad beans, pasteurized light and pale beers, and ripe avocados) and are often termed the *cheese reaction*. These indirectly acting agents are usually metabolized by MAO-A in the gut. When MAO-A is inhibited, tyramine absorption is unregulated, enters into the portal circulation, and causes release of stored catecholamines with resultant hypertensive response [67,68].

CLINICAL TOXICITY

The onset of symptoms from cyclic antidepressant overdose is rapid. Most patients who die from overdose do so before arriving at the hospital and after having ingested large (>1 g) amounts of drug [66]. Signs and symptoms usually occur within the first 6 hours after ingestion. Patients who survive the first 24 hours without hypoxic insult generally do well [66]. The progression of toxicity is rapid and unpredictable, with patients capable of deteriorating from an awake, alert state to seizures, hypotension, and dysrhythmias within 30 to 60 minutes and with minimal warning signs [6,69–75]. Cardiac arrest due to cyclic antidepressant poisoning may sometimes respond to prolonged resuscitative efforts. One case reports a patient who survived after a resuscitation of approximately 70 minutes [76].

Vital signs on presentation usually include tachycardia, although patients taking beta-blockers or those with underlying conduction blocks, or those in a premorbid state may present with bradycardia. Cyclic antidepressants without major antimuscarinic effects, such as trazodone, nefazodone, and the SSRIs, may not cause significant tachycardia. Bupropion-toxic patients almost always have vital signs reflecting a hyperadrenergic state [77–79]. Initial blood pressure may be elevated but can rapidly change to hypotension. The respiratory rate and body temperature may be elevated. If marked myoclonus or seizures develop, severe hyperthermia may result [39,43,71]. Cyclic antidepressants with prominent antimuscarinic effects may cause mydriasis, urinary retention, ileus, and cutaneous vasodilation (Table 123.2). Absence of these signs does not rule out cyclic antidepressant ingestion.

Dependent on the ingested agent, progression of toxicity may be precipitous and lead to coma, hypotension, seizures, dysrhythmia, and death. The newer agents (e.g., nefazodone, trazodone, the SSRIs) are more likely to be sedating and less likely to exhibit cardiovascular toxicity [69,70,73–75]. Maprotiline, venlafaxine, amoxapine, and loxapine tend to cause CNS toxicity before cardiovascular toxicity [71,80–92]. Bupropion may cause seizures in therapeutic dosing and exhibits a dose-dependent increase in toxicity (greater than 450 mg) [77,93,94]. With the cyclic antidepressants, it is unusual for patients to have significant cardiovascular disturbances without an altered mental status [10].

Cyclic antidepressant-induced seizures are generally single or brief flurries of motor activity. However, status epilepticus may occur without any prodrome, and this is especially true with amoxapine, loxapine, or bupropion. Status epilepticus may be difficult to treat; if prolonged, it leads to overall deterioration in the patient's condition, particularly with cyclic agents [25,77,93–102].

Signs of cardiovascular toxicity may exist even with therapeutic dosing of classic cyclic antidepressants. A prolonged QTc interval and sinus tachycardia may be observed on the electrocardiogram (ECG) in non-overdose states [103]. Sinus tachycardia is frequently the presenting dysrhythmia; aberrancy and ventricular tachycardia develop with increasing toxicity. As cardiovascular toxicity progresses, the frontal plane axis shifts rightward. This is gradually followed by repolarization abnormalities, intraventricular conduction delays, ventricular dysrhythmia, high-grade atrioventricular blocks, profound bradycardias, and asystole [40,104–108]. Trazodone, citalopram, and escitalopram may cause marked QTc interval prolongation and torsades de pointes (polymorphous) ventricular tachycardia in the absence of other ECG abnormalities [109].

Many of the cyclic antidepressants show early changes to the ECG axis. The terminal 40 milliseconds of the frontal plane QRS complex shifts to a rightward vector of 130 to 270 degrees. If computerized vector analysis is not available, a widened slurred S wave in leads I and aVL and an R wave in aVR represent this vector. Looking for these changes in overdosed or comatose patients may help in establishing a diagnosis. However, a small portion of the population normally has this unusual vector. Patients with extreme leftward axis deviation as a baseline may not show the rightward change with cyclic antidepressant toxicity [70,74,99,110–113]. The absence of this finding does not rule out a classic cyclic antidepressant poisoning; its presence with coma, seizures, dysrhythmias, or hypotension is very suggestive of cyclic antidepressant toxicity [69].

The serotonin syndrome varies from mild to life threatening. Classic manifestations are altered mental status, autonomic dysfunction, and neuromuscular irritability. Signs and symptoms include tachycardia, unstable blood pressure, hyperthermia, mydriasis, diaphoresis, blurred vision, nausea, vomiting, diarrhea, shivering, tremor, incoordination, hyperreflexia, myoclonus, rigidity, agitation, confusion, delirium, seizure, and coma. Lactic acidosis, rhabdomyolysis, myoglobinuria, and multiorgan failure may develop in severe cases [101,114,115].

SSRIs, except for venlafaxine, citalopram, and escitalopram [101,109], are expected to have minimal cardiac effects. Citalopram, escitalopram, and ritanserin may significantly affect the QTc with at least one case of arrhythmia reported from citalopram [109]. Overdoses with extremely large amounts of fluoxetine and citalopram have caused atrial fibrillation and bradycardias. Evidence of Na^+ and Ca^{2+} channel blockade has been shown at extremely high serum levels [89]. Animal experiments with paroxetine required much larger doses, compared to amitriptyline, to induce dysrhythmias [6,7,82–89,91].

The onset of MAOI and food or drug interaction usually occurs within 30 to 60 minutes of ingesting the offending substance. Signs and symptoms of this type of reaction include hypertension, tachycardia or reflex bradycardia, severe (occipital) headache, nausea and vomiting, hyperthermia, altered mental status, seizures, intracranial hemorrhage, and death.

Patients with acute MAOI overdoses may be asymptomatic on presentation. Signs and symptoms typically develop within 6 to 12 hours of ingestion if the person is on the medication chronically but may be delayed for 24 hours if this is a new medication for the patient. An initial stage of neuromuscular excitation such as agitation, tremors, myoclonus, and hyperreflexia with hypertension usually occurs. The face may be flushed. As toxicity progresses, the mental status deteriorates, and there is a general elevation of all vital signs. Seizures may develop. As monoamine neurotransmitters become depleted, hypotension and cardiovascular collapse may ensue. Respiratory depression may occur and the mental status will deteriorate. If the patient survives this progression, there may be secondary complications from rhabdomyolysis, electrolyte abnormalities, lactic acidosis, and multiple organ system failure. Toxicity may last for up to 72 hours [66]. MAOI ingestions can be very challenging to manage as the patient can variably show either a hyperadrenergic state or a catecholamine depleted state. The swings in the vital signs can be rapid, unexpected, and uncontrolled [116–118].

Secondary complications, such as noncardiogenic pulmonary edema, aspiration pneumonia, and rhabdomyolysis, frequently develop in patients with antidepressant overdoses. Overdoses with agents that have prominent antimuscarinic properties (e.g., amitriptyline) may cause urinary retention, ileus, and abdominal distention. Although rare, tardive dyskinesia, neuroleptic malignant syndrome, and the syndrome of inappropriate antidiuretic hormone secretion all have been reported in association with cyclic antidepressant overdose [39,119–122]. In addition to causing seizures and cardiovascular toxicity, venlafaxine may cause direct muscle toxicity leading to severe rhabdomyolysis [123].

In therapeutic doses, cyclic antidepressant agents and SSRIs may interact with other medications, increasing the effect of one or both agents. This effect may be magnified after an overdose. Drug interactions may alter metabolism, elimination, or the free fraction of the drug. Most antidepressants are metabolized through the CYP 2D6 microsomal agents and as such, are subject to induction and interference. Agents that stimulate the hepatic P450 microsomal system (phenobarbital, carbamazepine, phenytoin, and rifampin, and cigarette smoking) increase the clearance of cyclic antidepressants. Cimetidine, as a competitor for the hepatic microsomal enzymes, leads to an increase in cyclic antidepressant levels. The coadministration of cyclic antidepressants and antipsychotic agents may lead to competitive inhibition of the metabolism of both drugs. Other medications that increase the steady-state levels of cyclic antidepressants include chloramphenicol and disulfiram, whereas erythromycin decreases the level. Acute ethanol intoxication may decrease cyclic antidepressant metabolism, resulting in markedly prolonged serum drug half-life [106].

Patients taking MAOIs should avoid any agents that have serotonergic effects or act as indirect sympathomimetics (e.g., amphetamine, ephedrine, dopamine, phenylpropanolamine, meperidine, tramadol, dextromethorphan, and St. John's wort) [124–126]. Similar effects have been reported with paroxetine with the use of phenobarbital, cimetidine, and phenytoin. The potential exists for the potentiation of warfarin effect when they are administered in conjunction with paroxetine. The interaction of fluoxetine and cyclic antidepressants causes an increase in serum levels of the cyclic antidepressant and can lead to cyclic antidepressant toxicity. Therapeutic administration of an SSRI and a cyclic antidepressant with strong serotonergic effects (e.g., clomipramine) or two SSRIs may induce the serotonergic syndrome. The interaction of MAOIs and cyclic antidepressants may lead to significant and life-threatening toxicity, particularly with those antidepressants that have predominantly serotonergic effect (trazodone, clomipramine, and the SSRIs) [29]. The administration of the selective MAO-B inhibitor selegiline with an SSRI or a cyclic antidepressants does not appear to have as strong a serotonergic effect but still may cause drug interactions [127].

Although the differential diagnosis includes many substances that share some of the effects of cyclic antidepressants, duplicating the entire constellation of signs and symptoms is relatively unusual. Like cyclic antidepressants, anticholinergic and antihistaminic medications can cause dilated pupils, GI hypomotility, confusion, and seizures. Phenothiazines also cause these effects and may increase the QTc. Thioridazine and mesoridazine, two phenothiazines, prolong the QRS and QTc. The atypical neuroleptics (risperidone and olanzapine) have similar sedative, cardiac, and movement effects. Other drugs that affect QRS width include type IA antiarrhythmics (quinidine, procainamide, and disopyramide) and type IC antiarrhythmics (flecainide, encainide, and propafenone). Hyperkalemia and hypocalcemia also widen the QRS complex, and the latter can cause muscle twitching and myoclonus. Beta-blockers, particularly propranolol, cause seizures and conduction abnormalities in overdose. Tramadol, an opiate analgesic that also causes biogenic amine reuptake inhibition, may cause opioid and serotonergic toxicity, especially when given in conjunction with an SSRI or MAOI. Cyclobenzaprine, a muscle relaxant, and carbamazepine share the cyclic antidepressant structure and can cause a similar picture with sedation, hypotension, and prolonged QTc interval.

DIAGNOSTIC EVALUATION

Patients with suspected cyclic antidepressant overdose should have routine blood analyses. Stress leukocytosis may occur with any antidepressant overdoses, especially if seizures have occurred. Electrolyte, blood urea nitrogen, creatinine, and glucose levels should be determined, with special attention to the anion gap. Because rhabdomyolysis may occur, most frequently with seizures, creatinine kinase should be followed [39,119]. Urinalysis is also useful in the diagnosis of rhabdomyolysis and possible myoglobinuric renal failure. Frequent ECGs are a necessity and should be done any time that the patient has a change in status. Arterial blood gas and chest radiograph should be obtained as clinically indicated. Since repetitive arterial sampling may be extremely painful and is sometimes

TABLE 123.5

DRUGS THAT MAY INTERFERE WITH THE TRICYCLIC ANTIDEPRESSANT QUALITATIVE DRUG SCREEN

Drugs	Minimal serum concentration level
Carbamazepine	Therapeutic range
Chlorpromazine	Therapeutic range
Cyclobenzaprine	10 to 20 μg/L
Cyproheptadine	390 to 400 μg/L
Diphenhydramine	>120 μg/L
Quetiapine	Therapeutic range
Thioridazine	Therapeutic range

associated to complications such as infection, injury, and thrombosis [128], and since venous pH has shown to strongly correlate that of an arterial sample in cyclic antidepressant overdose [128], using venous blood for the serial measurement of serum pH is recommended.

Quantitative tricyclic antidepressant levels rarely if ever contribute to the clinical patient management. Although total tricyclic levels of more than 1,000 ng per mL have been associated with significant toxicity [33,36,69,105,108], there is poor correlation between toxicity and serum level. Repeated levels during resolution of toxicity may be misleading; physical signs of toxicity abate before a significant drop in serum levels because of the prolonged elimination half-life and extensive protein binding [36]. A qualitative screen using a tricyclic antidepressant immunoassay is usually sufficient. However, other drugs that have structural similarity can produce a false-positive result (Table 123.5) [129–135] and if clinical findings are inconsistent with immunoassay results, it may be necessary to perform a more specific test such as gas chromatography with mass spectrometry. Although a toxicology testing is discretionary, acetaminophen and salicylate levels and a pregnancy test in a woman of childbearing age should always be checked.

MANAGEMENT

Patients who have ingested cyclic antidepressants require immediate evaluation and stabilization. Those who are awake and alert should receive an oral dose of activated charcoal. Patients who have ingested a classic agent (amitriptyline, nortriptyline, imipramine, desipramine, clomipramine, doxepin, dothiepin, protriptyline, and maprotiline) can be safely observed in the emergency department if they are asymptomatic. An asymptomatic patient implies one with a normal ECG throughout the observation period, a mild sinus tachycardia that resolves within the first 1 to 2 hours, clear mental status, and a nontoxic acetaminophen level. This observation period is defined as a 6-hour interval during which the patient is on continuous ECG monitoring and has intravenous access in place [49,105,119,120,136,137,139,141]. In addition, these patients must have had adequate GI decontamination and, preferably, have passed a charcoal stool. Patients should always be referred for psychiatric evaluation and pregnant women should be directed to prenatal counseling.

No consensus has been reached on emergency department observation for patients with ingestions of bupropion, trazodone, nefazodone, venlafaxine, and the SSRIs because of the paucity of overdose data for these medications [80,82,141,142]. Observation of asymptomatic patients for 6 to 8 hours or until the ECG returns to normal or baseline is reasonable. Any patient with signs or symptoms of toxicity should be admitted to the intensive care unit. Admission (or prolonged observation) is also prudent for patients with sustained-release bupropion overdose, as seizures have been reported as far as 12 to 16 hours after ingestion [141].

Symptomatic patients should have a rapid evaluation of the airway and, if obtunded or hypoventilating, be immediately intubated. Because cyclic antidepressant toxicity increases with acidemia, an ABG demonstrating a pH <7.4 or hypercarbia should prompt intubation and hyperventilation even in the patient who is able to protect his or her airway. Once an airway is established, the patient should be appropriately ventilated to prevent respiratory acidosis and subsequent deterioration of his or her condition. If the patient has an altered mental status, a rapid bedside determination of serum glucose or administration of 25 to 50 g dextrose (0.5 to 1.0 g per kg), 2 mg naloxone, and 100 mg thiamine should be given intravenously [34].

GI decontamination for severely ill patients should consist of activated charcoal with or without gastric lavage. Because some cyclic antidepressants have a small enterohepatic circulation, an additional one to two doses of aqueous charcoal (25 g) may be considered [36,138–140]. This dose should not be administered in the presence of an ileus or gastric distention. Because the majority of these agents are extensively protein bound, hemodialysis and hemoperfusion are not effective in reducing the toxic effects of cyclic antidepressants [143–146].

Single or brief flurries of seizures should be treated with a benzodiazepine [26,45,143]. Seizures are frequently isolated, and the additional use of an anticonvulsant is not indicated in this situation. Status epilepticus should be aggressively managed to prevent the development of acidosis, hyperthermia, and rhabdomyolysis [26]. As cardiotoxicity worsens dramatically in the presence of acidemia, rapid control of seizures is mandatory. Status epilepticus should be managed with large doses of benzodiazepines [143]. Failing this, management becomes controversial. Administering a nondepolarizing short-acting neuromuscular blocking agent such as vecuronium along with a barbiturate anticonvulsant (e.g., phenobarbital, 15 to 20 mg per kg, or thiopental, 3 to 5 mg per kg) is one option [146,148]. Chemical paralysis helps treat or prevent hyperthermia, rhabdomyolysis, acidosis, and further deterioration. If available, continuous electroencephalographic monitoring should be used. If the patient continues to have seizure activity once the paralytic has worn off, an additional dose of vecuronium should be given and an alternative anticonvulsant or general anesthesia should be administered [26,81,146–149]. Propofol may be useful since it has both GABA and NMDA activity but there are no data on its use in this setting. Serum alkalinization does not affect seizure activity [146].

Hypotension often responds to fluid resuscitation. Because concomitant acidosis or abnormal cardiac conduction is often present, a sodium bicarbonate solution can be used for both fluid resuscitation and serum alkalinization. A solution of 1,000 mL dextrose 5% in water with 150 mEq $NaHCO_3$ (roughly equivalent to 0.9% NaCl) is suggested. The rate of fluid administration should be adjusted to maintain a serum pH of 7.45 to 7.55 without causing hypernatremia. In an adult, an initial rate of approximately 200 to 300 mL per hour (1.5 to 2.0 times maintenance fluids) is usually adequate. Many clinicians give boluses of sodium bicarbonate (44 to 50 mEq per bolus) to achieve the same effect.

In the event of refractory hypotension, invasive monitoring (arterial line, central venous pressure, or Swan–Ganz catheterization) may be necessary. Pressor therapy with direct-acting sympathomimetics, such as NE (Levophed™), phenylephrine (Neo-Synephrine™), or epinephrine, has been shown to be more effective than indirect-acting agents, such as dopamine [26,142,150,151]. In experimental rat models, the combination of epinephrine and sodium bicarbonate increased survival and decreased the frequency of arrhythmias [142]. Moreover, this duo drug regimen was found to be more efficacious than the combination of sodium bicarbonate and norepinephrine [152]. If hypotension remains refractory, an inotropic agent such as dobutamine may be required [142,150,151]. If the patient still persists with severe hypotension, then the use of vasopressin in addition to the use of fluids, bicarbonate, and vasopressors may be warranted. Vasopressin has been shown to sustain blood pressure and improve organ perfusion in several critical care settings, including once case study that showed immediate success in a patient who overdosed on amitriptyline [152,153]. Unlike other conventional treatments that are dependent on the catecholamine receptors, vasopressin works directly on the smooth muscle causing an influx of calcium into the cell, resulting in vasoconstriction [154]. This mechanism is mediated via the G-receptor protein, called V1. The dose required to see significant improvement is still unclear, but most authors suggest dose <0.4 U per minute to minimize the possible adverse effects such as end organ vasoconstriction and platelet aggregation [155].

Abnormal conduction (QRS complex >100 milliseconds in the limb leads) and ventricular dysrhythmias are treated with alkalinization. A combination of sodium bicarbonate infusion and hyperventilation may be more useful than either alone, although hyperventilation is effective if the patient cannot tolerate the sodium load [51,58,60,62,150]. By combining the two modalities, the arterial partial pressure of carbon dioxide can be maintained at approximately 30 to 35 mm Hg, which prevents cerebral vasoconstriction, while serum sodium is kept within reasonable limits. Optimal arterial pH is between 7.45 and 7.55. Ventricular dysrhythmias that are not responsive to alkalinization may respond to lidocaine or hypertonic saline. Other than β-adrenergic blockers, no antidysrhythmics have been studied; although phenytoin has been used anecdotally (see the Controversies section). In animal studies, propranolol was effective in improving conduction but led to intractable hypotension [51,58,59]. Other type IA and IC antidysrhythmics are contraindicated because they worsen cardiotoxicity. Amiodarone, a class III antidysrhythmic, was found to be of no benefit in TCA-poisoned animal models. In addition, it was felt that the use of amiodarone may have been detrimental because it can further prolong the QTc interval and cause negative inotropy [156]. The successful use of magnesium sulfate was reported in a 23-month-old child who presented with ventricular tachycardia after ingesting unknown amounts of amitriptyline. The child had received normal saline, lidocaine, bicarbonate infusion, and cardioversion without effect. Subsequent magnesium sulfate resulted in normalization of the cardiac rhythm and clinical improvement [76]. Overdrive pacing is another option, but controlled studies are lacking [54].

More recently, the use of intralipids in the clinical scenario of lipid-soluble drug toxicity such as local anesthetics and calcium channel blockers, have been gaining wide acceptance in the practice of critical care and emergency medicine [144,157–160]). Numerous studies have demonstrated significant cardiovascular improvement with severe lipid-soluble drug toxicity when infused with lipid emulsions. Most cyclic antidepressants are lipid soluble and produce significant cardiovascular instability and collapse that may be refractory to standard measures and sodium bicarbonate therapy. In animal models, infusion with intralipids proved to be more potent in reversing cardiac arrest and hypotension and also preventing further cardiovascular collapse [144,157]. Currently, there are two theories that explain why lipid emulsions may be effective. The first theory is based on the fact that the intralipids create a lipid basin that sequesters lipid-soluble drugs away from their site of action. The second theory is that lipid emulsions provide relief to a stressed myocardium by providing high energy to the heart [157,158]. This concept is similar to the use of high-dose insulin regimen for calcium channel blockers toxicity. In conclusion, intralipid infusion should be strongly considered when conventional treatments such as oxygen therapy, fluids, vasopressors, and sodium bicarbonate have failed to provide significant results.

Treatment of the serotonin syndrome is primarily supportive. Sedation, paralysis, intubation and ventilation, anticonvulsants, antihypertensives, and aggressive rapid cooling may all be necessary. Some success has been achieved with the nonspecific serotonin antagonist cyproheptadine (4 to 12 mg every 8 hours orally or 4 mg per hour) [114,115]. Dopamine-2-receptor antagonists, such as haloperidol, have occasionally been effective, but safety and efficacy data are lacking. Bromocriptine increases brain serotonin levels and is contraindicated, and dantrolene may enhance brain 5-HT metabolism and should not be used.

Any patient with an acute MAOI overdose or persistent signs and symptoms from food or drug interactions should be admitted to an intensive care setting for at least 24 hours. Therapy for food or drug interactions is aimed at lowering the blood pressure. A rapidly direct-acting agent that is easy to titrate is recommended (e.g., nitroprusside or nitroglycerine).

Treatment of MAOI overdose is entirely supportive. Muscular hyperactivity and seizures are treated with high-dose benzodiazepines. Hyperthermia that does not respond to benzodiazepine therapy and cooling requires rapid-sequence intubation and paralysis with a nondepolarizing agent to completely shut down muscle activity. Bromocriptine should not be used, as it has drug interactions and is an uncontrolled D_2 agonist and stimulant. Dantrolene is ineffective as it works peripherally and does not affect the central causes of hyperthermia [66,161–163]. Symptomatic or severe cardiovascular (sympathetic) hyperactivity should be treated with agents that have readily reversible effects and can be titrated to response. Agents such as nitroprusside, nitroglycerine, and esmolol are recommended. Nicardipine can also be used. For cardiovascular depression, direct-acting agents, such as epinephrine, norepinephrine, and isoproterenol, are preferred. Although MAO inhibition may prolong their effects, these agents are also metabolized by catechol-*O*-methyltransferase.

With the exception of MAOI overdosed patients, those who survive the first 24 hours without major complications (hypoxia, prolonged seizures, profound acidosis, and hyperthermia) generally do well. Most patients show some improvement within 24 hours. Once cardiac conduction improves (narrowing of QRS complex to 100 milliseconds), alkalinization can be discontinued (usually within 12 hours) and the pH allowed to normalize. If the QRS complex again widens, alkalinization should be resumed and the weaning process repeated. Once the ECG has normalized without alkalinization, the patient should be monitored for an additional 12 to 24 hours in the intensive care unit. The patient should be awake and alert and have passed a charcoal stool before transfer out of the unit. All overdose patients should be referred for psychiatric evaluation before discharge [6,104–106].

OTHER MANAGEMENT CONSIDERATIONS

Controversial or investigational therapies for cyclic antidepressant poisoning include phenytoin, physostigmine, prophylactic alkalinization, mechanical cardiovascular support, antibody therapy, and adenosine antagonists. Although phenytoin binds to voltage-dependent Na^+ channels and prevents propagation of seizures, it has no GABA effect and does not prevent toxic seizures. Some animal studies suggested that phenytoin was effective but others did not [151,164]. Studies using phenytoin to improve cardiac conduction were poorly controlled and not reproducible [105,147,164–166]. Canine data showed that phenytoin transiently facilitates conduction but then increases the incidence and duration of ventricular tachycardia and does not improve survival, suggesting that phenytoin is potentially detrimental [164].

Physostigmine (see Chapter 121) has been used to antagonize the antimuscarinic effects of cyclic antidepressants such as agitated delirium [147,167–169]. However, bradycardia and asystole have been reported with physostigmine in the presence of aberrant conduction, and as a carbamate, it may precipitate seizures [65]. Thus, physostigmine is not advocated to treat acute cyclic antidepressant overdose [169] and is contraindicated in those with cardiac conduction disturbances.

No studies have been done regarding prophylactic alkalinization in patients with normal cardiac condition. Because altering the pH alters the reliability of the QRS width as a predictor of cardiotoxicity, such therapy is not recommended. Alkalinization is also not without risks, including hyperosmolality, cerebral vasoconstriction, and alterations in ionized calcium concentrations. There is no evidence that it affects the seizure threshold.

In moribund patients in whom conventional therapy has failed, the use of mechanical circulatory support, such as intraaortic balloon pump assist or partial cardiac bypass, may be life-saving. In this situation, the use of extracorporeal measures supports myocardial, hepatic, and cerebral perfusion while allowing the liver endogenously to detoxify the cyclic antidepressant [170].

Adenosine receptors may be involved in cyclic antidepressant-induced cardiovascular toxicity. Adenosine receptor activation has been shown to cause peripheral vasodilation, decrease in cardiac output, and degranulation of mast cells [171]. In animals with cyclic antidepressant poisoning, adenosine receptor antagonists have reversed hypotension and QRS prolongation [171].

References

1. Bronstein AC, Spyker DA, Cantilena LR Jr, et al: 2007 Annual Report of the American Association of Poison Control Centers' National Poison Data System (NPDS): 25th Annual Report. *Clin Toxicol (Philadelphia)* 46(10):927–1057, 2008.
2. Kosten TR, Rounsaville BJ, Babor TF, et al: A preliminary study of desipramine in the treatment of cocaine abuse in methadone maintenance patients. *Br J Psychiatry* 151:834–843, 1987.
3. Richardson JW III, Richelson E: Antidepressants: a clinical update for medical practitioners. *Mayo Clin Proc* 59(5):330–337, 1984.
4. Richelson E: Antimuscarinic and other receptor-blocking properties of antidepressants. *Mayo Clin Proc* 58(1):40–46, 1983.
5. Cole JO: Where are those new antidepressants we were promised? *Arch Gen Psychiatry* 45(2):193–194, 1988.
6. Hayes PE, CA: Kristoff, Adverse reactions to five new antidepressants. *Clin Pharm* 5(6):471–480, 1986.
7. Stark P, Fuller RW, Wong DT: The pharmacologic profile of fluoxetine. *J Clin Psychiatry* 46(3 Pt 2):7–13, 1985.
8. Kulig K: Management of poisoning associated with "newer" antidepressant agents. *Ann Emerg Med* 15(9):1039–1045, 1986.
9. Knudsen K, Heath A: Effects of self poisoning with maprotiline. *Br Med J (Clin Res Ed)* 288(6417):601–603, 1984.
10. Settle E: Bupropion: a novel antidepressant—update 1989. *Int Drug Ther News* 24:29, 1989.
11. Richelson E: Pharmacology of antidepressants. *Psychopathology* 20[Suppl 1]:1–12, 1987.
12. Richelson E: The newer antidepressants: structures, pharmacokinetics, pharmacodynamics, and proposed mechanisms of action. *Psychopharmacol Bull* 20(2):213–223, 1984.
13. Wander TJ, Nelson A, Okazaki H, et al: Antagonism by antidepressants of serotonin S1 and S2 receptors of normal human brain in vitro. *Eur J Pharmacol* 132(2–3):115–121, 1986.
14. Snyder SH, Yamamura HI: Antidepressants and the muscarinic acetylcholine receptor. *Arch Gen Psychiatry* 34(2):236–239, 1977.
15. Tetrud JW, Langston JW: The effect of deprenyl (selegiline) on the natural history of Parkinson's disease. *Science* 245(4917):519–522, 1989.
16. Collis MG, Shepherd JT: Antidepressant drug action and presynaptic alpha-receptors. *Mayo Clin Proc* 55(9):567–572, 1980.
17. Follmer CH, Lum BK: Protective action of diazepam and of sympathomimetic amines against amitriptyline-induced toxicity. *J Pharmacol Exp Ther* 222(2):424–429, 1982.
18. Richelson E, Nelson A: Antagonism by antidepressants of neurotransmitter receptors of normal human brain in vitro. *J Pharmacol Exp Ther* 230(1):94–102, 1984.
19. Schwartz R, Esler M: Catecholamine levels in tricyclic antidepressant self-poisoning. *Aust N Z J Med* 4(5):479, 1974.
20. Blackwell B: Adverse effects of antidepressant drugs. Part 1: monoamine oxidase inhibitors and tricyclics. *Drugs* 21(3).201–219, 1981.
21. Blackwell B, Marley E: Interactions of cheese and of its constituents with monoamine oxidase inhibitors. *Br J Pharmacol Chemother* 26(1):120–141, 1966.
22. Smith C: The role of monoamine oxidase in the intraneuronal metabolism of norepinephrine released by indirectly acting sympathomimetic amines or by adrenergic nerve stimulation. *J Pharmacol Exp Ther* 151:207, 1966.
23. Hill S, Yau K, Whitwam J: MAOIs to RIMAs in anaesthesia—a literature review. *Psychopharmacology (Berl)* 106[Suppl]:S43–S45, 1992.
24. Olson KBN, Pentel P: Survey of causes and consequences of seizures during drug intoxication. *Vet Hum Toxicol* 24:23, 1982.
25. Rudorfer MV: Cardiovascular changes and plasma drug levels after amitriptyline overdose. *J Toxicol Clin Toxicol* 19(1):67–78, 1982.
26. Roszkowski AP, Schuler ME, Schultz R: Augmentation of pentylenetetrazol induced seizures by tricyclic antidepressants. *Mater Med Pol* 8(2):141–145, 1976.
27. Weinberger J, Nicklas WJ, Berl S: Mechanism of action of anticonvulsants. Role of the differential effects on the active uptake of putative neurotransmitters. *Neurology* 26(2):162–166, 1976.
28. Leonard BE: Pharmacological differences of serotonin reuptake inhibitors and possible clinical relevance. *Drugs* 43[Suppl 2]:3–9; discussion 9–10, 1992.
29. Dechant KL, Clissold SP: Paroxetine. A review of its pharmacodynamic and pharmacokinetic properties, and therapeutic potential in depressive illness. *Drugs* 41(2):225–253, 1991.
30. Baldessarini R: Drugs and treatment of psychiatric disorders, in Hardman J, Limbird LE, Molinoff PB (eds.): *Goodman and Gilman's The Pharmacological Basis of Therapeutics.* 1st ed. New York, Mc-Graw Hill, 1996, p 1.
31. Wells DG, Bjorksten AR: Monoamine oxidase inhibitors revisited. *Can J Anaesth* 36(1):64–74, 1989.
32. Mahmood I: Clinical pharmacokinetics and pharmacodynamics of selegiline. An update. *Clin Pharmacokinet* 33(2):91–102, 1997.
33. Perry PJ, Pfohl BM, Holstad SG: The relationship between antidepressant response and tricyclic antidepressant plasma concentrations. A retrospective analysis of the literature using logistic regression analysis. *Clin Pharmacokinet* 13(6):381–392, 1987.
34. Alvan G: Effect of activated charcoal on plasma levels of nortriptyline after single dose in man. *Eur J Clin Pharmacol* 5:236, 1973.
35. Bickel MH, Baggiolini M: The metabolism of imipramine and its metabolites by rat liver microsomes. *Biochem Pharmacol* 15(8):1155–1169, 1966.
36. Gard H, Knapp D, Walle T, et al: Qualitative and quantitative studies on the disposition of amitriptyline and other tricyclic antidepressant drugs in man as it relates to the management of the overdosed patient. *Clin Toxicol* 6(4):571–584, 1973.
37. Gram LF, Bjerre M, Kragh-Sørensen P, et al: Imipramine metabolites in blood of patients during therapy and after overdose. *Clin Pharmacol Ther* 33(3):335–342, 1983.
38. Seaberg DC, Weiss LD, Yealy DM, et al: Effects of alpha-1-acid glycoprotein on the cardiovascular toxicity of nortriptyline in a swine model. *Vet Hum Toxicol* 33(3):226–230, 1991.
39. Rosenberg J, Pentel P, Pond S, et al: Hyperthermia associated with drug intoxication. *Crit Care Med* 14(11):964–969, 1986.
40. Langou RA, Van Dyke C, Tahan SR, et al: Cardiovascular manifestations of tricyclic antidepressant overdose. *Am Heart J* 100(4):458–464, 1980.
41. Janowsky D, Curtis G, Zisook S, et al: Trazodone-aggravated ventricular arrhythmias. *J Clin Psychopharmacol* 3(6):372–376, 1983.
42. Kulig K, Rumack BH, Sullivan JB Jr, et al: Amoxapine overdose. Coma and seizures without cardiotoxic effects. *JAMA* 248(9):1092–1094, 1982.
43. Lesar T, Kingston R, Dahms R, et al: Trazodone overdose. *Ann Emerg Med* 12(4):221–223, 1983.
44. Dallos V, Heathfield K: Iatrogenic epilepsy due to antidepressant drugs. *Br Med J* 4(675):80–82, 1969.
45. Ellison DW, Pentel PR: Clinical features and consequences of seizures due to cyclic antidepressant overdose. *Am J Emerg Med* 7(1):5–10, 1989.
46. Pratt GD, Bowery NG: Repeated administration of desipramine and a GABAB receptor antagonist, CGP 36742, discretely up-regulates GABAB receptor binding sites in rat frontal cortex. *Br J Pharmacol* 110(2):724–735, 1993.
47. Malatynska E, Miller C, Schindler N, et al: Amitriptyline increases GABA-stimulated 36Cl-influx by recombinant (alpha 1 gamma 2) GABAA receptors. *Brain Res* 851(1–2):277–280, 1999.

48. Malatynska E, Giroux ML, Dilsaver SC, et al: Chronic treatment with amitriptyline alters the GABA-mediated uptake of 36Cl- in the rat brain. *Pharmacol Biochem Behav* 39(2):553–556, 1991.
49. Connolly SJ, Mitchell LB, Swedlow CD, et al: Clinical efficacy and electrophysiology of imipramine for ventricular tachycardia. *Am J Cardiol* 53(4):516–521, 1984.
50. Glassman AH: Cardiovascular effects of tricyclic antidepressant. *Annu Rev Med* 35:503, 1984.
51. Nattel S, Keable H, Sasyniuk BI: Experimental amitriptyline intoxication: electrophysiologic manifestations and management. *J Cardiovasc Pharmacol* 6(1):83–89, 1984.
52. Sasyniuk BI, Jhamandas V, Valois M: Experimental amitriptyline intoxication: treatment of cardiac toxicity with sodium bicarbonate. *Ann Emerg Med* 15(9):1052–1059, 1986.
53. Byrne JE, Gomoll AW: Differential effects of trazodone and imipramine on intracardiac conduction in the anesthetized dog. *Arch Int Pharmacodyn Ther* 259(2):259–270, 1982.
54. Davison ET: Amitriptyline-induced Torsade de Pointes. Successful therapy with atrial pacing. *J Electrocardiol* 18(3):299–301, 1985.
55. Herrmann HC, Kaplan LM, Bierer BE: Q-T prolongation and torsades de pointes ventricular tachycardia produced by the tetracyclic antidepressant agent maprotiline. *Am J Cardiol* 51(5):904–906, 1983.
56. Vlay SC, Friedling S: Trazodone exacerbation of VT. *Am Heart J* 106(3): 604, 1983.
57. Nattel S: Frequency-dependent effects of amitriptyline on ventricular conduction and cardiac rhythm in dogs. *Circulation* 72(4):898–906, 1985.
58. Nattel S, Mittleman M: Treatment of ventricular tachyarrhythmias resulting from amitriptyline toxicity in dogs. *J Pharmacol Exp Ther* 231(2):430–435, 1984.
59. Freeman JW, Loughhead MG: Beta blockade in the treatment of tricyclic antidepressant overdosage. *Med J Aust* 1(25):1233–1235, 1973.
60. Bajaj AK, Woosley RL, Roden DM: Acute electrophysiologic effects of sodium administration in dogs treated with O-desmethyl encainide. *Circulation* 80(4):994–1002, 1989.
61. Bessen HA, Niemann JT: Improvement of cardiac conduction after hyperventilation in tricyclic antidepressant overdose. *J Toxicol Clin Toxicol* 23 (7–8):537–546, 1985.
62. Bessen HA, Niemann JT, Haskell, et al: Effect of respiratory alkalosis in tricyclic antidepressant overdose. *West J Med* 139(3):373–376, 1983.
63. Tobis JM, Aronow WS: Cardiotoxicity of amitriptyline and doxepin. *Clin Pharmacol Ther* 29(3):359–364, 1981.
64. Bellet S, Hamdan G, Somlyo A, et al: The reversal of cardiotoxic effects of quinidine by molar sodium lactate: an experimental study. *Am J Med Sci* 237:165, 1959.
65. Kingston M: Hyperventilation in tricyclic antidepressant poisoning. *Crit Care Med* 7(12):550, 1979.
66. Linden CH, Rumack BH, Strehlke C: Monoamine oxidase inhibitor overdose. *Ann Emerg Med* 13(12):1137–1144, 1984.
67. McCabe BJ: Dietary tyramine and other pressor amines in MAOI regimens: a review. *J Am Diet Assoc* 86(8):1059–1064, 1986.
68. Norberg KA: Drug-induced changes in monoamine levels in the sympathetic adrenergic ganglion cells and terminals. A histochemical study. *Acta Physiol Scand* 65(3):221–234, 1965.
69. Caravati EM, Bossart PJ: Demographic and electrocardiographic factors associated with severe tricyclic antidepressant toxicity. *J Toxicol Clin Toxicol* 29(1):31–43, 1991.
70. Groleau G, Jotte R, Barish R: The electrocardiographic manifestations of cyclic antidepressant therapy and overdose: a review. *J Emerg Med* 8(5):597–605, 1990.
71. Wedin GP, Oderda GM, Klein-Schwart W, et al: Relative toxicity of cyclic antidepressants. *Ann Emerg Med* 15(7):797–804, 1986.
72. Hulten B-A, Adams R, Askenasi VD, et al: Predicting severity of tricyclic antidepressant overdose. *J Toxicol Clin Toxicol* 30(2):161, 1992.
73. Rasmussen J: Amitriptyline and imipramine poisoning. *Lancet* 2(7417): 850, 1965.
74. Shannon M: Duration of QRS disturbances after severe tricyclic antidepressant intoxication. *J Toxicol Clin Toxicol* 30(3):377, 1992.
75. Hulten BA, Heath A, Knudsen K, et al: Severe amitriptyline overdose: relationship between toxicokinetics and toxicodynamics. *J Toxicol Clin Toxicol* 30(2):171, 1992.
76. Citak A, Soysal DD, Ucsel R, et al: Efficacy of long duration resuscitation and magnesium sulphate treatment in amitriptyline poisoning. *Eur J Emerg Med* 9(1):63–66, 2002.
77. Shepherd G: Adverse effects associated with extra doses of bupropion. *Pharmacotherapy* 25(10):1378–1382, 2005.
78. Shepherd G, Velez LI, Keyes DC: Intentional bupropion overdoses. *J Emerg Med* 27(2):147–151, 2004.
79. Isbister GK, Balit CR: Bupropion overdose: QTc prolongation and its clinical significance. *Ann Pharmacother* 37(7–8):999–1002, 2003.
80. Bateman DN, Chaplin S, Ferner RE: Safety of mianserin. *Lancet* 2(8607):401–402, 1988.
81. Bender AS, Hertz L: Evidence for involvement of the astrocytic benzodiazepine receptor in the mechanism of action of convulsant and anticonvulsant drugs. *Life Sci* 43(6):477–484, 1988.
82. Burrows GD, Davies B, Hamer A, et al: Effect of mianserin on cardiac conduction. *Med J Aust* 2(2):97–98, 1979.
83. Burrows GD, Norman TR, Dennerstein L, et al: Antidepressant therapy: benefits and risks in perspective. *Acta Psychiatr Scand Suppl* 320:43–47, 1985.
84. Curtis RA, Giacona N, Burrows D, et al: Fatal maprotiline intoxication. *Drug Intell Clin Pharm* 18(9):716–720, 1984.
85. Juvent M, Douchamps J, Delcourt E, et al: Lack of cardiovascular side effects of the new tricyclic antidepressant tianeptine. A double-blind, placebo-controlled study in young healthy volunteers. *Clin Neuropharmacol* 13(1):48–57, 1990.
86. Lemberger L, Bergstrom RF, Wolen RL, et al: Fluoxetine: clinical pharmacology and physiologic disposition. *J Clin Psychiatry* 46(3 Pt 2):14–19, 1985.
87. Maguire KP, Norman TR, Burrows GD, et al: A pharmacokinetic study of mianserin. *Eur J Clin Pharmacol* 21(6):517–520, 1982.
88. Munger MA, Effron BA: Amoxapine cardiotoxicity. *Ann Emerg Med* 17(3):274–278, 1988.
89. Pacher P, Ungvari Z: Speculations on difference between tricyclic and selective serotonin reuptake inhibitor antidepressants on their cardiac effects. Is there any? *Curr Med Chem* 6(6):469–480, 1999.
90. Steinberg MI, Smallwood JK, Holland DR, et al: Hemodynamic and electrocardiographic effects of fluoxetine and its major metabolite, norfluoxetine, in anesthetized dogs. *Toxicol Appl Pharmacol* 82(1):70–79, 1986.
91. Nilsson B: Adverse reactions in connection with zimeldine treatment—a review. *Acta Psychiatr Scand Suppl* 308:115, 1983.
92. Lijeqvist J, Edvardsson N: Torsade de pointes, tachycardia, induced by overdose of zimedine. *J Clin Pharmacol* 14:666, 1989.
93. Balit CR, Lynch CN, Isbister GK: Bupropion poisoning: a case series. *Med J Aust* 178(2):61–63, 2003.
94. Jepsen F, Matthews J, Andrews FJ: Sustained release bupropion overdose: an important cause of prolonged symptoms after an overdose. *Emerg Med J* 20(6):560–561, 2003.
95. Taboulet P, Michard F, Muszynski J, et al: Cardiovascular repercussions of seizures during cyclic antidepressant poisoning. *J Toxicol Clin Toxicol* 33(3):205–211, 1995.
96. White CM, Gailer RA, Levin GM, et al: Seizure resulting from a venlafaxine overdose. *Ann Pharmacother* 31(2):178–180, 1997.
97. Curran S, de Pauw K: Selecting an antidepressant for use in a patient with epilepsy. Safety considerations. *Drug Safety* 18(2):125–133, 1998.
98. Schlienger RG, Klink MH, Eggenberger C, et al: Seizures associated with therapeutic doses of venlafaxine and trimipramine. *Ann Pharmacother* 34(12):1402–1405, 2000.
99. Graudins A, Dowsett RP, Liddle C: The toxicity of antidepressant poisoning: is it changing? A comparative study of cyclic and newer serotonin-specific antidepressants. *Emerg Med (Fremantle)* 14(4):440–446, 2002.
100. Pisani F, Oteri G, Costa C, et al: Effects of psychotropic drugs on seizure threshold. *Drug Saf* 25(2):91–110, 2002.
101. Kelly CA, Dhaun N, Laing WJ, et al: Comparative toxicity of citalopram and the newer antidepressants after overdose. *J Toxicol Clin Toxicol* 42(1):67–71, 2004.
102. Montgomery SA: Antidepressants and seizures: emphasis on newer agents and clinical implications. *Int J Clin Pract* 59(12):1435–1440, 2005.
103. Borganelli M, Forman MB: Simulation of acute myocardial infarction by desipramine hydrochloride. *Am Heart J* 119(6):1413–1414, 1990.
104. Salzman C: Clinical use of antidepressant blood levels and the electrocardiogram. *N Engl J Med* 313(8):512, 1985.
105. Boehnert MT, Lovejoy FH Jr: Value of the QRS duration versus the serum drug level in predicting seizures and ventricular arrhythmias after an acute overdose of tricyclic antidepressants. *N Engl J Med* 313(8):474–479, 1985.
106. Bramble MG, Lishman AH, Purdon J, et al: An analysis of plasma levels and 24-hour ECG recordings in tricyclic antidepressant poisoning: implications for management. *Q J Med* 56(219):357–366, 1985.
107. Pentel P, Sioris L: Incidence of late arrhythmias following tricyclic antidepressant overdose. *Clin Toxicol* 18(5):543–548, 1981.
108. Emerson T: Inaccuracy of QRS interval as TCA toxicity indicator. *Ann Emerg Med* 16(11):1312, 1987.
109. Catalano G, Catalano MC, Epstein MA, et al: QTc interval prolongation associated with citalopram overdose: a case report and literature review. *Clin Neuropharmacol* 24(3):158–162, 2001.
110. Niemann JT, Bessen HA, Rothstein RJ, et al: Electrocardiographic criteria for tricyclic antidepressant cardiotoxicity. *Am J Cardiol* 57(13):1154–1159, 1986.
111. Wolfe TR, Caravati EM, Rollins DE: Terminal 40-ms frontal plane QRS axis as a marker for tricyclic antidepressant overdose. *Ann Emerg Med* 18(4):348–351, 1989.
112. Liebelt EL, Francis PD, Woolf AD: ECG lead aVR versus QRS interval in predicting seizures and arrhythmias in acute tricyclic antidepressant toxicity. *Ann Emerg Med* 26(2):195–201, 1995.
113. Bailey B, Buckley NA, Amre DK: A meta-analysis of prognostic indicators to predict seizures, arrhythmias or death after tricyclic antidepressant overdose. *J Toxicol Clin Toxicol* 42(6):877–888, 2004.
114. Graudins A, Stearman A, Chan B: Treatment of the serotonin syndrome with cyproheptadine. *J Emerg Med* 16(4):615–619, 1998.
115. Horowitz BZ, Mullins ME: Cyproheptadine for serotonin syndrome in an accidental pediatric sertraline ingestion. *Pediatr Emerg Care* 15(5):325–327, 1999.

116. Giroud C, Horisberger B, Eap C, et al: Death following acute poisoning by moclobemide. *Forensic Sci Int* 140(1):101–107, 2004.
117. Hilton SE, Maradit H, Moller HJ: Serotonin syndrome and drug combinations: focus on MAOI and RIMA. *Eur Arch Psychiatry Clin Neurosci* 247(3):113–119, 1997.
118. Erich JL, Shih RD, O'Connor RE: "Ping-pong" gaze in severe monoamine oxidase inhibitor toxicity. *J Emerg Med* 13(5):653–655, 1995.
119. Jennings AE, Levey AS, Harrington JT: Amoxapine-associated acute renal failure. *Arch Intern Med* 143(8):1525–1527, 1983.
120. Roy TM, Ossorio MA, Cipolla LM, et al: Pulmonary complications after tricyclic antidepressant overdose. *Chest* 96(4):852–856, 1989.
121. Tao GK, Harada DT, Kootsikas ME, et al: Amoxapine-induced tardive dyskinesia. *Drug Intell Clin Pharm* 19(7–8):548–549, 1985.
122. Taylor NE, Schwartz HI: Neuroleptic malignant syndrome following amoxapine overdose. *J Nerv Ment Dis* 176(4):249–251, 1988.
123. Pascale P, Odd M, Pacher P, et al: Severe rhabdomyolysis following venlafaxine overdose. *Ther Drug Monit* 27(5):562–564, 2005.
124. Asch DA, Parker RM: The Libby Zion case. One step forward or two steps backward? *N Engl J Med* 318(12):771–775, 1988.
125. Chen DT, Ruch R: Safety of moclobemide in clinical use. *Clin Neuropharmacol* 16[Suppl 2]:S63–S68, 1993.
126. Cuthbert MF: Monoamine oxidase inhibitors. *Br Med J* 2(602):433, 1968.
127. Izumi T, Nobuyuki I, Kitaichi AK, et al: Effects of co-administration of a selective serotonin reuptake inhibitor and monoamine oxidase inhibitors on 5-HT-related behavior in rats. *Eur J Pharmacol* 532(3):258–264, 2006.
128. Eizadi-Mood N, Moein N, Saghaei M: Evaluation of relationship between arterial and venous blood gas values in the patients with tricyclic antidepressant poisoning. *Clin Toxicol (Philadelphia)* 43(5):357–360, 2005.
129. Fleischman A, Chiang VW: Carbamazepine overdose recognized by a tricyclic antidepressant assay. *Pediatrics* 107(1):176–177, 2001.
130. Matos ME, Burns MM, Shannon MW: False-positive tricyclic antidepressant drug screen results leading to the diagnosis of carbamazepine intoxication. Pediatrics 105(5): E66, 307–310, 2000.
131. Sorisky A, Watson DC: Positive diphenhydramine interference in the EMIT-st assay for tricyclic antidepressants in serum. *Clin Chem* 32(4):715, 1986.
132. McAlpine SB, Calabro JJ, Robinson MD, et al: Late death in tricyclic antidepressant overdose revisited. *Ann Emerg Med* 15(11):1349–1352, 1986.
133. Wians FH Jr, Norton JT, Wirebaugh SR: False-positive serum tricyclic antidepressant screen with cyproheptadine. *Clin Chem* 39(6):1355–1356.
134. Pentel P, Olson KR, Becker CE, et al: Late complications of tricyclic antidepressant overdose. *West J Med* 138(3):1355–1356, 423–424, 1983.
135. Van Hoey N: Effect of cyclobenzaprine on tricyclic antidepressant assays. The annals of pharmacotherapy 39:1314–1317, 2005.
136. Callaham M: Admission criteria for tricyclic antidepressant ingestion. *West J Med* 137(5):425–429, 1982.
137. Greenland P, Howe TA: Cardiac monitoring in tricyclic antidepressant overdose. *Heart Lung* 10(5):856–859, 1981.
138. Crome P, Adams R, Ali C, et al: Activated charcoal in tricyclic antidepressant poisoning: pilot controlled clinical trial. *Hum Toxicol* 2(2):205–209, 1983.
139. Hultén BA, Adams R, Askenasi R, et al: Activated charcoal in tricyclic antidepressant poisoning. *Hum Toxicol* 7(4):307–310, 1988.
140. Goldberg MJ, Park GD, Spector R: Lack of effect of oral activated charcoal on imipramine clearance. *Clin Pharmacol Ther* 38(3):307–310, 350–353, 1985.
141. Tokarski GF, Young MJ: Criteria for admitting patients with tricyclic antidepressant overdose. *J Emerg Med* 6(2):121–124, 1988.
142. Knudsen K, Abrahamsson J: Effects of epinephrine and norepinephrine on hemodynamic parameters and arrhythmias during a continuous infusion of amitriptyline in rats. *J Toxicol Clin Toxicol* 31(3):461–471, 1993.
143. Pentel PR, Bullock ML, DeVane CL: Hemoperfusion for imipramine overdose: elimination of active metabolites. *J Toxicol Clin Toxicol* 19(3):239–248, 1982.
144. Asbach HW, Holz F, Mohring K, et al: Lipid hemodialysis versus charcoal hemoperfusion in imipramine poisoning. *Clin Toxicol* 11(2):121–124, 211–219, 1977.
145. Comstock TJ, Watson WA, Jennison TA: Severe amitriptyline intoxication and the use of charcoal hemoperfusion. *Clin Pharm* 2(1):85–88, 1983.
146. Bartholini G: GABA receptor agonists: pharmacological spectrum and therapeutic actions. *Med Res Rev* 5(1):55–75, 1985.
147. Beaubien AR, Carpenter DC, Mathieu LF, et al: Antagonism of imipramine poisoning by anticonvulsants in the rat. *Toxicol Appl Pharmacol* 38(1):1–6, 1976.
148. Blake KV, Massey KL, Hendeles L, et al: Relative efficacy of phenytoin and phenobarbital for the prevention of theophylline-induced seizures in mice. *Ann Emerg Med* 17(10):1024–1028, 1988.
149. Hagerman G, Hanashiro PK: Reversal of tricyclic-antidepressant-induced cardiac conduction abnormalities by phenytoin. *Ann Emerg Med* 10(2):82–86, 1981.
150. Hoffman JR, Votey SR, Bayer M, et al: Effect of hypertonic sodium bicarbonate in the treatment of moderate-to-severe cyclic antidepressant overdose. *Am J Emerg Med* 11(4):336–341, 1993.
151. Teba L, Schiebel F, Dedhia HV, et al: Beneficial effect of norepinephrine in the treatment of circulatory shock caused by tricyclic antidepressant overdose. *Am J Emerg Med* 6(6):566–568, 1988.
152. Knudsen K, Abrahamsson J: Epinephrine and sodium bicarbonate independently and additively increase survival in experimental amitriptyline poisoning. *Crit Care Med* 25(4):669–674, 1997.
153. Barry J, Durkovich D, Williams S: Vasopressin treatment for cyclic antidepressant overdose. *J Emerg Med* 31:65–68, 2006.
154. Holmes CL, Patel BM, Russel JA, et al: Physiology of vasopressin relevant to management of septic shock. *Chest* 120:989–1002, 2001.
155. Mutlu GM, Factor P: Role of vasopressin in the management of septic shock. *Intensive Care Med* 30:1276–1291, 2004.
156. Barrueto F, Chuang A, Cotter BW, et al: Amiodarone fails to improve survival in amitriptyline-poisoned mice. *Clin Toxicol (Philadelphia)* 43(3):147–149, 2005.
157. Harvey M, Cave G: Intralipid outperforms sodium bicarbonate in a rabbit model of clomipramine toxicity. *Ann Emerg Med* 49:178–185, 2007.
158. Weinberg G, Ripper R, Feinstein DL, et al: Lipid emulsion infusion rescues dogs from bupivacaine induced cardiac toxicity. *Reg Anesth Pain Med* 28:198–2002, 2003.
159. Yoav G, Odelia G, Shaltiel C, et al: A lipid emulsion reduces mortality from clomipramine overdose in rats. *Vet Hum Toxicol* 44:30, 2002.
160. Tebbut S, Harvey M, Nicholson T, et al: Intralipid prolongs survival in a rat model of a verapamil toxicity. *Acad Emerg Med* 13:134–139, 2006.
161. Guze BH, Baxter LR Jr: Current concepts. Neuroleptic malignant syndrome. *N Engl J Med* 313(3):163–166, 1985.
162. Sheehan DV, Claycomb JB, Kouretas N: Monoamine oxidase inhibitors: prescription and patient management. *Int J Psychiatry Med* 10(2):99–121, 1980.
163. Vassallo SU, Delaney KA: Pharmacologic effects on thermoregulation: mechanisms of drug-related heatstroke. *J Toxicol Clin Toxicol* 27(4–5): 199–224, 1989.
164. Callaham M, Schumaker H, Pentel P: Phenytoin prophylaxis of cardiotoxicity in experimental amitriptyline poisoning. *J Pharmacol Exp Ther* 245(1):216–220, 1988.
165. Mayron R, Ruiz E: Phenytoin: does it reverse tricyclic-antidepressant-induced cardiac conduction abnormalities? *Ann Emerg Med* 15(8):876–880, 1986.
166. Kulig K, Bar-Or D, Marx J, et al: Phenytoin as treatment for tricyclic antidepressant cardiotoxicity in a canine model. *Vet Hum Toxicol* 26(5): A-2, 1984.
167. Burks JS, Walker J, Rumack BH, et al: Tricyclic antidepressant poisoning. Reversal of coma, choreoathetosis, and myoclonus by physostigmine. *JAMA* 230(10):1405–1407, 1974.
168. Goldberger AL, Curtis GP: Immediate effects of physostigmine on amitriptyline-induced QRS prolongation. *J Toxicol Clin Toxicol* 19(5):445–454, 1982.
169. Pentel P, Peterson CD: Asystole complicating physostigmine treatment of tricyclic antidepressant overdose. *Ann Emerg Med* 9(11):588–590, 1980.
170. Southall DP, Kilpatrick SM: Imipramine poisoning: survival of a child after prolonged cardiac massage. *Br Med J* 4(5943):508, 1974.
171. Kalkan S, Aygoren O, Akgun A, et al: Do adenosine receptors play a role in amitriptyline-induced cardiovascular toxicity in rats? *J Toxicol Clin Toxicol* 42(7):945–954, 2004.

CHAPTER 124 ■ ANTIPSYCHOTIC POISONING

MICHAEL J. BURNS AND CHRISTOPHER H. LINDEN

Antipsychotic agents, sometimes termed *neuroleptics* and *major tranquilizers*, are primarily used to treat schizophrenia, the manic phase of bipolar disorder, and agitated behavior. They are also used as preanesthetics and to treat drug-associated delirium and hallucinations, nausea, vomiting, headaches, hiccups, pruritus, Tourette's syndrome, and a variety of extrapyramidal movement disorders (e.g., chorea, dystonias, hemiballismus, spasms, tics, torticollis). Antipsychotics are a structurally diverse group of heterocyclic compounds; more than 50 different drugs are available for clinical use worldwide with numerous others in various stages of development. Classes include benzamide, benzepine, butyrophenone (phenylbutylpiperidine), dibenzo-oxepino pyrrole, diphenylbutylpiperidine, indole, phenothiazine, quinolinone, rauwolfia alkaloid, and thioxanthene derivatives (Table 124.1). The phenothiazine and thioxanthene classes are further subdivided into three groups (aliphatic, piperazine, and piperidine) based on central ring side-chain substitution.

Although traditionally classified by structure, antipsychotics are more ideally classified by pharmacologic profile. Each agent has a unique receptor-binding profile (Table 124.2), and this profile can be used to predict adverse effects in both therapeutic and overdose situations [1–3]. Clinical toxicity is the result of exaggerated pharmacologic activity. Antipsychotics are also classified as *typical* or *atypical* (Tables 124.1 and 124.2). Traditional or conventional antipsychotics, which readily produce extrapyramidal signs and symptoms (EPS) at antipsychotic doses, are considered typical. Newer agents that have minimal extrapyramidal side effects at clinically effective antipsychotic doses are effective for treating the negative symptoms (e.g., alogia, avolition, social withdrawal, flattened affect) of schizophrenia and have a low propensity to cause tardive dyskinesia with long-term treatment are considered atypical [1–4]. The characterization of antipsychotics as typical or atypical is ultimately determined by receptor binding. One or more of several different receptor-binding characteristics are associated with drug atypia, and each agent is atypical for different reasons [4,5]. Understanding how specific receptor-binding characteristics produce clinical effects has facilitated the development of antipsychotics that separate antipsychotic activity from other activity, thus minimizing adverse effects and maximizing patient compliance.

Antipsychotic toxicity may occur as an idiosyncratic reaction during therapeutic use or following accidental or intentional overdose. Central nervous system (CNS) and cardiovascular disturbances are the most common dose-related toxic manifestations, but other effects include the anticholinergic syndrome (see Chapter 121) and various extrapyramidal syndromes. Therapeutic use has been associated with agranulocytosis, aplastic anemia, diabetes mellitus, hepatotoxicity, hypertriglyceridemia, fatal myocardial infarction, myocarditis, neuroleptic malignant syndrome (see Chapter 66), pancreatitis, seizures, sleep apnea, sudden infant death syndrome, sudden adult death, venous thromboembolism, and vasculitis [21–29]. Most deaths are the consequence of suicidal overdose by psychotic or depressed adults and frequently involve mixed ingestions or ingestion of the agents chlorpromazine, loxapine, mesoridazine, quetiapine, or thioridazine [30,31]. Because of a large toxic to therapeutic ratio for most antipsychotics, fatalities rarely occur. In 2007, there were 46,239 antipsychotic exposures reported to United States poison centers, of which 41,607 (90%) were due to atypical agents and 4,632 (10%) were due to phenothiazines [32]. Major toxicity and death occurred in 1.1% and 0.02% of atypical agent exposures, and in 0.8% and 0.04% of phenothiazine exposures. From this data, death occurred in less than four patients for every 1,000 antipsychotic agent toxic exposures. Quetiapine was most commonly associated with fatality in both mixed and single substance ingestions but this may reflect usage pattern and not individual agent toxicity [32]. From another study, the most toxic antipsychotics result in death from poisoning for every 100 patient-years of use [30]. Dose-related effects are most pronounced in nonhabituated patients at the extremes of age.

Recent data has demonstrated that users of antipsychotic drugs have higher rates of sudden cardiac than do nonusers and former users of antipsychotic drugs [6]. The increased risk of sudden cardiac death is similar in magnitude for both typical and atypical agents, with adjusted incidence-rate ratios of 1.99 and 2.26, respectively, when compared with nonusers. For both classes of drugs, the risk of sudden cardiac death increases significantly with an increasing dose. Users of clozapine and thioridazine had the greatest increased of sudden cardiac death, with an adjusted incidence rate that was more than three times that for nonusers.

PHARMACOLOGY

Antipsychotics bind to and antagonize presynaptic (autoreceptors) and postsynaptic type 2 dopamine (D_2) receptors in the CNS and peripheral nervous system [7]. Initially, dopamine neurons increase the synthesis and release of dopamine in response to autoreceptor antagonism. With repeated dosing, however, depolarization inactivation of the neuron occurs, and decreased synthesis and release of dopamine occur despite ongoing postsynaptic receptor blockade [7,8].

All antipsychotics produce their therapeutic antipsychotic effect from mesolimbic D_2-receptor antagonism. D_2-receptor affinity (potency) in this region strongly correlates with the daily therapeutic dose (see Table 124.1) [1,4,9]. Simultaneous antagonism of other D_2 receptors produces additional clinical effects, the majority of which are undesirable. Mesocortical receptor blockade appears to create cognitive impairment and further worsens the negative symptoms of schizophrenia [10]. Excessive D_2-receptor blockade in mesocortical and mesolimbic areas, as occurs after neuroleptic overdose, may partly mediate CNS depression from these agents. Antagonism of nigrostriatal D_2-receptors produces EPS (e.g., acute dystonia, akathisia, parkinsonism). D_2-receptor potency in nigrostriatal relative to mesolimbic areas correlates with the likelihood of developing EPS [1,2,4,11,12]. Typical antipsychotics antagonize basal ganglia D_2 receptors in the same dose range necessary for limbic D_2-receptor blockade, thus creating high EPS liability [11,12]. The high-potency or typical agents (i.e., fluphenazine,

TABLE 124.1

CLASSIFICATION AND DOSING OF NEUROLEPTIC AGENTS

Structural class	Generic name (trade name)	Affinity of neuroleptic agent for dopamine (D_2) receptor (potency)[a]	Daily dose range (mg)
Typical agents			
Butyrophenone (phenyl-butylpiperidine)	Droperidol (Inapsine)	3+	1.25–30
	Haloperidol (Haldol)	2+	1–30
	Other: benperidol, bromperidol, melperone, pipamperone, trifluperidol[c]		
Diphenylbutylpiperidine	Pimozide (Orap)	2+	1–20
	Other: fluspirilene, penfluridol[c]		
Indole	Molindone (Moban)	1+	15–225
	Other: oxypertine[c]		
Phenothiazine			
Aliphatic	Chlorpromazine (Thorazine)	2+	25–2,000
	Promazine (Sparine)[b]	—	50–1,000
	Promethazine (Phenergan)	2+	25–150
	Triflupromazine (Vesprin)	—	5–90
Piperazine	Acetophenazine (Tindal)	—	40–400
	Fluphenazine (Prolixin)	3+	0.5–30
	Perphenazine (Trilafon)	3+	4–64
	Prochlorperazine (Compazine)	2+	10–150
	Trifluoperazine (Stelazine)	3+	2–40
	Thiethylperazine (Torecan)	—	10–30
Piperidine	Mesoridazine (Serentil)	2+	30–400
	Thioridazine (Mellaril, Millazine)	2+	20–800
	Other: diethazine, ethopropazine, levomepromazine, perazine, pipotiazine thiopropazate, thioproperazine, pericyazine[c]		
Thioxanthene	Chlorprothixene (Taractan)	2+	30–600
	Clopenthixol[c]	—	—
	Flupenthixol[c]	3+	4
	Thiothixene (Navane)	3+	6–60
	Zuclopenthixol (Cisordinol, Clopixol)[c]	3+	10–50
Atypical agents			
Benzamides	Amisulpride[c]	2+	100–1,200
	Raclopride[c]	3+	5–8
	Remoxipride[c]	1+	150–600
	Sulpiride[c]	2+	100–1,600
	Sultopride[c]	2+	100–1,200
	Trimethobenzamide (Tigan)[b]	—	100–600
	Other: epidepride, eticlopride levosulpiride, nemonapride, tiapride[c]		
Benzepine			
Dibenzodiazepine	Clozapine (Clozaril, Leponex)	1+	150–900
Dibenzo-oxazepine	Loxapine (Loxitane)	1+	20–250
Thienobenzodiazepine	Olanzapine (Zyprexa)	2+	5–20
Dibenzothiazepine	Quetiapine (Seroquel)	1+	300–600
Dibenzothiazepine	Zotepine[c]	2+	100–300
	Other: butaclamol, fluperlapine, clothiapine, metiapine, savoxepine[c]		
Indole			
Benzisoxazole	Risperidone (Risperdal)	3+	2–16
	Paliperidone (Invega)	3+	3–12
Imidazolidinone	Sertindole (Serlect)[c]	3+	12–24
Benzisothiazole	Ziprasidone (Zeldox)	3+	40–160
	Other: iloperidone[c]		
Pyrrole	Asenapine (Saphris)	3+	10–20
Quinolinone	Aripiprazole (Abilify, Abitat)	3+	10–30
	Bifeprunox[c]		

[a] A higher numerical value indicates greater binding affinity (greater antagonism) at D_2 receptor. Binding affinity (potency) at D_2 receptor correlates with daily dose range.
[b] Antiemetic only.
[c] Not available for clinical use in the United States.
0, minimal to none; 1+, low; 2+, moderate; 3+, high to very high.

TABLE 124.2

RELATIVE NEURORECEPTOR AFFINITIES FOR NEUROLEPTICS[a]

Neuroleptic agent	Receptor					
	H_1 Histaminergic	α_1-Adrenergic	α_2-Adrenergic	M_1 muscarinic	5-HT_{2A} serotonergic	EPS risk[b]
Typical agents						
Chlorpromazine	2+	3+	0	1+	3+	1+
Fluphenazine	0	0	0	0	0	3+
Haloperidol	0	1+	0	0	1+	3+
Loxapine	3+	3+	0	2+	3+	1+
Mesoridazine	3+	3+	–	1+	–	1+
Molindone	0	0	1+	0	0	3+
Perphenazine	1+	1+	0	0	–	3+
Pimozide	0	1+	–	0	1+	3+
Prochlorperazine	1+	1+	0	0	0	3+
Thioridazine	2+	3+	0	3+	2+	1+
Thiothixene	0	0	0	0	0	3+
Trifluoperazine	0	1+	0	0	1+	3+
Atypical agents						
(Ami)sulpiride	0	0	0	0	0	1+
Asenapine	3+	2+	2+	0	3+	1+
Aripiprazole	2+	2+	0	0	3+	0
Clozapine	3+	3+	3+	3+	3+	0
Olanzapine	2+	2+	0	3+	3+	0
Paliperidone	1+	2+	1+	0	3+	1+[c]
Quetiapine	3+	3+	0	3+	1+	0
Remoxipride	0	0	0	0	0	1+
Risperidone	1+	2+	1+	0	3+	1+[c]
Sertindole	0	1+	0	0	3+	0
Ziprasidone	0	3+	0	0	3+	1+
Zotepine	2+	0	2+	0	3+	1+

[a]Relative neuroreceptor affinity [neuroreceptor affinity at receptor X/dopamine (D_2)-receptor affinity] indicates relative receptor antagonism at therapeutic (D_2-blocking) antipsychotic doses.
[b]A higher M_1 and 5-HT_2 relative neuroreceptor affinity confers a lower EPS risk.
[c]Dose-dependent incidence of extra EPS.
Adapted from references [1–20].
0, minimal to none; 1+, low; 2+, moderate; 3+, high; 4+, very high; EPS, extrapyramidal side effects.

haloperidol, perphenazine, thiothixene, and trifluoperazine) are most commonly associated with EPS [1]. Atypical agents have low D_2-receptor potency and occupancy (i.e., clozapine, olanzapine, quetiapine) at therapeutic doses, are partial D_2-receptor agonists (e.g., aripiprazole), or are more site selective (i.e., sulpiride, raclopride) and preferentially antagonize limbic D_2 receptors [2–4,8,13]. Thus, they are less likely to cause EPS or worsen negative symptoms of schizophrenia at therapeutic doses.

D_2-receptor blockade in the anterior hypothalamus (preoptic area) may alter core temperature set point and block thermosensitive neuronal inputs and thermoregulatory responses [7]. Hypothermia or hyperthermia may result. D_2-receptor blockade in the pituitary (tuberoinfundibular pathway) results in sustained elevated prolactin secretion, which may cause galactorrhea, gynecomastia, menstrual changes, and sexual dysfunction (impotence in men) [1,11]. The antiemetic activity of antipsychotics results from similar inhibition of dopaminergic receptors in the chemoreceptor trigger zone (area postrema) of the medulla oblongata [7]. Antagonism of dopamine receptors present on peripheral sympathetic nerve terminals and vascular smooth muscle cells may produce autonomic dysfunction (i.e., tachycardia, hypertension, diaphoresis, pallor) [7,33–35]. Simultaneous blockade of D_2 receptors in the hypothalamus, striatum, mesocortical and mesolimbic areas, peripheral sympathetic nerve terminals, and vasculature mediate the neuroleptic malignant syndrome in susceptible individuals (see Chapter 66).

In addition to D_2 receptors, antipsychotics are competitive antagonists at a wide range of neuroreceptors; varied binding affinities exist at α-adrenergic ($\alpha_{1,2}$), dopaminergic (D_{1-5}), histaminergic (H_{1-3}), muscarinic (M_{1-5}), and serotonergic (5-HT_{1-7}) receptors (see Table 124.2) [1,4,12]. The neuroreceptor-binding profile for each agent predicts clinical effects. The ratio of other neuroreceptor-binding affinities to D_2-receptor–binding affinity (relative binding affinity) predicts the likelihood of producing those receptor-mediated effects at clinically effective antipsychotic (D_2-blocking) doses and in overdose [1,12]. A ratio similar to or greater than 1 makes other receptor-mediated effects likely. High relative α_1-adrenergic antagonism (i.e., aliphatic and piperidine phenothiazines, asenapine, clozapine, olanzapine, risperidone, ziprasidone) correlates with the incidence and severity of orthostatic hypotension, reflex tachycardia, nasal congestion, and miosis [11]. Significant relative α_2-adrenergic blockade, as occurs with asenapine, clozapine, paliperidone, and risperidone, may result in sympathomimetic effects (e.g., tachycardia). High relative H_1-receptor blockade (e.g., aliphatic and piperidine phenothiazines, asenapine, clozapine, olanzapine, quetiapine) produces sedation, appetite stimulation, and hypotension [1,11]. Relative potency at M_1 receptors correlates directly with anticholinergic effects (i.e., tachycardia, hypertension, mydriasis, blurred vision, ileus, urinary retention, dry skin and mucous membranes, cutaneous flushing, sedation, memory dysfunction, hallucinations, agitation, delirium, and hyperthermia) and inversely with the incidence of extrapyramidal reactions [1]. Olanzapine, clozapine, and aliphatic and piperidine phenothiazines are associated with clinically significant anticholinergic effects. The ability of clozapine to produce sialorrhea is likely mediated by its partial agonism at M_1 and M_4 receptors [1]. High relative antagonism at 5-HT_{1A} and 5-HT_{2A} receptors appears to predict a low EPS risk [1,7,36,37]. The clinical effects that occur with other neuroreceptor subtype binding are not well understood.

The advent of atypical agents, which provide an improved motor side effect profile, marks significant progress in neuroleptic development. Atypical agents may be subdivided into four functional groups: (a) the D_2-, D_3-receptor antagonists (i.e., amisulpride, raclopride, remoxipride, and sulpiride); (b) the D_2-, 5HT_{2A}-, and α_1-receptor antagonists (i.e., paliperidone, risperidone and ziprasidone); (c) the broad-spectrum, multireceptor antagonists (i.e., asenapine, clozapine, olanzapine, quetiapine); and (d) the D_2-, 5-HT_{1A}-receptor partial agonists (i.e., aripiprazole, bifeprunox), also known as dopamine and serotonin system stabilizers [3] (see Table 124.2). One or more of several different pharmacologic mechanisms define drug atypia. Low D_2-receptor potency (high-milligram dosing), low (less than 70%) D_2-receptor occupancy in mesolimbic and nigrostriatal areas at therapeutic drug doses, partial agonist activity at D_2 receptors, selective mesolimbic D_2-receptor antagonism, and high D_1-, D_4-, M_1-, 5HT_{1A}-, 5HT_{2A}-receptor potencies relative to D_2-receptor–binding are pharmacologic characteristics that alone or in combination may be responsible for the atypical nature of these agents [1–3,7,13,36,37]. Conversely, typical antipsychotics are characterized by high D_2-receptor potency (low-milligram dosing) and a narrow receptor profile in the brain [1]. Unlike typical agents, atypical agents also appear to have a minimal propensity to elevate serum prolactin concentrations.

Serotonin antagonism enhances antipsychotic efficacy and reduces the incidence of EPS [36,37]. 5HT_{2A}-receptor antagonism in the striatum and prefrontal cortex offsets neuroleptic-induced D_2-receptor blockade and reduces EPS and negative symptoms of schizophrenia, respectively [7,10,36–38]. 5HT_{2A}-receptor antagonism also increases serotonin levels in the limbic system, which may have a direct antipsychotic effect [7,10]. Drugs with high relative 5HT_{2A}-receptor antagonism as compared to D_2-receptor antagonism (i.e., amperozide, asenapine, clozapine, olanzapine, paliperidone, risperidone, ziprasidone) can be given in smaller clinically effective antipsychotic doses and thus have a smaller risk of inducing EPS [1,11,38,39]. In addition, antipsychotics that stimulate 5HT_{1A} autoreceptors in the striatum (i.e., aripiprazole, clozapine, ziprasidone) reduce striatal D_2-receptor blockade, thereby decreasing the likelihood of EPS [8,36,37].

Aliphatic and piperidine phenothiazines (e.g., chlorpromazine, thioridazine, mesoridazine) have local anesthetic, quinidine-like (type Ia) antiarrhythmic, and myocardial depressant effects [7]. These agents block both fast-sodium channels responsible for myocardial membrane depolarization [40]. Sodium channel blockade is voltage and frequency dependent; blockade is augmented at less negative membrane potentials and faster heart rates [40]. Thus, the anticholinergic properties (e.g., tachycardia) and tissue acidemia-producing effects (e.g., seizures, hypotension) of these drugs potentiate their sodium channel blocking effects. Although specifically demonstrated for sertindole and thioridazine only, all neuroleptics appear to variably antagonize delayed-rectifier, voltage-gated, potassium channels responsible for myocardial membrane repolarization; antagonism occurs specifically at the potassium channel encoded by the human ether-a-go-go (*hERG*) gene [41,42]. Potassium-channel blockade is concentration-, voltage-, and reverse-frequency dependent; blockade is increased at higher tissue concentrations, less negative membrane potentials, and slower heart rates [41,42]. Potassium channel blockade may result in early after depolarizations and subsequent torsade de pointes (TdP)–type ventricular tachycardia. Haloperidol, mesoridazine, thioridazine, and pimozide share an added property of calcium channel blockade [43,44].

Electrophysiologic effects variably include a depressed rate of phase 0 depolarization, depressed amplitude and duration of phase 2, and prolongation of phase 3 repolarization. Ventricular repolarization abnormalities, such as T-wave changes (blunting, notching, inversion), increased U-wave amplitude, and prolongation of the QT interval, are the earliest and most consistent electrocardiographic changes produced by neuroleptics [45–48]. Dose-related prolongation of the QT interval has been described with droperidol, haloperidol, loxapine, phenothiazines, pimozide, quetiapine, risperidone, sertindole, and ziprasidone [31,41,42,45–57]. Conduction disturbances (i.e., bundle-branch, fascicular, intraventricular, and atrioventricular [AV] blocks) and supraventricular and ventricular tachyarrhythmias (i.e., monomorphic and polymorphic TdP ventricular tachycardia, ventricular fibrillation) have been reported [31,49,57–61]. Cardiac effects are dose and concentration dependent but can occur with therapeutic as well as toxic doses. Ventricular tachyarrhythmias and asphyxia (due to seizures, aspiration, or respiratory depression) have been postulated as etiologies of sudden death for patients taking therapeutic doses of antipsychotics, particularly phenothiazines [29,62].

Antipsychotics produce dose-related electroencephalographic changes, and some agents have been shown to lower the seizure threshold [26,27,63–66]. The risk of seizures is dose related, and thus, greatest after overdose [27,65,66]. Chlorpromazine, clozapine, and loxapine are the most likely agents to produce seizures [26,27,54,63–66]. Most other agents, however, are uncommonly associated with seizures, even after overdose. The mechanism by which antipsychotics produce seizures is not well understood but likely involves dose-related blockade of norepinephrine reuptake, antagonism of gamma-aminobutyric acid type A receptors, and altered neuronal transmembrane ionic currents.

Antipsychotics have a relatively flat dose-response curve. Effective therapeutic doses vary over a wide range (see Table 124.1). The optimal dose is determined by the clinical response, not by serum drug levels. Pharmacologic effects generally last 24 hours or more, allowing for once-daily dosing. Tablet, capsule, and liquid oral preparations, suppository, and injectable immediate-release and sustained-release (depot) solutions are available [7]. Oral preparations include both rapidly disintegrating (sublingual absorption) and sustained-release formulations. Paliperidone, the active metabolite of risperidone, is commercially available in an extended-release oral preparation (Invega®). Following a single dose, plasma concentrations gradually rise and do not peak until approximately 24 hours after dosing [67]. Slow-release, highly lipophilic depot formulations (i.e., fluphenazine enanthate and decanoate, haloperidol decanoate, paliperidone palmitate) for intramuscular injection are created by esterifying the hydroxyl group of an antipsychotic with a long-chain fatty acid and dissolving it in a sesame oil vehicle. A long-acting formulation of risperidone (Risperdal Consta®) is available that contains an aqueous suspension of risperidone mixed with a biodegradable carbohydrate copolymer.

Antipsychotic pharmacokinetics are complex and incompletely understood [7]. When administered orally, they are well absorbed, but bioavailability is unpredictable (range: 10% to 70%) due to large interindividual variability and presystemic (hepatic and intestinal) metabolism [7,68,69]. After parenteral administration, drug bioavailability is 4 to 10 times greater than with oral dosing because of the absence of first-pass metabolism [7,68,69]. Hence, therapeutic intravenous (IV) or intramuscular (IM) doses are substantially less than oral ones. Plasma concentrations peak 1 to 6 hours after therapeutic oral and sublingual dosing, 30 minutes to 1 hour after immediate-release IM injection, and within 24 hours after oral dosing of extended-release preparations. After a single intramuscular dose of a depot preparation, plasma concentrations peak variably from a few days to over 2 weeks after initial injection. [67–69]. After oral overdose, absorption should occur more rapidly (first-order kinetics), but peak plasma concentrations are delayed, as more time is required for complete absorption. As a result, clinical effects are expected to occur sooner and last longer. Erratic absorption may occur after ingestion of agents with significant anticholinergic effects.

After absorption, antipsychotics are highly bound to plasma proteins (75% to 99%) [7,68,69]. However, because they are also highly lipophilic, volumes of distribution are large (10 to 40 L per kg) and serum drug levels after therapeutic doses are quite low (one to several hundred ng per mL). These pharmacokinetic characteristics make extracorporeal removal by hemodialysis or hemoperfusion impractical. Antipsychotics tend to accumulate in the brain, easily cross the placenta, and are found in breast milk [7]. Elimination occurs slowly and extensively by hepatic metabolism, with serum concentration half-lives averaging 20 to 40 hours. Depot antipsychotics have an apparent elimination half-life of 1 to 3 weeks due to slow tissue absorption [68]. Small amounts (1% to 3%) are excreted unchanged by the kidney. As a rule, hepatic metabolism yields multiple metabolites, some of which are pharmacologically active and likely to extend parent drug effects after therapeutic or toxic dosing [70,71]. Metabolites are eliminated by urinary and biliary excretion and can be detected in the urine for several days after a single ingestion and for a month or more after cessation of long-term therapy [7,69]. Large interindividual variations in the metabolism of neuroleptics result in significant differences in steady-state plasma concentrations with fixed, therapeutic dosing [7,68,69,72]. There is often little correlation between neuroleptic dose, serum concentrations, and clinical effects.

Renal insufficiency may rarely result in drug accumulation and toxicity [73]. Renal excretion accounts for a significant proportion of total drug elimination for the benzamide (e.g., remoxipride, sulpiride) and benzisoxazole derivatives (e.g., paliperidone, risperidone) [67–69]. Thus, dose alteration is recommended for patients with renal insufficiency who regularly take these agents. Other neuroleptics, however, do not routinely require dose alteration for patients with renal impairment. Dose adjustment is also recommended for those patients who have a diminished ability to clear neuroleptics, such as the elderly and those with significant hepatic disease or specific cytochrome P450 enzyme deficiencies (i.e., CYP2D6, CYP1A2) [7,69]. Most antipsychotics are pregnancy category C and should be used in pregnancy only if the potential benefit justifies the potential risk to the fetus. Breast feeding is not recommended for women taking neuroleptics because most neuroleptics are secreted into breast milk, and their safety in infants is not established.

The majority of patients who take an accidental or intentional overdose of an antipsychotic agent remain asymptomatic or develop only mild toxicity [5,32]. Toxic effects result from exaggerated pharmacologic activity and include CNS and consequent respiratory depression, miosis or mydriasis, cardiovascular abnormalities, agitation, confusion, delirium, anticholinergic stigmata, seizures, EPS, and myoclonic jerking. Hypothermia and, less commonly, hyperthermia have occurred. Hypothermia may result from α_1-adrenergic–mediated peripheral vasodilation at low ambient temperature, hypotension, coma, loss of shivering capabilities, and disrupted hypothalamic thermoregulation. Peripheral vasodilation at high ambient temperature, seizures, neuromuscular agitation, loss of sweating capabilities, and hypothalamic dysfunction may contribute to hyperthermia. Seizures are uncommon and occur mainly in patients with underlying epilepsy and those with clozapine and loxapine overdoses. In one study of 299 patients with neuroleptic overdose, the incidence of seizure was only 1% [31]. Rhabdomyolysis, myoglobinuria, and acute renal failure may occur after prolonged convulsions [65,74]. CNS depression is the most frequent clinical finding after neuroleptic overdose [31,75–79]. Sinus tachycardia and orthostatic hypotension are the most frequent cardiovascular findings [31,75–79]. Other cardiovascular effects include hypertension, cardiac conduction disturbances, tachyarrhythmias, bradyarrhythmias, and, rarely, pulmonary edema [80,81]. Anticholinergic stigmata (see Chapter 121) may occur after overdose with aliphatic and piperidine phenothiazines, clozapine, and olanzapine [5,76,79,82–86].

Of the thousands of antipsychotic overdoses reported each year, less than 1% result in fatal toxicity [30,32]. Fatality is most often due to respiratory arrest before medical intervention, arrhythmias, or aspiration-induced respiratory failure [5,7,29,32]. Toxic and lethal doses are highly variable and are influenced by the agent ingested, the presence of coingestants and comorbid illness, the age and habituation of the patient, and the time to treatment. Nonhabituated patients at the extremes of age are more sensitive to the toxic effects of these drugs than those who have taken this drug chronically before an acute overdose. The ingestion of a single tablet of chlorpromazine, clozapine, loxapine, mesoridazine, olanzapine, quetiapine, or thioridazine may cause CNS and respiratory depression in young children [5,73,74,84]. Death of an infant was reported after the ingestion of only 350 mg of chlorpromazine. Adult fatalities have been reported after ingestions of 2.0 g of clozapine and chlorpromazine, 2.5 g of loxapine and mesoridazine, 1.5 g of thioridazine, and 600 mg of olanzapine [87,88]. Many patients, however, have survived much higher ingestions. In general, acute ingestion of greater than twice a maximal therapeutic dose is potentially serious.

Unintended adverse effects that occur during therapeutic use may be idiosyncratic or dose related, occur early or late during the course of therapy, or result from interactions with other drugs, and are often due to receptor antagonism. The major adverse side effect, both in terms of prevalence and in terms of the distress that it causes, is the tendency to induce extrapyramidal dysfunction.

Extrapyramidal syndromes are a group of movement disorders that result from the interference with neurotransmitter (primarily D_2-receptor blockade) function in the basal ganglia. EPS occur in up to 75% of patients treated with low-milligram, high-potency traditional agents (e.g., fluphenazine, haloperidol, thiothixene), but an incidence not significantly different from placebo ($<5\%$) has been described with newer atypical agents (e.g., aripiprazole, clozapine, olanzapine, quetiapine) [89–91]. EPS may occur early (i.e., within a few hours to days), at an intermediate stage (i.e., a few days to months) or late (i.e., after >3 months) in the course of therapy. Early EPS include acute dyskinesia (acute dystonic reactions), intermediate syndromes include akathisia and parkinsonism, and late disorders include tardive dyskinesia, tardive dystonia, and focal perioral tremor (rabbit syndrome). EPS are more commonly associated with therapeutic doses of neuroleptics but may follow acute overdose (e.g., acute dystonic reactions [ADRs]), particularly in children [5,75,92]. Only ADRs, the acute syndrome most likely to develop in the intensive care unit, are discussed.

ADRs are reversible motor disturbances consisting of sustained, uncoordinated, and involuntary spasmodic movements of various muscle groups. Although ADRs most often occur after administration of therapeutic doses of antipsychotics [93], they have also been described after administration of antihistamines (both H_1- and H_2-blockers), anticholinergics (e.g., benztropine, diphenhydramine), anticonvulsants (e.g., carbamazepine, phenytoin), calcium channel blockers (e.g., nifedipine, verapamil), metoclopramide, cyclic antidepressants (e.g., amitriptyline, amoxapine, doxepin, imipramine), selective serotonin reuptake inhibitors (e.g., fluoxetine, sertraline), monoamine oxidase inhibitors (e.g., phenelzine, tranylcypromine), anesthetic induction agents (e.g., ketamine, etomidate, thiopental), cholinergics (e.g., bethanechol, insecticides), and cocaine. ADRs can also occur as a primary (non–drug-related) disorder [94].

The pathophysiology of ADRs is not fully elucidated but involves a disruption of cholinergic (interstriatal) and dopaminergic (nigrostriatal) pathways in the basal ganglia. Normally, dopamine is an excitatory neurotransmitter and acetylcholine is an inhibitory neurotransmitter [95]. Normal balance between these closely linked pathways is necessary for coordinated muscular activity. Dopaminergic D_1-, gamma-aminobutyric acid- (striatonigral), glutaminergic- (corticostriatal), noradrenergic-, $5HT_{1A}$- and $5HT_{2A}$- (raphe-striatal and raphe-nigral), and sigma (σ)- (red nucleus, substantia nigra, and cranial nerve motor nuclei) receptor inputs modulate this balance [7,8,36,37,96,97]. Blockade of striatal D_2 receptors by high-potency neuroleptics disrupts the dopaminergic–cholinergic balance in favor of cholinergic excess, and dystonia results [98,99]. Agents that balance D_2-receptor antagonism with D_1-, M_1-, or $5HT_{2A}$-receptor antagonism or $5HT_{1A}$-receptor agonism prevent striatal cholinergic excess and are less likely to precipitate acute dystonia [1,14,36,37,100]. Gamma-aminobutyric acid–receptor affinity correlates inversely, whereas σ- and *N*-methyl-D-aspartate-glutamate receptor–binding affinities correlate directly with the clinical incidence of acute dystonia [8,96,97].

Paradoxically, ADRs may also result from hyperdopaminergic function induced by D_2-receptor blockade in the basal ganglia [101,102]. Acute D_2-receptor blockade may stimulate increased dopamine synthesis and release from nigrostriatal neurons and postsynaptic receptor upregulation (supersensitivity). As brain concentration of drug declines hours to days after a dose, a state of dopamine excess develops, and dystonia results [101,102].

ADRs usually occur soon after initiation of therapy or after an increase in dose. Fifty percent of ADRs occur within 48 hours of initiating therapy, and 90% within 5 days [103–105]. Peak incidence occurs when drug levels are declining in the serum. Although the absolute incidence of ADRs is unknown, they are estimated to occur in 25% of patients treated with IM depot preparations, 16% of patients who have been given haloperidol, 8% of patients treated with thiothixene, 2% to 12% of all patients who take phenothiazines, 3.5% of patients treated with chlorpromazine, and 1% or less in patients taking atypical agents [11,88,98,103,104]. Phenothiazines that contain a piperazine side chain (i.e., prochlorperazine, trifluoperazine, perphenazine, fluphenazine, and acetophenazine) are associated with a higher incidence of dystonic reactions than are other phenothiazines [103]. Atypical agents (particularly clozapine) are unequivocally associated with a reduced incidence of ADRs [11]. The likelihood of an ADR is more dependent on individual susceptibility than on neuroleptic structure, potency, dose, and duration of therapy [106]. ADRs most commonly occur in men, patients 5 to 45 years of age (particularly those younger than 15 years old), and those with a personal or family history of dystonia or a recent history of drug (i.e., cocaine) or alcohol abuse [103–105,107].

Seizures are an uncommon side effect of certain antipsychotics (e.g., clozapine, chlorpromazine, loxapine). They typically occur at higher therapeutic doses and after overdose in susceptible patients. Seizures are usually generalized and of the major motor type. Clozapine, the most epileptogenic agent at therapeutic dosing, is associated with a seizure rate of approximately 1% at doses lower than 300 mg per day, a rate of 2.7% at doses between 300 and 600 mg per day, and a rate of 4.4% with doses larger than 600 mg per day [64,65]. A cumulative seizure risk of 10% after 3.8 years of treatment has been demonstrated with clozapine [79,80]. Newer, atypical agents show no increase in seizure risk when compared with haloperidol or placebo [26]. Other risk factors for seizures include a history of organic brain disease, epilepsy, electroconvulsive therapy, abnormal baseline electroencephalogram, polypharmacy, and initiation and rapid dose titration of neuroleptics [26,66]. After overdose, the incidence of seizures is as high as 60% and 10% for loxapine and clozapine, respectively, whereas the incidence for most other neuroleptics is approximately 1% [5,31,54,76].

Agranulocytosis (absolute neutrophil count <500 cells per mm^3) is a serious idiosyncratic side effect of clozapine and phenothiazine therapy. It is rare (0.1 to 1.0 per 1,000 persons) with phenothiazines and usually occurs in the first 12 weeks of therapy [108,109]. A cumulative risk of 0.91% (9 per 1,000 persons) at 18 months is reported with clozapine; more than 80% of cases occur in the first 3 months [21,110]. Initial mortality rates associated with agranulocytosis ranged from 30% to 85%, but with regular white blood cell count monitoring and treatment with granulocyte colony stimulating factor (G-CSF), mortality rates have dropped to 3% to 4% [21,110,111]. The mechanism underlying clozapine-induced agranulocytosis may be both immune-mediated and the result of direct myelotoxicity from the drug [112]. Granulocyte colony-stimulating factor has been useful in treatment, halving recovery time from 16 to 8 days [113,114]. Agranulocytosis has not been reported after acute overdose. Neutropenia has also been associated with the therapeutic use of olanzapine, quetiapine, and risperidone [115–117].

Hepatic transaminitis is an adverse side effect of most antipsychotics [11,23]. Hepatotoxicity is idiosyncratic, often occurs within the first 3 months of treatment, and is usually mild and self-limiting (most patients remain asymptomatic). The patterns of hepatoxicity are both hepatitic (including nonalcoholic steatohepatitis) and cholestatic [118,119].

Most atypical neuroleptics result in an increased appetite and weight gain. More importantly, and perhaps causally related, the therapeutic use of atypical agents has been associated with an increased risk of developing type II diabetes mellitus [107–124]. Several cases of fatal diabetic ketoacidosis and hyperglycemia hyperosmolar nonketotic coma have been reported in patients taking clozapine and olanzapine [124–126]. Pancreatitis has been associated with the use of clozapine, and hypertriglyceridemia has been reported in patients treated with clozapine, olanzapine, and quetiapine [106,127–130].

Allergic dermatitis, cholestatic jaundice, irreversible pigmentary retinopathy, photosensitivity reactions, and priapism are uncommon idiosyncratic reactions associated with phenothiazine therapy [11,23,131–134]. Myocarditis and cardiomyopathy have been rarely associated with the use of clozapine; these conditions are idiosyncratic, frequently fatal, often occur within the first 2 weeks of treatment, and are likely the result of acute hypersensitivity [25,135,136].

Drug interactions and adverse effects may be pharmacodynamic (i.e., receptor or channel mediated) or pharmacokinetic (i.e., altered absorption, metabolism, or protein binding) [137,138]. Combining antipsychotics with other CNS depressants (i.e., antihistamines, cyclic antidepressants, ethanol, opiates, sedative–hypnotics) may produce enhanced CNS and respiratory depression. Respiratory depression and arrest has been reported with the coadministration of clozapine and lorazepam or diazepam [139–142]. Exaggerated anticholinergic effects may occur with concurrent use of tricyclic antidepressants, certain skeletal muscle relaxants, antihistamines, and antiparkinson agents. The combination of antipsychotics with significant α_1-adrenergic blockade and certain antihypertensive agents (e.g., hydralazine, prazosin) may precipitate hypotension. Enhanced cardiotoxicity may occur when mesoridazine or thioridazine is combined with type IA antiarrhythmic agents or tricyclic antidepressants. High-dose droperidol, haloperidol, sertindole, thioridazine, and ziprasidone may potentiate QT prolongation produced by other cardioactive agents.

Most antipsychotic agents are extensively metabolized by the hepatic cytochrome P450 (CYP) enzyme system, particularly the CYP2D6 and CYP1A2 isoenzymes. Other drugs that are substrates (i.e., cyclic antidepressants), inhibitors (i.e., cimetidine, erythromycin, selective serotonin reuptake inhibitors), or inducers (i.e., anticonvulsants) of similar CYP isoenzymes may alter antipsychotic metabolism and precipitate adverse effects. These interactions often go unnoticed, but they may be clinically significant. Cimetidine, erythromycin, and fluvoxamine have precipitated clinical clozapine toxicity from hepatic CYP1A2 isoenzyme inhibition [143–146]. Paroxetine may precipitate risperidone toxicity from CYP2D6 isoenzyme inhibition. Knowledge of antipsychotic-associated drug interactions facilitates recognition and treatment of these increasingly common iatrogenic events.

CLINICAL TOXICITY

Acute overdose may result in nausea and vomiting soon after ingestion. CNS and cardiovascular effects, however, usually dominate the clinical picture [5,31,55–58,61,75–79]. In mild intoxication, findings include ataxia, confusion, lethargy, slurred speech, tachycardia, and hypertension or orthostatic hypotension. Anticholinergic signs (e.g., dry skin and mucosa, decreased bowel sounds, urinary retention) and hyperreflexia may also be present. Although usually considered an idiosyncratic reaction, EPS (e.g., ADRs) have been described after acute neuroleptic overdose, particularly in children [5,75,92]. Electrocardiographic changes such as prolonged PR and QT intervals, ST-segment depression, T-wave abnormalities (biphasic, blunting, inversion, notching, widening), and increased U waves may be seen [31,45–48]. Other than sinus tachycardia, repolarization abnormalities are the earliest and most common electrocardiographic findings associated with neuroleptic poisoning [31,45–48,52,147].

Signs and symptoms of moderate poisoning include low-grade coma (see Chapter 117), respiratory depression, and hypotension. Miosis or mydriasis may occur. Miosis is more likely to occur following overdose of both atypical and typical agents; it has been described in 75% of adults and 72% of children after phenothiazine overdose [5,77,79,84,148]. Internuclear ophthalmoplegia has been reported [149]. Paradoxical agitation, delirium, hallucinations, psychosis, myoclonic jerking, and tachypnea may occur [5,76,79,82–86,150]. Central and peripheral anticholinergic stigmata frequently occur after overdose with chlorpromazine, clozapine, mesoridazine, olanzapine, and thioridazine [5,76,79,82–86].

In severe poisoning, high-grade coma with loss of most or all reflexes, apnea, hypotension, seizures, and a variety of cardiac conduction disturbances and arrhythmias may develop. Conduction disturbances include all degrees of AV block, bundle-branch and fascicular block, and nonspecific intraventricular conduction delay [31,46,48,49,54,58–61,147]. Bradyarrhythmias occur uncommonly and, when present, may signify impending respiratory arrest. Tachyarrhythmias include sinus and supraventricular tachycardias, supraventricular and ventricular premature beats, ventricular tachycardia and fibrillation, and TdP [5,31,45–49,57–61,151]. The latter arrhythmia typically occurs in the setting of QT-interval prolongation and has been described with amisulpride, droperidol, haloperidol, mesoridazine, pimozide, and thioridazine [152]. TdP has also been described when critically ill patients are given haloperidol for sedation. In one study, TdP occurred in 3.6% of such patients; the incidence was 64% in those given greater than 35 mg of haloperidol in less than 6 hours and 84% when given to those with a corrected QT (QTc) interval greater than 500 milliseconds [153]. TdP has been rarely associated with therapeutic (usually large) doses of droperidol [49,50,154]. Discovery of this association prompted the Federal Drug Administration to issue a "black box" warning to U.S. health care personnel for droperidol in 2001 [155]. Serious cardiovascular toxicity occurs more commonly when piperidine phenothiazines have been ingested [31]. In one study of 299 patients with neuroleptic overdose, thioridazine was associated with a significantly greater incidence of prolonged QRS, prolonged QTc, and arrhythmia as compared to other neuroleptics [31]. Electrocardiographic abnormalities or obvious cardiotoxicity should be evident within several hours of overdose. Newer agents alter cardiac conduction less frequently but are not entirely void of cardiotoxicity. Prolonged QRS and QT intervals and hypotension have been described after risperidone overdose, and ventricular tachycardia has occurred after remoxipride overdose [61]. The new drug approval application for sertindole was withdrawn in the United States due to dose-related prolongation of the QT interval that occurred during premarketing trials with the drug [53].

Although the overall seizure incidence is about 1% for patients that overdose on neuroleptics, the incidence is much greater following ingestion of chlorpromazine, clozapine, loxapine, mesoridazine, and thioridazine [5,30,31,54,76]. Occasionally, hypothermia or hyperthermia may be seen [156]. Pulmonary edema has been reported rarely as a complication of overdose with chlorpromazine, clozapine, haloperidol, and perphenazine [5,80,81]. Neuroleptic malignant syndrome (NMS) is an idiosyncratic reaction that rarely occurs after acute overdose. Acute overdose, however, may infrequently produce a clinical picture (i.e., the presence of hyperthermia, autonomic instability, neuromuscular hyperreactivity, and hypertonia) that could be misinterpreted as NMS [15]. Agents that produce anticholinergic effects (e.g., clozapine, mesoridazine, olanzapine, thioridazine) would be more likely to do this.

Loxapine poisoning results in an atypical clinical picture. Cardiovascular effects are mild or absent, but convulsions are common and often lead to rhabdomyolysis and subsequent renal failure [54,157].

Following overdose, toxic effects (e.g., CNS depression) begin within 1 to 2 hours, maximal severity is usually evident by 2 to 6 hours, and resolution usually occurs by 24 to 48 hours after ingestion. The presentation is the same regardless of age and whether the overdose is acute or chronic. Early deaths are due to respiratory arrest, arrhythmias, shock, or aspiration-associated respiratory failure. Later complications include cerebral and pulmonary edema, disseminated intravascular coagulation, rhabdomyolysis, myoglobinuric renal failure, and infection.

ADRs are characterized by abrupt onset, intermittent and repetitive nature, normal physical examination except for muscular findings, a history of recent neuroleptic use, and rapid response to anticholinergic drug therapy [98,103–105]. Muscle contractions may sometimes be sustained but usually last from seconds to minutes. They may be focal at the onset and then spread to contiguous muscles; occasionally, they are generalized [158]. Patients remain alert and oriented during these reactions.

Although dystonia may occur in any striated muscle, one of five areas is typically affected [98,103–105,159–161]. ADRs involving the muscles of the eye (oculogyric crisis) cause upward gazing, rotation of the eyes, and spasm of the lids. Those involving muscles of the tongue and jaw (buccolingual crisis) produce trismus, protrusion of the tongue, dysphagia, dysarthria, and facial grimacing. Contractions of muscles of the neck or back result in abnormal head positioning (torticollic reactions) or arching and twisting of the torso (opisthotonic posturing), respectively. When muscles of the abdominal wall are involved, patients present with abdominal wall pain and spasm, bizarre gait patterns, kyphosis, and lordosis (tortipelvic and gait crises). Buccolingual and torticollic ADRs are the most common [103–105].

Although ADRs are rarely life threatening, those involving the tongue, jaw, neck, and chest can result in upper airway compromise and impaired respiratory mechanics [162,163]. Stridor can occur in those with buccolingual and torticollic reactions. Death from respiratory failure has been reported [162,164].

DIAGNOSTIC EVALUATION

The diagnosis of antipsychotic poisoning is made from a history of exposure, physical findings, and supporting evidence from electrocardiographic, laboratory, and other ancillary studies. A complete history should be obtained from the patient as well as the person(s) who found or brought the patient (to corroborate the patient's history). As with all drug ingestions, the name, quantity, and time of ingestion of the drug(s) should be determined. For patients who become toxic during chronic therapy, a recent medication or dose change or an illness may be responsible. Patients and family members should be specifically questioned about the possibility of antipsychotic exposure when signs of an EPS are present.

Physical examination should focus on the vital signs, respiratory function, and neurologic status. Physical findings that suggest neuroleptic poisoning include CNS and respiratory depression, sinus tachycardia, miosis, anticholinergic stigmata, orthostatic hypotension, and the presence of EPS. The patient should be examined for evidence of coexisting trauma. An initial rhythm strip and subsequent 12-lead electrocardiogram (ECG) should be evaluated. Arterial blood gas determinations and a chest radiograph should be ordered in patients with significant CNS depression. An abdominal radiograph showing radiopaque densities in the gastrointestinal (GI) tract may suggest butyrophenone or phenothiazine poisoning if the etiology of symptoms is unknown. The absence of this finding, however, does not rule out poisoning by these agents. Routine laboratory evaluation should include a complete blood cell count and electrolyte count and blood urea nitrogen, creatinine, and glucose tests. Measurements of serum acetaminophen and salicylate should be performed on all patients with intentional overdose. In patients with seizures, hyperthermia, and severe poisoning, laboratory evaluation should include urinalysis (routine and for myoglobin); creatinine phosphokinase, calcium, magnesium, and phosphate tests; and a coagulation profile. Women of childbearing age should have a pregnancy test performed.

Toxicologic analysis of the urine and serum by immunoassay and chromatography–mass spectrometry may be performed to confirm the identity of the offending agent and to rule out other ingestants [165]. Quantitative drug levels are not helpful in predicting clinical toxicity or guiding treatment [7,68,69,72]. Although neither sensitive nor specific, or readily available, the Forrest, Mason, and Phenistix (Ames Company, Inc., Elkhart, IN) colorimetric tests are rapid urine screens that may be positive with phenothiazine ingestions [166]. These tests, however, do not detect nonphenothiazine neuroleptic agents. Certain neuroleptics (e.g., chlorpromazine, mesoridazine, quetiapine, and thioridazine) will commonly produce false positive results for tricyclic antidepressants on most commercially available immunoassay screens used by hospitals to test for drugs of abuse [167].

Patients with ADRs should be questioned regarding current medications, previous ADRs, recreational drug use, and change in the dose of a neuroleptic or other medication associated with this syndrome. The diagnosis is made on the basis of history of drug exposure and the physical examination.

A complete blood cell count should be performed on patients who develop a fever or infection while taking clozapine or phenothiazines.

Agents that cause CNS and cardiovascular effects similar to those resulting from antipsychotic poisoning include antiarrhythmic, anticholinergic, anticonvulsant, antidepressant, antihistamine, opioid, other psychotropic agents (e.g., lithium, bupropion) and sedative–hypnotics, and skeletal muscle relaxants. It may be impossible to distinguish cyclic antidepressant or type IA antiarrhythmic agent poisoning from poisoning due to chlorpromazine, thioridazine, or mesoridazine without toxicologic analysis. CNS infection, cerebrovascular accident, occult head trauma, and metabolic abnormalities should also be considered in the differential diagnosis.

The differential diagnosis of an ADR includes primary dystonias, seizures, cerebrovascular accident, encephalitis, tetanus, hypocalcemia, drug intoxication (especially anticholinergic, anticonvulsant, and strychnine), hysterical conversion reactions, joint dislocations, meningitis, hypomagnesemia, torticollis, and alkalosis.

MANAGEMENT

All patients who are symptomatic after acute overdose should be observed until they are alert. Those with mild toxicity can often be managed in the emergency department or a similarly equipped observation unit. Those with protracted hypotension, significant CNS depression or agitation, seizures, acid-base disturbances, nonsinus arrhythmias, and cardiac conduction disturbances should be admitted to an intensive care unit. Patients with ECG abnormalities (e.g., prolonged QRS or QTc intervals) who are otherwise asymptomatic should be admitted to a cardiac monitored bed; such findings have been implicated in sudden death.

Treatment is primarily supportive. The tempo and sequence of interventions depend on the clinical severity. Advanced life support measures should be instituted as necessary, and underlying metabolic abnormalities corrected. All patients require cardiac and respiratory monitoring. Vital signs should be obtained frequently. Endotracheal intubation for airway protection or ventilatory support may be required. Patients with seizures or hyperthermia should have continuous (rectal probe) temperature monitoring. Those with altered mental status should receive supplemental oxygen and be given a diagnostic trial of naloxone (2 mg IV), dextrose (25 g IV), and thiamine (100 mg IV). Although reversal of CNS depression after naloxone administration has been reported [168], such a response is inconsistent with the pharmacology of neuroleptics and should not be expected.

Hypotension should be initially treated with Trendelenburg's position and several liters (10 to 40 mL per kg IV) of normal saline. α_1-adrenergic agonists (i.e., norepinephrine, phenylephrine) are first-line agents for treating refractory hypotension, particularly in patients who have been poisoned by antipsychotics with significant α_1-adrenergic blockade. Central venous, intra-arterial, and pulmonary artery pressure monitoring may be necessary for optimal management of patients who are hemodynamically unstable.

Sinus and supraventricular tachycardias rarely require specific treatment. If they are associated with hypotension, correction of this abnormality is often all that is necessary. Sodium bicarbonate (1 to 2 mEq per kg IV) may be effective and is strongly recommended for patients who have wide QRS complexes or ventricular tachyarrhythmias. Lidocaine (1 to 1.5 mg per kg IV) and electrical cardioversion are alternative treatments for patients with ventricular tachyarrhythmias, depending on hemodynamic stability. Type IA (i.e., disopyramide, quinidine, procainamide), type IC (i.e., propafenone), and type III (i.e., amiodarone) antiarrhythmic drugs are not recommended and are potentially dangerous; they may worsen cardiac conduction abnormalities [169]. TdP ventricular tachycardia should be treated with magnesium (50 to 100 mg per kg

IV over 1 hour); or an increase in heart rate (overdrive pacing) should be treated using isoproterenol or electricity [170–172]. Increasing the heart rate may shorten a prolonged QT interval and thus facilitate conversion of this arrhythmia. The blood pressure should be carefully monitored during isoproterenol administration, as it may cause or worsen hypotension. A search for and correction of hypokalemia, hypomagnesemia, and other electrolyte disturbances is requisite to the management of TdP. Bradyarrhythmias associated with hemodynamic compromise should be treated with atropine, epinephrine, dopamine, and isoproterenol according to current advanced cardiac life support protocols. Complete heart block may require temporary cardiac pacing.

Recent literature supports the antidotal use of intravenous fat emulsions (IFE) for severe central nervous system or cardiovascular toxicity from highly lipophilic drugs [173]. IFE infusions may create a "lipid sink" whereby lipophilic drugs are sequestered in a newly created intravascular lipid compartment, thereby reducing tissue binding. Alternatively, IFE infusions may restore myocardial function by providing exogenous fatty acid substrate or by increasing intracellular calcium for myocyte function [173]. In a rabbit model of chlorpromazine toxicity, IFE treatment decreased free drug available for tissue toxicity and increased survival in poisoned animals [174]. In human case reports, IFE administration has been temporally associated with attenuation of QTc prolongation and CNS depression from quetiapine overdose [175,176]. The overwhelming majority of antipsychotic-overdose patients do well with good supportive care and would not necessitate IFE infusion therapy. ILE treatment, however, should be strongly considered and is recommended for patients with severe and refractory cardiovascular or CNS toxicity from antipsychotic drugs. IFE is commonly administered an IV bolus followed by a 3 to 24 hour continuous infusion. A reasonable dosing algorithm for both adults and children is a 1 to 2 mL per kg IV bolus of 20% IFE over 1 minute followed by 0.25 to 0.5 mL per kg per minute continuous IV infusion (total dose 2 g per kg per day IFE) [173].

Seizures are often self-limited and may not require specific treatment. If prolonged or recurrent, seizures should be treated with incremental doses of diazepam or lorazepam (initial dose, 0.05 to 0.10 mg per kg IV). A short-acting barbiturate (e.g., amobarbital, 10 to 15 mg per kg IV at a maximal rate of 100 mg per minute) or a long-acting one (e.g., phenobarbital, 20 mg per kg IV at a maximal rate of 30 mg per minute) may sometimes be necessary. The effectiveness of phenytoin is not established for neuroleptic-associated seizures. Refractory convulsions, as seen in loxapine poisoning [54,157], may require the use of a paralyzing agent to prevent complications such as hyperthermia and rhabdomyolysis. A nondepolarizing neuromuscular blocker, such as pancuronium (0.06 to 0.10 mg per kg IV) or vecuronium (0.08 to 0.10 mg per kg IV) is recommended over succinylcholine. Continued treatment of seizures, as indicated by electroencephalogram monitoring, is necessary during therapeutic paralysis. Diuresis and alkalinization of urine may be useful in preventing myoglobinuric renal failure for patients with rhabdomyolysis (see Chapter 73).

Physostigmine may be used safely and effectively in poisoned patients who have significant peripheral or central anticholinergic stigmata (i.e., agitated delirium) and normal PR and QRS intervals on ECG (see Chapter 121) [99]. Its use has been described with chlorpromazine, clozapine, olanzapine, and thioridazine poisoning [83,85,86]. Physostigmine should be given slowly intravenously (0.02 mg per kg in children or 2 mg in adults) over 3 minutes. Alternatively, agitated delirium from the anticholinergic syndrome may be treated with benzodiazepines.

After stabilization, GI decontamination should be performed for patients with acute ingestions. Oral activated charcoal (1 g per kg) with or without a cathartic is the preferred method for the majority of patients. Although gastric lavage may benefit comatose patients who present within 1 hour of drug ingestion, it is not routinely recommended for neuroleptic overdose for which the mortality rate is very low [177]. If performed, gastric lavage should always be followed with activated charcoal administration. Because of decreased GI tract motility resulting from poisoning, decontamination (activated charcoal administration) may be of benefit many hours after overdose.

Although clinical improvement was reported during combined hemodialysis and charcoal hemoperfusion [178], the effect was transient, and measures to enhance the elimination of neuroleptic agents, such as diuresis, dialysis, and hemoperfusion, have not been shown to be pharmacokinetically effective [179,180]. Repeated oral doses of activated charcoal are of potential but unproved benefit. Use of multidose charcoal is not recommended and potentially harmful for patients who have developed an ileus.

The vast majority of patients with neuroleptic poisoning recover completely within several hours to several days, depending on severity. Patients with intentional overdosage require psychiatric evaluation before discharge.

Patients with respiratory distress secondary to ADRs should be given supplemental oxygen. Those with buccolingual and torticollic crises should be given nothing by mouth, because doing so could precipitate choking. Because ADRs rarely result from an overdose, GI tract decontamination is usually not indicated and may, in fact, be hazardous because of the potential for airway complications.

Administration of an anticholinergic agent readily reverses ADRs, presumably by restoring the balance between cholinergic and dopaminergic pathways in the basal ganglia [98]. Benztropine mesylate, 1 to 2 mg, or diphenhydramine, 50 to 100 mg, given intravenously over 1 to 2 minutes, can be used. Reversal of signs and symptoms usually occurs within a few minutes. In some cases, a second dose is needed for complete resolution. Benztropine appears to be more effective and is less likely to cause sedation and hypotension than diphenhydramine and is the preferred agent in adults [105,181]. Although benztropine is contraindicated in children younger than 3 years of age because of its anticholinergic effects [182], this is precisely the desired effect, and its administration in small doses (e.g., 0.25 to 0.50 mg) is appropriate in this situation. As an alternative, diphenhydramine (1 mg per kg IV) can be used. Benztropine and diphenhydramine can also be given intramuscularly, but it may take 30 to 90 minutes for the ADR to resolve when this route is used. Cases resistant to anticholinergic agents may respond to diazepam (0.1 mg per kg IV) or lorazepam (0.05 to 0.10 mg per kg IV).

Subsequent therapy with an oral anticholinergic agent should be continued for 48 to 72 hours. Without such therapy, the ADR may recur because it may take several days to eliminate completely the agent that caused it and the duration of action of drugs used to treat it is much shorter. In addition to benztropine and diphenhydramine, biperiden (2 mg 1 to 3 times a day), trihexyphenidyl (2 mg twice per day), or amantadine (100 to 200 mg twice per day) can be used for oral therapy. For reasons already noted, benztropine (1 to 2 mg twice per day) is the preferred agent for adults. Children younger than 3 years can be given diphenhydramine (1 mg per kg orally three or four times per day). Although patients who have had an ADR are at increased risk for future ADRs, those requiring continued antipsychotic therapy can usually continue or resume taking the offending agent provided they are also maintained on anticholinergic therapy. As an alternative, they can be switched to atypical antipsychotic with less dopaminergic-blocking activity.

References

1. Richelson E: Receptor pharmacology of neuroleptics: relation to clinical effects. *J Clin Psychiatry* 60[Suppl 10]:5–14, 1999.
2. Jibson MD, Tandon R: New atypical antipsychotic medications. *J Psychiatr Res* 32:215–228, 1998.
3. Blin O: A comparative review of new antipsychotics. *Can J Psychiatry* 44:235–244, 1999.
4. Tandon R, Milner K, Jibson MD: Antipsychotics from theory to practice: integrating clinical and basic data. *J Clin Psychiatry* 60[Suppl 8]:21–28, 1999.
5. Burns MJ: The pharmacology and toxicology of atypical antipsychotic agents. *J Tox Clin Toxicol* 39(1):1–14, 2001.
6. Ray WA, Chung CP, Murray KT, et al: Atypical antipsychotic drugs and the risk of sudden cardiac death. *NEJM* 360:225–235, 2009.
7. Baldessarini RJ, Tarazi FI: Pharmacotherapy of psychosis and mania, in Brunton LL, Lazo JS, Parker KL (eds): *Goodman & Gilman's The Pharmacological Basis of Therapeutics*. 11th ed. New York, McGraw-Hill Companies, Inc, 2006 pp 461–500.
8. Kinon BJ, Lieberman JA: Mechanisms of action of atypical antipsychotic drugs: a critical analysis. *Psychopharmacology* 124:2–34, 1996.
9. Seeman P, Lee T, Chau-Wong M, et al: Antipsychotic drug doses and neuroleptic dopamine receptors. *Nature* 261:717–719, 1976.
10. Risch SC: Pathophysiology of schizophrenia and the role of newer antipsychotics. *Pharmacotherapy* 16[Suppl]:11–14, 1996.
11. Casey DE: The relationship of pharmacology to side effects. *J Clin Psychiatry* 58[Suppl 10]:55–62, 1997.
12. Black JL, Richelson E: Antipsychotic drugs: prediction of side effect profiles based on neuroreceptor data derived from human brain tissue. *Mayo Clin Proc* 62:369–372, 1987.
13. Farde L, Nordstrom A, Wiesel F, et al: Positron emission tomographic analysis of central D_1 and D_2 dopamine receptor occupancy in patients treated with classical neuroleptics and clozapine. *Arch Gen Psychiatry* 49:538–544, 1992.
14. Meltzer HY, Matsubara S, Lee JC: Classification of typical and atypical antipsychotic drugs on the basis of dopamine D-1, D-2 and serotonin$_2$ pK_i values. *J Pharmacol Exp Ther* 251:238–246, 1989.
15. Burris KD, Molski FR, Xu C, et al: Aripiprazole, a novel antipsychotic, is a high-affinity partial agonist at human dopamine D2 receptors. *J Pharmacol Exp Ther* 302:381–389, 2002.
16. Goren JL, Levin GM: Quetiapine, an atypical antipsychotic. *Pharmacotherapy* 18:1183–1194, 1998.
17. Markowitz JS, Brown CS, Moore TR: Atypical antipsychotics part I. pharmacology, pharmacokinetics, and efficacy. *Ann Pharmacother* 33:73–85, 1999.
18. Pickar D: Prospects for pharmacotherapy of schizophrenia. *Lancet* 345: 557–562, 1995.
19. Seeger TF, Seymour PA, Schmidt AW, et al: Ziprasidone (CP-88,059): a new antipsychotic with combined dopamine and serotonin receptor antagonist activity. *J Pharmacol Exp Ther* 275:101–113, 1995.
20. Bymaster FP, Perry KW, Nelson DL, et al: Olanzapine: a basic science update. *Br J Psychiatry* 174[Suppl 37]:36–40, 1999.
21. Alvir J, Lieberman J, Safferman A, et al: Clozapine-induced agranulocytosis: incidence and risk factors in the United States. *N Engl J Med* 329:162–167, 1993.
22. Laidlaw ST, Snowden JA, Brown MJ: Aplastic anemia and remoxipride. *Lancet* 342:1245, 1993.
23. Selim K, Kaplowitz N: Hepatotoxicity of psychotropic drugs. *Hepatology* 29:1347–1351, 1999.
24. Thorogood M, Cowen P, Mann J, et al: Fatal myocardial infarction and use of psychotropic drugs in young women. *Lancet* 340:1067–1068, 1992.
25. Grenade LL, Graham D, Trontell A: Myocarditis and cardiomyopathy associated with clozapine use in the United States [letter]. *N Engl J Med* 345(3):224, 2001.
26. Cold JA, Wells BG, Froemming JH: Seizure activity associated with antipsychotic therapy. *DICP* 24:601–606, 1990.
27. Logothetis J: Spontaneous epileptic seizures and electroencephalographic changes in the course of phenothiazine therapy. *Neurology* 17:869–877, 1967.
28. Kahn A, Blum D: Phenothiazines and sudden infant death syndrome. *Pediatrics* 70:75–78, 1982.
29. Mehtonen OP, Aranko K, Malkonen L, et al: A survey of sudden death associated with the use of antipsychotic or antidepressant drugs: 49 cases in Finland. *Acta Psychiatr Scand* 84:58–64, 1991.
30. Buckley N, McManus P: Fatal toxicity of drugs used in the treatment of psychotic illnesses. *Br J Psychiatry* 172:461–464, 1998.
31. Buckley NA, Whyte IM, Dawson AH: Thioridazine has greater cardiotoxicity in overdose than other neuroleptics. *J Toxicol Clin Toxicol* 33:199–204, 1995.
32. Bronstein AC, Spyker DA, Cantilena LR, et al: 2007 Annual report of the American Association of Poison Control Centers' National Poison Data System (NPDS): 25th annual report. *Clin Toxicol* 46:927–1057, 2008.
33. Goldberg LI, Rajkes SI: Dopamine receptors: applications in clinical cardiology. *Circulation* 72:245–248, 1985.
34. Stoof JC, Kebabian JW: Two dopamine receptors: biochemistry, physiology and pharmacology. *Life Sci* 34:2281–2286, 1984.
35. Lindvall O, Bjorklung A, Skagerberg G: Dopamine-containing neurons in the spinal cord: anatomy and some functional aspects. *Ann Neurol* 14:255–260, 1983.
36. Huttunen M: The evolution of the serotonin-dopamine antagonist concept. *J Clin Psychopharmacol* 15:4S–10S, 1995.
37. Lieberman JA, Mailman RB, Duncan G, et al: Serotonergic basis of antipsychotic drug effects in schizophrenia. *Biol Psychiatry* 44:1099–1117, 1998.
38. Leysen JE, Janssen PMF, Schotte A, et al: Interaction of antipsychotic drugs with neurotransmitter receptor sites in vitro and in vivo in relation to pharmacologic and clinical effects: role of 5-HT_2 receptors. *Psychopharmacol (Berl)* 112[Suppl 1]:S40–S54, 1993.
39. Shahid M, Walker GB, Zorn SH, Wong EHF: Asenapine: a novel psychopharmacologic agent with a unique human receptor signature. *J Psychopharmacol* 23:65–73, 2009.
40. Ogata N, Narahashi T: Block of sodium channels by psychotropic drugs in single guinea-pig cardiac myocytes. *Br J Pharmacol* 97:905–913, 1989.
41. Drolet B, Vincent F, Rail J, et al: Thioridazine lengthens repolarization of cardiac ventricular myocytes by blocking the delayed rectifier potassium current. *J Pharm Exp Ther* 288:1261–1268, 1999.
42. Rampe D, Murawsky K, Grau J, et al: The antipsychotic agent sertindole is a high affinity antagonist of the human cardiac potassium channel hERG. *J Pharm Exp Ther* 286:788–793, 1998.
43. Gould RJ, Murphy KMM, Reynolds IJ, et al: Antischizophrenic drugs of the diphenylbutylpiperidine type act as calcium channel antagonists. *Proc Natl Acad Sci USA* 86:5122–5125, 1983.
44. Gould RJ, Murphy KMM, Reynolds IJ, et al: Calcium channel blockade: possible explanation for thioridazine's peripheral side effects. *Am J Psychiatry* 141:352–357, 1984.
45. Wendkos MH: The significance of electrocardiogenic changes produced by thioridazine. *J New Drugs* 4:322–332, 1964.
46. Fowler ND, McCall D, Chou T, et al: Electrocardiographic changes and cardiac arrhythmias in patients receiving psychotropic drugs. *Am J Cardiol* 37:223–230, 1981.
47. Flugelman MY, Tal A, Pollack S, et al: Psychotropic drugs and long QT syndromes: case reports. *J Clin Psychiatry* 46:290–291, 1985.
48. Elkayam U, Frishman W: Cardiovascular effects of phenothiazines. *Am Heart J* 100:397–401, 1980.
49. Lawrence KR, Nasraway SA: Conduction disturbances associated with administration of butyrophenone antipsychotics in the critically ill: a review of the literature. *Pharmacotherapy* 17:531–537, 1997.
50. Frye MA, Coudreaut MF, Hakeman SM, et al: Continuous droperidol infusion for management of agitated delirium in an intensive care unit. *Psychosomatics* 36:301–305, 1995.
51. Riker RR, Fraser GL, Cox PM: Continuous infusion of haloperidol controls agitation in critically ill patients. *Crit Care Med* 22:433–440, 1994.
52. Fulop G, Phillips RA, Shapiro AK, et al: ECG changes during haloperidol and pimozide treatment of Tourette's disorder. *Am J Psychiatry* 144:673–675, 1987.
53. Lee AM, Knoll JL, Suppes R: The atypical antipsychotic sertindole: a case series. *J Clin Psychiatry* 58:410–416, 1997.
54. Peterson C: Seizures induced by acute loxapine overdose. *Am J Psychiatry* 138:1089–1091, 1981.
55. Hustey FM: Acute quetiapine poisoning. *J Emerg Med* 17:995–997, 1999.
56. Kopala LC, Day C, Dillman B, et al: A case of risperidone overdose in early schizophrenia: a review of potential complications. *J Psychiatry Neurosci* 23:305–308, 1998.
57. Krahenbuhl SI, Sauter B, Kupferschmidt H, et al: Reversible QT prolongation with torsades de pointes in a patient with pimozide intoxication. *Am J Med Sci* 309:315–316, 1995.
58. Marris-Simon P, Zell-Kanter M, Kendzlerski D, et al: Cardiotoxic manifestations of mesoridazine overdose. *Ann Emerg Med* 17:1074–1078, 1988.
59. Hulisz DT, Dasa SL, Black LD, et al: Complete heart block and torsades de pointes associated with thioridazine poisoning. *Pharmacotherapy* 14:239–245, 1994.
60. Wilt JL, Minnema AM, Johnson RF, et al: Torsades de pointes associated with the use of intravenous haloperidol. *Ann Intern Med* 119:391–394, 1993.
61. Palatnick W, Meatherall R, Tenenbein M: Ventricular tachycardia associated with remoxipride overdose [abstract]. *J Toxicol Clin Toxicol* 33:492, 1995.
62. Hollister LE, Kosek JV: Sudden death during treatment with phenothiazine derivatives. *JAMA* 192:1035–1038, 1965.
63. Marks RC, Luchins DJ: Antipsychotic medications and seizures. *Psychiatr Med* 9:37–52, 1991.
64. Devinsky O, Honigfeld G, Patin J: Clozapine-related seizures. *Neurology* 41:369–371, 1991.
65. Devinsky O, Honigfeld G, Pacia SV: Seizures during clozapine therapy. *J Clin Psychiatry* 55[Suppl B]:153S–156S, 1994.

66. Alldredge BK: Seizure risk associated with psychotropic drugs: clinical and pharmacokinetic considerations. *Neurology* 53[Suppl 2]:S68–S75, 1999.
67. Invega® [serial online]. Janssen®, Division of Ortho-McNeil-Janssen Pharmaceuticals, Inc. Titusville, NJ, [cited September 25, 2009]. Available at: http://www.invega.com/invega/shared/pi/invega.pdf#zoom = 100.
68. Javaid JI: Clinical pharmacokinetics of antipsychotics. *J Pharmacol* 34:286–295, 1994.
69. Ereshefsky L: Pharmacokinetics and drug interactions: update for new antipsychotics. *J Clin Psychiatry* 57[Suppl 11]:12–25, 1996.
70. Heath A, Svensson C, Martensson E: Thioridazine toxicity: an experimental cardiovascular study of thioridazine and its major metabolites in overdose. *Vet Hum Toxicol* 27:100–105, 1985.
71. Axelsson R, Martensson E: Side effects of thioridazine and their relationship with the serum concentrations of the drug and its main metabolites. *Curr Ther Res* 28:463, 1980.
72. Fang J, Gorrod JW: Metabolism, pharmacogenetics, and metabolic drug-drug interactions of antipsychotic drugs. *Cell Mol Neurobiol* 19:491–510, 1999.
73. Bond GR, Thompson JD: Olanzapine pediatric overdose [letter]. *Ann Emerg Med* 34:292–293, 1999.
74. Parsons M, Buckley NA: Antipsychotic drugs in overdose: practical management guidelines. *CNS Drugs* 6:427–441, 1997.
75. Acri AA, Henretig FM: Effects of risperidone in overdose. *Am J Emerg Med* 16:498–501, 1998.
76. LeBlaye I, Donatini B, Hall M, et al: Acute overdosage with clozapine: a review of the available clinical experience. *Pharmaceutical Med* 6:169–178, 1992.
77. O'Malley GF, Seifert S, Heard K, et al: Olanzapine overdose mimicking opioid intoxication. *Ann Emerg Med* 34:279–281, 1999.
78. Harmon TJ, Benitez JG, Krenzelok EP, et al: Loss of consciousness from acute quetiapine overdosage. *J Toxicol Clin Toxicol* 36:599–602, 1998.
79. Barry D, Meyskens FL, Becker CE: Phenothiazine poisoning: a review of 48 cases. *Calif Med* 118:1–5, 1973.
80. Mahutte CK, Nakassuto SK, Light RW: Haloperidol and sudden death due to pulmonary edema. *Arch Intern Med* 142:1951–1952, 1982.
81. Li C, Gefter WB: Acute pulmonary edema induced by overdosage of phenothiazines. *Chest* 101:102–104, 1992.
82. McAllister CJ, Scowden EB, Stone WJ: Toxic psychosis induced by phenothiazine administration in patients with chronic renal failure. *Clin Nephrol* 10:191–195, 1978.
83. Schuster P, Gabriel E, Luefferie B, et al: Reversal by physostigmine of clozapine-induced delirium. *Clin Toxicol* 10:437–441, 1977.
84. Yip L, Dart RC, Graham K: Olanzapine toxicity in a toddler [letter]. *Pediatrics* 102:1494, 1998.
85. Burns MJ, Linden CH, Graudins A, et al: A comparison of physostigmine and benzodiazepines for the treatment of anticholinergic poisoning. *Ann Emerg Med* 35:374–381, 2000.
86. Ferraro KK, Burkhart KK, Donovan JW, et al: A retrospective review of physostigmine in olanzapine overdose [abstract]. *J Toxicol Clin Toxicol* 39(5):474, 2001.
87. Meeker JE, Herrmann PW, Som SW: Clozapine tissue concentrations following an apparent suicidal overdose of Clozaril. *J Anal Toxicol* 16:54–56, 1992.
88. Elian AA: Fatal overdose of olanzapine. *Forensic Sci Int* 91:231–235, 1998.
89. Casey DE: Neuroleptic-induced acute extrapyramidal syndromes and tardive dyskinesia, in Hirsch S, Weinberger DR (eds): *Schizophrenia*. Oxford, UK, Blackwell Science, 1995, p 546.
90. Cortese L, Pourcher-Bouchard E, Williams R: Assessment and management of antipsychotic-induced adverse events. *Can J Psychiatry* 43[Suppl 1]:15S–20S, 1998.
91. Balestrieri M, Vampini C, Bellantuono C: Efficacy and safety of novel antipsychotics: a critical review. *Hum Psychopharmacol Clin Exp* 15:499–512, 2000.
92. Bonin MM, Burkhart KK: Olanzapine overdose in a 1-year-old male. *Ped Emerg Care* 15:266–267, 1999.
93. McGeer PL, Boulding JE, Gibson WC, et al: Drug-induced extrapyramidal reactions. *JAMA* 177:665–670, 1961.
94. Stahl SM, Berger PA: Bromocriptine, physostigmine, and neurotransmitter mechanisms in the dystonias. *Neurology* 32:889–892, 1982.
95. Young AB, Albion RL, Penney JB: Neuropharmacology of basal ganglia function: relationship to pathophysiology of movement disorders, in Grossman AR, Sambrook MA (eds): *Neural Mechanisms in Disorders of Movement*, London, Libbey, 1989, p 17.
96. Carlsson A, Walters N, Carlsson ML: Neurotransmitter interactions in schizophrenia—therapeutic implications. *Biol Psychiatry* 46:1388–1395, 1999.
97. Jeanjean AP, Laterre C, Maloteaux JM: Neuroleptic binding to sigma receptors: possible involvement in neuroleptic-induced dystonia. *Biol Psychiatry* 41:1010–1019, 1997.
98. Rupniak NMJ, Jenner P, Marsden CD: Acute dystonia induced by neuroleptic drugs. *Psychopharmacol* 88:403–419, 1986.
99. Baldessarini RJ, Tarsy D: Dopamine and the pathophysiology of dyskinesia induced by antipsychotic drugs. *Annu Rev Neurosci* 3:23–41, 1980.
100. Stockmeier CA, DiCarlo JJ, Zhang Y, et al: Characterization of typical and atypical antipsychotic drugs based on in vivo occupancy of $serotonin_2$ and $dopamine_2$ receptors. *J Pharmacol Exp Ther* 266:1374–1384, 1993.
101. Kolbe H, Clow A, Jenner P, et al: Neuroleptic-induced acute dystonic reactions may be due to enhanced dopamine release or to supersensitive postsynaptic receptors. *Neurology* 31:434–439, 1981.
102. Marsden CD, Jenner P: The pathophysiology of extrapyramidal side-effects of neuroleptic drugs. *Psychol Med* 10:55–72, 1980.
103. Swett C: Drug-induced dystonia. *Am J Psychiatry* 132:532–534, 1982.
104. Ayd FJ: A survey of drug-induced extrapyramidal reactions. *JAMA* 175:1054–1060, 1961.
105. Lee AS: Treatment of drug-induced dystonic reactions. *JACEP* 8:453–457, 1979.
106. Kingsbury SJ, Fayek M, Trufasiu D: The apparent effects of ziprasidone on plasma lipids and glucose. *J Clin Psychiatry* 62:347–349, 2001.
107. Lebovitz HE: Metabolic consequences of atypical antipsychotic drugs. *Psychiatr Q* 74:277–290, 2003.
108. Litvak R, Kaelbling R: Agranulocytosis, leukopenia and psychotropic drugs. *Arch Gen Psychiatry* 24:265–267, 1971.
109. Trayle WH: Phenothiazine-induced agranulocytosis [letter]. *JAMA* 256:1957, 1986.
110. Safferman A, Lieberman JA, Kane JM, et al: Update on the clinical efficacy and side effects of clozapine. *Schizophr Bull* 17:247–261, 1991.
111. Iqbal MM, Rahman A, Husain K, et al: Clozapine: a clinical review of adverse effects and management. *Ann Clin Psychiatry* 15:33–48, 2003.
112. Lorenz M, Evering WE, Provencher A, et al: Atypical antipsychotic-induced neutropenia in dogs. *Toxicol Appl Pharmacol* 155:227–236, 1999.
113. Geibig CB, Marks LW: Treatment of clozapine- and molindone-induced agranulocytosis with granulocyte colony-stimulating factor. *Pharmacotherapy* 27:1190–1194, 1993.
114. Gerson SL: G-CSF and the management of clozapine-induced agranulocytosis. *J Clin Psychiatry* 55[Suppl B]:139–142, 1994.
115. Steinwachs A, Grohmann R, Pedrosa F, et al: Two cases of olanzapine-induced reversible neutropenia. *Pharmacopsychiatry* 32:154–156, 1999.
116. Ruhe HG, Becker HE, Jessurun P: Agranulocytosis and granulocytopenia associated with quetiapine. *Acta Psychiatr Scand* 104:311–313, 2001.
117. Dernovsek Z, Tavcar: Risperidone-induced leucopenia and neutropenia. *Br J Psychiatry* 171:393–394, 1997.
118. Whitworth AB, Liensberger D, Fleischhacker WW: Transient increase of liver enzymes induced by risperidone: two case reports [letter]. *J Clin Psychopharmacol* 19:475–476, 1999.
119. Haberfellner EM, Honsig T: Nonalcoholic steatohepatitis: a possible side effect of atypical antipsychotics. *J Clin Psychiatry* 64:851, 2003.
120. Liebzeit KA: New onset diabetes and atypical antipsychotics. *Eur Neuropsychopharmacol* 11:25–32, 2001.
121. Gianfrancesco F, White R, Ruey-hua W, et al: Antipsychotic-induced type 2 diabetes: evidence from a large health plan database. *J Clin Psychopharmacol* 23:328–335, 2003.
122. Citrone LL, Jaffe AB: Relationship of atypical antipsychotics with development of diabetes mellitus. *Ann Pharmacother* 37:1849–1857, 2003.
123. Torrey EF, Swalwell CI: Fatal olanzapine-induced ketoacidosis. *Am J Psychiatry* 160:2241, 2003.
124. Koller EA, Doraiseamy PM: Olanzapine-associated diabetes mellitus. *Pharmacotherapy* 22:841–852, 2002.
125. Meatherall R, Younes J: Fatality from olanzapine-induced hyperglycemia. *J Forensic Sci* 47:893–896, 2002.
126. Wehring HJ, Kelly DL, Love RC, et al: Deaths from diabetic ketoacidosis after long-term clozapine treatment. *Am J Psychiatry* 160:2241–2242, 2003.
127. Koller EA, Cross JT, Doraiswamy PM: Pancreatitis associated with atypical antipsychotics: from the Food and Drug Administration's Med Watch surveillance system and published reports. *Pharmacotherapy* 23:1123–1130, 2003.
128. Haupt DW, Newcomer JW: Hyperglycemia and antipsychotic medications. *J Clin Psychiatry* 62[Suppl 27]:15–26, 2001.
129. Meyer JM: Novel antipsychotics and severe hyperlipidemia. *J Clin Psychopharmacol* 21:369–374, 2001.
130. Domon SE, Webber JC: Hyperglycemia and hypertriglyceridemia secondary to olanzapine. *J Clin Adolesc Psychopharmacol* 11:285–288, 2001.
131. Horio T: Chlorpromazine photoallergy: co-existence of immediate and delayed type. *Arch Dermatol* 111:1469–1471, 1975.
132. Fishbain DA: Priapism resulting from fluphenazine hydrochloride treatment reversed by diphenhydramine. *Ann Emerg Med* 14:600–602, 1985.
133. Gomez EA: Neuroleptic-induced priapism. *Tex Med* 81:47–48, 1985.
134. Derby L, Gutthann SP, Jick H, et al: Liver disorders in patients receiving chlorpromazine or isoniazid. *Pharmacotherapy* 13:354–358, 1993.
135. Anonymous: Clozapine and myocarditis. *WHO drug information* 8:212–213, 1994.
136. Merrill DB, Dec GW, Goff DC: Adverse cardiac effects associated with clozapine. *J Clin Psychopharmacol* 25:32–41, 2005.
137. DeVane CL: Drug interactions and antipsychotic therapy. *Pharmacotherapy* 16[Suppl]:15–20, 1996.
138. Goff DC, Baldessarini RJ: Drug interactions with antipsychotic agents. *J Clin Psychopharmacol* 13:57–67, 1993.
139. Cobb CD, Anderson CB, Seidel DR: Possible interaction between clozapine and lorazepam [letter]. *Am J Psychiatry* 148:1606–1607, 1991.
140. Grohmann R, Ruther E, Sassim N, et al: Adverse effects of clozapine. *Psychopharmacology* 99[Suppl]:S101–S104, 1989.

141. Edge SC, Markowitz JS, DeVane CL: Clozapine drug interactions: a review of the literature. *Hum Psychopharmacol* 12:5–20, 1997.
142. Klimke A, Klieser E: Sudden death after intravenous application of lorazepam in a patient treated with clozapine [letter]. *Am J Psychiatry* 151:780, 1994.
143. Szymanski S, Liberman JA, Picou D, et al: A case report of cimetidine-induced clozapine toxicity. *J Clin Psychiatry* 52:21–22, 1991.
144. Cohen LG, Chesley S, Eugenio L, et al: Erythromycin-induced clozapine toxic reaction. *Arch Intern Med* 156:675–677, 1996.
145. Funderberg LG, Vertrees JE, True JE, et al: Seizure following addition of erythromycin to clozapine treatment. *Am J Psychiatry* 151:1840–1841, 1994.
146. Stevens I, Gaertner HJ: Plasma level measurement in a patient with clozapine intoxication. *J Clin Psychopharmacol* 16:86–87, 1996.
147. Axelsson R, Aspenstrom G: Electrocardiographic changes and serum concentrations in thioridazine-treated patients. *J Clin Psychiatry* 43:332–335, 1982.
148. Mitchell AA, Lovejoy FH, Goldman P: Drug ingestions associated with miosis in comatose children. *J Pediatr* 89:303–305, 1976.
149. Cook FF, Davis RG, Russo LS: Internuclear ophthalmoplegia caused by phenothiazine intoxication. *Arch Neurol* 38:465–466, 1981.
150. Knight ME, Roberts RJ: Phenothiazine and butyrophenone intoxication in children. *Pediatr Clin North Am* 33:299–309, 1986.
151. Zee-cheng CS, Mueller CE, Seifert CF, et al: Haloperidol and torsades de pointes [letter]. *Ann Intern Med* 102:418, 1985.
152. Isbister GK, Murray L, John S, et al: Amisulpride deliberate self-poisoning causing severe cardiac toxicity including QT prolongation and torsades de pointes. *Med J Aust* 184(7):354–356, 2006.
153. Sharma ND, Rosman HS, Padhi D, et al: Torsades de pointes associated with intravenous haloperidol in critically ill patients. *Am J Cardiol* 81:238–240, 1998.
154. Lischke V, Behne M, Doelken P, et al: Droperidol causes a dose-dependent prolongation of the QT interval. *Anesth Analg* 79:983–986, 1994.
155. MedWatch 2001 Safety Information Summaries: Inapsine (Droperidol). Available at: http://www.fda.gov/medwatch/safety/2001/safety01.htm#inapsi. Accessed January 16, 2005.
156. Baker PB, Merigian KS, Roberts JR, et al: Hyperthermia, hypotension, hypertonia, and coma in a massive thioridazine overdose. *Am J Emerg Med* 6:346–349, 1988.
157. Tam CW, Olin BR, Ruiz AE: Loxapine-associated rhabdomyolysis and acute renal failure. *Arch Intern Med* 140:975–976, 1980.
158. Hoffman AS, Schwartz HI, Novick RM: Catatonic reaction to accidental haloperidol overdose: an unrecognized drug abuse risk. *J Nerv Ment Dis* 174:428–430, 1986.
159. Fahn S: The varied clinical expressions of dystonia. *Neurol Clin* 2:541–554, 1984.
160. Jeste DV, Wisniewski AA, Wyatt RJ: Neuroleptic-associated tardive syndromes. *Psychiatr Clin North Am* 9:183–192, 1986.
161. Jankovic J: Drug-induced and other orofacial-cervical dyskinesias. *Ann Intern Med* 94:788–793, 1981.
162. Pollera CF, Cognetti F, Nardi M, et al: Sudden death after acute dystonic reactions to high-dose metoclopramide [letter]. *Lancet* 2:460–461, 1984.
163. Newton-John H: Acute upper airway obstruction due to supraglottic dystonia inducted by a neuroleptic. *BMJ* 297:964–965, 1988.
164. Koek RJ, Edmond HP: Acute laryngeal dystonic reactions to neuroleptics. *Psychosomatics* 30:359–364, 1989.
165. Baselt RC (ed): *Disposition of Toxic Drugs and Chemicals in Man*. 7th ed. Foster City, CA, Biomedical Publications, 2004.
166. Forrest FM, Forrest IS, Mason AS: Review of rapid urine tests for phenothiazine and related drugs. *Am J Psychiatry* 118:300–307, 1961.
167. Sloan KL, Haver VM, Saxon AJ: Quetiapine and false-positive urine drug testing for tricyclic antidepressants [letter]. *Am J Psychiatr* 157:148–149, 2000.
168. Chandavasu O, Chatkupt S: Central nervous system depression from chlorpromazine poisoning: successful treatment with naloxone. *J Pediatr* 106:515–516, 1985.
169. Kawamura T, Kodama I, Toyama J, et al: Combined application of class I antiarrhythmic drugs causes "additive," "reductive," or "synergistic" sodium channel block in cardiac muscles. *Cardiovasc Res* 24:925–931, 1990.
170. Lumpkin J, Watanabe AS, Rumack BH, et al: Phenothiazine-induced ventricular tachycardia following acute overdose. *JACEP* 8:476–478, 1979.
171. Pietro DA: Thioridazine-associated ventricular tachycardia and isoproterenol [letter]. *Ann Intern Med* 94:411, 1981.
172. Kemper A, Dunlop R, Pietro D: Thioridazine-induced torsades de pointes successful therapy with isoproterenol. *JAMA* 249:2931–2934, 1983.
173. Turner-Lawrence DE, Kerns II W: Intravenous fat emulsion: a potential novel antidote. *J Med Toxicol* 4:109–114, 2008.
174. Krieglstein J, Meffert A, Niemeyer HD: Influence of emulsified fat on chlorpromazine availability in rabbit blood. *Experimentia* 30:924–926, 2008.
175. Finn SDH, Uncles DR, Willers J, et al: Early treatment of a quetiapine and sertraline overdose with Intralipid®. *Anaesthesia* 64:191–194, 2009.
176. Lu JJ, Hast HA, Erickson TB: Dramatic QTc narrowing after Intralipid administration in quetiapine overdose [abstract]. *Clin Toxicol* 47:740, 2009.
177. Kulig K, Bar-Or D, Cantrill SV, et al: Management of acutely poisoned patients without gastric emptying. *Ann Emerg Med* 14:562–567, 1985.
178. Koppel C, Schirop T, Ibe K, et al: Hemoperfusion in chlorprothixene overdose. *Intensive Care Med* 13:358–360, 1987.
179. Donlon PT, Tupin JP: Successful suicides with thioridazine and mesoridazine. *Arch Gen Psychiatry* 34:955–957, 1977.
180. Hals PA, Jacobsen D: Resin hemoperfusion in levomepromazine poisoning: evaluation of effect on plasma drug and metabolite levels. *Hum Toxicol* 3:497–503, 1984.
181. Bailie GR, Nelson MV, Krenzelok EP, et al: Unusual treatment response of a severe dystonia to diphenhydramine. *Ann Emerg Med* 16:705–708, 1987.
182. Merck and Company, Inc: Cogentin, in *Physicians' Desk Reference*. Montvale, NJ, Medical Economics, 2002 pp 2055–2056.

CHAPTER 125 ■ BETA-BLOCKER POISONING

SHAN YIN AND JAVIER C. WAKSMAN

Since 1958, when dichloroisoprenaline, the first β-adrenergic blocker, was synthesized, more than a dozen beta-blockers have been introduced into the international pharmaceutical market. Originally developed for the treatment of angina pectoris and dysrhythmias, beta-blockers are now used in a wide variety of disorders. Intoxication may result from oral, parenteral, and even ophthalmic use [1].

PHARMACOLOGY

Beta-blockers act by competitively inhibiting the binding of epinephrine and norepinephrine to β-adrenergic neuroreceptors in the heart (β_1), blood vessels, bronchioles (β_2), and other organs (Table 125.1). Binding to the β receptor (G-protein–coupled receptor) activates phosphodiesterase and increases cytoplasmic cyclic adenosine monophosphate (cAMP). This in turn leads to modification of cellular processes and changes in ionic channel conductance. By reducing the activity of β receptors, the production of cAMP is decreased and β effect is diminished [2].

Beta-blockers are usually rapidly absorbed after oral administration. The beta-blocker dose required to produce a toxic effect is variable, depending on the sympathetic tone and metabolic capacity of the person and the pharmacologic properties of the particular beta-blocker [2]. The first signs of toxicity may appear 20 minutes after ingestion, with peak effects typically occurring 1 to 2 hours after an immediate-release preparation overdose. Absorption of modified-release formulations may be erratic after an overdose, however, and clinical

TABLE 125.1

DISTRIBUTION AND FUNCTION OF β-RECEPTORS

Receptor subtype	Location	Response to stimulation
β_1	Eye	Aqueous humor production
	Heart	Increased automaticity, conduction velocity, contractility, and refractory period
β_2	Kidney	Renin production
	Blood vessels	Smooth muscle contraction
	Bronchioles	Smooth muscle contraction
	Fat	Lipolysis
	Liver	Gluconeogenesis, glycogenolysis
	Pancreas	Insulin release
	Skeletal muscle	Increased tone, potassium uptake
	Uterus	Smooth muscle relaxation

toxicity may be significantly delayed. The duration of toxicity may be several days [2].

The pharmacologic and pharmacokinetic properties of beta-blockers are variable (Table 125.2). Cardioselectivity tends to be lost at high doses, and membrane-stabilizing effects, which are minimal at therapeutic doses, assume a more important role [2]. Membrane dysfunction may account for many of the central nervous system (CNS) and myocardial depressant effects in patients poisoned by membrane-active drugs such as propranolol. The half-life may be significantly prolonged in patients with decreased hepatic and renal perfusion [2]. Intrinsic heart, kidney, and liver disease as well as the concomitant use of drugs with similar activity increase the risk of toxicity.

CLINICAL TOXICITY

The major manifestations relate to the cardiovascular system and CNS. Respiratory, peripheral vascular, and metabolic (hypoglycemic and hyperkalemic) effects have been infrequently reported [2,3].

Patients with severe poisoning frequently present with hypotension and bradycardia. Tachycardia and hypertension have been reported with agents possessing intrinsic sympathomimetic activity, however, particularly pindolol [2]. Congestive heart failure and pulmonary edema have infrequently been reported and mainly occur in patients with underlying heart disease [4]. Electrocardiographic manifestations may include prolonged PR interval, intraventricular conduction delay, progressive atrioventricular heart block, nonspecific ST-segment and T-wave changes, early repolarization, prolonged corrected QT (QTc) interval, and asystole [5–7]. Sotalol poisoning may result in ventricular tachycardia, torsade de pointes, ventricular fibrillation, and multifocal ventricular extrasystoles [8,9]. Labetalol, which also has mild β-receptor–blocking properties, may cause profound hypotension, possibly from decreased peripheral resistance.

Depression in the level of consciousness, ranging from drowsiness to coma with seizures, is another common feature of beta-blocker poisoning. Significant CNS depression has been reported in the absence of cardiovascular compromise [2] or hypoglycemia and may be due to direct membrane effects [10]. Cerebral hypoperfusion, hypoxia, and metabolic or respiratory acidosis frequently contribute to CNS toxicity. Beta-blockers with high lipid solubility (e.g., propranolol, penbutolol, metoprolol) appear more likely to cause CNS effects than those with low lipid solubility (e.g., atenolol) [11,12].

Bronchospasm is a relatively rare consequence of beta-blocker poisoning and usually occurs more frequently in patients with preexisting reactive airway disease. In most instances, respiratory depression appears to be secondary to a CNS effect [13–16].

Although it does occur, hypoglycemia is not a common complication of beta-blocker poisoning [17]. It appears to be more common in diabetics, children, and uremic patients and it is the consequence of impaired glycogenolysis and hepatic gluconeogenesis [18]. A blunted tachycardic response to hypoglycemia may occur in patients with beta-blocker toxicity, although other symptoms of hypoglycemia appear unaffected.

Oliguric renal failure has been reported as a complication of labetalol poisoning [19]. Mesenteric ischemia and subsequent cardiovascular collapse have occurred after propranolol overdose [20].

Sudden discontinuation of long-term beta-blocker therapy may precipitate angina pectoris and myocardial infarction. This is the result of the "beta-blocker withdrawal phenomenon," explained by the theory that long-term beta-blocker therapy not only diminishes receptor occupancy by catecholamines but also increases the number of receptors sensitive to adrenergic stimulation. When beta-blockers are suddenly withdrawn, the increased pool of sensitive receptors responds more readily to the stimulation of circulating catecholamines [17].

DIAGNOSTIC EVALUATION

The history should include the time, amount, and formulation of drugs ingested; the circumstances involved; time of onset and nature of any symptoms; and treatments rendered before arrival, as well as underlying health problems. Beta-blocker poisoning may be difficult to recognize, especially when multiple drugs have been ingested [2]. Beta-blocker poisoning should be suspected in a patient in whom hypotension or seizures suddenly develop or who has bradycardia resistant to the usual doses of chronotropic drugs [21]. Evaluation of patients with suspected beta-blocker poisoning should begin with a complete set of vital signs, continuous cardiac rhythm monitoring, and a 12-lead electrocardiogram. Physical examination should focus on the cardiovascular, pulmonary, and neurologic systems. Vital signs and physical examination should be frequently repeated.

Serum drug levels may help confirm the diagnosis but are rarely available quickly enough to be clinically useful. In addition, differences in individual patient metabolism and sympathetic tone may make interpretation of blood levels difficult [2,3]. A serum and urine specimen can be saved for later analysis in forensic cases. Continuous cardiac rhythm monitoring, interpretation of 12-lead electrocardiograms, and measurement of oxygen saturation should be routine. Laboratory evaluation of symptomatic patients should include electrolytes, blood urea nitrogen, creatinine, bicarbonate, and glucose. Arterial blood gas and a chest film should be obtained as clinically indicated. Serum acetaminophen and aspirin levels should be obtained in patients with suicidal ideation.

The differential diagnosis of beta-blocker toxicity includes antidysrhythmic drugs, calcium channel blockers, cholinergic agents, clonidine, digitalis, narcotics, sedative hypnotics, and tricyclic antidepressants. Anaphylactic, cardiogenic, hypovolemic, and septic shock should also be considered.

The prognosis associated with beta-blocker intoxication is generally positive. A review of two regional poison control centers [22] found that 15% of patients developed cardiac toxicity, and only 1.4% died. The only factor associated with increased

TABLE 125.2

PHARMACOLOGIC AND PHARMACOKINETIC PROPERTIES OF β-ADRENERGIC BLOCKING AGENTS

Agent	Adrenergic receptor blocking activity	Intrinsic sympathomimetic activity	Lipid solubility	Extent of absorption (%)	Absolute oral bioavailability (%)	Half-life (h)	Protein binding (%)	Metabolism/excretion
Acebutolol	$\beta_1{}^a$	+	Low	90	20–60	3–4	26	Hepatic, renal excretion 30%–40%, nonrenal 50%–60%
Atenolol	$\beta_1{}^a$	0	Low	≈50	≈50	5–8	<5	≈75% excreted unchanged in urine and feces
Betaxolol	$\beta_1{}^a$	0	Low	≅100	89	14–22	≈50	Hepatic; >80% recovered in urine
Bisoprolol	$\beta_1{}^a$	0	Low	≥90	80	9–12	≈30	≈50% excreted unchanged in urine, remainder as inactive metabolites
Esmolol	$\beta_1{}^a$	0	Moderate	NA	NA	0.15	55	Rapid metabolism by esterases in cytosol of red blood cells
Metoprolol, long-acting	$\beta_1{}^a$	0	Moderate	95	40–50	3–7	12	Hepatic, renal excretion, <5% unchanged
Carteolol	β_1, β_2	++	Low	80	85	6	23–30	50%–70% unchanged in urine
Nadolol	β_1, β_2	0	Low	30	30–50	20–24	30	Urine, unchanged
Penbutolol	β_1, β_2	+	High	≈100	≈100	5	80–98	Hepatic (conjugation and oxidation); renal excretion of metabolites
Pindolol	β_1, β_2	+++	Moderate	95	≈100	3–4[b]	40	Urinary excretion of metabolites (60%–74%) and unchanged drug (35%–40%)
Propranolol, long-acting	β_1, β_2	0	High	90	30	3–5	90	Hepatic; <1% excreted unchanged in urine
Sotalol	β_1, β_2	0	Low	No data	90–100	12	0	Not metabolized; excreted unchanged in urine
Timolol	β_1, β_2	0	Low to moderate	90	75	4	10	Hepatic; urinary excretion of metabolites and unchanged drug
Carvedilol	β_1, β_2, α_1	0	High	NA	25–35	6–10	95–98	Hepatic (aromatic ring oxidation and conjugation), 16% renal excretion
Labetalol	β_1, α_1	0	Moderate	100	30–40	5.0–5.8	50	55%–60% excreted in urine as conjugates or unchanged drug

[a]Inhibits β_2 receptors (bronchial and vascular) at higher doses.
[b]In elderly hypertensive patients with normal renal function, $t^1/_2$ is variable (7–15 h).
0, none; +, low; ++, moderate; +++, high; NA, not applicable (available intravenously only).
Reprinted from Olin BR, Hebel SK (eds): *Drug Facts and Comparisons*. St. Louis, Facts and Comparisons, Inc, 1997; Hardman J, Limbird L, Molinoff P, et al. (eds): *Goodman and Gilman's Pharmacological Basis of Therapeutics*. 9th ed. New York, McGraw-Hill, 1996.

morbidity was coingestion of cardioactive drugs such as calcium channel blockers, cyclic antidepressants, and neuroleptics [22].

MANAGEMENT

Treatment is primarily supportive. This may include prompt endotracheal intubation and mechanical ventilation and management of life-threatening bradydysrhythmias, hypotension, bronchospasm, and seizures. These attempts should precede any measures (as described later) used to prevent or reduce drug absorption. A bedside glucose measure or, alternatively, an intravenous bolus of glucose (50 mL of $D_{50}W$ in adults; 4 mL per kg of $D_{25}W$ in children) as well as naloxone (2 mg in adults and children) should be given to patients with altered mental status (Fig. 125.1).

Activated charcoal is the preferred methods for gastrointestinal decontamination [14]. Gastric lavage has not been shown to improve outcome after poisoning and should not be used routinely, but considered for recent life-threatening ingestions in patients who have not already vomited [23]. Lavage may cause bradycardia from vagal effects. Thus, atropine should be given prior to initiation, and lavage should be withheld in patients with existing bradycardia and conduction abnormalities. Whole-bowel irrigation with polyethylene glycol (Golytely^{TM}) at a rate of 2 L per hour until the rectal effluent is clear may be considered for gastrointestinal decontamination in modified-release preparation overdoses.

Hypotension should be first treated with judicious intravenous crystalloid fluids. Because hypotension seldom responds solely to this treatment and because administration of high volumes (greater than 2 L) of intravenous fluids may pose a risk to develop pulmonary edema, the prompt use of inotropic drugs such as dopamine, dobutamine, epinephrine, norepinephrine, and phenylephrine is usually required [24]. Bradycardia from β-adrenergic antagonist poisoning seldom responds to atropine.

Calcium

The goal of calcium therapy is to increase extracellular calcium concentrations thus increasing calcium influx through any unblocked calcium channels. Calcium has demonstrated effectiveness in animal models [25] and improvement reported in human cases [26]. However, responses are variable and often short-lived, and patients with significant toxicity usually fail to improve with calcium alone. Conduction disturbances, contractility, and blood pressure, may be improved, but generally there is no increase in heart rate. Optimum dosing has yet to be established.

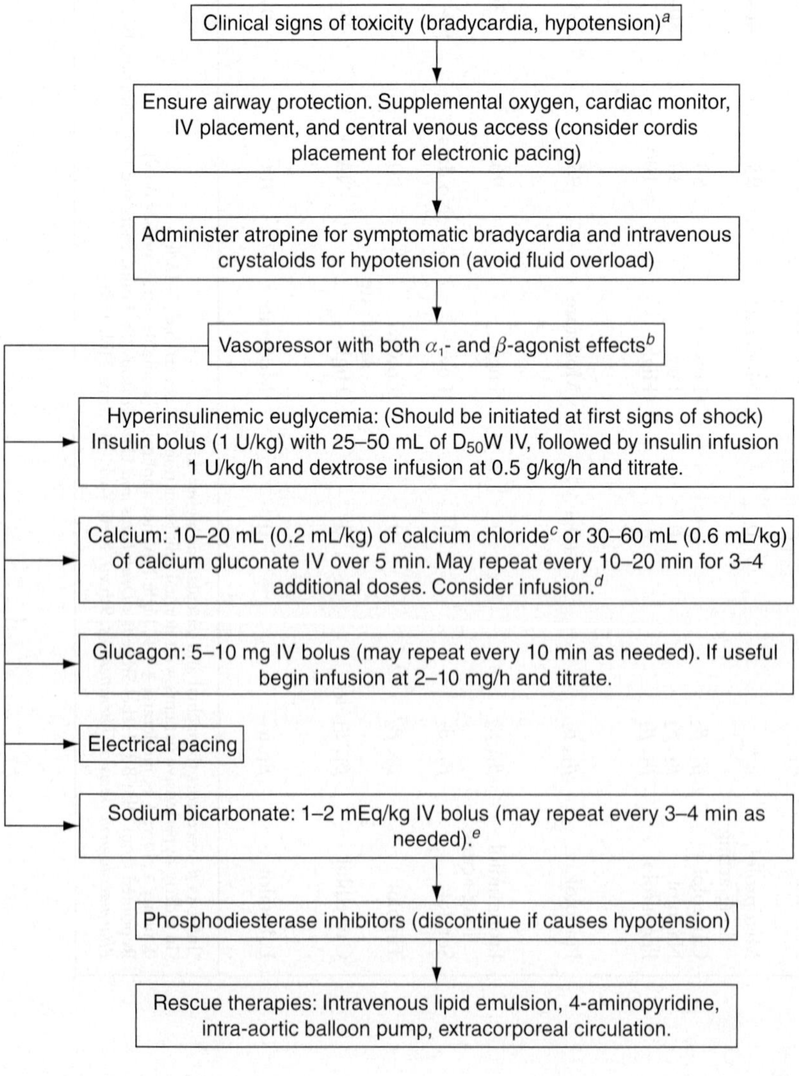

FIGURE 125.1. Suggested algorithm for treatment of beta-blocker poisoning. [a]Patients with significant toxicity will often require multiple therapies and the initiation of these simultaneously. In less severely poisoned patients, therapies can be added sequentially depending on clinical response. Decontaminate on a case-by-case basis, but preservation of vital signs takes precedence over decontamination. [b]May need multiple pressors at very high doses. [c]Administer calcium chloride via a central venous catheter. [d]Calcium infusion: 0.4 mL/kg/h of calcium chloride or 1.2 mL/kg/h of calcium gluconate. May allow higher doses and permissive hypercalcemia depending on response. [e]Administer sodium bicarbonate for wide complex conduction defects caused by beta-blocking agents with membrane stabilizing activity.

Calcium chloride compared to calcium gluconate contains three times the amount of elemental calcium on a milliequivalent basis (10% calcium chloride: 272 mg elemental calcium or 13.6 mEq per 1 g ampule; 10% calcium gluconate: 90 mg elemental calcium or 4.5 mEq per 1 g ampule). However, it is recommended to only give calcium chloride via a central venous catheter. Calcium gluconate can be given via a peripheral line.

Optimum calcium dosing is not well established. Initial doses are generally given as boluses (10 to 20 mL of 10% calcium chloride or 30 to 60 mL of 10% calcium gluconate). Additional boluses may be given every 10 to 20 minutes. Boluses should be given over a 5-minute period in conjunction with cardiac monitoring as rapid infusions have resulted in hypotension, atrioventricular dissociation, and ventricular fibrillation. The effects of boluses may be transient, and a constant infusion required. Infusions can be started at 0.4 mL per kg per hour for calcium chloride and 1.2 mL per kg per hour for calcium gluconate and titrated to effect. Additional boluses can be given as needed. Calcium levels should be monitored. Raising serum ionized calcium to 2 to 3 mEq per L improves canine cardiac performance in verapamil poisoning, and is a reasonable goal to attain. It may be necessary to continue therapy despite high serum calcium levels if the patient is only responding to calcium administration. Hypercalcemia can lead to renal failure and limb or mesenteric ischemia. It is recommended to stop calcium infusions if no beneficial effect is observed.

Glucagon

Although there are no controlled trials of glucagon for beta-blocker overdose in humans, glucagon has served as an effective agent for reversing hypotension and bradycardia in multiple case reports [14,27–29]. Glucagon has a half-life of 20 minutes, so a continuous intravenous infusion of 1 to 10 mg per hour is recommended after an initial bolus of 3 to 10 mg for adults. In children, an initial intravenous dose of 0.05 mg per kg should be followed by a continuous infusion of 0.07 mg per kg per hour [2,3,27]. This dose is titrated to patient response, and large total doses may be required. The dose should be tapered once the patient's clinical condition improves. The mechanism by which glucagon produces a positive inotropic and chronotropic effect on the heart is believed to be activation of the adenyl cyclase pathway, which converts adenosine triphosphate to cAMP through an independent receptor, changing membrane ion conductivity, altering calcium influx, and augmenting contractility even in the presence of complete β-adrenergic blockade [28]. It is recommended that glucagon be reconstituted in a solution of 5% dextrose in water or in preservative-free saline, rather than the diluent provided by the manufacturer, as the latter contains phenol that might be toxic in the large doses often needed to treat beta-blocker toxicity [27,30]. Severe phenol toxicity is usually manifested as chemical burns, lethargy, coma, cardiac dysrhythmias, and death [31]. Non–phenol-containing, high-dose glucagon preparations are now available [32].

Phosphodiesterase Inhibitors

The simultaneous use of multiple agents may be effective when a single agent fails. Although theoretically promising, phosphodiesterase inhibitors such as amrinone and milrinone, which inhibit the breakdown of cAMP to AMP, have not proven to be superior to glucagon in reversing the hemodynamic effects of beta-blocker overdose in a canine model [33,34]. Other studies using dogs have shown no additional benefit of combining a phosphodiesterase inhibitor with glucagon [35,36]. It has been suggested that phosphodiesterase inhibitors might be used in cases of beta-blocker poisoning when adequate doses of glucagon are not available [33]. The phosphodiesterase inhibitor enoximone has been successfully used in cases of beta-blocker overdoses [37].

Sodium Bicarbonate

A number of beta-blockers (propranolol, carvedilol, pindolol, and acebutolol) also affect cardiac sodium channels producing membrane stabilizing effects which may result in quinidine-like dysrhythmias (e.g., wide QRS complexes). This effect may respond to intravenous boluses of sodium bicarbonate albeit in a canine model; sodium bicarbonate was ineffective in treating propranolol toxicity that resulted in bradycardia, hypotension, and wide QRS intervals [38]. In a case report, sodium bicarbonate appeared to reverse QRS widening following an acebutolol overdose [39]. The recommended dose is 1 to 2 mEq per kg given as a rapid infusion over several minutes.

Hyperinsulin–Euglycemia Treatment

High-dose insulin while maintaining euglycemia has been proposed as an antidote for beta-blocker poisoning [40]. Insulin is an inotropic agent which may enhance response to catecholamines and reverse metabolic acidosis. Although results in animals remain encouraging [41–43], further studies are needed in humans. Several case reports described successful insulin–euglycemia therapy for calcium channel blocker toxicity [44] (one patient also ingested a beta-blocker). Therefore, this treatment should be considered an option in patients with refractory beta-blocker toxicity as both classes bear similarities in the clinical manifestation and mechanism of toxicity [45]. The recommended doses are 0.5 to 1.0 IU per kg per hour [40]. A second intravenous infusion of $D_{10}W$ or $D_{25}W$ containing potassium chloride should be simultaneously administered to the insulin infusion at a rate sufficient to maintain the serum glucose and potassium concentrations in the normal range.

Vasopressin

The use of vasopressin in beta-blocker toxicity has been suggested. In one animal trial which compared vasopressin with glucagon in the treatment of beta-blocker toxicity, vasopressin was neither found to increase survival nor had a significant effect on any of the cardiac parameters tested relative to glucagon [46]. High-dose insulin treatment also improved survival when compared to vasopressin with epinephrine in a swine model [43].

Lipid Emulsion

The use of lipid emulsion has been suggested in the treatment of the cardiotoxic effects of local anesthetics. Various animal models of bupivacaine toxicity have demonstrated faster return of spontaneous circulation following treatment with lipid emulsion therapy [47,48] as well as improved cardiodynamic parameters when compared with epinephrine [49]. However, a pig model did not show any improvement in survival when compared to saline controls [50]. Positive outcomes with the use of lipid emulsion were described in human case reports of bupivacaine [51–53], bupropion and lamotrigine [54], and quetiapine and sertraline overdoses [55]. Lipid emulsion was also investigated for the treatment of beta-blockers toxicity; however, there is currently no experience in humans. In a rabbit model, lipid emulsion successfully improved hypotension induced by propranolol when compared with placebo [56]. In a separate study on rats, pretreatment with lipid emulsion resulted in a significant reduction in QRS duration and a nonsignificant improvement in bradycardia induced by propranolol when compared to placebo [57]. The mechanism of how lipid emulsion may be beneficial is not completely understood. The possible explanations include the creation of lipid sink for fat-soluble drugs, augmentation of cardiac energy substrates, or the improvement of myocardial function by increasing intracellular calcium [58]. No standard dosing regimen exists. However, a loading dose of 1.5 mL per kg administered over 1 minute, repeated one or two times every 3 to 5 minutes as needed is often used. If hemodynamic improvement is noted, the loading dose should be followed by a continuous infusion at a rate of 0.25 to 0.5 mL per kg per minute. Further information can be found at www.lipidrescue.org.

Extracorporeal Removal

Although the efficacy of hemodialysis in acute beta-blocker poisoning has not been studied in controlled clinical trials, it is theoretically useful in removing beta-blockers that have a low volume of distribution, are not significantly protein bound, and are hydrophilic. This would include acebutolol, atenolol, nadolol, sotalol, and timolol. Hemodialysis appeared to be clinically useful in a number of case reports involving atenolol, acebutolol, sotalol, and nadolol poisoning [59,60] and in cases of refractory torsade de pointes due to sotalol [61,62]. Charcoal hemoperfusion has also been suggested as an adjunctive therapy in patients severely poisoned with beta-blockers, although experience is limited [63]. Continuous venovenous hemodiafiltration was also successfully used in the treatment of a combined atenolol/nifedipine overdose [64]. The molecular adsorbent recirculating system (MARS) is a blood purification system that may be effective in removing protein bound toxins. There are case reports describing its successful use in theophylline [65] and phenytoin [66] MARS may theoretically be helpful in removing highly protein bound beta-blockers such as propranolol and carvedilol.

Other Interventions

Transient blood pressure elevations caused by pindolol usually require no specific treatment. Short-acting agents such as nitroprusside should be used if marked blood pressure elevation occurs, especially if it is accompanied by organ ischemia. Ventricular dysrhythmias induced by sotalol have been treated with lidocaine, isoproterenol, magnesium, and cardioversion defibrillation [6]. Electrical cardiac pacing may be needed if bradycardia, hypotension, and heart block fail to respond to pharmacologic therapy [2], or if ventricular tachydysrhythmias associated with a prolonged QTc interval are difficult to control [6]. In severe overdoses, a pacemaker may not capture. If capture occurs, the increased heart rate may not increase blood pressure. Heart rates greater than 90 to 100 beats per minute significantly decrease diastolic filling time and may adversely affect inotropy. Intra-aortic balloon pump counterpulsation [32] and extracorporeal circulation [67,68] have been successfully used for cardiovascular support.

Patients with beta-blocker overdose who have abnormal vital signs, altered mental status, or dysrhythmias on presentation should be admitted to an intensive care unit. If vital signs can be supported, complete recovery should be expected within 24 to 48 hours. Patients may be discharged after at least 6 hours of emergency department observation if they have ingested an immediate-release product, present with mild to absent toxicity and remain or become asymptomatic, have normal vital signs on discharge, and have received activated charcoal. These patients should be referred for psychiatric evaluation in the event of an intentional overdose or discharged in the care of a reliable observer after an accidental overdose. Any other symptoms mandate longer observation or admission. Because of the potential for delayed toxicity, prolonged observation is recommended after modified-release preparation overdose.

References

1. Fraunfelder FT: Ocular beta-blockers and systemic effects. *Arch Intern Med* 146:1073–1074, 1986.
2. Frishman W, Jacob H, Eisenberg E, et al: Clinical pharmacology of the new beta-adrenergic blocking drugs. Part 8. Self-poisoning with beta-adrenoceptor blocking agents: recognition and management. *Am Heart J* 98:798–811, 1979.
3. Prichard BN, Battersby LA, Cruickshank JM: Overdosage with beta-adrenergic blocking agents. *Adverse Drug React Acute Poisoning Rev* 3:91–111, 1984.
4. Richards DA, Prichard BN: Self-poisoning with beta-blockers. *Br Med J* 1:1623–1624, 1978.
5. Lagerfelt J, Matell G: Attempted suicide with 5.1 g of propranolol. A case report. *Acta Med Scand* 199:517–518, 1976.
6. Khan A, Muscat-Baron JM: Fatal oxprenolol poisoning. *Br Med J* 1:552, 1977.
7. Gwinup GR: Propranolol toxicity presenting with early repolarization, ST segment elevation, and peaked T waves on the ECG. *Ann Emerg Med* 17:171–174, 1988.
8. Totterman KJ, Turto H, Pellinen T: Overdrive pacing as treatment of sotalol-induced ventricular tachyarrhythmias (torsade de pointes). *Acta Med Scand Suppl* 668:28–33, 1982.
9. Baliga BG: Beta-blocker poisoning: prolongation of Q-T interval and inversion of T wave. *J Indian Med Assoc* 83:165, 1985.
10. Frishman W, Kostis J, Strom J, et al: Clinical pharmacology of the new beta-adrenergic blocking drugs. Part 6. A comparison of pindolol and propranolol in treatment of patients with angina pectoris. The role of intrinsic sympathomimetic activity. *Am Heart J* 98:526–535, 1979.
11. Turner P: Fatal oxprenolol poisoning. *Br Med J* 1:1084, 1977.
12. Buiumsohn A, Eisenberg ES, Jacob H, et al: Seizures and intraventricular conduction defect in propranolol poisoning. A report of two cases. *Ann Intern Med* 91:860–862, 1979.
13. Mattingly PC: Oxprenolol overdose with survival. *Br Med J* 1:776–777, 1977.
14. Shore ET, Cepin D, Davidson MJ: Metoprolol overdose. *Ann Emerg Med* 10:524–527, 1981.
15. Wallin CJ, Hulting J: Massive metoprolol poisoning treated with prenalterol. *Acta Med Scand* 214:253–255, 1983.
16. Weinstein RS, Cole S, Knaster HB, et al: Beta blocker overdose with propranolol and with atenolol. *Ann Emerg Med* 14:161–163, 1985.
17. Frishman W, Silverman R: Clinical pharmacology of the new beta-adrenergic blocking drugs. Part 2. Physiologic and metabolic effects. *Am Heart J* 97:797–807, 1979.
18. Bressler P, DeFronzo RA: Drugs and Diabetes. *Diabetes Rev* 2:53–84, 1994.
19. Korzets A, Danby P, Edmunds ME, et al: Acute renal failure associated with a labetalol overdose. *Postgrad Med J* 66:66–67, 1990.
20. Pettei MJ, Levy J, Abramson S: Nonocclusive mesenteric ischemia associated with propranolol overdose: implications regarding splanchnic circulation. *J Pediatr Gastroenterol Nutr* 10:544–547, 1990.
21. Bekes CE, Scott WE: Occult metoprolol overdose. *Crit Care Med* 13:870–871, 1985.
22. Love JN, Howell JM, Litovitz TL, et al: Acute beta blocker overdose: factors associated with the development of cardiovascular morbidity. *J Toxicol Clin Toxicol* 38:275–281, 2000.
23. Toxicology AAoC: Position paper: gastric lavage. *J Toxicol Clin Toxicol* 42(7):933–943, 2004.
24. Critchley JA, Ungar A: The management of acute poisoning due to beta-adrenoceptor antagonists. *Med Toxicol Adverse Drug Exp* 4:32–45, 1989.
25. Vick JA, Kandil A, Herman EH, et al: Reversal of propranolol and verapamil toxicity by calcium. *Vet Hum Toxicol* 25:8–10, 1983.
26. O'Grady J, Anderson S, Pringle D: Successful treatment of severe atenolol overdose with calcium chloride. *CJEM* 3:224–227, 2001.
27. Illingworth RN: Glucagon for beta-blocker poisoning. *Practitioner* 223:683–685, 1979.
28. Kosinski EJ, Malindzak GS: Glucagon and isoproterenol in reversing propranolol toxicity. *Arch Intern Med* 132:840–843, 1973.

29. Robson RH: Glucagon for beta-blocker poisoning. *Lancet* 1:1357–1358, 1980.
30. Mofenson HC, Caraccio TR, Landano J: Glucagon for propranolol overdose. *JAMA* 255:2025, 1986.
31. Spiller HA, Quadrani-Kushner DA, Cleveland P: A five year evaluation of acute exposures to phenol disinfectant (26%). *J Toxicol Clin Toxicol* 31:307–313, 1993.
32. Lane AS, Woodward AC, Goldman MR: Massive propranolol overdose poorly responsive to pharmacologic therapy: use of the intra-aortic balloon pump. *Ann Emerg Med* 16:1381–1383, 1987.
33. Love JN, Leasure JA, Mundt DJ, et al: A comparison of amrinone and glucagon therapy for cardiovascular depression associated with propranolol toxicity in a canine model. *J Toxicol Clin Toxicol* 30:399–412, 1992.
34. Sato S, Tsuji MH, Okubo N, et al: Milrinone versus glucagon: comparative hemodynamic effects in canine propranolol poisoning. *J Toxicol Clin Toxicol* 32:277–289, 1994.
35. Love JN, Leasure JA, Mundt DJ: A comparison of combined amrinone and glucagon therapy to glucagon alone for cardiovascular depression associated with propranolol toxicity in a canine model. *Am J Emerg Med* 11:360–363, 1993.
36. Sato S, Tsuji MH, Okubo N, et al: Combined use of glucagon and milrinone may not be preferable for severe propranolol poisoning in the canine model. *J Toxicol Clin Toxicol* 33:337–342, 1995.
37. Hoeper MM, Boeker KH: Overdose of metoprolol treated with enoximone. *N Engl J Med* 335:1538, 1996.
38. Love JN, Howell JM, Newsome JT, et al: The effect of sodium bicarbonate on propranolol-induced cardiovascular toxicity in a canine model. *J Toxicol Clin Toxicol* 38:421–428, 2000.
39. Donovan KD, Gerace RV, Dreyer JF: Acebutolol-induced ventricular tachycardia reversed with sodium bicarbonate. *J Toxicol Clin Toxicol* 37:481–484, 1999.
40. Megarbane B, Karyo S, Baud FJ: The role of insulin and glucose (hyperinsulinaemia/euglycaemia) therapy in acute calcium channel antagonist and beta-blocker poisoning. *Toxicol Rev* 23:215–222, 2004.
41. Reikeras O, Gunnes P, Sorlie D, et al: Metabolic effects of low and high doses of insulin during beta-receptor blockade in dogs. *Clin Physiol* 5:469–478, 1985.
42. Kerns W, Schroeder D, Williams C, et al: Insulin improves survival in a canine model of acute beta-blocker toxicity. *Ann Emerg Med* 29:748–757, 1997.
43. Holger JS, Engebretsen KM, Fritzlar SJ, et al: Insulin versus vasopressin and epinephrine to treat beta-blocker toxicity. *Clin Toxicol (Phila)* 45:396–401, 2007.
44. Yuan TH, Kerns WP, Tomaszewski CA, et al: Insulin-glucose as adjunctive therapy for severe calcium channel antagonist poisoning. *J Toxicol Clin Toxicol* 37:463–474, 1999.
45. DeWitt CR, Waksman JC: Pharmacology, pathophysiology and management of calcium channel blocker and beta-blocker toxicity. *Toxicol Rev* 23:223–238, 2004.
46. Holger JS, Engebretsen KM, Obetz CL, et al: A comparison of vasopressin and glucagon in beta-blocker induced toxicity. *Clin Toxicol (Phila)* 44:45–51, 2006.
47. Weinberg GL, VadeBoncouer T, Ramaraju GA, et al: Pretreatment or resuscitation with a lipid infusion shifts the dose-response to bupivacaine-induced asystole in rats. *Anesthesiology* 88:1071–1075, 1998.
48. Weinberg G, Ripper R, Feinstein DL, et al: Lipid emulsion infusion rescues dogs from bupivacaine-induced cardiac toxicity. *Reg Anesth Pain Med* 28:198–202, 2003.
49. Weinberg GL, Di Gregorio G, Ripper R, et al: Resuscitation with lipid versus epinephrine in a rat model of bupivacaine overdose. *Anesthesiology* 108:907–913, 2008.
50. Hicks SD, Salcido DD, Logue ES, et al: Lipid emulsion combined with epinephrine and vasopressin does not improve survival in a swine model of bupivacaine-induced cardiac arrest. *Anesthesiology* 111:138–146, 2009.
51. Rosenblatt MA, Abel M, Fischer GW, et al: Successful use of a 20% lipid emulsion to resuscitate a patient after a presumed bupivacaine-related cardiac arrest. *Anesthesiology* 105:217–218, 2006.
52. Warren JA, Thoma RB, Georgescu A, et al: Intravenous lipid infusion in the successful resuscitation of local anesthetic-induced cardiovascular collapse after supraclavicular brachial plexus block. *Anesth Analg* 106:1578–1580, 2008.
53. Foxall G, McCahon R, Lamb J, et al: Levobupivacaine-induced seizures and cardiovascular collapse treated with Intralipid. *Anaesthesia* 62:516–518, 2007.
54. Sirianni AJ, Osterhoudt KC, Calello DP, et al: Use of lipid emulsion in the resuscitation of a patient with prolonged cardiovascular collapse after overdose of bupropion and lamotrigine. *Ann Emerg Med* 51:412–415, 5 e1, 2008.
55. Finn SDH, Uncles DR, Willers J, et al: Early treatment of a quetiapine and sertraline overdose with Intralipid. *Anaesthesia* 64:191–194, 2009.
56. Harvey MG, Cave GR: Intralipid infusion ameliorates propranolol-induced hypotension in rabbits. *J Med Toxicol* 4:71–76, 2008.
57. Cave G, Harvey MG, Castle CD: The role of fat emulsion therapy in a rodent model of propranolol toxicity: a preliminary study. *J Med Toxicol* 2:4–7, 2006.
58. Turner-Lawrence DE, Kerns Ii W: Intravenous fat emulsion: a potential novel antidote. *J Med Toxicol* 4:109–114, 2008.
59. Snook CP, Sigvaldason K, Kristinsson J: Severe atenolol and diltiazem overdose. *J Toxicol Clin Toxicol* 38:661–665, 2000.
60. Rooney M, Massey KL, Jamali F, et al: Acebutolol overdose treated with hemodialysis and extracorporeal membrane oxygenation. *J Clin Pharmacol* 36:760–763, 1996.
61. Singh SN, Lazin A, Cohen A, et al: Sotalol-induced torsades de pointes successfully treated with hemodialysis after failure of conventional therapy. *Am Heart J* 121:601–602, 1991.
62. Zebuda C, Majlesi N, Greller HA, et al: Sotalol-induced tosades de pointes treated with hemodialysis. *Clin Toxicol* 46:603, 2008.
63. Anthony T, Jastremski M, Elliott W, et al: Charcoal hemoperfusion for the treatment of a combined diltiazem and metoprolol overdose. *Ann Emerg Med* 15:1344–1348, 1986.
64. Pfaender M, Casetti PG, Azzolini M, et al: Successful treatment of a massive atenolol and nifedipine overdose with CVVHDF. *Minerva Anesthesiol* 74:97–100, 2008.
65. Korsheed S, Selby NM, Fluck RJ: Treatment of severe theophylline poisoning with the molecular adsorbent recirculating system (MARS). *Nephrol Dial Transplant* 22:969–970, 2007.
66. Sen S, Ratnaraj N, Davies NA, et al: Treatment of phenytoin toxicity by the molecular adsorbents recirculating system (MARS). *Epilepsia* 44:265–267, 2003.
67. Kolcz J, Pietrzyk J, Januszewska K, et al: Extracorporeal life support in severe propranolol and verapamil intoxication. *J Intensive Care Med* 22:381–385, 2007.
68. Rygnestad T, Moen S, Wahba A, et al: Severe poisoning with sotalol and verapamil. Recovery after 4 h of normothermic CPR followed by extra corporeal heart lung assist. *Acta Anaesthesiol Scand* 49:1378–1380, 2005.

CHAPTER 126 ■ CALCIUM CHANNEL ANTAGONIST POISONING

CHRISTOPHER R. DEWITT

INTRODUCTION

Calcium channel antagonists (CCA) effectively treat a variety of medical conditions. Yet, accidental and intentional overdoses of theses agents can be life threatening. CCAs consistently top the list of cardiovascular medications with the greatest proportion of deaths per exposure [1–3]. Severely poisoned patients demonstrate cardiovascular collapse as well as metabolic derangements similar to diabetic acidosis. Cardiovascular instability is often refractory to typical cardiotonic therapies and medication doses. There is no antidote for CCAs, and no controlled clinical studies to guide therapy. Treatment recommendations are therefore based on case series, case reports, animal studies, and extrapolation. Simultaneous use of multiple therapies is often required and should be tailored to the patient's cardiovascular and metabolic responses. Overall goals of treatment are to provide supportive care, optimize cardiovascular and metabolic function, and decrease drug absorption. If vital signs can be supported until the drug is metabolized or eliminated, most patients will survive without sequelae.

PHYSIOLOGY AND PATHOPHYSIOLOGY

Available CCAs antagonize calcium influx through L-type voltage sensitive channels [4], a specific type of calcium channel found in the heart, vascular smooth muscle, and pancreatic β-islet cells. Multiple physiologic functions are dependent on this calcium influx.

In the cardiovascular system, calcium influx through L-type channels is responsible for the spontaneous pacemaker activity of the sinoatrial (SA) node and depolarization of the atrioventricular (AV) node [4,5]. Other myocardial cells rely on sodium influx for initial depolarization [5,6], but calcium entry via L-type channels contributes to the plateau phase of their action potential [5,7]. Calcium entering during the plateau phase signals the release of additional calcium from the sarcoplasmic reticulum into the cytosol, allowing contraction to occur [5,8,9]. The magnitude and duration of sarcoplasmic calcium release and myocardial contraction is proportional to the magnitude and duration of calcium entry via L-type channels [8]. Vascular smooth muscle tone is also maintained by a similar mechanism [8]. Thus, therapeutic clinical effects of CCAs arise from blockade of L-type channels resulting in decreased cytosolic calcium levels. Depending on the class of CCA administered (see Pharmacology section), the clinical result is depression of SA node automaticity, AV node conduction, myocardial contractility, and vasodilation. The pathophysiologic effects of CCA overdose are essentially an exaggeration of pharmacologic effects that lead to cardiovascular shock. In canines, shock ensues despite a 14-fold or greater increase in endogenous catecholamine concentrations [10–12].

In addition to cardiovascular effects, CCA poisoning also produces a diabetogenic effect of hyperglycemia and acidosis. Insulin secretion is dependent on calcium influx into pancreatic β-islet cells. Although generally not a concern at therapeutic doses, CCBs decrease insulin secretion [13–16]. In canine models of verapamil-induced shock, systemic insulin levels fail to increase in response to an intact glucogenic response and hyperglycemia [10,12,17]. Experimentally, verapamil toxicity also produces systemic [12,18] and myocardial [10] resistance to insulin-mediated carbohydrate uptake. The cause of this resistance may be multifactorial involving decreased substrate delivery from poor perfusion, interference with calcium-dependent cellular insulin responsiveness and glucose uptake, and inhibition of calcium-stimulated mitochondrial dehydrogenases (i.e., pyruvate dehydrogenase) and glucose catabolism [12]. More recent evidence suggests CCAs interfere with cellular signaling, specifically recruitment of glucose transporter proteins (GLUTs) from the intracellular space to cell membranes [19]. These GLUTs are responsible for normal cellular uptake of glucose.

Verapamil toxicity also produces a state of hyperlacticacidemia due to a combination of tissue hypoperfusion and probably a defect in carbohydrate metabolism [12]. In stressed states such as CCA toxicity, the heart switches from preferentially using free fatty acids to carbohydrates (glucose and lactate) for energy production [10,11,17]. Although there is an abundance of circulating carbohydrates (e.g., glucose and lactate), they are essentially unavailable for use because of insulin resistance and decreased insulin availability.

In essence, CCAs decrease cytosolic calcium levels resulting in desirable cardiovascular effects at therapeutic doses, and at toxic doses an exaggeration of those effects. Additionally, toxicity produces a vicious cycle where the myocardium is preferentially metabolizing carbohydrates yet carbohydrate utilization is hindered by impaired insulin release and insulin resistance.

PHARMACOLOGY

In the United States, available CCAs fall into one of three classes: phenylalkylamine (verapamil), benzothiazepine (diltiazem), and dihydropyridines (nifedipine and all other agents). At therapeutic doses, each class has differing affinities for myocardial tissues and vascular smooth muscle. Verapamil and diltiazem are potent inhibitors SA node automaticity, AV node conduction, myocardial contractility, and cause modest vasodilation [20,21]. Verapamil affects the SA node, contractility, and vasodilation more than diltiazem [20,21]. This is probably why verapamil generally causes more deaths than other CCAs [1–3]. Dihydropyridines are far more selective for vascular smooth muscle, and at therapeutic doses have very little effect on cardiac pacemaker cells or contractility [9,20,21]. In significant poisoning this selectivity is lost however.

Pharmacologic properties of CCAs make extracorporeal removal of limited or no value as demonstrated in several cases [22–24], although plasmapheresis was believed to be beneficial in several cases [25–27]. Therapeutic half-lives of CCBs are variable, but in overdose can be prolonged [22,28–31]. The duration of toxicity in most cases is less than 24 hours, but has been reported to last 48 hours with sustained release (SR) verapamil [32] and for more than 5 days with amlodipine [33].

Verapamil, diltiazem, nifedipine, and several of the newer dihydropyridines are available in both immediate release (IR) and SR formulations. This information becomes important when considering how long to observe asymptomatic patients after an overdose. Immediate-release preparations produce signs or symptoms of toxicity within 6 hours of ingestion [34] whereas toxicity with SR products may be delayed 6 to 12 hours [34–37] or rarely longer [38]. Amlodipine, a dihydropyridine, has unique pharmacokinetics however. It is not a sustained release product, but has a late onset of peak effect and long half-life allowing for delayed and prolonged toxicity.

There is no accurate definition of a toxic dose, and patients have demonstrated significantly different effects at similar doses. Unintentional overdoses are common, but uncommonly result in significant effect. However, several adult patients have developed toxicity and death at doses less than maximum recommended daily doses [39]. Factors that could have contributed to this are advanced age, underlying medical conditions, additional medications, and chewing and swallowing SR preparations—essentially changing the pharmacokinetics into an IR formulation [39]. In general, the most significant poisonings are large intentional ingestions, but patients with significant underlying medical diseases, or advanced age can have significant effects at lower doses.

CLINICAL MANIFESTATIONS

Cardiovascular effects are the primary manifestation of CCA poisoning. Alterations in mental status without significant hypotension should not be attributed to CCA ingestion. Minimally intoxicated patients, or those who present soon after ingestion, may demonstrate no signs of toxicity. All CCAs can cause hypotension in overdose. However, the cause of the hypotension is typically an extension of the drugs' therapeutic effects. (i.e., dihydropyridines causing significant vasodilation with reflex tachycardia where verapamil and diltiazem slow

SA and AV node conduction, decrease contractility, and cause vasodilation) Thus, in overdose normal sinus rhythm or reflex tachycardia is commonly seen with nifedipine [34,37,40], where sinus bradycardia, AV nodal blocks, and junctional rhythm are common with verapamil and diltiazem [34,37,41]. This selectivity may be lost in large overdoses so that dihydropyridine poisoning results in bradycardia and/or impaired cardiac conduction [33,34,37,42–47]. Although overdose experience with dihydropyridines other than nifedipine is limited [33,45–48], they would be expected to have effects similar to nifedipine. The exception may be amlodipine where toxic effects may be delayed [46].

Severe poisoning is characterized by hypotension and bradycardia [34,37,40,49,50], hyperglycemia [37,38,40,42,45–47, 49–59] and metabolic acidosis [17,33,42,46,47,49,52,53,56, 59]. Hyperglycemia is due to aforementioned alterations in insulin and carbohydrate homeostasis (see Physiology and Pathophysiology section). In fact, in a recent review of 40 CCA overdoses the degree of hyperglycemia was the best predictor of the composite end points of death, pacemaker requirement, or vasopressor requirement [60]. Dysfunctional carbohydrate metabolism and tissue hypoperfusion result in hyperlacticacidemia. In addition, tissue hypoperfusion can result in cerebrovascular accidents, seizures, renal failure, myocardial infarction, and noncardiogenic pulmonary edema [61].

DIFFERENTIAL DIAGNOSIS

CCA poisoning should be considered in any patient presenting with hypotension and bradycardia. Suspicions that the patient is poisoned with a CCA should be raised even further if there is associated hyperglycemia and acidosis. However, the differential diagnosis of a patient with hypotension and bradycardia includes other toxicologic causes such as beta-blockers, digoxin and other cardiac glycosides, antidysrhythmics, and clonidine. However, nontoxicologic causes such as myocardial disease, hyperkalemia, sepsis, and hypothyroidism should also be considered.

MANAGEMENT

General

Management of a patient with CCA poisoning begins with airway management and maintenance of vital signs. Vascular access should be obtained and continuous blood pressure and cardiac monitoring initiated. Preemptive intubation should strongly be considered in patients with significant ingestions or signs of toxicity due to the potential for rapid deterioration. In bradycardic patients, administration of atropine before intubation may prevent vagal responses from laryngoscopy. An electrocardiogram (ECG) should be obtained. The presence of dysrhythmias or conduction disturbances, which may be as subtle as PR prolongation in some patients, should be noted. Measurements of renal function, electrolytes, complete blood counts, liver function tests, arterial blood gases, and acetaminophen, salicylate, and digoxin levels should be guided by the clinical picture and medical history.

Serum CCA levels are not routinely available and do not help with patient management, but may be necessary for confirmation of the diagnosis. In patients with severe or refractory hypotension, urinary catheterization and central venous catheterization are recommended to guide fluid and vasopressor therapy. Finally, early consultation with a medical toxicologist, regarding medical therapy, and a cardiologist, regarding pacemaker or intra-aortic balloon pump placement, is recommended.

Gastrointestinal Decontamination

Definitive data regarding the utility of gastrointestinal decontamination in overdoses are lacking, and all forms of decontamination carry potential risks. However, CCA overdoses can result in serious morbidity and mortality, so that potential benefits of decontamination may outweigh risks in significant ingestions. Risks and benefits should be considered on a case-by-case basis, and interventions necessary to maintain vital signs take precedence over decontamination. Aspiration is one of the main risks associated with decontamination. Thus, assurance of airway control prior to decontamination is necessary.

Activated charcoal should be administered to all significant ingestions. The greatest benefit of charcoal administration occurs within the first 2 hours after ingestion [62]. However, it may hold benefit, especially for SR preparations, up to 4 hours after ingestion [63]. Gastric lavage should not be used routinely, but considered for recent life-threatening ingestions in patients who have not already vomited [64]. Like laryngoscopy, lavage may theoretically cause bradycardia from vagal effects. Thus, atropine should be given prior to initiation, and lavage should be withheld in patients with existing bradycardia and conduction abnormalities [20].

Large ingestions of SR preparations may provide a gastrointestinal depot of drug causing recurrent cardiovascular compromise, or rise in serum drug levels up to 18 hours after initial decontamination [35,38,49,53,58,65,66]. A rise in serum amlodipine levels has been demonstrated 24.5 hours after ingestion—approximately 22 hours after decontamination [47]. Therefore repeat charcoal doses or whole bowel irrigation (WBI) with polyethylene glycol should be considered for large ingestions of SR products in patients with functioning gastrointestinal tracts [61]. Repeat charcoal dosing has also been recommended in large overdoses of IR products [29]. One or two additional doses of activated charcoal (0.5 g per kg without cathartic) separated by 2 to 4 hours may be sufficient. Because of the large volumes necessary, polyethylene glycol WBI should be administered via nasogastric tube (0.5 L per hour for small children and 1 to 2 L per hour for adults). However, it may be prudent to withhold WBI in patients with hemodynamic compromise [67].

Cardiovascular Support

Hypotension can initially be treated with intravenous crystalloids with close monitoring for fluid overload. Although usually ineffective in severe poisoning [34,38,40,41,58], atropine should be given for symptomatic bradycardia. Treatment beyond general supportive care, intravenous fluids, and atropine will depend on the clinical situation. Seriously poisoned patients may require rapid simultaneous administration of multiple therapies. Transvenous pacing may be attempted, but in significant poisoning there may be failure to capture, and blood pressure may not improve despite an increase in heart rate [34,38].

Vasopressors

The exact sequence of pharmacologic therapies has not been studied. However, healthcare providers generally have the greatest familiarity with dosing and administration of vasopressor agents. Thus, these agents can often be initiated rapidly and may improve cardiovascular instability. Ideally and agent with both α_1- and β-agonist effects should be instituted. Improvements have been noted with dopamine, dobutamine, norepinephrine, isoproterenol, and epinephrine [34,37,49,50, 52,68]. However, no specific agent has demonstrated superiority so it is reasonable for clinicians to start with the agent they are most familiar with. There is scant information regarding vasopressin utility in CCA poisoning, but based on available data it should not be used as monotherapy in CCA poisoning. Animal models have demonstrated either no improvement in mean arterial pressure [69] or decreased survival [70] with vasopressin compared to saline controls. However, there was improvement in systemic vascular resistance and blood pressure after vasopressin was administered to two patients unresponsive to multiple other therapies [71].

Multiple simultaneous vasoactive agents may be required depending on the hemodynamic response, and require doses much higher than ACLS-based doses [72]. Because vasopressors can result in tachydysrhythmias, increased myocardial oxygen consumption and vasospastic events, these agents should be the first to be weaned from a patient who has stabilized.

Hyperinsulinemic Euglycemia

Hyperinsulinemic euglycemia (HIE) refers to the administration of high-dose regular insulin while maintaining normal serum glucose levels. HIE is thought to overcome the CCA-induced compromise of cardiovascular carbohydrate uptake thus improving hemodynamic embarrassment. The exact mechanisms underlying these actions still remain controversial [73], but may be best described in the following animal studies.

Four animal studies (mongrel dogs) of HIE in verapamil poisoning [10,11,17,74] have been rated as very good to excellent quality by an expert panel [72]. Where survival from poisoning was measured, 100% of animals treated with insulin survived [74]. However, survival with epinephrine [17,74], glucagon [17,74], and calcium [17] was 33%, 0%, and 17%, respectively. Insulin also increased the mean lethal dose of verapamil and time to death compared to epinephrine and glucagon [11]. In these studies HIE improved and sustained cardiac contractility, systolic and diastolic function, and systemic and cardiac blood flow compared to calcium, glucagon, and epinephrine [10,11,17,74]. Insulin improved myocardial metabolism and function without increasing myocardial oxygen consumption [10,11]. Epinephrine, glucagon, and calcium however contribute to oxygen wasting [17].

The first report of HIE therapy, published in 1999, included five CCA-poisoned patients who failed to respond to other therapies [48]. The benefit of HIE was striking. Insulin dosing included a 10 to 20 IU bolus with a 25-g bolus of glucose followed by an infusion of 0.1 to 1.0 IU per kg per hour (mean 0.5 IU per kg per hour) and dextrose 10 to 75 g per hour (mean 28.4 g per hour). One patient failed to improve with respiratory support, crystalloids, atropine, calcium, and glucagon. After initiation of HIE blood pressure improved, complete heart block resolved, and echocardiographically measured ejection fraction increased from 10% to 30%. Many other cases have been published and the clinical data supporting HIE have recently been reviewed [73,75]. The data provides multiple examples of CCA-poisoned patients improving with HIE therapy after failing treatments such as atropine, pacing, vasopressors, calcium, glucagon, and phosphodiesterase inhibitors.

Clinical improvement is gradual and may take 30 minutes or more. However, one patient who failed to respond to dopamine, norepinephrine, calcium, and glucagon showed a dramatic response within 15 minutes of receiving a 10-fold dosing error of insulin (1,000 IU) [76]. Patients responding to insulin therapy demonstrate improved blood pressure, myocardial contractility, and metabolic acidosis, whereas effects on bradycardia and cardiac conduction are variable [73].

Failures of HIE therapy have also been reported [77]. Our lack of knowledge regarding optimum dosing of insulin has been suggested as a reason for failures with HIE [78]. Canine studies of verapamil toxicity employed insulin doses of up to 16 IU per kg per hour, but a dose–response relationship for insulin has not been determined [78]. The timing of HIE administration may also be a consideration. In several failures HIE was initiated multiple hours after ingestion when significant hemodynamic compromise was already present. This suggests a threshold point in CCA poisoning where there may be no beneficial intervention once that threshold is crossed. Therefore, HIE should be instituted well before profound shock supervenes. Although an optimal dosing scheme has yet to be established, a rational starting point is an initial insulin bolus of 1 IU per kg with 25 g of dextrose, followed by an infusion at 1 U per kg per hour and 0.5 g per kg per hour of dextrose [61,73]. It is believed supraphysiologic insulin doses are required to overcome CCA inhibition of insulin responsive GLUTs (see Physiology and Pathophysiology section) [19]. Increasing the insulin dose may be of benefit if response is insufficient. Serum glucose should be monitored closely and dextrose infusions adjusted to maintain normal ranges.

Hypoglycemia and hypokalemia, expected adverse effects of HIE, can be easily detected and treated. The safety of HIE therapy was recently demonstrated in a prospective observational study [79]. Serum glucose and potassium were monitored every 30 minutes until stable and then 1 to 2 hourly thereafter. Out of seven patients only one episode of hypoglycemia (43.5 mg per dL) occurred (occurring 33.5 hours after ingestion when the maximal effects of CCA-induced insulin resistance would be waning). Hypokalemia (2.5 to 3.5 mmol per L) occurred in two patients without any clinical significance. However, it has been suggested that mild hypokalemia may provide a beneficial effect in CCA poisoning [48,59].

Hypoglycemic effects of insulin last for hours after infusions are discontinued which requires continued monitoring of blood glucose during this period. Aggressive correction of insulin-induced hypokalemia is unnecessary unless the patient is symptomatic, or potassium level falls below an arbitrarily suggested level of 2.5 mEq per L [48].

Calcium

The goal of calcium therapy is to increase extracellular calcium concentrations thus increasing calcium influx through any unblocked calcium channels. Calcium has demonstrated effectiveness in animal models [80–83], and improvement reported in human cases [37,38,41,44,56,84,85]. However, responses are variable and often short-lived, and patients with significant toxicity often fail to improve with calcium alone [28,34,40,43,49]. Conduction disturbances, contractility, and blood pressure, may be improved, but generally, there is no increase in heart rate [34,40,49,58]. Optimum dosing has yet to be established, and 4.5 to 95.3 mEq were used in one case series without an identifiable dose–response [34].

Calcium chloride compared to calcium gluconate contains three times the amount of elemental calcium on a milliequivalent basis (10% calcium chloride: 272 mg elemental calcium or 13.6 mEq per 1 g ampule; 10% calcium gluconate: 90 mg elemental calcium or 4.5 mEq per 1 g ampule). However, it is recommended to only give calcium chloride via a central venous catheter [84]. Calcium gluconate can be given via a peripheral line.

Optimum calcium dosing is not well established. Initial doses are generally given as boluses (10 to 20 mL of 10% calcium chloride, or 30 to 60 mL of 10% calcium gluconate) [46,86–88]. Additional boluses may be given every 10 to 20 minutes. Some authors suggest more aggressive dosing of 1 g every 2 to 3 minutes until clinical response is seen [37]. Boluses should be given over a 5-minute period in conjunction with cardiac monitoring as rapid infusions have resulted in hypotension, atrioventricular dissociation, and ventricular fibrillation [89,90]. The effects of boluses may be transient, and a constant infusion required [37,46,86,87]. Infusions can be started at 0.4 mL per kg per hour for calcium chloride and 1.2 mL per kg per hour for calcium gluconate and titrated to effect. Additional boluses can be given as needed. Calcium levels should be monitored. One author recommends maintaining serum ionized calcium levels approximately twice normal [91]. Raising serum ionized calcium to 2 to 3 mEq per L improves canine cardiac performance in verapamil poisoning [17,80] and is a reasonable goal to attain. It may be necessary to continue therapy despite high serum calcium levels if the patient is only responding to calcium administration. Significantly poisoned patients have tolerated high serum calcium levels without untoward effect [35,37,44,66], including one patient who obtained a peak serum calcium level of 23.8 mg per dL [38]. However, a patient in another report achieved a peak calcium level of 32.3 mg per dL and developed anuric renal failure and eventually died [92]. It has been recommended to stop calcium infusions if no beneficial effect is observed [93]. In addition, calcium should not be administered to a patient with proven or potential digoxin toxicity.

Glucagon

Glucagon possesses both inotropic and chronotropic effects [94], and experimentally increases heart rate, cardiac output, and reverses AV nodal blocks in CCA poisoning [95]. Several case reports noted improvement with glucagon therapy [50,51,65,96], but failures are also reported [52,58,59,97]. Five to ten milligrams (150 μg per kg) given intravenously over 1 to 2 minutes is a typical starting dose [95]. Cardiovascular effects of glucagon last only 10 to 15 minutes [98,99], so repeat boluses may be required every 5 to 10 minutes followed by a continuous infusion of 2 to 10 mg per hour (50–100 μg per kg per hour) [20,95]. Glucagon is a potent emetic [98], so airway control should be ensured before administration. Hyperglycemia and hypokalemia may also be observed with glucagon administration [98].

Phosphodiesterase Inhibitors

Phosphodiesterase inhibitors (PDI) such as inamrinone (amrinone) and milrinone increase cytosolic calcium and improve inotropy. Phosphodiesterase inhibitors have been used in combination with other therapies to treat CCA-poisoned patients [54,55], and appear to be effective in animal models [100,101]. However, they can be difficult to titrate and cause vasodilation and hypotension.

RESCUE AND EXPERIMENTAL THERAPIES

Nonpharmacologic Therapies

If available, intra-aortic balloon counterpulsation [57], or cardiopulmonary bypass [58,102] may provide a bridge to survival in patients unresponsive to other therapies.

Pharmacologic Therapies

4-Aminopyridine

4-Aminopyridine is an orphan drug used to treat spinal cord injury and multiple sclerosis. It improves contractility by indirectly increasing intracellular calcium levels and has shown benefit in animal studies of verapamil toxicity [103,104] and in one human case report [24]. Unfortunately, it causes seizures and has a narrow therapeutic index. It may be considered if all other treatments are failing.

Intravenous Lipid Emulsion

Perhaps, the most promising new therapy for CCA poisoning is intravenous lipid emulsion (ILE). Intravenous lipids have traditionally been used as a source of free fatty acids in parenteral nutrition. A chance observation led to the finding that ILE is beneficial in the treatment of local anesthetic-induced cardiac arrest [105]. Multiple animal studies followed demonstrating dramatic results with ILE for local anesthetic toxicity. This led to the incorporation of ILE into anesthesiology guidelines for the treatment of local anesthetic cardiotoxicity [106].

Intravenous lipids have recently been investigated in verapamil toxicity. In a rat model, ILE significantly prolonged survival and doubled the median lethal dose of verapamil [107]. Intravenous lipid emulsion dramatically improved blood pressure and survival rate compared with saline in dogs pretreated with atropine and calcium chloride [108]. The two case reports of ILE for CCA poisoning have suggested a benefit [109,110].

Proposed mechanisms of ILE therapy include creation of a "lipid sink" where lipid soluble toxins are sequestered, augmenting cardiac energy supplies, and increasing intracellular calcium in cardiac myocytes [111]. In addition, ILE is inexpensive and readily available. The main safety concern regarding ILE therapy is pulmonary fat emboli. The one study to specifically examine this failed to demonstrate signs of fat emboli with ILE therapy [112].

Although experimental evidence for ILE for CCA poisoning is currently limited, it should be considered for patients who are failing other more traditional therapies. Dosing recommendations can be found at www.lipidrescue.org.

DISPOSITION

Patients with signs or symptoms of toxicity require ICU admission. Disposition of symptomatic patients depends on the formulation ingested. Patients with large or intentional ingestions of SR products or amlodipine should undergo appropriate decontamination and 24 hours of observation in a closely monitored setting. Patients with small unintentional ingestions of SR products may be medically cleared after appropriate decontamination if they remain asymptomatic with normal vital signs and ECGs for 8 to 12 hours. Close attention should be paid to subtle ECG signs of toxicity such as PR prolongation. Patients ingesting non-SR products may be cleared after 6 to 8 hours of observation if normal vital signs and ECGs are maintained.

References

1. Lai M, Klein-Schwartz W, Rodgers G, et al: 2005 Annual Report of the American Association of Poison Control Centers' national poisoning and exposure database. *Clin Toxicol* 44(6):803–932, 2006.
2. Bronstein A, Spyker D, Cantilena Jr L, et al: 2006 Annual Report of the American Association of Poison Control Centers' National Poison Data System (NPDS). *Clin Toxicol* 45(8):815–917, 2007.
3. Bronstein A, Spyker D, Cantilena Jr L: 2007 Annual Report of the American Association of Poison Control Centers' National Poison Data System (NPDS): 25th Annual Report. *Clin Toxicol* 46(10):927–1057, 2008.
4. Katz A: Cardiac ion channels. *N Engl J Med* 328(17):1244–1251, 1993.

5. Antman E, Stone P, Muller J, et al: Calcium channel blocking agents in the treatment of cardiovascular disorders. Part I: Basic and clinical electrophysiologic effects. *Ann Intern Med* 93(6):875–885, 1980.
6. Katz A: Basic cellular mechanisms of action of the calcium-channel blockers. *Am J Cardiol* 55(3):2B–9B, 1985.
7. Katz A: Selectivity and toxicity of antiarrhythmic drugs: molecular interactions with ion channels. *Am J Med* 104(2):179–195, 1998.
8. Rasmussen H: The calcium messenger system (1). *N Engl J Med* 314(17): 1094–1101, 1986.
9. Stone P, Antman E, Muller J, et al: Calcium channel blocking agents in the treatment of cardiovascular disorders. Part II: Hemodynamic effects and clinical applications. *Ann Intern Med* 93(6):886–904, 1980.
10. Kline J, Leonova E, Williams T, et al: Myocardial metabolism during graded intraportal verapamil infusion in awake dogs. *J Cardiovasc Pharmacol* 27(5):719–726, 1996.
11. Kline J, Raymond R, Leonova E, et al: Insulin improves heart function and metabolism during non-ischemic cardiogenic shock in awake canines. *Cardiovasc Res* 34(2):289–298, 1997.
12. Kline J, Raymond R, Schroeder J, et al: The diabetogenic effects of acute verapamil poisoning. *Toxicol Appl Pharmacol* 145(2):357–362, 1997.
13. Yamaguchi I, Akimoto Y, Nakajima H, et al: Effect of diltiazem on insulin secretion. I. Experiments in vitro. *Jpn J Pharmacol* 27(5):679–687, 1977.
14. Devis G, Somers G, Van Obberghen E, et al: Calcium antagonists and islet function. I. Inhibition of insulin release by verapamil. *Diabetes* 24(6): 247–251, 1975.
15. Ohta M, Nelson J, Nelson D, et al: Effect of Ca++ channel blockers on energy level and stimulated insulin secretion in isolated rat islets of Langerhans. *J Pharmacol Exp Ther* 264(1):35–40, 1993.
16. De Marinis L, Barbarino A: Calcium antagonists and hormone release. I. Effects of verapamil on insulin release in normal subjects and patients with islet-cell tumor. *Metabolism* 29(7):599–604, 1980.
17. Kline J, Leonova E, Raymond R: Beneficial myocardial metabolic effects of insulin during verapamil toxicity in the anesthetized canine. *Crit Care Med* 23(7):1251–1263, 1995.
18. Ten Harmsel A, Holstege C, Louters L: High dose insulin reverses verapamil inhibition of glucose uptake in mouse striated muscle [abstract]. *Ann Emerg Med* 46(3):S77, 2005.
19. Bechtel L, Haverstick D, Holstege C: Verapamil toxicity dysregulates the phosphatidylinositol 3-kinase pathway. *Acad Emerg Med* 15(4):368–374, 2008.
20. Salhanick S, Shannon M: Management of calcium channel antagonist overdose. *Drug Safety* 26(2):65–79, 2003.
21. Michel M: Chapter 31. Pathophysiology of Ischemic Heart Disease, in Brunton L, Parker K, Murri N, Blumenthal D (eds): *Goodman & Gilman's The Pharmacologic Basis of Therapeutics online edition*. 11th ed. McGraw Hill, 2006. Available at: http://www.accessmedicine.com/content.aspx?aID = 944592 [Accessed July 27, 2009].
22. Luomanmaki K, Tiula E, Kivisto K, et al: Pharmacokinetics of diltiazem in massive overdose. *Ther Drug Monit* 19(2):240–242, 1997.
23. Williamson K, Dunham G: Plasma concentrations of diltiazem and desacetyldiltiazem in an overdose situation. *Ann Pharmacother* 30(6):608–611, 1996.
24. ter Wee P, Kremer Hovinga T, Uges D, et al: 4-Aminopyridine and haemodialysis in the treatment of verapamil intoxication. *Hum Toxicol* 4(3):327–329, 1985.
25. Kuhlmann U, Schoenemann H, Muller T, et al: Plasmapheresis in life-threatening verapamil intoxication. *Artif Cells Blood Substit Immobil Biotechnol* 28(5):429–440, 2000.
26. Ezidiegwu C, Spektor Z, Nasr M, et al: A case report on the role of plasma exchange in the management of a massive amlodipine besylate intoxication. *Ther Apher Dial* 12(2):180–184, 2008.
27. Kolcz J, Pietrzyk J, Januszewska K, et al: Extracorporeal life support in severe propranolol and verapamil intoxication. *J Intensive Care Med* 22(6):381–385, 2007.
28. Roberts D, Honcharik N, Sitar D, et al: Diltiazem overdose: pharmacokinetics of diltiazem and its metabolites and effect of multiple dose charcoal therapy. *J Toxicol Clin Toxicol* 29(1):45–52, 1991.
29. Buckley C, Aronson J: Prolonged half-life of verapamil in a case of overdose: implications for therapy. *Br J Clin Pharmacol* 39(6):680–683, 1995.
30. Kivisto K, Neuvonen P, Tarssanen L: Pharmacokinetics of verapamil in overdose. *Hum Exp Toxicol* 16(1):35–37, 1997.
31. Ferner R, Monkman S, Riley J, et al: Pharmacokinetics and toxic effects of nifedipine in massive overdose. *Hum Exp Toxicol* 9(5):309–311, 1990.
32. Barrow P, Houston P, Wong D: Overdose of sustained-release verapamil. *Br J Anaesth* 72(3):361–365, 1994.
33. Adams B, Browne W: Amlodipine overdose causes prolonged calcium channel blocker toxicity. *Am J Emerg Med* 16(5):527–528, 1998.
34. Ramoska E, Spiller H, Winter M, et al: A one-year evaluation of calcium channel blocker overdoses: toxicity and treatment. *Ann Emerg Med* 22(2):196–200, 1993.
35. Spiller H, Meyers A, Ziemba T, et al: Delayed onset of cardiac arrhythmias from sustained-release verapamil. *Ann Emerg Med* 20(2):201–203, 1991.
36. Tom P, Morrow C, Kelen G: Delayed hypotension after overdose of sustained release verapamil. *J Emerg Med* 12(5):621–625, 1994.
37. Howarth D, Dawson A, Smith A, et al: Calcium channel blocking drug overdose: an Australian series. *Hum Exp Toxicol* 13(3):161–166, 1994.
38. Buckley N, Dawson A, Howarth D, et al: Slow-release verapamil poisoning. Use of polyethylene glycol whole-bowel lavage and high-dose calcium. *Med J Aust* 158(3):202–204, 1993.
39. Olson K, Erdman A, Woolf A, et al: Calcium channel blocker ingestion: an evidence-based consensus guideline for out-of-hospital management. *Clin Toxicol (Philadelphia)* 43(7):797–822, 2005.
40. Ramoska E, Spiller H, Myers A: Calcium channel blocker toxicity. *Ann Emerg Med* 19(6):649–653, 1990.
41. Erickson F, Ling L, Grande G, et al: Diltiazem overdose: case report and review. *J Emerg Med* 9(5):357–366, 1991.
42. Herrington D, Insley B, Weinmann G: Nifedipine overdose. *Am J Med* 81(2):344–346, 1986.
43. Lee D, Greene T, Dougherty T, et al: Fatal nifedipine ingestions in children. *J Emerg Med* 19(4):359–361, 2000.
44. Haddad L: Resuscitation after nifedipine overdose exclusively with intravenous calcium chloride. *Am J Emerg Med* 14(6):602–603, 1996.
45. Boyer E, Shannon M: Treatment of calcium-channel-blocker intoxication with insulin infusion [letter]. *NEJM* 344(22):1721–1722, 2001.
46. Rasmussen L, Husted S, Johnsen S: Severe intoxication after an intentional overdose of amlodipine. *Acta Anaesthesiol Scand* 47(8):1038–1040, 2003.
47. Koch A, Vogelaers D, Decruyenaere J, et al: Fatal intoxication with amlodipine. *J Toxicol Clin Toxicol* 33(3):253–256, 1995.
48. Yuan T, Kerns W, Tomaszewski C, et al: Insulin-glucose as adjunctive therapy for severe calcium channel antagonist poisoning. *J Toxicol Clin Toxicol* 37(4):463–474, 1999.
49. Hofer C, Smith J, Tenholder M: Verapamil intoxication: a literature review of overdoses and discussion of therapeutic options. *Am J Med* 95(4):431–438, 1993.
50. Ashraf M, Chaudhary K, Nelson J, et al: Massive overdose of sustained-release verapamil: a case report and review of literature. *Am J Med Sci* 310(6):258–263, 1995.
51. Walter F, Frye G, Mullen J, et al: Amelioration of nifedipine poisoning associated with glucagon therapy. *Ann Emerg Med* 22(7):1234–1237, 1993.
52. Proano L, Chiang W, Wang R: Calcium channel blocker overdose. *Am J Emerg Med* 13(4):444–450, 1995.
53. Isbister G: Delayed asystolic cardiac arrest after diltiazem overdose; resuscitation with high dose intravenous calcium. *Emerg Med J* 19(4):355–357, 2002.
54. Goenen M, Col J, Compere A, et al: Treatment of severe verapamil poisoning with combined amrinone-isoproterenol therapy. *Am J Cardiol* 58(11):1142–1143, 1986.
55. Wolf L, Spadafora M, Otten E: Use of amrinone and glucagon in a case of calcium channel blocker overdose. *Ann Emerg Med* 22(7):1225–1228, 1993.
56. da Silva O, de Melo R, Jorge Filho J: Verapamil acute self-poisoning. *Clin Toxicol* 14(4):361–367, 1979.
57. Frierson J, Bailly D, Shultz T, et al: Refractory cardiogenic shock and complete heart block after unsuspected verapamil-SR and atenolol overdose. *Clin Cardiol* 14(11):933–935, 1991.
58. Hendren W, Schieber R, Garrettson L: Extracorporeal bypass for the treatment of verapamil poisoning. *Ann Emerg Med* 18(9):984–987, 1989.
59. Marques M: Treatment of calcium channel blocker intoxication with insulin infusion: case report and literature review. *Resuscitation* 57(2):211–213, 2003.
60. Levine M, Boyer E, Pozner C, et al: Assessment of hyperglycemia after calcium channel blocker overdoses involving diltiazem or verapamil. *Crit Care Med* 35(9):2071–2075, 2007.
61. DeWitt C, Waksman J: Pharmacology, pathophysiology and management of calcium channel blocker and beta-blocker toxicity. *Toxicol Rev* 23(4):223–238, 2004.
62. Bond G: The role of activated charcoal and gastric emptying in gastrointestinal decontamination: a state-of-the-art review. *Anns Emerg Med* 39(3):273–286, 2002.
63. Laine K, Kivisto K, Neuvonen P: Effect of delayed administration of activated charcoal on the absorption of conventional and slow-release verapamil. *J Toxicol Clin Toxicol* 35(3):263–268, 1997.
64. American Academy of Clinical Toxicology E, Toxicologists C: Position Paper: Gastric Lavage. *J Toxicol Clin Toxicol* 42(7):933–943, 2004.
65. Doyon S, Roberts J: The use of glucagon in a case of calcium channel blocker overdose. *Ann Emerg Med* 22(7):1229–1233, 1993.
66. Luscher T, Noll G, Sturmer T, et al: Calcium gluconate in severe verapamil intoxication. *N Engl J Med* 330(10):718–720, 1994.
67. Cumpston K, Aks S, Sigg T, et al: Whole bowel irrigation and the hemodynamically unstable calcium channel blocker overdose: Primum non nocere. *J Emerg Med* Ahead of print. 2008.
68. Chimienti M, Previtali M, Medicia A, et al: Acute verapamil poisoning: successful treatment with epinephrine. *Clin Cardiol* 5(3):219–222, 1982.
69. Sztajnkrycer M, Bond G, Johnson S, et al: Use of vasopressin in a canine model of severe verapamil poisoning: a preliminary descriptive study. *Acad Emerg Med* 11(12):1253–1261, 2004.
70. Barry J, Durkovich D, Cantrell L, et al: Vasopressin treatment of verapamil toxicity in the porcine model. *J Med Toxicol* 1(1):3–10, 2005.

71. Kanagarajan K, Marraffa J, Bouchard N, et al: The use of vasopressin in the setting of recalcitrant hypotension due to calcium channel blocker overdose. *Clin Toxicol* 45(1):56–59, 2007.
72. Albertson T, Dawson A, de Latorre F, et al: TOX-ACLS: toxicologic-oriented advanced cardiac life support. *Ann Emerg Med* 37[4, Suppl]:S78–S90, 2001.
73. Lheureux P, Zahir S, Gris M, et al: Bench-to-bedside review: hyperinsulinaemia/euglycaemia therapy in the management of overdose of calcium-channel blockers. *Crit Care* 10(3):212, 2006.
74. Kline J, Tomaszewski C, Schroeder J, et al: Insulin is a superior antidote for cardiovascular toxicity induced by verapamil in the anesthetized canine. *J Pharmacol Exp Ther* 267(2):744–750, 1993.
75. Megarbane B, Karyo S, Baud F: The role of insulin and glucose (hyperinsulinaemia/euglycaemia) therapy in acute calcium channel antagonist and beta-blocker poisoning. *Toxicol Rev* 23(4):215–222, 2004.
76. Place R, Carlson A, Leiken J, et al: Hyperinsulin therapy in the treatment of verapamil overdose [abstract]. *J Toxicol Clin Toxicol* 38:576–577, 2000.
77. Herbert J, O'malley C, Treacey J, et al: Verapamil therapy unresponsive to dextrose/insulin therapy [abstract]. *J Toxicol Clin Toxicol* 39:293–294, 2001.
78. Cumpston K, Mycyk M, Pallasch E, et al: Failure of hyperinsulinemia/euglycemia therapy in severe diltiazem overdose [abstract]. *J Toxicol Clin Toxicol* 40:618, 2002.
79. Greene S, Gawarammana I, Wood D, et al: Relative safety of hyperinsulinaemia/euglycaemia therapy in the management of calcium channel blocker overdose: a prospective observational study. *Intensive Care Med* 33(11):2019–2024, 2007.
80. Hariman R, Mangiardi L, McAllister R, et al: Reversal of the cardiovascular effects of verapamil by calcium and sodium: differences between electrophysiologic and hemodynamic responses. *Circulation* 59(4):797–804, 1979.
81. Martin T, Menegazzi H, Perel H, et al: Extraordinary medical therapy for severe verapamil overdose [abstract]. *Ann Emerg Med* 21(5):627, 1992.
82. Strubelt O, Diederich K: Experimental investigations on the antidotal treatment of nifedipine overdosage. *J Toxicol Clin Toxicol* 24(2):135–149, 1986.
83. Vick J, Kandil A, Herman E, et al: Reversal of propranolol and verapamil toxicity by calcium. *Vet Hum Toxicol* 25(1):8–10, 1983.
84. Lam Y, Tse H, Lau C: Continuous calcium chloride infusion for massive nifedipine overdose. *Chest* 119(4):1280–1282, 2001.
85. Woie L, Storstein L: Successful treatment of suicidal verapamil poisoning with calcium gluconate. *Eur Heart J* 2(3):239–242, 1981.
86. Kenny J: Treating overdose with calcium channel blockers. *BMJ* 308(6935):992–993, 1994.
87. Newton C, Delgado J, Gomez H: Calcium and beta receptor antagonist overdose: A review and update of pharmacological principles and management. *Semin Respir Crit Care Med* 23(1):19–25, 2002.
88. Pearigen P, Benowitz N: Poisoning due to calcium antagonists. Experience with verapamil, diltiazem and nifedipine. *Drug Saf* 6(6):408–430, 1991.
89. Carlon G, Howland W, Goldiner P, et al: Adverse effects of calcium administration. Report of two cases. *Arch Surg* 113(7):882–885, 1978.
90. Chin R, Garmel G, Harter P: Development of ventricular fibrillation after intravenous calcium chloride administration in a patient with supraventricular tachycardia. *Ann Emerg Med* 25(3):416–419, 1995.
91. Kerns W: Management of beta-adrenergic blocker and calcium channel antagonist toxicity. *Emerg Med Clin North Am* 25(2):309–331; abstract viii. 2007.
92. Sim M, Stevenson F: A fatal case of iatrogenic hypercalcemia after calcium channel blocker overdose. *J Med Toxicol* 4(1):25–29, 2008.
93. Kline J: Calcium Channel Antagonists, in Ford M, Delaney K, Ling L, Erickson T (eds): *Clin Toxicol*. Philadelphia, PA, W.B. Saunders, 2001 p 370–378.
94. Lucchesi B: Cardiac actions of glucagon. *Circ Res* 22(6):777–787, 1968.
95. Bailey B: Glucagon in beta-blocker and calcium channel blocker overdoses: a systematic review. *J Toxicol Clin Toxicol* 41(5):595–602, 2003.
96. Mahr N, Valdes A, Lamas G: Use of glucagon for acute intravenous diltiazem toxicity. *Am J Cardiol* 79(11):1570–1571, 1997.
97. Anthony T, Jastremski M, Elliott W, et al: Charcoal hemoperfusion for the treatment of a combined diltiazem and metoprolol overdose. *Ann Emerg Med* 15(11):1344–1348, 1986.
98. Parmley W: The role of glucagon in cardiac therapy. *N Engl J Med* 285(14):801–802, 1971.
99. Parmley W, Glick G, Sonnenblick E: Cardiovascular effects of glucagon in man. *N Engl J Med* 279(1):12–17, 1968.
100. Alousi A, Canter J, Fort D: The beneficial effect of amrinone on acute drug-induced heart failure in the anaesthetised dog. *Cardiovasc Res* 19(8):483–494, 1985.
101. Koury S, Stone C, Thomas S: Amrinone as an antidote in experimental verapamil overdose. *Acad Emerg Med* 3(8):762–767, 1996.
102. Holzer M, Sterz F, Schoerkhuber W, et al: Successful resuscitation of a verapamil-intoxicated patient with percutaneous cardiopulmonary bypass. *Crit Care Med* 27(12):2818–2823, 1999.
103. Agoston S, Maestrone E, van Hezik E, et al: Effective treatment of verapamil intoxication with 4-aminopyridine in the cat. *J Clin Invest* 73(5):1291–1296, 1984.
104. Tuncok Y, Apaydin S, Gelal A, et al: The effects of 4-aminopyridine and Bay K 8644 on verapamil-induced cardiovascular toxicity in anesthetized rats. *J Toxicol Clin Toxicol* 36(4):301–307, 1998.
105. Brent J: Poisoned patients are different—sometimes fat is a good thing. *Crit Care Med* 37(3):1157–1158, 2009.
106. Picard J, Ward S, Zumpe R, et al: Guidelines and the adoption of 'lipid rescue' therapy for local anaesthetic toxicity. *Anaesthesia* 64(2):122–125, 2009.
107. Tebbutt S, Harvey M, Nicholson T, et al: Intralipid prolongs survival in a rat model of verapamil toxicity. *Acad Emerg Med* 13(2):134–139, 2006.
108. Bania T, Chu J, Perez E, et al: Hemodynamic effects of intravenous fat emulsion in an animal model of severe verapamil toxicity resuscitated with atropine, calcium, and saline. *Acad Emerg Med* 14(2):105–111, 2007.
109. Dolcourt B, Aaron C: Intravenous fat emulsion for refractory verapamil and atenolol induced shock: a human case report. *Clin Toxicol* 46(7):619–620, 2008.
110. Young A, Velez L, Kleinschmidt K: Intravenous fat emulsion therapy for intentional sustained-release verapamil overdose. *Resuscitation* 80(5):591–593, 2009.
111. Turner-Lawrence D, Kerns Ii W: Intravenous fat emulsion: a potential novel antidote. *J Med Toxicol* 4(2):109–114, 2008.
112. Bania T, Medlej K, Chu J, et al: Does the Pulmonary Fat Emboli Syndrome Occur with Intravenous Fat Emulsion Therapy? *Acad Emerg Med* 15[5, Suppl 1]:S94, 2008.

CHAPTER 127 ■ CARDIAC GLYCOSIDE POISONING

MARK A. KIRK AND BRYAN S. JUDGE

Cardiac glycosides (CGs) are naturally occurring substances whose medicinal benefits have been recognized for centuries [1]. Digoxin is the major CG used for medicinal purposes today. It is most widely used in the treatment of congestive heart failure and acute atrial fibrillation associated with a rapid ventricular response rate [2]. Although digoxin is responsible for most cases of CG poisoning, exposure to plant (i.e., dogbane, foxglove, lily of the valley, oleander, red squill, and Siberian ginseng) and animal (i.e., *Bufo* toad species) sources and topical aphrodisiacs can also result in serious toxicity [3–5].

PHARMACOLOGY

Digoxin exerts a positive inotropic effect, thereby enhancing the force of myocardial contraction. Direct effects of digoxin include prolongation of the effective refractory period in the atria and the atrioventricular (AV) node, which diminishes the conduction velocity through those regions. CGs are readily absorbed through the gastrointestinal tract; digoxin has up to 80% bioavailability [6]. Digoxin has a volume of distribution (V_d) of 5.1 to 7.4 L per kg [7] and a half-life of 36 to 48 hours [2]. The generally accepted therapeutic serum concentration range for digoxin is 0.8 to 2.0 ng per mL for inotropic support in patients with left ventricular dysfunction. Higher concentrations (1.5 to 2.0 ng per mL) may be needed for ventricular rate control in patients with atrial dysrhythmias. Digoxin is primarily eliminated by the kidneys. In patients with renal dysfunction, digoxin clearance is reduced. Serum digoxin concentrations can be altered by numerous drug interactions [8–10].

Toxicity results from an exaggeration of therapeutic effects [6]. Cardiac glycosides bind to and inactivate the sodium–potassium adenosine triphosphatase pump (Na^+–K^+-ATPase) on cardiac cell membranes. This pump maintains the electrochemical membrane potential, vital to conduction tissues, by concentrating Na^+ extracellularly and K^+ intracellularly. When Na^+–K^+-ATPase is inhibited, the Na^+–calcium exchanger removes accumulated intracellular sodium in exchange for calcium. This exchange increases sarcoplasmic calcium and is the mechanism responsible for the positive inotropic effect of digitalis. Intracellular calcium overload causes delayed after depolarizations and gives rise to triggered dysrhythmias. Increased vagal tone and direct AV depression may produce conduction disturbances. The decreased refractory period of the myocardium increases automaticity.

CLINICAL PRESENTATION

Differences between the presentations of patients with CG poisoning due to a single acute ingestion and those with chronic toxicity resulting from excessive therapeutic doses are illustrated in Table 127.1. Diagnosing chronic CG toxicity is more difficult because the presentation may mimic more common illnesses, such as influenza or gastroenteritis. Patients with chronic CG toxicity may present with constitutional, gastrointestinal, psychiatric, or visual complaints that may not be recognized as signs of digitalis toxicity. Symptoms most commonly reported include fatigue, weakness, nausea, anorexia, and dizziness [11]. Neuropsychiatric signs and symptoms include headache, weakness, vertigo, syncope, seizures, memory loss, confusion, disorientation, delirium, depression, and hallucinations [12]. The most frequently reported visual disturbances are cloudy or blurred vision, loss of vision, and yellow-green halos or everything appearing "washed in yellow" (xanthopsia) [13].

Cardiac manifestations of CG toxicity are common and potentially life threatening. An extremely wide variety of dysrhythmias has been reported [14,15]. Dysrhythmias frequently associated with CG toxicity include premature ventricular contractions, paroxysmal atrial tachycardia or atrial fibrillation with a conduction block, junctional tachycardia, sinus bradycardia, AV nodal blocks, ventricular tachycardia, and ventricular fibrillation. Atrial tachycardia (enhanced automaticity) with variable AV block (impaired conduction), atrial fibrillation with an accelerated or slow junctional rhythm (regularization of atrial fibrillation), and fascicular tachycardia are highly suggestive of CG toxicity [16,17]. Bidirectional ventricular tachycardia, a narrow-complex tachycardia with right bundle-branch morphology, is highly specific, but not pathognomonic for digitalis toxicity [14].

True end-organ digoxin sensitivity is seen with myocardial disease, myocardial ischemia, and metabolic or electrolyte disturbances [18]. Hypokalemia, hypomagnesemia, and hypercalcemia predispose to toxicity [2]. The elderly are at increased risk, whereas renal impairment, hepatic disease, hypothyroidism, chronic obstructive pulmonary disease, and drug interactions alter sensitivity to CGs [1].

DIAGNOSTIC EVALUATION

Essential laboratory tests include serum digoxin concentrations, electrolytes, blood urea nitrogen, creatinine, calcium, magnesium, and electrocardiogram. Additional laboratory tests should be obtained as clinically indicated. Serum digoxin concentrations can assist in the diagnosis of CG poisoning but often are unreliable indicators of toxicity [17]. A therapeutic concentration does not exclude poisoning, as predisposing factors can cause an individual to become poisoned despite a concentration within the therapeutic range. Conversely, high serum

TABLE 127.1

CHARACTERISTICS OF ACUTE AND CHRONIC CARDIAC GLYCOSIDE TOXICITY

Clinical finding	Acute toxicity	Chronic toxicity
Gastrointestinal toxicity	Nausea, vomiting	Nausea, vomiting
Central nervous system toxicity	Headache, weakness, dizziness, confusion, and coma	Confusion, coma
Cardiac toxicity	Bradydysrhythmias, supraventricular dysrhythmias with AV block; ventricular dysrhythmias are uncommon	Virtually any dysrhythmia (ventricular or supraventricular dysrhythmias with or without AV block); ventricular dysrhythmias are common
Serum potassium	Elevated but may be normal (high concentrations correlated with toxicity)	Low or normal (hypokalemia secondary to concomitant diuretic use)
Serum digoxin concentration	Markedly elevated	May be within "therapeutic" range or minimally elevated

AV, atrioventricular.
Adapted and combined from references [1,11,12,14,32].

digoxin concentrations after an acute ingestion are not always indicative of toxicity [19]. Digoxin follows a two-compartment model of distribution, with relatively rapid absorption into the plasma compartment and then slow redistribution into the tissue compartment [2]. Serum digoxin concentrations most reliably correlate with toxicity when obtained after distribution is complete, which occurs 6 hours or more after oral or intravenous digoxin administration.

Naturally occurring digitalis glycosides from plants and animals can cross-react with the digoxin assay. The degree of cross-reactivity is unknown, and no good correlation has been established between serum concentrations of these glycosides and toxicity [5]. A false-positive digoxin assay (usually less than 3 ng per mL), may occur in neonates and patients with renal insufficiency, liver disease, and pregnancy [20–22] because of endogenous digoxin-like immunoreactive factors.

Hyperkalemia may be a better indicator of end-organ toxicity than the serum digoxin concentration in the acutely poisoned patient [23]. In contrast, hypokalemia and hypomagnesemia are commonly seen in the chronically intoxicated patient, presumably as a result of concomitant diuretic use.

MANAGEMENT

The management of CG poisoning includes supportive care, prevention of further drug absorption, antidotal therapy, and safe disposition. Meticulous attention to supportive care and a search for easily correctable conditions, such as hypoxia, hypoventilation, hypovolemia, hypoglycemia, and electrolyte disturbances, are top priorities. All patients should have vascular access established and continuous cardiac monitoring. Patients with clinical toxicity or elevated serum digoxin concentrations should be admitted to the intensive care unit.

Prevention of further drug absorption should be addressed after life support measures have been initiated. Gastric lavage has little if any benefit in the management of digoxin toxicity. Activated charcoal effectively binds cardiac glycosides, and multiple doses of activated charcoal enhance intestinal digoxin elimination after oral and intravenous digoxin administration [24,25]. A recent study demonstrated that activated charcoal favorably impacts the pharmacokinetic profile of CGs in patients self-poisoned with seeds from the yellow oleander tree [26]. However, further research is necessary to clarify whether patients poisoned with yellow oleander will benefit from activated charcoal since clinical outcomes reported in previous studies have been conflicting [27,28].

Conventional treatment of bradydysrhythmia includes the use of atropine, isoproterenol, and cardiac pacing. However, atropine sulfate has been used with variable success in patients with digitalis toxicity exhibiting AV block [29], isoproterenol may increase ventricular ectopy and cardiac tissue may be unresponsive to electrical pacing, the fibrillation threshold may be lowered, and the pacing wire itself may induce ventricular fibrillation [30]. Digoxin-specific antibody fragments (Fab) are now considered first-line therapy in patients with symptomatic bradycardia [31].

Digoxin-specific antibody Fab is also the treatment of choice for life-threatening ventricular dysrhythmias. If this therapy is not immediately available, phenytoin and lidocaine, which depress increased ventricular automaticity without slowing AV nodal conduction, should be the initial therapy [17,32]. Amiodarone was successful in two cases refractory to other antidysrhythmics [33,34]. Intravenous magnesium, 2 to 4 g (10 to 20 mL of a 20% solution) over 1 minute, may also be useful [35]. Quinidine and procainamide are contraindicated in digitalis toxicity because they depress AV nodal conduction and may worsen cardiac toxicity [1]. Electrical cardioversion of the digitalis-toxic patient should be performed with extreme caution and considered a last resort. A low-energy setting (e.g., 10 to 25 W per second) should be used and preparations made to treat potential ventricular fibrillation [32].

Hyperkalemia is common in patients with acute digoxin poisoning, and empiric administration of supplemental potassium should be avoided [36]. This increase in serum potassium concentration reflects a change in potassium distribution and not an increase in total body potassium stores. Significant hyperkalemia due to acute overdose is another indication for digoxin-specific antibody Fab. If digoxin-specific antibody Fab are not immediately available and the patient has hyperkalemia with associated electrocardiogram changes, intravenous glucose and insulin, sodium bicarbonate, continuous inhaled β agonists such as albuterol (if there is no tachydysrhythmia or ectopy), and sodium polystyrene sulfonate should be administered. The use of intravenous calcium to treat hyperkalemia in CG toxic patients remains controversial and has been previously avoided by many clinicians because additional calcium has been reported to enhance cardiac toxicity [18]. However, some authors have questioned this dogma—citing animal studies and human case reports that document no untoward effects when calcium is administered in the setting of CG toxicity—and recommend the use of intravenous calcium in those patients with CG toxicity who have life-threatening hyperkalemia with significant changes on the electrocardiogram such as loss of P waves or widening of the QRS [37]. Hemodialysis may be of benefit in a CG-poisoned patient with renal failure and hyperkalemia.

Supplemental potassium may be beneficial in chronic digitalis toxicity when diuretic-induced hypokalemia is a factor. Potassium should be administered cautiously, as renal dysfunction may be the cause of digitalis toxicity. Hypomagnesemia is common in patients with chronic CG toxicity, and supplemental magnesium is recommended for such patients [38].

Digoxin-specific antibody Fab therapy is indicated for patients with dysrhythmias that threaten or result in hemodynamic compromise and patients with serum potassium greater than 5.0 to 5.5 mEq per L after acute CG overdose [39,40]. Chronically poisoned patients who are asymptomatic can often be managed with discontinuation of digoxin and close observation. The threshold for treatment with digoxin-specific antibody Fab should be lower in those patients with signs of cardiac toxicity or who have predisposing conditions such as chronic pulmonary disease, hypokalemia, hypothyroidism, renal dysfunction, or underlying cardiac disease [11]. Animal studies and case reports suggest digoxin-specific antibody Fab may be an effective treatment for patients poisoned by plant or animal sources of CG [3,5].

Digoxin-specific antibody Fab can reverse digitalis-induced dysrhythmias, conduction disturbances, myocardial depression, and hyperkalemia. In a multicenter study, 90% of patients with digoxin or digitoxin toxicity had a complete or partial response to digoxin-specific antibody Fab therapy [39]. Complete resolution of toxicity occurred in 80% of the patients, and partial response occurred in 10%. The time to initial response from end of digoxin-specific antibody Fab infusion was within 1 hour (mean 19 minutes), and the time to complete response was 0.5 to 6.0 hours (mean: 1.5 hours). Treatment failures have been attributed to inadequate or delayed dosing, moribund clinical state before digoxin-specific antibody Fab therapy, pacemaker-induced dysrhythmias, and incorrect diagnosis of digitalis toxicity [39,41].

Digoxin-specific antibody Fab dosage (number of vials) calculations are based on the serum digoxin concentration or estimated body load of digoxin. It is assumed that equimolar doses of antibody fragments are required to achieve neutralization [42]. A 40-mg dose of digoxin-specific antibody Fab (one vial) binds 0.6 mg of digoxin. The number of vials required can be calculated by dividing the total body burden by 0.6. The body burden can be estimated from the milligram amount of an acute ingestion or by multiplying the serum digoxin concentration (ng per mL) by the volume of distribution of digoxin (=5.6 L per kg times the body weight in kg) and dividing by 1,000.

In the largest study of Fab for digoxin poisoning ($n = 150$, mean serum concentration of 8 ng per mL), the dose of Fab required to reverse digoxin toxicity was five vials with a range from 3 to 20 vials [39]. A severely toxic patient in whom the quantity ingested acutely is unknown should be given 5 to 10 vials at a time and the clinical response observed. If cardiac arrest is imminent or has occurred, the dose can be given as a bolus. Otherwise, it should be infused over 30 minutes. In contrast, patients with chronic therapeutic overdose often have only mildly elevated digoxin concentrations and respond to one to two vials of digoxin-specific antibody Fab. The recommended dose for a given patient can be determined using the tables in the package insert or by contacting a regional poison center or toxicology consultant.

The dose of digoxin-specific antibody Fab needed to treat nondigoxin CG poisoning is unknown but likely to be greater than that necessary for digoxin poisoning. Starting with 5 to 10 vials and repeating this dose as necessary is a reasonable approach.

Free digoxin concentrations are decreased to zero within 1 minute of digoxin-specific antibody Fab therapy, but total serum digoxin concentrations are markedly increased [39,43]. Because most assay methods measure total (bound and free) digoxin, very high digoxin concentrations are seen after digoxin-specific antibody Fab treatment, but they have no correlation with toxicity [43]. Serum concentrations may be unreliable for several days after digoxin-specific antibody Fab therapy [44].

The digoxin–Fab complex is excreted in the urine and has a half-life of 16 to 20 hours [45]. In patients with renal failure, elimination of the digoxin–Fab complex is prolonged and free digoxin concentrations gradually increase over 2 to 4 days after digoxin-specific antibody Fab administration [46]. In one report of 28 patients with renal impairment given digoxin-specific antibody Fab, only one patient had recurrent toxicity, which occurred 10 days after digoxin-specific antibody Fab treatment and persisted for 10 days [47]. Monitoring of free digoxin concentrations may be beneficial for titrating effect in those patients reliant on the inotropic action of digoxin, detecting rebound toxicity in patients with renal impairment, assessing the need for further treatment with digoxin-specific antibody Fab, or in guiding the reinstitution of digoxin therapy [48]. Hemodialysis has not been reported to enhance digoxin–Fab complex elimination.

Digoxin-specific antibody Fab therapy has been associated with mild adverse drug events such as rash, flushing, and facial swelling [39,41]. However, neither acute anaphylaxis nor serum sickness has been described [41]. Before digoxin-specific antibody Fab administration, an asthma and allergy history should be obtained. Intradermal skin testing should be considered in high-risk patients. If a patient with a positive skin test is dying, however, the risk–benefit ratio obviously favors treatment [41]. A precipitous drop in the serum potassium, recurrence of supraventricular tachydysrhythmias previously controlled by digoxin, and development of cardiogenic shock in a patient dependent on digoxin for inotropic support have all been associated with digoxin-specific antibody Fab therapy [39]. Recurrent toxicity has been observed in 3% of patients [41]. In most, it was attributed to inadequate initial dose of digoxin-specific antibody Fab dosing and reversed with a repeat dose.

Patients who receive digoxin-specific antibody Fab require continued monitoring in an intensive care unit for at least 24 hours. Those with elevated drug concentrations resulting from chronic therapy who are hemodynamically stable can be observed on a telemetry unit. Discontinuing the use of digoxin or decreasing the dose, modifying predisposing factors, and closely monitoring subsequent therapy are necessary to avert further toxic episodes. Patients with suicidal ingestions should have a psychiatric evaluation before discharge.

References

1. Smith TW, Antman EM, Friedman PL, et al: Digitalis glycosides: mechanisms and manifestations. *Prog Cardiovasc Dis* 26:413, 1984.
2. Smith TW: Pharmacokinetics, bioavailability and serum levels of cardiac glycosides. *J Am Coll Cardiol* 5:43A, 1985.
3. Shumaik GM, Wu AW, Ping AC: Oleander poisoning: treatment with digoxin-specific Fab antibody fragments. *Ann Emerg Med* 17:732, 1988.
4. Rich SA, Libera JM, Locke RJ: Treatment of foxglove extract poisoning with digoxin-specific Fab fragments. *Ann Emerg Med* 22(12):1904–1907, 1993.
5. Brubacher JR, Ravikumar PR, Bania T, et al: Treatment of toad venom poisoning with digoxin-specific Fab Fragments. *Chest* 110(5):1282–1288, 1996.
6. Smith TW: Digitalis: Mechanisms of action and clinical use. *N Engl J Med* 318:358, 1988.
7. Baselt RC: *Disposition of Toxic Drugs and Chemicals in Man.* 6th ed. Foster City, CA, Biomedical Publications, 2003, p 1146.
8. Marcus FI: Pharmacokinetic interactions between digoxin and other drugs. *J Am Coll Cardiol* 5:82A–90A, 1985.
9. Humphries TJ, Merritt GJ: Review article: drug interactions with agents used to treat acid-related diseases. *Aliment Pharmacol Ther* 13[Suppl 3]:18–26, 1999.
10. Izzo AA, Di Carlo G, Borrelli F, et al: Cardiovascular pharmacotherapy and herbal medicines: the risk of drug interaction. *Int J Cardiol* 98:1–14, 2005.
11. Wofford JL, Ettinger WH: Risk factors and manifestations of digoxin toxicity in the elderly. *Am J Emerg Med* 9:11–15, 1991.
12. Huffman JC, Stern T: Neuropsychiatric consequences of cardiovascular medications. *Dialogues Clin Neurosci* 9(1):29–45, 2007.
13. recognizing the varied visual presentations. *J Clin Neuroophthalmol* 13:275–280, 1993.
14. Moorman JR, Pritchett EL: The arrhythmias of digitalis intoxication. *Arch Intern Med* 145:1289, 1985.
15. Mahdyoon H, Battilana G, Rosman H, et al: The evolving pattern of digoxin intoxication: observations at a large urban hospital from 1980 to 1988. *Am Heart J* 120:1189–1194, 1990.
16. Marchlinski FE, Hook BG, Callans DJ: Which cardiac disturbances should be treated with digoxin immune Fab (Ovine) antibody? *Am J Emerg Med* 9:24–28, 1991.
17. Kelly RA, Smith TW: Recognition and management of digitalis toxicity. *Am J Cardiol* 69:108G–119G, 1992.
18. Akera T, Ng Y: Digitalis sensitivity of Na,K-ATPase, myocytes and the heart. *Life Sci* 48:97–106, 1991.
19. Offhaus JM, Judge BS: Massive unintentional digoxin ingestion successfully managed without the use of activated charcoal or digoxin-specific antibody fragments. *Clin Toxicol* 43(6):650, 2005.
20. Gervais A: Digoxin-like immunoreactive substance (DLIS) in liver disease: Comparison of clinical and laboratory parameters in patients with and without DLIS. *Drug Intell Clin Pharm* 21:540, 1987.
21. Graves SW, Brown B, Valdes R: An endogenous digoxin-like substance in patients with renal impairment. *Ann Intern Med* 99:604, 1983.
22. Stone J, Bentur Y, Zalstein E, et al: Effect of endogenous digoxin-like substances on the interpretation of high concentrations of digoxin in children. *J Pediatr* 117:321–325, 1990.
23. Bismuth C, Gaultier M, Conso F, et al: Hyperkalemia in acute digitalis poisoning: prognostic significance and therapeutic implications. *Clin Toxicol* 6:153, 1973.
24. Lalonde RL, Deshpande R, Hamilton PP, et al: Acceleration of digoxin clearance by activated charcoal. *Clin Pharmacol Ther* 37(4):367–371, 1985.
25. Critchley JA, Critchley LA: Digoxin toxicity in chronic renal failure: treatment by multiple dose activated charcoal intestinal dialysis. *Hum Exp Toxicol* 16(12):733–735, 1997.

26. Roberts DM, Southcott E, Potter JM, et al: Pharmacokinetics of digoxin cross-reacting substances in patients with acute yellow oleander (*Thevetia peruviana*) poisoning, including the effect of activated charcoal. *Ther Drug Monit* 28(6):784–792, 2006.
27. de Silva HA, Fonseka MM, Pathmeswaran A, et al: Multiple-dose activated charcoal for treatment of yellow oleander poisoning: a single-blind, randomised, placebo-controlled trial. *Lancet* 361(9373):1935–1938, 2003.
28. Eddleston M, Juszczak E, Buckley NA, et al: Randomised controlled trial of routine single or multiple dose superactivated charcoal for self-poisoning in a region with high mortality. *Clin Toxicol* 43(5):442–443, 2005.
29. Duke M: Atrioventricular block due to accidental digoxin ingestion treated with atropine. *Am J Dis Child* 124:754, 1972.
30. Bismuth C, Motte G, Conso F, et al: Acute digitoxin intoxication treated by intracardiac pacemaker: experience in sixty-eight patients. *Clin Toxicol* 10:443, 1977.
31. Lapostolle F, Borron SW, Verdier C, et al: Digoxin-specific Fab fragments as single first-line therapy in digitalis poisoning. *Crit Care Med* 36(11):3014–3018, 2008.
32. Sharff JA, Bayer MJ: Acute and chronic digitalis toxicity: Presentation and Treatment. *Ann Emerg Med* 11:327, 1982.
33. Nicholls DP, Murtagh JG, Holt DW: Use of amiodarone and digoxin specific Fab antibodies in digoxin overdosage. *Br Med J* 53:462, 1985.
34. Maheswaran R, Bramble MG, Hardisty CA: Massive digoxin overdose—successful treatment with intravenous amiodarone. *Br Med J* 287:392, 1986.
35. French JH, Thomas RG, Siskind AP, et al: Magnesium therapy in massive digoxin intoxication. *Ann Emerg Med* 13:562, 1984.
36. Springer M, Olsen KR, Feaster W: Acute massive digoxin overdose: survival without use of digitalis-specific antibodies. *Am J Emerg Med* 4:364, 1986.
37. Erickson CP, Olson KR: Case files of the medical toxicology fellowship of the California poison control system—San Francisco: calcium plus digoxin—more taboo than toxic? *J Med Toxicol* 4(1):33–39, 2008.
38. Beller GA, Hood WB Jr, Smith TW, et al: Correlation of serum magnesium levels and cardiac digitalis intoxication. *Am J Cardiol* 33:225, 1974.
39. Antman EM, Wenger TL, Butler VP Jr, et al: Treatment of 150 cases of life-threatening digitalis intoxication with digoxin-specific Fab antibody fragments: final report of a multicenter study. *Circulation* 81:1744–1752, 1990.
40. Woolf AD, Wenger TL, Smith TW, et al: Results of multicenter studies of digoxin-specific antibody fragments in managing digitalis intoxication in the pediatric population. *Am J Emerg Med* 9:16–20, 1991.
41. Hickey AR, Wenger TL, Carpenter VP, et al: Digoxin immune Fab therapy in the management of digitalis intoxication: safety and efficacy results of an observational surveillance study. *J Am Coll Cardiol* 17:590–598, 1991.
42. Smolarz A, Roesch E, Lenz H, et al: Digoxin specific antibody (Fab) fragments in 34 cases of severe digitalis intoxication. *Clin Tox* 23:327, 1985.
43. Smith TW, Haber E, Yeatman L, et al: Reversal of advanced digoxin intoxication with Fab fragments of digoxin-specific antibodies. *N Engl J Med* 294:797, 1976.
44. Gibbs I, Adams PC, Parnham AJ, et al: Plasma digoxin: assay anomalies in Fab-treated patients. *Br J Clin Pharmacol* 16:445, 1983.
45. Smith TW, Lloyd BL, Spicer N, et al: Immunogenicity and kinetics of distribution and elimination of sheep digoxin-specific IgG and Fab fragments in the rabbit and baboon. *Clin Exp Immunol* 36:384, 1979.
46. Allen NM, Dunham GD, Sailstad JM, et al: Clinical and pharmacokinetic profiles of digoxin immune Fab in four patients with renal impairment. *Drug Intell Clin Pharm* 25:1315–1320, 1991.
47. Wenger TL: Experience with digoxin immune Fab (Ovine) in patients with renal impairment. *Am J Emerg Med* 9:21–23, 1991.
48. Ujhelyi MR, Robert S: Pharmacokinetic aspects of digoxin-specific Fab therapy in the management of digitalis toxicity. *Clin Pharmacokinet* 28:483–493, 1995.

CHAPTER 128 ■ CHOLINERGIC POISONING

CYNTHIA K. AARON

Cholinergic (acetylcholinesterase inhibitor) agents are used in medicine, as insecticides, and as "nerve agent" chemical weapons. Most poisonings are accidental dermal contamination during agricultural use of pesticides [1]. The majority of suicide attempts are ingestions [2]. Food-borne exposures have produced epidemics such as "Ginger Jake paralysis" (delayed neuropathy) due to contamination of an alcoholic drink with triorthocresyl phosphate [3] and a large epidemic of mild-to-moderate symptoms related to use of the insecticide aldicarb on watermelons [4].

PHARMACOLOGY

Cholinesterase inhibitors act by blocking the active site of acetylcholinesterase (AChE). Organophosphates form a covalent phosphate linkage at the enzyme active site. Enzyme regeneration occurs by either de novo synthesis, hydrolysis of the serine–organophosphorus bond, or oxime regeneration. However, over 24 to 48 hours, most phosphorylated molecules *age* or become resistant to reactivation by oxime therapy. Carbamates are reversible inhibitors of AChE, occupying (but not modifying) the catalytic region of the enzyme. AChE activity is restored when the carbamate spontaneously leaves the enzyme's active site [5]. AChE inhibitors such as tacrine, rivastigmine, donepezil, and galantamine have been used for treatment of Alzheimer's dementia. The characteristics and treatment of exposure to these products is covered at the end of this chapter.

Inhibition of AChE allows the neurotransmitter acetylcholine to accumulate and remain active in the synapse, resulting in sustained depolarization of the postsynaptic neuron or effector organ. This effect occurs in the central nervous system (CNS) as well as at muscarinic sites in the peripheral nervous system, nicotinic sites in the sympathetic and parasympathetic ganglia, and nicotinic sites at the neuromuscular junction. In general, effects at muscarinic sites are sustained, whereas nicotinic sites are stimulated and then depressed (hyperpolarization block). Signs and symptoms of cholinergic toxicity typically appear when 60% to 80% of cholinesterase activity has been inhibited [6]. The pharmacologic and toxicologic effects of acetylcholinesterase inhibitor are an extension of their mechanism of action (Table 128.1).

In addition to acute cholinergic effects, organophosphates cause two other toxic effects. Intermediate syndrome (IMS) is a recurrence of weakness that occurs hours to days after a serious organophosphate exposure [7]. Some authors have suggested that IMS is caused by inadequate oxime therapy when serum organophosphate concentrations remain elevated due to redistribution, altered metabolism, or decreased clearance [8]. It is also possible that IMS is due to desensitization block with downregulation and eventual decrease in the nicotinic receptor activity. Since the nicotinic receptor has five subunits, there is probably significant polymorphism at this receptor affecting clinical response [9].

TABLE 128.1

PHARMACOLOGIC EFFECTS OF CHOLINESTERASE INHIBITION RECEPTOR TYPE

Location	Effects
Muscarinic (increased stimulation)	
Pupils	Miosis (constriction)
Ciliary body	Blurred vision
Exocrine glands	Increased secretions
Lacrimal	Tearing
Salivary	Salivation
Respiratory	Bronchorrhea, rhinorrhea
Heart	Bradycardia
Smooth muscle	Contraction
Bronchial	Bronchoconstriction
Gastrointestinal	Nausea, vomiting, abdominal cramps, diarrhea
Bladder	Incontinence, frequency
Sphincter of Oddi	Pancreatitis
Central nervous system	Variable[a]
Nicotinic (stimulation; then depression)	
Skeletal muscle	Weakness, cramps, fasciculation, paralysis
Sympathetic ganglia	Tachycardia, hypertension; then hypotension
Central nervous system	Variable symptoms from anxiety and restlessness to confusion, obtundation, coma, and seizures[a]

[a]Relative contributions of nicotinic and muscarinic receptors to central nervous system effects are unclear.

The second noncholinergic effect is organophosphorus-induced delayed peripheral neuropathy (OPIDN). This is a delayed peripheral neuropathy, which appears to be mediated by a membrane-bound specific "neuropathy target esterase." Organophosphates that have been associated with OPIDN are aryl organophosphorus esters that contain either a pentavalent phosphorus atom (type I, including derivatives of phosphoric, phosphonic, and phosphoramidic acids, or phosphorofluoridates) or a trivalent phosphorus atom (type II or phosphorus acid derivatives). This neuropathy primarily involves motor fibers. Histologic analysis shows progressive neuronal degeneration, beginning with axonal swelling followed by demyelination, axonal degeneration, and neuronal cell body death and Wallerian degeneration or "dying back" phenomenon [10].

CLINICAL MANIFESTATIONS

Excessive acetylcholine produces symptoms of muscarinic and nicotinic excess. These clinical effects are outlined in Table 128.2. One mnemonic used to describe the muscarinic toxidrome is DUMBELS (*d*iarrhea, *u*rination, *m*iosis, *b*ronchospasm, *e*mesis, *l*acrimation, *s*alivation). Miosis may be the most sensitive marker for moderate or severe exposure to a acetylcholinesterase inhibitor [11]. Lacrimation, rhinorrhea, salivation, and profuse sweating are common in moderate to severe poisoning. Abdominal cramping, diarrhea, and vomiting are very common with severe poisoning. Fasciculations are typically observed in severe overdoses.

Respiratory failure is a common cause of death from acetylcholinesterase inhibitor poisoning [2]. Cholinergic excess has direct deleterious effects on the respiratory center; causes bronchial muscle spasm and noncardiogenic pulmonary edema with exuberant mucus production; and severe respiratory muscle impairment. Respiratory failure may be further complicated by aspiration.

Cardiac toxicity has been increasingly described as a complication of organophosphate poisoning. There are three phases of reported toxicity including a brief period of intense sympathomimetic tone, a period of enhanced parasympathetic activity, and corrected QT (QTc) interval prolongation with potential for torsade de pointes. Prolongation of the QTc is a marker of severity and patients with a QTc greater than 440 milliseconds require higher doses of atropine and have a higher mortality than those a QTc less than 440 milliseconds [12]. Electrocardiographic abnormalities including nonspecific ST-T changes, tachydysrhythmias, bradydysrhythmias, and polymorphic (torsade de pointes) ventricular tachycardia have been reported [13]. The effect on blood pressure is variable. Patients poisoned with dimethoate have an initial benign course but develop refractory hypotension and cardiogenic shock within 36 to 48 hours [2].

The CNS effects of cholinergic poisoning include altered mental status seizures and coma [2]. Dystonias and choreoathetoid movements have also been observed [14]. Less severe

TABLE 128.2

SYMPTOMS OF CHOLINERGIC POISONING

Exposure only	Mild poisoning	Moderate poisoning	Severe poisoning
No symptoms	Can walk	Cannot walk	Unconscious
	Fatigue	Weakness	Unreactive pupils
	Headache	Difficulty speaking	Fasciculations
	Dizzy	Fasciculations	Flaccid paralysis
	Nausea	Miosis	Secretions mouth/nose
	Vomiting	ChE 10%–20% of normal	Moist rales
	Numbness		Respiratory distress
	Sweating		Seizures
	Salivation		ChE <10% of normal
	Chest tightness		
	Abdominal cramps		
	Diarrhea		
	ChE 20%–50% of normal		

ChE, RBC cholinesterase.

acute manifestations include anxiety, agitation, emotional lability, headaches, insomnia, tremor, difficulty in concentrating, slurred speech, ataxia, and hyperreflexia or hyporeflexia. In some cases, acute organophosphate poisoning may produce longer-lasting neuropsychiatric sequelae [15]. This has been labeled the chronic organophosphorus-induced neuropsychiatric disorder (COPIND). These problems seem most severe after serious acute intoxications and usually resolve within 1 year [15].

Cholinergic signs and symptoms typically begin minutes to hours after exposure [2]. Symptom onset is rarely more than 12 hours after exposure. Onset may be delayed for lipophilic compounds (e.g., fenthion, dichlofenthion, leptophos) [2] or compounds that require hepatic metabolism to a more toxic intermediate (e.g., parathion is metabolized to paraoxon) [16]. Progressive or prolonged symptoms raise the suspicion of continued absorption of the poison.

Life-threatening cholinergic symptoms from organophosphate toxicity generally abate within 1 to 3 days, although many cases requiring weeks of intensive care are reported [17]. Symptoms usually resolve within 12 to 48 hours after exposure to carbamates and other reversible cholinesterase inhibitors [18].

The intermediate syndrome, characterized by weakness of neck muscles, motor cranial nerves, proximal limb muscles, and respiratory muscles, but without prominent muscarinic findings beginning 24 to 96 hours after the onset of poisoning and lasting 4 to 18 days has been described [8]. An early clinical indication of this syndrome is that affected patients are unable to lift their heads up from their beds [17].

Delayed neuropathy occurs 1 to 3 weeks after the acute cholinergic crises. Patients may initially recover then show progressive signs and symptoms of OPIDN. Since this is a dying back axonopathy that usually spares the neuronal cell body, the peripheral neuropathy is characterized by both paresthesias and motor dysfunction occurring first in the longest skeletal nerves with development of foot drop and a high-stepping gait. Symptoms develop slowly and can be divided into three phases: progressive, stationary, and improvement. During the progressive phase, patients have a peripheral sensory neuropathy with complaints of burning, tightness, or pain in the legs and feet. This is followed by numbness and tingling. Subsequently, motor weakness develops, with weakness and atrophy of the peroneal muscles causing a foot drop. After approximately 1 week, the paresis may ascend symmetrically into the upper extremities. The sensory loss may occur in a stocking–glove distribution, and the patient loses proprioception. With time, a positive Romberg's sign and loss of lower-extremity deep tendon reflexes may develop. Flaccid paralysis may occur in severe cases. During the stationary phase, paresis may persist or resolve within 2 to 9 weeks, and motor findings may cease to progress. This may occur over 3 to 12 months. The improvement phase may begin 6 to 18 months after exposure. Partial or complete motor function returns in reverse order of loss. During this phase, central cord or brain lesions may be unmasked and spasticity may develop [19].

DIAGNOSTIC EVALUATION

The diagnosis of the cholinergic poisoning is based on a history of exposure, clinical findings (toxidrome), and improvement after appropriate antidotal therapy. The primary laboratory studies for evaluating anticholinesterase poisoning are plasma cholinesterase (also known as butyrylcholinesterase or pseudocholinesterase) and red blood cell (RBC) acetylcholinesterase. These tests are not rapidly available in most clinical settings. Both may be used to confirm the clinical diagnosis. RBC acetylcholinesterase has a similar structure to synaptic acetylcholinesterase and it has been validated as a surrogate for synaptic acetylcholinesterase [20].

Plasma cholinesterase is synthesized in the liver. It falls and recovers more rapidly than RBC cholinesterase. Only transient decreases of RBC and plasma cholinesterase occur with carbamate poisoning, because inactivated AChE spontaneously reactivates with plasma elimination half-lives of 1 to 2 hours [21].

In suspected cholinesterase inhibitor poisoning, plasma and RBC acetylcholinesterase levels should be sent for laboratory determination initially and repeated if the clinical course is atypical [22]. Blood for cholinesterase determination should be drawn into a fluoride free tube as fluoride inactivates enzyme systems. Samples should be spun down and frozen for storage. The assaying laboratory should be contacted to obtain specific drawing and storing instructions.

Acute exposures are usually classified based on the degree of depression of RBC cholinesterase: mild (20% to 50% of baseline), moderate (10% to 20% of baseline), and severe (less than 10% of baseline) (see Table 128.2). An EMG using repetitive tetanic nerve stimulation can be done to characterize the block and to estimate the amount of enzyme inhibition [23]. Since there is a wide range for normal RBC cholinesterase level (substantial interindividual variation), a person's baseline needs to be established if return to working with pesticides is a consideration. [24] Workers should be removed from exposure until RBC cholinesterase is at least 75% of their baseline values [25]. Workers who do not have an established RBC cholinesterase baseline should not return to work until their RBC cholinesterase levels have reached a plateau.

Several organophosphates are metabolized to *p*-nitrophenol that can be easily detected in the urine soon after poisoning [26]. Organophosphate concentrations can be measured in serum [27], but contribute little to patient management. These measurements can be useful in determining residual organophosphate residue in a patient with prolonged signs of toxicity and perhaps whether oxime therapy needs to be continued, particularly when combined with the ability to reactivate the AChE [23]. Supplemental studies include serum electrolytes, blood urea nitrogen, creatinine, glucose, calcium, magnesium, lipase, arterial blood gases, electrocardiography, and chest radiography.

The intermediate syndrome is diagnosed by clinical findings associated with a reproducible EMG-nerve conduction study using repeated submaximal tetanic nerve stimulation and measuring compound muscle action potentials [28]. No specific laboratory studies are available for evaluating OPIDN. Electromyography (EMG) may help to determine the extent of the peripheral neuropathy, and there are specific EMG findings associated with OPIDN [29].

Toxicologic differential diagnosis for cholinergic toxicity includes nicotine, carbachol, methacholine, arecoline, bethanechol, pilocarpine, and Inocybe or Clitocybe mushrooms. Nontoxicologic diagnoses that may be mistaken for cholinergic toxicity include myasthenia gravis and Eaton–Lambert syndrome.

MANAGEMENT

Patients with all but the mildest symptoms should be admitted to an intensive care unit for careful observation and antidotal therapy as clinically indicated. The initial priorities are managing the patient's airway, breathing, and circulation. All personnel who are involved in the resuscitation and decontamination process should wear masks or respirators, aprons, and nitrile or butyl rubber gloves to avoid secondary contamination.

Most patients with severe cholinergic poisoning will require airway management and ventilatory assistance for respiratory failure. Succinylcholine should be used with caution to aid intubation because prolonged (hours to days) paralysis may result [30]. A reasonable alternative is to use a double-dose of a nondepolarizing neuromuscular blocker (such as vecuronium) Airway and bronchial secretions are treated with atropine. The initial adult dose is 1 to 2 mg parenterally, which is doubled every 5 minutes (pediatric dose, 0.05 mg per kg) as needed until pulmonary secretions are controlled [31].

Initial resuscitation with IV fluids is needed because of significant gastrointestinal (GI) fluid losses Blood pressure support may require direct-acting pressors such as norepinephrine, phenylephrine, epinephrine and cardiac depression may require the use of dobutamine [2]. Patients should be treated with atropine (using the dosing scheme describe in the previous paragraph) until the systolic blood pressure is greater than 80 mm Hg and urine output exceeds 0.5 mL per kg per hour [31]. Electrical pacing is rarely needed to treat ventricular dysrhythmias. Potassium and magnesium should be normalized to minimize QTc prolongation.

Seizures should be treated with IV atropine and a benzodiazepine (diazepam, 0.2 to 0.4 mg per kg or an equivalent). Animal studies suggest that both atropine and benzodiazepine are efficacious [32]. Given the potential benefits of benzodiazepines in severe organophosphate poisonings to mitigate neuropsychiatric sequelae, it is reasonable to administer a benzodiazepine even if seizures are not apparent.

Decontamination can limit absorption and prevent re-exposure. All of the patient's clothing should be removed and discarded, and the body should be thoroughly washed with mild soap and water. If the ingestion is recent, nasogastric suction can used to attempt to aspirate any product remaining in the stomach [33]. Although single and multidose charcoal did not change outcome in one trial [34], many of the subjects in this trial had long delays before treatment and it is possible that early treatment may limit toxicity. Dilute hypochlorite solution (household bleach) inactivates the organophosphorus ester and can be used to decontaminate equipment but should not be used on skin [35].

Antidotal therapy is comprised of two complementary agents, atropine and an oxime such as pralidoxime (North America, India, and Asia) or obidoxime (Europe and Middle East). Atropine is a competitive antagonist of acetylcholine at the muscarinic receptors but has no effect on muscle weakness or paralysis and does not affect the AChE regeneration rate. As noted above, atropine is primarily indicated for control of pulmonary secretions and bronchospasm. It has a secondary role in helping to control seizures and CNS manifestations of poisoning [36]. Careful titration of atropine to the individual patient is required, with frequent clinical reevaluation to prevent atropine toxicity [33]. Atropine therapy should be restarted at the first signs of cholinergic excess. A continuous atropine infusion may be necessary to stabilize the patient, after which the infusion can be titrated back while close observation is maintained. Most patients will respond to 3 to 5 mg per hour [33]. In general, higher doses of atropine are required during the first 24 hours with organophosphate pesticides than with nerve agents. Tachycardia is not a contraindication to atropine therapy; it may reflect hypoxia or sympathetic stimulation. Mydriasis may be an early response but is a poor marker for adequate atropinization. A common pitfall is inadequate atropine dosing during serious cholinergic agent overdoses. High doses of atropine are commonly needed for control of secretions. Daily doses in excess of 100 mg are occasionally required for several days [37]. Glycopyrrolate is an antimuscarinic agent that does not penetrate the CNS. It can be substituted for atropine when isolated peripheral cholinergic toxicity is present. The recommended dose is 0.05 mg per kg. One study suggested that a combination of atropine and glycopyrrolate may improve outcomes [38].

Pralidoxime (2-PAM) and obidoxime are nucleophilic oximes that regenerate AChE at muscarinic and nicotinic synapses by reversing the AChE active site phosphorylation. Although pralidoxime does not enter the CNS well, rapid improvement in coma or termination of seizures has been observed after pralidoxime administration [39]. The antidotal effect of atropine and oximes is synergistic.

Although oximes remain a standard therapy for organophosphate poisoning, recent studies have highlighted our limited understanding of their role. Although one recent randomized controlled trial showed a dramatic treatment effect with pralidoxime [40], a second trial found no benefit and a trend toward worse outcomes [41]. There are several possible explanations for these discrepant results, including differences in the lipophilicity, side chains (O′-dimethyl vs. O′-diethyl organophosphates), rate of aging, and interaction between inhibition/re-inhibition and spontaneous reactivation of the parent and oxime-bound compounds. Future studies will have to address these differences.

Although the optimal treatment protocol for pralidoxime is not known, there is consensus that many older protocols used insufficient doses [42]. Animal studies suggested that a serum concentration of 4 mg per mL were effective [43], and earlier pharmacokinetic studies suggested the use of 1 to 2 g IV pralidoxime followed by 1 g every 6 to 12 hours would produce a serum level of 4 mg per mL [44,45]. Subsequent studies in poisoned patients have shown that the amount of circulating inhibitor (parent or metabolite of the original organophosphate) determines the need for oxime [46]. Patients who have ingested massive amounts of an organophosphate may have prolonged high levels of circulating inhibitor for days after ingestion and the pralidoxime blood level of 4 mg per mL is too low to allow for continued reactivation of the acetylcholinesterase. Ideally, poisoned patients should be followed by serial evaluation of the ability to reactivate their cholinesterase in vitro [6]. Since this is not feasible for most patients, the following suggestions can be made. The World Health Organization recommends an initial pralidoxime dose of 30 mg per kg IV followed by 8 mg per kg per hour or alternatively, 30 mg per kg every 4 hours if a continuous infusion is not possible [42]. The appropriate dose of obidoxime 250 mg initially followed by 750 mg over 24 hours [47]. Muscle fasciculation and weakness should show a response within 60 minutes after dosing and the dose titrated upwards if the patient has breakthrough signs and symptoms. In mass casualty situations, the intramuscular route of administration may be more practical. The duration of therapy is based on clinical response and is usually 24 to 48 hours. Under ideal conditions, serum samples can be assayed for acetylcholinesterase reactability and this can be used to guide oxime therapy [48]. Some patients may require continuous treatment for greater than 1 week, depending on the body burden of organophosphate and reinhibition of reactivated acetylcholinesterase.

Although hemoperfusion can enhance the elimination of anticholinesterase agents [49], the availability of specific antidotes for organophosphates and the relatively short course of carbamate intoxications make this procedure unnecessary.

Carbamate poisonings are expected to have a good prognosis because the duration of serious signs and symptoms is limited. Severe organophosphate poisonings may require prolonged respiratory support, with its attendant complications. Death from acute organophosphate poisonings usually occurs within 24 hours in untreated cases, although exposures to fenthion and dimethoate may lead to death within 72 hours even if treated [2]. Aggressive respiratory management, timely antidotal therapy, and intensive supportive care are expected to improve morbidity and mortality. Recovery from OPIDN may be gradual or not at all. CNS anoxic sequelae have the worse prognosis and are not specific to cholinesterase inhibitors but rather a consequence of prolonged hypoxia.

Toxicity of AChE Inhibitors Used to Treat Alzheimer's Disease

With the increasing use of AChE inhibitors to treat dementia, there has been an increasing number of exposures to these medications. Symptoms can range from general weakness [50] to salivation and GI effects [51] but are generally milder than pesticides. However, one case of deliberate ingestion of 288 mg of rivastigmine results in seizures, respiratory muscle weakness and bronchial secretions [52]. Muscarinic effects should be treated with atropine and one report has suggested that isolated CNS effects without peripheral muscarinic symptoms can be treated with pralidoxime alone [53].

NERVE AGENTS USED IN WARFARE

Since the Persian Gulf War and in the aftermath of the terrorist attacks of September 11, 2001, there has been increasing concern about the potential use of nerve agents such as GA (Tabun), GB (Sarin), GD (Soman), and VX. These chemicals are similar in structure and function to the organophosphate insecticides but have a much greater potency. Please see Chapter 214 for a complete discussion of this topic.

References

1. Kahn E: Pesticide related illness in California farm workers. *J Occup Med* 18:693–696, 1976.
2. Eddleston M, Eyer P, Worek F, et al: Differences between organophosphorus insecticides in human self-poisoning: a prospective cohort study. *Lancet* 366:1452–1459, 2005.
3. Morgan JP: The Jamaica ginger paralysis. *JAMA* 248:1864–1867, 1982.
4. Centers for Disease Control (CDC): Aldicarb food poisoning from contaminated melons—California. *MMWR Morb Mortal Wkly Rep* 35:254–258, 1986.
5. Lotti M: Clinical toxicology of anticholinesterase agents in humans, in: Krieger R, ed: *Handbook of pesticide toxicology. Agents*. Vol 2. 2nd ed. San Diego: Academic Press, 2001, pp 1043–1085.
6. Thiermann H, Worek F, Eyer P, et al: Obidoxime in acute organophosphate poisoning. 2—PK/PD relationships. *Clin Toxicol (Philadelphia)* 47:807–813, 2009.
7. Senanayake N, Karalliedde L: Neurotoxic effects of organophosphorus insecticides. An intermediate syndrome. *N Engl J Med* 316:761–763, 1987.
8. Senanayake N, Johnson MK: Acute polyneuropathy after poisoning by a new organophosphate insecticide. *N Engl J Med* 306:155–157, 1982.
9. Karalliedde L, Baker D, Marrs TC: Organophosphate-induced intermediate syndrome: aetiology and relationships with myopathy. *Toxicol Rev* 25: 1–14, 2006.
10. Jokanovic M, Stukalov PV, Kosanovic M: Organophosphate induced delayed polyneuropathy. *Curr Drug Targets CNS Neurol Disord* 1:593–602, 2002.
11. Okumura T, Takasu N, Ishimatsu S, et al: Report on 640 victims of the Tokyo subway sarin attack. *Ann Emerg Med* 28:129–135, 1996.
12. Shadnia S, Okazi A, Akhlaghi N, et al: Prognostic value of long QT interval in acute and severe organophosphate poisoning. *J Med Toxicol* 5:196–199, 2009.
13. Yurumez Y, Yavuz Y, Saglam H, et al: Electrocardiographic findings of acute organophosphate poisoning. *J Emerg Med* 36:39–42, 2009.
14. Moody SB, Terp DK: Dystonic reaction possibly induced by cholinesterase inhibitor insecticides. *Drug Intell Clin Pharm* 22:311–312, 1988.
15. Rosenstock L, Keifer M, Daniell WE, et al: Chronic central nervous system effects of acute organophosphate pesticide intoxication. The Pesticide Health Effects Study Group. *Lancet* 338:223–227, 1991.
16. Buratti FM, Volpe MT, Meneguz A, et al: CYP-specific bioactivation of four organophosphorothioate pesticides by human liver microsomes. *Toxicol Appl Pharmacol* 186:143–154, 2003.
17. Eddleston M, Roberts D, Buckley N: Management of severe organophosphorus pesticide poisoning: *Crit Care* 6:259–259, 2002.
18. Lifshitz M, Shahak E, Bolotin A, et al: Carbamate poisoning in early childhood and in adults. *J Toxicol Clin Toxicol* 35:25–27, 1997.
19. Lotti M, Moretto A: Organophosphate-induced delayed polyneuropathy. *Toxicol Rev* 24:37–49, 2005.
20. Thiermann H, Szinicz L, Eyer P, et al: Correlation between red blood cell acetylcholinesterase activity and neuromuscular transmission in organophosphate poisoning. *Chem Biol Interact* 157–158:345–347, 2005.
21. Lifshitz M, Rotenberg M, Sofer S, et al: Carbamate poisoning and oxime treatment in children: a clinical and laboratory study. *Pediatrics* 93:652–655, 1994.
22. Abdullat IM, Battah AH, Hadidi KA: The use of serial measurement of plasma cholinesterase in the management of acute poisoning with organophosphates and carbamates. *Forensic Sci Int* 162:126–130, 2006.
23. Thiermann H, Zilker T, Eyer F, et al: Monitoring of neuromuscular transmission in organophosphate pesticide-poisoned patients. *Toxicol Lett* 191:297–304, 2009.
24. Coye MJ, Lowe JA, Maddy KT: Biological monitoring of agricultural workers exposed to pesticides: I. Cholinesterase activity determinations. *J Occup Med* 28:619–627, 1986.
25. Agency Paetsooehhacep: Guidelines for physicians who supervise workers exposed to cholinesterase-inhibiting pesticides. Available at: http://www.oehha.ca.gov/pesticides/pdf/docguide2002.pdf. Accessed December 27, 2009.
26. Barr DB, Turner WE, DiPietro E, et al: Measurement of p-nitrophenol in the urine of residents whose homes were contaminated with methyl parathion. *Environ Health Perspect* 110[Suppl 6]:1085–1091, 2002.
27. Inoue S, Saito T, Mase H, et al: Rapid simultaneous determination for organophosphorus pesticides in human serum by LC-MS. *J Pharm Biomed Anal* 44:258–264, 2007.
28. Jayawardane P, Dawson AH, Weerasinghe V, et al: The spectrum of intermediate syndrome following acute organophosphate poisoning: a prospective cohort study from Sri Lanka. *PLoS Med* 5(7):e147, 2008.
29. Wadia RS, Chitra S, Amin RB, et al: Electrophysiological studies in acute organophosphate poisoning. *J Neurol Neurosurg Psychiatry* 50:1442–1448, 1987.
30. Selden BS, Curry SC: Prolonged succinylcholine-induced paralysis in organophosphate insecticide poisoning. *Ann Emerg Med* 16:215–217, 1987.
31. Eddleston M, Buckley NA, Eyer P, et al: Management of acute organophosphorus pesticide poisoning: *Lancet* 371:597–607, 2008.
32. McDonough JH Jr, Jaax NK, Crowley RA, et al: Atropine and/or diazepam therapy protects against soman-induced neural and cardiac pathology. *Fundam Appl Toxicol* 13:256–276, 1989.
33. Eddleston M, Dawson A, Karalliedde L, et al: Early management after self-poisoning with an organophosphorus or carbamate pesticide – a treatment protocol for junior doctors. *Crit Care* 8:R391–R397, 2004.
34. Eddleston M, Juszczak E, Buckley NA, et al: Multiple-dose activated charcoal in acute self-poisoning: a randomised controlled trial. *Lancet* 371:579–587, 2008.
35. Holstege CP, Kirk M, Sidell FR: Chemical warfare. Nerve agent poisoning. *Crit Care Clin* 13:923–942, 1997.
36. Eddleston M, Singh S, Buckley N: Acute organophosphorus poisoning. *Clin Evidence* (10):1652–1663, 2003.
37. Golsousidis H, Kokkas V: Use of 19 590 mg of atropine during 24 days of treatment, after a case of unusually severe parathion poisoning. *Hum Toxicol* 4:339–340, 1985.
38. Arendse R, Irusen E: An atropine and glycopyrrolate combination reduces mortality in organophosphate poisoning. *Hum Exp Toxicol* 28:715–720, 2009.
39. Lotti M, Becker CE: Treatment of acute organophosphate poisoning: evidence of a direct effect on central nervous system by 2-PAM (pyridine-2-aldoxime methyl chloride). *J Toxicol Clin Toxicol* 19:121–127, 1982.
40. Pawar KS, Bhoite RR, Pillay CP, et al: Continuous pralidoxime infusion versus repeated bolus injection to treat organophosphorus pesticide poisoning: a randomised controlled trial. *Lancet* 368:2136–2141, 2006.
41. Eddleston M, Eyer P, Worek F, et al: Pralidoxime in acute organophosphorus insecticide poisoning–a randomised controlled trial. *PLoS Med* 6:2009.
42. Buckley NA, Eddleston M, Szinicz L: Oximes for acute organophosphate pesticide poisoning. *Cochrane Database Syst Rev* CD005085, 2005.
43. Sundwall A: Minimum concentrations of *N*-methylpyridinium-2-aldoxime methane sulphonate (P2 S) which reverse neuromuscular block. *Biochem Pharmacol* 8:413–417, 1961.
44. Medicis JJ, Stork CM, Howland MA, et al: Pharmacokinetics following a loading plus a continuous infusion of pralidoxime compared with the traditional short infusion regimen in human volunteers. *J Toxicol Clin Toxicol* 34:289–295, 1996.
45. Schexnayder S, James LP, Kearns GL, et al: The pharmacokinetics of continuous infusion pralidoxime in children with organophosphate poisoning. *J Toxicol Clin Toxicol* 36:549–555, 1998.
46. Eyer P, Worek F, Thiermann H, et al: Paradox findings may challenge orthodox reasoning in acute organophosphate poisoning. *Chem Biol Interact* 187(1-3):270–278, 2009.

47. Eyer F, Worek F, Eyer P, et al: Obidoxime in acute organophosphate poisoning: 1—clinical effectiveness. *Clin Toxicol (Phila)* 47:798–806, 2009.
48. Eyer P: The role of oximes in the management of organophosphorus pesticide poisoning. *Toxicol Rev* 22:165–190, 2003.
49. Peter JV, Moran JL, Pichamuthu K, et al: Adjuncts and alternatives to oxime therapy in organophosphate poisoning–is there evidence of benefit in human poisoning? A review. *Anaesth Intensive Care* 36:339–350, 2008.
50. Lai MW, Moen M, Ewald MB: Pesticide-like poisoning from a prescription drug. *N Engl J Med* 353:317–318, 2005.
51. Sener S, Ozsarac M: Case of the month: rivastigmine (Exelon) toxicity with evidence of respiratory depression. *Emerg Med J* 23:82–85, 2006.
52. Brvar M, Mozina M, Bunc M: Poisoning with rivastigmine. *Clin Toxicol (Phila)* 43:891–892, 2005.
53. Hoffman RS, Manini AF, Russell-Haders AL, et al: Use of pralidoxime without atropine in rivastigmine (carbamate) toxicity. *Hum Exp Toxicol* 28:599–602, 2009.

CHAPTER 129 ■ COCAINE POISONING

RICHARD D. SHIH AND JUDD E. HOLLANDER

Cocaine (benzoylmethylecgonine) is an alkaloid compound derived from the South American plant *Erythroxylon coca*. Its use as an illicit drug of abuse has reached epidemic proportions. Thirty-four million US citizens have used cocaine at least once; 5.9 million have used cocaine in the past year; and 2.1 million have used cocaine in the past month [1]. Among drug-related emergency department visits, cocaine is the most commonly used illicit substance seen [2]. Of all drug-related emergency department visits in the United States, cocaine is involved in approximately 20% [2].

PHARMACOLOGY

The pharmacologic effects of cocaine are complex, and they include direct blockade of the fast sodium channels, increase in norepinephrine release for the adrenergic nerve terminals, interference with neuronal catecholamine reuptake, and increase in excitatory amino acid concentration in the central nervous system (CNS). Blockade of the fast sodium channels stabilizes axonal membranes, producing a local anesthetic-like effect and a type I antidysrhythmic effect on the myocardium. The increase in catecholamine levels produces a sympathomimetic effect. The result of increased excitatory amino acid concentration in the CNS is increased extracellular dopamine concentration.

Cocaine is well absorbed through the mucosa of the respiratory, gastrointestinal, and genitourinary tract, including less common routes of absorption such as the urethra, bladder, and vagina. The cocaine hydrochloride salt is the form most often abused nasally or parenterally. Crack cocaine and cocaine freebase are alkaloid forms of cocaine that are produced by an extraction process. These forms are heat stable, can be smoked, and are absorbed through the pulmonary system. When intravenously administered or inhaled, cocaine is rapidly distributed throughout the body and CNS, with peak effects in 3 to 5 minutes. With nasal insufflation, absorption peaks in 20 minutes.

Cocaine has a half-life of 0.5 to 1.5 hours. It is rapidly hydrolyzed to the inactive metabolites ecgonine methyl ester and benzoylecgonine, which account for 80% of cocaine metabolism. These compounds have half-lives of 4 to 8 hours, with effects similar to those of cocaine. Minor cocaine metabolites include ecgonine and norcocaine. Urinary toxicology screens for recreational drugs typically assess for the presence of benzoylecgonine, which is usually present for 48 to 72 hours after cocaine use [3].

Cocaine is frequently abused in combination with other drugs. In particular, ethanol is a frequent coingestant [2]. This may be a popular combination because ethanol antagonizes cocaine's stimulatory effects. The metabolism of cocaine in the presence of ethanol produces cocaethylene, which has additional cardiovascular and behavioral effects [4]. Cocaethylene and cocaine are similar with regard to behavioral effects. However, cocaethylene has been more likely to result in death in animal studies. Human studies demonstrate that cocaethylene produces milder subjective effects and similar hemodynamic effects when compared with cocaine. Cocaethylene also has a direct myocardial depressant effect [4].

Cocaine toxicity is due to an exaggeration of its pharmacologic effects, resulting in myriad consequences that have an impact on every organ system. The widespread effects of cocaine are related to its ability to stimulate the peripheral and central sympathetic nervous systems, in addition to local anesthetic-like effects. Cocaine-induced seizures are most likely due to excess catecholamine stimulation.

Cocaine causes vascular effects through multiple pathophysiologic mechanisms that have been best described in the heart [5–7]. These include arterial vasoconstriction, in situ thrombus formation, platelet activation, and inhibition of endogenous fibrinolysis. In addition, myocardial oxygen demand is increased by cocaine-induced tachycardia and hypertension [5–8]. The direct local anesthetic-like effect of cocaine or secondary cocaine-induced myocardial ischemia [5,9] may be responsible for cardiac conduction disturbances [9] and dysrhythmias.

CLINICAL PRESENTATION

Clinical manifestations of acute cocaine toxicity may occur in a number of different organ systems. Most severe cocaine-related toxicity and cocaine-related deaths are manifested by signs of sympathomimetic overdrive (e.g., tachycardia, hypertension, dilated pupils, and increased psychomotor activity). This increased psychomotor activity causes increased heat production and can lead to severe hyperthermia and rhabdomyolysis [10].

Cocaine-induced cardiovascular effects are common. Of cocaine-related emergency department visits, chest pain is the most common complaint. Although most of these patients do not have serious underlying etiology, myocardial infarction due to cocaine is a well-established entity and needs to be excluded [11,12]. It occurs in 6% of patients presenting with cocaine-associated chest pain [13]. The risk of myocardial infarction is increased 24-fold in the hour after cocaine use. In patients aged 18 to 45 years, 25% of myocardial infarctions are attributed to cocaine use [14]. Cocaine-associated myocardial infarction typically occurs in patients aged 18 to 60 years without apparent massive cocaine exposure or without evidence of cocaine toxicity. Patients with cocaine-associated myocardial infarctions frequently have atypical chest pain or chest pain that is delayed hours to days after their most recent cocaine use [5,11].

Cardiac conduction disturbances (e.g., prolonged QRS and QTc) and cardiac dysrhythmias (e.g., sinus tachycardia, atrial fibrillation/flutter, supraventricular tachycardias, idioventricular rhythms, ventricular tachycardia, torsade de pointes, and ventricular fibrillation) may occur after cocaine use [15–17]. Aortic dissection and endocarditis associated with cocaine abuse are uncommon [18].

The neurologic effects of cocaine may be manifested in a number of ways. Altered mental status and euphoria are typically short lived and without serious sequelae. The stimulatory effects of cocaine can lead to seizures, cerebral infarction, intracerebral bleeding, subarachnoid hemorrhage, transient ischemic attacks, migraine-type headache syndromes, cerebral vasculitis, anterior spinal artery syndrome, and psychiatric manifestations [19–21]. Cocaine is associated with a sevenfold increased risk of stroke in women [22].

Cocaine-induced seizures are typically single, brief, generalized, self-limited, and not associated with permanent neurologic deficit. These seizures may occur in the presence or absence of concurrent structural disease, such as infarction or hemorrhage. Multiple or focal seizures are usually associated with concomitant drug use or an underlying seizure disorder [19].

Cocaine has a number of direct and indirect effects on the lungs, and they are associated with how the drug is used [23]. These effects include asthma exacerbations, pneumothorax, pneumomediastinum, noncardiogenic pulmonary edema, alveolar hemorrhage, pulmonary infarction, pulmonary artery hypertrophy, and acute respiratory failure [24,25]. Asthma exacerbations are more common with crack cocaine usage, most likely due to particulate by-products of combustion [26]. Inhalation of cocaine is typically associated with deep Valsalva maneuvers to maximize drug delivery and can cause pneumothorax, pneumomediastinum, and noncardiogenic pulmonary edema.

The intestinal vascular system is particularly sensitive to cocaine effects because the intestinal walls have a wide distribution of α-adrenergic receptors. Acute intestinal infarction has been associated with all routes of cocaine administration [27].

The most deadly gastrointestinal manifestation of cocaine usage is seen in the patient who presents after ingesting packets filled with cocaine. These patients have been termed *body packers* or *body stuffers*. Body packers are patients who swallow carefully prepared condom or latex packets filled with large quantities of highly purified cocaine for the purposes of smuggling this drug into the country. In contrast, body stuffers are typically "street" drug dealers who swallow packets of cocaine while fleeing the police. These packets were generally prepared for distribution to individual customers and not to protect the body stuffer from absorbing cocaine. It was previously thought that cocaine ingested orally was metabolized in the gastrointestinal track and did not lead to systemic toxicity. This is clearly not the case and toxicity can develop in body stuffers and packers from cocaine leaking out of the swallowed packets. The dosage of cocaine exposure in body stuffers is generally substantially less than that of a body packer. However, toxicity is more likely to occur in the setting of body stuffers. Although massive exposure to leakage from a condom or latex-filled packet of a body packer can occur, most body packers identified by airport immigration officers, do not develop clinical toxicity. However, any patient identified as a body packer who has developed any signs of systemic cocaine toxicity (tachycardia, hypertension, diaphoresis, etc.) can rapidly develop worsening symptoms including life-threatening ones. These patients, when identified, have a high potential for progressively worsening toxicity and mortality [28].

Premature atherosclerosis can develop in chronic cocaine users. Further, cocaine-induced left ventricular hypertrophy can lead to hypertrophic and eventually a dilated cardiomyopathy and congestive heart failure [5]. Cocaine-associated dilated cardiomyopathy appears to have a reversible component, and some patients have demonstrated improvement after cessation of cocaine use [5].

Chronic severe cocaine users can present with lethargy and a depressed mental status that is not attributable to any other etiology (diagnosis of exclusion), the "cocaine washout syndrome." This self-limited syndrome usually abates within 24 hours but can last for several days and is thought to result from excessive cocaine usage that depletes essential neurotransmitters [29].

Chronic inhalational use of cocaine does not appear to lead to long-term pulmonary effects. Spirometry and lung mechanics are typically normal even in heavy chronic users [30].

Chronic cocaine usage during pregnancy increases the chance for premature delivery and abruptio placentae [31]. Maternal cocaine usage is associated with low birth weight, small head circumference, developmental problems, and birth defects in the neonate [32–34]. Neonates exposed to cocaine in utero may develop cocaine withdrawal syndrome, which typically begins 24 to 48 hours after birth and is characterized by irritability, jitteriness, and poor eye contact.

DIAGNOSTIC EVALUATION

Patients manifesting cocaine toxicity should have a complete evaluation focusing on the history of cocaine use, signs and symptoms of sympathetic nervous system excess, and evaluation of specific organ system complaints. It is of paramount importance to determine whether signs and symptoms are due to cocaine itself, underlying structural abnormalities, or cocaine-induced structural abnormalities.

Friends or family of patients with altered mental status should be questioned about a history of cocaine usage and the events before presentation. Many patients deny cocaine use. Urine drug testing may be helpful in establishing recent cocaine use [35,36].

When the history is clear and symptoms are mild, laboratory evaluation is usually unnecessary. In contrast, if the patient manifests moderate or severe toxicity, routine laboratory evaluation should include a complete blood cell count, serum electrolytes, glucose, blood urea nitrogen, creatinine, creatine kinase (CK), cardiac marker determinations, arterial blood gas analysis, and urinalysis. Sympathetic excess may result in hyperglycemia and hypokalemia. Elevated CK is associated with rhabdomyolysis. Cardiac markers are elevated in myocardial infarction. However, false elevations of CK–MB fraction are common [12]. In the setting of an elevated absolute CK–MB, caution should be placed on the use of the CK–MB relative index, because it may be falsely low when there is concurrent myocardial infarction and rhabdomyolysis. Cardiac troponin I is the preferred method to distinguish true- from false-positive CK–MB determinations [12].

Chest radiography and electrocardiography (ECG) should be obtained in patients with chest pain or cardiovascular complaints. The initial ECG is a less useful diagnostic tool than for patients with chest pain that is unrelated to cocaine. Many young cocaine-using patients have ST-segment elevation in the absence of acute myocardial infarction. This is due to early repolarization changes [15,16].

Observation for a 9- to 12-hour period is also a useful tool for the evaluation of patients presenting with cocaine-associated chest pain. Patients without new ischemic changes on ECG, a normal troponin test, and no cardiovascular complications during this observation (dysrhythmias, acute myocardial infarction or recurrent symptoms) can safely be sent home with follow up and planned outpatient workup [17,37]. Recent data also suggests that a strategy using coronary computerized angiographic tomography might identify patients safe for discharge in a slightly more rapid time frame [38].

A brief seizure temporally related to cocaine use in an otherwise healthy person should be evaluated with a head computed tomography (CT). Further workup in an otherwise asymptomatic patient may not be necessary [19]. Patients with concurrent headache, suspected subarachnoid hemorrhage, or other neurologic manifestations may necessitate lumbar puncture after head CT to rule out serious pathology. Patients who are suspected of body stuffing should be evaluated by abdominal radiographs and cavity searches (digital or visual examination of the rectum or vagina).

MANAGEMENT

The initial management of cocaine-toxic patients should focus on airway, breathing, and circulation. Treatments are directed at a specific sign, symptom, or organ system affected and are summarized in Table 129.1.

Patients who present with sympathetic excess and psychomotor agitation are at risk for hyperthermia and rhabdomyolysis. Management should focus on lowering core body

TABLE 129.1

TREATMENT SUMMARY FOR COCAINE-RELATED MEDICAL CONDITIONS

Medical condition	Treatments
Cardiovascular	
Dysrhythmias	
Sinus tachycardia	Observation Oxygen Diazepam or lorazepam
Supraventricular tachycardia	Oxygen Diazepam or lorazepam Consider diltiazem, verapamil or adenosine If hemodynamically unstable: cardioversion
Ventricular dysrhythmias	Oxygen Diazepam or lorazepam Consider Sodium bicarbonate and/or lidocaine If hemodynamically unstable: defibrillation
Acute coronary syndrome	Oxygen Aspirin Diazepam or lorazepam Nitroglycerin Heparin For ST segment elevation (STEMI): Percutaneous intervention (angioplasty and stent placement) preferred. Consider fibrinolytic therapy. Consider morphine sulfate, phentolamine, verapamil or glycoprotein IIb/IIIa inhibitors
Hypertension	Observation Diazepam or lorazepam Consider nitroglycerin, phentolamine and nitroprusside
Pulmonary edema	Furosemide Nitroglycerin Consider morphine sulfate or phentolamine
Hyperthermia	Diazepam or lorazepam Cooling methods If agitated, consider paralysis and intubation
Neuropsychiatric	
Anxiety and agitation	Diazepam or lorazepam
Seizures	Diazepam or lorazepam Consider phenobarbital
Intracranial hemorrhage	Surgical consultation
Rhabdomyolysis	IV hydration Consider sodium bicarbonate or mannitol If in acute renal failure: hemodialysis
Cocaine washout syndrome	Supportive care
Body packers	Activated charcoal Whole-bowel irrigation Laparotomy or endoscopic retrieval

TABLE 129.2

SUMMARY OF RECOMMENDATIONS BASED ON RANDOMIZED CONTROLLED CLINICAL TRIALS

Reference	Population	Intervention	Control	Primary outcome	Design	Effect measure	Summary
Baumann et al., 2000	40 patients with potential cocaine-associated acute coronary syncrome	Diazepam plus placebo nitroglycerin ($N = 12$), nitroglycerin and placebo diazepam ($N = 13$), or diazepam and nitroglycerin arms were used ($N = 15$). Diazepam was administered 5 mg intravenously every 5 minutes for a total dose of 15 mg. Nitroglycerin, 0.4 mg, was administered sublingually every 5 minutes for up to a total of 3 doses.	No patients received placebo diazepam and placebo nitroglycerin	Chest pain resolution, and changes in blood pressure, pulse rate, cardiac output, cardiac index, stroke volume, and stroke index over the 15-minute treatment period.	Prospective, randomized, double-blind trial	Chest pain severity improved similarly in the three groups and there were no differences in response of cardiac measures to the therapies administered.	No difference in treatment between diazepam only, nitroglycerin only or combined therapy.
Honderick et al., 2003	27 patients with cocaine-associated chest pain	Nitroglycerin (group I, $N = 15$) of nitroglycerin plus lorazepam (group II, $N = 12$) was utilized. The nitroglycerin was administered sublingually and the lorazepam was administered intravenously, 1 mg every 5 minutes for a total of two doses.	No patients received placebo	Chest pain score (0–10 scale) measured at 5 minutes after each medication administration.	Prospective, randomized, single-blind trial	5 minutes after initial treatment, there was no difference in the mean chest pain scores. 5 minutes after the second treatment, the mean scores were 4.6 and 1.5, respectively that was statistically significant.	Lorazepam with nitroglycerin appears to be more efficacious than nitroglycerin alone in the treatment of cocaine-associated chest pain

temperature, halting further muscle damage and heat production, and ensuring good urinary output. The primary agents used for muscle relaxation are benzodiazepines [11].

The use of antipsychotic agents for cocaine-induced neurobehavioral agitation is controversial [39]. In mild cases, antipsychotics may be useful. In cases of severe cocaine-induced agitation, few data exist on antipsychotics' safety and efficacy. In these cases, benzodiazepines are preferred and supranormal cumulative doses may be necessary. Core body temperatures may be highly elevated. This should be treated aggressively with iced water baths or cool water mist with fans. Some cases of severe muscle overactivity may require general anesthesia with nondepolarizing neuromuscular blockade. Succinylcholine, a depolarizing neuromuscular-blocking agent, may increase the risk of hyperkalemia in the setting of severe cocaine-induced rhabdomyolysis. In addition, plasma cholinesterase is responsible for the metabolism of both succinylcholine and cocaine. When these two agents are used simultaneously, prolonged clinical effects of either or both agents might result. Therefore, nondepolarizing agents are preferred.

Patients with severe hypertension can usually be safely treated with benzodiazepines. When benzodiazepines are not effective, nitroglycerin, nitroprusside, or phentolamine can be used. Beta-blockers are contraindicated. Their use in this setting can lead to unopposed alpha stimulation with paradoxic exacerbation of hypertension and worsening coronary vasoconstriction [40,41].

Patients with chest pain and suspected cocaine-induced ischemia or myocardial infarction should be treated with aspirin, benzodiazepines, and nitroglycerin as first-line agents. Benzodiazepines decrease the central stimulatory effects of cocaine, thereby indirectly reducing its cardiovascular toxicity [11]. Benzodiazepines have been shown to have a comparable and possibly an additive effect to nitroglycerin with respect to chest pain resolution and hemodynamic and cardiac functional parameters (cardiac output) for patients with cocaine-associated chest pain [42,43] (Table 129.2). Weight-adjusted unfractionated heparin or enoxaparin would be reasonable to use in patients with documented ischemia. Patients who do not respond to these initial therapies can be treated with phentolamine or calcium channel blocking agents [44,45]. The International Guidelines for Emergency Cardiovascular Care recommend α-adrenergic antagonists (phentolamine) for the treatment of cocaine-associated acute coronary syndrome [46]. Beta-blockers are contraindicated, as they can exacerbate cocaine-induced coronary artery vasoconstriction [40].

Primary reperfusion therapy is best done with percutaneous interventions, when available [47]. Fibrinolytic therapy in this setting is somewhat controversial. The mortality from cocaine-associated myocardial infarction is low. Patients with cocaine-associated chest pain have a high prevalence of "false-positive ST-segment elevations," up to 43% in one study [48]. Therefore, treatment of all patients with cocaine-associated chest pain who meet standard ECG thrombolysis in myocardial infarction criteria would result in fibrinolytic administration to more patients without acute myocardial infarction than with acute myocardial infarction.

Supraventricular dysrhythmias may be difficult to treat. Initially, benzodiazepines should be administered. Adenosine can be given, but its effects may be temporary. Use of calcium channel blockers in association with benzodiazepines appears to be most beneficial. Beta-blockers should be avoided [46].

Ventricular dysrhythmias should be managed with benzodiazepines, lidocaine, or sodium bicarbonate [46]. Bicarbonate is preferred in patients with QRS widening and ventricular dysrhythmias that occur soon after cocaine use. In this setting, the dysrhythmias are presumably related to sodium channel blocking effects of cocaine. Lidocaine can be used when dysrhythmias appear to be related to cocaine-induced ischemia [9,46].

Seizures should be treated with benzodiazepines and phenobarbital. Phenytoin is not recommended in cases associated with cocaine. Although no studies have compared barbiturates to phenytoin for control of cocaine-induced seizures, barbiturates are theoretically preferable because they also produce CNS sedation and are generally more effective for toxin-induced convulsions. If these agents are not rapidly effective, nondepolarizing neuromuscular blockade and general anesthesia are indicated.

Patients with cerebrovascular complications or focal neurologic findings should be managed as usual. However, the utility of fibrinolytic agents in cocaine-associated cerebrovascular infarction is unknown.

Cocaine body stuffers who are asymptomatic should be given activated charcoal [49]. Whole-bowel irrigation with subsequent radiologic verification of passage of all drug-filled containers should be considered [28]. Body stuffers who manifest clinical signs of toxicity should be treated similarly to other cocaine-intoxicated patients. Body packers who develop any signs of cocaine toxicity, need to be identified as quickly as possible and treated very aggressively. These individuals have a high likelihood of developing worsening toxicity and life-threatening symptomatology. Initial use of activated charcoal and surgical removal of ruptured cocaine packets is warranted in almost all cases and can be life saving [29].

References

1. National Survey on Drug Use and Health, 2007. Available at http://www.samhsa.gov.
2. SAMHSA: Drug Abuse Warning Network, 2004: National Estimates of Drug-Related Emergency Department Visits. Available at http://www.samhsa.gov or at http://www.health.org.
3. Kolbrich EA, Barnes AJ, Gorelick DA, et al: Major and minor metabolites of cocaine in human plasma following controlled subcutaneous cocaine administration. *J Anal Toxicol* 30:501, 2006.
4. Patel MB, Opreanu M, Shah AJ, et al: Cocaine and alcohol: a potential lethal duo. *Am J Med* 122:e5, 2009.
5. Hollander JE: Management of cocaine associated myocardial ischemia. *N Engl J Med* 333:1267, 1995.
6. Lange RA, Hillis RD: Cardiovascular complications of cocaine use. *N Engl J Med* 345:351, 2001.
7. Pozner CN, Levine M, Zane R: The cardiovascular effects of cocaine. *J Emerg Med* 29:173, 2005.
8. Lange RA, Cigarroa RG, Yancy CW, et al: Cocaine-induced coronary-artery vasoconstriction. *N Engl J Med* 321:1557, 1989.
9. Shih RD, Hollander JE, Hoffman RS, et al: Clinical safety of lidocaine in cocaine associated myocardial infarction. *Ann Emerg Med* 26:702, 1995.
10. Singhal PC, Rubin RB, Peters A, et al: Rhabdomyolysis and acute renal failure associated with cocaine abuse. *J Toxicol Clin Toxicol* 28:321, 1990.
11. Hollander JE: Cocaine Intoxication and Hypertension. *Ann Emerg Med* 51:S18, 2008.
12. McCord J, Jneid H, Hollander JE, et al: Management of cocaine-associated chest pain and myocardial infarction: a scientific statement from the American Heart Association Acute Cardiac Care Committee of the Council on Clinical Cardiology. *Circulation* 117:1897, 2008.
13. Weber JE, Chudnofsky C, Wilkerson MD, et al: Cocaine associated chest pain: how common is myocardial infarction? *Acad Emerg Med* 7:873, 2000.
14. Qureshi AI, Suri FK, Guterman LR, et al: Cocaine use and the likelihood of nonfatal myocardial infarction and stroke. Data from the third National Health and Nutrition Examination Survey. *Circulation* 103:502, 2001.
15. Hollander JE, Lozano M Jr, Fairweather P, et al: "Abnormal" electrocardiograms in patients with cocaine-associated chest pain are due to "normal" variants. *J Emerg Med* 12:199, 1994.
16. Hamad A, Khan M: ST-segment elevation in patients with cocaine abuse and chest pain: is there a pattern? *Am J Cardiol* 86:1054, 2000.
17. Weber JE, Shofer FS, Larkin GL, et al: Validation of a brief observation period for patients with cocaine-associated chest pain. *N Engl J Med* 348:510, 2003.

18. Hsue PY, Salinas CL, Bolger AF, et al: Acute aortic dissection related to crack cocaine. *Circulation* 105:1592–1595, 2002.
19. Shih RD, Majlesi N, Hung O, et al: Cocaine-associated seizures and incidence of status epilepticus. *Ann Emerg Med* 50:S27, 2007.
20. Bolla KI, Funderburk FR, Cadet JL: Differential effects of cocaine and cocaine alcohol on neurocognitive performance. *Neurology* 54:2285, 2000.
21. Kaye BR, Fainstat M: Cerebral vasculitis associated with cocaine abuse. *JAMA* 258:2104, 1987.
22. Petitti DB, Sidney S, Quesenberry C, et al: Stroke and cocaine or amphetamine use. *Epidemiology* 9:956, 1998.
23. Wilson KC, Saukkonen JJ: Acute respiratory failure from abused substances. *J Intensive Care Med* 19:183, 2004.
24. Restrepo CS, Carrillo JA, Martínez S, et al: Pulmonary complications from cocaine and cocaine-based substances: imaging manifestations. *Radiographics* 27:941, 2007.
25. Wolff AJ, O'Donnell AE: Pulmonary effects of illicit drug use. *Clin Chest Med* 25:203, 2004.
26. Rome LA, Lippman ML, Dalsey WC, et al: Prevalence of cocaine use and its impact on asthma exacerbation in an urban population. *Chest* 117:1324, 2000.
27. Linder JD, Monkemuller KE, Raijman I, et al: Cocaine-associated ischemic colitis. *South Med J* 93:909, 2000.
28. Gill JR, Graham SM: Ten years of "body packers" in New York City: 50 deaths. *J Foren Sci* 47:843, 2002.
29. Sporer KA, Lesser M: Cocaine washed out syndrome. *Ann Emerg Med* 21:112, 1992.
30. Kleerup EC, Koyal SN, Marques-Magallanes JA, et al: Chronic and acute effects of "crack" cocaine on diffusing capacity, membrane diffusion, and pulmonary capillary blood volume in the lung. *Chest* 122:629, 2002.
31. Dombrowski MP, Wolfe HM, Welch RA, et al: Cocaine abuse is associated with abruptio placentae and decreased birth weight, but not shorter labor. *Obstet Gynecol* 77:139, 1991.
32. Bada HS, Das A, Bauer CR, et al: Low birth weight and preterm births: Etiologic fraction attributable to prenatal drug exposure. *J Perinatol* 25, 631, 2005.
33. Eyler FD, Behnke M, Conlon M, et al: Birth outcome from a prospective, matched study of prenatal crack/cocaine use: I. Interactive and dose effects on health and growth. *Pediatrics* 101:229, 1998.
34. Chavez GF, Mulinare J, Cordero JF: Maternal cocaine use during early pregnancy as a risk factor for congenital urogenital anomalies. *JAMA* 262:795, 1989.
35. Perrone J, De Roos F, Jayaraman S, et al: Drug screening versus history in detection of substance use in ED psychiatric patients. *Am J Emerg Med* 19:49, 2001.
36. Steele MT, Westdorp EJ, Garza AG, et al: Screening for stimulant use in adult emergency department seizure patients. *J Toxicol Clin Toxicol* 38:609, 2000.
37. Cunningham R, Walton MA, Weber JE, et al: One-Year medical outcomes and emergency department recidivism after emergency department observation for cocaine-associated chest pain. *Ann Emerg Med* 53:310, 2009.
38. Walsh KM, Chang AM, Perrone J, et al: Coronary computerized tomography angiography for rapid discharge of low risk patients with cocaine associated chest pain. *J Med Toxicol* 5:111, 2009.
39. Cleveland NJ, Dewitt CD, Heard K: Ziprasidone pretreatment attenuates the lethal effects of cocaine in a mouse model. *Acad Emerg Med* 12:385, 2005.
40. Lange RA, Cigarroa RG, Flores ED, et al: Potentiation of cocaine-induced coronary vasoconstriction by beta-adrenergic blockade. *Ann Intern Med* 112:897, 1990.
41. Sand IC, Brody SL, Wrenn KD, et al: Experience with esmolol for the treatment of cocaine associated cardiovascular complications. *Am J Emerg Med* 9:161, 1991.
42. Baumann BM, Perrone J, Hornig SE, et al: Randomized controlled double blind placebo controlled trial of diazepam, nitroglycerin or both for treatment of patients with potential cocaine associated acute coronary syndromes. *Acad Emerg Med* 7:878, 2000.
43. Honderick T, Williams D, Seaberg D, et al: A prospective, randomized, controlled trial of benzodiazepines and nitroglycerine or nitroglycerine alone in the treatment of cocaine-associated acute coronary syndromes. *Am J Emerg Med* 21:39, 2003.
44. Chan GM, Sharma R, Price D, et al: Phentolamine therapy for cocaine-association acute coronary syndrome (CAACS). *J Med Toxicol* 2:108, 2006.
45. Negus BH, Willard JE, Hillis LD, et al: Alleviation of cocaine induced coronary vasoconstriction with intravenous verapamil. *Am J Cardiol* 73:510, 1994.
46. Albertson TE, Dawson A, de Latorre F, et al: TOX-ACLS: toxicologic-oriented advanced cardiac life support. *Ann Emerg Med* 37:S78, 2001.
47. Hollander JE, Burstein JL, Shih RD, et al: Cocaine Associated Myocardial Infarction Study (CAMI) Group. Cocaine associated myocardial infarction: clinical safety of thrombolytic therapy. *Chest* 107:1237, 1995.
48. Gitter MJ, Goldsmith SR, Dunbar DN, et al: Cocaine and chest pain: clinical features and outcome of patients hospitalized to rule out myocardial infarction. *Ann Intern Med* 115:277, 1991.
49. Tomaszewski C, McKinney P, Phillips S, et al: Prevention of toxicity from oral cocaine by activated charcoal in mice. *Ann Emerg Med* 22:1804, 1993.

CHAPTER 130 ■ CORROSIVE POISONING

ROBERT P. DOWSETT AND CHRISTOPHER H. LINDEN

Initially referring to acids, the term *corrosives* is now used synonymously with *caustics*, a term originally applied to alkalis. In solution, acids and bases donate or accept a proton altering the hydrogen ion concentration. This is measured as pH, the negative logarithm of the H^+ ion concentration (M/L) Water, at 25°C, has a pH of 7 and is considered neutral. Solutions with a pH of less than 2 or greater than 12 are considered strongly acidic or basic. The pH levels of some common solutions are listed in Table 130.1.

Corrosives cause injury by reacting with organic molecules and disrupting cell membranes. They also cause thermal burns if heat is generated by dissolution and neutralization reactions. Reactions between strong acids and strong bases are usually highly exothermic. Metallic lithium, sodium, potassium, some aluminum and lithium salts, and titanium tetrachloride react violently when placed in water, producing large amounts of heat. Chlorine reacts with water in an exothermic reaction to form hydrochloric and hypochlorous acids, elemental chlorine, and free oxygen radicals. Similar reactions occur with bromine. Ammonia combines with water to form ammonium hydroxide in a reaction that liberates heat; the hydroxide formed is then responsible for corrosive effects. Nitrogen dioxide reacts with water to release heat and produce nitric and nitrous acid. Hydrogen peroxide liberates oxygen on contact with water.

The mixing of chemicals can result in reactions that liberate caustic gases. Mixing ammonia with hypochlorite (household bleach) generates chloramine gases (NH_2Cl and $NHCl_2$), which are highly irritating to mucosal epithelia. Combining bleach with acid (acid toilet bowl or drain cleaners) produces chlorine gas. A number of metallic compounds react with acids, resulting in the liberation of potentially explosive hydrogen gas. Hydrogen sulfide and sulfur oxide gas result from the action of acids on sulfur-containing compounds such as orthopedic plaster casting material in sink drains [1]. Zinc hydroxide, present in soldering flux, is corrosive in an acidic environment such as the stomach [2].

TABLE 130.1

APPROXIMATE pH OF COMMON SOLUTIONS

Solution	pH
1.0 M hydrochloric acid	0
1 M hydrochloric acid solution	0
1 M nitric acid solution	0
0.1 M sulfuric acid	0.96
Battery acid (1% solution)	1.4
Gastric juice	1.2–3.0
Lemon juice	2
Domestic toilet cleaner (1%)	2.0
1 M acetic acid solution	2.37
1 M carbonic acid	5.7
Rain water	6.5
Water (pure, at 25°C)	7.0
Bleach (1% solution)	9.5–10.2
Automatic dishwasher detergents	10.4–13.0
Laundry detergents	11.6–12.6
Domestic ammonium cleaners	11.9–12.4
Ammonia 10%	12.5
Oven cleaner	13
Drain cleaner	13.3–14.0
1.0 M potassium hydroxide	14
1.0 M NaOH	14
Saturated ammonia solution	15

During 2007, 147,703 exposures to corrosive chemicals were reported by U.S. poison centers; actual exposures are estimated to be several times greater [3]. Lethal exposures constituted 1.9% of all reported deaths due to poisoning [3]. Exposures to chemicals accounted for 7.6% of poisonings in children younger than 6 years of age. Only a few of these cases resulted in serious injury, with only three deaths. Adults, usually by deliberate intent, ingest a larger amount of corrosive [4]. Deaths most commonly result from intentional exposure to drain cleaners and acidic cleaners [3].

Concentrated lye (sodium or potassium hydroxide) solutions used for laundering and plumbing purposes caused most of the serious injuries due to corrosive ingestions before 1970 [5]. Currently available liquid lye drain cleaners are less concentrated (less than 10%) but are still responsible for the largest number of severe gastrointestinal injuries; however, acid bowl cleaners now account for almost as many deaths [3]. Severe alkali injuries can result from the ingestion of powdered automatic dishwasher detergents and oven cleaners [6,7]. Household ammonia and bleaches, and hydrogen peroxide solutions are in general much less potent than industrial ones but can cause significant injury if ingested in large amounts [4,6].

PATHOPHYSIOLOGY

Alkalis cause liquefaction necrosis, a process resulting from the saponification of fats, dissolution of proteins, and emulsification of lipid membranes. The resultant tissue softening and sloughing may allow the alkali to penetrate to deeper levels. Tissue injury progresses rapidly over the first few minutes but can continue for several hours [8]. Over the ensuing 4 days, bacterial infection and inflammation cause additional injury. Granulation tissue then develops, but collagen deposition may not begin until the second week. The tensile strength of healing tissue is lowest during the first 2 weeks. Epithelial repair may take weeks to months. Scar retraction begins in the third week and continues for months.

Acid burns are characterized by coagulation necrosis. Protein is denatured, resulting in the formation of a firm eschar [9]. The release of heat is typically higher than for alkali reactions [10]. Subsequent responses are similar to those seen with alkalis.

Hydrocarbons can produce injury by dissolving lipids in cell membranes and coagulating proteins. Significant damage may occur with ingestion or after prolonged dermal contact [11]. Ingestion of a toluene containing glue can cause caused corrosive esophagitis [12]

Alkaline solutions with a pH of greater than 12.5 are likely to cause mucosal ulceration, with deeper tissue necrosis resulting if the pH approaches 14 [13]. However, solutions with a pH of less than 12.5 can still cause significant injury, and solutions of different chemicals but the same pH produce different degrees of tissue damage [13].

The physical state of a chemical also influences its toxicity. Corrosives that are gases at room temperature primarily affect the skin, eyes, and airways. Saturated acid solutions may liberate significant amounts of acid fumes, particularly if heated. Solid compounds tend to produce highly concentrated solutions on contact with body fluids and cause more severe injuries [14]. Solutions with a high viscosity tend to cause deeper burns [13].

Most systemic effects that occur after exposure to corrosives are secondary to inflammation, acidosis, infection, and necrosis [15]. Fluid and electrolyte shifts occur, resulting in hypovolemia, acidosis, and organ failure. Some chemicals, such as phenol, hydrazine, and chromic acid, can be absorbed after dermal exposure or ingestion and cause systemic toxicity [16,17].

CLINICAL MANIFESTATIONS

Chemical burns to the eye range from irritation to severe and permanent damage [18]. Eye pain, blepharospasm, conjunctival hemorrhages, and chemosis are seen in all grades of injury. Decreased visual acuity may result from excessive tearing, corneal edema and ulceration, anterior chamber clouding, or lens opacities. Roper-Hall's classification of injury predicts severity of subsequent vision loss [19] (Table 130.2).

TABLE 130.2

GRADING OF SEVERITY OF OCULAR CHEMICAL BURNS

Grade	Cornea	Limbal ischemia	Prognosis
I	Epithelial loss	None	Good
II	Stromal haze, iris details visible	$<1/3$ of vessels affected	Good
III	Total epithelial loss, iris details obscured	$1/3$–$1/2$ of vessels affected	Doubtful, vision reduced
IV	Opaque, no view of iris or pupil	$>1/2$ of vessels affected	Poor

Severe burns can result in increased intraocular pressure, anterior chamber clouding, lens opacities, and perforation of the globe [18]. Severity can be assessed by the extent of ischemia of conjunctival vessels at the limbus of the eye. If more than half of these vessels are obliterated, the prognosis is poor [19].

Significant differences exist between thermal and chemical burns of the skin. Although pain usually occurs immediately, it may be delayed several hours after corrosive exposure [20]. Assessing the depth of dermal injury can be difficult. Chemical burns rarely blister, and the affected skin is usually dark, insensate, and firmly attached regardless of the burn depth [21]. Healing usually takes longer than for thermal burns.

Some chemical warfare agents cause severe dermal injury. Sulfur mustard, the most common antipersonnel agent used, and lewisite (chlorovinylarsine dichloride) are potent alkylating agents, resulting in severe vesiculation of the skin 4 to 12 hours after exposure. Phosgene oxide has a similar action, but its effects are almost immediate. Respiratory burns are nearly always associated with sulfur mustard exposure [22]. White phosphorus is used in incendiary devices and in the manufacture of fertilizers and insecticides. It ignites spontaneously when exposed to air.

Ingested corrosives typically injure the oropharynx, esophagus, and stomach but may cause damage as distal as the proximal jejunum [23,24]. Areas most commonly affected are those of anatomic narrowing: the cricopharyngeal area, diaphragmatic esophagus, and antrum and pylorus of the stomach [23]. Multiple sites are affected in up to 80% of patients [24]. Esophageal lesions are seen predominantly in the lower half, and gastric burns are usually most severe in the antrum [24]. In the presence of food, gastric injuries tend to be less severe and involve the lesser curve and pylorus [10]. Vomiting is associated with a higher incidence of severe esophageal injuries [25].

Ingestion of alkali is associated with a higher incidence and severity of esophageal lesions than ingestion of acid, which typically causes stomach injury although this is not a consistent finding [4,25]. Alkaline agents have little taste, but acids are extremely bitter and more likely to be expelled if accidentally ingested.

Alkaline solids may adhere to mucosa of the oropharynx and cause oral pain that limits the quantity swallowed, thus sparing the esophagus [26]. If alkaline solids are swallowed, severe upper esophageal burns are seen [27]. Shallow ulcers may result when tablets become lodged in the esophagus (pill esophagitis). Hemorrhage and stricture formation may occur after esophageal impaction of potassium chloride, iron, quinidine, etidronate, antibiotics, and anti-inflammatory agents [28].

Common symptoms from corrosive ingestion are oropharyngeal pain, dysphagia, abdominal pain, vomiting, and drooling [29]. Less commonly, stridor, hoarseness, hematemesis, and melena are seen. Patients who are asymptomatic are unlikely to have significant injuries, although this may be difficult to assess in children who may appear to have no or minimal symptoms [29]. Vomiting, drooling, and stridor appear to be predictive of more severe injuries [29].

The absence of burns in the oropharynx does not exclude burns further along the gastrointestinal tract, and it is not predictive of less severe distal injuries [29]. Patients with laryngeal burns have a greater incidence and severity of esophageal lesions [25].

Hemorrhage, perforation, and fistula formation may occur in patients with full-thickness esophageal necrosis [24]. Untreated, perforations rapidly progress to septic shock, organ failure, and death. Some gastric perforations may become walled to form an abscess around the liver or in the lesser sac.

Severe gastric burns may extend to adjacent organs [30]. Perforation of the anterior esophageal wall may lead to formation of a tracheoesophageal fistula and tracheobronchial necrosis [31,32]. Tracheoesophageal–aortic and aortoesophageal fistulas, rare and uniformly fatal complications, are suggested by hemoptysis or hematemesis, which develops into torrential bleeding [33,34].

Burns to the larynx occur in up to 50% of patients and are the most common cause of respiratory distress [25]. Typically, the epiglottis and aryepiglottic folds are edematous, ulcerated, or necrotic. The absence of respiratory symptoms on presentation does not exclude the presence of laryngeal burns that may eventually require intubation [25]. Respiratory distress may also be due to the aspiration of corrosives [35].

Esophageal strictures develop in up to 70% of burns that result in deep ulceration, whether discrete or circumferential, and nearly all burns resulting in deep necrosis [24]. Strictures do not develop after superficial mucosal ulceration [35]. Strictures may become symptomatic as early as the end of the second week; half develop during initial hospitalization, and 80% are evident within 2 months [36]. Those that develop early often progress rapidly and require urgent intervention. Gastric outlet strictures may also occur, but only 40% become symptomatic [24]. Strictures can develop in the mouth and pharynx [25].

Esophageal pseudodiverticulum may occur in patients with esophageal stricture as early as 1 week after corrosive ingestions. It appears to result from incomplete destruction of the esophageal wall and usually resolves with dilation of associated strictures [37].

Deaths that occur are in patients who have extensive necrosis in the upper gastrointestinal tract. Sepsis secondary to perforation is the most common cause of death; severe hemorrhage or aspiration may also contribute [24].

Esophageal carcinoma, usually squamous cell, is a well-documented complication of alkali burns [38]. It occurs most commonly at the level of the tracheal bifurcation and is estimated to occur 1,000 times more frequently in patients who have had corrosive injuries than in the general population. Symptoms can develop 22 to 81 years after the initial insult.

Systemic toxicity has occurred with burns caused by arsenic and other heavy metals, cyanide, acetic acid, formic acid, fluoride, hydrazine, hydrochloric acid, nitrates, sulfuric acid, and phosphoric acid [39–43]. Severe acid burns may be accompanied by a metabolic acidosis and hypotension. The anion gap is usually elevated, although a hyperchloremic acidosis may be seen in hydrochloric acid and ammonium chloride ingestion. After hydrochloric acid ingestion, cardiovascular collapse is the most common cause of early death; myocardial infarction has occurred after large ingestions. Other findings associated with severe acid injuries include hemolysis, hemoglobinuria, nephrotoxicity, and pulmonary edema [40,41,43].

Acute hemolysis, hyperkalemia, hypoxia, and cardiorespiratory arrest have occurred after the use of dialysis equipment and syringes sterilized with bleach [44]. Vascular oxygen embolization can occur after the ingestion of concentrated hydrogen peroxide [45]

DIAGNOSTIC EVALUATION

Resuscitation and decontamination should take priority over completing a detailed history and physical examination. Medical staff should wear protective clothing to avoid becoming secondary casualties. The duration of exposure, symptoms, and details of prehospital treatment should be noted. Identification of the compounds involved and any measures required for their safe handling can be established by a number of means: Container labeling, material safety data sheets and safety officers in cases of workplace exposure, fire department hazardous materials units, and regional poison information centers. Measuring the pH of a product may be helpful.

If the exposure is the result of an industrial or transportation accident, the patient should be evaluated for traumatic injuries. Suicidal patients should be evaluated for other possible toxic exposures (e.g., ingestion of alcohol or medications). Pulmonary exposures should be evaluated as outlined in Chapter 64.

After decontamination, assessment of eye exposures should include measurement of visual acuity and conjunctival pH and a slit-lamp examination. Chemosis, conjunctival hemorrhages, corneal epithelial defects, stromal opacification, and loss of limbic vessels should be noted. If injury to the anterior chamber is suspected, intraocular pressure should be measured.

Assessment of dermal injury is similar to that for thermal burns. Location, size, color, texture, and neurovascular status should be noted. If the affected area is greater than 15% of total body surface area or if systemic toxicity is possible, a complete physical examination with appropriate monitoring and laboratory testing should be performed.

With ingestions, the ability to swallow secretions and findings on examination of the oropharynx, neck, chest, and abdomen should be noted. Particular attention should be given to assessing the patency of the airway. Patients with signs and symptoms suggestive of significant injuries should have an electrocardiogram, arterial blood gas analysis, complete blood cell count, type and cross-match, coagulation profile, and biochemistry testing, including electrolytes, glucose, and liver and renal function. Radiologic studies should include a chest radiograph and an upright abdominal film. Upper gastrointestinal endoscopy should be performed in symptomatic patients or those with visible burns in the mouth or throat. Although the absence of symptoms or signs does not preclude the presence of gastrointestinal burns, in patients with accidental ingestions, such injuries are always of a minor nature and endoscopy is not necessary [23]. Minor symptoms or grade I visible burns following the accidental ingestion of substances shown to have low toxicity, such as sodium hypochlorite household bleach (less than 10% solution) and hair relaxer gel, do not necessarily require endoscopy, as significant injuries are rare in this setting [46–48]. However, endoscopy is still recommended if excessive drooling or dysphagia or significant mucosal burns occur after ingestion of these products or if there is doubt about the exact composition of the ingested substance [46,47]. In contrast, in those with ingestions of strong acids or bases, significant injuries may be present in the absence of clinical findings, and endoscopy is indicated. The optimal timing of endoscopy appears to be 6 to 24 hours after exposure. Because injuries may progress over several hours, endoscopy performed earlier may not detect the full extent of injury and therefore may need to be repeated [2]. If performed later, the risk of perforation is increased [24].

In the past, it was recommended that the endoscope not be passed beyond the first circumferential or full-thickness lesion because of the risk of iatrogenic perforation [48]. This complication was a significant problem in the days when rigid endoscopes were used. It is extremely rare with flexible endoscopy. Not examining beyond the first significant lesion results in failure to detect more distal lesions of the stomach or duodenum [49]. Flexible endoscopy, preferably using a small-diameter (e.g., pediatric) endoscope, of the entire upper gastrointestinal tract is safe and usually well tolerated [24]. The endoscope should be advanced across the cricopharynx under direct vision to assess for the presence of laryngeal burns [24]. If laryngeal edema or ulceration is noted, the airway should be intubated before endoscopy is continued. Examination should be done gently with minimal air insufflation, avoiding retroversion or retroflexion, and the procedure terminated if the endoscope cannot be easily passed through a narrowed area. Therapeutic dilation of the esophagus on initial endoscopy carries a high risk of perforation and should be avoided [23]. It should also be avoided during the subacute phase (5 to 15 days after ingestion), when the tensile strength of tissues is lowest [24].

TABLE 130.3

EXAMPLES OF CLASSIFICATIONS FOR GRADING SEVERITY OF GASTROINTESTINAL CORROSIVE INJURY

Grade I	Mucosal inflammation
Grade II	A. Hemorrhages, erosions, and superficial ulceration
	B. Deep discrete or circumferential ulceration
Grade III	A. Small, scattered areas of necrosis
	B. Extensive necrosis involving the whole esophagus
First degree	Mucosal inflammation, edema, or superficial sloughing
Second degree	Damage extends to all layers of, but not through, the esophagus
Third degree	Ulceration through to periesophageal tissues

A number of different systems for grading gastrointestinal burns have been proposed [23,24]. Some parallel grading systems used for thermal skin burns; others differentiate several levels of ulceration and necrosis (Table 130.3). The important findings are depth of ulceration and presence of necrosis. Injuries that consist only of mucosal inflammation or superficial ulceration and do not involve the muscularis are not at risk for stricture formation [24]. Patients with full-thickness circumferential burns and extensive necrosis are at high risk for perforation and stricture formation. Deep ulceration, whether transmural or not, and discrete areas of necrosis can sometimes lead to stricture formation.

Contrast esophagography is less sensitive than endoscopy in visualizing ulceration but has a role in the detection of suspected perforation [50]. A water-soluble contrast agent should be used. Cineesophagography can detect esophageal motility disorders, the pattern of which may predict the likelihood of stricture formation. Strictures can be expected to develop in all patients with an atonic dilated or rigid esophagus and in some individuals with abnormal, uncoordinated contractions [51]. Endoscopic ultrasonography can accurately grade corrosive injuries and predict complications [52]. Esophageal motility studies may predict the risk of stricture formation in those patients with no peristaltic response; these motility abnormalities persist for at least 3 months [53].

Evaluation of patients with symptoms and signs of systemic toxicity should include routine monitoring and ancillary testing. The extent and type of testing depend on the nature and severity of clinical abnormalities and the chemical involved. Patients with significant exposure to some phenols (e.g., nitrophenol and pentachlorophenol) and to hydrazine should have methemoglobin level determination.

MANAGEMENT

Advanced life support measures should be instituted as appropriate. Decontamination is the next priority; procedures are specific to the route of exposure. Treatment of systemic poisoning is primarily supportive; in some cases, antidotal therapy may also be necessary.

Irrigation should be performed immediately for eye exposures. The procedure is described in Chapter 117. The persistence of eye pain despite irrigation for at least 15 minutes indicates significant injury or incomplete decontamination. Failure to irrigate the eye adequately or remove particles after chemical exposure is associated with chronic complications [54]. Up to one third of patients with lime burns still have particles present in the eye on presentation [54]. All cases in which injury is detected or symptoms persist require ophthalmologic evaluation. Management may consist of topical antibiotics, mydriatics, steroids, and eye patching. The role of neutralization of chemical burns is currently under investigation. Ascorbic acid had been used to treat alkali burns, but its effectiveness has not been well studied, and it cannot be recommended [18].

The initial treatment of dermal exposure is prompt irrigation with copious amounts of water for at least 15 minutes for acid exposures and 30 minutes for alkali exposures (see Chapter 119). Longer irrigation is recommended for alkalis because they have detergent properties [20]. Although tissue neutralization occurs within 10 minutes with acids and 1 hour with alkalis in experimental studies, delayed irrigation may be beneficial [55]. Clothes act as a reservoir, and failure to remove them may result in full-thickness burns developing from even mildly corrosive chemicals [20]. Neutralization has been used [56], but because data on its efficacy are lacking, such therapy cannot be recommended.

Water irrigation may sometimes be dangerous or ineffective. Metallic lithium, sodium, potassium and cesium, titanium tetrachloride, and organic salts of lithium and aluminum react violently with water; burns caused by these agents should be inspected closely and any particles removed and placed in an anhydrous solution (oil) before the area is irrigated. Alternatively, the area can be wiped with a dry cloth to remove particles and the skin then deluged with water to dissipate any heat. Phenol is not water soluble, and dilution with water may aid its penetration into tissues, increasing systemic absorption [16]. Soaking experimental phenol burns with isopropyl alcohol or polyethylene glycol in mineral oil is superior to rinsing with water [57]. Isopropyl alcohol and polyethylene glycol may be absorbed by burns, and their use should be followed by liberal washing with water. Ready-mixed concrete can be easily removed from skin by soaking or irrigating with 50% dextrose in water [58].

Application of a copper sulfate solution has been suggested to assist in identification and neutralization of white phosphorus particles on the skin, but systemic absorption of copper sulfate can result in massive hemolysis with acute renal failure and death [59]. The use of a Wood's lamp to detect fluorescent phosphorus particles is safer [16]. Such burns should be kept wet because phosphorus ignites in dry air. Because sulfur mustard is poorly water soluble, a mild detergent should be used for its removal. Military decontamination kits contain chloramine wipes, which inactivates sulfur mustard [60]. British antilewisite, or dimercaprol, is an effective chelator of lewisite and can be applied topically to the skin or eye [22].

Patients with second- or third-degree skin burns should be referred to a surgeon. Definitive management is the same as for thermal burns, although more aggressive use of early débridement and grafting has been suggested [21].

Despite the rapidity of tissue injury following ingestion, decontamination should be considered. Rinsing with water or saline is recommended for mouth exposures. Dilution by drinking up to 250 mL (120 mL for a child) water or milk is recommended for particulate ingestion, because the corrosive may adhere to the esophageal wall. Although this procedure exposes the stomach to the corrosive agent, it further dilutes the substance. As the efficacy of dilution is greatest if performed within 5 minutes of exposure and declines rapidly thereafter, it is reasonable to use any drinkable beverage, except carbonated ones, if water or milk is not immediately available. The role of dilution for liquid ingestion is less clear, but it is usually recommended. It may, however, promote emesis and may not be effective in limiting tissue damage unless undertaken within minutes of injury. Emesis is contraindicated because of the risk of aspiration and its association with an increased severity of esophageal and laryngeal burns [25].

The administration of weak acids or bases can neutralize, as well as dilute, ingested corrosives [61]. Although weak acids are more effective than milk or water in neutralizing the pH, neutralization, which is accompanied by the production of heat, could lead to thermal injury in addition to corrosive effects. The heat generated by in vitro neutralization is small (less than 3°C) for liquid alkali but may be greater for solid forms [61]. The benefit of such therapy is unknown and not recommended [62].

Using a nasogastric tube for gastric aspiration, dilution, or lavage is another subject of debate [9]. Esophageal perforation is a potential complication, but no cases of nasogastric tube perforation have been reported. Placement of a gastric tube with fluoroscopic or endoscopic guidance has been suggested, but the blind, gentle introduction of a small-bore tube in a cooperative patient, particularly for an ingested acid, also appears to be safe [23]. If inserted, the tube should be firmly taped in place to avoid motion. Gastric contents should be aspirated. Dilution or lavage with small aliquots (120 to 250 mL) of water can then be performed.

Activated charcoal does not adsorb inorganic acids or alkali. In addition, because it interferes with endoscopic evaluation, unless a corrosive that has significant systemic toxicity and is known to be bound by activated charcoal has been ingested, this agent should be avoided. Symptomatic patients should otherwise be given nothing by mouth before endoscopy.

Corticosteroids have been used to reduce the incidence and severity of esophageal strictures after alkali burns. Such therapy is based on studies showing a decrease stricture formation in animals pretreated with steroids [63]. Because strictures do not develop in patients with first-degree esophageal burns, steroids are not indicated in those with such findings [64]. Similarly, steroids do not appear to influence the development of esophageal strictures after extensive deep ulceration or necrosis [64], and hence they are not recommended in patients with these injuries. Studies on the efficacy of steroids in patients with injuries of moderate severity have yielded conflicting results (Table 130.4). Most have been retrospective and poorly controlled [65–67]. Three analyses of pooled data from retrospective and prospective studies concluded a lower incidence of stricture formation with steroids in one study, but no difference in the other two [68–70]. There have been three prospective controlled studies of steroid use [71–73]. Two studies came to different conclusions; one showing a benefit with steroids, the other not [71,72] A criticism of the negative study was the delay to commencing steroids [74]. In an unpublished prospective randomized controlled trial of 362 patients, steroids did not show a benefit (73).

If steroids are administered, the recommended dose is 1 to 2 mg per kg per day prednisolone or methylprednisolone for 3 weeks followed by gradual tapering [74]. One comparative study suggested improved burn healing and reduced the need for dilatations with dexamethasone (1 mg per kg per day) compared with prednisolone (2 mg per kg per day) [75]. To approximate experimental conditions showing a beneficial effect, the initial dose of steroids should be given on presentation. Active bleeding and perforation are contraindications to steroid use.

Prophylactic antibiotics have also been advocated for patients with significant gastrointestinal injuries. Their benefits have not been studied in humans, and opinions differ as to their value. Controlled animal experiments have shown a combination of steroids and antibiotics to give the best outcome with respect to stricture formation and mortality [76] and suggest that a broad-spectrum antibiotic (e.g., a second-generation

TABLE 130.4

RESULTS OF CONTROLLED TRIALS OF STEROIDS FOR ESOPHAGEAL STRICTURES FOLLOWING CORROSIVE ESOPHAGEAL BURNS

Intervention	Year	Study	No. of patients	Findings	Reference
Prednisolone 25 mg 6 hourly (children 1.5 mg/kg/d for 2 weeks then tapered	1970	Retrospective controlled trial	21	Esophageal stricture rate: 27% in study group; 0% in controls	[64]
Methylprednisolone 125 mg IM, two doses 6 hours apart, then 40 mg 6 hourly for 5 days followed by reducing Depo-Medrol until healed	1980	Prospective randomized controlled trial	20	Esophageal stricture rate: 22% in study group; 36% in controls	[72]
Prednisolone 2 mg/kg/d IV until oral intake: 2.5 mg/kg/d for 21 days	1990	Prospective randomized controlled trial	25	Esophageal stricture rate: 7% in study group; 0% in controls	[71]
Steroid (not specified) 2 mg/kg/d (max. 30 mg/d) for 3 weeks	2005	Prospective randomized controlled trial	223	Esophageal stricture rate: 12% in study group; 19% in controls (NS)	[73]

cephalosporin) should be administered, particularly in those treated with steroids.

If initiated, the decision to continue or cease steroid and antibiotic therapy should be based on endoscopic findings. Patients with no injury or mucosal inflammation or small areas of superficial ulceration are not at risk for strictures or perforation and require supportive therapy only. Symptomatic relief can be provided with antacids, sucralfate, histamine-2–blockers (H_2-blockers), or analgesics. Patients with persistent symptoms or inconclusive findings on endoscopy should be admitted for observation. If symptoms persist, endoscopy should be repeated. Patients can commence oral fluids when they are able to swallow their own secretions. They can be discharged when tolerating oral fluids.

Patients with deep discrete ulcerations, circumferential or extensive superficial ulcerations, or small isolated areas of necrosis are at risk for stricture formation and should be given nothing by mouth. Fluids, analgesics, and H_2-blockers should be administered parenterally. Intravenous steroids and antibiotics should also be considered in those with alkali burns. Patients with deep transmural ulceration or necrosis are at risk for perforation as well as stricture formation. Although the use of steroids in this group is potentially hazardous and not recommended, antibiotics should be given along with other supportive measures. Hyperalimentation, either parenteral or by jejunostomy feeding tube, may be required.

Surgical exploration is indicated if perforation or penetration into surrounding tissues is suspected by findings such as fever, progressive abdominal or chest pain, hypotension, or signs of peritonitis or proved by endoscopic or radiographic findings. Tracheoesophageal fistulas are usually fatal unless recognized early and repaired, although one case reported successful conservative treatment [32]. Laparotomy and early excision have been suggested for patients with extensive full-thickness necrosis, but an advantage of this approach over more conservative treatment is not clear [77]. The mortality for patients who have major emergency surgery is 9% to 66% [77,78].

Stricture formation is usually treated with endoscopic dilatation beginning 3 to 4 weeks after ingestion. An average of eight sessions is required, but recurrence is common in the first 12 months [79]. In a group of 195 patients with corrosive-induced esophageal strictures, the risk of perforation for each dilatation session was 1.3%, but, because of the requirement for multiple dilations, the risk per patient was 17% [79]. Perforations were most likely to occur during the first three dilations. Features of perforation include dyspnea, malaise, tachycardia, fever, and subcutaneous crepitations. The majority are detected during the procedure or by the presence of pneumomediastinum, or pneumothorax or hydrothorax on chest radiograph, but occasionally contrast esophagography or esophagoscopy is required for confirmation. The death rate from perforation is 16% to 23% [79]. Early or prophylactic bougienage is of unclear benefit and has been associated with an increased risk of perforation. One study has shown a decrease in the number of dilatations required following interlesional steroid injection [80].

Placement of specialized nasogastric tubes or stents has lowered the rate of stricture formation in uncontrolled clinical trials and is superior to steroids in animal experiments [81]. An additional benefit of combining the use of a stent with systemic steroids has been suggested [81]. Oral sucralfate and H_2-blockers have no proven benefit in increasing tissue healing or reducing complications [82].

Surgery may ultimately be required if there is complete or near-complete obliteration of the esophageal lumen for more than 3 cm, if dysphagia recurs within a few weeks after successful dilation, or if perforation occurs during dilation [74]. Occasionally, resection and end-to-end anastomosis are possible, but usually extensive reconstruction, with colonic interposition, is necessary. The overall mortality from colonic replacement surgery is 2.0% to 3.6% and commonly results from sepsis secondary to anastomosis leakage or colonic graft necrosis [83]. Gastrectomy or gastrojejunostomy may also be required if gastric outlet obstruction develops [84]. Early definitive surgery for gastric outlet obstruction appears to be more advantageous than staged surgery [85]. Endoscopic balloon dilation may be an acceptable alternative procedure [86]. Diode laser-assisted radial lysis using a rigid endoscope has also been used to treat strictures successfully [87].

Supportive management is the mainstay of treatment for systemic toxicity. Heavy metal, cyanide, and hydrogen sulfide poisoning may require antidotal therapy (see Chapter 133). Neurologic toxicity due to hydrazine may respond to intravenous pyridoxine, administered at an initial dose of 25 mg per kg repeated in several hours, if necessary [42] (see Chapter 137). Methemoglobinemia may require treatment with methylene blue (see Chapter 117). Hemodialysis may enhance the elimination of heavy metals and dichromate, particularly if renal failure develops [88].

References

1. Peters JW: Hydrogen sulfide poisoning in a hospital setting. *JAMA* 246:1588, 1981.
2. Wit J, Noack L, Gdanietz K, et al: Experimental studies on caustic burns of the stomach by aggressive chemicals. *Prog Pediatr Surg* 25:68, 1990.
3. Bronstein AC, Spyker DA, Cantilena LR, et al: AAPCC 2007 Annual Report of the American Association of Poison Control Centers' National Poison Data System: 25th Annual Report. *Clin Toxicol (Philadelphia)* 46:927, 2008.
4. Arevalo-Silva C, Eliashar R Wohlgelernter J, et al: Ingestion of Caustic Substances: a 15-Year Experience. *Laryngoscope* 116:1422, 2006.
5. Leape LL, Ashcraft AW, Scarpelli DG, et al: Hazard to health: liquid lye. *N Engl J Med* 284:578, 1971.
6. Dogan Y, Erkan T, Çokugras FC, et al: Caustic gastroesophageal lesions in childhood: an analysis of 473 cases. *Clin Pediatr (Philadelphia)* 45:435, 2006.
7. Bertinelli A, Hamill J, Mahadevan M, et al: Serious injuries from dishwasher powder ingestions in small children. *J Paediatr Child Health* 42:129, 2006.
8. Kirsh MM, Ritter F: Caustic ingestion and subsequent damage to the oropharyngeal and digestive passages. *Ann Thorac Surg* 21:74, 1976.
9. Ashcraft KW, Padula RT: The effect of dilute corrosives on the esophagus. *Pediatrics* 53:226, 1974.
10. Penner GE: Acid ingestion: toxicology and treatment. *Ann Emerg Med* 9:374, 1980.
11. Papini RP: Is all that's blistered burned? A case of kerosene contact burns. *Burns* 17:415, 1991.
12. Pace F, Greco S, Pallotta S, et al: An uncommon cause of corrosive esophageal injury. *World J Gastroenterol* 14:636 2008.
13. Vancura EM, Clinton JE, Ruiz E, et al: Toxicity of alkaline solutions. *Ann Emerg Med* 9:118, 1980.
14. Crain EF, Gershel JC, Mezey AP: Caustic ingestions: symptoms as predictors of esophageal injury. *Am J Dis Child* 138:863, 1984.
15. Okonek S, Bierbach H, Atzpodien W: Unexpected metabolic acidosis in severe lye poisoning. *Clin Toxicol* 18:225, 1981.
16. Mozingo DW, Smith AA, McManus WF, et al: Chemical burns. *J Trauma-Injury Infect Crit Care* 28:642, 1988.
17. McKinney PE, Brent J, Kulig K: Acute zinc chloride ingestion in a child: local and systemic effects. *Ann Emerg Med* 23:1383, 1994.
18. Beare JD: Eye injuries from assault with chemicals. *Br J Ophthalmol* 74:514, 1990.
19. Roper-Hall MJ: Thermal and chemical burns. *Trans Ophthalmol Soc U K* 85:631, 1965.
20. Wilson GR, Davidson PM: Full thickness burns from ready-mixed cement. *Burns Incl Therm Inj* 12:139, 1985.
21. Sawhney CP, Kaushish R: Acid and alkali burns: considerations in management. *Burns* 15:132, 1989.
22. Mellor SG, Rice P, Cooper GJ: Vesicant burns. *Br J Plast Surg* 44:434, 1991.
23. Sugawa C, Lucas CE: Caustic injury of the upper gastrointestinal tract in adults: a clinical and endoscopic study. *Surgery* 106:802, 1989.
24. Zargar SA, Kochhar R, Mehta S, et al: The role of fiberoptic endoscopy in the management of corrosive ingestion and modified endoscopic classification of burns. *Gastrointest Endosc* 37:165, 1991.
25. Vergauwen P, Moulin D, Buts JP, et al: Caustic burns of the upper digestive and respiratory tracts. *Eur J Pediatr* 150:700, 1991.
26. Madarikan BA, Lari J: Ingestion of dishwasher detergent by children. *Br J Clin Pract* 44:35, 1990.
27. Einhorn A, Horton L, Altieri M, et al: Serious respiratory consequences of detergent ingestions in children. *Pediatrics* 84:472, 1989.
28. Bott S, Prakash C, McCallum RW: Medication induced esophageal injury: survey of the literature. *Am J Gastroenterol* 82:758, 1987.
29. Gorman RL, Khin-Maung-Gyi MT, Klein-Schwartz W, et al: Initial symptoms as predictors of esophageal injury in alkaline corrosive ingestions. *Am J Emerg Med* 10:189, 1992.
30. Purucker EA, Sudfeld S, Matern S: Gastrobronchial fistula after caustic injury due to lye ingestion. *Endoscopy* 35:252, 2003.
31. Sarfati E, Jacob L, Servant JM, et al: Tracheobronchial necrosis after caustic ingestion. *J Thorac Cardiovasc Surg* 103:412, 1992.
32. Restrepo S, Mastrogiovanni L, Kaplan J, et al: Tracheoesophageal fistula caused by ingestion of a caustic substance. *Ear Nose Throat J* 82:349, 2003.
33. Rabinovitz M, Udekwu AO, Campbell WL, et al: Tracheoesophageal-aortic fistula complicating lye ingestion. *Am J Gastroenterol* 85:868, 1990.
34. Yegane RA, Bashtar R, Bashashati M: Aortoesophageal fistula due to caustic ingestion. *Eur J Vasc Endovasc Surg* 35:187, 2008.
35. Cheng HT, Cheng CL, Lin CH, et al: Caustic ingestion in adults: the role of endoscopic classification in predicting outcome. *BMC Gastroenterol* 8:31, 2008.
36. Kikendall JW: Caustic ingestion injuries. *Gastroenterol Clin North Am* 20:847, 1991.
37. Kochhar R, Mehta SK, Nagi B, et al: Corrosive acid-induced esophageal intramural pseudodiverticulosis: a study of 14 patients. *J Clin Gastroenterol* 13:371, 1991.
38. Kochhar R, Sethy PK, Kochhar S, et al: Corrosive induced carcinoma of esophagus: Report of three patients and review of literature. *J Gastroenterol Hepatol* 21:777, 2006.
39. Caravati EM: Metabolic abnormalities associated with phosphoric acid ingestion. *Ann Emerg Med* 16:904, 1987.
40. Greif F, Kaplan O: Acid ingestion: another cause of disseminated intravascular coagulation. *Crit Care Med* 14:990, 1986.
41. Jefferys DB, Wiseman HM: Formic acid poisoning. *Postgrad Med* 56:761, 1980.
42. Harati Y, Naikan E: Hydrazine toxicity, pyridoxine therapy, and peripheral neuropathy. *Ann Intern Med* 104:728, 1986.
43. Wang XW, Davies JWL, Sirvent RLZ, et al: Chromic acid burns and acute chromium poisonings. *Burns Incl Therm Inj* 11:181, 1985.
44. Hoy RH: Accidental systemic exposure to sodium hypochlorite during hemodialysis. *Am J Hosp Pharm* 38:1512, 1981.
45. Pritchett S, Green D, Rossos P: Accidental ingestion of 35% hydrogen peroxide. *Can J Gastroenterol* 21:665, 2007
46. Harley EH, Collins MD: Liquid household bleach ingestion in children: a retrospective review. *Laryngoscope* 107:122, 1997.
47. Rauch DA: Hair relaxer misuse: don't relax. *Pediatrics* 105:1154, 2000.
48. Graeber GM, Murray GF: Injuries of the esophagus. *Semin Thorac Cardiovasc Surg* 4:247, 1992.
49. Previtera C: Caustic ingestions [letter]. *Pediatr Emerg Care* 7:126, 1991.
50. Muhletaler CA, Gerlock AJ, de Soto L, et al: Acid corrosive esophagitis: radiographic findings. *Am J Roentgenol* 134:1137, 1980.
51. Kuhn JR, Tunell WP: The role of initial cine-esophagography in caustic esophageal injury. *Am J Surg* 146:804, 1983.
52. Chiu HM, Lin JT, Huang SP, et al: Prediction of bleeding and stricture formation after corrosive ingestion by EUS concurrent with upper endoscopy. *Gastrointest Endosc* 60:827, 2004.
53. Genc A, Mutaf O: Esophageal motility changes in acute and late periods of caustic esophageal burns and their relation to prognosis in children. *J Pediatr Surg Surg* 37:1526, 2002.
54. Rozenbaum D, Baruchin AM, Dafna Z: Chemical burns of the eye with special reference to alkali burns. *Burns* 17:136, 1991.
55. Yano K, Hata Y, Matsuka K, et al: Experimental study on alkaline skin injuries: periodic changes in subcutaneous tissue pH and the effects exerted by washing. *Burns* 19:320, 1993.
56. Woodard D: Irrigation with acetic acid [letter]. *Ann Emerg Med* 18:911, 1989.
57. Hunter DM, Timerding BL, Leonard RB, et al: Effects of isopropyl alcohol, ethanol, and polyethylene glycol/industrial methylated spirits in the treatment of acute phenol burns. *Ann Emerg Med* 21:1303, 1992.
58. Cuomo MD, Sobel RM: Concrete impaction of the external auditory canal. *Am J Emerg Med* 7:32, 1989.
59. Eldad A, Simon GA: The phosphorous burn: a preliminary comparative experimental study of various forms of treatment. *Burns* 17:198, 1991.
60. Borak J, Sidell FR: Agents of chemical warfare: sulfur mustard. *Ann Emerg Med* 21:303, 1992.
61. Homan CS, Singer AJ, Thomajan C, et al: Thermal characteristics of neutralization therapy and water dilution for strong acid ingestion: an in-vivo canine model. *Acad Emerg Med* 5:286, 1998.
62. Smilkstein MJ: Should we add acid to an alkali injury? For now, let's remain neutral. *Acad Emerg Med* 2:945, 1995.
63. McNeil RA, Wellborn RB: Prevention of corrosive stricture of the esophagus of the rat. *J Laryngol* 80:346, 1966.
64. Webb WR, Koutras P, Eckker RR, et al: An evaluation of steroids and antibiotics in caustic burns of the esophagus. *Ann Thorac Surg* 9:95, 1970.
65. Ferguson MK, Migliore M, Staszak VM, et al: Early evaluation and therapy for caustic esophageal injury. *Am J Surg* 157:116, 1989.
66. Gundogdu HZ, Tanyel FC, Buyukpamukcu N, et al: Conservative treatment of caustic esophageal strictures in children. *J Pediatr Surg* 27:767, 1992.
67. Ulman I, Mutaf O: A critique of systemic steroids in the management of caustic esophageal burns in children. *Eur J Pediatr Surg* 8:71, 1998.
68. Howell JM, Dalsey WC, Hartsell FW, et al: Steroids for the treatment of corrosive esophageal injury: a statistical analysis of past studies. *Am J Emerg Med* 10:421, 1992.
69. Oakes DD, Sherck JP, Mark JB: Lye ingestion: clinical patterns and therapeutic implications. *J Thorac Cardiovasc Surg* 83:194, 1982.
70. Fulton JA, Hoffman RS: Steroids in second degree caustic burns of the esophagus: a systematic pooled analysis of fifty years of human data: 1956–2006. *Clin Toxicol* 45:402, 2007.
71. Anderson KD, Rouse TM, Randolph JG: A controlled trial of corticosteroids in children with corrosive injury of the esophagus. *N Engl J Med* 323:637, 1990.
72. Hawkins DB, Demeter MJ, Barness TE: Caustic ingestions: controversies in management: a review of 214 cases. *Laryngoscope* 90:98, 1980.
73. Dogan Y, Gulcan M, Urganci N, et al: The effect of steroid therapy on severe corrosive oesophageal burns in children; a multicentric prospective study [abstract]. *J Pediatr Gastroenterol Nutr* 40:656, 2005.
74. Wason S, Stephan M: Corticosteroids in children with corrosive injury of the esophagus [letter]. *N Engl J Med* 324:418, 1991.
75. Bautista A, Varela R, Villanueva A, et al: Effects of prednisolone and dexamethasone in children with alkali burns of the oesophagus. *Eur J Pediatr Surg* 6:198, 1996.

76. Haller JR, Bachman K: The comparative effect of current therapy on caustic burns of the esophagus. *Pediatrics* 34:236, 1964.
77. Berthet B, Castellani P, Brioche MI, et al: Early operation for severe corrosive injury of the upper gastrointestinal tract. *Eur J Surg* 162:951, 1996.
78. Wu MH, Lai WW: Surgical management of extensive corrosive injuries of the alimentary tract. *Surg Gynecol Obstet* 177:12, 1993.
79. Karnak I, Tanyel FC, Buyukpamukcu N, et al: Esophageal perforations encountered during the dilation of caustic esophageal strictures. *J Cardiovasc Surg* 39:373, 1998.
80. Kochhar R, Makharia GK: Usefulness of intralesional triamcinolone in treatment of benign esophageal strictures. *Gastrointest Endosc* 56:829, 2002.
81. De Peppo F, Zaccara A, Dall'Oglio L, et al: Stenting for caustic strictures: esophageal replacement replaced. *J Pediatr Surg* 33:54, 1998.
82. Reddy AN, Budraja M: Sucralfate therapy for lye-induced esophagitis. *Am J Gastroenterol* 83:71, 1988.
83. Mutaf O, Ozok G, Avanoglu A: Oesophagoplasty in the treatment of caustic oesophageal strictures in children. *Br J Surg* 82:644, 1995.
84. Chaudhary A, Puri AS, Dhar P, et al: Elective surgery for corrosive-induced gastric injury. *World J Surg* 20:703, 1996.
85. Hwang TL, Chen MF: Surgical treatment of gastric outlet obstruction after corrosive injury—can definitive surgery be used instead of staged operation? *Int Surg* 81:119, 1996.
86. Kochhar R, Sethy PK, Nagi B, et al: Endoscopic balloon dilatation of benign gastric outlet obstruction. *J Gastroenterol Hepatol* 19:418, 2004.
87. Saetti R, Silvestrini M, Cutrone C, et al: Endoscopic treatment of upper airway and digestive tract lesions caused by caustic agents. *Ann Otol Rhinol Laryngol* 112:29, 2003.
88. Kaufman DB, DiNicola W, McIntosh R: Acute potassium dichromate poisoning. Treated by peritoneal dialysis. *Am J Dis Child* 119:374, 1970.

CHAPTER 131 ■ SALICYLATE AND OTHER NONSTEROIDAL ANTI-INFLAMMATORY DRUG POISONING

MARCO L.A. SIVILOTTI AND CHRISTOPHER H. LINDEN

Nonsteroidal anti-inflammatory drugs (NSAIDs) include aspirin, related salicylates (Table 131.1), and a variety of other drugs (e.g., ibuprofen, indomethacin, phenylbutazone, and ketorolac), which modulate inflammation by inhibiting cyclooxygenase (COX). In clinical use for 100 years, aspirin still enjoys widespread popularity in the adult population, both by self-medication and by physician-recommended usage.

While the institution of child-resistant packaging and concerns about Reye's syndrome resulted in a dramatic decline in pediatric overdose, aspirin remains a leading cause of death due to pharmaceutical overdose [1–3]. Reducing the amount of aspirin available over the counter was associated with a fewer overdose deaths in the United Kingdom [4]. Nevertheless, vigilance remains necessary because chronic salicylate intoxication, particularly in the elderly, is commonly unrecognized or mistaken for other conditions, such as dehydration, dementia, sepsis, and multiorgan failure. In contrast, most other NSAIDs have a substantially greater safety margin than aspirin in overdose. Although availability without prescription has resulted in increased use and frequency of overdose, significant acute toxicity is uncommon [1,5,6].

PHARMACOLOGY

All NSAIDs have analgesic and antipyretic as well as anti-inflammatory activity. These effects are due to inhibition of COX, also known as *prostaglandin G/H synthase*, the enzyme responsible for the conversion of arachidonic acid to prostaglandins and thromboxanes [7,8]. The analgesic dose of most NSAIDs is approximately one-half the anti-inflammatory dose. For some NSAIDs, such as aspirin, ibuprofen, and fenoprofen, this gap is larger, whereas the converse is true for sulindac and piroxicam [9]. Antipyretic effects appear to be due to decreased pyrogen production peripherally as well as to a central hypothalamic effect. The existence of central nervous system (CNS) sites of action mediating analgesic activity has been postulated [10].

Two isoforms of COX have been characterized: COX-1, constitutionally present in platelets, endothelium, gastric mucosa, and the kidneys; and COX-2, induced by a variety of inflammatory mediators (e.g., cytokines, endotoxin, growth factors, hormones, and tumor promoters) but suppressed by glucocorticoids [8,11]. The anti-inflammatory and analgesic properties of NSAIDs appear to be primarily due to the inhibition of COX-2. Their adverse effects on gastric mucosa (e.g., hemorrhage, ulceration, and perforation) and kidney function (e.g., decreased renal blood flow and glomerular filtration rate), and their effects on platelet function appear to be mediated primarily by COX-1, but COX-2 inhibition may also be involved [8,12,13].

NSAIDs can be classified on the basis of their selectivity for COX-2. In particular, the coxibs rofecoxib, valdecoxib, and celecoxib were developed specifically for their COX-2 selectivity and the promise of improved safety. However, an increased risk of thrombotic events, primarily myocardial infarction and stroke, was identified in clinical trials and led to regulatory restrictions on the selective COX-2 inhibitors [14,15]. These adverse cardiovascular effects appear to be due to a relative excess of COX-1–generated thromboxane A2, which is vasoconstrictive and platelet-activating (i.e., prothrombic), and a relative lack of COX-2–generated prostaglandin I_2 (prostacyclin), which is vasodilatory and platelet inhibitory (i.e., antithrombotic) [8,14]. It is important to note that traditional NSAIDS diclofenac, meloxicam, and nabumetone exhibit partial COX-2 selectivity, and that other traditional, nonselective NSAIDs may also contribute to adverse cardiovascular events. Thus, selectivity is relative, and all NSAIDs inhibit both COX isoforms in a dose-dependent manner.

Inhibition of COX-1 may result in increased lipoxygenation of arachidonic acid to leukotrienes. This alternate metabolic pathway seems to be responsible for the sometimes fatal allergic reactions to NSAIDs especially prevalent in adults with asthma

TABLE 131.1

SALICYLATE PREPARATIONS

Compound	Common/trade names	Percentage salicylate
Acetylsalicylic acid	Aspirin	75
Bismuth subsalicylate	In Pepto-Bismol	37
Choline salicylate	Arthropan	56
Choline and magnesium salicylate	Trilisate	76
Difluorophenyl salicylic acid	—	—
Diflunisal	Dolobid	—[a]
Homomenthyl salicylate	In sunscreens	51
Magnesium salicylate	Doan's Caplets, Magan	90
Methyl salicylate	Oil of wintergreen	89
Salicylic acid	In topical keratolytics	100
Salicylsalicylic acid	Salsalate, Disalcid	96
Sodium salicylate	Pabalate	84
Trolamine salicylate	Aspercreme	48

[a]Not hydrolyzed to salicylic acid but may cause screening tests for salicylate to be falsely positive.

and nasal polyps [16,17]. The expression or upregulation of COX-2 may be involved in the pathogenesis of Alzheimer's disease and some cancers (e.g., colon).

Aspirin (acetylsalicylic acid) is unique in that it acetylates a serine residue near the active site of COX, thereby irreversibly inhibiting its catalytic function. In contrast, the inhibition of COX by other NSAIDs is reversible and transient. This difference in activity is most notable in platelets, in which thromboxane A_2 is essential for normal function [18]. Even in low doses (80 mg), aspirin inhibits platelet aggregation and prolongs the bleeding time for up to 1 week (pending the production of new platelets), whereas other NSAIDs do not have clinically significant platelet effects [19].

In high doses, aspirin and other salicylates also inhibit the hepatic synthesis of clotting factor VII and, to some degree, factors IX and X, thereby prolonging the prothrombin time. This effect appears to be due to interference with the activity of vitamin K and can be reversed by administration of phytonadione (vitamin K_1). In contrast, other NSAIDs have insignificant effects on clotting-factor synthesis [19].

Salicylates

Salicylates are available in oral, rectal, and topical formulations. Enteric-coated and sustained-release aspirin tablets are also marketed. Aspirin preparations frequently contain other drugs such as anticholinergics, antihistamines, barbiturates, caffeine, decongestants, muscle relaxants, and opioids. The recommended pediatric dose of aspirin is 10 to 20 mg per kg of body weight every 6 hours, up to 60 mg per kg per day; for adults, the recommended dose is 1,000 mg initially, followed by 650 mg every 4 hours for anti-inflammatory effect. Therapeutic doses of other salicylate salts are similar but depend on their salicylate content (see Table 131.1) and formulation. After a single oral dose of aspirin, therapeutic effects begin within 30 minutes, peak in 1 to 2 hours, and last approximately 4 hours.

Being a weak acid (pK_a, 3.5), aspirin is predominantly nonionized at gastric pH and, therefore, theoretically well absorbed in the stomach. However, gastric acidity reduces the solubility of aspirin, thereby slowing the dissolution of tablets. Hence, despite its higher pH, most absorption actually occurs in the small intestine, probably because of its much larger surface area. Peak serum salicylate levels of 10 to 20 mg per dL (0.7 to 1.4 mmol per L) occur 1 to 2 hours after ingestion of a single therapeutic dose. Levels up to 30 mg per dL can occur with long-term therapy and may be necessary for maximal anti-inflammatory effects in some patients. Absorption is delayed or prolonged after ingestion of enteric-coated or sustained-release preparations and suppository use [20]. With overdose, slow pill dissolution, and delayed gastric emptying due to aspirin-induced pylorospasm may lead to absorption continuing for 24 hours or longer after ingestion [21].

During absorption, aspirin is rapidly hydrolyzed by plasma esterases to its active metabolite, salicylic acid. At physiologic pH, salicylic acid (pK_a: 3.0) is more than 99.9% ionized to salicylate, which, in contrast to nonionized salicylic acid, diffuses poorly across cell membranes. The drug may become sequestered preferentially in inflamed tissue due to this pH-dependent ionization.

The apparent volume of distribution of salicylate at pH 7.4 is only 0.15 L per kg, in part due to its extensive protein binding. Only free (i.e., unbound) salicylate is pharmacologically active. However, salicylate is unique in that its apparent volume of distribution is not constant. High drug levels (e.g., as a result of chronic therapeutic dosing or acute overdose), low albumin levels, and the presence of other drugs that bind to albumin increase the amount and fraction of free drug [22]. When this occurs, the apparent volume of distribution may increase to 0.60 L per kg [23]. Acidemia, as a consequence of either concomitant illness or severe poisoning, may additionally increase the fraction of nonionized, diffusible drug, promote its tissue penetration, and increase the apparent volume of distribution even more.

After single therapeutic doses, salicylate is metabolized in the liver to the inactive metabolites salicyluric acid (the glycine conjugate; 75% of the dose), salicyl phenolic glucuronide (10%), salicyl acyl glucuronide (5%), and gentisic acid (less than 1%). The remaining 10% of the dose is excreted unchanged in the urine. When serum concentrations exceed 20 mg per dL, the two main pathways of metabolism become saturated, and elimination changes from first order (i.e., proportional to the serum level) to zero order (constant), as described by Michaelis–Menton kinetics. Hence, the apparent half-life of salicylate is 2 to 3 hours after a single therapeutic dose, 6 to 12 hours with chronic therapeutic dosing (i.e., serum levels of 20 to 30 mg per dL), and 20 to 40 hours with overdose (i.e., when levels exceed 30 mg per dL) [24]. Because of saturable metabolism, a small increase in the daily dose can lead to a large increase in serum drug levels, with the potential for unintentional poisoning [25]. Depletion of glycine stores may reduce the capacity of the salicyluric acid pathway and further slow elimination in overdose [26].

Renal excretion of salicylate becomes the most important route of elimination when hepatic transformation becomes saturated. The rate of excretion is determined by the glomerular filtration, active proximal tubular secretion of salicylate, and passive distal tubular reabsorption of salicylic acid. Alkalinization of the urine decreases the passive reabsorption of salicylic acid by converting it to ionized, nondiffusible salicylate and thereby increases drug excretion. Similarly, increasing the rate of urine flow increases drug clearance by increasing the glomerular filtration and decreasing the distal tubular reabsorption of salicylic acid (by diluting its concentration in the tubular lumen). Combined alkalinization and diuresis can augment the renal elimination of salicylate by 20-fold or more [27,28]. Conversely, dehydration and aciduria perhaps due to preexisting illness or to salicylate poisoning itself decrease salicylate excretion, and increase the duration of toxicity once it develops.

Salicylates readily cross the placenta and enter breast milk. Salicylate elimination in the fetus or infant may be prolonged because of immature metabolic pathways and renal function [29]. It may also be prolonged in patients with liver or renal disease.

The pathophysiology of salicylate poisoning is multifactorial [30–35]. Initially and in mild poisoning, direct stimulation of the respiratory center in the medulla by toxic salicylate concentrations results in a respiratory alkalosis, unless blunted by concomitant ingestion of CNS depressants [31]. Direct stimulation of the medullary chemoreceptor zone and irritant effects on the gastrointestinal tract are responsible for nausea and vomiting. Exaggerated antipyretic effects involving the hypothalamus may cause vasodilation and sweating [36]. Dehydration results from gastrointestinal, skin, and insensible fluid losses. The osmotic diuresis that occurs as bicarbonate is excreted in response to alkalemia also contributes to dehydration. Sodium and potassium depletion result from excretion of these electrolytes along with bicarbonate (in exchange for hydrogen ion reabsorption). A functional hypocalcemia (decreased ionized calcium) may accompany alkalemia and cause or contribute to cardiac arrhythmias, tetany, and seizures.

Subsequently, in moderate poisoning, the accumulation of salicylate in cells causes uncoupling of mitochondrial oxidative phosphorylation, inhibition of the Krebs cycle, inhibition of amino acid metabolism, and stimulation of gluconeogenesis, glycolysis, and lipid metabolism [37,38]. These derangements result in increased but ineffective metabolism, with increased glucose, lipid, and oxygen consumption and increased amino acid, carbon dioxide, glucose, ketoacid, lactic acid, and pyruvic acid production. High serum levels of organic acids contribute to an increased anion-gap metabolic acidosis, and the renal excretion of these acids results in aciduria. However, increased carbon dioxide production further stimulates the respiratory center, and the respiratory alkalosis persists, resulting in alkalemia with paradoxical aciduria. An osmotic diuresis further accentuates fluid and electrolyte losses.

In severe poisoning, progressive dehydration and impaired cellular metabolism cause multisystem organ dysfunction. Metabolic acidosis with acidemia becomes the dominant acid–base disturbance. Respiratory acidosis, lactic acidosis, and impaired renal excretion of organic acids due to dehydration and acute tubular necrosis contribute to the acidemia. Acidemia increases the fraction of nonionized salicylate in serum, thereby promoting its tissue penetration and toxicity, and rapid clinical deterioration may ensue with increasing brain salicylate levels. Impaired cellular metabolism can cause increased capillary permeability [39] leading to cerebral edema and noncardiogenic pulmonary edema or acute respiratory distress syndrome. Coma and seizures may result from impaired cellular metabolism, cardiovascular depression, cerebral edema, acidemia, hypoglycemia, and acute white matter damage due to myelin disintegration and activation of glial caspase-3 [41,42]. Respiratory alkalosis may be replaced by respiratory acidosis if coma or seizures cause respiratory depression. Tissue hypoxia resulting from pulmonary edema, impaired perfusion, or seizures may lead to anaerobic metabolism and concomitant lactic acidosis.

Hemorrhagic diathesis may result from increased capillary fragility, decreased platelet adhesiveness, thrombocytopenia, and coagulopathy secondary to liver dysfunction. It occurs primarily in patients with chronic poisoning.

Other Nonsteroidal Anti-inflammatory Drugs

Despite their structural diversity, the pharmacokinetics of traditional NSAIDs are quite similar. Like aspirin, they are weak acids, with pK_a ranging from 3.5 to 5.6 and pH-dependent ionization being the major determinant of tissue distribution and sequestration. They are rapidly absorbed after ingestion, have small volumes of distribution (0.08 to 0.20 L per kg), and are 90% to 99% protein bound (principally to albumin). Most have half-lives of less than 8 hours, with low non–flow-dependent hepatic clearance, primarily by the CYP2C subfamily of cytochrome P450 enzymes, to inactive metabolites that are then conjugated, mostly with glucuronic acid, and excreted in the urine. Sulindac is one exception in that its sulfide metabolite is the active form of the drug and has a half-life of 16 hours [42]. Nabumetone is also a prodrug, and its active metabolite, 6-methoxy-2-naphthylacetic acid, has a half-life of more than 20 hours (and even longer in the elderly) [43]. Phenylbutazone, oxyphenbutazone, and piroxicam are notable for half-lives of longer than 30 hours. Diflunisal, like aspirin, has a dose-dependent half-life of 5 to 20 hours. Indomethacin, sulindac, etodolac, piroxicam, carprofen, and meloxicam undergo enterohepatic recirculation [42,44,45]. Small amounts (less than 10%) of nonsalicylate NSAIDs are excreted unchanged in the urine, limiting the effect of urine pH on clearance. The coxibs are nonacidic drugs [13], highly protein bound and primarily metabolized in the liver.

In contrast to salicylates, the metabolism of most nonsalicylate NSAIDs is not saturable or prolonged in overdose, and elimination follows first-order kinetics. An exception is phenylbutazone, whose elimination may follow Michaelis–Menton kinetics.

Toxic effects of NSAIDs appear to be primarily due to exaggerated pharmacologic effects, with gastric irritation and renal dysfunction resulting from the inhibition of prostaglandin synthesis [46]. In contrast to salicylate poisoning, the acidosis that sometimes occurs with large overdoses of these agents appears to be due to high levels of parent drug and metabolites rather than to disruption of metabolism [47]. Mechanisms responsible for their CNS toxicity remain to be defined.

CLINICAL TOXICITY

Salicylates

Salicylate poisoning may occur with acute as well as chronic overdose [30–35,48–55]. It most commonly results from ingestion, but poisoning due to topical use [56] and rectal self-administration [57] has been reported. The ingestion of topical preparations of methyl salicylate (oil of wintergreen, also present in Chinese propriety medicines) can result in

TABLE 131.2

SEVERITY OF SALICYLATE POISONING

Severity grade	Serum pH	Underlying acid–base abnormality
Mild	>7.45	Respiratory alkalosis
Moderate	7.35–7.45	Combined respiratory alkalosis and metabolic acidosis
Severe	<7.35	Metabolic acidosis with or without respiratory acidosis

rapid-onset poisoning, due to its concentration, rapid absorption kinetics, and higher lipid solubility [58]. Infants may become poisoned by ingesting the breast milk of women chronically taking therapeutic doses of salicylate [59]. Intrauterine fetal demise resulting from poisoning during pregnancy [60] and neonatal poisoning resulting from the transplacental diffusion of therapeutic doses of salicylate taken before delivery [61] have also been described. Delays to presentation, diagnosis, and chronicity each increase the severity and mortality [50,62,63] and with severe poisoning, the fatality rate may be as high as 50% [51,55].

Regardless of whether poisoning is acute or chronic, it can be characterized as mild, moderate, or severe on the basis of the serum pH and underlying acid–base disturbance (Table 131.2). This approach was first described in the classic papers by Done [48,64], who also developed a nomogram that attempted to correlate the severity of poisoning with a timed salicylate level after acute ingestion. Although Done's nomogram has subsequently been shown to have poor predictive value in acute poisoning [49] and is not applicable to chronic poisoning, to acute poisoning by enteric-coated aspirin and nonaspirin salicylates, or to patients with acidemia [62] his observation that the clinical severity of poisoning correlates with acid–base status remains undisputed.

Mild poisoning is characterized by alkalemia (serum pH greater than 7.45) and a pure respiratory alkalosis. It may develop 2 to 8 hours after acute ingestion of 150 to 300 mg per kg of aspirin [48,64] or any time during chronic therapy. Associated signs and symptoms include nausea, vomiting, abdominal pain, headache, tinnitus, tachypnea (or subtle hyperpnea), ataxia, dizziness, agitation, and lethargy. The anion gap (see Chapter 71) is normal until late in this stage, when compensatory renal bicarbonate excretion eventually lowers the serum bicarbonate level. Serum glucose, potassium, and sodium values may be high, low, or normal. Despite total body fluid and electrolyte depletion and clinical dehydration, laboratory evidence of dehydration (e.g., hemoconcentration, increased serum blood urea nitrogen [BUN] and creatinine, increased urine specific gravity) may be absent.

Moderate poisoning is characterized by a near normal serum pH (7.35 to 7.45) with an underlying metabolic acidosis as well as respiratory alkalosis. It can occur 4 to 12 hours after an acute overdose of 300 to 500 mg per kg of aspirin [48,64]. It may also occur in patients with chronic ingestion who delay seeking medical care for symptoms of mild poisoning and continue to take salicylate. Electrolyte analysis demonstrates a low serum bicarbonate value with an increased anion gap. Gastrointestinal and neurologic symptoms are more pronounced. There may be agitation, fever, asterixis, diaphoresis, deafness, pallor, confusion, slurred speech, disorientation, hallucinations, tachycardia, tachypnea, and orthostatic hypotension. Coma and seizures can also occur. Leukocytosis, thrombocytopenia, increased or decreased serum glucose and sodium values, hypokalemia, and increased serum BUN, creatinine, and ketones may be present.

Severe poisoning is defined by the presence of acidemia (serum pH less than 7.35) with underlying metabolic acidosis and respiratory alkalosis or acidosis and a high anion gap. It can occur 6 to 24 hours or more after the acute ingestion of more than 500 mg per kg of aspirin [48,64] or in unrecognized or untreated chronic poisoning. Severe dehydration and marked sinus tachycardia are often present. Other findings may include coma, seizures, papilledema, hypotension, dysrhythmias, congestive heart failure, oliguria, hypothermia or hyperthermia, rhabdomyolysis and multiple organ failure [55,63,65,66]. Laboratory abnormalities are similar to those seen in moderate poisoning but are more pronounced. Hypoglycemia, pulmonary edema and cerebral edema or hemorrhage may be present [54,67]. Asystole is the most common terminal dysrhythmia, but ventricular tachycardia and ventricular fibrillation can also occur [54,55,68,69]. When cardiac arrest occurs, death appears to be inevitable. Successful resuscitation in this situation has yet to be reported [69].

Although an increased anion-gap metabolic acidosis is often said to be a hallmark of salicylate poisoning, in reality a variety of acid-base disturbances may be seen depending on the delay to presentation and severity of poisoning. As noted earlier, the anion gap may be normal and acidosis absent in early or mild intoxication. In addition, the anion gap is rarely above 20 mEq per L, even in advanced poisoning [31]. It is, therefore, more appropriate to say that an abnormal acid–base status is the hallmark of salicylate poisoning. In adults, combined respiratory alkalosis and metabolic acidosis is the most common finding (50% to 61%), followed by pure respiratory alkalosis (20% to 25%), pure metabolic acidosis (15% to 20%), and a combined respiratory and metabolic acidosis (5%) [31,55]. Metabolic acidosis is more common and respiratory alkalosis less common (and often absent) in children than in adults [50,55] suggesting that children progress more rapidly from mild-to-moderate to severe poisoning, perhaps because of more rapid and extensive tissue distribution of drug [70]. Metabolic acidosis is also more common in patients with large acute ingestions, chronic intoxication, and delayed presentation or treatment [31,50,51,55,71]. The onset and progression of toxicity may be delayed after overdose with enteric-coated or sustained-release formulations [20].

Potential complications of both therapeutic and toxic doses of salicylate include gastrointestinal tract bleeding, increased prothrombin time, hepatic toxicity, pancreatitis, proteinuria, and abnormal urinary sediment. Significant bleeding, gastrointestinal tract perforation, blindness, and inappropriate secretion of antidiuretic hormone are rare complications of acute poisoning.

Other Nonsteroidal Anti-inflammatory Drugs

With the exception of mefenamic acid and phenylbutazone, significant toxicity from acute overdose is unusual. Manifestations typically include nausea, vomiting, abdominal pain, headache, confusion, tinnitus, drowsiness, and hyperventilation [5,72,73]. Glycosuria, hematuria, and proteinuria are also common. Occasionally, acute renal failure (acute tubular necrosis or interstitial nephritis) can develop. Symptoms rarely last more than several hours, and acute renal toxicity is almost always reversible over a period of a few days to a few weeks. Experience with selective COX-2 inhibitor overdose is limited, but acute toxicity appears to be similar [74].

Muscle twitching and grand mal seizures have been reported in 30% of mefenamic acid overdoses [75]. Apnea, coma, and cardiac arrest can also occur [75]. Metabolic acidosis, coma, seizures, hepatic dysfunction, hypotension, and cardiovascular collapse are relatively frequent after phenylbutazone overdose [72,73,76–78]. Uncommonly, coma, hyperactivity, hypothermia, seizures, metabolic acidosis, acute renal insufficiency, thrombocytopenia, acute respiratory distress syndrome, upper gastrointestinal tract bleeding, and respiratory depression are seen in ibuprofen poisoning [47,78–87]. Death can result from ibuprofen alone or combined with other drugs [1,88–90], but despite the frequency of overdose, it is extremely rare [1,5,6]. Seizures and metabolic acidosis have also been reported in ketoprofen and naproxen poisoning [91,92].

Minimum toxic and lethal doses are not well defined. Little correlation was found between the amount of ibuprofen reportedly ingested and symptoms in adults [77]. In the pediatric population, however, the mean amount ingested was much greater in symptomatic patients (440 mg per kg) than asymptomatic ones (114 mg per kg) [79]. The spectrum of toxicity appears to be the same in children and adults [90]. Elderly patients are at increased risk of developing toxicity with both therapeutic doses and overdoses [93]. Even with severe poisoning, complete recovery usually occurs within 24 to 48 hours.

DIAGNOSTIC EVALUATION

The history should include the time or times of ingestion, the specific product and formulation, the amount ingested, and any concomitant ingestion or medication use. Physical examination should focus on vital signs, neurologic and cardiopulmonary function, and assessment of the state of hydration. Vital signs should include an accurate temperature and respiratory rate and, if possible, orthostatic measurements of pulse and blood pressure. The fundi should be examined for papilledema. Stool and urine should be tested for occult blood. Peritoneal signs should be sought on abdominal examination.

Salicylates

Laboratory evaluation of patients with salicylate poisoning should include arterial or venous blood gases, complete blood cell count, serum electrolyte, glucose, BUN, creatinine, and salicylate levels, and urinalysis. Patients with moderate-to-severe salicylate poisoning should also have serum calcium, magnesium, and ketones, liver function tests, coagulation profile, electrocardiogram; and chest radiograph. Because patients often confuse aspirin and acetaminophen, testing should be performed for both.

The ferric chloride spot test can be used to rapidly detect the presence of salicylate in urine or commercial products [94]. Several drops of 10% ferric chloride added to urine turn purple if salicylate is present. A positive urine test indicates exposure but not overdose because positive results are seen with therapeutic dosing. False-positive reactions may be caused by acetoacetic acid, phenylpyruvic acid, phenothiazines, and phenylbutazone. A quantitative serum salicylate level is necessary to confirm the diagnosis of poisoning. Diflunisal may result in falsely elevated salicylate levels when measured by fluorescence polarization immunoassay or the Trinder colorimetric assay [95].

Salicylate levels must be interpreted with respect to the duration (i.e., acute vs. chronic overdose) and time of ingestion. At similar salicylate levels, patients with chronic poisoning tend to be more ill than those with acute poisoning [32,54,55]. Soon after an acute overdose, levels can be quite high (e.g., greater than 60 mg per dL) in the absence of significant toxicity. Conversely, with chronic overdosage and late in the course of an acute overdose, moderate or severe toxicity may be present despite serum salicylate concentrations in the high therapeutic range. At similar salicylate levels, children, the elderly, and those with underlying disease tend to be more ill than otherwise healthy adults [32,52,70,96]. Poisoning in such patients, particularly if chronic, can occasionally be seen with therapeutic salicylate levels. Hence, as noted previously, the severity of poisoning is ultimately determined by acid–base status and clinical findings.

Serial salicylate levels are necessary for confirming the efficacy of gastrointestinal tract decontamination and enhanced elimination procedures but do not obviate the need for continued clinical and metabolic monitoring. Depending on the severity and course of poisoning, drug levels and other laboratory tests should be repeated at 2- to 6-hour intervals. Monitoring of drug levels for at least 12 hours is necessary to exclude significant ongoing absorption after overdose.

Historically, at least 25% of patients with chronic salicylate poisoning are initially undiagnosed [31,51,71]. These patients are typically elderly, have a variety of presenting complaints and underlying illnesses, and have been medicating themselves with aspirin. To avoid missing the diagnosis, all patients should be asked specifically about the use of nonprescription drugs. Asking about tinnitus or hearing distortion, which occurs with salicylate levels in the high end of the therapeutic range (i.e., 20 to 30 mg per dL), may also suggest the diagnosis in patients with unknown ingestions or unexplained complaints. Occult salicylate poisoning should be considered in any patient with an unexplained acid–base disturbance, altered mental status, fever, diaphoresis, dyspnea, vomiting, and pulmonary edema [31,71].

The differential diagnosis of salicylate poisoning includes infection (particularly meningitis); CNS trauma and tumors; congestive heart failure; chronic obstructive pulmonary disease; carbon monoxide, isoniazid, lithium, and valproate intoxication; toxic gas inhalation; and other toxic causes of an elevated anion-gap acidosis, particularly methanol and ethylene glycol (see Chapters 71 and 119). Hemodynamic, autonomic, and laboratory manifestations of severe poisoning resemble the systemic inflammatory response syndrome and may be mistaken for sepsis [61,65,66,97]. Salicylate poisoning has also been misdiagnosed as alcohol intoxication, alcohol withdrawal, dementia, diabetic ketoacidosis, impending myocardial infarction, nonspecific asterixis and encephalopathy, and viral encephalitis.

In infants and children, salicylate poisoning may be confused with inborn errors of metabolism. It may be particularly difficult to distinguish from Reye's syndrome, because they are not only similar in presentation but appear to be interrelated [98,99]. Fatty infiltration of the liver on pathologic examination of a biopsy specimen, low (i.e., subtherapeutic) cerebrospinal fluid salicylate levels, and high alanine, glutamine, and lysine levels indicate Reye's syndrome rather than salicylate poisoning. Radiopaque densities in the stomach on abdominal radiograph suggest the possibility of an enteric-coated or sustained-release formulation or a magnesium or bismuth salt of salicylate [100].

Other Nonsteroidal Anti-inflammatory Drugs

The initial evaluation of patients with nonsalicylate-NSAID overdose is similar to that for salicylates. Evaluation of acid–base, electrolyte, and renal parameters is particularly important. Additional ancillary testing is dictated by clinical severity. Quantitative serum levels of nonsalicylate NSAIDs are neither routinely available nor necessary for treatment.

Many medical conditions and other intoxications cause signs and symptoms similar to those seen in nonsalicylate NSAID poisoning. In the absence of a history of ingestion, the diagnosis is made by exclusion of other etiologies.

MANAGEMENT

Salicylates

Supportive care, limiting drug absorption, and enhancing drug elimination are the goals of therapy. Resuscitative measures should be instituted as necessary. It is critically important to remember that, should endotracheal intubation be necessary, hyperventilation must be accomplished before, during, and after this procedure to prevent worsening acidemia, which increases the fraction of nonionized salicylic acid available for tissue distribution, thereby enhancing toxicity. The administration of respiratory depressants or failure to adequately hyperventilate unconscious or paralyzed patients can result in rapid deterioration and death of severely poisoned patients [62,68,101]. Because an increase in the partial pressure of carbon dioxide (PCO_2) is almost inevitable following intubation and mechanical ventilation, it is recommended that patients with arterial PCO_2 values below 20 mm Hg be given an intravenous bolus of 1 to 2 mEq per kg sodium bicarbonate at the time of intubation.

Arterial blood gases should always be checked after intubation and after bicarbonate therapy.

Because CNS hypoglycemia may occur despite a normal serum glucose value [101], 50 mL of 50% dextrose in water should be given intravenously to any patient with an altered mental status whose capillary glucose concentration is not already elevated [49]. Anticonvulsants (e.g., benzodiazepines, propofol, and barbiturates) as well as supplemental glucose should be given to patients with seizures. It is also prudent to treat seizures with $NaHCO_3$, as acidemia is likely to worsen. Hyperthermia should be treated with cooling blankets, ice packs, and evaporative methods (see Chapter 66).

Central venous pressure monitoring may be necessary for optimal treatment of hypotension, especially if there is evidence of heart failure or pulmonary edema. Patients with noncardiac pulmonary edema should be treated with positive pressure ventilation rather than diuretics. Again, maintaining hyperventilation and reducing acidemia are critical in patients with compromised pulmonary function.

Additional supportive measures are directed at correction of dehydration and metabolic derangements. The degree of dehydration parallels the severity of poisoning [64], but it is often unappreciated, underestimated, or undertreated. Patients with mild, moderate, or severe poisoning typically have volume deficits of 1 to 2, 3 to 4, or 5 to 6 L (20, 40, and 60 mL per kg in children), respectively. In the presence of acidemia, hypokalemia is more severe than indicated by the serum potassium level (by approximately 0.6 mEq per L for each 0.1 unit of decrease in pH) and should be treated aggressively.

Acidemia should also be treated aggressively with intravenous $NaHCO_3$. Since the respiratory alkalosis is a concomitant primary acid–base disturbance and not just a compensatory response, the administration of bicarbonate is unlikely to blunt the respiratory drive and increase the PCO_2, which might otherwise limit the change in serum pH. In addition, the goal of therapy is to limit the tissue distribution of salicylates by increasing the serum pH. The dose of bicarbonate needed may be substantial, and is typically 4 to 5 ampules or 200 to 300 mEq in an adult with severe poisoning.

As with repleting volume, at least half of the $NaHCO_3$ deficit should be given during the first hour either by continuous infusion or by 0.5 to 1.0 mEq per kg boluses every 10 minutes. Arterial blood gases should be reevaluated during after such therapy. Potential complications of $NaHCO_3$ administration include excessive alkalemia, hypokalemia, hypocalcemia, hypernatremia, and fluid overload. Relative contraindications to hypertonic $NaHCO_3$ include oliguric renal failure, congestive heart failure, and cerebral or pulmonary edema.

Tetany should be treated with intravenous calcium chloride or calcium gluconate (10 mL of a 10% solution over 5 to 10 minutes). Fresh-frozen plasma, red blood cell, and platelet transfusions may be required for patients with active bleeding or significant blood loss. Asymptomatic increases in international normalized ratio can be treated with subcutaneous vitamin K.

Gastrointestinal decontamination should be performed in all patients with intentional overdoses and those with accidental ingestions of greater than 150 mg per kg. Because of delayed absorption, decontamination may be effective for as long as 24 hours after overdose, even in patients with spontaneous vomiting [21]. Considerable diversity in opinion exists, however, regarding the optimal method of decontamination [103].

Activated charcoal is effective in preventing salicylate absorption in simulated overdose [104] and, therefore, it is recommended for all significant ingestions, regardless of delay in presentation. Multiple oral doses of charcoal [105] or gastric lavage preceded and followed by another dose of activated charcoal may be the more effective for preventing the absorption of large overdoses [106]. Many grams of aspirin have been recovered by lavage up 24 hours after ingestion [21]. Repeated doses of activated charcoal or whole-bowel irrigation may be effective for patients who have ingested enteric-coated or sustained-release formulations and those with serum drug levels that continue to rise despite other decontamination measures [107].

The efficacy of multiple-dose charcoal therapy in enhancing salicylate elimination may depend on the formulation. Increases in serum salicylate elimination reported using an effervescent preparation containing bicarbonate [108] could not be replicated with multiple doses of noneffervescent charcoal in simulated overdose (i.e., less than 3 g) in humans [109–112]. Oral charcoal does not substantially accelerate the elimination of intravenously administered salicylic acid in pigs, discounting the role of gut dialysis or enterohepatic circulation [113]. If multiple-dose charcoal is used, sorbitol should not be included with the subsequent doses [114,115].

Salicylate elimination can be enhanced by urine alkalinization and diuresis [27,28,32–34,116], extracorporeal removal [117], and perhaps by glycine administration [52]. It should be emphasized that serum and urine alkalinization and establishing a urine output of 1 to 2 mL per kg per hour are equally important goals in the management of patients with salicylate toxicity [35,118,119]. Moreover, alkalinization of the urine is difficult to achieve in patients with acidemia and aciduria (i.e., severe clinical toxicity) [64]. Theoretical concerns regarding pulmonary or cerebral edema should not preclude aggressive fluid therapy, as administering only maintenance fluids intravenously is insufficient treatment for a patient with salicylate poisoning.

Indications for urine alkalinization and alkaline diuresis include acid-base abnormalities and systemic symptoms with a salicylate level that is greater than 30 mg per dL after an acute overdose. Patients with chronic overdoses may be symptomatic and require treatment, despite lower salicylate levels. The goal is to achieve a urine pH of 7.5 or greater. All patients treated with alkaline diuresis need close monitoring in an intensive care unit or similar setting. Bladder catheterization is essential in those with moderate or severe poisoning, in whom hourly monitoring of urine output and pH is required. Arterial or venous blood gases, electrolytes, BUN, creatinine, glucose, and salicylate concentrations should initially be rechecked at 2- to 4-hour intervals, depending on the severity of poisoning, the results of previous testing, and the response to therapy. Cardiac monitoring and frequent reevaluations of vital signs, mental status, and pulmonary function are also necessary during alkaline diuresis.

Alkalinization of the urine may be impossible to achieve in the presence of dehydration and hypokalemia because hydrogen ions are excreted in exchange for reabsorbed sodium and potassium, respectively [62,120]. Therefore, correction of fluid and potassium deficits is critical.

The amount of bicarbonate and supplementary potassium necessary to achieve and maintain an alkaline urine depends on the severity of poisoning (Table 131.2). For example, the initial intravenous fluids for a moderately poisoned patient could be 1 L of 5% dextrose in one-half normal saline to which 75 mEq of sodium bicarbonate (i.e., 1.5 ampules of 8.4% sodium bicarbonate) and 40 mEq of potassium chloride have been added. In severe poisoning, however, 150 mEq of sodium bicarbonate (i.e., 3 ampules of 8.4% sodium bicarbonate) and 60 mEq of potassium chloride should be added to each liter of 5% dextrose in water initially, and adjusted as necessary. In patients with hypernatremia, a more hypotonic solution should be used. Again, the use of a dextrose-containing solution is important because of the potential for occult CNS hypoglycemia. Although forced diuresis (e.g., 500 mL per hour urine output in adults) is no longer recommended [121], a moderate rate of fluid administration (3 to 4 mL per kg per hour) is recommended. Although counterintuitive, even patients with mild poisoning (i.e., alkalemia) should be given bicarbonate (and fluids); this is necessary to replace ongoing renal losses and prevent deterioration. The onset of diuresis may be delayed an hour or two after the institution of therapy.

Carbonic anhydrase inhibitors (e.g., acetazolamide) should never be used to alkalinize the urine (especially without concomitant bicarbonate therapy) because the resultant systemic acidosis may promote tissue distribution of salicylate and result in clinical deterioration [122,123]. Similarly, the use of tris-hydroxymethyl aminomethane, an organic H^+ buffer that increases serum and urine pH, is not recommended. Although tris-hydroxymethyl aminomethane has been suggested for the treatment of acidemia and aciduria refractory to bicarbonate administration, it has not been studied in human salicylate poisoning and has a number of potential adverse effects (e.g., hypoglycemia, extravasation necrosis, phlebitis, respiratory depression, and increased intracellular pH leading to decreased pH gradients with increased tissue distribution and intracellular trapping of salicylate) [124].

As with $NaHCO_3$ therapy for acidemia, complications of alkaline diuresis include excessive alkalemia, hypokalemia, hypocalcemia, hypernatremia, and fluid overload [52,119,121]. Young children, the elderly, and those with severe poisoning are most susceptible to such complications. Alkaline diuresis is contraindicated in patients with oliguric renal failure, congestive heart failure, and cerebral or pulmonary edema. Such therapy should be withheld or discontinued if the serum pH exceeds 7.55.

Hemodialysis is indicated in patients with severe poisoning and those with moderate poisoning who fail to improve with alkaline diuresis [34–36,51,52,62]. Hemodialysis is essential for successful outcome in patients with coma, seizures, cerebral or pulmonary edema, and renal failure [36,55]. Whether the term *coma*, as used here, should include altered mental status (e.g., confusion and disorientation) and any impairment in the level of consciousness as well as unresponsiveness is controversial. Erring on the side of treatment is recommended. Acidemia and temperature greater than 38°C are associated with high mortality [55] and should also be considered potential indications for hemodialysis, particularly if the patient is resistant to bicarbonate and fluid therapy. Similarly, patients with moderate poisoning who have liver dysfunction and, hence, impaired ability to eliminate salicylate may also benefit from hemodialysis.

A high salicylate level is often cited as an indication for hemodialysis but recommendations vary widely with cutoffs ranging from 40 to 200 mg per dL (100 mg per dL being the most common) for acute ingestions and 60 to 80 mg per dL for chronic exposures [124]. In one study [51], salicylate levels in fatal cases ranged from 34 to 193 mg per dL and in another [54], some patients died with drug levels in the therapeutic range. Moreover, drug levels do not discriminate patients who die from survivors [54,55]. Clearly, the salicylate level should not be used as the sole indication for hemodialysis. Instead, the severity of poisoning is determined by clinical findings, which reflect tissue drug concentration and effect, depend on factors that influence tissue distribution, and do not necessarily correlate with blood levels, particularly when acidemia is present [122]. Moreover, a serum salicylate concentration should be interpreted in the context of a simultaneous measurement of serum pH. Hence, hemodialysis is appropriate for patients with high drug levels who have severe clinical toxicity (particularly acidemia), but it may not be necessary in those without such manifestations [55]. Conversely, patients with low salicylate levels, particularly those with significant underlying cardiorespiratory disease, should be treated with hemodialysis if they exhibit clinical or laboratory manifestations of severe toxicity. Because of delays inherent in the turnaround time for salicylate determinations and in preparing for hemodialysis, the projected clinical course should also be considered. Waiting for the salicylate level to reach some predetermined level before initiating hemodialysis in patients who are severely poisoned or deteriorating despite other treatments is ill-advised.

Hemodialysis is preferred over continuous renal replacement therapy or hemoperfusion due to the rapid clearances and correction of fluid, electrolyte and acid–base abnormalities achieved [117,126,127]. A high-bicarbonate (e.g., up to 40 mEq per L) dialysate solution (bath) should be used, and potassium should usually be added to the dialysate solution. Peritoneal dialysis and exchange transfusion are also less effective [128].

Failure to adequately correct fluid deficits prior to initiating hemodialysis can result in disastrous consequences. In contrast to the typical dialysis (i.e., renal failure) patient who is fluid overloaded, those with salicylate poisoning are typically hypovolemic. Uncorrected or occult hypovolemia can result in cardiovascular decompensation with hemodynamic instability and even cardiac arrest when dialysis is started because of the acute decrease in intravascular volume that occurs when blood is removed and used to prime the dialysis tubing and pump at the beginning of dialysis. This complication can be prevented or minimized by ensuring adequate volume resuscitation, giving a bolus of saline, and priming the tubing and pump with saline (rather than blood) prior to initiating dialysis.

Oral administration of glycine or *N*-glycylglycine has been used in overdose patients to promote drug clearance [26,129]. Because the conjugation of salicylic acid with glycine to form salicyluric acid becomes saturated and glycine levels decrease in overdose patients, supplemental glycine can enhance the formation and excretion of this metabolite. To date, clinical experience with this therapy is limited, its comparative efficacy is unknown, and the side effects of nausea and vomiting with glycine have been problematic. Doses used ranged from 8 g dissolved in water initially, followed by 4 g every 4 hours for 16 hours, to 20 g followed by 10 g every 2 hours for 10 hours for glycine. The dose for *N*-glycylglycine was 8 g dissolved in water followed by 2 to 4 g every 2 hours for 16 hours.

Other Nonsteroidal Anti-inflammatory Drugs

The treatment of nonsalicylate NSAID poisoning is supportive and symptomatic. Although most patients require only observation, airway protection, mechanical ventilation, and fluid resuscitation, use of anticonvulsants for seizures, bicarbonate for acidosis, vitamin K or fresh-frozen plasma for coagulopathy, antacids and histamine$_2$–receptor antagonists for gastritis, and blood products for gastrointestinal tract bleeding may occasionally be required. Naloxone has been reported to reverse CNS depression in a toddler with ibuprofen toxicity [81]. Renal function should be monitored carefully in patients with abnormal urinalysis, underlying renal disease, or advanced age. Liver function tests should be followed in patients with severe phenylbutazone and piroxicam poisoning [78].

Gastrointestinal decontamination with activated charcoal should be considered for patients who present soon after a significant ingestion, defined as greater than ten therapeutic doses in adults and more than five adult doses in children [72,73]. Although charcoal hemoperfusion has been used to treat a patient with severe phenylbutazone poisoning who had impaired renal and hepatic function [76], extracorporeal elimination measures are unlikely to be effective because of the high-protein binding and rapid intrinsic elimination of these agents. Multiple-dose charcoal therapy enhances the elimination of therapeutic doses of phenylbutazone by 30% [130] and may be similarly effective for other agents, but the clinical benefit of such therapy after overdose is likely to be limited.

References

1. Watson WA, Litovitz TL, Rodgers GC, et al: 2004 annual report of the American Association of Poison Control Centers Toxic Exposure Surveillance System. *Am J Emerg Med* 23:589, 2005.
2. Brigden M, Smith RE: Acetylsalicylic-acid-containing drugs and nonsteroidal anti-inflammatory drugs available in Canada. *Can Med Assoc J* 156:1025, 1997.
3. McLoone P, Crombie IK: Hospitalisation for deliberate self-poisoning in Scotland from 1981 to 1993: trends in rates and types of drugs used. *Br J Psychiatry* 169:81, 1996.
4. Hawton K, Simkin S, Deeks J, et al: UK legislation on analgesic packs: before and after study of long term effect on poisonings. *BMJ* 329:1076–1081, 2004.
5. Smolinske SC, Hall AH, Vandenberg SA, et al: Toxic effects of nonsteroidal anti-inflammatory drugs in overdose: an overview of recent evidence on clinical effects and dose-response relationships. *Drug Saf* 5:252, 1990.
6. Veltri JC, Rollins DE: A comparison of the frequency and severity of poisoning cases for ingestion of acetaminophen, aspirin, and ibuprofen. *Am J Emerg Med* 6:104, 1988.
7. Vane JR: Inhibition of prostaglandin synthesis as a mechanism of action for the aspirin-like drugs. *Nature* 231:232, 1971.
8. Patrono C, Garcia Rodriguez LA, Landolfi R, et al: Low-dose aspirin for the prevention of atherothrombosis. *N Engl J Med* 353:2373, 2005.
9. Jungnickel PW: Selection of non-steroidal anti-inflammatory drugs. *Fam Pract Res J* 16:33, 1984.
10. Bannwarth B, Demotes-Mainard F, Schaeverbeke T: Central analgesic effects of aspirin-like drugs. *Fundam Clin Pharmacol* 9:1, 1995.
11. Masferrer JL, Zweifel BS, Seibert K, et al: Selective regulation of cellular cyclooxygenase by dexamethasone and endotoxin in mice. *J Clin Invest* 86:1375, 1990.
12. Jouzeau J-Y, Terlain B, Abid A, et al: Cyclo-oxygenase isoenzymes. *Drugs* 53:563, 1997.
13. FitzGerald GA, Patrono C: The coxibs, selective inhibitors of cyclooxygenase-2. *N Engl J Med* 345:433, 2001.
14. Fitzgerald GA: Coxibs and cardiovascular disease. *N Engl J Med* 351:1709, 2004.
15. Cairns JA: The coxibs and traditional nonsteroidal anti-inflammatory drugs: a current perspective on cardiovascular risks. *Can J Cardiol* 23:125–131, 2007.
16. Arm JP, Auten KF: Leukotriene receptor and aspirin sensitivity. *N Engl J Med* 347:1524, 2002.
17. Gollapaudi RR, Teirstein PS, Stevenson DD, et al: Aspirin sensitivity: implications for patients with coronary artery disease. *JAMA* 292:3017, 2004.
18. Buchanan MR: Biological basis and clinical implications of acetylsalicylic acid resistance. *Can J Cardiol* 22:149–151, 2006.
19. Romsing J, Walther-Larsen S: Peri-operative use of nonsteroidal anti-inflammatory drugs in children: analgesic efficacy and bleeding. *Anaesthesia* 52:673, 1997.
20. Wortzman DJ, Grunfeld A: Delay absorption following enteric-coated aspirin overdose. *Ann Emerg Med* 16:434, 198.
21. Matthew H, Mackintosh TF, Tompsett SL, et al: Gastric aspiration and lavage in acute poisoning. *BMJ* 1:1333, 1966.
22. Alvan G, Bergman U, Gustaffson LL: High unbound fraction of salicylate in plasma during intoxication. *Br J Clin Pharmacol* 11:625, 1981.
23. Rubin GM, Tozer TN, Oie S: Concentration-dependence of salicylate distribution. *J Pharm Pharmacol* 35:115, 1983.
24. Snodgrass W, Rumack BH, Peterson RG, et al: Salicylate toxicity following therapeutic doses in young children. *Clin Toxicol* 18:247, 1981.
25. Levy G, Tsuchiya T: Salicylate accumulation kinetics in man. *N Engl J Med* 287:430, 1972.
26. Patel DK, Ogunbona A, Notarianni LJ, et al: Depletion of plasma glycine and effect of glycine by mouth on salicylate metabolism during aspirin overdose. *Hum Exp Toxicol* 9:389, 1990.
27. Morgan AG, Polak A: The excretion of salicylate in salicylate poisoning. *Clin Sci* 41:475, 1971.
28. Levy G: Pharmacokinetics of salicylate in man. *Drug Metab Rev* 9:3, 1979.
29. Garretson LK, Procknal JA, Levy G: Fetal acquisition and neonatal elimination of a large amount of salicylate. *Clin Pharmacol Ther* 17:98, 1975.
30. Segar WE, Holliday MA: Physiologic abnormalities of salicylate intoxication. *N Engl J Med* 259:1191, 1958.
31. Gabow PA, Anderson RJ, Potts DE, et al: Acid base disturbances in the salicylate intoxicated adult. *Arch Intern Med* 138:1481, 1978.
32. Temple AR: Acute and chronic effects of aspirin toxicity and their treatment. *Arch Intern Med* 141:364, 1981.
33. Proudfoot AT: Toxicity of salicylates. *Am J Med* 75:99, 1983.
34. Brenner BE, Simon RR: Management of salicylate intoxication. *Drugs* 24:335, 1987.
35. O'Malley GF. Emergency department management of the salicylate-poisoned patient. *Emerg Med Clin North Am* 25(2):333–346, 2007.
36. Lovejoy F: Aspirin and acetaminophen: a comparative view of their antipyretic and analgesic activity. *Pediatrics* 62[Suppl]:904, 1978.
37. Miyahara J, Karle R: Effect of salicylate on oxidative phosphorylation of mitochondrial fragments. *Biochem J* 97:194, 1965.
38. Smith M: The metabolic basis of the major symptoms in acute salicylate intoxication. *Clin Toxicol* 1:387, 1968.
39. Hormaechea E, Carlson RW, Rogove H, et al: Hypovolemia, pulmonary edema, and protein changes in severe salicylate poisoning. *Am J Med* 66:1046, 1979.
40. Kuzak N, Brubacher JR, Kennedy JR: Reversal of salicylate-induced euglycemic delirium with dextrose. *Clin Toxicol* 45:526–529, 2007.
41. Rauschka H, Aboul-Enein F, Bauer J, et al: Acute white matter damage in lethal salicylate intoxication. *Neurotoxicology* 28:33–37, 2007.
42. Davies NM, Watson MS: Clinical pharmacokinetics of sulindac: a dynamic old drug. *Clin Pharmacokinet* 32:437, 1997.
43. Roth SH: Nabumetone: a new NSAID for rheumatoid arthritis and osteoarthritis. *Orthop Rev* 21:223, 1992.
44. Laufen H, Leitold M: The effect of activated charcoal on the bioavailability of piroxicam in man. *Int J Clin Pharm Ther Toxicol* 24:48, 1986.
45. Turck D, Roth W, Busch U: A review of the clinical pharmacokinetics of meloxicam. *Br J Rheumatol* 35[Suppl 1]:13, 1996.
46. Murray MD, Brater DC: Renal toxicity of the nonsteroidal anti-inflammatory drugs. *Annu Rev Pharmacol Toxicol* 32:435, 1993.
47. Linden CH, Townsend PL: Metabolic acidosis after acute ibuprofen overdosage. *J Pediatr* 111:922, 1987.
48. Done AK: Salicylate intoxication: significance of measurements of salicylates in blood in cases of acute ingestion. *Pediatrics* 26:800, 1960.
49. Dugandzic RM, Tierney MG, Dickinson GE, et al: Evaluation of the validity of the Done nomogram in the management of acute salicylate intoxication. *Ann Emerg Med* 18:1186, 1989.
50. Goudrealt P, Temple AR, Lovejoy FH: The relative severity of acute versus chronic salicylate poisonings in children: a clinical comparison. *Pediatrics* 70:566, 1982.
51. McGuigan MA: A two-year review of salicylate deaths in Ontario. *Arch Intern Med* 147:510, 1987.
52. Notarianni L: A reassessment of the treatment of salicylate poisoning. *Drug Saf* 7:292, 1992.
53. Winters RW, White JS, Hughes MC, et al: Disturbances of acid base equilibrium in salicylate intoxication. *Pediatrics* 23:260, 1959.
54. Thisted B, Krantz T, Shrom J, et al: Acute salicylate poisoning in 177 consecutive patients treated in ICU. *Acta Anaesthesiol Scand* 31:312, 1987.
55. Chapman BJ, Proudfoot AT: Adult salicylate poisoning: deaths and outcome in patients with high plasma salicylate concentrations. *Q J Med* 72:699, 1989.
56. Brubacher JR, Hoffman RS: Salicylism from topical salicylate: review of the literature. *Clin Toxicol* 34:431, 1996.
57. Watson JE, Tagupa ET: Suicide attempt by means of aspirin enema. *Ann Pharmacother* 28:467, 1994.
58. Chan TY: The risk of severe salicylate poisoning following the ingestion of topical medicaments or aspirin. *Postgrad Med J* 72:109, 1996.
59. Clark JH, Wilson WG: A 16-day-old breast-fed infant with metabolic acidosis caused by salicylate. *Clin Pediatr* 20:53, 1981.
60. Palatnick W, Tenebein M: Aspirin poisoning during pregnancy: increased fetal sensitivity. *Am J Perinatol* 15:39, 1998.
61. Buck ML, Grebe TA, Bond GR: Toxic reaction to salicylate in a newborn infant: similarities to neonatal sepsis. *J Pediatr* 122:955, 1993.

62. Yip L, Dart RC, Gabow PA: Concepts and controversies in salicylate toxicity. *Emerg Med Clin North Am* 12:351, 1994.
63. Leventhal LJ, Kuritsky L, Ginsberg R, et al: Salicylate-induced rhabdomyolysis. *Am J Emerg Med* 7:409, 1989.
64. Done AK: Aspirin overdosage: incidence, diagnosis and management. *Pediatrics* 62[Suppl]:890, 1978.
65. Leatherman JW, Schmitz PG: Fever, hyperdynamic shock, and multiple system organ failure. *Chest* 100:1391, 1991.
66. Montgomery H, Porter JC, Bradley RD: Salicylate intoxication causing a severe systemic inflammatory response and rhabdomyolysis. *Am J Emerg Med* 12:531, 1994.
67. Heffner JE, Sahn SA: Salicylate-induced pulmonary edema. *JAMA* 95:405, 1981.
68. Berk WA, Anderson JC: Salicylate-associated asystole: report of two cases. *Am J Med* 86:505, 1989.
69. Kent K, Ganetsky M, Cohen J, et al: Non-fatal ventricular dysrhythmias associated with severe salicylate toxicity. *Clin Toxicol* 46:297–299, 2008.
70. Nigogi SK, Rieders R: Salicylate poisoning: differences in tissue levels and distribution between children and adults. *Eur J Toxicol* 2:234, 1969.
71. Anderson RJ, Potts DE, Gabow PA: Unrecognized adult salicylate intoxication. *Ann Intern Med* 85:745, 1976.
72. Vale JA, Meredith TS: Acute poisoning due to non-steroidal anti-inflammatory drugs: clinical features and management. *Med Toxicol* 1:12, 1986.
73. Court H, Volans GN: Poisoning after overdose with nonsteroidal anti-inflammatory drugs. *Adverse Drug React Acute Poison Rev* 3:1, 1984.
74. Forrester MB. Celecoxib exposures reported to Texas poison control centres from 1999 to 2004. *Hum Exp Toxicol* 25:261–266, 2006.
75. Balali-Mood M, Proudfoot AT, Critchley JAJH, et al: Mefenamic acid overdose. *Lancet* 1:1354, 1981.
76. Berlinger WG, Spector R, Flanigan MJ: Hemoperfusion for phenylbutazone poisoning. *Ann Intern Med* 96:334, 1982.
77. Strong JE, Wilson J, Douglas JF, et al: Phenylbutazone self-poisoning treated by charcoal haemoperfusion. *Anaesthesia* 34:1038, 1979.
78. Virji MA, Venkataraman SK, Lower DR, et al: Role of laboratory in the management of phenylbutazone poisoning. *Clin Toxicol* 41:1013–1024, 2003.
79. Hall AH, Smolinske SC, Conrad FL, et al: Ibuprofen overdose: 126 cases. *Ann Emerg Med* 15:1308, 1986.
80. Ritter A, Eskin B: Ibuprofen overdose presenting with severe agitation and hypothermia. *Am J Emerg Med* 16:549, 1998.
81. Easley RB, Altemeier WA: Central nervous system manifestations of an ibuprofen overdose reversed by naloxone. *Pediatric Emerg Care* 16:39, 2000.
82. Oker EE, Hermann L, Baum CR, et al: Serious toxicity in a young child due to ibuprofen. *Acad Emerg Med* 7:821, 2000.
83. Seifert SA, Brownstein AC, McGuire T: Massive ibuprofen ingestion with survival. *Clin Toxicol* 38:55, 2000.
84. Lee CY, Finkler A: Acute intoxication due to ibuprofen overdose. *Pathol Lab Med* 110:747, 1986.
85. Kim J, Gazarian M, Verjee Z: Acute renal insufficiency in ibuprofen overdose. *Pediatr Emerg Care* 11:107, 1995.
86. Sanders LR: Exercise-induced acute renal failure associated with ibuprofen, hydrochlorothiazide, and triamterene. *J Am Soc Nephrol* 5:2020, 1995.
87. Mattana J, Perinbasekar S, Brod-Miller C: Near-fatal but reversible acute renal failure after massive ibuprofen ingestion. *Am J Med Sci* 313:117, 1997.
88. Barry WS, Meinzinger MM, Howse CR: Ibuprofen overdose and exposure in utero: results from a postmarketing voluntary reporting system. *Am J Med* 77:35, 1984.
89. Court H, Streete P, Volans GN: Acute poisoning with ibuprofen. *Hum Toxicol* 2:381, 1983.
90. Hall AH, Smolinske SC, Kulig KW, et al: Ibuprofen overdose: a prospective study. *West J Med* 148:653, 1988.
91. Bond GR, Curry SC, Arnold-Capell PA, et al: Generalized seizures and metabolic acidosis after ketoprofen overdose. *Vet Hum Toxicol* 31:369, 1989.
92. Martinez R, Smith DW, Frankel LR: Severe metabolic acidosis after acute naproxen sodium ingestion. *Ann Emerg Med* 18:1102, 1989.
93. Woodhouse KW, Wynne H: The pharmacokinetics of non-steroidal anti-inflammatory drugs in the elderly. *Clin Pharmacokinet* 12:111, 1987.
94. Duffens KR, Smilkstein MJ, Bessen HA, et al: Falsely elevated salicylate levels due to diflunisal overdose. *J Emerg Med* 5:499, 1987.
95. Hoffman RJ, Nelson LS, Hoffman RS: Use of ferric chloride to identify salicylate-containing products. *Clin Toxicol* 40:547, 2002.
96. Bailey RB, Jones SR: Chronic salicylate intoxication: a common cause of morbidity in the elderly. *J Am Geriatr Soc* 37:556, 1989.
97. Chalasani N, Roman J, Jurado RL: Systemic inflammatory response syndrome caused by chronic salicylate intoxication. *South Med J* 89:479, 1996.
98. Quint PA, Allman FD: Differentiation of chronic salicylism for Reye's syndrome. *Pediatrics* 74:1117, 1984.
99. Osterloh J, Cunningham W, Dixon A, et al: Biochemical relationships between Reye's and Reye's-like metabolic and toxicological syndromes. *Med Toxicol Adverse Drug Exp* 4:272, 1989.
100. Wason S, Dalsey W, Billmire ME: Play-Doh in the gastrointestinal tract: modify CHIP to CHIPPED. *Am J Dis Child* 139:1149, 1985.
101. Greenberg MI, Hendrickson RG, Hoffman M: Deleterious effects of endotracheal intubation in salicylate poisoning. *Ann Emerg Med* 41:583, 2003.
102. Thurston J, Pollock PG, Warren SK, et al: Reduced brain glucose with normal plasma glucose in salicylate poisoning. *J Clin Invest* 49:2130, 1970.
103. Juurlink DN, McGuigan MA: Gastrointestinal decontamination for enteric-coated aspirin overdose: what to do depends on who you ask. *J Toxicol Clin Toxicol* 38:465, 2000.
104. Curtis RA, Barone J, Giacon N: Efficacy of ipecac and activated charcoal/cathartic: prevention of salicylate absorption in a simulated overdose. *Arch Intern Med* 144:48, 1984.
105. Filippone G, Fish SS, Laconture PG, et al: Reversible adsorption (desorption) of aspirin from activated charcoal. *Arch Intern Med* 147:1390, 1987.
106. Burton GT, Bayer MJ, Barron L, et al: Comparison of activated charcoal and gastric lavage in the prevention of aspirin absorption. *J Emerg Med* 1:411, 1984.
107. Kirshenbaum LA, Mathews SC, Sitar DS, et al: Whole-bowel irrigation versus activated charcoal for the ingestion of modified-release pharmaceuticals. *Clin Pharmacol Ther* 46:264, 1989.
108. Hillman RJ, Prescott LF: Treatment of salicylate poisoning with repeated activated charcoal. *BMJ* 291:1472, 1985.
109. Ho JL, Tierney MG, Dickinson GE: An elevation of the effect of repeated doses of oral activated charcoal on salicylate elimination. *J Clin Pharmacol* 29:366, 1989.
110. Kirshenbaum LA, Matthew SC, Sitar DS, et al: Does multiple-dose charcoal therapy enhance salicylate excretion? *Arch Intern Med* 150:1281, 1990.
111. Mayer AL, Sitar DS, Tenenbein M: Multiple-dose charcoal and whole bowel irrigation do not increase clearance of absorbed salicylate. *Arch Intern Med* 152:393, 1992.
112. Barone JA, Raia JJ, Huang YC: Evaluation of the effects of multiple-dose activated charcoal on the absorption of orally administered salicylate in a simulated toxic ingestion model. *Ann Emerg Med* 17:34, 1988.
113. Johnson D, Eppler J, Giesbrecht E, et al: Effect of multiple-dose activated charcoal on the clearance of high-dose intravenous aspirin in a porcine model. *Ann Emerg Med* 26:569, 1995.
114. Keller RE, Schwab RA, Krenzelok EP: Contribution of sorbitol combined with activated charcoal in prevention of salicylate absorption. *Ann Emerg Med* 19:654, 1990.
115. Gren J, Woolf A: Hypermagnesemia associated with catharsis in a salicylate-intoxicated patient with anorexia nervosa. *Ann Emerg Med* 18:200, 1989.
116. Prescott LF, Balali-Mood M, Critchley JAJH, et al: Diuresis or urinary alkalinization for salicylate poisoning? *BMJ* 285:1383, 1982.
117. Winchester JF, Gelfand MC, Helliwell M, et al: Extracorporeal treatment of salicylate or acetaminophen poisoning: is there a role? *Arch Intern Med* 141:370, 1981.
118. Coppack SW, Higgins CS: Algorithm for modified alkaline diuresis in salicylate poisoning. *BMJ* 289:1452, 1984.
119. Elenbaas RM: Critical review of forced alkaline diuresis in acute salicylism. *Crit Care Q* 3:89, 1982.
120. Robin ED, Davis RP, Rees SB: Salicylate intoxication with special reference to the development of hypokalemia. *Am J Med* 26:869, 1959.
121. Lawson AAH, Proudfoot AT, Brown SS, et al: Forced diuresis in the treatment of acute salicylate poisoning in adults. *Q J Med* 38:31, 1969.
122. Hill JB: Experimental salicylate poisoning: observations on the effects of altering blood pH on tissue and plasma salicylate concentrations. *Pediatrics* 47:658, 1971.
123. Sweeney K, Chapron D, Brandt L, et al: Toxic interaction between acetazolamide and salicylate: case reports and a pharmacokinetic explanation. *Clin Pharmacol Ther* 40:518, 1986.
124. Yip L, Jastremski MS, Dart RD: Salicylate intoxication. *J Intensive Care Med* 12:66, 1997.
125. Spritz N, Fahey TJ, Thompson DD, et al: The use of extracorporeal hemodialysis in the treatment of salicylate intoxication in a 2-year-old child. *Pediatrics* 24:540, 1959.
126. Jacobsen O, Wiik-Larsen E, Bredesen JE: Haemodialysis or haemoperfusion in severe salicylate poisoning? *Hum Toxicol* 7:161, 1988.
127. Goodman JW, Goldfarb DS: The role of continuous renal replacement therapy in the treatment of poisoning. *Semin Dialysis* 19:402–407, 2006.
128. Schlegel RJ, Altstatt LB, Canales L, et al: Peritoneal dialysis for severe salicylism: an evaluation of indications and results. *J Pediatr* 69:553, 1966.
129. Muhlebach S, Steger P, Conen D, et al: Successful therapy of salicylate poisoning using glycine and activated charcoal. *Schweizer Med Wochen J Suisse Med* 126:2127, 1996.
130. Neuvonen PJ, Elonen E: Effect of activated charcoal on absorption and elimination of phenobarbitone, carbamazepine, and phenylbutazone in man. *Eur J Clin Pharmacol* 17:51, 1980.

CHAPTER 132 ■ ENVENOMATIONS

ROBERT L. NORRIS

"Their supreme arrogance, developed over millions of years as masters of their environment, commands respect out of all proportions to their size" [1].

Although made in reference to snakes, this statement could easily apply to any of the vast numbers of venomous creatures on the planet. Few areas of medicine are immersed in such controversy and misperception as the management of envenomations. This chapter provides guidance for the evaluation and management of bites and stings of venomous snakes, spiders, and scorpions indigenous to North America. While the general principles of management of envenomations outlined here may be applicable to other regions of the world, specific approaches, such as indications for and types and doses of antivenoms, vary by region, and local experts should be consulted for advice.

SNAKE ENVENOMATION

All of the terrestrial American venomous snakes belong to one of two families: Viperidae (subfamily Crotalinae, or pit vipers) and Elapidae (or coral snakes). Venomous snakes are native to every state of the United States except Alaska, Hawaii, and Maine.

Pit Viper Envenomation

At least 99% of venomous snakebites in the United States are inflicted by pit vipers [2]. The pit vipers of North America include the rattlesnakes (genera *Crotalus* and *Sistrurus*), and the cottonmouth water moccasins, copperheads, and cantils (*Agkistrodon* spp). These snakes are characterized by paired, pitlike heat receptors (foveal organs) located on the anterolateral aspects of the head. These receptors aid the snake in aiming its strike and likely function in determining the quantity of venom to be injected [3,4].

Pit viper venoms contain numerous enzymatic components and a number of nonenzymatic, low-molecular-weight polypeptides [3–5]. Venom compositions vary not only from species to species, but from snake to snake within a species, and even in an individual snake depending on its age, size, health, and other factors [3,4]. In general, the most serious envenomations in North America are caused by the rattlesnakes (particularly *Crotalus* spp), with cottonmouth water moccasin (*Agkistrodon piscivorus* ssp) bites being less severe and copperhead (*A. contortrix* ssp) bites causing predominantly local findings with little serious systemic toxicity.

The major enzymes in pit viper venoms include hyaluronidase (spreading factor), phospholipase A (responsible for cell membrane disruption), and various proteases (causing local tissue destruction) [4,5]. Venom metalloproteinases, termed *disintegrins*, result in disruption of vascular integrity [6]. Despite the impressive toxicity of such enzymes, the nonenzymatic, low-molecular-weight polypeptide fractions appear to be up to 20 times more lethal, on a weight-for-weight basis, than crude venom [7]. The toxicity of pit viper venom is enhanced by release of various autopharmacologic compounds from damaged tissue (e.g., histamine, bradykinin, and serotonin) [4].

Clinical Manifestations

Envenomated patients typically experience moderate-to-severe pain at the bite site within 5 to 10 minutes. The pain is often described as burning and may radiate along the bitten extremity. Swelling at the bite site soon follows and may progress along the entire extremity within hours. There is often local ecchymosis because of disruption of blood vessels. A persistent bloody effluent from the wound suggests the presence of snake venom anticoagulants. Rapid lymphatic absorption of venom may lead to impressive, early lymphangitis and regional adenopathy [3].

Within the first 24 to 36 hours, hemorrhagic bullae or serum-filled vesicles may develop at the bite site and along the bitten extremity. These are less common in bites treated early with adequate amounts of antivenom [4,7]. Petechiae or purpura may also be present.

Systemic manifestations of pit viper envenomation can involve virtually any organ system. Nausea and vomiting are common and may appear early with severe bites [7]. Weakness, diaphoresis, fever and chills, dizziness, and syncope may also occur [3,4]. Some patients experience a minty, rubbery, or metallic taste in their mouth and hypersalivation [4,7]. Muscle fasciculations or paresthesias of the scalp, face, tongue, or digits indicate a moderate-to-severe envenomation. Systemic coagulopathy can lead to bleeding at any anatomic site, including the gastrointestinal, respiratory, genitourinary, and central nervous systems, although clinically significant bleeding is uncommon following bites in North America [3,7].

Alterations in heart rate and blood pressure may occur. Early hypotension is usually due to pooling of blood in the pulmonary and splanchnic vascular beds, whereas delayed shock is due to blood loss, third spacing of intravascular volume, and hemolysis [3,4,8]. Pulmonary edema can occur in severe envenomations, and is secondary to disruption of pulmonary vasculature intimal linings and pooling of pulmonary blood [3,5].

Multifactorial renal failure may occur, but is uncommon. Contributing factors include hypotension; hemoglobin, myoglobin, and fibrin deposition in renal tubules; and direct venom nephrotoxicity [3,7].

Muscle weakness may be seen after bites by some rattlesnakes that possess phospholipase A_2 neurotoxins in their venoms, such as the eastern diamondback rattlesnake (*Crotalus adamanteus*) [9] or some specimens of the Mohave rattlesnake (*Crotalus scutulatus*) [10]. Neuromuscular respiratory failure is rare, but can occur in severe bites by the Mohave rattlesnake in certain geographic locations [7].

Snake venoms do not appear to cross the blood–brain barrier to any significant extent, and rare findings such as seizures and coma are secondary to hypotension, hypoxia, or intracranial bleeding [2].

Diagnostic Evaluation

Important aspects of the history include details of the incident (such as type and size of snake if known, time and number of bites, and methods of first aid applied) and the patient's medical

TABLE 132.1

CLINICAL GRADING SCALE AND RECOMMENDED CROFAB® DOSAGES FOR NORTH AMERICAN PIT VIPER ENVENOMATION[a]

Severity grade	Nonenvenomation	Mild	Moderate	Severe
Fang marks	±	+	+	+
Pain	None	Mild to moderate	Severe	Severe
Edema (proximal extent)	None	Minimal (0–15 cm)	Moderate (15–30 cm)	Severe (>30 cm)
Erythema	None	+	+	+
Ecchymosis	None	±	+	+
Systemic signs or symptoms	None	None	Mild	Moderate to severe
Laboratory values	Normal	Normal	Mildly abnormal	Very abnormal
Initial CroFab dose (number of vials)[b]	0	0 (if no progression) 4–6 (if progressing)	4–6	6[c]

[a]Not applicable to coral snake envenomations or envenomation by snakes outside of North America.
[b]CroFab® (BTG International Inc., West Conshohocken, PA)—If findings of envenomation progress during the first hour following the initial dose, the dose should be repeated. Once stabilization occurs, two vials are given every 6 hours for three additional doses (see text).
[c]Larger doses may be required in some cases with acute, life-threatening envenomation.

history (including any prior snakebites, medications, allergies, and tetanus immunization status).

Pit viper envenomation is a true emergency with potential for multisystem involvement. The severity of the bite must be assessed, and the clinical severity grading scale in Table 132.1 may be useful in evaluating most pit viper bites [4]. Approximately 20% of bites by U.S. pit vipers result in no envenomation ("dry bites") [4,7,11]. It must be understood, however, that severity can progress rapidly, and the patient must be frequently reevaluated for a worsening clinical condition. Good clinical judgment is more important than overreliance on grading scales. Consultation with an authority in the area of toxinology is prudent.

Puncture-wound patterns can be misleading in the diagnosis of snakebite. Occasionally, there is only a single puncture wound or many tiny punctures [12]. A dry bite may or may not have fang puncture marks, but there is no more pain than would be expected from simple puncture wounds. Envenomation is confirmed by the presence of local tissue effects (particularly progressive swelling), systemic effects, and/or laboratory abnormalities.

Essential laboratory studies include a complete blood cell count, serum electrolytes, blood urea nitrogen, creatinine, prothrombin time or international normalized ratio, fibrinogen, fibrin degradation products, and urine analysis. Blood for type and screening should also be sent for evaluation as soon as possible as direct venom effects and antivenom effects may interfere with this process later [13]. Also helpful are creatine phosphokinase as a measure of muscle damage and intracompartmental pressure measurements in patients with suspected compartment syndrome. Obtain a chest radiograph, arterial blood gases, and an electrocardiogram as clinically indicated.

Occasionally, the history and diagnosis may be unclear, especially in children [14]. When patients present without having seen a snake and have no findings other than puncture wounds and mild pain, the differential diagnosis includes a dry bite, bite by other animal or arthropod (e.g., nonvenomous snake, centipede, or spider), and puncture wounds from inanimate objects (e.g., thorns).

Management

First-aid efforts are best limited to reassuring the victim, immobilizing and splinting the extremity at heart level, and transporting the victim as quickly as possible to a hospital.

Previously recommended first-aid measures including incision, suction, constriction bands pressure immobilization, tourniquets, packing of the extremity in ice, or application of electric shocks should be avoided as they are ineffective and may result in further complications [15–17].

Two large-bore intravenous (IV) lines infusing normal saline should be established, preferably in sites other than the bitten extremity, and blood work sent to the laboratory. Continuous cardiac and pulse oximetry monitoring are indicated, and oxygen is administered if hemoglobin saturation is low or if the patient is experiencing any respiratory distress. Any devices applied in the field in an attempt to limit venom spread should be left in place until an IV line is established.

Management of significant pit viper envenomation centers on the judicious use of an appropriate antivenom. In North America, antivenom therapy is indicated for victims with progressive local tissue findings or systemic abnormalities (significant systemic symptoms or signs, or laboratory abnormalities [e.g., paresthesias, hypotension, prolongation of prothrombin time or international normalized ratio, hypofibrinogenemia, or thrombocytopenia]) (see Fig. 132.1). Controversy exists, however, on the use of antivenom for copperhead (*A. contortrix*) bites presenting with progressive soft-tissue swelling in the absence of systemic abnormalities. Given that most such bites do well with conservative therapy alone [7], the cost–benefit ratio of giving antivenom in these cases is currently unclear and requires further research [18,19].

Antivenom Administration

If possible, informed consent should be obtained before antivenom administration. Antivenom should be administered in a closely monitored setting. Epinephrine and endotracheal intubation equipment should be immediately available at the bedside during antivenom administration, and a physician should be in attendance to observe and manage any acute adverse drug effects that may develop.

In the United States there is currently a single commercially available antivenom for pit viper bites—CroFab® Crotalidae Polyvalent Immune Fab, Ovine (BTG International Inc., West Conshohocken, PA). This antiserum contains purified Fab immunoglobulin fragments from sheep immunized with one of four different pit viper venoms. It comes in a lyophilized state and is effective against all North American pit vipers.

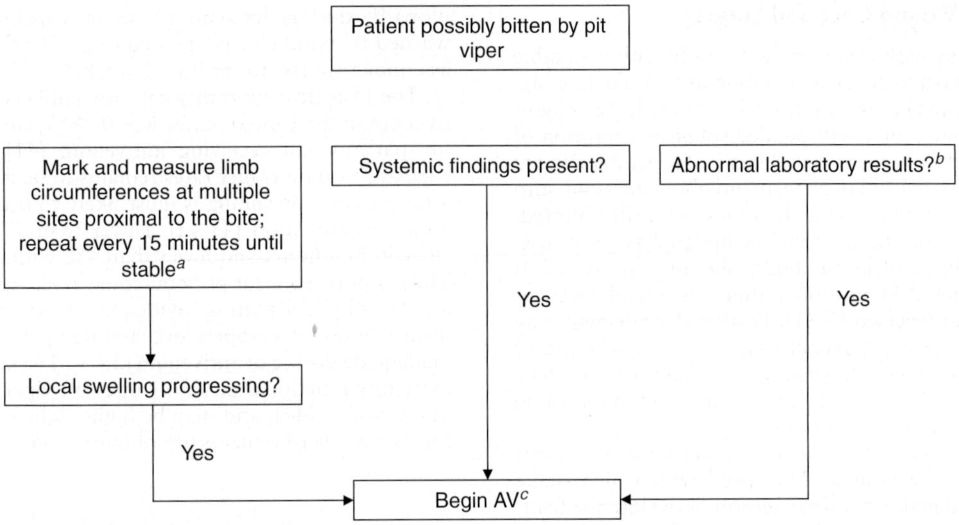

FIGURE 132.1. Guidelines for beginning antivenom therapy for victims of pit viper bite in the United States (see text for details). [a]Keep extremity at heart level, being careful to differentiate redistribution of edema (with changing limb position) from progression of severity of swelling. [b]Repeat normal lab work every hour for 4–6 hours until AV is started or the decision is made that AV is not necessary (i.e., the bite resulted in no envenomation or a mild, nonprogressive envenomation). [c]Abnormal coagulation studies may not return to normal for 4–6 hours after antivenom administration—time necessary for the body to replete coagulation factors after neutralization of venom. AV, antivenom.

Antivenom should be started as soon as possible after indications for administration are met. Although there are no defined end points in terms of time or dosage for when to withhold antivenom, antivenom is beneficial for treating only findings directly related to continued presence of unbound venom in the circulation (e.g., ongoing coagulopathy). It is ineffective in reversing end-organ damage that has resulted from prior venom effects (e.g., renal failure). The efficacy of antivenom in preventing local wound necrosis is limited, as it cannot reverse local cellular damage once it has been initiated by rapidly acting venom enzymes and nonenzymatic polypeptides [14,20,21]. Any ability to reduce necrosis depends on early administration.

Dosing of CroFab® is based on severity of the bite (see Table 132.1), not on age or size of the patient. The initial dose is four to six vials for patients with signs or symptoms of systemic toxicity or evidence of progressive local venom effects. Each CroFab® vial should be reconstituted with 10 mL of warm sterile water or saline. The total dose to be administered is diluted in 250 mL of crystalloid and infused over 1 hour (starting slowly at the onset of infusion and gradually increasing the rate). During the hour after the initial dose is completed, the patient is monitored for further progression of local effects and systemic symptoms, and laboratory studies are repeated [13]. The starting dose of CroFab® is repeated if venom effects continue to progress. This pattern is continued until the patient stabilizes. Coagulation studies may not normalize after the initial dose, as time is required for repletion of coagulation factors after venom neutralization, but they should show evidence of improvement [22,23]. After stabilization, two vials of CroFab® are administered every 6 hours for three additional doses. Further doses may be needed at the physician's discretion.

Adverse effects of antivenoms, as heterologous serum products, are divided into three major groups: acute allergic and nonallergic anaphylaxis, and delayed serum sickness. Acute reactions most commonly manifest with hives and/or bronchospasm [24], though hypotension and angioedema can also occur. Serum sickness is characterized by pruritus, fever, arthralgias, lymphadenopathy, and malaise, which can occur 1 to 2 weeks after antivenom therapy [3]. The incidence of acute reactions to CroFab® is approximately 15% and serum sickness occurs in approximately 3% of patients [25]. Management of acute reactions centers on rapid diagnosis, temporarily halting the infusion and treating with epinephrine, antihistamines, and steroids (see Chapter 194). Generally, once the reaction is controlled, the antivenom infusion can be restarted, possibly in a more dilute state and at a slower rate. Serum sickness is relatively benign and easily treated with steroids, antihistamines, and nonsteroidal anti-inflammatory drugs until symptoms resolve [26]. Most cases do well with oral prednisone (1 to 2 mg per kg per day) until symptoms resolve, followed by a taper over another week.

Supportive Measures

Venom-induced hypotension should be treated with antivenom and volume expansion. If organ perfusion fails to respond promptly with crystalloid infusion (1 to 2 L in an adult and 20 to 40 mL per kg in a child), administration of albumin is advisable as this agent is likely to stay in the leaky vascular system for longer periods of time [4,8]. Pressors should be used as a last resort [4].

Although pit viper envenomation can result in significant coagulopathies, the incidence of clinically significant bleeding in the United States is low [13,27]. Management of coagulopathy in patients with evidence of clinically significant bleeding, other than microscopic hematuria or minor gingival bleeding, may require administration of packed red blood cells, platelets, fresh-frozen plasma, and/or cryoprecipitate [4,28]. There is limited experience using recombinant factor VIIa for severe coagulopathy following rattlesnake bite [29]. It is important to begin antivenom therapy before the infusion of such products to avoid adding fuel to an unabated consumptive coagulopathy.

Therapy to prevent acute renal failure includes ensuring adequate hydration and monitoring urinary output. Hemoglobinuria and myoglobinuria are treated in standard fashion. If renal failure occurs, dialysis may be required, although it does not remove circulating venom components [4,7].

Although steroids are useful in the management of adverse reactions to antivenom (see previous discussion), there is no role for them in the primary management of snake envenomation.

Wound Care and Surgery

Wound care begins with cleaning the bite site with a suitable germicidal solution and covering it with a dry, sterile dressing. As soon as antivenom has been started, if indicated, the extremity should be elevated in a well-padded splint in a position of function with cotton between the digits [3,4]. Antibiotics are unnecessary unless field management involved incisions into the bite site [30] or the wound becomes clinically infected. Tetanus immunization status should be updated as necessary.

Intact hemorrhagic blebs and bullae should be protected. If ruptured, they should be unroofed after any attendant coagulopathy has been reversed [7,31]. Further debridement may be necessary if there is significant tissue necrosis. The use of hyperbaric oxygen therapy to treat these wounds has yet to be fully studied [4,32]. Physical therapy is important in returning the extremity to functional capacity.

The role of surgery in the primary management of pit viper envenomation is very limited. The speed with which snake venom is absorbed makes routine excision of the bite site fruitless [33], and routine exploration of the site does nothing to mitigate systemic effects of venom, may worsen the overall outcome by adding surgical trauma, and prolongs hospitalization [4].

The incidence of compartment syndrome after snake envenomation appears low despite the frequently impressive local findings of bitten extremities [34,35]. Myonecrosis that occurs is usually due to direct venom effects and rarely vascular compromise from elevated intracompartmental pressures [21,34,35]. In combined series of nearly 2,000 victims of pit viper envenomation, only 4 patients required fasciotomy; each of these patients received inappropriate ice treatment or inadequate antivenom [34,35]. If there is concern about an impending compartment syndrome, intracompartmental pressures should be checked using any standard technique. If pressures exceed 30 to 40 mm Hg and remain elevated for more than 1 hour despite appropriate antivenom administration, limb elevation and possibly mannitol infusion (1 to 2 g per kg in a normotensive patient), fasciotomy may be required [35,36]. While some evidence suggests that fasciotomy may actually worsen local myonecrosis [37], unabated elevation of intracompartmental pressures can have disastrous effects, such as debilitating neuropathy [38], and fasciotomy may still be required. Whenever possible, informed consent should be obtained prior to proceeding with fasciotomy.

Disposition and Outcome

Patients with apparent dry bites can be discharged from the emergency department if they remain asymptomatic with normal laboratory values (repeated prior to discharge) after 8 hours of observation [39]. The envenomated patient can be discharged from the hospital when all venom effects have begun to resolve and when antivenom therapy is complete, which is usually within 48 hours after admission. At the time of discharge, every patient should have appropriate follow-up arranged for continued wound care and physical therapy, and should be warned about the symptoms of serum sickness. If such symptoms occur, the patient should seek medical care promptly.

Venom-induced coagulopathy and thrombocytopenia may recur anytime up to 14 days after the last dose of antivenom [40]. Therefore, patients should be followed closely for this phenomenon after discharge from the hospital. If there is evidence of clinically significant bleeding on follow-up or if the laboratory coagulopathy is severe, additional antivenom can be considered, although its efficacy at reversing delayed recurrence of coagulopathy appears to be reduced and the need to treat asymptomatic coagulopathy during recovery is controversial [22,23,40]. Nevertheless, patients who developed coagulopathy during the acute phase of envenomation should be warned to avoid elective procedures and risky activities (such as contact sports) for at least 2 weeks.

The historical mortality rate for patients treated with antivenom in the United States was 0.28%, compared to 2.61% for patients not receiving antivenom [41]. The impact of CroFab® on mortality rates remains to be determined. Death after pit viper poisoning is most likely to occur 6 to 48 hours after envenomation [41,42]. Fewer than 17% of deaths occur within 6 hours and fewer than 4% within 1 hour [41,42]. The major reasons for poor outcome in pit viper envenomation are delay in presentation, inadequate fluid resuscitation, inappropriate use of vasopressors, and delay in administration or inadequate dosing of antivenom [2,43]. The incidence of upper-extremity functional disability after pit viper envenomation is at least 32% [44], and may be higher when careful, objective functional measurements are obtained [45].

Coral Snake Envenomation

There are fewer than 100 coral snake bites reported in the United States each year [46]. The U.S. coral snakes include the eastern coral snake (*Micrurus fulvius*), the Texas coral snake (*Micrurus tener*), and the Sonoran coral snake (*Micruroides euryxanthus*). Mexico boasts 15 *Micrurus* species as well as the Sonoran coral snake [47]. Native U.S. coral snakes can be identified by a characteristic red, yellow, and black banding pattern, with the red and yellow bands contiguous and the bands completely encircling the body. This color pattern does not, however, reliably identify coral snakes south of Mexico City [48]. Coral snakes lack the pitlike heat-receptor organs of pit vipers. While only 40% of coral snake bites result in envenomation because of their much less effective venom-delivery mechanism (small fangs fixed in an upright position on the anterior maxillae) [4,49], it has been estimated that one large coral snake is capable of delivering enough venom to kill four to five humans [50,51]. In the United States, it appears that the severity of envenomation tends to be greatest with the eastern coral snake (*M. fulvius*), less with the Texas coral snake (*M. tener*) and least with the Sonoran coral snake (*Micrur. euryxanthus*) [4,52].

Clinical Manifestations

Coral snake venoms are primarily neurotoxic; low-molecular-weight polypeptides in the venom are capable of inducing nondepolarizing, postsynaptic blockade at neuromuscular junctions [3,53]. There are few local findings at the bite site, and the onset of systemic symptoms may be delayed for many hours [3,49,54]. Fang marks may be small and difficult to detect [55], with variable pain and little swelling at the site [54]. The patient may experience local paresthesias that may radiate proximally and be associated with muscle fasciculations [54,56]. The earliest systemic findings may include alteration of mental status [3,57]. Nausea and vomiting may occur, along with increased salivation [3,49]. Bulbar-type paralysis can occur as early as 90 minutes after the bite and progress to peripheral paralysis [4]. Findings may include extraocular muscle paresis, ptosis, pinpoint pupils, dysphagia, dysphonia, slurred speech, and laryngeal spasm [49,54,56]. Death from coral snake envenomation has been reported because of respiratory failure or cardiovascular collapse [4].

Diagnostic Evaluation

The important history is similar to that obtained in victims of pit viper bites. In areas where coral snakes coexist with harmless coral snake mimics, it is helpful if the color pattern of the offending snake can be recalled.

The clinical grading scale outlined for pit viper envenomation does not apply to coral snake bites because of the paucity of local findings and the potential delay in the onset of systemic symptoms [4]. There are no characteristic changes in routine laboratory tests in coral snake envenomation [2].

The differential diagnosis of coral snake envenomation is usually limited to bites by other brightly colored snakes, such as milk snakes (*Lampropeltis* sp). With these harmless coral snake mimics, the red and yellow bands are separated by black bands, and the bands do not completely encircle the body. The simple rhyme "red on yellow, kill a fellow; red on black, venom lack" is applicable only to snakes found north of Mexico City [48]. The remainder of the differential diagnosis is the same as for pit vipers.

Management

Rapid transportation to a hospital is of utmost priority following coral snake bites [2]. In Australia, where all native venomous snakes are elapid relatives of the coral snake, a potentially beneficial first-aid intervention is use of a pressure-immobilization wrap. In this technique, the entire bitten extremity is firmly wrapped with an elastic or crepe bandage and splinted [58]. The wrap is applied snuggly—as tightly as for a sprained ankle [58]—and it is important that the extremity be kept as immobile as possible and the patient carried to medical care [59]. One small animal study has demonstrated apparent benefit of the technique in prolonging survival following coral snake venom injection [60].

As with pit viper bites, attention is initially directed to the patient's airway, breathing, and circulatory status. Supplemental oxygen should be administered, cardiac and pulse oximetry monitoring established, and at least one IV line should be started. Impending respiratory failure is suggested by cyanosis, trismus, laryngeal or pharyngeal spasm, increased salivation, or any sign of cranial nerve paralysis [54]. If any of these findings is present, prophylactic intubation is indicated to prevent aspiration. Once the airway and respiratory status are addressed, a more complete physical examination is performed. Any swelling should be documented and observed for progression.

Antivenom Therapy

As with most venomous snakebites, definitive management of significant *Micrurus* bites should center on the use of appropriate antivenom. However, the only approved antivenom for coral snake bites in the U.S., Antivenin (*Micrurus fulvius*) (Wyeth Laboratories Inc., Marietta, PA) has been discontinued with remaining stocks due to expire in October 2011. It is possible that another pharmaceutical company may resume coral snake antivenom production for the U.S. Research into the use of an alternative foreign-produced antivenom for U.S. coral snake bites is also under way. (Updates on this topic can be obtained by contacting regional poison control centers.) If an effective coral snake antivenom is available, it should be administered in a monitored setting (with epinephrine available), in consultation with an expert in snake venom poisoning, and with informed consent if possible. Antivenom administration to any patient clearly bitten by a positively identified *Micrurus* specimen, even in the absence of signs or symptoms, has been recommended given that once signs or symptoms begin to appear, it may be difficult to reverse or halt their progression [49,54]. This is likely unnecessary, however, if the offending snake was a Texas coral snake (*M. tener*) [52].

There is no antivenom for the Sonoran coral snake (*Micruroides. euryxanthus*), but the venom of this snake is much less toxic, and there have been no reported deaths after its bite [4,57]. Management of any coral snake bite, in the absence of available antivenom, is entirely supportive. Airway protection and ventilatory support may be required for days following *Micrurus* bites [54], but with modern intensive care, the prognosis should be good nonetheless.

Wound Care

The wounds from a coral snake bite should be washed with a germicidal solution and tetanus prophylaxis updated as necessary. Prophylactic antibiotics are not indicated.

Disposition and Outcome

All patients with potential coral snake bites should be admitted to an intensive care unit for at least 24 hours for close monitoring regardless of symptoms or antivenom requirement [61]. The projected case-fatality rate in untreated cases is up to 10% [49]. Total resolution of all signs or symptoms (e.g., weakness) may take several weeks [54,56].

Exotic (Imported) Snake Envenomation

Exotic venomous snakes are commonly kept in zoos, museums, and sometimes by private individuals in "underground zoos." Occasionally, they may be inadvertently found in imported goods and produce. If the setting of a victim of exotic venomous snakebite, every effort should be made to correctly identify the snake. This can be done by contacting available zoo personnel or biologists. The treating physician should then call a regional poison control center for assistance (1-800-222-1222). These centers have access to a national listing of available sources of exotic antivenoms in stock in the United States. Antivenoms tend to be quite specific for the species against which they protect, and should be used only if there is clear evidence of their efficacy against the offending species. Sound supportive care, combined with an appropriate antivenom when available, should offer the best chances of an optimal outcome.

SPIDER ENVENOMATION

While many spiders are capable of biting humans, only two types are medically significant in North America: the widow spiders (*Latrodectus* sp) and the recluse spiders (*Loxosceles* sp).

Widow Spider Envenomation

Of five known species of widow spider in the United States, the black widows (*Latrodectus mactans*, *Latrodectus hesperus*, and *Latrodectus variolus*) are the best known [62]. The female black widow is dark black and oval shaped, with a characteristic ventral red, orange, or yellow (hourglass-shaped) marking on the abdomen. The body is approximately 1.5 cm long and the leg span up to 4 cm. The other two species in the United States are the red-legged widow or red widow (*Latrodectus bishopi*) and the brown widow (*Latrodectus geometricus*) [62]. Widow spiders are found in all of the 48 contiguous states and Hawaii [63], and are responsible for most of the very rare spider-related deaths in North America. Only the female is dangerous to humans; the male, a nondescript and much smaller brown spider, is incapable of delivering a bite through human skin [64].

The venom of all species of widow spiders is similar in composition and toxic effects [65]. The most deleterious venom component is alpha-latrotoxin, a potent neurotoxin that acts primarily at the neuromuscular junction [64]. The venom initially stimulates the release of neurotransmitters (acetylcholine, epinephrine, and norepinephrine) and then blocks neurotransmission by depleting synaptic vesicles [64–66]. It does not cause dermonecrosis or hemolysis [67].

Clinical Manifestations

The widow spider bite may be unnoticed by the patient or may be felt as a pinprick [65]. The bite site may be visible, with tiny fang marks approximately 1 mm apart, and the area may be slightly warm and blanched with a surrounding erythematous, indurated zone [68]. Swelling is minimal [69].

Significant symptoms usually appear 10 minutes to 2 hours after envenomation [42,68]. The most prominent symptom is pain. It begins at the bite site as a dull ache and spreads first to local muscle groups and then to larger regional muscle groups of the abdomen, back, chest, pelvis, and lower extremities. Muscle spasms and rigidity are classically present [68,70,71]. Spasms of abdominal musculature can mimic an acute abdomen, though rebound tenderness is absent. Chest muscle rigidity may produce respiratory distress [70,71]. The respiratory rate increases, and there may be associated tachycardia and hypertension. Pain severity typically peaks after several hours [72]. In patients at risk, the hypertension can lead to cerebrovascular accidents, exacerbation of congestive heart failure, and myocardial ischemia [64,65,73]. Cardiac dysrhythmias and priapism have been reported [68,74].

Associated signs or symptoms include diaphoresis, fever, headache, nausea and vomiting, restlessness and anxiety, periorbital edema, and skin rash [68,70]. Deep tendon reflexes may be increased [71].

Diagnostic Evaluation

The history surrounding a widow spider bite is confusing if a spider was not seen. A high index of suspicion should be maintained in patients presenting with compatible complaints. It is important to obtain a medical history, such as hypertension, pregnancy status, allergies, and tetanus immunization status. The physical examination entails a general screening with particular attention to the vital signs, which should be checked at frequent intervals. Close examination for a bite site may be productive.

There are no diagnostic changes in routine laboratory tests in widow spider envenomation. An elevation in white blood cell count and serum creatine phosphokinase values may be seen [75], and proteinuria has been reported [76]. An electrocardiogram and chest radiograph should be obtained as clinically indicated. A pregnancy test should be obtained in women of childbearing age as widow spider venom is a potent abortifacient.

The differential diagnosis includes envenomations by other arthropods, such as neurotoxic scorpions (see the section "Scorpion Envenomation"), and systemic disorders, such as acute rhabdomyolysis, heat cramps, heat stroke, neuroleptic malignant syndrome, tetanus, and strychnine poisoning. Various causes of abdominal pain and rigidity should be considered.

Management

Although there are no specific first-aid measures effective in widow spider bites, temporary application of ice to the bite site may reduce pain [64]. Adequate airway, respiration, and circulatory status should be ensured. After providing oxygen, cardiac and pulse oximetry monitoring, and starting an IV line, attention should be directed to alleviating painful muscle spasms. Although there are anecdotal reports of successful treatment of painful muscle spasms with IV calcium gluconate [69,70], larger case series have found it completely ineffective [62]. Similarly, methocarbamol has met with only limited anecdotal success [69]. Benzodiazepines and opioids can be administered in usual doses and are often most effective when administered in combination [62].

Hypertension usually responds to bed rest, muscle relaxants, analgesics, and sedation [64]. Specific antihypertensive agents can be used if necessary [64].

Antivenom

A specific, equine, whole-immunoglobulin widow spider antivenom, Antivenin (*L. mactans*) (manufactured by Merck & Co., Inc., West Point, PA) is effective regardless of which *Latrodectus* species is involved [77]. Indications for antivenom use remain controversial [78], but are generally accepted to include a patient who is severely envenomated, is pregnant or in labor, or has a history of cardiovascular disease or other major medical problems and evidence of significant envenomation despite benzodiazepine and opioid therapy [68,71,72]. Antivenom is very effective in relieving pain, but its use solely for this purpose is controversial [69,79]. *Latrodectus* antivenoms manufactured by other countries appear to be effective in managing bites by widow spiders native to the United States [80,81].

As with snake antivenom administration, informed consent should be obtained and antivenom administered in a monitored setting with epinephrine available at the bedside. Prior to antivenom administration, the patient can be premedicated with IV antihistamines (H_1 and H_2 blockers), though the benefit of such an approach is unproven. The antivenom can be given intravenously (one reconstituted vial further diluted in 50 to 100 mL of normal saline, administered over 30 minutes) or intramuscularly (one reconstituted vial in the anterolateral thigh) [82], with the physician in immediate attendance to observe for any sign of adverse drug events. The IV route is preferred if the patient is in shock or younger than 12 years [82]. The dosage is the same for children [64,70]. One vial is generally adequate, but a second vial can be administered if necessary [70,72]. Signs or symptoms should completely resolve within a few hours of antivenom administration [70,72].

The types of adverse drug events seen with widow spider antivenom are the same as for snake antivenoms, but the risk of serum sickness may be less because of the smaller total amount of foreign protein infused [72].

The clinical course of most patients with widow spider envenomation is benign [68], but significant pain and spasms can persist for 2 to 3 days [72,79]. Most healthy adults do well with supportive measures and adequate administration of parenteral benzodiazepines and opioids [68].

Disposition and Outcome

Patients can be discharged from the hospital when signs or symptoms of envenomation have been significantly controlled, though it may be best to admit and observe younger children. Patients should be given analgesics and muscle relaxants, prescribed bed rest, and instructed to return if they worsen. The mortality rate from widow spider envenomation in the United States is less than 1% [65,68]. Recovery from widow spider envenomation may sometimes be slow, with weakness, fatigue, paresthesias, headache, and insomnia persisting for several months [64].

Recluse Spider Envenomation

Of the 13 species of recluse spider (*Loxosceles* spp) found in the United States [83], the brown recluse (*Loxosceles reclusa*) is best known [84]. It is characterized by a violin-shaped marking on the dorsal aspect of the cephalothorax and three pairs of eyes, in contrast to the four pairs found in most spiders. The adult body is 10 to 15 mm long and the legs span 2 to 3 cm. Both the male and female spiders are dangerous [72].

The brown recluse is found throughout the southern, south-central, and midwestern United States; other species are found in the western part of the country [62]. While recluse spiders may cause severe dermonecrosis (necrotic arachnidism), the majority of bites actually result in insignificant lesions [85].

The venoms of the different species of recluse spider have similar toxic effects [86]. They contain a number of different proteins, most of which demonstrate enzymatic activity [87]. Sphingomyelinase D is likely responsible for the venom's cytotoxic and hemolytic effects [88–90]. Venom activation of the complement cascade induces a series of autopharmacologic changes that amplify toxicity to a variable degree in victims [91].

The cutaneous changes seen after a recluse spider bite are initiated by venom-induced endothelial damage in small dermal vessels that become occluded with microthrombi, producing vascular stasis and infarction [92]. Polymorphonuclear leukocytes are attracted to the site via a chemotactic response and propagate the inflammatory, necrotic reaction [92,93]. Accumulation of polymorphonuclear leukocytes at the site appears to be a vital component of the dermonecrotic response and is related to complement activation [93].

Clinical Manifestations

The clinical course of recluse spider envenomation varies from a mild temporary irritation at the bite site to a rare, severe, potentially fatal outcome [84]. The bite is occasionally felt as a mild stinging sensation, although it may go completely unnoticed [94]. During the next several hours, there may be pruritus, tingling, mild swelling, and redness or blanching at the bite site [95]. Variable degrees of local pain and tenderness due to local vasospasm and ischemia occur within 2 to 8 hours [95,96]. At 12 to 18 hours, a small central vesicle (clear or hemorrhagic) often develops at the site and is surrounded by an irregular zone of erythema or ecchymosis and edema, which may have a distinct gravitational distribution around the central lesion [97]. The vesicle ruptures, and the erythema gives way to violaceous discoloration [96]. In 5 to 7 days, the bite site undergoes aseptic necrosis (i.e., dry, gangrenous slough), with the center becoming depressed below the normal level of the skin, and a black eschar forms. The eschar later sloughs, leaving an open ulcer that heals in weeks to months [96]. Bites to fatty regions of the body tend to be more severe, with undermining of the skin and more extensive scarring [96]. Necrosis rarely involves deeper structures such as nerves, muscles, tendons, or ligaments [98]. Lesions destined to develop significant necrosis usually demonstrate early evidence of local ischemia [95].

Systemic (viscerocutaneous) loxoscelism is rare, but can be rapidly progressive and severe, particularly in children [72]. Systemic symptoms generally start 24 to 72 hours after the bite and occasionally occur before cutaneous findings become impressive [99]. Symptoms are often flulike, with fever, chills, headache, malaise, weakness, nausea and vomiting, myalgias, and arthralgias [96]. Hemolytic anemia with hemoglobinemia, hemoglobinuria, jaundice, thrombocytopenia, disseminated intravascular coagulation, acute renal failure, seizures, and coma have been reported [72]. The severity of systemic symptoms is directly related to the quantity of venom deposited, but does not necessarily correlate with the severity of cutaneous changes [97].

Diagnostic Evaluation

It is rare for a victim of a *Loxosceles* bite to see the offending spider because the bite is relatively painless and a large percentage of bites occur while the victim is asleep [85]. Because the spider is rarely available for identification, determining the cause of early lesions is difficult [97], and the diagnosis of spider bite is usually presumptive. The working diagnosis should be cutaneous necrosis if the precise cause is unknown and necrotic arachnidism if a biting spider was seen but not identified.

An examination for evidence of systemic loxoscelism should be performed. The severity of any lesion present should be assessed and any evidence of secondary infection noted. There are no characteristic changes in routine laboratory tests in recluse spider envenomation. In patients with severe envenomation, laboratory studies should include a complete blood cell count and urinalysis [96]. If there is any evidence of consumptive coagulopathy, hemolysis, or hemoglobinuria, further studies should include prothrombin time and partial thromboplastin time, electrolytes, blood urea nitrogen, and creatinine, and a specimen should be sent for blood typing and screening. The white blood cell count may be as high as 20,000 to 30,000 per mm^3, and the hemoglobin may fall to as low as 4 g per dL [67,72,96]. Serial complete blood cell counts and urinalyses should be obtained in patients with significant lesions or systemic loxoscelism [96].

There is no commercially available test to definitively diagnose recluse spider envenomation. The differential diagnosis for *Loxosceles* envenomation includes bites or stings by other arthropods (e.g., other spiders, ticks, scorpions, ants, fleas, kissing bugs, and biting flies), superficial skin infections (especially methicillin-resistant *Staphylococcus aureus*), cutaneous anthrax, diabetic ulcers, plant puncture wounds, sporotrichosis, toxic epidermal necrolysis, pyoderma gangrenosum, erythema nodosum, erythema migrans, herpes zoster, herpes simplex, erythema multiforme, purpura fulminans, and contact dermatitis.

Management

No commercial antivenoms exist for *Loxosceles* bites in the United States. The majority of cases require only local wound care, including cleansing of the bite site, application of a sterile dressing, immobilization with a well-padded splint, and tetanus prophylaxis as necessary [67]. Frequent local application of ice or cold packs during the first 72 hours to reduce sphingomyelinase D activity is probably beneficial [84]. If an ulcer develops, it should be cleaned several times each day with hydrogen peroxide or povidone–iodine solution [96]. Pruritus can be treated with antihistamines. Antibiotics to prevent secondary cellulitis may be beneficial [84] and should include coverage for methicillin-resistant *S. aureus* [100].

It is important to emphasize to patients that nothing has been proven to decrease the extent of dermonecrosis after these bites and that most lesions heal quite satisfactorily with conservative management alone [67,96,101]. Controversial modalities for managing the wound include the use of steroids, dapsone, colchicine, surgery, hyperbaric oxygen therapy, and topical nitroglycerine application [78,87,102–105]. Routine use of these agents should be avoided until prospective controlled studies prove that benefits outweigh risks.

Early excision of the wound site is contraindicated because it is impossible to predict the ultimate extent and severity of the lesion [87]. Severe-appearing lesions commonly involute and regress spontaneously to leave minimal defects [106]. Surgical procedures that might be required, such as skin grafting, should be postponed at least 6 to 8 weeks to ensure that the necrotic process has been completed and to improve chances of healing [87]. Hyperbaric oxygen therapy may be useful in particularly severe wounds, but this remains unproven [87,107].

Initial management of systemic loxoscelism includes adequate hydration, maintaining electrolyte balance, and administering nonsalicylate antipyretics and analgesics [67,96]. Although the use of systemic corticosteroids to stabilize red blood cell membranes has yet to be studied in a controlled fashion, an early, short course of therapy may be beneficial in patients with hemolysis. The recommended dose is 1 mg per kg per day of prednisone orally for 2 to 4 days [67]. Blood products are used as indicated to treat anemia or thrombocytopenia [67]. If hemoglobinuria occurs, hydration becomes critically important, and urine output should be maintained at 2 to 3 mL per kg per hour [96]. If renal failure develops, dialysis may be indicated [67,96]. Dialysis does not remove venom or hemoglobin from the circulation, however [96].

Disposition and Outcome

Patients may be discharged from the hospital when systemic effects have resolved. Close follow-up (daily wound checks) should be provided to patients with cutaneous lesions. Although there have been no reports of deaths in patients bitten by positively identified recluse spiders in the United States [72,96], there is risk of death from systemic loxoscelism, especially in children.

SCORPION ENVENOMATION

The only scorpion species of major medical importance that is native to the United States is the bark scorpion (*Centruroides sculpturatus* [formerly *C. exilicauda*]) [108]. This species is found throughout Arizona and immediately surrounding regions of neighboring states [109]. Other closely related *Centruroides* scorpions of medical importance are found in Mexico. The bark scorpion is 13 to 75 mm long and yellow brown in color, with variable striping on the dorsum [109–111], and has a small subaculear tubercle at the base of the stinger [112].

The venom of *C. sculpturatus* is complex. It contains at least five distinct neurotoxins that cause release of neurotransmitters from the autonomic nervous system and adrenal medulla and stimulate depolarization of neuromuscular junctions [113,114]. Its venom contains no major enzymatic components [115].

Clinical Manifestations

Most *C. sculpturatus* stings are minor, with the most serious envenomations occurring in children [116]. The sting usually produces intense pain at the site, although local pain may be absent in children younger than 10 years [110]. Pain or numbness may radiate up the extremity [110]. Soft-tissue swelling and ecchymosis are notably absent [115].

Systemic symptoms may include restlessness or anxiety, uncoordinated neuromotor hyperactivity, oculomotor dysfunction, and respiratory distress related to excess secretions, airway obstruction, and in some cases, noncardiogenic pulmonary edema [116,117]. Hyperactivity may be mistaken for seizures [118]. Supraventricular tachycardia and hypertension have been reported [113], and severe hyperthermia may occur [111]. The duration of symptoms appears to be inversely proportional to age and may persist for up to 30 hours [110].

Local consequences after envenomation by other scorpions in the United States consist of immediate, brief, intense pain; mild soft-tissue swelling; and mild ecchymosis [119]. Systemic manifestations are uncommon, and allergic reactions are rare [77].

Diagnostic Evaluation

Patients stung by scorpions frequently see the offending organism. A general medical history should be obtained, symptoms assessed, and prehospital treatments noted. Vital signs should be frequently monitored. The sting site should be inspected and the patient examined for signs of systemic toxicity.

There are currently no commercial laboratory tests of diagnostic benefit in patients suspected of *C. sculpturatus* envenomation. The white blood cell count and serum glucose may be elevated [113]. Increases in serum amylase, creatine phosphokinase, and renal function studies, mild abnormalities in coagulation parameters, and cerebral spinal fluid pleocytosis have been reported [117].

The diagnosis is usually not difficult because adults often relate the history of a scorpion sting; in children, the clinical picture after a *C. sculpturatus* sting is rarely confused with other diagnoses [110]. The differential diagnosis includes central nervous system infection, widow spider envenomation, tetanus, dystonic drug reaction, intoxication (e.g., pesticides, anticholinergics, sympathomimetics, xanthines, propoxyphene, and strychnine), drug withdrawal, anaphylaxis, and seizure disorder.

Management

The majority of *C. sculpturatus* stings can be treated with cold compresses and analgesics [113]. Patients with more severe envenomations should receive oxygen and have an IV line established, along with continuous cardiac and pulse oximetry monitoring. The airway should be secured if there are signs of respiratory failure or inability to handle secretions [117]. Anxiety, restlessness, muscular hyperactivity, and moderate hypertension can initially be treated with parenteral benzodiazepines and bed rest [109]. β-Adrenergic–blocking agents have been recommended for hemodynamically significant supraventricular tachycardia [113,114], though caution must be used to ensure that hypertension is not exacerbated because of unopposed α-adrenergic effects. A combined beta-/alpha-blocking agent has theoretical advantages in such scenarios. Antihypertensive agents can be used for severe blood pressure elevation. Narcotics should be avoided because they appear to have a synergistic neurotoxic effect with the venom [120].

At the time of this writing, there were no commercially available antivenoms for scorpion stings in the United States. Recent work, however, demonstrates significant efficacy in the use of scorpion-specific $F(ab')_2$ antivenom (Anascorp, *Centruroides* [scorpion] immune $F(ab')_2$ intravenous [equine], Instituto Bioclon, Mexico) in rapidly reversing the neurotoxic effects, benzodiazepine requirements, and serum venom levels in children stung by bark scorpions in Arizona [116]. The University of Arizona Poison and Drug Information Center should be contacted for updates and availability of this product (phone: 1–800-222–1222). In the absence of available antivenom, the treating physician faced with a severely envenomated victim must rely on sound supportive care in an intensive care setting. Such care may be required for several days [116].

Deaths after a *C. sculpturatus* sting are exceptionally rare [109,113], but the potential for a fatal outcome should not be underestimated, especially in small children and the infirm.

SUMMARY (Table 132.2)

TABLE 132.2

SUMMARY OF HOSPITAL MANAGEMENT RECOMMENDATIONS FOR ENVENOMATIONS IN NORTH AMERICA

Syndrome	Management
Pit viper	
Rattlesnake (*Crotalus* or *Sistrurus* spp), cottonmouth water moccasin, or copperhead (*Agkistrodon* spp)	■ ABCs, O_2, cardiac/pulse oximetry monitoring, two large-bore IV lines, physiologic saline infusion ■ Measure extremity circumferences every 15 minutes during acute phase ■ Laboratory assessment (see text) ■ Update tetanus immunization status as needed ■ No evidence of envenomation—monitor for a minimum of 8 hours [39] ■ Mild envenomation without evidence of progression—no antivenom, admit for monitoring [24] ■ Mild envenomation with progression or moderate-to-severe envenomation (evidence of systemic toxicity [systemic signs or symptoms, or laboratory abnormalities])—administer antivenom (see text) [24] ■ Shock management includes IV physiologic saline boluses (10–20 mL/kg) and antivenom; if refractory, consider albumin [8] and, as last resort, vasopressors [4] ■ Blood products uncommonly required after administration of adequate antivenom [28] ■ If concerned re: compartment syndrome, measure intracompartmental pressures (see text); fasciotomy only for documented increase in pressures unresponsive to elevation of the extremity and antivenom [36] ■ Antibiotics only for evidence of secondary infection (uncommon) [30]
Coral snake	
Texas or Eastern coral snake (*Micrurus* spp)	■ ABCs, O_2, cardiac/pulse oximetry monitoring, at least one large-bore IV line, physiologic saline infusion ■ Early intubation and respiratory support if any evidence of difficulty with breathing or handling secretions [54] ■ Update tetanus immunization status as needed ■ No evidence of envenomation—admit for monitoring (minimum of 24 hours) [61] ■ Evidence of neurotoxicity—administer antivenom if available (see text); if no antivenom available, supportive care only; admit for monitoring until recovered
Sonoran coral snake (*Micruroides euryxanthus*)	■ ABCs, O_2, cardiac/pulse oximetry monitoring, at least one large-bore IV line, physiologic saline infusion ■ Update tetanus immunization status as needed ■ No evidence of envenomation—admit for monitoring (minimum of 24 hours) ■ Evidence of neurotoxicity—admit for monitoring until recovered, supportive care only
Widow spider (*Latrodectus* spp)	■ ABCs, O_2, cardiac/pulse oximetry monitoring, at least one large-bore IV line, physiologic saline infusion ■ Update tetanus immunization status as needed ■ No evidence of envenomation—monitor for 6–8 hours) ■ Evidence of envenomation Mild: analgesics and muscle relaxants (narcotics and benzodiazepines) [62] More severe or high-risk patient (see text): consider antivenom administration with informed consent (see text) [68]
Recluse spider (*Loxosceles* spp)	■ Laboratory assessment (see text) ■ Conservative wound care (cleansing, splinting, debride only clearly necrotic tissue) ■ Update tetanus immunization status as needed ■ Any evidence of infection: broad-spectrum antibiotics (include MRSA coverage) [84,100] ■ Daily wound checks until progressive healing ■ Delay any required skin grafts for 6–8 weeks (see text) [87] ■ If evidence of systemic toxicity: admit, IV fluids, steroids (see text); blood product transfusion and dialysis for renal failure as needed [67,96]
Scorpion	
Neurotoxic scorpion (e.g., *Centruroides sculpturatus*)	■ ABCs, O_2, cardiac/pulse oximetry monitoring, at least one large-bore IV line, physiologic saline infusion ■ Analgesics (nonnarcotic), benzodiazepines [109,120] ■ Update tetanus immunization status as needed ■ If severe: consider antivenom if available, otherwise conservative care [116]
Nonneurotoxic scorpion	■ Analgesics as needed ■ Update tetanus immunization status as needed

ABCs, airway, breathing, circulation assessment and management as needed; O_2, oxygen; IV, intravenous; MRSA, methicillin-resistant *Staphylococcus aureus.*

References

1. Mattison C: *Snakes of the World.* New York, Facts on File, 1986.
2. Parrish HM: Incidence of treated snakebites in the United States. *Public Health Rep* 81:269, 1966.
3. Wingert WA, Wainschel J: Diagnosis and management of envenomation by poisonous snakes. *South Med J* 68:1015, 1975.
4. Russell FE: *Snake Venom Poisoning.* 2nd ed. New York, Scholium, 1983.
5. Russell FE, Puffer HW: Pharmacology of snake venoms, in Minton SA (ed): *Snake Venoms and Envenomation.* New York, Marcel Dekker Inc, 1971, p 87.
6. Gutierrez JM, Rucavadoa R, Escalantea T, et al: Hemorrhage induced by snake venom metalloproteinases: biochemical and biophysical mechanisms involved in microvessel damage. *Toxicon* 45:997, 2005.
7. Russell FE, Carlson RW, Wainschel J, et al: Snake venom poisoning in the United States: experiences with 550 cases. *JAMA* 233:341, 1975.
8. Schaeffer RC, Carlson RW, Puri VK, et al: The effects of colloidal and crystalloidal fluids on rattlesnake venom shock in the rat. *J Pharmacol Exp Ther* 206:687, 1978.
9. Bonilla CA, Fiero K, Frank LP: Isolation of a basic protein neurotoxin from *Crotalus adamanteus* venom. I. purification and biological properties. *Toxicon* 8:123, 1970.
10. Jansen PW, Perkin RM, Van Stralen D: Mojave rattlesnake envenomation: prolonged neurotoxicity and rhabdomyolysis. *Ann Emerg Med* 21:322, 1992.
11. Parrish HM, Goldner JC, Silberg SL: Poisonous snakebites causing no venenation. *Postgrad Med* 39:265, 1966.
12. Norris RL: Fang marks and the diagnosis of venomous snakebite. *Wilderness Environ Med* 6:159, 1995.
13. Banner W: Bites and stings in the pediatric patient. *Curr Probl Pediatr* 18:9, 1988.
14. LoVecchio F, DeBus DM: Snakebite envenomation in children: a 10-year retrospective review. *Wilderness Environ Med* 12:184, 2001.
15. Hardy DL: A review of first aid measures for pitviper bite in North America with an appraisal of Extractor™ suction and stun gun electroshock, in Campbell JA, Brodie ED (eds): *Biology of the Pitvipers.* Tyler, TX, Selva, 1992, p 405.
16. Bush SP, Hegewald KG, Green SM, et al: Effects of a negative pressure venom extraction device (Extractor™) on local tissue injury after artificial rattlesnake envenomation in a porcine model. *Wilderness Environ Med* 11:180, 2000.
17. Bucknall NC: Electrical treatment of venomous bites and stings. *Toxicon* 29:397, 1991.
18. Lavonas EJ, Gerardo CJ, O'malley G, et al: Initial experience with Crotalidae polyvalent immune Fab (ovine) antivenom in the treatment of copperhead snakebite. *Ann Emerg Med* 43:200, 2004.
19. Campbell BT, Corsi JM, Boneti C, et al: Pediatric snakebites: lessons learned from 114 cases. *J Pediatr Surg* 43:1338, 2008.
20. Dart RC, Seifert SA, Carroll L, et al: Affinity-purified, mixed monospecific crotalid antivenom ovine Fab for the treatment of crotalid venom poisoning, *Ann Emerg Med* 30:33, 1997.
21. Garfin SR, Castilonia RR, Mubarak SJ, et al: The effect of antivenin on intramuscular pressure elevations induced by rattlesnake venom. *Toxicon* 23:677, 1985.
22. Ruha A-M, Curry SC, Beuhler M, et al: Initial postmarketing experience with Crotalidae polyvalent immune Fab for treatment of rattlesnake envenomation. *Ann Emerg Med* 39:609, 2002.
23. Yip L: Rational use of Crotalidae polyvalent immune Fab (ovine) in the management of crotaline bite. *Ann Emerg Med* 39:648, 2002.
24. CroFab full prescribing information. Available at: http://www.crofab.com/pdf/CroFab_PI.pdf. Protherics, Inc. Brentwood, TN, 2010. Accessed: March 21, 2011.
25. Dart RC, McNally J: Efficacy, safety, and use of snake antivenoms in the United States. *Ann Emerg Med* 37:181, 2001.
26. Corrigan P, Russell FE, Wainschel J: Clinical reactions to antivenin. *Toxicon* 16[Suppl 1]:457, 1978.
27. Van Mierop LH, Kitchens CS: Defibrination syndrome following bites by the Eastern diamondback rattlesnake. *J Fla Med Assoc* 67:21, 1980.
28. Burgess JL, Dart RC: Snake venom coagulopathy: use and abuse of blood products in the treatment of pit viper envenomation. *Ann Emerg Med* 20:795, 1991.
29. Ruha AM, Curry SC: Recombinant factor VIIa for treatment of gastrointestinal hemorrhage following rattlesnake envenomation. *Wild Environ Med* 20:156, 2009.
30. Clark RF, Selden BS, Furbee B: The incidence of wound infection following crotalid envenomation. *J Emerg Med* 11:583, 1993.
31. Tanen DA, Ruha AM, Graeme KA, et al: Epidemiology and hospital course of rattlesnake envenomations cared for at a tertiary referral center in central Arizona. *Acad Emerg Med* 8:177, 2001.
32. Stolpe MR, Norris RL, Chisholm CD, et al: Preliminary observations on the effects of hyperbaric oxygen therapy on western diamondback rattlesnake (*Crotalus atrox*) venom poisoning in the rabbit model. *Ann Emerg Med* 18:871, 1989.
33. Allen FM: Observations of local measures in the treatment of snake bite. *Am J Trop Med* 19:393, 1939.
34. Curry SC, Kraner JC, Kunkel DB, et al: Noninvasive vascular studies in management of rattlesnake envenomations to extremities. *Ann Emerg Med* 14:1081, 1985.
35. Garfin SR: Rattlesnake bites: current hospital therapy. *West J Med* 137:411, 1982.
36. Dart R, Russell FE: Animal poisoning, in Hall J, Schmidt G, Wood L (eds): *Principles of Critical Care.* New York, McGraw-Hill, 1992, p 2163.
37. Tanen DA, Danish DC, Grice GA, et al: Fasciotomy worsens the amount of myonecrosis in a porcine model of crotaline envenomation. *Ann Emerg Med* 44:99, 2004.
38. Hardy DL, Zamudio KR: Compartment syndrome, fasciotomy and neuropathy after a rattlesnake envenomation: aspects of monitoring and diagnosis. *Wild Environ Med* 17:36, 2006.
39. Gomez HF, Dart RC: Clinical toxicology of snakebite in North America, in Meier J, White J (eds): *Handbook of Clinical Toxicology of Animal Venoms and Poisons.* Boca Raton, FL, CRC Press, 1995, p 619.
40. Boyer LV, Seifert SA, Clark RF, et al: Recurrent and persistent coagulopathy following pit viper envenomation. *Arch Intern Med* 159:706, 1999.
41. Parrish HM: *Poisonous Snakebites in the United States.* New York, Vantage Press, 1980.
42. Parrish HM: Analysis of 460 fatalities from venomous animals in the United States. *Am J Med Sci* 245:129, 1963.
43. Hardy DL: Fatal rattlesnake envenomation in Arizona: 1969–1984. *Clin Toxicol* 24:1, 1986.
44. Grace TG, Omer GE: The management of upper extremity pit viper wounds. *Am J Hand Surg* 5:168, 1980.
45. Simon TL, Grace TG: Envenomation coagulopathy from snake bites. *New Engl J Med* 305:1347, 1981.
46. Watson WA, Litovitz TL, Klein-Schwartz W, et al: 2003 annual report of the American Association of Poison Control Centers Toxic Exposure Surveillance System. *Am J Emerg Med* 22:333, 2004.
47. Campbell JA, Lamar WW: *Venomous Reptiles of the Western Hemisphere,* Ithaca, NY, Cornell University Press, 2004, p 1.
48. Minton SA: Identification of poisonous snakes, in Minton SA (ed): *Snake Venoms and Envenomation.* New York, Marcel Dekker Inc, 1971, p 1.
49. Parrish HM, Khan MS: Bites by coral snakes: report of 11 representative cases. *Am J Med Sci* 253:561, 1967.
50. Fix JD: Venom yield of the North American coral snake and its clinical significance. *South Med J* 73:737, 1980.
51. Minton SA, Minton MR: *Venomous Reptiles.* New York, Scribner's, 1969.
52. Morgan DL, Borys DL, Stanford R, et al: Texas coral snake (*Micrurus tener*) bites. *South Med J* 100:152, 2007.
53. Lee CY: Elapid neurotoxins and their mode of action. *Clin Toxicol* 3:457, 1970.
54. Kitchens CS, Van Mierop LHS: Envenomation by the Eastern coral snake (*Micrurus fulvius*): a study of 39 victims. *JAMA* 258:1615, 1987.
55. Norris RL, Dart RC: Apparent coral snake envenomation in a patient without fang marks. *Am J Emerg Med* 7:402, 1989.
56. Pettigrew LC, Glass JP: Neurologic complications of a coral snake bite. *Neurology* 35:589, 1985.
57. McCollough NC, Gennaro JF: Treatment of venomous snakebite in the United States. *Clin Toxicol* 3:483, 1970.
58. White J: Snakebite: an Australian perspective. *J Wilderness Med* 2:219, 1991.
59. Sutherland SK: Pressure immobilization for snakebite in southern Africa remains speculative. *South Afr Med J* 85:1039, 1995.
60. German BT, Hack JB, Brewer K, et al: Pressure-immobilization bandages delay toxicity in a porcine model of eastern coral snake (*Micrurus fulvius fulvius*) envenomation. *Ann Emerg Med* 45:603, 2005.
61. Gaar GG: Assessment and management of coral and other exotic snake envenomations. *J Fla Med Assoc* 83:178, 1996.
62. Russell FE, Madon NB: New names for the brown recluse and the black widow. *Postgrad Med* 70:31, 1981.
63. Brown KS, Necaise JS, Goddard J: Additions to the known U.S. distribution of *Latrodectus geometricus* (Araneae: Theridiidae). *J Med Entomol* 45:959, 2008.
64. Kobernick M: Black widow spider bite. *Am Fam Physician* 29:241, 1984.
65. Maretic Z: Latrodectism: variations in clinical manifestations provoked by *Latrodectus* species of spiders. *Toxicon* 21:457, 1983.
66. Baba A, Cooper JR: The action of black widow spider venom on cholinergic mechanisms in synaptosomes. *J Neurochem* 34:1369, 1980.
67. Anderson PC: Necrotizing spider bites. *Am Fam Physician* 26:198, 1982.
68. Moss HS, Binder LS: A retrospective review of black widow spider envenomation. *Ann Emerg Med* 16:188, 1987.
69. Reeves JA, Allison EJ, Goodman PE: Black widow spider bite in a child. *Am J Emerg Med* 14:469, 1996.
70. Russell FE: Muscle relaxants in black widow spider (*Latrodectus mactans*) poisoning. *Am J Med Sci* 243:159, 1962.
71. Russell FE, Marcus P, Streng JA: Black widow spider envenomation during pregnancy: report of a case. *Toxicon* 17:188, 1979.

72. Wong RC, Hughes SE, Voorhees JJ: Spider bites. *Arch Dermatol* 123:98, 1987.
73. Erdur B, Turkcuer I, Bukiran A, et al: Uncommon cardiovascular manifestations after a *Latrodectus* bite. *Am J Emerg Med* 25:232, 2007.
74. Hoover NG, Fortenberry JD: Use of antivenin to treat priapism after a black widow spider bite. *Pediatrics* 114:e128, 2004.
75. Clark RF, Wethern-Kestner S, Vance MV, et al: Clinical presentation and treatment of black widow spider envenomation: a review of 163 cases. *Ann Emerg Med* 21:782, 1992.
76. Sherman RP, Groll JM, Gonzalez DI, et al: Black widow spider (*Latrodectus mactans*) envenomation in a term pregnancy. *Curr Surg* 57:346, 2000.
77. King LE, Rees RS: Spider bites and scorpion stings, in Rakel RE (ed): *Conn's Current Therapy*. 39th ed. Philadelphia, WB Saunders, 1987, p 970.
78. Vetter RS, Isbister GK: Medical aspects of spider bites. *Annu Rev Entomol* 53:409, 2008.
79. Allen RC, Norris RL: Delayed use of antivenin in black widow spider (*Latrodectus mactans*) envenomation. *J Wilderness Med* 2:187, 1991.
80. Daly F, Hill RE, Bogdan GM, et al: Neutralization of *Latrodectus mactans* and *L. hesperus* venom by redback spider (*L. hasseltii*) antivenom. *Clin Toxicol* 39:119, 2001.
81. Graudins A, Padula M, Broady K, et al: Red-back spider (*Latrodectus hasselti*) antivenom prevents the toxicity of widow spider venoms. *Ann Emerg Med* 37:154, 2001.
82. Antivenin (Latrodectus mactans) (Black Widow Spider Antivenin) Equine Origin. Whitehouse Station, NJ, Merck & Co, Inc., 2005. Available at: http://www.merck.com/product/usa/pi_circulars/a/antivenin/antivenin_pi.pdf. Accessed June 14, 2009.
83. Gertsch WJ, Ennik F: The spider genus *Loxosceles* in North America, Central America, and the West Indes, Aranie (Loxoscelidae). *Bull Am Museum Nat History* 175:264, 1983.
84. Wilson DC, King LE: Spiders and spider bites. *Dermatol Clin* 8:277, 1990.
85. Berger RS, Millikan LE, Conway F: An *in vitro* test for *Loxosceles reclusa* spider bites. *Toxicon* 11:465, 1973.
86. Smith CW, Micks DW: A comparative study of the venom and other components of three species of *Loxosceles*. *Am J Trop Med Hyg* 17:651, 1968.
87. Wasserman GS: Wound care of spider and snake envenomations. *Ann Emerg Med* 17:1331, 1988.
88. Rees RS, Nanney LB, Yates RA, et al: Interaction of brown recluse spider venom on cell membranes: the inciting mechanism? *J Invest Dermatol* 83:270, 1984.
89. Forrester LJ, Barrett JT, Campbell BJ: Red blood cell lysis induced by the venom of the brown recluse spider: the role of sphingomyelinase D. *Arch Biochem Biophys* 187:355, 1978.
90. Kurpiewski G, Forrester LJ, Barrett JT, et al: Platelet aggregation and sphingomyelinase D activity of a purified toxin from the venom of *Loxosceles reclusa*. *Biochim Biophys Acta* 678:467, 1981.
91. Jansen GT, Morgan PN, McQueen JN, et al: The brown recluse spider bite: Controlled evaluation of treatment using the white rabbit as a model. *South Med J* 64:1194, 1971.
92. Berger RS, Adelstein EH, Anderson PC: Intravascular coagulation: the cause of necrotic arachnidism. *J Invest Dermatol* 61:142, 1973.
93. Smith CW, Micks DW: The role of polymorphonuclear leukocytes in the lesion caused by the venom of the brown spider, *Loxosceles reclusa*. *Lab Invest* 22:90, 1970.
94. Hershey FB, Aulenbacher CE: Surgical treatment of brown spider bites. *Ann Surg* 170:300, 1969.
95. Rees R, Campbell D, Rieger E, et al: The diagnosis and treatment of brown recluse spider bites. *Ann Emerg Med* 16:945, 1987.
96. Wasserman GS, Anderson PC: Loxoscelism and necrotic arachnidism. *J Toxicol Clin Toxicol* 21:451, 1983–1984.
97. Arnold RE: Brown recluse spider bites: five cases with a review of the literature. *JACEP* 5:262, 1976.
98. Fardon DW, Wingo CW, Robinson DW, et al: The treatment of brown spider bite. *Plast Reconstr Surg* 40:482, 1967.
99. Dillaha CJ, Jansen GT, Honeycutt WM, et al: North American loxoscelism. *JAMA* 188:153, 1964.
100. Frithsen IL, Vetter RS, Stocks IC: Reports of envenomation by brown recluse spiders exceed verified specimens of *Loxosceles* spiders in South Carolina. *J Am Board Fam Med* 20:483, 2007.
101. Berger RS: Management of brown recluse spider bite. *JAMA* 251:889, 1984.
102. Berger RS: A critical look at therapy for the brown recluse spider bite. *Arch Dermatol* 107:298, 1973.
103. Hansen RC, Russell FE: Dapsone use for *Loxosceles* envenomation treatment. *Vet Hum Toxicol* 26:260, 1984.
104. Burton KG: Nitroglycerine patches for brown recluse spider bites. *Am Fam Physician* 51:1401, 1995.
105. Lowry BP, Bradfield JF, Carroll RG, et al: A controlled trial of topical nitroglycerine in a New Zealand white rabbit model of brown recluse spider envenomation. *Ann Emerg Med* 37:161, 2001.
106. Anderson PC: What's new in loxoscelism 1978? *J Missouri State Med Assoc* 74:549, 1977.
107. Maynor ML, Moon RE, Klitzman B, et al: Brown recluse spider envenomation: a prospective trial of hyperbaric oxygen therapy. *Acad Emerg Med* 4:184, 1997.
108. Valdez-Cruz NA, Dávila S, Licea A, et al: Biochemical, genetic and physiological characterization of venom components from two species of scorpions: *Centruroides exilicauda* Wood and *Centruroides sculpturatus* Ewing. *Biochimie* 86:387, 2004.
109. Likes K, Banner W, Chavez M: *Centruroides exilicauda* envenomation in Arizona. *West J Med* 141:634, 1984.
110. Rimsza ME, Zimmerman DR, Bergeson PS: Scorpion envenomation. *Pediatrics* 66:298, 1980.
111. Stahnke HL: Arizona's lethal scorpion. *Ariz Med* 29:490, 1972.
112. Arakelian G: Arizona bark scorpion (*Centruroides sculpturatus*). Los Angeles County Agricultural Commissioner/Weights and Measures Department. 2008. Available at: http://www.cdfa. ca.gov/phpps/PPD/PDF/Centruroides_sculpturatus.pdf. Accessed June 13, 2009.
113. Rachesky IJ, Banner W, Dansky J, et al: Treatments for *Centruroides exilicauda* envenomation. *Am J Dis Child* 138:1136, 1984.
114. Simard JM, Watt DD: Venoms and toxins, in Polis GA (ed): *The Biology of Scorpions*. Stanford, CA, Stanford University Press, 1990, p 414.
115. Curry SC, Vance MV, Ryan PJ, et al: Envenomation by the scorpion *Centruroides sculpturatus*. *J Toxicol Clin Toxicol* 21:417, 1983–1984.
116. Boyer LV, Theodorou AA, Berg RA, et al: Antivenom for critically ill children with neurotoxicity from scorpion stings. *N Engl J Med* 360:2090, 2009.
117. Berg RA, Tarantino MD: Envenomation by the scorpion *Centruroides exilicauda* (*C. sculpturatus*): severe and unusual manifestations. *Pediatrics* 87:930, 1991.
118. Bond GR: Antivenin administration for *Centruroides* scorpion sting: risks and benefits. *Ann Emerg Med* 21:788, 1992.
119. Ellis MD: *Dangerous Plants, Snakes, Arthropods and Marine Life of Texas*. Washington DC, U.S. Department of Health, Education, and Welfare, Public Health Service, U.S. Government Printing Office. 1975.
120. Stahnke HL, Dengler AH: The effect of morphine and related substances on the toxicity of venoms: 1. *Centruroides sculpturatus* Ewing scorpion venom. *Am J Trop Med* 13:346, 1964.

CHAPTER 133 ■ HEAVY METAL POISONING

LUKE YIP*

This chapter focuses on the aspects of acute poisoning by arsenic, lead, and mercury that are potentially life threatening or may lead to permanent organ damage and hence require immediate, usually intensive, medical care. Reviews of the evaluation and management of asymptomatic exposures and nonacute poisoning can be found elsewhere [1,2].

ARSENIC

Exposure to arsenic may come from natural sources, industrial processes, commercial products, food, or intentionally

*The views expressed do not necessarily represent those of the agency or the United States.

administered sources either with a benevolent (acute promyelocytic leukemia [APL] treatment, folk and naturopathic remedies) [3,4] or malevolent intent. Today, acute arsenic poisoning is most commonly the result of an accidental ingestion or the result of a suicidal or homicidal intent.

Pharmacology

Arsenic compounds can be classified into three major groups: inorganic, organic, and arsine gas (AsH_3). The latter is discussed separately. Arsenic compounds can also be classified by their valence state. The three most common valence states are the metalloid (elemental [0] oxidation state), arsenite (trivalent [+3] state), and arsenate (pentavalent [+5] state). In general, the arsenic compounds can be arranged in their order of decreasing toxicity: inorganic trivalent compounds, organic trivalent compounds, inorganic pentavalent compounds, organic pentavalent compounds, and elemental arsenic. Trivalent arsenic is generally two- to tenfold more toxic than pentavalent arsenic. The minimum oral lethal human dose of arsenic trioxide (trivalent) is probably between 10 and 300 mg. Some marine organisms and algae contain large amounts of organic arsenic in the form of arsenobetaine—a trimethylated arsenic compound—and arsenocholine. Arsenobetaine and arsenocholine are excreted unchanged in the urine, with total clearance in about 2 days, and exert no known toxic effects in humans.

The major routes of entry into the human body are ingestion and inhalation. Soluble forms of ingested arsenic are 60% to 90% absorbed from the gastrointestinal (GI) tract. The amount of arsenic absorbed by inhalation is also thought to be in this range. Toxic systemic effects have been reported from rare occupational accidents in which arsenic trichloride or arsenic acid was splashed on worker's skin.

After absorption, arsenic is bound to proteins in the blood and redistributed to the liver, spleen, kidneys, lungs, and GI tract within 24 hours. Clearance from these tissues is dose dependent. Two to four weeks after exposure ceases, most of the arsenic remaining in the body is found in keratin-rich tissues (e.g., skin, hair, and nails).

Both forms of arsenic, arsenite and arsenate, undergo biomethylation in the liver to monomethylarsonic acid (MMA) and dimethylarsinic acid (DMA). The methylation process may represent detoxification because the metabolites exert less acute toxicity in experimental lethality studies. The liver's efficiency in methylation decreases with increasing arsenic dose. When the methylating capacity of the liver is exceeded, exposure to excess concentrations of inorganic arsenic results in increased retention of arsenic in soft tissues.

Arsenic is eliminated from the body primarily by renal excretion. Urinary arsenic excretion begins promptly after absorption, and depending on the amount of arsenic ingested, urinary arsenic excretion may remain elevated for 1 to 2 months. After acute intoxication by inorganic arsenic, arsenic is excreted in the urine as inorganic arsenic, MMA and DMA, but their proportion varies with time [5]. During the first 2 to 4 days after the intoxication, arsenic is excreted mainly in the inorganic form. This is followed by a progressive increase of the proportion excreted as MMA and DMA. The time at which arsenic is primarily excreted as its methylated metabolites depends on the severity and duration of the intoxication. Pentavalent arsenic is cleared more rapidly than trivalent arsenic. Because arsenic is quickly cleared from the blood, blood concentrations may be normal, while urine concentrations remain markedly elevated. Renal dysfunction may be a major impediment to normal elimination of arsenic compounds.

Inorganic arsenic can cross the human placenta. This was evident by the high arsenic concentrations found in a neonate following acute maternal arsenic intoxication [6].

There are two major mechanisms by which arsenic compounds appear to produce injury involving multiorgan systems. It is believed that arsenic's overt toxicity is related to its reversible binding with sulfhydryl enzymes, leading to the inhibition of critical sulfhydryl-containing enzyme systems. Trivalent arsenite is particularly potent in this regard. The pyruvate and succinate oxidation pathways are particularly sensitive to arsenic inhibition. Dihydrolipoate, a sulfhydryl cofactor, appears to be a principal target. Normally, dihydrolipoate is oxidized to lipoate via a converting enzyme, dihydrolipoate dehydrogenase. Arsenic reacts with both dihydrolipoate and dihydrolipoate dehydrogenase, preventing the formation of lipoate. Lipoate is involved in the formation of key intermediates in the Krebs cycle. As a result of lipoate depletion, the Krebs cycle and oxidative phosphorylation are inhibited. Without oxidative phosphorylation, cellular energy stores (adenosine triphosphate [ATP]) are depleted, resulting in metabolic failure and cell death.

The other major mechanism by which arsenic is believed to produce cellular injury is termed *arsenolysis*. Pentavalent arsenate can competitively substitute for phosphate in biochemical reactions. During oxidative phosphorylation, energy is produced and stored in the form of ATP. The stable phosphate ester bond in ATP can be replaced by an arsenate ester bond. However, the high energy stored in the arsenate ester bond is wasted because it is unstable and rapidly hydrolyzed. Cellular respiration is stimulated in a futile attempt to restore this wasted energy. In effect, trivalent arsenic compounds inhibit critical enzymes in the Krebs cycle, leading to inhibition of oxidative phosphorylation, and pentavalent arsenic compounds uncouple oxidative phosphorylation by arsenolysis. This results in the disruption of cellular oxidative processes, leading to endothelial cellular damage. The fundamental lesion seen clinically is loss of capillary integrity, resulting in increased permeability of blood vessels and tissue hypoxia, leading to generalized vasodilation, transudation of plasma, hypovolemia, and shock.

In vitro, the effects of arsenic trioxide on repolarizing cardiac ion currents appear to be one of antagonism on both I_{Kr} and I_{Ks} as well as activation of I_{K-ATP}, which maintains normal repolarization [3]. In addition, arsenic trioxide increases cardiac calcium currents and reduces surface expression of the cardiac potassium channel human ether-a-go-go-related gene. The variability in QTc interval prolongation and the onset of ventricular dysrhythmias during arsenic therapy may represent these competing effects.

Clinical Toxicity

The most prominent clinical findings associated with acute arsenic poisoning are related to the GI tract. Some arsenic is corrosive. Acute ingestion may lead to oral irritation and a burning sensation in the mouth and throat. A metallic taste and/or a garlicky odor to the breath have been described, but often are not present. Nausea, vomiting, and abdominal pain are common. The toxic effects of arsenic on the GI tract are manifested as increased peristalsis and profuse watery stools and bleeding. In serious cases, hemorrhagic gastroenteritis may ensue within minutes to hours after acute ingestion. Nausea, vomiting, and severe hemorrhagic gastroenteritis can all lead to profound intravascular volume loss resulting in hypovolemia shock, which is the major cause of mortality and morbidity.

Noncardiogenic pulmonary edema may occur from increased capillary permeability, and cardiogenic pulmonary edema may occur from myocardial depression. Electrocardiogram (ECG) changes associated with arsenic poisoning consist of nonspecific ST- and T-wave changes, sometimes mimicking ischemia or hyperkalemia and QTc prolongation [7–9]. These

TABLE 133.1

ADVERSE DRUG EVENTS ASSOCIATED WITH ARSENIC TRIOXIDE INDUCTION THERAPY

Cardiovascular	QTc prolongation ($\geq$500 msec), torsades de pointes, sudden death, tachycardia
Hematologic	Hyperleukocytosis (10,000–170,000 cells/μL)
Nervous system	Peripheral neuropathy, headache
Metabolic	Hypokalemia, hypomagnesemia, hyperglycemia
APLDS	Fever, pleural or pericardial effusion, pleural infiltrates, respiratory distress, weight gain, musculoskeletal pain
GI	Nausea, vomiting, diarrhea
Dermatologic	Skin rash

APLDS, acute promyelocytic leukemia differentiation syndrome; GI, gastrointestinal.

ECG abnormalities are reported to occur in half the patients with arsenic poisoning, and these ECG changes may be evident from 4 to 30 hours postingestion, persisting for up to 8 weeks.

At least five cases of arsenic-induced polymorphic ventricular tachycardias consistent with torsades de pointes have been reported [8,9]. In all these cases, QTc prolongation was evident on the admission ECG. Except in the case of the patient who presented with cyanosis and cardiorespiratory arrest, peripheral neuropathy was a prominent finding on physical examination at the time of hospital admission, and the polymorphic ventricular tachydysrhythmias were ultimately self-limited. Although these cases were able to document as to when during the hospital course torsades de pointes were observed, the time between arsenic exposure and the onset of cardiac dysrhythmias can only be speculated.

Arsenic was abandoned 30 years ago as an anticancer medicinal, but has attracted renewed attention as a treatment for APL on the basis of impressive results from clinical studies in China and the United States [3]. Arsenic trioxide is licensed for use in patients with relapsed or refractory APL. Induction therapy in APL patients receiving daily median arsenic trioxide infusions of 0.15 mg per kg (range, 0.06 to 0.2 mg per kg) during 1 to 2 hours until bone marrow remission or for a maximum of 60 days has been associated with adverse drug events (Table 133.1) [3]. In patients receiving multiple courses of arsenic trioxide therapy, their QTc intervals returned to pretreatment values before their second course, signifying that arsenic trioxide may not permanently prolong the QTc interval.

Both acute and chronic arsenic poisoning may affect the hematopoietic system. A reversible bone marrow depression with pancytopenia, particularly leukopenia, may occur. However, it is the chronic form that is usually associated with severe hematopoietic derangements. A wide variety of hematologic abnormalities have been described with arsenic poisoning, including anemia, absolute neutropenia, thrombocytopenia, eosinophilia, and basophilic stippling [10]. Anemia is, in part, due to an increase in hemolysis and disturbed erythropoiesis/myelopoiesis with reticulocytosis and predominant normoblastic erythropoiesis. Accelerated pyknosis of the normoblast nucleus, karyorrhexis, is characteristic of arsenic poisoning, and the typical "cloverleaf" nuclei may be evident [11]. Hematologic findings may appear within 4 days after acute arsenic ingestion, and in the absence of any specific therapy, erythrocytes, leukocytes, and thrombocytes were reported to return to normal values within 2 to 3 weeks after discontinuing arsenic exposure.

Neurologic manifestations of arsenic poisoning have included confusion, delirium, convulsions, encephalopathy, and coma [12]. Neuropathy is usually not the initial complaint associated with acute arsenic poisoning. Arsenic-induced polyneuropathy has traditionally been described as an axonal-loss sensorimotor polyneuropathy (low-amplitude/unelicitable sensory and motor conduction responses, often with preserved motor conduction velocities). The first symptoms of neuropathy have been reported to appear 1 to 3 weeks after the presumptive arsenic exposure [12,13]. Clinical involvement spans the spectrum from mild paresthesia with preserved ambulation to distal weakness, quadriplegia, and respiratory muscle insufficiency. Arsenic neuropathy is a symmetrical sensorimotor neuropathy, with the sensory component being more prominent in a "stocking-and-glove" distribution [13,14]. This polyneuropathy may progress in an ascending fashion to involve proximal arms and legs. Dysesthesias begin in the lower extremities, with severe painful burning sensation occurring in the soles of the feet. There is loss of vibration and positional sense, followed by the loss of pinprick, light touch, and temperature sensation. Motor dysfunction is characterized by the loss of deep tendon reflexes and muscle weakness. In severe poisoning, ascending weakness and paralysis may occur and involve the respiratory muscles, resulting in neuromuscular respiratory failure [15,16]. It has been reported that many of the patients with arsenic neuropathy were initially thought to have Landry–Guillain–Barré disease [12,16].

Because the fundamental lesion in arsenic toxicity is the loss of capillary integrity, increased glomerular capillary permeability may result in proteinuria. However, the kidneys are relatively spared from the direct toxic effects of arsenic. Hypovolemic shock associated with the prominent GI symptoms may lead to hypoperfusion of the kidneys, resulting in oliguria, acute tubular necrosis, and renal insufficiency or failure. The kidneys are the main route of excretion for arsenic compounds. Normal-functioning kidneys can excrete more than 100 mg of arsenic in the first 24 hours [17]. Because of shock and decreased glomerular filtration rate and depending on the dose of arsenic ingested, peak urinary arsenic excretion may often be delayed by 2 to 3 days. Hemodialysis contributes minimally to arsenic clearance compared with the normal-functioning kidneys [18].

Dermal changes occurring most frequently in arsenic-exposed humans are hyperpigmentation, hyperkeratosis, and skin cancer [19]. The lesions usually appear 1 to 6 weeks after the onset of the illness. In most cases, a diffuse, branny desquamation develops over the trunk and extremities; it is dry, scaling, and nonpruritic. Patchy hyperpigmentation—dark-brown patches with scattered pale spots, sometimes described as "raindrops on a dusty road"—occurs particularly on the eyelids, temples, axillae, neck, nipples, and groin. Arsenic hyperkeratosis usually appears as cornlike elevations, less than 1 cm in diameter, occurring most frequently on the palms of the hands and on the soles of the feet. Most cases of arsenic keratoses remain morphologically benign for decades, and in other cases, marked atypia (precancerous) develops and appears indistinguishable from Bowen's disease—an in situ squamous cell carcinoma. Skin lesions take several years to manifest the characteristic pigmented changes and hyperkeratoses, whereas it takes up to 40 years before skin cancer becomes evident. Brittle nails with transverse white bands (leukonychia striata arsenicalis transversus) appearing on the nails have been associated with arsenic poisoning and are known as Reynolds–Aldrich–Mees lines [20–22]. It reflects transient disruption of nail plate growth during acute poisoning. Leukonychia striata arsenicalis transversus takes about 5 to 6 weeks to appear over the lunulae after an acute poisoning. Thinning of the hair and patchy or diffuse alopecia are also associated with arsenic poisoning [12,23].

Diagnostic Evaluation

The temporal sequence of organ system injury may suggest acute arsenic intoxication. After a delay of minutes to hours, severe hemorrhagic gastroenteritis becomes evident, which may be accompanied by cardiovascular collapse or death. Bone marrow depression with leukopenia may appear within 4 days of arsenic ingestion and usually reaches a nadir at 1 to 2 weeks. Encephalopathy, congestive cardiomyopathy, noncardiogenic pulmonary edema, and cardiac conduction abnormalities may occur several days after improvement from the initial GI manifestation. Sensorimotor peripheral neuropathy may become apparent several weeks after resolution of the initial signs (gastroenteritis or shock) of intoxication resulting from ingestion.

The differentiation between arsenic neuropathy and Landry–Guillain–Barré disease is based on clinical and laboratory findings in that arsenic neuropathy rarely involves the cranial nerves, sensory manifestations are more prominent, weakness in the distal portions of the extremities is more severe, and the cerebrospinal fluid protein concentrations are usually less than 100 mg per dL [12,13].

Laboratory investigation should include complete blood count with peripheral smear, electrolytes, liver enzymes, creatine phosphokinase, arterial blood gas, renal profile with urine analysis, ECG, chest radiograph, and blood and urine arsenic concentrations. Nerve conduction velocity studies may be indicated if peripheral neurologic symptoms are present. Some arsenic compounds, particularly those of low solubility, are radiopaque, and if ingested, they may be visible on an abdominal radiograph.

The most important diagnostic test is urinary arsenic measurement. Urine arsenic concentrations may be measured as "spot," that is, the concentration in a single-voided urine specimen, reported in μg per L. Urine arsenic concentrations may also be measured as a timed urine collection, or the concentration in urine collected during a 12- to 24-hour period, reported in micrograms per 12 or 24 hours. The quantitative 24-hour urine collection is considered the most reliable. In an emergency situation, the spot urine sample may be of value. Normal total urinary arsenic values are less than 50 μg per L or less than 25 μg per 24 hours. In the first 2 to 3 days following acute symptomatic intoxications, total 24-hour urinary arsenic excretion is typically in excess of several thousand micrograms, with spot urine concentration greater than 1,000 μg per L, and depending on the severity, it may not return to background for weeks. Recent ingestion of seafood may markedly elevate urinary arsenic values for the next 2 days. Therefore, it is important to take a careful dietary history of the past 48 hours when only total urinary arsenic is measured. Speciation of the urinary arsenic can be performed in some laboratories. Otherwise, the urinary arsenic test should be repeated in 2 to 3 days. Whole blood arsenic, normally less than 1 μg per dL, may be elevated early on in acute intoxication. However, blood concentrations decline rapidly to normal values despite elevated urinary arsenic excretion and continuing symptoms. Elevated arsenic content in hair and nail segments, normally less than 1 part per million, may persist for months after urinary arsenic values have returned to background. However, caution should be exercised when interpreting the arsenic content obtained from hair and nails because the arsenic content of these specimens may be increased by external exposure.

Management

The management of acute arsenic poisoning relies on supportive care and chelation therapy. Treatment begins with eliminating further exposure to the toxin and providing basic and advanced life support. Anyone with arsenic intoxication necessitating hospitalization should initially be admitted to an intensive care unit (ICU).

Gastric lavage should be performed following an acute ingestion and should be considered if the ingestion has been within the past 24 hours, as some arsenic compounds of low solubility may be retained in the stomach for a prolonged period of time. Frequently, seriously poisoned patients will have already vomited, evacuating some of their stomach contents. Activated charcoal and cathartics may be used, but their efficacy is unclear [24]. When there is evidence of a heavy metal burden on an abdominal radiograph, whole-bowel irrigation (WBI) with a polyethylene glycol electrolyte solution may rapidly help clear the GI tract of the metallic load. However, the absence of radiopacities on the abdominal radiograph is nondiagnostic and WBI should still be considered when there is a definite history that a poorly soluble arsenic compound has been ingested.

Intravascular volume depletion may require aggressive replacement with crystalloids, colloids, and blood products. Vasopressors are recommended for refractory hypotension. Invasive monitoring of the patient's hemodynamic status may be necessary.

In acute arsenic poisoning, extended cardiac monitoring for ventricular dysrhythmias is indicated for all patients who have prolonged QTc on their ECG. Electrolyte abnormalities—in particular, hypokalemia and hypomagnesemia—should be aggressively corrected, and concomitant QTc interval–prolonging drugs should be avoided. Serum potassium concentrations should be maintained at more than 4.0 mmol per L and magnesium concentrations at more than 1.8 mg per dL (0.74 mmol per L). There are no good data to indicate that suppression of ventricular dysrhythmias decreases mortality rates. If dysrhythmias occur, they should be treated according to current advanced cardiac life support guidelines. Type IA antidysrhythmic cardiac medications should be avoided because these drugs may themselves cause further QTc prolongation and worsen the polymorphic ventricular tachycardia. Lidocaine, magnesium, and isoproterenol have been used with limited success in the management of arsenic-induced torsades de pointes. A transvenous pacemaker for overdrive pacing may be necessary. Noncardiogenic and cardiogenic pulmonary edema should be managed according to current guidelines. In patients receiving arsenic trioxide induction therapy who develop prolonged QTc of more than 500 milliseconds on ECG, the risk/benefits of continuing therapy should be considered.

Hematologic effects of arsenic poisoning should be managed symptomatically with blood product transfusions and antibiotics as necessary for severe anemia, bleeding, or infections.

Patients with arsenic polyneuropathy should be given analgesics for pain and physical therapy for rehabilitation. Patients with polyneuropathy associated with severe arsenic poisoning should be observed closely for respiratory dysfunction. Neuromuscular respiratory failure may be delayed 1 to 2 months after the initial presentation. In cases in which there is progressive sensorimotor dysfunction, particularly ascending weakness, respiratory muscle function should be monitored carefully. When there is evidence of impending neuromuscular respiratory failure, aggressive supportive measures should be initiated in a timely fashion.

Patients with renal failure may benefit from hemodialysis. However, hemodialysis has limited use when normal renal function is present. Hemodialysis (initiated 24 to 96 hours postingestion) has been reported to remove about 4 mg of arsenic during a 4-hour period in patients with established renal failure [18]. It should not be surprising that only small amounts of arsenic are removed by dialysis as minimal amounts of arsenic are left in the central compartment once tissue distribution and equilibration is complete.

The principle behind chelation therapy is to increase excretion of the metal and decrease the target organ's metal burden. A chelator is an organic compound that has a selective affinity for heavy metals. It competes with tissues and other compounds containing thiol groups for metal ions, removes metal ions that previously have been bound, and binds with the metal ion to form a stable complex (chelate), rendering the metal less reactive and less toxic. The metal–chelator complex is water soluble and can be excreted in the urine, bile, or both, and to some extent, it can be removed by hemodialysis.

Dimercaprol (2,3-dimercapto-1-propanol [British anti-Lewisite, BAL]) is the traditional chelating agent that has been used clinically in arsenic poisoning. In humans and animal models, the antidotal efficacy of BAL has been shown to be most effective when it was promptly administered (i.e., minutes to hours) after acute arsenic exposure [25]. In cases of suspected acute symptomatic intoxication, treatment should not be delayed while waiting for specific laboratory confirmation. BAL is administered parenterally as a deep intramuscular (IM) injection. The initial dose is 3 to 5 mg per kg every 4 hours, gradually tapering to every 12 hours during the next several days. As the patient improves, this may be switched to 2,3-dimercaptosuccinic acid (DMSA; succimer) (see section "Lead" of this chapter). In the United States, DMSA is available only in an oral formulation. This precludes its use in acute severe arsenic intoxication when shock, vomiting, gastroenteritis, and splanchnic edema limit GI absorption. For patients with stable GI and cardiovascular status, a dose regimen of 10 mg per kg every 8 hours for 5 days, reduced to every 12 hours for another 2 weeks, may be employed. D-Penicillamine has also been reported to be successful adjunct treatment in cases of acute pediatric arsenic toxicity [26]. Oral D-penicillamine, 25 mg per kg every 6 hours (maximum of 1 g per day), should be used if BAL or DMSA is unavailable or if the patient is unable to tolerate these medications. Disadvantages in using D-penicillamine include that it is administered only by the oral route, it is usually not well tolerated, it should be used with caution in patients who are allergic to penicillin, and it entails potential enhanced absorption of arsenic–chelate complex. Adverse drug events associated with long-term D-penicillamine treatment include fever, pruritus, leukopenia, thrombocytopenia, eosinophilia, and renal toxicity. A complete blood count and renal function tests should be monitored weekly during D-penicillamine therapy.

BAL and its metal chelate dissociate in an acid medium and maintenance of an alkaline urine may protect the kidneys during chelation therapy [27]. BAL should be administered with caution in patients with glucose-6-phosphate dehydrogenase deficiency because it may cause hemolysis. The adverse drug events of BAL appear to be dose dependent, with an incidence of greater than 50% at a dose of 5 mg per kg [28]. The reported adverse drug events include pain at the injection site; systolic and diastolic hypertension with tachycardia; nausea; vomiting; headache; burning or constricting sensation in the mouth, throat, and eyes; lacrimation; salivation; rhinorrhea; muscle aches; tingling of the extremities; pain in the teeth; sense of constriction in the chest; abdominal pain; sterile or pyogenic abscesses at the site of injection; and a feeling of anxiety or unrest. In addition to these adverse drug events, a febrile reaction may occur in children. These signs and symptoms are most severe within 30 minutes after administration of BAL and usually dissipate within 1 to 1.5 hours. The adverse drug events may be lessened by the use of epinephrine or by pretreatment with antihistamine or ephedrine [28].

The therapeutic end points of chelation are poorly defined. Usually 24-hour urinary arsenic excretion is followed before, during, and after chelation with continued chelation therapy until the urinary arsenic excretion is less than 25 μg per 24 hours. Alternatively, when it can be demonstrated that more than 90% of the total arsenic excreted in the urine is in the form of MMA and DMA, endogenous biomethylation and detoxification may obviate the need for continued chelation [5]. This is likely to occur during the recovery period when urinary inorganic arsenic concentration has declined to less than 100 μg per 24 hours or total blood arsenic concentration is less than 200 μg per L [5].

Chelation therapy may not reverse neuropathy [12–14,29]. Early treatment may prevent incipient peripheral neuropathy in some, but not all, patients. However, the value of chelation in the treatment of an established arsenic neuropathy has not been demonstrated. In cases of chronic symptomatic arsenic intoxication with high urinary arsenic excretion, an empiric course of chelation may be warranted.

ARSINE GAS

Arsine (AsH_3) is a colorless, nonirritating, inflammable gas with a garlicky odor. It is considered to be the most toxic of the arsenic compounds. The garlic-like odor is not a reliable indicator of exposure as hazardous effects may occur below the odor threshold [30]. Exposure usually occurs in industrial/occupational settings, such as smelting and refining of metals and ores, galvanizing, soldering, etching, lead plating, metallurgy, burning fossil fuels, and the microelectronic/semiconductor industry [31]. (Computer chips made of gallium arsenide are etched with strong acids.)

Pharmacology

Arsine binds to red blood cells (RBCs) causing a rapid and severe Coombs' negative hemolytic anemia. The exact mechanism by which arsine is lytic to the RBC has not been definitively elucidated [31,32]. In vitro and animal studies indicate that hemolysis requires the presence of oxygen, there is a reduction in the RBCs' glutathione concentration, which is time- and concentration dependent on arsine gas exposure, and there is an inverse correlation between the reduced glutathione concentration and the extent of hemolysis. These findings are consistent with a mechanism of oxidative stress-induced damages to the RBCs, resulting in hemolysis.

Toxic concentrations of arsine appear to have deleterious effect on the kidneys. Acute renal failure was often a common cause of death prior to advent of hemodialysis [31,33,34]. Postulated mechanisms of arsine-induced renal failure include direct toxic effects of arsine on renal tubular cell respiration, hypoxia due to the hemolytic anemia, and the massive release of the "arsenic–hemoglobin–haptoglobin complex" precipitating in the tubular lumen, resulting in a toxic effect on the nephron [35]. Depending on the severity, renal failure may be evident by 72 hours from the time of exposure [31].

Clinical Toxicity

The severity and time to manifestation of arsine poisoning depend on the concentration and duration of the exposure. After an acute massive exposure, death may occur without the classic signs and symptoms of arsine poisoning. It is believed that after low-concentration exposures, arsine is rapidly and efficiently cleared from plasma into the RBCs. However, high concentrations of arsine may exceed the binding capacity of the erythrocytes, and the gas may directly damage vital organs. In cases in which signs and symptoms of arsine poisoning develop over time, the associated morbidity and mortality is partly related to the consequences of its hematologic and renal effects. In general, after a significant exposure to arsine, there is usually a delay of 2 to 24 hours before symptoms of arsine poisoning become apparent [31].

Initial complaints include dizziness, malaise, weakness, dyspnea, nausea, vomiting, diarrhea, headache, and abdominal pain [31,36]. Dark-red discoloration of the urine, hemoglobinuria, and/or hematuria frequently appear 4 to 12 hours after inhalation of arsine. Depending on the severity of the exposure, reddish staining of the conjunctiva and duskily bronzed skin may become apparent within 12 to 48 hours [36]. However, the sensitivity of this sign is unclear. The conjunctival and skin discoloration is due to the presence of hemoglobin. This should be distinguished from true jaundice due to the presence of bilirubin. The triad of abdominal pain, hematuria, and bronze-tinted skin is recognized as a characteristic clinical feature of arsine poisoning [31].

In one study, ECG changes associated with arsine poisoning included peaked T waves, particularly in the precordial leads [30]. The most pronounced T-wave changes occurred between the second and the twelfth day after exposure. The severity of illness did not correlate with the height of the T wave. There was no delay in atrioventricular or intraventricular conduction times. There was progressive normalization of the T-wave amplitude evident on the weekly follow-up ECG. The exact cause of the ECG change remains speculative.

Management

All patients hospitalized for arsine poisoning should be admitted in the ICU. The management of arsine poisoning should be directed at preventing further exposure to the gas, restoring the intravascular RBC concentration, monitoring the serum potassium, preventing further renal insult, and providing aggressive supportive care. In cases of acute and severe arsine poisoning, exchange transfusion or plasma exchange may be an efficient and effective means of management [31,34,37]. It is important to maintain good urine output (2 to 3 mL per kg per hour) at all times. Alkalinization of the urine has been recommended to prevent deposition of RBC breakdown products in the kidneys. In situations in which there is evidence of renal insufficiency or failure, both exchange transfusion and hemodialysis may be required. There are practical and theoretic considerations for using exchange transfusion. It restores the intravascular RBC concentration and removes erythrocyte debris and arsenic–hemoglobin complexes [34]. Hemolysis due to arsine poisoning can be a dynamic process; there is one report of ongoing hemolysis for at least 4 days in patients not selected for exchange transfusion [38]. Theoretic support for the use of exchange transfusion came from animal studies where a large proportion of the fixed arsenic in the blood of animals poisoned with arsine was in a nondialyzable form, and adequate removal of arsine and its associated toxic complexes would be a problem with hemodialysis alone. It has been suggested that with early diagnosis of arsine poisoning and prompt institution of exchange transfusion, the incidence of renal damage and long-term renal insufficiency may be reduced [33,38].

The results of using BAL in the treatment of acute arsine poisoning have been disappointing [36,39]. BAL does not appear to afford protection against arsine-induced hemolysis. It remains speculative whether BAL would be of benefit in subacute or chronic arsine poisoning [31].

LEAD

The use of lead and its environmental contamination has increased dramatically since the beginning of the Industrial Revolution. However, for the past 20 years, environmental and occupational exposure to lead as well as the severity of lead poisoning have decreased because of government regulations and increased public health awareness of the problems associated with lead, especially at low-concentration exposures.

The major environmental sources of lead include vehicle exhaust, paint, food, and water. Combustion of leaded gasoline by motor vehicles produced lead in automobile emissions, which is the main source of airborne lead. Airborne lead can be inhaled directly or deposited in the environment (soil, water, and crops). The content of lead in residential paint was not regulated until 1977. More than half of the older residential and commercial structures built prior to 1960 have been painted with lead-based paints. With time, flaking, chipping, peeling, and chalking of the paint occurs—a potential source of lead exposure. Industrial use of corrosion-resistant lead paint continues. High-concentration exposure may result from renovation, sandblasting, torching, or demolition of older applications. Food may contain lead that has been deposited in the soil or water. Food may be contaminated with lead when it is harvested, transported, processed, packaged, and prepared. Lead exposure may occur from use of lead-glazed pottery or ceramic ware for cooking and eating as well as from the consumption of food from lead-soldered cans. Water from leaded pipes, soldered plumbing, and water coolers is also a potential source of lead exposure. Some traditional Hispanic, Asian, and Middle Eastern folk medicine has been shown to contain significant amounts of lead. Mexican folk remedies, "azarcon" and "greta," are prescribed by the local folk healers (curanderos) to treat nonspecific GI symptoms collectively known as "empacho." Azarcon is a bright-orange powder and greta is a fine yellowish powder. Other names such as alarcon, coral, liga, Maria Luisa, and rueda have been given to these lead-containing folk remedies. In Asian communities, lead-containing folk remedies include bali goli, chuifong tokuwan, ghasard, knadu, payloo-ah, and Po Ying Tan. Middle Eastern lead-containing folk medicines include alkohl, cebagin, kohl, saoott, and surma.

The most significant way in which children are exposed to lead is through inhalation and ingestion. Children can ingest chips from lead-painted surfaces, or by mouthing items contaminated with lead from dust, soil, or paint. Some children are given folk remedies containing large quantities of lead. Another potential source of lead exposure in children is the preparation of infant formulas in vessels with lead solder.

Aside from the environmental sources, lead exposure in adults primarily comes from the occupational setting, particularly for electricians; cable splicers; plumbers; lead, copper, zinc, and silver miners; printers; lead smelters and refiners; steel welders and cutters; painters; auto repairers (radiator repair mechanics); sandblasting, demolition, and construction workers; battery manufacturers; solderers; bricklayers; silversmiths; glass manufacturers; and ship builders. One source of lead exposure that is not often considered is retained lead bullets, especially those that are near synovial surfaces.

Hobbies and related activities such as home remodeling, target shooting at indoor firing ranges, stained glass making, glazed pottery making, lead soldering, and making illicitly distilled whiskey ("moonshine") can potentially subject adults and their families to high concentrations of lead.

Pharmacology

In adults, about 10% of an ingested dose is absorbed, whereas in children, up to 50% may be absorbed. GI absorption may be increased by iron or calcium deficiency and varies directly with the solubility of the lead compound ingested and inversely with particle size. The oral dose associated with the lowest observable effect level in humans is uncertain. Acute human ingestion of 15 g of lead oxide has resulted in fatality.

Inhalation of lead is a significant route of exposure as lead particles (e.g., dust) and fumes can potentially reach the alveoli, where absorption from the lower respiratory tract is nearly complete. Airborne lead particles are usually too large to enter the alveoli of small children. These particles (when inhaled) are returned to the posterior pharynx through ciliary action and swallowed. Dermal absorption of lead is rapid and extensive for alkyl lead compounds, but minimal for inorganic lead.

After absorption, almost all lead in the blood is located within the RBCs [40]. RBC lead has a half-life of 30 to 40 days and is circulated and distributed into soft tissues and bones. The half-life of lead in the soft tissues is about 40 days, whereas the half-life in bones is 20 to 30 years. Hence, blood lead concentration may be declining as the soft tissue and bone burdens are rising. Equilibration between bone and blood lead does occur. The major depot for lead in the body is the skeletal system, which contains more than 90% in adults and more than 70% in children, in terms of the total body lead burden [41]. The primary sources of lead that cause clinical and subclinical symptoms are the blood and soft tissues. Lead that is deposited and incorporated into the matrix of bone can be mobilized during pregnancy, lactation, osteoporosis, and prolonged immobilization [42]. In addition, lead that is deposited in bone may have some toxic effects on bone growth and function.

The kidneys filter lead unchanged (with some active tubular transport at high concentrations), and the excretion rate depends on the glomerular filtration rate and renal blood flow. The kidneys account for about 75% of daily lead loss [40]. However, elimination of lead from the body is influenced by the relative concentration of lead in the various body compartments.

Common forms of inorganic lead are generally devoid of significant irritant or corrosive effects. However, alkyl lead compounds may be moderately irritating. The multisystemic toxicity of lead is mediated by at least two primary mechanisms: the inhibition of enzymatic processes, sometimes as a result of sulfhydryl group binding, and interaction with essential cations, in particular calcium, zinc, and ferrous iron. Pathologic alterations in cellular and mitochondrial membranes, neurotransmitter biosynthesis and function, heme biosynthesis, and nucleotide metabolism may also occur.

One of the principal toxic effects of lead is inhibition of enzymes along the heme biosynthesis pathway. Specifically, lead inhibits the enzymes δ-aminolevulinic acid (ALA) dehydrase and ferrochelatase. As a result, δ-ALA cannot be converted to porphobilinogen and iron cannot be incorporated into protoporphyrin IX. This is reflected by a measurable increase in serum ALA and protoporphyrin concentrations. The increase in protoporphyrin forms the basis of the erythrocyte protoporphyrin (EP) test, which has been used to screen for chronic lead exposure. Lead also inhibits the nonenzymatic mobilization of iron stores, which further contributes to the effect of anemia. Impaired heme biosynthesis may have widespread effects because of its impact on the cytochrome systems. In addition, lead appears to shorten erythrocyte survival time by interfering with the sodium-potassium–adenosine triphosphatase pump mechanism and by attaching to RBC membranes, causing increased mechanical fragility and cell lysis. Decreased heme synthesis and increased RBC destruction results in reticulocytosis. Inhibition of pyrimidine-5′-nucleotidase by lead results in accumulation of ribonucleic acid degradation products and aggregation of ribosomes in RBCs, which produce punctate basophilic stippling. However, neither anemia nor basophilic stippling is a sensitive or specific indicator of lead intoxication. Lead-induced anemia results from either a prolonged exposure or a concentrated short-term exposure with a latent period of several weeks.

Lead toxicity produces anatomic lesions in the proximal tubule and loops of Henle, which is characterized by round acidophilic intranuclear inclusion bodies. Most often, lead-induced renal injury is associated with prolonged exposure to large amounts of lead, resulting in progressive renal insufficiency.

The toxic effects of lead involve both the peripheral nervous system and the central nervous system (CNS). Peripheral nervous system toxicity is known as lead palsy and is due to the degenerative changes in the motoneurons and their axons, with secondary effects involving the myelin sheaths [43]. Lead palsy is usually a pure motor neuropathy and is the result of advanced chronic lead poisoning. Both adults and children can present with CNS dysfunction; however, children are the ones who present with encephalopathy [44,45]. Although lead encephalopathy is rare today, it is the most serious consequence of lead poisoning and is probably due to inhibition of the intracellular enzyme systems within the CNS.

Clinical Toxicity

Poisoning is usually the result of continued exposure to small amounts of lead rather than a single acute event. However, acute ingestion can produce lead toxicity [44, 46]. Usually the clinical presentation of acute lead toxicity appears to be associated with a sharp incremental rise in the concentration of lead in various soft tissues, and this often occurs against the background of chronic lead poisoning.

The multisystemic toxicity of lead presents a spectrum of clinical findings ranging from overt, life-threatening intoxication to subtle, subclinical deficits. Acute ingestion of very large quantities of lead (gram quantities) may cause abdominal pain, toxic hepatitis, and anemia (usually hemolytic).

Subacute or chronic exposure causes nonspecific constitutional symptoms such as fatigue, arthralgias, decreased libido, irritability, impotence, depression, anorexia, malaise, myalgias, weight loss, and insomnia [47]. GI symptoms include nausea, constipation or diarrhea, and intestinal spasm. The intestinal spasm, "lead colic," can cause severe, excruciating, paroxysmal, abdominal pain. CNS findings range from impaired concentration, visual–motor coordination, and headache, to severe, life-threatening encephalopathy characterized by vomiting, tremors, hyperirritability, ataxia, confusion, delirium, lethargy, obtundation, convulsions, coma, and death. A peripheral motor neuropathy, predominantly affecting the upper extremities, may result in extensor weakness. In rare instances, severe cases may produce frank "wrist drop." Decreased intelligence, impaired neurobehavioral development, decreased stature or growth, and diminished auditory acuity may occur. Hematologic manifestations include normochromic or microcytic anemia. This may be accompanied by basophilic stippling of the erythrocytes. Nephrotoxic effects include overt reversible acute tubular dysfunction, in particular, Fanconi-like aminoaciduria in children, and chronic progressive renal interstitial fibrosis following heavy long-term exposure in lead workers. Sometimes hyperuricemia, with or without evidence of gout, may be associated with the renal insufficiency [48]. An association between lead exposure and hypertension may exist in susceptible populations.

Repeated, intentional inhalation of leaded gasoline may result in ataxia, myoclonic jerking, hyperreflexia, delirium, and seizures.

Diagnostic Evaluation

Although encephalopathy and abdominal colic following a suspect activity may readily suggest the diagnosis of severe lead intoxication, the nonspecific nature of mild-to-moderate intoxication frequently presents a diagnostic challenge.

Exposure is often not suspected, and symptoms are commonly attributed to a "nonspecific viral illness." Lead intoxication should be considered in patients presenting with multisystem findings including headache, abdominal pain, and anemia, and less commonly, motor neuropathy, gout, and renal insufficiency. Lead encephalopathy should be considered in any child with delirium or seizures, and milder degrees of intoxication should be considered in children with neurobehavioral deficits or developmental delays. Lead encephalopathy has usually been associated with blood lead concentrations of 100 μg per dL or more [49]. Blood lead concentrations greater than 80 μg per dL are occasionally associated with acute severe illness.

Whole blood lead concentration and EP are the two methods most commonly used in testing for lead intoxication. Whole blood lead concentration is the most useful screening and diagnostic test for acute or recent lead exposure. This test does not measure total body lead burden, but it does reflect abrupt changes in lead exposure. Elevation in EP (>35 μg per dL) reflects lead-induced inhibition of heme biosynthesis. Because only actively forming erythrocytes are affected, elevations in EP will typically lag behind lead exposure by 2 to 6 weeks. EP value may help distinguish between recent and remote lead exposure. An extremely high whole blood lead concentration in the presence of a normal EP concentration would suggest a recent lead exposure. An elevated EP concentration is not specific for lead exposure, and may also occur with iron deficiency. EP is not a sensitive screening tool for low-concentration (<30 μg per dL) lead poisoning. EP and blood lead concentrations should be used as complementary methods of testing for lead intoxication.

EP, free EP, and zinc EP measure the same basic process and have very similar interpretations, but are not identical. EP is the most precise terminology. Because lead blocks (ferrochelatase) the final step in heme biosynthesis, it was originally thought that "free" EP was formed. However, it was subsequently shown that other porphyrins were measured in minute amounts, and most protoporphyrin had nonenzymatically bound zinc and was therefore not "free" [50].

Relationships between blood lead concentrations and clinical findings have generally been based on subacute and chronic exposure, and not on transiently high values that may result immediately following exposure prior to tissue equilibration (Table 133.2). Interindividual variability in response is extensive.

Measurement of urinary lead excretion is not very useful in the diagnosis of lead exposure. Urinary lead excretion reflects the plasma lead concentration, which increases and decreases more rapidly than blood lead concentration.

Nonspecific laboratory criteria consistent with lead toxicity include normochromic or microcytic anemia, basophilic stippling of RBC on peripheral smear, increased urinary ALA, and coproporphyrin. Liver transaminases may be elevated in acute intoxication. Low-molecular-weight proteinuria and enzymuria may precede elevations in serum creatinine. Radiopacities on abdominal radiograph may be evidence of lead in the GI tract following recent ingestion. This is especially true for lead-based ceramic glazes [46].

Management

Acute lead encephalopathy is a medical emergency that requires intensive care and monitoring of the patient. Prompt consultation with a toxicologist should be obtained to assist in the management. Because up to 25% of the children who survive an acute episode of encephalopathy sustain permanent CNS damage [49], medical treatment should be instituted before its onset. It has long been recommended that any child who is symptomatic from lead poisoning or has a whole blood lead concentration greater than 80 μg per dL should be hospitalized immediately and treated as a medical emergency [49]. More recently, the Centers for Disease Control has issued a statement that children with blood lead concentrations of 70 μg per dL or greater require immediate chelation therapy [51].

Although present-day recommendations for the treatment of lead encephalopathy were derived from experiences in managing children [49,52–54], they have been extrapolated to adults. The basic treatment plan consists of supportive measures and the use of chelating agents. As with any potential life-threatening emergency, assessment and aggressive management of the airway, breathing, and circulation should be paramount.

GI decontamination, beginning with gastric lavage, is indicated following acute ingestion of virtually any lead-containing substances because even small quantities of paint chip or a sip of lead-containing glaze may contain several hundred milligrams of lead. The use of activated charcoal has been suggested; however, its efficacy is unknown. Abdominal radiograph may reveal radiopaque foreign bodies in the GI tract following recent ingestion of lead-containing substances such as paint chips, lead weights, and lead-based ceramic glazes [46]. WBI with polyethylene glycol solution has been suggested as a means of decontaminating the GI tract when the presence of lead is evident on radiographic examination of the abdomen [46]. The effectiveness of WBI can be followed by serial abdominal radiographs. Although it is important to eliminate the source of continued lead absorption, therapy should not be delayed by attempts at GI decontamination, especially in cases

TABLE 133.2

WHOLE BLOOD LEAD CONCENTRATION AND ASSOCIATED CLINICAL FINDINGS

Whole blood lead concentration (μg/dL)	Associated clinical findings
<25	Decreased intelligence and impaired neurobehavioral development among children with in utero or early childhood exposure; generally without demonstrable toxic effects in adults
20–60	Mild overt effects such as headache, irritability, difficulty concentrating, slowed reaction time, and impaired visual–motor coordination, and insomnia may emerge Anemia may begin to appear Reversible, subclinical slowing of motor nerve conduction velocity may be detected
60–80	Subclinical effects on renal function GI symptoms (e.g., anorexia, constipation, and/or diarrhea, and abdominal colic) may emerge
>80	Serious overt intoxication, including abdominal pain (colic), and nephropathy
>100	Encephalopathy and overt neuropathy

of encephalopathy. Ultimately, the chief priority is to identify and eradicate the source of lead exposure and institute control measures to prevent repeated intoxication. In addition, other possibly exposed persons should be promptly evaluated.

Lead-containing buckshot, shrapnel, or bullets in or adjacent to synovial spaces should be surgically removed if possible, especially if associated with evidence of systemic lead absorption.

In a child presenting with encephalopathy, immediate treatment should begin with establishing an adequate urine output [49]. This can be accomplished by intravenous (IV) infusion (10 to 20 mL per kg) of 10% dextrose in water during 1 to 2 hours. If this fails to produce a urine output, infusion of a 20% mannitol solution (1 to 2 g per kg) is recommended at 1 mL per minute. Once urine output has been established, IV fluids should be restricted to the calculated basal water and electrolyte requirements plus a careful assessment of continuing losses. An indwelling Foley catheter should be used to monitor the rate of urine formation. IV fluids should be adjusted hourly in order to maintain urine flow that is within the basal metabolic limits, which is 0.35 to 0.50 mL of urine secreted per calorie metabolized per 24 hours or 350 to 500 mL per m^2 per 24 hours. Such management is designed to avoid excessive fluid administration and prevent further development of cerebral edema. Severe lead encephalopathy can occur without cerebral edema [52]. However, when cerebral edema occurs in the presence of encephalopathy, there is further insult to the brain, and it may be the immediate cause of death. Children with encephalopathy may exhibit syndrome of inappropriate antidiuretic hormone [54].

Benzodiazepines should be used for immediate control of seizures. If paralysis with sedation or general anesthesia is required for controlling seizure activities, a bedside electroencephalogram should be obtained to rule out electrical status. Because high doses of phenytoin and phenobarbital were required to control the initial seizures in lead encephalopathy, paraldehyde was formerly used [54]. However, barbiturates were recommended in the prevention of seizures during the early convalescent phase of lead encephalopathy [49]. Repeated seizures and hypoxia can exacerbate cerebral edema [49,54], so it was suggested that anticonvulsants be administered when there is evidence of increased muscle tone or muscle twitching; one should not wait for obvious seizure activity [49].

Computed tomography scan of the head should be performed in patients presenting with encephalopathy to rule out cerebral edema. If there is evidence of cerebral edema, intracranial pressure (ICP) monitoring should be performed (with neurosurgical consultation) to assist with the management of the patient. Avoid performing a lumbar puncture when there is increased ICP associated with cerebral edema. Measures advocated to control cerebral edema and increased ICP include careful sedation and neuromuscular paralysis, elevation of the head of the bed, hyperventilation, restriction of fluid therapy, ventricular drainage, diuretics (e.g., mannitol or furosemide), and steroids. These measures are "borrowed" from the neurosurgical experience in managing increased ICP. Restriction of fluids and the use of mannitol have been discussed previously. Maintaining the arterial partial pressure of carbon dioxide between 25 and 30 mm Hg by controlled hyperventilation has been shown to result in cerebral vasoconstriction and reduced ICP. The benefit of glucocorticoids in treating perifocal vasogenic edema due to an intrinsic intracranial mass lesion is well established. However, glucocorticoids have not been proved beneficial in models of intracellular cytotoxic edema, and neurologic outcome studies do not support the routine use of glucocorticoids following head injury, global brain ischemia, and cerebral vascular accidents [55]. If the cerebral edema associated with lead encephalopathy is believed to be vasogenic in origin, the empiric use of dexamethasone should be considered. Surgical attempts to relieve ICP by flap craniotomy have not been shown to be beneficial [56]. However, ventricular drainage (via the intracranial bolt placed for ICP monitoring) may effectively reduce a rising ICP.

Chelating agents have been shown to decrease blood lead concentrations and increase urinary lead excretion. Chelation has also been associated with improvement in symptoms and decreased mortality. However, controlled clinical trials demonstrating therapeutic efficacy is lacking, and treatment recommendations have been largely empiric. Although there appears to have been a sharp reduction in pediatric mortality due to acute lead encephalopathy with the advent of chelation treatment, there were concomitant advances in the management of elevated ICP, and the decline in mortality cannot necessarily be attributed to the use of chelation alone. BAL and calcium disodium edetate (CaEDTA) are the two chelators used in the treatment of lead encephalopathy. DMSA is used for less severe poisoning.

BAL increases both fecal and urinary excretion of lead. It is distributed widely throughout all body tissues, including the brain and RBCs. Because BAL is excreted in the urine and to some extent in the bile, patients with renal failure are not precluded from the use of BAL, whereas patients with hepatic insufficiency may have a lower tolerance to BAL [57]. Details regarding the use of this agent are discussed in section "Arsenic" of this chapter. BAL and medicinal iron can form a toxic complex that is a potent emetic, but the treatment of anemia with iron should be delayed until BAL therapy has been completed. If severe anemia requires prompt intervention during chelation therapy, transfusion would be preferable.

CaEDTA enhances the elimination of lead and, to a lesser extent, the elimination of endogenous metals (e.g., zinc, manganese, iron, and copper). Increased urinary lead excretion begins within 1 hour and is followed by a decrease in whole blood lead concentration over the course of treatment. CaEDTA diffuses rapidly and uniformly throughout the body, but it does not appear to enter RBCs and very slowly diffuses across the blood–brain barrier [58]. CaEDTA mobilizes lead (primarily) from soft tissues and from a fraction of the larger lead stores present in bone. CaEDTA is not metabolized; rather, it is cleared from the body by urinary excretion. It can be administered IV or IM, with the former being the preferred and most effective route. Oral administration of CaEDTA has been known to increase absorption of lead from the GI tract; therefore, it should not be given by this route. The principal toxic effect of CaEDTA is on the kidneys, which can result in renal tubular necrosis [59]. The renal toxicity is dose related and reversible. Because CaEDTA increases renal excretion of lead and its accumulation increases the risk of nephrotoxicity, anuria would be a contraindication in its use. An adequate urine flow should be established before initiating CaEDTA therapy.

In the management of patients with lead encephalopathy, some clinicians would advocate the use of BAL and CaEDTA beginning with a priming dose of BAL at the same time that an adequate urine output is being established. The priming dose of BAL is 75 mg per m^2 (3 to 5 mg per kg) IM and is administered every 4 hours. After 4 hours have elapsed since the priming dose of BAL, a continuous slow IV infusion of CaEDTA 1,500 mg per m^2 per day (30 mg per kg per day) is started. In cases where there is evidence of cerebral edema and/or increased ICP associated with encephalopathy, CaEDTA (same dosage) should be given by deep IM injection in two to three divided doses every 8 to 12 hours. When the IM route is preferred, procaine (0.5%) should be given along with CaEDTA because IM administration of CaEDTA is extremely painful. BAL and CaEDTA are usually continued for 5 days. In patients with high body lead burdens, cessation of chelation is often followed by a rebound in blood lead concentration as bone stores equilibrate with lower soft-tissue concentrations.

A second course of chelation may be considered on the basis of whole blood lead concentration after 2 days of interruption of BAL and CaEDTA treatment, and the persistence or recurrence of symptoms. A third course may be required if the whole blood concentration rebounds to 50 μg per dL or greater within 48 hours after the second chelation treatment. If chelation is required for the third time, it should begin a week after the last dose of BAL and CaEDTA.

In the management of symptomatic patients with lead poisoning who are not overtly encephalopathic, most clinicians would advocate the same course of treatment as for those with encephalopathy, but with lower doses of BAL and CaEDTA. The priming dose of BAL is 50 mg per m^2 (2 to 3 mg per kg) IM and is administered every 4 hours. After 4 hours have elapsed since the priming dose of BAL, a continuous slow IV infusion of CaEDTA 1,000 mg per m^2 per day (20 to 30 mg per kg per day) is started. Alternatively, CaEDTA may be given in two to three divided doses every 8 to 12 hours by continuous infusion or deep IM injection. BAL and CaEDTA should be continued for 5 days with daily monitoring of whole blood lead concentrations. BAL may be discontinued any time during these 5 days if the whole blood lead concentration decreases to less than 50 μg per dL, but CaEDTA treatment should continue for 5 days. A second or third course of chelation may be considered on the basis of the same guidelines as discussed in the previous paragraph.

In the management of asymptomatic patients with whole blood lead concentrations 70 g per dL or greater, some clinicians would advocate the use of BAL and CaEDTA in the same doses and with the same guidelines as for treatment of symptomatic lead poisoning without encephalopathy. A second course of chelation with CaEDTA alone may be necessary if the whole blood lead concentration rebounds to 50 μg per dL or more within 5 to 7 days after chelation has ceased. Some clinicians prefer DMSA.

A water-soluble analogue of BAL, DMSA enhances the urinary excretion of lead, mercury, and arsenic. It has an insignificant effect on elimination of the endogenous minerals calcium, iron, and magnesium. Minor increases in zinc and copper excretion may occur. Oral DMSA is rapidly but variably absorbed, with peak blood concentrations occurring between 1 and 2 hours. The drug is predominantly cleared by the kidneys, with peak urinary elimination of the parent drug and its metabolites occurring between 2 and 4 hours. DMSA is approved for use in lead and mercury intoxications, in which it is associated with increased urinary excretion of the metals, and concurrent reversal of metal-induced enzyme inhibition. Oral DMSA is comparable to parenteral CaEDTA in decreasing whole blood lead concentration during treatment. Although treatment with DMSA has been associated with subjective clinical improvement, controlled clinical trials demonstrating therapeutic efficacy have not been reported. Reported adverse drug events of DMSA include GI disturbances (anorexia, nausea, vomiting, and diarrhea), mercaptan-like (sulfur) odor to the urine, rashes, mild-to-moderate neutropenia, and mild, reversible increases in hepatic transaminases.

Although DMSA is officially approved for use only in children with whole blood concentration in excess of 45 μg per dL, it has similar ability to lower whole blood lead concentration in adults. Treatment is initiated at an oral dose of 10 mg per kg (350 mg per m^2) every 8 hours for 5 days. Treatment is then continued at the same dose every 12 hours for an additional 2 weeks. An additional course of treatment may be considered on the basis of posttreatment whole blood lead concentrations and the persistence or recurrence of symptoms. Whole blood lead concentration may decline by more than 50% during treatment, but patients with large body burdens may experience rebound to within 20% of pretreatment concentrations as bone body stores reequilibrate with tissue concentrations. An interval of 2 or more weeks may be indicated to assess the extent of posttreatment rebound in whole blood lead concentration. Experience with oral DMSA in severe lead intoxication (e.g., lead encephalopathy or lead colic) is very limited, and consideration should be given to parenteral chelation therapy in such cases.

MERCURY

Mercury (Hg) is a naturally occurring metal that is mined chiefly as mercuric sulfate (HgS) in cinnabar ore. It is converted into three primary forms, each with a distinct toxicology: elemental (Hg^0) mercury, inorganic (mercurous [Hg^{+1}] and mercuric [Hg^{2+}]) mercury salts, and organic (alkyl and phenyl) mercury. The pattern and severity of toxicity are highly dependent on the form of mercury and route of exposure, mostly because of different pharmacokinetic profiles.

Elemental Mercury

Elemental mercury is the only metal that exists in liquid form at standard temperature and pressure. As such, metallic mercury can evaporate slowly at room temperature or rapidly when heated, and can contribute to the partial pressure of the ambient air that is breathed. A small spill in an enclosed space (e.g., a bedroom) can also produce high concentrations of mercury in the air because of its high vapor pressure. Various instruments contain elemental mercury including thermometers, manometers, barometers, switches, pumps, and special surgical tubes (such as Miller-Abbott, Canter, and Kaslow). Dental amalgam is prepared with elemental mercury and contains approximately 50% elemental mercury by weight.

Personnel in occupational settings who are potentially exposed include chlor-alkali mercury cell operation workers, electroplaters, explosives manufacturers, laboratory personnel, pesticide/fungicide production and application workers, manufacturers of batteries or mercury vapor lamps, metallurgists, and miners and processors of cinnabar, gold, silver, copper, and zinc. Exposure to mercury vapor from elemental mercury spill, work hazard, home gold ore purification, accidental heating of metallic mercury, and vacuum cleanup of a mercury spill have also been reported [60].

Pharmacology

When ingested, elemental mercury is poorly absorbed (<0.01%) from the healthy, intact, and normal-functioning GI tract. In contrast, inhaled mercury vapor is believed to cross the alveolar membranes rapidly because of its high diffusibility and high lipid solubility. About 75% of the inhaled dose is retained [61]. The absorbed elemental mercury vapor rapidly diffuses into the RBCs, where it undergoes oxidation to the mercuric ion and binds to ligands in the RBC. However, a certain amount of the dissolved vapor persists in the plasma to reach the blood–brain barrier, which it crosses readily [62]. Once in the brain tissue, the dissolved mercury vapor is oxidized to mercuric ion, trapping it within the CNS, where it is available for binding tissue ligands. Elemental mercury vapor is also easily transported across the placenta [63].

Elemental mercury vapor is eliminated from the body mainly as mercuric ion by urinary and fecal routes. Exhalation of mercury vapor and secretion of mercuric ions in saliva and sweat do occur and contribute to the elimination process. The rate of excretion is dose dependent. Elemental mercury follows a biphasic elimination rate, initially rapid and then slow, with a biologic half-life in humans of about 60 days.

Mercuric ion has an affinity to bind and react with sulfhydryl moieties of proteins, leading to nonspecific inhibition of enzyme systems and pathologic alteration of cellular membranes.

The pulmonary and central nervous systems bear the brunt of the insult in elemental mercury vapor poisoning. Damage to the respiratory system results from acute inhalation exposure to high concentrations of elemental mercury vapor, which acts as a direct airway irritant and a cellular poison [60,64]. Pulmonary toxicity is characterized by exudative alveolar and interstitial edema, erosive bronchitis and bronchiolitis with interstitial pneumonitis, and desquamation of the bronchial epithelium. The ensuing obstruction results in alveolar dilatation, interstitial emphysema, pneumatocele formation, pneumothorax, and mediastinal emphysema.

In the CNS, a cumulative toxic effect occurs as the inhaled elemental mercury vapor is oxidized to mercuric ion, leading to progressive CNS dysfunction. As would be expected, CNS toxicity is typically the result of chronic elemental mercury vapor exposure.

Clinical Toxicity

The ingestion of elemental mercury usually causes no adverse effects [65]. However, systemic absorption of mercury is possible in the presence of any bowel abnormality affecting mucosal integrity or impeding normal motility and transit. In addition, inflammatory bowel disease or enteric fistula allowing for prolonged elemental mercury exposure and the conversion of metallic mercury to an inorganic absorbable ion has been reported [66]. Elemental mercury that is retained in the appendix can result in local inflammation, perforation, and the consequent possibility of systemic mercury intoxication. Signs of appendiceal inflammation or systemic mercury absorption and toxicity should be appropriately monitored and treated. Prophylactic appendectomy in the absence of signs and symptoms of appendicitis should be avoided because of the risk of mercury extravasation through the surgical anastomosis and intra-abdominal suppurative complications [67].

Subcutaneous injection of elemental mercury may cause a local fibrous reaction, local abscess, granuloma formation, and systemic embolization, and systemic absorption with toxic manifestations has been reported [68,69].

IV injected elemental mercury has been reported to cause pulmonary and systemic mercury embolization, associated with an elevated blood mercury concentration, and sequelae may include tremor, lower extremity weakness, and reduced carbon monoxide diffusing capacity [68,70,71]. Mercury extravasation at the injection site can produce a severe local inflammatory reaction. Granuloma formation with fibrosis and inflammation with systemic mercury absorption has also been reported.

Acute intense inhalation of mercury vapor in a confined or poorly ventilated space may result in death. Initial symptoms usually occur within several hours following exposure and include fever, chills, headache, dyspnea, gingivostomatitis, nausea, vomiting, metallic taste in the mouth, paroxysmal cough, tachypnea, chest tightness, diarrhea, and abdominal cramps [64]. These symptoms may subside or, in severe cases, may progress to interstitial pneumonitis, bilateral infiltrates, atelectasis, noncardiogenic pulmonary edema, interstitial pulmonary fibrosis, and death [64]. In addition, complications such as subcutaneous emphysema, pneumomediastinum, and pneumothorax may occur. Children younger than 30 months seem to be particularly susceptible to such exposures [72].

Aspiration of elemental mercury may cause no acute respiratory symptoms, cough and mild dyspnea, acute pneumonitis, or progressive cough with copious amounts of frankly bloody sputum production, leading to respiratory compromise and death [73]. Most patients remain asymptomatic or recover without any significant sequelae. In two cases, systemic absorption of the aspirated elemental mercury was suggested by elevations in the 24-hour urinary mercury concentrations, but neither patient became symptomatic. Elemental mercury was consistently evident on chest radiographs obtained on follow-up examination, which varied from 1 month to 20 years. One case with postmortem findings from the lungs 22 years later included globules of elemental mercury surrounded by extensive fibrosis and granuloma formation. Subclinical changes in peripheral nerve function and renal function have been reported, but symptomatic neuropathy and nephropathy are rare.

Diagnostic Evaluation

Diagnosis depends on integration of characteristic findings with a history of known or potential exposure, and the presence of elevated whole blood mercury concentration and urinary mercury excretion. Abdominal radiographs may be used to document the extent of the GI contamination following elemental mercury ingestion. Radiographs of the injection site may help to define the extent of the infiltrated mercury. Chest radiograph and computed axial tomography scan may be useful in determining the location of systemic embolization.

Whole blood and urinary mercury concentrations are useful in confirming exposure. In most people without occupational exposure, whole blood mercury concentration is less than 2 μg per dL and "spot" or single-voided urine mercury concentration is less than 10 μg per L. A quantitative 24-hour urinary mercury excretion, usually less than 50 μg per 24 hours, is probably the most useful tool in diagnosing acute exposure (Table 133.3).

Management

Any patient requiring hospitalization because of acute elemental mercury inhalation or aspiration should be admitted to the ICU. As with any potential life-threatening emergency, assessment and aggressive management of the airway, breathing, and circulation should be paramount. Treatment is primarily supportive. Another priority is to identify and eradicate the source of elemental mercury exposure and to identify and evaluate other possibly exposed persons.

In cases in which elemental mercury ingestion has been documented, WBI with polyethylene glycol electrolyte solution or surgical removal may be necessary, depending on radiographic evidence of mercury retention, elevated blood urine mercury concentrations, and the patient's clinical status. Repeat abdominal radiographs may be used to document the effectiveness of WBI or to follow the progress of the ingested metallic mercury.

Aggressive local wound management of the injection site(s) should include prompt excision of all readily accessible

TABLE 133.3

ELEMENTAL MERCURY VAPOR EXPOSURE

Urine mercury concentration (μg/L)	Associated clinical findings
30–50	Subclinical neuropsychiatric effects
50–100	Early subclinical tremor
>100	Overt neuropsychiatric disturbances
>200	True tremors

subcutaneous areas in which metallic mercury is demonstrated, copious saline irrigation to remove metallic mercury droplets, and suction removal of the mercury [74]. Surgical excision of mercury granulomas has also been recommended [68]. Injection of dimercaprol BAL into the wound is not recommended as it may delay wound healing [75].

Patients acutely exposed to elemental mercury vapor should be monitored closely for respiratory symptoms. Chest radiographs, arterial blood gases, and pulmonary function should be followed in symptomatic patients. Oxygen and bronchodilators should be administered as needed. Progressive deterioration of respiratory function may require aggressive airway management with tracheal intubation, mechanical ventilation, and positive end-expiratory pressure. Early treatment with corticosteroids has been used in an attempt to reduce the complication of pulmonary fibrosis. However, neither corticosteroids nor prophylactic antibiotics have proved to be beneficial in the management of elemental mercury vapor-induced pulmonary complications.

Patients who have aspirated elemental mercury should be managed in a similar fashion. Vigorous suctioning, postural drainage, and good pulmonary toilet may assist the patient in expectorating some of the aspirated mercury. In addition, bronchoscopy may be indicated.

Chelating agents that are commercially available in the United States for use in the treatment of mercury poisoning include BAL, DMSA, and D-penicillamine (see sections "Arsenic" and "Lead" of this chapter). The choice of chelator depends on the form of mercury involved and the presenting signs and symptoms of the patient. DMSA and D-penicillamine may facilitate the absorption of mercury from the GI tract and should not be given when there is still evidence of mercury present in the gut. Because animal studies show that BAL may redistribute mercury to the brain from other tissue sites [76–78] and the brain is a target organ in elemental mercury poisoning, it would seem prudent not to use BAL for the treatment of inhalational exposures. DMSA appears to be associated with fever adverse events and more efficient mercury excretion when compared with D-penicillamine and is preferred for mercury vapor poisoning. DMSA may enhance urinary mercury excretion and reduce nephrotoxicity after GI absorption of elemental mercury [79]. The initial recommended dose of DMSA is 10 mg per kg every 8 hours, tapering to every 12 hours during the next several days. DMSA can be administered via nasogastric tube in severe poisoning cases in which endotracheal intubation is required.

The therapeutic end points of chelation are poorly defined. Probably the only objective measurable effectiveness of chelation therapy is enhanced urinary excretion of mercury. A potential end point for chelation may be when the patient's urinary mercury concentration approaches normal. Although the use of chelators is recommended to increase excretion and relieve target organs of metal burden, the use of BAL has not been proved to affect the course of elemental mercury-induced respiratory failure, and the effect of DMSA on clinical outcome has not yet been fully studied.

There is no role for multiple-dose activated charcoal, hemoperfusion, or hemodialysis in removing elemental mercury.

Inorganic Mercury

Acute inorganic mercury poisoning is usually the result of intentional or accidental ingestion. Most of the literature on inorganic mercury poisoning deals with mercuric chloride (mercuric bichloride [$HgCl_2$]), with the lethal adult dose estimated to be between 1 and 4 g.

Mercurials are available in medications (antiparasitic, antihelminthic, vermifuge, antiseptic, antipruritic, and disinfectant), paints, stool fixatives, permanent-wave solutions, teething powder, button batteries, fungicides/biocides, folk remedies (Mexican-American treatments for "empacho," a chronic stomach ailment; Asian, particularly Chinese, herbal or patent medications), and occult practices (Latin American and Caribbean natives). Although mercurial medications have largely been replaced by less toxic drugs, topical antiseptics containing mercury are still being used.

Pharmacology

Absorption of inorganic mercury salt from the GI tract is probably dose dependent. After absorption, the salt dissociates into the ionic form and is initially distributed between RBCs and plasma. Distribution of mercury within the body and within the organs varies widely. It has been demonstrated by animal autoradiographic study that mercuric ion is accumulated predominantly in the renal cortex [80]. Mercury ions do not appear to significantly cross the blood–brain barrier or the placental barrier. However, on the basis of the autoradiographic study, the brain does take up mercury slowly and retains it for a relatively longer period of time [80]. Mercury ions are eliminated from the body mainly by the urinary and fecal routes. The rate of excretion is dose dependent. Inorganic mercury follows a biphasic elimination rate, initially rapid and then slow, with a biologic half-life of about 60 days in humans.

Mercury ions have an affinity to bind and react with sulfhydryl moieties of proteins, leading to nonspecific inhibition of enzyme systems and pathologic alteration of cellular membranes. In addition, inorganic mercurials are highly corrosive substances.

The target organs of inorganic mercury poisoning are the GI tract and kidneys. The caustic property of the inorganic mercurials could potentially cause damage throughout GI tract, including corrosive stomatitis, necrotizing esophagitis, gastritis, and ulcerative colitis. A report of postmortem examination of patients who died within 48 hours postingestion showed severe hemorrhagic necrosis of the upper GI wall [81]. Nephrotoxicity following inorganic mercury poisoning from acute tubular necrosis of the distal portions of the proximal convoluted tubules resulted in acute oliguric renal failure and uremia [81,82]. The CNS is usually spared because only small amounts of mercuric ion can cross the blood–brain barrier. However, cases of CNS toxicity have been described with chronic mercury ingestion.

Clinical Toxicity

The clinical effects of acute inorganic mercury poisoning can be divided into the initial local corrosive effect on the GI tract followed by the injury that occurs at the site of excretion, which is the kidneys.

Inorganic mercury is a highly caustic substance. Depending on the amount ingested, the GI symptoms that follow may vary from mild gastritis to severe necrotizing ulceration of the intestinal mucosa, which can be fatal within a few hours [83]. Ingestion of 100 mg of inorganic mercury has been reported to be associated with a bitter metallic taste in the mouth, a sense of constriction about the throat, substernal burning, gastritis, abdominal pains, nausea, and vomiting [82]. A serious acute inorganic mercury ingestion may cause the abrupt onset of hematemesis, hemorrhagic gastroenteritis, and abdominal pain. Intestinal necrosis may ensue. In addition, massive bleeding from the colon has been reported to occur as late as 8 to 9 days postingestion [81]. Most of the bleeding came from the rectum, which was the most severely involved section of the colon. Such injuries to the GI tract can lead to massive fluid, electrolyte, and blood loss, resulting in shock and death.

Acute inorganic mercury ingestion may lead to acute oliguric renal failure because of acute tubular necrosis. Invariably, those patients who develop renal involvement initially have severe GI symptoms [83]. Typically, oliguric renal failure occurs within 72 hours postingestion, and as such, the initial GI symptoms may be resolving while renal toxicity may not yet be [81,83]. Spontaneous resolution of acute toxic anuria with renal tubular regeneration may be expected to occur between 8 to 12 days [84], with clinical recovery (if it occurs) between 9 and 14 days [81,83]. Chronic exposure may result in CNS toxicity.

Diagnostic Evaluation

Diagnosis depends on integration of characteristic findings with a history of known or potential exposure and presence of elevated whole blood mercury concentration and urinary mercury excretion. Inorganic mercury may be visualized on an abdominal radiograph as radiopaque foreign bodies in the GI tract. A positive radiograph would support the diagnosis, but a negative one would not exclude it.

Whole blood and urinary mercury concentrations (see section "Elemental Mercury" of this chapter) are useful in confirming exposure. Whole blood mercury concentration greater than 50 μg per dL in acute inorganic mercury poisoning is often associated with gastroenteritis and acute renal tubular necrosis.

Management

General management considerations are the same as for elemental mercury poisoning. In patients with acute ingestion, GI decontamination should be performed as soon as possible to minimize absorption and decrease the corrosive effect of the ingested inorganic salt. As with the ingestion of any corrosive substance, inducing emesis is to be discouraged. Elective tracheal intubation may be prudent prior to attempting GI decontamination. Gastric lavage should be performed with caution as the GI tract may have already been severely damaged. Endoscopy is recommended if corrosive injury (drooling, dysphagia, and abdominal pain) is suspected. Although theoretically reasonable but not rigorously studied, the use of a protein gastric lavage solution (1 pint of skim milk with 50 g of glucose, 20 g of sodium bicarbonate, and three eggs beaten into a mixture) to bind the mercury has been suggested, along with rinsing the stomach with egg white or concentrated human albumin after the lavage [82]. Activated charcoal may be considered as 1 g of charcoal is capable of binding 850 mg of mercuric chloride [82].

In cases in which there is radiographic evidence of radiopaque foreign bodies in the GI tract and if there is no evidence of gastroenteritis, WBI with polyethylene glycol electrolyte solution should be considered. Repeat abdominal radiographs may be used to document the effectiveness of WBI.

GI injury may result in severe fluid, electrolyte, and blood loss, and attention should be given to monitoring the patient's volume status. Replace intravascular and GI losses by the appropriate administration of crystalloid, colloid, and blood product. An indwelling Foley catheter should be placed to carefully monitor the urine output, which should be maintained at 2 to 3 mL per kg per hour. It is important to distinguish between oliguria due to inadequate volume resuscitation and oliguria due to toxic nephropathy resulting in renal failure. Invasive hemodynamic monitoring may be necessary.

It should be remembered that inorganic mercury is a highly corrosive substance. Aggressive surgical intervention may be required in cases in which there is severe gastric necrosis or when hemorrhagic ulcerative colitis becomes life threatening [81,85]. It has been suggested that the rectum should be resected at the time of colectomy when it is indicated for controlling hemorrhage from the colon [81].

BAL and DMSA (see sections "Arsenic" and "Lead" of this chapter) are the chelating agents of choice. The effectiveness of BAL depends on the promptness of its administration and the administration of an adequate dose. BAL is most effective if given within 4 hours of ingestion [86]. Prompt intervention is paramount in reducing renal injury, so expedient chelation therapy would be prudent in suspected cases of acute inorganic mercury poisoning. Chelation should not be withheld while waiting for laboratory confirmation of mercury poisoning. DMSA is also effective, but the capacity of the GI tract to absorb orally administered DMSA may be very much impaired in cases of severe inorganic mercury poisoning when hemorrhagic gastroenteritis, hemodynamic instability, and splanchnic edema are present. Once the GI and cardiovascular status has been stabilized, chelation with DMSA may be substituted for BAL.

Once renal damaged has occurred from inorganic mercury poisoning, therapy should be directed at the acute renal failure that may ensue. Hemodialysis should be used to support the patient through the oliguric or anuric renal failure period. A potential problem arises with continued BAL therapy in patients who develop renal insufficiency because the kidneys are one of the main routes by which BAL-Hg is eliminated. In such circumstances, BAL therapy may be judiciously continued as there is some evidence from animal studies that a significant fraction of BAL-Hg is also excreted in the bile. Some studies indicate that hemodialysis may contribute to the elimination of BAL-Hg in patients with renal failure [87–89]. In a patient who has renal failure but is otherwise stable and has a functional GI tract, DMSA may be an alternative to BAL.

Organic Mercury

The organomercurials are compounds in which the mercury atom is joined to a carbon atom via a covalent bond. It is the relative stability of this covalent bond that determines the toxicology of the organic mercury compounds. The organomercurials can be classified as short-chain alkyl (methyl-, ethyl-, and propylmercury), long-chain alkyl, and aryl (phenyl) mercury compounds. In general, the short-chain alkyl group, particularly methylmercury, is considered the most toxic. Acute ingestion of 10 to 60 mg per kg of methylmercury may be lethal, and chronic daily ingestion of 10 μg per kg may be associated with adverse neurologic and reproductive effects.

Potential sources of exposure to organic mercury include herbicide, fungicide, germicide, and timber preservative. In the general population, the major source of exposure to methylmercury is through the consumption of predacious fish (e.g., pike, tuna, and swordfish). Major incidents of human poisoning with methylmercury have occurred (Minamata and Iraq epidemics) with devastating outcomes.

Pharmacology

Organic mercury antiseptics undergo limited skin penetration; however, in rare cases, such as topical application to an infected omphalocele, dermal absorption can occur.

Methylmercury is well absorbed after inhalation, ingestion, and probably dermal exposure. It is widely distributed throughout the body [90]. In the blood, more than 90% is found in the

RBCs, with whole blood-to-plasma ratios of 200:1 to 300:1 [91]. Methylmercury is present in the body as water-soluble complexes mainly attached to thiol ligands and is highly mobile. It enters the endothelial cells of the blood–brain barrier as a specific complex with L-cysteine. This L-complex is structurally similar to the large neutral amino acid L-methionine and carried across the cell membrane on the large neutral amino acid carrier [92]. Methylmercury is transported out of mammalian cells as a complex with reduced glutathione and is secreted into bile as a glutathione complex. The glutathione moiety is degraded in the bile duct and gallbladder and finally to the L-cysteine complex. It is reabsorbed and returned to the liver, thereby completing the enterohepatic cycle [93–95]. In humans, about 10% of the body's methylmercury burden is in the CNS and the biologic half-life of methylmercury is 45 to 70 days [96]. Methylmercury readily passes the blood–brain barrier as well as the placenta barrier [97]. In animal studies, the dissociation between the carbon and mercury bond of methylmercury is very slow [91], and phenylmercury undergoes rapid breakdown to inorganic mercury within 24 hours [90,98]. In humans, the major route of excretion of methylmercury is in the feces, with less than 10% appearing in the urine [99]. Extensive enterohepatic recirculation in the GI tract has been demonstrated to occur with methylmercury [100].

Mercury has an affinity to bind and react with sulfhydryl moieties of proteins, leading to nonspecific inhibition of enzyme systems and pathologic alteration of cellular membranes. The CNS is particularly vulnerable to the toxic effects of methylmercury and is a potent teratogen and reproductive toxin. Methylmercury has been shown to alter brain ornithine decarboxylase, an enzyme associated with cellular maturity, and neurotransmitter uptake at the pre- and postsynaptic adrenergic receptor sites [101].

Clinical Toxicity

Most of the detailed information regarding toxicity has been derived from methylmercury poisoning cases. Methylmercury is a cumulative poison, primarily affecting the CNS. There does not appear to be a distinct difference between acute and chronic methylmercury poisoning. Following acute methylmercury intoxication, symptoms are usually delayed for several weeks or months. The classic triad of methylmercury poisoning is dysarthria, ataxia, and constricted visual fields [102]. Other signs and symptoms include paresthesias, hearing impairment, progressive incoordination, loss of voluntary movement, and mental retardation. Perinatal exposure to methylmercury has caused mental retardation and a cerebral palsy type of syndrome in offspring. Ethylmercury compounds may also cause gastroenteritis. Phenylmercury compounds produce a pattern of toxicity intermediate between alkyl and inorganic mercury.

Diagnostic Evaluation

Diagnosis depends on integration of characteristic findings with a history of known or potential exposure, and presence of elevated whole blood mercury concentration, which may reflect recent exposure. Whole blood mercury concentrations greater than 20 μg per dL have been associated with symptoms. Hair concentrations have been used to document remote exposure. Urinary mercury concentrations are not useful.

Management

General management considerations are the same as for elemental mercury poisoning. Following acute ingestion of organic mercurials, gastric lavage should be performed. Administration of activated charcoal may be of benefit. A successful way to increase the rate of methylmercury excretion is to introduce a nonabsorbable mercury-binding substance (polythiol resin) into the GI tract so as to interrupt the enterohepatic recirculation of methylmercury [103,104]. Repeated oral administration of a polythiol resin in methylmercury intoxication may be beneficial.

Limited data suggest that oral neostigmine may improve motor strength in patients with moderate-to-severe chronic methylmercury intoxication [104]. DMSA is the preferred chelating agent. BAL has been ineffective in treating neurologic symptoms because of methylmercury poisoning [105]. In addition, animal studies show that BAL may redistribute mercury to the brain from other tissue sites [76–78]. In contrast, DMSA was effective in reducing the brain concentration of methylmercury [106], and DMSA prevented the development of cerebellar damage in methylmercury-poisoned animals [107]. However, in humans, the effect of DMSA on clinical outcome has not yet been fully studied.

Hemodialysis is of little value because methylmercury has a large volume of distribution, and a considerable amount of methylmercury resides within the RBCs.

References

1. Sullivan JB, Krieger GR (eds): *Hazardous Materials Toxicology: Clinical Principles of Environmental Health*. Baltimore, MD, Williams & Wilkins, 1992.
2. Rom WN, Markowitz S (eds): *Environmental and Occupational Medicine*. 4th ed. Philadelphia, Wolters Kluwer/Lippincott Williams & Wilkins, 2007.
3. Au WY, Kwong YL: Arsenic trioxide: safety issues and their management. *Acta Pharmacol Sin* 29:296–304, 2008.
4. Litzow MR: Arsenic trioxide. *Expert Opin Pharmacother* 9:1773–1785, 2008.
5. Mahieu P, Buchet JP, Roels HA, et al: The metabolism of arsenic in humans acutely intoxicated by As_2O_3. Its significance for the duration of BAL therapy. *Clin Toxicol* 18:1067, 1981.
6. Lugo G, Cassady G, Palmisano P: Acute maternal arsenic intoxication with neonatal death. *Am J Dis Child* 117:328, 1969.
7. Gousios AG, Adelson L: Electrocardiographic and radiographic findings in acute arsenic poisoning. *Am J Med* 27:659, 1959.
8. Little RE, Kay GN, Cavender JB, et al: Torsade de points and T-U wave alternans associated with arsenic poisoning. *Pacing Clin Electrophysiol* 13:164, 1990.
9. Beckman KJ, Bauman JL, Pimental PA, et al: Arsenic-induced torsade de pointes. *Crit Care Med* 19:290, 1991.
10. Ringenberg QS, Doll DC, Patterson WP, et al: Hematologic effects of heavy metal poisoning. *South Med J* 81:1132–1139, 1988.
11. Limarzi LR: The effects of arsenic (Fowler's solution) on erythropoiesis. *Am J Med Sci* 206:334, 1943.
12. Heyman A, Pfeiffer JB, Willett RW, et al: Peripheral neuropathy caused by arsenical intoxication. *N Engl J Med* 254:401, 1956.
13. Jenkins RB: Inorganic arsenic and the nervous system. *Brain* 89:479, 1966.
14. Chhuttani PN, Chawla LS, Sharma TD: Arsenic neuropathy. *Neurology* 17:269, 1967.
15. Greenberg C, Davies S, McGowan T, et al: Acute respiratory failure following severe arsenic poisoning. *Chest* 76:596, 1979.
16. Donofrio PD, Wilbourn AJ, Albers JW, et al: Acute arsenic intoxication presenting as Guillain-Barre-like syndrome. *Muscle Nerve* 10:114, 1987.
17. Fesmire FM, Schauben JL, Roberge RJ: Survival following massive arsenic ingestion. *Am J Emerg Med* 6:602, 1988.
18. Vaziri ND, Upham T, Barton CH: Hemodialysis clearance of arsenic. *Clin Toxicol* 17:451, 1980.
19. Shannon RL, Strayer DS: Arsenic-induced skin toxicity. *Hum Toxicol* 8:99, 1989.
20. Reynolds ES: An Account of the epidemic outbreak of arsenical poisoning occurring in beer drinkers in the North of England and the Midland Counties in 1900. *Med Chir Trans* 84:409–452, 1901.
21. Aldrich CJ: Leuconychia striata arsenicalis transversus. *Am J Med Sci* 127:702, 1904.
22. Mees RA: The nails with arsenical polyneuritis. *JAMA* 72:1337, 1919.

23. Ayres S Jr, Anderson NP: Cutaneous manifestations of arsenic poisoning. *Arch Dermatol* 30:33, 1934.
24. Al-Mahasneh QM, Rodgers GC, Benz FW, et al: Activated charcoal as an adsorbent for inorganic arsenic. *Vet Hum Toxicol* 32:351, 1990.
25. Eagle M, Magnuson HJ: The systemic treatment of 227 cases of arsenic poisoning (encephalitis, dermatitis, blood dyscrasias, jaundice, fever) with 2,3 dimercaptopropanol (BAL). *Am J Syph Gonor Ven Dis* 30:420, 1946.
26. Peterson RG, Rumack BH: D-penicillamine therapy of acute arsenic poisoning. *J Pediatr* 91:661, 1977.
27. Klaassen CD: Heavy metals and heavy metal antagonists, in Gilman AG, Goodman LS, Rall TW, Murad F (eds): *The Pharmacological Basis of Therapeutics*. 7th ed. New York, Macmillan, 1985, p 1605.
28. Tye M, Siegel JM: Prevention of reaction to BAL. *JAMA* 134:1477, 1947.
29. Le Quesne PM, McLeod JG: Peripheral neuropathy following a single exposure to arsenic. *J Neurol Sci* 32:437, 1977.
30. Josephson CJ, Pinto SS, Petronella SJ: Arsine: electrocardiographic changes produced in acute human poisoning. *Arch Ind Hyg* 4:43, 1951.
31. Fowler BA, Weissberg JB: Arsine poisoning. *N Engl J Med* 291:1171, 1974.
32. Thomas R, Young R: Arsine: acute exposure guideline levels. *Inhal Toxicol* 13[Suppl]:43–77, 2001.
33. Uldall PR, Khan HA, Ennis JE, et al: Renal damage from industrial arsine poisoning. *Br J Ind Med* 27:372, 1970.
34. Hesdorffer CS, Milne FJ, Terblanche J, et al: Arsine gas poisoning: the importance of exchange transfusions in severe cases. *Br J Ind Med* 43:353, 1986.
35. Muehrcke RC, Pirani CL: Arsine-induced anuria: a correlative clinicopathological study with electron microscopic observations. *Ann Intern Med* 68:853, 1968.
36. Macaulay DB, Stanley DA: Arsine poisoning. *Br J Ind Med* 13:217, 1956.
37. Song Y, Wang D, Li H, et al: Severe acute arsine poisoning treated by plasma exchange. *Clin Toxicol* 45:721–727, 2007.
38. Teitelbaum DT, Kier LC: Arsine poisoning: report of five cases in the petroleum industry and a discussion of the indications for exchange transfusion and hemodialysis. *Arch Environ Health* 19:133, 1969.
39. Pino SS, Petronella SJ, Johns DR, et al: Arsine poisoning: a study of thirteen cases. *Arch Ind Hyg* 1:437, 1950.
40. Rabinowitz MB, Wetherill GW, Kopple JD: Kinetic analysis of lead metabolism in healthy humans. *J Clin Invest* 58:260, 1976.
41. Barry PSI: A comparison of concentrations of lead in human tissues. *Br J Ind Med* 32:119, 1975.
42. Markowitz ME, Weinberger HL: Immobilization-related lead toxicity in previously lead-poisoned children. *Pediatrics* 86:455, 1990.
43. Thomson RM, Parry GJ: Neuropathies associated with excessive exposure to lead. *Muscle Nerve* 33:732–741, 2006.
44. Alexander FW, Delves HT: Deaths from acute lead poisoning. *Arch Dis Child* 47:446–448, 1972.
45. Lin-Fu JS: Vulnerability of children to lead exposure and toxicity. *N Engl J Med* 289:1229, 1973.
46. Roberge RJ, Martin TG, Dean BS, et al: Ceramic lead glaze ingestions in nursing home residents with dementia. *Am J Emerg Med* 12:77–81, 1994.
47. Cullen MR, Robins JM, Eskenazi B: Adult inorganic lead intoxication: presentation of 31 new cases and a review of recent advances in the literature. *Medicine (Baltimore)* 62:221, 1983.
48. Ball GV, Sorensen LB: Pathogenesis of hyperuricemia in saturnine gout. *N Engl J Med* 280:1199, 1969.
49. Chisolm JJ Jr: Treatment of lead poisoning. *Modern Treat* 8:593, 1971.
50. Piomelli S: The diagnostic utility of measurements of erythrocyte porphyrins. *Hematol Oncol Clin North Am* 1:419, 1987.
51. Centers for Disease Control and Prevention (CDC): *Managing Elevated Blood Lead Levels Among Young Children: Recommendations from the Advisory Committee on Childhood Lead Poisoning Prevention. March 2002*. Atlanta, GA, CDC. Available at: www. cdc.gov/nceh/lead/CaseManagement/caseManage_main.htm. Accessed July 4. 2006.
52. Coffin R, Phillips JL, Staples WI, et al: Treatment of lead encephalopathy in children. *J Pediatr* 69:198, 1966.
53. Chisolm JJ Jr: The use of chelating agents in the treatment of acute and chronic lead intoxication in childhood. *J Pediatr* 73:1, 1968.
54. Chisolm JJ Jr, Kaplan E: Lead poisoning in childhood-comprehensive management and prevention. *J Pediatr* 73:942, 1968.
55. Jastremski M, Sutton-Tyrrell K, Vaagenes P, et al: Glucocorticoid treatment does not improve neurological recovery following cardiac arrest. *JAMA* 262:3427, 1989.
56. Greengard J, Voris DC, Hayden R: The surgical therapy of acute lead encephalopathy. *JAMA* 180:660, 1962.
57. Stocken LA, Thompson RM: Reactions of British anti-lewisite with arsenic and other metals in living systems. *Physiol Rev* 29:168, 1949.
58. Foreman H, Trujillo TT: The metabolism of C^{14}-labeled ethylenediaminetetraacetic acid in human beings. *J Lab Clin Med* 43:566, 1954.
59. Foreman H, Finnegan C, Lushbaugh CC: Nephrotoxic hazards from uncontrolled edathamil calcium disodium therapy. *JAMA* 160:1042, 1956.
60. Clarkson TW, Magos L: The toxicology of mercury and its chemical compounds. *Crit Rev Toxicol* 36(8):609–662, 2006.
61. Cherian MG, Hursh JB, Clarkson TW, et al: Radioactive mercury distribution in biological fluids and excretion in human subjects after inhalation of mercury vapor. *Arch Environ Health* 33:109, 1978.
62. Magos L: Mercury-blood interaction and mercury uptake by the brain after vapor exposure. *Environ Res* 1:323, 1967.
63. Clarkson TW, Magos L, Greenwood MR: The transport of elemental mercury into fetal tissues. *Biol Neonate* 21:239, 1972.
64. Asano S, Eto K, Kurisaki E, et al: Acute inorganic mercury vapor inhalation poisoning. *Pathol Int* 50:169–174, 2000.
65. Wright N, Yeoman WB, Carter GF: Massive oral ingestion of elemental mercury without poisoning. *Lancet* 1:206, 1980.
66. Bredfeldt J, Moeller D: Systemic mercury intoxication following rupture of a Miller-Abbott tube. *Am J Gastroenterol* 69:478, 1978.
67. Rusyniak DE, Nanagas KA: Conservative management of elemental mercury retained in the appendix. *Clin Toxicol* 46(9):831–833, 2008.
68. Bradberry SM, Feldman MA, Braithwaite RA, et al: Elemental mercury-induced skin granuloma: a case report and review of the literature. *Clin Toxicol* 34(2):209–216, 1996.
69. Zillmer EA, Lucci KA, Barth JT, et al: Neurobehavioral sequelae of subcutaneous injection with metallic mercury. *J Toxicol Clin Toxicol* 24:91, 1986.
70. Deschamps F, Strady C, Deslee G, et al: Five years of follow-up after elemental mercury self-poisoning. *Am J Forensic Med Pathol* 23(2):170–172, 2002.
71. Torres-Alanis O, Garza-Ocanas L, Pineyro-Lopez A: Intravenous self-administration of metallic mercury: report of a case with a 5-year follow-up. *Clin Toxicol* 35:83, 1997.
72. Jaffe KM, Shurtleff DB, Robertson WO: Survival after acute mercury vapor poisoning. *Am J Dis Child* 137:749, 1983.
73. Janus C, Klein B: Aspiration of metallic mercury: clinical significance. *Br J Radiol* 55:675, 1982.
74. Bleach N, McLean LM: The accidental self-injection of mercury: a hazard for glass-blowers. *Arch Emerg Med* 4:53, 1987.
75. Baruch AD, Hass A: Injury to the hand with metallic mercury. *J Hand Surg* 9 A:446, 1984.
76. Berlin M, Ullrebg S: Increased uptake of mercury in mouse brain caused by 2,3-dimercaptopropanol. *Nature* 197:84, 1963.
77. Berlin M, Lewander T: Increased brain uptake of mercury caused by 2,3-dimercaptopropanol (BAL) in mice given mercuric chloride. *Acta Pharmacol* 22:1, 1965.
78. Canty AJ, Kishimoto R: British anti-lewisite and organomercury poisoning. *Nature* 253:123, 1972.
79. Kosnett M, Dutra C, Osterloh J, et al: Nephrotoxicity from elemental mercury: protective effects of dimercaptosuccinic acid. *Vet Hum Toxicol* 31:351, 1989.
80. Berlin M, Ullrebg S: Accumulation and retention of mercury in the mouse. *Arch Environ Health* 6:589, 1963.
81. Sanchez-Sicilia L, Seto DS, Nakamoto S, et al: Acute mercurial intoxication treated by hemodialysis. *Ann Intern Med* 59:692, 1963.
82. Schreiner GE, Maher JF: Toxic nephropathy. *Am J Med* 38:409, 1965.
83. Troen P, Kaufman SA, Katz KH: Mercuric bichloride poisoning. *N Engl J Med* 244:459, 1951.
84. Fishman AP, Kroop IG, Leiter HE, et al: A management of anuria in acute mercurial intoxication. *NY State J Med* 48:2363, 1948.
85. Sauder PH, Livardjani F, Jaeger A, et al: Acute mercury chloride intoxication. Effects of hemodialysis and plasma exchange on mercury kinetic. *J Toxicol Clin Toxicol* 26:189, 1988.
86. Longcope WT, Luetscher JA Jr, Calkins E, et al: Clinical uses of 2,3 dimercaptopropanol (BAL). *J Clin Invest* 25:557, 1946.
87. Doolan PD, Hess WC, Kyle LH: Acute renal insufficiency due to bichloride of mercury. *N Engl J Med* 249:273, 1953.
88. Maher JF, Schreiner GE: The dialysis of mercury and mercury-BAL complex. *Clin Res* 7:298, 1959.
89. Leumann EP, Brandenberger H: Hemodialysis in a patient with acute mercuric cyanide intoxication. Concentrations of mercury in blood, dialysate, urine, vomitus, and feces. *J Toxicol Clin Toxicol* 11:301, 1977.
90. Gage JC: Distribution and excretion of methyl and phenyl mercury salts. *Br J Ind Med* 21:197, 1964.
91. Norseth T, Clarkson TW: Studies on the biotransformation of 203 Hg-labeled methyl mercury chloride in rats. *Arch Environ Health* 21:717, 1970.
92. Kerper LE, Ballatori N, Clarkson TW: Methylmercury transport across the blood-brain barrier by an amino acid carrier. *Am J Physiol* 262:R761, 1992.
93. Ballatori N, Clarkson TW: Biliary secretion of glutathione and glutathione-metal complexes. *Fundam Appl Toxicol* 5:816, 1985.
94. Dutczak WJ, Ballatori N: γ-Glutamyl transferase dependent biliary-hepatic recycling of methyl mercury in the guinea pig. *J Pharmacol Exp Ther* 262:619, 1992.
95. Dutczak WJ, Ballatori N: Transport of the glutathionemethyl mercury complex across liver canalicular membranes on reduced glutathione carriers. *J Biol Chem* 269:9746, 1994.
96. Aberg B, Ekman L, Falk R, et al: Metabolism of methylmercury (^{203}Hg) compounds in man, excretion and distribution. *Arch Environ Health* 19:478, 1969.
97. Suzuki T, Matsumoto N, Miyama T, et al: Placental transfer of mercuric chloride, phenylmercuric acetate and methylmercury acetate in mice. *Ind Health* 5:149, 1967.

98. Miller VL, Klavano PA, Csonka E: Absorption, distribution and excretion of phenyl mercuric acetate. *Toxicol Appl Pharmacol* 2:344, 1960.
99. Eckman L, Greitz V, Magi A, et al: Metabolism and retention of methyl-203-mercury nitrate in man. *Nord Med* 79:450, 1968.
100. Norseth T, Clarkson TW: Intestinal transport of 203 Hg-labeled methylmercury chloride. *Arch Environ Health* 22:568, 1971.
101. Slotkin TA, Bartolome J: Biochemical mechanisms of developmental neurotoxicity of methyl mercury. *Neurotoxicology* 8:65, 1987.
102. Hunter D, Bonford RR, Russell DS: Poisoning by methylmercury compounds. *Q J Med* 9:193, 1940.
103. Clarkson TW, Small H, Norseth T: The effect of a thiol containing resin on the gastrointestinal absorption and fecal excretion of methylmercury compounds in experimental animals. *Fed Proc* 30:543, 1971.
104. Bakir F, Damluji SF, Amin-Zaki L, et al: Methylmercury poisoning in Iraq. An interuniversity report. *Science* 181:230, 1973.
105. Hay WJ, Rickards AG, McMenemey WH, et al: Organic mercurial encephalopathy. *J Neurol Neurosurg Psychiatry* 26:199, 1963.
106. Aaseth J: Recent advance in the therapy of metal poisoning with chelating agents. *Hum Toxicol* 2:257, 1983.
107. Magos L, Peristianis GC, Snowden RT: Postexposure preventive treatment of methylmercury intoxication in rats with dimercaptosuccinic acid. *Toxicol Appl Pharmacol* 45:463, 1978.

CHAPTER 134 ■ HYDROCARBON POISONING

WILLIAM J. LEWANDER AND ALFRED ALEGUAS JR

Hydrocarbons are a group of organic compounds composed primarily of hydrogen and carbon. Although often mixtures, hydrocarbons may be divided into four basic types: aliphatic, halogenated, aromatic, and terpene.

Hydrocarbon exposures are frequent and account for an inordinate number of health care visits and hospital admissions. The American Association of Poison Control Centers reported 54,766 hydrocarbon exposures in 2007 [1,2]. Twenty-two percent were seen in a health care facility, and there were seven deaths. Nearly 32% of total exposures occurred in children younger than 6 years of age and involved ingestions, and most of these were accidental.

Storage in unmarked, readily accessible containers and an attractive color or aroma account for the high percentage of exposures in young children. In adolescents and adults, poisoning generally results from inhalational abuse, occupational exposure, intentional ingestion, or accidental aspiration during the siphoning of fuels. Cutaneous and even intravenous exposures have also been described. Ingestions in adults usually involve larger volumes, and there is a much greater likelihood of other coingested drugs or toxins. The majority of deaths are due to intentional inhalation abuse.

ALIPHATIC HYDROCARBONS

Aliphatic hydrocarbons, known as petroleum distillates, are straight-chain compounds produced from the fractional distillation of natural petroleum (Table 134.1). They are the most common cause of hydrocarbon poisoning.

After ingestion, the major toxicity of petroleum distillates is their potential to cause a fulminant, and sometimes fatal, chemical pneumonitis. Aspiration of even small amounts may produce severe pulmonary toxicity. Although vomiting often precedes and precipitates aspiration, lack of vomiting does not preclude the possibility that aspiration has occurred. Little or no systemic toxicity occurs even with intragastric administration of large doses (12 to 18 mL per kg) [3,4].

The risk of aspiration increases with low viscosity, low surface tension, and high volatility. Viscosity, the tendency to resist flow, is the most important property determining aspiration potential [5]. Substances with low viscosity (e.g., gasoline, mineral seal oil, and kerosene) have a high aspiration potential, whereas those with high viscosity (e.g., mineral oil and fuel oil) have a low potential for aspiration. Reduced surface tension may also allow a substance to spread rapidly from the upper gastrointestinal (GI) tract to the trachea. High volatility (tendency of a liquid to become a gas) increases the likelihood of pulmonary absorption.

Aspirated petroleum distillates inhibit surfactant, resulting in alveolar collapse, ventilation–perfusion mismatch, and subsequent hypoxemia. In addition, bronchospasm and direct capillary damage lead to a chemical pneumonitis and hemorrhagic bronchitis–alveolitis [2,5,6]. In animals exposed to kerosene, acute alveolitis peaked at 3 days and resolved by 10 days [7]. Histologically, a chronic proliferative process occurred, peaking at 10 days and resolving over several weeks. When highly viscous petroleum distillates are aspirated, a less inflammatory but more localized and indolent lipoid pneumonia may occur [8].

TABLE 134.1

COMMON PETROLEUM DISTILLATES

Product	Synonym	Main use
Gasoline	Petroleum spirits	Fuel
Petroleum naphtha fluid	Ligroin	Cigarette lighter
VM and P naphtha thinner	Varnish naphtha	Paint or varnish
Mineral spirits	Painter's naphtha Stoddard solvent White spirits Varsol Mineral turpentine Petroleum spirits	Dry cleaner Solvent Paint thinner
Kerosene fluid	Coal oil	Charcoal lighter Solvent Fuel for stoves, lamps
Fuel oil	Home heating oil	Fuel
Diesel oil	Gas oil	Furniture polish

Central nervous system (CNS) manifestations result principally from hypoxia and acidosis caused by pulmonary toxicity [9]. Although systemic toxicity is uncommon, it may be seen if the petroleum distillate is a vehicle for more toxic substances (e.g., heavy metal and pesticide), if it contains additives, or if a concomitant or massive ingestion has occurred [10]. Cardiovascular, hepatic, renal, and hematologic toxicities depend on the specific toxic substance involved.

Use of aliphatic hydrocarbons as volatile substances of abuse (VSA) is a serious and growing problem. It is most often seen in adolescents who use VSA as an easily available, legal, and affordable substitute for other intoxicants [11,12]. The most common aliphatic VSA are *n*-hexane, *n*-butane, isobutane, and propane—seen in adhesives, aerosols, liquefied petroleum gas (i.e., cigarette lighter refills and camp stoves), and gasoline. Inhalation may involve sniffing, "huffing" (spraying the solvent onto a cloth held to the mouth and nose), "bagging" (spraying the solvent into a paper or plastic bag and repeatedly inhaling the vapors), or a variant of these techniques [11]. These highly lipid-soluble substances are rapidly absorbed through the lungs and distributed to the CNS and fatty tissues [13]. The onset of symptoms occurs in seconds to minutes, with peak effects occurring somewhat later due to slower diffusion into tissues. Elimination of aliphatic hydrocarbon VSA is primarily by pulmonary excretion, and successive oxidation and metabolism by hepatic cytochrome P450 mixed-function oxidases [13].

Aliphatic VSA toxicity includes acute and chronic neurologic dysfunction; asphyxia; cardiovascular abnormalities; and pulmonary, GI, and cutaneous irritation. CNS toxicity ranges from stimulation at initial or low doses to a depressant effect, with general inhibition of cortical function at high doses [14]. Peripheral neuropathy and irreversible CNS damage have been reported [15–18]. Inhaled aliphatic hydrocarbons are asphyxiants (as well as pulmonary irritants) and may cause hypoxemia by decreasing the concentration of oxygen in inspired air. Their arrhythmogenic effects are thought to be due to their potentiation of endogenous catecholamines ("cardiac sensitization"), which may promote dysrhythmias (e.g., ventricular tachycardia or fibrillation) [19]. Additional factors such as hypoxia, acidosis, electrolyte abnormalities, and underlying cardiac conditions may contribute to arrhythmias. Dermal and mucosal irritation is due to their ability to dissolve lipids after prolonged or high-dose exposure [20]. Deaths associated with inhalational abuse may result from coma with respiratory depression, aspiration, or injuries incurred while intoxicated as well as from cardiac arrhythmias [21].

Clinical Manifestations

The clinical course after the ingestion of petroleum distillates primarily depends on the presence or absence of concomitant aspiration and its severity. Patients who aspirate generally demonstrate symptoms within 30 minutes; those who do not have symptoms within 6 hours of exposure remain asymptomatic [22]. Presenting signs and symptoms usually involve three main organ systems: pulmonary, CNS, and GI. Cardiovascular, renal, hematologic, and cutaneous toxicity have also been reported [23,24]. In most cases, symptoms resolve during the next 2 to 5 days with supportive care [22,25].

Initial coughing, gasping, and choking may progress and peak during the first 24 to 48 hours to tachypnea with grunting respirations, nasal flaring, retractions, and cyanosis [10,22]. The odor of petroleum distillates may be apparent on the breath. Wheezing, rhonchi, and rales may be heard on auscultation. In severe cases, pulmonary edema and hemoptysis occur. Arterial blood gases may demonstrate hypoxemia from ventilation–perfusion mismatch and early hypocarbia, which progresses to hypercarbia and acidosis. Abnormalities on chest radiographs occur in up to 75% of hospitalized patients, appearing within 2 hours in 88% of patients and by 12 hours in 98% [10,26], but may be delayed up to 72 hours. Early radiographic abnormalities include unilateral, but more commonly bilateral, basilar infiltrates and fine punctate perihilar densities. Localized areas of atelectasis are often present, whereas pleural effusions, pneumatoceles, and pneumothoraces occur infrequently [25,26]. Pneumatoceles generally occur 3 to 15 days after ingestion and resolve during 15 days to 21 months [2,27]. Radiographic findings correlate poorly with clinical symptoms and may persist for several days to weeks after symptoms have resolved [25–27]. Asymptomatic patients may have abnormal chest radiographs, whereas symptomatic patients may have minimal or no radiographic abnormalities early in the course [10].

Within the first 24 to 48 hours, fever (38°C to 39°C) and leukocytosis are common [22]. The persistence of fever beyond 48 hours suggests bacterial superinfection.

CNS involvement may occur in those with aspiration-induced hypoxemia, large intentional ingestions, or ingestions of mixtures that contain other toxic agents (e.g., aromatic hydrocarbons). Symptoms range from dizziness and lethargy (91%) to somnolence (5%) and, rarely, coma (3%) and convulsions (1%) [10,28]. The severity of CNS dysfunction often correlates with the severity of aspiration.

GI symptoms, such as local irritation of the oropharynx (e.g., burning), nausea, vomiting, and abdominal pain, are commonly reported. Hematemesis and melena occur rarely [10]. Vomiting appears to increase the likelihood of aspiration [25,29]. Cardiovascular toxicity is uncommon, but dysrhythmias and sudden death after gasoline siphoning have been reported [30].

Inhalation abuse may result in a range of acute CNS manifestations, including dizziness, incoordination, restlessness, excitement, euphoria, confusion, hallucinations, slurred speech, and coma with respiratory depression [31]. Peripheral neuropathy has been reported after chronic exposure [15,16]. Pulmonary toxicity may present as respiratory distress with cyanosis, or syncope with tachycardia or bradycardia. GI irritation may cause nausea, vomiting, and abdominal pain. Dermatologic manifestations range from perioral frost or pigmentation (after direct inhalation from a container) to local skin irritation [10].

Cases of acute renal tubular necrosis [32,33], hemoglobinuria secondary to intravascular hemolysis [34,35], severe burns after prolonged immersion in gasoline [36], and supraglottitis [37] have been reported. Aliphatic hydrocarbons are highly flammable, especially gasoline, and accidental thermal burns may occur during recreational use [38]. Therefore, patients with unexplained burns should be questioned regarding possible inhalation abuse. Chronic gasoline inhalation may also be accompanied by organo-lead poisoning [20,21,39]. Parenteral administration of petroleum distillates has caused local cellulitis, thrombophlebitis, and necrotizing myositis, with resultant compartment syndromes. Associated systemic effects include febrile reactions, hemorrhagic pneumonitis, pulmonary edema, seizures, and CNS depression [23,40,41].

Diagnostic Evaluation

After ingestion, diagnostic evaluation includes a thorough history (e.g., identity, amount, and concentration of toxin; time of ingestion; and symptoms before presentation at health care facility) and a physical examination (focusing on vital signs and the respiratory, CNS, and GI systems). Pulse oximetry should be monitored and a chest radiograph obtained in all symptomatic patients and in cases in which aspiration is suspected.

In symptomatic patients or those who have ingested concomitant toxins or toxic additives, laboratory evaluation should include an arterial blood gas determination; complete blood cell count; electrolyte, blood urea nitrogen, creatinine, and glucose measurements; liver function tests; and urinalysis.

Management

Patients with ingestions who remain or become asymptomatic with a normal chest radiograph (obtained 2 hours or more after exposure) may be discharged after 6 hours of observation. All symptomatic patients, those with abnormal chest radiographs, arterial blood gases, or pulse oximetry, and patients with suicidal intent should be hospitalized. Gastric decontamination is not recommended in petroleum distillate ingestion because absorption and systemic toxicity are minimal, and spontaneous or induced vomiting increases the risk of aspiration and pneumonitis [28,42]. Gastric decontamination is recommended only if potentially toxic amounts of aromatic or halogenated hydrocarbons, pesticides, heavy metals, or other substances have been ingested. Ipecac syrup is not recommended for GI decontamination. Patients who are unconscious, unable to protect the airway (e.g., poor or absent gag reflex), or deteriorating should be intubated with a cuffed endotracheal tube (in patients older than 6 years of age) and then have gastric aspiration or lavage performed. Activated charcoal and cathartic are indicated only if a toxic additive is present or concomitant ingestion has occurred. If cutaneous exposure has occurred, contaminated clothing should be removed and the skin thoroughly washed with soap and water [10].

All patients with respiratory symptoms should be given oxygen, placed on a cardiac monitor, and have intravenous access established. An arterial blood gas determination and chest radiograph should be obtained. The need for intubation should be based on clinical assessment of respiratory distress and objective data from arterial blood gases or pulse oximetry. Chest radiographs do not always correlate with clinical status and should not be used as the sole determinant for respiratory interventions. Continuous positive airway pressure may be necessary to maintain oxygenation, but the patient should be carefully monitored for the development of a pneumothorax. Bronchospasm should be treated with β_2-agonist bronchodilators because of potential myocardial sensitization to catecholamines [43].

Supportive care of pneumonitis includes careful monitoring of acid–base, fluid, and electrolyte balance (e.g., cautious hydration to avoid pulmonary edema), serial arterial blood gases or pulse oximetry, and chest radiograph evaluation. Complete blood cell counts with differential, serial sputum, or tracheal aspirate Grams stains and cultures assist in determining if bacterial superinfection has occurred. Baseline renal and liver function studies and a toxic screen should be obtained if toxic additives or concomitant ingestion is suspected. Animal and clinical investigations have failed to demonstrate any beneficial effect of steroid treatment [44,45]. Two animal studies indicate that they may be harmful [46–48]. In addition, prophylactic antibiotics have not been shown to be helpful [42,45,46]. Fever and leukocytosis secondary to chemical pneumonitis are common during the first 24 to 48 hours in the absence of superimposed bacterial pneumonia [10]. Antibiotics (e.g., penicillin or clindamycin) should be given only to patients with documented bacterial pneumonias (e.g., Grams stain or culture of sputum or tracheal aspirate) or worsening chest radiograph, leukocytosis, and fever after the first 40 hours [10]. Successful use of high-frequency jet ventilation and extracorporeal membrane oxygenation for the treatment of respiratory failure has been reported [49–51]. Other measures such as cardiopulmonary bypass, partial liquid fluorocarbon ventilation, and exogenous surfactant have been suggested for refractory cases, but the data to support their use are limited. [52,53].

Most patients with petroleum distillate poisoning recover fully with supportive care. Because minor pulmonary function abnormalities have been detected in as many as 82% of patients with aspiration pneumonitis who subsequently become asymptomatic [54], follow-up care with pulmonary function testing should be considered. When appropriate, the patient should receive psychiatric evaluation and poison-prevention education before final disposition.

HALOGENATED HYDROCARBONS

Halogenated hydrocarbons are aliphatic and aromatic derivatives that contain one or more atoms of chlorine, bromine, fluorine, or iodine. Although dozens of halogenated hydrocarbons are currently recognized, relatively few account for the majority of the toxic exposures. Like the aliphatic agents, halogenated hydrocarbons pose an aspiration risk. However, they are more readily absorbed from the GI tract and can cause systemic toxicity, most notably of the CNS, cardiovascular system, and hepatic and renal systems.

Halogenated hydrocarbons are used in the household and industry. They are frequently used as solvents, degreasers, dry-cleaning agents, refrigerants, aerosol propellants, and fumigants. Toxic exposures occur most commonly through inhalation, and several halogenated hydrocarbons (e.g., trichloroethylene, methylene chloride, and fluorocarbons) are intentionally inhaled for recreational purposes [55]. Bagging and huffing have been associated with a number of solvent-abuse deaths.

After absorption from the GI tract and occasionally through the skin, halogenated hydrocarbons are concentrated in adipose tissue, liver, and kidney. Metabolism and elimination vary according to the individual substance, with most undergoing at least some excretion through the lungs as unchanged parent compound and nearly all undergoing some degree of metabolism in the liver, with subsequent excretion of metabolites by the lungs and/or kidneys. Carbon tetrachloride (CCl_4), methylene chloride, and trichloroethane are prototypes of this class.

Carbon Tetrachloride

Previously used as a dry-cleaning agent and antihelminthic, CCl_4 is now restricted to industrial use, primarily in the production of refrigerants, aerosol propellants, and solvents. It is well absorbed through the skin [56], lungs, and GI tract, and it is concentrated in adipose tissue [57]. Approximately 50% of an absorbed dose is excreted unchanged by the lungs. Most of the remainder is metabolized by the liver to reactive intermediates or free radicals, or both, which covalently bind to proteins and induce lipid peroxidation, resulting in hepatocellular damage [58]. Ethanol, methanol, and isopropyl alcohol all increase CCl_4 hepatotoxicity, presumably through enzyme induction [59]. At lower doses, fatty degeneration of the liver occurs; at higher concentrations, centrilobular necrosis results [60]. In addition to hepatic damage, CCl_4 produces acute tubular necrosis of the kidney, affecting the proximal tubules and Henle's loop [61]. Although a direct nephrotoxic effect is likely [62], volume contraction may contribute to renal failure in some patients [63].

Inhalation exposure to CCl_4 may produce symptoms ranging from mild CNS depression to coma and death [64]. Although the estimated lethal dose of orally ingested CCl_4 is 90 to 100 mL, deaths have occasionally been reported after much smaller doses.

Nausea, vomiting, abdominal pain, diarrhea, drowsiness, and light-headedness usually occur within a few hours of exposure, regardless of route of exposure. Although liver enzymes may start to rise on the first day after exposure, clinical hepatotoxicity generally occurs on days 2 to 4, with fever, liver tenderness and enlargement, and jaundice [64]. Decline in renal function may occur concomitantly with hepatic dysfunction, although renal failure occasionally appears in the absence of hepatic failure [65]. Rarely, CCl_4 toxicity is accompanied by coma, convulsions, or myocarditis.

Early fatalities are the result of respiratory depression or cardiac dysrhythmias caused by cardiac sensitization to circulating catecholamines. Later deaths occur as the result of hepatic or renal failure, generally within the first week. In nonfatal cases, liver function tests generally return to normal within 2 weeks; recovery is usually complete.

Treatment initially involves stabilization and monitoring for respiratory depression and cardiac dysrhythmias. Exposure should be interrupted by removing victims of inhalation from the exposure site; in dermal exposures, contaminated clothing should be removed and the skin washed thoroughly. Patients who ingest more than 0.3 mL per kg should undergo gastric aspiration or lavage, preferably within 3 to 4 hours of ingestion [66]. Abdominal radiographs may be helpful in confirming suspected ingestions because CCl_4 is radiopaque [67]. There is no evidence regarding the use of activated charcoal in adsorbing CCl_4. Laboratory evaluation should include a complete blood cell count, routine serum chemistries, liver function tests, and urinalysis. Patients with respiratory symptoms or altered mental status should also be evaluated for possible aspiration pneumonitis, as described for aliphatic hydrocarbon exposures. Although CCl_4 appears not to be well removed by hemodialysis, dialysis may be required in cases of renal failure [68].

Animal studies suggest that hyperbaric oxygen may increase survival after intragastric administration of CCl_4 [69], although little human data exist on this topic [70,71]. Additional experimental work is being conducted to examine the utility of *N*-acetylcysteine in the reduction of CCl_4-induced hepatotoxicity. Because toxic intermediates of hepatic P450 are thought to be responsible for CCl_4 toxicity, it is thought that *N*-acetylcysteine may help prevent the development of liver failure [72,73]. Although human experience with this therapy is extremely limited in this setting and still considered experimental, a dosage schedule identical to that for acetaminophen is generally used.

Methylene Chloride

Methylene chloride is a colorless, volatile liquid commonly used as a solvent in aerosol products and as a degreaser and paint remover. It is well absorbed through the lungs and GI tract, but absorption through intact skin appears to be minimal. The majority of a dose is metabolized by the liver to carbon dioxide and carbon monoxide with small amounts exhaled unchanged [74].

The main toxicity of methylene chloride is CNS depression, which results from direct effects and from cellular asphyxia due to elevated levels of carboxyhemoglobin [75,76]. An 8-hour exposure to 250 ppm of methylene chloride resulted in carboxyhemoglobin fractions greater than 8% [77], and with large exposures, carboxyhemoglobin fractions up to 50% have been reported. In the few cases of methylene chloride ingestion that have been reported, CNS depression, tachypnea, and corrosive injury to the GI tract were the most common findings [78]. When the carboxyhemoglobin fraction is elevated, signs and symptoms of carbon monoxide poisoning may also be evident [79,80]. Nephrotoxicity and hepatotoxicity have also been reported [81,82].

Treatment involves stabilization, evaluation, and monitoring for aspiration, CNS and cardiovascular depression, dysrhythmias, corrosive injury, carbon monoxide poisoning, and hepatic and renal dysfunction. The patient should be removed from the source of inhalation exposure, and contaminated clothing should be removed. Exposed skin should be washed with soap and water. In cases of ingestion, gastric aspiration or lavage should be considered. The role of activated charcoal in methylene chloride ingestions is unclear [83]. In all cases, the carboxyhemoglobin fraction as well as complete blood cell count, routine serum chemistries, liver function tests, and urinalysis should be determined and supplemental oxygen provided.

Although hyperbaric oxygen is commonly used in cases of severe carbon monoxide poisoning, its role in methylene chloride toxicity is still being delineated [84,85]. It would appear reasonable to institute hyperbaric therapy when elevated carboxyhemoglobin levels are documented. Management is otherwise supportive.

Trichloroethane

1,1,1-Trichloroethane has been widely marketed as a safer alternative to CCl_4 for use as a cleaning agent and degreaser. It is also present in typewriter correction fluid and aerosol hairsprays, water repellents, and furniture polishes. In spite of its relative safety, death can occur, usually as a result of occupational or recreational inhalation exposure [86,87].

Trichloroethane is rapidly absorbed through the lungs and GI tract. Under most circumstances, significant cutaneous absorption is unlikely. Distribution is greatest to tissues with a high concentration of lipid, including the CNS. Most of an absorbed dose is excreted unchanged through the lungs, with smaller quantities metabolized in the liver and excreted by the kidneys [10].

Toxicity primarily involves the CNS, with signs and symptoms ranging from dizziness, headache, fatigue, and ataxia with mild-to-moderate exposures to seizures, coma, apnea, and death at higher vapor concentrations [88].

As with the aliphatic hydrocarbons, trichloroethane-induced cardiac sensitization to the effects of circulating catecholamines is thought to be responsible for sudden death associated with inhalational exposure [89,90]. Premature ventricular contractions and ST depression have been observed after acute inhalation [91], and myocarditis has been reported after chronic inhalation abuse [92]. Hepatic and renal toxicities are rare.

Management involves evaluation and treatment for aspiration, CNS and cardiovascular depression, and dysrhythmias. Decontamination measures may also be appropriate. In the absence of sudden death, recovery is generally rapid and complete.

AROMATIC HYDROCARBONS

Aromatic hydrocarbons contain one or more benzene rings. They include benzene, toluene, xylene, diphenyl, phenol, and styrene. Aromatic hydrocarbons are common constituents of glues, paints, paint removers, lacquers, degreasers, and adhesives. Although the aromatic hydrocarbons have aspiration risks similar to those of the other hydrocarbons, they also exhibit potentially severe systemic toxicity. Exposure is primarily through inhalation (occupational or abuse) or from ingestion. Benzene, toluene, and xylene are the three most commonly encountered agents.

Benzene

Benzene is a colorless liquid used widely in the chemical industry and less commonly as a solvent. It is well absorbed through the lungs and GI tract, but absorption through the skin is limited [93]. The lungs excrete up to 50% of an absorbed dose unchanged, whereas most of the remaining amount is metabolized by hepatic P450 enzymes to potentially cytotoxic metabolites [61,94]. Elimination of the parent compound and its metabolites generally occurs within 48 hours.

Benzene has acute and chronic toxicity [95]. Acute exposure primarily causes CNS depression [10]. Initial euphoria is rapidly followed by nausea, dizziness, and headache; subsequent progression to ataxia, seizures, and coma may occur. Persistent symptoms may include insomnia, anorexia, and headache.

Inhalation of high concentrations may lead to development of pulmonary edema; as with other hydrocarbons, aspiration and cardiac dysrhythmias may develop. Long-term exposure to benzene may result in a depression of bone marrow elements, which may progress to aplastic anemia [64,96]. Epidemiologic studies also suggest an increased risk of acute myelocytic and monocytic leukemia in workers with prolonged exposure to benzene [97,98].

Management should focus on stabilizing the patient and evaluation and monitoring for aspiration, CNS and cardiovascular depression, and dysrhythmias. It is generally agreed that amounts in excess of 1 to 2 mL per kg should be removed from the GI tract (via gastric aspiration or lavage), although some sources recommend removal of virtually any amount. The role of activated charcoal in this setting is unproved [10,99]. Subsequent therapy is supportive.

Toluene

Toluene is a colorless, volatile, sweet-smelling liquid that is a common ingredient in paints, paint thinners, lacquers, and glues (e.g., airplane model glue). Although toxicity may occur accidentally in industry or in the household, toluene is one of the most commonly abused solvents [100,101]. It is highly lipid soluble, and peak blood concentrations occur within 15 to 30 minutes with inhalation [64]. Animal studies suggest that ingested toluene is well absorbed from the GI tract, with 1 to 2 hours after exposure. Absorption through intact skin is slow.

Approximately 20% of an absorbed dose is exhaled unchanged. Most of the remainder is metabolized by the liver's cytochrome P450 system. Elimination is biphasic, with an initial alpha-phase having a half-life of 4 to 5 hours [102] and representing exhalation combined with distribution to fatty tissues [13]. The beta-phase has an apparent half-life of 15 to 20 hours and represents hepatic metabolism.

Toxic effects involve the CNS and peripheral nervous system as well as the kidney and heart [103]. Electrolyte and metabolic disturbances may also result. Acute exposure to toluene has variable effects on the CNS, depending on the concentration and duration of exposure [101,104,105]. Initially, toluene causes intoxication, which can progress to coma with prolonged exposure to high concentrations. Chronic abuse may also lead to persistent signs and symptoms of acute toxicity, including neuropsychiatric symptoms, weakness, nausea, vomiting, peripheral neuropathy, rhabdomyolysis [101], and abdominal pain [11]. Toluene toxicity is associated with a high incidence of renal dysfunction, particularly renal tubular acidosis (i.e., bicarbonate wasting) [101,106,107]. Laboratory findings include metabolic acidosis (with or without an increased anion gap), electrolyte disturbances (e.g., hypokalemia, hypocalcemia, hypophosphatemia, and hyperchloremia), and hematuria, proteinuria, and pyuria [106]. These abnormalities are the result of tubulointerstitial damage and are generally reversible on cessation of exposure. As with other hydrocarbons, acute toluene inhalation has also been associated with sudden cardiorespiratory arrest [108,109].

The diagnosis of toluene poisoning is generally made on the basis of the history, with known exposure or solvent abuse the prominent features. Toluene toxicity should also be considered in any individual with altered mental status and metabolic acidosis of unclear cause [110]. Management includes evaluation and treatment for aspiration; CNS and cardiovascular depression; dysrhythmias; renal dysfunction; fluid, electrolyte, and acid–base disturbances; and rhabdomyolysis. Laboratory testing should include calcium and phosphate levels. Gastric aspiration or lavage may be appropriate in cases of ingestion (with recognition of the aspiration risk).

Xylene

Xylene is a clear liquid that is widely used as a solvent in paints and lacquers, degreasers, adhesives, cleaning agents, and aviation fuel. It is rapidly absorbed by the pulmonary and GI systems and, to some extent, through the skin. The highest concentrations are found in the adrenal gland, bone marrow, spleen, brain, and blood [64]. Small amounts are excreted unchanged through the lungs; most of the remainder is metabolized in the liver and metabolites excreted in the urine. Ethanol consumption causes delays to metabolic clearance of xylene.

Xylene primarily affects the CNS [111]. As with other hydrocarbons, inhalation has been associated with sudden death, presumably secondary to cardiac dysrhythmia [112]. At low doses, headache, nausea, light-headedness, and ataxia may develop; at higher doses, confusion, coma, and respiratory depression may develop. Hepatic damage, Fanconi's syndrome, and pulmonary edema have also been described [112–114]. The evaluation and treatment of xylene exposure is similar to that described for other aromatic hydrocarbons.

TERPENES

Terpenes are aliphatic cyclic hydrocarbons. They include turpentine, pine oil, and camphor. Camphor is discussed elsewhere [10,115]. As its name suggests, pine oil is the product of pine trees and composed primarily of terpene alcohols. It is a component in household cleaners (e.g., Pine-Sol, Clorox Company, Oakland, CA), normally present in concentrations of 20% to 35%, but occasionally in concentrations exceeding 60%. Turpentine is a pine tree distillate commonly used as a solvent for paint and varnish.

Toxicity almost always results from ingestion. The aspiration risk appears to be somewhat less than that of other aliphatic hydrocarbons, presumably because of the lower volatility of terpenes; CNS and GI effects are more pronounced, however. Ingestions of more than 2 mL per kg of turpentine are considered potentially toxic [116]. Although 60 to 120 g of pine oil is commonly cited as the lethal dose in adults, survival has been reported after ingestion of 400 to 500 g [117]. The minimal lethal dose of pine oil reported in children is 14 g [118].

Turpentine is well absorbed through the lungs and GI tract [116] and distributed throughout the body, with highest concentrations in the liver, spleen, brain, and kidney [116]. Although the specifics of its metabolism are unclear, turpentine or its metabolites are largely excreted through the kidney. Pine oil is also well absorbed from the GI tract, and after absorption, it is metabolized by the epoxide pathway and excreted in the urine [117]. Although the volume of distribution is unknown, it is thought to be quite large, with high concentrations in the brain, kidney, and lung.

Manifestations of toxicity include nausea, vomiting, diarrhea, weakness, somnolence, or agitation. In severe cases, stupor or coma may result, although seizures appear to be uncommon [119]. Systemic toxicity, when it occurs, usually develops within 2 to 3 hours of ingestion. In mild and moderate cases, GI and CNS symptoms generally resolve within 12 hours. Turpentine ingestion has been associated with hemorrhagic cystitis, with dysuria and hematuria occurring 12 hours to 3 days after exposure [120].

Management includes evaluation and treatment for aspiration, gastroenteritis, and CNS depression. The distinctive odors of turpentine and pine oil may provide a clue to diagnosis. Gastric aspiration or lavage is recommended for patients who present within 2 hours of ingesting greater than 2 mL per kg of turpentine or 5 mL of pure pine oil [121]. Because of the risk of aspiration, airway protection should be considered in all but the most alert patients.

Patients who remain asymptomatic or have only mild GI or CNS symptoms 6 hours after ingestion are unlikely to develop serious complications. Patients with pulmonary complications or severe CNS depression require intensive care unit admission and often require ventilatory support.

References

1. Annual report of the American Association of Poison Control Centers National Poison Data System, VA, 2007.
2. Gerarde HW: Toxicological studies in hydrocarbons vs kerosene. *Toxicol Appl Pharmacol* 1:462, 1959.
3. Wolfe B, Brodeur A, Shields J: The role of gastrointestinal absorption of kerosene in producing pneumonitis in dogs. *Pediatrics* 76:867, 1970.
4. Dice WH, Ward G, Kelley J, et al: Pulmonary toxicity following gastrointestinal ingestions of kerosene. *Ann Emerg Med* 11:138, 1982.
5. Gerarde HW: Toxicologic studies on hydrocarbons IX. The aspiration hazard and toxicity of hydrocarbons and hydrocarbon mixtures. *Arch Environ Health* 6:329, 1963.
6. Giammona ST: Effects of furniture polish on pulmonary surfactant. *Am J Dis Child* 13:658, 1967.
7. Gross P, McNemey JM, Babyale MA: Kerosene pneumonitis: an experimental study with small doses. *Am Rev Respir Dis* 88:656, 1963.
8. Beermann B, Christensson T, Moller P, et al: Lipoid pneumonia: an occupational hazard of fire-eaters. *Br Med J* 289:1728, 1984.
9. Wolfsdorf J: Kerosene intoxication: an experimental approach to the etiology of the CNS manifestations in primates. *J Pediatr* 88:1037, 1976.
10. Shannon MW, Borron SW, Burns MJ: *Haddad and Winchester's Clinical Management of Poisoning and Drug Overdose, Petroleum Distillates*. 4th ed. pp 1343–1346, 2007.
11. Linden CH: Volatile substances of abuse. *Emerg Med Clin North Am* 3:559, 1990.
12. Fishman M, Bruner A, Adger H Jr: Substance abuse among children and adolescents. *Pediatr Rev* 11:394, 1997.
13. Baselt RC, Caravey RH: *Disposition of Toxic Drugs and Chemicals in Man*. 5th ed. Foster City, CA, Chemical Toxicology Institute, 1995, p 235.
14. Sandmeyer EE: Aliphatic hydrocarbons, in Clayton GD, Clayton FE (eds): *Patty's Industrial Hygiene and Toxicology*. 5th ed. New York, John Wiley and Sons, 2000, p 3175.
15. Greenes D: Volatile substance abuse. *Clin Toxicol Rev* 18:7, 1996.
16. Altenkirch H, Stoltenburg G, Wagner HM: Experimental studies on hydrocarbon neuropathies induced by methyl-ethyl-ketone (MEK). *J Neurol* 219:159, 1978.
17. Hormes J, Filley C, Rosenberg N: Neurologic sequelae of chronic solvent vapor abuse. *Neurology* 36:698, 1986.
18. Jorgensen NK, Cohr KH: N-hexane and its toxicologic effects: a review. *Scand J Work Environ Health* 7:157, 1987.
19. Boon N: Solvent abuse and the heart. *BMJ* 294:722, 1977.
20. Fortenberry JD: Gasoline sniffing. *Am J Med* 79:740, 1985.
21. Anderson HR, Dick B, MacNair RS, et al: An investigation of 140 deaths associated with volatile substance abuse in the United Kingdom (1971–1981). *Hum Toxicol* 1:207, 1982.
22. Anas N, Namasonthia V, Ginsburg CM: Criteria for hospitalizing children who have ingested products containing hydrocarbons. *JAMA* 246:840, 1981.
23. Wason S, Greiner PT: Intravenous hydrocarbon abuse. *Am J Emerg Med* 4:543, 1986.
24. Anene O, Castello FV: Myocardial dysfunction after hydrocarbon ingestion. *Crit Care Med* 22:528, 1994.
25. Foley JC, Dreyer NB, Soule AB Jr, et al: Kerosene poisoning in young children. *Radiology* 62:817, 1954.
26. Eade NR, Taussig LM, Marks MI: Hydrocarbon pneumonitis. *Pediatrics* 54:351, 1974.
27. Bergeson PS, Hales SW, Lustgarten MD, et al: Pneumatoceles following hydrocarbon ingestion. *Am J Dis Child* 129:49, 1975.
28. Press E, Adams WC, Chittenden RF, et al: Report of the subcommittee on accidental poisoning: co-operative kerosene poisoning study. *Pediatrics* 29:648, 1962.
29. Bratton L, Haddow JE: Ingestion of charcoal lighter fluid. *J Pediatr* 87:633, 1974.
30. Bass M: Death from sniffing gasoline [letter]. *N Engl J Med* 299:203, 1978.
31. Flanagan RJ, Ives RJ: Volatile substance abuse. *Bull Narc* 46:49, 1994.
32. Barrientos A, Ortuno MT, Morales JM, et al: Acute renal failure after use of diesel fuel as shampoo. *Arch Intern Med* 137:1217, 1977.
33. Crisp AJ, Bhalla AK, Hoffbrand BI: Acute tubular necrosis after exposure to diesel oil. *BMJ* 2:177, 1979.
34. Adler R, Robinson RG, Bindin NJ: Intravascular hemolysis: an unusual complication of hydrocarbon ingestion. *J Pediatr* 89:679, 1976.
35. Stockman JA: More on hydrocarbon-induced hemolysis. *J Pediatr* 90:848, 1977.
36. Walsh WA, Scarpa FJ, Brown RS, et al: Gasoline immersion burn case report. *N Engl J Med* 291:830, 1974.
37. Grufferman S, Walker FW: Supraglottitis following gasoline ingestion. *Ann Emerg Med* 11:368, 1982.
38. Cole M, Herndon HN, Desai MH, et al: Gasoline explosions, gasoline sniffing: an epidemic in young adolescents. *J Burn Care Rehabil* 7:532, 1986.
39. Chessare JD, Wodarcyk K: Gasoline sniffing and lead poisoning in a child. *Am Fam Physician* 38:181, 1988.
40. Neeld EM, Limacher MC: Chemical pneumonitis after the intravenous injection of hydrocarbons. *Radiology* 129:36, 1978.
41. Tenenbein M: Pediatric toxicology: current controversies and recent advances. *Curr Probl Pediatr* 16:185, 1986.
42. Litovitz T, Green AE: Health implications of petroleum distillate ingestion. *Occup Med* 3:555, 1988.
43. James FW, Kaplan S, Benzing G: Cardiac complications following hydrocarbon ingestion. *Am J Dis Child* 121:431, 1971.
44. Schwartz SI, Breslau RC, Kutner F, et al: Effects of drugs and hyperbaric oxygen environment on experimental kerosene pneumonitis. *Dis Chest* 47:353, 1965.
45. Steele RW, Conklin RH, Mark HM: Corticosteroids and antibiotics for the treatment of fulminant hydrocarbon aspiration. *JAMA* 219:1424, 1972.
46. Brown J, Burke B, Dajani AS: Experimental kerosene pneumonia: evaluation of some therapeutic regimens. *J Pediatr* 84:396, 1974.
47. Zieserl E: Hydrocarbon ingestion and poisoning. *Comp Ther* 5:35, 1979.
48. Marks MI, Chicoine L, Legere G, et al: Adrenocorticosteroid treatment of hydrocarbon pneumonia in children. A cooperative study. *J Pediatr* 81:366, 1972.
49. Liebelt EI, DeAngelis CD: Evolving trends and treatment advances in pediatric poisoning. *JAMA* 282:1113, 1999.
50. Bysani GK, Rucoba RJ, Noah ZL: Treatment of hydrocarbons pneumonitis. High frequency jet ventilation as an alternative to extracorporeal membrane oxygenation. *Chest* 106:300, 1994.
51. Chyka PA: Benefits of extracorporeal membrane oxygenation for hydrocarbon pneumonitis. *J Toxicol Clin Toxicol* 34:357, 1996.
52. Willson DF, Thomas NJ, Markovitz BP, et al: Effect of exogenous surfactant (Calfactant) in pediatric acute lung injury: a randomized controlled trial. *JAMA* 293(4):470–476, 2005.
53. Widner LR, Goodwin SR, Berman LS, et al. Artificial surfactant for therapy in hydrocarbon-induced lung injury in sheep. *Crit Care Med* 24:9, 1996.
54. Gurwitz D, Kattan M, Levison H, et al: Pulmonary function abnormalities in asymptomatic children after hydrocarbon pneumonitis. *Pediatrics* 62:789, 1978.
55. Kurtzman TL, Otsuka KN, Wahl RA: Inhalant abuse by adolescents. *J Adolesc Health* 28:170, 2001.
56. Javier Perez A, Courel M, Sobrado J, et al: Acute renal failure after topical application of carbon tetrachloride. *Lancet* 1:515, 1987.
57. Sanzgiri UY, Srivatsan V, Muralidhara S, et al: Uptake, distribution, and elimination of carbon tetrachloride in rat tissues following inhalation and ingestion exposures. *Toxicol Appl Pharmacol* 143:120, 1997.
58. Castro GD, Diaz Gomez MI, Castro JA: DNA bases attack by reactive metabolites produced during carbon tetrachloride biotransformation and promotion of liver microsomal lipid peroxidation. *Res Commun Mol Pathol Pharmacol* 95:253, 1997.
59. Cornish HH, Adefuin J: Potentiation of carbon tetrachloride toxicity by aliphatic alcohols. *Arch Environ Health* 14:447, 1967.

60. Plaa GL: Chlorinated methanes and liver injury: highlights of the past 50 years. *Annu Rev Pharmacol Toxicol* 40:42, 2000.
61. Ehrenreich T: Renal disease from exposure to solvents. *Ann Clin Lab Sci* 7:6, 1977.
62. Koren G: The nephrotoxic potential of drugs and chemicals. Pharmacological basis and clinical relevance. *Med Toxicol Adverse Drug Exp* 4:59, 1989.
63. Sinicrope RA, Gordon JA, Little JR, et al: Carbon tetrachloride nephrotoxicity: a reassessment of pathophysiology based upon the urinary diagnostic indices. *Am J Kidney Dis* 3:362, 1984.
64. Bergman K: Application and results of whole-body autoradiography in distribution studies of organic solvents. *Crit Rev Toxicol* 12:59, 1983.
65. Alston WC: Hepatic and renal complications arising from accidental carbon tetrachloride poisoning in the human subject. *Clin Pathol* 23:249, 1970.
66. Fogel RP, Davidman M, Poleski MH, et al: Carbon tetrachloride poisoning treated with hemodialysis and total parenteral nutrition. *Can Med Assoc J* 128:560, 1983.
67. McGuigan MA: Carbon tetrachloride. *Clin Toxicol Rev* 9:1, 1987.
68. Spiegel SM, Hyams BB: Radiographic demonstration of a toxic agent. *J Can Assoc Radiol* 34:204, 1984.
69. Burk RF, Reiter R, Lane JM: Hyperbaric oxygen protection against carbon tetrachloride hepatotoxicity in rats: association with altered metabolism. *Gastroenterology* 90:812, 1986.
70. Truss CD, Killenberg PG: Treatment of carbon tetrachloride poisoning with hyperbaric oxygen. *Gastroenterology* 82:767, 1982.
71. Burkhart KK, Hall AH, Gerace R, et al: Hyperbaric oxygen treatment for carbon tetrachloride poisoning. *Drug Saf* 6:332, 1991.
72. Simko V, Michael S, Katz J, et al: Protective effect of oral acetylcysteine against the hepatorenal toxicity of carbon tetrachloride potentiated by ethyl alcohol. *Alcohol Clin Exp Res* 16:795, 1992.
73. Valles EG, de Castro CR, Castro JA: *N*-acetyl cysteine is an early but also a late preventive agent against carbon tetrachloride-induced liver necrosis. *Toxicol Lett* 71:87, 1994.
74. Jonsson F, Bois F, Johanson G: Physiologically based pharmacokinetic modeling of inhalation exposure of humans to dichloromethane during moderate to heavy exercise. *Toxicol Sci* 59:209, 2001.
75. Rioux JP, Myers RA: Methylene chloride poisoning: a paradigmatic review. *J Emerg Med* 6:227, 1988.
76. Dhillon S, Von Burg R: Methylene chloride. *J Appl Toxicol* 15:329, 1995.
77. Lawwerys RR: *Industrial Chemical Exposure: Guidelines for Biological Monitoring.* Davis, CA, Biomedical, 1983, p 83.
78. Chang YL, Yang CC, Deng JF, et al: Diverse manifestations of oral methylene chloride poisoning: report of 6 cases. *J Toxicol Clin Toxicol* 37:497, 1999.
79. Fagin J, Bradley J, Williams D: Carbon monoxide poisoning secondary to inhaling methylene chloride. *BMJ* 281:1461, 1980.
80. Agency for Toxic Substances and Disease Registry: Methylene chloride toxicity. *Am Fam Physician* 47:1159, 1993.
81. Miller L, Pateras V, Friederici H, et al: Acute tubular necrosis after inhalation exposure to methylene chloride. *Arch Intern Med* 145:145, 1985.
82. Kim H: A case of acute toxic hepatitis after suicidal chloroform and dichloromethane ingestion. *Am J Emerg Med* 26(9):1073.e3–1073.e6, 2008.
83. Soslow A: Methylene chloride. *Clin Toxicol Rev* 9:1, 1987.
84. Rioux JP, Myers RA: Hyperbaric oxygen for methylene chloride poisoning: report on two cases. *Ann Emerg Med* 18:691, 1989.
85. Rudge FW: Treatment of methylene chloride induced carbon monoxide poisoning with hyperbaric oxygenation. *Mil Med* 155:570, 1990.
86. King GS, Smialek JE, Troutman WG: Sudden death in adolescents resulting from the inhalation of typewriter correction fluid. *JAMA* 253:1604, 1985.
87. Jones RD, Winters DP: Two case reports of deaths on industrial premises attributed to 1,1,1-trichloroethane. *Arch Environ Health* 38:59, 1983.
88. Laine A, Seppalainen AM, Savolainen K, et al: Acute effects of 1,1,1-trichloroethane inhalation on the human central nervous system. *Int Arch Occup Environ Health* 69:53, 1996.
89. Adgey AA, Johnston PW, McMechan S: Sudden cardiac death and substance abuse. *Resuscitation* 29:219, 1995.
90. Bailey B, Loebstein R, Lai C, et al: Two cases of chlorinated hydrocarbon-associated myocardial ischemia. *Vet Hum Toxicol* 39:298, 1997.
91. Herd PA, Lipsky M, Martin HF: Cardiovascular effects of 1,1,1-trichloroethane. *Arch Environ Health* 28:227, 1974.
92. McLeod AA, Margot R, Monaghan MJ, et al: Chronic cardiac toxicity after inhalation of 1,1,1-trichloroethane. *BMJ* 294:727, 1987.
93. Susten AS, Dames BL, Burg JR, et al: Percutaneous penetration of benzene in hairless mice: an estimate of dermal absorption during tire-building operations. *Am J Ind Med* 7:323, 1985.
94. Lovern MR, Cole CE, Schlosser PM: A review of quantitative studies of benzene metabolism. *Crit Rev Toxicol* 31:285, 2001.
95. Snyder R: Overview of the toxicology of benzene. *J Toxicol Environ Health A* 61:339, 2000.
96. Smith MT: Overview of benzene-induced aplastic anaemia. *Eur J Haematol Suppl* 60:107, 1996.
97. Snyder R, Kalf GF: A perspective on benzene leukemogenesis. *Crit Rev Toxicol* 24:177, 1994.
98. Ireland B, Collins JJ, Buckley CF, et al: Cancer mortality among workers with benzene exposure. *Epidemiology* 8:318, 1997.
99. Laass W: Therapy of acute oral poisonings by organic solvents: treatment by activated charcoal in combination with laxatives. *Arch Toxicol* 4[Suppl]:406, 1980.
100. Burgnone F, DeRosa E, Perbellini L, et al: Toluene concentrations in the blood and alveolar air of workers during the workshift and the morning after. *Br J Ind Med* 43:56, 1986.
101. Flanagan RJ, Ruprah M, Meredith TJ, et al: An introduction to the clinical toxicology of volatile substances. *Drug Saf* 5:359, 1990.
102. Von Burg R: Toluene. *J Appl Toxicol* 13:441, 1993.
103. Greenberg MM: The central nervous system and exposure to toluene: a risk characterization. *Environ Res* 72:1, 1997.
104. Stollery BT, Flindt MLH: Memory sequelae of solvent intoxication. *Scand J Work Environ Health* 14:45, 1988.
105. Voigts A, Kaufman CE: Acidosis and other metabolic abnormalities associated with paint sniffing. *South Med J* 76:443, 1983.
106. Fischman CM, Oster JR: Toxic effects of toluene. A new cause of high anion gap metabolic acidosis. *JAMA* 241:1713, 1979.
107. Bass M: Sudden sniffing death. *JAMA* 212:2075, 1970.
108. Carder JR, Fuerst RS: Myocardial infarction after toluene inhalation. *Pediatr Emerg Care* 13:117, 1997.
109. Shannon M: Toluene. *Clin Toxicol Rev* 9:1, 1987.
110. Fay M, Eisenmann C, Diwan S, et al: ATSDR evaluation of health effects of chemicals. V. Xylenes: health effects, toxicokinetics, human exposure, and environmental fate. *Toxicol Ind Health* 14:571, 1998.
111. Morley R, Eccleston DW, Douglas CP, et al: Xylene poisoning: a report of one fatal case and two cases of recovery after prolonged unconsciousness. *BMJ* 3:442, 1970.
112. Rastogi SP, Gold RM, Arruda JAL: Fanconi's syndrome associated with carburetor fluid intoxication. *Am J Clin Pathol* 82:124, 1984.
113. Abu Al Ragheb S, Salhab AS, Amr SS: Suicide by xylene ingestion: a case report and review of literature. *Am J Forensic Med Pathol* 7:327, 1986.
114. Lahoud CA, March JA, Proctor DD: Campho-Phenique ingestion: an intentional overdose. *South Med J* 90:647, 1997.
115. McGuigan MA: Turpentine. *Clin Toxicol Rev* 8:1, 1985.
116. Koppel C, Tenczer J, Tennesmann U, et al: Acute poisoning with pine oil: metabolism of monoterpenes. *Arch Toxicol* 49:73, 1981.
117. Hill RM, Barer J, Hill LL, et al: An investigation of recurrent pine oil poisoning in an infant by the use of gas chromatographic-mass spectrometric methods. *J Pediatr* 87:115, 1975.
118. Troulakis G, Tsatsakis AM, Tzatzarakis M, et al: Acute intoxication and recovery following massive turpentine ingestion: clinical and toxicological data. *Vet Hum Toxicol* 39:155, 1997.
119. Klein FA, Hackler RH: Hemorrhagic cystitis associated with turpentine ingestion. *Urology* 16:187, 1980.
120. Brook MP, McCarron MM, Mueller JA: Pine oil cleaner ingestion. *Ann Emerg Med* 18:391, 1989.
121. Scalzo AJ, Weber TR, Jaeger RW, et al: Extracorporeal membrane oxygenation for hydrocarbon aspiration. *Am J Dis Child* 144:867, 1990.

CHAPTER 135 ■ HYDROFLUORIC ACID POISONING

KENNON HEARD

INTRODUCTION

Hydrofluoric acid (HF) is a commonly encountered industrial reagent that is available in concentrations from 6% to 90%. It is used for the production of fluorocarbons, etching glass, and silicone, and as a household rust-removal agent. Sodium fluoride is used as a rodenticide and also as a preservative in blood collection tubes. A related compound, ammonium bifluoride is used in rust removers, commonly found in commercial car washes.

MECHANISM OF ACTION

HF (pK_a = 3.8) is a weak acid. Hence, compared with other acids, it is relatively less ionized at any given pH. This allows HF to penetrate more deeply into tissue and to be more readily absorbed into the systemic circulation than other acids. Once absorbed, it disassociates and the fluoride anion binds to divalent cations, forming insoluble salts (primarily calcium fluoride, fluorapatite, and magnesium fluoride). This results in tissue and systemic hypocalcemia and hypomagnesemia. Fluoride also directly poisons several enzymes and cellular transport proteins. High-concentration HF exposures result in rapid onset of local pain and tissue injury with or without systemic toxicity, whereas low-concentration exposures can result in life-threatening hypocalcemia and hypomagnesemia, with minimal or absent local corrosive effect.

DERMAL EXPOSURE

Clinical Manifestations

While most dermal exposures will result in minor symptoms or superficial chemical burns, systemic toxicity may occur following dermal exposure. Symptoms may be delayed for 24 hours or more following low-concentration (<20% HF) exposure, and there is often severe pain with minimal skin abnormalities. Symptoms can develop within several hours of exposure to medium concentrations (20% to 50% HF). While the initial injury is not always visible, patients exposed to medium-concentration products often go on to have erythema, blanching, or necrosis of the involved area. High-concentration (>50% HF) exposures result in the immediate injury expected after exposure to concentrated acids. Patients may develop full- or partial-thickness injury that includes tissue necrosis and eschar formation [1].

Evaluation and Treatment

Laboratory studies are not indicated for small, low-concentration dermal exposures. However, exposure to products containing more than 50% HF that involve more than 1% of the skin or exposure to any HF product that affects more than 5% of the skin can cause hypocalcemia, so patients with these burns should have serum calcium levels monitored, as described in the systemic toxicity section below [2].

The most important step in treatment is decontamination by irrigating the affected area for at least 15 minutes as quickly as possible. In one large case series of exposures, many of which involved concentrations of greater than 40% HF, immediate irrigation produced excellent outcome in the majority of patients [3]. Hexafluoride, an irrigating solution developed to bind fluoride, does not appear to offer any improvement over water irrigation [4].

After irrigation, apply a 2.3% to 2.5% calcium gluconate preparation in a water-soluble gel to the exposed areas for at least 30 minutes or until symptoms resolve [5]. This treatment often remains effective if it is delayed several hours after symptoms develop [6]. The role of topical therapy following high-concentration exposures is less well defined, but it is recommended [7].

If pain is not relieved by topical therapy, regional intra-arterial or intravenous calcium perfusion should be initiated. The major drawback of intra-arterial perfusion is the requirement for arterial catheterization. Brachial, radial, and femoral catheterization have all been described. Following cannulation, monitor arterial waveform to assure that the catheter remains patent and properly placed within the artery. If there is any question as to adequate placement, perform arteriography prior to infusing calcium. Flushing the catheter with heparin may help keep the catheter patent [2]. The largest case series reported infusion of 50 mL of 2.5% calcium gluconate in saline over 4 hours [2]. It is not uncommon to have to repeat the dose several times over a 12- to 24-hour period.

Regional perfusion using a Bier block may allow treatment without arterial cannulization. Some clinicians advocate this technique before proceeding to intra-arterial administration. This technique requires venous cannulation in the affected extremity. The extremity is exsanguinated by elevation and compression with an Esmarch bandage. The blood pressure cuff should be inflated to a pressure 100 mm Hg above systolic pressure and remain up for 15 to 20 minutes following calcium administration. The usual dose is 40 mL of a 2.5% calcium gluconate solution [8]. The cuff is then gradually deflated over 5 minutes. Pain is usually relieved within minutes of the calcium administration.

If the affected area is not an extremity, calcium can be directly injected into the burn. The most common method is injection of 0.3 to 0.5 mL per cm^2 of 2.5% calcium gluconate. Calcium chloride should not be used as it can cause tissue injury. Excision of exposed tissue is not recommended.

OCULAR EXPOSURE

Clinical Manifestations

While most human reports describe good outcomes following ocular HF exposure, animal studies have demonstrated that severe injury is possible. Although most patients have rapid onset of pain, HF can penetrate the eye and cause severe and delayed injury.

Evaluation and Treatment

Immediate irrigation is the most important treatment. Irrigation with calcium salts appears to offer no benefit over saline in animal models, and may increase the incidence of ulceration [9]. Following irrigation, the pH should be measured and a fluorescein examination should be performed. All patients with persistent symptoms or obvious corneal damage should have immediate evaluation by an ophthalmologist. Some will require admission for continuous irrigation. Patients who are asymptomatic after irrigation should have next-day follow-up with an ophthalmologist. Routine therapy for corneal burns from HF has included mydriatics, topical antibiotics, and steroids [10–12]. Treatment of these burns with calcium gluconate eyedrops has been suggested, but no systematic human studies have been reported [12].

INHALATION

Clinical Manifestations

Inhalation of HF may result in severe airway injury, pulmonary injury, and systemic fluoride poisoning. Patients may present with severe or minimal symptoms and go on to develop complications over time [13]. While systemic fluoride poisoning may occur [14], the major mechanism of pulmonary injury is acute lung injury.

Evaluation and Treatment

Following inhalation of HF, patients should have chest radiographs, evaluation of oxygenation, and monitoring for hypocalcemia. Treatment is supportive, and early airway intervention may be required for patients with symptoms of upper airway obstruction. There are several uncontrolled reports of good outcomes following treatment with nebulized calcium gluconate solution (2.5% to 5.0%) [15,16].

INGESTION

Clinical Manifestations

Oropharyngeal burns are rarely noted, even in fatal poisonings [17]. While gastrointestinal symptoms such as nausea, vomiting, and gastritis may occur, the primary manifestation of oral HF exposures is systemic fluoride toxicity (see below). Following accidental sip ingestions, patients who are able to swallow should be given 30 to 60 mL of water to drink to dilute any HF still in contact with the esophageal mucosa. While it is commonly recommended to administer calcium or magnesium antacids, animals studies have found that very high doses are required to affect mortality [18,19]. Patients with accidental ingestion of products containing more than 7% HF or deliberate ingestion of any HF or ammonium fluoride product are at risk for systemic poisoning and require continuous cardiac monitoring, reliable vascular access, and close monitoring of serum calcium levels, as described in the next section.

Systemic Toxicity

Systemic fluoride toxicity may occur following inhalation and dermal or oral exposure to HF-containing products. While the exact mechanism of fluoride toxicity requires continued research [20], human cases of fatal HF toxicity consistently demonstrate profound hypocalcemia) [21]. Other manifestations include hypomagnesemia, acidosis, and hyperkalemia. Minimally symptomatic patients may progress rapidly to cardiovascular collapse [22].

Because successful resuscitation from cardiac arrest following systemic fluoride poisoning is rare, treatment should be started early to prevent cardiac dysrhythmias and arrest. Patients should have continuous cardiac monitoring, reliable vascular access, and frequent measurement of serum calcium and magnesium. If the history suggests that there has been a significant exposure, prophylactic calcium should be initiated at a rate of 1 g over 30 minutes [20]. Patients who have normal vital signs and remain stable should have serum calcium levels monitored every 30 minutes for the first 2 to 3 hours. Calcium chloride 1-g boluses should be repeated as needed to maintain the serum calcium in the high normal range. Patients with hypocalcemia, dysrhythmias, or hypotension should receive 2 to 3 g of calcium every 15 minutes, and central venous access should be obtained. Successful treatment of cardiac arrest has generally been associated with administration of large doses (>10 g) of calcium. Intravenous magnesium sulfate 2 to 6 g over 30 minutes followed by a continuous 1- to 4-g infusion has also been suggested.

Beyond calcium and magnesium administration, fluoride-poisoned patients require excellent supportive care. Patients with symptoms of airway involvement should be intubated. Similarly, ventilation and oxygenation problems are rare but should be treated aggressively if present. Successful electrical cardioversion for dysrhythmias following calcium and magnesium therapy has been reported [23].

A therapy that is unproven but has theoretical benefit is serum and urine alkalinization. One animal study showed that systemic alkalosis increased the fatal fluoride dose in rats [24]. While this study has obvious limitations, serum alkalinization should be considered in critically ill patients. However, over-alkalinization may worsen hypocalcemia; therefore, serum pH should be maintained between 7.4 and 7.5. While fluoride is cleared by hemodialysis, patients with severe poisoning will be too unstable to be dialyzed.

References

1. Division of Industrial Hygiene: National Institute of Health hydrofluoric acid burns. *Ind Med* 12:634, 1943.
2. Siegel DC, Heard JM: Intra-arterial calcium infusion for hydrofluoric acid burns. *Aviat Space Environ Med* 63(3):206–211, 1992.
3. Hamilton M: OH Congress. Hydrofluoric acid burns. *Occup Health (Lond)* 27(11):468–470, 1975.
4. Hojer J, Personne M, Hulten P, et al: Topical treatments for hydrofluoric acid burns: a blind controlled experimental study. *J Toxicol Clin Toxicol* 40(7):861–866, 2002.
5. Trevino MA, Herrmann GH, Sprout WL: Treatment of severe hydrofluoric acid exposures. *J Occup Med* 25(12):861–863, 1983.
6. El Saadi MS, Hall AH, Hall PK, et al: Hydrofluoric acid dermal exposure. *Vet Hum Toxicol* 31(3):243–247, 1989.
7. Sadove R, Hainsworth D, Van Meter W: Total body immersion in hydrofluoric acid. *South Med J* 83(6):698–700, 1990.
8. Graudins A, Burns MJ, Aaron CK: Regional intravenous infusion of calcium gluconate for hydrofluoric acid burns of the upper extremity [see comments]. *Ann Emerg Med* 30(5):604–607, 1997.

9. Beiran I, Miller B, Bentur Y: The efficacy of calcium gluconate in ocular hydrofluoric acid burns. *Hum Exp Toxicol* 16(4):223–228, 1997.
10. McCulley JP, Whiting DW, Petitt MG, et al: Hydrofluoric acid burns of the eye. *J Occup Med* 25(6):447–450, 1983.
11. McCulley JP: Ocular hydrofluoric acid burns: animal model, mechanism of injury and therapy. *Trans Am Ophthalmol Soc* 88(1):649–684, 1990.
12. Rubinfeld RS, Silbert DI, Arentsen JJ, et al: Ocular hydrofluoric acid burns. *Am J Ophthalmol* 114(4):420–423, 1992.
13. Kirkpatrick JJ, Enion DS, Burd DA: Hydrofluoric acid burns: a review. *Burns* 21(7):483–493, 1995.
14. Watson AA, Oliver JS, Thorpe JW: Accidental death due to inhalation of hydrofluoric acid. *Med Sci Law* 13(4):277–279, 1973.
15. Lee DC, Wiley JF II, Synder JW II, et al: Treatment of inhalational exposure to hydrofluoric acid with nebulized calcium gluconate. *J Occup Med* 35(5):470, 1993.
16. Kono K, Watanabe T, Dote T, et al: Successful treatments of lung injury and skin burn due to hydrofluoric acid exposure. *Int Arch Occup Environ Health* 73[Suppl]:S93–S97, 2000.
17. Bost RO, Springfield A: Fatal hydrofluoric acid ingestion: a suicide case report. *J Anal Toxicol* 19(6):535–536, 1995.
18. Kao WF, Deng JF, ChiangSC, et al: A simple, safe, and efficient way to treat severe fluoride poisoning—oral calcium or magnesium. *J Toxicol Clin Toxicol* 42(1):33–40, 2004.
19. Heard K, Delgado J: Oral decontamination with calcium or magnesium salts does not improve survival following hydrofluoric acid ingestion. *J Toxicol Clin Toxicol* 41(7):789–792, 2003.
20. McIvor ME: Acute fluoride toxicity: pathophysiology and management. *Drug Saf* 5(2):79–85, 1990.
21. Rabinowitch IM: Acute fluoride poisoning. *Can Med Assoc J* 52(2):345–349, 1945.
22. Kao WF, Dart RC, Kuffner E, et al: Ingestion of low-concentration hydrofluoric acid: an insidious and potentially fatal poisoning. *Ann Emerg Med* 34(1):35–41, 1999.
23. Stremski ES, Grande GA, Ling LJ: Survival following hydrofluoric acid ingestion. *Ann Emerg Med* 21(11):1396–1399, 1992.
24. Reynolds KE, Whitford GM, Pashley DH: Acute fluoride toxicity: the influence of acid-base status. *Toxicol Appl Pharmacol* 45(2):415–427, 1978.

CHAPTER 136 ■ IRON POISONING

MILTON TENENBEIN

Historically, iron poisoning is the most common cause of poisoning death in children younger than 6 years [1]; however, morbidity and mortality have decreased secondary to unit-dose packaging of iron supplements [2]. Notably, a clinically important proportion of iron overdoses is purposeful, involves adolescents and adults, and results in significant morbidity and mortality [3].

Iron occurs naturally in the body. It is highly reactive, and there are complex mechanisms for its absorption, transport, and storage. The capacity of these systems to cope with an acute overdose is unknown; it likely varies from individual to individual and with the state of iron stores. Incomplete understanding of iron toxicokinetics is primarily responsible for controversies regarding (a) the toxic dose; (b) the optimal method of gastrointestinal decontamination; (c) the efficacy of intragastric complexation therapies; and (d) the indications, dose, duration, and efficacy of deferoxamine therapy.

PHARMACOLOGY

Iron is readily available as ferrous salts, either alone or in combination with other minerals and vitamins. Its common salts are ferrous gluconate, sulfate, fumarate, and succinate, which are 12%, 20%, 33%, and 35% elemental iron, respectively. These fractions are important because toxicity is related to the amount of elemental iron ingested. Iron is marketed in both conventional and delayed-release formulations. Product labels may not specify the tablet formulation, an important determinant of the onset and duration of toxicity. Carbonyl iron is a highly purified form of metallic iron. It is uncharged and not a salt [4].

Iron absorption, transport, and storage are well reviewed elsewhere [5]. Because there is no endogenous mechanism for iron excretion, total body iron is a function of the absorptive process. Absorption occurs in the proximal small bowel, with approximately 10% of the ingested dose absorbed, but with tenfold variations depending on iron stores and the amount ingested. The actual mechanism of iron absorption is not well understood, but it is believed to be an active process. Iron can also be passively absorbed once the active process is saturated, such as after a massive overdose [6]. Even in such a situation, a relatively small amount (15%) is actually absorbed [6].

Peak serum iron concentrations occur within 4 to 6 hours after an overdose of conventional tablets. The time to peak serum concentration is not known for delayed-release products. The half-life after therapeutic dosing is approximately 6 hours [5], with rapid decline because of tissue distribution. In plasma, iron is bound to transferrin, a specific β_1-globulin responsible for iron transport throughout the body. In iron overdose, transferrin-binding capacity is exceeded, but free plasma iron does not truly exist. Iron complexes with other plasma proteins and organic ligands and is referred to as *nontransferrin-bound plasma iron* [7]. However, it is only loosely bound and is quite available to produce tissue damage and organ dysfunction.

There are two typical overdose scenarios: innocent overdose by young children and purposeful overdose by adolescents and adults. Serious iron overdose in young children frequently involves the ingestion of a product intended for adults, typically a prenatal iron supplement. Ingestion of pediatric preparations, such as multivitamin plus iron tablets, is more common [8]; such preparations are unlikely to result in significant toxicity because of their low elemental iron content (as little as 4 mg per tablet). Although liquid iron preparations are often found in homes with infants and toddlers, there are no published cases of clinically important iron poisoning because of these products. Iron overdose is less common among teenagers and adults, but when it occurs, it is typically more severe. Of particular note is the high incidence of deliberate iron overdose in pregnant women [9].

Iron exerts both local and systemic effects. The local irritant effect on the gastrointestinal tract results in nausea, vomiting, abdominal cramps, and diarrhea. These symptoms are produced by relatively small doses (20 mg per kg of elemental iron). The degree of systemic toxicity is, however, dose related. Because most published data are anecdotal, specific values have not been established. In the pediatric literature, more than 60 mg per kg of elemental iron produces significant systemic toxicity [10], with a lethal dose being 200 to 250 mg per kg [10]. Both the figures are likely overestimates; more realistic figures are probably half as much. The lowest reported lethal dose for a toddler is approximately 75 mg per kg of elemental iron [11]. The author's own experience and that of others [12] suggests that the range of toxicity in adults is similar to that in children. An ingestion of 1.5 g of elemental iron by an adult should be cause for concern. Adults have died after ingestion of as little as 2 [13] and 5 g [12] of elemental iron; the former patient had significant hepatic disease and the latter ingested 70 mg per kg. There have been no published reports of serious or fatal poisoning from the ingestion of carbonyl iron products [4]. Although its bioavailability after therapeutic dosing is similar to ferrous salts, its absorption is limited after an overdose. Single doses of 10 g (140 mg per kg) have been tolerated in humans.

Poor, unpredictable absorption of iron and its unknown capacity for binding by ferritin and as hemosiderin contribute to uncertainty regarding the toxic dose. As reflected by serum iron concentrations, which are measured in micrograms per deciliter, the size of the potentially toxic iron pool is likely to be small—on the order of milligrams—even after gram quantities of iron have been ingested. That the body burden of iron is relatively small after an overdose is not well appreciated, but it has important implications for the dose and duration of deferoxamine therapy.

Iron itself is neither caustic nor corrosive. It is a potent catalyst of free radical formation, which results in highly reactive species that attack many intracellular molecules [14]. Iron-generated free radical formation is thought to contribute to acute iron toxicity [15] and to be responsible for much of the damage and dysfunction of chronic iron overload [7].

Free radicals produce damage at their site of origin. Because of local protective mechanisms, a significant concentration of free radicals is required to cause damage. Sites exposed to high iron concentrations are most susceptible to injury. One such area is the gastrointestinal tract. Gastrointestinal mucosal necrosis and bleeding [16] may occur without systemic toxicity. Notably, gut toxicity can occur distally with proximal sparing [16] and may be absent in the face of fatal systemic poisoning [6].

Systemic toxicity results when the absorbed iron is transported to target organs, such as the liver and heart. Nontransferrin-bound iron is rapidly cleared by the liver [17], putting this organ at risk for toxicity [18].

CLINICAL TOXICITY

Traditionally, acute iron intoxication is divided into five clinical stages [19]: gastrointestinal toxicity, relative stability, circulatory shock, hepatic necrosis, and gastrointestinal scarring. An orderly progression through all these stages may not occur. Fatalities are possible without significant gastrointestinal involvement [6], and hepatotoxicity may be absent in otherwise severe poisoning. Presenting signs and symptoms depend on the time since ingestion.

The most common time of presentation is during the first stage (gastrointestinal toxicity), when abdominal pain, vomiting, diarrhea, hematemesis, and hematochezia are seen. Gastrointestinal toxicity usually occurs within the first few hours of overdose. If enteric-coated tablets have been ingested, gastrointestinal toxicity can be delayed as long as 12 hours. The severity of this stage is variable. Life-threatening hypovolemic shock may occur, especially if initial symptoms were severe or ignored. Occasionally, segmental intestinal infarction may occur, necessitating bowel resection [16]. Isolated hepatotoxicity or gastrointestinal obstruction would be an unlikely presentation of iron poisoning.

The second stage, a period of relative stability, follows initial gastrointestinal symptoms. Apparent improvement in the patient's clinical status should not lead to complacency. Patients are not completely asymptomatic; careful assessment and repeated monitoring should document some degree of hypovolemia, circulatory shock, and acidosis.

The third stage, circulatory shock, can occur within several hours of iron overdose and may persist up to 48 to 72 hours. Its pathogenesis is complex and poorly understood and is based on the results of limited experimental animal data [20–23]. Circulatory shock may be hypovolemic, distributive, or cardiogenic. The time of onset can be somewhat helpful in elucidating its cause, but there is considerable overlap. Shock occurring within a few hours of the overdose suggests hypovolemia secondary to fluid and, rarely, blood loss from the gastrointestinal tract. Hyperferremia-associated coagulopathy may contribute to bleeding [24]. Distributive shock depends on iron absorption and begins within the first 24 hours. Suggested mechanisms include direct effects of iron or ferritin or an effect mediated by release of vasoactive substances, resulting in decreased vascular tone or increased vascular permeability [22]. Cardiogenic shock usually occurs 1 to 3 days after overdose [25].

The occurrence of metabolic acidosis in iron poisoning usually precedes circulatory shock. Acidosis is a direct toxic effect of iron that occurs after the plasma's capacity to bind the absorbed ferric ion has been exceeded. When this occurs, the ferric ion becomes hydrated and protons are released [$Fe^{3+} + 3H_2O \rightarrow Fe(OH)_3 + 3H^+$]. Thus, each unbound ferric ion generates three protons. The acidosis can be quite profound, requiring large amounts of bicarbonate for treatment [23]. Other factors contributing to acidosis include the generation of organic acids resulting from iron's interference with intracellular oxidative metabolism and lactate production secondary to shock.

The fourth stage, hepatotoxicity, is second only to shock as a cause of death [18]. It may occur any time during the first 48 hours after overdose. The pathogenesis of hepatic necrosis is believed to be iron-catalyzed free radical production and subsequent lipid peroxidation of hepatic mitochondrial membranes [15].

The fifth stage, gastrointestinal scarring, is the consequence of iron's local action on the gut and usually occurs 2 to 4 weeks after overdose. Ongoing and protracted abdominal pain during the first week is associated with the later development of this complication [16]. Most cases involve the gastric outlet, but isolated strictures of distal intestine have been reported [16].

The consequences of iron poisoning in pregnant women are no different from those in other patients, but because transplacental iron passage is an energy-requiring saturable process, the fetus is relatively protected [26]. Although deferoxamine in animals is associated with potential harm to the fetus, its risk in humans is overemphasized [26]. The health of the fetus depends on its mother, and treatment should be no different from that given to a nonpregnant woman.

DIAGNOSTIC EVALUATION

Essential laboratory tests include abdominal radiographs, serum iron and bicarbonate concentrations, and blood gas determinations. Because iron tablets are radiopaque, an abdominal radiograph can be used to verify an overdose and quantify the amount ingested [27–29]. However, iron tablets may not be visible if they have dissolved or been chewed, a liquid preparation has been ingested, or there is only a small amount of iron in each tablet (e.g., pediatric iron-containing multivitamins) [30]. If tablets are visible, serial abdominal radiographs may be used to judge the effectiveness of gastrointestinal decontamination.

Serum iron concentration is the single most important test. It verifies the ingestion, guides management, and provides prognostic information. A peak serum concentration of less than 500 μg per dL (90 μmol per L) is usually associated with negligible-to-mild systemic toxicity; however, there may be significant gastrointestinal symptoms. Moderate systemic toxicity is expected with a peak concentration of 500 to 1,000 μg per dL (90 to 180 μmol per L). A peak serum concentration greater than 1,000 μg per dL (180 μmol per L) is associated with severe toxicity, such as profound acidosis, shock, hepatotoxicity, coma, and death. Mortality approaches 100% when serum concentration is greater than 10,000 μg per dL (1,800 μmol per L). The time of blood sampling to estimate peak serum iron concentration should be 4 to 6 hours after an overdose of conventional tablets and several hours later for an overdose of delayed-release formulations. However, the type of preparation ingested is usually unknown at the time a patient seeks treatment and is difficult to establish even after the fact [31]. Serial serum iron concentration determinations are recommended during the early hours after overdose, especially when the first value is 300 to 500 μg per dL (55 to 90 μmol per L). Determinations should be obtained every 2 hours until a definite downward trend is established. A concurrent abdominal radiograph may be helpful. If many tablets are visible, the subsequent serum iron level will likely be higher. However, a negative radiograph does not guarantee that peak serum iron level has occurred. It is desirable to obtain blood specimens before initiating deferoxamine therapy because it can confound the laboratory determination of serum iron concentration, resulting in falsely lower levels [32]. When clinically indicated, deferoxamine therapy should not be delayed because of blood sampling issues.

Blood gas or serum bicarbonate determinations should be done early because acidosis is the first objective indicator of systemic toxicity. Frequency of blood gas determinations is guided by previous values, the need for bicarbonate therapy, and clinical course. A pH of less than 7.30 is indicative of significant toxicity.

Recommended laboratory tests include blood coagulation panels and hepatic and renal function tests. Blood coagulation panels should be done early and repeated throughout the first few days in patients with significant toxicity because a biphasic coagulopathy may develop [24]. Blood should be typed and cross-matched as clinically indicated. Hepatic function should be monitored daily during the first 72 hours and longer if values remain significantly abnormal. Renal function tests should be obtained regularly, especially during deferoxamine therapy, because of the risk for acute renal failure [33].

The total iron-binding capacity (TIBC) is not recommended in the assessment or management of patients with iron overdose [34]. Routine methods for TIBC determination are unreliable during hyperferremic states and are time consuming [34]. The TIBC becomes falsely elevated in the presence of high serum iron concentrations, and it has yet to be demonstrated that iron toxicity occurs only when the serum iron concentration exceeds the TIBC [34]. A serum iron concentration that is less than the TIBC does not rule out acute iron poisoning.

One retrospective study of acute iron overdose showed that vomiting was a highly sensitive predictor of a serum iron concentration greater than 300 μg per dL (54 μmol per L). In addition, a white blood cell count greater than 15,000 per μL or a serum glucose concentration greater than 150 mg per dL (8.3 mmol per L) has a positive predictive value of 100% for a serum iron level greater than 300 μg per dL (54 μmol per L) [35]. However, these tests have unacceptably low sensitivity and negative predictive value. Although such surrogate markers may be helpful when serum iron concentrations are not readily available, these associations have not been confirmed in subsequent studies [36,37]. The absence of vomiting, a white blood cell count less than 15,000 per μL, or a serum glucose concentration of less than 150 mg per dL (8.3 mmol per L) should not be relied on as a surrogate marker for a serum iron level of less than 300 μg per dL (54 μmol per L).

It is difficult to accurately predict outcomes because the published literature chiefly consists of anecdotal reports. Survival is expected with peak serum iron concentrations of less than 1,000 μg per dL (180 μmol per L) and appropriate supportive care. The chief causes of death are shock and hepatic failure. Acute renal failure may result from shock or deferoxamine therapy without adequate volume replacement [33]. *Yersinia septicemia* has been reported in patients treated with deferoxamine [27,38].

Differential diagnosis becomes an issue only when the history of iron overdose is unknown. In such situations, diagnosis can be quite problematic because of the multiple and varied clinical features at presentation (e.g., abdominal pain, gastrointestinal hemorrhage, shock, and coma). From the poisoning perspective, corrosive ingestion and acute heavy metal poisoning are the main considerations.

MANAGEMENT

The initial management of a patient with an iron overdose presents a challenge because the patient often presents before the peak of clinical toxicity. Many patients, especially young children, may be asymptomatic or only mildly ill. The challenge lies in identifying those who are at risk for significant toxicity in order to place them in an appropriate setting for the required level of care. The decision for the iron-overdosed critically ill patient is straightforward. Table 136.1 provides guidelines for intensive care unit admission for those patients who are not critically ill.

TABLE 136.1

SUGGESTED CRITERIA FOR ADMISSION OF THE NONCRITICALLY ILL IRON-OVERDOSED PATIENT TO AN INTENSIVE CARE UNIT

	Admit to ICU	Strongly consider admission to ICU
Amount of elemental iron ingested		
Child (<6 y)	>60 mg/kg	45–60 mg/kg
Adult (all others)	>3.0 g	2.0–3.0 g
Tablets seen in radiograph[a]		
Child (<6 y)	1/kg	0.75–1.00/kg
Adult (all others)	>50	33–50
Peak serum iron concentrations	>1,000 μg/dL (>180 μmol/L)	750–1,000 μg/dL (135–180 μmol/L)
Arterial pH	<7.30	7.30–7.35

[a] Assuming 60-mg elemental iron/tablet.
Note: Not all criteria need to be present.

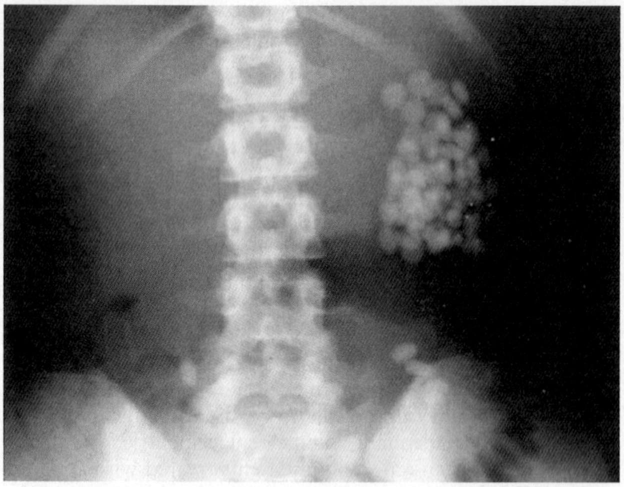

FIGURE 136.1. Abdominal radiograph of a 16-year-old girl with a potentially lethal iron overdose after syrup of ipecac-induced emesis and gastric lavage. Gastroscopy ruled out adherence of iron to the stomach wall and medication concretion. She subsequently underwent whole-bowel irrigation. Her peak serum iron concentration was 253 μg per dL (46 μmol per L), and she was not treated with deferoxamine.

Because activated charcoal does not adsorb iron [28], whole-bowel irrigation (WBI; Fig. 136.1) is recommended as the decontamination procedure of choice for the iron-overdosed patient [29]. WBI should be initiated when there is radiographic documentation of iron ingestion and considered when there is a history of elemental iron ingestion greater than 60 mg per kg in children and 1.5 g per kg in adults. If emesis hampers effective WBI, consider metoclopramide (1 mg per kg intravenously in adults and 0.1 mg per kg in children) or ondansetron (8 mg per kg intravenously in adults or 0.1 to 0.2 mg per kg in children).

Iron can become adherent to the gastrointestinal mucosa or may form tablet bezoars [39]. The latter is primarily a problem with conventional iron tablets and not with the enteric-coated varieties. Radiographs in three planes (flat, upright, and decubitus) should identify these two situations. A computed tomographic (CT) scan is another consideration. Barium studies are unlikely to be helpful because of the anticipated lack of contrast between barium and iron. If WBI is ineffective, removal of iron via gastrotomy should be considered [39,40]. For surgical intervention to be effective, it should be done before the iron is absorbed and most tablets must be in a localized area rather than scattered throughout the gastrointestinal tract. A combined approach of gastrotomy for tablet retrieval followed by WBI after surgery has been described [40]. The former removed the iron from the stomach and the latter removed it from the intestinal tract. Endoscopic removal of an iron bezoar from the stomach has been reported [41].

The oral administration of bicarbonate, phosphate, or deferoxamine is not recommended. These agents have been advocated as a way to decrease iron absorption by precipitating it as an insoluble salt or by chelating it. In vitro [42] and animal [43] studies do not support bicarbonate or phosphate administration, and the latter therapy has resulted in hypocalcemia and hypovolemia in iron-overdosed patients [44]. Oral deferoxamine is not recommended. It is neither appreciably toxic nor absorbed from the gastrointestinal tract, but the same is not true of its chelate, ferrioxamine [19,21,45]. The latter has been shown to be lethal in animals [21,46].

Supportive care should be provided concurrently with gastrointestinal decontamination. In patients with severe poisoning, two intravenous (IV) lines are required: one for fluid resuscitation and bicarbonate administration and the other for deferoxamine therapy. Very large amounts of crystalloid and bicarbonate may be required [23], and occasionally, colloid or blood may be necessary. Because of the complex nature of shock in iron poisoning, early placement of a Swan-Ganz catheter may be needed to assist in diagnosis and monitor the effectiveness of therapy. Early shock should respond to vigorous volume resuscitation; occasionally, pressor therapy may be needed. Late shock usually requires inotropic support. Failure of inotropic support suggests the need for afterload reduction [25]; once a patient has reached this point, the prognosis is grave. An arterial catheter for frequent blood gas determinations and a Foley catheter for monitoring urine output are essential in all critically ill patients.

Parameters requiring serial monitoring include arterial blood gas, hematocrit, serum electrolytes, renal and hepatic function, and blood coagulation. The frequency of these determinations depends on previous results and the patient's clinical condition and response to the therapy.

Acute hepatic failure is managed by standard protocols. Acute renal failure may be a consequence of shock or deferoxamine therapy in the setting of hypovolemia [33]. Hemodialysis may be required in such situations, especially if deferoxamine therapy is continued, to remove the toxic chelate, ferrioxamine. Coagulopathy during the first few hours after overdose is related to serum iron concentration and is transient. Specific therapy is unnecessary. Deferoxamine lowers the serum iron concentration and may hasten its resolution [24]. Coagulopathy occurring many hours to a few days after overdose is a manifestation of hepatic failure. Administration of fresh-frozen plasma is recommended, as vitamin K_1 is unlikely to be helpful.

Hemodialysis or hemoperfusion is not recommended for iron removal because of the rapid extravascular distribution of the iron and its binding to plasma proteins as nontransferrin-bound iron [7]. However, hemodialysis is indicated for patients with renal failure.

Deferoxamine, the specific treatment of choice for acute iron poisoning [15,19], is a naturally occurring siderophore isolated from *Streptomyces pilosus*. Its pharmacology was described in the early 1960s [47,48]. Its binding constant for ferric iron is 10^{31}, which compares with 10^{27} to 10^{29} for transferrin. It is capable of removing iron from ferritin and hemosiderin and, to a very minor degree, from transferrin, but not at all from cytochromes, hemoglobin, or myoglobin.

Although deferoxamine is regarded as the treatment of choice, its effectiveness has been questioned because it has limited chelating capacity and only small amounts of iron are recovered in the urine after its administration to iron-poisoned patients [49]. The manufacturer's recommended daily deferoxamine dosage of 6 g is capable of chelating 510 mg of iron or 8.5 ferrous sulfate tablets. Although this would seem to be insignificant in the patient who has ingested 50 tablets, the poor absorption of iron and the body's large storage capacity for it result in only a relatively small amount being responsible for toxicity. Therefore, the chelation of small amounts of iron may be quite beneficial. Alternatively, 510 mg of iron is approximately 10% of the total amount of iron and approximately 35% of the nonheme iron in a 70-kg man [50].

Historically, therapy was based on the deferoxamine chelation challenge test and relied on visual detection of a change in urine color to rusty orange (vin rosé) caused by the presence of ferrioxamine after intramuscular administration of deferoxamine. This test has never been validated and is not recommended.

Traditional indications for deferoxamine therapy have been based on the peak serum iron concentration, the serum iron concentration relative to the TIBC, the results of a chelation challenge test, and the patient's clinical condition. The therapy has been recommended for those with peak serum iron concentrations ranging from 300 to 500 μg per dL (55 to 90 μmol per L) [51]. Significant morbidity is unlikely with peak concentrations of less than 500 μg per dL (90 μmol per L). Values at the lower end of the above range are based on the upper limit of normal for TIBC, which, as discussed earlier, is invalid. Hence, a serum iron concentration of 500 μg per dL (90 μmol per L) or greater is recommended as an indication for deferoxamine therapy in an otherwise asymptomatic patient. Deferoxamine therapy is indicated when toxic signs and symptoms are present, regardless of the serum iron concentration. Such symptoms include acidosis, shock, and decreased level of consciousness or coma. Although some toxicologists also advocate deferoxamine therapy for those with recurrent vomiting or diarrhea, these symptoms can be seen in patients who do not develop systemic toxicity.

Deferoxamine can be given intravenously or intramuscularly. The manufacturer recommends intramuscular therapy unless the patient is in shock, presumably because of concern for hypotension, which is associated with rapid IV administration. The patient should be fluid resuscitated, and IV deferoxamine therapy should be initiated slowly and gradually increased to 15 mg per kg per hour during 20 to 30 minutes. Continuous IV infusion is the recommended method for administering deferoxamine. This is based on studies in patients with transfusion-induced iron overload, demonstrating that IV deferoxamine results in greater urinary iron elimination, higher peak deferoxamine serum concentrations, and more stable serum deferoxamine levels [52].

The optimal dose of deferoxamine is uncertain. The manufacturer recommends a daily maximum dose of 6 g given in divided doses. A continuous infusion protocol of 15 mg per kg per hour until 24 hours after the urine returns to its normal color has also been recommended [15]. The latter protocol exceeds the manufacturer's guidelines for patients heavier than 17 kg. Neither recommendation is evidence based. Only two patients treated with 15 mg per kg per hour over a prolonged course have been well described in the literature [53,54]. Furthermore, continuous IV deferoxamine therapy in patients with acute iron poisoning for longer than 24 to 48 hours has been associated with the development of adult respiratory distress syndrome [55]. Four patients with mild-to-moderate iron poisoning without evidence of shock, acidosis, or sepsis who received 15 mg per kg per hour of deferoxamine intravenously for 2 to 3 days died of noncardiogenic pulmonary edema [55]. Continuous IV deferoxamine therapy should not routinely exceed the first 24 hours. If prolonged chelation therapy is deemed necessary, interrupting therapy for 12 of every 24 hours to allow excretion of ferrioxamine can be considered. Careful monitoring of pulmonary status is required during prolonged therapy.

Indications for discontinuing deferoxamine therapy include resolution of the signs and symptoms of systemic iron toxicity and correction of acidosis. Deferoxamine therapy is rarely needed beyond 24 hours and should be used with caution for periods longer than this.

Adverse drug events from short-term deferoxamine therapy are few, but significant. Rapid IV administration is associated with tachycardia, hypotension, shock, a generalized beet-red flushing of the skin, blotchy erythema, and urticaria. Acute renal failure can result when deferoxamine is administered to patients with hypovolemia [33]. Pulmonary toxicity and acute respiratory distress syndrome are associated with continuous IV therapy over several days [55]. Patients receiving deferoxamine may be at increased risk for *Yersinia* infections [27,38].

Before discharge, a psychiatric assessment is indicated for all patients with purposeful ingestions. Those who have required deferoxamine therapy should have a follow-up visit approximately 1 month after discharge. At this time, the patient's iron status and gastrointestinal tract should be assessed. He or she should also be advised of the symptoms of gastrointestinal obstruction and to return immediately if they occur. Chronic hepatic or cardiac dysfunction has not been reported after acute iron overdose.

References

1. Litovitz T, Manoguerra A: Comparison of pediatric poisoning hazards: an analysis of 38 million exposure incidents. *Pediatrics* 89:999, 1992.
2. Tenenbein M: Unit-dose packaging of iron supplements and reduction of iron poisoning in young children. *Arch Pediatr Adolesc Med* 159:557, 2005.
3. Litovitz TL, Klein-Schwartz W, White S, et al: 1999 Annual report of the American Association of Poison Control Centers Toxic Exposure Surveillance System. *Am J Emerg Med* 18:517, 2000.
4. Madiwale T, Liebelt E: Iron: not a benign therapeutic drug. *Curr Opin Pediatr* 18:174, 2006.
5. Harju E: Clinical pharmacokinetics of iron preparations. *Clin Pharmacokinet* 17:69, 1989.
6. Reissman KR, Coleman TJ, Budai BS, et al: Acute intestinal iron intoxication. I. Iron absorption, serum iron and autopsy findings. *Blood* 10:35, 1955.
7. Hershko C, Peto TE: Non-transferrin plasma iron. *Br J Haematol* 66:149, 1987.
8. Krenzelok EP, Hoff JV: Accidental childhood iron poisoning: a problem of marketing and labeling. *Pediatrics* 63:591, 1979.
9. Rayburn W, Aronow R, DeLancey B, et al: Drug overdose during pregnancy: an overview from a metropolitan poison control center. *Obstet Gynecol* 64:611, 1984.
10. Henretig FM, Temple AR: Acute iron poisoning in children. *Emerg Med Clin North Am* 2:121, 1984.
11. Smith RP, Jones CW, Cochran EW: Ferrous sulfate toxicity. *N Engl J Med* 243:641, 1950.
12. Olenmark M, Biber B, Dottori O, et al: Fatal iron intoxication in late pregnancy. *J Toxicol Clin Toxicol* 25:347, 1987.
13. Lavender S, Bell SA: Iron intoxication in an adult. *BMJ* 2:406, 1970.
14. Halliwell B, Gutteridge JMC: Oxygen free radicals and iron in relation to biology and medicine: some problems and concepts. *Arch Biochem Biophys* 246:501, 1986.
15. Robotham JL, Lietman PS: Acute iron poisoning. *Am J Dis Child* 134:875, 1980.
16. Tenenbein M, Littman C, Stimpson RE: Gastrointestinal pathology in adult iron overdose. *J Toxicol Clin Toxicol* 28:311, 1990.
17. Wright TL, Brissot P, Ma W, et al: Characterization of non-transferrin-bound iron clearance by rat. *J Biol Chem* 261:10909, 1986.
18. Robertson A, Tenenbein M: Hepatotoxicity in acute iron poisoning. *Hum Exp Toxicol* 24:559, 2005.
19. Banner W Jr, Tong TG: Iron poisoning. *Pediatr Clin North Am* 33:393, 1986.
20. Reissmann KR, Coleman TJ: Acute intestinal iron intoxication. II. Metabolic, respiratory and circulatory effects of absorbed iron salts. *Blood* 10:46, 1955.
21. Whitten CF, Chen Y, Gibson GW: Studies in acute iron poisoning: further observations on desferrioxamine in the treatment of acute experimental iron poisoning. *Pediatrics* 38:102, 1966.
22. Whitten CF, Chen YC, Gibson GW: Studies in acute iron poisoning: the hemodynamic alterations in acute experimental iron poisoning. *Pediatr Res* 2:479, 1968.
23. Vernon DD, Banner W, Dean JM: Hemodynamic effects of experimental iron poisoning. *Ann Emerg Med* 18:863, 1989.
24. Tenenbein M, Israels SJ: Early coagulopathy in severe iron poisoning. *J Pediatr* 113:695, 1988.
25. Tenenbein M, Kopelow ML, deSa DJ: Myocardial failure and shock in iron poisoning. *Hum Toxicol* 7:281, 1988.
26. Tenenbein M: Poisoning in pregnancy, in Koren G (ed): *Maternal-Fetal Toxicology: A Clinician's Guide*. New York, Marcel Dekker Inc, 1990, p 89.
27. Mofenson HC, Caraccio TR, Sharieff N: Iron sepsis. *Yersinia enterocolitica* septicemia possibly caused by an overdose of iron. *N Engl J Med* 316:1092, 1987.
28. Decker WJ, Combs HF, Corby DG: Adsorption of drugs and poisons by activated charcoal. *Toxicol Appl Pharmacol* 13:454, 1968.
29. Tenenbein M: Position statement: whole bowel irrigation. American Academy of Clinical Toxicology; European Association of Poison Centres and Clinical Toxicologists. *J Toxicol Clin Toxicol* 35:753, 1997.
30. Everson GW, Oudjhane K, Young LW, et al: Effectiveness of abdominal radiographs in visualizing chewable iron supplements following overdose. *Am J Emerg Med* 7:459, 1989.
31. Boggs DR: Fate of a ferrous sulfate prescription. *Am J Med* 82:124, 1987.
32. Gevirtz NR, Wasserman LR: The measurement of iron and iron-binding capacity in plasma containing deferoxamine. *J Pediatr* 68:802, 1966.
33. Koren G, Bentur Y, Strong D, et al: Acute changes in renal function associated with deferoxamine therapy. *Am J Dis Child* 143:1077, 1989.

34. Tenenbein M, Yatscoff RW: The TIBC in iron poisoning: is it useful? *Am J Dis Child* 145:437, 1990.
35. Lacouture PG, Wason S, Temple AR, et al: Emergency assessment of severity of iron overdose by clinical and laboratory methods. *J Pediatr* 99:89, 1981.
36. Knansel AL, Collins-Barrow MD: Applicability of early indicators of iron toxicity. *J Natl Med Assoc* 78:1037, 1986.
37. Palatnick W, Tenenbein M: Leukocytosis, hyperglycemia, vomiting and positive x-rays are not indicators of severity of iron overdose in adults. *Am J Emerg Med* 14:454, 1996.
38. Melby K, Slordahl S, Gutteberg TJ, et al: Septicemia due to *Yersinia enterocolitica* after oral overdoses of iron. *BMJ* 285:467, 1982.
39. Foxford R, Goldfrank L: Gastrotomy: a surgical approach to iron overdose. *Ann Emerg Med* 14:1223, 1985.
40. Tenenbein M, Wiseman N, Yatscoff RW: Gastrotomy and whole bowel irrigation in iron poisoning. *Pediatr Emerg Care* 7:286, 1991.
41. Ng HW, Tse ML, Lau FL, et al: Endoscopic removal of iron bezoar following acute overdose. *Clin Toxicol* 46:913, 2008.
42. Czajka PA, Konrad JD, Duffy JP: Iron poisoning: an in vitro comparison of bicarbonate and phosphate lavage solutions. *J Pediatr* 98:491, 1981.
43. Dean BS, Krenzelok EP: In vivo effectiveness of oral complexation agents in the management of iron poisoning. *J Toxicol Clin Toxicol* 25:221, 1987.
44. Bachrach L, Correa A, Levin R, et al: Iron poisoning: complications of hypertonic phosphate lavage therapy. *J Pediatr* 94:147, 1979.
45. Whitten CF, Gibson GW, Good MH, et al: Studies in acute iron poisoning. I. Deferoxamine in the treatment of acute iron poisoning: clinical observations, experimental studies and theoretical considerations. *Pediatrics* 36:322, 1965.
46. Adamson IY, Sienko A, Tenenbein M: Pulmonary toxicity of deferoxamine in iron-poisoned mice. *Toxicol Appl Pharmacol* 120:13, 1993.
47. Moeschlin S, Schnider U: Treatment of primary and secondary hemochromatosis and acute iron poisoning with a new potent iron-eliminating agent (desferrioxamine B). *N Engl J Med* 269:57, 1963.
48. Keberle H: The biochemistry of desferrioxamine and its relation to iron metabolism. *Ann N Y Acad Sci* 119:758, 1964.
49. Proudfoot AT, Simpson D, Dyson EH: Management of acute iron poisoning. *Med Toxicol* 1:83, 1986.
50. Worwood M: The clinical biochemistry of iron. *Semin Hematol* 14:3, 1977.
51. Bosse GM: Conservative management of patients with moderately elevated serum iron levels. *J Toxicol Clin Toxicol* 33:135, 1995.
52. Propper RD, Shurin SB, Nathan DG: Reassessment of the use of desferrioxamine B in iron overload. *N Engl J Med* 294:1421, 1976.
53. Peck MG, Rogers JF, Rivenbark JF: Use of high doses of deferoxamine (Desferal) in an adult patient with acute iron overdosage. *J Toxicol Clin Toxicol* 19:865, 1982.
54. Henretig FM, Karl SR, Weintraub WH: Severe iron poisoning treated with enteral and intravenous deferoxamine. *Ann Emerg Med* 12:306, 1983.
55. Tenenbein M, Kowalski S, Sienko et al: Pulmonary toxic effects of continuous desferrioxamine administration in acute iron poisoning. *Lancet* 339:699, 1992.

CHAPTER 137 ■ ISONIAZID POISONING

JAMES B. MOWRY AND R. BRENT FURBEE

Isoniazid (isonicotinic acid hydrazide [INH]) is the cornerstone of treatment and prevention of tuberculosis. It is available under a variety of brand names in 50-, 100-, and 300-mg tablets; as an oral syrup (50 mg per 5 mL); as an injectable solution (100 mg per mL); and in powder form. It is also available in combination with rifampin, pyridoxine, and other antitubercular drugs.

In 2007, the American Association of Poison Control Centers reported 330 cases with exposure to INH, including 228 single exposures [1]; 33% of the cases involved adults, with 34% being intentional. No deaths were reported, but 33% of the cases exhibited moderate-to-severe toxicity.

PHARMACOLOGY

As a bactericidal agent, INH interferes with lipid and nucleic acid biosynthesis in the growing *Mycobacterium* organism. It is rapidly and nearly completely absorbed after oral administration, with peak plasma concentrations occurring within 1 to 2 hours [2]. The rate and extent of absorption are decreased by food. The volume of distribution of INH approximates total body water (0.67 ± 0.15 L per kg), with cerebrospinal fluid concentrations 90% of those of serum [3]. INH passes into breast milk and through the placental barrier. There is little protein binding.

Between 75% and 95% of an INH dose is metabolized in the liver within 24 hours by acetylation to acetylisoniazid and hydrolysis to isonicotinic acid and hydrazine [2]. Genetic variation in its metabolism significantly alters plasma concentration, elimination half-life, and toxicity [4]. The elimination half-life in rapid acetylators (e.g., Asians, Eskimos, and American Indians) is 0.5 to 1.5 hours, whereas it is 2 to 4 hours in slow acetylators (e.g., people of African descent and Caucasians) [5]. The elimination half-life can be prolonged in people with liver disease. Rapid acetylators excrete 2.5% of INH as unchanged drug, compared with 10% in slow acetylators [2]. In addition, slow acetylators may have a higher percentage of the dose metabolized to hydrazine, a potential hepatotoxin [6]. INH exhibits dose-dependent inhibition of the mixed-function oxidases CYP2C19 and CYP3A, increasing the risk of adverse drug reactions in slow acetylators during the coadministration of drugs metabolized by these enzymes (e.g., phenytoin, carbamazepine, and diazepam) [7].

The usual adult INH dose is 5 mg per kg per day (maximum, 300 mg). The dose is increased to 15 mg per kg (maximum, 900 mg) when INH is used in combination with other antitubercular drugs and administered twice weekly. Acute ingestion of 1.5 to 3.0 g in adults may be toxic, with 6 to 10 g uniformly associated with severe toxicity and significant mortality [8]. The pediatric INH dose is 10 to 15 mg per kg per day (maximum, 300 mg) and is increased to 20 to 30 mg per kg (maximum, 900 mg) when concurrent INH and other antitubercular drugs are administered twice weekly. When INH is used in combination with rifampin, limiting the INH dose to 10 mg per kg per day and the rifampin dose to 15 mg per kg per day may minimize hepatotoxicity in children [9]. In patients with preexisting seizure disorders, convulsions have occurred with doses as low as 14 mg per kg per day; 19 mg per kg per day resulted in seizures in a 7-year-old child [8].

Daily therapeutic INH doses produce peak serum concentrations between 1 and 7 μg per mL. Intermittent INH therapy may produce concentrations between 16 and 32 μg per mL. Serum INH concentrations in acute ingestions have ranged from 20 μg per mL to more than 710 μg per mL, with little correlation to severity of intoxication [10–13].

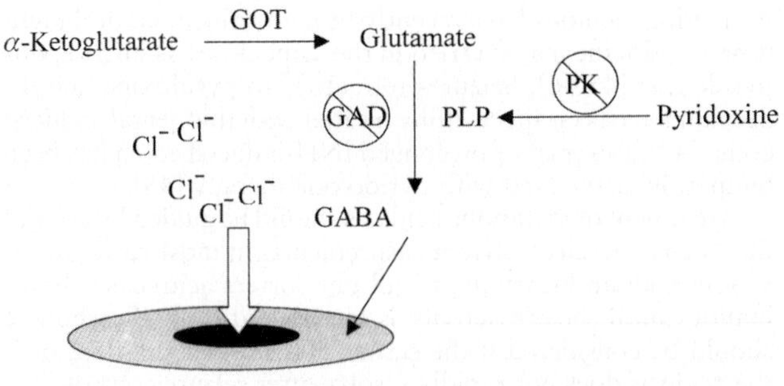

FIGURE 137.1. Role of isoniazid in the reduction of γ-aminobutyric acid (GABA) concentration. Cl^-, chloride ions; GAD, glutamic acid decarboxylase; GOT, glutamic oxaloacetic transaminase; PK, pyridoxine kinase; PLP, pyridoxal 5′-phosphate; ⊘, inhibited by isoniazid.

The central nervous system toxicity of INH and its metabolites is believed to be due to a decrease in the concentration of γ-aminobutyric acid, an inhibitory neurotransmitter that suppresses neuronal depolarization by opening chloride ionophores (Fig. 137.1). INH combines with pyridoxine (vitamin B_6) and is excreted in the urine as pyridoxal isonicotinylhydrazine [14]. It also competes with pyridoxine for pyridoxine kinase, the enzyme that converts pyridoxine to pyridoxal 5′-phosphate, the cofactor for glutamic acid decarboxylase–mediated conversion of glutamate to γ-aminobutyric acid [15]. In addition, INH inhibits glutamic acid decarboxylase activity. Its metabolism results in metabolites such as hydrazides and hydrazones, which inhibit pyridoxal 5′-phosphate and pyridoxine kinase, respectively [16].

INH causes a peripheral neuropathy that may be responsive to pyridoxine supplementation [17]. Wallerian degeneration of the myelin sheath and axon with blockade of fast axoplasmic transport is noted, with sensory nerves affected more than motor nerves [18–22]. Peripheral neuropathy is most commonly associated with chronic INH use in slow acetylators but may occur after acute massive overdose [23,24].

The mechanism of INH-induced hepatic injury is not understood. Hepatitis occurs in 0.1% to 1.1% of patients receiving INH, especially those with advanced age and alcohol consumption [25–28]. Concurrent rifampin therapy increases the incidence of hepatitis to 2.7% in adults and 6.9% in children [9,25–28]. It is unclear whether this effect is due to an influence of rifampin on INH metabolism or to the additive effect of two hepatotoxic drugs [28]. The histopathologic pattern of hepatic injury closely resembles viral hepatitis. Hypersensitivity seems unlikely, as rechallenge often fails to produce recurrence. Hepatic damage may be due to hydrazine metabolites of INH, covalently binding to liver macromolecules and producing necrosis [29]. Both rapid and slow acetylators have been described as having a greater risk for hepatotoxicity, although other researchers failed to find an association with acetylator status [26,30]. More recent work suggests that slow acetylators may be more susceptible to antitubercular drug–induced hepatitis and may develop more severe hepatotoxicity than do rapid acetylators [31].

The severe metabolic acidosis seen in acute INH intoxication is almost entirely due to seizure activity [32]. Although INH may interfere with nicotinamide adenine dinucleotide–mediated conversion of lactate to pyruvate, acidosis was not observed in animal studies until seizures occurred and lactic acidosis resolved within 2 hours after seizures ceased [32]. β-Hydroxybutyric acid production has also been reported after INH overdose, but does not appear responsible for INH-induced acidosis [33].

Hyperglycemia may result from disruptions of the Krebs cycle that require nicotinamide adenine dinucleotide and from stimulation of glucagon secretion [12].

CLINICAL PRESENTATION

Signs and symptoms usually appear within 30 minutes to 2 hours after acute INH overdose. Nausea, vomiting, dizziness, slurred speech, blurred vision, and visual hallucinations (e.g., bright colors, spots, and strange designs) are among the first manifestations [8,10]. Stupor and coma can develop rapidly, followed by intractable tonic–clonic generalized or localized seizures, hyperreflexia or areflexia, and cyanosis [8,10]. In severe cases, cardiovascular and respiratory collapse results in death. Oliguria progressing to anuria has been reported [8]. The metabolic alterations are striking and include severe metabolic acidosis, hyperglycemia, glycosuria, ketonuria, and hyperkalemia [8,10,12]. The triad of metabolic acidosis refractory to sodium bicarbonate therapy, seizures refractory to anticonvulsants, and coma suggests INH toxicity.

Hepatotoxicity usually presents as elevated serum aspartate aminotransferase values within the first few months of therapy. Fatalities from INH-induced hepatitis during chemoprophylaxis are between 4.2 and 7.0 per 100,000 persons [34]. When peripheral neuropathy occurs, it is within 3 to 35 weeks of initiating the therapy [22]. Other chronic effects include dysarthria, irritability, seizures, dysphoria, and inability to concentrate [25]. Optic neuritis and optic atrophy have also been reported, but their occurrence is often associated with the administration of ethambutol as well [35,36].

DIAGNOSTIC EVALUATION

Initial laboratory evaluation should include serum electrolytes, blood urea nitrogen, creatinine, glucose, calcium, and magnesium levels. Laboratory workup for anion-gap metabolic acidosis (e.g., serum methanol, ethylene glycol, salicylate, and acetaminophen levels) should also be considered. Arterial blood gases, electrocardiogram, chest radiograph, head computed tomography, and lumbar puncture should be obtained as clinically indicated.

Qualitative INH identification in urine using reagent-impregnated paper strips or a point-of-care testing device sensitive to INH metabolites [37,38] and quantitative serum INH identification are not widely enough available to be clinically useful to confirm diagnosis.

Acute INH intoxication should be considered in the differential diagnosis of any patient presenting with unexplained neurologic symptoms, particularly intractable seizure activity [8,13]. Conditions that may resemble INH toxicity include (a) central nervous system tumors and infections; (b) electrolyte abnormalities; (c) thyroid dysfunction; (d) hypoglycemia; (e) poisoning by anticholinergic, cholinergic, and sympathomimetic agents, or by tricyclic antidepressants (e.g., amoxapine), theophylline, organophosphates, meperidine (normeperidine), propoxyphene (norpropoxyphene), carbon monoxide, or cyanide; and (f) withdrawal syndromes [39]. Other causes of an anion-gap metabolic acidosis such as diabetic ketoacidosis, uremia, ethylene glycol, methanol, and salicylates should also be considered.

Ingestion of rifampin–INH combination products may produce, in addition to the symptoms of INH poisoning, (a) a striking red-orange discoloration of the skin, urine, sclera, and mucus membranes; (b) periorbital or facial edema; (c) pruritus; and (d) nausea, vomiting, or diffuse abdominal tenderness [40]. Transient elevations in total bilirubin and alkaline phosphatase, indicating cholestasis, may also be noted.

MANAGEMENT

The initial management of a patient with acute INH overdose focuses on protection of airway, support of respiration, treatment of seizures, correction of metabolic acidosis, minimization of drug absorption, and in selected cases, enhancement of INH elimination.

Gastrointestinal decontamination, if performed, should consist of the administration of activated charcoal. In severely ill patients, gastric lavage should be considered. Emesis is contraindicated because of the potential for rapid and unpredictable onset of seizures and coma.

Patients who have ingested a potentially toxic INH dose should be observed for at least 6 hours [8]; those who remain asymptomatic after gastrointestinal decontamination may be referred for psychiatric evaluation. All symptomatic patients should be admitted to an intensive care setting.

Seizures are often refractory to most conventional anticonvulsants [41]. Diazepam appears to be the most effective single agent, but its efficacy may be limited and large doses may be required. Animal data suggest sodium valproate may be effective [42]. Pyridoxine has dose-related effectiveness against convulsions and prevents lethality at doses from 75 to 300 mg per kg in canine models of INH toxicity [43]. In animal studies, when single-anticonvulsant regimens of pyridoxine, phenobarbital, pentobarbital, phenytoin, and diazepam were compared with the latter four anticonvulsants in combination with pyridoxine; pyridoxine was the only single agent that reduced the severity of convulsions and prevented death [41,43]. The combination of each of the other anticonvulsants with pyridoxine also prevented both convulsions and death. Therefore, pyridoxine, in conjunction with a benzodiazepine such as diazepam or lorazepam, is the preferred treatment for neurologic toxicity.

Intravenous pyridoxine therapy should be administered at the first sign of neurologic toxicity in milligram doses equal to the amount of INH ingested [8,10,44]. INH-overdosed patients treated with such pyridoxine doses exhibited no recurrent seizure activity, a decreased duration of coma, and prompt resolution of their metabolic acidosis [13]. If the amount of INH ingested is unknown, at least 5 g of pyridoxine should be administered [8,10]. In patients without seizures, the pyridoxine dose may be administered over 30 to 60 minutes. In those with seizure activity, it may be given as a bolus during 3 to 5 minutes. The pyridoxine dose should be repeated if seizures persist or recur. Intravenous diazepam or lorazepam should also be given [8,41]. As inadequate intravenous stores of pyridoxine in treating facilities have recently been documented, oral high-dose pyridoxine may be tried in the same doses as intravenous pyridoxine [45,46]. Seizures refractory to pyridoxine and diazepam have been successfully treated with thiopental-induced coma [47]. Reversal of prolonged INH-induced coma has been temporally associated with pyridoxine therapy [48].

Treatment of metabolic acidosis should be guided by arterial blood gas and electrolyte measurements. In most cases, intravenous sodium bicarbonate will not correct acid–base abnormalities until seizure activity is terminated [13]. Bicarbonate should be considered if the serum pH is lower than 7.2 or if the acidosis does not rapidly resolve after seizure control.

The role of forced diuresis in the management of INH overdose is unclear. Large amounts of INH recovered in the urine of some patients (43% to 58% of ingested doses) are offset by those reporting minimal recovery (6 to 144 mg) [11,49,50]. Peritoneal dialysis is somewhat effective but inefficient, whereas exchange transfusion is ineffective [49,51]. Hemodialysis and charcoal hemoperfusion increase the clearance of INH and decrease its half-life by 50%, but they have not been reported to remove significant quantities of INH (90 to 340 mg) [50,52].

Considering the rapid elimination half-life of INH and the efficacy of pyridoxine and benzodiazepine therapy, measures to enhance INH elimination are of limited use in the routine management of INH toxicity. However, patients with intractable acid–base disturbances, persistent seizures, or liver or renal dysfunction should be considered candidates for hemodialysis or charcoal hemoperfusion (if available). Unless the patient has experienced significant anoxia as a result of coma or seizures, neurologic recovery may be expected within 24 to 48 hours.

Prevention of peripheral neuropathy during chronic INH therapy can be accomplished by the administration of pyridoxine, 15 to 50 mg per day, in high-risk patients [19]. Peripheral neuropathy that develops during INH therapy is generally reversible on withdrawal of INH and treatment with high-dose pyridoxine (100 to 200 mg per day) [19]. However, the neuropathy may take months to a year or more to resolve, and in some cases, it may be permanent.

The management of INH-induced hepatotoxicity includes supportive care and cessation or reduction of INH administration. It is recommended that INH be discontinued in patients whose transaminase concentrations have risen to three times the upper limit of normal in the presence of jaundice or hepatitis symptoms or greater than five times the upper limit of normal if asymptomatic [27,30].

References

1. Bronstein AC, Spyker DA, Cantilena LR, et al: 2007 Annual report of the American Association of Poison Control Centers' National Poison Data System (NPDS): 25th Annual report. *Clin Toxicol* 46:927, 2008.
2. Ellard G, Gammon P: Pharmacokinetics of isoniazid metabolism in man. *J Pharmacokinet Biopharm* 4:83, 1976.
3. Thummel KE, Shen DD, Isoherranen N, et al: Appendix II. Design and optimization of dosage regimens: pharmacokinetic data, in Brunton LL et al (eds): *Goodman & Gilman's the Pharmacological Basis of Therapeutics*. 11th ed. New York, McGraw-Hill, 2006, p 1787.
4. Parkin DP, Vandenplas S, Botha FJ, et al: Trimodality of isoniazid elimination. Phenotype and genotype in patients with tuberculosis. *Am J Respir Crit Care Med* 155:1717, 1997.
5. Jeanes C, Schaefer O, Eidus L: Inactivation of isoniazid by Canadian Eskimos and Indians. *Can Med Assoc J* 106:331, 1972.
6. Sarma G, Immanuel C, Kailasam S, et al: Rifampin-induced release of hydrazine from isoniazid: a possible cause of hepatitis during treatment of tuberculosis with regimens containing isoniazid and rifampin. *Am Rev Respir Dis* 133:1072, 1986.
7. Desta Z, Soukhova NV, Flockhart DA: Inhibition of cytochrome P450 (CYP450) isoforms by isoniazid: potent inhibition of CYP2C19 and CYP3 A. *Antimicrob Agents Chemother* 45:382, 2001.
8. Sievers ML, Kerrier RN: Treatment of acute isoniazid toxicity. *Am J Hosp Pharm* 32:202, 1975.
9. O'Brien R, Long M, Cross F, et al: Hepatotoxicity from isoniazid and rifampin among children treated for tuberculosis. *Pediatrics* 72:491, 1983.
10. Brown C: Acute isoniazid poisoning. *Am Rev Respir Dis* 105:206, 1972.
11. Sitprija V, Holmes J: Isoniazid intoxication. *Am Rev Respir Dis* 90:248, 1964.
12. Terman D, Teitelbaum D: Isoniazid self-poisoning. *Neurology* 20:299, 1970.
13. Wason S, Lacouture P, Lovejoy F: Single high-dose pyridoxine treatment for isoniazid overdose. *JAMA* 246:1102, 1981.
14. Sah P: Nicotinyl and isonicotinyl hydrazones of pyridoxal. *J Am Chem Soc* 76:300, 1954.
15. Williams H, Killah M, Jenny E: Convulsant effects of isoniazid. *JAMA* 152:1317, 1953.
16. Biehl J, Vilter R: Effects of isoniazid on pyridoxine metabolism. *Proc Soc Exp Biol Med* 85:389, 1954.
17. Schröder JM: Isoniazid, in Spencer PS, Schaumberg HH (eds): *Experimental and Clinical Neurotoxicology*. 2nd ed. New York, Oxford University Press, 2000, p 690.
18. Beuche W, Friede RL: Remodeling of nerve structure in experimental isoniazid neuropathy in the rat. *Brain* 109:759, 1986.

19. Chua CL, Ohnishi A, Tateishi J, et al: Morphometric evaluation of degenerative and regenerative changes in isoniazid-induced neuropathy. *Acta Neuropathol* 60:183, 1983.
20. Ohnishi A, Chua CL, Kuroiwa Y: Axonal degeneration distal to the site of accumulation of vesicular profiles in the myelinated fiber axon in experimental isoniazid neuropathy. *Acta Neuropathol* 67:195, 1985.
21. Schmued LC, Albertson CM, Andrews A, et al: Evaluation of brain and nerve pathology in rats chronically dosed with ddI or isoniazid. *Neurotoxicol Teratol* 18:555, 1996.
22. Ochoa J: Isoniazid neuropathy in man: quantitative electron microscope study. *Brain Res* 93:831, 1970.
23. Yamamoto M, Sobue G, Mukoyama M, et al: Demonstration of slow acetylator genotype of *N*-acetyltransferase in isoniazid neuropathy using an archival hematoxylin and eosin section of a sural nerve biopsy specimen. *J Neurol Sci* 135:51, 1996.
24. Gurnani A, Chawla R, Kundra P, et al: Acute isoniazid poisoning. *Anaesthesia* 47:781, 1992.
25. Blumberg H, Burman W, Chaisson R, et al: American Thoracic Society/Centers for Disease Control and Prevention/Infectious Diseases Society of America: treatment of tuberculosis. *Am J Respir Crit Care Med* 167:603, 2003.
26. Tostmann A, Boeree M, Aarnoutse R, et al: Antituberculosis drug-induced hepatotoxicity: concise up-to-date review. *J Gastroenterol Hepatol* 23:192, 2008.
27. Dickinson D, Bailey W, Hirschowitz B, et al: Risk factors for isoniazid (INH)-induced liver dysfunction. *J Clin Gastroenterol* 3:271, 1981.
28. Steele MA, Burk RF, DesPrez RM: Toxic hepatitis with isoniazid and rifampin. A meta-analysis. *Chest* 99:465, 1991.
29. Timbrell J, Mitchell J, Snodgrass W, et al: Isoniazid hepatotoxicity: the relationship between covalent binding and metabolism in vivo. *J Pharmacol Exp Ther* 213:364, 1980.
30. Saukkonen JJ, Cohn DL, Jasmer RM, et al: An official ATS statement: hepatotoxicity of antituberculosis therapy. *Am J Respir Crit Care Med* 174:935, 2006.
31. Huang YS, Chern HD, Su WJ, et al: Polymorphism of the *N*-acetyltransferase 2 gene as a susceptibility risk factor for antituberculosis drug-induced hepatitis. *Hepatology* 35:883, 2002.
32. Chin L, Sievers M, Herrier R, et al: Convulsions as the etiology of lactic acidosis in acute isoniazid toxicity in dogs. *Toxicol Appl Pharmacol* 49:377, 1979.
33. Pahl M, Vaziri N, Ness R, et al: Association of beta hydroxybutyric acidosis with isoniazid intoxication. *J Toxicol Clin Toxicol* 22:167, 1984.
34. Millard P, Wilcosky T, Reade-Christopher S, et al: Isoniazid-related fatal hepatitis. *West J Med* 164:486, 1996.
35. Boulanouar A, Abdallah E, el Bakkali M, et al: Severe toxic optic neuropathies caused by isoniazid. Apropos of 3 cases. *J Fr Ophtalmol* 18:183, 1995.
36. Polak BC, Tutein Nolthenius PA, Rietveld E, et al: Visual impairment due to optic neuropathy in 2 patients on amiodarone therapy, i.e. ethambutol and isoniazide. *Ned Tijdschr Geneeskd* 145:922, 2001.
37. Kilburn J, Beam R, David H, et al: Reagent-impregnated paper strip for detection of metabolic products of isoniazid in urine. *Am Rev Respir Dis* 106:923, 1972.
38. Whitfield R, Cope GF: Point-of-care test to monitor adherence to antituberculous treatment. *Ann Clin Biochem* 41:411, 2004.
39. Olson K, Pentel P, Kelly M: Physical assessment and differential diagnosis of the poisoned patient. *Med Toxicol Adverse Drug Exp* 2:52, 1987.
40. Holdiness M: A review of the Redman syndrome and rifampin overdosage. *Med Toxicol Adverse Drug Exp* 4:444, 1989.
41. Chin L, Sievers M, Herrier R, et al: Potentiation of pyridoxine by depressants and anticonvulsants in the treatment of acute isoniazid intoxication in dogs. *Toxicol Appl Pharmacol* 58:504, 1981.
42. Biggs C, Pearce B, Fowler L, et al: Effect of isonicotinic acid hydrazide on extracellular amino acids and convulsions in the rat: reversal of neurochemical and behavioural deficit by sodium valproate. *J Neurochem* 63:2197, 1994.
43. Chin L, Sievers M, Laird H, et al: Evaluation of diazepam and pyridoxine as antidotes to isoniazid intoxication in rats and dogs. *Toxicol Appl Pharmacol* 45:713, 1978.
44. Wood J, Peesker S: The effect on GABA metabolism in brain of isonicotinic acid hydrazide and pyridoxine as a function of time after administration. *J Neurochem* 190:1527, 1972.
45. Burda AM, Sigg T, Haque D, et al: Inadequate pyridoxine stock and its effect on patient outcome. *Am J Ther* 14:262, 2007.
46. Hira HS, Ajmani A, Jain SK, et al: Acute isoniazid poisoning: role of single high oral dose of pyridoxine. *J Assoc Physicians India* 35:792, 1987.
47. Bredemann J, Krechel S, Eggers G: Treatment of refractory seizures in massive isoniazid overdose. *Anesth Analg* 71:554, 1990.
48. Brent J, Vo N, Kulig K, et al: Reversal of prolonged isoniazid-induced coma by pyridoxine. *Arch Intern Med* 150:1751, 1990.
49. Cocco A, Pazourek L: Acute isoniazid intoxication: management by peritoneal dialysis. *N Engl J Med* 269:852, 1963.
50. Konigshausen T, Atrogge G, Hein D, et al: Hemodialysis and hemoperfusion in the treatment of most severe INH poisoning. *Vet Hum Toxicol* 21[Suppl]:12, 1979.
51. Katz B, Carver M: Acute poisoning with isoniazid treated by exchange transfusion. *Pediatrics* 18:72, 1956.
52. Jorgensen H, Weith J: Dialysable poisons: hemodialysis in the treatment of acute poisoning. *Lancet* 1:81, 1963.

CHAPTER 138 ■ LITHIUM POISONING

KENT R. OLSON AND THANJIRA JIRANANTAKAN

Lithium was introduced in the nineteenth century for the treatment of gout. Apparently, toxicity was rarely encountered because of low recommended doses. In the 1940s, lithium chloride was briefly marketed as a salt substitute, but was withdrawn after several cases of serious intoxication and death resulted from its use. In 1949, its antimanic properties were reported, and lithium has found increasingly wide psychiatric use since its approval by the U.S. Food and Drug Administration in 1970 [1,2].

In patients with mania, lithium reduces hyperactivity, irritability, pressured speech, assaultive behavior, and sleeplessness. These effects may require several days of therapy, during which time alternate medications are used. Lithium is very effective in reducing the recurrence of episodes of manic–depressive bipolar disorder and is used to treat some patients with unipolar depression and schizophrenia. It induces neutrophilia (up to 1.5 to 2.0 times the normal leukocyte counts) by enhanced production of G-CSF (granulocyte colony-stimulating factor) and stimulation of pluripotential stem cell production. Lithium has been used to treat a variety of causes of neutropenia [1,3,4].

Lithium is available in conventional tablets or capsules containing 300 mg (8.12 mEq) of lithium carbonate or in sustained-release preparations containing 450 mg (12.18 mEq) of lithium carbonate. Liquid solutions of lithium citrate containing 8 mEq per 5 mL are also available [3].

PHARMACOLOGY

Lithium is the lightest alkali metal, occupying the same column in the periodic table as sodium and potassium, elements with which it shares some properties. However, it has no known normal physiologic role. The exact mechanisms of its therapeutic and toxic effects remain to be determined. Lithium affects ion transport and cell membrane potential by competing with sodium and potassium and possibly other cations. However, unlike sodium and potassium, lithium does not produce a large distribution gradient and, therefore, cannot maintain a significant membrane potential. It is believed to enhance serotonin and acetylcholine effects, resulting in an indirect effect on the central nervous system (CNS). In addition, its inhibitory effects on second messengers, such as inositol phosphates, may reduce neuronal responsiveness to some neurotransmitters [1].

Lithium is readily absorbed from the gastrointestinal tract. The bioavailability of conventional tablets and capsules and the liquid solution is 95% to 100%; bioavailability is not affected by food. Normally, absorption is complete within 1 to 6 hours; peak levels are reached in 2 to 4 hours [1,3]. Sustained-release preparations are less predictably absorbed (60% to 90%), and peak levels may be delayed by more than 4 to 12 hours [3]. Overdose has resulted in delayed peak levels or secondary peak levels as long as 148 hours after ingestion [5]. In one case, esophagoscopy at 84 hours revealed a 5- to 6-cm tablet and hair bezoar in the stomach [6].

Lithium initially occupies an apparent volume of distribution of 0.3 to 0.4 L per kg (approximately that of intracellular water), but further distribution into various intracellular tissue compartments occurs during 6 to 10 hours, with the final volume of distribution being 0.7 to 1.0 L per kg. This explains why initial serum lithium levels may be very high, with few or no signs of toxicity. After a single dose, the equilibrium serum lithium concentration can be expected to increase by 1.0 to 1.5 mEq per L for each 1.0 mEq of lithium per kilogram of body weight. Steady-state tissue levels are achieved after 3 to 4 days of the therapy. Tissue distribution is uneven; whereas the cerebrospinal fluid lithium concentration is only 40% to 60% that of plasma, the saliva concentration may be two to three times greater than that of plasma. Lithium is not bound to serum proteins and freely crosses the placenta [1,3].

Lithium is not metabolized. More than 95% of absorbed lithium is excreted by the kidneys, with 4% to 5% eliminated in sweat and 1% in the feces. It is also excreted in breast milk. Eighty percent of renally filtered lithium is reabsorbed in the proximal tubule against a concentration gradient that does not distinguish lithium from sodium. Sodium depletion can result in as much as a 50% increase in lithium reabsorption. The usual renal clearance is 10 to 40 mL per minute, but it may be 10 to 15 mL per minute or less in the elderly and in patients with renal dysfunction or dehydration [3,7,8]. However, lithium excretion rate may be different in different types of renal failure. Some study demonstrated increased fractional excretion of lithium in patients with prerenal failure, but decreased fractional excretion in acute tubular necrosis (ATN) renal failure [9]. The elimination half-life averages 20 to 24 hours; in patients with chronic intoxication, it may be as long as 47.6 hours [10]. The very slow terminal elimination phase may last up to 10 to 14 days because of gradual lithium release from tissue storage sites such as a bone and the brain [1].

Therapeutic serum lithium concentrations are usually considered to be 0.80 to 1.25 mEq per L; prophylaxis against recurrent manic–depressive illness may be achieved with levels of 0.75 to 1.00 mEq per L. Drug levels should be drawn at least 10 to 12 hours after the last dose to allow for complete tissue distribution. Onset of therapeutic effects usually requires 5 to 21 days after initiation of daily drug administration. Therapeutic levels are achieved by administration of 600 to 1,200 mg of lithium carbonate (16 to 32 mEq of lithium) per day. Careful monitoring of lithium levels is essential because of its low toxic-to-therapeutic ratio [3].

Lithium intoxication primarily involves the CNS and kidneys, although a variety of other organ systems are also affected (Table 138.1). Lithium intoxication may follow an acute overdose or result from chronic accumulation because of either an increase in dosage or a decrease in lithium elimination by the kidneys. Most serious toxicity occurs in patients with chronic intoxication, especially in older patients and patients with renal insufficiency [11].

Acute ingestion of at least 1 mEq per kg (40 mg per kg of lithium carbonate) in a person not previously taking lithium would be required to produce a potentially toxic serum lithium level. The acute toxic dose in a patient already taking lithium ("acute-on-chronic" overdose) depends on the prior lithium level (due to tissue soaking). The dose required to produce chronic intoxication depends on the individual's rate of renal elimination of lithium.

TABLE 138.1

COMMON FEATURES OF LITHIUM INTOXICATION

Feature	Number	Percentage of total
Confusion	19[a]	68
Agitation	17	61
Drowsiness	16[a]	57
Mutism	5	18
Coma (grades III–IV)	1	4
Convulsions	4	14
Hyperreflexia	22	79
Increased tone	16	57
Ankle clonus	4	14
Extensor plantar responses	3	11
Tremor	18	64
Ataxia	14	50
Dysarthria	10	36
Myoclonus	7	25
Vomiting	7	25
Diarrhea	4	14
Acute diabetes insipidus	3	11
Acute renal failure	2	7

[a]Excludes one patient who also took temazepam in overdose.
Reprinted from Dyson EH, Simpson D, Prescott LF, et al: Self-poisoning and therapeutic intoxication with lithium. *Hum Toxicol* 6:326, 1987, with permission.

CLINICAL MANIFESTATIONS

Signs and symptoms of mild lithium intoxication include nausea, vomiting, lethargy, fatigue, memory impairment, and fine tremor. Moderate signs and symptoms of toxicity include confusion, agitation, delirium, coarse tremor, hyperreflexia, hypertension, tachycardia, dysarthria, nystagmus, ataxia, muscle fasciculations, extrapyramidal syndromes, and choreoathetoid movements. Patients with severe toxicity may also exhibit bradycardia, complete heart block, Brugada syndrome, coma, seizures, nonconvulsive status epilepticus, hyperthermia, neuroleptic malignant syndrome, serotonin syndrome, and hypotension [12–15]. Permanent sequelae include choreoathetosis, tardive dystonia, tremor, peripheral neuropathy, scanning speech, dysarthria, muscle rigidity, cognitive deficits, nystagmus, and ataxia [16–20].

Neurotoxic effects of lithium usually develop gradually and may become progressively severe over several days. Neurologic manifestations may worsen even as serum lithium levels are falling and may persist for days to weeks after cessation of the therapy, in part because of slow movement of lithium into and out of intracellular brain sites and possibly brain damage, such as demyelination caused by lithium [19].

Cardiovascular manifestations are nonspecific. The electrocardiogram changes are often similar to those seen with hypokalemia and may result from displacement of intracellular potassium by lithium; U waves and flattened, biphasic, or inverted T waves can be seen with therapeutic doses and mild overdoses. Sinus and junctional bradycardia, sinoatrial and first- degree AV block, and QRS and QTc interval prolongation may be seen with severe intoxication [20,21]. Life-threatening dysrhythmias are rare. Patients with complete heart block during lithium treatment have been reported [12,13]. This lithium-associated cardiac toxicity is more common in patients older than 65 years with baseline EKG abnormalities, conduction abnormalities, use of renal toxic medication, and concomitant use of AV nodal–blocking agents [13]. Brugada syndrome precipitated by lithium has been reported [14]. Pulse and blood pressure abnormalities may be seen in moderate or severe poisoning, but they are usually not pronounced. Hypotension is more often due to dehydration, which can be a cause and a complication of lithium intoxication, than direct cardiotoxicity [20,21].

Chronic lithium therapy has several important effects on renal function, including impaired urinary concentrating ability, nephrogenic diabetes insipidus (NDI), and a sodium-losing nephritis [2]. These effects appear to be dose related and usually correct within several weeks of discontinuing the therapy [20]. Excessive water and sodium loss lead to increased proximal tubular reabsorption of lithium by transport mechanisms designed for sodium reabsorption. The accumulation of lithium may be enhanced by illnesses that result in decreased glomerular filtration rate, such as fever with sweating, gastroenteritis, and heart failure, or by diuretic drugs that enhance distal tubular sodium and fluid loss. Rising lithium levels may further aggravate nephrotoxicity. A patient who has remained stable with a satisfactory lithium serum level at a constant daily dosage for years may suddenly develop life-threatening intoxication within days of entering such a vicious cycle [2].

Metabolic abnormalities associated with lithium use include hypercalcemia, hypermagnesemia, nonketotic hyperglycemia, transient diabetic ketoacidosis, and goiter. Hypothyroidism is rare [20].

Lithium is teratogenic in rats, mice, and rabbits, and human fetal malformations have been described, including cardiac defects such as Ebstein's anomaly [22].

Several drugs may interact with lithium to alter its pharmacokinetics or directly enhance its toxicity. Diuretics may promote fluid and sodium depletion, leading to enhanced tubular lithium reabsorption. This effect appears to be much less apparent with furosemide than with thiazide diuretics. Aminophylline, urea, bicarbonate, and acetazolamide may decrease serum lithium levels by increasing the glomerular filtration rate. Nonsteroidal anti-inflammatory drugs, including the selective cyclooxygenase-2 inhibitor rofecoxib [23], may decrease the glomerular filtration rate and lithium elimination. Antipsychotic medications may have additive CNS depressant effects; in addition, lithium may enhance their dopamine-blocking and serotonergic effects and induce or aggravate rigidity and hyperthermia, possibly inducing neuroleptic malignant syndrome and serotonin syndrome [15,20]. Angiotensin-converting enzyme inhibitors (ACEIs) increase steady-state lithium concentrations by 36.1% and reduced lithium clearance by 25.5% resulting patients presented with lithium toxicity [24].

DIAGNOSTIC EVALUATION

The history should include the type of lithium preparation ingested, the amount(s) and time(s) of ingestion, and the nature of the symptoms. It is important to differentiate patients with acute lithium overdose from those with chronic intoxication resulting from excessive daily doses or impaired renal elimination.

The physical examination should focus on the vital signs, neurologic function, and cardiovascular status. All patients should have an electrocardiogram and laboratory evaluation, including serum electrolytes, glucose, blood urea nitrogen, creatinine, and serum lithium level. Lithium levels should be repeated at frequent (i.e., 2- to 4-hour) intervals after acute overdose until peak levels are observed. If the levels are elevated, they should be repeated until they fall below the toxic range and the patient becomes asymptomatic. Electroencephalography should be considered in patients who presented with coma to evaluate nonconvulsive status epilepticus [15].

Patients with chronic intoxication are typically brought to medical attention by a family member or therapist because of neurologic symptoms. There is usually a recent history of excessive fluid loss caused by gastroenteritis, other flulike illness, or excessive urination. The severity of chronic intoxication generally correlates with the serum lithium level [2,20]. In patients undergoing chronic therapy, mild neurotoxic effects may occur with serum lithium concentrations of less than 1.5 mEq per L. Steady-state concentrations of 1.5 to 3.0 mEq per L are associated with mild or moderate toxicity. Severe poisoning and death may occur with serum concentrations greater than 3 to 4 mEq per L [2,10,20].

After acute overdose, the predominant initial symptoms are nausea and vomiting [2]. Patients do not usually have significant neurologic manifestations despite high serum lithium levels during the first 12 hours or more after ingestion because lithium is taken up slowly by the brain and other tissues [10]. Serum lithium concentrations as high as 10.6 mEq per L without significant toxicity have been reported after acute overdose [25–27]. However, intoxication may develop during the subsequent 24 to 48 hours, even as serum levels fall [19,20,28]. Levels drawn shortly after acute or acute-on-chronic overdose cannot be used reliably to predict toxicity or guide therapy (Fig. 138.1) [2,10]. There does not appear to be any clinical variable that accurately predicts which patients will deteriorate. The use of cerebrospinal fluid levels to estimate brain concentrations more closely has been advocated [29]. However, cerebrospinal fluid concentrations do not reflect intracellular brain tissue levels or predict the level of coma (Fig. 138.2) [2,25,30].

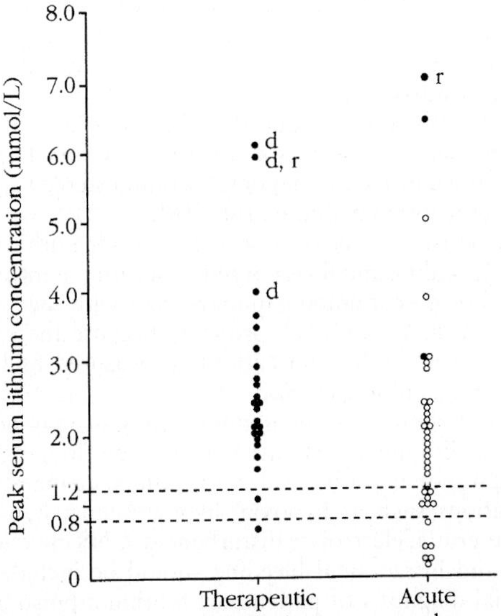

FIGURE 138.1. Lack of correlation between serum levels and toxic manifestations in patients with acute intoxication. d, diabetes insipidus; r, renal failure. [Reprinted from Dyson EH, Simpson D, Prescott LF, et al: Self-poisoning and therapeutic intoxication with lithium. *Hum Toxicol* 6:326, 1987, with permission.]

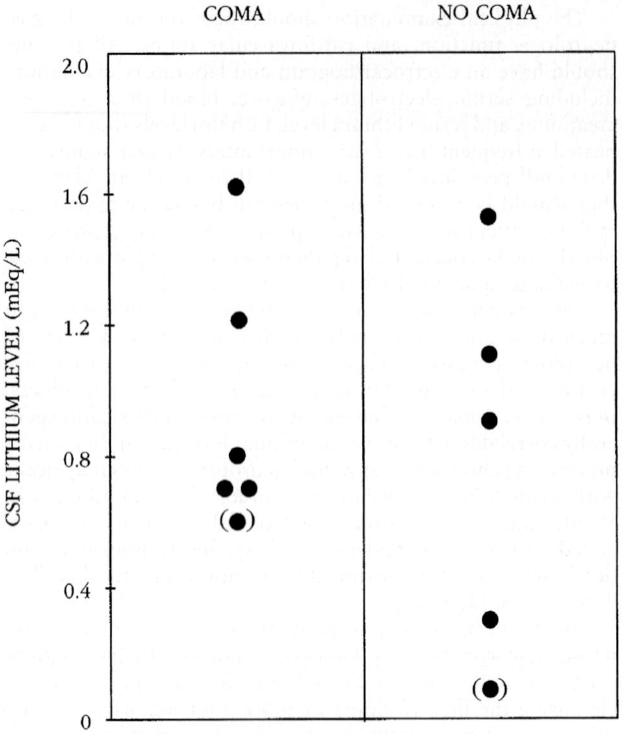

FIGURE 138.2. Cerebrospinal fluid (CSF) levels in patients with and without coma. [Reprinted from Lee BL, Brown CR, Becker CE, et al: Lithium overdose: factors that predict outcome in poisoned patients. *Vet Hum Toxicol* 28:505, 1986, with permission.]

Patients with acute-on-chronic overdose usually have a clinical course similar to those with acute ingestions. However, a smaller total dose may produce severe intoxication, depending on the preingestion therapeutic serum level.

Elevated blood urea nitrogen and creatinine reflect renal insufficiency and suggest that intoxication results from gradual accumulation of lithium rather than acute ingestion. Elevated creatinine may also be caused by cross-reactivity of the assay with creatine from muscle destruction and should prompt the measurement of serum creatine phosphokinase and urinalysis for myoglobinuria.

Patients with lithium-induced NDI usually have dilute urine with a low-measured osmolality relative to serum. The diagnosis is confirmed by lack of response to administered vasopressin by the inappropriately dilute urine [16].

Leukocytosis may be seen in patients taking lithium. It is a nonspecific finding and does not reflect severity of intoxication. A reduced or absent anion gap may occur with severe lithium carbonate intoxication [31], probably because the carbonate anion (but not the lithium cation) is measured and used in calculating the anion gap [32].

Plain radiographs of the abdomen may or may not reveal radiopaque lithium tablets after acute ingestion. A negative radiograph should not be used to rule out acute ingestion [33].

Conditions such as hypoxia, hypoglycemia, hypothermia or hyperthermia, electrolyte disturbances, CNS infection, head trauma, and intracranial bleeding should be included in the differential diagnosis of patients with lithium poisoning. In a patient with hyperthermia and rigidity who is also taking antipsychotic medications, neuroleptic malignant syndrome and serotonin syndrome should be considered (see Chapter 68). Other drug intoxications should be considered (see Chapter 68), especially if CNS symptoms appear shortly after an acute overdose.

MANAGEMENT

In patients with altered mental status, initial management should include (a) assessment and stabilization of the airway; (b) administration of oxygen; (c) assisted ventilation, if needed; (d) vascular access; and (e) administration of dextrose, naloxone, and thiamine. Diazepam or barbiturates should be administered to patients with seizures. Patient with nonconvulsive status epilepticus should be monitored by electroencephalography to confirm the resolution of seizure activity. If hyperthermia is present, immediate cooling measures should be instituted, including tepid sponging and fanning and neuromuscular paralysis, if needed. Hypovolemia, if present, should be treated with intravenous crystalloids. Cardiac dysrhythmias do not usually require treatment, but should respond to usual agents.

Asymptomatic patients with acute or acute-on-chronic overdose should be observed for a minimum of 6 hours after ingestion. Serial lithium levels should be obtained to confirm lack of significant absorption. Patients with mild overdoses can often be monitored and treated in the emergency department. Symptomatic patients, patients with a massive acute ingestion, and those whose levels continue to rise beyond 6 hours after ingestion should be admitted to an intensive care setting.

Lithium-induced NDI does not respond to vasopressin, but it has been reported to improve with hydrochlorothiazide, amiloride, carbamazepine, and indomethacin [20]. However, the gradual onset and the duration required of hydrochlorothiazide, carbamazepine, and amiloride therapy would limit their clinical usefulness. One case report suggests indomethacin may be acutely effective in treating lithium-induced NDI [34].

After acute ingestion, the gastrointestinal tract should be decontaminated as soon as possible to prevent continued absorption of lithium. Ipecac-induced emesis is not recommended because it yields poor return of gastric contents [35]. Gastric lavage can be performed, although there is little evidence for benefit [36]. Activated charcoal does not effectively bind lithium and should be given only if coingestion of another drug is suspected [37]. Whole-bowel irrigation (see Chapter 117) has been successful for large ingestions, especially if they involve sustained-release tablets [38]. If a tablet mass or concretion is suspected because of sustained high levels after 2 to 3 days, radiographic contrast studies, ultrasound, or gastroduodenal endoscopy and endoscopic removal should be considered [6]. Preliminary evidence in animals and human volunteers suggests that sodium polystyrene sulfonate (Kayexalate) binds lithium and may enhance its elimination [39,40]. One case report describes its use in a patient with acute-on-chronic lithium overdose [41]. There is no consensus at this point as to whether the administration of potassium with the polystyrene sulfonate enhances or decreases lithium excretion.

In most patients with mild or moderate intoxication, intravenous fluid therapy is effective in restoring and maintaining renal elimination of lithium. A crystalloid solution (half-normal or normal saline) aiming for urine output of 1 to 3 mL per kg per hour should be administered after an initial saline bolus (10 to 20 mL per kg), depending on the degree of dehydration. Serum electrolytes should be followed closely because hypernatremia may occur. To estimate the effectiveness of renal elimination, the lithium clearance can be estimated by obtaining simultaneous urine and serum lithium levels [42]:

Approximate renal lithium clearance = urine flow rate (mL/min) × urine lithium (mEq/L) / serum lithium (mEq/L).

Normal lithium clearance is 10 to 40 mL per minute. If the clearance is below normal in a patient without underlying cardiac or renal dysfunction, the rate of fluid administration should be increased because this suggests low renal perfusion secondary to dehydration. In human studies, water loading, furosemide, thiazide, ethacrynic acid, ammonium chloride, and spironolactone did not increase lithium clearance. Sodium bicarbonate, acetazolamide, urea, and aminophylline were effective. However, clinical studies in patients with lithium intoxication treated by these agents have not been reported [7].

Hemodialysis is the most efficient method for removing lithium, achieving clearance rates of up to 100 to 150 mL per minute [2,30,42]. However, lithium is only slowly removed from intracellular tissue compartments, especially the brain, and rebound increases of serum lithium levels often occur within several hours after dialysis. Hemodialysis should be repeated frequently until the serum level drawn 6 to 8 hours after the last dialysis is 1 mEq per L or less [2]. However, despite repeated dialyses, patients with significant neurologic toxicity do not promptly improve. Recovery, if it occurs, may take several days to weeks [2,29,30].

The indications for hemodialysis are not well established. It is generally agreed that patients with severe clinical toxicity and those with renal dysfunction should undergo dialysis. Asymptomatic patients or those with mild-to-moderate intoxication who are otherwise healthy may be managed with intravenous fluids as long as they remain clinically stable or are improving and satisfactory lithium clearance (>15 to 20 mL per minute) is achieved. Patients with chronic serum levels exceeding 2.5 mEq per L accompanied by symptoms and those with acute poisoning and peak levels exceeding 10 mEq per L (in which significant toxicity is expected to occur with subsequent tissue distribution) should also be considered for hemodialysis. However, some clinicians advocate hemodialysis for patients who have acute ingestion without prior lithium body burden and a serum lithium concentration greater than 4 mEq per L [43].

Continuous renal replacement therapy (e.g., venovenous or arteriovenous hemodiafiltration) has been reported to successfully remove lithium without the need for hemodialysis [44–47]. In one case, 14 hours of continuous arteriovenous hemodiafiltration was estimated to achieve lithium elimination equivalent to 5.75 hours of hemodialysis [48]. In another case report, clearances of up to 38 mL per minute were achieved with continuous venovenous hemodiafiltration [46]. Continuous renal replacement therapy removes lithium slowly, without rebound rises in levels seen with intermittent hemodialysis, and can also be performed in facilities without full dialysis capabilities.

References

1. Baldessarini RJ: Drugs used in the treatment of psychiatric disorders, in Gilman AG, Goodman LS, Rall TW, et al (eds): *Goodman and Gilman's the Pharmacological Basis of Therapeutics*. 7th ed. New York, Macmillan, 1985, p 387.
2. Amdisen A: Clinical features and management of lithium poisoning. *Med Toxicol* 3:18, 1988.
3. McEvoy GK, McQuarrie GM (eds): *Drug Information 86*. Bethesda, MD, American Hospital Formulary Service, American Society of Hospital Pharmacists, 1986, p 1099.
4. Focosi D, Azzara A, Kast RE, et al: Lithium and hematology: established and proposed uses. *J Leukoc Biol* 85:20, 2009.
5. Friedberg RC, Spyker DA, Herold DA: Massive overdoses with sustained-release lithium carbonate preparations: pharmacokinetic model based on two case studies. *Clin Chem* 37:1205, 1991.
6. Thornley-Brown D, Galla JH, Williams PD, et al: Lithium toxicity associated with a trichobezoar. *Ann Intern Med* 116:739, 1992.
7. Thomsen K, Schou M: Renal lithium excretion in man. *Am J Physiol* 215:823, 1968.
8. Okusa MD, Jovita L, Crystal T: Clinical manifestations and management of acute lithium intoxication. *Am J Med* 97:383, 1994.
9. Steinhauslin F, Bumier M, Magnin JL, et al: Fractional excretion of trace lithium and uric acid in acute renal failure. *J Am Soc Nephrol* 4:1429, 1994.
10. Dyson EH, Simpson D, Prescott LF, et al: Self-poisoning and therapeutic intoxication with lithium. *Hum Toxicol* 6:326, 1987.
11. Oakley PW, Whyte IM, Carter GL: Lithium toxicity: an iatrogenic problem in susceptible individuals. *Aust NZ J Psychiatry* 35:703, 2001.
12. Shiraki T, Kohno K, Saito D, et al: Complete atrioventricular block secondary to lithium therapy. *Circ J* 72:847, 2008.
13. Serinken S, Karcioglu O, Korkmaz A: Rarely seen cardiotoxicity of lithium overdose: complete heart block. *Int J Cardiol* 132:276, 2008.
14. Pirotte MJ, Mueller JG, Popraski T: A case report of Brugada-type electrocardiographic changes in a patient taking lithium. *Am J Emerg Med* 26:113.e1, 2008.
15. Kaplan PW, Birbeck G: Lithium-induced confusional states: nonconvulsive status epilepticus or triphasic encephalopathy. *Epilepsia* 47:2071, 2006.
16. Chakrabarti S, Chand PK: Lithium induced tardive dystonia. *Neurol India* 50:473, 2002.
17. Bartha L, Marksteiner J, Bauer G, et al: Persistent cognitive deficits associated with lithium intoxication: a neuropsychological case description. *Cortex* 38:743, 2002.
18. Apte SN, Langston JW: Permanent neurological deficits due to lithium toxicity. *Ann Neurol* 13:453, 1983.
19. Adityanjee, Munshi KR, Thampy A: The syndrome of irreversible lithium-effectuated neurotoxicity. *Clin Neuropharmacol* 28:38, 2005.
20. Simard M, Gumbiner B, Lee A, et al: Lithium carbonate intoxication: a case report and review of the literature. *Arch Intern Med* 149:36, 1989.
21. Mitchell JE, MacKenzie TB: Cardiac effects of lithium therapy in man: a review of the literature. *J Clin Psychiatry* 43:47, 1982.
22. Weinstein MR, Goldfield MD: Cardiovascular malformations with lithium use during pregnancy. *Am J Psychiatry* 132:529, 1975.
23. Ratz Bravo AE, Egger SS, Crespo S, et al: Lithium intoxication as a result of an interaction with rofecoxib. *Ann Pharmacother* 38:1189, 2004.
24. Finley PR, O'Brien JG, Coleman RW: Lithium and angiotensin-converting enzyme inhibitors: evaluation of a potential interaction. *J Clin Psychopharmacol* 16:68, 1996.
25. Lee BL, Brown CR, Becker CE, et al: Lithium overdose: factors that predict outcome in poisoned patients. *Vet Hum Toxicol* 28:505, 1986.
26. Genser AS, Smith P, Honcharuk L, et al: Lithium overdose: when to dialyze? A report of 28 consecutive cases. *Vet Hum Toxicol* 30:355, 1988.
27. Nagappan R, Parkin WG, Holdsworth SR: Acute lithium intoxication. *Anaesth Intensive Care* 30:90, 2002.
28. Rose SR, Klein-Schwartz W, Oderda GM, et al: Lithium intoxication with acute renal failure and death. *Drug Intell Clin Pharm* 22:691, 1988.
29. Clendenin NJ, Pond SM, Kaysen G, et al: Potential pitfalls in the evaluation of the usefulness of hemodialysis for the removal of lithium. *Clin Toxicol* 19:341, 1982.
30. Jaeger A, Sauder P, Kopferschmitt J, et al: Toxicokinetics of lithium intoxication treated by hemodialysis. *Clin Toxicol* 23:501, 1985.
31. Kelleher SP, Raciti A, Arbeit LA: Reduced or absent anion gap as a marker of severe lithium carbonate intoxication. *Arch Intern Med* 146:1839, 1986.
32. Leon M, Graeber C: Absence of high anion gap metabolic acidosis in severe ethylene glycol poisoning: a potential effect of simultaneous lithium carbonate ingestion. *Am J Kidney Dis* 23:313, 1994.
33. Savitt DL, Hawkins HH, Roberts JR: The radiopacity of ingested medications. *Ann Emerg Med* 16:331, 1987.
34. Martinez EJ, Sinnott JT, Rodriguez-Paz G, et al: Lithium induced nephrogenic diabetes insipidus treated with indomethacin. *South Med J* 86:971, 1993.
35. Krenzelok EP, McGuigan M, Lheur P: Position statement: ipecac syrup. American Academy of Clinical Toxicology; European Association of Poisons Centres and Clinical Toxicologists. *J Toxicol Clin Toxicol* 35:699, 1997.
36. Teece S, Crawford I: Best evidence topic report: no clinical evidence for gastric lavage in lithium overdose. *Emerg Med J* 22:43, 2005.
37. Favin FD, Klein-Schwartz W, Oderda GM, et al: In vitro study of lithium carbonate adsorption by activated charcoal. *J Toxicol Clin Toxicol* 26:443, 1988.
38. Smith SW, Ling LJ, Halstenson CE: Whole-bowel irrigation as a treatment for acute lithium overdose. *Ann Emerg Med* 20:536, 1991.
39. Tomaszewski C, Musso C, Pearson JR, et al: Lithium absorption prevented by sodium polystyrene sulfonate in volunteers. *Ann Emerg Med* 21:1308, 1992.
40. Linakis JG, Hull KM, Lacouture PG, et al: Enhancement of lithium elimination by multiple-dose sodium polystyrene sulfonate. *Acad Emerg Med* 4:175, 1997.
41. Roberge RJ, Martin TG, Schneider SM: Use of sodium polystyrene sulfonate in a lithium overdose. *Ann Emerg Med* 22:1911, 1993.
42. Jacobsen D, Aasen G, Frederichsen P, et al: Lithium intoxication: pharmacokinetics during and after terminated hemodialysis in acute intoxications. *Clin Toxicol* 25:81, 1987.
43. Jaeger A, Sauder P, Kopeferschmidtt J, et al: When should dialysis be performed in lithium poisoning? A kinetic study in 14 cases of lithium toxicity. *J Toxicol Clin Toxicol* 31:429, 1993.
44. Beckmann U, Oakley PW, Dawson AH, et al: Efficacy of continuous venovenous hemodialysis in the treatment of severe lithium toxicity. *J Toxicol Clin Toxicol* 39:393, 2001.

45. Hazouard E, Ferrandiere M, Rateau H, et al: Continuous veno-venous hemofiltration versus continuous veno-venous hemodialysis in severe lithium self-poisoning: a toxicokinetics study in an intensive care unit. *Nephrol Dial Transplant* 14:1605, 1999.
46. van Bommel EF, Kalmeijer MD, Ponssen HH: Treatment of life-threatening lithium toxicity with high-volume continuous venovenous hemofiltration. *Am J Nephrol* 20:408, 2000.
47. Menghini VV, Albright RC Jr: Treatment of lithium intoxication with continuous venovenous hemodiafiltration. *Am J Kidney Dis* 36:E21, 2000.
48. Bellomo R, Kearly Y, Parkin G, et al: Treatment of life-threatening lithium toxicity with continuous arterio-venous hemodiafiltration. *Crit Care Med* 19:836, 1991.

CHAPTER 139 ■ METHYLXANTHINE POISONING

MICHAEL W. SHANNON†

The methylxanthines most commonly used in the clinical setting are theophylline and its ethylenediamine salt, aminophylline. Until recently, theophylline was used exclusively as a bronchodilator for the management of reversible obstructive pulmonary diseases and as a respiratory stimulant for the treatment of apnea of prematurity in neonates. During the 1980s, its use fell dramatically as more effective therapies for recurrent bronchospasm became available [1]. However, there has been renewed interest in theophylline as the scope of its pharmacologic benefits broadens. Potential uses for theophylline now include preconditioning of cardiac ischemia [2], treatment of bradycardia [3], amelioration of perinatal asphyxia [4], acute mountain sickness [5], bradycardia after spinal cord injury [6], protection from contrast-induced nephropathy [7], and treatment of attention-deficit hyperactivity disorder [8]. Recent clinical trials of theophylline for asthma have demonstrated substantial benefit, restoring interest in the drug for this indication [9–16]. Despite its renewed popularity, theophylline, with its potent pharmacologic actions, variable metabolic disposition in humans, and narrow therapeutic-to-toxic ratio, is a common cause of intoxication [1,17].

Caffeine and theobromine are other widely used methylxanthines. Caffeine is found in many pharmaceutical preparations (e.g., antisleep drugs), as well as in dietary supplements, including guarana and kola nut. Although severe toxicity from caffeine ingestion is uncommon, case reports of serious poisoning in children and adults are well documented [18–20]. Because caffeine and other xanthine derivatives are structurally similar to theophylline, signs and symptoms of toxicity resemble those seen in theophylline intoxication, and the approach to management is identical.

Three clinical circumstances account for most cases of theophylline poisoning: unintentional ingestions by children, intentional ingestions (suicide attempts) by adolescents or adults, and medication errors (miscalculation of dose, change in frequency of administration, lack of serum drug level monitoring, or an unrecognized drug–drug or drug–disease interaction) [1,21,22]. Most cases of theophylline intoxication result from chronic, unintentional overmedication.

PHARMACOLOGY

Theophylline is available commercially as a liquid, tablet, sustained-release capsule, or solution for intravenous administration. Overdose of sustained-release theophylline can lead to a marked delay in complete absorption, with peak serum theophylline concentrations occurring as long as 15 to 24 hours after ingestion [23]. Therapeutic serum theophylline concentrations range from 10 to 20 μg per mL.

A loading dose of 5 to 6 mg per kg of intravenous aminophylline should produce a serum theophylline level of 10 μg per mL in patients not currently taking theophylline. Maintenance dosages vary with age and underlying conditions (Table 139.1). For patients taking theophylline regularly, a loading dose increases the steady-state serum theophylline level. Typically, administration of 1 mg per kg of theophylline raises the serum drug concentration by 2 μg per mL. This relationship can also be used to predict the theophylline concentration after an overdose; the maximum possible drug concentration (in micrograms per milliliter) should be no more than twice the ingested or administered dose (in milligrams per kilogram).

Theophylline has a volume of distribution of 0.4 L per kg and is 40% to 65% bound to plasma proteins [24]. Its metabolism is almost exclusively by hepatic cytochrome P450 system; it is oxidized or demethylated in the liver by at least two isoenzymes (CYP1A2 and CYP3A4) [24]. Less than 15% of the drug is excreted unchanged in urine. At therapeutic doses, hepatic metabolism generally occurs by first-order elimination kinetics [25]. The drug exhibits saturable (Michaelis–Menten) kinetics in overdose leading to prolonged, unpredictable elimination rates. The elimination half-life of theophylline also varies widely with age: typical half-lives are 20 to 30 hours in

TABLE 139.1

INTRAVENOUS AMINOPHYLLINE MAINTENANCE DOSES

Age group	Infusion rate (mg/kg/h)
Newborn	0.3–0.4
1–6 mo	0.5–0.6
6 mo–9 y	1.0–1.2
9–16 y	0.9–1.1
Smoker age 12–50 y	1.0
Nonsmoker age 16–50 y	0.5–0.7
Older than 50 y	0.4–0.6
Cor pulmonale	0.3–0.5
Liver failure	0.1–0.5
Congestive heart failure	0.1–0.5

† Deceased.

TABLE 139.2

FACTORS AFFECTING SERUM THEOPHYLLINE CONCENTRATIONS

Drugs that *increase* theophylline clearance
Barbiturates
Carbamazepine
Cigarette smoke
Phenytoin
Rifampin
Drugs that *decrease* theophylline clearance
Cimetidine
Ciprofloxacin
Clarithromycin
Fluvoxamine
Erythromycin
Norfloxacin
Ofloxacin
Zafirlukast
Conditions that *increase* theophylline clearance
Cigarette smoking
Cystic fibrosis
Hyperthyroidism
Conditions that *decrease* theophylline clearance
Hepatitis/cirrhosis
Congestive heart failure
Some viral infections

premature infants, 4 to 7 hours in newborns, 3 to 4 hours in children 6 months to 18 years of age, and 8 to 9 hours in adults [24–27]. Many drugs, chemicals, and medical conditions affect the steady-state serum concentration and elimination half-life of theophylline (Table 139.2). The drugs that inhibit theophylline clearance are those that inhibit CYP1A2 and CYP3A4, including erythromycin, clarithromycin, ciprofloxacin, and cimetidine [24,28]. Drugs that increase theophylline clearance include barbiturates, carbamazepine, and the polyaromatic hydrocarbons of cigarette smoke (including passive smoke inhalation) [29,30]. Enzyme induction by these drugs can be temporary; if patients who smoke quit abruptly, theophylline clearance can fall to normal within days, leading to inadvertent theophylline intoxication unless dose is adjusted accordingly. Several disease states are also associated with a reduction in theophylline clearance, including congestive heart failure and liver disease [24,31]. Both hyperthyroidism and cystic fibrosis are associated with increased elimination of theophylline [32].

Theophylline has a variety of physiologic effects in therapeutic doses (Table 139.3). These effects include smooth muscle relaxation, mild central nervous system (CNS) excitation, and diuresis. Intoxication is associated with an array of other metabolic and clinical consequences. Although the effects of theophylline have been well characterized, their pharmacologic and pathophysiologic mechanisms remain poorly understood. Three primary cellular mechanisms of theophylline action have been theorized: inhibition of cyclic guanosine monophosphate or cyclic adenosine monophosphate (cAMP) activity, adenosine receptor antagonism, and adrenergic hyperstimulation (particularly at the beta-receptor) secondary to elevated levels of circulating plasma catecholamines [33–36]. Inhibition of calcium translocation and leukotriene production has also been postulated to be a fourth mechanism.

The physiologic changes seen with therapeutic doses of theophylline, including tachycardia, diuresis, bronchodilation, and CNS excitation, were thought to result from theophylline's inhibition of phosphodiesterase, the intracellular enzyme that inactivates cAMP, an important "second messenger" [37]. Such enzyme inhibition would lead to elevated intracellular cAMP concentrations, affecting a broad range of physiologic responses. However, this theory has been brought into question; in vitro data indicate that phosphodiesterase inhibition does not occur at therapeutic serum concentrations of theophylline, suggesting that increased cAMP activity is not a major mechanism of its therapeutic effects [38]. Whether the increased theophylline concentrations seen in the intoxicated patient are sufficient to inhibit phosphodiesterase activity is unknown.

TABLE 139.3

PHYSIOLOGIC EFFECTS OF THEOPHYLLINE

Central nervous system
Stimulation of cortical centers
Stimulation of medullary respiratory center
Nausea and emesis
Cerebral vasoconstriction and decreased cerebral blood flow
Cardiovascular
Positive inotropic and chronotropic effects
Vascular smooth muscle relaxation
Pulmonary
Bronchial smooth muscle relaxation
Increased ventilation
Stimulation of diaphragmatic and intercostal muscles
Gastrointestinal
Increased gastric acid and pepsin secretion
Relaxation of esophageal smooth muscle and possible reflux
Renal
Increased blood flow and glomerular filtration rate
Increased diuresis (<48 h)
Endocrine
Increased plasma catecholamines
Augmented dopamine β-hydroxylase and rennin
Metabolic
Lipolysis
Gluconeogenesis and glycogenolysis
Musculoskeletal
Augmented contractility
Disturbances in depolarization (e.g., tremor)

Investigation has also been directed at the role of adenosine receptor antagonism as a mechanism of theophylline action. Adenosine is a nucleoside that promotes smooth muscle constriction, slows cardiac conduction, and acts as an endogenous anticonvulsant. With the structure of theophylline being similar to that of adenosine and with the drug having opposite physiologic actions, theophylline may be a simple competitive antagonist at bronchial and vascular smooth muscle, cardiac, and CNS sites. However, adenosine antagonism alone does not provide a complete explanation for theophylline's pharmacologic effects [39,40].

Additional data suggest that many of theophylline's actions can be accounted for by its stimulation of plasma catecholamines release [32,41]. Plasma concentrations of epinephrine, norepinephrine, and dopamine all rise significantly after theophylline administration [40]. With therapeutic doses, plasma catecholamine activity typically increases four- to sixfold. After theophylline intoxication, plasma catecholamine activity may rise to 30-fold [33,35]. Increased plasma catecholamines provide a ready explanation for many of the effects of theophylline seen after therapeutic doses and potentially mediate many of the effects of theophylline intoxication. In all probability, the combined effects of adenosine receptor antagonism and catecholamine release are responsible for the predominant effects of theophylline intoxication.

Plasma catecholamines, particularly epinephrine, are capable of inducing hypokalemia, hyperglycemia, and metabolic acidosis. Epinephrine-induced hypokalemia appears to result from β_2-adrenergic receptor–linked stimulation of Na^+/K^+ adenosine triphosphatase. This leads to increased intracellular transport of potassium with preservation of total body potassium content [42]. Consistent with the theories of plasma catecholamine activity is the observation that theophylline-induced hypokalemia can be inhibited by pretreatment with propranolol or reversed by propranolol administration [43].

The CNS effects of theophylline intoxication include respiratory stimulation, vomiting, and seizures. These may result from disturbances in CNS cyclic guanosine monophosphate activity, adenosine antagonism, or adrenergic excess. Changes in neuronal transmembrane potentials by any of these mechanisms would lower excitation thresholds. Additionally, there are theories that theophylline inhibits CNS γ-aminobutyric acid receptor activity and stimulates *N*-methyl-D-aspartate and other excitatory neurotransmitters production. Theophylline administration has been associated with an abnormal electroencephalogram pattern in 34% of children and 12% of adults [44,45]. Cerebral vascular effects are also significant with theophylline and other methylxanthines because they are potent cerebral vasoconstrictors. This is the presumed mechanism of the efficacy of caffeine in the treatment of migraine headache. However, decreases in cerebral blood flow can be extreme, particularly during inhalational anesthetics administration [46]. In animal models, theophylline amplifies brain damage induced by seizures [47].

CLINICAL TOXICITY

Manifestations of theophylline intoxication can be classified into five categories: cardiac, CNS, gastrointestinal, musculoskeletal, and metabolic [1,17]. The cardiovascular effects of theophylline intoxication consist of rhythm and vascular disturbances. The hallmark (and first sign) of theophylline poisoning is sinus tachycardia, which occurs in more than 95% of cases. With more severe intoxication, unstable supraventricular tachydysrhythmias and ventricular dysrhythmias may occur. A common cause of death with severe theophylline intoxication is intractable ventricular dysrhythmias.

Blood pressure disturbances are also common. At lower ranges of intoxication, a mildly elevated blood pressure may be present, although severe hypertension is unusual in isolated theophylline poisoning. In severe cases of theophylline poisoning, hypotension with a widened pulse pressure is seen in the face of an increased cardiac index. Hypotension is caused by a marked fall in systemic vascular resistance [34].

The CNS effects of theophylline poisoning become prominent in severe overdose. The stimulatory actions of theophylline first produce hyperventilation with mild respiratory alkalosis. Significantly intoxicated patients develop agitation and anxiety. Vomiting, which can be severe, partly results from stimulation of the vomiting center of the medullary chemoreceptor trigger zone.

The most severe CNS manifestation of theophylline intoxication is seizures; these are a poor prognostic sign. Theophylline-induced seizures are typically tonic–clinic in nature and may be focal; they may be single, but are commonly multiple and typically resistant to conventional anticonvulsants. Seizures after theophylline intoxication are associated with a high frequency of adverse neurologic outcomes and a mortality that approaches 50% in elderly patients [48,49].

The gastrointestinal effects of theophylline poisoning consist of vomiting, diarrhea, and hematemesis. Vomiting results in part from hypersecretion of gastric acid and the enzymes gastrin and pepsin [50]. These acids and digestive enzymes are gastric irritants that can produce mucosal hemorrhage with hematemesis. Finally, theophylline is a potent relaxer of lower esophageal sphincter resting tone; this action facilitates the reflux of gastric contents.

Skeletal muscle tremor is a common feature of theophylline poisoning. These tremors are coarse; myoclonic jerks may also be present. Muscular hypertonicity also appears to be linked to theophylline's actions as a β_2-adrenoreceptor; this is evidenced by a similar syndrome occurring after excess administration of potent β_2-agonists (e.g., terbutaline).

A number of metabolic disturbances accompany theophylline intoxication: metabolic acidosis, hypokalemia, hyperglycemia, hypophosphatemia, hypomagnesemia, and hypercalcemia [26,51–55]. The resulting clinical picture can mimic diabetic ketoacidosis [56]. Metabolic acidosis may appear late and is typically modest; acidemia may not occur because of a superimposed respiratory alkalosis. Hypokalemia and hyperglycemia correlate strongly with the degree of intoxication after acute theophylline poisoning [57]. However, there are no obvious clinical consequences of hypokalemia. Hypercalcemia and hypophosphatemia are common, but not invariable, disturbances. Their cause is unclear, although theophylline (and epinephrine) has been shown to increase concentrations of parathyroid hormone, and correction of theophylline-induced hypercalcemia has been reported after propranolol administration [58].

Several studies have suggested that the metabolic and clinical consequences of theophylline intoxication vary, depending on whether the poisoning occurs through a single ingestion (or single intravenous overdose), chronic overmedication, or acute-on-therapeutic intoxication, in which the patient has maintained serum theophylline concentrations in the therapeutic range but then received a single toxic dose [18,22]. With *acute theophylline intoxication*, the patient ingests a single toxic dose of theophylline or inadvertently receives a toxic dose of intravenous aminophylline. The clinical course of acute theophylline intoxication strongly correlates with serum theophylline concentration. Serum theophylline concentrations of 20 to 40 μg per mL are associated with nausea, vomiting, and tachycardia. When theophylline concentrations are 40 to 70 μg per mL, premature ventricular contractions, agitation, and tremor appear. At theophylline concentrations greater than 80 μg per mL, life-threatening events, including severe cardiac dysrhythmias and intractable seizures, occur [16,59,60]. Hypokalemia can be profound after acute intoxication, with serum potassium concentrations falling to as low as 2.1 mEq per L. Serum glucose can be as high as 300 to 350 mg per dL.

In *chronic theophylline overmedication*, the patient ingests theophylline for at least 24 hours in doses or under conditions that exceed theophylline clearance. The result is a relatively slow rise in body "theophylline burden"-to-toxic concentrations. Victims of chronic overmedication are more likely to be neonates or elderly patients who have underlying cardiac disease or are taking/receiving medications that inhibit theophylline metabolism. These factors contribute to greater morbidity and mortality after chronic theophylline overmedication [18,30]. Signs of severe intoxication may occur with steady-state serum theophylline concentrations as low as 20 to 30 μg per mL. Seizures have occurred in patients with concentrations as low as 17 μg per mL. Patients with chronic theophylline overmedication are also less likely to have hypokalemia and hyperglycemia. The most striking feature of chronic theophylline overmedication is that there is *no significant correlation* between serum theophylline concentration and the appearance of life-threatening events [1,22,61,62]. Seizures and dysrhythmias may appear with serum theophylline concentrations in the therapeutic or mildly toxic range [22,61]. As a result, serum theophylline concentration *should not be used* to predict the appearance of these events.

Patients who are chronically receiving theophylline in appropriate doses and then take or receive an acute overdose of theophylline develop *acute-on-therapeutic theophylline intoxication*. In these patients, clinical and metabolic consequences have features that are intermediate between those found with acute intoxication and chronic overmedication. Clinical manifestations are somewhat predicted by peak serum theophylline concentration, with life-threatening events usually not appearing until serum theophylline concentrations exceed 60 μg per mL. Metabolic disturbances are not as severe and have little or no correlation with serum theophylline concentration [1,21,22].

Patient age appears to be a significant risk factor for the development of life-threatening events after theophylline intoxication with those at extremes of age (i.e., neonates and elderly patients) [1,62]. For example, after chronic overmedication, patients older than 75 years have an almost 10-fold greater risk of a life-threatening event than do adolescents with comparable serum theophylline concentration [1,62]. There is evidence that in patients with chronic theophylline intoxication, age is a better predictor of major toxicity than serum theophylline concentration. Potential explanations for this observation include the differing pharmacokinetics found at extremes of age or the higher prevalence of significant underlying multisystem disease and use of multiple drugs in these patients.

DIAGNOSTIC EVALUATION

Essential laboratory studies to obtain in the patient with theophylline intoxication include serum theophylline concentration, serum electrolytes, blood urea nitrogen, creatinine, glucose, calcium, magnesium, phosphorus, liver function panel, and creatinine phosphokinase. Urine should be frequently evaluated for evidence of myoglobinuria. An electrocardiogram should be obtained; all patients with theophylline intoxication should be placed on continuous electrocardiogram monitoring. Arterial blood gas and complete blood cell count should be obtained as clinically indicated.

Sequential serum theophylline concentrations should be obtained every 1 to 2 hours until a plateau and subsequent substantive decline have been documented because delayed peaks in serum theophylline concentration may occur after an overdose. All abnormal laboratory studies should be serially monitored until all values have returned to normal.

MANAGEMENT

The management of theophylline intoxication consists of stabilization, decreasing absorption, and enhancing elimination. After acute ingestion, decreasing absorption is a primary concern. Treatment of chronic intoxication or intoxication after intravenous administration of theophylline generally focuses more on enhancing elimination.

Airway protection is paramount, and the threshold for tracheal intubation in the patient with seizures or other alterations in consciousness should be low. Assisted ventilation may be necessary if there is coingestion of a CNS depressant or if medications that depress respiratory drive, such as diazepam for seizures, are required for management.

If hypotension does not respond to an initial intravenous fluid bolus, propranolol may have a positive effect on blood pressure stabilization. If a vasopressor is also required, α-adrenergic agents such as phenylephrine or norepinephrine may be more efficacious; dopamine, which has some vasodilating properties at low doses, may be relatively ineffective.

Although no controlled clinical studies are available, there have been reports of success in treating tachydysrhythmias, particularly supraventricular tachycardias, with β-adrenergic antagonists, such as propranolol. Propranolol counters tachycardia, restores coronary blood flow, and interrupts the reentry phenomena that often underlie theophylline-induced dysrhythmias [33]. A potential hazard of propranolol administration is drug-induced bronchospasm; therefore, it should be used cautiously, if at all, in patients with significant reactive airways disease. Esmolol, an ultrashort-acting β_1-selective antagonist, has also been shown to be effective for select theophylline-induced tachydysrhythmias [63].

The antidysrhythmic agent adenosine has become the treatment of choice for supraventricular tachycardias and may be an important therapeutic addition in the management of theophylline-induced tachyarrhythmias. Having a significant effect on atrioventricular node conduction, adenosine can promptly reverse supraventricular tachycardias. Moreover, because of the evidence that adenosine and theophylline compete for the same receptor, adenosine may be a specific antidote for theophylline-induced supraventricular tachycardia. However, published clinical data in this regard are limited [64–66]. Amiodarone or lidocaine is the recommended treatment of ventricular irritability associated with hemodynamic compromise.

Seizures should be treated aggressively. High-dose benzodiazepine may be necessary for seizure termination. Phenytoin may be ineffective for theophylline-induced seizures [67], and in animal studies, it appears to contribute to theophylline-induced seizures. If seizures become prolonged, general anesthesia with a rapid-acting barbiturate, such as thiopental or pentobarbital, may be necessary. Neuromuscular blockade should be considered for seizures that are unresponsive to these modalities because significant morbidity may result from the rhabdomyolysis, hyperthermia, and acidosis of status epilepticus. There is some evidence that propranolol may help prevent or control theophylline-induced seizures [68].

Vomiting can be treated with the H_2-antagonist ranitidine, which reduces gastric acid hypersecretion [69,70]. Cimetidine administration is relatively contraindicated in theophylline poisoning because it inhibits theophylline metabolism. The dose of ranitidine is 50 to 100 mg given intravenously for adults and 0.1 to 0.5 mg per kg in children. Doses can be repeated every 6 to 8 hours. Metoclopramide also is an effective antiemetic that stimulates upper gastrointestinal motility and increases lower esophageal tone, without affecting theophylline clearance. The initial dose of metoclopramide is 0.5 to 1.0 mg per kg given intravenously for adults or 0.1 mg per kg for children (maximum, 1.0 mg per kg), although the risk of dystonia increases with increasing dose. Ondansetron is an alternative antiemetic, offering the advantage of effective antiemesis with no alterations in mental status and no risk of dystonic reaction. The phenothiazine antiemetics prochlorperazine and promethazine can lower seizure threshold and should not be administered.

Treatment of metabolic acidosis is aimed at maintaining a normal serum pH. For hypokalemia, it is important to emphasize that because hypokalemia's origin is predominantly the intracellular shift of potassium with minimal losses of total body potassium content through urine or vomitus, reversal of hypokalemia is best accomplished by lowering the theophylline concentration. Aggressive replacement of potassium may result in "overshoot" hyperkalemia [71]. Intravenous infusions of potassium chloride or potassium phosphate at 40 mEq per L in a saline solution should be adequate; intravenous boluses are usually not indicated. Hypophosphatemia, hypomagnesemia, hypercalcemia, and hyperglycemia rarely require correction.

Because vomiting is such a prominent feature of theophylline intoxication, there is rarely a need to perform gastric emptying. However, activated charcoal (see Chapter 117) is highly effective in reducing the absorption of theophylline and should be administered to all patients with recent ingestions. Whole-bowel irrigation (see Chapter 117) may be effective, particularly for sustained-release formulations, but its role in the treatment of theophylline intoxication remains undefined.

The repeated administration of activated charcoal (multiple-dose activated charcoal [MDAC]; see Chapter 117) is a valuable therapeutic measure for enhancing theophylline elimination [26,72–74]. Moreover, because MDAC acts through the principle of "gastrointestinal dialysis," it is effective even if theophylline intoxication occurs after intravenous administration of aminophylline [75]. MDAC is potentially as effective as hemodialysis in accelerating theophylline clearance [76,77]. However, it is not a substitute for hemodialysis in situations where rapid reduction in body theophylline burden is essential. All patients with significant theophylline intoxication should receive MDAC until the theophylline level is less than 15 μg per mL. Typical dosing is 1 g per kg charcoal every 4 hours (maximum, 50 g per dose). An effective alternative is 20 g every 2 hours [74]. Another alternative to bolus serial charcoal is administration via continuous nasogastric infusion at a rate of 0.25 to 0.50 g per kg per hour. Repeated vomiting, present in up to 80% of patients with theophylline intoxication [78], may delay or prevent successful MDAC administration. Aggressive antiemetic therapy is usually necessary.

In severely intoxicated patients or patients with moderate toxicity who are unable to tolerate MDAC, rapid removal of theophylline is essential. This is best accomplished by hemodialysis or hemoperfusion. If the need for extracorporeal drug removal is anticipated, a nephrologist should be involved early in management. Because of the time and personnel required to initiate extracorporeal drug removal, early notification can expedite the process once the decision has been made. Morbidity and mortality may be significantly lower if these procedures are undertaken before the onset of life-threatening disturbances. Indications for extracorporeal drug removal include hemodynamic instability or repeated seizures (regardless of serum theophylline concentration) and acute intoxication with a serum theophylline concentration greater than 80 μg per mL. Extracorporeal measures should be considered in patients younger than 6 months or older than 60 years with chronic intoxication and a theophylline concentration greater than 30 μg per mL.

Charcoal hemoperfusion has traditionally been considered the extracorporeal drug-removal method of choice for theophylline intoxication [79,80]. It reduces the elimination half-life of theophylline to as low as 0.7 to 2.1 hours [77], increasing clearance four- to sixfold [79]. However, hemoperfusion has significant risks, including hypotension, thrombocytopenia, red cell destruction, bleeding diathesis, and hypocalcemia. Also, there are few medical centers with the equipment and personnel needed to perform this procedure. The combination of scarce access to the procedure, increasing efficiency of hemodialysis, and the comparable efficacy of the two procedures has made hemodialysis the preferred procedure for treatment of severe theophylline intoxication [81].

Hemodialysis has many advantages over hemoperfusion. First, it is a technique that is widely available and relatively simple to perform. The need for administration of blood products is considerably less with hemodialysis. Dialysis can also increase theophylline clearance substantially, depending on the blood flow rates achieved by the device. Also, hemodialysis does not require the same degree of anticoagulation required by hemoperfusion, which lowers the risk of bleeding diathesis. Finally, the overall rate of complications is lower for hemodialysis than for hemoperfusion.

Peritoneal dialysis is an ineffective mode of drug removal in theophylline intoxication and is not recommended. Exchange transfusion, formerly thought to have no role in theophylline poisoning, has been used successfully in neonates with severe intoxication [82]. Other extracorporeal drug-removal methods, such as hemofiltration and plasmapheresis, have not been sufficiently evaluated, although there are case reports that these procedures have therapeutic value [83,84]. Hemofiltration, because it is a slow, passive, cardiac output-dependent technique, is unlikely to effect the rapid removal of theophylline that is necessary in severe intoxications.

CAFFEINE

Caffeine is a component of the three most popular beverages in the world: coffee, tea, and carbonated soft drinks. It is also used therapeutically as an antisleep aid and in many headache medications. Having a wide margin of safety and a relatively short elimination half-life—3 hours in adults, but 1 to 6 days in neonates—caffeine can be ingested daily in amounts as high as 1 g [85]. However, daily doses in this range are associated with unwanted adverse effects, including anxiety, jitteriness, and tachycardia.

The pharmacokinetic profile of caffeine resembles theophylline, with an important exception: whereas metabolism of theophylline (1,3-dimethylxanthine) produces inactive metabolites, caffeine (1,3,7-trimethylxanthine) undergoes 7-demethylation to form theophylline. Therefore, caffeine ingestion is invariably associated with measurable serum theophylline concentrations. After caffeine intoxication, serum theophylline concentration is a useful measure of toxicity. Many of the clinical manifestations of caffeine intoxication may in fact result from the effects of theophylline at its susceptible end organs.

The single ingestion of more than 1.5 g of caffeine (30 to 50 mg per kg in children) can produce serious adverse effects with the same manifestations found in acute theophylline intoxication [86]. Ingestions of more than 100 to 200 mg per kg are potentially lethal [85]. The five major disturbances occurring after caffeine intoxication are gastrointestinal, neurologic, metabolic, cardiac, and musculoskeletal [19]. Nausea and vomiting, with occasional hematemesis, predominate. CNS excitation may be manifested by anxiety, agitation, and seizures in severe cases. The same hypokalemia, hyperglycemia, and metabolic acidosis that appear after severe acute theophylline intoxication occur with caffeine poisoning. The most common cause of death after caffeine intoxication is intractable cardiac dysrhythmias [87]; severe acute overdoses have led to myocardial infarction [88]. Musculoskeletal effects can be prominent with caffeine intoxication; one feature is the appearance of severe rhabdomyolysis [89]. Life-threatening events after acute caffeine intoxication are associated with serum concentrations of more than 100 to 150 μg per mL. However, seizures after caffeine intoxication have occurred at serum concentrations as low as 50 μg per mL. Death has been reported with serum concentrations as low as 80 μg per mL. However, serum caffeine concentrations as high as 385 μg per mL have been associated with survival [90].

Management of caffeine intoxication follows the same principles as theophylline intoxication. Patient stabilization includes treatment of life-threatening seizures and cardiac dysrhythmias. Activated charcoal should be administered as soon as possible to provide gastrointestinal decontamination. Aggressive antiemetic therapy should be administered. MDAC is presumed to be equally effective for caffeine intoxication. Caffeine can be eliminated via hemodialysis; this procedure should be considered in those with seizures, cardiac dysrhythmias, or serum caffeine concentrations in excess of 100 μg per mL.

References

1. Shannon M: Life-threatening events after theophylline overdose. A 10-year prospective analysis. *Arch Intern Med* 159:989, 1999.
2. Schaefer S, Correa SD, Valente RJ, et al: Blockade of adenosine receptors with aminophylline limits ischemic preconditioning in human beings. *Am Heart J* 142:E4, 2001.
3. Cawley M, Al-Jazairi A, Stone E: Intravenous theophylline—an alternative to temporary pacing in the management of bradycardia secondary to AV nodal block. *Ann Pharmacother* 35:303, 2001.
4. Jenik A, Ceriani Cernadas JM, Gorenstein A, et al: A randomized double-blind, placebo-controlled trial of the effects of prophylactic theophylline on renal function in term neonates with perinatal asphyxia. *Pediatrics* 105:E45, 2000.
5. Fischer R, Lang SM, Steiner U, et al: Theophylline improves acute mountain sickness. *Eur Respir J* 15:123, 2000.
6. Schulz-Stubner S: The use of small-dose theophylline for the treatment of bradycardia in patients with spinal cord injury. *Anesth Anal* 101:1809, 2005.
7. Bagshaw S, Ghali W: Theophylline for prevention of contrast-induced nephropathy: a systematic review and meta-analysis. *Arch Intern Med* 165:1087, 2005.
8. Mohammadi MR, Kashani L, Akhondzadeh S, et al: Efficacy of theophylline compared to methylphenidate for the treatment of attention-deficit hyperactivity disorder in children and adolescents: a pilot double-blind randomized trial. *J Clin Pharm Ther* 29:139, 2004.
9. Ream R, Loftis LL, Albers GM, et al: Efficacy of IV theophylline in children with severe status asthmaticus. *Chest* 119:1480, 2001.
10. Derks M, Koopmans RP, Oosterhoff E, et al: Prevention by theophylline of beta-2-receptor down regulation in healthy subjects. *Eur J Drug Metab Pharmacokinet* 25:179, 2000.
11. Kawai M, Kato M: Theophylline for the treatment of bronchial asthma: present status. *Methods Find Exp Clin Pharmacol* 22:309, 2000.
12. Weinberger M, Hendeles L: Theophylline in asthma. *N Engl J Med* 334:1380, 1996.
13. Szefler SJ, Bender BG, Jusko WJ, et al: Evolving role of theophylline for treatment of chronic childhood asthma. *J Pediatr* 127:176, 1995.
14. Wheeler D, Jacobs BR, Kenreigh CA, et al: Theophylline versus terbutaline in treating critically ill children with status asthmaticus—a prospective, randomized, controlled trial. *Pediatr Crit Care Med* 6:237, 2005.
15. Shah A: Which is more steroid sparing in persistent bronchial asthma? Montelukast or theophylline. *J Allergy Clin Immunol* 113:S34, 2004.
16. Holimon TD, Chafin C, Self T: Nocturnal asthma uncontrolled by inhaled corticosteroids: theophylline or long-acting [beta]2 agonists? *Drugs* 61:391, 2001.
17. Adinoff A: Life-threatening events after theophylline overdose: a 10-year prospective analysis. *Pediatrics* 106:467, 2000.
18. Nagesh R, Murphy K: Caffeine poisoning treated by hemoperfusion. *Am J Kidney Dis* 12:316, 1988.
19. Zimmerman P, Pulliam J, Schwengels J, et al: Caffeine intoxication: a near fatality. *Ann Emerg Med* 14:1227, 1985.
20. Garriott J, Simmons LM, Poklis A, et al: Five cases of fatal overdose from caffeine-containing "look alike" drugs. *J Anal Toxicol* 9:141, 1985.
21. Shannon M, Lovejoy F: Effect of acute versus chronic intoxication on clinical features of theophylline poisoning in children. *J Pediatr* 121:125, 1992.
22. Shannon M: Predictors of major toxicity after theophylline overdose. *Ann Intern Med* 119:1161, 1993.
23. Robertson NJ: Fatal overdose from a sustained-release theophylline preparation. *Ann Emerg Med* 14:154, 1985.
24. Hendeles L, Jenkins J, Temple R: Revised FDA labeling guidelines for theophylline oral dosage forms. *Pharmacotherapy* 15:409, 1995.
25. Gaudreault P, Guay J: Theophylline poisoning—pharmacological considerations and clinical management. *Med Toxicol* 1:169, 1986.
26. Shannon M: Theophylline and caffeine, in Haddad L, Winchester J, Shannon M (eds): *Clinical Management of Poisoning and Drug Overdose*. Philadelphia, WB Saunders, 1998, p 1093.
27. Lowry J, Jarrett RV, Wasserman G, et al: Theophylline toxicokinetics in premature newborns. *Arch Pediatr Adolesc Med* 155:934, 2001.
28. Faber MS, Jetter A, Fuhr U: Assessment of CYP1A2 activity in clinical practice: Why, how, and when? *Basic Clin Pharmacol Toxicol* 97(3):125–134, 2005.
29. Khan MI, Khan S: Smoking causes an upwards shift of the narrow therapeutic window of xanthine derivatives, theophylline (XD, T), resulting in an underestimation of its effective therapeutic dose, and may result in treatment failure. *Chest* 122:83S, 2002.
30. Mayo PR: Effect of passive smoking on theophylline clearance in children. *Ther Drug Monit* 23:503, 2001.
31. Orlando R, Padrini R, Perazzi M, et al: Liver dysfunction markedly decreases the inhibition of cytochrome P450 1A2-mediated theophylline metabolism by fluvoxamine. *Clin Pharm Ther* 79:489, 2006.
32. Self T, Chafin C, Soberman J: Effect of disease states on theophylline serum concentrations: are we still vigilant? *Am J Med Sci* 319:177, 2000.
33. Curry SC, Vance MV, Requa R, et al: The effects of toxic concentrations of theophylline on oxygen consumption, ventricular work, acid base balance and plasma catecholamine levels in the dog. *Ann Emerg Med* 14:554, 1985.
34. Curry SC, Vance MV, Requa R, et al: Cardiovascular effects of toxic concentrations of theophylline in the dog. *Ann Emerg Med* 14:547, 1985.
35. Shannon M: Hypokalemia, hyperglycemia and plasma catecholamine activity after severe theophylline intoxication. *Clin Toxicol* 32:41, 1991.
36. Vestal RE, Eiriksson CE Jr, Musser B, et al: Effect of intravenous aminophylline on plasma levels of catecholamines and related cardiovascular and metabolic responses in man. *Circulation* 67:162, 1983.
37. Lipworth B: Phosphodiesterase type inhibitors for asthma: a real breakthrough or just expensive theophylline? *Ann Allergy Asthma Immunol* 96:640, 2006.
38. Polson JB, Kranowski JJ, Goldman AL, et al: Inhibition of human pulmonary phosphodiesterase activity by therapeutic levels of theophylline. *Clin Exp Pharmacol Physiol* 5:535, 1978.
39. Li H, Henry J: Adenosine receptor blockade reveals *N*-methyl-D-aspartate receptor- and voltage-sensitive dendritic spikes in rat hippocampal CA1 pyramidal cells in vitro. *Neuroscience* 100:21, 2000.
40. Martinez-Tica J, Zornow M: Effects of adenosine agonists and an antagonist on excitatory transmitter release from the ischemic rabbit hippocampus. *Brain Res* 872:110, 2000.
41. Higbee MD, Kumar M, Galant SP: Stimulation of endogenous catecholamine release by theophylline: a proposed additional mechanism of action for theophylline effects. *J Allergy Clin Immunol* 70:377, 1982.
42. DeFronzo RA, Bia M, Birkhead G: Epinephrine and potassium homeostasis. *Kidney Int* 20:83, 1981.
43. Amin DN, Henry JA: Propranolol administration in theophylline overdose. *Lancet* 1:520, 1985.
44. Miura T, Kimura K: Theophylline-induced convulsions in children with epilepsy. *Pediatrics* 105:920, 2000.
45. Richards W, Church JA, Brent DK: Theophylline-associated seizures in children. *Ann Allergy* 54:276, 1985.
46. Muhling J, Dehne MG, Sablotzki A, et al: Effects of theophylline on human cerebral blood flow velocity during halothane and isoflurane anaesthesia. *Eur J Anaesthesiol* 16:380, 1999.
47. Pinard E, Riche D, Puiroud S, et al: Theophylline reduces cerebral hyperaemia and enhances brain damage induced by seizures. *Brain Res* 511:303, 1990.
48. Nakada T, Kwee IL, Lerner AM, et al: Theophylline-induced seizures: clinical and pathophysiologic aspects. *West J Med* 138:371, 1983.
49. Phung ND: Theophylline toxicity in ambulatory elderly patients. *Immunol Allergy Pract* 8:17, 1986.
50. Fredholm BB: On the mechanism of action of theophylline and caffeine. *Acta Med Scand* 217:149, 1985.
51. Charytan D, Jansen K: Severe metabolic complications from theophylline intoxication. *Nephrology* 8:239, 2003.
52. de Galan B, Tack CJ, Lenders JW, et al: Effect of 2 weeks of theophylline on glucose counterregulation in patients with type 1 diabetes and unawareness of hypoglycemia. *Clin Pharmacol Ther* 74:77, 2003.
53. Sawyer WT, Caravati EM, Ellison MJ, et al: Hypokalemia, hyperglycemia, and acidosis after intentional theophylline overdose. *Am J Emerg Med* 3:408, 1985.
54. Shannon M, Lovejoy F: Hypokalemia after theophylline intoxication. The effects of acute vs. chronic poisoning. *Arch Intern Med* 149:2725, 1989.
55. Hall KW, Dobson KE, Dalton JG, et al: Metabolic abnormalities associated with intentional theophylline overdose. *Ann Intern Med* 101:457, 1984.
56. Polak M, Rolon MA, Chouchana A, et al: Theophylline intoxication mimicking diabetic ketoacidosis in a child. *Diabetes Metab* 25:513, 1999.
57. Shannon MW, Lovejoy FH, Woolf A: Prediction of serum theophylline concentration after acute theophylline intoxication [abstract]. *Ann Emerg Med* 19:627, 1990.
58. McPherson ML, Prince SR, Atamer ER, et al: Theophylline-induced hypercalcemia. *Ann Intern Med* 105:52, 1986.
59. Gaudreault P, Guay J: Theophylline and caffeine poisoning, in Harwood-Nuss A, Linden CH, Luten RC, et al (eds): *The Clinical Practice of Emergency Medicine*. Philadelphia, PA, Lippincott-Raven, 1996, p 1425.
60. Baker MD: Theophylline toxicity in children. *J Pediatr* 109:538, 1986.
61. Bertino JS, Walker JW: Reassessment of theophylline toxicity-serum concentrations, clinical course, and treatment. *Arch Intern Med* 147:757, 1987.
62. Shannon M, Lovejoy F: The influence of age vs. peak serum concentration of life-threatening events after chronic theophylline intoxication. *Arch Intern Med* 150:2045, 1990.
63. Gaar GG, Banner W, Laddu AR: The effects of esmolol on the hemodynamics of acute theophylline toxicity. *Ann Emerg Med* 16:1334, 1987.
64. Berul CI: Higher adenosine dosage required for supraventricular tachycardia in infants treated with theophylline. *Clin Pediatr* 32:167–168, 1993.
65. Biery JC, Kauflin MJ, Mauro VF: Adenosine in acute theophylline intoxication. *Ann Pharmacother* 29:1285–1288, 1995.
66. Giagounidis AA, Schäfer S, Klein RM, et al: Adenosine is worth trying in patients with paroxysmal supraventricular tachycardia on chronic theophylline medication. *Eur J Med Res* 3(8):380–382, 1998.
67. Blake KV, Massey KL, Hendeles L, et al: Relative efficacy of phenytoin and phenobarbital for the prevention of theophylline-induced seizures in mice. *Ann Emerg Med* 17:1024, 1988.

68. Schneider SM, Zea B, Michelson EA: Beta-blockade for acute theophylline-induced seizures. *Vet Hum Toxicol* 29:451, 1987.
69. Sessler CN: Poor tolerance of oral activated charcoal with theophylline overdose. *Am J Emerg Med* 5:492, 1987.
70. Amitai Y, Yeung AC, Moye J, et al: Repetitive oral activated charcoal and control of emesis in severe theophylline toxicity. *Ann Intern Med* 105:386, 1986.
71. D'Angio R, Sabatelli F: Management considerations in treating metabolic abnormalities associated with theophylline overdose. *Arch Intern Med* 147:1837, 1987.
72. Kulig KW, Bar-Or D, Rumack BH: Intravenous theophylline poisoning and multiple-dose charcoal in an animal model. *Ann Emerg Med* 16:842, 1987.
73. Shannon MW, Amitai Y, Lovejoy FH: Role of multiple-dose activated charcoal in young infants with theophylline intoxication. *Pediatrics* 80:368, 1987.
74. Park GD, Radomski L, Goldberg MJ, et al: Effect of size and frequency of oral doses of charcoal on theophylline clearance. *Clin Pharmacol Ther* 34:663, 1983.
75. Levy G: Gastrointestinal clearance of drugs with activated charcoal. *N Engl J Med* 307:676, 1982.
76. Rutten J, van den Berg B, van Gelder T, et al: Severe theophylline intoxication: a delay in charcoal haemoperfusion solved by oral activated charcoal. *Nephrol Dial Transplant* 20:2868, 2005.
77. Heath A, Knudsen K: Role of extracorporeal drug removal in acute theophylline poisoning—a review. *Med Toxicol* 2:294, 1987.
78. Paloucek FP, Rodvold KA: Evaluation of theophylline overdoses and toxicities. *Ann Emerg Med* 17:135, 1988.
79. Russo ME: Management of theophylline intoxication with charcoal-column hemoperfusion. *N Engl J Med* 300:24, 1979.
80. Sahney S, Abarzua J, Sessums L: Hemoperfusion in theophylline neurotoxicity. *Pediatrics* 71:615, 1983.
81. Shannon M: Comparative efficacy of hemodialysis and hemoperfusion in severe theophylline intoxication. *Acad Emerg Med* 4:674, 1997.
82. Shannon M, Wernovsky B, Morris C: Exchange transfusion in the treatment of severe theophylline poisoning. *Pediatrics* 89:145, 1992.
83. Okada S, Teramoto S, Matsuoka R: Recovery from theophylline toxicity by continuous hemodialysis with filtration. *Ann Intern Med* 133:922, 2000.
84. Laussen P, Shann F, Butt W, et al: Use of plasmapheresis in acute theophylline toxicity. *Crit Care Med* 19:288, 1991.
85. Dalvi RR: Acute and chronic toxicity of caffeine: a review. *Vet Hum Toxicol* 28:144, 1986.
86. Benowitz N, Osterloh J, Goldschlager N: Massive catecholamine release from caffeine poisoning. *JAMA* 248:1097, 1982.
87. Strubelt O, Diederich KW: Experimental treatment of the acute cardiovascular toxicity of caffeine. *Clin Toxicol* 37:29, 1999.
88. Forman J, Aizer A, Young CR: Myocardial infarction resulting from caffeine overdose in an anorectic woman. *Ann Emerg Med* 29:178, 1997.
89. Kamijo Y, Soma K, Asari Y, et al: Severe rhabdomyolysis following massive ingestion of oolong tea: Caffeine intoxication with coexisting hyponatremia. *Vet Hum Toxicol* 41(6):381–383, 1999.
90. Dietrich AM, Mortensen M: Presentation and management of an acute caffeine overdose. *Pediatr Emerg Care* 6:296, 1990.

CHAPTER 140 ■ OPIOID POISONING

ROBERT P. DOWSETT AND LUKE YIP*

Natural opioids (e.g., morphine and codeine) are harvested from the seedpods of the poppy plant *Papaver somniferum*. Semisynthetic opioids (e.g., dextromethorphan, heroin, hydrocodone, hydromorphone, oxycodone, and oxymorphone) are derivatives of morphine, whereas synthetic opioids (e.g., buprenorphine, butorphanol, diphenoxylate, fentanyl, meperidine, methadone, nalbuphine, pentazocine, propoxyphene, and tramadol) are not.

Clandestine laboratories have produced potent opioids as new manufacturing methods have been developed to circumvent the use of controlled or unavailable precursor compounds. Because these drugs may contain a wide variety of active ingredients, adulterants, and contaminants, the clinical syndromes seen in the abuser may be only partly related to the opioid component.

PHARMACOLOGY

Opioids interact with central nervous system (CNS) receptors to produce their analgesic, euphoric, and sedative effects. Historically, on the basis of animal studies, three major opioid receptors designated *mu*, *kappa*, and *sigma* have been proposed [1]. The *sigma* receptor is no longer considered an opioid subtype because it is insensitive to naloxone, has dextrorotatory stereochemistry binding, and has no endogenous ligand. The International Union on Receptor Nomenclature recommends a change from the Greek alphabet to one similar to other neurotransmitter systems; receptors are denoted by their endogenous ligand (opiates *p*eptides) with a subscript denoting their order of discovery: *delta* to OP_1 *kappa* to OP_2, and *mu* to OP_3 [2] (Table 140.1).

Most opioid analgesics are well absorbed after parenteral administration, from the pulmonary capillaries and mucosal sites. Analgesia is promptly achieved after parenteral administration and within 15 to 30 minutes after oral dosing. Peak plasma levels are generally attained within 1 to 2 hours after therapeutic oral doses. However, acute overdose may produce decreased intestinal peristalsis, resulting in delayed and prolonged absorption. Therapeutic and toxic serum drug concentrations are not well established.

All opioids undergo hepatic biotransformation, including hydroxylation, demethylation, and glucuronide conjugation. Considerable first-pass metabolism accounts for the wide variations in oral bioavailability noted with drugs such as morphine and pentazocine. Only small fractions of the parent drug are excreted unchanged in the urine. Active metabolites can contribute to the toxicological profile of specific drugs.

All opioids elicit the same overall physiologic effects as morphine, the prototype of this group. A typical morphine dose (5 to 10 mg) usually produces analgesia without altering mood or mental status in a patient. Sometimes dysphoria rather than euphoria is manifest, resulting in mild anxiety or a fear reaction. Nausea is frequently encountered, and vomiting is occasionally observed. Morphine and most of its congeners cause miosis in humans. This effect is exacerbated after an overdose, resulting in profound pupillary constriction, predominantly a central effect. Cerebral circulation does not appear to be altered by therapeutic doses of morphine unless respiratory depression and carbon dioxide retention result in cerebral vasodilation.

Respiratory failure is the most serious consequence of opiate overdose. Opioid agonists reduce the sensitivity of the medullary chemoreceptors in the respiratory centers to an increase in carbon dioxide tension and depress the ventilatory

*The views expressed do not necessarily represent those of the agency or the United States.

TABLE 140.1

OPIATE RECEPTOR SYSTEM AND CLINICAL EFFECTS

μ Opioid receptors (OP_3)	κ Opioid receptors (OP_2)	δ Opioid receptors (OP_1)
Supraspinal/spinal analgesia	Supraspinal/spinal analgesia	Supraspinal/spinal analgesia
Peripheral analgesia	Dysphoria	Modulation of OP_3 function
Sedation	Psychotomimesis	Respiratory depression
Euphoria	Diuresis	
Respiratory depression	Miosis	
Miosis		
Constipation		
Pruritus		
Bradycardia		
Prolactin release		
Growth hormone release		
Physical dependence		

response to hypoxia. Even small doses of morphine depress respiration, decreasing minute and alveolar ventilation [3]. The peak respiratory-depressant effect is usually noted within 7 minutes of intravenous (IV) morphine administration, but may be delayed up to 30 minutes if the drug is intramuscularly administered. Normal carbon dioxide sensitivity and minute volume usually return 5 to 6 hours after a therapeutic dose [3].

Therapeutic opiate doses cause arteriolar and venous dilation and may result in a mild decrease in blood pressure. This change in blood pressure is clinically insignificant while the patient is supine, but significant orthostatic changes are common [4]. Hypotension appears to be mediated by histamine release [5]. Myocardial damage (necrotizing angiitis) in opiate overdose associated with prolonged hypoxic coma may be mediated by cellular components released during rhabdomyolysis, direct toxic effects, or hypersensitivity to the opioids or adulterants [6].

Heroin (diacetylmorphine) has two to five times the analgesic potency of morphine [7]. Virtually all street heroin in the United States is produced in clandestine laboratories and adulterated before distribution (Table 140.2). The purity of street heroin is between 5% and 90%. Physiologically, the effects of heroin are identical to those described for morphine [8]. Heroin can be administered intravenously, intranasally, or inhaled as a volatile vapor, and can be mixed with other drugs of abuse, typically amphetamine or cocaine ("speed ball"). The plasma half-life of heroin is 5 to 15 minutes. Heroin is initially deacetylated in the liver and plasma, and then renally excreted as a conjugate, with small amounts of morphine, diacetylmorphine, and 6-monoacetylmorphine [8]. Individual variation in sensitivity and tolerance makes correlation of serum levels with clinical symptoms difficult.

TABLE 140.2

HEROIN ADULTERANTS

Mannitol	Antipyrine
Dextrose	Boric acid
Lactose	Mercurous salts
Talc	Animal manure
Sodium bicarbonate	Cocaine
Quinine	Amphetamine
Strychnine	Methamphetamine
Caffeine	Barbiturates
Phenacetin	Flour
Procaine	Magnesium sulfate
Lidocaine	Antihistamines
Benzocaine	Phencyclidine
Tetracaine	Scopolamine

The initial heroin rush is probably due to its high lipid solubility and rapid penetration into the CNS [8]. The majority of its lasting effects are attributable to its metabolites 6-monoacetylmorphine and morphine [8]. Fatal overdoses with heroin have been reported with serum morphine concentrations of 0.1 to 1.8 μg per mL [9].

Codeine (methylmorphine) is formulated as a sole ingredient and in combination with aspirin or acetaminophen. Codeine is rapidly absorbed by the oral route, producing a peak plasma level within 1 hour of a therapeutic dose [10]. Usually 10% of codeine is metabolized to morphine by CYP2D6; this may be greatly increased in patients with duplicated or amplified CYP2D6 genes, resulting in opioid toxicity [11]. This pathway may be inhibited by quinidine [12]. Clearance of codeine by CYP3A4 may be inhibited by clarithromycin and voriconazole [11]. Codeine and morphine appear in the urine within 24 to 72 hours. However, only morphine is detected in the urine at 96 hours [10]. The effect of codeine on the CNS is comparable with, but less pronounced than that of, morphine. Fatal ingestions with codeine alone are rare. The estimated lethal dose in a nontolerant adult is 800 mg, with a serum codeine concentration of 0.14 to 4.8 mg per dL [13].

Fentanyl, a phenylpiperidine derivative, has a potency 200 times that of morphine. Legitimate use is limited to anesthesia, and it is known to be commonly abused by hospital personnel. Rapid IV administration may result in acute muscular rigidity primarily involving the trunk and chest wall, which impairs respiration. Although motor activity resembling seizures has been associated with fentanyl use, simultaneous electroencephalogram recording during fentanyl induction of general anesthesia failed to show epileptiform activity [14]. This suggests a myoclonic rather than epileptic nature of the observed muscle activity [14].

Fentanyl is available as a transdermal delivery system that establishes a depot of drug in the upper skin layers, where it is available for systemic absorption. After removal of the patch, drug absorption from the dermal reservoir continues with an apparent half-life of 17 hours, versus 2 to 4 hours with IV administration [15].

By manipulating the chemical structure of fentanyl, α-methylfentanyl (China white), 3-methylfentanyl, and para-fluoro-fentanyl have been produced and distributed on the street as heroin substitutes. They are 200 to 3,000 times more potent than heroin [16]. α-Methyl-acetyl-fentanyl, α-methylfentanyl acrylate, and benzylfentanyl are 6,000 times more potent than morphine [17].

Meperidine, another phenylpiperidine derivative, is less than half as effective when given orally as compared to the parenteral route [18]. It appears to be a common drug of abuse among medical personnel, yet there are few reports of meperidine poisoning or fatalities [19]. Peak plasma levels are 30 minutes after intramuscular administration, and 1 to 2 hours after an oral dose [18]. The duration of action is 2 to 4 hours [18]. Meperidine is metabolized primarily by *N*-demethylation to normeperidine, an active metabolite with half the analgesic and euphoric potency of its parent and twice the convulsant property [20]. Excretion is primarily through the kidneys as conjugated metabolites [21]. Meperidine and normeperidine may be detected in either urine or serum [21]. The seizures reported with meperidine toxicity have been attributed to the accumulation of normeperidine, which has an elimination half-life of 14 to 24 hours [18,22].

A synthetic meperidine analog, methyl-phenyl-propionoxypiperidine has been used as a heroin substitute. Methyl-phenyl-tetrahydropyridine, a contaminant produced during the clandestine synthesis of this agent, led to an epidemic of Parkinsonism among IV drug abusers within days of repeated injections [23].

Diphenoxylate is structurally similar to meperidine. Diphenoxylate (2.5 mg) is formulated with 0.025 mg atropine sulfate (Lomotil) and used in the treatment of diarrhea. In therapeutic doses, the drug has no significant CNS effects. Symptoms arising from a toxic ingestion may be delayed because of decreased gastrointestinal (GI) motility and accumulation of the hepatic metabolite difenoxin, a potent opioid with a long serum half-life [24]. The ingestion of only six to eight Lomotil tablets may cause serious toxicity in children [24].

Methadone is used for chronic pain conditions and maintenance of opiate addicts. It is well absorbed orally, producing a peak plasma level within 2 to 4 hours [25]. It has a prolonged but variable duration of action; the half-life averages 25 hours, but may be as long as 52 hours during long-term maintenance therapy [25]. As little as 40 to 50 mg may produce coma and respiratory depression in a nontolerant adult [26]. A protracted clinical course is expected after an overdose [27].

Propoxyphene is structurally related to methadone. It is available alone or in combination with aspirin or acetaminophen. Oral administration is followed by rapid absorption, with peak serum levels occurring in 1 hour [28]. The plasma half-life of propoxyphene and its main active metabolite, norpropoxyphene, is 6 to 12 hours and 37 hours, respectively. Norpropoxyphene is the primary metabolite excreted in the urine [29]. It is believed to play a role in the prolonged clinical course after an overdose [30]. Blood levels in fatal overdose cases range from 0.028 to 42.7 mg per L [31].

Pentazocine is a synthetic analgesic in the benzomorphan class and has been involved in the drug abuse trade [32]. It has agonist as well as weak antagonist activity at the opioid receptors. It has one third the analgesic potency of morphine [32]. Orally administered, pentazocine achieves peak plasma levels within 1 hour and is extensively metabolized in the liver with the parent compound and metabolites detectable in either urine or plasma [32]. Pentazocine (Talwin), in combination with the antihistamine tripelennamine, was known on the street as *T's and Blues* and was used as a heroin substitute [33].

In an attempt to curtail pentazocine abuse, the oral preparation was reformulated to contain 0.5 mg naloxone (Talwin-NX). When Talwin-NX is parenterally administered, the effects of pentazocine are antagonized by naloxone, which has precipitated withdrawal in opiate-dependent individuals. Because the duration of action of pentazocine exceeds that of naloxone, delayed respiratory depression may occur.

Dextromethorphan, an analogue of codeine, is found in a large number of nonprescription cough and cold remedies. It is available as a single ingredient but usually formulated in combination with sympathomimetic and antihistamine drugs. Dextromethorphan is well absorbed from the GI tract, with peak plasma levels occurring 2.5 and 6.0 hours after ingestion of regular and sustained-release preparations, respectively. The therapeutic effect is 3 to 6 hours, with a corresponding plasma half-life of 2 to 4 hours. The predominant antitussive effect is attributed to the active metabolite dextrorphan [34]. Within the therapeutic dose, dextromethorphan lacks analgesic, euphoric, and physical dependence properties [35].

Hydromorphone and oxycodone are orally administered opioids used in the treatment of chronic pain conditions. A number of sustained-release formulations are available, and can result in prolonged poisoning in overdose. A formulation of hydromorphone has recently been withdrawn from the market because alcohol could accelerate the release of the drug [36]. The sustained-release properties of some formulations of oxycodone can be circumvented by crushing or dissolving the tablet, resulting in fatal narcotic overdoses in drug abusers [37].

Tramadol is structurally similar to morphine. It is a centrally acting analgesic with moderate affinity for *mu* receptors. The metabolite *O*-demethyl-tramadol appears to have a higher affinity than the parent compound. Most of the analgesic effects are attributed to nonopioid properties of the drug, probably by blocking the reuptake of biogenic amines (e.g., norepinephrine and serotonin) at synapses in the descending neural pathways, which inhibits pain responses in the spinal cord [38].

Buprenorphine is a partial agonist activity with high affinity to, and slow dissociation from, the *mu* receptor. It displaces other opioids and its dose–response curve has a ceiling effect, resulting in less respiratory depression in overdose, although apnea may still occur [39,40]. It has poor oral bioavailability and is administered sublingually. It is also formulated with naloxone that is active only if administered intravenously [41]. Other partial agonists include butorphanol and nalbuphine. They can precipitate opioid withdrawal (see Chapter 145) in those taking other opioids.

CLINICAL PRESENTATION

Miosis, respiratory depression, and coma are the hallmarks of opiate intoxication, with the magnitude and duration of toxicity dependent on the dose and degree of tolerance. The clinical effects of an overdose with any one of the agents in this class are similar. However, there are important differences between certain drugs. Overdoses resulting in toxicity often have a prolonged clinical course, in part because of opiate-induced decreased GI motility when taken orally and prolonged half-life of the drug or its active metabolite(s). Miosis is considered a pathognomonic finding in opiate poisoning, with the exception of meperidine, propoxyphene, pentazocine, and dextromethorphan use, in the case of a mixed overdose with an anticholinergic or sympathomimetic drug, or when severe acidemia, hypoxemia, hypotension, or CNS structural disorder is present.

CNS depression occurs in most severely intoxicated patients. However, codeine, meperidine, and dextromethorphan intoxications are remarkable for CNS hyperirritability, resulting in a mixed syndrome of stupor and delirium. In addition, patients with meperidine toxicity may also have tachypnea, dysphoric and hallucinogenic episodes, tremors, muscular twitching, and spasticity, whereas patients with dextromethorphan toxicity may also manifest restlessness, nystagmus, and clonus [22,42].

Pulmonary edema may complicate the clinical course of opioid overdose and appears more prevalent with heroin, morphine, codeine, methadone, and propoxyphene [13,43,44]. Pulmonary edema has occurred in postoperative patients who received naloxone and after naloxone therapy in overdose patients [45,46]. However, naloxone does not appear to alter the

TABLE 140.3

PULMONARY COMPLICATIONS ASSOCIATED WITH OPIATE ABUSE

Pulmonary arteritis (cotton)	Bacterial pneumonia
Pulmonary thrombosis (talc)	Aspiration pneumonitis
Pulmonary hypertension (talc)	Pulmonary edema
Septic emboli	Atelectasis
Lung abscess	Respiratory arrest

vascular permeability of the lung directly [47]. Typically, the patient has a depressed consciousness and respiration. After naloxone administration, the patient awakens and over minutes to hours is noted to become hypoxic and develop pulmonary edema. Acute naloxone-induced withdrawal has been associated with massive CNS sympathetic discharge, which may be a precipitating factor in the development of neurogenic pulmonary edema [48]. It appears that the pulmonary injury is at the alveolar–capillary membrane, resulting in manifestations consistent with acute respiratory distress syndrome [49]. It does not appear to be an immune-mediated mechanism [50]. Pulmonary edema may present within 2 hours of parenteral heroin use, up to 4 hours after intranasal heroin use, and up to 24 hours after methadone overdose [51].

Patients with heroin-induced pulmonary edema typically have normal capillary wedge pressures and elevated pulmonary arterial pressures [52]. In contrast, elevated systemic, pulmonary arterial, and pulmonary capillary wedge pressures and total systemic vascular resistance are seen with pentazocine intoxication [53]. This effect is believed to result from transient endogenous catecholamine release [54]. Persistent pulmonary symptoms beyond 24 to 48 hours may indicate aspiration or bacterial pneumonitis, with atelectasis, fibrosis, bronchiectasis, granulomatous disease, or pneumomediastinum [55]. Adulterants in street drugs are potential pulmonary toxins [56]. Dyspnea, hypoxemia, and the presence of multiple reticulonodular infiltrates on chest radiograph may be caused by adulterants in the IV mixture. A summary of the potential pulmonary complications associated with opioid abuse is provided in Table 140.3.

Heroin toxicity may be associated with cardiac conduction abnormalities and dysrhythmias, which may be the result of metabolic derangements associated with hypoxia, a direct effect of the abused agent, or adulterants (e.g., quinine) in street drugs [57–59].

Leukoencephalopathy associated with inhalational abuse of heroin ("chasing the dragon") typically progresses for several weeks. Initially, cerebellar ataxia and motor restlessness may be followed by the development of pyramidal tract lesions, pseudobulbar reflexes, spastic paresis, myoclonic jerks, and choreoathetoid movements. A quarter of patients may progress to hypotonic paresis, akinetic mutism, and death [60].

Seizures and focal neurologic signs are usually absent after opiate intoxication [61] unless precipitated by severe hypoxia, an intracranial process (e.g., brain abscess and subarachnoid hemorrhage), proconvulsive adulterants, meperidine, propoxyphene, pentazocine (T's and Blues), or tramadol use [33,62–65]. Meperidine- and propoxyphene-related seizures may become more frequent in chronic drug abusers with renal insufficiency.

Disabling myoclonus has been reported after several days of fentanyl therapy by the transdermal delivery system [17].

The clinical course after propoxyphene overdose may be severe and rapidly progressive, with cardiac dysrhythmias, circulatory collapse, seizures, and respiratory arrest developing within 45 minutes [66]. Seizure may be focal or generalized [62]. Propoxyphene appears to be responsible for CNS toxicity (respiratory depression and seizures) and cardiac toxicity (QRS prolongation and dysrhythmias) [67], whereas norpropoxyphene contributed only to the cardiotoxicity in one animal study [68]. Cardiotoxicity may be exacerbated by hypoxia or adulterants (e.g., quinine) in street drugs. The minimum toxic dose reported is 10 mg per kg, and 20 mg per kg is considered potentially fatal, but tolerance develops with chronic use [69]. Doses of 1,000 to 2,000 mg can be ingested or injected, with minimal signs of intoxication in chronic propoxyphene abusers and heroin addicts [70].

Anxiety, dysphoria, and hallucinations are more common with pentazocine than with other opiate derivatives [32]. Acute toxicity in combination with tripelennamine results in the typical opiate intoxication syndrome as well as dyspnea, hyperirritability, hypertension, and seizures. It is believed that these effects may be directly related to tripelennamine [33].

Hypotension may occur after opiate overdose, although pentazocine intoxication may result in hypertension [33]. Heroin and propoxyphene toxicity may be associated with nonspecific ST-segment and T-wave changes, first-degree atrioventricular block, atrial fibrillation, prolonged QTc intervals, and ventricular dysrhythmias [57]. Cardiovascular findings may be exacerbated by hypoxia or adulterants (e.g., quinine) in street drugs.

Dextromethorphan abuse seems to be self-limiting because of adverse drug events, such as lethargy, somnambulism, and ataxia [71]. It is associated with a psychologic rather than physiologic dependence syndrome [72]. Recreation dextromethorphan abusers report increased perceptual awareness, altered time perception, euphoria, and visual hallucinations [71]. Long-term use may result in bromide toxicity [73]. Because dextromethorphan frequently appears in combination products, the contribution of these coingestants should be considered.

Methadone can produce bradycardia, QTc prolongation, and torsades de pointes. Bradycardia has been reported infrequently and is postulated to be because of methadone's structural similarity to verapamil [74,75]. QTc prolongation and torsades de pointes have been associated with mean daily methadone dose 397 $\pm$ 238 mg; mean QTc interval on presentation was 615 $\pm$ 77 ms. In one case series, the majority of patients were receiving a potentially QT-prolonging drug, 41% of the patients had hypokalemia, and 18% of the patients were found to have structural heart disease [76]. A proposed mechanism is inhibition of the cardiac potassium channel by the nontherapeutic (S)-methadone isomer [77]. This isomer is metabolized by CYP2B6; 6% of the population are slow metabolizers, resulting in elevated levels of (S)-methadone and increased QTc intervals [77,78].

The onset of anticholinergic and opioid effects may be significantly delayed after a diphenoxylate overdose [79]. Atropine effects (CNS excitement, hypertension, fever, and flushed dry skin) occur before, during, or after opioid effects. However, opioid effects (CNS and respiratory depression with miosis) may predominate or occur without any signs of atropinism. Cardiopulmonary arrest has been reported to occur 12 hours after ingestion of diphenoxylate [80].

Patients presenting after a tramadol overdose may exhibit lethargy, nausea, tachycardia, agitation, seizures, coma, hypertension, respiratory depression metabolic acidosis, acute hepatic failure, and acute renal failure [81]. Tramadol-associated seizures are brief, and significant respiratory depression is uncommon [65].

Interaction between meperidine and monoamine oxidase inhibitors (MAOIs), dextromethorphan and MAOIs, and tramadol and selective serotonin reuptake inhibitors may result in the serotonin syndrome [82–84]. Patients with severe serotonin syndrome exhibit rapid onset of altered mental status, muscle rigidity, hyperthermia, autonomic dysfunction, coma, seizures, and death.

Rhabdomyolysis, hyperkalemia, myoglobinuria, and acute renal failure may complicate the clinical course of an acute opioid overdose [85]. Acute renal failure may be due to direct insult by the abused substance, adulterants in street drugs, and prolonged coma [58,85]. Chronic parenteral drug use may result in glomerulonephritis and renal amyloidosis and has been associated with concurrent bacterial infections [86]. Potential lethal acute infections have been linked to clostridia contamination [87].

Body packers or "mules" are people who transport large numbers of concentrated heroin packets in their GI tract from one country to another. If one of these packets ruptures, the amount of drug released can cause severe and prolonged toxicity [88]. They may also develop features of intestinal obstruction and, occasionally, intestinal perforation and peritonitis [89].

DIAGNOSTIC EVALUATION

Laboratory studies such as complete blood cell count, serum electrolytes, blood urea nitrogen, creatinine and creatine phosphokinase, urinalysis, arterial blood gas, electrocardiography, chest and abdominal radiography, head computed tomography, and lumbar puncture should be obtained as clinically indicated. Arterial blood gas usually reflects hypoventilation, respiratory acidosis, and metabolic acidosis [90]. If pulmonary edema develops, chest radiographs typically reveal bilateral fluffy alveolar infiltrates, occasionally unilateral in nature, and echocardiograms show normal cardiac function [43]. A markedly negative anion gap with hyperchloremia should raise the suspicion of bromide poisoning from chronic dextromethorphan use [73]. Chest radiographic findings of pulmonary edema usually resolve within 24 to 48 hours.

It is recommended that an ECG be obtained prior to commencing methadone therapy and within 30 days of commencement and then yearly to monitor the QTc interval [91].

Leukoencephalopathy associated with inhalational abuse of heroin appears as hypoattenuation in the affected white matter, although this may not be apparent until late in the disease. Magnetic resonance imaging typically demonstrates white matter hyperintensity on T2-weighted sequences. Affected areas are initially the occipital and cerebellar white matter, followed by involvement of the parietal, temporal, and frontal lobes. The cerebellar peduncles, splenium of the corpus callosum, posterior limb of the internal capsules, corticospinal tract, medial lemniscus, and tractus solitarius may also be involved [60].

TABLE 140.4

INFECTIOUS COMPLICATIONS IN INTRAVENOUS DRUG ABUSERS

Endocarditis	Lymphadenitis
Aspergillosis	Epidural abscess
Bacterial meningitis	Phlebitis
Cutaneous abscess	Viral hepatitis
Mycotic aneurysm	Wound botulism
Cellulitis	Tetanus
Brain abscess	Osteomyelitis
Lymphangitis	Septicemia
Subdural abscess	HIV/AIDS

AIDS, acquired immunodeficiency syndrome; HIV, human immunodeficiency virus.

Quantitative serum opiate levels do not contribute to patient management. A urine toxicology screen may confirm the diagnosis, but is rarely necessary for acute patient management. Commercial opioid assays are unlikely to detect synthetic opioids. The metabolites of naloxone are chemically related to oxymorphone, but naloxone is not known to give false-positive immunoassay urine screens for opioid substances [92]. False-positive serology tests for syphilis have been reported among drug addicts [93]. Laboratory investigation should also include tests for infection in patients with fever (Table 140.4).

MANAGEMENT

A diagnosis of opioid poisoning should be considered in all comatose patients. However, the classic triad of opiate toxicity (coma, miosis, and respiratory depression) may not be apparent after a mixed overdose. Respiratory support is paramount in the management of patients with opioid toxicity; one should secure the airway and ventilate with 100% oxygen. Vascular access should be established. The patient should be placed on continuous pulse oximetry and cardiac monitoring. Vital signs should be monitored frequently.

Naloxone is a specific opiate receptor antagonist and can reverse the analgesia, respiratory depression, miosis, hyporeflexia, and cardiovascular effects of opiate toxicity [94,95]. The goal of naloxone therapy is to reestablish adequate spontaneous ventilation. The initial IV naloxone dose should be 0.1 mg if the patient is possibly opioid dependent; larger doses may precipitate acute opioid-withdrawal syndrome. Otherwise, an initial 2 mg dose can be administered. If there is history of an opiate exposure, a strong suspicion based on presenting signs and symptoms, or a partial response to the initial naloxone dose, repeated IV naloxone boluses up to 10 mg should be administered because methadone, pentazocine, propoxyphene, diphenoxylate, and sustained-release preparations of oxycodone and hydromorphone may not respond to the usual naloxone doses [96,97]. Despite its strong affinity to *mu* receptors, buprenorphine overdose can be treated effectively with normal doses of naloxone [40].

Intramuscular, intralingual, endotracheal, intraosseous, and intranasal routes of naloxone administration are acceptable alternatives when IV access is not readily available [96,98–100]. Repeat naloxone boluses may be required every 20 to 60 minutes because of its short elimination half-life (60 to 90 minutes). A continuous naloxone infusion should be considered in patients who have a positive response but require repeated bolus doses because of recurrent respiratory depression [100,101]. A therapeutic continuous naloxone infusion can be made by administering two third of the effective naloxone bolus dose per hour. The infusion is titrated to maintain adequate spontaneous ventilation without precipitating acute opioid withdrawal and empirically continued for 12 to 24 hours. The patient should be admitted to an intensive care or high-dependency setting for continuous monitoring. After the naloxone therapy is discontinued, the patient should be carefully observed for 4 hours for recurrent respiratory depression.

Naloxone is effective in reversing diphenoxylate-induced opioid toxicity. However, recurrence of respiratory and CNS depression is common [79]. All patients with significant diphenoxylate overdose should be observed in an intensive care setting for at least 24 hours.

Hypotension may respond to naloxone therapy but may require fluid resuscitation and vasopressors. Overzealous fluid resuscitation should be avoided because of the risk of pulmonary edema.

The management of seizures should follow present treatment guidelines and include benzodiazepines or barbiturates.

Adjunct naloxone therapy may be effective in propoxyphene, but not in meperidine- or tramadol-related seizures [102]. Seizures have been reported after naloxone administration for tramadol overdose [65].

The management of serotonin syndrome is primarily supportive (see Chapters 66 and 124). Sedation, paralysis, intubation and ventilation, anticonvulsants, antihypertensives, and aggressive rapid cooling may all be necessary. Some success has been obtained with the nonspecific serotonin antagonist cyproheptadine (4 to 8 mg every 8 hours orally) or olanzapine (sublingual 10 mg) [103,104].

GI decontamination should be considered for orally administered opioids after vital signs have been stabilized. The clinical benefits of multiple oral doses of activated charcoal are unproven, but it is potentially beneficial because of the prolonged absorption phase that is typically encountered with opiate overdoses. Repeat charcoal doses should not be used in the absence of active bowel sounds.

The management of pulmonary edema should include adequate ventilation, oxygenation, and positive-pressure ventilation as needed [105]. Inotropic agents and diuretics are of little value.

Bradycardia secondary to methadone administration responds to ceasing the drug; atropine has not been utilized [75]. If patients receiving methadone develop a QTc interval of more than 500 milliseconds, consideration should be given to reducing the dose or discontinuing the drug [91].

Asymptomatic body packers should be conservatively managed when the condition of packaging does not appear to be compromised. One proposed guideline involves the oral administration of a water-soluble contrast solution followed by serial abdominal radiographs (Table 140.5) [106]. Whole-bowel irrigation (WBI) with polyethylene glycol electrolyte lavage solution (PEG-ELS) has also been advocated on the basis of case reports [107].

Pruritus is a common opioid adverse drug event. It may be localized or general, and ranges from mild to severe. Antihistamines are usually ineffective, but naloxone has frequently been found to offer relief. Ondansetron has been reported to provide relief in refractory cases [108].

TABLE 140.5

MEDICAL MANAGEMENT FOR ASYMPTOMATIC BODY PACKERS

1. Administer an oral dose of water-soluble contrast (e.g., Gastrografin): 1 mL/kg[a]
2. Perform abdominal radiographs (supine and upright) at least 5 h after oral contrast administration
3. If radiographs are positive, perform daily abdominal radiographs, and after a spontaneous bowel movement
4. All bowel movements are checked for drug packets
5. The patient may be discharged after passage of two packet-free bowel movements *and* negative abdominal radiographs

[a]Patients are permitted to feed normally, and vascular access should be maintained.

Leukoencephalopathy associated with inhalational abuse of heroin has been reported to improve following the antioxidant ubiquinone (coenzyme Q10) administration in doses of 30 to 300 mg QID [109].

Nalmefene is also effective for the reversal of opioid-induced CNS effects and can be administered orally or intravenously. Its half-life and dose-dependent duration of action are 4 to 8 hours after IV administration [110]. The initial adult dose is 0.5 mg for those who are not opioid dependent and 0.1 mg for those suspected of having opioid dependency. If there is an incomplete response or no response, additional doses can be given at 2- to 5-minute intervals. A total dose of 1.5 mg may be necessary to exclude the possibility of opioid poisoning. The principal advantage over naloxone is its considerably longer duration of antagonistic action however; withdrawal syndromes precipitated by nalmefene use would also be prolonged.

Naltrexone is a potent, long-acting pure opiate antagonist that is effective orally. Its use is primarily limited as adjunctive therapy for opioid detoxification. Naltrexone may induce a withdrawal syndrome that lasts up to 72 hours.

References

1. Brill JE: Control of pain. *Crit Care Clin* 8:203, 1992.
2. Dhawan BN, Cesselin F, Raghubir R, et al: International Union of Pharmacology. XII. Classification of opioid receptors. *Pharmacol Rev* 48:567, 1996.
3. Romberg R, Olofsen E, Sarton E, et al: Pharmacodynamic effect of morphine-6-glucuronide versus morphine on hypoxic and hypercapnic breathing in healthy volunteers. *Anesthesiology* 99:788, 2003.
4. Zelis R, Mansour EJ, Capone RJ, et al: The cardiovascular effects of morphine: the peripheral capacitance and resistance vessels in human subjects. *J Clin Invest* 54:1247, 1974.
5. Fahmy NR, Sunder N, Soter NA: Role of histamine in the hemodynamic and catecholamine responses to morphine. *Clin Pharmacol Ther* 33:615, 1983.
6. Melandri R, Re G, Lanzarini C, et al: Myocardial damage and rhabdomyolysis associated with prolonged hypoxic coma following opiate overdose. *J Toxicol Clin Toxicol* 34:199, 1996.
7. Lasagna L: The clinical evaluation of morphine and its substitute as analgesic. *Pharmacol Rev* 16:47, 1964.
8. Sporer KA: Acute heroin overdose. *Ann Int Med* 130:584, 1999.
9. Nakamura GR: Toxicologic assessments in acute heroin fatalities. *Clin Toxicol* 13:75, 1978.
10. Soloman MD: A study of codeine metabolism. *Clin Toxicol* 7:255, 1974.
11. Gasche Y, Daali Y, Fathi M, et al: Codeine intoxication associated with ultrarapid CYP2D6 metabolism. *N Engl J Med* 351:2827, 2004.
12. Desmeules J, Gascon MP, Dayer P, et al: Impact of environmental and genetic factors on codeine analgesia. *Eur J Clin Pharmacol* 41:23, 1991.
13. Peat MA, Sengupta A: Toxicological investigations of cases of death involving codeine and dihydrocodeine. *Forensic Sci* 9:21, 1977.
14. Smith NT, Benthuysen JL, Bickford RG, et al: Seizures during opioid anesthetic induction—are they opioid-induced rigidity? *Anesthesiology* 71:852, 1989.
15. Duragesic, fentanyl [package insert]. Piscataway, NJ, Janssen Pharmaceutica, 1991.
16. Buchanan JF, Brown C: Designer drugs: a problem in clinical toxicology. *Med Toxicol Adverse Drug Exp* 3:1, 1988.
17. Hibbs J, Perper J, Winek CL: An outbreak of designer drug-related deaths in Pennsylvania. *JAMA* 265:1011, 1991.
18. Stambaugh JE, Wainer IW, Sanstead JK, et al: The clinical pharmacology of meperidine: comparison of routes of administration. *J Clin Pharmacol* 16:245, 1976.
19. Ward CF, Ward GC, Saidman CJ: Drug abuse in anesthesia training programs: a survey, 1970–1980. *JAMA* 250:922, 1983.
20. Hershley LA: Meperidine and central neurotoxicity. *Ann Intern Med* 98:548, 1983.
21. Mather LE, Tucker GT, Pflug AE, et al: Meperidine kinetics in man—intravenous injection in surgical patients and volunteers. *Clin Pharmacol Ther* 17:21, 1977.
22. Morisy L, Platt D: Hazards of high dose meperidine. *JAMA* 255:467, 1986.
23. Langston JW, Irwin I, Langston EB, et al: Chronic Parkinsonism in humans due to a product of meperidine-analog synthesis. *Science* 219:979, 1983.
24. Thomas TJ, Pauze D, Love JN: Are one or two dangerous? Diphenoxylate-atropine exposure in toddlers. *J Emerg Med* 34:71, 2008.
25. Berkowitz BA: The relationship of pharmacokinetics to pharmacological activity: morphine, methadone and naloxone. *Clin Pharmacokinet* 1:219, 1976.
26. Kreek MJ: Medical complications in methadone patients. *Ann N Y Acad Sci* 311:110, 1978.
27. Norris JV, Don HF: Prolonged depression of respiratory rate following methadone analgesia. *Anesthesiology* 45:361, 1976.
28. Wolen RL, Guber CM, Kiplinger GF, et al: Concentration of propoxyphene in human plasma following oral, intramuscular and intravenous infusion. *Toxicol Appl Pharmacol* 19:480, 1971.

29. Verbely K, Inturrisi CE: Disposition of propoxyphene and norpropoxyphene in man after a single oral dose. *Clin Pharmacol Ther* 15:302, 1973.
30. Bellville JW, Seed JC: A comparison of the respiratory depressant effects of dextropropoxyphene and codeine in man. *Clin Pharmacol Ther* 9:428, 1968.
31. Hawton K, Simkin S, Gunnell D, et al: A multicentre study of coproxamol poisoning suicides based on coroners' records in England. *Brit J Clin Pharmacol* 59:207, 2005.
32. Brogden RN, Speight TM, Avery GS: Pentazocine: a review of its pharmacological properties, therapeutic efficacy and dependence liability. *Drugs* 5:6, 1973.
33. Debard ML, Jagger JA: "T's and B's": Midwestern heroin substitute. *Clin Toxicol* 18:1117, 1981.
34. Silvasti M, Karttunen P, Tukiainen H, et al: Pharmacokinetics of dextromethorphan and dextrorphan: a single dose comparison of three preparations in human volunteers. *Int J Clin Pharmacol Ther Toxicol* 25:493, 1987.
35. Bem JL, Peck R: Dextromethorphan: an overview of safety issues. *Drug Saf* 7:190, 1992.
36. Murray S, Wooltorton E: Alcohol-associated rapid release of a long-acting opioid. *Can Med Assoc J* 173:756, 2005.
37. Charatan F: Time-release analgesic drug causes fatal overdoses in United States. *West J Med* 175:82, 2001.
38. Raffa RB, Friderichs E, Reimann W, et al: Opioid and nonopioid components independently contribute to the mechanism of action of tramadol, an "atypical" opioid analgesic. *J Pharmacol Exp Ther* 260:275, 1992.
39. Carrieri MP, Amass L, Lucas GM, et al: Buprenorphine use: The international experience. *Clin Infect Dis* 15:S197, 2006.
40. Boyd J, Randell T, Luurila H, et al: Serious overdoses involving buprenorphine in Helsinki. *Acta Anaesthesiol Scand* 47:1031, 2003.
41. Robinson SE: Buprenorphine-containing treatments: place in the management of opioid addiction. *CNS Drugs* 20:697, 2006.
42. Pender ES, Parks BR: Toxicity with dextromethorphan-containing preparations: a literature review and report of two additional cases. *Pediatr Emerg Care* 7:163, 1991.
43. Jaffe RB, Koschmann EB: Intravenous drug abuse: pulmonary, cardiac and vascular complications. *Am J Roentgenol Radium Ther Nucl Med* 109:107, 1970.
44. Zyroff J, Slovis TL, Nagler J: Pulmonary edema induced by oral methadone. *Radiology* 112:567, 1974.
45. Brimacombe J, Archdeacon J, Newell S, et al: Two cases on naloxone-induced pulmonary oedema: the possible use of phentolamine in management. *Anaesth Intensive Care* 19:578, 1991.
46. Schwartz JA, Koenigsberg MD: Naloxone-induced pulmonary edema. *Ann Emerg Med* 16:1294, 1987.
47. Silverstein JH, Gintautas J, Tadoori P, et al: Effects of naloxone on pulmonary capillary permeability. *Prog Clin Biol Res* 328:389, 1990.
48. Pallasch TJ, Gill CJ: Naloxone-associated morbidity and mortality. *Oral Surg* 52:602, 1981.
49. Sklar J, Timms RM: Codeine-induced pulmonary edema. *Chest* 72:230, 1977.
50. Dettmeyer R, Schmidt P, Musshoff F, et al: Pulmonary edema in fatal heroin overdose: immunohistological investigations with IgE, collagen IV and laminin—no increase of defects of alveolar-capillary membranes. *Forensic Sci Int* 110:87, 2000.
51. Presant S, Knight L, Klassen G: Methadone-induced pulmonary edema. *Can Med Assoc J* 113:966, 1975.
52. Gopiathan K, Sajoja J, Speare R, et al: Hemodynamic studies in heroin induced acute pulmonary edema. *Circulation* 61[Suppl 3]:44, 1970.
53. Lee G, DeMaria AN, Amsterdam EA, et al: Comparative effects of morphine, meperidine and pentazocine on cardiocirculatory dynamics in patients with acute myocardial infarction. *Am J Med* 60:949, 1976.
54. Tammisto T, Jaattela A, Nikki P, et al: Effect of pentazocine and pethidine on plasma catecholamine levels. *Ann Clin Res* 3:22, 1971.
55. Pare JA, Fraser RG, Hogg JC, et al: Pulmonary mainline granulomatosis: talcosis on intravenous methadone abuse. *Medicine* 58:229, 1979.
56. Glassroth J, Adams GD, Schnoll S: The impact of substance abuse on the respiratory system. *Chest* 91:596, 1987.
57. Glauser FL, Downie RL, Smith WR: Electrocardiographic abnormalities in acute heroin overdosage. *Bull Narc* 29:85, 1977.
58. Pearce CJ, Cox JGC: Heroin and hyperkalemia. *Lancet* 2:923, 1980.
59. Perry DC: Heroin and cocaine adulteration. *Clin Toxicol* 8:239, 1975.
60. Hagel J, Andrews G, Vertinsky T, et al: "Chasing the dragon"—imaging of heroin inhalation leukoencephalopathy. *Canadian Assoc Radiologists J* 56:199, 2005.
61. Sternbach G, Moran J, Eliastam M: Heroin addiction: acute presentation of medical complications. *Ann Emerg Med* 9:161, 1980.
62. Tennant FS: Complication of propoxyphene abuse. *Arch Intern Med* 132:191, 1973.
63. Amine ARL: Neurosurgical complications of heroin addiction: brain abscess and mycotic aneurysm. *Surg Neurol* 7:385, 1977.
64. Citron BP, Halpern M, Haverback BJ: Necrotizing angiitis associated with drug abuse: a new clinical entity. *Clin Res* 19:181, 1971.
65. Spiller HA, Gorman SE, Villalobos D, et al: Prospective multicenter evaluation of tramadol exposure. *J Toxicol Clin Toxicol* 35:361, 1997.
66. Sloth Madsen P, Strom J, Reiz S, et al: Acute propoxyphene self-poisoning in 222 consecutive patients. *Acta Anaesthesiol Scand* 28:661, 1984.
67. Lund-Jacobsen H: Cardio-respiratory toxicity of propoxyphene and norpropoxyphene in conscious rabbits. *Acta Pharmacol Toxicol* 42:171, 1978.
68. Afshari R, Maxwell S, Dawson A, et al: ECG abnormalities in coproxamol (paracetamol/dextropropoxyphene) poisoning. *J Toxicol Clin Toxicol* 43:255, 2005.
69. Strom J: Acute propoxyphene self-poisoning with special reference to propoxyphene cardiotoxicity and treatment. *Dan Med Bull* 36:316, 1989.
70. Woody GE, McLellan AT, O'Brien CP, et al: Lack of toxicity of high dose propoxyphene napsylate when used for maintenance treatment of addiction. *J Toxicol Clin Toxicol* 16:473, 1980.
71. McCarthy JP: Some less familiar drugs of abuse. *Med J Aust* 20:1078, 1971.
72. Murray S, Brewerton T: Abuse of over-the-counter dextromethorphan by teenagers. *South Med J* 86:1151, 1993.
73. Ng YY, Lin WL, Chen TW, et al: Spurious hyperchloremia and decreased anion gap in a patient with dextromethorphan bromide. *Am J Nephrol* 12:268, 1992.
74. Wheeler AD, Tobias JD: Bradycardia during methadone therapy in an infant. *Pediatr Crit Care Med* 7:83, 2006.
75. Ashwath ML, Ajjan M, Culclasure T: Methadone-induced bradycardia. *J Emerg Med* 29:73, 2005.
76. Krantz MJ, Lewkowiez L, Hays H, et al: Torsade de pointes associated with very-high-dose methadone. *Ann Intern Med* 137:501, 2002.
77. Eap CB, Crettol S, Rougier JS, et al: Stereoselective block of hERG channel by (S)-methadone and QT interval prolongation in CYP2B6 slow metabolizers. *Clin Pharmacol Ther* 81:719, 2007.
78. Crettol S, Deglon JJ, Besson J, et al: ABCB1 and cytochrome P450 genotypes and phenotypes: influence on methadone plasma levels and response to treatment. *Clin Pharmacol Ther* 80:668, 2006.
79. McCarron MM, Challoner KR, Thompson GA: Diphenoxylate-atropine (Lomotil) overdose in children: an update (report of eight cases and review of the literature). *Pediatrics* 87:694, 1991.
80. Cutler EA, Barrett GA, Craven PW, et al: Delayed cardiopulmonary arrest after Lomotil ingestion. *Pediatrics* 65:157, 1980.
81. De Decker K, Cordonnier J, Jacobs W, et al: Fatal intoxication due to tramadol alone: case report and review of the literature. *Forensic Sci Int* 175:79, 2008.
82. Rivers N: Possible lethal reaction between Nardil and dextromethorphan. *Can Med Assoc J* 103:85, 1970.
83. Kesavan S, Sobala GM: Serotonin syndrome with fluoxetine plus tramadol. *J R Soc Med* 92:474, 1999.
84. Sternbach H: The serotonin syndrome. *Am J Psychiatry* 148:705, 1991.
85. Schwatzfarb D, Singh G, Marcus D: Heroin-associated rhabdomyolysis with cardiac involvement. *Arch Intern Med* 137:1255, 1977.
86. Dubrow A, Mittman N, Ghali V, et al: The changing spectrum of heroin-associated nephropathy. *Am J Kidney Dis* 5:36, 1985.
87. Finn SP, Leen E, English L, et al: Autopsy findings in an outbreak of severe systemic illness in heroin users following injection site inflammation: an effect of Clostridium novyi exotoxin? *Arch Pathol Lab Med* 127:1465, 2003.
88. Utecht MJ, Facinelli Stone A, McCarron MM: Heroin body packers. *J Emerg Med* 11:33, 1993.
89. Hutchins KD, Pierre-Louis PJ, Zaretski L, et al: Heroin body packing: three fatal cases of intestinal perforation. *J Forensic Sci* 45:42, 2000.
90. Duberstein JL, Kaufman DM: A clinical study of an epidemic of heroin intoxication and heroin-induced pulmonary edema. *Am J Med* 51:704, 1971.
91. Krantz MJ, Martin J, Stimmel B, et al: QTc interval screening in methadone treatment. *Ann Intern Med* 150;387, 2009.
92. Storrow AB, Wians FH, Mikkelsen SL, et al: Does naloxone cause a positive urine opiate screen? *Ann Emerg Med* 24:1151, 1994.
93. Cushman P Jr, Sherman C: Biologic false-positive reactions in serologic tests for syphilis in narcotic addiction. Reduced incidence during methadone maintenance treatment. *Am J Clin Pathol* 61:346, 1974.
94. Handal KA, Schauben JL, Salamone FR: Naloxone. *Ann Emerg Med* 12:438, 1983.
95. Hanston P, Evenepoel M, Ziade D, et al: Adverse cardiac manifestations following dextropropoxyphene overdose: can naloxone be helpful? *Ann Emerg Med* 25:263, 1995.
96. Goldfrank LR: The several uses of naloxone. *Emerg Med* 30:105, 1984.
97. Schneir AB, Vadeboncoeur TF, Offerman SR, et al: Massive OxyContin ingestion refractory to naloxone therapy. *Ann Emerg Med* 40:425, 2002.
98. Maio RF, Gaukel B, Freeman B: Intralingual naloxone injection for narcotic-induced respiratory depression. *Ann Emerg Med* 16:572, 1987.
99. Tandberg D, Abercrombie D: Treatment of heroin overdose with endotracheal naloxone. *Ann Emerg Med* 11:443, 1982.
100. Kelly AM, Kerr D, Dietze P, et al: Randomised trial of intranasal versus intramuscular naloxone in prehospital treatment for suspected opioid overdose. *Med J Aust* 182:24, 2005.
101. Goldfrank LR, Weisman RS, Errick JK, et al: A dosing nomogram for continuous infusion intravenous naloxone. *Ann Emerg Med* 15:566, 1986.
102. Fiut RE, Picchioni AL, Chin L: Antagonism of convulsive and lethal effects induced by propoxyphene. *J Pharm Sci* 55:1085, 1966.
103. Graudins A, Stearman A, Chan B: Treatment of the serotonin syndrome with cyproheptadine. *J Emerg Med* 16:615, 1998.

104. Boddy R, Dowsett RP, Jeganathan D: Sublingual olanzapine for the treatment of serotonin syndrome. *Clin Toxicol* 44:439, 2006.
105. Sporer KA, Dorn E: Heroin-related noncardiogenic pulmonary edema: a case series. *Chest* 120:1628, 2001.
106. Marc B, Baud FJ, Aelion MJ, et al: The cocaine body-packer syndrome: evaluation of a method of contrast study of the bowel. *J Forensic Sci* 35:345, 1990.
107. Traub SJ, Hoffman RS, Nelson LS: Body packing – The internal concealment of illicit drugs. *N Engl J Med* 349:2519, 2003.
108. Larijani GE, Goldberg ME, Rogers KH: Treatment of opioid-induced pruritus with ondansetron: report of four patients. *Pharmacotherapy* 16:958, 1996.
109. Gacouin A, Lavoue S, Signouret T, et al: Reversible spongiform leucoencephalopathy after inhalation of heated heroin. *Intensive Care Med* 29:1012, 2003.
110. Gal TJ, Difazio CA: Prolonged antagonism of opioid action with intravenous nalmefene in man. *Anesthesiology* 64:175, 1986.

CHAPTER 141 ■ PESTICIDE POISONING

WILLIAM K. CHIANG AND RICHARD Y. WANG

A pesticide is as an agent intended for killing, preventing, repelling, or mitigating any pest. With the increasing use, environmental contamination and reports of epidemic pesticide poisoning are inevitable [1–3]. The health consequences from the long-term and low-level exposure to these chemicals, such as carcinogenesis [4,5], teratogenicity [6], fertility [7], and neurologic sequelae [8,9], may be significant and immeasurable. In many countries in which there are limited regulations on pesticide usage, pesticide ingestion is one of the leading forms of suicide, and pesticide exposure is a major occupational risk [10–12]. Even in the United States, pesticide exposures remain a major public health problem [13]. The World Health Organization estimated that accidental and occupational pesticide poisonings worldwide account for 1.5 million cases and 28,000 deaths annually [14].

This chapter focuses on selected pesticides that are most clinically important. Some of the common pesticides are provided in Table 141.1. Organophosphate insecticides are covered in Chapter 128. Further information on the identification and toxicity of pesticide products may be obtained from sources such as material data safety sheets, *Hayes' Handbook of Pesticide Toxicology, Farm Chemicals Handbook*, and the pesticide label database (http://www.cdpr.ca.gov/docs/label/labelque.htm).

ORGANOCHLORINES

Organochlorines are commonly used as insecticides, soil fumigants, solvents, and herbicides. Human toxicity can result from either acute or chronic exposure. Contamination typically occurs during production and application of these agents. Infants and toddlers are at risk for toxicity from bioaccumulation in foodstuffs, excretion in breast milk, and concentration in fetal tissues [15–17]. These toxicants can cause a variety of systemic manifestations, but are most notable for their central nervous system (CNS) effects. Organochlorines can be divided into four structural categories: dichlorodiphenyltrichloroethane (DDT) and related agents, hexachlorocyclohexanes, cyclodienes, and toxaphenes.

DDT is a well-known organochlorine. It was a popular insecticide in the agricultural industry during the 1960s. The many environmental concerns related to the use of DDT, including carcinogenesis, bioaccumulation, and other health risks to humans and animals, led to the banning of its use in the United States as of 1972. DDT is no longer being produced in the United States. Dicofol (a miticide) and methoxychlor are structurally related to DDT. The cyclodienes include chlordane, heptachlor, endrin, aldrin, and dieldrin. The use of several of these insecticides in the United States was discontinued between 1988 and 1990. Some of the other organochlorines that are structurally related to the cyclodienes include endosulfan, chlordecone, kelevan, and mirex. Endosulfan is considered highly toxic and is registered for agricultural, but not residential, use in the United States [18]. Mirex and chlordecone (Kepone) are no longer being used in the United States.

Pharmacology

The organochlorines are well absorbed from the gastrointestinal (GI) tract. For example, death can occur within 2 hours of intentionally ingesting endosulfan, and most deaths associated with chlordane have been from oral exposures in children. The serum half-lives of these chemicals are long, varying from days to months, because of their high lipid solubility. This allows these agents to be stored in fatty tissues (e.g., brain), with the resultant delay in total body clearance. The organochlorines are known to concentrate in breast milk and fetal tissue. At delivery, it has been shown that fetal blood and tissue had higher concentrations of lindane (γ-hexachlorocyclohexane, Kwell) than maternal samples [16,17]. However, teratogenic effects have not been demonstrated in the limited number of animal studies performed [19].

Organochlorines are metabolized by the microsomal enzymes in the liver. Toxaphene, chlordane, DDT, and lindane can induce microsomal enzyme activity and affect not only their own metabolism but also the effects of coadministered medications [20].

Chlordane has several metabolites, such as heptachlor, oxychlordane, and heptachlor epoxide. Most of the available information on chlordane and metabolite tissue distribution is from case reports of accidental and suicidal exposures. Depending on the source, the elimination half-life of chlordane varies from 21 to 88 days [21,22]. Most of the chlordane and metabolites are excreted by the biliary system. On absorption into the body, aldrin is rapidly metabolized to the epoxide derivative, dieldrin. Because very little of aldrin remains, its toxicity is attributed to dieldrin. Dieldrin is stored in fatty tissues, and its elimination half-life in humans is approximately 369 days [23]. Endrin, an isomer of dieldrin, is rapidly metabolized in both humans and animals, with an elimination half-life of 2 to 6 days [24].

TABLE 141.1

COMMON PESTICIDES

Inorganic and organometal pesticides	**Herbicides**	Dicrotophos
Aluminum phosphide	Amitrole	Dimefox
Antimony potassium tartrate	Atrazine	Dioxathion
Arsenical pesticides	Bromoxynil	Edifenphos
Barium carbonate	Cycloate	Endothion
Boric acid	Dicamba	Fenitrothion
Calcium chloride	Dichlobenil	Fensulfothion
Copper sulfate	2,4-Dichlorophenoxyacetic acid	Fenthion
Elemental mercury	Diquat	Fonofos
Elemental sulfur	Diuron	Formothion
Lead arsenate	Ioxynil	Jodfenphos
Mercuric chloride	MCPA	Leptophos
Methylmercury	Mecoprop	Malathion
Phosphorus	Molinate	Merphos
Sodium chlorate	Phenmedipham	Methidathion
Sodium dichromate	Paraquat	Mevinphos
Thallium sulfate	Propanil	Mipafox
Zinc chloride	Propazine	Monocrotophos
Zinc phosphide	Pyrazon	Naled
Pyrethrins, pyrethroids, and plant-derived pesticides	Silvex	Oxydemeton-methyl
	Simazine	Parathion
Anabasine	TCA	Parathion-methyl
Barthrin	2,3,5-Trichlorophenoxyacetic acid	Phenthoate
Blasticidin S	**Fungicides and biocides**	Phorate
Cartap	Benomyl	Phosalone
Chlordecone	Captafol	Phosphamidon
Cyfluthrin	Captan	Phoxim
Cyfluthrinate	1-Chloro dinitrobenzene	Pirimiphos-methyl
Cyhalothrin	Dichloran	Schradan
Cypermethrin	Diphenyl	Temephos
Decamethrin	Maneb	Thiometon
Deltamethrin	Organotins (tributyltin)	Trichlorfon
Fluvalerate	Quintozene	**Carbamates**
Fluvalinate	Tetrachlorophthalide	Aldicarb
Nicotine	Thiabendazole	Bendiocarb
Phenothrin	Thiram	4-Benxiothielyn-*N*-methylcarbamate
Pyrethrins	Thiophanate-methyl	Bufencarb
Resmethrin	Zineb	Carbaryl
Ricin	Ziram	Carbofuran
Rotenone	**Organochlorine insecticides**	Dioxacarb
Sabadilla	Aldrin	Isolan
Strychnine	Chlordane	3-Isopropyl phenyl-*N*-methylcarbamate
Tralocythrin	Chlorobenzilate	Landrin
Tralomethrin	Chlordecone	Methomyl
Fumigants and nematocides	DDT	Mexacarbate
Acrylonitrile	Dicofol	Oxamyl
Aluminum phosphide	Dieldrin	Phencyclocarb
Boron trifluoride	Endrin	Promecarb
Carbon disulfide	Endosulfan	Propoxur
Carbon tetrachloride	Ethylan	**Miscellaneous pesticides**
Chloropicrin	Heptachlor	Azoxybenzene
1,2-Dibromoethane	Hexachlorobenzene	Busulfan
1,2-Dichloroethane	Isobenzan	Chlorambucil
p-Dichlorobenzene	Kelevan	Chlordimeform
1,2-Dichloropropane	Kelthane	Chlorfenxon
1,3-Dichloropropene	Lindane (γ-hexachlorocyclohexane)	DEET
Epoxyethane	Mirex	5-Fluorouracil
Hydrogen cyanide	Methoxychlor	Hexamethylmelamine
Methylbromide	TDE	Metaldehyde
Naphthalene	Toxaphene	Methotrexate
1,1,1-Trichloroethane	**Organophosphate insecticides**	Porfiromycin
Trichloroethylene	Azinphos-methyl	Propargite
Synthetic organic rodenticides	Carbophenothion	Thiotepa
ANTU	Carejin	**Nitro compounds and related phenolic pesticides**
Brodifacoum	Chlorfenvinphos	Binapacryl
Chloralose	Chlorphoxim	Dinocap
Difenacoum	Chlorpyrifos	2,4-Dinitrophenol
Diphacinone	Demeton	Dinoseb
Fluoroacetamide	Demeton-methyl	Pentachlorophenol
Fluoroethanol	Dialifos	TCDD
Norbormide	Diazinon	
Pyriminil	Dicapthon	
Sodium fluoroacetate	Dichlofenthion	
Warfarin	Dichlorvos	

ANTU, α-naphthylthiourea; DDT, dichlorodiphenyltrichloroethane; DEET, *N-N*-diethyl-*m*-toluamide; MCPA, 4-chloro-2-methylphenoxyacetic acid; TCA, trichloroacetic acid; TCDD, tetrachlorodibenzodioxin; TDE, 1,1-dichloro-2,2-bis(4-chlorophenyl)ethane.
Classifications adapted from Hayes WJ Jr, Laws ER (eds): *Handbook of Pesticide Toxicology.* San Diego, Academic, 1991.

TABLE 141.2

ORGANOCHLORINE LEVELS OF TOXICITY

High	Endrin, dieldrin, aldrin, endosulfan
Moderate	Chlordecone, heptachlor, chlordane, toxaphene, dichlorodiphenyltrichloroethane, hexachlorobenzene
Low	Methoxychlor, perthane, kelthane, chlorobenzilate, mirex

Organochlorines have several mechanisms of action. They alter sodium- and potassium channel movement across the neuronal membranes and can be considered axonal toxins. With DDT, sodium ion transport is facilitated and potassium transport is inhibited. This results in the spontaneous firing and prolongation of action potentials and repetitive firing after a stimulus. DDT also inhibits Na^+/K^+ adenosine triphosphatase and calmodulin activities, which reduces the rate of neuronal repolarization. This may account for some of the neurologic manifestations such as paresthesias, thought disturbances, myoclonus, and seizures. Cyclodienes, hexachlorocyclohexanes, and toxaphenes manifest neurotoxicity by inhibiting γ-aminobutyric acid receptor function in the CNS [25]. In the limbic system, lindane can directly excite neurons and result in agitation and seizures [25,26]. Abnormalities in respiratory rate patterns can result from direct medullary toxicity or pulmonary aspiration. The level of toxicity of the various organochlorines can be categorized into high, moderate, and low (Table 141.2).

Clinical Toxicity

Poisoning can result from ingestion, dermal absorption, or inhalation. Inadvertent human exposures to aldrin and dieldrin have resulted from pesticide spraying, which causes dermal and inhalational absorption. The use of lindane in home vaporizers has resulted in significant inhalation toxicity [27]. Agents such as dieldrin, lindane, and Kepone have good dermal penetration. Workers who directly handled lindane had health complaints of headaches, paresthesias, tremors, confusion, and memory impairment [28]. Also, seizures have been reported in occupational surveys among sprayers and applicators of aldrin and dieldrin [29,30]. As little as two total body applications on two successive days of 1% lindane (Kwell), a common scabicide, resulted in seizures in an 18-month-old child [31]. The peak concentration of lindane occurs 6 hours after dermal application; thus, delayed and prolonged manifestations of toxicity may occur from dermal absorption. Dermatitis can occur from the topical exposure to dicofol and methoxychlor [24]. Intradermal and subcutaneous injections of these agents can result in chemical dermatitis and sterile abscesses [32]. Dicofol and methoxychlor have minimal toxicity. Human volunteers ingesting up to 2 mg per kg per day of methoxychlor for 8 weeks did not demonstrate any ill effects [33].

Seizures are the most prominent CNS effect of these agents. The seizures occur soon after exposure, may present without a prodrome, and can be quite protracted in frequency [24,34–38]. Late-onset seizures may result from delayed GI or dermal absorption. Acute exposures to DDT present initially with tremors, nausea, vomiting, muscle weakness, and confusion, which may progress to seizures [39]. Among the organochlorines, both psychomotor agitation and CNS depression have been described. Chlordecone, mirex, and endosulfan are more likely to cause tremors and agitation than seizures. Kelthane, perthane, methoxychlor, and lindane are more likely to cause CNS sedation than excitation. Endrin is considered one of the most toxic of the chlordienes, with reports of hyperthermia and decerebrate posturing [24]. In 1984, an outbreak of endrin toxicity from contaminated foodstuffs occurred in Pakistan, where seizures resulted in a 10% mortality rate [36].

Neurologic symptoms resolve quickly because of rapid distribution of the organochlorines from blood to lipid stores. Because redistribution back into the blood pool can occur at a later time, continual observation of the patient for delayed toxicity may be warranted. Some of the long-term CNS effects (i.e., thought disturbances) after significant exposures may be due to direct chemical toxicity or anoxic encephalopathy from sustained seizures [40]. Chlordecone is a recognized neurotoxin, causing peripheral neuropathies [41].

Nausea, vomiting, and diarrhea may occur after ingestions, especially if petroleum distillates are part of the preparation. Pulmonary aspiration of these agents can cause tachypnea and significant respiratory distress, with resultant pulmonary edema [40]. When dicofol is heated or comes in contact with an acid, it decomposes to hydrogen chloride, which causes respiratory irritation [24]. Hypersensitivity pneumonitis may result from inhalational exposures when the organochlorine is mixed with pyrethrins.

Cardiac dysrhythmias, including ventricular fibrillation, have been reported from organochlorine exposure [42]. Halogenated hydrocarbons sensitize the myocardium to catecholamines, which results in a variety of rhythm disturbances. Cardiotoxicity can be exacerbated by either stress-provoking events or the exogenous administration of catecholamines. In severely ill patients, other causes of cardiac dysrhythmias, such as hypoxia and acidemia, should be considered.

Significant elevations in liver enzymes were reported in a group of 19 workers with a 10-year lindane exposure [43]. Animal studies with acute oral exposures to lindane have demonstrated fatty degeneration and necrosis of the liver [44]. From the few reports of human exposures to chlordane, there is little evidence of hepatotoxicity from this agent [21,45,46]. Microsomal enzyme induction has been demonstrated in animals that were orally administered chlordane. Long-term exposure among 233 workers with aldrin, dieldrin, endrin, and telodrin for 4 to 12 years was not associated with any significant elevation of hepatic enzymes or hepatic enzyme induction.

Hematologic dyscrasias, including aplastic anemia, leukopenia, leukocytosis, granulocytopenia, granulocytosis, eosinophilia, thrombocytopenia, and pancytopenia, have been reported after repeated lindane exposures [27,47]. However, all of the involved preparations also contained benzene, which can account for such findings. Megaloblastic anemia and bone marrow depression have been associated with chlordane exposures. DDT and toxaphene are suspected human carcinogens [48,49]. The risks for aldrin and dieldrin as human carcinogens could not be determined by the International Agency for Research on Cancer because of insufficient human and animal data [48].

Diagnostic Evaluation

Serum and urine concentrations of these organochlorines are commonly measured by gas chromatography or mass spectrometry. In an obvious exposure, these measurements are academic and would not alter clinical management. There are no correlations between concentrations in body tissues and specific health effects. If the diagnosis is in doubt, these measurements can at least confirm or rule out the insecticide exposure. Although blood is commonly sampled for the detection of these chemicals, adipose tissue or human milk may be used as well [50]. The laboratory should be consulted regarding the availability of analytical methods for biological specimens other than blood. An acute exposure can be determined by a quantitative comparison of parent compound to metabolite. Because DDT and aldrin are rapidly metabolized on systemic absorption, their elevated concentrations in the blood would support a recent exposure.

Chlorinated hydrocarbons are radiopaque, and their radiopacity is directly related to the number of chlorine atoms per molecule. Thus, radiographs can assist in demonstrating aspiration pneumonia and gut burden.

Management

Rescue workers and health care providers must use proper equipment, such as gloves and gowns, to prevent unnecessary exposure to these chemicals when providing assistance to these patients [51]. Initial treatment of organochlorine exposure involves limiting further chemical absorption by the patient. The patient should be removed from the scene, disrobed, and thoroughly and repeatedly washed with soap and water. Washing should include hair and fingernails. The patient's clothing and leather goods must be placed in a plastic bag and discarded because of the tenacious binding of these agents to leather. All wash water should be contained and discarded in a secure fashion.

The role of gastric decontamination depends on the clinical presentation. Immediately after an intentional ingestion and in asymptomatic patients without spontaneous emesis, gastric aspiration should be carefully performed with a small nasogastric tube. Activated charcoal should be administered soon after ingestion (preferably within 1 hour) because it can limit further gut absorption and enhance elimination by interrupting enterohepatic or enteroenteric circulation [27]. Also, cholestyramine may interrupt enteric circulation and enhance elimination. Chlordecone and chlordane undergo enterohepatic circulation, and cholestyramine is indicated in symptomatic patients. In a controlled trial, cholestyramine was administered as 16 g per day to symptomatic factory workers exposed to chlordane. After 5 months, chlordane fecal elimination was shown to increase by 3.3 to 17.8 times, with neurologic symptoms improving as concentrations declined. Milk- and oil-based cathartics should be avoided because their high lipid solubility can enhance gut absorption. Hemodialysis is not effective in enhancing elimination of these chemicals because of their high volume of distribution and protein binding [52]. Hemoperfusion is probably of no benefit [52].

Organochlorine-induced seizures are managed with benzodiazepines and barbiturates. Phenytoin has not been demonstrated to be more effective as an anticonvulsant than barbiturates and it may actually increase the incidence of these seizures [53,54]. For uncontrolled status epilepticus, muscle paralysis and general anesthesia may be necessary. Aggressive seizure control is warranted to limit further development of CNS damage, metabolic acidosis, hyperthermia, rhabdomyolysis, and myoglobinuric renal failure.

Respiratory distress due to bronchospasm is managed with humidified oxygen and nebulized bronchodilators. Parenteral administration of adrenergic amines is not recommended because it may potentiate myocardial irritability. Early administration of steroids and prophylactic use of antibiotics for pulmonary aspiration have not been demonstrated to improve patient outcome. The early use of antibiotics may predispose to the selective growth of other bacterial organisms.

After appropriate decontamination, asymptomatic patients with an oral exposure can be observed for 6 hours and then discharged if their clinical status remains unchanged. Patients presenting with cardiovascular, CNS, or persistent respiratory manifestations should be admitted for further therapy and observation.

PYRETHROIDS

Pyrethrum is a collection of naturally occurring insecticide esters from the chrysanthemum flower. The pyrethrin I ester has the greatest insecticidal activity and is subject to rapid environmental degradation. To enhance its effectiveness in commercial use, synthetic alternatives known as pyrethroids were developed that are more resistant to decay. These compounds are present in consumer products, from flea and tick removers for pets to topical pediculicides.

Pharmacology

The pyrethroids (including pyrethrins) delay closure of the sodium channel during the end of depolarization, with resultant insect paralysis. Piperonyl butoxide is commonly added to commercial preparations to inhibit insects' ability to metabolize the pyrethroid and prolong activity. In mammals, these agents are relatively nontoxic because of the low concentrations and rapid mammalian metabolism. However, people who are allergic to ragweed may have hypersensitivity reactions to pyrethroids. The degree of this cross-sensitization has been reported to be as high as 46%. Pyrethroids have no effects on cholinesterase activity, and atropine and pralidoxime are not indicated in therapy.

Pyrethroids are readily absorbed from the GI tract. Dermal absorption varies depending on the type of agent and additive organic solvents. Systemic absorption is enhanced in the presence of petroleum distillates. These compounds are highly lipid soluble and largely metabolized by the mixed-function oxidase enzymes in the liver.

Clinical Toxicity

Poisoning from pyrethroids can result from inhalational, dermal, or oral exposures [42,44,55–57]. Nausea, vomiting, and diarrhea may occur after ingestion [44,57]. Neurologic manifestations and hypersensitivity reactions, including anaphylaxis, are the most common forms of systemic toxicity. Neurologic findings depend on the type and concentration of the pyrethroid and include paresthesias, muscle fasciculations, coma, and seizures [44,55,57]. Patients with an intentional ingestion of a mixture containing an organophosphate and a pyrethroid can present with predominant cholinergic manifestations [58].

Management

Treatment is very similar to that described for organochlorines (see previous discussion). GI decontamination may be appropriate, but there is no role for repeat-dose–activated charcoal and cholestyramine therapy because enterohepatic circulation has not been demonstrated for the pyrethroids. Hypersensitivity reactions, including anaphylaxis, should be managed with epinephrine, steroids, antihistamines, bronchodilators, and vasopressors, as indicated.

Asymptomatic patients with oral exposures can be observed for 6 hours and medically cleared of toxicity if their clinical status remains unchanged. Patients presenting with cardiovascular, CNS, or persistent respiratory manifestations should be admitted for further therapy and observation.

ANTICOAGULANTS

Bishydroxycoumarin (dicumarol), the first anticoagulant, was isolated as the hemorrhagic agent in *sweet clover disease*, a bleeding disorder that resulted from the ingestion of spoiled clover silage. Numerous congeners, such as warfarin (3-α-acetonylbenzyl-4-hydroxycoumarin), have since been synthesized and used as a rodenticide. Typically, for the bait to be effective, the rodent must consume it for 3 to 10 days; however, continuous feeding for 21 days may be necessary to achieve 100% mortality. As rodents became increasingly resistant, warfarin derivatives were introduced and have supplanted warfarin. These "superwarfarins," or long-acting anticoagulants, include brodifacoum, difenacoum, and indanedione derivatives. The long-acting anticoagulants are 100 times more potent than warfarin and have a much longer half-life. Most anticoagulant rodenticide is packaged with cereal or other food products as bait, with the amount of rodenticide in the product varying from 0.025% to 0.005% per weight. Acute accidental or suicidal ingestion of a minimal amount of bait containing long-acting anticoagulants is unlikely to cause toxicity [59]. However, a "mouthful" of a long-acting anticoagulant ingestion in an adult human has been reported to cause significant coagulopathy [60–62].

Pharmacology

Warfarin and its derivatives are oxidized by mixed-function oxidases into inactive metabolites in the liver [63]. The plasma half-life of warfarin is 42 hours, with duration of action of 2 to 5 days [63]. The long-acting anticoagulants are concentrated in the liver and have extremely long half-lives; brodifacoum has a half-life of 120 days in dogs, 61 hours in rabbits, and 156 hours in rats [64–66]. The half-life of long-acting anticoagulants may be affected by the dose. The exact half-life of long-acting anticoagulants in humans is unknown, and because of significant interspecies variation, animal data cannot be extrapolated to humans. Case reports in human exposures have reported half-lives of 6 to 23 days for chlorophacinone and 16 to 39 days for brodifacoum [60,67–70]. Clinical coagulopathy may persist as long as 42 to 300 days [67–69,71–74].

These anticoagulants inhibit vitamin K 2,3-epoxide reductase and, to a lesser extent, vitamin K reductase. These enzymes are responsible for the cyclic regeneration of vitamin K [75,76]. Vitamin K is the active coenzyme responsible for activation of clotting factors II, VII, IX, and X, as well as anticoagulant factors protein C and protein S, by hepatic γ-carboxylation of the *N*-terminal glutamate residual of these proteins [75]. Once activated, vitamin K–dependent clotting factors can interact with calcium and phospholipids in the coagulation cascade [70]. Inhibition of vitamin K 2,3-epoxide reductase and vitamin K reductase depletes vitamin K and vitamin K–dependent clotting factors, resulting in coagulopathy and bleeding. The half-lives of vitamin K–dependent clotting factors are 7 hours for factor VII, 24 hours for factor IX, 36 hours for factor X, and 50 hours for factor II [63]. Because factor VII has the shortest half-life of the vitamin K–dependent clotting factors, increases in prothrombin time or international normalized ratio (INR) are not seen until 50% to 70% of factor VII is depleted. In a healthy person, this change occurs 24 to 48 hours after ingestion [59]. Clinical coagulopathy may not be evident for several days when the other vitamin K–dependent factors are also depleted, however [77,78].

Clinical Toxicity

The primary manifestation of poisoning is coagulopathy. The most common signs are cutaneous bleeding, soft-tissue ecchymosis, gingival bleeding, epistaxis, hematuria, and increased menstrual bleeding [61,79]. Gross hematuria, GI bleeding, hemoptysis, and peritoneal and diffuse alveolar bleeding may occur in patients with more serious poisoning [80–83]. Fatalities are uncommon and usually result from complications of intracranial hemorrhage [82,84].

Management

Gastric decontamination with activated charcoal should be initiated for acute ingestions. The most important laboratory studies are the prothrombin time and INR. Soon after an acute ingestion, values are expected to be normal; assays must be repeated at least 48 hours after exposure because of delayed coagulopathy [59]. Prophylactic vitamin K therapy can delay the onset of coagulopathy, but is not recommended as it may obscure the diagnosis and mandate prolonged coagulation profile monitoring, which might otherwise be unnecessary. Clotting factor analysis, particularly for factor VII, is a more sensitive and earlier indicator of coagulopathy [59]. Factor analysis does not offer more useful information in most patients with minimal ingestions, however. Occasionally, serum detection for warfarin and its derivatives has demonstrated unsuspected exposures in patients with coagulopathy of unknown cause [62,71]. In patients with coagulopathy, serial monitoring of warfarin derivative concentrations can assist in predicting the duration of coagulopathy and therapy [67].

The primary treatment of anticoagulant toxicity is vitamin K replacement [85,86]. Warfarin and its congeners have much less effect on human than on rat vitamin K reductase, thus allowing vitamin K rescue therapy for anticoagulant toxicity in humans. Because a single dose of vitamin K therapy cannot affect the prolonged toxicity of the long-acting anticoagulants, empiric vitamin K therapy is not recommended unless the patient has a coagulopathy. Vitamin K is not immediately effective in reversing coagulopathy; fresh-frozen plasma (FFP) administration is indicated in patients with significant bleeding diathesis (Table 141.3). Factor-specific concentrates have been demonstrated to decrease the time to correction of the INR in patients with a coagulopathy from warfarin toxicity faster than FFP [87]. The experience with these agents in the treatment of long-acting anticoagulant rodenticides, such as brodifacoum, is limited. Activated factor VII (FVIIa), FFP, and vitamin K have been used to treat brodifacoum toxicity [88,89]. In one of these instances, a product containing FVIIa and prothrombin complex concentrates (factor II, IX, and X) was used [88]. Some advantages of factor-specific concentrates over FFP include improved consistency in correction of the INR and decreased amount of fluid administered.

Only vitamin K_1 (phytonadione) should be used because the other forms (K_2, K_3, and K_4) are ineffective in the treatment of anticoagulant toxicity. Vitamin K_1 can be administered orally, subcutaneously, intramuscularly, and intravenously. Intravenous administration has been associated with anaphylactoid reactions and death [90–92]. Furthermore, it offers no real advantage over other routes of administration. Intramuscular injection may cause hematoma formation in patients with coagulopathy. Subcutaneous administration of vitamin K_1 is safe and effective. Oral vitamin K_1 may be simpler and just as efficacious [93]. The oral vitamin K_1 dose required to reverse coagulopathy is variable, but typically ranges from 100 to 300 mg per day, divided three to four times per day [61,66,80]. The amount

TABLE 141.3

TREATMENT GUIDELINES FOR COAGULOPATHY FROM LONG-ACTING WARFARIN-LIKE RODENTICIDES IN PATIENTS WITH NO UNDERLYING RISKS FOR THROMBOEMBOLISM

Active bleeding, major and life threatening

1. Factor replacement
   Fresh-frozen plasma (15 mL/kg)
   and
   Factor-specific concentrates, such as prothrombin complex concentrates (50 units/kg) or activated factor VII
   and
2. Vitamin K_1 intravenous (adult 10 mg, pediatrics 100 μg/kg by slow infusion)
3. Packed red blood cells for significant bleeding (i.e., anemia and hypotension)

No active bleeding and international normalized ratio (INR) $\geq$4.0

1. Vitamin K_1 intravenous (adult 10 mg, pediatrics 100 μg/kg by slow infusion)

Adapted from Leissinger CA, Blatt PM, Hoots WK, et al: Role of prothrombin complex concentrates in reversing warfarin anticoagulation: a review of the literature. *Am J Hematol* 83:137–143, 2008; and Watt BE, Proudfoot AT, Bradberry SM, et al: Anticoagulant rodenticides. *Toxicol Rev* 24:259–269, 2005.

of vitamin K therapy must be titrated to clinical response, however. The duration of vitamin K therapy and coagulopathy is also highly variable, ranging from 40 to 300 days. When the patient's INR has remained normal for several days after stopping the treatment, vitamin K therapy can be discontinued. The trend of the patient's concentration of clotting factors during this period may assist the determination of this clinical endpoint. Various methods have been proposed to decrease the duration of coagulopathy, including administration of hepatic enzyme inducers such as phenobarbital [64,66]. There is no good evidence to support any of these therapies, however.

STRYCHNINE

The use of strychnine as a pesticide dates back to the sixteenth century, when an extract of the Filipino St. Ignatius bean (*Strychnos ignatii*) was introduced as a rodenticide in Europe. Strychnine was used as a tonic, cathartic, and aphrodisiac as late as 1970, and resulted in numerous deaths [94]. It is also found as an adulterant in illicit drugs, such as cocaine and heroin. The only "legitimate" uses of strychnine today are as a pesticide and in research study of neural transmission [94,95].

Pharmacology

Strychnine is rapidly absorbed through the nasal mucosa and orally in the small intestine. It undergoes hepatic oxidative transformation to unknown metabolites [96], and only 10% to 20% is excreted unchanged in the urine within 24 hours. The half-life of strychnine in humans is 10 to 16 hours, and the volume of distribution is 13 L per kg [97,98].

Strychnine competitively antagonizes postsynaptic glycine receptors at the spinal cord and, to a lesser degree, at the brain stem, cerebral cortex, and hippocampus [95,99,100]. Strychnine-binding sites overlap, but are distinct from glycine-binding sites at the glycine receptor [100,101]. Glycine receptors at the cerebral cortex and hippocampus are of a subtype insensitive to strychnine and are minimally affected [95]. The action of glycine is similar to that of γ-aminobutyric acid in that it enhances chloride ionic channel conduction, resulting in hyperpolarization of postsynaptic membrane and an increased threshold for neurologic transmission [95,102]. The highest concentration of glycine receptors is found at the ventral horn motor neurons in the spinal cord [102]. Glycine antagonism reduces neuromuscular inhibition, including reciprocal inhibition between antagonistic muscles, resulting in contraction of both flexor and extensor muscle groups [103]. The pharmacologic effect of strychnine is quite similar to that of tetanus toxin, which inhibits the release of glycine at postsynaptic neurons in the spinal cord [102,104].

Clinical Toxicity

The onset of toxicity is usually within 15 to 30 minutes of exposure. The lethal dose in adults is typically 50 to 100 mg, but it may be as little as 5 to 10 mg in children [94,105]. Diffuse muscle contractions and spasms are the primary manifestations of strychnine toxicity. Facial muscle spasms result in risus sardonicus (the "sardonic smile") and trismus. Opisthotonos, abdominal muscle contractions, and tonic movements of the extremities may resemble convulsions. Because glycine has limited effects in the higher CNS centers, seizures are unlikely and mental status is normally preserved until the patient is hypoxic or moribund [94,105]. The extensor muscles appear to be more affected than the flexor muscles because they are the antigravity muscles and generally stronger [94,105]. Muscle contractions can be triggered or amplified by any stimulations, including auditory, tactile, and visual stimuli, and may lead to lactic acidosis, rhabdomyolysis, and hyperthermia [103,106]. Respiratory depression results from sustained chest and diaphragmatic muscle contractions and brain-stem depression. Death is related to respiratory depression, anoxia, and complications from significant muscle contractions [97,105]. The clinical manifestations of strychnine toxicity differ from tetanus infection in that the onset of symptoms in tetanus infection is more gradual and the duration of illness is more prolonged [104].

Management

Securing the airway, assisting breathing, and maintaining the circulatory system are the immediate goals in symptomatic patients. Electrolytes, acid–base changes, oxygenation saturation, renal function, urine output, and temperature must be monitored carefully in any symptomatic patient. GI decontamination should be performed in any case of suspected strychnine ingestion. Enhanced elimination by urinary manipulation has no effect because of minimal renal elimination [96]. Hemodialysis or charcoal hemoperfusion is ineffective because of the large volume of distribution.

Termination of muscle contractions prevents or reverses lactic acidosis, rhabdomyolysis, hyperthermia, and respiratory depression. Benzodiazepines are the initial agents of choice in attenuating musculoskeletal signs and symptoms [107–109]. Benzodiazepines enhance γ-aminobutyric acid effects in the spinal cord and may displace strychnine binding to glycine receptors [100,110,111]. Barbiturates also are reported to be useful in the treatment of strychnine toxicity. These agents may not be completely effective in patients with severe strychnine poisoning, however, and other agents such as propofol and adjunct nondepolarizing neuromuscular blockade may be required [98,105]. Strychnine toxicity usually resolves within

12 to 24 hours [96,103,112]. Supportive therapy should be continued until the patient is asymptomatic.

SODIUM MONOFLUOROACETATE

Sodium monofluoroacetate is frequently referred to as "compound 1080," the number assigned to the compound during its initial development. It is the primary toxic constituent in the South African gifblaar (*Dichapetalum cymosum*), but it is also present in other plants in South America and Australia. Fluoroacetate is highly toxic to all mammals, and its use was banned in the United States in 1972 because of human fatalities and indiscriminate extermination of nontarget species. The congener sodium fluoroacetamide (compound 1081), also used as a pesticide, has mechanisms and effects similar to those of fluoroacetate. Prior to compound 1080's ban in the United States in 1972, it was mostly used in livestock protection collars (tubular collars filled with pesticide, which is released when bitten by predators).

Pharmacology

Fluoroacetate appears to be minimally absorbed through skin but rapidly absorbed from the GI tract. It is metabolized to fluorocitrate in the tricarboxylic acid (TCA) cycle, with 12% of the ingested dose excreted in the urine [113]. In animals with relative resistance to monofluoroacetate, a hepatic defluorination system cleaves the carbon–fluoride bond to detoxify the compound [114].

Fluoroacetate is structurally similar to acetate and is incorporated into the TCA cycle with the assistance of acetyl coenzyme A. Fluoroacetate combines with citrate to form fluorocitrate in the TCA cycle [115]. Fluorocitrate inhibits aconitase and succinate dehydrogenase and disrupts the TCA cycle, halting cellular respiration and causing cell death [108,115,116]. Organs with high metabolic demands, such as the brain and heart, are immediately affected [117]. The lethal dose of sodium monofluoroacetate is 2 to 10 mg per kg [116].

Clinical Toxicity

The onset of poisoning occurs within 1 to 2 hours of exposure. Nausea and vomiting are followed by CNS and cardiovascular manifestations, which are the primary toxicities in humans [116,117]. The patient may present with agitation, lethargy, seizures, and coma [117–119]. Cardiovascular manifestations include tachycardia, premature ventricular contractions, ST-segment abnormalities, hypotension, ventricular tachycardia, and ventricular fibrillation [116]. Acute renal failure may be related to hypotension, rhabdomyolysis, and the direct toxic effects of monofluoroacetate on the kidney [117]. Fatality is related to CNS and cardiovascular toxicities [120,121]. Laboratory abnormalities include significant metabolic acidosis and hypocalcemia from the fluoride ion.

Management

General supportive measures are paramount and aimed at maintaining the airway, breathing, and circulation. Activated charcoal should be administered in all suspected oral exposures presenting within 1 to 2 hours after ingestion. Seizures should be treated with benzodiazepines or barbiturates. Hypocalcemia and prolonged QTc intervals may require calcium and magnesium supplementation. Various treatments have been tested in animals [122,123]. The most useful agent appears to be glyceryl monoacetate, which provides excess acetate as a substrate for the TCA cycle [122,124]. The clinical use of glyceryl monoacetate remains unproven, however.

ALUMINUM AND ZINC PHOSPHIDES

Aluminum and zinc phosphides are highly toxic insecticides and rodenticides commonly used as solid fumigants and grain preservatives. They are considered to be ideal pesticides for grain preservation because of the simplicity of application, low cost, and high efficacy without grain contamination. Although highly restricted in the United States, aluminum phosphide is widely available and commonly used for home grain storage in Asia and the Middle East. Typically, each pellet contains 3 g of 56% aluminum phosphide [125]. Aluminum phosphide has become one of the most common suicidal agents in India and other developing countries [10,125–128]. As little as 0.5 g can be fatal to an adult [129]. Phosphides are widely used in grain freighters and have emerged as the major maritime occupational health hazard [130]. Phosphine is slowly liberated when phosphides react with moisture in the environment.

Pharmacology

Phosphides react with water to form phosphine; the reaction is exothermic and it may be accelerated in the acidic environment of the stomach [126,131]. Phosphine is then readily absorbed in the stomach. Phosphine itself can also be absorbed through the lungs. There is limited information on the pharmacokinetics and metabolism of phosphine, although it is known to be partly eliminated through the lungs [131].

The exact mechanisms of toxicity have not been elucidated; the most likely mechanism is related to noncompetitive inhibition of cytochrome C oxidase. Also, phosphine increases the production of superoxide dismutase and lipid peroxidation [132]. As a cellular toxin, phosphine has deleterious effects on multiple organ systems, particularly organs with high metabolic demands.

Clinical Toxicity

Inhalation of phosphine gas results in immediate eye and mucus membrane irritation and early onset of pulmonary symptoms [126,129]. Oral ingestion of phosphides causes profound GI symptoms, including nausea, vomiting, and abdominal pain [125,129]. In these instances, esophageal lesions, such as ulcers, perforations, and strictures, can occur and they are typically associated with the ingestion of undiluted pellets [133,134]. Respiratory symptoms include cough, dyspnea, and chest tightness. Pulmonary edema and respiratory failure may be delayed for several hours after oral exposure to phosphides [125,135,136]. Hypotension and shock are expected within 6 hours in serious exposures. Fatalities are related to cardiovascular collapse from vasodilation and myocardial damage [137–139]. Various electrocardiographic changes have been reported, including ST-segment elevation and depression, QRS prolongation, bundle-branch blocks, atrioventricular nodal blockade, and supraventricular and ventricular tachycardia [140–142]. CNS effects lead to headache, lethargy, and encephalopathy [134]. Other manifestations include severe metabolic acidosis, hepatitis, and renal failure [137]. Mortality rates vary from 38% to 77% in suicidal ingestions [125,129,135,138,139].

Management

The patient should be immediately removed from the contaminated environment after the rescuer is adequately protected. Airway, breathing, and circulatory support are important in the immediate management. Activated charcoal should be mixed with sorbitol or magnesium citrate, rather than plain water, to reduce further liberation of phosphine in the GI tract [126]. Careful lavage with sodium bicarbonate (3% to 5% solution) or antacid has been advocated [143], but has not been adequately studied.

Cardiac monitoring and electrocardiography should be performed in suspected phosphine toxicity. Respiratory status should be monitored by continued clinical evaluation. Hypo- and hypermagnesemia have been reported with aluminum phosphide poisoning. Chest radiography, pulse oximetry, and arterial blood gases should be obtained as clinically indicated. The diagnosis may be suggested from a decaying fish odor released by substituted phosphines and diphosphines [126]. Silver nitrate–impregnated paper blackens in the presence of phosphine in the gastric fluid [144].

There is no antidote for phosphine poisoning. The mainstay of therapy is supportive care. Although intravenous magnesium therapy has been successful in treating various dysrhythmias [145–149], it has not been uniformly effective [150]. Magnesium therapy in phosphide poisoning should be considered in patients with dysrhythmias or hypomagnesemia.

METHYL BROMIDE

Methyl bromide (CH_3Br) is a colorless halogenated hydrocarbon gas primarily used as a fumigant for the control of nematodes, insects, rodents, fungi, and weeds. Methyl bromide has become one of the most widely used pesticides in the United States and worldwide since the abandonment of chlordane and acrylonitrile as fumigants [151,152]. Because methyl bromide causes ozone depletion in the stratosphere, the Montreal Protocol restricted its use in most developed countries since 2005. The United Nations proposed complete elimination of methyl bromide use worldwide by 2015. Methyl bromide was particularly popular in the food industry because it is extremely effective, is able to diffuse into any empty spaces, and does not leave any residues after proper ventilation. Space fumigation of fruits and tobacco can be performed in an airtight (fumigation) chamber. For soil fumigation, methyl bromide can be applied underground and sealed with an overlying tent or polyethylene cover. For structural fumigation, gas-proof tarpaulins are applied over the structure before the application of methyl bromide [153]. Methyl bromide is still used for the manufacture of chemicals such as aniline dyes. It has a musty and chloroform-like odor at high concentrations, but it is odorless at lower, but still very toxic, concentrations [154]. Because methyl bromide is heavier than air, it is particularly dangerous in an enclosed environment. Inadvertent exposures from accidents or inadequate ventilation have caused significant toxicities and fatalities [120,151,155–157].

Pharmacology

Methyl bromide is primarily absorbed through the lungs. Cutaneous absorption is minimal. Methyl bromide easily penetrates and is retained in cloth, rubber, and leather [153,158]. It is eliminated unchanged in the lungs, but a small proportion is metabolized to 5-methylcysteine and inorganic bromide; these are excreted in the urine [159].

The mechanism of toxicity is probably related to the methylation of sulfhydryl groups in different intracellular enzymes, as in heavy metal intoxication. Low concentrations of bromide can be detected in the serum after significant exposure to methyl bromide, but they do not correlate well with toxicity [151]. The symptoms of methyl bromide toxicity are distinctly different from those of bromide salt toxicity [160].

Toxic effects primarily involve the central nervous and pulmonary systems [151]. Although exposures to concentrations of 2,000 ppm or greater may produce immediate CNS depression and respiratory failure, symptoms may be delayed for 1 to 6 hours or longer with exposure to lower concentrations [153,157]. The current Occupational Safety and Health Administration permissible exposure limit for methyl bromide is 20 ppm [161].

Clinical Toxicity

Patients with mild toxicity may manifest dizziness, headache, confusion, weakness, nausea, vomiting, and dyspnea [120]. Initial or mild symptoms are frequently dismissed as viral symptoms [156]. Skin irritation and burns commonly underlie clothes and rubber gloves, where the methyl bromide gas is trapped [158]. After a significant exposure, the patient may present with tremor, myoclonus, and behavioral changes [121,162,163]. Severe toxicity may result in bronchitis, pulmonary edema, convulsions, and coma [151,157]. Fatality is related to pulmonary and CNS toxicities, although damage to different internal organs has been demonstrated [151,160,164]. Prolonged exposure to low concentrations of methyl bromide may cause subacute neurologic effects, such as headaches, confusion, behavioral changes, visual disturbance, and motor and sensory deficits [160,165–167]. Residual neurologic deficits may remain after significant acute or chronic exposure [160,164,168].

The essential laboratory studies in patients with methyl bromide intoxication are arterial blood gas or pulse oximetry monitoring. Chest radiography is useful in evaluating patients with pulmonary symptoms. Serum bromide concentrations may confirm exposure, but do not correlate with the severity of exposure. Serum bromide concentrations varied from 4.0 to 65.6 mg per dL in methyl bromide fatalities [151,160,169]. When the serum bromide concentration is significantly elevated, an elevated chloride concentration may be observed because of cross-reactivity in the analytical method [168].

Management

Treatment consists of supportive therapy, particularly of the airway, breathing, and circulation. Because methyl bromide is a gas, GI decontamination is not relevant. Clothing should be completely removed and the skin washed with soap and water to eliminate potential methyl bromide residues. Various compounds with sulfhydryl groups, such as dimercaprol and *N*-acetylcysteine, have been suggested as potential antidotes [158,162], but have not been demonstrated to be effective.

N,*N*-DIETHYL-*M*-TOLUAMIDE

N,*N*-diethyl-*m*-toluamide (diethyltoluamide, or DEET) was initially synthesized in 1954 and marketed as an insect repellent. Currently, DEET is the most effective and one of the most widely used insect repellents [170]. Use of DEET continues to increase with increasing public concern over Lyme disease and West Nile virus transmission. The concentration of DEET in the various products varies from 5% to 100%.

Pharmacology

DEET is well absorbed through the skin, with 48% of the applied dose absorbed within 6 hours. The plasma concentration peaks 1 hour after dermal application [171]. DEET is primarily metabolized in the liver, and 70% of the absorbed dose is excreted as metabolites within the first 24 hours. Another 10% to 15% is excreted unchanged in the urine [171]. DEET and its metabolites may accumulate in the fatty tissue, particularly after repeated applications.

The mechanism of DEET toxicity is unknown. Animals develop CNS symptoms similar to those reported in humans. Most reports of human poisoning involve children, likely because children absorb a higher ratio of DEET relative to their body weight. The initial theory suggested that patients with ornithine-carbamoyltransferase deficiency might be particularly susceptible to DEET toxicity [172]. However, recent reports have refuted this theory [173,174].

Clinical Toxicity

DEET may cause toxicity that is limited to skin irritation, contact dermatitis, skin necrosis, and urticaria [174–176]. Anaphylactic reactions have occasionally been reported with cutaneous application [176]. Manifestations of systemic poisoning vary from anxiety to behavioral changes, tremors, lethargy, ataxia, confusion, seizures, and coma [172–174,177–179]. Almost all of these case reports are related to application of concentrated DEET preparations or repeated application of lower concentration preparations [140,172,173,180].

Management

Treatment is largely supportive. Patients with dermal exposure should have their skin washed with soap and water to prevent further systemic absorption. Seizures may be treated with benzodiazepines. Neurologic workup may be required in many patients. The symptoms of DEET toxicity should be distinguished from those of Reye syndrome [172]. There is no antidote, and extracorporeal removal procedures are not helpful. Measures to prevent DEET toxicity may be the most important treatment. These include avoidance of concentrated DEET preparations. Products containing 20% to 30% DEET are adequate and safer than those with higher concentrations; concentrations of 10% or less are recommended for children. DEET should be applied only to exposed skin. An additional agent, such as permethrin, can be applied to clothing and may decrease the need of DEET [170]. The skin should be washed with soap when the insect repellent is no longer required, and the number of repeat applications should be limited.

PENTACHLOROPHENOL

Pentachlorophenol was first synthesized in 1841 and first used as a pesticide in 1936 [141]. It is primarily used as a wood preservative, however. Unlike other types of pesticide toxicity in adults, pentachlorophenol poisoning usually results from occupational exposure [142]. Occupational exposures to pentachlorophenol at wood-treating facilities frequently result from improper ventilation and inadequate engineering controls. Low-concentration, prolonged exposures to pentachlorophenol have been reported in log home residents from pentachlorophenol-treated wood [181]. Epidemics of infant poisoning have resulted from diapers improperly laundered with pentachlorophenol-containing antimicrobial soaps [182].

Pharmacology

Pentachlorophenol can be absorbed by the respiratory, oral, and dermal routes, although pulmonary absorption is the most efficient route. The volume of distribution is 0.35 L per kg and the pK_a is 5.0 [183]. Pentachlorophenol is primarily (74%) eliminated unchanged in the urine. A small proportion is oxidized to chlorohydroquinone, which is then eliminated in the urine. After a single oral exposure, the plasma half-life of pentachlorophenol is 27 to 35 hours [183]. Because of the low pK_a and significant renal elimination, pentachlorophenol elimination can be enhanced by urinary alkalinization [184].

The mechanism of toxicity of pentachlorophenol is similar to that of dinitrophenol: these agents uncouple oxidative phosphorylation by interfering with electron transport between flavoprotein and cytochrome P450.

Clinical Toxicity

Acute exposure results in headache, diaphoresis, nausea, vomiting, weakness, abdominal pain, and fever. With severe toxicity, significant hyperthermia (up to 108°F or 42.2°C), coma, convulsions, cerebral edema, and cardiovascular collapse may occur [141,185–187]. Laboratory studies may reveal a respiratory alkalosis and metabolic acidosis from significant exposures. Chronic exposures to pentachlorophenol have been reported to cause aplastic anemia, intravascular hemolysis, and pancreatitis [188–190]. Chloracne has also been reported from these exposures because of dioxin contamination in the product [186].

Management

Initial treatment includes oxygen supplementation, airway support, fluid resuscitation, and cardiac monitoring. Core temperature should be frequently monitored, and external cooling should be initiated immediately for significant hyperthermia. Seizures should be treated immediately with benzodiazepines or barbiturates to prevent further temperature increase and rhabdomyolysis. Fluid administration should be adequate to maintain a urine output of 1 to 2 mL per minute. Gastric decontamination (see Chapter 117) should be performed for oral exposure. The skin should be decontaminated with soap and water. Urinary alkalinization should be considered in patients with significant pentachlorophenol toxicity, although its clinical efficacy remains unproven [184].

PARAQUAT

Paraquat (1,1-dimethyl,4,4-bipyridyl dichloride) was developed in 1882 and for many years was used as an oxidation–reduction indicator. An electron donation to the compound forms a blue free radical; hence, paraquat was commonly called *methyl viologen*. The herbicidal properties of paraquat were discovered in 1955, and it was marketed as an herbicide in 1962. Today, paraquat is most commonly used as a nonselective contact herbicide in many countries. Paraquat can be applied safely when used according to the manufacturer's guidelines [191]. Typically, it is available as a 10% to 30% concentrated solution for agricultural use or as a 5% powder for domestic use. Once diluted, paraquat has limited absorption through the skin [192] and by aerosolization into the respiratory system [193]. Paraquat is naturally inactivated in the soil and leaves little active residue in the environment. Despite its many desirable properties, however, the consequences of ingesting concentrated paraquat products are deadly. The median lethal dose of paraquat is 3 to 5 g in adults [194]. As little as a mouthful (10 to 15 mL) of a 20% solution of paraquat is fatal. Paraquat ingestion is a prevalent method of suicide in countries such as Taiwan, Japan, Malaysia, the West Indies, and Samoa [10].

Pharmacology

Although oral exposure to paraquat is the most common route of toxicity, less than 5% of the ingested amount is actually absorbed [195]. Any recent food ingestion may decrease the amount of systemic absorption. The peak plasma concentration is reached within 1 to 2 hours after ingestion. Paraquat is almost completely eliminated unchanged by the renal system [195]. Plasma paraquat concentrations decline rapidly after peak absorption because of tissue distribution. The terminal plasma half-life of paraquat is 12 hours with normal renal function, but it may be as long as 120 hours as renal function deteriorates [196]. The volume of distribution of paraquat estimated from kinetic study in one patient is 2.75 L per kg. Paraquat is particularly sequestered in the lungs and kidneys [195].

Dermal absorption of paraquat is minimal unless the exposure is prolonged with concentrated solutions [192]. Aerosolized paraquat particles have a diameter greater than 5 μm and do not reach the lower respiratory tree [193]. Concern about paraquat absorption from smoking marijuana is unfounded because much of the paraquat is pyrolyzed during the smoking process [197]. Paraquat toxicity from marijuana smoking has not been reported.

The primary organ of toxicity is the lung because of selective accumulation of paraquat. Paraquat is actively transported into type I and II alveolar cells through an existing transport system for endogenous polyamines. Paraquat and polyamines share a common structural property: they have two positively charged quaternary nitrogen atoms separated by a distance of 6 to 7 nm [198]. Diquat, another related herbicide with different structural features, is not selectively taken up and does not cause pulmonary toxicity [198,199]. Inside the cell, paraquat undergoes a single-electron reduction into paraquat free radical. This free radical reacts with oxygen to form superoxide free radicals, which then deplete nicotinamide adenine dinucleotide phosphate, leading to lipid peroxidation and subsequent cellular destruction [200,201]. Also, this mechanism of action is responsible for the phytotoxic property of paraquat. There is also evidence for direct inhibition of electron chain transfers in mitochondria [200].

Clinical Toxicity

The onset and severity of poisoning is largely determined by the amount of exposure. Patients who ingest more than 40 mg per kg usually die within hours to a few days [202]. These patients experience multiple organ failure, including acute respiratory distress syndrome, cerebral edema, myocardial necrosis, and hepatic and renal failure [202–205]. Death can be dramatic and may occur even before the development of significant chest radiographic abnormalities [202]. Patients who ingest 20 to 40 mg per kg of paraquat are most likely to die from pulmonary fibrosis, which progresses after a few days to a few weeks [206,207]. Ingestion of less than 20 mg per kg may lead to mild toxicity [202,206].

Paraquat is extremely corrosive to mucus membranes, and patients frequently complain of pain in the mouth, throat, esophagus, and abdomen [203,206]. The absence of significant ulcerations in the esophagus or stomach within the first 24 hours of exposure is a good prognostic indicator [203]. The development of renal failure is a poor prognostic indicator [196,203,208]. This phenomenon cannot be fully explained by the decreased elimination of paraquat in the body because most of the paraquat dose is eliminated within the first 24 hours, even in the setting of renal failure [196,209]. Conversely, renal failure may signify a large paraquat exposure. Almost all patients with renal failure from paraquat have significant pulmonary toxicity, but there are occasional reports of renal failure without significant pulmonary toxicity [205]. The prognosis for a patient with paraquat ingestion can be determined by the measurement of plasma paraquat concentration and its relation to time of ingestion [210]. The nomogram initially was presented by Proudfoot et al. [211] and subsequently refined by Hart et al. [210]. The availability of paraquat measurements depends on regional practice because the laboratory analysis is not routine. Although it is generally accepted that paraquat is not absorbed through the skin, it can be corrosive to the skin and nails [192]. Occasionally, dermal absorption and systemic toxicity may occur from prolonged exposure or exposure to concentrated products [212].

Management

It is critical to prevent systemic absorption of paraquat. Once ingested, it is rapidly absorbed and sequestered, frequently leading to death [205]. GI decontamination should be performed in any suspected paraquat ingestion. Orogastric lavage should be performed if the ingestion is within 1 to 2 hours. Fuller's earth (1 to 2 g per kg) or activated charcoal should be administered with a cathartic agent as soon as possible to bind any residual paraquat in the GI tract [213–215]. Multiple doses of oral adsorbents should be continued until there is evidence of adsorbent in the stool. This is done to prevent desorption of the paraquat. Any dermal exposure should be thoroughly washed with soap. Plasma and urine analytical methods to detect paraquat are useful to confirm the diagnosis and assess the prognosis; they are generally not useful in direct management of the patient. A rapid qualitative screen for paraquat exposure may be performed by the addition of sodium dithionite to urine under alkaline condition, however. A change in color to blue confirms paraquat's absorption [216]. Furthermore, prognosis may be predicted by the degree of color change: dark blue for poor prognosis and light blue for moderate-to-severe poisoning [217].

The treatment of paraquat toxicity consists of supportive care, particularly respiratory monitoring and support. Chest radiographs, judicious administration of supplemental oxygen, and monitoring for acute respiratory distress syndrome and impending respiratory failure are important in patients with significant exposure. Excessive oxygen supplementation may increase the formation of paraquat free radicals and worsen pulmonary toxicity [218]. Supplemental oxygen should be administered only when it is necessary and should be maintained at the minimal required level.

Experimental therapies for paraquat toxicity have been formulated using various strategies [200,208]. Forced diuresis does not have significant effects on paraquat elimination. Hemodialysis and charcoal hemoperfusion can increase elimination. In an animal model, the institution of charcoal hemoperfusion within 2 hours after paraquat ingestion decreased the fatality rate [219], and institution of hemoperfusion 2 hours after paraquat administration did not alter the paraquat concentration in the central compartment [220,221]. Clinically, hemodialysis, charcoal hemoperfusion, and continuous arteriovenous hemofiltration have not altered mortality rates. There are significant limitations in applying extracorporeal procedures. Because the volume of distribution of paraquat is relatively large and paraquat is rapidly sequestered into tissue compartments, extracorporeal removal must be performed during peak absorption (within 2 hours after ingestion) to significantly decrease the paraquat body load. Because most patients present a number of hours after ingestion and the logistics of extracorporeal removal typically translate into an additional 1- to 2-hour delay, the amount of paraquat removed in most instances is insignificant.

Immunotherapy with monoclonal antibody fragments (Fab, Fv) against paraquat or against the active transport mechanism in the cells is intriguing [222,223]. More research is required to assess the value of this therapy, however. Various agents such as putrescine and spermidine [224,225] and β-adrenergic receptor blockers have been demonstrated to prevent active transport of paraquat into lung tissues but failed to provide any benefits in vivo.

Various antioxidants and free radical scavengers, such as vitamins C and E [201,208,226], deferoxamine [227], superoxide dismutase [228], clofibrate [208], selenium [229], glutathione peroxide, and *N*-acetylcysteine [230,231], have been tested against paraquat toxicity. To date, there has been no or insignificant improvement in animal models. A recent study using inhaled nitric oxide in rats demonstrated benefits in preventing pulmonary injuries and survival. Several studies have demonstrated increased patient survival with corticosteroids and cyclophosphamide therapy [232–238]. The use of methylprednisolone and cyclophosphamide to limit the acute inflammatory response from paraquat toxicity appears to decrease mortality in patients with moderate-to-severe poisoning from ingested paraquat on the basis of prospective controlled trials [237,238]. In a randomized-controlled trial, paraquat-poisoned patients with a predicted mortality of 50% or greater and less than 90% and treated with pulse-dose methylprednisolone and cyclophosphamide (Table 141.4) were less likely to die at 6 weeks than those who did not receive the treatment (mortality rate: 5/16, 31.3% vs. 6/7, 85.7%) (Table 141.5)

TABLE 141.4

TREATMENT GUIDELINES FOR PULSE-DOSE METHYLPREDNISOLONE AND CYCLOPHOSPHAMIDE IN PATIENTS WITH PARAQUAT TOXICITY [237][a]

Initial pulse-dose therapy
Cyclophosphamide 15 mg/kg/d administered as an infusion in 200 mL D5NS over 2 h for 2 d
Methylprednisolone 1 g/d administered as an infusion in 200 mL D5NS over 2 h for 3 d
After initial pulse-dose therapy
Dexamethasone 5 mg IV every 6 h until $PaO_2 \geq 80$ mm Hg or death
If $PaO_2 < 60$ mm Hg after initial pulse therapy, repeat pulse-dose therapy with
Methylprednisolone 1 g/d administered as an infusion in 200 mL D5NS over 2 h for 3 d, and
If WBC >3,000 per μL at >2 wk after initial pulse-dose therapy, add
Cyclophosphamide 15 mg/kg/d administered as an infusion in 200 mL D5NS over 2 h for 1 d

[a]Initiated after gastrointestinal decontamination and two sessions of charcoal hemoperfusion within 24 h of ingesting paraquat in patients with moderate-to-severe toxicity.

[237]. All patients received GI decontamination and two sessions of charcoal hemoperfusion within 24 hours of hospitalization, which were completed prior to the initiation of the pulse-dose therapy. Methylprednisolone and cyclophosphamide do not appear to affect the mortality rate in patients with mild and fulminant paraquat poisonings [217,236]. Cyclophosphamide can cause a transient leukopenia (WBC <3,000 per μL) in patients treated with the protocol [233,237]. Additional clinical trials at other centers are needed to verify that pulse-dose therapy with methylprednisolone and cyclophosphamide improves survival in patients with paraquat toxicity.

Other agents that may alter pulmonary fibrosis, such as colchicine [239], nonsteroidal anti-inflammatory agents, collagen synthesis inhibitors [240], and angiotensin-converting enzyme inhibitors [241], also require further study. Niacin, which increases nicotinamide adenine dinucleotide phosphate synthesis, has some protective effects in rats, but it is unclear if it is applicable to human toxicity [242].

Early lung transplantation has been unsuccessful because of toxicity to the transplanted lung from paraquat distributing from tissue stores [243,244]. A successful case of lung transplantation was performed in a patient 44 days after paraquat poisoning, however [245].

DIQUAT

Diquat (1,1′-ethylene-2,2′-dipyridylium ion) is a contact herbicide with action and structure similar to that of paraquat. Diquat and paraquat liberate hydrogen peroxide and oxygen free radicals, resulting in toxicity to plants and animals. The use of diquat is more limited and hence results in fewer intoxications than paraquat. Diquat is often formulated with paraquat.

Pharmacology

The kinetics of diquat are unknown in humans. In animal models, less than 10% of the oral dose is absorbed. More than 90% of the absorbed dose is eliminated unchanged by the kidneys. There are no known metabolites of diquat.

Although diquat is less toxic than paraquat, human fatalities have been reported with ingestion of 20 to 50 mL of a 20% solution [246]. Similar to paraquat, diquat causes multiple organ damage. Diquat normally spares the pulmonary system, however [246]. This is because diquat is not actively transported to and concentrated in the alveolar cells of the lungs [199].

Clinical Toxicity

Symptoms of diquat toxicity may be delayed several hours to 2 days [247]. Vomiting, abdominal pain, GI tract erosions, and paralytic ileus are common manifestations of toxicity [246,248,249]. Acute renal failure may be related to hypovolemia and the direct toxic effects. The effects of diquat on the CNS may result in lethargy, seizures, and coma [248,250]. Brain stem infarctions may be specific to diquat toxicity. All patients who die have significant CNS manifestations before cardiovascular collapse [246,249].

Management

Treatment is largely supportive and similar to that for paraquat. Gastric lavage should be performed for any potential diquat ingestion within 2 hours. Fuller's earth or activated charcoal should be administered as soon as possible. Hemodialysis or

TABLE 141.5

SUMMARY OF RECOMMENDATIONS BASED ON RANDOMIZED-CONTROLLED CLINICAL TRIAL FOR THE USE OF CYCLOPHOSPHAMIDE AND METHYLPREDNISOLONE IN PATIENTS WITH PARAQUAT POISONING

Reference	Population	Intervention	Control	Primary outcome	Design	Effect measure	Summary
Lin et al, 2006 [237]	23 paraquat-poisoned patients admitted to a single facility within 24 h of exposure with a predictive mortality ≥50% and <90%, a dark-blue or navy-blue urine dithionite test, and >15 y in age; patients with other routes of exposure and significant comorbidities, such as cancer, were excluded; 100% intentional self-harm; mean times to initiation of gastrointestinal decontamination and charcoal hemoperfusion since exposure in interventional and control groups were ≤7.5 h; mean plasma paraquat concentration (mg/L): control 6.4 ± 5.4, interventional 5.9 ± 4.9; prevalence of predictive mortality ≥80% and <90% was 42.9% in control group and 50% in interventional group	*Initial pulse-dose therapy:* Cyclophosphamide 15 mg/kg/d IV in 200 mL D5NS over 2 h for 2 d Methylprednisolone 1 g/d IV in 200 mL D5NS over 2 h for 3 d *Second pulse-dose therapy:* If PaO_2 <60 mm Hg, methylprednisolone 1 g/d IV in 200 mL D5NS over 2 h for 3 d, *and* If WBC >3,000 per μL at >2 wk after initial pulse-dose therapy, cyclophosphamide 15 mg/kg/d IV in 200 mL D5NS over 2 h for 1 d	Dexamethasone 5 mg IV every 6 h until PaO_2 ≥80 mm Hg or death	Mortality at the end of 6 wk	Randomized-controlled trial; blinded during data analysis	Mortality rate, *n* (%): 6/7 (85.7%) control group, 5/16 (31.3%) intervention group, $P = 0.272$	Pulse-dose therapy with cyclophosphamide and methylprednisolone appeared to decrease the mortality rate in patients with moderate-to-severe poisoning from the ingestion of paraquat

hemoperfusion has not been demonstrated to be effective for the treatment of diquat toxicity [246,249,251,252].

CHLOROPHENOXY HERBICIDES

Chlorophenoxy herbicides are used to control broad-leaf weeds and woody plants. They exert their effects by mimicking the action of auxins (plant growth hormones) and cause overstimulation of plant growth. Numerous derivatives are available for agricultural and domestic use [253]. The most commonly used agents include 2,4-dichlorophenoxyacetic acid (2,4-D), 2,4,5-trichlorophenoxyacetic acid (2,4,5-T), and 2-methyl-4-chlorophenoxypropionic acid. Many preparations contain more than one chlorophenoxy herbicide or other types of herbicides. Despite extensive use of these agents, fatality and significant toxicity are limited. The chlorophenoxy herbicides are notorious because of dioxin contamination in Agent Orange, a 1-to-1 mixture of 2,4-D and 2,4,5-T used extensively in the Vietnam War, so named for the color of the drums used to store it. Agent Orange contained dioxin (2,3,7, 9-tetrachlorodibenzodioxin), a contaminant in the synthesis of chlorophenoxy compounds and a potent teratogen in animals [254,255].

Pharmacology

In general, chlorophenoxy herbicides are well absorbed orally. They have small volumes of distribution, large renal excretion, and a low pK_a [253]. 2,4-D has a volume of distribution of 0.1 to 0.3 L per kg and a pK_a of 2.6 to 3.5 [256]. Oral doses of 5 mg per kg in human volunteers produce no ill effects. The peak serum concentration is achieved within 4 to 12 hours [257], 80% of the absorbed dose is eliminated unchanged in the urine, and 13% is eliminated as acid-labile conjugates. The plasma half-life is 18 to 40 hours and varies with urine pH; it may range from 4 to 220 hours [258]. The volume of distribution of 2,4,5-T is 6.1 L per kg. It is exclusively excreted unchanged in the urine, and the plasma half-life is 11 to 23 hours [259].

Various mechanisms of toxicity in humans are postulated. Uncoupling of oxidative phosphorylation has been demonstrated in vitro and may be responsible for a mild heat exhaustion syndrome [260,261]. Chlorophenoxy herbicides can interfere with the TCA cycle and cellular metabolism by forming analogues with acetyl coenzyme A [259,260]. There may be other direct toxic effects on skeletal muscles and peripheral nerves [262].

Clinical Toxicity

GI symptoms are common, and patients frequently experience nausea, vomiting, diarrhea, and abdominal pain [261,263, 264]. Ulcerations may occur at the mouth and pharynx, but are uncommon elsewhere in the GI tract [260]. A mild heat exhaustion syndrome consisting of fever, diaphoresis, and hyperventilation can be seen [261,263]. The CNS is particularly affected, and patients may present with confusion, lethargy, convulsions, and coma [263,265]. Prolonged coma (up to 4 days) has been reported with 2,4-D toxicity [266]. Myotonia, rhabdomyolysis, and chronic muscle weakness are also reported [264]. Renal complications may result from rhabdomyolysis and myoglobinuria [267]. Hypocalcemia may occasionally be seen as a result of rhabdomyolysis and hyperphosphatemia [265,268]. Fatality is uncommon, and the cause of death remains unclear [258,260,264,268–270].

Management

Gastric decontamination with lavage should be performed within 1 to 2 hours of ingestion. Skin should be decontaminated with soap and water. Basic supportive therapies include the maintenance of good urine output (1 to 2 mL per kg per hour) with fluid resuscitation and external cooling for hyperthermia. Because of the low pK_a and renal elimination of chlorophenoxy herbicides, urinary alkalinization can significantly enhance renal excretion and decrease the plasma half-life of various chlorophenoxy herbicides [263]. Thus, it should be initiated in patients with significant toxicity by using a sodium bicarbonate infusion to titrate the urinary pH to 7.50 to 8.0. The patient's fluid status should be closely monitored because renal dysfunction may develop from chlorophenoxy herbicide toxicity. Although the utility of extracorporeal elimination of chlorophenoxy herbicides in poisoned patients has not been studied, hemodialysis may be useful for 2,4-D because of its small volume of distribution. Patients with renal insufficiency and significant toxicity would gain the most benefit from hemodialysis.

CHLORATE SALTS

Chlorate salts (sodium chlorate [$NaClO_3$] and potassium chlorate [$KClO_3$]) are nonspecific herbicides. They are also used in the manufacture of explosives, dyestuffs, tanning agents, and matches.

Pharmacology

Chlorates are strong oxidizing agents that result in hemolysis and methemoglobinemia. They have direct toxic effects on the kidneys and indirect nephrotoxicity from hemoglobinuria. Because chlorates are primarily eliminated by the kidneys, nephrotoxicity further enhances their toxicity. The acute lethal dose is 25 to 35 g [271].

Clinical Toxicity

GI symptoms are prominent within hours after an acute exposure and include nausea, vomiting, diarrhea, and abdominal pain [271–273]. Hemolytic anemia and methemoglobinemia result from the oxidizing effects. Both entities may result in a significantly decreased oxygen-carrying capacity and cellular hypoxia [272,274]. Cyanosis may be evident with significant methemoglobinemia. Acute renal failure typically develops within 48 hours after exposure [271,273,275]. Significant hyperkalemia from hemolysis is another potential fatal complication.

Management

Initial supportive care should be directed at the airway, breathing, and maintenance of circulation. Continuous cardiac monitoring should be initiated. Gastric decontamination should be performed within 2 hours after ingestion unless the patient already has significant vomiting. Laboratory studies should include hemoglobin, serum electrolytes, blood urea nitrogen, creatinine, and methemoglobin concentrations. Electrocardiogram and arterial blood gas should be obtained as clinically indicated. Intravenous or oral sodium thiosulfate (2 to 5 g) has been advocated to inactivate the chlorate ion, but its efficacy has not been clinically proven [276]. Methylene blue should be administered for clinically significant methemoglobinemia, but it may not be effective in the setting of significant hemolysis because intact intracellular enzymes are required for its therapeutic effect [277]. Methylene blue is indicated in patients with a methemoglobin concentration of more than 20% or at a lower value in symptomatic patients with anemia. The initial dose is 1 to 2 mg per kg administered IV over 5 minutes and a response is anticipated within 30 minutes. Subsequent doses of methylene blue can be administered if there is an initial success, but it is withheld if no response is observed. Exchange transfusion may be required for refractory methemoglobinemia or significant hemolysis. Hemodialysis can remove chlorates and is recommended in patients with associated renal dysfunction [271,276].

ACKNOWLEDGMENT

This chapter was written by Richard Y. Wang in his private capacity. No official support or endorsement by the Centers for Disease Control and Prevention (CDC) is intended or should be inferred. The views expressed in this chapter do not necessarily represent the views of CDC or the United States.

References

1. Ferrer A, Cabral JP: Epidemics due to pesticide contamination of food. *Food Addit Contam* 6[Suppl 1]:S95–S98, 1989.
2. Hayes WJ: Introduction, in Hayes WJ, Laws ER (eds): *Handbook of Pesticide Toxicology*. San Diego, Academic Press, 1991, p 1.
3. Turnbull GJ: Pesticide residues in food—a toxicological view: discussion paper. *J R Soc Med* 77:932–935, 1984.
4. Pearce NE, Sheppard RA, Smith AH, et al: Non-Hodgkin's lymphoma and farming: an expanded case-control study. *Int J Cancer* 39:155–161, 1987.
5. Wiklund K, Dich J, Holm LE: Risk of malignant lymphoma in Swedish pesticide appliers. *Br J Cancer* 56:505–508, 1987.
6. Wilson J: Environmental chemicals, in Wilson JG, Fraser FC (eds): *Handbook of Teratology General Principles and Etiology*. New York, Plenum Press, 1977, p 357.
7. Donat H, Matthies J, Schwarz I: Fertility of workers exposed to herbicides and pesticides. *Andrologia* 22:401–407, 1990.
8. Semchuk KM, Love EJ, Lee RG: Parkinson's disease and exposure to agricultural work and pesticide chemicals. *Neurology* 42:1328–1335, 1992.
9. Tanner CM, Langston JW: Do environmental toxins cause Parkinson's disease? A critical review. *Neurology* 40[Suppl 17–30]; discussion 30–11, 1990.
10. Eddleston M: Patterns and problems of deliberate self-poisoning in the developing world. *Q J Med* 93:715–731, 2000.
11. Jeyaratnam J: Acute pesticide poisoning: a major global health problem. *World Health Stat Q* 43:139–144, 1990.
12. Levine RS, Doull J: Global estimates of acute pesticide morbidity and mortality. *Rev Environ Contam Toxicol* 129:29–50, 1992.
13. Centers for Disease Control and Prevention: National Center for Environmental Health/Fact Sheet/Pesticides, 2004. Available at: http://www.cdc.gov/nceh/hsb/pesticides/activities.htm, June 25, 2009.
14. Bodeker W: Suicidal pesticide poisoning. *World Health Forum* 12:208–209, 1991.
15. Chao HR, Wang SL, Lin TC, et al: Levels of organochlorine pesticides in human milk from central Taiwan. *Chemosphere* 62:1774–1785, 2006.
16. Roncevic N, Pavkov S, Galetin-Smith R, et al: Serum concentrations of organochlorine compounds during pregnancy and the newborn. *Bull Environ Contam Toxicol* 38:117–124, 1987.
17. Saxena MC, Siddiqui MK, Agarwal V, et al: A comparison of organochlorine insecticide contents in specimens of maternal blood, placenta, and umbilical-cord blood from stillborn and live-born cases. *J Toxicol Environ Health* 11:71–79, 1983.
18. U.S. Environmental Protection Agency: Reregistration eligibility decision for endosulfan, 2002. Available at: http://www.epa.gov/oppsrrd1/reregistration/REDs/endosulfan_red.pdf, June 25, 2009.
19. Palmer AK, Cozens DD, Spicer EJ, et al: Effects of lindane upon reproductive function in a 3-generation study in rats. *Toxicology* 10:45–54, 1978.
20. Conney AH, Welch RM, Kuntzman R, et al: Effects of pesticides on drug and steroid metabolism. *Clin Pharmacol Ther* 8:2–10, 1967.
21. Kutz FW, Strassman SC, Sperling JF, et al: A fatal chlordane poisoning. *J Toxicol Clin Toxicol* 20:167–174, 1983.
22. Olanoff LS, Bristow WJ, Colcolough J Jr, et al: Acute chlordane intoxication. *J Toxicol Clin Toxicol* 20:291–306, 1983.
23. Hunter CG, Robinson J, Roberts M: Pharmacodynamics of dieldrin (HEOD). Ingestion by human subjects for 18 to 24 months, and postexposure for eight months. *Arch Environ Health* 18:12–21, 1969.
24. Hayes W: Chlorinated hydrocarbon insecticides, in Hayes WJ (ed): *Pesticides Studied in Man*. Baltimore, Williams & Wilkins, 1982, p 172.
25. Shankland DL: Neurotoxic action of chlorinated hydrocarbon insecticides. *Neurobehav Toxicol Teratol* 4:805–811, 1982.
26. Matsumura F, Ghiasuddin SM: DDT sensitive Ca ATPase in the axonic membrane, in Narahashi T (ed): *Neurotoxicology of Insecticides and Pheromones*. New York, Plenum, 1979, p 245.
27. Morgan DP, Roberts RJ, Walter AW, et al: Anemia associated with exposure to lindane. *Arch Environ Health* 35:307–310, 1980.
28. Nigma SK, Karnik AB, Majumber SK, et al: Serum hexachlorocyclohexane residues in workers engaged at a HCH manufacturing plant. *Int Arch Occup Environ Health* 57:315, 1986.
29. Kazantzis G, McLaughlin AI, Prior PF: Poisoning in Industrial Workers by the Insecticide Aldrin. *Br J Ind Med* 21:46–51, 1964.
30. Patel TB, Rao VN: Dieldrin poisoning in man; a report of 20 cases observed in Bombay State. *Br Med J* 1:919–921, 1958.
31. Telch J, Jarvis DA: Acute intoxication with lindane. *Can Med Assoc J* 127:821, 1982.
32. Goldberg LH, Shupp D, Weitz HH, et al: Injection of household spray insecticide. *Ann Emerg Med* 11:626–629, 1982.
33. Wills J: Effects of chlorinated hydrocarbons on smaller animals as guides in the design of experiments with human volunteers, in Miller MW, Berg GG (eds): *Chemical Fallout; Current Research on Persistent Pesticides*. Springfield, Thomas, 1969, p 461.
34. Centers for Disease Control and Prevention: Unintentional topical lindane ingestions—United States, 1998–2003. *MMWR Morb Mortal Wkly Rep* 54:533–535, 2005.
35. Eyer F, Felgenhauer N, Jetzinger E, et al: Acute endosulfan poisoning with cerebral edema and cardiac failure. *J Toxicol Clin Toxicol* 42:927–932, 2004.
36. Rowley DL, Rab MA, Hardjotanojo W, et al: Convulsions caused by endrin poisoning in Pakistan. *Pediatrics* 79:928–934, 1987.
37. Runhaar EA, Sangster B, Greve PA, et al: A case of fatal endrin poisoning. *Hum Toxicol* 4:241–247, 1985.
38. Wells WL, Milhorn HT Jr: Suicide attempt by toxaphene ingestion: a case report. *J Miss State Med Assoc* 24:329–330, 1983.
39. Ozucelik DN, Karcioglu O, Topacoglu H, et al: Toxicity following unintentional DDT ingestion. *J Toxicol Clin Toxicol* 42:299–303, 2004.
40. Shemesh Y, Bourvine A, Gold D, et al: Survival after acute endosulfan intoxication. *J Toxicol Clin Toxicol* 26:265–268, 1988.
41. Taylor JR: Neurological manifestations in humans exposed to chlordecone: follow-up results. *Neurotoxicology* 6:231–236, 1985.
42. He F, Sun J, Han K, et al: Effects of pyrethroid insecticides on subjects engaged in packaging pyrethroids. *Br J Ind Med* 45:548–551, 1988.
43. Kashyap SK: Health surveillance and biological monitoring of pesticide formulators in India. *Toxicol Lett* 33:107–114, 1986.
44. Poulos L, Athanaselis S, Coutselinis A: Acute intoxication with cypermethrin (NRDC 149). *J Toxicol Clin Toxicol* 19:519–520, 1982.
45. Aldrich FD, Holmes JH: Acute chlordane intoxication in a child. Case report with toxicological data. *Arch Environ Health* 19:129–132, 1969.
46. Barnes R: Poisoning by the insecticide chlordane. *Med J Aust* 1:972–973, 1967.
47. Berry DH, Brewster MA, Watson R, et al: Untoward effects associated with lindane abuse. *Am J Dis Child* 141:125–126, 1987.
48. International Agency for Research on Cancer: IARC Monographs. Available at: http://monographs.iarc.fr/ENG/Classification/index.php, June 25, 2009.
49. *National Toxicology Program: Report on Carcinogens*. 11th ed. Research Triangle Park, U.S. Department of Health and Human Services, Public Health Service, 2004. Available at: http://ntp.niehs.nih.gov/ntp/roc/toc11.html, June 25, 2009.
50. Frank R, Braun HE, Stonefield KI, et al: Organochlorine and organophosphorus residues in the fat of domestic farm animal species, Ontario, Canada 1986–1988. *Food Addit Contam* 7:629–636, 1990.
51. Nitsche K, Lange M, Bauer E, et al: Quantitative distribution of locally applied lindane in human skin and subcutaneous fat in vitro. Dependence of penetration on the applied concentration, skin state, duration of action and nature and time of washing. *Derm Beruf Umwelt* 32:161–165, 1984.

52. Daerr W, Kaukel E, Schmoldt A: Hemoperfusion—a therapeutic alternative to early treatment of acute lindane poisoning. *Dtsch Med Wochenschr* 110:1253–1255, 1985.
53. Tilson HA, Hong JS, Mactutus CF: Effects of 5,5-diphenylhydantoin (phenytoin) on neurobehavioral toxicity of organochlorine insecticides and permethrin. *J Pharmacol Exp Ther* 233:285–289, 1985.
54. Tilson HA, Shaw S, McLamb RL: The effects of lindane, DDT, and chlordecone on avoidance responding and seizure activity. *Toxicol Appl Pharmacol* 88:57–65, 1987.
55. He F, Wang S, Liu L, et al: Clinical manifestations and diagnosis of acute pyrethroid poisoning. *Arch Toxicol* 63:54–58, 1989.
56. Wax PM, Hoffman RS: Fatality associated with inhalation of a pyrethrin shampoo. *J Toxicol Clin Toxicol* 32:457–460, 1994.
57. Yang PY, Lin JL, Hall AH, et al: Acute ingestion poisoning with insecticide formulations containing the pyrethroid permethrin, xylene, and surfactant: a review of 48 cases. *J Toxicol Clin Toxicol* 40:107–113, 2002.
58. Tripathi M, Pandey R, Ambesh SP, et al: A mixture of organophosphate and pyrethroid intoxication requiring intensive care unit admission: a diagnostic dilemma and therapeutic approach. *Anesth Analg* 103:410–412, table of contents, 2006.
59. Smolinske SC, Scherger DL, Kearns PS, et al: Superwarfarin poisoning in children: a prospective study. *Pediatrics* 84:490–494, 1989.
60. Burucoa C, Mura P, Robert R, et al: Chlorophacinone intoxication. A biological and toxicological study. *J Toxicol Clin Toxicol* 27:79–89, 1989.
61. Chow EY, Haley LP, Vickars LM, et al: A case of bromadiolone (superwarfarin) ingestion. *CMAJ* 147:60–62, 1992.
62. Weitzel JN, Sadowski JA, Furie BC, et al: Surreptitious ingestion of a long-acting vitamin K antagonist/rodenticide, brodifacoum: clinical and metabolic studies of three cases. *Blood* 76:2555–2559, 1990.
63. Baselt RC: Brodifacoum, in Baselt RC (ed): *Disposition of Toxic Drugs and Chemicals in Man.* 7th ed. Foster City, Biomedical Publications, 2004, p 124.
64. Bachmann KA, Sullivan TJ: Dispositional and pharmacodynamic characteristics of brodifacoum in warfarin-sensitive rats. *Pharmacology* 27:281–288, 1983.
65. Breckenridge AM, Cholerton S, Hart JA, et al: A study of the relationship between the pharmacokinetics and the pharmacodynamics of the 4-hydroxycoumarin anticoagulants warfarin, difenacoum and brodifacoum in the rabbit. *Br J Pharmacol* 84:81–91, 1985.
66. Lipton RA, Klass EM: Human ingestion of a "superwarfarin" rodenticide resulting in a prolonged anticoagulant effect. *JAMA* 252:3004–3005, 1984.
67. Bruno GR, Howland MA, McMeeking A, et al: Long-acting anticoagulant overdose: brodifacoum kinetics and optimal vitamin K dosing. *Ann Emerg Med* 36:262–267, 2000.
68. Hollinger BR, Pastoor TP: Case management and plasma half-life in a case of brodifacoum poisoning. *Arch Intern Med* 153:1925–1928, 1993.
69. Lewis-Younger C, Horowitz Z: Elimination of brodifacoum [abstract]. *J Toxicol Clin Toxicol* 39:474, 2001.
70. Wessler S, Gitel SN: Warfarin. From bedside to bench. *N Engl J Med* 311:645–652, 1984.
71. Jones EC, Growe GH, Naiman SC: Prolonged anticoagulation in rat poisoning. *JAMA* 252:3005–3007, 1984.
72. Watts RG, Castleberry RP, Sadowski JA: Accidental poisoning with a superwarfarin compound (brodifacoum) in a child. *Pediatrics* 86:883–887, 1990.
73. Murdoch DA: Prolonged anticoagulation in chlorphacinone poisoning. *Lancet* 1:355–356, 1983.
74. Chong LL, Chau WK, Ho CH: A case of "superwarfarin" poisoning. *Scand J Haematol* 36:314–315, 1986.
75. Fasco MJ, Hildebrandt EF, Suttie JW: Evidence that warfarin anticoagulant action involves two distinct reductase activities. *J Biol Chem* 257:11210–11212, 1982.
76. Furie B, Furie BC: Molecular basis of vitamin K-dependent gamma-carboxylation. *Blood* 75:1753–1762, 1990.
77. Hirsh J: Oral anticoagulant drugs. *N Engl J Med* 324:1865–1875, 1991.
78. Majerus PW, Tollefsen DM: Blood coagulation and anticoagulant, thrombolytic, and antiplatelet drugs, in Goodman LS, Gilman A, Brunton LL, et al (eds): *Goodman & Gilman's the Pharmacological Basis of Therapeutics.* 11th ed. New York, McGraw-Hill, 2006.
79. Greeff MC, Mashile O, MacDougall LG: "Superwarfarin" (bromodialone) poisoning in two children resulting in prolonged anticoagulation. *Lancet* 2:1269, 1987.
80. Barnett VT, Bergmann F, Humphrey H, Chediak J: Diffuse alveolar hemorrhage secondary to superwarfarin ingestion. *Chest* 102:1301–1302, 1992.
81. Hoffman RS, Smilkstein MJ, Goldfrank LR: Evaluation of coagulation factor abnormalities in long-acting anticoagulant overdose. *J Toxicol Clin Toxicol* 26:233–248, 1988.
82. Kruse JA, Carlson RW: Fatal rodenticide poisoning with brodifacoum. *Ann Emerg Med* 21:331–336, 1992.
83. Ross GS, Zacharski LR, Robert D, et al: An acquired hemorrhagic disorder from long-acting rodenticide ingestion. *Arch Intern Med* 152:410–412, 1992.
84. Basehore LM, Mowry JM: Death following ingestion of superwarfarin rodenticide: a case report. *Vet Hum Toxicol* 29:459, 1987.
85. Spahn DR, Tucci MA, Makris M: Is recombinant FVIIa the magic bullet in the treatment of major bleeding? *Br J Anaesth* 94:553–555, 2005.
86. Wallace S, Worsnop C, Paull P, et al: Covert self poisoning with brodifacoum, a "superwarfarin." *Aust N Z J Med* 20:713–715, 1990.
87. Leissinger CA, Blatt PM, Hoots WK, et al: Role of prothrombin complex concentrates in reversing warfarin anticoagulation: a review of the literature. *Am J Hematol* 83:137–143, 2008.
88. Kapadia P, Bona R: Acquired deficiency of vitamin K-dependent clotting factors due to brodifacoum ingestion. *Conn Med* 72:207–209, 2008.
89. Zupancic-Salek S, Kovacevic-Metelko J, Radman I: Successful reversal of anticoagulant effect of superwarfarin poisoning with recombinant activated factor VII. *Blood Coagul Fibrinolysis* 16:239–244, 2005.
90. de la Rubia J, Grau E, Montserrat I, et al: Anaphylactic shock and vitamin K1. *Ann Intern Med* 110:943, 1989.
91. Labatut A, Sorbette F, Virenque C: Shock states during injection of vitamin K. *Therapie* 43:58, 1988.
92. Rich EC, Drage CW: Severe complications of intravenous phytonadione therapy. Two cases, with one fatality. *Postgrad Med* 72:303–306, 1982.
93. Crowther MA, Douketis JD, Schnurr T, et al: Oral vitamin K lowers the international normalized ratio more rapidly than subcutaneous vitamin K in the treatment of warfarin-associated coagulopathy. A randomized, controlled trial. *Ann Intern Med* 137:251–254, 2002.
94. Van Heerden PV, Edibam C, Augustson B, et al: Strychnine poisoning—alive and well in Australia! *Anaesth Intensive Care* 21:876–877, 1993.
95. Hayes WJ, Laws ER: Botanical rodenticides, in Hayes WJ, Laws ER (eds): *Handbook of Pesticide Toxicology.* San Diego, Academic Press, 1991, p 615.
96. Baselt RC: Strychnine, in Baselt RC (ed): *Disposition of Toxic Drugs and Chemicals in Man.* 7th ed. Foster City, Biomedical Publications, 2004, p 1039.
97. Heiser JM, Daya MR, Magnussen AR, et al: Massive strychnine intoxication: serial blood levels in a fatal case. *J Toxicol Clin Toxicol* 30:269–283, 1992.
98. Palatnick W, Meatherall R, Sitar D, et al: Toxicokinetics of acute strychnine poisoning. *J Toxicol Clin Toxicol* 35:617–620, 1997.
99. Halsey MJ, Little HJ, Wardley-Smith B: Systemically administered glycine protects against strychnine convulsions, but not the behavioural effects of high pressure, in mice. *J Physiol* 408:431–441, 1989.
100. Ruiz-Gomez A, Morato E, Garcia-Calvo M, et al: Localization of the strychnine binding site on the 48-kilodalton subunit of the glycine receptor. *Biochemistry* 29:7033–7040, 1990.
101. O'Connor V, Phelan PP, Fry JP: Interactions of glycine and strychnine with their receptor recognition sites in mouse spinal cord. *Neurochem Int* 29:423–434, 1996.
102. Westfall TC, Westfall DP: Neurotransmission: the autonomic and somatic motor nervous systems, in Goodman LS, Gilman A, Brunton LL, Lazo JS, Parker KL (eds): *Goodman & Gilman's the Pharmacological Basis of Therapeutics.* 11th ed. New York, McGraw-Hill, 2006, p 267.
103. Boyd RE, Brennan PT, Deng JF, et al: Strychnine poisoning. Recovery from profound lactic acidosis, hyperthermia, and rhabdomyolysis. *Am J Med* 74:507–512, 1983.
104. Bleck TP: Pharmacology of tetanus. *Clin Neuropharmacol* 9:103–120, 1986.
105. Perper JA: Fatal strychnine poisoning—a case report and review of the literature. *J Forensic Sci* 30:1248–1255, 1985.
106. Yamarick W, Walson P, DiTraglia J: Strychnine poisoning in an adolescent. *J Toxicol Clin Toxicol* 30:141–148, 1992.
107. Jackson G, Ng SH, Diggle GE, et al: Strychnine poisoning treated successfully with diazepam. *Br Med J* 3:519–520, 1971.
108. Lambert JR, Byrick RJ, Hammeke MD: Management of acute strychnine poisoning. *Can Med Assoc J* 124:1268–1270, 1981.
109. O'Callaghan WG, Joyce N, Counihan HE, et al: Unusual strychnine poisoning and its treatment: report of eight cases. *Br Med J (Clin Res Ed)* 285:478, 1982.
110. Peng YB, Lin Q, Willis WD: Effects of GABA and glycine receptor antagonists on the activity and PAG-induced inhibition of rat dorsal horn neurons. *Brain Res* 736:189–201, 1996.
111. Young AB, Zukin SR, Snyder SH: Interaction of benzodiazepines with central nervous glycine receptors: possible mechanism of action. *Proc Natl Acad Sci U S A* 71:2246–2250, 1974.
112. Maron BJ, Krupp JR, Tune B: Strychnine poisoning successfully treated with diazepam. *J Pediatr* 78:697–699, 1971.
113. Baselt RC: Fluoroacetate, in Baselt RC (ed): *Disposition of Toxic Drugs and Chemicals in Man.* 7th ed. Foster City, Biomedical Publications, 2004, p 470.
114. Kostyniak PJ, Bosmann HB, Smith FA: Defluorination of fluoroacetate in vitro by rat liver subcellular fractions. *Toxicol Appl Pharmacol* 44:89–97, 1978.
115. Peters R, Wakelin RW: Biochemistry of fluoroacetate poisoning; the isolation and some properties of the fluorotricarboxylic acid inhibitor of citrate metabolism. *Proc R Soc Lond B Biol Sci* 140:497–507, 1953.
116. Egekeze JO, Oehme FW: Sodium monofluoroacetate (SMFA, compound 1080): a literature review. *Vet Hum Toxicol* 21:411–416, 1979.
117. Chung HM: Acute renal failure caused by acute monofluoroacetate poisoning. *Vet Hum Toxicol* 26[Suppl 2]:29–32, 1984.
118. Brockmann JL, McDowell AV, Leeds WG: Fatal poisoning with sodium fluoroacetate; report of a case. *J Am Med Assoc* 159:1529–1532, 1955.

119. Gajdusek DC, Luther G: Fluoroacetate poisoning a review and report of a case. *Am J Dis Child* 79:310–320, 1950.
120. Polkowski J, Crowley MS, Moore AM, et al: Unintentional methyl bromide gas release Florida, 1988. *J Toxicol Clin Toxicol* 28:127–130, 1990.
121. Wyers H: Methyl bromide intoxication. *Br J Ind Med* 2:24, 1945.
122. Chenoweth MB: Monofluoroacetic acid and related compounds. *Pharmacol Rev* 1:383, 1949.
123. Omara F, Sisodia CS: Evaluation of potential antidotes for sodium fluoroacetate in mice. *Vet Hum Toxicol* 32:427–431, 1990.
124. Chenoweth MB, Kandel A, Johnson LB, et al: Factors influencing fluoroacetate poisoning; practical treatment with glycerol monoacetate. *J Pharmacol Exp Ther* 102:31–49, 1951.
125. Chugh SN, Dushyant, Ram S, et al: Incidence & outcome of aluminium phosphide poisoning in a hospital study. *Indian J Med Res* 94:232–235, 1991.
126. Chugh SN: Aluminium phosphide poisoning: present status and management. *J Assoc Physicians India* 40:401–405, 1992.
127. Singh D, Jit I, Tyagi S: Changing trends in acute poisoning in Chandigarh zone: a 25-year autopsy experience from a tertiary care hospital in northern India. *Am J Forensic Med Pathol* 20:203–210, 1999.
128. Abder-Rahman HA, Battah AH, Ibraheem YM, et al: Aluminum phosphide fatalities, new local experience. *Med Sci Law* 40:164–168, 2000.
129. Siwach SB, Yadav DR, Arora B, et al: Acute aluminum phosphide poisoning—an epidemiological, clinical and histo-pathological study. *J Assoc Physicians India* 36:594–596, 1988.
130. Wilson R, Lovejoy FH, Jaeger RJ, et al: Acute phosphine poisoning aboard a grain freighter. Epidemiologic, clinical, and pathological findings. *JAMA* 244:148–150, 1980.
131. Baselt RC: Phosphine, in Baselt RC (ed): *Disposition of Toxic Drugs and Chemicals in Man.* 7th ed. Foster City, Biomedical Publications, 2004, p 907.
132. Hsu CH, Chi BC, Liu MY, et al: Phosphine-induced oxidative damage in rats: role of glutathione. *Toxicology* 179:1–8, 2002.
133. Misra SP, Dwivedi M: Aluminum phosphide-induced esophageal strictures: a new cause of benign esophageal strictures. *J Clin Gastroenterol* 43:405–409, 2009.
134. Darbari A, Tandon S, Chaudhary S, et al: Esophageal injuries due to aluminum phosphide tablet poisoning in India. *Asian Cardiovasc Thorac Ann* 16:298–300, 2008.
135. Chopra JS, Kalra OP, Malik VS, et al: Aluminium phosphide poisoning: a prospective study of 16 cases in one year. *Postgrad Med J* 62:1113–1115, 1986.
136. Chugh SN, Ram S, Mehta LK, et al: Adult respiratory distress syndrome following aluminium phosphide ingestion. Report of 4 cases. *J Assoc Physicians India* 37:271–272, 1989.
137. Chugh SN, Jaggal KL, Sharma A, et al: Magnesium levels in acute cardiotoxicity due to aluminium phosphide poisoning. *Indian J Med Res* 94:437–439, 1991.
138. Katria R, Eihence GP, Mehrotta ML: A study of aluminium phosphide poisoning with special references to electrocardiographic changes.. *J Assoc Physicians India* 38:471, 1990.
139. Singh S, Singh D, Wig N, et al: Aluminum phosphide ingestion—a clinico-pathologic study. *J Toxicol Clin Toxicol* 34:703–706, 1996.
140. Zadikoff CM: Toxic encephalopathy associated with use of insect repellant. *J Pediatr* 95:140–142, 1979.
141. Wood S, Rom WN, White GL Jr, et al: Pentachlorophenol poisoning. *J Occup Med* 25:527–530, 1983.
142. Gasiewicz TA: Nitro compounds and related phenolic pesticides, in Hayes WJ, Laws ER (ed): *Handbook of Pesticide Toxicology*. San Diego, Academic Press, 1991, p 1207.
143. Gupta S, Ahlawat SK: Aluminum phosphide poisoning—a review. *J Toxicol Clin Toxicol* 33:19–24, 1995.
144. Chugh SN, Ram S, Chugh K, et al: Spot diagnosis of aluminium phosphide ingestion: an application of a simple test. *J Assoc Physicians India* 37:219–220, 1989.
145. Raman R, Dubey M: The electrocardiographic changes in quick phos poisoning. *Indian Heart J* 37:193–195, 1985.
146. Chugh SN, Jaggal KL, Ram S, et al: Hypomagnesaemic atrial fibrillation in a case of aluminium phosphide poisoning. *J Assoc Physicians India* 37:548–549, 1989.
147. Ram A, Srivastava SSL, Ehlence GP, et al: A study of aluminium phosphide poisoning with special reference to therapeutic efficacy of magnesium sulphate. *J Assoc Physicians India* 36:23, 1988.
148. Suresh V: Magnesium sulphate in aluminium phosphide poisoning. *J Assoc Physicians India* 37:482, 1989.
149. Chugh SN, Kolley T, Kakkar R, et al: A critical evaluation of anti-peroxidant effect of intravenous magnesium in acute aluminium phosphide poisoning. *Magnes Res* 10:225–230, 1997.
150. Siwach SB, Singh P, Ahlawat S, et al: Serum & tissue magnesium content in patients of aluminium phosphide poisoning and critical evaluation of high dose magnesium sulphate therapy in reducing mortality. *J Assoc Physicians India* 42:107–110, 1994.
151. Marraccini JV, Thomas GE, Ongley JP, et al: Death and injury caused by methyl bromide, an insecticide fumigant. *J Forensic Sci* 28:601–607, 1983.
152. Kurtz PJ, Deskin R, Harrington RM: Pesticides, in Hayes AW (ed): *Principles and Methods of Toxicology.* 2nd ed. New York, Raven Press, 1989, p 173.
153. Lowe J, Sullivan JBJ: Fumigants, in Sullivan JB, Krieger GR (eds): *Hazardous Materials Toxicology: Clinical Principles of Environmental Health.* Baltimore, Williams & Wilkins, 1992, p 1053.
154. Ruth JH: Odor thresholds and irritation levels of several chemical substances: a review. *Am Ind Hyg Assoc J* 47:A142–A151, 1986.
155. Fuortes LJ: A case of fatal methyl bromide poisoning. *Vet Hum Toxicol* 34:240–241, 1992.
156. Goldman LR, Mengle D, Epstein DM, et al: Acute symptoms in persons residing near a field treated with the soil fumigants methyl bromide and chloropicrin. *West J Med* 147:95–98, 1987.
157. Bishop CM: A case of methyl bromide poisoning. *Occup Med (Lond)* 42:107–109, 1992.
158. Zwaveling JH, de Kort WL, Meulenbelt J, et al: Exposure of the skin to methyl bromide: a study of six cases occupationally exposed to high concentrations during fumigation. *Hum Toxicol* 6:491–495, 1987.
159. Baselt RC: Methyl bromide, in Baselt RC (ed): *Disposition of Toxic Drugs and Chemicals in Man.* 7th ed. Foster City, Biomedical Publications, 2004, p 711.
160. Hine CH: Methyl bromide poisoning. A review of ten cases. *J Occup Med* 11:1–10, 1969.
161. Occupational Safety and Health Administration: Methyl bromide: Safety and Health topics. U.S. Department of Labor, 2004. Available at: http://www.osha.gov/dts/chemicalsampling/data/CH_251900.html, December 16, 2009.
162. Rathus EM, Landy PJ: Methyl bromide poisoning. *Br J Ind Med* 18:53–57, 1961.
163. Shield LK, Coleman TL, Markesbery WR: Methyl bromide intoxication: neurologic features, including simulation of Reye syndrome. *Neurology* 27:959–962, 1977.
164. Viner N: Methyl bromide poisoning: a new industrial hazard. *CMAJ* 53:43, 1945.
165. Collins RP: Methyl bromide poisoning; a bizarre neurological disorder. *Calif Med* 103:112–116, 1965.
166. Drawneek W, O'Brien MJ, Goldsmith HJ, et al: Industrial methyl-bromide poisoning in fumigators. A case report and field investigation. *Lancet* 2:855–856, 1964.
167. Chavez CT, Hepler RS, Straatsma BR: Methyl bromide optic atrophy. *Am J Ophthalmol* 99:715–719, 1985.
168. Zatuchni J, Hong K: Methyl bromide poisoning seen initially as psychosis. *Arch Neurol* 38:529–530, 1981.
169. Behrens RH, Dukes DC: Fatal methyl bromide poisoning. *Br J Ind Med* 43:561–562, 1986.
170. Insect repellents. *Med Lett Drugs Ther* 31:45, 1989.
171. Lur'e AA, Gleiberman SE, Tsizin Iu S: Pharmacokinetics of insect repellent, *N,N*-diethyltoluamide. *Med Parazitol (Mosk)* 47:72–77, 1978.
172. Heick HM, Shipman RT, Norman MG, James W: Reye-like syndrome associated with use of insect repellent in a presumed heterozygote for ornithine carbamoyl transferase deficiency. *J Pediatr* 97:471–473, 1980.
173. Centers for Disease Control and Prevention: Seizures temporally associated with use of DEET insect repellent—New York and Connecticut. *MMWR Morb Mortal Wkly Rep* 38:678–680, 1989.
174. Lipscomb JW, Kramer JE, Leikin JB: Seizure following brief exposure to the insect repellent *N,N*-diethyl-*m*-toluamide. *Ann Emerg Med* 21:315–317, 1992.
175. Reuveni H, Yagupsky P: Diethyltoluamide-containing insect repellent: adverse effects in worldwide use. *Arch Dermatol* 118:582–583, 1982.
176. Miller JD: Anaphylaxis associated with insect repellent. *N Engl J Med* 307:1341–1342, 1982.
177. Tenenbein M: Severe toxic reactions and death following the ingestion of diethyltoluamide-containing insect repellents. *JAMA* 258:1509–1511, 1987.
178. Roland EH, Jan JE, Rigg JM: Toxic encephalopathy in a child after brief exposure to insect repellents. *Can Med Assoc J* 132:155–156, 1985.
179. Edwards DL, Johnson CE: Insect-repellent-induced toxic encephalopathy in a child. *Clin Pharm* 6:496–498, 1987.
180. Gryboski J, Weinstein D, Ordway NK: Toxic encephalopathy apparently related to the use of an insect repellent. *N Engl J Med* 264:289–291, 1961.
181. Centers for Disease Control and Prevention: Follow-up on pentachlorophenol in log homes. *MMWR Morb Mortal Wkly Rep* 31:170–171, 1982.
182. Brown BW: Fatal phenol poisoning from improperly laundered diapers. *Am J Public Health Nations Health* 60:901–902, 1970.
183. Baselt RC: Pentachlorophenol, in Baselt RC (ed): *Disposition of Toxic Drugs and Chemicals in Man.* 7th ed. Foster City, Biomedical Publications, 2004, p 855.
184. Uhl S, Schmid P, Schlatter C: Pharmacokinetics of pentachlorophenol in man. *Arch Toxicol* 58:182–186, 1986.
185. Gordon D: How dangerous is pentachlorophenol? *Med J Aust* 2:485, 1956.
186. Exon JH: A review of chlorinated phenols. *Vet Hum Toxicol* 26:508–520, 1984.
187. Gray RE, Gilliland RD, Smith EE, et al: Pentachlorophenol intoxication: report of a fatal case, with comments on the clinical course and pathologic anatomy. *Arch Environ Health* 40:161–164, 1985.

188. Roberts HJ: Aplastic anemia due to pentachlorophenol. *N Engl J Med* 305:1650–1651, 1981.
189. Cooper RG, Macauley MB: Pentachlorophenol pancreatitis. *Lancet* 1:517, 1982.
190. Hassan AB, Seligmann H, Bassan HM: Intravascular haemolysis induced by pentachlorophenol. *Br Med J (Clin Res Ed)* 291:21–22, 1985.
191. Hart TB: Paraquat—a review of safety in agricultural and horticultural use. *Hum Toxicol* 6:13–18, 1987.
192. Smith JG: Paraquat poisoning by skin absorption: a review. *Hum Toxicol* 7:15–19, 1988.
193. Chester G, Ward RJ: Occupational exposure and drift hazard during aerial application of paraquat to cotton. *Arch Environ Contam Toxicol* 13:551–563, 1984.
194. Smith LL: The toxicity of paraquat. *Adverse Drug React Acute Poisoning Rev* 7:1–17, 1988.
195. Baselt RC: Paraquat, in Baselt RC (ed): *Disposition of Toxic Drugs and Chemicals in Man.* 7th ed. Foster City, Biomedical Publications, 2004, p 844.
196. Bismuth C, Scherrmann JM, Garnier R, et al: Elimination of paraquat. *Hum Toxicol* 6:63–67, 1987.
197. Landrigan PJ, Powell KE, James LM, et al: Paraquat and marijuana: epidemiologic risk assessment. *Am J Public Health* 73:784–788, 1983.
198. Gordonsmith RH, Brooke-Taylor S, Smith LL, et al: Structural requirements of compounds to inhibit pulmonary diamine accumulation. *Biochem Pharmacol* 32:3701–3709, 1983.
199. Rose MS, Smith LL: Tissue uptake of paraquat and diquat. *Gen Pharmacol* 8:173–176, 1977.
200. Smith LL: Mechanism of paraquat toxicity in lung and its relevance to treatment. *Hum Toxicol* 6:31–36, 1987.
201. Yasaka T, Okudaira K, Fujito H, et al: Further studies of lipid peroxidation in human paraquat poisoning. *Arch Intern Med* 146:681–685, 1986.
202. Pond SM: Manifestations and management of paraquat poisoning. *Med J Aust* 152:256–259, 1990.
203. Bismuth C, Garnier R, Dally S, et al: Prognosis and treatment of paraquat poisoning: a review of 28 cases. *J Toxicol Clin Toxicol* 19:461–474, 1982.
204. Russell LA, Stone BE, Rooney PA: Paraquat poisoning: toxicologic and pathologic findings in three fatal cases. *Clin Toxicol* 18:915–928, 1981.
205. Florkowski CM, Bradberry SM, Ching GW, et al: Acute renal failure in a case of paraquat poisoning with relative absence of pulmonary toxicity. *Postgrad Med J* 68:660–662, 1992.
206. Vale JA, Meredith TJ, Buckley BM: Paraquat poisoning: clinical features and immediate general management. *Hum Toxicol* 6:41–47, 1987.
207. Hudson M, Patel SB, Ewen SW, et al: Paraquat induced pulmonary fibrosis in three survivors. *Thorax* 46:201–204, 1991.
208. Bismuth C, Garnier R, Baud FJ, et al: Paraquat poisoning. An overview of the current status. *Drug Saf* 5:243–251, 1990.
209. Hawksworth GM, Bennett PN, Davies DS: Kinetics of paraquat elimination in the dog. *Toxicol Appl Pharmacol* 57:139–145, 1981.
210. Hart TB, Nevitt A, Whitehead A: A new statistical approach to the prognostic significance of plasma paraquat concentrations. *Lancet* 2:1222–1223, 1984.
211. Proudfoot AT, Stewart MS, Levitt T, et al: Paraquat poisoning: significance of plasma-paraquat concentrations. *Lancet* 2:330–332, 1979.
212. Tungsanga K, Chusilp S, Israsena S, et al: Paraquat poisoning: evidence of systemic toxicity after dermal exposure. *Postgrad Med J* 59:338–339, 1983.
213. Gaudreault P, Friedman PA, Lovejoy FH Jr: Efficacy of activated charcoal and magnesium citrate in the treatment of oral paraquat intoxication. *Ann Emerg Med* 14:123–125, 1985.
214. Nokata M, Tanaka T, Tsuchiya K, et al: Alleviation of paraquat toxicity by Kayexalate and Kalimate in rats. *Acta Pharmacol Toxicol (Copenh)* 55:158–160, 1984.
215. Meredith TJ, Vale JA: Treatment of paraquat poisoning in man: methods to prevent absorption. *Hum Toxicol* 6:49–55, 1987.
216. Braithwaite RA: Emergency analysis of paraquat in biological fluids. *Hum Toxicol* 6:83–86, 1987.
217. Lin JL, Leu ML, Liu YC, et al: A prospective clinical trial of pulse therapy with glucocorticoid and cyclophosphamide in moderate to severe paraquat-poisoned patients. *Am J Respir Crit Care Med* 159:357–360, 1999.
218. Keeling PL, Pratt IS, Aldridge WN, et al: The enhancement of paraquat toxicity in rats by 85% oxygen: lethality and cell-specific lung damage. *Br J Exp Pathol* 62:643–654, 1981.
219. Widdop BM, Medd RK, Braithwaite RA: Charcoal haemoperfusion in the treatment of paraquat poisoning. *Proc Eur Soc Toxicol* 18:156, 1976.
220. Hampson EC, Effeney DJ, Pond SM: Efficacy of single or repeated hemoperfusion in a canine model of paraquat poisoning. *J Pharmacol Exp Ther* 254:732–740, 1990.
221. Pond SM, Rivory LP, Hampson EC, et al: Kinetics of toxic doses of paraquat and the effects of hemoperfusion in the dog. *J Toxicol Clin Toxicol* 31:229–246, 1993.
222. Wright AF, Green TP, Robson RT, et al: Specific polyclonal and monoclonal antibody prevents paraquat accumulation into rat lung slices. *Biochem Pharmacol* 36:1325–1331, 1987.
223. Pond SM, Chen N, Bowles MR: Prevention of paraquat toxicity in alveolar type II cells by paraquat-specific antibodies [abstract]. *Vet Hum Toxicol* 35:332, 1993.
224. Dunbar JR, DeLucia AJ, Acuff RV, et al: Prolonged, intravenous paraquat infusion in the rat. II. Paraquat-induced alterations in lung polyamine metabolism. *Toxicol Appl Pharmacol* 94:221–226, 1988.
225. Smith LL: The identification of an accumulation system for diamines and polyamines into the lung and its relevance to paraquat toxicity. *Arch Toxicol Suppl* 5:1–14, 1982.
226. Redetzki HM, Wood CD, Grafton WD: Vitamin E and paraquat poisoning. *Vet Hum Toxicol* 22:395–397, 1980.
227. Osherrof MR, Schaich KM, Drew RT, et al: Failure of deferoxamine to modify the toxicity of paraquat in rats. *J Free Radical Biol Med* 1:71, 1985.
228. Frank L: Superoxide dismutase and lung toxicity. *Trends Pharmacol Sci* 14:124, 1983.
229. Glass M, Sutherland MW, Forman HJ, et al: Selenium deficiency potentiates paraquat-induced lipid peroxidation in isolated perfused rat lung. *J Appl Physiol* 59:619–622, 1985.
230. Shum S, Hale TW, Habasang R: Reduction of paraquat toxicity by *N*-acetylcysteine. *Vet Hum Toxicol* 6:31, 1982.
231. Cramp TP: Failure of *N*-acetylcysteine to reduce renal damage due to paraquat in rats. *Hum Toxicol* 4:107, 1985.
232. Addo E, Poon-King T: Leucocyte suppression in treatment of 72 patients with paraquat poisoning. *Lancet* 1:1117–1120, 1986.
233. Lin JL, Wei MC, Liu YC: Pulse therapy with cyclophosphamide and methylprednisolone in patients with moderate to severe paraquat poisoning: a preliminary report. *Thorax* 51:661–663, 1996.
234. Vieira RJ, Zambrone FAD, Madureira PR, et al: Treatment of paraquat poisoning using cyclophosphamide and dexamethasone [abstract]. *J Toxicol Clin Toxicol* 35:515, 1997.
235. Botella de Maglia J, Belenguer Tarin JE: Paraquat poisoning. A study of 29 cases and evaluation of the effectiveness of the "Caribbean scheme." *Med Clin (Barc)* 115:530–533, 2000.
236. Perriens JH, Benimadho S, Kiauw IL, et al: High-dose cyclophosphamide and dexamethasone in paraquat poisoning: a prospective study. *Hum Exp Toxicol* 11:129–134, 1992.
237. Lin JL, Lin-Tan DT, Chen KH, et al: Repeated pulse of methylprednisolone and cyclophosphamide with continuous dexamethasone therapy for patients with severe paraquat poisoning. *Crit Care Med* 34:368–373, 2006.
238. Afzali S, Gholyaf M: The effectiveness of combined treatment with methylprednisolone and cyclophosphamide in oral paraquat poisoning. *Arch Iran Med* 11:387–391, 2008.
239. Vincken W, Huyghens L, Schandevyl W, et al: Paraquat poisoning and colchicine treatment. *Ann Intern Med* 95:391–392, 1981.
240. Akahori F, Oehme FW: Inhibition of collagen synthesis as a treatment for paraquat poisoning. *Vet Hum Toxicol* 25:321–327, 1983.
241. Mohammadi-Karakani A, Ghazi-Khansari M, Sotoudeh M: Lisinopril ameliorates paraquat-induced lung fibrosis. *Clin Chim Acta* 367:170–174, 2006.
242. Brown OR, Heitkamp M, Song CS: Niacin Reduces Paraquat Toxicity in Rats. *Science* 212:1510–1512, 1981.
243. Kamholz S, Veith FJ, Mollenkopf F, et al: Single lung transplantation in paraquat intoxication. *N Y State J Med* 84:82–84, 1984.
244. Toronto Lung Transplant group: sequential bilateral lung transplantation for paraquat poisoning. *J Thorac Cardiovasc Surg* 89:734–742, 1985.
245. Walder B, Brundler MA, Spiliopoulos A, et al: Successful single-lung transplantation after paraquat intoxication. *Transplantation* 64:789–791, 1997.
246. Vanholder R, Colardyn F, De Reuck J, et al: Diquat intoxication: report of two cases and review of the literature. *Am J Med* 70:1267–1271, 1981.
247. Baselt RC: Diquat, in Baselt RC (ed): *Disposition of Toxic Drugs and Chemicals in Man.* 7th ed. Foster City, Biomedical Publications, 2004, p 368.
248. Manoguerra AS: Full thickness skin burns secondary to an unusual exposure to diquat dibromide. *J Toxicol Clin Toxicol* 28:107–110, 1990.
249. McCarthy LG, Speth CP: Diquat intoxication. *Ann Emerg Med* 12:394–396, 1983.
250. Stancliffe TC, Pirie A: The production of superoxide radicals in reactions of the herbicide diquat. *FEBS Lett* 17:297–299, 1971.
251. Okonek S, Hofmann A: On the question of extracorporeal hemodialysis in diquat intoxication. *Arch Toxicol* 33:251–257, 1975.
252. Powell D, Pond SM, Allen TB, et al: Hemoperfusion in a child who ingested diquat and died from pontine infarction and hemorrhage. *J Toxicol Clin Toxicol* 20:405–420, 1983.
253. Arnold EK, Beasley VR: The pharmacokinetics of chlorinated phenoxy acid herbicides: a literature review. *Vet Hum Toxicol* 31:121–125, 1989.
254. Klaassen CD: Toxic effects of pesticides, in Casarett LJ, Doull J, Klaassen CD (eds): *Casarett and Doull's Toxicology: the Basic Science of Poisons.* 6th ed. New York, McGraw-Hill Medical Pub. Division, 2001, p 791.
255. Centers for Disease Control and Prevention: Serum 2,3,7, 8-tetrachlorodibenzo-p-dioxin levels in US Army Vietnam-era veterans. The Centers for Disease Control Veterans Health Studies. *JAMA* 260:1249–1254, 1988.
256. Baselt RC: 2,4-Dichlorophenoxyacetic acid, in Baselt RC (ed): *Disposition of Toxic Drugs and Chemicals in Man.* 7th ed. Foster City, Biomedical Publications, 2004, p 323.
257. Kohli JD, Khanna RN, Gupta BN, et al: Absorption and excretion of 2,4-dichlorophenoxyacetic acid in man. *Xenobiotica* 4:97–100, 1974.
258. Dudley AW Jr, Thapar NT: Fatal human ingestion of 2,4-D, a common herbicide. *Arch Pathol* 94:270–275, 1972.

259. Baselt RC: 2,4,5-Trichlorophenoxyacetic acid, in Baselt RC (ed): *Disposition of Toxic Drugs and Chemicals in Man.* 7th ed. Foster City, Biomedical Publications, 2004, p 1147.
260. Dickey W, McAleer JJ, Callender ME: Delayed sudden death after ingestion of MCPP and ioxynil: an unusual presentation of hormonal weedkiller intoxication. *Postgrad Med J* 64:681–682, 1988.
261. Flanagan RJ, Meredith TJ, Ruprah M, et al: Alkaline diuresis for acute poisoning with chlorophenoxy herbicides and ioxynil. *Lancet* 335:454–458, 1990.
262. Friesen EG, Jones GR, Vaughan D: Clinical presentation and management of acute 2,4-D oral ingestion. *Drug Saf* 5:155–159, 1990.
263. Prescott LF, Park J, Darrien I: Treatment of severe 2,4-D and mecoprop intoxication with alkaline diuresis. *Br J Clin Pharmacol* 7:111–116, 1979.
264. Roberts DM, Seneviratne R, Mohammed F, et al: Intentional self-poisoning with the chlorophenoxy herbicide 4-chloro-2-methylphenoxyacetic acid (MCPA). *Ann Emerg Med* 46:275–284, 2005.
265. Meulenbelt J, Zwaveling JH, van Zoonen P, et al: Acute MCPP intoxication: report of two cases. *Hum Toxicol* 7:289–292, 1988.
266. O'Reilly JF: Prolonged coma and delayed peripheral neuropathy after ingestion of phenoxyacetic acid weedkillers. *Postgrad Med J* 60:76–77, 1984.
267. Berwick P: 2,4-dichlorophenoxyacetic acid poisoning in man. Some interesting clinical and laboratory findings. *JAMA* 214:1114–1117, 1970.
268. Kancir CB, Andersen C, Olesen AS: Marked hypocalcemia in a fatal poisoning with chlorinated phenoxy acid derivatives. *J Toxicol Clin Toxicol* 26:257–264, 1988.
269. Fraser AD, Isner AF, Perry RA: Toxicologic studies in a fatal overdose of 2,4-D, mecoprop, and dicamba. *J Forensic Sci* 29:1237–1241, 1984.
270. Osterloh J, Lotti M, Pond SM: Toxicologic studies in a fatal overdose of 2,4-D, MCPP, and chlorpyrifos. *J Anal Toxicol* 7:125–129, 1983.
271. Jackson RC, Elder WJ, Mc DH: Sodium-chlorate poisoning complicated by acute renal failure. *Lancet* 2:1381–1383, 1961.
272. Jansen H, Zeldenrust J: Homicidal chronic sodium chlorate poisoning. *Forensic Sci* 1:103–105, 1972.
273. Stavrou A, Butcher R, Sakula A: Accidental self-poisoning by sodium chlorate weed-killer. *Practitioner* 221:397–399, 1978.
274. Cunningham NE: Chlorate poisoning—two cases diagnosed at autopsy. *Med Sci Law* 22:281–282, 1982.
275. Steffen C, Wetzel E: Pathologic aspects of chlorate poisoning. *Hum Toxicol* 4:541, 1985.
276. Helliwell M, Nunn J: Mortality in sodium chlorate poisoning. *Br Med J* 1:1119, 1979.
277. Curry S: Methemoglobinemia. *Ann Emerg Med* 11:214–221, 1982.

CHAPTER 142 ■ PHENCYCLIDINE AND HALLUCINOGEN POISONING

FRANK F. DALY AND LUKE YIP*

PHENCYCLIDINE

Phencyclidine (phenyl-cyclohexyl-piperidine, or PCP) is a dissociative anesthetic chemically related to ketamine. PCP is a synthetic compound developed in the 1950s as an anesthetic–analgesic for animals and was used as a general anesthetic in man. However, there was an unacceptably high incidence of postoperative delirium and adverse drug events were not a deterrent for PCP abuse. Tables 142.1 and 142.2 show the slang, or street names, for both PCP and ketamine.

Pharmacology

PCP has acid and alkaloid forms. Both are odorless, nonvolatile, sold as "angel dust," and may be ingested or injected intravenously. PCP acid is a white crystalline substance sold as or incorporated into tablets. It deteriorates when heated and is not suitable for smoking. PCP alkaloid is a grayish-white amorphous powder smoked after incorporation into marijuana (e.g., "super grass," "super weed") or tobacco (e.g., "clickers," "primos") cigarettes. More often, the alkaloid is dissolved in a liquid hydrocarbon and applied to the wrapper of a tobacco cigarette. The ether-like or formaldehyde odor surrounding some patients who have used PCP is the smell of the volatile hydrocarbon used to dissolve PCP alkaloid.

Several analogs of PCP are occasionally used as street drugs (Table 142.3). Their pharmacologic actions are similar to those of PCP and cannot be distinguished clinically. In addition, street PCP samples may be contaminated with 1-piperidinocyclohexane-carbonitrile, a precursor of PCP that is more potent than PCP and capable of generating cyanide [1], although the clinical significance of this is unknown.

PCP has multiple mechanisms of action (Table 142.4), which helps to explain the varied signs and symptoms associated with PCP intoxication. It is well absorbed from the gastrointestinal (GI) and respiratory tracts. PCP is a weak base (pK_a 8.5), has a volume of distribution 6.2 L per kg, and is extensively protein-bound (65%) [2]. PCP concentrates in the brain, lungs, adipose tissue, and liver. The average serum half-life in controlled studies is 17 hours [2]. PCP is metabolized by the liver and excreted predominantly as inactive compounds [2–5]. Small amounts of PCP are excreted in perspiration, saliva, and gastric juice. PCP has been detected in umbilical and infant blood, amniotic fluid, and breast milk [6,7].

Clinical Toxicity

Drinking PCP, injecting intravenous PCP, or swallowing the remnants of a PCP-soaked cigarette has resulted in severe

TABLE 142.1

SLANG TERMS (STREET NAMES) FOR PHENCYCLIDINE

Cyclone	KJ
DOA	Mist
Dust	Rocket fuel
Elephant tranquilizer	Scuffle
Goon	Sernyl
Hog	

*The views expressed do not necessarily represent those of the agency or the United States.

TABLE 142.2

SLANG TERMS (STREET NAMES) FOR KETAMINE

Green	Special K
Jet	Special LA coke
K	Super acid
Mauve	Super C
Purple	

intoxication within 1 hour. Clinical experience with PCP intoxication is derived from case reports [8–15] and small clinical series [16–20]. The hallmarks of PCP intoxication are nystagmus and hypertension. Nystagmus may be horizontal, vertical, or rotary. Patients may have systolic or diastolic hypertension. Hypertension usually resolves within 4 hours, but a significant number of patients may remain hypertensive for more than 24 hours.

Tachycardia is common, but heart rates more than 120 per minute are unusual. Hypothermia (<36.7°C), hyperthermia (>38.9°C), respiratory compromise, tachypnea, hypotension, and cardiac arrest are reported, but are uncommon.

Patients may present with delirium or normal sensorium. Lethargy, stupor, and unconsciousness are uncommon presentations. The most common behavioral effects are violent and agitated behavior, which may result in severe penetrating or blunt trauma. Patients may exhibit bizarre behavior such as driving less than 10 mph on the freeway, "playing bumper cars" on the freeway, sleeping on top of cars that are blocking traffic, lying down in a busy street, and wandering or acting wildly in public. Only 20% of PCP users report hallucinations or delusions. The visual hallucinations are typically concrete and realistic (e.g., blue fish). Patients may appear mute or may stare blankly.

The most common neuromuscular finding is rigidity of all extremities. It is often associated with jerky or thrashing movements, tremors, or twitching. Other musculoskeletal disturbances include oculogyric crisis, trismus, facial grimacing, circumoral muscle twitching, lip smacking or chewing movements, torticollis, tongue spasms, opisthotonos, and catalepsy. Patients may exhibit self-limited slow, writhing movements of the extremities or body. Athetosis and muscle stiffness may appear simultaneously. Intermittent athetoid movements may last for more than 10 hours. Rhabdomyolysis may occur, even in calm-appearing patients. Grand mal seizures and status epilepticus are uncommon.

The major autonomic effects are profuse diaphoresis, copious oral or pulmonary secretions, and urinary retention. Bronchospasm has been reported in patients who smoked or sniffed PCP. Pupillary size is usually normal, but miosis or mydriasis may be evident.

Clinically, acute PCP intoxication can be divided into major and minor clinical syndromes [20]. Major syndromes, representing moderate-to-severe PCP intoxication, are delirium, toxic psychosis, catatonic syndrome, and coma. They may include any of the effects previously discussed. Minor syndromes are lethargy or stupor, bizarre behavior, violent behavior, agitation, and euphoria. They represent mild PCP intoxication, and complications are rare.

TABLE 142.3

PHENCYCLIDINE ANALOGS USED AS STREET DRUGS

PCE (cyclohexamine)
PCPP (phenylcyclopentylpiperidine)
PHP (phenylcyclohexylpyrrolidine)
TCP (thienylcyclohexylpiperidine)

TABLE 142.4

PHENCYCLIDINE PHARMACOLOGY

Sites	Actions
N-methyl-D-aspartate receptor	Glutamate antagonist
D_2 dopamine receptor	Blocks dopamine reuptake Interferes with dopamine release
Serotonergic receptor	Antagonist
Cholinesterase	Antagonist
Nicotinic receptor	Antagonist
Muscarinic receptor	Anticholinergic effects may include tachycardia, mydriasis and urinary Cholinergic effects may include miosis salivation and diaphoresis Binds to receptors in the heart
Na^+ and K^+ channels	Antagonist
Presynaptic brain neurons	Increase catecholamine release

Data from references [53–63].

Delirium is the most common presentation of PCP intoxication. Patients may be found wandering in traffic or appear intoxicated with ethanol. Patients exhibit signs and symptoms such as slurred, bizarre, or repetitive speech; ataxia; disorientation; confusion; poor judgment; inappropriate affect; amnesia of recent events; bizarre behavior; agitation; and violence. The duration of this syndrome often lasts for a few hours and rarely lasts more than 3 days, but has been reported to persist for 1 to 3 weeks.

Patients presenting with toxic psychosis often have a history of chronic PCP use (e.g., smoking) during the week before admission. This psychosis is characterized primarily by hallucinations, delusions, and paranoid ideation. Hallucinations may be auditory or visual, or both, and may involve seeing brilliantly colored objects, but objects are not distorted and there are no kaleidoscopic effects. Patients may be preoccupied with religious thoughts or have religious delusions. It is common for patients to have pressured speech, scream, or make animal sounds. Signs and symptoms persist for a median of 3 days (range, 1 to 30 days).

The catatonic syndrome manifests primarily as a combination of signs: posturing, catalepsy, rigidity, mutism, staring, negativism, nudism, impulsiveness, agitation, violence, and stupor. Stereotypies, mannerisms, grimacing, and verbigeration may also be present. Patients are typically mute, staring blankly, motionless, stiff, standing with extremities or head in bizarre positions, and unresponsive to noxious stimuli. Catatonic syndrome usually does not persist for more than 24 hours (range, 2 to 6 days), and most patients recover within 4 to 6 hours. The majority of patients emerging from catatonic syndrome are agitated or combative for several hours; the other patients emerge with delirium, lethargy, psychosis, bizarre behavior, or normal sensorium.

Patients with delirium and violent or bizarre behavior may subsequently lapse into coma. Coma may also occur abruptly and may last up to 6 days. Patients emerging from coma may exhibit delirium, catatonic syndrome, toxic psychosis, stupor, agitation, violence, bizarre behavior, or normal sensorium. The duration of the emergent phenomenon is variable.

Violent, agitated, and euphoric patients typically have a clear sensorium. Patients with euphoria may report a sense of well being or feeling "spaced out," "freaked out," or "tingling all over." Such behavior usually lasts several hours.

Neonatal jitteriness, hypertonicity, and vomiting have been associated with maternal PCP abuse [21]. Chronic PCP intoxication has not been described, and there is no documentation of PCP flashbacks.

Diagnostic Evaluation

PCP intoxication is a clinical diagnosis. It is based on a history of possible PCP exposure associated with clinical findings consistent with PCP intoxication and the exclusion of other neuropsychiatric or behavioral disorders. The drug history should include the type of product, method of use, time of exposure, circumstances surrounding intoxication, and description of any effects witnessed by others or experienced by the patient. Particular attention should be paid to any abnormal behavior that might have resulted in occult trauma (e.g., jumps or falls).

The physical examination should focus on the vital signs, sensorium, behavior, and musculoskeletal, autonomic, and neurologic findings. A thorough examination should be performed to exclude occult trauma. Explosions in clandestine laboratories may lead to smoke or chemical inhalation, thermal or chemical burns, and blunt or penetrating trauma.

Laboratory tests should include complete blood cell count, serum electrolytes, blood urea nitrogen, creatinine, glucose, creatine phosphokinase (CPK), liver function tests, and urine analysis to include myoglobin. Common abnormal test results associated with PCP intoxication include hypoglycemia, elevated white blood cell count, serum CPK, serum glutamic oxaloacetic transaminase/serum glutamic pyruvic transaminase, and uric acid. Chest radiograph, electrocardiogram, arterial blood gas, computed tomography of the head, and lumbar puncture should be obtained as clinically indicated.

Serum or urine PCP levels can confirm the diagnosis of PCP intoxication but neither contributes to the patient management nor correlates with the severity of intoxication [22]. Rapid urine qualitative drug screens that detect PCP should be interpreted with caution. Dextromethorphan use may lead to false-positive PCP results on urine qualitative drug screens [23]. Diphenhydramine may interfere with PCP determination by gas–liquid chromatography [24].

Management

The immediate management is to assess and treat acute threats to the airway, breathing, and circulation. Close monitoring of the patient in a quiet area with limited stimuli may reduce the need for physical restraint or sedation and provide a safe environment for the patient, attending staff, and other patients. Routine gastric decontamination is not recommended.

Patients with major PCP intoxication syndrome or complicated minor PCP intoxication syndrome should be managed in an intensive care unit. These patients should receive supplemental oxygen, secure vascular access, and have their vital signs and cardiac rhythm continuously monitored. A core temperature should be obtained in all patients.

Hemodynamic effects of PCP usually do not require specific treatment. Abnormal vital signs should be managed in the context of the overall clinical status of the patient. Mild sinus tachycardia or hypertension not associated with psychomotor agitation or evidence of end organ damage usually does not require pharmacologic treatment. Treatment of psychomotor agitation using benzodiazepine sedation often results in improvement or resolution of sinus tachycardia and hypertension. Persistent significant hypertension despite resolution of psychomotor agitation, or if there is evidence of end organ damage, should be treated with intravenous nitroprusside or nitroglycerin titrated to effect. The use of β-adrenergic or calcium-channel antagonists to treat drugs of abuse-induced tachycardia or hypertension is not routinely recommended and may have deleterious effects.

Patients with hypotension should receive fluid resuscitation while alternative causes are considered (e.g., occult trauma). Persistent hypotension refractory to fluids necessitates a vasopressor such as norepinephrine or epinephrine. Pulmonary artery catheter hemodynamic monitoring may provide important data to guide pharmacologic intervention. Cardiac dysrhythmias should be managed according to current Advanced Cardiac Life Support guidelines.

Core temperature approaching or exceeding 104°F (40°C) is immediately life threatening and warrants aggressive management. Rapid-sequence induction, intubation, and ventilation may be required. Completely undress the patient, begin continuous monitoring of the patient's core temperature, and initiate active cooling measures. Active cooling should be terminated when the patient's core temperature approaches 101°F (38.3°C). Antipyretics (e.g., acetaminophen, aspirin, non-steroidal anti-inflammatory drugs) are not useful, and there is no good evidence that dantrolene, bromocriptine, or amantadine enhances the cooling process in patients with life-threatening hyperthermia.

The initial management of a patient with altered mental status should include assessment and treatment of all readily reversible causes such as hypoxia, hypoglycemia, opioid toxicity, and thiamine deficiency. Imaging studies of the head should be performed on patients with persistent altered mental status, followed by lumbar puncture as clinically indicated. Antibiotic and antiviral medications should be administered as soon as the diagnosis of meningitis or encephalitis is entertained.

Mild psychomotor agitation usually does not require active intervention, but sedation becomes necessary for patients whose behavior poses a danger to themselves or others. Haloperidol and chlorpromazine have been reported to be safe and effective in the management of patients with PCP intoxication who exhibit violent or bizarre behavior [20,25–27]. Benzodiazepines may be preferred treatment for patients with major or minor PCP syndromes; however, benzodiazepines lack anticholinergic and extrapyramidal side effects, do not lower seizure threshold, and have not been associated with hyperthermia or neuroleptic malignant syndrome. The dose of benzodiazepine should be titrated to achieve moderate sedation to obviate physical restraints. Occasionally, large doses (e.g., >100 mg of diazepam) may be necessary to achieve safe gentle sedation. The patient's ability to protect the airway should be carefully monitored. Intubation and ventilation are rarely necessary.

Seizures should be treated with incremental doses of intravenous benzodiazepine. Cumulative high-dose benzodiazepine may be required. If seizure activity is not rapidly controlled, intravenous propofol or phenobarbital is indicated. Seizures refractory to sedative hypnotic drugs should be managed with non-depolarizing neuromuscular blockade and general anesthesia, along with continuous electroencephalogram monitoring.

Fluid management should address any electrolyte and acid–base abnormalities. Management of rhabdomyolysis should include treatment of psychomotor agitation and generous intravenous crystalloid fluids to maintain urine output of at least 2 to 3 mL per kg per hour to minimize the risk of acute tubular necrosis. The role of alkalinizing the urine to provide renal protection when rhabdomyolysis is present is controversial. As serum myoglobin levels are not usually rapidly available, serum CPK may be monitored noting that the clinically important myoglobin serum peak may precede the CPK peak by several hours. Care should be taken to prevent dependent muscle injury.

Although urinary acidification can increase renal PCP excretion [9], the risks associated with urinary acidification outweigh potential benefits [10]. Hemodialysis is not indicated for enhanced drug elimination but may be necessary in patients with acute renal failure.

Patients with persistent suicidal ideation or psychosis should be referred to the psychiatric service.

HALLUCINOGENS

Psychedelic hallucinogens are primarily composed of synthetic indolamines (derivatives of tryptamine), phenethylamines (derivatives of amphetamine, see Chapter 144), and plant products. The psychedelic experience may precipitate homicidal acts [28–30], self-destructive behavior [31], accidental injuries, and acute or chronic psychosis. Physiologic effects vary from mild flushing to life-threatening alterations in vital signs, coma, seizures, and coagulopathy.

Pharmacology

Synthetic hallucinogens are sold as liquid, powder, tablets, capsules, microdots (dried drug residue) on printed paper, liquid-impregnated blotter paper, and as windowpanes (translucent 3 × 3 mm gelatin squares).

The routes of administration are oral, intranasal, sublingual, conjunctival, smoking, or intravenous injection. Blotter paper is chewed and swallowed, whereas microdot paper is usually licked. Windowpanes are usually placed under the tongue or in the conjunctival sac, and may also be swallowed.

The mechanisms of action for psychedelic hallucinogens are presumed to involve various neurotransmitters in the central nervous system. Psychedelic hallucinogen effects on thought and perception appear to primarily involve serotonin (5-hydroxytryptamine) neurotransmission. Serotonin modulates psychological and physiological processes such as affect, mood, personality, sexual activity, appetite, motor function, pain perception, sleep induction, and temperature regulation [32]. Serotonin causes vasoconstriction in all vascular beds except for coronary arteries and skeletal muscles, in which it causes vasodilation.

Tryptamine derivatives have been shown to act at presynaptic type 2 serotonin receptors (i.e., serotonin reuptake sites) [33]. Some of these compounds appear to be partial agonists or agonist–antagonists at these receptors.

Hallucinogens are readily absorbed from the GI tract, metabolized by the liver, and excreted predominately as pharmacologically inactive compounds. The clinical effects produced by different agents are very similar.

Lysergic acid (LSD, or "acid"), the most widely abused tryptamine derivative, was originally synthesized from an ergot alkaloid. The usual street form is a 1 cm^2 piece of blotter paper ("tabs"). At doses of 100 μg, LSD produces perceptual distortions and hallucinations.

Morning glory (*Ipomoea* and *Rivea* genera) seeds contain lysergic acid derivatives that are one tenth as potent as LSD. Users report that to achieve the desired hallucinogenic effect requires ingestion of 200 to 300 macerated seeds.

Psilocybin and psilocin are tryptamine derivatives found in *Psilocybe* and other hallucinogenic fungi ("magic mushrooms"). It is usually sold in the form of dried mushroom, capsules, or paper packets of brown powder. Pure psilocybin is available in capsules of white powder. The effective psilocybin dose is 5 to 15 mg, which is equivalent to ingestion of one to five large mushrooms. However, the clinical effects are dependent on a number of factors, including dose, method of preparation, and individual patient factors [34].

The toads of the genus *Bufo* secrete a mixture of hallucinogenic tryptamine derivatives and cardioactive compounds on their skin [35,36]. Toad licking has been popularized by the belief that hallucinogenic effects may be achieved by licking the skin of live toads.

Dimethyltryptamine (DMT) is an endogenous serotonin metabolite and is also found in the Yakee plant (*Virola calophylla*), which is native to the Amazon basin. Street DMT is available as liquid or yellow-tan powder that is sprinkled on tobacco, marijuana, or parsley and smoked. DMT is broken down in the GI tract; there is minimal systemic absorption after ingestion.

Mescaline, another amphetamine congener, is the psychedelic constituent of peyote (North American dumping cactus, *Lophophora williamsii*) and other cacti. Small segments of the crown of the cactus, known as "buttons" or "moons," may be swallowed whole or chopped into small pieces. Ground peyote may be smoked. The hallucinogenic dose of mescaline is 300 mg, corresponding to 6 to 12 buttons.

Clinical Toxicity

Acute psychedelic effects ("trip" or "tripping") are characterized by changes in sensory perception. They include euphoria or dysphoria; an increase in the intensity of sensory perception; distortions of time, place, and body image; visual hallucinations; synesthesias (i.e., "seeing sounds" and "hearing colors"); illusions; loss of spatial sense; and feelings of unreality. The visual hallucinations are characteristically nebulous, rapidly changing, and unreal (e.g., streaks and blobs of color or kaleidoscopic, multicolored shifting patterns). Visions and mystical experiences have been described [37]. Hallucinogenic drug effects may be variable, even in the same individual on different occasions. The person is usually awake and may appear hyperalert, but is often quiet, calm, withdrawn, depressed, uncommunicative, and oblivious to surroundings or preoccupied with internal stimuli. For some people, the psychedelic experience may be frightening or terrifying, which results in anxiety, agitation, violence, or panic (e.g., a "bad trip" or "bummer"). In general, tryptamine, amphetamine derivatives, and mescaline have clinical effects similar to those of LSD. The most common presentation is acute panic reactions. Patients typically present with anxiety, apprehension, a sense of loss of self-control, and frightening illusions.

The effects of LSD typically begin within 30 to 60 minutes, peak at 2 to 4 hours, and return to baseline within 12 hours. Accidental LSD ingestion by children has resulted in hyperactivity, tachycardia, and hyperventilation [38]; in one case, the reaction was described as "stark terror" [39]. The initial effects of morning glory seeds are listlessness, apathy, and irritability, followed by mild LSD-type effects. Severe psychedelic reactions have been reported [40–42]. Psilocybin effects usually last less than 4 hours but prolonged psychedelic effects have been reported after ingestion of 200 psilocybin mushrooms [43]. The effects of DMT are milder, occur sooner, and have shorter duration than those of LSD [44].

Hallucinogenic mushroom abuse has been associated with facial flushing, salivation, lacrimation, tachycardia, hypertension, mydriasis, nausea, vomiting, diarrhea, and hyperreflexia. Chills and myalgias may also occur [45].

Severe or life-threatening autonomic effects following hallucinogenic intoxication are rare and usually occur only after large doses. Manifestations include stupor or coma, bradycardia or tachycardia, shock or hypertension, severe hyperthermia, seizures, muscle rigidity, and coagulopathy.

No deaths directly attributable to the toxic effects of LSD have been reported. However, massive LSD overdose has resulted in severe autonomic effects such as coma, toxic psychosis, hyperventilation, respiratory arrest, hypertension, hyperthermia, tachycardia, athetosis, dystonic movements, and coagulopathy [46,47]. Serotonin syndrome has been associated with LSD use [48,49].

Intravenous injection of *Psilocybe* mushroom extract has resulted in systemic autonomic effects [45,50].

Persistent LSD effects rarely include prolonged psychotic reactions, depression, exacerbation of preexisting psychiatric illness, and hallucinogen-persisting perception disorder (flashbacks). Hallucinogen-persisting perception disorder is a chronic disorder that occurs after cessation of the acute intoxication and is characterized by recurrence of intrusive images. It can be triggered by stress, illness, and exercise. Flashbacks have been reported after LSD [51], morning glory seeds [41,42], and psilocybin [43] intoxication.

Diagnostic Evaluation

Psychedelic hallucinogen intoxication is a clinical diagnosis. It is based on a history of possible psychedelic hallucinogen exposure associated with clinical findings consistent with psychedelic hallucinogen intoxication. The drug history should include a history of prior drug abuse and psychiatric illness. Often, the name of the drug is not given but the route of intoxication and dosage form are described (e.g., "ate a paper," "chewed a button," "put acid in my eye"). Sometimes the only history is "on a trip."

Physical examination should focus on eliciting signs of autonomic disturbances, synesthesias, illusions, hallucinations, delusions, and abnormal behavior. Laboratory tests should include serum electrolytes, blood urea nitrogen, creatinine, glucose, CPK, and urinalysis. Urine toxicology screen may confirm the diagnosis of psychedelic hallucinogen intoxication and may be useful in patients with unexplained hallucinations. Quantitative hallucinogen drug levels are not clinically useful and do not contribute to patient management. Although laboratory tests are available for LSD and its metabolite [52], it is not part of most standard drug abuse screens. Electrocardiogram, arterial blood gas, imaging studies, and lumbar puncture should be obtained as clinically indicated.

Management

Management of psychedelic tryptamine is the same as for PCP. Patients should be placed in a quiet area with limited stimuli accompanied by a patient advocate. The advocate should provide reality testing and reassure the patient that it is a drug-induced experience and the adverse drug event will resolve within a few hours. This approach may not be practical or effective for severely disturbed or uncommunicative patients, and liberal intravenous benzodiazepine doses should be administered to achieve the desired effect. Depressed or withdrawn patients are unpredictable and should be kept under close observation. GI decontamination is unlikely to benefit a symptomatic patient and is not indicated. Cyproheptadine may be considered in patients exhibiting serotonin syndrome (see Chapters 66 and 124). Patients are expected to completely recover within 24 hours. Persistent signs and symptoms may be due to a psychiatric condition precipitated by the psychedelic drug, and the patient should be referred to the psychiatric service.

References

1. Soine WH, Vincek WC: Phencyclidine contaminant generates cyanide. *N Engl J Med* 301:439, 1979.
2. Cook CE, Brine DR, Jeffcoat AR, et al: Phencyclidine disposition after intravenous and oral doses. *Clin Pharmacol Ther* 31:625, 1982.
3. Syracuse CD, Kuhnert BR, Golden NL, et al: Measurement of the amino acid metabolite of phencyclidine by selected ion monitoring. *Biomed Environ Mass Spectrom* 13:113, 1986.
4. Wall ME, Brine DR, Jeffcoat AR, et al: Phencyclidine metabolism and disposition in man following a 100 μg intravenous dose. *Res Comm Substance Abuse* 2:161, 1981.
5. Wong LK, Beimann K: Metabolites of phencyclidine. *Clin Toxicol* 9:583, 1976.
6. Kaufman KR, Petrucha RA, Pitts FN, et al: PCP in amniotic fluid and breast milk: a case report. *J Clin Psychol* 44:269, 1983.
7. Kautman KR, Petrucha RA, Pitts FN, et al: Phencyclidine in umbilical cord blood: preliminary data. *Am J Psychol* 140:450, 1983.
8. Armen R, Kanel G, Reynolds T: Phencyclidine-induced malignant hyperthermia causing submassive liver necrosis. *Am J Med* 77:167, 1984.
9. Aronow R, Done AK: Phencyclidine overdose: an emerging concept of management. *JACEP* 7:56, 1978.
10. Barton CH, Sterling ML, Vaziri ND: Rhabdomyolysis and acute renal failure associated with phencyclidine intoxication. *Arch Intern Med* 140:568, 1980.
11. Burns RS, Lerner SE: Perspectives: acute phencyclidine intoxication. *Clin Toxicol* 9:477, 1976.
12. Eastman JW, Cohen SN: Hypertensive crisis and death associated with phencyclidine poisoning. *JAMA* 231:1270, 1975.
13. Rainey JM, Crowder MK: Prolonged psychosis attributed to phencyclidine: report of three cases. *Am J Psychiatry* 132:1076, 1975.
14. Rosen A: Case report: symptomatic mania and phencyclidine abuse. *Am J Psychiatry* 136:118, 1979.
15. Tong TG, Benowitz NL, Becker CE, et al: Phencyclidine poisoning. *JAMA* 234:512, 1975.
16. Barton CH, Sterling ML, Vaziri ND: Phencyclidine intoxication: clinical experience in 27 cases confirmed by urine assay. *Ann Emerg Med* 10:243, 1981.
17. Cravey RH, Reed D, Ragle JL: Phencyclidine-related deaths: a report of nine fatal cases. *J Anal Toxicol* 3:199, 1979.
18. Liden CB, Lovejoy FH, Costello CE: Phencyclidine: nine cases of poisoning. *JAMA* 234:513, 1975.
19. McCarron MM, Schulze BW, Thompson GA, et al: Acute phencyclidine intoxication: incidence of clinical findings in 1,000 cases. *Ann Emerg Med* 10:237, 1981.
20. McCarron MM, Schulze BW, Thompson GA, et al: Acute phencyclidine intoxication: clinical patterns, complications, and treatment. *Ann Emerg Med* 10:290, 1981.
21. Strauss AA, Modaniou HD, Bosu SK: Neonatal manifestations of phencyclidine (PCP) abuse. *Pediatrics* 68:550, 1981.
22. Walberg CB, McCarron MM, Schulze BW: Quantitation of phencyclidine in serum by enzyme immunoassay: results in 405 patients. *J Anal Toxicol* 7:106, 1983.
23. Schier J: Avoid unfavorable consequences: dextromethorphan can bring about a false positive phencyclidine urine drug screen. *J Emerg Med* 18:379, 2000.
24. Ragan FA, Samuels MS, Hite SA, et al: Diphenhydramine interferes with determination of phencyclidine by gas-liquid chromatography. *Clin Chem* 26:785, 1980.
25. Giannini AJ, Eighan MS, Loiselle RH, et al: Comparison of haloperidol and chlorpromazine in the treatment of phencyclidine psychosis. *J Clin Pharmacol* 24:202, 1984.
26. Luisada PV: The phencyclidine psychosis, phenomenology and treatment, in Peterson RC, Stillman RC (eds): *Phencyclidine (PCP) Abuse: An Appraisal.* Washington, DC, NIDA Research Monograph 21, 1978, p 241.
27. Schwarz BE, Bickford RB: Reversibility of induced psychosis with chlorpromazine. *Proc Staff Meet Mayo Clin* 30:407, 1955.
28. Klepfisz A, Racy J: Homicide and LSD. *JAMA* 223:429, 1973.
29. Knudsen K: Homicide after treatment with lysergic acid diethylamide. *Acta Psychiatr Scand Suppl* 180:389, 1965.
30. Reich P, Hepps R: Homicide during a psychosis induced by LSD. *JAMA* 219:869, 1972.
31. Thomas R, Fuller D: Self-inflicted ocular injury associated with drug use. *J S C Med Assoc* 68:202, 1972.
32. Feldberg W: The monoamines of the hypothalamus as mediators of temperature responses, in Robson JM, Stacey RS (eds): *Recent Advances in Pharmacology*. 4th ed. London, Churchill Livingstone, 1968, p 349.
33. Haigler HJ, Aghajanian GK: Lysergic acid diethylamide and serotonin: a comparison of effects on serotonergic neurons and neurons receiving a serotonergic input. *J Pharmacol Exp Ther* 188:688, 1974.

34. Benjamin DR: *Mushrooms Poisons and Panaceas: A Handbook for Naturalists, Mycologists and Physicians*. New York, NY, W. H. Freeman and Company, 1995.
35. Chilton WS, Bigwood J, Jensen RE: Psilocin, bufotenine, and serotonin: historical and biosynthetic observations. *J Psychedelic Drugs* 11:61, 1979.
36. Lyttle T: Misuse and legend in the toad licking phenomenon. *Int J Addict* 28:521, 1993.
37. Pahnke WN, Jurland AA, Unger S, et al: The experimental use of psychedelic (LSD) psychotherapy. *JAMA* 212:1856, 1970.
38. Ianzito BM, Liskow B, Stewart MA: Reaction to LSD in a two-year-old child. *J Pediatr* 80:643, 1972.
39. Milman DH: An untoward reaction to accidental ingestion of LSD in a 5-year-old girl. *JAMA* 201:143, 1967.
40. Cohen S: Suicide after ingestion of morning glory seeds. *Am J Psychiatry* 120:1024, 1964.
41. Fink PJ, Goldman MJ, Lyons I: Morning glory seed psychosis. *Arch Gen Psychiatry* 15:209, 1966.
42. Ingram AL: Morning glory seed reaction. *JAMA* 190:1133, 1964.
43. Dewhurst K: Psilocybin intoxication. *Br J Psychiatry* 137:303, 1980.
44. Rosenberg DE, Isbell H, Miner EJ: Comparison of a placebo, N-dimethyltryptamine, and 6-hydroxy-N-dimethyltryptamine in man. *Psychopharmacologia* 4:39, 1963.
45. Sivyer C, Dorrington L: Intravenous injection of mushrooms [letter]. *Med J Aust* 140:182, 1984.
46. Friedman SA, Hirsch SE: Extreme hyperthermia after LSD ingestion. *JAMA* 217:1549, 1971.
47. Klock JC, Boerner U, Becker CE: Coma, hyperthermia and bleeding associated with massive LSD overdose. *West J Med* 120:183, 1974.
48. Heard K, Daly FF, O'Malley G, et al: Respiratory distress after use of droperidol for agitation. *Ann Emerg Med* 34:410, 1999.
49. Mills K: Serotonin syndrome: a clinical update. *Crit Care Clin* 13:763, 1997.
50. Curry SC, Rose MC: Intravenous mushroom poisoning. *Ann Emerg Med* 14:900, 1985.
51. Horowitz MJ: Flashbacks: recurrent intrusive images after the use of LSD. *Am J Psychiatry* 126:565, 1969.
52. McCarron MM, Walberg CB, Baselt RC: Confirmation of LSD intoxication by analysis of serum and urine. *J Anal Toxicol* 14:165, 1990.
53. Boyorh MA, Zukowska-Grojec Z, Palkovits M, et al: Effect of phencyclidine (PCP) on blood pressure and catecholamine levels in discrete brain nuclei. *Brain Res* 321:315, 1984.
54. Fosset M, Renaud JF, Lenoie MC, et al: Interaction of molecules of phencyclidine series with cardiac cells: association with the muscarinic receptor. *FEBS Lett* 103:133, 1979.
55. Haring R, Kloog Y, Sokolovsky M: Localization of phencyclidine binding sites on alpha and beta subunits of the nicotinic acetylcholine receptor from *Torpedo ocellata* electric organ using azido phencyclidine. *J Neurosci* 4:627, 1984.
56. Johnson SW, Haroldsen PE, Hoffer BJ, et al: Presynaptic dopaminergic activity of phencyclidine in rat caudate. *J Pharmacol Exp Ther* 229:322, 1984.
57. Paster Z, Maayani S, Weinstein H, et al: Cholinolytic action of phencyclidine derivatives. *Eur J Pharmacol* 25:270, 1974.
58. Quirion R, Hammer RP, Herkenham M, et al: Phencyclidine (angel dust) sigma opiate receptor: visualization by tritium-sensitive film. *Proc Natl Acad Sci USA* 78:5881, 1981.
59. Smith RC, Meltzer HY, Arora RC, et al: Effects of phencyclidine on catecholamines and serotonin uptake in synaptosomal preparations from rat brain. *Biochem Pharmacol* 26:1436, 1977.
60. Tourneur Y, Romey G, Lazdunski M: Phencyclidine blockade of sodium and potassium channels in neuroblastoma cells. *Brain Res* 245:154, 1982.
61. Vincent JP, Cavey D, Kamenk JM, et al: Interaction of phencyclidines with the muscarinic and opiate receptors in the central nervous system. *Brain Res* 152:176, 1978.
62. Vincent JP, Vignon J, Kartalovski B, et al: Compared properties of central and peripheral binding sites for phencyclidine. *Eur J Pharmacol* 68:79, 1980.
63. Wong EHF, Kemp JA: Sites for antagonism of *N*-methyl-D-aspartate receptor channel complex. *Annu Rev Pharmacol Toxicol* 31:401, 1991.

CHAPTER 143 ■ SEDATIVE–HYPNOTIC AGENT POISONING

ANDIS GRAUDINS

Sedative–hypnotics include benzodiazepines (BZDs), barbiturates, non-BZD nonbarbiturate agents (NBNBs), and some muscle relaxants. The barbiturates and "bromides" were the first to become available. In the 1960s, the NBNBs, such as meprobamate (Miltown), were introduced and became popular. NBNBs have been mostly supplanted by the BZDs, which have greater efficacy and a larger therapeutic ratio, and are currently one of the most widely prescribed classes of drugs (Table 143.1). BZDs and their derivatives are used to treat anxiety, depression, panic disorders, insomnia, musculoskeletal disorders, seizures, and alcohol withdrawal, and are used as adjuncts for anesthesia and procedural sedation.

BENZODIAZEPINES

Pharmacology

BZDs exert their therapeutic effect at specific BZD receptor sites in the central nervous system (CNS) [1]. The BZD receptor is located within the γ-aminobutyric acid-A (GABA-A) receptor supramolecular complex (GRSMC). Binding of GABA or GABA plus a BZD causes an allosteric change in the GRSMC. This results in an alteration in chloride-channel permeability, with an increase in chloride flux and hyperpolarization. GABA is an inhibitory neurotransmitter, and its receptors form an inhibitory bidirectional system with connections within many areas of the CNS. Once neurotransmission has been altered, there is a secondary effect on neurotransmitter release from the internuncial neurons. For the most part, activation of a GABA neuron leads to changes in dopamine release, although norepinephrine and acetylcholine may be involved. Serotonin effect is minimal except for neurons in the dorsal raphe [2]. Activation of GRSMC by a BZD potentiates synaptic GABA-mediated inhibition [3,4]. The GRSMCs are located throughout the brain and the spinal cord area. The BZD receptors are categorized as omega 1, omega 2, and omega 3. Each of the omega subtypes tends to cluster in particular areas of the CNS [2,5–7]. The omega-1 subtype predominates in the sensorimotor cortex and is predominantly sedative–hypnotic. The omega-2 subtype is concentrated in the limbic areas of the brain with mainly anxiolytic and anticonvulsant properties [2,3].

BZD absorption from the gastrointestinal (GI) tract depends on the properties and pharmaceutical formulation of each drug. Peak levels occur within 3 hours post-ingestion; intramuscular absorption can be erratic and delayed. Duration of action is dependent on the lipophilicity of each compound; the more

TABLE 143.1

SEDATIVE–HYPNOTIC AGENTS

Benzodiazepines	Nonbenzodiazepine nonbarbiturates
Alprazolam	Alpidem
Bromazepam	Baclofen
Brotizolam	Buspirone
Chlordiazepoxide	Chloral hydrate
Clobazam	Chlormethiazole
Clorazepate	Ethinamate
Diazepam	Ethchlorvynol
Estazolam	Glutethimide
Flunitrazepam	Meprobamate
Flurazepam	Methaqualone
Halazepam	Methyprylon
Lorazepam	Paraldehyde
Midazolam	Zolpidem
Nitrazepam	
Oxazepam	
Quazepam	
Triazolam	
Barbiturates	
Amobarbital	
Aprobarbital	
Butalbital	
Mephobarbital	
Pentobarbital	
Phenobarbital	
Secobarbital	
Thiopental	

lipophilic, the shorter the duration of action. BZDs are highly protein-bound (85% to 99%). Their volume of distribution depends on lipid solubility and varies from 0.26 to 0.58 L per kg for chlordiazepoxide to 0.95 to 2.00 L per kg for diazepam. BZDs are metabolized by hepatic microsomal oxidation (N-dealkylation) and then glucuronidation [8,9]. They can be classified on the basis of elimination half-life (Table 143.2).

Fatality from pure BZD overdose is rare. Toxicity may vary between individual agents. Alprazolam overdose was found to result in more frequent intensive care unit admission, mechanical ventilation, and flumazenil use than other benzodiazepines [10]. A retrospective review of 1,239 overdose cases from one medical examiner's office revealed only two deaths solely related to diazepam overdose [11]. In chronic abusers, rapid clinical recovery after BZD overdose is believed to result from adaptation or tolerance to the depressant effect [12].

Clinical Presentation

Overdose commonly occurs as a part of polydrug ingestions. BZDs alone produce slurred speech, lethargy, ataxia, nystagmus, and coma. Loss of deep tendon reflexes and apnea are unusual except with a massive overdose. There are rare case reports of coma, cardiac arrest, acute respiratory distress syndrome, and pulmonary edema [12–15]. Abrupt cessation of BZDs after long-term use may result in a withdrawal syndrome [16,17] (see Chapter 145).

Diagnostic Evaluation

Recommended laboratory studies include serum electrolytes, blood urea nitrogen, creatinine, and glucose. Because BZDs may be involved in polydrug overdoses, serum acetaminophen levels and a 12-lead electrocardiogram (ECG) results should

TABLE 143.2

DURATION OF ACTION AND ELIMINATION HALF-LIFE ($T^1/_2$) OF BENZODIAZEPINES

Agent	Duration (h)	Elimination $t^1/_2$(h)	Peak effect (h)	Active metabolites
Ultra-short–acting	<10			
Midazolam (Versed)		2–5	0.3–0.8	–
Temazepam (Restoril)		10	2–3	–
Triazolam (Halcion)		1.7–3.0	0.5–1.5	+
Brotizolam		5	1	–
Short-acting	10–24			
Alprazolam (Xanax)		11–14	0.7–1.6	+
Lorazepam (Ativan)		10–20	2	–
Oxazepam (Serax)		3–21	1–2	–
Bromazepam		8–20	1–2	–
Flunitrazepam		20–30	2–8	+
Estazolam		10–24	1	–
Long-acting	>24	5–30	2–4	+
Chlordiazepoxide (Librium)		36–200	1.0–2.5	+
Clorazepate (Tranxene)		10–50	1–4	–
Clonazepam (Klonopin)		20–50	1–2	+
Diazepam (Valium)		50–100	3–6	+
Flurazepam (Dalmane)		26–200	6	+
Quazepam		11–77	1–3	+
Clobazam		14	1–3	+
Halazepam		Metabolites: 50–100		+
Prazepam (Centrax)		25–41 Metabolites: 40–114	6	+

also be obtained. Creatine phosphokinase (CPK), urine analysis, arterial blood gas, imaging studies, serum salicylate concentrations, and lumbar puncture should be obtained as clinically indicated. Quantitative BZD levels are not useful in the clinical management of overdose cases.

Management

The most important aspect of BZD overdose management is supportive care. Airway management should precede all interventions, and intubation is indicated if the patient cannot adequately maintain spontaneous ventilation or protect the airway. Vascular access should be established. The patient should be placed on continuous pulse oximetry and cardiac monitoring. Activated charcoal (1 g per kg) may be considered in awake patients if the presentation is within 1 hour of ingestion, but there is currently no evidence to suggest that administration changes outcome following simple BZD overdose and may in fact be harmful in patients who subsequently become sedated if the airway is unprotected. Charcoal administration is often not practical as many adult patients, presenting with deliberate self-poisoning, do so more than 2 hours post-ingestion [18]. Additionally, the risks of charcoal administration in a sedated patient with isolated benzodiazepine ingestion must be weighed against the low risk of morbidity and mortality seen with this type of poisoning. There is no evidence to suggest that repeat-dose charcoal enhances BZD elimination [19].

Flumazenil (Romazicon, Anexate) is a BZD antagonist that binds to the GRSMC omega-1 and -2 subtypes, competitively inhibiting BZD binding and thereby reversing BZD sedative and anxiolytic effects [20]. It may also reverse BZD-induced respiratory depression, obviating the need for intubation, but this effect is inconsistent. It does not fully reverse the amnestic effects of BZDs. Patients may appear awake and alert, but subsequent recall (e.g., of instructions) may be poor [21,22].

For most patients with pure benzodiazepine poisoning, supportive care with attention to airway and ventilatory status is all that is required to manage their overdose. It is uncommon for patients to require administration of flumazenil to treat sedation alone. This agent should never be considered in place of airway intervention in compromised patients. Adverse drug events associated with flumazenil use include anxiety, nausea, agitation, and crying. It should be avoided in patients who are suspected to be BZD-tolerant [23]. Flumazenil may precipitate an abrupt withdrawal syndrome with potential for seizures in these patients. This may occur after short-term use of benzodiazepines [24]. Flumazenil should also be avoided in patients with polypharmacy overdoses in whom reversal of BZD effect may unmask the epileptogenic effects of the other drugs (e.g., cyclic antidepressants, isoniazid, and cocaine). Flumazenil is contraindicated in patients with electrocardiographic evidence of cyclic antidepressant toxicity (e.g., prolonged QRS duration), as this finding is associated with a high risk of seizures [25]. Patients with a history of epilepsy are also at increased risk for seizures. Flumazenil has been suggested for both diagnostic purposes in undifferentiated coma and therapeutic purposes. Despite this, its role and indications remain unclear in the management of the BZD-poisoned patient [23]. Flumazenil does not reduce hospital length of stay or need for high-dependency monitoring. If administering flumazenil, the initial dose should be 0.05 to 0.1 mg. This can be repeated at 30-second intervals. In general, if there has not been any response after a total dose of 1 to 2 mg, the diagnosis of benzodiazepine poisoning is unlikely. In the uncommon situation where it may be used to reverse toxicity in deliberate self-poisoning, the aim is to titrate a flumazenil dose such that the patient is moderately drowsy and easily aroused, and *not* to have the patient completely awake, alert, and keen to self-discharge from hospital. Because flumazenil has a short half-life (approximately 50 minutes), it may be administered as an infusion in severe BZD poisoning, in a similar fashion to naloxone in severe opioid poisoning [26]. Seizures that result from flumazenil therapy may require treatment with large doses of BZDs or barbiturates (e.g., thiopental or phenobarbital).

Treatment of BZD withdrawal is similar to that for barbiturates and other nonbarbiturate sedative–hypnotics (see later discussion here and Chapter 145).

BARBITURATES

Barbiturates were the cornerstone of sedative–hypnotic therapy until the 1970s. Since then, the incidence of barbiturate overdose has declined, coincident with their diminishing use [27].

Pharmacology

Barbiturates depress the activity of all excitable tissues. They enhance GABA postexcitatory inhibition at the nerve terminal and appear to have a binding site on the GRSMC, leading to increased chloride flux. The CNS is most sensitive, with skeletal and smooth muscle depression evident at higher doses.

Barbiturates are available in all forms, although most toxicity results from ingestion. Barbiturates are divided into groups based on their duration of action. Ultra-short–acting barbiturates are highly lipid soluble and rapidly partition into the CNS, with subsequent redistribution to all tissues. When parenterally administered, they have rapid onset with less than 1-hour duration of effect; their predominant role is in induction of anesthesia.

Short- and intermediate-acting barbiturates are intermediate in lipid solubility and are used as anxiolytics and sedatives. Long-acting barbiturates have relatively low lipid solubility and are mainly used as anticonvulsants. Systemic toxicity tends to be a function of the drug's elimination half-life (Table 143.3).

Barbiturates are well absorbed from the GI tract; serum levels and symptoms are detectable within 30 minutes, and their peak effect occurs by 4 hours. Barbiturates are variably metabolized by the liver, with most of the highly lipid-soluble group excreted after glucuronidation. The longer-acting barbiturates rely more on urinary excretion for elimination (phenobarbital, 25% to 33%; barbital, 95%; primidone, 15% to 42%; phenylethylmalonamide a metabolite of primidone, 95%) [28]. As they are weak acids, renal elimination can be enhanced by urinary alkalinization. The kinetics of barbiturate elimination are mixed: first order at low concentrations and zero order at high ones [29]. Therapeutic serum drug levels are 10 to 40 μg per mL for phenobarbital and 1 to 5 μg per mL for the short-acting barbiturates. Toxic dosages are in the range of 6 to 10 g for the long-acting barbiturates and 3 to 6 g for the short-acting ones. Most patients demonstrate some degree of sedation with levels of 8 mg per kg. Tolerance rapidly develops, and chronic users may require 5 to 10 times the normal dose for sedation. Depending on the degree of tolerance, drug levels associated with coma range from 80 to 120 μg per mL for phenobarbital and 15 to 50 μg per mL for short-acting agents. Other sedatives (e.g., ethanol) have an additive effect and can result in toxicity at lower doses and blood concentrations [30].

Clinical Manifestations

The most common toxic scenario results from accidental or intentional oral barbiturate ingestion by a seizure patient or family member. Barbiturates may be involved in polypharmacy overdoses, particularly butalbital, a component of several common headache medications (e.g., Fiorinal).

TABLE 143.3

DURATION OF ACTION AND ELIMINATION HALF-LIFE ($t^1/_2$) OF BARBITURATES

Barbiturate	Duration (h)	Elimination $t^1/_2$ (h)
Ultra-short–acting	<1/2	
Thiopental (Pentothal)		6–46
Thiamylal (Surital)		NA
Methohexital (Brevital)		1–2
Short-acting	3	
Hexobarbital (Sombulex)		3–7
Pentobarbital (Nembutal)		15–48
Secobarbital (Seconal)		19–34
Intermediate-acting	3–6	
Amobarbital (Amytal)		8–42
Aprobarbital (Alurate)		14–34
Butabarbital (Butisol)		34–42
Butalbital (Fiorinal, Esgic)		NA
Long-acting	6–12	
Barbital		48
Mephobarbital (Mebaral)		48–52
Phenobarbital (Luminal)		24–144
Primidone (Mysoline)		10–12

NA, not available.
Adapted from Harves SC: Hypnotics and sedatives, in Goodman L, Gilman A (eds): *The Pharmacological Basis of Therapeutics*. 8th ed. New York, Macmillan, 1990, p 357.

Most patients present with some degree of sedation, which is evident within 30 minutes after ingestion of the agent. This may rapidly progress to coma, respiratory collapse, and hypotension. The patient may be mildly hypothermic from loss of autonomic function and decrease in overall muscle activity. The CNS depression is generalized, although there are many reports of focal findings [30,31]. Cardiovascular collapse with severe hypotension is believed to be due to direct myocardial suppression and vascular dilation, an indicator of serious toxicity. Dysrhythmias are rare. The gut becomes atonic, producing delayed absorption or ileus, which may then progress to bowel necrosis. Bullous skin lesions over pressure points occur in 6% of patients within 24 hours of ingestion [32,33]. The lesions are tense clean bullae surrounded by erythema, and the bullae fluid has detectable amounts of barbiturate. The presence of bullae is not pathognomonic for barbiturate poisoning. Bullae formation has also been reported following other sedative–hypnotics, tricyclic antidepressants, methadone, and carbon monoxide poisoning. Crystalluria has been reported [34].

Withdrawal symptoms may occur after 1 to 2 months of chronic use. Symptoms usually present after 2 to 7 days of abstinence or four to five elimination half-lives. Agitation, hyperreflexia, anxiety, and tremor are the most common symptoms, followed by confusion and hallucinations. In early withdrawal, up to 75% of patients experience seizures. Barbiturate withdrawal seizures appear to be more severe than ethanol withdrawal seizures. Transplacental tolerance occurs, with neonatal irritability noted for months after birth [35].

Diagnostic Evaluation

Serum phenobarbital concentration should be determined in situations where phenobarbital or primidone overdose is suspected. However, results of other serum barbiturate concentrations are generally not available in a clinically meaningful time. Recommended laboratory studies include complete blood cell count, serum electrolytes, blood urea nitrogen, creatinine, glucose, and liver function tests. Because barbiturates may be involved in polydrug overdoses, serum acetaminophen concentration, to exclude occult ingestion, and an ECG should also be obtained. CPK, urine analysis, arterial blood gas, imaging studies, and lumbar puncture should be obtained as clinically indicated.

Management

The most important aspect of barbiturate overdose management is supportive care. Early airway management is imperative, as up to 40% of patients may suffer from pulmonary aspiration. Frequent monitoring of all vital signs, including rectal temperature, is indicated. Vascular access should be obtained. The patient should be placed on continuous pulse oximetry and cardiac monitoring. A single dose of activated charcoal (1 g per kg) should be considered in large ingestions with appropriate airway protection.

Multiple-dose activated charcoal (MDAC) and urinary alkalinization can enhance the elimination of phenobarbital and possibly other barbiturates [36–38]. In a human volunteer study, MDAC was superior to urinary alkalinization in enhancing elimination of intravenously administered phenobarbital [39]. MDAC is recommended for all barbiturate overdoses, and urinary alkalinization is recommended for those involving long-acting agents such as phenobarbitone.

Hypotension should initially be treated with intravenous normal saline. Because its etiology is multifactorial, hypotension unresponsive to intravenous crystalloids challenge should be treated with dopamine or norepinephrine. Invasive hemodynamic monitoring and supportive therapy should be considered in severe or refractory cases. Cardiovascular instability unresponsive to conservative measures is also an indication for extracorporeal drug removal. Hemoperfusion (clearance, 100 to 300 mL per minute for phenobarbital) removes more drug than hemodialysis (clearance, 60 to 75 mL per minute), but more modern high-flow hemodialysis has the potential to be as effective as hemoperfusion, especially if combined with multiple-dose oral charcoal [40–42]. On completion of treatment, serum drug concentrations may rebound because of redistribution, and repeat hemodialysis/hemoperfusion may be necessary. Hypothermia requires rewarming. The patient should be monitored for development of aspiration pneumonia, acute respiratory distress syndrome, and electrolyte derangement.

Barbiturates suppress brain electrical activity, and an isoelectric electroencephalogram is not necessarily an indicator of poor prognosis; full recovery has been reported in patients with an isoelectric tracing.

Barbiturate withdrawal should be managed in a controlled environment with adequate resuscitation equipment available because seizures and cardiovascular collapse may occur. Because almost all sedative–hypnotic agents are cross-tolerant, barbiturate withdrawal can be treated with reinstitution of the same drug or another sedative–hypnotic (e.g., BZDs) in equipotent doses (Table 143.4). The goal in therapy is to suppress signs and symptoms of withdrawal. Patients should initially be given sufficient amounts of drug to induce sedation. Using an agent with a long duration of action (e.g., phenobarbital) maintains the serum concentrations, thereby limiting the side effects and cravings associated with falling levels. The dose is decreased by 10% every 3 days. If the equivalent phenobarbital dose is unknown, 120 mg can be administered orally or intravenously every 1 to 2 hours until withdrawal symptoms resolve or drowsiness ensues [17,43].

TABLE 143.4

SEDATIVE–HYPNOTIC EQUIVALENTS

Diazepam, 5 mg, is equivalent to	
Oxazepam	30 mg
Chlordiazepoxide	25 mg
Flurazepam	15 mg
Clorazepate	3.75 mg
Lorazepam	1 mg
Triazolam	0.5 mg
Alprazolam	0.25 mg
Phenobarbital, 30 mg, is equivalent to	
Pentobarbital	100 mg

Adapted from references [43,99].

Tolerance can be ascertained by the pentobarbital suppression test. The patient is given phenobarbital, 200 mg, every 2 hours until sedation occurs. If the initial 200 mg does not cause sedation, tolerance is present. If more than 1,200 mg is required to produce sedation, the patient will most likely experience withdrawal symptoms.

NONBENZODIAZEPINE, NONBARBITURATE SEDATIVE–HYPNOTICS

NBNB sedative–hypnotics include glutethimide (Doriden), ethchlorvynol (Placidyl), meprobamate (Miltown), chloral hydrate (Noctec), and the antispasmodic–muscle relaxants carisoprodol (Soma) and baclofen (Lioresal). Toxic effects and overdoses can be seen from legitimate and illicit use. Newer agents have also been introduced that vary in their toxicity in overdose. These include buspirone, an azaspirodecanedione that binds to 5-hydroxytryptamine receptors; zopiclone, a cyclopyrrolone with sedative–hypnotic activity; and zolpidem and alpidem, which are imidazopyridine sedative–hypnotic and anxiolytic agents, respectively. Many of these medications have a high abuse potential secondary to their ability to induce tolerance and dependence. In addition, a large percentage of those who use and abuse these medications have a history of psychiatric disorders and concurrent ethanol abuse.

Chloral Hydrate

Chloral hydrate was first introduced in 1869 and is still used for sedation in pediatric patients [44]. It is rapidly absorbed from the GI tract, with onset of action within 30 minutes. Chloral hydrate undergoes hepatic biotransformation by alcohol dehydrogenase. The principal metabolite trichloroethanol (TCE) has a longer half-life (4 to 12 hours) than the parent compound. When alcohol dehydrogenase is inhibited by 4-methylpyrazole, increased sedation is seen in 4-methylpyrazole–treated rats after chloral hydrate administration [45]. This suggests that the parent compound is more sedating than TCE and that the previously held belief that acute ethanol ingestion enhances TCE production and sedation may not be the case. However, acute chloral hydrate metabolism inhibition by ethanol may explain the additive effect of ethanol on chloral hydrate sedation ("Mickey Finn") [45]. The metabolism of chloral hydrate to TCE is age-related, with an increasing elimination half-life as the neonate ages to toddler [46]. In neonates, the glucuronidation pathway is still immature and chloral hydrate competes with bilirubin. In addition, renal clearance is limited due to immature kidney function. This can lead to direct hyperbilirubinemia in the neonate [46–48]. Saturation kinetics leading to prolonged elimination has been demonstrated in cases of overdose [49].

There has been a number of reports regarding pediatric chloral hydrate toxicity [49,50]. The lethal dose in adults is 5 to 10 g, but as little as 1.25 g has been fatal. Patients have survived reported doses as high as 36 g [51,52]. Toxicity develops within 3 to 4 hours after ingestion and is manifested by significant GI irritation, ranging from gastritis to perforation [53]. Other findings include CNS depression, pinpoint pupils, hypothermia, hypotension, and respiratory depression. Paradoxic CNS excitation, particularly in children, has been reported coinciding with peak plasma levels (1 to 3 hours) [48]. Myocardial depression results from decreased myocardial contraction and decreased refractory period. Cardiac dysrhythmias such as multifocal premature ventricular contractions, supraventricular dysrhythmias, and ventricular tachycardia have been reported [54].

Tolerance and addiction can develop in chronic abusers. The addicted patient may take very large doses of the drug and can suffer a withdrawal syndrome similar to that from alcohol [55]. Because this drug is hepatotoxic, the abuser may experience unexpected liver failure, leading to acute intoxication and death at doses that were previously tolerated [56].

The treatment of chloral hydrate poisoning is primarily supportive. All patients with a suspected ingestion should have an established intravenous line and continuous pulse oximetry and cardiac monitoring. Activated charcoal (1 g per kg) should be considered in symptomatic patients presenting early post-ingestion with appropriate airway protection. As chloral hydrate is radiopaque, large ingested amounts may be seen on abdominal radiographs.

Cardiac dysrhythmias may not respond to standard antidysrhythmics, such as lidocaine. Beta-blockers (e.g., propranolol 1.0 mg IV) may be of benefit [57]. Ventricular dysrhythmias may be partly due to TCE sensitization of myocardium to endogenous catecholamines similar to other halogenated hydrocarbons. Hypothermia can generally be treated with passive rewarming. Hemoperfusion may be considered in patients with prolonged coma, refractory dysrhythmias, or hypotension [58]. TCE clearance by hemodialysis varies between 120 and 162 mL per minute. In one patient who ingested 38 g, the half-life decreased from 35 to 6 hours after hemodialysis [58].

Ethchlorvynol

Ethchlorvynol is a hypnotic with muscle relaxant and anticonvulsant activities. Clinical effects are apparent within 15 to 30 minutes, and peak levels are seen in 1 to 2 hours. Ethchlorvynol is highly lipid-soluble and is stored in adipose tissue and the brain. It has a unique half-life, being 10 to 25 hours in therapeutic ingestions but up to 100 hours in very large overdoses. Ninety percent of the drug is metabolized by the liver. The patient may present with an altered sensorium ranging from dizziness to facial tingling, giddiness, excitement, dysarthria, ataxia, mydriasis, nystagmus, or areflexia after smaller doses. Severe overdose is characterized by profound and prolonged coma (more than 1 week), hypothermia, respiratory depression, hypotension, and bradycardia [59]. Comatose patients may have an isoelectric electroencephalogram. Seizures may occur after acute ethchlorvynol ingestion. A sometimes clinically useful property of ethchlorvynol is its aromatic and quite pungent odor, described as similar to that of a new car or plastic shower curtain. It may be detected on the patient's breath.

As in other medications of this group, chronic abuse of ethchlorvynol resulted in tolerance and dependence. Sudden withdrawal can be confused with delirium tremens or an acute psychotic reaction [60].

Treatment is supportive. Hemoperfusion effectively clears the drug [61]. However, lipid redistribution of the drug means that repeated hemoperfusion may be necessary.

Glutethimide

The toxic dose of glutethimide is more than 3.0 g, with a usual fatal dose being 10 to 20 g. Glutethimide is highly lipid-soluble and displays two-compartment kinetics, with rapid intake in the brain followed by systemic distribution. Gastrointestinal glutethimide absorption is erratic, but its onset of action is 20 to 30 minutes [62]. Glutethimide is metabolized in the liver to an active metabolite, 4-hydroxy-2-ethyl-2-phenylglutarimide [62], which has a longer duration of action and is more potent than the parent compound [63]. It also stimulates the hepatic microsomal enzyme system and has considerable anticholinergic activity.

Acute glutethimide overdose is similar to that seen with barbiturates. Profound and prolonged coma is similar to that seen with ethchlorvynol. Glutethimide has been reported to produce thick and tenacious bronchial secretions. The most unique aspect of acute glutethimide intoxication is the fluctuating level of consciousness [63]. The reason for this is unclear, but theories include enterohepatic recirculation of the drug and its metabolites, prolonged absorption of the parent compound from an anticholinergic-induced paralytic ileus, and redistribution from adipose stores. Increased intracranial pressure, seizures, areflexia, and muscular twitching may be evident. Hypotension, hypothermia, persistent acidosis, and cardiac arrest have all been reported [63]. The chronic use of glutethimide leads to tolerance and addiction.

Glutethimide was frequently abused as a combination drug with codeine. Most preparations containing codeine also contained acetaminophen. This combination of glutethimide and Tylenol No. 3 or Tylenol No. 4 was called "loads" or "fours and doors."

The mainstay of treatment for glutethimide poisoning is supportive care. Because there may be significant anticholinergic-induced delay in gastric emptying, late administration of activated charcoal may be effective. Treatment with MDAC may increase glutethimide and 4-hydroxy-2-ethyl-2-phenylglutarimide elimination because of its known enterohepatic circulation. Case reports suggest that charcoal hemoperfusion may hasten recovery from coma, but this has never been examined in a controlled fashion [64].

Meprobamate and Carisoprodol

Meprobamate (e.g., Equanil, Miltown, Bamate, Neuramate) is an unusual member of this class of medications. It has antianxiety and muscle-relaxant effects in addition to sedative properties. Meprobamate is available in regular and sustained-release formulation. Toxicity can be seen in ingestions as small as 2.0 g and fatalities with as little as 12 g [65]. Survival has been documented with doses as high as 40 g.

Meprobamate is rapidly and completely absorbed after an oral dose [65]. Peak effect is seen in 3 hours, with a half-life of 10 hours. Most patients feel an effect for up to 36 hours. The drug is largely metabolized in the liver, induces microsomal enzymes, and its inactive metabolites are excreted in the urine. Very little of the drug is plasma protein-bound.

The clinical picture of meprobamate poisoning is similar to that of the other medications in this class, with predominately CNS and respiratory function impairment [65]. Hypotension is primarily mediated by a fall in systemic vascular resistance dysrhythmias, and palpitations [66]. Persistently elevated serum levels may indicate ongoing drug absorption from bezoar formation. Levels more than 20.5 mg per dL have been associated with CNS depression and coma. A withdrawal-abstinence syndrome beginning 1 to 2 days after cessation can occur even after chronic daily ingestions of as little as 1.6 g. Treatment of meprobamate poisoning is similar to that for the other medications in this class. MDAC may be of value after large ingestions because of potential for gastric concretion formation [67]. Hemoperfusion hastens drug clearance and should be considered in patients with cardiovascular compromise or failure to improve despite aggressive supportive treatment [68].

Carisoprodol (Soma, Rela) is a congener of meprobamate used as a muscle relaxant. Carisoprodol is metabolized in the liver and excreted in the urine, with an elimination half-life of 4 to 6 hours. Some of the ingested dose is metabolized to meprobamate by CYP2C19 [69]. The predominant side effect of the drug is drowsiness. Rarely seen idiosyncratic reactions include asthenia, transient quadriplegia, dizziness, ataxia, diplopia, agitation, confusion, and disorientation. Its toxicity and treatment are otherwise similar to those of meprobamate [70].

Baclofen

Although usually not considered a sedative or hypnotic drug, baclofen (Lioresal) toxicity may mimic that of sedative–hypnotics, and treatment is similar. Baclofen is a potent GABA-B agonist. Its primary use is as an antispasmodic agent, decreasing flexor tone and spasm in certain neurologic diseases. Therapeutic doses of baclofen are 15 to 60 mg per day. Baclofen is cleared by the kidney, with only a small portion hepatically transformed. Baclofen is well absorbed from the GI tract. Elimination is by first-order elimination kinetics, with a half-life of 2 to 6 hours after therapeutic dosing. Intrathecal baclofen is being used increasingly to treat intractable spasticity in children and in patients with spinal cord injury. Complications such as baclofen overdose and withdrawal syndrome may be related to pump malfunction, refilling mistakes, and programming mistakes related to adjustment of pump flow rate [71,72].

Hypotension and hypertension have been reported with baclofen toxicity [73]. Coma, seizures, severe myoclonus, apnea, and hypothermia may be evident [74]. Cardiac effects include prolonged PR and QTc intervals, junctional escape beats, premature atrial contractions with block, supraventricular tachycardia, and bradycardia [73]. Myoclonus and hyporeflexia have also been reported as well as seizure activity documented on EEG monitoring [71].

Management following baclofen either by the oral or intrathecal route intoxication is primarily supportive. Mechanical ventilatory support is often required after overdose [73]. Baclofen, in a large overdose, is more slowly absorbed from the GI tract than after a single therapeutic dose, suggesting that the administration of activated charcoal may be of benefit. Symptomatic bradycardia responds to atropine [75]. Hypotension commonly responds to intravenous fluids. Ventilatory assistance may be required for prolonged periods, averaging 3 to 7 days [76]. Patients have been observed to be persistently symptomatic up to 60 hours post-ingestion even when serum baclofen levels are undetectable [77]. Benzodiazepines should be used to control seizure activity or myoclonus.

Baclofen withdrawal syndrome (Chapter 145) may result after sudden cessation of oral baclofen therapy or in patients being treated with intrathecal baclofen where there may be pump failure and reduced baclofen delivery. Withdrawal may present with mental status changes, delirium, hallucinations, hypertension, hyperthermia, myoclonus, hyperreflexia, seizure activity, and may mimic signs of serotonin syndrome or neuroleptic malignant syndrome in some cases [71,78]. A close evaluation of the baclofen pump is essential in these cases to identify any potential dosing errors or malfunction with the pump system. Treatment includes supportive care and reinstitution of baclofen therapy as soon as practicable, but may also require the acute use of high-dose parenteral benzodiazepines to attenuate symptoms and signs of neuromuscular hyperexcitability and seizure activity [78,79].

Buspirone

Buspirone is a serotonergic and dopaminergic active drug with minimal sedative–hypnotic effects during therapeutic dosing. It also has central acetylcholine and norepinephrine effects. Its mechanism of action is not fully understood, but it appears to interact with exogenous and endogenous BZD, binding at the GRSMC as well as 5-hydroxytryptamine receptors. At low doses, it is predominately anxiolytic, although it may take several weeks to reach this effect. At high doses, it can cause sedation similar to that seen with BZDs (20 mg per day), but the sedation is much less than that seen with an equivalent dose of the BZD. It is well absorbed orally, and peak serum levels occur within 1 to 2 hours. It is hepatically metabolized, with an elimination half-life of 2 to 3 hours.

Adverse drug events reported during therapeutic dosing include weakness, GI distress, dysphoria, headache, and dizziness. It may cause a withdrawal syndrome after prolonged use but does not cross-react with BZDs in treating BZD withdrawal. Flumazenil does not reverse buspirone effect.

Buspirone has been an uncommon drug in overdose settings. Serotonin syndrome has rarely been reported when buspirone has been added to therapy in patients prescribed selective serotonin reuptake inhibitor medications such as fluoxetine, fluvoxamine, and sertraline [80–82]. Supportive care is the mainstay of therapy after an overdose.

Zopiclone

Zopiclone is a non-BZD agent with sedative–hypnotic, anxiolytic, and muscle-relaxant properties but is predominately marketed as a hypnotic agent. It appears to bind to the GRSMC, possibly with its own binding site. It has been found to displace diazepam and flunitrazepam from their BZD binding sites. It is well absorbed orally, with peak plasma concentration within 30 to 90 minutes. It undergoes first-order kinetics of distribution and is extensively metabolized. Elimination occurs by the kidneys and lungs. Absorption is significantly affected by gastric emptying. Adverse drug events include a bitter taste in the mouth, and there is carryover sedation into the next day. There may be a morning-after amnesic effect. After chronic dosing, physical dependency and withdrawal have been reported. It may also potentiate the sedative effects of ethanol.

Isolated zopiclone poisoning commonly follows a similar benign course to that of benzodiazepine poisoning [83]. Patients with concurrent ethanol or other sedative ingestion may develop significantly greater sedation. Observation and supportive care is the mainstay of therapy. Isolated reports have noted mild to moderate and delayed onset (14 to 16 hours post-ingestion) methemoglobinemia (10 to 23%) following zopiclone overdose [84]. This may be related to production of large amounts of an N-oxide metabolite of the parent drug [84]. Zopiclone poisoning has been reported to respond to flumazenil [85].

Zolpidem and Alpidem

Zolpidem and alpidem are imidazopyridine agents used as hypnotic and anxiolytic agents, respectively. Both bind to the GRSMC, zolpidem at the omega-1 and alpidem at the omega-1/omega-3 receptor binding sites. Both agents are rapidly absorbed orally, highly protein-bound, and hepatically metabolized. Zolpidem has an elimination half-life of 2.5 to 5.0 hours and alpidem of 8 to 20 hours. Adverse drug events associated with zolpidem use include anxiety, dizziness, drowsiness, fatigue, headache, diplopia, diarrhea, tremor, and hangover effect with anterograde amnesia. Alpidem use has been associated with adverse drug events such as sedation, headache, dizziness, insomnia, nausea, and vomiting. Alpidem has been reported to increase serum hepatic transaminase levels. Tolerance, dependency, and subsequent withdrawal are possible. Coingestion with other sedative agents, including alcohol, will result in increased sedation.

The most common findings seen after zolpidem overdose include sedation and respiratory depression. Cardiovascular or ECG changes do not occur in isolated zolpidem toxicity. Death has been reported with the combination of overdose with zolpidem and other CNS depressants, although no deaths have been reported with zolpidem overdose alone [86]. Treatment of overdose is predominately supportive. Flumazenil has been used to reverse the effects of zolpidem in overdose [87].

γ-Hydroxybutyrate

γ-Hydroxybutyrate (GHB) was originally used as an anesthetic induction agent and subsequently found to be a naturally occurring GABA metabolite in the CNS. It does not interact with GABA-A receptors, and as a result, its effects are not antagonized by flumazenil [88]. The mechanism of action of GHB may result from its interaction with specific GHB receptors, GABA-B receptors, and by elevation of CNS dopamine and endorphin levels [88]. GHB can be administered orally or parenterally with clinical effects occurring within 30 minutes of ingestion. Metabolism is by succinate semialdehyde to succinate, which enters the Krebs cycle and is eventually metabolized to carbon dioxide and water. GHB is also excreted (2% to 5%) unchanged in urine [89].

γ-Hydroxybutyrate can be obtained illicitly by mail order in powder form and reconstituted to a liquid. GHB is commonly produced in illicit backyard laboratories in the United States. Recipes for its production can be found on the Internet. Production begins with γ-butyrolactone, which is treated with an alkali such as sodium hydroxide to open the lactone ring to produce GHB when heated. If the pH of the solution is not back-titrated with acid, it may result in a highly alkaline solution. Esophageal burns and subsequent stricture formation has been reported after ingestion of an alkali GHB solution [90]. GHB is abused for its hypnotic and euphoric effects recreationally and may also have been used as a date-rape drug. Many states in the United States have categorized GHB as a Schedule-1 controlled substance.

"Pine needle oil" contains 1,4-butanediol and has been reported to induce a similar toxicity to GHB. Alcohol and aldehyde dehydrogenase catalyze the conversion of 1,4-butanediol to GHB, resulting in a clinical syndrome similar to GHB toxicity. This reaction can be inhibited by ethanol, 4-methylpyrazole, and disulfiram [91]. Butanediol and γ-butyrolactone are freely available for legal purchase over the Internet in many countries. As both are metabolized to GHB when ingested and result in similar toxicity, they are often purchased instead of GHB to avoid legal prosecution [92].

Symptoms of GHB toxicity occur rapidly after ingestion and may be potentiated by alcohol and other sedative agents, including opioids. Death has resulted from mixed intoxication with opioids [93]. Drowsiness, euphoria, hallucinations, delirium, nausea, vomiting, hypothermia, seizures, and coma can be seen. Recovery from pure GHB poisoning is typically rapid with return of consciousness within a few hours of ingestion [94]. Mass exposures have been reported in the popular press, usually in the setting of a dance rave, party, or nightclub [95]. Chronic use can lead to tolerance and physical dependence. A withdrawal syndrome comprising anxiety, agitation, paranoia, and visual and auditory hallucinations has been reported [96].

Management of GHB intoxication is supportive. Airway protection and ventilatory support are the mainstay of therapy. Prolonged sedation may indicate coingestion of other sedative agents. Flumazenil (GABA-A receptor antagonist) and physostigmine (short-acting acetylcholinesterase) do *not* reverse sedation [97,98] and may result in unwanted toxic effects of the respective antidotal agent. Because GHB is usually ingested as a liquid formulation and has a rapid onset of action, activated charcoal is unlikely to be beneficial.

ACKNOWLEDGMENT

Professor Cynthia Aaron contributed to the writing of this chapter in previous editions.

References

1. Tallman JF, Paul PM, Skolnick P: Receptors for the age of anxiety: pharmacology of the benzodiazepines. *Science* 207:274, 1980.
2. Perrault G, Morel E, Sanger DJ, et al: Differences in pharmacological profiles of a new generation of benzodiazepine hypnotics. *Eur J Pharmacol* 187:487, 1990.
3. Dennis TD, Benavides J, Scatton B: Distribution of central omega 1 (benzodiazepine1) and omega 2 (benzodiazepine2) receptor subtypes in the monkey and human brain: an autoradiographic study with [3 H] flunitrazepam and the omega 1 selective ligand [3 H] zolpidem. *J Pharmacol Exp Ther* 247:309, 1988.
4. Study RE, Barker JL: Cellular mechanisms of benzodiazepine action. *JAMA* 247:2147, 1982.
5. Ruano D, Benavides J, Machado A, et al: Regional differences in the enhancement by GABA of [3 H] zolpidem binding to omega sites in rat membranes and sections. *Brain Res* 600:134, 1993.
6. Langer SZ, Arbilla S: Imidazopyridines as a tool for the characterization of benzodiazepine receptors: a proposal for a pharmacological classification of omega receptor subtypes. *Pharm Biochem Behav* 29:763, 1988.
7. Benavides J, Peny B, Ruano D, et al: Comparative autoradiographic distribution of central omega (benzodiazepine) modulatory site subtypes and high, intermediate, and low affinity for zolpidem and alpidem. *Brain Res* 604:240, 1993.
8. Greenblat DJ, Shader RI, Abernathy DR: Current status of benzodiazepines. *N Engl J Med* 309:410, 1983.
9. Greenblat DJ, Shader RI, Abernathy DR, et al: Current status of benzodiazepines (first of two parts). *N Engl J Med* 3009:354, 1983.
10. Isbister GK, O'Regan L, Sibbritt D, et al: Alprazolam is relatively more toxic than other benzodiazepines in overdose. *Br J Clin Pharmacol* 8:88, 2004.
11. Finkle BS, McCloskey KL, Goodman LS, et al: Diazepam and drug associated deaths: a survey in the United States and Canada. *JAMA* 242:429, 1979.
12. Olson KR, Yin L, Osterloh J, et al: Coma caused by trivial triazolam overdose. *Am J Emerg Med* 3:210, 1985.
13. Berger R, Green G, Melnick A, et al: Cardiac arrest caused by oral diazepam intoxication. *Clin Pediatr* 14:842, 1975.
14. Stringer MD: Adult respiratory distress syndrome associated with flurazepam overdose. *J Roy Soc Med* 78:74, 1985.
15. Richman S: Acute pulmonary edema associated with Librium use. *Radiology* 103:57, 1979.
16. Sellers EM: Alcohol, barbiturate and benzodiazepine withdrawal syndromes: clinical management. *Can Med Assoc J* 139:113, 1988.
17. Sellers EM, Busto U, Sellers EM, et al: Withdrawal reaction after long-term therapeutic use of benzodiazepines. *N Engl J Med* 315:854, 1986.
18. Karim A, Ivatts S, Dargan P, et al: How feasible is it to conform to the European guidelines on administration of activated charcoal within one hour of an overdose? *Emerg Med J* 18(5):390–392, 2001.
19. Anonymous: Position statement and practice guidelines on the use of multidose activated charcoal in the treatment of acute poisoning. American Academy of Clinical Toxicology; European Association of Poisons Centres and Clinical Toxicologists. *J Toxicol Clin Toxicol* 37(6):731–751, 1999.
20. Benavides J, Peny B, Durand A, et al: Comparative in vivo and in vitro ω(benzodiazepine) site ligands in inhibiting [3 H] flumazenil binding in the rat central nervous system. *J Pharmacol Exp Ther* 263:884, 1992.
21. Sanders LD, Piggott SE, Issac PA, et al: Reversal of benzodiazepine sedation with the antagonist flumazenil. *Br J Anaesth* 66:445, 1991.
22. Hommer D, Weingartner H, Breier A: Dissociation of benzodiazepine-induced amnesia from sedation by flumazenil pretreatment. *Psychopharmacol* 112:455, 1993.
23. Seger DL: Flumazenil—treatment or toxin? *J Toxicol Clin Toxicol* 42:209, 2004.
24. Mintzer MZ, Griffiths RR: Flumazenil-precipitated withdrawal in healthy volunteers following repeated diazepam exposure. *Psychopharmacol* 178: 259, 2005.
25. Haverkos GP, DiSalvo RP, Imhoff TE: Fatal seizures after flumazenil administration in a patient with mixed overdose. *Ann Pharmacother* 28(12):1347–1349, 1994.
26. Maxa JL, Ogu CC, Adeeko MA: Continuous-infusion flumazenil in the management of chlordiazepoxide toxicity. *Pharmacotherapy* 23:1513, 2003.
27. Watson WA, Litovitz TL, Rodgers GC, et al: 2004 Annual Report of the American Association of Poison Control Centers Toxic Exposure Surveillance System. *Am J Emerg Med* 23(5):589–666, 2005.
28. Sumner DJ, Kalk J, Whiting B: Metabolism of barbiturate after over-dosage. *Br Med J* 1:335, 1975.
29. McCarron MM, Schulze BW, Walberg CB, et al: Short acting barbiturate overdosage. *JAMA* 248:55, 1982.
30. Wilber GS, Coldwell BB, Trenholm HL: Toxicity of ethanol-barbiturate mixtures. *J Pharm Pharmacol* 21:232, 1969.
31. Carroll BJ: Barbiturate overdosage: presentation with focal neurological signs. *Med J Aust* 1:1133, 1969.
32. Anonymous: Barbiturate coma and blisters. *Lancet* 1:733, 1972.
33. Beveridge GW, Lawson AAH: Occurrence of bullous lesions in acute barbiturate poisoning. *Br Med J* 1:835, 1965.
34. Van Heijst ANP, deJong W, Seldenrijk R, et al: Coma and crystalluria: a massive primidone intoxication treated with hemoperfusion. *J Toxicol Clin Toxicol* 20:307, 1983.
35. Desmond MM, Schwanecte RP, Wilson GS, et al: Maternal barbiturate utilization and neonatal withdrawal symptomatology. *J Pediatr* 80:190, 1972.
36. Berg MJ, Berlinger WG, Goldber MJ, et al: Acceleration of the body clearance of phenobarbital by oral activated charcoal. *N Engl J Med* 307:642, 1982.
37. Boldy DAR, Vale JA, Prescott PI: Treatment of phenobarbitone poisoning with repeat oral administration of activated charcoal. *Q J Med* 235:997, 1986.
38. Wakabayashi Y, Maruyama S, Hachimura K, et al: Activated charcoal interrupts enteroenteric circulation of phenobarbital. *J Toxicol Clin Toxicol* 32:419–424, 1994.
39. Frenia ML, Schauben JL, Wears RL, et al: Multiple-dose activated charcoal compared to urinary alkalinization for the enhancement of phenobarbital elimination. *J Toxicol Clin Toxicol* 34:169–175, 1996.
40. DeBroc ME, Bismuth C, DeGroot G, et al: Haemoperfusion: A useful therapy for the severely poisoned patient? *Hum Toxicol* 5:11, 1986.
41. Jacobsen D, Wiik-Larsen E, Dahl T, et al: Pharmacokinetic evaluation of haemoperfusion in phenobarbital poisoning. *Eur J Clin Pharmacol* 26:109, 1984.
42. Zawada ET, Nappi J, Done G, et al: Advances in the hemodialysis management of phenobarbital overdose. *South Med J* 76:6, 1983.
43. Smith DE, Wesson DR: A new method for treatment of barbiturate dependence. *JAMA* 213:294, 1970.
44. Brow AM, Cade JF: Cardiac arrhythmias after chloral hydrate overdose. *Med J Aust* 1:28, 1980.
45. Hung O, Kaplan J, Hoffman R, et al: Improved understanding of the ethanol-chloral hydrate interaction using 4-MP. *J Toxicol Clin Toxicol* 35:507, 1997.
46. Mayers DJ, Hindmarsh KW, Sankaran D, et al: Chloral hydrate disposition following single-dose administration to critically ill neonates and children. *Dev Pharmacol Ther* 16:71, 1991.
47. Lambert GH, Muraskas J, Anderson CL, et al: Direct hyperbilirubinemia associated with chloral hydrate administration in the newborn. *Pediatrics* 86:277, 1990.
48. Reimche LD, Sankara K, Hindmarsh KW, et al: Chloral hydrate sedation in neonates and infants: clinical and pharmacologic considerations. *Dev Pharmacol Ther* 12:57, 1989.
49. Anyebuno MA, Rosenfeld CR: Chloral hydrate toxicity in a term infant. *Dev Pharmacol Ther* 17:116, 1991.
50. Jastak JT, Pallasch T: Death after chloral hydrate sedation: report of a case. *J Am Dent Assoc* 116:345, 1988.

51. Bowyer K, Glasser SP: Chloral hydrate overdose and cardiac arrhythmias. *Chest* 77(2):232–235, 1980.
52. Gaulier JM, Merle G, Lacassie E, et al: Fatal intoxications with chloral hydrate. *J Forensic Sci* 46(6):1507–1509, 2001.
53. Lee DC, Vassalluzzo C: Acute gastric perforation in a chloral hydrate overdose. *Am J Emerg Med* 16(5):545–546, 1998.
54. Sing K, Erickson T, Amitai Y, et al: Chloral hydrate toxicity from oral and intravenous administration. *J Toxicol Clin Toxicol* 34:101–106, 1996.
55. Leuschner J, Zimmermann T: Examination of the dependence potential of chloral hydrate by oral administration to normal monkeys. *Arzneimittelforschung* 46(8):751–754, 1996.
56. Ramdhan DH, Kamijima M, Yamada N, et al: Molecular mechanism of trichloroethylene-induced hepatotoxicity mediated by CYP2E1. *Toxicol Appl Pharmacol* 231(3):300–307, 2008.
57. Zahedi A, Grant MH, Wong DT: Successful treatment of chloral hydrate cardiac toxicity with propranolol. *Am J Emerg Med* 17(5):490–491, 1999.
58. Buur T, Larsson R, Norlander B: Pharmacokinetics of chloral hydrate poisoning treated with hemodialysis and hemoperfusion. *Acta Med Scand* 223(3): 269–274, 1988.
59. Yell RP: Ethchlorvynol overdose. *Am J Emerg Med* 8(3):246–250, 1990.
60. Flemenbaum A, Gunby B: Ethchlorvynol (Placidyl) abuse and withdrawal (review of clinical picture and report of 2 cases). *Dis Nerv Syst* 32(3):188–192, 1971.
61. Kathpalia SC, Haslitt JH, Lim VS: Charcoal hemoperfusion for treatment of ethchlorvynol overdose. *Artif Organs* 7(2):246–248, 1983.
62. Crow JW, Lain P, Bochner F, et al: Glutethimide and pharmacokinetics in man. *Clin Pharmacol Ther* 22:458, 1977.
63. Hansen AR, Kennedy KA, Ambre JJ, et al: Glutethimide poisoning. A metabolite contributes to morbidity and mortality. *N Engl J Med* 292(5): 250–252, 1975.
64. Vale JA, Rees AJ, Widdop B, et al: Use of charcoal haemoperfusion in the management of severely poisoned patients. *Br Med J* 1(5948):5–9, 1975.
65. Bailey DN: Meprobamate ingestion: a five year review of cases with serum concentrations and clinical findings. *Am J Clin Pathol* 75:102, 1981.
66. Landier C, Lanotte R, Legras A, et al: State of shock during acute meprobamate poisoning. 6 cases. *Ann Fr Anesth Reanim* 13(3):407–411, 1994.
67. Hassen E: Treatment of meprobamate overdose with repeated oral doses of activated charcoal. *Ann Emer Med* 15:73, 1986.
68. Jacobsen D, Wiik-Larsen E, Saltvedt E, et al: Meprobamate kinetics during and after terminated hemoperfusion in acute intoxications. *J Toxicol Clin Toxicol* 25(4):317–331, 1987.
69. Dalen P, Alvan G: Formation of meprobamate from carisoprodol is catalysed by CYP2C19. *Pharmacogenetics* 6:387–394, 1996.
70. Siddiqi M, Jennings CA: A near-fatal overdose of carisoprodol (SOMA): case report. *J Toxicol Clin Toxicol* 42:239, 2004.
71. Darbari FP, Melvin JJ, Piatt JH Jr, et al: Intrathecal baclofen overdose followed by withdrawal: clinical and EEG features. *Pediatr Neurol* 33(5):373–377, 2005.
72. Yeh RN, Nypaver MM, Deegan TJ, et al: Baclofen toxicity in an 8-year-old with an intrathecal baclofen pump. *J Emerg Med* 26(2):163–167, 2004.
73. Nugent S, Katz MD, Little TE: Baclofen overdose with cardiac conduction abnormalities: case report and review of the literature. *Clin Toxicol* 24:321.1986.
74. Yassa RY, Iskandar HL: Baclofen induced psychosis: two cases and a review. *J Clin Psych* 49:318, 1988.
75. Cohen MD, Gaily RA, McCoy GC: Atropine in the treatment of baclofen overdose. *Am J Emerg Med* 4:552, 1986.
76. Rushman S, McLaren I: Management of intra-thecal baclofen overdose. *Intensive Care Med* 25(2):239, 1999.
77. Perry H, Shannon M, Wright R, et al: Baclofen overdose: a pediatric mass exposure. *J Toxicol Clin Toxicol* 35:549, 1997.
78. Shirley KW, Kothare S, Piatt JH Jr, et al: Intrathecal baclofen overdose and withdrawal. *Pediatr Emerg Care* 22(4):258–261, 2006.
79. Samson-Fang L, Gooch J, Norlin C: Intrathecal baclofen withdrawal simulating neuroepileptic malignant syndrome in a child with cerebral palsy. *Dev Med Child Neurol* 42(8):561–565, 2000.
80. Baetz M, Malcolm D: Serotonin syndrome from fluvoxamine and buspirone [letter]. *Can J Psychiatry* 40:428–429, 1995.
81. Bonin B, Vandel P, Vandel S, et al: Serotonin syndrome after sertraline, buspirone and loxapine? *Therapie* 54(2):269–271, 1999.
82. Manos GH: Possible serotonin syndrome associated with buspirone added to fluoxetine. *Ann Pharmacother* 34(7–8):871–874, 2000.
83. Harry P: Intoxications aigues par les nouveaux psychotropes. *Rev Prat* 47(7):731–735, 1997.
84. Fung HT, Lai CH, Wong OF, et al: Two cases of methemoglobinemia following zopiclone ingestion. *Clin Toxicol (Philadelphia, Pa)* 46(2):167–170, 2008.
85. Cienki JJ, Burkhart KK, Donovan JW: Zopiclone overdose responsive to flumazenil. *Clin Toxicol (Philadelphia, Pa)* 43(5):385–386, 2005.
86. Wyss PA, Radovanovic D, Meier-Abt PJ: Akute Uberdosierungen mit Zolpidem (Stilnox). *Schweiz Med Wochenschr* 126(18):750–756, 1996.
87. Burton JH, Lyon L, Dorfman T, et al: Continuous flumazenil infusion in the treatment of zolpidem (Ambien) and ethanol coingestion. *J Toxicol Clin Toxicol* 36(7):743–746, 1998.
88. Carter LP, Koek W, France CP: Behavioral analyses of GHB: receptor mechanisms. *Pharmacol Ther* 121(1):100–114, 2009.
89. Ragg M: Gamma hydroxybutyrate overdose. *Emerg Med* 9:29–31, 1997.
90. Dyer JE, Reed JH: Alkali burns from illicit manufacture of GHB (abstract). J *Toxicol Clin Toxicol* 5:553, 1997.
91. Dyer JE, Galbo MJ, Andrews KM: 1,4-butanediol, "Pine Needle Oil": Overdose mimics toxic profile of GHB (abstract). *J Toxicol Clin Toxicol* 5:554, 1997.
92. Persson SA, Eriksson A, Hallgren N, et al: GHB–farlig, beroendeframkallande och svarkontrollerad "partydrog." *Lakartidningen* 98(38): 4026–4031, 2001.
93. Ferrara SD, Tedechi L, Frison G, et al: Fatality due to gamma hydroxybutyrate (GHB) and heroin intoxication. *J Forensic Sci* 4:501–504, 1995.
94. Van Sassenbroeck DK, De Neve N, De Paepe P, et al: Abrupt awakening phenomenon associated with gamma-hydroxybutyrate use: a case series. *Clin Toxicol (Philadelphia, Pa)* 45(5):533–538, 2007.
95. Brown TC: Epidemic of gamma-hydroxybutyrate (GHB) ingestion. *Med J Aust* 181(6):343, 2004.
96. Bennett WR, Wilson LG, Roy-Byrne PP: Gamma-hydroxybutyric acid (GHB) withdrawal: a case report. *J Psychoactive Drugs* 39(3):293–296, 2007.
97. Bania TC, Chu J: Physostigmine does not effect arousal but produces toxicity in an animal model of severe gamma-hydroxybutyrate intoxication. *Acad Emerg Med* 12(3):185–189, 2005.
98. Zvosec DL, Smith SW, Litonjua R, et al: Physostigmine for gamma-hydroxybutyrate coma: inefficacy, adverse events, and review. *Clin Toxicol (Philadelphia, Pa)* 45(3):261–265, 2007.
99. Harrison M, Busto U, Naranjo CA, et al: Diazepam tapering in detoxification for high-dose benzodiazepine abuse. *Clin Pharmacol Ther* 36:527, 1984.

CHAPTER 144 ■ AMPHETAMINES

MICHAEL C. BEUHLER

INTRODUCTION

The term "amphetamine" includes a wide range of amine compounds with sympathetic-like effects. The simplest member of this group is amphetamine, but there are hundreds of molecules with related chemical structures that have similar clinical effects. This chapter will focus on the more important and commonly used licit and illicit members of this group.

Amphetamine and methamphetamine are the most well-known members of this class. **Amph**etamine or alpha-methyl **phe**nylethylamine was first synthesized over 120 years ago, and it was widely used by many (including the U.S. military) as the stimulant Benzedrine, beginning in the 1930s. Restricting to prescription decreased use slightly, but it has been continued to be used for both licit (Attention deficit hyperactivity disorder [ADHD], narcolepsy, and weight loss) and illicit reasons. Currently, Adderall® (a mixture of *l* and *d* amphetamine) and Vyvanse® (Lisdexamfetamine; metabolized to *d*-amphetamine) are two commonly used medicinal amphetamine preparations.

Methamphetamine (or N-methyl amphetamine) is undergoing a surge in United States and worldwide popularity. One reason for its popularity over amphetamine is its longer duration of action. Another reason is that the Drug Enforcement Agency has taken actions to limit the availability of precursor compounds for the synthesis of amphetamine, including the unrelated removal of phenylpropanolamine from the OTC market. Finally, synthesis can be conducted by individuals without specialized training using materials that are not difficult to obtain, resulting in a relatively pure product. Currently, Desoxyn® is a methamphetamine containing prescription preparation used for ADHD and obesity.

There are several other medicinal compounds that have clinical effects similar to amphetamines, with a select few discussed here. Ritalin® (methylphenidate) is commonly used in children for ADHD and is occasionally abused. Phenylpropanolamine (Dexatrim®) was used more extensively in the past as a decongestant and weight loss agent; in 2005 the FDA removed it from OTC sales due to concerns about increased stroke risk and it is no longer available as an Rx [1]. Ephedrine has been used extensively in the past in herbal weight loss/energy preparations as well as a decongestant in cough/cold preparations; but in 2004, the FDA prohibited the sale of dietary supplements containing ephedra (ephedrine and pseudoephedrine) over safety concerns. Additionally, in 2006, requirements regulating the sale of ephedrine were enacted in an attempt to limit its diversion for methamphetamine synthesis. Phentermine is an amphetamine derivative that is used for appetite suppression. Selegiline is an amphetamine derivative with selective monoamine oxidase inhibitor (MAOI)-B effects that is metabolized to l-methamphetamine. Propylhexedrine (Benzedrex® nasal inhaler), although not a true amphetamine, has sympathomimetic and vasoconstrictor properties and is occasionally abused.

Some amphetamine analogs with aromatic ring substitutions have direct affinity for serotonin receptors as well as increased inhibition of serotonin uptake, thereby exerting both sympathomimetic and serotonergic effects manifested by hallucinatory properties. One of the more popular compounds in this group is 3,4-methylenedioxy-methamphetamine (MDMA or Ecstasy). Other similar ring-substituted amphetamine compounds include 3,4-methylenedioxy amphetamine (MDA), 3,4-methylenedioxy-*N*-ethylamphetamine (MDEA or Eve), 2,5-dimethoxy-4-bromo-phenethylamine (2-CB; not strictly an amphetamine), para-methoxy amphetamine (PMA), 2,5-dimethoxy-4-methyl-amphetamine (DOM), and 2,5 dimethoxy-4-bromo-amphetamine (DOB; also the similar chlorine and iodine derivatives DOC and DOI exist). The 2,5 dimethoxy halogenated amphetamine derivatives (DOB, DOC, DOI) are common substitutions for LSD found on blotter paper in the United States [2].

Recent increases in clandestine methamphetamine production facilities ("meth labs") have resulted in concern for environmental contamination and bystander toxicity from laboratory chemicals. The vast majority of illicit amphetamine laboratories currently produce methamphetamine by reductive dehydroxylation of ephedrine or pseudoephedrine. Methamphetamine laboratories are often discovered after a chemical mishap or explosion and are a health risk due to the chemicals used, which include respiratory irritants and caustics [3]. Methcathinone is a potent, occasionally used amphetamine-like substance produced from the *oxidation* of ephedrine in amateur labs, instead of the usual *reduction* to methamphetamine; toxicity is similar except that cases of Parkinson-like neurotoxicity from manganese in the impure product have been reported.

There are two methods most commonly being utilized for methamphetamine synthesis. The one resulting in the cleanest product probably the more dangerous one is the Birch or "Nazi" method, which utilizes lithium metal as the reducing agent dissolved in anhydrous ammonia. The other method is the hydriodic acid method, which usually utilizes red phosphorus and iodine, as the availability of hydriodic acid is restricted.

Depending upon the illicit amphetamine purchased, there is a chance that it will contain one or more contaminants, or possibly be substituted by another sympathomimetic. Street purchased methamphetamine tends to be of better purity than cocaine, while MDMA is very commonly substituted or combined with other psychoactive substances. The exact "contaminants" or other chemicals present in street purchased amphetamines are highly variable based on drug, year, and location. Previously reported substitutions include acetaminophen, anesthetics (benzocaine, lidocaine, procaine), cocaine, caffeine, ephedrine, ketamine, lead (rare), talc, phencyclidine, piperazine compounds (benzylpiperazine and others), phenylpropanolamine, pseudoephedrine, strychnine, and quinine [4]. Depending on the quantity of the adulterant, it may contribute to the effect or toxicity of the sympathomimetic drugs.

Occasionally, an individual will ingest an amphetamine while it is wrapped in plastic or other non-permeable material. Body *packers* or "mules," are people who transport large quantities of specially prepared drug packets in their gastrointestinal (GI) tract. Each packet usually contains drugs in sufficient quantity and purity to cause life-threatening toxicity if rupture occurs. Body *stuffers* are people who quickly swallow ("stuff") drug-containing packets in an attempt to get rid of evidence and avoid arrest by the police. These packets are usually poorly prepared and are at increased risk of leakage and rupture, but often contain far less drug than a packet from a body packer. Rarely, individuals will ingest a plastic bag containing a drug with holes or a corner of the bag cut off in an attempt to produce a sustained release effect [5].

PHARMACOLOGY

Amphetamine and methamphetamine are similar in their pharmacokinetic properties and have similar physiological effects in humans [6]. They do not have significant direct effects at adrenergic or dopamine receptors; rather their effects are mediated by an increase in the concentration of synaptic dopamine and to a lesser extent, serotonin and norepinephrine. This increase occurs by several mechanisms. Amphetamine and methamphetamine enter the presynaptic cytoplasm by passive diffusion and uptake by biogenic amine uptake transporters. Amphetamine moves into the synaptic vesicles by diffusion and by the vesicular monoamine transporters (VMATs), subsequently causing release of stored dopamine and norepinephrine, most likely by collapsing the proton gradient as well as an effect on VMAT. This increases the cytosolic levels of these biogenic amines, which then results in increased synaptic levels due to increased reverse transport activity by the amine transporters, especially the dopamine transporter. Part of the mechanism of action of amphetamines' raising synaptic levels is also due to competitive inhibition of biogenic amines reuptake from the synapse into the presynaptic terminal. Finally, some amphetamines have MAOI activity, which inhibits the breakdown of dopamine, serotonin, and norepinephrine, with some (PMA for example) having significant MAOI activity [7,8].

The mechanism of action of MDMA toxicity includes a direct effect at some serotonin receptors, as well as some of the indirect effects described above mediated by a release of serotonin. Additionally, human and animal studies have shown that MDMA produces a dose-related depletion of serotonin and serotonin transporter activity, and produces serotonergic neuronal degeneration [9]. Methamphetamine causes dopamine and serotonergic neuronal toxicity as well as a decrease in dopamine, VMAT, and serotonin transporter activity in the brain, at least in part by free radical injury [10,11].

Peak plasma concentrations of methamphetamine are reported within 4 hours for an insufflated dose, within 2 to 3 hours for a smoked dose and nearly immediate for an IV dose [12,13]; however levels do not correlate with the degree of clinical toxicity [14]. Methamphetamine and amphetamine have an *l* and *d* isomer; the *d* form is more potent in causing pleasurable CNS stimulation and persistent cardiovascular activation than the *l* form [15]. Most abused methamphetamine is the *d* isomer, having been synthesized from ephedrine or pseudoephedrine. However, the *d* form of methamphetamine has a shorter half-life (10 to 11 hours) than the *l* form (13 to 15 hours) [15,13]. The α-carbon on the amphetamine molecule protects it against MAO degradation. The majority of methamphetamine is either eliminated unchanged, N-demethylated to amphetamine (active) or hydroxylated to p-hydroxymethamphetamine (active) with contribution from cytochrome 2D6 [16,17]; amphetamine undergoes a similar metabolism, except that it is deaminated to an inactive metabolite as well as hydroxylated to p-hydroxyamphetamine (active). Excretion of both is increased in acidic urine, but this fact has no clinical utility as the risks of urinary acidification outweigh any potential benefits. Urine usually remains positive for 24 hours or longer in high dose chronic abusers [18]. The serotonergic amphetamine and amphetamine-like compounds (MDMA, PMA, 2-CB) are not metabolized to amphetamine or methamphetamine.

CLINICAL PRESENTATION

Methamphetamine toxicity has been reported following ingestion, inhalation (smoking), insufflation (intranasal), rectal, subcutaneous, intramuscular, and intravenous exposure [19]. The onset and duration of methamphetamine toxicity depends on factors such as dose, route of exposure, individual tolerance, pattern of use, ambient temperature, and crowding/stimulation level. Most people develop signs and symptoms within a few minutes of parenteral drug use, whereas signs and symptoms may be delayed for hours after ingestion with body packers and body stuffers. In most patients, the majority of sympathomimetic effects are expected to resolve within 24 to 36 hours post exposure [19]. Life-threatening toxicity is more common in drug abusers and in people who overdose with suicide intent, and it can also occur in body packers and body stuffers.

Methamphetamine toxicity usually results in a group of signs and symptoms known as the "sympathomimetic toxidrome," including hypertension, tachycardia, tachypnea, hyperthermia, diaphoresis, mydriasis, hyperactive bowel sounds, agitation, anxiety, and toxic psychosis. This pattern of symptoms is seen for other members of the amphetamine group as well as other sympathomimetics like cocaine and caffeine; but this pattern of symptoms can be variable depending on the sympathomimetic agent involved. For example, phenylpropanolamine has peripheral alpha vasoconstrictive effects that can result in a reflex bradycardia.

Airway and breathing abnormalities are uncommon with ingestion. Transient cough, pleuritic chest pain, and shortness of breath are common after insufflation or smoking. People present in illicit drug laboratory fires and explosions may have thermal injury to their oropharyngeal or upper airway. Insufflation or smoking methamphetamine may result in bronchospasm, pneumothorax, pneumomediastinum, pneumonitis, and noncardiogenic pulmonary edema. Noncardiogenic pulmonary edema and acute respiratory distress syndrome may be associated with multisystem organ failure. Tachypnea is common secondary to agitation or metabolic acidosis. Hypoventilation is rare but may occur secondary to intracranial pathology or the end stage of multisystem organ failure.

Many of the adverse cardiovascular effects result from increases in peripheral catecholamines, which result in a mismatch of oxygen consumption and delivery; there may be a direct cardiotoxic effect of methamphetamine as well. Palpitations and chest pain are common complaints. Acute myocardial infarction due to vasospasm, plaque rupture, and/or thrombosis can occur [20]. Life-threatening atrial or ventricular dysrhythmias, sudden death, and aortic dissection have been reported, with potential synergy if cocaine is also present [21,20]. Coronary artery disease and cardiomyopathy have been reported with chronic amphetamine abuse [14,22,23]. Peripheral vascular ischemia can result from oral sympathomimetic abuse but is uncommon unless an inadvertent intra-arterial injection occurs. Hypotension is unusual but may be secondary to dehydration, myocardial depression, intestinal ischemia, or sepsis.

There are several important findings that may be apparent on the Head-Eyes-Ears-Nose-Throat exam. Mydriasis is common and various forms of nystagmus have been reported. Patients who abuse and binge on sympathomimetic agents are often dehydrated and have dry mucous membranes. Nasal mucosal abnormalities, including nasal septal perforations, are well reported in patients who chronically insufflate cocaine and are possible with insufflation of other sympathomimetics. An increase in dental pathology has been noted in users of methamphetamines, manifested by a distinctive pattern of caries on the buccal smooth surfaces of the posterior teeth and the interproximal surfaces of the anterior teeth. The teeth may be loose, rotting, or crumbling, and are usually beyond salvage. The pathology of these changes is uncertain, but is believed to be due to a combination of decrease in salivation (xerostomia) along with increased ingestion of sugar- and acid-containing sodas, poor hygiene, poor nutrition, localized vasospasm, and bruxism, a side effect especially seen with MDMA. [24,25,26].

Central nervous system effects are the reason for abuse as well as often the reason for seeking care. Methamphetamine produces a euphoric and anorexic effect, with smoked and injected administration producing a greater "rush." The most common presenting symptoms include agitation and altered mental status; other symptoms include headache, hyperactivity, agitation, toxic psychosis, loss of consciousness, focal neurologic deficits, and seizures [27,19]. Hyperthermia may be more common and worse in patients with uncontrolled psychomotor agitation, especially when patients are physically but not chemically restrained. Altered mental status may be secondary to hypoglycemia or an acute intracranial process. Headache may be secondary to intracranial or subarachnoid hemorrhage [21,14,28,29]. Focal neurological deficit may be secondary to cerebral ischemia or infarction, vasospasm, or direct injection trauma. On arteriography, multiple occlusions or "beading" has been observed of the arteries; this is thought to represent some combination of local vasospasm or vasculitis [30,1,28]. Seizures may occur in association with and independent of intracranial hemorrhage or cerebral infarction. Prolonged methamphetamine (and probably MDMA) use may lead to cognitive decline represented by attention and memory changes [11].

Some abusers develop stereotyped, compulsive behavior such as cleaning or buttoning shirts; in some cases it has been observed that addicts compulsively take apart appliances, usually without reassembly. Psychosis from amphetamines is not uncommon and can present as paranoid delusions and perceptual disturbances; these may persist long after the drug has been stopped and can result in homicidal or self-destructive behavior [31,32,19]. After binge use, patients may develop a withdrawal pattern of symptoms consisting of generalized fatigue, dysphoria, decreased level of consciousness, and profound lethargy.

One occasionally sees choreiform, ballistic, bruxism, torticollis, or athetoid involuntary movements with amphetamine and methamphetamine abuse [33]. These movements can be fast or slow and they can involve the facial, extremity, or trunk muscles. Ataxia may result if the trunk or limb movements are severe enough. These movements usually begin after prolonged abuse of amphetamine or methamphetamine and may become worse or reoccur with additional drug abuse. Usually, the symptoms resolve over several hours to a week following abstinence. However, they may only diminish in magnitude and persist for months or even rarely, years. The movements may be diminished with voluntary motor activity or during sleep. The mechanism for these movements is not well understood, and may involve a disruption of the normal dopamine neurotransmitter system [34].

Abdominal findings may include increased bowel sounds, bowel obstruction from body packing, and abdominal pain due to intestinal ischemia or bowel perforation [35,36]. Psychomotor agitation and seizures can result in rhabdomyolysis [37]. Hyperthermia and multisystem organ failure may result in coagulopathy and disseminated intravascular coagulation (DIC). Hepatic injury progressing to fatal fulminant liver failure can occur from MDMA without any preceding hyperthermia. Dehydration, increased anion gap metabolic acidosis associated with increased lactate, and hypokalemia are common in patients with significant sympathomimetic toxicity. Urinary retention has been reported from amphetamine toxicity. Acute tubular necrosis may occur secondary to hyperthermia, hypovolemia, hypotension, and rhabdomyolysis.

Diaphoresis with either warm or cool skin is common. Scarring and hyperpigmentation ("track marks") in areas above veins suggest chronic intravenous drug use. Skin popping, or subcutaneous injection of the drug can result in scabs, circular scars, and lesions in a variety of areas. Additional excoriations and rashes can result from skin picking and scratching. Abscesses and infection are not uncommon.

Medical complications from drug abuse include endocarditis, hepatitis, human immunodeficiency virus infection, cellulitis, septic emboli, abscesses, tetanus, and wound botulism. Methamphetamine abuse is associated with an increased risk of HIV infection both because of increase in risk taking behavior (IVDA, unprotected intercourse, untreated STDs) and probable enhancement of HIV infectivity [38].

Most of the time, the toxicity observed in the methamphetamine using patient is due to the drug and not from any adulterants. Adulterants are not usually present in large enough amounts, and methamphetamine is relatively pure and sufficiently toxic in its own right. However, some important exceptions should be noted. The addition of benzocaine has caused methemoglobinemia [39]. Intra-arterial injection of a drug may cause injury, possibly potentiated by any talc present. Talc pulmonary emboli have been reported as well, which probably contribute to pulmonary hypertension. Lastly, substitution is more of a problem with the ring-modified amphetamines (MDMA); the real substance present in the street purchased product is likely to be contaminated with or entirely be a piperazine (BZP and others), caffeine, methamphetamine, or some other substituted amphetamine such as PMA.

In addition to having some sympathomimetic qualities, nearly all of the ring-substituted amphetamines (MDMA, DOM) also have hallucinogenic properties likely due to their direct and indirect effect at serotonin receptors. The route of abuse for methylenedioxymethamphetamine (MDMA) is usually ingestion. Methylenedioxyamphetamine (MDA) is an analog of MDMA and has similar effects as MDMA. Serious autonomic reactions include many of the sympathomimetic symptoms discussed above as well as seizures, rigidity, dysrhythmias, and profound hyperthermia with grave consequences (rhabdomyolysis, renal failure, DIC) [40]. Given the increased serotonin levels produced, at least part of this toxicity should be characterized as serotonin toxicity/syndrome.

Some of the ring-substituted amphetamines have specific toxicities. There are several reports of hepatoxicity resulting in hepatomegaly, jaundice, and death caused by MDMA that did not stem from hyperthermia or shock liver; this probably resulted from an immunological component [41,40]. Hyperthermia is more common with the ring-substituted amphetamines, likely from contribution from serotonin toxicity and possibly from mitochondrial uncoupling [42]. Hyponatremia resulting in altered mental status, coma, seizures, cerebral edema, and death is also sometimes seen following MDMA use. This probably results from some combination of inappropriate antidiuretic hormone secretion (SIADH) and from excessive water drinking. SIADH may possibly be more commonly observed in young women from MDMA use, as there seem to be an inappropriately large number of cases in this group. The observed clinical toxicity from PMA or "death" includes hyperthermia, hypoglycemia, hyperkalemia, and prolonged QRS; the effects are similar to MDMA but may be more severe because its dose response curve is steep regarding elevating brain serotonin levels, PMA exposures are often unintentional, and it has significant MAOI activity [43,7,44]. Bromodimethoxyamphetamine (DOB) is highly potent, enough so that a dose (2 to 5 mg) can be found on a small piece of paper possibly being sold as LSD. Large doses of DOB have been reported to result in significant vasospasm that has resulted in seizures and deaths [45].

DIAGNOSTIC EVALUATION

Patients with amphetamine toxicity (sympathomimetic toxicity) should have frequent vital sign determinations including core or rectal temperature measurement, intravenous access, and continuous cardiac monitoring. Those with abnormal vital signs or mental status should have an electrocardiogram, complete blood cell count, electrolyte, blood urea nitrogen, creatinine, glucose, and arterial blood gas determinations. Patients with chest pain, dysrhythmias, or persistent pulse or blood pressure abnormalities should be evaluated for acute coronary or vascular syndromes. Patients with prolonged immobilization, uncontrolled psychomotor agitation, or hyperthermia should have serial CPKs to evaluate for rhabdomyolysis. Those that either have or have had significant hyperthermia or shock should also have liver injury and function tests (lactate dehydrogenase, aspartate aminotransferase, alanine aminotransferase, and coagulation profile) to evaluate for multisystem organ failure and DIC.

Several imaging studies may be warranted for an amphetamine toxic patient, depending on their clinical presentation. Those with respiratory symptoms or chest pain should have a chest radiograph and possibly a chest CT if there is concern for aortic dissection. Patients with headache or seizures should be evaluated for intracranial hemorrhage with computed tomography of the brain. Those with continued suspicion for subarachnoid hemorrhage with a negative CT scan should also have a lumbar puncture [28]. Plain and oral contrast abdominal radiographs may be helpful in detecting drug-containing packets in the GI tract of body packers, but their sensitivity is quite low for stuffers. Experience with abdominal CT and abdominal ultrasound for detection of stuffer packets is limited. A negative imaging study cannot be used to rule out drug packets in the GI tract.

The results of toxicology screening for most drugs of abuse rarely contribute to or alter patient management. However, in the case of sympathomimetic toxicity, the urine drug screen is reasonably sensitive to the recent use of methamphetamine/amphetamine as well as cocaine and can assist in differentiating these syndromes that can be important in management. If toxicology drug screening is essential, health care providers should contact their clinical laboratory to determine included substances as well as causes of false–positive and false–negative results. For example, the ability for immunologically based drug screens to detect MDMA (or similar ring-substituted amphetamines) is highly variable, but there are specific immunologically-based MDMA drug screens available.

A positive drug screen can confirm the presence of amphetamine or similar structured drug, whereas a negative drug screen is non-diagnostic. For amphetamines, the screen is typically reasonably sensitive for use within the last few days, but has terrible specificity. A sampling of some common substances that may cause a positive amphetamine screen are bupropion, chloroquine, clobenzorex, ephedrine, methylphenidate, phenelzine, phentermine, phenylpropanolamine, pseudoephedrine, selegiline, tranylcypromine, trazodone, and Vicks® inhaler [46,47,48]. One should remember that if the result of a toxicology screen is to be used for forensic purposes, the chain of custody should be maintained, and results will need to be confirmed using a more rigorous analytical method such as gas chromatography/mass spectrometry.

Toxicologic and nontoxicologic conditions that may have a similar presentation or that present concomitantly (Table 144.1) should be evaluated for and excluded. A serum lactate level may be helpful in patients with increased anion gap metabolic acidosis of unclear cause. An elevated lactate level would be expected in patients with compromised tissue perfusion (e.g., occurring with shock and intestinal or limb ischemia), in those with hypermetabolic states in which metabolic demands exceed available substrates, or in those with cellular dysfunction in whom normal substrates cannot be used. Other causes of increased anion gap metabolic acidosis (e.g., ethylene glycol, methanol, iron, salicylate) should be investigated when the lactate level is normal or near normal. The possibility of concomitant poisoning with by-products or impurities related to the illicit synthesis of methamphetamine (e.g., phenethylamine derivatives, caffeine, ephedrine, mercury, strychnine, or lead) would be rare, but should also be considered.

TABLE 144.1

DIFFERENTIAL DIAGNOSIS OF AMPHETAMINE TOXICITY

Toxicologic
β-Agonists toxicity (clenbuterol and others)
Black widow envenomation
Cocaine
Dextromethorphan
Methylxanthine toxicity (caffeine, theophylline)
Monamine oxidase inhibitor toxicity
Neuroleptic malignant syndrome
Piperazine compounds (benzylpiperazine and others)
Phencyclidine toxicity (PCP)
Bark scorpion envenomation (found mostly in AZ)
Salicylates
Serotonin toxicity
Strychnine
Withdrawal from sedative–hypnotics, including baclofen, barbiturates, benzodiazepines, clonidine, chloral hydrate, ethanol, γ-hydroxybutyrate, γ-butyrolactone, meprobamate, as well as from β-antagonists such as propofol
Nontoxicologic
Endocarditis
Encephalitis and meningitis
Heat stroke
Intracranial bleed or mass lesion
Pheochromocytoma
Sepsis
Thyrotoxicosis

MANAGEMENT

Patients who present with life-threatening effects from amphetamine toxicity or those that are at increased risk for developing them (such as a packer) should be managed in an intensive care unit (Table 144.2). The overall approach to these patients is aggressive supportive care with supplemental oxygen, sedation, fluid administration, and close monitoring while addressing the specific myriad complications that can occur.

The hemodynamic effects of amphetamines are primarily caused by release of catecholamines and not by a direct effect at receptors. Mild sinus tachycardia and hypertension not associated with psychomotor agitation or evidence of end organ damage usually do not require pharmacologic treatment. Treatment of psychomotor agitation utilizing appropriate benzodiazepine doses will often result in improvement or resolution of tachycardia and hypertension. If benzodiazepines do not provide adequate improvement, rate-related cardiac ischemia may be treated with a beta-blocker, preferably a short-acting and easily titratable agent such as esmolol, or a calcium-channel blocker, being cautious to exclude cocaine toxicity if a beta-blocker is being used. Patients with life-threatening dysrhythmias who are hemodynamically unstable should be cardioverted or defibrillated. Persistent hypertension, especially if there is evidence of end organ damage or hyperthermia, should be treated with benzodiazepines as well as phentolamine, nitroprusside, or nitroglycerin with careful dose titration.

Patients presenting with chest pain should be evaluated for acute coronary syndromes and managed accordingly [23]. Thrombolytic therapy or procedural coronary intervention may be indicated as per current guidelines. In these circumstances, cardiology consultation is recommended, especially since coronary vasospasm is a possibility. Other important potential causes of chest pain such as pneumothorax, pneumomediastinum, infection, septic emboli, and aortic dissection should be ruled out.

Hypotension should be treated with fluids, and patients assessed for comorbid potential life-threatening conditions such as dysrhythmias, acute coronary syndromes, pneumothorax, aortic dissection, hyperkalemia, GI hemorrhage, and sepsis. Persistent symptomatic hypotension that is refractory to

TABLE 144.2

INDICATIONS FOR ADMITTING PATIENTS TO AN INTENSIVE CARE UNIT

Acute coronary syndromes	Multisystem organ failure
Aortic dissection	Peripheral ischemia
Body packer or body stuffer	Persistent psychomotor agitation
Cerebral ischemia or infarction	Pneumothorax
Dysrhythmias	Rhabdomyolysis
Hyperthermia	Seizure
Intracranial bleed	
Myocardial infarction	

fluids necessitates treatment with a direct acting vasopressor such as norepinephrine, epinephrine, or phenylephrine. At times, the choice and dose of vasopressor should be guided by pulmonary artery catheter hemodynamic monitoring or bedside ultrasound.

Management of bronchospasm should include nebulized β_2 agonists (such as albuterol) and anticholinergic agents (such as ipratropium bromide). Noncardiogenic pulmonary edema and acute respiratory distress syndrome should be managed according to current guidelines. The benefit of corticosteroids in patients with sympathomimetic-induced bronchospasm, pneumonitis, and noncardiogenic pulmonary edema has not been well studied, but may be considered in patients with severe or persistent symptoms. Occasionally, pneumomediastinum and pneumothorax following smoking methamphetamine is observed. Patients with pneumothorax may require tube thoracostomy depending on the size of the pneumothorax. For a pneumomediastinum, the work up usually involves an oral contrast imaging study to rule out esophageal perforation, but surprisingly these commonly have a completely benign course.

The initial management of a patient with an altered mental status includes assessing and treating all readily reversible causes such as hypoxia, hypoglycemia, electrolyte abnormalities (especially hyponatremia), opioid toxicity, and thiamine deficiency. Imaging studies of the head should be performed on patients with persistent altered mental status, potentially followed by lumbar puncture if indicated. Mild agitation or anxiety may be treated with oral benzodiazepines. Psychomotor agitation that poses a danger to the patient or others requires more aggressive sedation. Incremental doses of intravenous benzodiazepine should be used to achieve the desired effect, noting that significant doses of benzodiazepines may be required. The role of antipsychotics for controlling agitation should be as an adjunctive therapy and not the primary means of control, but does appear to be safe and efficacious in adult and pediatric populations [19,49,50]. One should recognize the other clinical precautions that accompany the use of this pharmaceutical drug class (EKG changes, NMS, etc.). If agitation is severe, more aggressive measures such as sedation and paralysis may be required to protect the patient and the staff. Restraints should only be used during the relatively short time of gaining control of the agitation using pharmaceutical methods, as the restrained agitated patient is at risk for several adverse outcomes, including sudden death.

Patients presenting with seizures should be treated with incremental doses of intravenous benzodiazepines. If seizures are not rapidly controlled, intravenous propofol or phenobarbital is indicated usually along with intubation to secure the airway. The role for phenytoin is limited in the patient with toxicological causes of seizures and usually should be avoided. Seizures refractory to sedative–hypnotic drugs should be managed with non-depolarizing neuromuscular blockade and general anesthesia along with continuous electroencephalogram monitoring. The work up of seizures should include a CT scan to evaluate for potential physical causes. Patients with intracranial hemorrhage or cerebral infarction should have neurosurgery or neurology consultation as appropriate. As the etiology of the "beading" seen on angiography is uncertain, the role of calcium channel blockers (e.g., nimodipine) and/or steroids for such patients is equally uncertain.

Patients with peripheral vascular ischemia should be managed in conjunction with a vascular service. Intra-arterial administration of α-adrenergic receptor antagonists such as phentolamine may relieve localized arterial vasospasm; if multiple areas of vasospasm are observed, there may be a role for intravenous nitroprusside. This adverse effect may be observed more typically with some of the substituted hallucinogenic amphetamines such as DOB [45]. Accidental intra-arterial injection during intravenous abuse may lead to significant tissue destruction through emboli (e.g., talc and the other cutting agents), thrombosis, and vasoconstriction. There is no consensus on managing these patients although adequate fluid resuscitation, acetylsalicylate, and heparin appear to be reasonable; other interventions that have been used for intra-arterial injection accidents with heroin include intra-arterial phentolamine, thrombolytics, and dexamethasone.

Core temperature approaching or more than 104°F (40°C) should be aggressively managed, as the risk for multisystem organ failure exponentially rises with the temperature. One should undress the patient, initiate active cooling measures, and continuously monitor the patient's core temperature. Active cooling techniques include spraying the patient with cool water, draping with cold water soaked sheets along with large fans for evaporation, ice packs in the axilla and groin, or a cooling blanket possibly used *under* the patient while utilizing evaporative cooling from above. Active cooling should be terminated when the patient's core temperature approaches 101°F (38.3°C). Benzodiazepines are useful in decreasing motor agitation contributing to the hyperthermia. Paralysis and intubation would be a last resort to treating persistent rigidity associated hyperthermia. Antipyretics (e.g., acetaminophen, aspirin, nonsteroidal anti-inflammatory drugs) are not useful, and there is no evidence that dantrolene, bromocriptine, or amantadine enhance the cooling process in these patients with life-threatening hyperthermia.

Fluid management should address any electrolyte and acid–base abnormalities. Management of rhabdomyolysis should include generous intravenous crystalloid fluids to maintain urine output of at least 2 to 3 mL per kg per hour to minimize the risk of acute tubular necrosis. The role of alkalinizing the urine to provide renal protection when rhabdomyolysis is present is controversial, but may be performed if desired. As serum myoglobin levels are not usually rapidly available, serum CPK may be monitored instead. Although no longer recommended for amphetamine toxicity, urinary acidification would increase the urinary excretion of amphetamine but the risks outweigh any potential benefits.

The serotonergic amphetamines MDMA and like compounds can cause significant serotonin toxicity when combined with other pharmaceuticals that have serotonin effects such as SSRIs, MAOIs, and cocaine. Differentiating the degree of concomitant serotonin toxicity can be difficult, but the physical examination findings of myoclonus and hyperreflexia with the lower extremity reflexes more pronounced than the upper extremity reflexes would be strongly suggestive of serotonin toxicity. Treatment is benzodiazepines and supportive care, although cyproheptadine may be of some benefit; an adult dose for serotonin toxicity is 8 mg orally every few hours to a maximum of 32 mg/day. The hyponatremia arising from SIADH should be treated with water restriction and may require hypertonic 3% normal saline. These fluid requirements should be balanced with other fluid issues such as the possible presence of rhabdomyolysis.

The involuntary abnormal choreiform and athetoid movements following abuse may be the reason for presentation and can be a source of great anxiety for the patient. When the symptom onset is rapid and not present for a long period of time, antipsychotics such as haloperidol have theoretical benefit and may be efficacious [33]. When the involuntary movements have lasted for a long time, antipsychotics may be less effective. Sedatives have been observed to increase the movements in some patients. There has been some success in alleviating symptoms using centrally acting antimuscarinic drugs (e.g., benztropine) [34].

There is no consensus on management of asymptomatic body stuffers. Sometimes individuals claim to have ingested drug packets in an attempt to avoid going to jail, a technique which often works in the short term. The count of the number of packets or the amount of drugs in the packet is usually unreliable. Even when bags or packets are ingested, they are rarely seen on imaging studies. An abdominal CT scan is more reliable than plain abdominal imaging, but false negatives do occur. GI decontamination using activated charcoal (AC) at a dose of 1 to 2 gram per kg should be considered for these patients. Multiple doses of AC have no proven benefit and may be harmful in potentially causing obstruction. The risks of forced AC administration usually outweigh any potential benefit when a patient will not voluntarily drink the AC. However, this risk/benefit ratio should be reassessed should a patient clinically deteriorate to the point of requiring intubation. Occasionally, whole bowel irrigation is also employed for these patients (see below). Given the lack of endpoint (i.e., passed packets) in most of these patients, they will require a period of sufficient observation. The safest approach to these patients would be admission for a minimum of 24 hours of close hemodynamic observation, with additional observation time should any unexplained increase in pulse or blood pressure occur. Note this observation period may not be sufficient for all patients; cases of toxicity have resulted from more than 36 hours from ingestion of a sealed baggie [5].

Asymptomatic body packers should also be conservatively managed. One proposed guideline involves the oral administration of a water-soluble contrast solution followed by serial abdominal radiographs (see Chapter 140, Table 140.5). Whole bowel irrigation (WBI) with isotonic polyethylene glycol electrolyte solution has also been advocated for GI decontamination based on case reports. Some clinicians advocate administering polyethylene glycol solution, 1 L per hour, to adults until there is no longer significant concern for retained packets in the GI tract. This is usually signaled by a clear rectal effluent, no radiographic evidence of drug packets in the GI tract, a negative rectal examination for any packets, and an accurate accounting of the number of ingested packets. It does appear that the packet count for body packers is sometimes more reliable than for body stuffers, but still may not be correct. Administration of multiple doses of cathartics is not considered whole-bowel irrigation and may result in severe fluid and electrolyte abnormalities [51,52,53,54].

Body packers and body stuffers who develop sympathomimetic toxicity should be suspected of having leakage or rupture of the drug packets in their GI tract [55]. In the case of a body packer, this is an absolute indication for emergent surgical intervention due to the massive amount of drug present. Surgical intervention is also indicated for patients with intestinal obstruction, ischemia, or perforation and may be indicated when packets fail to progress through the GI tract after conservative management. Endoscopic retrieval of packets retained in the stomach is rarely performed due to risk of rupture, but if implemented, it should be by an experienced endoscopist.

The proper management of patients exposed to methamphetamine laboratories varies depending on the exposure scenario and the type of laboratory. Many times, the only treatment required is adequate burn care as many of these patients present with thermal burns from a laboratory fire. The most dangerous components to a methamphetamine laboratory (besides the occasional armed psychotic inhabitant) are the possible gases: anhydrous ammonia, hydrochloric acid (HCl), and phosphine. Generally, the HCl and phosphine levels are only present in high enough levels to cause injury during the process of the "cook" [56,57]. All can cause significant pulmonary edema with the injury from phosphine potentially being delayed by several hours and anhydrous ammonia causing significant ocular and dermal injury as well. Methamphetamine laboratories also use caustics and solvents that on contact with skin or eyes can cause significant injury [3]. Variations in the synthesis methods, exposure duration, and preexisting conditions as well as chapter space make it difficult to give further exacting treatment recommendations. It should be noted that despite the subjective complaints, a minor transient exposure to a methamphetamine laboratory is unlikely to cause significant injury, and that unless gross contamination is present, a gentle cleaning with soap and water is adequate for nearly all exposures [58].

ACKNOWLEDGMENT

Dr. Edwin K. Kuffner, MD, contributed to previous versions of this chapter.

References

1. Cantu C, Arauz A, Murillo-Bonilla LM, et al: Stroke associated with sympathomimetics contained in over-the-counter cough and cold drugs. *Stroke* 34:1667, 2003.
2. *Microgram Bulletin*, U.S. Department of Justice, Drug Enforcement Administration, Office of Forensic Sciences. Issues 4/09, 3/09, 6/08, 3/08, 12/07, 12/06, 11/06, and 5/06.
3. Farst K, Duncan JM, Moss M, et al: Methamphetamine exposure presenting as caustic ingestions in children. *Ann Emerg Med* 49(3):341–343, 2007.
4. Klatt EC, Montgomery S, Nemiki T, et al: Misrepresentation of stimulant street drugs: a decade of experience in analysis program. *J Toxicol Clin Toxicol* 24:441, 1986.
5. Hendrickson RG, Horowitz Z, Norton RL: "Parachuting" meth: a novel delivery method for methamphetamine and delayed-onset toxicity from "body stuffing." *Clin Tox* 44:379–382, 2006.
6. Lamb RJ, Henningfield JE: Human D-amphetamine drug discrimination: methamphetamine and hydromorphone. *J Exp Anal Behav* 61:169–180, 1994.
7. Green AL, El Hait MAS: p-Methoxyamphetamine, a potent reversible inhibitor of type A-monoamine oxidase in vitro and in vivo. *J Pharm Pharmacol* 32:262–266, 1980.
8. Sulzer D, Sonders MS, Poulsen NW, et al: Mechanisms of Neurotransmitter release by amphetamines: a review. *Progress Neurobio* 75:406–433, 2005.
9. Ricaurte GA, Forno LS, Wilson MA, et al: 3,4-Methylenedioxymethamphetamine selectively damages central serotonergic neurons in nonhuman primates. *JAMA* 260:51, 1988.
10. Sekine Y, Ouchi Y, Takei N, et al: Brain serotonin transporter density and aggression in abstinent methamphetamine abusers. *Arch Gen Psychiatry* 63:90–100, 2006.
11. McCann UD, Kuwabara H, Kumar A, et al: Persistent cognitive and dopamine transporter deficits in abstinent methamphetamine users. *Synapse* 62:91–100, 2008.
12. Harris DS, Boxenbaum H, Everhart ET, et al: The bioavailability of intranasal and smoked methamphetamine. *Clin Pharmacol Ther* 74:475–486, 2003.
13. Hart CL, Gunderson EW, Perez A, et al: Acute physiological and behavioral effects on intranasal methamphetamine in humans. *Neuropsychopharmacology* 33(8):1847–1855, 2008.
14. Karch SB, Stephens BG, Ho CH: Methamphetamine-related deaths in San Francisco: demographic, pathologic and toxicologic profiles. *J For Sci* 44(2): 359–367, 1999.
15. Mendelson J, Uemura N, Harris D, et al: Human pharmacology of the methamphetamine stereoisomers. *Clin Pharmacol Ther* 80:403–420, 2006.
16. Baselt RC: Disposition of toxic drugs and chemicals in Man. 8th ed. Biomedical Publications, Foster City, California, 2008.
17. Lin LY, Di Stefano EW, Schmitz DA, et al: Oxidation of methamphetamine and methylenedioxymethamphetamine by CYP 2D6. *Drug Met Disposition* 25(9):1059–1064, 1997.
18. Shults TF. The medical review officer handbook. 8th ed. Quadrangle Research, LLC, North Carolina, 2002.
19. Derlet RW, Rice P, Horowitz BZ, et al: Amphetamine toxicity: experience with 127 cases. *J Emerg Med* 7:157, 1989.
20. Kaye S, McKetin R, Duflou J, et al: Methamphetamine and cardiovascular pathology: A review of the evidence. *Addiction* 102:1204–1211, 2007.
21. Davis GG, Swalwell CI: Acute aortic dissections and ruptured berry aneurysms associated with methamphetamine abuse. *J Forensic Sci* 39:1481, 1994.
22. Shao-hua Y, Ren L, Yang T, et al: Myocardial lesions after long term administration of methamphetamine in rats. *Chin Med Sci J* 23(4):239–243, 2008.
23. Turnipseed SD, Richards JR, Kirk JD, et al: Frequency of acute coronary syndrome in patients presenting to the emergency department with chest pain after methamphetamine use. *J Emerg Med* 24(4):369–373, 2003.

24. Klasser GD: The methamphetamine epidemic and dentistry. *Gen Den* 54(6): 431–439, 2006.
25. Shaner JW, Kimmes N, Saini T, et al: "Meth mouth": rampant caries in methamphetamine abusers. *AIDS Patient Care and STDs* 20(3):146–150, 2006.
26. Hamamoto DT, Rhodus NL: Methamphetamine abuse and dentistry. *Oral Diseases* 15:27–35, 2009.
27. Kolecki P: Inadvertent methamphetamine poisoning in pediatric patients. *Pediatr Emerg Care* 14(6):385–387, 1998.
28. Buxton N, McConachie NS: Amphetamine abuse and intracranial haemorrhage. *J R Soc Med* 93:472–477, 2000.
29. Delaney P, Estes M: Intracranial hemorrhage with amphetamine abuse. *Neurology* 30:1125–1128, 1980.
30. Rothrock JF, Rubenstein R, Lyden PD: Ischemic stroke associated with methamphetamine inhalation. *Neurology* 38:589, 1988.
31. Mahoney JJ III, Kalechstein AD, De La Garza R II, et al: Presence and persistence of psychotic symptoms in cocaine versus methamphetamine-dependent participants. *Am J Addict* 17:83–98, 2008.
32. Kratofil PH, Baberg HT, Dimsdale JE: Self-mutilation and severe self-injurious behavior associated with amphetamine psychosis. *Gen Hosp Psychiatry* 18:117–120, 1996.
33. Rhee KJ, Albertson TE, Douglas JC: Choreoathetoid disorder associated with amphetamine-like drugs. *Am J Emerg Med* 6:131, 1988.
34. Lundh H, Tunving K: An extrapyramidal choreiform syndrome caused by amphetamine addiction. *J Neurol Neurosurg Psychiatry* 44:728–730, 1981.
35. Herr RD, Caravati EM: Acute transient ischemic colitis after oral methamphetamine ingestion. *Am J Emerg Med* 9:406, 1991.
36. Brannan TA, Soundararajan S, Houghton BL: Methamphetamine-associated shock with intestinal infarction. *Med Gen Med* 6:6, 2004.
37. Kendrick WC, Hull AR, Knochel JP: Rhabdomyolysis and shock after intravenous amphetamine administration. *Ann Intern Med* 86:381, 1977.
38. Liang, H, Wang X, Chen H, et al: Methamphetamine enhances HIV infection of macrophages. *Am J Pathol* 172(6):1467–1470, 2008.
39. McKinney CK, Postiglione KF, Herold DA: Benzocaine-adulterated cocaine in association with methemoglobinemia. *Clin Chem* 38(4):596–597, 1992.
40. Henry JA, Jeffreys KJ, Dawling S: Toxicity and deaths from 3,4-methylenedioxymethamphetamine ("ecstasy"). *Lancet* 340:384, 1992.
41. Brauer RB, Heidecke CD, Nathrath W, et al: Liver Transplantation for the treatment of fulminant hepatic failure induced by the ingestion of ecstasy. *Transpl Int* 10:229–233, 1997.
42. RuRusyniak DE, Tandy SL, Hekmatyar SK, et al: The role of mitochondrial uncoupling in 3,4-methylenedioxymethamphetamine-mediated skeletal muscle hyperthermia and rhabdomyolysis. *J Pharmacol Exp Ther* 313:629–639, 2005.
43. Felgate HE, Felgate PD, James RA, et al: Recent paramethoxyamphetamine deaths. *J Analyt Toxicol* 22:169, 1998.
44. Ling LH, Marchant C, Buckley NA, et al: Poisoning with the recreational drug paramethoxyamphetamine ("death"). *MJA* 174(7):453–455, 2001.
45. Bowen JS, Davis GB, Kearney TE, et al: Diffuse vascular spasm associated with 4-bromo-2,5-dimethoxyamphetamine ingestion. *JAMA* 249:1477, 1983.
46. von Mach MA, Weber C, Meyer M, et al: Comparison of urinary on-site immunoassay screening and gas chromatography-mass spectrometry results of 111 patients with suspected poisoning presenting at an emergency department. *Ther Drug Monit* 29(1):27–39, 2007.
47. Lora-Tamayo C, Tena T, Rodriquez A, et al: High concentration of chloroquine in urine gives positive result with amphetamine CEDIA reagent. *J Anal Toxicol* 26:58, 2002.
48. Weintraub D, Linder MW: Amphetamine positive toxicology screen secondary to bupropion. *Depress Anxiety* 12:53–54, 2000.
49. Ruha AM, Yarema MC: Pharmacologic treatment of acute pediatric methamphetamine toxicity. *Pediatr Emerg Care* 22(12):782–785, 2006.
50. Richards JR, Derlet RW, Duncan DR: Methamphetamine toxicity: treatment with a benzodiazepine versus a butyrophenone. *Eur J Emerg Med* 4:130–135, 1997.
51. Marc B, Baud FJ, Aelion MJ, et al: The cocaine body-packer syndrome: evaluation of a method of contrast study of the bowel. *J Forensic Sci* 35:345–355, 1990.
52. Hoffman RS, Smilkstein MJ, Goldfrank LR: Whole bowel irrigation and the cocaine body-packer: a new approach to a common problem. *Am J Emerg Med* 8:523–527, 1990.
53. Farmer JW, Chan SB: Whole bowel irrigation for contraband body packers. *J Clin Gastroenterol* 37(2):147–150. 2003.
54. Traub SJ, Hoffman RS, Nelson LS: Body packing–the internal concealment of illicit drugs. *N Engl J Med* 349:2519–2526, 2003.
55. Watson CJE, Thompson HJ, Johnston PS: Body-packing with amphetamines—an indication for surgery. *J R Soc Med* 84:311, 1991.
56. Van Dyke M, Erb N, Arbuckle S, et al: A 24 hour study to investigate persistent chemical exposures associated with clandestine methamphetamine laboratories. *J Occ Env Hyg* 6:82–89, 2009.
57. Willers-Russo LJ: Three fatalities involving phosphine gas, produced as a result of methamphetamine manufacturing. *J Forensic Sci* 44(3):647–652, 1999.
58. Burgess JL, Barnhart S, Checkoway H: Investigating clandestine drug laboratories: adverse medical effects in law enforcement personnel. *Am J Indust Med* 30:488–494, 1996.

CHAPTER 145 ■ WITHDRAWAL SYNDROMES

PAUL M. WAX AND JENNIFER SMITH

As many as 25% of hospitalized adult patients at a university hospital may have a history of ethanol dependence and abuse [1]. Anticipation and recognition of early signs of sedative–hypnotic withdrawal in the sedative–hypnotic abuser allows timely treatment and prevents development of serious withdrawal manifestations, such as seizures, hyperthermia, and delirium. The management of withdrawal syndromes from γ-hydroxybutyrate (GHB) and baclofen may be particularly challenging. Recognition and treatment of the less life-threatening signs and symptoms of opioid withdrawal avoid unnecessary investigation of the frequently severe gastrointestinal symptoms and make the patient more comfortable and able to cooperate. Because ethanol and other sedative–hypnotic withdrawal may have life-threatening manifestations, patients with signs of significant withdrawal should be admitted to the intensive care unit (ICU) for stabilization and monitoring. In addition, drug-dependent patients admitted to the ICU for management of other serious medical or surgical problems may subsequently enter withdrawal in this substance-free environment [2].

Clinical withdrawal implies the presence of physical tolerance and dependency. Factors contributing to the development of dependency include dose of the drug, duration of effect, frequency of administration, and duration of abuse. Shorter-acting drugs require more frequent administration to produce dependency and are associated with more acute and severe withdrawal symptoms than longer-acting drugs. *Tolerance* is defined as a decreased physiologic response elicited by a given dose of the drug. A patient who chronically ingests large amounts of ethanol may not be sedated by a dose that would render a nondrinker comatose. A heroin abuser who has been drug-free during a year's imprisonment may suffer fatal respiratory depression from a dose of heroin that previously would have provided only mild sedation. This physiologic tolerance to drug effect that occurs with chronic use may arise from changes in drug metabolism, such as increased activity of hepatic microsomal enzyme systems and changes in drug effect at the cellular level [3]. Cross-tolerance occurs when the chronic ingestion of one substance decreases the response to a second substance. Cross-dependency allows one drug to be substituted for another to prevent withdrawal symptoms. Ethanol, the barbiturates, and nonbarbiturate sedative–hypnotic agents are cross-tolerant and cross-dependent with one another but not with other sedating drugs such as opioids, neuroleptics, or antihistamines. These factors have important therapeutic implications.

ETHANOL WITHDRAWAL

Pathophysiology

Ethanol produces its toxic effects (relaxation, euphoria, disinhibition, slurred speech, ataxia, sedation, stupor, coma, and respiratory depression; see Chapter 119) through modulation of a variety of neuroreceptors and ion channels [4]. It acts, in part, by interacting with the γ-aminobutyric acid ($GABA_A$) receptor complex, potentiating inhibitory GABAergic receptor function by inducing chloride flux through the chloride channels of the receptor complex [5]. Ethanol also inhibits excitatory *N*-methyl-D-aspartate (NMDA) glutamate receptor function, contributing to impaired cognition and blackouts associated with chronic ethanol use [6]. Inhibition of NMDA receptor function changes intracellular calcium levels and, as a result, affects cell-signaling cascades, including phosphorylation [7]. Other neurotransmitter systems affected by ethanol include dopamine and serotonin [8]. Ethanol has been found to affect 5-hydroxytryptamine receptor function by increasing the potency with which agonists bind this receptor [4]. Ethanol consumption may also result in an increase in endogenous opiates, contributing to its euphoric effect [9]. In addition, ethanol may exert its effect by altering the lipid matrix of cell membranes [10]. Although it was not recognized until the 1950s that delirium was a manifestation of ethanol withdrawal rather than toxicity, it is now clear that the hallmarks of ethanol and other sedative–hypnotic intoxication are distinctly different from the manifestations of withdrawal from these agents [11,12].

Ethanol withdrawal produces a hyperadrenergic state characterized by intense sympathetic nervous system activation. This may be due in part to compensatory central nervous system (CNS) mechanisms that counteract the depressant effects of ethanol intoxication. During withdrawal, these compensatory mechanisms are unopposed, resulting in increased neural stimulation [13]. In support of this theory, elevated levels of plasma and urinary catecholamines have been associated with tachycardia, elevated blood pressure, and tremors observed in withdrawing patients [14]. A decrease in the inhibitory activity of presynaptic α_2-receptors has been demonstrated and may explain, in part, the increase in norepinephrine levels [15]. In addition, an increase in β-adrenergic receptors during withdrawal has been demonstrated [16]. One study showed an increase in plasma levels of the dopamine metabolite homovanillic acid in patients presenting with delirium tremens [17].

Compensatory changes in number and function of inhibitory $GABA_A$ receptors and excitatory NMDA glutamate receptors during chronic ethanol use may contribute to the CNS stimulation brought on by the cessation of ethanol. The abrupt withdrawal of the GABA-potentiating effects of ethanol leads to a disinhibition of neural pathways in the CNS [18]. During withdrawal, ethanol's enhancing effect on chloride flux is lost, resulting in a decrease in GABAergic functioning. Tachycardia, diaphoresis, tremors, anxiety, and seizures have been associated with this reduction in GABA-induced chloride flux [19]. Upregulation in NMDA glutamate receptors and changes in their receptor subunit composition increases calcium flux through these receptors [20]. This likely contributes to the excitotoxic neuronal cell death associated with ethanol withdrawal [21]. Repeated episodes of withdrawal increase the propensity for ethanol withdrawal seizures through altered $GABA_A$ and NMDA receptor function [22,23]. Because NMDA receptors mediate dopaminergic transmission, the increased NMDA receptor function that occurs during withdrawal may also lead to decreased dopaminergic and serotonergic transmission, contributing to alcohol craving [7].

Ethanol withdrawal occurs when a dependent patient suddenly stops drinking or drinks at a slower rate than previously. In either case, a significant drop in the serum ethanol level occurs. In chronic alcoholics, signs of withdrawal are commonly present even when their serum ethanol concentrations are higher than 100 mg per dL [24]. Patients admitted to the ICU with ethanol withdrawal often have a significant underlying disease that has led to an inability to maintain an ethanol intake adequate to prevent withdrawal. Alcoholic gastritis, hepatitis, pancreatitis, and pneumonia commonly precipitate decreased ethanol use and withdrawal. These patients typically present to the hospital after 24 to 48 hours of abdominal pain or fever and may be tremulous or have had a withdrawal seizure. Another type of ICU patient prone to withdrawal is one who has continued to imbibe ethanol nearly to the moment of arrival at the hospital. Intoxicated patients are prone to experience traumatic events and arrive in the operating room, recovery room, or ICU still intoxicated. A history of ethanol abuse or previous withdrawal may not be available in the postoperative or intubated patient when initial signs of withdrawal occur. Failure to recognize ethanol withdrawal in the seriously ill or injured patient may lead to prolonged complications [13].

Clinical Manifestations

Ethanol withdrawal results in a variety of signs and symptoms that vary in severity and duration. In their landmark article, Victor and Adams [12] described withdrawal as a tremulous–hallucinating–epileptic–delirious state. Although this description is often used to divide ethanol withdrawal syndrome into four stages, it is important to remember that the various manifestations of ethanol withdrawal form a progressive continuum of severity. A patient in ethanol withdrawal may exhibit one or more of these manifestations. The sequence of clinical events may be inconsistent. The severity of the withdrawal is often dose-dependent, with more severe reactions associated with heavier and longer periods of drinking [24]. It has been suggested that repeated withdrawal episodes produce a kindling effect, such that each subsequent withdrawal elicits increasingly more severe reactions [15,23,24].

Tremulousness and seizures are the most common clinical manifestations of ethanol withdrawal. They tend to occur early and are generally considered mild-to-moderate ethanol withdrawal symptoms. Delirium tremens is a late manifestation of ethanol withdrawal and constitutes the most serious clinical presentation. Although dramatic and life threatening, delirium tremens is but one aspect of ethanol withdrawal and affects 5% of withdrawal patients [25].

Mild ethanol withdrawal is usually characterized by a period of acute tremulousness (the "shakes"). It begins 6 to 8 hours after a reduction in ethanol intake [24,26]. Patients usually complain of tremulousness, nausea, vomiting, anorexia, anxiety, and insomnia. Physical examination reveals evidence of mild CNS and autonomic hyperactivity, which includes tachycardia, mild hypertension, hyperreflexia, irritability, and a resting tremor. Occasionally, significant tremor may not be appreciated despite the patient's complaint of feeling "shaky inside." Despite the fact that patients in delirium tremens have evidence of significant disorientation, this milder form of withdrawal is characterized by a clear sensorium, although the patient may have a minor disorientation to time. Symptoms of mild ethanol withdrawal usually peak between 24 and 36 hours, and 75% to 80% of these patients recover uneventfully in a few days. Approximately 20% to 25% of patients presenting with mild ethanol withdrawal progress to serious withdrawal manifestations, which include seizures, hallucinations, or delirium tremens. However, it is impossible to reliably predict which patients will deteriorate [24].

Seizures that occur in alcoholics may or may not be due to ethanol withdrawal. Although ethanol withdrawal accounts for many of these seizures, other common causes include preexisting idiopathic and post-traumatic epilepsy [11,12]. Other complications of ethanol abuse not necessarily associated with withdrawal, such as hypoglycemia, hypomagnesemia, and hyponatremia, may also precipitate seizure activity [27]. Ethanol intoxication itself is not thought to be proconvulsant [28]. Alcoholic patients with a history of epilepsy appear to have a greater incidence of seizures than those without a preexisting seizure disorder. Failure to comply with anticonvulsant regimens may, in part, account for this. Brief abstinence (even overnight) may also lower the seizure threshold sufficiently to provoke seizures in susceptible patients. Because management strategies differ depending on whether the patient has a history of previous seizure disorder unrelated to ethanol withdrawal, differentiating between them becomes important [29].

Early studies showed that as many as 25% to 33% of patients in ethanol withdrawal demonstrate seizure activity [11,12]. Most ethanol withdrawal seizures ("rum fits") occur between 7 and 48 hours after cessation or relative abstinence from drinking [30]. Mild-to-moderate signs of withdrawal may precede the seizures, or the seizure may herald the onset of ethanol withdrawal. They are short, generalized, tonic–clonic seizures, 40% of which are limited to a single isolated event. Often a short burst of two to six seizures with normal sensorium between seizures occurs over a few hours. Patients with ethanol withdrawal seizures usually have normal baseline electroencephalograms, in contrast to those with underlying seizure disorders. Status epilepticus or recurrent seizure activity lasting longer than 6 hours is distinctly uncommon in ethanol withdrawal and suggests another diagnosis [31].

Ethanol-related seizures may foreshadow the development of delirium tremens. In one series of patients with ethanol withdrawal seizures, delirium tremens developed in 33% [32]. In some patients, postictal confusion blended imperceptibly into delirium tremens. Approximately 40% of patients in whom delirium tremens subsequently developed exhibited an initial clearing followed by the onset of delirium tremens 12 hours to 5 days later.

Disordered perceptions characterized by hallucinations and nightmares were noted in 25% of tremulous patients in early withdrawal by Victor and Adams [12]. The hallucinations were predominantly visual in nature, auditory only in 20% of cases, and rarely tactile or olfactory. Commonly described visual phenomena in this setting may include the graphic depiction of bugs crawling on the walls or bed [32].

A subset of hallucinating patients does not demonstrate tremulousness or other signs of sympathetic hyperactivity. Known as *acute alcoholic hallucinosis*, this uncommon clinical presentation (occurring in 2% of the patients of Victor and Adams) is a distinct manifestation of ethanol withdrawal that usually begins within 8 to 48 hours of cessation of drinking [12]. It is characterized by disabling auditory hallucinations, often of a persecutory nature. These patients display no evidence of formal thought disorder, have no personal or family history of schizophrenia, and are usually oriented to person and place. In most cases, symptoms last for 1 to 6 days, although they may persist for months and come to resemble chronic paranoid schizophrenia. These symptoms usually respond to therapy with cross-tolerant agents such as benzodiazepines [33].

Delirium tremens is characterized by a significant alteration of sensorium associated with dramatic autonomic and CNS hyperactivity. Only 5% of patients who exhibit any of the previously discussed manifestations of ethanol withdrawal progress to delirium tremens. Delirium tremens appears to be more common in patients with a history of significant withdrawal and a long history of ethanol use. Patients in whom delirium tremens develops may not have demonstrated earlier signs of withdrawal. Other patients who have had ethanol withdrawal seizures or hallucinations may deceptively improve before the onset of delirium tremens, which is rarely seen before 48 to 72 hours after cessation or reduction in drinking and may be delayed for as long as 5 to 14 days [12,26]. These patients are truly delirious, exhibiting disorientation, global confusion, hallucinations, and delusions. Speech is unintelligible. Psychomotor disturbances, such as picking at bedclothes, significant restlessness, and agitation, are common and often require the use of physical restraints. Autonomic disturbances, such as tachycardia, hypertension, tachypnea, hyperpyrexia, diaphoresis, and mydriasis, are present. Cardiac dysrhythmias may also occur [34]. Seizures rarely occur during delirium tremens [26]. Concomitant illness, trauma, seizures, or therapeutic drugs may mask or modify the typical presentation.

Mortality for delirium tremens varies with the presence of underlying disease. Higher mortality is associated with superimposed pneumonia, meningitis, pancreatitis, gastrointestinal bleeding, and major trauma. In the untreated patient without serious coexisting medical disease, mortality usually is a consequence of severe dehydration or hyperthermia, or both, precipitating cardiovascular collapse [35]. Before adequate therapeutic agents were available, a mortality rate of 24% to 35% was cited in the literature [36]. This had decreased to 5% to 10% with the use of barbiturates and paraldehyde [37]. The use of benzodiazepines and intensive supportive care and earlier recognition of withdrawal should further reduce mortality in the absence of significant underlying disease [18].

Diagnostic Evaluation

The differential diagnosis of ethanol withdrawal includes other causes of a hyperadrenergic state. Most importantly, ethanol-related hypoglycemia needs to be differentiated from withdrawal. Clinically, these two conditions may appear remarkably similar, although only hypoglycemia rapidly improves after intravenous (IV) glucose administration [38].

Intoxication with sympathomimetic agents such as cocaine or amphetamine shares many features with ethanol withdrawal, including signs and symptoms of adrenergic excess. Overdose of monamine oxidase inhibitors, phencyclidine, anticholingergic agents, and lithium, as well as neuroleptic malignant syndrome and serotonin syndrome, may all demonstrate marked agitation and confusion [39]. In the elderly patient, almost any therapeutic drug may be associated with delirium [40]. Withdrawal from other sedative–hypnotics, such as benzodiazepines, barbiturates, GHB, and baclofen, may precipitate a delirium-tremens-like state (see following discussion).

Significant underlying metabolic, traumatic, and infectious disorders should be excluded in the patient with altered mental status associated with ethanol withdrawal. Differentiation may require lumbar puncture, laboratory tests, and computed tomographic scan. These include CNS emergencies, such as intracranial bleeds, meningitis, and encephalitis; metabolic causes, including hypoxia, hypercarbia, sepsis, thiamine deficiency, and sodium and calcium abnormalities; and endocrine disturbances, such as thyroid storm and pheochromocytoma. Distinguishing between delirium tremens and hepatic encephalopathy may be difficult, especially because these conditions often coexist [41].

Management

A successful strategy in treating ethanol withdrawal must address several key goals: alleviation of symptoms, prevention of progression of withdrawal to a more serious stage, avoidance of complications, treatment of coexisting medical problems, and planning for long-term rehabilitation and drug independence [26]. Initial management involves securing the airway, breathing, and circulation. Patients with an altered level of consciousness require oxygen and IV administration of at least 100 mg thiamine and 50 g glucose. The latter two substrates are particularly important, as Wernicke's encephalopathy and hypoglycemia may be confused or coexist with ethanol withdrawal. Severely agitated patients may initially require physical restraints to prevent injury and facilitate sedation. Prolonged use of physical restraints without adequate sedation, however, may be detrimental because agitated patients quite often continue to struggle against their restraints. Such activity perpetuates the risk for hyperthermia, muscle destruction, and resultant myoglobinuric renal failure. Volume resuscitation, correction of electrolyte abnormalities, and vigilance in the diagnosis and treatment of coexisting medical and surgical disorders are vital in reducing morbidity and mortality in the patient with delirium tremens [37,42].

Achievement of adequate sedation is the cornerstone of successful treatment of ethanol withdrawal [43]. Sedation alleviates the excitatory manifestations of withdrawal, prevents progression to delirium tremens, and prevents common complications of agitation, including trauma, rhabdomyolysis, and hyperthermia. Although many agents have been used over the years, benzodiazepines have proved the most effective [43–47]. Benzodiazepines, unlike the neuroleptics, are cross-tolerant with ethanol and function as a replacement drug for the short-acting ethanol, increasing the affinity of GABA for the $GABA_A$ receptor [48].

Diazepam (Valium), chlordiazepoxide (Librium), and lorazepam (Ativan) are the most commonly used parenteral agents. All three drugs can easily be given intravenously to facilitate rapid sedation and titration of effect. Of these agents, only lorazepam has reliable intramuscular (IM) absorption [24,49]. Diazepam and chlordiazepoxide are long-acting agents with active metabolites that prolong their therapeutic effect, avoiding the need for frequent dosing that is associated with shorter-acting agents. Lorazepam, a shorter-acting agent, has no active metabolites and is better tolerated in the elderly and in patients with hepatic dysfunction, producing less sedation. Prolonged therapy (e.g., >1 month) with high-dose IV lorazepam, however, has also been associated with acute tubular necrosis secondary to the polyethylene glycol used as the lorazepam diluent [50]. Continuous IV infusion of midazolam, a short-acting agent, has also been recommended in the treatment of delirium tremens [51]. However, this approach requires more vigilant monitoring and does not provide the advantages of a long-acting benzodiazepine that is gradually eliminated over several days. Midazolam infusion is also considerably more expensive than therapy with longer-acting agents [52].

The benzodiazepine of choice in the treatment of ethanol withdrawal remains controversial [53,54]. Although many investigators have suggested that lorazepam may be the preferred agent [13,37,55], long-acting benzodiazepines such as diazepam may be more effective in preventing ethanol withdrawal seizures and contributing to smoother withdrawal with less breakthrough or rebound symptoms [56,57].

Symptom-triggered benzodiazepine treatment for alcohol withdrawal is strongly encouraged [58]. The Clinical Institute Withdrawal Assessment for Alcohol (CIWA-A) scale is a reliable, validated scale to assess severity of alcohol withdrawal so treatment can be appropriately titrated and individualized. It includes subjective parameters such as anxiety, auditory and visual disturbances, headache, and nausea as well as objective parameters such as tremor, sweating, agitation, and clouding of sensorium. [59] The dose of benzodiazepines needed to achieve adequate sedation varies considerably depending on the patient's tolerance. Although oral therapy may be appropriate in patients with mild withdrawal, those with significant signs of withdrawal require IV treatment. Therapy with an IV benzodiazepine is titrated to the patient's needs by the use of frequent boluses until withdrawal symptoms subside. Using such a front-loading technique helps avoid undertreatment or excessive sedation [60,61]. For example, 5 to 20 mg of diazepam can be administered to the patient every 5 minutes until he or she is quietly asleep but can be easily awakened. Initial safe titration of benzodiazepines requires continual reevaluation by an observer at the bedside. In patients with moderate withdrawal symptoms, a study showed that using a symptom-triggered approach, instead of a fixed-schedule approach, resulted in the administration of less total medication and fewer hours of medication (9 hours vs. 68 hours) [62,63]. A recent study in a surgical ICU demonstrated that this symptom-orientated bolus-titrated approach decreases the severity and duration of alcohol withdrawal symptoms, resulting in reduced medication requirements, fewer days of ventilation, lower incidence of pneumonia, and shorter ICU stay [64].

Failure to obtain adequate sedation with standard doses of the chosen agent should not prompt a switch to an alternative benzodiazepine. Some patients require very high doses to achieve sedation; cases of patients receiving more than 1,000 mg diazepam during 24 hours have been reported [62]. Recent research into GABA receptor physiology suggests that resistance to large doses of benzodiazepines in some patients with alcohol withdrawal may be due to alterations in $GABA_A$ receptor subunits [65]. Chronic ethanol exposure produces upregulation of $GABA_A$ receptor α_4 subunits that are insensitive to benzodiazepines, and downregulation of benzodiazepine-sensitive α_1 subunits. If a patient with severe alcohol withdrawal does not respond to large doses of a benzodiazepine, administration of an alternative agent may be warranted. A drug such as a barbiturate, which acts on the $GABA_A$ receptor regardless of its specific α subunit composition, would be appropriate.

Recent research also suggests that changes in NMDA glutamate receptor physiology may be important in both clinical signs and symptoms of ethanol withdrawal and the excitotoxic neuronal cell death that may occur. In animal studies, NMDA receptor antagonists may attenuate the development of ethanol dependence if administered concomitantly, and may prevent withdrawal seizures and neuronal excitotoxicity if given during periods of withdrawal [20]. Patients who are refractory to high dose $GABA_A$ agonists may potentially benefit from addressing the glutaminergic as well as the GABergic manifestations of ethanol withdrawal. Options here are limited, but drugs such as propofol, which possess both GABA agonist and NMDA antagonist properties, may be particularly helpful.

Adequate early treatment with benzodiazepines usually suppresses significant manifestations of withdrawal and prevents progression to delirium tremens. If delirium tremens is already manifest, sedation with a benzodiazepine does not completely reverse mental status abnormalities. This may be a consequence of the incomplete cross-tolerance of benzodiazepine with ethanol or perhaps the lack of immediate reversibility of some of the CNS effects of withdrawal [66].

Barbiturates, particularly intermediate and long-acting agents such as pentobarbital and phenobarbital, are an alternative class of cross-tolerant sedative–hypnotic agents that can be used in the treatment of ethanol withdrawal [67]. Although excess sedation and a greater tendency to produce respiratory depression may be more of a concern with barbiturates as compared with benzodiazepines, the drugs are still titrated until the patient is quietly asleep but easily awakened [68]. Phenobarbital dosages more than 20 mg per kg may be required. Withdrawal patients with idiopathic or post-traumatic epilepsy who require maintenance anticonvulsant levels may particularly benefit from this alternative strategy. Phenobarbital may also be useful for those patients who are resistant to benzodiazepine therapy.

Propofol, a sedative–hypnotic agent used for induction and maintenance of anesthesia, has been used successfully for treatment of severe ethanol withdrawal that is resistant to large doses of benzodiazepines (>1,000 mg per day) [69–71]. Like ethanol, it acts as an agonist at the $GABA_A$ receptor and also inhibits the NMDA receptor. Its onset of action is rapid, it is easily titratable, and sedative effects wear off quickly after short-term use (<72 hours). The fact that it addresses the glutaminergic as well as the GABAergic aspects of ethanol withdrawal may be one reason for its increased apparent effectiveness in patients resistant to standard therapy with benzodiazepines. Disadvantages of its use include high cost and prolonged sedation when it is used for extended periods [72]. No controlled trials have compared propofol and benzodiazepines for treatment of ethanol withdrawal.

Intravenous and oral ethanol have been used to suppress withdrawal and continue to be used by some medical practitioners, especially surgeons [73,74]. However, IV ethanol intensifies the biochemical abnormalities associated with ethanol metabolism, shifting energy production toward lactate and ketogenesis [75]. The use of ethanol in the treatment of ethanol withdrawal is not recommended [76].

The use of phenothiazines and butyrophenones to treat ethanol withdrawal has been associated with excessive fatalities [42,75,77]. These agents have been shown to lower the seizure threshold, induce hypotension, impair thermoregulation, and precipitate dystonic reactions [78–80]. These drugs have no role in the management of sedative–hypnotic withdrawal [81].

Beta-blockers and central adrenergic agonists have also been promoted as primary agents and as adjuncts to sedative–hypnotics in the treatment of ethanol withdrawal [82]. These agents do not prevent agitation, hallucinations, confusion, and seizures [46,67]. α_2-Receptor agonists such as clonidine and lofexidine act centrally to attenuate sympathetic outflow from the locus ceruleus [15,24]. Although α_2 agonists may help relieve mild withdrawal symptoms such as tremor, diaphoresis, and tachycardia [83,84], there is no evidence that they prevent delirium tremens [85]. A double-blind study comparing oral benzodiazepines (diazepam or alprazolam) to clonidine in the treatment of mild ethanol withdrawal showed that the benzodiazepines were significantly more efficacious in decreasing withdrawal symptoms [48]. A role for sympatholytic agents in management of seriously ill patients has not been demonstrated.

Valproate has been suggested as an alternative or adjunctive treatment for ethanol withdrawal. It appears to potentiate GABAergic neural transmission through a variety of mechanisms, including activation of glutamic acid decarboxylase. Although there is evidence that valproate may be effective in alleviating withdrawal symptoms, further research is needed before it can be recommended for use in ethanol withdrawal [86].

Baclofen is a $GABA_B$ agonist that appears to have a role in the treatment of alcohol withdrawal. In a randomized, controlled trial, it was comparable to benzodiazepines in relieving symptoms of moderate alcohol withdrawal in an outpatient setting [81]. It has also been shown to be more effective than placebo in controlling craving and in inducing abstinence from alcohol. The mechanism for this effect may be due to the influence of $GABA_B$ agonist on the mesolimbic dopamine pathway [82]. Baclofen has not been studied for use in the treatment of alcohol withdrawal in the intensive care setting.

Gamma-hydroxybutyric acid (GHB) is another $GABA_B$ agonist which recent research has suggested may have a role in the treatment of alcohol withdrawal. In randomized, controlled trials, it was comparable to benzodiazepines and clomethiazole in relieving symptoms of moderate alcohol withdrawal in an outpatient setting. Transient vertigo was the most commonly reported side effect, but also occurred with clomethiazole and benzodiazepine treatment. GHB may resolve withdrawal-associated symptoms of anxiety, agitation, and depression more quickly than benzodiazepines, possibly due to its action on dopaminergic and serotonergic neurotransmitter systems [87,88]. This method of treatment is not commonly used, and further study is warranted.

Magnesium sulfate has been suggested as a potential therapy for alcohol withdrawal, but no sound studies have been able to confirm that magnesium supplementation helps alleviate signs or symptoms of alcohol withdrawal, either in normomagnesemic or hypomagnesemic patients [89].

Adequate sedation of the patient with early signs of withdrawal prevents the development of ethanol withdrawal seizures and progression to delirium tremens. Patients who have had an ethanol withdrawal seizure are at risk for progression to delirium tremens and should be sedated with benzodiazepines or barbiturates, as previously discussed. A randomized, controlled trial evaluating patients presenting to the emergency department with ethanol withdrawal seizures and lacking other signs of moderate alcohol withdrawal showed that a one-time dose of lorazepam, 2 mg IV, was more effective than placebo in preventing recurrent ethanol withdrawal seizures [90]. No evidence has been shown to prove that phenytoin is efficacious in the treatment or prevention of ethanol withdrawal seizures [26,91]. Clinical studies failed to show any significant benefit of IV phenytoin when compared with placebo in the prevention of subsequent ethanol withdrawal seizures [92–94].

The use of anticonvulsants to prevent or treat ethanol withdrawal seizures should be limited to patients with an underlying seizure disorder who require maintenance anticonvulsant therapy [29]. These patients often seize at the onset of mild withdrawal secondary to poor compliance with their anticonvulsant regimen and require restoration of adequate serum levels with an anticonvulsant such as phenytoin. Patients who present with an apparent ethanol withdrawal seizure but do not have a history of either underlying seizure disorder or previous ethanol withdrawal seizures require a full seizure workup. For those rare patients in ethanol withdrawal in whom status epilepticus develops, aggressive anticonvulsant treatment is indicated and phenobarbital or phenytoin, or both, can be used in addition to the benzodiazepines. Because status epilepticus and seizures during delirium tremens are rare sequelae of ethanol withdrawal, their occurrence requires a search for underlying traumatic injuries and infection, regardless of any previous history of ethanol withdrawal seizures.

BENZODIAZEPINE WITHDRAWAL

Since their introduction in the early 1960s, benzodiazepines have replaced the barbiturates as the most widely prescribed sedative–hypnotic agents. Initially, these newer agents were not thought to have the same serious withdrawal problems associated with the barbiturates [95]. Subsequent experience has shown that withdrawal from benzodiazepines may be as severe as withdrawal from barbiturates or ethanol. It is estimated that 10% to 20% of adults in the United States use benzodiazepines on a regular basis [96]. The early signs of withdrawal from benzodiazepines are the same as those of ethanol withdrawal. Differences include delayed time of onset, depending on the duration of action of the agent involved, and the presence or absence of active metabolites. When delayed tachycardia, hypertension, and irritability develop in a hospitalized patient, prior benzodiazepine abuse should be suspected.

Pathophysiology

Signs and symptoms of benzodiazepine withdrawal occur when tolerant patients experience a decline in brain benzodiazepine levels. Individuals who have not developed tolerance do not experience symptoms of withdrawal. Patients who have taken therapeutic amounts of these drugs over an extended period may experience withdrawal (therapeutic dose withdrawal) [97,98], although more commonly it occurs in those who have been regularly taking higher than recommended antianxiety doses. A high daily dose and long duration of benzodiazepine use correlate with a greater risk of developing a moderate-to-severe withdrawal syndrome [96,99]. Although withdrawal usually occurs after abrupt discontinuation of these medications, it may occur to a lesser extent during drug tapering [95]. Iatrogenic benzodiazepine withdrawal has also been described in patients following discontinuation of midazolam-induced sedation in the ICU [100].

Although the mechanisms for benzodiazepine tolerance and withdrawal are not fully understood, it appears that changes in $GABA_A$ receptor subunits, similar to those that occur with chronic ethanol use, may be responsible [101]. Ultimately, a decrease in the availability of exogenous benzodiazepine results in unopposed nervous system stimulation and an increase in agitation and anxiety.

Variability in the time course and severity of withdrawal among the various benzodiazepines can be explained by their differing pharmacokinetics [102]. Drug half-life and the presence of active metabolites correlate with the onset, frequency, and severity of withdrawal symptoms. The onset of withdrawal from shorter-acting agents without active metabolites, such as lorazepam or alprazolam, may be precipitous, with marked symptoms as early as 24 hours after cessation of the drug [103]. Signs of withdrawal from longer-acting agents, such as diazepam, which have a long elimination half-life in addition to active metabolites, may be delayed for 8 days or longer. Withdrawal symptoms from long-acting benzodiazepines may persist for months [104,105]. Concurrent use of other cross-tolerant sedative–hypnotic substances, such as ethanol, barbiturates, chloral hydrate, glutethimide, ethchlorvynol, or meprobamate, along with benzodiazepines increases the probability of developing withdrawal on abrupt discontinuation of these substances.

Administration of the competitive benzodiazepine antagonist flumazenil can result in iatrogenic benzodiazepine withdrawal. Flumazenil is used to reverse sedation in the settings of benzodiazepine overdose, IV conscious sedation, and general anesthesia [106] and was suggested as an adjunct in the weaning of patients from mechanical ventilation [107]. However, flumazenil has not been proved effective in the treatment of benzodiazepine-induced respiratory depression [106]. A history of benzodiazepine use and dependence may not be available when unconscious patients are admitted to the ICU, and benzodiazepine withdrawal with seizures and death has been reported after the use of flumazenil [108–110]. Hence, flumazenil should be used with caution (see Chapter 143).

Clinical Manifestations

Benzodiazepine withdrawal is characterized by CNS excitation and autonomic hyperactivity. Mild early manifestations of withdrawal include psychological symptoms such as anxiety, apprehension, irritability, mood swings, dysphoria, and insomnia. Somatic complaints commonly include nausea, palpitations, tremor, diaphoresis, and muscle twitching.

More severe signs of withdrawal include vomiting, cramps, tachycardia, postural hypotension, and hyperthermia. Significant neuromuscular hyperactivity may be manifested as fasciculations, myoclonic jerks, and seizures [111]. Agitated delirium accompanied by hallucinations and paranoid delusions, and catatonia, have been described [112,113].

In patients taking clonazepam, withdrawal symptoms may develop 3 to 4 days after cessation of therapy. Clonazepam withdrawal may be precipitated or accentuated, or both, by concomitant neuroleptic therapy [114,115].

Diagnostic Evaluation

Benzodiazepine withdrawal may be difficult to distinguish from an underlying anxiety disorder [112]. The time course of the symptoms helps distinguish these two diagnoses. Withdrawal symptoms often worsen rapidly in the early period, followed by gradual improvement and resolution. Unmasked anxiety disorders tend not to deteriorate significantly and persist with time. Perceptual disturbances, not generally associated with underlying anxiety disorders, are commonly found during early withdrawal and may also help distinguish withdrawal from the return of anxiety [104]. These disturbances include paresthesia, tinnitus, visual abnormalities, vertigo, metallic taste, depersonalization, and derealization [98].

Management

Treatment strategies for benzodiazepine withdrawal are similar to those used for ethanol withdrawal. Reinstitution of the drug at a dose that relieves withdrawal symptoms followed by slow withdrawal during 2 to 4 weeks minimizes symptoms and affects the desired decrease in CNS tolerance. Alternatively, a similar cross-tolerant agent can be used. A long-acting benzodiazepine such as diazepam or chlordiazepoxide is preferred. Short-acting agents are disadvantageous because maintenance of therapeutic serum drug levels requires frequent drug administration. In patients with moderate-to-severe symptoms (e.g., seizures, delirium), small IV boluses, such as 5 mg of diazepam, should be given until adequate sedation is achieved. Patients experiencing milder symptoms can be treated by the oral route. Barbiturates such as pentobarbital and phenobarbital can also be used in the treatment of benzodiazepine withdrawal [116,117].

Beta-blockers and clonidine have also been used in the treatment of benzodiazepine withdrawal [118]. Propranolol (10 to 40 mg every 6 hours) may help ameliorate tremor, muscle twitching, tachycardia, and hypertension. However, it has little effect on anxiety, agitation, and dysphoria [96]. Clonidine use has also been advocated, although its efficacy in modulating the intensity, severity, and duration of withdrawal has been questioned [119]. As with ethanol withdrawal, it is important to realize that treating peripheral manifestations of withdrawal may obscure early signs of impending delirium and impedes the assessment of adequate sedation. Phenothiazines and butyrophenones exhibit no cross-tolerance to the benzodiazepines and do not have a role in the treatment of benzodiazepine withdrawal, for the same reasons seen in ethanol withdrawal [120].

Limited data are available on the treatment of flumazenil-induced benzodiazepine withdrawal. Because flumazenil has a relatively short half-life (approximately 1 hour), supportive care should be sufficient in the treatment of mild withdrawal symptoms. The precipitation of seizure activity may require treatment with a benzodiazepine or barbiturate. Due to flumazenil receptor blockade, higher doses of GABAergic agonists may be required.

γ-HYDROXYBUTYRATE WITHDRAWAL

Withdrawal from the commonly abused street drugs GHB or its congeners γ-butyrolactone and 1,4-butanediol (see Chapter 143) may be dramatic and potentially life threatening [121,122]. The pathophysiology is similar to that for benzodiazepine withdrawal. Heavy users of these chemicals report using multiple daily doses (as frequent as every 1 to 3 hours) around the clock [123]. GHB acts as an agonist at GHB and $GABA_B$ receptors. Withdrawal symptoms may include agitation, mental status changes, hypertension, and tachycardia. Other findings are tremulousness, diaphoresis, tachypnea, rigidity, irritability, paranoia, insomnia, and auditory and visual hallucinations [124,125]. High-frequency users appear to be at greatest risk for developing withdrawal delirium after abrupt discontinuation of these agents. Onset of symptoms may begin as early as 1 to 6 hours after the last dose [126]. Severe withdrawal symptoms may persist from 5 to 15 days onward and require prolonged ICU care. Many of these patients require physical restraints and heavy sedation [126]. The use of IV benzodiazepine and other cross-tolerant agents is recommended in the management of these patients. As use and abuse of GHB and its precursors becomes more common, more cases of withdrawal are being reported, including cases in which patients are refractory to large doses of benzodiazepines. Successful treatment of this subset of patients with pentobarbital [127,128] and baclofen [129] has been reported. Barbiturates such as pentobarbital may be helpful because unlike benzodiazepines, they are capable of opening $GABA_A$ chloride channels independently of GABA's presence. Pentobarbital dosages used in case series were 1 to 2 mg per kg IV every 30 to 60 minutes, titrated to improvement in vital signs and altered sensorium. Baclofen's usefulness may stem from the fact that like GHB, it is an agonist at $GABA_B$ receptors, whereas benzodiazepines act only on the $GABA_A$ receptor. One case report describes dosing of 10 mg orally three times daily successfully prevented seizures which occurred every time GHB was withdrawn from a dependent patient.

BACLOFEN WITHDRAWAL

Baclofen is a $GABA_B$ receptor agonist used to treat spasticity resulting from multiple sclerosis or CNS injury. It can be taken orally or delivered by an intrathecal pump, which allows higher CNS levels without the side effects associated with large oral doses. An abrupt discontinuation or decrease in baclofen dose may result in a withdrawal syndrome [130]. The pathophysiology is similar to that for benzodiazepine withdrawal. There are many scenarios in which an intrathecal drug delivery system may fail, including errors in programming the pump or filling the reservoir, development of kinks or occlusions in the tubing, and battery failure.

Onset of withdrawal symptoms may occur within a few hours to a few days after a decrease in baclofen dose. Mild-to-moderate withdrawal symptoms may include increased spasticity, tachycardia, hypertension, fever, neuromuscular rigidity, hyperreflexia, psychosis, and delirium. Severe withdrawal, particularly from intrathecal baclofen, may result in coma, seizures, rhabdomyolysis, hyperthermia, disseminated intravascular coagulation, circulatory failure, delirium, and coma [131–134]. Occasionally, patients may develop a reversible cardiomyopathy. In the most severe cases, multiorgan failure and death may occur [120,121]. The delirium observed with baclofen withdrawal may resemble the altered mental status caused by baclofen intoxication, and baclofen intoxication should always be considered along with withdrawal in the differential diagnosis of delirium in a patient on baclofen. The severe withdrawal syndrome may also mimic other conditions such as infection, serotonin syndrome, and neuroleptic malignant syndrome. In cases such as these, the diagnosis may be easy to miss, and evaluation for pump failure should always be considered. Pump integrity and function may be assessed by plain films, dye studies, nuclear medicine flow studies, port aspirations, or if necessary, operative exploration. Cautiously administering a bolus of baclofen by the pump, by way of lumbar puncture, or by a lumbar drain, and assessing for improvement in 30 to 60 minutes may help confirm the diagnosis. Oral baclofen may also be used, though large doses may be needed and clinical improvement may be delayed by several hours [134].

In addition to supportive care, the most important step in management of baclofen withdrawal is the replacement of the baclofen. Patients who were receiving oral therapy may have the drug administered by nasogastric tube if they are unable to take it by mouth secondary to their withdrawal symptoms. Patients withdrawing from intrathecal baclofen may require high doses of oral baclofen, or may not respond to oral replacement therapy [135]. Replacement oral baclofen doses for intrathecal baclofen withdrawal often range between 10 and 30 mg orally, every 4 to 8 hours [134]. In patients not responding to oral replacement, the reason for pump failure should be identified and remedied, with the previous intrathecal baclofen dose reinstituted [136]. Bolus dosing of baclofen by the pump, by way of lumbar puncture, or by a lumbar drain may be required to initially reverse severe manifestations. If there is any delay in administering baclofen intrathecally in these patients, other sedative medications such as benzodiazepines, barbiturates, or propofol should be provided intravenously. As with oral baclofen dosing and with benzodiazepine treatment of severe ethanol withdrawal, large doses of these agents may be necessary to control severe symptoms, with attention to airway support if the patient is not already intubated. Cyproheptadine (4 to 8 mg orally every 6 to 8 hours) has been suggested as a useful adjunctive therapy in patients with intrathecal baclofen withdrawal who are well enough to take oral medications. More study is needed before this can be definitively recommended. [137].

OPIOID WITHDRAWAL

Opioid withdrawal occurs when a tolerant individual experiences a decline in CNS levels of a chronically used opioid. Unlike withdrawal from sedative–hypnotic agents [138], the manifestations of opioid withdrawal are not usually life-threatening. Recognition of the problem facilitates optimum management of the critically ill patient.

Pathophysiology

Opioid receptors in the locus ceruleus bind exogenous opioids, such as heroin, methadone, or codeine, as well as endogenous opioid-like substances known as *endorphins* and *enkephalins*. Stimulation of opioid receptors reduces the firing rate of locus ceruleus noradrenergic neurons, resulting in the inhibition of catecholamine release [139,140]. The stimulation of inhibitory adrenergic receptors, also found in the locus ceruleus, causes a similar reduction in sympathetic outflow. Chronic opioid use may produce an increase or upregulation of these adrenergic receptors. Subsequent withdrawal of opioids results in increased sympathetic discharge and noradrenergic hyperactivity.

The time course of the withdrawal syndrome depends on pharmacokinetic parameters of the individual opioids [139]. Withdrawal symptoms usually appear about the time of the next expected dose [141]. Withdrawal from heroin, which has a short half-life, begins 4 to 8 hours after the last dose, whereas withdrawal from methadone, with a long half-life, is delayed until 36 to 72 hours after the last dose. Withdrawal symptoms are more intense if the opioid has a shorter half-life, whereas symptoms are less dramatic but often more prolonged if the abused opioid has a long half-life. Typically, heroin withdrawal peaks at 36 to 72 hours, with symptoms subsiding by 7 to 10 days. Methadone withdrawal may not peak until the sixth day of abstinence and may persist for weeks.

Because prolonged opioid use may be required to facilitate ventilator management in intensive care patients, iatrogenic opioid withdrawal may complicate ventilator weaning [142,143]. Methadone administered by nasogastric tube or subcutaneously has been successfully used to treat these withdrawal symptoms. The use of methadone may shorten the phase of ventilator weaning in these patients.

Clinical Manifestations

Early signs of opioid withdrawal include mydriasis, lacrimation, rhinorrhea, diaphoresis, yawning, piloerection, anxiety, and restlessness [144]. With time, these symptoms may worsen and be accompanied by mild elevation in pulse, blood pressure, and respiratory rate. Myalgias, vomiting, diarrhea, anorexia, abdominal pain, and dehydration accompany more severe withdrawal. Although these patients may become extremely restless, fever and central agitation such as seizures (except in cases of neonatal withdrawal) and mental status alteration are not part of opioid withdrawal. An intense craving for the drug accompanies withdrawal. Recognition of these signs and symptoms in the ICU patient obviates the need for extensive evaluation of the gastrointestinal symptoms and puts clinically puzzling pain complaints in perspective. Appropriate therapy alleviates the patient's discomfort and facilitates management of more pressing ICU problems. After the resolution of most of the objective signs of withdrawal, subjective symptoms, especially dysphoria, may persist for weeks [140].

Opioid withdrawal may occur suddenly in the opioid-dependent patient given naloxone [145]. This iatrogenic withdrawal often occurs after naloxone is given to a patient who is lethargic or comatose and has unrecognized opioid dependency. Naloxone-induced withdrawal may also occur in dependent patients after use of naloxone to reverse the effects of an opioid used during procedural sedation. Vomiting and subsequent aspiration in the unconscious patient are the major complications arising from this problem. This abstinence syndrome is of brief duration due to the short half-life of naloxone, lasting 20 to 60 minutes, and treatment with opioids to reverse the unwarranted effects of naloxone is not indicated. Naloxone, if required, should not be withheld in the dependent patient. A starting dose of 0.04 to 0.10 mg should be used, titrated until the desired effect is achieved or mild signs of withdrawal occur. Coma or hypoventilation that persists after the onset of withdrawal signs is not reversed by administration of additional naloxone.

Naltrexone, an orally active opioid antagonist, induces withdrawal symptoms for up to 48 hours. Nalmefene, another opioid antagonist, may also cause prolonged withdrawal symptoms in the opioid-tolerant patient. A less commonly recognized cause of opioid withdrawal is the use of agonist-antagonist in the opioid-dependent person. Drugs with agonist-antagonist activity include pentazocine (Talwin), nalbuphine (Nubain), and butorphanol (Stadol).

Management

Treatment of opioid withdrawal is a two-tier approach, using cross-tolerant opioid replacement or sympatholytic therapy (e.g., clonidine), or both. The benzodiazepines are not cross-tolerant with opioids. Their role is limited to the management of significant anxiety associated with opioid withdrawal.

Substitution of long-acting methadone for heroin has played a prominent role in the management of opioid addiction [138]. First used in the 1960s for the treatment of heroin addiction [146], methadone was chosen for its chemical similarity to heroin, oral availability, and long half-life (24 to 36 hours). Although the use of methadone for the outpatient treatment of opioid dependence is tightly regulated, physicians do not need special licensing to prescribe methadone to hospitalized patients.

Methadone may be useful in treating the uncomfortable symptoms in patients who depend on any opioid. The dose should be judiciously titrated to relieve symptoms but avoid oversedation. A safe initial dose is 20 mg orally or 10 mg IM. The IM route guarantees absorption in the vomiting patient [144]. Relief of symptoms usually occurs within 30 to 60 minutes when the drug is given parenterally and longer when it is given orally. A second 10 mg IM dose can be given if significant relief is not achieved 1 hour after the first IM dose. Administering 10 to 20 mg by IM route blocks most manifestations of physiologic withdrawal, although some patients may require 20 to 40 mg daily or divided twice per day to avoid psychological withdrawal. In general, dosing to prevent withdrawal symptoms requires considerably less drug than dosing for methadone maintenance. Although withdrawal from opioids should not be attempted during an acute medical illness, once they are medically stabilized, heroin-dependent patients can be tapered with methadone over 1 week. Methadone-dependent patients require 4 weeks or more of gradually decreasing dosages. Notable drugs that interact with methadone, lowering its plasma concentration and potentially precipitating opioid withdrawal, include rifampin and phenytoin [147,148].

For those patients enrolled in methadone maintenance programs, considerably larger doses of methadone are often employed. Some of these patients, particularly early in treatment, may continue to abuse heroin. Higher methadone doses, as much as 150 mg a day or more, have been recommended as a means to reduce concurrent heroin use and retain patients in treatment programs [149,150]. Some community clinics use doses as high as 200 to over 300 mg per day in select patients.

The treatment of pain in patients receiving methadone may require the use of additional opioid analgesia, such as morphine, codeine, or oxycodone. In patients on methadone maintenance, the established maintenance dose may not provide adequate analgesia because of tolerance to the analgesic effects of methadone. Successful pain relief requires the continuation of the methadone maintenance dose supplemented by additional analgesics [151].

Every attempt should be made to minimize significant withdrawal manifestations in the opioid-dependent pregnant patient. Withdrawal in these patients may adversely affect the developing fetus, causing fetal distress and even intrauterine death [152]. Oral methadone maintenance is more compatible with maternal and fetal well-being than continued heroin abuse [153,154] and would likely also decrease the risk of intrauterine acquisition of acquired immunodeficiency syndrome. Cautious treatment of these patients with sufficient methadone to avoid withdrawal may avert these additional complications. After delivery, the neonate must be hospitalized and withdrawn from the drug. In selected pregnancies, lowering the maternal methadone dosage may lead to decreased incidence and severity of neonatal withdrawal [155].

While methadone has been extensively used for decades to help opiate addicted patients circumvent the health problems associated with illicit intravenous drug abuse, there are valid concerns about its safety as well. Methadone is known to cause dose-related respiratory depression and sleep apnea, which varies greatly based on an individual patient's underlying tolerance. The risk of this increases when methadone is combined with other depressant drugs [156]. Other concerns have increasingly come to light in recent years. Disproportionate numbers of patients on methadone were found to have suffered sudden cardiac death, often without underlying structural heart disease [156]. Though the majority of methadone associated sudden deaths are likely due to respiratory depression, it was also discovered that methadone is a potent potassium channel blocker, especially at higher doses. This prolongs cardiac repolarization (lengthening the QTc interval and predisposing to Torsades de Pointe) [156]. While it is unknown how clinically significant this finding may be, some experts suggest that QTc intervals be checked prior to initiating methadone therapy and be followed during chronic therapy to watch for lengthening of the QTc [156–158].

In recent years, buprenorphine, a partial mu-opioid agonist and K-opioid antagonist, has been increasingly advocated as an alternative to methadone for both maintenance and short-term management of opioid withdrawal [159]. Buprenorphine can be given orally, sublingually, intramuscularly, or intravenously [160,161]. Because of its partial agonist activity, it causes less CNS and respiratory depression and has a ceiling effect, so is less likely to be dangerous in overdose than methadone (though respiratory depression may still occasionally be seen, especially at higher doses, and deaths have been reported). This characteristic also renders it able to block the euphoric effects of heroin and morphine. It produces only a mild withdrawal syndrome when treatment is ceased, but care should be taken when initiating therapy in opioid dependent patients as it may precipitate withdrawal [161]. Of interest, a recent case of deliberate buprenorphine overdose resulted not in respiratory depression but severe opioid withdrawal lasting 4 days [162]. Compared to methadone, opioid withdrawal symptoms may resolve more quickly with buprenorphine but the latter is no more effective when used in the maintenance treatment of heroin dependence [163,164]. Buprenorphine does not seem to have the same propensity to prolong the QT interval as methadone [158]. Buprenorphine has a long half-life (~40 hours), so an additional benefit is that it may be administered every other day or even three times a week as maintenance therapy for opioid addicted patients. Special training and licensing are required for physicians who wish to prescribe buprenorphine or methadone (when used as treatment for opioid dependence) on an outpatient basis.

Sublingual buprenorphine tablets and solution are available as monotherapies as well as in combination with naloxone in a 4:1 (buprenorphine: naloxone) ratio (Suboxone). The naloxone is poorly absorbed sublingually and therefore does not interfere with buprenorphine's effects when taken as directed. Naloxone is added to the buprenorphine to block buprenorphine's euphorigenic effects if an attempt is made to divert the drug for illicit intravenous use (crushing and dissolving tablets etc.).

Sublingual dosing of buprenorphine for opioid dependence maintenance therapy starts with an introductory dose of 2 to 8 mg, based on the patient's degree of neuroadaptation to opioids. Dosing may be to be advanced to 4 to 16 mg on the second day. Over time the dose may be individualized to a range of 4 to 24 mg daily, every other day, or three times a week (though currently this dosing regimen is not recommended) [165]. When initiating buprenorphine therapy, physicians must be alert to the possibility of precipitated withdrawal, and patients should always be prepared for this. Because buprenorphine binds more tightly to the mu-opioid receptor than does heroin or methadone, it knocks any residual drug off the receptor and blocks its agonist effects since buprenorphine itself is only a partial agonist). To minimize this risk, the first dose of buprenorphine should be given at least 6 hours after the last heroin use (ideally once if the patient is already experiencing mild withdrawal symptoms). If the patient is on methadone, the first dose of buprenorphine should be given as long as possible after the last methadone dose (at least 24 hours, longer if the baseline methadone dose is higher) [165]. Precipitated withdrawal symptoms usually start 1 to 4 hours after the buprenorphine dose and last about 12 hours. These symptoms are worst during the first day, but patients transitioning to buprenorphine from methadone may experience mild discomfort and dysphoria for up to 1 to 2 weeks, depending on how much methadone they were using previously. Symptomatic treatment with medication such as clonidine may be employed during this period as needed.

When transitioning from methadone maintenance to buprenorphine, it is recommended that the patient be stabilized on as small a methadone dose as possible (preferably <30 mg daily) prior to initiating transfer. This minimizes risk of withdrawal and improves success. It is not recommended that patients on 60 mg or more of methadone daily be transitioned. While starting on too low a buprenorphine dose may be insufficient to manage withdrawal, too high a dose increases the risk of precipitated withdrawal. An average starting dose for patients on 20 to 40 mg methadone daily is 4 mg of buprenorphine, with reassessments later in the day or the next day to titrate dose [165]. In addition to maintenance therapy, various tapering opioid detoxification regimens using buprenorphine exist, with starting doses ranging from 1 to 8 mg daily. Therapy may be tapered over 5 to 14 days [161].

Clonidine, a central α_2-adrenergic agonist that binds to the α_2-receptors in the locus ceruleus, is also used to treat opioid withdrawal [166,167]. Stimulation of central α_2-receptors results in feedback inhibition of the norepinephrine activity, decreasing the firing rate of the noradrenergic neurons. These noradrenergic neurons also possess opioid receptors whose stimulation produces a similar reduction in sympathetic activity through the same intracellular messenger system [141]. Clonidine used without the addition of a replacement opioid has been found to be as effective as methadone in treating medically ill hospitalized patients in opioid withdrawal [168]. Clonidine may be administered in doses of 0.1 to 0.2 mg every 4 to 6 hours. Treatment is often continued for 5 to 10 days and then slowly tapered by 0.2 mg per day. Clonidine transdermal patches provide steady-state clonidine levels and may also be useful [151]. Tachyphylaxis to the effects of clonidine may develop by 10 to 14 days [139]. The most concerning side effect of clonidine is hypotension, especially with the first dose. This requires close monitoring. In one study, patients administered buprenorphine–naloxone were more likely to complete a short-term detoxification program and report fewer withdrawal and craving symptoms than those treated with clonidine [169]. The long-term success of this approach is unclear.

Combination therapy with clonidine and naltrexone has also been used for rapid opioid detoxification. Proponents of this approach emphasize the shortened period of withdrawal associated with the addition of naltrexone [170]. Continuing naltrexone as deterrent therapy after opioid withdrawal (akin to the use of disulfiram with alcoholics) has also been advocated, but this approach has a high attrition rate [171]. Delirium has been reported during rapid opioid detoxification of methadone maintenance patients [172].

Administering high doses of opioid antagonists to addicted individuals while under anesthesia has been suggested as a method of achieving detoxification from opiates within 24 to 48 hours. This method, known as ultrarapid detoxification, has been associated with pulmonary and renal failure as well as other complications, including death [173]. Additionally, long-term follow-up has demonstrated relapse of drug abuse in many of these patients [174]. This approach is not recommended.

References

1. Moore RD, Bone LR, Geller G, et al: Prevalence, detection, and treatment of alcoholism in hospitalized patients. *JAMA* 261:403, 1989.
2. Fruensgaard K: Withdrawal psychosis: a study of 30 consecutive cases. *Acta Psychiatr Scand* 53:105, 1976.
3. Tabakoff B, Cornell N, Hoffman PL: Alcohol tolerance. *Ann Emerg Med* 15:1005, 1986.
4. Narahashi T, Kuriyama K, Illes P, et al: Neuroreceptors and ion channels as targets of alcohol. *Alcohol Clin Exp Res* 25:182S, 2001.
5. Charness ME, Simon RP, Greenberg DA: Ethanol and the nervous system. *N Engl J Med* 321:442–454, 1989.
6. Tsai G, Gastfriend DR, Coyle JT: The glutamatergic basis of human alcoholism. *Am J Psychiatry* 152:332, 1995.
7. Davis KM, Wu JY: Role of glutamatergic and GABAergic systems in alcoholism. *J Biomed Sci* 8:7, 2001.
8. Saitz R, O'Malley SS: Pharmacotherapies for alcohol abuse. Withdrawal and treatment. *Med Clin North Am* 81:881, 1997.
9. Gianoulakis C, Angelogianni P, Meany M, et al: Endorphins in individuals with high and low risk for development of alcoholism, in Reids LD (ed): *Opioids, Bulimia, and Alcohol Abuse and Alcoholism*. New York, Springer-Verlag, 1990, p 229.
10. Goldstein DB: Effect of alcohol on cellular membranes. *Ann Emerg Med* 15:1013, 1986.
11. Isbell H, Fraser HF, Wikler A, et al: An experimental study of the etiology of rum fits and delirium tremens. *Q J Stud Alcohol* 16:1, 1955.
12. Victor M, Adams RD: The effects of alcohol on the nervous system. *Proc Assoc Res Nerv Ment Dis* 32:526, 1953.
13. Koch-Weser J, Sellers EM, Kalant H: Alcohol intoxication and withdrawal. *N Engl J Med* 294:757, 1976.
14. Hawley RJ, Major LF, Schulman EA, et al: Cerebrospinal fluid 3-methoxy-4-hydroxyphenylglycol and norepinephrine levels in alcohol withdrawal. Correlations with clinical signs. *Arch Gen Psychiatry* 42:1056, 1985.
15. Linnoila M, Mefford I, Nutt D, et al: NIH conference. Alcohol withdrawal and noradrenergic function. *Ann Intern Med* 107:875, 1987.
16. Hawley RJ, Major LF, Schulman EA, et al: CSF levels of norepinephrine during alcohol withdrawal. *Arch Neurol* 38:289, 1981.
17. Sano H, Suzuki Y, Ohara K, et al: Circadian variation in plasma homovanillic acid level during and after alcohol withdrawal in alcoholic patients. *Alcohol Clin Exp Res* 16:1047, 1992.
18. Adinoff B, Bone GH, Linnoila M: Acute ethanol poisoning and the ethanol withdrawal syndrome. *Med Toxicol Adverse Drug Exp* 3:172, 1988.
19. Frye GD: Gamma aminobutyric acid in alcohol withdrawal, in Porter RJ, Mattson RH, Cramer JA, et al (eds): *Alcohol and Seizures Basic Mechanisms and Clinical Concepts*. Philadelphia, FA Davis Co, 1990, p 87.
20. Nagy J, Kolok S, Boros A, et al: Role of altered structure and function of NMDA receptors in development of alcohol dependence. *Curr Neuropharmacol* 3:281, 2005.
21. Dodd P: Neural mechanisms of adaptation in chronic ethanol exposure and alcoholism. *Alcohol Clin Exp Res* 20:151A, 1996.
22. Gonzalez LP, Veatch LM, Ticku MK, et al: Alcohol withdrawal kindling: mechanisms and implications for treatment. *Alcohol Clin Exp Res* 25:197S, 2001.
23. Becker HC: The alcohol withdrawal "kindling" phenomenon: clinical and experimental findings. *Alcohol Clin Exp Res* 20:121A, 1996.
24. Mendelson JH, Mello NK: Medical progress. Biologic concomitants of alcoholism. *N Engl J Med* 301:912, 1979.
25. Lerner WD, Fallon HJ: The alcohol withdrawal syndrome. *N Engl J Med* 313:951, 1985.
26. Brown CG: The alcohol withdrawal syndrome. *Ann Emerg Med* 11:276, 1982.
27. Johnson R: Alcohol and fits. *Br J Addict* 80:227, 1985.
28. Simon RP: Alcohol and seizures. *N Engl J Med* 319:715, 1988.
29. Morris JC, Victor M: Alcohol withdrawal seizures. *Emerg Med Clin North Am* 5:827, 1987.
30. Victor M, Brausch C: The role of abstinence in the genesis of alcoholic epilepsy. *Epilepsia* 8:1, 1967.
31. Thompson WL: Management of alcohol withdrawal syndromes. *Arch Intern Med* 138:278, 1978.
32. Turner RC, Lichstein PR, Peden JG Jr, et al: Alcohol withdrawal syndromes: a review of pathophysiology, clinical presentation, and treatment. *J Gen Intern Med* 4:432, 1989.
33. Surawicz FG: Alcoholic hallucinosis: a missed diagnosis. Differential diagnosis and management. *Can J Psychiatry* 25:57, 1980.
34. Fisher J, Abrams J: Life-threatening ventricular tachyarrhythmias in delirium tremens. *Arch Intern Med* 137:1238, 1977.
35. Tavel ME, Davidson W, Batterton TD: A critical analysis of mortality associated with delirium tremens. *Am J Med Sci* 242:58, 1961.
36. Moore M, Gray MG: Delirium tremens: a study of cases at the Boston City Hospital 1915–1936. *N Engl J Med* 220:953, 1939.
37. Rosenbloom A: Emerging treatment options in the alcohol withdrawal syndrome. *J Clin Psychiatry* 49:28, 1988.
38. Victor M, Adams RD, Collins GH: *The Wernicke-Korsakoff Syndrome*. Philadelphia, FA Davis Co, 1971.
39. Goldfrank LR, Delaney KA, Flomenbaum NE: Substance withdrawal, in Goldfrank LR, Flomenbaum NE, Lewin NA, et al (eds): *Goldfrank's Toxicologic Emergencies*. Norwalk, CT, Appleton & Lange, 1994, p 905.
40. Anonymous: Drugs that cause psychiatric symptoms. *Med Lett Drugs Ther* 31:113, 1989.
41. Lichtigfeld FJ: Hepatic encephalopathy and delirium tremens–double jeopardy. *S Afr Med J* 67:880, 1985.
42. Delaney KA, Goldfrank L: Delirium assessment and management in the critical care environment. *Probl Crit Care* 1:78, 1987.
43. Mayo-Smith MF, Beecher LH, Fischer TL, et al: Management of alcohol withdrawal delirium. An evidence-based practice guideline. *Arch Intern Med* 164:1405, 2004.
44. Moskowitz G, Chalmers TC, Sacks HS, et al: Deficiencies of clinical trials of alcohol withdrawal. *Alcohol Clin Exp Res* 7:42, 1983.
45. Thompson WL, Johnson AD, Maddrey WL: Diazepam and paraldehyde for treatment of severe delirium tremens. A controlled trial. *Ann Intern Med* 82:175, 1975.
46. Liskow BI, Goodwin DW: Pharmacological treatment of alcohol intoxication, withdrawal and dependence: a critical review. *J Stud Alcohol* 48:356, 1987.
47. Ntais C, Pakos E, Kyzas P, et al: Benzodiazepines for alcohol withdrawal. *Cochrane Database Syst Rev* 2:2, 2006.
48. Adinoff B: Double-blind study of alprazolam, diazepam, clonidine, and placebo in the alcohol withdrawal syndrome: preliminary findings. *Alcohol Clin Exp Res* 18:873, 1994.
49. Wartenberg AA: Treatment of alcohol withdrawal syndrome. *JAMA* 250:1271, 1983.
50. Laine GA, Hossain SM, Solis RT, et al: Polyethylene glycol nephrotoxicity secondary to prolonged high-dose intravenous lorazepam. *Ann Pharmacother* 29:1110, 1995.
51. Lineaweaver WC, Anderson K, Hing DN: Massive doses of midazolam infusion for delirium tremens without respiratory depression. *Crit Care Med* 16:294, 1988.
52. Hoey LL, Nahum A, Vance-Bryan K: A prospective evaluation of benzodiazepine guidelines in the management of patients hospitalized for alcohol withdrawal. *Pharmacotherapy* 14:579, 1994.
53. Bird RD, Makela EH: Alcohol withdrawal: what is the benzodiazepine of choice? *Ann Pharmacother* 28:67, 1994.
54. Shaw GK: Detoxification: the use of benzodiazepines. *Alcohol Alcoholism* 30:765, 1995.
55. Miller WC Jr, McCurdy L: A double-blind comparison of the efficacy and safety of lorazepam and diazepam in the treatment of the acute alcohol withdrawal syndrome. *Clin Ther* 6:364, 1984.
56. Mayo-Smith MF: Pharmacological management of alcohol withdrawal. A meta-analysis and evidence-based practice guideline. American Society of Addiction Medicine Working Group on Pharmacological Management of Alcohol Withdrawal. *JAMA* 278:144, 1997.
57. Ritson B, Chick J: Comparison of two benzodiazepines in the treatment of alcohol withdrawal: effects on symptoms and cognitive recovery. *Drug Alcohol Depend* 18:329, 1986.
58. Daeppen JB, Gache P, Landry U, et al: Symptom-triggered vs fixed-schedule doses of benzodiazepine for alcohol withdrawal: a randomized treatment trial. *Arch Intern Med* 162:1117, 2002.
59. Sullivan JT, Sykora K, Schneiderman J, et al: Assessment of alcohol withdrawal: the revised clinical institute withdrawal assessment for alcohol scale. *Br J Addict* 84:1353–1357, 1989.
60. Sellers EM, Naranjo CA, Harrison M, et al: Diazepam loading: simplified treatment of alcohol withdrawal. *Clin Pharmacol Ther* 34:822, 1983.
61. Wartenberg AA, Nirenberg TD, Liepman MR, et al: Detoxification of alcoholics: improving care by symptom-triggered sedation. *Alcohol Clin Exp Res* 14:71, 1990.
62. Nolop KB, Natow A: Unprecedented sedative requirements during delirium tremens. *Crit Care Med* 13:246, 1985.
63. Saitz R, Mayo-Smith MF, Roberts MS, et al: Individualized treatment for alcohol withdrawal. A randomized double-blind controlled trial. *JAMA* 272:519, 1994.
64. Spies CD, Otter HE, Huske B, et al: Alcohol withdrawal severity is decreased by symptom-orientated adjusted bolus therapy in the ICU. *Intensive Care Med* 29:2230, 2003.
65. Enoch M: The role of $GABA_A$ receptors in the development of alcoholism. *Pharmacol Biochem Behav* 90:95, 2008.
66. Aaronson LM, Hinman DJ, Okamoto M: Effects of diazepam on ethanol withdrawal. *J Pharmacol Exp Ther* 221:319, 1982.
67. Young GP, Rores C, Murphy C, et al: Intravenous phenobarbital for alcohol withdrawal and convulsions. *Ann Emerg Med* 16:847, 1987.
68. Holloway HC, Hales RE, Watanabe HK: Recognition and treatment of acute alcohol withdrawal syndromes. *Psychiatr Clin North Am* 7:729, 1984.
69. McCowan C, Marik P: Refractory delirium tremens treated with propofol: a case series. *Crit Care Med* 28:1781, 2000.
70. Coomes TR, Smith SW: Successful use of propofol in refractory delirium tremens. *Ann Emerg Med* 30:825, 1997.

71. Takeshita J: Use of propofol for alcohol withdrawal delirium: a case report. *J Clin Psychiatry* 65:134, 2004.
72. Barr J, Egan TD, Sandoval NF, et al: Propofol dosing regimens for ICU sedation based upon an integrated pharmacokinetic-pharmacodynamic model. *Anesthesiology* 95:324, 2001.
73. Faillace LA, Flamer RN, Imber SD, et al: Giving alcohol to alcoholics. An evaluation. *Q J Stud Alcohol* 33:85, 1972.
74. Rosenbaum M, McCarty T: Alcohol prescription by surgeons in the prevention and treatment of delirium tremens: historic and current practice. *Gen Hosp Psychiatry* 24:257, 2002.
75. Golbert TM, Sanz CJ, Rose HD, et al: Comparative evaluation of treatments of alcohol withdrawal syndromes. *JAMA* 201:99, 1967.
76. Hodges B, Mazur JE: Intravenous ethanol for the treatment of alcohol withdrawal syndrome in critically ill patients. *Pharmacotherapy* 24:1578, 2004.
77. Thomas DW, Freedman DX: Treatment of the alcohol withdrawal syndrome: comparison of promazine and paraldehyde. *JAMA* 188:316, 1964.
78. Blum K, Eubanks JD, Wallace JE, et al: Enhancement of alcohol withdrawal convulsions in mice by haloperidol. *Clin Toxicol* 9:427, 1976.
79. Greenblatt DJ, Gross PL, Harris J, et al: Fatal hyperthermia following haloperidol therapy of sedative-hypnotic withdrawal. *J Clin Psychiatry* 39:673, 1978.
80. Sereny G, Kalant H: Comparative clinical evaluation of chlordiazepoxide and promazine in treatment of alcohol withdrawal syndrome. *BMJ* 1:92, 1965.
81. Gillman MA, Lichtigfeld FJ: The drug management of severe alcohol withdrawal syndrome. *Postgrad Med J* 66:1005, 1990.
82. Horwitz RI, Gottlieb LD, Kraus ML: The efficacy of atenolol in the outpatient management of the alcohol withdrawal syndrome. Results of a randomized clinical trial. *Arch Intern Med* 149:1089, 1989.
83. Wilkins AJ, Jenkins WJ, Steiner JA: Efficacy of clonidine in treatment of alcohol withdrawal state. *Psychopharmacology (Berl)* 81:78, 1983.
84. Bjorkqvist SE: Clonidine in alcohol withdrawal. *Acta Psychiatr Scand* 52:256, 1975.
85. Anonymous: Treatment of alcohol withdrawal. *Med Lett Drugs Ther* 28:75, 1986.
86. Harris JT, Roache JD, Thornton JE: A role for valproate in the treatment of sedative-hypnotic withdrawal and for relapse prevention. *Alcohol Alcoholism* 35:319, 2000.
87. Addolorato G, Balducci G, Capristo E, et al: Gamma-hydroxybutyric acid (GHB) in the treatment of alcohol withdrawal syndrome: a randomized comparative study versus benzodiazepine. *Alcohol Clin Exp Res* 23(10):1596–1604, 1999.
88. Nimmerrichter AA, Walter H, Gutierrez-Lobos KE, et al: Double-blind controlled trial of gamma-hydroxybutyrate and clomethiazole in the treatment of alcohol withdrawal. *Alcohol Alcoholism* 37(1):67–73, 2002.
89. Wilson A, Vulcano B: A double-blind, placebo-controlled trial of magnesium sulfate in the ethanol withdrawal syndrome. *Alcohol Clin Exp Res* 8(6):542–545, 1984.
90. D'Onofrio G, Rathlev NK, Ulrich AS, et al: Lorazepam for the prevention of recurrent seizures related to alcohol. *N Engl J Med* 340(12):915–921, 1999.
91. Gessner PK: Is diphenylhydantoin effective in treatment of alcohol withdrawal? *JAMA* 219:1072, 1972.
92. Alldredge BK, Lowenstein DH, Simon RP: Placebo-controlled trial of intravenous diphenylhydantoin for short-term treatment of alcohol withdrawal seizures. *Am J Med* 87:645, 1989.
93. Chance JF: Emergency department treatment of alcohol withdrawal seizures with phenytoin. *Ann Emerg Med* 20:520, 1991.
94. Rathlev NK, D'Onofrio G, Fish SS, et al: "The lack of efficacy of phenytoin in the prevention of recurrent alcohol-related seizures." *Ann Emerg Med* 23(3):513–518, 1994.
95. Tyrer P, Owen R, Dawling S: Gradual withdrawal of diazepam after long-term therapy. *Lancet* 1:1402, 1983.
96. MacKinnon GL, Parker WA: Benzodiazepine withdrawal syndrome: a literature review and evaluation. *Am J Drug Alcohol Abuse* 9:19, 1982.
97. Winokur A, Rickels K, Greenblatt DJ, et al: Withdrawal reaction from long-term, low-dosage administration of diazepam. A double-blind, placebo-controlled case study. *Arch Gen Psychiatry* 37:101, 1980.
98. Petursson H, Lader MH: Withdrawal from long-term benzodiazepine treatment. *BMJ* 283:643, 1981.
99. Lukas SE, Griffiths RR: Precipitated diazepam withdrawal in baboons: effects of dose and duration of diazepam exposure. *Eur J Pharmacol* 100:163, 1984.
100. Van Engelen BG, Gimbrere JS, Booy LH: Benzodiazepine withdrawal reaction in two children following discontinuation of sedation with midazolam. *Ann Pharmacother* 27:579, 1993.
101. Scharf MB, Feil P: Acute effects of drug administration and withdrawal on the benzodiazepine receptor. *Life Sci* 32:1771, 1983.
102. Benzer D, Cushman P Jr: Alcohol and benzodiazepines: withdrawal syndromes. *Alcohol Clin Exp Res* 4:243, 1980.
103. Noyes R Jr, Clancy J, Coryell WH, et al: A withdrawal syndrome after abrupt discontinuation of alprazolam. *Am J Psychiatry* 142:114, 1985.
104. Busto U, Sellers EM, Naranjo CA, et al: Withdrawal reaction after long-term therapeutic use of benzodiazepines. *N Engl J Med* 315:854, 1986.
105. Ashton H: Benzodiazepine withdrawal: an unfinished story. *BMJ* 288:1135, 1984.
106. *Mazicon Product Monograph*. Nutley, NJ, Hoffmann-La Roche, 1992.
107. Kleinberger G, Grimm G, Laggner A, et al: Weaning patients from mechanical ventilation by benzodiazepine antagonist Ro15-1788. *Lancet* 2:268, 1985.
108. Lopez A, Rebollo J: Benzodiazepine withdrawal syndrome after a benzodiazepine antagonist. *Crit Care Med* 18:1480, 1990.
109. Burr W, Sandham P, Judd A: Death after flumazenil. *BMJ* 298:1713, 1989.
110. Lheureux P, Vrankx M, Askenasi R: Administration of flumazenil. *Ann Emerg Med* 20:592, 1991.
111. Owen RT, Tyrer P: Benzodiazepine dependence. A review of the evidence. *Drugs* 25:385, 1983.
112. De Bard ML: Diazepam withdrawal syndrome: a case with psychosis, seizure, and coma. *Am J Psychiatry* 136:104, 1979.
113. Rosebush PI, Mazurek MF: Catatonia after benzodiazepine withdrawal. *J Clin Psychopharmacol* 16:315, 1996.
114. Ghadirian AM, Gauthier S, Wong T: Convulsions in patients abruptly withdrawn from clonazepam while receiving neuroleptic medication. *Am J Psychiatry* 144:686, 1987.
115. Jaffe R, Gibson E: Clonazepam withdrawal psychosis. *J Clin Psychopharmacol* 6:193, 1986.
116. Preskorn SH, Denner LJ: Benzodiazepines and withdrawal psychosis. Report of three cases. *JAMA* 237:36, 1977.
117. Wikler A: Diagnosis and treatment of drug dependence of the barbiturate type. *Am J Psychiatry* 125:758, 1968.
118. Abernethy DR, Greenblatt DJ, Shader RI: Treatment of diazepam withdrawal syndrome with propranolol. *Ann Intern Med* 94:354, 1981.
119. Goodman WK, Charney DS, Price LH, et al: Ineffectiveness of clonidine in the treatment of the benzodiazepine withdrawal syndrome: report of three cases. *Am J Psychiatry* 143:900, 1986.
120. Dysken MW, Chan CH: Diazepam withdrawal psychosis: a case report. *Am J Psychiatry* 134:573, 1977.
121. Craig K, Gomez HF, McManus JL, et al: Severe gamma-hydroxybutyrate withdrawal: a case report and literature review. *J Emerg Med* 18:65, 2000.
122. McDaniel CH, Miotto KA: Gamma hydroxybutyrate (GHB) and gamma butyrolactone (GBL) withdrawal: five case studies. *J Psychoactive Drugs* 33:143, 2001.
123. Miotto K, Darakjian J, Basch J, et al: Gamma-hydroxybutyric acid: patterns of use, effects and withdrawal. *Am J Addict* 10:232, 2001.
124. Bowles TM, Sommi RW, Amiri M: Successful management of prolonged gamma-hydroxybutyrate and alcohol withdrawal. *Pharmacotherapy* 21:254, 2001.
125. Wojtowicz J, Yarema M, Wax P: Withdrawal from gamma-hydroxybutyrate, 1,4, butanediol, and gamma-butyrolactone: a case report and systematic review. *CJEM* 10:69, 2008.
126. Dyer JE, Roth B, Hyma BA: Gamma-hydroxybutyrate withdrawal syndrome. *Ann Emerg Med* 37:147, 2001.
127. Sivilotti ML, Burns MJ, Aaron CK, et al: Pentobarbital for severe gamma-butyrolactone withdrawal. *Ann Emerg Med* 38:660, 2001.
128. McDonough M, Kennedy N, Glasper A, et al: Clinical features and management of gamma-hydroxybutyrate (GHB) withdrawal: a review. *Drug Alcohol Depend* 75:3, 2004.
129. Le Tourneau J, Hagg DS, Smith SM, et al: Baclofen and gamma-hydroxybutyrate withdrawal. *Neurocrit Care* 8:430, 2008.
130. Kao LW, Amin Y, Kirk MA, et al: Intrathecal baclofen withdrawal mimicking sepsis. *J Emerg Med* 24:423, 2003.
131. Turner MR, Gainsborough N: Neuroleptic malignant-like syndrome after abrupt withdrawal of baclofen. *J Psychopharmacol* 15:61, 2001.
132. Alden TD, Lytle RA, Park TS, et al: Intrathecal baclofen withdrawal: a case report and review of the literature. *Childs Nerv Syst* 18:522, 2002.
133. Samson-Fang L, Gooch J, Norlin C: Intrathecal baclofen withdrawal simulating neuroepileptic malignant syndrome in a child with cerebral palsy. *Dev Med Child Neurol* 42:561, 2000.
134. Zuckerbraun NS, Ferson SS, Albright AL, et al: Intrathecal baclofen withdrawal: emergency recognition and management. *Pediatr Emerg Care* 20:759, 2004.
135. Greenberg MI, Hendrickson RG: Baclofen withdrawal following removal of an intrathecal baclofen pump despite oral baclofen replacement. *J Toxicol Clin Toxicol* 41:83, 2003.
136. Coffey RJ, Edgar TS, Francisco GE, et al: Abrupt withdrawal from intrathecal baclofen: recognition and management of a potentially life-threatening syndrome. *Arch Phys Med Rehabil* 83:735, 2002.
137. Meythaler JM, Roper JF, Brunner RC: Cyproheptadine for intrathecal baclofen withdrawal. *Arch Phys Med Rehabil* 84:638, 2003.
138. Khantzian EJ, McKenna GJ: Acute toxic and withdrawal reactions associated with drug use and abuse. *Ann Intern Med* 90:361, 1979.
139. Freitas PM: Narcotic withdrawal in the emergency department. *Am J Emerg Med* 3:456, 1985.
140. George CF, Robertson D: Clinical consequences of abrupt drug withdrawal. *Med Toxicol Adverse Drug Exp* 2:367, 1987.
141. Flemenbaum A, Boza R, Slater VL, et al: Clonidine opiate withdrawal. *Res Staff Physician* 35:111, 1989.
142. Bohrer H, Schmidt H, Bach A, et al: Methadone treatment of opioid withdrawal in intensive care patients. *Lancet* 341:636, 1993.

143. Tobias JD, Schleien CL, Haun SE: Methadone as treatment for iatrogenic narcotic dependency in pediatric intensive care unit patients. *Crit Care Med* 18:1292, 1990.
144. Fultz JM, Senay EC: Guidelines for the management of hospitalized narcotics addicts. *Ann Intern Med* 82:815, 1975.
145. Goldfrank LR: The several uses of naloxone. *Emerg Med* 16:105, 1984.
146. Dole VP, Nyswander M: A medical treatment of diacetylmorphine (heroin) addiction. *JAMA* 193:80, 1965.
147. Kreek MJ, Garfield JW, Gutjahr CL, et al: Rifampin-induced methadone withdrawal. *N Engl J Med* 294:1104, 1976.
148. Tong TG, Pond SM, Kreek MJ, et al: Phenytoin-induced methadone withdrawal. *Ann Intern Med* 94:349, 1981.
149. Donny EC, Walsh SL, Bigelow GE, et al: High-dose methadone produces superior opioid blockade and comparable withdrawal suppression to lower doses in opioid-dependent humans. *Psychopharmacology (Berl)* 161:202, 2002.
150. Faggiano F, Vigna-Taglianti F, Versino E, et al: Methadone maintenance at different dosages for opioid dependence. *Cochrane Database Syst Rev* 2:2, 2006.
151. Zweben JE, Payte JT: Methadone maintenance in the treatment of opioid dependence. A current perspective. *West J Med* 152:588, 1990.
152. Zuspan FP, Gumpel JA, Mejia-Zelaya A, et al: Fetal stress from methadone withdrawal. *Am J Obstet Gynecol* 122:43, 1975.
153. Fraser AC: Drug addiction in pregnancy. *Lancet* 2:896, 1976.
154. Kandall SR: Managing neonatal withdrawal. *Drug Ther* 6:47, 1976.
155. Dashe JS, Sheffield JS, Olscher DA, et al: Relationship between maternal methadone dosage and neonatal withdrawal. *Obstet Gynecol* 100:1244, 2002.
156. Chugh SS, Socoteanu C, Reinier K, et al: A community-based evaluation of sudden death associated with therapeutic levels of methadone. *Am J Med* 121:66, 2008.
157. Andrews CM, Krantz MJ, Wedam EF, et al: Methadone-induced mortality in the treatment of chronic pain: Role of QT prolongation. *Cardiol J* 16:210, 2009.
158. Anchersen K, Clausen T, Gossop M, et al: Prevalence and clinical relevance of corrected QT interval prolongation during methadone and buprenorphine treatment: a mortality assessment study. *Addiction* 104: 993, 2009.
159. Lintzeris N, Bell J, Bammer G, et al: A randomized controlled trial of buprenorphine in the management of short-term ambulatory heroin withdrawal. *Addiction* 97:1395, 2002.
160. Welsh CJ, Suman M, Cohen A, et al: The use of intravenous buprenorphine for the treatment of opioid withdrawal in medically ill hospitalized patients. *Am J Addict* 11:135, 2002.
161. Robinson SE: Buprenorphine-containing treatments: place in the management of opioid addiction. *CNS Drugs* 20:697, 2006.
162. Clark NC, Lintzeris N, Muhleisen PJ: Severe opiate withdrawal in a heroin user precipitated by a massive buprenorphine dose. *Med J Aust* 176:166, 2002.
163. Gowing L, Ali R, White JM: Buprenorphine for the management of opioid withdrawal. Cochrane Database of Systematic Reviews 2009, Issue 3. Art. No.: CD002025. DOI: 10.1002/14651858.CD002025.pub4.
164. Mattick RP, Kimber J, Breen C, et al: Buprenorphine maintenance versus placebo or methadone maintenance for opioid dependence. *Cochrane Database Syst Rev* 2:2, 2006.
165. http://www.health.vic.gov.au/dpu/downloads/bupguide.pdf.
166. Gold MS, Redmond DE Jr, Kleber HD: Clonidine blocks acute opiate-withdrawal symptoms. *Lancet* 2:599, 1978.
167. Gold MS, Pottash AC, Sweeney DR, et al: Opiate withdrawal using clonidine. A safe, effective, and rapid nonopiate treatment. *JAMA* 243:343, 1980.
168. Umbricht A, Hoover DR, Tucker MJ, et al: Opioid detoxification with buprenorphine, clonidine, or methadone in hospitalized heroin-dependent patients with HIV infection. *Drug Alcohol Depend* 69:263, 2003.
169. Ling W, Amass L, Shoptaw S, et al: A multi-center randomized trial of buprenorphine-naloxone versus clonidine for opioid detoxification: findings from the national Institute on Drug Abuse Clinical trials network. *Addiction* 100(8):1090, 2005.
170. Stine SM, Kosten TR: Use of drug combinations in treatment of opioid withdrawal. *J Clin Psychopharmacol* 12:203, 1992.
171. Warner EA, Kosten TR, O'Connor PG: Pharmacotherapy for opioid and cocaine abuse. *Med Clin North Am* 81:909, 1997.
172. Golden SA, Sakhrani DL: Unexpected delirium during Rapid Opioid Detoxification (ROD). *J Addict Dis* 23:65, 2004.
173. Hamilton RJ, Olmedo RE, Shah S, et al: Complications of ultrarapid opioid detoxification with subcutaneous naltrexone pellets. *Acad Emerg Med* 9:63, 2002.
174. Pfab R, Hirtl C, Zilker T: Opiate detoxification under anesthesia: no apparent benefit but suppression of thyroid hormones and risk of pulmonary and renal failure. *J Toxicol Clin Toxicol* 37:43, 1999.

SECTION XI ■ SURGICAL PROBLEMS IN THE INTENSIVE CARE UNIT

FRED A. LUCHETTE

CHAPTER 146 ■ EPISTAXIS

AVINASH V. MANTRAVADI, CHAD A. ZENDER AND LOUIS G. PORTUGAL

Epistaxis is a common occurrence in the general population and most frequently is minor and self-limiting. In the intensive care setting, however, epistaxis may further destabilize an already unstable patient and may be life-threatening. Appropriate management of epistaxis requires careful evaluation and management of the patient's hemodynamic status and prompt control of the source of bleeding.

BLOOD SUPPLY OF THE NOSE

The internal and external carotid arteries, with frequent free anastomoses within the nasal mucosa, provide a rich blood supply to the nose, and venous drainage parallels the arterial supply.

The internal carotid artery (ICA) supplies the nasal mucosa through the ethmoid branches of the ophthalmic artery. The ophthalmic artery, the first branch off of the ICA, enters the orbit through the optic canal and divides into anterior and posterior ethmoidal branches. Both anterior and posterior ethmoidal arteries exit the orbit through the medial orbital wall at the level of the frontoethmoid suture line, an important landmark in the operative management of epistaxis originating from these vessels. These arteries then pass medially through the roof of the ethmoid sinuses and enter the anterior cranial fossa, from which they descend through the cribriform plate to enter the nose. The anterior ethmoidal artery, the larger of the two, supplies the anterior nasal septum and lateral nasal wall. The posterior ethmoidal artery supplies the region of the superior turbinate and corresponding portion of the septum.

The external carotid artery (ECA) supplies the nose through two of its terminal branches, the facial artery and the internal maxillary artery. The facial artery, a major branch of the external carotid system, providing blood supply to most of the lower face and lips, supplies the superior labial artery, which enters the nose lateral to the anterior nasal spine and supplies the anterior nasal septum (Figs. 146.1 and 146.2).

The maxillary segment of the internal maxillary artery (IMA) is the primary contributor to the nasal blood supply, crossing the infratemporal fossa to the pterygopalatine fossa. At this point, it divides into multiple terminal branches that supply the nasal cavity primarily by the sphenopalatine artery (SPA). The SPA enters the nasal cavity through the sphenopalatine foramen at the lateral nasal wall posterior to the horizontal portion of the middle turbinate, and divides into multiples branches that supply the posterior septum, lateral nasal wall, and sinuses (Fig. 146.3).

On the anterior nasal septum lies *Kiesselbach's plexus* or *Little's area*, an abundant plexus of vessels consisting of the most prominent anastomoses between the external and internal carotid artery systems. It is at this region that anterior epistaxis most frequently originates, reported in up to 90% of cases [1,2]. Posterior epistaxis, on the other hand, most frequently occurs near the sphenopalatine foramen from branches of the SPA, frequently a result of prior surgery or trauma.

CAUSES OF EPISTAXIS

Risk factors and causes of epistaxis may be divided into local and systemic etiologies (Table 146.1).In the intensive care unit (ICU) setting, epistaxis usually results from a combination of these etiologies; however, direct nasal trauma still plays a central role in its development. Trauma may result from digital manipulation by the patient or nasal fractures with subsequent mucosal disruption; however, in the ICU, nasal trauma is often iatrogenic from nasal oxygen, continuous positive airway pressure (CPAP), or particularly from nasal tube placement (nasogastric feeding tubes, nasal endotracheal tubes, etc.). Nasal cannulas in particular cause bleeding as a result of mucosal abrasions or mucosal drying from non-humidified high flow oxygen. A humidified face mask or face tent is preferred in particularly high-risk patients (history of epistaxis, long-term anticoagulation). Simply moving a nasal tube to the contralateral side may minimize or prevent progression of traumatic epistaxis resulting from tube placement.

Other causes of mucosal dryness include overuse of nasal decongestants or cocaine. Alterations in nasal airflow with subsequent drying may result from congenital or acquired anatomic abnormalities such as septal spurs and deviations, as well as septal perforations (which can themselves be caused by the potent vasoconstrictive effects of drugs such as cocaine). Epistaxis occurs more frequently during the winter months, presumably because of the lower humidity in ambient air. Because factors such as mucosal dryness and trauma most frequently affect the anterior nose, most epistaxis is anterior in nature.

Systemic factors and preexisting conditions place ICU patients at particularly high risk for epistaxis. Studies show that up to 45% of patients admitted for epistaxis have a comorbid condition that could cause or exacerbate bleeding [3]. Literature has identified patients older than 50 years as being particularly predisposed to severe epistaxis refractory to local measures of control, likely due to the effects of endothelial degeneration, atherosclerotic changes, and other systemic conditions. These include hypertension, atherosclerotic vascular disease, coagulopathies, and conditions requiring antiplatelet or anticoagulative medications (aspirin, clopidogrel, heparin, warfarin) such as deep vein thrombosis (DVT), pulmonary embolus (PE), cardiac arrhythmias, coronary artery disease (CAD), and vascular stent placement. Medications such as these all affect coagulation and may subsequently result in recurrent or refractory episodes of nasal bleeding. However, the conditions for which these agents are used present a particular challenge, as stoppage of these medications can be life-threatening.

Coagulopathies such as von Willebrand disease and hemophilia must be considered in patients with recurrent or refractory disease. Failure to identify these conditions may result in a delay in administration of medical therapies such as factor VIII or desmopressin acetate that can aid in reversing the underlying disease process.

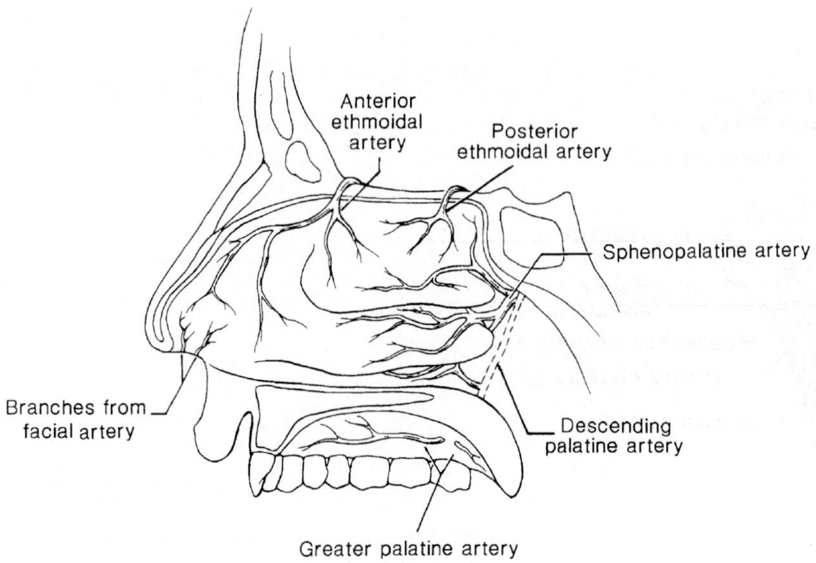

FIGURE 146.1. Blood supply of the lateral nasal wall.

In the ICU setting, it is most often a combination of a number of the above factors that results in epistaxis. Identifying and addressing the various contributing factors is of central importance when managing epistaxis in the ICU.

MANAGEMENT

Initial evaluation of the ICU patient with epistaxis should first and always be guided by the rules of *A*irway, *B*reathing, and *C*irculation, with a quick determination of the severity of the bleed. In case of a severe bleed in an unstable patient, the airway should be secured (by intubation) and two large bore intravenous (IV) lines should be placed if not already established. If the patient already has a tracheostomy tube in place, the cuff should be inflated to prevent passage of blood products and protect the airway. Frequent suctioning of the pharynx can assist in reducing aspiration. Once the airway is secured and hemodynamic status addressed, efforts can be focused on the control of bleeding. Typically, most patients are hemodynamically stable and are able to protect their airway, allowing for a more thorough examination.

In patients who are hemodynamically stable, a short and focused history, including information regarding nasal trauma, duration, and amount of blood loss is invaluable. After the severity has been assessed, one can discern laterality, history of coagulation and hemodynamic disorders, and iatrogenic factors that may be contributing. In the ICU setting, patients are frequently unable to provide a history such that nursing, family members, and other ancillary staff are needed to provide crucial information. It is also necessary to determine if a bleed is originating anteriorly in the nasal vault or more posteriorly (e.g., copious amounts of expectorated blood, hematemesis), which is typically more severe and is not easily stopped with local pressure or topical cauterization. One must exercise caution when suctioning the nasopharynx to avoid dislodgment of clot into the hypopharynx and larynx, which may result in airway compromise.

Vital signs should be assessed and hypertension controlled to reduce the bleeding. The nasal examination may then be undertaken, best accomplished with good lighting, a nasal speculum, and suction. If a discrete source of bleeding is easily visualized, then local coagulation with silver nitrate applicators may suffice. However, diffuse bleeding is often noted, and a vasoconstrictive agent such as oxymetazoline or phenylephrine may be sprayed to decrease bleeding and improve visualization.

The first step in attempted control of epistaxis should consist of a topical vasoconstrictive agent (oxymetazoline or phenylephrine) sprayed liberally on the side of bleeding (if localized) or bilaterally, followed by uninterrupted external digital pressure for 15 to 20 minutes. Pressure should be applied with a tight pinch, compressing the nasal alae against the nasal septum in such a manner as to prevent passage of nasal airflow. During this time, the oropharynx should be examined to evaluate for

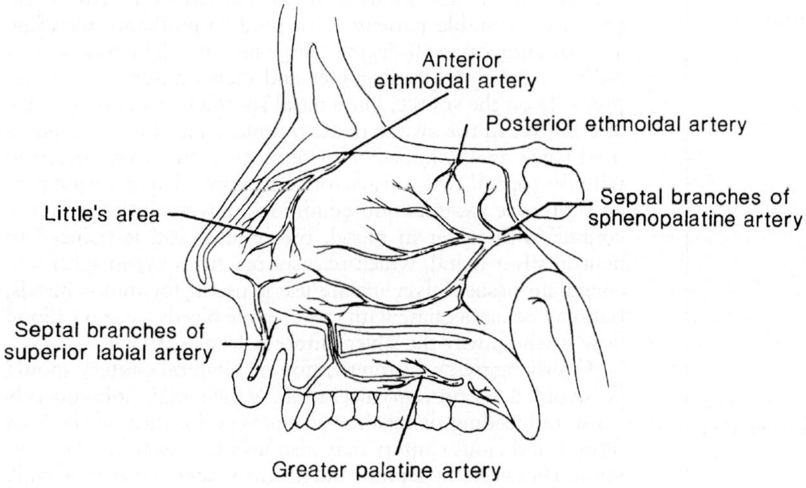

FIGURE 146.2. Blood supply of the nasal septum.

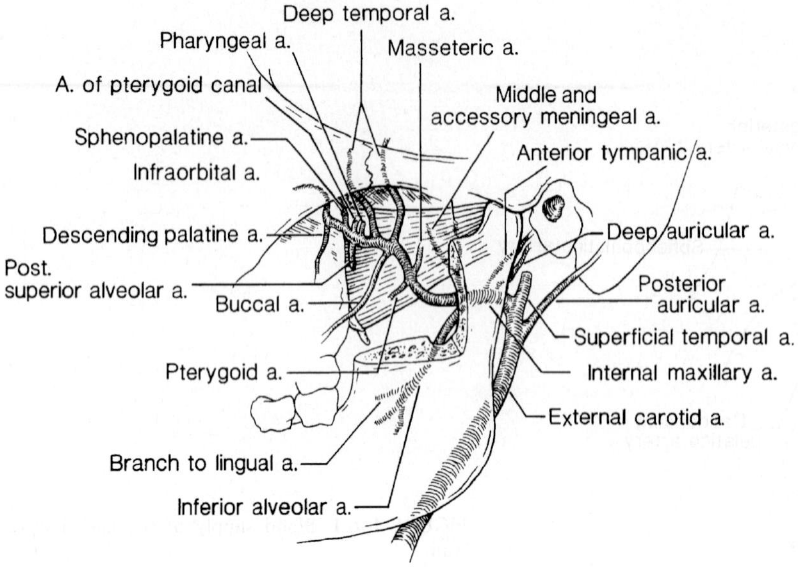

FIGURE 146.3. Course and branches of the internal maxillary artery.

continued bleeding, which may raise suspicion for a posterior source. One should be aware that only minimal anterior bleeding may occur with significant posterior epistaxis.

Because the majority of bleeding is anterior on the septum, a topical vasoconstrictive agent and external pressure will frequently achieve hemostasis and is sometimes all that is necessary. Krempl et al. found that up to 65% of cases of epistaxis were controlled with a topical vasoconstrictor and pressure alone [4]. If these measures are successful, measures should be taken to decrease mucosal drying and subsequent recurrence, including placement of a humidified face tent, topical vasoconstrictive agent twice daily for a maximum of 5 days (to prevent complications such as rebound nasal congestion and septal perforation), frequent topical saline sprays, application of lubricating ointment (e.g., neomycin/polymyxin) to the nasal septum twice daily, and control of hypertension.

Laboratory tests should be considered in patients with significant or recurrent epistaxis. A complete blood cell count, coagulation studies, and a bleeding time should be performed. In patients with severe bleeding or those who are severely anemic, one should consider a crossmatch with the initial blood draw due to the time necessary to prepare blood products. Liver function tests may help elucidate the cause and identify patients with coagulopathies as a result of impaired hepatic function.

TABLE 146.1

ETIOLOGIES OF EPISTAXIS

Local factors	Systemic factors
Anatomic Septal deviation, Septal spur Septal perforation	Hypertension[a]
Trauma[a] Digital/nose-picking Nasal/facial fractures Nasal tube placement (nasogastric, nasotracheal, etc.)	Coagulopathy[a] Hepatic dysfunction Disorders of platelet function/aggregation (e.g., von Willebrand disease) Hematologic malignancy Hemophilia
Mucosal dryness[a] Cold weather Nasal cannula use CPAP Chronic intranasal corticosteroid use Nasal decongestant overuse Cocaine abuse	Medication effect[a] ASA Clopidogrel Warfarin Heparin
Sinonasal infection/ inflammation	Vascular disorders Wegener's granulomatosis Churg-Strauss syndrome Hereditary hemorrhagic telangiectasia
Nasal polyposis	Drug abuse (e.g., cocaine)
Intranasal mass Arteriovenous malformation Malignancy	Alcohol abuse
Foreign body	Renal failure
Recent nasal/facial surgery	Malnutrition

[a]In ICU patients, epistaxis most commonly results from a combination of these factors.

Cautery

The majority of nosebleeds arise from Kiesselbach's plexus on the anterior nasal septum, and cauterization may be performed either with silver nitrate applicators or electrocautery to the bleeding site if unresponsive to topical vasoconstrictors and pressure. In stable patients with mild to moderate bleeding, a nasal endoscope (0-degree telescope with light source) can aid in visualizing bleeding sites and focus cauterization more precisely on the source, but a nasal speculum remains a viable alternative. In the awake patient, topical anesthesia should be used (such as 4% lidocaine or tetracaine) that may be mixed with the topical vasoconstrictor being applied, to decrease pain and improve examination conditions. Silver nitrate, when in contact with water in blood, precipitates and is reduced to neutral silver metal, which releases reactive oxygen species to coagulate tissue. Silver nitrate use is useful for minor bleeds, but may be inadequate with more severe bleeds as heavy blood flow washes away the silver nitrate before it can act.

Overly aggressive cauterization or bilateral cautery should be avoided to prevent ulceration, which may subsequently cause re-bleeding or result in a septal perforation in the long term. Injudicious cautery may also lead to synechia (scar) formation between the septum and the turbinate/lateral nasal wall, which can later impair the patient's breathing and result in abnormal airflow.

An additional tool in initial control in patients with evidence of significant posterior bleeding includes transpalatal vasoconstriction of the sphenopalatine artery, utilizing a 25-gauge needle bent at 2.5 cm and injecting 1 to 2 mL of 1% lidocaine with epinephrine (1:100,000) in the descending palatine foramen, located just medial to the upper second molar. This procedure may slow bleeding enough to allow for improved examination [5].

Nasal Packing

Nasal packing, which is typically described as anterior or posterior, should be considered as the next step in management after failure of local and medical measures such as external pressure and cautery. Packing can also be used in cases where the source of bleeding is not evident on physical examination, or when the bleeding is severe and must be temporized until further definitive management can be performed.

Anterior Nasal Packing

Anterior nasal packing is generally performed for epistaxis originating from the anterior nasal cavity to tamponade the vessel at the source, as well as to provide coverage of the bleeding site, allowing the primary stages of healing to occur in the absence of further local trauma and desiccation that can result in re-bleeding. As most epistaxis occurs anteriorly, this form of packing is usually sufficient. Many different types of packs are now available, utilizing a variety of both absorbable and nonabsorbable materials. The choice of anterior packing material is based on clinician preference and comfort level, as well as product availability in the hospital.

Common absorbable materials used for anterior packing include gelatin foam (e.g., GelFoam®-Pfizer, Inc, New York, NY) and oxidized cellulose (e.g., Surgicel®-Ethicon, Inc, Somerville, NJ), which encourage platelet aggregation and protect bleeding sites from further trauma and desiccation. Other materials include microfibrillar collagen (e.g., Avitene©-Davol Inc, Cranston, RI) and thrombin-gelatin combinations (Floseal®-Baxter International, Deerfield, IL) that can be instilled in the nasal cavity as a slurry. The advantages of these products include their ease of use, decreased patient pain, elimination of the need for pack removal, and improved conformity to the irregular contours of the nasal cavity. However, these products may not be effective in control of brisk arterial bleeding as they apply only low pressure to the nasal mucosa, and they are significantly more expensive than traditional packs.

Traditional nasal packing has involved the use of 0.5-in by 72.0 petroleum jelly strip gauze, layered with a bayonet forceps from inferior to superior along the length of the nasal cavity (Fig. 146.4). Over the years, the use of nonabsorbable sponges composed of hydroxylated polyvinyl acetate that expands when wet (e.g., Merocel® Medtronic Inc, Mystic, CT) has gained popularity due to their ease of use and applicability by hand without the need for additional instruments. The sponge is coated in antibiotic ointment prior to placement primarily for lubrication to ease application and decrease further septal trauma, but there is no published evidence to support a decrease in infectious complications [5,6]. Using a bayonet forceps or by hand, the sponge is then placed in the nasal cavity on the side of bleeding, sliding along the nasal septum to avoid the turbinates and ensure tamponade of the septal bleeding source. The packing should slide easily and should not require a high degree of force to decrease further mucosal trauma. Once in place, the sponge is copiously impregnated with a vasoconstrictive agent or sterile saline. Subsequent swelling of the sponge provides high pressure against the site of bleeding resulting in hemostasis. At this point, the oropharynx should be inspected to evaluate for continued bleeding posteriorly. Persistent anterior bleeding around the pack may necessitate repositioning or augmenting the pack. Anterior nasal packing has been shown in randomized, controlled trials to successfully control bleeding in up to 80% of cases [7,8]. The use of the Merocel® has published success rates up to 92% [9].

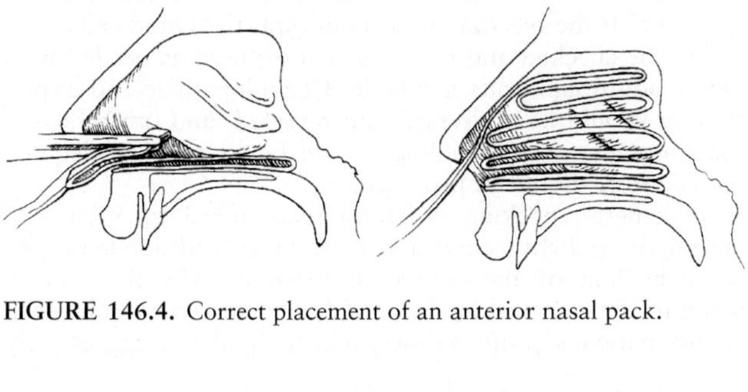

FIGURE 146.4. Correct placement of an anterior nasal pack.

Posterior Packing

After anterior packing is applied, continued postnasal bleeding should necessitate placement of a posterior pack. Posterior epistaxis is seen more frequently in elderly patients and patients with a history of prior sinus surgery or craniofacial trauma, systemic disorders, and prior nosebleeds [10]. The incidence of posterior epistaxis is, therefore, greater in ICU patients. Because of the often severe nature of the bleeding and relative inaccessibility of the source, conservative measures with pressure and cauterization as well as anterior packing have a limited role in the control of posterior epistaxis. The sphenopalatine artery is a large-caliber vessel, and the blood loss from an episode of posterior epistaxis is often significant, such that consideration should be given to blood transfusion as indicated. Posterior packing is also used as a temporizing measure to slow bleeding in anticipation of surgical management.

The classic posterior nasal packing consists of rolled gauze or tonsil packs secured in the posterior choanae by inserting the pack through the oral cavity and then into the nasopharynx by sutures through the nose (Fig. 146.5). Although very effective, this is difficult to perform, time consuming, and painful for the patient, and it is rarely performed today.

A more commonly used method of posterior nasal packing utilizes a Foley catheter (12 or 14 French) with a 30-mL balloon, readily available in the ICU setting. The nose is first cleared of any previously placed packs, debris, or clots, and topical anesthesia with a vasoconstrictor is applied. With the balloon deflated, the Foley catheter is inserted through the involved nares into the nasopharynx. One may examine the posterior oropharynx to confirm that the tip of the catheter has been placed entirely through the nasal cavity. The catheter is inflated with 10 to 20 mL saline and then pulled anteriorly to wedge the balloon snugly into the posterior nasal cavity and choanae (Fig. 146.6). The oropharynx is again examined to ensure that the soft palate is not displaced or engaged by the balloon, as this may lead to palatal necrosis. While the catheter is held under tension, anterior nasal packing is placed as above. The Foley catheter is then secured against the anterior nasal packing (extending out of the involved nares) using an umbilical cord clamp to maintain pressure and prevent posterior migration of the balloon into the pharynx. The clamp should be rotated periodically to reduce the occurrence of alar and columellar necrosis (additional padding may be placed), and the area must be checked frequently for this complication.

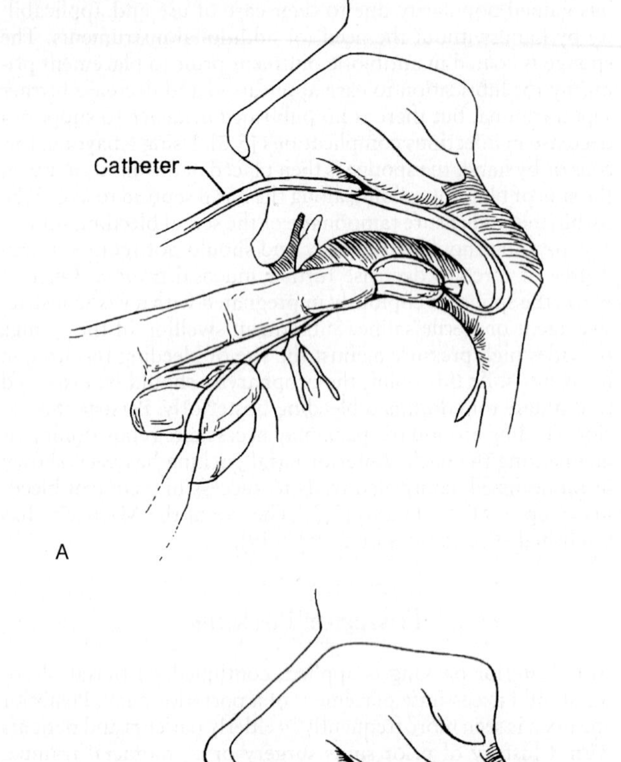

FIGURE 146.5. A,B: Insertion of a nasopharyngeal (posterior) pack (traditional method).

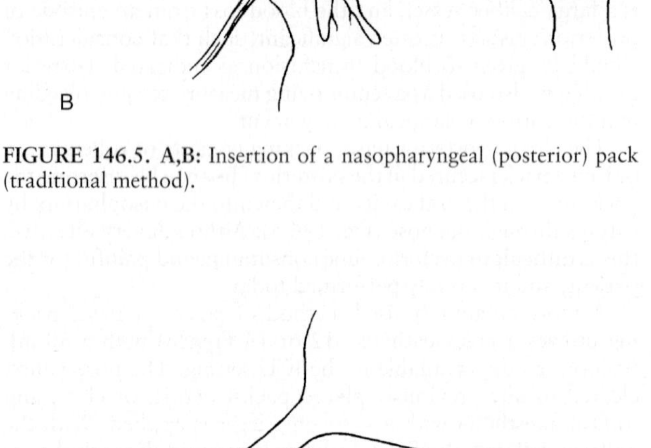

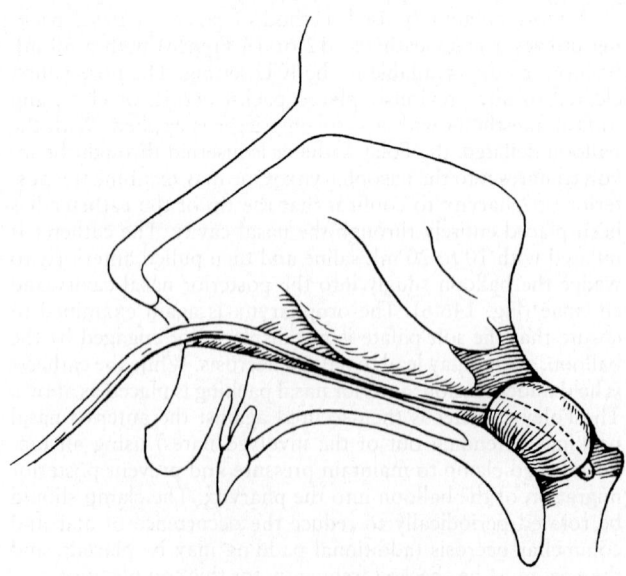

FIGURE 146.6. Foley catheter with balloon inflated.

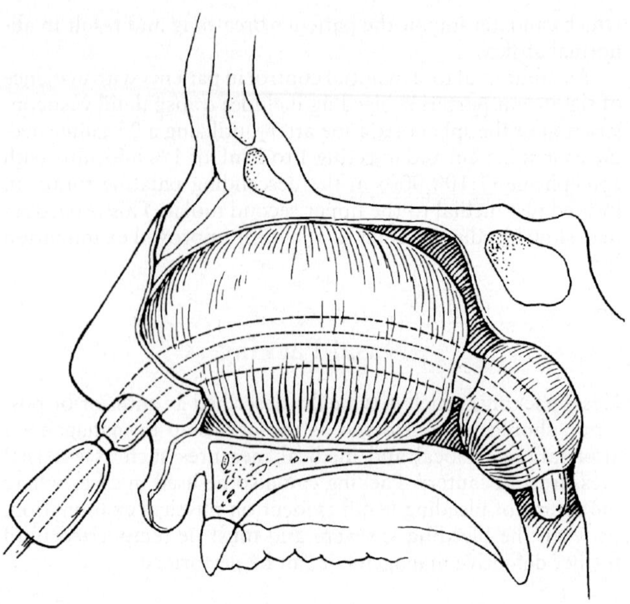

FIGURE 146.7. Balloon tampons in place.

Additional options for posterior nasal packing include balloon tampons designed for this purpose (Fig. 146.7). These devices consist of a catheter with two balloons: one that inflates in the choanae and a second that inflates in the nasal cavity. Although easy to insert, the balloons do not conform to the contour of the nasal cavity and consequently may fail. If bleeding persists, a classic posterior pack should be placed.

Complications associated with the posterior nasal pack may be serious, and all of these patients should remain hospitalized and monitored. Pulmonary compliance may be impaired through a postulated "nasopulmonary reflex" ("diving reflex"), of questionable clinical significance, which may result in apnea, hypoxia, and dysrhythmias [11,12]. All patients with posterior packs are hospitalized and monitored, and unstable or unhealthy patients should be admitted to the ICU. Eating is impaired by a posterior pack, and strong consideration should be given to keeping the patient NPO. The airway may become compromised, and intubation or rarely tracheostomy may be necessary. In addition, the procedure is often painful due to pressure on the posterior septum and choanae, and alar necrosis may result from pressure anteriorly. Posterior nasal packing alone has been shown to have a success rate of up to 70% for control of bleeding, a modest figure considering the aforementioned risks and potential complications [13,14]. As a result, additional measures have gained support in the treatment of posterior epistaxis, as later described.

MANAGEMENT AFTER PACKING

Once the patient's condition has been stabilized and bleeding controlled, attention should be redirected to the patient's general state. If the bleeding was significant, the blood cell count should be checked and the patient transfused as needed with ample additional units available. Coagulopathies and hypertension should be addressed and reversed, and other factors that may aggravate bleeding should be corrected. Adequate pain control should be provided.

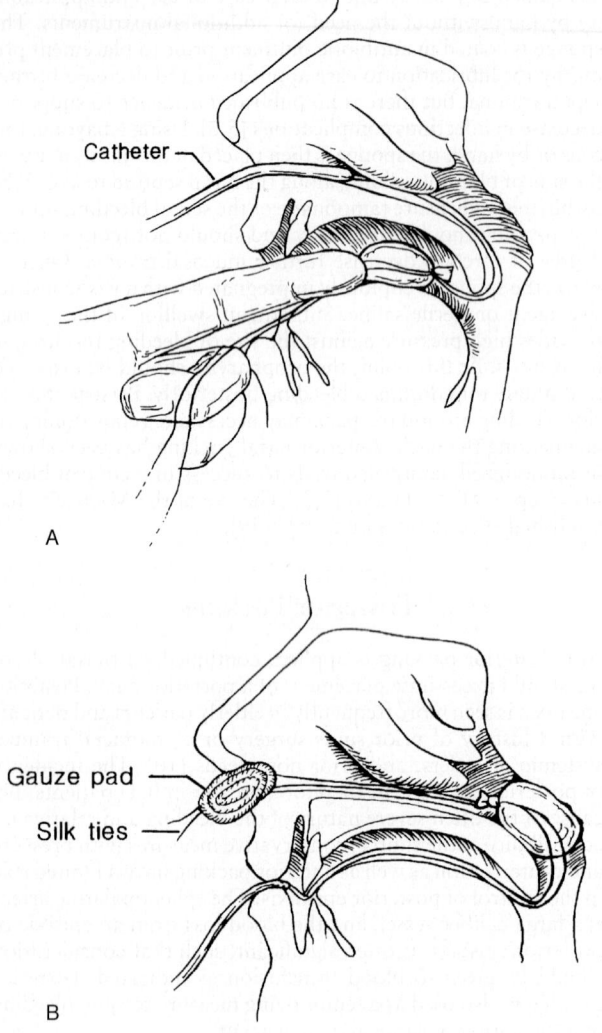

In general, packing is left in place for 3 to 5 days to permit the patient's condition to stabilize and adequate primary healing of the source of bleeding. The decision of when to remove packing in an ICU patient is also influenced by the patient's comorbidities, which should be aggressively controlled/minimized. Antibiotics with adequate *S. Aureus* coverage (e.g., cephalexin, clindamycin if penicillin allergy) should be used while nasal packing is in place to decrease the bacterial load that accumulates on the packing and prevent a life-threatening toxic shock syndrome. If antibiotic-impregnated gauze packing is used, the incidence of clinically significant secondary infections is quite low, and antibiotics may not be needed in immunocompetent, stable patients [12]. It is also important to minimize the amount of time that packing is used in immunocompromised individuals because of their increased susceptibility for infections.

If a posterior nasal pack is used, utilizing a balloon in the choanae, it should be slowly deflated prior to removal. If bleeding recurs, the balloon can be reinflated and left in place longer. If repeated attempts at removing nasal packing are unsuccessful, arterial ligation or embolization must be considered. Endoscopic-guided cauterization may be effective in controlling persistent localized bleeding [15].

ARTERIAL LIGATION

If nasal packing fails to achieve control of bleeding, or if the patient has had multiple episodes of epistaxis, arterial ligation may be warranted. In an extreme situation in which a patient is having life-threatening epistaxis, ligation of the external carotid artery decreases the nasal blood flow and can be life saving but does not result in long-term control of bleeding [16]. If the bleeding is localized to the anterior/superior nasal cavity, consideration should be given to ligation of the ethmoidal arteries. Most often, the bleeding is diffuse, and the ethmoidal arteries are ligated together with the sphenopalatine artery.

Angiographic arterial embolization of the ethmoidal arteries is not advised due to the risk of blindness and stroke, and they must therefore be ligated surgically, which drastically reduces these risks [17]. The ethmoidal arteries are approached through the external ethmoidectomy ("Lynch") incision made halfway between the medial canthus and the nasal dorsum. The vessels are identified along the frontoethmoid suture line as they leave the orbit and enter the ethmoid sinus. Once identified, the arteries are ligated with clips or suture [18]. The relationship of these vessels to the lacrimal crest and optic nerve is critical because the posterior ethmoidal artery lies just a few millimeters from the optic nerve, and severe iatrogenic complications can result if the anatomy is not respected.

Ligation of the sphenopalatine artery in the treatment of posterior epistaxis may be performed using an open or endoscopic approach. However, endoscopic techniques are being performed with greater frequency due to its equal efficacy and decreased morbidity when compared to the open Caldwell-Luc procedure. It has even been shown to have a role in treating patients with severe epistaxis and coagulopathies [19]. Transnasal endoscopic sphenopalatine artery ligation (TESPAL) is performed under general or local anesthesia using a nasal endoscope to identify the sphenopalatine artery and its branches at the sphenopalatine foramen. Endonasally, an incision is made with a sickle knife just anterior to the crista ethmoidalis under the middle turbinate, and a mucoperiosteal flap is raised. As the crista ethmoidalis is encountered, the vessels are identified leaving the sphenopalatine foramen posteriorly, and vascular clips and/or cautery are applied under direct vision. Complications include palatal numbness, sinusitis, decreased lacrimation, and septal perforation; however, control rates are reported up to 87% to 100% [20,21].

The traditional open approach involves clipping the internal maxillary artery (prior to the SPA) in the pterygopalatine foramen through the maxillary antrum. A Caldwell-Luc approach is undertaken (intraoral sublabial incision for access to the anterior face of the maxillary sinus), and the anterior wall of the maxillary sinus is partially removed. The posterior wall of the sinus is then breached and the pterygopalatine fossa entered. The internal maxillary artery and its branches are identified and locking clips placed. The vessels themselves are not transected. Complications of this procedure include facial and buccal numbness and discomfort (from potential infraorbital nerve transection), sinusitis, oroantral fistula, and chronic pain. Failures can occur in up to 40% of cases due to difficulty in identifying the internal maxillary artery, incomplete vessel ligation, formation of anastomoses distal to the ligation (e.g., in the descending palatine artery), and persistent hypertension [14].

After the arteries are ligated, any nasal packing is removed and the nasal cavity is examined for persistent bleeding. If bleeding is present, endoscopic cauterization should be attempted, as well as further medical evaluation for an uncorrected coagulopathy.

ARTERIAL EMBOLIZATION

Selective angiography with embolization of source vessels has compared well in the literature with other invasive techniques for management of refractory epistaxis, with success rates reported from 80% to 90% [20,22]. It may be performed prior to or after surgical management in the event of failure, and presents a treatment option for patients who are very poor operative candidates. However, the procedure is dependent on the availability of an experienced interventional neuroradiologist. As noted earlier, embolization cannot be performed for epistaxis in the superior nasal cavity in the region supplied by the ethmoidal arteries, as these vessels arise from the ICA and ligation could have devastating consequences including blindness or stroke. The internal maxillary artery, however, arises from the ECA, and embolization is a viable option. The procedure is performed using a single femoral puncture, usually under local anesthesia. After diagnostic carotid angiography is performed, the catheter is advanced into the IMA, and embolization is performed with Gelfoam®, coils, or polyvinyl alcohol particles. Often the vessels are embolized bilaterally to decrease the likelihood of development of collateral circulation and re-bleeding, reported in 10% to 20% of cases. Complications are similar to those for any cerebral angiography and include stroke (reported in up to 4% of cases), blindness, temporofacial pain, and renal abnormalities due to contrast loads.

SURGERY, EMBOLIZATION, OR PACKING?

Data remains controversial regarding which is the superior treatment modality for epistaxis: arterial ligation or embolization, both of which are employed when local cautery or nasal packing has failed. Patients with bleeding from the ethmoidal artery region (anterior epistaxis) are better served by surgery due to the risks associated with embolization of the internal carotid artery system. However, bleeding from the SPA/IMA region (posterior epistaxis) may be treated by either or both modalities.

Although both approaches have been shown to control bleeding in up to 85% of patients [23–25], multiple case series reports have found surgical arterial ligation to be equal to or better than embolization in terms of success rate [20,22]. Patients not stable enough to tolerate general anesthesia may benefit from embolization, which does not require general anesthetic but does expose the patient to the risks of angiography. Skilled personnel are required for either technique. Goddard and Reiter showed that there were no differences in length of

TABLE 146.2

SUMMARY OF EVIDENCE-BASED TREATMENT RECOMMENDATIONS IN THE MANAGEMENT OF EPISTAXIS

Intervention	Year	Study	No. of patients	Findings	Reference
A. Medical/nonsurgical management					
Hold warfarin (if applicable)	1997	Prospective	20	No decrease in bleeding or effect on hospital stay	Srinivasan, et al. [41]
Oral ice pack placement	1991	Prospective	16	Decreased nasal mucosal blood flow	Porter, et al. [42]
Intranasal topical antiseptic	1999	RCT	22	Topical is equal to silver nitrate cautery in control	Murthy, et al. [43]
Intranasal topical lubricant + steroid	1999	Prospective	100	Resolution of symptoms in 89% of chronic bleeds	London, et al. [44]
Oxymetazoline as initial therapy	1995	Retrospective	60	Effective as sole therapy in 65% of patients	Krempl, et al. [4]
Oxymetazoline for posterior epistaxis	1999	Retrospective	36	All cases resolved with initial or repeat doses only	Doo, et al. [45]
Iodoform gauze pack versus Merocel	1995	RCT	50	No significant difference in controlling epistaxis, Merocel more comfortable and easier to insert	Corbridge, et al. [46]
Merocel as initial therapy	1996	Retrospective	83	Effective in controlling epistaxis in 91.5% alone	Pringle, et al. [9]
B. Surgical management					
Endoscopic electrocautery for posterior epistaxis	2005	Prospective	43	Effective localization of source and control	Thornton, et al. [47]
TESPAL for control of refractory bleed	2003	Retrospective	127	98% control rate with no further therapy	Kumar, et al. [20]
TESPAL versus packing for recurrent epistaxis	2006	RCT	19	TESPAL superior for control, comfort, hospital stay and cost	Moshaver, et al. [28]
TESPAL +/− ant. ethmoid ligation for refractory bleeding	2000	Retrospective	287	TESPAL +/− ant. Ethmoid ligation equally effective as conventional measures, but improved cost and shorter stay	Srinivasan, et al. [17]
Embolization for refractory epistaxis	2008	Retrospective	70	Effective for control but increased cost	Christensen, et al. [48]
IMA ligation versus embolization for refractory posterior epistaxis	1998	Retrospective	39	IMA ligation more effective, but increased minor complications	Cullen, et al. [22]
Surgery versus packing versus embolization for posterior epistaxis	2002	Retrospective	203	Both surgery and embolization more effective for control; Surgery decreases hospital stay and cost	Klotz, et al. [26]

IMA, internal maxillary artery; TESPAL, transnasal endoscopic sphenopalatine artery ligation; RCT, Randomized Control Trial.

stay, transfusions, complications, or deaths between packing, embolization, and surgery, but the study did show a significant decrease in hospital charges in the packing group as compared to the embolization and surgery groups. However, Klotz et al. showed that early intervention with invasive measures results in a shorter hospital course, improved control of bleeding, decreased discomfort as associated with packing, and ultimately *less* cost [26,27]. In a randomized, prospective trial, Moshaver et al. further added support to early surgical intervention, demonstrating that health care costs were decreased by more than 50% and earlier hospital discharge was facilitated when posterior epistaxis was treated with temporizing packing followed by early TESPAL [28].

In the ICU setting in a patient population with multiple comorbidities, it is often the overall stability of the patient, ability to tolerate general anesthesia (for surgical intervention), or ability to tolerate angiography (e.g., no history of severe atherosclerosis, ability to lay flat, adequate renal functio) that dictates the most appropriate course of care for a patient with severe epistaxis. An in-depth knowledge of the treatment modalities available is critical to the clinician responsible for the direction of therapy (Table 146.2).

References

1. Viehweg TL, Roberson JB, Hudson JW: Epistaxis: diagnosis and treatment. *J Oral Maxillofac Surg* 64:511–518, 2006.
2. Douglas R, Wormald PJ: Update on epistaxis. *Curr Opin Otolaryngol Head Neck Surg* 15:180–183, 2007.
3. Awan MS, Iqbal M, Imam SZ: Epistaxis: when are coagulation studies justified? *Emerg Med J* 25:156–157, 2008.
4. Krempl GA, Noorily AD: Use of oxymetazoline in the management of epistaxis. *Ann Otol Rhinol Laryngol* 104:704–706, 1995.
5. Schlosser RJ: Epistaxis. *N Engl J Med* 360(8):784–789, 2009.
6. Jacobson JA, Kasworm EM: Toxic shock syndrome after nasal surgery: case reports and analysis of risk factors. *Arch Otolaryngol Head Neck Surg* 112:329–332, 1986.

7. Badran K, Malik TH, Belloso A, et al: Randomized controlled trial comparing Merocel and RapidRhino packing in the management of anterior epistaxis. *Clin Otolaryngol* 30(4):333–337, 2005.
8. Mathiasen RA, Cruz RM: Prospective, randomized, controlled clinical trial of a novel matrix hemostatic sealant in patients with acute anterior epistaxis. *Laryngoscope* 115:899–902, 2005.
9. Pringle MB, Beasley P, Brightwell AP: The use of Merocel nasal packs in the treatment of epistaxis. *J Laryngol Otol* 110:543, 1996.
10. Viducich RA, Blanda MP, Gerson LW: Posterior epistaxis: clinical features and acute complications. *Ann Emerg Med* 25:592, 1995.
11. Loftus BC, Blitzer A, Cozine K: Epistaxis, medical history, and the nasopulmonary reflex: what is clinically relevant? *Otolaryngol Head Neck Surg* 110:363, 1994.
12. Derkay CS, Hirsch BE, Johnson JT, et al: Posterior nasal packing. Are intravenous antibiotics really necessary? *Arch Otolaryngol Head Neck Surg* 115:439, 1989.
13. Viducich RA, Blanda MP, Gerson LW: Posterior epistaxis: clinical features and acute complications. *Ann Emerg Med* 25:592–596, 1995.
14. Gifford TO, Orlandi RR: Epistaxis. *Otolaryngol Clin North Am* 41:525–536, 2008.
15. Elwany S, Abdel-Fatah H: Endoscopic control of posterior epistaxis. *J Laryngol Otol* 110:432, 1996.
16. Waldron J, Stafford N: Ligation of the external carotid artery for severe epistaxis. *J Otolaryngol* 21:249, 1992.
17. Srinivasan V, Sherman IW, O'Sullivan G: Surgical management of intractable epistaxis: audit of results. *J Laryngol Otol* 114:697–700, 2000.
18. Kirchner JA, Yanagisawa E, Crelin ES Jr: Surgical anatomy of the ethmoidal arteries. *Arch Otolaryngol* 74:382, 1961.
19. Shah AG, Stachler RJ, Krouse JH: Endoscopic ligation of the sphenopalatine artery as a primary management of severe posterior epistaxis in patients with coagulopathy. *Ear Nose Throat* 84(5):296, 2005.
20. Kumar S, Shetty A, Rockey J, et al: Contemporary surgical treatment of epistaxis: what is the evidence for sphenopalatine artery ligation? *Clin Otolaryngol* 28:360–363, 2003.
21. Coel MN, Janon EA: Angiography in patients with intractable epistaxis. *Am J Roentgenol Radium Ther Nucl Med* 116:37, 1972.
22. Cullen MM, Tami TA: Comparison of internal maxillary artery ligation versus embolization for refractory posterior epistaxis. *Otolaryngol Head Neck Surg* 118:636–642, 1998.
23. Strong EB, Bell DA, Johnson LP, et al: Intractable epistaxis: transnasal ligation vs. embolization: efficacy review and cost analysis. *Otolaryngol Head Neck Surg* 113:674, 1995.
24. Spafford P, Durham JS: Epistaxis: efficacy of arterial ligation and long-term outcome. *J Otolaryngol* 21:252, 1992.
25. Elden L, Montanera W, Terbrugge K, et al: Angiographic embolization for the treatment of epistaxis: a review of 108 cases. *Otolaryngol Head Neck Surg* 111:44, 1994.
26. Klotz DA, Winkle MR, Richmon J, et al: Surgical management of posterior epistaxis: a changing paradigm. *Laryngoscope* 112:1577–1582, 2002.
27. Goddard JC, Reiter ER: Inpatient management of epistaxis: outcomes and cost. *Otolaryngol Head Neck Surg* 132(5):707, 2005.
28. Moshaver A, Harris JR, Liu R, et al: Early operative intervention versus conventional treatment in epistaxis: randomized prospective trial. *J Otolaryngol* 33:185–188, 2004.
29. Ogura JH, Unno T, Nelson JR: Baseline values in pulmonary mechanics for physiologic surgery of the nose: preliminary report. *Ann Otol Rhinol Laryngol* 78:369, 1968.
30. Budrovich R, Saetti R: Microscopic and endoscopic ligature of the sphenopalatine artery. *Laryngoscope* 102(12):1391–1394, 1992.
31. Elahi MM, Parnes LS, Fox AJ, et al: Therapeutic embolization in the treatment of intractable epistaxis. *Arch Otolaryngol Head Neck Surg* 121:65, 1995.
32. Andersen PJ, Kjeldsen AD, Nepper-Rasmussen J: Selective embolization in the treatment of intractable epistaxis. *Acta Otolaryngol* 125(3):293, 2005.
33. Metson R, Lane R: Internal maxillary artery ligation for epistaxis: an analysis of failures. *Laryngoscope* 98:760, 1988.
34. Pearson BW, MacKenzie RG, Goodman WS: The anatomical basis of transnasal ligation of the maxillary artery in severe epistaxis. *Laryngoscope* 79:969, 1969.
35. Durr DG: Endoscopic electrosurgical management of posterior epistaxis: shifting paradigm. *J Otolaryngol* 33(4):211, 2004.
36. McGarry GW, Aitken D: Intranasal balloon catheters: how do they work? *Clin Otolaryngol* 16:388, 1991.
37. Taylor MT: Avitene—its value in the control of anterior epistaxis. *J Otolaryngol* 9:468, 1980.
38. Wurtele P: How I do it: emergency nasal packing using an umbilical cord clamp to secure a Foley catheter for posterior epistaxis. *J Otolaryngol* 25:46, 1996.
39. O'Leary-Stickney K, Makielski K, Weymuller EA Jr: Rigid endoscopy for the control of epistaxis. *Arch Otolaryngol Head Neck Surg* 118:966, 1992.
40. Massick D, Tobin E: Epistaxis, in Haughey BH, Thomas JR (eds): *Cummings Otolaryngology—Head and Neck Surgery.* Philadelphia, Elsevier-Mosby, 942–961, 2005.
41. Srinivasan V, Patel H, John DG, et al: Warfarin and epistaxis: should warfarin always be discontinued? *Clin Otolaryngol* 22:542–544, 1997.
42. Porter M, Marais J, Tolly N: The effect of ice packs upon nasal mucosal blood flow. *Acta Otolaryngol* 111(6):1122–1125, 1991.
43. Murthy P, Nilssen EL, Roa S, et al: A randomised clinical trial of antiseptic nasal carrier cream and silver nitrate cautery in the treatment of recurrent anterior epistaxis. *Clin Otolaryngol Allied Sci* 24(3):228–231, 1999.
44. London SD, Lindsey WH: A reliable medical treatment for recurrent mild anterior epistaxis. *Laryngoscope* 109(9):1535–1537, 1999.
45. Doo G, Johnson DS: "Oxymetazoline in the treatment of posterior epistaxis." *Hawaii Med J* 58(8):210–212, 1999.
46. Corbridge RJ, Djazaeri B, Hellier WPL, et al: A prospective randomized controlled trial comparing the use of Merocel nasal tampons and BIPP in the control of acute epistaxis. *Clin Otolaryngol* 20:305–307, 1995.
47. Thornton MA, Mahesh BN, Lang J: Posterior epistaxis: identification of common bleeding sites. *Laryngoscope* 115:588–590, 2005.
48. Christensen NP, Smith DS, Barnwell SL, et al: Arterial embolization in the management of posterior epistaxis. *Otolaryngol Head Neck Surg* 133(5): 748–753, 2005.

CHAPTER 147 ■ ESOPHAGEAL PERFORATION AND ACUTE MEDIASTINITIS

JASON W. SMITH, CHRISTOPHER H. WIGFIELD AND ROBERT B. LOVE

ESOPHAGEAL PERFORATION

Introduction

Esophageal perforation is both a highly lethal disease and primarily a surgical problem, and has remained such since nearly 4,000 BC as documented in the Edwin Smith Papyrus. Boerhaave then recorded his classical description of spontaneous rupture of the esophagus in 1724 [1]. Recently, there has been a shift in the etiology of esophageal perforation such that iatrogenic injury from instrumentation is the most common cause of esophageal perforation accounting for 40% of cases, while trauma represents 20%, spontaneous rupture (Boerhaave's) 15%, and tumor, foreign bodies, and operative injury collectively represent the remaining 25% of cases, leaving the two

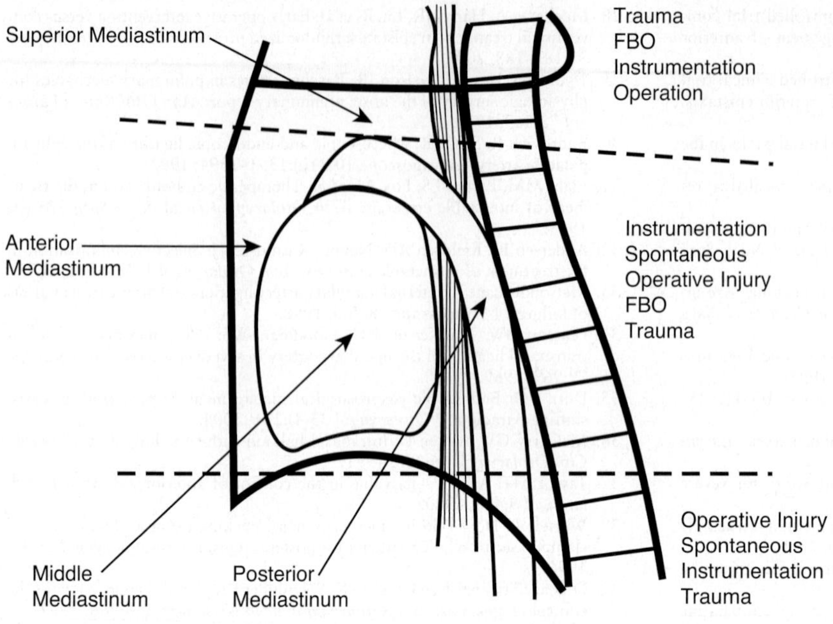

FIGURE 147.1. Zones of the mediastinum: these are identified on the left-hand side of the diagram. The superior mediastinum contains the thymic remnants, brachiocephalic veins, superior vena cava, aortic arch, trachea, phrenic nerve, vagus nerve, and the left recurrent laryngeal nerve. The anterior mediastinum contains primarily adipose and lymphatic tissue. The middle mediastinum is composed of the heart, pericardium, pulmonary trunk, aortic root, phrenic nerve, and tracheal bifurcation. The posterior mediastinum holds the descending thoracic aorta, azygos vein, esophagus, sympathetic chains, splanchnic nerves, and the thoracic duct. The right side of the diagram depicts each region of the esophagus, cervical, thoracic, and abdominal, and the injuries that occur there in decreasing order.

most common causes in the modern era as endoscopy related injury and anastomotic leakage [2]. The mortality associated with perforation of the esophagus remains high despite the most modern surgical and medical care, and ranges from 10% for early diagnosis to 75% for cases with late presentation.

Esophageal Anatomy

The esophagus is a muscular tube that extends from the pharynx to the stomach and is between 23 and 27 cm in length. It has three anatomic narrowings at the upper esophageal sphincter, at the level of the aortic arch and crossing of the left mainstem bronchus, and at the lower esophageal sphincter. The wall of the esophagus is comprised of the outer longitudinal muscle and the thicker inner layer of circular muscle. The innermost layer is the epithelial mucosa of the esophagus. The blood supply to the esophagus in the cervical region is primarily derived from the inferior thyroid artery. The thoracic esophagus receives its primary blood supply from the bronchial arteries and also receives branches directly from the descending thoracic aorta. The left gastric artery and the inferior phrenic arteries supply the abdominal portion of the esophagus. These arteries form a rich submucosal network of anastomoses that permit extensive mobilization and resection without fear of devascularization. The innervation of the esophagus is primarily from the vagus. Injury to the recurrent laryngeal branch of the vagus is well known for resulting in vocal cord paralysis, but less well known is the fact that significant functional impairment also occurs in the cricopharyngeal constrictor and motility of the cervical esophagus, contributing to the risk of aspiration after such an injury.

Pathophysiology

The most common locations for perforation of the esophagus to occur are at the narrowest portions of the organ but they can and do occur at any point. The absolute narrowest area in most people is at the cricopharyngeus muscle at the level of C5–C6, which corresponds to the upper esophageal sphincter (UES). This represents the portion of the esophagus most often injured during endoscopy and the risk is increased with hyperextension of the neck and in patients with bone spurs on the anterior surface of the vertebral bodies secondary to the presence of minimal tissue in the posterior cervical compartment between the posterior wall of the esophagus and the spine. The incidence of perforation during flexible endoscopy is about 0.03%; this is markedly improved over the era of routine rigid endoscopy which carried a much higher incidence of injury in the 0.11% range. Other iatrogenic causes of injury at the UES is transesophageal echocardiography performed during cardiac surgery and has a slightly higher incidence at 0.18% and other manipulations of the hypopharynx as in endotracheal intubation or nasogastric tube placement (Fig. 147.1).

The next narrow portion is at the level of the aortic arch and left mainstem bronchus and this is a common site for foreign body obstruction and ultimate perforation. Fish and chicken bones are the most common offenders in adults, while children tend to have a much wider variety of culprit objects such as safety pins, parts of toys, plastic elements. In the elderly, oral hardware such as dentures account for the majority of ingested items.

The gastroesophageal junction (GEJ) is the third region of narrowing and is most often perforated iatrogenically during dilations of the distal esophagus for achalasia or distal esophageal strictures. Perforation also results from biopsies in this area during evaluations for metaplasia. The GEJ is the most severely injured area of the esophagus in patients with accidental or intentional ingestion of chemical substances. The relaxation of the LES in response to injury along with intense pylorospasm results in continued reflux of caustic substances into the distal esophagus. This prolongs contact with the mucosa resulting in more severe injuries. Alkaline substances tend to create a more severe injury to the esophagus due to the liquefactive necrosis and the slow transit time, while acids tend to move more quickly through the esophagus and create a coagulative necrosis limiting the depth of injury.

Spontaneous perforation of the esophagus (Boerhaave's) is most commonly discovered in the distal left posterior lateral aspect about 2 to 3 cm from the GEJ. This area has a less developed muscular layer to accommodate the exit of neurovascular structures and tapering of the muscle as to spread out onto the stomach wall, allowing the increased pressure during retching to result in rupture into the left chest. The cervical esophagus is much more vulnerable to external trauma than

TABLE 147.1

CAUSES OF ESOPHAGEAL PERFORATION

Spontaneous (Boerhaave's syndrome)
Iatrogenic
Endoscopy (esp. with sclerotherapy or biopsy)
Dilation with bougie or balloon
Naso/orogastric tubes
Endotracheal intubation
Operative injury
Trauma
Caustic ingestion
Infections (tuberculosis, herpes simplex, CMV)
Malignancy
Zollinger–Ellison syndrome

Note: The percentages of each etiologies will vary depending on the location of the perforation and time period studied.
CMV, cytomegalovirus.

the thoracic esophagus and up to 6% of penetrating injuries to the neck may have a concomitant esophageal perforation, whereas only 0.7% of penetrating thoracic injuries result in an injury to the esophagus. Blunt traumatic injury to the esophagus is extremely rare and is almost always located in the cervical esophagus (Table 147.1).

Presentation

Delay in diagnosing an injury to the esophagus is the most important determinant of mortality in this disease and thus a high index of suspicion should be maintained whenever injury to the esophagus is a possibility in a differential diagnosis. Perforation of the esophagus leads to contamination of the surrounding tissues in the neck, mediastinum, or abdomen and localized sepsis due to the degree of aerobic and anaerobic bacterial contamination. Chief complaints are therefore related to the effects of local tissue inflammation and the systemic inflammatory response. The most common presenting symptom in patients with esophageal perforation is pain followed by other common signs including fever, dyspnea, and subcutaneous emphysema, which may extend into the head and neck. Auscultation of the heart tones may reveal a crunching sound that is related to air in the mediastinum and is a classic sign of esophageal perforation. Pain resulting from esophageal perforation is dependent on the location. A cervical perforation tends to cause less pain and more vague symptoms of neck stiffness, headache, and backache. Symptoms with more distal perforation in the thoracic esophagus tend to be substernal and can lateralize to the side of perforation with proximal esophageal perforations tending to be on the right side and more distal perforations on the left side. This must be differentiated from acute coronary syndromes and should be considered in patients with severe chest pain after an acute myocardial infarction has been eliminated as the etiology.

Presenting signs of perforation may be subtle and nonspecific in the early phase with tachycardia being the most well recognized, and persistent tachycardia in a patient who has undergone an endoscopic evaluation or a surgical procedure involving the esophagus should warrant an evaluation for rupture. As the course progresses, these patients rapidly develop systemic sepsis with hypotension and tachycardia, tachypnea and worsening respiratory distress, renal failure, and mental status alterations. Failure to recognize septic shock and intervene early in this patient population may lead to death within 12 to 24 hours.

Diagnostic Evaluation

A chest radiograph is often one of the first tests obtained in patients with pain in the chest or neck. The presence of a pleural effusion, pneumothorax, or pneumomediastinum, in the setting of a suspicious history, is highly suggestive of an esophageal perforation. A contrast esophagram, however, is the gold standard for diagnosis of perforation. It has a high sensitivity and specificity and is relatively easy to obtain in any facility. Following an initial evaluation with water-soluble contrast, a barium contrast study should be done to rule out a leak. The false negative rate for esophageal perforation utilizing water-soluble contrast is 20% to 25%, even when digital subtraction imaging techniques are used [3,4]. Therefore, a negative study with water-soluble contrast does not complete the evaluation [5]. Concern over the inflammatory reaction associated with barium extravasation in the setting of bacterial contamination is warranted if an intra-abdominal perforation is suspected and the patient is presenting with peritonitis [6]. Such a response has not been demonstrated in the mediastinum and barium should be used to increase the sensitivity of the imaging [7]. Patients who cannot perform a swallowing test or are in extremis are most often imaged with computed tomography with oral contrast administered by nasogastric tube, which must be positioned in the proximal esophagus to provide diagnostic value. The key finding on a computed tomography (CT) scan for diagnosing a perforation is an extraluminal collection of gas or subcutaneous emphysema. Periesophageal fluid collections with air-fluid interfaces, esophageal wall thickening effacement of fat planes, extravasation of oral contrast and pleural effusions are other radiographic findings consistent with a perforation. Computed tomography is also useful in the evaluation for abscess or empyema formation with a long-standing leak [8–11] (Fig. 147.2).

The role of esophagoscopy in the diagnosis of esophageal perforation has been established in the setting of traumatic injuries with a high sensitivity for detecting injury [12–14]. In non-traumatic settings, the sensitivity has not been established and the use of endoscopy remains as an adjunct to imaging modalities. This may be related to the difficulty in locating sites of perforation in the esophageal mucosa when there are no attendant signs of trauma [15].

Treatment

There is a paucity of reliable data regarding the treatment of esophageal perforation. This is partly a result of the fact that patients present with a wide variety of symptoms, differing severity of injury and are treated by several different specialties. Several principles in the management of esophageal perforation are paramount: control of ongoing soilage by closure of the leak, management of sepsis with adequate drainage and support of the patient with fluids, nutrition, and appropriate antibiotics.

After goal-directed resuscitation and initiation of broad-spectrum antibiotic therapy, the treatment of choice for most patients with perforations of the esophagus remains surgical. For early perforations less than 24 hours in hemodynamically stable patients, consideration may be given to direct primary repair of the injury. This is generally possible in cases where there is a small injury with little soilage or devitalized tissue in a surgically accessible location and early detection has been achieved. Access to the cervical esophagus is generally obtained through an anterior neck incision along the anterior border of the left sternocleidomastoid muscle. The carotid sheath and its contents are retracted laterally and the thyroid and trachea retracted medially to expose the esophagus. In the mediastinum,

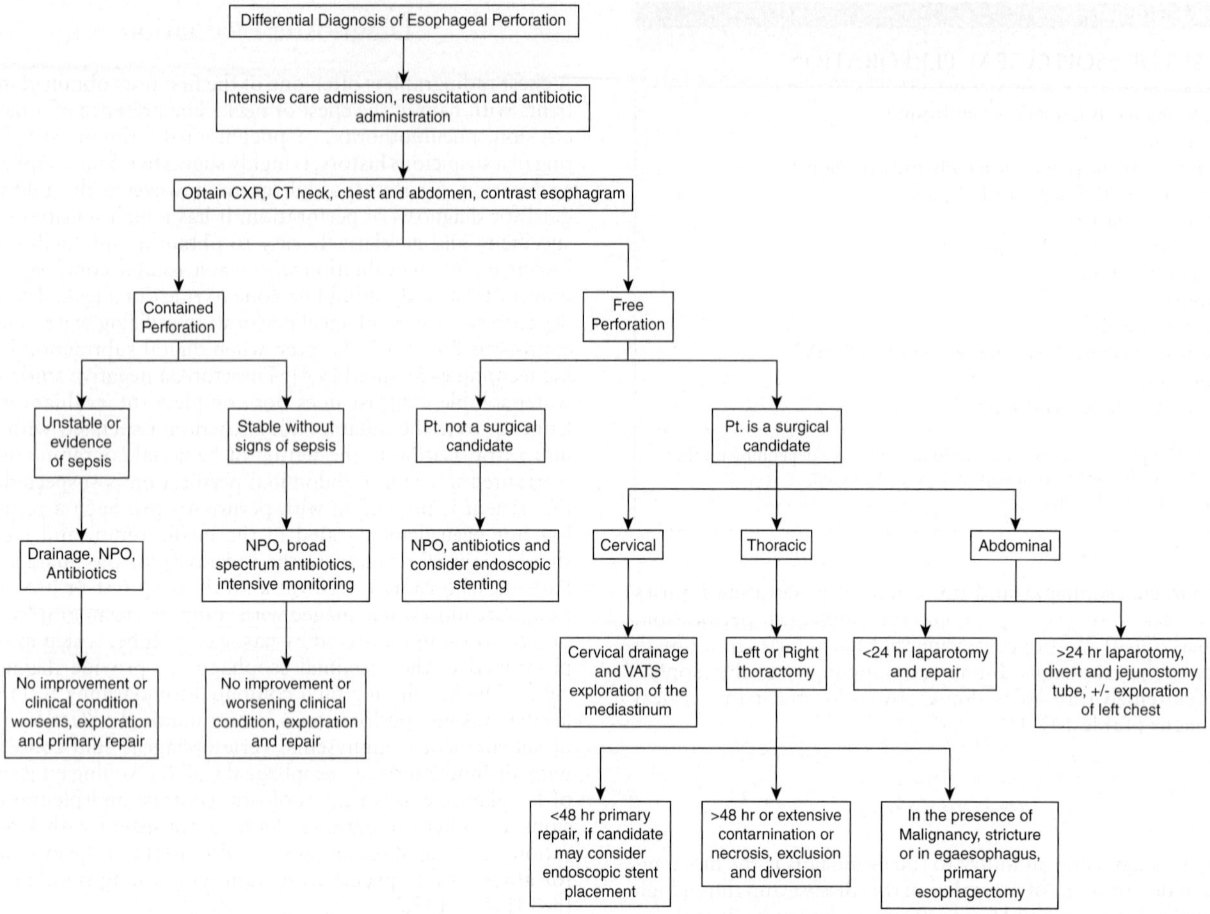

FIGURE 147.2. Algorithm for the diagnosis and management of a perforation of the esophagus. Early diagnosis followed by resuscitation and surgical consultation are the keys to decreasing the mortality from this highly lethal condition.

a right posterolateral thoracotomy is used to access lesions in the middle third of the esophagus and a left posterolateral thoracotomy provides exposure for the distal third of the thoracic esophagus. Upper midline laparotomy or left thoracotomy may be used to access the gastroesophageal junction. If amenable to repair, the esophagus is usually closed with a single layer of interrupted full thickness sutures and the anastomosis is reinforced with a well-vascularized local tissue flap from the latissimus dorsi muscle, pericardium, or omentum.

In cases where the diagnosis has been delayed for more than 24 hours, there is extensive tissue injury, or intense local sepsis, primary repair is ill-advised. In this situation, it is prudent to perform a resection of the esophagus or proximal diversion with a cervical esophagostomy and exclusion of the injured esophagus with creation of enteral feeding access. After the resolution of sepsis and once the patient is nutritionally repleted, reestablishment of intestinal continuity can be achieved with a gastric pull-up or intestinal interposition techniques. If there is a coexisting underlying esophageal pathology such as megaesophagus, achalasia, esophageal stricture, or carcinoma, esophagectomy with or without reconstruction is the operation of choice. In patients who cannot tolerate a definitive repair, surgical management should be limited to placement of an esophageal T-tube for drainage and creation of a controlled esophageal fistula.

Patients who have a small contained perforation, stable vital signs and no ongoing sepsis may be candidates for nonoperative management. This includes radiographic demonstration that ongoing soilage is absent and drainage of intrathoracic fluid collections is amenable to interventional radiology or by the placement of thoracostomy tubes. These patients should also be placed on a substantial course of culture directed antibiotic therapy, and be started on parenteral nutrition with complete rest of the upper gastrointestinal tract.

Given the high mortality associated with surgical repair of esophageal perforations, it is not surprising that innovation continues in this complex disease process. The development of even more advanced endoscopic therapeutic modalities has provided some new options in the management of these patients, including endoscopic closure and stenting. There are several small series which have been published recently that suggest that endoscopic stenting of spontaneous or iatrogenic esophageal perforations can be effective as initial or definitive therapy [16]. There is experimental evidence demonstrating the efficacy of endoluminal closure devices for management of esophageal perforation. There appears to be a faster rate of healing and return to normal function with the use of clipping devices over endoluminal suturing techniques [17]. Clinical evidence is limited to case reports and series, but does appear feasible. Although there is a clear selection bias favoring patients with less severe disease and more favorable prognosis, it is appealing to consider a therapy with a much less invasive approach and potentially less severe dysregulation of systemic inflammation. The other major endoluminal therapy in use is the esophageal stent. Endoscopically placed occlusive stents have been used to close perforations and quickly restore intestinal continuity with good effect. A recent series reported that 23 patients were treated with endoluminal stents and they had no resultant mortality and only 10% went on to require surgical intervention [16]. This may represent a new paradigm in the management of this disease process that will have a less profound effect on the counter regulatory cytokine response and immune function.

Follow-up

In addition to the operative mortality, there is a high risk of anastomotic complications after repair of esophageal perforations approaching 40% to 50%. This includes stricture and disruption of the esophageal anastomosis [18]. In the immediate postoperative period, these patients should remain in the intensive care setting or in a specialized surgical unit where early signs of anastomotic complications can be identified and addressed in a timely fashion. Thoracostomy tubes are generally left in place until the first feeding to identify an early anastomotic dehiscence. Once the patient is discharged from the hospital, the most important chronic problem is stricture of the anastomosis and complaints of dysphagia should prompt a contrast imaging study of the esophagus.

MEDIASTINITIS

Introduction

Since the time of Boerhaave, physicians have recognized mediastinitis as a highly lethal disease for which treatments have only been developed in the very recent past [1]. The incidence of mediastinitis after coronary artery bypass grafting (CABG) ranges from 0.5% to 1.25% and carries an in-hospital mortality up to 14% compared to 1.1% in CABG patients who do not develop sternal wound infections [19,20]. Mediastinitis is also associated with a significant increase in long-term mortality after coronary artery bypass grafting with patients survival at 1 year dropping from 95% to 78% [19]. We now recognize a number of causes of mediastinitis in addition to the original description of spontaneous esophageal rupture. These include the acute causes of mediastinitis, iatrogenic perforation of the esophagus, post-sternotomy, head and neck infections, pulmonary infection, abdominal infections, chest wall osteomyelitis, or direct posttraumatic. Chronic causes of mediastinitis include granulomatous diseases, fibrotic diseases, autoimmune diseases, and drug reactions [21].

The mediastinum is divided into the superior and inferior regions, and the inferior mediastinum includes the anterior, middle, and posterior compartments [22]. The superior mediastinum is bounded by the pleura laterally, the thoracic inlet superiorly and inferiorly by a line extending from the sternal angle to the intervertebral disc between the fourth and fifth thoracic vertebral bodies. Structures contained in the superior mediastinum include the thymic remnants, brachiocephalic vein, superior vena cava, aortic arch and the branch vessels, the trachea and the phrenic, vagus and recurrent laryngeal nerves. The anterior mediastinum is defined by the posterior surface of the sternum and the anterior pericardium, the inferior margin of the superior mediastinum and the diaphragm. The anterior mediastinum is devoid of major anatomical structures and is primarily occupied by adipose, connective, and lymphatic tissue. The middle mediastinum consists of the heart and pericardium, the pulmonary trunk, phrenic nerves, and the distal trachea including the bifurcation into the right and left mainstem bronchi. The posterior mediastinum extends from the posterior surface of the pericardium to the spinal column. The major contents of this compartment are the descending aorta, azygos vein, esophagus, sympathetic chains, splanchnic nerves, thoracic duct, and lymphatics.

Acute Mediastinitis

The most common cause of acute mediastinitis is post sternotomy. The Centers for Disease Control and Prevention define mediastinitis as a deep sternal incisional surgical site infection [23]. The incidence of mediastinitis after sternotomy ranges from 0.4% to 5.0% in the literature with most series reporting 1% to 2%, and an associated mortality of 10% to 20% [19,24]. Risk factors associated with the development of a deep sternal wound infection can be divided into preoperative, intraoperative, and postoperative risks. Preoperative factors are male gender, presence of hypertension, chronic obstructive pulmonary disease, diabetes, obesity, large breast size, history of smoking, and older than 70 years [20,25–31]. Intraoperative variables include an extended cardiopulmonary bypass pump time, the use of autotransfused shed mediastinal blood, and harvest of both internal mammary arteries [32–34]. Postoperative risk factors include reexploration for bleeding, prolonged intubation, and tracheostomy [35–37]. Recognition of the importance of these predictors allows the intensivist to maintain a high index of suspicion in the immediate postoperative period for the development of this devastating complication (Table 147.2).

The next most common cause of acute mediastinitis is descending cervical infection generally from odontologic procedures or disease, tonsillitis, or pharyngitis. Infections of the head and neck region can reach the mediastinum by three primary pathways from the cervical fascial planes. The pretracheal, perivascular, and retropharyngeal spaces have all been implicated as routes for spread of descending infections to gain access through the thoracic inlet into the mediastinum [38]. Based on the report by Pearse in 1938, the retropharyngeal space was once thought to be the culprit in the majority (70%) of descending cervical infections, however, a small recent study suggests that the perivascular space may be more important and that the carotid sheath may need to be opened and drained in a majority of cases [39,40].

Presentation

Acute mediastinitis usually presents within the first 7 to 10 days after surgery with fever, leukocytosis, chest pain, dysphagia, or respiratory distress [41]. Other presenting symptoms

TABLE 147.2

RISK FACTORS FOR POSTOPERATIVE MEDIASTINITIS

Diabetes
COPD
Harvest of bilateral internal thoracic arteries
Tobacco use
Prolonged ventilation
Obesity
Advanced age
Renal failure
Prolonged bypass pump time
Extensive use of electrocautery
Bleeding requiring reexploration

COPD, chronic obstructive pulmonary disease.

include drainage or erythema in the sternal wound, presence of a sternal click or dehiscence of the sternum, and subcutaneous emphysema.

When the source of infection is the neck, the primary symptoms are neck and/or throat pain in the early phases followed by edema, dysphagia, and odynophagia which is generally easily recognized. Although fever and leukocytosis are relatively nonspecific findings, in the presence of chest pain in the postoperative period it should raise the suspicion for diagnosis. One must be alert to the possibility of acute airway obstruction in the case of descending infection secondary to airway edema or epiglottitis [42].

Diagnosis

The initial evaluation, especially in cases with respiratory compromise, usually includes a chest radiograph, which is often nondiagnostic, but may show alterations in the normal tissue planes with edema, fluid, or air [42]. Chest x-ray may demonstrate diffuse mediastinal widening or air-fluid interfaces in the mediastinum in advanced cases. With esophageal perforation pneumothorax, pneumomediastinum and pleural effusion are common findings.

Computed tomography imaging of the chest with both oral and intravenous contrast is generally the next study evaluating pathologic processes in the thorax and has the most utility in identifying major infections in the mediastinum. CT allows the easy evaluation of both the neck and the abdomen to assess the relationship of any fluid collections in the chest to other potential sources of infection. It also allows precise localization of the fluid collection and possible intervention in selected cases. CT is also an important element in the preoperative planning of surgical drainage procedures and should not be omitted in the work up of this highly lethal disease. In cases where esophageal perforation is suspected, a contrast esophagram with Gastrografin is indicated as discussed in the previous section.

The diagnosis of mediastinitis is defined by the Centers for Disease Control as an infection in a patient who has one of the following conditions: (i) organisms cultured from mediastinal tissue or fluid, obtained during a surgical operation or needle aspiration; (ii) evidence of mediastinitis seen during a surgical operation or histologic examination; (iii) a patient with fever, chest pain, or sternal instability with no cause and at least one of the following: (a) purulent discharge from mediastinal area, (b) organisms cultured from blood or discharge from mediastinal area, or (c) mediastinal widening on chest x-ray [43].

Treatment

The treatment of mediastinitis is directed toward the primary pathological process, but initial measures include the administration of broad-spectrum antibiotic therapy, fluid resuscitation, and surgical drainage for control of the source. Mediastinitis tends to be a polymicrobial infection, however, antimicrobial therapy can be directed toward likely organisms depending on the etiology of the infection. Cultures from patients with descending cervical mediastinitis secondary to an odontologic or oropharyngeal process are likely to grow Gram-negative aerobes and anaerobes, including anaerobic *Streptococcus* and *Bacteroides* species. Deep sternal wound infections in postoperative mediastinitis most often grow *Staphylococcus aureus*, aerobic *Streptococcus*, *Pseudomonas aeruginosa*, and *Enterococcus* spp. When the origin of the septic focus is within the chest wall, periosteum of the ribs, or pleural space, the infected tissues may harbor tuberculosis or fungi.

Patients with mediastinitis will often present late in the course of the disease due to the nonspecific and misleading nature of the early symptoms. Because of this they often have clinical signs of sepsis with significant third space fluid losses and vasodilatory shock. Volume resuscitation should be started early with emphasis on goal-directed resuscitation to restore hemodynamic parameters. Most of these patients will ultimately require surgical intervention and adequate cardiac preload is essential for successful anesthesia induction. Once volume expansion is adequate, consideration can be given to the addition of vasoactive agents to increase the systolic blood pressure if vasodilation is an element of the patient's presentation.

Surgical drainage is the standard definitive therapy in all forms of mediastinitis. Descending cervical infections will require the primary oral process to be addressed in addition to incision and drainage of the neck through either a vertical incision along the anterior border of the sternocleidomastoid muscle, and thoracotomy or thoracoscopy for mediastinal drainage and placement of thoracostomy tubes for continued chest drainage. Incisions in the neck should be allowed to heal by the secondary intention to prevent ongoing sources of infection. Occasionally, infections limited to the superior mediastinum may be adequately addressed by the cervical incision, however, these patients must be carefully selected to avoid leaving the patient with ongoing septic foci as nearly 50% of patients treated by the cervical approach alone go on to require thoracotomy for unrecognized mediastinal disease [44].

Poststernotomy mediastinitis requires an aggressive approach to reduce the morbidity and mortality associated with this complication. Exploration of the mediastinum by reopening the median sternotomy incision is the standard approach. All necrotic tissue and bone are widely debrided, and tissue is mobilized as a flap to fill the dead space left by the debridement. Reclosure of the sternum by direct rewiring has been reported to carry a mortality up to 45%, which is unacceptably high [45]. Tissue flaps may be created with various rotational techniques or omental harvest, but the most common is medialization of bilateral pectoralis major muscles as local flaps. Using omentum has the disadvantage of requiring a laparotomy and opening of an additional body cavity, but has the distinct advantage of being simple and performed quickly in the unstable patient. Vacuum closure of the mediastinum is gaining acceptance as an alternative to immediate flap closure. Reports indicate that mortality is comparable when used as definitive therapy or as a bridge to a delayed myocutaneous flap closure [46].

Chronic Mediastinitis

Granulomatous infections like histoplasmosis, syphilis, tuberculosis, and coccidiomycosis as well as noninfectious processes like sarcoidosis cause a subacute prolonged mediastinal inflammation called chronic mediastinitis. The primary pathologic process is one of diffuse fibrosis of the mediastinum. This may also result from prolonged acute mediastinitis. Risk factors for development of chronic mediastinitis include the presence of autoimmune diseases such as lupus erythematosus, rheumatoid arthritis, and Raynaud's phenomenon, or the presence of mediastinal foreign bodies. Symptoms are generally low grade and well tolerated in the early stages and include cough, dyspnea, wheezing, chest pain, or dysphagia. Compression or obstruction of major vascular structures such as the superior vena cava (SVC) may lead to SVC syndrome. Radiographic studies may demonstrate widening of the mediastinum resulting from diffuse fibrosis or calcifications of involved lymph nodes and granulomas. Contrast CT of the chest is particularly helpful in the evaluation of vascular compression but will also clarify the extent of the mediastinal involvement in the fibrotic process and evaluate the lung parenchyma and associated thoracic viscera. There is no single accepted or effective treatment for chronic mediastinitis. Antibiotics are indicated for documented bacterial or fungal infection, while chemotherapeutic regimens have had limited success in modulating the ongoing inflammatory process, and surgical therapy is generally limited to tissue biopsy for diagnosis. For vascular compression, endovascular stenting may have an increasing role in palliation of SVC syndrome.

Esophageal perforation and mediastinitis represent relatively rare disease processes that often present as acute life threatening illnesses. As such they are not particularly amenable to well designed randomized controlled trials in the evaluation of different therapeutic options. A review of the literature does not demonstrate any class I data related to therapies for the treatment of these diseases and such data is not likely to be forthcoming. Further advances are likely to continue to come from retrospective analysis of innovative approaches to these complex problems.

References

1. Derbes VJ, Mitchell RE Jr: Hermann Boerhaave's Atrocis, nec descripti prius, morbi historia, the first translation of the classic case report of rupture of the esophagus, with annotations. *Bull Med Libr Assoc* 43(2):217–240, 1955.
2. Amrani L, Menard C, Berdah S, et al: From iatrogenic digestive perforation to complete anastomotic disunion: endoscopic stenting as a new concept of "stent-guided regeneration and re-epithelialization." *Gastrointest Endosc* 69:1282–1287, 2009.
3. Foster JH, Jolly PC, Sawyers JL, et al: Esophageal perforation: diagnosis and treatment. *Ann Surg* 161:701–709, 1965.
4. Wychulis AR, Fontana RS, Payne WS: Instrumental perforations of the esophagus. *Dis Chest* 55:184–189, 1969.
5. Buecker A, Wein BB, Neuerburg JM, et al: Esophageal perforation: comparison of use of aqueous and barium-containing contrast media. *Radiology* 202:683–686, 1997.
6. Cochran DQ, Almond CH, Shucart WA: An experimental study of the effects of barium and intestinal contents on the peritoneal cavity. *Am J Roentgenol Radium Ther Nucl Med* 89:883–887, 1963.
7. Vessal K, Montali RJ, Larson SM, et al: Evaluation of barium and Gastrografin as contrast media for the diagnosis of esophageal ruptures or perforations. *Am J Roentgenol Radium Ther Nucl Med* 123:307–319, 1975.
8. Young CA, Menias CO, Bhalla S, et al: CT features of esophageal emergencies. *Radiographics* 28:1541–1553, 2008.
9. White CS, Templeton PA, Attar S: Esophageal perforation: CT findings. *AJR Am J Roentgenol* 160:767–770, 1993.
10. Backer CL, LoCicero J III, Hartz RS, et al: Computed tomography in patients with esophageal perforation. *Chest* 98:1078–1080, 1990.
11. Maher MM, Lucey BC, Boland G, et al: The role of interventional radiology in the treatment of mediastinal collections caused by esophageal anastomotic leaks. *AJR Am J Roentgenol* 178:649–653, 2002.
12. Horwitz B, Krevsky B, Buckman RF Jr, et al: Endoscopic evaluation of penetrating esophageal injuries. *Am J Gastroenterol* 88:1249–1253, 1993.
13. Arantes V, Campolina C, Valerio SH, et al: Flexible esophagoscopy as a diagnostic tool for traumatic esophageal injuries. *J Trauma* 66:1677–1682, 2009.
14. Dissanaike S, Shalhub S, Jurkovich GJ: The evaluation of pneumomediastinum in blunt trauma patients. *J Trauma* 65:1340–1345, 2008.
15. Pasricha PJ, Fleischer DE, Kalloo AN: Endoscopic perforations of the upper digestive tract: a review of their pathogenesis, prevention, and management. *Gastroenterology* 106:787–802, 1994.
16. Freeman RK, Van Woerkom JM, Vyverberg A, et al: Esophageal stent placement for the treatment of spontaneous esophageal perforations. *Ann Thorac Surg* 88:194–198, 2009.
17. Raju GS: Endoscopic closure of gastrointestinal leaks. *Am J Gastroenterol* 104:1315–1320, 2009.
18. Fischer A, Thomusch O, Benz S, et al: Nonoperative treatment of 15 benign esophageal perforations with self-expandable covered metal stents. *Ann Thorac Surg* 81:467–472, 2006.
19. Braxton JH, Marrin CA, McGrath PD, et al: Mediastinitis and long-term survival after coronary artery bypass graft surgery. *Ann Thorac Surg* 70:2004–2007, 2000.
20. Salehi Omran A, Karimi A, Ahmadi SH, et al: Superficial and deep sternal wound infection after more than 9000 coronary artery bypass graft (CABG): incidence, risk factors and mortality. *BMC Infect Dis* 7:112, 2007.
21. Ronson RS, Duarte I, Miller JI: Embryology and surgical anatomy of the mediastinum with clinical implications. *Surg Clin North Am* 80:157–169, x–xi, 2000.
22. Moore KL: *Clinically Oriented Anatomy*. 3rd ed. Baltimore, MD, Williams and Wilkins, 1992.
23. Mangram AJ, Horan TC, Pearson ML, et al: Guideline for prevention of surgical site infection, 1999. Hospital Infection Control Practices Advisory Committee. *Infect Control Hosp Epidemiol* 20:250–278; quiz 79–80, 1999.
24. Fowler VG Jr, O'Brien SM, Muhlbaier LH, et al: Clinical predictors of major infections after cardiac surgery. *Circulation* 112:1358–1365, 2005.
25. Baskett RJ, MacDougall CE, Ross DB: Is mediastinitis a preventable complication? A 10-year review. *Ann Thorac Surg* 67:462–465, 1999.
26. Gummert JF, Barten MJ, Hans C, et al: Mediastinitis and cardiac surgery–an updated risk factor analysis in 10,373 consecutive adult patients. *Thorac Cardiovasc Surg* 50:87–91, 2002.
27. Robicsek F: Postoperative sterno-mediastinitis. *Am Surg* 66:184–192, 2000.
28. Abboud CS, Wey SB, Baltar VT: Risk factors for mediastinitis after cardiac surgery. *Ann Thorac Surg* 77:676–683, 2004.
29. Hollenbeak CS, Murphy DM, Koenig S, et al: The clinical and economic impact of deep chest surgical site infections following coronary artery bypass graft surgery. *Chest* 118:397–402, 2000.
30. Copeland M, Senkowski C, Ulcickas M, et al: Breast size as a risk factor for sternal wound complications following cardiac surgery. *Arch Surg* 129:757–759, 1994.
31. Copeland M, Senkowski C, Ergin MA, et al: Macromastia as a factor in sternal wound dehiscence following cardiac surgery: management combining chest wall reconstruction and reduction mammoplasty. *J Card Surg* 7:275–278, 1992.
32. Borger MA, Rao V, Weisel RD, et al: Deep sternal wound infection: risk factors and outcomes. *Ann Thorac Surg* 65:1050–1056, 1998.
33. Milano CA, Kesler K, Archibald N, et al: Mediastinitis after coronary artery bypass graft surgery. Risk factors and long-term survival. *Circulation* 92:2245–2251, 1995.
34. Dial S, Nguyen D, Menzies D: Autotransfusion of shed mediastinal blood: a risk factor for mediastinitis after cardiac surgery? Results of a cluster investigation. *Chest* 124:1847–1851, 2003.
35. Grossi EA, Culliford AT, Krieger KH, et al: A survey of 77 major infectious complications of median sternotomy: a review of 7,949 consecutive operative procedures. *Ann Thorac Surg* 40:214–223, 1985.
36. Lu JC, Grayson AD, Jha P, et al: Risk factors for sternal wound infection and mid-term survival following coronary artery bypass surgery. *Eur J Cardiothorac Surg* 23:943–949, 2003.
37. Curtis JJ, Clark NC, McKenney CA, et al: Tracheostomy: a risk factor for mediastinitis after cardiac operation. *Ann Thorac Surg* 72:731–734, 2001.
38. Singhal P, Kejriwal N, Lin Z, et al: Optimal surgical management of descending necrotising mediastinitis: our experience and review of literature. *Heart Lung Circ* 17:124–128, 2008.
39. Pearse HE: Mediastinitis following cervical suppuration. *Ann Surg* 108:588–611, 1938.
40. Moriwaki Y, Sugiyama M, Matsuda G, et al: Approach for drainage of descending necrotizing mediastinitis on the basis of the extending progression from deep neck infection to mediastinitis. *J Trauma* 53:112–116, 2002.
41. Athanassiadi KA: Infections of the mediastinum. *Thorac Surg Clin* 19:37–45, vi, 2009.
42. Kiernan PD, Hernandez A, Byrne WD, et al: Descending cervical mediastinitis. *Ann Thorac Surg* 65:1483–1488, 1998.
43. Horan TC, Andrus M, Dudeck MA: CDC/NHSN surveillance definition of health care-associated infection and criteria for specific types of infections in the acute care setting. *Am J Infect Control* 36:309–332, 2008.
44. Wheatley MJ, Stirling MC, Kirsh MM, et al: Descending necrotizing mediastinitis: transcervical drainage is not enough. *Ann Thorac Surg* 49:780–784, 1990.
45. El Oakley RM, Wright JE: Postoperative mediastinitis: classification and management. *Ann Thorac Surg* 61:1030–1036, 1996.
46. Luckraz H, Murphy F, Bryant S, et al: Vacuum-assisted closure as a treatment modality for infections after cardiac surgery. *J Thorac Cardiovasc Surg* 125:301–305, 2003.

CHAPTER 148 ■ MANAGEMENT OF THE POSTOPERATIVE CARDIAC SURGICAL PATIENT

SAJID SHAHUL, CATHY DUDICK AND ALAN LISBON

The management of the postoperative cardiac surgical patient is a dynamic process that requires modern intensive care unit (ICU) technology and sharp clinical skills. Early detection of acute complications has a significant impact on morbidity and mortality. The postoperative care of cardiac surgical patients is best handled using a systematic approach [1,2].

MONITORING

The restoration and maintenance of physiologic homeostasis without further injury to the heart and other organs represent the most important goal in the care of the postoperative cardiac surgical patient and requires proper patient monitoring. An arterial cannula, usually in the radial artery, permits easy access to blood for various laboratory tests (see Chapter 3) and provides the ability to measure systemic blood pressure continuously, mean arterial pressure (MAP) being the value of most interest. The MAP is the least dependent on site or technique of measurement and the least affected by measurement damping; it also determines tissue blood flow by autoregulation [3].

At least one lead of the surface electrocardiogram also should be displayed, with several leads being monitored for ST-segment changes. Pulse oximetry allows assessment of oxygen saturation and reduces the need for arterial blood gases.

A triple-lumen pulmonary artery catheter (PAC) inserted through an internal jugular vein permits measurement of the right atrial, pulmonary artery, and pulmonary artery occlusion (PAOP) pressures and the determination of cardiac output (CO) and mixed venous saturation. Pulmonary artery catheters with an oximeter probe at the distal end allow continuous monitoring of mixed venous oxygen saturation and cardiac index. However, based on multiple, randomized controlled clinical trials in a variety of settings, the routine use of pulmonary artery catheterization does not lead to improved clinical outcomes [4–9]. Although the PAC-Man trial, an open randomized trial involving 65 UK ICUs and over 1,000 patients, demonstrated no clear benefit or harm in using a PAC [4], the use of a PAC carries attendant risks such as infection, pulmonary artery rupture, and arrhythmia.

Transesophageal echocardiography is now used both as a monitoring and a diagnostic tool, both in the operating room and the ICU. It allows real-time evaluation of intracardiac blood flow, anatomy, and function. It may be superior to invasive monitoring [10], particularly in the setting of valvular disease or respiratory disease when pressure-based readings may not accurately reflect volume status. In both cardiac and noncardiac patient populations, several studies demonstrated that TEE provided unexpected information that significantly altered the therapeutic plan, even in patients with an indwelling PAC [10]. The therapeutic management decisions gleaned from TEE ranges from 10% to 69%, with the majority of studies demonstrating the 60% to 65% range. The diagnostic yield of TEE approaches 78% [11].

INITIAL ASSESSMENT

A brief but systematic physical examination of the patient is mandatory on arrival in the ICU. Inspection of the skin and extremities may reveal intraoperative injuries, infiltration or disconnection of intravenous (IV) infusions, absence of pulses, signs of drug or transfusion reactions, or evidence of hypoperfusion. Auscultation of the chest may reveal unilateral absence of breath sounds due to malposition of the endotracheal tube or pneumothorax. The abdomen should be inspected to ensure that no abdominal distention is present. Mediastinal and chest tubes should be examined for drainage.

Initial laboratory studies should include arterial blood gas, hematocrit, sodium, potassium, glucose, calcium, magnesium, prothrombin time (PT), partial thromboplastin time (PTT), and platelet count. A portable chest radiograph and a 12-lead electrocardiogram with atrial electrograms should be obtained immediately on admission to the ICU. The postoperative chest radiograph should be inspected with specific attention to the following: (a) pneumothorax and mediastinal shift; (b) position of the endotracheal tube, nasogastric tube, and intravascular catheters; (c) size and contour of the mediastinal silhouette; and (d) pleural and extrapleural fluid collections.

PHYSIOLOGIC PRINCIPLES OF CARDIAC FUNCTION

Cardiac function is determined by intrinsic myocardial properties as well as by ambient loading conditions. The inotropic state (contractility) of the myocardium during systole is a determinant of systolic stroke volume (SV). Systolic function is also determined by ambient hemodynamic conditions (heart rate [HR], preload, and afterload). The conceptual framework that provides maximal information about intrinsic myocardial properties, as well as the interrelationships between systolic contractility, preload, and afterload, is represented by the ventricular pressure–volume (PV) relationship (Fig. 148.1). The cardiac cycle has four phases: (a) passive ventricular filling during diastole (which, in Fig. 148.1, has been extended as a curvilinear line to describe the distensibility of the ventricle beyond the range of the illustrated cardiac cycle), (b) isovolemic systole (before aortic valve opening), (c) systolic ejection, and (d) isovolemic relaxation.

The SV for an individual cardiac cycle can be obtained by subtracting end-systolic ventricular volume from the end-diastole volume (EDV). The systolic ejection fraction can be determined from the fractional relationship between SV and EDV. This framework aids in conceptualizing and predicting the effects of changes in loading conditions and contractility on measurable hemodynamic parameters.

Left atrial pressure can be measured, or its mean can be estimated by the measurement of PAOP pressure or pulmonary diastolic pressure. These three pressures are equal only under

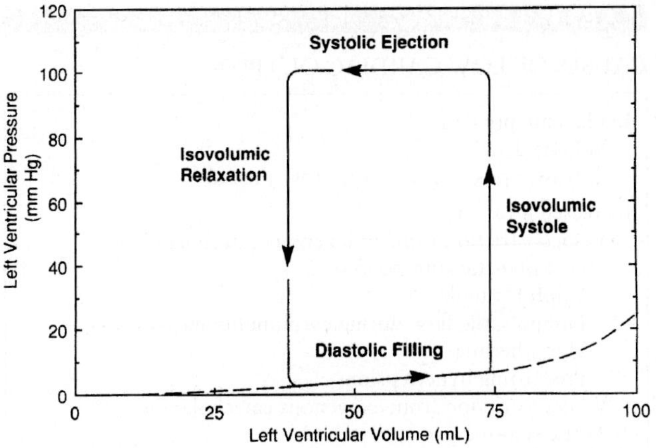

FIGURE 148.1. The left ventricular pressure-volume diagram. Phases of the cardiac cycle.

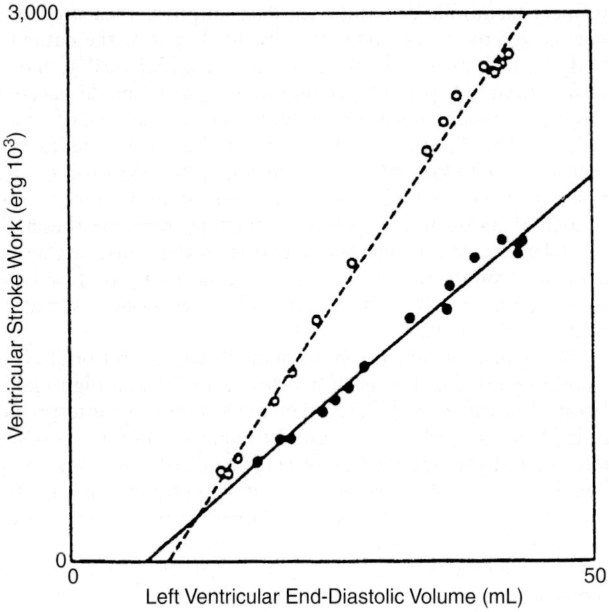

FIGURE 148.2. The preload recruitable stroke work relationship for the left ventricle. The slope of this relationship is sensitive to inotropic interventions and is increased by the infusion of calcium. [Reprinted from Glower DD, Spratt JA, Snow ND, et al: Linearity of the Frank-Starling relationship in the intact heart: the concept of preload recruitable stroke work. *Circulation* 71:994, 1985, with permission.]

ideal circumstances. Generally, pulmonary diastolic pressure exceeds pulmonary artery occlusion pressure, which exceeds mean left atrial pressure. These differences are determined by gravitational effects related to pulmonary artery catheter position and by diastolic pressure gradients in the pulmonary vasculature.

Although the systolic SV of the left ventricle is not measured directly, it can be determined from measurements of CO and HR. If LV systolic ejection fraction (EF) has been determined, the end-diastolic volume (EDV) and end-systolic volume (ESV) of the left ventricle can be determined: EDV = SV/EF and ESV = EDV − SV.

Preload is an estimation of average end-diastolic myocardial fiber length and correlates best with ventricular EDV. As the left ventricle distends, EDV, rather than end-diastolic pressure, is a highly predictive determinant of systolic function. Mechanical interaction between the two ventricles and between each ventricle and the surrounding mediastinal and thoracic structures can also influence ventricular distensibility. LV end-diastolic pressure (rather than EDV) can be used to monitor preload only when those factors that alter ventricular distensibility are constant. When ventricular distensibility is changing (due to, for example, the loss of myocardial compliance that occurs with transient ischemia), the measurements or estimates of ventricular diastolic pressure do not accurately represent preload.

The term *afterload* usually is used to describe the forces that retard the ventricular ejection of blood. The afterload of the right and left ventricles is determined primarily by the resistive and capacitive characteristics of the pulmonary and systemic circulations. As blood is ejected from the ventricle, the actual afterload forces that oppose the shortening of myocardial fibers are distributed as stresses throughout the ventricular walls.

The Frank-Starling principle is useful in predicting the hemodynamic outcome of therapeutic interventions. This is illustrated by the curvilinear relationship between ventricular stroke work (y-axis) and ventricular end-diastolic pressure (x-axis). When preload is represented by EDV, rather than by end-diastolic pressure, this relationship becomes linear and is minimally affected by afterload and HR [12]. The slope of this relationship is a sensitive indicator of intrinsic myocardial performance and responds appropriately to inotropic interventions. The augmentation of stroke work by increases in preload is referred to as *preload recruitable stroke work* (Fig. 148.2).

Increases in CO, afterload, preload, inotropic state, and HR are all achieved with increased myocardial oxygen demand. Intraoperatively, myocardial oxygen demand is eliminated by hypothermia and chemical cardioplegia. Postoperatively, if the myocardial work is too intense or the blood supply is too small, myocardial ischemia, failure, and infarction may result. An important feature of myocardial oxygen consumption is that oxygen extraction is nearly maximal at rest, so that increases in myocardial oxygen consumption can only be achieved by increases in coronary blood flow. Increased afterload is, to a degree, self-compensatory in that increased diastolic coronary perfusion pressure tends to increase coronary blood flow. Increases in inotropic activity may also be associated with increases in myocardial blood flow and a correspondent increase in diastolic aortic pressure.

Maximizing cardiac function to meet metabolic demands, therefore, involves the manipulation of volumes and pressures that affect preload and afterload and the support and enhancement of myocardial contractility. Andre and DelRossi [13] note that the postoperative myocardium is cold and stiff and generally behaves as a pressure-overloaded system. Volume may be needed despite high measured filling pressures. As the patient recovers and the myocardium warms, compliance improves and the relationship of filling pressures to ventricular volumes changes.

Initial Status

On arrival to the ICU, a systematic assessment should include preoperative history with attention to medications and cardiac function, intraoperative history, vital signs, and physical examination. Immediate goals and short-term goals need to be established. Many patients arrive hypothermic with temperatures ranging from 34°C to 36°C as a result of deliberate systemic cooling during cardiopulmonary bypass. Persistent peripheral vasoconstriction can be the result of elevated angiotensin levels [14]. Shivering during rewarming increases metabolic and circulatory demands, increases carbon dioxide production, and complicates ventilator management. Shivering can be eliminated with paralyzing agents and sedation [15,16]. The patient is generally maximally warm by 4 to 6 hours after operation.

As the patient rewarms and awakens, the goal is to support the recovering myocardium until it is independently able to meet metabolic demands. Cardiac output is measured and normalized to cardiac index (CI) by dividing it by the patient's body surface area. Efforts to correct an initial cardiac index of less than 2 L per m^2 per minute should be made because low cardiac index is associated with an increased risk of death [17,18]. The clinical correlates of reduced cardiac index are pale and cool skin, cyanotic mottling of the skin (occurring first over the knees), decreased urine output, and deterioration of mental status or slowness in awakening from anesthesia. A low CI and decreased peripheral perfusion also cause metabolic acidosis (from lactic acid accumulation in poorly perfused tissues; see Chapter 71), which, to a mild degree, occurs even after routine operations.

Normally, the mixed venous hemoglobin saturation (SvO_2) should be 60% or higher. If it is less than 50%, a high likelihood of death exists [17,19]. The SvO_2 should be interpreted in light of the cardiac index and hemoglobin. In the worst situation, and the one that often leads to death, the SvO_2 may be adequate only because so much of the peripheral tissues are underperfused [17]. In this case, however, the cardiac index also is reduced. The value of SvO_2 is limited because it does not describe the balance of oxygen in those tissues with fixed oxygen extraction. The kidney, skin, and resting muscle can maintain viability during reduced blood flow by augmenting oxygen extraction. The heart and brain, on the other hand, extract oxygen nearly maximally at rest, and their vulnerability to ischemia is not reflected by widened oxygen extraction.

Postoperative hypertension is common and may be a consequence of several factors, such as inadequate sedation, hypoxemia, hypercarbia, activation of cardiogenic reflexes, vasoactive drug administration, and withdrawal of beta-blocking agents; however, intense vasoconstriction accounts for most of the hypertension. Failure to control the blood pressure increases the risk of aortic tear, elevates myocardial oxygen demand, leading to the possibility of decreased subendocardial perfusion and ischemia.

As a consequence of fluid administration, the patient seen in the ICU just after an operation on cardiopulmonary bypass usually weighs 2 to 5 kg more than preoperatively. Urine output is typically high in patients with good LV function. If urine output is low, intravascular volume or CO may be low. Inappropriate antidiuretic hormone excretion commonly exists as a consequence of operative trauma. The patient is frequently treated with IV nitroglycerin and other afterload-reducing and venodilating agents. These agents shift blood volume to the periphery and consequently decrease preload. These factors tend to reduce urine output.

TABLE 148.1

CAUSES OF LOW CARDIAC OUTPUT

- Inadequate preload
  - Volume deficit
  - Excessive positive end-expiratory pressure
- Increased afterload
  - Vasoconstriction from endogenous catecholamines
    - (sympathetic stimulation)
    - Painful stimuli
    - Nonpulsatile flow during cardiopulmonary bypass
    - Hypothermia
    - Preexisting hypertension
  - Vasoconstriction from exogenous catecholamines
  - Aortic stenosis
  - Idiopathic hypertrophic subaortic stenosis
- Myocardial depression
  - Uncorrected mechanical lesions
    - Incomplete coronary revascularization
    - Valvular stenosis or insufficiency
    - Mechanical valve malfunction
  - Functional depression (lasts ~24 h)
  - Coronary spasm
  - Inadequate myocardial protection intraoperatively
    - Myocardial edema
    - Myocardial ischemia
    - Myocardial necrosis-infarct
- Metabolic derangement
  - Hypocalcemia
  - Hypomagnesemia
  - Hypoxia
  - Acidosis
- Arrhythmias
- Conduction defects
- Tamponade
- Pharmacologic depression
  - Anesthetic agents
  - Quinidine
  - Procainamide
  - Lidocaine
  - Beta-blockers
  - Calcium channel blockers

Treatment of Low Cardiac Output

Low CO in the postoperative period is associated with a higher incidence of respiratory, renal, hepatic, and neurologic failure. Treatment of low CO first requires an analysis of possible causes (Table 148.1). Operative complications, such as coronary graft closure, inadequate revascularization, poor myocardial protection, valve malfunction, or paravalvular leak, can cause pump dysfunction. Graft closure or acute coronary occlusion can have immediate hemodynamic effects (a fall in CO and a rise in left-sided filling pressures). Early graft failures are usually due to technical factors, but perioperative myocardial infarction due to coronary spasm can also occur in operated or in nonoperated vessels [20]. When the diagnosis of spasm is entertained and ST-segment changes as well as wall motion abnormalities occur, aggressive management with nitroglycerin and diltiazem should be instituted [21]. If these drugs are unsuccessful in reversing the hemodynamic deterioration, cardiac catheterization or reexploration, or both, inspection of the grafts should be considered [22]. Myocardial depression can be seen in the first 24 hours as a result of the operation. Common causes of perioperative pump dysfunction include arrhythmias, tamponade, hypovolemia, myocardial infarction, systemic acidosis, electrolyte imbalance, and hypoxia.

Early graft patency is an important determinant of postoperative ventricular function and performance on stress tests. On the other hand, the occurrence of perioperative myocardial infarction without hemodynamic compromise has not been shown to be significantly related to graft patency, late survival, or cardiac performance status [23]. The treatment of perioperative infarction consists of therapy to maintain CO, including afterload reduction, especially with nitroglycerin and beta-blockade, if tolerated.

If an obvious cause of low CO is not identified, a systematic approach toward optimizing pump function should be undertaken (Table 148.2). An easy way to organize this approach is by examining preload, afterload, rate, contractility, and rhythm. Because CO is the product of SV and HR ($CO = SV \infty HR$), either can be increased.

On arrival to the ICU, many patients exhibit intravascular volume depletion, despite an increase in total body water. The rewarming that is actively done during the early postoperative period causes progressive peripheral vasodilatation and relative

TABLE 148.2

TREATMENT OF LOW CARDIAC OUTPUT

Treat or exclude complications
Valve malfunction (reoperate)
Coronary graft occlusion (reoperate)
Tamponade (reoperate)
Bleeding (reoperate)
Coronary spasm (nifedipine, 10 mg sublingually)
Treat arrhythmias by optimizing heart rate
Increase rate to 90–100 beats/min
Atrial pacing if no heart block
Atrioventricular pacing if heart block
BP (systolic) ≥100, or BP (MAP) ≥85
Low LAP (<15 mm Hg)
Give volume (packed cells) if Hct <25%
Give Ringer's lactate or hetastarch if Hct ≥25%
Continue stepwise treatment with volume and dilators until cardiac index adequate (≥2.5); do not allow LAP to remain >15 mm Hg or BP to remain <100
High LAP (≥15 mm Hg): Begin nitroprusside[a] or nitroglycerin, 0.2–0.6 μg/kg/min and increase until desired effect obtained
BP (systolic) <100 or BP (MAP) <85
Low LAP (<15 mm Hg)
Give volume (packed cells) if Hct <25%
Give Ringer's lactate or hetastarch if Hct ≥25%
High LAP (≥15 mm Hg): if BP still low
Give epinephrine 2–5 μg/min; increase gradually to 10 μg/min maximum; dobutamine, milrinone
When BP ≥100, begin nitroprusside,[a] 0.2–0.6 μg/kg/min; increase until desired effect obtained

[a]See text for alternative drugs.
Note: If BP and cardiac output still low, insert intra-aortic balloon pump.
BP, blood pressure; Hct, hematocrit; LAP, left atrial pressure; MAP, mean arterial pressure.

hypovolemia. The goal MAP is 70 to 80 mm Hg [13]. Normovolemia is essential and can be accomplished with autotransfusion, normal saline, lactated Ringer's solution, albumin (25% solution), or hydroxyethyl starch (hetastarch). In the Saline versus Albumin Fluid Evaluation (SAFE) study involving almost 7,000 patients, albumin had no proven advantage over crystalloids in critically ill patients, although a larger volume of crystalloid is necessary compared to colloid [24]. Hetastarch can provide volume expansion for more than 24 hours. At doses more than 20 mL per kg, it can cause a decrease of factor VIII levels and platelets. Urticarial and anaphylactoid reactions as well as pancreatitis can occur with the use of this product [25].

In addition to ensuring adequate volume resuscitation, clinician should optimize cardiac rate and rhythm. Ventricular filling occurs during diastole and is augmented by a properly timed atrial contraction. If the heart rate is excessive to the extent that there is inadequate time for ventricular filling, cardiac output will be affected. This is particularly true of the hypertrophied or pressure overloaded ventricle and a heart rate of 90 to 100 beats per minute is optimal [13]. After cardiac surgery, atrial fibrillation, sinus bradycardia, and varying degrees of heart blockage can occur. These arrhythmias are usually transient and may be related to perioperative beta-blockade, hyperkalemic damage during the administration of cardioplegia, or unprotected ischemia of the conduction system [26]. Permanent injury to the conduction system is usually the result of surgically induced trauma.

Temporary atrial and ventricular wires are placed at the time of surgery and can be used to maintain CO. Simple atrial pacing (at a rate of 80 to 100 beats per minute) for the treatment of sinus bradycardia may effectively augment CO. Atrial pacing can aggravate a first-degree heart blockage and introduce an atrioventricular dyssynchrony. In this situation, atrioventricular sequential pacing should be attempted. The optimal atrioventricular interval is usually in the range of 100 to 175 milliseconds, depending on the HR. The advantage of atrial pacing over atrioventricular sequential pacing is the maintenance of the normal anatomic pattern of ventricular activation. Loss of the normal sequence of activation depresses ventricular function by approximately 10% to 15%.

Although a low MAP is most common, occasionally one must lower excessive afterload to improve cardiac output. Decreasing systemic vascular resistance (SVR) decreases the heart's oxygen demand. In patients with relatively normal LV function, nitroprusside reliably decreases SVR and increases CO, whereas nitroglycerin may lower CO, perhaps as a result of too great a decrease in cardiac preload (left atrial pressure).

The PV relationship of the left ventricle can be used to predict improvements in stroke volume secondary to reductions in afterload. The therapeutic results depend on the inotropic state of the ventricle. Ventricles with the poorest contractility benefit the most from afterload reduction. If the ventricle is operating on an end-systolic PV relationship with a shallow slope (depressed contractility), reducing afterload (and end-systolic pressure) results in a relatively large increase in SV (Fig. 148.3).

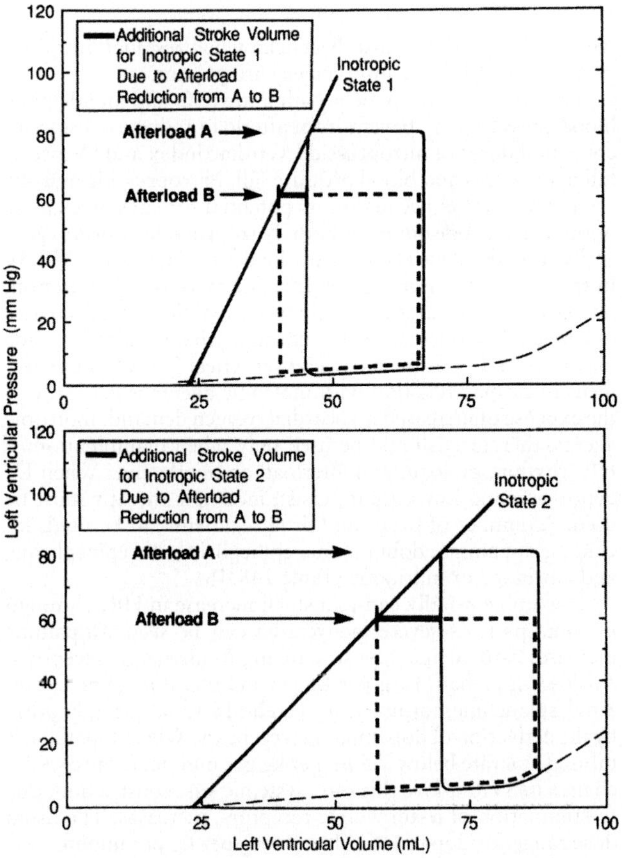

FIGURE 148.3. The improvement in stroke-volume that can be achieved with a reduction in afterload (and consequently, a reduction in end-systolic pressure) depends on the inotropic state of the myocardium. There is more to be gained by afterload reduction in a ventricle with depressed inotropic state (a smaller slope of the end-systolic pressure-volume relationship).

TABLE 148.3

VASODILATORS USED IN POSTOPERATIVE CARDIAC SURGERY PATIENTS

Drug	Dosage range[a]	Activity: Arterial	Activity: Venous	Onset	Duration	Mechanism	Comments	Toxicity
Nitroprusside (Nipride)	0.2–5.0 μg/kg/min	+3	+2	Immediate	Immediate	Direct vasodilator	May increase myocardial ischemia	Cyanide and thiocyanate
Nitroglycerin	0.3–5.0 μg/kg/min	+1	+4	Immediate	30 min	Direct vasodilator	Improves myocardial ischemia	—
Clevidipine	2–6 mg/h	+3	–	Immediate	Immediate	Direct vasodilator	Low incidence of side effects in comparison to other vasodilators	
Hydralazine	5–10 mg IV 10–20 mg IM	+4	0	15–30 min 20–80 min	2–6 h	Direct vasodilator	Reflex increases cardiac output and heart rate; may cause angina in ischemic heart	None short term
Enalaprilat	0.625–1.25 mg IV	+4	0	15 min	4–6 h	Angiotensin-converting enzyme inhibition	Use cautiously with renal impairment	May cause hyperkalemia; rare angioedema

[a]Initiate treatment at low end of dosage range.

Afterload reduction is also beneficial when residual mitral regurgitation and aortic insufficiency are present.

The postoperative patient with a low CO and an adequate blood pressure may benefit from afterload reduction using incremental doses of nitroprusside. Cardiac index and SV rise as filling pressures and blood pressure fall. Nitroprusside must be used with caution because of its potential for causing cyanide or thiocyanate poisoning, or both. Nitroprusside infusions generally should not exceed 8 μg per kg per minute (Table 148.3). In the presence of ischemia or an acute myocardial infarction, nitroglycerin increases regional myocardial flow and decreases ischemic ST segments toward normal, whereas nitroprusside may have an opposite and deleterious effect [27,28]. Improvement in cardiac function with inotropic agents is generally at the expense of increased myocardial oxygen demand. Inotropic agents, therefore, should be used only when manipulation of HR, rhythm, preload, and afterload are ineffective. When LV depression and low output persist, inotropic therapy must be used. A number of drugs and drug regimens can be used, including dopamine, dobutamine, epinephrine, norepinephrine, and amrinone or milrinone (Table 148.4).

Dopamine usually causes a small increase in HR, although in some patients severe tachycardia can be seen. Dopamine increases cardiac index by stimulating β-adrenergic receptors. At doses less than 3 μg per kg per minute, dopamine causes renal, splanchnic, coronary, and cerebral arterial vasodilatation by the activation of dopaminergic receptors. When dopamine is infused at a rate below 7.5 μg per kg per minute, it causes little change in SVR; above this rate, systemic vasoconstriction, due to stimulation of α-adrenergic receptors, increases. The usual dose range for dopamine is 1 to 20 μg per kg per minute.

Dobutamine is a synthetic catecholamine with minimal α-adrenergic activity but pronounced β_1- and β_2-adrenergic activity. It increases CO by increasing ventricular contractility and rate as well as causing peripheral vascular dilatation. For patients with a low CO and marked peripheral vasoconstriction, dobutamine is preferable to dopamine when the latter is used alone. Nevertheless, because dobutamine is a vasodilator, use of this drug in the presence of hypotension may lead to further hypotension. The usual doses for dobutamine are 5 to 20 μg per kg per minute.

Epinephrine is an α-, β_1-, and β_2-receptor agonist. It increases myocardial contractility and rate. It also increases ventricular irritability. Peripherally, its β-mediated effects (vasodilation) predominate at low doses, whereas α-mediated effects (vasoconstriction) predominate at high doses. The usual epinephrine dose is 1 to 10 μg per minute (0.015 to 0.15 μg per kg per minute).

Norepinephrine has α- and β-adrenergic activity. It increases systemic and pulmonary blood pressure myocardial contractility and CO. Internal mammary grafts remain innervated and are responsive to vasoactive drugs; saphenous vein grafts are not. Norepinephrine has been shown to decrease flow in internal mammary grafts less than phenylephrine in the early postoperative period [29]. The usual dosage is 4 to 10 μg per minute (0.06 to 0.150 μg per kg per minute).

Milrinone is an "inodilator," producing a positive inotropic independent of adrenergic stimulation and causing a reduction in systemic and pulmonary vascular resistance. Milrinone is a phosphodiesterase inhibitor that increases intracellular concentrations of cyclic adenosine monophosphate. Milrinone is a bipyridine derivative that is 20 times more potent than amrinone [30,31]. They are usually used as a second-line medication when a low CO persists despite catecholamines. Concomitant use of catecholamines usually offsets any associated vasodilation. The usual dosage of milrinone is a loading dose of 50 μg per kg over 10 minutes, followed by an infusion of 0.375 to 0.75 μg per kg per minute. Administration of milrinone over a period of 10 minutes prevents the vasodilation that is observed with rapid loading [32–34].

Arginine vasopressin may be helpful if hypotension persists despite adequate cardiac output, despite use of vasoactive

TABLE 148.4

INOTROPIC AGENTS USED IN POSTOPERATIVE CARDIAC SURGERY PATIENTS

		Activity					
Drug	Dose range	Alpha	Beta	Onset	Offset (min)	Heart rate[a]	Comments
Dopamine	1–3 μg/kg/min	Plus renal and mesenteric vasodilatation, dopaminergic	Same as alpha	Immediate	Few	Increase of 20%–30% non-dose related (rate: idiopathic increase to 50%–70%)	Minimal PVR at dose <10 μg/kg/min; renal blood flow at low dose[b]
	1–10 μg/kg/min	+2	+2				
	>10 μg/kg/min		+2				
Dobutamine	1–10 μg/kg/min	0	+4	Immediate	2–3	25%–30%	Very similar to isoproterenol; tachyphylaxis[b]
Epinephrine	1–2 μg/min	0	+2	Immediate	2–3	+1	Predominant effect varies with dose, marked vasoconstriction at high doses
	2–10 μg/min	+2	+2				
	>10 μg/min	+2	0				
Norepinephrine	2–16 μg/min	+4	+2	Immediate	2–3	0	Pronounced vasoconstriction increases myocardial work; valuable in vasodilated patient or in use with vasodilator; may reduce renal perfusion, especially at higher doses[b]
Amrinone	10–30 μg/kg/min[c]			2–10 min	60–90	0	Increases output and decreases SVR; no tachyphylaxis; may cause thrombocytopenia
Milrinone	0.375–0.75 μg/kg/min[d]			5 min	2–4 h	+10%	Increases output; decreases SVR, PVR; may increase ventricular ectopic activity
Calcium chloride ($CaCl_2$)	100–200 mg	Restores ionized Ca^{2+} and acts synergistically with inotropic catecholamines	Same as alpha	Immediate	15	0	
Vasopressin	0.1–0.4 U/min			Immediate	Few	0	Works by V1 and V2 receptors to offset vasoplegia

[a]Depends on balance of direct cardiac effect versus reflex effects.
[b]May all decrease endocardial ratio (diastolic pressure time index/systolic pressure time index).
[c]Initiate amrinone with 0.75-mg/kg bolus over 5 min; repeat up to 2 times if necessary. Next, titrate infusion to increase cardiac index 25% to 40%.
[d]Initiate with 50-μg/kg bolus over 5 min.
PVR, pulmonary vascular resistance; SVR, systemic vascular resistance.

substances like epinephrine; "vasoplegia" or autonomic failure may be present. Vasopressin levels are low in normotensive patients after cardiac surgery and disproportionately low in patients with "vasodilatory shock." Acting on vascular V1 and renal V2 receptors, in doses ranging from 0.1 to 0.4 U per min, vasopressin can be effective in improving vascular tone. Care in its use must be taken in patients with marginal cardiac output as vasopressin may further compromise splanchnic blood flow [13].

Myocardial depression can occur as a result of excess citrate administration, as seen during massive blood transfusions. Administration of calcium chloride (100 to 200 mg IV) can augment contractility.

Occasionally, CO remains inadequate even after preload, afterload, and contractility are optimized. Additional energy can be added to the system by mechanical support. The most common method to achieve this is by the insertion of an intra-aortic balloon pump (IABP), through a femoral artery. By raising aortic diastolic pressure, the IABP increases diastolic pressure time index (DPTI). Because the IABP decreases afterload, it allows better ventricular emptying, which decreases LV diastolic pressure, thus further increasing DPTI. Coronary blood flow and CO increase. Proper balloon pump function requires synchronization with the cardiac cycle using the electrocardiogram or intra-arterial pressure tracing. The IABP is inflated with helium (40 mL) at the onset of diastole and deflated at the onset of systole. Weaning is usually accomplished by gradually reducing the proportion of augmented beats from 1:1 to 1:3 or by reducing balloon volume.

The insertion of the IABP is done preoperatively typically for unstable angina, LV failure, or cardiogenic shock. The balloon is inserted intraoperative mainly because of an inability to wean from bypass. The IABP has a high complication rate; these complications include aortic dissection, arterial perforation, femoral artery occlusion or thrombosis with leg ischemia, arterial emboli, and wound infection [35]. Although extremely rare, spinal cord ischemia resulting in paraplegia has been reported [36]. Blood seen in the lumen of the IABP signals rupture of the balloon and requires immediate removal.

Rarely, patients require even more mechanical assistance than can be provided with the IABP. In these cases, an option is the use of an LV-assist device [37,38]. This device pumps blood around the injured left ventricle, something that the IABP cannot do.

Hypotension

Causes of hypotension (MAP less than 70) include those for low CO (see Table 148.1). Therapeutic interventions for hypotension must prevent a catastrophic outcome. Untreated hypotension results in coronary hypoperfusion, arrhythmias, ventricular dysfunction, and death. Other possible causes of decreased afterload include pharmacologic vasodilatation or sepsis. Immediate treatment consists of norepinephrine (approximately 4 to 10 μg per minute) and volume repletion.

Evaluation of hypotension should include measurements of cardiac index, HR, and right and left atrial filling pressures. Hypovolemia presents with low filling pressures and low CO. LV depression presents with high left atrial and, sometimes, right atrial pressures and a very low CO. Bradycardia, especially in the presence of a poorly compliant postoperative ventricle, causes hypotension because the ventricle is unable to compensate by augmenting SV. Treatment of hypotension begins with optimization of rate (Table 148.5). If the rate is too slow, atrial (or, in the presence of complete heart block, atrioventricular) pacing should be used to bring the rate up to 90 to 100, depending on the response. Arrhythmias should be treated promptly (see "Arrhythmias" section of this chapter and Chapters 41–43). Intravascular volume should be optimized. Ventricular filling pressures in the early postoperative patient routinely need to be higher than normal to maximize SV, because the ventricle is stiff and dysfunctional after cardiopulmonary bypass.

TABLE 148.5

MANAGEMENT OF BRADYCARDIA

Diagnosis	Treatment
Sinus or nodal	Atrial pacing at 80–100 beats/min
AV block	AV sequential pacing at 80–100 beats/min (? digoxin toxic)
Atrial fibrillation	Ventricular pacing

AV, atrioventricular.

Echocardiography provides for a real time measure of the filling status of the ventricles. It avoids the pitfalls of a Swan as it can measure volume and does not use pressures as a surrogate for volume. Also right and left sided outputs can be calculated. It provides for a very reliable and quick way to evaluate and treat hypotension.

Tamponade

Cardiac tamponade results from the accumulation of fluid or clotted blood within the mediastinum, creating a restriction for diastolic filling of both ventricles. The findings associated with tamponade in the immediate postoperative period include: (a) elevation and equalization of the central venous pressure, pulmonary diastolic pressure, left atrial pressure (pulmonary artery capillary wedge pressure), and right ventricular diastolic pressure (central venous pressure); (b) low urine output; (c) excessive chest tube drainage; (d) mediastinal widening on chest radiograph; and (e) low CO and hypotension. Echocardiographic findings of tamponade include RV diastolic collapse, right atrial systolic collapse, IVC plethora, and respirophasic changes in transmitral filling.

The treatment for cardiac tamponade is early reoperation. The patient may temporarily respond to some simple supportive measures such as reducing airway pressure, infusing intravascular volume expanders, and providing inotropic support. Myocardial dysfunction and myocardial edema reduce the amount of space occupied by fluid and clot required to cause tamponade physiology [39].

Although cardiac tamponade usually presents within the first 24 hours postoperatively, it can present as a subacute syndrome as late as several weeks following surgery. The symptoms are often nonspecific and can include malaise, low-grade fever, diaphoresis, dyspnea, chest pain, and anorexia. Transesophageal or transthoracic echocardiography may demonstrate retained clot and blood or wall abnormalities characteristic of tamponade (diastolic collapse of the right atrium and right ventricle). On occasion, right-sided heart catheterization may be necessary to establish the diagnosis (equalization and elevation of filling pressures).

Hypertension

Postoperative hypertension frequently occurs after coronary artery bypass grafting in patients with good LV function, or after corrective surgery for aortic stenosis or idiopathic hypertrophic subaortic stenosis. Postoperative hypertension is a common problem in patients with a history of hypertension. Other causes of hypertension may also involve hypoxemia, hypercarbia, shivering, or anxiety. Hypertension is deleterious because it increases myocardial work and it increases wall tension that may result in rupture of aortic suture lines. The treatment of choice for systolic blood pressures higher than 150 mm Hg is nitroprusside. Beta-blockers can be added for additional blood pressure reduction.

In some patients with a hyperdynamic left ventricle (normal SV and increased peripheral resistance), sodium nitroprusside treatment may be ineffective. In this group, nitroprusside reduces peripheral vascular resistance, which causes reflex sympathetic stimulation. This unmasks the underlying hyperdynamic heart, and SV, pulse pressure, and HR increase [40,41].

Beta-blockers are also effective in controlling hypertension in the cardiac surgical patient; esmolol can be given as a 500 μg per kg loading dose and an infusion of 50 to 300 μg per kg per minute [41]. Enalaprilat, 0.625 to 1.25 mg IV, can also be effective. Diuretics are valuable for managing patients with difficult-to-control hypertension. If the hypertension existed preoperatively, long-term antihypertensive agents should be restarted.

Arrhythmias

Arrhythmias primarily affect CO and blood pressure. At Beth Israel Deaconess Medical Center in Boston, most cardiac surgical patients undergo placement of temporary epicardial pacing wires—two ventricular and two atrial electrodes. The wires are used diagnostically or therapeutically in approximately 80% of patients.

Atrial wires facilitate the diagnosis or conversion of supraventricular tachycardia, especially atrial flutter. By pacing at a rate faster than the intrinsic atrial rate, the atrium becomes entrained. The critical entrainment rate is evidenced by lead II P waves changing from negative to positive. When the critical entrainment rate has been reached for the critical duration (usually 10 to 20 seconds), the atrial pacer may be slowed and then stopped; the atrial rhythm follows the slowing and then converts to sinus rhythm mechanism. The atrial electrical activity can be recorded on a unipolar precordial (V) lead while standard limb leads are in place; the atrial wires can be attached to the right and left arm leads (with standard leg leads in place) and the electrical signals recorded on a bipolar lead (I) or unipolar leads (II or III). Homogeneous atrial flutter with an atrial rate of 240 to 340 breaks more easily than a more rapid atrial flutter [37,38].

The primary use of the pacing wires postoperatively is to increase a slow HR (see Table 148.5). For sinus bradycardia, atrial pacing should be used. For a junctional slow rhythm, atrial pacing should be tried, but if any atrioventricular block exists, sequential atrial and ventricular pacing are necessary. For complete heart block, sequential atrial and ventricular pacing should be used. Postoperatively, CO is higher with atrial than with ventricular pacing. In patients with LV hypertrophy, the difference may be as great as 40% [42], because these patients have a greater need for atrial systole to fill the poorly compliant, hypertrophied ventricle.

TREATMENT OF SPECIFIC ARRHYTHMIAS

Ventricular arrhythmias can be caused by myocardial ischemia, hypokalemia, hypomagnesemia, hypoxia, acidosis, sympathetic stimulation, or irritation related to malpositioned intracardiac catheters. Initial treatment should be directed at eliminating any of the triggering factors. Atrial pacing at a more rapid rate may exceed the rate of firing of an ectopic ventricular focus and then suppress its emergence. In the early postoperative period, ventricular ectopy often occurs when the serum potassium concentration is in the low normal range. Keeping the potassium concentration between 4.5 and 5.0 mEq per L and the magnesium more than 2 mEq per L tends to suppress ectopic beats [43,44]. It is not necessary to treat isolated premature ventricular contractions (PVCs) because they are most likely benign. However, if PVCs are more than six per minute, multifocal, or present in salvos of three or more consecutive beats, treatment is then necessary. The easiest therapy for PVCs is atrial pacing at a rate faster than the patient's baseline. Amiodarone bolus IV, followed by an IV infusion usually suppresses them. Among the risks of treatment are the proarrhythmic effects of most available agents [45].

Ventricular tachycardia (VT) can occur at a relatively slow rate and depress blood pressure minimally, or it can occur at a rapid rate, leading to severe LV depression. In either case, VT can degenerate into ventricular fibrillation. When VT markedly depresses blood pressure, direct current cardioversion should be performed immediately. Cardioversion should be performed using a synchronized (with the QRS) mode with 200 J, escalating if necessary to 400 J. In hemodynamically stable patients, lidocaine or amiodarone sometimes terminates VT and obviates the need for cardioversion (see Chapter 6).

Ventricular fibrillation is fatal if not treated immediately. This arrhythmia mandates immediate electrical defibrillation (asynchronous mode) using the same energy levels mentioned above (see Chapter 6). An overall approach to ventricular arrhythmias in the postoperative cardiac surgery patient is found in Table 148.6. Amiodarone by IV administration may be useful in the treatment and prophylaxis of ventricular fibrillation or tachycardia.

Supraventricular tachycardias occur commonly during the first few postoperative days. They develop in 11% to 40% of patients after coronary bypass grafting and more than 50% of patients after valvular surgery [46]. Premature atrial contractions may progress to either atrial flutter or atrial fibrillation. These arrhythmias occur in 25% to 33% of postoperative cardiac surgical patients and may be due to unprotected atrial ischemia, atrial stretch, administration of hyperkalemic cardioplegic solutions, or pericarditis secondary to surgery [47]. Prophylactic treatment of all post–heart surgery patients with beta-blockers reduces the incidence of atrial fibrillation [48–50]. Patients who were taking beta-blocking agents preoperatively benefit more from beta-blocker prophylaxis than do those who were not taking beta-blockers before operation. Most recently, the Prophylactic Oral Amiodarone for the Prevention of Arrhythmias That Begin Early After Revascularization, Valve Replacement, or Repair (PAPABEAR) data demonstrated that oral amiodarone prophylaxis of atrial tachyarrhythmias after cardiac surgery is effective [51].

Atrial fibrillation is the most common arrhythmia affecting patients in the postoperative period and is more common in the elderly and those undergoing valvular surgery. Other supraventricular tachycardias can also affect the patient during the first 24 to 36 hours after surgery. When junctional tachycardia occurs, the rapid rate causes inadequate ventricular diastolic filling. In addition, the lack of a normal atrioventricular delay causes mitral and tricuspid regurgitation, because the ventricles contract before the mitral and tricuspid valves have closed. For atrial fibrillation, the class I recommendation of the American College of Cardiology practice guidelines is to administer AV

TABLE 148.6

MANAGEMENT OF VENTRICULAR ARRHYTHMIAS

Diagnosis	Treatment
Premature ventricular contractions	Atrial pacing to suppress automatic focus; Amiodarone bolus, plus drip; keep K^+ 4.5–5.0; eliminate acidosis; $Mg^{2+} > 2$
Ventricular tachycardia	If BP adequate: Amiodarone bolus plus lidocaine drip; keep K^+ 4.5–5.0; eliminate acidosis ischemia; if tachycardia persists, electrical cardioversion $Mg^{2+} > 2$ If BP low: immediate electrical cardioversion, followed by lidocaine; maintain K^+ 4.5–5.0; amiodarone, 150 mg IV over 10 min
Ventricular fibrillation	Immediate defibrillation

BP, blood pressure.

nodal blocking agents [52], such as diltiazem or a beta-blocker. Use of beta-blockers must be done with care particularly in the immediate postoperative period when myocardial function is still compromised. Despite the current recommendation, the mainstay of treatment is conversion to and maintenance of sinus rhythm with amiodarone (150 mg IV over 10 minutes followed by an infusion of 1 mg per minute for 6 hours and then 0.5 mg per minute for 6 hours) (13 IV ibutilide, a class III potassium channel blocker, can also acutely convert atrial fibrillation or flutter after cardiac surgery) [49].

Atrial flutter often can be treated effectively with atrial overdrive pacing, using the atrial epicardial electrodes (usually at rates of 350 to 400 beats per minute). Atrial fibrillation ordinarily cannot be treated using overdrive pacing. Indeed, atrial fibrillation can be induced when these techniques fail to convert atrial flutter to sinus rhythm. The ventricular response to atrial fibrillation, however, is sometimes slower and better tolerated than that of the ventricular response to atrial flutter. Pharmacologic therapy for atrial flutter has two goals: (a) blockade of the atrioventricular node to decrease ventricular response and (b) conversion to sinus rhythm. IV diltiazem (10 to 20 mg, followed by 5 to 15 mg per hour) or esmolol (500 μg per kg loading dose and an infusion of 50 to 300 μg per kg per minute) slows the rate by increasing the degree of atrioventricular block. Esmolol may be more effective in restoring sinus rhythm [53]. Beta-blockers and calcium channel blockers should not be used concomitantly. Procainamide (see Chapter 42) may convert the rhythm to sinus mechanism. If pharmacologic therapy fails to convert atrial flutter, electrical cardioversion can be used [54]. An overall approach to supraventricular and ventricular arrhythmias as well as common drug therapy for rate control in the postoperative cardiac surgery patient is found in Table 148.7.

Respiratory System

Respiratory dysfunction can complicate the postoperative course in approximately 8% of cardiac patients. Cardiac surgery reduces functional residual capacity, causes atelectasis [55], increases shunting, and decreases arterial oxygenation. The alveolar–arterial oxygen tension gradient typically widens on the day of and the day after surgery, but then the gradient usually narrows. A positive end-expiratory pressure (PEEP) of 5 cm H_2O helps to restore functional residual capacity toward normal [56].

Most cardiac surgical patients arrive in the cardiac surgical ICU requiring mechanical ventilation (see Chapter 58). The initial ventilator settings are typically as follows: rate, 8 to 10 breaths per minute; fractional inspired oxygen (FIO_2) concentration, 1.0; tidal volume, 6 ml per kg predicted body weight. Lung protective ventilation is recommended in patients with established acute lung injury [57]. After the first set of arterial blood gas measurements returns, the FIO_2 is decreased to maintain the oxygen pressure at 80 to 100 mm Hg; minute volume is regulated to keep carbon dioxide pressure at approximately 40 mm Hg. Oxygen consumption and carbon dioxide increase as the patient warms. PEEP is added as needed to keep FIO_2 below 0.5. High levels of PEEP may be necessary when there is a large intrapulmonary shunt.

Patients should be extubated in the first 6 hours post routine cardiac surgery, unless specific hemodynamic concerns apply. Sato and colleagues have demonstrated extubation within is feasible (9.5%) with low complications in on pump CABG'S. Extubation within the first few hours postoperatively can be done in most patients with good LV function without significant valvular disease and uneventful weaning from cardiopulmonary bypass. If hemodynamic instability is present, controlled ventilation allows better control of arterial pH and carbon dioxide pressure as well as more vigorous fluid administration without as much worry about adverse pulmonary effects. In the presence of excessive mediastinal bleeding, continued mechanical ventilation permits a smoother return to the operating room if re-exploration is necessary (see the section Bleeding).

A complete discussion of management of mechanical ventilation (e.g., initiation and discontinuation) can be found in Chapters 58, 59, and 60. Contraindications to weaning from mechanical ventilation include unstable hemodynamics, excessive bleeding, severe acid–base abnormalities, unstable arrhythmias, and patients who are still warming. In patients who are doing well from cardiac and respiratory standpoints, the presence of an IABP is not a contraindication to weaning and extubation.

Some patients arriving in the cardiac surgical ICU may have undergone minimally invasive procedures such as single-vessel bypass grafting through a small anterior thoracotomy [59]. These patients typically have been extubated in the operating room. They may have more pain than patients who have undergone a standard median sternotomy and have a need for careful balance of pain relief against respiratory depression. They may also have areas of myocardium that have not been revascularized.

Rarely, the postoperative course is complicated by fulminant, noncardiogenic pulmonary edema. Left atrial pressures are low, and the protein content of the edema fluid is high—70% to 96% that of plasma [60]. Some patients may present with "postpump syndrome." In its most severe form, these individuals have a coagulopathy, pulmonary dysfunction with hypoxia, renal and cerebral insufficiency, and a diffuse inflammatory response that is characterized by increased capillary permeability and leakage of fluid into the interstitial space with diffuse edema, fever, and leukocytosis. The cause of these derangements may be activation of complement (C3 and C5) during cardiopulmonary bypass [61,62]. Various drugs have been implicated, including protamine and plasma protein fractions [62].

The phrenic nerve may be injured at the time of surgery by surgical manipulation and by cooling [63]. In a patient with good pulmonary function preoperatively, the postoperative course is not affected. However, in the patient with marginal

TABLE 148.7

MANAGEMENT OF SUPRAVENTRICULAR ARRHYTHMIAS

Diagnosis	Treatment
Premature atrial contractions	Atrial pacing at faster rate
Atrial flutter	If markedly BP or ischemia: DC cardioversion, followed by Amiodarone If BP adequate and no ischemia: Amiodarone overdrive pacing; if heart rate >120 beats/min; diltiazem or esmolol to slow
Atrial fibrillation	If markedly ↓ BP or ischemia: DC cardioversion, followed by Amiodarone If BP adequate and no ischemia Amiodarone; if heart rate >120 beats/min, diltiazem or esmolol

↓, low; BP, blood pressure; DC, direct current.

reserves, prolonged ventilatory support may be necessary. Poor diaphragmatic function must be suspected if there is paradoxic breathing when weaning, elevated diaphragm on chest radiograph, or decreased vital capacity. The diagnosis can usually be made with fluoroscopy.

Renal System

Renal function is, in many respects, a reflection of cardiac function. The risk factors commonly seen in acute renal failure include: (a) preoperative renal failure, (b) diabetes mellitus, (c) postoperative hypotension, (d) old age, and (e) prolonged operation. With adequate CO, most post-cardiac surgical patients have a high urine output, usually more than 50 mL per hour.

Many patients exhibit a marked diuresis in the immediate postoperative period with urine outputs of 200 to 500 mL per hour. The cause of this diuresis is multifactorial. Hypothermia diminishes flow to the outer renal cortex, decreases the free water clearance, and increases the filtration fraction [64]. Atrial distention may promote the release of atrial natriuretic factor and inhibit the release of vasopressin. A marked diuresis is generally not seen in those patients who have acute reductions in chronically elevated left atrial pressures [65].

Salt and water, accumulated during the intraoperative and early postoperative periods, are excreted over the first several days postoperatively. In patients who have good LV function, the diuresis usually begins on the second postoperative day.

Renal failure following heart surgery occurs in approximately 7% of post-cardiac patients. It carries a high mortality rate—27% to 47% [66,67]. Factors that increase the risk of perioperative renal failure include exposure to contrast media, perioperative use of aminoglycosides, nonsteroidal anti-inflammatory agents, or angiotensin-converting enzyme inhibitors.

Bleeding

Bleeding is a common problem after cardiac surgery and can be surgical or nonsurgical in nature. Persistent surgical bleeding may require reoperation. Nonsurgical bleeding can be multifactorial. Common causes include residual heparin activity, abnormal clotting factors, uncontrolled fibrinolysis, and thrombocytopenia. A careful history provides the best clue to intrinsic bleeding problems. Patients taking aspirin or anti-inflammatory drugs usually have some degree of platelet dysfunction. Screening tests include PT, PTT, platelet count, and bleeding time. Specific abnormalities require further evaluation and correction before elective heart surgery is performed (see Chapters 108 to 109).

Intraoperative factors can predispose to bleeding. Inadequate heparin administration results in excessive consumption of clotting factors. Inadequate neutralization of heparin with protamine leaves residual heparin activity. Improved titration of heparin and protamine can be achieved by assaying heparin activity either indirectly with an activated clotting time or directly with a heparin analyzer [68,72]. Prolonged cardiopulmonary bypass causes platelet dysfunction and depletion and dilution of clotting factors. Disseminated intravascular coagulation occurs rarely, whereas a substantial body of evidence suggests that some primary fibrinolysis occurs routinely during cardiopulmonary bypass (see Chapter 108). We routinely use Tranexamic acid—intraoperatively at our institution.

A standard battery of screening tests enables an assessment of postoperative clotting mechanisms. For abnormal bleeding workup, we routinely obtain a PT, PTT, platelet count, and thrombin time (TT). When the TT is prolonged, a reptilase time distinguishes between excess heparin and fibrinolysis or consumption. A systematic analysis of clotting disorders may be based on the information given in Table 148.8. Platelets may

TABLE 148.8

EXCESSIVE BLEEDING FROM CLOTTING ABNORMALITIES IN THE POSTOPERATIVE CARDIAC SURGERY PATIENT

	Tests							
Cause	PT	PTT	TT	Platelet count	RT	FIB	FSP	Treatment
Heparin excess	N			N	N	N	N	Protamine sulfate titrated with activated clotting time or heparin assay
Excessive primary fibrinolysis		N–Sl		N		N		EACA, 4–8 g IV over 10 min followed by 1 g/h infusion for 5–8 h (until clotting factors N); FFP to regulate clotting factors
Compensated[a]	N							
Uncompensated[a]			N					
Excessive consumption[b]								Treat cause: FFP, cryoprecipitate, platelets
Thrombocytopenia or platelet dysfunction[c]	N	N	N		N	N	N	Platelets
Undefined[d]	Sl		Sl	N	N	N	N	FFP, cryoprecipitate, ? EACA

[a] *Compensated* refers to a minor fibrinolysis under which the body can keep up with the deficiencies; *uncompensated* refers to a rapid process under which the body cannot keep up with the fibrinolysis.
[b] Rare excessive consumption (also known as *disseminated intravascular coagulation*) always has associated secondary fibrinolysis.
[c] Platelets may be reduced in function as well as number.
[d] This group, probably of mixed etiology, occurs frequently.
EACA, epsilon-aminocaproic acid; FFP, fresh-frozen plasma; FIB, fibrinogen; FSP, fibrin-split products; N, normal; PT, prothrombin time; PTT, partial thromboplastin time; RT, reptilase time; Sl, slightly; TT, thrombin time.

be deficient in function as well as in number; cardiopulmonary bypass causes both defects [69].

Treatment is based on the diagnosis, although the diagnosis may not be straightforward because the pathogenesis of abnormal clotting may be mixed. Residual heparin effect is a common problem. Although heparin is fully reversed after the operation, heparin rebound can occur as heparin that was stored in body fat elutes into the blood. Heparin rebound is the most common cause of prolonged PTT and TT [70–72]. A normal reptilase time establishes this diagnosis, and additional protamine treats it.

Excessive primary fibrinolysis and excessive consumption may be indistinguishable by the tests listed, although the latter condition is usually characterized by a lower platelet count. Treatment of disseminated intravascular coagulation should be aimed at its cause. Treatment of primary fibrinolysis consists of repleting clotting factors and infusing an antifibrinolytic agent, epsilon–aminocaproic acid. Cryoprecipitate is the cold insoluble protein fraction of plasma that is rich in factor V, factor VIII, von Willebrand factor, and fibrinogen. It is more concentrated than fresh-frozen plasma, but, because it is a pooled product, it carries a higher risk of transfusion-related infection.

When platelet dysfunction is suspected, either on the basis of preoperative aspirin intake or prolonged cardiopulmonary bypass, platelets should be transfused. Platelet transfusion should be considered in any patient with a platelet count of 100,000 per mm^3 who continues to bleed despite aggressive procoagulant therapy [71,72].

In some centers, PEEP is used to help control bleeding after cardiac surgery. Some studies have shown a marked diminution of bleeding with levels of PEEP from 10 to 20 cm H_2O [73,74]; others have not [75].

The definition of *excessive bleeding* varies with each patient. As a general guideline, however, bleeding is excessive when drainage from chest tubes is more than 400 mL per hour for the first hour, 300 mL per hour for the first 2 hours, 200 mL per hour for the first 3 consecutive hours, or 100 mL per hour over the first 6 hours. A sudden increase in bleeding suggests an arterial source and mandates re-exploration. Bleeding that is sufficient to cause marked hypotension or tamponade also requires re-exploration. Massive bleeding necessitates emergency re-exploration, regardless of any clotting abnormalities [76,77].

When bleeding is so rapid that cardiac arrest is imminent, the patient should *not* be brought back to the operating room to control bleeding. Instead, the sternotomy should be reopened immediately in the ICU and digital pressure must be applied on the obvious site of bleeding. Transfusions are administered to increase blood volume and blood pressure. Then the patient is transferred to the operating room for definitive control of the bleeding [76,77].

The use of autotransfusion has reduced requirements for transfusing homologous blood. Blood for autotransfusion can be collected in a removable chamber that is part of the standard chest drainage system and is reinfused by gravity drainage, much like a homologous transfusion. It has been demonstrated that autotransfused blood is extensively defibrinated [77].

Fever and Antibiotics

Temperature fluctuations are expected after cardiac surgery. Systemic warming before the termination of cardiopulmonary bypass brings the core temperature to 37°C, but cooling subsequently occurs as heat transfers to the cool extremities. Patients routinely have temperatures in the 34°C to 36°C range when they arrive in the ICU. Warming, shivering, and vasodilatation occur during the first several hours. Temperatures in the 38°C to 39°C range should be expected at this time and require no further evaluation. However, fever during subsequent days is abnormal and requires the usual investigation (see Chapter 76).

Prophylactic antibiotics are widely recommended because of the seriousness of infections of the mediastinum, sternum, cardiac suture lines, and prosthetic valves. Although staphylococcal infections are the greatest concern, antibiotics with broad-spectrum coverage are generally used in preference to specific antistaphylococcal antibiotics [78,79]. Antibiotics should be stopped within 2 days; administration for a longer period offers no advantage [80].

One third of all hospital-acquired bacteremias and most candidemias are associated with vascular catheters [80]. Positive cultures are yielded in 1.5% of vascular catheters, and pulmonary artery catheters have the highest rate of colonization (2.1%) [81]. Catheter-related sepsis is most commonly due to coagulase-negative staphylococci and cannot be treated successfully with antibiotics unless the catheter is removed. A 7- to 10-day course of systemic antibiotics is then usually sufficient, although 4 to 6 weeks is necessary for cases of septic venous thrombosis.

Mediastinal infections are seen in approximately 1% of postoperative cardiac surgical patients. Risk factors include long operation, reoperation, low CO, and prolonged mechanical ventilation [82].

Psychological and Neurologic Dysfunction

Severe neurologic dysfunction occurs in 0.5% to 2.0% of coronary artery bypass graft operations. The incidence is higher in open chamber operations (4% to 10%). More commonly, subtle changes occur, such as cognitive dysfunction and ophthalmologic abnormalities. Central and peripheral nervous system dysfunction occur postoperatively. These events may be caused by emboli of air, clot, or other particulate matter [83].

Peripheral neuropathies can occur in the lower extremities and involve the femoral and peroneal nerves. Both neuropathies are preventable. Injuries of the brachial plexus can occur during sternal retraction secondary to compression or penetration of bone fragments [84,85]. Postoperative psychological dysfunction occurs in 40% to 60% of patients. Three types have been described: (a) an organic syndrome, which corresponds to the central metabolic neurologic dysfunction described above, (b) a postcardiotomy delirium, occurring after a lucid interval, and (c) a postcardiotomy depressive syndrome. Multiple risk factors for the latter two syndromes have been identified, including increased use of anticholinergic drugs, elevated preoperative blood urea nitrogen or decreased body weight, decreased body temperature while on cardiopulmonary bypass, and increased magnitude of overall preoperative sickness. Patients undergoing valve operations are affected more commonly than are patients undergoing coronary revascularization. The incidence seems to be higher in the elderly. Postulated pathogenic mechanisms include cerebral microemboli, cerebral red cell sludging, and sensory deprivation [85–88].

Treatment of the depressed patient begins with frequent reassurance and antidepressant therapy. In patients with postcardiotomy delirium, helpful measures include family support, general reassurance, and adequate sleep. Removing the patient from the ICU is desirable. Administration of small doses of IV haloperidol (1 to 2 mg or more) is very helpful in postcardiotomy delirium.

Gastrointestinal Complications

Gastrointestinal complications occur in approximately 1% of patients undergoing cardiac surgery. Patients with low CO and multiple organ failure are more prone to developing gastric and duodenal bleeding (see Chapters 91, 92). Other gastrointestinal complications include cholecystitis, pancreatitis, intestinal obstruction, or ischemia. These complications can occur anytime from 2 days to 4 weeks after operation. A nasogastric tube is placed in the operating room and used routinely to prevent postoperative gastric distention. In most cases, the tube can be removed on the first postoperative day after endotracheal extubation.

Bowel ischemia and bowel infarction can be caused by embolism or low mesenteric flow. Emboli can originate from the heart, from an atherosclerotic aorta, or from suture lines communicating with the systemic circulation. Atrial fibrillation predisposes to the formation of atrial thrombi and embolization. Low CO, α-adrenergic pressors, and digoxin all increase the risk of low mesenteric flow (see Chapter 151). When bowel ischemia or infarction is suspected, laparotomy should be performed urgently.

To prevent upper gastrointestinal ulceration and bleeding, the gastric pH should be maintained above 4.0. Histamine-2–blockers or proton pump inhibitors and antacids may be required. Sucralfate is an effective prophylactic agent, and because it does not reduce acidity, it may decrease colonization of the upper gastrointestinal tract with Gram-negative organisms [89]. The early institution of enteral feedings may also reduce the incidence of gastrointestinal bleeding and complications. During low CO states, intestinal absorption is not totally suppressed, only delayed [90].

Pancreatitis is a potentially lethal complication of cardiac surgery. Its occurrence is probably related to decreased splanchnic blood flow, and therefore it tends to occur in patients who have associated cardiac complications. In approximately one third of cardiac surgical patients, there is a significant rise in the level of serum amylase (>300 IU per L) by the second postoperative day [91]. However, clinically overt pancreatitis occurs in only approximately 2% of patients. Nonpancreatic hyperamylasemia is associated with increased mortality. The cause is unknown [92].

Endocrine Complications

Hyperglycemia is the most common endocrine abnormality requiring postoperative management and occurs frequently whether or not there was preexisting diabetes. Van de Berge et al. [93] published data from a mixed medical/surgical patient population of which a majority had undergone cardiac surgery demonstrating a significant reduction in morbidity and mortality for those who had tight glycemic control (at or below 110 mg per dL). However, in a recent study published by the NICE sugar study investigators, it was found that intensive glucose control increased mortality among adults in the ICU: a blood glucose target of 180 mg or less per deciliter resulted in lower mortality than did a target of 81 to 108 mg per deciliter [94]. During cardiac operations, insulin requirements under hypothermia are low but increase dramatically during rewarming. Insulin requirements usually decrease by the third postoperative day as the stress of surgery diminishes. However, intensive management of diabetes may be necessary when the patient resumes an oral diet. It is not uncommon for non–insulin-dependent diabetics to require insulin at the time of discharge.

Thyroid dysfunction can occur in seriously ill patients who were euthyroid preoperatively. The perioperative determination of thyroid function is difficult because of abnormalities in thyroxine binding and the fact that thyroid-stimulating hormone responds sluggishly to decreased triiodothyronine and thyroxine levels in critically ill patients. Advances in the care of the postoperative cardiac surgery patient, based on randomized controlled trials or meta-analyses of such trials, are summarized in Table 148.9.

TABLE 148.9

SUMMARY OF ADVANCES IN MANAGEMENT OF POSTOPERATIVE CARDIAC PATIENT

- Albumin has no proven advantage over crystalloids for resuscitation in critically ill patients [24].
- Prophylactic use of beta-blockers reduces the incidence of atrial fibrillation [42,49,50].
- The rapid shallow breathing index (RSBI) predicts success in weaning from mechanical ventilation [95].
- Hyperamylasemia occurs in one third of cardiac surgical patients but only 2% develop overt pancreatitis [91].
- Tight glycemic control increases morbidity and mortality [94].
- The routine use of pulmonary artery catheterization does not lead to improved clinical outcomes [5–9].

References

1. Kirklin J, Barratt-Boyes B: Postoperative care, in Kirklin J, Barratt-Boyes B (eds): *Cardiac Surgery*. New York, Churchill Livingstone, 1993, p 167.
2. Lisbon A, Vander Salm TJ, Visner MS: Management of the postoperative cardiac surgical patient, in Irwin RS, Cerra FB, Rippe JM (eds): *Intensive Care Medicine*. Philadelphia, PA, Lippincott–Raven Publishers, 1999, p 1637.
3. Bersten AD, Soni N, Oh T (eds): *Oh's Intensive Care Manual*. 5th ed. Edinburgh, Butterworth-Heinemann, 2003, p 79.
4. Harvey S, Harrison DA, Singer M, et al: Assessment of the clinical effectiveness of pulmonary artery catheters in management of patients in intensive care (PAC-Man): a randomised controlled trial. *Lancet* 366(9484):472, 2005.
5. Richard C, Warszawski J, Anguel N, et al: Early use of the pulmonary artery catheter and outcomes in patients with shock and acute respiratory distress syndrome: a randomized controlled trial. *JAMA* 290:2713, 2003.
6. Sandham JD, Hull RD, Brant RF, et al: A randomized, controlled trial of the use of pulmonary-artery catheters in high-risk surgical patients. *N Engl J Med* 348:5, 2003.
7. The ESCAPE Trial Investigators and ESCAPE Study Coordinators: Evaluation study of congestive heart failure and pulmonary artery catheterization effectiveness: the ESCAPE trial. *JAMA* 294:1625, 2005.
8. Shah MR, Hasselblad V, Stevenson LW, et al: Impact of the pulmonary artery catheter in critically ill patients: meta-analysis of randomized clinical trials. *JAMA* 294:1664, 2005.
9. The National Heart, Lung, and Blood Institute Acute Respiratory Distress Syndrome (ARDS) Clinical Trials Network: Pulmonary-artery versus central venous catheter to guide treatment of acute lung injury. *N Engl J Med* 354:2213, 2006.
10. Wake PJ, Ali M, Carroll J, et al: Clinical and echocardiographic diagnoses disagree in patients with unexplained hemodynamic instability after cardiac surgery. *Can J Anaesth* 48(8):778, 2001.
11. Porembka DT: Importance of transesophageal echocardiography in the critically *ill and injured patient. Crit Care Med* 35[8, Suppl]:S414–S430, 2007.
12. Glower DD, Spratt JA, Snow ND, et al: Linearity of the frank-starling relationship in the intact heart: the concept of preload recruitable stroke work. *Circulation* 71:994, 1985.
13. Andre AD, DelRossi A: Hemodynamic management of patients in the first 24 hours after cardiac surgery. *Crit Car Med* 33:2082, 2005.
14. Taylor KM, Morton JJ, Brown JJ, et al: Hypertension and the renin-angiotensin system following open-heart surgery. *J Thorac Cardiovasc Surg* 74:840, 1977.
15. Rodriguez JL, Weissman C, Damask MC, et al: Physiologic requirements during rewarming: suppression of the shivering response. *Crit Care Med* 11:490, 1983.
16. Ralley FE, Wynando JE, Rams JG, et al: The effects of shivering on oxygen consumption and carbon dioxide production in patients rewarming from hypothermic cardiopulmonary bypass. *Can J Anaesth* 35:332, 1988.
17. Ferraris VA, Ferraris SP: Risk factors for postoperative morbidity. *J Thorac Cardiovasc Surg* 111:731, 1996.
18. Dietzman RH, Ersek RA, Lillehei CW, et al: Low output syndrome. Recognition and treatment. *J Thorac Cardiovasc Surg* 57:138, 1969.

19. Higgins T, Estafanous F, Lloyd F, et al: Stratification of morbidity and mortality outcome by preoperative risk factors in coronary artery bypass patients: a clinical severity score. *JAMA* 207:2344, 1994.
20. Berger PB, Alderman EL, Nadel A, et al: Frequency of early occlusion and stenosis in a left internal mammary artery to left anterior descending artery bypass graft after surgery through a median sternotomy on conventional bypass: benchmark for minimally invasive direct coronary artery bypass. *Circulation* 100:2353, 1999.
21. Bojar RM: *Manual of Perioperative Care in Cardiac and Thoracic Surgery.* 2nd ed. Boston, Blackwell Science, 1994.
22. Lemmer JH Jr, Kirsch MM: Coronary artery spasm following coronary artery surgery. *Ann Thorac Surg* 46:108, 1988.
23. Force T, Hibberd P, Weeks G, et al: Perioperative myocardial infarction after coronary artery bypass surgery. *Circulation* 82:903, 1990.
24. The SAFE Study Investigators: A comparison of albumin and saline for fluid resuscitation in the intensive care unit. *N Engl J Med* 350:2247, 2004.
25. Smith PK, Buhrman WC, Ferguson TB Jr, et al: Conduction block following cardioplegic arrest: prevention by augmented atrial hypothermia. *Circulation* 68[Suppl]:II1, 1983.
26. Kajani M, Waxman H: Hematologic problems after open heart surgery, in Kotler M, Alfieri A (eds): *Cardiac and Noncardiac Complications of Open Heart Surgery: Prevention, Diagnosis, and Treatment.* Mt. Kisco, NY, Futura, 1992, p 219.
27. Flaherty JT, Magee PA, Gardner TL, et al: Comparison of intravenous nitroglycerin and sodium nitroprusside for treatment of acute hypertension developing after coronary bypass surgery. *Circulation* 65:1072, 1982.
28. Kaplan JA, Finlayson DC, Woodward S: Vasodilator therapy after cardiac surgery: a review of the efficacy and toxicity of nitroglycerin and nitroprusside. *Can Anaesth Soc J* 27:254, 1980.
29. Dinardo JA, Bert A, Schwartz MJ, et al: Effects of vasoactive drugs on flows through internal mammary artery and saphenous vein grafts in man. *J Thorac Cardiovasc Surg* 102:730, 1991.
30. Bojar RM: *Manual of Perioperative Care in Adult Cardiac Surgery.* 4th ed. Malden, MA, Blackwell, 2005, p 363.
31. Rathmell JP, Prielipp RC, Butterworth JF, et al: A multicenter, randomized, blind comparison of amrinone with milrinone after elective cardiac surgery. *Anesth Analg* 86:683, 1998.
32. Feneck RO: Effects of variable dose milrinone in patients with low cardiac output after cardiac surgery. *Am Heart J* 121:1995, 1991.
33. Prielipp RC, Butterworth JF, Zaloga GP, et al: Effects of amrinone on cardiac index, mixed venous oxygen saturation and venous admixture in patients recovering from cardiac surgery. *Chest* 99:820, 1991.
34. Feneck RO: Effects of variable dose milrinone in patients with low cardiac output after cardiac surgery. European Multicenter Trial Group. *Am Heart J* 121:1995, 1991.
35. Reichert CL, Koolen JJ, Visser GA: Transesophageal echocardiographic evaluation of left ventricular function during intraaortic balloon pump counterpulsation. *J Am Soc Echocardiogr* 6:490, 1993.
36. Tatar H, Cacek S, Demirkilic U, et al: Vascular complications of intraaortic balloon pumping: unsheathed versus sheathed insertion. *Ann Thorac Surg* 55:1518, 1993.
37. Lee WA, Gillinov AM, Cameron DE, et al: Centrifugal ventricular assist device for support of the failing heart after cardiac surgery. *Crit Care Med* 21:1186, 1993.
38. Oz M, Rose E, Levin H: Selection criteria for placement of left ventricular assist devices. *Am Heart J* 129:173, 1995.
39. Chuttani K, Tischler MD, Pandian NG, et al: Diagnosis of cardiac tamponade after cardiac surgery: relative value of clinical, echocardiographic, and hemodynamic signs. *Am Heart J* 127:913, 1994.
40. Wake PJ, Cheng DCH: Postoperative intensive care in cardiac surgery. *Curr Opin Anaesthesiol* 14:41, 2001.
41. Gray RJ, Bateman TM, Czer LSC, et al: Comparison of esmolol and nitroprusside for acute postsurgical hypertension. *Am J Cardiol* 59:887, 1987.
42. Friesen WG, Woodson RD, Ames AW, et al: A hemodynamic comparison of atrial and ventricular pacing in postoperative cardiac surgical patients. *J Thorac Cardiovasc Surg* 55:271, 1968.
43. England MR, Gordon G, Salem M, et al: Magnesium administration and dysrhythmias after cardiac surgery; a prospective controlled, double blind, randomized trial. *JAMA* 68:2395, 1992.
44. Johnson RG, Goldberger AL, Thurer RL, et al: Lidocaine prophylaxis in coronary revascularization patients: a randomised, prospective trial. *Ann Thorac Surg* 55:1180, 1993.
45. Zipes DP: Proarrhythmic events. *Am J Cardiol* 61:70A, 1988.
46. Ommen SR, Odell JA, Standon MS: Atrial arrhythmias after cardiothoracic surgery. *N Engl J Med* 336:1429, 1997.
47. Smith PK, Buhrman WC, Levett JM, et al: Supraventricular conduction abnormalities following cardiac operations: a complication of inadequate atrial preservation. *J Thorac Cardiovasc Surg* 85:105, 1983.
48. Andrews TC, Reimold SC, Berlin JA, et al: Prevention of supraventricular arrhythmias after coronary artery bypass surgery. A meta-analysis of randomized controlled trials. *Circulation* 84[Suppl III]:III236, 1991.
49. Chung MK: Cardiac surgery: postoperative arrhythmias. *Crit Care Med* 28[Suppl]:N136, 2000.
50. Lauer M, Eagle K: Arrhythmias following cardiac surgery, in Podrid P, Kowey P (eds): *Cardiac Arrhythmia. Mechanisms, Diagnosis, and Management.* Baltimore, Williams & Wilkins, 1995, p 1206.
51. Mitchell LB, Exner DV, Wyse DG, et al: Prophylactic oral amiodarone for the prevention of arrhythmias that begin early after revascularization, valve replacement, or repair (PAPABEAR). *JAMA* 294:3093, 2005.
52. Fuster V, Ryden LE, Asinger RW, et al: ACC/AHA/ESC guidelines for the management of patients with atrial fibrillation: a report of the American College of Cardiology/American Heart Association Task Force on practice guidelines and the European Society of Cardiology Committee for practice guidelines and policy conferences. *J Am Coll Cardiol* 38:1231, 2001.
53. Platia EV, Michelson EL, Porterfield JK, et al: Esmolol versus verapamil in the acute treatment of atrial fibrillation or atrial flutter. *Am J Cardiol* 63:925, 1989.
54. Lauer MS, Eagle KA: Atrial fibrillation following cardiac surgery, in Falk RH, Podrid PJ (eds): *Atrial Fibrillation: Mechanisms and Management.* New York, Raven Press, 1992, p 127.
55. Ramsay J: The respiratory, renal and hepatic systems: effects of cardiac surgery and cardiopulmonary bypass, in Mora CT (ed): *Cardiopulmonary Bypass.* New York, Springer, 1995, p 147.
56. Downs JB, Mitchell LA: Pulmonary effects of ventilatory pattern following cardiopulmonary bypass. *Crit Care Med* 4:295, 1976.
57. International Consensus Conferences in Intensive Care Medicine: Ventilator-associated lung injury in ARDS. *Am J Respir Crit Care Med* 160:2118, 1999.
58. Gajic O, Dara S, Mendez JL, et al: Ventilator-associated lung injury in patients without lung injury at the onset of mechanical ventilation. *Crit Care Med* 32:1817, 2004.
59. Landreneau RJ, Mack MJ, Magovern JA, et al: "Keyhole" coronary artery bypass surgery. *Ann Surg* 224:453, 1996.
60. Culliford AT, Thomas S, Spencer FC: Fulminating noncardiogenic pulmonary edema. A newly recognized hazard during cardiac operations. *J Thorac Cardiovasc Surg* 80:868, 1980.
61. Cameron D: Initiation of white cell activation during cardiopulmonary bypass: cytokines and receptors. *J Cardiovasc Pharmacol* 27[Suppl 1]:S1, 1996.
62. Moore FD Jr, Warner KG, Assousa S, et al: The effects of complement activation during cardiopulmonary bypass. *Ann Surg* 208:95, 1988.
63. Espositio RA, Spencer FC: The effect of pericardial insulation on hypothermic phrenic nerve injury during open-heart surgery. *Ann Thorac Surg* 43:303, 1987.
64. Utley JR, Wachtel C, Cain RB, et al: Effects of hypothermic, hemodilution, and pump oxygenation on organ water content, blood flow and oxygen delivery, and renal function. *Ann Thorac Surg* 31:121, 1981.
65. Shannon RP, Libby E, Elahi D, et al: Impact of acute reduction in chronically elevated left atrial pressure on sodium and water excretion. *Ann Thorac Surg* 46:430, 1988.
66. Kobrin S, Tobias S: Renal complications of open heart surgery, in Kotlet M, Alfieri A (eds): *Cardiac and Noncardiac Complications of Open Heart Surgery: Prevention, Diagnosis and Treatment.* Mt. Kisco, NY, Futura, 1992, p 311.
67. Kellerman PS: Perioperative care of the renal patient. *Arch Intern Med* 154:1674, 1994.
68. Kaul TK, Crow MJ, Rajah SM, et al: Heparin administration during extracorporeal circulation. Heparin rebound and postoperative bleeding. *J Thorac Cardiovasc Surg* 78:95, 1979.
69. Van Oeveren W, Kazatchkine MD, Descamps-Latsha B, et al: Deleterious effects of cardiopulmonary bypass. A prospective study of bubble versus membrane oxygenation. *J Thorac Cardiovasc Surg* 89:888, 1985.
70. Pifarre R, Babka R, Sullivan HJ, et al: Management of postoperative heparin rebound following cardiopulmonary bypass. *J Thorac Cardiovasc Surg* 81:378, 1981.
71. Levi M, Cromheecke ME, de Jonge E, et al: Pharmacological strategies to decrease excessive blood loss in cardiac surgery: a meta-analysis of clinically relevant end points. *Lancet* 354:1940, 2000.
72. Levy JH, Buckley MJ, D'Ambra MN, et al: Symposium: pharmacologic control of bleeding in patients undergoing open heart surgery. *Contemp Surg* 48:175, 1996.
73. Ilabaca PA, Ochsner JL, Mills NL: Positive end-expiratory pressure in the management of the patient with a postoperative bleeding heart. *Ann Thorac Surg* 30:281, 1980.
74. Hoffman WS, Tomasello DN, MacVaugh H: Control of postcardiotomy bleeding with PEEP. *Ann Thorac Surg* 34:71, 1982.
75. Zurick AM, Ursua J, Ghattas M, et al: Failure of positive end-expiratory pressure to decrease postoperative bleeding after cardiac surgery. *Ann Thorac Surg* 34:608, 1982.
76. Fairman RM, Edmunds LH Jr: Emergency thoracotomy in the surgical intensive care unit after open cardiac operation. *Ann Thorac Surg* 32:386, 1981.
77. Hartz RS, Smith JA, Green D: Autotransfusion after cardiac operation. *J Thorac Cardiovasc Surg* 96:178, 1988.
78. Kreter B, Woods M: Antibiotic prophylaxis for cardiothoracic operations. Meta-analysis of thirty years of clinical trials. *J Thorac Cardiovasc Surg* 104:590, 1992.
79. Hall J, Christiansen K, Carter M, et al: Antibiotic prophylaxis in cardiac operations. *Ann Thorac Surg* 56:916, 1993.
80. Maki DG: Infections associated with intravascular lines, in Remington JS, Swartz MN (eds): *Current Clinical Topics in Infectious Diseases.* New York, McGraw-Hill, 1982.

81. Damen J, Verhoef J, Bolton DT, et al: Microbiologic risk of invasive hemodynamic monitoring in patients undergoing open-heart operations. *Crit Care Med* 13:548, 1985.
82. Grossi EA, Culliford AT, Krieger KH, et al: A survey of 77 major infectious complications of median sternotomy: a review of 7,949 consecutive operative procedures. *Ann Thorac Surg* 40:214, 1985.
83. Puskas JD, Winston AD, Wright CE, et al: Stroke after coronary artery operation: incidence, correlates, outcome, and cost. *Ann Thorac Surg* 69:1053, 2000.
84. Vander Salm TJ, Cereda JM, Cutler BS: Brachial plexus injury following median sternotomy. *J Thorac Cardiovasc Surg* 80:447, 1980.
85. Seyfer AE, Grammer NY, Bogumill GP, et al: Upper extremity neuropathies after cardiac surgery. *J Hand Surg (Am)* 10:16, 1985.
86. Kuroda Y, Uchimoto R, Kaieda R, et al: Central nervous system complications after cardiac surgery: a comparison between coronary artery bypass grafting and valve surgery. *Anesth Analg* 76:222, 1993.
87. Smith LW, Dimsdale JE: Postcardiotomy delirium: conclusions after 25 years? *Am J Psychiatry* 146:452, 1983.
88. Summers WK: Psychiatric sequelae to cardiotomy. *J Cardiovasc Surg* 20:471, 1979.
89. Egleston CV, Wood AE, Gorey TF, et al: Gastrointestinal complications after cardiac surgery. *Ann R Coll Surg Engl* 75:52, 1993.
90. Berger MM, Berger-Gryllaki M, Wiesel PH, et al: Intestinal absorption in patients after cardiac surgery. *Crit Care Med* 28:2217, 2000.
91. Svenson LG, Decker G, Kinsley RB: A prospective study of hyperamylasemia and pancreatitis after cardiopulmonary bypass. *Ann Thorac Surg* 39:409, 1985.
92. Rattner DW, Guz Y, Vlahakes GJ: Hyperamylasemia after cardiac surgery. Incidence, significance, and management. *Ann Surg* 209:279, 1989.
93. Van den Berge G, Wouters P, Weekers F, et al: Intensive insulin therapy in critically ill patients. *N Engl J Med* 345:1359, 2001.
94. NICE-SUGAR Study Investigators, Finfer S, Chittock DR, Su SY. Intensive versus conventional glucose control in critically ill patients. *N Engl J Med* 360:1283, 2009.
95. Tobin MJ, Yang KL: A prospective study of indexes predicting the outcome of trials of weaning from mechanical ventilation. *N Engl J Med* 324:1445, 1991.

CHAPTER 149 ■ NONCARDIAC SURGERY IN THE CARDIAC PATIENT

STEVEN B. EDELSTEIN AND SCOTT W. BYRAM

Much has been written regarding the management of the patient with significant coronary artery disease presenting for noncardiac surgery. As the patient population in the United States continues to age, the issues surrounding risk assessment, perioperative optimization of drug regimens, and evidence-based improvement in overall outcome will persist. This chapter will focus on the issues of risk assessment and the current state of perioperative medical management for the cardiac patient presenting for intermediate- to high-risk surgical procedures.

PATHOPHYSIOLOGY OF PERIOPERATIVE CARDIAC COMPLICATIONS

It is well known that nonfatal perioperative myocardial infarction (MI) is an independent risk factor for subsequent MI and cardiac death within 6 months [1]. It has also been reported that those patients who have cardiac arrest after noncardiac surgery have a significantly elevated hospital mortality rate that has been reported as high as 65% [2].

Much research has been performed to elucidate the etiology of cardiac complications. A recent review of the subject matter by Grayburn and Hillis [3] identified some of the major issues and pathophysiologic changes that surround perioperative cardiac complications. It has become clear that plaque rupture occurs in about half of all perioperative myocardial infarctions [4]. Autopsy series also indicate that acute coronary thrombosis contributes to approximately one third of perioperative ischemic morbidity [5]. In fact, a study that involved patients who underwent coronary angiography prior to vascular surgery revealed that the majority of nonfatal myocardial infarctions occurred in arteries without high-grade stenosis [6].

The remainder of ischemic events appears to be the result of an imbalance between myocardial oxygen supply and consumption in the presence of existing coronary artery disease. It is well known that myocardial supply/demand can be adversely affected by anemia, hypotension leading to tachycardia, hypertension (resulting from postoperative pain or withdrawal of anesthesia), or shifts in intravascular volume. Also, alterations in the inflammatory and coagulation cascades can ultimately play a role in the development of myocardial ischemic events [3,7,8].

Obviously, the causes of perioperative myocardial infarction/ischemia are complex and not clearly elucidated. Devereaux et al. [9] have developed a summary of potential triggers for perioperative elevation in troponin levels, arterial thrombosis, and fatal myocardial infarction. It is also important to note that the majority of perioperative myocardial infarctions occur 1 to 4 days following noncardiac surgery [10] (Fig. 149.1).

DIAGNOSIS OF PERIOPERATIVE MYOCARDIAL INFARCTION IN NONCARDIAC SURGERY

A problem exists when discussing the issues of myocardial infarction and noncardiac surgery. Currently there is no consensus on diagnostic criteria as to what constitutes a perioperative MI in patients undergoing noncardiac surgery. Devereaux et al. [11], to overcome this issue, formulated a proposed diagnostic criterion for perioperative MI. The criteria were adapted from a consensus document of the European Society of Cardiology/American College of Cardiology (ESC/ACC) [12]. These criteria have been summarized in Table 149.1. The criteria rely on biochemical markers such as cardiac troponin, creatine kinase MB (CK-MB), and other objective measures such as

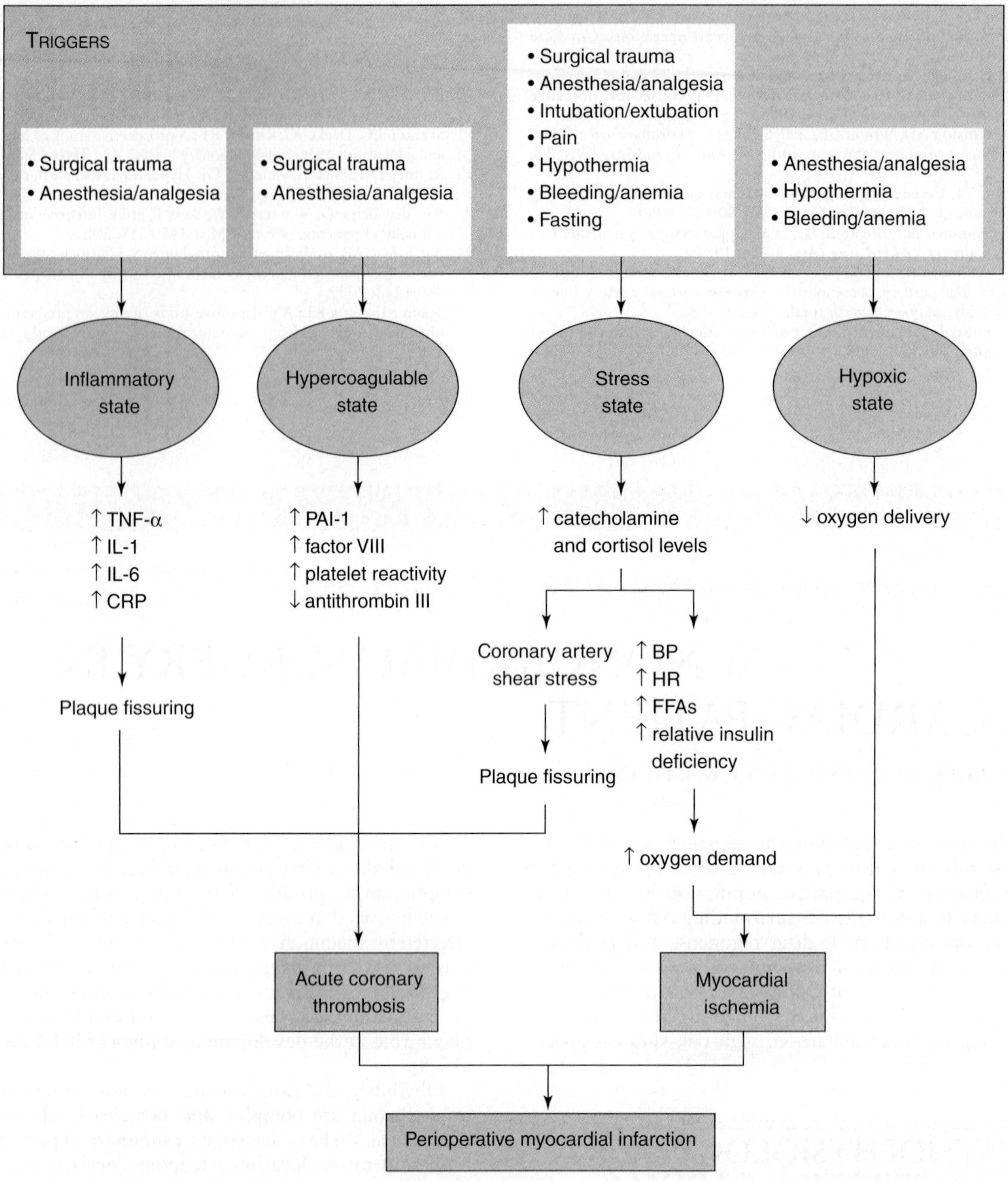

FIGURE 149.1. Potential triggers of states associated with perioperative elevations in troponin levels, arterial thrombosis, and fatal myocardial infarction. BP, blood pressure; CRP, C-reactive protein; FFAs, free fatty acids; HR, heart rate; IL, interleukin; PAI-1, plasminogen activator inhibiter-1; TFN-*α*, tumor necrosis factor-*α*. [Reprinted from Devereaux PJ, Goldman L, Cook DJ, et al: Perioperative cardiac events in patients undergoing noncardiac surgery: a review of the magnitude of the problem, the pathophysiology of the events and methods to estimate and communicate risk. *CMAJ* 173(6):627–634, with permission. © 2000 CMA Media Inc.]

electrocardiogram (ECG) changes and echocardiographic evidence of ischemia.

HISTORY OF RISK ASSESSMENT

For many years, the goal has been to identify a risk assessment tool that would help to identify patients at risk for perioperative cardiac complications. Once identification of this patient subset has been made, interventions could then be performed to reduce the incidence of perioperative myocardial ischemia and infarction [13].

Dripps Index of the American Society of Anesthesiologists

Since the 1960s, the desire to find the optimal tool of risk assessment has been present. The American Society of Anesthesiologists (ASA) developed the Dripps Index as a way not only to identify risk among patient groups, but also to provide a common framework and communication device that could easily be distributed among differing medical specialties [14]. In 1970, Vacanti et al. [15] used the index to predict cardiac death within 48 hours of surgery. Within the five physical status

TABLE 149.1

PROPOSED DIAGNOSTIC CRITERIA FOR PERIOPERATIVE MYOCARDIAL INFARCTION IN PATIENTS UNDERGOING NONCARDIAC SURGERY

The diagnosis of perioperative MI requires any one of the following criterion:

Criterion 1: A typical rise in the troponin level or a typical fall of an elevated troponin level detected at its peak after surgery in a patient without documented alternative explanation for an elevated troponin level (e.g., pulmonary embolism); or a rapid rise and fall of CK-MB only if troponin measurement is unavailable.[a]

This criterion requires that one of the following criteria must also exist:

- Ischemic signs of symptoms (e.g., chest, arm, or jaw discomfort, shortness of breath, pulmonary edema)
- Development of pathological Q waves on ECG
- ECG changes indicative of ischemia
- Coronary artery intervention
- New or presumed new cardiac wall motion abnormality on ECG, or new or presumed new fixed defect on radionuclide imaging

Criterion 2: Pathological findings of an acute or healing MI

Criterion 3: Development of new pathological Q waves on an ECG if troponin levels were not obtained or were obtained at times that could have missed the clinical event

[a]Because CK-MB is both less sensitive and less specific in the perioperative setting compared with other settings and compared with troponin levels, it should be used for diagnostic purposes only when troponin levels are not obtainable.
CK-MB, creatine kinase; MB, isoenzyme; ECG, electrocardiogram; MI, myocardial infarction.
From Devereaux PJ, Goldman L, Yusef S, et al: Surveillance and prevention of major perioperative ischemic cardiac events in patients undergoing noncardiac surgery: a review. *CMAJ* 173(7):779–788, with permission. © 2000 CMA Media Inc.

grades identified, perioperative mortality rates range from 0% for ASA status 1 to 9.4% for ASA status 5. However, some of the major drawbacks to the utilization of the ASA score are that it was developed prior to multivariate clinical prediction rules, has limited utility, is very subjective, and is not uniformly reproducible [16].

Goldman Risk Assessment Tool

One of the original cardiac risk assessment tools developed in the 1970s by Goldman was an elaborate attempt to identify those patients at undue risk [17]. Risk assessment was based on several clinical variables. Goldman identified nine independent variables associated with perioperative cardiac events. These are included in Table 149.2, and consist of variables ranging from advanced age to the presence of significant valvular heart disease.

Each variable was assigned specific points and the patients were divided into risk class depending on the number of points generated. The highest classification—class IV (more than 26 points) was associated with a 78% incidence of major cardiac complications in the perioperative period. However, the drawback to use of the tool was the cumbersome nature, making the utilization of the Goldman risk assessment tool somewhat impractical.

TABLE 149.2

GOLDMAN'S NINE INDEPENDENT VARIABLES ASSOCIATED WITH PERIOPERATIVE CARDIAC EVENTS

- Age over 70 years
- Myocardial infarction in the preceding 6 months
- Preoperative third heart sound or jugular venous distention
- Significant valvular aortic stenosis
- Emergency surgery
- Intraperitoneal, intrathoracic, or aortic operation
- More than 5 premature ventricular beats per minute documented at any time before operation
- Rhythm other than sinus or the presence of atrial premature contractions on preoperative electrocardiogram
- One or more markers of poor general medical condition

From Goldman L, Caldera DL, Nussbaum SR, et al: Multifactorial index of cardiac risk in noncardiac surgical procedures. *N Engl J Med* 297:845–850, 1977.

Detsky Modification of the Goldman Risk Assessment Tool

In 1986 Detsky attempted to modify the Goldman risk assessment tool by the addition of angina severity and a history of recent pulmonary edema [18]. Broad categories included the variables of coronary artery disease, Canadian Cardiovascular Society Angina Classification, alveolar pulmonary edema, suspected critical aortic stenosis, arrhythmias, poor general medical status, emergency surgery, and age 70 or older. However, just as with Goldman, this risk assessment tool was viewed to be exceedingly cumbersome. It appears that both indices may not have sufficient discriminate power to identify significant coronary artery disease in patients at the lower end of the spectrum of clinical risk [19] and both indices have been refuted or supported by an equal number of studies [20].

Adding to the controversy has been a prospective cohort study that compared the varying risk indices for patients undergoing noncardiac surgery. Gilbert et al. [16] compared 2,035 patients referred for consultation prior to noncardiac surgery and four risk indices: the Dripps Index of the ASA, the original cardiac risk index described by Goldman, the modified Detsky (which had been modified in 1997 by the American College of Physicians by stratifying patients into three risk groups) [21], and the Canadian Cardiovascular Society (CCS) Index for angina level [22]. The most striking finding of the study was that existing cardiac risk prediction methods had a generally poor degree of accuracy.

Eagle Criteria

Eagle et al. [23], while assessing the validity of dipyridamole-thallium stress testing in vascular patients, developed another set of risk criteria for patients undergoing major vascular surgery. The group found five clinical predictors of postoperative cardiac events. These included: presence of Q waves on resting ECG, history of angina, history of ventricular ectopy requiring treatment, diabetes mellitus requiring medical treatment, and age above 70 years. Also on logistic regression, the group noted two independent dipyridamole thallium test predictors of ischemic events that included thallium redistribution and ischemic ECG changes during or after pharmacologic stressing.

Lee Revised Cardiac Risk Index Stratification System

In an attempt to simply the Goldman index, Lee et al. [24] developed the Revised Cardiac Risk Index (RCRI) Stratification System. The RCRI for the first time identified six independent risk predictors associated with cardiac morbidity and noncardiac surgery. These included: high-risk surgery (examples included intraperitoneal, intrathoracic, or suprainguinal vascular reconstruction), a history of ischemic heart disease (excluding previous revascularization), a history of congestive heart failure (CHF), a history of cerebrovascular disease, preoperative treatment with insulin, and a preoperative serum creatinine level more than 2.0 mg per dL (greater than 177 μmol per L).

Cardiac events were determined to be myocardial infarction, cardiac arrest, pulmonary edema, or complete heart block. Four classifications were noted in which risk factors ranged from 0 to 3 or more and correlated to event rate:

- Class I (0 risk factors)—event rate 0.4% (95% confidence interval)
- Class II (1 risk factor)—rate 0.9%
- Class III (2 risk factors)—rate 6.6%
- Class IV (3 or more risk factors)—rate 11.0%

The RCRI has been the most widely accepted risk index, and Romero and de Virgilio [20] have proposed utilizing the RCRI to identify patients who should be treated with strategies to reduce oxygen consumption rather than undergo additional noninvasive testing. They based their recommendations on comments elicited by Bodenheimer [25], who felt that improved outcomes were more likely a result from controlling postoperative myocardial oxygen demand than additional risk stratification.

Miscellaneous Risk Assessment Tools

Other attempts at risk stratification and adjustment are mentioned in the literature. In 2004, Atherly et al. [26] compared the National Surgical Quality Improvement Program (NSQIP), the DxCG, and the Charlson Comorbidity Index. The NSQIP [27] is based on a medical record abstraction of 45 preoperative and 17 intraoperative factors. Factors are multiplied by weights drawn from a model developed using 41,360 patients from the Veteran Affairs Health Care System. Some of the major components of the NSQIP specific to mortality include: ASA class, ventilator dependence, emergency case, age, abnormal albumin, ascites, complexity score, and contaminated wound [28]. In addition to those mentioned earlier, functional status, a history of chronic obstructive pulmonary disease, anemia (hematocrit 38% or less), and elevated white blood cell counts (11,000 or more) are important predictors of morbidity. The ultimate risk score represents the probability of individual patient mortality.

The DxCG uses *International Classification of Disease* (ICD-9) codes, sex, and age to assign a continuous risk score, and the Charlson Comorbidity Index (CCI) was developed to predict empirically the probability of 1-year mortality. The CCI contains 19 categories of comorbidities drawn from the ICD-9 codes. Each of the categories has a weight, which indicates an increase in the risk for 1-year mortality and scores range from 0 to 6.

Atherly et al. [26] found substantial disagreement in the risk assessment calculated by the three methodologies. A weak association was noted between the CCI and DxCG, but neither correlated well with the NSQIP. Overall, the NSQIP was felt to be the best predictor of surgical mortality.

AMERICAN COLLEGE OF CARDIOLOGY/AMERICAN HEART ASSOCIATION TASK FORCE: PRACTICE GUIDELINES ON PERIOPERATIVE CARDIOVASCULAR EVALUATION FOR NONCARDIAC SURGERY

Practice guidelines serve the purpose of putting forth recommendations based on critically evaluated studies with special emphasis on blinded, randomized, placebo-controlled trial studies. The American College of Cardiology/American Heart Association (ACC/AHA) Practice Guidelines on Perioperative Cardiovascular Evaluation for Noncardiac Surgery [29], most recently revised in 2007 (30), begins with the opening statement that the overriding theme of the guidelines was that preoperative intervention was rarely necessary simply to lower the risk of surgery unless such intervention was indicated irrespective of the preoperative context. The desire of the guideline was also to integrate the clinical determinants of risk, the risk of the surgical procedure, and the role of testing into a cohesive format. In addition, the goal of the preoperative consultation was to provide short- and long-term assessment of cardiac risk and avoid unnecessary testing.

Clinical Predictors

One of the major changes in the 2007 revision of the ACC/AHA guidelines is the manner in which risk is assessed. In the 2002 version of the guidelines, risk factors were divided into three groups: major, intermediate, and minor clinical predictors [29]. With the new revision, the minor clinical predictors were removed from the algorithm because, although they may signify risk for coronary disease, they have not been shown to independently increase risk for perioperative cardiac complication [30].

Also changed in 2007, the *major clinical predictors* have been renamed *active cardiac conditions* (Table 149.3). Because of the increasing use of the Revised Cardiac Risk Index created by Lee et al. [24], the committee chose to replace the *intermediate clinical predictors* with five of six risk factors identified by Lee's group. These five risk factors are: history of ischemic heart disease, compensated heart failure, history of cerebrovascular disease, diabetes mellitus, and renal insufficiency. The sixth risk factor identified by Lee et al., type of surgery, is addressed elsewhere in the new guidelines.

Functional Capacity

The guidelines also focused significantly on the concept of functional capacity. Functional capacity is best expressed in metabolic equivalent (MET) levels that correlate with specific activities. Basic energy expenditure for activities of daily living (e.g., eating, walking) are around 1 to 4 METs, while strenuous exercise is often more than 10 METs [31]. It has been shown in prior studies that patients unable to obtain a 4-MET demand do poorly in the perioperative period [32] as well as in the long term [33].

Risk of Surgical Procedure

Different surgical procedures are clearly associated with varying amounts of hemodynamic stress. For example, application and release of an aortic cross clamp during abdominal aortic aneurysm repair induces far more physiologic insult than

TABLE 149.3

ACTIVE CARDIAC CONDITIONS FOR WHICH THE PATIENT SHOULD UNDERGO EVALUATION AND TREATMENT BEFORE NONCARDIAC SURGERY (CLASS I, LEVEL OF EVIDENCE: B)

Condition	Examples
Unstable coronary syndromes	Unstable or severe angina[a] (CCS class III or IV[b])
	Recent MI[c]
Decompensated HF (NYHA functional class IV; worsening or new-onset HF)	
Significant arrhythmias	High-grade atrioventricular block Mobitz II atrioventricular block Third-degree atrioventricular heart block Symptomatic ventricular arrhythmias Supraventricular arrhythmias (including atrial fibrillation) with uncontrolled ventricular rate (HR >100 beats per minute at rest) Symptomatic bradycardia Newly recognized ventricular tachycardia
Severe valvular disease	Severe aortic stenosis (mean pressure gradient >40 mm Hg, aortic valve area <1.0 cm^2, or symptomatic) Symptomatic mitral stenosis (progressive dyspnea on exertion, exertional presyncope, or HF)

[a]According to Campeau.[9]
[b]May include "stable" angina in patients who are unusually sedentary.
[c]The American College of Cardiology National Database Library defines recent MI as more than 7 days but less than or equal to 1 month (within 30 days).
CCS indicates Canadian Cardiovascular Society; HF, heart failure; HR, heart rate; MI, myocardial infarction; NYHA, New York Heart Association.
Reprinted from Fleisher et al: ACC/AHA 2007 Guidelines on Perioperative Cardiovascular Evaluation and Care for Noncardiac Surgery: Executive Summary. *J Am Coll Cardiol* 50(17):1714, 2007, with permission from Elsevier.

cataract surgery does. Furthermore, recent evidence suggests that major vascular surgery (excluding carotid endarterectomy) may be associated with more than 5% risk for perioperative cardiac death or nonfatal myocardial infarction [30]. With this in mind, the most recent revision of the ACC/AHA guidelines classifies vascular surgery separately as the highest risk group [30] (Table 149.4). Procedures associated with a 1% to 5% cardiac risk, such as orthopedic and intraperitoneal surgeries, are classified as intermediate risk. Most ambulatory surgeries are associated with less than 1% cardiac risk and are classified as low risk.

TABLE 149.4

CARDIAC RISK STRATIFICATION FOR NONCARDIAC SURGERY[a]

Risk stratification	Procedure examples
Vascular (reported cardiac risk often >5%)	Aortic and other major vascular surgery Peripheral vascular surgery
Intermediate (reported cardiac risk generally 1%–5%)	Intraperitoneal and intrathoracic surgery Carotid endarterectomy Head and neck surgery Orthopedic surgery Prostate surgery
Low[b] (reported cardiac risk generally <1%)	Endoscopic procedures Superficial procedure Cataract surgery Breast surgery Ambulatory surgery

[a]Combined incidence of cardiac death and nonfatal myocardial infarction.
[b]These procedures do not generally require further preoperative cardiac testing.
Reprinted from Fleisher et al: ACC/AHA 2007 Guidelines on Perioperative Cardiovascular Evaluation and Care for Noncardiac Surgery: Executive Summary. *J Am Coll Cardiol* 50(17):1717, 2007, with permission from Elsevier.

American College of Cardiology/American Heart Association Five Step Algorithm

In the 2007 revision, the authors generated a five-step algorithm for preoperative risk assessment (Fig. 149.2). This was a definite improvement from the somewhat confusing 3-part, 8-step algorithm published in 2002. The simplified recommendations were necessary considering the abysmal (as low as 21%) implementation of the 2002 guidelines [34]. These new guidelines reflect the authors' sentiment in their opening statement that cardiac intervention is not indicated unless it would be performed regardless of a preoperative context. In addition, the algorithm offers recommendations for noninvasive testing and treatment with beta-blockers for selected patients.

Despite these improvements, many authors are still critical of the algorithm. Brett argues that the guidelines are still too ambiguous, referring to the final point of the decision tree: "consider testing if it will change management" [35]. He also makes a point that sometimes noninvasive testing helps patients weigh the risks and benefits of truly elective surgery. In any case, the new algorithm will likely decrease the number of noninvasive test ordered, thus reducing cost and delay in performing elective procedures.

Preoperative Screening ECG

Not long ago it was commonplace to see electrocardiograms in the chart for most surgical patients as part of a preoperative workup. Because these extensive workups were often fruitless, and some testing caused more harm than good, the ASA assembled a task force to develop a practice advisory for

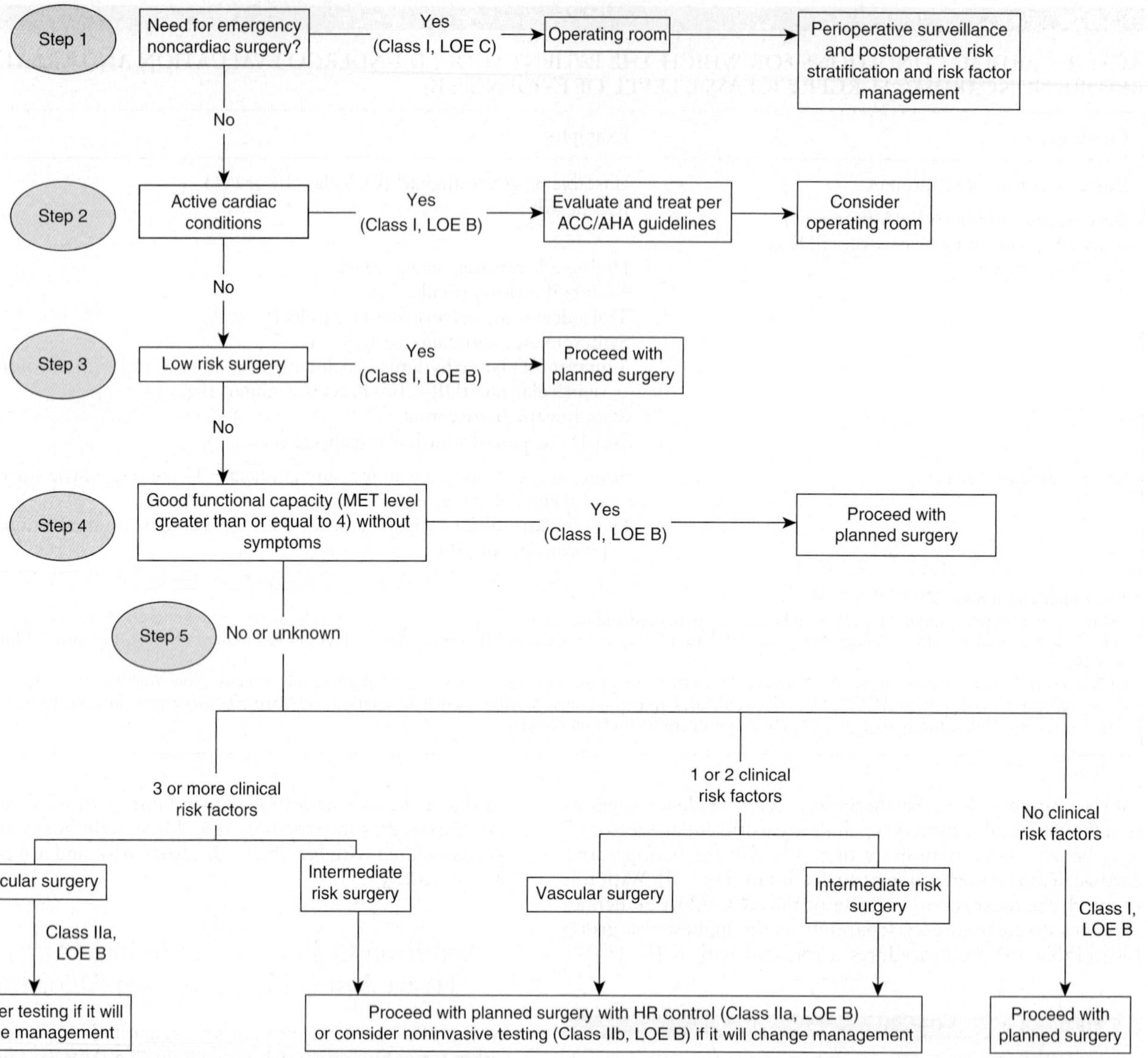

FIGURE 149.2. Cardiac evaluation and care algorithm for noncardiac surgery based on active conditions, known cardiovascular disease, or cardiac risk factors for patients 50 years of age or older. (Reprinted from Fleisher et al: ACC/AHA 2007 Guidelines on Perioperative Cardiovascular Evaluation and Care for Noncardiac Surgery: Executive Summary. *J Am Coll Cardiol* 50(17):1716, 2007, with permission from Elsevier.)

preanesthetic evaluation [36]. The task force cited that few screening ECG findings resulted in changes in clinical management. They also stated that based on evidence, age alone may not be an indication for ECG. Proponents of screening ECGs argue that these studies may identify patients with coronary disease not recognized by clinical history. Moreover, these newly identified patients could then be further tested or medically managed with beta-blockade. However, this argument may be flawed for several reasons. First of all, a positive ECG in an asymptomatic patient would not alter further testing if the practitioner uses the ACC/AHA algorithm [30]. Second, according to van Klei et al., ECG abnormalities, including left and right bundle branch blocks, were no more predictive of postoperative MI than history alone [37]. Finally, starting beta-blocker therapy is probably not indicated in otherwise asymptomatic patients [30]. Fleisher, however, does make one argument that may be valid for obtaining preoperative ECG [38]. Without a preoperative ECG, the first occasion that the ECG may be seen as abnormal is when the patient is in the operating room prior to induction. Under these circumstances, it may be beneficial to compare the new findings with an old ECG to identify the acuity of the changes and determine whether or not to proceed. Currently, however, the ACC/AHA states that preoperative screening ECGs are indicated only for vascular surgeries and for certain patient populations having intermediate-risk surgery (Table 149.5) [30].

PREOPERATIVE NONINVASIVE CARDIAC TESTING

As mentioned earlier, part of the ACC/AHA guidelines [29] was to help direct the clinician as to which patients should undergo preoperative testing. The guidelines, however, did not elucidate which noninvasive testing regimen should be undertaken. Exactly which method of evaluation is chosen is again another source of controversy. Testing the low-risk patient undergoing low-risk surgery is ultimately an exercise in futility and an overall waste of time and resources. High-risk patients undergoing high-risk surgery will most likely benefit from invasive testing [39]. The question arises as to what to do with the patient

TABLE 149.5

INDICATIONS FOR PREOPERATIVE RESTING ECG

Benefit >>> Risk (class I)
1. Patients with at least one clinical risk factor (coronary heart disease, history of CVA, renal insufficiency, diabetes mellitus) who are undergoing vascular surgery
2. Patients with known coronary heart disease, peripheral arterial disease, or cerebrovascular disease who are undergoing intermediate-risk surgery

Benefit >> Risk (class IIa)
1. Patients with no clinical risk factors who are undergoing vascular surgery

Benefit ≥ Risk (class IIb)
1. Patients with at least one clinical risk factor who are undergoing intermediate-risk surgery

Risk > Benefit (class III)
1. Asymptomatic patients undergoing low-risk surgery

Reprinted from Fleisher et al: ACC/AHA 2007 Guidelines on Perioperative Cardiovascular Evaluation and Care for Noncardiac Surgery: Executive Summary. *J Am Coll Cardiol* 50(17):1711, 2007, with permission from Elsevier.

with intermediate clinical predictors and needs intermediate- to high-risk surgery [40].

The purpose of noninvasive testing is to accrue information that adds to that already provided by whichever cardiac risk index was implemented. Ideally, it will not lead to harmful delays but rather to proven therapy to reduce risk [3].

There are some generally accepted principles regarding what exactly is an effective screening test [36]. These principles should be kept in mind when assessing any test:

1. Accuracy of test: The test must be able to detect the target condition earlier than without screening and with sufficient accuracy to avoid producing large numbers of false–positive and false–negative results.
2. Effectiveness of early detection: Screening for and testing persons who have early disease should improve the likelihood of favorable health outcomes (e.g., reduced disease-specific morbidity and mortality) compared to treating patients when they present with signs and symptoms of the disease.

Exercise Stress Testing

Exercise stress testing is a well-established mechanism of assessment that allows the identification or absence of myocardial ischemia while the patient is undergoing physical exertion. The purpose of the examination is to elevate the myocardial oxygen consumption to a rate in which demand outweighs supply, leading to ischemic changes on ECG. The inherent drawback of this method of assessment is that it relies on patient participation. At times, due to deconditioning or medical issues, such as claudication, the patient cannot reach target heart rate and thus ischemic episodes may be missed.

Unfortunately in meta-analysis, the mean sensitivity of exercise ECG testing for the prediction of multivessel coronary artery disease has been reported to be 81% (range 40% to 100%) with a mean specificity of 66% (range 17% to 100%) [41]. The meta-analysis also reconfirmed that the sensitivity of the examination was adversely affected in patients who could not reach maximal heart rate, especially vascular surgery patients in which approximately 50% could not reach the target rate.

In addition to the failure to reach target heart rate, other limitations of exercise testing exist. These include ECG changes on resting ECG, the presence of left bundle branch block, failure in determining the extent of myocardial ischemia, and lack of information regarding left ventricular function [42].

Myocardial Perfusion Imaging

To overcome some of the inherent problems of exercise stress testing, pharmacologic stress myocardial perfusion imaging was developed [43]. This examination consists of the administration of a vasodilating agent such as adenosine or dipyridamole to induce vasodilation that would parallel the effect of exercise on coronary anatomy. In addition, a radionuclide is administered, such as thallium-201. Images are obtained over time and positive examinations are those in which areas of initial filling defects resolve, or undergo redistribution of thallium, during the rest phase.

Several complications and contraindications exist with the use of adenosine and dipyridamole. Since they are potent vasodilators, these agents are obviously contraindicated in those patients with preexisting hypotension and ongoing symptoms of unstable angina. Other relative contraindications to administration of adenosine include high-degree atrioventricular block, bronchospastic disease, and atrial arrhythmia disorders such as sick sinus syndrome.

Eagle et al. found that patients with one or two risk factors for coronary artery disease, and redistribution on dipyridamole thallium had a 29% cardiac event rate versus a 3.2% rate in patients without redistribution. The sensitivity of the examination, however, appears to be in detecting the presence or absence or coronary artery disease, not ischemia [23].

In addition it has been reported that the accuracy and positive likelihood ratio for dipyridamole thallium stress testing is low and that the examination does not provide independent prognostic value beyond clinical risk stratification [44]. Other prospective blinded studies confirmed a lack of association between reversible defects on dipyridamole thallium and adverse cardiac events in patients undergoing elective vascular surgery (of note, these studies excluded low-risk patients undergoing vascular surgery) [45,46].

In the study by de Virgilio et al. [46], the adverse cardiac event rate was 13.8% for patients with a reversible defect on thallium testing versus 9.8% for those who did not have a reversible defect ($p = 0.70$). The adverse event rate in patients with two or more reversible defects was 12.5% versus 11.1% in patients with fewer than two reversible defects. Sensitivity with two or more defects was 11%, with a specificity of 90%. The overall positive and negative predictive values were 12.5% and 89%, respectively. The authors concluded that since there was no demonstrable correlation between dipyridamole thallium and perioperative adverse cardiac events, one could not recommend the test as a screening tool prior to vascular surgery.

Another imaging study is dipyridamole technetium-99m sestamibi testing. Technetium-99m sestamibi is a radiotracer that differs from thallium-201 and ultimately allows for acquisition of higher resolution tomographic cardiac images. Stratmann et al. [47] studied 229 patients scheduled for vascular surgery who underwent sestamibi testing. Of those enrolled, 197 underwent surgery within 3 months of the initial examination with an overall cardiac event rate of 5%. The perioperative cardiac event rate between those with normal, abnormal, or reversible sestamibi images was not clinically significant; however, abnormal and reversible sestamibi images were independent multivariable predictors of increased risk of late cardiac events.

Dobutamine Stress Echocardiography

Dobutamine stress echocardiography (DSE) was developed as a tool for assessing the presence of coronary artery disease and was reported by Berthe et al. [48] in 1986. Essentially the examination is composed of the administration of a pharmacologic inotropic agent (e.g., dobutamine), which is designed to increase heart rate and myocardial contractility, thus increasing myocardial oxygen consumption. In the presence of coronary artery disease, demand will overcome supply and myocardial dysfunction will be present. Myocardial dysfunction will be evident by echocardiography, manifested by areas of hypokinesis, akinesis, or dyskinesis. The development of new wall motion abnormalities following dobutamine administration is considered an indication of significant coronary artery disease [49].

When dobutamine stress echocardiography and dipyridamole-thallium testing were compared in the same patient population, they appeared to have comparable specificity and sensitivity [50]. A subsequence meta-analysis study revealed a 9% incidence of perioperative myocardial infarction in patients with reversible ischemia or regional wall abnormalities in one or more areas [51].

The Dutch Echocardiographic Cardiac Risk Evaluation Applying Stress Echocardiography (DECREASE) Study Group performed a large retrospective study with results released in 2001. The study noted that the adverse event rate was 10.6% in patients with three or more cardiac risk factors and five or more segments of new wall motion abnormalities (NWMAs) versus a 2% adverse event rate in patients without NWMAs. It is also interesting to note that the study reported perioperative death and myocardial infarction rates of 6.5%, 10%, and 16% in patients with respective scores on a modified Revised Cardiac Index of 3, 4, and 5 who were treated with beta-blockade but also had ischemia on DSE [52]. A drawback to the utilization of echocardiography was that the study showed that DSE did not add incremental value in low- or medium-risk patients (score of 0 to 2 on Revised Cardiac Risk Index) [3].

Although the results of this retrospective study were encouraging, there are other studies that tend to question the validity of DSE for preoperative evaluation. It appears that echocardiography has limited prognostic value as a routine test. Rohde et al. [53] reported that an abnormal echocardiogram with any degree of systolic dysfunction, moderate to severe left ventricle hypertrophy, moderate to severe mitral regurgitation, or aortic gradient of 20 mm Hg or higher provided a sensitivity of 80%, specificity of 52%, positive predictive value of 12%, and negative predictive value of 97%. However, severe left ventricular (LV) dysfunction compared to mild–moderate LV dysfunction did not have a strong association with cardiogenic pulmonary edema and MI. Thus, given the heterogeneity of findings, it appears that echocardiography adds little to risk models.

Another retrospective study in 2002 by Morgan et al. [54] examined the utility of dobutamine stress echocardiography in 85 preoperative patients in accordance with the ACC/AHA guidelines. The DSE was positive in 4 patients (4.7%), negative in 74 (87.1%), and nondiagnostic in 7 (8.2%). The DSE obtained in 48 patients with a history of diabetes mellitus (DM), mild angina, or "minor clinical predictors" produced only negative results. Of the four positive patients, three underwent angiography and one underwent coronary artery bypass grafting (CABG) prior to surgery. No patient had any perioperative morbidity related to myocardial ischemia. Morgan et al. [54] went further to recommend that DSE is recommended in patients with:

1. Intermediate clinical predictors (one or more) [prior MI, compensated CHF, DM with mild angina] with poor functional capacity less than 4 METs
2. Intermediate clinical predictors (one or more) with moderate to excellent functional capacity greater than 4 METs and high surgical risk and unable to perform exercise stress test

Grayburn and Hillis [3] went on to state more strongly that the test had limited value given that the likelihood ratio of a positive test report was low and thus had a low positive predictive value. The authors strongly felt that patients with positive test results are often subjected to further evaluation that may cause an unnecessary delay in noncardiac surgery.

A recent study by Kertai et al. [55] used a meta-analytic approach adjusting for reported variability in test performance between the individual studies. The results revealed that there was clinical utility for the use of dobutamine stress echo in perioperative risk assessment. Overall sensitivity and specificity of the test were found to be high, 85% and 70%, respectively. The conclusion by the authors was that the predictive value of a positive DSE for the composite endpoint of cardiac death and myocardial infarction was significantly increased. However, much work is still in progress regarding the overall utility of DSE and cardiac risk assessment.

So is DSE better than nuclear scintigraphy (thallium imaging)? Beattie et al. [56] addressed this question with a recent meta-analysis. The authors felt that the meta-analysis contained the statistical power to demonstrate that DSE had better negative predictive characteristics than thallium imaging (TI). Although a moderate to large perfusion defect by either DSE or TI predicted postoperative MI and death, they concluded that DSE was superior to TI in predicting postoperative cardiac events.

What about the patient with a negative examination? The meta-analysis [56] also revealed that a negative DSE reduced the probability of MI or death. It was evident that there were fewer false negative DSE results. And what about the patient with moderate or multiple defects? Moderate or multiple defects on DSE were noted to be at least as accurate as the demonstration of a large perfusion defect on TI. However, the group's final conclusion was that a negative test did not reliably confirm less risk of a perioperative cardiac event, although a positive DSE was two times more predictive than a positive TI.

Invasive Cardiac Evaluation

Once a decision has been made regarding preoperative invasive cardiac evaluation, either based on clinical history or noninvasive testing, several questions remain. Namely, what is to be done with the information obtained? Is a surgical or percutaneous intervention warranted? Will it make a difference?

There are clearly some indications in which invasive testing are warranted. These include recent myocardial infarction with residual angina, angina unresponsive to medical therapy, unstable angina, and proposed intermediate-risk or high-risk noncardiac surgery after equivocal noninvasive test results [39].

Essentially, the original ACC/AHA guidelines [29] did not recommend coronary angiography as risk stratification in patients undergoing noncardiac surgery; however, they did recommend angiography if indications for angiography independent of planned surgery were present [40]. However, confusion persists regarding the role of preoperative angiography and subsequent preoperative intervention to reduce risk of noncardiac surgery.

Role of Coronary Artery Bypass Grafting Prior to Noncardiac Surgery

In the 1980s, an initial study by Hertzer et al. [57] revealed that the cumulative cardiac mortality rate at 10 years was markedly increased for patients with suspected but uncorrected coronary artery disease as compared with those patients without evidence of coronary artery disease or those patients who had undergone myocardial revascularization. This ultimately led to the belief that aggressive coronary revascularizations prior to vascular operations were warranted.

A series of studies by Gagnon et al. [58] and Allen et al. [59] also recommended prophylactic CABG or angioplasty prior to noncardiac surgery. Nielsen et al. [60] found in the early 1990s that patients who had a CABG operation appeared to have a low rate of perioperative cardiac complications. This observation was further enhanced by Eagle et al. [61] who used the Coronary Artery Surgery Study (CASS) registry. After reviewing the data, the group found that patients who underwent major vascular, abdominal, thoracic, or head/neck surgery after previous CABG had fewer perioperative deaths and myocardial infarctions than patients receiving medical therapy.

Ultimately, these observational studies became the basis for the ACC/AHA guideline recommendations that invasive testing for risk stratification was not indicated in patients who had a CABG surgery within 5 years and were currently without symptoms [29]. Grayburn and Hillis [3] have strongly voiced opposition to the utilization of CABG in the *asymptomatic* patient. They felt that the morbidity and mortality associated with the CABG procedure, which includes nonfatal MI, death, stroke, and cognitive dysfunction, outweighed any benefit.

The group also held the valid viewpoint that recovery from CABG would cause a significant delay in obtaining the noncardiac surgery. In fact, as indicated by Mason et al. [62], coronary angiography appears to carry a 0.3% risk of mortality, while CABG has been reported to have an operative risk of 3% overall and approximately 5% in the patient with peripheral vascular disease.

One of the stronger studies in support of avoiding coronary artery revascularization before noncardiac surgery was published from the CARP (Coronary Artery Revascularization Prophylaxis) trial [63]. This was a multicenter trial that randomly assigned patients who were at increased risk and had clinically significant coronary artery disease to either undergo revascularization or no revascularization before elective major vascular surgery. The major end point of the study was long-term mortality. A group of 510 patients out of 5,859 were deemed eligible, with 258 assigned to preoperative revascularization (CABG or percutaneous angioplasty) and 240 assigned to medical management.

The study revealed that at 2.7 years, mortality in the revascularization group was 22% and in the nonrevascularization group 23%. Positive postoperative myocardial infarction (as documented by elevated troponin levels) was 12% in revascularization group and 14% in nonrevascularization group. One problem with the study was that it lacked the power to detect a beneficial effect on the intervention in the short term; however, the group felt that there appeared to be no reduction in the number of postoperative myocardial infarctions, deaths, or days in the hospital. Another criticism of the study has been that the selection of patients was based on intermediate or minor clinical predictors and as such may have selected a lower risk patient population. The study also did not account for patients with left main disease, aortic stenosis, or severe left ventricular dysfunction [64].

A recent review of the role of preoperative coronary revascularization was performed by Kertai [65]. Within the review, Kertai noted that though CABG provided more complete revascularization as compared to percutaneous coronary intervention, the CARP trial and subsequent studies with subgroup analyses found that coronary revascularization preoperatively did not improve perioperative and long-term mortality rates.

The Role of Preoperative Coronary Angioplasty

As evident from the previous section there appears to be little support for prophylactic CABG in the asymptomatic patient presenting for noncardiac surgery. However, what about the patient who has received a percutaneous coronary intervention (PCI)? Does preoperative PCI reduce the operative risk of the patient undergoing noncardiac surgery?

Several studies have addressed this question. In a retrospective cohort study by Posner et al. [66], adverse outcomes after noncardiac surgery among patients with a prior PCI, patients with nonrevascularized coronary artery disease (CAD), and normal controls were compared. They ultimately compared the risk for developing adverse cardiac outcomes within 30 days (notably death, myocardial infarction, angina, CHF, malignant dysrhythmias, cardiogenic shock, coronary artery bypass graft after angioplasty). The results of the study revealed that patients who underwent PCI had twice the risk of adverse cardiac outcome as normal controls and half the risk of adverse outcomes as patients with CAD. Compared to the group with uncorrected CAD, the PCI group exhibited no difference in myocardial infarction rates or death.

Timing between the PCI and noncardiac surgery was also important in this study. It was revealed that patients who had a PCI more than 90 days from the noncardiac surgery seemed to have a lower risk of poor outcome as compared to the nonrevascularized patients with CAD. But of note, the study revealed that those who underwent recent PCI had a threefold increase in risk compared to normal controls.

Posner et al. felt that the most surprising result of the study was the similarity of outcome between patients with recent PCI and uncorrected CAD. The group also felt that this helped to substantiate earlier work by Lauperta et al. [67] and Seeger et al. [68] who found similar noncardiac surgery outcomes between patients who underwent prophylactic revascularization and patients without intervention.

Adding to the controversy is a retrospective study performed by Landesberg et al. [69] who reviewed patients who underwent coronary revascularization prior to noncardiac surgery based on the results of a preoperative positive stress thallium examination. His group concluded that long-term survival after major vascular surgery was significantly improved in patients undergoing coronary revascularization. However, Godet et al. [70] were highly critical of this provocative study, deeming it importantly flawed on several points:

1. The study lacked adequate power.
2. Propensity score analysis, which balances all the observed covariants associated with exposure to PCI [71], did not take into account important variables occurring during or after the procedure that may be associated with poor outcomes.
3. The goodness of fit of the propensity score was significant, indicating inappropriate fit of the model.

Godet et al. ultimately performed their own study that analyzed a cohort of 1,152 patients after abdominal aortic aneurysm repair, in which 78 underwent PCI. The study revealed five variables that independently predicted severe postoperative coronary events: age over 75 years, blood transfusion, repeated surgery, preoperative hemodialysis, and previous cardiac failure. The study also revealed five variables that independently predicted postoperative death: age over 75 years, repeated surgery, previously abnormal ST segment/T waves, previous hypertension, and previous cardiac failure. In their conclusions, the group stated that in the PCI group, the observed percentages of patients with a severe postoperative coronary event (9%) were not significantly different from the expected percentages (8.2% and 6.9%, respectively). Of note, when all patients were pooled together, the odds ratios of PCI were not significant and the propensity score analysis provided a similar conclusion.

In the Bypass Angioplasty Revascularization Investigation (BARI) trial, a prospective, randomized trial was designed to compare PCI to CABG on risks of subsequent noncardiac surgery [72]. The results ultimately indicated that the rates of myocardial infarction and death between the two groups PCI and CABG after noncardiac surgery were similar, thus failing to favor one intervention versus another.

In 2007 the COURAGE trial research group reported the results of a multicenter, randomized trial of 2287 patients with multivessel coronary artery disease. The study noted that PCI compared with optimal medical therapy did not reduce the risk of death, myocardial infarction, or other major cardiovascular events during an average observation period of 4.6 years [73]. Though this study was not directed to the patient undergoing noncardiac surgery, it makes the point that interventions in medically optimized, cardiac stable patients may have little value in reducing overall morbidity and mortality.

Obviously, the question regarding the value of PCI or coronary bypass grafting prior to major vascular surgery has not been definitively answered. Complicating the situation is the observation that both the risk of surgery and PCI are substantially higher in patients with peripheral artery disease. This, as noted by Saw et al. [74], may be due to systemic atherosclerotic burden that ultimately leads to increased cardiovascular and cerebrovascular complications.

Considerations for the Patient with Recent Percutaneous Coronary Intervention

An important clinical situation to consider is what to do with the patient who has undergone recent PCI. It is conceivable that during the noninvasive preoperative screening of the intermediate- to high-risk patient, a clinically significant coronary artery lesion is noted. The decision to correct the lesion is usually undertaken by the invasive cardiologist, sometimes during a diagnostic angiography [75]. Balloon angioplasty has given way to more definite treatments such as the placement of bare metal or drug-eluting coronary artery stents. Exactly when and which intervention was made has tremendous implication if these patients present for noncardiac surgery.

Complications from stent placement usually arise from the nature of the thrombogenicity of the stent at the blood-tissue interface leading to thrombosis or embolization. There appear to be multifactorial causes for these events, namely, the type of stent, its length, the size of the final lumen diameter, and the presence of persistent dissection at the time of implantation. Cutlip et al. [76] have reported a 50% incidence of acute myocardial infarction that carries an overall 20% mortality rate in the patient who has had thrombosis with recent stent placement. These concerns have also caused many to recommend caution when dealing with patients and recent PCI [77].

The 2002 ACC/AHA recommendations regarding the patient who has a coronary artery stent suggested at least 2 weeks and ideally 4 to 6 weeks between stent implantation and noncardiac surgery [29]. This would include a full 4 weeks of dual antiplatelet therapy (aspirin and a thienopyridine, such as clopidogrel or ticlopidine) during stent reendothelialization and 2 weeks for restoration of normal platelet function.

Interestingly, the recommendations by the 2002 ACC/AHA committee arose not from randomized controlled trials, but from two retrospective studies [29]. Kaluza et al. [78] noticed that 40 patients who underwent noncardiac surgery within 2 weeks of implantation had a high incidence of severe, catastrophic complications. Of the patients evaluated, 18% had myocardial infarctions, 20% died, and 28% had major bleeding. In a larger series, Wilson et al. [79] noted that 4% of patients undergoing noncardiac surgery within 6 weeks of stent placement suffered a myocardial infarction in which 2.9% of this group ultimately died. They noted that there were no complications seen in patients who were 7 weeks after implantation.

A retrospective study reviewing the risks of noncardiac surgery after coronary stenting was performed by Reddy and Vaitkus [80]. In their small patient population, they noted that of the patients who had major adverse cardiovascular events (MI, stent thrombosis, major bleeding, or death), 38% had undergone noncardiac surgery within 14 days of stent placement and 62% had undergone noncardiac surgery 15 to 42 days after implantation. No patient developed major adverse cardiovascular events after 42 days, leading the authors to suggest that a patient should be considered high-risk if surgery was performed up to 6 weeks following stent placement.

Drug-Eluting Cardiac Stents

It is also important to note that the 2002 ACC/AHA guidelines [29] were only for bare metal stents and not for drug-eluting coronary stents or patients who are under brachytherapy. The presence of paclitaxel or sirolimus may delay endothelialization of the coronary stent and may necessitate a longer period of antiplatelet therapy [81]. A case report by Auer et al. [82] discusses a patient who had the simultaneous placement of a bare metal stent in the right coronary artery and two paclitaxel-eluting stents in the left circumflex 12 weeks prior to noncardiac surgery. Interestingly, 2 hours after surgery the patient had an acute myocardial infarction and catheterization revealed patency of only the RCA-bare metal stent.

In an editorial, Berger et al. [83] recommended that if a patient was scheduled to have noncardiac surgery within 2 months of PCI and the surgery/surgeon did not permit continuation of aspirin and clopidogrel throughout the perioperative period, then bare-metal stents should be used. Mendoza et al. [84] recommended at least a 3-month delay from time of implantation of a drug-eluting stent and noncardiac surgery. This recommendation was based on observations and extrapolation of case reports.

However, a new set of recommendations has been issued regarding the discontinuation of antiplatelet therapy in patients with coronary artery stents. The American Heart Association Scientific Statement by the AHA/ACC/ACS/ADA in February 2007 stated that elective surgical procedures in patients receiving drug-eluting stents should be delayed for at least 12 months. During that time, the patient should receive an entire course of dual antiplatelet therapy composed of aspirin and thienopyridines. However, if surgery cannot be delayed, then the consensus of the group was to recommend the implantation of bare metal stents or balloon angioplasty or continuation of aspirin throughout the perioperative period [85]. This recommendation was also incorporated into the 2007 ACC/AHA guidelines [30]. A summary of the recommendations regarding percutaneous coronary interventions is noted in Figure 149.3.

Heart Failure and Noncardiac Surgery

Definition

As mentioned earlier, one of the high-risk clinical predictors for a postoperative complication is the history of heart failure (HF). The question arises as to how to approach the patient with a history of HF and how best to manage these patients as they present for noncardiac surgery. In 2003, the Framingham Heart Study estimated that there are approximately 550,000 new cases of HF each year with a prevalence of 5 million patients [86].

Heart failure patients presenting for noncardiac surgery are known to have a twofold higher mortality and readmission rate than those patients with CAD alone or no disease. This has been noted to be the case across all types of surgeries. In

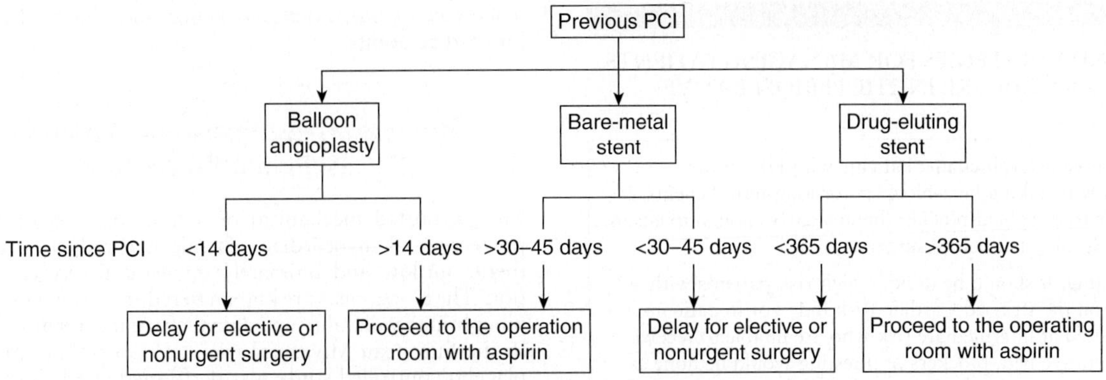

FIGURE 149.3. Proposed approach to the management of patients with previous percutaneous coronary intervention who require noncardiac surgery, based on expert opinion. (Reprinted from Fleisher et al: ACC/AHA 2007 Guidelines on Perioperative Cardiovascular Evaluation and Care for Noncardiac Surgery: Executive Summary. *J Am Coll Cardiol* 50(17):1720, 2007, with permission from Elsevier.)

fact, there is a two- to fourfold increase in mortality for HF patients compared with all others [87]. In evaluating outcomes of Medicare HF patients undergoing noncardiac surgery, Hernandez et al. [88] used a multivariable logistic regression model to assess mortality and readmission rates in the presence of preexisting HF. The group noted that the risk-adjusted operative mortality (defined as death before discharge or within 30 days of surgery) was 11.7% in the HF group versus 6.2% in the control group and 6.6% in the group with isolated CAD. The risk-adjusted 30-day readmission rate in the HF group was as high as 20% and with control, it was approximately 11%. The patients with CAD without the presence of HF had a readmission rate of 14.2%.

Defining exactly which signs and symptoms constitute CHF can be somewhat controversial. However, the ACC/AHA have developed a definition of heart failure that includes various stages, each with their own specific treatment regimen (Table 149.6). It is also important to remember that patients with left ventricular dysfunction may present with a variety of syndromes, notably, a syndrome of decreased exercise tolerance, a syndrome of fluid retention, or those who have no symptoms and incidentally discovered left ventricular dysfunction [89].

TABLE 149.6

ACC/AHA STAGES OF EVOLUTION HEART FAILURE

Stage A: High risk for heart failure, but without structural heart disease or symptoms of heart failure (e.g., hypertension, coronary artery disease, diabetes mellitus, utilizing cardiotoxins, or family history of cardiomyopathy)
Stage B: Structural heart disease but without symptoms of heart failure (e.g., patients with previous MI, LV systolic dysfunction, asymptomatic valvular disease)
Stage C: Structural heart disease with prior or current symptoms of heart failure (e.g., patients with known structural heart disease, shortness of breath and fatigue, reduced exercise tolerance)
Stage D: Refractory heart failure requiring specialized interventions (e.g., patients who have marked symptoms at rest despite maximal medical therapy)

LV, left ventricular; MI, myocardial infarction.
From Hunt SA, Baker DW, Chin MH, et al: ACC/AHA Guidelines for the evaluation and management of congestive heart failure in the adult: executive summary. *Circulation* 104:2996–3007, 2001, with permission.

Evaluation of the Patient with Heart Failure

The Lee Revised Cardiac Risk Index does not take into account changes in the patient's clinical status over time. Hernandez et al. [90] gives the following example of a common clinical conundrum. For example, if a patient has decompensated HF on the day of surgery, the surgery is subsequently cancelled for the patient to clinically improve. We can assume that improvement has been made over time and the patient presents again for noncardiac surgery. The patient's calculated risk remains the same, which may or may not reflect reality. This situation is similar to the patient who has a recent acute coronary syndrome who returns for surgery after being delayed for months to undergo coronary revascularization.

Are there specific noninvasive tests that have particular value when assessing the patient with CHF presenting for noncardiac surgery? Numerous studies have shown value in diagnostic and prognostic markers of HF such as natriuretic peptides. With commercial assays of B-type natriuretic peptide and N-terminal pro-B-type natriuretic peptide being more widespread, it may be possible to improve both the preoperative classification of HF and diagnosis of HF as a postoperative complication by incorporating markers in routine assessment [90–92].

Echocardiography has been found to have a limited prognostic value as a routine test in the presence of heart failure. Rohde et al. [53] addressed this issue regarding the value of transthoracic echocardiography as a tool for risk stratification and found that an abnormal echocardiogram with any degree of systolic dysfunction, moderate to severe left ventricle hypertrophy, moderate to severe mitral regurgitation, or aortic gradient of 20 mm Hg or higher provided a sensitivity of 80%, specificity of 52%, a positive predictive value of 12%, and negative predictive value of 97%. However, severe LV dysfunction compared to mild to moderate LV dysfunction did not have a strong association with cardiogenic pulmonary edema and MI. Because of the heterogeneity of findings, the authors concluded that transthoracic echocardiography added little to risk models.

Right Heart Catheterizations in the Heart Failure Patient

The utilization of right heart catheterization (RHC) in patients having noncardiac surgery has also been evaluated. Obviously, intraoperative hemodynamic changes are associated with increased perioperative complication rates [10]. However, in a

TABLE 149.7

TESTS AND STRATEGIES FOR MANAGING PATIENTS WITH HEART FAILURE IN THE PERIOPERATIVE SETTING

Perioperative beta-blockade: Patients with HF should normally be taking beta-blockers for long-term benefits. If not, try to start beta-blocker therapy early enough to ensure it is well tolerated before surgery.
Stress testing: It should be done in high-risk patients with ≥3 points on the Revised Cardiac Risk Index or in patients considered at intermediate risk who are unable to receive perioperative beta-blockers of if testing would be done as normal clinical care for long-term goals.
Degree of HF compensation: Currently requires clinical judgment. No objective testing strategies have been evaluated in the perioperative setting.
Echocardiography: Routine use of echocardiography does not add information for risk stratification or potential changes in management. It should be reserved for evaluation of clinical changes as done for routine management of HF.
Right heart catheterization and monitoring: Current evidence does not support its routine use. If needed, measurement of central venous pressure is adequate for perioperative management of volume status.

HF, heart failure.
Adapted from Hernandez AF, Newby LK, O'Connor CM: Preoperative evaluation for major noncardiac surgery—focusing on heart failure. *Arch Intern Med* 164:1729–1736, 2004. Copyright © 2004, American Medical Association. All rights reserved.

recent randomized controlled trial of elderly patients undergoing major noncardiac surgery, Sandham et al. [93] showed no benefit for the utilization of perioperative RHC. Within the study, 2,000 patients over the age of 60 with ASA classifications of III and IV were randomized to RHC-directed care versus usual care. Results revealed no improvement in the perioperative course of the RHC-directed therapy over those receiving standard care. There was a slightly higher incidence of pulmonary embolism in the catheter group that was not explained. A reported limitation of this study was that the patients with a NYHA class III or IV HF comprised only 13% of study population. Thus, it is clearly unknown whether RHC is of value in this subpopulation. The study also noted that there was a higher use of inotropes (48.9% vs. 32.8%) in the RHC-directed group, which the authors felt may be the reason for the overall lack of benefit of the invasive monitors.

The appropriate management for this patient population includes risk assessment by the previously mentioned tools. This goes along with constant surveillance and reevaluation of clinical scenarios as they arise. Hernandez et al. [90] suggested a template for tests and strategies for the management of patients with heart failure in the perioperative period (Table 149.7). Again, tailoring to each specific patient is warranted.

Pharmacologic Interventions to Reduce Risk During Noncardiac Surgery

It is obvious that many patients with coronary artery disease will continue to present for noncardiac surgery. Interventions such as coronary stent placement and CABG appear to be of value only if the patient is symptomatic prior to coming for surgery. As such, there is a strong interest in developing pharmacologic regimens that may help reduce the incidence of major cardiac events.

Role of α_2-Agonists and Myocardial Ischemia Prevention

The purported mechanism of action for α_2-agonists in the prevention of myocardial ischemia is a reduction in sympathetic outflow and ultimately myocardial oxygen consumption. The α_2-agonists are known to reduce postganglionic norepinephrine availability and spinal efferent sympathetic output. In the European Mivazerol trial, a double-blind, randomized placebo controlled study was performed at 61 European centers utilizing intravenous mivazerol, an α_2-agonist [94]. Patients either had documented coronary artery disease or were at high-risk for the disease. The drug was administered for 72 hours from induction of anesthesia into the postoperative period. There was a mix of perceived high-risk or intermediate-risk surgeries including vascular surgery or nonvascular thoracic, abdominal, and orthopedic procedures. The conclusions of the study revealed no alterations in the rates of myocardial infarction or cardiac death in patients with known disease.

Two further studies seemed to substantiate the protective properties of α_2-agonists, specifically clonidine. Maekawa et al. [95], in a meta-analysis of the literature, noted that in subgroup analysis, clonidine reduced the incidence of myocardial ischemia in patients undergoing cardiac or noncardiac surgery. Rates of bradycardia were similar in the clonidine and the placebo groups. Wallace et al. [96] performed a prospective, double-blind, clinical trial with patients with documented coronary artery disease or who were at-risk for coronary artery disease. Oral clonidine plus patch therapy was used, and patch therapy was maintained for 4 days. There was a noted decrease in the incidence of perioperative myocardial ischemia with clonidine, intraoperatively and postoperatively. Also of interest, there was a marked reduction in the incidence of postoperative mortality for up to 2 years.

In a quantitative systematic review, six trials utilizing α_2-agonists were reviewed [97]. The group noted that α_2-agonists decreased the incidence of myocardial ischemia during surgery (19.4% vs. 32.8%) compared with placebo. Of note, there was not a significant decrease in myocardial infarction rates (6.1% vs. 7.3%) compared with placebo. Also of significance, the α_2-agonist decreased the risk of cardiac death from 2.3% to 1.1% as compared to placebo.

Statin Therapy

Statins have recently gained favor as medications used to possibly alter perioperative myocardial ischemia. These low-density lipoprotein lowering agents are well known to attenuate coronary artery plaque inflammation. Statins also contain pleiotropic properties that possibly affect plaque stability by the inhibition of anti-thrombogenic, antiproliferative, and leukocyte anti-adhesive properties [98] (Table 149.8).

Early work has shown a decrease in risk of a major coronary event in the presence of statin therapy [99]. In a relatively recent case–control study, Poldermans et al. [104,105] have shown that the utilization of statin therapy has been associated with a fourfold reduced risk in perioperative mortality. This result was seen consistently within subgroups according to the type of surgery, cardiac risk factors, and cardioprotective medication use including aspirin and beta-blockers. These results were also later substantiated in a randomized trial by Durazzo et al. [106], which also noted a reduction in perioperative myocardial infarction rates.

TABLE 149.8

PROPOSED MECHANISM OF STATINS IN THE PRESENCE OF CORONARY ARTERY DISEASE

Inhibition of neovascularization [99–101]
Inflammatory modulation [99–101]
↑ Atherosclerotic plaque stabilization by decreasing the size of the lipid core [101]
↓ Endothelial basement membrane degradation [101]
↓ Smooth muscle apoptosis by decreasing macrophage infiltration [100,102]
↓ The release of matrix metalloproteinases [100,102]
↓ Interferon-Γ release and leukocyte adhesion [100–102]
↓ Complement mediated injury by decreasing C-reactive protein [100–103]
↑ Decay-accelerating factor [100]
↑ The expression of the vasodilator eNOS and ↓ the vasoconstrictor endothelin-1 [100,101]
↓ Thrombogenic response to plaque rupture by inhibiting platelet activation (by increasing eNOS and decreasing thromboxane A2 production) [100,102]

eNOS, endothelial nitric oxide synthetase.
Adapted from Biccard BM, Sear JW, Foex P: Statin therapy: a potential useful perioperative intervention in patients with cardiovascular disease. *Anaesthesia* 60:1106–1114, 2005.

In a review of the literature by Biccard et al. [107], it was evident that a majority of studies have shown statins to be beneficial in the surgical patient, especially in regard to all-cause mortality, cardiovascular mortality, and myocardial infarction. The group ultimately recommended that statins be administered preoperatively in high-risk patient populations, but recognized the fact that larger studies would need to be performed to verify this position.

Assuming patients present for noncardiac surgery while on statin drugs, is it acceptable to discontinue therapy? Lindenauer et al. [108] noted that temporarily discontinuing statin therapy for approximately 24 hours appears to be safe. However, Heeschen et al. [109] noted that in high-risk patients, if the drug is discontinued for more than 3 days, these patients appear to be at increased risk for a major cardiac complication. It would appear to be prudent to reinstitute the utilization of lipid-lowering agents as soon as feasibly possible.

Beta-Blocker Therapy

The utilization of beta-blocker therapy to reduce perioperative morbidity and mortality in the cardiac patient undergoing noncardiac surgery has gained much favor. The initial study by Mangano et al. [7] noted that with the use of atenolol, the postoperative mortality rate was reduced from 14% to 3% during the first year and 21% to 10% the second year after noncardiac surgery. This study was ultimately substantiated by Poldermans et al. [110] in a retrospective study, which confirmed the benefit of beta-blockade, bisoprolol, in intermediate risk patients.

However, the study revealed that beta-blockers failed to lower the cardiac event rate in patients who were at very high risk (three or more clinical risk factors and five or more new wall motion abnormalities on echocardiography).

Another study supportive of the use of beta-blocker therapy was that of the previously cited DECREASE (Dutch Echocardiographic Cardiac Risk Evaluation Applying Stress Echocardiography Study Group) study [52]. The DECREASE supported the merits of beta-blocker therapy and was a controlled trial study in which 112 patients were randomized to standard care or bisoprolol. The results revealed that 3.4% of the bisoprolol group compared with 34% of the standard group experienced the study's primary end point of either death from cardiac causes or nonfatal myocardial infarction.

Stevens et al. [97], on systemic review, revealed that the utilization of beta-blockers in the noncardiac surgical patient resulted in a reduction of ischemic episodes during surgery (7.6% vs. 20.2%) as compared with placebo. Beta-blockers also appeared to decrease ischemic episodes after surgery and reduced the risk of myocardial infarction and cardiac death. Important to note was that only two trials were performed with high-risk groups.

However, recently, the effectiveness of beta-blocker therapy in the perioperative period has come under question [111,112]. In a large systematic review and meta-analysis of randomized controlled trials, Devereaux et al. [113] came to some interesting conclusions. Perioperative outcomes for the study included total mortality, cardiovascular mortality, nonfatal MI, nonfatal cardiac arrest, nonfatal stroke, congestive heart failure, hypotension needing treatment, bradycardia needing treatment, and bronchospasm within 30 days of surgery.

In 22 trials that were reviewed, approximately 2,437 patients were randomized. The utilization of perioperative beta-blockers did not show any statistically significant beneficial effects on any of the individual outcomes, only nominally statistically significant beneficial relative risk for the composite outcome of cardiovascular mortality, nonfatal MI, and nonfatal cardiac arrest. There was also a relative risk in regard to bradycardia requiring treatment and only a nominally significant risk for hypotension needing treatment.

Some of the problems identified in this systematic review were that only a moderate number of events occurred in the perioperative beta-blocker trials. In addition, the meta-analyses revealed a large treatment effect, which is inconsistent with the beta-blocker trials in myocardial infarction and congestive heart failure [114,115]. More importantly, the authors felt that the nominally statistically significant beneficial result of decreased major perioperative cardiovascular events with beta-blocker treatment showed moderate heterogeneity that ultimately weakened the reliability of this finding.

In 2006, the Metoprolol after Vascular Surgery (MaVS) was associated with a reduction in cardiovascular events, but also, treated patients were found to have lower postoperative heart rates and more intraoperative hypotension. Overall, there was not a substantial difference in cardiac events when compared to placebo on 6-month follow-up [116]. The incidence of hypotension and bradycardia was also substantiated in the DIPOM (diabetic postoperative mortality and morbidity) trial [117]. The trial failed to show a reduction in cardiac events in diabetic patients without coronary artery disease undergoing vascular surgery but noted significant hypotension and bradycardia.

Data from the recently concluded POISE (Perioperative Ischemic Evaluation) trial has also added to the controversy [118]. The result of this large, randomized controlled trial in which perioperative metoprolol was utilized, revealed fewer nonfatal myocardial infarction rates and fewer nonfatal cardiac arrests in the treatment group. However, it was also noted that more deaths were in the metoprolol treated group, though they were noncardiac in nature. In addition, more patients in the metoprolol group developed ischemic stroke (41 vs. 19) compared with placebo and for every 1200 patients treated, metoprolol appeared to prevent 15 myocardial infarctions at a cost of eight excess deaths and five disabling strokes.

On a recent analysis of noncardiac surgical randomized trials by Beattie et al. [119], it was recognized that effective control of heart rate is important for achieving improved cardiac outcomes. The cardioprotective effects of heart rate control appear to be evident, but beta-blockers do not appear to reliably

TABLE 149.9

CLINICAL RECOMMENDATIONS FOR IMPLEMENTING BETA-BLOCKERS IN THE PERIOPERATIVE SETTING

Recommendations	Description and rationale
Monitor perioperative heart rate and blood pressure	Serially assess hemodynamic measures at pre-specified intervals. Withhold or administer beta-blocker according to preset thresholds/criteria. Such an approach may help detection of issues such as hypovolemia, infection, sepsis.
Implement a "run-in" phase for perioperative beta-blockade	Initiate therapy at least 7 days before operative intervention. Allows for both acute (hemodynamic) and delayed (anti-inflammatory) effects of beta-blockers. Promotes early recognition of adverse effects (e.g., bradycardia, hypotension, bronchospasm).
Adjust dose to achieve target heart rate of 60 beats per minute, avoiding hypotension	Heart rate control remains the major mechanism of beta-blocker benefit. Helps identify and prevent perioperative bradycardia and intraoperative hypotension. Can require variable doses of drug and thus allows for individualization of therapy.
Recognize that beta-blockers differ considerably	Short vs. long-acting agents, varying clinical effects based on receptor agonism. IV vs. PO route of administration important as IV route can rapidly precipitate side effects. Tailor therapy to maintain same agent/dose (s) as in the preoperative setting.
Continue beta-blockers if already on therapy	Sudden withdrawal of beta-blockers known to cause upregulated beta-receptor state. Class I ACC/AHA recommendation, especially if an original indication already exists. Strive to maintain same agent as the preoperative setting.

Reprinted from Chopra V, Plasiance B, Cavsooglu E, et al: Perioperative beta-blockers for major noncardiac surgery: Primum Non Nocere. *Am J Med* 122(3):228, 2009, with permission from Elsevier.

decrease heart rate in all patients and may be associated with more significant side effects. As such, other medications may be necessary to achieve the goal of heart rate control.

So what to recommend? A recent review by Chopra et al. [120] recognized that though there was a benefit from perioperative beta-blockers, the widespread implementation of perioperative beta-blockade to lower risk groups was probably unwarranted. The group strongly recommended caution when using beta-blockers in patients with low to moderate cardiovascular risk profiles (Table 149.9).

Anesthetic Management and Cardiac Outcome

Currently little is known about the long-term effects of anesthetic management on the cardiac patient presenting for noncardiac surgery. What is known is that there are some well-known predictors of perioperative morbidity and mortality: presence of clinical comorbidities, nature of surgical procedure, and clinical management [121]. Overall, Arbous et al. [122] and Sigurdsson and McAteer [123] have reported that the risk of anesthesia in the immediate perioperative period is remarkably small with a frequency of death attributed to anesthesia to be less than 1 in 200,000 anesthetics. To date there has been no study that has shown a definitive difference regarding the choice of anesthetic technique (e.g., regional vs. general anesthesia) and perioperative outcome.

Monk et al. [124] tried to address the issue of long-term outcomes and anesthesia. The group performed a prospective observational study in which 1,065 patients underwent general anesthesia for major noncardiac surgery. There were no protocols that regulated the type of anesthetic agents used, except for the utilization of Bispectral Index (Aspect Medical Systems, Inc., Norwood, MA) monitoring and electroencephalogram electrode montage. The study revealed that the following preoperative clinical indicators were significant univariate predictors of 1-year mortality: Charlson Comorbidity Score 3 or higher, ASA status III or IV, age 65 or older, history of hypertension, history of coronary artery disease, history of hepatic disease, and history of myocardial infarction. Perioperative factors that were significant predictors of 1-year mortality included: long surgical procedure, intracavitary surgery, longer duration of intraoperative systolic hypotension, and increased cumulative deep hypnotic time (BIS less than 45). Interestingly enough, protective factors that were deemed to be important were advanced education level, larger values of BMI (body mass index), increased preoperative diastolic blood pressure, and high performance on the preoperative Mini-Mental Status Examination.

The results of this study have not been universally accepted, with several criticisms regarding design and data interpretation. Especially difficult to accept were the results surrounding anesthetic depth, cumulative deep hypnotic time, and interpretation of BIS data [125]. Ultimately, studies that are better designed to address these concerns will need to be performed to validate the position of Monk et al.

There is, however, some evidence to support use of inhaled volatile anesthetics over total intravenous anesthesia. Recent studies have suggested a cardioprotective effect of volatile anesthetics. In fact, in the most recent revision of the ACC/AHA guidelines, the authors acknowledge the benefit of volatile anesthetic use in patients at risk for myocardial ischemia [30]. The mechanisms for the cardioprotection are not completely known, but are likely to involve a preconditioning effect, a post-conditioning effect, and an anti-apoptotic effect [126]. These recommendations may help the practitioner decide how to provide anesthesia if general anesthesia is planned; however, they do not aid with the decision between general and regional anesthesia.

SUMMARY

The care of the cardiac patient presenting for noncardiac disease will continue to be challenging. Risk assessment and risk modification continue to evolve, and currently no examination

TABLE 149.10

SUMMARY OF ADVANCES FOR REDUCING PERIOPERATIVE CARDIAC MORBIDITY AND MORTALITY FOR NONCARDIAC PROCEDURES

- Perioperative beta-blockers reduce incidence of cardiac events, however, are associated with complications of perioperative hypotension and bradycardia and possibly stroke [7,110–119].
- Identification of at risk patients continues to evolve [24,29,30].
- Dobutamine stress echocardiography is preferred to noninvasive screening test for identifying patients at risk for postoperative cardiac events [56].
- Routine use of pulmonary artery catheters in high-risk surgical patients is controversial but may be of value [93].
- Myocardial ischemia is reduced with α_2-agonists and statins [94,96,105–108].
- Anesthetic agents may play a cardioprotective role in high risk populations [30,126]

or biochemical marker appears to meet all the criteria necessary. Each of the noninvasive tests previously mentioned have their supporters and detractors, but all have the same goal, that is, to identify the patient at risk who would benefit from further medical optimization prior to undergoing the stress of surgery.

The role for preoperative coronary artery bypass and coronary angioplasty continues to appear to be limited; however, definitive trials are yet to be performed. The utilization of pharmacologic agents such as beta-blockers and statins continue to show great promise but questions also continue to arise, especially when focusing on the risk versus benefits of these therapies. Results of the large, multicenter trials such as the POISE trial have refocused attention to the need of balancing the risk of instituting therapy without regard to the possible detrimental side effects of such medications.

Advances in noncardiac surgery in the cardiac patient, based on randomized, controlled trials or meta-analyses of such trials, are summarized in Table 149.10.

References

1. Jonsdottir LS, Sigfusson N, Sigvaldason H, et al: Incidence and prevalence of recognized and unrecognized myocardial infarction in women. The Reykjavik Study. *Eur Heart J* 19:1011–1018, 1998.
2. Sheifer SE, Gersh BJ, Yanez ND III, et al: Prevalence, predisposing factors, and prognosis of clinically unrecognized myocardial infarction in the elderly. *J Am Coll Cardiol* 35:119–126, 2000.
3. Grayburn PA, Hillis LD: Cardiac events in patients undergoing noncardiac surgery: shifting the paradigm from noninvasive risk stratification to therapy. *Ann Intern Med* 138(6):506–511, 2003.
4. Cohen MC, Artez TH: Histological analysis of coronary artery lesions in fatal postoperative myocardial infarction. *Cardiovasc Pathol* 8:133–139, 1999.
5. Dawood MM, Gutpa DK, Southern J, et al: Pathology of fatal perioperative myocardial infarction: implications regarding pathophysiology and prevention. *Int J Cardiol* 57:37–44, 1996.
6. Ellis SG, Hertzer NR, Young JR, et al: Angiographic correlates of cardiac death and myocardial infarction complication major nonthoracic vascular surgery. *Am J Cardiol* 77:1126–1128, 1996.
7. Mangano DT, Layug EL, Wallace A, et al: Effect of atenolol on mortality and cardiovascular morbidity after noncardiac surgery [published correction appears in N Engl J Med 336:1039, 1997]. *N Engl J Med* 335:1713–1720, 1996.
8. Mangano DT, Hollenberg M, Fegert G, et al: Perioperative myocardial ischemia in patients undergoing noncardiac surgery: I. Incidence and severity during the 4-day perioperative period. *J Am Coll Cardiol* 17:843–850, 1991.
9. Devereaux PJ, Goldman L, Cook DJ, et al: Perioperative cardiac events in patients undergoing noncardiac surgery: a review of the magnitude of the problem, the pathophysiology of the events and methods to estimate and communicate risk. *CMAJ* 173(6):627–634, 2005.
10. Mangano DT, Browner WS, Hollenberg M, et al: Association of perioperative myocardial ischemia with cardiac morbidity and mortality in men undergoing noncardiac surgery. The Study of the Perioperative Ischemia Research Group. *N Engl J Med* 323:1781–1788, 1990.
11. Devereaux PJ, Goldman L, Yusuf S, et al: Surveillance and prevention of major perioperative ischemic cardiac events in patients undergoing noncardiac surgery: a review. *CMAJ* 173(7):779–788, 2005.
12. Alpert JS, Thygesen K, Antman E, et al: Myocardial infarction redefined: a consensus document of the Joint European Society of Cardiology/American College of Cardiology Committee for the redefinition of myocardial infarction. *J Am Coll Cardiol* 36:959–969, 2000.
13. Wilson R, Crouch EA: Risk assessment and comparisons: an introduction. *Science* 236:267–270, 1987.
14. ASA: New classification of physical status. *Anesthesiology* 24:111, 1963.
15. Vacanti CJ, Van Houten RJ, Hill RC: A statistical analysis of the relationship of the physical status to postoperative mortality in 68,388 cases. *Anesth Analg* 49:564–566, 1970.
16. Gilbert K, Larocque BJ, Patrick LT: Prospective evaluation of cardiac risk indices for patients undergoing noncardiac surgery. *Ann Intern Med* 133(5):356–359, 2000.
17. Goldman L, Caldera DL, Nussbaum SR, et al: Multifactorial index of cardiac risk in noncardiac surgical procedures. *N Engl J Med* 297:845–850, 1977.
18. Detsky AS, Abrams HB, Forbath N, et al: Cardiac assessment for patients undergoing noncardiac surgery: a multifactorial clinical risk index. *Arch Intern Med* 146:2131–2134, 1986.
19. Younis LT, Miller DD, Chaitman BR: Preoperative strategies to assess cardiac risk before noncardiac surgery. *Clin Cardiol* 18:447–454, 1995.
20. Romero L, de Virgilio C: Preoperative cardiac risk assessment—an updated approach. *Arch Surg* 136:1370–1376, 2001.
21. Guidelines for assessing and managing the perioperative risk from coronary artery disease associated with major noncardiac surgery. American College of Physicians. *Ann Intern Med* 127:309–312, 1997.
22. Campeau L: Grading of angina pectoris [letter]. *Circulation* 54:522–523, 1976.
23. Eagle K, Coley C, Newell J, et al: Combining clinical and thallium data optimizes preoperative assessment of cardiac risk before major vascular surgery. *Ann Intern Med* 110:859–866, 1989.
24. Lee TH, Marcantonio ER, Mangione CM, et al: Derivation and prospective validation of a simple index for prediction of cardiac risk of major noncardiac surgery. *Circulation* 100:1043–1049, 1999.
25. Bodehemier M: Noncardiac surgery in the cardiac patient: what is the question? *Ann Intern Med* 123:763–764, 1996.
26. Atherly A, Fink A, Campbell DC, et al: Evaluating alternative risk-adjustment strategies for surgery. *Am J Surg* 188:566–570, 2004.
27. Khuri SF, Daley J, Henderson W, et al: The Department of Veterans Affairs' NSQIP. the first national, validated, outcome-based, risk-adjusted, and peer-controlled program for the measurement and enhancement of the quality of surgical care. *Ann Surg* 228(4):491–507, 1998.
28. Fink A, Campbell D, Mentzer R, et al: The National Surgical Quality Improvement Program in non-veterans administration hospitals. *Ann Surg* 236(3):344–354, 2002.
29. Eagle KA, Berger PB, Calkins H, et al: ACC/AHA Guideline update for perioperative cardiovascular evaluation for noncardiac surgery—executive summary: a report of the American College of Cardiology/American Heart Association Task Force on practice guidelines (Committee to update the 1996 Guidelines on Perioperative Cardiovascular Evaluation for Noncardiac Surgery). *Circulation* 105:1257–1267, 2002.
30. Fleisher LA, Beckman JA, Brown KA, et al: ACC/AHA 2007 Guidelines on Perioperative Cardiovascular Evaluation and Care for Noncardiac Surgery: Executive Summary. *J am Coll Cardiol.* 50(17):1707–1732, 2007.
31. Fletcher GF, Balady G, Froelicher VR, et al: Exercise standards. A statement for healthcare professionals from the American Heart Association. *Circulation* 91:580–615, 1995.
32. Reilly DF, McNeely MJ, Doerner D, et al: Self-reported exercise tolerance and the risk of serious perioperative complications. *Arch Intern Med* 159:2185–2192, 1999.
33. Morris CK, Ueshima K, Kawaguchi T, et al: The prognostic value of exercise capacity: a review of the literature. *Am Heart J* 122:1423–1431, 1991.
34. Hoeks SE, Scholte op Reimer WJ, Lenzen MJ, et al: Guidelines for cardiac management in noncardiac surgery are poorly implemented in clinical practice. *Anesthesiology* 107:537–544, 2007.
35. Brett AS. Are the current perioperative risk management strategies for myocardial infarction flawed? *Circulation* 117:3145–3151, 2008.
36. Pasternak LR, Arens JF, Caplan RA, et al: Practice advisory for preanesthesia evaluation. *Anesthesiology* 96:485–496, 2002.

37. van Klei WA, Bryson GL, Yang H, et al: The value of routine preoperative electrocardiography in predicting myocardial infarction after noncardiac surgery. *Annals of Surgery* 246:165–170, 2007.
38. Fleisher, L. The preoperative electrocardiogram: what is the role in 2007? *Annals of Surgery* 246:171–172, 2007.
39. Mukherjee D, Eagle K: Perioperative cardiac assessment for noncardiac surgery: eight steps to the best possible outcome. *Circulation* 107:2771–2774, 2003.
40. Eagle KA, Brundage BH, Chaitman BR, et al: Guidelines for perioperative cardiovascular evaluation for noncardiac surgery. Report of the American College of Cardiology/American Heart Association Task Force on Practice Guidelines. *J Am Coll Cardiol* 27:910–948, 1996.
41. Gianrossi R, Detrano R, Mulvihill D, et al: Exercise-induced ST depression in the diagnosis of coronary artery disease: a meta-analysis. *Circulation* 80:87–98, 1989.
42. Cardiovascular stress testing: a description of various types of stress tests and indications for their use: Mayo Clinic Cardiovascular Working Group on Stress Testing. *Mayo Clin Proc* 71:43–52, 1996.
43. Zaret BL, Wackers FJ: Nuclear cardiology (1). *N Engl J Med* 329:775–783, 1993.
44. Baron JF, Mundler O, Bertrand M, et al: Dipyridamole-thallium scintigraphy and gated radionuclide angiography to assess cardiac risk before abdominal aortic surgery. *N Engl J Med* 330:663–669, 1994.
45. Mangano D, London M, Tubau J, et al: Dipyridamole thallium 201 scintigraphy as a preoperative screening test: a reexamination of its predictive potential. *Circulation* 84:493–502, 1991.
46. De Virgilio C, Toosie K, Elbassir M, et al: Dipyridamole-thallium/sestamibi before vascular surgery: a prospective blinded study in moderate risk patients. *J Vasc Surg* 32:77–89, 2000.
47. Stratmann H, Younis L, Wittry M, et al: Dipyridamole technetium-99m sestamibi myocardial tomography in patients evaluated for elective vascular surgery: prognostic value for perioperative and late cardiac events. *Am Heart J* 131:923–929, 1996.
48. Berthe C, Pierard LA, Hiernaux M, et al: Predicting the extent and location of coronary artery disease in acute myocardial infarction by echocardiography during dobutamine infusion. *Am J Cardiol* 58:1167–1172, 1986.
49. Sawada SG, Segar DS, Ryan T, et al: Echocardiographic detection of coronary artery disease during dobutamine infusion. *Circulation* 83:1605–1613, 1991.
50. Kontas MC, Akosah KO, Brath LK, et al: Cardiac complications in noncardiac surgery: value of dobutamine stress echocardiography versus dipyridamole-thallium imaging. *J Cardiothorac Vasc Anesth* 10:329–335, 1996.
51. Shaw LJ, Eagle KA, Gersh BJ, et al: Meta-analysis of intravenous dipyridamole-thallium-201 imaging (1985–1994) and dobutamine echocardiography (1991–1994) for risk stratification before vascular surgery. *J Am Coll Cardiol* 27:787–798, 1996.
52. Boersma E, Poldermans D, Bax JJ, et al: Predictors of cardiac events after major vascular surgery: role of clinical characteristics, dobutamine echocardiography, and β-blocker therapy. *JAMA* 285:1865–1873, 2001.
53. Rohde LE, Polanczyk CA, Goldman L, et al: Usefulness of transthoracic echocardiography as a tool for risk stratification of patients undergoing major noncardiac surgery. *Am J Cardiol* 87:505–509, 2001.
54. Morgan PB, Panomitros GE, Nelson AC, et al: Low utility of dobutamine stress echocardiograms in the preoperative evaluation of patients scheduled for noncardiac surgery. *Anesth Analg* 95:512–516, 2002.
55. Kertai MD, Boersma E, Bax JJ, et al: A meta-analysis comparing the prognostic accuracy of six diagnostic tests for predicting perioperative cardiac risk in patients undergoing major vascular surgery. *Heart* 89:1327–1334, 2003.
56. Beattie WS, Abdelnaem E, Wijeysundera DN, et al: A meta-analytic comparison of preoperative stress echocardiography and nuclear scintigraphy imaging. *Anesth Analg* 102:8–16, 2006.
57. Hertzer NR, Young JR, Beven EG, et al: Late results of coronary bypass in patients with infrarenal aortic aneurysms. The Cleveland Clinic Study. *Ann Vasc Surg* 205:360–367, 1987.
58. Gagnon RM, Dumont G, Sestier F, et al: The role of coronary angioplasty in patients with associated noncardiac medical and surgical conditions. *Can J Cardiol* 6:287–292, 1990.
59. Allen JR, Helling TS, Hartzler GO: Operative procedures not involving the heart after percutaneous transluminal coronary angioplasty. *Surg Gynecol Obstet* 173:285–288, 1991.
60. Nielsen JL, Page CP, Mann C, et al: Risk of major elective operation after myocardial revascularization. *Am J Surg* 164:423–436, 1992.
61. Eagle KA, Charanjit SR, Mickel MC, et al: Cardiac Risk of Noncardiac Surgery: Influence of Coronary Disease and Type of Surgery in 3368 Operations. *Circulation* 96:1882–1887.
62. Mason JJ, Owens DK, Harris RA, et al: The role of coronary angiography and coronary revascularization before noncardiac surgery. *JAMA* 273:1919–1925, 1995.
63. McFalls EO, Ward HB, Moritz TE, et al: Coronary-artery revascularization before elective major vascular surgery. *N Engl J Med* 351(27):2795–2804, 2004.
64. Landesberg G, Berlatzky Y, Bocher M, et al: A clinical survival score predicts the likelihood to benefit from preoperative thallium scanning and coronary revascularization before major vascular surgery. *Eur Heart J* 2006;533–9.
65. Kertai M: Preoperative Coronary Revascularization in High-risk patients undergoing vascular surgery: a core review. *Anesth Analg* 106:751–758, 2008.
66. Posner KL, Van Norman GA, Chan V: Adverse cardiac outcomes after noncardiac surgery in patients with prior percutaneous transluminal coronary angioplasty. *Anesth Analg* 89:553–560, 1999.
67. Lapuerta P, L'Italien GL, Paul S, et al: Neural network assessment of perioperative cardiac risk in vascular surgery patients. *Med Decis Making* 18:70–75, 1998.
68. Seeger JM, Rosenthal GR, Self SB, et al: Does routine stress-thallium cardiac scanning reduce postoperative cardiac complications? *Ann Surg* 219:654–661, 1994.
69. Landesberg G, Mosseri M, Wolf YG, et al: Preoperative thallium scanning, selective coronary revascularization and long-term survival after major vascular surgery. *Circulation* 108:177–183, 2003.
70. Godet G, Riou B, Bertrand M, et al: Does preoperative coronary angioplasty improve perioperative cardiac outcome? *Anesthesiology* 102(4):739–746, 2005.
71. Joffe MM, Rosenbaum PR: Propensity scores. *Am J Epidemiol* 150:327–333, 1999.
72. Hassan SA, Hlatky MA, Boothroyd DB, et al: Outcomes of noncardiac surgery after coronary bypass surgery or coronary angioplasty in the bypass angioplasty revascularization investigation. *Am J Med* 110:260–266, 2001.
73. Boden WE, O'Rourke RA, Teo KK, et al: COURAGE Trial Research Group. Optimal medical therapy with or without PCI for stable coronary disease. *N Engl J Med* 356:1–14, 2007.
74. Saw J, Bhatt DL, Moliterno DJ, et al: The influence of peripheral arterial disease on outcomes. A pooled analysis of mortality in eight large randomized percutaneous coronary intervention trials. *J Am Coll Cardiol* 48:1567–1572, 2006.
75. Rankin JM, Spinelli JJ, Carere RG, et al: Improved clinical outcome after widespread use of coronary-artery stenting in Canada. *N Engl J Med* 341:1957–1965, 1999.
76. Cutlip DE, Baim DS, Ho KK, et al: Stent thrombosis in the modern era. A pooled analysis of multicenter coronary stent clinical trails. *Circulation* 103:1967–1971, 2001.
77. Van Norman GA, Posner K: Coronary stenting or percutaneous transluminal coronary angioplasty prior to noncardiac surgery increases adverse perioperative cardiac events: the evidence is mounting. *J Am Coll Cardiol* 36:2351–2352, 2000.
78. Kaluza GL, Joseph J, Lee JR, et al: Catastrophic outcomes of noncardiac surgery soon after coronary stenting. *J Am Coll Cardiol* 35:1288–1294, 2000.
79. Wilson SH, Fasscas P, Orford JL, et al: Clinical outcomes of patients undergoing non-cardiac surgery in the two months following coronary stenting. *J Am Coll Cardiol* 42:234–240, 2003.
80. Reddy PR, Vaitkus PT: Risks of noncardiac surgery after coronary stenting. *Am J Cardiol* 95:755–757, 2005.
81. Dupuis JY, Labinaz M: Noncardiac surgery in patients with coronary artery stent: what should the anesthesiologist know? *Can J Anesth* 52(4):356–361, 2005.
82. Auer J, Berent R, Weber T, et al: Risk of noncardiac surgery in months following placement of a drug-eluting coronary stent [letter]. *J Am Coll Cardiol* 43:713, 2004.
83. Berger PB, Wilson SH, Fasseas P, et al: Reply to "Clinical outcomes of patients undergoing noncardiac surgery in the two months following coronary stenting." *J Am Coll Cardiol* 43(4):714–715, 2004.
84. Mendoza CE, Virani SS, Shah N, et al: Noncardiac surgery following percutaneous coronary interventions. *Catheter Cardiovasc Interv* 63:267–273, 2004.
85. Grines CL, Bonow RO, Casey DE, et al: Prevention of premature discontinuation of dual antiplatelet therapy in patients with coronary artery stents. *Circulation* 115:813–818, 2007.
86. American Heart Association: *2003 Heart and Stroke Statistical Update*. Dallas, AHA, 2003.
87. Rich MW: Epidemiology, pathophysiology, and etiology of congestive heart failure in older adults. *J Am Geriatr Soc* 45:968–974, 1997.
88. Hernandez AF, Whellan DJ, Stroud S, et al: Outcomes in heart failure patients after noncardiac surgery. *J Am Coll Card* 44(7):1446–1453, 2004.
89. Hunt SA, Baker DW, Chin MH, et al: ACC/AHA Guidelines for the evaluation and management of congestive heart failure in the adult: executive summary. *Circulation* 104:2996–3007, 2001.
90. Hernandez AF, Newby LK, O'Connor CM: Preoperative evaluation for major noncardiac surgery—focusing on heart failure. *Arch Intern Med* 164:1729–1736, 2004.
91. Levin ER, Gardner DG, Samson WK: Natriuretic peptides. *N Engl J Med* 339:321–328, 1998.
92. Maisel AS, Krishnaswamy P, Nowak RM, et al: Rapid measurement of B-type natriuretic peptide in the emergency diagnosis of heart failure. *N Engl J Med* 347:161–167, 2002.
93. Sandham J, Hull R, Brant FB, et al: A randomized, controlled trial of the use of pulmonary artery catheters in high-risk surgical patients. *N Engl J Med* 348:5–14, 2003.
94. Oliver MF, Goldman L, Julian DG, et al: Effect of mivazerol on perioperative cardiac complications during noncardiac surgery in patients with coronary heart disease—the European mivazerol trial. *Anesthesiology* 91(4):951–961, 1999.

95. Maekawa M, Kamae I, Nishi N: Efficacy of clonidine for prevention of perioperative myocardial ischemia—a critical appraisal and meta-analysis of the literature. *Anesthesiology* 96(2):323–329, 2002.
96. Wallace AW, Galindez D, Salahieh A, et al: Effect of clonidine on cardiovascular morbidity and mortality after noncardiac surgery. *Anesthesiology* 101(2):284–293, 2004.
97. Stevens R, Burri H, Tramer MR: Pharmacologic myocardial protection in patients undergoing noncardiac surgery: a quantitative systematic review. *Anesth Analg* 97:623–633, 2003.
98. van Haelst PL, van Doormall JJ, May JF, et al: Secondary prevention with fluvastatin decreases levels of adhesion molecules, neopterin and C-reactive protein. *Eur J Intern Med* 12:503–509, 2001.
99. The Long-Term Intervention with Pravastatin in Ischemic Disease (LIPID) Study Group. Prevention of cardiovascular events and death with pravastatin in patients with coronary heart disease and a broad range of initial cholesterol levels. *N Engl J Med* 339:1349–1357, 1998.
100. Mason JC: Statins and their role in vascular protection. *Clin Sci* 105:251–266, 2003.
101. Libby P: Inflammation in atherosclerosis. *Nature* 420:868–874, 2000.
102. Laws PE, Spark JI, Cowled PA, et al: The role of statins in vascular disease. *Eur J Vasc Endovasc Surg* 27:6–16, 2004.
103. Albert MA, Danielson E, Rifai PM, et al: Effect of statin therapy on C-reactive protein levels. The Pravastatin Inflammation/CRP Evaluation (PRINCE): a randomized trial and cohort study. *JAMA* 286:64–70, 2001.
104. Kertai MD, Poldermans D: The utility of dobutamine stress echocardiography for perioperative and long-term cardiac risk assessment. *J Cardiothorac Vasc Anesth* 19(4):520–528, 2005.
105. Poldermans D, Bax JJ, Kertai MD, et al: Statins are associated with a reduced incidence of perioperative mortality in patients undergoing major noncardiac vascular surgery. *Circulation* 107:1848–1851, 2003.
106. Durazzo AE, Machado FS, Ikeoka DT, et al: Reduction in cardiovascular events after vascular surgery with atorvastatin: a randomized trial. *J Vasc Surg* 39:967–975, 2004.
107. Biccard BM, Sear JW, Foex P: Statin therapy: a potential useful perioperative intervention in patients with cardiovascular disease. *Anaesthesia* 60:1106–1114, 2005.
108. Lindenauer PK, Keow P, Wang K, et al: Lipid-lowering therapy and in-hospital mortality following major noncardiac surgery. *JAMA* 291:2092–2099, 2004.
109. Heeschen C, Hamm CW, Laufs U, et al: Withdrawal of statins in patients with acute coronary syndromes. *Circulation* 105:1446–1452, 2002.
110. Poldermans D, Boersma E, Bax JJ, et al: The effect of bisoprolol on perioperative mortality and myocardial infarction in high-risk patients undergoing vascular surgery. *N Engl J Med* 341:1789–1794, 1999.
111. Yang H, Raymer K, Butler R, et al: Metoprolol after vascular surgery (MaVS) [abstract]. *Can J Anesth* 51:A7, 2004.
112. Giles JW, Sear JW, Foex P: Effect of chronic β-blockade on perioperative outcome in patients undergoing noncardiac surgery: an analysis of observational and case control studies. *Anaesthesia* 59:574–583, 2004.
113. Devereaux PJ, Beattie WS, Choi PT-L, et al: How strong is the evidence for the use of perioperative beta blockers in non-cardiac surgery? Systematic review and meta-analysis of randomized controlled trials. *BMJ* 331(7512):313–321, 2005.
114. Yusuf S, Peto R, Lewis J, et al: β-blockade during and after myocardial infarction: an overview of the randomized trials. *Prog Cardiovasc Dis* 27:335–371, 1985.
115. MERIT-HF Study Group: Effect of metoprolol CR/XL in chronic heart failure: metoprolol CR/XL randomized intervention trial in congestive heart failure (MERIT-HF). *Lancet* 353:2001–2007, 1999.
116. Yang H, Raymer K, Butler R, et al: The effects of perioperative beta-blockade: results of the Metoprolol after Vascular Surgery (MaVS) study, a randomized controlled trial. *Am Heart J*. 152:983–990, 2006.
117. Juul AB, Wetterslev J, Gluud C; DIPOM Trial Group. Effect of perioperative beta blockade in patients with diabetes undergoing major non-cardiac surgery: randomized placebo controlled blinded multicentre trial. *BMJ* 332:1482, 2006.
118. Devereaux PJ, Yang H, Yusuf S, et al: Effects of extended-release metoprolol succinate in patients undergoing non-cardiac surgery (POISE trial): a randomized controlled trial. For the POISE Study Group. *Lancet* 371:1839–1847, 2008.
119. Beattie WS, Wijesundera DN, Karkouti K, et al: Does tight heart-rate control improve beta blocker efficacy? An updated analysis of the noncardiac surgical randomized trials. *Anesth Analg* 106:1039–1048, 2008.
120. Chopra V, Plasiance B, Cavsooglu E, Flanders S, Eagle K. Perioperative Beta-blockers for major noncardiac surgery: Primum Non Nocere, *Am J Med* 122(3):222–229, 2009.
121. Fleisher LA, Anderson GF: Perioperative risk: how can we study the influence of provider characteristics? *Anesthesiology* 96:1039–1041, 2002.
122. Arbous MS, Grobbee DE, van Kleef JW, et al: Mortality associated with anaesthesia: a qualitative analysis to identify risk factors. *Anaesthesia* 56:1141–1153, 2001.
123. Sigurdsson GH, McAteer E: Morbidity and mortality associated with anesthesia. *Acta Anaesthesiol Scand* 40:1057–1063, 1996.
124. Monk T, Saini V, Weldon BC, et al: Anesthetic management and one-year mortality after noncardiac surgery. *Anesth Analg* 100:4–10, 2005.
125. Cohen NH: Anesthetic depth is not (yet) a predictor of mortality! *Anesth Analg* 100:1–3, 2005.
126. De Hert SG, Preckel B, Schlack WS: Updated on inhalational anaesthetics. *Curr Opin Anesthesiol* 22:491–495, 2009.

CHAPTER 150 ■ DIAGNOSIS AND MANAGEMENT OF INTRA-ABDOMINAL SEPSIS

DENNIS I. SONNIER, SHRAWAN G. GAITONDE, PATRICK D. SOLAN AND THOMAS L. HUSTED

INTRODUCTION

The intensive care unit is home to a diversity of patients suffering from intra-abdominal sepsis. Patients may be undergoing treatment for a cardiac or pulmonary condition and may develop an intra-abdominal process as an additional insult, or abdominal distention or peritonitis may arise in a patient recently transported from the operating room after an abdominal procedure, and some patients may be new admissions to the hospital with the signs and symptoms of an intra-abdominal infection.

Several principles are crucial to the management of these patients, such as aggressive resuscitation and monitoring, early administration of antibiotics, and careful consideration of an expanded list of differential diagnoses. Also required are thorough assessments of the patient's ability to tolerate various interventions, the importance of gaining source control, and the need for multidisciplinary teams made of intensivists, surgeons, interventional radiologists, and gastroenterologists among others. With the ubiquitous presence of drug resistant organisms, it is imperative to prescribe antimicrobial medications with the mind-set of antibiotic stewardship.

New paradigms are developing in the management of these diseases, such as molecular targets of therapy, delivery of advanced care at the bedside, damage control strategies, and minimally invasive techniques alone or in combination with a definitive surgical procedure.

PATHOPHYSIOLOGY OF THE LOCAL AND SYSTEMIC RESPONSE TO INTRA-ABDOMINAL INFECTIONS

Patients with intra-abdominal infections can be viewed as a unique subset of sepsis syndrome patients. The defense mechanisms of the peritoneal cavity help explain the specific pattern of response seen. Well-defined systems are available for rapid mechanical clearance of foreign particulates and solutes from the intraperitoneal space. Diaphragmatic lymphatic channels provide a means for the entry of peritoneal fluid (and any bacteria or proinflammatory mediators) through the thoracic duct into the venous circulation. Lymphatic capillaries are distributed in the subperitoneal connective tissue of the diaphragm. Mesothelial cells are organized into two discrete populations: cuboidal cells and flattened cells. Gaps (stomas) between neighboring cells are abundant in the peritoneal mesothelium and found only among cuboidal cells [1,2]. The average area of a stoma is approximately 102 μm. Peritonitis increases the diameter of these stomas [3]. Inspiration decreases intrathoracic pressure relative to intra-abdominal pressure, creating a pressure gradient favoring fluid movement across the diaphragm and out of the abdomen. Entry of proinflammatory substances into the lymphatic channels and subsequently the vascular space would be expected to produce many of the hemodynamic and respiratory signs of severe sepsis. Positive-pressure ventilation likely attenuates this process but has not been well studied as a therapeutic maneuver [4].

Other peritoneal defense mechanisms include resident peritoneal macrophages and large recruitable pools of circulating neutrophils and monocytes. These cell types participate in bacterial isolation and abscess formation. Ingestion of microorganisms by these cells may result in secretion of a variety of proinflammatory mediators, including chemokines, cytokines, lipid derivatives, oxidants, and lysosomal enzymes. Manipulation of the number and function of these resident and recruited cells is now possible through the use of colony-stimulating factors, but has not been examined in clinical trials. Similarly, manipulation of the expression of proinflammatory mediators from these inflammatory cells has been postulated to modulate the sepsis response, but clinical trials have been disappointing to date.

The release of proinflammatory products of peritoneal origin into mesenteric, lymphatic, and vascular channels, and this contribution to the systemic septic response has not been fully addressed. Liver dysfunction is common during the course of intra-abdominal infection and occasionally progresses to fatal hepatic failure [5,6]. Considerable evidence supports the notion that various macrophage products, including interleukins-1 and -6 and tumor necrosis factor-α, substantially alter hepatocyte function [7]. In addition to conversion of hepatic synthetic function to acute-phase reactants, serum chemistries reveal evidence of ductal epithelial cytotoxicity, including elevated alkaline phosphatase levels and elevated bilirubin levels. The large number of fixed tissue phagocytes (Kupffer cells) in the liver that are capable of responding to endotoxin absorbed from systemic or mesenteric blood vessels represents a potentially important source of chemokines, cytokines, and other hepatocyte regulatory substances, although portal endotoxemia has not been detected in humans [8,9].

The bacteriology of mixed flora infections, encompassing aerobic, anaerobic, and facultative Gram-negative organisms, explains at least part of the local histopathology of intra-abdominal infection. Facultative and aerobic Gram-negative organisms express and release endotoxin and endotoxin-associated proteins spontaneously, and such shedding is likely intensified by administration of antibiotics [10]. Aside from the potential for inducing the release of cytokines and other inflammatory mediators, these substances induce local thrombosis through a variety of endothelial and macrophage-mediated processes. Synergistic interactions between certain anaerobes, most notably *Bacteroides fragilis*, and endotoxin-bearing Gram-negative organisms suppress local host defense mechanisms and facilitate the establishment of infection [11–13]. *B. fragilis* produces a capsular polysaccharide that interferes with complement activation and inhibits leukocyte function [14]. These phenomena are thought to restrict the delivery of phagocytes to the site of infection, permitting a more rapid rate of bacterial growth than would otherwise be seen.

CLINICAL ASPECTS OF CARE FOR PATIENTS WITH INTRA-ABDOMINAL INFECTIONS

Initial Therapeutic Goals

For the critically ill patient with an intra-abdominal infection, perforation, or ischemic process, timely resuscitation is crucial to their survival. Resuscitative efforts should begin when the patient enters the hospital, rather than waiting for admission to the ICU. During a thorough diagnostic workup with a history and physical, laboratory values and imaging, findings such as severe peritonitis, portal venous gas, or free intraperitoneal air may be discovered that necessitate immediate intervention. In these cases, the need for intervention supersedes the need for ICU admission. Without source control, peritoneal soiling will continue, and the patient's condition will continue to deteriorate. The patient should be prepared for the operating room. Due to the global vasodilatory effects of anesthesia, the patient should receive rapid volume loading. Resuscitative efforts can continue intraoperatively, led by a combined effort of the surgeon and anesthesiologist.

In patients not requiring immediate operative intervention, resuscitation should begin rapidly. Supplemental oxygen should be provided, with a secure airway by endotracheal intubation, if indicated. Lung protective ventilatory strategy should also be employed to prevent volutrauma, with tidal volumes of approximately 6 ml per kg of ideal body weight [15]. Adequate venous and arterial access should be gained to infuse fluids and blood products as well as provide invasive hemodynamic monitoring and easy blood sampling. Pulmonary artery catheters should be carefully considered, but have proven to be of marginal assistance when the patient is unresponsive to fluid resuscitation [16].

Appropriate resuscitative goals must be established and pursued for each patient, starting by using crystalloid solution to achieve a central venous pressure of 8 to 12 mm Hg. Vasopressors, namely, norepinephrine, should be used to achieve a mean arterial pressure of 65 mm Hg, with supplemental low dose vasopressin use, if necessary. Transfusion of packed red cells should be considered in patients with active bleeding or with hemoglobin less than 7 g per dL, to augment oxygen delivery. In addition to the standard hemodynamic parameters, oxygen delivery parameters such as continuous mixed venous oxygen saturation (SvO2) or mixed central venous oxygen saturation (ScvO2) may be followed. ScvO2 of more than 70% is desirable, with transfusion or pressor therapy to achieve this endpoint. Arterial lactate clearance is another useful parameter. A lactate clearance of at least 10%, measured at 2-hour intervals, has been recently demonstrated to be equal to ScvO2 as an indicator of response to resuscitation. More traditional endpoints should also be considered, such as adequate urine

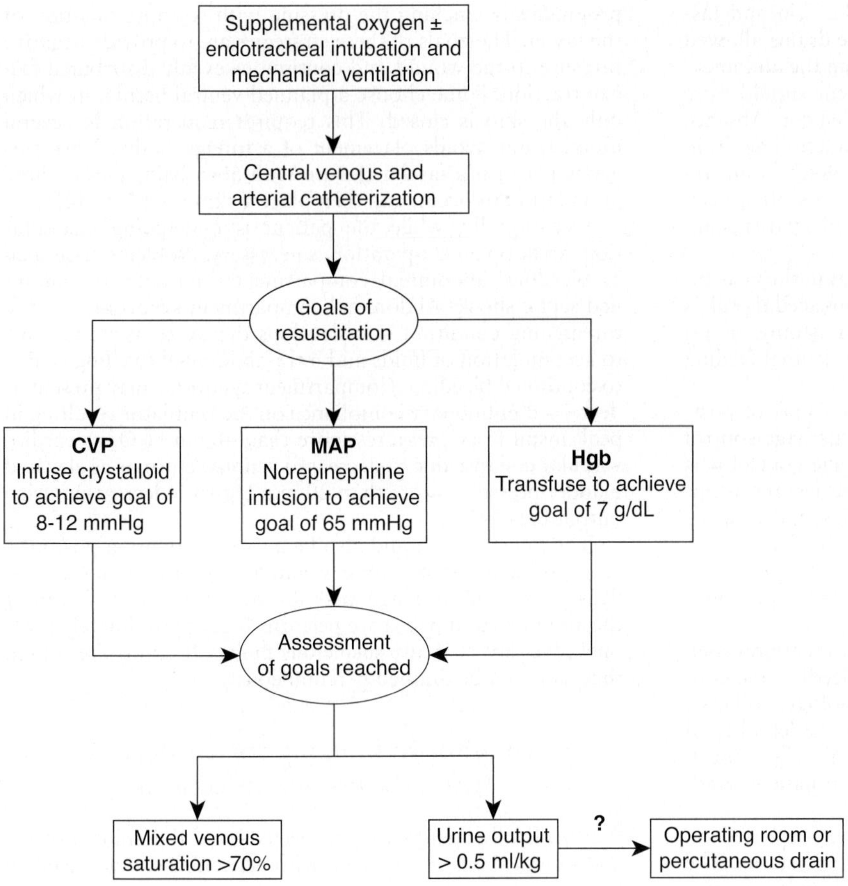

FIGURE 150.1. Algorithm for resuscitation of patients with suspected intra-abdominal infections. Crystalloid or packed red blood cells are infused to achieve goals of resuscitation, while end points are assessed by means of urine output and mixed venous saturation from a superior vena caval sample. Patient responsiveness to resuscitation will dictate whether operative or radiographic intervention is warranted. CVP, central venous pressure; MAP, mean arterial pressure; Hgb, serum hemoglobin level.

output and serial physical exam, specifically extremity warmth and level of consciousness. Newer measures such as tissue oxygen saturation measured by near infrared spectroscopy are being studied and may be beneficial as additional noninvasive means of guiding resuscitative efforts [16–22].

Blood cultures should be obtained upon admission, ideally before administration of intravenous antibiotics. Antibiotic therapy should be started immediately. Broad-spectrum antibiotics against Gram-positive, Gram-negative, and anaerobic bacterial organisms should be chosen. Antifungal coverage should be considered, especially if there is an upper gastrointestinal source, in those on long-term antibiotics or in an immunosuppressed patient [17,23].

Sepsis may be complicated by coagulopathy and DIC. For the patient about to undergo an operation, coagulopathy should be reversed with FFP and/or cryoprecipitate, and platelets should be transfused if counts are less than 50,000 per mm^3. Thromboelastography (TEG) is being increasingly used in ICUs and may prove beneficial for patients with intra-abdominal sepsis [24–26] (see Fig. 150.1).

Surgical Management of Diffuse Peritonitis

First of the surgical concerns during management of any intra-abdominal infection is achieving source control. The infectious or inflammatory process should be removed. All compartments of the abdomen should be explored, including the subphrenic, subhepatic, pelvic, and interloop spaces. All abscesses are drained, all inflamed or perforated bowel is resected, and the abdomen is irrigated with copious amounts of warm saline. The mantra "drainage, debridement, diversion then drugs" expresses the surgeon's opinion about the importance of gaining source control.

After source control is achieved, the surgeon turns their attention to intra-abdominal reconstruction. Primary anastomosis is nearly always performed after resection of small bowel segments. Large intestinal reconstruction is not as straight forward. The majority of data regarding restoring intestinal continuity in the setting of diffuse peritonitis is taken from the treatment of diverticulitis. A two-stage procedure is the default operative mode in sick patients. After resection of all inflamed bowel, this involves creation of an end colostomy proximally and leaving a rectal stump distally, with the intention of restoration of intestinal continuity at a future date. The goal of a two-stage procedure is to avoid anastomotic dehiscence. This procedure is associated with its own morbidities, including stoma complications, abscess formation, and leakage. Primary anastomosis, with on-table colonic washout is increasingly used in perforated diverticulitis, with the goal of avoiding morbidity of stoma complications and need for future laparotomy. Mortality and complications have been shown to be similar to two-stage procedure, with similar operative times. These studies involve heavy selection bias, thus primary anastomosis is still not universally accepted as an alternative to two-stage procedure. The most important factors for the surgeon to consider are the amount of peritoneal soilage and the hemodynamic status of the patient. Patients with perioperative shock, especially those on vasopressors, should not undergo primary anastomosis of small or large bowel [27–30].

In the patient with diffuse peritonitis, after a stoma or anastomosis is created, a drain is usually placed. Closed suction drains (Jackson-Pratt or Blake type) are preferred to open drains (Penrose type). Drain tips are positioned near the inflamed organ, in paracolic gutters or another dependent portion of the abdomen and exit through the skin and fascia, away from the laparotomy incision. These drains allowed continued efflux of contaminated material from the abdomen. Change in character or quantity of the effluent should raise suspicions of leak or need for further debridement. Absence of drainage, though, may be a sign of a nonfunctioning drain rather than a sign of lack of continued pathology. Drain removal is a variable and stepwise process. Patients often keep drains until enteral diet is tolerated. Occasionally, patients are discharged with drains in place.

A critically ill patient who is likely not to eat in the near future should have a feeding tube placed. Various feeding tubes are used, including nasogastric, gastric, jejunostomy, or g-j tubes, allowing for gastric decompression and jejunal feeding simultaneously.

Though the open abdomen has long been a part of postoperative management of patients, the term "damage control surgery" has only recently been coined. Damage control was first used in the management of traumatic injuries, but is applicable in the setting of inflammatory, infectious, and vascular pathology in the abdomen of a patient in extremis. This process is now the subject of extensive study as a deliberate process in management. The intensivist's role in this strategy is paramount [31].

Damage control surgery (DCS) is defined as an abbreviated laparotomy, consisting of gaining control of bleeding and contamination in a patient on the verge of physiologic collapse. DCS is designed to help solve the problem of the lethal triad of acidosis, coagulopathy, and hypothermia. This triad continues to develop intraoperatively and can lead to patient death despite a technically correct operation [31,32].

Selecting the proper patient for this strategy is based on criteria involving disease process and physiologic status. The decision is made early in the preoperative or intraoperative phase of care by the surgeon, with constant communication with the anesthesiologist. These criteria have been defined by multiple authors. The disease based criteria consist of an inaccessible injury, multiple severe injuries, severe contamination, need for a time consuming procedure, need for a second look to reevaluate the intra-abdominal contents or inability to close abdominal fascia. The physiologic criteria include hypothermia ($<35°C$), metabolic acidosis (<7.30), nonmechanical bleeding, and poor response to resuscitation [33].

Three general phases of damage control are described. In the initial phase, the abbreviated laparotomy involves a thorough exploration and control of bleeding, and then contamination. No reconstruction efforts are made at this time. The abdomen is closed with towel clamps, a running nylon skin suture, or a layered vacuum assisted closure.

Second is the resuscitative phase. This involves establishing clean IV access and removing femoral lines if possible. A ventilation strategy should have the goal of oxygenation and ventilation while avoiding volutrauma from excess tidal volumes and careful use of Positive End-Expiratory Pressure (PEEP) to avoid diminishing venous return. Fluid and product resuscitation should be used to correct acidosis, restore normal tissue perfusion, and optimize oxygen delivery. This should all be done in a warm ICU room with warm IV fluids to correct hypothermia. Twelve to 48 hours should be allowed for the completion of resuscitation [31–34].

Third is the definitive operation, when packs are removed, the abdomen is reexplored, reconstruction is undertaken, and the abdomen is irrigated [31–34]. Abdominal closure is also part of the definitive operation. Frequently a tension free closure of fascia is not possible. In this case, surgeons often elect for replacing the suction assisted closure in conjunction with a progressive closure strategy. Several strategies exist but all involve changing abdominal dressings every 2 to 3 days and progressively cinching the dressing with re-approximation of the fascia. The goals of these strategies are to provide negative pressure to the wound and continuous evenly distributed fascial traction. Some choose a planned ventral hernia, in which only the skin is closed. This requires reoperation in several months, but avoids placement of a foreign body. Other surgeons perform a fascial closure with absorbable mesh, allow granulation to occur, and then place a skin graft [35–42].

Occasionally, while the patient is undergoing resuscitation, an unplanned operation is necessary. Problems arise such as bleeding, abdominal compartment syndrome, or continued septic shock. Abdominal compartment syndrome is a life threatening condition that develops during resuscitation due to accumulation of fluids and intra-abdominal swelling or due to continued bleeding. Compartment syndrome may present as decreased pulmonary compliance on the ventilator resulting in peak inspiratory pressures more than 40 cm H_2O, as cardiovascular collapse due to decreased venous return or as elevated bladder pressures more than 20 mm Hg with decreasing urine output [31–34].

The intensivist should also be aware of common postoperative problems, namely abscess and fistula formation. If fevers, ileus, or wound drainage arise during this phase, CT scan of the abdomen and pelvis are performed at approximately postoperative day 7. If any suspicious fluid collections are found, they can then be drained percutaneously.

Diagnostic Imaging for Suspected Intra-abdominal Infections

A critically ill patient with a suspected intra-abdominal process and a clinical exam consistent with peritonitis should be taken to the operating room for exploration and treatment. Without such findings on exam, diagnostic imaging is the next important step in the management of these patients.

Routinely, plain abdominal X-rays are obtained. They are easily acquired, have minimal radiation exposure, and can be done at the bedside. The acute abdominal series routinely consists of upright chest, upright abdominal, and supine abdominal films. Plain films have shown the most utility in the diagnosis of the perforated viscous and acute intestinal obstruction. For proper detection of free air, 5 to 10 minutes in the upright position are necessary before performing the study, to allow air to move to a visible location under the diaphragms. If the patient is unable to maintain an upright position, left lateral decubitus position is the next best. Plain films may demonstrate an obstructive process, showing distended bowel loops, step ladder air–fluid levels, and a paucity of distal bowel gas. Frequently however, critically ill patients are unable to sit upright or in a decubitus position for any amount of time. In addition, plain films lack the diagnostic accuracy to discover most intra-abdominal infections, and another mode is needed [43–45].

Computed tomography (CT) is the gold standard for the diagnosis of intra-abdominal processes, their locations and complications, with superior sensitivity and specificity for a range of life threatening diseases including, but not limited to, mesenteric ischemia, hernia, pancreatitis, diverticular abscess, and aneurysmal disease. Helical CT technology has improved both the quality and ease of administration of CT scans. Despite its diagnostic superiority, CT is not without its problems, especially in the ICU setting. Many critically ill patients are unable to be transferred to the radiology suite. Some morbidly obese patients are unable to fit into conventional scanners. CT scans obtained for suspected intra-abdominal infection should be performed with intravenous, oral, and sometimes rectal contrast. Failure to use contrast can significantly decrease diagnostic accuracy. Many ICU patients are unable to receive contrast, due to renal insufficiency or inability to tolerate orally administered contrast. Decisions about the use of contrast should be made with careful consideration weighing the input from surgeons and radiologists alike [43–45].

Ultrasound (US) is the workhorse of the ICU. In addition to its use as a tool in obtaining central and arterial access, echocardiography, bladder scans, focused abdominal sonogram for trauma (FAST), thoracentesis, and the detection of DVTs, ultrasound is a portable technology with applications in diagnosis and treatment of many intra-abdominal processes at the bedside in the ICU. US is the diagnostic procedure of choice in the setting of right upper quadrant diseases such as acalculous cholecystitis and hepatic lesions, as well as in pelvic diseases including ovarian torsion, PID, and ectopic pregnancy. US is also used at the bedside by the interventional radiologist to percutaneously drain abdominal fluid collections. In addition, US techniques are expanding to include natural orifice transluminal endoscopic surgery (NOTES) procedures for endoscopic ultrasound (EUS) guided drainage of collections in the chest, abdomen, and pelvis. Limitations of ultrasound include poor imaging with increased body wall thickness and bowel gas interference [44–49].

In the era of increasing use of minimally invasive technologies, bedside laparoscopy in the ICU is increasingly common and safe. Bedside laparoscopy can be performed by an abdominal drain tract or new port site. In addition, new devices are being developed that can be used without general anesthesia or pneumoperitoneum. The utility of bedside laparoscopy lies in its ability to diagnose various conditions such as mesenteric ischemia and cholecystitis or for use in trauma, while avoiding the morbidity of an exploratory laparotomy in a critically ill patient [50–53].

MANAGEMENT OF SPECIFIC INTRA-ABDOMINAL INFECTIONS

Management of Abscesses

Once intra-abdominal infection is recognized, and resuscitation and antibiotics have been started, a decision must be made regarding the most appropriate avenue for gaining source control. Percutaneous abscess drainage (PAD) has replaced the need for emergent operative intervention in the management of many intra-abdominal processes [20]. In some patients who become asymptomatic after drainage, PAD provides definitive therapy. In those with ultimately fatal diseases, palliation is provided, and the morbidity of subsequent surgical drainage may be avoided. In other situations, it allows for initial source control and medical stabilization so that an elective one stage operation can be performed. PAD and operative intervention are best viewed as complementary rather than competitive techniques.

Inflammation may manifest as a phlegmon, seen as a viable inflamed mass around the affected tissue, a liquefied abscess, necrotic tissue, or a combination. Liquefied abscesses are drainable, whereas phlegmon and necrotic tissue are not. Decisions regarding which mode of intervention to use are largely based on CT findings and require experience, clinical judgment, and careful consideration of underlying and coexistent disease processes. Close cooperation between the surgeon, interventional radiologist, and other physicians involved in the patient's care is mandatory.

The basic requirements for catheter drainage include a safe route of percutaneous access and a fluid collection of drainable viscosity. Specific indications for PAD have expanded significantly and now include many conditions that were previously thought undrainable, such as multiple or multiloculated abscesses, abscesses with enteric communication, infected hematomas, and deep pelvic abscesses [54,55]. In fact, for abdominal collections that require drainage, PAD is considered the standard, unless a hard indication for an operation exists [54,55]. Advances in endoluminal ultrasound techniques have facilitated advanced drainage procedures. Those abscesses in contact with the rectum or vagina can be treated with catheter drainage through these organs. These ultrasound-guided transrectal and transvaginal drainage procedures are effective and well tolerated [47,56,57].

It is generally possible to distinguish drainable fluid from phlegmon or necrotic tissue using a combination of imaging and fine-needle aspiration. Not all fluid collections require drainage, but intervention is required for those that are infected and for sterile collections that cause symptoms due to mass effect.

It is important to consider the possibility of underlying neoplastic disease in the setting of enteric perforation, especially in elderly patients. Significant soft tissue thickening of the bowel wall, especially if localized and non-circumferential, should raise the possibility of an underlying tumor, as should the demonstration of potential metastatic disease such as adenopathy or liver lesions. A "target" appearance, with circumferential low-attenuation submucosal thickening sandwiched between the enhancing mucosa and submucosa, is believed to be specific for inflammatory disease. To exclude the possibility of neoplasia fully, follow-up imaging is needed to document resolution, or confirmatory tests such as barium contrast studies or endoscopy can be performed.

Technical Aspects of Drainage Procedures for Intra-abdominal Abscesses

Excellent imaging is a key element for successful PAD. Imaging permits precise localization and characterization of disease, appropriate access route planning, and immediate assessment of technical success. Imaging is also needed for adequate follow-up to identify problems and gauge outcome. It is important that the drainage route not cross a sterile fluid collection or other infected space because of the risk of cross-contamination. Crossing the pleural space for thoracic and upper abdominal drainage carries the risk of empyema formation. Thus, collections in the upper abdomen often require an angled subcostal or low intercostal approach [58]. It is acceptable to cross the peritoneal space to drain an extraperitoneal abscess. Placement of a catheter through the small bowel or colon should always be avoided. Transgastric drainage of lesser sac pseudocysts has been advocated by some authors and appears to be safe, although this approach remains controversial [55]. Lesser sac collections also can be approached transhepatically through the left lobe of the liver [59], although traversing solid organs should be avoided whenever possible. Obviously, it is important to be aware of, and avoid, major vascular structures.

In most cases, drainage is performed following fine-needle (18- to 22-gauge) aspiration with the aspirate being used to document infection and gauge the viscosity of the fluid. In some situations, single-step aspiration of the fluid may suffice, without the need for tube placement. Examples include clearly aseptic collections, small abscesses (2 to 3 cm) into which tube placement would be difficult and relatively nonviscous collections that can be completely evacuated. However, for most collections, a drain should be placed to ensure complete evacuation and to minimize the chance of recurrence. If the patient is not already receiving antimicrobial therapy, this should be instituted before the drainage procedure to minimize the infectious complications of contaminating sterile tissue, although continued antibiotic coverage will be dictated by the contents of the fluid collection.

A multitude of catheters are available for percutaneous insertion. The choice of catheter size is determined primarily by the viscosity of the fluid to be drained. In the majority of cases, 8 to 12 French drains are sufficient [60,61]. Larger drains may be needed for collections that contain debris or more viscous fluid. Drains of larger caliber can be placed at a later time, if needed, by exchange over a guidewire. Although most abscesses can be drained with a single catheter, there should be no hesitation in placing as many drains as are needed to evacuate the abscesses effectively.

After catheter placement, the cavity should be evacuated as completely as possible and irrigated with saline until the fluid is clear. Initial manipulation of the catheter(s) and irrigation should be done as gently as possible to minimize the induction of transient bacteremia and subsequent potential hemodynamic instability. For cavities that are completely evacuated at the initial drainage and for which there are no abnormal communications to viscera, simple gravity drainage generally suffices. For larger or more viscous collections and those with ongoing output due to fistulous connections, suction drainage with sump catheters is more effective [59,61,62]. Thoracic drains should always be placed to water-seal suction to avoid the complication of simple or tension pneumothorax.

Proper catheter management following the initial placement is a critical determinant of success and requires the interventional radiologist to become an active member of the management team [63]. Drains should be checked regularly (at least daily) to monitor the volume and nature of the output, ensure adequate function and clinical response, and quickly recognize and correct any catheter-related problems. Periodic irrigation of the drains is recommended, once or several times per day, with sterile saline [64]. This can be performed by either physicians or trained nurses. Fibrinolytic agents may be useful for evacuation of fibrinous or hemorrhagic collections. Repeat imaging studies and catheter injections are frequently used to document progress and identify problems. Occasionally, it is necessary to add, replace, or reposition drain catheters.

Catheters should be removed when criteria for abscess resolution are met. Clinical criteria of success include resolution of symptoms and indicators of infection. Catheter-related criteria include a decrease in daily drainage to less than 10 mL and a change in the character of the drainage from purulent to serous. Radiographic criteria include abscess resolution and closure of any fistulous communications. If catheters are maintained until these criteria are satisfied, the likelihood of recurrence of the abscess is minimized. For sterile fluid collections, the drain should be removed as soon as possible, generally within 24 to 48 hours, to minimize the risk of superinfection [64].

In evaluating the causes of PAD failure, a number of factors are consistently identified, namely a fluid collection too viscous for drainage and the presence of phlegmon or necrotic debris. Technical modifications such as increasing the drain size and irrigation can salvage some of these drainage procedures. Recognition of phlegmon or necrotic tissue on follow-up imaging studies may lead to cessation of attempts at PAD. Multiloculated collections and multiple abscesses are another cause of failure that can be minimized by using an adequate number of catheters along with mechanical disruption of adhesions with a guidewire. Fistulous communications, either unrecognized or persistent, are yet another potential cause of failure, as is drainage of a necrotic tumor mistaken by imaging to represent an abscess.

Recognition of a significant soft tissue component, maintenance of a high index of suspicion, and the use of percutaneous biopsies can minimize the risk of failing to appreciate the presence of tumor. Suspicious fluid also can be sent for cytologic assessment. The success rate for PAD tends to be lower in immunocompromised patients (53%) patients, as compared to immunocompetent patients (73%) [65].

Appendicitis

Inflammation and infection of the vermiform appendix is the most common intra-abdominal infection requiring surgical intervention [66]. Though the highest incidence is during the first two decades of life, acute appendicitis affects all age groups.

Appendicitis results from obstruction of the appendiceal lumen due to fecalith, lymphadenopathy, foreign body or mass, which initially results in increased luminal pressure, stasis of luminal contents, and soft tissue edema. An intense inflammatory reaction ensues, causing neutrophil infiltration. Venous outflow obstruction develops followed by arterial inflow insufficiency, ultimately resulting in gangrene and perforation.

Classic appendicitis presents with migratory abdominal pain. Initially dull and poorly localized in the periumbilical region, the pain changes to a sharper quality located in the right lower quadrant over McBurney's point. Anorexia is present early and a mild fever is often present. Nausea and vomiting may also be seen, but if they appear early, before development of pain, suspicion should arise for gastroenteritis. Exam reveals focal peritonitis, often evidenced by rebound tenderness, though a cadre of different signs may be elicited [66]. Leukocytosis, if present at all, is mild. Clinical signs of perforation include intense pain, prolonged symptoms, high fever, significant leukocytosis, tachycardia, and severe tenderness [67].

If the diagnosis cannot be made confidently or if perforation is suspected, contrast enhanced CT scan of the abdomen and pelvis may be ordered and has a 95% positive predictive value for acute appendicitis. CT scan may demonstrate appendiceal dilation and wall thickening, periappendiceal fat stranding, appendicolith, phlegmon, abscess, gross perforation, or free fluid [44,68]. Ultrasound is slightly less reliable for diagnosis and demonstration of complications, but is most useful in evaluating for alternate diagnoses, especially gynecologic disorders [68]. Care should be taken to distinguish periappendiceal changes with those around the terminal ileum that may represent inflammatory bowel disease.

Management is started by early administration of intravenous antibiotics covering against Gram-negative bacteria and anaerobes [69]. In acute non-perforated appendicitis, operative intervention should proceed as quickly as possible. Laparoscopic appendectomy is now the procedure of choice, though in thin males open appendectomy is acceptable. Laparoscopic approach provides superb visualization and allows evaluation of other pelvic and abdominal organs [66]. If perforation is found at laparoscopy, the appendix is resected, irrigation is performed, and antibiotics are continued for an extended course of 7 days.

Periappendiceal masses found on imaging may be a phlegmon or an abscess, representing a contained perforation. If feasible, percutaneous drainage of discrete abscesses is standard. If adequate drainage is achieved, management without appendectomy in the acute setting is safe and effective. Less than 10% of patients will fail this approach and require emergent appendectomy [70].

Current controversy exists concerning the need for interval appendectomy (IA) after initial nonsurgical management. Standard for many years was to perform an IA after a resolution phase of 6 to 8 weeks. IA is often a technically difficult operation due to adhesions and distorted anatomy, and many surgeons will elect not to perform IA. This strategy may be most appropriate, as risk of recurrence of appendicitis or related complication is low, only 5% to 9% in current studies [69–72]. Accurate predictors of recurrence are needed. Also of concern is the risk of malignancy. Appendiceal neoplasm is present in 1.7% of surgical specimens [73,74]. In 1.2% of patients managed nonoperatively, a malignancy was discovered at follow up [70]. Careful consideration of the patient's physiologic status and risk factors must be made.

Diverticulitis

Diverticulitis is an inflammation of colonic diverticula, while these are actually pseudodiverticula – small herniations of colonic mucosa and submucosa through the muscularis [75]. Diverticula develop from a combination of increased intracolonic pressure and mural weakness at the site of blood vessel penetration into the colon [76,77]. The diverticula become occluded with fecal matter. Local ischemia and bacterial overgrowth result in microperforation and the start of the inflammatory cascade [29].

Diverticulitis presents as a constellation of signs and symptoms, most commonly a triad of fever, lower abdominal pain, and leukocytosis. It is typically a disease of older patients, and very rare in patients younger than 40 [78]. Patients also report constipation, recent hematochezia, nausea, vomiting, and dysuria. Pneumaturia and fecaluria are rare, but indicate colovesicular fistula [79]. Diverticulitis is primarily a clinical diagnosis, but contrast enhanced CT is usually performed to assess the location and severity of disease. CT shows colonic wall thickening and fat stranding around an area with diverticula [80]. Masses, fistulas, abscesses, and perforation may also be visualized.

Management is based upon severity of symptoms, number of recurrences, and presence of any complications of diverticulitis. For those with minor symptoms, oral antibiotics can be given, with a gentle resumption of a regular diet. Complicated disease is defined as having a pericolic or pelvic abscess, fistula, stricture, obstruction, hemorrhage, perforation, or diffuse peritonitis [29,81]. For those with complicated diverticulitis, with more severe symptoms or with signs of systemic inflammation, hospital admission, bowel rest, and parenteral antibiotics are mandated after immediate fluid resuscitation [79]. Length of therapy is variable, but usually is continued until leukocytosis is improved, the patient is afebrile, and has decreased abdominal tenderness [29,75,79].

Emergent surgical intervention may be required. Any patient with diffuse peritonitis, obstruction, severe perforation, or not responding to antibiotics alone mandates an immediate surgical exploration and washout with any necessary interventions for repair of colonic perforation [75,81]. Abscesses as a result of complicated diverticulitis are treated similarly as all other intra-abdominal abscesses. In the abscess of generalized peritonitis and hemodynamic instability, well-circumscribed abscesses should be drained percutaneously [75,82,83]. After hospital discharge, patients should undergo colonoscopy, especially in cases of right-sided diverticulitis and those cases with perforation. It is imperative to rule out a potential malignancy. Typically, a 6-week cooling off period is allowed before endoscopy.

Elective surgical intervention is indicated in several circumstances. Those patients with numerous recurrences are at risk for multiple hospital admissions, future complicated disease, and associated colostomy. Elective resection may spare them this morbidity. Complicated disease is much more likely on first presentation, however, and better predictors are needed to determine who will have a recurrence of complicated disease [81]. Any patient having an attack complicated by abscess, stricture, fistula, or contained perforation should undergo elective resection. Patients in whom an underlying colon cancer cannot be successfully ruled out should also undergo interval elective resection [84].

Operative intervention in the elective setting is usually a resection of the affected colon, with colorectal anastomosis. Technique in emergent operations can range from resection of the grossly inflamed tissue and end colostomy (Hartmann's procedure) to resection and primary anastomosis. Both approaches have been shown to be safe, and the decision depends on extent of inflammation and soilage [27,28,30]. The resection of all areas containing diverticula is not necessary, as often they can be scattered about the entirety of the colon [80].

Acute Pancreatitis

Pancreatitis continues to be a difficult disease to treat, despite numerous attempts to clarify and standardize treatment algorithms [85]. The leading causes of acute pancreatitis in North America are biliary disease and alcohol use [86]. The diagnosis of acute pancreatitis is often not difficult – the combination of acute abdominal pain, elevated serum pancreatic enzymes, and nausea and vomiting strongly suggest the diagnosis. The controversy arises in the treatment of complicated acute pancreatitis.

Complicated acute pancreatitis is a disease often encountered in the modern ICU. Patients with pancreatitis often require massive fluid resuscitation and are at increased risk for organ failure [86]. Initial consideration should be given to adequate resuscitation, preserving organ function, providing enteral nutrition, and possibly antibiotics. Although controversy exists for each therapy, the consensus is to resuscitate patients with crystalloid to preserve organ function. Urine output remains the most reliable parameter. Enteral nutrition should be established through gastric feeds to preserve gut immune function and attempt to reverse the catabolic state [86]. Antibiotics directed to Gram-negative and anaerobic flora are reserved for patients with proven infection or prophylactic treatment for those with worsening clinical condition and developing organ failure [87].

Acute pancreatitis is frequently plagued by one of four possible complications – pancreatic pseudocyst, pancreatic abscess, pancreatic necrosis, and infected pancreatic necrosis. Pancreatic pseudocyst is rarely a cause of intra-abdominal sepsis and the natural history of pseudocyst is usually self-limited. If a pseudocyst becomes infected it is classified and treated as an abscess. Percutaneous drainage of infected fluid collections is the treatment of choice and should be undertaken expeditiously once the collections are discovered [88]. Pancreatic necrosis is diagnosed by contrast-enhanced CT scan. Absence of enhancement of the organ strongly suggests necrosis. Necrosis can be missed if CT scan is performed too soon after admission [89]. Treatment strategy is determined by whether the necrosis is sterile or infected. Patients with pancreatic necrosis exhibiting neither organ failure nor hemodynamic instability likely have sterile necrosis. Conversely, patients with worsening clinical conditions despite maximum therapy likely have infected necrosis. Any doubt may be answered by percutaneous image-guided biopsy for culture. The distinction is important since markedly different treatments are employed.

Pancreatic necrosis which remains sterile does not require any additional antimicrobial therapy. Should clinical deterioration occur, it is best to initiate treatment for infected pancreatic necrosis. The treatment for infected pancreatic necrosis is as drastic as it is controversial. Antibiotic therapy should be initiated immediately; a carbapenem such as imipenem/cilastin is recommended [87]. Prophylactic antibiotic coverage for sterile pancreatic necrosis has been proposed to prevent infection, but meta-analysis has not shown this to be true. Sterile pancreatic necrosis should not receive antimicrobial therapy [87].

In addition to antimicrobial therapy for infected pancreatic necrosis, surgical intervention should be considered. The timing and approach of surgical intervention is often debated. Consensus is that if clinically possible, delayed debridement is optimal, resulting in decreased mortality. Pancreatic necrosectomy in the acute stages of necrotizing pancreatitis may become necessary in the clinically worsening patient, but mortality remains exceedingly high [88]. Interest has developed in a minimally invasive approach to pancreatic debridement, using a combination of retroperitoneal nephroscopic debridement, percutaneous drainage, and endoscopic drainage and debridement. These approaches will require further study and have not reached the standard of care in North America [90,91].

Biliary Tract Infections

Acute Acalculous Cholecystitis

Acute cholecystitis in the intensive care setting is a different disease than the stone related disease found in ambulatory patients. Acute acalculous cholecystitis (AAC) is seen in patients suffering from diverse disease processes such as cardiac ischemia, burns, hemorrhage, pneumonia, or severe volume depletion. These patients may be undergoing such treatments as vasopressor support, transfusion, prolonged ventilatory support, high levels of PEEP, prolonged NPO status, and TPN. All of these conditions and treatments are risk factors for development of AAC [92–94]. Acalculous cholecystitis is the gallbladder's reaction to severe systemic illness, rather than a local process as occurs in gallstone related disease.

Decreased digestive stimulation causes stasis, gallbladder distention, and increased intraluminal pressure with associated bile infiltration into the mucosal and muscular layers. There is lymphatic distention and tissue edema [95]. Transfusion of packed red blood cells leads to changes in bile composition and increased sludge [92]. Gut hypoperfusion results in microvascular occlusion and leukocyte recruitment [95–99]. Thus gallbladder empyema, gangrene, and perforation may occur.

Critically ill patients are often obtunded or sedated and are unable to exhibit right upper quadrant tenderness. Hepatic transaminase and alkaline phosphatase levels are often normal and not helpful for diagnosis. A new leukocytosis or fever in a patient with appropriate risk factors should prompt radiographic evaluation, as a delay in diagnosis substantially increases mortality [100,101].

As in all cases of suspected right upper quadrant disease, ultrasound is the initial test of choice. Findings on ultrasound consistent with AAC are pericholecystic fluid, gallbladder distention or elongation, wall thickening, mucosal sloughing, and especially intramural gas [102,103]. Concern exists about the poor accuracy of US in the setting of acalculous disease as there are no standards for the normal gallbladder appearance in critical illness and diagnosis may be missed [104,105]. Since US is quick, portable, and repeatable, accuracy improves upon repeating the exam or using US in conjunction with cholescintigraphy [103,106]. CT scan is most useful in its ability to evaluate the entire abdomen, therefore it is ordered when AAC is not foremost of differential diagnoses. CT is still able to detect AAC in many cases, with findings similar to ultrasound [103,107–109]. Cholescintigraphy, a type of HIDA scan, visualizes injected intravenous radionucleotide buildup in the gallbladder. With intravenous morphine to augment the biliary secretion of the radionucleotide and CCK to visualize gallbladder emptying, superior diagnostic accuracy is achieved [103,105,106]. The large drawbacks of cholescintigraphy is that it is a time consuming test performed in the radiology suite and thus may not be appropriate for critically ill patients.

Antibiotics against Gram-negative rods should begin immediately after the diagnosis is made [69]. Definitive therapy for AAC is cholecystectomy, but treatment strategy is guided by the physiologic status of the patient. ICU patients already suffering complications from their primary, non-gallbladder illness are often unable to tolerate anesthesia and operative intervention. In this setting, percutaneous cholecystostomy under US or CT guidance is safe and effective. With a low failure rate, it can provide adequate source control [110–112]. Open cholecystostomy was performed in the past, but is obsolete in settings where image guided percutaneous drainage is available. When the patient physiologically improves, definitive therapy may be administered by laparoscopic cholecystectomy, on an elective rather than emergent basis [101,103,113]. Only in extremely ill or elderly patients, may cholecystectomy be avoided and cholecystostomy be considered definitive therapy [114].

Ascending Cholangitis

Since Charcot described the elements of "hepatic fever" in 1877, ascending cholangitis (AC) has been consistently defined as having two main features: common bile duct (CBD) obstruction and bactibilia [115]. Today, many of the critically ill patients presenting with AC have recently undergone manipulation of the biliary tract or stent placement. In patients without recent instrumentation, choledocholithiasis, benign or malignant stricture, adenopathy, and postoperative anastomotic stricture are important causes of cholangitis [116–118].

Partial obstruction of the hepatobiliary tract results in higher levels of bactibilia, but any acute obstruction will result in increased intraductal pressures. The increased pressure distends the ducts and increases wall permeability. Translocation of bacteria and toxins occurs and causes systemic toxicity, bacteremia, and hepatic abscesses [118].

The diagnosis of ascending cholangitis is clinical. Charcot described a triad of fever with rigors, right upper quadrant abdominal pain, and jaundice. Reynold's pentad also includes hypotension and altered mental status [119]. These clinical findings are still commonly seen in AC today; however, the classic triad and pentad are only seen in late disease. Patients presenting earlier often have right upper quadrant pain, fever without chills, and hyperbilirubinemia. Elevated transaminases and alkaline phosphatase may also be present due to biliary obstruction and hepatic injury and should not be confused with acute viral hepatitis [115,116].

In the patient with ascending cholangitis, imaging serves several functions—especially confirming diagnosis. Cross-sectional imaging is important for defining the level of obstruction. Etiology and treatment of a proximal CBD obstruction would be quite different than that of a periampullary obstruction. Imaging will also serve to elucidate associated pathology such as hepatic metastasis or abscess. As in all patients with right upper quadrant pain, the initial study of choice is ultrasound [120]. Both ultrasound and CT can accurately detect a dilated CBD and extrahepatic biliary obstruction, but neither can determine the cause and exact level of obstruction, compared to direct cholangiography [121,122]. MRCP is comparable to direct cholangiography in its ability to determine cause and level of obstruction and is noninvasive. Unfortunately, MRCP has a minimal role in the management of acute AC, since these patients will need an invasive procedure for treatment [115,122].

Once a diagnosis of cholangitis is made, prompt initiation of antibiotics and drainage of the biliary tree is required. ICU admission is needed in moderate and severe cases, and aggressive supportive care should ensue. Antibiotic profile should be selected to cover enteric organisms, including *E. coli, Klebsiella, Pseudomonas, and Enterococcus* [115,116]. The preferred method for complete visualization and decompression of the biliary tree is endoscopic retrograde cholangiopancreatography (ERCP). Bile samples should be sent for culture. If the patient is unstable or all stones are unable to be cleared, a nasobiliary drain should be placed. Nasobiliary drains allow for subsequent imaging and sampling. In a stable patient, after successful removal of all stones, an internally draining stent should be placed [115,123,124]. If malignancy is suspected, brushings and cytology should be performed. If a gallstone is lodged at the ampulla or multiple impacted stones are present, papillotomy is required. Percutaneous transhepatic cholangiography (PTC) may be performed if ERCP provides inadequate decompression, if obstruction is proximal, or if the patient is too unstable to tolerate sedation needed for ERCP. If all interventions should fail, the final and definitive solution may be operative drainage of the bile ducts. After cholangitis resolves, patients will require a definitive operation. Laparoscopic cholecystectomy should be performed for gallstone related disease. Advanced imaging or laboratory studies may be needed for workup and planning for resection of malignant disease [115–118, 125].

Colonic Disease

Clostridium difficile Pseudomembranous Colitis

Initially named because of the difficulty in cultivating the bacterium [126], *Clostridium difficile* infection is an increasingly common and severe problem in modern intensive care units. With abundant use of broad-spectrum antibiotics and frequent colonization, *C. diff* associated diarrhea or pseudomembranous colitis is the most common nosocomial infectious diarrhea in adults [127–131].

C. Diff colitis is an opportunistic infection. During antimicrobial therapy for various infections, intestinal flora is destroyed, leaving ample resources for *C. difficile* to multiply. *C. difficile* is a Gram-positive, anaerobic, spore-forming bacillus. This microbe produces two exotoxins, toxin A and toxin B, which are responsible for causing diarrhea, colitis, and systemic illness. Recently, a hypervirulent strain has emerged, BI/NAP1/027, which produces "binary toxin" and increased levels of toxins A and B. This strain has been associated with increased disease severity and recurrence [132–134].

C. difficile infection can manifest in several forms. The most common *C. diff* presentation is colitis with diarrhea, though as many as 20% to 37% [135–137] of patients may have such severe colonic dysmotility that diarrhea is absent. Severe enteritis has been described, and though it is rare, it is capable of producing profound illness [138]. Patients presenting with signs and symptoms of systemic illness are labeled as having severe or fulminant colitis, carrying a mortality rate of 35% [139].

Multiple modalities may be implemented in the diagnosis of fulminant pseudomembranous colitis. In the critically ill patient, the presence of diarrhea is often the first clue. The presence of abdominal distention or peritonitis on physical exam, as well as profound leukocytosis and bandemia are all significant in *C. diff* infection. The gold standard for diagnosis of *C. diff* infection is the notoriously slow cytotoxin assay, which takes 1 to 3 days to result. Most commonly, hospitals use an ELISA to detect the presence of toxin A or B, but these assays have been criticized as having a high false negative rate [135]. Many institutions have established the practice of repeating the test at the next episode of diarrhea to improve diagnostic accuracy. New assays are being tested, which are both rapid and highly accurate [140].

Presence of pseudomembranes, disseminated yellow punctuate mural plaques on endoscopy, can assure the diagnosis. Flexible sigmoidoscopy is commonly performed, but studies have shown poor accuracy in the setting of disease limited to the ascending colon. Colonoscopy of the entire colon may be performed, but would require bowel prep and carries greater risk of colonic perforation in a patient already suffering from severe illness [135,137,141].

In patients with a clinical picture consistent with fulminant colitis, computed tomography (CT) has been found to be the most sensitive measure of colonic inflammation [137]. CT scan may show perforation, colonic thickening, colonic distention, pericolonic inflammation, or free abdominal fluid. CT can localize disease as right or left side predominant or can confirm presence of pancolitis. Though the predictive nature of CT scan is debated, diagnosis made by CT scan, as compared to endoscopy or toxin assay, has been shown to predict survival in patients undergoing colectomy for pseudomembranous colitis [135,141,142].

The mainstay of *C. diff* colitis treatment is medical. When feasible, patients with moderate disease should be discontinued from other antimicrobial therapy. Narcotics, loperamide, Lomotil, or other antimotility agents should also be discontinued, as they promote retention of toxins. Patients should receive general supportive therapy.

Moderate disease is treated with oral metronidazole, with oral vancomycin reserved for recurrent disease. Other antibiotic usage, as well as the duration of therapy is frequently debated. Ten days of therapy after cessation of other antibiotics is considered sufficient [143].

For initial recurrent disease, another round of metronidazole is given, followed by oral vancomycin therapy for a second recurrence. For patients with inability to tolerate oral medications, a nasogastric tube should be used to deliver the medications or vancomycin may be given rectally. Intravenous metronidazole may be added in this scenario, but independently is not as effective as oral therapy [144]. Adjunctive medical therapies may be considered for recurrent disease. Probiotics are frequently used to repopulate gut flora. *Saccharomyces boulardii* is thought to have anti-inflammatory effects on the colon [145]. In small, randomized controlled trials, probiotics have shown a favorable effect. Probiotic cocktails have been shown to both prevent and decrease recurrence of *C. diff* infections [146].

Cutting-edge therapies target the toxin-mediated mechanism of *C. diff* colitis. IVIG administration [147] and treatment with monoclonal antibodies [133] are currently being used in clinical trials. *C. difficile* infections progress to fulminant disease in 3% to 8% of patients [132]. Fulminant or complicated disease is defined variably throughout the literature. Definitions generally include such parameters as need for ICU admission, need for surgery, and presence of shock, respiratory failure, or renal failure.

Physicians and researchers have struggled to find adequate predictors of disease severity. Many recent studies have sought to elucidate exactly which factors predict a patient's risk of mortality. Profound leukocytosis is often seen in *C. diff* infections and several studies show increase in mortality associated with a WBC count more than 20,000 per μL. High band percentage or leukopenia were also associated with poor survival. Patient age more than 70 years, ASA score of 4 or 5, low diastolic blood pressures are all factors frequently associated with poor survival in fulminant disease [50,128,132,139]. Length of stay preceding diagnosis of *C. diff* colitis was associated with decreased survival, both in surgically and medically treated groups [50].

Development of fulminant colitis is a surgical concern, and colectomy can be curative in many patients. The true difficulty for the clinician is discovering a window in which patients with fulminant disease will benefit from colectomy, without exposing excess numbers of patients to the morbidity of surgery. Overall, the mortality associated with colectomy in the setting of fulminant *C. diff* colitis is between 35% and 57%. Several studies call for early surgical management and even a surgical opinion in all cases of severe disease [128,132,135,136,141,148,149].

Need for preoperative vasopressors was associated with increase in perioperative mortality from 14% to 65% [135]. Similarly, in another study, patients requiring preoperative vasopressors or intubation had an increase in mortality from 16% to 84% [141]. Preoperative presence of acute respiratory failure and acute renal failure have been identified as independent predictors of mortality after colectomy [149]. However, patients having a recent surgical procedure had improved mortality after colectomy (77%), compared to those that did not have a recent procedure (23%) [141].

Though several operative approaches have been described for fulminant pseudomembranous colitis, the operation of choice is total colectomy with end ileostomy. In series where left hemicolectomy was performed, mortality increased from 11% to 14% after total colectomy to 100% after left hemicolectomy [136,150]. The exception to this finding is in right-side only disease, identified on endoscopy. Patients undergoing right hemicolectomy had no decrease in survivals [135]. These data highlight the need for early diagnosis of *C. difficile* infection and early surgical intervention, before the development of organ failure.

Toxic Megacolon

Toxic megacolon (TM) has been recognized as a clinical entity for over 60 years, and is defined as an inflammation of the colon causing progressive dilation in the presence of systemic toxicity [151]. Initially described in patients with complicated ulcerative colitis (UC) or Crohn's disease, it is seen more recently as a complication of many various conditions of the colon. Due to improved management techniques of inflammatory bowel disease (IBD) and increased awareness of associated complications, the incidence of TM has decreased in these conditions. TM is still frequently diagnosed as the initial presentation of previously unknown UC [152–154]. TM caused by *C. diff* colitis is on the rise in modern hospitals due to the increasing severity and incidence of *C. diff* infections. Associated with immunosuppression due to AIDS, CMV colitis is also increasingly common. Salmonella, *E. coli* 0157, Shigella, Campylobacter, amoeba, and other infectious diarrheal illnesses have each been recognized as a cause of TM. TM has also developed after various chemotherapy treatments, bowel ischemia, and treatment with antimotility drugs [155–163]. During a workup for possible TM, it is also important to consider intestinal pseudo-obstruction and actual bowel obstruction, though these patients do not exhibit the systemic illness of TM patients.

On gross pathologic specimens, IBD related TM shows dilation, mural thinning, and deep ulcerations while microscopic examination shows myocyte degeneration, abundant granulation tissue with intact Auerbach and Meissner's plexuses. *C. diff* related disease shows the yellow plaques consistent with that disease. CMV related disease shows inclusion bodies on microscopic specimens [151]. The etiology of toxic megacolon lies in the induction of nitric oxide (NO) in the inflamed colonic tissue. NO has been shown to decrease smooth muscle activity. NO synthase was upregulated in surgical specimens of TM as well as in animal models, which also demonstrated colonic dilation and decreased contractile activity [164,165].

Diagnosis of toxic megacolon first involves key elements in the patient's history. Especially important are a personal or family history of inflammatory bowel disease, symptoms of extraintestinal manifestations of IBD, timing of symptoms of diarrhea, abdominal pain and blood per rectum, recent antibiotic use or hospitalization, HIV status and sexual history, recent travel, recent meals as well as any recent starting or stopping of any medications. Next, determining the level of systemic illness is important. Classic criteria require three of the following: fever >38°C, HR >120 per minute, leukocytosis >10,500 per μL, anemia. In addition, one of the following is needed: dehydration, altered consciousness, electrolyte disturbances, or hypotension. The severity of each of these criteria is not specifically defined [154]. These criteria pre-date modern definitions of SIRS/sepsis, which could be used alternatively. Coupled with these above criteria, radiographic evidence of colonic dilation is required.

Classically plain films have been used to diagnose and follow progression of colonic dilation. Typically, a colon dilated to 6 cm was worrisome of an impending perforation, although large variability is seen. Plain films are also able to demonstrate colonic perforation. Recently, CT scan has been found to be superior to plain films. CT scans of TM patients demonstrate dilation in the right and transverse more than left colon. Diameter of 6 to 10 cm with abnormal haustral patterns is the typical finding. Frequently target or accordion signs are visible. Also, significant ascites and pleural effusions are present. CT does not demonstrate superiority in diagnosing the underlying etiology of the TM, but CT is able to detect complications of the disease that were missed on plain films. These findings include small perforations, abscesses, ascending phlebitis, and septic emboli [151,166]. CT scans should be performed upon diagnosis if possible, but are unnecessary in the severely ill patient.

Management of TM involves aggressive medical treatment from the moment of diagnosis and early surgical consultation. Patients should receive supportive ICU therapies and monitoring. Nasogastric tubes should be placed for decompression. Broad-spectrum antibiotics should be started. Treatment of the specific etiology of the TM should begin promptly. Steroids have been given for patients with diagnosis of toxic megacolon due to Crohn's disease or ulcerative colitis, but extreme caution should be used to ensure that an infectious cause is not present and avoid steroids in such cases. Salicylates should also be avoided in the setting of TM [151,159]. An adjunct to medical therapy is postural therapy. Benefit has been shown to patient rolling or a knee-elbow posture. This is presumed to reduce distention by allowing colonic gas to move distally and be more easily expelled [167,168].

Surgical consultation should be obtained as soon as the diagnosis of toxic megacolon is established. Though medical therapy has been shown to be effective in some cases, many patients will not respond and will need a timely, life saving colectomy. Certain indications for an operation include signs of peritonitis, free air, uncontrollable rectal bleeding, and failure of medical therapy. There is no specific size for colon diameter that necessitates colectomy, rather the overall clinical picture should determine therapy. Controversy exists as to the timing of surgery and the definition of medical failure. Medical failure should be viewed as continued clinical deterioration or progressive colonic dilation. Some patients exhibit marked improvement with medical therapy. Others exhibit prompt deterioration and should be taken to the operating room. Often patients show variable degrees of toxicity and questionable response to therapy (i.e., improvement in heart rate but continue to have fever). These patients may undergo a short trial of medical therapy, lasting 24 to 36 hours, with close examination by critical care and surgical teams. Any sign of complication or worsening condition should be managed operatively [152,153,156,169].

Several procedures are proposed for operative management of toxic megacolon. Overall operative mortality for TM is in the range of 7% to 30%, depending on the timing and type of procedure performed. The procedure of choice in modern surgical care is the subtotal colectomy with end ileostomy, leaving a rectal stump or creating a sigmoid mucous fistula. This procedure removes the diseased colon and leaves adequate tissue for future resection or reconstruction. It can be performed safely and quickly [151–153,156,169].

Postoperative Peritonitis

Postoperative peritonitis (PP) is primarily a consequence of anastomotic leakage (66%), intra-abdominal abscess (13%), or perforated viscous (7%) [170]. Local tissue ischemia, infected hematoma, and bile leakage are also common causes of PP and all have an iatrogenic component [171].

PP is a highly lethal condition, with a mortality rate of 30% [172], in part because it is often diagnosed late, due to ascribing clinical deterioration to other possible primary processes, or the reluctance to admit the possibility of a suture-line dehiscence. Malnourished patients, those with resistant organisms, those with multiple organ failures, and the elderly are all at risk for PP [173].

This diagnosis should be considered in any patient with signs of sepsis who has undergone a recent abdominal procedure, particularly those that included a gastrointestinal anastomosis or diffuse soilage. Laparotomy itself introduces free air into the abdominal cavity, thus pneumoperitoneum is a nonspecific finding in patients during the first few days after operation. Diffuse tenderness may not be uniformly present, as it can be masked by incisional pain. Intra-abdominal fluid is to be expected in the recent postoperative period. However, if US or CT reveals large amounts of fluid or persistent peritoneal fluid, image-guided aspiration should be considered for diagnostic purposes. A Gram's stain that reveals white cells, bacteria, or enteric contents is an indication for immediate laparotomy.

Surgical treatment should include either re-anastomosis in small bowel leaks or end-colostomy in colonic leaks, depending upon the degree of fecal contamination and the patient's condition. Postoperative abscesses should be percutaneously drained with image guidance. Patients suffering from PP who have been hospitalized for several days may be infected with resistant organisms. Cultures should be followed closely and therapy extended if the patient is without clinical improvement [174]. The postoperative patient deserves the highest degree of suspicion for anastomotic leak upon any suggestion that an intra-abdominal process has developed.

Enteric Fistula

Gastrointestinal fistulas are among the most dreaded and difficult to manage complications treated by surgeons and intensivists. A fistula is defined as an abnormal communication between two epithelialized surfaces. Enterocutaneous fistulas (ECFs), connections between bowel and skin, are associated with mortality rates of up to 21% [175] and long, expensive hospital stays. Patients suffering from ECFs are also frequently plagued with such problems as severe fluid and electrolyte imbalances, malnutrition, anemia, sepsis, and difficult wound care issues.

More recently, open-air fistulas, or enteroatmospheric fistulas (EAF) are increasingly common, as a consequence of damage control surgery and the open abdomen. EAFs involve spillage of intestinal contents into an open laparotomy wound, rather than to the skin. This combination of a large open wound and continuing peritonitis leads to a profoundly catabolic state. This is a dire situation, with mortality approaching 65%, considerable patient suffering, and huge demands on resources and clinicians to provide adequate nursing and wound care [175,176].

Enteric fistulas have numerous antecedent causes, including trauma, foreign body, infection, inflammatory bowel disease, radiation treatment, vascular insufficiency, anastomotic leak, inadvertent enterotomy, and other iatrogenic injury. Fistulas are classified as high output (>500 mL per day), moderate output (200 to 500 mL per day), or low output (<200 mL per day). It is also important to classify a fistula according to its site of origin (e.g., gastrocutaneous, colocutaneous). EAFs are classified as superficial or deep, depending on if they drain outward onto the exposed bowel or inward into the peritoneal cavity [175,176].

ECFs typically present as occult sepsis in a postoperative patient, who has a continued postoperative ileus, a distended abdomen, late postoperative fevers, or increasing leukocytosis. Often there are signs of a wound infection followed by the appearance of intestinal contents through the wound. Diagnosis of fistula is a clinical one, made at the bedside, though laboratory and imaging studies are useful in fistula characterization and management. Fistulogram, that is, contrast injected into the fistula or drain under fluoroscopy, is the prime means of characterizing the fistula, providing information about its location and most importantly can show presence or absence of obstruction distal to the fistula, which precludes spontaneous closure in all instances. CT scan is most useful in elucidating intra-abdominal abscess or other pathology and allows for percutaneous drainage [175,177]. Studying the fistula is the clinician's lowest priority among management goals. Stabilization of the patient, protection of the skin, and ramping nutrition up to goal should all be accomplished first.

Management of patients with fistula disease demands aggressive supportive care. Volume replacement and maintenance is paramount, as patients may lose several liters of fluid daily from intestinal contents measured by drains and bags, as well as large amounts of insensate losses from open wounds and increased respiratory rates. Fluid losses should be measured and replaced. Hypokalemia can be a lethal problem commonly seen with high output fistulas, and should be meticulously managed. Patients should be placed on strict NPO status, gastric secretions should be minimized with a proton pump inhibitor and initially a nasogastric tube should be inserted to prevent distal transit of gastric secretions. Octreotide is often used to decrease fistula output by inhibiting pancreatic and intestinal secretions and decreasing intestinal motility [175,176,178].

Wound management is crucial to timely healing of ECFs and requires a thoughtful and imaginative approach by a team including senior surgeons and wound care/stoma specialists. Goals of wound management include protection of surrounding skin, measuring the effluent, and avoiding desiccation of the exposed bowel. Careful efforts should be made to avoid worsening of the fistula or creation of a new fistula in the surrounding area. Skin should be kept clean and dry. Skin protection can be accomplished with duoderm and ostomy glue placed around the wound edges. Effluent can be collected in a standard ostomy pouch or by intubating the fistula opening with a sump or "whistle-tip" catheter on low suction [175,177]. Recent reports show that with painstaking wound care, 37% to 46% of ECFs may close spontaneously [179,180].

Wound management in patients with open-air fistulas is considerably more complex, due to exposed intra-abdominal contents. Approximately 12 to 14 days postoperatively, dense adhesions form between exposed bowel loops, and they become fused. If a deep EAF is present, and the opening is unable to be drained with sumps, free soiling of the peritoneal cavity will continue. Negative pressure wound therapies are now being employed with some success in this situation, as they allow for continuous drainage. Caution should be used to protect exposed bowel from direct suction with plastic sheeting [176,180]. Superficial EAFs can be functionally converted into an ECF by placing a skin graft onto the granulation tissue of the fused, exposed bowel. Once the skin graft heals, an ostomy pouch may be placed over the fistula [175,176]. Patients with EAF may have a difficult, open wound for months.

Prolonged intestinal failure is the hallmark of severe fistula disease and aggressive nutritional support is a chief principle in the management of ECFs. Ongoing inflammatory processes result in increased nutritional need and inefficient use of supplied nutrients. Draining intestinal secretions result in major protein losses. Patients with high output fistulas have substantially increased nutritional requirements, often more than double their baseline calculated calorie and protein requirements. Additionally, patients will require much higher doses of vitamins and trace elements [175]. Patients with fistula disease may also benefit from immunonutrition supplementation. Glutamine supplementation is thought to normalize intestinal immunology and cytokine profiles as well as reversing intestinal villus atrophy. Other nutrients such as arginine and fish oil are associated with improved outcomes in critically ill patients [181–183].

Patients with low output fistulas should be able to receive the majority of their nutrition enterally, by a low residue, easily absorbable formula. High output fistulas can also be managed with enteral nutrition. Using a feeding tube in the proximal jejunum, sufficient absorption should occur if at least 4 feet of normal intestine exists between the ligament of Treitz and the fistula. If insufficient length is present here, then enteral feeding may be provided with the tip of the feeding tube distal to the fistula. Another alternative for enteral feeding is fistuloclysis, feeding directly into the fistula itself. When enteral nutrition is provided, it is best given in elemental or semi-elemental formulations, which facilitate absorption. Enteral nutrition is believed by many to have equal efficacy in fistula closure to parenteral nutrition, is able to prevent intestinal mucosal atrophy and reduce incidence of other nosocomial infections [175,184–188]. Full enteral nutritional support is not always possible, due to distal obstruction, sepsis, hypotension, or poor absorptive capacity, and additional support is needed.

The widespread use of parenteral nutrition (TPN) has improved fistula management dramatically, allowing patients' nutritional needs to be met when it is not possible to do so enterally. TPN is thought to reduce overall patient mortality and result in increased rates of fistula closure. Parenteral nutrition also allows for custom replacement of micronutrients and trace elements. Unfortunately, TPN carries risks of central venous catheter insertion, increased expense, catheter related sepsis, thrombosis, and TPN associated cholestasis, and liver dysfunction [175,185–188].

Surgical mantra dictates that if ECFs do not heal spontaneously by 6 weeks, then they will ultimately require operative management. Timing of surgical repair is crucial, since early in the postoperative process, patients develop dense adhesions intra-abdominally that prevent access into the abdomen. Most surgeons describe a waiting period of several months before attempting surgical repair. This delay is to allow time for maturation of these adhesions, for resolution of any infectious processes, and for optimization of nutrition.

CONCLUSION

Intensive care unit patients can have primary intra-abdominal infections leading to sepsis or the abdomen may be a source of secondary sepsis in the previously physiologically compromised patient. Regardless of the circumstances, intra-abdominal sepsis requires a stepwise approach that includes prompt and judicious resuscitation, adequate source control, and broad-spectrum antibiotic coverage. Equally important as fluid and medical therapy is an overall design to preserve and restore gastrointestinal function and continuity. A multidisciplinary team approach to essential to succeed in the intensive care unit caring for patients with intra-abdominal infections.

References

1. Li JC, Yu SM: Study on the ultrastructure of the peritoneal stomata in humans. *Acta Anat (Basel)* 141(1):26–30, 1991.
2. Oya M, Shimada T, Nakamura M, et al: Functional morphology of the lymphatic system in the monkey diaphragm. *Arch Histol Cytol* 56(1):37–47, 1993.
3. Levine S, Saltzman A: Postinflammatory increase of lymphatic absorption from the peritoneal cavity: role of diaphragmatic stomata. *Microcirc Endothelium Lymphatics* 4(5):399–413, 1988.
4. Elk JR, Adair T, Drake RE, et al: The effect of anesthesia and surgery on diaphragmatic lymph vessel flow after endotoxin in sheep. *Lymphology* 23(3):145–148, 1990.
5. Banks JG, Foulis AK, Ledingham IM, et al: Liver function in septic shock. *J Clin Pathol* 35(11):1249–1252, 1982.
6. Gimson AE: Hepatic dysfunction during bacterial sepsis. *Intensive Care Med* 13(3):162–166, 1987.
7. Cerra FB: Multiple organ failure syndrome. *Dis Mon* 38(12):843–947, 1992.
8. Moore FA, Moore EE, Poggetti R, et al: Gut bacterial translocation via the portal vein: a clinical perspective with major torso trauma. *J Trauma* 31(5):629–636; discussion 636–638, 1991.
9. van Deventer SJ, Knepper A, Landsman J, et al: Endotoxins in portal blood. *Hepatogastroenterology* 35(5):223–225, 1988.
10. Shenep JL, Flynn PM, Barrett FF, et al: Serial quantitation of endotoxemia and bacteremia during therapy for gram-negative bacterial sepsis. *J Infect Dis* 157(3):565–568, 1988.
11. Boland G, Lee MJ, Mueller PR: Acute cholecystitis in the intensive care unit. *New Horiz* 1(2):246–260, 1993.
12. Onderdonk AB, Bartlett JG, Louie T, et al: Microbial synergy in experimental intra-abdominal abscess. *Infect Immun* 13(1):22–26, 1976.
13. Salacata A, Chow JW: Cephalosporin therapeutics for intensive care infections. *New Horiz* 1(2):181–186, 1993.
14. Frazee RC, Nagorney DM, Mucha P Jr: Acute acalculous cholecystitis. *Mayo Clin Proc* 64(2):163–167, 1989.
15. Ventilation with lower tidal volumes as compared with traditional tidal volumes for acute lung injury and the acute respiratory distress syndrome. The Acute Respiratory Distress Syndrome Network. *N Engl J Med* 342(18):1301–1308, 2000.
16. Rivers E, Nguyen B, Havstad S, et al: Early goal-directed therapy in the treatment of severe sepsis and septic shock. *N Engl J Med* 345(19):1368–1377, 2001.
17. Dellinger RP, Levy MM, Carlet JM, et al: Surviving Sepsis Campaign: international guidelines for management of severe sepsis and septic shock: 2008. *Crit Care Med* 36(1):296–327, 2008.
18. Hebert PC, Wells G, Blajchman MA, et al: A multicenter, randomized, controlled clinical trial of transfusion requirements in critical care. Transfusion Requirements in Critical Care Investigators, Canadian Critical Care Trials Group. *N Engl J Med* 340(6):409–417, 1999.
19. Jones AE, Shapiro NI, Trzeciak S, et al: Lactate clearance vs central venous oxygen saturation as goals of early sepsis therapy: a randomized clinical trial. *JAMA* 303(8):739–746, 2010.
20. Marshall JC, Innes M: Intensive care unit management of intra-abdominal infection. *Crit Care Med* 31(8):2228–2237, 2003.
21. Russell JA, Walley KR, Singer J, et al: Vasopressin versus norepinephrine infusion in patients with septic shock. *N Engl J Med* 358(9):877–887, 2008.
22. Tisherman SA, Barie P, Bokhari F, et al: Clinical practice guideline: endpoints of resuscitation. *J Trauma* 57(4):898–912, 2004.
23. Blot S, De Waele JJ: Critical issues in the clinical management of complicated intra-abdominal infections. *Drugs* 65(12):1611–1620, 2005.
24. Daudel F, Kessler U, Folly H, et al: Thromboelastometry for the assessment of coagulation abnormalities in early and established adult sepsis: a prospective cohort study. *Crit Care* 13(2):R42, 2009.
25. Hoffmann JN, Schick K: Antithrombin and hypercoagulability in sepsis: insights from thrombelastography? *Crit Care* 11(1):115, 2007.
26. Sivula M, Pettila V, Niemi TT, et al: Thromboelastometry in patients with severe sepsis and disseminated intravascular coagulation. *Blood Coagul Fibrinolysis* 20(6):419–426, 2009.
27. Abbas S: Resection and primary anastomosis in acute complicated diverticulitis, a systematic review of the literature. *Int J Colorectal Dis* 22(4):351–357, 2007.
28. Constantinides VA, Tekkis PP, Athanasiou T, et al: Primary resection with anastomosis vs. Hartmann's procedure in nonelective surgery for acute colonic diverticulitis: a systematic review. *Dis Colon Rectum* 49(7):966–981, 2006.
29. Jacobs DO: Clinical practice. Diverticulitis. *N Engl J Med* 357(20):2057–2066, 2007.
30. Regenet N, Tuech JJ, Pessaux P, et al: Intraoperative colonic lavage with primary anastomosis vs. Hartmann's procedure for perforated diverticular disease of the colon: a consecutive study. *Hepatogastroenterology* 49(45): 664–667, 2002.
31. Sagraves SG, Toschlog EA, Rotondo MF: Damage control surgery—the intensivist's role. *J Intensive Care Med* 21(1):5–16, 2006.
32. Jaunoo SS, Harji DP: Damage control surgery. *Int J Surg* 7(2):110–113, 2009.
33. Hoey BA, Schwab CW: Damage control surgery. *Scand J Surg* 91(1):92–103, 2002.

34. Kushimoto S, Miyauchi M, Yokota H, et al: Damage control surgery and open abdominal management: recent advances and our approach. *J Nippon Med Sch* 76(6):280–290, 2009.
35. Campbell A, Chang M, Fabian T, et al: Management of the open abdomen: from initial operation to definitive closure. *Am Surg* 75[11, Suppl]:S1–S22, 2009.
36. Cothren CC, Moore EE, Johnson JL, et al: One hundred percent fascial approximation with sequential abdominal closure of the open abdomen. *Am J Surg* 192(2):238–242, 2006.
37. Koss W, Ho HC, Yu M, et al: Preventing loss of domain: a management strategy for closure of the "open abdomen" during the initial hospitalization. *J Surg Educ* 66(2):89–95, 2009.
38. Mentula P, Leppaniemi A: Prophylactic open abdomen in patients with postoperative intra-abdominal hypertension. *Crit Care* 14(1):111, 2010.
39. Miller PR, Meredith JW, Johnson JC, et al: Prospective evaluation of vacuum-assisted fascial closure after open abdomen: planned ventral hernia rate is substantially reduced. *Ann Surg* 239(5):608–614; discussion 614–616, 2004.
40. Perathoner A, Klaus A, Muhlmann G, et al: Damage control with abdominal vacuum therapy (VAC) to manage perforated diverticulitis with advanced generalized peritonitis-a proof of concept. *Int J Colorectal Dis* 25:767–774, 2010.
41. Tieu BH, Cho SD, Luem N, et al: The use of the Wittmann Patch facilitates a high rate of fascial closure in severely injured trauma patients and critically ill emergency surgery patients. *J Trauma* 65(4):865–870, 2008.
42. Wondberg D, Larusson HJ, Metzger U, et al: Treatment of the open abdomen with the commercially available vacuum-assisted closure system in patients with abdominal sepsis: low primary closure rate. *World J Surg* 32(12):2724–2729, 2008.
43. Gupta H, Dupuy DE: Advances in imaging of the acute abdomen. *Surg Clin North Am* 77(6):1245–1263, 1997.
44. Stoker J, van Randen A, Lameris W, et al: Imaging patients with acute abdominal pain. *Radiology* 253(1):31–46, 2009.
45. Vijayaraghavan G, Kurup D, Singh A: Imaging of acute abdomen and pelvis: common acute pathologies. *Semin Roentgenol* 44(4):221–227, 2009.
46. Beaulieu Y, Marik PE: Bedside ultrasonography in the ICU: part 2. *Chest* 128(3):1766–1781, 2005.
47. Galasso D, Voermans RP, Fockens P: Role of endosonography in drainage of fluid collections and other NOTES procedures. *Best Pract Res Clin Gastroenterol* 23(5):781–9.
48. Nakamoto DA, Haaga JR: Emergent ultrasound interventions. *Radiol Clin North Am* 42(2):457–478, 2004.
49. Piraka C, Shah RJ, Fukami N, et al: EUS-guided transesophageal, transgastric, and transcolonic drainage of intra-abdominal fluid collections and abscesses. *Gastrointest Endosc* 70(4):786–792, 2009.
50. Dudukgian H, Sie E, Gonzalez-Ruiz C, et al: *C. difficile* colitis—predictors of fatal outcome. *J Gastrointest Surg.* 14(2):315–322, 2010.
51. Gagne DJ, Malay MB, Hogle NJ, et al: Bedside diagnostic minilaparoscopy in the intensive care patient. *Surgery* 131(5):491–496, 2002.
52. Nassar AH, Htwe T, Hefny H, et al: The abdominal drain. A convenient port for second-look laparoscopy. *Surg Endosc* 10(11):1114–1115, 1996.
53. Peris A, Matano S, Manca G, et al: Bedside diagnostic laparoscopy to diagnose intra-abdominal pathology in the intensive care unit. *Crit Care* 13(1):R25, 2009.
54. Maher MM, Gervais DA, Kalra MK, et al: The inaccessible or undrainable abscess: how to drain it. *Radiographics* 24(3):717–735, 2004.
55. vanSonnenberg E, D'Agostino HB, Casola G, et al: Percutaneous abscess drainage: current concepts. *Radiology* 181(3):617–626, 1991.
56. Alis H, Soylu A, Dolay K, et al: Endoscopic transcolonic catheter-free pelvic abscess drainage. *Can J Gastroenterol* 22(12):983–986, 2008.
57. Sailer M, Bussen D, Fuchs KH, et al: Endoscopic ultrasound-guided transrectal aspiration of pelvic fluid collections. *Surg Endosc* 18(5):736–740, 2004.
58. Neff CC, Mueller PR, Ferrucci JT, Jr., et al: Serious complications following transgression of the pleural space in drainage procedures. *Radiology* 152(2):335–341, 1984.
59. Mueller PR, Ferrucci JT, Jr., Simeone JF, et al: Lesser sac abscesses and fluid collections: drainage by transhepatic approach. *Radiology* 155(3):615–618, 1985.
60. Gobien RP, Stanley JH, Schabel SI, et al: The effect of drainage tube size on adequacy of percutaneous abscess drainage. *Cardiovasc Intervent Radiol* 8(2):100–102, 1985.
61. vanSonnenberg E, Mueller PR, Ferrucci JT, Jr., et al: Sump catheter for percutaneous abscess and fluid drainage by trocar or Seldinger technique. *AJR Am J Roentgenol* 139(3):613–614, 1982.
62. Golden GT, Roberts TL, 3rd, Rodeheaver G, et al: A new filtered sump tube for wound drainage. *Am J Surg* 129(6):716–717, 1975.
63. Goldberg MA, Mueller PR, Saini S, et al: Importance of daily rounds by the radiologist after interventional procedures of the abdomen and chest. *Radiology* 180(3):767–770, 1991.
64. vanSonnenberg E, Ferrucci JT, Jr., Mueller PR, et al: Percutaneous drainage of abscesses and fluid collections: technique, results, and applications. *Radiology* 142(1):1–10, 1982.
65. Lambiase RE, Deyoe L, Cronan JJ, et al: Percutaneous drainage of 335 consecutive abscesses: results of primary drainage with 1-year follow-up. *Radiology* 184(1):167–179, 1992.
66. Humes DJ, Simpson J: Acute appendicitis. *BMJ* 333(7567):530–534, 2006.
67. Prystowsky JB, Pugh CM, Nagle AP: Current problems in surgery. Appendicitis. *Curr Probl Surg* 42(10):688–742, 2005.
68. Birnbaum BA, Wilson SR: Appendicitis at the millennium. *Radiology* 215(2):337–348, 2000.
69. Solomkin JS, Mazuski JE, Bradley JS, et al: Diagnosis and management of complicated intra-abdominal infection in adults and children: guidelines by the Surgical Infection Society and the Infectious Diseases Society of America. *Clin Infect Dis* 50(2):133–164, 2010.
70. Andersson RE, Petzold MG: Nonsurgical treatment of appendiceal abscess or phlegmon: a systematic review and meta-analysis. *Ann Surg* 246(5):741–748, 2007.
71. Kaminski A, Liu IL, Applebaum H, et al: Routine interval appendectomy is not justified after initial nonoperative treatment of acute appendicitis. *Arch Surg* 140(9):897–901, 2005.
72. Tekin A, Kurtğlu HC, Can I, et al: Routine interval appendectomy is unnecessary after conservative treatment of appendiceal mass. *Colorectal Dis* 10(5):465–468, 2008.
73. Bucher P, Mathe Z, Demirag A, et al: Appendix tumors in the era of laparoscopic appendectomy. *Surg Endosc* 18(7):1063–1066, 2004.
74. Murphy EM, Farquharson SM, Moran BJ: Management of an unexpected appendiceal neoplasm. *Br J Surg* 93(7):783–792, 2006.
75. Spirt MJ: Complicated intra-abdominal infections: a focus on appendicitis and diverticulitis. *Postgrad Med* 122(1):39–51, 2010.
76. Bassotti G, Chistolini F, Morelli A: Pathophysiological aspects of diverticular disease of colon and role of large bowel motility. *World J Gastroenterol* 9(10):2140–2142, 2003.
77. Commane DM, Arasaradnam RP, Mills S, et al: Diet, ageing and genetic factors in the pathogenesis of diverticular disease. *World J Gastroenterol* 15(20):2479–2488, 2009.
78. Jun S, Stollman N: Epidemiology of diverticular disease. *Best Pract Res Clin Gastroenterol* 16(4):529–542, 2002.
79. Stollman N, Raskin JB: Diverticular disease of the colon. *Lancet* 363(9409):631–639, 2004.
80. Bordeianou L, Hodin R: Controversies in the surgical management of sigmoid diverticulitis. *J Gastrointest Surg* 11(4):542–548, 2007.
81. Chapman J, Davies M, Wolff B, et al: Complicated diverticulitis: is it time to rethink the rules? *Ann Surg* 242(4):576–581; discussion 581–583, 2005.
82. McLoughlin RF, Mathieson JR, Cooperberg PL, et al: Peritoneal abscesses due to bowel perforation: effect of extent on outcome after percutaneous drainage. *J Vasc Interv Radiol* 6(2):185–189, 1995.
83. Pai PR, Supe AN, Bapat RD, et al: Intraperitoneal abscesses: diagnostic dilemmas and therapeutic options. *Indian J Gastroenterol* 14(1):3–7, 1995.
84. Makela JT, Kiviniemi HO, Laitinen ST: Elective surgery for recurrent diverticulitis. *Hepatogastroenterology* 54(77):1412–1416, 2007.
85. Stevens T, Parsi MA, Walsh RM: Acute pancreatitis: problems in adherence to guidelines. *Cleve Clin J Med* 76(12):697–704, 2009.
86. Talukdar R, Vege SS: Recent developments in acute pancreatitis. *Clin Gastroenterol Hepatol* 7[11 Suppl]:S3–S9, 2009.
87. Pezzilli R: Pharmacotherapy for acute pancreatitis. *Expert Opin Pharmacother* 10(18):2999–3014, 2009.
88. Harrison S, Kakade M, Varadarajula S, et al: Characteristics and outcomes of patients undergoing debridement of pancreatic necrosis. *J Gastrointest Surg* 14(2):245–251, 2009.
89. Koo BC, Chinogureyi A, Shaw AS: Imaging acute pancreatitis. *Br J Radiol* 83(986):104–112, 2010.
90. Navaneethan U, Vege SS, Chari ST, et al: Minimally invasive techniques in pancreatic necrosis. *Pancreas* 38(8):867–875, 2009.
91. Tang LJ, Wang T, Cui JF, et al: Percutaneous catheter drainage in combination with choledochoscope-guided debridement in treatment of peripancreatic infection. *World J Gastroenterol* 16(4):513–517, 2010.
92. Theodorou P, Maurer CA, Spanholtz TA, et al: Acalculous cholecystitis in severely burned patients: incidence and predisposing factors. *Burns* 35(3):405–411, 2009.
93. Wang AJ, Wang TE, Lin CC, et al: Clinical predictors of severe gallbladder complications in acute acalculous cholecystitis. *World J Gastroenterol* 9(12):2821–2823, 2003.
94. Hamp T, Fridrich P, Mauritz W, et al: Cholecystitis after trauma. *J Trauma* 66(2):400–406, 2009.
95. Laurila JJ, Ala-Kokko TI, Laurila PA, et al: Histopathology of acute acalculous cholecystitis in critically ill patients. *Histopathology* 47(5):485–492, 2005.
96. Orlando R III, Gleason E, Drezner AD: Acute acalculous cholecystitis in the critically ill patient. *Am J Surg* 145(4):472–476, 1983.
97. Hakala T, Nuutinen PJ, Ruokonen ET, et al: Microangiopathy in acute acalculous cholecystitis. *Br J Surg* 84(9):1249–1252, 1997.
98. Warren BL: Small vessel occlusion in acute acalculous cholecystitis. *Surgery* 111(2):163–168, 1992.
99. McChesney JA, Northup PG, Bickston SJ: Acute acalculous cholecystitis associated with systemic sepsis and visceral arterial hypoperfusion: a case series and review of pathophysiology. *Dig Dis Sci* 48(10):1960–1967, 2003.
100. Gajic O, Urrutia LE, Sewani H, et al: Acute abdomen in the medical intensive care unit. *Crit Care Med* 30(6):1187–1190, 2002.
101. Laurila J, Syrjala H, Laurila PA, et al: Acute acalculous cholecystitis in critically ill patients. *Acta Anaesthesiol Scand* 48(8):986–991, 2004.
102. Cohan RH, Mahony BS, Bowie JD, et al: Striated intramural gallbladder lucencies on US studies: predictors of acute cholecystitis. *Radiology* 164(1):31–35, 1987.

103. Huffman JL, Schenker S: Acute acalculous cholecystitis: a review. *Clin Gastroenterol Hepatol* 8(1):15–22, 2010.
104. Boland GW, Slater G, Lu DS, et al: Prevalence and significance of gallbladder abnormalities seen on sonography in intensive care unit patients. *AJR Am J Roentgenol* 174(4):973–977, 2000.
105. Puc MM, Tran HS, Wry PW, et al: Ultrasound is not a useful screening tool for acute acalculous cholecystitis in critically ill trauma patients. *Am Surg* 68(1):65–69, 2002.
106. Mariat G, Mahul P, Prév t N, et al: Contribution of ultrasonography and cholescintigraphy to the diagnosis of acute acalculous cholecystitis in intensive care unit patients. *Intensive Care Med* 26(11):1658–1663, 2000.
107. Bennett GL, Rusinek H, Lisi V, et al: CT findings in acute gangrenous cholecystitis. *AJR Am J Roentgenol* 178(2):275–281, 2002.
108. Fidler J, Paulson EK, Layfield L: CT evaluation of acute cholecystitis: findings and usefulness in diagnosis. *AJR Am J Roentgenol* 166(5):1085–1088, 1996.
109. Singh AK, Sagar P: Gangrenous cholecystitis: prediction with CT imaging. *Abdom Imaging* 30(2):218–221, 2005.
110. Basaran O, Yavuzer N, Selcuk H, et al: Ultrasound-guided percutaneous cholecystostomy for acute cholecystitis in critically ill patients: one center's experience. *Turk J Gastroenterol* 16(3):134–137, 2005.
111. Tsuyuguchi T, Takada T, Kawarada Y, et al: Techniques of biliary drainage for acute cholecystitis: Tokyo Guidelines. *J Hepatobiliary Pancreat Surg* 14(1):46–51, 2007.
112. Welschbillig-Meunier K, Pessaux P, Lebigot J, et al: Percutaneous cholecystostomy for high-risk patients with acute cholecystitis. *Surg Endosc* 19(9):1256–1259, 2005.
113. Akyurek N, Salman B, Yuksel O, et al: Management of acute calculous cholecystitis in high-risk patients: percutaneous cholecystotomy followed by early laparoscopic cholecystectomy. *Surg Laparosc Endosc Percutan Tech* 15(6):315–320, 2005.
114. Griniatsos J, Petrou A, Pappas P, et al: Percutaneous cholecystostomy without interval cholecystectomy as definitive treatment of acute cholecystitis in elderly and critically ill patients. *South Med J* 101(6):586–590, 2008.
115. Lillemoe KD: Surgical treatment of biliary tract infections. *Am Surg* 66(2):138–144, 2000.
116. Bornman PC, van Beljon JI, Krige JE: Management of cholangitis. *J Hepatobiliary Pancreat Surg* 10(6):406–414, 2003.
117. Hanau LH, Steigbigel NH: Acute (ascending) cholangitis. *Infect Dis Clin North Am* 14(3):521–546, 2000.
118. Kimura Y, Takada T, Kawarada Y, et al: Definitions, pathophysiology, and epidemiology of acute cholangitis and cholecystitis: Tokyo Guidelines. *J Hepatobiliary Pancreat Surg* 14(1):15–26, 2007.
119. Reynolds BM, Dargan EL: Acute obstructive cholangitis; a distinct clinical syndrome. *Ann Surg* 150(2):299–303, 1959.
120. Blackbourne LH, Earnhardt RC, Sistrom CL, et al: The sensitivity and role of ultrasound in the evaluation of biliary obstruction. *Am Surg* 60(9):683–690, 1994.
121. Balthazar EJ, Birnbaum BA, Naidich M: Acute cholangitis: CT evaluation. *J Comput Assist Tomogr* 17(2):283–289, 1993.
122. Magnuson TH, Bender JS, Duncan MD, et al: Utility of magnetic resonance cholangiography in the evaluation of biliary obstruction. *J Am Coll Surg* 189(1):63–71; discussion 71–72, 1999.
123. Lee JK, Lee SH, Kang BK, et al: Is it necessary to insert a nasobiliary drainage tube routinely after endoscopic clearance of the common bile duct in patients with choledocholithiasis-induced cholangitis? A prospective, randomized trial. *Gastrointest Endosc* 71(1):105–110, 2010.
124. Sharma BC, Kumar R, Agarwal N, et al: Endoscopic biliary drainage by nasobiliary drain or by stent placement in patients with acute cholangitis. *Endoscopy* 37(5):439–443, 2005.
125. Nagino M, Takada T, Kawarada Y, et al: Methods and timing of biliary drainage for acute cholangitis: Tokyo Guidelines. *J Hepatobiliary Pancreat Surg* 14(1):68–77, 2007.
126. Bartlett JG: *Clostridium difficile* infection: historic review. *Anaerobe* 15(6):227–229, 2009.
127. Gerding DN: *Clostridium difficile* 30 years on: what has, or has not, changed and why? *Int J Antimicrob Agents* 33[Suppl 1]:S2–S8, 2009.
128. Lamontagne F, Labbe AC, Haeck O, et al: Impact of emergency colectomy on survival of patients with fulminant *Clostridium difficile* colitis during an epidemic caused by a hypervirulent strain. *Ann Surg* 245(2):267—272, 2007.
129. Kelly CP, Pothoulakis C, LaMont JT: *Clostridium difficile* colitis. *N Engl J Med* 330(4):257–262, 1994.
130. Wiesen P, Van Gossum A, Preiser JC: Diarrhoea in the critically ill. *Curr Opin Crit Care* 12(2):149–154, 2006.
131. Leclair MA, Allard C, Lesur O, et al: *Clostridium difficile* infection in the intensive care unit. *J Intensive Care Med* 25(1):23–30, 2010.
132. Jaber MR, Olafsson S, Fung WL, et al: Clinical review of the management of fulminant *clostridium difficile* infection. *Am J Gastroenterol* 103(12):3195–3203; quiz 3204, 2008.
133. Lowy I, Molrine DC, Leav BA, et al: Treatment with monoclonal antibodies against *Clostridium difficile* toxins. *N Engl J Med* 362(3):197–205, 2010.
134. Warny M, Pepin J, Fang A, et al: Toxin production by an emerging strain of *Clostridium difficile* associated with outbreaks of severe disease in North America and Europe. *Lancet* 366(9491):1079–1084, 2005.
135. Dallal RM, Harbrecht BG, Boujoukas AJ, et al: Fulminant *Clostridium difficile*: an underappreciated and increasing cause of death and complications. *Ann Surg* 235(3):363–372, 2002.
136. Koss K, Clark MA, Sanders DS, et al: The outcome of surgery in fulminant *Clostridium difficile* colitis. *Colorectal Dis* 8(2):149–154, 2006.
137. Longo WE, Mazuski JE, Virgo KS, et al: Outcome after colectomy for *Clostridium difficile* colitis. *Dis Colon Rectum* 47(10):1620–126, 2004.
138. Lavallee C, Laufer B, Pepin J, et al: Fatal *Clostridium difficile* enteritis caused by the BI/NAP1/027 strain: a case series of ileal C. difficile infections. *Clin Microbiol Infect* 15(12):1093–1039, 2009.
139. Sailhamer EA, Carson K, Chang Y, et al: Fulminant *Clostridium difficile* colitis: patterns of care and predictors of mortality. *Arch Surg* 144(5):433–439; discussion 439–440, 2009.
140. Quinn CD, Sefers SE, Babiker W, et al: C. Diff Quik Chek complete enzyme immunoassay provides a reliable first-line method for detection of Clostridium difficile in stool specimens. *J Clin Microbiol* 48(2):603–605, 2010.
141. Hall JF, Berger D: Outcome of colectomy for *Clostridium difficile* colitis: a plea for early surgical management. *Am J Surg* 196(3):384–388, 2008.
142. Ash L, Baker ME, O'Malley CM, Jr., et al: Colonic abnormalities on CT in adult hospitalized patients with *Clostridium difficile* colitis: prevalence and significance of findings. *AJR Am J Roentgenol* 186(5):1393–400, 2006.
143. Bartlett JG: Clinical practice. Antibiotic-associated diarrhea. *N Engl J Med* 346(5):334–339, 2002.
144. Maroo S, Lamont JT: Recurrent *Clostridium difficile*. *Gastroenterology* 130(4):1311–1316, 2006.
145. Pothoulakis C: Review article: anti-inflammatory mechanisms of action of *Saccharomyces boulardii*. *Aliment Pharmacol Ther* 30(8):826–833, 2009.
146. McFarland LV: Evidence-based review of probiotics for antibiotic-associated diarrhea and *Clostridium difficile* infections. *Anaerobe* 15(6):274–280, 2009.
147. Salcedo J, Keates S, Pothoulakis C, et al: Intravenous immunoglobulin therapy for severe *Clostridium difficile* colitis. *Gut* 41(3):366–370, 1997.
148. Gash K, Brown E, Pullyblank A: Emergency subtotal colectomy for fulminant *Clostridium difficile* colitis—is a surgical solution considered for all patients? *Ann R Coll Surg Engl* 92(1):56–60, 2010.
149. Seder CW, Villalba MR, Jr., Robbins J, et al: Early colectomy may be associated with improved survival in fulminant *Clostridium difficile* colitis: an 8-year experience. *Am J Surg* 197(3):302–307, 2009.
150. Lipsett PA, Samantaray DK, Tam ML, et al: Pseudomembranous colitis: a surgical disease? *Surgery* 116(3):491–496, 1994.
151. Sheth SG, LaMont JT: Toxic megacolon. *Lancet* 351(9101):509–513, 1998.
152. Fazio VW: Toxic megacolon in ulcerative colitis and Crohn's colitis. *Clin Gastroenterol* 9(2):389–407, 1980.
153. Grieco MB, Bordan DL, Geiss AC, et al: Toxic megacolon complicating Crohn's colitis. *Ann Surg* 191(1):75–80, 1980.
154. Jalan KN, Sircus W, Card WI, et al: An experience of ulcerative colitis. I. Toxic dilation in 55 cases. *Gastroenterology* 57(1):68–82, 1969.
155. Anderson JB, Tanner AH, Brodribb AJ: Toxic megacolon due to Campylobacter colitis. *Int J Colorectal Dis* 1(1):58–59, 1986.
156. Ausch C, Madoff RD, Gnant M, et al: Aetiology and surgical management of toxic megacolon. *Colorectal Dis* 8(3):195–201, 2006.
157. Beaugerie L, Ngo Y, Goujard F, et al: Etiology and management of toxic megacolon in patients with human immunodeficiency virus infection. *Gastroenterology* 107(3):858–863, 1994.
158. Bellary SV, Isaacs P: Toxic megacolon (TM) due to Salmonella. *J Clin Gastroenterol* 12(5):605–607, 1990.
159. Chaudhuri A, Bekdash BA., Toxic megacolon due to Salmonella: a case report and review of the literature. *Int J Colorectal Dis* 17(4):275–279, 2002.
160. McGregor A, Brown M, Thway K, et al: Fulminant amoebic colitis following loperamide use. *J Travel Med* 14(1):61–62, 2007.
161. Nayar DM, Vetrivel S, McElroy J, et al: Toxic megacolon complicating Escherichia coli O157 infection. *J Infect* 52(4):e103–e106, 2006.
162. Upadhyay AK, Neely JA: Toxic megacolon and perforation caused by Shigella. *Br J Surg* 76(11):1217, 1989.
163. Hayes-Lattin BM, Curtin PT, Fleming WH, et al: Toxic megacolon: a life-threatening complication of high-dose therapy and autologous stem cell transplantation among patients with AL amyloidosis. *Bone Marrow Transplant* 30(5):279–285, 2002.
164. Mourelle M, Vilaseca J, Guarner F, et al: Toxic dilatation of colon in a rat model of colitis is linked to an inducible form of nitric oxide synthase. *Am J Physiol* 270(3, Pt 1):G425–G430, 1996.
165. Mourelle M, Casellas F, Guarner F, et al: Induction of nitric oxide synthase in colonic smooth muscle from patients with toxic megacolon. *Gastroenterology* 109(5):1497–502, 1995.
166. Imbriaco M, Balthazar EJ: Toxic megacolon: role of CT in evaluation and detection of complications. *Clin Imaging* 25(5):349–354, 2001.
167. Panos MZ, Wood MJ, Asquith P: Toxic megacolon: the knee-elbow position relieves bowel distension. *Gut* 34(12):1726–1727, 1993.
168. Present DH, Wolfson D, Gelernt IM, et al: Medical decompression of toxic megacolon by "rolling." A new technique of decompression with favorable long-term follow-up. *J Clin Gastroenterol* 10(5):485–490, 1988.
169. Gan SI, Beck PL: A new look at toxic megacolon: an update and review of incidence, etiology, pathogenesis, and management. *Am J Gastroenterol* 98(11):2363–2371, 2003.

170. Roehrborn A, Thomas L, Potreck O, et al: The microbiology of postoperative peritonitis. *Clin Infect Dis* 33(9):1513–1519, 2001.
171. Hutchins RR, Gunning MP, Lucas DN, et al: Relaparotomy for suspected intraperitoneal sepsis after abdominal surgery. *World J Surg* 28(2):137–141, 2004.
172. Lamme B, Boermeester MA, Reitsma JB, et al: Meta-analysis of relaparotomy for secondary peritonitis. *Br J Surg* 89(12):1516–1524, 2002.
173. Malangoni MA: Evaluation and management of tertiary peritonitis. *Am Surg* 66(2):157–161, 2000.
174. Augustin P, Kermarrec N, Muller-Serieys C, et al: Risk factors for multidrug resistant bacteria and optimization of empirical antibiotic therapy in postoperative peritonitis. *Crit Care* 14(1):R20, 2010.
175. Dudrick SJ, Maharaj AR, McKelvey AA: Artificial nutritional support in patients with gastrointestinal fistulas. *World J Surg* 23(6):570–576, 1999.
176. Schecter WP, Hirshberg A, Chang DS, et al: Enteric fistulas: principles of management. *J Am Coll Surg* 209(4):484–491, 2009.
177. Osborn C, Fischer JE: How I do it: gastrointestinal cutaneous fistulas. *J Gastrointest Surg* 13(11):2068–2073, 2009.
178. Hesse U, Ysebaert D, de Hemptinne B: Role of somatostatin-14 and its analogues in the management of gastrointestinal fistulae: clinical data. *Gut* 49[Suppl 4]:iv11–iv21, 2001.
179. Martinez JL, Luque-de-Leon E, Mier J, et al: Systematic management of postoperative enterocutaneous fistulas: factors related to outcomes. *World J Surg* 32(3):436–443; discussion 444, 2008.
180. Wainstein DE, Fernandez E, Gonzalez D, et al: Treatment of high-output enterocutaneous fistulas with a vacuum-compaction device. A ten-year experience. *World J Surg* 32(3):430–435, 2008.
181. Bower RH, Cerra FB, Bershadsky B, et al: Early enteral administration of a formula (Impact) supplemented with arginine, nucleotides, and fish oil in intensive care unit patients: results of a multicenter, prospective, randomized, clinical trial. *Crit Care Med* 23(3):436–449, 1995.
182. Calder PC: Immunonutrition in surgical and critically ill patients. *Br J Nutr* 98[Suppl 1]:S133–S139, 2007.
183. de Aguilar-Nascimento JE, Caporossi C, Dock-Nascimento DB, et al: Oral glutamine in addition to parenteral nutrition improves mortality and the healing of high-output intestinal fistulas. *Nutr Hosp* 22(6):672–676, 2007.
184. Becker HP, Willms A, Schwab R: Small bowel fistulas and the open abdomen. *Scand J Surg* 96(4):263–271, 2007.
185. Kelly DA: Intestinal failure-associated liver disease: what do we know today? *Gastroenterology* 130[2, Suppl 1]:S70–S77, 2006.
186. Lloyd DA, Gabe SM, Windsor AC: Nutrition and management of enterocutaneous fistula. *Br J Surg* 93(9):1045–1055, 2006.
187. Meguid MM, Campos AC: Nutritional management of patients with gastrointestinal fistulas. *Surg Clin North Am* 76(5):1035–1080, 1996.
188. Visschers RG, Olde Damink SW, Winkens B, et al: Treatment strategies in 135 consecutive patients with enterocutaneous fistulas. *World J Surg* 32(3): 445–453, 2008.

CHAPTER 151 ■ MESENTERIC ISCHEMIA

TAKKI MOMIN AND JOHN RICOTTA

Mesenteric ischemia is a rare, life-threatening condition characterized by compromise of the splanchnic circulation resulting in bowel ischemia. Recognition of this disorder has been increasing, and it is estimated to occur in 1 of every 1,000 hospital admissions [1]. It is often encountered in association with other critical illnesses and has a wide spectrum of clinical presentation, making the diagnosis difficult to establish. In mild cases, asymptomatic reversible mucosal ischemia may ensue, whereas frank bowel necrosis and perforation may follow prolonged malperfusion. The classic finding of pain out of proportion to physical examination is often present, but some patients may have only vague abdominal complaints [2]. Frank bowel necrosis with peritonitis portends a poor prognosis with a mortality rate that can reach 90% [3]. Associated cellular injury often induces a systemic inflammatory response that triggers a cascade of events leading to multiorgan failure and death, even after successful intestinal resection. Effective treatment of this disease requires prompt diagnosis, rapid restoration of circulation, surgical resection of nonviable bowel, and supportive care [4].

ANATOMY OF THE MESENTERIC CIRCULATION

The small bowel and colon are principally supplied by the celiac artery (CA), superior mesenteric artery (SMA), and inferior mesenteric artery (IMA). These arteries communicate through an extensive network of collateral blood vessels that can preserve arterial perfusion to the splanchnic organs when one or more of the main arteries occludes or becomes stenotic due to atherosclerotic disease. The gastroduodenal artery and pancreaticoduodenal arcades provide an important source of collateral flow between the CA and SMA. The SMA and IMA communicate through several collateral vessels including the marginal artery of Drummond and the meandering artery also known as the arc of Riolan. The hypogastric artery can provide collateral flow to the IMA through the hemorrhoidal and sacral arteries in the pelvis [5,6] (Fig. 151.1).

ETIOLOGY

Mesenteric ischemia can occur acutely, resulting in rapid development of bowel ischemia, or chronically, producing postprandial pain, fear of eating, and weight loss. Acute ischemia may result from acute arterial occlusion due to thrombosis or embolism, acute occlusion of intestinal venous outflow, or ischemia from impaired flow without fixed obstruction in the setting of sepsis and shock. Chronic ischemia is usually the result of progressive atherosclerotic narrowing of multiple mesenteric arteries.

Acute Mesenteric Insufficiency

Arterial insufficiency accounts for approximately 95% of cases of acute mesenteric insufficiency (AMI) and may be embolic (50%), thrombotic (25%), or nonocclusive (20%). The remaining 5% of cases of AMI are due to mesenteric venous thrombosis [7]. The most common source of arterial emboli is the heart. Patients will typically have a history of atrial fibrillation, myocardial infarction, left ventricular aneurysm, or a prosthetic heart valve [8]. The SMA is the most frequent site of embolization because of the preferential flow pattern established at the origin of the artery where it takes an oblique angle [9]. More than half of the emboli will lodge at or near the branch point of the middle colic artery, a point of anatomic narrowing in the SMA. When this occurs, flow through the proximal jejunal branches continues, producing a distinct pattern of bowel ischemia with preservation of proximal jejunum [10].

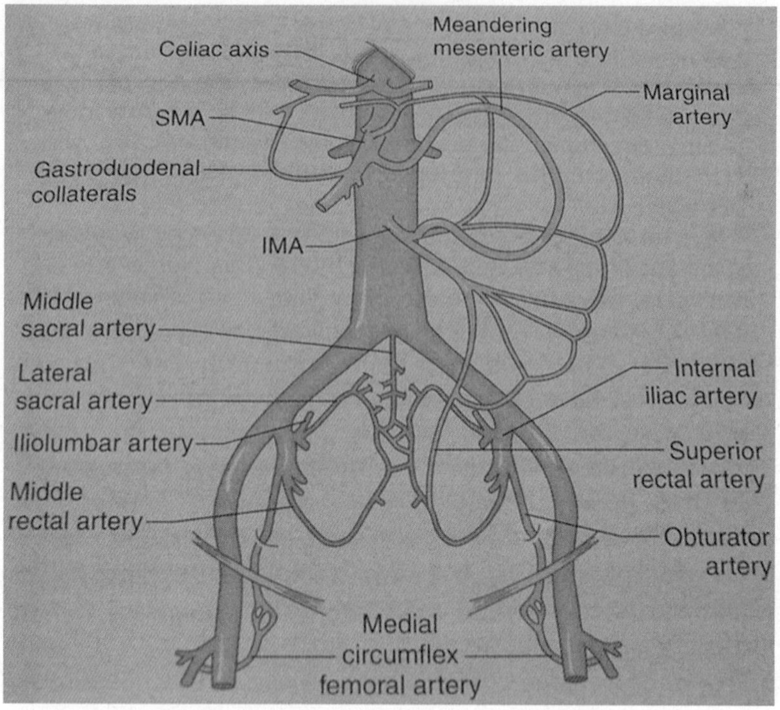

FIGURE 151.1. Schematic of splanchnic circulation. Rutherford Vascular Surgery. Abdominal and Iliac Aneurysms, 1431–1436, Copyright Elsevier (2005).

Acute thrombosis is usually superimposed on chronic coexisting atherosclerotic occlusive disease. The thrombus develops within the proximal SMA or CA in close proximity to the origin of the vessel where it is affected by atherosclerotic disease. In patients with asymptomatic, compensated mesenteric occlusive disease, acute ischemia develops from abrupt thrombosis of a diseased but patent artery (usually the SMA) as a consequence of plaque disruption or flow disturbance beyond a high-grade orificial stenosis [11].

In nonocclusive mesenteric ischemia, the reduction in blood flow usually occurs from low cardiac output or splanchnic vasoconstriction. This is often seen in the intensive care setting, associated with a number of underlying medical conditions such as congestive heart failure, cardiogenic shock, renal disease, hypovolemia, and sepsis [10,12,13]. In addition, vasoactive agents like digitalis and α-adrenergic agonists can induce mesenteric ischemia by splanchnic arteriolar vasoconstriction [13]. Intestinal hypoperfusion can also result from the release of inflammatory mediators associated with severe systemic illness such as pancreatitis, sepsis, trauma, and burns [14,15]. Abdominal compartment syndrome should also be considered as a potential cause of mesenteric ischemia. Excessive intra-abdominal pressure, measured as a bladder pressure more than 25 mm Hg, leads to direct compression of the inferior vena cava and portal vein as well as decreased flow in the inferior vena cava and superior vena cava [16].

Acute mesenteric ischemia may also result from extrinsic mechanical compression of either the arterial or the venous supply to the bowel when local blood supply becomes compromised by a strangulated hernia or intussusception [17]. Sacrifice of a major visceral branch or surgical interruption of the collateral circulatory pathways in the setting of prior visceral artery occlusion may, on rare occasions, result in acute mesenteric ischemia [18]. A well recognized example is ischemia to the sigmoid colon following ligation of the inferior mesenteric artery during aortic resection, or left colectomy, in a patient who has an asymptomatic SMA occlusion and relies on the IMA for visceral perfusion. Aortic dissection may occasionally cause mesenteric ischemia by creating a static or dynamic obstruction at the origin of one or more of the visceral vessels [19]. In this circumstance, perfusion to the mesenteric arteries may be established by either a fenestration procedure or surgical revascularization [19,20].

Mesenteric venous thrombosis (MVT) is an infrequent cause of bowel ischemia. Over 80% of patients diagnosed with MVT are associated with an underlying identifiable coagulation disorder that predisposes them to venous thrombosis. These include both inherited hypercoagulable disorders such as protein C or S deficiency, antithrombin III deficiency, factor V Leiden mutation, and methylenetetrahydrofolate reductase mutations and acquired hypercoagulable states such as malignancy, oral contraceptive use, polycythemia vera, thrombocytosis, trauma, or critical illness [21–23]. The presentation of patients with MVT varies depending on the extent and location of thrombus. Patients typically present with anorexia and nonspecific, vague abdominal pain that may be acute, but is more commonly insidious. Peritonitis is rarely seen and restricted to patients with frank bowel necrosis. The triad of thrombus within the SMV, thickened small bowel wall, and free fluid in the peritoneal cavity as identified on CT maybe an early indication of bowel infarction and the subsequent need for laparotomy [24].

Chronic Mesenteric Insufficiency

Chronic mesenteric ischemia (CMI) results from atherosclerotic disease of the mesenteric arteries and usually requires stenosis or occlusion of two or more mesenteric vessels. Stenosis or occlusion of a single mesenteric vessel will rarely result in abdominal pain; when it does, the SMA is usually the vessel involved. Progression to occlusion most often occurs gradually and allows development of robust collaterals in the splanchnic circulation to compensate for inflow disease. The basal circulation to the intestine is sufficient to maintain adequate blood flow at rest, but when metabolic demands increase, such as in the postprandial state, the higher resistance collateral circulation is inadequate to meet the increased oxygen requirements and symptoms of vascular insufficiency develop. The classic presentation includes a preexistent history of postprandial abdominal pain that results in food avoidance and significant weight loss. Abdominal pain without weight loss is unusual for mesenteric ischemia and suggests an alternate diagnosis [25].

PATHOPHYSIOLOGY

Mesenteric ischemia occurs when there is inadequate delivery of oxygenated blood to satisfy the metabolic demands of the intestines. The presence of an extensive collateral network in the splanchnic circulation maintains intestinal viability even with as much as a 75% reduction in normal blood flow [25,26]. Under normal conditions, the splanchnic circulation maintains regional blood flow to compensate for systemic changes in hemodynamics through autoregulatory mechanisms. This is achieved by altering the vasomotor tone of the arteriolar resistance vessels. Under circumstances of decreased perfusion pressure, the precapillary arterioles reflexively vasodilate to enhance regional blood flow by lowering mesenteric vascular resistance. A combination of local, humoral, and neural factors mediate the vasomotor tone of these resistance vessels in response to various pathologic conditions [25–27].

In the setting of acute mesenteric thrombosis or embolus, reflexive vasodilation initially occurs and transiently enhances blood flow through existing collateral circulatory pathways. As intestinal ischemia progresses, paradoxical vasoconstriction results and local blood flow is critically reduced to a point where secondary arteriolar thrombosis ensues [28].

Intestinal ischemia from mesenteric venous thrombosis results from venous outflow obstruction leading to venous hypertension resulting in reduction of capillary and arteriolar flow. The thrombosis initially begins in the small veins out in the periphery and extends proximally toward the superior mesenteric vein. Vasospasm of the mesenteric arterioles is also believed to play a major role in ischemia associated with venous thrombosis [28–33].

Early histologic evidence of intestinal ischemia can be observed after only 5 to 10 minutes of arterial occlusion [34–38]. When the ischemic insult is not severe and perfusion can be rapidly restored, these changes are reversible. If ischemic cellular injury persists, tissue infarction will occur, starting from the mucosal surface of the intestine where blood supply is most tenuous. With prolonged ischemia, the bowel wall becomes edematous from increased vascular permeability. Hemorrhage of the mucosal and submucosal layers follows. As infarction extends transmurally, the integrity of the intestinal wall is destroyed and risk of perforation increases. During advanced stages of ischemia, the intestine loses its protective barrier function, resulting in passage of inflammatory cells and translocation of enteric organisms into the portal circulation. Locally produced mediators are released into the circulation along with bacterial endotoxin, triggering an intense systemic inflammatory response. The resulting sepsis and physiologic stress imposed by systemic inflammatory response often leads to multiorgan dysfunction and possibly death [15,39].

CLINICAL PRESENTATION

Mesenteric ischemia can manifest itself in a variety of ways depending on etiology and degree of intestinal ischemia. The signs and symptoms may be subtle, nonspecific, and insidious, especially in chronic and subacute forms of mesenteric ischemia. When ischemia develops acutely, the most common predominant symptom is sudden onset of severe abdominal pain that is often out of proportion to physical findings. However, pain is absent in 25% of individuals with acute nonocclusive ischemia [39]. Symptoms may be nonspecific, including nausea, vomiting, diarrhea, and abdominal distension. Gastrointestinal symptoms may not always dominate the clinical presentation. Acute mental status changes have been reported in 30% of elderly patients with intestinal ischemia [40].

DIAGNOSTIC EVALUATION

Leukocyte count, serum lactic acid level, and arterial blood gas are the most common tests routinely ordered to screen patients for mesenteric ischemia. In patients with acute intestinal ischemia, 75% will have a leukocytosis greater than 15,000 cells per mm^3 and 50% will present with a metabolic acidosis [41]. Unfortunately, abnormalities in these studies accompany other abdominal pathologies, making them nonspecific [42–47].

Plain radiographs lack specificity, and in some cases, abdominal films may even appear normal in the presence of bowel infarction [48]. Some common radiographic features observed in intestinal ischemia include presence of bowel wall thickening, intramural gas (pneumatosis), bowel distention, and mesenteric or portal venous air [49,50]. None of these findings, however, are sensitive or specific to intestinal ischemia. Pneumatosis, when present, is often a sign of advanced ischemia with bowel infarction, although it may also be associated with other acute abdominal conditions such as peptic ulcer and inflammatory bowel disease [51]. The most practical purpose of obtaining plain films in the workup of mesenteric ischemia is often to exclude other causes of acute abdominal pain, most notably gastrointestinal perforations.

Computed tomography (CT) has emerged as one of the most accurate and expeditious methods of diagnosing abdominal pathologies (Fig. 151.2). It is often the first and most common imaging modality employed in the initial evaluation of abdominal pain. Computed tomography is more sensitive than plain films in detecting abnormalities associated with intestinal ischemia such as bowel edema, pneumatosis, and portal venous gas [52]. With intravenous contrast enhancement, CT scanning can assess the mesenteric arterial and venous circulation, permitting detection of both arterial occlusion and venous thrombosis [53,54]. CT angiography (CTA) is the best imaging technique for diagnosis of mesenteric venous occlusion (Fig. 151.3). CTA, however, is not useful in the diagnosis of nonocclusive mesenteric ischemia, and the absence of findings on CT imaging does not exclude the diagnosis of mesenteric ischemia. In recent years, the use of magnetic resonance imaging (MRI) in the detection of intestinal ischemia has been investigated [55–57]. Limited availability, longer scanning time, and higher expense limits the utility of MRI, and it has not been widely accepted in the routine workup of a patient with abdominal pain suspected of having acute mesenteric ischemia [58].

Angiography is used when CTA is inconclusive and when an endovascular intervention is contemplated. Arteriography not only permits endoluminal intervention in select cases of arterial or venous thrombosis, but also allows for selective arterial administration of vasodilating agents like papaverine to counteract vasospasm in patients with nonocclusive mesenteric ischemia [59]. Both lateral and anterior–posterior projections of the mesenteric arteries should be obtained to allow optimal imaging of the proximal and distal SMA and celiac artery [60]. Although effective in identifying arterial pathology, arteriography cannot assess the extent of bowel ischemia or infarction.

Nonocclusive mesenteric ischemia produces a characteristic irregular pruning pattern on arteriography related to segmental vasoconstriction of the arterial branches [60,61] (Fig. 151.4). Acute arterial embolus often demonstrates an abrupt luminal cutoff sign with a meniscus where the clot lodges [62]. In the SMA, the embolus frequently lodges at or just distal to the origin of the middle colic artery and is best visualized on arteriography in the lateral projection. Thrombosis of the mesenteric artery typically occurs at the origin of the vessel where there is underlying arteriosclerotic occlusive disease precipitating the

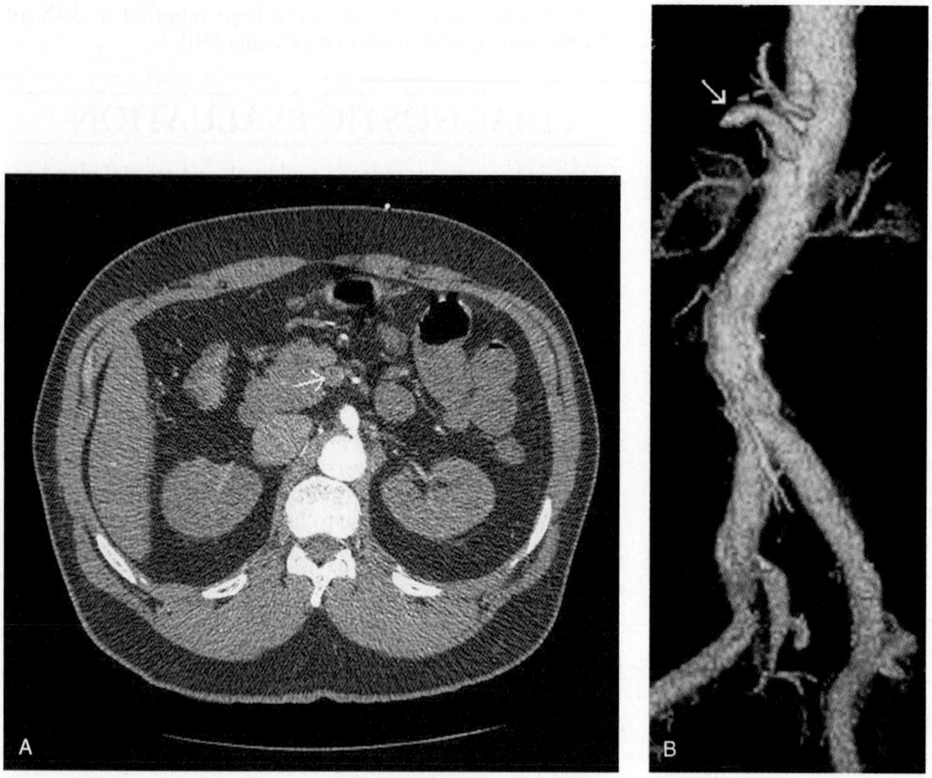

FIGURE 151.2. CTA of patient with mesenteric occlusion axial (A), 3D reconstruction (B).

thrombotic process [60]. There are exceptions to these observations but differentiating embolic from thrombotic disease on arteriography has important clinical implications in planning therapeutic interventions [41,63,64].

Duplex ultrasonography of the mesenteric vessels can be an accurate and cost-effective method of assessing the proximal celiac and superior mesenteric arteries. Ultrasonography can identify the presence of occlusive disease and quantify the degree of stenosis based on velocity criteria [65,66] (Table 151.1). Ultrasound is commonly employed as an initial screening study in the vascular evaluation of symptomatic patients suspected of having chronic mesenteric arterial disease. In addition, ultrasonography can identify nonspecific abnormalities including bowel wall edema, absent peristalsis, and even hepatic portal venous gas [67,68]. Duplex ultrasonography, however, has limited application in the diagnosis of acute mesenteric ischemia due to limitations in its ability to visualize beyond the proximal mesenteric circulation and to insonate through distended bowel.

In the intensive care setting, endoscopy may provide diagnostic alternative in the critically ill patient avoiding the danger of patient transport [69,70]. Endoscopic findings in ischemic colitis can be quite varied. Friable edematous mucosa or patchy areas of mucosal ischemia requires repeat endoscopy and supportive care, while frank intestinal necrosis mandates immediate surgical intervention. Endoscopy is unable to accurately

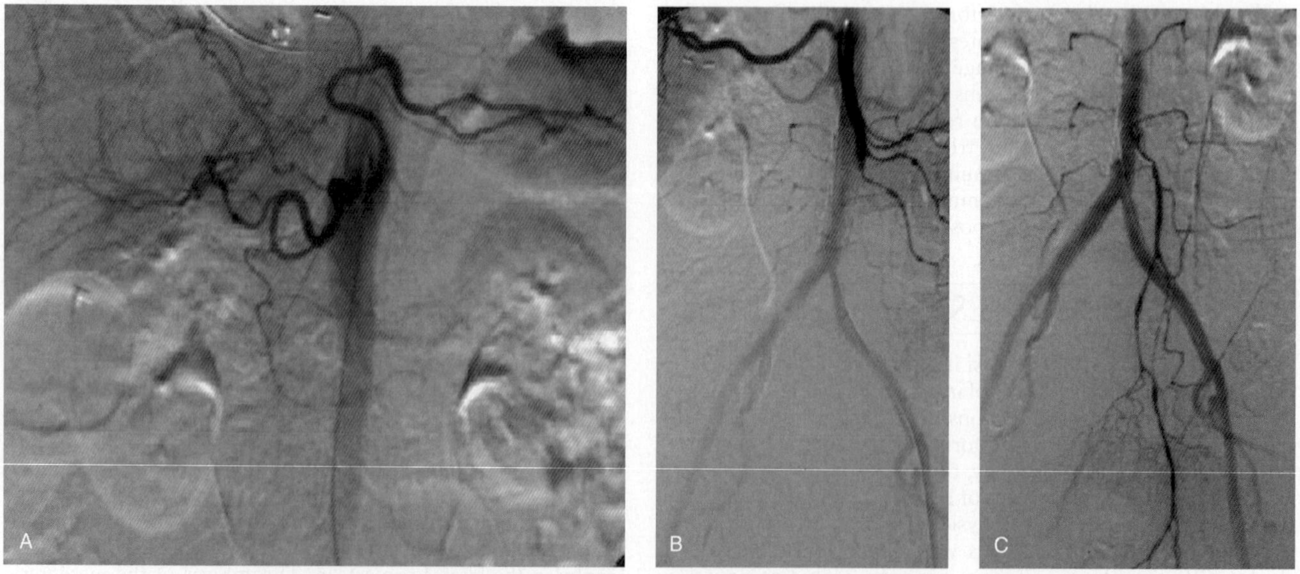

FIGURE 151.3. Beaded appearance of celiac artery (A), superior mesenteric artery (B), and inferior mesenteric artery (C) in a patient with nonocclusive mesenteric ischemia.

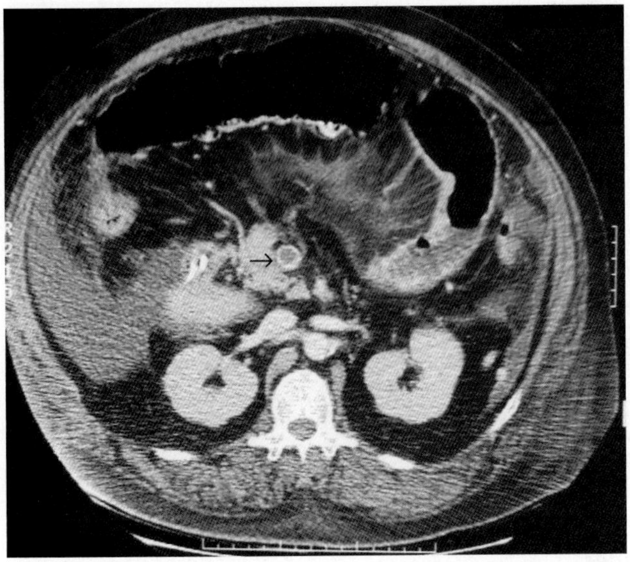

FIGURE 151.4. CT scan showing SMV thrombosis.

assess the depth of ischemic involvement beyond the mucosal surface [71–76], and most of the intestine supplied by the SMA is not readily accessible by conventional endoscopy.

TREATMENT

The treatment of mesenteric ischemia is largely determined by its specific etiology, the duration of ischemic insult, and the extent of infarcted bowel. It is critical to make the diagnosis accurately and expeditiously, initiate treatment to minimize ischemic injury, and preserve intestinal length to avoid the sequelae of short gut syndrome [77,78]. The initial management of patients with mesenteric ischemia involves resuscitation to optimize perfusion and physiologically prepare the patient for possible surgery. Broad-spectrum antibiotics should be initiated for potential infection along with systemic anticoagulation to minimize propagation of the thrombotic process [79]. If symptoms are mild, patients may be considered for immediate arteriography to elucidate the cause of ischemia with consideration of simultaneous catheter-based therapeutic intervention [79,80]. Patients presenting with peritonitis or bowel infarction require immediate laparotomy in lieu of time-consuming diagnostic evaluation that can risk further ischemic injury. The surgical management entails resection of grossly necrotic or nonviable intestine along with embolectomy or arterial revascularization to restore perfusion.

SMA embolus requires surgical extraction of the obstructing clot with assessment of distal perfusion to affected bowel. The arterial vasoconstriction that occurs distal to the embolus can be treated by direct intra-arterial administration of papaverine [81]. Pharmacologic thrombolysis using endovascular techniques has been reported for treating select patients with early mesenteric ischemia without bowel infarction [81–86]. In most cases of acute mesenteric thrombosis, however, severe atherosclerotic occlusive disease is present in the proximal vessel and open revascularization with a bypass is recommended over a percutaneous approach [87,88].

Patients with nonocclusive mesenteric ischemia are initially treated medically to optimize perfusion. The underlying systemic illness is aggressively treated while avoiding any aggravating agents like vasopressors. The diagnosis of nonocclusive ischemia is best made angiographically, which also allows for catheter-based intervention with intra-arterial infusion of papaverine to reverse vasospasm [81]. Patients who have nonocclusive mesenteric disease may still require surgical intervention if the ischemia results in bowel infarction.

Treatment of mesenteric venous thrombosis is focused on systemic anticoagulation with bowel rest. The underlying specific condition or coagulation disorder responsible for causing the thrombotic event should be identified, and the patient should be vigorously resuscitated since considerable third space loss can occur. Surgical thrombectomy of the venous circulation is rarely effective and should be reserved for cases of acute thrombosis without establishment of effective collaterals for venous drainage [89–92]. Patients require systemic anticoagulation in the postoperative period and many may need lifelong therapy due to a hypercoagulable state. Intestinal infarction may be present in the acute form, but the mortality rate and length of involved bowel is less than in acute arterial disease [93]. Preexisting liver disease and previous abdominal surgery, most commonly splenectomy, are two strongly associated risk factors for patients who develop mesenteric venous thrombosis [93].

Patients with chronic mesenteric ischemia have classically been treated with surgical revascularization through either an aortomesenteric bypass or transaortic endarterectomy. More than 90% of the patients will have occlusions in both the SMA and CA [94]. An arteriogram is necessary to determine the location of inflow occlusion and to assess the status of the distal mesenteric circulation for operative planning. Considerable controversy exists regarding the method of revascularization, the number of vessels to revascularize, and the best suited conduit [94]. The two commonly employed methods of revascularization include antegrade supraceliac aortomesenteric bypass and retrograde infrarenal aortomesenteric bypass. In general, antegrade bypass is preferred as the flow is more hemodynamically optimal and the supraceliac aorta is more likely to be disease free. Antegrade bypass, however, involves some degree of renal and visceral ischemia, in addition to increased afterload on the heart. In patients with renal insufficiency or significant underlying cardiac disease, a retrograde bypass, from the aorta or the iliac vessels, may be preferred. However, the rate of symptomatic recurrence is not definitely related to either the method of revascularization or the number of vessels revascularized [12,94]. The goal of multiple visceral revascularization therefore must be balanced against the operative risks entailed in a more extensive procedure.

The endovascular approach for patients with chronic mesenteric ischemia is emerging as a first line treatment option [95–99]. The objective in management of patients with chronic mesenteric ischemia is to relieve symptoms, prevent bowel infarction, and enable weight gain. Total mesenteric arterial occlusions are considered a relative contraindication to endovascular therapy due to fear of distal embolization. Comparisons of open versus endoluminal treatment for mesenteric arterial insufficiency suggest lower periprocedural complications associated with endoluminal techniques, but a higher incidence of late failure [96–99].

In patients with bowel ischemia, determining bowel viability can be the most challenging aspect of the operation. Accurate

TABLE 151.1

DUPLEX CRITERIA FOR MESENTERIC ARTERIAL STENOSIS

Vessel	Peak systolic velocity	Stenosis (%)
Superior mesenteric artery	≥275 cm/sec	70–100
Celiac artery	≥200 cm/sec	70–100

differentiation between viable and nonviable bowel determines the limits of resection and maximizes the residual absorptive reserve of the digestive tract. Determination of bowel viability involves visual and Doppler inspection and if needed a fluorescein-assisted tissue perfusion scan [100]. When bowel viability is indeterminate at initial exploration, a "second-look" procedure to reassess intestinal viability within 24 to 48 hours is used to avoid extensive resection at the first operation [100]. During the initial exploration, grossly nonviable bowel is resected and the intestinal tract is left in discontinuity. The abdomen is closed with drapes or a plastic bag, and the patient is transferred to the critical care unit for aggressive resuscitation and optimization. A second operation is performed in 18 to 24 hours after the patient's condition has been rendered optimal, or earlier in cases of deterioration.

The high mortality rate traditionally associated with intestinal ischemia has decreased in recent years with advancements in surgical revascularization and postoperative critical care. Contemporary studies on survival rates in patients with acute mesenteric ischemia have identified several factors associated with higher mortality: advanced age, inadequate intestinal resection, and presence of nonocclusive mesenteric disease [12]. An aggressive approach to diagnosis and treatment, employing liberal use of arteriography and minimally invasive techniques combined with traditional surgical intervention increases survival [95]. Open surgical revascularization is associated with lower rates of symptom recurrence compared to percutaneous treatment [96]. The most common cause of postoperative death is multiorgan failure followed by cardiovascular complications. Even with successful treatment, long-term survival for patients with acute mesenteric ischemia is generally poor with the majority of deaths related to coronary artery disease, short bowel syndrome, or recurrent mesenteric ischemia [12].

References

1. Stoney RJ, Cunningham CG: Acute mesenteric ischemia. *Surgery* 114:489–490, 1993.
2. Stamatakos M, Stefanaki C, Mastrokalos D, et al: Mesenteric Ischemia: still a deadly puzzle for the Medical Community. *Tohoku J Exp Med* 216:197–204, 2008.
3. Ernst CB: Bypass procedures for chronic mesenteric ischemia, in Ernst CB, Stanley JC (eds): *Current Therapy in Vascular Surgery*. 4th ed. St. Louis, Mosby, 2001, pp 682–685.
4. Eltarawy IG, Etman Y, Zenati M, et al: Acute mesenteric ischemia: the importance of early surgical consultation. *Am Surg* 75(3):212–219, 2009.
5. Safioleas MC, Moulakakis KG, Papavassiliou VG, et al: Acute mesenteric ischaemia, a highly lethal disease with a devastating outcome. *Vasa* 35(2):106–111, 2006.
6. Lin PH, Chaikof EL: Embryology, anatomy, and surgical exposure of the great abdominal vessels. *Surg Clin North Am* 80:417–433, 2000.
7. Lock G: Acute mesenteric ischemia: classification, evaluation and therapy. *Acta Gastroenterol Belg* 65(4):220–225, 2002. Review
8. Abboud B, Daher R, Boujaoude J: Acute mesenteric ischemia after cardio-pulmonary bypass surgery. *World J Gastroenterol* 14(35):5361–5370, 2008.
9. Bingol H, Zeybek N, Cingoz F, et al: Surgical therapy for acute superior mesenteric artery embolism. *Am J Surg* 188(1):68–70, 2004.
10. Chang JB, Stein TA: Mesenteric Ischemia: acute and chronic. *Ann Vasc Surg* 17:323–328. 2003.
11. Wain RA, Hines G: Surgical management of mesenteric occlusive disease; a contemporary review of invasive and minimally invasive techniques. *Cardiol Rev* 16:69–75, 2008.
12. Park WM, Gloviczki P, Cherry KJ, et al: Contemporary management of acute mesenteric ischemia: factors associated with survival. *J Vasc Surg* 35:445–452, 2002.
13. Trompeter M, Brazda T, Remy CT: Non-occlusive mesenteric ischemia: etiology, diagnosis, and interventional therapy. *Eur Radiol* 12(5):1179–1187, 2002.
14. Endean ED, Barnes SL, Kwolek CJ, et al: Surgical management of thrombotic acute intestinal ischemia. *Ann Surg* 233:801–808, 2001.
15. Deitch EA: Bacterial translocation or lymphatic drainage of toxic products from the gut: what is important in human beings? *Surgery* 131:241–244, 2002.
16. Carlotti AP, Carvalho WB: Abdominal compartment syndrome: a review. *Pediatr Crit Care Med* 10(1):115–120, 2009.
17. Candrlic K, Sego K, Kovacic B, et al: Abdominal angina caused by kinking of the superior mesenteric artery. *Coll Antropol* 32(4):1271–1273, 2008.
18. Tollefson DFJ, Ernst CB: Colon ischemia following aortic reconstruction. *Ann Vasc Surg* 5:485–490, 1991.
19. Cambria RP, Brewster DC, Gertler J, et al: Vascular complications associated with spontaneous aortic dissection. *J Vasc Surg* 7:199–209, 1988.
20. Lauterbach SR, Cambria RP, Brewster DC, et al: Contemporary management of aortic branch compromise resulting from acute aortic dissection. *J Vasc Surg* 33:1185–1192, 2001.
21. Abdu RA, Zakhour BJ, Dallis DJ: Mesenteric venous thrombosis—1911 to 1984. *Surgery* 101:383–388, 1987.
22. Harvard TRS, Green D, Bergan JJ, et al: Mesenteric venous thrombosis. *J Vasc Surg* 9:328–333, 1989.
23. Kumar S, Sarr MG, Kamath PS: Mesenteric venous thrombosis. *N Engl J Med* 345:1683–1688, 2001.
24. Aschoff AJ, Stuber G, Becker B, et al: Evaluation of acute mesenteric ischemia: accuracy of biphasic mesenteric multi-detector CT angiography. *Abdom Imaging* 34:345–357, 2009.
25. Patel A, Kaleya R, Sammartano RJ: Pathophysiology of mesenteric ischemia. *Surg Clin North Am* 72:31–41, 1992.
26. Ceppa EP, Fuh KC, Bulkey GB: Mesenteric hemodynamic response to circulatory shock. *Curr Opin Crit Care* 9:127–132, 2003.
27. Jacobson ED, Pawlik WW: Adenosine regulation of mesenteric vasodilation. *Gastroenterology* 107:1168–1180, 1994.
28. Toung T, Reilly PM, Fuh KC, et al: Mesenteric vasoconstriction in response to hemorrhagic shock. *Shock* 13:267–273, 2000.
29. Bailey RW, Bulkley GB, Hamilton SR, et al: Protection of the small intestine from nonocclusive mesenteric ischemic injury due to cardiogenic shock. *Am J Surg* 153:108–115, 1987.
30. Bailey RW, Bulkley GB, Hamilton SR, et al: The fundamental hemodynamic mechanism underlying gastric "stress ulceration" in cardiogenic shock. *Ann Surg* 205:597–611, 1987.
31. McNeill JR, Wilcox WC, Pang CCY: Vasopressin and angiotensin: reciprocal mechanism controlling mesenteric conductance. *Am J Physiol* 232:H260–H266, 1977.
32. Arvidsson D, Rasmussen I, Almqvist P, et al: Splanchnic oxygen consumption in septic and hemorrhagic shock. *Surgery*. 109:190–197, 1991.
33. Faroog MM, Freischlag JA: Skeletal muscle ischemia and reperfusion: mechanisms of injury and intervention, in Siadawy AN, Sumpio BE, DePalma RG (eds): *The Basic Science of Vascular Disease*. 1st ed. Armonk, NY, Futura Publishing Company, 1997, pp 775–795.
34. Granger DN: Role of xanthine oxidase and granulocytes in ischemia-reperfusion injury. *Am J Physiol* 255:H1269–H1275, 1988.
35. Zimmerman BJ, Granger DN: Reperfusion injury. *Surg Clin North Am* 72:65–83, 1992.
36. Korthuis RJ, Smith JK, Carden DL: Hypoxic reperfusion attenuates postischemic microvascular injury. *Am J Physiol* 256:H315–H319, 1989.
37. Perry MA, Wadhwa SS: Gradual introduction of oxygen reduces reperfusion injury in cat stomach. *Am J Physiol* 254:G366–G372, 1988.
38. Mitsudo S, Brandt LJ: Pathology of intestinal ischemia. *Surg Clin North Am* 72:43–63, 1992.
39. Gray BH, Sullivan TM: Mesenteric vascular disease. *Curr Treat Options Cardiovasc Med* 3:195–206, 2001.
40. Ozden N, Gurses B: Mesenteric ischemia in the elderly. *Clin Geriatric Medicine*. 23(4):871–887, vii–viii, 2007.
41. Bassiouny H: Nonocclusive mesenteric ischemia. *Surg Clin North Am* 77(2):319–326. 1997.
42. Kurland B, Brandt LJ, Delany HM: Diagnostic tests for intestinal ischemia. *Surg Clin North Am* 72:85–105, 1992.
43. Barnett S, Davidson E, Bradley E: Intestinal alkaline phosphatase and base deficit in mesenteric occlusion. *J Surg Res* 20:243–246, 1976.
44. Graeber G, Cafferty P, Reardon M, et al: Changes in serum total creatinine phosphokinase (CPK) and its isoenzymes caused by experimental ligation of the superior mesenteric artery. *Am J Surg* 193:499–505, 1981.
45. Calman C, Hersey F, Skaggs J: Serum lactic dehydrogenase in the diagnosis of the acute surgical abdomen. *Surgery* 44:43–51, 1958.
46. Barth K, Alderson P, Strandberg J, et al: Early imaging of experimental intestinal infarction with 99 m Tc-pyrophosphate. *Radiology* 133:459–462, 1979.
47. Kosloske A, Goldthorn J: Paracentesis as an aid to the diagnosis of intestinal gangrene: experience in 50 infants and children. *Arch Surg* 117:571–575, 1982.
48. Smerud MJ, Johnson CD, Stephens DH: Diagnosis of bowel infarction: a comparison of plain films and CT scan in 23 cases. *Am J Roentgenol* 154:99–103, 1990.

49. Liebman PR, Patten MT, Manny J, et al: Hepatic-portal venous gas in adults: etiology, pathophysiology and clinical significance. *Ann Surg* 187:281–287, 1978.
50. Tomchick FS, Wittenberg J, Ottinger LW: The roentgenologic spectrum of bowel infarction. *Radiology* 96:249–260, 1970.
51. Wolf EL, Sprayregen S, Bakal CW: Radiology in intestinal ischemia: plain film, contrast, and other imaging studies. *Surg Clin North Am* 72:107–124, 1992.
52. Klein HM, Lensing R, Klosterhalfen B, et al: Diagnostic imaging of mesenteric infarction. *Radiology* 197:79–92, 1995.
53. Federle MP, Chun G, Jeffrey RB, et al: Computed tomographic findings in bowel infarction. *Am J Roentgenol* 142:91–95, 1984.
54. Rosen A, Korobkin M, Silverman PM, et al: Mesenteric vein thrombosis: CT identification. *Am J Roentgenol* 143:83–86, 1984.
55. Chan FP, Li KC, Heiss SG, et al: A comprehensive approach using MR imaging to diagnose acute segmental mesenteric ischemia in a porcine model. *Am J Roentgenol* 173:523–529, 1999.
56. Hricak H, Amparao E, Fisher MR, et al: Abdominal venous system: assessment using MR. *Radiology* 156:415–422, 1985.
57. Wilkerson DK, Mezvich R, Drake C: Magnetic resonance imaging of acute occlusive intestinal ischemia. *Journal of Vascular Surgery* 11:567–571, 1990.
58. Pedrosa Ivan, Rofsky NM: MR imaging in abdominal emergencies. *Rad Clin North Am* 41:1243–1273, 2003.
59. Wilcox MG, Howard TJ, Plaskon LA, et al: Current theories of pathogenesis and treatment of nonocclusive mesenteric ischemia. *Dig Dis Sci* 40:709, 1995.
60. Clark RH, Gallant TE: Acute mesenteric ischemia: angiographic spectrum. *Am J Roentgenol* 142:555–562, 1984.
61. Siegelman SS, Sprayregen S, Boley SJ: Angiographic diagnosis of mesenteric arterial vasoconstriction. *Radiology* 112:533–542, 1974.
62. Boley SJ, Freinstein FR, Sammartano R, et al: New concepts in the management of emboli of the superior mesenteric artery. *Surg Gynecol Obstet* 153:561–569, 1981.
63. Ottinger L: The surgical management of acute occlusion of the superior mesenteric artery. *Ann Surg* 188:721–731, 1978.
64. Clavian PA, Huber O, Mirescu D, et al: CT scan as a diagnostic procedure in mesenteric ischemia due to mesenteric venous thrombosis. *Br J Surg* 76:93–94, 1989.
65. Mitchell EL, Chang EY, Landry GJ, et al: Duplex criteria for native superior mesenteric artery stenosis overestimate stenosis in stented superior mesenteric arteries. *J Vasc Surg* 335–340, 2009.
66. Harward TRS, Smith S, Seeger JM: Detection of celiac axis and superior mesenteric artery occlusive disease with use of abdominal duplex scanning. *J Vasc Surg* 17:738–745, 1993.
67. Fleischer AC, Muhletaler CA, James AE Jr: Sonographic assessment of the bowel wall. *Am J Roentgenol* 136:887–891, 1981.
68. Kreigshauer JS, Reading CC, King BF, et al: Combined systemic and portal venous gas: sonographic and CT detection in two cases. *Am J Roentgenol* 154:1219–1221, 1990.
69. Barba CA: The intensive care unit as an operating room. *Surg Clin North Am* 80:957–973, 2000.
70. Orlando R III, Crowell KL: Laparoscopy in the critically ill. *Surg Endosc* 11:1072–1074, 1997.
71. Iberti TJ, Salky BA, Onofrey D: Use of bedside laparoscopy to identify intestinal ischemia in postoperative cases of aortic reconstruction. *Surgery* 105:686–689, 1989.
72. Anadol AZ, Ersoy E, Taneri F, et al: Laparoscopic "second-look" in the management of mesenteric ischemia. *Surg Laparosc Endosc Percuta Tech* 14:191–193, 2004.
73. Regan F, Karstad RR, Magnuson TH: Minimally invasive management of acute superior mesenteric artery occlusion: combined urokinase and laparoscopic therapy. *Am J Gastroenterol* 91:1019–1021, 1996.
74. Safran D, Orlando R III: Physiologic effects of pneumoperitoneum. *Am J Surg* 167:281, 1994.
75. Brandt CP, Priebe PP, Eckhauser ML: Diagnostic laparoscopy in the intensive care patient. *Surg Endosc* 7:168–172, 1993.
76. Toursarkissian B, Thompson RW: Ischemic colitis. *Surg Clin North Am* 77:461–470, 1997.
77. Thompson JS, DiBaise JK, Iyer KR, et al: Postoperative short bowel syndrome. *J Am Coll Surg* 201:85–89, 2005.
78. Scolapio JS, Fleming CR: Short bowel syndrome. *Gastroenterol Clin North Am* 27:467–479, 1998.
79. Chang RW, Chang JB, Longo WE: Update in management of mesenteric ischemia. *World J Gastroenterol* 12(20):3243–3247, 2006.
80. Schermerhorn ML, Giles KA, Hamdan AD, et al: Mesenteric revascularization: management and outcomes in the United States, 1988–2006. *J Vasc Surg* 50:341–348, 2009.
81. Klotz S, Vestring T, Rotker J, et al: Diagnosis and treatment of non occlusive mesenteric ischemia after heart surgery. *Ann Thorac Surg* 72:1583–1586. 2001.
82. McBride KD, Gaines PA: Thrombolysis of a partially occluding superior mesenteric artery thromboembolus by infusion of streptokinase. *Cardiovasc Intervent Radiol* 17:164–166, 1994.
83. Schoots IG, Levi MM, Reekers JA, et al: Thrombolytic therapy for acute superior mesenteric artery occlusion. *J Vasc Interv Radiol* 16:317–329, 2005.
84. Herbert GS, Steele SR: "Acute and chronic mesenteric ischemia." *Surg Clin North Am* 87:1115–1134, 2007.
85. VanDeinse WH, Zawacki JK, Phillips D: Treatment of acute mesenteric ischemia by percutaneous transluminal angioplasty. *Gastroenterology* 91:475–478, 1986.
86. Hallisey MJ, Deschaine J, Illescas FF, et al: Angioplasty for the treatment of visceral ischemia. *J Vasc Intervent Radiol* 6:785–791, 1995.
87. Whitehill T, Rutherford R: Acute mesenteric ischemia caused by arterial occlusions: optimal management to improve survival. *Semin Vasc Surg* 3:149–155, 1990.
88. Wyers M, Powell R, Nolan B, et al: Retrograde mesenteric stenting during laparotomy for acute occlusive mesenteric ischemia. *J Vasc Surg* 45:269–275, 2007.
89. Boley SJ, Kaleya RN, Brandt LJ: Mesenteric venous thrombosis. *Surg Clin North Am* 72:183–201, 1992.
90. Bergentz S, Ericsson B, Hedner U, et al: Thrombosis in the superior mesenteric and portal veins: report of a case treated with thrombectomy. *Surgery* 76:286–290, 1974.
91. Lopera JE, Correa G, Brazzini A, et al.: Percutaneous transhepatic treatment of symptomatic mesenteric venous thrombosis. Journal of Vascular Surgery 36:1058–61. 2002.
92. Henao EA, Bohannon TW, Silva MB: Treatment of portal venous thrombosis with selective superior mesenteric artery infusion of recombinant tissue plasminogen activator. *J Vasc Surg* 38:1411–1415, 2003.
93. Abu-Daff S, Abu-Daff N, Al-Shahed M: "Mesenteric venous thrombosis and factors associated with mortality: a statistical analysis with five-year follow-up." *J Gastrointest Surg* 13:1245–1250, 2009.
94. Park WM, Cherry KJ, Chua HK, et al: Current results of open revascularization for chronic mesenteric ischemia: a standard for comparison. *J Vasc Surg* 35:853–859, 2002.
95. Berland T, Oldenburg WA: Acute mesenteric Ischemia. *Curr Gastroenterol Rep* 10(3):341–346, 2008.
96. Karthikeshwar K, O'Hara PJ, Gray BH, et al: Chronic mesenteric ischemia: open surgery versus percutaneous angioplasty and stenting. *J Vasc Surg* 33:63–71, 2001.
97. Kougias P, El Sayed HF, Zhou W, et al: Management of chronic mesenteric ischemia. The role of endovascular therapy. *J Endovasc Ther* 14(3):395–405, 2007.
98. Zerbib P, Lebuffe G, Sergent-Baudson G, et al: Endovascular versus open revascularization for chronic mesenteric ischemia: a comparative study. *Langenbecks Arch Surg* 393:865–870, 2008.
99. Oderich GS, Bower TC, Sullivan TM, et al: Open versus endovascular revascularization for chronic mesenteric ischemia: risk-stratified outcomes. *J Vasc Surg* 49:1472–1479, 2009.
100. Shaw RS: The "second-look" after superior mesenteric arterial embolectomy or reconstruction for mesenteric infarction, in Ellison EH, Friesen JR, Kulholland JH (eds): *Current Surgical Management.* Philadelphia, WB Saunders, 1965, p 509.

CHAPTER 152 ■ COMPARTMENT SYNDROME OF THE ABDOMINAL CAVITY

AJAI K. MALHOTRA AND RAO R. IVATURY

ABDOMINAL COMPARTMENT SYNDROME

Introduction

The association of elevated intra-abdominal pressure (IAP) and organ system dysfunction was described as early as the mid-nineteenth century [1]. However, the acceptance of this association as a distinct nosologic entity—abdominal compartment syndrome (ACS)—happened only in the late twentieth century. Even now, more than 20 years after the phrase was coined by Kron et al. [2], there is disagreement as to whether ACS is a distinct clinicopathologic entity in which the organ system dysfunction is causally related to the elevation in IAP or whether the elevated IAP is merely an epi-phenomenon observed in some critically ill patients, especially those receiving large volume crystalloid resuscitation [3]. The reasons for this are many and include (1) the variability of normal IAP [4], (2) lack of agreement as to the best method of measuring IAP [5], (3) lack of agreement about the level of IAP that is well tolerated and any elevation beyond which leads to pathologic consequences in the form of organ system dysfunction (Fig. 152.1) [6], (4) lack of agreement as to when intervention is necessary—in the prodromal phase to prevent development of organ system dysfunction or only after there is evidence of organ system dysfunction [7], and (5) the ideal intervention. These reasons not withstanding, the sheer volume of literature published about all aspects of this condition over the last two decades has reduced the army of skeptics to a corporal's guard. The current chapter focuses on the current understanding of ACS and attempts to provide a practical approach to the diagnosis, and management of this potentially devastating condition.

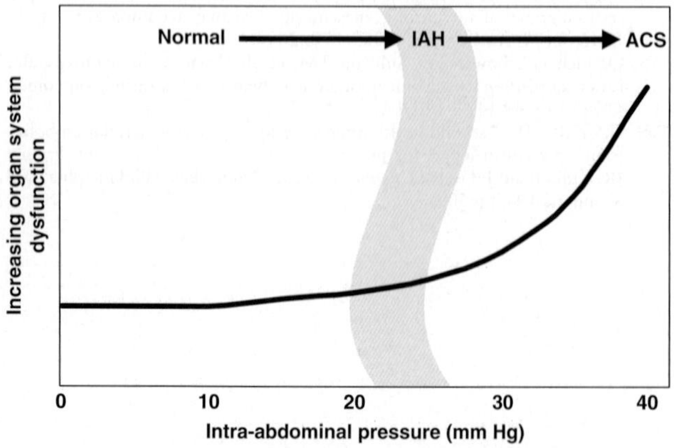

FIGURE 152.1. The continuum of normal intra-abdominal pressure to intra-abdominal hypertension (IAH). As the level of IAH increases organ dysfunction appears and the condition is called abdominal compartment syndrome. Note that the boundaries of normal IAP/IAH and IAH/ACS are wavy (grey zone). These boundaries are different in different individuals and also under different physiological state in the same individual.

The abdominal cavity is a space defined partly by rigid and inflexible structures—pelvis, spine, and coastal arches—and partly by more flexible structures—the musculoaponeurotic abdominal wall and the diaphragm. The total volume that can be accommodated within the confines of the abdomen is limited by these anatomical boundaries. Whenever there is a discrepancy between the available space, defined by the anatomical limits of the abdominal cavity, and the sum total volume of intra-abdominal structures—fluids and intra-abdominal organs—the pressure within the abdominal cavity tends to rise. This situation may arise from any condition that leads to increase in the total volume of structures—accumulation of fluid or swelling of organs—or decreased space—vigorous muscle contraction, loss of domain, etc. Initially the discrepancy is well tolerated by stretching of the flexible boundaries. However, as the limits of this accommodation are reached, even small increments in the intra-abdominal volume lead to large increases in IAP [6]. The elevated IAP affects organ system function in multiple ways. In the initial stages there is a purely mechanical effect best observed in the respiratory system, with embarrassment of ventilation due to elevation of the diaphragm, and in the kidneys where there is a fall in the glomerular filtration pressure affecting renal function. As the IAP continues to rise, there is decreased venous return to the heart affecting cardiac function and resulting in decreased cardiac output (CO). This reduction in CO has profound effects on every cell within the body as it globally decreases tissue perfusion. Finally, there is evidence that the elevated IAP in and of itself acts as a potent pro-inflammatory stimulus augmenting the systemic inflammation already set in motion by (1) the primary process that initiated the elevation of IAP and (2) tissue hypoperfusion caused by the diminished CO.

Definitions

As already mentioned earlier, there are no uniformly accepted definitions of the terms used in the context of ACS. Often, ACS and elevated IAP are used interchangeably, and the units of pressure measurement vary between mm Hg and cm H_2O. At the first World Congress on Abdominal Compartment Syndrome held at Noosa, Australia, in December 2004, attempts were made to develop consensus definitions of these terms and also to standardize the units and methodology used for measuring IAP. The definitions that follow are those that were developed at that conference and are used throughout the chapter. The units used are mm Hg unless otherwise specified. The method used to measure IAP, unless otherwise specified, is by the well-described technique of measuring bladder pressure, where the level of the pubic symphysis is considered 0 mm Hg [8].

Normal IAP: IAP varies between subatmospheric to a mean of 6.5 mm Hg [4]. It is affected by body habitus (chronically elevated in morbid obesity) [4], phase of respiration (higher during inspiration), and body position (elevated in the erect position) [5].

Consensus definition: IAP to be considered normal should be measured in the supine position, at end expiration and should have a value <10 mm Hg [7].

Elevated IAP—intra-abdominal hypertension (IAH): Brief elevations of IAP are fairly common and seen during sneezing, coughing etc and are of little clinical significance. Even in critically ill patients, brief elevations maybe observed during changes in body positions etc and are likewise clinically unimportant [4]. For IAP to be considered elevated, in a clinically significant fashion the elevation has to be sustained. The value at which IAP is considered elevated is a matter of debate; however, since alterations in physiology maybe observed even at relatively mild elevations to about 12 mm Hg, this value is the one supported by consensus.

Consensus definition: IAH should be defined as peak measured IAP of ≥ 12 mm Hg on two measurements 1 to 6 hours apart [7].

ACS: The point at which IAH develops into ACS remains controversial. Although it is generally agreed that ACS is the association of IAH, causing one or more organ system dysfunction, how the organ system dysfunction should be identified is not as well defined. When very sensitive and often invasive measures of organ system dysfunction are used, even minor elevations of IAP have been shown to affect function (Fig. 152.2) [9]. Also organ system function maybe affected at a certain IAP in one individual whereas the same level of IAP may not significantly alter organ system function in another individual [4]. Second, the level of IAH that is well tolerated can be different under differing physiologic states even in the same individual. For example, the threshold at which IAH leads to organ system dysfunction is significantly lowered posthemorrhagic shock as compared with baseline conditions [10]. Last, there is evidence that primary ACS (caused by an intra-abdominal pathology—see later) is less well tolerated than secondary ACS [11] (caused by resuscitation in the absence of significant intra abdominal pathology—see below).

Consensus definition: ACS should be diagnosed in the presence of (1) peak IAP of ≥ 20 mm Hg on two measurements 1 to 6 hours apart and (2) one or more organ system failure that was not previously present as defined by sequential organ failure assessment (SOFA) score of ≥ 3 (or an equivalent scoring system) [7].

Types of ACS: Initially ACS was described after intra-abdominal catastrophe—traumatic or inflammatory—and termed primary ACS [2]. More recently, it has been recognized that ACS can also develop in the absence of abdominal injury/pathology. This is usually observed in patients requiring massive volume resuscitation for any form of shock, usually traumatic or septic. It is believed that this form of ACS, termed secondary ACS, is due to leakage of fluid from within the capillaries resulting in massive edema of the intra-abdominal organs causing increased volume [11,12]. At times, the two conditions may coexist as in a patient with an intra-abdominal injury/pathology who during the recovery phase develops pneumonia and sepsis resulting in leaky capillaries. Recurrent ACS may be observed following therapy for either primary or secondary ACS, and this has been called tertiary ACS [13]. Finally, a very early hyperacute form of secondary ACS has been recognized that develops while repair of extra-abdominal injuries is being carried out simultaneous with massive volume resuscitation required for the hemorrhagic shock produced by the extra-abdominal injury [11]. Previously, hyperacute ACS was used to describe physiologic, transient, clinically insignificant elevations of IAP observed during sneezing, coughing, etc [14].

Consensus definitions

Primary ACS: Primary ACS is defined as ACS developing in a person where the proximate cause of the ACS is intra-abdominal/pelvic pathology that usually requires abdominal surgery and/or angio-radiologic intervention. The pathology may be traumatic, and/or inflammatory in nature [7].

Secondary ACS: Secondary ACS is defined as ACS developing due to increased volume of intra-abdominal contents from accumulation of fluid and/or visceral swelling, and where the proximate cause of the increase in volume is not any intra-abdominal/pelvic pathology requiring abdominal surgery and/or angio-radiologic therapy. Secondary ACS is usually observed during massive volume resuscitation for major nonabdomino/pelvic injuries, burns, severe acute pancreatitis, septic shock from a nonabdomino/pelvic infective source, etc [7].

Tertiary ACS: Tertiary ACS solely refers to ACS that develops or persists despite previous attempts to prevent or treat primary or secondary ACS [7].

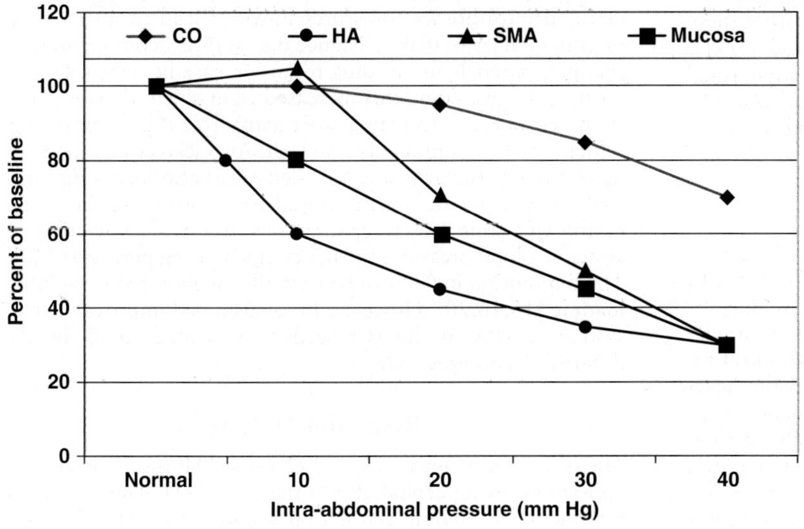

FIGURE 152.2. Effect of increasing intra-abdominal pressure on cardiac output (CO), hepatic artery flow (HA), superior mesenteric artery flow (SMA), and gastrointestinal mucosal flow (mucosa). Note that the splanchnic and mucosal flows start to decrease even at fairly low levels of intra-abdominal hypertension and even when global CO has not been affected.

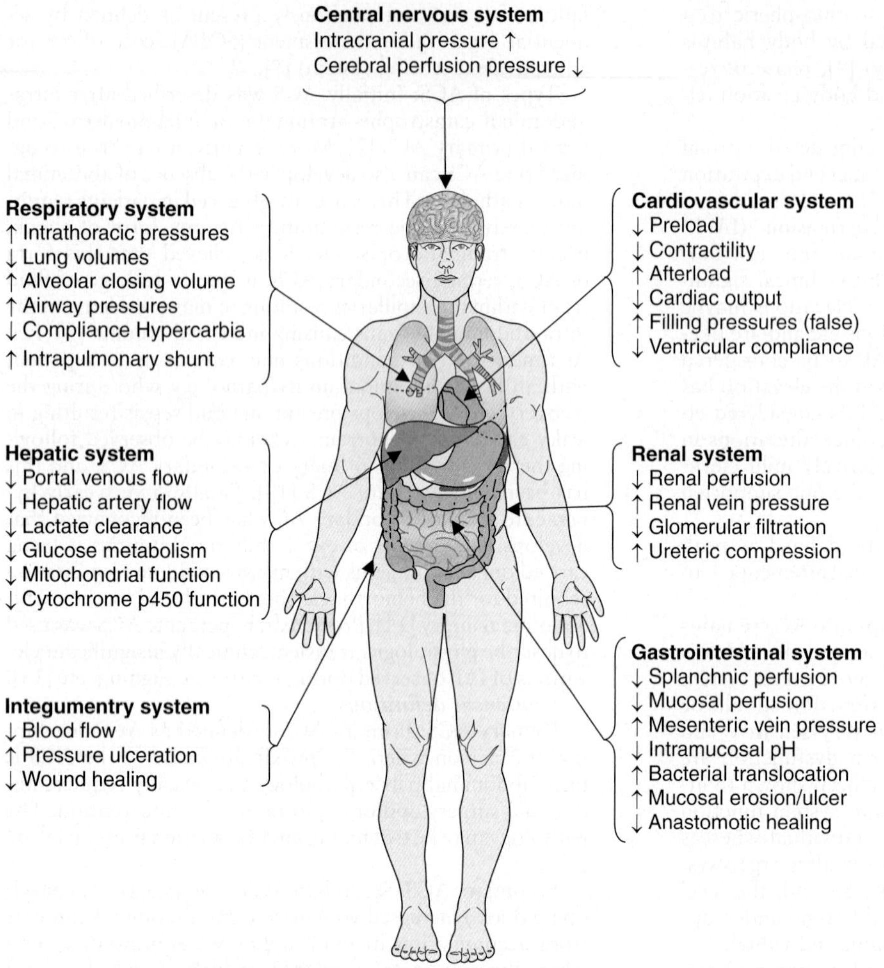

FIGURE 152.3. Effect of abdominal compartment syndrome on various body systems.

Hyperacute ACS: The term should be reserved for a very early form of secondary ACS that develops while surgical and/or angio-radiologic control of an injury is being carried out simultaneous with massive volume resuscitation for the shock caused by the same injury [11].

Impact of ACS on the Body

ACS has profound and far reaching effects on every major organ system of the body (Fig. 152.3). As mentioned earlier, these effects are related to (i) the mechanical pressure caused by IAH, (ii) the reduced perfusion to the tissues caused by diminished CO, and (iii) ACS amplifying the systemic inflammatory response already in motion due to the primary pathology, its treatment and tissue hypoperfusion.

Cardiovascular Effects

ACS affects each of the three determinants of cardiac function—preload, contractility, and afterload. IAH leads to compression of the inferior vena cava decreasing venous return from the lower half of the body [15]. In addition, elevated IAP raises the diaphragm leading to increased intrathoracic pressure, further impeding venous return to the heart [16]. Paradoxically, the central venous and the pulmonary capillary wedge pressures actually rise leading to a dissociation between the commonly used measures of cardiac filling and true cardiac end diastolic volumes. This increase in the filling pressure is merely the transmission of increased intrathoracic pressure to the measured intravascular pressure and not a true reflection of intravascular volume and cardiac filling [17]. Other techniques that directly measure cardiac end diastolic volumes tend to give a more accurate picture of cardiac filling [18]. The decreased venous return and cardiac filling negatively impact cardiac contractility. In addition, ACS directly leads to a decrease in ventricular compliance further affecting cardiac filling and contractility [15]. The effects of elevated intrathoracic pressures are more prominent on the right ventricle. Normally the right ventricle acts more as a conduit than as a pump. The elevated intrathoracic pressures however lead to an increase in pulmonary vascular resistance due to direct compression of the lung parenchyma leading to an increase in right-sided afterload. To overcome this increased right-sided afterload, the right ventricle has to play a more active role if left ventricular filling is to be maintained [19]. Last, ACS leads to an increase in systemic vascular resistance—left-sided afterload—that initially may cause the mean arterial pressure to rise; however, as the CO continues to fall, the net result is a lowering of systemic blood pressure, further compromising perfusion [20]. The diminution in CO can be partially ameliorated by volume loading [15,16,20]. However, for a sustained improvement in systemic perfusion, the ACS needs to be treated usually by abdominal decompression.

Respiratory Effects

The direct mechanical effect of elevated IAP results in the diaphragm moving cephalad into the chest [21]. This results in a reduction in minute ventilation leading to hypercarbia and respiratory acidosis. The compressive effect also leads to an increase in pulmonary closing volume and decrease in functional residual capacity and lung compliance [16]. The effect of these later changes is a mismatch between ventilation and perfusion and increased right to left shunting causing hypoxia. Clinically the earliest observed change is an increase in peak airway pressure, or if the patient is on a pressure limited ventilatory mode, a decrease in tidal volume [16]. If the ACS is not treated at this stage, the full effects on the respiratory system are observed with hypoxia, hypercarbia, and respiratory acidosis [16]. The hypoxia caused by the respiratory system effects adds to the tissue hypoxia produced by the diminished tissue perfusion due to the cardiovascular effects of ACS.

Renal Effects

ACS causes direct compression of the renal parenchyma causing elevation of renal venous pressure and increased renal vascular resistance [22–24]. In addition, the reduction in CO leads to diminished perfusion to the kidneys [20]. The end result is a reduction in urine production and, if left untreated, overt renal failure. Decreased urine output is often the first sign of developing ACS. Increasing CO only partially compensates for the reduction in glomerular filtration pressure, and insertion of ureteric stents offers no benefit [25].

Splanchnic and Hepatic Effects

While difficult to observe clinically, animal studies have demonstrated profound reductions in mesenteric and hepatic blood flow occurring with ACS. The reduction in flow is disproportionate, that is, it is observed whenever IAH is present even in the absence of significant hypotension and decrease in CO (Fig. 152.2) [26]. Within the bowel, the mucosa seems to be the most sensitive to these reductions. Initially, the reduced flow leads to increasing mucosal hypoxia and acidosis [27]. In later stages frank mucosal ulceration maybe observed. The net effect of these changes is loss of the selective absorptive function of the mucosa causing increased bacterial translocation and production of oxygen free radicals [28]. The exact consequences of bacterial translocation into the mesenteric venous and lymphatic systems are not clear. Some continue to believe that bacterial translocation may be responsible for driving the systemic inflammatory response [29]. Besides increased translocation, there is evidence that ACS, by decreasing mesenteric perfusion, may negatively impact healing of intestinal anastomosis [30].

Central Nervous System Effects

Elevated IAP leads to elevations in central venous pressures that are directly transmitted to the venous outflow from the cranial cavity leading to increased intracranial pressure (ICP) and reduction in cerebral perfusion pressure (CPP) [31]. Although these effects may be well tolerated by the uninjured brain, there is concern that ACS may contribute to secondary brain injury by its effect on CPP. Although not uniformly accepted as a therapy, there are some reports of head injured patients with elevated ICP, unresponsive to other measures for reduction of ICP, being treated by abdominal decompression [32,33].

Effects on the Integument

The effects of reduction in CO are particularly prominent in the integumentary blood flow. Profound reductions in flow to the abdominal wall have been observed. The reduction in integumentary flow may lead to problems with wound healing and higher risk of decubitus ulcers.

ACS, Systemic Inflammation, and Multiple Organ Dysfunction Syndrome

The large majority of patients that develop ACS are in a state of systemic inflammation and due to this are at a high risk for developing multiple organ dysfunction syndrome (MODS). The systemic inflammatory state in these patients is caused by (1) the primary pathology and its treatment causing ACS and (2) the tissue hypoperfusion and hypoxia caused by the cardiovascular and respiratory effects of ACS. Studies have clearly demonstrated an association of ACS and MODS [34]. What is less clear is whether MODS is caused or contributed to by ACS or whether the primary condition and its treatment that led to the development of ACS, independently caused MODS also. In animal models, ACS is associated with a disproportionate reduction in mesenteric flow, even when the mean pressure and CO are maintained [26]. In a human study of patients requiring high-volume resuscitation it was shown that patients resuscitated to a supraphysiologic oxygen delivery of 600 mL per minute per m^2 by volume loading required significantly larger volume as compared with a matched group resuscitated to only 500 mL per minute per m^2. As expected, the supraphysiologic group with the higher volume resuscitation had a higher incidence of ACS. The unexpected finding however was that the supraphysiologic group that developed ACS also had a higher incidence of gut ischemia, as measured by gastric mucosal pH, and worse outcomes [35]. The authors opined that the mesenteric ischemia, present despite higher systemic oxygen delivery in the supraphysiologic group, was caused by the ACS and was responsible for the worse outcomes. A large animal (swine) study examined the cytokine response to ACS alone, shock alone, or sequential shock resuscitation and ACS. It demonstrated that when ACS follows shock and resuscitation the cytokine response and neutrophil-mediated end organ injury are amplified as compared to either of the states occurring alone [36]. Another small animal study examined the effect of ACS at different time periods following shock and resuscitation. That study demonstrated that ACS was associated with worse outcomes in terms of end organ damage, and mortality when it occurred at the time when the neutrophils were maximally primed by the preceding shock and resuscitation [37]. Putting all of these studies together the hypothesis gaining acceptance is that the ACS acts as a second inflammatory stimulus—second hit in a two hit model—precipitating MODS in patients already primed by the primary condition that led to the development of ACS [38]. If this hypothesis is accepted, then the mechanism by which ACS acts as a second inflammatory stimulus needs further study. Some believe that increased bacterial translocation is the mechanism by which ACS acts as a second inflammatory stimulus leading to MODS. Some [28,39,40], though not all [41], animal studies of ACS have demonstrated increased bacterial translocation from the gut.

TECHNIQUE OF MEASURING IAP

A number of techniques have been used to measure IAP. Some are more invasive than others. IAP can be measured directly by accessing the peritoneal cavity. This method has been used during laparoscopic procedures, but is impractical due to the invasiveness and risk of infection outside of the operating room. Other techniques depend upon indirectly measuring IAP by measuring the pressure within the lumen of a hollow structure to which the IAP is directly transmitted—urinary bladder, stomach, rectum, or inferior vena cava. Of all the techniques, the most commonly used one is measuring pressure within the urinary bladder via a bladder catheter. The technique is simple and noninvasive since virtually all patients that may or do develop ACS have an indwelling bladder catheter. The setup consists of a three-way stop cock connected to (1) the aspiration port of the urine collection bag tube via pressure tubing and an 18-gauge needle, (2) a 50-mL syringe with sterile saline, and (3) pressure transducer tubing. The actual technique consists of emptying the bladder, clamping the tube of the collection bag distal to the aspiration port, and instilling 50 mL of sterile saline into the bladder. After instillation of the saline, the clamp should be briefly loosened to empty the tubing toward the patient's side of air, and reapplied without loosing the saline. After emptying the air, the pressure within the bladder is measured and recorded. The level of the pubic symphysis is considered 0 mm Hg [8]. Studies have shown excellent correlation between the true IAP and the bladder pressure measured by this technique. Like all techniques however, the accuracy of the measured pressure depends on how meticulously it is performed. The greatest source of error comes from incomplete emptying of the air. Air in the system anywhere from the transducer through the three-way connection into the pressure tubing, urine collection bag tubing, and the bladder catheter can dampen the pressure and give an erroneously low reading. Also in patients with very small bladders or those having bladder spasms the pressure recording maybe falsely high. If the above sources of error are kept in mind and care taken to avoid them, bladder pressure measurement is an excellent technique of monitoring patients for ACS, and is by far the commonest one used for this purpose.

MONITORING FOR AND INCIDENCE AND PREVALENCE OF ACS IN THE ICU

Patients at risk of developing ACS may broadly be classified into five categories: (1) patients with severe systemic sepsis from any source, especially those where the source is within the abdomen; (2) patients undergoing massive fluid resuscitation for shock usually septic or traumatic, especially where the source of hemorrhage is within the abdomen; (3) patients undergoing abdominal damage control surgery; (4) patients with an intra-abdominal catastrophe, for example, severe pancreatitis, bowel necrosis, etc; and (5) patients undergoing large-volume resuscitation for major burn injuries. All such patients should be monitored for the development of ACS usually by intermittent bladder pressure measurements. It should be borne in mind that even patients that are being managed with the open abdomen technique for the prevention or treatment of ACS can develop recurrent ACS—tertiary ACS—and should be monitored for it. In addition, any critically ill patient with acute cardiorespiratory deterioration should be evaluated for the development of ACS.

The exact prevalence of ACS in the ICU population is difficult to determine since (1) it is different in differing patient populations, so if the ICU manages trauma, surgical and burn patients the incidence and prevalence will be higher as opposed to a medical ICU, with the mixed ICU falling somewhere in between and (2) differing definitions of IAP, IAH and ACS used by different investigators. In a prospective multicenter study examining the prevalence of IAH and ACS, where IAH was defined as IAP >12 mm Hg, and ACS was defined as IAP >20 mm Hg with at least one organ system failure, 59% of patients had IAH and 8% had ACS. As expected, the prevalence was higher in surgical, trauma and burn patients as compared to medical patients. Also in burn patients the development of ACS was correlated to the size of the burn [42]. Another multicenter study with similar definitions of IAH and ACS was conducted in fourteen ICUs. That study enrolled 250 consecutive patients and followed them to discharge, death, or for 28 days and recorded the cumulative incidence of IAH and ACS. The cumulative incidence for the period of study was 32% for IAH and 4% for ACS, although only one patient required decompression. In this later study however, medical patients that tend to have a lower incidence of ACS accounted for 46% of the study population. The same study also examined the risk factors for the development of IAH and also it's effect on outcomes. It concluded that the development of IAH was an independent predictor of mortality, and the independent predictors of IAH on day one were liver dysfunction, abdominal surgery, fluid resuscitation with >3,500 mL over the preceding 24 hours, and ileus [43].

TREATMENT THRESHOLD

Although all agree that if a patient has severely elevated IAP with multiple organ system dysfunction, the patient should be treated for ACS. What is less clear is whether to treat patients much earlier in the process where the IAP is only moderately elevated and there is borderline dysfunction of only one organ system, or even earlier when the IAP is barely above 12 mm Hg. Since in the large majority of patients the treatment entails surgery and leaving the abdomen open, there are potential risks to the therapy. On the other hand there is evidence to suggest that earlier the treatment is initiated better is the final outcome [11,12,44]. In balance, all patients at risk of developing ACS should be monitored by frequent bladder pressure measurements. Patients that develop organ system dysfunction that, in the judgment of the treating physician, can be causally related to IAH should have therapy initiated. If the patient has increasing IAP but does not have any organ system dysfunction then the monitoring should continue with close observation for the development of organ system dysfunction, so that therapy can be initiated at the earliest sign of dysfunction. Finally almost all patients with IAP >20 mm Hg and rising, even without evidence of organ system dysfunction, should have therapy for impending ACS.

TREATMENT OF ACS

Therapy for ACS or impending ACS is aimed at reducing IAP. In the large majority of patients, this entails surgical decompression by performance of a laparotomy, and leaving the abdomen open till the visceral swelling and/or the fluid accumulation within the abdomen is diminished to a point that the IAP will not rise to pathological levels on abdominal closure. As this is fairly radical therapy with significant morbidity less invasive medical therapy has been attempted.

Medical (Minimally Invasive) Management

Medical management of ACS has limited application at best. It is possible that with more study, medical management may become the modality of choice for the patients in the prodromal phase where there is impending organ system dysfunction. Medical therapy consists of one or more of (1) neuromuscular blockade; (2) needle/tube drainage of intra-abdominal fluid; and (3) continuous external negative pressure therapy by special custom made devices.

Neuromuscular blockade is attractive in theory but no studies have been performed to evaluate it as sole therapy for ACS. It is often used in situations where abdominal closure was desirable and hence was performed but due to many factors, the closure was "tight." Two case reports are available where neuromuscular blockade was used for the treatment of acute ACS. One report however cautioned that surgical decompression may still be necessary after treatment with neuromuscular-blocking agents [45,46]. Aside from these case reports no studies are available that have adequately tested this form of therapy for acute ACS.

A small proportion of patients develop ACS not due to swelling of the viscera, rather due to accumulation of large volume of fluid and/or blood within the abdominal cavity. This is more often observed in patients with secondary ACS especially when caused by volume resuscitation for major burns. Such patients can be treated by placing a needle or small catheter within the peritoneal cavity. Case reports of successful management are present in the burn literature [47].

Continuous external negative pressure therapy is performed using custom made devices that surround the abdomen and create a negative pressure outside of the abdominal wall. Such devices have been used successfully in morbidly obese patients with chronic ACS [48,49]. There application in patients with acute ACS has not been reported, but in animal studies of acute ACS, they have shown potential [50].

Surgical Therapy

Surgical therapy in the form of decompressive laparotomy with the abdomen left open is the most often used treatment modality for impending or actual ACS. There is a large body of literature to support that such therapy, when performed early, rapidly reduces IAH and reverses organ system dysfunction. However, it should be pointed out that there have been no randomized trials to prove the benefits. The available evidence in favor of its use is class-II at best and is based on expert opinion and case control studies.

Surgical decompression of the abdomen for the treatment of ACS is performed by a generous midline laparotomy. After the laparotomy, the abdomen is left in the open state—fascia is not reapproximated. There are a number of methods available for managing the open abdomen. The method of management should be such that it can be performed rapidly, prevent heat loss from the internal viscera, protect the swollen viscera, and allow relatively free egress of the large amount of fluid that may accumulate within the cavity with continued resuscitation. In addition, the method should not damage the fascia and skin so that formal closure can be achieved later. In the authors' current practice, a large plastic sheet is laid over the bowel, and tucked deep in the paracolic gutters laterally, over the stomach/spleen and liver superiorly, and deep in the pelvis inferiorly. This sheet not only protects the internal viscera, and prevents heat loss, it also prevents adhesion formation between the bowel surface, and the abdominal wall, allowing for formal fascial closure at a later date. Small perforations are made in this sheet to allow fluid egress. Moistened gauze bandage is placed on top of this plastic sheet, and drains—Jackson Pratt or large (20 Fr) red rubber with multiple holes—are placed within the bandage. A Steridrape large enough to cover the bandage and adhere to the surrounding skin is placed over the bandage. The drains are connected, through collecting buckets, to wall suction at about 100 mm Hg. This system is easy to manage for the nursing staff, and allows for the fluid to be measured.

There are multiple problems associated with the open abdomen. In the absence of normal biological coverage, the body loses heat, the exposed viscera can desiccate, fistula can form from the mechanical trauma of dressing changes, and the large open wound is a major metabolic drain to the body. In addition to these short-term problems, in the longer term, in the absence of a complete fascio-muscular envelope, it is difficult to perform many physical actions for gainful employment. Because of these factors, how the open abdominal wound is managed has both long- and short-term consequences. There is no single method that will be suitable for all patients, and some tailoring to the need of the individual patient will be necessary to optimize functional outcome, and minimize complications.

Patients, in whom recovery progresses rapidly with brisk diuresis, and resolution of bowel edema, it may be possible to achieve fascial closure within 5 to 7 days. In many instances, however, this does not happen, or the patient develops some septic complication and the bowel becomes swollen again. After about a week in the open situation two factors prevent fascial closure. First, the fascial edges retract laterally, and second, adhesions form between the external surface of the bowel, and the abdominal wall. A plastic sheet interposed between the bowel surface and abdominal wall serves to prevent adhesion formation, and the VAC apparatus (KCI USA, Texas) can help medial mobilization of the retracted fascial edge. Using these techniques fascial reapproximation has been achieved up to 3 weeks after decompressive surgery [51].

Patients in whom, despite all measures, fascial closure is not possible, skin flaps can be mobilized, and closed over the bowel. In situations where skin flaps cannot be mobilized, the bowel surface can be allowed to granulate over, and then covered with split thickness skin graft. While waiting for adequate granulation tissue to form, extreme care is necessary, with minimum dressing changes performed very delicately so that mechanical trauma to the bowel surface is minimized, and fistula formation is prevented. After skin coverage is achieved, either by medial mobilization of skin flaps or by split thickness skin grafts over the granulated bowel, patients are left with a large ventral hernia that will require repair at a later date. The repair is usually carried out 6 to 9 months later to allow the inflammatory reaction to subside, and adhesions to become less vascular. A good way to check if a patient with split thickness skin graft is ready to have it taken off and hernia repaired is to try and pinch the skin off the bowel. In the initial stages, the skin graft is tightly adherent to the bowel wall, not allowing the skin to be pinched up. With the passage of time, and resolution of the inflammatory adhesions, the skin can be pinched off the bowel. Multiple techniques are used to repair the ventral hernia and reconstruct the abdominal wall. An innovative approach involves separating the various layers of the abdominal wall and instead of the patient having an incomplete multilayered abdominal wall the patient ends up with a single layered, but complete, fascio-muscular abdominal wall [52]. This approach allows native tissue to be used and avoids the need of prosthetic meshes, with their attendant complications. Good long-term functional results have been reported with this technique [53]. Alternatively, permanent prosthetic mesh may be used to bridge the gap in fascia, or a combination of techniques can be used. Preoperative use of tissue expanders to facilitate tension-free repair of these large ventral hernias has also been reported [54].

PREVENTION OF ACS

The best method of preventing the development of ACS is prompt recognition by frequent bladder pressure measurements and early action to prevent rising IAP turning into frank ACS with organ system dysfunction. In some surgical patients however, it may be possible to recognize that the patient has a high likelihood of developing ACS postoperatively. In such patients, surgeons are leaning toward preventing the development of ACS by leaving the abdomen in the open state. An interesting study was performed on patients with ruptured abdominal aortic aneurysms, in whom outcomes of patients with early placement of mesh (avoiding tight fascial reapproximation and possible ACS) were compared with outcomes from similar patients in whom tight closure was performed only later to be replaced by mesh due to the development of ACS. The incidence of multiorgan system failure was significantly lower in the patients where a tight closure and possible ACS were avoided [44]. In patients undergoing laparotomy and who fall into the high-risk category for the development of ACS, strong consideration should be given to leave the abdomen open and prevent ACS.

The other major group of patients that is likely to develop ACS are those receiving large volume crystalloid resuscitation. Although early and rapid volume resuscitation is in many situations the only therapy that will rapidly reverse hypoperfusion, it is an independent risk factor for the development of ACS. Careful and frequent reevaluations should be performed on all patients receiving large volume resuscitation so that as soon as the need for the large volume diminishes, the infusion is turned down to minimize the chances of developing ACS [55].

OUTCOMES FOLLOWING ACS THERAPY

Patients requiring therapy for, or prevention from, ACS tend to be critically ill and have high morbidity and mortality. However, the development of ACS tends to increase mortality [34]. The reported mortality of patients requiring abdominal decompression for ACS is 29% to 62% [56]. In addition, patients with open abdomens pose significant management challenges if the morbidity of the treatment—open abdomen—is to be kept low. The most significant source of morbidity is the development of enterocutaneous fistula with rates reported as high as 18% [57]. To avoid this, dressing changes should be kept to a minimum and the exposed bowel should not be allowed to desiccate by placing nonadherent dressings over it. Besides this, the open abdomen is a significant metabolic drain to the body. This large open wound, coupled with the inflammation from the condition leading to the development of ACS, can rapidly lead to a state of severe malnutrition. Patients should be given adequate nutritional support, enteral if possible, and parenteral if not. By using evidence-based practices and continuously evolving clinical practice as knowledge becomes available, certain ICUs have shown a remarkable improvement in outcomes. Cheatham et al. in a recent study demonstrated that although the patient population remained the same, survival to hospital discharge improved from 50% to 72% and same admission primary fascial closure improved from 59% to 81% [58].

Despite improvements, the short-term in-hospital mortality and morbidity of patients managed with the open-abdomen technique for ACS remains high. However, patients that survive to discharge do surprisingly well. A prospective study examining the physical and mental states and employability of patients that had undergone management of ACS by the open-abdomen technique, demonstrated that within 18 months of abdomen closure, these indices were equivalent to a comparable cohort that did not have the open abdomen [59].

THE FUTURE

Despite the large body of literature about ACS, there are a significant number of intensivists and a small number of surgeons who continue to discount the existence of this disease entity. It is important to continue to educate these clinicians for the benefit of their patients. Further research needs to be carried out to define exactly which patients are likely to develop ACS so that prophylactic measures can be performed and ACS prevented. In addition, there needs to be a better understanding of the threshold at which therapy is the most beneficial so that only the patients that are likely to benefit from the therapy are subjected to the risks of the therapy. Finally, research in other modalities of resuscitation that can reduce the large volumes necessary will help in preventing ACS. A better understanding of the systemic inflammatory response with the attendant capillary leak may allow therapies to be developed that can attenuate the "runaway" systemic inflammation or at least reduce the capillary leak thereby reducing the chance of developing ACS.

CONCLUSION

Raised IAP leads to IAH that can cause organ system dysfunction and this combination of IAH and organ system dysfunction is termed ACS. There remain many areas of confusion in terms of terminology, diagnosis, appropriate treatment threshold, and the best treatment. The recent World Congress on ACS has helped clarify some of these issues. Any patient with organ system dysfunction or impending dysfunction in association with IAH should have prompt therapy. Although there are some medical therapies that show some promise, the best therapy to rapidly decrease IAP and reverse the organ system dysfunction remains surgical decompressive laparotomy and leaving the abdomen open. The open abdomen can be associated with significant morbidity hence extreme care is necessary in the management of such patients. As soon as the patient's condition improves attempts to close the abdomen or at least provide biological coverage should be initiated. In patients who are left with a large hernia, delayed repair with component separation or prosthetic mesh offers excellent long-term functional results.

References

1. Emerson H: Intra-abdominal pressures. *Arch Int Med* 7:754–784, 1911.
2. Kron IL, Harman PK, Nolan SP: The measurement of intra-abdominal pressure as a criterion for abdominal reexploration. *Ann Surg* 199:28–30, 1984.
3. Balogh Z, McKinley BA, Cox Jr CS, et al: Abdominal compartment syndrome: the cause or effect of postinjury multiple organ failure. *Shock* 20:483–492, 2003.
4. Sanchez NC, Tenofsky PL, Dort JM, et al: What is normal intra-abdominal pressure? *Am Surg* 67:243–248, 2001.
5. Malbrain ML: Different techniques to measure intra-abdominal pressure (IAP): time for a critical reappraisal. *Intensive Care Med* 30:357–371, 2004.
6. Malbrain ML: Abdominal pressure in the critically ill: measurement and clinical relevance. *Intensive Care Med* 25:1453–1458, 1999.
7. Muckart DJJ, Ivatury RR, Leppaniemi A, et al: Definitions, in Ivatury RR, Cheatham ML, Malbrain MLNG, Sugrue M, (eds): *Abdominal Compartment Syndrome*. Georgetown, TX, Landes Bioscience, 2006, also available at Eurekah.com.
8. Iberti TJ, Lieber CE, Benjamin E: Determination of intra-abdominal pressure using a transurethral bladder catheter: clinical validation of the technique. *Anesthesiol* 70:47–50, 1989.
9. Schein M, Ivatury R: Intra-abdominal hypertension and the abdominal compartment syndrome. *Br J Surg* 85:1027–1028, 1998.
10. Simon RJ, Friedlander MH, Ivatury, RR, et al: Hemorrhage lowers the threshold for intra-abdominal hypertension-induced pulmonary dysfunction. *J Trauma* 42:398–403, 1997.
11. Rodas EB, Malhotra AK, Chhitwal R, et al: Hyperacute abdominal compartment syndrome: an unrecognized complication of massive intraoperative resuscitation for extra-abdominal injuries. *Am Surg* 71:977–981.
12. Maxwell RA, Fabian TC, Croce M, et al: Secondary abdominal compartment syndrome: an underappreciated manifestation of severe hemorrhagic shock. *J Trauma* 47:995–999, 1999.
13. Gracias VH, Braslow B, Johnson J, et al: Abdominal compartment syndrome in the open abdomen. *Arch Surg* 137:1298–1300, 2002.
14. Malbrain MLNG, Deeren D, DePotter TJR: Intra-abdominal hypertension in the critically ill: is it time to pay attention. *Curr Opin Crit Care* 11:156–171, 2005.
15. Kashtan J, Green JF, Parson EQ, et al: Hemodynamic effects of increased abdominal pressure. *J Surg Res* 30:249–255, 1981.
16. Richardson JD, Trinkle JK: Hemodynamic and respiratory alterations with increased intra-abdominal pressure. *J Surg Res* 20:401, 1976.

17. Hering R, Rudolph J, Spiegel TV, et al: Cardiac filling pressures are inadequate for estimating circulatory volume in states of elevated intraabdominal pressure. *Intensive Care Med* 24:S409, 2003.
18. Diebel LN, Wilson RF, Tagett MG, et al: End-diastolic volume: a better indicator of preload in the critically ill. *Arch Surg* 127:817–822, 1992.
19. Eddy AC, Rice CL, Anasdi DM: Right ventricular dysfunction in multiple trauma victims. *Am J Surg* 155:712–715, 1988.
20. Ridings PC, Bloomfield GL, Blocher CR, et al: Cardiopulmonary effects of raised intra-abdominal pressure before and after volume expansion. *J Trauma* 39:1071–1075, 1995.
21. Williams H, Simms H: Abdominal compartment syndrome: case reports and implications for management in critically ill patients. *Am Surg* 63:555–558, 1997.
22. Doty JM, Saggi BH, Sugerman HJ, et al: Effect of increased renal venous pressure on renal function. *J Trauma* 47:1000–1003, 1999.
23. Doty JM, Saggi BH, Blocher CR, et al: Effects of increased renal parenchymal pressure on renal function. *J Trauma* 48:874–877, 2000.
24. Platell CF, Hall J, Clarke G, et al: Intra-abdominal pressure and renal function after surgery to the abdominal aorta. *Aust NZ J Surg* 60:213–216, 1990.
25. Lindstrom P, Wadstorm J, Ollerstram A, et al: Effects of increased intra-abdominal pressure and volume expansion on renal function in the rat. *Nephrol Dial Transplant* 18:2269–2277, 2003.
26. Diebel LN, Dulchavsky SA, Wilson RF: Effect of increased intra-abdominal pressure on mesenteric arterial and intestinal mucosal blood flow. *J Trauma* 33:45–49, 1992.
27. Bongard FB, Ryan M, Dubecz: Adverse consequences of increased intraabdominal pressure on bowel tissue oxygen. *J Trauma* 39:519–525, 1995.
28. Diebel LN, Dulchavsky SA, Brown HJ: Splanchnic ischemia and bacterial translocation in the abdominal compartment syndrome. *J Trauma* 43:852–855, 1997.
29. Hassoun HT, Kone BC, Mercer DW, et al: Post-injury multiple organ failure: the role of the gut. *Shock* 15:1–10, 2001.
30. Kologlu M, Sayek I, Kologlu LB, et al: Effect of persistently elevated intraabdominal pressure on healing of colonic anastomosis. *Am J Surg* 178:293–297, 1999.
31. Josephs LG, Este-McDonald JR, Birkett DH, et al: Diagnostic laparoscopy increases intracranial pressure. *J Trauma* 36:815–818, 1994.
32. Bloomfield GL, Dalton JM, Sugerman HJ, et al: Treatment of increasing intracranial pressure secondary to the acute abdominal compartment syndrome in a patient with combined abdominal and head trauma. *J Trauma* 39:1168–1170, 1995.
33. Joseph DK, Dutton RP, Aarabi B, et al: Decompressive laparotomy to treat intractable intracranial hypertension after traumatic brain injury. *J Trauma* 57:687–695, 2004.
34. Raeburn CD, Moore EE, Biffl WL, et al: The abdominal compartment syndrome is a morbid complication of postinjury damage control surgery. *Am J Surg* 182:542–546, 2001.
35. Balogh Z, McKinley BA, Cocanour CS, et al: Supranormal trauma resuscitation causes more cases of abdominal compartment syndrome. *Arch Surg* 138:637–643, 2003.
36. Oda J, Ivatury RR, Blocher CR, et al: Amplified cytokine response and lung injury by sequential hemorrhagic shock and abdominal compartment syndrome in a laboratory model of ischemia-reperfusion. *J Trauma* 52:625–632, 2002.
37. Rezendo-Neto JB, Moore EE, Masuno T, et al: The abdominal compartment syndrome as a second insult during systemic neutrophil priming provokes multiple organ injury. *Shock* 20:303–308, 2003.
38. Bathe OF, Chow AW, Phang PT: Splanchnic origin of cytokines in a porcine model of mesenteric ischemia-reperfusion. *Surgery* 123:79–88, 1998.
39. Eleftheriadis E, Kotzampassi K, Papanotas K, et al: Gut ischemia, oxidative stress, and bacterial translocation in elevated abdominal pressure in rats. *World J Surg* 20:11–16, 1996.
40. Gargiulo NJ III, Simon RJ, Leon W, et al: Hemorrhage exacerbates bacterial translocation at low levels of intra-abdominal pressure. *Arch Surg* 133:1351–1355,1998.
41. Doty JM, Oda J, Ivatury RR, et al: The effects of hemodynamic shock and increased intra-abdominal pressure on bacterial translocation. *J Trauma* 52:13–17, 2002.
42. Malbrain ML: Is it wise not to think about intraabdominal hypertension in the ICU? *Curr Opin Crit Care* 10:132–145, 2004.
43. Malbrain ML, Chiumello D, Pelosi P, et al: Incidence and prognosis of intraabdominal hypertension in a mixed population of critically ill patients: a multi-center epidemiological study. *Crit Care Med* 33:315–322, 2005.
44. Rasmussen TE, Hallett JW Jr, Noel AA, et al: Early abdominal closure with mesh reduces multiple organ failure after ruptured abdominal aortic aneurysm repair: guidelines from a 10-year case control study. *J Vasc Surg* 35:246–253, 2002.
45. Macalina JU, Goldman RK, Mayberry JC: Medical management of abdominal compartment syndrome: case report and a caution. *Asian J Surg* 25:244–246, 2002.
46. DE Waele JJ, Benoit D, Hoste E, et al: A role for muscle relaxation in patients with abdominal compartment syndrome? *Intensive Care Med* 29:332, 2003.
47. Latenser BA, Kova-Vern A, Komball D, et al: A pilot study comparing percutaneous decompression with decompressive laparotomy for acute abdominal compartment syndrome in thermal injury. *J Burn Care Rehab* 23:190–195, 2002.
48. Saggi BH, Bloomfield GL, Sugerman HJ, et al: Treatment of intracranial hypertension using non-surgical abdominal decompression. *J Trauma* 46:646–651, 1999.
49. Sugerman HJ, Felton WL III, Sismanins A, et al: Continuous negative abdominal pressure device to treat pseudotumor cerebri. *Int J Obes Relat Metab Disord* 25:486–490, 2001.
50. Adams J, Osiovich H, Goldberg R, et al: Hemodynamic effects of continuous negative extrathoracic pressure and continuous positive airway pressure in piglets with normal lungs. *Biol Neonate* 62:69–75, 1992.
51. Garner GB, Ware DN, Cocanour CS, et al: Vacuum-assisted wound closure provides early fascial reapproximation in trauma patients with open abdomens. *Am J Surg* 2001;182:630–632.
52. Ramirez OM, Ruas E, Dellon AL: "Components separation" method for closure of abdominal-wall defects: an anatomic and clinical study. *Plast Reconstr Surg* 86:519, 1990.
53. Fabian TC, Croce MA, Pritchard E, et al: Planned ventral hernia. Staged management for acute abdominal wall defects. *Ann Surg*. 219:643, 1994.
54. Livingston DH, Sharma PK, Glantz AI: Tissue expanders for abdominal wall reconstruction following severe trauma. Technical note and case reports. *J Trauma* 32:82, 1992.
55. Ivatury RR: Supranormal trauma resuscitation and abdominal compartment syndrome. *Arch Surg* 139:225–226, 2004.
56. Decker G. Abdominal compartment syndrome. *J Chir* 138:270–276, 2001.
57. Nicholas JM, Rix EP, Easley A, et al: Changing patterns in the management of penetrating abdominal trauma: the more things change the more they are the same. *J Trauma* 55:1095–1110, 2003.
58. Cheatham ML, Safcsak K: Is the evolving management of intra-abdominal hypertension and abdominal compartment syndrome improving survival? *Crit Care Med* 38:402–407, 2010.
59. Cheatham ML, Safcsak K: Long term impact of abdominal decompression: a prospective comparative analysis. *J Am Coll Surg* 207:573–579, 2008.

CHAPTER 153 ■ NECROTIZING SOFT TISSUE INFECTIONS

RICHARD L. GAMELLI AND JOSEPH A. POSLUSZNY JR

Necrotizing soft tissue infections (NSTIs) include a spectrum of diseases ranging from necrotizing fasciitis to gas gangrene and Fournier's gangrene. These infections occur within the soft tissue compartment from the dermis to the fascia and deep to the muscle layer, are associated with necrotizing changes, progress rapidly and can occur at any location in the body. Although many terms have been used to describe these infections, NSTI encompasses all necrotizing infections of the soft tissue compartment as they share common clinical, pathophysiologic, microbial, treatment, and outcome characteristics [1].

Most of the clinical information for NSTIs stems from large retrospective reviews [2–6]. Few prospective studies have been performed given the high morbidity and mortality associated with these infections. However, these retrospective reviews have been surprisingly similar, each confirming previous data on risk factors, inciting events, microbiology, diagnosis, prognosis, and management while providing unique findings about their populations, NSTI, and its management.

EPIDEMIOLOGY AND RISK FACTORS

Surveillance of NSTIs in the United States no longer occurs, but the incidence can be estimated from epidemiologic studies [7]. Using a statewide database, Mulla et al. estimated an incidence of NSTI of 1.3/100,000 people with a total of 216 patients in Florida treated for NSTI in 2001 [8]. Demonstrating the frequent occurrence of cellulitis and rare incidence of NSTI, using an insurance claims database in Utah, Ellis Simonsen et al. estimated an incidence rate of cellulitis of 24.6/1,000 person years with an incidence rate for NSTI of only 0.04/1,000 person years [9]. NSTI is found in all age groups but most commonly in adults [10].

NSTIs occur in a wide range of patients who almost always possess preexisting conditions. More than 80% to 90% of patients with NSTIs possess comorbidities [2,3,11], whereas 62% may have three or more preexisting conditions [11]. Diabetes is the most frequent preexisting condition. In two large retrospective reviews, diabetes was present in 56% and 70% of the patients, respectively [2,4]. Other common preexisting conditions include obesity, hypertension, cirrhosis/chronic liver failure, peripheral vascular disease, HIV, and immunosuppressive therapy [2,3,12,13]. Behaviors like intravenous drug abuse (IVDA) and alcoholism leading to chronic liver disease also increase the risk of developing a NSTI [2,6,11,14]. Preexisting disease is not only a risk factor for NSTI but also for mortality [15]. When totaling comorbidities, patients who died had an average of 1.5 comorbidities versus 1.0 for survivors [3]. Preexisting conditions that correlated with mortality include cardiac disease, pulmonary disease, carcinoma, malnutrition, and IVDA [4].

Although preexisting conditions may increase the risk of developing a NSTI and mortality from NSTI, time to surgical debridement is the main risk factor for mortality. Since 1985, we have known that both prompt and radical surgical debridement of all devitalized tissue improves mortality [16]. Since then, many studies have supported early and aggressive surgical therapy for NSTI. Bilton et al. showed that delay in therapy increased mortality (38% mortality) when compared with early and aggressive surgical debridement (4% mortality) [12]. McHenry et al. found an average time to debridement of 25 hours in survivors but 90 hours for nonsurvivors [5]. Elliott et al. showed an average time to debridement of 1.2 days for survivors and 3.1 days for nonsurvivors [4]. On multivariate analysis, Wong et al. found that a delay in surgery of more than 24 hours was the only variable to correlate with increased mortality [2].

Although the incidence of NSTI is relatively low, the mortality is high at approximately 25% [17,18]. Early and radical surgical debridement is the key to successful treatment.

INCITING EVENTS

Many patients report an insect bite, blister, abscess, or the feeling of a pulled muscle several days prior to presenting with a NSTI. Although some (15% to 52%) cases of NSTI are idiopathic in origin, the remainder have an identifiable source [3,5,11,15]. Abscesses, foot ulcers, traumatic wounds, burns, surgical wounds, IVDA, decubitus ulcers, perforated viscus, and strangulated hernia were all identified as inciting events by Elliott et al. [4]. Endorf et al. also reported liposuction, an infected arteriovenous graft, invasive rectal cancer, a percutaneous gastrostomy tube site, and an enterocutaneous fistula as suspected causes of NSTI [3]. Anaya et al. found inciting events to include subcutaneous/IV injection, trauma, postoperative wound infection, boils, chronic wounds/ulcers, bites, and perirectal abscesses [11].

PATHOPHYSIOLOGY

Regardless of the inciting event, the pathophysiology of NSTIs is quite similar. NSTIs are a specific disease process in which entry of organisms through a compromised skin barrier results in a soft tissue infection that rapidly spreads along the superficial fascia of the subcutaneous tissue but initially spares the overlying skin and underlying muscle [19]. The rapidly spreading infection causes thrombosis of penetrating vessels, which in turn causes necrosis of overlying tissues supplied by those vessels. Histologic examination reveals necrosis of the superficial fascia, thrombosis and suppuration of veins traversing the fascia and microorganisms proliferating in the destroyed fascia [2]. Systemic spread of infection causes overwhelming sepsis or toxic shock syndrome if associated with streptococcal exotoxin of group A streptococcus (GAS) [20,21]. When muscle is involved early, the pathogen is commonly a clostridial species [22].

MICROBIOLOGY

The microbial causes of NSTIs can be polymicrobial or monomicrobial. The majority of NSTIs (53% to 85%) are polymicrobial [2,4,5]. Organisms in polymicrobial NSTIs include anaerobes and aerobes, Gram-positive and Gram-negatives and rarely fungi (<5%) [3,4,5]. In Elliott et al., the organisms recovered from NSTIs included streptococci, staphylococci, enterococci, *E. coli*, *Proteus*, *Klebsiella*, *Enterobacter*, *Pseudomonas*, *Acinetobacter*, *Eikenella*, *Citrobacter*, peptostreptococci, *Bacteroides*, clostridia, and fungal species [23]. In a similar analysis, Wong et al. identified streptococcal species, staphylococcal species, enterococci, *Escherichia coli*, *Acinetobacter*, *Pseudomonas*, and *Klebsiella* as the most common isolates with *Bacteroides* being the most frequent anaerobe [2]. In Elliott et al., four or more organisms grew from the initial wound culture almost 50% of the time [4].

Monomicrobial NSTI occurs in approximately 15% to 29% of cases and over 50% of these monomicrobial NSTI are attributable to GAS [2,4,5]. Occasionally, monomicrobial NSTIs are caused by clostridia species [22], methicillin-resistant *Staphylococcus aureus* (MRSA) [24–28], and even group B streptococcus [20]. Tissue cultures have been found to not yield any organisms in 9% to 18% of debrided tissue samples [2,3]. In cases in which no organism is cultured and GAS is suspected, polymerase chain reaction can be used to amplify the streptococcal pyrogenic exotoxin B gene in tissue samples [29]. Although this may not be necessary for immediate management, it may aid in subsequent antibiotic therapy, prophylaxis of other close personal contacts, and for epidemiologic studies.

Attempts have been made to classify NSTIs based on microbial characteristics and to correlate the infectious organism to an inciting event, risk factor, or anatomic location [2,30,31]. Given the lack of uniformity and consistency in this classification system and the need to still treat all NSTIs initially

TABLE 153.1

MICROBIAL CLASSIFICATION OF NECROTIZING SOFT TISSUE INFECTIONS

Type I	Polymicrobial
Type II	Group A Streptococcus ± additional organisms
Type III	Unique and emerging pathogens (CA-MRSA, *Acinetobacter*, *Clostridia*, *Vibrio*)

CA-MRSA, community-acquired methicillin-resistant *Staphylococcus aureus*.

with prompt diagnosis, early surgical debridement, broad-spectrum antimicrobials, adequate nutrition and critical care support, labeling an NSTI based on the type of organism present should be used only to guide later antimicrobial choice and for research purposes. Therefore, we supply a slightly modified table listing the historical classification of Type I (polymicrobial) and II (GAS ± additional organisms) NSTIs with an additional classification of Type III (community-acquired MRSA, *Acinetobacter*, *Clostridial*, and *Vibrio* species) to include emerging or unique pathogens which require consideration when NSTI is suspected (Table 153.1) [30,31]. These unique NSTI pathogens are discussed in more detail later. Although some classifications consider Type I to be polymicrobial and Type II to be monomicrobial, given the virulent nature and incidence of GAS, these infections remain as their own group.

DIAGNOSIS

The diagnosis of NSTI is not difficult when obvious signs of tissue necrosis are present. However, this is rare. Wong et al. found that only 14.6% of their patients eventually diagnosed with NSTI had the diagnosis of NSTI or a suspicion of NSTI on admission [2]. Most often, patients were diagnosed with cellulitis or an abscess. Hard clinical signs of NSTI (bullae, skin necrosis, crepitance, gas on radiograph) are present on admission for only 44% of patients with NSTI [14]. The difficulty with diagnosing NSTI is determining when NSTI is present before these obvious signs present as delay is detrimental to patient outcome. If distinguishing nonnecrotizing infection from NSTIs is not possible, then close monitoring of physical examination changes is required to avoid further progression of the disease process. Therefore, the majority of this section focuses the physical examination features common to NSTI and measures that can be employed to earlier diagnose NSTI and thus, prompt more expeditious treatment.

Physical Exam

Signs shared by both nonnecrotizing and necrotizing soft tissue infections include pain, erythema, induration, and swelling. The hard signs of NSTI which may help to differentiate it from nonnecrotizing infection include crepitus, blistering, and skin necrosis, all of which occur at later stages of the disease process. In Elliott et al., on admission, crepitus was present in 36% of patients, skin necrosis in 31% and blistering in 23% [4]. Similarly, Faucher et al. found an open wound in 39%, crepitus in 32%, and vesicles in 23% of patients on admission. However, symptoms common to nonnecrotizing and necrotizing soft tissue infections (pain 89%, edema 84% and erythema 74%) were predominant on admission [11]. If a patient presents with tenderness, erythema and warmth, the development of bullae may be the first sign leading to a higher suspicion of NSTI [2]. NSTI has also been described as having poorly defined and indistinct margins of tissue involvement, tenderness beyond the area of cutaneous involvement and pain out of proportion to physical findings [2,4]. In an attempt to earlier differentiate benign soft tissue infections from NSTI, Wang et al. developed a staging system for the progression of NSTI using only cutaneous manifestations. Stage 1 included tenderness to palpation beyond the apparent area of skin involvement, erythema, swelling, and calor. Stage 2 included blister or bullae formation and later, Stage 3 included crepitus, skin anesthesia, and skin necrosis with dusky coloration. By Day 4 of hospitalization, 68% of their patients with NSTI displayed Stage 3 cutaneous manifestations whereas only 5% did at time of admission. Although this system helps to describe the cutaneous manifestations of NSTI, absence of these cutaneous manifestations does not exclude NSTI [32]. Waiting for the presence of Stage 3 cutaneous manifestations may be detrimental to the patient.

Imaging

Plain radiography, ultrasound, CT and MRI have all been studied as adjuncts to physical exam in cases of suspected NSTI. Classically, air or gas between the muscle and soft tissue layer is diagnostic of NSTI and very often, clostridial NSTI. However, gas is found on x-ray in only a small percentage (16–19%) of cases [2,14]. The soft tissue changes seen with both complex cellulitis and NSTI are indistinguishable on plain radiograph. Therefore, plain radiography is only valuable in the rare cases in which air is present between the tissues. Ultrasound may benefit these patients in that it is quick, noninvasive and can be performed at the bedside. However, there are few studies on ultrasound use to distinguish NSTI from cellulitis [33,34]. Yen et al. showed that ultrasound had 88% sensitivity and 93% specificity for NSTI in a limb using diffuse thickening of the subcutaneous tissue accompanied by a layer of fluid accumulation more than 4 mm in depth along the deep fascial layer when compared with the contralateral limb [33]. Ultrasound is limited by the need for operator experience, the interpretation of the images, and its use in body areas aside from limbs. CT can be used as an adjunct to an equivocal physical exam. Similar to the findings on plain radiograph, gas in the subcutaneous tissues is characteristic of NSTI on CT. Since gas is not seen in all cases of NSTI, other features include thickened, asymmetrical fascia, fluid and gas collections along the deep fascial sheaths, and extension of edema into the intermuscular septa and muscles [35,36]. MRI has also been studied in the differentiation between NSTI and simple/complex cellulitis using fascial inflammatory changes as the indicator of NSTI [37,38]. MRI was found to have a sensitivity of 100% and specificity of 86% in a small cohort [37]. However, whether NSTI could have been diagnosed prior to MRI or if the delay needed for MRI altered patient outcome were not identified. If an imaging modality is deemed necessary to confirm NSTI due to equivocal physical examination findings, it may be prudent to start with the least invasive plain radiograph to look for gas and then progress to CT if necessary. Ultrasound can be used in centers if the technician and radiologist are comfortable with the exam and its interpretation. Operative debridement should not be delayed in cases in which NSTI can be confirmed on physical exam.

Laboratory

Laboratory values may aid physical examination in differentiating nonnecrotizing from necrotizing soft tissue infections.

Wall et al. used admission white blood cell count greater than 15.4×10^9 per L and serum sodium less than 135 mmol per L to help differentiate necrotizing infections from simple cellulitis [39]. Their model had a sensitivity of 90% and specificity of 76%. Positive predictive value was only 26%, but negative predictive value was 99%. This model was particularly effective in the absence of hard signs of NSTI. Wong et al. proposed another scoring system entitled the Laboratory Risk Indicator for Necrotizing Fasciitis (LRINEC) [40]. This model consists of point values assigned for C-reactive protein (above or below 150 mg per L), white cell count per mm^3 (less than 15, 15 to 25, or more than 25), hemoglobin (more than 13.5, 11 to 13.5, or less than 11), sodium (more or less than 135 mmol per L), creatinine (more or less than 141 μmol per L), and glucose (more or less than 10 mmol per L). With a possible total score of 13, they conclude that anyone with a score of 6 or greater should be carefully evaluated for NSTI, and a score of 8 or greater is highly predictive of NSTI (positive predictive value 93%). Careful physical examination and clinical suspicion should trump any score based on laboratory values, but these may be useful adjuncts in questionable cases.

Combined Diagnostic Modalities

Although adjunctive diagnostic modalities may help differentiate necrotizing from nonnecrotizing soft tissue infections, studies on their effectiveness are singular; little is known about the effectiveness of these modalities when combined [13]. In an attempt to combine physical exam and laboratory findings, Chan et al. prospectively studied the diagnosis and management decisions of surgery residents when presented patients with suspicion of NSTI using first only physical examination findings and then a combination of physical examination and serum WBC and Na values. Only 43% of patients had hard signs of NSTI on presentation. 90% of NSTI patients met one of these laboratory criteria (WBC count of >15,400 and Na level of <135) whereas 81% met both. Prior to knowing the laboratory values, residents felt that only 43% of patients had an NSTI. After reviewing these laboratory values and correlating their physical exam findings, suspicion of NSTI increased to 86%. Combining physical exam and radiographic data, Elliot et al. found crepitus, blistering or radiographic evidence of soft tissue gas in 85.3% of NSTI patients on admission [4]. Unfortunately, 20% of their NSTI patients did not have any of these three findings, leaving a large percentage of patients needing additional methods for diagnosing NSTI. As diagnosis of NSTI remains clinical, prospective trials incorporating multiple modalities for diagnosing NSTI will be essential to providing clinicians with a more reliable means of early diagnosis.

Others

Frozen-section biopsies have been effective in the diagnosis of NSTI. Again, the delay in waiting for pathologic review, the morbidity and high rate of negative tissue biopsies, and other logistical problems make frozen section somewhat unwieldy in the practical setting. Others have proposed a "finger test" consisting of a small incision under local anesthesia with digital probing. Lack of bleeding or presence of dishwater pus prompts exploration in the operating room [41]. Wang and Hung used tissue oxygen-saturation monitoring to diagnose NSTI [42]. In their series, a tissue oxygen saturation of less than 70% had a sensitivity of 100% and specificity of 97%. However, they excluded patients with peripheral vascular disease, venous stasis, shock, and hypoxia, while these subgroups may make up a significant portion of patients with NSTI.

Definitive Diagnosis

Histologic examination of involved tissue provides a definitive diagnosis but is not practical as infection may significantly progress during the time required for pathologic review. There are no consensus criteria for determining whether an infection is necrotizing in nature, but several common signs and symptoms are seen. Intraoperative findings of a NSTI include graying necrotic fascia, lack of resistance of muscular fascia to blunt dissection, lack of bleeding during dissection and the presence of foul-smelling dishwater pus [32].

SURGICAL MANAGEMENT

The mainstay of therapy for NSTI is surgery. Early surgical intervention has been shown to improve outcomes in patients with these infections [2,4,12,14,16]. The primary principle in operative debridement of NSTIs is expeditious removal of all necrotic or infected skin and subcutaneous tissue. Confirmatory findings include necrosis of the superficial fascia, thrombosis of superficial vessels, and foul-smelling discharge. There may be little or no resistance to blunt dissection along normally adherent superficial fascial planes [41]. Complete debridement of all necrotic tissue to areas of healthy, bleeding tissue is essential to allow delivery of antibiotics to the area as delivery cannot occur through the thrombosed vessels. Fluid and tissue cultures should be sent for immediate Gram's stain and aerobic and anaerobic culture and sensitivities. Deep fascia and muscle should be inspected; if muscle is involved, this may signal a clostridial infection. Dire circumstances necessitate amputation and can occur in 18% to 27% of cases [2,4,5]. Peripheral vascular disease and/or diabetes may predispose to amputation [2,5]. Colostomies may be necessary to temporarily control fecal flow in patients with large perineal defects [4] although it can be delayed if the infectious process is suspected to spread along the anterior abdominal wall.

Despite the obvious need for swift radical excision, incisions may be planned along geometric lines with an eye on eventual wound closure. Clearly viable skin should be preserved if possible to aid in future definitive wound coverage. Once hemostasis has been achieved, the wounds should be packed open, and a dilute Betadine solution in saline can be used for the initial dressing. Repeat debridements may be necessary, but it is preferable to attempt complete debridement at the initial setting to prevent further spread of infection. Large retrospective reviews have reported 2.7 to 3.8 debridements per patient [2–6]. Frequent wound examination is prudent, and any signs of ongoing spread of infection, including failure to respond to resuscitation, should prompt a return trip to the operating room for a second look. Bedside intervention may be necessary in the unstable patient and can be accomplished with sharp debridement and portable electrocautery.

Although prompt surgical management is key to decreasing morbidity and mortality, patients in septic shock on admission are an interesting challenge. The question is whether it is better to treat these patients with supportive care, antibiotics, and pressors and wait until hemodynamic stabilization for debridement or to continue resuscitation and supportive care while debriding the necrotic tissue. Boyer et al. showed that waiting >14 hours for surgical treatment in patients with NSTI and septic shock significantly decreased survival [43].

Clearly, early surgical debridement of necrotic tissue is beneficial to patient outcomes. Easily identifying patients with an NSTI early in their course remains a clinical challenge, but relies on experienced physical exam and if needed, additional diagnostic modalities.

ANTIBIOTICS AND PHARMACOTHERAPY

Prompt empiric broad-spectrum antibiotic therapy is an important adjunct to operative debridement. Antibiotic choice should cover Gram-positive, Gram-negative, and anaerobic organisms. The most common antibiotic regimens consist of Gram-positive coverage with penicillin or an extended-spectrum penicillin derivative (or vancomycin in penicillin-allergic patients), Gram-negative coverage with aminoglycosides, cephalosporins or carbapenems, and anaerobic coverage with clindamycin or metronidazole [4]. The use of vancomycin, linezolid, daptomycin, or quinupristin/dalfopristin should be considered until MRSA has been ruled out [31,44]. Clindamycin has had particular success in the pediatric population [45] and may be of most benefit in blocking exotoxin and M protein production, leading to decreased tissue inflammation and sepsis [44,46]. The duration of antibiotic use has not been prospectively studied. Antibiotics should continue until at least all surgical debridement has taken place.

The use of intravenous immunoglobulin and activated protein C has been explored, but their usefulness remains undefined. Intravenous polyspecific immunoglobulin G has been used in combination with antibiotics in patients with accompanying toxic shock syndrome from invasive GAS infection [47]. Recombinant activated protein C/drotrecogin alpha has been used in critically ill patients with severe sepsis [48]. One case report identifies a potential benefit in the use of drotrecogin alpha in a patient with NSTI [44]. However, the use of drotrecogin alpha should be used with caution given the high risk of bleeding associated with its use combined with the typical need for repeated operative debridement and grafting.

Starting with broad-spectrum antibiotic coverage for Gram-positive, Gram-negative, and anaerobes with the addition of coverage for community-acquired (CA)-MRSA is essential. Once the pathogen(s) has been isolated, narrowing the antibiotic coverage is appropriate.

WOUND MANAGEMENT

After surgical debridement of NSTIs, patients may have extremely large soft tissue defects. Definitive wound coverage may require multiple modalities. Repetitive dressing changes should be used in the initial days following debridement until the wound is clean and there are no signs of recurrent or ongoing infection. Many surgeons advise saline wet-to-dry or wet-to-wet dressing changes. The use of 5% mafenide acetate solution applied to postgraft NSTI wounds has been shown to increase the success of first-time wound closure [49]. Additional topical antimicrobials that can be used include bacitracin, polymyxin, vancomycin, nystatin, and Betadine based on the culture and sensitivities of the pathogen [3].

A vacuum-assisted closure (VAC) device (Kinetic Concepts, Inc., San Antonio, TX) can be employed to reduce chronic edema, increase local blood flow, enhance the formation of granulation tissue, and promote contraction of the wound edges [50,51]. The VAC has also been useful in secondary wound infection after debridement of large areas of NSTI [52]. A small study by Huang et al. showed that a VAC may reduce wound size and decrease overall nursing care time, but was more expensive per day than conventional wet-to-dry dressings [53]. Any surrounding erythema, excessive pain or fevers should prompt removal of the VAC and examination of the wound. Regardless of the methods used, after the appearance of adequate granulation tissue, further surgical closure of the wound may be contemplated. In these often obese patients, redundant skin and subcutaneous tissue may allow for primary closure of the wounds, particularly in those involving the groin and perineal areas. Wounds not amenable to primary closure require coverage with split-thickness skin grafts and have been found to be necessary in 36% to 46% of patients [3,14].

The use of hyperbaric oxygen (HBO) has been advocated as a postsurgery adjunct in the treatment of NSTI as a means of decreasing morbidity, mortality and time to wound closure. However, a consensus on the benefit from HBO has not been established [4,54–56]. A recent retrospective review of hyperbaric oxygen therapy for NSTI showed a small, but not statistically significant decrease in mortality with HBO therapy [57]. A survival benefit may exist for the use of HBO in clostridial myonecrosis [4,56].

Following surgical debridement, operative wounds should be managed with frequent dressing changes with topical antimicrobial solutions until the area is free of infection and necrotic tissue. The use of a VAC device or HBO therapy may be employed based on a center's familiarity with these techniques.

NUTRITIONAL SUPPORT

These often critically ill patients will inevitably need nutritional supplementation to meet their increased metabolic state. Graves et al. found that 94% of their patients with necrotizing fasciitis needed either total enteral or parenteral nutrition for a mean of 24 days [58]. They used indirect calorimetry to determine individual energy requirements in this population, and found that these patients required caloric intake at 124% of their basal energy expenditure, or roughly 25 kcal per kg per actual weight per day. However, there were wide variations in energy requirements between patients, and they recommend routine indirect calorimetry to better provide appropriate nutritional supplementation.

Concomitant with ensuring adequate nutrition in patients recovering from an NSTI is proper glycemic control. Although no studies connecting poorer outcomes and hyperglycemia exist for patients with NSTIs, the depth of literature promoting the benefits of glycemic control in critical care can reasonably be extrapolated to the NSTI patient. Reduced morbidity and mortality in surgical ICU patients with tight glycemic control was first demonstrated in 2001 with the van den Berghe study [59]. Since then, control of blood glucose levels with algorithm or computer program assistance has become the standard of care in all ICUs [17]. Although preventing hyperglycemia is a priority so to is preventing hypoglycemia from overaggressive insulin use. Recently, the NICE-SUGAR study has demonstrated the side effects of hypoglycemic events with intensive insulin therapy; the safest and most beneficial glucose range has not yet been established [18]. Regardless, prevention of hyper- and hypoglycemia should improve patient outcomes. With the high prevalence of diabetes in patients with NSTI, glycemic control is an even more challenging task in this patient population.

OUTCOMES

Mortality

Mortality rates for NSTI range from 6% to 76% [5]. A recent review summarizing 67 outcome studies on NSTI since 1980 shows an average mortality of 23.5% [60], while another recent review reports a similar mortality rate of 25% [61]. As mentioned earlier, the greatest risk factor for mortality is time to surgical debridement [4,5,12,16,62]. In a more recent examination of time to surgical debridement influencing outcome, Gunter et al. was able to reduce time from presentation to OR to 8.6 hours and thus decrease overall mortality to 9% by using an emergency general surgery service [63].

Various parameters have been used to predict mortality. In Yilmazlar et al., an APACHE II score of <13 was associated with a mortality of 21% while an APACHE II score of ≥14 was associated with an 86% mortality [57]. APACHE II scores of >20 have been associated with 100% mortality [57], and a 14.2-fold increased risk of death [62]. A LRINEC score of ≥6 was associated with increased amputation and mortality rates [64]. Bacteremia on admission has been associated with a 5.2-fold increased risk for death [19]. Preexisting conditions associated with higher mortality rates include IVDA, chronic renal insufficiency, and heart disease [62]. As expected, nonsurvivors have more body surface area involvement (13 vs. 6%), are obtunded (62%), have elevated serum lactate and creatinine on admission [4] and are older (age >60) [19].

Function, Disposition, and Cost

Given the high mortality rates associated with NSTI, the majority of studies focus on mortality outcomes. However, knowledge of functional outcome, hospital length of stay, and cost are important for the health care provider, patient, and families in terms of predicting physical, social, and economic support after recovery from the acute illness. Commonly, patients who survive an NSTI are left with a permanent physical disability. Retrospective reviews have shown that 15% to 28% [2,4,5,14,62] of patients with an NSTI will have an extremity amputated. Pham et al. retrospectively reviewed survivors of NSTI and found that, as expected, extremity involvement was associated with more functional limitations [65]. More long-term studies are necessary to assess the physical disability and therapy needs for these patients once their acute illness has resolved to properly maximize outcomes.

Almost half of all patients requiring radical surgical debridement will require further hospitalization or transfer to an inpatient rehabilitation facility after resolution of acute treatment [3]. Endorf et al. found the average length of hospital stay was 32 days for survivors and the overall ICU length of stay was 21 days [3]. Other studies report the average duration of hospitalization ranging from 29 to 41 days for all survivors [2,11].

Given the number of surgical interventions, length of hospital stay and use of critical care services, the cost of treating a patient with NSTI is quite high. Faucher et al. estimated a cost of $5,202 per patient day in 1999 for an average total of $153,803 per survivor [11]. Mulla et al. found that the median total patient charges for NSTI in 2001 were $54,533 [8]. With escalating health care costs both in and out of the hospital, an updated analysis of the long-term cost of NSTIs is necessary.

EMERGING PATHOGENS

Pathogens with unique antimicrobial resistance patterns and that specifically affect certain patient populations have recently been identified as causes of NSTIs. These pathogens should be considered when a patient is not improving despite adequate debridement and administration of broad-spectrum antibiotics.

MRSA

MRSA has been classified as either hospital-acquired (HA) or CA. Of NSTIs caused by MRSA, the majority of cases are CA [14,25–28]. The emergence of CA-MRSA may lie in its increased virulence and potential for necrosis. CA-MRSA manifests its virulence via Panton-Valentine leukocidin, a cytotoxin against leukocytes. These CA-MRSA infections are similar in presentation to other bacterial causes of NSTI. Unique inciting events or preexisting conditions leading to CA-MRSA susceptibility have not been identified. In a retrospective review, Lee et al. found MRSA in 39% of their NSTIs with at least 80% of these being CA-MRSA [27] Interestingly, 86% to 93% of CA-MRSA NSTI are monomicrobial [27,28]. Also, their antibiotic susceptibility profiles differ based on region. In Lee et al., from Houston, TX, they found that their MRSA were 100% susceptible to vancomycin or rifampin, 93% to trimethoprim-sulfamethoxazole, and 62% to clindamycin [27]. However, Miller et al. in Los Angeles, CA found their MRSA from NSTIs to be 100% susceptible to vancomycin, rifampin, clindamycin, gentamicin, and trimethoprim-sulfamethoxazole, 71% to tetracycline, 36% to levofloxacin, and 14% to erythromycin [28].

Acinetobacter

Acinetobacter baumannii as the cause for NSTI is rare but presents a clinical challenge in that it is resistant to most antibiotics, possesses unique virulence factors that may increase the speed at which necrosis occurs and is difficult to diagnosis given its pleomorphic appearance on Gram stain. *Acinetobacter* NSTIs are common in United States soldiers with wartime wounds sustained in Iraq and/or Afghanistan [66–68]. Antibiotic choice with an *Acinetobacter* infection may be the most challenging decision. In several case series and reports, *A. baumannii* strains were found to be sensitive to only amikacin, tobramycin, ampicillin/sulbactam [69], carbapenems [68], and possibly colistin [66,67] or were found to be resistant to all tested antibiotics [66,67,69]. Colistin should be used with caution due to its nephrotoxicity.

Clostridia

Clostridial myonecrosis, also known as "gas gangrene," is an aggressive infection of skeletal muscle. It is often associated with skeletal muscle trauma or recent surgery, but may be found with IVDA [70] and malignancy [22]. The most common organism seen is *Clostridium perfringens*, although it may be caused by *Clostridium novyi*, *Clostridium septicum*, *Clostridium histolyticum*, *Clostridium sordelli*, or *Clostridium fallax*. These organisms produce more than 12 toxins that may rapidly

TABLE 153.2

SUMMARY OF ADVANCES IN REDUCING MORBIDITY AND MORTALITY FROM NSTIs

- Early surgical debridement and management reduces morbidity and mortality [2,4,5,12,16].
- Laboratory values and imaging may help in the diagnosis of NSTIs when physical examination is equivocal [33–40].
- Empiric broad-spectrum antibiotics are critical adjunctive therapy [4,44–46].
- Prolonged nutritional support is needed for increased metabolic needs [58].
- CA-MRSA and *Acinetobacter* are new pathogens in NSTIs [14,25–28,57,64–66].

CA-MRSA, community-acquired methicillin-resistant *Staphylococcus aureus*; NSTIs, necrotizing soft tissue infections.

cause systemic shock. Symptoms may be similar to NSTI but gas in skeletal muscle or involved muscle at surgery can signal a clostridial infection. Antibiotic coverage is also similar, with penicillin, clindamycin, and metronidazole being the most common combination. Surgical exploration of superficial and deep muscle compartments is mandatory, and severe limb infection may require amputation [7]. Trunk involvement is associated with a worse outcome than limb infection (63% vs. 12% mortality) [71].

SUMMARY

NSTIs, albeit somewhat rare, can be rapidly lethal. The mainstays of management are prompt diagnosis, aggressive use of empiric antibiotics, and, most importantly, early radical debridement of affected tissue.

Advances in diagnosing and treating NSTIs are summarized in Table 153.2.

References

1. Anaya D, Dellinger EP: Necrotizing soft-tissue infection: diagnosis and management. *Clin Infect Dis* 44:705–710, 2007.
2. Wong C, Chang H, Pasupathy S, et al: Necrotizing fasciitis: clinical presentation, microbiology, and determinants of mortality. *J Bone Joint Surg* 85:1454, 2003.
3. Endorf FE, Supple KG, Gamelli RL: The evolving characteristics and care of necrotizing soft-tissue infections. *Burns* 31:269, 2005.
4. Elliott DC, Kufera JA, Myers RAM: Necrotizing soft tissue infections: risk factors for mortality and strategies for management. *Ann Surg* 224:672, 1996.
5. McHenry CF, Piotrowski JJ, Petrinic D, et al: Determinants of mortality for necrotizing soft-tissue infections. *Ann Surg* 221(5):558–565, 1995.
6. Tillou A, St. Hill CR, Brown C, et al: Necrotizing soft tissue infections: improved outcomes with modern care. *Am Surg* 70:841–844, 2004.
7. Chapnick EK, Abter EI: Necrotizing soft-tissue infections. *Infect Dis Clin North Am* 10:835, 1996.
8. Mulla ZD, Gibbs SG, Aronoff DM: Correlates of length of stay, cost of care, and mortality among patients hospitalized for necrotizing fasciitis. *Epidemiol Infect* 135(5):868–876, 2007.
9. Ellis Simonsen SM, Van Orman ER, Hatch BE, et al: Cellulitis incidence in a defined population. *Epidemiol Infect* 134:293–299, 2006.
10. Fustes-Morales A, Gutierrez-Castrellon P, Duran-McKinster C, et al: Necrotizing fasciitis: report of 39 pediatric cases. *Arch Dermatol* 138:893, 2002.
11. Faucher LD, Morris SE, Edelman LS, et al: Burn center management of necrotizing soft-tissue surgical infections in unburned patients. *Am J Surg* 182:563, 2001.
12. Bilton BD, Zibari GB, McMillan RW, et al: Aggressive management of necrotizing fasciitis serves to decrease mortality: a retrospective study. *Am Surg* 64:397, 1998.
13. Chan T, Yaghoubian A, Rosing D, et al: Low sensitivity of physical examination findings in necrotizing soft tissue infection is improved with laboratory values: a prospective study. *Am J Surg* 196:926–930, 2008.
14. Yaghoubian A, de Virgilio C, Dauphine C, et al: Use of admission serum lactate and sodium levels to predict mortality in necrotizing soft-tissue infections. *Arch Surg* 142(9):840–846, 2007.
15. Childers BJ, Potyondy LD, Nachreiner R, et al: Necrotizing fasciitis: a fourteen-year retrospective study of 163 consecutive patients. *Am Surg* 68:109, 2002.
16. Freischlag JA, Ajalat G, Busuttil RW: Treatment of necrotizing soft tissue infections: the need for a new approach. *Am J Surg* 149(6):751–755, 1985.
17. Dellinger RP, Levy MM, Carlet JM, et al: Surviving sepsis campaign: international guidelines for management of severe sepsis and septic shock: 2008. *Crit Care Med* 36:296–327, 2008.
18. NICE-SUGAR Study Investigators: Intensive versus conventional glucose control in critically ill patients. *N Engl J Med* 360:1283–1297, 2009.
19. Barillo DJ, McManus AT, Cancio LC, et al: Burn center management of necrotizing fasciitis. *J Burn Care Rehab* 24:127, 2003.
20. Stevens DL: Streptococcal toxic shock syndrome associated with necrotizing fasciitis. *Annu Rev Med* 51:271, 2000.
21. Gardam MA, Low DE, Saginur R, et al: Group B streptococcal necrotizing fasciitis and streptococcal toxic shock-like syndrome in adults. *Arch Intern Med* 158:1704, 1998.
22. Abella BS, Kuchinic P, Hiraoka T, et al: Atraumatic Clostridial myonecrosis: case report and literature review. *J Emerg Med* 24:401, 2003.
23. Elliott D, Kufera JA, Myers RAM: The microbiology of necrotizing soft-tissue infections. *Am J Surg* 179:361, 2000.
24. Wong CH, Tan SH, Kurup A, et al: Recurrent necrotizing fasciitis caused by methicillin-resistant staphylococcus aureus. *Eur J Clin Microbiol Infect Dis* 23:909, 2004.
25. Young LM, Price SC: Community-acquired methicillin-resistant Staphylococcus aureus emerging as an important cause of necrotizing fasciitis. *Surg Infect* 9(4):469–474, 2008.
26. Wibbenmeyer LA, Kealey GP, Latenser BA, et al: Emergence of the USA300 strain of methicillin-resistant Staphylococcus aureus in a burn-trauma unit. *J Burn Care Res* 29:790–797, 2008.
27. Lee TC, Carrick MM, Scott BG, et al: Incidence and clinical characteristics of methicillin-resistant Staphylococcus aureus necrotizing fasciitis in a large urban hospital. *Am J Surg* 194:809–813, 2007.
28. Miller LG, Perdreau-Remington F, Reig G, et al: Necrotizing fasciitis caused by community-associated methicillin-resistant *Staphylococcus aureus* in Los Angeles. *N Engl J Med* 352:1445–1453, 2005.
29. Louie L, Simor AE, Louie M, et al: Diagnosis of group A streptococcal necrotizing fasciitis by using PCR to amplify the streptococcal pyrogenic exotoxin B gene. *J Clin Microbiol* 36:1769, 1998.
30. Bisno AL, Stevens DL: Streptococcal infections of skin and soft tissues. *New Engl J Med* 334:240–245, 1996.
31. Sarani B, Strong M, Pascual J, et al: Necrotizing fasciitis: current concepts and review of the literature. *J Am Coll Surg* 208(2):279–288, 2009.
32. Wang YS, Wong CH, Tay YK: Staging of necrotizing fasciitis based on the evolving cutaneous features. *Int J Derm* 46:1036–1041, 2006.
33. Yen ZS, Wang HP, Ma HM, et al: Ultrasonographic screening of clinically-suspected necrotizing fasciitis. *Acad Emerg Med* 9(12):1448–1451, 2002.
34. Chao HC, Kong MS, Lin TY: Diagnosis of necrotizing fasciitis in children. *J Ultrasound Med* 18:277–281, 1999.
35. Fayad LM, Carrino JA, Fishman EK: Musculoskeletal infection: role of CT in the emergency department. *Radiographics* 27:1723–1736, 2007.
36. Wysoki MG, Santora TA, Shah RM, et al: Necrotizing fasciitis: CT characteristics. *Radiology* 203:859–863, 1997.
37. Schmid MR, Kossmann T, Duewell S: Differentiation of necrotizing fasciitis and cellulitis using MR imaging. *Am J Roent* 170:615–620, 1998.
38. Brothers TE, Tagge DU, Stutley JE: Magnetic resonance imaging differentiates between necrotizing and non-necrotizing fasciitis of the lower extremity. *J Am Coll Surg* 187:416–421, 1998.
39. Wall DB, Klein SR, Black S, et al: A simple model to help distinguish necrotizing fasciitis from nonnecrotizing soft tissue infection. *J Am Coll Surg* 191:227, 2000.
40. Wong CH, Khin LW, Heng KS, et al: The LRINEC (Laboratory Risk Indicator for Necrotizing Fasciitis) score: a tool for distinguishing necrotizing fasciitis from other soft tissue infections. *Crit Care Med* 32:1535, 2004.
41. Wong CH, Wang YS: The diagnosis of necrotizing fasciitis. *Curr Opin Infect Dis* 18:101, 2005.
42. Wang TL, Hung CR: Role of tissue oxygen saturation monitoring in diagnosing necrotizing fasciitis of the lower limbs. *Ann Emergency Med* 44:222, 2005.
43. Boyer A, Vargas F, Coste F, et al: Influence of surgical treatment timing on mortality from necrotizing soft tissue infections requiring intensive care management. *Int Care Med* 35:847–853, 2009.
44. Bland CM, Frizzi JD, Reyes A: Use of drotrecogin alfa in necrotizing fasciitis: a case report and pharmacologic review. *J Intensive Care Med* 23(5):342–346, 2008.
45. Zimbelman J, Palmer A, Todd J: Improved outcome of clindamycin compared with beta-lactam antibiotic treatment for invasive *Streptococcus pyogenes* infection. *Pediatr Infect Dis J* 18:1096, 1999.
46. Stevens DL: The flesh-eating bacterium: what's next? *J Infect Dis* 179:S366–S374, 1999.
47. Norrby-Teglund A, Muller MP, Mcgeer A, et al: Successful management of severe group A streptococcal soft tissue infections using an aggressive medical regimen including intravenous polyspecific immunoglobulin together with a conservative surgical approach. *Scand J Infect Dis* 37:166, 2005.
48. Bernard GR, Vincent JL, Laterre PF, et al: Efficacy and safety of recombinant human activated protein C for severe sepsis. *N Engl J Med* 344:699, 2001.
49. Heinle EC, Dougherty WR, Garner WL, et al: The use of 5% mafenide acetate solution in the postgraft treatment of necrotizing fasciitis. *J Burn Care Rehab* 22:35, 2001.
50. Argenta LC, Morykwas MJ: Vacuum-assisted closure: a new method for wound control and treatment: clinical experience. *Ann Plast Surg* 38:563, 1997.
51. Mullner T, Mrkonjic L, Kwasny O, et al: The use of negative pressure to promote the healing of tissue defects: a clinical trial using the vacuum sealing technique. *Br J Plast Surg* 50:194, 1997.
52. De Geus HRH, Van der Klooster JM: Vacuum-assisted closure in the treatment of large skin defects due to necrotizing fasciitis. *Intensive Care Med* 31:601, 2005.
53. Huang WS, Hsieh SC, Hsieh CS, et al: Use of vacuum-assisted wound closure to manage limb wounds in patients suffering from acute necrotizing fasciitis. *Asian J Surg* 29(3):135–139, 2006.

54. Riseman JA, Zamboni WA, Curtis A, et al: Hyperbaric oxygen therapy for necrotizing fasciitis reduces mortality and the need for debridements. *Surgery* 108:847, 1990.
55. Korhonen K: Hyperbaric oxygen therapy in acute necrotizing infections. With a special reference to the effects on tissue gas tensions. *Ann Chirur Gyn* 89:7, 2000.
56. George ME, Rueth NM, Skarda DE, et al: Hyperbaric oxygen does not improve outcome in patients with necrotizing soft tissue infection. *Surg Infect* 10(1):21–28, 2009.
57. Yilmazlar T, Ozturk E, Alsoy A, et al: Necrotizing soft tissue infections: APACHE II score, dissemination and survival. *World J Surg* 31:1858–1862, 2007.
58. Graves C, Saffle J, Morris S, et al: Caloric requirements in patients with necrotizing fasciitis. *Burns* 31:55, 2005.
59. van den Berghe G, Wouters P, Weekers F, et al: Intensive insulin therapy in the critically ill patients. *N Engl J Med* 345:1359, 2001.
60. May AK: Skin and soft tissue infections. *Surg Clin N Am* 89:403–420, 2009.
61. Cuschieri J: Necrotizing soft tissue infection. *Surg Infect* 9(6):559–562, 2008.
62. Anaya DA, McMahon K, Nathens AB, et al: Predictors of mortality and limb loss in necrotizing soft tissue infections. *Arch Surg* 140:151–157, 2005.
63. Gunter OL, Guillamondegui OD, May AK, et al: Outcome of necrotizing skin and soft tissue infections. *Surg Infect* 9(4):443–450, 2008.
64. Su YC, Chen HW, Hong YC, et al: Laboratory risk indicator for necrotizing fasciitis score and the outcomes. *ANZ J Surg* 78:968–972, 2008.
65. Pham TN, Moore ML, Costa BA, et al: Assessment of functional limitation after necrotizing soft tissue infection. *J Burn Care Res* 30:301–306, 2009.
66. Scott PT, Peterson K, Fishbain J, et al: *Acinetobacter baumannii* infections among patients at military medical facilities treating injured U.S. service members, 2002–2004. *Morb Mortal Wkly Rep* 53(45):1063–1066, 2004.
67. Aronson NE, Sanders JW, Moran KA: In harm's way: infections in deployed American military forces. *Clin Infect Dis* 43:1045–1051, 2006.
68. Sebeny PJ, Riddle MS, Petersen K: *Acinetobacter baumannii* skin and soft-tissue infection associated with war trauma. *Clin Infect Dis* 47:444–449, 2008.
69. Charnot-Katsikas A, Dorafshar AH, Aycock JK, et al: Two cases of necrotizing fasciitis due to *Acinetobacter baumannii*. *J Clin Micro* 47(1):258–263, 2009.
70. Kimura AC, Higa JI, Levin RM, et al: Outbreak of necrotizing fasciitis due to *clostridium sordelli* among black-tar heroin users. *Clin Infect Dis* 38:87, 2004.
71. Nichols RL, Smith JW: Anaerobes from a surgical perspective. *Clin Infect Dis* 18[Suppl]:S280, 1991.

CHAPTER 154 ■ ACUTE LIMB ISCHEMIA: ETIOLOGY, DIAGNOSIS, AND TREATMENT STRATEGIES

PEGGE M. HALANDRAS AND ROSS MILNER

INTRODUCTION

Acute limb ischemia (ALI) occurs in the setting of inadequate blood flow and therefore, oxygen delivery to an extremity. This state of hypoperfusion leads to systemic acid–base abnormalities and electrolyte disturbances that ultimately affect cardiopulmonary and renal function in patients managed in the intensive care unit (ICU). Revascularization of an ischemic limb leads to an additional host of metabolic problems as toxic byproducts that build up in the ischemic tissue bed and inflammatory mediators are released. ALI is a vascular emergency with 30-day mortality rates of 15% and amputation rates of 10% to 30% reported in the literature [1]. This chapter outlines common etiologies, diagnosis, and treatment strategies to manage acute lower extremity ischemia in patients that are often critically ill.

ETIOLOGY

The most common etiologies of ALI can be separated into two categories consisting of either embolism or thrombosis. Embolic events result from the detachment of thrombus or atherosclerotic plaques from proximal sources and often result in extreme peripheral ischemia as emboli may become lodged in a previously normal artery without significant collateral vasculature. Cardiac sources of emboli constitute 80% to 90% of peripheral emboli [2]. Myocardial infarction and cardiac arrhythmias such as atrial fibrillation lead to stasis and dilation of the left atrium and ventricle resulting in the formation of a cardiac thromboembolic source [3,4]. The presence of valvular heart disease and prosthetic heart valves are additional sources of cardiac emboli. Noncardiac sources of emboli include arterial aneurysms, ulcerated atherosclerotic plaque, and paradoxic emboli from venous thrombi. Additional noncardiac sources of emboli may occur with recent vascular interventions such as aortic surgery, percutaneous interventions with the passage of wires and catheters or balloon pump placement. The contribution of noncerebral emboli to the development of acute limb ischemia is illustrated by the observance that two-thirds of emboli travel to the lower extremity vasculature. One-half of these emboli obstruct iliofemoral arteries and the remaining half obstructs the popliteal and tibial vessels [5].

Thrombotic occlusions may occur in either native arteries or bypass grafts. Thrombosis of a native artery occurs with progression of an atherosclerotic lesion or rupture of an unstable plaque. Thrombotic occlusions occur most frequently at the site of arterial bifurcations or at areas of anatomic compression such as the superficial femoral artery at the level of the adductor canal [6]. Arterial trauma from fractures, dislocations, blunt injury, bullet wounds, or catheter access may result in pseudoaneurysms, intimal flaps, or dissections and may progress to acute thrombosis of a native artery. Femoral or popliteal aneurysms may also be responsible for ALI by either embolism of thrombus from the aneurysm or thrombosis of the aneurysm itself and occlusion of distal perfusion in the setting of inadequate collateral formation. More commonly, thrombosis in situ occurs with occlusion of bypass grafts. Occlusion of a bypass graft in the immediate postoperative period is typically secondary to a technical defect. Occlusions of bypass grafts at later time periods may be due to intimal hyperplasia, progression of distal disease, low flow states experienced by critically ill patients, or acquired hypercoagulable states. In general, ALI secondary to thrombosis in situ or bypass graft occlusion may manifest as an acute-on-chronic process with less profound ischemia due to collateral formation not seen with acute embolic events. Therefore, management may not require immediate surgical revascularization and it is possible to proceed with initial nonoperative management including preoperative imaging such as angiography and thrombolytic therapy.

Other etiologies of ALI include aortic dissection creating malperfusion, intense vasospasm resulting from drugs such as cocaine, ergots or vasopressors, and hypercoagulable disorders. Alterations in coagulability have been attributed to both venous and arterial thromboembolism. Increases in coagulation activity in the arterial system in the ICU population have been observed in multitrauma victims, septic patients, and in the setting of heparin-induced thrombocytopenia (HIT) and disseminated intravascular coagulation (DIC) [7,8]. Likewise, inherited coagulation disorders are associated with arterial occlusions. Circulating antiphospholipids (lupus anticoagulant and anticardiolipin antibodies), gene mutations (prothrombin, factor V Leiden, methylene tetrahydrofolate reductase), alterations in activity levels of protein C and S, deficiencies of antithrombin III, and protein C&S have all been shown to contribute to the pathogenesis of arterial thrombosis [9].

EVALUATION

A careful history and physical examination is important in determining the etiology, establishing the extent of ischemia, and determining appropriate treatment of patients with acute lower extremity ischemia. Frequently, patients in the ICU are unable to provide valuable history regarding possible comorbidities that may contribute to the acute onset of their ischemia, coexistence of chronic arterial ischemia, and information concerning the onset of symptoms. Therefore, a careful review of the patient's medical history including a history of atrial fibrillation, coagulation disorders, recent percutaneous interventions, imaging demonstrating mural thrombus or aneurysmal disease, history of claudication or rest pain, and past lower extremity revascularization procedures should be performed. Risk factors including coronary artery disease, hypertension, diabetes mellitus, hyperlipidemia and history of tobacco use should also be assessed.

A thorough physical examination is necessary to determine the duration and extent of ischemia that will ultimately determine the most suitable algorithm for treatment. Both lower extremities should be evaluated for signs of chronic disease including sparse hair growth, elevation pallor, dependent rubor, dystrophic nail growth, or chronic ulcers. Identifying the 6 "Ps" of acute ischemia including paresthesia, pain, pallor, pulselessness, poikilothermia, and paralysis is a useful tool to help establish the diagnosis and duration of acute ischemia. Initially, patients may experience pain in an ischemic limb that may progress to sensory deficit and eventually to paralysis. In addition, the level of pallor, coolness, or mottling may assist in determining the level of arterial injury of obstruction. Frequently, ischemic findings are most severe one joint distal to the level of obstruction.

A pulse exam may provide important clues about the underlying pathology but may also be misleading secondary to the subjectivity of this physical examination finding. Findings such as a "water-hammer" pulse indicating pulsation against an occlusion may be present following embolism or early thrombosis. A palpable thrill, audible bruit, or hematoma may indicate pseudoaneurysm or arteriovenous fistula in the setting of noniatrogenic or iatrogenic trauma seen with percutaneous interventions. If used correctly, continuous wave Doppler is a crucial tool in the bedside evaluation of the ischemic limb. A normal triphasic signal consists of forward systolic, reverse systolic and forward diastolic flow. A monophasic signal is characterized as a signal without pulsatile variability and signifies a proximal obstruction. Ankle–brachial indices (ABI) may also be obtained at the bedside and consist of calculating a ratio of ankle-to-brachial pressure. Abnormal results (<0.9) must be interpreted with caution as medial calcification of vessels frequently observed in diabetics yield an ABI >1. This occurs as calcifications prevent vessels from being compressed by a pneumatic cuff. ABIs may also be decreased at baseline in those patients with chronic lower extremity ischemia. Therefore, in a situation of suspected acute ischemia, ABIs should be compared between limbs and to ABIs obtained before the event if this value was recorded.

Further diagnostic testing may be required for operative planning but institution limitations and the urgency of revascularization should be considered when obtaining additional tests. Arterial duplex ultrasound is valuable for determining occlusive lesions, bypass graft occlusions, and the presence of distal and proximal arterial disease. This noninvasive test is operator dependent but has been shown to correlate with contrast angiography findings [10]. Digital subtraction angiography is considered the gold standard for diagnostic imaging in the acute setting. This testing modality provides anatomical detail concerning the offending lesion, presence of chronic atherosclerotic disease, and the status of distal arterial targets. Findings will assist in planning operative intervention including thrombectomy, bypass, or further percutaneous intervention. In addition to its diagnostic advantages, angiography may also be used as a therapeutic modality with the institution of catheter directed therapies. Adverse effects of contrast angiography include nephrotoxicity from contrast administration, embolization, and access site complications including dissection, pseudoaneurysm, arteriovenous fistula, and bleeding. Further imaging with CT or MRI may be necessary if aortic dissection or aortoiliac occlusion is suspected. Otherwise, these tests are time consuming and may not supply information regarding distal arterial runoff that cannot be obtained by angiography in the patient requiring urgent revascularization.

TREATMENT

Planning revascularization of the acutely ischemic limb requires consideration of the patient's overall medical condition, likely etiology and the viability of the ischemic limb. If the patient is not medically stable to proceed to the operating room or angiography suite, revascularization may be postponed in the interest of preserving "life over limb." In addition, revascularization of an ischemic limb with permanent ischemic nerve or muscle damage may result in a nonfunctional limb and primary amputation may be the most effective treatment strategy. Predicting the urgency of revascularization required to salvage an acutely ischemic limb is a difficult task and treatment paradigms have evolved with the advent of catheter directed thrombolytic therapy. The goal of the revised Rutherford Criteria proposed by The Society for Vascular Surgery and International Society for Cardiovascular Surgery (SVS/ISCVS) is to stratify levels of severity of ALI (Table 154.1). Category I limbs are considered viable with no sensory or muscle deficits. This category includes limbs that are not immediately threatened and may be managed either without an intervention or after a thorough evaluation. Class II limbs have been stratified into two subcategories. Class IIa limbs are marginally threatened

TABLE 154.1

CLINICAL CATEGORIES OF ACUTE LIMB ISCHEMIA

Category	Description/prognosis	Sensory loss	Muscle weakness	Doppler signal (arterial)	Doppler signal (venous)
I. Viable	Not immediately threatened	None	None	Audible	Audible
II. Threatened					
a. Marginally	Salvageable if promptly treated	Minimal (toes) or None	None	Inaudible	Audible
b. Immediately	Salvageable with immediate revascularization	More than toes, associated with rest pain	Mild, moderate	Inaudible	Audible
III. Irreversible	Major tissue loss or permanent nerve damage inevitable	Profound, anesthetic	Profound paralysis (rigor)	Inaudible	Inaudible

Modified from reporting criteria recommended by the Society for Vascular Surgery and the International Society for Cardiovascular Surgery [11], Vascular Surgery, and the NORTH American Chapter.

with minimal sensory loss. This category of ischemic limbs can be salvaged with appropriate revascularization directed by further studies such as angiography. Class IIb limbs are immediately threatened with more profound sensory loss and mild-to-moderate muscle weakness. Salvage of Class IIb limbs should be managed with emergent revascularization efforts [11].

The main treatment modalities of acute limb ischemia include anticoagulation, open surgical management, percutaneous intervention, and primary amputation. A combination of both open surgery and percutaneous management are often required. Once the decision to proceed to either the operating room or angiography suite has been made, the patient should be systemically heparinized if no contraindications to anticoagulation exist. Full intravenous anticoagulation with heparin prevents further propagation of thrombus and recurrent emboli until definitive management is instituted [5]. Heparin bolus should routinely be 100 to 150 U per kg and a drip of 60 to 80 U per kg per hour should be started to achieve an activated partial clotting of greater than two times control.

Surgical Revascularization

Open surgical treatment includes Fogarty balloon thromboembolectomy, endarterectomy with patch angioplasty, and surgical bypass. If the diagnosis of an embolus to the femoral bifurcation is suspected, patients may be expediently managed by the passage of thromboembolectomy catheters via a groin incision in a retrograde and antegrade fashion. Femoral artery exposure may suffice but exposure of the below-knee trifurcation vessels may also be needed for adequate tibial–peroneal thrombectomy. Preoperative testing such as angiography or other imaging studies may be bypassed to avoid prolonged ischemic time. Focal femoral artery occlusions have become more common with frequent percutaneous interventions and the subsequent use of arterial closure devices. This complication can also be effectively managed by open surgical techniques such as foreign body removal, thromboembolectomy, endarterectomy with patch angioplasty, or interposition bypass. If after thrombectomy, an occluded outflow signal is detected or there is an absent pedal signal, an intraoperative arteriogram should be performed to identify native arterial lesions or residual thrombus. If the arteriogram reveals adequate inflow and distal target, and an appropriate conduit is available, surgical bypass may be the most appropriate option for revascularization. Long segment occlusions and thrombosed popliteal aneurysms with patent distal targets are indications for proceeding with surgical bypass.

Thrombolysis

Catheter-directed thrombolytic therapy has emerged as an alternative to open surgical treatment for ALI. Patients with Rutherford category I and IIa ischemia or with a high likelihood of thrombosis (in situ or bypass graft in the setting of inadequate conduit) are candidates for thrombolysis. Therapy includes performing an arteriogram to identify an acute occlusion and percutaneously crossing the lesion with a guidewire. Thrombus is then infused with thrombolytic agents through an infusion catheter. Infusion catheters typically allow for saturation of the entire thrombus with a lytic agent through a multi-sideport design or infusion guidewire. The effectiveness of thrombolytic therapy is typically monitored by reimaging with angiography at 6- to 12-hour intervals after initiation. Patients should also undergo serial neurologic, vascular and laboratory examinations. CBCs and fibrinogen levels should be followed to identify hemorrhagic trends and because fibrinogen levels less than 100 mg per dL have been associated with systemic fibrinolysis and an increased risk of bleeding, including intracranial hemorrhage [12]. Restoration of flow within a thrombosed artery or bypass graft will assist with unmasking the causative lesion and assist in planning future interventions to maintain patency. Percutaneous interventions may include angioplasty or stenting of native or anastomotic stenoses and open surgical interventions may include a new surgical bypass or surgical bypass revision.

Common thrombolytic agents used include streptokinase (produced by cultures of β-hemolytic streptococci), urokinase (extracted from human urine), and recombinant tissue-type plasminogen activator (rt-PA). Currently, there is no consensus regarding the superiority of one agent in terms of efficacy and safety. One open trial comparing intra-arterial streptokinase with intra-arterial and intravenous rt-PA confirmed 100% angiographic success with intra-arterial rt-PA as compared with intra-arterial streptokinase (80%) and intravenous rt-PA (45%). Thirty-day limb salvage rates were 80%, 60%, and 45%, respectively [13]. In contrast, a randomized trial comparing rt-PA to urokinase (UK) confirmed a faster 24-hour lysis rate with rt-PA but similar 30-day clinical success rates [14]. A secondary end point of the randomized Surgery versus Thrombolysis for Ischemia of the Lower

Extremity (STILE) study compared patency rates and safety between rt-PA and UK. No difference in efficacy or bleeding complications was reported between the two treatment groups [12]. In contrast, a randomized study treating thrombotic infrainguinal arterial occlusions with either UK or rt-PA showed slightly improved lysis in the rt-PA group with an increase in the rate of local hematomas [15]. A newer alternative is the concurrent use of abciximab, the platelet glycoprotein IIb–IIIa antagonist, with UK. A randomized trial in which patients received UK plus abciximab versus UK plus placebo showed a trend toward amputation-free survival at 90-days in the combination group as compared to the placebo group. Thrombolysis occurred at a faster rate but a higher risk of nonfatal major bleeding was seen in the combination group [16].

Several multicenter randomized control trials have compared open surgical revascularization with catheter directed thrombolysis. The Thrombolysis or Peripheral Arterial Surgery (TOPAS) study randomized patients with acute arterial obstruction (less than or equal to 14 days) to catheter-directed intra-arterial thrombolysis with UK or bypass surgery. Patients had both embolic and thrombotic etiologies including occluded bypass grafts. There were no significant differences between the two groups with regards to amputation-free survival at 6 months and mortality rates at discharge, 6 months and a year after randomization. At 6 months, the thrombolysis group underwent fewer open surgical procedures without a significant increased risk of amputation or death when compared to the surgical group [17]. The STILE trial randomized patients with nonembolic native artery or bypass occlusions (bypass within the past 6 months) to either treatment group. Composite outcomes of death, major amputation, and ongoing or recurrent ischemia were higher in the thrombolysis versus surgery group (61.7% vs. 36.1%). A secondary stratification of patients with regards to duration of ischemia confirmed that in patients with acute ischemia of <14 days, amputation-free survival at 6 months and shorter hospital stays were improved in those patients treated with thrombolysis [12]. In summary, the findings in these trials are difficult to generalize as different etiologies (embolism, thrombosis, and occluded bypass grafts), different durations of pretreatment ischemia and different thrombolytic agents were analyzed. Therefore, a working party reached a consensus proposal on the use of thrombolysis in the management of lower-limb arterial occlusion [18]. Recommendations included the following:

1. Thrombolysis followed by correction of the causative lesion in patients with native artery occlusions with ischemia <14 days is recommended. Immediate surgical revascularization should be a priority if thrombolysis will lead to an unacceptable delay in reperfusion.
2. Primary amputation is indicated in patients with irreversible ischemia.
3. Occluded bypass grafts may be managed by thrombectomy and surgical revision, catheter-directed thrombolysis, or insertion of a new graft. The age and type of bypass, duration, and degree of ischemia and availability of venous conduit should be considered when deciding on a treatment strategy.

Advances in percutaneous treatment of ALI include the adjuncts of mechanical thrombectomy and aspiration thrombectomy. These treatment modalities may be used alone in patients with contraindications to thrombolytic therapy, to debulk occlusive thrombus and thereby reduce the time needed for effective thrombolysis, or to remove residual thrombus following thrombolysis. Mechanical thrombectomy is performed with two FDA-approved devices in the infrainguinal arterial system. AngioJet relies on the Venturi effect in which saline is directed at high pressure in a retrograde fashion within the inflow lumen of the thrombectomy catheter. This creates a negative pressure zone at the tip of the catheter and results in thrombus fragmentation and aspiration. A pulse-spray of thrombolytic agent within the thrombus followed by mechanical thrombectomy, termed pharmacomechanical thrombolysis, is an additional treatment strategy employed with the AngioJet system. The Trellis Thrombectomy System is an additional mechanical thrombectomy device. This device allows isolation of a treatment segment by proximal and distal occlusion balloons. A dispersion catheter infuses thrombolytic agent within the treatment zone and an oscillating dispersion wire exposes the thrombus to the agent and fragments the thrombus. The fragmented thrombus is then aspirated via a port distal to the proximal balloon. Finally, mechanical thrombectomy may also be achieved with the use of percutaneous aspiration thrombectomy catheters. This technique involves a large-bore catheter connected to a syringe to aspirate thrombus.

TABLE 154.2

ABSOLUTE AND RELATIVE CONTRAINDICATIONS TO TREATMENT WITH THROMBOLYTIC THERAPY

Contraindications to thrombolytic therapy

Absolute
1. Established cerebrovascular event (including TIAs within last 2 months)
2. Active bleeding diathesis
3. Recent gastrointestinal bleeding (<10 days)
4. Neurosurgery (intracranial, spinal) within last 3 months
5. Intracranial trauma within last 3 months

Relative major
1. Cardiopulmonary resuscitation with last 10 days
2. Major nonvascular surgery or trauma within last 10 days
3. Uncontrolled hypertension: >180 mm Hg systolic or >110 mm Hg diastolic
4. Puncture of noncompressible vessel
5. Intracranial tumor
6. Recent eye surgery

Relative minor
1. Hepatic failure, particularly those with coagulopathy
2. Bacterial endocarditis
3. Pregnancy
4. Diabetic hemorrhagic retinopathy

Modified from Working Party on Thrombolysis in the Management of Limb Ischemia: Thrombolysis in the management of lower limb peripheral arterial occlusion—consensus document. *J Vasc Interv Radiol* 7:S337–S349, 2003.

Contraindications to management of ALI with thrombolysis include category IIb ischemic limbs requiring immediate revascularization or category III ischemic limbs best treated with primary amputation. Contraindications to the use of thrombolytic agents are patients with a hemorrhagic disorder or an anatomic lesion with the potential to cause hemorrhage [18]. Table 154.2 lists both absolute and relative contraindications to thrombolytic therapy. Intracranial hemorrhage is one of the most devastating complications of thrombolytic therapy and may be fatal in some instances.

Finally, revascularization of an acutely ischemic limb may create significant tissue edema. The ischemia-reperfusion theory of cellular injury proposes that reperfusion of ischemic muscle results in multiple events causing cellular swelling and the formation of excessive interstitial fluid. This creates an environment in which extravascular pressure exceeds capillary pressure within a confined muscle compartment. Consequently, nutrient blood flow is restricted and will ultimately result in tissue infarction [19]. Therefore, four-compartment fasciotomy to prevent compartmental hypertension and further morbidity may be necessary. The decision to perform a fasciotomy is frequently clinically based but may also be objectively guided by the measurement of compartment pressures.

CONCLUSION

In summary, ALI is associated with significant morbidity and mortality. ALI has multiple etiologies with the most common being embolism and thrombosis. Effective management demands that a clinician critically evaluate a patient to determine the patient's overall medical condition, contributing comorbidities and degree of ischemia. Careful physical examination will reveal clues regarding an acute embolic event in the setting of healthy lower extremity vasculature versus acute ischemia in the setting of chronic lower extremity ischemia. Open thromboembolectomy may offer the most expedient and effective revascularization of an acute embolic ischemic event. In contrast, catheter-directed thrombolytic therapy provides a mechanism for clearance of thrombus from distal runoff and unmasking of lesions responsible for an ischemic event. Correction of responsible lesions may proceed with percutaneous or open management. In general, revascularization with thrombolysis requires a longer time to revascularization and patients that have a contraindication to thrombolytic therapy may be excluded. Therefore, the management of ALI is most successful with a logical protocol that allows for the institution of multiple treatment modalities.

References

1. Dormandy J, Heeck L, Vig S: Acute limb ischemia. *Semin Vasc Surg* 12:148–153, 1999.
2. Elliot JP Jr, Hageman J, Szilagyi D, et al: Arterial embolization: Problems of source, multiplicity, recurrence, and delayed treatment. *Surgery* 88:833–845, 1980.
3. Asinger RW, Mikell FL, Elsperger J, et al: Incidence of left-ventricular thrombosis after acute transmural myocardial infarction. Serial evaluation by two-dimensional echocardiography. *N Engl J Med* 305(6):297–302, 1991.
4. Menke J, Luthje L, Kastrup A, et al: Thromboembolism in atrial fibrillation. *Am J Cardiol* 105:502–510, 2010.
5. Clagett GP, Sobel M, Jackson MR, et al: Antithrombotic therapy in peripheral arterial occlusive disease: The seventh ACCP Conference on antithrombotic and thrombolytic therapy. *Chest* 126:609S–626S, 2004.
6. Zarins CK, Weisenberg E, Kolettis G, et al: Differential enlargement of artery segments in response to enlarging atherosclerotic plaques. *J Vasc Surg* 7:386–394, 1988.
7. Engelmann DT, Gabram SGA, Allen L, et al: Hypercoagulability following multiple trauma. *World J Surg* 20:5–10, 1996.
8. Boldt J, Papsordf M, Rothe A, et al: Changes of the hemostatic network in critically ill patients – is there a difference between sepsis, trauma, and neurosurgery patients? *Crit Care Med* 28(2):445–450, 2000.
9. Kim RJ, Becker RC: Association between factor V Leiden, prothrombin G20210 A and methylenetetrahydrofolate reductase C677 T mutations and events of the arterial circulatory system: a meta-analysis of published studies. *Am Heart J* 146(6):948–957, 2003.
10. Grassbaugh JA, Nelson PR, Rzucidlo EM, et al: Blinded comparison of preoperative duplex ultrasound scanning and contrast arteriography for planning revascularization at the level of the tibia. *J Vasc Surg* 37(6):1186–1190, 2003.
11. Rutherford RB, Baker JD, Ernst C, et al: Recommended standards for reports dealing with lower extremity ischemia: Revised version. *J Vasc Surg* 26:517–538, 1997.
12. The STILE Investigators. Results of a prospective randomized trial evaluating surgery versus thrombolysis for ischemia of the lower extremity. *Ann Surg* 220(3):251–268, 1994.
13. Berridge DC, Gregson RH, Hopkinson BR, et al: Randomized trial of intra-arterial recombinant tissue plasminogen activator, intravenous recombinant tissue plasminogen activator and intra-arterial streptokinase in peripheral arterial thrombolysis. *Br J Surg* 78(8):988–995, 1991.
14. Meyerovitz MF, Goldhaber SZ, Reagan K, et al: Recombinant tissue-type plasminogen activator versus urokinase in peripheral arterial and graft occlusions: a randomized trial. *Radiology* 175:75–78, 1990.
15. Schweizer J, Altmann E, Florek HJ, et al: Comparison of tissue plasminogen activator and urokinase in the local infiltration thrombolysis of peripheral arterial occlusions. *Eur J Radiol* 23:64–73, 1996.
16. Duda SH, Tepe G, Luz O: Peripheral artery occlusion: treatment with abciximab plus urokinase versus with urokinase alone—a randomized pilot trial (the PROMPT Study). Platelet receptor antibodies in order to manage peripheral artery thrombosis. *Radiology* 221(3):689–696, 2001.
17. Ouriel K, Veith FJ, Sasahara AA: A comparison of recombinant urokinase with vascular surgery as initial treatment for acute arterial occlusion of the legs. *N Engl J Med* 338:1105–1111, 1998.
18. Working Party on Thrombolysis in the Management of Limb Ischemia: Thrombolysis in the management of lower limb peripheral arterial occlusion—consensus document. *J Vasc Interv Radiol* 7:S337–S349, 2003.
19. Walker PM: Ischemia/reperfusion injury in skeletal muscle. *Ann Vasc Surg* 5:399–402, 1991.

CHAPTER 155 ■ PRESSURE SORES: PREVENTION AND TREATMENT

VICTOR G. CIMINO, WELLINGTON J. DAVIS III AND SAMIR R. SHAH

PATHOPHYSIOLOGY

Pressure sores develop secondary to unrelieved pressure exerted on soft tissue overlying bony prominences. The National Pressure Ulcer Advisory Panel defines pressure ulcers as localized areas of tissue necrosis that develop when soft tissue is compressed between a bony prominence and an external surface for a prolonged period of time [1]. Clinicians frequently use the terms *decubitus ulcer* and *pressure sore* interchangeably. The word *decubitus* has its origin from the Latin word decumbre, which means to lie down [2]. The term decubitus ulcer therefore only applies to ulcers that occur in a lying position; it fails to describe ulcers that may occur in seated or other positions. Pressure sore is the preferred term because it describes all ulcers that result from pressure over weight-bearing areas regardless of position.

Landis [3] in 1930 suggested that constant pressure greater than the normal arterial capillary pressure, 32 mm Hg, can impair local perfusion. This is the most important determinant in the development of pressure sores. The distribution of pressure in healthy patients in supine, prone, and various sitting positions has been extensively documented by various authors [4,5]. It is well accepted that the sacrum, buttocks, heels, and occiput are subject to the highest pressures in the supine position, with a range of 40 to 60 mm Hg. In the sitting position, pressures in excess of 75 mm Hg have been recorded over the ischial tuberosities [6]. The majority of pressure sores occur below the umbilicus, two-thirds in the hip and buttock region, and one-fourth to one-third in the lower extremities.

Studies of pressure tolerance in various tissue types by Husain [7] have demonstrated that muscle has a lower pressure tolerance when compared with skin and subcutaneous tissue. Le et al. [8] demonstrated that pressure applied to the soft tissue over bony prominences can cause infarction of muscle and subcutaneous tissue without skin necrosis. This explains the "tip of the iceberg" phenomenon not infrequently seen in clinical pressure sores. One of the most important studies regarding pressure tolerance was performed by Kosiak [9]. He demonstrated irreversible changes in dog muscle and skin when subjected to a pressure of 70 mm Hg applied continuously for 2 hours. More importantly, he showed that no changes occurred if pressure was relieved every 5 minutes. These findings illustrate the mechanism of pressure sore formation as well as reveal the major key to prevention.

There are multiple additional factors that contribute to the formation of pressure sores outside the local effects of unrelieved pressure. As suggested by the multifactorial hypothesis of Enis and Sarmiento [10], the intrinsic factors of malnutrition, advanced age, hypotension, impaired mobility, impaired sensation, and sepsis predispose critically ill patients to the development of pressure sores. Skin contamination with stool, excess moisture, and shear forces are extrinsic factors that further increase the risk of pressure sore formation.

EPIDEMIOLOGY

In the early twentieth century, pressure sores were most commonly observed in young patients with chronic diseases such as tuberculosis, osteomyelitis, and chronic renal disease. This changed in the mid-1940s with improved early and late mortality rates after spinal cord injury. Spinal cord injury patients became the largest high-risk group for the development of pressure sores. Today, the elderly citizens have become the fastest growing segment in the American population. Residents in nursing homes and chronic care facilities are now recognized as the largest high-risk group for the development of pressure sores.

In an acute care hospital, the prevalence of pressure sores ranges from 3% to 11% of all admissions. It increases to 28% when subpopulations of high-risk patients are studied. The average cost of treating an established pressure ulcer ranges from \$4,000 to \$40,000. This does not include medicolegal liability costs, which are an increasing concern and focus.

Patients in the intensive care unit (ICU) often have multiple risk factors for the development of pressure sores: restricted mobility, impaired sensation and/or mental status, impaired perfusion, fecal and urinary incontinence, poor nutrition, advanced age, shear forces, and friction. In addition, ICU patients have various other physiologic impairments. A study by Eachempati et al. [11] has revealed emergent admission, age, days in bed, and days without nutrition as independent predictors of pressure sore formation. Even more recently, Feuchtinger et al. [12] have found in the cardiac surgery population temperature manipulation, vasoactive agents, hypotensive periods, anemia, operating room time, steroids, and low albumin levels to be significant risk factors for the development of pressure sores. Diabetes mellitus and high acute physiology and chronic health evaluation (APACHE II) scores also identify high-risk patients [13]. Spinal cord injury patients continue to be a challenging subgroup. Improved awareness of the risk factors as well as knowledge of the options for prevention and treatment of pressure sores will improve patient care and allow for more efficient use of healthcare resources. Once pressure sores develop. There are few patients who will be candidates for definitive surgical closure because of their concurrent medical disabilities. The pressure sore then becomes a costly chronic medical problem. In any debilitated patient population, pressure sores are extremely difficult to heal.

RISK, EVALUATION, AND PREVENTION

Prevention of pressure sores in the ICU begins with education of the entire hospital staff. Identification of patients at high risk is the initial step. All patients should be routinely screened on admission for risk factors that may predispose them to the development of pressure sores. The basic tenets of prevention include pressure reduction over bony prominences, alternation of weight-bearing surfaces, good skin hygiene, and the maintenance or restoration of adequate nutrition. At this time, there is no universally accepted screening tool for quantifying risk for pressure sore development, but the risk factors are well known. Considering the cost of managing an established pressure sore, it is likely that excess prevention is less costly than nonaction. The Braden scale is one of the most widely used risk assessment tools. It has six subscales: sensory perception, skin moisture, activity, mobility, friction and shear, and nutritional status. Regardless of the screening tool, the most important factor is starting preventive measures as soon as patients at risk are identified [14]. Inattention to previously noted risk factors or early signs of skin breakdown can result in a clinically significant pressure sore in less time than the standard 8-hour nursing shift.

Dispersion of pressure is a vital component of preventive measures and management. Before the 1960s, frequent patient body positioning for avoidance of skin maceration was the mainstay of pressure sore prevention. This is still considered the basic tenet in preventive measure. Patients confined to bed should be turned every 2 hours. Alternating 30-degree oblique supine positions are best [15]. The 90-degree lateral position should be avoided. More importantly, patients in a sitting position should have their weight shifted several times every hour [6].

In the 1960s, pressure-reduction technology using the principle of dispersion became available to improve local blood flow and minimize tissue ischemia. These devices are based on the concept of suspension or buoyancy [16]. The greater the body surface area supported by the surface, the greater the distribution of the patient's weight against the mattress and the lower the effective contact pressure on the skin. The available devices achieve buoyancy through the use of water, air, gel, foam, or circulating ceramic beads. The cost of these various systems ranges from \$35 to \$140 per day of use.

It has been well demonstrated in the literature that transcutaneous oxygen tension can be maintained in an acceptable range in the supine position with the use of air-fluidized and low-air–loss beds in comparison to standard hospital mattresses [17]. Only with the use of air-fluidized systems is this maintained in the lateral decubitus position. Inman et al. [18] studied 100 consecutive patients who were at risk for pressure ulcer development and randomly assigned half to receive care on a standard ICU bed and half to a low-air–loss surface.

The patient groups were comparable, and all other treatment measures were standardized. The low-air–loss patient group developed fewer and less severe pressure ulcers than those who were treated on the standard surface. Taking into account the cost of the low-air–loss surface and the treatment of an established pressure sore, low-air–loss therapy is not only effective in preventing pressure sores from occurring, but it is also cost-effective. The low-air–loss mattress is a highly valuable preventive measure for the critically ill patient while not interfering with the patient's care.

Good skin care is another important adjunctive component of pressure sore prevention. This involves keeping the bed free of particulate matter and solid objects that may cause abrasions or lacerations. Daily skin assessments should be a part of routine nursing care to screen for the development of pressure sores, especially heel ulcers. Daily application of creams and lotions to the feet is inexpensive and can be vital to heel ulcer prevention. Control of both urinary and fecal incontinence and diarrhea are also important. As discussed previously, excess moisture may increase the possibility of pressure sore formation. Bacterial contamination can delay wound healing and extend the zone of tissue necrosis. Enterostomal therapists or wound care nurses can be invaluable resources in the management of these wounds. Colostomies are occasionally necessary to obtain control of the fecal stream with complex sacral or perineal wounds and open pelvic fractures. This decision should be made in conjunction with plastic and general surgical consultation.

Heel ulcers are a clinical problem that warrants special attention. A national pressure ulcer prevalence study by Meehan [19] identified the heel as the second most common site for the development of pressure ulcers. With the introduction of pressure-reduction surfaces, the incidence of sacral ulcers decreased, but there was a concomitant increase in heel ulcers. A study by Blaszczyk et al. [20] developed a useful heel pressure ulcer risk assessment tool to identify patients at risk for the development of heel ulcers.

The patient specific variables include; age over 70 years, diabetes mellitus, mental status changes (agitation, confusion, stupor, unresponsiveness), and immobility of the lower extremity. These specific risk factors are added up and the activity level is then assessed; this determines the risk factor level. Ambulatory patients should get universal heel precautions only. Patients who walk with assistance with one or no risk factors receive universal precautions only, two risk factors yield preventive precautions, and three or more risk factors yield strict precautions. Nonambulatory patients without any risk factors receive universal precautions, one risk factor yields preventive precautions, and patients with two or more risk factors receive strict precautions [20].

Universal heel precautions include daily assessment of feet, daily skin care (creams or lotions), turning every 2 hours, standard hospital pressure-reduction mattress, mobilization out of bed three times a day, and active range of motion. Preventive heel precautions additionally include assessment of feet two times a day, friction reduction (creams or lotions twice daily, socks or support hose, transparent films, or hydrocolloid to heels every week), and pressure reduction (pillow support keeping heels off bed, heel roll or heel cushion, passive range of motion exercises). Strict heel precautions additionally include foot assessment three times a day, creams or lotions three times a day, and heel protection (heel lift, heel cushion). This protocol resulted in a decrease of heel pressure ulcers in the medical ICU patient population [20].

Prior to surgical intervention for heel ulcers, including debridement, patients should be evaluated for vascular insufficiency by obtaining an ankle–brachial pressure index. If this is abnormal, a formal vascular surgery consultation should be obtained.

An effort should be made to remove trauma patients from spine boards and also remove rigid cervical collars as quickly as possible. Patients who require a cervical collar for an extended period should be assessed so that the collar fits properly. Blaylock [21] reported a successful routine for care that significantly reduced pressure ulceration from cervical collars. In patients with an unstable cervical spine, an oscillating support surface may reduce the risk of developing pressure sores. These low-air-loss mattresses also oscillate continuously from side-to-side up to 62 degrees to redistribute pressure on the skin. Selection of this surface should be made after consultation with a spine surgeon.

Nutritional assessment and support are obvious integral components in the care of every critically ill patient. It is well known that malnutrition impairs wound healing. A serum albumin less than 2.5 g per dL has been correlated with the development of pressure sores. It is important that a patient's nutritional status is optimized prior to any reconstructive surgical intervention needed to close a chronic pressure sore. Weekly monitoring of the visceral protein prealbumin can be used to assess the adequacy of the patient's nutritional status and response to dietary supplementation. A more detailed discussion of nutritional assessment and management is beyond the scope of this chapter.

Other patient specific issues to consider are anemia of chronic disease, spasticity in spinal cord injury patients, and long-standing contractures.

WOUND CLASSIFICATION AND MANAGEMENT

According to the National Pressure Ulcer Advisory Panel, wounds are generally classified as follows [1]:

Grade I: Nonblanchable erythema of the skin with the lesion being limited to the epidermis and dermis. Heralds skin ulceration. (Persistent skin erythema.)

Grade II: Any partial-thickness skin loss. Full-thickness ulceration of the skin extending through to the subcutaneous adipose tissue at any level above muscle fascia. (Ranges from abrasion, blister to shallow crater clinically.)

Grade III: Ulceration extending down through the subcutaneous tissue to the underlying muscle. Muscle fascia exposed but not violated.

Grade IV: Ulceration extending through muscle to bone or involving any joint space or supporting structures (such as tendon).

There are two other classification systems, Shea and Yarkony-Kirk, with parameters similar to those of the National Pressure Ulcer Advisory Panel classification. None of these classifications takes into account presence of infection, amount of necrotic tissue, or size of the ulcer.

Wound management is based on awareness of the acute, chronic, local, and systemic factors that resulted in wound formation. The premorbid status, with particular attention to nutritional history and ambulatory status, is critical to management.

The principles of pressure sore management are the following:

- Prevention
  - Education of staff
  - Identification of high-risk patients
  - Precautions
- Early identification of skin impairment
- Debridement
- Treatment of infection
- Local wound care

- Pressure dispersion
- Optimization of global medical status
- Definitive wound closure

Pressure sores are best evaluated by history and physical. Clinical findings can guide the initial management of most pressure sores without costly additional studies. Initial management should focus on the identification of active infection. This is suspected when wound edge cellulitis, purulent discharge, and/or foul odor are present [6]. The gold standard for a diagnosis of osteomyelitis is bone biopsy. More recently, though, magnetic resonance imaging has become a useful noninvasive tool that is very sensitive for the diagnosis of osteomyelitis. The overall clinical condition of the patient should determine the aggressiveness of workup and surgical intervention. Most often, the diagnosis can be made by physical examination, and other studies rarely provide more information. Debridement is probably best limited to infected and obviously necrotic tissue until nutritional status has been optimized.

Most grade I and II pressure sores respond well to debridement, control of infection, and pressure dispersion if the patient is stable medically. Nonetheless, these sores require careful attention despite their initial, relatively innocuous appearance. As discussed previously, the skin is more resistant to pressure than the underlying muscle and subcutaneous fat; this may result in necrotic tissue beneath intact skin. Not infrequently, what may initially appear to be a grade I or II ulcer may actually be a grade III or IV lesion before the eventual loss of the overlying skin.

Ideally, wound debridement will consist of the removal of all necrotic tissue and evacuation of pus and any infected material. This can be performed by sharp debridement or with enzymatic agents with the additional assistance of frequent dressing changes. Extent and aggressiveness of debridement at the authors' institution is often tempered by the clinical status of the wound (infected or noninfected, wet vs. dry necrotic tissue) and the clinical status of the patient (severity of anemia, hemodynamic stability, severity of malnutrition, presence of sepsis). Decisions about wound management are made on a case-by-case basis in conjunction with the ICU and infectious disease teams.

Debridements can commonly be performed at the patient's bedside with appropriate lighting and instruments. Most patients require little or no anesthetic for the debridement of frankly necrotic material. Wound cultures will provide data regarding bacterial colonization. Colonization of pressure sores is polymicrobial. *Bacteroides, Pseudomonas, Proteus, Staphylococcus,* and *Streptococcus* species as well as other enteric flora are the most commonly cultured organisms.

Fortunately, invasive sepsis from a pressure sore is rare. Anecdotally, most cases of sepsis are secondary to abscess formation under an unroofed dry eschar. Sepsis more commonly results from a urinary tract infection or pneumonia. In cases in which the source of sepsis is unclear, computed tomography scanning of the soft tissue or surgical exploration of pressure sores may be mandated. When sepsis is attributed to a pressure sore, the mortality rate is high [22]. Parenteral antibiotics are administered only in the presence of sepsis or if wound closure is planned.

Currently, it is recognized that most topically applied antimicrobial agents and detergents have a toxic effect on human fibroblasts and keratinocytes [15,21–29]. Detergents are used for cleansing the skin surrounding the ulcer. Topical antibiotics such as dilute Dakin's solution or neomycin irrigant help control bacterial colonization in highly contaminated wounds with minimal adverse effect on fibroblasts and keratinocytes [30].

A moist environment with minimal bacterial contamination is desirable for the optimization of reepithelialization. Wet-to-moist dressings with normal saline are recommended as the initial treatment of most grade III and IV pressure ulcers. If the wound is limited to the skin or superficial subcutaneous tissue, an occlusive hydrocolloid dressing may be used as an alternative to wet gauze dressings if the wound has been adequately debrided [31]. Xakellis and Chrischilles [32] performed a prospective randomized study comparing hydrocolloid versus saline gauze dressings in the treatment of pressure ulcers in the long-term care setting. Hydrocolloid treatment required one-eighth the nursing time required by saline gauze treatment. There was no statistically significant difference in the healing time between the study groups; however, the cost was 3.3 times greater in the hydrocolloid group. The value of reducing the time nurses spend on dressing changes may translate into improved overall care of the patient. If an occlusive dressing is applied, fecal contamination under the dressing must be prevented.

Grade III and IV ulcers are treated, in principle, the same as grade I and II ulcers. In the case of exposed or devitalized bone, debridement of all necrotic tissue is necessary. Plain films, bone scans, and erythrocyte sedimentation rates are very nonspecific and generally provide little useful information to support the diagnosis of osteomyelitis. One must rely on clinical suspicion, magnetic resonance imaging, or bone biopsy to confirm the diagnosis. Again, the treatment is focused on adequate debridement, local wound care, pressure dispersion, and nutritional support. Prolonged parenteral antibiotics for bone exposure alone are not recommended unless a definitive debridement and wound closure are contemplated. Some patients may require multiple serial debridements until the wound is controlled.

At the authors' institution, the management of eschars is primarily dictated by the clinical status of the eschar. If the eschar is dry, firm, immobile, and shows no evidence of infection, the eschar is often dressed with silver sulfadiazine twice a day to lower bacterial counts and serially reevaluated until it begins to soften and slough. The necrotic tissue is then debrided at that time. This is done to allow time for healing and allow nonviable tissue to clearly demarcate itself, thereby minimizing the amount of healthy tissue that will be excised at the time of debridement. Eschars that are soft, soupy, mobile, or have evidence of infection are debrided early. On rare occasion, a computed tomography scan may assist in making the decision to observe what may appear to a stable ulcer, when there is a concern of underlying infection that is not apparent on physical examination.

After initial sharp wound debridement, subsequent debridement may be facilitated with the use of topical enzymes. Collagenase ointment facilitates eschar separation and is most applicable in chronic conditions. It works well at removing fibrinous exudate overlying healthy tissue in the base of grade III and IV pressure sores. Enzymatic debridement is particularly useful in patients with intact sensation, in whom surgical debridement at the wound margins may be painful. Collagenase is generally applied once a day with a topical antibiotic powder. Once all eschar is separated and fibrinous exudate removed, the collagenase ointment should be discontinued. Calcium alginate products minimize bacterial contamination and are highly absorbent. They may be useful in treating wounds with a high exudative component after adequate debridement. Enzymatic debridement is a good adjuvant therapy in pressure sores but should not be considered a substitute for sharp debridement. Clinical judgment and experience should dictate its use and application.

An increasingly utilized option in the management of Stage III/IV pressure ulcers is the use of negative pressure wound therapy (NPWT) known as the vacuum-assisted closure (V.A.C.®). This device applies subatmospheric pressure to the wound bed through a secured foam dressing [33]. The V.A.C.® is thought to improve the status of chronic "unsalvageable" wounds in four ways: decreased time for granulation tissue and wound contracture, reduced bacterial colonization, decreased edema, and minimized dressing changes [33,34].

Several studies have focused on the use of the V.A.C.® for pressure sores. Isago et al. treated 10 patients with Stage IV pressure ulcers for 5 weeks. They demonstrated that after V.A.C.® therapy the wound area and depth was reduced by an average of 55% and 61% respectively [35]. Other studies have compared the V.A.C.® with saline, hydrocolloid, or alginate dressings. Overall, patients with V.A.C.® treatment had evidence of more healthy tissue growth [34,36]. Healthpoint system (HP) products offer enzymatic ointments (Accuzyme, Iodosorb, and Panafil) to manage pressure sores. In an article by Ford et al., the NPWT group versus the HP had a decreased number of polymorphonuclear cells and lymphocytes per high-powered field. This translates to increased rates of wound healing and reduced inflammatory changes [37].

Negative pressure therapy has maximum benefits with large wounds with high exudates, tunneling, or undermining [33]. Prior to use, wounds must be adequately prepared. The end points of treatment with wound V.A.C.® therapy depend on whether a patient is a surgical candidate. In such an instance, the V.A.C.® may be used as an adjunct modality until nutritional status is optimized, appropriate antibiotics are instituted, and comorbidities are stabilized. This may allow progression to the point that wound closure is achieved or a lesser surgical procedure may be performed [33].

Once the wound is determined that it will re-epithelialize, V.A.C.® may be discontinued. Nonetheless, it is imperative to assess the wound frequently and document volume changes. If there is no progress or worsens after 2 to 4 weeks of therapy, then it is reasonable to reassess the appropriateness of VAC therapy [33]. Also, it is paramount that patients adhere to strict off loading regimen, maintain an adequate seal, and tolerate dressing changes all of which may be problems in the ICU setting.

Pressure ulcers are a costly healthcare problem and it is estimated that over 1.6 million wounds develop each year, with a cost of $2.2 to $3.6 billion [33]. There is literature to support early initiation of NPWT which may be associated with reduced length of stay at long-term care facilities leading to overall reduced healthcare costs [38]. Philbeck et al. surmised that there would be approximately $9,000 in savings for pressure sores with NPWT versus saline-soaked gauze over a period of 97 days [39].

Nonetheless, there is a paucity of prospective randomized studies evaluating the cost-effectiveness of the wound V.A.C.® with pressure sores. In the future, we need data that will ascertain the role of NPWT in reducing costs. In addition, we need to determine the role of NPWT as an adjunctive therapy in advanced pressure ulcers management.

Newer technologies such as topical growth factors and cultured skin material are evolving, but their current use is still experimental. When the roles of these treatments are defined, they will not substitute conventional measures of wound care. With appropriate treatment, Conway and Griffith [40] found that 30% to 80% of pressure sores healed without surgical intervention during 3 to 6 months.

OPERATIVE TREATMENT

Patients are considered candidates for surgical closure of pressure sores if they have failed the previously described treatment and are otherwise in reasonably good health. The majority of ICU patients with pressure sores do not meet the general criteria for definitive wound closure during their ICU stay. Chronic malnutrition, poor neurologic status, and noncompliance with postoperative protocol are a few of the relative contraindications to definitive wound closure. The wounds of most ICU patients that do require closure will not be closed for weeks to months after the patients' initial ICU admission. At the time of closure, it is critical that the patient's medical condition is stable and has been restored as close as possible to the premorbid state. The wound must also be well controlled. The lack of enthusiasm of surgeons for primary flap closure is related to the high recurrence rate. Evans and Dufresne [41] reviewed their experience with the surgical therapy of pressure sores and found that 82% recurred at the same site in paraplegic patients. Overall, there was a 91% recurrence rate in the same group. The average time to pressure sore recurrence was 18.2 months and pressure sore recurrence was unaffected by the type of closure that was performed. The authors concluded that the physician and the patient must be willing to accept the inevitability of recurrence at the same or other location. Surgical flap closure is reserved for patients in whom healing has plateaued after maximizing all factors. They must also demonstrate the personal and social support necessary to participate in a comprehensive wound care program.

Prior to surgery, nutritional status is optimized. Bowel preparation is based on the surgeon's preference and is individualized according to the wound and the patient. All nonviable tissue is debrided and bony prominences are reduced. This is frequently a staged procedure to minimize hematoma formation and acute blood loss. The goals of wound closure are to eliminate dead space and to provide wound approximation with minimal tension while the patient is positioned in a normal resting posture. The most common reasons for early failure of flap closure are inadequate debridement, hematoma formation, wound tension, and postoperative positioning. Other reasons for failure are uncontrolled spasm, unaddressed limb contracture, infection, and noncompliance with postoperative protocols.

A myriad of options are available for the flap closure of pressure sores. At the authors' institution, rotation advancement flaps based on the gluteal muscles are preferred for sacral ulcer closure due to the ability to safely readvance the flap if a recurrence should occur. Posterior thigh flaps are preferred for the closure of ischial ulcers, and the traditional tensor fascia lata flap is generally used for trochanteric ulcer closure. Patients with trochanteric ulcers should be evaluated for hip joint stability because they may require a Girdlestone arthroplasty if hip dislocation is contributing to pressure sore formation.

Surgery is usually not necessary for definitive wound closure in ICU patients who were previously ambulating and who in the long term will maintain the ability to ambulate. Even grade III and IV ulcers usually heal with local wound care, good nutritional support, and alleviation of the pressure in ambulators. In the rare instance of a refractory sacral pressure ulcer in an ambulatory patient, use of the gluteus muscle should be tempered to minimize the significant disability caused by the sacrifice of this muscle.

POSTOPERATIVE MANAGEMENT

The critical principles of postoperative management are avoidance of compression of the vascular pedicle, minimization of tension on wound edges, obliteration of dead space, adequate drainage, minimization of shear forces, and pressure dispersion. Air-fluid beds are generally used a minimum of 3 weeks postoperatively. This helps to reduce the likelihood of secondary pressure sores. At the authors' institution, air-fluidized beds are used postoperatively in all patients who undergo flap

TABLE 155.1

SUMMARY OF ADVANCES FOR REDUCING RISK OF PRESSURE SORES

- Early identification of patients at risk using standardized risk assessment tools reduces the incidence of skin breakdown [14,38].
- Pressure-reducing bedding maintains transcutaneous oxygen tension [16,17].
- Hydrocolloid dressing reduces nursing time but increases cost compared with saline dressings for pressure sores [30].
- Negative-pressure wound therapy promotes angiogenesis, new tissue growth, and reduced bacterial growth [31–34].

closure of pressure sores. Jackson-Pratt drains are left in place for a minimum of 2 weeks to facilitate the evacuation of any fluid collections and to obliterate dead space underlying the flap. Parenteral antibiotics are continued for an additional 4 to 6 weeks for all patients diagnosed with osteomyelitis. Bone cultures are sent routinely in all cases in which reduction of bony prominences is performed. Attention to urinary and fecal diversion should be maintained. Recently, at the authors' institution, the V.A.C.® has proved a useful tool postoperatively for edema control, wound drainage, and the obliteration of dead space with good success in place of or as an adjunct to Jackson-Pratt drains. It has been used in selected cases immediately after wound closure and on a few occasions after reexploration for hematoma evacuation.

After flap closure, patients are instructed to remain off the flap surface for a minimum of 5 weeks postoperatively. At 5 weeks, a progressive program of gradual return of weight-bearing tolerance on the operative site is started. The greatest challenge is a life-long commitment to self-care that minimizes the risks of the development of pressure sores in patients with long-standing risk factors.

Advances in reducing risks in pressure sores, based on randomized, controlled trials or meta-analyses of such trials as well as prospective studies, are summarized in Table 155.1.

References

1. National Pressure Ulcer Advisory Panel: *Pressure Ulcer Treatment: Clinical Practice Guideline*. Washington, DC, US. Department of Health and Human Services, 1994, p 15.
2. Woolf HB (ed): *Webster's New Collegiate Dictionary*. Springfield, MA, G & C Merriman, 1974.
3. Landis DM: Studies of capillary pressure in human skin. *Heart* 15:209, 1930.
4. Lindan O, Greenway RM, Piazza JM: Pressure distribution on the surface of the body. *Arch Phys Med Rehabil* 46:378, 1965.
5. Dansereau JG, Conway H: Closure of decubiti in paraplegics. *Plast Reconstr Surg* 33:474, 1964.
6. Culliford AT, Levine JP: *Pressure Sores. Current Therapy in Plastic Surgery*. Philadelphia, PA, Saunders-Elsevier, 2006.
7. Husain T: An experimental study of some pressure effects on tissues with reference to the bed-sore problem. *J Pathol Bacteriol* 66:347, 1953.
8. Le KM, Madsen BL, Barth PW, et al: An in-depth look at pressure sores using monolithic silicon pressure sensors. *Plast Reconstr Surg* 74:745, 1984.
9. Kosiak M: Etiology and pathology of ischemic ulcers. *Arch Phys Med Rehabil* 40:62, 1959.
10. Enis J, Sarmiento A: The pathophysiology and management of pressure sores. *Orthop Rev* 2:26, 1973.
11. Eachempati SR, Hydo LJ, Barie PS: Factors influencing the development of decubitus ulcers in critically ill surgical patients. *Crit Care Med* 29:1678, 2001.
12. Feuchtinger J, Halfens RJ, Dassen T: Pressure ulcer risk in cardiac surgery: a review of the research literature. *Heart Lung* 34:375, 2005.
13. Keller BP, Wille J, van Ramshorst B, et al: Pressure ulcers in intensive care patients: a review of risks and prevention. *Intensive Care Med* 28:1379, 2002.
14. Bergstrom N, Braden BJ, Laguzza A: The Braden Scale for predicting pressure sore risk. *Nurs Res* 36:205, 1987.
15. Seiler WO, Stahelin HB: Recent findings on decubitus ulcer pathology: implications for care. *Geriatrics* 41:47, 1986.
16. Tallon R: Support surfaces—a technology review. *Nurs Manage* 27:58, 1996.
17. Feldman DL, Sepka RS, Klitzman B: Tissue oxygenation and flow on specialized and conventional hospital beds. *Ann Plast Surg* 30:441, 1993.
18. Inman KJ, Sibbald WJ, Rutledge FS, et al: Clinical utility and cost-effectiveness of an air suspension bed in the prevention of pressure ulcers. *JAMA* 269:1139, 1993.
19. Meehan M: National pressure ulcer prevalence survey. *Adv Wound Care* 7:27, 1994.
20. Blaszczyk J, Majewski M, Sato F: Make a difference: standardize your heel care practice. *Ostomy Wound Manage* 44:32, 1998.
21. Blaylock B: Solving the problem of pressure ulcers resulting from cervical collars. *Ostomy Wound Manage* 42:26, 1996.
22. Galpin JE, Chow AW, Bayer AS, et al: Sepsis associated with decubitus ulcers. *Am J Med* 61:346, 1976.
23. Hellewell TB, Major DA, Foresman PA, et al: A cytotoxicity evaluation of antimicrobial and non-microbial wound cleansers. *Wounds* 9:1, 1997.
24. Cooper ML, Laxer JA, Hansbrough JF: The cytotoxic effects of commonly used topical microbial agents on human fibroblasts and keratinocytes. *J Trauma* 31:775, 1991.
25. Lineaweaver W, McMorris S, Soucy D, et al: Cellular and bacterial toxicities of topical antimicrobials. *Plast Reconstr Surg* 75:394, 1985.
26. Boyce ST, Warden GD, Holder IA: Noncytotoxic combinations of topical antimicrobial agents for use with cultured skin substitutes. *Antimicrob Agents Chemother* 39:1324, 1995.
27. Boyce ST, Warden GD, Holder IA: Cytotoxicity testing of topical antimicrobial agents on human keratinocytes and fibroblasts for cultured skin grafts. *J Burn Care Rehabil* 16:97, 1995.
28. Boyce ST, Holder IA: Selection of topical antimicrobial agents for cultured skin for burns by combined assessment of cellular toxicity and antimicrobial activity. *Plast Reconstr Surg* 92:493, 1993.
29. Cooper ML, Boyce ST, Hansbrough JF, et al: Cytotoxicity to cultured human keratinocytes to topical anti-microbial agents. *J Surg Res* 48:190, 1990.
30. Mc Kenna PJ, Lehr GS, Leist P, et al: Antiseptic effectiveness with fibroblast preservation. *Ann Plast Surg* 27:265, 1991.
31. Choucair M, Phillips T: A review of wound healing and dressing materials. *Wounds* 8:165, 1996.
32. Xakellis GC, Chrischilles EA: Hydrocolloid versus saline-gauze dressings in treating pressure ulcers: a cost effectiveness analysis. *Arch Phys Med Rehabil* 73:463, 1992.
33. Gupta S, Baharestani M, Baranoski S, et al: Guidelines for managing pressure ulcers with negative pressure wound therapy. *Adv Skin Wound Care* 17[Suppl 2]:1–16, 2004.
34. Smith N: The benefits of VAC therapy in the management of pressure ulcers. *Br J Nurs* 13(22):1359–1365, 2005.
35. Isago T, Nozaki M, Kikuchi Y, et al: Negative-pressure dressings in the treatment of pressure ulcers. *J Dermatol* 30(4):299–305, 2003.
36. Joseph E, Hamori CA, Bergman S, et al: A prospective randomization trial of vacuum assisted closure versus standard therapy of chronic non healing wounds. *Wounds* 12:60, 2000.
37. Ford CN, Reinhard ER, Yeh D, et al: Interim analysis of a prospective, randomized trial of vacuum-assisted closure versus the healthpoint system in the management of pressure ulcers. *Ann Plast Surg* 49(1):55–61, 2002; discussion 61.
38. Baharestani MM, Houliston-Otto DB, Barnes S: Early versus late initiation of negative pressure wound therapy: examining the impact on home care length of stay. *Ostomy Wound Manage* 54(11):48–53, 2008.
39. Philbeck TE Jr, Whittington KT, Millsap MH, et al: The clinical and cost effectiveness of externally applied negative pressure wound therapy in the treatment of wounds in home healthcare medicare patients. *Ostomy Wound Manage* 45(11):41–50, 1999.
40. Conway H, Griffith BH: Plastic surgery for closure of decubitus ulcers in patients with paraplegia based on experience with 1,000 cases. *Ann Surg* 91:946, 1956.
41. Evans GR, Dufresne CR, Manson PN: Surgical correction of pressure ulcers in an urban center: is it efficacious? *Adv Wound Care* 7:40, 1994.

CHAPTER 156 ■ MANAGEMENT OF THE OBSTETRICAL PATIENT IN THE INTENSIVE CARE SETTING

JOHN G. GIANOPOULOS AND JONATHAN F. CRITCHLOW

Pregnancy is a common occurrence in everyday life. Yet, many women suffer significant risk and even death from the normal physiologic phenomenon of pregnancy. The United States enjoys one of the lowest maternal mortality levels in the world. However, for every 100,000 live births 10 to 12 women die secondary to medical or obstetric complications of pregnancy. It is not uncommon for the intensive care team to care for pregnant patients with critical conditions. Improvements in obstetric, anesthetic, and intensive care have led to the decline in maternal mortality and the shifting of responsible causes [1,2]. Today there are fewer pregnant patients with septic causes for their critical illness and more patients with hypertension and concurrent medical illness admitted to the intensive care setting [3].

The approach to the pregnant patient in the intensive care setting requires a thorough knowledge of the normal maternal adaptations to pregnancy, the potential fetal effects of any diagnostic or therapeutic modalities needed, and the potential for obstetric complication of any procedures. This chapter reviews the maternal anatomic and physiologic adaptations to pregnancy, considerations of potential harm from diagnostic studies, selected therapeutic interventions, and specific pregnancy disease states that may complicate the care of the critically ill pregnant patient such as preeclampsia, eclampsia, obstetric hemorrhage, and trauma. Specifics related to the diagnosis and treatment of respiratory failure in pregnancy is discussed elsewhere in the text (see Chapter 51).

MATERNAL PHYSIOLOGIC ADAPTATION TO PREGNANCY

Cardiovascular System

The cardiovascular system undergoes significant alteration under the influence of the altered hormonal milieu of pregnancy. Cardiac output begins to rise in the first trimester and continues a steady rise peaking at 30% to 50% of preexisting levels by 32 weeks' gestation [4]. The rise in cardiac output is produced by increases in both heart rate and stroke volume which are in response to an increase in endogenous circulating catecholamines, which affect both an inotropic and a chronotropic response [5,6]. Peripheral vascular resistance is reduced secondary to a direct effect of progesterone relaxing the smooth muscle intima of the precapillary resistance vessels, resulting in vasodilatation [6]. The arterial–venous shunt of the placenta also contributes to decreased vascular resistance. In the third trimester, the enlarged uterus may compress the vena cava (particularly in the supine position) leading to decreased venous return to the heart and a decrease in cardiac output. The third-trimester pregnant patient is best positioned so that the uterus is displaced to the left, allowing adequate venal caval flow and venous return to avoid hypotension. There is a slight drop in mean arterial pressure in normal pregnancy beginning during the second trimester secondary to the reduction in peripheral resistance. Blood volume increases in pregnancy, peaking at 50% above prepregnancy levels. The maximal increase in blood volume occurs at about 32 weeks' gestation [7,8]. This increased blood volume leads to normalization of mean arterial pressures by term.

The pulmonic and systemic circulations undergo similar alterations. There is vasodilatation with an increased volume to capacitance. However, in the pulmonic circulation the volume and capacitance changes almost equal each other. Therefore, there is virtually no change in mean pulmonic pressures [9,10]. When the pulmonic circulation is evaluated by central catheterization, no changes in pulmonary artery pressures or wedge pressures can be attributed to pregnancy [9,11]. The increased pulmonic volume with increased capacitance renders the pregnant patient susceptible to fluid overload and pulmonary edema. Pulmonary edema will occur much more readily in pregnancy secondary to these specific maternal adaptations.

Respiratory Adaptations

Progesterone affects the hypothalamic apneustic center. Carbon dioxide sensitivity is reduced to 30 mm Hg. This results in an increased respiratory rate and an increased tidal volume. The pregnant patient is in a chronic state of respiratory alkalosis. The kidneys compensate by excreting bicarbonate to maintain normal acid–base equilibrium [12]. The normal blood gas of pregnancy is a compensated respiratory alkalosis. The normal pH is 7.44 and the bicarbonate decreases 4 mEq per L [12]. Vital capacity and maximum voluntary ventilation are not altered. The functional residual capacity is reduced as the diaphragm is elevated. The reduced bicarbonate level renders the pregnant patient much more susceptible to the development of metabolic acidosis in response to a variety of conditions [12,13].

Hematologic Adaptations

Plasma volume in pregnancy increases by 50% for prepregnancy levels. The red cell mass will increase in pregnancy by 30% over prepregnancy levels. This leads to a dilutional effect, decreasing hemoglobin concentrations (lower normal: 10.5 to 11 g per dL) and hematocrit levels (30% to 35%). This phenomenon has been termed the *physiologic anemia* of pregnancy [8,14].

Increased catecholamine and steroid levels in pregnancy cause a demargination of mature leukocytes from the endothelium. This leads to a physiologic leukocytosis of pregnancy, with the white blood cell count increasing by 5,000 to 10,000 cells per mL [8,14].

Estrogen stimulates the hepatocyte endoplasmic reticulum, leading to an increased protein production. There is also increased synthesis of several clotting factors (VII, VIII, IX, and X) throughout pregnancy. Fibrinogen increases by 20%, with an average level during gestation of 400 mg. These increases render the pregnant woman hypercoagulable [15]. Critically ill pregnant patients rendered immobile require some form of prophylaxis to prevent venous thromboembolic events as they are at higher risk secondary to the hypercoagulability of pregnancy.

Renal Adaptations

Renal plasma blood flow and glomerular filtration rate increase by approximately 30% to 50% from prepregnant levels resulting in an increased creatinine, urea, and uric acid clearance, with a decrease in serum creatinine (normal: 0.5 to 0.9 mg per dL), blood urea nitrogen (normal: 10 to 15 mg per dL), and uric acid (normal: 2.5 to 3.5 mEq per L) levels [15–17]. When drugs with renal clearance are used in pregnancy, their dose needs to be adjusted to account for increased renal clearance. Progesterone relaxes the renal collecting system. The muscularis of the bladder is relaxed and urinary stasis occurs. The angle of the urethra to the vagina is altered, making urinary tract infections common in pregnancy. If bladder catheterization is required for more than 12 hours, antibiotic prophylaxis is needed to prevent urinary tract infection (Table 156.1).

DIAGNOSTIC RADIATION EXPOSURE

Diagnostic radiographic procedures are essential in the management of the critically ill patient. These procedures may be undertaken with care in the pregnant patient. Adverse fetal effects are reported with ionizing radiation exposure to the fetus in excess of 10 cGy [18–20]. Microcephaly, intrauterine growth restriction, and poor fetal development have all been reported [18–20]. Direct radiation exposure to the pelvis of 10 cGy or greater in the first trimester may result in intrauterine fetal death. Direct fetal exposure of 5 cGy or less has not been shown to increase fetal malformation. However, a very small risk of increased childhood malignancy has been reported. Direct doses of 1 cGy or less have not been shown to produce any significant fetal effect [18–20]. Single-shot examinations such as chest radiographs, abdominal images, or imaging of long bones expose the fetus to very little risk. Fluoroscopic examinations are to be avoided in pregnancy because of the significant amount of radiation exposure [19,20].

Computed tomography (CT) of the head and thorax produces little direct radiation to the pelvis (0.05 to 0.1 cGy) and may be undertaken with relative safety [21]. Abdominal and pelvic CT scanning delivers 3 to 10 cGy to the pelvis and should be avoided in the first trimester. In the second and third trimester, abdominal and pelvic CT examinations may be done with caution [21,22]. If a significant alteration in management is to be undertaken as a result of the information obtained from the procedure, the potential fetal risk should be considered. Magnetic resonance scanning has not been extensively studied in pregnancy. However, this technology is considered extremely safe in pregnancy and may be an alternative to CT scanning in the first trimester [23,24]. Magnetic resonance imaging examinations are used as an adjunct to ultrasound in the second and third trimesters to aid in the diagnosis of certain fetal anomalies. Contrast agents should be avoided in the first trimester [23,24].

Radionuclide procedures may be done in pregnancy. The overall radiation dose to fetus with most procedures is low. Most of the contrast agents used in these examinations are renally cleared. It is important to place an indwelling bladder catheter to reduce total radiation dose to the fetus because retained urine in the maternal bladder could expose the fetus to larger radiation doses than the initial pass through the placental circulation [19,25–27].

TABLE 156.1

PHYSIOLOGIC MATERNAL ADAPTATION TO PREGNANCY

System	Alternations
Cardiovascular	Cardiac output, HR × SV = CO Increased 20%–30% Both heart rate and stroke volume increased
Peripheral vascular resistance	Decreased as resistance vessels with vasodilatation
Blood flow	Increased to Uterus Skin Kidney Breast
Pulmonic circulation	Blood volume increases equal capacitance increase No change in pulmonary artery pressures
Pulmonary system	Tidal volume increased Respiratory rate increased Functional residual capacity reduced Compensated respiratory alkalosis
Renal system	Renal artery perfusion increased Glomerular filtration rate increased Creatinine clearance increased BUN, serum creatinine, serum uric acid decreased Renal clearance of drugs increased Bladder muscularis relaxation Urinary stasis infection risk Dilated renal pelvises and ureters
Gastrointestinal system	Decreased gastric motility Aspiration risk with anesthesia Decreased colonic motility Constipation complaints
Hematologic system	Plasma volume increases 40%–50% Red cell mass increases 20%–30% "Physiologic anemia" Leukocytosis Increased liver-produced clotting factors Increased fibrinogen Hypercoagulable state

BUN, blood urea nitrogen; CO, cardiac output; HR, heart rate; SV, stroke volume.
From Gianopoulos JG: Establishing the criteria for anesthesia and other precautions for surgery during pregnancy. *Surg Clin North Am* 75:33, 1995, with permission.

TABLE 156.2

RADIATION DOSE AND FETAL EFFECT

Radiation dose to fetus (cGy)	Theoretical or actual fetal effect
0–5	No reported malformation; potential for oncogenesis and increased cancer risk
5–10	Potential for oncogenesis; potential for IUGR
10–20	Microcephaly, IUGR, 2.4% mental retardation
20–50	Microcephaly, IUGR, fetal death, mental retardation
50–100	Microcephaly, IUGR, 18% mental retardation, fetal death

IUGR, intrauterine growth retardation.
From Gianopoulos JG: Breast disease in pregnancy, in Isaccs JH (ed): *Textbook of Breast Disease*. Philadelphia, Mosby-Year Book, 1992, p 131, with permission.

If excessive radiation doses to the pelvis are inadvertently administered, it is important to calculate the fetal isodose radiation exposure. If an excess of 10 cGy has been delivered to the fetus, there may be significant fetal effect. Table 156.2 outlines potential fetal effects of radiation exposure.

MEDICATIONS AND PREGNANCY

Analgesic Agents

Opiate narcotic agents administered for short periods of time have been shown to be safe in pregnancy. Morphine and meperidine administered intravenously, intramuscularly, or in patient-controlled pumps, have demonstrated no adverse fetal effects. Chronic opiate use in pregnancy has been associated with intrauterine growth restriction. Intrauterine fetal addiction with withdrawal may occur [28–30]. Intrauterine fetal withdrawal has been associated with intrauterine fetal demise. Oral opiates may be used with similar cautions.

Codeine-containing compounds should be avoided in the first trimester because they have a small teratogenic potential [30]. These compounds may be used in the second and third trimesters for short intervals with little fetal risk. Nonsteroidal anti-inflammatory agents may decrease fetal renal blood flow, leading to oligohydramnios. They also will lead to the in utero closure of the ductus arteriosus, producing fetal pulmonary hypertension after 32 weeks' gestation. Short courses of indomethacin may be used with caution prior to 32 weeks' gestation. Benzodiazepines may be used; they have not been shown to exert an adverse fetal effect. High doses near the time of delivery may lead to neonatal depression [30,31].

Antibiotics

Penicillin, penicillin derivatives, as well as cephalosporins have no known adverse fetal effect. Erythromycin, clindamycin, and vancomycin are considered safe in pregnancy. There is some concern regarding renal toxicity with vancomycin. Aminoglycosides have been implicated with fetal ototoxicity [30]. However, only streptomycin and kanamycin have been implicated. Gentamicin has not been reported to have significant ototoxicity. Gentamicin may be used in life-threatening infections while carefully monitoring levels. Sulfonamides complete with

TABLE 156.3

ANTIBIOTICS IN PREGNANCY

Penicillin/cephalosporin
No adverse effect in nonallergic patient
Aminoglycosides
Renal toxicity and ototoxicity
Use in life-threatening infections
Tetracycline
Contraindicated
Staining of teeth
Bone demineralization
Sulfa drugs
Avoid first trimester
Third trimester use with bilirubin displacement
Kernicterus
Chloramphenicol
Grey baby syndrome
Fluoroquinolones
Fetal effect—avoid use

From Gianopoulos JG: Establishing the criteria for anesthesia and other precautions for surgery during pregnancy. *Surg Clin North Am* 75:33, 1995, with permission.

bilirubin-binding sites and may lead to neonatal kernicterus if administered in the third trimester. Tetracycline is teratogenic, leading to brown teeth and abnormal long bone development [30,32,33] (Table 156.3).

Anticoagulants

Unfractionated heparin, because of its molecular size and ionic negative charge, has been shown not to cross the placental membrane [34]. Therefore, it is the anticoagulant of choice in all trimesters of pregnancy and may be used with relative fetal safety. Fractionated heparins also have been shown not to cross the placental membrane. They may be used throughout pregnancy as well. If fractionated heparins are used in pregnancy, it is advised to change to unfractionated heparin late in the third trimester. If surgical intervention is needed, unfractionated heparin may be reversed with protamine sulfate and the activated partial thromboplastic time is a more reliable monitor for anticoagulant effect than the activated factor Xa assessment needed to assess the activity of fractionated heparins [35,36]. Warfarin and its derivatives are contraindicated in the first trimester as these agents are teratogenic, producing midline defects such as clefts, cardiac septal defect, and limb bud abnormalities. In all trimesters, warfarin crosses the placenta and may lead to spontaneous fetal bleeding [37–39]. In some select cardiac patients (particularly those with mechanical valves), warfarin may be used in the second and early third trimesters. Fetal intracranial bleeding has been observed with warfarin use in the late third trimester.

Antihypertensives

Pregnant patients will require acute antihypertensive intervention when the systolic blood pressure exceeds 160 mm Hg or the diastolic blood pressure exceeds 110 mm Hg. Preservation of the fetal circulation must be kept in mind when treating these conditions. For the acute management of hypertensive crisis in pregnancy, hydralazine has been recommended [40,41]. A test dose of 5 mg intravenous (IV) is given, followed by 10-mg doses. However, recent data show labetalol may be a superior antihypertensive in acute situations, as it does not increase the maternal pulse rate. A 10-mg test dose is given IV, followed by a 20-mg dose at 10 minutes if no response is observed. If still no response in blood pressure is observed, the dose may be increased to 40 mg in 10 minutes and followed by 80 mg in 10 minutes. The 80 mg dose may be repeated one time. The total dose should not exceed 220 mg. Labetalol may also be administered as a continuous IV drip at 2 to 4 mg per minute [42,43]. Nifedipine may be used in less acute conditions with caution due to paradoxical hypotension. Hydrating the patient with IV fluids will reduce the incidence of a decrease in blood pressure

Sodium nitroprusside should be avoided if possible. This agent is converted in the fetus to sodium thiocyanate, which cannot be metabolized because the fetus lacks the necessary hepatic cytochrome. In extreme situations when other agents have not been effective, it may be used with caution [44–46]. Angiotensin-converting enzyme inhibitors and angiotensin receptor blocker agents are contraindicated in pregnancy. They have been associated with fetal anomalies and intrauterine fetal death secondary to fetal cardiovascular collapse [30].

Vasoconstrictor and Inotropic Agents

Profound hypotension unresponsive to postural change and fluid resuscitation may require vasoconstrictor therapy. Phenylephrine has been shown to be safe in treating hypotension secondary to spinal or epidural anesthesia. Its excessive alpha activity makes it less effective in treating critically ill patients. Dopamine and isoproterenol alter uterine blood flow less than phenylephrine. In situations in which vasoconstrictor therapy is needed in a critically ill patient, dopamine is recommended. At low doses, 2 to 4 μg per minute, uterine blood flow is increased [46,47].

SPECIFIC PREGNANCY DISORDERS

Hypertensive Disorders of Pregnancy

Hypertension complicates 8% to 10% of all pregnancies, yet despite modern medical management it continues to be a leading cause of maternal mortality. Hypertension during pregnancy is classified as preexisting chronic hypertension, preeclampsia/eclampsia, chronic hypertension with superimposed preeclampsia, and gestational hypertension [42].

Preeclampsia is defined as proteinuric hypertension after the 20th week of gestation. Hypertension is defined as a sustained blood pressure of 140 mm Hg systolic and/or 90 mm Hg diastolic. Proteinuria must exceed 300 mg in 24 hours. A dipped urine sample of 1+ repeated in 6 hours or a single 3+ or 4+ dip also will meet the criteria to make the diagnosis. Preeclampsia may lead to significant maternal end organ damage, secondary to vasospasm [42,48]. The organ dysfunction leads to with renal failure, liver compromise, intravascular coagulopathy, thrombocytopenia, pulmonary edema, hemolysis, and cardiac failure. Preeclampsia is classified as mild or severe. Severe preeclampsia occurs when any of the following criteria are met: blood pressure 160/110 mm Hg, thrombocytopenia, elevated liver enzymes, oliguria, proteinuria in excess of 5 g in 24 hours, hyperreflexia, scotomata, epigastric pain, renal failure, pulmonary edema, disseminated intravascular coagulopathy, and fetal compromise. Mild preeclampsia is preeclampsia without any criteria met to classify as severe. Eclampsia is defined as preeclampsia with the onset of maternal seizure in a patient without previous seizure disorder.

The specific etiology of pre-eclampsia remains a medical enigma. However, much is known regarding the underlying pathophysiology of this disease. Arteriolar vasospasm with intravascular volume depletion is the primary pathologic alteration leading to preeclampsia. Precipitating pathologic factors include failure of prostacyclin-mediated vasodilatation in the vascular system, endothelial damage leading to the release of endothelins, thromboxane, and vasoactive proteins [49–51]. Placental vascular growth factor inhibitory proteins have been implicated in the etiology.

These intravascular changes lead to the loss of catecholamine insensitivity of normal pregnancy and angiotensin hypersensitivity. The increase in peripheral vascular resistance leads to hypertension, diminished blood flows to vital organs, and microangiopathy. Albumin concentrations decrease in the blood secondary to proteinuria which contributes to a decrease in plasma oncotic pressure. This, along with endothelial damage, leads to generalized edema, ascites, and in severe cases, pulmonary edema. Renal blood flow is decreased and fibrin deposition occurs in the glomeruli. Renal endothelial cells swell and the filtration function of the kidney is impaired, allowing large protein molecules to enter the collecting tubules [52]. Hyperreflexia is common. The mechanism responsible for central nervous system dysfunction is not totally understood. Hypertensive encephalopathy, cerebral vasospasm, and cerebral edema contribute to the pathologic milieu, which may lead to an area of localized cerebral irritability leading to an epileptic focus resulting in seizure activity.

A syndrome of hemolysis, elevated liver enzymes, and low platelets is sometimes seen in patients suffering from preeclampsia and is termed the HELLP syndrome [53]. This constellation of end organ abnormalities may be seen in 2% to 12% of patients with preeclampsia. As many as 30% to 50% of these patients may not manifest hypertension or proteinuria. This syndrome is a severe form of preeclampsia and is life threatening. The exact pathogenesis is not known; however, vasospasm, endothelial damage, and microangiopathic hemolysis all contribute. Platelet consumption and fibrin deposition in the liver lead to areas of necrosis. Rarely, subcapsular hematoma may occur. The diagnosis is made by the observation of hemolysis on peripheral blood smear, elevations in lactate dehydrogenase, alanine aminotransferase, and thrombocytopenia (platelet count less than 100,000 per mm^3) [53]. Occasionally, in very preterm gestations, one may treat this condition conservatively with IV steroids (dexamethasone, 10 mg IV every 6 hours). However, a randomized trial assessing this therapy failed to show any improvement in most cases. There was a minimal effect in the most severe cases however. This therapy may be used with very preterm infants [54,55]. In most cases, especially in the mid-to-late third trimester, delivery is warranted [42].

Management

The definitive treatment of preeclampsia is delivery. At term, patients should be stabilized and delivery effected. A preterm pregnancy may be treated conservatively if no signs of severe preeclampsia are observed [42,48]. In select cases of severe preeclampsia, remote from term patients may be followed in a tertiary care setting conservatively. The agents of choice for the treatment of hypertension are hydralazine or labetalol. Labetalol acts on both alpha- and beta-receptors without increasing the heart rate [54]. Patients remote from term should be given steroids to enhance fetal pulmonary maturity (betamethasone, 12 mg intramuscularly [IM] every 24 hours for two doses or dexamethasone, 6 mg IM every 12 hours for four doses). Tests of fetal well-being with ultrasound and fetal monitoring (nonstress test) should be performed. In severe cases (particularly with oliguria or pulmonary edema), invasive maternal hemodynamic monitoring may be beneficial. Diuretics should not be used unless pulmonary edema is present, as intravascular volume is already depleted. At the time of labor or in severe cases, IV magnesium sulfate is the analeptic of choice. It has been shown to be superior to other agents in randomized trials at preventing eclamptic seizures [56–59]. A loading dose of 2 to 4 g is given IV slowly during 15 to 20 minutes. This is then followed by a maintenance dose of 1 to 2 g per hour. Magnesium levels may become toxic, leading to respiratory or cardiac arrest [56,57]. These patients require intensive monitoring of their respiratory function, cardiovascular function, and neurologic status. As magnesium is renally cleared, adequate urine output must be maintained. If patients manifest oliguria, a decrease or discontinuation of magnesium is indicated. Magnesium toxicity may be reversed with the administration of IV calcium (10 mL of a 10% solution of calcium gluconate given slowly IV over 10 minutes).

Eclamptic seizures are treated with IV magnesium. In cases unresponsive to magnesium, benzodiazepines may be used, such as diazepam (5 to 10 mg IV). When the seizure activity persists, the next agent of choice is phenytoin (10 to 20 mg per kg IV during 20 minutes). If the seizure still continues, IV amobarbital in 50-mg increments to a total dose of 200 mg is administered. In severe refractory cases, muscle paralysis with general anesthesia and ventilatory support is needed [57,59,60].

Patients with severe disease during weeks 24 to 28 of pregnancy are treated conservatively with aggressive maternal support and steroids for fetal lung development. An attempt should be made to achieve a gestational age of 28 weeks, if the maternal and fetal condition remains stable. From 28 to 34 weeks, steroids are given and delivery should be undertaken within 48 hours, if the maternal and fetal conditions remain stable. When severe pre-eclampsia presents after 34 weeks of gestation, delivery should occur after maternal stabilization [59]. The route of delivery should be determined by obstetric factors and vaginal delivery may be undertaken.

Rarely, patients may rupture a subcapsular liver hematoma. This manifests with severe right upper quadrant and shoulder pain. If shock ensues, immediate operation is needed. In more stable patients, the diagnosis may be confirmed with ultrasound or CT scan.

Obstetric Hemorrhage

Despite medical interventions, obstetric hemorrhage remains a significant cause of maternal morbidity, mortality, and fetal loss. Physiologic changes in the uterine blood flow increase uterine artery blood flow to 500 to 600 mL per minute at term. Patients in the third trimester with placental disruptions such as placenta previa or abruption may suffer rapid and significant blood loss, leading to hemodynamic compromise. Hemorrhage in the third trimester of pregnancy is an acute medical emergency.

There is a normal physiologic blood loss at the time of delivery. In an average vaginal delivery, the patient may lose 300 to 500 mL, and this increases to 1,000 to 1,500 mL with cesarean section [14]. When significant hemorrhage occurs, prompt medical or surgical intervention is needed.

Antepartum Hemorrhage

First and second trimester conditions such as spontaneous abortion and ectopic pregnancy may lead to significant blood loss. Patients treated for spontaneous abortion or ruptured ectopic gestation need continuous hemodynamic monitoring and aggressive fluid and blood product replacement to avoid hemodynamic compromise and hypovolumic shock. Third trimester bleeding is most often placental in nature, such as abnormal placental location, placenta previa or premature placental separation from the uterine wall (abruption placenta).

Placenta Previa

The placenta is located over the cervical os in 1 in 150 to 200 pregnancies. These patients usually present with painless vaginal bleeding and may have multiple sporadic episodes of bleeding. The diagnosis is made ultrasonically with observation of the placenta covering all or part of the cervical os [60,61]. The bleeding episodes are usually self-limiting, although sometimes the bleeding will not remit and immediate cesarean section is warranted. Once the diagnosis is made, these patients are treated with conservative management. Bed rest, blood replacement, and close surveillance of maternal and fetal well-being are the mainstays of therapy [61]. In stable cases remote from term, patients with good family support at home, may be treated as outpatients. Most cases near term require hospitalization and close monitoring. If stable, patients are assessed for fetal lung maturity with an amniocentesis at 35 to 36 weeks and cesarean section is preformed if fetal lung maturity is documented [61]. Rarely, the placenta may invade the myometrium (accreta abutting the myometrium, increta invading partially into the myometrium, and percreta invading through the myometrium). These conditions often will require hysterectomy at the time of cesarean operation. These procedures incur significant blood loss and these patients need close postoperative monitoring for hemodynamic status [61].

Abruption Placenta

Placental abruption, the premature separation of the placenta from the uterine wall, complicates up to 1% of all pregnancies. This condition may lead to severe vaginal bleeding or may be concealed within the uterus. These patients have a significant risk of coagulopathy, and coagulation studies are indicated. The therapy consists of maternal stabilization with fluid and blood product replacement, if necessary, and fetal monitoring since fetal mortality rates may be as high as 25% to 40%. Fetal loss is more likely if fetal maternal hemorrhage has occurred, and assessment of fetal blood in the maternal circulation with Kleihauer–Betke testing is indicated. If coagulopathy ensues (as is seen in 15% to 30% of these cases), resuscitation with blood-replacement products such as fresh-frozen plasma or cryoprecipitate is necessary [62]. At term, delivery is indicated. With preterm presentation, if the abruption is not severe and maternal and fetal status are stable, an attempt at conservative management with intensive surveillance may be undertaken. In these cases, steroids are given to enhance fetal lung maturity. At the time of delivery, bleeding may be vigorous and operative interventions such as uterine artery ligation, hypogastric artery ligation, radiographic directed embolization, or hysterectomy may be necessary [62].

Postpartum Hemorrhage

Significant hemorrhage postpartum occurs in 2% to 5% of deliveries. The most common cause is uterine atony in the immediate postpartum period. Retained placental fragments, lacerations of the cervix and vagina, and unrecognized coagulopathies are other potential causes [63]. Blood loss of more than 500 mL at vaginal delivery or 1,000 mL at cesarean section is classified as postpartum hemorrhage [16]. Delayed hemorrhage, 3 to 7 days postpartum, most often is due to retained placental fragments or unrecognized congenital coagulopathies [63].

The immediate management consists of an investigation for the cause. Careful examination of the cervix and vagina to assess for unrecognized lacerations is warranted. Assessment of the contractile status of the uterus is also performed. In cases of atony, uterine oxytocic agents are administered. Oxytocin solutions are given IV (20 to 40 units added to 1 liter IV solutions and administered at 200 to 300 mL per hour) [63–65]. Vigorous external uterine massage is also used. In most cases, this is all that is necessary to resolve the problem. If atony persists, ergot-containing agents such as Methergine, 0.2 mg IM, may be used. These compounds are contraindicated in patients with hypertension as significant elevations in blood pressure may occur and rarely may lead to intracerebral hemorrhage. Prostaglandin agents of the F2 alpha class (Hemabate, 250 μg) may be given intramuscularly [65,66]. These agents may cause significant bronchospasm and are contraindicated in patients with asthma. Assessment for coagulopathy is warranted in unresponsive cases [66,67].

If medical management is unsuccessful, surgical intervention is needed. An intrauterine examination under anesthesia for retained products and dilatation and uterine curettage may be performed. If still unresponsive, angiographic uterine artery embolization or surgical intervention with uterine artery or hypogastric artery ligation is needed. In cases of unresponsive atony, uterine-constricting suture of the B Lynch type may be employed. If all measures have failed to resolve the bleeding, hysterectomy may be employed as a last resort [68,69].

Amniotic Fluid Embolism

Amniotic fluid embolism presents as a sudden and acute cardiovascular and respiratory collapse at or around the time of delivery. In the past, this condition had an 80% to 100% maternal mortality. Most cases follow vaginal births, but cases have been associated with abruption, ruptured uterus, and second and early third trimester abortions. Today, with rapid identification and maternal cardiovascular and respiratory support, the mortality rate has been reduced to 50% [70,71]. Amniotic fluid contains many vasoactive and fibrinolytic compounds that, if extravasated into the vascular space, may cause an immediate cardiovascular collapse, with respiratory failure. Immediate and aggressive intervention is necessary to save the mother's life. Intubation and mechanical ventilation with positive end-expiratory pressure is employed. Inotropic and vasoconstrictor agents are needed for cardiac and vascular support. Invasive right-sided cardiac monitoring is also indicated. Blood from the pulmonary artery should be assessed for fetal squamous cells. If found, the diagnosis is confirmed, although the absence of these cells does not preclude the diagnosis [72]. These patients will often experience a rapid and fulminant disseminated intravascular coagulation, requiring resuscitation with fresh-frozen plasma and cryoprecipitate. These patients require intensive monitoring and support (see Chapter 51). If the patient survives the initial insult, most will survive [72–74].

Hemolytic Uremic Syndrome/Thrombotic Thrombocytopenic Purpura

Hemolytic uremic syndrome/thrombotic thrombocytopenic purpura rarely occurs in pregnancy. It is often confused with preeclampsia. Renal failure, thrombocytopenia, and hemolysis are observed in the hemolytic uremic syndrome. If neurologic symptoms are observed, thrombotic thrombocytopenic purpura is diagnosed. This rare condition carries a high maternal mortality if not recognized and rapidly treated. It occurs late in the third trimester or in the immediate postpartum period [75]. Thrombotic occlusion of the microvasculature with platelets leads to hemolysis, producing the findings of this syndrome [75,76,77]. Plasma exchange should be initiated immediately, as it is the most effective treatment for this condition. In some patients as an adjunct to plasma exchange, high-dose IV steroids have sometimes been used with some positive effect on outcome. Patients will usually recover if aggressive therapy and support through their renal failure phase is undertaken early in the course of the disease [77–79].

Burn Injuries

Pregnancy does not alter the acute management of the patient suffering from burn injuries. Aggressive fluid replacement therapy, antibiotics, and oxygen therapy are the mainstays of treatment. The fetal outcome is related to the severity of the maternal burn injury and the development of any maternal complications [80]. If maternal burn injury exceeds 50%, the fetal mortality approaches 100%. In the third trimester, if maternal burn injury is greater than 50%, delivery is indicated. If the maternal burn is 30% or less, fetal survival approaches 80% [80]. Fetal death usually occurs in the first week flowing the burn injury. If the fetus is remote from term, steroids for fetal lung maturity are indicated. If preterm labor ensues and the maternal burn injury is less than 30%, uterine-relaxant tocolytic agents are indicated. Septic complications of burn wound and frank maternal sepsis may lead to labor or fetal amnionitis. Broad-spectrum antibiotics, tetanus toxoid, and immunoglobulin therapy are not contraindicated in pregnancy. Prompt and aggressive therapy for the maternal burn injury produces the best pregnancy outcomes [81].

Trauma Complicating Pregnancy

Trauma is the most common cause of death in pregnancy not related to obstetric factors. Six percent to 7% of pregnant patients will suffer a traumatic injury during their pregnancy. However, less than 1% will require hospitalization [82].

The physiologic alterations of pregnancy, particularly the increased blood volume, make the pregnant trauma patient less likely to immediately manifest signs of shock, although uterine blood flow may be compromised early and fetal compromise is common. The abdominal position of the uterus in the third trimester makes this organ more susceptible to both blunt and penetrating trauma. As the uterus grows, the bladder is pulled superior and rendered more susceptible to traumatic injury in pregnancy.

Motor vehicle accidents with either deceleration forces or blunt trauma are the most common mechanisms occurring during pregnancy. They account for 60% of injuries in pregnancy. The pregnancy outcome is directly related to the severity of the maternal injuries. The most common cause of fetal death is maternal death [83,84].

Following blunt injury secondary to a motor vehicle accident, placental abruption is the most common complication associated with the pregnancy. Abruptions occur in 2% to 4% of patients with these injuries. Ultrasound to detect abruptions is not sensitive, having only 20% to 30% sensitivity [84–86]. Fetal contraction monitoring is a sensitive measure for the diagnosis of abruptions. Contraction monitoring has a high negative predictive value. Most abruptions will occur in the first 4 to 8 hours postinjury. No consensus exists as to the length of the post-trauma monitoring interval, but at least 4 hours is recommended [87,88]. Rarely, a delayed abruption up to 48 hours postinjury may occur. There is no sensitive test to predict delayed abruption. However, if fetal maternal hemorrhage is observed, the incidence is higher. All patients should be screened with a Kleihauer–Betke assay to assess for fetal–maternal bleeding [89]. If positive, a longer period of observation is warranted. As small amounts of fetal blood may enter the maternal circulation, all patients require blood typing and assessment of Rh status. All Rh-negative patients should receive prophylaxis with Rh immunoglobulin, 300 μg, to prevent isoimmunization. The mother and fetus require continuous monitoring. The usual markers of severity of maternal illness—blood pressure, heart rate, hematocrit, and arterial partial pressure of carbon dioxide—are not predictive of fetal outcome. All maternal injuries need to be treated as they normally would be, regardless of the pregnancy. Pneumatic antishock devices should be avoided in the pregnant patient, as uterine blood flow is dramatically decreased by these devices. Imaging studies with ultrasound are the first line for assessment. In the second and third trimesters, CT scans of the abdomen and pelvis may be undertaken but they expose the fetus to 5 to 7 cGy of radiation. If peritoneal lavage is necessary, it may be performed with care taken to avoid the uterus during catheter insertion; either an open technique or using ultrasonic guidance are preferable. In severe cases, cesarean section may improve maternal outcome, by removing the placental arteriovenous shunt [90].

Penetrating Trauma

Penetrating injuries to pregnant patients most commonly are gunshot wounds or knife wounds. Pregnant patients have a better prognosis after penetrating abdominal trauma as the large muscular uterus protects maternal vital organs. Maternal visceral injuries complicate 19% of penetrating abdominal trauma with a 3.9% maternal mortality rate [91]. The anterior and central location of the uterus subjects the fetus to significant risk with penetrating wounds. The fetus is injured in 66% of these cases, with a high 40% to 70% fetal mortality rate [92]. The management of these injuries remains controversial. Many experts advocate surgical exploration. Conservative management with imagining and observation also may be considered. Lower abdominal penetrating injuries have a less likely chance of producing maternal organ injury, but carry a significant risk of fetal injury. The best management is to individualize assessment with aggressive surgical intervention when fetal or maternal indicators warrant. A coordinated effort between the trauma surgeon and obstetrician will provide the best outcome for both mother and fetus [91–93].

Advances in management of critically ill pregnant patients, based on randomized controlled trials or meta-analyses of such trials, are summarized in Table 156.4.

TABLE 156.4

SUMMARY OF ADVANCES IN MANAGEMENT OF THE CRITICALLY ILL PREGNANT PATIENT AS IDENTIFIED IN RANDOMIZED CONTROL TRIAL DATA

- Magnetic resonance imaging is used in the second and third trimesters to aid with fetal diagnosis [25,26].
- Magnesium sulfate is preferred treatment for preeclamptic seizures at the time of labor [57,59].
- Coagulopathy associated with abruption placenta should be managed with replacement blood products [64].
- Dexamethasone to treat HELLP syndrome only has minimal affect in the most severe cases [55].

References

1. Kaunitz AM, Hughes JM, Grimes D, et al: Causes of maternal mortality in the United States. *Obstet Gynecol* 65:605, 1985.
2. Varner MW: Maternal mortality in Iowa from 1952 to 1986. *Surg Gynecol Obstet* 168:555, 1989.
3. Maternal Mortality and Morbidity Review Committee: Pregnancy-associated mortality—medical causes of death 1995–1998. *Matern Mortal Morb Rev Mass* 1:1, 2000.
4. Adams JQ, Alexander AM: Alterations in cardiovascular physiology during labor. *Am J Obstet Gynecol* 12:542, 1958.
5. Metcalf J, Veland K: Maternal cardiovascular adjustments to pregnancy. *Prog Cardiovasc Dis* 16:363, 1974.
6. Christianson RE: Studies on blood pressure during pregnancy. Influence of parity and age. *Am J Obstet Gynecol* 125:509, 1976.
7. Caton WL, Roby EC, Reed DE, et al: The circulating red cell volume and body hematocrit in normal pregnancy and the puerperium. *Am J Obstet Gynecol* 61:1207, 1951.
8. Lund CS, Donovan JC: Blood volume during pregnancy. *Am J Obstet Gynecol* 98:393, 1967.
9. Veland K, Novy M, Paterson EN, et al: Maternal cardiovascular dynamics. *Am J Obstet Gynecol* 104:856, 1969.
10. ElKayam V, Gleicher N: Cardiovascular physiology of pregnancy, in Elkayam V, Gleicher N (eds): *Cardiac Problems in Pregnancy*. New York, Alan R. Liss, 1982.
11. Barton WM: The pregnant surgical patient. Medical evaluation and management. *Ann Intern Med* 101:633, 1987.
12. Weinberger SE, Weiss ST, Cohen WR, et al: Pregnancy and the lung. *Am Rev Respir Dis* 127:559, 1980.
13. Awe RJ, Nicotra MB, Newsom TD, et al: Arterial oxygenation and alveolar—arterial gradients in term pregnancy. *Obstet Gynecol* 53:182, 1979.
14. Pritchard JA, Rowland RC: Blood volume changes in pregnancy and the puerperium. *Am J Obstet Gynecol* 88:391, 1964.
15. Barron WM: Medical evaluation of the pregnant patient requiring non-obstetric surgery. *Clin Perinatol* 12:481, 1985.
16. Lindheimer MD, Katz AL: The renal response to pregnancy, in Brenner BM, Rector RC (eds): *The Kidney*. Philadelphia, WB Saunders, 1986.
17. Barron WM, Lindheimer MD: Renal sodium and water handling in pregnancy. *Obstet Gynecol Ann* 13:35, 1984.
18. Brent RL: The effects of embryonic and fetal exposure to x-rays, microwaves, and ultrasound. *Clin Obstet Gynecol* 26:484, 1983.
19. Houston CS: Diagnostic, irradiation of women during the reproductive period. *Can Med Assoc J* 117:648, 1977.
20. Mossman KL, Heil RT: Radiation risks in pregnancy. *Obstet Gynecol* 60:237, 1982.
21. Wagner LK, Archer BR, Zeck OT: Conceptus dose from two state of the art CT scanners. *Radiology* 159:787, 1986.
22. Forsted DH, Kalbhon CL: CT of pregnant women for urinary tract calculi, pulmonary thromboembolism and acute appendicitis. *AJR Am J Roentgenol* 178:1285, 2002.
23. Shellock FG, Kanal E: Bioeffects and safety of MRI procedures, in Edelman RR, Hesselink JR, Zlatkin MB (eds): *Clinical Magnetic Resonance Imaging*. 4th ed. Philadelphia, WB Saunders, 2000, p 935.
24. Wienreb JC, Lowe TW, Santos-Ramos R, et al: Magnetic resonance imaging in obstetric diagnosis. *Radiology* 154:157, 1985.
25. Baker J, Amjad A, Groth M, et al: Bone scanning in pregnant patients with breast carcinoma. *Clin Nucl Med* 12:519, 1987.
26. Husak V, Wiedermann M: Radiation absorbed dose estimated to the embryo from some nuclear medicine procedures. *Eur J Nucl Med* 5:205, 1980.
27. Smith EM, Warner GG: Estimates of radiation dose to the embryo from nuclear medicine procedures. *J Nucl Med* 17:836, 1976.
28. Kalter H, Warkany J: Congenital malformations. *N Engl J Med* 308:491, 1983.
29. Abboud JK, Raya J, Noveshed R, et al: Intrathecal morphine for relief of labor pain in a parturient with severe pulmonary hypertension. *Anesthesiology* 59:477, 1983.
30. Briggs GG, Bodendoter TW, Freeman RK, et al: *Drugs in Pregnancy and Lactation: A Reference Guide to Fetal and Neonatal Risk*. Baltimore, Williams & Wilkins, 1994.
31. Pedersen H, Finster M: Anesthetic risk in the pregnant surgical patient. *Anesthesiology* 51:439, 1979.
32. Shepard TF: Human teratogenicity. *Adv Pediatr* 33:225, 1986.
33. Chow AW, Jewesson RJ: Pharmacokinetics and safety of antimicrobial agents in pregnancy. *Rev Infect Dis* 7:278, 1985.
34. Flessa HC, Klapstrom AB, Glueck MJ, et al: Placental transport of heparin. *Am J Obstet Gynecol* 93:570, 1965.
35. Sanson BJ, Lensing AW, Prins ML, et al: Safety of low molecular weight heparin in pregnancy: a systematic review. *Thromb Haemost* 81:668, 1999.
36. Forestier F, Daffos F, Capella-Pavlousky M: Low molecular weight heparin (PK 10169) does not cross the placenta during the second trimester of

pregnancy: study by direct fetal blood sampling under ultrasound. *Thromb Res* 34:507, 1984.
37. Ginsberg B, Hirsch J, Turner C, et al: Risks to the fetus of anticoagulant therapy during pregnancy. *Thromb Haemost* 61:197, 1989.
38. Hall JG, Pavi RM, Wilson KM: Maternal and fetal sequelae of anticoagulants during pregnancy. *Am J Med* 68:122, 1978.
39. Vitale N, DeFeo M, DeSanto LS, et al: Dose dependant fetal complications of warfarin in pregnant women with mechanical heart valves. *J Am Coll Cardiol* 33:1642, 1999.
40. Magee LA, Cham C, Waterman ES, et al: Hydralazine for the treatment of severe hypertension in pregnancy: meta-analysis. *BMJ* 327:555, 2003.
41. Magee LA, Ornstein MP, Von Dadelszen P: Fortnightly review: management of hypertension in pregnancy. *BMJ* 318:1332, 1999.
42. *Working Group Report on High Blood Pressure in Pregnancy*. Washington, DC, National Institutes of Health, 2000.
43. Duley L, Henderson-Smart DJ: Drugs for treatment of very high blood pressure during pregnancy. *Cochrane Database Syst Rev* 4:CD001449, 2002.
44. O'Mailia JJ, Sander GE, Giles TD: Nifedipine associated myocardial ischemia or infarction in the treatment of hypertensive emergencies. *Ann Intern Med* 107:185, 1987.
45. Navity J, Cefalo RC, Lewis PE: Fetal toxicity of nitroprusside in the pregnant ewe. *Am J Obstet Gynecol* 139:708, 1981.
46. Wheeler AJ, James FM III, Melo PS, et al: Effect of nitroglycerin and nitroprusside in the uterine vasculature of gravid ewes. *Anesthesiology* 52:390, 1980.
47. Ralston DH, Shreider SM, deLorimer AA: Effect of equipotent ephedrine, metaraminol, mephentermine and methoxamine on uterine blood flow in the pregnant ewe. *Anesthesiology* 40:354, 1974.
48. Sibai BM: Pitfalls in diagnosis and management of pre-eclampsia. *Am J Obstet Gynecol* 159:1, 1988.
49. Everitt RB, Worliy RJ, MacDonald J, et al: Effect of prostaglandin synthetic inhibitors on pressor response to angiotensin II in human pregnancy. *J Clin Endocrinol Metab* 46:1007, 1978.
50. Gant NF, Chand S, Whalley PG, et al: The nature of pressor responsiveness to angiotensin II in human pregnancy. *Obstet Gynecol* 43:854, 1974.
51. Mastrogiannis DS, O'Brien WF, Krammer K, et al: Potential role of endothelial in normal and hypertensive pregnancies. *Am J Obstet Gynecol* 165:1771, 1997.
52. Meyer NL, Mercer BM, Friedman SA, et al: Urinary dipstick protein: a poor predictor of absent or severe proteinuria. *Am J Obstet Gynecol* 170:137, 1994.
53. Weinstein L: Syndrome of hemolysis, elevated liver enzymes and low platelet count a severe consequence of hypertension in pregnancy. *Am J Obstet Gynecol* 142:159, 1982.
54. Mabie W, Gonzalez AR, Sibas BM, et al: A comprehensive trial of labetalol and hydralazine in the acute management of severe hypertension complicating pregnancy. *Obstet Gynecol* 70:328, 1987.
55. Fonseca JE, Mendez F, Catano C, et al: Dexamethasone treatment does not improve the outcome of women with HELLP syndrome: a double-blind, placebo-controlled, randomized clinical trial. *Am J Obstet Gynecol* 193:1591, 2005.
56. Lucas MJ, Leveno KJ, Cunningham FG: A comparison of magnesium sulfate with phenytoin for the prevention of eclampsia. *N Engl J Med* 333:201, 1995.
57. Witlin AG, Sibai B: Magnesium sulfate therapy in preeclampsia and eclampsia. *Obstet Gynecol* 92:883, 1998.
58. The Magpie Trial Collaborative Group: Do women with pre-eclampsia, and their babies, benefit from magnesium sulfate? The Magpie Trial: a randomized placebo controlled trial. *Lancet* 359:1877, 2002.
59. Sibai B: Diagnosis, prevention, and management of eclampsia. *Obstet Gynecol* 105:402, 2005.
60. Clark S: Placenta previa accreta and prior cesarean section. *Obstet Gynecol* 66:89, 1985.
61. Brenner WE, Edelmar DA, Hendricks CA: Characteristics of patients with placenta previa and results of expectant management. *Am J Obstet Gynecol* 132:180, 1978.
62. Hurd WW, Meodornik M, Hertzberg V, et al: Selective management of abruptio placentae: a prospective study. *Obstet Gynecol* 61:467, 1983.
63. Luea WE: Post partum hemorrhage. *Clin Obstet Gynecol* 23:637, 1980.
64. Cassidy GN, Moore DL, Bridenbaugh D: Postpartum hypertension after use of vasoconstrictor and oxytocin drugs: etiology incidences, complications and treatment. *JAMA* 172:101, 1960.
65. Hayashi RH, Castello MS, Noah ML: Management of severe postpartum hemorrhage due to uterine atony using an analogue of prostaglandin F_2. *Obstet Gynecol* 58:426, 1981.
66. Leary AM: Severe bronchospasm and hypotension after 15 methyl prostaglandin F_2 & in atonic postpartum hemorrhage: *J Obstet Anesth* 3:42, 1994.
67. Schwartz PE: The surgical approach to severe postpartum hemorrhage, in Bereowitz RL (ed): *Critical Care of the Obstetric Patient*. New York, Churchill Livingstone, 1983, p 285.
68. Pais SO, Glickman M, Schwartz P, et al: Embolization of pelvic arteries for control of postpartum hemorrhage. *Obstet Gynecol* 53:754, 1980.
69. Ferguson JE II, Bourgesis FJ, Underwood P: B-Lynch suture for postpartum hemorrhage. *Obstet Gynecol* 95:1020, 2000.
70. Clark SL, Hankins GD, Dudley DA, et al: Amniotic fluid: analysis of the national registry. *Am J Obstet Gynecol* 172:1158, 1995.
71. Gilbert W, Danielsen B: Amniotic fluid embolism: decreased mortality in a population based study. *Obstet Gynecol* 93:973, 1999.
72. Lee W, Gensberg KA, Cotton DB, et al: Squamous and trophoblastic cells in the maternal pulmonary circulation identified by invasive hemodynamic monitoring during the postpartum period. *Am J Obstet Gynecol* 155:159, 1986.
73. Davies S: Amniotic fluid embolism and isolated disseminated intravascular coagulation. *Can J Anaesth* 46:456, 1999.
74. Gilmore DA, Wakins J, Secrest J, et al: Anaphylactoid syndrome of pregnancy: a review of the literature with latest management and outcome data. *AANA J* 71:120, 2003.
75. Esplin MS, Branch DW: Diagnosis and management of thrombotic microangiopathies during pregnancy. *Clin Obstet Gynecol* 42:360, 1999.
76. Von Baeyer H: Plasmapheresis in thrombotic microangiopathy-associated syndromes: review of outcome data derived from clinical trials and open studies. *Ther Apher* 6:320, 2002.
77. Wyllie BF, Garg AX, Macnab J, et al: Thrombotic thrombocytopenic purpura/haemolytic uraemic syndrome: a new index predicting response to plasma exchange. *Br J Haematol* 132:204, 2006.
78. Michael M, Elliott EJ, Ridley GF, et al: Interventions for haemolytic uraemic syndrome and thrombotic thrombocytopenic purpura. *Cochrane Database Syst Rev* CD003595, 2009.
79. Bell WR, Braine HG, Ness PM, et al: Improved survival in thrombotic thrombocytopenia purpura hemolytic uremic syndrome. *N Engl J Med* 325:398, 1991.
80. Amy B, McManus W, Goodwin C, et al: Thermal injury in the pregnant patient. *Surg Gynecol Obstet* 161:209, 1985.
81. Rayburn W, Smith B, Feller I, et al: Major burns during pregnancy: effects on fetal well-being. *Obstet Gynecol* 63:392, 1984.
82. Lavery J, Staton-McCormick M: Management of moderate to severe trauma in pregnancy. *Obstet Gynecol Clin North Am* 22:69, 1995.
83. Peckham AF, King RA: A study of intercurrent conditions observed during pregnancy. *Am J Obstet Gynecol* 87:609, 1963.
84. Drost RF, Rosemary AS, Sherman HF, et al: Major trauma in pregnant women: maternal/fetal outcome. *J Trauma* 30:576, 1990.
85. Rothenberger D, Quattlebaum F, Perry J, et al: Blunt maternal trauma, a review of 103 cases. *J Trauma* 18:173, 1978.
86. Goodwin T, Breen M: Pregnancy outcome and fetal maternal hemorrhage after non-catastrophic trauma. *Am J Obstet Gynecol* 162:665, 1990.
87. Dahmus M, Sebai B: Blunt abdominal trauma, are there any predictive factors for abruptio placentae or maternal fetal distress? *Am J Obstet Gynecol* 169:1054, 1993.
88. Connolly A, Katz V, Bash K, et al: Trauma and pregnancy. *Am J Perinatol* 14:331, 1997.
89. Pearlman M, Tintinalli J, Lorenz R: A prospective controlled study of outcome after trauma during pregnancy. *Am J Obstet Gynecol* 162:1502, 1990.
90. Pearlman M, Tintinalli J, Lorenz R: Blunt trauma during pregnancy. *N Engl J Med* 323:1609, 1990.
91. Committee on Trauma, American College of Surgeons: *Advanced Trauma Life Support Program for Physicians*. Chicago, American College of Surgeons, 1997.
92. Buchsbaum H (ed): *Penetrating Injury of the Abdomen. Trauma in Pregnancy.* Philadelphia, Saunders, 1979, p 82.
93. Awwad J, Azar G, Seoud M, et al: High velocity penetrating wounds of the gravid uterus: review of 16 years of civil war. *Obstet Gynecol* 83:259, 1994.

ARTHUR L. TRASK • STEPHEN L. BARNES

CHAPTER 157 ■ SHOCK: AN OVERVIEW

MICHAEL L. CHEATHAM, ERNEST F.J. BLOCK, HOWARD G. SMITH,
MATTHEW W. LUBE AND JOHN T. PROMES

Shock is one of the most complex conditions encountered in the critically ill patient. The term "shock" encompasses a broad range of pathologic processes that may require diametrically opposed methods of treatment. The underlying cause may be quite evident, as in traumatic hemorrhage, or occult, as in severe sepsis due to infection. Delayed shock resuscitation is associated with significant morbidity and mortality. Therapy must commonly be initiated before all clinical information and diagnostic studies are available. As a result, the intensivist must possess a solid understanding of the common shock states, their clinical presentation, and the necessary therapeutic interventions. Although mortality remains high, increasing application of early goal-directed resuscitation to achieve defined physiologic endpoints has significantly improved patient outcome from shock [1–3].

Over the centuries, shock has been defined in various ways. In 1534, Ambrose Pare wrote that shock was caused by "toxins in the blood" and recommended phlebotomy as the treatment, a practice that persisted until the early 1800s. By that time, shock-associated hypotension was well recognized as was the detrimental impact of bloodletting on systemic perfusion [4]. Although subsequent early definitions of shock lack scientific terminology, they compensate for this in their simplicity. John Collins Warren described shock as "a momentary pause in the act of death," whereas Samuel David Gross defined shock as "a rude unhinging of the machinery of life" [5]. In the 1930s, Alfred Blalock published his classic series of investigations into shock confirming that hypotension was due to loss of blood and plasma into the tissues (so called "third-space losses" due to increased capillary permeability) [6]. Blalock found that the hypotension and high mortality of shock were reversible through the infusion of crystalloid solutions to replace lost intravascular and interstitial fluid, and that simple reinfusion of lost blood was not sufficient. Shock was thus identified as a systemic disorder caused by increased vascular permeability, interstitial edema, and intravascular volume depletion with the classic signs of hypotension, decreased urinary output, and multiple organ failure.

The importance of regional end-organ perfusion, rather than simply systemic blood flow alone, is the singular concept for recognizing and improving patient outcome from shock. Perfusion may be decreased either systemically (as in hemorrhagic or cardiogenic shock) or only regionally (as in septic shock) with global perfusion being normal or even elevated. Regardless of cause or severity, all forms of shock have the commonality of perfusion inadequate to meet metabolic demands at the cellular level. Decreased organ perfusion leads to tissue hypoxia, anaerobic metabolism, activation of the inflammatory cascade, and eventually organ dysfunction. The ultimate consequences of shock depend on the degree and duration of hypoperfusion, the number of organs affected, and the presence of prior organ dysfunction. The challenges to the intensivist are identifying the hypoperfused state, diagnosing its cause, and rapidly restoring cellular perfusion.

PHYSIOLOGY

Significant progress has been made in elucidating the cellular basis for shock. Although low blood pressure and other vital sign derangements were previously thought to be sufficient to cause shock, they are now recognized as being signs of a complex physiologic cascade of events. The delivery and consumption of oxygen at the mitochondrial level, as well as the adequate removal of cellular waste products, is of paramount importance to survival. Cellular hypoxia leads to local vasoconstriction, thrombosis, anaerobic glycolysis, release of superoxide radicals, accumulation of pyruvate and lactate, and intracellular acidosis. The severity of a patient's acidemia, demonstrated by elevated base deficit or lactate levels, correlates with the lethality of shock [7].

In patients who experience such an anaerobic insult, injured tissues and damaged cells release a variety of intracellular mediators which initiate the proinflammatory cascade. Cytokines are small polypeptides and glycoproteins produced by a variety of immunologic cells that are responsible for many of the sequelae seen during shock. Tumor necrosis factor alpha (TNF-α) is one of the earliest cytokines released and is a product of monocytes, macrophages, and T-cells. TNF-α levels rise after a variety of cellular insults and cause hypotension, procoagulant activity, muscle breakdown, catabolism and cachexia. TNF-α levels have been seen to correlate with mortality in animal models of hemorrhagic shock [8]. Produced by macrophages and endothelial cells, interleukin-1 (IL-1) has similar effects, producing fever and anorexia. Activated T-cells produce interleukin-2 which augments cell mediated immunity. Interleukin-6, together with IL-1, mediates the acute phase response to injury and may have a role in the development of acute lung injury. Interleukin-8 is chemotactic for neutrophils and interleukin-12 has a role in cell-mediated immunity by promoting the differentiation of T-helper 1 cells. A variety of "anti-inflammatory" cytokines such as growth hormone interleukin-4, interleukin-10, interleukin-13, soluble TNF receptors (sTNFR), and IL-1 receptor antagonists (IL-1ra) are simultaneously released in an attempt to counterbalance the proinflammatory cascade.

These proinflammatory and counter-regulatory substances may lead to processes that may not be in the best interest of the patient in shock. The body's (mal)adaptive response to the primary injury or inciting event may cause secondary injury to previously unaffected cells and organs leading to impaired perfusion, cellular death, and organ dysfunction. This systemic inflammatory response syndrome, if left unabated, may result in the multiple organ dysfunction syndrome, a common cause of shock-related morbidity and mortality.

IL-1 also activates the patient's hypothalamopituitary axis (HPA) as well as the neuroendocrine response to critical illness. HPA activation releases adrenocorticotrophic hormone (ACTH) that acts on the adrenal gland to stimulate glucocorticoid (cortisol) production. Appropriate adrenocortical response to shock is essential for patient survival. Relative adrenal insufficiency during critical illness is a commonly underappreciated reason for a patient's failure to respond to resuscitative interventions [9]. Vasopressin (antidiuretic hormone [ADH]) is cosecreted from the posterior pituitary and potentiates the effect of ACTH. In addition to its primary osmoregulatory role in resorption of water from the nephron's collecting duct, ADH is also a potent vasoconstrictor, improving systemic perfusion, and promoting gluconeogenesis and glycolysis to provide much needed metabolic substrates.

The neuroendocrine response to shock involves many counter-regulatory substances. Epinephrine and norepinephrine are produced from the adrenal medulla and synapses of the sympathetic nervous system respectively. β-Adrenergic stimulation results in increased heart rate and contractility, and α-adrenergic stimulation increases systemic vascular resistance and blood pressure through peripheral vasoconstriction. Blood is thus shunted from less essential organs preserving flow to the heart and brain. Sympathetic stimulation also causes venoconstriction accelerating venous return to the central circulation. Through their metabolic effects, catecholamine secretion contributes to stress induced hyperglycemia, a common problem during critical illness. The renin angiotensin system is activated resulting in the release of angiotensin-II (AT-II), another potent vasoconstrictor and stimulus for aldosterone secretion. Aldosterone promotes salt and water conservation at the level of the distal renal tubule in an attempt to preserve intravascular volume. It also regulates acid-base and potassium homeostasis. Glucagon is produced by the pancreatic alpha islet cells and, unlike insulin, has a catabolic role. Release of many of these substances also leads to decreased levels of circulating insulin. The resultant catabolic state characterized by insulin resistance, hyperglycemia, lipolysis, free fatty acid formation, ketogenesis, erosion of lean body mass and negative nitrogen balance may last for weeks to months.

CLASSIFICATION

Shubin and Weil's classic paper distinguished the various forms of shock with respect to cardiovascular parameters [10]. Four categories of inadequate systemic perfusion were described: (a) hypovolemic, (b) obstructive, (c) cardiogenic, and (d) distributive. Although new etiologies of shock (e.g., adrenal insufficiency of critical illness) have recently received significant attention, they are easily placed into one of these physiologic descriptions.

Hypovolemic Shock

Hypovolemic shock is the most common form of shock. Almost all forms include some component of hypovolemia as a result of decreased intravascular volume or "preload." The sympathetic response to reduced preload is arterial vasoconstriction, diverting blood from the splanchnic viscera, skin, and skeletal muscle. Physical findings include cold clammy skin, tachypnea, tachycardia, and low urinary output, all a result of either hypovolemia or compensatory mechanisms.

Hypovolemic shock is stratified into four classes based on the degree of circulating volume loss (Table 157.1). It is important to recognize that significant blood volume may be lost in the absence of any clinical signs. Compensatory mechanisms allow systemic blood pressure to be maintained and a well-compensated patient may display tachycardia as the only objective clinical abnormality, even with a blood volume loss of up to 30%. Hypovolemic shock may be further subclassified as either hemorrhagic or nonhemorrhagic. Hemorrhagic shock may be visibly apparent (external blood loss from traumatic injury) or occult (chronic gastrointestinal hemorrhage). Emphasis on hemorrhage control rather than simply volume replacement is an essential difference in the management of hemorrhagic shock [11,12]. Nonhemorrhagic hypovolemic shock is seen in a number of pathologic states and may be caused by absolute loss of total body fluid volume and/or migration of acellular fluid from the intravascular to the interstitial compartment (third spacing). Third spacing of fluid occurs predictably in severe illnesses such as pancreatitis, small bowel obstruction, and burns. Volume depletion may also occur as a consequence of uncompensated gastrointestinal, urinary, or evaporative losses. It is imperative that the intensivists focus on resuscitation of the patient's intravascular volume as opposed to total body volume. Failure to do so will uniformly result in under-resuscitation and poor patient outcome.

Obstructive Shock

Obstructive forms of shock are those in which the underlying pathology is a mechanical obstruction to normal cardiac output (CO) with a resulting diminution in systemic perfusion. Cardiac tamponade is an example of obstructive shock. A small amount of fluid (usually less than 200 mL) within a noncompliant pericardium may produce significant myocardial compression [13]. Clinical signs of tamponade include jugular venous distention and a central venous pressure (CVP) waveform

TABLE 157.1

CLASSIFICATION OF SHOCK[a]

	Class I	Class II	Class III	Class IV
Blood loss (mL)	Up to 750	750–1,500	1,500–2,000	≥2,000
Blood loss (% blood volume)	Up to 15	15–30	30–40	≥40
Pulse rate	<100	>100	>120	≥140
Blood pressure	Normal	Normal	Decreased	Decreased
Pulse pressure	Normal/increased	Decreased	Decreased	Decreased
Capillary refill	Normal	Decreased	Decreased	Decreased
Respiratory rate	14–20	20–30	30–40	>35
Urinary output (mL/h)	30 or more	20–30	5–15	Negligible
Central nervous system	Slightly anxious	Anxious	Anxious, confused	Confused, lethargic
Fluid replacement	Crystalloid	Crystalloid	Crystalloid + blood	Crystalloid + blood

[a]Estimates based on a 70-kg male.
Modified from Committee on Trauma of the American College of Surgeons: *Advanced Trauma Life Support for Doctors*. Chicago, American College of Surgeons, 2008, p 61.

demonstrating a rapid "x" descent and a blunted "y" descent due to inability of the heart to fill during diastole. Pulsus paradoxus, an exaggerated fluctuation in arterial pressure caused by changes in intrathoracic pressure during respiration, may be present. Formal echocardiography is helpful in making the diagnosis although recent advances in the use of bedside ultrasonography by noncardiologists have demonstrated excellent sensitivity and rapid performance of the examination [14].

Pulmonary venous thromboembolism is another example of obstructive shock and may present as profound circulatory collapse. CO is restricted either by mechanical obstruction of the pulmonary arterial tree or by pulmonary hypertension induced by release of secondary mediators. Additional findings include elevated CVP and pulmonary hypertension, but normal pulmonary artery occlusion pressure (PAOP). Through similar mechanisms, venous air embolism can completely obstruct pulmonary arterial blood flow, with ensuing cardiac arrest. Central hemodynamics mimic those of pulmonary embolism. Although numerous causes exist, of greatest concern are the placement and removal of central venous catheters and surgical procedures in which the operative site is more than 5 cm above the right atrium [15]. Venous air embolism is diagnosed by auscultation of the classic "mill wheel" heart murmur. Immediate placement of the patient in a head-down, left lateral decubitus position is advocated, as are attempts to aspirate air from the right ventricle through a central venous catheter.

Finally, tension pneumothorax may cause shock through obstruction of venous return. Elevated intrapleural pressure collapses intrathoracic veins resulting in inadequate venous filling. Tension pneumothorax should be diagnosed by physical examination and not by radiography. Needle decompression often restores venous filling sufficiently until a thoracostomy tube can be placed.

Cardiogenic Shock

In cardiogenic shock, the underlying defect is primary ventricular pump failure, the most common cause of coronary artery disease related mortality. The foundations of ventricular failure include (a) myocardial infarction with loss of myocardium, (b) reduced contractility (cardiomyopathy), (c) ventricular outflow obstruction (aortic stenosis or dissection), (d) ventricular filling anomalies (atrial myxoma, mitral stenosis), (e) acute valvular failure (aortic or mitral regurgitation), (f) cardiac dysrhythmias, and (g) ventriculoseptal defects. Most often, cardiogenic shock is a direct or indirect consequence of acute myocardial infarction.

Cardiogenic shock due to left ventricular infarction suggests that more than 40% of the left ventricle is involved [16]. On physical examination, signs of peripheral vasoconstriction are evident and oliguria is common. The typical hemodynamic profile includes systemic hypotension with decreased CO and elevated PAOP. Physical examination findings of pulmonary and peripheral edema as well as hepatomegaly may suggest volume overload, but are commonly due to third spacing of fluid due to shock with relative intravascular volume depletion being present. In such situations, hemodynamic monitoring using echocardiography or a volumetric pulmonary artery catheter may provide additional diagnostic information clarifying the patient's true volume status.

Right ventricular dysfunction as a consequence of inferior wall myocardial infarction carries a better prognosis than left-sided failure. Diagnosis may be suggested by elevated right ventricular diastolic pressure with decreased pulmonary artery pressure [17]. Hypotension caused by right-sided heart failure must be distinguished from left-sided failure because of the significant differences in their management. Shock from right-sided failure is corrected by volume resuscitation to maintain right ventricular preload while left-sided failure is treated by volume restriction to reduce myocardial work. If inotropes are indicated, agents that do not increase pulmonary vascular resistance should be chosen [18].

Dysrhythmias are another source of cardiogenic shock. In addition to malignant dysrhythmias, such as ventricular fibrillation, atrial dysrhythmias such as atrial fibrillation or flutter as well as supraventricular tachycardia are common in the critically ill and may result in shortened diastolic filling time with a profound decrease in CO.

Distributive Shock

The classic hemodynamic profile of septic shock (high CO and systemic hypotension) has prompted some clinicians to institute antimicrobial therapy and search for an infectious source in any patient who exhibits these cardiac parameters. Such hyperdynamic patterns, however, are seen in non-infectious conditions as well including anaphylaxis, spinal cord injury, and severe liver dysfunction. The term distributive shock, rather than septic shock, is therefore used to account for these dissimilar diseases with a common hemodynamic picture.

The management of septic shock remains a major challenge to the intensivist [1–3]. A milieu of inflammatory cytokines, bacterial factors, and complement and coagulation activation combine to induce the complex hemodynamic pattern characteristic of septic shock. In most forms of shock, illness leads to a low CO state with elevated systemic vascular resistance (SVR) and reduced mixed venous oxygen saturation (SvO_2). Early septic shock, however, is manifested by normal-to-low cardiac filling pressures, increased CO, decreased SVR, and increased SvO_2 [19]. Despite elevated systemic blood flow and oxygen delivery (DO_2), abnormalities exist in tissue oxygen extraction at the cellular level, perhaps through disruption of normal mitochondrial metabolic pathways [20,21]. Sepsis-induced myocardial depression may be demonstrated through decreased ejection fraction, right ventricular dysfunction, and left ventricular dilation. In the later stages of septic shock, cardiac function deteriorates with the patient's hemodynamic status mimicking that of cardiogenic shock with decreased CO and increased SVR [22].

Anaphylaxis represents another form of distributive shock in which histamine-mediated vasodilatation occurs. The most common causes are medications, insect envenomations, blood products, radiographic contrast media, and food allergies [23]. Reactions severe enough to result in shock occur shortly after exposure to the offending agent. Physical findings include a dermatologic reaction (erythema, urticaria) and obstructive respiratory processes. Occasionally, the reaction is severe enough to produce shock through myocardial depression.

Neurogenic shock, another form of distributive shock, occurs as a result of upper thoracic spinal cord injury with hypotension, bradycardia, and warm, dry skin due to loss of sympathetic vascular tone. Although euvolemic, patients demonstrate relative hypovolemia due to vasodilatation of the intravascular space. If hypotension does not respond to volume resuscitation, it may be treated with vasopressors and any bradycardia may be corrected with atropine. In the trauma patient, hemorrhage should always be excluded before attributing shock to a neurogenic source [24].

Over the last decade, endocrine insufficiency as a result of critical illness has been recognized as an underappreciated cause of distributive shock. This relative adrenal insufficiency may worsen the impact of the various shock states as the patient is unable to respond appropriately to the stress of their critical illness [25,26]. Corticosteroid supplementation in such patients can significantly improve systemic perfusion as well as reduce the patient's requirement for vasopressor support.

PHYSIOLOGIC MONITORING

Vital sign derangements are typically the first indication that a shock state is present. Normalization of such parameters signifies that the patient is appropriately responding to resuscitative therapy. Physiologic monitoring is thus essential to both the diagnosis and management of shock. Such monitoring typically begins with the use of routine vital signs, but may progress to the application of invasive monitoring techniques.

Vital Signs

The diagnosis of shock was originally based on abnormalities in a patient's vital signs. Until the late 1960s, the presence of tachycardia and hypotension was considered synonymous with shock. Over time, it became apparent that normalization of heart rate, blood pressure, temperature, and urinary output was not necessarily sufficient to reverse a patient's shock state. Critically ill patients continued to have a high incidence of multiple organ failure and mortality despite seemingly adequate resuscitation based on restoration of vital signs to "normal." Shock is therefore defined by the adequacy of end-organ perfusion rather than derangements in vital signs alone. Nevertheless, these physiologic parameters remain the foundation for the initial recognition that shock is present.

Heart Rate

Alterations in heart rate are common during shock. Tachycardia is most common and is usually a direct effect of intravascular volume loss in where heart rate increases to maintain adequate CO and DO_2 to tissues. These increases may become pathologic if inadequate diastolic filling time results in decreased stroke volume. Tachycardia can be used to predict the presence of intravascular volume depletion and its resolution to suggest volume resuscitation adequacy [27]. Decreased heart rate, in response to a volume challenge, can be a simple and useful test for diagnosing hypovolemia.

Bradycardia is usually representative of severe physiologic derangement and impending cardiovascular collapse. Its presence in a critically ill patient demands immediate attention. Patients receiving beta-blocker therapy or with high spinal cord injuries or pacemakers may not be able to increase their heart rate and compensate for their shock. Patients with an inappropriately low heart rate and inadequate CO will benefit from increasing heart rate by withholding beta-blocker therapy, use of chronotropic medications, or reprogramming their pacemakers to a higher rate.

Blood Pressure

Hypertension is an uncommon finding in shock. Patients are typically hypotensive due to the presence of hypovolemia, decreased cardiac contractility, or systemic vasodilatation. Normotension should be restored as quickly as possible to improve tissue perfusion and oxygen delivery at the cellular level. Blood pressure may be measured either noninvasively or invasively. Both techniques are subject to certain mechanical and physiologic measurement errors, or "dynamic response artifacts," that can result in inappropriate therapy if unrecognized by the clinician [28]. Because of these intrinsic monitoring errors, systolic blood pressure (SBP) and diastolic blood pressure (DBP) measurements may vary widely from one measurement technique to another. The mean arterial pressure (MAP), however, will remain fairly consistent regardless of the measurement method and any artifact present. As a result, MAP should be used to titrate resuscitative therapies rather than SBP or DBP. MAP is calculated as

$$\text{MAP} = [\text{SBP} + 2(\text{DBP})]/3$$

Temperature

Patient temperature, although not indicative of either the presence or absence of shock, may help define the cause and can have significant prognostic value [29,30]. The presence of hypothermia (core body temperature less than 96.8°F or 36.0°C) suggests severe physiologic derangement and has a significant impact on patient survival [31]. Hypothermia places the patient at risk for cardiac dysrhythmias, acute renal failure, and refractory coagulopathy [32]. Although hypothermia reduces metabolic activity of the body, rewarming significantly increases global metabolic demands and oxygen consumption ($\dot{V}O_2$). Such demands may exceed the patient's capacity to deliver oxygen to the cells, resulting in an oxygen transport imbalance. Care must be taken to ensure adequate DO_2 and tissue perfusion during rewarming. Because of its significant morbidity and mortality, nontherapeutic hypothermia should be avoided or rapidly corrected in most critically ill patients [29,30].

Urine Output

Inadequate renal blood flow results in decreased urinary output. Oliguria is one of the earliest signs of inadequate perfusion at the tissue level. Worsening renal function is an important indicator of the presence of shock. Decreases in urine output as a result of hypovolemia are seen before changes in heart rate or blood pressure (Table 157.1). Improvements in urine volume in response to fluid loading can guide shock resuscitation as long as confounding factors are not present (e.g., diabetes insipidus, diabetic ketoacidosis, and diuretic therapy).

Pulse Oximetry

Technologic advances in the 1970s and 1980s led to the widespread introduction of pulse oximetry as the "fifth" vital sign [33]. Pulse oximetry is now routinely used in the critically ill as a noninvasive method of continuously monitoring arterial oxygen saturation. This addition to the traditional four vital signs serves two purposes. First, it provides an early warning of hypoxemia, allowing corrective interventions to be made. Second, it can be used as an endpoint in the resuscitation of patients and in the assessment of oxygen transport balance.

Hemodynamic Monitoring

In 1970, Swan and Ganz introduced the flow-directed pulmonary artery catheter, allowing clinicians to measure pulmonary artery pressures at the bedside [34]. In 1972, addition of a temperature thermistor provided the ability to calculate CO. These advancements provided clinicians with the ability to assess a variety of new hemodynamic parameters evaluating patient preload, contractility, and afterload. In the 1980s, continuous mixed venous oximetry was added as the importance of DO_2, $\dot{V}O_2$, and oxygen transport balance in the diagnosis and management of the shock states became clear. By the early 1990s, catheters capable of calculating right ventricular volumes became available, further improving preload assessment. Current pulmonary artery catheters continuously assess hemodynamic and oxygen transport variables providing the clinician with minute-by-minute assessments of cardiopulmonary function by which to guide resuscitation. Although pulmonary artery catheterization is performed with much less frequency than in years past, it remains an important monitoring technology for the most critically ill patients with shock and has recently been demonstrated to improve patient outcome when used in a goal-directed fashion [35,36]. A variety of other hemodynamic monitoring techniques have been developed including arterial pressure wave contour analysis, esophageal Doppler, and transesophageal echocardiography among others. Regardless of the method by which hemodynamic data is obtained, a thorough understanding of the available hemodynamic and oxygenation variables is essential if resuscitative therapy is to improve patient outcome from shock (Tables 157.2 and 157.3) [37].

Pressure and Pressure-Derived Variables

Pressure variables form the foundation for physiologic monitoring in shock assessment. It is important to recognize, however, that the absolute value of any single pressure variable is not as important as the trend, calculated variables, and perfusion pressures that may be identified using this pressure.

TABLE 157.2

HEMODYNAMIC VARIABLES

Variable (abbreviation)	Unit	Normal range
Measured variables		
Systolic blood pressure (SBP)	mm Hg	90–140
Diastolic blood pressure (DBP)	mm Hg	50–90
Systolic pulmonary artery pressure (PAS)	mm Hg	15–30
Diastolic pulmonary artery pressure (PAD)	mm Hg	4–12
Pulmonary artery occlusion pressure (PAOP)	mm Hg	2–15
Central venous pressure (CVP)	mm Hg	0–8
Heart rate (HR)	beats/min	Varies by patient
Cardiac output (CO)	L/min	Varies by patient
Stroke volume (SV)	mL/beat	Varies by patient
Right ventricular ejection fraction (RVEF)	Fraction	0.40–0.60
Calculated variables		
Mean arterial pressure (MAP)	mm Hg	70–105
Mean pulmonary artery pressure (MPAP)	mm Hg	9–16
Cardiac index (CI)	L/min/m^2	2.8–4.2
Stroke volume index (SVI)	mL/min/m^2	30–65
Systemic vascular resistance index (SVRI)	Dyne/sec/cm^5	1,600–24,00
Pulmonary vascular resistance index (PVRI)	Dyne/sec/cm^5	250–340
Left ventricular stroke work index (LVSWI)	g × m/m^2	43–62
Right ventricular stroke work index (RVSWI)	g × m/m^2	7–12
Coronary perfusion pressure (coronary PP)	mm Hg	>50
Cerebral perfusion pressure (cerebral PP)	mm Hg	50–70
Abdominal perfusion pressure (APP)	mm Hg	>60
Right ventricular end-diastolic volume index (RVEDVI)	mL/m^2	80–120
Global end-diastolic volume index (GEDVI)	mL/m^2	600–800
Stroke volume variation (SVV)	%	<10
Pulse pressure variation (PPV)	%	<10
Body surface area (BSA)	m^2	Varies by patient

TABLE 157.3

OXYGENATION VARIABLES

Variable (abbreviation)	Unit	Normal range
Measured variables		
Arterial oxygen tension (PaO_2)	mm Hg	70–100
Arterial carbon dioxide tension ($PaCO_2$)	mm Hg	35–50
Arterial oxygen saturation (SaO_2 or SpO_2)	Fraction	0.92–0.98
Mixed venous oxygen saturation (SvO_2)	Fraction	0.65–0.75
Mixed central venous oxygen saturation ($ScvO_2$)	Fraction	0.70–0.80
Mixed venous oxygen tension (PvO_2)	mm Hg	35–40
Hemoglobin (Hgb)	g/dL	13–17
Calculated variables		
Oxygen delivery index (DO_2I)	mL/min/m^2	500–650
Oxygen consumption index ($\dot{V}O_2I$)	mL/min/m^2	110–150
Arterial oxygen content (CaO_2)	mL O_2/dL blood	16–22
Venous oxygen content (CvO_2)	mL O_2/dL blood	12–17
Arterial–venous oxygen content difference ($Ca–vO_2$)	mL O_2/dL blood	3.5–5.5
Oxygen utilization coefficient (OUC)	Fraction	0.25–0.35

Mean Arterial and Mean Pulmonary Arterial Pressure. MAP has been discussed previously. Mean pulmonary arterial pressure (MPAP) is the equivalent pressure for the pulmonary circuit (Fig. 157.1) and is calculated using pulmonary arterial systolic (PAS) and diastolic (PAD) pressure:

$$MPAP = [PAS + 2(PAD)]/3$$

Mean pressures should be used to guide decision making and resuscitative therapy whenever possible as they are less

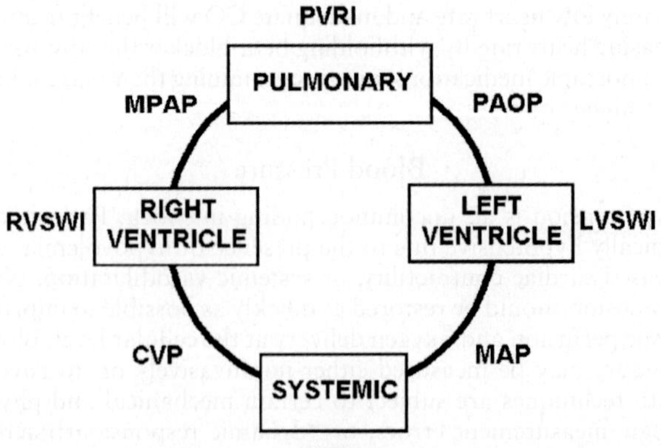

FIGURE 157.1. Hemodynamic calculations. PAOP, pulmonary artery occlusion pressure; CVP, central venous pressure; MAP, mean arterial pressure; MPAP, mean pulmonary artery pressure; SVRI, systemic vascular resistance index; PVRI, pulmonary vascular resistance index; LVSWI, left ventricular stroke work index; RVSWI, right ventricular stroke work index.

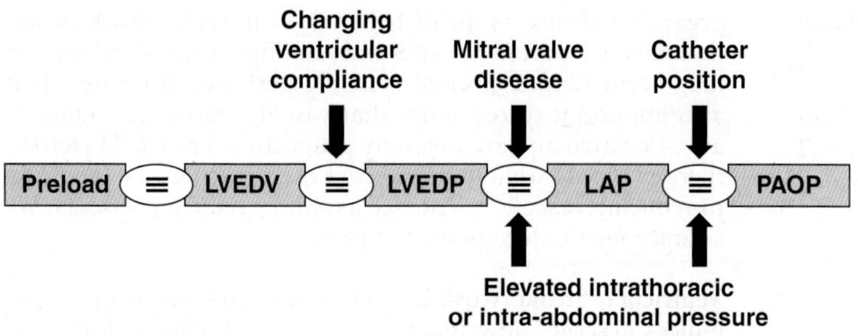

FIGURE 157.2. The "PAOP assumption": Why intracardiac filling pressures do not accurately estimate preload status? LVEDV, left ventricular end-diastolic volume; LVEDP, left ventricular end-diastolic pressure; LAP, left atrial pressure; PAOP, pulmonary artery occlusion pressure. [Adapted from Cheatham ML: Right ventricular end-diastolic measurements in the resuscitation of trauma victims. *Int J Crit Care* 7:165–176, 2000, with permission.]

subject to monitoring artifacts. They are also essential components to calculate vascular resistance and cardiac work.

Pulmonary Artery Occlusion and Central Venous Pressure. Fluid administration is an essential element in the initial resuscitation of almost all forms of shock. Intracardiac-filling pressure measurements such as PAOP or "wedge" and CVP are commonly used to estimate intravascular volume or "preload." Preload, by the Frank–Starling Law, is defined in terms of myocardial fibril length at end-diastole. Because this is clinically immeasurable, several assumptions are made to use PAOP to clinically assess the preload status of the left ventricle (Fig. 157.2). These assumptions are frequently invalid in critically ill patients due to changing ventricular compliance caused by a variety of factors. As a result, PAOP measurements should be carefully considered as estimates of intravascular volume status in the patient with shock [38–40]. In fact, reliance on PAOP measurements for preload assessment in critically ill patients may lead to inappropriate interventions in more than 50% of patients [41]. The trend rather than the absolute value of such measurements in response to therapeutic interventions is of greater value. The optimal PAOP is that value which, through careful evaluation of the patient's hemodynamic status, is determined to optimize systemic perfusion (CO) and cellular oxygenation (DO_2, $\dot{V}O_2$). For similar reasons, absolute CVP measurements do not accurately portray left ventricular volume status or ventricular function [38–41]. As with PAOP, the trend of CVP measurements in response to therapeutic measures may be of value.

Perfusion Variables

The importance of adequate end-organ perfusion in correcting the shock state cannot be overemphasized. The following perfusion variables are easily calculated and represent important resuscitation endpoints in the critically ill.

Coronary Perfusion Pressure. Maintaining adequate coronary perfusion pressure (PP) should be a primary goal in the resuscitation of any patient in shock. Patients with preexisting coronary artery disease may have marginal myocardial blood flow, which is only worsened by inadequate systemic perfusion during shock. Coronary PP is calculated as the pressure change across the coronary artery during maximal blood flow:

$$\text{coronary perfusion} = \text{pressure change across the coronary artery}$$
$$\text{coronary PP} = \text{DBP} - \text{PAOP}$$

The goal should be to maintain coronary PP greater than 50 mm Hg. Failure to maintain this level of perfusion increases the risk for myocardial ischemia and infarction. Note that DBP and not SBP is the critical determinant of coronary perfusion as maximal myocardial blood flow occurs during diastole. PAOP estimates myocardial wall tension and resistance to perfusion by approximating end-diastolic pressure in the left ventricle.

Cerebral Perfusion Pressure. Monitoring cerebral perfusion pressure is important in the head-injured patient with increased intracranial pressure (ICP) [42]. Because the brain is enclosed within the skull with little room for expansion, increases in ICP and development of cerebral edema can have significant and detrimental effects on cerebral blood flow and oxygenation. Monitoring of ICP is an important component of the hemodynamic monitoring of patients with brain injury and shock. Cerebral PP is calculated as the pressure change across the brain:

$$\text{cerebral perfusion} = \text{pressure change across the brain}$$
$$\text{cerebral PP} = \text{MAP} - \text{ICP (or CVP, whichever is higher)}$$

The goal should be to maintain a cerebral PP of 50 to 70 mm Hg [42]. This may be accomplished by either increasing MAP (using a vasopressor such as norepinephrine) or decreasing intracerebral volume (through the use of mannitol or hypertonic fluids), thereby decreasing ICP. Maintenance of a cerebral PP >70 mm Hg does not appear to provide a survival benefit and may lead to potentially detrimental over-resuscitation.

Abdominal Perfusion Pressure. Analogous to coronary and cerebral PP, abdominal perfusion pressure (APP) has been identified as a valuable parameter in the resuscitation of patients with elevated intra-abdominal pressure (IAP), a condition present in over half of all ICU patients [43,44]. IAP is most commonly determined as intravesicular or "bladder" pressure by transducing the patient's indwelling urinary catheter [45,46]. APP is calculated as the pressure change across the abdominal organs:

$$\text{abdominal perfusion} = \text{pressure change across the abdominal organs}$$
$$\text{APP} = \text{MAP} - \text{IAP}$$

Failure to maintain APP ≥60 mm Hg has been found to discriminate between survivors and nonsurvivors [43]. Maintenance of adequate APP through a balance of judicious fluid resuscitation and application of vasoactive medications has been demonstrated to reduce the incidence of acute renal failure [47].

Blood Flow and Flow-Derived Variables

Critically ill patients with shock and systemic malperfusion frequently benefit from calculation of blood flow-related variables such as CO and stroke volume (SV). Flow-related variables are used with pressure variables to calculate vascular resistance and estimate the work performed by the left and right ventricles. Such advanced hemodynamic monitoring should be implemented whenever a patient fails to respond to resuscitation as expected.

Interpatient variability makes it difficult to assign a normal range to flow-derived variables. What might be an adequate CO for a 50-kg woman is inadequate for a 150-kg man. To normalize these measurements and allow comparison from patient to patient, flow-derived variables are indexed to body surface area (BSA), obtained from a nomogram. Indexed variables, such as cardiac index (CI) and stroke volume index (SVI), are more meaningful because normal ranges aid in interpretation.

All flow-derived hemodynamics should be indexed to facilitate comparison with accepted normal ranges.

Cardiac Index and Stroke Volume Index. CI is the total blood flow from the heart (in liters per minute) divided by BSA. SVI is the volume of blood ejected from the heart per beat, divided by BSA:

$$\text{CI} = \text{cardiac output/BSA}$$
$$\text{SVI} = \text{CI/heart rate}$$

Most shock states have a decreased CI as a result of intravascular volume depletion, poor underlying cardiac pump function, increased vascular resistance, or a combination of these factors. To maintain CI, tachycardia is the usual response to inadequate preload and a low SVI. Appropriate therapy is to restore intravascular volume and increase SVI, thus improving CI. An increased CI may be seen in early septic shock, but may also be seen with other nonshock hyperdynamic states, such as cirrhosis, pregnancy, and high-performance athletes.

Systemic Vascular Resistance Index/Pulmonary Vascular Resistance Index. According to Ohm's law, the resistance of an electrical circuit is equal to the voltage difference across the circuit divided by the current. A simplified view of the circulatory system can be likened to an electrical circuit in which the resistance across the systemic or pulmonary vascular beds is calculated using Ohm's law (Fig. 157.1):

Resistance = voltage difference/current
Vascular resistance = pressure change/total blood flow
SVRI = change in pressure across the systemic circuit (mm Hg)/total blood flow (L/min/m^2)
SVRI (in dynes/sec/cm^5) = (MAP − CVP)(79.9)/CI
PVRI = change in pressure across the pulmonary circuit (mm Hg)/total blood flow (L/min/m^2)
PVRI (in dynes/sec/cm^5) = (MPAP − PAOP)(79.9)/CI

The constant, 79.9, is used to convert mm Hg · L per minute to the more physiologic units of dynes per seconds per · cm^5.

Increased SVRI is commonly seen in obstructive, hypovolemic, late septic, and cardiogenic shock. Systemic resistance may also rise in nonshock states such as pheochromocytoma (secondary to increased endogenous catecholamine output). Decreased SVRI is common in distributive shock states (neurogenic, early septic, endocrine shock). Vasodilators such as sodium nitroprusside, nitroglycerin, and other antihypertensives reduce SVRI.

Increased PVRI is indicative of pulmonary hypertension and may be classified as being either primary or secondary. Primary pulmonary hypertension is an intrinsic lung disease developing over many years and typically refractory to treatment. Secondary pulmonary hypertension may develop as a result of acute respiratory distress syndrome, application of positive end-expiratory pressure (PEEP), or development of mitral or aortic stenosis. Treatment of pulmonary hypertension begins with institution of increased inspired oxygen fractions due to oxygen's effect as a potent pulmonary vasodilator. Nitroglycerin and morphine sulfate also are helpful in the acute treatment of pulmonary hypertension. Decreased PVRI occurs in the setting of various shock states. Treatment is rarely instituted to specifically increase PVRI alone.

Perfusion pressure and vascular resistance determine total blood flow to an organ, but absolute values of these determining factors do not define the shock state. For example, a high vascular resistance is commonly compensatory for reduced systemic perfusion pressure. The same numeric value of high resistance may contribute to organ dysfunction when it is so high that perfusion pressure cannot overcome it. When organ blood flow is maldistributed, as in septic shock or abdominal compartment syndrome, multiple organ dysfunction may occur despite normal systemic perfusion pressures. It is also important to recognize that vascular resistance numbers are calculated and are inversely proportional to CI. Therefore, therapy should usually be directed at enhancing CI in addition to reducing vascular resistance as simply reducing vascular resistance may reduce perfusion pressure.

Ventricular Stroke Work Indices. The ventricular stroke work indices describe how much work the ventricles perform and can identify patients with poor cardiac function. They may also be useful to construct ventricular function curves to assess a patient's response to therapy. As with vascular resistance, the work performed by the heart can also be calculated using the laws of physics. Work is calculated as the force generated multiplied by the distance over which the work is performed. Clinically, the force generated (per area) by each side of the heart is the change in pressure it creates across the ventricle. The distance (per area) is the volume of blood ejected with each beat (SVI) normalized for patient size. Therefore,

Ventricular stroke work index = change in pressure × change in volume
Left ventricular stroke work index (LVSWI) = (MAP − PAOP) (SVI) (0.0136) (g · m/m^2)
Right ventricular stroke work index (RVSWI) = (MPAP − CVP) (SVI) (0.0136) (g · m/m^2)
The constant (0.0136) converts mm Hg · L/beat · m^2 to g · m/m^2.

Increased LVSWI/RVSWI is relatively uncommon, but may be encountered in patients with ventricular hypertrophy, pulmonary hypertension, or in athletes. Decreased LVSWI/RVSWI is much more common and may be seen in various shock states; heart failure; aortic or mitral stenosis; myocardial depression, ischemia, or infarction; or advanced age. When evaluating decreased ventricular stroke work, it is important to keep in mind that the decreased function may be due to decreased intravascular volume (decreased SVI), changes in vascular resistance (increased MAP or MPAP), or decreased contractility. If preload and afterload remain constant, decreases in stroke work indicate decreases in ventricular contractility.

Volumetric Variables

The clinical accuracy of pressure-based monitoring techniques is limited by a variety of factors including proper catheter positioning, pressure transducer calibration, and pressure waveform interpretation. By the Frank–Starling principle, ventricular preload is defined as myocardial muscle fiber length at end-diastole with the appropriate clinical correlate being end-diastolic volume. As ventricular chamber volume cannot be directly measured, intracardiac filling pressures such as PAOP and CVP have been used as estimates of end-diastolic volume under the erroneous assumption that ventricular compliance remains constant. Ventricular compliance, however, is *constantly* changing in the critically ill, resulting in a variable relationship between pressure and volume. Further, PAOP and CVP must be measured relative to an arbitrary reference point (typically the perceived position of the right atrium) and are subject to the impact of increased intrathoracic and intra-abdominal pressure (as may occur with acute lung injury, PEEP, intra-abdominal hypertension, abdominal compartment syndrome, etc.) (Fig. 157.2). Although attempts may be made to calculate transmural PAOP and CVP values, these estimates are inexact and the level of precision necessary to measure CVP accurately at the bedside is rarely performed [48]. As a result, changes in PAOP and CVP as commonly measured do not directly reflect changes in intravascular volume in the critically ill and may lead to inappropriate clinical interventions and under-resuscitation [41].

In the 1990s, a new generation of monitoring technologies were introduced that provide volumetric as opposed to pressure-based estimates of hemodynamic function. These included continuous CO, right ventricular ejection fraction (RVEF), and right ventricular end-diastolic volume index (RVEDVI), via a modified pulmonary artery catheter, or global ejection fraction (GEF), global end-diastolic volume index (GEDVI), intrathoracic blood volume index (ITBVI), and extravascular lung water (EVLW) via an arterial catheter using the arterial pulse contour analysis technique. Continuous volumetric monitoring provides a minute-by-minute assessment of patient response to therapeutic interventions, potentially allowing more rapid and effective resuscitation compared to traditional pressure-based monitoring techniques [27,49–52]. Both RVEDVI and GEDVI have been demonstrated to be superior to PAOP and CVP as predictors of preload recruitable increases in CI during shock resuscitation [27,40,41,49–52]. Further, several studies have demonstrated either significantly improved organ perfusion and function or increased patient survival when volumetric resuscitation endpoints are employed [27,49,50]. More recently, arterial pulse contour analysis has been used to measure stroke volume variation (SVV), the variation in beat-to-beat stroke volume during a single respiratory cycle, as well as pulse pressure variation (PPV), the beat-to-beat difference between SBP and DBP. Both of these parameters have been suggested to be valuable predictors of hypovolemia and fluid responsiveness [53]. These advanced hemodynamic monitoring techniques are appropriate for patients with shock who fail to respond appropriately to initial attempts at resuscitation using conventional endpoints.

Oxygen Transport Variables

With recognition of the importance of oxygen delivery (DO_2) and oxygen consumption ($\dot{V}O_2$) in the treatment of the various shock states, monitoring of a patient's oxygen transport balance has become commonplace (Table 157.3). The foremost question in critical care is whether oxygen transport to the tissues is sufficient to meet the demand for oxygen at the cellular level.

Oxygen transport represents the balance between supply and demand. When supply exceeds demand, the cellular oxygen requirements of the body are being met, and normal metabolic processes proceed uninhibited. When oxygen supply equals demand, vital functions may progress normally, but with little physiologic reserve, such that a relatively minor insult can upset the oxygen transport balance. In such a situation, organs that possess a high baseline oxygen extraction, such as the heart, are at significant risk for ischemia. When shock-induced systemic or regional malperfusion exists, oxygen demand exceeds supply, and the available cellular oxygen is inadequate to support normal physiology. Energy must therefore be produced via anaerobic metabolism with production of lactic acid as a by-product. As lactic acid cannot be reutilized in the absence of oxygen, it accumulates leading to metabolic acidosis, cellular injury, and cellular death. Left unchecked, this imbalance in oxygen transport will result in the development of multisystem organ failure and patient death. The role of the intensivist is to recognize oxygen supply imbalances at the cellular level, initiate therapeutic interventions to increase oxygen delivery, prevent further organ dysfunction, ensure adequate physiologic oxygen reserve to cope with acute increases in oxygen demand, and improve patient outcome from shock.

Knowledge of the oxygen transport equations is essential to understanding the pathophysiology and appropriate treatment for the various shock states. Any assessment of oxygen transport begins with the calculation of DO_2 and $\dot{V}O_2$. To accomplish this, the oxygen content of the blood at various points in the systemic and pulmonary circulation must be identified (Fig. 157.3). Central to these calculations are the recognition that (1) oxygen may be either "bound" or "unbound" to erythrocytes, (2) each gram of hemoglobin (Hgb) can carry up to 1.34 mL of oxygen, (3) the solubility of oxygen in blood is 0.0031 mL per dL, and (4) the amount of oxygen carried by Hgb depends upon its saturation.

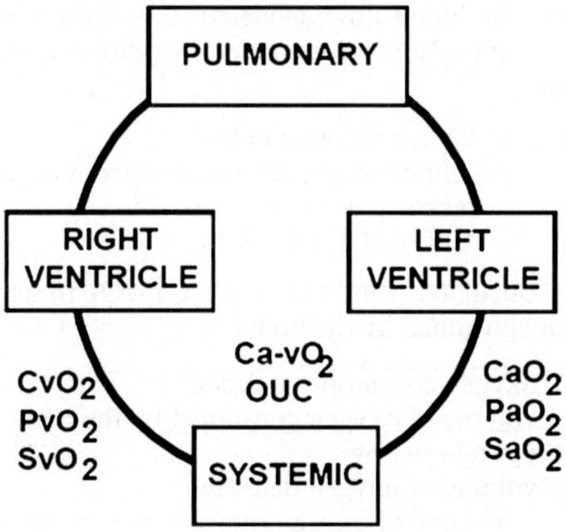

FIGURE 157.3. Oxygenation calculations. CaO_2, arterial oxygen content; PaO_2, arterial oxygen tension; SaO_2, arterial oxygen saturation; CvO_2, venous oxygen content; PvO_2, venous oxygen tension; SvO_2, mixed venous oxygen saturation; $Ca\text{–}vO_2$, arterial–venous oxygen content difference; OUC, oxygen-utilization coefficient.

The oxygen content of arterial blood as it leaves the heart may be calculated as:

$$\begin{aligned} CaO_2 &= \text{oxygen bound to arterial Hgb} + \text{oxygen dissolved in arterial blood} \\ &= (1.34 \times \text{Hgb} \times SaO_2) + (PaO_2 \times 0.0031) \end{aligned}$$

In a similar fashion, the oxygen content of venous blood as it returns to the heart may be calculated as:

$$\begin{aligned} CvO_2 &= \text{oxygen bound to venous Hgb} + \text{oxygen dissolved in venous blood} \\ &= (1.34 \times \text{Hgb} \times SvO_2) + (PvO_2 \times 0.0031) \end{aligned}$$

The partial pressure of oxygen in venous blood (PvO_2) is typically 35 to 40 Torr. As a result, for most purposes, the contribution of dissolved oxygen in venous blood is so small as to be clinically insignificant and is often disregarded. The arterial–venous oxygen content difference ($Ca\text{–}vO_2$) therefore represents the amount of oxygen extracted by the tissues and organs of the body. It is frequently elevated in shock, due to the increased oxygen demands of injured tissue, and represents an important resuscitation endpoint. The $Ca\text{–}vO_2$ is calculated as:

$$\begin{aligned} Ca\text{–}vO_2 &= \text{arterial–venous oxygen content difference} \\ &= CaO_2 - CvO_2 \end{aligned}$$

$Ca\text{–}vO_2$ is an important indicator of the relative balance between CI and $\dot{V}O_2$. A $Ca\text{–}vO_2$ in excess of 5.5 mL per dL of oxygen suggests that CI is inadequate to meet cellular oxygen demands and that anaerobic metabolism and lactic acidosis may result. Maneuvers to improve CI and DO_2 should be performed to meet the patient's cellular oxygen demand and reduce $Ca\text{–}vO_2$ to a normal range.

The volume of oxygen delivered from the left ventricle (DO_2) and the amount of oxygen consumed by the organs ($\dot{V}O_2$) provide the clinician with vital information by which to assess the patient's overall oxygen transport balance. DO_2 is determined by two factors: the volume of oxygen in blood

(CaO_2) and the blood flow delivered (CI). Values indexed to BSA allow comparison across patients of differing body habitus, so that

$$\begin{aligned} DO_2I &= \text{oxygen delivery index} \\ &= \text{volume of oxygen pumped from the left ventricle per minute per m}^2 \\ &= (CaO_2)\,(CI)\,(10\ \text{dL/L}) \end{aligned}$$

$\dot{V}O_2$ is calculated similarly, using $Ca\text{–}vO_2$ to account for the oxygen consumed by the body:

$$\begin{aligned} \dot{V}O_2I &= \text{oxygen consumption index} \\ &= \text{volume of oxygen consumed by the body per min per m}^2 \\ &= \text{volume of oxygen delivered} \\ &\quad - \text{volume of oxygen returned per minute per m}^2 \\ &= (Ca\text{–}vO_2)\,(CI)\,(10\ \text{dL/L}) \end{aligned}$$

One of the most important determinants of tissue DO_2I is Hgb concentration. The optimal Hgb concentration during shock resuscitation remains a topic of significant debate. Although previous clinical trials concluded that a Hgb concentration of 7 g per dL is sufficient and that transfusion to higher levels provides no survival benefit, it must be remembered that hemodynamically unstable patients, including hemorrhagic shock victims, were excluded from the study [54]. Further, patients with recent acute myocardial infarction or unstable angina were felt to require a higher Hgb concentration to ensure adequate DO_2I. More recent studies in hemorrhagic shock patients, however, have demonstrated significantly improved survival among patients resuscitated to a Hgb >11 g per dL [55]. Recent evidence-based medicine guidelines have advocated higher Hgb levels in patients with myocardial ischemia, severe hypoxemia, acute hemorrhage, cyanotic heart disease, lactic acidosis, or closed head injury [2]. Although a subject of continued controversy, the optimal Hgb concentration can appropriately be considered the level that restores a patient's oxygen transport balance while minimizing the potentially detrimental infectious and immunosuppressive effects of allogeneic blood.

Shock Resuscitation Adequacy

Resuscitation of the critically ill patient who has developed one of the shock states is an ongoing process. It requires constant assessment of the patient's response to resuscitative therapy. In the patient whose shock state and oxygen transport balance fail to improve, the administered therapies must be reconsidered and adjusted as necessary to achieve the desired outcome. To guide this dynamic resuscitation, "resuscitation adequacy" endpoints may be employed.

Mixed Venous Oximetry

Continuously measured SvO_2 correlates well with calculated oxygen extraction ratios and represents a valuable endpoint for assessing the adequacy of shock resuscitation [56]. The four factors affecting SvO_2 are (1) SaO_2, (2) Hgb concentration, (3) CO, and (4) $\dot{V}O_2$. Increases in any of the three variables affecting DO_2 (SaO_2, Hgb concentration, and CO) result in an increase in SvO_2, whereas uncompensated increases in $\dot{V}O_2$ result in a decrease in SvO_2. The SvO_2 measured in the proximal pulmonary artery is a global flow-weighted average of the effluent blood from all perfused vascular beds. SvO_2 does not reflect the oxygenation of nonperfused tissues; thus, a normal SvO_2 does not mean that all organs are adequately oxygenated. In the absence of a pulmonary artery catheter, the mixed central venous oxygen saturation ($ScvO_2$) may be measured either intermittently using a venous blood gas drawn from a central venous catheter whose tip is located in the superior vena cava or continuously via a special oximetric central venous catheter [1]. It should be recognized that SvO_2 and $ScvO_2$ are not equivalent measurements with normal $ScvO_2$ values being 0.05 to 0.1 higher than SvO_2.

A low SvO_2 (less than 0.65) virtually always indicates an unfavorable disturbance in the normal balance between DO_2 and $\dot{V}O_2$. Normal or high values of SvO_2 are more difficult to interpret. A normal SvO_2 in a patient with otherwise normal hemodynamics generally indicates a stable condition with a satisfactory oxygen transport balance. A high SvO_2 (greater than 0.75) is difficult to interpret and implies a either a maldistribution of peripheral blood flow, providing some vascular beds with DO_2 in excess of consumption, or the presence of "shunting" in which oxygenated blood is returned to the heart without releasing its bound oxygen. This state of vaso-deregulation is often associated with high-flow states such as cirrhosis, sepsis, pregnancy, and inflammation.

Arterial Lactate

As discussed previously, shock is hypoperfusion resulting in inadequate DO_2 to meet tissue oxygen demand at the cellular level. The resulting oxygen debt forces cells to switch to anaerobic metabolism to make adenosine triphosphate by the inefficient method of glycolysis. The by-products of glycolysis are hydrogen ion, pyruvate, and lactate. If aerobic metabolism is restored through resuscitation and improved tissue DO_2, the excess hydrogen ion is buffered, and both pyruvate and lactate are metabolized to yield adenosine triphosphate. Under continued anaerobic conditions, however, hydrogen ion and lactate accumulate within the cell, resulting in acidosis, injury, and cellular death. Serum lactate levels therefore provide the clinician with an excellent laboratory marker of the presence of anaerobic metabolism as well as resuscitation adequacy.

Elevated serum lactate levels indicate that the patient has sustained a period of inadequate perfusion and oxygenation within the past 6 to 12 hours with the severity of lactic acidosis directly correlating with the severity of the shock insult. If such levels are rising, anaerobic metabolism remains ongoing and the magnitude of resuscitative therapy should be increased. A decreasing lactate level suggests that resuscitation has been adequate and anaerobic metabolism has resolved. Although serum lactate levels identify the presence of anaerobic metabolism, they are not specific in identifying the location of abnormal regional perfusion. Further, profound hypoperfusion can exist despite normal lactate levels when there is inadequate blood flow to ischemic tissues. Some septic patients have increased lactate levels in the absence of hypoperfusion as a result of increased aerobic glycolysis. In this situation, the elevated lactate continues to be significant despite resuscitation and is an indicator of a potentially severe pathologic process. Patients with significant hepatic dysfunction do not clear lactate normally, and will therefore manifest higher lactate levels in the absence of anaerobic metabolism [57].

Elevated lactate concentrations predict an increased mortality rate. The magnitude and duration of the elevation correlate with mortality and reversal of hyperlactatemia suggests a better prognosis. Mortality rates of 24% to 86% are seen if lactate has not normalized by 48 hours [57–61].

Base Deficit

The presence of an elevated base deficit correlates directly with the presence and severity of shock [61–63]. It predicts fluid resuscitation requirements and is a rapidly obtainable monitor of resuscitation adequacy [62]. Further, base deficit normalizes rapidly with restoration of aerobic metabolism, making it a useful physiologic marker by which to guide resuscitation. Base deficit must be interpreted with caution in the patient who has received exogenous sodium bicarbonate as it will no longer be useful as a predictor of resuscitation adequacy.

Rutherford et al. identified that patients younger than 55 years of age without a head injury who demonstrate a base deficit of −15 mmol per L have a 25% mortality rate [63]. Patients with a head injury or patients older than 55 years without a head injury have a 25% mortality at a base deficit of −8 mmol per L. These authors suggested that base deficit could be used to identify patients in severe shock who might benefit from having operative procedures terminated early (so-called "damage control laparotomy").

Treatment Principles

Patient morbidity and mortality after development of one of the shock syndromes correlates directly with the duration and severity of malperfusion. The intensivist must therefore rapidly diagnose the presence and cause of shock, restore systemic and regional perfusion to prevent ongoing cellular injury, and prevent the development of end-organ failure. The intensivist must command a strong understanding of the various therapeutic options for each of the shock states. Using the hemodynamic variables and calculations previously described, shock resuscitation should focus on assessment of preload, contractility, afterload, and oxygen transport balance with the intent to optimize the patient's end-organ perfusion and cellular oxygenation. In addition, the etiology for the shock state should be investigated to treat and/or correct the underlying cause. This may be simple, as in needle decompression for a tension pneumothorax, or may be complex, as in the treatment of sepsis.

Preload

In almost all shock states, a component of diminished preload, either relative or absolute, exists. Therefore, the initial therapeutic intervention for almost all patients in shock should be a crystalloid bolus of 20 mL per kg with subsequent resuscitation guided by signs of improved organ perfusion: reduction in tachycardia, restoration of normotension, maintenance of adequate urinary output, return of normal mentation, improvement in systemic oxygenation, and/or correction of abnormalities in serum lactate or base deficit. In patients with preexisting cardiopulmonary disease or those who do not respond to resuscitation as expected, invasive hemodynamic monitoring may be of value in achieving these goals.

Over-resuscitation with intravenous fluids should be avoided and can cause acute lung injury, intra-abdominal hypertension, and abdominal compartment syndrome. Although some authors have suggested the use of colloid-based resuscitation to avoid such complications, large-scale clinical trials and meta-analyses have failed to demonstrate a survival advantage to such an approach [64,65]. A subset analysis of the SAFE trial demonstrated an increased mortality in head injured patients who received colloid-based resuscitation [66]. A balanced resuscitation using a combination of crystalloid and colloid reduces the required resuscitation volume and appears to be associated with decreased organ dysfunction and failure [65].

In patients with hemorrhagic shock, blood product transfusions should be considered early in the volume resuscitation phase as increasing evidence from the battlefield has demonstrated improved survival with early, aggressive blood, plasma, and platelet transfusions to restore adequate hemoglobin concentration and normal coagulation [55]. Current evidence suggests that a 1:1:1 ratio of packed red blood cells/plasma/platelets reduces the morbidity and mortality of hemorrhagic shock [67,68].

Contractility

Resuscitative therapy should optimize the patient's heart rate. Although tachycardia may partially compensate for low perfusion, further increases in heart rate may only decrease diastolic filling of the heart and reduce CO. Treatment of pain and anxiety as well as control of supraventricular tachyarrhythmias in the volume-resuscitated patient can improve CO. In bradycardia from neurogenic shock, atropine-induced blockage of parasympathetic stimulation may help ameliorate the hypoperfusion by raising heart rate and CO. Patients taking beta-blockers who have inappropriately low heart rates may benefit from administration of both calcium and glucagon. Those with pacemakers who are unable to raise their own heart rates in response to shock will frequently benefit from resetting their pacemakers to a more physiologically appropriate higher rate.

Contractility agents should be considered only after adequate attempts to improve preload have been made. Dopamine, a naturally occurring catecholamine that is the immediate precursor of norepinephrine, is a widely used agent with a variable dose response. Classically, low rate (0 to 3 μg per kg per minute) or so-called "renal dose" dopamine was advocated to increase glomerular filtration rate, renal blood flow, and urinary output. The clinical benefit of such therapy, however, has been disproven and dopamine's use in this fashion has largely been abandoned [69]. In moderate doses (5 to 10 μg per kg per minute), cardiac contractility and heart rate are increased through stimulation of cardiac beta-receptors. High-dose dopamine therapy (10 μg per kg per minute and higher) results in stimulation of α-adrenergic receptors, elevating systemic blood pressure. Although a valuable tool in improving cardiac performance, dopamine should be used with caution in patients with coronary artery stenosis because of the potential risk of tachycardia and increased myocardial oxygen demand.

Dobutamine is a synthetic catecholamine that also acts on β_1-receptors, but, unlike dopamine, does not directly release norepinephrine. Dobutamine has both chronotropic and systemic vasodilatory effects, reducing afterload and increasing CO in the weakened heart. However, it should be used with caution in hypovolemic, vasodilated states, as it may decrease blood pressure and increase heart rate, leading to reduced systemic perfusion [70].

Norepinephrine is a naturally occurring catecholamine with both α- and β-adrenergic activity. As a potent vasoconstrictor, there is some reluctance to use this agent because of its possible effects on mesenteric and renal blood flow. However, in the setting of an appropriately volume-repleted patient who remains hypotensive, norepinephrine has been shown to be effective and safe and may have beneficial effects on renal function [71]. It should be considered the vasopressor of choice of all but the cardiogenic shock states [2].

Amrinone is a noncatecholamine intravenous inotrope that, like dobutamine, has vasodilatory effects. Its mechanism of action is as a phosphodiesterase-III inhibitor, raising intracellular cyclic adenosine monophosphate levels. In patients with shock due to congestive heart failure, amrinone increases stroke volume without an effect on heart rate. In some patients with hypovolemic shock, its vasodilatory properties preclude its use because of dramatic hypotension.

Afterload

If preload is optimized and hemodynamic goals have still not been met, afterload should be assessed and corrected as needed. The persistently hypotensive patient should not be considered a candidate for afterload reduction. In patients with hypertension or even normotension, however, afterload reduction may allow for improved CO and, hence, improved resuscitation especially in patients with decreased contractility.

Sodium nitroprusside is a commonly used agent with the advantages of rapid onset and short duration, making it ideal for titration in the hemodynamically labile patient. Nitroprusside acts as both a venous and arterial vasodilator, in essentially equal amounts. However, it should be used with caution in patients with coronary artery disease when concerns of coronary steal and myocardial ischemia exist. Alternatively, intravenous nitroglycerin may be used. Although primarily affecting venous capacitance, nitroglycerin also decreases arterial resistance and may improve CO. Angiotensin-converting enzyme–inhibiting agents may also be of significant value in reducing afterload in the normovolemic patient with poor cardiac function.

Afterload may also be reduced mechanically, using a percutaneously placed intra-aortic balloon counterpulsation pump (IABP). IABP is most commonly used in myocardial infarction and in the immediate postoperative period following coronary artery bypass. IABP provides mechanical afterload reduction and improves coronary artery perfusion. IABP demonstrates survival benefit primarily in myocardial infarction patients who have reversible pathology and has been used successfully in high-risk patients undergoing noncardiac surgery [72].

Although afterload reduction may be beneficial in improving cardiac performance, the patient with aortic stenosis leading to shock may be harmed by use of these agents. In this disease, left ventricular wall tension remains high, and afterload reduction only serves to reduce coronary perfusion by reducing coronary perfusion pressure.

In septic and neurogenic shock, it will often be necessary to counteract the vasodilatory effects of the underlying disease process. Recent studies suggest that norepinephrine should be used as the first-line agent and vasopressin in low doses (0.01 to 0.04 U per minute) should be added when patients fail to respond to norepinephrine. Vasopressin should be used with caution in patients with poor cardiac function [2]. Studies in Europe with terlipressin, a synthetic vasopressin analogue with theoretical advantages over arginine vasopressin, are ongoing [73].

Oxygen Transport

The goal of shock resuscitation is to improve tissue oxygenation so that oxygen delivery meets the demand of cells to function aerobically. Beginning in 1977, Shoemaker et al. suggested in a series of clinical trials that resuscitation to achieve "supranormal" CI (>4.5 L per minute per m^2), DO_2I (>600 mL per minute per m^2), and $\dot{V}O_2I$ (>170 mL per minute per m^2) levels was associated with improved high-risk patient survival following operative procedures [74,75]. Subsequent trials, however, identified that it is a patient's ability to spontaneously reach such supranormal levels of oxygen transport that is predictive of survival and not the applied intervention itself [74–79]. In fact, Balogh et al. have demonstrated that supranormal resuscitation is associated with a higher incidence of over-resuscitation, intestinal malperfusion, abdominal compartment syndrome, multiple system organ failure, and death [80]. They concluded that traumatic shock patients should be resuscitated to achieve a DO_2I of 500 mL per minute per m^2 during the first 24 hours of resuscitation and that maintaining such a level beyond 24 hours is rarely beneficial unless evidence of ongoing shock is present. The potential benefits of adequate sedation and analgesia as a method to reduce oxygen demand must always be considered in any patient who presents with shock.

SYSTEMATIC APPROACH TO THE TREATMENT OF SHOCK

Perhaps most noteworthy in the recent literature on the treatment of shock are multiple studies demonstrating that a proactive, systematic, evidence-based approach to shock resuscitation improves patient outcome (Table 157.4) [1–3]. The Surviving Sepsis Campaign is a multimodality approach to timely resuscitation of the septic patient encompassing diagnosis, source control, fluid resuscitation, vasoactive medications, appropriate antimicrobial therapy, correction of oxygen transport inequalities, low-dose steroid administration for relative adrenal insufficiency, selective use of recombinant human activated protein C, targeted blood product administration, mechanical ventilation strategies geared at reducing barotrauma, sedation, and neuromuscular blocking protocols that include daily interruption, glycemic control, deep venous thrombosis prophylaxis, and stress ulcer prophylaxis [2,3]. This comprehensive approach to the critically ill patient has also been applied with marked success outside the ICU setting using the "rapid response team" concept to treat nonseptic shock patients as well [81]. Many of these same tenets of shock resuscitation are also applicable to the other shock states that may be encountered.

Shock resuscitation continues to evolve as new research identifies the pathophysiology of the various shock states. Numerous treatments for shock are currently being evaluated

TABLE 157.4

SUMMARY OF ADVANCES IN MANAGING SHOCK BASED ON RANDOMIZED CONTROLLED CLINICAL TRIALS

- Patients with hypotension or evidence of anaerobic metabolism should receive immediate early goal-directed resuscitation to restore systemic perfusion and oxygenation within six hours [1,2]
- Fluid resuscitation using either 0.9% normal saline or 4% albumin may be considered equivalent with similar outcomes in 28-day mortality [64].
- Patients in shock should be resuscitated to maintain a mean arterial pressure ≥65 mm Hg [2,3]
- Centrally administered norepinephrine or dopamine should be considered the vasopressors of choice for noncardiogenic shock resuscitation [2]
- Dobutamine is the inotropic agent of choice for cardiogenic shock [2]
- Low-dose dopamine infusions should not be used for renal protection [69]
- Resuscitation to achieve supranormal levels of oxygen delivery or consumption do not improve patient outcome [78,80]
- Recombinant human activated Protein C should not be administered to septic patients with an APACHE-II <25 [2]
- Corticosteroids should not be used to treat septic shock unless the patient demonstrates evidence of symptomatic adrenal insufficiency [2]
- Transfuse packed red blood cells when hemoglobin decreases to <7.0 gm/dL. A higher hemoglobin level is appropriate in patients with myocardial ischemia, severe hypoxemia, acute hemorrhage, cyanotic heart disease, lactic acidosis, or closed head injury [2,54].
- A 1:1:1 red blood cell/plasma/platelet transfusion strategy should be utilized in patients with massive hemorrhagic shock (≥4 units of packed red blood cells over 1 h or ≥10 units over 24 h [more than one total blood volume]) [67].
- Hypothermia should be rapidly corrected in any patient with shock [30].
- Patients resuscitated to elevated levels of preload have significantly improved visceral perfusion than those resuscitated to normal preload with additional inotropes. Elevated preload levels do not affect pulmonary function [49].

including nitric oxide therapy, levosimendan, intravenous immunoglobulin, continuous hemodiafiltration, factor VIIa, and statin therapy among others [82–86]. Time will determine whether these therapies provide a survival benefit to the patient with shock.

SUMMARY

Shock is a common and highly lethal condition that is commonly encountered in the critically ill patient. Its cause is varied and complex. It may present in a spectrum from subclinical laboratory abnormalities to complete cardiovascular collapse. A high degree of clinical suspicion and thorough evaluation are essential to both making the diagnosis and initiating timely resuscitative therapy. Inadequate tissue perfusion that is unresponsive to initial treatment should lead to early, goal-directed therapy. Correction of abnormalities in ventricular preload, contractility, afterload, and oxygen transport are the first steps to breaking the cycle of cellular injury and microcirculatory failure. Correction of the precipitating, underlying condition is essential for patient survival. Early treatment to predefined physiologic endpoints reduces the potentially devastating complication of end-organ dysfunction and failure.

References

1. Rivers E, Nguyen B, Havstad S, et al: Early goal-directed therapy in the treatment of severe sepsis and septic shock. *N Engl J Med* 345:1368, 2001.
2. Dellinger RP, Levy MM, Carlet JM, et al: Surviving Sepsis Campaign: international guidelines for management of severe sepsis and septic shock: 2008. *Crit Care Med* 36:296, 2008.
3. Levy MM, Dellinger RP, Townsend SR, et al: The Surviving Sepsis Campaign: Results of an international guideline-based performance improvement program targeting severe sepsis. *Crit Care Med* 38:367, 2010.
4. Cheatham ML: The death of George Washington: An end to the controversy? *Am Surg* 74:770, 2008.
5. Gross S: *A System of Surgery: Pathologic, Diagnostic, Therapeutic and Operative*. Philadelphia, Lea and Febiger, 1872.
6. Brooks B, Blalock A: Shock with particular reference to that due to hemorrhage and trauma to muscles. *Ann Surg* 100:728, 1934.
7. Kaplan LJ, Kellum JA: Initial pH, base deficit, lactate, anion gap, strong ion difference, and strong ion gap predict outcome from major vascular injury. *Crit Care Med* 32:1120, 2004.
8. Jiang J, Bahrami S, Leichtfried G, et al: Kinetics of endotoxin and tumor necrosis factor appearance in portal and systemic circulation after hemorrhagic shock in rats. *Ann Surg* 221:100, 1995.
9. Annane D, Sebille V, Charpentier C, et al: Effect of treatment with low doses of hydrocortisone and fludrocortisone on mortality in patients with septic shock. *JAMA* 288:862, 2002.
10. Weil MH, Shubin H: Shock following acute myocardial infarction. Current understanding of hemodynamic mechanisms. *Prog Cardiovasc Dis* 11:1, 1968.
11. Bickell WH, Wall MJ Jr, Pepe PE, et al: Immediate versus delayed fluid resuscitation for hypotensive patients with penetrating torso injuries. *N Engl J Med* 331:1105, 1994.
12. Dutton RP, Mackenzie CF, Scalea TM: Hypotensive resuscitation during active hemorrhage: Impact on in-hospital mortality. *J Trauma* 52:1141, 2002.
13. Shabetai R: Cardiac tamponade, in Shaberai R (ed): *The Pericardium*. New York, Grune & Sutton, 1981, p 224.
14. Rozycki GS, Feliciano DV, Schmidt JA, et al: The role of surgeon-performed ultrasound in patients with possible cardiac wounds. *Ann Surg* 223:737, 1996.
15. Pronovost PJ, Wu AW, Sexton JB: Acute decompensation after removing a central line: practical approaches to increasing safety in the intensive care unit. *Ann Intern Med* 140:1025, 2004.
16. Alonso DR, Scheidt S, Post M, et al: Pathophysiology of cardiogenic shock: quantification of myocardial necrosis: clinical, pathologic and electrocardiographic correlation. *Circulation* 48:588, 1973.
17. Shah PK, Maddahi J, Berman DS, et al: Scintigraphically detected predominant right ventricular dysfunction in acute myocardial infarction: clinical, hemodynamic correlates and implications for therapy and prognosis. *J Am Coll Cardiol* 6:1264, 1985.
18. Babaev A, Frederick PD, Pasta DJ, et al: Trends in management and outcomes of patients with acute myocardial infarction complicated by cardiogenic shock. *JAMA* 294:448, 2005.
19. Wilson RF, Sarver EJ, Leblanc PL: Factors affecting hemodynamics in shock with sepsis. *Ann Surg* 174:939, 1971.
20. Ruokonen E, Takala J, Kari A, et al: Regional blood flow and oxygen transport in septic shock. *Crit Care Med* 21:1296, 1993.
21. Crouser ED, Julian MW, Blaho DV, et al: Endotoxin induced mitochondrial damage correlates with impaired respiratory activity. *Crit Care Med* 30:276, 2002.
22. Parker MM, McCarthy KE, Ognibene FP, et al: Right ventricular dysfunction and dilatation, similar to left ventricular changes, characterize the cardiac depression of septic shock in humans. *Chest* 97:126, 1990.
23. Sampson HA, Munoz-Furlong A, Bock SA: Symposium on the definition and management of anaphylaxis: summary report. *J Allergy Clin Immunol* 115:584, 2005.
24. Zipnick RI, Scalea TM, Trooskin SZ, et al: Hemodynamic responses to penetrating spinal cord injuries. *J Trauma* 35:578, 1993.
25. Marik P, Zaloga G: Adrenal insufficiency during septic shock. *Crit Care Med* 31:141, 2003.
26. Gannon TA, Britt RC: Adrenal insufficiency in the critically Ill trauma population. *Am Surg* 72:373, 2006.
27. Chang MC, Meredith JW: Cardiac preload, splanchnic perfusion, and their relationship during resuscitation in trauma patients. *J Trauma* 42:577, 1997.
28. Poelaert J: Haemodynamic monitoring. *Curr Opin Anaesthesiol* 14:27, 2001.
29. Shafi S, Elliot AC, Gentillelo L: Is hypothermia simply a marker of shock and injury severity or an independent risk factor for mortality in trauma patients? Analysis of a large national trauma registry. *J Trauma* 59:1081, 2005.
30. Clemner TP, Fisher CJ Jr, Bone RC, et al: The Methylprednisolone Severe Sepsis Study Group: hypothermia in the sepsis syndrome and clinical outcome. *Crit Care Med* 20:1395, 1992.
31. Zell SC, Kurtz KJ: Severe exposure hypothermia: a resuscitative protocol. *Ann Emerg Med* 14:339, 1985.
32. Weinberg AD: Hypothermia. *Ann Emerg Med* 22:370, 1993.
33. Neff TA: Routine oximetry: a fifth vital sign? *Chest* 94:227, 1998.
34. Swan HJC, Ganz W, Forrester J, et al: Catheterization of the heart in man with use of a flow-directed balloon-tipped catheter. *N Engl J Med* 283:447, 1970.
35. Friese RS, Shafi S, Gentilello LM: Pulmonary artery catheter use is associated with reduced mortality in severely injured patients: A National Trauma Databank analysis of 53,312 patients. *Crit Care Med* 34:1597, 2006.
36. Giglio MT, Marucci M, Testini M, et al: Goal-directed haemodynamic therapy and gastrointestinal complications in major surgery: a meta-analysis of randomized controlled trials. *Br J Anaesth* 103:637, 2009.
37. Rhodes A, Grounds RM: New technology for measuring cardiac output: the future. *Curr Opin Crit Care* 11:224, 2005.
38. Calvin JE, Driedger AA, Sibbald WJ: Does the pulmonary capillary wedge pressure predict left ventricular preload in critically ill patients? *Crit Care Med* 9:437, 1981.
39. Packman MI, Rackow EC: Optimum left heart filling pressure during fluid resuscitation of patients with hypovolemic and septic shock. *Crit Care Med* 11:165, 1983.
40. Cheatham ML: Right ventricular end-diastolic volume measurements in the resuscitation of trauma victims. *Int J Crit Care* 7:165, 2000.
41. Diebel LN, Wilson RF, Tagett MG, et al: End-diastolic volume: a better indicator of preload in the critically ill. *Arch Surg* 127:817, 1992.
42. Bratton SL, Chestnut RM, Ghajar J, et al: Guidelines for the management of severe traumatic brain injury. IX. Cerebral perfusion thresholds. *J Neurotrauma* 24:S59–S64, 2007.
43. Cheatham ML, Malbrain MLNG: Abdominal perfusion pressure. In: Ivatury RR, Cheatham ML, Malbrain MLNG, Sugrue M (eds): *Abdominal Compartment Syndrome*. Landes Biomedical, Georgetown, 2006.
44. Malbrain MLNG, Chiumello D, Pelosi P, et al: Prevalence of intra-abdominal hypertension in critically ill patients: a multicentre epidemiological study. *Intensive Care Med* 30:822–829, 2004.
45. Malbrain MLNG, Jones F: Intra-abdominal pressure measurement techniques, in Ivatury RR, Cheatham ML, Malbrain MLNG, Sugrue M (eds): *Abdominal Compartment Syndrome*. Landes Biomedical, Georgetown, 2006.
46. Cheatham ML, De Waele J, De Keulenaer B, et al: The effect of body position on intra-abdominal pressure measurement: a multicenter analysis. *Crit Care Med* 37:2187, 2009.
47. Dalfino L, Tullo L, Donadio I, et al: Intra-abdominal hypertension and acute renal failure in critically ill patients. *Intensive Care Med* 34:707, 2008.
48. Magder, Sheldon MD: Central venous pressure: a useful but not so simple measurement. *Crit Care Med* 34:2224, 2006.
49. Miller PR, Meredith JW, Chang MC: Randomized, prospective comparison of increased preload versus inotropes in the resuscitation of trauma patients: effects on cardiopulmonary function and visceral perfusion. *J Trauma* 44:107, 1998.
50. Cheatham ML, Safcsak K, Block EF, et al: Preload assessment in patients with an open abdomen. *J Trauma* 46:16, 1999.
51. Cheatham ML, Nelson LD, Chang MC, et al: Right ventricular end-diastolic volume index as a predictor of preload status in patients on positive end-expiratory pressure. *Crit Care Med* 26:1801, 1998.

52. Chaney JC, Derdak S: Minimally invasive hemodynamic monitoring for the intensivist: current and emerging technology. *Crit Care Med* 30(10):2338–2345, 2002.
53. Wiesenack C, Prasser C, Rodig G, et al: Stroke volume variation as an indicator of fluid responsiveness using pulse contour analysis in mechanically ventilated patients. *Anesth Analg* 96:1254, 2003.
54. Hébert PC, Wells G, Blajchman MA, et al: A multicenter, randomized, controlled clinical trial of transfusion requirements in critical care. *N Engl J Med* 340:409, 1999.
55. Spinella PC, Perkins JG, Grathwohl KW, et al: Warm fresh whole blood is independently associated with improved survival for patients with combat-related traumatic injuries. *J Trauma* 66[Suppl]:S69, 2009.
56. Nelson LD, Rutherford EJ: Monitoring mixed venous oxygen. *Respir Care* 92:154, 1992.
57. Kruse JA, Zaidi SAJ, Carlson RW: Significance of blood lactate levels in critically ill patients with liver disease. *Am J Med* 83:77, 1987.
58. Abramson D, Scalea TM, Hitchcock R, et al: Lactate clearance and survival following injury. *J Trauma* 35:584, 1993.
59. Kruse JA, Haupt MT, Puri VK, et al: Lactate levels as predictors of the relationship between oxygen delivery and consumption in ARDS. *Chest* 98:959, 1990.
60. Mizock BA, Falk JL: Lactic acidosis in critical illness. *Crit Care Med* 20:80, 1992.
61. Husain FA, Martin MJ, Mullenix PS, et al: Serum lactate and base deficit as predictors of mortality and morbidity. *Am J Surg* 185:485, 2003.
62. Davis JW, Shackford SR, Mackersie RC, et al: Base deficit as a guide to volume resuscitation. *J Trauma* 28:1464, 1998.
63. Rutherford EJ, Morris JA, Reed G, et al: Base deficit stratifies mortality and determines therapy. *J Trauma* 33:417, 1992.
64. Finfer S, Bellomo R, Boyce N, et al: A comparison of albumin and saline for fluid resuscitation in the intensive care unit. *N Engl J Med* 350:2247, 2004.
65. Vincent JL, Navickis RJ, Wilkes MM: Morbidity in hospitalized patients receiving human albumin: a meta-analysis of randomized, controlled trials. *Crit Care Med* 32:2029, 2004.
66. SAFE Study Investigators: Saline or albumin for fluid resuscitation in patients with traumatic brain injury. *N Engl J Med* 357:874, 2007.
67. Borgman MA, Spinella PC, Perkins JG, et al: The ratio of blood products transfused affects mortality in patients receiving massive transfusions at a combat support hospital. *J Trauma* 63:805, 2007.
68. Ketchum L, Hess JR, Hiippala S: Indications for early fresh frozen plasma, cryoprecipitate, and platelet transfusion in trauma. *J Trauma* 60(Suppl):S51, 2006.
69. Bellomo R, Chapman M, Finfer S, et al: Low-dose dopamine in patients with early renal dysfunction: a placebo-controlled randomised trial. *Lancet* 356:2112, 2000.
70. Rude RE, Izquierdo C, Buja LM: Effects of inotropic and chronotropic stimuli on acute myocardial ischemic injury. I. Studies with dobutamine in the anesthetized dog. *Circulation* 65:1321, 1982.
71. Marin C, Eon B, Saux P, et al: Renal effects of norepinephrine used to treat septic shock patients. *Crit Care Med* 18:282, 1990.
72. Grotz RL, Yeston NS: Intra-aortic balloon counterpulsation in high-risk cardiac patients undergoing noncardiac surgery. *Surgery* 106:1, 1989.
73. Singer M: Arginine vasopressin vs. terlipressin in the treatment of shock states. Best Practice & Research. *Clin Anaesthesiol* 22:359, 2008.
74. Shoemaker WC, Appel PL, Kram HB, et al: Prospective trial of supranormal values of survivors as therapeutic goals in high-risk surgical patients. *Chest* 94:1176, 1998.
75. Bland RD, Shoemaker WC, Abraham E, et al: Hemodynamic and oxygen transport patterns in surviving and nonsurviving postoperative patients. *Crit Care Med* 13:85, 1985.
76. Tuchschmidt J, Fired J, Astiz M, et al: Elevation of cardiac output and oxygen delivery improves outcome in septic shock. *Chest* 102:216, 1992.
77. Yu M, Levy MM, Smith P, et al: Effect of maximizing oxygen delivery on morbidity and mortality rates in critically ill patients: a prospective, randomized, controlled study. *Crit Care Med* 21:830, 1993.
78. Velmahos GC, Demetriades D, Shoemaker WC, et al: Endpoints of resuscitation of critically injured patients: normal or supranormal? a prospective randomized trial. *Ann Surg* 232:409, 2000.
79. McKinley BA, Kozar RA, Cocanour CS, et al: Normal versus supranormal oxygen delivery goals in shock resuscitation: the response is the same. *J Trauma* 53:825, 2002.
80. Balogh Z, McKinley BA, Cocanour CS, et al: Supranormal trauma resuscitation causes more cases of abdominal compartment syndrome. *Arch Surg* 138:637, 2003.
81. Sebat F, Musthafa AA, Johnson D, et al: Effect of a rapid response system for patients in shock on time to treatment and mortality during 5 years. *Crit Care Med* 35:2568, 2007.
82. Lamontagne F, Meade M, Ondiveeran HK, et al: Nitric oxide donors in sepsis: a systemic review of clinical and in vivo preclinical data. *Shock* 30:653, 2008.
83. Pinto BB, Rehberg S, Ertmer C, et al: Role of levosimendan in sepsis and septic shock. *Curr Opin Anaesthesiol* 21:168, 2008.
84. Kreymann KG, de Heer G, Nierhaus A, et al: Use of polyclonal immunoglobulins as adjunctive therapy for sepsis or septic shock. *Crit Care Med* 35:2677, 2007.
85. Dutton RP, Stein DM: The use of factor VIIa in haemorrhagic shock and intracerebral bleeding. *Injury* 37:1172, 2006.
86. Kopterides P, Falagas ME: Statins for sepsis: a critical and updated review. *Clin Microbiol Infect* 15:325, 2009.

CHAPTER 158 ■ RESUSCITATION FROM SHOCK FOLLOWING INJURY

DONALD H. JENKINS, JOHN B. HOLCOMB, PHILLIP A. LETOURNEAU, DUSTIN L. SMOOT AND STEPHEN L. BARNES

After the initial evaluation and operative management of the surgical/trauma patient, many patients require further resuscitation, support, and care in an intensive care unit (ICU) setting. This chapter provides a brief outline of considerations, priorities, treatment algorithms, and the newest innovations that may assist any intensivist tasked with managing such critically ill surgical patients.

STATEMENT OF THE PROBLEM

Surgical patients die from shock abruptly through lack of oxygen delivery to the heart and brain, or subacutely through development of multiple organ dysfunction from late recognition of shock or inadequate resuscitation. Unlike the typical nonsurgical critically ill patient, exsanguination is often the cause of death in the surgical/trauma patient, second only to central nervous system injuries as the cause of death of trauma victims in the United States [1–3]. The control of hemorrhage has been identified as a priority in modern trauma patient care, second in importance only to adequate ventilation [4]. Advanced Trauma Life Support teaches a schema that incorporates the vital signs, skin color, capillary refill, and mentation to alert the physician to how severely injured the patient may be and help to quantify how much blood the patient may have lost [4]. By the time the blood pressure falls, the patient has lost 30% to 40% of his or her blood volume, or approximately 2,000 mL. This situation demands rapid action, but action should not wait until this point has been reached.

One classification system defines four types of shock: *Hypovolemic* (such as dehydration, diarrhea, and hemorrhage, the most common form of shock following major trauma), *distributive* (such as septic shock, the most common form of shock in the late phase of recovery—5 days or more—after major surgery/trauma), *cardiogenic* (such as from massive myocardial infarction or arrhythmia), and *obstructive* (such as from tension pneumothorax, pulmonary embolus, or pericardial tamponade). By far, hemorrhagic shock is the most common form following major surgery/trauma and the major focus of this chapter (although the astute physician should always keep tension pneumothorax in the differential diagnosis). Therefore, in most instances, the ICU physician faced with a surgical patient in shock should direct initial efforts toward correction of hypovolemia.

Without obvious external bleeding, vital signs and evidence of organ hypoperfusion are assessed to evaluate the patient for significant or ongoing hemorrhage. A falling hematocrit may be a sign, but as hemorrhage causes loss of cells and fluid in equal proportion, an isolated normal hematocrit should not be reassuring to the clinician. With very rapid hemorrhage, a patient can die with a normal hematocrit. A fall in central venous oxygen saturation when the cardiac output remains the same may be one of the earliest signs of hemorrhage in the ICU setting as the body begins to extract more oxygen from the remaining blood.

PHYSIOLOGY OF EFFECTS OF HEMORRHAGE

The physiologic responses to hemorrhage can be broken into three categories: Hemostasis, oxygen delivery, and immunology.

Hemostasis

If bleeding does not stop, then no intervention can prevent death. It is this concept that has led to some of the most heated debates in the resuscitation literature: "Does resuscitation promote tissue perfusion and cellular metabolism, thus increasing survival, or does the increase in blood pressure destroy clot, promote rebleeding, and decrease survival?" [5]. The astute physician recognizes that both concepts are true. Cellular metabolism must be ensured, without overwhelming the clotting mechanism.

After injury, the body attempts to stop hemorrhage by clotting at the site of vascular injury. This is accomplished by the interaction of circulating clotting factors, platelets, and tissue factors from the injured cells. These factors work primarily to form a "plug" initiated by the physical presence of the platelets and augmented by the cross-linking of fibrin to form a more permanent seal. The tissue injury factors released may also lead to constriction of the local blood vessels to decrease the blood flow to the leaking area concurrently with platelet plug formation and is mediated both locally by tissue factors as well as centrally. Finally, when the blood loss leads to a fall in the blood pressure, the clotting efforts are aided by a smaller vessel diameter, decreased wall tension, and lower pressure head.

Oxygen Delivery

In 1872, Gross called shock a "rude unhinging of the machinery of life." Although this definition is accurate, it is not precise. It is at the level of cellular oxygen delivery and utilization that the understanding of shock is defined. Without oxygen, the cells may survive briefly using anaerobic metabolism. Many of the physiologic defense mechanisms work to augment this delivery and depend on oxygen-carrying capacity, cardiac output, and oxygen delivery to and utilization by the cell.

The oxygen-carrying capacity of blood depends on the amount of circulating hemoglobin, which diminishes continually during hemorrhage. Although erythropoietin stimulates the production of new red blood cells (RBCs) and eventually restores hemoglobin over weeks, this response does not acutely restore oxygen-carrying capacity [6]. As hemorrhage proceeds, the body becomes incapable of supporting metabolic need. The primary defense, however, is the extra capacity inherent in the human system: only approximately 25% to 30% of the transported oxygen is normally used, leaving central venous or mixed venous oxygen saturations in the range of 70%. When fully stressed, extraction improves as anaerobic metabolism leads to lactic acidosis, which shifts the oxygen dissociation curve to favor release of oxygen at the tissue level. This allows much more oxygen to be removed from the hemoglobin, and much lower central venous oxygen saturations.

Cardiac output is the product of heart rate and stroke volume. There is reserve built into the heart rate, in that most people use only approximately two-thirds of their maximal heart rate. Pain, fear, and a variety of baroreceptors release catecholamines and other factors in response to hemorrhage. These lead to an increased heart rate, and thus increased cardiac output and oxygen delivery. With a few exceptions, in the elderly or those with heart disease, this response is maximally achieved by the body, in an unaided fashion.

The stroke volume can be increased by increased contractility through the direct effects of many of the same substances that increase heart rate. In hemorrhage, however, the primary component of cardiac output is the volume of blood coming into the heart (preload). During hemorrhage, the preload falls. As the blood pressure falls, oncotic forces predominate and fluid begins to shift into the vascular space. This "borrowing" of fluid from the interstitial, and ultimately from the intracellular, space is gradual, with a gradual restoration of the blood pressure—often not to normal—which allows time for the clotting mechanisms to stop the bleeding and stabilize the clot.

Other factors that restore the preload include the prevention of further fluid loss via the kidney. A lower blood pressure leads to less filtration and less fluid removed in urine. In addition, antidiuretic hormone and the renin–angiotensin systems act to augment this response. Catecholamines and large proteins circulate as part of the defense signaling systems. These augment the oncotic pull. The glucose that increases with the release of corticosteroids also acts to pull fluid into the vascular space. Finally, the body is willing to shunt blood away from most areas of the body to support cardiac preload and the brain. This shunting is very evident in the pale clammy skin of hemorrhagic shock. Initially it is less evident in the relative ischemia that occurs in every other organ of the body.

Oxygen delivery (DO_2) to the tissues includes the variables of cardiac output, arterial oxygen content (CaO_2, the total amount of oxygen in the blood), which includes the amount of hemoglobin that is present. During hemorrhage, these components are altered, and oxygen delivery may be decreased. Cardiac output can be indexed to body surface area and expressed as cardiac index, which when multiplied by CaO_2 yields an oxygen delivery index (DO_{2I}). Normal DO_{2I} is roughly 450 mL per minute per m^2 and it may increase by as much as 30% in response to injury. The primary goal of shock resuscitation is the early establishment of "adequate" oxygen delivery (DO_2) to vital organs; however, adequate is subject to ongoing debate.

The complications of a "successful" resuscitation that should be watched for are related to ischemia and reperfusion injury. These may manifest as multiple organ dysfunction syndrome or individual organ dysfunction. Hepatic dysfunction may present as jaundice and coagulopathy. Pulmonary dysfunction and acute respiratory distress syndrome may be seen as renal failure, with rising blood urea nitrogen and creatinine. Compromise of intestinal mucosa may lead to sepsis, bleeding, or perforation.

Immunology

Hemorrhagic shock alone, without tissue injury, was once thought to have minimal consequences [7]. Hemorrhagic shock alone has been shown to result in a multitude of responses, however, especially in the immune system. The immune system is intended to protect the body from infectious invaders and remove aberrant cells to prevent cancer. During shock, cells produce messengers or mediators that signal for the help of this system [8]. During reperfusion, these mediators are released widely into the systemic circulation.

Currently, a focus in hemorrhagic shock research is the effect of resuscitation on the immune and coagulation system. Extensive research in the last decade has shown that hemorrhagic shock from trauma activates both the inflammatory and coagulation system, resulting in profound perturbations in both. This is often manifested by a spectrum of clinical problems starting from acute lung injury, progressing to acute respiratory distress syndrome, systemic inflammatory response syndrome, hypo- or hypercoagulation, bleeding or diffuse thrombosis, and even multiple organ dysfunction syndrome [9]. One of the major areas of study involves the activated immune response that results in enhanced activation and increased adhesion of leukocytes. During this activated stage, neutrophils can release harmful reactive oxygen species, which are thought to play a major role in loss of capillary integrity. This leads to edema and the sequestration of fluid in the tissues outside the vascular space.

Although it has been clear that the immune response occurs in response to shock and reperfusion, it now seems that some of the resuscitation fluids used to treat the shock may trigger this altered immune and coagulation response. The immunologic response to various resuscitation fluids is now an area of intense research [10,11].

HEMORRHAGIC SHOCK MANAGEMENT

The first goal in hemorrhagic shock, following assessment of the ABCs (airway, breathing, and circulation), is to stop ongoing bleeding. In the surgical/trauma patient reaching the ICU, this has generally been accomplished in the emergency department (ED), interventional suite, and/or operating room. During the ICU phase, resuscitation is continued, and can last 24 to 48 hours. The goal of resuscitation is to restore normal perfusion to all body organ systems, using the components of oxygen delivery: hemoglobin, cardiac output, and oxygenation. In hemorrhagic shock, this primarily involves hemorrhage control, reversal of coagulopathy, and then administration of sufficient volumes of blood products and crystalloid fluid volume to restore normal aerobic metabolism.

Confirmation of a hypoperfusion state (shock) is obtained through simple examination and a single blood test. Shock is diagnosed by the effect of hypoperfusion on the body's organ systems: low blood pressure, tachycardia, oliguria, tachypnea, decreased mental status or agitation, skin cyanosis, pallor, decreased pulse character, or mottling. Equivocal cases can be confirmed by obtaining an arterial blood gas and looking for a base deficit exceeding 6 or a serum lactate assay (more than 2 mmol per L). Hypoperfusion implies inadequate delivery of oxygen to the body's cells. Oxygen delivery is a function of cardiac performance, arterial hemoglobin content, and arterial oxygen saturation. All attempts to correct shock involve optimizing these three variables. Hypotension is not synonymous with shock, which can be present in a normotensive patient. Conversely, not all hypotensive patients are in shock. Hypotension, like many other physical findings, is but one sign helpful in the overall clinical picture of shock diagnosis. As detailed below, reestablishment of normal heart rate, blood pressure and urine output does not equate to resolution of shock; resolution of tissue hypoperfusion as manifested by lactate clearance does.

Resuscitation of the patient in shock should be approached in two phases, based on the end points of the resuscitative effort. In the first phase, the patient should be resuscitated to a systolic blood pressure of 80 to 100 mm Hg or mean arterial pressure of 55 to 65 mm Hg, a urine output of 0.5 mL per kg per hour, and an arterial oxygen saturation of 93% or higher. These end points are pursued to prevent imminent death from hypoperfusion to the heart and brain, and should be achieved optimally within 1 hour.

In the second phase, resuscitation is continued with fluid, as well as inotropic and vasopressor agents, as needed, to the goal of eliminating the base deficit of metabolic acidosis, or, if available, restoring the serum lactate or base deficit to a normal level. This end point is important in reversing systemic anaerobic metabolism, which, if unrelieved, leads inexorably to multiple organ failure (MOF). This goal should be accomplished within 12 to 24 hours.

Lessons Learned from War

The modern-day trauma system owes a large debt to combat casualty care. Techniques from system development to operating room procedures have their roots in battlefield medicine. Resuscitation as well, is no stranger to advancement during wartime. To understand the advancements made and differences that exist with modern combat resuscitation strategies it is important to understand the history of combat resuscitation.

A modern ATLS resuscitation strategy of 2 L of crystalloid owes its roots to strategies developed during the Vietnam War. Based on research by Shires [12,13], Dillon [14], and others, the need for volume resuscitation was brought to the forefront to replace an interstitial volume debt secondary to intravascular movement in hemorrhagic shock. High volume crystalloid resuscitation strategies were used to replace volume loss encountered by the bleeding soldier in ratios of 3:1 to as high as 8:1. The physiology was sound, but disappointingly when outcomes were examined, clinical efficacy in the way of improved survival was not seen over previous war efforts with Killed in Action rates of 16% for the US Civil War, 19.6% for World War I, 19.8% for World War II, and 20.2% for the Vietnam War [15]. In fact, the adopted strategy of IV fluid administration would spawn its own set of complications, most notably the emergence of Da Nang lung known more widely now as acute respiratory distress syndrome. Initially felt to be the result of the volume of resuscitation, eventually its mechanisms linked to immunologic effects would come to be understood by Ashbaugh et al. in their case series of 12 patients (seven with trauma) published in the Lancet in 1967 [16].

High-volume crystalloid resuscitation strategies were further supported by Shoemakers early prospective study of 67 patients with greater than 2,000 mL of blood loss. Supranormal endpoints of resuscitation, defined as a cardiac index >4.52 L per minute per m^2, oxygen delivery $\geq$670 mL per minute per m^2, and oxygen consumption $\geq$166 mL per minute per m^2 were assessed against "standard" therapy. Survival was nearly double in the supranormal group as well as statistically significant decreases in length of ICU stay, mean number of organ failures, and days of ventilation [17]. Despite these promising results, several other groups failed to achieve similar findings. More importantly with an ever increasing understanding of the immunology of intravenous fluids and resulting proinflammatory properties the complications of high-volume crystalloid resuscitation for combat casualties came into question.

If aggressive crystalloid resuscitation was not the answer, then what would the optimal resuscitation strategy be? A report by the Institute of Medicine in 1999 as well as two consensus conferences held by Office of Naval Research, the US Army Medical Research and Material Command and the Uniformed Services University of Health Sciences in 2001 and 2002 tried to answer the question.

The IOM report was the first to recognize the several inadequacies of the then standard fluid therapy. First noted was the paucity of good Level I and II data to support the then standard of care. Second, the immunologic activity of common intravenous fluids used and deleterious effects of high-volume resuscitation was better defined as it related to complications [17]. This report would mark a significant paradigm shift. Initial recommendations were to remove the racemic mixture of D and L Lactated Ringers (still clinically available) in favor of L-isomer only. Replacement of lactate with ketones was advocated. Finally, the report supported the initial battlefield use of low volume hypertonic saline (HTS) resuscitation [18]. A 250-mL bolus of HTS was chosen based on research showing decreased neutrophil activation as well as increased oncotic properties as well as the battlefield logistics of less fluid to carry for frontline medics.

The 2001 consensus conference took it one step further by defining what the endpoints of resuscitation would be on the battlefield [19]. Triggers for fluid resuscitation would be systolic blood pressure less than 80 mm Hg or absence of palpable radial pulse, decreasing blood pressure, or altered mental status with no confounding brain injury [19]. This protocol allowed for "permissive hypotension" during resuscitation until definitive hemorrhage control. The goal was not to return blood pressure to normal, but rather to target clinical goals of mentation and palpable pulse. These protocols were developed with several civilian trauma studies in mind.

The first by Bickel and Mattox done at the Ben Taub in which 598 adult patients sustaining penetrating torso trauma with a systolic blood pressure less than 90 were assigned to either standard fluid therapy with Lactated Ringers or IV cannulation with no fluid infusion. Although controversies with study design and protocol surround the results, a significant survival benefit 70% versus 62% was seen for the delayed resuscitation arm [20].

Second were several studies that suggested early aggressive fluid resuscitation before hemorrhage control may have a deleterious effect. As early as 1964, Shaftan et al. published data showing the effects of aggressive volume correction slowed spontaneous control of arterial bleeding [21]. This was followed by military research data done in swine by Bickell et al. Adult swine had their infrarenal aorta cannulated with a stainless steel wire. The wire was pulled creating a 5-mm aortotomy and free intraperitoneal hemorrhage. Eight pigs received 80 mL per kg of Lactated Ringers where the control group received nothing. Hemorrhage was significantly higher in the intravenous fluid group (2,142 $\pm$ 178 mL vs. 783 $\pm$ 85 mL, $p < 0.05$) as well as mortality (8 of 8 vs. 0 of 8, $p < 0.05$) [22]. This ultimately culminated in a complete 180-degree shift from the high volume crystalloid resuscitation seen in the Vietnam War.

If awake, alert, and having a palpable pulse, a soldier sustaining a penetrating wound should have an IV placed, but no fluids would be infused. PO fluids would be encouraged and evacuation undertaken to the next level of care. If resuscitation had to be undertaken, again recognizing a low-volume strategy the recommendation of the panel was for 500 mL hetastarch (Hespan or Hextend) as FDA approval for HTS was lacking. The hetastarch bolus could be repeated at which point a reassessment was done and if no response the possibility of futility was entertained [23].

Expanding on this the 2002 consensus conference held in conjunction with the Canadian Defense and Civil Institute for Environmental Medicine reexamined prehospital requirements for fluid therapy. The "hypotensive" strategy was again approved, but the recommendation for initial battlefield fluid was changed to hypertonic saline dextran (HTS-D) based on then current research showing a favorable volume expansion profile of the dextran with the inflammatory inhibition of the HTS component [24,25].

Current strategies in the Iraq and Afghanistan wars are very similar. First and foremost, the problem had to be defined with the unique set of circumstances that are present in live fire situations. The first point of care would be the battlefield medic. It was recognized that logistical problems exist in bringing care to the wounded at the point of injury. Hemorrhage control still remains the first priority in resuscitating the injured patient, for if quick, effective hemostasis cannot be achieved fluid therapy has no hope of working in austere environments where definitive therapy may be hours away [23]. This has led to the reintroduction of vascular tourniquets, the use of Battlefield hemostatic dressings, and newer therapies such as Factor VII to arrest hemorrhage so that resuscitation efforts can be effective, a discussion of which is beyond the scope of this chapter.

As recognized in the previous consensus conferences, if medics are to be mobile and effective on the battlefield they need the ability to carry their supplies with them [18,19,23,24]. This makes low-volume intravascular expansion much more attractive. For this reason, colloid solutions, specifically Hespan or Hextend, continue to be the fluid of choice for military applications [23]. HTS-D has fallen out of favor due to more current civilian prehospital data that has shown an increase in mortality in trauma patients during interim analysis of the recent ROC trial [26].

With the choice of fluids now made (Hespan or Hextend), the next decision point is how to get those fluids into an injured soldier. Trauma providers know the key tenet of ATLS "two large-bore IVs in the antecubital fossa." This principle becomes increasingly difficult in combat conditions. To this end, the US military takes a different approach. If awake, alert and having a palpable radial pulse, a wounded soldier with a palpable radial pulse have a single 18-gauge peripheral IV placed (chosen for ease of cannulation versus a larger bore IV) and PO fluids encouraged [23]. If IV access cannot be obtained or conditions will not allow access, a sternal intraosseous device is placed. Sternum was chosen as the reproducible target as extremity injuries prevail in current warfare and the trunk remains relatively protected with modern armor. The sternal IO can be placed with reproducible landmarks quickly and in low- or no-light conditions making it extremely beneficial in modern combat [23].

Resuscitation then continues as appropriate with evacuation to the next level of care. It is at this level that the paradigm has shifted dramatically. The emphasis now is on damage control. This pertains not only to the way in which the operations are done (quick procedures leaving abdominal wounds open, temporary packing for hemorrhage control, and temporary vascular shunts) but also to the way in which resuscitation is continued. The use of early blood and coagulation component therapy as well as fresh whole blood (FWB) is emphasized. Again logistics dictate limited storage capabilities in far forward treatment centers. This continues to promote a walking blood bank using fellow combat troops as donors, a luxury not afforded by the civilian trauma provider.

Clinically, FWB has been demonstrated to reverse dilutional coagulopathy, with evidence that a single unit of FWB has a hemostatic effect similar to 10 units of platelets [27–34]. In a retrospective study of the results of the FWB procedures for one U.S. Combat Support Hospital in 2004, 87 patients received 545 units. In that experience the FWB drive was called for only after the patient had received a massive transfusion, yet the transfusion of FWB resulted in significant improvements in both hemoglobin concentration and coagulation parameters [32].

The nature of military medical logistics frequently limits the availability of FFP, platelets, and cryoprecipitate for transfusion in theaters, giving the battlefield physician few options in the treatment of traumatic coagulopathy. However, the use of FWB in massively transfused patients may circumvent the problem of dilutional coagulopathy. Consider the usual mixture of one packed RBC unit (335 mL) with a hematocrit of 55%, one unit of platelet concentrate (50 mL) with 5.5×10^{10} platelets, and one unit of FFP (275 mL) with 80% coagulation factor activity. This combination results in 660 mL of fluid with a hematocrit of 29%, 88,000 platelets per μL, and 65% coagulation factor activity. By definition, transfusion of these standard components will only serve to further dilute critical factors in a bleeding casualty. In contrast, FWB is replete with functional platelets as well as fully functional clotting factors. A 500-mL unit of FWB has a hematocrit of 38% to 50%, 150,000 to 400,000 platelets per μL, and 100% activity of clotting factors diluted only by the 70 mL of anticoagulant [35]. In addition, the viability and flow characteristics of fresh RBC are better than their stored counterparts that have undergone metabolic depletion and membrane loss.

Initial retrospective studies by Holcomb found higher 24-hour (96% vs. 88%, $p = 0.018$) and 30-day (95% vs. 82%, $p = 0.020$) survival in a group of combat casualties when FWB was used [36]. The immunology and pathophysiology of improved clinical outcomes continues to be an active area of research. Also reported from military and civilian evidence is that higher ratio FFP to PRBC improves outcomes [37–39]. The exact ratio is still part of ongoing research, with some evidence suggesting that there may be a survival bias in those patients receiving higher ratios. Despite these controversies, the early and aggressive use of blood and coagulation factors forms the cornerstone of damage control resuscitation.

DAMAGE CONTROL RESUSCITATION

The concept of damage control resuscitation or hemostatic resuscitation has rapidly evolved on the modern battlefield. This concept is philosophically derived from the widely practiced damage control surgery approach to severely injured patients. Understanding the epidemiology of combat casualties is paramount to devising a logical resuscitation strategy. Most deaths (80%) in combat operations are not preventable [40,41]. Of the remaining 20% of potentially preventable deaths in combat casualties, two-thirds are from hemorrhage. Furthermore, the killed in action rate is lower than at any time in history, while the died of wounds rate has increased, largely due to improved body armor, rapid evacuation, improved extremity hemorrhage control, and medic training [40]. With the recent widespread use of tourniquets and hemostatic dressings for compressible hemorrhage control, the current unmet need is for rapid, effective interventions for noncompressible hemorrhage from the neck, axilla, thorax, abdomen, groin, and pelvis.

Fortunately, most casualties receive at most one to four units of packed RBCs after injury and are not at high risk of presenting or developing a coagulopathy and subsequently dying [42]. Only 5% to 10% of all combat casualties require massive transfusion (10 or more units of packed RBCs) and this group constitutes those at risk for hemorrhagic death [43]. These same patients are those who will benefit from early use of recombinant activated factor VII (rFVIIa), as described in the Clinical Practice Guideline (Table 158.1).

The 5% to 10% of all combat casualties that require massive transfusion fall into two broad categories. Group 1 patients are the wounded who are clearly in profound shock, arrive moribund, and are resuscitated with heroic efforts. These casualties do not pose a diagnostic dilemma; rather, they require immediate hemorrhage control and very rapid resuscitation with the optimal ratio of all available products. Surgically, the only question is what cavity to enter first, as they usually have multiple significant injuries. Frequently, these casualties have severely injured extremities, requiring life-saving tourniquets and delayed completion amputations after successful truncal hemorrhage control. These casualties, if surviving the initial 10 to 15 minutes resuscitation in the ED, require the full massive transfusion protocol and surgical intervention described in the following sections.

Group 2 patients are more difficult to recognize. They are typically the young soldier with incredible physiologic reserve who arrive "talking and looking good," who are actually in shock, have had significant blood loss, and soon progress to cardiovascular collapse. This classic presentation occurs once a week at a busy combat hospital. The challenge is rapidly separating these critical casualties from those who are really hemodynamically stable. These casualties require rapid and accurate diagnosis of their hemorrhagic injury. This group needs immediate hemorrhage control, as fast as group 1; however, they are much more difficult to initially diagnose. Traditional reliance on mental status, blood pressure and pulse rate is notoriously inaccurate for individual risk stratification [44–47].

Fortunately, there are five risk factors that are easily identified very early in the hospital course of severely injured casualties, each of which independently predicts the need for massive transfusion and/or increased risk of death. These simple variables are now available within 2 to 5 minutes after presentation in every ED and each of these variables is independently associated with massive transfusion or death after trauma; any one of them should prompt activation of the massive transfusion protocol (discussed later).

First, an initial international normalized ratio (INR) of 1.5 or more reliably predicts those military casualties who will require massive transfusion [48–50] Patients who have a significant injury present with a coagulopathy as a marker of severe injury. Severity of injury and mortality is linearly associated with the degree of the initial coagulopathy [35,47–50]. Second, a base deficit of 6 or more is strongly associated with the need for massive transfusion and mortality in both civilian and military trauma. Patients have an elevated base deficit before their blood pressure drops to classic "hypotension" levels [51–53]. Third, a temperature of 96°F or less is associated with an increase in mortality. Trauma patients who are hypothermic are in shock, not perfusing their mitochondria, and are not generating heat fast enough to keep up with their ongoing heat loss [52–54]

Fourth, a hemoglobin of 11 mg per dL or less on presentation to the ED is associated with massive transfusion and a mortality rate of 39% [43]. Otherwise, young healthy soldiers who present with a low hemoglobin have only one reason for their anemia, namely, acute blood loss [43,55]. Lastly, a systolic blood pressure of 90 mm Hg or less is indicative casualties who have lost more than 40% of their blood volume (2,000 mL in an adult), are experiencing impending cardiovascular collapse, and have a significantly increased mortality [56,57].

The current resuscitation protocol for combat casualties not only has an affect on current military outcomes (initial reports show Case Fatality Rates dropping from a historic 20% to close to 10%), but has provided exciting tools for civilian trauma providers [40,58].

TABLE 158.1

U.S. CENTRAL COMMAND CLINICAL PRACTICE GUIDELINE FOR USE OF RECOMBINANT FACTOR VIIA (RFVIIA) AND THAWED PLASMA

1. Background: The most critically injured casualties present hypothermic (T ≤96°F) acidemic (BD ≤6), with a coagulopathy (INR ≥1.5), hypotensive (SBP ≤90 mm Hg) or with a Hgb ≤11). Interventions aimed at reversing the coagulopathy starting as soon after arrival as possible may improve survival.
2. Recombinant factor VIIa is FDA-approved for use during critical bleeding or surgery in hemophilic patients with inhibitors to factor VIII or IX. rFVIIa has been shown to be safe and decreases transfusion requirements in humans with life-threatening hemorrhage, including patients with hypothermia (30°C–33°C, pH >7.1). In a total of seven prospective randomized surgical trials, the drug causes no increase in any complication.
3. Plasma used in a 1:1 ratio with PRBCs has been shown to improve survival in combat casualties.
4. In the combat surgical setting, rFVIIa and plasma should be used in patients who are
   (a) Hypotensive from blood loss (SBP ≤90 mm Hg)
   (b) Have a base deficit ≥6
   (c) Hypothermic (*T* ≤96°F)
   (d) Coagulopathic (clinically or an INR ≥1.5)
   (e) Have a Hgb ≤11
   (f) Have weak or absent radial pulse character
   (g) Have more than one major amputation
   (h) Have major truncal injury with a positive FAST examination
   (i) Abnormal mental status from trauma or CT scan with intracranial injury
   (j) Have >1,000 mL immediately out of a chest tube or >200 mL/h
   (k) Anticipated and actual transfusion of >four units of PRBCs
   (l) Require damage control maneuvers
   (m) Require fresh whole blood
5. Guidelines for administration
   (a) Protocol for use
      (i) Infuse rFVIIa at dose of three vials (2.4 mg) or 90–120 μg/kg IV push.
      (ii) If coagulopathic bleeding continues 20 min after infusion
         (1) Administer two additional units fresh whole blood or four units FFP, 10 packs of cryoprecipitate and 6 packs of platelets
         (2) Redose rFVIa 90–120 μg/kg rFVIIa IV push.
   (b) Administration limits
      (i) Four doses (typically 12 vials) within a 6-h period.
      (ii) If bleeding persists after four doses, there should be attention to conservation of resources. Consult the senior surgeon before administering more rFVIIa.

BD, base deficit; CT, computed tomography; FAST, focused abdominal sonogram for trauma; FDA, Food and Drug Administration; Hgb, hemoglobin; INR, international normalized ratio; PRBC, packed red blood cell; SBP, systolic blood pressure; T, temperature.

Emphasis on early hemorrhage control and damage control resuscitation through aggressive replacement of blood component and coagulation factors still needs further study, but remains one of the positive hallmarks of modern combat medicine. From the point of injury on the battlefield to the arrival at definitive care facilities the current combat casualty enters into a well thought out system of multiphasic resuscitation with specific goals to be achieved at each level; early hemorrhage control, limited intravascular replacement until definitive control is available, and the early use of blood and coagulation factors in a damage control resuscitative strategy.

Civilian Experience

Damage control resuscitation defines a new philosophy of acute traumatic resuscitation. Its tenants define a number of important maneuvers during the resuscitation. First is permissive relative hypotension, with a goal systolic blood pressure slightly below normal. Next is prevention and treatment of hypothermia, acidosis, and hypocalcemia, while avoiding hemodilution with crystalloid fluids. Early surgical control of bleeding is also tantamount to damage control resuscitation. Lastly, hemostatic resuscitation with blood products in high ratios of fresh frozen plasma (FFP) and platelets to packed red blood cells, with appropriate use of adjuvants like factor VIIa, and fibrinogen containing compounds, is considered fundamental to this approach to the hemorrhaging patient [59].

There has been ongoing controversy in the surgical literature concerning the optimal use of resuscitative fluids. Questions of type, amount, and timing dominate the ongoing discussion. In addition, some authors maintain that the differences between civilian and military mechanisms of injury limit the applicability of military data to the civilian practice patterns. There is some belief that combat-related injuries result in a distinct patient population, and that lessons learned there may not be translatable to the civilian population [60,61]. However, multiple civilian studies in Europe and in the United States demonstrate similar results to wartime casualties and the benefits to aggressively resuscitating these patients with plasma and platelets versus excessive crystalloid. The evidence in these studies is all retrospective, and is subject to survivor bias and multiple other confounding variables. Unfortunately, no prospective randomized trials have been conducted examining any resuscitation strategy, including damage control resuscitation.

The early coagulopathy of trauma, identified by as early as 1969 by Simmons and Borowiecki, and highlighted separately by Brohi and MacLeod is a common and dangerous condition that many patients manifest upon admission to the emergency department [50]. Brohi defines coagulopathy as prothrombin time (PT) over 18 seconds, activated partial thromboplastin time (aPTT) over 60 seconds, or thrombin time over 15 seconds. This London study found a significant coagulopathy in 24.4% of patients admitted to their ED. This coagulopathic cohort had a much greater mortality (46% vs. 10.9%, $p < 0.001$) compared with those with normal coagulation studies. Contradicting previous suspicions about the contribution of fluids to coagulopathy, Brohi found that the early coagulopathy of trauma was not linked to amount of IV fluids (crystalloid and colloid) administered [49].

Adding to this observation, Gonzalez et al. demonstrated that patients that arrived to the emergency department in a coagulopathic state (INR = 1.8 ± 0.2) and received primarily PRBCs and crystalloid fluids were persistently coagulopathic on admission to the ICU (INR = 1.6 ± 0.1). Ninety-one patients were identified who received >10 units of PRBCs in the first 24 hours of admission. According to the massive transfusion protocol at that time, FFP was not transfused until the patients received six units of PRBCs. Once admitted to the ICU, patients received a ratio of FFP/PRBC 1:1. Using univariate logistic regression analysis, the authors concluded that risk of mortality was increased with higher initial ICU INR. This study highlighted the potential importance of earlier administration of FFP and its possible benefits in the form of improved patient survival [34].

Recent civilian studies have demonstrated benefits in survival with high FFP to PRBC ratios, as well as platelets to PRBCs. A study by Holcomb et al.included 466 massively transfused (≥10 units PRBCs in 24 hours). This retrospective multicenter study demonstrated that patients who received a high ratio of FFP to PRBCs (≥1:2) had increased survival (59.6%) compared with those who received a low ratio (<1:2) of FFP to PRBCs (40.4%, $p = <0.01$). This effect was also seen in patients who received a high ratio (≥1:2) of platelets to PRBCs. Those patients had 59.9% survival compared with those in the low (<1:2) platelet to PRBCs group, who demonstrated only 40.1% survival at 30 days ($p = <0.01$) [37]. Another paper with the same cohort of patients highlighted the importance of early (within 6 hours) administration of high FFP ratios. This study showed that a transfusion ratio of ≥1:1 FFP/PRBCs in the first 6 hours of admission decreased mortality at 6 hours (2% vs. 15.2% and 37.3% for ratios ≥1:1, 1:4 to 1:1, and <1:4, $p = <0.001$) and in hospital mortality (25% vs. 41.1% and 54.9% for the same groups, $p = <0.04$). Patients receiving high platelet/PRBC ratios also had improved survival [62].

Another large single-center retrospective study examined 383 patients that received greater than 10 units of PRBCs in the first 24 hours of admission. This group, from Los Angeles, demonstrated survival benefit with higher ratios of FFP to PRBCs. Patients that received ≤1:3 FFP to RBC had 25% mortality, whereas those that received >1:3 had 49% mortality. Further analysis demonstrated that the mean FFP/PRBC ratio for survivors was 1:2.1. Nonsurvivors received 1:3.7 FFP/PRBC ($p < 0.001$). They concluded that higher FFP/PRBC ratios improve survival, but unlike the Holcomb study, no benefit was shown when ratios were more aggressive than 1:3 [63].

Two recent studies from New Orleans also examine FFP/PRBC ratios and survival. Both are retrospective single center-studies. The first study reports that 135 patients, suffering 72% penetrating injuries, received >10 units of PRBCs during the first 24 hours of treatment. All of these patients received surgical intervention. In this population they report a dramatic improvement in survival for patients that received >1:2 FFP to PRBC compared with those who received 1:4, 26% versus 87.5% ($p = 0.0001$) [37]. The second study also examines patients who underwent emergency surgery for trauma and received >10 units of PRBCs. The population of 135 patients were coagulopathic, as defined by INR >1.2, PT >16 seconds, and partial thromboplastin time > 50 seconds. A statistically significant improvement in survival was demonstrated in patients receiving 1:1 ratio of FFP to PRBCs compared with those who received 1:4, 28% compared with 51% ($p = 0.03$). This study also demonstrated an improvement in ICU days (10 vs. 23, $p = <0.01$) in the 1:1 group versus 1:4 [64].

Other studies have demonstrated improved survival with aggressive use of FFP associated with massive transfusion protocols. One study, from Nashville, is a retrospective study with a historical control before implementation of a massive transfusion protocol that specified a ratio of 2:3 FFP to PRBC and 1:5 platelets to PRBCs. The study included 264 total patients, with 125 in the protocol group and 141 in the historical group. The authors demonstrated an improvement in survival from 37.6% to 56.8% ($p = 0.001$) after implementation of the protocol. The transfusion protocol cohort also protected against MOF in univariate and logistic regression analysis. The authors attribute the protection from multiorgan failure to the overall decrease in number of blood product units that patients received as a result of enrollment into the transfusion protocol [65].

Two recent European studies also demonstrate benefits to early plasma transfusion both in trauma patients and in other surgical patients. Maegele et al.demonstrate survival benefit for trauma patients at <6 hours, 24 hours, and 30 days in groups that received high (1:1 and <0.9) ratios of FFP/PRBC. This study included a multicenter retrospective review of 713 patients who received >10 units PRBCs in 24 hours. Patients who received >1:1 FFP to PRBCs had 6-hour mortality equal to 24.6%, 24-hour mortality at 32.6%, and 30-day morality at 45.5%. The mortality rates for 1:1 ratio were 9.6%, 16.7%, and 35.1% at the same time points ($p < 0.005$ for all values). However, these increases in survival came with the cost of increase septic-related complications. The incidence of multiorgan failure in the 1:1 FFP/PRBC group was the greatest at 67% [66].

A group of investigators in Denmark have assessed the principles of damage control resuscitation outside of trauma. A review of 832 surgical patients, including abdominal surgery, cardiovascular, orthopedic surgery, and trauma patients, demonstrated improved survival for patients receiving a ratio of FFP/PRBC equal to 1:1.3 compared with those who received 1:1.6. Mortality at 30 days was 20.4% for the high ratio group compared with 31.5% ($p = 0.0002$). Higher FFP/PRBC ratios did increase ICU days and hospital stay [67]. This study suggests that aggressive use of plasma may be indicated in all bleeding patients, regardless of traumatic etiology.

One recent multicenter study from the Glue grant project demonstrates a lower risk of mortality with a high FFP/PRBC ratio, but also highlights risks associated with transfusion. This study, by Sperry et al., included 415 patients and did not show a crude improvement in mortality, but did reveal a significant difference in 24-hour mortality (high FFP/PRBC 3.9% vs. low FFP/PRBC 12.8%, $p = 0.012$). Their high ratio group received ≥1:1.5 FFP to PRBCs. On Cox regression analysis, the group demonstrated a 52% reduced risk in mortality if patients received the higher FFP/PRBC ratio ($p = 0.002$). Although there was no increase in multiorgan failure or infection, the high FFP/PRBC group did have an increased (2×) risk of acute respiratory distress syndrome ($p = 0.004$) [68].

Watson et al. demonstrate an association between plasma and MOF in an examination of 1,175 patients in a prospective multicenter study. Using Cox proportional hazard regression, the researchers found a 2.1% increased risk of MOF with every unit of FFP transfused. The risk of ARDS increased 2.5% with each unit of FFP. However, the group also reported that each unit of FFP decreased the risk of mortality by 2.9% [69].

Other civilian studies that do not find a survival benefit to high FFP/PRBC ratios. Kashuk et al., report a single-center retrospective study that examined 133 patients who received >10 units of PRBCs in the first 6 hours. This study presented data that patients receiving FFP/PRBC ratios of 1:2 to 1:3 had the lowest predicted probability of mortality. However, the study did note improvement in coagulopathy with higher ratios of FFP/PRBC. However, because of small study size, this was not statistically significant. Also, of important note, the number of patients receiving FFP/PRBC at a 1:1 ratio was only 11 [61]. Another paper, from Baltimore, also fails to demonstrate a survival benefit from high (1:1) FFP/PRBC ratios. However, their massive transfusion subgroup was underpowered, at 81 patients, to demonstrate a survival benefit [60]. A previous study from the same group also highlighted the increased risk of infection and mortality associated with transfusion of PRBCs and FFP [70].

In summary, much like the recent military experience, the preponderance of civilian experience suggest that early and increased use of FFP and platelets in trauma resuscitation results in an overall reduction in early and late mortality. By decreasing early hemorrhagic death, there may be an association with increased risk of infection, ARDS, and multiorgan failure, but patients will survive to suffer these events.

RESUSCITATIVE FLUIDS

In hemorrhagic shock, the choice of intravenous fluid has been long debated and is beyond the scope of this chapter. Historically, a crystalloid solution such as normal saline or lactated Ringer's solution was used in the initial resuscitation. Recent evidence suggests that a more aggressive use of blood and blood products, a so-called damage control resuscitation encompassing "hemostatic resuscitation" may be more beneficial (see Damage Control Resuscitation section). Traditional regimens call for using crystalloids while awaiting blood products from the blood bank, with a rate of infusion of 500 mL to 1,000 mL bolus during 15 to 20 minutes and repeated as necessary. Certainly by the time 2 L of crystalloid have been used for resuscitation, blood product replacement should be given at similar rates of infusion. All fluids should be infused via a warming device to alleviate or prevent hypothermia. Unfortunately, this approach may worsen the coagulopathy present in the most severely injured trauma patients.

Our current recommendations are to minimize the amount of crystalloid a patient receives. Physicians in the ED have little control over what fluids a patient may receive before arrival to the hospital. Blood is the fluid of choice to resuscitate the surgical patient from hemorrhage. Although hemorrhage as the cause of shock had been debated for many years, the treatment of hemorrhage by returning blood to the body seemed logical. The first successful animal transfusion was by Richard Lower in 1665. In 1667, he transfused the blood of a lamb into a human to treat melancholy [71]. Because of transfusion reactions, blood transfusions were infrequently used before the 1900s. During this period, however, the use of autotransfusion emerged. The first American use of autotransfusion was in 1916 after a splenectomy. World War I saw the widespread use of blood banks. Brown, in 1931, was the first to autotransfuse the blood obtained from a hemothorax [72]. World War II demonstrated that truly massive use of blood across multiple theaters of war was possible. With the advent of cardiac surgery in the 1950s, autotransfusion became more common [73]. Its usefulness for the trauma victim was firmly established in the late 1960s and the early 1970s [74–78]. Complications from autotransfusion such as thrombocytopenia, disseminated intravascular coagulopathy (DIC), hypofibrinogenemia, infection, and air embolism have been well documented [78]. Improvement of delivery systems with filters and air monitors, as well as a limit to the amount of blood autotransfused, has kept these problems to a minimum. Because autotransfusion has restrictions on its use, autotransfusion alone will never be adequate for resuscitation, but the value of its use should not be overlooked.

Whole blood contains all of the factors lost by the bleeding patient; this includes plasma proteins, clotting factors, platelets, and white blood cells, as well as erythrocytes. Although FWB is a superb resuscitation fluid, it has a short storage life [36]. Infectious disease testing and blood banking inventory management issues have made FWB largely unavailable in civilian trauma centers. However, whole blood is used in many centers and clinical studies on whole blood are planned for civilian trauma patients. Prospective data collected in these studies may present an impetus for change in blood banking and provide access to this resuscitative fluid.

Usually, oxygen-carrying capacity is gained by giving RBCs. These should be typed and cross-matched to the patient to avoid transfusion reactions. In severe hemorrhage, time may not be available for cross-matching, so type-specific or even O-negative blood should be administered. PRBCs can be stored for 42 days according to current FDA standards. However, detrimental effects of stored PRBCs can be related to their age. Hyperkalemia is a well-known problem with red cell storage. Potassium is lost into the PRBC supernatant at a rate of 1 mEq a day [79]. Cardiac events have been attributed to PRBCs stored for less than a week [80]. Also multiple studies have documented increased infection risk, multiorgan failure and decreased survival associated with older RBCs [81–85]. Despite safeguards, clerical errors lead to mismatched blood administrations, with a rate of fatal major ABO blood group reactions of between 1 in 500,000 and 1 in 2 million. Currently, the risk of infection from a transfused unit is 1 in 30,000 to 1 in 150,000 for hepatitis C, and 1 in 200,000 to 1 in 2,000,000 for human immunodeficiency virus [86].

Thawed plasma is FFP that is stored for up to 5 days at 1°C to 6°C. This storage timeline is based on similar red blood cell storage guidelines and preservation of factors V and VIII, however clinical data is lacking [59,87]. It is unknown what the biologic effect is of storing thousands of proteins at 4°C for 5 days and then administrating them to patients who are in shock. As more centers are using earlier and increased amounts of plasma, thawed plasma is now routinely available at many trauma centers, and increasingly stored in emergency departments. Type AB plasma, the universal donor for plasma, is chosen initially before cross-matched product is available. Having thawed plasma available in the ED allows for identification of severely injured patients requiring massive transfusion and initiation of a protocol driven high ratio of FFP to PRBCs. Primary risks associated with plasma are transfusion-related lung injury (TRALI), infection, and multiorgan failure [69,70]. As described earlier, the risk of infection and MOF was increased 2.1% with each unit of plasma [69]. However, these observations have been made in the context of higher survival in patients that received high ratios of FFP, suggesting that those patients survived with the potential cost of developing sepsis and multiorgan failure.

Platelets are transfused in two different formulations. Pooled whole blood-derived platelets are generally transfused in six unit increments from five to six different blood donors. Apheresis platelet units are derived from a single donor and are transfused in volumes approximately equal to five to six units of pooled whole blood-derived platelets. Both types of platelets are stored at room temperature for up to 5 days. Bacterial contamination from skin flora remains the greatest risk of platelet transfusion. However, apheresis platelet units have been shown to have lower risk of infection in the United States. This risk is derived from a decreased number of venipunctures of donors. European studies have failed to demonstrate a similar benefit [88].

Cryoprecipitate is a product of FFP that contains factor VIII, von Willebrand factor, fibrinogen, fibronectin, factor XIII, and platelet microparticles. Cryoprecipitate is made after centrifuging thawed plasma and removing the supernatant. It has a shelf life of one year when frozen at −20°C [89]. The American Association of Blood Banks mandates a minimum of 150 mg of fibrinogen per unit. Cryoprecipitate is customarily transfused in 10 unit bags, although this is highly variable. As a result of this practice, patients generally receive 2.5 g of cryoprecipitate per transfusion. Its indications for use and benefits derived from it are controversial. Two studies from the military demonstrate improved survival in patients who received relatively high doses of cryoprecipitate [90,91]. Fibrinogen concentrate, a product licensed for use in many European countries, has also been investigated. Fries et al., in Austria, have demonstrated that blood loss is decreased after administration of fibrinogen in coagulopathic swine with a liver injury [92]. Ex vivo experiments also demonstrated improved clot characteristics after administration of fibrinogen concentrate [93,94]. However, the data for this product are limited and this is a potential area of clinical investigation.

HTS is any sodium chloride solution that is more concentrated than normal saline. Solutions of 3.0%, 5%, and 7.5% are commercially available. However, 7.5% HS is not approved for use in the United States. High concentrations of sodium chloride in the vascular system favor the flux of water from the interstitial space and from the cells to augment the blood volume. This results in a rapid restoration of intravascular volume. Infusions of small amounts of these solutions lead to hemodynamic responses equivalent to much larger volumes of crystalloid solutions. This is advantageous because of the rapidity of the response. In some military and wilderness environments, the smaller and much lighter volume of fluid is a significant advantage logistically. Recent work suggests that these fluids decrease the activation of neutrophils, so they may offer an advantage in preventing multiple organ dysfunction syndrome [95]. The proponents of these fluids believe that the smaller volumes lead to less tissue edema and associated potential complications. Once fluid is drawn into the vascular space, the sodium chloride is diluted, so it then equilibrates across the fluid spaces of the body. As this happens, the effect of the HTS is gradually lost. Increases in mean arterial pressure are short-lived, with hemodynamic effects lasting only 15 to 75 minutes [96]. The largest potential danger with hypertonic solutions is hypernatremia. This may be accentuated in the previously dehydrated patient without additional extravascular fluid to donate to the vascular system. Although some rapid and transient hypernatremia seems to be tolerated, caution in administration and careful monitoring of sodium levels are important in the safe use of these solutions [97].

Vasopressor agents can be useful for achieving a minimal acceptable blood pressure, but typically only after adequate resuscitation. Phenylephrine, dopamine, norepinephrine, and vasopressin are the preferred agents, starting in the lower dose range. If blood pressure and intravascular volume status are acceptable but there is evidence of ongoing hypoperfusion (elevated lactate or base deficit), an inotropic agent such as dobutamine or dopamine can be used. Recent work suggests that adrenal insufficiency is much more common than previously thought, especially in conjunction with etomidate use, and responds well to 2 to 3 days of steroids and vasopressin [98].

In general, the intensivist should approach cardiovascular support in the surgical and trauma patient using the four parameters of hemodynamic performance: (a) preload (best index: pulmonary artery occlusion pressure, "wedge"), (b) afterload (best index: calculated systemic vascular resistance = (mean arterial pressure − central venous pressure [CVP])/cardiac output × 80), (c) cardiac contractility (best index: stroke volume = cardiac output/heart rate), and (d) heart rate. All but heart rate traditionally require invasive monitoring with a pulmonary artery catheter for accurate measurement.

For intravascular volume depletion, hypovolemia, and cardiovascular instability due to sepsis, this manipulation of variables should proceed in the order listed, assuring adequate preload (wedge of 15 to 18 mm Hg) by volume repletion before adjusting other variables (such as adding inotropes for diminished cardiac output). There is, however, a certain cohort of surgical patients who are "nonresponders" to ongoing volume resuscitation. These patients do not vasodilate with initial volume loading. Additional volume loading in the setting of persistent high systemic vascular resistance sets the stage for a problematic tissue edema entity called secondary abdominal compartment syndrome (ACS) wherein intra-abdominal pressure reaches deleterious levels due to "third-spacing" of resuscitation fluid in the abdomen. This occurs in patients without intra-abdominal injuries who require massive resuscitation for injuries in which hemorrhage control is difficult or delayed (e.g., pelvic fractures, mangled extremities). These are the patients who receive 10 to 20 L of crystalloid. In contrast, primary ACS occurs in patients with abdominal injury and the ACS is directly attributed to hemorrhage and tissue response within the abdomen to the primary trauma. Formation of secondary ACS in this group of nonresponders led Balogh and colleagues [99] to decrease DO_2 goal from 600 or more to 500 mL per minute per m^2. The cardiac index and SvO_2 response to this ICU resuscitation protocol and clearance of metabolic acidosis were similar to historic matched controls. The DO_2 600 or more cohort received significantly more crystalloid, had greater incidence of intra-abdominal pressure more than 20 mm Hg (42%* vs. 20%; $^*p < 0.05$), ACS (16%* vs. 8%), MOF (22%* vs. 9%), and death (27%* vs. 11%). The use of plasma has also been linked to avoiding ACS. Cotton et al. demonstrate a significant decrease (from 9.9% to 0%, $p < 0.001$) in the incidence of ACS after implementation of a massive transfusion protocol [65].

MANAGEMENT OF COAGULOPATHY

Ideally decisions regarding management of coagulopathy in trauma, the operating room, or the ICU ideally should be based on laboratory data. Unfortunately, this ideal situation is rarely achieved. Although point-of-care coagulation testing is commercially available via devices designed for home use monitoring of INR, most EDs and ICUs do not have this capability, and they have not been validated in critically injured patients. Patients who have received large amounts of crystalloids, colloids, and/or packed RBCs or other blood components should have a coagulation panel performed that includes PT, activated partial thromboplastin time, INR, and platelet count. When suspicion of consumption and/or dilutional coagulopathy exists, a more complete coagulopathy panel should be performed to include fibrinogen, D-dimer, and fibrin split products. The bleeding patient with thrombocytopenia, hypofibrinogenemia, elevated fibrin split products, and D-dimer should be considered to have a dilutional coagulopathy. We have recently added thromboelastography (TEG) to our coagulation panel.

A recent study by Hess et al. describes the relationship of abnormal coagulation studies and mortality. This paper highlights the connection between injury severity score and coagulopathy, with a linear correlation between the two values. The authors find that an abnormal INR increases the risk of death from 4.2% to 26.4%. Abnormal aPTT increases the risk from 4.0% to 43.2%. These laboratory values are therefore cheap and reliable indicators of mortality risk, and suggest that early and aggressive treatment of coagulopathy may impact survival [100].

TEG, a simple test developed in 1948 and used primarily in cardiac and transplant surgery, provides a rapid and comprehensive analysis of coagulation status and can likely be used in place of a DIC panel [101–104]. Use of the thrombelastography test is occurring more frequently in trauma patients. In swine TEG has been shown to be a more sensitive test than PT and aPTT, and may be a better test than traditional laboratory tests [105]. TEG has been shown to be better in certain circumstances as it allows testing of blood in its in vivo state temperature rather than warming it up in the laboratory. Watts et al. [106] showed enzyme slowing and decreased platelet function each individually contribute to hypothermic coagulopathy in trauma patients, particularly at body temperatures <34°C, whereas such changes were not evident on standard coagulation testing. TEG will likely become more widely used as clinicians become more aware of its usefulness and limitations.

Because prolonged hypotension is a known predisposing factor for the development of coagulopathy after trauma, aggressive resuscitation is the most critical factor in prevention of coagulopathy in the injured patient [107]. Platelets and coagulation factors are consumed with ongoing bleeding. In addition, intravascular volume replacement with crystalloid, colloid, or packed RBCs results in dilution of coagulation factors and platelets, with dilutional thrombocytopenia being the most frequent coagulopathy in trauma patients [108,109]. DCR concepts describe replacing lost intravascular volume with plasma and platelet proteins and minimizing ongoing dilution with excessive crystalloids. Various formulas exist regarding whether to begin with platelets, cryoprecipitate, or FFP when correcting dilutional coagulopathies and regarding when to begin this replacement (e.g., after *n* units of packed RBCs).

Recent studies have investigated the role of activated protein C in traumatic coagulopathy. Brohi et al. describe indirect evidence for consumption of activated protein C as a result of hypoperfusion [110]. Another study by Brohi correlates D-dimer levels, as a corollary of fibrinolysis, with degree of shock and hypoperfusion. This relationship between shock and the anticoagulant and fibrinolytic pathways suggests the need to decrease the severity and duration of shock as a method to manage coagulopathy [111].

If laboratory data are available, they can be used to guide therapy. However in most rapidly bleeding patient's laboratory data returns far too slowly to make intelligent decisions for optimal care. It is this reason that ratio driven transfusion is likely optimal while the patient is bleeding. Once bleeding is controlled, transfusion therapy can convert to laboratory driven parameters. Platelet counts can be obtained to assess need for platelet transfusion (see later discussion), PT/activated partial thromboplastin time to assess need for FFP (if PT or activated partial thromboplastin time are greater than 1.5 times normal), and fibrinogen levels to assess need for FFP (below normal fibrinogen level) and/or cryoprecipitate (fibrinogen levels less than 100 mg per dL). A panel of the aforementioned tests plus fibrin split products and D-dimer demonstrate whether dilutional coagulopathy or fibrinolysis is present. [112]. Conversely, if TEG is available (especially rapid TEG), it likely can be used to drive optimal use of blood products, although these guidelines have not been prospectively validated [113].

Acute hemolytic transfusion reactions, although rare, remain a cause of coagulopathy (from compatibility mismatch). The physician must consider this as a possible inciting cause for DIC, especially when no other cause is apparent. The physician must also be familiar with other less common coagulopathies in the trauma patient (and treatment) such as primary fibrinolysis (epsilon–aminocaproic acid), uremia (desmopressin/1-deamino-8-D-arginine vasopressin), and primary liver disease (FFP and vitamin K). With wider spread of the use of TEG early in trauma resuscitation, the incidence of fibrinolysis is likely to increase.

Platelet counts of less than 20,000 per μL should always be corrected in any bleeding trauma patient being resuscitated, whether or not a life-threatening injury has been identified. If the patient has a known history of aspirin use within the preceding 7 days, ibuprofen or other nonsteroidal anti-inflammatory drug use within the last 2 to 3 days, or an unknown history, it may be necessary to transfuse platelets despite a platelet count greater than 50,000 per μL, particularly in those patients with head injury or those being managed nonoperatively for significant liver or other solid organ injury. Platelet counts of less than 100,000 per μL are a relative indication for platelet transfusion in the head-injured patient with evidence of intracranial hemorrhage, whether as a single-system injury or as part of multisystem injuries. Each unit of platelets transfused can be expected to raise the platelet count by at least 5,000. It is possible that we have been overly restrictive in the use of platelet transfusions, as recent data suggests that increased and early use improves survival, and that keeping platelet counts >100,000 are associated with improved outcomes [66,89].

Recombinant factor VIIa (rFVIIa) has emerged as an adjuvant to plasma and platelets in the military and has also been extensively studied in civilian trauma centers. However, there exists controversy on timing, appropriate doses, and indications for the use of recombinant factor VIIa [114]. One Level I study on rFVIIa has been published. The primary endpoint for this randomized double-blind clinical trial was blood product use. In blunt trauma patients, a decreased need for RBC transfusion was seen in patients who received rFVIIa (14% vs. 33% required >20 units of PRBCs, $p = 0.02$). In penetrating trauma, a similar trend was demonstrated, but it did not decrease statistical significance. There were no differences in thrombotic complications between groups and mortality differences were not seen [115]. One military study did demonstrate a survival benefit in patients who received rFVIIa compared to those that did not (14% vs. 35%, $p = 0.01$). Other retrospective studies have demonstrated decreased transfusion requirements with rFVIIa use and no increase in thromboembolic events when matched to controls [116]. Timing of administration has also been studied. The dose of rFVIIa seems to be most effective when given early in a massive transfusion protocol [117]. The use of rFVIIa remains controversial and may be considered as an adjuvant to massive transfusion, based on individual physician preference, although no improvement in survival has been seen.

The early use of plasma and platelets has been demonstrated to improve coagulopathy, although it is unclear why this happens. It seems simplistic to think a minimally improved INR could account for changes in survival or be based on replacing a small percentage of lost coagulation factors. Dente et al.demonstrated an improvement in PT and INR (15.1 ± 0.26 and 1.31 ± 0.29 compared with 17.5 ± 1.1 and 1.72 ± 0.17, $p = 0.04$) with their massive transfusion protocol compared with a historical control group. These benefits were demonstrated on admission to the ICU [118]. Subjectively, using the concepts of DCR has decreased the incidence of coagulopathic bleeding, allowing easier control of surgical bleeding [119]. By identifying patients with coagulopathy secondary to injury, early implementation of an evidenced-based massive transfusion protocol should decrease coagulopathy and improve the possibility of survival. Our recommendation marries the use of a massive transfusion protocol to the tenants of damage control resuscitation. This approach to the severely injured trauma patient will improve survival, but also may present more risk to infection and multi-organ failure. Patients will, however, suffer those complications with the benefit of survival. Critics of this approach have wisely and appropriately noted the pitfalls of retrospective studies and the potential for survivorship bias. To address these concerns, prospective observational trials are ongoing and randomized control trials are being planned.

PRACTICING DAMAGE CONTROL RESUSCITATION

Damage control resuscitation consists of two components: Hypotensive resuscitation and hemostatic resuscitation [120,121]. Hypotensive resuscitation is a military concept that dates from World Wars I and II, and was resurrected in the early 1990s in Houston. The key is to maximize the resuscitation benefit to the mitochondria while at the same time minimizing rebleeding by not "popping the clot," a strategy that is supported by a significant body of scientific data. This not only preserves the resuscitation fluid within the vascular system but is also logistically sound by preventing needless waste of blood and fluids [20,46,122–127].

Hemostatic resuscitation is a concept centered on the surgical judgment inherent in damage control surgery, namely, "staying out of trouble rather than getting out of trouble" [120,121,128]. By focusing on restoring normal physiology, rather than normal anatomy, this surgical approach has decreased mortality in severely injured trauma patients and has become standard surgical teaching. From a resuscitation viewpoint, the damage control philosophy can be extended to resuscitation, focusing on restoring normal coagulation and minimizing crystalloid and even initial packed RBC resuscitation in the severely injured casualty. Both traditional resuscitation products further dilute the already deficient coagulation factors and can increase MOF [129–139]. The aggressive hemostatic resuscitation techniques described herein should be performed in parallel with equally aggressive and definitive control of bleeding.

PROCESS OF DAMAGE CONTROL RESUSCITATION

The first element of damage control resuscitation is the rapid diagnosis and surgical control of named vessels and gauze packing (standard damage control surgery) in the operating room. Damage control surgery has improved outcomes in severely injured trauma patients [125,128].

Thawed plasma is used as a primary resuscitative fluid, and is started in the ED. This product is shelf-stable for 5 days and thus is available on casualty arrival. This approach not only addresses the metabolic abnormality of shock, but also reverses the coagulopathy present on arrival in the ED. Storing plasma for 5 days does not significantly impair the labile factors (V and VIII), and allows this product to be immediately available for transfusion [140]. The Office of the U.S. Army Surgeon General Blood Bank consultant has recommended use of thawed plasma in theaters and the only two Level 1 trauma centers in the Department of Defense have this product available for their trauma patients [47,120,121].

The packed RBC to plasma ratio of 1:1, early transfusion of platelets, and cryoprecipitate are indicated [141,142]. Coagulopathy is not only present on presentation to the ED but is exacerbated by the "bloody vicious cycle" of hemorrhage leading to crystalloid resuscitation, then hemodilution and hypothermia, followed by further hemorrhage, and so on [48,49,52]. Furthermore, transfusion of large amounts of preserved RBCs contributes to a dilutional coagulopathy, which is primarily the result of thrombocytopenia and poor platelet function [129–131]. In addition, compared to fresh blood cells, stored platelets demonstrate decreased thrombotic function, primarily due to a decrease in expression of high-affinity thrombin receptors during platelet storage [143].

End Points of Resuscitation

The search has been to find this "holy grail" of resuscitation: a better end point of adequate resuscitation than heart rate, blood pressure, or urine output. Cardiac output, venous return, low perfusion, and acidosis were all observed in Cannon's original shock experiments [122,144]. Urine output is often used as a surrogate marker of adequate resuscitation of an end organ, but has several drawbacks as a lone marker of adequacy of resuscitation. Resuscitation to normal levels of oxygen delivery and oxygen consumption were seen as possible goals of resuscitation, but even using these parameters, a significant number of patients proceeded to organ failure and death.

Lactate that accumulates with a lack of tissue oxygenation correlates with base deficit in hemorrhagic shock. Correction of an elevated serum lactate or base deficit is viewed as a better, if not the best, end point for resuscitation of hemorrhagic shock [145]. One criticism of using the base deficit is that its recovery lags behind resuscitation, it is complicated by excess chloride, and its continued pursuit of a normal value leads to overresuscitation. Serum lactate elevation has also been criticized as being too broad a test, and it does not portray what goes on at the cellular level.

Therefore, other techniques that include subcutaneous or intraluminal oxygen tension probes and gastric or luminal wall pH probes have all been described to show end-organ resuscitation [146–148]. Most recently, the use of near-infrared spectroscopy has shown promise in identifying patients in shock, but it remains to be seen if these indices can be used to judge adequacy of resuscitation from shock [149,150]. They all have their benefits, but they are variously invasive and expensive in relation to serum base deficit and lactate. At this time, their impracticality precludes their generalized use [151].

CONCLUSIONS

The thoughtful intensivist balances all needs of the patient when using blood products, fluids, and drugs in the resuscitation of patients in shock. Volume replacement is given for lost volume. Oxygen-carrying capacity replaces lost RBCs, and coagulopathy is reversed with hemostatic replenishment. Judicious use of steroids, pressors, and metabolic control are

TABLE 158.2

SUMMARY OF ADVANCES IN MANAGING RESUSCITATION BASED ON RANDOMIZED CONTROLLED CLINICAL TRIALS

- A restrictive transfusion strategy is at least as effective and possibly superior to a liberal transfusion strategy in critically ill patients, with the possible exception of acute myocardial infarction and unstable angina patients [5].
- Factor VIIa decreased transfusions with *trends* toward decreased mortality and critical complications [115].
- Gastric mucosal pH may be an important marker of resuscitation and may provide an early warning for systemic complications in the postresuscitative period [148].
- Etomidate use results in temporary and reversible adrenal insufficiency, responsive to vasopressin and steroids [98].

the order of the day. The effect of each treatment is carefully monitored for its impact on the patient in a stepwise fashion, all the while monitoring indicators of tissue perfusion. Interventions are crisply applied and then removed on the basis of critically and serially evaluated data.

Research must continue to focus on rapid surgical control of hemorrhage and the use of hemostatic adjuncts. Research should also consider the immunologic and coagulation response of the body when creating a better fluid for initial resuscitation, such as an oxygen-carrying product, and the identification of accurate measurements of adequate resuscitation. The overarching metabolic milieu, including adrenal function, glucose control, and response to vasoactive medications, must also be carefully studied for best practices and best combination therapies, including dose–response effects. Finally, identifying the best marker or, better yet, combination of markers to prove adequacy of resuscitation deserve thorough study. The risks and benefits of given therapies must be thoughtfully balanced, given the needs of the patient in a particular situation.

Advances in managing resuscitation, based on randomized controlled trials or meta-analyses of such trials, are summarized in Table 158.2.

ACKNOWLEDGMENTS

The authors would like to acknowledge the outstanding contributions to this chapter by Dr. David G. Burris, Dr. Christoph R. Kaufmann, Dr. David Elliot, and all the brave men and women of the 10th Combat Support Hospital and the 332nd Expeditionary Medical Group, Iraq.

References

1. Baker CC, Oppenheimer L, Stephens B, et al: Epidemiology of trauma deaths. *Am J Surg* 140:144, 1980.
2. Bellamy RF: The causes of death in conventional land warfare: implications for combat casualty care research. *Mil Med* 149:55, 1984.
3. Sauaia A, Moore FA, Moore EE, et al: Epidemiology of trauma deaths: a reassessment. *J Trauma* 38:185, 1995.
4. Committee on Trauma: *Advanced Trauma Life Support Program for Doctors*. Chicago, American College of Surgeons, 1997.
5. Herbert PC, Wells G, Blajchman MA, et al: A multicenter, randomized, controlled clinical trial of transfusion requirements in critical care. *N Engl J Med* 340:409, 1999.
6. Hobisch-Hagen P, Wiederman F, Mayr A, et al: Blunted erythropoietic response to anemia in multiply traumatized patients. *Crit Care Med* 29:743, 2001.
7. Trunkey D: Hypovolemic and traumatic shock, in Geller E (ed): *Shock and Resuscitation*. New York, McGraw-Hill, 1993, p 321.
8. Chaudry IH, Ayala A: Mechanism of increased susceptibility to infection following hemorrhage. *Am J Surg* 165[Suppl]:59s, 1993.
9. Peitzman AB, Billiar TR, Harbrecht BG, et al: Hemorrhagic shock. *Curr Probl Surg* 32:927, 1995.
10. Alam HB, Sun L, Ruff P, et al: E- and P-selectin expression depends on the resuscitation fluids used in hemorrhaged rats. *J Surg Res* 94:145, 2000.
11. Alam HB, Austin B, Koustova E, et al: Resuscitation induced pulmonary apoptosis and intracellular adhesion molecule-1 expression in rats are attenuated by the use of ketone Ringer's solution. *J Am Coll Surg* 193:255, 2001.
12. Shires GT, Carrico CJ, Baxter CR, et al: Principles in treatment of severely injured patients. *Adv Surg* 4:255–324, 1970.
13. Shires GT, Coln D, Carrico J, et al: Fluid therapy in hemorrhagic shock. *Arch Surg* 88:688–693, 1964.
14. Dillon J, Lunch LJ, Meyers R, et al: A bioassay of treatment of hemorrhagic shock. *Arch Surg* 93:537–555, 1966.
15. Alam HB, Rhee P: New developments in fluid resuscitation. *Surg Clin North Am* 87:55–72, 2007.
16. Ashbaugh DG, Bigelow DB, Petty TL, et al: Acute respiratory distress in adults. *Lancet* 12:319–323, 1967.
17. Fleming A, Bishop M, Shoemaker W, et al: Prospective trial of supranormal values as goals of resuscitation in severe trauma. *Arch Surg* 127:1175–1181, 1992.
18. Fluid Resuscitation: State of the Science for Treating Combat Casualties and Civilian Injuries. Washington DC, Institute of Medicine, 1999.
19. Fluid Resuscitation in pre-hospital trauma care: a consensus view. *J R Army Med Corps* 147:147–152, 2001.
20. Bickel WH, Wall MJ, Pepe PE, et al: Immediate versus delayed fluid resuscitation for hypotensive patient with penetrating torso injuries. *N Engl J Med* 331:1105–1109, 1994.
21. Shaftan GW, Chiu CJ, Grosz CS, et al: The effect of transfusion and of certain hemodynamic factors on the spontaneous control of arterial hemorrhage. *J Cardiovasc Surg* 5:251–256, 1964.
22. Bickell WH, Bruttig SP, Millnamow GA, et al: The detrimental effects of intravenous crystalloid after aortotomy in swine. *Surgery* 110:529–536, 1991.
23. *Prehospital Trauma Life Support Military Edition*. 6th ed. Philadelphia, PA, Mosby, 2007.
24. *Fluid Resuscitation in Combat*. Toronto, Ontario, Canada, Defense and Civil Institute of Environmental Medicine, 2001.
25. Santry HP, Alam HB: Fluid resuscitation: past, present, and the future. *Shock* 33:229–241, 2010.
26. The NHLBI halts study of concentrated saline for patients with shock due to lack of survival benefit. NIH news. Cited March 2009. Available at: http://www.nih.gov/news/health/mar2009/nhlbi-26.htm.
27. Lozano ML, Rivera J, Gonzalez-Conejero R, et al: Loss of high-affinity thrombin receptors during platelet concentrate storage impairs the reactivity of platelets to thrombin. *Transfusion* 37:368, 1997.
28. Mohr R, Goor DA, Yellin A, et al: Fresh blood units contain large potent platelets that improve hemostasis after open heart operations. *Ann Thorac Surg* 53:650, 1992.
29. Mabry RL, Holcomb JB, Baker AM, et al: United States Army Rangers in Somalia: an analysis of combat casualties on an urban battlefield. *J Trauma* 49:515, 2000.
30. Loong ED, Law PR, Healey JN: Fresh blood by direct transfusion for haemostatic failure in massive haemorrhage. *Anaesth Intensive Care* 9:371, 1981.
31. Manno CS, Hedberg KW, Kim HC, et al: Comparison of the hemostatic effects of fresh whole blood, stored whole blood, and components after open heart surgery in children. *Blood* 77:930, 1991.
32. Spinella PC, Grathwohl K, Holcomb JB, et al: Fresh warm whole blood use during combat. *Crit Care Med* 33:146S, 2006.
33. Davis JW, Parks SN, Kaups KL, et al: Admission base deficit predicts transfusion requirements and risk of complications. *J Trauma* 41:769, 1996.
34. Gonzalez EA, Moore FA, Holcomb JB, et al: Fresh frozen plasma should be given earlier to patients requiring massive transfusion. *J Trauma* 62:112, 2006.
35. Armand R, Hess JR: Treating coagulopathy in trauma patients. *Transfus Med Rev* 17:223, 2003.
36. Spinella PC, Perkins JG, Grathwohl KW, et al: Warm fresh whole blood is independently associated with improved survival for patients with combat-related traumatic injuries. *J Trauma* 66:S69–S76, 2009.
37. Holcomb JB, Wade CE, Michalek JE, et al: Increased plasma and platelet to red blood cell ratios improves outcome in 466 massively transfused civilian trauma patients. *Ann Surg* 248:447–458, 2008.
38. Borgman MA, Spinella PC, Perkins JG, et al: The ratio of blood products transfused affects mortality in patients receiving massive transfusions at a combat support hospital. *J Trauma* 63:805–813, 2007.
39. Duchesne JC, Hunt JP, Wahl G, et al: Review of current blood transfusions strategies in a mature level I trauma center: were we wrong for the last 60 years? *J Trauma* 65:272–276, 2008.
40. Holcomb JB, Stansbury LG, Champion HR, et al: Understanding combat casualty statistics. *J Trauma* 60:397–401, 2006.
41. Holcomb JB, McMullin NR, Pearce L, et al: Causes of death in U.S. special operations forces in the Global War on Terrorism: 2001–2004. *Ann Surg* 245(6):986–991, 2007.
42. Como JJ, Dutton RP, Scalea TM, et al: Blood transfusion rates in the care of acute trauma. *Transfusion* 44:809, 2004.
43. Schreiber MA, Perkins JP, Kiraly L, et al: Early predictors of massive transfusion in combat casualties. *J Trauma* 205(4):541–545, 2006.
44. Cooke WH, Ryan KL, Convertino VA: Lower body negative pressure as a model to study progression to acute hemorrhagic shock in humans. *J Appl Physiol* 96:1249, 2004.
45. Cooke WH: Heart rate variability and its association with mortality in prehospital trauma patients. *J Trauma* 60:363, 2006.
46. Carrico CJ, Holcomb JB, Chaudry IH; PULSE Trauma Work Group: Post resuscitative and initial utility of life saving efforts. Scientific priorities and strategic planning for resuscitation research and life saving therapy following traumatic injury: report of the PULSE Trauma Work Group. *Acad Emerg Med* 9:621, 2002.
47. Damage Control Resuscitation: *Optimal Correction of the Coagulopathy of Trauma Clinical Guideline*. Office of the Surgeon General. Army Medical Department, March 3, 2006.
48. MacLeod JB, Lynn M, McKenney MG, et al: Early coagulopathy predicts mortality in trauma. *J Trauma* 55:39–44, 2003.

49. Brohi K, Singh J, Heron M, et al: Acute traumatic coagulopathy. *J Trauma* 54:1127–1130, 2003.
50. MacLeod J, Lynn M, McKenney MG, et al: Predictors of mortality in trauma patients. *Am Surg* 70:805, 2004.
51. Eastridge BJ, Owsley J, Sebesta J, et al: Admission physiology criteria after injury on the battlefield predict medical resource utilization and patient mortality. *J Trauma* 61:820, 2006.
52. Cosgriff N, Moore EE, Sauaia A, et al: Predicting life-threatening coagulopathy in the massively transfused trauma patient: hypothermia and acidoses revisited. *J Trauma* 42:857, 1997.
53. Martini WZ, Pusateri AE, Uscilowicz JM, et al: Independent contributions of hypothermia and acidosis to coagulopathy in swine. *J Trauma* 58:1002, 2005.
54. Martin RS, Kilgo PD, Miller PR, et al: Injury-associated hypothermia: an analysis of the 2004 National Trauma Data Bank. *Shock* 24:114, 2005.
55. Beale E, Zhu J, Chan L, et al: Blood transfusion in critically injured patients: a prospective study. *Injury* 37:455, 2006.
56. Holcomb JB, Salinas J, McManus JM, et al: Manual vital signs reliably predict need for life-saving interventions in trauma patients. *J Trauma* 59:821, 2005.
57. Franklin GA, Boaz PW, Spain DA, et al: Prehospital hypotension as a valid indicator of trauma team activation. *J Trauma* 48(6):1034, 2000.
58. Gwande A: Casualties of war: military care for the wounded from Iraq and Afghanistan. *N Engl J Med* 351:2471–2475, 2004.
59. Spinella PC, Holcomb JB: Resuscitation and transfusion principles for traumatic hemorrhagic shock. *Blood Rev* 2009 [Epub ahead of print].
60. Scalea TM, Bochicchio KM, Lumpkins K, et al: Early aggressive use of fresh frozen plasma does not improve outcome in critically injured trauma patients. *Ann Surg* 248:578–584, 2008.
61. Kashuk JL, Moore EE, Johnson JL, et al: Postinjury life threatening coagulopathy: is 1:1 fresh frozen plasma the answer? *J Trauma* 65:261–271, 2008.
62. Zink KA, Sambasivan CN, Holcomb JB: A high ratio of plasma and platelets to packed red blood cells in the first 6 hours of massive transfusion improves outcomes in a large multicenter study. *Am J Surg* 197:565–570, 2009.
63. Teixeira P, Inaba K, Shulman I, et al: Impact of plasma transfusion in massively transfused trauma patients. *J Trauma* 66:693–697, 2009.
64. Duchesne JC, Islam TM, Stuke L, et al: Hemostatic resuscitation during surgery improves survival in patients with traumatic-induced coagulopathy. *J Trauma* 67:33–39, 2009.
65. Cotton BA, Au BK, Nunez TC, et al: Predefined massive transfusion protocols are associated with a reduction in organ failure and postinjury complications. *J Trauma* 66:41–49, 2009.
66. Maegele M, Lefering R, Paffrath T, et al: Red blood cell to plasma ratios transfused during massive transfusion are associated with mortality in severe multiply injury: a retrospective analysis from the trauma registry of the Deutsche Gesellschaft fur unfallchirugie. *Vox Sang* 95:112–119, 2008.
67. Johansson PI, Stensballe J: Effect of haemostatic control resuscitation on mortality in massively bleeding patients: a before and after study. *Vox Sang* 96:111–118, 2009.
68. Sperry JL, Ochoa JB, Gunn SR, et al: An FFP:PRBC transfusion ratio $\geq$1:1.5 is associated with a lower risk of mortality after massive transfusion. *J Trauma* 65:986–993, 2008.
69. Watson GA, Sperry JL, Rosengart MR, et al: Fresh frozen plasma is independently associated with a higher risk of multiple organ failure and acute respiratory distress syndrome. *J Trauma* 67:221–227, 2009.
70. Bochicchio GV, Napolitano L, Joshi M, et al: Outcome analysis of blood product transfusion in trauma patients: a prospective, risk-adjusted study. *World J Surg* 32:2185–2189, 2008.
71. Kendrick DB: *Blood Program in World War II*. Washington, DC, U.S. Government Printing Office, 1964.
72. Brown AL, Debenham MW: Autotransfusion: use of blood from hemothorax. *JAMA* 96:1223, 1931.
73. Cuello L, Vazquez E, Rios R, et al: Autologous blood transfusion in thoracic and cardiovascular surgery. *Surgery* 62:814, 1967.
74. Symbas PN: Autotransfusion from hemothorax: experimental and clinical studies. *Am J Surg* 12:689, 1972.
75. Klebanoff G: Early clinical experience with a disposable unit for the intraoperative salvage and reinfusion of blood loss (intraoperative autotransfusion). *Am J Surg* 120:718, 1970.
76. Dowling J: Autotransfusion, its use in the severely injured patient, in *Proceedings of the First Annual Bently Autotransfusion Seminar*. San Francisco, CA, 1972, p 11.
77. Reul GJ Jr, Solis RT, Greenberg SD, et al: Experience with autotransfusion in the surgical management of trauma. *Surgery* 76:546, 1974.
78. Mattox KL, Walker LE, Beall AC, et al: Blood availability for the trauma patient. *J Trauma* 15:663, 1975.
79. McClatchey KD (ed): *Clinical Laboratory Medicine*. Philadelphia, Lippincott Williams & Wilkins, 2002.
80. Baz EMK, Kanazi GE, Mahfouz RAR, et al: An unusual case of hyperkalaemia-induced cardiac arrest in a paediatric patient during transfusion of a "fresh" 6-day-old blood unit. *Transfus Med* 12:383–386, 2002.
81. Bernard AC, Davenport DL, Chang PK, et al: Intraoperative transfusion of 1 U to 2 U packed red blood cells is associated with increased 30-day mortality, surgical-site infection, pneumonia, and sepsis in general surgery patients. *J Am Coll Surg* 208:931–937, 2009.
82. Taylor RW, Manganaro L, O'Brien J, et al: Impact of allogenic packed red blood cell transfusion on nosocomial infection rates in the critically ill patient. *Crit Care Med* 30:2249–2254, 2002.
83. Sadjadi J, Cureton EL, Twomey P, et al: Transfusion, not just injury severity, leads to posttrauma infection: a matched cohort study. *Am Surg* 75:307–312, 2009.
84. Escobar GA, Cheng AM, Moore EE, et al: Stored packed red blood cells transfusion up-regulates inflammatory gene expression in circulating leukocytes. *Ann Surg* 246:129–134, 2007.
85. Murrell Z, Haukoos JS, Putnam B, et al: The effect of older blood on mortality, need for ICU care, and length of ICU stay after major trauma. *Am Surg* 71:781–785, 2005.
86. Goodnough LT, Brecher ME, Kanter MH, et al: Transfusion medicine: first of two parts—blood transfusion. *N Engl J Med* 340:438, 1999.
87. Lamboo M, Poland DC, Eikenboom JC, et al: Coagulation parameters of thawed fresh-frozen plasma during storage at different temperatures. *Transfus Med* 17:182–186, 2007.
88. Vamvakas EC: Relative safety of pooled whole-blood derived versus single-donor (apheresis) platelets in the United States: a systematic review of disparate risks. *Transfusion* 2009. Epub ahead of print.
89. Callum JL, Karkouti K, Lin Y: Cryoprecipitate: the current state of knowledge. *Transfus Med Rev* 23:177–188, 2009.
90. Perkins KG, Andrew CP, Spinella PC, et al: An evaluation of the impact of apheresis platelets used in the setting of massively transfused trauma patients. *J Trauma* 66:S77–S85, 2009.
91. Stinger HK, Spinella PC, Perkins JG: The ratio of fibrinogen to red cells transfused affects survival in casualties receiving massive transfusions at an army combat support hospital. *J Trauma* 64:S79–S85, 2008.
92. Fries D, Krismer A, Klingler A, et al: Effect of fibrinogen on reversal of dilutional coagulopathy: a porcine model. *Br J Anaesth* 95:172–177, 2005.
93. Fenger-Eriksen C, Anker-Moller E, Heslop J, et al: Thrombelastographic whole blood clot formation after ex vivo addition of plasma substitutes: improvements of the induced coagulopathy with fibrinogen concentrate. *Br J Anaesth* 94:324–329, 2005.
94. Fries D, Innerhofer P, Reif C, et al: The effect of fibrinogen substitution on reversal of dilutional coagulopathy: an in vitro model. *Anesth Analg* 102:347–351, 2006.
95. Rhee P, Burris D, Kaufmann C, et al: Lactated ringers resuscitation causes neutrophil activation after hemorrhagic shock. *J Trauma* 44:313, 1998.
96. Tyagi R, Donaldson K, Loftus CM, et al: Hypertonic saline: a clinical review. *Neurosurg Rev* 30:277–290, 2007.
97. Vassar MJ, Fischer RP, O'Brien PE, et al: A multicenter trial for resuscitation of injured patients with 7.5% sodium chloride. *Arch Surg* 128:1003, 1993.
98. Hildreth AN, Mejia VA, Maxwell RA, et al: Adrenal suppression following a single dose of etomidate for rapid sequence induction: a prospective randomized study. *J Trauma* 65:573–579, 2008.
99. Balogh Z, McKinley BA, Cocanour CS, et al: Supra-normal trauma resuscitation causes more cases of abdominal compartment syndrome. *Arch Surg* 138:637, 2003.
100. Hess JR, Lindell AL, Stansbury LG, et al: The prevalence of abnormal results of conventional coagulation tests on admission to a trauma center. *Transfusion* 49:34–39, 2009.
101. Mallett SV, Cox DJA: Thromboelastography. *Br J Anaesth* 69:307, 1992.
102. Spiess BD, Gillies BSA, Chandler W, et al: Changes in transfusion therapy and reexploration rate after institution of a blood management program in cardiac surgical patients. *J Cardiothorac Vasc Anesth* 9:168, 1995.
103. Tuman KJ, Spiess BD, McCarthy RJ, et al: Effects of progressive blood loss on coagulation as measured by thrombelastography. *Anesth Analg* 66:856, 1987.
104. McNicol PL, Liu G, Harley ID, et al: Patterns of coagulopathy during liver transplantation: experience with the first 75 cases using thromboelastography. *Anaesth Intensive Care* 22:659, 1994.
105. Martini WZ, Cortez DS, Dubick MA, et al: Thromboelastography is better than PT, aPTT, and activated clotting time in detecting clinically relevant clotting abnormalities after hypothermia, hemorrhagic shock and resuscitation in pigs. *J Trauma* 65:535–543, 2008.
106. Watts D, Trask A, Soeken K, et al: Hypothermic coagulopathy in trauma: effect of varying levels of hypothermia on enzyme speed, platelet function, and fibrinolytic activity. *J Trauma* 44:846–854, 1998.
107. Harke H, Rahman S: Haemostatic disorders in massive transfusion. *Bibl Haematol (Switzerland)* 46:179, 1980.
108. Moore EE, Dunn E, Brestich DJ, et al: Platelet abnormalities associated with massive autotransfusion. *J Trauma* 20:1052, 1980.
109. Faringer PD, Mullins RJ, Johnson RL, et al: Blood component supplementation during massive transfusion of AS-1 cells in trauma patients. *J Trauma* 34:481, 1993.
110. Brohi K, Cohen MJ, Ganter MT, et al: Acute traumatic coagulopathy: initiated by hypoperfusion, modulated through the protein C pathway? *Ann Surg* 245:812–818, 2007.
111. Brohi K, Cohen MJ, Ganter MT, et al: Acute coagulopathy of trauma: hypoperfusion induces systemic anticoagulation and hyperfibrinolysis. *J Trauma* 64:1211–1217, 2008.
112. Kaufmann CR, Dwyer KM, Crews JD, et al: Usefulness of thrombelastography in assessment of trauma patient coagulation. *J Trauma* 42:716, 1997.

113. Kashuk JL, Moore EE, Le T, et al: Noncitrated whole blood is optimal for evaluation of postinjury coagulopathy with point-of-care rapid thrombelastography. *J Surg Res* 156:133–138, 2009.
114. Duchesne JC, Mathew KA, Marr AB, et al: Current evidence based guidelines for factor VIIa use in trauma: the good, the bad, and the ugly. *Am Surg* 74:1159–1165, 2008.
115. Boffard K, Riou B, Warren B, et al: Recombinant factor VIIa as adjunctive therapy for bleeding control in severely injured trauma patients: two parallel randomized, placebo-controlled, double-blind clinical trials. *J Trauma* 59:8, 2005.
116. O'Keeffe T, Refaai M, Tchorz K, et al: A massive transfusion protocol to decrease blood component use and costs. *Arch Surg* 143:686–691, 2008.
117. Perkins JG, Schreiber MA, Wade CE, et al: Early versus late recombinant factor VIIa in combat trauma patients requiring massive transfusion. *J Trauma* 62:1095–1101, 2007.
118. Dente CJ, Shaz BH, Nicholas JM, et al: Improvements in early mortality and coagulopathy are sustained better in patients with blunt trauma after institution of a massive transfusion protocol in a civilian level I trauma center. *J Trauma* 66:1616–1624, 2009.
119. Holcomb JB, Jenkins D, Rhee P, et al: Damage control resuscitation: directly addressing the early coagulopathy of trauma. *J Trauma* 62:307–310, 2007.
120. McMullin NR, Holcomb JB, Sondeen J: Hemostatic resuscitation, in *Yearbook of Intensive Care and Emergency Medicine 2006*. Berlin, Springer-Verlag, 2006, p 265.
121. Hess JR, Holcomb JB, Hoyt DB: Damage control resuscitation: the need for specific blood products to treat the coagulopathy of trauma. *Transfusion* 46:685, 2006.
122. Cannon W, Frawer J, Cowell E: The preventive treatment of wound shock. *JAMA* 70:618, 1918.
123. Holcomb JB: Fluid resuscitation in modern combat casualty care: lessons learned from Somalia. *J Trauma* 54[5, Suppl]:S46, 2003.
124. Sondeen JL, Coppes VG, Holcomb JB: Blood pressure at which rebleeding occurs after resuscitation in swine with aortic injury. *J Trauma* 54[5, Suppl]:S110, 2003.
125. Bellamy R, Lounsbury D (ed): *NATO Emergency War Surgery Handbook*. 3rd ed. Washington, DC, Borden Institute, 2004.
126. Dutton RP, Mackenzie CF, Scalea TM: Hypotensive resuscitation during active hemorrhage: impact on in-hospital mortality. *J Trauma* 52:1141, 2002.
127. Wade CE, Holcomb JB: Endpoints in clinical trials of fluid resuscitation of patients with traumatic injuries. *Transfusion* 45[Suppl]:4S, 2005.
128. Holcomb JB, Hirshberg A, Helling TS: Military, civilian, and rural application of the damage control philosophy. *Mil Med* 166:490, 2001.
129. Lim RC Jr, Olcott CT, Robinson AJ, et al: Platelet response and coagulation changes following massive blood replacement. *J Trauma* 13:577, 1973.
130. Miller RD, Robbins TO, Tong MJ, et al: Coagulation defects associated with massive blood transfusions. *Ann Surg* 174:794, 1971.
131. Counts RB, Haisch C, Simon TL, et al: Hemostasis in massively transfused trauma patients. *Ann Surg* 190:91, 1979.
132. Davis RW, Patkin M: Ultrafresh blood for massive transfusion. *Med J Aust* 1:172, 1979.
133. Simmons RL, Collins JA, Heisterkamp CA, et al: Coagulation disorders in combat casualties. I. Acute changes after wounding. II. Effects of massive transfusion. 3. Post-resuscitative changes. *Ann Surg* 169:455, 1969.
134. Kiraly LN, Differding JA, Enomoto TM, et al: Resuscitation with normal saline (NS) vs. lactated ringers (LR) modulates hypercoagulability and leads to increased blood loss in an uncontrolled hemorrhagic shock swine model. *J Trauma* 61:57, 2006.
135. Todd AR, Malinoski D, Muller PJ, et al: Hextend attenuates hypercoagulability after severe liver injury in swine. *J Trauma* 59:589, 2005.
136. Alam HB, Stanton K, Koustova E, et al: Effect of different resuscitation strategies on neutrophil activation in a swine model of hemorrhagic shock. *Resuscitation* 60:91, 2004.
137. Malone DL, Dunne J, Tracy JK, et al: Blood transfusion, independent of shock severity, is associated with worse outcome in trauma. *J Trauma* 54:898, 2003.
138. Chen H, Alam HB, Querol RI, et al: Identification of expression patterns associated with hemorrhage and resuscitation: integrated approach to data analysis. *J Trauma* 60(4):701–723; discussion 723-4, 2006.
139. Ayuste EC: Hepatic and pulmonary apoptosis after hemorrhagic shock in swine can be reduced through modifications of conventional Ringer's solution. *J Trauma* 60:52, 2006.
140. Downes KA, Wilson E, Yovian R, et al: Serial measurement of clotting factors in thawed plasma stored for 5 days. *Transfusion* 41:570, 2001.
141. Repine TB, Perkins JG, Kauvar DS, et al: The use of fresh whole blood in massive transfusion. *J Trauma* 60[6, Suppl]:S59, 2006.
142. Ketchum L, Hess JR, Hiippala S: Indications for early FFP, cryoprecipitate and platelet transfusion in trauma. *J Trauma* 60[6, Suppl]:S51, 2006.
143. Malone DL, Hess JR, Fingerhut A: Massive transfusion practices around the globe and a suggestion for a common massive transfusion protocol. *J Trauma* 60[6, Suppl]:S91, 2006.
144. Cannon WB: Wound shock, in Weed F, McAfee L (eds): *The Medical Department of the United States Army in the World War*. Washington, DC, Government Printing Office, 1927, p 185.
145. Davis JW, Shackford SR, Mackersie RC, et al: Base deficit as a guide to volume resuscitation. *J Trauma* 28:1464, 1988.
146. Powell CC, Schultz SC, Burris DG, et al: Subcutaneous oxygen tension: a useful adjunct in assessment of perfusion status. *Crit Care Med* 23:867, 1995.
147. Knudson MM, Bermudez KM, Doyle CA, et al: Use of tissue oxygen tension measurements during resuscitation from hemorrhagic shock. *J Trauma* 42:608, 1997.
148. Ivatury RR, Simon RJ, Havriliak D, et al: Gastric mucosal pH and oxygen delivery and oxygen consumption indices in the assessment of adequacy of resuscitation after trauma: a prospective randomized study. *J Trauma* 39:128, 1995.
149. Taylor JH, Mulier KE, Myers DE, et al: Use of ear-infrared spectroscopy in early determination of irreversible hemorrhagic shock. *J Trauma* 58:1119, 2005.
150. Crookes BA, Cohn SM, Bloch S, et al: Can near-infrared spectroscopy identify the severity of shock in trauma patients? *J Trauma* 58:806, 2005.
151. Irwin RS, Rippe JM (eds): *Intensive Care Medicine*. 5th ed. Philadelphia, PA, Lippincott, Williams & Wilkins, 2003.

CHAPTER 159 ■ THE MANAGEMENT OF SEPSIS

PAUL E. MARIK

Sepsis is among the most common reasons for admission to medical ICUs throughout the world. Over the last two decades, the incidence of sepsis in the United States has trebled and is now the 10th leading cause of death [1,2]. Advances in medical technologies, the increasing use of immunosuppressive agents, and the aging of the population have contributed to the exponential increase in the incidence of sepsis. In the United States alone, approximately 750,000 cases of sepsis occur each year, at least 225,000 of which are fatal [1,2]. Septic patients are generally hospitalized for extended periods, rarely leaving the ICU before 2 to 3 weeks. Despite the use of antimicrobial agents and advanced life support, the case fatality rate for patients with sepsis has remained between 20% and 30% over the last two decades [1,2]. This chapter provides an overview of this vast topic with particular emphasis on the management of severe sepsis and septic shock.

DEFINITIONS

Sepsis originally meant "putrefaction," a decomposition of organic matter by bacteria and fungi. Since then, a wide variety of definitions have been applied to sepsis, including sepsis syndrome, severe sepsis, septicemia, and septic shock [3]. In 1991, the American College of Chest Physicians/Society of Critical Care Medicine developed a new set of terms and definitions to define "sepsis" in a more precise manner [4]. The definitions take into account the findings that sepsis may result from a multitude of infectious agents and microbial mediators and may not be associated with actual bloodstream infection. Although the use of these criteria has been criticized and a "newer" diagnostic schema has been suggested (PIRO, which stands for predisposition, insult infection, response, organ dysfunction), these criteria still provide a useful framework to approach patients with infectious diseases [5]. The term "systemic inflammatory response syndrome" (SIRS) was coined to describe the common systemic response to a wide variety of insults. It is characterized by two or more of the following clinical manifestations: (a) a body temperature of >38°C or <36°C; (b) a heart rate greater than 90 beats per minute; (c) tachypnea, as manifested by a respiratory rate of greater than 20 breaths per minute; (d) an alteration of the WBC count of greater than 12,000 cells per mm^3, less than 4,000 cells per mm^3 or the presence of greater than 10% immature neutrophils. When the SIRS is the result of a confirmed infectious process, it is termed "sepsis." Severe sepsis is defined as sepsis plus either organ dysfunction or evidence of hypoperfusion or hypotension. Septic shock is best defined as systolic pressure less than 90 mm Hg (or a fall in systolic pressure of >40 mm Hg) or a mean arterial pressure less than 65 mm Hg after a crystalloid fluid challenge of 30 mL per kg body weight (approximately 2,000 mL) in patients with sepsis and in the absence of other causes for hypotension [6]. In a patient previously known to have a low baseline blood pressure, septic shock is defined as a 30% or greater drop in the mean arterial pressure.

Three stages in the hierarchy of the host's response to infection was therefore recognized, namely, sepsis, severe sepsis and septic shock, with sepsis having the best prognosis and septic shock the worst. Data from recently published trials support this postulate, with the mortality from sepsis ranging from 10% to 15%, severe sepsis from 17% to 20% and septic shock from 43 to 54% [6]. The distinction between severe sepsis and septic shock is critically important as it stratifies patients into groups with a low and high risk of dying respectively. It also suggests that a more aggressive treatment strategy may be indicated in patients with septic shock (see Fig. 159.1).

In patients with shock, the serum lactate has long been recognized to be a marker of disease severity and to be useful for disease stratification [7,8]. Septic patients with a lactate above 4 mmol per L are at an increased risk of death and warrant a more aggressive approach to resuscitation [9–11]. In addition the rate of lactate clearance has been demonstrated to be a good prognostic marker [12].

SITES OF INFECTION AND BACTERIOLOGY

The microbiology and primary sources of infection have undergone a remarkable transition over the past 30 years. The predominant pathogens responsible for sepsis in the 1960s and 1970s were Gram-negative bacilli; however, over the last few decades there has been a progressive increase in the incidence of sepsis caused by Gram-positive and opportunistic fungal pathogens [1]. Data from the large sepsis trials published during the last decade indicate that Gram-positive and Gram-negative pathogens are responsible for about 25% of infections each, with a further 15% due to mixed Gram-positive, Gram-negative organisms, with fungal pathogens accounting for between 5% and 10% of cases. This evolution in the spectrum of pathogens has been associated with an increase in the incidence of multiresistant organisms. Although the abdomen was the major source of infection from 1970 to 1990, in the last two decades pulmonary infections have emerged as the most frequent site of infection.

PATHOGENESIS OF SEPSIS

The pathogenesis of sepsis is exceeding complex and involves an interaction between multiple microbial and hosts factors. Indeed, after exposure to both Gram-negative and Gram-positive bacteria, macrophages upregulate the expression of over 1,000 genes (and proteins) and downregulate an excess of 300 genes, the net result depending on the complex interrelated interaction of these factors [13]. With advances in molecular biology many of the mysteries of sepsis are being unraveled; however, we have only just embarked on our journey along the "sepsis superhighway." The reader is referred to many excellent reviews on this topic [14–19]. Essentially as noted by William Osler in 1921 "*except on a few occasions the patient appears to die from the body's response to infection rather than from it*" [20]. Sepsis can be viewed as an excessively exuberant proinflammatory response with increased production of proinflammatory mediators with activation of leukocytes, mononuclear cells, and the coagulation cascade. The end result is widespread microvascular and cellular injury. The cellular injury results in alteration of cellular and subcellular membranes and receptors, activation of intracellular enzymes, increased apoptosis, mitochondrial dysfunction, and sepsis-related immunosuppression. The excessive proinflammatory responses together with activation of the coagulation cascade are believed to be fundamental events resulting in a systemic microvascular injury. The systemic microvascular injury is a defining characteristic of sepsis and is believed to play a major pathophysiologic role in the progressive organ dysfunction of sepsis.

ORGAN SYSTEM INVOLVEMENT IN SEPSIS

The Hemodynamic Derangements of Sepsis

Sepsis is characterized by a complex combination of cardiovascular derangements, including vasodilation, hypovolemia, myocardial depression, and altered microvascular flow. In volume resuscitated patients with septic shock, systemic vascular resistance is usually low, contractility and biventricular ejection fractions are reduced while ventricular dimensions and heart rate are increased. Despite these changes, volume resuscitated patients typically have a hyperdynamic circulation with a high cardiac output. However, recent data suggest that up to 60% of patients with septic shock may have a hypodynamic circulation with a deceased ejection fraction (<45%) and global left ventricular (LV) hypokinesia [21]. Furthermore, increasing evidence suggests that patients with sepsis develop structural injury to the contractile apparatus of the heart that may contribute to the myocardial dysfunction in sepsis. This is evident by elevated levels of troponin and B-type natriuretic peptide in patients with sepsis [22–24]. Estimates of LV ejection fraction correlate negatively with increased levels of cardiac troponin in patients with septic shock. These data suggest that all patients with sepsis should undergo serial echocardiography to characterize the hemodynamic pattern, as this impacts on the approach to the use of vasopressor and inotropic agents [21]. In addition, cardiac troponin should be measured to assess the degree of myocardial injury.

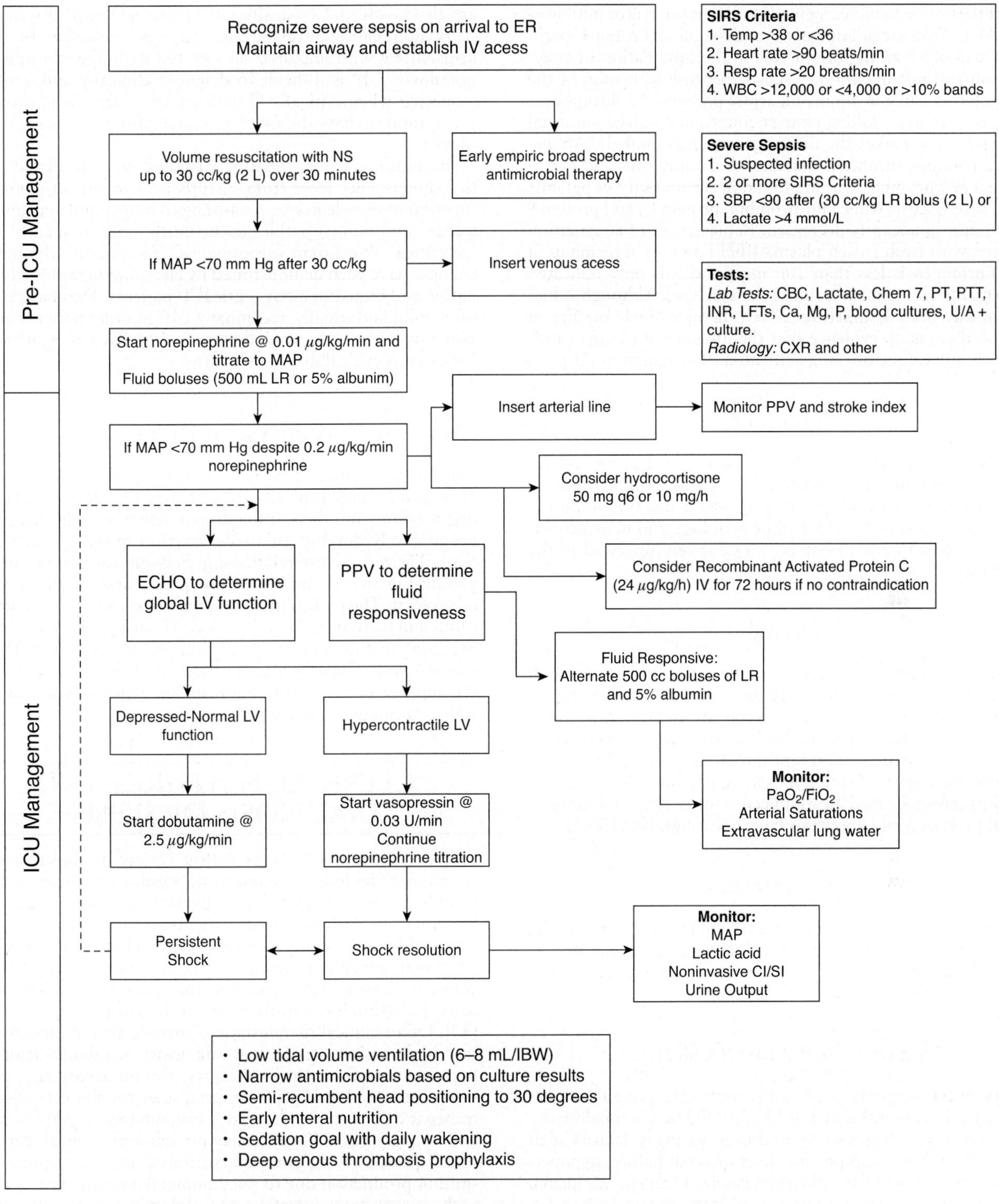

FIGURE 159.1. Suggested approach to the management of patients with severe sepsis and septic shock. CBC, complete blood cell count; CI, cardiac index; CXR, chest x-ray; ER, emergency room; IBW, ideal body weight; ICU, intensive care unit; IV, intravenous; LFTs, liver function tests; LR, lactated Ringer's solution; LV, left ventricle; MAP, mean arterial pressure; NS, normal saline; PPV, pulse pressure variation; PT, prothrombin time; SBP, systolic blood pressure; SI, stroke index; SIRS, systemic inflammatory response syndrome; PTT, partial thromboplastin time; WBC, white blood cell.

Coagulation Activation

Activation of the coagulation cascade with the generation of fibrin is a pathologic and physiologic hallmark of sepsis that occurs in both the intravascular and extravascular compartments [25]. Intravascular coagulation is characterized by diffuse microvascular thrombosis that contributes to widespread ischemic organ damage. Activation of coagulation during sepsis is primarily driven by the tissue factor pathway. Fibrin formation in sepsis likely results from both increased fibrin generation and impaired fibrin degradation. Inhibition of fibrinolysis is primarily due to increases in plasminogen activator inhibitor-1 (PAI-1). Downregulation of the anticoagulant Protein C pathway also plays an important role in the modulation of coagulation and inflammation in sepsis. Because activation of the coagulation cascade almost all septic patients are thrombocytopenic (or have a falling platelet count), and indeed a normal platelet count makes the diagnosis of sepsis unlikely. An elevated D-dimer, thrombin–antithrombin complexes and a prolonged prothrombin time are found in the majority of patients with severe sepsis while antithrombin, protein C, and protein S levels are significantly decreased. Replacement of coagulation factors with fresh frozen plasma ([FFP] and cryoprecipitate if the fibrinogen is less than 100 mg per dL) is only indicated in patients with clinical evidence of bleeding. Although it had previously been assumed that such therapy "fuels the fire of DIC," there is no evidence that the infusion of plasma products stimulates the ongoing activation of coagulation [26].

Pulmonary

Sepsis is by far the most common cause of the acute respiratory distress syndrome (ARDS) [27–29]. The mortality rate for patients with sepsis complicated by ARDS has been reported to be as high as 60%. The pathophysiology and management of patients with ARDS has been extensively reviewed in the literature.

Renal

Acute renal failure is a serious complication in patients with sepsis. Despite improvements in the support of these patients, the mortality rate remains consistently above 50%. It is, therefore, essential that all patients with sepsis be aggressively resuscitated in an attempt to prevent this complication. The pathogenetic mechanisms leading to ARF in patients with sepsis are unclear ;however, mediator-induced cytotoxicity, alterations in renal perfusion and apoptosis have been suggested [30,31].

Gastrointestinal

The most important gastrointestinal complications occurring in patients with sepsis include gastric stress ulceration, a diffuse splanchnic mucosal injury with increased intestinal permeability and intrahepatic cholestasis.

Nervous and Musculoskeletal

Septic encephalopathy is an acute, reversible, generalized disturbance in cerebral function [32,33]. Septic encephalopathy is essentially a diagnosis by exclusion as many factors such as sedative drugs, encephalitis, liver or renal failure, hypoperfusion, fever, adrenal insufficiency, cerebral vascular accidents, and drug fever either alone or in combination may result in disturbed cerebral function. Electroencephalography is useful in confirming the diagnosis of septic encephalopathy and allows assessment of the severity of the encephalopathy. Treatment is essentially supportive.

Critical illness polyneuropathy (CIP), as initially described by Bolton et al. in 1984, is a sensorimotor polyneuropathy that is often a complication of sepsis and multiorgan failure, occurring in 70% of such patients [34–36]. Postmortem examination of peripheral nerve specimens from patients with CIP has shown primary degeneration of motor and sensory nerves that supply the limbs and respiratory system. Although this denervation is more widespread and severe in the distal muscle groups, the phrenic nerve, diaphragm, and intercostals muscles are also involved. Classically, CIP is associated with a symmetric predominantly distal paresis, with legs involved worse than arms, along with impaired sensory testing in the feet and hyporeflexia. CIP is difficult to diagnose clinically and is often suspected when critically ill patients are otherwise improving yet continue to have difficulty in weaning from mechanical ventilation.

In addition to neuropathy, weakness in critically ill septic patients may stem from disturbances in the structure or function of muscle per se. According to biopsy and neurophysiologic studies, myopathies occur much more frequently during critical illness than was previously recognized. Myopathic changes have been demonstrated by electromyographic examination and biopsy in many septic ICU patients. The changes are often mild and usually accompany CIP. In other patients however, myopathy is the predominant finding. This myopathy has been called critical illness myopathy.

Sepsis and Multisystem Organ Dysfunction

The ultimate cause of death in patients with sepsis is multiple organ failure. Typically, patients will first develop a single organ failure and then, if the disease remains unchecked, will progressively develop failure/dysfunction of other organ systems. There is a close relationship between the severity of organ dysfunction on admission to an ICU and the probability of survival. The pathogenesis of organ dysfunction is multifactorial and incompletely understood. Tissue hypoperfusion and hypoxia are dominant factors. Multisystem organ dysfunction has an extraordinarily high mortality and, for many patients, the support of this syndrome does not improve survival but rather prolongs the dying process.

CLINICAL FEATURES AND DIAGNOSIS OF SEPSIS

Sepsis is a systemic process with a variety of clinical manifestations. The initial symptoms of sepsis are nonspecific and include malaise, tachycardia, tachypnea, fever, and sometimes hypothermia. Although most patients with sepsis have an elevated white cell count, some patients present with a low white cell count, which in general, is a poor prognostic sign. A band count in excess of 10% has been reported to have a high specificity (92%) but low sensitivity for the diagnosis of sepsis (43%) [37]. Other clinical manifestations include altered mental status, hypotension, respiratory alkalosis, metabolic acidosis, hypoxemia with acute lung injury, thrombocytopenia, consumptive coagulopathy, proteinuria, acute tubular necrosis, intrahepatic cholestasis, elevated transaminases, hyperglycemia, and hypoglycemia. Patients may present with clinical features of a localized site of infection, such as cough, tachypnea and sputum production due to pneumonia; flank pain and dysuria with urinary tract infection and abdominal pain with intra-abdominal infection.

The manifestations of sepsis can sometimes be quite subtle, particularly in the very young, the elderly, and those patients with chronic debilitating or immunosuppressing conditions. These patients may present with normothermia or hypothermia. The failure to generate a temperature greater than 99.6°F (37.5°C) in the first 24 hours of clinical illness, has been associated with an increased mortality rate. An altered mental state or an otherwise unexplained respiratory alkalosis may be the presenting feature of sepsis.

The signs and symptoms of systemic inflammation are not useful in distinguishing infectious from noninfectious causes of SIRS. Furthermore, a bacterial pathogen is not isolated in all patients with sepsis. Consequently, a number of biomarkers have been evaluated as more specific indicators of infection, including procalcitonin (PCT) and triggering receptor expressed on myeloid cells (TREM-1). PCT, a propeptide of calcitonin, is normally produced in the C-cells of the thyroid. In healthy individuals, PCT levels are very low (<0.1 ng per mL). In patients with sepsis, however, PCT levels increase dramatically, sometimes to more than several hundred nanograms per milliliter. The exact site of PCT production during sepsis is uncertain; however, mononuclear leukocytes and the liver seem to be the major sources of PCT. TREM-1 is a monocyte receptor that is upregulated by bacterial and fungal pathogens [38]. The ligand for TREM-1 is unknown. A soluble form of TREM-1 (sTREM-1) is released from activated phagocytes and can be found in body fluids. The use of these biomarkers has not gained widespread acceptance presumable due to the cost of the tests and the uncertain diagnostic accuracy.

Blood cultures are considered to provide the clinical gold standard for the diagnosis of bacterial infections. However, blood cultures are only positive in between 20% and 30% of patients with sepsis; moreover, it takes 2 to 3 days before the results become available. Molecular methods based on polymerase chain reaction (PCR) technology have been developed for infection diagnosis and pathogen identification. These methods offer a new approach based on detection and recognition of pathogen DNA in the blood, or indeed other clinical samples, with the potential to obtain results in a much shorter time frame (hours) than is possible with conventional culture. PCR based pathogen detection depends on the ability of the reaction to selectively amplify specific regions of DNA, allowing even minute amounts of pathogen DNA in clinical samples to be detected and analyzed. This technique holds great promise and may revolutionize our approach to the diagnosis of bacterial, fungal, and viral infections.

MANAGEMENT OF SEPSIS

The management of patients with severe sepsis and septic shock is complex requiring multiple concurrent interventions with close monitoring and frequent re-evaluations. These patients are best managed in intensive care units by physicians experienced in the management of critically ill septic patients. The reader is referred to the "*Surviving Sepsis Campaign guidelines for the management of severe sepsis and septic shock*"; these guidelines were developed by a number of international critical care organizations and should serve as the framework for the management of patients with sepsis [10].

The current strategy for the management of patients with sepsis is largely based on treating or eliminating the source of infection, timely and appropriate usage of antimicrobial agents, hemodynamic optimization, and other physiologic organ supportive measures (see Table 159.1). Attempts at downregulating the proinflammatory response with novel agents directed at specific proinflammatory mediators has uniformly met with failure. However, both activated protein C (APC) and glucocorticoids (low dose) are immunomodulators that have been demonstrated to improve the outcome of patients at high risk of death.

TABLE 159.1

SUGGESTED FLUID RESUSCITATION ALGORITHM FOR HEMODYNAMIC INSTABILITY OF SEVERE SEPSIS AND SEPTIC SHOCK

1 L Normal Saline 15–20 minutes
1 L 30 minutes
Start Norepinephrine if MAP ≤70 mm Hg
1 L 500 cc 5% albumin over 30–40 minutes
1 L Ringers 30–40 minutes
1 L 500 cc 5% albumin over 30–40 minutes
Ringers lactate 200 cc/h
Bolus 500 cc 5% albumin or Ringers Lactate

It has become increasingly apparent that in many patients there is a long delay in both the recognition of sepsis and the initiation of appropriate therapy. This has been demonstrated to translate into an increased incidence of progressive organ failure and a higher mortality. Kumar et al. investigated the relationship between the duration of hypotension prior to antimicrobial administration in 2600 patients with sepsis induced hypotension [39]. They reported that the risk of dying increased progressively with time to receipt of the first dose of antibiotic. Furthermore, there was a 5% to 15% decrease in survival with every hour delay over the first 6 hours. In the ENHANCE study, the mortality was 33% if drotrecogin alpha-activated (APC) was given within the first 24 hours of admission as compared to 52% if it was given on day 3 of hospitalization [40].

Levy et al. retrospectively analyzed the Sequential Organ Failure Assessment scores during the first 48 hours in 1,036 severely septic patients [41]. From baseline to day 1, the direction of change in cardiovascular, renal, respiratory, hematologic, and hepatic functions independently predicted 28-day mortality. The implications of this study is that if organ dysfunction is not improving during the first day of severe sepsis, the mortality risk is significantly increased, underscoring the importance of early recognition and therapeutic intervention to prevent sequential organ dysfunction [42]. Similarly, Rivers et al. demonstrated that early (within 6 hours) clearance of lactate is associated with improved outcome in severe sepsis and septic shock [12].

The concept that early aggressive treatment (within the first 6 hours of admission to hospital) of patients with severe sepsis and sepsis shock reduces sequential organ failure and improves survival has been demonstrated in the "landmark" study by Rivers et al. [43]. In this study, *early aggressive therapy* that optimized cardiac preload, afterload, and contractility in patients with severe sepsis and septic shock improved survival. The patients in the early-therapy group received, on average, approximately 1,500 mL more in total fluids in the first 6 hours of treatment than did the standard-therapy group and had a significantly higher mean arterial pressure (mean [±SD], 95 ± 19 vs. 81 ± 18 mm Hg; $p < 0.001$). Mortality was 30.5% in the group receiving early goal-directed treatment, as compared with 46.5% in the control group ($p = 0.009$). This strategy for managing patients with severe sepsis and septic shock has been called "early goal-directed therapy (EGDT)."

While the concept of early, as opposed to delayed, volume resuscitation and the timely initiation of appropriate antibiotics in patients suffering from severe sepsis and septic shock is a scientifically sound concept, the author believes that the major pillars on which EGDT is based (central venous pressure [CVP] >8 mm Hg, $ScvO_2$ >70% and blood transfusion) may be flawed (see later) [44]. A more evidence-based approach is provided in Figure 159.1.

Identification and Eradication of the Source of Infection

One of the most challenging features of the sepsis syndrome is that of identifying and eradicating, as early as possible, the source of infection. The majority of patients presenting with severe sepsis usually have a pulmonary, genitourinary, primary blood stream, intra-abdominal, or intravenous catheter as a source of infection. Recent studies have demonstrated that in approximately 75% of patients with presumed sepsis, an etiological agent can be isolated, these being equally divided amongst Gram-positive and Gram-negative organisms. It has been known for centuries that, unless the source of the infection is controlled, the patient cannot be cured of his or her infective process and that death will eventually ensue. Surgical control or percutaneous drainage of the infective process is therefore essential in most patients with severe intra-abdominal infections; recovery will not occur without them. Infected central venous catheters must be removed from patients with catheter related sepsis [45].

Antimicrobial Agents

Antimicrobial therapy remains the cornerstone of treatment in patients with sepsis. Empiric intravenous antibiotic therapy should be started within the first hour of recognition of severe sepsis, after appropriate cultures have been obtained. The choice of antibiotics is largely determined by the source or focus of infection, the patient's immunologic status, whether the infection is nosocomial or community acquired as well as knowledge of the local microbiology and sensitivity pattern. Initial empirical anti-infective therapy should include one or more drugs that have activity against the likely pathogens (bacterial or fungal) and that penetrate into the presumed source of sepsis. Because the identity of the infecting pathogen(s) and its sensitivity pattern(s) are unknown at the time of initiation of antibiotics, patients with severe sepsis and septic shock the initial regimen should include two or more antibiotics or an extended spectrum β-lactam antibiotic. A number of studies have demonstrated that appropriate initial antimicrobial therapy, defined as the use of at least one antibiotic active in vitro against the causative bacteria reduced mortality when compared with patients receiving inappropriate therapy [45,46]. Once a pathogen is isolated, monotherapy is adequate for most infections; this strategy of initiating broad-spectrum cover with two or more antibiotics and then narrowing the spectrum to a single agent when a pathogen is identified is known as "antimicrobial de-escalation." The indications for continuation of double-antimicrobial therapy include enterococcal infections and severe intra-abdominal infections. The role of double-antimicrobial therapy with a β-lactam antibiotic and aminoglycoside in patients with suspected or proven *Pseudomonas aeruginosa* infections is unclear; however, double coverage is prudent in immunocompromised patients [47,48]. In patients with culture-negative sepsis, continuation of the initial empiric combination is warranted. Additional antibiotics or a change in antibiotics may be required in patients with culture-negative sepsis who do not appear to be responding to the initial empiric regimen.

Although monotherapy is considered standard for community-acquired pneumonia, a survival benefit of a combination β-lactam and macrolide has been suggested. Waterer et al. found that patients with bacteremic pneumococcal disease who receive at least two effective antibiotic agents within the first 24 hours after presentation to hospital had a significantly lower mortality than patients who received only one effective antibiotic agent [49]. The most common combination was a third-generation cephalosporin with a macrolide or quinolone. Using a large hospital database, Brown et al. demonstrated a lower mortality, shorter length of stay and lower hospital charges for patients with community-acquired pneumonia treated with dual therapy using macrolides as the second agent [50].

To rapidly achieve adequate blood and tissue concentrations, antibiotics should be given intravenously, at least initially. Dosing regimens should take into account whether the antibiotic "kills" by time-dependent kinetics (e.g., β-lactam antibiotics, vancomycin) or concentration-dependent kinetics (e.g., aminoglycoside) [51,52]. The clinical effectiveness of β-lactam antibiotics and vancomycin is optimal when the concentration of the antimicrobial agent in the serum exceeds the minimum inhibitory concentration of the infecting organism for at least 40% of the dosing interval. In addition, antibiotic dosing should also take into account the patient's hepatic and renal function.

Chastre et al. performed a study in which patients with ventilator associated pneumonia were randomized to receive either 8 or 15 days of antibiotics [53]. Those treated for 8 days had neither excess mortality nor more recurrent infections, although those with nonfermenting Gram-negative bacilli did have a higher pulmonary infection recurrence rate. Antibiotics should therefore be continued until clinical improvement is noted and ordinarily should not be continued for more than 10 days (14 days for *P. aeruginosa* and Acinetobacter species), except in cases of osteomyelitis and endocarditis.

Hemodynamic Support

Fluid Resuscitation: Initial Versus Late

In the first hours of severe sepsis, venodilatation, transudation of fluid from the vascular space into the tissues, reduced oral intake and increased insensible loss combine to produce hypovolemia. Along with ventricular dysfunction, and arteriolar dilation volume depletion contributes to impaired global perfusion and organ function. Treating hypovolemia is the most important component of the early management of severe sepsis. However, once the patient has received an adequate fluid challenge (3 to 5 L) further fluid challenges may not increase cardiac output and global perfusion. Additional fluid may increase interstitial edema and further comprise the microvascular dysfunction that characterizes severe sepsis. The current paradigm of fluid management in patients with sepsis is one of adequate initial fluid resuscitation followed by conservative late fluid management. Conservative late fluid management is defined as even-to-negative fluid balance measured on at least two consecutive days during the first 7 day after septic shock onset. In a retrospective cohort study, Murphy et al. demonstrated that an approach that combines both adequate initial fluid resuscitation followed by conservative late fluid management was associated with improved survival [54]. Additional studies have demonstrated that those patients who have a smaller cumulative fluid balance have improved clinical outcomes [55–57].

Although the type of fluid used in the resuscitation of patients with sepsis has not been definitively shown to affect outcome, subgroup analysis of the SAFE study suggested a trend towards a more favorable outcome in patients who received albumin [58]. This finding is supported by experimental studies [59] and patients with malaria (similar pathophysiology to Gram-negative sepsis) [60]. Albumin has a number of properties that may be advantageous in patients with sepsis including the maintenance of the endothelial glycocalyx and endothelial function as well as having antioxidant and anti-inflammatory properties that may translate into less "third" space fluid loss. Hydroxyethyl starch solutions were previously recommended in patients with sepsis; however, these synthetic colloids have recently been demonstrated to be associated with an increased risk of renal failure (and death) and should therefore be avoided in patients with sepsis [61]. Despite differences in composition, normal saline (NS) and Lactated Ringer's solution (LR) are frequently considered equivalent and lumped under the term "balanced salt solution." However, both experimental and clinical data have demonstrated that these fluids are not equivalent. Studies have demonstrated the development of a hyperchloremic metabolic acidosis in human volunteers and patients resuscitated with normal saline [62–65]. Although the clinical implications of this finding are unclear, the additional loss (renal) of HCO_3 in the setting of reduced buffering capacity only adds to the acid–base burden characteristic of hypoperfused states [63]. Furthermore, resuscitation with normal saline may produce a "dilutional acidosis." Many erroneously believe that LR may worsen or cause a "lactic acidosis." This is impossible as lactate (the base) has already donated H+ ions; indeed, LR is converted to glucose (mainly in the liver). This reaction consumes hydrogen ions, thereby generating HCO_3 [66]. Although, the lactate concentration (base) may increase with LR, this increase is associated with an increase in HCO_3 and an increase in pH (even with liver disease). This observation was elegantly demonstrated by Phillips et al. in a swine hemorrhagic shock model; the results demonstrated a significantly higher pH (7.41 vs. 7.17) in animals resuscitated with LR as compared to normal saline [67]. In addition to its effects on acid–base balance, solutions high in chloride have been shown both experimentally and clinically to reduce the glomerular filtration rate (GFR) (due to tubuloglomerular feedback) [68]. The effects of normal saline on acid–base balance and renal function may be dose related. These data suggest that in patients with sepsis (except those with hyperkalemia), LR may be preferable to normal saline. There is however, no outcome data to support this recommendation. Furthermore, it should be noted LR solution is a racemic mixture containing both the L- and D-isomer of lactate. Small animal hemorrhagic shock models have suggested that the D-isomer is proinflammatory and increases apoptotic cell death [69–71]. The clinical implications of these findings are unclear.

On the synthesis of these data, we recommend initial resuscitation with NS (30 mL per kg). Normal saline is preferred until renal function tests and potassium are known. Patients who respond poorly to this initial bolus (±2 L) may best be fluid resuscitated with alternating boluses (500 mL) of albumin and LR until the hemodynamic goals are achieved (see "The Endpoints of Resuscitation" section and Fig. 159.1). The goal of this approach is to maintain normal acid–base balance, achieve adequate intravascular volume, and yet limit the total amount of fluid given.

Vasopressors, Inotropes, and Cardiac Function

The optimal time to initiate vasopressor agents has not been rigorously studied. Many patients with severe sepsis will respond to a 2-L fluid challenge and require little additional hemodynamic support. Others will remain hypotensive despite 10 L of fluid (fluid does not increase vascular tone!). The goal of fluid resuscitation is the rapid early restoration of intravascular volume followed by a conservative fluid strategy. We have therefore recommended that a vasopressor agent (norepinephrine) be started once the patient has received 2 L of crystalloid [6,72]. At this point, the norepinephrine (starting at 0.01 μg per kg per minute) should be titrated upwards while fluid resuscitation continues (albumin and LR). Ongoing fluid resuscitation should be guided by mean arterial pressure, pulse pressure variation, urine output, oxygenation as well as cardiac output (determined noninvasively), and extravascular lung water measurement [73,74]. Bedside echocardiography is very useful to determine LV size and function. The CVP neither intravascular volume nor does it predict fluid responsiveness and therefore has no place in the resuscitation of patients with sepsis [75].

Although there are little data to suggest that one vasopressor results in better outcomes than another (norepinephrine, epinephrine, vasopressin) [76–78], we favor norepinephrine as the first-line agent followed by dobutamine or epinephrine in patients with poor LV function and vasopressin (fixed dose of 0.03 U per minute) in patients with "preserved" LV function and a low systemic vascular resistance (see Fig. 159.1). In patients with sepsis, norepinephrine increases blood pressure, as well as cardiac output, renal, splanchnic, cerebral blood flow, and microvascular blood flow while minimally increasing heart rate [79,80]. Norepinephrine would therefore appear to be the ideal fist-line agent for the management of septic shock; additional agents should be considered in patients who remain hypotensive or display evidence of inadequate tissue or organ perfusion despite doses of norepinephrine up to 0.2 μg per kg per minute. The second/third-line agents should be chosen based on the patient's hemodynamic profile as determined by ECHO and noninvasive assessment of cardiac output.

Dopamine has a number of theoretical disadvantages in patients with sepsis. It tends to increase heart rate that increases myocardial oxygen demand and is associated with splanchnic mucosal ischemia. In addition, dopamine inhibits T and B lymphocytes and decreases secretion of prolactin, growth hormone, and TSH. The SOAP study suggested that septic patients who received dopamine had an increased mortality when compared with other vasopressors [81]. This drug should therefore be avoided in patients with sepsis. Similarly phenylephrine is not recommended, as in experimental models it decreases cardiac output as well as renal and splanchnic blood flow [82]. Furthermore, these agents have not been rigorously tested in randomized controlled studies.

The Endpoints of Resuscitation

The optimal "hemodynamic" endpoint of resuscitation in patients with sepsis is unknown. Similarly, the target mean arterial pressure (MAP) is controversial. Traditional teaching suggests that we should achieve a MAP above 60 mm Hg. However, this pressure is below the autoregulatory range of a number of organs, particularly in elderly patients with atherosclerotic disease. The *Surviving Sepsis Campaign* Guidelines suggest targeting a MAP above 65 mm Hg [10]. In a dose escalation study, Jhanji et al. incrementally increased the dose of norepinephrine to achieve a MAP of 60, then 70, then 80, and lastly 90 mm Hg [80]. In this study, global oxygen delivery, cutaneous microvascular flow, and tissue oxygenation increased with each sequential increase in MAP. However, LeDoux et al. demonstrated that increasing the MAP from 65 to 85 mm Hg with norepinephrine did not significantly affect systemic oxygen metabolism, skin microcirculatory blood flow, urine output, or splanchnic perfusion [83]. Dubin demonstrated that increasing mean arterial pressure from 65 to 75 and 85 mm Hg did not improve microcirculatory blood flow [84]. Similarly, Bourgoin et al. demonstrated that increasing MAP from 65 to 85 mm Hg with norepinephrine neither affected metabolic variables nor improved renal function [85]. However, Derudre et al. demonstrated that in patients with septic shock when the MAP was increased from 65 to 75 mm Hg, urinary output increased significantly while the renal resistive index significantly decreased [86]. These data suggest that although the endpoint of resuscitation should be individualized, a MAP of 65 to 70 mm Hg may be a reasonable initial target.

Central venous oxygen saturation ($ScvO_2$) is used as the endpoint of resuscitation in the EGDT algorithm [43]. This is problematic for a number of reasons. Septic patients usually have a normal or increased $ScvO_2$ due to reduced oxygen extraction [87,88]. A normal $ScvO_2$ therefore does not exclude tissue hypoxia [89]. A low $ScvO_2$ is an important sign of inadequate oxygen delivery to meet systemic oxygen demands. However, it provides no information for the reason for this inadequacy, nor does it provide guidance as to the optimal therapeutic approach. It is noteworthy that in the Rivers study the mean $ScvO_2$ was 49% with 65% of patients having a $ScvO_2$ less than 70%. To our knowledge, no other sepsis study has reproduced this finding, with the mean $ScvO_2$ (on presentation) in most sepsis studies being approximately 70% [89–91]. This suggests that other factors may have been in play to account for the low $ScvO_2$ in the Rivers study [92,93]. These factors include the delayed presentation to hospital (possibly due to socioeconomic factors), greater number of patients with comorbid medical conditions and a high incidence of alcohol use [93]. Thus the combination of significant comorbidities (including heart disease) and a more delayed arrival of patients to the Emergency Department in the River's study may have led to a low cardiac output state, and in turn, to the very low $ScvO_2$ values.

ADJUNCTIVE THERAPIES

While antibiotics, fluid resuscitation, vasopressors/inotropic agents and source control form the basic elements of the management of severe sepsis/septic shock, a number of adjunctive agents have been demonstrated to improve outcome or hold promise in improving the outcome of patients with sepsis. These agents should be considered in patients with severe sepsis/septic shock. The benefit of these agents is, however, time dependent and should be started as soon as possible and always within the first 24 hours of ICU admission

Corticosteroids

While the role of hydrocortisone in patients with septic shock is controversial, hydrocortisone should be considered in patients who require in excess of 0.2 μg per kg per minute of norepinephrine [94,95]. Adrenal function testing is not required in these patients. Evolving data suggest that increased levels of inflammatory mediators persist long after clinical resolution of sepsis [96,97]. Furthermore, abruptly stopping steroids results in a rebound phenomenon with worsening lung inflammation and hypotension These data suggest that the duration of therapy should be guided by the length of the immune dysregulation and should then be followed by a slow taper. Furthermore, the risk/benefit ratio of treatment with glucocorticoids is tightly linked to the dosage used. Although high doses of glucocorticoids blunt all arms of the immune system, stress-doses (200 to 300 mg hydrocortisone Eq per day) inhibit systemic inflammation; yet, maintain innate and Th1 immune responsiveness and prevent an overwhelming compensatory anti-inflammatory response [98,99]. Similarly, although myopathy is common in patients treated with high-dose corticosteroids, this complication is uncommon with stress-doses of corticosteroids. On the basis of these data, we suggest treatment with hydrocortisone in a dose of 50 mg every 6 hourly or a 100 mg bolus followed by an infusion at 10 mg per hour for 10 to 14 days followed by a slow taper.

Activated Protein C

The PROWESS study demonstrated a significant reduction in mortality in patients with severe sepsis and septic shock who were treated with activated protein C (APC) within 24 hours of hospital admission [100]. APC should be considered in patients with septic shock and those with sepsis and at least one organ failure, who are at a high risk of death, particularly patients with severe community-acquired pneumonia [101]. The use of APC in patients with sepsis has, however, become a very controversial and charged issue. This is largely driven by the high rate of serious bleeding that has been reported in retrospective cohort studies [102]. APC should be avoided in patients at high risk of bleeding, including patients with a platelet count of <30,000 per mL^3. Although APC increases the partial thromboplastin time (PTT) in vitro, the PROWESS study demonstrated an increased risk of bleeding when the PTT increased above 75 seconds. On the basis of these data, we monitor the PTT in patients on APC and hold the infusion (for a few hours) and transfuse FFP when the PTT exceeds 80 seconds (anecdotal experience only). Disseminated intravascular coagulation (DIC) is not a contraindication to APC; indeed in PROWESS the risk reduction was greater in patients with overt DIC than those without DIC (RR of 0.6 vs. 0.85) [103].

Patients with purpura fulminans and multiorgan failure due to meningococcal infection have significantly higher plasma PAI-1 levels as well as lower protein C levels than patients with meningococcal infection, but without purpura or organ failure [104]. In view of the low protein C levels in purpura fulminans, numerous case reports as well as open label studies have been published suggesting a benefit of treatment with APC [104–106]. Many of these patients concomitantly received FFP, fibrinogen, and platelets. APC has also been used for the treatment of purpura fulminans associated with Streptococcal and Staphylococcal infections [107].

Enteral Nutrition Supplemented with Omega-3 Fatty Acids

Three randomized controlled trials have demonstrated that in patients with sepsis and ARDS an enteral nutritional formula high in omega-3 fatty acids was associated with an increase in ventilator-free days, a shorter ICU stay, and a lower morality than patients fed a diet with a low omega-3 to omega-6 fatty acid ratio [108]. On the basis of these data, an enteral nutritional formula high in omega-3 fatty acids should be initiated within 24 hours of admission to the ICU. Patients are best fed gastrically via an oral or nasogastric tube. The use of vasopressors agents is not a contraindication to the use of enteral nutrition; indeed, enteral nutrition reduces the risk of gastric stress ulceration and bowel ischemia [109,110].

Polyclonal Immunoglobulins

Two meta-analyses have demonstrated that polyclonal immunoglobulins particularly those preparations enriched with IgA and IgM (IgGAM) reduce the mortality in patients with septic shock [111,112]. It is not clear which patient subgroups would benefit from this therapy; clearly asplenic patients should receive IgGAM as well as those patients at high risk of death.

ADJUNCTIVE THERAPIES OF POSSIBLE BENEFIT

Statins

HMG-CoA reductase inhibitors (statins) are a group of drugs with anti-inflammatory, immunomodulating, antioxidant, antiproliferative, antiapoptotic, antithrombotic, and endothelial stabilizing effects. Statins increase expression of endothelial nitric oxide (eNOS) while downregulating inducible nitric oxide (iNOS) [113]. Furthermore, statins interfere with leucocyte–endothelial interactions by decreasing expression of adhesion molecules and have antithrombotic effects. Experimental sepsis studies have demonstrated improved outcome with the use of statins and clinical studies have demonstrated that patients taking statins have a better outcome when they become septic [113–115]. We recommend the use of high-dose statins (e.g., atorvastatin/simvastatin 80 mg daily) in patients with severe sepsis; statins should however be avoided in patients taking azole antifungal as well as calcineurin inhibitors. The clinician should monitor for rhabdomyolysis.

Selenium

Sepsis is associated with an increase in reactive oxygen species and low endogenous antioxidative capacity. The selenium dependent glutathione-peroxidases (GPx) as well as thioredoxin reductases are important compounds responsible for the maintenance of the redox system in all cells including the immune-competent cells. The activity of these enzymes is mainly regulated by the availability of selenium. The selenium in intensive care (SIC) study demonstrated that high-dose intravenous selenium improved the outcome of patients with severe SIRS, sepsis, and septic shock [116]. Selenium supplementation should be considered in patients with severe sepsis and septic shock. Although the optimal dose and route remain to be established, we recommend a dose of 400 to 600 μg PO daily.

Zinc

Zinc is required for normal function of both the innate and acquired immune systems. Zinc deficiency results in marked abnormalities of immune function with zinc supplementation restoring natural killer cell activity, lymphocyte production, mitogen responses, wound healing, and resistance to infection. Stress, trauma, and sepsis have been associated with very low serum zinc levels [117,118]. In an experimental sepsis model, mortality was significantly increased with zinc deficiency, while zinc supplementation normalized the inflammatory response, diminished tissue damage and reduced mortality [119]. The benefit of zinc supplementation in patients with sepsis has yet to be determined.

CONCLUSION

The last two decades has seen a remarkable growth in our understanding of sepsis and the complex interconnection of multiple biological pathways involved in the septic process. This increased knowledge has opened the door to new therapeutic approaches to sepsis, and it is likely that these new approaches will lead to a reduction in the morbidity and mortality of patients with sepsis.

References

1. Martin GS, Mannino DM, Eaton S, et al: The epidemiology of sepsis in the United States from 1979 through 2000. *N Engl J Med* 348:1546–1554, 2003.
2. Angus DC, Linde-Zwirble WT, Lidicker J, et al: Epidemiology of severe sepsis in the United States: analysis of incidence, outcome and associated costs of care. *Crit Care Med* 29:1303–1310, 2001.
3. Bone RC: Sepsis, the sepsis syndrome, multiorgan failure: a plea for comparable definitions. *Ann Intern Med* 114:332–333, 1991.
4. Society of Critical Care Medicine Consensus Conference Committee: American College of Chest Physicians/Society of Critical Care Medicine Consensus Conference: Definitions for sepsis and organ failure and guidelines for the use of innovative therapies in sepsis. *Crit Care Med* 20:864–874, 1992.
5. Levy MM, Fink MP, Marshall JC, et al: 2001 SCCM/ESICM/ACCP/ATS/SIS International Sepsis Definitions Conference. *Crit Care Med* 31:1250–1256, 2003.
6. Marik PE, Lipman J: The definition of septic shock: implications for treatment. *Crit Care Clin* 9:101–103, 2007.
7. Cady LD Jr, Weil MH, Afifi AA, et al: Quantitation of severity of critical illness with special reference to blood lactate. *Crit Care Med* 1:75–80, 1973.
8. Weil MH, Afifi AA: Experimental and clinical studies on lactate and pyruvate as indicators of the severity of acute circulatory failure (shock). *Circulation* 41:989–1001, 1970.
9. Varpula M, Tallgren M, Saukkonen K, et al: Hemodynamic variables related to outcome in septic shock. *Intensive Care Med* 31:1066–1071, 2005.
10. Dellinger RP, Levy MM, Carlet JM, et al: Surviving sepsis campaign: international guidelines for management of severe sepsis and septic shock: 2008. *Crit Care Med* 36:296–327, 2008.
11. Howell MD, Donnino M, Clardy P, et al: Occult hypoperfusion and mortality in patients with suspected infection. *Intensive Care Med* 33:1892–1899, 2007.
12. Nguyen HB, Rivers EP, Knoblich BP, et al: Early lactate clearance is associated with improved outcome in severe sepsis and septic shock. *Crit Care Med* 32:1637–1642, 2004.
13. Nau GJ, Richmond JF, Schlesinger A, et al: Human macrophage activation programs induced by bacterial pathogens. *Proc Natl Acad Sci U S A* 99:1503–1508, 2002.
14. Cinel I, Opal SM: Molecular biology of inflammation and sepsis: a primer. *Crit Care Med* 37:291–304, 2009.
15. O'Brien JM Jr, Ali NA, Aberegg SK, et al: Sepsis. *Am J Med* 120:1012–1022, 2007.
16. Mackenzie I, Lever A: Management of sepsis. *BMJ* 335:929–932, 2007.
17. Abraham E, Singer M: Mechanisms of sepsis-induced organ dysfunction. *Crit Care Med* 35:2408–2416, 2007.
18. Singer M: Mitochondrial function in sepsis: acute phase versus multiple organ failure. *Crit Care Med* 35:S441–S448, 2007.
19. Russell JA: Management of sepsis. *N Engl J Med* 355:1699–1713, 2006.
20. Osler W: The evolution of modern medicine. New Haven, CT: Yale University Press; 1921.
21. Vieillard-Baron A, Caille V, Charron C, et al: Actual incidence of global left ventricular hypokinesia in adult septic shock. *Crit Care Med* 36:1701–1706, 2008.
22. McLean AS, Huang SJ, Hyams S, et al: Prognostic values of B-type natriuretic peptide in severe sepsis and septic shock. *Crit Care Med* 35:1019–1026, 2007.
23. Favory R, Neviere R: Significance and interpretation of elevated troponin in septic patients. *Crit Care* 10:224, 2006.
24. Mehta NJ, Khan IA, Gupta V, et al: Cardiac troponin I predicts myocardial dysfunction and adverse outcome in septic shock. *Int J Cardiol* 95:13–17, 2004.
25. Wang L, Bastarache JA, Ware LB: The coagulation cascade in sepsis. *Curr Pharm Des* 14:1860–1869, 2008.
26. Levi M, Toh CH, Thachil J, et al: Guidelines for the diagnosis and management of disseminated intravascular coagulation. British Committee for Standards in Haematology. *Br J Haematol* 145:24–33, 2009.
27. Leaver SK, Evans TW: Acute respiratory distress syndrome. *BMJ* 335:389–394, 2007.
28. Calfee CS, Matthay MA: Nonventilatory treatments for acute lung injury and ARDS. *Chest* 131:913–920, 2007.
29. Girard TD, Bernard GR: Mechanical ventilation in ARDS: a state-of-the-art review. *Chest* 131:921–929, 2007.
30. Groeneveld ABJ, Tra DD, van der Meulen J: Acute renal failure in the medical intensive care unit: predisposing, complicating factors and outcome. *Nephron* 59:602–610, 1991.
31. Schrier RW, Wang W: Acute renal failure and sepsis. *N Engl J Med* 351:159–169, 2004.
32. Streck EL, Comim CM, Barichello T, et al: The septic brain. *Neurochemical Research* 33:2171–2177, 2008.
33. Papadopoulos MC, Davies DC, Moss RF, et al: Pathophysiology of septic encephalopathy: a review. *Crit Care Med* 28:3019–3024, 2000.
34. Bolton CF, Laverty DA, Brown JD, et al: Critically ill polyneuropathy: electrophysiological studies and differentiation from Guillain-Barre syndrome. *J Neurol Neurosurg Psychiatry* 49:563–573, 1986.
35. Bolton CF, Gilbert JJ, Hahn AF, et al: Polyneuropathy in critically ill patients. *J Neurol Neurosurg Psychiatry* 47:1223–1231, 1984.
36. Bolton CF: Sepsis and the systemic inflammatory response syndrome: neuromuscular manifestations. *Crit Care Med* 24:1408–1416, 1996.
37. Cavallazzi R, Bennin CL, Hirani A, et al: Is the band count useful in the diagnosis of infection? An accuracy study in critically ill patients. *J Intensive Care Med* (in press): 2010.
38. Bouchon A, Facchetti F, Weigand MA, et al: TREM-1 amplifies inflammation and is a crucial mediator of septic shock. *Nature* 410:1103–1107, 2001.

39. Kumar A, Kazmi M, Roberts D, et al: Duration of shock prior to antimicrobial administration is the critical determinant of survival in human septic shock. *Crit Care Med* 32[Suppl]:41, 2004.
40. Bernard GR, Margolis BD, Shanies HM, et al: Extended evaluation of recombinant human activated protein C United States Trial (ENHANCE US): a single-arm, phase 3B, multicenter study of drotrecogin alfa (activated) in severe sepsis. *Chest* 125:2206–2216, 2004.
41. Levy MM, Macias WL, Russell JA, et al: Failure to improve during the first day of therapy is predictive of 28-day mortality in severe sepsis. *Chest* 124[Suppl]:120S, 2004.
42. Guidet B, Aegerter P, Gauzit R, et al: Incidence and impact of organ dysfunctions associated with sepsis. *Chest* 127:942–951, 2005.
43. Rivers E, Nguyen B, Havstad S, et al: Early goal-directed therapy in the treatment of severe sepsis and septic shock. *N Engl J Med* 345:1368–1377, 2001.
44. Marik PE, Varon J: Early goal directed therapy (EGDT): on terminal life support? *Am J Emerg Med* 28(2):243–245, 2010.
45. Mermel LA, Farr BM, Sherertz RJ, et al: Guidelines for the management of intravascular catheter-related infections. *CID* 32:1249–1272, 2001.
46. Kollef MH, Napolitano LM, Solomkin JS, et al: Health care-associated infection (HAI): a critical appraisal of the emerging threat-proceedings of the HAI Summit. *Clin Infect Dis* 47[Suppl 2]:S55–S99, 2008.
47. Paul M, Benuri-Silbiger I, Soares-Weiser K, et al: Beta lactam monotherapy versus beta lactam-aminoglycoside combination therapy for sepsis in immunocompetent patients: systematic review and meta-analysis of randomised trials. *Br Med J* 328:668, 2004.
48. Leibovici L, Paul M, Poznanski O, et al: Monotherapy versus beta-lactam-aminoglycoside combination treatment for gram-negative bacteremia: a prospective, observational study. *Antimicrob Agents Chemother* 41:1127–1133, 1997.
49. Waterer GW, Somes GW, Wunderink RG: Monotherapy may be suboptimal for severe bacteremic pneumococcal pneumonia. *Arch Intern Med* 161:1837–1842, 2001.
50. Brown RB, Iannini P, Gross P, et al: Impact of initial antibiotic choice on clinical outcomes in community-acquired pneumonia: analysis of a hospital claims-made database. *Chest* 123:1503–1511, 2003.
51. Marik PE, Lipman J, Kobilski S, et al: A prospective randomized study comparing once- versus twice-daily amikacin dosing in critically ill adult and pediatric patients. *J Antimicrob Chemother* 28:753–764, 1991.
52. Prins JM, Buller HR, Kuijper EJ, et al: Once versus thrice daily gentamicin in patients with serious infections. *Lancet* 341:335–339, 1993.
53. Chastre J, Wolff M, Fagon JY, et al: Comparison of 8 vs 15 days of antibiotic therapy for ventilator-associated pneumonia in adults: a randomized trial. *JAMA* 290:2588–2598, 2003.
54. Murphy CV, Schramm GE, Doherty JA, et al: The importance of fluid management in acute lung injury secondary to septic shock. *Chest* 136:102–109, 2009.
55. Alsous F, Khamiees M, DeGirolamo A, et al: Negative fluid balance predicts survival in patients with septic shock: a retrospective pilot study. *Chest* 117:1749–1754, 2000.
56. Vincent JL, Sakr Y, Sprung CL, et al: Sepsis in European intensive care units: results of the SOAP study. *Crit Care Med* 34:344–353, 2006.
57. Comparison of two fluid-management strategies in acute lung injury. *N Engl J Med* 354:2564–2575, 2006.
58. Finfer S, Bellomo R, Boyce N, et al: A comparison of albumin and saline for fluid resuscitation in the intensive care unit. *N Engl J Med* 350:2247–2256, 2004.
59. Walley KR, McDonald TE, Wang Y, et al: Albumin resuscitation increases cardiomyocyte contractility and decreases nitric oxide synthase II expression in rat endotoxemia. *Crit Care Med* 31:187–194, 2003.
60. Maitland K, Pamba A, English M, et al: Randomized trial of volume expansion with albumin or saline in children with severe malaria: preliminary evidence of albumin benefit. *Clin Infect Dis* 40:538–545, 2005.
61. Brunkhorst FM, Engel C, Bloos F, et al: Intensive insulin therapy and pentastarch resuscitation in severe sepsis. *N Engl J Med* 358:125–139, 2008.
62. Scheingraber S, Rehm M, Sehmisch C, et al: Rapid saline infusion produces hyperchloremic acidosis in patients undergoing gynecologic surgery. *Anesthesiol* 90:1265–1270, 1999.
63. Kellum JA, Bellomo R, Kramer DJ, et al: Etiology of metabolic acidosis during saline resuscitation in endotoxemia. *Shock* 9:364–368, 1998.
64. Waters JH, Gottlieb A, Schoenwald P, et al: Normal saline versus lactated Ringer's solution for intraoperative fluid management in patients undergoing abdominal aortic aneurysm repair: an outcome study. *Anesth Analg* 93:817–822, 2001.
65. Reid F, Lobo DN, Williams RN, et al: (Ab)normal saline and physiological Hartmann's solution: a randomized double-blind crossover study. *Clin Sci (Lond)* 104:17–24, 2003.
66. White SA, Goldhill DR, White SA, et al: Is Hartmann's the solution? *Anaesthesia* 52:422–427, 1997.
67. Phillips CR, Vinecore K, Hagg DS, et al: Resuscitation of hemorrhagic shock with normal saline vs. lactated Ringer's effects on oxygenation, extravascular lung water and hemodynamics. *Crit Care* 13:R30, 2009.
68. Wilcox CS: Regulation of renal blood flow by plasma chloride. *J Clin Invest* 71:726–735, 1983.
69. Deb S, Martin B, Sun L, et al: Resuscitation with lactated Ringer's solution in rats with hemorrhagic shock induces immediate apoptosis. *J Trauma* 46:582–588, 1999.
70. Ayuste EC, Chen H, Koustova E, et al: Hepatic and pulmonary apoptosis after hemorrhagic shock in swine can be reduced through modifications of conventional Ringer's solution. *J Trauma* 60:52–63, 2006.
71. Alam HB, Rhee P: New developments in fluid resuscitation. *Surg Clin North Am* 87:55–72, 2007.
72. Raghavan M, Marik PE: Management of sepsis during the early golden hours. *J Emerg Med* 31:185–199, 2006.
73. Marik PE, Cavallazzi R, Vasu T, et al: Dynamic changes in arterial waveform derived variables and fluid responsiveness in mechanically ventilated patients. A systematic review of the literature. *Crit Care Med* 37:2642–2647, 2009.
74. Marik PE: Techniques for assessment of intravascular volume in critically ill patients. *J Intensive Care Med* 24(5):329–337, 2009.
75. Marik PE, Baram M, Vahid B: Does the central venous pressure predict fluid responsiveness? A systematic review of the literature and the tale of seven mares. *Chest* 134:172–178, 2008.
76. Annane D, Vignon P, Renault A, et al: Norepinephrine plus dobutamine versus epinephrine alone for management of septic shock: a randomised trial. *Lancet* 370:676–684, 2007.
77. Myburgh JA, Higgins A, Jovanovska A, et al: A comparison of epinephrine and norepinephrine in critically ill patients. *Int Care Med* 34:2226–2234, 2008.
78. Russell JA, Walley KR, Singer J, et al: Vasopressin versus norepinephrine infusion in patients with septic shock. *N Engl J Med* 358:877–887, 2008.
79. Treggiari MM, Romand JA, Burgener D, et al: Effect of increasing norepinephrine dosage on regional blood flow in a porcine model of endotoxin shock. *Crit Care Med* 30:1334–1339, 2002.
80. Jhanji S, Stirling S, Patel N, et al: The effect of increasing doses of norepinephrine on tissue oxygenation and microvascular flow in patients with septic shock. *Crit Care Med* 37:1961–1966, 2009.
81. Sakr Y, Reinhart K, Vincent JL, et al: Does dopamine administration in shock influence outcome? Results of the Sepsis Occurrence in Acutely Ill Patients (SOAP) Study. *Crit Care Med* 34:589–597, 2006.
82. Malay MB, Ashton JL, Dahl K, et al: Heterogeneity of the vasoconstrictor effect of vasopressin in septic shock. *Crit Care Med* 32:1327–1331, 2004.
83. Ledoux D, Astiz M, Carpati CM, et al: Effects of perfusion pressure on tissue perfusion in septic shock. *Crit Care Med* 28:2729–2732, 2000.
84. Dubin A, Pozo M, Casabella CA, et al: Increasing arterial pressure with norepinephrine does not improve microcirculatory blood flow: a prospective study. *Crit Care* 13:R92, 2009.
85. Bourgoin A, Leone M, Delmas A, et al: Increasing mean arterial pressure in patients with septic shock: effects on oxygen variables and renal function. *Crit Care Med* 33:780–786, 2005.
86. Deruddre S, Cheisson G, Mazoit JX, et al: Renal arterial resistance in septic shock: effects of increasing mean arterial pressure with norepinephrine on the renal resistive index assessed with Doppler ultrasonography. *Int Care Med* 33:1557–1562, 2007.
87. Krafft P, Steltzer H, Hiesmayr M, et al: Mixed venous oxygen saturation in critically ill septic shock patients. The role of defined events. *Chest* 103:900–906, 1993.
88. Liu NK, Zhang YP, Titsworth WL, et al: A novel role of phospholipase A2 in mediating spinal cord secondary injury. *Ann Neurol* 59:606–619, 2006.
89. Marik PE, Bankov A: Sublingual capnometry versus traditional markers of tissue oxygenation in critically ill patients. *Crit Care Med* 31:818–822, 2003.
90. van Beest PA, Hofstra JJ, Schultz MJ, et al: The incidence of low venous oxygen saturation on admission to the intensive care unit: a multi-center observational study in the Netherlands. *Crit Care* 12:R33, 2008, doi:10.1186/cc6811.
91. Shapiro NI, Howell MD, Talmor D, et al: Implementation and outcomes of the Multiple Urgent Sepsis Therapies (MUST) protocol. *Crit Care Med* 34:1025–1032, 2006.
92. Bellomo R, Reade MC, Warrillow SJ: The pursuit of a high central venous oxygen saturation in sepsis: growing concerns. *Crit Care* 12:130, 2008, doi:10.1186/cc6841.
93. Perel A: Bench-to-bedside review: the initial hemodynamic resuscitation of the septic patient according to surviving sepsis campaign guidelines-does one size fit all? *Crit Care* 12:223, 2008.
94. Marik PE: Critical illness related corticosteroid insufficiency. *Chest* 135:181–193, 2009.
95. Marik PE, Pastores SM, Annane D, et al: Recommendations for the diagnosis and management of corticosteroid insufficiency in critically ill adult patients: consensus statements from an international task force by the American College of Critical Care Medicine. *Crit Care Med* 36:1937–1949, 2008.
96. Kellum JA, Kong L, Fink MP, et al: Understanding the inflammatory cytokine response in pneumonia and sepsis: results of the Genetic and Inflammatory Markers of Sepsis (GenIMS) Study. *Arch Intern Med* 167:1655–1663, 2007.
97. Yende S, D'Angelo G, Kellum JA, et al: Inflammatory markers at hospital discharge predict subsequent mortality after pneumonia and sepsis. *Am J Respir Crit Care Med* 177:1242–1247, 2008

98. Keh D, Boehnke T, Weber-Cartens S, et al: Immunologic and hemodynamic effects of "low-dose" hydrocortisone in septic shock: a double-blind, randomized, placebo-controlled, crossover study. *Am J Respir Crit Care Med* 167:512–520, 2003.
99. Kaufmann I, Briegel J, Schliephake F, et al: Stress doses of hydrocortisone in septic shock: beneficial effects on opsonization-dependent neutrophil functions. *Int Care Med* 34:344–349, 2008.
100. Bernard GR, Vincent JL, Laterre PF, et al: Efficacy and safety of recombinant human activated protein C for severe sepsis. *N Engl J Med* 344:699–709, 2001.
101. Laterre PF, Garber G, Levy H, et al: Severe community-acquired pneumonia as a cause of severe sepsis: data from the PROWESS study. *Crit Care Med* 33:952–961, 2005.
102. Eichacker PQ, Natanson C: Increasing evidence that the risks of rhAPC may outweigh its benefits. *Int Care Med* 33:396–399, 2007.
103. Dhainaut JF, Yan SB, Joyce DE, et al: Treatment effects of drotrecogin alfa (activated) in patients with severe sepsis with or without overt disseminated intravascular coagulation. *J Thromb Haemost* 2:1924–1933, 2004.
104. White B, Livingstone W, Murphy C, et al: An open-label study of the role of adjuvant hemostatic support with protein C replacement therapy in purpura fulminans-associated meningococcemia. *Blood* 96:3719–3724, 2000.
105. Wcisel G, Joyce D, Gudmundsdottir A, et al: Human recombinant activated protein C in meningococcal sepsis. *Chest* 121:292–295, 2002.
106. Hasin T, Leibowitz D, Rot D, et al: Early treatment with activated protein C for meningococcal septic shock: case report and literature review. *Int Care Med* 31:1002–1003, 2005.
107. Rintala E, Kauppila M, Seppala OP, et al: Protein C substitution in sepsis-associated purpura fulminans. *Crit Care Med* 28:2373–2378, 2000.
108. Pontes-Arruda A, DeMichele S, Srth A, et al: The use of an inflammation modulating diet in patients with acute lung injury or acute respiratory distress syndrome: a meta-analysis evaluation of outcome data. *JPEN J Parenter Enteral Nutr* 32(6):596–605, 2008.
109. Zaloga GP, Roberts PR, Marik PE: Feeding the hemodynamically unstable patient: a critical evaluation of the evidence. *Nutr Clin Pract* 18:285–293, 2003.
110. Marik PE, Vasu T, Hirari A, et al: Stress ulcer prophylaxis in the new millennium: a systematic review and meta-analysis. *Crit Care Med* 38:2222–2228, 2010.
111. Kreymann KG, de HG, Nierhaus A, et al: Use of polyclonal immunoglobulins as adjunctive therapy for sepsis or septic shock. *Crit Care Med* 35:2677–2685, 2007.
112. Laupland KB, Kirkpatrick AW, Delaney A: Polyclonal intravenous immunoglobulin for the treatment of severe sepsis and septic shock in critically ill adults: a systematic review and meta-analysis. *Crit Care Med* 35:2686–2692, 2007.
113. Terblanche M, Almog Y, Rosenson RS, et al: Statins: panacea for sepsis? *Lancet Infect Dis* 6:242–248, 2006.
114. Novack V, Terblanche M, Almog Y: Do statins have a role in preventing or treating sepsis? *Crit Care* 10:113, 2006.
115. Merx MW, Liehn EA, Janssens U, et al: HMG-CoA reductase inhibitor simvastatin profoundly improves survival in a murine model of sepsis. *Circulation* 109:2560–2565, 2004.
116. Angstwurm MW, Engelmann L, Zimmermann T, et al: Selenium in Intensive Care (SIC): results of a prospective randomized, placebo-controlled, multiple-center study in patients with severe systemic inflammatory response syndrome, sepsis, and septic shock. *Crit Care Med* 35:118–126, 2007.
117. Gaetke LM, McClain CJ, Talwalkar RT, et al: Effects of endotoxin on zinc metabolism in human volunteers. *Am J Physiol* 272:E952-E956, 1997.
118. Wong HR, Shanley TP, Sakthivel B, et al: Genome-level expression profiles in pediatric septic shock indicate a role for altered zinc homeostasis in poor outcome. *Physiological Genomics* 30:146–155, 2007.
119. Knoell DL, Julian MW, Bao S, et al: Zinc deficiency increases organ damage and mortality in a murine model of polymicrobial sepsis. *Crit Care Med* 37:1380–1388, 2009.

CHAPTER 160 ■ MULTIPLE ORGAN DYSFUNCTION SYNDROME

ANDREW C. BERNARD AND TIMOTHY A. PRITTS

Care of the critically ill has advanced substantially in the past 50 years to the point that patients who previously succumbed to illness or injury may now survive their initial insult. Unfortunately, this places them at risk for multiple organ dysfunction syndrome (MODS), with subsequent failure of organ systems and increased mortality [1]. A thorough understanding of the pathophysiology and treatment of MODS is necessary to attempt to mitigate associated secondary morbidity and mortality.

MODS can be defined as "the inability of one or more organs to support its activities spontaneously without intervention" [2]. Initial recognition of MODS came from combat casualty care during World War II as resuscitation strategies advanced sufficiently to allow casualties to survive the initial hemorrhagic shock insult, but rendered them vulnerable to subsequent acute renal failure [3]. Improved intensive care and resuscitation strategies subsequently led to the recognition of pulmonary failure in the form of ARDS during the Vietnam conflict [4]. Basic science and clinical research has increased our insight into the role of cellular hypoxia in the development of organ dysfunction and failure. Although advances in support for failing organs, including continuous dialysis and advanced ventilator care, have potentially increased survival, MODS remains a common cause of death in the intensive care unit.

DIAGNOSTIC CRITERIA AND SCORING SYSTEMS

MODS severity determines mortality [5]. Organ failure severity scoring was initially described by Knaus in 1985 [6]. Modern scoring systems consider grade and severity and are intended to serve as predictors of outcome. Among the most commonly used scoring systems are the multiple organ dysfunction score (MODS), sequential organ failure assessment (SOFA) and logistic organ dysfunction score (LODS) [7–9]. All include clinical and laboratory data for six organs: respiratory, cardiovascular, hematologic, hepatic, renal, and central nervous system (Table 160.1) [10]. The Denver Multiple Organ Failure (MOF) score is a simpler 4-point scale that has similar or superior specificity [11]. A "cellular injury score" based on measures of cellular dysfunction has also been described [12]. No single scoring system has been proven superior but all predict outcome more accurately than health care resource utilization [11,13]. The acute physiology and chronic health evaluation (APACHE), originally described by Knaus in 1985, is a scoring system that considers patient factors unrelated to the acute illness as well as acute illness severity [14]. APACHE considers many variables and is therefore not as easily calculable at

TABLE 160.1

CRITERIA USED IN COMMON ORGAN DYSFUNCTION SCORING SYSTEMS

Organ	Variable	Denver MOF [11]	SOFA [8]	LODS [9]	MODS [7]
Respiratory	PaO_2/FIO_2	Yes	Yes	Yes	Yes
	MV		Yes		
Hematology	Platelets		Yes	Yes	Yes
	WBC			Yes	
Hepatic	Bilirubin	Yes	Yes	Yes	Yes
	Prothrombin time			Yes	
Cardiovascular	MAP		Yes		
	SBP			Yes	
	Heart rate			Yes	
	PAR [(HR*CVP)/MAP]				Yes
	Dopamine		Yes		
	Dobutamine		Yes		
	Epinephrine		Yes		
	Norepinephrine		Yes		
	Any inotrope	Yes			
CNS	GCS		Yes	Yes	Yes
Renal	Creatinine	Yes	Yes	Yes	Yes
	BUN			Yes	
	Urine output		Yes	Yes	

Denver MOF, Denver multiple organ failure score; SOFA, sequential organ failure assessment; LODS, logistic organ dysfunction score; MODS, multiple organ dysfunction score; PaO_2, blood partial pressure of oxygen; FIO_2, fraction of inspired gas which is oxygen; MV, mechanical ventilation requirement; WBC, elevated white blood count; PAR, pressure adjusted heart rate; HR, heart rate; CVP, central venous pressure; MAP, mean arterial pressure; SBP, systolic blood pressure; CNS, central nervous system; GCS, Glasgow Coma Scale score; BUN, blood urea nitrogen.
Modified from Mizock BA: The multiple organ dysfunction syndrome. *Dis Mon* 55(8):476–526, 2009.

the bedside as MODS, SOFA, LODS, or Denver, but it reliably predicts both outcome and resource utilization, has been refined to its current version, APACHE IV, and may be useful for benchmarking ICU performance [15].

EPIDEMIOLOGY

Incidence of MODS varies based on primary diagnosis and the scoring system used to determine organ dysfunction. Seventy-one percent of ICU patients have some organ dysfunction [16] and about half have MODS [17], depending on the criteria used. For example, in one adult trauma ICU 47% had MODS, defined by SOFA ≤ 3 in two or more systems [18]. Septic patients are more likely to have organ dysfunction and more organ failures than nonseptic patients and mortality is higher if sepsis is present (31% vs. 21%) [16].

ETIOLOGY

MODS is most often the result of shock, sepsis, and trauma but there are many causes (Table 160.2) [19]. Forty-one percent of those patients with organ dysfunction have sepsis [16]. Sepsis most commonly originates in the lung (68%) and abdomen (22%) but there are many causes of sepsis-induced MODS [16].

MECHANISMS OF MULTIORGAN DYSFUNCTION SYNDROME

The systemic inflammatory response syndrome (SIRS) is frequently viewed as a predecessor to MODS and these syndromes represent a continuum of dysfunction. Components of the SIRS response are seen in virtually all patients following operation or injury. This response is usually self-regulating and rarely progresses to MODS. MODS may be viewed as a result of an ongoing and dysregulated SIRS response with progressive organ system derangement.

Despite extensive efforts, the pathophysiology of MODS is not fully understood and remains an area of intensive investigation [20]. Several mechanisms for the onset and propagation of MODS have been proposed, including an initial insult leading immediately to organ failure, a "two hit" model, where an initial stimulus primes the immune system to respond to a subsequent insult with an exuberant reaction, and the concept that a continuous ongoing insult contributes to MODS [20]. In clinical practice, each of these scenarios may result in MODS.

A common theme in the onset and propagation of MODS is the presence of a disordered immune response. It is likely that ongoing tissue hypoxia leads to activation of the acute inflammatory response and to dysregulation of the immune system [21]. Although the inflammatory response is an important component of normal recovery from injury and illness, organ failure appears to result from a loss of the balance between the pro- and anti-inflammatory cascades [22]. The proinflammatory response to a stimulus predominates initially, with increased release of proinflammatory mediators, increased capillary permeability, macrophage and neutrophil activation with tissue invasion and damage, disordered apoptosis, and microvascular thrombosis [23]. This initial response is normally tempered by the anti-inflammatory response, but this relationship may become dysfunctional. Together, these processes lead to early onset of MODS. If the organism survives the initial insult and onset of MODS, a period of immunosuppression follows. During this period, the patient becomes highly susceptible to nosocomial infection, with a normally survivable event such as pneumonia representing a life-threatening "second hit" [24].

TABLE 160.2

RISK FACTORS FOR MODS

Infection
Peritonitis and intra-abdominal infection
Pneumonia
Necrotizing soft tissue infections
Tropical infections (e.g., falciparum malaria, typhoid fever, dengue fever)
Inflammation
Pancreatitis
Ischemia
Ruptured aortic aneurysm
Hemorrhagic shock
Mesenteric ischemia
Immune reactions
Autoimmune disease
Reactive hemophagocytic syndrome
Antiphospholipid antibody syndrome
Transplant rejection
Graft versus host disease
Iatrogenic causes
Delayed or missed injury
Blood transfusion
Injurious mechanical ventilation
Treatment associated increased intra-abdominal pressure
Intoxication
Drug reactions (anticonvulsants, carboplatin, antiretrovirals, colchicines, propofol, amiodarone, monoclonal antibodies)
Arsenic
Drug intoxication (ecstasy, cocaine, salicylates, acetaminophen)
Endocrine
Adrenal crisis
Pheochromocytoma
Thyroid storm
Myxedema coma

Reproduced from Mizock BA: The multiple organ dysfunction syndrome. *Dis Mon* 55(8):476–526, 2009.

Extensive research continues to examine the potential role of the intestine in the onset and propagation of SIRS and MODS. From this work, it is hypothesized that acute injury damages the intestinal mucosa, leading to increased cytokine production from the intestinal epithelium and lamina propria with resultant systemic inflammatory response, and organ injury [25,26]. Under these circumstances, the intestinal barrier fails, leading to organ dysfunction. More recent studies have begun to examine the gut as a source of mediators that directly lead to organ damage [27]. These studies suggest that substances in the gut-derived mesenteric lymph directly lead to pulmonary dysfunction during shock states [28]. Full characterization of these mediators remains elusive.

CURRENT MANAGEMENT STRATEGIES

Course of MODS

Outcome in MODS partly depends upon host factors including genetics. Some patients are genetically predisposed to enhanced immune reactivity [29]. In most patients, MODS progression follows a typical sequence first described by Don Fry in 1980, beginning with lung failure, followed by the liver, gastric mucosa, and kidney [30]. Lung dysfunction was recently reaffirmed as the initial manifestation of MODS in the majority of patients [31]. Although a typical sequence of organ dysfunction usually occurs, the timing and rate of progression vary. MODS follows a bimodal onset with early and late MODS characterized by different patient characteristics and mechanisms of death [32]. An important distinction must also be made with early organ dysfunction during resuscitation, which is often reversible, and not necessarily the same as early MODS [33].

Respiratory organ dysfunction is the most common early manifestation of MODS but is often not associated with death [34]. Renal, central nervous and hematologic system impairments characterize MODS progression and are more strongly associated with mortality. Treatment of MODS therefore is focused on early recognition of those at risk, removing the source, and preventing MODS progression [35]. Clinicians should move briskly to optimize cardiorespiratory function, remove catabolic foci, and provide nutrition while using antimicrobials selectively and avoiding transfusion. Key advances in the treatment of patients with severe critical illness and MODS based on randomized controlled trials are summarized in Table 160.3.

TABLE 160.3

ADVANCES IN MANAGEMENT OF MULTIPLE ORGAN DYSFUNCTION SYNDROME BASED ON RANDOMIZED CONTROLLED CLINICAL TRIALS

Advance	Reference	Remarks
Early goal-directed therapy using venous oxygen saturation as a target.	[35]	Included as one of the Surviving Sepsis Guidelines.
Digestive tract or oropharynx decontamination with antimicrobials reduces 28-day mortality in ICU patients	[40]	Not widely practiced in the United States, as it conflicts with principles of antimicrobial stewardship
Lung protective ventilation strategies are associated with reduced mortality and increased ventilator-free days	[43]	Lung protective strategies are commonly utilized in ICU settings
Aggressive enteral nutrition is associated with improved immune function and less mortality in burned children	[49]	Landmark study suggested that protein repletion is essential in critically ill patients
Adjuvant treatment of patients with severe sepsis and septic shock with selenium is associated with decreased mortality	[53]	Mechanism of effect is unknown

Resuscitation

The Surviving Sepsis Guidelines summarize current best practice regarding resuscitation as of 2008 [36]. One major strategy to reduce MODS is to ensure optimal initial resuscitation. Resuscitation should target adequate oxygen delivery evidenced by oxygen saturation in mixed venous blood (SvO_2-saturation in mixed venous blood obtained from a pulmonary artery catheter or $ScvO_2$-saturation in central venous blood obtained from a central venous catheter in superior vena cava). Rivers et al. showed that by using oxygen delivery as a target for resuscitation with fluid, blood, and inotropes, lactic acidemia was less severe and outcomes were improved [37]. Inadequate initial resuscitation contributes to MODS [38]. For a comprehensive discussion of this topic, see Chapter 159.

Preventing MODS Progression

Source control is critical to prevent perpetuation of the inflammatory response [36]. Antimicrobials should be used as above, with tailored therapy and de-escalation [13]. On the basis of the possible role of the gut and enteric bacteria as a "motor" for MODS, several groups have proposed cleansing the bowel of bacteria to disrupt this relationship, but studies have yielded conflicting results and this practice remains controversial [27–29,39]. Although a recent European study supports parenteral and topical oropharyngeal antibiotics in reducing mortality, this is not widely accepted in the United States because it seemingly goes against the principle of antimicrobial stewardship [40]. Transfusion is a risk factor for MODS, suggesting that a conservative approach to blood transfusion is appropriate [41].

Mechanical ventilation contributes to distant organ dysfunction in acute lung injury (ALI) and acute respiratory distress syndrome (ARDS) [42]. In the ARDSNet trial, the "lung protective strategy" of plateau $\leq$30 cm H_2O and tidal volumes $\leq$6 mL per kg body weight was associated with a reduction in all cause mortality of 9% compared with conventional ventilation with plateau pressures $\leq$50 cm H_2O and tidal volumes $\leq$12 mL per kg body weight [43]. A European study affirmed that use of a ventilation strategy with volumes greater than ARDSNet (>7.4 mL tidal volume per kg body weight) increased mortality [44]. For a comprehensive discussion of this topic, see Chapters 47 and 58.

Although Van den Berghe initially reported reduced mortality with intensive insulin therapy and the mortality reduction was in septic MODS [45], unacceptably high rates of hypoglycemia have since been reported [46] without a mortality benefit.

Steroid therapy in patients with sepsis and MODS may be used for select indications. For a comprehensive discussion of this topic, see Chapter 159.

Nutrition

There are data to suggest that early initiation of enteral nutrition improves outcome in patients with severe trauma, surgery, sepsis, and MODS. MODS is attenuated in patients receiving enteral nutrition within 24 hours as opposed to initiation later [47,48]. Recent retrospective data support early enteral feeding to reduce ICU and hospital mortality [49]. Both the American and European Societies of Parenteral and Enteral Nutrition (ASPEN and ESPEN) recommend enteral nutrition in ventilated patients if hemodynamics are adequate and gastrointestinal function is present and the gut works [50,51]. Arginine has been shown to be beneficial in surgical and trauma patients but cannot be recommended in septic medical patients because of immunoinflammatory characteristics [50]. However, omega fatty acids do appear beneficial in shortening length of stay, ventilator days, and mortality in septic patients. Serum selenium is depleted in trauma and surgical patients and some evidence suggests that selenium depletion contributes to MODS. Selenium repletion reduced MODS in a multi-institutional prospective randomized trial [52]. For a comprehensive discussion of this topic, see Chapters 159 and 192.

Recombinant human activated protein C was initially shown to reduce mortality in septic patients though its benefit has been questioned in recent studies [13]. rhAPC remains indicated in adults with high risk of death [36]. For a comprehensive discussion of this topic, see Chapter 159.

Continuous renal replacement therapy has been associated with reduction of MODS severity, theoretically due to modulation of elevated pro- and anti-inflammatory cytokines [53], but no large studies currently support its use for this purpose. Other novel therapies include pharmacologic manipulation of the microcirculation or augmentation of mitochondrial oxidative metabolism to enhance oxygen delivery [13].

PROGNOSIS AND ICU LENGTH OF STAY

Up to 20% of patients admitted to intensive care units develop aspects of MODS, with significantly increased morbidity and mortality [54]. MODS severity is decreasing but ICU mortality remains stable, perhaps because overall acuity is increasing [35,55]. In an epidemiologic study of sepsis in 2001, Angus determined that dysfunction of one, two, or three organ systems conveys 1%, 4.7%, and 20.7% mortality, respectively [19]. Four-organ dysfunction was associated with 65% to 74% mortality [16,19]. A more recent study examining the outcomes of critically ill patients reported ICU mortality of 10% for failure of three systems or less, increasing to 25% and 50% for four- and five-organ system failure, respectively. Mortality of seven-system failure was 100% [56]. In addition to mortality, MODS also affects long-term functional outcome [18].

MODS is the most common reason for prolonged stays in the intensive care unit, exceeding single organ system failure and simply the need for ventilatory support [54]. The onset of MODS is associated with a markedly increased length of ICU stay and risk of mortality [17]. Determining prognosis for individual patients with MODS remains challenging. Severity of organ dysfunction at the time of ICU admission or during the ICU stay correlates well with mortality, with the highest scores suggestive of a nonsurvivable situation, but does not allow accurate bedside prediction of an individual patient's outcome [7]. The strongest independent risk factors for death appear to be CNS failure (RR = 16.06) and cardiovascular failure (RR = 11.83) [56].

CONCLUSIONS

MODS is largely a result of medical progress and modern ICU care. A common denominator in the pathogenesis of MODS appears to be cellular hypoperfusion, leading to an imbalanced immune response, with resultant organ damage and failure. Treatment of patients at risk for MODS is supportive, ensuring adequate resuscitation, nutrition, source control, and support of individual organ systems as they fail. Despite modern critical care, MODS remains a common cause of death in critically ill patients.

References

1. Levine JH, Durham RM, Moran J, et al: Multiple organ failure: is it disappearing? *World J Surg* 20(4):471–473, 1996.
2. Baue AE: Multiple organ failure—the discrepancy between our scientific knowledge and understanding and the management of our patients. *Langenbecks Arch Surg* 385(7):441–453, 2000.
3. Churchill ED: *Surgeon to Soldiers: Diary and Records of the Surgical Consultant, Allied Force Headquarters, World War 2*. Philadelphia, PA: Lippincott, 1972.
4. Ashbaugh DG, Bigelow DB, Petty TL, et al: Acute respiratory distress in adults. *Lancet* 2(7511):319–323, 1967.
5. Barie PS, Hydo LJ: Influence of multiple organ dysfunction syndrome on duration of critical illness and hospitalization. *Arch Surg* 131(12):1318–1323, 1996; discussion 1324.
6. Knaus WA, Draper EA, Wagner DP, et al: Prognosis in acute organ-system failure. *Ann Surg* 202(6):685–693, 1985.
7. Marshall JC, Cook DJ, Christou NV, et al: Multiple organ dysfunction score: a reliable descriptor of a complex clinical outcome. *Crit Care Med* 23(10):1638–1652, 1995.
8. Vincent JL, Moreno R, Takala J, et al: The SOFA (sepsis-related organ failure assessment) score to describe organ dysfunction/failure. On behalf of the Working Group on Sepsis-Related Problems of the European Society of Intensive Care Medicine. *Intensive Care Med* 22(7):707–710, 1996.
9. Le Gall JR, Klar J, Lemeshow S, et al: The logistic organ dysfunction system. A new way to assess organ dysfunction in the intensive care unit. ICU Scoring Group. *JAMA* 276(10):802–810, 1996.
10. Afessa B, Gajic O, Keegan MT: Severity of illness and organ failure assessment in adult intensive care units. *Crit Care Clin* 23(3):639–658, 2007.
11. Sauaia A, Moore EE, Johnson JL, et al: Validation of postinjury multiple organ failure scores. *Shock* 31(5):438–447, 2009.
12. Oda S, Hirasawa H, Sugai T, et al: Cellular injury score for multiple organ failure severity scoring system. *J Trauma* 45(2):304–310; discussion 310–311, 1998.
13. Mizock BA: The multiple organ dysfunction syndrome. *Dis Mon* 55(8):476–526, 2009.
14. Knaus WA, Draper EA, Wagner DP, et al: APACHE II: a severity of disease classification system. *Crit Care Med* 13(10):818–829, 1985.
15. Zimmerman JE, Kramer AA, McNair DS, et al: Acute Physiology and Chronic Health Evaluation (APACHE) IV: hospital mortality assessment for today's critically ill patients. *Crit Care Med* 34(5):1297–1310, 2006.
16. Vincent JL, Sakr Y, Sprung CL, et al: Sepsis in European intensive care units: results of the SOAP study. *Crit Care Med* 34(2):344–353, 2006.
17. Barie PS, Hydo LJ: Epidemiology of multiple organ dysfunction syndrome in critical surgical illness. *Surg Infect (Larchmt)* 1(3):173–185, 2000; discussion 185–186.
18. Ulvik A, Kvale R, Wentzel-Larsen T, et al: Multiple organ failure after trauma affects even long-term survival and functional status. *Crit Care* 11(5):R95, 2007.
19. Angus DC, Linde-Zwirble WT, Lidicker J, et al: Epidemiology of severe sepsis in the United States: analysis of incidence, outcome, and associated costs of care. *Crit Care Med* 29(7):1303–1310, 2001.
20. Barie PS, Hydo LJ, Pieracci FM, et al: Multiple organ dysfunction syndrome in critical surgical illness. *Surg Infect (Larchmt)* 10(5):369–377, 2009.
21. Rittirsch D, Flierl MA, Ward PA: Harmful molecular mechanisms in sepsis. *Nat Rev Immunol* 8(10):776–787, 2008.
22. Ward NS, Casserly B, Ayala A: The compensatory anti-inflammatory response syndrome (CARS) in critically ill patients. *Clin Chest Med* 29(4):617–625, 2008, viii.
23. Lenz A, Franklin GA, Cheadle WG: Systemic inflammation after trauma. *Injury* 38(12):1336–1345, 2007.
24. Tschoeke SK, Hellmuth M, Hostmann A, et al: The early second hit in trauma management augments the proinflammatory immune response to multiple injuries. *J Trauma* 62(6):1396–1403, 2007; discussion 1403–1404.
25. Pritts T, Hungness E, Wang Q, et al: Mucosal and enterocyte IL-6 production during sepsis and endotoxemia–role of transcription factors and regulation by the stress response. *Am J Surg* 183(4):372–383, 2002.
26. Clark JA, Coopersmith CM: Intestinal crosstalk: a new paradigm for understanding the gut as the "motor" of critical illness. *Shock* 28(4):384–393, 2007.
27. Senthil M, Brown M, Xu DZ, et al: Gut-lymph hypothesis of systemic inflammatory response syndrome/multiple-organ dysfunction syndrome: validating studies in a porcine model. *J Trauma* 60(5):958–965, 2006; discussion 965–967.
28. Magnotti LJ, Upperman JS, Xu DZ, et al: Gut-derived mesenteric lymph but not portal blood increases endothelial cell permeability and promotes lung injury after hemorrhagic shock. *Ann Surg* 228(4):518–527, 1998.
29. Villar J, Maca-Meyer N, Perez-Mendez L, et al: Bench-to-bedside review: understanding genetic predisposition to sepsis. *Crit Care* 8(3):180–189, 2004.
30. Fry DE, Pearlstein L, Fulton RL, et al: Multiple system organ failure. The role of uncontrolled infection. *Arch Surg* 115(2):136–140, 1980.
31. Ciesla DJ, Moore EE, Johnson JL, et al: The role of the lung in postinjury multiple organ failure. *Surgery* 138(4):749–757, 2005; discussion 757–758.
32. Moore FA, Sauaia A, Moore EE, et al: Postinjury multiple organ failure: a bimodal phenomenon. *J Trauma* 40(4):501–510, 1996; discussion 510–512.
33. Ciesla DJ, Moore EE, Johnson JL, et al: Multiple organ dysfunction during resuscitation is not postinjury multiple organ failure. *Arch Surg* 139(6):590–594, 2004; discussion 594–595.
34. Russell JA, Singer J, Bernard GR, et al: Changing pattern of organ dysfunction in early human sepsis is related to mortality. *Crit Care Med* 28(10):3405–3411, 2000.
35. Barie PS, Hydo LJ, Shou J, et al: Decreasing magnitude of multiple organ dysfunction syndrome despite increasingly severe critical surgical illness: a 17-year longitudinal study. *J Trauma* 65(6):1227–1235, 2008.
36. Dellinger RP, Levy MM, Carlet JM, et al: Surviving sepsis campaign: international guidelines for management of severe sepsis and septic shock: 2008. *Crit Care Med* 36(1):296–327, 2008.
37. Rivers E, Nguyen B, Havstad S, et al: Early goal-directed therapy in the treatment of severe sepsis and septic shock. *N Engl J Med* 345(19):1368–1377, 2001.
38. Levy B, Sadoune LO, Gelot AM, et al: Evolution of lactate/pyruvate and arterial ketone body ratios in the early course of catecholamine-treated septic shock. *Crit Care Med* 28(1):114–119, 2000.
39. Marshall JC, Christou NV, Meakins JL: The gastrointestinal tract. The "undrained abscess" of multiple organ failure. *Ann Surg* 218(2):111–119, 1993.
40. de Smet AM, Kluytmans JA, Cooper BS, et al: Decontamination of the digestive tract and oropharynx in ICU patients. *N Engl J Med* 360(1):20–31, 2009.
41. Napolitano LM, Kurek S, Luchette FA, et al: Clinical practice guideline: red blood cell transfusion in adult trauma and critical care. *Crit Care Med* 37(12):3124–3157, 2009.
42. Slutsky AS, Tremblay LN: Multiple system organ failure. Is mechanical ventilation a contributing factor? *Am J Respir Crit Care Med* 157(6 Pt 1):1721–1725, 1998.
43. Ventilation with lower tidal volumes as compared with traditional tidal volumes for acute lung injury and the acute respiratory distress syndrome. The acute respiratory distress syndrome network. *N Engl J Med* 342(18):1301–1308, 2000.
44. Sakr Y, Vincent JL, Reinhart K, et al: High tidal volume and positive fluid balance are associated with worse outcome in acute lung injury. *Chest* 128(5):3098–3108, 2005.
45. van den Berghe G, Wouters P, Weekers F, et al: Intensive insulin therapy in the critically ill patients. *N Engl J Med* 345(19):1359–1367, 2001.
46. Treggiari MM, Karir V, Yanez ND, et al: Intensive insulin therapy and mortality in critically ill patients. *Crit Care* 12(1):R29, 2008.
47. Moore FA, Moore EE: The evolving rationale for early enteral nutrition based on paradigms of multiple organ failure: a personal journey. *Nutr Clin Pract* 24(3):297–304, 2009.
48. Alexander JW, MacMillan BG, Stinnett JD, et al: Beneficial effects of aggressive protein feeding in severely burned children. *Ann Surg* 192(4):505–517, 1980.
49. Artinian V, Krayem H, DiGiovine B: Effects of early enteral feeding on the outcome of critically ill mechanically ventilated medical patients. *Chest* 129(4):960–967, 2006.
50. Kreymann KG, Berger MM, Deutz NE, et al: ESPEN Guidelines on enteral nutrition: Intensive care. *Clin Nutr* 25(2):210–223, 2006.
51. McClave SA, Martindale RG, Vanek VW, et al: Guidelines for the provision and assessment of nutrition support therapy in the adult critically Ill patient: Society of Critical Care Medicine (SCCM) and American Society for Parenteral and Enteral Nutrition (A.S.P.E.N.). *JPEN J Parenter Enteral Nutr* 33(3):277–316, 2009.
52. Angstwurm MW, Engelmann L, Zimmermann T, et al: Selenium in Intensive Care (SIC): results of a prospective randomized, placebo-controlled, multiple-center study in patients with severe systemic inflammatory response syndrome, sepsis, and septic shock. *Crit Care Med* 35(1):118–126, 2007.
53. Ratanarat R, Brendolan A, Piccinni P, et al: Pulse high-volume haemofiltration for treatment of severe sepsis: effects on hemodynamics and survival. *Crit Care* 9(4):R294–R302, 2005.
54. Martin CM, Hill AD, Burns K, et al: Characteristics and outcomes for critically ill patients with prolonged intensive care unit stays. *Crit Care Med* 33(9):1922–1927, 2005; quiz 1936.
55. Ciesla DJ, Moore EE, Johnson JL, et al: A 12-year prospective study of postinjury multiple organ failure: has anything changed? *Arch Surg* 140(5):432–438, 2005; discussion 438–440.
56. Mayr VD, Dunser MW, Greil V, et al: Causes of death and determinants of outcome in critically ill patients. *Crit Care* 10(6):R154, 2006.

CHAPTER 161 ■ TRAUMA SYSTEMS

CHRISTOPH R. KAUFMANN AND KEVIN DWYER

INTRODUCTION

The number of people who die from injuries worldwide is tremendous, numbering in the millions annually. Trauma also constitutes a public health crisis in the United States and is responsible for 150,000 lives lost annually. Trauma is the fifth leading cause of death in the United States by 2006 statistics published by the Center for Disease Control (CDC). It is the leading cause of death in the young, ages 1 to 44. Trauma is responsible for more years of productive life lost than cancer and heart disease combined. On average 36 life years (productive years) are lost per one trauma death compared with 12 life years lost for a heart disease death and 16 life years for cancer. For every death from trauma, there are three individuals who suffer permanent disability and 75 who suffer temporary disability. The cost of injuries in terms of lost wages, direct and indirect medical expenses, and property damage is over $400 billion [1,2].

BACKGROUND

Trauma is a time-sensitive disease, perhaps more so than any other. Indeed, half of all injury deaths occur before any intervention. Patients who are bleeding have only minutes to live unless the hemorrhage can be controlled. This control often involves operative intervention. This time-sensitive nature is best described by the "Golden Hour" concept. Severely injured trauma patients have a "golden hour" during which they should be transported to a trauma center and their injuries addressed.

Baron Dominique Jean Larrey, Napoleon's surgeon-in-chief, created the concept of the flying ambulance or "ambulance volantes." The important concept was that soldiers injured on the battlefield should be treated in the field and evacuated for surgical treatment as soon as possible. To achieve this goal, Larrey instituted the use of a horse-drawn cart on the battlefield—the flying ambulance.

Trauma systems today are focused on the rapid transport of injured patients to the appropriate level of care. This should be a verified trauma center rather than simply the closest hospital with an emergency department. The goal of trauma systems is quite simple: get the right patient to the right facility at the right time. Delay in care may result in early effects such as hemorrhagic shock or late effects such as sepsis from open fractures.

DEFINITIONS

Typically, trauma patients are individuals suffering from penetrating, blunt, or thermal trauma. Clearly combinations of mechanisms may occur, as well as special circumstances such as blast injury. Trauma patients should be triaged to the most appropriate facility for care. Triage should be based both on severity of injuries identified as well as on risk of severe injury. This is because the total sum of injuries is not known until the patient has been fully evaluated at the appropriate trauma center. Just because a patient is hemodynamically normal at a given point in time does not imply that he or she will remain that way.

Trauma centers are hospitals that have been designated by the state or other designating authority as qualified to care for injured patients. There are usually a limited number of trauma centers in a certain geographic area so that each receives an adequate volume of patients required to maintain clinical expertise. Most frequently, trauma centers are designated as Level I through Level IV (some states have also designated Level V trauma centers). Level I trauma centers provide the highest level of care, plus have research and teaching responsibilities. Level II trauma centers are intended to also provide for the full spectrum of trauma care, but do not have the research and teaching requirements. Level III facilities do not provide the full spectrum of trauma care; they usually do not provide neurosurgical services. Level IV trauma centers provide trauma care commensurate with their existing resources.

HISTORY

In 1966, the National Academy of Sciences and the National Research Council published "Accidental Death and Disability: The Neglected Disease of Modern Society," which highlighted trauma as a major public health problem and made specific recommendations to reduce accidental death and disability. This led to national and state legislation including the Highway Safety Act and the National Traffic and Motor Vehicle Safety Act that was the first effort to regulate traffic safety and reduce automobile related death and injuries. The Emergency Medical Systems (EMS) program was also established. Later, in 1973, the EMS Systems Act identified trauma systems as one of 15 essential components of an EMS system and appropriated federal funds [3].

VERIFICATION AND DESIGNATION

The trauma system encompasses the complete care of the injured patient from the point of injury prehospital to the completion of the rehabilitative process. Important activities of that system include injury prevention, education, research, and financial viability. For this, there needs to be a lead agency established by each state that has the authority to create and execute policy for the injured patients, as well as designate the trauma centers to manage the injured patients. In order to receive a designation, a hospital or medical center has to demonstrate the standards of care established by the designating authority to achieve the level of trauma center, I, II, III, or IV desired. The trauma center is then evaluated and verified by either an internal team or an external reviewer, such as the American

College of Surgeons (ACS), as meeting the necessary criteria to be a trauma center in the system. This verification is then recommended to the lead agency of the state for designation of a trauma center. The lead agency regulates the quality of trauma systems components and establishes trauma triage guidelines.

The American College of Surgeons Committee on Trauma wrote the "Optimal Hospital Resources for Care of the Seriously Injured" in 1976 and there is presently the fifth edition called the Resources for Optimal Care of the Injured Patient 2006. The ACS established this document and his since added greatly to it as a resource for quality of care and standards of both trauma centers and trauma systems. The ACS verification process consists of hospital site reviews to determine quality of care and appropriateness of the trauma PI process. This verification process can then be accepted by the state as the designating authority to either designate or maintain designation of the trauma center. The ACS-COT also reviews statewide trauma systems to make recommendations to the system as a whole [4–8].

QUALITY OF CARE

Early studies, such as those done in Orange County and San Diego County, California, refined the preventable mortality concept. These studies were able to clearly identify a group of trauma patients that died from inadequate care—preventable mortalities. This concept provided a tool that could be used to examine quality of trauma care in any region or system. Teaching local and state legislators about the shortcomings of existing systems of care resulted in improved funding for trauma system components in many of the areas examined. Publication of these studies provided a necessary stimulus to many parts of the United States to begin to improve trauma care and develop trauma care systems.

As it became appreciated that data was important for determining quality of care, trends, and preventable mortality, trauma registries became a required part of trauma center work. Aggregations of these hospital-based trauma registries then developed as a result of State-sponsored trauma registries and research-oriented databases (such as the Major Trauma Outcome Study). Being able to examine populations of trauma patients led to developing mathematical formulas calculating the probability of survival of an individual trauma patient and comparing quality of care at trauma centers based on patient survival.

In 1990, the U.S. federal government passed Federal Law 101–590, Title XII of Public Health Service Act, which provided for grants to states to develop statewide trauma care systems. One of the products developed during the time the program was active (1992 to 1995) was the Model Trauma Care System Plan. The MTCSP was written to be a guide for states to implement a trauma system. The grant funds were modest (approximately $5 million per year), but resulted in states developing legislation, designating trauma centers, and establishing state trauma offices and procedures. Unfortunately, this Health Resources and Services Administration program underwent rescission of program funds in 1995 and was closed. In 1998, the program was again appropriated for several years, as before. During this time, a new State trauma system template was developed based on the public health model. Benchmarks, indicators, and scores were included in this federal document to permit states to score their own progress in developing an inclusive statewide trauma system.

The ACS-COT also helped develop the prototype Advanced Trauma Life Support Course in Nebraska in 1978 [9]. The course was then adopted and managed by the College as one of the most successful educational programs for doctors worldwide. ATLS lays the groundwork for the initial assessment and resuscitation of the injured patient. Every physician and medical student and perhaps all healthcare workers are familiar with the principles of the ATLS approach to trauma patients. These are the primary survey with the concept of ABCDE, and the secondary survey. In the primary survey, A is for airway, B is for breathing, C is for circulation, D is for disability, and E is for exposure. The secondary survey is a head-to-toe physical exam as well as pertinent history. The concept of the primary survey is to identify life-threatening problems and begin treatment within 15 to 30 seconds. The remainder of the ATLS teaches diagnostic and life-saving interventions as well as emphasizing the need to transfer a seriously injured patient to a trauma center. ATLS has been introduced in over 50 countries worldwide.

The ACS-COT also has developed a trauma system consultation process that can be applied to states, multistate jurisdictions, and even single-county systems.

As one examines the challenges and successes of trauma systems over the past 25 years, it remains clear that all phases of care are equally important to the successful outcome desired. In the context of critical care, let us examine each phase of care.

A. Identification/recognition of incident: Should the system fail to identify that an injury has occurred, the patient may succumb before medical care can be started. This happens not infrequently in rural and remote parts of our country. Even if the patient is found and transported to an appropriate trauma center, the delay in care may result in sepsis from open fractures not cared for in a timely manner or organ failure from delay in resuscitation. Some locations in our nation are so remote that even when the injured patient is recognized immediately, it can take more than 24 hours for him or her to arrive in a definitive care facility. The risk for poor outcomes is the same in either case.
B. EMS care and transport: The prehospital care systems are extremely variable across the United States. These systems range from volunteer to fire-based to government-employed professionals to contracted professionals. Again, the timely and vigorous resuscitation required by trauma patients can tax even the most experienced crew. Indeed, what quality EMS providers do is provide intensive care in the prehospital setting. Inadequate or delayed resuscitation can have profound immediate and late effects, similar to those already mentioned. The single greatest cause of mortality among trauma patients is head injury. If the patient is not rapidly and adequately resuscitated, the brain may never recover from even minor insult. The most severe brain insults may be rapidly fatal, even near the most capable institutions. Some brain injury patients appear to be awake at first but then drop their GCS score dramatically. The most classic of these is the epidural hematoma—the "talk and die" injury. As the epidural hematoma increases in size, herniation will occur unless the intracranial blood is rapidly evacuated. This entity is a good test of system performance; the patient must quickly get to a trauma center where a neurosurgeon is rapidly available. If this is the case, this is a readily survivable injury. Otherwise, it will result in death or permanent disability. Head-injured patients are among the most demanding in intensive care medicine. Early surgical intervention is much preferred over long-term care.
C. Emergency Department (ED) care: Many clinicians feel that the battle is won or lost by the time the patient arrives in the trauma center ED. This is not correct. Again, inadequate or delayed resuscitation may contribute to a poor outcome. This may happen many ways: too slow a resuscitation may result in prolonged hypotension with potential for organ damage—the brain being particularly susceptible. Too slow

to the operating room for care of open fractures may result in infection and sepsis.

Conversely, overaggressive resuscitation in the face of some injuries such as brain injury or pulmonary contusion may also cause problems. In these cases, too much resuscitation fluid may result in unnecessary tissue edema. This will cause increased intracranial pressure and poor perfusion in the closed space of the skull. With the lungs, the leaky capillaries associated with pulmonary contusion will cause the contusion to blossom more than necessary, with potential for more difficulty in ventilating the patient and weaning him or her from the ventilator.

D. Operating room (OR) care: Prior to intensive care unit (ICU) admission, many trauma patients will have required operative intervention. Inadequate correction of coagulopathy during the operation may contribute to later difficulties in ICU care. More hemorrhage into the tissues may cause pressure problems in fascial compartments, ongoing hemorrhage in the abdomen or chest causing abdominal compartment syndrome or thoracic compartment syndrome. All these compartment syndromes can also be caused by inadequate fluid resuscitation. Tissue hypoxemia and injury with later swelling and edema can result in any of these compartment syndromes. A modern massive transfusion protocol is a must for each trauma center today.

E. ICU care: Each of the issues mentioned above may also occur in the ICU setting. Just because the patient is now in the ICU does not mean that preventable problems will not arise. The burden remains for each care provider involved in the care of an individual trauma patient to make sure that care is provided in a thoughtful, timely, and expert manner. Under- or over-resuscitation can still occur. Delay in identification of injuries, such as bowel injuries may result in sepsis. Inattention to the need to decompress the stomach of a trauma patient with a gastric tube may lead to aspiration and pneumonia. Inattention to a small "CT" pneumothorax may lead to a complete or even a tension pneumothorax, particularly in the face of positive pressure ventilation. Patients can die of a tension pneumothorax even in an ICU setting. Intravenous catheters placed in the field under less-than-ideal circumstances may be contaminated and lead to sepsis if not replaced in a timely manner. Other chapters in this section give detail for the care of shock, resuscitation, management of sepsis, multiple organ dysfunction syndrome, traumatic brain injury, spinal cord injury, thoracic and cardiac trauma, abdominal trauma, burn management, and orthopedic injuries.

F. Ward care after leaving the ICU—these critical care trauma patients will need close follow up on the trauma center wards. Often sepsis may occur on the floor and MOD syndrome as well. The physicians following these patients must be capable of early recognition of these problems and institute immediate therapy when such problems are recognized.

G. Rehabilitation: Though many think the rehabilitative process begins after leaving the hospital, it should begin on the first full hospital day. Patients need to be mobilized early, and physical and occupational therapy consults should be on the admission orders. All patients with even minor head injuries need cognitive testing and evaluation by speech therapists. Any patients with head or spinal cord injuries or with a cluster of serious injuries need a physical medicine and rehabilitation physician involved with their care early in their hospitalization. The discharge plan needs to be formulated early and the resources of the patient and families need to be understood so the maximum benefit of rehabilitation and recovery can be realized. Trauma patients may also have been injured while using drugs or alcohol. Some trauma patients may have suicidal or depressive motives related to their injuries. All seriously injured patients may suffer from posttraumatic stress. It is the obligation of the trauma service to address these issues and have social services, counselors, and psychiatric services as part of the team so that the patient has the opportunity for the best possible outcome.

H. Performance Improvement, Research, Education, and Injury Prevention: An essential mission of any trauma service is quality assurance of care and performance improvement (PI). Opportunities for improvement in patient care from specific events or trends in complications must be recognized, discussed, and acted upon to promote the quality of care of trauma patients and the function of the trauma team. It is essential that all trauma centers have a current, thorough trauma registry to record all the clinical information from every trauma patient. As part of the trauma system, this information needs to be shared with the state trauma registry and the National Trauma Data Bank at the ACS. The information obtained from the trauma center registry feeds an effective PI program. The information from the trauma registry as well as those registries of the state and the NTDB also promote research and injury prevention. It is essential for the trauma center to be involved in injury prevention. The knowledge of which injuries are prevalent in that region will direct the focus of the injury prevention program. Research activity is encouraged at all trauma centers but is essential for a level one center. Finally, ongoing educational programs of all care givers involved with trauma care, including prehospital and rehabilitative services as an essential duty of a trauma center, and the trauma system.

I. Special Considerations in Trauma Systems

DISASTER MANAGEMENT

Most disasters are major incidents such as plane crashes, explosions in chemical factories, natural disasters such as hurricanes, or results of war and terrorist activities such as the events of 9/11/2001. An effective trauma system should be primed to manage these disasters. To successfully manage a disaster with many victims, there needs to be preplanning and organization of resources. There needs to be training done within the trauma system, stockpiling of supplies, an effective communication and triage system, and a clear understanding of the resources of each hospital and trauma center in the area. Without a trauma system, the wrong facilities would end up with the wrong patients (i.e., a seriously injured patient to a small hospital). The trauma system needs to predefine the triage of patients of a disaster according to severity of injury and volume of patients. This planning needs to have the trauma centers and trauma medical directors involved as they are the experts in the management of trauma patients. The most important principle is triage of the most seriously injured to the higher level of care in the fastest amount of time, and to avoid overtriage of minor injuries to the major trauma center. Triage guidelines should include re-triage to the trauma facilities. In a wider scope, there needs to be disaster planning between neighboring trauma systems in the event the trauma centers in a system are also damaged or unable to manage the load of injured patients [10,11].

RURAL TRAUMA

The establishment of a trauma system is of even greater necessity in a rural environment to improve the outcomes of the injured patients. In 9 of the 10 categories of injury for both urban and rural hospitals, the mortality rate is higher in the rural facility, and it is double for motor vehicle crashes.

Most of the problems with rural trauma relate to the time to definitive care at a trauma center. There is increased discovery time, time for the prehospital personnel to get to the patient, transportation over great distances and hard terrain, and transfer to the highest level of medical center. To decrease the mortality and morbidity of these patients, the trauma system needs to be firmly established and designate and train lower level trauma centers in areas of sparse population, provide consistent training of the volunteer prehospital personnel, and establish effective communication and transport systems between the prehospital and level III and IV trauma centers as well as to the regional Level II or I trauma center [12].

The American College of Surgeons sponsors specific courses for training in both rural trauma and disaster management, the Rural Trauma Team Development Course (RTTDC), and the Disaster Management and Emergency Preparedness course (DMEP).

In summary, trauma systems provide for early recognition, prehospital care, resuscitation and operative care critical care management, long-term care, and rehabilitation. Performance improvement remains an essential trauma system function.

References

1. Ten Leading Causes of Death and Injury (Chart): Centers for Disease Control and Prevention.
2. Accidental Death and Disability: *The Neglected Disease of Modern Society*. Washington, DC: National Academy of Sciences, 1966.
3. West JG, Trunkey DD, Lim RC: Systems of trauma care. A study of two counties. *Arch Surg* 114(4):455–460, 1979.
4. Committee on Trauma, American College of Surgeons: Resources for optimal care of the injured patient 2006. Chicago, American College of Surgeons, 2006.
5. Mann NC, Mullins RJ, MacKenzie EJ, et al: Systematic review of published evidence regarding trauma system effectiveness. *J Trauma* 47[3, Suppl]:s25–s33, 1999.
6. Mullins RJ, Mann NC: Population-based research assessing the effectiveness of trauma systems. *J Trauma* 47[3, Suppl]:s59–s66, 1999.
7. Jurkovich GJ, Mock C: Systematic review of trauma system effectiveness based on registry comparisons. *J Trauma* 47[3 Suppl]:s46–s55, 1999.
8. Celso B, Tepas J, Langland-Orban B, et al: A systematic review and meta-analysis comparing outcome of severely injured patients treated in trauma centers following the establishment of trauma systems. *J Trauma* 60(2):371–378, 2006.
9. American College of Surgeons. *Advanced Trauma Life Support for Doctors*. 8th ed. Chicago: American College of Surgeons, 2009.
10. Frykberg ER: Medical management of disasters and mass casualties from terrorist bombings: How can we cope. *J Trauma* 53(2):201–212, 2002.
11. Lennquist S: Management of major accidents and disasters: An important responsibility for the trauma surgeons. *J Trauma* 62(6):1321–1329, 2007.
12. Rogers FB, Shackford SR, Osler TM, et al: Rural trauma: The challenge for the next decade. *J Trauma* 47(4):802, 1999.

CHAPTER 162 ■ TRAUMATIC BRAIN INJURY

TODD W. TRASK AND ARTHUR L. TRASK

When Dr. Rosner first published his recommendations that were to change the management of traumatic brain injury (TBI), he recommended using cerebral perfusion pressure (CPP = mean arterial pressure [MAP]—intracranial pressure [ICP]) as a better way to manage severe TBI patients than just using the level of ICP [1,2]. This was the beginning of the changes in TBI management. Dr. Marion and Spiegel have published the article "Changes in the Management of Severe TBI: 1991–1997" [3]. Recommendations to change severe TBI management, based on evidence, developed by The Brain Trauma Foundation, in combination with the Trauma committee of the American Association of Neurological Surgeons (AANS), the Congress of Neurological Surgeons (CNS), and AANS/CNS Joint Section on Neurotrauma & Critical Care have been updated several times with the latest version in 2007 [4]. Neurosurgeons were surveyed by the Brain Trauma Foundation in 1991 and 1997 to determine if they were changing their management of severe TBI patients. The use of steroids was significantly reduced from 1991 to 1997 and hyperventilation was also discontinued. In 2004, we published our results of an evidence-based medicine protocol [5]. Our results showed a decrease in hospital intensive care stay by 1.8 days ($p = 0.021$). The Glasgow Outcome Scores (GOS) of good or moderate from 1991 to 1995 were 43.3%. For the period 1997 to 2000, our patients' GOS of good or moderate were 61.5% ($p = <0.001$). The overall mortality rate decreased from 17.8% for the early group compared to 13.8% for the later group [6–8].

We recommend that the intensive (ICU) care of severe TBI patients be driven by institutional protocols developed by key participants, that is, ICU care providers, using current recommendations for managing these patients [4]. Each hospital has different approaches to critical care and the reason we suggest assembling this key group of individuals is to assure that the plan for care fits into the way things are done in each hospital.

Above all, we recommend an evidence-based approach to the care of these critically ill patients. New evidence will be presented each year and adopting what has high credibility to that protocol makes good sense. We recommend keeping a TBI patient database to know with certainty how your results compare with other trauma centers in the USA and the world. By having a TBI database, you might also consider doing a prospective study using different techniques for similar TBI problems or management [9–13].

IDENTIFICATION

Identification of severe traumatic brain injury requires two criteria to be met. First, the Glasgow Coma Score (GCS) must be 8 or less. The GCS was first described in 1974 by Graham Teasdale and Bryan J. Jennett, professors of neurosurgery at the University of Glasgow, Scotland. In 1981, they approached F.A. Davis, the author of a textbook *Management of Head Injuries* who included the scoring system for identification of different levels of TBI.

The next criteria for a severe TBI is an abnormal brain computed tomography (CT) with findings such as contusion, hematoma, diffuse axonal injury (DAI), compressed basal cistern, subarachnoid hemorrhage (SAH), and/or other clear signs of brain injury. When only an abnormal GCS is present, it is possible to be due to something other than TBI. When an injured patient arrives in an emergency department (ED), these two assessments are done to identify a severe TBI patient. When these criteria are met, the patient should be moved to a Neurotrauma ICU, a part of the recognized Trauma Center, as soon as possible, provided other types of operative treatment are not more urgently needed. Placement of an intracranial pressure monitor should be considered in the multiple-injured TBI patient, simultaneously with the non-neurosurgical operative procedures.

MONITORS

We recommend intracranial pressure (ICP) monitors for assessing the moment-to-moment status of your patient. Generally, a ventriculostomy type monitor is superior to an intraparenchymal (Bolt) monitor. The ventriculostomy can accurately determine the intracranial pressure but also allows the neurophysicians to drain cerebrospinal fluid (CSF). The latest recommendation for ICP monitors is to have an electronic continuous record with instantaneous alerts for significant increases to allow immediate interventions per protocol. Many devices are available for measuring brain oxygen levels as well as oxygen from the jugular bulb. The value of these measurements is yet to be determined by the BTF and AANS [14–19].

An understanding of the Monro-Kellie doctrine is essential. In 1783, Alexander Monro deduced that the cranium was a "rigid box" filled with a "nearly incompressible brain" and that its total volume tends to remain constant. The doctrine states that any increase in the volume of the cranial contents (e.g., brain, blood, or cerebrospinal fluid), will elevate intracranial pressure. Furthermore, if one of these three elements increases in volume, it must occur at the expense of the volume of the other two elements. In 1824, George Kellie confirmed many of Monro's early observations. If as a result of trauma a hematoma forms on the outside of the brain (epidural hematoma), under the dura (subdural hematoma), or within the brain itself, the space occupied by the hematoma must result in a commensurate decrease of the intracranial blood or CSF volume. Once these compensatory mechanisms are exhausted, intracranial pressure will rise rapidly, and brain herniation may occur. Cerebral edema can mimic an expanding mass lesion, with similar pathophysiology, and potential for the irreversible damage associated with uncal and/or tonsillar herniation (see graph in Fig. 162.1).

In general, the reaction to an intracranial mass or cerebral edema is to reduce the amount of venous blood and CSF within the skull. The body's response to the injury is to keep the pressure inside the skull as close to normal as possible by reducing those volumes that can be reduced. When a sudden increase of ICP occurs and the patient has a ventriculostomy, the neurointensivist may drain additional CSF from this closed box. This in turn helps to keep the ICP under control while other measures are taken to reduce the ICP in a more lasting fashion. We will discuss more about this under patient management.

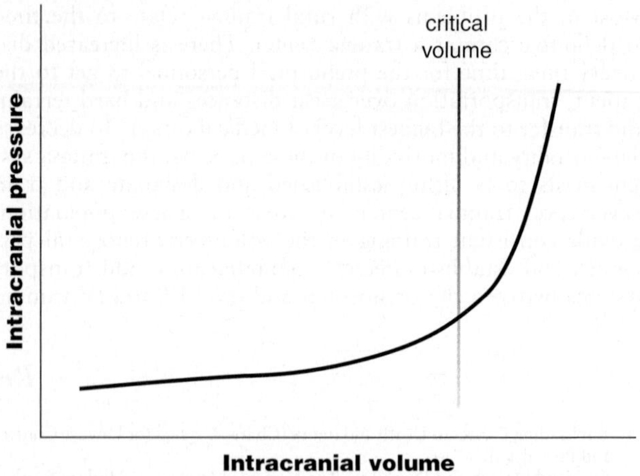

FIGURE 162.1. As the Monro-Kellie doctrine indicates, the skull is a closed box. When intracranial volume increases to the *critical volume* due to traumatic brain injury, that is, subdural hematoma (SDH), epidural hematoma (EDH), or massive cerebral edema, note the dramatic vertical increase in intracranial pressure. If this occurs and the volume is not reduced, brain herniation will occur.

The next consideration for the severe TBI patient is determining what other injuries the patient might have. A qualified trauma surgeon must be involved to assist the neurointensivist with the fluid/blood product management. For example, a patient with a class III anterior posterior pelvic fracture will lose huge amounts of blood even if managed by a trauma orthopedist with pelvic circumference reduction. This is an indication for a pulmonary artery catheter (PAC) (or one of the newer devices for monitoring pressures and cardiac output) to monitor the resuscitation as closely as possible. The goal is maintaining the patient's systolic pressure at or above 90 torr. In the book, *Management and Prognosis of Severe Traumatic Brain Injury*, a joint project of the Brain Trauma Foundation and American Association of Neurological Surgeons, class two evidence states that allowing the systolic BP to drop below 90 torr will likely produce secondary brain injury. The BTF class two evidence criteria are clinical studies in which the data was collected prospectively or retrospective analyses that were based on clearly reliable data. Types of studies so classified include: observational studies, cohort studies, prevalence studies, and case control studies. Class two evidence shows that post injury hypotension has dramatic impact on the brain injury outcome. We recommend using the PAC data to assist in fluid/blood product management to maintain a PCWP between 10 to 15 mm Hg and a CI of 2.6 L per minute per m^2. Invasive hemodynamic monitoring may also help avoid fluid overload and possibly associated increases in cerebral edema. A new monitoring device is now being evaluated for these multiply-injured patients. The use of The InSpectra^{TM} StO_2 Tissue Oxygenation Monitor will provide continuous, real-time information for perfusion status monitoring and a new hemodynamic parameter (StO_2) to assist clinicians in the early detection of inadequate tissue perfusion (hypoperfusion). This device would noninvasively monitor hemodynamic status and tissue oxygenation, both of which are critical for severe TBI patients [19].

The oxygen saturation level and the PCO_2 level are also extremely important for the ICU management of these patients. The Brain Trauma Foundation has gone to great lengths to provide training to prehospital providers so that they recognize the importance of keeping the O_2 saturation more than 90%. This same standard must be maintained in the ICU as well. Patients with severe TBI should have endotracheal intubation as early as possible after the traumatic event. Once the patient arrives in the Trauma Bay, the ventilator must be set to assure adequate oxygenation and also to maintain the PCO_2 level around 38 to 40 mm Hg. Most intensivists/respiratory care physicians recommend keeping the head of the bed elevated to 30°. In addition to aiding respiratory function, elevation also provides some slight assistance in maintaining the ICP in the desired range.

Major trauma accompanied with significant blood loss often will result in coagulopathy. The American College of Surgeons Committee on Trauma in their Advanced Trauma Life Support Course™ classifies shock into four classes. Primarily, class III (1,500 to 2,000 mL blood loss) and class IV (>2,000 mL blood loss) are frequently associated with coagulopathy. In addition, we also know that certain severe TBI cases may present or develop coagulation abnormalities. Using a device called a Thromboelastogram™ (TEG) will assess the coagulation status of these patients and offers a rapid technique for identification of coagulation problems. A TEG is also useful for identifying hypercoagulability, and the associated risk of venous thromboembolism [20–26]. Electroencephalography (EEG) monitoring and Ultrasound monitors are being used more frequently today and are very useful for those patients being treated with pharmacological coma.

It is necessary to observe closely for impending Diabetes Insipidus (DI) by frequent serum Na determinations, urine output >200 cc per hour and urine specific gravity <1.005. This is considered Central DI and is due to a lack or an inadequate amount of ADH (vasopressin). Treatment is with subcutaneous vasopressin (ADH) or intravenous deamino-8-D-arginine (DDAVP).

Cerebral microdialysis is possible with a ventriculostomy in place. During periods of metabolic stress with TBI, many neurointensivists are using this technique to measure changes in lactate, excitatory amino acids, glycerol, glucose, and pyruvate as well as other metabolic compounds during periods of metabolic stress of TBI. The future of patient management may be augmented by these studies, but at present no recommendations are evidence based.

PATIENT MANAGEMENT

Avoiding seizures is a key management endeavor. This activity may exacerbate metabolic derangements already present, and result in secondary injury. Loading severe TBI patients with phenytoin is recommended provided adequate hemodynamic stability exists. The loading dose we recommend is 18 mg per kg at a rate of 25 mg per minute. The maintenance dose is 100 mg every 8 hours IV. Maintenance dosing for 7 days is indicated. Class II evidence shows that prophylactic anticonvulsants have no benefit after 7 days, provided there have been no seizures. We recommend obtaining a free phenytoin level 72 hours after the loading dose [27–29].

The syndrome of inappropriate antidiuretic hormone (SIADH) may occur. This usually appears late in the course of TBI and appears as hyponatremia since the hormone causes water retention diluting the plasma electrolytes. If early in the care for mild hyponatremia, water restriction is usually sufficient but, the CPP should not be allowed to drop as a result of the restriction. This syndrome needs to be distinguished from the cerebral salt wasting syndrome which is thought to be caused by a brain-secreted natriuretic peptide. The difference can usually be elicited by measuring urine sodium levels that are inappropriately elevated in cerebral salt-wasting syndrome. Treatment for this syndrome is salt and volume replacement. For an in-depth discussion of this subject, readers are referred to Chapter 72.

Attempting to keep the brain activity at a minimum is another management activity. Fast acting drugs are suggested during the first 48 hours after injury to allow the neurospecialists to reexamine the patient frequently to determine deterioration or improvements in coma scoring. Use of propofol and fentanyl for this period is suggested. When the status of the patient has been well established, we suggest switching to longer acting (less expensive) medications. We recommend using lorazepam and morphine to keep the Richmond Agitation Sedation Scale (RASS) score @ −2 to −3 (see Fig. 162.2). The RASS has been shown to be a useful adjunct in the management of the severe TBI patient [30].

Another adjunct in the management is temperature control. While a study has been suggested using hypothermia (to 32°C) for patients aged less than 45 years, normovolemia and with a GCS >4, the multicenter trial did not confirm this hypothesis and was terminated [31]. Nonetheless, it is essential to avoid temperature elevations. Anticipating temperature elevations and monitoring closely will allow the management team to use cooling techniques and/or medications such as acetaminophen to keep the temperature ≤38°C.

Gastric mucosal protection is necessary to prevent stress ulcers. We suggest prophylaxis using a histamine receptor antagonist, a proton pump inhibitor. Once a feeding program is started the problem of stress ulcers decreases.

The nursing staff must play an important role in the management of these critical ill patients. They should repeat the motor score and eye score to detect improvement or deterioration. They must assume responsibility for frequent checks of urine output, temperature, ICP, CPP, Hb, electrolytes, and graphing trends for the neurointensivist to review during reexaminations.

When the nurse documents an elevated ICP of ≥20 for more than 10 minutes, (these are suggested criteria and each hospital will need to decide what early criteria they will use) we suggest immediate drainage of CSF by the ventriculostomy. Next optimize temperature control, increase sedation, and paralyze patient. The next step is again a decision each hospital should make. Hyperosmolar therapy with mannitol or hypertonic saline should be considered. Nicole Forster in her publication suggests that mannitol is the first choice for pharmacological ICP reduction [31]. Cruz, Battison, Valadka, Shackford, Ware, and White all believe some form of hypertonic saline should be used to reduce the ICP [32–38]. There are considerable differences of opinion on this topic. At this time, each facility should review these articles and the ICU team must decide on what hyperosmolar therapy to use. Repeat imaging should always be considered in the event of unexpected ICP changes.

If the ICP rises to ≥25 for 30 minutes the neurology team should discuss the use of pentobarbital coma or consider performing an early decompressive craniectomy as recent literature suggests a role for this procedure in some patients [39–42]. The best results are observed when the craniectomy is performed early and before significant deterioration has occurred.

Hopefully, with all of the above strategies, patients will gradually improve showing better motor scores and improved CT scan. The criteria for discontinuing the major TBI protocol should be (a) when the patient is requiring less sedation with the RASS being −2 to −3, (b) the paralytics have been discontinued, (c) temperature control is no longer a problem, (d) recent CT scan shows stability and/or improvement, and (e) the ICP has been ≤20 for at least 24 hours and the neurosurgeon has discontinued the ventriculostomy.

During this critical period, nutritional support should be initiated. Assessment of the metabolic needs of these patients is crucial and nutritional support plays a major role in recovery. A consultation with a physiatrist, who in collaboration with the neurointensivist team, will suggest the physical therapy, occupational therapy, and speech therapy. These therapies will be started to aid in the long-term recovery of these patients.

Score	Term	Description
+4	Combative	Overly combative, violent, immediate danger to staff
+3	Very agitated	Pulls or removes tube(s) or catheter(s), aggressive
+2	Agitated	Frequent nonpurposeful movement, fights ventilator
+1	Restless	Anxious but movements not aggressive, vigorous
0	Alert & calm	
−1	Drowsy	Not fully alert, but has sustained awakening (eye opening/eye contact) to voice (≥10 sec)
−2	Light sedation	Briefly awakens with eye contact to voice (<10 sec)
−3	Moderate sedation	Movement or eye opening to voice (but no eye contact)
−4	Deep sedation	No response to voice, but movement or eye opening to physical stimulation
−5	Unarousable	No response to voice or physical stimulation

Procedure for RASS Assessment

1. Observe patient
   a. Patient is alert, restless, or agitated. (score 0 to +4)
2. If not alert, state patient's name and say to open eyes and look at speaker
   b. Patient awakens with sustained eye opening and eye contact. (score −1)
   c. Patient awakens with eye opening and eye contact, but not eye contact. (score −2)
   d. Patient has any movement in response to voice but no eye contact. (score −3)
3. When no response to verbal stimulation, physically stimulate patient by shaking shoulder and/or rubbing sternum.
   e. Patient has any movement to physical stimulation (score −4)
   f. Patient has no response to any stimulation (score −5)

FIGURE 162.2. The Richmond Agitation Sedation Scale (RASS). [Adapted from Sessler CN, Gosnell MS, Grap MJ, et al. The Richmond Agitation-Sedation Scale: validity and reliability in adult intensive care unit patients. *Am J Respir Crit Care Med* 166:1338–1344, 2002.]

FUTURE POTENTIAL TREATMENT OPTIONS

a. A multicenter trial: Citicoline Brain Injury Treatment Trial (COBRIT). This is a phase 3 double-blind, randomized, prospective clinical trial to determine if treating head injured patients (severe, moderate, and complicated mild) with citicoline will improve recovery. Citicoline, also known as cytidine diphosphate-choline (CDP-choline) is a psychostimulant/nootropic. It is an intermediate stage in the generation of phosphatidylcholine from choline and increases dopamine receptor densities. The patients are randomized to citicoline or placebo. The reason for this compound being tested is that several meta-analyses indicate a benefit of this compound in stroke and dementia. Eight sites are participating.
b. Spreading Depressions (formerly COSBID) is in the study preparation phase. Cortical Spreading Depression (CSD) is a wave of mass neuronal firing, neuronal, and glial depolarization. It propagates through gray matter at a rate of between 1 and 5 mm per minute and depletes energy stores and may activate cell death cascades. Spreading Depressions (SD) are seizure like waves that actively propagate a breakdown of ion homeostasis and may alter blood flow through injured, but potentially salvageable brain tissue. The objective of this study will be to determine if SD actually causes secondary brain injury after TBI. If the answer is yes, then a method to block the SD waves will be developed. The results of this study are eagerly awaited.
c. Another study, labeled SOLVAY, is designed to study SLV334 in a phase 2a randomized, placebo-controlled, double-blind pharmacokinetic and safety study. If shown to be safe, a phase 3 trial of this drug which has a new mechanism—endothelin antagonism, matrix metalloprotease inhibition, and "anti-apoptotic effect"—will be developed with multiple centers.
d. A phase 3 prospective randomized multicenter clinical trial is underway with an expectation of about 1,400 patients over a 5-year period. Titled the *B*rain *O*xygen and *O*utcome in *S*evere *T*raumatic Brain Injury (BOOST) Study, it is designed to compare the standard management of ICP/CPP versus brain oxygen-based therapy to determine which category of patients will have the best long-term outcome.

Much progress in treating TBI has occurred. Careful management of the CPP, ICP, cardiac output, tissue oxygenation, PCO_2, temperature, and the other body parameters that support brain metabolism and recovery is indicated. Much opportunity for improving the management of TBI patients still exists when given by well-trained critical care teams resulting in more updates on management sequelae in this ever-encouraging field of emergency trauma care.

References

1. Rosner MJ, Daughton S: Cerebral perfusion pressure management in head injury. *J Neurosurgery* 30:933–941, 1990.
2. Rosner MJ, Rosner SD, Johnson AH: Cerebral perfusion pressure: Management protocol and clinical results. *J Neurosurgery* 83:949–962, 1995.
3. Marion DW, Spiegel TP: Changes in the management of severe traumatic brain injury: 1991–1997. *Crit Care Med* 28(1):16–18, 2000.
4. Brain Trauma Foundation Guidelines. Available at: http://www.braintrauma.org. Accessed 2007.
5. Fakhry SM, Trask AL, Waller MA, et al: Management of brain-injured patients by an evidence-based protocol improves outcomes and decreases *hospital* charges. *J Trauma* 56(3):492–500, 2004.
6. Spain DA, McIlvoy LH, Fix SE, et al: Effect of a clinical pathway for severe traumatic brain injury on resource utilization. *J Trauma* 45:101–105, 1998.
7. Faul M, Wald MM, Rutland-Brown W, et al: Using a cost-benefit analysis to estimate outcomes of a clinical treatment guideline: testing the brain trauma

foundation guidelines for the treatment of severe traumatic brain injury. *J Trauma* 63:1271–1278, 2007.
8. Palmer S, Bader MK, Qureshi A, et al: The impact on outcomes in a community hospital setting of using the AANS traumatic brain injury guidelines. *J Trauma* 50:657–664, 2001.
9. Marion DW, Spiegel TP: Changes in the management of severe traumatic brain injury: 1991–1997. *Crit Care Med* 28(1):16–18, 2000.
10. Marik PE, Varon J, Trask T, et al: Management of head trauma. *Chest* 122(2):699–711, 2002.
11. Valadka AB, Andrews BT, Bullock MR, et al: How well do neurosurgeons care for trauma patients? A survey of AAST members. *Neurosurgery* 48(1):17–25, 2001.
12. Hesdorffer DC, Ghajar J, Iacono L: Predictors of compliance with the evidence-based guidelines for TBI care: a survey of US trauma centers. *J Trauma* 52(6):1202–1209, 2002.
13. Espinosa-Aguilar A, Reyes-Morales H, Huerta-Posada CE, et al: Design and validation of a critical pathway for hospital management of patients with severe traumatic brain injury. *J Trauma* 64(5):1327–1341, 2008.
14. Cohn SM, Nathens AB, Moore FA, et al: Tissue oxygen saturation predicts the development of organ dysfunction during traumatic shock resuscitation. *J Trauma* 62:44–55, 2007.
15. Cruz J: The first decade of continuous monitoring of jugular bulb oxyhemoglobin saturation: management strategies and clinical outcome. *Crit Care Med* 26(2):344–355, 1998.
16. Valadka AB, Gopinath SP, et al: Relationship of brain tissue PO_2 to outcome after severe head injury. *Crit Care Med* 26(9):1576–1585, 1998.
17. Vespa P: Perfusing the brain after traumatic brain injury: what clinical index should we follow? *Crit Care Med* 32(7):1621–1623, 2004.
18. Kirkness CJ, Thompson HJ, et al: Brain tissue oxygen monitoring in traumatic brain injury: Cornerstone of care or another brick in the wall? *Crit Care Med* 37(1):371–372, 2009.
19. Stewart C, Haitsma I, et al: The new Licox combined brain tissue oxygen and brain temperature monitor: assessment of in vitro accuracy and clinical experience in severe traumatic brain injury. *Neurosurgery* 63(6):1159–1165, 2008.
20. Kaufman CR, Dwyer KM, Crews JD, et al: Usefulness of thromboelastography in assessment of trauma patient coagulation. *J Trauma* 42:716–722, 1997.
21. Watts DD, Trask A, Soeken F, et al: Hypothermic coagulopathy in trauma: effect of varying of hypothermia on enzyme speed, platelets function and fibrinolytic activity. *J Trauma* 44:846–854, 1998.
22. Rugeri L, Levrat A, David JS, et al: Diagnosis of early coagulation abnormalities in trauma patients by rotational thromboelastography. *J Thromb Haemost* 5:289–295, 2007.
23. Levrat A, Gros A, Rugeri L: Evaluation of rotation thromboelastography for the diagnosis of hyperfibrinolysis in trauma patients. *Br J Anaesth* 100:792–797, 2008.
24. Bartal C, Yitzhak A: The role of thromboelastometry and recombinant factor VIIa in trauma. *Curr Opin Anesthesiol* 22(2):281–288, 2009.
25. Stein DM, Dutton R, et al: Reversal of coagulopathy in critically ill patients with traumatic brain injury: recombinant factor VIIa is more cost effective than plasma. *J Trauma* 66(1):63–75, 2009.
26. Talving P, Benfield R, et al: Coagulopathy in severe traumatic brain injury: A prospective study. *J Trauma* 66(1):55–62, 2009.
27. Temkin NR, Dikmen SS, Wilensky AJ, et al: A randomized, double-blind study of phenytoin for the prevention of post-traumatic seizures. *N Engl J Med* 323(8):497–502, 1990.
28. Neurosurgical panel. Antiseizure prophylaxis for penetrating brain injury. *J Trauma* 51(2):S41–S43, 2001.
29. Chang BS, Lowenstein DH: Practice parameter: antiepileptic drug prophylaxis in severe traumatic brain injury. *Neurology* 60(11):10–16, 2003.
30. Ely EW, Truman B, Shintani A, et al: Monitoring sedation status over time in ICU patients: reliability and validity of the Richmond Agitation-Sedation Scale (RASS). *JAMA* 289(22):2983–2991, 2003.
31. Clifton G, Drever P, Valadka A, et al: Multicenter trial of early hypothermia in severe brain injury. *J Neurotrauma* 26(3):393–397, 2009.
32. Forster N, Engelhard K, et al: Managing elevated intracranial pressure. *Curr Opin Anesthesiol* 17(5):371–376, 2004.
33. Cruz J, Minoja G, et al: Successful use of the new high-dose mannitol treatment in patients with GCS scores of 3 and bilateral abnormal pupillary widening: a randomized trial. *J Neurosurg* 100:376–383, 2004.
34. Battison C, et al: Randomized, controlled trial on the effect of a 20% mannitol solution and a 7.5% saline/6% dextran solution on increased intracranial pressure after brain injury. *Crit Care Med* 33(1):196–202, 2005.
35. Valadka A, Robertson C: Should we be using hypertonic saline to treat intracranial hypertension? *Crit Care Med* 28(4):1245–1246, 2000.
36. Shackford S, Bourguignon P, et al: Hypertonic saline resuscitation of patients with head injury: a prospective, randomized clinical trial. *J Trauma* 44(1):50–58, 1998.
37. Ware ML, Nemanl V, et al: Effects of 23.4% NaCl solution in reducing intracranial pressure in patients with TBI: a preliminary study. *Neurosurgery* 57(4):727–736, 2005.
38. White H, Cook D, et al: The use of hypertonic saline for treating intracranial hypertension after TBI. *Anesth Analg* 102:1836–1846, 2006.
39. Polin RS, Shaffrey ME, Bogaev CA, et al: Decompressive bifrontal craniectomy in the treatment of severe refractory post-traumatic cerebral edema. *Neurosurgery* 41(1):84–94, 1997.
40. Ziai WC, Port JD, Cowan JA, et al: Decompressive craniectomy for intractable cerebral edema: experience of a single center. *J Neurosurg Anesthesiol* 15(1):25–32, 2003.
41. Hutchinson P, Kirkpatrick P: Decompressive craniectomy in head injury. *Curr Opin Crit Care* 10:101–104, 2004.
42. Cooper JD, Rosenfeld J, et al: Early decompressive craniectomy for patients with severe traumatic brain injury and refractory intracranial hypertension—a pilot randomized trial. *J Crit Care* 23(3):387–393, 2008.

CHAPTER 163 ■ SPINAL CORD TRAUMA

HOWARD B. LEVENE, MICHAEL Y. WANG AND BARTH A. GREEN

INTRODUCTION

"The Spine" is often thought of a single unit, as is "the liver" or "the intestines," but the concept is somewhat misleading. "The Spine" is really a structure with two parts. The first part, the bony spine, serves dually to support the body and to protect the vulnerable neurological structures inside. The second of the two parts of the spine, the neurological spine, is more than just a "coaxial cable" connecting the brain to the remainder of the body. The neurological spine, the spinal cord, is a complex extension of the central nervous system, capable of learning and adapting. When the bony protection fails, the spinal cord (and possibly the cervical-medullary brainstem or the cauda equina) is traumatized with multiple systemic consequences. These consequences may result in a catastrophic injury. To better develop treatments for spinal cord injury, the pathophysiology of the injury continues to be thoroughly studied [1–8]. In this chapter, traumatic forces are emphasized, but the reader should keep in mind that vascular, infectious, or toxic/metabolic/ischemic damage to the spinal cord may present in a patient with a similar profile of deficits and clinical challenges.

Injury to the spine can be thought of in two phases. The first phase called "Primary Injury" is the moment when excessive kinetic energy is transmitted to the spinal cord in the moment of trauma. The "Secondary Injury" follows immediately after that as the damage from the primary injury creates biologic sequelae. Secondary injury in spinal cord injury (SCI) is believed to involve the release of neurotoxic chemicals, creation of free radicals, recruitment/activation of macrophages, disruption of the blood-spinal cord barrier, generation of lipid peroxidation, presence of oxidative cell stress, and other events [9]. Even without a complete understanding of all of the variety of events in spinal cord injury, it is believed that secondary injury can be modulated with appropriate therapeutic interventions. These include, but are not limited to, decompressive surgery [10,11] steroids [12–17], hypothermia [18–23], immunomodulation [24–26], nutrition [27,28], and other therapies.

Given the tremendous socioeconomic and psychosocial impact of spinal cord injury, there have been several human clinical trials [12,15,29–32] to date in an effort to limit the secondary injury, but there is no one therapeutic strategy that is clearly effective in affecting outcome.

Surgical management of spinal cord injury is also still under debate, especially in terms of the timing and utility of the surgical intervention [11,33,34]. Fortunately, there are treatments available for the spinal cord injured patients such as physical therapy, outpatient therapy, and adaptive therapies [35–40].

The future of treatment for spinal cord injured patients will likely involve a combination of techniques, such as applying neurotrophic factors, nerve grafting, cellular injection, hypothermia, tissue engineering, neuromodulation, and other innovative approaches. This chapter addresses the many problems unique to the management of a spinal cord-injured patient. The specific surgical treatments for each pathologic entity are beyond the scope of this chapter.

HISTORY

The Edward Smith Papyrus [41–43] represents one of the earliest records of spinal cord injury. Dating back approximately to 2500 B.C.E., there is a case report by Imhotep, a physician and architect to the Pharoh Zoser III. In this Papyrus, he describes 48 trauma cases, 6 of which involve vertebral column injury. In the most famous case, Imhotep describes a case of "crushed vertebra" where "incontinence, paralysis, and loss of sensation" follow. In his medical opinion, treatment was not to be pursued. The Greek Physician Galen, some 3000 years later, conducted animal experiments noting the difference in effects between longitudinal and horizontal cord transactions [41]. Only 500 years after Galen, the laminectomy was introduced by Paulus. In 1543, Vesalius then introduced remarkably detailed anatomical drawings of human anatomy. In the early twentieth century, despite significant scientific and engineering advancements, the opinion of Imhotep still reigned true and traumatic SCI was felt to be a terminal condition.

The recognition that spinal cord injury should not be viewed as a terminal condition owes much to the insights of Sir Ludwig Guttmann (UK) and Sir George Bedbrook (Australia). In the aftermath of World War II, these two physicians were at the forefront of refusing to accept the inevitable prognosis for SCI [44,45]. They pioneered the idea that the sequelae of SCI do not need to be fatal and that an intensive regiment of physical therapy and care may be life-saving and life-improving.

EPIDEMIOLOGY

There are more than 200,000 people in the United States living with a chronic SCI. Each year, approximately 11,000 Americans are afflicted with this condition [46]. More than half of the people who sustain SCIs are 15 to 29 years old (CDC data: http://www.cdc.gov/ncipc/factsheets/scifacts.htm). Approximately 80% of the injured are male [46]. There is a growing trend of seeing SCI among middle-aged and elderly patients due to improved lifestyle habits and improved survivability of injuries. Data collected from North America, Europe, and Australia confirm similar results [47]. The cervical spine is the most commonly injured site, with the remaining injury sites divided between thoracic, thoracolumbar, and lumbosacral levels [48].

The mechanism of injury can be blunt (e.g., motor vehicle accident, fall, assault) or penetrating (e.g., gunshot wound, knife, and other sharp object). Approximately 50% of the injuries derive from a motor vehicle accident, with the remainder primarily from falls (23%), violence (14%), and sports (9%) [46].

NEUROLOGIC INJURY

As a trauma patient is assessed through the initial "ABCDE" of Advanced Trauma Life Support, the physician must perform a neurologic examination. The neurologic examination is of paramount importance localizing the probable site of injury as well as to assess the severity of injury to the spinal cord. Once the SCI is identified, the physician can classify the injury by mechanism (e.g., penetrating vs. blunt), level (cervical, thoracic, lumbar), and degree of neurological impairment (often through the American Spinal Injury Association [ASIA] scale).

To assess the degree of neurologic injury, particular attention is paid to the motor, sensory, reflex, and rectal examinations. Based on the degree of functional impairment, the ASIA has proposed an easily used scoring system (Table 163.1). The neurologic injury is categorized using this score and by noting lowest normal segmental level. (When referring to the "level" of injury, it is important to note that the level is the corresponding "neurological level" or dermatological level and not the "bony level." For example, consider a patient shot in the spine. A neurosurgeon evaluates the patient and states that the patient has a complete neurological injury at the "L4" level. This means that the lowest spinal level with completely normal function is at the L4 neurons of the spinal cord. The bony disruption, however, may be at approximately T12, which corresponds to the locations of neurons that innervate L5 and below.)

In this classification scheme, the severity of injury is denoted by Grade, followed by letters A-E. The letters serve as shorthand to classify the severity of injury as it relates to sensory and motor function. Grade A (complete) denotes a complete injury with no sensory or motor function preserved in sacral segments S4–5. Grade B (incomplete) denotes sensory, but not motor function preserved below the neurologic level and extends through sacral segments S4–5. Grade C (incomplete) denotes motor function preserved below the neurologic level with muscle strength graded below antigravity strength. Grade D (incomplete) denotes motor function preserved below neurologic level with muscle strength graded more than or equal to antigravity strength, but not normal. Grade E denotes a normal

TABLE 163.1

AMERICAN SPINAL INJURY ASSOCIATION GRADING SCALE FOR SPINAL CORD INJURY

Clinical grade	Neurologic examination
A	No motor or sensory function preserved
B	Sensory but no motor function preserved
C	Nonuseful motor function preserved (less than antigravity strength)
D	Motor function preserved but weak
E	Normal motor and sensory function

sensory and motor exam [49,50]. The grades have a prognostic feature. Complete recovery of function after a Grade A injury is unlikely. However, improvement of one or two grades is seen in more than 10% of patients. Some recovery is most likely to occur in Grade D injuries [51].

SCI may be also classified as complete or incomplete. In complete SCI, there is no preservation of motor function and/or sensation for three spinal segments below the level of injury. Complete injuries above T6 are usually associated with spinal shock. Spinal shock is characterized by: hypotension from interruption of sympathetics, bradycardia from unopposed vagal (parasympathetic) output, hypothermia, and transient loss of all neurologic function resulting in a flaccid paralysis and areflexia. Incomplete SCI may be further subclassified into specific neurological symptoms based on the anatomy of the injury.

SPECIFIC NEUROLOGIC SYNDROMES

Specific neurologic syndromes have been described for particular incomplete spinal cord injuries [52,53]. These syndromes include the anterior cord syndrome, the central cord syndrome, the posterior cord syndrome, Brown-Sequard (hemisection cord syndrome), conus medullaris syndrome, cauda equina syndrome, and cord concussion syndrome.

The **anterior cord syndrome** is characterized by complete paralysis and hypoalgesia (to pain and temperature) from damage to anterior and anterolateral column function below the level of injury, with preservation of proprioception (vibration and position sense) and light touch from posterior column function. This syndrome occurs most commonly after trauma focused at the anterior spinal cord as well as ischemia in the territory supplied by the anterior spinal artery, which supplies the corticospinal and spinothalamic tracts in the anterior 2/3 of the spinal cord. It is classified as an ASIA B injury.

The **central cord syndrome** is characterized by motor dysfunction more pronounced in the distal upper extremities than in the lower extremities ("man in a barrel"), accompanied by varying degrees of sensory loss and bladder dysfunction. The injury occurs characteristically after a hyperextension injury in elderly patients with acquired cervical stenosis from spondylosis or in athletes with congenital cervical stenosis. The injury can be seen in the absence of any clear radiographic disruption of the bones or ligaments. Most patients recover the ability to walk, with partial restoration of upper-extremity strength. It is associated with severe allodynia of the hands. (Allodynia is pain from stimuli that are not normally painful.)

The **posterior cord syndrome** is an uncommon presentation in which position sense, vibration sense, and crude touch are impaired due to injury to the dorsal columns or injury directed to the posterior of the spinal cord.

The **Brown-Sequard syndrome,** or **hemisection cord syndrome,** presents with ipsilateral paresis and loss of proprioception, touch, and vibration below the level of the lesion and the contralateral loss of pain and temperature sensation. This can be the result of penetrating injuries or asymmetrical lateral closed injuries resulting in a spinal cord hemisection, and is usually not seen in the pure form. Asymmetrical, lateral closed injuries are often confused with an ipsilateral brachial plexus injury.

The **conus medullaris syndrome** occurs with injuries at the thoracolumbar junction. This syndrome has components of both spinal cord and nerve root injury due to the dense population of nerve roots emerging from the caudal end of the spinal cord. Symmetric lower-extremity motor impairment and anesthesia with bowel, bladder, and sexual dysfunction are typically seen. There is typically a symmetric "saddle" area loss of sensory function. Spinal cord function recovery from this syndrome is less likely than recovery from nerve root injury. In cases of the **cauda equina syndrome,** partial recovery is possible with decompression [54]. Cauda equina injuries occur at spinal levels below the termination of the cord, typically at L1 or below.

Cord concussions present with transient neurologic symptoms followed by rapid resolution. These injuries are seen most commonly in athletes with low velocity hyperflexion or extension injuries of the cervical spine. Complete recovery is the rule; however, patients should be evaluated meticulously for severe stenosis or occult spinal instability and intraspinal hematomas. This is in contrast to "stingers or burners" that involve cervical nerve roots only. The issue of "return to play" [55–60] is especially important in the field of athletics. Currently, there is no agreed upon measure to predict which athletes are most at risk of further injury. However, "functional" stenosis [61] and anatomic measurements [56] may both play a role.

PATHOPHYSIOLOGY

The injury to the spinal column and spinal cord involves the transfer of energy sufficient to disrupt the cell membranes and mechanical attachments of the ligaments, muscles, and joints. This results from movement and stressing of the spine beyond its biomechanical/physiological limits in hyperflexion/hyperextension, rotation, compression, or a combination thereof. Injury may result in retropulsion of materials (e.g., bone, cartilage, blood, foreign body) into the spinal canal. Disruption of the vertebral column may also damage the spinal cord within the canal (e.g., dislocation injuries) by reducing the spinal column diameter and compressing the spinal cord. The spinal cord may also be injured by direct laceration or transaction of the cord (e.g., bullet or knife injury). Direct crush, stretch, and shear injury to neurons within the spinal cord leads to immediate cell death.

Secondary injury occurs as the body responds to the damage from the primary injury. There are many mechanisms that initiate secondary injury. These include systemic hypoxia (e.g., hypotension from neurogenic shock or hypovolemic shock, hypoperfusion, etc), local vascular insufficiency (local hypoxia) from trauma, direct penetrating trauma, and spinal compression.

The secondary injury involves biochemical changes and the release of neurotoxic substances. Toxic substances, such as glutamate and free radicals contribute to cell damage and death. These biochemical changes lead to excitotoxicity, neurotransmitter accumulation, arachidonic acid release, free radical production, eicosanoid production, and lipid peroxidation. There are electrolytic shifts such as increased intracellular calcium, increased extracellular potassium, and increased intracellular sodium. The disruption in electrolytes is compounded with the loss of energy metabolism, as the neurons are unable to produce adenosine triphosphate (ATP). Within minutes to hours, oxidative stress leads to cell necrosis. Apoptosis follows further depletion of cells. Over the following days to months, demyelination occurs with the loss of oligodendrocytes. Glial scar formation and axonal degeneration/retraction follow [9]. The damage of the cord may be visualized as edema.

Because spinal cord-injured patients frequently also suffer polytrauma, they are susceptible to derangements of homeostasis. Cardiovascular and pulmonary compromise may affect perfusion and oxygen delivery to the spinal cord, exacerbating the damage. Recent work in animal models of SCI suggests that SCI itself may further disrupt homeostasis. There is evidence from animal models of SCI for a systemic inflammatory response capable of disrupting the cardiopulmonary and renal system [62]. Vasoactive substances released by injured cells and endothelin released from damaged capillaries may also disrupt the spinal cord microcirculation. Ischemia may thus cause neurologic deficits to extend rostrally beyond the initially injured area [63,64].

Because cell death due to secondary injury is an ongoing process, it is believed that early pharmacologic intervention and maintenance of adequate tissue perfusion can salvage these neurons. Given that only 5% to 10% of the descending pathways are necessary for retention of some neurological function [4], even a modest preservation of axons during an injury could have a profound impact on the life of a person with spinal cord injury.

ACUTE MANAGEMENT

Care of the spinal injury patient begins in the field with Emergency Medical Services personnel. The "ABCDE" (**A**irway, **B**reathing, **C**irculation, **D**isability, **E**xposure) of Advanced Trauma Life Support are followed. Attention to maintaining a patent airway and the management of shock take precedence. The patient is immobilized with a rigid cervical collar and backboard for transportation to a trauma center. Intubation and helmet removal should be attempted only with strict attention to maintaining neck alignment. This is particularly important in unresponsive patients, as 3% to 5% of comatose patients have a coexisting cervical spine injury. Additionally, there may be a second site spinal injury, which occurs in 15% of SCI patients.

In the trauma center, the priority remains the maintenance of tissue oxygenation and perfusion, with particular attention to maintaining an adequate mean arterial blood pressure. In this regard, the spinal injury patient presents particular challenges. Immobilization of the cervical spine during intubation is essential and is best accomplished with fiberoptic or awake nasotracheal maneuvers. Mechanical respiratory efforts may be minimal when the injury level is C5 or higher. In these patients, muscular expansion of the rib cage is absent and diaphragmatic breathing may be weakened. Thus, intubation with in-line stabilization using two physicians may be the only option to quickly establish airway control and ventilation. Caution should be exercised in suctioning the oropharynx, as this may stimulate autonomic reflex arcs, causing profound bradycardia and even cardiac arrest. The emergent cricothyroidotomy for airway access must also be considered.

Cervical and high thoracic injuries may result in spinal shock, which can severely complicate the management of a patient already in hypovolemic shock. The clinical picture is hypotension with an associated bradycardia and often hypothermia. Treatment is with mild fluid resuscitation and continuous intravenous inotropic infusions possessing alpha-adrenergic properties to increase the heart rate, cardiac output, and vasomotor tone. Dopamine, because of its mixed alpha-and beta-adrenergic effects, is a useful medication to treat spinal shock. Acutely symptomatic bradycardia should be treated with intravenous atropine. Monitoring with pulmonary atrial catheters (e.g., Swan-Ganz catheters) can help determine the adequacy of perfusion and cardiac output.

Associated extraspinal injuries are common and must also be ruled out. This would be assessed in the "D" and "E" sections of the assessment. Because spinal column injuries are typically the result of severe traumatic mechanisms, the incidence of associated cranial, thoracic, abdominal, and orthopedic injuries is high. Priority must be given to the most life-threatening injuries. If the patient is stable and cooperative, an exam to determine the level of injury (e.g., the ASIA scale) is performed.

The diagnosis of a spinal column injury is based on the clinical examination and radiologic investigations. In an awake, non-intoxicated patient, the absence of pain along the spinal axis is useful to rule out injury. In these patients, a low-velocity injury may require no x-rays, and a high-velocity injury requires only limited plain x-rays. It is essential that radiographic evidence of spinal column injury be correlated with the clinical examination, as 15% of patients have injuries at multiple spinal segments. X-ray, computed tomography, and magnetic resonance imaging investigations are needed in patients who are not able to fully cooperate with the neurologic examination.

Radiographs are useful not only for the detection of but also for the classification of injuries. The fracture types, as well as the degree of cord compression, are particularly important aspects of the injury that determine the management strategy. For the cervical spine, plain lateral x-rays must include the C7-T1 junction, as 31% of injuries occur between C6 and T1. In large, bulky patients, downward traction on the shoulders, a swimmer's view, or a computed tomography scan of the cervical spine may be needed to properly visualize the cervicothoracic junction. Lateral x-rays allow evaluation of vertebral alignment (>3 mm subluxation suggests instability), canal diameter (normal is >12 mm), angulation of the intervertebral space (normal is <11°), width of the interspinous gap, and the atlantodental interval (the distance between the anterior margin of the dens and the closest point on the anterior arch of C1, which should be 3 mm in adults). Soft tissue swelling in the prevertebral space is an indirect indicator of cervical spine injury (maximum prevertebral space in adults at C1 is 10 mm, C2–4 is 5 to 7 mm, and C5–7 is 22 mm).

In the thoracic and lumbar spine, anterior compression fractures and fracture dislocations are usually clearly visible on lateral x-rays. Splaying of the interspinous ligaments is indicative of disruption of the posterior tension band, comprised of the spinous processes and the interspinous ligament. Burst fractures may be difficult to detect on a lateral x-ray but are evident from an abnormally increased intrapedicular space when compared to adjacent levels. Computed tomography is particularly useful in burst fractures for assessing the degree of canal compromise by retropulsed bone fragments from the vertebral body.

If the patient is otherwise systemically stable, cervical traction using a halo frame or Gardner-Wells tongs may be used to restore alignment of the cervical spine and to reduce neural compression. Traction must be initiated with caution, however, as neurologic deterioration can occur from overdistraction or movement of acutely herniated disk material [65]. Before traction is initiated, a full set of x-rays and a magnetic resonance imaging scan help to reduce the likelihood of worsening deficits. In the subaxial spine, it is prudent to begin with 10 lbs and to add weight until reduction is achieved or a total of 5 lbs per cervical level has been used. Serial lateral x-rays or fluoroscopic images should be taken and repeat physical exams performed after each addition of weight to ensure that the neck and spine have not been overdistracted. Of note, not all spine surgeons advocate the routine use of MRI in all cervical spine injuries [66]. Care should be also taken to avoid traction when possible in patients with ankylosing spondylitis because further fracture and·distraction of the vertebral column is likely.

Early intervention to prevent delayed sequelae should also be initiated at this point. This would include use of good respiratory therapy (e.g., incentive spirometry), GI prophylaxis (e.g., H-blockers), and pulmonary embolism prophylaxis (e.g., heparin derivatives, supportive stockings, and sequential compression devices).

ANATOMY

The human vertebral column consists of 7 cervical, 12 thoracic, 5 lumbar, and 1 fused sacrococcygeal vertebrae. A plum line

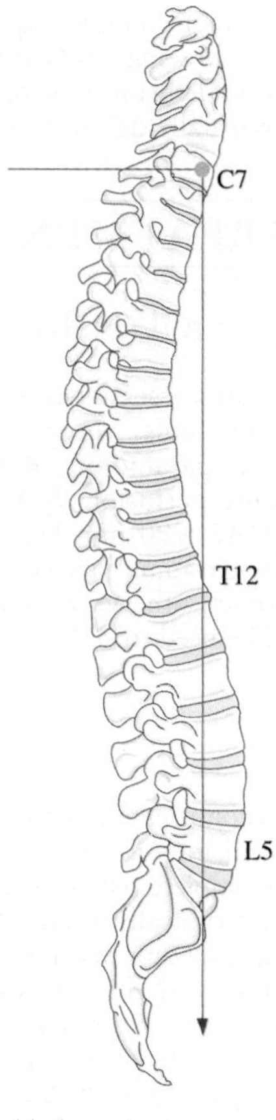

FIGURE 163.1. Sagittal balance image.

dropped from the C7 vertebra, tracing an imaginary line of gravity, runs anterior to the vertebral column in the thoracic and somewhat posterior in the lumbar regions. The line should normally fall near the sacral promontory. This is known as "sagittal balance" (Fig. 163.1).

The cervical canal is wider at the Cl and C2 levels, below which the canal diameter slowly tapers caudally. The lumbar canal is slightly wider than the thoracic canal. The greatest degree of flexion and extension occurs at the atlanto-occipital junction, and the greatest rotatory capability occurs at the atlantoaxial joint. Cervical vertebrae have transverse foramina that transmit the vertebral artery, which usually enters between C6 and C7.

The rib cage and costovertebral ligaments afford an additional element of stability compared with either the cervical or the thoracolumbar junction. Therefore, more force is required to produce a fracture in the mid thoracic spine region than the cervical or lumbar region. By the same token, less mobility is afforded in the thoracic spine [67]. The facet joint plane in the thoracic region is more sagittal than the cervical spine, but more coronal than the typical lumbar spine. The combination of these factors protects against rotational injury and allows somewhat more axial rotation.

The vascular supply of the spinal cord comprises the single anterior spinal artery, the paired posterior spinal arteries, and the segmental radicular arteries. The anterior spinal artery supplies the anterior two thirds of the cord, and the posterior spinal arteries supply the posterior third of the cord. In the cervical cord, the main vascular supplies come from the spinal arteries, but in the thoracic and lumbar regions, the segmental radicular arteries are the major contributors of blood supply. In the upper thoracic cord, the vascular supply may be sparse, especially between the fourth and eighth vertebrae, creating the watershed zone [68], which may be prone to hypotensive and hypoxic insults. The artery of Adamkiewicz (artery of lumbar enlargement) usually arises from T8 to T12 on the left side, most commonly arising from T10 to T12 on the left.

At the thoracolumbar junction and distally, the vertebral bodies allow a greater degree of motion. The lack of rib cage support, the increased room for flexion-extension, and the change in disc size and shape may all contribute to the relatively greater mobility of the lumbar spine. However, the additional degree of mobility at the thoracolumbar junction, especially from Tll to L2, makes this region more susceptible to injury than other adjacent portions of the spine. Because the middle and upper thoracic regions are relatively fixed, the thoracolumbar junction acts as a zone of mechanical stress concentration. The conus medullaris usually resides between the Tll and the Ll-2 disc space, and could be compromised by injuries at this level.

BIOMECHANICS OF INJURY AND STABILITY

Because the neural and musculoskeletal components of the human spine are intimately associated, any discussion regarding blunt traumatic spinal cord injury requires an understanding of the vertebral column. Concepts of stability in the vertebral column are complex. This reflects the intricate nature of the arrangements of joints in the spinal column. Each vertebra has multiple sites of articulation and interaction with the neighboring vertebra (intervertebral disks, facet joints, connecting ligaments). To maintain the stability of this naturally flexible structure, the body must incorporate a complex array of muscles and ligaments.

The vertebral column serves to transmit loads, to permit motion, and to protect the spinal cord. Instability of the spinal column may then be defined as its failure to perform any of these functions under physiologic levels of mechanical loading. This failure may occur acutely or in a progressive, delayed manner. In cases of traumatic spinal cord injury, the vertebral column acutely fails to shield the neural elements from external forces as a result of being stressed beyond its mechanical tolerances.

Various classification schemes have been devised to predict if the spine is unstable. The most common of these is the

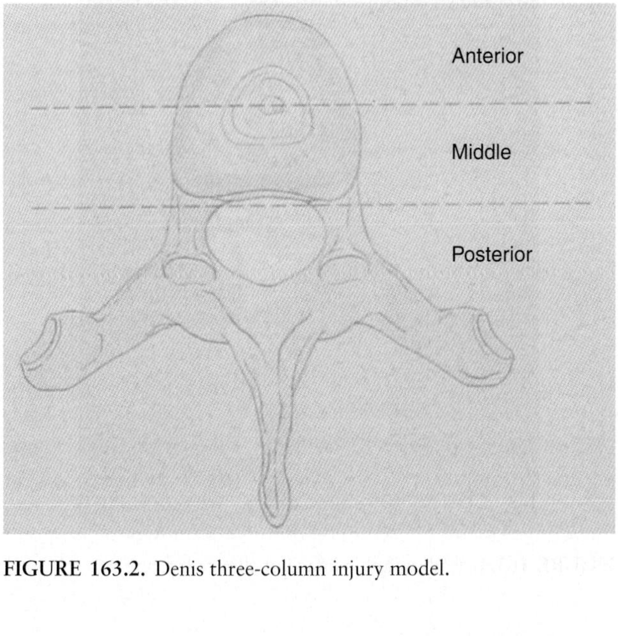

FIGURE 163.2. Denis three-column injury model.

three-column theory introduced by Denis [69,70] (Fig. 163.2). Although these concepts were originally based on studies of thoracolumbar fractures, these principles have been applied successfully to other regions of the spine. This classification system divides the spine into anterior, middle, and posterior columns. The anterior column consists of the anterior half of the vertebral body, the anterior half of the intervertebral disk, and the anterior longitudinal ligament. The middle column consists of the posterior half of the vertebral body, the posterior half of the intervertebral disk, and the posterior longitudinal ligament. The posterior column consists of the posterior arch, the facet joint complex, the interspinous ligament, the supraspinous ligament, and the ligamentum flavum. The diagnosis of instability is made if two or more of the columns are compromised.

External forces placed on the spine include axial compression, distraction, flexion, extension, and translation. Axial compression in the cervical spine results in disruptions of the ring of Cl and burst fractures of the remaining vertebrae. Axial compression in the thoracolumbar spine results in burst fractures. When compressive forces are applied anterior to the spinal column and result in a component of flexion, anterior compression fractures result. Severe flexion is the most common injury mechanism in the cervical spine. This can cause odontoid fractures, teardrop fractures of the vertebral bodies, dislocations of the vertebral bodies, and jumped facets. In the thoracolumbar spine, severe flexion results in compression of the anterior vertebral body. If the fulcrum of force is anterior to the vertebral column, as occurs when a seat-belted passenger is involved in a motor vehicle accident, a flexion-distraction injury of the thoracolumbar junction may result. If the injury passes through the disk space or through the vertebral body, a "chance fracture" may occur (Fig. 163.3).

White and Panjabi [67] recommended a systematic approach to stability, and devised a checklist to determine it. In an adult cervical spine, horizontal subluxation more than 3 mm or an angulation more than 11 degrees is considered unstable [71]. Fractures or alignment patterns that suggest substantial disruption of the bony/ligamentous structures on radiographs suggest injury. Other more complex systems to measure spine stability have also been developed [72].

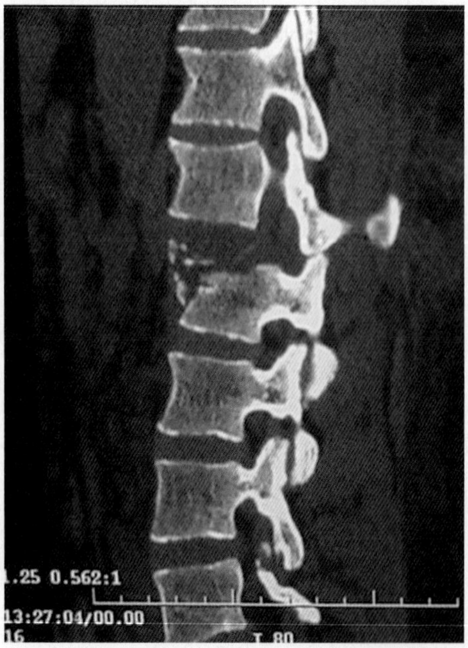

FIGURE 163.3. Radiographic image of chance fracture.

Instability of the spinal column requires maintenance of spinal precautions and bracing. In many instances, surgical realignment, fixation, and fusion will be necessary. Of note, missile injuries do not usually destabilize the spine.

TREATMENT

Initial (Field)

As the ABCDEs of trauma assessment are completed, the surgeon must reach certain goals. Maintaining an airway while stabilizing the spine is paramount. Blood pressure should be maintained to assure perfusion. Suggested levels are SBP >120 mm Hg and MAP >90 mm Hg. All unconscious patients (e.g., major blunt trauma victims) must be assumed to have an SCI until proven otherwise. A rigid backboard and cervical collar should be used to stabilize the spine.

Surgical

Radiologically proven compression of the spinal cord and nerve roots mandates surgical intervention for decompression and stabilization in the incomplete patient (e.g., ASIA B, C, or D).

Neural compression typically results from acute displacement of bone fragments, disruption of ligaments, and disk herniation. Delayed spinal cord compression may also develop from an expanding hematoma within the spinal canal or an inadequately immobilized spine where a prolapsed disk or bone could dynamically compress the cord. Late deterioration of motor or sensory function would prompt a clinician to search for a cause such as post-traumatic syringomyelia and/or progressive deformity. Overall, loss of neurologic function when compared to admission occurs in approximately 3% of patients [51].

Surgery for patients with complete loss of neurologic function remains controversial. Early surgical stabilization within the days after injury has more recently become popular because of the increasing safety of general anesthesia. Early stabilization allows for safe mobilization of the patient, physical and occupational therapy, and improved pulmonary toilet. Surgery for patients who have suffered severe injuries to vital organs may have to have their surgeries delayed. In these cases, maintenance of spinal precautions with a cervical collar and strict "log rolling" for nursing care should prevent deterioration.

The question of whether emergent surgery to the spinal cord improves the neurologic outcome remains controversial [11,33,34,65,73–76]. To directly answer this question, the STASCIS trial (Surgical Treatment of Acute Spinal Cord Injury Study) has been initiated. In this ongoing study, patients with cervical SCI, ASIA scores A, B, C, D, are identified and enrolled in this multicenter study. Patients were stratified into "early" (<24 hours) or "delayed" (>24 hours) groups based on time to decompression. (Decompression occurred by either cervical traction or surgery). At a 1-year follow up, 25% of patients in the early decompression group had a 2 or more grade improvement in ASIA score as compared to the delayed group, with 0% ($p = 0.009$). These results suggest that early decompression (within 24 hours of injury) is the most favorable course of action to treat traumatic SCI [77]. However, there are criticisms of the study. The study has a significant selection bias as the groups are noncontrolled. However, experimental models in animals do suggest that earlier decompression maximizes recovery [78].

Reviews of patients from the National Inpatient Sample allow comparisons between conservative treatment and laminectomy and/or fusion for patients with SCI. When compared to nonsurgical SCI patients, patients with surgery had longer lengths of hospital stay (14 days vs. 9 days), but had lower mortality rates (3% vs. 7%) [10]. Other reviews of the literature provide somewhat contradictory conclusions regarding lengths of stay and neurological improvement [74].

PHARMACOLOGIC THERAPY FOR SPINAL CORD INJURY

Animal models of spinal cord injury have offered the hope that damage caused by secondary injury can be mitigated by early pharmacologic intervention. Three large, randomized, multicenter clinical trials have investigated the use of high dose methylprednisolone for spinal cord injury [13,79]. The standard dose is 30 mg per kg intravenous (IV) methylprednisolone over 1 hour, then 5.4 mg per kg per hour over the next 24 hours.

There has been a great deal of controversy surrounding the quality of the NASCIS trials, leading some authors to conclude that any possible benefits from high-dose methylprednisolone are outweighed by the increased incidence of steroid-related complications [15,16,80,81]. The authors of this chapter no longer use steroids for the treatment of acute spinal cord injury.

Trials of novel pharmacologic interventions for spinal cord injury are currently underway in both clinical and animal models. The therapies include using pharmaceuticals such as riluzole [1,30,82], minocycline [1,30,33,83], polyethylene glycol [1,30,84], erythropoietin [1,30], hypertonic saline [24,85–89], and Cethrin® [1,33]. Injections of autologous macrophages [90–93] and the application of hypothermia [18,19,20,22,23,94,95] are also being investigated. None of these therapies have been shown to be completely safe or effective for the treatment of acute spinal cord injury as of the date of this publication, although several are under clinical trial investigations.

MEDICAL MANAGEMENT OF SPINAL CORD-INJURED PATIENTS

The SCI patient presents unique challenges for the medical team providing both acute and chronic care. As with many other patients, those SCI patients with multiple comorbidities and advanced age are more likely to have poorer outcomes [10]. Several medical problems are frequently associated with a vertebral fracture or spinal cord injury. Some are related to the systemic effect of spinal cord injury, and the others are related to paralysis and prolonged immobilization. The concepts of kinetic therapy and the Roto-Rest treatment table (or similar devices) is endorsed by these authors as a means of minimizing the high morbidity associated with the effects of paralysis and immobility in all of the body systems following acute spinal cord injury.

Cardiovascular

Hypotension and bradycardia from spinal shock may be present. Management with titrated dopamine to support BP and atropine to increase heart rate are recommended. The patient may demonstrate autonomic hyperreflexia or dysreflexia, which is periodic autonomic instability triggered by stimuli such as bladder filling or catheterization when the injury occurs at or above the T6 level. The patients often describe exaggerated autonomic responses, including headache, flushing, diaphoresis, and paroxysmal hypertension. The effects of autonomic hyperreflexia may be life threatening if associated with hypertension. The treatment is to remove offending stimuli, such as by bladder decompression or bowel disimpaction. If a patient is in crisis, sublingual Procardia may be used to help avert a hemorrhagic stroke while one searches for the aggravating factors.

Pulmonary

The risk of pulmonary complications clearly increases with higher-level injuries due to the loss of phrenic nerve innervations (C3–5). For patients with injuries at C1–4, tracheostomy and prolonged mechanical ventilation are probably required. In patients with lower-level injuries, however, all attempts should be made to avoid a tracheostomy. For high cervical injury, one could consider a diaphragmatic pacemaker [96–98]. All injuries above T5 will have significant loss of inspiratory/expiratory force and volume given intercostals denervation.

Respiratory diseases account for 28% of deaths and are the leading cause of mortality in the first year after spinal cord injury [99]. Spinal injury patients are at high risk for pulmonary infection for a number of reasons. Prolonged poor pulmonary toilet, an inability to clear upper airway secretions, poor respiratory capacity, nosocomial exposure, weakened immune responses, and any accompanying chest trauma all increase the risk of pneumonia. The judicious use of aggressive suctioning, pulmonary toilet (e.g., incentive spirometry), chest physiotherapy, bronchodilators, positive-pressure ventilation, and bronchoscopic airway clearance helps prevent infection. Severe atelectasis can also cause respiratory distress in the absence of infection. The authors of this chapter advocate kinetic therapy (the Roto-Rest treatment table) to minimize the risks of pulmonary complications. The placement of an abdominal binder can minimize paradoxical respiratory effort and increase respiration.

Upper Gastrointestinal and Nutrition

All patients should have a nasogastric tube placed to suction drainage in the emergency room, as immobilization predisposes the patient to aspiration. Post-traumatic ileus is also common in this patient population. An indwelling gastric or duodenal tube also allows for early feeding as soon as any ileus has resolved. This supplementation is critical after trauma, as the energy demand of the patients is roughly 150% of their basal requirement. Special attention must also be directed at meeting the patient's increased protein requirements. Proper nutritional support prevents catabolism, supplements wound healing, and maximizes immune protection [27,100]. Parenteral appropriate until the ileus resolves, but tube feeding should begin as early as possible. Even small feeds through a nasogastric tube ("trophic feeding") may reduce the risk of sepsis through enterocyte nutrition.

Gastric ulcers are common in spinal cord injury patients, and this risk is increased with the use of high-dose methylprednisolone. Gastrointestinal hemorrhage is less common and occurs in 3% of patients [101]. H_2-blockers, proton-pump inhibitors, and sucralfate appear to be similarly effective in reducing the risk of gastrointestinal hemorrhage. GI protection is also especially important in patients receiving high-dose steroids. Pancreatitis and acalculous cholecystitis can also occur, especially if parenteral nutrition is used for prolonged periods of time. These disorders can be diagnosed by elevated amylase and bilirubin levels, respectively. Early recognition of these disorders depends on a high level of clinical vigilance. Since the SCI patient may have lost sensation of the abdomen, cardinal signs of acute abdomen e.g., rebound) may not be present.

Lower Gastrointestinal and Genitourinary

Immediately after a complete spinal cord injury the bladder is acontractile. Indwelling catheterization allows bladder drainage and measurements of fluid balance. Intermittent catheterization every 4 to 6 hours should commence as soon as possible to reduce the risk of urinary tract infections. These infections are common and should be treated aggressively to prevent urosepsis. The presence of urea-splitting organisms also increases the incidence of renal stone formation [101]. In addition, clinicians should be aware of autonomic dysreflexia, where an out of proportion sympathetic response may be elicited from a distended bladder or distended bowel. The person with SCI (often a T2 or higher injury) who presents to the emergency department with tachycardia, hypertension, severe headache, and so on, needs to be properly diagnosed rapidly. Often a simple treatment (bladder catheterization, bowel disimpaction) may be what is primarily required [102]. Other causes include decubitus ulcers, undiagnosed fistulae, or other infectious lesions. Sublingual Procardia may provide quick relief of hypertension. This relief can be life sparing.

After severe spinal injury, rectal tone is most often flaccid in lower motor neuron injuries. Constipation can easily occur unless manual evacuation is carried out on a regular basis. The liberal use of rectal suppositories stimulates bowel emptying, and regular doses of stool softener should also be used. New surgical procedures to restore manual bladder control are available [40,103]. Devices to aid in defecation are also being investigated and developed [38].

Clinicians should be aware of the systemic effects that SCI has on the reproductive system, especially in men [104–106] and should be prepared to counsel the patient on his options.

Infectious Disease/Fever

The "5 W's" of fever workup are relevant for the SCI patient: Wind (atelectasis), Water (urinary infection), Wound (wound infection), Walk (DVTs), and Weird (drug reactions.) Routine lab analysis should be part of the initial workup for fever. These include erythrocyte sedimentation rate (ESR) and C-reactive protein as infection markers. One should also order tests such as urine analysis and culture for UTI, duplex ultrasound for DVTs, blood cultures for sepsis, skin inspection for breakdown or infection, liver function tests (LFTs) including total and direct bilirubin, amylase, and lipase for hepatitis, acalculous cholecystitis, or pancreatitis. Again, it is important to note that SCI patients may be unable to alert physicians to common signs (e.g., leg pain, abdominal pain) due to their injuries.

Cutaneous and Musculoskeletal

Pressure ulcers are common after spinal cord injury and occur in up to 25% to 30% of patients (101). Transport on hard backboards, prolonged immobilization, loss of cutaneous sensation, and reduced skin perfusion all predispose to skin breakdown. The sacrum, heels, ischium, and occiput are most commonly involved.

Prevention of pressure ulcers begins in the emergency room. Patients should be removed from the backboard and any hard surfaces as soon as possible, as pressure necrosis of the skin can occur in less than 1 hour on these surfaces. In the acute care setting, the patient should be turned in a "log roll" fashion every 2 hours until the spine is proven to be stable or until the spine is stabilized surgically. Alternatively, an electrically driven kinetic bed such as the Roto-Rest (Kinetic Concepts, San Antonio, TX) or other pressure relieving beds or mattress overlays can be used [107].

Stage I lesions can be managed with aggressive mobilization and adhesive barrier dressings. Once the dermis has been compromised, however, daily sterile dressing may be needed for wound debridement. Deeper lesions may require debridement and skin grafting in the operating room. Proper management of even mild lesions prevents devastating late sequelae such as sepsis from infected ulcers. The development of the "VAC" aided healing of severe decubitus ulcers provides gentle suction which debrides and reduces the size of the ulcer. Relief of the pressure source and debridement and cleaning of the wound is essential. The patient must be given a high protein diet to facilitate decubitus ulcer healing. In the subacute and chronic setting, muscle denervation leads to atrophy, spasticity, and contracture formation. Passive range of motion exercises and splinting forestall the formation of contractures. Etidronate sodium and increasing mobility may reduce heterotopic ossifications [108]. Proper nutritional support is essential.

Thromboembolism

The combination of trauma, paralysis, and immobility places paralyzed patients at high risk of developing deep venous thrombosis and pulmonary embolism. The incidence of lower-extremity venous thrombosis varies widely in literature reports depending on the test used (fibrinogen scanning, clinical, impedance plethysmography, venography). Rates ranging from 12% to 81% have been reported. The highest reported frequency of PE was approximately 5% [109]. PE is responsible for 10% of all deaths after SCI [99]. The risk of PE peaks at 2 to 3 weeks after injury.

These authors advocate the use of the Roto-Rest kinetic treatment table (or similar devices) for all acute spinal cord injury to combat pulmonary emboli. Routine use of pneumatic compression devices and subcutaneous heparin (or similar drugs) can reduce the risk of thromboembolism [110–112]. For example, 5,000 units of subcutaneous heparin can be administered twice daily within the first 2 days of injury. The prophylactic use of a vena cava filter is advocated by some, but controversy exists [113,114]. For patients who are not able to utilize to pneumatic compression devices and prophylactic heparin, vena cava (temporary or permanent) filters are a recommended option [115–118].

Psychosocial

All acute spinal cord injury patients experience psychological sequelae to their catastrophic injury. Most often, family and friends experience similar effects including denial, depression, anger, and finally coping. The coping phase is when the person decides to deal with the realities of their disability, although not to accept that their paralysis is "forever." A team of caring physicians and other health professionals including rehabilitation psychologists is essential for a number of psychosocial actions. Antidepressants can also be helpful in certain cases.

The spinal cord injured community has unique needs. This community is not a homogenous group, as different levels of injury will leave the person with SCI with different amounts of residual function. As such, the immediate needs of the person with SCI are also not uniform. When asked what problems if addressed would lead to the greatest increase in quality of life, the people with high cervical injuries (quadriplegics) identified restoration of hand and arm use as the most important. People with lower injuries (paraplegics) identified bladder, bowel, autonomic dystrophy, and sexual function as the most important issues to address [35]. Listening to the needs of this community will help researchers develop practical improvements to help the SCI community.

SPINAL CORD INJURY IN CHILDREN

By adolescence the spine is well developed and the patterns of injury resemble those of adults. Perhaps because of the increased mobility of the developing spine, pediatric spinal cord injuries are rare [119]. Because of the greater proportional mass of the head, however, children are more susceptible to atlanto-occipital injuries. The hypermobility of the pediatric spine also accounts for cases of spinal cord injury without radiographic abnormality (SCIWORA). This represents 15% to 20% of all pediatric spinal cord injuries [120,121].

The principles in managing pediatric spinal cord injuries are similar to that of adults. Because children cannot cooperate fully with the physical examination, it is important to recognize subtle physical and radiologic signs. As such, an increased reliance must often be placed on radiographic studies. Many of the standard measurements used to evaluate cervical x-rays need to be adjusted for the pediatric spine.

In young children, the increased relative size of the head compared to body results in neck flexion when placed on a rigid backboard. This malalignment can accentuate deformity in cervical spine and should be avoided. Equipment tailored

TABLE 163.2

COMPLETED PROSPECTIVE RANDOMIZED CONTROLLED SCI CLINICAL TRIALS[a]

Trial name	Year	No. of patients	Study design	SCI type, treatment window (h)	Treatment arms	Conclusions
NASCIS I	1984	330	Phase III RCT	I, 48	MPSS 100 mg × 10 d MPSS 1000 mg × 10 d	No difference
NASCIS II	1990	487	Phase III RCT	C/I, 12	MPSS (24 h) Naloxone Placebo	Negative primary analysis; secondary analysis showed improved recovery if treated w/MPSS win 8 h of injury; naloxone negative
Maryland GM-1	1991	34	Phase II RCT—pilot study	I, 72	GM-1 Placebo	Improved neurological recovery w/GM-1 in this small pilot study
Otani et al.	1994	158	Nonblinded RCT	?, 8	MPSS (NASCIS II 24 h) Placebo	Significantly more steroid-treated patients had some sensory improvement, no motor differences
TRH	1995	20	Phase II RCT—pilot study	C/I, 2	TRH Placebo	Suggestion of improved neurological recovery w/TRH in this small pilot study
NASCIS III	1997	499	Phase III RCT	I, 12	MPSS (24 h) MPSS (48 h) MPSS bolus then TM	Improved neurological recovery w/ MPSS if administered early (w/in 3 h after SCI); TM not superior to MPSS
Nimodipine	1998	100	Phase III RCT	C/I, 6	Pimodipine MPSS (24 h) Nimodipine + MPSS (24 h) Placebo	No difference; study likely underpowered to detect a difference
Gacyclidine	1999	280	Phase II RCT	C/I, 2	Gacyclidine (0.005 mg/kg) Gacyclidine (0.01 mg/kg) Gacyclidine (0.02 mg/kg) Placebo	Negative study; trend to improved motor recovry w/imcomplete cervical injuries
Pointillart et al.	2000	106	Blinded RCT	?, 8	MPSS (NASCIS II 24 h) Nimodipine MPSS & nimodipine Placebo	No neurological differences between groups; trend to increased infections in groups receiving MPSS
Sygen (GM-1)	2001	797	Phase III RCT	I, 72	MPSS & low-dose GM-1 MPSS & high-dose GM-1 MPSS & placebo	Negative primary outcomes; trend to improved secondary outcomes

[a]Further trials are not planned for any of the agents presented in this table, to the knowledge of the authors.
C, complete; I, incomplete; RCT, randomized controlled clinical trial; TM, tirilizad mesylate; ?, unpublished or unclear data.

TABLE 163.3

SUMMARY OF RECENTLY PUBLISHED AND ONGOING, WELL-DOCUMENTED, UNPUBLISHED EXPERIMENTAL TRIALS FOR ACUTE AND SUBACUTE SC[a]

Trial name	Intervention	Lead center organization	Date of initiation	Proposed no. of patients	Complete, published phases	Current study type	Registration information[b]
Recently published studies							
OEF stimulation	Device implantation	Indiana U Medical Center	?	20	10 patients, Phase I	Phase I/II	NR
Australian OEC trial	OEC transplantation	Australia	Pre-2005	6	Phase I, single-blinded w/control	?	NR
PROCORD (enrollment suspended)	Activated Autologous Macrophages	Proneuron	2005	61, suspended at 50	Phase I	Phase II, randomized, multicenter controlled trial	NR
Prague BMSC transplantation	BMSC transplantation	Prague	?	20	?	?	NR
Korean BMSC transplantation	BMSC transplantation	Intra U Hospital	2001	35	Phase I/II nonrandomized	?	NR
Ongoing, unpublished studies							
STASCIS	Timing of surgical decompression	U of Toronto, Thomas Jefferson U, Spine Trauma Study Group	2003	450	NA	Nonrandomized prospective observational	NR
Early & late surgery for traumatic central cord syndrome	Surgical decompression	U of Maryland	May 2007	30	?	Phase II	NCT00475748
Systemic hypothermia	Hypothermia (cooled to 33°C at 0.5°C/h maintained for 48 h)	Miami	January 2007	100	NA	Phase I/II	NR
Minocycline	250 mg IV bid × 7 d	Calgary	?	?	Phase I	Phase II	NR
Riluzole	Na+ channel blockade, antiglutamatergic 50 mg PO bid	U of Toronto North American Clinical Trials Network	Late 2007	36	NA	Phase I	NR
ATI-355	Nago-blockade	Novartis	May 2006	16	NA	Phase I	NCT00406016
Cethrin	Rho inhibition	BioAxone Therapeutics/ Alseres Pharmaceutical	February 2005	47	NA	Phase I/II	NCT00500812
CSF drainage	72 h of CSF drainage	U of British Columbia	March 2008	22 enrolled to date	NA	Phase I	NCT00135278

[a]To the authors' knowledge, all therapies presented here are currently being investigated in clinical trials, or further trials are planned.
[b]At http://www.clinicaltrials.gov.
bid, twice daily administration; IV, intravenous; NA, not applicable; NR, not registered; OEF, oscillating electrical field; PO, by mouth; U, university.

for pediatric spine immobilization should be used whenever possible. Unlike adults, the majority of these injuries can be treated nonsurgically with bracing [122].

FUTURE ADVANCES

Approximately 100 years ago at the beginning of the 20th century, Dr. Alfred Reginald Allen induced a spinal cord injury in an animal model for the purpose of understanding SCI [123]. His advancements were not alone, as the 20th century was remarkable for incredible advances in science, medicine, engineering, and technology. Many of these advances have helped to make the opening years of the 21st century, 2001 to 2010, the "decade of the spine."

In the realm of Basic Science research, there have been great advances in understanding the pathophysiology of SCI [1,5,6,82]. Understanding of the mechanisms of inflammation, cell migration, immunology, and cell death allow for basic scientists to identify pathways that can be directly targeted in future clinical investigations. Understanding biochemical environment of the region of the SCI allows scientists to better engineer biological repair strategies. For example, understanding the inhibitory properties of the glial scar after an injury may allow scientists to target and overcome these obstacles [9].

The surgical realm continues to advance, with improvements in spine fusion techniques and hardware. Clinical studies, like STASCIS [33,77,76] also allow the clinician to best judge the optimal time to initiate treatment. New and innovative devices are coming to market to stabilize and repair the bony, ligamentous, and disk injuries that often accompany SCI [124–131].

Additional studies into autologous (e.g., macrophage, oligodendrocyte, Schwann) and stem cell transplantation, tissue engineering, and hypothermia are being actively pursued to further develop methods to preserve function or to restore function to the person living with an SCI [1,9,19,33,41,45,93,132–138]. Hypothermia research suggests that cooling patients with SCI may protect neural tissue from secondary injury by increasing tissue tolerance to reduced blood flow and oxygenation. Efficacy and safety studies of moderate hypothermia (32°C to 34°C) are currently under investigation [19].

New medical therapies are being tested. Minocycline is being tested in a Canadian trial [83,139,140] as a treatment to reduce oligodendrocyte and microglial apoptosis. Riluzole, a sodium channel inhibitor, is also in multicenter trials [1,104,139]. Rho inhibitors are also being investigated. This includes Nogo, a critical inhibitor of neural regeneration by inhibition of guanosine triphosphatase (GTPase). Local injection of anti-Rho antibodies is in a phase II study [141].

Oscillating field stimulation to promote axonal regrowth along the cranial/caudal plane (as opposed to random orientation) is being studied as well [142,143].

There have been studies to bypass the injured CNS and to tap directly into the brain, allowing a person with SCI to control simple machines [144–150]. These are adaptive strategies such as Functional Electrical Stimulation (FES), Robotics and Brain Machine Interfaces.

The hope of neural restoration remains the focus of intense basic science research. Whether through stem cell transplantation, molecular manipulation, or modulation of the local cytokine milieu, the aim is to restore function to cells that have already been damaged or destroyed. Because reinnervation of the spinal cord is the best way to fully restore neurologic function, research in this area remains the primary goal at the Miami Project to Cure Paralysis.

Despite all of the exciting advances forthcoming in the field of spinal cord injury, prevention of injury remains a top priority. Programs such as the Think First initiative in Florida have already dramatically reduced the incidence of diving-related cervical spine injuries. Physicians, who are most acutely aware of the devastating consequence of spinal cord injury, must assume a key role in educating the public on how to avoid these catastrophic injuries.

SUMMARY OF RECOMMENDATIONS BASED UPON RANDOMIZED CONTROLLED CLINICAL TRIALS

A recent review of completed clinical trials has been published by Dr. Fehling's group. Completed trials are reproduced as Table 163.2, and ongoing clinical trials are reproduced as Table 163.3 [139].

Unfortunately, there is no consensus on the single best treatment available for a spinal cord injury. At present, there are multiple options available for treatments that include hypothermia, reduction by traction, and surgical decompression. Fortunately, there are ongoing clinical trials to aid clinicians in future decision making and with evidence-based medicine. One such example comes from our department at the University of Miami. Allan Levi and colleagues have been investigating hypothermia in treating Spinal Cord Injury in clinical settings [94,95].

References

1. Baptiste DC, Fehlings MG: Pharmacological approaches to repair the injured spinal cord. *J Neurotrauma* 23:318–334, 2006.
2. Fehlings MG, Agrawal S: Role of sodium in the pathophysiology of secondary spinal cord injury. *Spine* 20:2187–2191, 1995.
3. Fehlings MG, Nashmi R: Assessment of axonal dysfunction in an in vitro model of acute compressive injury to adult rat spinal cord axons. *Brain research* 677:291–299, 1995.
4. Fehlings MG, Tator CH: The relationships among the severity of spinal cord injury, residual neurological function, axon counts, and counts of retrogradely labeled neurons after experimental spinal cord injury. *Exp Neurol* 132:220–228, 1995.
5. Hulsebosch CE: Recent advances in pathophysiology and treatment of spinal cord injury. *Adv Physiol Educ* 26:238–255, 2002.
6. Sharma HS: Pathophysiology of blood-spinal cord barrier in traumatic injury and repair. *Curr Pharm Des* 11:1353–1389, 2005.
7. Wood PL: *Neuroinflammation: mechanisms and management.* Totowa, NJ, Humana Press, 2003.
8. Young W: Spinal cord contusion models. *Prog Brain Res* 137:231–255, 2002.
9. Eftekharpour E, Karimi-Abdolrezaee S, Fehlings MG: Current status of experimental cell replacement approaches to spinal cord injury. *Neurosurg Focus* 24:E19, 2008.
10. Boakye M, Patil CG, Santarelli J, et al: Laminectomy and fusion after spinal cord injury: national inpatient complications and outcomes. *J Neurotra* 25:173–183, 2008.
11. Fehlings MG, Sekhon LH, Tator C: The role and timing of decompression in acute spinal cord injury: what do we know? What should we do? *Spine* 26:S101–S110, 2001.
12. Bracken MB: Methylprednisolone and acute spinal cord injury: an update of the randomized evidence. *Spine* 26:S47–S54, 2001.
13. Bracken MB, Shepard MJ, Holford TR, et al: Administration of methylprednisolone for 24 or 48 hours or tirilazad mesylate for 48 hours in the treatment of acute spinal cord injury. Results of the third national acute spinal cord injury randomized controlled trial. National acute spinal cord injury study. *JAMA* 277:1597–1604, 1997.
14. Ducker TB, Zeidman SM: Spinal cord injury. Role of steroid therapy. *Spine* 19:2281–2287, 1994.

15. Hurlbert RJ: The role of steroids in acute spinal cord injury: an evidence-based analysis. *Spine* 26:S39–S46, 2001.
16. Lammertse DP: Update on pharmaceutical trials in acute spinal cord injury. *J Spinal Cord Med* 27:319–325, 2004.
17. Merola A, O'Brien MF, Castro BA, et al: Histologic characterization of acute spinal cord injury treated with intravenous methylprednisolone. *J Orthop Trauma* 16:155–161, 2002.
18. Cappuccino A: Moderate hypothermia as treatment for spinal cord injury. *Orthopedics* 31:243–246, 2008.
19. Dietrich WD III: Therapeutic hypothermia for spinal cord injury. *Crit Care Med* 37:S238–S242, 2009.
20. Garza M: "Cool" new treatment: NFL uses hypothermia for spinal cord injury. *JEMS* 32:20, 2007.
21. Herold JA, Kron IL, Langenburg SE, et al: Complete prevention of postischemic spinal cord injury by means of regional infusion with hypothermic saline and adenosine. *J Thorac Cardiovasc Surg* 107:536–541; discussion 541–532, 1994.
22. Kwon BK, Mann C, Sohn HM, et al: Hypothermia for spinal cord injury. *Spine J* 8(6):859–874, 2008.
23. Yoshitake A, Mori A, Shimizu H, et al: Use of an epidural cooling catheter with a closed countercurrent lumen to protect against ischemic spinal cord injury in pigs. *J Thorac Cardiovasc Surg* 134:1220–1226, 2007.
24. Levene HB, Erb CJ, Gaughan JP, et al: Hypertonic saline as a treatment for acute spinal cord injury: effects on somatic and autonomic outcomes as observed in a mouse model. *Clin Neurosurg* 54:213–219, 2007.
25. Popovich PG, Jones TB: Manipulating neuroinflammatory reactions in the injured spinal cord: back to basics. *Trends Pharmacol Sci* 24:13–17, 2003.
26. Tyagi R, Donaldson K, Loftus CM, et al: Hypertonic saline: a clinical review. *Neurosurg Rev* 30:277–289; discussion 289–290, 2007.
27. Nutritional support after spinal cord injury. *Neurosurgery* 50:S81–S84, 2002.
28. Hausmann ON, Fouad K, Wallimann T, et al: Protective effects of oral creatine supplementation on spinal cord injury in rats. *Spinal Cord* 40:449–456, 2002.
29. Baptiste DC, Fehlings MG: Emerging drugs for spinal cord injury. *Expert Opin Emerg Drugs* 13:63–80, 2008.
30. Fehlings MG, Baptiste DC: Current status of clinical trials for acute spinal cord injury. *Injury* 36[Suppl 2]:B113–B122, 2005.
31. Fehlings MG, Bracken MB: Summary statement: the sygen(GM-1 ganglioside) clinical trial in acute spinal cord injury. *Spine* 26:S99–S100, 2001.
32. Tator CH, Fehlings MG: Review of clinical trials of neuroprotection in acute spinal cord injury. *Neurosurg Focus* 6:e8, 1999.
33. Baptiste DC, Fehlings MG: Update on the treatment of spinal cord injury. *Prog Brain Res* 161:217–233, 2007.
34. Fehlings MG, Perrin RG: The role and timing of early decompression for cervical spinal cord injury: update with a review of recent clinical evidence. *Injury* 36[Suppl 2]:B13–B26, 2005.
35. Anderson KD: Targeting recovery: priorities of the spinal cord-injured population. *J Neurotrauma* 21:1371–1383, 2004.
36. Behrman AL, Nair PM, Bowden MG, et al: Locomotor training restores walking in a nonambulatory child with chronic, severe, incomplete cervical spinal cord injury. *Phys Ther* 88:580–590; discussion 590–585, 2008.
37. Harness ET, Yozbatiran N, Cramer SC: Effects of intense exercise in chronic spinal cord injury. *Spinal Cord* 46(11):733–737, 2008.
38. Uchikawa K, Takahashi H, Deguchi G, et al: A washing toilet seat with a CCD camera monitor to stimulate bowel movement in patients with spinal cord injury. *Am J Phys Med Rehabil* 86:200–204, 2007.
39. Van Houtte S, Vanlandewijck Y, Kiekens C, et al: Patients with acute spinal cord injury benefit from normocapnic hyperpnoea training. *J Rehabil Med* 40:119–125, 2008.
40. Xiao CG, Du MX, Dai C, et al: An artificial somatic-central nervous system-autonomic reflex pathway for controllable micturition after spinal cord injury: preliminary results in 15 patients. *J Urol* 170:1237–1241, 2003.
41. Anderberg L, Aldskogius H, Holtz A: Spinal cord injury—scientific challenges for the unknown future. *Ups J Med Sci* 112:259–288, 2007.
42. Goodrich JT: History of spine surgery in the ancient and medieval worlds. *Neurosurg Focus* 16:E2, 2004.
43. Rahimi SY, McDonnell DE, Ahmadian A, et al: Medieval neurosurgery: contributions from the Middle East, Spain, and Persia. *Neurosurg Focus* 23:E14, 2007.
44. Donovan WH: Donald Munro Lecture. Spinal cord injury—past, present, and future. *J Spinal Cord Med* 30:85–100, 2007.
45. Kakulas BA: Neuropathology: the foundation for new treatments in spinal cord injury. *Spinal Cord* 42:549–563, 2004.
46. Spinal cord injury. Facts and figures at a glance. *J Spinal Cord Med* 28:379–380, 2005.
47. Wyndaele M, Wyndaele JJ: Incidence, prevalence and epidemiology of spinal cord injury: what learns a worldwide literature survey? *Spinal Cord* 44:523–529, 2006.
48. Sekhon LH, Fehlings MG: Epidemiology, demographics, and pathophysiology of acute spinal cord injury. *Spine* 26:S2–S12, 2001.
49. Kirshblum SC, Memmo P, Kim N, et al: Comparison of the revised 2000 American spinal injury association classification standards with the 1996 guidelines. *Am J Phys Med Rehabil* 81:502–505, 2002.
50. Maynard FM Jr, Bracken MB, Creasey G, et al: International standards for neurological and functional classification of spinal cord injury. American spinal injury association. *Spinal Cord* 35:266–274, 1997.
51. Marino RJ, Ditunno JF Jr, Donovan WH, et al: Neurologic recovery after traumatic spinal cord injury: data from the model spinal cord injury systems. *Arch Phys Med Rehabil* 80:1391–1396, 1999.
52. Benzel EC, Tator CH, AANS Publications Committee: *Contemporary management of spinal cord injury.* Park Ridge, IL, American Association of Neurological Surgeons, 1995.
53. McKinley W, Santos K, Meade M, et al: Incidence and outcomes of spinal cord injury clinical syndromes. *J Spinal Cord Med* 30:215–224, 2007.
54. Harrop JS, Hunt GE Jr, Vaccaro AR: Conus medullaris and cauda equina syndrome as a result of traumatic injuries: management principles. *Neurosurg Focus* 16:e4, 2004.
55. Cantu RC: Stingers, transient quadriplegia, and cervical spinal stenosis: return to play criteria. *Med Sci Sports Exerc* 29:S233–S235, 1997.
56. Cantu RV, Cantu RC: Current thinking: return to play and transient quadriplegia. *Curr Sports Med Rep* 4:27–32, 2005.
57. Levene HB, Harrop J: Athletics and spinal cord injury: cervical stenosis definition may hold key to consensus. *Neurotrauma & Critical Care News* (Spring), 2006.
58. Morganti C, Sweeney CA, Albanese SA, et al: Return to play after cervical spine injury. *Spine* 26:1131–1136, 2001.
59. Vaccaro AR, Harrop JS, Daffner SD, et al: Acute cervical spine injuries in the athlete. *International Sport Med Journal* 4(1), 2003.
60. Vaccaro AR, Klein GR, Ciccoti M, et al: Return to play criteria for the athlete with cervical spine injuries resulting in stinger and transient quadriplegia/paresis. *Spine J* 2:351–356, 2002.
61. Kim DH, Vaccaro AR, Berta SC: Acute sports-related spinal cord injury: contemporary management principles. *Clin Sports Med* 22:501–512, 2003.
62. Gris D, Hamilton EF, Weaver LC: The systemic inflammatory response after spinal cord injury damages lungs and kidneys. *Exp Neurol* 211:259–270, 2008.
63. Harrop JS, Sharan AD, Vaccaro AR, et al: The cause of neurologic deterioration after acute cervical spinal cord injury. *Spine* 26:340–346, 2001.
64. Tator CH, Fehlings MG: Review of the secondary injury theory of acute spinal cord trauma with emphasis on vascular mechanisms. *J Neurosurg* 75:15–26, 1991.
65. Tator CH, Fehlings MG, Thorpe K, et al: Current use and timing of spinal surgery for management of acute spinal surgery for management of acute spinal cord injury in North America: results of a retrospective multicenter study. *J Neurosurg* 91:12–18, 1999.
66. Vaccaro AR, Nachwalter RS: Is magnetic resonance imaging indicated before reduction of a unilateral cervical facet dislocation? *Spine* 27:117–118, 2002.
67. Panjabi MM, White AA: *Biomechanics in the musculoskeletal system.* New York, Churchill Livingstone, 2001.
68. Louis R: *Surgery of the spine: surgical anatomy and operative approaches.* Berlin, New York, Springer-Verlag, 1983.
69. Denis F: The three column spine and its significance in the classification of acute thoracolumbar spinal injuries. *Spine* 8:817–831, 1983.
70. Denis F: Spinal instability as defined by the three-column spine concept in acute spinal trauma. *Clin Orthop Relat Res* (189):65–76, 1984.
71. White AA, Panjabi MM: *Clinical biomechanics of the spine.* Philadelphia, PA, Lippincott, 1990.
72. Patel AA, Vaccaro AR, Albert TJ, et al: The adoption of a new classification system: time-dependent variation in interobserver reliability of the thoracolumbar injury severity score classification system. *Spine* 32:E105–E110, 2007.
73. Albert TJ, Kim DH: Timing of surgical stabilization after cervical and thoracic trauma. Invited submission from the joint section meeting on disorders of the spine and peripheral nerves, March 2004. *J Neurosurg* 3:182–190, 2005.
74. Fehlings MG, Perrin RG: The timing of surgical intervention in the treatment of spinal cord injury: a systematic review of recent clinical evidence. *Spine* 31:S28–S35; discussion S36, 2006.
75. Fehlings MG, Tator CH: An evidence-based review of decompressive surgery in acute spinal cord injury: rationale, indications, and timing based on experimental and clinical studies. *J Neurosurg* 91:1–11, 1999.
76. Ng WP, Fehlings MG, Cuddy B, et al: Surgical treatment for acute spinal cord injury study pilot study #2: evaluation of protocol for decompressive surgery within 8 hours of injury. *Neurosurg Focus* 6:e3, 1999.
77. Fehlings MG, Vaccaro AR, Aarabi B, et al: A prospective, multicenter trial to evaluate the role and timing of decompression in patients with cervical spinal cord injury: initial one year results of the STASCIS study *AANS.* Chicago, 2008.
78. Rabinowitz RS, Eck JC, Harper CM Jr, et al: Urgent surgical decompression compared to methylprednisolone for the treatment of acute spinal cord injury: a randomized prospective study in beagle dogs. *Spine (Phila Pa 1976)* 33:2260–2268, 2008.
79. Bracken MB, Shepard MJ, Collins WF Jr, et al: Methylprednisolone or naloxone treatment after acute spinal cord injury: 1-year follow-up data. Results of the second national acute spinal cord injury study. *J Neurosurg* 76:23–31, 1992.
80. Pharmacological therapy after acute cervical spinal cord injury. *Neurosurgery* 50:S63–S72, 2002.

81. Bracken MB: Steroids for acute spinal cord injury. *Cochrane Database Syst Rev* CD001046, 2002.
82. Schwartz G, Fehlings MG: Secondary injury mechanisms of spinal cord trauma: a novel therapeutic approach for the management of secondary pathophysiology with the sodium channel blocker riluzole. *Prog Brain Res* 137:177–190, 2002.
83. Wells JE, Hurlbert RJ, Fehlings MG, et al: Neuroprotection by minocycline facilitates significant recovery from spinal cord injury in mice. *Brain* 126:1628–1637, 2003.
84. Ditor DS, John SM, Roy J, et al: Effects of polyethylene glycol and magnesium sulfate administration on clinically relevant neurological outcomes after spinal cord injury in the rat. *J Neurosci Res* 85:1458–1467, 2007.
85. Legos JJ, Gritman KR, Tuma RF, et al: Coadministration of methylprednisolone with hypertonic saline solution improves overall neurological function and survival rates in a chronic model of spinal cord injury. *Neurosurgery* 49:1427–1433, 2001.
86. Spera PA, Arfors KE, Vasthare US, et al: Effect of hypertonic saline on leukocyte activity after spinal cord injury. *Spine* 23:2444–2448; discussion 2448–2449, 1998.
87. Spera PA, Vasthare US, Tuma RF, et al: The effects of hypertonic saline on spinal cord blood flow following compression injury. *Acta Neurochir (Wien)* 142:811–817, 2000.
88. Sumas ME, Legos JJ, Nathan D, et al: Tonicity of resuscitative fluids influences outcome after spinal cord injury. *Neurosurgery* 48:167–172; discussion 172–163, 2001.
89. Tuma RF, Vasthare US, Arfors KE, et al: Hypertonic saline administration attenuates spinal cord injury. *J Trauma* 42:S54–S60, 1997.
90. Hauben E, Nevo U, Yoles E, et al: Autoimmune T cells as potential neuroprotective therapy for spinal cord injury. *Lancet* 355:286–287, 2000.
91. Popovich PG, Guan Z, McGaughy V, et al: The neuropathological and behavioral consequences of intraspinal microglial/macrophage activation. *J Neuropathol Exp Neurol* 61:623–633, 2002.
92. Schwartz M, Hauben E: T cell-based therapeutic vaccination for spinal cord injury. *Prog Brain Res* 137:401–406, 2002.
93. Schwartz M, Lazarov-Spiegler O, Rapalino O, et al: Potential repair of rat spinal cord injuries using stimulated homologous macrophages. *Neurosurgery* 44:1041–1045; discussion 1045–1046, 1999.
94. Levi AD, Casella G, Green BA, et al: Clinical outcomes using modest intravascular hypothermia after acute cervical spinal cord injury. *Neurosurgery* 66(4):670–677, 2010.
95. Levi AD, Green BA, Wang MY, et al: Clinical application of modest hypothermia after spinal cord injury. *J Neurotrauma* 26:407–415, 2009.
96. Krieger LM, Krieger AJ: The intercostal to phrenic nerve transfer: an effective means of reanimating the diaphragm in patients with high cervical spine injury. *Plast Reconstr Surg* 105:1255–1261, 2000.
97. Miller JI, Farmer JA, Stuart W, et al: Phrenic nerve pacing of the quadriplegic patient. *J Thorac Cardiovasc Surg* 99:35–39; discussion 39–40, 1990.
98. Winter A, Weierman RJ, Laing J: Diaphragm pacer for high spinal cord injury. *J Med Soc N J* 80:121–122, 1983.
99. DeVivo MJ, Krause JS, Lammertse DP: Recent trends in mortality and causes of death among persons with spinal cord injury. *Arch Phys Med Rehabil* 80:1411–1419, 1999.
100. Apelgren KN, Wilmore DW: Nutritional care of the critically ill patient. *Surg Clin North Am* 63:497–507, 1983.
101. Chen D, Apple DF Jr, Hudson LM, et al: Medical complications during acute rehabilitation following spinal cord injury—current experience of the model systems. *Arch Phys Med Rehabil* 80:1397–1401, 1999.
102. Karlsson AK: Autonomic dysreflexia. *Spinal Cord* 37:383–391, 1999.
103. Xiao CG, de Groat WC, Godec CJ, et al: "Skin-CNS-bladder" reflex pathway for micturition after spinal cord injury and its underlying mechanisms. *J Urol* 162:936–942, 1999.
104. Anderson KD, Borisoff JF, Johnson RD, et al: Long-term effects of spinal cord injury on sexual function in men: implications for neuroplasticity. *Spinal Cord* 45:338–348, 2007.
105. Kafetsoulis A, Brackett NL, Ibrahim E, et al: Current trends in the treatment of infertility in men with spinal cord injury. *Fertil Steril* 86:781–789, 2006.
106. Patki P, Hamid R, Shah J, et al: Fertility following spinal cord injury: a systematic review. *Spinal Cord* 45:187, 2007.
107. Green BA, Green KL, Klose KJ: Kinetic nursing for acute spinal cord injury patients. *Paraplegia* 18:181–186, 1980.
108. Stover S: Heterotopic ossification, in Bloch RF, Basbaum M (eds): *Management of spinal cord injuries*. Baltimore, Williams & Wilkins, 1986, pp xvii, 462p.
109. Furlan JC, Fehlings MG: Role of screening tests for deep venous thrombosis in asymptomatic adults with acute spinal cord injury: an evidence-based analysis. *Spine* 32:1908–1916, 2007.
110. Prevention of venous thromboembolism in the acute treatment phase after spinal cord injury: a randomized, multicenter trial comparing low-dose heparin plus intermittent pneumatic compression with enoxaparin. *J Trauma* 54:1116–1124; discussion 1125–1116, 2003.
111. Hebbeler SL, Marciniak CM, Crandall S, et al: Daily vs twice daily enoxaparin in the prevention of venous thromboembolic disorders during rehabilitation following acute spinal cord injury. *J Spinal Cord Med* 27:236–240, 2004.
112. Slavik RS, Chan E, Gorman SK, et al: Dalteparin versus enoxaparin for venous thromboembolism prophylaxis in acute spinal cord injury and major orthopedic trauma patients: 'DETECT' trial. *J Trauma* 62:1075–1081; discussion 1081, 2007.
113. Johns JS, Nguyen C, Sing RF: Vena cava filters in spinal cord injuries: evolving technology. *J Spinal Cord Med* 29:183–190, 2006.
114. Maxwell RA, Chavarria-Aguilar M, Cockerham WT, et al: Routine prophylactic vena cava filtration is not indicated after acute spinal cord injury. *J Trauma* 52:902–906, 2002.
115. Deep venous thrombosis and thromboembolism in patients with cervical spinal cord injuries. *Neurosurgery* 50:S73–S80, 2002.
116. Velmahos GC, Kern J, Chan L, et al: Prevention of venous thromboembolism after injury. *Evid Rep Technol Assess (Summ)* (22):1–3, 2000.
117. Velmahos GC, Kern J, Chan LS, et al: Prevention of venous thromboembolism after injury: an evidence-based report–part I: analysis of risk factors and evaluation of the role of vena caval filters. *J Trauma* 49:132–138; discussion 139, 2000.
118. Velmahos GC, Kern J, Chan LS, et al: Prevention of venous thromboembolism after injury: an evidence-based report—part II: analysis of risk factors and evaluation of the role of vena caval filters. *J Trauma* 49:140–144, 2000.
119. Durkin MS, Olsen S, Barlow B, et al: The epidemiology of urban pediatric neurological trauma: evaluation of, and implications for, injury prevention programs. *Neurosurgery* 42:300–310, 1998.
120. Brown RL, Brunn MA, Garcia VF: Cervical spine injuries in children: a review of 103 patients treated consecutively at a level 1 pediatric trauma center. *J Pediatr Surg* 36:1107–1114, 2001.
121. Grabb PA, Pang D: Magnetic resonance imaging in the evaluation of spinal cord injury without radiographic abnormality in children. *Neurosurgery* 35:406–414; discussion 414, 1994.
122. Eleraky MA, Theodore N, Adams M, et al: Pediatric cervical spine injuries: report of 102 cases and review of the literature. *J Neurosurg* 92:12–17, 2000.
123. Allen AR: Surgery of experimental lesion of spinal cord equivalent to crush injury of fracture dislocation of spinal column. A preliminary report. *JAMA* 57:878–880, 1911.
124. Artificial intervertebral disc arthroplasty for treatment of degenerative disc disease of the cervical spine. *Technol Eval Cent Asses Program Exec Summ* 22:1–4, 2008.
125. Bartels RH, Donk RD, Pavlov P, et al: Comparison of biomechanical properties of cervical artificial disc prosthesis: a review. *Clin Neurol Neurosurg* 110(10):963–967, 2008.
126. Kim SW, Shin JH, Arbatin JJ, et al: Effects of a cervical disc prosthesis on maintaining sagittal alignment of the functional spinal unit and overall sagittal balance of the cervical spine. *Eur Spine J* 17:20–29, 2008.
127. Rabin D, Pickett GE, Bisnaire L, et al: The kinematics of anterior cervical discectomy and fusion versus artificial cervical disc: a pilot study. *Neurosurgery* 61:100–104; discussion 104–105, 2007.
128. Rohlmann A, Zander T, Bock B, et al: Effect of position and height of a mobile core type artificial disc on the biomechanical behaviour of the lumbar spine. *Proc Inst Mech Eng G J Aerosp Eng* 222:229–239, 2008.
129. Sasso RC, Best NM: Cervical kinematics after fusion and bryan disc arthroplasty. *J Spinal Disord Tech* 21:19–22, 2008.
130. Sasso RC, Smucker JD, Hacker RJ, et al: Artificial disc versus fusion: a prospective, randomized study with 2-year follow-up on 99 patients. *Spine* 32:2933–2940; discussion 2941–2932, 2007.
131. Yang YC, Nie L, Cheng L, et al: Clinical and radiographic reports following cervical arthroplasty: a 24-month follow-up. *Int Orthop* 33(4):1037–1042, 2008.
132. Cummings BJ, Uchida N, Tamaki SJ, et al: Human neural stem cells differentiate and promote locomotor recovery in spinal cord-injured mice. *Proc Natl Acad Sci U S A* 102(39):14069-14074, 2005.
133. Lu J, Ashwell K: Olfactory ensheathing cells: their potential use for repairing the injured spinal cord. *Spine* 27:887–892, 2002.
134. Nomura H, Tator CH, Shoichet MS: Bioengineered strategies for spinal cord repair. *J Neurotrauma* 23:496–507, 2006.
135. Phinney DG, Isakova I: Plasticity and therapeutic potential of mesenchymal stem cells in the nervous system. *Curr Pharm Des* 11:1255–1265, 2005.
136. Rapalino O, Lazarov-Spiegler O, Agranov E, et al: Implantation of stimulated homologous macrophages results in partial recovery of paraplegic rats. *Nat Med* 4:814–821, 1998.
137. Sykova E, Jendelova P: Magnetic resonance tracking of implanted adult and embryonic stem cells in injured brain and spinal cord. *Ann N Y Acad Sci* 1049:146–160, 2005.
138. Xiang S, Pan W, Kastin AJ: Strategies to create a regenerating environment for the injured spinal cord. *Curr Pharm Des* 11:1267–1277, 2005.
139. Hawryluk GW, Rowland J, Kwon BK, et al: Protection and repair of the injured spinal cord: a review of completed, ongoing, and planned clinical trials for acute spinal cord injury. *Neurosurg Focus* 25:E14, 2008.
140. McPhail LT, Stirling DP, Tetzlaff W, et al: The contribution of activated phagocytes and myelin degeneration to axonal retraction/dieback following spinal cord injury. *Eur J Neurosci* 20:1984–1994, 2004.
141. Rossignol S, Schwab M, Schwartz M, et al: Spinal cord injury: time to move? *J Neurosci* 27:11782–11792, 2007.

142. Bohnert DM, Purvines S, Shapiro S, et al: Simultaneous application of two neurotrophic factors after spinal cord injury. *J Neurotrauma* 24:846–863, 2007.
143. Shapiro S, Borgens R, Pascuzzi R, et al: Oscillating field stimulation for complete spinal cord injury in humans: a phase 1 trial. *J Neurosurg* 2:3–10, 2005.
144. Hoffmann U, Vesin JM, Ebrahimi T, et al: An efficient P300-based brain-computer interface for disabled subjects. *J Neurosci Methods* 167:115–125, 2008.
145. Lebedev MA, Carmena JM, O'Doherty JE, et al: Cortical ensemble adaptation to represent velocity of an artificial actuator controlled by a brain-machine interface. *J Neurosci* 25:4681–4693, 2005.
146. Moxon KA, Hallman S, Aslani A, et al: Bioactive properties of nanostructured porous silicon for enhancing electrode to neuron interfaces. *J Biomater Sci Polym Ed* 18:1263–1281, 2007.
147. Ojemann JG, Leuthardt EC, Miller KJ: Brain-machine interface: restoring neurological function through bioengineering. *Clin Neurosurg* 54:134–136, 2007.
148. Patil PG, Turner DA: The development of brain-machine interface neuroprosthetic devices. *Neurotherapeutics* 5:137–146, 2008.
149. Stieglitz T: Neural prostheses in clinical practice: biomedical microsystems in neurological rehabilitation. *Acta Neurochir (Wien)* 97:411–418, 2007.
150. Utsugi K, Obata A, Sato H, et al: Development of an optical brain-machine interface. *Conf Proc IEEE Eng Med Biol Soc* 2007:5338–5341, 2007.

CHAPTER 164 ■ THORACIC AND CARDIAC TRAUMA

SCOTT B. JOHNSON AND JOHN G. MYERS

INTRODUCTION

Thoracic trauma is responsible for 20% to 25% of the estimated 150,000 trauma related deaths per year in the United States and is the leading cause of death in the first four decades of life. Two thirds of thoracic-related deaths occur in the prehospital setting, usually due to significant cardiac, great vessel, or tracheobronchial injuries. In a study of over 1,300 patients presenting to a level I trauma center with thoracic trauma, Kulshrestha and colleagues reported an overall mortality rate of 9.4%, with 56% of these occurring within the initial 24 hours. While the two strongest determinants of increased mortality were a low GCS and increased age, penetrating injury, liver or spleen injury, long bone fracture, and more than five rib fractures also adversely affected mortality [1]. In a study of trauma-related hospital deaths at an urban level I trauma center, Demetriades and colleagues found a penetrating mechanism, age more than 60, and chest AIS >3 to be significant variables associated with patients who had no vital signs on admission [2].

Overall, motor vehicle collisions account for 70% to 80% of all thoracic injuries. The incidence of penetrating injuries varies widely but is usually more prevalent in urban centers. The majority of thoracic injuries can be treated with careful observation or tube thoracostomy. It is historically reported that 12% to 15% of patients with thoracic injury will require thoracotomy. In a Western Trauma Association multicenter review, only 1% of all trauma patients required nonresuscitative thoracotomy [3]. With the improvements in prehospital care and transport, more of the severely injured patients who would have previously died at the scene are making it to the hospital alive. Success in the management of these injuries rests in having a high index of suspicion for the life-threatening thoracic injuries, prompt recognition and treatment of associated injuries, and aggressive management of coexisting pulmonary dysfunction.

INDICATIONS FOR URGENT SURGICAL INTERVENTION

Bleeding

Hemothorax is second only to rib fractures as the most common associated finding in thoracic trauma, being present in approximately 25% of patients with thoracic trauma. Bleeding can arise from the chest wall, lung parenchyma, major thoracic vessels, heart, or diaphragm. A small or moderate-size hemothorax that stops bleeding immediately after placement of a tube thoracostomy can usually be managed conservatively. However, if the patient continues to bleed at a rate of more than 200 cc per hour, exploration is indicated. The accumulation of more than 1,500 cc of blood within a pleural space is considered a massive hemothorax and is an indication for exploration. If the patient becomes hemodynamically unstable at anytime and an intrathoracic source is suspected, emergent thoracotomy should be performed irrespective of chest tube drainage. A chest radiograph should always be obtained after placing a tube thoracostomy to ensure proper position of the tube and complete drainage of the pleural space. Video-assisted thoracoscopic surgery (VATS) can be considered in the stable patient with retained hemothorax or in a stable patient who continues to bleed at a slow but steady rate; however, the surgeon should not hesitate to convert to open thoracotomy if visualization is inadequate or drainage and evacuation of the pleural space is incomplete.

Cardiovascular Collapse

The indications for resuscitative emergency department thoracotomy (EDT) continue to be debated. Our indications, which are considered to be fairly liberal, include (1) loss of vitals in the Emergency Department for both blunt and penetrating trauma and (2) loss of vitals en route, with less than 10 minutes of prehospital CPR, with some sign of life upon arrival, or a suspected intrathoracic etiology. Penetrating thoracic injuries, specifically stab wounds, have the highest rate of survival. Data for blunt trauma are much less encouraging but should not be used as a deterrent, as there are several functional survivors in most reported series. A retrospective study of 959 patients undergoing resuscitative thoracotomy concluded that EDT in blunt trauma with more than 5 minutes or penetrating trauma with more than 15 minutes of prehospital CPR is futile care [4]. When performed, resuscitative thoracotomy should be performed early. Discovered tamponade should be released; massive pulmonary bleeding should be quickly controlled with staplers, clamping, or manual compression; and cardiac wounds should be controlled. With no intrathoracic source, the aorta should be clamped and internal cardiac massage continued.

Massive Air Leak

Findings on initial presentation of significant subcutaneous emphysema, a subsequent large or persistent air leak, or persistent pneumothorax should alert the clinician to the presence of a major tracheobronchial injury. This injury is potentially lethal but relatively rare, found in only 2% to 5% of patients with thoracic trauma. Significant tracheobronchial injuries may result in a massive air leak, leading to hypoventilation. Maneuvers to stabilize the patient should include decreasing airway pressures. Contralateral mainstem intubation can also be attempted. Major tracheobronchial injuries generally should be repaired as early as the patient's condition allows.

Tamponade

Cardiac tamponade results when fluid or air collects within an intact pericardial sac, resulting in compression of the right heart with subsequent obstruction of venous return and cardiovascular collapse. Potential findings upon presentation include tachycardia and hypotension, cervical cyanosis, jugular venous distension, muffled heart sounds, and pulsus paradoxus. The diagnosis is confirmed with echocardiography, pericardial window, or at the time of emergent thoracotomy. Treatment requires prompt resuscitation and decompression of the pericardium, followed by repair of the bleeding source.

DIAGNOSTICS

Diagnostic imaging plays a key role in the management of patients after chest trauma and has considerable impact on therapeutic decision-making. The information generated by diagnostic imaging procedures not only serves to tailor therapy to the individual needs of the patient, but also helps to determine overall prognosis and outcome. Radiologic imaging plays an important role in the workup of any patient with suspected chest trauma. The chest radiograph is the initial imaging study of choice to be obtained in patients with suspected chest injury. Chest Computed Tomography (CT), however, is being used with increasing frequency in the evaluation of patients with chest trauma. CT can be useful in assessing suspected traumatic aortic, pulmonary, airway, skeletal, and diaphragmatic injuries. Magnetic resonance imaging (MRI) on the other hand has a limited role in the initial evaluation of any patient with suspected chest trauma. To undergo an MRI, the patient must be stable, and many trauma patients cannot be scanned because of bulky, mechanical supportive equipment. However, in selected patients who are hemodynamically stable, MRI may be particularly useful for the evaluation of spine and diaphragm injuries. Other imaging modalities available to the clinician include echocardiography, angiography, and VATS, which can be both diagnostic and therapeutic when appropriately indicated.

Plain Chest Radiograph

The frontal chest radiograph is the most appropriate initial radiographic study to obtain for the evaluation of patients with suspected chest injury. This study is particularly useful in helping to rule out major injury. Ideally, the radiograph should be obtained with the patient in the upright position because of mediastinal widening that is typically seen in the supine position. Chest radiography has a 98% negative predictive value and is therefore quite useful when normal. However, abnormal findings may be subtle and quite nonspecific. Radiographic findings that may indicate mediastinal injury, such as major aortic disruption, include abnormal contour or indistinctness of the aortic knob, apical pleural cap, rightward deviation of the nasogastric tube, thickening of the right paratracheal stripe, downward displacement of the left mainstem bronchus, rightward deviation of the trachea, and, not uncommonly, nonspecific mediastinal widening. Most life-threatening injuries can be screened by the plain chest radiograph and a careful physical exam. Blunt thoracic injuries detected by CT alone infrequently require immediate therapy. If immediate therapy is needed, findings will usually be visible on plain radiographs or obvious on clinical exam. Although a plain upright chest radiograph remains one of the basic imaging studies routinely performed on initial screening, it may be over-utilized. A recent study suggests that in the presence of a normal physical exam in the hemodynamically stable patient, obtaining a routine chest radiograph is actually unnecessary, since it rarely, if ever, changes clinical care [5].

Chest Computed Tomography

CT is highly sensitive in detecting thoracic injuries after blunt chest trauma and is superior to routine CXR in visualizing lung contusions, pneumothorax, and hemothorax, and it can often alter initial therapeutic management in a significant number of patients with suspected chest trauma. It has also been shown to detect unexpected injuries and abnormalities, resulting in altered management in a substantial number of patients when applied appropriately [6]. It can be particularly useful in screening for major intrathoracic aortic injury. In one study, contrast-enhanced CT scanning was 100% sensitive in detecting major thoracic aortic injury based on clinical follow-up and was 99.7% specific, with 89% positive and 100% negative predictive values for an overall diagnostic accuracy of 99.7% [7]. An unequivocally normal mediastinum at CT, with no hematoma and a regular aorta surrounded by a normal fat pad, has essentially a 100% negative predictive value for aortic injury [7–10]. It has also been shown that CT scanning detects 11% of thoracic aortic injuries that are not detected by routine, plain chest radiography alone [11].

CT scanning can also be useful in detecting hemopericardium and/or hemothorax from any cause, injury to the brachiocephalic vessels, pneumothorax, rib fractures, pulmonary parenchymal contusion, and sternal fractures. It can also be useful in detecting pneumomediastinum caused by pulmonary interstitial emphysema, bronchial or tracheal rupture (commonly associated with pneumothorax), esophageal rupture, or iatrogenic injury from over-ventilation or traumatic intubation. In addition, CT scanning can detect injuries otherwise missed by routine plain radiograph. In one study comparing CT scanning with plain radiography, CT scanning detected serious injuries in 65% of those patients not found to have injury on plain film. These injuries included (in decreasing order of frequency) lung contusions, pneumothoraces, hemothoraces, diaphragmatic ruptures, and myocardial ruptures [12]. Even in those patients without suspected chest trauma, CT scanning of the abdomen, which commonly includes the lower portion of the thorax, often yields important information regarding possible intrathoracic injury. In one study, hematoma surrounding the intrathoracic aorta near the level of the diaphragmatic crura seen on intra-abdominal CT scanning was found to be a relatively insensitive but highly specific sign for thoracic aortic injury after blunt trauma. Therefore, the presence of this sign seen on abdominal CT imaging should prompt more specific imaging of the thoracic aorta to evaluate potential thoracic aortic injury [13]. CT scanning has also been shown to be useful to help define the extent of pulmonary contusion and identify those patients at high risk for acute pulmonary failure in those patients with PaO_2/FIO_2 lower than 300. 3-D CT scanning has also been shown to be useful in diagnosing and determining the severity of sternal fractures [14]. With the advent of high resolution CT scanners that can reconstruct axial, coronal, and sagittal images, even penetrating diaphragmatic injuries, which are difficult to image preoperatively, can be diagnosed with a relatively high sensitivity and specificity [15]. Despite its usefulness however, thoracic CT scanning is not necessarily routinely indicated for all patients with chest wall trauma. In addition, although there has been a dramatic increase in the utilization of CT scanning in the last decade, its usefulness in detecting clinically relevant injury has recently come into question, especially in those patients with a normal screening plain chest radiograph [16].

Ultrasound

Transesophageal echocardiography (TEE) is rapidly gaining acceptance as an important diagnostic tool available to the trauma surgeon and is showing particular promise in diagnosing traumatic intrathoracic aortic injuries. Although somewhat invasive, its portability makes it a diagnostic procedure of choice in looking at the heart and great vessels in multiply injured trauma patients. In one particular study of 58 patients with thoracic trauma, TEE demonstrated its usefulness in diagnosing thoracic aortic injury and permitted the identification of small lesions not detectable by CT scanning or angiography [17]. TEE has shown to be an important diagnostic tool for examining the thoracic aorta and is valuable in identifying aortic injury in high-risk trauma patients who are too unstable to undergo transport to the aortography suite. Nienaber et al. prospectively compared TEE with aortogram in evaluation of nontraumatic aortic dissection and found the technique to be a safe and highly sensitive method of diagnosing lesions of the descending aorta, with accuracy approaching 100% [18]. When an aortic injury is present, typical findings on the TEE can include aortic wall hematomas, intimal flaps, or disruptions. Several groups have shown TEE to be accurate in identifying aortic pathology after trauma, with its diagnostic efficacy mainly limited by the experience of the person performing the exam [19–21]. In addition, it has been shown to be useful in diagnosing blunt cardiac rupture, when other diagnostic modalities have failed, as well as in diagnosing severe valvular regurgitation intraoperatively following foreign body removal [22,23].

Numerous studies report that transthoracic echocardiography (TTE) is emerging as an effective noninvasive screening examination for pericardial effusion in the trauma setting. Although subxiphoid pericardial window is currently considered the gold standard to confirm the diagnosis of pericardial tamponade, conventional 2-dimensional TTE has been shown to reveal as little as 50 mL of blood within the pericardium and can show cardiac pseudoaneurysms and the location of foreign bodies [24–27]. Lopez et al. [28] showed that TTE can detect and distinguish hemopericardium from other effusions of lower echogenicity. In prospective studies of patients sustaining penetrating precordial injuries, TTE demonstrated sensitivities of 56% to 90%, with specificities of 93% to 97%. Its overall accuracy was 90% to 96% [29,30]. Because TTE is an examination that can be performed at the bedside, it can be performed rapidly and may decrease the time to diagnosis versus pericardial window (15.5 minutes vs. 42.4 minutes in one study by Meyer et. al.) [30]. It has also been shown that earlier therapeutic intervention facilitated by TTE may be associated with improved survival [31]. In addition, TTE has been shown to be able to identify cardiac sources for hemodynamic instability in the operating room unrelated to tamponade, such as the relatively rare case of atrioventricular valve rupture, which would otherwise be difficult to diagnose, therefore allowing for expeditious repair using cardiopulmonary support [32]. Thus, both TTE and TEE are emerging as useful screening modalities that can be used to evaluate both penetrating and blunt cardiac injuries.

Angiography

Thoracic aortography historically has been the gold standard for diagnosing thoracic aortic injury and for defining the extent of the injury and involvement of branch disease, if present. Aortography usually requires approximately 40 mL of a nonionic iodinated contrast material injected at a rate of 18 to 20 mL per sec. At least two views are obtained—one in the anteroposterior plane and another usually at a 45 degree left anterior oblique projection. If these do not accurately visualize the areas of concern, then additional views may be necessary, either from a lateral or a right anterior oblique projection. Diagnosis of aortic injury angiographically is usually made by finding one or more of the following: an irregular or discontinued contour of the aortic lumen, an intimal flap, an aortic dissection, and/or a luminal outpouching (i.e., pseudoaneurysm). Thoracic aortography can detect blunt traumatic aortic injuries with 96% sensitivity and 98% specificity. False negative examinations are usually related to incomplete or inadequate injections or projections. To be an adequate study, the aortic root as well as the distal descending thoracic aorta should be visualized since these locations are involved, respectively, with 8% and 2% of all blunt thoracic aortic injuries. False positives usually relate to a prominent ductus diverticulum or from an ulcerated atheromatous plaque. A ductus diverticulum can be seen in up to 9% of thoracic aortograms and is related to a remnant of the enlarged mouth of the ductus arteriosus. It appears as a localized bulge of the anterior wall of the aorta and can be differentiated from a pseudoaneurysm due to its usually smooth, regular, symmetrical borders; intimal disruption is typically absent. In addition, the aortic lumen adjacent to the diverticulum is not narrowed, and there is absence of retention of contrast upon the washout phase of the angiogram, which is often typical of pseudoaneurysms. Ulcerated atheromas usually are small, isolated outpouchings of the aortic wall with a collar button appearance. They are typically located in the mid-descending aorta rather that at the aortic isthmus. It is not uncommon for them to occur in individuals that demonstrate widespread atherosclerotic disease and should, therefore, be suspected on angiograms obtained in clinically relevant individuals. Angiography is invasive and can have associated complications. The complications associated with arteriography include allergic reactions, renal failure, local puncture site problems, stroke, and even death. Radiographic contrast media cause severe anaphylactic reactions in less than 2% of cases. A prior history of allergic reaction to intravascular contrast material increases the risk for a subsequent reaction, even after premedication with histamine blockers and steroids. Patients with preexisting comorbidities, such as renal disease, diabetes mellitus, congestive heart failure, or who are elderly (over 70 years of age) have the highest risk for acute renal dysfunction following contrast administration. The reported incidence of contrast-induced nephropathy varies from less than 1% in the general patient population to as high as 92% among patients with comorbidities that predispose to renal insults, such as diabetes and renal insufficiency [33].

Arteriography requires arterial puncture with cannulation, usually percutaneously. Possible entry sites include not only the femoral artery (most common) but also the axillary and brachial arteries. Possible puncture site complications include hematoma, pseudoaneurysm, arteriovenous fistula, hemorrhage, arterial thrombosis, and femoral neuralgia. Fortunately, clinically significant local arterial complications occur in only 0.1% to 5% of cases. The risk of complications is also related to the indication for arteriography. Fortunately, the lowest risk for complications occur in trauma patients and the complication rates quoted in older studies may not accurately reflect current risk.

Video-Assisted Thoracoscopic Surgery

The role of thoracoscopy in trauma has been explored by a number of investigators in the literature. Prior to the modern video era, Jones et al. described management of 36 patients with thoracoscopy under local anesthesia as a diagnostic tool to define intrathoracic injuries and to visualize ongoing hemorrhage [34] Four patients in their series were spared abdominal exploration when the diaphragm was found devoid of injury. More recently, Ochsner et al. [35] and Mealy et al. [36] have demonstrated the usefulness of VATS as a diagnostic tool in the assessment of diaphragmatic integrity in cases of penetrating and blunt thoracic injuries respectively. VATS has become an acceptable surgical modality in the diagnostic evaluation of suspected diaphragmatic injury and has been shown to have therapeutic benefit when evacuation of clotted hemothoraces is able to be performed in stable patients with penetrating chest injures [37]. Main indications for VATS include diagnosis and treatment of diaphragmatic injuries, diagnosis of persistent hemorrhage, management of retained thoracic collections, assessment of cardiac and mediastinal structures, diagnosis of bronchopleural fistulas, and diagnosis and treatment of persistent posttraumatic pneumothorax. VATS has been shown to be a useful alternative to an open thoracotomy in selected patients. Because lung deflation with single-lung ventilation is a critical component of the technique, VATS is relatively contraindicated in patients unable to tolerate this. Caution should be used in patients with suspected obliteration to their pleural cavity secondary to previous infection ("pleurisy") or surgery. VATS should have no role in the management of unstable patients or in those patients unable to tolerate formal thoracotomy for any reason. Whether VATS should be considered as the initial approach in evaluation of all stable chest trauma patients when an intrathoracic injury is suspected is still debated, and appropriate patient selection remains important.

SPECIFIC INJURIES

Chest Wall

Rib Fractures

Rib fractures are a common injury and are often associated with other injuries. Rib fractures themselves usually cause only minor problems; however, they may be a marker of more severe injury, and it may be the underlying pulmonary contusion that often accompanies the rib fracture that may be more clinically relevant. A study by Flagel et al. showed that 13% of those patients in the National Trauma Data Bank who had one or more rib fractures ($n = 64{,}750$) developed complications including pneumonia, acute respiratory distress syndrome, pulmonary embolus, pneumothorax, aspiration pneumonia, empyema, and the need for mechanical ventilation. They also showed that increasing number of rib fractures correlated directly with increasing pulmonary morbidity and mortality. The overall mortality rate for patients with rib fractures was 10%. The mortality rate increased ($p < 0.02$) with each additional rib fracture, independent of patient age. This ranged from 5.8% for a single rib fracture to 10% in the case of 5 fractured ribs. The mortality rate increased dramatically for the groups with 6, 7, and 8 or more fractured ribs to 11.4%, 15.0%, and 34.4%, respectively [38]. Interestingly, in their study epidural analgesia was associated with a reduction in mortality for all patients sustaining rib fractures, particularly those with more than four fractures. Since this was not a prospective randomized study, it is difficult to tell if there was a correlation between patients that received epidural catheters having an overall lower injury severity score. However, in one prospective randomized trial by Bulger et al., trauma patients with rib fractures were randomized to either receive epidural anesthesia or intravenous opioids for pain relief, and it was shown that those patients with epidural anesthesia had a lower incidence of nosocomial pneumonia and shorter duration of mechanical ventilation [39]. The number of patients that could receive epidural anesthesia was limited, however, due to strict inclusion criteria. The age of the patient sustaining rib fractures should be taken into account, as well as the location of the fractures. It has been shown that rib fractures occurring in the very young should alert the clinician to possible nonaccidental trauma (NAT). In one study by Barsness et al., rib fractures in children under 3 years of age had a positive predictive value of NAT of 95%, and rib fracture was the only skeletal manifestation of NAT in 29% of the children [40]. With regards to the elderly, it has been shown that there is a linear relationship between age and complications, including mortality. It has been shown that elderly patients with rib fractures have up to twice the mortality of younger patients with similar injuries [41]. In addition, this increase in mortality may begin to be seen in patients as early as 45 years of age when more than four ribs are involved [42]. The location of the rib fracture(s) is also important, as it has been shown that left-sided rib fractures are associated with splenic injuries, and right-sided rib fractures are associated with liver injuries. While isolated rib fractures have an associated incidence of vascular injury of only 3%, first rib fractures in association with multiple rib fractures have a 24% incidence of associated vascular injury. A first rib fracture along with findings of a widened mediastinum, upper extremity pulse deficit, brachial plexus injury, and/or expanding hematoma should prompt work-up for a possible subclavian arterial injury.

Flail Chest

Flail chest occurs when multiple adjacent ribs are broken in two locations, thereby allowing that portion of the chest wall to move independently with respiration. The strict definition of flail chest is the fracture of at least four consecutive ribs in two or more places; however, the functional definition is an incompetent segment of chest wall large enough to impair the patient's respiration. Major mortality and morbidity of flail chest can be attributed to the usual underlying associated pulmonary contusion and the hypoventilation/hypoxia that results from the paradoxical movement of the chest wall. This is a mechanical problem in which negative pressure generated during inspiration within the thorax is dissipated by movement of the flail segment inward. This movement equalizes the intrathoracic pressure, which would normally be accomplished by the movement of air into the lungs. In addition, the underlying pulmonary contusion usually leads to a ventilation perfusion mismatch, contributing to the hypoxia; the pain associated with multiple rib fractures can lead to splinting and contribute to hypoventilation. As a result, both oxygenation as well as ventilation is compromised. Usually a large number of ribs have to be involved to be clinically significant. Fortunately, this occurs relatively rarely with rib fractures. Flagel et al. showed an overall incidence of flail chest of 3.95% in patients with 6 rib fractures; 4.84% in those with 7 rib fractures; and 6.42% in those with 8 or more rib fractures [38].

The basic treatment for flail chest injury has not changed appreciably over the last several decades. Ventilatory support in the form of mechanical, positive pressure ventilation remains the gold standard against which all other forms of treatment are measured. Avery et al. coined this type of treatment "internal pneumatic stabilization" in 1956 [43]. Positive pressure ventilation, which effectively forces the flail segment to rise and fall normally with inspirations, effectively allows stabilization of the flail segment with respect to the remainder of the chest wall. Surgical stabilization of the chest wall has been shown to be of some benefit with regard to shorter length of ventilator dependency, lower rates of pneumonia, and shorter intensive care unit stays, although this form of therapy is not yet widely practiced [44]. Pain control continues to be an important adjunct in any treatment regimen.

Sternal Fracture

Sternal fractures have been shown to decrease the stability of the thorax in cadavers [45]. They usually occur as a deceleration force during traffic accidents together with blunt force trauma from foreign objects, such as steering wheels, although they have been reported as a complication of CPR, which interestingly was found in 14% of medical autopsy cases that had received chest compressions prior to death [46]. Traffic accidents are the cause of sternal fractures in almost 90% of cases, with approximately 25% of fractures graded as moderately to severely displaced. Approximately 30% of patients will have associated injuries, with craniocerebral trauma and rib fractures being the most commonly associated injuries [47]. Displaced fractures are more likely to have associated thoracic and cardiac injuries and are more likely to require surgical fixation.

However, the majority of patients can be safely observed and even discharged home as long as the following criteria are met: (1) the injury is not one of high-velocity impact, (2) the fracture is not severely displaced, (3) there are no clinically significant associated injuries, and (4) complex analgesic requirements are not required. Most serious complications and deaths that occur in patients with sternal fractures are not due to the fracture itself but rather are related to the associated injuries, such as flail chest, head injury, or pulmonary or cardiac contusion. Although approximately 22% of patients will exhibit electrocardiographic changes, elevated creatine kinase MB isoenzymes, or echocardiographic abnormalities, only approximately 6% of patients will exhibit a clinically significant myocardial contusion. In addition to myocardial contusion, other complications of sternal fracture such as mediastinal abscess, mediastinitis, and acute tamponade have all been reported. Indications for operative sternal fixation are certainly not absolute and should be judged individually. Generally accepted criteria include severe pain, sternal instability causing respiratory compromise, and severe displacement. Only a small percentage of patients (2% in one series) actually require sternal fixation [48]. A lack of consensus among surgeons on how to treat these injuries, in addition to a lack of randomized trials concerning their optimal approach, continues to prevail.

Scapular Fracture

Scapular fractures are relatively rare and were once presumed to be an indicator of severe underlying trauma and subsequent higher mortality. They occur in only approximately 1% to 4% of blunt trauma patients who present to a level I trauma center and are associated with a higher incidence of thoracic injury compared to those patients who sustain blunt trauma without a scapular fracture. However, more recent studies have indicated that although patients with scapular fractures tend to have more severe chest injuries and a higher overall injury severity score, their length of intensive care unit stay, length of hospital stay, and overall mortality is not necessarily increased [49,50]. Treatment is usually conservative and, most of the time, necessarily aimed at the associated injuries that are commonly present.

Scapulothoracic Dissociation

Scapulothoracic dissociation is an infrequent injury with a potentially devastating outcome. Scapulothoracic dissociation results from massive traction injury to the anterolateral shoulder girdle with disruption of the scapulothoracic articulation. Identification of this injury requires a degree of clinical suspicion, based upon the injury mechanism and physical findings. Assessment of the degree of trauma to the musculoskeletal, neurologic, and vascular structures should be made. Based upon clinical findings, a rational diagnostic approach can be navigated and appropriate surgical intervention planned. Scapulothoracic dissociation frequently is associated with acromioclavicular separation, a displaced clavicular fracture, subclavian or axillary vascular disruption, and a sternoclavicular disruption. Clinically, patients usually present with a laterally displaced scapula, a flail extremity, an absent brachial pulse, and massive swelling of the shoulder. Vascular injury occurs in 88% of patients and severe neurologic injuries occur in 94% of patients. Many of these patients have a poor outcome and present with a flail, flaccid extremity that usually results in early amputation and have an overall mortality of 10%. One of the most devastating aspects of scapulothoracic dissociation is the brachial plexus injuries that occur, which are typically proximal, involving the roots and cords—brachial plexus avulsions are not unusual. Attempts at repair of complete brachial plexus injuries with grafts or nerve transfers have generally been unsuccessful [51]. Treatment includes arterial and venous ligation to stop exsanguination if present, orthopedic stabilization and consideration for above elbow amputation electively, if brachial plexus avulsion is present, to allow for a more useful extremity. Overall prognosis for limb recovery is poor.

Traumatic Asphyxia

Traumatic asphyxia occurs as a result of a sudden or severe compression injury of the thorax or upper abdomen. It is most often associated with blunt trauma secondary to a crush injury. Entrapment of children under automatic garage doors is a prime example, as reported by Kriel et al. [52]. The true incidence of traumatic asphyxia is unknown, but it is considered to be a relatively rare event. The diagnosis is usually made based on the mechanism of injury and physical examination. Associated injuries are common and therefore should be investigated. The usual physical findings consist of facial edema, cyanosis, and petechial hemorrhages of the upper torso, neck, and face. The petechiae usually occur within the conjunctiva and oral mucosa and become most prominent a few hours after the initial injury. Neurologic findings are not rare and are thought to be secondary to anoxic injury, as well as possible cerebral edema and hemorrhage. The exact pathophysiology is thought to be due to a crushing injury applied to the mediastinum, which causes the heart to force blood out of the right atrium retrograde into the valveless innominate and jugular venous system. In addition, a sudden reflexive inspiration is thought to occur against a closed glottis, which may elevate the intrathoracic pressures to high levels. This results in a sudden and rapid increase in the pressure of the small veins of the face and neck, resulting in the typical petechial hemorrhages that are observed.

Treatment is generally supportive. Specific therapy for traumatic asphyxia is based on physiologic techniques to decrease intracranial pressure, including elevation of the head of the bed and oxygen therapy. The need to treat possible associated injuries may take priority. Commonly associated injuries include rib fractures, pulmonary contusions, extremity fractures, pneumothorax, hemothorax, flail chest, and blunt pelvic and intra-abdominal injuries (i.e., splenic and/or liver lacerations). The prognosis of patients with traumatic asphyxia is generally good, as long as the patient did not sustain prolonged apnea or hypoxia. The majority of fatalities are usually from associated injuries and their complications. When death does occur, it usually occurs in patients who have sustained a prolonged compression, causing massive irreversible neurologic insult from the resultant apnea and hypoxia.

Pleural Space

Pneumothorax

This section will only focus on pneumothoraces associated with trauma. For further general discussion of pneumothorax in the critically ill, readers are referred to Chapter 57. For in depth discussion of imaging studies on the topic of pneumothorax, readers are referred to Chapters 57 and 63. A traumatic pneumothorax occurs from either blunt or penetrating trauma, with resultant direct injury to the pleural barrier. Rib fractures may or may not be present. Mechanical ventilation can also be considered a traumatic cause of pneumothorax and has an overall associated incidence of 5%. This incidence increases dramatically in patients with underlying lung diseases, such as COPD and acute respiratory distress syndrome (ARDS). Iatrogenic causes of pneumothorax are also prevalent within the hospital setting. Central-line insertions are associated with a 3% to 6% incidence of pneumothorax.

All types of pneumothorax may progress to tension pneumothorax, which occurs in 1% to 3% of spontaneous pneumothoraces and can occur at any stage of treatment. As tension pneumothorax is a rapidly progressive condition, early identification is essential and immediate decompression should be performed when suspected on clinical grounds.

Tension pneumothorax is a clinical diagnosis, and treatment should never be delayed to obtain a confirmatory radiograph. Open pneumothorax is caused when a penetrating chest injury opens the pleural space to the atmosphere. Open pneumothorax may also occur with massive blunt trauma that literally rips open the chest. This leads to a collapsed lung and a "sucking" chest wound. Open pneumothorax is an injury commonly seen on the battlefield. In civilian life, impalement by objects is a common cause. In injuries where the chest wall wound diameter approaches two thirds of the diameter of the trachea, air will preferentially enter the pleural space through the wound during respiration, thereby inhibiting normal ventilation through the upper airway, leading to profound hypoventilation and subsequent hypoxia. Changes in venous return can occur similar to that seen in a tension pneumothorax, which in turn can lead to hemodynamic instability. The presence of a "sucking" chest wound makes the diagnosis obvious. External wound size may not correlate with the degree of compromise, as it is the size of the atmospheric-pleural connection that is most correlative.

Treatment includes appropriate resuscitative maneuvers, including securing the airway, adequate ventilation, and locating the wound and placing a sterile occlusive dressing over it to allow negative pressure ventilation to resume. If this does not suffice, intubation and positive pressure mechanical ventilation may be necessary. A standard method of coverage involves placing a nonporous dressing over the wound and taping it on three sides, allowing it to act as a one-way valve, allowing air to escape during expiration but occlusive during negative pressure inspiration. A chest tube is routinely sterilely inserted at a separate site away from the site of injury to treat any possible tension pneumothorax that may arise. The wound should be cared for locally and associated injuries should be sought and treated appropriately.

Hemothorax

After rib fractures, hemothorax is the second most common complication of chest trauma. It can be caused by bleeding from anywhere in the chest cavity, including the chest wall, lung parenchyma, major thoracic vessels, heart, or diaphragm. It presents in approximately 25% of patients with chest trauma. Patients with hemothorax typically have decreased breath sounds and dullness to percussion over the affected side with associated dyspnea and tachypnea. Depending on the amount of blood loss, they may be in hemodynamic shock. The major cause of significant hemothorax is usually due to a laceration to the lung or bleeding from an injured intercostal vessel or internal mammary artery. Radiographic films may not reveal a fluid collection of less than 300 mL. Small hemothoraces usually seal themselves within a few days. Accumulation of more than 1,500 mL of blood within a pleural space is considered massive, is more commonly seen on the left side, and is usually due to aortic rupture (blunt trauma) or pulmonary hilar or major vessel injury (penetrating trauma). Massive hemothorax can lead to hemodynamic instability including hypotension and circulatory collapse. Neck veins may be flat or distended, depending on whether or not blood loss or increased intrathoracic pressure predominates. A mediastinal shift with tracheal deviation is typically away from the side of blood accumulation.

Treatment of acute hemothorax includes supplemental oxygen therapy and, in most cases, the insertion of a large bore (i.e., 36 French) tube thoracostomy anterior to the midaxillary line at the fifth or sixth intercostal space. A moderate-size hemothorax (500 to 1,500 mL) that stops bleeding immediately after a tube thoracostomy can usually be managed conservatively with a closed drainage system. Bleeding from pulmonary parenchymal injuries that do not involve the hilum usually will stop on their own because of the low pulmonary pressures and high concentrations of tissue thromboplastin within the lung [53]. If, however, the patient continues to bleed at a rate of 100 to 200 mL per hour, then exploration is indicated. Likewise, if the patient bleeds out more than 1,500 mL initially through the chest tube, exploration is indicated. If the patient is hemodynamically unstable at any time, and intrathoracic bleeding is suspected as the cause, emergent thoracotomy should be done regardless of chest tube output. A chest radiograph should always be obtained after placing a tube thoracostomy to check position of the tube and to make sure that the pleural space is adequately drained. If a large amount of retained blood and clot remains within the pleural space despite tube thoracostomy, exploration with open evacuation should be considered. VATS is an option in the stable patient with retained hemothorax or in a stable patient that continues to bleed at a slow but steady rate; however, the surgeon should not hesitate to convert to open thoracotomy if visualization is inadequate or drainage and evacuation of the pleural space is incomplete. If the retained hemothorax is not massive, nonoperative therapy can be considered as these may lyse with time. Alternatively, it has been shown that a retained hemothorax can be successfully treated with instillation of thrombolytics into the pleural space. This has been deemed safe even in patients who have sustained multiple trauma [54].

Lung

Contusion

Pulmonary contusion is a common injury found in patients sustaining blunt chest trauma, with an approximate incidence of 30% to 75%. Mortality is between 10% and 25%. Hemorrhage and interstitial edema result from injury to the lung. This can lead to alveolar collapse and the typical parenchymal consolidation seen on radiograph. Injury to the parenchyma from blunt force trauma is thought to be caused by a combination of events that include alveolar stretching, parenchymal tearing, and concussive forces. Lung injury in the absence of identifiable rib fractures typically exhibits diffuse injury; whereas rib fractures and flail chest are associated with more localized injury. The extravasation of blood into the alveolar space causes subsequent consolidation which can then lead to an intrapulmonary shunt. A flail chest may be associated with pulmonary contusion in approximately three fourths of the time, which more than doubles the morbidity and mortality. Hypoxemia, although nonspecific, is the most common clinical finding associated with pulmonary contusion and should raise the suspicion of its diagnosis. Typical chest radiographic findings in the appropriate clinical setting remain the mainstay of diagnosis. Typical findings usually demonstrate a focal or diffuse consolidative process that does not typically follow anatomical segments or lobes. Rib fractures are the most common bony injuries seen and should raise suspicion for the diagnosis of pulmonary contusion, even if other clinical signs are absent at the time. Pulmonary contusion may not become radiographically apparent for up to 48 hours postinjury, with an average delay of 6 hours. On the other hand, CT scanning of the chest has been shown to be able to demonstrate the presence of pulmonary contusion almost immediately postinjury [55–58]. In addition, it can help estimate the total volume of injured lung present. This can be helpful in predicting the need for eventual ventilatory support. It has been shown that when pulmonary contusion involves 28% or more of the total lung volume, essentially all patients eventually require mechanical ventilation; whereas when 18% or less of the lung volume is involved, the need for mechanical ventilatory support is unlikely [59]. Treatment of pulmonary contusion is generally supportive. Close respiratory monitoring and frequent clinical examination is important, as approximately half of all respiratory failures secondary to pulmonary contusion occur usually within the first few hours postinjury. Once diagnosed and coexistent injuries are treated, and the need for emergent surgery is ruled out or performed as required, the patient should be transferred to a monitored bed. Good pulmonary toilet should be employed and may be achieved through several mechanisms, including nasotracheal suction, chest physiotherapy, and postural drainage. This helps to minimize atelectasis and expel bronchial secretions. If patients are still unable to clear their secretions adequately, bronchoscopy can be helpful. Adequate analgesia is also important in maintaining good pulmonary toilet. This can be achieved through nerve blocks, systemic opioids, or epidural anesthesia. Mechanical ventilation can minimize edema and increase functional residual capacity, which in turn can decrease shunting and reduce hypoxemia. Positioning patients with the injured lung in the nondependent position may also improve oxygenation, especially in those patients refractory to other measures. Fluid administration should be done judiciously, as hypervolemia may worsen fluid extravasation into the alveolar spaces and worsen parenchymal consolidation, especially since capillary permeability is already compromised. However, under-resuscitation should also be avoided, as this may lead to thickened secretions, possibly worsening cardiac output and shunt fraction. Obviously, fluid administration in these patients can be a difficult balancing act, and good clinical judgment is important. Positive end expiratory pressure (PEEP) should be maintained at the minimum value necessary to ensure adequate oxygenation, since excessive PEEP may actually worsen gas exchange and can actually extend the area of injury. Atelectasis can lead to infectious pneumonia, which typically begins to contribute more to the hypoxia after the initial couple of days postinjury. Pulmonary infections may develop in up to 50% of patients with pulmonary contusion. Furosemide, in addition to its diuretic affect, can be useful in the treatment of patients with pulmonary contusion. Acute respiratory distress syndrome (ARDS) can complicate pulmonary contusion in 5% to 20% of cases, and respiratory dysfunction is a common sequela that can be found in a majority of patients in the long term. Dyspnea may affect as many as 90% of patients during the first 6 months postinjury. In addition, functional reserve capacity has been found to be diminished as late as 4 years after injury, with the majority of patients demonstrating subtle changes on CT [60].

Tracheobronchial Injury/Lung Laceration

Tracheobronchial injury can be a challenge to diagnose, manage, and definitively treat. The true incidence of tracheobronchial injury is difficult to establish, as a large proportion (30% to 80%) of these patients will die before reaching the hospital. It is estimated on the basis of autopsy reports that 2.5% to 3.2% of patients who die as a result of trauma may have associated tracheobronchial injury [61,62]. More than 80% of tracheobronchial injury due to blunt trauma is located within 2.5 cm of the carina. Resuscitation of a patient with tracheobronchial injury can be difficult, since obtaining adequate ventilation may require novel approaches to secure the airway. Patients with tracheal or bronchial injuries make this initial assessment particularly challenging. The majority of patients with tracheobronchial injury seen in the emergency department have some degree of respiratory difficulty, and these patients may require emergent measures to secure and control the airway. Orotracheal intubation is the most common method used. Patients with cervical injuries and open neck wounds can be intubated through the open wound to secure the airway if necessary. The initial physical findings in patients with tracheobronchial injury can be subtle. However, several abnormalities can alert the physician to the diagnosis. Tachypnea and subcutaneous emphysema are common. Pneumothorax may or may not be seen on a plain radiograph. The liberal use of bronchoscopy is mandatory in identifying tracheobronchial injuries and constitutes the gold standard in diagnosis. Findings that can typically be seen on bronchoscopy include obstruction of the airway with blood and inability to visualize the more distal lobar bronchi because of collapsed proximal bronchi. Visualization of a bronchial tear is confirmatory. Associated injuries are common and are usually related to the mechanism and location of the tracheobronchial injury. The most commonly associated injury related to penetrating tracheobronchial injury is esophageal perforation. Most repairs of cervical tracheal injuries are approached through a collar incision. In patients with injuries high in the mediastinal trachea or with suspected great-vessel injury, a median sternotomy may be necessary. When the injury is associated with a unilateral pneumothorax or a bronchial injury is diagnosed preoperatively, an ipsilateral posterolateral thoracotomy is the incision of choice. For injuries to the mediastinal trachea, an approach by a right posterolateral thoracotomy (usually high through the fourth intercostal space) is reasonable. Since the initial report by Shaw and colleagues, primary repair of the injured tracheobronchial tree has been encouraged [61,63–67]. Most patients can undergo primary repair of their tracheobronchial injury using tailored surgical techniques specific to the injury. When a major bronchus is disrupted, lobectomy is the preferred method of treatment, with closure of the bronchial stump debrided back to healthy tissue. With injuries to the mainstem bronchi, primary repair is preferred over pneumonectomy whenever possible, due to the higher mortality associated with pneumonectomy, especially in the trauma setting. Injury to the trachea can be either primarily repaired or converted to a tracheostomy if necessary for airway control. Nonoperative management of tracheobronchial injury has been reported to be successful in selected cases. Those patients that seem most appropriate for this approach are those with membranous injuries. Patients that have cartilaginous injuries are more likely to require operative repair. Tracheobronchial injury encompasses a heterogeneous group of injuries that requires skillful airway management, careful diagnostic evaluation, and operative repairs that are often creative and necessarily unique to the given injury.

Heart

Cardiac Contusion/Blunt Cardiac Rupture

Most blunt cardiac injuries are not serious. However, moderately severe cardiac injuries may cause arrhythmias or result in low-output cardiac failure. The clinical significance of myocardial contusion following blunt thoracic trauma is still largely unknown. In one study by Lindstaedt et al., approximately 20% of patients who were admitted to a surgical intensive care unit because of their injuries met the criteria for diagnosis of myocardial contusion [68]. Their criteria include exclusion of pathologic findings on ECG known to be present prior to injury; echocardiographic evidence of akinetic wall motion abnormalities; combination of regional wall motion abnormality, significant isoenzyme elevation (CK-MB >7%), and ECG abnormality; regional wall motion abnormality in the baseline echocardiogram and in the control echocardiogram at follow-up; or confirmation of myocardial contusion at autopsy or intraoperatively. Even though the prevalence of the injury was significant in their population, the overall prognosis was excellent, and the authors recommend that specific diagnostic and therapeutic measures should be limited to cases where cardiac complications develop. The combination of a normal ECG and normal serum troponin levels, drawn at the time of presentation and 8 hours later, essentially rule out significant myocardial contusion and is sufficient, in the absence of other reasons for hospitalization, to discharge such patients safely home. However, patients with an abnormal ECG and elevated troponin should be monitored for at least 24 hours. Cardiac contusion may lead to cardiogenic shock resistant to inotropic support. The use of intra-aortic balloon counterpulsation as a mechanical means of augmenting cardiac function following cardiac contusion has been reported with success even in elderly patients [69]. Severe injuries to the heart can result in cardiac rupture. Atrial and/or ventricular rupture can occur, leading to profound hemodynamic compromise. Rapid recognition of such injuries is necessary for successful treatment. Associated injuries are common and include closed head injury, pulmonary contusion and/or laceration, multiple rib fractures, liver and spleen injury, and traumatic aortic injury; these account for approximately 25% of fatalities seen in patients with blunt cardiac injury. The usual clinical presentation of cardiac rupture is cardiac tamponade secondary to hemopericardium, although less than 15% of these patients actually manifest physiological evidence of tamponade. Associated pericardial tears may allow for decompression of intrapericardial hemorrhage through the pleural space, preventing the development of cardiac tamponade but leading to hemothorax. Pericardial rupture is rare, but can occur in isolation or with associated injuries such as blunt cardiac or diaphragmatic rupture, which has a high mortality. Hypotension is usually present, and the diagnosis of cardiac rupture should be considered in any patient who has hypotension in the absence of overt blood loss. The chest radiograph may not show evidence of cardiac injury, even in the face of tamponade and hemodynamic compromise, since a rapid accumulation of blood into the pericardial space can occur without significantly altering the cardiac silhouette. Echocardiography can be useful in diagnosing pericardial tamponade. Diagnosis of blunt cardiac rupture should be strongly suspected when hemopericardium is seen by ultrasound in the setting of blunt trauma. The diagnostic dependability of pericardiocentesis is limited in the assessment of traumatic hemopericardium and potential cardiac rupture because of significant false negative and false positive results. Performing a pericardial window in the operating room, however, can be both diagnostic and therapeutic, and it can confirm hemopericardium and allow for rapid decompression and median sternotomy. Nevertheless, the diagnosis of blunt cardiac rupture requires a fair degree of clinical suspicion, particularly in the setting of hypotension that does not respond to adequate volume resuscitation. Perchinsky et al. reviewed a consecutive series of 27 patients seen between 1984 and 1993 with blunt cardiac rupture. Overall survival rate was 41%. Of note was that three out of nine (33%) patients presenting to the emergency department with no identifiable blood pressure or viable electrical heart rhythm survived resuscitation, surgery, and initial hospital care. No patient survived rupture of two or more cardiac chambers in their series, however [70]. Although cardiac exploration should be performed with cardiopulmonary bypass support nearby, repair of cardiac rupture does not necessarily require its use.

Cardiac Valvular Injuries

Blunt cardiac injury may result in valvular insufficiency. The right ventricle is immediately behind the sternum, which makes it particularly vulnerable to injury. Acute severe elevation of right intraventricular pressures has been shown to result in injury of the tricuspid valvular apparatus [71]. The most common injury is chordal rupture, followed by rupture of the anterior papillary muscle and leaflet tears. Posttraumatic aortic valve regurgitation has also been reported and affects all ages and is often found in association with sternal or multiple rib fractures [72]. Traumatic mitral valve insufficiency has been shown to present with either complete papillary muscle avulsion from its ventricular attachment or with chordal tears and/or leaflet damage. Those with papillary muscle avulsion typically present with severe regurgitation. Those patients with less severe injuries to the mitral valve, such as chordal tears and/or leaflet damage, usually present with less severe symptoms and may even be asymptomatic. Not only can blunt cardiac injury cause acute valvular incompetence, but it can also predispose patients to delayed valvular dysfunction. In a study performed by Ismailov et al. looking at hospital patient discharges, patients who sustained blunt cardiac injury had an associated 12-fold increased risk for developing tricuspid valve insufficiency and a 3.4-fold increased risk of developing aortic valvular insufficiency later in life, which appeared to be independent of age, race, sex, and injury severity score [73]. There was no correlation found with increased risk for mitral valve insufficiency, however. Traumatic valve insufficiency, depending on severity and valve involved, may necessitate surgical treatment.

Penetrating Cardiac Injury

The clinical presentation of penetrating cardiac injury ranges from one of hemodynamic stability to complete cardiopulmonary arrest. Beck's Triad represents the classical presentation of the patient arriving in the emergency department in pericardial tamponade and includes venous hypertension, arterial hypotension, and muffled heart sounds. Kussmaul's sign, jugular venous distention seen with expiration, is another classic sign attributed to pericardial tamponade. The physiology of pericardial tamponade is related to the relative inelastic and noncompliant pericardium. Sudden acute loss of intracardiac blood volume into the pericardial sac leads to an acute pressure rise and compression of the thin-walled right ventricle and atria. This decreases the heart's ability to fill, resulting in decreased left ventricular filling and ejection fraction, thus decreasing cardiac output. Subxiphoid pericardial window remains the gold standard for the diagnosis of cardiac injury. It can also be therapeutic and can be done under local anesthesia in the operating room to allow release of tamponade prior to the induction of general anesthesia. If blood is found, then the surgeon can proceed immediately to median sternotomy and cardiorrhaphy. In relatively stable patients who do not require emergency room thoracotomy, median sternotomy is the incision of choice to repair penetrating cardiac wounds [74,75]. TTE has clearly emerged as the technique of choice for the diagnosis of penetrating cardiac injuries. Jimenez et al. showed that TTE had 90% accuracy, 97% specificity, and 90% sensitivity in detecting penetrating cardiac injuries [29]. The usefulness of echocardiography may be in its ability to identify obvious hemopericardium, thereby allowing the trauma surgeon to proceed directly to median sternotomy and thus eliminating the need for a subxiphoid pericardial window in many cases. Indications to perform EDT include loss of vital signs with suspected pericardial tamponade, especially in the case of suspected penetrating trauma to the heart. An anterolateral thoracotomy is typically performed in between chest compressions and should be extended through all of the subcutaneous tissues, as well as the anterior chest wall muscles, until the intercostal space is identified. Typically, the patient's vital signs quickly return to acceptable levels. Internal defibrillation may be necessary, as the heart is often found to be in ventricular fibrillation. Epinephrine and similar drugs should specifically be avoided, as release of the tamponade is usually more than sufficient to allow the patient's vital signs to return. Epinephrine can increase chronotropy, inotropy, and intraventricular pressures, which can potentially extend ventricular injuries and make repair difficult and unnecessarily challenging. If sinus rhythm cannot be restored despite all attempts, the prognosis is grave and the outcome is invariably poor. Once vital signs are reestablished, attention can then be given to repairing the cardiac injury. Definitive cardiac repair does not necessarily have to be done immediately, however, and in some cases may be ill-advised when performing an emergency room thoracotomy, since it is the tamponade and not the blood loss per se that causes hemodynamic collapse. Once the tamponade is released, digital pressure can be directly applied to the cardiac wound which is often all that is needed once vital signs are restored to maintain relative hemostasis until definitive repair can be done in an operating room. In the authors' opinion, the use of adjunct measures, such as balloon tamponade with a Foley catheter, can be fraught with creating more injuries or extending existing myocardial lacerations and should be avoided if possible. Vascular clamps can be placed on bleeding right atrial wounds but usually are not necessary and may cause more harm than not, extending small injuries into larger ones. In addition, cross-clamping of the thoracic aorta is generally not necessary and ill-advised with isolated penetrating cardiac wounds. If necessary, it can be temporarily occluded digitally against the bodies of the thoracic vertebrae until adequate resuscitation has taken place. An attempt should be made to trace the trajectory of the wounding agent, as missiles often enter into one thorax and then enter the contralateral hemithorax. Once the tamponade has been released, and the patient has regained a rhythm and a blood pressure and the bleeding sites are identified and digitally controlled, the experienced surgeon can then attempt closure of the cardiac wound in an appropriate equipped operating room. Total inflow occlusion of the heart can be done if the blood loss is substantial through the wound and proper placement of sutures difficult in the face of on-going blood loss without the aid of cardiopulmonary bypass. This maneuver is performed by placing caval tapes around both the superior and inferior vena cavae within the pericardium, which, when tethered, results in immediate emptying of the heart. The tolerance of the injured heart to this maneuver is limited, however, and should be used only for short periods if found to be necessary. This procedure can result in cardiopulmonary arrest and ventricular fibrillation, and appropriate plans should be made prior to caval occlusion should this happen. Atrial injuries can be repaired with running 2-0 Prolene. Ventricular wounds may be repaired while digitally occluding the laceration while placing a horizontal mattress stitch with a pledget surrounding the wound, usually with 2-0 Prolene. Repairing cardiac injuries resulting from gunshot wounds can be more challenging when compared with stab wounds, since they tend to have associated blast defects, which can make repair difficult. The repair of ventricular wounds adjacent to or involving coronary arteries can be challenging. If the coronary artery is injured itself but is quite distal (e.g., distal 1/3 of the left anterior descending artery), simple ligation can be done without serious consequences. However, if the injury is more proximal than this, ligation of the injury with distal bypass using a segment of saphenous vein or mammary artery is recommended. This can be done on or off cardiopulmonary bypass but usually requires the expertise of an experienced cardiac surgeon to perform. If the injury does not involve the coronary artery but is in close proximity, suturing of the injury may require placement of a horizontal U-stitch underneath the bed of the coronary artery, thereby closing the injury without compromising coronary blood flow. Patients who have sustained injury to their coronary artery that has already sustained irreversible myocardial damage may require intra-aortic balloon counterpulsation as part of their resuscitation.

Esophagus

Iatrogenic injuries to the esophagus are the most common, particularly those of iatrogenic esophageal perforation. Traumatic injury and Boerhaave's syndrome account for most of the rest.

Flexible endoscopy is associated with an extremely low risk of perforation. However, when flexible endoscopy is paired with a therapeutic intervention, such as dilatation or stent placement, the risk of perforation dramatically increases. As a result, most patients with iatrogenic perforation occur in patients undergoing therapeutic maneuvers in response to treating an underlying esophageal problem. Almost any form of esophageal instrumentation can cause perforation. Examples include nasogastric tube placement and performance of TEE. Common sites for perforation of the esophagus occur at areas of narrowing, such as in the pyriform fossa, at the aortic arch, near the carina, or at the lower esophageal junction. Perforation of an existing diverticulum can also occur, but this occurs rarely and is usually associated with blind passage of an endoscope when no antecedent barium swallow was obtained. The esophagus may also perforate at the site of a malignant stricture during forceful dilation or, more commonly, in the area of the esophagus just proximal to the stricture. Pneumatic dilatation for achalasia carries an increased risk compared with routine esophageal dilatation, since this requires an uncontrolled tear of the lower esophageal sphincter to affect a myotomy. The risk of perforation with pneumatic balloon dilatation of the lower esophageal sphincter for achalasia ranges from 2% to 6%. Risk of perforation when performing esophageal dilation increases when dealing with long strictures or ones with poor blood supply, such as with radiation-induced strictures. Caustic strictures are usually transmural associated with extensive esophageal wall fibrosis and usually require repeated dilations, thereby multiplying the risk of perforation over time. Stent placement for the palliation of esophageal cancer is associated with a perforation rate of 7% to 15%. The incidence of perforation following sclerotherapy for esophageal varices is approximately 1% to 3% and typically occurs several days after the procedure, presumably due to tissue necrosis.

Patients who present with esophageal perforation usually complain of pain. Findings may include fever and subcutaneous or mediastinal air. Crepitus in the neck is relatively common following perforations of the cervical esophagus and can be detected on physical exam in approximately 60% of patients. Pleural effusions are present in more than 50% of patients with perforations of their thoracic esophagus. Radiologic studies are important in diagnosing patients with esophageal perforation. A plain chest radiograph may show subcutaneous emphysema, pneumomediastinum, pleural effusion, mediastinal air–fluid levels, or pneumothorax. Radiographic abnormalities can be found in as many as 90% of patients on plain film. Contrast studies are performed to confirm the diagnosis of perforation and to define the exact site. Water-soluble contrast agents such as Gastrografin have been the preferred agents of choice, at least initially. However, Gastrografin can cause severe pneumonitis if aspirated into the lungs, and its use may not demonstrate small leaks. Because of this, it is the authors' preference to use thin barium, because it is more inert and is better at detecting smaller leaks. CT scanning can be particularly helpful in showing mediastinal findings when the perforation has already sealed.

The optimal management of esophageal perforation is patient-specific and should take into account the clinical setting. This includes consideration of the patient's underlying disease process, the degree of sepsis, if any, the location of the perforation, and whether or not the perforation is contained. A nonoperative approach may be considered in patients with minimal symptoms and physical findings who do not appear septic and have a small, contained leak. Nonoperative management should include the use of broad-spectrum intravenous antibiotics and nothing to eat or drink by mouth (NPO). A nasogastric tube should be specifically avoided. There is no clear consensus as to generally how long a patient with a contained leak should be left NPO or how long intravenous antibiotics should be continued. However, clear liquids can usually be safely started within a few days and the diet advanced cautiously, especially when no further extravasation is seen on repeat contrast study.

Surgery should be performed if the patient appears septic, the leak freely communicates with either the peritoneal or thoracic cavities, or there is an associated mediastinal abscess. Primary repair can be done regardless of the timing of the injury, as long as the tissues appear healthy at the time of surgery. Drainage alone can be done for cervical perforations, especially if the perforation cannot be found at the time of operation, which is not infrequent. Primary repair with drainage is the preferred method when possible; however, if the esophageal tissues do not appear viable to hold sutures, then esophagectomy with proximal diversion may be necessary. It is important when primarily repairing the esophagus that the mucosal edges are defined, as the injury seen in the muscle layer is often only the "tip of the iceberg," and closure of the entire mucosal defect is necessary if adequate healing is to occur. As a general rule, esophageal reconstruction should not be done at the time of esophageal resection if the patient is septic, as it can usually be done at a later date once the patient heals and is beyond the acute event. In these cases, it is better to create an end cervical esophagostomy and oversew the gastric stump with the placement of enteral feeding catheters. If a cancer is perforated during instrumentation, then resection over primary repair is the preferred surgery of choice. Obviously, if the patient has widespread metastatic disease, then good clinical judgment needs to be used in deciding whether an operation should be done at all. Management of a perforation following achalasia dilatation should consist of primary closure of the perforation in addition to performing a surgical myotomy 180 degrees away from the site of perforation. An antireflux procedure consisting of a partial wrap to cover the area of repair can also be done to buttress the repair. This type of surgery is most commonly approached through the chest.

Spontaneous perforation of the esophagus usually can be related to forceful vomiting and retching. Boerhaave's syndrome has been reported following a variety of activities including straining, weightlifting, coughing, and emesis. The clinical features of Boerhaave's syndrome are similar to that of iatrogenic perforation, in that pain is the most common presenting symptom. Many patients with Boerhaave's syndrome do not have the classic antecedent history of forceful vomiting. The vast majority of these patients develop perforations in the distal esophagus on the left side, and the workup and treatment of patients with Boerhaave's syndrome is similar to those with iatrogenic perforations. Operation is usually indicated.

A Mallory-Weiss tear is a mucosal laceration, usually near the gastroesophageal junction, caused by forceful vomiting, and a hiatal hernia is found in more than 75% of patients. Most tears occur within 2 cm of the gastroesophageal junction on the lesser curvature of the stomach. Majority of the patients present with gastrointestinal bleeding. The classic presentation in up to 80% of patients is that of forceful emesis followed by hematemesis. Massive bleeding occurs in 10% of patients. Upper endoscopy usually confirms the diagnosis. The management of Mallory-Weiss tears is generally supportive, since the bleeding is usually self-limited. Occasionally gastric embolization may be necessary; surgical over-sewing of the tear is rarely necessary.

Esophageal injuries due to penetrating trauma are rare, with most series averaging only a handful [76–78]. They result most commonly from transmediastinal gunshot wounds. Asensio et al. reported their experience consisting of 43 penetrating esophageal injuries managed over a period of 6 years. Overall, 28 of their 32 survivors (88%) were managed by primary repair alone [79]. The overall mortality for their series was 26%. The authors also reported that these mortality figures were consistent with others reported in the literature, which have remained high and relatively stable approximately for the last 20 years, thus attesting to the critical nature of these injuries. Only Symbas et al. (48 cases) and Defore et al. (77 cases) have reported larger experiences but over much longer spans of time–15 and 22 years, respectively [76,77]. Penetrating esophageal injuries are not easily detected and require a high index of suspicion. Delay in diagnosis is associated with higher mortality. However, mortality can exceed 20% even for patients who are promptly diagnosed. Esophagoduodenoscopy (EGD) is a sensitive and safe diagnostic test for the detection of esophageal injury. A study by Flowers et al. showed that EGD had a sensitivity of 100%, a specificity of 96%, and an accuracy of 97% in detecting penetrating esophageal injuries [80]. There was no morbidity related to the examination, and, most importantly, no esophageal injuries were missed. The authors commented that the most significant potential weakness of flexible EGD for esophageal trauma is that it actually may be too sensitive. EGD is most helpful in excluding esophageal injury in patients who require a surgical procedure for another injury. When found, prompt primary repair is the treatment of choice.

Caustic Injuries of the Esophagus

Caustic injuries of the esophagus can be very challenging to manage. They are most frequently due to suicide attempts in adults and accidental ingestion in children. The degree of injury to the esophagus is directly proportional to the amount of caustic substance ingested. Lye causes transmural liquefaction necrosis of the esophagus and therefore is most injurious. Diagnosis is usually from history, although patients attempting suicide may present with no history at all or, even worse, an inaccurate one. Examination of the buccal mucosa, mouth, tongue, and gums can often show chemical burns and suggest the diagnosis. Endoscopy should be performed to document the proximal extent of the injury only; there is no need to pass the endoscope further, since it may actually be harmful and potentially lead to perforation. Passage of an NGT is controversial, although it may actually help to "stent" the esophagus open and be associated with lower rates of stricture formation. Arterial blood gases should be obtained with particular attention paid to the base deficit, as this can be a marker for severity of injury. Signs and symptoms of perforation and sepsis should be carefully monitored. The patient should be made NPO, and broad spectrum intravenous antibiotics should be given. Steroids are controversial but have been associated with lower rates of stricture formation in some series [81,82]. Intravenous fluids should be given and consideration given to performing esophagectomy, if signs of perforation and mediastinal sepsis are present. Intra-abdominal perforations can also occur, as well as injury to surrounding structures (e.g., spleen, colon). If esophageal resection becomes clinically indicated due to sepsis, immediate reconstruction is ill-advised. Esophagectomy can be performed either transhiatally or transthoracically, with creation of an end cervical esophagostomy. Intra-abdominal feeding tubes should be placed for enteral access. Delayed reconstruction can then be performed electively once the sepsis clears and the patient heals, usually several months later. Late stricture formation is common and can be difficult to manage. In addition, the pharyngeal phase of swallowing can be affected, leading to debilitating problems with speech and swallowing. It is not uncommon to require serial dilations or even late esophagectomy if stricture formation develops. It typically involves long segments of the esophagus and is panmural in depth, often making dilation impossible or at best marginally effective. Overall prognosis is variable depending on the degree of injury.

Thoracic Aortic Injury

Traumatic disruption of the thoracic aorta immediately leads to death in majority of the patients. These horizontal acceleration/deceleration injuries usually result from a disruption of the integrity of the aortic wall just distal to the ligamentum arteriosum. Patients fortunate enough to survive initial injury usually do so because the aortic adventitial tissues are able to tamponade the tear, thereby preventing fatal intrathoracic exsanguination. The risk of rupture is dependent on multiple factors, including the ability of the adventitial tissues to contain the leak, the patient's systemic blood pressure, and the size of the contained pseudoaneurysm.

The entire surgical treatment section is confusing and needs to be rewritten. It jumps back and forth to operate and then not operate. It can be summarized and your opinion then given.

While emergent operative repair of thoracic aortic tears had become the standard of care, after 1997 there has been emerging evidence that not all thoracic aortic tears should be treated equally. In addition, associated injuries such as pulmonary contusions, intracranial hemorrhage, and/or intra-abdominal hemorrhage (which are common in these patients) may take precedence over the aortic injury. In these cases, the aortic injury can be acutely managed medically and definitive treatment delayed, so long as certain criteria are met. With careful medical management (strict blood pressure control, minimization of dP/dT), it has been shown that many thoracic aortic injuries can undergo delayed repair, perhaps resulting in superior outcomes when compared with those patients undergoing emergent repair [83,84]. A recent prospective, observational study sponsored by the American Association for the Surgery of Trauma (AAST) looked at the subgroup of patients that underwent immediate repair versus those that underwent delayed repair [85]. Those patients that underwent delayed repair of stable thoracic aortic injury actually had improved survival regardless of the presence of major associated injuries, although their length of ICU stay was longer. It should be noted that patients with no major associated injuries who underwent delayed repair had a significantly higher complication rate when compared to those patients undergoing immediate repair. Although there has not been a randomized, controlled trial of early versus delayed repair, these results probably reflect selection bias. However, selection bias, which reflects the "art" of clinical treatment planning, should not be underscored when making decisions regarding these often multiply injured patients. In addition, successful nonoperative therapy of descending thoracic aortic injury has been reported [86]. Justification for nonoperative therapy includes favorable anatomy of the injury (contained, small injury, hemodynamic stability) as well as the presence of coexisting injuries, which would render the operative risk prohibitively high. These include patients with spinal cord injury that might make lateral decubitus positioning dangerous; patients with pulmonary contusions that may make single lung ventilation difficult; and patients with closed head injury, solid abdominal organ injury, or major fractures in which systemic heparinization would be ill-advised. One accepted method of operative repair is the "clamp-and-sew" technique, in which the proximal and distal aorta are simply clamped, thereby isolating the injury so that either primary repair or interposition grafting can be performed. Operative mortality is generally reported to be 10% to 20% in most series, with major morbidity including renal failure and paraplegia, which appears to increase with prolonged (i.e., >30 minutes) clamp times [87]. Another accepted method of operative repair utilizes bypass of the injured segment during repair, either with partial left heart bypass or with proximal to distal aortic shunt placement (i.e., Gott shunt). Partial left heart bypass (with cannulae in the left atrium and distal aorta) allows controlled off-loading of the left heart in addition to maintaining distal aortic perfusion, especially to the kidneys, that may decrease (but not negate) the incidence of paraplegia, especially when prolonged clamp times are anticipated. Since there has not been a randomized controlled trial comparing the two techniques, and there is no conclusive evidence that one technique is superior over the other in terms of outcome, both methods are acceptable, and their performance is usually based on surgeon preference. The need for operative repair, however, which was once considered the gold standard, is now coming into question. There have been many reports showing that endovascular stent grafting of selected patients may actually be superior to that of "mandatory" operative repair. A prospective, multicenter study sponsored by the AAST was recently published that clearly shows the early efficacy and safety of endovascular stent grafting in selected patients with traumatic thoracic aortic injuries [88]. The patients who underwent stent grafting had a significantly lower mortality (adjusted odds ratio: 8.42; 95% CI: [2.76 to 25.69]; adjusted p value <0.001) and fewer blood transfusions (adjusted mean difference: 4.98; 95% CI [0.14 to 9.82]; adjusted p value <0.046) compared to those patients that underwent operative repair. In addition, among the patients with major extrathoracic injuries, a significantly higher mortality and pneumonia rate were found in the operative group (adjusted p values 0.04 and 0.03, respectively). The major drawback seen in patients undergoing stent grafting were device-related complications, which developed in 20% of the patients. Their conclusion was that stent grafting of thoracic aortic injuries is now more commonly chosen by surgeons as the preferred method of repair and is associated with significantly lower mortality but that there is a considerable risk of serious device-related complications.

CARDIOPULMONARY CRITICAL CARE

Overview

It is not uncommon for severely injured patients to require cardiac and/or pulmonary support. This may be independent of whether or not they have sustained direct thoracic trauma. Pharmacologic drug therapy may be required to sustain adequate cardiac output and maintain necessary end-organ perfusion. In severe cases, cardiac failure may require mechanical support in the form of intra-aortic balloon pump counterpulsation. Respiratory support may be provided simply with supplemental oxygen administration; however, intubation and mechanical ventilation may be required. Unique ventilatory strategies such as high frequency oscillatory ventilation are sometimes required. In extreme cases, extracorporeal membrane oxygenation (ECMO) can be used and is potentially lifesaving in a certain subset of selected patients. Due to both the severity of injury as well as the need for ventilatory support, it is not unusual for these patients to develop acute lung injury as well as ventilator-associated pneumonia.

Pharmacologic Drug Therapy

Pharmacologic agents are usually used early in the treatment of cardiogenic shock. For an in depth discussion of this topic, readers are referred to Chapter 58–60. Perfusion of vital organs is dependent on adequate oxygen and nutrient delivery to the tissues. This delivery is dependent on an adequate blood pressure (perfusion pressure), cardiac output, and intravascular volume including hemoglobin. If cardiac output and perfusion is maintained and yet there is not adequate oxygen-carrying capacity (i.e., hemoglobin), oxygen delivery to the tissues will be limited. There continues to be controversy and debate regarding what is considered to be an adequate hemoglobin level. However, many centers now use a hemoglobin level of <7 g per dL as a transfusion trigger for patients without evidence of ischemic cardiac disease, signs and symptoms of impaired tissue perfusion, shock, or ongoing blood loss [89].

In addition, intravascular volume status, especially in chronically ill patients, is sometimes confusing. In fact, only half of ICU patients with hemodynamic instability will actually respond to fluid loading with a significant increase in their cardiac output [90]. This is because it is sometimes difficult to assess clinically exactly where the patient's heart is working on the Frank-Starling curve. If it is on the initial rise of the curve, the stroke volume is highly and directly dependent on the preload, and administering fluid will result in an increase in stroke volume. In contrast, however, if the heart is working on the top, more flat (and possibly even declining) portion of the Frank-Starling curve, fluid administration will not increase stroke volume and may actually worsen heart failure and pulmonary edema and, therefore, oxygen delivery to the tissues. Passive leg raise, which auto-transfuses volume to the patient, may be a reliable and simple predictor of responsiveness to volume administration. Measurements of cardiac output and responsiveness to fluid challenges can be obtained through the use of traditional, invasive pulmonary arterial catheter monitoring or, more recently, through less invasive means, such as esophageal Doppler monitoring, pulse contour analysis, indicator dilution, thoracic bioimpedance, and partial nonrebreathing systems.

Intra-Aortic Balloon Pump

When pharmacologic treatment is inadequate and cardiogenic shock becomes refractory due to pump failure, mechanical devices may be indicated. One such device is the intra-aortic balloon pump (IABP). For an in depth discussion of this topic, readers are referred to Chapter 45.

Metabolic support of the critically ill patient is important. For an in depth discussion of this topic, readers are referred to Chapter 190.

Mechanical Ventilation

For a complete discussion of mechanical ventilatory support, readers are referred to Chapter xx.

EXTRACORPOREAL MEMBRANE OXYGENATION

In patients who fail standard ventilatory strategies, rescue modalities such as ECMO may be a life-saving alternative. ECMO provides oxygenation of blood outside of the body (hence its extracorporeal nature) by membrane oxygenators similar to those used in cardiopulmonary bypass circuits. It requires placement of catheters within the vascular tree that allows deoxygenated blood to be drained and delivered to the membrane oxygenators; it then allows oxygenated blood to be delivered back to the patient. A certain degree of heparinization is usually required to prevent clotting of both the bypass circuits as well as the oxygenators. Typically, a catheter is strategically placed to drain the venous system to maximize the increase in O_2 content that can be achieved, which provides inflow into the oxygenators, which then oxygenate the blood and sweep off the excess carbon dioxide. The blood is then transfused back into the arterial system (venoarterial ECMO) or venous system (venovenous ECMO) depending on the setup. Given the low pressure characteristics of the venous system as well as its overall easier accessibility, venovenous ECMO is becoming increasingly more common. In addition, with the advent of newer catheters, a single catheter can now be used for both inflow and outflow which can be placed into the jugular vein and positioned such that deoxygenated blood drains from the superior and inferior vena cava (outflow) to the oxygenator, which is then returned directly to the right atrium (inflow). There is generally some mixing of the oxygenated and deoxygenated blood, but this type of system obviates the needs to access the arterial system and is still quite effective at oxygenating blood.

Several recent articles have suggested the usefulness of ECMO in the surgical intensive care unit, but its exact role is yet to be determined [91–93].

Respiratory Complications

As a result of either primary lung contusion or from the treatment necessary to treat generalized traumatic injury (e.g., massive transfusions, mechanical ventilation, etc.), the lungs are susceptible to acute injury. Complications which can develop include transfusion related lung injury (TRALI), ventilator associated pneumonia (VAP), or ARDS. For an in depth discussion of these three complications, readers are referred to Chapters 47, 68, and 114.

SUMMARY

In summary, most thoracic trauma can be managed without surgery or, at most, with minimally invasive interventions. Multiply injured patients with thoracic injuries need to be comprehensively evaluated and their injuries prioritized and as a result, their successful care often requires a multidisciplinary approach. The treatment of thoracic injuries is evolving and requires a working knowledge of a number of both diagnostic and therapeutic modalities. As with almost all other traumatic injuries, the key to optimal treatment and outcome is dependent upon having a high index of suspicion for the injury and to identify it early. The ability to competently manage all aspects of a critically injured patient is also important in effecting a successful overall outcome.

References

1. Kulshrestha P, Munshi I, Wait R: Profile of chest trauma in a level I trauma center. *J Trauma* 57(3):576–581, 2004.
2. Demetriades D, Murray J, Charalambides K, et al: Trauma fatalities time and location of hospital deaths. *J Am Coll Surg* 198(1):20–26, 2004.
3. Karmy-Jones R, Jurkovich GJ, Shatz DV, et al: Management of traumatic lung injury: a Western Trauma Association multicenter review. *J Trauma* 51(6):1049–1053, 2001.
4. Martin SK, Shatney CH, Sherck JP, et al: Blunt trauma patients with prehospital pulseless electrical activity (PEA): poor ending assured. *J Trauma* 53(5):876–881, 2002.
5. Wisbach GG, Sise MJ, Sack DI, Swanson SM et al: What is the role of chest x-ray in the initial assessment of stable trauma patients? *J Trauma* 62(1): 74–79, 2007.
6. Deunk J, Dekker HM, Brink M, et al: The value of indicated computed tomography scan of the chest and abdomen in addition to the conventional radiologic work-up for blunt trauma patients. *J Trauma* 63(4):757–763, 2007.
7. Mirvis SE, Shanmuganathan K, Buell J, et al: Use of spiral computed tomography for the assessment of blunt trauma patients with potential aortic injury. *J Trauma* 45(5):922–930, 1998.
8. Wicky S, Wintermark M, Schnyder P, et al: Imaging of blunt chest trauma. *Eur Radiol* 10:1524–1538, 2000.
9. Patel NH, Stephens KE Jr, Mirvis SE, et al: Imaging of acute thoracic aortic injury due to blunt trauma: a review. *Radiology* 209:335–348, 1998.
10. Gavant ML: Helical CT grading of traumatic aortic injuries: impact on clinical guidelines for medical and surgical management. *Radiol Clin North Am* 37:553–574, 1999.
11. Ekeh AP, Peterson W, Woods RJ, et al: Is chest X-Ray an adequate screening tool for the diagnosis of blunt thoracic aortic injury? *J Trauma* 65(5):1088–1092, 2008.
12. Chen MY, Miller PR, McLaughlin CA, et al: The trend of using computed tomography in the detection of acute thoracic aortic and branch vessel injury after blunt thoracic trauma: single-center experience over 13 years. *J Trauma* 56(4):783–785, 2004.
13. Wong H, Gotway MB, Sasson AD, et al: Periaortic hematoma at diaphragmatic crura at helical CT: sign of blunt aortic injury in patients with mediastinal hematoma. *Radiology* 231(13):185–189, 2004.
14. Kehdy F, Richardson JD: The utility of 3-D CT scan in the diagnosis and evaluation of sternal fractures. *J Trauma* 60(3):635–636, 2006.
15. Stein DM, Gregory B, York GB, et al: Accuracy of computed tomography (CT) scan in the detection of penetrating diaphragm injury. *J Trauma* 63(3):538–543, 2007.
16. Plurad D, Green D, Demetriades D, et al: The Increasing use of chest computed tomography for trauma: is it being overutilized? *J Trauma* 62(3):631–635, 2007.
17. Goarin JP, Catoire P, Jacquens Y, et al: Use of transesophageal echocardiography for diagnosis of traumatic aortic injury. *Chest* 112:71–80, 1997.
18. Nienaber C, Spielmann R, Kodolitsch Y, et al: Diagnosis of thoracic aortic dissection magnetic resonance imaging versus transesophageal echocardiography. *Circulation* 85:434, 1992.
19. Brooks SW, Young JC, Cmolik B, et al: The use of transesophageal echocardiography in the evaluation of chest trauma. *J Trauma* 32:761, 1992.
20. Goarin JP, Le Bret F, Riou B, et al: Early diagnosis of traumatic thoracic aortic rupture by transesophageal echocardiography. *Chest* 103:618, 1993.
21. Wolfenden H, Newman DC: Transesophageal echocardiography: an increasing role in the diagnosis of traumatic aortic rupture. *J Thorac Cardiovasc Surg* 106:757, 1993.
22. Yoon D, Hoftman N, Ren W, et al: Intraoperative transesophageal echocardiography in chest trauma. *J Trauma* 65(4):924–926, 2008.
23. Wong SSF: Penetrating thoracic injuries: the use of transesophageal echocardiography to monitor for complications after intracardiac nail removal. *J Trauma* 64(5):E69–E70, 2008.
24. Choo MH, Chia BL, Chia FK, et al: Penetrating cardiac injury detected by two-dimensional echocardiography. *Am Heart J* 108:417–420, 1984.
25. Hassett A, Moran J, Sabiston DC, et al: Utility of echocardiography in the management of patients with penetrating missile wounds of the heart. *Am J Cardiol* 7:1151–1156, 1987.
26. Horowitz MS, Schultz CS, Stinson EB, et al: Sensitivity and specificity of echocardiographic diagnosis of pericardial effusion. *Circulation* 50:239–247, 1974.
27. Miller FA, Seward JB, Gersh BJ, et al: Two-dimensional echocardiographic findings in cardiac trauma. *Am J Cardiol* 50:1022–1027, 1982.
28. Lopez J, Garcia MA, Coma I, et al: Identification of blood in the pericardial cavity in dogs by two-dimensional echocardiography. *Am J Cardiol* 53:1194–1197, 1984.
29. Jimenez E, Martin M, Krukenkamp I, et al: Subxiphoid pericardiotomy versus echocardiography: A prospective evaluation of the diagnosis of occult penetrating cardiac injury. *Surgery* 108:676–680, 1990.
30. Meyer D, Jessen M, Grayburn P: Use echocardiography to detect occult cardiac injury after penetrating thoracic trauma: a prospective study. *J Trauma* 39:902–909, 1995.
31. Plummer D, Bunette D, Asinger R, et al: Emergency department echocardiography improves outcome in penetrating cardiac injury. *Ann Emerg Med* 21:709–712, 1992.
32. Petkov MP, Napolitano CA, Tobler HG, et al: A rupture of both atrioventricular valves after blunt chest trauma: the usefulness of transesophageal echocardiography for a life-saving diagnosis. *Anesth Analg* 100:1256–1258, 2005.
33. Berkseth RO, Kjellstrand CM: Radiologic contrast induced nephropathy. *Med Clin North Am* 68, 351–370, 1984.
34. Jones JW, Kitahama A, Webb WR, et al: Emergency thoracoscopy: a logical approach to chest trauma management. *J Trauma* 21:280–284, 1981.
35. Ochsner MG, Rozycki CS, Lucente F, et al: Prospective evaluation of thoracoscopy for diagnosing diaphragmatic injury in thoracoabdominal trauma: a preliminary report. *J Trauma* 34:704–709, 1993.
36. Mealy K, Murphy M, Broe P: Diagnosis of traumatic rupture of the right hemidiaphragm by thoracoscopy. *Br J Surg* 80:210–211, 1993.
37. Abolhoda A, Livingston DH, Donahoo JS, et al: Diagnostic and therapeutic video assisted thoracic surgery (VATS) following chest trauma. *Eur J Card Thor Surg* 12:356–360, 1997.
38. Flagel BT, Luchette FA, Reed RL, et al: Half-a-dozen ribs: the breakpoint for mortality. *Surgery* 138:717–725, 2005.
39. Bulger EM, Edwards T, Klotz P, et al: Epidural analgesia improves outcome after multiple rib fractures. *Surgery* 136:426–430, 2004.
40. Katherine BA, Cha ES, Bensard DD, et al: The positive predictive value of rib fractures as an indicator of nonaccidental trauma in children. *J Trauma* 54:1107–1110, 2003.
41. Bulger EM, Arneson MA, Mock CN, et al: Rib fractures in the elderly. *J Trauma* 48:1040–1047, 2000.
42. Holcomb JB, McMullin NR, Kozar RA: Morbidity from rib fractures increases after age 45. *J Am Coll Surg* 196:549–555, 2003.
43. Avery EE, Morch ET, Benson DW: Critically crushed chest: a new method of treatment with continuous mechanical hyperventilation to produce alkalotic apnea and internal pneumatic stabilization. *J Thorac Cardiovasc Surg* 32:291–311, 1956.
44. Tanaka H, Yukioka T, Yamaguti Y, et al: Surgical stabilization of internal pneumatic stabilization? a prospective randomized study of management of severe flail chest patients. *J Trauma* 52:727–732, 2002.
45. Watkins R IV, Watkins R III, Williams L, et al: Stability provided by the sternum and rib cage in the thoracic spine. *Spine* 30(11):1283–1286, 2005.
46. Black CJ, Busuttil A, Robertson C: Chest wall injuries following cardiopulmonary resuscitation. *Resuscitation* 63:339–343, 2004.
47. Garrel TV, Ince A, Junge A, et al: The sternal fracture: radiographic analysis of 200 fractures with special reference to concomitant injuries. *J Trauma* 57:837–844, 2004.
48. Athanassiadi K, Gerazounis M, Moustardas M, et al: Sternal fractures: retrospective analysis of 100 cases. *World J Surg* 26:1243–1246, 2002.

49. Weening B, Walton C, Cole PA, et al: Lower mortality in patients with scapular fractures. *J Trauma* 59:1477–1481, 2005.
50. Veysi VT, Mittal R, Agarwal S, et al: Multiple trauma and scapula fractures: so what? *J Trauma* 55:1145–1147, 2003.
51. Sedel L: The results of surgical repair of brachial plexus lesions. *J Bone Joint Surg Br* 64:54–66, 1982.
52. Kriel RL, Gormley ME, Krach LE, et al: Automatic garage door openers: hazards for children. *Pediatrics* 98:770–773, 1996.
53. Sherwood SF, Hartsock RL: Thoracic injuries, in McQuillian KA, Von Rueden KT, Hartstock RL, Flynn MB, Whalen E (eds): *Trauma Nursing From Resuscitation Through Rehabilitation.* 3rd ed. Philadelphia, PA, Saunders, 2002 p 543–590.
54. Kimbrell BJ, Yamzon J, Petrone P, et al: Intrapleural thrombolysis for the management of undrained traumatic hemothorax: a prospective observational study. *J Trauma* 62(5):1175–1179, 2007.
55. Toombs BD, Sandlet SV, Lester RG: Computed tomography of chest trauma. *Radiology* 140:733–738, 1981.
56. Shin B, McAlslan TC, Hankins JR: Management of lung contusion. *Am Surg* 45:168–179, 1979.
57. Schild HH, Strunk H, Weber W: Pulmonary contusion: CT vs plain radiograms. *J CAT* 13:417–420, 1989.
58. Hankins JR, Attar S, Turney SZ: Differential diagnosis of pulmonary parenchymal changes in thoracic trauma. *Am Surg* 39:309–318, 1973.
59. Wagner RB, Jamieson PM: Pulmonary contusion: evaluation and classification by computed tomography. *Surg Clin N Am* 69:211–224, 1989.
60. Kishikawa M, Yoshioka T, Shimazu T: Pulmonary contusion causes long-term respiratory dysfunction with decreased functional residual capacity. *J Trauma* 31:1203–1210, 1991.
61. Roxburgh JC: Rupture of the tracheobronchial tree. *Thorax* 42:681–688, 1987.
62. Lynn RB, Iyengar K: Traumatic rupture of the bronchus. *Chest* 61:81–83, 1972.
63. Edwards WH Jr, Morris JA Jr, de Lozier JB III, et al: Airway injuries: the first priority in trauma. *Am Surg* 53:192–197, 1987.
64. Grover FL, Ellestad C, Arom KV, et al: Diagnosis and management of major tracheobronchial injuries. *Ann Thorac Surg* 28:384–391, 1979.
65. Flynn AE, Thomas AN, Schecter WP: Acute tracheobronchial injury. *J Trauma* 29:1326–1330, 1989.
66. Baumgartner F, Sheppard B, de Virgilio C, et al: Tracheal and main bronchial disruptions after blunt chest trauma: presentation and management. *Ann Thorac Surg* 50:569–574, 1990.
67. Shaw RR, Paulson DL, Kee KL Jr: Traumatic tracheal rupture. *J Thorac Cardiovasc Surg* 42:281–297, 1961.
68. Lindstaedt M, Germing A, Lawo T, et al: Acute and long-term clinical significance of myocardial contusion following blunt thoracic trauma: results of a prospective study. *J Trauma* 52(3):479–485, 2002.
69. Penney DJ, Bannon PG, Parr MJ: Intra-aortic balloon counterpulsation for cardiogenic shock due to cardiac contusion in an elderly trauma patient. *Resuscitation* 55:337–340, 2002.
70. Perchinsky MJ, Long WB, Hill JG: Blunt cardiac rupture. The Emanuel Trauma Center experience. *Arch Surg* 130(8):852–856; discussion 856–857, 1995.
71. Perlroth MG, Hazan E, Lecompte Y, et al: Chronic tricuspid regurgitation and bifascicular block due to blunt chest trauma. *Am J Med Sci* 291(2):119–125, 1986.
72. Lundevall J: Traumatic rupture of the aorta, with special reference to road accidents. *Acta Pathol Microbiol Scand* 62:29–33, 1964.
73. Ismailov RM, Weiss HB, Ness RB, et al: Blunt cardiac injury associated with cardiac valve insufficiency: trauma links to chronic disease. *Injury* 36(9):1022–1028, 2005.
74. Asensio JA, Stewart BM, Murray J, et al: Penetrating cardiac injuries. *Surg Clin North Am* 76:685–725, 1996.
75. Duval P: Le incision median thoraco-laparotomy: Bull Et Mem Soc De Chir De Paris, xxxiii: 15. As quoted by Ballana C (1920) Bradshaw lecture. The surgery of the heart. *Lancet* CXCVIII:73–79, 1907.
76. Symbas PN, Hatcher CR, Vlasis SE: Esophageal gunshot injuries. *Ann Surg* 191:703, 1980.
77. Defore WW, Mattox KL, Hansen HA, et al: Surgical management of penetrating injuries of the esophagus. *Am J Surg* 134:734, 1977.
78. Cheadle W, Richardson JD: Options in management of trauma to the esophagus. *Surg Gynecol Obstet* 155:380, 1982.
79. Asensio JA, Berne J, Demetriades D, et al: Penetrating esophageal injuries: time interval of safety for preoperative evaluation-how long is safe? *J Trauma* 43(2):319–324, 1997.
80. Flowers JL, Graham SM, Ugarte MA, et al: Flexible endoscopy for the diagnosis of esophageal trauma. *J Trauma* 40(2):261–265; discussion 265–266, 1996.
81. Mamede RC, De Mello Filho FV: Treatment of caustic ingestion: an analysis of 239 cases. *Dis Esophagus* 15(3):210–213, 2002.
82. Bautista A, Varela R, Villanueva A, et al: Effects of prednisolone and dexamethasone in children with alkali burns of the esophagus. *Eur J Pediatr Surg* 6:198–203, 1996.
83. Pacini D, Angeli E, Fattor R, et al: Traumatic rupture of the thoracic aorta: ten years of delayed management. J *Thorac Cardiovasc Surg* 129:880–884, 2005.
84. Kwon CC, Gill IS, Fallon WF, et al: Delayed operative intervention in the management of traumatic descending thoracic aortic rupture. *Ann Thorac Surg* 74:S1888–S1891, 2002.
85. Demetriades D, Velmahos GC, Scalea TM, et al: Blunt traumatic thoracic aortic injuries: early or delayed repair—results of an American association for the surgery of trauma prospective study. *J Trauma* 66(4):967–973, 2009.
86. Hirose H, Gill IS, Malangoni MA: Nonoperative management of traumatic aortic injury. *J Trauma* 60(3):597–601, 2006.
87. Von Oppell UO, Dunne TT, De Groot MK, et al: Traumatic aortic rupture: twenty-year meta-analysis of mortality and risk for paraplegia. *Ann Thorac Surg* 58:585–593, 1994.
88. Demetriades D, Velmahos GC, Scalea TM, et al: Operative repair or endovascular stent graft in blunt traumatic thoracic aortic injuries: results of an American Association for the Surgery of Trauma Multicenter Study. *J Trauma* 64(3):561–571, 2008.
89. Earley AS, Gracias VH, Haut E, et al: Anemia management program reduces transfusion volumes, incidence of ventilator-associated pneumonia, and cost in trauma patients. *J Trauma* 61(1):1–7, 2006.
90. Michard F, Teboul JL: Predicting fluid responsiveness in ICU patients: a critical analysis of the evidence. *Chest* 121:2000–2008, 2002.
91. Brederlau J, Anetseder M, Schoefinius A, et al: Arteriovenous extracorporeal lung assist and high frequency oscillatory ventilation in post-traumatic acute respiratory distress syndrome. *J Trauma* 64(4):E65–E68, 2008.
92. Yuan KC, Fang JF, Chen MF: Treatment of endobronchial hemorrhage after blunt chest trauma with extracorporeal membrane oxygenation (ECMO). *J Trauma* 65(5):1151–1154, 2008.
93. Liao CH, Huang YK, Tseng CN, et al: Successful use of extracorporeal life support to resuscitate traumatic inoperable pulmonary hemorrhage. *J Trauma* 64(2):E15–E17, 2008.

CHAPTER 165 ■ CRITICAL CARE OF THE PATIENT WITH ABDOMINAL TRAUMA

JUSTIN L. REGNER AND JOHN B. CONE

In many ways the care of the abdominal trauma patient in the intensive care unit (ICU) is similar to that of other patients with abdominal pathology and as such should be familiar to the intensivists. This chapter will focus on those common aspects of abdominal trauma care that are sufficiently rare in the nontrauma patients that many intensivists may have little experience in recognizing or managing them.

One possible origin of the word abdomen is the Latin *abdere*, meaning to conceal. Few areas of the human body are as difficult to assess following injury or to monitor subsequently as is the abdomen. Much of the morbidity and mortality due to abdominal injury results from delay in recognizing conditions that are easily corrected once identified. Improvements in resuscitation and modern high-speed imaging have done much to improve the initial management of abdominal trauma. However, after the patient reaches the ICU, the ability to follow changes occurring within the abdomen deteriorates substantially.

ICU ADMISSION

In previous years, trauma patients arriving in the ICU were assumed to have had their injuries identified and repaired prior to arrival, and therefore the ICU was for monitoring and support. Today the ICU plays a larger role in the care of trauma patients. Many patients with abdominal injuries are managed nonoperatively. Many operated patients have their surgery performed in stages with interposed additional resuscitation in the ICU. The management of the abdominal injuries is now known to have an impact on the function of remote organs such as the lung and the brain, thus there must be close cooperation and shared knowledge between the trauma surgeon and the intensivist.

Trauma surgeons have traditionally divided injured patients into those injured by penetrating mechanisms such as gunshot wounds or stab wounds and those injured by blunt mechanisms such as car crashes and falls. Clearly, some patients manifest components of both types of injury but this classification has been a useful way to divide and compare trauma patients for years. Despite this long tradition and its advantages, for our purposes, it may be more useful to think of abdominal trauma patients coming into the ICU as those who have been operated upon and those who have not.

Operative trauma patients will have had a laparotomy and their injuries should have been defined. There will be a tendency for the intensivist to consider them identical to the elective general surgical patient who has undergone a comparable operation. While there are certainly areas of commonality, there are critical differences that must be considered. The elective general surgical patient will not, in all probability, have had a period of shock preoperatively and intraoperatively. The general surgical patient will usually have only a single acute problem unlike the trauma patient who may have sustained multiple organ system injuries including more than one in the abdomen. These differences often lead to management problems and complications that would not be expected in the general surgical patient and to more frequent complications such as infections.

Many blunt injury patients and some penetrating injury patients are now managed with the intention of not operating on them. This approach has grown out of the recognition that many trauma laparotomies are nontherapeutic as opposed to negative. For example, a laparotomy for hemoperitoneum that identifies a small liver laceration and a minor tear in the mesentery is certainly not a negative laparotomy but if both injuries have stopped bleeding spontaneously, it is difficult to argue that the surgery was therapeutic. Nontherapeutic laparotomies are not without consequences. They are painful, they expose the patient to early risks of wound infection, pneumonia, DVT, and so on, and the late risks of incisional hernia and bowel obstruction [1,2]. These risks are statistically small but significant. However, avoiding them by attempting to manage injured patients nonoperatively is only sensible if it can be done without a significant increase in the incidence of missed injures that do need intervention.

NONOPERATIVE MANAGEMENT

Nonoperative management of intra-abdominal injury is so widely practiced that trauma surgeons often feel they have to attempt nonoperative management or justify why they want to operate on a splenic or liver laceration. Nonoperative management of abdominal organ injury is appropriate only for hemodynamically stable patients whose injuries are identified by imaging. Hemodynamic stability is a nonspecific state but generally implies a systolic blood pressure more than 90 mm Hg without the rapid infusion of fluid, blood products, or the use of pressors. Significant tachycardia or metabolic acidosis if present would also preclude a state of hemodynamic stability. Other factors beyond hemodynamic stability also deserve consideration before a decision to attempt nonoperative management is made. Are there multiple injuries that may increase the risk of failure? Are there medical conditions such as portal hypertension or the use of anticoagulants? Patients with severe head injuries or ischemic heart disease are often considered a high operative risk but a failure of nonoperative management also poses a high risk mortality. Other factors also play a role. Older patients are less likely to undergo successful nonoperative management [3,4].

As imaging has improved, trauma surgeons have been given a more precise determination of the anatomic location and severity of the injury prior to deciding whether or not to operate. This information has allowed the construction of a number of models intended to predict the success of nonoperative management [5]. CT based injury grading systems do show a positive correlation with clinical outcomes but like most scoring systems work better for analyzing populations than for predicting the outcome of individual patients [6,7].

One of the most useful CT findings is the presence of extravasated vascular contrast. This contrast blush usually represents either active bleeding or a pseudoaneurysm of a parenchymal artery. Such patients have a higher probability of failing nonoperative management. Angiographic embolization of the injured vessel may help to restore them to the nonoperative pathway [8].

Spleen

The current practice of managing splenic injury without surgery grew out of a desire to protect children from post-splenectomy sepsis. It was discovered that most children's injured spleens stop bleeding without surgery. This practice was gradually extended into the adult population where the results are not as good but still approach 80% among stable patients. Multiple studies have been conducted in an attempt to more accurately predict which patients will succeed and which will fail attempts at nonoperative management. They have focused on combinations of patient factors such as age and vital signs and CT factors such as contrast blush and depth of laceration [3,4,6]. Failure of nonoperative management not only delays effective therapy and consumes resources, but patients who fail attempted nonoperative management have greater morbidity and mortality [8]. Advanced age, portal hypertension, and coagulopathy increase the probability of the failure of nonoperative management.

The nonoperative management of a ruptured spleen must be a joint effort between the surgical team and the ICU team. The parameters that will default the patient to the operative pathway should be agreed upon in advance between those who will be monitoring and supporting and those who will operate. In general, any indication of hemodynamic instability should lead to immediate surgery and splenectomy. If the patient experiences a steadily falling hemoglobin level but never manifests any change in vital signs, there should be prior agreement regarding the number of units of packed red blood cells (PRBCs) to be transfused prior to resorting to surgery. The absolute number will vary with the estimated operative risk, other factors predicting success or failure, and the patient's preference but should rarely exceed four units of PRBCs for an isolated splenic injury.

Splenic embolization may be an option in some facilities for those patients whose CT demonstrates a contrast blush within the spleen. If embolization is to be utilized, it should be performed by a team that is readily available and has demonstrated success with the procedure.

Patients admitted to the ICU for nonoperative management of an isolated splenic injury should receive their planned immunizations including pneumococcal, meningococcal, and Hemophilus influenza vaccine since there is evidence that these vaccines are more effective with the spleen *in situ* [9].

When the splenic injury is successfully managed nonoperatively, there are still potential complications. Delayed bleeding of a lacerated spleen is a well-recognized complication of splenic injury. Many programs will follow elaborate algorithms specifying when patients may increase physical activity and participate in activities such as physical therapy since such activity is perceived to play a role in delayed rupture. However, there is no convincing evidence that, short of avoiding a blow to the flank, one regimen is superior to another. Pain associated with either capsular distention or infracted splenic tissue may eventually necessitate splenectomy, particularly if the spleen is embolized. The other major complication is an infection involving the injured splenic parenchyma or the perisplenic hematoma resulting in either splenic or subphrenic abscess [10]. Unexplained fever, leukocytosis, pleural effusion, or hiccoughs should necessitate an abdominal CT scan looking for evidence of infection. Most such infections can be effectively treated with antibiotics and percutaneous drainage but failure to respond promptly should result in exploration, evacuation of the infected hematoma, and splenectomy.

Liver

The other commonly injured organ in blunt abdominal trauma is the liver. The injured liver differs from the injured spleen in two significant ways. First, removal of the injured organ is not a treatment option. Second, the liver secretes bile directly into the GI tract so that liver injuries have a more complex range of complications including bile leak, hemobilia, obstructive jaundice, and so on. While the surgical options differ from the spleen, the decision to operate should be based on similar considerations. The first criterion for successful nonoperative management is hemodynamic stability. A patient who does not meet this condition should be taken to the OR, explored, and if necessary, packed, since the organ cannot be totally removed. Experienced trauma or hepatic surgeons will more often be able to perform a definitive procedure initially but the lack of such surgeons should rarely lead to an attempt to manage an unstable patient nonoperatively. Perihepatic packing followed by either angiography with embolization, reexploration when more experienced personnel are available, or transfer to a more capable facility are all preferable to attempting to manage an unstable patient nonoperatively. Conversely, surgical exploration in the face of hemodynamic stability by an inexperienced team is a recipe for disaster and should be avoided.

Patients with solitary liver injuries admitted to the ICU for nonoperative management should first be evaluated for hemodynamic stability and if stable should next be evaluated to determine whether they are likely to benefit from angiography and embolization. Patients with contrast extravasation or severe lacerations extending deep into the hepatic parenchyma are candidates for angiography with embolization. Liver injuries in the face of cirrhosis, portal hypertension, or coagulopathy are much more likely to fail nonoperative management than comparable injuries lacking these comorbidities.

Complications of nonoperative management are primarily the result of bleeding, infection, bile leak, hepatic necrosis, and jaundice. Delayed bleeding from a liver laceration may occur but sudden unrelenting hemorrhage from the liver necessitating emergency surgery is rare beyond 24 hours postinjury. Steadily falling hemoglobin levels in an otherwise stable patient are an indication for either repeat CT scanning to verify that the bleeding is coming from the liver or angiography in an attempt to identify a vessel suitable for embolization.

Bile leaks from the injured liver may result in either contained collections known as bilomas or more diffuse biliary ascites. Bilomas may cause compression of adjacent structures producing jaundice or gastric outlet obstruction in the subhepatic location but the more common problem resulting from bile leak is secondary infection. Small bile leaks occur commonly after liver injury but most are of no clinical significance. Elevated liver function tests after liver injury are an indication for hepatobiliary imaging, or hepatobiliary iminodiacetic acid (HIDA) scan to evaluate for a bile leak. Signs and symptoms of infection are usually better evaluated with a CT scan. Patients in whom a fluid collection is identified should undergo percutaneous drainage if they show evidence of infection. If the drained fluid shows a bilirubin level significantly above that of serum, the patient should then undergo HIDA scanning. Most such bile leaks will seal with adequate drainage of the fluid collection. If bilious drainage persists, they should be evaluated for endoscopic retrograde cholangiopancreatogram (ERCP) with stent placement.

High fevers, often exceeding 39°C, may be seen in patients with liver injury typically beginning 48 to 72 hours postinjury. These fevers have been blamed on atelectatic lung immediately above the diaphragm or on areas of hepatic necrosis. Solid evidence to firmly establish the cause of such fevers is not available. Patients who sustain severe liver injuries but remain hemodynamically stable may nonetheless harbor significant areas of devitalized liver. In the vast majority, this necrotic liver does not require resection. However, if the necrotic liver becomes infected or if the patient deteriorates, resectional debridement of the necrotic material may be necessary.

Hemobilia is a rare complication of hepatic injury. The classic triad of gastrointestinal hemorrhage, jaundice, and right upper quadrant pain should suggest the diagnosis. It may present anytime from the first few days postinjury to months later. Diagnosis is often difficult and delayed. The bleeding is usually intermittent so that diagnostic endoscopy may demonstrate no source for the bleeding. Any patient with a history of hepatic trauma, either immediate or more remote, who has evidence of unexplained gastrointestinal hemorrhage, should undergo diagnostic angiography coupled with therapeutic embolization if a hepatic pseudoaneurysm is identified [11].

Kidney

Renal injury is most often the result of blunt trauma and frequently occurs in conjunction with other injuries. Right renal injury most frequently occurs in conjunction with hepatic injury and left renal injury in conjunction with splenic injury. Renal injury is almost always associated with hematuria but the severity of the hematuria and the degree of the renal injury are often discordant. Gross hematuria may appear dramatic but most renal bleeding diminishes spontaneously within a few hours of injury. Even impressive perinephric hematomas on CT often have little impact on management decisions [12,13].

The kidney has two possible responses to injury that may require monitoring and or intervention, contrast extravasation from bleeding or a urine leak. Rarely will the hemodynamically stable patient continue to bleed from a lacerated kidney. In such cases, the management is similar to the other solid organs with appropriate imaging to confirm the source of bleeding followed either by embolization or surgical exploration. Usually, extravasation of urine from an injured kidney will resolve spontaneously [12,13]. Extravasated contrast that is confined within Gerota's fascia does not mandate immediate intervention since it will frequently resolve spontaneously or respond to minimally invasive methods. Leakage of urine as demonstrated by delayed contrast extravasation outside of Gerota's fascia may still resolve but is more likely to benefit from percutaneous drainage of the renal collecting structures. Persistent urine leakage often indicates ureteral obstruction from either urinoma or retroperitoneal hematoma and may benefit from ureteral stenting.

Renal vascular injury is most often recognized on CT with intravenous contrast as an area of renal parenchyma that does not enhance. This injury may involve a single segment of the kidney or the entire kidney. Although gross hematuria may occur, it is typically of very short duration and may be absent altogether. Microscopic hematuria is virtually always present. The arterial injury may be either complete disruption or thrombosis. However, even with complete disruption, significant hemorrhage into the retroperitoneum is rare. Revascularization is rarely of benefit since in most cases, the time required for diagnosis, surgical exposure, and repair is beyond the warm ischemia tolerance of the kidney. Segmental infarction or even infarction of one entire kidney is usually well tolerated if the other kidney is healthy. Sequelae such as pain, abscess, bleeding, or hypertension are rare. Compression of the kidney by either hematoma or urinoma with subsequent renovascular hypertension (Page kidney) is extremely rare.

Pancreas

Blunt pancreatic injury is typically the result of high energy impact to the epigastrium. Because the pancreas is well protected by the costal margin and is located deep in the retroperitoneum, isolated pancreatic injury is rare. Physical findings are usually minimal and laboratory and imaging studies are often nondiagnostic. As a result of the difficulty in early diagnosis, isolated pancreatic injuries are rarely the cause of ICU admission. However, patients with injuries to liver, spleen, or kidney may show some abnormality associated with the pancreas during the course of their nonoperative management. Elevations in serum amylase or nonspecific findings on CT scan will not usually change the plan to manage the patient nonoperatively. However, it is important to insure that the duodenum is not injured. Duodenal perforation and pancreatic injury are often difficult to differentiate.

Serum amylase values are commonly relied upon to evaluate the pancreas following injury but the sensitivity and specificity of serum amylase leaves much to be desired in the early postinjury period. Serum amylase values determined within 3 hours of injury appear to be particularly unreliable [14]. A normal serum amylase value later in the patient's course appears reliable in excluding a significant pancreatic injury. An elevated serum amylase value is much less specific, particularly in the setting of head injury [15]. Certainly, an elevated amylase should raise the level of suspicion sufficiently to pursue further evaluation of the pancreas. CT findings may also be less than diagnostic. Suggestive CT findings include visualization of a fracture of the pancreas, intrapancreatic hematoma, fluid in the lesser sac, retroperitoneal hematoma or fluid, and so on. As with the serum amylase value, CT scans obtained very early postinjury may be falsely negative [16]. These findings should not be interpreted as suggesting that a delayed work up is the preferred method but rather these results emphasize the importance of repeating both the amylase and if necessary the CT scan in cases where suspicion of pancreatic injury remains.

The critical determinant of whether pancreatic injuries can be managed nonoperatively is the integrity of the pancreatic duct. If pancreatic ductal disruption is present, distal resection or internal drainage produces much less morbidity than simple drainage or noninvasive management [17]. If no definitive reason for surgical exploration exists but there is reason to suspect or diagnose a pancreatic injury, it is imperative to evaluate the ductal integrity. If there is any suggestion of instability or peritoneal signs, this should be performed at the time of abdominal exploration. Otherwise, the patient may be a candidate for magnetic resonance cholangiopancreatography (MRCP) or even the more invasive ERCP. Delay in diagnosing and providing definitive therapy for a ductal injury may have devastating consequences.

Pelvic Fracture

Pelvic fractures represent the exception to the rule that nonoperative management is only suitable for hemodynamically stable patients. Surgical exploration of the pelvic hematoma is usually not an effective way to control the hemorrhage from a pelvic fracture. Thus, once other sources of bleeding have been excluded, even hemodynamically unstable patients may be managed in the ICU.

Although the focus of pelvic fracture management in the ICU is on dealing with the blood loss into the pelvis, it is important not to lose sight of the abdominal distention, and limitation of diaphragmatic excursion that can occur. Patients with significant bleeding into the pelvis should be monitored very carefully for respiratory compromise. This is particularly true during any transport out of the ICU to sites such as radiology. If there is any doubt of the patient's ability to maintain adequate spontaneous ventilation, the airway should be secured electively and the patient placed on positive pressure ventilation.

A great deal of force is required to fracture the pelvis. Therefore, it is not surprising that associated injuries are common. Abdominal injuries and lower extremity fractures are both common in patients with pelvic fractures. These associated injuries often make it difficult to ascertain the site of bleeding. It is essential to evaluate the CT scan for the presence of intraperitoneal blood and solid organ injury as well as the size of the pelvic hematoma and the type of pelvic fracture. Lower extremities should be examined and x-rayed if any question exists of fracture. The type and location of pelvic fracture can provide valuable information regarding the likelihood of bleeding. Fractures or ligamentous disruptions of the posterior pelvis are more likely to be associated with severe hemorrhage than anterior fractures, acetabular fractures, or fractures of the iliac wing [18]. So called vertical shear fractures of the pelvis are particularly likely to be associated with arterial bleeding from the superior gluteal artery or other branches of the internal iliac system [19].

It is imperative to carefully examine the perineum for lacerations that may suggest an open pelvic fracture. This includes a careful rectal examination and a vaginal examination for females. If there is any indication of blood in the rectum or vagina, an endoscopic or speculum examination is required. An adequate examination is likely to be extremely painful with the pelvic fracture and often fractured lower extremities that make positioning very difficult. The examination should not be compromised even if it requires airway control and deep sedation. It may also require the assistance of the orthopedist to minimize fracture movement during the examination. The consequences of missing an open pelvic fracture may be disastrous.

Imaging of the abdomen and pelvis can provide a tremendous amount of information to assist the physician in deciding whether the ongoing blood loss is coming from the pelvic fracture or the abdominal viscera. However, the old adage, "Death begins in radiology" remains true today. Patients with pelvic fractures are at risk for both massive hemorrhage and the respiratory compromise often associated with a massively distended abdomen. They should be accompanied by personnel capable of dealing with these problems whenever they leave the ICU.

If there is a significant increase in the free blood within the peritoneal cavity on repeat focused assessment with sonography for trauma (FAST) examination or repeat CT scan, it may be impossible to be certain whether the bleeding is coming from a decompressed pelvic hematoma or from an abdominal site. In such cases, the patient should be explored. If the only source of the blood loss is found to be the pelvis, the hematoma should be left intact, the abdomen closed, and the patient's pelvic fracture managed in the appropriate manner based on the fracture and hematoma. If the pelvic hematoma is significantly disrupted the only option is packing of the pelvis to achieve tamponade of the bleeding. If the patient has not already been studied angiographically, this should also be completed urgently.

Once the bleeding has been determined to be arising from the pelvic fracture, the first priority as with any other trauma patient, is the maintenance of intravascular volume, hemoglobin concentration, and the correction of coagulation abnormalities. The blood bank should be notified to keep adequate quantities of PRBCs, plasma, and platelets available. The fracture should be stabilized since continued movement of fracture fragments leads to further bleeding. This may be accomplished by one or more of several techniques depending on the fracture and the pelvic geometry [20]. Close consultation between the orthopedic trauma service, the general surgical trauma service, and the ICU is vital. If the pelvic volume is enlarged by the expanding hematoma, every effort should be made to reduce the volume toward normal thus compressing the hematoma. This may be accomplished by external fixation devices or some form of pelvic binder [21]. If stabilization of the fracture and compression do not promptly control the hemorrhage, the patient should undergo angiography of the pelvis with the plan to embolize any bleeding vessels arising from the internal iliac system and stent any injury to the common or external iliac systems. Severe vertical shear pelvic fractures even when managed appropriately may frequently require up to 20 units of PRBCs and the accompanying plasma and platelets. If all the other options have been exhausted or are unavailable, consideration may be give to retroperitoneal exploration for the purpose of packing or ligation of the internal iliac vessels [22].

The complications of pelvic fracture are primarily the result of massive blood loss and transfusion and of increased intra-abdominal pressure from the hematoma leading to respiratory compromise, renal failure, and acidosis that will be discussed in more detail under the abdominal compartment syndrome.

Other

Nonoperative management of abdominal injuries is usually confined to the so-called solid organs. There are two exceptions to this generalization. Intramural hematoma of the duodenum and extraperitoneal rupture of the urinary bladder are commonly and effectively managed nonoperatively.

Blunt duodenal injuries are primarily the result of a direct blow to the epigastrium such as from the steering wheel or seat belt in a motor vehicle crash. In the American Association for the Surgery of Trauma (AAST) grading system, duodenal hematomas are either Grade I or II injuries depending on the length of the duodenum involved [23]. This injury is commonly thought of as an injury of childhood, particularly from child abuse, but it does occur in adults as well. Symptoms, when present, will be those of gastric outlet obstruction. Diagnosis is made from a CT scan with oral contrast or an upper GI study. The patient should be carefully evaluated for any evidence of a concomitant pancreatic injury. Such patients are best managed conservatively if there are no associated injuries. Gastric decompression and nutrition support should be employed and the patient reevaluated radiographically at weekly intervals. The obstruction usually resolves in 2 to 3 weeks. If it has not resolved in this time period, surgical exploration for possible stricture repair should be considered.

Approximately 80% of bladder injuries occur in the setting of pelvic fracture although only about 5% of pelvic fractures are associated with bladder injuries [24]. Bladder injuries are most often extraperitoneal and result from perforation of the bladder by bone fragments from fractures of the parasymphyseal pelvis. This may occur even though the final position of the bone fragments as demonstrated on radiographs does not appear near the bladder. Radiographs taken in the hospital do not reflect the location of the bone fragments at the point of maximal displacement during the crash. Bladder injury is also suggested by the inability to void or the incomplete return of catheter irrigation into the bladder. Any pelvic fracture associated with gross hematuria requires imaging of the bladder. Diagnosis requires retrograde contrast injection into the bladder with images taken in both the AP and lateral views and postvoiding. CT scan with IV contrast can give a high quality image of the bladder if the Foley catheter is clamped early enough to produce distention of the bladder or extravasation. Extraperitoneal rupture is demonstrated by the leakage of contrast with the contrast confined to the area around the base of the bladder. Extraperitoneal injuries typically resolve with simple catheterization in 7 to 10 days. Prior to removal of the catheter, a repeat cystogram should be obtained to confirm closure. Persistent extravasation often requires surgical repair of the bladder.

PENETRATING INJURY

The majority of the patients admitted to the ICU for nonoperative management will have sustained blunt trauma but in some institutions selected cases of penetrating trauma may be admitted to the ICU for close monitoring. As with blunt trauma, the fundamental requirement for nonoperative management is hemodynamic stability and the absence of peritonitis. Any change toward hemodynamic instability or the development of peritoneal signs should mandate exploration.

Stab wounds are much more likely to be monitored nonoperatively than gunshot wounds. This is because knife wounds not only have a lower incidence of actually penetrating the posterior abdominal fascia but even if penetration occurs, they have a lower risk of producing an injury that requires repair. In addition to frequent serial abdominal examination and serial laboratory studies, any of the several techniques may be employed in an effort to determine the need for subsequent surgical exploration. These may include local wound exploration looking for evidence of posterior fascial penetration, diagnostic peritoneal lavage, FAST examination, or CT scan [25]. These modalities will most commonly have been employed in the emergency department but the intensivist should be familiar with the results and the possibility that they may need to be repeated while the patient is in the ICU.

Gunshot wounds are rarely managed nonoperatively if they enter the peritoneal cavity because of the much higher probability of visceral, particularly hollow viscus, injury. However, the advent of high-resolution CT imaging is now allowing the nonoperative management of highly selected abdominal gunshot wounds. These cases are primarily patients in whom the entire tract of the missile appears to be visible within the liver [26] and who are considered high-risk operative candidates either because of multiple previous abdominal operations or serious medical comorbidities. Such patients should be monitored in a manner similar to blunt trauma patients with the added concern that hollow viscus injury is still a concern.

MISSED INJURIES

No matter how careful the initial evaluation of the trauma patient, almost all series report a 10% to 20% incidence of missed injuries that are discovered in a delayed fashion [27]. Most of these are minor fractures discovered as the patient begins to increase activity and reports pain. The consequences of these delays in diagnosis are generally minor. However, a delay in the diagnosis of a hollow viscus injury may have serious repercussions. Avoiding delays in diagnosis requires the cooperation of the entire trauma team including emergency physicians, surgeons, intensivists, and radiologists. The initial examination should be complete and take into account mechanism of injury, bruises and abrasions, patient complaints, and laboratory and radiographic studies. In spite of such a thorough evaluation, additional information will often become available over the first 24 to 48 hours. Bruises, abrasions, seat belt marks, and so on will often be more apparent the next day. Laboratory and even imaging studies are less sensitive when the patient arrives at the trauma center within an hour or two of injury. Although not a formal component of the Advanced Trauma Life Support (ATLS) course, these facts have led many trauma centers to institute a formal tertiary survey at 24 of injury after admission [28]. During the tertiary survey, the patient should be carefully reexamined looking for new evidence of traumatic injury, such as seat belt abrasions that were not apparent initially. The abdomen should be reevaluated for evidence of peritoneal irritation. Radiographs should be reexamined and compared with the formal radiology interpretation. Such tertiary surveys are even more important when the patient is initially unstable and examiners may be distracted by urgency of the situation. Although there is no evidence to suggest the routine use of repeat imaging, a repeat FAST or even CT scan should be obtained if there is any question of change in the initial evaluation. Some injuries such as pancreatic or duodenal injury may be more apparent on a CT scan performed at 24 hours postinjury than on the initial scan. Even the sensitivity of procedures such as peritoneal lavage increases with time.

Bowel

The major concern with missed abdominal injury is the possibility of a missed bowel perforation. A patient who has a bowel perforation with significant spillage will manifest signs of peritoneal irritation quickly if the examination is not compromised by head injury, intoxication, or distracting injuries. Small perforations with minimal spillage may show little in the way of physical findings for several hours. Such injuries are often missed on preoperative imaging and can be easily missed at the time of surgical exploration. Both the patient arriving in the ICU with negative abdominal imaging studies and the patient admitted following abdominal exploration must be reevaluated for bowel injury if they show signs of intra-abdominal infection, unexplained sepsis, prolonged ileus, glucose intolerance, and so on.

With typical 20–20 hindsight it is the knee-jerk reaction to ask how an injury could have been missed at the time of surgical exploration but unfortunately it is easy to be misled at the time of exploration. Urgency of hemorrhage control may lead to oversight. An apparently straight missile tract may not have been so straight. Bowel may have been in a different configuration at the time of penetration. Areas that did not appear injured such as the retroperitoneum may not have been explored. Areas of bowel injury that did not appear transmural may have been deeper than was realized. It is incumbent upon the operating surgeon to explore the abdomen thoroughly but in spite of this, injuries will at times be missed. Neither the operating surgeon nor the intensivist caring for the patient in the ICU should dismiss the possibility if the patient is not recovering as anticipated.

Patients admitted to the ICU for planned nonoperative management are at particular risk. The sensitivity and specificity of CT scanning leave much to be desired for hollow viscus injury [29]. Spillage of oral contrast into the peritoneal cavity is a relatively infrequent finding, even with significant bowel injury. The segmental ileus resulting from the injury tends to obstruct the flow of contrast proximal to the site of injury. Free air may be demonstrated but its absence certainly cannot exclude bowel injury. An area of localized thickening of the bowel wall is suggestive of injury, while a diffuse thickening is more compatible with either excess fluid administration or poor perfusion. The CT finding that causes the most confusion is free fluid in the peritoneal cavity without evidence of a solid organ injury to account for the bleeding. Some consider this sufficient evidence for exploration, while others disagree [30].

Injuries of the mesentery are usually detected on CT due to the associated hemoperitoneum and mesenteric hematoma. It is much more difficult on CT to recognize which mesenteric rents will be associated with intestinal ischemia and delayed perforation. Any mesenteric injury that is not explored surgically must be monitored carefully in the postinjury period to allow the recognition of ischemic bowel prior to perforation. The development of a rising WBC, glucose intolerance, persistent ileus, or signs of peritoneal irritation should prompt investigation if not exploration.

Even bowel injuries that are transmural may show little in the way of physical findings for several days. The localized area of ileus associated with the injury, the diffuse ileus from injury, edema, and narcotic administration may limit the degree of spillage. This same process will often prevent the spillage of CT contrast delaying the diagnosis initially. The physician caring for such patients should remember that an ileus is not a diagnosis but a sign. If it persists, it is important for the intensivist to search for the cause. This may require repeat imaging.

Pancreas

Injuries to the pancreas are easy to miss. CT scans and serum amylase determinations performed in the first 3 hours after injury may be normal [14,16]. The accuracy of both tests increases with time. With isolated pancreatic injury, a missed injury is most likely to result in the leakage of pancreatic secretions but since the enzymes are not activated this is usually well tolerated. Most often the fluid is confined to the lesser sac and unless it becomes infected will resolve spontaneously assuming it does not arise from a major ductal injury. If a major duct is injured the fluid may eventually organize into a pseudocyst requiring internal drainage. Less frequent is the development of pancreatic ascites.

Renal Collecting System

Injuries to the renal collecting system including the renal pelvis, ureters, and bladder may present as a rising blood urea nitrogen (BUN) without obvious explanation, as new onset ascites without evidence of portal hypertension, as drainage of serosanguineous fluid from the incision, or as a mass in the flank or pelvis. In the presence of urinary tract infection, this may lead to the serious complication of an infected pelvic hematoma. The diagnosis is usually not difficult as long as a urine leak is considered. CT with intravenous contrast will usually establish the diagnosis. Any unexplained fluid collection in the abdomen that is aspirated should be analyzed for creatinine and compared to a simultaneous serum level. Most injuries that are diagnosed late can be managed with decompression or stenting although complete transection of a ureter will require reimplantation.

Solid Organs

The probability of missing a solid organ injury if the patient has received a CT scan with intravenous contrast is low. Such scans identify approximately 98% of solid organ injuries. However, if the patient does not receive such a scan on the basis of what is perceived to be a normal physical examination with or without a FAST examination, such errors are then more likely. As already discussed, there are many reasons for an erroneous physical examination. Blood in the peritoneal cavity does not always produce peritoneal irritation immediately. There may be associated intoxication, head injury, or distracting injuries. FAST examinations are intended to assess the quantity of free fluid in the abdomen, not the integrity of the organs. Many liver, spleen, or kidney lacerations produce little or no free fluid on initial examination. Patients admitted to the ICU without abdominal CT scanning or if no contrast was employed should be monitored with both vital signs and serial laboratory studies at a frequency appropriate for their overall condition. Any unexplained deterioration in either should prompt an immediate FAST examination if the patient is unstable and both a FAST and a CT if the patient is sufficiently stable to transport to radiology.

ABDOMINAL COMPARTMENT SYNDROME

The abdominal compartment syndrome (ACS) is a well-recognized complication of abdominal trauma but despite widespread familiarity among intensivists, the diagnosis is often delayed or missed all together. There are reports in the medical literature dating back to the 1800s describing the deleterious results of intra-abdominal hypertension but the clinical diagnosis was imprecise, unreliable, and infrequently made. With the report by Kron et al. [31] in the 1980s describing the indirect measurement of intra-abdominal pressure by the bladder, the bedside diagnosis became more precise and easily quantifiable. The pathophysiology and treatment became well defined. Abdominal compartment syndrome assumed even greater importance with the widespread use of damage control surgical techniques. A complete review of abdominal compartment syndrome is presented in Chapter 156, including current definitions, pathophysiology, systemic consequences, measuring techniques, and management. We discuss it briefly here as it relates specifically to abdominal trauma.

Pathophysiology

The fundamental physiology of ACS does not differ from any other compartment syndrome, whether in the leg, the cranium, or elsewhere. It may occur as a result of bleeding, edema, or packing within the abdomen; referred to as primary compartment syndrome, or as a result of ischemia-reperfusion and capillary leak associated with other disease processes such as major burns or systemic sepsis. This is referred to as secondary compartment syndrome. Pressure within the relatively rigid abdominal compartment increases until the perfusion pressure is inadequate to meet the oxygen and nutrient needs of the tissues within the compartment.

$$APP = MAP - IAP \quad (1)$$

where APP, abdominal perfusion pressure; MAP, mean arterial pressure; IAP, intra-abdominal pressure.

However, unlike the more rigid bony cranium, the abdominal compartment is only semirigid. As IAP increases, the abdomen distends and a portion of the pressure is transmitted to the surrounding structures. To have a reproducible diagnosis we must standardize the measurement technique. While the most direct technique involves the insertion of a fluid filled catheter directly into the peritoneal cavity, this is often not practical in injured patients. The accepted clinical technique is an indirect measurement by the bladder although IAP can also be measured through the stomach or the inferior vena cava (IVC).

TABLE 165.1

GRADING SCALE FOR INTRA-ABDOMINAL HYPERTENSION [32]

Grade	IAP (mm Hg)	Recommendations
I	10–15	Monitor, maintain intravascular volume
II	16–25	Sedation, muscle relaxants, increase cardiac output, often with volume expansion
III	26–35	Decompression
IV	>35	Decompression and reexploration, especially if organ dysfunction is present

Intra-abdominal hypertension is usually defined as an IAP >12 mm Hg or an APP <60 mm Hg.

When IAP rises to a critical level it not only compromises blood flow to intra-abdominal organs, it also produces deleterious effects on the respiratory, cardiovascular, and central nervous systems. Various grading scales of intra-abdominal hypertension have been proposed such as the one shown in Table 165.1.

Abdominal compartment syndrome (ACS) may be defined as an abdominal pressure more than 25 mm Hg, APP less than 50 mm Hg, or with one or more organs showing signs of dysfunction at IAP >20 mmHg [31a,b].

Clinical Manifestations

Increases in IAP impact virtually every system in the body. Often the first measurable findings involve the respiratory system where increased IAP is often the cause of increased $PaCO_2$ due to altered distribution of ventilation. This is usually followed by increased airway pressure and decreased pulmonary compliance, both static and dynamic [32,33]. These changes are often not correctly attributed to increased IAP because there are a multitude of other possible explanations such as pulmonary edema, acute lung injury, and so on.

Increased IAP increases renal vein pressure with elevations in plasma rennin and aldosterone as well as decreased renal blood flow, glomerular filtration, and urine output [34]. The fall in urine output may briefly be offset by volume expansion but as the pressure in the abdomen rises, this ceases to be effective and BUN and creatinine increase.

The increase in IAP results in an elevated CVP and pulmonary capillary wedge pressure as the volume is shifted into the thoracic cavity. In spite of this, actual venous return and cardiac output decrease and systemic and pulmonary vascular resistance increase. This compromise in venous return is transmitted to the CNS with resulting increase in intracranial pressure and decrease in cerebral perfusion pressure.

Management of Intra-abdominal Hypertension

In patients judged to be at high risk for the development of ACS, the risk may be reduced by leaving the abdomen open at the time of surgery. Similarly, a patient who is very difficult to close due to edematous bowel or pelvic hematoma may be better managed as an open abdomen from the beginning (Fig. 165.1). Anytime there is a suspicion of ACS, the initial diagnostic step should be the measurement of IAP, usually by the bladder. If IAP is elevated to harmful levels the only

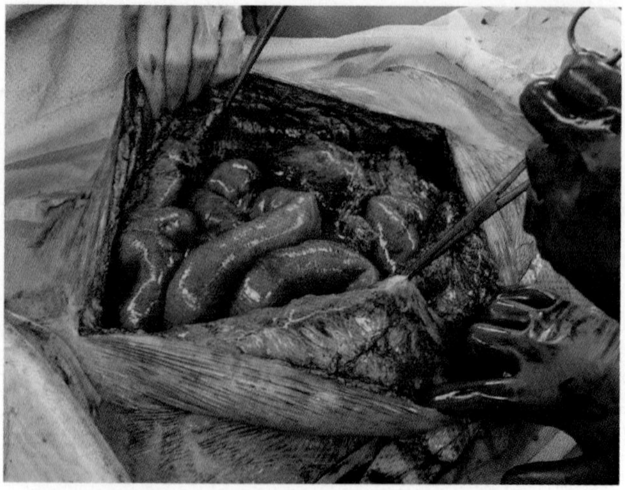

FIGURE 165.1. Massive bowel edema following damage control surgery for a gunshot wound to the abdomen preventing its closure.

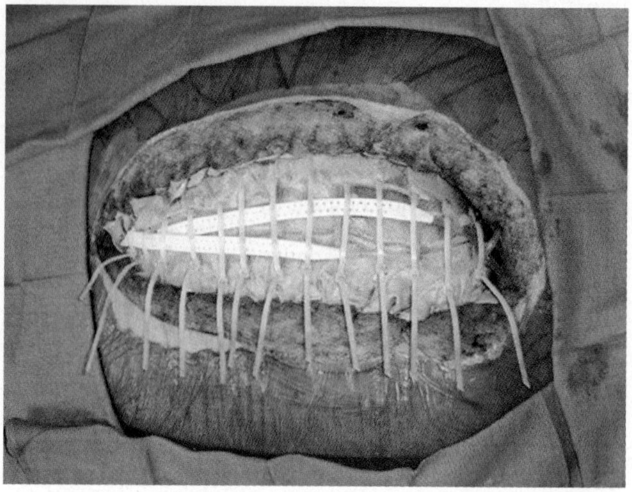

FIGURE 165.2. Homemade vacuum pack dressing for temporary closure of a damage control abdomen.

therapeutic choices are to either remove a portion of the contents or to enlarge the compartment. The next step is a determination of what is causing the increased pressure if this is not already known. Bedside ultrasound will allow the determination of whether there is a large quantity of free fluid in the abdomen. If so, either simple paracentesis or the insertion of a drain may resolve the problem. Large quantities of fluid within distended bowel loops may be reduced with a nasogastric tube. IAP may also be reduced in some patients with the use of improved analgesia and/or pharmacologic muscle relaxation. While these few special cases should not be overlooked, most cases of ACS will require surgical decompression and some form of temporary abdominal closure.

Open Abdomen

Patients whose abdomen is opened to prevent or treat ACS will require some alternative method of closure to prevent evisceration, to reduce fluid and heat loss, and to minimize loss of domain of the abdominal viscera. One of the easiest forms of closure that allows expansion of the abdominal cavity is the towel clip closure. This technique is based on the rapid closure of the skin only with multiple surgical towel clips [35]. The success of this technique depends on the elasticity of the skin to allow expansion of the visceral compartment. While it is simple and fast, towel clip closure has largely been abandoned in recent years as it has been recognized that a significant number of patients developed a recurrent compartment syndrome as the elastic limits of the skin were reached and exceeded. The gap in the *linea alba* has also been bridged with absorbable mesh or simple gauze packing [36]. Other popular techniques have been based on the silo idea similar to that used for newborns with gastroschisis [35]. Several materials have been utilized for the silo from 3 liter bags of fluid to adhesive drapes to sterile silastic sheets.

Currently the most popular management of the open abdomen is some form of vacuum pack dressing [37] (Fig. 165.2). The fundamental principal is the application of a nonadherent barrier over the bowel followed by some form of negative pressure connection and then a closed, sealed covering over the abdomen. The benefits of such a negative pressure dressing include the more rapid removal of fluid from the peritoneal cavity and the collapse of any free space in the abdomen. The negative pressure should also assist with the more rapid mobilization of edema from the bowel and abdominal walls and possibly minimize the contracture of the abdominal wall muscles. A number of homemade devices have been described and a commercial system is now also available.

When the bleeding has been controlled, the edema is resolving, and the packing has been removed, the next priority is abdominal closure. The longer the abdomen remains open, the greater will be the difficulty in achieving closure. Efforts to reduce the volume of the abdominal contents will include dieresis, removal of packing, and removal of fluid collections or hematoma. Actual re-approximation of the midline fascia may be facilitated by frequent "reefing" of the closure in a manner analogous to that employed in neonates with a silo, by the use of pharmacologic muscle relaxants or by more complex surgical techniques such as component separation [38]. In some patients, the bowel may heal into a solid mass prior to achieving closure. In these cases, a planned ventral hernia is the best option available with skin closure accomplished by either elevating skin flaps directly over bowel or by performing a split thickness skin graft directly onto bowel.

Prolonged exposure of the bowel by any of these techniques results in a substantial risk of enterocutaneous fistula formation. Fistula formation into such large open wounds almost never allows spontaneous fistula closure and greatly complicates the wound management as well as fluid and nutritional management. The primary goal of this phase of open abdominal management is to achieve some form of wound closure before fistula formation occurs.

DAMAGE CONTROL SURGERY

Historically trauma surgeons were taught that all bleeding must be stopped, all sources of contamination repaired or exteriorized, and other injuries definitively repaired prior to closing the abdomen regardless of the duration of the operation. However, with a better understanding and improved recognition of the metabolic failure that accompanies the so-called "bloody vicious cycle" of hypothermia, acidosis, and coagulopathy, current practice calls for a more abbreviated surgical technique referred to as damage control surgery [39]. These techniques should be employed only in the small percentage of patients with life threatening injuries complicated by profound shock. Damage control surgery as generally practiced consists of three phases:

I. Limited operative intervention to control hemorrhage, usually by ligation, shunting, or packing and to control contamination usually by ligation or stapling.

Little or no repair or reconstruction is performed at this stage. Closure is rapid and temporary.

II. Resuscitation to include aggressive correction of volume and hemoglobin deficits, replacement of coagulation factors, correction of acidosis, and restoration of body temperature usually carried out in the ICU.

III. Planned return to the operating room to complete definitive repairs, remove packs, and look for additional injuries. Definitive closure may be accomplished at this time or delayed for a later time. This phase should take place only when the deficits described above have been corrected.

Inability to correct the deficits described above may reflect continued bleeding. It is not difficult to overlook a surgical bleeding site when it is obscured by diffuse nonsurgical bleeding. Despite this fact, making the decision to return to the OR before correction of the deficits is a difficult one. Various criteria have been described for emergent return to the OR [40] but in practice the decision is often based on progress or the lack thereof. If the temperature, the pH, the coagulation studies, and the vital signs are getting better, it is usually worth persisting with the resuscitation efforts. If over a predefined time period of 2 to 3 hours of maximal effort most of these parameters are not improving, it is worth the risk of transporting the patient back to the OR for another look. Another indication for cutting short the resuscitation period is the development of an abdominal compartment syndrome that is limiting ventilation or cardiac output.

Acidosis

Hypovolemic shock in the severely injured patient produces a metabolic derangement that will not have disappeared with the restoration of normal vital signs. One manifestation of this metabolic failure is a persistent lactic acidosis. A variety of endpoints for resuscitation have been proposed including CVP, wedge pressure, oxygen delivery, oxygen consumption, and right ventricular volume but none have been shown to be more reliable than resolution of the lactic acidosis. Although crystalloid undoubtedly has a place in this resuscitation, recent data suggests that more of the resuscitation should be based on PRBCs, fresh frozen or thawed plasma, and platelets [41]. The traditional ratio has been one unit of plasma for each four units of PRBCs but current information suggests that a ratio closer to 1:1 may be advantageous. Spontaneous resolution of the acidosis with resuscitation suggests that the oxygen debt incurred during the shock phase is being repaid and serves as a marker of adequate resuscitation. However, during severe acidosis the patient is at increased risk for cardiac arrhythmias and becomes unresponsive to catecholamines either endogenous or exogenous. Coagulopathy is made worse by severe acidosis. Thus, it may be appropriate to use alkalinizing agents such as sodium bicarbonate or THAM (trishydroxymethylaminomethane) to raise the pH to approximately 7.2 [42]. Although the use of such agents is widely practiced, their use is largely based on *in vitro* data and theory. There is no clinical proof that they are beneficial. Evidence of supranormal oxygen delivery or consumption during resuscitation have been proposed as appropriate goals of resuscitation but current evidence suggests that they should be considered as predictors of improved outcome rather than therapeutic goals [43].

Hypothermia

If a patient's last body temperature prior to leaving the OR was less than 35°C, the risk of death is more than 40× greater than for patients with final body temperature more than 35°C. [44]. Hypothermia in the abdominal trauma patient is a multifactorial problem. Many patients arrive hypothermic due to exposure and shock prior to presentation to the trauma center. This problem is often compounded by further exposure to cold environments in the ED or the OR, the infusion of cold fluids, and the open body cavity. Inadequate oxygen delivery leads to inadequate oxygen consumption and a failure of heat production. This may be worsened by vasodilation from either intoxicants or anesthetic agents and loss of shivering ability from muscle relaxants. It is critical to prevent the development of hypothermia since it is very difficult to correct once present.

However, despite efforts in the ED and the OR, many damage control patients will be delivered to the ICU already hypothermic. In this circumstance, aggressive efforts must be employed including warming all fluids, raising the room temperature to uncomfortable levels, covering all body regions including the head, and the use of warming systems such as the Bair Hugger®. Lavage of the NG tube or chest tube with warm saline solution may also be utilized. In severe cases of hypothermia, it may be appropriate to utilize continuous arteriovenous rewarming as described by Gentilello et al. [45]. The inability to correct hypothermia if these measures have been employed usually indicates a failure of adequate resuscitation and that oxygen consumption is still inadequate.

Coagulopathy

The coagulation abnormalities associated with severe trauma include dilution of clotting factors and platelets from crystalloid infusion, consumption of clotting factors, hypothermia, and the anticoagulant effects of fibrin degradation products. In addition, there is the increasing use of anticoagulants and antiplatelet agents in patients with underlying comorbidities. Current data suggests that the coagulopathy of trauma and shock can be minimized by the use of blood component therapy with ratios closer to those of whole blood [41].

Upon arrival in the ICU from the initial phase of damage control surgery, blood should immediately be sent to the laboratory for clotting studies including prothrombin time, activated partial thromboplastin time, platelet count, and fibrinogen level. Hypothermia and acidosis impair the coagulation process and should be the initial focus of ICU care since factor replacement will have limited benefit in a patient who is hypothermic and acidotic.

Patients with prolonged clotting times should have aggressive replacement of clotting factors with fresh frozen or thawed plasma, while those with low levels of fibrinogen should also receive cryoprecipitate. Platelets should be replaced to achieve levels of more than 100,000 per μL.

Patients with nonsurgical bleeding who are judged to have adequate factor replacement and who are not extremely acidotic or hypothermic should be considered for the administration of recombinant Factor VIIa (rFVIIa). Although not formally approved for use in trauma patients, rFVIIa has shown benefit in two clinical trials of bleeding from trauma patients and while expensive, does appear to be safe in the injured patient [46].

SUMMARY

There are a host of similarities between the abdominal trauma patient and the general abdominal surgery patient and it has been assumed for the purposes of this chapter that the intensivist is familiar with managing these general surgical patients. This chapter has attempted to focus on the areas of abdominal trauma infrequently seen in general surgery or nonsurgical patients. The elective abdominal surgery patient will usually have a single defined problem and will generally begin in a hemodynamically stable state. The abdominal trauma patient has an unknown number of injuries on presentation and the physiologic disruption resulting from the injury and the period of shock may compromise the ability to locate or repair all of them prior to arrival in the ICU. The trauma surgeon and the trauma intensivist must work in close cooperation since diagnosis, resuscitation, and treatment are a continuum beginning in the ED and extending seamlessly into the OR and the ICU. There should be no rigidly defined rules regarding who identifies the injuries or resuscitates the patient. Nowhere is the concept of the trauma team more important than in the ICU management of abdominal trauma patients.

References

1. Hasaniya N, Demetriades D, Stephen A, et al: Early morbidity and mortality of non-therapeutic operations for penetrating trauma. *Am Surg* 60:744–747, 1994.
2. Morrison JE, Wisner DH, Bodai BI: Complications after negative laparotomy for trauma: Long term follow-up in a health maintenance organization. *J Trauma* 41:509–513, 1996.
3. Peitzman AB, Heil B, Rivera L, et al: Blunt splenic rupture in adults: multi-institutional study of the eastern association for the surgery of trauma. *J Trauma* 49:177–87, 2000.
4. Godley CD, Warren RL, Sheridan RL, et al: Non-operative management of blunt splenic injury in adults: Age over 55 years as a powerful indicator for failure. *J Am Coll Surg* 183:133–139, 1996.
5. Malhotra AK, Fabian TC, Croce MA, et al: Blunt hepatic injury: a paradigm shift from operative to non-operative management in the 1990s. *Ann Surg* 231:804–813, 2000.
6. Cohn SM, Arango JI, Myers JG, et al: Computed tomography grading systems poorly predict the need for intervention after spleen and liver injury. *Am Surg* 75:133–139, 2009.
7. MacLean AA, Durso A, Cohn SM, et al: A clinically relevant liver injury grading system by CT, preliminary report. *Emerg Radiol* 12:34–37. 2005.
8. Davis KA, Fabian TC, Croce MA, et al: Improved success in nonoperative management of blunt splenic injuries: Embolization of splenic artery pseudoaneurysms. *J Trauma* 44:1008–1013, 1998.
9. Howdieshell TR, Heffernan D, Dipiro JT, et al: Surgical infection society guidelines for vaccination after traumatic injury. *Surg Infect (Larchmt)* 7:275–303, 2006.
10. Sekikawa T, Shatney CH: Septic sequelae after splenectomy for trauma in adults. *Am J Surg* 145:667–673, 1983.
11. Cyret P, Baumer R, Roche A: Hepatic hemobilia of traumatic or iatrogenic origin. Recent advances of diagnosis and therapy. Review of the literature for 1976–1981. *World J Surg* 8:2–8, 1984.
12. McAninch JW, Carroll PR: Renal exploration after trauma: indications and reconstruction techniques. *Urol Clin North Am* 16:203–212, 1989.
13. Husmann DA, Gilling PJ, Perry MO, et al: Major renal lacerations with devitalized fragments following blunt abdominal trauma. A comparison between non-operative (expectant) versus surgical management. *J Urol* 150:1774–1777, 1993.
14. Takishima T, Sugimoto K, Hirata M, et al: Serum amylase levels on admission in the diagnosis of blunt injury to the pancreas: its significance and limitations. *Ann Surg* 226:70–76, 1997.
15. Liu KJ, Lichtor T, Cho MJ, et al: Serum amylase and lipase elevation is associated with intracranial events. *Am Surg* 67:215–219, 2001.
16. Jeffrey R, Federle M, Creass R: Computed tomography of pancreatic trauma. *Radiology* 147:491–494, 1983.
17. Olah A, Issekutz A, Haulik L, et al: Pancreatic transaction from blunt abdominal trauma: early versus delayed diagnosis and surgical management. *Dig Surg* 20:408–414, 2003.
18. Magnussen RA, Tressler MA, Obremskey WT, et al: Predicting blood loss in isolated pelvic and acetabular high energy trauma. *J Orthop Trauma* 21:603–607, 2007.
19. Eastridge BJ, Starr A, Minei JP, et al: The importance of fracture pattern in guiding therapeutic decision making in patients with hemorrhagic shock and pelvic ring disruption. *J Trauma* 53:446–450, 2002.
20. Friese G, LaMay G: Emergency stabilization of unstable pelvic fractures. *Emerg Med Serv* 34:65–71, 2005.
21. Ghanayem AJ, Stover MD, Goldstein JA, et al: Emergent treatment of pelvic fractures comparison of methods for stabilization. *Clin Orthop Rel Res* 318:75–80, 1995.
22. Totterman A, Madsen JE, Skaga NO, et al: Extraperitoneal pelvic packing: a salvage procedure to control massive traumatic pelvic hemorrhage. *J Trauma* 62:843–852, 2007.
23. Moore EE, Cogbill T, Malangoni M, et al: Organ injury scaling II: Pancreas, duodenum, small bowel, colon and rectum. *J Trauma* 30:1427–1429, 1990.
24. Cass AS: The multiple injured patient with bladder trauma. *J Trauma* 24:731–734, 1984.
25. Oreskovich MR, Carrico CJ: Stab wounds to the anterior abdomen. Analysis of a management plan using local wound exploration and quantitative peritoneal lavage. *Ann Surg* 198:411–419, 1983.
26. Demetriades D, Gomez H, Chahwan S, et al: Gunshot injuries to the liver: The role of selective non-operative management. *J Am Coll Surg* 188:343, 1999.
27. Buduhan G, McRitchie DI: Missed injuries in patients with multiple trauma. *J Trauma* 49:600–605, 2000.
28. Biffl WL, Harrington DT, Cioffi WG: Implementation of a tertiary trauma survey decreases missed injuries. *J Trauma* 54:38–43, 2003.
29. Malhotra AK, Fabian TC, Katsis SB, et al: Blunt bowel and mesenteric injuries: the role of screening computed tomography. *J Trauma* 48:991–998, 2000.
30. Livingston DH, Lavery RF, Passannante MR, et al: Free fluid on abdominal computed tomography without solid organ injury after blunt abdominal does not mandate celiotomy. *Am J Surg* 182:6–9, 2001.
31. Kron IL, Harman PK, Nolan SP: The measurement of intra-abdominal pressure as a criterion for re-exploration. *Ann Surg* 199:28–30, 1984.

31a. Malbrain ML, Cheatham ML, Kirkpatrick A, et al: Results from the international conference of experts on intra-abdominal hypertension and abdominal compartment syndrome. I. Definitions. *Intensive Care Med* 32:1722–1732, 2006.

31b. Cheatham ML, Malbrain ML, Kirkpatrick A, et al: Results from the international conference of experts on intra-abdominal hypertension and abdominal compartment syndrome. II. Recommendations. *Intensive Care Med* 33:951–962, 2007.

32. Meldrum DR, Moore FA, Moore EE, et al: Prospective characterization and selective management of the abdominal compartment syndrome. *Am J Surg* 174:667–672, 1997.
33. Cullen DJ, Coyle JP, Teplich R, et al: Cardiovascular, pulmonary, and renal effects of massively increased intra-abdominal pressure in critically ill patients. *Crit Care Med* 17:118–121, 1989.
34. Harman PK, Kron IL, McLachlan HD, et al: Elevated intra-abdominal pressure and renal function. *Ann Surg* 196:594–597, 1982.
35. Feliciano DV, Burch JM: Towel clips, silos, and heroic forms of wound closure, in Maull KI, Cleveland HC, Feliciano DV, et al. (eds): *Advances in Trauma and Critical Care*, Vol 6. Chicago, Year Book, 1991, p 231–250.
36. Saxe JM, Ledgerwood AM, Lucas CE: Management of the difficult abdominal closure. *Surg Clin North Am* 73:243–251, 1993.
37. Barker DE, Kaufman HJ, Smith LA, et al: Vacuum pack technique of temporary abdominal closure: a 7 year experience with 112 patients. *J Trauma* 48:201–206, 2000.
38. Ramirez OM, Ruas E, Dellon AL: "Components separation" method for closure of abdominal wall defects: an anatomic and clinical study. *Plast Reconst Surg* 86:519–526, 1990.
39. Rotondo MF, Schwab CW, McGonigal MD, et al: "Damage control": an approach for improved survival in exsanguinating penetrating abdominal injury. *J Trauma* 35:375–382, 1993.
40. Morris JA Jr, Eddy VA, Rutherford EF: The trauma celiotomy: the evolving concepts of damage control. *Curr Prob Surg* 33:611–700, 1996.
41. Holcomb JB, Wade CE, Michalek JE, et al: Increased plasma and platelet to red blood cell ratio improves outcome in 466 massively transfused civilian trauma patients. *Ann Surg* 248:447–458, 2008.
42. Lier H, Krep H, Schroeder S, et al: Preconditions of hemostasis in trauma. A review. The influence of acidosis, hypocalcemia, anemia and hypothermia on functional hemostasis in trauma. *J Trauma* 65:951–960, 2008.
43. Durham RM, Neunaber K, Mazuski JE, et al: The use of oxygen consumption and delivery as endpoints for resuscitation in critically ill patients. *J Trauma* 41:32–39, 1996.
44. Cushman JG, Feliciano DV, Renz BM, et al: Iliac vascular injury: operative physiology related to outcome. *J Trauma* 42:1033–1040, 1997.
45. Gentilello LM, Cobean RA, Offner PJ, et al: Continuous arteriovenous rewarming: rapid reversal of hypothermia in critically ill patients. *J Trauma* 32:316–325, 1992.
46. Boffard KD, Riou B, Warren B, et al: Recombinant factor VIIa as adjunctive therapy for bleeding control in severely injured trauma patients: two parallel, randomized, placebo-controlled, double blind clinical trials. *J Trauma* 59:8–15, 2005.

CHAPTER 166 ■ BURN MANAGEMENT

PHILIP FIDLER

DEFINITION AND GENERAL CONSIDERATIONS

A burn is a tissue injury resulting from excessive exposure to thermal, chemical, electrical, or radioactive agents [1]. The transfer of thermal energy over time is proportional to tissue damage.

In the United States, 60,000 to 80,000 people are hospitalized annually for burn care, but only 1,500 to 2,000 people sustain more than 40% total body surface area (TBSA) burns [2]. The elderly population is growing and contributes significantly to the increase in burn related hospitalizations. Among elderly victims, two thirds are flame burned, half have impaired judgment, and three fourths have a concomitant medical condition [2,3]. This population, typically debilitated by limited mobility, is particularly susceptible to large scald injuries, which can be devastating despite their clean appearance [4].

While all human tissue can be burned, the skin is most susceptible and is composed of essentially two distinct layers; the superficial epidermis, which is attached by a basement membrane to the foundation layer—dermis. The epidermis is of ectodermal origin and is invaluable for its vapor barrier, pigment, and immunological functions. While biologically very active, at approximately seven cell layers of keratinocytes, it has little mechanical integrity—the role of the dermis. Fortunately, the epidermis for practical purposes is "immortal" and when mechanically disrupted, will recover anew, without scar. In contrast, the dermis is derived from mesenchymal cells and provides the mechanical integrity to the skin, our "leather" so to speak, and has no native regenerative qualities. Dermis, when injured, repairs by way of scarring. Therefore, the essence of acute burn wound care is to sustain dermal viability.

The term burn will mean "burned skin of partial or full thickness depth." It is essential to discern between partial thickness and full thickness injuries of the dermis (commonly called second and third degree burns), as the latter requires operative interventions [2,3]. Pale, leathery, and insensate skin are features of full thickness injury, while blistering, weeping, pink and painful burns characterize partial thickness injury. Currently, no technology supersedes clinical experience in making this distinction, however, laser Doppler imaging has been validated in some centers [5]. Furthermore, the injury is dynamic and partial thickness injuries can worsen ("convert") to full thickness injuries for a variety of reasons.

When the burn injury coincides with blunt trauma, an evaluation for internal hemorrhage, closed head trauma, and long bone fractures is mandatory; the burned skin becomes a secondary concern [6]. Victim extrication from a closed space fire, such as in a bedroom, should make one expect an inhalational injury (see "Inhalation Injury"). The TBSA involved as partial and full thickness skin injury, age, comorbidities, and inhalational injury contributes to the morbidity and mortality of burn victims. Burns involving over 20% TBSA and those with inhalational injury of any burn size are at risk for burn shock (see "Burn Shock" section).

By the 1980s, a paradigm shift toward "early" (within 5 days) operative excision occurred because of the realization that the presence of burned tissue drives "burn shock" [6,7]. During the first half of the twentieth century burn wounds were treated with topical antibiotics and allowed to suppurate from the viable margin; subsequently, bacterial infections causing burn wound sepsis were commonplace [3,7]. The diminution of burn wound sepsis and advances in critical care borrowed from all disciplines have contributed to a remarkable LD50 for 90% TBSA burned in young people and 40% TBSA burned in the elderly [3,8] (Pruitt diagram; Fig. 166.1). Three clinical data points: age more than 60 years, TBSA burned more than 40%, and inhalational injury confer mortality rates over 90% when all three are present and 33% when two factors are present [8]. A rule of thumb with larger burns is a day in the ICU for each percentage of TBSA burned. Mortality usually occurs from multisystem organ failure secondary to sepsis. The substantial reduction in mortality at major burn centers has prompted research focus on improvement in quality of life [7]. Early transfer of patients to regional burn centers as per the guidelines of the American Burn Association has been shown to confer best outcomes [2,9].

BURN SHOCK

Burn shock is a form of vasodilatory shock, akin to "systemic inflammatory response," and creates an astounding volume requirement for the burned patient. It occurs most commonly with burns of at least 20% TBSA and is essentially universal in larger surface area burns. Increased vascular permeability and decreased capillary oncotic pressure combine to create severe edema, even in non-burned tissues. Kinins, serotonin, histamine, prostaglandins, and oxygen radicals are some of the vasoactive mediators released in response to burn injury and stimulate vascular permeability. Albumin is functionally lost into the interstitium thereby increasing extravascular oncotic pressure compounding the edema [3,10]. Unresuscitated patients perish from hypovolemic shock, historically likened to the demise from cholera; this association contributed to the understanding of the profound dehydration following burn injury [11].

While the resuscitation in burn shock may be conceptualized as optimizing the viability of the partial thickness (second degree) component of the burn injury, treatment is focused on intravascular volume repletion. Central shunting of blood compensates for the anhydremia, yet deprives the injured tissue of perfusion. Under perfusion deprives the partial thickness injury of essential nutrient delivery and gas exchange resulting in conversion of partial thickness injury to full thickness injury—which requires operative repair. Excessive resuscitation compounds tissue edema resulting in the same demise. It seems evolutionary biology has not accounted for intravenous fluid resuscitation, hence the response is maladaptive [12].

The patient's TBSA burn and weight dictates their fluid requirements for the first 24 hours. A number of methods to calculate the TBSA burned exist. The "rule of nines" and the Lund-Browder scales are useful for contiguous injury, while the palmer surface of the patient's hand, representing 1% TBSA, is used as a guide in noncontiguous injuries [3] (Fig. 166.2).

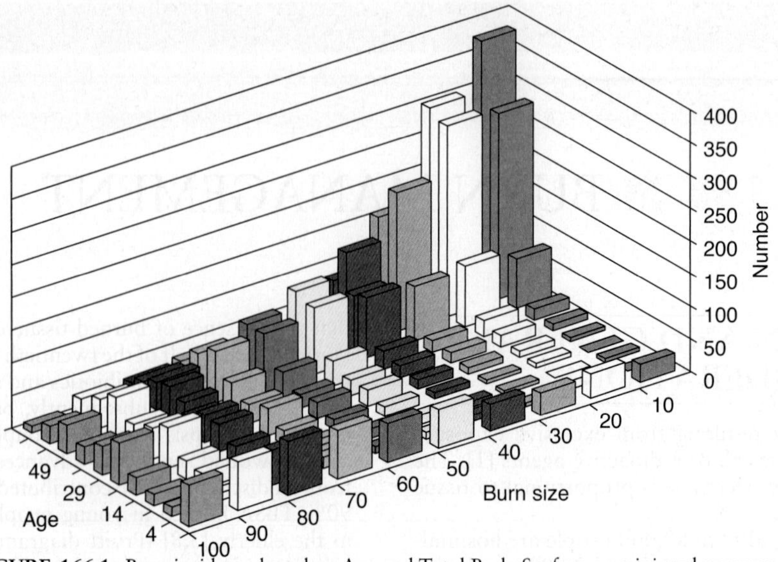

FIGURE 166.1. Burn incidence based on Age and Total Body Surface area injured per year in the United States.

Fluid "requirement" should be thought of as that volume needed to optimize organ function; debate continues over appropriate endpoints of resuscitation—most clinicians accept ½ cc per kg per hour of urine output. If the urine output is more than 1 mL per kg per hour, then the rate of infusion should be decreased, this typically occurs by the third post burn day with the return of vascular integrity (See Fig. 166.4 Parkand formula). Thereafter, it is sufficient to limit the infusion and allow the concurrent insensible losses to correct volume overload—judicious diuresis with a loop diuretic may be employed. The timing and use of pressors requires clinical judgment in the face of hypotension despite adequate intravascular volume repletion. In patients with persistent oliguria, preexisting renal failure, or congestive heart failure, a pulmonary artery catheter is advised. While oliguria bodes poorly, excessive urine output should not be admired. If urine output is exceeding expectations, it is good practice to check the urine electrolytes, particularly for glycosuria and treat hyperglycemia accordingly [13]. Tight glucose control between 80 to 120 mg per dL with insulin is advocated [13].

The biological basis of burn wound conversion has not been fully elucidated. It is known that necrosis occurring from direct cellular damage and ischemia is not the only pathway. With cell death in evidence, the presence of apoptotic populations has been identified [14]. Macrophage inducible nitric oxide synthase may be an inciting factor in such apoptosis and its inhibition seems to limit apoptosis in animal models [14,15].

Central venous access is generally necessary because extremity edema makes peripheral access tenuous and is ideally, but not essentially, placed through non-burned tissue.

A number of resuscitative regimens have been advocated, none proven superior to date. Most are iterations of an isotonic solution in the first 12 hours of shock [3,11,15,16].

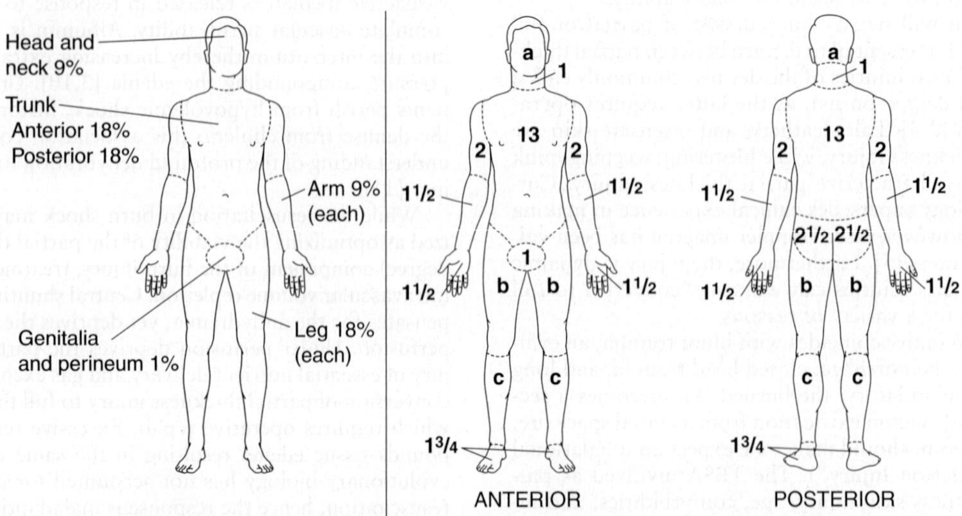

FIGURE 166.2. The Rule of Nines has been the primary method used to identify the percent of body surface burn. The Lund-Browder Diagram is a newer way of estimating the percent of body burn.

The use of colloid seems ill advisable in the first 12 hours after injury, as it seems to aggravate water loss into the pulmonary interstitium and potentiates pulmonary edema [3,15,16]. The commonest colloids are albumin, the most popular, and fresh frozen plasma (FFP). Proponents of albumin value its high oncotic pressure and maintenance of intravascular volume. Those against, argue that albumin is lost into the interstitium worsening edema there, possibly aggravating pulmonary edema. Again, the evidence suggests this risk is most pronounced within the first 12 hours post injury. Albumin is generally not used in patients with serum concentrations above 2.5 mg per dL. While FFP has less oncotic potential than albumin it may have a favorable immunomodulatory benefit, resulting in a truncation of the capillary leak associated with burn shock [3]. Both groups state that the use of colloid reduces the total volume of resuscitation and consequently protects against the detriments of excessive water administration. No level I evidence exists for the resuscitative fluid of choice [10]. A prospective, multicenter trial is needed to answer this question [10].

The pathophysiological similarities between septic shock, systemic inflammatory response, and burn shock may have a common pathway that could be interrupted to improve outcomes [17]. Beta blockade, antihistamines, FFP, generous narcosis, nonsteroidal anti-inflammatory agents, glucocorticosteroids and recently, drotrecogin alfa are amongst the many approaches investigated to mitigate this cellular "hysteria" [2,17]. None of these approaches have proven superiority in multicenter prospective trials to date.

The GI tract is an underutilized resuscitative venue and enteral hydration seems to have been forgotten with the advent of improved intravenous therapy [18]. Enteral nutrition and resuscitation may begin on the day of injury with the caution that patients in shock, requiring vasopressors, can develop bowel ischemia and enteral feeds may increase the metabolic needs of the gut, contributing to bowel ischemia and necrosis. Patient's not tolerating enteral feeds or those with abdominal hypertension (see "Abdominal Compartment Syndrome" section) should be given TPN; this is uncommonly necessary.

Adrenal insufficiency should be suspected when volume repleted hypotension persists despite pressors and is further suggested by concurrent hyponatremia and hyperkalemia. While the characterization of adrenal insufficiency is more expansive in the septic shock literature, numerous case reports and some prospective data support its presence in thermally injured patients. A high mortality exists when disturbances in the hypothalamic-pituitary-adrenal axis are found early in a patient's burn shock course [19,20]. One need not await the results of a corticotropin stimulation test in the face of circulatory collapse and glucocorticoid supplementation should be initiated. In questionable cases, a corticotropin stimulation test is confirmatory and not skewed by Decadron, which enhances vascular tone but has no mineral corticoid activity unlike hydrocortisone. A single blood cortisol of less than 15 μg/dL, in a stressed patient, is suggestive of insufficiency, and it is probably wise to supplement. Glucocorticoids are known to unfavorably affect skin engraftment, and this risk must be weighed against the patients' circulatory failure. Vitamin A supplementation seems to limit the unfavorable wound healing delays and atrophy seen with glucocorticosteroid therapy [20,21].

INHALATION INJURY

Burn victims have two unique pulmonary disorders: restrictive respiratory failure secondary to burn eschar involving the anterior torso and inhalational injury. Torso eschar needs to be divided (see "Escharotomy" section).

An inhalational injury occurs when toxic combustants have been inhaled, and cause a severe inflammatory response in the bronchial pulmonary tree and systemically [22,23]. Extrication from a smoke filled room and findings of singed facial structures, carbonaceous sputum, and respiratory distress corroborate the diagnosis but are not exclusionary. Approximately 30% of adult burn admissions have inhalational injury, which increases mortality rate for like burn size [8,9]. Concurrent inhalational injury intensifies burn shock and may require up to 50% more fluid for adequate resuscitation [3,24,25]. This component of the inhalational injury cascade seems driven mainly by the sensory neuronal pathway, as it can be truncated by capsaicin blockade in an experimental ovine model. Histamine, cyclooxygenase, and atropine blockade do not decrease the response [23,26,27]. Neutrophils invade alveolar spaces via the pulmonary vasculature and likely contribute to O_2 radical production and injury [27,28].

Airway management is paramount. One needs to be particularly observant for signs of upper airway obstruction, secondary to edema, which often develops hours after initial injury. Stridorous patients should be intubated urgently; preferably with an 8 fr endotracheal tube to allow for bronchoscopy and toilet. Immediate threats to life are, in particular, carbon monoxide (CO) poisoning and cyanide (CN^-) toxicity. Generally the lethal level is >60% COHgb and 100% mask O_2 should bring the half-life of COHgb to normal within an hour's time [29]. CN^- poisoning causes cytochrome oxidase inhibition and loss of hypoxic pulmonary vasoconstriction increasing dead space. CN^- is lethal in levels over 1 μg per mL, while 0.02 μg per mL occurs in healthy nonsmokers [25,29]. It would seem rare to have an increased CN^- level without corresponding increase in COHgb; thus, it is fair to say that a normal COHgb, for practical purposes, rules out CN^- toxicity [22,29].

Inhalational injury may best be thought of as a syndrome with a number of sequelae, including endobronchial and interstitial edema, alveolar damage, mucociliary dysfunction, endobronchial slough with cast formation, functional pulmonary shunting, and decreased compliance. Increased bronchial blood flow causes increased interstitial edema [23]. In time, the bronchial epithelium sloughs and combines with exudates and fibrin to form aggregates ("plugs") that support bacterial growth. The tenacious plugs create subsequent mechanical airway obstructions. While there is a dearth of prospective data, aerosolized heparin in conjunction with *N*-Acetyl-cysteine, is advocated in some centers to prevent cast formation and seems particularly helpful in the pediatric population where the narrower airways are at greater risk for obstruction [30]. Burn victims are susceptible to pneumonia because of their immunocompromised state, their immobility, and inability to clear secretions.

Ongoing study of the mechanisms of this form of shock and pharmacological interventions are being intensely investigated. Currently, no objective scale of severity for inhalational injury exists. Bronchoscopy is most useful to characterize the presence or absence of tracheobronchial inflammation and provide toilet.

Prophylactic antibiotics are not recommended. Pneumonia and tracheobronchitis should be treated by culture directed therapy, utilizing Gram's stain, culture of sputum, or bronchoscopy specimens, and local biograms [30,31]. Goals to minimize incidence revolve around proper toilet, limiting aspiration, utilizing lung protective ventilator management, and frequent surveillance [3,30,31]. Patients' overall condition and pulmonary performance by way of usual weaning parameters dictate extubation time. The risk of upper airway obstruction prior to extubation should be assessed by deflating the balloon and audible appreciation of air leak, "no air leak, no extubation." Laryngoscopy may reveal glottic swelling. Glucocorticoid steroids may be considered for the treatment of upper airway edema in lieu of an early extubation but are not indicated for the pulmonary component of inhalational injury and not recommended when a large surface area burn is present. Healing time for patients with lower respiratory injury is longer [23]. The timing of tracheostomy has not been standardized but is probably beneficial in patients expected to be intubated beyond 3 weeks particularly for the benefits of oral hygiene, positioning, and earlier weaning.

SURGICAL CONSIDERATIONS FOR THE ICU

The decision to operate or manage partial thickness injuries expectantly is complex and depends on the location of injuries, patient condition, and survivability (see introduction).

Escharotomy

Full thickness burned skin (eschar) is a restrictive entity; its noncompliance, especially when circumferential, in the face of growing interstitial pressure deprives limb perfusion. This mandates operative release termed escharotomy, which is often limb saving. It may be performed at the bedside, ideally but not essentially, with electrocautery. Incisions are made through the eschar to relieve the underlying pressure. When eschar is involved around the chest wall, incisions are made along the bilateral anterior axillary lines craniocaudally and intercepted transversely joining these incisions at the approximate level of the second rib and xiphoid (Fig. 166.3). This maneuver releases the chest wall, enhancing tidal volume and decreasing airway pressure. If involving the neck region, incisions are made to allow jugular venous drainage. Rarely, lateral canthotomies, which are incisions through the lateral orbital skin and tendon of the canthus, are needed to release ocular pressure in the instance of retrobulbar edema. Although vigilance is the rule, the areas in question are typically apparent within the first 12 hours of injury.

Burn Wound Sepsis

Burn victims develop multiple defects in their immune system that predispose them to an increased risk of infection. Primary treatment is surgical excision and tissue coverage with autograft, skin substitute, or topical antibiotics, alone or in combination. This immunocompromised state combined with loss of the skin barrier can lead to severe infections. Topical antimicrobials (e.g., silver sulfadiazine or mafenide acetate), as well as local wound care, help decrease the amount of burn wound infections [2,6,7]. However, they cannot eradicate burn wound sepsis. Mafenide acetate penetrates eschar and is most effective against Gram negative organisms. It is known to cause metabolic acidosis as a carbonic anhydrase inhibitor and may select for fungal overgrowth.

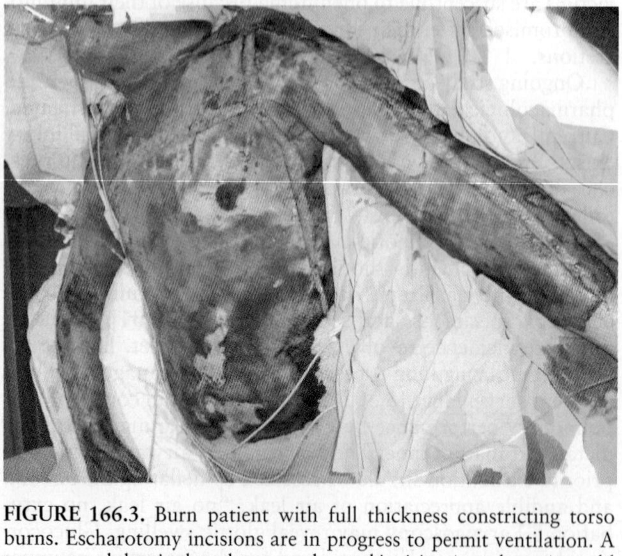

FIGURE 166.3. Burn patient with full thickness constricting torso burns. Escharotomy incisions are in progress to permit ventilation. A transverse abdominal or chevron subcostal incision (not shown) would complete the release.

The signs of burn wound sepsis are diffuse, typically a greenish grey discoloration of the burn, purulent fluid from the wound, and eschar separation along with cellulitis in the surrounding unburned skin. If not treated at the earliest possible time, systemic sepsis will develop. Diagnosis can be confirmed by biopsy of the wound but should not preclude total and urgent excision. Systemic antibiotics are started if infection is suspected and altered or stopped once burn biopsies for quantitative bacterial counts and blood culture results are obtained and negative for infection.

Abdominal Compartment Syndrome

By transducing a transurethral catheter, the urinary bladder pressure is obtained as an indirect measure of intra-abdominal pressure. A measurement more than 20 cm H_2O is loosely defined as abdominal hypertension, which may develop into organ dysfunction, namely renal failure, respiratory embarrassment, and bowel ischemia and denotes abdominal compartment syndrome. Extrinsic renal vein compression leads to progressive oliguria, and respiratory failure is secondary to restrictive airway dynamics. The definitive treatment is celiotomy, although lesser interventions such as peritoneal drainage and or continuous venovenous hemodialysis (CVVHD) are under investigation [32,33].

Cardiovascular Response

Unresuscitated burn victims die of hypovolemic shock. An untreated victim would show progressively decreasing preload and cardiac output. Unfortunately, during the initial 12 to 36 hour postinjury period, even "adequate" volume repletion will not maintain cardiac output. Decreased cardiac contractility and diastolic dysfunction prevail. Animal data suggests a pro inflammatory mediated mechanism *vis-a-vis* the CD-14 and Toll-like–receptor 4 complexes–as seen with endotoxic shock; it is corroborated by echocardiographic abnormalities in burn victims [34,35]. This decrease in contractility is more pronounced in those with inhalational injury and is, in part, nitric oxide mediated [36]. This temporary, seemingly maladaptive cardiac dysfunction passes with time and is followed by a hyperdynamic cardiac performance, which is maintained, often for weeks, post burn [34].

Naturally, the elderly, particularly those with pre-injury cardiac compromise, are more susceptible to congestive heart failure. The quest to rule out an acute myocardial ischemic event will often reveal elevations in cardiac enzymes, both CPK and Troponin-I. Heart muscle is obviously compromised in burn shock, and serum levels of cardiac enzymes are often found within the range attributed to myocardial infarction in the "acute chest pain" setting [35,37]. This quandary is common—what to do about it? Surprisingly, the actual occurrence of a coronary artery thrombosis has rarely been reported. Cardiac stress or "Troponin leak" is seen in many shock states. Emergent cardiac catheterization based on these enzyme elevations may be more harmful than helpful in that traveling long distances throughout a hospital with a critically ill burn victim has substantial inherent risks [38]. A 12-lead EKG should be obtained, and if regional ischemic pattern is present or is suggestive of coronary artery thrombosis or spasm, then a cardiac catheterization is prudent [35]. The lab value of Troponin-I or CPK-MB alone in the course of early burn shock should not dictate emergent catheterization.

Metabolic and Nutritional Considerations

The insensible fluid and protein losses from burn wounds are extraordinary. We know that protein catabolism, compounded by losses through the wound bed and the interstitium, results in severe hypoproteinemia. The hypermetabolic response that occurs, after a thermal injury is more than that observed after any form of trauma or sepsis [3,8]. The magnitude of the response parallels the severity of the burn to a maximum at a burn size of 60%. An increase in temperature of 2°F to 3°F occurs with this response. Patients are kept in a warm environment to help decrease the total energy expenditure [39]. The loss of vasomotor tone autoregulation, possibly in an effort to provide maximal nutrient delivery and gas exchange to the wounded tissues, results in significant evaporative heat loss. Hypothermia from weeping wounds and dwindling energy supplies from the catabolic, muscle wasting condition of burn shock is easily avoided with external warming. Burn centers often keep patients' rooms 90°F to 100°F in the hopes of shunting caloric needs away from thermostasis toward needed wounded repair [40].

Early surgical excision of the burn wound is the most effective means to this end; it truncates the shock state. Clearly, the presence of burned tissue drives the inflammation in the early post injury period, not to be confused with supervening bacterial sepsis, which often occurs days later or in neglected burn wounds.

Muscle wasting, a seemingly unavoidable complication of the hypermetabolism associated with burn wounds, can be ameliorated through anabolic enhancement [41,42]. The two most common approaches are recombinant Human Growth Hormone (HGH) and Oxandrolone. HGH is associated with hyperglycemia, often requiring insulin support and has largely been supplanted by Oxandrolone, which must be given enterally at 10 mg b.i.d., and so the effect is limited in the face of ileus [42,43]. A major thermal injury is characterized by increased muscle proteolysis, lipolysis, and gluconeogenesis. Burn wounds use glucose in greatly increased quantities. Hyperglycemia is common in burn catabolism and may exacerbate muscle wasting. Nonetheless, the known benefits of glucose control from other disease entities in the critically ill are likely to be beneficial in burn victims, and insulin supplementation is recommended [44]. Severe loss of nitrogen, which also occurs, needs to be replaced to combat the muscle wasting and to enhance the immune system. This replacement is absolutely necessary to fight infection and for wound healing. Burn patients need two to three times the basal energy expenditure. Significant burn injuries require 2 g per kg protein. Glucose should contribute 50% to 60% of the calories and the calorie-to-nitrogen ratio should approach 100:1 [43]. All attempts should be made to feed the patient enterally, as enteral feeding decreases the risk of infection. Nutrition may be started on the day of injury.

Infection and Immunity

Patients with significant burns are at high risk for infection, and this is often the precipitating cause of late deaths. The pulmonary tree and the wound beds themselves are the commonest sites and foci for fatal infection. Burn wounds, particularly devitalized full thickness eschar, provide fertile ground for bacterial growth. Early wound infections, within the first 10 days, are typically Gram positive organisms. Later, Pseudomonas is a common and potentially lethal organism, and even later, fungal infections may occur and portend an ominous sign [45]. When surgical excision is not an option, topical antibiotics are the mainstay. Other sites of infection include central lines and Foley catheters. A strong belief exists that the intestine may be a source of unexplained bacteremia by bacterial translocation. This risk may be decreased by enteral feedings. Immunoenhancing regimens are an area of intense study [43,46]. The integrity of the atrophied GI tract is compromised, leading to translocation of bacteria, toxins, or both, putting the burn victim at risk. Evidence demonstrating the presence of bacteria and endotoxin in the lymphatic system makes a plausible case for concern.

ELECTRICAL INJURY

Electrical injuries are divided into high voltage (more than 1,000 volts) or low-voltage injuries (less than 1,000 volts). Low-voltage injuries present as thermal burns, with injuries to the tissue from the outside in. High-voltage injuries may present with little injury to the skin, but significant injuries to the muscle, vasculature, and the bone underneath [47]. Very high voltage injuries occur with obvious disruption of the soft tissue common in electrical line workers. Electrical injuries vary with the source voltage, contact time, and current pathway [2,47,48].

Immediate threats to life are dysrhythmias and spinal cord injury, from either direct nerve injury or tetany resulting in spinal column fracture and cord injury [49,50]. The latter can cause mechanical respiratory failure and paralysis [47,48]. The cutaneous lesions may be subtle and efforts should be made to find entrance and exit lesions, as these will direct the practitioner to focus on the intervening tissues. Compartment syndromes from myonecrosis are common, particularly in the upper extremities, and compartment releases by fasciotomy should be pursued. Often nonviable muscle needs resection. Fluid resuscitation must be initiated quickly; frequently, these patients require a higher volume of fluid due to the underlying tissue injury. Myonecrosis will lead to myoglobinuria, which can lead to renal failure. Serum levels of creatinine phosphokinase into the tens of thousands are often present, and the risk of renal failure is reduced by maintaining a high urine output of 100 mL per hour. Mannitol may be added once resuscitation is well underway. Alkalinizing the urine is advocated by some with the theoretical benefit of preventing heme pigment sedimentation; however, at present, it is by no means mandatory. Pyrophosphate scanning can be used to find occult myonecrosis [51]. One may find serial daily monitoring of the CPK helpful to assess the extent of muscle damage and recovery. Persistent elevations are suggestive of skeletal muscle necrosis and surgical debridement is likely to be beneficial [47].

CHEMICAL INJURY

Acids, "burn" by coagulation necrosis, creating an eschar that limits deeper penetration, whereas alkali, "burn" by liquefaction necrosis in the subcutaneous fat, creating vascular thrombosis and subsequent dermal ischemia. Hydrofluoric acid (HF) burns carry the unique concern of calcium and magnesium chelation and risk cardiac arrest secondary to severe hypocalcemia; intra-arterial infusion of calcium gluconate has been met with some success and may limit digital ischemia and intravenous calcium repletion is necessary. A calcium gluconate slurry may be massaged into the exposed area to potentiate systemic absorption of HF.

PSYCHIATRIC AND ANALGESIC CONSIDERATIONS

Theoretically, those with altered thought processes or coping skills are accident prone. Suicide attempts by self-immolation account for as many as 5% of seriously burned adults. The concurrence of a serious psychiatric comorbid condition is alarmingly high in burn victims and is estimated between 30% and 70% [3].

Burns are commonly known to be one of the most painful medical conditions. No single analgesia regimen can possibly characterize the needs of all burn victims, and suffice to say, the uninitiated practitioner may find the dosing of narcotics multiples of what is commonly used post surgery. Generally, narcotics and benzodiazepines are given as continuous drips; it is common to have moderately burned patients on morphine drips of 10 to 20 mg per hour and benzodiazepines coinciding at 1 to 4 mg per hour. Overtime, the large doses require large volumes of distribution and tolerance lead to even higher dosing. Unlike other critically ill patients, it is not prudent to eliminate these medications for frequent "full" neurological assessment. The physiological benefit of "successful" doses of these medications goes far beyond simple mercy, but portends toward decreased catabolism, cardiovascular stress, and reduced risk of posttraumatic stress disorder [4]. Once the patient's burn wounds have been managed adequately, and wound closure and burn shock are resolving, a stepwise weaning of these agents is done to permit ventilator weaning and to avoid sequelae of withdrawal.

Parkland Formula: Total Fluids for 24 hours
Ringers Lactate = 4 cc × kg × % BSA
Example: A 70-kg man with a 50% TBSA burn would thus have a total deficit of 14 L (4 cc × 70 kg × 50% BSA = 14,000) in 24 h. Half the 24-h deficit should be repleted in the first 8 h, due to the high risk of hypovolemic shock early in the course. In this example that is 7 L within the first 8 h would mean a rate of 875 cc/h for the first 8 h. It is important to note that this recommendation starts at the time of injury, and often, patients are brought in hours after injury, often necessitating an increase or decrease in the rate to insure that this amount is given within the first 8 h. The rate would subsequently be decreased to **438 cc/h** for the next 16 h. The formulas are used to determine how much fluid should be given to the burn victim in the first 24 hours. Both formulas are being used today. The Brooke formula is the military formula and our service personnel will be resuscitated using this formula. Many of the other burn centers use the Parkland formula which was developed at the Parkland Trauma Center in Dallas, Texas.

FIGURE 166.4. Modified Brooke Formula:
Total Fluids for 24 hours
Ringers Lactate = 1.5 mL × kg × % BSA
Plasma = 0.5 mL × kg × % BSA
D5W = 2,000 mL

References

1. Venes D, Thomas CL, Taber CW: Taber's Online vs 2.0. Retrieved June 16, 2004, from www.tabers.com.
2. Herndon DN (ed): *Total Burn Care*. 2nd ed. London, Saunders, 2002.
3. Sheridan RL, Tompkins RG, Burns. in Greenfield LJ, Mulholland MW, Oldham KT, Zelenock GB, Lillemoe KD (eds): *Surgery: Scientific Principles and Practice*. 2nd ed. Philadelphia, Lippincott-Raven, 1997 p 420–437.
4. Cerovac S, Roberts AH: Burns sustained by hot bath and shower water. *Burns* 26(3):251–259, 2000.
5. JC Jeng A, Bridgeman L, Shivnan PM: Laser Doppler imaging determines need for excision and grafting in advance of clinical judgment: a prospective blinded trial. *Burns* 29(7):665–670, 2003.
6. Still JM, Law EJ: Primary excision of the burn wound. *Clin Plast Surg* 27(1):23–47, 2000.
7. Jaskille AD, Shupp JW, Pavlovich AR, et al: Outcomes from Burn Injury—should decreasing mortality continue to be our compass? *Clin Plast Surg* 36(4):701–708, 2009.
8. Ryan CM, Schoenfeld DA, Cassem EH, et al: Estimates of the probability of death from burn injuries. *N Engl J Med* 338(25):1848–1850, 1998.
9. Sheridan RL, Tompkins RG: What's new in burns and metabolism. *J Am Coll Surg* 198(2):243–263, 2004.
10. American Burn Association: Practice guidelines for burn care. *J Burn Care Rehabil* 1S–69S, 2001.
11. Buhl: Mitteilungen aus der pfeuferschen klinik: epidemische cholera. *Z Rationaelle Med* 6:1–105, 1855.
12. Fidler PE: Can Dermal Regeneration Template be Enhanced by Meshing, "V. A.C'ing" and Stacking? John A. Boswick M.D., Memorial Burn and Wound Symposium Maui, Hawaii February 25th, 2005.
13. Hemmila MR, Taddonio MA, Arbabi S, et al: Intensive insulin therapy is associated with reduced infectious complications in burn patients. *Surgery* 144(4):629–635; discussion 635–637, 2008.
14. Evers LH, Lassen A, Bhavsar D, et al: Reduction of apoptosis after I-NOS inhibition in full thickness burn wound. *J Burn Care Res* 30(2):S44, 2009.
15. Mcleod BC: Therapeutic apheresis: use of human serum albumin, fresh frozen plasma and cryosupernatant plasma in therapeutic plasma exchange. *Best Pract Clin Haematol* 19(1):157–167, 2006.
16. Pruitt BA: Does hypertonic burn resuscitation make a difference? *Crit Care Med* 28(1):277–278, 2000.
17. Agarwal N, Petro J, Salisbury RE: Physiologic profile monitoring in burned patients. *J Trauma* 23(7):577–583, 1983.
18. Kramer GC, Michell MW, Oliveira H, et al: Oral and enteral resuscitation of burn shock the historical record and implications for mass casualty care. *J Burns Surg Wound Care* [serial online] 2003;2(1):19. Retrieved June 18, 2004, from www.journalofburns.com.
19. Fuchs PC, Groger A, Bozkurt A: Cortisol in severely burned patients: investigations on disturbance of the hypothalamic-pituitary-adrenal axis. *Shock* 28(6):662–667, 2007.
20. Hunt TK, Ehrlich HP, Garcia JA, et al: Effect of vitamin a on reversing the inhibitory effect of cortisone on healing of open wounds in animals and man. *Ann Surg* 170:633–641, 1969.
21. Wicke C, Halliday B, Allen D, et al: Effects of steroids and retinoids on wound healing. *Arch Surg* 135:1265–1270, 2000.
22. Thiessen JL, Herndon LD, Traber HA, et al: Smoke inhalation and pulmonary blood flow. *Prog Resp Res* 26:77–84, 1990.
23. Tasaki O, Mozingo DW, Ishihara S, et al: Effect of Sulfo Lewis C on smoke inhalation injury in an ovine model. *Crit Care Med* 26(7):1238–1243, 1998.
24. Konigova R: Factors influencing survival and quality of life in burns. *Acta Chir Plast* 38(4):116–118, 1996.
25. Prien T: Toxic smoke compounds and inhalation injury—a review. *Burns* 14(6):451–460, 1998.
26. Cox RA, Soejima K, Burke AS, et al: Enhanced pulmonary expression of endothelin-1 in an ovine model of smoke inhalation injury. *J Burn Care Rehabil* 22(6):375–383, 2001.
27. Herndon DN, Traber DL, Niehaus GD, et al: The pathophysiology of smoke inhalation injury in a sheep model. *J Trauma* 24(32):1044–1051, 1984.
28. Rawlingson A: Nitric oxide, inflammation and acute burn injury. *Burns* 29:631–640, 2003.
29. Clark CJ, Campbell D, Reid WH: Blood carboxyhaemoglobin and cyanide levels in fire survivors. *Lancet* 1:1332–1335, 1981.
30. Murakami K, McGuire R, Cox RA, et al: Heparin nebulization attenuates acute lung injury in sepsis following smoke inhalation in sheep. *Shock* 18(3):236–241, 2002.
31. Tasaki O, Mozingo DW, Dubick MA, et al: Effects of heparin and lisofylline on pulmonary function after smoke inhalation injury in an ovine model. *Crit Care Med* 30(3):637–643, 2002.
32. Ivy ME, Possenti PP, Kepros J, et al: Abdominal compartment syndrome in patients with burns. *J Burn Care Rehabil* 20(5):351–353, 1999.
33. Ivy ME, Atweh NA, Palmer J, et al: Intra-abdominal hypertension and abdominal compartment syndrome in burn patients. *J Trauma* 49(3):387–391, 2000.
34. Kuwagata Y, Sugimoto H, Yoshioka T, et al: Left ventricular performance in patients with thermal injury or multiple trauma: a clinical study with echocardiography. *J Trauma* 32(2):158–165, 1992.

35. Gregg SC, Fidler PE, Atweh NA: Coronary stenting during burn shock: diagnostic and treatment considerations. *J Burn Care Rehabil* 27(6):905–909, 2006.
36. Bak Z, Sjöberg F, Eriksson O, et al: Cardiac dysfunction after burns. *Burns* 34(5):603–609, 2008.
37. Svensson L, Nordlander R, Axelsson C: Are predictors for myocardial infarction the same for women and men when evaluated prior to hospital admission? *Int J Cardiol* 109(2):241–247, 2006.
38. Voigt LP, Pastores SM, Raoof ND, et al: Review of a large clinical series: intrahospital transport of critically ill patients. *J Intensive Care Med* 24:108–115, 2009.
39. Kelemen JJ, Cioffi WG, Mason AD, et al: Effect of ambient temperature on metabolic rate after thermal injury. *Ann Surg* 223(4):406–412, 1996.
40. Oda J, Kasai K, Noborio M: Hypothermia during burn surgery and postoperative acute lung injury in extensively burned patients. *J Trauma* 66(6):1525–1530, 2009.
41. Botfield C, Hinds CJ: Growth hormone in catabolic illness. *Curr Opin Clin Nutr Metab Care* 3(2):139–144, 2000.
42. Pham TN, Klein MB, Gibran NS, et al: Impact of oxandrolone treatment on acute outcomes after severe burn injury. *J Burn Care Res* 29(6):902–906, 2008.
43. Peng X, Yan H, You Z, et al: Effects of enteral supplementation with glutamine granules on intestinal mucosal barrier function in severe burned patients. *Burns* 30:135–139, 2004.
44. Gibson B, Galiatsatos P, Rabiee A, et al: Intensive insulin therapy confers a similar survival benefit in the burn intensive care unit to the surgical intensive care unit. *Surgery* 146(5):922–930, 2009.
45. Tredget EE: Pseudomonas infections in the thermally injured patient. *Burns* 30:3–26, 2004.
46. Deitch EA, Rutan RL, Rutan TC: Burn management, in Irwin RS, Cerra FB, Rippe JM (eds): *Intensive Care Medicine*. 4th ed. Philadelphia, Lippincott-Raven, 1999.
47. Rai J, Jeschke M, Barrow RE, et al: Electrical injuries: a 30-year review. *J Trauma* 46(5):933–936, 1999.
48. Koumbourlis AC: Electrical injuries. *Crit Care Med* 30(11):S424–S430, 2002.
49. Zack F, Hammer U, Klett I, et al: Myocardial injury due to lightning. *Int J Legal Med* 110:326–328, 1997.
50. Lee RC, Zhang D, Hannig J: Biophysical injury mechanisms in electrical shock trauma. *Annu Rev Biomed Eng* 2:477–509, 2000.
51. Affleck DG, Edelman L, Morris SE: Assessment of tissue viability in complex extremity injuries: utility of the pyrophosphate nuclear scan. *J Trauma* 50(2):263–269, 2001.

CHAPTER 167 ■ ORTHOPEDIC INJURY

GREGORY J. DELLA ROCCA AND SEAN E. NORK

EPIDEMIOLOGY

Blunt and penetrating trauma kills more than 100,000 people in the United States each year, is the leading cause of death in Americans younger than 45 years of age, and results in staggering losses of health in surviving trauma patients, with associated losses of economic productivity [1]. Trauma evacuation systems have improved dramatically over the past few decades, and patients are much more likely to survive injuries that would have resulted in early mortality only 30 to 40 years ago. Many polytraumatized patients sustain orthopedic injuries, such as extremity fractures, pelvic fractures, or dislocations. These need to be recognized and addressed appropriately to minimize consequent morbidity and mortality. A dedicated orthopedic trauma service, specifically constructed to manage patients with complex fractures and dislocations in the setting of other systemic injuries, may be associated with improved outcomes for trauma patients. The orthopedic traumatologist is not only trained in the surgical management of the individual orthopedic injuries, but is also comfortable with functioning as a member of a multidisciplinary team that, of necessity, also includes emergency physicians, abdominal and chest surgeons, neurosurgeons, urologists, and plastic surgeons, to name a few.

Musculoskeletal injuries in trauma patients come in many varieties. Articular (joint) fractures represent complex injuries requiring prolonged reconstruction; although they routinely occur in polytraumatized patients, their management is beyond the scope of this discussion. Long bone (femur, tibia, humerus, forearm) fractures can have direct impact upon a patient's early mortality and late morbidity. Pelvic fractures are associated with early mortality, and their recognition and acute management is vital as part of the life-saving efforts of the trauma team. Open fractures are associated with the development of sepsis if not properly addressed. Compartment syndrome, a sequela of severe extremity trauma, is a soft-tissue condition that can result in early morbidity, associated with the impact of myonecrosis on renal function, as well as late disability, associated with fibrosis of one or more muscles important for activities of daily living. Venous thromboembolic (VTE) disease is a danger for all trauma patients, and the risk of VTE has been shown to be increased significantly in patients with pelvic and hip fractures. Finally, lesser fractures can have dramatic implications on future function for trauma patients; it has been shown that failure to identify and/or address complex injuries of the foot, for example, is associated with poor long-term outcomes in patients who survive major trauma [2,3].

In this chapter, we will introduce challenges and knowledge associated with multiple problems that affect trauma patients: open fractures, pelvic fractures, long bone fractures, knee dislocations, compartment syndrome, deep venous thrombosis, and neurological injury. It is our goal to discuss orthopedic treatment considerations for all of these trauma sequelae such that they can be integrated into the management of the patient who is the victim of multiple trauma.

OPEN FRACTURES

Open fractures, or fractures with associated skin wounds allowing communication of the external environment with the fractured bone surfaces, are present in a high percentage of polytraumatized patients. Frequently, the open fracture wound contains gross contamination, including dirt or vegetable matter, clothing, or glass. These wounds historically are at high risk of infection without adequate and early treatment of the open wound. Management protocols for open fractures are different from those for closed fractures, and considerations regarding timing of definitive stabilization of both types of fractures may differ. The basic treatment protocol for open fractures includes antibiotic administration, wound debridement, wound irrigation, fracture stabilization, and wound closure or coverage.

The Gustilo-Anderson classification scheme is the most widely utilized classification for open fractures. It was initially published in 1976 [4]. Type I open fractures are fractures with a clean wound measuring less than 1 cm in length. Type II open fractures are fractures with a laceration measuring more than 1 cm in length and without extensive soft tissue damage. Type III open fractures are fractures with extensive soft tissue damage or an open segmental fracture (a two-level fracture of the same long bone). "Special categories" were created for open fractures associated with vascular injuries, farm injuries, and high-velocity gunshot wounds. Type III fractures, therefore, represented a highly heterogeneous group of severe open fractures; a modification of the classification scheme for type III open fractures, published in 1981, was therefore developed [5]. Type IIIA open fractures have extensive soft tissue damage but adequate soft tissue coverage, or are the result of high-energy trauma irrespective of laceration size. Type IIIB open fractures entail extensive soft tissue loss, periosteal stripping, bone exposure, and massive contamination. No mention of requirement for muscle flap fracture coverage is made by the authors (despite the fact that many of these wounds indeed do require flap coverage); this is a bastardization of the classification that has been propagated over the years [6], although it was suggested by Gustilo himself in a subsequent letter to the editors of the *Journal of Bone and Joint Surgery* [7]. Type IIIC open fractures are those associated with a vascular injury that (importantly) requires repair; those open fractures associated with arterial injuries that are not repaired do not fall into this type. An important point must be made about this classification scheme: it is best utilized during operative debridement of the open fracture. The presence of a small open wound in the skin may belie the extensive soft tissue injury underneath, leading to a misclassification of the open fracture. However, this may be of relative unimportance, as the reliability of this classification scheme has been questioned [8–10].

Antibiotic administration has been shown to be highly effective in decreasing infection rates after open fractures [11]. Short courses of first generation cephalosporins (typically, cefazolin), initiated as soon as possible after injury, appear to be beneficial in limiting infections after open fracture [12]. Aminoglycosides and penicillins are often utilized in the treatment of type III open fractures and highly contaminated open fractures [13], respectively. Older studies have demonstrated that administration of broad-spectrum antibiotics lead to decreased infection rates [14]. However, the scientific evidence for this practice is limited [12]. Administration of aminoglycosides for the treatment of open fractures must be accomplished judiciously to minimize risk of oto- and nephrotoxicity. Quinolone antibiotics, effective against gram-negative bacteria, have been shown to be effective at reducing infection rates for type I and type II open fractures [15], but they may have an adverse effect on fracture healing; this effect has been shown in animal studies [16,17]. Duration of antibiotic administration is a matter of debate. Older recommendations included 72 hours of antibiotic treatment for types I and II open fractures and 120 hours for type III open fractures [18]. However, Dellinger et al. published in 1988 that a single day of antibiotics is as effective as 5-day regimens for preventing infection after open fracture, in a prospective randomized trial [19].

Surgical debridement of open fracture wounds in a complete and expeditious manner is likely the most important factor in successful management. Sharp debridement should be meticulous and methodical. All foreign material is removed. Bone ends should be delivered into the wound, and complete exploration of the injury zone is necessary. Often, long longitudinal extensions of the traumatic wound are necessary for adequate exploration. All tissue which is completely devitalized, including bone fragments devoid of soft tissue attachments, should be removed [20,21]. Judgments related to the removal of large articular (i.e., joint surface) fragments may be required to balance the risk of severe disability with loss of said fragments *versus* risk of infection with their retention. Devitalized extra-articular fragments can be cleaned and used as a reduction aid intraoperatively if fixation is proceeding immediately, or they may be stored and utilized later if fixation is delayed; these fragments are ultimately discarded [22]. In general, therefore, it is better not to discard bone fragments from open fractures until the patient has arrived in the operating room for definitive management of the open fracture by the orthopedic surgeon.

Wound irrigation generally follows sharp debridement. Little data exists on the type of irrigant, the amount of irrigant, and the method of irrigation that is the best. Irrigation solutions generally are based upon normal saline (0.9% NaCl). Additives historically have included bacitracin, cefazolin, neomycin, soaps, bleach, Betadine, and other antiseptics (such as benzalkonium chloride). Some of these, such as antiseptics, have been shown to be detrimental to wound viability [23]. Antibiotics appear to offer no benefit over normal saline alone [24]. A prospective, randomized study revealed that a nonsterile soap solution demonstrated decreased wound complications and equal efficacy at reducing infection after open fracture as compared to a sterile saline solution containing bacitracin [25]. A recent survey of nearly 1,000 orthopedic surgeons revealed a high preference for saline irrigant [26]. High *versus* low-pressure lavage for open fracture wounds has also been a source of debate. Although high-pressure lavage has been thought historically to be better for removal of surface bacteria and inorganic material from soft tissues, it is damaging to both soft tissues and bone, and there is some evidence that it can *increase* bacterial penetration of bone in an animal model [27]. The same survey of 984 orthopedic surgeons who revealed a preference for saline irrigant also revealed a preference for low-pressure lavage for open fracture wounds [26]. No consensus exists on the volume of irrigant. Protocols vary between institutions and even within institutions, based upon surgeon preference. Up to 9 liters of irrigant are utilized in some centers, but there is no scientific evidence upon which a recommendation can be based. Ultimately, it is the opinion of most surgeons that wound debridement is the most critical aspect of treating open fracture wounds, and that the irrigation component of this treatment is of relatively less importance.

Methods of fixation for open fractures are variable. Historically, acute open reduction and internal fixation of open fractures was contraindicated, without good scientific evidence. However, the Harborview group in Seattle demonstrated that acute open reduction and internal fixation of open ankle fractures is a safe and effective method of treatment [28]. External fixation is relatively rapid and fixation points can be kept out of the zone of injury. Mobilization of fracture ends can be accomplished at the time of future debridement, if necessary, and staged open reduction and internal fixation with external fixator removal is safe and effective [29–31]. Plate or nail fixation at the time of irrigation and debridement is also safe and effective [28,32], but limits the surgeon's ability to re-displace bone ends for wound exploration if repeat debridement is indicated.

Early wound closure or coverage is preferred, as this appears to limit the infection of open fracture wounds [33]. Acute primary closure of open fracture wounds after debridement and fixation, if possible, has been shown to be a safe method of treatment [34]. Early coverage of open fracture wounds that are unable to be closed primarily has also been shown to be safe and effective [35]. Adjuncts to wound closure, especially in the setting of skin tension, include "pie-crusting" of skin about the wound(s) [36] or performing open wound management with a vessel loop closure technique to re-approximate wound edges [37] and/or use of negative pressure wound dressings [38,39]. Also, if doubts about the safety of closure at the time of initial debridement and fixation persist, then open wound management and repeat debridement are appropriate until closure or coverage is considered safe. This may be a consideration for significantly contaminated wounds at the time of presentation, or open fracture wounds in polytraumatized patients [33]. Negative pressure wound dressings can be utilized successfully for open fracture wounds as a bridge to delayed closure with successful reduction of infection rates in some series [40], or as a bridge to delayed free tissue transfer with reduction of infection rates as compared to traditional dressings [41], perhaps allowing for a possible reduction in need for free tissue transfer [42]. However, this may be a limited process, and earlier wound closure or flap coverage may reduce infection rates over late wound closure or coverage, despite utilization of the negative pressure dressing [43].

An ongoing source of debate in the management of open fractures relates to the timing of debridement. A standard benchmark that has been propagated internationally is that open fractures should undergo urgent irrigation and debridement procedures within 6 hours. However, this benchmark has recently been questioned, as it appears to have little scientific evidence supporting it. In a seminal article on treatment of open fractures, Patzakis and Wilkins demonstrated no relationship between time from injury to surgical debridement of open fractures and subsequent development of infection [14]. A recent prospective, observational study of open fracture patients across eight trauma centers in the United States also failed to show a correlation between time to surgical debridement and the risk of infection of open fracture wounds [44]. Although urgency of treatment for open fractures associated with massive contamination, vascular injury, and/or limb crush is evident, routine emergent management does not appear to be required for open fractures, and after-hours surgery done in a hurried fashion by under-experienced practitioners and teams may result in an increased rate of minor complications [45]. However, it is generally accepted by orthopedic surgeons internationally that open fracture treatment does not represent an elective practice [46].

The polytraumatized patient who sustains high-energy open fractures of the extremities occasionally is a candidate for amputation. Properly indicated, a well-executed amputation can be a life-saving procedure which has the potential to shorten rehabilitation times associated with prolonged reconstruction of the mangled extremity. The debate often centers on whether a limb might be amenable to salvage *versus* amputation at the time of the trauma patient's arrival to the hospital. Errors in judgment regarding this problem have the potential to affect a patient's outcome significantly, both physiologically and psychologically. It should be noted that short-term and intermediate-term outcomes reveal similar levels of disability between limb salvage patients and amputees after major lower extremity trauma [47,48], perhaps indicating that one practice is not routinely better than another. Multiple assessment tools have been developed to assist surgeons with making decisions regarding limb salvage *versus* amputation, including the Mangled Extremity Severity Score (MESS) [49,50] (Table 167.1). However, many of these tools are mediocre at best with regard to their predictive value, as demonstrated by the Lower Extremity Assessment Project (LEAP) [51,52]. A historically held indication for acute amputation in the setting of a mangled extremity, the lack of plantar foot sensation, has been refuted

TABLE 167.1

MANGLED EXTREMITY SEVERITY SCORE (MESS)

Type	Characteristics	Injuries	Points
Skeletal/soft tissue group			
1	Low energy	Stab wound, simple closed fracture, small-caliber GSW	1
2	Medium energy	Open or multilevel fractures, dislocations, moderate crush injury	2
3	High energy	Shotgun blast, high-velocity GSW	3
4	Massive crush	Logging, railroad, oil rig accidents	4
Shock group			
1	Normotensive	BP stable in field and OR	0
2	Transiently hypotensive	BP unstable in field, responsive to IV fluids	1
3	Prolonged hypotension	Systolic BP <90 in field and unresponsive to IV fluids	2
Ischemia group			
1	None	Pulsatile limb, no sign of ischemia	0[a]
2	Mild	Diminished pulses, no sign of ischemia	1[a]
3	Moderate	No pulse via U/S, sluggish CR, paresthesia, diminished motor	2[a]
4	Advanced	Pulseless, cool, paralyzed, numb limb without CR	3[a]
Age group			
1	<30 years		0
2	30–50 years		1
3	>50 years		2

[a]Points ×2 if ischemic time >6 hours.
Note: MESS equals sum of scores for each of the group types; minimum score is 1, maximum score is 14.
BP, blood pressure; CR, capillary refill; GSW, gunshot wound; IV, intravenous; OR, operating room.
Adapted from Helfet DL, Howey T, Sanders R, et al: Limb salvage versus amputation: preliminary results of the Mangled Extremity Severity Score. *Clin Orthop* 256:80–86, 1990.

by the LEAP study team; many patients presenting with absent plantar foot sensation recovered it completely over time, indicating that the most tibial nerve injuries are neurapraxias (as opposed to complete disruptions) [53]. Ultimately, each injured patient must be carefully scrutinized, and no particular physical examination finding or trauma scale has been shown to be absolutely predictive of the success or failure of attempts at limb salvage. Therefore, thoughtful interpretation of trauma scores is imperative prior to making the choice between salvage and amputation for the mangled extremity in the traumatized patient.

PELVIC FRACTURES

Evaluation

The pelvic ring, functionally, is a rigid ring, despite the fact that it comprises three bones—two hipbones and the sacrum—with three articulations—two sacroiliac joints and the pubic symphysis. It is designed to distribute the weight of the torso, arms, and head onto the legs for normal bipedal ambulation. The pelvis contains the acetabulae, which represent the articulations with the lower extremities, and the lumbosacral junction, representing the articulation with the spine. The sacroiliac joints and pubic symphysis are thought to have minimal motion, and are connected by stout ligaments. In some cases, incompetence of these joints can lead to laxity and chronic pain, which may occur after trauma, complicated vaginal birth in females, or in an idiopathic manner [54,55]. Further ligamentous connection between the posterior and anterior pelvis is provided by the sacrospinous and sacrotuberous ligaments. The transverse processes of the fifth lumbar vertebra are attached to the posterior iliac crests by the iliolumbar ligaments.

Disruption of the pelvic ring in young patients requires a high-energy mechanism, such as a motor vehicle crash or fall from a significant height. As the pelvis functionally is a rigid ring, the discovery of a single break in that ring should prompt careful scrutiny for at least one other break. For example, pubic ramus fractures, in the anterior aspect of the pelvic ring, may be obvious on plain radiographs, but associated sacral fractures may not be readily apparent on plain radiographs due to the overlying bowel gas, radio-opaque contrast agents in the bowel or bladder, or bony anatomy. They may be visible on CT scanning. A high index of suspicion must be maintained. It should also be emphasized that acetabular fractures of a transverse nature (not isolated wall or column fractures) often represent a component of a pelvic ring disruption, and suspicion that such disruption has occurred should be maintained when these acetabular fracture types are present.

Multiple classification schemes exist that describe various aspects of pelvic ring injuries. The Young and Burgess classification is perhaps the most commonly utilized descriptive scheme for pelvic ring injuries, in which they are classified as anteroposterior compression (APC) injuries, lateral compression (LC) injuries, vertical shear (VS) injuries, and "complex patterns" [56]. The Young and Burgess classification can be helpful for identification of other problems that can be associated with the pelvic ring injury, such as increased incidence of head trauma with LC injuries and of abdominal and chest trauma with APC injuries [57], and it can be somewhat predictive of transfusion requirements in trauma patients [58]. Other commonly utilized classification schemes include the Tile classification [59] and the AO/Orthopedic Trauma Association classification [60]. No pelvic fracture classification scheme, however, possesses all seven of the following requisites for universally applicable schemes: ease of use, prognostic value (outcomes), descriptive value (describe the injury), therapeutic value (direct treatment), research value (allows direct comparison between groups), intra-observer reliability, and inter-observer reliability.

Orthopedic examination of the pelvic fracture patient is similar to the orthopedic examination of all polytraumatized patients, covering the entire musculoskeletal system in a methodical manner. Focused examination of the pelvis includes observation of limb deformity; abnormal limb rotation or shortening in the setting of pelvis injury may be secondary either to pelvic deformity or to hip dislocation (with or without associated acetabular fracture), or to extra-pelvic lower extremity fracture. Skin about the pelvis, including about the perineum, must be carefully examined for lacerations that can be associated with open pelvic fractures. Open wounds may be present within folds of skin, and a thorough examination is necessary. Lacerations may lurk within the fold of skin inferior to the scrotum in males, and examination of this area cannot be neglected. Extensive ecchymoses should be noted; these may be indicative of degloving injuries. Digital rectal examination is also required to detect occult open fractures into the rectum, and (chaperoned) vaginal examination is also required in women to detect open fractures violating the vaginal vault. Speculum examination is not generally performed in the trauma bay. Blood emanating from the anus or vagina can be an indicator of open pelvic fracture. Urethral disruptions can also occur with pelvic fracture, and blood at the urethral meatus can be indicative of such an injury. Manual palpation of the pelvis and gentle compression of the iliac crests may detect abnormal motion or crepitus associated with an unstable disruption of the pelvic ring, although this manipulation lacks sensitivity and specificity [61]. Pelvic manipulations must be undertaken judiciously; unstable pelvic ring disruptions can cause life-threatening hemorrhage, which can be exacerbated by repeated examinations. Repeated examinations also can induce severe patient discomfort. A neurovascular examination of both legs, as well as examination of anal sphincter tone and of the bulbocavernosus reflex, is routine.

Standard radiography of the pelvis begins with the anteroposterior view. The inlet radiograph, with the beam tilted approximately 40° caudad, can detect anteroposterior translation of the hemipelvis and rotational hemipelvic deformities. The outlet radiographs, with the beam tilted approximately 40° cephalad, can detect "vertical" translation (more often, a flexion deformity) of the hemipelvis and is useful for visualizing sacral fractures. Judet radiographs, with the patient or x-ray beam tilted approximately 45° to either side, are reserved for patients with acetabular fractures detected on anteroposterior radiographs. Computed tomography (CT) has become routine for polytraumatized patients, and provides extensive information regarding the bony anatomy of a pelvic fracture and/or dislocation. In the setting of pelvic and acetabular fractures, CT scanning is also invaluable for planning of the surgical reconstruction. The CT scan is of limited utility, however, for acetabular fractures if the hip remains dislocated during the scan. Therefore, it is desirable to reduce fracture-dislocations of the hip (acetabulum) prior to CT scanning of the pelvis for adequate delineation of fracture anatomy and for preoperative planning.

Acute Management

Pelvic fracture patients often have multiple associated injuries, all of which may contribute to the overall physiological condition of the patient. Early mortality of patients with pelvic fractures may be related to patient age and occurs as a result of catastrophic hemorrhage, head injury, or multiple organ system failure [62,63]. As the pelvic fracture may contribute directly to morbidity and mortality, early stabilization is preferred. This stabilization may be performed at the scene of the injury by emergency medical personnel, by the application of a circumferential sheet, pelvic binder, or other compressive garment. Sheets are readily available, inexpensive, and easy to apply [64]. The personnel applying the sheet should do their best to avoid wrinkling the sheet, which may cause skin compromise [65]. Overcompression of the pelvic ring is avoided, as the exact nature of the pelvic injury is unknown; overcompression of certain types of unstable fracture patterns may lead to laceration of the bladder, rectum, vagina, or other intrapelvic structures. Although circumferential pelvic wraps may assist with patient transport and comfort and can successfully reduce some types of pelvic ring disruptions [66], a recent study failed to demonstrate decreases in mortality, transfusion requirements, or the need for pelvic angiography by their use [67].

Upon arrival at the trauma center, all circumferential clothing (including pelvic wraps/binders) is removed to allow for examination of the lower abdomen and pelvis. Binders or wraps can easily be re-applied after examination. Large-bore intravenous access is necessary for fluid resuscitation. Keeping patients warm avoids coagulopathy. Although pelvic fractures may be associated with catastrophic hemorrhage, ongoing hemodynamic instability can arise from a number of causes unrelated to the specific pelvic injury. A full assessment of the patient is required. "Open book" (i.e., anteroposterior compression) injuries of the pelvis can be treated with reapplication of a circumferential wrap. Grossly unstable pelvic injuries can be treated provisionally with the application of skeletal traction, on the same side(s) of the pelvic injury(ies), through either the distal femur or the proximal tibia as the side of pelvic instability. Skeletal traction is also used routinely in the provisional stabilization of acetabular fractures prior to definitive treatment in the operating room; traction can minimize contact of the femoral head with rough acetabular fracture edges.

Pelvic external fixation can be utilized in a resuscitative fashion. External fixator application is difficult, but possible, in the trauma bay. An experienced orthopedic surgeon should perform external fixation of the pelvis, if indicated, to avoid inaccurate pin placement and associated cutout of pins from the iliac crests or injury to the intrapelvic or gluteal structures [68]. Factors that increase difficulty for the application of anteriorly based external fixators can be the rotational deformity and/or instability of one or both hemipelves. Anteriorly based pelvic external fixators are not good at controlling completely unstable posterior pelvic ring disruptions, and reduction of the anterior pelvic ring may be associated with further displacement of the posterior pelvic ring in some circumstances [69]. The antishock "C-clamp" has also been utilized successfully for emergent stabilization of the unstable pelvic ring disruptions [70]. It was designed to be placed posteriorly, with the clamp engaging the posterolateral ilia and exerting compression. The connecting frame can be rotated out of the way to allow for access to the abdomen or perineum. Dangers of application of the C-clamp, especially by inexperienced practitioners, can include fracture and/or penetration of one or both ilia or aberrant placement of one or both ends of the clamp through the greater sciatic notch(es) [71]. The C-clamp has also been applied successfully to the anterior pelvic ring as a resuscitative aid [72].

Patients with pelvic ring disruptions may demonstrate hemodynamic instability that is refractory to volume resuscitation. An ongoing search for sources of blood loss is vital. A recent publication demonstrated that, at a single trauma center, 21% of patients with pelvic fractures and hemodynamic instability (systolic blood pressure <90 mm Hg) refractory to a 2 L bolus of saline ultimately expired, and 75% of those patients expired as a result of exsanguination [73]. Unstable pelvic fractures are more highly associated with pelvic hemorrhage than are stable pelvic fractures. Therefore, investigation of other potential sources of hemorrhage is vital, especially in the hemodynamically unstable trauma patient with a stable pelvic fracture pattern [74]. Patients with unstable anteroposterior compression injuries have been demonstrated to require massive transfusions, followed by those patients with vertical shear or complex mechanism pelvic ring disruptions, and lastly by those with lateral compression injuries [58,75]. However, fracture pattern may not always be indicative of transfusion requirements or the need for angiographic arterial embolization [76].

The hemodynamically unstable patient with a pelvic ring disruption may have significant fracture-associated hemorrhage. Pelvic fracture-associated bleeding comes from three sources: fracture surfaces, lacerated or ruptured veins, or lacerated or ruptured arteries. Fracture surfaces may not be a source of ongoing massive blood loss, and therefore may contribute negligibly to hemodynamic instability [77]. Distinguishing between major sources of pelvic hemorrhage—arterial or venous—represents a challenging but important task, and prior studies have examined multiple factors that may be associated with successful angiographic embolization, used for arterial hemorrhage, including patient age, trauma scores, shock on arrival to the trauma center, and fracture pattern [78]. Venous hemorrhage after pelvic fracture can be adequately treated with pelvic stabilization, either by circumferential pelvic wrap or by external fixation, while arterial hemorrhage can be addressed with angiographic embolization [79]. Transient response to initial resuscitation, lack of response to provisional pelvic stabilization, and presence of a contrast blush on pelvic CT scanning are all thought to be indicative of arterial hemorrhage that may be amenable to angiographic embolization [80,81].

Pelvic packing has been used for control of severe hemorrhage in hemodynamically unstable patients. It has been proposed that packing may be a more reliable method of treating severe pelvic fracture-associated hemorrhage than angiographic embolization with regard to controlling continued hemorrhage and limiting patient death due to exsanguination [82]. Angiography may also be delayed, and emergency stabilization of the fracture along with or without pelvic packing may be more reliable at controlling severe fracture-associated hemorrhage [83]. Another recent series documented a 30-day survival rate for pelvic fracture patients treated with extraperitoneal pelvic packing of 72%, and subsequent angiography was successful in detecting arterial hemorrhage in 80% of the patients after packing. Immediate increases in systolic blood pressure after packing were also noted [84]. Importantly, both angiography and pelvic packing must be used in a judicious fashion; this will help minimize complications related to both (such as gluteal necrosis).

Genitourinary injuries occur in a small subset of patients with pelvic fracture. This frequency has been shown to approximate 4.6% in a recent study of the U.S.A. National Trauma Data Bank [85]. Another recent study estimated a genitourinary injury rate of 6.8% in pelvic fractures; importantly, 23% of these injuries were missed at the time of initial evaluation [86]. Bladder injuries can also be seen in conjunction with acetabular fractures [87]. Urological injuries most commonly take the form of urethral disruption, extraperitoneal bladder rupture, or intraperitoneal bladder rupture. Diagnosis is often by retrograde cystourethrogram, with careful attention to post-drainage images to detect bladder ruptures not detectable when the bladder is filled with contrast [88]. Urethral disruption appears to occur distal to the urogenital diaphragm, contrary to classical teaching [89]. Primary realignment, when possible, is accomplished endoscopically followed by threading of the urinary catheter by the Seldinger technique [90]. This repair may be accomplished at the time of pelvic fracture repair, using a team approach [91]. Routine use of suprapubic catheters in the management of urethral disruptions is discouraged, as it may increase the rate of infection, especially in the setting of open reduction and internal fixation of anterior pelvic ring injuries [92]. Bladder injuries are more commonly extraperitoneal. Nearly all present with gross hematuria. Intraperitoneal bladder ruptures are generally treated with surgical exploration, to delineate the extent of injury fully, and with Foley (preferred if open reduction and internal fixation of the pelvic ring fractures will be accomplished) or suprapubic catheters. Extraperitoneal ruptures may be managed with Foley catheters; the bulk of these require no formal repair [93]. However, if open reduction and internal fixation of the pelvic fracture is planned, then primary repair of the extraperitoneal rupture is also accomplished at the same time, with a low infection rate [91]. Use of suprapubic catheters is not required if large-bore Foley catheters are employed after repair of bladder ruptures.

Open pelvic fractures represent a subset of severe injuries with a historically high mortality rate. A recent systematic review calculated the total mortality rate in open pelvic fracture patients across multiple published series prior to 1991 as 30%, and since 1991 as 18%, with the decrease likely owing to aggressive management of the pelvic fracture, selective diversion of the fecal stream, and advances in critical care medicine [94]. These open fractures may be occult, localized within the rectum or vagina. Visual as well as digital exploration is mandatory in these patients. Examination of bowel contents for gross or occult blood is also necessary. Diversion of the fecal stream may be indicated in patients with extensive or posterior wounds associated with their pelvic fractures, but routine use of fecal diversion does not appear to reduce infection rates in patients with open pelvic fractures [95]. Selective fecal diversion, however, does appear beneficial in open pelvic fracture patients with perineal wounds [96].

LONG BONE FRACTURES

Femoral Shaft Fractures

Femoral shaft fractures often occur in conjunction with other injuries after high-velocity blunt or penetrating trauma. Fracture of the femur is associated with significant morbidity in the polytraumatized patient; significant hemorrhage can occur, even in the absence of open wounds. Bilateral femoral shaft fractures are associated with higher mortality rates than are seen in patients with unilateral femoral shaft fractures [97]. Open femoral shaft fractures are unusual and require significant energy to create the situation where the fracture fragment(s) travel(s) through the robust soft tissue envelope of the thigh. Thorough evaluation of any femur fracture patient for associated injuries is necessary.

Initial management of femoral shaft fractures often entails placement of traction devices in the field. These devices are meant to be portable, and they rest against the ischial tuberosity, against which they provide traction through the ankle or the foot. Splinting of femoral shaft fractures is marginally effective at best, as it requires a splint to include the trunk for effective immobilization. The portable traction devices should be removed as quickly as possible to prevent sciatic nerve pressure injury or skin ulceration. Skin or, more commonly, skeletal traction is routinely applied in the emergency department, as a temporizing measure prior to transport to the operating room and to allow for continued evaluation of the patient for other injuries. This traction provides patient comfort, provides immobilization for the fracture, and limits fracture shortening. It can also function as a temporary treatment modality in the setting of operating room unavailability. Evaluation of the patient prior to transport to the operating room should include an investigation of the ipsilateral femoral neck with thorough radiographic imaging. A high percentage of femoral neck fractures are missed in the setting of ipsilateral femoral shaft fractures, and CT scans do not appear to be 100% sensitive for their diagnosis [98].

Operative management is the mainstay of therapy for fractures of the femoral shaft. In the United States, definitive treatment of the femoral shaft fracture patient in skeletal traction is of historical interest only. A distinct advantage of femur fracture stabilization includes the ability to mobilize the patient, thereby avoiding complications associated with prolonged bed rest in critically injured patients, such as pneumonia, pressure ulcers, and deep vein thrombosis. The gold standard for treatment of closed fractures of the femoral shaft is reamed, statically locked, antegrade (from the hip region) medullary nailing. This method of treatment has been demonstrated to be highly effective in numerous studies [99–101], and it can allow for early unprotected weight bearing [102]. Open fractures of the femoral shaft are also effectively treated with medullary nailing, after appropriate irrigation and debridement [10]. Entry portal—piriformis fossa *versus* trochanteric—seems to make little difference in healing rates [101]. Early dynamic locking can be associated with shortening of the fracture, and is generally not utilized in trauma [103]. Retrograde nailing (entry point through the knee) is also effective [104]. Reaming prior to nailing appears to improve healing rates of femoral shaft fractures [105,106], although this may come at the expense of increased pulmonary injury in the setting of chest-injured patients [107].

Other methods of fixation for femoral shaft fractures include open reduction and internal fixation with a plate-and-screw construct and external fixation. Plate fixation is often, but not always, reserved for extremely proximal or extremely distal femoral shaft fractures and for fractures in which intramedullary fixation is contraindicated (e.g., the presence of device, such as a total hip arthroplasty stem, within the femoral canal). Plate fixation has been employed successfully in polytraumatized patients with femoral shaft fractures [108]. External fixation can also be used in the acute setting to stabilize femoral shaft fractures in a minimally invasive and rapid fashion. Although femoral shaft fractures can heal with definitive external fixation, this method of treatment is rarely utilized. Conversion of external fixation to medullary nail fixation for femoral shaft fractures has been demonstrated to be effective and safe [29–31].

Early femoral shaft stabilization is associated with improved outcomes in polytraumatized patients [109]. The method of stabilization is unimportant for these early outcomes; medullary nailing, plate and screw fixation, or external fixation all provide similar benefit. Controversy remains regarding the optimal method of early femur fracture stabilization in the polytraumatized patient, including chest- and head-injured patients. The Hannover group has published extensively regarding the second-hit phenomenon of femoral nailing in polytraumatized patients, and has made recommendations that pulmonary- and head-injured patients perhaps undergo acute "damage-control orthopedic surgery" with external fixation of a femoral shaft fracture, followed by staged conversion from external fixation to medullary nailing when the patient's condition has improved and resuscitation has been completed [107,110–112]. However, some recent studies have demonstrated that reduced rates of acute respiratory distress syndrome (ARDS) can be achieved with acute nailing of femoral shaft fractures, instead of with damage control orthopedics, in polytraumatized patients [113–115]. Adequate resuscitation has been shown to be important prior to nailing [114]. Also, the utilization of reaming has been shown not to create increased rates of ARDS in polytraumatized patients undergoing medullary nailing of femur fractures, as compared to patients undergoing nailing without reaming [114].

Tibial Shaft Fractures

Fractures of the tibial shaft are very common in polytraumatized individuals and after high-velocity trauma. Tibial fractures have a higher likelihood of being open [116,117], perhaps secondary to the thin soft tissue envelope surrounding the human tibia. This soft tissue envelope may also play a role in the increased likelihood of infection and nonunion for tibial fractures treated operatively; infected nonunion is more common after tibial fracture than after any other fracture of a long bone [118]. Compartment syndrome is also common after high-energy fractures of the tibia, even when the fractures are open [10].

Principles of treatment of tibial shaft fractures are similar to those of femoral shaft fractures; to provide comfort, restore length, alignment, and rotation, and allow for early mobilization. Tibial fractures are commonly treated with medullary nailing techniques, unless there are fracture extensions into the knee and/or ankle joint. Nailing of tibia fractures can provide sufficient stability to allow for full weight bearing after surgery [119]. Plating of tibia fractures is more often done for those fractures with involvement of the articular surfaces of the tibia, and normally weight bearing is restricted in those patients until some evidence of radiographic healing is present. External fixation is most often utilized in a temporary fashion, especially with large open wounds requiring repeat debridement, in complex fractures involving the tibial plateau or tibial plafond, or in patients with significant physiological instability. Conversion of external fixation to nailing is safe, when the patient's condition permits [30,31].

Tibia fractures in patients sustaining multisystem trauma can be stabilized in a delayed fashion, after the physiological condition of the patient has improved. Unlike femoral shaft fractures, tibia fractures can be effectively treated temporarily with long-leg splints. This allows for patients to be gotten out of bed and to sit up in bed or a chair, with improvements in pulmonary function. However, splinted tibia fractures must be carefully monitored for skin breakdown from the splinting material, compartment syndrome, and impending skin compromise from unstable fracture ends.

Humeral Shaft Fractures

Fractures of the humeral shaft are a source of morbidity in polytraumatized patients. They have implications for early rehabilitation as well as for future function. Injuries associated with humeral shaft fractures that have profound consequences on outcomes include brachial artery injuries and nerve injuries; the radial nerve is particularly susceptible to concomitant injury with humeral shaft fracture. Management of humeral shaft fractures and their sequelae are based upon the overall condition of the patient and on the personality of the injury.

Humeral shaft fractures, when they occur in isolation, are particularly amenable to closed management. Splinting, casting, and fracture bracing have all been noted to be highly successful in achieving union of humerus fractures [120,121], and long-term outcomes (at a minimum of 1 year) are thought to be as good as those after surgical repair [122]. Critically, these results were obtained in isolated humeral shaft fractures. Considerations for the management of humerus fractures in polytraumatized patients, however, likely are different.

Polytraumatized patients often require the use of both arms for effective mobilization and rehabilitation. They often are subjected to prolonged bed rest, and may be incapable of the frequent fracture brace adjustment that is advocated by Sarmiento and colleagues [120]. As fracture braces are not generally utilized in the acute phase after fracture (delay of 1 to 3 weeks prior to application is common), early splints can be cumbersome for patients and caregivers, can be unwieldy, and are not generally removable for the purposes of skin monitoring and vascular access. Obtunded patients also cannot complain about pressure points beneath a non-removable splint, and they do not routinely change position in an effort to alleviate pressure points. Skin necrosis can be a danger in this setting. For all of these reasons, management of humeral shaft fractures in polytraumatized patients is normally operative.

Humerus fractures can be treated either with open reduction and internal fixation, utilizing a plate-and-screw construct, or with medullary nailing. Advocates of plate-and-screw fixation cite the ability of humeral shaft fracture patients to utilize their arms for assistance with ambulation (i.e., weight-bearing on crutches or a walker) after fixation [123]. Advocates of medullary nailing for humeral shaft fractures have demonstrated good outcomes [124], although no literature exists that provides evidence regarding immediate weight bearing after nailing of humerus fractures. Some literature exists that appears to favor plating *versus* nailing for humeral shaft fractures, as shoulder impingement and reoperation risk appear to be lower with plating [125–127], although a definitive answer regarding optimal surgical treatment of humeral shaft fractures is not available. In the setting of radial nerve palsy, present between 8% and 11% of the time [128,129], nerve exploration can also occur at the time of surgery. However, radial nerve palsy is not an indication for operative exploration of the nerve [130]; the bulk of radial nerve palsies appear to be neurapraxias, and a recent study reported that 89% recover normal distal neurological function after closed humeral shaft fracture management [131]. Even secondary radial nerve palsies (those occurring later, such as after fracture manipulation) appear to have a high rate of complete recovery despite nonoperative management [129].

Forearm Fractures

Forearm fractures, while not often a contributing factor to mortality in the polytraumatized patient, are a source of long-term morbidity if not properly addressed. The forearm functions as a mobile unit which is dependent upon the anatomy of the radius and the ulna. The radius and ulna are "parallel" but curved bones, and this anatomy is vital for the maintenance of proper forearm rotation (pronation and supination). The maximal radial bow has been shown, in anatomical studies, to be approximately 16 mm and located near the junction between the middle and distal one thirds of the forearm length [132]. Encroachment of either bone or of foreign material into this region may have adverse consequences on forearm rotation, and may create limitations of pronation, supination, or both.

Fracture of one bone of the adult forearm often leads to injury associated with the other bone, whether it is fracture or dislocation of the other bone, with dislocation of the other bone; dislocation, when it occurs, is either at the elbow (radius) or wrist (ulna). The anatomical connections between the radius and ulna include the proximal and distal radioulnar joints and the interosseous ligaments; deformation of one bone, due to fracture, that is not "compensated" by fracture of the other bone will cause the other bone to be drawn in the direction of the deformation, causing dislocation. Typical patterns include displaced proximal ulnar shaft fractures associated with dislocations of the radial head from the capitellum (the "Monteggia" fracture–dislocation) and displaced distal radial shaft fractures associated with dislocations of the ulnar head from the distal radioulnar joint (the "Galeazzi" fracture–dislocation).

Careful scrutiny of the elbow, forearm, and wrist is vital for the detection of these injuries, which may be overlooked in the setting of multiple trauma. Failure to recognize these injuries acutely can result in increased difficulty with surgical reconstruction (if accomplished late) or significant disability (if reconstruction is never accomplished). Forearm fractures tend to shorten, due to the powerful investing musculature of the forearm, and surgical repair is often more straightforward when it can be undertaken within a few days of injury. Perfect anatomical reconstruction is associated with the best outcomes. Early motion is encouraged to minimize the likelihood of excessive bone formation within the injured tissues between the radius and ulna, which can lead to encroachment of the two bones and restriction of forearm rotation. The repaired forearm is often protected and weight bearing is restricted for a number of weeks. However, "platform" walkers or crutches may be utilized for assistance with ambulation in many cases; the weight of assisted ambulation is borne through the elbow (as opposed to the wrist and forearm) with these devices.

Although forearm fractures may not be a direct cause of early mortality in most patients who succumb to the sequelae of severe trauma, it can be a contributing factor. Forearm fractures can result in lacerations of the ulnar and/or radial arteries, which can contribute to blood loss. Forearm compartment syndrome can also develop in the patient with severe forearm fractures; unrecognized compartment syndrome can result in myonecrosis with resultant myoglobinuria and potential contribution to renal insufficiency (see below), let alone future disability. Open fractures of the forearm should not be thought to decompress the compartments of the forearm adequately; a heightened index of suspicion of compartment syndrome should be maintained in all patients with high-energy fractures of the forearm, whether they are closed or open fractures.

COMPARTMENT SYNDROME

Muscle groups are divided into compartments by layers of fascia, which are noncompliant. Injury to a particular muscular compartment can induce edema and/or hemorrhage within the compartment, leading to increased intracompartmental pressures due to the noncompliant nature of the surrounding fascia. Increased intracompartmental pressure can lead to venous congestion and resultant muscle ischemia within the involved compartment(s). This scenario is termed "compartment syndrome." As nerves traverse the muscular compartments, they are also susceptible to compartment pressure-related compromise.

The absolute intracompartmental pressure at which a compartment syndrome exists continues to be a matter of debate. Some authors have previously advocated threshold intracompartmental pressures, such as absolute values of 30 mm Hg or 40 mm Hg, as diagnostic of compartment syndrome. However, a differential between intracompartmental pressure and diastolic blood pressure is thought to be a more reliable indicator of evolving compartment syndrome. The pressure differential (referred to as ΔP or "delta-P") thought to be diagnostic of compartment syndrome is commonly accepted to be 30 mm Hg or less [133]. The improved reliability of ΔP measurements, as opposed to absolute measurements of intracompartmental pressures alone, was recently illustrated in a series of 101 tibial fracture patients. In this series, 41 patients had continuous leg intramuscular compartment pressures more than 30 mm Hg for over 6 hours in the setting of a satisfactory ΔP (defined as $\geq$30 mm Hg). No difference in outcome regarding return to function and muscle strength was noted, as compared to a control group of 60 patients without elevated intramuscular pressures [134].

The number of muscle compartments is variable based upon location in the body. The brachium has two muscular compartments (anterior and posterior), the forearm has three muscular compartments (dorsal, volar, and mobile wad), the thigh has three muscular compartments (anterior, posterior, and adductor), and the leg has four muscular compartments (anterior, lateral, superficial posterior, and deep posterior). The exact number of muscular compartments in the hand and the foot are a matter of debate. Hand compartments include the interosseous compartments as well as the thenar and hypothenar compartments, and foot compartments include the interosseous compartments as well as the abductor and adductor compartments. The gluteal muscles are also contained within fascial compartments, and gluteal compartment syndromes have been documented in obtunded trauma patients as well as intoxicated patients (and others with an altered level of consciousness), with the gluteal muscles in a dependent position, who do not change their position for an extended period of time [135].

Compartment syndrome is a problem that can arise in polytraumatized patients who have sustained high-energy injuries. Younger patients may be more susceptible [136]. Typical injuries associated with development of compartment syndrome include fractures, dislocations, crush injuries, and prolonged episodes of limb ischemia. The syndrome can also develop after reperfusion of a dysvascular limb that occurs after a revascularization procedure or simply after a manipulative reduction of a fracture that reduces kinking and occlusion of vessels. Isolated soft-tissue injury (without fracture) was the second most common cause of compartment syndrome in a large series of patients reviewed over an eight-year period [137]. Another study examined a cohort of 38 patients without fracture who developed compartment syndrome at a single trauma unit in Great Britain. Frank muscle necrosis was noted in 20% of patients without fracture, as compared to 8% of patients with fracture, indicating that a high index of suspicion for compartment syndrome in trauma patients must be maintained, even in patients without fractures [138]. Penetrating injuries, such as gunshot and stab wounds, can lacerate arteries within a single compartment or multiple compartments, leading to hemorrhage under pressure into a confined environment and creating a compartment syndrome. The presence of a penetrating injury or open fracture (which results in fascial disruption) should ***not*** create a false sense that compartment syndrome will not develop; compartment syndromes have been documented to occur in the setting of penetrating injury or open fracture [139].

Compartment syndrome can also develop after stabilization of a fracture, such as after nailing a tibia fracture, once the compartment has been returned to its pre-injury length and its available volume is thereby diminished. This "finger-trap" phenomenon was initially described in the literature by Matsen and Clawson [140]. More recent mathematical and experimental analyses indicate that the available volume within a given muscular compartment varies inversely with acute changes in the length of the limb [141]. Tibial traction or fracture reduction in the setting of tibial shaft fractures raises compartment pressures [142]. A fracture situation in which excessive shortening is corrected, or vigorous traction is required to maintain reduction, should perhaps prompt increased vigilance for the development of compartment syndrome. This risk must be balanced, however, during staged management of severe fractures, as the consequence of initial inadequate limb-length restoration may be increased difficulty of the definitive reconstructive procedure at the time of formal open reduction and internal fixation. Also, a recent report revealed that in tibial plateau fractures, application of an external fixator device which spans the knee and fracture may lead to transient elevations of intracompartmental pressure, but does not appear to cause a compartment syndrome [143].

Missed compartment syndromes can lead to significant morbidity. Frank muscle necrosis is a normal sequela of compartment syndrome, and associated joint contractures have been extensively described in the literature. Elevated levels of serum creatine phosphokinase (CPK) or the appearance of myoglobinuria (which can be misinterpreted as hematuria) are associated with muscle necrosis, and have been utilized in the past as diagnostic tools for evolving compartment syndromes [144,145]. Delayed treatment of compartment syndrome is fraught with complications [146]. Infection rates are dramatically increased when fasciotomy for compartment syndrome is delayed [147]. Fasciotomy revision, performed in a delayed fashion for inadequate index fasciotomy (and failure to relieve compartment syndrome), has been associated with increased rates of mortality and major amputation [148]. Often, it is not possible to determine the exact time of onset for a compartment syndrome. Therefore, the recommendation is that fasciotomy be undertaken as expeditiously as possible after diagnosis of compartment syndrome, and that a high index of suspicion for the development of compartment syndrome should be maintained in patients with high-energy trauma or trauma patients who are obtunded.

Compartment syndromes should be diagnosed during the evolution phase. A high clinical suspicion should be maintained in any patient who has sustained a high-energy injury. Pain out of proportion to the injury should alert the examiner to the possibility of impending compartment syndrome. Orthopedic injuries are very painful by their nature, and patients often have differing pain tolerances (sometimes affected by chronic narcotic use/abuse), so the examiner should be sensitive to *changes* in pain level as reported by the injured patient. Traditionally, the "five P's" have been utilized in the awake, responsive patient for examination of the leg and ruling out compartment syndrome: pain with palpation of the compartment, pallor, paresthesia, pain with passive stretch, and pulselessness are commonly quoted as signs of compartment syndrome. Pulselessness should not be included in this list, as it requires excessive pressures to occlude arteries–in excess of systolic pressure–and should this scenario arise, it would likely be associated with complete myonecrosis within compartments involved. Excessive pain with passive stretch of muscles within each compartment should alert the examiner to evolving compartment syndrome. Awareness of the patient's injuries and their direct contribution to pain with the motion of a joint (e.g., intra-articular fracture) should be considered. All compartments in a traumatized extremity should be examined. Muscle compartments tend to be very firm in the setting of evolving compartment syndrome.

Direct monitoring of intracompartmental pressure is possible utilizing the wick catheter technique, an arterial pressure line setup, or a variety of commercially available devices. These methods provide direct measurements of intracompartmental pressures in mm Hg. It should be emphasized, however, that compartment syndrome is primarily a diagnosis based upon physical examination. Physical examination findings consistent with evolving compartment syndrome should prompt surgical intervention, even in the setting of compartment pressure measurements that indicate normal ΔP, as the consequences of missed compartment syndrome include frank myonecrosis and irreversible neurological injury. Complete reliance upon direct intracompartmental measurements may result in undertreatment or overtreatment of compartment syndrome. Intracompartmental pressure measurements have been shown to be highest within 5 cm of fracture, and measurements taken outside of this zone may be spuriously low and lead to undertreatment [149]. Also, there is a documented decrease in diastolic blood pressure after induction of general anesthesia; intracompartmental pressure measurements obtained in a patient under anesthetic must be interpreted cautiously as the ΔP value may be spuriously low and lead to overtreatment [150]. Diagnosis of compartment syndrome is variably difficult, even at large trauma centers [151], and high indices of suspicion need to be maintained to prevent undertreatment (and overtreatment) of compartment syndromes.

Obtunded patients should be monitored serially. The examiner should note compartment firmness and proceed appropriately. Significant degrees of subcutaneous edema can mask tense compartments. Compartment pressure monitoring with commercially available devices or with an arterial pressure line setup may be utilized for diagnosis in the obtunded patient, especially if the patient exhibits no response to painful stimuli and if physical examination of compartment tightness is impeded by extensive surrounding edema (e.g., with anasarca).

Open fractures do not necessarily decompress compartments through which the fracture fragments or projectiles have penetrated. An approximately 9% rate of compartment syndrome has been reported with open fractures of the tibial shaft [139]. The degree of soft tissue injury appeared to be directly proportional to the incidence of compartment syndrome in this population. Therefore, compartment syndrome should be suspected in all patients with appropriate symptomatology, and the presence of open wounds does not negate the possibility that compartment syndrome may be evolving.

Techniques of fasciotomy have been described extensively. Adequate decompression of all compartments in the affected portion of the extremity is the goal. During fasciotomy, nonviable muscle is debrided. Following fasciotomy, closure of the fascia is not indicated (this would re-create the compartment syndrome). Skin closure should be undertaken cautiously. Use of vessel loops to assist with skin reapproximation has been described [152]. Negative-pressure wound therapy devices may also be beneficial in promoting growth of granulation tissue on a fasciotomy bed, in anticipation of skin grafting, or in maintaining smaller wound dimensions, in anticipation of delayed primary closure [153,154]. Most fasciotomy patients will require return to the operating room for further irrigation and debridement procedures, followed by delayed primary skin closure or skin grafting.

The greatest risk of fasciotomy in patients with evolving compartment syndrome is incomplete fasciotomy technique. It is imperative to verify that all compartments in the affected extremity have been released, regardless of surgical approach utilized. Anatomy may be distorted due to fracture deformity, excessive hematoma, or soft tissue avulsion, and it occasionally can be difficult to discern fascial planes. Also, visualization can be impaired by "minimally invasive" or "cosmetic" incisions, and therefore it is inappropriate to perform fasciotomy in the urgent to emergent situation on a traumatized extremity through anything but full-length incisions. Small incisions for fasciotomy are described and often are used for the treatment of exertional compartment syndrome, but their utility in trauma is questionable at best. Visual verification of complete release of all four compartments should be made prior to the initiation of wound closure and departure from the operating room.

Fasciotomy can be associated with both acute and long-term morbidity. Multiple neurovascular structures can be injured during fasciotomy. Risk can be minimized by careful and meticulous dissection technique, maintaining nerves and vessels within a cutaneous flap (if possible), and assuring that neither is directly exposed to the environment (dressing) at the conclusion of the case. At least one case of profound hemorrhage after erosion of an artery beneath a negative-pressure wound therapy device has been reported [155]. Analysis of long-term outcomes related to fasciotomy is difficult in the trauma setting due to the concomitant injuries that have invariably occurred and which can have an effect upon function. Nevertheless, a retrospective analysis of 40 patients undergoing leg fasciotomy for a variety of reasons has been published [156]. Complications of leg fasciotomy were common, and included neurological injury in 15%, hemorrhage in 35%, and infection in 25%. Only 45% of legs healed with a good functional result, and 27.5% had a severely disabled leg at the time of final healing. Five of the patients (12.5%) ultimately required ipsilateral leg amputation, and six patients (15%) expired. Another report indicated frequent patient complaints related to fasciotomy wounds, including decreased sensation, tethering of tendons, and recurrent ulceration [157]. Other known side effects of compartment release include pruritus, reflex sympathetic dystrophy, temperature sensitivity, venous stasis, and chronic edema. Despite these concerns, the morbidity and potential mortality of an untreated compartment syndrome is likely to be much higher. Also, a number of published reports, reviewed by Bong et al. [158], indicate that outcomes of fasciotomy for chronic exertional compartment syndrome (in the absence of trauma) are reliably good. These reports, however, require cautious interpretation for their application to trauma, as they did not include patients who required fasciotomy for trauma-related compartment syndrome.

OTHER SEQUELAE OF ORTHOPEDIC TRAUMA

Deep Venous Thrombosis

Polytraumatized patients with lower extremity or pelvic fractures often are subjected to prolonged periods of immobilization or reduced mobility. They are at risk for development of deep venous thrombosis (DVT) and subsequent pulmonary thromboembolism (PE). Management of the orthopedic trauma patient must take into account the increased propensity for these patients to develop venous thromboembolic disease.

There has been much debate in the literature about appropriate methods of DVT prophylaxis in orthopedic trauma patients. The Eastern Association for the Surgery of Trauma (EAST) states that the greatest risk factors in trauma patients for development of venous thromboembolism (VTE) are spinal fractures and spinal cord injury. They also state that insufficient evidence exists regarding risk of VTE in trauma patients as it relates directly to long bone fracture or pelvic fracture [159]. Trauma patients with pelvic and acetabular fractures are thought to have an increased risk of VTE [160]. However, there is little evidence in the literature, apart from observational studies, regarding the best method of DVT prophylaxis for pelvic and acetabular fracture patients [161].

Prophylaxis of trauma patients, especially those with pelvic and acetabular fractures, is important to reduce the risk of DVT. Trauma patients have been shown to have lower rates of DVT when both chemical and mechanical means of prophylaxis are utilized [162]. Mechanical DVT prophylaxis can consist of foot pumps or pneumatic compression devices. Continuous passive motion for the knee in the injured extremity has also been shown to be helpful [163]. Chemical DVT prophylaxis often consists of low-molecular-weight heparin (LMWH) in hospital inpatients; warfarin is not commonly used acutely in the trauma patient (although it may be utilized for longer-term DVT prophylaxis when indicated). In patients thought to be at higher risk of VTE and who are awaiting surgical intervention for fracture repair, chemical prophylaxis does not need to be halted in anticipation of surgery [164]. Despite adequate prophylaxis, however, patients are still at risk for development of DVT [165].

Patients with pelvic, acetabular, and proximal femoral (hip) fractures are at risk of development of VTE [160]. Fractures below the hip are associated with lower risk of DVT; 8% of patients with below-the-hip fractures were demonstrated in one study to develop DVT [166]. Fractures below the knee (i.e., tibia, ankle, foot) do not seem to elevate the risk of VTE significantly; low rates of DVT have been found in patients with ankle fractures treated with cast immobilization [167], and a recent study demonstrated that DVT prophylaxis was of limited to no benefit in patients with fractures below the knee [168].

Routine screening for the presence of DVT in trauma patients is not commonly done. Methods of detecting DVT include compression Doppler ultrasound and venography. In patients with pelvic and acetabular fracture, known to be at a higher risk for DVT than other patients with lower extremity fractures, venography has not been shown to be an effective screening tool [169]. In general, routine screening for DVT is ineffective in trauma patients with pelvic and acetabular fractures, as demonstrated in a recent review of 973 patients [170].

Peripheral Nerve Injury

The bulk of peripheral nerve injuries that occur as a consequence of trauma are neurapraxias, which often will recover with time. Typical neurological injuries include radial nerve palsies in association with humeral shaft fractures, sciatic nerve palsies (peroneal branch, in particular) in association with pelvic and acetabular fractures, and brachial plexopathies in association with scapulothoracic dissociation.

Radial nerve palsies occur after approximately 12% of humeral shaft fractures [129]. An early description of radial nerve palsy in association with humeral shaft fracture was published by Holstein and Lewis, and describes the association with a spiral fracture of the humeral shaft located at the junction between the middle and distal one thirds of the diaphysis [171]. However, some more recent research has called the relationship between this particular humerus fracture pattern and radial nerve palsy into question [129]. The radial nerve supplies motor innervation to the extensors of the hand and wrist; patients with radial nerve motor palsies will lack the ability to extend the wrist or hyperextend the interphalangeal joint of the thumb, which is mediated by the extensor pollicis longus. The extensor digitorum communis (EDC), also supplied by the radial nerve, extends the metacarpophalangeal joints of the hand, but patients may recruit other muscles or perform other functions (such as wrist flexion) that will serve to extend the digits, even though the EDC is not functional. The interphalangeal joints of the fingers (index, long, ring, small) are extended by the intrinsic muscles of the hand, which are innervated by the median and ulnar nerves, and therefore are not affected by radial nerve palsy. Radial nerve-mediated sensation includes the dorsal surfaces of the forearm and hand; the most specific location for radial nerve sensation is the dorsum of the first web space on the hand.

Most radial nerve palsies are thought to be traction injuries (neurapraxias), as opposed to complete disruptions (neurotmesis) or impalings on bone edges [172]. Rarely, the radial nerve may become entrapped within the humeral fracture site, creating neurological deficits [129]. In the setting of high-velocity penetrating injury (gunshot wounds), a radial nerve palsy may be secondary to blast effect of the projectile (as opposed to nerve transaction). Radial nerve palsy at presentation in a patient with a humeral shaft fracture is not considered an indication for surgery, either for nerve exploration or humeral shaft fracture fixation. In the past, humeral shaft fracture patients presenting with intact radial nerve function which then is lost after manipulation of the fracture (e.g., for reduction) was considered an indication for operative nerve exploration; it has been shown, however, that the bulk of these "iatrogenic" radial nerve palsies resolve on their own, with no residual deficit, and that fracture fixation or nerve exploration is not indicated in these patients either [129]. Humeral shaft fracture fixation should be undertaken in patients who would benefit (or who specifically request fixation), after thorough risk and benefit discussions with the patients and/or their families, and should not be prompted by the presence of a radial nerve deficit. Electromyography and nerve conduction studies are not helpful in the acute setting, and have low sensitivity and specificity regarding the etiology of radial nerve palsy immediately after injury. Ultrasonic examination, however, can be beneficial to detect nerve laceration or entrapment, when utilized by experienced practitioners [173].

Although radial nerve palsies are most often transient, their recovery can take many weeks to months. During this time, flexion contractures of the wrist and digits can occur. Splinting and occupational therapy, with daily manual stretching exercises, are beneficial to minimize this problem. Electromyography and nerve conduction studies may be performed between 6 and 12 weeks following the onset of the radial nerve palsy if there has been absolutely no recovery of function after the injury [172]. Functional recovery is slow; rapid recovery should not be expected. A good rule of thumb is that nerve recovery progresses at approximately 1 mm per day [174]. Therefore, an injury to the radial nerve at the midshaft of the humerus should be expected to result in dorsal hand sensory deficits for many weeks.

Sciatic nerve palsies can occur in conjunction with pelvic or acetabular fractures. Acetabular fractures with posterior dislocation of the hip have an association with the development of sciatic nerve palsy [175]. Pelvic or acetabular fractures, with extensions of fracture lines into the sciatic buttress at the greater sciatic notch, can result in direct laceration of the sciatic nerve; this pattern of fracture can also result in catastrophic hemorrhage due to laceration of the superior and/or inferior gluteal arteries. Pelvic ring disruptions, with wide displacement of the hemipelvis, can also cause sciatic nerve palsies or lumbosacral plexopathies [176], perhaps due either to avulsion of nerve roots or to neurapraxia [177,178]. Nerve roots may be lacerated in association with sacral fractures [179]. The peroneal division of the sciatic nerve is more commonly affected than the tibial division [180]; it has been postulated that this has to do with more points at which the peroneal nerves are tethered down the lower extremity than the tibial nerves.

The bulk of sciatic nerve palsies are also neurapraxias [177]. Prognosis of these, however, is poorer than that for radial nerve palsy, perhaps secondary to the long distance across which recovery must occur (the nerve bud must travel from the pelvis to at least the superior leg, where innervation of the peroneal muscles and ankle and toe dorsiflexors occurs) [180]. Electromyography and nerve conduction studies are useful for characterizing the injury, and many patients with mild injuries regain good function [181].

Scapulothoracic dissociation, likened to a closed forequarter amputation [182], occurs when the shoulder girdle and upper extremity are pulled away from the midline [183]. Prompt recognition of this injury complex is vital. Significant degrees of scapulothoracic dissociation can result in the rupture of subclavian or axillary vessels [182,184]. The injury complex can have devastating effects upon the neurological function of the upper extremity, due to the stretch of nerves or brachial plexus, or due to the avulsion of nerve roots from the cervical spine [182]. Degree of neurological injury and prognosis for recovery correlates with the location of vascular injury; more proximal vascular injury correlates with more severe neurological compromise and poorer prognosis [185]. Evidence of expanding hematoma within the axilla of a patient with such an injury should prompt emergent vascular surgical consultation. Careful attention to the vascular status of the distal upper extremity must be paid to any patient with a distracted clavicular fracture, a significantly-displaced scapular fracture, or a clear increase in distance on anteroposterior chest radiograph between the thoracic spine and the medial border of the scapula, known as the scapular index [186]. Computed tomography is of questionable benefit for initial diagnosis, as the axis of the beam may not be perfectly perpendicular to the axial skeleton, and therefore determination of scapular index may be unreliable. Recovery of brachial plexus function after scapulothoracic dissociation is unreliable at best, especially after nerve root avulsion [184,185,187].

References

1. Anderson RN, Smith BL: Deaths: leading causes for 2001. *Natl Vital Stat Rep* 52:1–85, 2003.
2. Turchin DC, Schemitsch EH, McKee MD, et al: Do foot injuries significantly affect the functional outcome of multiply injured patients? *J Orthop Trauma* 13:1–4, 1999.
3. Stiegelmar R, McKee MD, Waddell JP, et al: Outcome of foot injuries in multiply injured patients. *Orthop Clin North Am* 32:193–204, 2001.
4. Gustilo RB, Anderson JT: Prevention of infection in the treatment of one thousand and twenty-five open fractures of long bones. *J Bone Joint Surg [Am]* 58:453–458, 1976.
5. Gustilo RB, Mendoza RM, Williams DN: Problems in the management of type III (severe) open fractures: a new classification of type III open fractures. *J Trauma* 24:742–746, 1981.
6. Anglen J: Letter to the editor. *J Orthop Trauma* 21:422, 2007.
7. Gustilo RB: Letter to the editor. *J Bone Joint Surg [Am]* 77:1291–1292, 1995.
8. Horn BD, Rettig ME: Interobserver reliability in the Gustilo and Anderson classification of open fractures. *J Orthop Trauma* 7:357–360, 1993.
9. Brumback RJ, Jones AL: Interobserver agreement in the classification of open fractures of the tibia: the results of a survey of two hundred and forty-five orthopedic surgeons. *J Bone Joint Surg [Am]* 76:1162–1166, 1994.
10. Giannoudis PV, Papakostidis C, Roberts C: A review of the management of open fractures of the tibia and femur. *J Bone Joint Surg [Br]* 88:281–289, 2006.
11. Gosselin RA, Roberts I, Gillespie WJ: Antibiotics for preventing infection in open limb fractures. *Cochrane Database Syst Rev* (1):CD003764, 2004.
12. Hauser CJ, Adams Jr CA, Eachempati SR, et al: Surgical Infection Society guideline: prophylactic antibiotic use in open fractures: an evidence-based guideline. *Surg Infect (Larchmt)* 7:379–405, 2006.
13. Zalavras CG, Patzakis MJ: Open fractures: evaluation and management. *J Am Acad Orthop Surg* 11:212–219, 2003.
14. Patzakis MJ, Wilkins J: Factors influencing infection rate in open fracture wounds. *Clin Orthop* 243:36–40, 1989.
15. Patzakis M, Bains RS, Lee J, et al: Prospective, randomized, double-blind study comparing single-agent antibiotic therapy, ciprofloxacin, to combination antibiotic therapy in open fracture wounds. *J Orthop Trauma* 14:529–533, 2000.
16. Huddleston PM, Steckelberg JM, Hanssen AD, et al: Ciprofloxacin inhibition of experimental fracture healing. *J Bone Joint Surg [Am]* 82:161–173, 2000.
17. Perry AC, Prpa B, Rouse MS, et al: Levofloxacin and trovafloxacin inhibition of experimental fracture-healing. *Clin Orthop* 414:95–100, 2003.
18. Wilkins J, Patzakis M: Choice and duration of antibiotics in open fractures. *Orthop Clin North Am* 22:433–437, 1991.
19. Dellinger EP, Caplan ES, Weaver LD, et al: Duration of preventive antibiotic administration for open extremity fractures. *Arch Surg* 123:333–339, 1988.
20. Templeman DC, Gulli B, Tsukayama DT, et al: Update on the management of open fractures of the tibial shaft. *Clin Orthop* 350:18–25, 1998.
21. Ficke JR, Pollak AN: Extremity war injuries: development of clinical treatment principles. *J Am Acad Orthop Surg* 15:590–595, 2007.
22. Barei DP, Taitsman LA, Beingessner D, et al: Open diaphyseal long bone fractures: a reduction method using devitalized or extruded osseous fragments. *J Orthop Trauma* 21:574–578, 2007.
23. Conroy BP, Anglen JO, Simpson WA, et al: Comparison of castile soap, benzalkonium chloride, and bacitracin as irrigation solutions for complex contaminated orthopedic wounds. *J Orthop Trauma* 13:332–337, 1999.

24. Anglen JO: Wound irrigation in musculoskeletal injury. *J Am Acad Orthop Surg* 9:219–226, 2001.
25. Anglen JO: Comparison of soap and antibiotic solutions for irrigation of lower-limb open fracture wounds: a prospective, randomized study. *J Bone Joint Surg [Am]* 87:1415–1422, 2005.
26. Petrisor B, Jeray K, Schemitsch E, et al: Fluid lavage in patients with open fracture wounds (FLOW): an international survey of 984 surgeons. *BMC Musculoskelet Disord* 9:7, 2008.
27. Draeger RW, Dirschl DR, Dahners LE: Debridement of cancellous bone: a comparison of irrigation methods. *J Orthop Trauma* 20:692–698, 2006.
28. Franklin JL, Johnson KD, Hansen ST Jr: Immediate internal fixation of open ankle fractures: report of thirty-eight cases treated with a standard protocol. *J Bone Joint Surg [Am]* 66:1349–1356, 1984.
29. Nowotarski PJ, Turen CH, Brumback RJ, et al: Conversion of external fixation to intramedullary nailing for fractures of the shaft of the femur in multiply injured patients. *J Bone Joint Surg [Am]* 82:781–788, 2000.
30. Bhandari M, Zlowodzki M, Tornetta P III, et al: Intramedullary nailing following external fixation in femoral and tibial shaft fractures. *J Orthop Trauma* 19:140–144, 2005.
31. Della Rocca GJ, Crist BD: External fixation versus conversion to intramedullary nailing for definitive management of closed fractures of the femoral and tibial shaft. *J Am Acad Orthop Surg* 14:S131–S135, 2006.
32. Henley MB, Chapman JR, Agel J, et al: Treatment of type II, IIIA, and IIIB open fractures of the tibial shaft: a prospective comparison of unreamed interlocking intramedullary nails and half-pin external fixators. *J Orthop Trauma* 12:1–7, 1998.
33. Okike K, Bhattacharyya T: Trends in the management of open fractures: a critical analysis. *J Bone Joint Surg [Am]* 88:2739–2748, 2006.
34. DeLong WG Jr, Born CT, Wei SY, et al: Aggressive treatment of 119 open fracture wounds. *J Trauma* 46:1049–1054, 1999.
35. Gopal S, Majumder S, Batchelor AG, et al: Fix and flap: the radical orthopedic and plastic treatment of severe open fractures of the tibia. *J Bone Joint Surg [Br]* 82:959–966, 2000.
36. Dunbar RP, Taitsman LA, Sangeorzan BJ, et al: Technique tip: use of "pie crusting" of the dorsal skin in severe foot injury. *Foot Ankle Int* 28:851–853, 2007.
37. Schnirring-Judge MA, Anderson EC: Vessel loop closure technique in open fractures and other complex wounds in the foot and ankle. *J Foot Ankle Surg* 48:692–699, 2009.
38. DeFranzo AJ, Argenta LC, Marks MW, et al: The use of vacuum-assisted closure therapy for the treatment of lower-extremity wounds with exposed bone. *Plast Reconstr Surg* 108:1184–1191, 2001.
39. Herscovici D Jr, Sanders RW, Scaduto JM, et al: Vacuum assisted wound closure (VAC therapy) for the management of patients with high energy soft tissue injuries. *J Orthop Trauma* 17:683–688, 2003.
40. Stannard JP, Volgas DA, Stewart R, et al: Negative pressure wound therapy after severe open fractures: a prospective randomized study. *J Orthop Trauma* 23:552–557, 2009.
41. Rinker B, Amspacher JC, Wilson PC, et al: Subatmospheric pressure dressing as a bridge to free tissue transfer in the treatment of open tibia fractures. *Plast Reconstr Surg* 121:1664–1673, 2008.
42. Dedmond BT, Kortesis B, Punger K, et al: The use of negative-pressure wound therapy (NPWT) in the temporary treatment of soft-tissue injuries associated with high-energy open tibial shaft fractures. *J Orthop Trauma* 21:11–17, 2007.
43. Bhattacharyya T, Mehta P, Smith M, et al: Routine use of wound vacuum-assisted closure does not allow coverage delay for open tibia fractures. *Plast Reconstr Surg* 121:1263–1266, 2008.
44. Pollak AN, Jones AL, Castillo RC, et al: The relationship between time to surgical debridement and incidence of infection after open high-energy lower extremity trauma. *J Bone Joint Surg [Am]* 92:7–15, 2010.
45. Ricci WM, Gallagher B, Brandt A, et al: Is after-hours orthopedic surgery associated with adverse outcomes? A prospective comparative study. *J Bone Joint Surg [Am]* 91:2067–2072, 2009.
46. Schmidt AH: Commentary & perspective on "The relationship between time to surgical débridement and incidence of infection after open high-energy lower extremity trauma" by Andrew N. Pollak, MD, et al: *J Bone Joint Surg [Am]* 92, 2010.
47. Bosse MJ, MacKenzie EJ, Kellam JF, et al: An analysis of outcomes of reconstruction or amputation after leg-threatening injuries. *N Engl J Med* 347:1927–1931, 2002.
48. MacKenzie EJ, Bosse MJ, Pollak AN, et al: Long-term persistence of disability following severe lower-limb trauma: results of a seven-year follow-up. *J Bone Joint Surg [Am]* 87:1801–1809, 2005.
49. Johansen K, Daines M, Howey T, et al: Objective criteria accurately predict amputation following lower extremity trauma. *J Trauma* 30:568–572, 1990.
50. Helfet DL, Howey T, Sanders R, et al: Limb salvage versus amputation: preliminary results of the Mangled Extremity Severity Score. *Clin Orthop* 256:80–86, 1990.
51. Bosse MJ, MacKenzie EJ, Kellam JF, et al: A prospective evaluation of the clinical utility of the lower-extremity injury-severity scores. *J Bone Joint Surg [Am]* 83:3–14, 2001.
52. Ly TV, Travison TG, Castillo RC, et al: Ability of lower-extremity injury severity scores to predict functional outcome after limb salvage. *J Bone Joint Surg [Am]* 90:1738–1743, 2008.
53. Bosse MJ, McCarthy ML, Jones AL, et al: The insensate foot following severe lower extremity trauma: an indication for amputation? *J Bone Joint Surg [Am]* 87:2601–2608, 2005.
54. Garras DN, Carothers JT, Olson SA: Single-leg-stance (flamingo) radiographs to assess pelvic instability: how much motion is normal? *J Bone Joint Surg [Am]* 90:2114–2118, 2008.
55. Siegel J, Templeman DC, Tornetta 3rd P: Single-leg-stance radiographs in the diagnosis of pelvic instability. *J Bone Joint Surg [Am]* 90:2119–2125, 2008.
56. Young JW, Burgess AR, Brumback RJ, et al: Pelvic fractures: value of plain radiography in early assessment and management. *Radiology* 160:445–451, 1986.
57. Dalal SA, Burgess AR, Siegel JH, et al: Pelvic fracture in multiple trauma: classification by mechanism is key to pattern of organ injury, resuscitative requirements, and outcome. *J Trauma* 29:981–1000, 1989.
58. Magnussen RA, Tressler MA, Obremskey WT, et al: Predicting blood loss in isolated pelvic and acetabular high-energy trauma. *J Orthop Trauma* 21:603–607, 2007.
59. Tile M: Pelvic fractures: operative versus nonoperative treatment. *Orthop Clin North Am* 11:423–464, 1980.
60. Marsh JL, Slongo TF, Agel J, et al: Fracture and dislocation classification compendium–2007: Orthopedic Trauma Association classification, database and outcomes committee. *J Orthop Trauma* 21:S1–S133, 2007.
61. Hak DJ, Smith WR, Suzuki T: Management of hemorrhage in life-threatening pelvic fracture. *J Am Acad Orthop Surg* 17:447–457, 2009.
62. Kregor PJ, Routt MLC Jr: Unstable pelvic ring disruptions in unstable patients. *Injury* 30:SB19–SB28, 1999.
63. Sathy AK, Starr AJ, Smith WR, et al: The effect of pelvic fracture on mortality after trauma: an analysis of 63,000 trauma patients. *J Bone Joint Surg [Am]* 91:2803–2810, 2009.
64. Routt ML Jr, Falicov A, Woodhouse E, et al: Circumferential pelvic antishock sheeting: a temporary resuscitation aid. *J Orthop Trauma* 16:45–48, 2002.
65. Schaller TM, Sims S, Maxian T: Skin breakdown following circumferential pelvic antishock sheeting: a case report. *J Orthop Trauma* 19:661–665, 2005.
66. Krieg JC, Mohr M, Ellis TJ, et al: Emergent stabilization of pelvic ring injuries by controlled circumferential compression: a clinical trial. *J Trauma* 59:659–664, 2005.
67. Ghaemmaghami V, Sperry J, Gunst M, et al: Effects of early use of external pelvic compression on transfusion requirements and mortality in pelvic fractures. *Am J Surg* 194:720–723, 2007.
68. Palmer S, Fairbank AC, Bircher M: Surgical complications and implications of external fixation of pelvic fractures. *Injury* 28:649–653, 1997.
69. Lindahl J, Hirvensalo E, Bostman O, et al: Failure of reduction with an external fixator in the management of injuries of the pelvic ring: long-term evaluation of 110 patients. *J Bone Joint Surg [Br]* 81:955–962, 1999.
70. Heini PF, Witt J, Ganz R: The pelvic C-clamp for the emergency treatment of unstable pelvic ring injuries: a report on clinical experience of 30 cases. *Injury* 27:SA38–SA45, 1996.
71. Pohlemann T, Braune C, Gansslen A, et al: Pelvic emergency clamps: anatomic landmarks for a safe primary application. *J Orthop Trauma* 18:102–105, 2004.
72. Richard MJ, Tornetta 3rd P: Emergent management of APC-2 pelvic ring injuries with an anteriorly placed C-clamp. *J Orthop Trauma* 23:322–326, 2009.
73. Smith W, Williams A, Agudelo J, et al: Early predictors of mortality in hemodynamically unstable pelvis fractures. *J Orthop Trauma* 21:31–37, 2007.
74. Eastridge BJ, Starr A, Minei JP, et al: The importance of fracture pattern in guiding therapeutic decision-making in patients with hemorrhagic shock and pelvic ring disruptions. *J Trauma* 53:446–450, 2002.
75. Burgess AR, Eastridge BJ, Young JW, et al: Pelvic ring disruptions: effective classification system and treatment protocols. *J Trauma* 30:848–856, 1990.
76. Sarin EL, Moore JB, Moore EE, et al: Pelvic fracture pattern does not always predict the need for urgent embolization. *J Trauma* 58:973–977, 2005.
77. Elzik ME, Dirschl DR, Dahners LE: Hemorrhage in pelvic fractures does not correlate with fracture length. *J Trauma* 65:436–441, 2008.
78. Starr AJ, Griffin DR, Reinert CM, et al: Pelvic ring disruptions: prediction of associated injuries, transfusion requirement, pelvic arteriography, complications, and mortality. *J Orthop Trauma* 16:553–561, 2002.
79. Miller PR, Moore PS, Mansell E, et al: External fixation or arteriogram in bleeding pelvic fracture: initial therapy guided by markers of arterial hemorrhage. *J Trauma* 54:437–443, 2003.
80. Stein DM, O'Toole RV, Scalea TM: Multidisciplinary approach for patients with pelvic fractures and hemodynamic instability. *Scand J Surg* 96:272–280, 2007.
81. Stephen DJ, Kreder HJ, Day AC, et al: Early detection of arterial bleeding in acute pelvic trauma. *J Trauma* 47:638–642, 1999.
82. Osborn PM, Smith WR, Moore EE, et al: Direct retroperitoneal pelvic packing versus pelvic angiography: a comparison of two management protocols for haemodynamically unstable pelvic fractures. *Injury* 40:54–60, 2009.
83. Gansslen A, Giannoudis P, Pape HC: Hemorrhage in pelvic fracture: who needs angiography? *Curr Opin Crit Care* 9:515–523, 2003.

84. Totterman A, Madsen JE, Skaga NO, et al: Extraperitoneal pelvic packing: a salvage procedure to control massive traumatic pelvic hemorrhage. *J Trauma* 62:843–852, 2007.
85. Bjurlin MA, Fantus RJ, Mellett MM, et al: Genitourinary injuries in pelvic fracture morbidity and mortality using the National Trauma Data Bank. *J Trauma* 67:1033–1039, 2009.
86. Ziran BH, Chamberlin E, Shuler FH, et al: Delays and difficulties in the diagnosis of lower urologic injuries in the context of pelvic fractures. *J Trauma* 58:533–537, 2005.
87. Porter SE, Schroeder AC, Dzugan SS, et al: Acetabular fracture patterns and their associated injuries. *J Orthop Trauma* 22:165–170, 2008.
88. Carroll PR, McAninch JW: Major bladder trauma: the accuracy of cystography. *J Urol* 130:887–888, 1983.
89. Mouraviev BV, Santucci RA: Cadaveric anatomy of pelvic fracture urethral distraction injury: most injuries are distal to the external urinary sphincter. *J Urol* 173:869–872, 2005.
90. Londergan TA, Gundersen LH, van Every MJ: Early fluoroscopic realignment for traumatic urethral injuries. *Urology* 49:101–103, 1997.
91. Routt ML, Simonian PT, Defalco AJ, et al: Internal fixation in pelvic fractures and primary repairs of associated genitourinary disruptions: a team approach. *J Trauma* 40:784–790, 1996.
92. Brandes S, Borrelli J Jr: Pelvic fracture and associated urologic injuries. *World J Surg* 25:1578–1587, 2001.
93. Kotkin L, Koch MO: Morbidity associated with nonoperative management of extraperitoneal bladder injuries. *J Trauma* 38:895–898, 1995.
94. Grotz MRW, Allami MK, Harwood P, et al: Open pelvic fractures: epidemiology, current concepts of management and outcome. *Injury* 36:1–13, 2005.
95. Woods RK, O'Keefe G, Rhee P, et al: Open pelvic fracture and fecal diversion. *Arch Surg* 133:281–286, 1998.
96. Pell M, Flynn WJ, Seibel RW: Is colostomy always necessary in the treatment of open pelvic fractures? *J Trauma* 45:371–373, 1998.
97. Nork SE, Agel J, Russell GV, et al: Mortality after reamed intramedullary nailing of bilateral femur fractures. *Clin Orthop* 415:272–278, 2003.
98. Cannada LK, Viehe T, Cates CA, et al: A retrospective review of high-energy femoral neck-shaft fractures. *J Orthop Trauma* 23:254–260, 2009.
99. Winquist RA, Hansen SV, Clawson DK: Closed intramedullary nailing of femoral fractures: a report of 520 cases. *J Bone Joint Surg [Am]* 66:529–539, 1984.
100. Wolinsky PR, McCarty E, Shyr Y, et al: Reamed intramedullary nailing of the femur: 551 cases. *J Trauma* 46:392–399, 1999.
101. Ricci WM, Schwappach J, Tucker M, et al: Trochanteric versus piriformis entry portal for the treatment of femoral shaft fractures. *J Orthop Trauma* 20:663–667, 2006.
102. Brumback RJ, Uwagie-Ero S, Lakatos RP, et al: Intramedullary nailing of femoral shaft fractures. Part II: fracture-healing with static interlocking fixation. *J Bone Joint Surg [Am]* 70:1453–1462, 1988.
103. Brumback RJ, Reilly JP, Poka A, et al: Intramedullary nailing of femoral shaft fractures. Part I: decision-making errors with interlocking fixation. *J Bone Joint Surg [Am]* 70:1441–1452, 1988.
104. Ostrum RF, Agarwal A, Lakatos R, et al: Prospective comparison of retrograde and antegrade femoral intramedullary nailing. *J Orthop Trauma* 14:496–501, 2000.
105. Tornetta P III, Tiburzi D: Reamed versus nonreamed anterograde femoral nailing. *J Orthop Trauma* 14:15–19, 2000.
106. Bhandari M, Guyatt GH, Tong D, et al: Reamed versus nonreamed intramedullary nailing of lower extremity long bone fractures: a systematic overview and meta-analysis. *J Orthop Trauma* 14:2–9, 2000.
107. Pape HC, Regel G, Dwenger A, et al: Influences of different methods of intramedullary femoral nailing on lung function in patients with multiple trauma. *J Trauma* 35:709–716, 1983.
108. Bosse MJ, MacKenzie EJ, Riemer BL, et al: Adult respiratory distress syndrome, pneumonia, and mortality following thoracic injury and a femoral fracture treated either with intramedullary nailing with reaming or with a plate: a comparative study. *J Bone Joint Surg [Am]* 79:799–809, 1997.
109. Bone LB, Johnson KD, Weigelt J, et al: Early versus delayed stabilization of femoral fractures: a prospective randomized study. *J Bone Joint Surg [Am]* 71:336–340, 1989.
110. Pape HC, Hildebrand F, Pertschy S, et al: Changes in the management of femoral shaft fractures in polytrauma patients: from early total care to damage control orthopedic surgery. *J Trauma* 53:452–461, 2002.
111. Harwood PJ, Giannoudis PV, van Griensven M, et al: Alterations in the systemic inflammatory response after early total care and damage control procedures for femoral shaft fracture in severely injured patients. *J Trauma* 58:446–452, 2005.
112. Pape HC, Rixen D, Morley J, et al: Impact of the method of initial stabilization for femoral shaft fractures in patients with multiple injuries at risk for complications (borderline patients). *Ann Surg* 246:491–499, 2007.
113. Anwar IA, Battistella FD, Neiman R, et al: Femur fractures and lung complications: a prospective randomized study of reaming. *Clin Orthop* 422:71–76, 2004.
114. Society COT: Reamed versus unreamed intramedullary nailing of the femur: comparison of the rate of ARDS in multiple injured patients. *J Orthop Trauma* 20:384–387, 2006.
115. O'Toole RV, O'Brien M, Scalea TM, et al: Resuscitation before stabilization of femoral fractures limits acute respiratory distress syndrome in patients with multiple traumatic injuries despite low use of damage control orthopedics. *J Trauma* 67:1013–1021, 2009.
116. Howard M, Court-Brown CM: Epidemiology and management of open fractures of the lower limb. *Br J Hosp Med* 57:582–587, 1997.
117. Khatod M, Botte MJ, Hoyt DB, et al: Outcomes in open tibia fractures: relationship between delay in treatment and infection. *J Trauma* 55:949–954, 2003.
118. Patzakis MJ, Zalavras CG: Chronic posttraumatic osteomyelitis and infected nonunion of the tibia: current management concepts. *J Am Acad Orthop Surg* 13:417–427, 2005.
119. Finkemeier CG, Schmidt AH, Kyle RF, et al: A prospective, randomized study of intramedullary nails inserted with and without reaming for the treatment of open and closed fractures of the tibial shaft. *J Orthop Trauma* 14:187–193, 2000.
120. Sarmiento A, Zagorski JB, Zych GA, et al: Functional bracing for the treatment of fractures of the humeral diaphysis. *J Bone Joint Surg [Am]* 82:478–486, 2000.
121. Koch PP, Gross DF, Gerber C: The results of functional (Sarmiento) bracing of humeral shaft fractures. *J Shoulder Elbow Surg* 11:143–150, 2002.
122. Ekholm R, Tidermark J, Tornkvist H, et al: Outcome after closed functional treatment of humeral shaft fractures. *J Orthop Trauma* 20:591–596, 2006.
123. Tingstad EM, Wolinsky PR, Shyr Y, et al: Effect of immediate weightbearing on plated fractures of the humeral shaft. *J Trauma* 49:278–280, 2000.
124. Rommens PM, Kuechle R, Bord T, et al: Humeral nailing revisited. *Injury* 39:1319–1328, 2008.
125. McCormack RG, Brien D, Buckley RE, et al: Fixation of fractures of the shaft of the humerus by dynamic compression plate or intramedullary nail. *J Bone Joint Surg [Br]* 82:336–339, 2000.
126. Chapman JR, Henley MB, Agel J, et al: Randomized prospective study of humeral shaft fracture fixation: intramedullary nails versus plates. *J Orthop Trauma* 14:162–166, 2000.
127. Bhandari M, Devereaux PJ, McKee MD, et al: Compression plating versus intramedullary nailing of humeral shaft fractures–a meta-analysis. *Acta Orthop* 77:279–284, 2006.
128. Ekholm R, Adami J, Tidermark J, et al: Fractures of the shaft of the humerus: an epidemiological study of 401 fractures. *J Bone Joint Surg [Br]* 88:1469–1473, 2006.
129. Shao YC, Harwood P, Grotz MRW, et al: Radial nerve palsy associated with fractures of the shaft of the humerus: a systematic review. *J Bone Joint Surg [Br]* 87:1647–1652, 2005.
130. Hak DJ: Radial nerve palsy associated with humeral shaft fractures. *Orthopedics* 32:111, 2009.
131. Ekholm R, Ponzer S, Tornkvist H, et al: Primary radial nerve palsy in patients with acute humeral shaft fractures. *J Orthop Trauma* 22:408–414, 2008.
132. Schemitsch EH, Richards RR: The effect of malunion on functional outcome after plate fixation of fractures of both bones of the forearm in adults. *J Bone Joint Surg [Am]* 74:1068–1078, 1992.
133. McQueen MM, Court-Brown CM: Compartment monitoring in tibial fractures: The pressure threshold for decompression. *J Bone Joint Surg [Br]* 78:99–104, 1996.
134. White TO, Howell GED, Will EM, et al: Elevated intramuscular compartment pressures do not influence outcome after tibial fracture. *J Trauma* 55:1133–1138, 2003.
135. Henson JT, Roberts CS, Giannoudis PV: Gluteal compartment syndrome. *Acta Orthop Belg* 75:147–152, 2009.
136. Park S, Ahn J, Gee AO, et al: Compartment syndrome in tibial fractures. *J Orthop Trauma* 23:514–518, 2009.
137. McQueen MM, Gaston P, Court-Brown CM: Acute compartment syndrome: who is at risk? *J Bone Joint Surg [Br]* 82:200–203, 2000.
138. Hope MJ, McQueen MM: Acute compartment syndrome in the absence of fracture. *J Orthop Trauma* 18:220–224, 2004.
139. Blick SS, Brumback RJ, Poka A, et al: Compartment syndrome in open tibial fractures. *J Bone Joint Surg [Am]* 68:1348–1353, 1986.
140. Matsen FA 3rd, Clawson DK: The deep posterior compartmental syndrome of the leg. *J Bone Joint Surg [Am]* 57:34–39, 1975.
141. Kenny C: Compartment pressures, limb length changes and the ideal spherical shape: a case report and in vitro study. *J Trauma* 61:909–912, 2006.
142. Kutty S, Laing AJ, Prasad CV, et al: The effect of traction on compartment pressures during intramedullary nailing of tibial-shaft fractures. A prospective randomised trial. *Int Orthop* 29:186–190, 2005.
143. Egol KA, Bazzi J, McLaurin TM, et al: The effect of knee-spanning external fixation on compartment pressures in the leg. *J Orthop Trauma* 22:680–685, 2008.
144. Velmahos GC, Toutouzas KG: Vascular trauma and compartment syndromes. *Surg Clin North Am* 82:125–141, 2002.
145. Olson SA, Glasgow RR: Acute compartment syndrome in lower extremity musculoskeletal trauma. *J Am Acad Orthop Surg* 13:436–444, 2005.
146. Sheridan GW, Matsen FA 3rd: Fasciotomy in the treatment of the acute compartment syndrome. *J Bone Joint Surg [Am]* 58:112–115, 1976.
147. Williams AB, Luchette FA, Papaconstantinou HT, et al: The effect of early versus late fasciotomy in the management of extremity trauma. *Surgery* 122:861–866, 1997.
148. Ritenour AE, Dorlac WC, Fang R, et al: Complications after fasciotomy revision and delayed compartment release in combat patients. *J Trauma* 64[Suppl 2]:S153–S162, 2008.

149. Heckman MM, Whitesides TE Jr, Grewe SR, et al: Compartment pressure in association with closed tibial fractures. The relationship between tissue pressure, compartment, and the distance from the site of the fracture. *J Bone Joint Surg* 76:1285–1292, 1994.
150. Kakar S, Firoozabadi R, McKean J, et al: Diastolic blood pressure in patients with tibia fractures under anaesthesia: implications for the diagnosis of compartment syndrome. *J Orthop Trauma* 21:99–103, 2007.
151. O'Toole RV, Whitney A, Merchant N, et al: Variation in diagnosis of compartment syndrome by surgeons treating tibial shaft fractures. *J Trauma* 67:735–741, 2009.
152. Asgari MM, Spinelli HM: The vessel loop shoelace technique for closure of fasciotomy wounds. *Ann Plast Surg* 44:225–229, 2000.
153. Zannis J, Angobaldo J, Marks M, et al: Comparison of fasciotomy wound closures using traditional dressing changes and the vacuum-assisted closure device. *Ann Plast Surg* 62:407–409, 2009.
154. Yang CC, Chang DS, Webb LX: Vacuum-assisted closure for fasciotomy wounds following compartment syndrome of the leg. *J Surg Orthop Adv* 15:19–23, 2006.
155. White RA, Miki RA, Kazmier P, et al: Vacuum-assisted closure complicated by erosion and hemorrhage of the anterior tibial artery. *J Orthop Trauma* 19:56–59, 2005.
156. Heemskerk J, Kitslaar P: Acute compartment syndrome of the lower leg: retrospective study on prevalence, technique, and outcome of fasciotomies. *World J Surg* 67:744–747, 2003.
157. Fitzgerald AM, Gaston P, Wilson Y, et al: Long-term sequelae of fasciotomy wounds. *Br J Plast Surg* 53:690–693, 2000.
158. Bong MR, Polatsch DB, Jazrawi LM, et al: Chronic exertional compartment syndrome: diagnosis and management. *Bull Hosp Jt Dis* 62:77–84, 2005.
159. Rogers FB, Cipolle MD, Velmahos G, et al: Practice management guidelines for the prevention of venous thromboembolism in trauma patients: the EAST practice management guidelines work group. *J Trauma* 53:142–164, 2002.
160. Buerger PM, Peoples JB, Lemmon GW, et al: Risk of pulmonary emboli in patients with pelvic fractures. *Am Surg* 59:505–508, 1993.
161. Slobogean GP, Lefaivre KA, Nicolaou S, et al: A systematic review of thromboprophylaxis for pelvic and acetabular fractures. *J Orthop Trauma* 23:379–384, 2009.
162. Stannard JP, Lopez-Ben RR, Volgas DA, et al: Prophylaxis against deep-vein thrombosis following trauma: a prospective, randomized comparison of mechanical and pharmacological prophylaxis. *J Bone Joint Surg [Am]* 88:261–266, 2006.
163. Fuchs S, Heyse T, Rudofsky G, et al: Continuous passive motion in the prevention of deep-vein thrombosis: a randomized comparison in trauma patients. *J Bone Joint Surg [Br]* 87:1117–1122, 2005.
164. Cothren CC, Smith WR, Moore EE, et al: Utility of once-daily dose of low-molecular-weight heparin to prevent venous thromboembolism in multisystem trauma patients. *World J Surg* 31:98–104, 2007.
165. Stannard JP, Singhania AK, Lopez-Ben RR, et al: Deep-vein thrombosis in high-energy skeletal trauma despite prophylaxis. *J Bone Joint Surg [Br]* 87:965–968, 2005.
166. Abelseth G, Buckley RE, Pineo GE, et al: Incidence of deep-vein thrombosis in patients with lower extremity fractures distal to the hip. *J Orthop Trauma* 10:230–235, 1996.
167. Patil S, Gandhi J, Curzon I, et al: Incidence of deep-vein thrombosis in patients with fractures of the ankle treated in a plaster cast. *J Bone Joint Surg [Br]* 89:1340–1343, 2007.
168. Goel DP, Buckley R, de Vries G, et al: Prophylaxis of deep-vein thrombosis in fractures below the knee: a prospective randomized controlled trial. *J Bone Joint Surg [Br]* 91:388–394, 2009.
169. Stover MD, Morgan SJ, Bosse MJ, et al: Prospective comparison of contrast-enhanced computed tomography versus magnetic resonance imaging venography in the detection of occult deep pelvic vein thrombosis in patients with pelvic and acetabular fractures. *J Orthop Trauma* 16:613–621, 2002.
170. Borer DS, Starr AJ, Reinert CM, et al: The effect of screening for deep vein thrombosis on the prevalence of pulmonary embolism in patients with fractures of the pelvis and acetabulum: a review of 973 patients. *J Orthop Trauma* 19:92–95, 2005.
171. Holstein A, Lewis GB: Fractures of the humerus with radial-nerve paralysis. *J Bone Joint Surg [Am]* 45:1382–1388, 1963.
172. Lowe 3rd JB, Sen SK, MacKinnon SE: Current approach to radial nerve paralysis. *Plast Reconstr Surg* 110:1099–1113, 2002.
173. Bodner G, Buchberger W, Schocke M, et al: Radial nerve palsy associated with humeral shaft fracture: evaluation with US–initial experience. *Radiology* 219:811–816, 2001.
174. Seddon HG: Nerve grafting. *J Bone Joint Surg [Br]* 45:447–461, 1963.
175. Cornwall R, Radomisli TE: Nerve injury in traumatic dislocation of the hip. *Clin Orthop* 377:84–91, 2000.
176. Helfet DL, Koval KJ, Hissa EA, et al: Intraoperative somatosensory evoked potential monitoring during acute pelvic fracture surgery. *J Orthop Trauma* 9:28–34, 1995.
177. Huittinen VM, Slatis P: Nerve injury in double vertical pelvic fractures. *Acta Chir Scand* 138:571–575, 1971.
178. Harris WR, Rathbun JB, Wortzman G, et al: Avulsion of lumbar roots complicating fracture of the pelvis. *J Bone Joint Surg [Am]* 55:1436–1442, 1973.
179. Denis F, Davis S, Comfort T: Sacral fractures: an important problem. *Clin Orthop* 227:67–81, 1988.
180. Schmeling GJ, Perlewitz TJ, Helfet DL: Chapter 39: Early complications of acetabular fractures, in Tile M, Helfet DL, Kellam JF (eds): *Fractures of the Pelvis and Acetabulum*. 3rd ed. Philadelphia, Lippincott Williams & Wilkins, 2003, p 734.
181. Fassler PR, Swiontkowski MF, Kilroy AW, et al: Injury of the sciatic nerve associated with acetabular fracture. *J Bone Joint Surg [Am]* 75:1157–1166, 1993.
182. Brucker PU, Gruen GS, Kaufmann RA: Scapulothoracic dissociation: evaluation and management. *Injury* 36:1147–1155, 2005.
183. Ebraheim NA, An HS, Jackson WT, et al: Scapulothoracic dissociation. *J Bone Joint Surg [Am]* 70:428–432, 1988.
184. Althausen PL, Lee MA, Finkemeier CG: Scapulothoracic dissociation: diagnosis and treatment. *Clin Orthop* 416:237–244, 2003.
185. Sen RK, Prasad G, Aggarwal S: Scapulothoracic dissociation: level of vascular insult, an indirect prognostic indicator for the final outcome? *Acta Orthop Belg* 75:14–18, 2009.
186. Oreck SL, Burgess A, Levine AM: Traumatic lateral displacement of the scapula: a radiographic sign of neurovascular disruption. *J Bone Joint Surg [Am]* 66:758–763, 1984.
187. Zelle BA, Pape HC, Gerich TG, et al: Functional outcome following scapulothoracic dissociation. *J Bone Joint Surg [Am]* 86:2–8, 2004.

DAVID A. DRACHMAN • DAVID PAYDARFAR

CHAPTER 168 ■ AN APPROACH TO NEUROLOGIC PROBLEMS IN THE INTENSIVE CARE UNIT

DAVID A. DRACHMAN

Neurologic problems present in the intensive care unit (ICU) in two modes: (a) primary neurologic problems, usually under the care of a neurologist or neurosurgeon, and (b) secondary neurologic complications, occurring in patients with other medical or surgical disorders. Only a handful of common clinical situations bring neurologists and patients together in the ICU, although they may be caused by myriad disease states [1]. These situations include:

1. Depressed state of consciousness; coma
2. Altered mental function
3. Required support of respirations or other vital functions
4. Monitoring of increased intracranial pressure (ICP), respirations, state of consciousness
5. Determination of brain death
6. Prevention of further damage to the central nervous system
7. Management of seizures or status epilepticus
8. Evaluation of a neurologic disease that occurs in the course of a severe medical disease
9. Management of a severe medical disease that develops in the course of a neurologic illness

Patients with primary neurologic problems most commonly have conditions with an identified cause, such as stroke, seizures, Guillain-Barré syndrome, head trauma, or myasthenia gravis. Such patients are admitted to the ICU for close observation and management of vital functions, such as respiration, control of ICP, or arrest of seizure activity. These patients represent the minority of neurologic problems seen in the ICU. Far more frequently the neurologist is called on to evaluate the neurologic complications of medical disease: impairment of consciousness in a patient who has undergone cardiopulmonary resuscitation, development of delirium in an elderly individual with a serious infection, or occurrence of focal neurologic deficits in a patient with a ponderous medical record that reveals long-standing diabetes, renal failure, hypertension, and pulmonary disease.

The questions posed to the neurologic consultant are often imperfectly framed. Background observations regarding the origin, onset, and course of the neurologic abnormality may be unavoidably sparse and the history unavailable. The classic neurologic methodology, which involves a comprehensive history and meticulous examination, is rarely possible in patients encumbered with endotracheal tubes, cardiac monitors, and indwelling arterial and venous lines. For these reasons, neurologists must adopt special strategies to function effectively in the ICU, focusing sharply on the specific question with which they are dealing.

INDICATIONS FOR NEUROLOGIC CONSULTATION IN THE INTENSIVE CARE UNIT

Depressed State of Consciousness

The patient with the most common of ICU neurologic problems—a depressed state of consciousness, ranging from lethargy to coma—raises a host of questions. Does the patient have a focal brainstem lesion or diffuse cerebral involvement? Is there an anatomic lesion or a metabolic disorder? Have vital brainstem functions been impaired? Is ICP increased?

The most common primary neurologic causes of depressed consciousness include head trauma, intracranial hemorrhage, post cardiac arrest anoxia-ischemia, and less commonly, inapparent seizures. The secondary conditions seen most often are metabolic, such as anoxia, drug intoxication, or diabetic acidosis. Sometimes the diagnosis is evident, as in head trauma; other times determination of the cause of depressed consciousness may present a diagnostic challenge, demanding a race against the clock to avoid irreversible changes. In every case, it is crucial to establish whether depressed consciousness is due to intrinsic brainstem damage, increased ICP, toxins, widespread anoxia or ischemia, or some other less common cause. It is particularly important to sort out rapidly the component(s) that may be treatable.

Examination of the patient with depressed consciousness exemplifies some of the difficulties of neurologic care in the ICU. Details of this examination are described elsewhere [2]. Like the standard neurologic examination, however, it includes evaluation of mental status, cranial nerve functions, motor functions and coordination, reflexes, sensation, and vascular integrity. The observations made must be used to answer the questions posed above, supplemented by appropriate laboratory studies when possible.

A detailed evaluation of memory and cognitive function is rarely possible in patients who are lethargic, and never possible in those who are stuporous or comatose. Instead, the physician must estimate the patient's responsiveness. Can the patient say any words or respond to commands? Does the patient open his or her eyes? Does the patient groan in response to a painful stimulus or attempt to remove it in a purposeful way? What is the status of the vital functions? Is the respiratory pattern disturbed? The Glasgow Coma Scale score is a simple, but useful, way to document the patient's sensorium [3].

Cranial nerve evaluations include determination of vision, done by observing how the patient follows a large object or a light, gazes toward right and left visual fields, or blinks to a visual threat. Pupillary size, equality, and responsiveness to light are assessed. Corneal reflexes, cough, and vibrissal (nasal) reflexes are evaluated. "Doll's eyes" (vestibulo-ocular) responses are determined by rotation of the head from side to side; if they are absent, ice water caloric testing can be carried out. Facial movements are assessed in response to painful supraorbital stimuli; the gag reflex is tested in the usual fashion.

Motor function is evaluated as completely as possible. All limbs are observed for spontaneous movement and symmetry as well as tremor or other adventitious movements. If no spontaneous movements take place, a pinch or other noxious stimulus can be used to observe purposeful defensive movements. Decerebrate (i.e., four-limb extensor) and decorticate (i.e., upper limbs flexor, lower limbs extensor) rigidity are observed. Tone is assessed passively for spasticity or rigidity. Deep tendon reflexes are checked in the usual way, working around restraints and intravenous tubing. Grasp, suck, snout, and plantar reflexes are evaluated.

Pain is often the only sensory modality that can be tested. The physician must determine whether withdrawal from pinch or pinprick is appropriately defensive or (in the lower extremities) merely part of an exaggerated extensor–plantar response with triple flexion (flexion at hip, knee, and great toe), which may be mistaken for purposeful withdrawal. Finally, the vascular status is evaluated by listening for bruits over the carotid and subclavian arteries, the vertebral arteries, and the orbits.

Such an examination reveals the patient's state of consciousness, the integrity of brainstem reflexes, and the presence or absence of lateralizing or focal neurologic deficits. The value of the systematic (if limited) neurologic examination cannot be overestimated. For example, in a comatose patient, the finding of decerebrate rigidity that points to significant damage at the level of the pons may be more valuable than many laboratory studies, and unilateral weakness of limbs with ipsilateral hyperreflexia indicates a focal brain disorder rather than a diffuse metabolic problem.

Neurodiagnostic studies are often critical in the analysis of comatose patients in the ICU, but the patient's immobility and dependence on life support systems present special difficulties. A neuroradiology suite that is distant from the ICU presents additional obstacles. It is frequently difficult to obtain a magnetic resonance imaging scan, computed tomographic scan, or arteriogram on a patient who is dependent on a respirator. Paradoxically, in patients with the most urgent problems, it is often least convenient to obtain the maximum amount of neurodiagnostic information. The decision that a patient is too sick to have the crucial study performed is often incorrect. In such desperate cases, risks must be taken to obtain life-saving information.

Management of the patient with depressed consciousness depends largely on the cause. Techniques for eliminating toxins, reducing ICP, and maintaining vital functions must be applied, depending on the diagnostic context (see Chapter 169).

Altered Mental Function

In patients who remain relatively alert, other organic disorders may affect mental function, producing an often perplexing variety of clinical patterns. These include confusion, delirium, aphasia, and isolated memory impairment. The first question for the physician is whether the patient's abnormal mental function represents a recent change that is part of the present illness, or instead is part of a long-standing problem. It is also critical to note whether the change developed abruptly (e.g., after surgery or cardiac arrest) or if there is no known precipitating event; and whether it is improving, worsening, or stable.

Confusion and delirium are commonly reversible and generally result from metabolic and toxic disorders (see Chapters 169 and 197). Persistent aphasia and isolated memory impairment suggest focal damage to the brain, and an anatomic lesion should be sought. Dementia—cognitive and memory impairment—cannot be accurately evaluated in patients who have a depressed state of consciousness or the other mental changes indicated above. When dementia occurs *de novo* in a patient with a clear sensorium, it may indicate either reversible conditions (e.g., drug-induced, depression-related) or irreversible damage (e.g., diffuse anoxia or ischemia; see Chapter 169).

Any recent change of mental status in a patient in the ICU requires *prompt* investigation. Whether it signals worsening of the underlying medical disorder or direct involvement of the brain, the change should be assessed by an experienced neurologist as early in its evolution as possible, before it is complicated by the passage of time, advance of disease, and effects of additional treatments.

Support of Respiration and Other Vital Functions

Respiratory support is needed for neurologic patients in two circumstances: loss of brainstem reflex control of respiration and impairment of effective transmission of reflex impulses to functioning respiratory muscles. Ischemia, anoxia, compression, hemorrhage, and toxic depression may alter brainstem control of respirations, producing characteristic respiratory patterns that depend on the site of damage [2], such as central neurogenic hyperventilation, Cheyne-Stokes or periodic breathing, or apnea. The intensivist and neurologist should be familiar with the use of positive end-expiratory pressure and other ventilatory regimens, operation and interpreting read-out of the hospital's respirators, and the endotracheal intubation equipment. Further, the neurologist must understand the neurologic significance of different respiratory patterns, which are as much a part of the ICU neurologic examination as is reflex testing.

Effective transmission of respiratory impulses may be impaired at the cervical spinal cord, anterior horn cells, peripheral nerves, neuromuscular junctions, or muscles of respiration. Cervical traumatic injuries, amyotrophic lateral sclerosis, Guillain-Barré syndrome, myasthenia gravis, and muscular dystrophy may interfere with breathing at the respective levels noted. Some of these conditions are transitory (e.g., Guillain-Barré syndrome) or treatable (e.g., myasthenia gravis), with complete recovery depending largely on the success of maintaining respiration. Even in incurable conditions (e.g., amyotrophic lateral sclerosis), sustaining respiration during periods of decompensation, such as respiratory infections, can prolong life significantly.

Monitoring of Intracranial Pressure and State of Consciousness

In a number of neurologic disorders, extremely close observation is needed to avoid the development of dangerous, often irreversible, further damage to the brain. The most common disorder requiring such monitoring is head trauma. The lethargic patient must be carefully observed for evidence of increasing ICP due to cerebral edema, intracranial (subdural, epidural, intracerebral) hemorrhage, or both [4].

The need for prompt recognition and early treatment of significantly increased ICP cannot be overemphasized. Once uncal or tonsillar herniation with brainstem compression and development of Duret hemorrhages has occurred, the consequences of this secondary effect of brain injury may far outweigh the initial damage. (The methods for monitoring ICP with pressure-detecting catheters or bolts and assessing consciousness and brainstem functions with the Glasgow Coma Scale are described in Chapters 28 and 169.)

Determination of Brain Death

With the recognition that death of the brain and brainstem is equivalent to death of the patient, even though the heart continues to beat and respirations are sustained by artificial ventilation, the need to ascertain brain death has become more critical [5]. Early identification of brain death has three important justifications: (a) the use of viable donor organs for transplantation, (b) the termination of the hopeless vigil of a distraught family, and (c) the freeing of ICU beds for patients who may be helped. When one or more of these conditions prevails, it is important to determine the occurrence of brain death promptly. When none of the conditions is present, there is no urgency in declaring the patient brain dead.

It should be emphasized that brain death is specifically a determination that the brain and the brainstem are already dead—not a prediction that useful recovery is unlikely. It is also true that the longer one waits in even marginally uncertain cases, the clearer the evidence of brain death becomes. (The criteria for brain death are discussed extensively in Chapters 169 and 185.) The "CADRE" mnemonic may be useful in recalling the established criteria for brain death, in the absence of sedative drugs: Coma; *A*pnea; *D*ilated, fixed pupils; *R*eflex (brainstem) absence; and *E*lectroencephalographic silence.

Prevention of Further Damage to the Central Nervous System

A variety of neurologic disorders have the potential to cause further damage to the central nervous system. Acute strokes, or stroke in evolution, for example, may be arrested by thrombolytic treatment [6], endovascular clot removal or angioplasty, and stenting. These modalities may limit or even reverse the underlying ischemic process; and neuroprotective agents may, in the foreseeable future, prevent further damage. Coma following cardiac arrest should be promptly treated with hypothermia to preserve neurological function [7]. Spinal cord compression by metastatic tumor urgently requires surgical decompression followed by radiation therapy to avoid irreversible complete cord transection [8]. Among the infectious diseases of the nervous system, bacterial meningitis and certain treatable encephalitides (e.g., herpes simplex) require the immediate institution of antibiotic or antiviral therapy; spinal epidural abscess requires prompt surgical decompression as well. Although much of neurologic practice involves disorders for which progress is measured in months or years, cerebral anoxia, ischemia, hemorrhage, increased ICP, spinal cord compression, infectious diseases, and other acute disorders require prompt institution of treatment to avoid extension of the initial process. It is useful to remember that, as a largely post-mitotic structure, the brain has limited capability of regeneration, and its ability to survive without a continuing supply of nutrients is measured in minutes. Only in the ICU, with its facilities for careful monitoring and adjustment of therapy, can many of these treatments be successfully carried out.

Management of Status Epilepticus

Unlike simple, brief seizures, status epilepticus threatens lasting deficits or death if not controlled (see Chapter 172). Any patient whose sequential seizures cannot be arrested promptly with routine management (e.g., intravenous benzodiazepines, phenytoin) must be observed in the ICU, where therapy ranging up to general anesthesia with artificial ventilation may be required.

Evaluation of Neurologic Disease Accompanying Severe Medical Disease

Neurologic signs or symptoms develop in many patients admitted to the ICU for myocardial infarction, subacute bacterial endocarditis, cardiac arrhythmia, pneumonia, acute respiratory distress syndrome, septic shock, renal disease, hepatic failure, and other similar disorders while they are under treatment for the primary medical problem. Numerous questions are raised: Is the neurologic finding a consequence of the underlying disease, or is it coincidental? Does it demand further investigation at once, or can it wait? Should therapy be changed, or should new therapy be started? These issues demand the attention of the neurologist.

Management of Severe Medical Disease Accompanying Neurologic Illness

In patients with severe medical disease accompanying neurologic illness, unrelated medical illness most often develops in the setting of a chronic neurologic disorder. The demented patient may experience a myocardial infarct, or septicemia may develop in the patient with multiple sclerosis. Indirect relationships should be sought. Does the demented patient have multiple cerebral emboli from underlying cardiac disease? Is the patient with multiple sclerosis septicemic from a bladder infection due to impaired urinary control? Early recognition of a change in the seriousness of the neurologic patient's condition is often difficult, but it may be critical to a successful outcome.

PROGNOSTIC AND ETHICAL CONSIDERATIONS

When severe damage involves the brain, either as a separate neurologic condition or as a secondary consequence of other medical disease, the physician who requested neurologic consultation and the family often need guidance regarding the probable outcome. There are three critical questions: Will the patient survive? Has irreversible brain damage occurred? What is the likely degree of residual disability?

There are few simple rules that can be applied infallibly to determine the prognosis in, for example, comatose patients, especially early in the course. The most important consideration is often whether irreversible damage has affected crucial areas of the brain, rather than the depth of impairment of consciousness. The patient with glutethimide poisoning, for example, may show no evidence of any neurologic function yet can recover fully if vital functions are maintained. In contrast, the comatose patient with head trauma resulting in pontine hemorrhage and decerebrate rigidity may have a far worse prognosis. The probability of neurologic recovery generally declines with advancing age, size and location of the lesion, and duration of deficit. A number of studies have provided statistical guidelines that are of value in gauging the probability of recovery [9,10]. Guidelines for the evaluation of prognosis following cardiac arrest and resuscitation are particularly well documented, and the absence of pupillary and corneal reflexes or motor response to pain, the occurrence of myoclonic status epilepticus, absence of somatosensory evoked potentials (N20), and elevated neuron-specific enolase are particularly useful in early determination of poor prognosis (9).

Early in the course of coma, the physician should not be hasty in abandoning hope and vigorous medical efforts to maintain survival and to limit neurologic damage. Late in the course, or as poor prognostic signs accumulate, it is important to recognize the outer limits of possible recovery and to assess the value of continuing life support accordingly. The patient's wishes, expressed in a living will or durable power of attorney for health care and as interpreted by close, responsible family members ("substituted judgment"), should combine with the physician's prognostic judgment to help determine a medical course of action. Although management in the ICU usually entails the unstinting use of every available means of life support and treatment, there must eventually be a transition either to recovery or to a permanent state of dependence, and the nature and extent of continued treatment should be adjusted accordingly. The technical means of maintaining survival almost indefinitely by the use of extraordinary measures is now available. It is important for the physician and the patient's family to consider whether, in the case of a patient with irreversible and severe neurologic damage, they are extending life or prolonging the process of dying [11].

It is clear that neurologic problems abound in the ICU. A successful approach to these disorders requires the physician to recognize the nature of the clinical situation prompting neurologic consultation or admission to the ICU. An analysis of which of the nine types of neurologic clinical situations is being encountered often guides the physician initially in diagnosis and management. The following chapters discuss some of the more common neurologic problems encountered in the ICU, with specific attention to management in the ICU and a broader view of the neurologic conditions in general.

References

1. Ropper AH, Gress DR, Mayer S, et al: *Neurological and Neurosurgical Intensive Care.* 4th ed. Philadelphia, Lippincott Williams & Wilkins, 2004.
2. Posner JB, Saper CB, Schiff ND, et al: *Plum and Posner's Diagnosis of Stupor and Coma.* 4th ed. New York, Oxford University Press, 2007.
3. Teasdale G, Jennett B: Assessment of coma and impaired consciousness. A practical scale. *Lancet* 2:81, 1974.
4. Jennett B, Teasdale G: *Management of Head Injury.* Philadelphia, FA Davis, 1981.
5. Wijdicks EF: The diagnosis of brain death. *N Engl J Med* 344(16):1215, 2001.
6. Cronin CA: Intravenous tissue plasminogen activator for stroke: a review of the ECASS III results in relation to prior clinical trials. *J. Emergency Med* 38(1): 99–105, 2010.
7. Arrich J, Holzer M, Herkner H, et al: Hypothermia for neuroprotection in adults after cardiopulmonary resuscitation. *Cochrane Database Syst Rev* 4: CD004128, 2009.
8. Patchell RA, Tibbs PA, Regine WF, et al: Direct decompressive surgical resection in the treatment of spinal cord compression caused by metastatic cancer: a randomised trial. *Lancet* 366:643, 2005.
9. Wijdicks EFM, Hijdra A, Young GB, et al: Practice parameter: prediction of outcome in comatose survivors after cardiopulmonary resuscitation (an evidence-based review). *Neurology* 67:203–210, 2006.
10. Zandbergen EG, Hijdra A, Koelman JHTM, et al: For the PROPAC study group. Prediction of poor outcome within the first three days of postanoxic coma. *Neurology* 66:62–68, 2006.
11. Wanzer SH, Federman DD, Adelstein SJ, et al: The physician's responsibility toward hopelessly ill patients: a second look. *N Engl J Med* 320:844, 1989.

CHAPTER 169 ■ EVALUATING THE PATIENT WITH ALTERED CONSCIOUSNESS IN THE INTENSIVE CARE UNIT

RAPHAEL A. CARANDANG, LAWRENCE J. HAYWARD AND DAVID A. DRACHMAN

The spectrum of disease that leads to acute impairment of consciousness is broad; the disorders are varied and potentially life threatening and may be treatable if recognized early. The clinician evaluating the patient with an altered level of consciousness must do so in a systematic and efficient fashion. The approach consists of (a) rapidly determining the type of mental status change, (b) administering life support measures where urgently needed, (c) obtaining a detailed history and physical examination directed at determining more precisely the cause of the nervous system disorder, (d) selecting appropriate and informative diagnostic and laboratory studies, and (e) initiating more definitive treatment based on this assessment.

As a practical matter, *consciousness* refers to a state of awareness of self and environment that depends on intact arousal and content [1,2]. Arousal is the level of attentive wakefulness and readiness to respond to relevant sensory information. Alerting stimuli activate the ascending reticular activating system (ARAS), which extends from the superior pons to the thalamus and projects to multiple cortical areas. Diminished arousal implies dysfunction of either the ARAS or both cerebral hemispheres; lesions of the brainstem sparing the ARAS (e.g., of the medulla) or of only one hemisphere do not affect wakefulness. This chapter defines altered states of consciousness and presents a systematic approach to bedside evaluation and prognostication of the comatose patient.

ALTERED STATES OF CONSCIOUSNESS

Neurologists are frequently consulted for evaluation of patients who appear unconscious, confused, or awake and alert but noncommunicative.

Patient Who Appears Unconscious

Patients who appear unconscious lie mostly motionless, usually with the eyes closed and seemingly unaware of their environment. The causes of this condition include normal sleep, depressed consciousness, psychogenic coma, locked-in state, vegetative states, minimally conscious state, and brain death.

Sleep

The normal unconsciousness of sleep is characterized by prompt reversibility on threshold sensory stimulation, and maintenance of wakefulness following arousal. The degree of stimulation required depends on the stage of sleep (stage IV non–rapid eye movement sleep is the deepest) and the sensory stimulation used.

Depressed Consciousness

Consciousness is deemed depressed when suprathreshold sensory stimulation is required for arousal and wakefulness cannot be maintained unless the stimulation is continuous [1,2]. Responsible specific lesions involve the ARAS or both cerebral hemispheres; the former by brainstem damage, or compression due to masses situated in other compartments, and the latter by multifocal insults or unilateral lesions with associated major mass effect. In addition, a wide array of metabolic derangements, toxins, or diffuse injuries may depress consciousness by affecting the ARAS, the cerebral hemispheres, or both. The spectrum of depressed states—lethargy, hypersomnolence, obtundation, stupor, and coma—is defined by the level of consciousness observed on examination. The etiologies are diverse (Table 169.1), with the degree of depression dependent on the nature of the insult, its duration, and the location and extent of the brain injury.

The first signs of brain dysfunction may be mild and barely noticeable. The patient may be described initially as confused or drowsy before progressing to *lethargy* or *hypersomnolence* and eventually to a more depressed state. Hypersomnolent patients maintain arousal only with vigorous and continuous sensory stimulation; while awake, however, they may be oriented and make appropriate responses. The most common cause of hypersomnolence in the hospital is sleep deprivation, mostly iatrogenic, especially in the around-the-clock care setting of the intensive care unit (ICU). Patients with discrete diencephalic or midbrain tegmentum lesions may also present with hypersomnolence [3,4]. Because these lesions affect the ARAS and spare the cerebral hemispheres, cognitive content is usually preserved. Rostral extension of a midline lesion may involve thalamic structures (especially the dorsomedial nuclei) and cause difficulties with the ability to store new memories. Other mesencephalic structures may be affected and cause abnormalities of pupillary function, internuclear ophthalmoplegia, and third nerve dysfunction.

TABLE 169.1

DIFFERENTIAL DIAGNOSIS OF DEPRESSED CONSCIOUSNESS

I. Depressed consciousness with lateralizing signs of brain disease: brain tumor, cerebral hemorrhage, cerebral thrombosis, cerebral embolism, contusion, subdural or epidural hemorrhage, brain abscess, hypertensive encephalopathy

II. Depressed consciousness with signs of meningeal irritation: meningitis, subarachnoid hemorrhage, leptomeningeal carcinoma, or lymphoma

III. Depressed consciousness without lateralizing or meningeal signs: alcohol, barbiturate, or opiate intoxication: carbon monoxide poisoning, neuroleptic malignant syndrome, anoxia, hyponatremia, hypoglycemia, diabetic coma, uremia, hepatic coma, hypercapnia, nonconvulsive status epilepticus, infectious encephalitis, acute hydrocephalus, concussion, diffuse axonal injury, hypothermia

Adapted from Adams RD, Victor M: *Principles of Neurology*. 4th ed. New York, McGraw-Hill, 1989.

Obtunded patients usually can be aroused by light stimuli but are mentally dulled and unable to maintain wakefulness. *Stuporous* patients can be aroused only with vigorous noxious stimulation. While awake, neither obtunded nor stuporous patients demonstrate a normal content of consciousness, but both may display purposeful movements, attempting to ward off painful stimuli or to remove catheters, endotracheal tubes, or intravenous lines.

Patients in *coma* are unresponsive to suprathreshold sensory stimulation, including noxious stimulation that is strong enough to arouse a deeply sleeping patient but not strong enough to cause physical injury. Although the patient usually lies motionless, movements such as stereotyped, inappropriate postures (decerebration and decortication) and spinal cord reflexes (triple flexion and Babinski responses) may occur. Whatever the etiology, the duration of coma is typically no longer than 2 to 4 weeks, after which one of the three conditions supervenes: arousal to full or partial recovery, a vegetative state, or death.

Most of the literature on prognosis of comatose patients comes from nontraumatic coma, largely anoxic–ischemic brain injury. A landmark paper by Levy, Plum, and associates from 1981 established the neurological examination – particularly brainstem reflexes including pupillary, corneal, and oculocephalic reflexes – as important predictors of poor outcome in nontraumatic coma [5]. Multiple studies followed which confirmed the importance of motor responses in addition to brainstem examination, and some diagnostic tests were established as useful in predicting outcomes; these are well summarized in the American Academy of Neurology Practice Parameter by Wijdicks et al., published in 2006 [6]. Given the life-or-death responsibility of the physician providing a prognosis, only clinical indicators or diagnostic tests that are highly specific with a near zero false–positive rate are utilized. A poor outcome is predicted by the absence of pupillary and corneal reflexes, absent or extensor motor responses, absent responses to caloric testing of the oculovestibular reflex at day 3 post-arrest, and the presence of myoclonic status epilepticus on day 1 post-arrest. The absence of N20 responses on somatosensory evoked potential (SSEP) testing, and the finding of serum neuron-specific enolase levels more than 33 μg per L on days 1 to 3 post-arrest also indicate a poor prognosis (Fig. 169.1). Prognostication must include consideration of the etiology of the disease process, the clinical examination findings, and radiological evidence of damage to the upper pons, midbrain, diencephalon, and other vital structures for arousal.

Psychogenic Coma

Patients in psychogenic coma appear comatose but have clinical and laboratory evidence of wakefulness [1]. Psychogenic unresponsiveness may be suggested by active resistance or rapid closure of the eyelids, pupillary constriction to visual threat, fast phase of nystagmus (i.e., a saccade) on oculovestibular or optokinetic testing, and avoidance of self-injury (e.g., by averting an arm dropped toward the patient's face) or annoying stimulation such as a nasal tickle (moving head away from stimulus). Caloric testing with ice water irrigation of the ear will elicit a

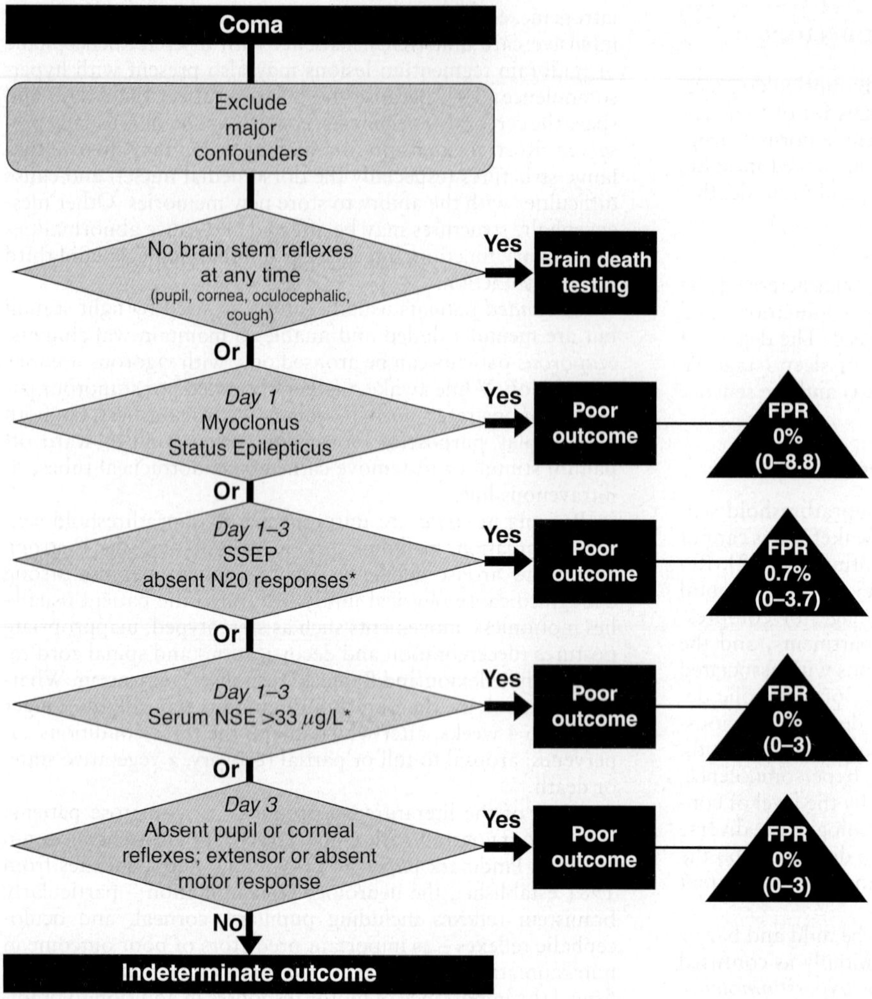

FIGURE 169.1. Algorithm for predicting outcome in comatose patients after cardiopulmonary arrest. FPR, false positive rate; NSE, neuron-specific enolase; SSEP, somatosensory evoked potential. [From Wijdicks EFM: The diagnosis of brain death. *N Engl J Med* 344:1215, 2001.]

normal nystagmoid response with the fast or corrective component directed away from the irrigated ear and possibly some nausea and vomiting. Deep tendon reflex examination is often normal but can be voluntarily suppressed. EEG alpha waves that attenuate with eye opening are inconsistent with coma or sleep. Most diagnostic tests will be unrevealing. Psychiatric conditions that may be associated with psychogenic coma are conversion reactions secondary to hysterical personality, severe depression, or acute situational reaction, catatonic schizophrenia, dissociative or fugue states, severe psychotic depression, and malingering.

Locked-in State

The locked-in state is a nearly total paralysis without loss of consciousness [7,8]. Because the most common cause of this state is destruction of the base of the pons, the patient is completely paralyzed except for muscles subserved by midbrain structures (i.e., vertical eye movements and blinking). Consciousness is preserved because the ARAS is located in the tegmentum of the pons, dorsal to the damaged area. The most frequent cause is cerebrovascular such as cerebral infarction from a basilar thromboembolism or pontine hemorrhage from uncontrolled hypertension; less frequent etiologies of the syndrome are acute polyneuropathy (Guillain-Barré syndrome), acute poliomyelitis, toxins that block transmission at the neuromuscular junction, and myasthenia gravis. It is important to note that locked-in patients are capable of hearing, seeing, and feeling external stimuli and pain. Adequate analgesia and anxiolysis should be provided despite the absence of external signs of pain and anxiety. A 5- to 10-year survival has been reported in as high as 80% of patients in some series and a surprising 58% of patients surveyed reported satisfaction with life despite their disability in a small case series [8].

Brain Death

The term *brain death* refers to a determination of physical death by brain-based, rather than cardiopulmonary-based, criteria [9]. Brain death is the irreversible destruction of the brain, with the resulting total absence of all cortical and brainstem function, although spinal cord reflexes may remain [10,11]. It is not to be confused with severe but incomplete brain damage with a poor prognosis or with a vegetative state, conditions in which some function of vital brain centers still remains. In brain death, support of other organs is futile for the patient, whereas when there is some residual brain or brainstem function, or a vegetative state, decisions regarding ongoing life support clearly depend on the wishes of the patient or his or her proxy.

In brain death, pupils are mid-position and round (not oval), and apnea persists even when arterial carbon dioxide tension (PCO_2) is raised to levels that should stimulate respiration. Table 169.2 summarizes the guidelines used in the United States. Brain death may be simulated by drug intoxications and cannot be evaluated when toxic drugs are present; depending on preserved renal and hepatic function most such toxic

TABLE 169.2

CRITERIA FOR BRAIN DEATH

Prerequisites

1. Clinical or neuroimaging evidence of an acute CNS catastrophe compatible with the clinical diagnosis of brain death
2. Exclusion of complicating medical conditions that may confound clinical assessment (no severe electrolyte, acid–base, or endocrine disturbance)
3. No drug intoxication or poisoning
4. Core temperature = 32°C (90°F)

1. Cerebral functions are absent.
   Coma, and absence of motor responses including decerebrate posturing, although spinal reflexes may be seen
2. Brainstem functions are absent.
   Absence of pupillary responses to light; pupils at mid-position and dilated
   Absent corneal reflexes, caloric reflexes, gag reflex, cough in response to tracheal suctioning, sucking and rooting reflexes
   Absence of respiratory drive at $PaCO_2$ 60 mm Hg, or 20 mm Hg above normal base-line values
   Interval between two separate examinations varies depending on the age of the patient if pediatric, but for adults is usually at least 6 hours
3. Ancillary Diagnostic tests:
   EEG showing electrocerebral silence
   Technetium Tc 99m hexametazime nuclear scan showing absence of activity in brain
   Cerebral angiography showing absence of blood flow in cerebral vessels
   Transcranial Doppler showing lack of diastolic or reverberating flow and small systolic peaks in early systole

Revised table from AAN Practice Guidelines. A Report of the Quality Standards Subcommittee of the American Academy of Neurology 1994; and Wijdicks EFM: The diagnosis of brain death. *N Engl J Med* 344:1215, 2001.

effects do not persist longer than 36 hours. Hypothermia also precludes a diagnosis of brain death, and the patient must be brought to normal temperature prior to declaring death. Brain death is a clinical diagnosis, but ancillary tests such as an EEG and blood flow studies (transcranial Doppler, technetium-99 m scan, or conventional cerebral angiography) may be useful where the clinical examination is compromised by sedating medications. Unresponsiveness that can mimic brain death may occur with extensive brainstem destruction, for example, after basilar artery thrombosis. Despite absent brainstem reflexes, continued cortical activity on the EEG and persistent cerebral blood flow would demonstrate that the patient is not brain dead.

The American Academy of Neurology has published practice parameters for the determination of brain death. The criteria take into account etiology, performance of two separate clinical examinations 6 hours apart, and include the method of apnea testing with preoxygenation and oxygen [11]. Since criteria for brain death vary from state to state, and procedures to determine brain death differ among institutions, it is important to be familiar with the guidelines in your institution [12]. The occurrence of brain death provides the opportunity for organ donation, and most institutions have a protocol that includes informing organ bank organizations to facilitate this.

Patient Who Appears Confused

Confusion is a general term used for patients who do not think with customary speed, clarity, or coherence. The causes of this condition include an acute confusional state, dementia, inapparent seizures, and receptive aphasia.

Acute Confusional State

When the cerebral hemispheres are insulted by toxic, metabolic, anoxic, structural, or infectious processes, the patient may appear acutely confused [13,14]. Poor arousal and an abnormal content of consciousness may contribute to the clinical presentation, and the etiologies are legion (Table 169.3). Patients with clouded consciousness are easily distracted or startled by environmental stimuli. Their processing of information is slow and effortful, arousal fluctuates from drowsiness to hyperexcitability, and poor attention span impairs recall and recent memory. If sensorial clouding becomes more advanced, sensory input is increasingly misinterpreted, daytime drowsiness alternates with nocturnal agitation, disorientation for place and time becomes apparent, and repeated prompting is required for a response to even the simplest commands.

Delirious patients typically manifest acutely fluctuating confusion, with psychomotor overactivity, agitation, autonomic instability, and often visual hallucinations. Clinical observations frequently suggest that the disturbance of cognition or perception is directly related to a potentially reversible general medical condition rather than to an evolving dementia. Hyperexcitability may alternate with periods of drowsiness or relative lucidity. Signs of autonomic overactivity include pupillary dilatation, diaphoresis, tachycardia, and hypertension. Patients with delirium may not sleep, sometimes for periods of several days; the success of treatment can be judged by the development of normal sleep. Delirium tremens, the most serious consequence of ethanol withdrawal, is perhaps the best-known example of this state. Because the routine Mini-Mental State Examination often cannot be administered to unstable, intubated patients, alternative screening tools have been developed for early detection and monitoring of delirium in the ICU [15,16]. Validated tools such as the Confusion Assessment Method, or CAM-ICU scale, have the advantage of being simple and easy to administer, highly reliable and applicable in patients who are intubated. Systematic screening may help detect early delirium and allow prompt, cost-effective treatment. Delirium has been linked to prolonged ICU stay and ventilator days, and is associated with postdischarge cognitive dysfunction and worse 6-month mortality outcomes [16,17]. The use of interventions that reduce delirium in the ICU include reduction and intermittent use of sedatives, or spontaneous awakening trials, as well as sedation with alpha adrenergic medications such as dexmedetomidine [18,19].

In beclouded dementia, confusion is superimposed on an underlying subacute or chronic cognitive disorder. The preexisting cerebral dysfunction may be mental retardation, dementia, or the deficits from a vascular, neoplastic, or demyelinative process. In some cases, the underlying disorder is not diagnosed until the confusion appears during an intercurrent illness (e.g., sepsis or infection, congestive heart failure, surgical procedures, anemia, drug overdose, or intolerance).

Dementia

Patients with dementia have subacute or chronic intellectual dysfunction unaccompanied by a reduction in arousal [20]. The patient exhibits a decline in multiple cognitive functions, including memory, language, spatial orientation, personality, abstract thinking, and insight. The ability to carry out testing requires relative preservation of attention and language

TABLE 169.3

CLASSIFICATION OF ACUTE CONFUSIONAL STATES

ACS not associated with focal or lateralizing neurologic signs and normal CSF
Metabolic disorders
Hepatic encephalopathy
Uremia
Hypercapnia
Hypoglycemia
Diabetic ketotic coma
Porphyria
Hypercalcemia
Infectious disorders
Septicemia[a]
Pneumonia[a]
Typhoid fever[a]
Rheumatic fever[a]
Drug intoxication
Opiates
Barbiturates
Tricyclic antidepressants
Other sedatives
Amphetamines[a]
Anticholinergic medications[a]
Abstinence states (i.e., withdrawal states)
Alcohol (delirium tremens)[a]
Barbiturates[a]
Benzodiazepines[a]
States that reduce cerebral blood flow or oxygen content
Hypoxic encephalopathy
Congestive heart failure
Cardiac arrhythmias
Situational psychoses (diagnoses)
Postoperative psychosis[a]
Posttraumatic psychosis[a]
Puerperal psychosis[a]
Intensive care unit psychosis[a]
ACS associated with focal or lateralizing neurologic signs and/or abnormal CSF
Cerebrovascular disease or space-occupying lesions (especially of the right parietal, inferofrontal, and temporal lobes)
Ischemic infarct[a]
Neoplasm[a]
Abscess[a]
Hemorrhage (intraparenchymal, subdural, epidural)[a]
Granuloma
Infectious disorders
Meningitis[a]
Encephalitis[a]
Subarachnoid hemorrhage[a]
Cerebral contusion and laceration[a]
ACS sometimes associated with focal or lateralizing neurologic signs
Postconvulsive delirium[a]
Acute hydrocephalus
Nonconvulsive status epilepticus
Nonketotic diabetic coma

[a]These disorders may be associated with signs of psychomotor overactivity or delirium.
ACS, acute confusional state; CSF, cerebrospinal fluid.
Adapted from Adams RD, Victor M: *Principles of Neurology*. 4th ed. New York, McGraw-Hill, 1989.

comprehension. The causes of dementia include degenerative processes (Alzheimer's disease, Pick's disease, Huntington's disease), metabolic and nutritional disorders (hypothyroidism, pellagra, vitamin B_{12} deficiency), infectious diseases (subacute spongiform encephalopathy, acquired immunodeficiency syndrome dementia, neurosyphilis, chronic meningitis, progressive multifocal leukoencephalopathy), cerebrovascular disorders (multi-infarct dementia, anoxia-ischemia), hydrocephalus with normal or increased intracranial pressure, and toxins.

Inapparent Seizures

Patients with nonconvulsive status epilepticus may appear disoriented, episodically unresponsive, or alternately lucid and confused; the EEG shows continuous or frequent epileptiform discharges [21,22]. Careful observation may alert the clinician to seizure phenomena, such as episodic staring, eye deviation or nystagmoid jerks, facial or hand clonic activity, and automatisms. The syndrome may be the result of a generalized (absence) status or a complex partial status. Complex partial status is the more common form seen in the ICU and may not be preceded by a history of complex partial seizures. The origin of the abnormal focal discharge may be from the temporal, frontal, or occipital lobes, and the EEG pattern during the ictus is variable. Inapparent seizures may occur in as many as 19% of all patients in the ICU, and 56% of patients who are comatose at the time of the monitoring. The yield of EEG monitoring is increased by continuous monitoring for 24 hours [23]. Nonconvulsive status epilepticus should be considered, and is the cause of otherwise unexplained coma in as many as 8% of patients [24]. A benzodiazepine, such as diazepam or lorazepam, may eliminate the discharge and improve the patient's confusion.

Receptive Aphasia

Patients with receptive aphasia often appear confused because they have a disorder of language comprehension [14]. The patient is awake and alert but unable to comprehend written or verbal commands despite voluminous (fluent) spontaneous speech. Paraphasias may be present (especially when the patient is asked to name objects) and consist of either inappropriately substituted words or nonsensical jargon. The responsible lesions are located in the dominant temporoparietal cortex and are often associated with subtle focal neurologic signs, including mild pronator drift of the right hand, right homonymous hemianopsia or superior quadrantanopsia, and right-sided sensory loss; gross hemiparesis is usually not found, as the frontal motor cortex is not affected.

Patient Who Appears Awake and Alert but Noncommunicative

Although sensory stimulation may arouse these patients, they seem unable or unwilling to speak. The causes of this condition include mutism, akinetic mutism, and the persistent vegetative state.

Mutism

Mutism is a manifestation of many clinical conditions, including aphonia, anarthria, oral-lingual apraxia, and aphasia. Only in aphasia, however, is written expression also impaired (i.e., agraphia).

Aphonia due to paralysis of the vocal cords and anarthria due to paralysis of the articulatory muscles are usually evident clinically in patients who are unable to make sounds but who mouth words appropriately. Oral-lingual (facial) apraxia is a disorder of learned mouth movements (e.g., speaking, blowing kisses, sucking through a straw, protruding the tongue to command) seen with isolated and discrete lesions involving the facial area of the dominant motor cortex [14,25].

Patients with expressive aphasia are unable to communicate normally by verbal or written language [1,13,14]. Nonfluent (Broca's) aphasia with diminished "telegraphic" output is usually intensely frustrating to the patient; occasionally, singing his or her words, rather than merely saying them, improves speech. Lesion location differs depending on whether comprehension is also affected or whether comprehension and repetition of words are relatively preserved or lost. At the least, the dominant frontal cortex is involved, and some degree of right hemiparesis is usually present.

Akinetic Mutism

Patients with akinetic mutism appear alert and exhibit sleep–wake cycles, but they show little evidence of cognitive function and do not meaningfully interact with the environment [1,14]. Brainstem function is intact, and patients may open their eyes to verbal stimuli or track moving objects. They have a paucity of movement even to noxious stimulation, despite little evidence of corticospinal or corticobulbar damage. Akinetic mutism is associated with large bilateral lesions of the basomedial frontal lobes, small lesions of the paramedian reticular formation in the posterior diencephalon and midbrain, and subacute communicating hydrocephalus.

Persistent Vegetative State

Patients in a persistent vegetative state are also akinetic and mute but lack outward manifestations of any significant brain activity other than reflex responses [1,14]. These may include decerebrate or decorticate posturing, deep tendon reflexes, Babinski or triple flexion reflexes, yawning, and so on. The term is usually reserved for the patient who has recovered only to this extent from coma due to a severe anoxic, metabolic, or traumatic brain injury, and has been in this condition for over a month. Neuropathologic findings in anoxic encephalopathy may include cortical pseudolaminar necrosis, cerebellar Purkinje cell loss, and necrosis of hippocampal cortex but relative sparing of brainstem structures [26]. Persistent vegetative state is considered permanent if the patient has been in this state for 3 months after nontraumatic or anoxic brain injury, and more than 12 months after traumatic brain injury [27].

Minimally Conscious State

These are patients who, similar to those in the vegetative state, have severely impaired consciousness, also manifest the posturing, reflexes, and diurnal cycles, but in addition show evidence of self and environmental awareness. They may follow simple commands, give gestural yes or no responses, verbalize intelligibly, and do other purposeful behaviors and visual tracking [1,13,14]. This is considered to be a transitional phase of recovery from coma after PVS, and patients with traumatic brain injury who are in a minimally conscious state have significantly better outcomes at 1 year than PVS patients. Many publicized reports of late recoveries from vegetative states were actually patients in MCS.

BEDSIDE EVALUATION OF THE COMATOSE PATIENT

Coma in the ICU is a medical emergency. The goal of each evaluation is to identify and treat promptly (if applicable) the cause of the comatose state; even if no definitive treatment is available, general medical and neurologic support is necessary. A neurologic consultation should be obtained early; the practice of obtaining imaging studies before a careful and systematic examination is often counterproductive when it delays focused evaluation and treatment. The proper approach requires (a) immediate administration of life-support measures, (b) completion of a general physical examination, (c) performance and interpretation of the neurologic examination, (d) selection of ancillary tests, and (e) institution of definitive treatment, based on the above observations.

Initial Measures

As in all emergencies, vital signs, respiration, and circulation are first stabilized and monitored; the comatose patient often requires an endotracheal tube for respiratory support and airway protection. A large-bore intravenous line is started, and the blood is drawn for a complete blood cell count, glucose, electrolytes (including Ca^{2+}), blood urea nitrogen, creatinine, liver transaminases, and a toxicology screen. Arterial blood is obtained for determination of oxygen tension, PCO_2, and pH. If there is any doubt about the etiology of coma, 100 mg thiamine, 50 g glucose, and 0.4 mg naloxone are administered intravenously.

General Physical Examination

In addition to the usual complete examination, several points warrant special attention [1,2,13]. Severe hypothermia (rectal temperature less than or equal to 32°C or 89.6°F) may cause coma (as in elderly patients exposed to the cold) or provide clues to other etiologies (e.g., overwhelming sepsis, drug or alcohol intoxication, hypothyroidism, hypoglycemia, Wernicke's encephalopathy) [28]. Severe hyperthermia may result from intracranial causes, including infection and anterior hypothalamic or pontine destruction. Meningeal signs (e.g., nuchal rigidity) may be absent in deeply comatose patients, even in the presence of overwhelming bacterial meningitis. This sign should never be sought if cervical spine fracture or dislocation is suspected.

The skin should be thoroughly inspected for signs of trauma. Basilar skull fractures may be signaled by blood behind the ear (Battle's sign), cerebrospinal fluid rhinorrhea, or otorrhea. Orbital fractures may cause bleeding into periorbital tissues ("raccoon eyes").

The breath odor may suggest metabolic derangement or intoxication. The spoiled fruit odor of diabetic coma, the uriniferous odor of uremia, and the musty fetor of hepatic encephalopathy sometimes can be recognized. Although the odor of alcohol is usually noted, its presence does not rule out superimposed structural causes of coma (e.g., subdural hematoma), and its absence does not rule out intoxication with odorless spirits (e.g., vodka).

Respiratory patterns in comatose patients are distinctive [1,13,14]. Bilateral hemispheric or diencephalic disturbances as well as systemic disorders may lead to periodic breathing in which increasing and then decreasing breaths (crescendo–decrescendo) alternate with apnea (Cheyne-Stokes respirations). Lesions of the midbrain-pontine tegmentum may give rise to tachypnea and a respiratory alkalosis unresponsive to oxygen (central neurogenic hyperventilation), but this is much less common than hyperpnea due to low oxygen tension, metabolic acidosis, or a primary respiratory alkalosis (e.g., salicylate poisoning). Lesions of the inferior pons may be associated with 2- to 3-second pauses following full inspiration (apneustic breathing). Compressive or intrinsic lesions of the medulla may cause chaotic breathing of varying rate and depth (Biot's breathing). Complete brainstem destruction results in apnea that is unresponsive to elevated PCO_2.

Neurologic Examination

The goal of the neurologic examination in the comatose patient is to determine the location of the lesion (ARAS or bilateral cerebral hemispheres) and its etiology (structural, causing destruction or compression of brain substance; toxic, metabolic, anoxic, or traumatic, affecting the nervous system in a diffuse or multifocal manner; subarachnoid blood or infection; or nonconvulsive status epilepticus). A critical part of this determination is the medical history, and heroic efforts to locate family members, witnesses, and medication lists are almost always rewarded. For example, truly sudden coma in a healthy person suggests drug intoxication, intracranial hemorrhage, meningoencephalitis, or an unwitnessed seizure.

Often an intubated patient with altered mental status will be on pharmacological sedation or anxiolysis for management of respiration, or safety in agitated or combative patients. Neurological examination should be performed after discontinuing any sedating medication that may alter the patient's responsiveness and significantly alter the examination findings.

Neurologic assessment must include a description of the level of consciousness, examination of the pupils, direct ophthalmoscopy, observation of spontaneous and induced ocular movements, elicitation of the corneal reflex, and tests of motor system function (including spontaneous and induced limb movements and asymmetries of tone), deep tendon reflexes, pathologic reflexes, and response to sensory stimulation—often pain. The importance of repeat examinations to document the temporal course of the patient's condition cannot be overemphasized.

Level of Consciousness

The level of consciousness is determined first by observing the patient undisturbed for several minutes. Any spontaneous (e.g., yawning, sneezing) or responsive (e.g., to ventilator noise) movements or postures are noted. A battery of graduated sensory stimuli is applied (whispered names, shouted names, loud noise, visual threat, noxious stimulation by supraorbital compression, vibrissal (nasal) stimulation, sternal rub, nail bed compression, or medial thigh pinch) and the response recorded (e.g., opens eyes, squeezes eyes shut, blinks symmetrically to visual threat, nods, turns head, groans, grimaces, purposefully withdraws, displays stereotyped posturing). Such careful documentation allows serial assessments of subtle changes over time by multiple examiners.

Serial documentation and accurate and reliable communication of findings can be facilitated by the use of standardized scales such as the Glasgow coma scale. While originally intended for use in traumatic brain injury, the Glasgow coma scale has become widely used and has been found to be predictive of outcomes, particularly in traumatic brain injury (Table 169.4). Because of its limitations, a more comprehensive coma scale called the Full Outline of Unresponsiveness, or FOUR score, incorporates brainstem reflexes and respiration [1,13,14,29]. These grading scales are helpful to standardize assessment, improve communication and serial monitoring, but are limited and cannot be substituted for a detailed bedside neurological examination.

Pupils

The pupils are examined for size, equality, and reactivity to light. Normal pupils confirm the integrity of a circuit involving the retina, optic nerve, midbrain, third cranial nerve, and pupillary constrictors. A strong flashlight and magnifying glass, or an ophthalmoscope, are usually necessary, and darkening the room is helpful.

TABLE 169.4

COMA GRADING SCALES

Glasgow Coma Scale
Eye response
4 = eyes open spontaneously
3 = eye opening to verbal command
2 = eye opening to pain
1 = no eye opening
Motor response
6 = obeys commands
5 = localizing pain
4 = withdrawal from pain
3 = flexion response
2 = extension response
1 = no motor response
Verbal response
5 = oriented
4 = confused
3 = inappropriate words
2 = incomprehensible words
1 = no verbal response
FOUR score
Eye response
4 = eyelids open or opened, tracking, or blinking to command
3 = eyelids open but not tracking
2 = eyelids closed but open to loud voice
1 = eyelids closed but open to pain
0 = eyelids remained closed with pain
Motor response
4 = thumbs up, fist or peace sign
3 = localizing to pain
2 = flexion response to pain
1 = extension response to pain
0 = no response to pain or generalized myoclonus
Brainstem reflexes
4 = pupils and corneals intact
3 = one pupil wide and fixed
2 = pupil or corneal absent
1 = pupil and corneal absent
0 = absent pupil, corneal and cough reflex
Respiration
4 = not intubated, regular breathing pattern
3 = not intubated, Cheyne-Stokes breathing
2 = not intubated, irregular breathing
1 = breathes above ventilator rate
0 = breathes at ventilator rate or apnea

Symmetrically small, light-reactive pupils (miosis) are normally seen in elderly and sleeping patients. Opiates, organophosphates, pilocarpine, phenothiazines, and barbiturates produce small pupils that may appear to be unreactive to light, whereas a large lesion of the pons (i.e., hemorrhage) characteristically produces tiny pinpoint pupils. Symmetrically large pupils (mydriasis) that do not react to light suggest midbrain damage, but they may also be seen following resuscitation when atropine has been used (in this case, the pupils do not constrict to 1% pilocarpine) [30], in cases of anoxia, following pressor doses of dopamine [31], and often in amphetamine or cocaine intoxication. Bilaterally fixed and midposition pupils indicate absent midbrain function, although severe hypothermia [28], hypotension, or intoxication with succinylcholine [32] or glutethimide [33] must be ruled out.

Pupillary asymmetry (anisocoria) suggests neurologic dysfunction if it is of recent onset, the inequality is more than

1 mm, and the degree of anisocoria changes with ambient lighting [34]. When the larger pupil is sluggishly reactive or fixed to light (but the contralateral consensual response is spared), uncal herniation due to an ipsilateral hemispheric mass compressing the third cranial nerve against the petroclinoid ligament must be considered. Unilateral pupillary dilatation may also indicate a mass in the cavernous sinus, aneurysm of the posterior communicating artery, focal seizure, or topical atropine-like drugs (e.g., used for ophthalmoscopic examination). On the other hand, with Horner's syndrome the affected pupil is smaller. In this condition, the pupillary asymmetry is increased in darkness and the smaller pupil is associated with partial ptosis of the upper eyelid, straightening of the lower eyelid, and facial anhidrosis. It may be caused by damage to descending sympathetic fibers anywhere from the hypothalamus to the upper thoracic cord, or to ascending sympathetic fibers in the cervical sympathetic chain, the superior cervical ganglion, the carotid artery, or the cavernous sinus.

Direct Ophthalmoscopy

Direct ophthalmoscopy may be limited by miosis or cataracts, but the pupils should never be pharmacologically dilated without clear documentation (with a large sign taped to the patient's bed), or if the patient's condition is uncertain or unstable. Obscuration of the disk margins, absent venous pulsations, and flame-shaped hemorrhages suggest early papilledema from an intracranial mass or systemic hypertension [35]. Subhyaloid and vitreous hemorrhages may be observed in the patient with subarachnoid hemorrhage or suddenly increased intracranial pressure.

Ocular Movements

Assessment of ocular movements begins by observing for tonic deviation of the eyes at rest [1]. The eyes may deviate toward the side of a lesion in the motor cortex (a gaze preference—away from the hemiparetic limbs) but usually can be induced to cross the midline. The eyes deviate away from the side of a pontine lesion (toward the hemiparetic limbs) and cannot be moved across the midline (a gaze paralysis). A seizure focus in the frontal (area 8) or supplementary motor (area 6) cortex can drive the eyes or cause nystagmoid jerks contralaterally (toward the side of the convulsing limbs) [36]. Tonic upward eye deviation may be seen after anoxia [37], and tonic downward deviation may be seen in thalamic hemorrhage, midbrain compression, and hepatic encephalopathy.

Spontaneous eye movements may have a localizing value. Roving eye movements (slow and random, usually conjugate and horizontal) and periodic alternating ("Ping-Pong") gaze (cyclic, conjugate excursions to the extremes of lateral gaze every 2 to 3 seconds) [38] are found in patients with intact brainstem function. Ocular bobbing consists of a rapid conjugate downward jerk followed by a slow upward drift (rate and rhythm are variable) and suggests a lesion in the posterior fossa, especially if horizontal eye movements are impaired [39]. The reverse movement, ocular dipping (slow downward, fast upward) can be seen after anoxia and in status epilepticus [40]. Conjugate spasmodic eye movements, rotating the eyes upward for minutes or longer (oculogyric crisis), in some patients may be an untoward effect of neuroleptic medications.

If spontaneous eye movements are absent or restricted to a particular direction, reflex movements should be tested by oculocephalic ("doll's eyes") and oculovestibular (caloric) stimulation [1,17,18,41]. Full eye movements induced by these maneuvers confirm the integrity of the brainstem tegmentum from the medullary-pontine junction to the midbrain. Oculocephalic testing is never done in patients with suspected cervical spine fracture or dislocation. The maneuver is performed by holding the patient's eyelids open and briskly rotating the head from one side to the other (for horizontal eye movements) and from flexion to extension (for vertical eye movements). In comatose patients with an intact brainstem, the eyes deviate to the side opposite the direction of head movement. If the oculocephalic response is not obtained or the movements are limited or asymmetric, the oculovestibular reflex should be tested. This is never done until the tympanic membrane is examined and seen to be intact. The patient's head is elevated to 30 degrees above horizontal, and up to 120 mL ice water is instilled slowly in the external auditory meatus with a large syringe and attached Teflon catheter. Each ear is tested separately for horizontal eye movements, with a 5-minute interval between right and left ears. In awake patients (or those in psychogenic coma), nystagmus with the fast phase away from the irrigated ear is induced. In comatose patients with an intact brainstem, a tonic conjugate eye deviation toward the irrigated ear is seen; a defective response implies brainstem damage. Vertical eye movements can be induced by irrigating both ears simultaneously with cold water (eyes deviate downward) and with warm (44°C) water (eyes deviate upward). Absent or deranged responses can be caused, in addition to various brainstem lesions, by previous vestibular (labyrinthine end-organ) lesions, vestibulosuppressant drugs (e.g., benzodiazepines, antihistamines, anticholinergics), hepatic encephalopathy, and neuromuscular blockers (e.g., succinylcholine). An ophthalmoplegia after intravenous phenytoin is well known [42].

Corneal Reflex

The corneal reflex is obtained by lightly touching the limbus of the cornea with a fine material (wisp of cotton, rolled corner of tissue paper, or a squirt of saline). Both eyes should blink to unilateral stimulation, confirming the integrity of a circuit involving the fifth cranial nerve, trigeminal sensory and facial motor nuclei in the pons, and both seventh cranial nerves. A blunted corneal response is commonly seen in chronic contact lens wearers. An absent blink on the stimulated side with an intact contralateral (consensual) response indicates ipsilateral motor damage.

Motor System

The examination of the motor system identifies whether limb movements are appropriate and purposeful or inappropriate and stereotyped. Left–right asymmetries or worsening of the motor response over time must be carefully noted. Appropriate movements include spontaneous turning in bed, drawing up the sheets, crossing the legs modestly, or rapid withdrawal (especially abduction) from noxious stimulation. Inappropriate movements include spontaneous or induced flexion–internal rotation of the arms with extension of the legs (decorticate posturing) or extension-adduction of all limbs (decerebrate posturing); whether flexor or extensor postures are induced depends partly on the position of the limbs [43]. These responses may occur occasionally in toxic-metabolic coma [44,45] but are more common with anatomic brainstem lesions. Facial grimaces or groans despite absent motor responses suggest that sensory pathways are grossly intact. Flexion of the leg at the hip, knee, and ankle (triple flexion response) is a spinally mediated exaggerated Babinski reflex that may persist in brain death.

Other spontaneous movements of the limbs and trunk have been observed in brain dead patients and are all forms of spinal reflexes, including myokymia, trunk flexion and the Lazarus sign, wherein the patient actually extends and pronates his or her arms forward and then crosses them over the chest [1,17,18,46]. These signs are easily misinterpreted by family members as well as medical practitioners who are not versed in the neurological examination.

INTERPRETATION OF THE NEUROLOGIC EXAMINATION

In general, focal neurologic signs suggest a structural cause of coma. Nevertheless, focal weakness is not unknown in hypoglycemia, hyperglycemia, hyponatremia, hyperkalemia, and rarely hepatic and uremic encephalopathies [47,48]; and continuous focal motor seizures (epilepsia partialis continua) may be a presenting sign of the hyperglycemic nonketotic hyperosmolar state [49]. Focal signs due to preexisting deficits may deceive even the ablest clinician. For example, if generalized seizures from a new metabolic imbalance develop in a patient with an old hemiplegia due to a cerebral infarction, apparently focal convulsions of the nonplegic limbs might falsely suggest a structural lesion of the intact cerebral hemisphere contralateral to the previously infarcted one. Other false localizing signs include sixth nerve palsies (due to transmitted increased intracranial pressure), visual field cuts (due to compression of the posterior cerebral artery), and hemiparesis ipsilateral to a third nerve palsy (due to compression of the contralateral cerebral peduncle against the tentorium [Kernohan's notch]).

Conversely, a nonfocal examination does not invariably indicate toxic-metabolic coma. Symmetric neurologic dysfunction may be caused by meningoencephalitis, subarachnoid hemorrhage, bilateral subdural hematomas, or thrombosis of the superior sagittal sinus. Multifocal seizures, myoclonus, asterixis, or fluctuation of the examination suggests a toxic or metabolic etiology, although periodic increases in intracranial pressure (plateau waves) and nonconvulsive seizures may lead to a waxing and waning mental status.

A preserved pupillary light reflex even in deep coma with absent oculovestibular and motor responses suggests a toxic or metabolic etiology. It is important to note that the pupils may be unreactive to light in severe hypothermia, deep barbiturate coma (the patient is usually apneic and hypotensive if the pupils are fixed), and glutethimide overdose. In addition, an expanding posterior fossa mass (e.g., cerebellar hemorrhage) may present with early signs of pontine compression and small, light-reactive pupils [50].

A useful rule is that toxic-metabolic coma usually has incomplete but symmetric dysfunction of neural systems affecting many levels of the neuraxis simultaneously while retaining the integrity of other functions at the same levels. Structural coma is characterized by regionally restricted anatomic defects [1,13,14]. For example, toxic-metabolic coma might present with intact pupillary reactivity and corneal reflexes but an absence of horizontal (pontine) and vertical (midbrain) reflex eye movements to oculovestibular testing. Such a presentation would be inconsistent with coma from a structural cause.

ANCILLARY TESTS

A computed tomographic (CT) scan without contrast infusion can reliably demonstrate intracranial bleeding such as intraparenchymal, epidural or subdural hematoma, or intraventricular hemorrhage. CT scans reveal hydrocephalus and may show anoxic–ischemic brain injury, with loss of grey–white differentiation, border-zone infarction from hypoperfusion, and diffuse cerebral edema (Fig. 169.2). Other coma-inducing lesions shown by CT scan include massive middle cerebral infarction, uncal herniation, and midline shift from large mass lesions with cerebral edema. Contrast enhancement may be required for suspected infectious or neoplastic masses. The CT scan does not reliably rule out inflammation, infection, subarachnoid blood, or early ischemia. CT angiography can be helpful in showing large vessel occlusion or dissection but has limited sensitivity and specificity. A CT scan can be considered the initial brain imaging study in patients with coma if lesions that require emergent surgical intervention, such as acute cerebellar hemorrhage, are considered [1,13,14].

Magnetic resonance imaging or MRI is clearly superior to CT scan in resolution, and special sequences are highly sensitive to acute ischemia and encephalitis. MRI is superior for anatomical detail and can produce excellent images of the posterior fossa, brainstem, and craniocervical junction. Diffusion weighted MRI studies, and particularly whole brain median apparent diffusion coefficient (ADC) imaging, is useful in assessing prognosis following anoxic/ischemic coma [51,52]. While it is not always logistically possible to perform MRI imaging on patients in the ICU, whenever possible it provides important information.

The cerebrospinal fluid must be examined if meningoencephalitis is suspected or if subarachnoid blood is not visualized on the CT scan. Occasionally, a sterile cerebrospinal fluid

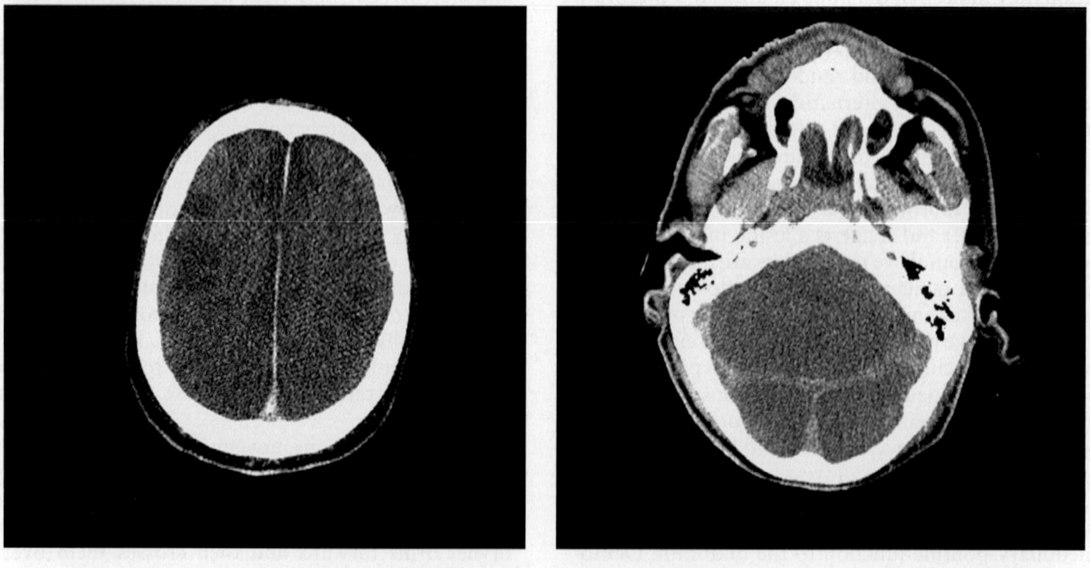

FIGURE 169.2. Noncontrast CT scan of patient with anoxic brain injury. Diffuse cerebral edema with loss of grey–white differentiation, obliteration of basal cisterns, multiple areas of hypodensity suggestive of anoxic–ischemic injury, and venous stasis with hyperdensity of the venous sinuses. This patient was brain dead clinically and by apnea testing.

pleocytosis follows status epilepticus [53]. The cerebrospinal fluid sent for protein 14–3-3 may also be useful for the diagnosis of Creutzfeldt-Jakob disease (CJD). Cytology and vascular endothelial growth factor (VEGF) levels can confirm the diagnosis of carcinomatous meningitis; and antibodies can be evaluated in paraneoplastic syndromes such as limbic encephalitis.

EEG provides a physiologic marker of brain function and may be helpful in nonconvulsive status epilepticus and psychogenic coma, and for documenting (but not primarily establishing) brain death by the presence of electrocerebral silence. In unresponsive patients, somatosensory or brainstem auditory evoked potentials may be very useful in evaluating the integrity of spinal, brainstem, or cortical pathways and, compared to EEG, are much less susceptible to drug effects and hypothermia. SSEPs are useful in prognostication of recovery from anoxic/ischemic coma during the first few days after cardiac arrest.

INITIATION OF EMERGENCY TREATMENT

Definitive treatment of altered consciousness depends on the underlying pathophysiologic process, but urgent therapeutic interventions may be required in life-threatening conditions or to prevent further central nervous system insult. Meticulous nursing care (fluid replacement, oxygenation and prevention of aspiration, nutrition, corneal protection, and conscientious skin, bowel, and bladder care) is essential. *Unnecessary sedation should be avoided*—it obscures evaluation of the patient's state of consciousness and makes assessment of any changes in the sensorium or cognition inaccessible to testing.

Recent and ongoing clinical trials are continuing to validate acute therapies that may protect the brain after insults such as cardiac arrest, traumatic brain injury, and stroke. For example, the induction of mild hypothermia (33°C for 12 to 24 hours) in comatose survivors of cardiac arrest improved the neurologic outcome in two randomized clinical trials [54,55]. Based on these studies, the American Heart Association and the International Liaison Committee on Resuscitation advised therapeutic mild hypothermia for unconscious victims of cardiac arrest [56]. Hypothermia appeared ineffective as an acute treatment for traumatic brain injury in one large randomized controlled trial [57] but may have been related to the delay in achieving goal temperature, duration of cooling, as well as other factors. A recent systematic review of 12 Randomized Controlled Trials that pooled 1,069 patients concluded that clinical mortality and outcome benefit may be derived from cooling patients with traumatic brain injury to a temperature of 32°C to 33°C for 48 hours and slowly rewarming them 24 hours after discontinuation of therapy [58]. A multicenter randomized clinical trial of early induced hypothermia for severe traumatic brain injury for 48 hours failed to show benefit but was terminated prematurely and was confounded by intracranial hypertension during rewarming [59]. There is a suggestion that hypothermia may benefit patients with acute stroke or refractory elevated intracranial pressure, but larger clinical trials are needed. Although prolonged or moderate hypothermia (28°C to 32°C) can be associated with complications of cardiac arrhythmia, coagulopathy, or infection, brief mild hypothermia appears relatively safe and effective [60,61]. If patients sustaining a neurologic insult are hypothermic upon admission to the ICU, it may be prudent to avoid aggressively warming them to normothermic levels. The benefit from mild hypothermia likely involves more complex biochemical mechanisms distinct from a simple reduction of oxygenation requirements. The deleterious effects of fever in brain injury are well documented in the laboratory and clinical outcome studies in a variety of diseases [62]. No large studies have prospectively addressed the effects of induced normothermia on outcomes. Comparison of endovascular and standard normothermia protocols to achieve a temperature of 36.5°C found no increase of adverse events, but was underpowered to show any benefit on neurologic outcome [63]. Further study in a larger sample of patients is warranted, and the development of protocols to control fever or induce normothermia is expected to benefit these patients.

CONCLUSION

Altered consciousness is common in patients in the ICU. A systematic and efficient approach is required to determine the location of the responsible lesion(s) or the cause(s) of impaired consciousness, both to allow institution of definitive therapies and to assess the prognosis accurately.

References

1. Posner JB, Saper CB, Schiff ND, et al: *Plum and Posner's Diagnosis of Stupor and Coma*. 4th ed. New York, Oxford University Press, 2007.
2. Fisher CM: The neurological examination of the comatose patient. *Acta Neurol Scand* 45[Suppl 36]:1, 1969.
3. Caplan LR: Top of the basilar syndrome. *Neurology* 30:72, 1980.
4. Bogousslvsky J, Regli F, Uske A: Thalamic infarcts: clinical syndromes, etiology, and prognosis. *Neurology* 38:837, 1988.
5. Levy DE, Bates D, Corona JJ et al: Prognosis in non-traumatic coma. *Ann Intern Med* 94:293–301, 1981.
6. Wijdicks EF, Hijdra A, Young GB, et al: Practice parameter: prediction of outcome in comatose survivors after cardiopulmonary resuscitation (an evidence-based review): report of the Quality Standards Subcommittee of the American Academy of Neurology. *Neurology* 67:203, 2006.
7. Patterson JR, Grabois M: Locked-in syndrome: a review of 139 cases. *Stroke* 17:758, 1986.
8. Doble JE, Haig AJ, Anderson C, et al: Impairment, activity, participation, life satisfaction and survival in persons with locked-in syndrome for over a decade: Follow up on a previously reported cohort. *J of Head Trauma Rehab* 18:435–444, 2003.
9. *President's Commission for the Study of Ethical Problems in Medicine and Biomedical and Behavioral Research: Defining Death: Medical, Legal, and Ethical Issues in the Determination of Death*. Washington, DC, US Government Printing Office, 1981.
10. Wijdicks EFM: The diagnosis of brain death. *N Engl J Med* 344:1215, 2001.
11. Quality Standards Subcommittee of the American Academy of Neurology: Practice parameters for determining brain death in adults [summary statement]. *Neurology* 45:1012, 1995.
12. Greer DM, Varelas PN, Haque S, et al: Variability of brain death determination guidelines in leading US neurologic institutions. *Neurology* 70:284–289, 2008.
13. Ropper AH, Gress DR, Diringer MN, (eds), et al: *Neurological and Neurosurgical Intensive Care*. 4th ed. Philadelphia, Lippincott Williams & Wilkins, 2004.
14. Ropper AH, Samuels MA: *Adams and Victor's Principles of Neurology*. 9th ed. New York: McGraw-Hill, 2009.
15. Bergeron N, Dubois MJ, Dumont M, et al: Intensive care delirium screening checklist: evaluation of a new screening tool. *Intensive Care Med* 27:859, 2001.
16. Ely EW, Inouye SK, Bernard G, et al: Delirium in Mechanically Ventilated Patients: Validity and Reliability of the Confusion Assessment Method for the Intensive Care Unit (CAM-ICU) *JAMA* 286:2703–2710, 2001.
17. Ely EW, Shintani A, Truman B, et al: Delirium as a predictor of mortality in mechanically ventilated patients in the intensive care unit. *JAMA* 291:1753–1762, 2004.
18. Girard TD, Kress JP, Fuchs BD, et al: Efficacy and safety of a paired sedation and ventilator weaning protocol for mechanically ventilated patients in intensive care (Awakening and Breathing Controlled trial): a randomised controlled trial. *Lancet*. 371:126–134, 2008.
19. Riker RR, Shehabi Y, Bokesch PM, et al: For the SEDCOM (Safety and Efficacy of Dexmedetomidine Compared With Midazolam) Study Group Dexmedetomidine vs Midazolam for Sedation of Critically Ill Patients: a Randomized Trial *JAMA* 301(5):489–499, 2009.
20. Strub RL, Black FW: *Neurobehavioral Disorders: A Clinical Approach*. Philadelphia, FA Davis, 1988.

21. Cascino GD: Nonconvulsive status epilepticus in adults and children. *Epilepsia* 34[Suppl 1]:S21, 1993.
22. Tomson T, Svangorg E, Wedlund JE: Nonconvulsive status epilepticus: high incidence of complex partial status. *Epilepsia* 27:276, 1986.
23. Claassen J, Mayer SA, Kowalski RG, et al: Detection of electrographic seizures with continuous EEG monitoring in critically ill patients *Neurology* 62:1743–1748, 2004.
24. Towne AR, Waterhouse EJ, Boggs JG, et al: Prevalence of nonconvulsive status epilepticus in comatose patients. *Neurology* 54:340, 2000.
25. Geschwind N: The apraxias: neural mechanisms of disorders of learned movement. *Am Sci* 63:188, 1975.
26. Kinney HC, Samuels MA: Neuropathology of the persistent vegetative state: a review. *J Neuropath Exp Neurol* 53:548, 1994.
27. Multi-Society Task Force on PVS. Medical aspects of the persistent vegetative state. *N Engl J Med* 330:1499–508, 1994.
28. Fischbeck KH, Simon RP: Neurological manifestations of accidental hypothermia. *Ann Neurol* 10:384, 1981.
29. Wijdicks EFM, Bamler WR, Maramattom BV, et al: Validation of a new coma scale: the FOUR score. *Ann Neurol.* 58:585–593, 2005
30. Thompson HS, Newsome DA, Loewenfeld IE: The fixed dilated pupils: sudden iridoplegia or mydriatic drops? A simple diagnostic test. *Arch Ophthalmol* 86:21, 1971.
31. Ong GL, Bruning HA: Dilated fixed pupils due to administration of high doses of dopamine hydrochloride. *Crit Care Med* 9:658, 1981.
32. Tyson RN: Simulation of cerebral death by succinylcholine sensitivity. *Arch Neurol* 30:409, 1974.
33. Brown DG, Hammill JF: Glutethimide poisoning: unilateral pupillary abnormalities. *N Engl J Med* 285:806, 1971.
34. Glaser JS: *Neuro-Ophthalmology*. Philadelphia: Lippincott Williams & Wilkins, 1999.
35. Neetens A, Smets RM: Papilledema. *Neuro-Ophthalmology* 9:81, 1989.
36. Wyllie E, Ludes H, Morris HH, et al: The lateralizing significance of versive head and eye movements during epileptic seizures. *Neurology* 36:606, 1986.
37. Keane JR: Sustained upgaze in coma. *Ann Neurol* 9:409, 1981.
38. Stewart JD, Kirkham TH, Mathieson G: Periodic alternating gaze. *Neurology* 29:222, 1979.
39. Mehler MF: The clinical spectrum of ocular bobbing and ocular dipping. *J Neurol Neurosurg Psychiatry* 51:725, 1988.
40. Ropper AH: Ocular dipping in anoxic coma. *Arch Neurol* 28:297, 1981.
41. Leigh RJ, Hanley DF, Munschauer FE, et al: Eye movements induced by head rotation in unresponsive patients. *Ann Neurol* 15:465, 1984.
42. Spector RH, Davidoff RA, Schwartzman RJ: Phenytoin-induced ophthalmoplegia. *Neurology* 26:1031, 1976.
43. Barolet-Romana G, Larson SJ: Influence of stimulus location and limb position on motor responses in the comatose patient. *J Neurosurg* 61:725, 1984.
44. Greenberg DA, Simon RP: Flexor and extensor postures in sedative drug-induced coma. *Neurology* 32:448, 1982.
45. Seibert DG: Reversible decerebrate posturing secondary to hypoglycemia. *Am J Med* 78:1036, 1985.
46. Saposnik G, Basile VS, Young GB: Movements in Brain Death: a Systematic Review. *Can J Neurol Sci.* 36:154–160, 2009.
47. Cadranel JF, Lebiez E, Di Martino et al: Focal Neurological signs in hepatic encephalopathy in cirrhotic patients: an underestimated entity? *Am J Gastroenterology* 96:515–518, 2001.
48. Palmer CA: Neurologic manifestations of renal disease. *Neurological Clinics* 20:23–34, 2002.
49. Singh BM, Strobos RJ: Epilepsia partialis continua associated with nonketotic hyperglycemia: clinical and biochemical profile of 21 patients. *Ann Neurol* 8:155, 1980.
50. Cuneo RA, Caronna JJ, Pitts L, et al: Upward transtentorial herniation. *Arch Neurol* 36:618, 1979.
51. Wijdicks EF, Campeau NG, Miller GM: MR imaging in comatose survivors of cardiac resuscitation. *Am J Neuroradiol* 22:1561–1565, 2001.
52. Wu O, Sorensen AG, Brenner T, et al: Comatose patients with cardiac arrest: predicting clinical outcome with diffusion weighted MRI imaging. *Radiology* 252:173–181, 2009.
53. Devinsky O, Nadi NS, Theodore WH, et al: Cerebrospinal fluid pleocytosis following simple, complex partial, and generalized tonic-clonic seizures. *Ann Neurol* 23:402, 1988.
54. The Hypothermia after Cardiac Arrest Study Group: Mild therapeutic hypothermia to improve the neurologic outcome after cardiac arrest. *N Engl J Med* 346:549, 2002.
55. Bernard SA, Gray TW, Buist MD, et al: Treatment of comatose survivors of out-of-hospital cardiac arrest with induced hypothermia. *N Engl J Med* 346:557, 2002.
56. Nolan JP, Morley PT, Vanden Hoek TL, et al: Therapeutic hypothermia after cardiac arrest: an advisory statement by the advanced life support task force of the International Liaison Committee on Resuscitation. *Circulation* 108:118, 2003.
57. Clifton GL, Miller ER, Choi SC, et al: Lack of effect of induction of hypothermia after acute brain injury. *N Engl J Med* 344:556, 2001.
58. McIntyre LA, Fergusson DA, Hebert PC, et al: Prolonged therapeutic hypothermia after traumatic brain injury in adults: a systematic review. *JAMA* 289:2992–2999, 2003.
59. Clifton GL, Valadka A, Zygun D, et al: Very early hypothermia induction in patients with severe brain injury. (the National Acute Brain Injury Study: Hypothermia II) A randomized trial. *Lancet Neurol* 10:131–139, 2011.
60. Polderman KH: Application of therapeutic hypothermia in the ICU. Opportunities and pitfalls of a promising treatment modality—Part 1: indications and evidence. *Intensive Care Med* 30:556, 2004.
61. Polderman KH: Application of therapeutic hypothermia in the intensive care unit: opportunities and pitfalls of a promising treatment modality—Part 2: practical aspects and side effects. *Intensive Care Med* 30:757, 2004.
62. Badjatia N: Hyperthermia and fever control in brain injury. *Crit Care Med* 37(7):s250–s257, 2009.
63. Broessner G, Beer R, Lackner P, et al: Prophylactic endovascularly based long-term normothermia in ICU patients with severe cerebrovascular disease: bicenter, prospective randomized trial. *Stroke* 40:e657–e665, 2009.

CHAPTER 170 ■ METABOLIC ENCEPHALOPATHY

PAULA D. RAVIN

Metabolic encephalopathy is a general term used to describe any process that affects global cortical function by altering the biochemical function of the brain. It is the most common cause of altered mental status in the intensive care unit (ICU) setting, either medical or surgical, and is also one of the most treatable. Early recognition of metabolic encephalopathy, therefore, is critical to the management of the ICU patient. The patients who are most at risk for development of a metabolic encephalopathy are those with single or multiple organ failure, the elderly (>60 years of age), those receiving multiple drugs with central nervous system (CNS) toxicity, and those with severe nutritional deficiencies such as cancer patients and alcoholics. Other risk factors include infection, temperature dysregulation (hypothermia or fever), chronic degenerative neurologic or psychiatric diseases such as dementia or schizophrenia, and endocrine disorders. Metabolic encephalopathy is always suspected when there is an altered cognitive status in the absence of focal neurologic signs or an obvious anatomic lesion such as an acute cerebrovascular accident or head injury. A patient may progress over days from intermittent agitation into depressed consciousness or quickly into coma without any antecedent signs (e.g., with hypoglycemia). In mild cases, it is easily mistaken for fatigue or psychogenic depression, whereas more severe cases may develop into coma and are life-threatening.

The altered mental status observed can start as mild confusion with intermittent disorientation to person, time, or place and difficulty attending to questions or tasks at hand. Delirium is a further change toward heightened arousal alternating with somnolence, often worse at night and fluctuating throughout the day. Finally, progression to lethargy, a state of sleepiness in which the person is difficult to arouse by vigorous stimulation, can lead into stupor or coma as impaired consciousness ensues.

TABLE 170.1

PATIENT PROFILE IN METABOLIC ENCEPHALOPATHY

Gradual onset over hours
Progressive if untreated
Waxing and waning level of consciousness
Patient treated with multiple CNS-acting drugs
Patient with organ failure, postoperative state, electrolyte disturbance, endocrine disease
No evidence of brain tumor or stroke on neurologic examination—usually nonfocal (except hypoglycemia)
Sometimes heralded by seizures—focal or generalized
Increased spontaneous motor activity—restlessness, asterixis, myoclonus, tremors, rigidity, and so forth
Abnormal blood chemistries, blood gases, anemia
Usually normal CNS imaging studies
Generalized electroencephalographic abnormalities—slowing, triphasic waves
Gradual recovery once treatment is initiated

CNS, central nervous system.

This sequence of events is often punctuated by focal or generalized tonic-clonic seizures and postictal somnolence as part of the overall clinical picture (Table 170.1).

Disorders that can be confused with metabolic encephalopathy include brain tumors, encephalitis, meningitis, closed head trauma, and brainstem cerebrovascular events. Brain tumors are usually recognizable because they produce focal neurologic deficits such as hemiplegia or hemianopsia, as do traumatic lesions of the brain and cortical strokes. Hypoglycemia can also present focally and is discussed further in the section on Hypoglycemic Encephalopathy. Brainstem stroke due to thrombosis of the basilar artery can be deceptive because there may be a gradual progression of signs and symptoms over several hours rather than a sudden presentation. Table 170.2 outlines some of the cardinal differences between brainstem stroke and metabolic encephalopathy.

EVALUATION

Clinical Examination

Initial observation of the patient's level of arousal, posture in bed, breathing pattern, vital signs, and behavioral fluctuations is highly suggestive of a metabolic disturbance in many cases. Waxing and waning levels of activity are the hallmark of metabolic encephalopathy and may occur over hours to days. Often signs of sympathetic overactivity (tachycardia, elevated blood pressure, tremulousness) and abnormal sleep patterns or "sun-downing" are present.

TABLE 170.3

EVALUATION FOR METABOLIC ENCEPHALOPATHY

Neurologic examination
Mental status
Pupillary responses
Oculomotor responses
Respiratory pattern
Motor activity, strength
Deep tendon reflexes, plantar responses
Initial laboratory tests
Blood sugar, electrolytes, lactate dehydrogenase, serum glutamic oxaloacetic transaminase, serum glutamic pyruvic transaminase, ammonia, blood urea nitrogen, creatinine, white blood cell count/differential, hemoglobin, hematocrit, blood gases
Electroencephalography
Neuroimaging
Head computed tomography or magnetic resonance imaging
± Lumbar puncture, toxicity screens, serum and urine osmolality, psychiatric examination

Mild *behavioral changes* are the earliest manifestations, such as lack of attentiveness to surroundings or a paucity of spontaneous speech, which may give the patient an apathetic or withdrawn appearance. The Mini-Mental State Examination easily reveals mild confusion and can be used to grade the patient's level of cognitive performance sequentially [1]. When there is impaired consciousness, however, this test is unreliable.

The *cranial nerve examination* is focused on pupillary responses, oculomotor function, and respiratory patterns (Table 170.3). As a rule, pupils are small, symmetric, and responsive to light in metabolic causes of obtundation or coma. Noteworthy exceptions to this are anticholinergic poisoning (e.g., atropine, scopolamine), which produces dilated sluggish pupils, and glutethimide (Doriden) poisoning, which results in mid- to large-sized sluggish or fixed pupils [2]. Ocular movements are usually unaffected initially, with eyes in midline position or slightly deviated outward and upward at rest (Bell's phenomenon). Doll's eye maneuvers produce conjugate deviation of the eyes opposite to the direction of head rotation. As the level of brainstem suppression progresses to coma, these responses may disappear completely, especially with an overdose of sedative drugs. In the face of hyperpnea and decerebrate

TABLE 170.2

SIGNS AND SYMPTOMS OF BRAINSTEM CEREBROVASCULAR ACCIDENT (CVA) AND METABOLIC ENCEPHALOPATHY

	Brainstem CVA	Metabolic encephalopathy
Patient profile	Known vascular disease Hypercoagulable state Acute onset (<8 h), usually >50 y	Organ failure Subacute onset(>8 h) except in hypoglycemia Any age, often >60 y
Motor involvement	Hemiplegic or paraplegic	Moving all limbs except for hypoglycemia
Sensory involvement	Unilateral facial sensory change, or hemianesthesia	No sensory symptoms
Mental status	Obtunded or agitated	Waxing and waning
Pupils	May have Horner's; may have fixed, dilated pupil	Small, normoactive
Eye movements	Disconjugate, skew deviation, cr N. III, IV, VI paresis	Conjugate, midline
Respirations	Apneustic, central hyperpnea, ataxic	Normal, hyperpneic + brief apnea

rigidity, the preservation of doll's eyes is a useful sign pointing to a metabolic, rather than anatomic, cause of coma.

Changes in the respiratory pattern are the next most important findings for the diagnosis of metabolic encephalopathy, also providing a clue as to its etiology. In the mildly confused patient, breathing may be normal, but lethargic or mildly obtunded patients tend to hyperventilate, with brief spells of apnea. This is due to transient lowering of the partial pressure of carbon dioxide (PCO_2) below 15 mm Hg without the appropriate CNS drive to breathe more rapidly at a lower tidal volume. After 12 to 30 seconds of apnea, the cycle of hyperventilation appears again, resulting in a pattern of "periodic respirations" [3]. Hypoventilation is usually seen with depressant drug overdoses, chronic pulmonary failure, and metabolic alkalosis of any cause. Cheyne-Stokes respiration, a rhythmic cycle of waxing and waning hyperpnea/apnea, is another pattern that is occasionally seen in metabolic encephalopathy caused by uremia or hypoxia, but more commonly this indicates bilateral structural lesions of the cortex. Other neurogenic respiratory patterns, such as constant or "central" neurogenic hyperventilation, cluster breathing, and ataxic breathing, are signs of brainstem dysfunction due to structural damage or suppression by barbiturates. These changes are seen only when the patient is stuporous or comatose.

Abnormal motor activity is characteristic of many metabolic encephalopathies and is quite varied in appearance; tremors, myoclonus, asterixis, rigidity, and choreoathetosis may be seen. Tremors are rhythmic, involuntary oscillatory movements seen in all limbs and often exaggerated during voluntary movement. Tremors occur most often in early hypoglycemic encephalopathy, thyrotoxicosis, acute uremia, chronic dialysis encephalopathy, hypercapnia, and drug intoxication, especially with sympathomimetic agents.

Myoclonus is multifocal, appearing as brief shock-like contractions of large muscle groups. Synchronous myoclonic jerks in all limbs can be seen in any patient who is slipping in and out of a drowsy sleep—also known as *sleep-onset myoclonus*. This is often seen in patients who are receiving large doses of narcotics. Multifocal myoclonus, in contrast, is seen in hypoxic–ischemic encephalopathy, chronic hepatic failure of all types, uremia, pulmonary failure, and intoxication with methaqualone and psychedelic agents [4].

Asterixis is a flapping movement produced by unsustained muscle contraction against gravity. Rhythmic extension and flexion of the outstretched limb is present, which disappears at rest. The most common setting for this is in hepatic encephalopathy of any cause, frequently with flapping of the hands, feet, jaw, and tongue. Subacute uremia and pulmonary failure produce asterixis accompanied by myoclonus, which presents a picture of almost constant muscular jerking movements.

Rigidity or generalized muscle spasms are states of constant muscle contraction that are seen when the degree of metabolic encephalopathy is more severe and leads to stupor or coma. This can be the result of end-stage hepatic failure, hypoglycemia (<25 mg glucose per dL) lasting more than a few minutes, acute renal failure, hyperthermia, and hypothermia below 92°F rectally. Rigidity with dystonic posturing is a clue to amphetamine or phenothiazine poisoning. Choreoathetosis, on the other hand, occurs in chronic hepatic failure, subacute bacterial endocarditis, post-hypoxic insult, Reye's syndrome, chronic dialysis, chronic hypoglycemia, and chronic hyperparathyroidism, appearing as a nonpatterned sequence of twisting or dance-like limb movements.

The *reflex examination* often reveals diffuse hyperreflexia, symmetric except in limbs that were previously affected by a structural lesion. Plantar responses, also known as the Babinski reflex, are typically extensor in both feet and can be elicited easily. In contrast, the sensory examination is usually not affected, but is unreliable if the patient is agitated or obtunded. Response to pinprick, painful pinch/pressure, or a cold stimulus on the limbs is the most useful in demonstrating a grossly intact sensory arc.

Abnormal autonomic responses in metabolic encephalopathy may demand intervention and can cause significant morbidity and mortality. Hypotension, unresponsive to volume expansion, points to intoxication with barbiturates or opiates, myxedema, or Addisonian crisis. In this setting, occult sepsis must always be ruled out before treating for specific metabolic derangements. Fever and leukocytosis may be absent in very debilitated patients. Examination of urine, blood cell counts and coagulation factors, blood and sputum cultures, chest x-ray, and a lumbar puncture are essential to rule out infection. If there remains any doubt about the cause of hypotension, empiric antibiotics, naloxone hydrochloride (Narcan) for possible opiate overdose, intravenous (IV) glucose (1 ampoule), and pressor agents should be added to other supportive measures acutely while the cause is being investigated.

Seizures are another significant symptom of metabolic encephalopathy, especially in uremia, hypoglycemia, pancreatic failure, and various types of metabolic acidosis (e.g., ethylene glycol, salicylates, and so forth). They occur most often at the onset of the metabolic disturbance, for example, as the blood urea nitrogen (BUN) is climbing acutely, and as a preterminal expression of severe neuronal injury in a comatose patient. Management of the seizures is typically ineffective until the underlying cause is corrected. In renal failure, however, one third to half of the standard loading doses of phenytoin or phenobarbital may be all that is needed to control seizures. The interictal electroencephalogram (EEG) serves as a guideline to the need for continued treatment once the encephalopathy has cleared or has become chronic and stable. A persistent focus of epileptiform activity warrants further investigation and anticonvulsant therapy.

The *laboratory investigation* of patients with delirium or coma is crucial in defining the cause of a metabolic encephalopathy. Blood tests for glucose, electrolytes, and blood gases should be drawn immediately along with a panel of hepatic function tests [ratio of serum alanine aminotransferase to serum aspartate aminotransferase, lactate dehydrogenase, ammonium ion (NH_4^+)], BUN, and creatinine. Serum and urine osmolality, cerebrospinal fluid (CSF) analysis, serum magnesium and phosphate levels, and specific hormone levels may be needed to define the cause of encephalopathy further. Careful review of all medications taken before and during hospitalization may direct attention to toxicology screens of blood and urine. The general toxicology screen should be sensitive to opiates, benzodiazepines, caffeine and salicylates, theophylline, barbiturates, and alcohol. Additional drug levels should be ordered if their use is known or suspected (e.g., digoxin, cocaine, phenytoin, and so forth). If there has been a sudden change in mental status, a bolus of 25 g glucose should be administered intravenously without hesitation to avoid prolonged hypoglycemia.

In general, the EEG in metabolic encephalopathy is abnormal; background slowing is the most common pattern found (<9 Hz) [5]. Other patterns can also be useful in identifying or corroborating the cause of the encephalopathy. Slow activity that is prominent frontally, with deep triphasic waves (in the 2- to 4-Hz range), is characteristic of hepatic encephalopathy but can be seen in renal failure too [6]. This has also been reported in levetiracetam toxicity [7], hyperammonemic states due to gastroplasty [8] and ureterosigmoidostomy [9], and rare metabolic disorders such as ornithine transcarbamylase deficiency [10]. Spreading of the slow activity toward the occipital leads is a sign of deepening coma in this setting. Bursts of high-voltage activity amidst normal background frequencies are also a sign of diffuse metabolic disturbance. More importantly, the EEG in a patient with an acute encephalopathy of unknown cause may reveal subclinical (electrical) status epilepticus, warranting urgent and aggressive anticonvulsant treatment. This is particularly common in the case of alcoholics and diabetics, who are at risk for multiple CNS insults.

Neuroimaging [computed tomography (CT) or magnetic resonance imaging (MRI)] scans are often crucial in situations in which there is rapid deterioration of mental status without focal signs or an obvious metabolic cause such as hypoglycemia. Most mass lesions, such as subdural hematomas or brain tumors, are evidenced clinically by a rostrocaudal progression of neurologic signs. The initial picture may be nonfocal with obtundation, but this is followed sequentially by flexor or extensor posturing on one or both sides and then the loss of pupillary or caloric responses. Later, medullary respiratory patterns or bradycardia appear. A noncontrast head CT or MRI is definitive in many cases but does not always distinguish a brainstem stroke. Early consultation by a neurologist is crucial, especially when the cause of impaired consciousness is not clearly due to a metabolic disorder. Transient changes in vascular permeability associated with Wernicke's encephalopathy can manifest as vasogenic edema in the brainstem periaqueductal and fourth ventricular areas along with contrast enhancement of the mammillary bodies [11].

Lumbar puncture is also indicated when there is a rapid onset of encephalopathy, especially with a fever, headache, or meningismus. Occult subarachnoid hemorrhage, infection, or elevated intracranial pressure may be found in the absence of funduscopic changes or clear-cut clinical history. Ideally, the lumbar puncture should be performed atraumatically with a small (22-gauge) spinal needle and a simultaneous sample of serum obtained to compare glucose and protein levels in the blood and CSF.

ETIOLOGY

Hepatic Failure

The clinical onset of *hepatic encephalopathy* may be subtle, with a blunting of affect and lethargy, or dramatic in 10% to 20%, with mania or an agitated delirium [12]. It is easy to recognize hepatic encephalopathy in an individual with the obvious stigmata of chronic liver disease, such as ascites, varices, or jaundice. In those without apparent liver disease, the mental changes may only appear after an additional metabolic demand on the liver. Such stressors are a high-protein meal, gastrointestinal bleeding with increased blood absorption from the gut, or hepatically metabolized drugs [13]. Sedatives and acetazolamide are particularly offensive in this situation.

Asterixis is the next most common clinical sign, appearing in all limbs, the jaw, and the tongue. As the patient progresses into a coma, it may be replaced by muscle spasticity and decorticate or decerebrate posturing to stimulation. The Babinski responses are present (extensor plantar reflexes), and gaze-evoked ocular movements are variable at this stage; pupillary responses are always preserved. Oculocephalic and vestibulo-ocular (caloric) responses remain until the patient is moribund. Hyperventilation is another consistent sign of hepatic encephalopathy and results in respiratory alkalosis. The ocular, pupillary, and respiratory patterns above help to distinguish severe hepatic encephalopathy from space-occupying lesions of the cortex and brainstem.

The pathophysiology of hepatic coma is not certain, but it is thought to be caused by portacaval shunting of neurotoxic substances. These putative toxins include excess ammonia, large molecules normally excluded by the blood–brain barrier [14], increased water, and the "false" neurotransmitter octopamine [15]. Hypoglycemia, as a result of decreased glycogen stores in the liver, may complicate the CNS picture.

The serum transaminases are usually elevated two- to threefold, and serum ammonia is at least in the high normal range once the patient is lethargic—with a linear correlation thereafter between higher laboratory values and lower cognitive state. The CSF remains normal until the serum bilirubin exceeds approximately 5 mg per dL, which tints the fluid yellow. The EEG characteristically shows progressive slowing from the frontal to the occipital leads as coma deepens. Triphasic waves are seen in most cases but are not pathognomonic.

Therapy for hepatic encephalopathy is directed toward decreasing the amount of toxic substances that are being shunted to the brain. Neomycin and lactulose help to sterilize and flush the gut. A protein-restricted diet and the exclusion of hepatically cleared drugs decrease the metabolic load, and IV glucose effectively maintains the serum glucose level. Neurologic recovery then depends on the capacity of the liver to regenerate at least 25% of its full function. With prolonged or repeated bouts of hepatic coma, there may be persistent, irreversible signs of basal ganglia dysfunction evidenced by chorea, postural tremors, or a parkinsonian picture (acquired hepatocerebral degeneration) [16].

Reye's Syndrome

Reye's syndrome is a unique and quite morbid form of acute hepatic encephalopathy seen in children, usually between ages 1 and 10 years. It occurs in the clinical setting of an acute viral infection, for example, chickenpox or influenza A or B, plus aspirin therapy [17]. Approximately 4 to 7 days after the viral symptoms start, the child becomes irritable, with vomiting and sometimes with headache or blurred vision. An agitated delirium, combativeness, and progressive obtundation rapidly ensue over hours, followed by hyperventilation, pupillary dilatation, and generalized seizures. Later in the course decerebrate rigidity, Babinski responses, and papilledema may develop as well.

The pathology of Reye's syndrome includes infiltration of the liver and other visceral organs with small fat droplets and diffuse cerebral edema. In cases that are complicated by severe hypoglycemia and seizures, anoxic damage with laminar necrosis of the cerebral cortex is also found. The cause of these changes is presumed to be mitochondrial poisoning, but the pathogenic agent has not yet been identified. Acetylsalicylic acid has consistently been implicated in this cellular damage. This has led to the standard practice of prescribing acetaminophen instead of aspirin for viral symptoms in children, thereby reducing the incidence of Reye's syndrome [18].

The differential diagnosis relies on measurement of liver function and a high index of suspicion in the appropriate setting. The serum transaminases rise three- to fivefold in the first 48 hours, and the serum ammonia is dramatically increased, sometimes into the 200 μmol per L range. Hypoglycemia is also an early sign, aggravating the lactic acidosis and respiratory alkalosis that are seen later in the course.

Treatment for Reye's syndrome is directed toward diminishing the cerebral edema, controlling seizures, and providing adequate electrolytes and glucose for support while the liver is effectively shut down with respect to oxidative metabolism. This is best achieved in an ICU with a standard protocol for Reye's disease using intracranial pressure monitoring and mannitol or glycerol for reduction of intracranial pressure [19].

The prognosis in recent years has improved markedly; mortality and morbidity are now 10% to 20%, as opposed to 40% to 50% two decades ago. Factors that contribute to a poor outcome are age less than 1 year, serum ammonia levels more than five times normal at their peak, and a prothrombin time more than 20 seconds. Other negative prognostic indicators are renal failure and a very rapid progression of liver failure in the first 48 hours. Early intervention is the key to a good outcome neurologically and systemically.

Renal Failure

Uremic encephalopathy may develop acutely, be superimposed on chronic renal insufficiency, or occur as a consequence of chronic dialysis. It is often a complication of systemic diseases that independently affect the kidneys and the CNS such as collagen-vascular disease, malignant hypertension, drug overdoses, diabetes, or bacterial sepsis. The clinical picture is initially variable and does not correlate directly with measures of renal failure such as BUN and creatinine.

The first sign of encephalopathy in uremia is delirium or a decrease in level of consciousness; hyperventilation and increased motor activity follow as the patient becomes obtunded. Also, there is a high frequency of generalized convulsions at the outset and a metabolic acidosis with low serum bicarbonate. The motor component is prominent in many patients with multifocal myoclonus, hypertonus or asterixis, and tremors, together producing a picture of "twitch-convulsif"—as if the patient had fasciculations [20]. Oculomotor function and pupillary responses are normal, but deep tendon reflexes may be asymmetric, and focal weakness often occurs, with shifting hemiparesis during a single period of encephalopathy. The variability of focal motor signs helps to rule out a structural lesion but does not obviate the need to look for multifocal seizures in a patient with overt twitching and depressed consciousness.

Studies of the effect of uremia on neuronal function have not been able to demonstrate a direct correlation between the cognitive state and levels of BUN or with any other biochemical or electrolyte markers. The EEG, although becoming slower with higher levels of BUN, also does not correlate with mental status changes, especially in chronic uremia [21]. Hence, the pathophysiology of uremic encephalopathy is not known.

The major diagnostic differential to consider is between a hypertensive crisis and uremic encephalopathy, because malignant hypertension often leads rapidly to renal failure and neurologic signs. Evidence of papilledema, retinal vasospasm, and cortical blindness or aphasia, with a diastolic blood pressure of more than 120 mm Hg, argues strongly for a hypertensive crisis. In contrast, a sudden rise of BUN alone is most consistent with uremic encephalopathy.

Two variants of this disorder are seen in patients on peritoneal dialysis or hemodialysis. The *acute dialysis dysequilibrium syndrome* is seen in children more often than in adults undergoing hemodialysis with large exchanges of dialysate. A sudden shift of solutes out of the vascular compartment produces a hyperosmolar state in the brain and subsequent water resorption intracerebrally. This results in water intoxication, with florid encephalopathy within 30 to 60 minutes. Slower dialysis obviates the problem in general [22].

Dialysis dementia is insidious by comparison and is evidenced by post-dialysis lethargy, asterixis, myoclonus, dysphasia, and progressive loss of cognitive abilities over years. This disorder has been linked to increased amounts of aluminum in the dialysate augmented by aluminum-containing antacids in the diet [23]. Although the brains of patients with this disorder do not contain excess aluminum compared to those of other dialysis patients, elimination of aluminum from these sources helps reverse the symptoms in the early stages. This syndrome is now relatively rare.

Pulmonary Failure

A combination of *hypoxemia* and *hypercarbia* can produce typical changes of a metabolic encephalopathy in patients with underlying pulmonary failure. Individuals with chronic obstructive pulmonary disease, for example, tolerate a PCO_2 of 50 to 60 mm Hg without mental status changes. However, a sudden increase of PCO_2 of up to 65 to 70 mm Hg due to hypoventilation, or impaired oxygen exchange, can lead to lethargy, headaches, and a rise in intracranial pressure. Associated signs are papilledema or retinal vein congestion, extensor Babinski signs, asterixis, myoclonus, and, often, generalized tremors. Seizures are rarely seen, and pupillary and oculomotor functions are preserved unless there is a concomitant hypoxic–ischemic insult [24].

This course of events may be precipitated by systemic infection with fatigue of ventilatory muscles, paralysis of these muscles by neuromuscular disease or Guillain-Barré syndrome, and sedative drugs with their depressant effect on the medullary respiratory center. In the well-compensated hypercarbic individual, oxygen therapy may be counterproductive by decreasing respiratory drive from the medulla. Rapid correction of hypercarbia by artificial ventilation, on the other hand, exacerbates the compensatory chronic metabolic alkalosis that these patients have, possibly resulting in a further depression of mental status plus seizures [25].

The critical factor in the development of pulmonary encephalopathy is a rapid increase in serum PCO_2. This may be complicated by the presence of sedatives, hypoxemia, cardiac failure, and renal hypoperfusion. Treatment is directed toward slow correction of hypercarbia while maintaining an adequate PO_2 and good cerebral blood flow. Prognosis for full neurologic recovery is good if the patient is not subjected to cerebral ischemia as well.

Hypoglycemic Encephalopathy

Hypoglycemia can occur as an isolated problem or as a complication of liver failure, of tumors producing insulin-like substances, or of urea cycle defects. The most common case is that of a diabetic with an accidental or deliberate overdose of insulin or oral hypoglycemic agents. An initial insulin reaction occurs when the serum glucose drops below approximately 40 mg per dL, producing flushing, sweating, faintness, palpitations, nausea, and anxiety. This persists for several minutes before the patient becomes confused and either agitated or drowsy [26]. Focal neurologic signs such as hemiparesis, cortical blindness, or dysphasia may appear at this point, mimicking an acute stroke [27]. If the serum glucose drops precipitously below 30 mg per dL, generalized convulsions may occur in flurries followed by a postictal coma. Prompt correction of the hypoglycemia at this point leads to reversal of the neurologic deficits, but repeated episodes can result in a subtle dementia evolving over many years [28].

When severe hypoglycemia is sustained for more than 10 minutes, stepwise progression of neurologic signs occurs. The first step is motor restlessness with frontal release signs such as sucking, grasping, and a tonic jaw jerk. Next, diffuse muscle spasms appear and sometimes myoclonic jerks. Finally, decerebrate rigidity is seen before the so-called medullary phase of hypoglycemia. The *medullary phase* describes a state of deep coma with dilated pupils, bradycardia, hypoventilation, and generalized flaccidity, much like hypoxic–ischemic coma. The pathologic changes associated with bouts of hypoglycemic encephalopathy are also similar to hypoxic–ischemic insults, although the cerebellum is relatively spared [29].

Differentiating hypoglycemic coma from a seizure disorder, a cerebrovascular accident, or a drug overdose is not possible at the outset unless stat serum glucose is obtained before IV fluids are administered. One should not delay treatment with a bolus of 50 mL 50% glucose (1 ampoule) if there is doubt about the cause of a rapidly evolving coma, because hypoglycemic encephalopathy can result in permanent neurologic deficits if not reversed in 20 minutes or less. The first bolus of glucose must be followed by close monitoring of blood glucose levels, because most agents that lead to symptomatic hypoglycemia are long acting [30].

Hyperglycemic Encephalopathy

Hyperglycemia that is severe enough to produce mental status changes rarely occurs in isolation from other metabolic disturbances. Hypokalemia and hypophosphatemia, hyperosmolality and ketoacidosis, or lactic acidosis often accompany serum glucose levels more than 300 mg per dL. In contrast, acidosis may be absent in nonketotic hyperglycemic hyperosmolar states, whereas the serum osmolality is often more than 350 mOsm per kg and serum glucose more than 800 mg per dL. The neurologic changes in any case appear to correlate best with abnormalities of serum osmolality and the rate at which it is corrected [31]. In juvenile or "brittle" diabetics, ketoacidosis develops after a dose of insulin is missed or an occult infection occurs. The first changes are mild confusion, lethargy, and deep regular inspirations (Kussmaul's breathing) in addition to signs of dehydration. Elderly patients are more prone to nonketotic hyperglycemia, especially when they have an inadequate diet, take medications that interfere with insulin metabolism [e.g., phenytoin (Dilantin), steroids], or take oral hypoglycemic agents [32]. Lactic acidosis may be present, in particular, with phenformin. These patients also tend to have focal or generalized seizures and transient or shifting hemiplegia as the level of coma deepens. The preservation of pupillary and oculocephalic responses helps to identify the clinical picture in such cases as being metabolic rather than structural.

The hyperosmolality occurring with hyperglycemia of any type causes a shift of water from the intracerebral to intravascular space with resulting brain shrinkage [33]. How this produces the neurologic changes observed is not known. More importantly, rapid correction of hyperosmolality by IV hydration and insulin results in cerebral water intoxication and signs of increased intracranial pressure. This is exemplified by the patient who begins to awaken from a hyperglycemic coma during IV therapy but later develops a headache and recurrent lethargy and seems to drift back into the previous state. Significant morbidity and mortality follow if these fluctuations are not observed and the IV treatment is modified appropriately [34]. Other details of the management of diabetic coma are addressed in Chapter 101.

Other Electrolyte Disturbances

Hyponatremia and *hypernatremia* cause fluid shifts and critical changes in serum osmolality, with the same effects on cerebral dysfunction as those described above. Mild to moderate *hyponatremia* (120 to 130 mEq per L) is evidenced by confusion or delirium with asterixis and multifocal myoclonus. If the serum sodium goes below 110 mEq per L, or drops at a rate more than 5 mEq per L per hour to 120 mEq per L and below, seizures and coma are likely to follow. This course of events portends permanent neurologic damage even after careful therapy [35]. Common causes of hyponatremia are (a) the syndrome of inappropriate antidiuretic hormone secretion (SIADH), with myriad etiologies; (b) excess volume expansion with hypotonic IV solutions; and (c) renal failure with a decreased glomerular filtration rate [36]. Other less common causes include psychogenic polydipsia, severe congestive heart failure, and Addison's disease.

The neurologic signs of hyponatremia are nonspecific, and the general approach to evaluation of an encephalopathy often identifies the problem. Treatment is directed toward the underlying cause with fluid restriction in mild cases, unless total body sodium is depleted. In moderate cases (i.e., a serum sodium of 105 to 115 mEq per L), PO sodium supplementation may be needed as well. A serum sodium below 100 mEq per L is life threatening. This requires judicious treatment with IV hypertonic saline at a rate calculated to replace about half of the total sodium deficit in 3 to 6 hours (averaging less than or equal to 0.5 mg Na^+ per hour). The remainder of the deficit should be administered in the next 24 to 48 hours [37]. Excessively rapid correction of severe hyponatremia, especially in alcoholic or malnourished individuals, can be associated with another serious neurologic complication known as *central pontine myelinolysis* [38]. Central pontine myelinolysis starts with a flaccid quadriparesis and inability to chew, swallow, or talk, or "locked-in syndrome" developing over a period of days. Patients who recover from the underlying systemic disorder are left with a spastic paraparesis and pseudobulbar speech; some may improve over several months.

Hypernatremia is not seen very often outside the hospital setting except in children with severe diarrhea and inadequate PO fluid intake. Excess diuretic therapy, hyperosmolar tube feedings, and restricted access to PO fluids are reflected in a serum sodium of more than 155 mEq per L in institutionalized patients. Clinically, one sees progressive confusion and obtundation in subacute cases. With levels of sodium more than 170 mEq per L developing acutely, the brain may shrink, and subdural hematomas can occur as a result of stretching of the dural vessels. These patients may complain of headache, develop seizures, or simply drift into a stupor. Catastrophic complications such as venous sinus thrombosis and irreversible coma are seen with a serum sodium level of more than 180 mEq per L due to the marked hyperosmolality that accompanies it.

The cause of profound hypernatremia is often diabetes insipidus, which may be secondary to head trauma. Impaired thirst mechanisms or depressed consciousness interfere with the polydipsia that is pathognomonic of diabetes insipidus [39]. The treatment of symptomatic hypernatremia depends on its cause: dehydration alone or complicated by additional sodium depletion due to hyperosmolar diuresis or excessive sweating. Fluid replacement is accomplished with 5% dextrose and water at a rate dependent on the total body water deficit—half of the water needed being administered IV in the first 12 to 24 hours and no faster. Saline solutions of half normal strength (0.45%) are used in most other cases. The exception is hyperosmolar diabetic coma, in which insulin and normal saline are both necessary to correct the severe serum hypertonicity.

Metabolic acidosis by itself produces only mild delirium or confusion [40] but may be accompanied by organ failure, direct CNS toxicity from drug metabolites, or volume depletion. The first sign of an encephalopathy caused by metabolic acidosis is hyperpnea followed by mental status changes and mild muscular rigidity. Ingestion of toxic doses of poisons such as methanol, ethylene glycol, and salicylates result in encephalopathy along with low serum bicarbonate levels (less than 15 mEq per L) [41]. Therapy must be directed toward vigorous correction of the metabolic acidosis while the specific cause is being elucidated.

Pancreatic Failure

Acute pancreatitis rarely leads to mental status changes during the initial bout. When recurrent or chronic, symptoms of encephalopathy may prominently wax and wane [42]. The clinical presentation is abdominal pain followed over 2 to 5 days by hallucinosis, delirium, focal or generalized seizures, and bilateral extensor Babinski responses. As the serum amylase continues to rise, the patient may lapse into a coma as a result of secondary hyperglycemia, hypocalcemia, and hypotension. The exact cause of the encephalopathy is unknown; the prognosis and treatment depend on the underlying cause and severity of the pancreatitis [43].

Endocrine Disorders

Adrenal disorders are an important consideration in acute encephalopathy, because hypo- and hyperadrenalism produce alterations in CNS function.

Addison's disease or *secondary adrenocortical deficiency* occurs acutely in the setting of septicemia, surgery, and, most frequently, sudden withdrawal of chronically administered steroids. In the latter, one does not see the stigmata of chronic adrenocorticotropic hormone deficiency but rather hypotension, a mild hyponatremia, hypoglycemia, and hyperkalemia, together with a delirium or stupor that fluctuates erratically [44]. The electrolyte disturbances in most cases are not severe enough to explain the encephalopathy; other pathologic mechanisms such as cerebral hypoperfusion or water intoxication have been suggested. Unlike many metabolic encephalopathies, adrenocortical insufficiency is associated with *decreased* muscle tone and deep tendon reflexes. Seizures and papilledema may appear when the patient has a profound adrenocorticotropic hormone deficiency and coma. The neurologic picture does not clear until cortisone replacement is given along with treatment of the electrolyte imbalances. These patients are also particularly sensitive to sedative medications and may lapse into coma with small doses of narcotics or barbiturates [45].

Excess steroids produce different forms of encephalopathy depending on whether the source is endogenous or exogenous. In Cushing's disease, psychomotor depression and lethargy are the norm, whereas high doses of prednisone usually cause elation, delirium, or frank psychosis [46]. The latter is not uncommon in the ICU setting due to the administration of stress levels of steroids and multiple other CNS toxins. The behavioral changes are key to recognizing this problem because there are no specific metabolic markers [47]. Treatment consists of withdrawal of the steroids and sometimes temporary use of tranquilizers or lithium for the psychiatric features as well. Full neurologic recovery may lag behind the treatment by several days to weeks.

Hypothyroidism is now a rare cause of encephalopathy and coma. It may be confused initially with other causes of hypotension, hypoventilation, and hyponatremia, such as septic shock, brainstem infarcts, or an overdose of sedatives. The diagnosis should be considered in any patient with hypothermia, pretibial edema, pseudomyotonic stretch reflexes (e.g., delayed relaxation of the knee jerk), and coarse hair or facies. Muscle enzymes, serum cholesterol, and lipids may be elevated along with the thyroid-stimulating hormone level [48]. Diagnostic confirmation is often delayed pending results of thyroid function tests, but replacement therapy should be initiated early with IV triiodothyronine or thyroxine. The constitutional symptoms may take several weeks to respond, but the neurologic picture clears promptly with proper treatment. Another form of hypothyroid associated encephalopathy is seen in Hashimoto's thyroiditis with a subacute subtle change in personality, memory deficits, and cerebellar ataxia accompanied by cerebellar atrophy on imaging studies. Confirmation of the diagnosis requires specific tests for antithyroglobulin and antithyroperoxidase antibodies along with an elevated TSH. Treatment with thyroid replacement therapy often results in recovery over a few months.

Thyrotoxicosis is more difficult to recognize because it can present in an apathetic form, as a thyroid storm, or in a subacute form. Elderly patients are more likely to appear depressed or stuporous and without evidence of hypermetabolism [49]. The key to the diagnosis in such cases is evidence of recent weight loss and atrial fibrillation, often with congestive heart failure and a proximal myopathy. In a thyroid storm, the patient with indolent hyperthyroidism may be stressed by an infection or surgery and responds with marked signs of hypermetabolism: tachycardia, fever, profuse sweating, and pulmonary or congestive heart failure. Neurologically, the individual becomes acutely agitated and delirious and then progresses into a stupor [50]. The subacute picture that precedes this is one of mild irritability, nervousness, tremors, and hyperactivity and is often misconstrued as an affective disorder rather than endocrine in origin. Ophthalmologic signs such as proptosis, chemosis, and periorbital edema are useful in identifying this form of thyrotoxicosis.

Therapy for thyrotoxic encephalopathy is aimed at ablation of the gland, but supportive care may require beta-blockers, digoxin, diuretics, and sometimes dexamethasone and sedatives for the associated hypermetabolic state. Encephalopathy is also seen in disorders of the pituitary gland and parathyroid gland, although rarely as a primary process. *Hypopituitarism* may result from radiation or surgery to the area of the sella and can present as a chronic encephalopathy with features of thyroid or adrenal insufficiency, or both. An acute coma due to infarction or hemorrhage of the pituitary gland, known as *pituitary apoplexy*, can be seen in acromegalics with large adenomas or in patients with postpartum hemorrhage and hypotension (Sheehan's syndrome) [51]. Subarachnoid blood and ocular abnormalities plus signs of increased intracranial pressure help to identify the lesion in such cases. Encephalopathy from *hyperpituitarism* reflects the specific neurohumoral substance that is being released in excess and does not represent a unique syndrome.

Hyperparathyroidism may be manifest neurologically with asthenia or a vague change in personality. The patient is mildly depressed, lacks energy, and fatigues easily. A serum calcium more than 12 mg per dL and elevated parathormone levels are important diagnostic findings. Occasionally, psychiatric symptoms predominate, starting with delirium and psychosis, or obtundation and coma when the serum calcium exceeds 15 mg per dL. Hypercalcemia caused by metastatic bone lesions, paraneoplastic parathormone-like substances, sarcoidosis, primary bone diseases, and renal failure are associated with a subacute or chronic encephalopathy similar to hyperparathyroidism. Treatment in these cases must be directed toward the underlying disease rather than addressing the hypercalcemia alone. Primary hyperparathyroidism is effectively managed by ablation of the overactive gland. This is not always possible, because the glands often are ectopic and may escape discovery on selective angiography or exploratory surgery.

Hypocalcemia due to *hypoparathyroidism* produces an encephalopathy that parallels the depression of serum calcium levels. At less than 4.0 mEq per L calcium, a blunted effect and seizures are common and may be confused with a dementing process or epilepsy. The motor signs of hypocalcemia, that is, tetany or neuromuscular irritability, should make one suspicious of a metabolic disturbance [39]. Another diagnostic dilemma is the occasional presentation of hypocalcemia with papilledema and headache. The opening pressure on lumbar puncture is elevated to the same degree as in pseudotumor cerebri, but a head CT is likely to show basal ganglia calcifications [48]. Furthermore, the presence of cataracts and mental dullness in a previously normal individual should lead one to check the serum calcium and parathormone levels.

The mechanism by which hypocalcemia and hypoparathyroidism produce these varied neurologic symptoms is not known. Replacement of serum calcium by dietary means is usually inadequate to correct the CNS disorder. Supplementation with vitamin D and calcitriol enhances the absorption and utilization of oral calcium.

Other Causes of Encephalopathy

The list of causes of diffuse or metabolic encephalopathies is so lengthy that the problem of diagnosis must be resolved by a process of elimination. Drugs and toxins lead all other possible causes, with a frequency of approximately 50% (see Chapters 117 through 145). Hepatic, renal, or pulmonary failure is causative in another 12% and endocrine or electrolyte disturbances in approximately 8%. Other less common etiologies include thiamine deficiency (Wernicke's encephalopathy), cardiac bypass surgery, subacute bacterial endocarditis, and hyperthermia. All of these disorders produce microembolic or microhemorrhagic/petechial lesions in specific areas of the brain.

Wernicke's encephalopathy develops acutely in the clinical setting of an alcoholic or a malnourished individual, especially when IV glucose solutions without vitamin supplementation are given. Because thiamine is a cofactor in the utilization of cerebral glucose, it is depleted by the IV infusion [52]; confusion, obtundation, and loss of short-term memory rapidly ensue. The hallmark of this entity is a striking impairment of ocular movements, causing an external ophthalmoplegia, nystagmus, and diminished oculocephalic responses. Prompt IV and PO administration of 100 mg thiamine restores ocular function completely. The cerebral symptoms resolve slowly with the addition of 100 mg PO thiamine daily for 3 days or more. If untreated, the patient may lapse into a coma due to autonomic failure with accompanying shock and hypothermia and often dies. Repeated or untreated episodes of Wernicke's disease may result in a chronic Korsakoff's psychosis with profound memory impairment [49].

More recently, recognition of autoantibodies to potassium channels (VGKC-Ab) and NMDA receptors presenting with a subacute limbic-type encephalopathy has led to exciting research into the role of channel blockade in reversible mental status changes. In many cases, there is no evidence of an occult cancer (e.g., testicular or ovarian in young people) and the prognosis with immunoglobulin or steroid therapy is good [50].

Hyperthermia due to heat stroke also has a characteristic clinical setting—young individuals experiencing excessive sweating caused by overactivity and elderly people receiving anticholinergics who are exposed to a hot environment [51]. In both cases, neurologic changes occur when the core body temperature reaches 42°C (107.6°F). The patient may become agitated and confused with intermittent generalized seizures or may immediately lapse into a coma as if due to a stroke. The presence of tachycardia, hot and dry skin, and diffuse hypertonus occurring in the appropriate circumstances identifies the likely etiology. Normal pupillary size and reflexes (except with anticholinergics) and oculocephalic responses, and the absence of focal motor signs also point to a nonstructural lesion. However, if the core body temperature is not lowered early in the course, the patient may be left with sequelae similar to those seen in hypoxic–ischemic encephalopathy. Other causes of temperature more than 42°C are rare and are not discussed here [53].

Up to 20% of patients with *bacterial or marantic endocarditis* can present with a subacute encephalopathy manifested by confusion and hyperpnea with or without fever [54]. It should be suspected in any patient with Gram-negative sepsis [37]; ovarian cancer; malignant melanoma; adenocarcinoma of the lung, breast, prostate, or pancreas; and an immunocompromised state. Definitive diagnosis rests on the blood culture results and an echocardiogram showing vegetations. Treatment is directed toward reducing or removing the cardiac source.

CONCLUSIONS

Metabolic encephalopathy is one of the most frequently seen neurologic disorders in the ICU arena. It is also one of the most diverse in its clinical presentations and requires a systematic approach to define the etiology and to institute effective treatment. The features that distinguish most metabolic encephalopathies from structural lesions are (a) a nonfocal neurologic examination, (b) increased motor activity, (c) intact ocular and pupillary reflexes, and (d) laboratory abnormalities that support the clinical picture. Additional tests such as an EEG, head CT, or toxicology screen are useful in ruling out other possible causes.

One should keep in mind that many patients in the ICU have an underlying chronic encephalopathy due to long-standing illness [56]. Therefore, they are more susceptible to minor metabolic perturbations induced by small doses of drugs, slight shifts of fluid balance, or worsening organ failure. Early recognition and correction of such factors improve the patient's prognosis for a full neurologic recovery. Toward this end, it is prudent to consult the neurologist before the complications of multiple treatments and further changes confound the clinical course.

References

1. Folstein MF, Folstein SE, McHugh PR: Mini-Mental State: a practical method for grading the cognitive state of patients for the clinician. *J Psycholinguist Res* 12:189, 1975.
2. Cohen PJ: Signs and stages of anesthesia, in Goodman LS, Gilman A (eds): *The Pharmacologic Basis of Therapeutics*. 5th ed. New York, Macmillan, 1975, p 60.
3. Posner JB, Saper CB, Schiff ND, et al: Examination of the comatose patient, in *Plum and Posner's Diagnosis of Stupor and Coma*. 4th ed. New York, Oxford University Press, 2007, p 46–53.
4. Celesia GG, Grigg MM, Ross E: Generalized status myoclonus in acute anoxic and toxic-metabolic encephalopathies. *Arch Neurol* 45(7):781, 1988.
5. Kaplan PW: The EEG in metabolic encephalopathy and coma. *J Clin Neurophys* 21(5):307–318, 2004.
6. Leonard JV: Acute metabolic encephalopathy: an introduction. *J Inherit Metab Dis* 28(3):403–406, 2005.
7. Vulliemoz S, Iwanowski P, Landis T, et al: Levetiracetam accumulation in renal failure causing myoclonic encephalopathy with triphasic waves. *Seizure* 18(5):376–378, 2009.
8. Cirignotta F, Manconi M, Mondini S, et al: Wernicke-Korsakoff encephalopathy and polyneuropathy after gastroplasty for morbid obesity: report of a case. *Arch Neurol* 49:653–656, 1992.
9. Edwards RH: Hyperammonemic encephalopathy related to ureterosigmoidostomy. *Arch Neurol* 41:1211–1212, 1984.
10. Hu W, Kantarci O: Ornithine transcarbamylase deficiency presenting as encephalopathy during adulthood following bariatric surgery. *Arch Neurol* 64:126–128, 2007.
11. Breningstall GN: Neurologic syndrome in hyperammonemic disorders. *Pediatr Neurol* 2(5):253–262, 1986.
12. Christensen E, Krintel JJ, Hansen SM, et al: Prognosis after the first episode of gastrointestinal bleeding or coma in cirrhosis. Survival and prognostic factors. *Scand J Gastroenterol* 24(8):999, 1989.
13. Laursen H, Westergaard G: Enhanced permeability to horseradish peroxidase across cerebral vessels in the rat after portacaval anastomosis. *Neuropathol Appl Neurobiol* 3:29, 1979.
14. James JH, Escourroule J, Fisher JE: Blood-brain neutral amino-acid transport activity is increased after portacaval anastomoses. *Science* 200:1395, 1978.
15. Klos KJ, Ahlskog J, Josephs JE, et al: Neurologic spectrum of chronic liver failure and basal ganglia T1 hyperintensity on magnetic resonance imaging: probable manganese neurotoxicity. *Arch Neurol* 62(9):1385–1390, 2005.
16. Hurwitz ES: Reye's syndrome. *Epidemiol Rev* 11:249, 1989.
17. Arrowsmith JB, Kennedy DL, Kuritsky JN, et al: National patterns of aspirin use and Reye syndrome reporting, United States, 1980–1985. *Pediatrics* 79(6):858, 1987.
18. Fishman RA: Brain edema and disorders of intracranial pressure, in Rowland LP (ed): *Merritt's Textbook of Neurology*. 8th ed. Philadelphia, Lea & Febiger, 1989, p 262.

19. Chadwick D, French AT: Uremic myoclonus: an example of reticular reflex myoclonus? *J Neurol Neurosurg Psychiatry* 42:52, 1979.
20. Kaplan PW: Stupor and coma: metabolic encephalopathies. *Suppl Clin Neurophysiol* 57:667–680, 2004.
21. Hagstam KE: EEG frequency content related to clinical blood parameters in chronic uremia. *Scand J Urol Nephrol* 19[Suppl 7]:1, 1971.
22. Raskin NH, Fishman RA: Neurologic disorders in renal failure. *N Engl J Med* 294:143, 204, 1976.
23. Alfrey AC: Dialysis encephalopathy syndrome. *Annu Rev Med* 29:93, 1978.
24. Glaser G, Pincus JH: Neurologic complications of internal disease, in Baker AB, Baker LH (eds): *Clinical Neurology*. Philadelphia, Harper & Row, 1983, p 17 (vol 4).
25. Rotherman EB, Safar P, Robin ED: CNS disorder during mechanical ventilation in chronic pulmonary disease. *JAMA* 189:993, 1964.
26. Fishbain DA, Rotundo D: Frequency of hypoglycemic delirium in a psychiatric emergency service. *Psychosomatics* 29(3):346, 1988.
27. Garty BZ, Dinari G, Nitzan M: Transient acute cortical blindness associated with hypoglycemia. *Pediatr Neurol* 3(3):169, 1987.
28. Malouf R, Brust JCM: Hypoglycemia: causes, neurological manifestations and outcome. *Ann Neurol* 17:421, 1985.
29. Foster JW, Hart RG: Hypoglycemic hemiplegia: two cases and a clinical review. *Stroke* 18(5):944, 1987.
30. Kitabchi EA, Goodman RC: Hypoglycemia, pathophysiology and diagnosis. *Hosp Pract* 22(11A):45, 59, 1987.
31. Wachtel TS, Silliman RA, Lamberton P: Predisposing factors for the diabetic hyperosmolar state. *Arch Intern Med* 147(3):499, 1987.
32. Arieff AI, Carroll HJ: Cerebral edema and depression of sensorium in nonketotic hyperosmolar coma. *Diabetes* 23:525, 1974.
33. Ryner MM, Fishman RA: Protective adaptation of brain to water intoxication. *Arch Neurol* 28:49, 1973.
34. Posner JB, Saper CB, Schiff ND, et al: Multifocal, diffuse and metabolic brain diseases causing stupor and coma, in *Plum and Posner's Diagnosis of Stupor and Coma*. 4th ed. New York, Oxford University Press, 2007, p 179–296.
35. Ayus JC, Krothapalli RK, Arieff AI: Treatment of symptomatic hyponatremia and its relation to brain damage. A prospective study. *N Engl J Med* 317(19):1190, 1987.
36. Streeton DH, Moses AM, Miller M: Disorders of the neurohypophysis, in Braunwald E, Isselbacher K, Petersdorf R, et al (eds): *Harrison's Principles of Internal Medicine*. 11th ed. New York, McGraw-Hill, 1987, p 1729.
37. Victor M: Neurologic disorders due to alcoholism and malnutrition, in Baker AB, Baker LH (eds): *Clinical Neurology*. Philadelphia, Harper & Row 1983, p 57 (vol 4).
38. Hattori S, Mochio S, Isogai Y, et al: Central pontine myelinolysis followed by frequent hyperglycemia and hypoglycemia—report of an autopsy case. *Brain Nerve* 41(8):795, 1989.
39. Adams RD, Victor M: Hypothalamic pituitary syndromes: diabetes insipidus, in Adams RD (ed): *Principles of Neurology*. 4th ed. New York, McGraw-Hill, 1989, p 448.
40. Levinsky N: Fluids and electrolytes: metabolic acidosis, in Braunwald E, Isselbacher K, Petersdorf R, et al (eds): *Harrison's Textbook of Internal Medicine*. 11th ed. New York, McGraw-Hill, 1987, p 210.
41. Perry S: Substance-induced organic mental disorders, in Hales RE, Yudofsky SC (eds): *Textbook of Neuropsychiatry*. Washington, DC, The American Psychiatric Press, 1987, p 214.
42. Sjaastad O, Gjessing L, Ritland S, et al: Chronic relapsing pancreatitis, encephalopathy with disturbance of consciousness and CSF amino acid aberration. *J Neurol* 220:83, 1979.
43. Johnson DA, Tong NT: Pancreatic encephalopathy. *South Med J* 70:165, 1977.
44. Kaminski HJ, Ruff RL: Neurologic complications of endocrine diseases. *Neurol Clin* 7(3):489, 1989.
45. Posner JB, Saper CB, Schiff ND, et al: Addison's Disease, in Plum and Posner's *Diagnosis of Stupor and Coma*. 4th ed. New York, Oxford University Press, 2007, p 234–235.
46. Whybrow P, Hurwitz TI: Psychological disturbances associated with endocrine disease and hormone therapy, in Sachar EJ (ed): *Hormones, Behavior and Pathophysiology*. New York, Raven Press, 1976.
47. Boston Collaborative Drug Surveillance Program: Acute adverse reactions to prednisone in relation to dosage. *Clin Pharmacol Ther* 13:694, 1997.
48. Greene R: The thyroid gland: its relationship to neurology, in Vinken PJ, Bruyn GW (eds): *The Handbook of Clinical Neurology*. New York, Elsevier North-Holland, 1976, p 253 (vol 27, pt 1).
49. Nemeroff CB: Clinical significance of psychoneuroendocrinology in psychiatry: focus on the thyroid and adrenal. *J Clin Psychiatry* 50[Suppl]:13–21, 1989.
50. Dalmau J: Limbic encephalitis and variants related to neuronal cell membrane autoantigens. *Rinsho Shinkeigaku* 48(11):871–874, 2008.
51. Tsementzis SA, Loizou LA: Pituitary apoplexy. *Neurochirurgie* 29(3):90, 1986.
52. Sommerfield AJ, Stimson R, Campbell IW: Hashimoto's encephalopathy presenting as an acute medical emergency. *Scott Med J* 49(4):155–156, 2004.
53. Delplace PO, Wery D, Lemort M, et al: A case of multiple brain calcifications associated with hypoparathyroidism. *J Belge Radiol* 72(4):263, 1989.
54. Goto I, Nagara H, Tateishi J, et al: Thiamine-deficient encephalopathy in rats: effects of deficiencies of thiamine and magnesium. *Brain Res* 372(1):31, 1986.
55. Muller PS: Diagnosis and treatment of neuroleptic malignant syndrome: a review. *Neuro View* 3(5):1, 1987.
56. Terpenning MS, Guggy BP, Kauffman CA: Infective endocarditis: clinical features in young and elderly patients. *Am J Med* 83:626, 1987.
57. Wilson JX, Young GB: Progress in clinical neurosciences: sepsis-associated encephalopathy: evolving concepts. *Can J Neurol Sci* 30(2):98–105, 2003.
58. Elie M, Cole MG, Primeau FJ, et al: Delirium risk factors in the hospitalized elderly. *J Gen Int Med* 13:204, 1998.

CHAPTER 171 ■ GENERALIZED ANOXIA/ ISCHEMIA OF THE NERVOUS SYSTEM

CAROL F. LIPPA AND MAJAZ MOONIS

Anoxic brain injury results from inadequate oxygen supply to the brain. The clinical picture ranges from mild confusion to deep coma with loss of brainstem responses. Anoxic damage can be caused by circulatory collapse, respiratory failure, or inadequate hemoglobin binding to oxygen. Prognosis and management of the anoxic patient depend in part on which of these mechanisms has caused the injury.

PATHOGENESIS

The brain is unique in that it uses almost exclusively aerobic metabolism of glucose. The continuous availability of oxygen is secured by the cerebral vasculature's autoregulatory mechanism [1], which controls the rate of blood flow over a wide range of blood pressures. If blood pressure drops too low for autoregulatory mechanisms to operate, oxygen extraction from the blood increases. Failure of this compensatory mechanism results in a changeover from aerobic to anaerobic metabolism.

In cardiac arrest, depletion of brain oxygen reserves occurs within 10 seconds, thereby eliminating the major source of neuronal energy from ATP (adenosine triphosphate) and phosphokinase. Excessive glutamate release and reduced reuptake lead to activation of the NMDA (*N*-methyl-D-aspartate) receptors and consequent ischemic cascade. The resulting intracellular (cytotoxic) edema leads to increased intracranial pressure.

The changeover to anaerobic metabolism results in neuronal catabolism. In cardiovascular collapse, loss of venous outflow leads to the accumulation of lactic acid and pyruvate, the end products of anaerobic metabolism. Buildup of these catabolites potentiates the cellular damage.

DIAGNOSIS

The first question to address when evaluating a comatose or obtunded patient with a possible hypoxic insult is whether the impaired consciousness is the result of a metabolic insult or a structural brain lesion. Coma caused by a mass lesion is usually associated with focal neurologic signs. Computed axial tomography (CT) or magnetic resonance imaging (MRI) scans usually reveal focal lesions in this setting. Metabolic causes, including anoxic encephalopathy, should be suspected when patients with impaired consciousness present with a non-focal examination.

The diagnosis is often suggested by the clinical setting (e.g., cardiac arrest in patients with arrhythmias or myocardial infarctions, or severe episodes of intraoperative hypotension). Arterial blood gas determination, if obtained during the causal event, can confirm the diagnosis. A partial pressure of oxygen of less than 40 mm Hg causes confusion and less than 30 mm Hg results in coma [2]. Associated abnormalities that potentiate anoxic damage include anemia, acidosis, hypercapnia, hyperthermia, and hypotension.

The internist or neurologist is often consulted to evaluate the patient who has impaired consciousness after well-documented cerebral hypoperfusion that has occurred during surgical operations requiring the use of extracorporeal circulation. The neurological examination is nonfocal. Because surgical patients with such a history often have preexisting illnesses (vascular disease, borderline renal function, hepatic impairment, diabetes), it is the obligation of the intensive care physician to determine new deficits due to anoxic encephalopathy, or other treatable conditions secondary to metabolic, infectious, and iatrogenic factors such as sedating medications. Intracerebral hemorrhage and subdural hematomas should also be sought, because they can occur spontaneously in the perioperative period, especially in anticoagulated patients.

CLINICAL COURSE AND PROGNOSIS

The clinical outcome of patients with anoxic injuries depends on the degree and duration of oxygen deprivation to the brain as well as the maintenance of blood flow. With complete cessation of blood flow to the brain, consciousness is lost after several seconds. If anoxia is moderately prolonged, the patient awakens but may have residual deficits, such as cognitive impairment, or later sequelae, including extrapyramidal movement disorders or seizures, which may not develop for days to weeks.

A delayed postanoxic syndrome may occur rarely in patients with anoxic insults after the initial coma. Three to 30 days following the initial anoxic insult, after the patient has regained consciousness and cognitive function, there is a secondary decline characterized by irritability, confusion, lethargy, clumsiness, and increased muscle tone; patients may become comatose again and die. This uncommon condition occurs most often in cases of carbon monoxide poisoning. Pathologically, widespread demyelination is seen without gray matter changes. The cause is unknown, but it may be due to alteration of enzymatic processes, edema, or damage to small blood vessels [2,3].

The overall prognosis for a meaningful recovery in patients with nontraumatic coma is guarded; the longer patients are in coma, the worse the outcome [4–6]. Most improvement occurs within the first 30 days. Non-anoxic metabolic coma carries the best prognosis, while anoxic coma has a better prognosis than coma resulting from structural lesions. A good outcome is seen in 50% of patients who awaken within 24 hours. Although infrequent seizures or myoclonus do not affect prognosis, myoclonic or nonconvulsive status epilepticus is a grave prognostic sign and is associated with poor recovery [4,7].

If consciousness is maintained during a hypoxic event, there is rarely permanent brain damage. Irreversible damage is rarely seen in healthy individuals if the duration of anoxia is less than 4 minutes, although it may be incurred in individuals with preexisting cerebrovascular disease in shorter periods.

In cases of nontraumatic coma, the most valuable prognostic information is obtained from the physical examination. Favorable prognostic indicators include

1. Recovery of multiple brainstem responses within 48 hours (pupillary, oculocephalic, and corneal) [4];
2. Return of purposeful responses to painful stimuli by 24 hours;
3. Primary pulmonary event leading to coma;
4. Hypothermia at the time of the anoxic event may be protective; patients who have experienced near-drowning, submerged in cold water up to 40 minutes may return to normal neurologic function [8];
5. Younger age (children and young adults) [9,10].

Poor prognostic indicators in persistent coma include

1. Absence of pupillary or corneal responses, and absent motor response to pain by the third day [11];
2. The loss of vestibulo-ocular responses at 12 hours and the presence of decerebrate or decorticate posturing at 24 hours [5,8];
3. Electroencephalogram (EEG) patterns: nonreactive EEG; burst suppression; alpha coma. Serial EEGs documenting improvement are associated with a better prognosis [12,13];
4. Short-latency somatosensory evoked potential tests are noninvasive tests of the sensory system that are absent in brain death but preserved in severe reversible comas, such as barbiturate coma that can mirror brain death [14,15]. Absent cortical N20 on somatosensory evoked response at 72 hours is associated with irreversible coma. N20 present at 8 hours has a 25% chance of recovery [15,16];
5. The presence of either diffuse edema or watershed infarctions on CT scans;
6. Loss of gray white matter distinction on CT scan and severe abnormalities on diffusion-weighted imaging [17,18];
7. Myoclonus or status epilepticus the first day.

A recent Academy of Neurology Practice Parameter by Wijdicks et al. [19] is an evidence-based review for predicting the outcome in survivors of cardiopulmonary resuscitation. The authors conclude that "Pupillary light response, corneal reflexes, motor response to pain, myoclonus status epilepticus, serum neuron-specific enolase and somatosensory evoked potential studies can reliably assist in accurately predicting poor outcome in comatose patients after cardiopulmonary resuscitation for cardiac arrest."

When prognosticating by the clinical criteria alone, one must be careful that no sedative, anesthetic, or anticonvulsant (Dilantin, phenobarbital) is being used, because these agents can suppress brainstem reflexes.

Respiratory insufficiency with maintained circulation carries a better prognosis. A low partial pressure of oxygen does not necessarily convey a bad prognosis in cases of isolated hypoxia [20] if circulation is carefully maintained [21].

Conversely, the presence of metabolic abnormalities, such as lactic acidosis, worsens prognosis.

In cases of out-of-hospital cardiac arrest, survival depends on the total time required to establish effective cerebral blood flow. The arrest time (AT) and the cardiopulmonary resuscitation (CPR) time to effective cardiac function represent a continuum from absence of cerebral blood flow to effective circulation, and together represent the total duration of ineffective cerebral blood flow. Short AT is compatible with good outcomes even after longer periods of CPR, whereas increasing lengths of AT reduce the time window for successful CPR. If AT is less than 6 minutes, prognosis for recovery is related to CPR time; over half of patients on whom CPR is successful within 30 minutes make a good neurologic recovery. When CPR time is longer, prognosis for neurologic recovery drops significantly. If AT exceeds 6 minutes, the chances of good neurologic outcome decrease [22]. Unsuccessful CPR before arrival at the emergency room predicts a poor prognosis [23]. Emergency crew–witnessed arrests, consciousness level on admission, and requirement for ventilation are independently useful to predict in-hospital outcome and mortality [24].

Magnetic resonance spectroscopy demonstrating elevated lactate and reduced *N*-acetyl acetate peaks is associated with a poor prognosis [25,26].

Cerebrospinal fluid (CSF) lactate levels [27], neuron-specific enolase, and brain-type creatine kinase isoenzyme levels may have predictive value 24 hours after cardiac arrest. Patients with either CSF neuron-specific enolase more than 33 μg per L at 24 hours or cerebrospinal fluid brain-type creatine kinase isoenzyme more than 50 U per L at 48 to 72 hours usually die. Creatine phosphokinase levels above 205 U per L are uniformly associated with a fatal outcome. A potentially useful laboratory screening test when lumbar puncture is not feasible is the serum neuron-specific enolase level, which has a fair correlation with outcome [28–30]. Similarly, S-100 protein, an astroglial marker, is elevated in anoxic arrest. Values of more than 0.2 mmol per L on day 2 are associated with 100% mortality, whereas values below this are associated with an 89% survival [31].

After out-of-hospital cardiac arrest, the overall probability of awakening is roughly 50% [32,33]. Much of this depends on the duration of coma. In cases of cardiac arrest, complete recovery occurs in 80% of patients in whom the coma resolves within 24 hours [32,33]. Others have shown that 72 hours is the upper limit for recovery of brain function sufficient to permit some degree of speech [34].

TREATMENT

Treatment approaches for cardiac arrest and perioperative hypoxic encephalopathy are similar. Optimal therapy is directed at preventing the recurrence of hypoxia. To ensure that the oxygen-carrying capacity of the blood is restored, excess oxygen administration is suggested for several hours after anoxic events. There is strong evidence that mild or moderate hypothermia may improve outcome after cardiac arrest [35,36]. Blood pressure is maintained at normotensive or mildly elevated levels. Mean arterial pressure should be 90 to 110 mm Hg in patients who are usually normotensive. The partial pressure of oxygen should be more than 100 mm Hg. The partial pressure of carbon dioxide is kept at the patient's baseline (usually 40 mm Hg), unless there are active signs of cerebral herniation; if herniation is suspected, the patient should be hyperventilated. Mild hypovolemia and elevation of the head of the bed to 30 degrees reduce intracranial pressure. Vital signs, hematocrit, electrolytes, blood sugar, and serum osmolality should be maintained in the normal range [12]. In all cases, a head CT or MRI scan and complete metabolic studies should be obtained to exclude structural and other functional causes. When any uncertainties exist, a neurologist should be consulted.

Seizures occur in 25% of patients in anoxic coma [4]. They are treated with loading and then maintenance doses of fosphenytoin (Cerebyx) (loading dose, 15 to 20 mg phenytoin equivalents per kg, rate not to exceed 100 mg phenytoin equivalents per minute; maintenance dose, 5 mg phenytoin equivalents per kg per day). Alternatively, intravenous phenytoin can be used (loading dose, 18 to 20 mg per kg; rate, 50 mg per minute; maintenance dose, 5 mg per kg). Patients with cardiac conduction abnormalities need to be carefully monitored while being loaded with fosphenytoin or phenytoin. Phenobarbital is usually avoided because of its sedative effects. If necessary, loading doses in adults are up to 500 mg intravenously, and maintenance doses are 2 to 4 mg per kg per day [37]. Because status epilepticus or frequent untreated seizures can further damage the brain, an EEG should be obtained if there is any question of subclinical epileptiform activity [10]. Some postanoxic patients develop delayed intention myoclonus. This can be distinguished from seizure activity because the latter is accompanied by an epileptiform discharge on the EEG, whereas myoclonus is not. Intention myoclonus can be treated with valproic acid.

Steroids, mannitol, and glycerol are ineffective and result in elevated serum blood glucose, which increase production of lactic acid, possibly potentiating preexisting damage. High dose barbiturates or calcium channel blockers have not demonstrated any improvement in outcome [38,39].

If the patient awakens, mobilization is initiated early to minimize the risk of bedsores and deep venous thrombosis. An empiric 7 to 10 days of bed rest may minimize the chance of developing postanoxic encephalopathy in cases of carbon monoxide poisoning [2,3].

Induced hypothermia may be protective. A randomized, controlled trial assessed the effects of moderate hypothermia and normothermia in patients who remained unconscious after resuscitation from out-of-hospital cardiac arrest. Of the 77 patients who were randomly assigned to treatment with hypothermia (core body temperature 33°C within 2 hours after the return of spontaneous circulation and maintained at that temperature for 12 hours) or normothermia, 21 of the 43 patients treated with hypothermia (49%) survived and had a good outcome, discharged home or to rehabilitation as compared with 9 of the 34 treated with normothermia (26%; $p = 0.046$). The odds ratio for a good outcome with hypothermia as compared with normothermia was 5.25 (95% confidence interval, 1.47 to 18.76; $p = 0.011$). Hypothermia was associated with a nonsignificant lower cardiac index, higher systemic vascular resistance, and hyperglycemia. The narrow inclusion criteria resulted in an international recommendation to cool only a restricted group of primary cardiac arrest survivors. In a broader retrospective study the efficacy and safety of endovascular cooling in unselected survivors of cardiac arrest was assessed. Consecutive comatose cardiac arrest survivors were either cooled to 33°C with endovascular cooling for 24 hours or treated with standard post-resuscitation therapy. Patients in the endovascular cooling group had twofold increased odds of survival (67/97 patients versus 466/941 patients; odds ratio 2.28, 95% CI, 1.45 to 3.57; $p < 0.001$). After adjustment for baseline imbalances, the odds ratio was 1.96 (95% CI, 1.19 to 3.23; $p = 0.008$). Bayesian analysis revealed odds ratios of 1.61 (95% credible interval, 1.06 to 2.44). In the endovascular cooling group, 51/97 patients (53%) survived with good outcome as compared with 320/941 (34%) in the control group (odds ratio 2.15, 95% CI, 1.38 to 3.35; $p = 0.0003$; adjusted odds ratio 2.56, 1.57 to 4.17). There was no difference in the rate of complications except for bradycardia. The investigators concluded that endovascular cooling improved survival when compared with standard treatment in comatose adult survivors of cardiac arrest [40].

CONCLUSION

The effects of oxygen deprivation depend on many factors; the degree and duration of hypoxia are the most important. In cases of cardiac arrest, brain damage is proportional to the amount of time without perfusion. The patient's age, underlying medical conditions, infection, and other metabolic imbalances also play a role in the body's ability to withstand oxygen deprivation.

Treatment strategies for the acute phase focus on supportive care. Elevation of the head of the bed, maintaining a relatively hypovolemic state, and avoidance of hypotension may be of benefit. A vigorous search should be made for concurrent metabolic abnormalities. Induced hypothermia improves outcome; administration of steroids, osmotic agents, neuroprotective agents, and prophylactic anticonvulsants are ineffective measures and may worsen the prognosis.

Prognosis is best determined by the early return of brainstem and cranial nerve function. Absence of brainstem functions 72 hours after the event is associated with irreversible coma [11]. Other poor prognostic signs include a brainstem auditory evoked response showing no cortical waves 8 hours after the arrest and a CT scan demonstrating diffuse edema, loss of gray–white matter distinction, or watershed infarcts. The overall functional recovery rate is approximately 13%. If a patient has not regained consciousness by 6 hours after the onset of coma, the chance of survival for 1 year is 10%, and many of these survivors remain in a vegetative state.

Data from recent studies of out-of-hospital cardiac arrest patients treated by induced hypothermia to 32°C suggest a better prognosis (survival increased threefold and neurological recovery almost 4.5 fold compared to patients who did not undergo hypothermia.) This better outcome was limited to patients with a primary cardiac arrest who had initiation of successful CPR within 15 minutes and had a stable circulation within 60 minutes. Patients with significant pretreatment hypothermia, bleeding disorders, terminal or other serious co-morbid conditions and unstable circulation after CPR were excluded. If one takes into account the retrospective nature of this study, the results are at best limited to the above population and can be considered hypothesis-generating data for future trials.

References

1. Dewey RC, Hunt WE: Cerebral hemodynamic crisis. Physiology, pathophysiology, and approach to therapy. *Am J Surg* 131:338, 1976.
2. Posner JB, Saper CB, Schiff ND, et al: Plum and Posner's diagnosis of stupor and coma, 4th Ed. Oxford University Press, 2007.
3. Plum F, Posner JB, Hain RF: Delayed neurological deterioration after anoxia. *Arch Intern Med* 110:56, 1962.
4. Levy DE, Bates D, Caronna JJ, et al: Prognosis in nontraumatic coma. *Ann Intern Med* 94:293, 1981.
5. Snyder BEAD, Ramirez-Lassepas M, Lippert DM: Neurologic status and prognosis after cardiopulmonary arrest: I. A retrospective study. *Neurology* 27:807, 1977.
6. Edgren E, Hedstrand U, Kelsy S, et al: Assessment of neurological prognosis in comatose survivors of cardiac arrest. BRCT1 study group. *Lancet* 343(8905):1055, 1994.
7. Wijdicks EF, Parisi JE, Sharbrough FW: Prognostic value of myoclonus in comatose survivors of cardiac arrest. *Ann Neurol* 38(4):697, 1994.
8. Mellion ML: Neurologic consequences of cardiac arrest and preventive strategies. *Med Health R I* 88:382, 2005.
9. Garcia JH: Morphology of cerebral ischemia. *Crit Care Med* 16:979, 1988.
10. Dickey W, Adgey AAJ: Resuscitation: mortality within hospital after resuscitation from ventricular fibrillation outside hospital. *Br Heart J* 67:334, 1992.
11. Zandbergen EGJ, de Haan RJ, Stoutenbeek CP, et al: Systemic review of early predictors of poor outcome in anoxic-ischemic coma. *Lancet* 352:1808, 1998.
12. Husain AM: Electrographic assessment of coma. *J Clin Neurophysiol* 23: 208, 2006.
13. Aichmer F, Bauer G: Cerebral anoxia. Clinical aspects, in Neidermeyer E, Lopes de Silva F (eds): *Electroencephalography: Basic Principles, Clinical Applications and Related Fields.* Baltimore, Urban & Schwarzenberg, 1987, p 445.
14. Facco E, Liviero MC, Munari M, et al: Short latency evoked potentials: new criteria for brain death? *J Neurol Neurosurg Psychiatry* 3:351, 1990.
15. Brunko E, Zegers de Beyl D: Prognostic value of early cortical somatosensory evoked potentials after resuscitation from cardiac arrest. *Electroencephalogr Clin Neurophysiol* 66:15, 1987.
16. Madl C, Krammer L, Yaganehfar W, et al: Detection of non traumatic comatose patients with no benefit of intensive care treatment by recording of sensory evoked potentials. *Arch Neurol* 53:512, 1996.
17. Arbelaez A: Diffusion weighted MR imaging of global cerebral anoxia. *AJNR Am J Neuroradiol* 20(6):999, 1999.
18. Roine RO, Raininko R, Erkinjuntti T, et al: Magnetic resonance imaging findings associated with cardiac arrest. *Stroke* 24:1005, 1993.
19. Wijdicks EF, Hijdra A, Young GB, et al: Practice parameter: prediction of outcome in comatose survivors after cardiopulmonary resuscitation (an evidence-based review): report of the Quality Standards Subcommittee of the American Academy of Neurology. *Neurology* 67:203, 2006.
20. Safar P, Bleyaert A, Nemoto EM, et al: Resuscitation after global brain ischemia-anoxia. *Crit Care Med* 6:215, 1978.
21. Pfeifer R, Borner A, Krack A, et al: Outcome after cardiac arrest: predictive values and limitations of the neuroproteins neuron-specific enolase and protein S-100 and the Glasgow Coma Scale. *Resuscitation* 65:49, 2005.
22. Abramson NS, Safar P, Detre KM: Neurologic recovery after cardiac arrest: effect of duration of ischemia. *Crit Care Med* 14:930, 1985.
23. Gray WA, Capone RJ, Most AS: Unsuccessful emergency medical resuscitation: are continued efforts in the emergency department justified? *N Engl J Med* 325:1393, 1991.
24. Grubb NR, Elton RA, Fox KA: In hospital mortality after out of hospital cardiac arrest. *Lancet* 346:417, 1995.
25. Lechleitner P, Felber S, Birbamer G, et al: Proton magnetic resonance spectroscopy of brain after cardiac resuscitation. *Lancet* 340:913, 1992.
26. Moonis M, Fisher M: Imaging of acute stroke. *Cerebrovasc Dis* 11:143, 2001.
27. Risto O, Somer H, Kaste M, et al: Neurologic outcome after out-of-hospital cardiac arrest: prediction by cerebrospinal fluid enzyme analysis. *Arch Neurol* 46:753, 1989.
28. Edgren E, Headstrand U, Nordin M, et al: Prediction of outcome after cardiac arrest. *Crit Care Med* 15:820, 1987.
29. Longstreth WT, Inui TS, Cobb LA, et al: Neurologic recovery after out-of-hospital cardiac arrest. *Ann Intern Med* 98:588, 1983.
30. Schoerkhuber W, Kittler H, Sterz F, et al: Time course of neuron-specific enolase. A predictor of neurological outcome after cardiac arrest. *Stroke* 30:1598, 1999.
31. Rosen H, Rosengren L, Herlitz J, et al: Increased serum levels of S-100 protein are associated with hypoxic brain damage after cardiac arrest. *Stroke* 29:473, 1998.
32. Ernest MP, Yarnell PR, Merrill SL, et al: Long-term survival and neurological status after resuscitation from out-of-hospital cardiac arrest. *Neurology* 30:1298, 1980.
33. Tweed WA, Thomassen A, Wernberg M: Prognosis after cardiac arrest based on age and duration of coma. *Can Med Assoc J* 126:1058, 1982.
34. Lowenstein DH, Aminoff MJ: Clinical and EEG features of status epilepticus in comatose patients. *Neurology* 42:100, 1992.
35. The Hypothermia after Cardiac Arrest Study Group: Mild therapeutic hypothermia to improve the neurologic outcome after cardiac arrest. *N Engl J Med* 346:549, 2002.
36. Bernard SA, Gray TW, Buist MD, et al: Treatment of comatose survivors of out-of-hospital cardiac arrest with induced hypothermia. *N Engl J Med* 346:557, 2002.
37. Simon RP, Aminoff MJ: Electrographic status epilepticus in fatal anoxic coma. *Ann Neurol* 20:351, 1986.
38. Rockoff MA, Marshall LF, Shapiro HM: High-dose barbiturate therapy in humans: a clinical review of 60 patients. *Ann Neurol* 6:194, 1979.
39. Brain Resuscitation Clinical Trial II Study Group: A randomized clinical study of a calcium-entry blocker (lidoflazine) in the treatment of comatose survivors of cardiac arrest. *N Engl J Med* 324:1225, 1991.
40. Holzer M, Mullner M, Sterz F, et al: Efficacy and safety of endovascular cooling after cardiac arrest: cohort study and Bayesian approach. *Stroke* 37: 1792–1797, 2006.

CHAPTER 172 ■ STATUS EPILEPTICUS

JAISHREE NARAYANAN AND CATHERINE A. PHILLIPS

DEFINITION AND CLASSIFICATION

Status epilepticus (SE) was originally defined as seizures lasting longer than 30 minutes, or 30 minutes of recurrent seizures without return to baseline neurologic status between events [1]. This has been largely replaced by an operational definition of SE, which is a 5-minute duration of continued seizure activity, or two or more seizures between which there is incomplete recovery. SE is considered to be a condition in which there is "a failure of the 'normal' factors that serve to terminate a typical generalized tonic-clonic seizure" [2,3]. This approach is more clinically appropriate and promotes early treatment with antiepileptic medication. SE is usually divided into: (a) convulsive SE, in which the patient does not regain consciousness between repeated generalized tonic-clonic attacks; (b) simple partial SE, characterized by continuous or repetitive focal seizures without loss of consciousness [4]; and (c) nonconvulsive SE (NCSE), such as absence or complex partial SE, characterized by a prolonged confusional state of 30 minutes or longer. NCSE is also used to describe continued seizure activity in patients who have few or no clinical signs other than coma.

Convulsive Status Epilepticus

Most generalized tonic-clonic SE consists of partial seizures that have secondarily generalized; primary generalized SE is less common [5]. Most patients do not convulse continuously. Instead, seizures of a few minutes' duration may be followed by a prolonged period of unconsciousness that leads to the next seizure. During convulsive SE, massive autonomic discharge occurs with tachycardia and hypertension. Corneal and pupillary reflexes are lost and plantar reflexes may be extensor. As SE continues, the motor manifestations may evolve into more subtle activity such as low-amplitude focal twitching, nystagmus, eye deviation, or recurrent pupillary hippus. This is sometimes called *subtle generalized SE* [4]. SE may also present in this more subtle form, without initial convulsive activity, in patients who are very encephalopathic; electroencephalography (EEG) is required to confirm the diagnosis. Myoclonic SE is often classified as a form of convulsive SE; it can occur in children with chronic epilepsy and mental retardation. It is characterized by repetitive, asynchronous myoclonus with variable clouding of consciousness and may evolve into generalized tonic-clonic SE. In adults, the myoclonic syndromes that occur are usually secondary to toxic or metabolic encephalopathies, most commonly severe cerebral anoxia [6]. The patients are usually comatose, and the prognosis is poor. In both forms of myoclonic SE, the EEG shows repetitive generalized epileptiform discharges.

Simple Partial Status Epilepticus

Simple partial status epilepticus is the second most common form of SE, after generalized tonic-clonic SE [4]. In partial motor SE, focal clonic or tonic-clonic activity is localized to the face or an extremity. This activity may spread, corresponding to the somatotopic organization of the motor cortex, known as a Jacksonian march. Alternatively, the partial motor seizures may be multifocal, in this case often precipitated by metabolic disorders, such as hyperglycemia with a hyperosmolar nonketotic state [7]. *Epilepsia partialis continua* refers to a form of partial motor SE characterized by continuous, highly localized seizures that do not secondarily generalize and in which consciousness is maintained.

Nonconvulsive Status Epilepticus

NCSE is an under-recognized cause of coma. In a recent study, NCSE was documented in 8% of all comatose patients, without signs of seizure activity [8]. In additional studies, 31% to 37% of patients with unexplained altered mental status in intensive care units were in NCSE. NCSE is more likely to occur in the setting of acute medical problems, both systemic and neurologic [8–10].

Nonconvulsive SE includes absence and complex partial SE [4]. Clinically, both absence and complex partial SE present with a prolonged period of altered behavior and can masquerade as a psychiatric fugue state. Absence SE involves a variable level of altered consciousness, which may be accompanied by subtle myoclonic movements of the face, eye blinking, and occasional automatisms of the face and hands. The EEG is diagnostic, revealing continuous or discontinuous generalized spike and slow-wave activity. Complex partial SE involves either a series of complex partial seizures with staring, unresponsiveness, and motor automatisms, separated by a confusional state, or a more prolonged state of partial responsiveness and semipurposeful automatisms. In both of these forms of SE, the patient is partially or totally amnestic for the episode.

ETIOLOGY

Some of the major underlying etiologies and precipitants of SE are shown in Table 172.1. Precipitants are factors that provoke SE where it otherwise would not have occurred, but they are not the underlying cause of the seizure disorder. Symptomatic SE, defined as SE resulting from an acute or chronic neurologic or metabolic insult, is typically more common than idiopathic SE (presumed genetic etiology for the seizures in an otherwise neurologically normal person) [5]. In most series, at least two-thirds of cases of SE are symptomatic. In adults, a major cause of SE is stroke, comprising more than 25% of the cases in one series [5]. Decreasing antiepileptic drugs was also a significant cause of SE in this same series, occurring in approximately 20% of the cases. Other major causes include alcohol withdrawal, anoxia, metabolic disease, viral encephalitis including Epstein–Barr virus or herpes simplex virus, HIV infection, and drug abuse [11,12]. The acute insults can cause SE in patients with or without epilepsy. Children younger than 1 year and adults older than 60 years represent the populations most at risk for developing SE [5].

TABLE 172.1

ETIOLOGIES AND PRECIPITANTS OF STATUS EPILEPTICUS

Etiologies
Structural brain lesion
Brain trauma
Brain tumors
Strokes
Hemorrhage
Central nervous system infections
Encephalitis
Meningitis
Toxic
Drugs (e.g., theophylline, lidocaine, penicillin)
Withdrawal states (e.g., alcohol, barbiturate)
Metabolic
Hypocalcemia
Hypomagnesemia
Hypoglycemia, hyperglycemia
Hyponatremia
Hyperosmolar state
Anoxia
Uremia
Precipitants
Changes in anticonvulsant blood levels
Errors in medication
Change in drug regimens
Altered drug absorption
Noncompliance
Intercurrent infection
Fever (e.g., upper respiratory or gastrointestinal infections)
Alcohol withdrawal

PROGNOSIS AND SEQUELAE OF STATUS EPILEPTICUS

Mortality in SE depends on the specific etiology, duration of the episode, and the age of the patient [13]. The acute insult triggering SE is one of the most important factors influencing mortality. Among the etiologic groups, anoxia has been associated with the highest mortality rate, followed by hemorrhage, tumor, metabolic disorders, and systemic infection. Alcohol withdrawal and antiepileptic drug discontinuation have been associated with a low mortality rate. Patients with idiopathic SE have a low mortality rate. The duration of SE strongly affects the ultimate prognosis. In one study, patients with seizure duration of longer than 60 minutes had a mortality of 32.0%, whereas patients with seizure duration of shorter than 60 minutes had a mortality of 2.7% [13]. Age is significantly associated with mortality, with patients above the age of 70 having a dramatically greater mortality [5,13,14]. Despite improved medical care, convulsive SE still has an overall mortality rate in the range of 7% to 25% [5,13–15]. The mortality of complex partial SE was 18% in one study [16]. Other adverse outcomes include intellectual deterioration, permanent neurologic deficits, and chronic epilepsy.

SE itself can produce profound neuronal damage. Neuropathologic studies of the brains of children and adults who died shortly after SE reveal ischemic neuronal changes in the hippocampus, middle layers of the cerebral cortex, cerebellum (Purkinje cells), basal ganglia, thalamus, and hypothalamus [17]. These changes mimic those of severe hypoxia or hypoglycemia. The degree of hyperthermia during an episode of SE has also been shown to correlate closely with the degree of central nervous system (CNS) damage [18].

The perpetuation of SE is most likely caused by an imbalance between excitotoxic (primarily mediated by glutamate) and inhibitory (primarily mediated by γ-aminobutyric acid [GABA]) mechanisms [15,16]. This can be related to downregulation in GABA receptors or excitotoxic mechanisms involving glutamate receptors—both NMDA(*N*-methyl-D-aspartate) and non-NMDA receptors [3,15,19]. Calcium influx during excitation appears to be a critical component of neuronal injury and cell death, with activation of proteases and lipases leading to degradation of intracellular elements [19].

Abnormal neuronal activity alone can cause permanent neurologic injury. This is supported by the observation that patients with complex partial or partial motor SE who do not have concomitant hypotension, hypoxia, or hyperpyrexia can still have subsequent neurologic injury in the region of the brain associated with the seizure. Chronic memory impairment may follow complex partial SE [20], and focal neuronal necrosis (and edema) in the region of the brain involved with seizure activity has been found after partial motor status [21,22]. Focal magnetic resonance imaging (MRI) changes can be seen after prolonged epileptic activity, particularly on diffusion-weighted and perfusion MRI [23].

The natural history of NCSE is not well defined, especially mortality and morbidity. This is partly due to methodological issues, such as the lack of a uniform accurate definition of NCSE, and not assigning appropriate significance to the underlying etiology, mental status changes, and associated complications [24–26]. Kaplan [27,28] reviewed the prognosis of NCSE and suggested that prognosis depends not only on detailed assessment of NCSE type, but also on level of consciousness. In another study designed specifically to determine the rate of morbidity and mortality, mortality was associated with an acute medical cause as the underlying etiology, severe mental status impairment, and development of acute complications, but not the type of EEG changes [10].

SYSTEMIC COMPLICATIONS

If convulsive SE is not terminated promptly, secondary metabolic and medical complications occur (Table 172.2). Cardiac arrhythmias occur due to autonomic overactivity, acidosis, and hyperkalemia. This can be further complicated by shock due to lactic acidosis or by pharmacologic intervention for the status itself. Respiratory dysfunction may be caused by mechanical impairment from tonic muscle contraction, disturbed respiratory center function, massive autonomic discharge producing increased bronchial constriction and secretions, aspiration pneumonia, and neurogenic pulmonary edema. Neurogenic pulmonary edema results from ictal increases in pulmonary circulation with transcapillary fluid flux [17]. Renal impairment may occur from a combination of rhabdomyolysis with myoglobinuria and hypotension with poor renal perfusion. Hyperthermia can result from excessive muscle activity and hypothalamic dysfunction; alternatively, it may be due to an underlying infection that is responsible for the initiation of SE. The distinction of hyperthermia from an infection or from SE itself can be complicated by the peripheral leukocytosis [17] that occurs with status epilepticus due to demargination. This can result in a white blood cell count in the range of 12,700 to 28,000 cells per mm^3. The differential may be normal or may show lymphocytic or polymorphonuclear predominance, but band forms are rarely present. In addition, a mild cerebrospinal fluid (CSF) pleocytosis can occur with SE [17]. The maximum cell count is usually less than 80 cells per mm^3, with an initial polymorphonuclear predominance that reverts to a lymphocytic predominance as the pleocytosis resolves over a

TABLE 172.2

MEDICAL COMPLICATIONS OF STATUS EPILEPTICUS

	Early	Late (after 30 min)
Cardiovascular system	Tachycardia Hypertension	Bradycardia Hypotension Cardiac arrest Shock
Respiratory system	Tachypnea Apnea with carbon dioxide retention	Apnea Cheyne–Stokes Aspiration pneumonia Neurogenic pulmonary edema
Renal system	—	Uremia Acute tubular necrosis Myoglobinuria
Autonomic nervous system	Mydriasis Salivary and tracheobronchial hypersecretion Excessive sweating Bronchial constriction	Hyperpyrexia
Metabolic	Lactic acidosis Hyperglycemia Hyperkalemia	Lactic acidosis Hypoglycemia Liver failure Elevated prolactin

few days. Mild transient elevations in CSF protein may also occur. However, lowering of the CSF glucose level does not occur, and reduced CSF glucose immediately suggests an underlying bacterial or fungal infection.

Increased lactate production from maximally exercised muscles results in metabolic acidosis within minutes after the start of SE. There is a variable respiratory contribution to the acidosis from carbon dioxide retention. The degree of acidosis does not correlate with the extent of neuropathologic damage [17]. After cessation of the seizure, lactate is rapidly metabolized, resulting in spontaneous resolution of the acidosis. Initially, hyperglycemia develops due to catecholamine and glucagon release; later, hypoglycemia occurs due to increased plasma insulin, increased cerebral glucose consumption, and excessive muscle activity.

INITIAL ASSESSMENT AND MEDICAL MANAGEMENT

SE is a medical emergency and must be treated immediately in a critical care setting. Pharmacologic intervention is more effective at an early stage of SE than after a delay [3,14,15,19,29,30]. Treatment must be fourfold: termination of seizures, prevention of recurrent seizures, identification of etiology, and treatment of complications. This discussion concentrates on generalized tonic-clonic SE, which is the most common form of status in adults and has the most harmful neurologic sequelae.

The initial step is to confirm the diagnosis. The patient must be carefully observed to be sure that generalized seizures are recurring without recovery of consciousness. A flurry of seizures separated by a normal level of consciousness does not constitute SE (although urgent treatment may still be required). In the intensive care unit, NCSE may present clinically with a change in mental status only. As mentioned earlier, in this setting NCSE appears to be greatly underdiagnosed. For diagnosis of NCSE, certain well-defined EEG criteria need to be met, including repetitive epileptiform activity at more than 3 per second, or repetitive epileptiform activity at less than 3 per second but with incrementing or decrementing onset for 10 seconds or more and/or clinical improvement after antiepileptic drug (AED) use. The EEG ictal episodes should be continuous or recurrent for more than 30 minutes without improvement in clinical state, or return to preictal EEG between seizures [27,28].

Once a diagnosis of SE is made, treatment must proceed rapidly but deliberately. For generalized SE, the initial assessment and treatment should begin within 5 to 10 minutes of the onset of seizure activity. Table 172.3 outlines a management protocol.

It is important to obtain as much history as possible within the first few minutes of assessment, including any history of a preexisting chronic seizure disorder and antiepileptic drug use, alcohol or drug abuse, or any recent neurologic insult. The examination should focus on signs of systemic illness (e.g., uremia, hepatic disease, and infection), illicit drug use, evidence of trauma, or focal neurologic abnormalities. After appropriate blood samples have been obtained, glucose administration is recommended. Hypoglycemia is a rare but easily reversible cause of SE and may result in irreversible CNS damage if left untreated. Because glucose administration may precipitate Wernicke–Korsakoff syndrome in some individuals with marginal nutrition, thiamine should also be given. Subsequent intravenous (IV) infusions should consist of saline solution, as some AEDs precipitate in glucose solutions. The patient must be assessed for other metabolic consequences of status. Hyperthermia should be treated and oxygenation must be maintained. The metabolic acidosis that occurs does not adversely affect neurologic outcome and does not need treatment with bicarbonate [14,31]. Blood pressure must be carefully monitored; the systemic hypertension and decreased cerebrovascular resistance of early SE provide adequate blood flow for the increased metabolic demand in the brain, but eventually hypotension may occur, making the brain vulnerable to inadequate perfusion. Pharmacologic intervention for the seizures can exacerbate any hypotension.

TABLE 172.3

MANAGEMENT GUIDELINES FOR GENERALIZED STATUS EPILEPTICUS IN ADULTS

0–9 min:
If diagnosis is uncertain, observe for: recurrence of generalized seizures without intervening recovery of consciousness; continuous seizure activity >5 min.

ABCs
Establish airway; pulse ox; administer 02; cardiac monitor.
Establish IV access (NS or saline lock), bedside rapid glucose determination.
Labs: CBC/diff, electrolytes, BUN/Cr/Glu, anticonvulsant drug levels, tox screen, other labs as indicated by history/examination.
If hypoglycemic give glucose (D50) 50–100 mL and thiamine 100 mg IV.

5–30 min:
Lorazepam 0.1 mg/kg IV (<2 mg/min), given 2 mg at a time (or diazepam 0.1–0.2 mg/kg, <2 mg/min).
Phenytoin 20 mg/kg IV at ≤50 mg/min (fosphenytoin 150 mg PE[a]/min), slower rate in elderly or if hypotension or bradycardia develop. Draw blood for level 10 min after infusion complete.
Cardiac monitoring, frequent BPs, careful observation of respiratory status, oximetry.
EEG monitoring, if possible.
Consider additional 5 mg/kg boluses of phenytoin to a maximum dose 30 mg/kg if seizures persist.
Lorazepam as needed for seizure during phenytoin load.

31–60 min:
If seizures persist: phenobarbital 20 mg/kg IV load, ≤100 mg/min. Or: induce coma, as below.
Anticipate respiratory depression and need for intubation.
If neuromuscular blockade required for intubation: EEG monitoring indicated.

>1 h:
For persistent status: induce coma. Intubate if not previously done.
Continuous EEG to monitor for seizures and level of anesthesia.
Pentobarbital 5 mg/kg IV load (give over 20 min); repeat as needed to produce burst-suppression pattern. EEG may need to be completely suppressed if seizure activity persists during the bursts. Maintenance infusion 0.5–10 mg/kg/h.
OR
Midazolam 0.2 mg/kg IV bolus, infusion 0.1–2.0 mg/kg/h (tolerance after 72 h);
OR
Propofol 3–5 mg/kg IV bolus, 1–15 mg/kg/h infusion
Monitor for hypotension, ileus. Continue maintenance doses of phenytoin and phenobarbital; maintain therapeutic levels.
Once burst-suppression pattern established, monitor EEG every 1–2 h. Review at least 5 min of EEG every hour. Adjust medication dose as needed.
Taper medication at 12 h. If seizures recur, resume infusion for 24 h, then taper again. Continue this process as necessary.

[a]Fosphenytoin dosing in "phenytoin equivalents" (PE).
BP, blood pressure; BUN, blood urea nitrogen; CBC, complete blood cell; Cr, creatine; EEG, electroencephalogram; Glu, glucose; IV, intravenous; NS, normal saline.

It is essential to determine whether a metabolic disorder is causing the SE; if this is the case, pharmacologic intervention for SE alone is not effective. Systemic and CNS infections must be excluded, and lumbar puncture is often necessary. A contrast-enhanced head CT scan can be useful after the patient has been medically stabilized and the SE has terminated. MRI is preferred for suspected small or subtle lesions but is often not practical in the emergent setting.

PHARMACOLOGIC MANAGEMENT

A variety of drugs are available to treat SE. It is important to understand the pharmacokinetics of these drugs to ensure effective use. Table 172.4 outlines some of these properties.

IV benzodiazepines are an appropriate initial treatment. The Veterans Affairs Status Epilepticus Cooperative Study Group trial suggested that phenobarbital is also effective as initial therapy, but phenytoin alone without a benzodiazepine may be less effective [29,32]. Diazepam and lorazepam are both effective in treating generalized SE [33], but lorazepam has a longer duration of action (2 to 24 hours), compared to diazepam (10 to 25 minutes) [34], and does not have extensive peripheral tissue uptake, unlike diazepam. Although lorazepam has slower CNS penetration than diazepam, the onset of action of less than 3 minutes is acceptable. For these reasons, lorazepam is the recommended first-line agent in status epilepticus. Both these drugs have significant and essentially the same cardiac, respiratory, and CNS depressant side effects [30]. Respiratory depression and apnea, which are potentiated by age and previous administration of sedative drugs, may occur abruptly with doses as small as 1 mg. Hypotension, which occasionally occurs, may be partially due to the propylene glycol solvent contained in the IV forms of diazepam and lorazepam.

If IV access is not available, rectal diazepam has been successful in achieving rapid therapeutic levels and effectively terminating prolonged generalized seizures. A commercially prepared diazepam rectal gel is available for this purpose [35]. Significant respiratory depression from rectal diazepam has not been reported [36]. Intramuscular (IM) administration is unsuitable for the treatment of status due to delayed peak levels [37]. Furthermore, the peak concentration after IM injection is much less than that after IV injection for both agents.

Phenytoin is usually given with benzodiazepines to control the SE and prevent recurrent seizures. A 20 mg per kg load is recommended, given at 50 mg per minute. If seizures continue,

TABLE 172.4

PROPERTIES OF DRUGS USED TO TREAT STATUS EPILEPTICUS

Drug	Route	Loading dose	Rate of administration	Time to enter brain	Time to peak brain concentration (min)	Minimum effective plasma concentration (μg/mL)	Side effects
Diazepam	IV, rectal	0.1–0.2 mg/kg, up to 20 mg	2 mg/min IV	<10 s	8	0.2–0.8	Respiratory depression/apnea (may be abrupt); hypotension; sedation, especially in combination with barbiturates
Lorazepam	IV	0.1 mg/kg	2 mg/min	<2–3 min	23	0.03–0.10	Same as diazepam; amnesia
Phenytoin	IV	20 mg/kg	50 mg/min	1–3 min	3–6	15–30	Hypotension and electrocardiogram changes during acute administration; sedation at high doses
Phenobarbital	IV	20 mg/kg	100 mg/min	3 min	5–15	10–40	Respiratory depression and sedation common with increasing doses, especially when benzodiazepines used; hypotension

IV, intravenous.

additional doses of up to another 10 mg per kg can be given. The serum level of phenytoin should be 15 to 30 μg per mL. IM administration should not be used because it results in precipitation at the injection site and has slow, erratic absorption. Hypotension, electrocardiogram changes, and respiratory depression can occur and may be due partly to the propylene glycol diluent [3]. Simultaneous cardiac monitoring should be performed, and slower infusion rates (25 mg per minute) should be considered in patients who are elderly or have a history of cardiac arrhythmias, compromised pulmonary function, or hypotension [38]. The most common adverse effect is hypotension, which is age related and much less common in patients younger than 40 years. Intravenous infusion of phenytoin carries a risk of medication extravasation into adjacent tissue. Tissue necrosis can rarely occur [39].

Fosphenytoin, a water-soluble prodrug of phenytoin, is rapidly converted enzymatically to phenytoin. Rapid and complete absorption occurs after IM administration [40,41]. Therapeutic phenytoin concentrations are attained in most patients within 10 minutes of rapid IV infusion (150 mg per minute) and within 30 minutes of slower IV infusion or IM injection [40,41]. Dosing for fosphenytoin is the same as for phenytoin, but needs to be given in "phenytoin equivalents." Cardiac monitoring is required during IV infusions of fosphenytoin. Maintenance doses of phenytoin or fosphenytoin should be started within 24 hours of the loading dose, with levels maintained in the high therapeutic range (15 to 25 μg per mL).

The antiepileptic effect of phenytoin or fosphenytoin is maximal within 10 minutes after the infusion is completed. SE persisting after this time is considered refractory SE (RSE). Treatment from this point on may vary. A loading dose of phenobarbital may be given, 10 mg per kg at a rate of 100 mg per minute, repeated as needed up to a total dose of 20 mg per kg. Target blood levels are 30 to 40 μg per mL. Respiratory depression is a major side effect, especially if benzodiazepines have been used. The response rate to a third-line agent such as phenobarbital may be very low [3], and because of this, some centers proceed at this point to a drug-induced coma rather than administering phenobarbital. For drug-induced coma, all patients must be intubated, as anesthetic doses of medication are required. Agents commonly used for RSE include pentobarbital, midazolam, and propofol [38]. All are extremely effective at suppressing clinical and electrographic seizures. Simultaneous EEG monitoring is mandatory during induction of coma. Phenobarbital is not used for this purpose, because it results in very prolonged coma. Pentobarbital is administered as a loading dose of 5 mg per kg, given slowly, and repeated as necessary with additional 5 mg per kg loads to stop electrographic seizure activity. The maintenance dose is 0.5 to 10 mg per kg per hour [3,30,38]. Cardiac depression is often produced, and careful hemodynamic monitoring is required. Vasopressors are frequently needed, and ileus is also common.

Treatment with midazolam is initiated with a 0.2 mg per kg IV bolus followed by an infusion of 0.1 to 2.0 mg per kg per hour [42,43]. Patients regain consciousness more rapidly after discontinuation of midazolam than with pentobarbital. The short elimination half-life of midazolam may be significantly prolonged in critically ill patients and can lead to accumulation of the drug [44]. Tolerance to the effects of midazolam also can develop after 36 to 48 hours, which can lead to escalating dose requirements. Because of this, if status is not terminated within 72 hours of midazolam treatment, changing to a pentobarbital infusion is recommended.

Propofol, a GABA agonist, has also been used as a potent antiepileptic agent. The loading dose is 3 to 5 mg per kg, with an infusion rate of 1 to 15 mg per kg per hour [30,45,46]. One significant disadvantage of this drug is the propofol infusion syndrome. This consists of profound hypotension, rhabdomyolysis, hyperlipidemia, cardiac arrhythmias, and metabolic acidosis. It has been described primarily in pediatric patients, and propofol is therefore not recommended for pediatric SE. Propofol has the advantage of rapid induction and elimination, but slow downward titration is important to avoid recurrent seizures [47].

There is relatively little prospective data to suggest that propofol, pentobarbital, or midazolam are dramatically different in efficacy for SE. Several studies seem to indicate that patients treated with pentobarbital have fewer treatment failures and breakthrough seizures, but more frequent episodes of hypotension. There is no clear difference in mortality among the three agents [48].

The dose of pentobarbital, midazolam, or propofol must be sufficient to terminate any seizure activity seen on the EEG. In many cases, the goal is to produce a burst-suppression EEG pattern, characterized by a flat background punctuated by bursts of mixed-frequency activity. If the bursts contain electrographic seizure activity, the coma should be deepened, at times to virtual electrocerebral silence. It is unclear if the coma needs to be deepened if only periodic sharp activity is seen on EEG. Further studies are needed to clarify fully what the appropriate EEG endpoint should be. During this time of drug-induced coma, maintenance doses of phenytoin and phenobarbital need to be continued and the serum levels kept in therapeutic range. Recently, propylene glycol toxicity has been reported in patients treated with barbiturate coma for refractory status epilepticus. These patients can develop hypotension and hepatic and renal failure. Hemodialysis is an option in these cases [49].

There is some evidence to suggest that intravenous valproate could be an appropriate second-line therapy. Intravenous valproate is well tolerated, with few adverse effects [50,51]. A loading dose of 25 mg per kg and an infusion rate of 3 to 6 mg per kg per minute have been used [52]. Studies have shown that it can be effective [53,54]. Although these early data appear promising, the overall role of IV valproate in the treatment of SE remains to be defined.

NCSE must be treated quickly, although the urgency is not as great as for convulsive SE. Diazepam and lorazepam are both effective in treating complex partial, partial motor, and absence SE. The response to benzodiazepines may be helpful in confirming the diagnosis if it is in question. The patient should also be started on antiepileptic medication appropriate for long-term management, given as a loading dose if appropriate. Valproic acid is an ideal drug for absence SE and can be given intravenously. The recommended starting dose is 15 mg per kg per day. Complex partial and partial motor SE both respond to phenytoin and phenobarbital, although epilepsia partialis continua can be notoriously resistant to treatment. Newer antiepileptic medications such as topiramate may also be effective, but need to be given orally [55]. The drug of choice for myoclonic status is valproate, but phenytoin and phenobarbital are also effective.

CONCLUSION

Status epilepticus is a true medical emergency and needs to be treated promptly and definitively. In convulsive SE, lorazepam is the drug of choice for immediate, short-term termination of ongoing seizure activity. A phenytoin loading dose should be administered simultaneously with the lorazepam. Phenytoin is safe and effective, has a rapid onset of seizure control, and may be used for maintenance therapy. If these drugs are ineffective, phenobarbital may be added, and if status still persists, a drug-induced coma should be induced. Physicians should be familiar with a treatment protocol, as appropriate therapy greatly reduces morbidity and mortality.

References

1. Working Group on Status Epilepticus: Treatment of convulsive status epilepticus. *JAMA* 270:855, 1993.
2. Lowenstein DH, Bleck T, MacDonald RL: It's time to revise the definition of status epilepticus. *Epilepsia* 40:120, 1999.
3. Lowenstein DH, Alldredge BK: Status epilepticus. *N Engl J Med* 338(14): 970, 1998.
4. Treiman DM: Status epilepticus, in Wyllie E (ed): *Treatment of Epilepsy: Principles and Practice*. Philadelphia, Lippincott Williams & Wilkins, 2001, p 681.
5. DeLorenzo RJ, Towne AR, Pellock JM, et al: Status epilepticus in children, adults, and the elderly. *Epilepsia* 33[Suppl 4]:15, 1992.
6. Hui AC, Cheng C, Lam A, et al: Prognosis following postanoxic myoclonus status epilepticus. *Eur Neurol* 54(1):10, 2005.
7. Cokar O, Aydin B, Ozer F: Nonketotic hyperglycemia presenting as epilepsia partialis continua. *Seizure* 13(4):264, 2004.
8. Towne AR, Waterhouse EJ, Boggs JG, et al: Prevalence of nonconvulsive status epilepticus in comatose patients. *Neurology* 54:340–345, 2000.
9. Claassen J, Mayer SA, Kowalski RG, et al: Detection of electrographic seizures with continuous EEG monitoring in critically ill patients. *Neurology* 62:1743–1748, 2004.
10. Shneker BF, Fountain NB: Assessment of acute morbidity and mortality in nonconvulsive status epilepticus. *Neurology* 61:1006, 2003.
11. Holtzman DM, Kaku DA, So YT: New-onset seizures associated with human immunodeficiency virus infection: causation and clinical features in 100 cases. *Am J Med* 87:173, 1989.
12. Lee KC, Garcia PA, Alldredge BK: Clinical features of status epilepticus in patients with HIV infection. *Neurology* 65(2):314, 2005.
13. Towne AR, Pellock JM, Ko D, et al: Determinants of mortality in status epilepticus. *Epilepsia* 35(1):27, 1994.
14. Sagduyu A, Tarlaci S, Sirin H: Generalized tonic-clonic status epilepticus: causes, treatment, complications and predictors of case fatality. *J Neurol* 245:640, 1998.
15. Payne TA, Bleck TP: Status epilepticus. *Crit Care Clin* 13(1):17, 1997.
16. Simon RP: Physiologic consequences of status epilepticus. *Epilepsia* 26[Suppl 1]:58, 1985.
17. Meldrum BS, Vigouroux RA, Brierley JB: Systemic factors and epileptic brain damage. *Arch Neurol* 29:82, 1973.
18. Alldredge BK, Lowenstein DH: Status epilepticus: new concepts. *Curr Opin Neurol* 12:183, 1999.
19. Lothman E: The biochemical basis and pathophysiology of status epilepticus. *Neurology* 40[Suppl 2]:13, 1990.
20. Krumholz A, Sung GY, Fisher RS, et al: Complex partial status epilepticus accompanied by serious morbidity and mortality. *Neurology* 45(8):1499, 1995.
21. Soffer D, Melamed E, Assaf Y, et al: Hemispheric brain damage in unilateral status epilepticus. *Ann Neurol* 20:737, 1986.
22. Fabene PF, Marzola P, Sbarbati A Bentivoglio M: Magnetic resonance imaging of chages elicited by status epilepticus in the rat brain: diffusion-weighted and T2-weighted images, regional blood volume maps and direct correlation with tissue and cell damage. *Neuroimage* 18:375, 2003.
23. Szabo K, Poepel A, Pohlmann-Eden B, et al: Diffusion weighted and perfusion MRI demonstrate parenchymal changes in complex partial status epilepticus. *Brain* 128(6):1369, 2005.
24. Tomson T, Lindbom U, Nilsson BY: Nonconvulsive status epilepticus in adults: thirty-two consecutive patients from a general hospital population. *Epilepsia* 33:829–835, 1992.
25. Young GB, Jordan KG, Doig GS: An assessment of nonconvulsive seizures in the intensive care unit using continuous EEG monitoring: an investigation of variables associated with mortality. *Neurology* 47:83–89, 1996.
26. Krumholz A: Epidemiology and evidence for morbidity of nonconvulsive status epilepticus. *J Clin Neurophysiol* 16(4):314–322, 1999.
27. Kaplan PW: Prognosis of nonconvulsive status epilepticus. *Epileptic Disord* 2:185–193, 2000a.
28. Kaplan PW: No, some types of nonconvulsive status epilepticus cause little permanent neurologic sequelae (or; "the cure may be worse than the disease." *Neurophysiol Clin* 30:377–382, 2000b.
29. Kaplan PW: Nonconvulsive status epilepticus. *Semin Neurol* 16:33–40, 1996.
30. Treiman DM, Meyers PD, Walton NY, et al: Veterans Affairs Status Epilepticus Cooperative Study Group: a comparison of four treatments for generalized convulsive status epilepticus. *N Engl J Med* 339(12):792, 1998.
31. Wijdicks EF, Hubmayr RD: Acute acid-base disorders associated with status epilepticus. *Mayo Clin Proc* 69:1044, 1994.
32. Shaner DM, McCurdy SA, Herring MO, et al: Treatment of status epilepticus: a prospective comparison of diazepam and phenytoin versus phenobarbital and optional phenytoin. *Neurology* 38:202, 1988.
33. Treiman DM: Pharmacokinetics and clinical use of benzodiazepines in the management of status epilepticus. *Epilepsia* 30[Suppl 2]:S4, 1989.
34. Greenblatt DJ, Divoll M: Diazepam versus lorazepam: relationship of drug distribution to duration of clinical action, in Delgado-Escueta AV, Wasterlain CG, Treiman DM, et al. (eds): *Advances in Neurology. Status Epilepticus*. Vol. 34. New York, Raven Press, 1983, p 487.
35. Cereghino JJ, Cloyd JC, Kuzniecky RI, et al: Rectal diazepam gel for treatment of acute repetitive seizures in adults. *Arch Neurol* 59(12):1915, 2002.
36. Pellock JM, Shinnar S: Respiratory adverse events associated with diazepam rectal gel. *Neurology* 64(10):1768, 2005.
37. Schmidt D: Benzodiazepines: diazepam, in Levy RH, Dreifuss FE, Mattson RH, et al. (eds): *Antiepileptic Drugs*. New York, Raven Press, 1989, p 735.

38. Manno EM: New management strategies in the treatment of status epilepticus. *Mayo Clin Proc* 78:508, 2003.
39. O'Brien TJ, Cascino GD, So E, et al: Incidence and clinical consequence of the purple glove syndrome in patients receiving intravenous phenytoin. *Neurology* 51:1034, 1998.
40. Browne TR, Kugler AR, Eldon MA: Pharmacology and pharmacokinetics of fosphenytoin. *Neurology* 46[Suppl 1]:3, 1996.
41. DeToledo JC, Ramsay RE: Fosphenytoin and phenytoin in patients with status epilepticus. *Drug Saf* 22(6):459, 2000.
42. Hanley DF, Kross JF: Use of midazolam in the treatment of refractory status epilepticus. *Clin Ther* 20(6):1093, 1998.
43. Koul RL, Raj Aithala G, Chacko A, et al: Continuous midazolam infusion as a treatment for status epilepticus. *Arch Dis Child* 76(5):445, 1997.
44. Naritoku DK, Sinha S: Prolongation of midazolam half-life after sustained infusion for status epilepticus. *Neurology* 54(6):1366, 2000.
45. Rossetti A, Reichhart M, Schaller M, et al: Propofol treatment of refractory status epilepticus: a study of 31 episodes. *Epilepsia* 45(7):757, 2004.
46. Stecker MM, Kramer TH, Raps EC, et al: Treatment of refractory status epilepticus with propofol: clinical and pharmacokinetic findings. *Epilepsia* 39(1):18, 1998.
47. Kalviainen R, Eriksson K, Parviainen I: Refractory generalised convulsive status epilepticus: a guide to treatment. *CNS Drugs* 19(9):759, 2005.
48. Claassen J, Hirsch LJ, Emerson RG, et al: Treatment of refractory status epilepticus with pentobarbital, propofol, or midazolam: a systematic review. *Epilepsia* 43(2):146, 2002.
49. Bledsoe KA, Kramer AH: Propylene glycol toxicity in barbiturate coma. *Neurocrit Care* 9(1):122–124, 2008.
50. Sinha S, Naritoku DK: Intravenous valproate is well tolerated in unstable patients with status epilepticus. *Neurology* 55(5):722, 2000.
51. Devinsky O, Leppik I, Willmore LJ, et al: Safety of intravenous valproate. *Ann Neurol* 38:670, 1995.
52. Venkataraman V, Wheless JW: Safety of rapid intravenous infusion of valproate loading doses in epilepsy patients. *Epilepsy Res* 35:147, 1999.
53. Limdi NA, Shimpi AV, Faught E, et al: Efficacy of rapid IV administration of valproic acid for status epilepticus. *Neurology* 64:353, 2005.
54. Peters CN, Pohlmann-Eden B: Intravenous valproate as an innovative therapy in seizure emergency situations including status epilepticus—experience in 102 adult patients. *Seizure* 14(3):164, 2005.
55. Towne AR, Garnett LK, Waterhouse EJ, et al: The use of topiramate in refractory status epilepticus. *Neurology* 60:332, 2003.

CHAPTER 173 ■ CEREBROVASCULAR DISEASE

MAJAZ MOONIS, JOHN P. WEAVER AND MARC FISHER

Cerebrovascular disease encompasses ischemic stroke from thrombosis or embolism, and hemorrhagic stroke including intracerebral hemorrhage (ICH) and subarachnoid hemorrhage. Many patients require management in the intensive care unit (ICU) due to the severity of disease or for monitoring after acute thrombolytic therapy. This chapter reviews the basic concepts of pathogenesis, diagnosis, evaluation, and management for patients with ischemic cerebrovascular disease (ICVD) and ICH. Subarachnoid hemorrhage is discussed in Chapter 78.

ISCHEMIC CEREBROVASCULAR DISEASE

ICVD comprises 85% of all strokes and is the most common neurologic problem that leads to acute hospitalization. Admission to the ICU is indicated in patients with (a) impaired consciousness; (b) associated comorbid conditions, particularly myocardial infarction; (c) stroke after coronary artery bypass grafting; (d) symptomatic secondary hemorrhagic conversion with neurologic deterioration; (e) for the initial 24 hours after administration of intravenous (IV) recombinant tissue plasminogen activator (rt-PA); and (f) after intra-arterial thrombolysis, angioplasty, stenting, or thrombectomy.

Pathophysiology

To ensure accurate diagnosis and appropriate therapy, ICVD is categorized along three axes: degree of completeness, anatomic territory, and underlying mechanism.

Degree of Completeness

Three degrees of completeness can be recognized: transient ischemic attack (TIA), stroke-in-evolution, and completed stroke. A TIA is an episode of temporary focal cerebral dysfunction occurring on a vascular basis. It typically resolves within minutes but may last up to 24 hours. A new definition was proposed and accepted when it was recognized that a significant percentage of patients whose deficits last up to 24 hours have minor stroke, not TIA. The new definition states TIA to be an acute vascular neurological deficit that is reversible within 60 minutes with no evidence of infarction on CT or MRI. A stroke-in-evolution is a neurovascular event that worsens over several hours to several days. In a completed stroke, the deficit remains fixed for at least 24 hours in the carotid system and for up to 72 hours in the vertebral-basilar system.

Anatomic Territory

Two broad clinical anatomic categories of ICVD syndromes are recognized, based on division of the cerebrovascular supply into those areas supplied by the carotid system (anterior circulation) and those supplied by the vertebral-basilar system (posterior circulation).

Symptoms commonly encountered in carotid system disease include aphasia, monoparesis or hemiparesis, monoparesthesias or hemiparesthesias, binocular visual field disturbance (hemianopia), or monocular visual loss. Symptoms that may be seen in vertebral-basilar system disease include hemianopia, cortical blindness, diplopia, vertigo, dysarthria, ataxia, and limb paresis or paresthesias, frequently with ipsilateral involvement of cranial nerve functions, and contralateral body involvement. Loss of consciousness or isolated vertigo rarely occurs without other vertebral-basilar symptoms. Other isolated symptoms, such as diplopia, amnesia, dysarthria, and light-headedness, usually do not serve as a basis for the diagnosis of vertebral-basilar disease; however, association with other brainstem symptoms may support this diagnosis [1].

Underlying Mechanism

Acute ICVD can be categorized as *large vessel thrombosis*, *small vessel thrombosis*, *cardioembolism*, or *stroke of*

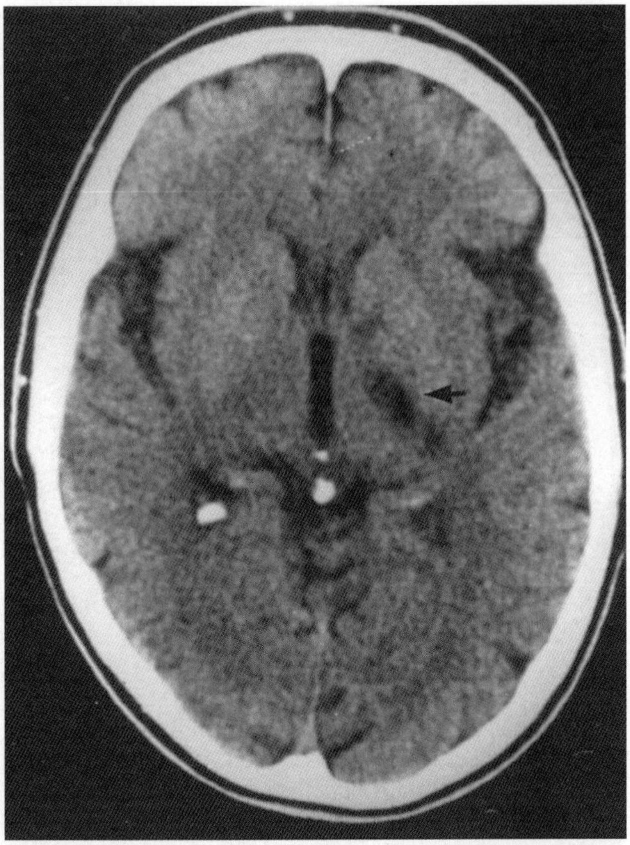

FIGURE 173.1. Lacunar infarct involving the left internal capsule seen on a computed tomography scan.

undetermined etiology. Large vessel atherothrombotic occlusion is due to atherosclerosis in the carotid or vertebral-basilar arteries and is a common cause of acute ICVD. The pattern and severity of the neurologic deficit depend on the arterial territory, completeness of occlusion, and collateral flow [1]. Small vessel occlusion occurs due to lipohyalinosis of the lenticulostriate arteries or basilar penetrators, and results in a small area of cerebral infarction called a *lacune* (Fig. 173.1). If a lacune is strategically placed in the internal capsule, thalamus, or basis pontis, substantial neurologic deficits occur. The most common lacunar syndromes are pure motor hemiparesis, pure sensory loss, ataxic hemiparesis, and dysarthria-clumsy hand syndrome [2].

The typical presentation of a cardioembolic stroke is with maximal deficit at onset, although a small minority may have a stuttering clinical course. Diagnosis may be difficult if the patient has coexistent large arterial lesions; as many as one third of patients with a cardiac embolic source have another potential explanation for their strokes [3]. The most common cardiac sources associated with cerebral embolic events are outlined in Table 173.1. Nonvalvular embolic source with atrial fibrillation is associated with a stroke risk of 4% to 5% per year, increasing with advancing age, the presence of paroxysmal/chronic atrial fibrillation, and an enlarged left atrium [4]. Transmyocardial infarction, atrial fibrillation, and mechanical valves are associated with a high risk, while the risk is lower in patients with bioprosthetic valves. Patent right-to-left cardiac shunts have been recognized by contrast echocardiography with increasing frequency in younger stroke patients. In the absence of a hypercoagulable state or atrial septal aneurysm, a patent foramen ovale (PFO) is not a significant risk factor for cardioembolic stroke, as up to 5% of the healthy population have a small PFO [5].

TABLE 173.1

CARDIAC SOURCES FOR CEREBRAL EMBOLI

Common
Nonvalvular atrial fibrillation
Acute anterior wall myocardial infarction
Ventricular aneurysms and dyskinetic segments
Rheumatic valvular disease
Prosthetic cardiac valves
Right-to-left shunts
Bacterial endocarditis
Less common
Mitral valve prolapse
Cardiomyopathy
Bicuspid aortic valve
Atrial myxoma
Nonbacterial endocarditis
Mitral annulus calcification
Idiopathic hypertrophic subaortic stenosis
Atrial septal aneurysm

Watershed infarction is due to globally diminished cerebral blood flow resulting from cardiac arrest or systemic hypotension, with focal infarction and deficits occurring in well-described patterns in the endarterial distribution between major vessels [6] (Fig. 173.2). In the carotid circulation, watershed infarcts occur between the distribution of the middle cerebral artery and either the anterior or posterior cerebral arteries. The usual anterior infarction causes contralateral weakness and sensory loss sparing the face; in posterior watershed infarcts, homonymous hemianopia with little or no weakness is most common. Quadriparesis, cortical blindness, or bilateral arm weakness (the "man-in-the-barrel" syndrome) may also be seen.

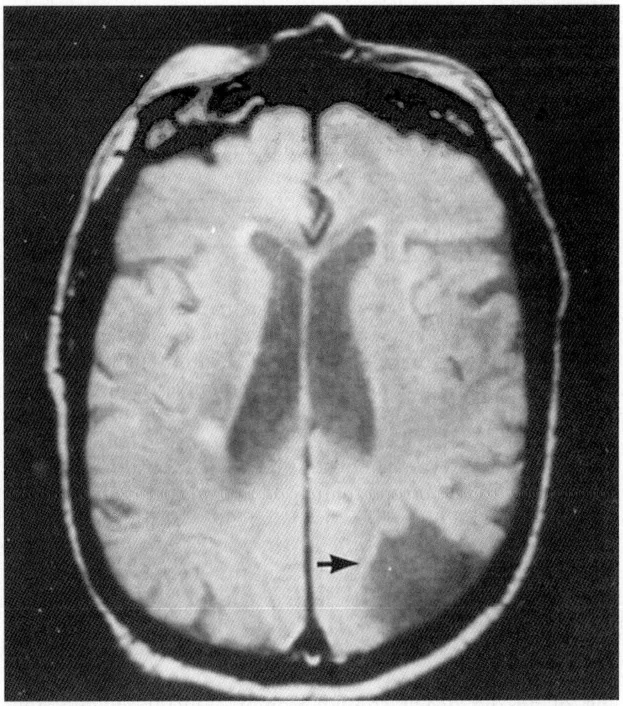

FIGURE 173.2. T1-weighted magnetic resonance imaging scan demonstrating a watershed infarction (*arrow*) in the border zone between the middle and posterior cerebral arteries.

Prognosis

The eventual prognosis of a completed stroke in either the carotid or vertebral-basilar distribution cannot be predicted with certainty during the initial phase of the ictus. The overall mortality varies from 3% to 20% in both vascular distributions [7]. Patients presenting with an altered level of consciousness, conjugate gaze paresis associated with contralateral dense hemiplegia, or decerebrate posturing have a poorer prognosis. However, functional outcome varies widely, with a favorable outcome observed in 20% to 70% of cases [8]. Lacunar syndromes are associated with very low 1-month mortality (approximately 1%) and good functional recovery in 75% to 80% of patients 1 to 3 months after stroke. The clinical course varies: One third of patients with large-artery atherothrombotic strokes have a progressive or fluctuating course, whereas less than one fifth of patients with cardioembolic disease follow a similar pattern [9]. More than 40% of patients with vertebral-basilar symptoms attributable to large-artery thrombosis have a progressive course.

Differential Diagnosis

The history and neurologic examination along with brain imaging enable the physician to differentiate among the major subtypes of ICVD: degree of completeness, territory involved, and ischemic mechanism. It is especially important to differentiate ICVD patients from those with primary ICH. Patients with cerebral hemorrhage typically have a progressive course, with evolution of symptoms over hours [10]. With recent improvement in imaging techniques (spiral computed tomography [CT], magnetic resonance imaging [MRI]), symptoms considered classic for ICH such as early obtundation, coma, seizures, headache, and vomiting are now known to be less reliable in making that diagnosis, since a similar presentation can be seen with ischemic stroke. Urgent imaging should remain the goal in all stroke patients presenting early within the first 3 hours of stroke onset, or those demonstrating worsening neurologic status. Conditions other than cerebrovascular events can occasionally cause acute focal neurologic deficits and must be considered. Primary or metastatic brain tumors with hemorrhage into the tumor may resemble a stroke (Fig. 173.3). Subdural hematomas may rarely present with acute focal neurologic deficits and must be considered in elderly patients, even without a history of head trauma. Patients with migraine headaches sometimes develop focal neurologic symptoms either before or during the early phase of the headache. Rarely, these deficits may occur in the absence of a headache (acephalgic migraine) or may persist (migrainous infarction). Patients with focal seizures may develop sensory, motor, and aphasic symptoms that can mimic ICVD, although they are usually stereotyped and transient. Occasionally, focal neurologic deficits may follow seizures and persist for 24 hours or longer (Todd's paralysis). In these cases, MR angiogram (MRA) or CT angiogram (CTA) can demonstrate arterial occlusion, making it more likely to be a stroke than Todd's paralysis. An important, uncommon, and reversible cause of acute neurological deficits is hypoglycemia, which should always be looked for before any aggressive treatment is initiated for a presumed ischemic stroke. Similarly in young patients or patients with a psychiatric history, objective neurological signs or corroborative radiological evidence must be established to avoid treating a functional paralysis with relatively aggressive therapy. Finally, worsening of an old deficit should prompt a metabolic/infectious evaluation, because the damaged cortex may act as a *locus minoris resistentiae*, with focal clinical worsening of a chronic deficit.

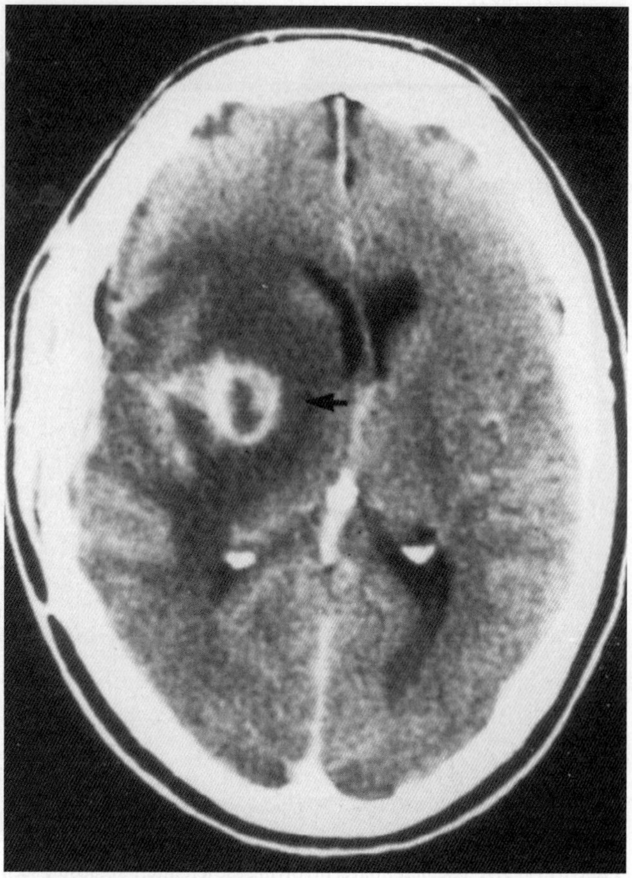

FIGURE 173.3. Malignant glioma with associated edema on a computed tomography scan in a patient who abruptly developed a pure motor deficit. The arrow points to the lacunar infarct.

Laboratory and Radiologic Evaluation

A comprehensive workup to determine stroke subtype, severity, and identification of possible multiple risk factors is important to determine effective treatment options. Early imaging in most ICVD patients helps in the differential diagnosis and is key in protocols for therapeutic intervention with rt-PA. Both CT and MRI scans are reliable and sensitive means of differentiating between ICVD, hemorrhage, and other mass lesions. MRI scans are more sensitive than CT scans for the identification of brain tumors, subarachnoid hemorrhage, and subdural hematomas, and MRI can identify ischemic infarction at an earlier stage (within 4 to 24 hours). MRI is probably more sensitive than CT in detecting intracerebral hemorrhage [11]. Newer MRI techniques, such as diffusion-weighted imaging (DWI) and perfusion imaging (PI), have important bearings on acute stroke diagnosis and treatment [12]. With DWI, ischemic lesions can be seen within minutes of onset. PI identifies areas of reduced blood flow, whereas in most cases, DWI hyperintensity indicates an area of irreversible ischemic injury. If the PI deficit is greater than the DWI area (DWI–PI mismatch), it demonstrates an ischemic tissue that is potentially reversible (ischemic penumbra). Magnetic resonance angiography (MRA), especially contrast-enhanced MRA (CEMRA), approaches the sensitivity of a four-vessel conventional angiogram. CEMRA has the added advantage of visualization of the vertebrobasilar system and the intracranial circulation with minimal increase in scan acquisition time. Early restoration of blood flow may result in normalization of this region, a reduced volume of infarction, and better stroke outcome. This is the basis of

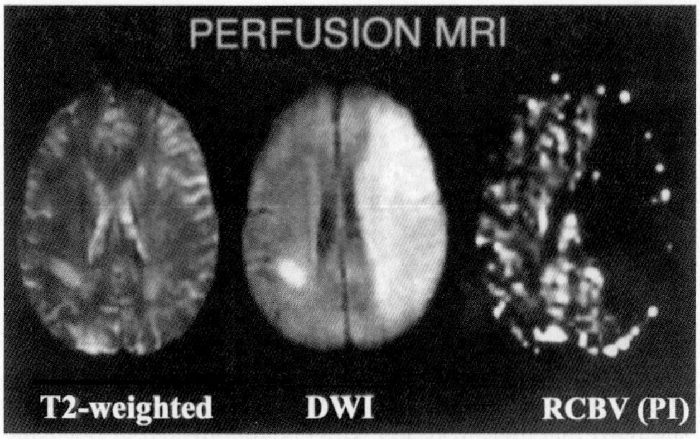

FIGURE 173.4. Magnetic resonance image of the brain with T2-weighted imaging, diffusion-weighted imaging (DWI), and perfusion imaging (PI) in a patient with acute ischemic stroke. Although T2 reveals very little change, there is a large DWI hyperintensity corresponding to a PI deficit (DWI-PI mismatch), demonstrating a completed infarct and a situation in which recombinant tissue plasminogen activator is not indicated. RCBV, regional cerebral blood volume.

thrombolytic therapy, and a persistent ischemic penumbra beyond 4.5 hours may be a reason to consider intra-arterial interventions [13,14] (Fig. 173.4).

An electrocardiogram should be obtained to assess possible underlying or concurrent cardiac rhythm or ischemic changes. Confusion may arise because T-wave, ST-segment, QRS complex changes, and rhythm disturbances may occur secondary to the cerebral ischemic event. Two-dimensional transthoracic, or transesophageal echocardiography, and telemetry/Holter monitoring should be done routinely because patients often have more than one potential underlying pathophysiology, and a cardiac structural or rhythm abnormality may change the treatment approach (Fig. 173.5). A transesophageal echocardiogram should especially be considered in younger patients, patients with an enlarged left atrium, and in cryptogenic stroke at all ages [14,15] (Fig. 173.6).

If an MRA has not been obtained to image the craniocervical vasculature, carotid artery ultrasound—a fast, reliable, and noninvasive technique—should be employed in suspected ischemic stroke of the carotid system as well as small vessel stroke, because of a high incidence of coexisting large vessel atherosclerotic stenosis. Transcranial Doppler ultrasound (TCD) can also provide information about the status of the intracranial vessels, both in the carotid and vertebral-basilar arterial territories [16,17]. Advances in CT angiography (CTA) provide high-resolution vascular imaging as well as the ischemic penumbra with perfusion CT (CTP) studies. With a combination of noncontrast CT (NCCT), CTA, and CTP, it is possible to rule out hemorrhage, assess the extent of early signs of infarction, and determine the site of arterial occlusion and ischemic penumbra. The latter two studies are important in making decisions in acute stroke management (i.e., to proceed with intravenous or intra-arterial interventions). This CT based combination allows a more rapid triage compared to MRI, since every minute wasted before thrombolysis is initiated results in a progressive reduction of salvageable tissue.

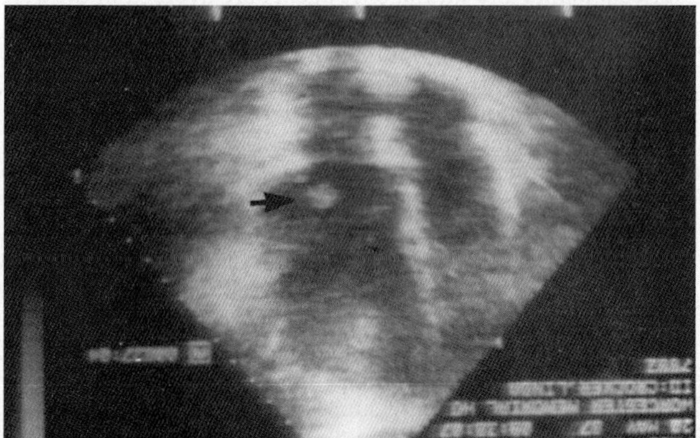

FIGURE 173.5. Echocardiogram in a patient with cardioembolic stroke, demonstrating a large thrombus (*arrow*) attached to the left mitral valve.

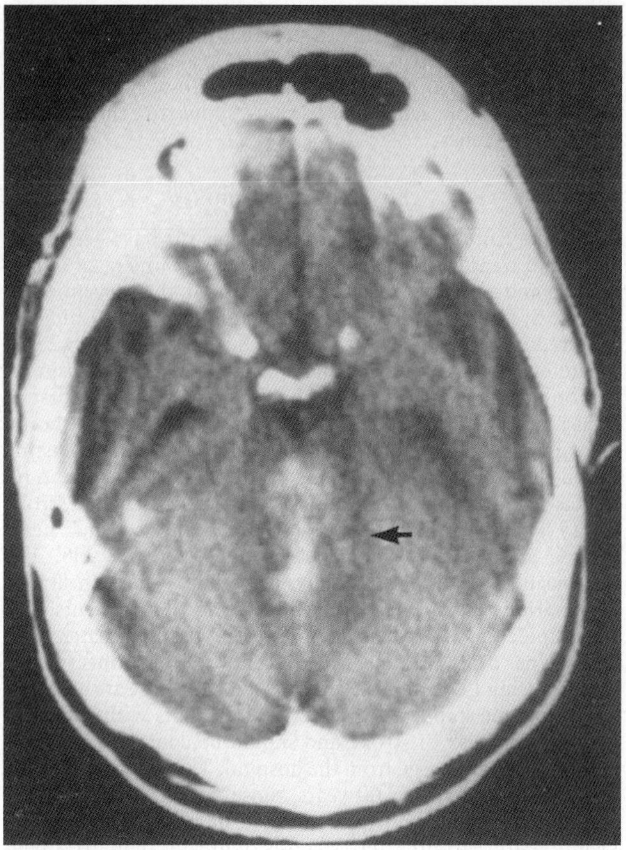

FIGURE 173.6. Midline cerebellar hemorrhage (*arrow*) seen on a computed tomography scan.

Complete blood count, partial thromboplastin time (PTT), prothrombin time (PT), comprehensive blood chemistry, chest radiograph, erythrocyte sedimentation rate, syphilis serology, and urinalysis should be obtained on day 1. Of these, if thrombolytic therapy is being contemplated, the blood glucose, PTT, PT, and platelet count should be obtained immediately. Fasting lipid profile, homocysteine, and C-reactive protein should be obtained by day 2 in all cases. Other blood studies, including anticardiolipin antibodies, hypercoagulable workup (protein S, protein C, antithrombin 3, factor V Leiden, prothrombin-2 gene mutation), serum viscosity, serum protein electrophoresis, and fibrinogen, should be completed in younger patients and in patients with a history of cancer, recurrent deep vein thrombosis, or a family history suggestive of an autosomal-dominant pattern of stroke. A lumbar puncture should be performed only if meningitis is suspected, in suspected vasculitis of the nervous system, or when aneurysm rupture is a consideration, despite a negative result in a brain imaging study (NCCT or MRI). Electroencephalography may be helpful when associated seizure activity is suspected.

Treatment

The treatment of ICVD can be divided into four major categories: prevention, acute interventions, supportive therapy, and newer approaches.

Stroke Prevention

Stroke prevention has improved as risk factors have been identified and treatments developed [18]. The treatment of hypertension and smoking cessation are helpful in the prevention of stroke. Systolic blood pressure reduction by 5 to 10 mm Hg may reduce relative risk of ischemic stroke by 20% to 25%. Angiotensin-converting enzyme inhibitors and angiotensin receptor blockers may offer additional protection against first or recurrent ischemic stroke. Patients with hyperglycemia should be aggressively treated to maintain euglycemic control (fasting blood glucose of less than 100 mg per dL). Use of HMG CoA reductase inhibitors (statins) reduces the risk of ischemic stroke by 25% to 30% in patients with underlying ischemic heart disease and possibly improves the outcome after AIS. The American College of Chest Physicians and American Stroke Association guidelines recommend starting all in-patients with hyperlipidemia (low-density lipoprotein [LDL] greater than 100 mg per dL) on statins. More recent trials of statins suggest that reducing LDL cholesterol to 70 mg per dL is safe and may have a plaque stabilization effect [19]. Patients with TIA have a substantial risk of stroke and should be completely investigated before discharge from the hospital. This is especially true for patients older than 60 years, those presenting with aphasia, motor deficits, or with associated diabetes. Patients with *symptomatic* carotid artery stenosis of greater than 70% benefit from carotid endarterectomy, provided the combined mortality and morbidity of the surgical procedure in the treating institution is less than 5.65% [20]. In nonsurgical TIA patients, antiplatelet therapy with aspirin, aspirin and extended-release dipyridamole (25/200 mg) twice daily, clopidogrel 75 mg once daily, or ticlopidine 250 mg twice daily is beneficial [21,22]. Indirect comparison of newer antiplatelet agents as compared to aspirin suggests that aspirin/extended-release dipyridamole (25/200 mg) (ERDP/ASA) twice daily is 23% more effective than aspirin alone, while clopidogrel offers no advantage over aspirin. However, the recently completed head-to-head comparative trial of clopidogrel vs ERDP/ASA failed to demonstrate a significant difference between the two medications. The combination of ERDP/ASA was associated with nonsignificantly fewer ischemic events, but with a greater number of intra- and extracerebral hemorrhages. On the other hand, there was a nonsignificant trend toward less congestive heart failure with this combination [23]. Atrial fibrillation with or without valvular heart disease is associated with a high stroke risk. Anticoagulation using warfarin reduces the absolute recurrent stroke relative risk by 8% in patients with nonvalvular atrial fibrillation. The annual risk of symptomatic hemorrhage is 1%, which can be minimized by keeping the international normalized ratio (INR) between 2 and 3 [15]. Ximelagatran, a thrombin inhibitor, in a head-to-head study with warfarin, failed to show noninferiority in reducing ischemic recurrent events and did not require INR monitoring, but the drug was not approved by the U.S. Food and Drug Administration (FDA) because of concerns of significant hepatic toxicity [24].

Supportive Therapy

Supportive therapy for ICVD patients should begin upon hospitalization. Elevated blood pressure should not be treated in the first 24 hours of an ischemic stroke unless malignant hypertension (>220 over 120 mm Hg) is present or other end-organ failure becomes evident (e.g., congestive heart failure, renal failure). The blood pressure typically returns to baseline with bed rest; if it remains substantially elevated, it should be carefully lowered by no more than 20% of the mean arterial pressure. Subcutaneous heparin therapy should be considered for immobilized ICVD patients to reduce the risk of pulmonary emboli. Indwelling urinary catheters and excessive IV lines should be avoided, as they can promote infection. Elevated temperature should be lowered, as hyperthermia is clearly deleterious. Aspiration pneumonia can be avoided by delaying oral feedings until swallowing is well performed. Early mobilization and rehabilitation should be attempted.

Acute Treatment

Standard therapies in ICVD patients are directed at reversing the neurologic deficit and preventing progression. The National Institute of Neurological Disorders and Stroke (NINDS) trial demonstrated that patients treated with rt-PA within 3 hours of stroke onset had a 10% to 12% absolute greater chance of being free of disability or being left with minor disability at 3 months. The benefit was greatest for those treated within the first 90 minutes of stroke onset compared to those treated between 90 and 180 minutes. There was a tenfold greater incidence of ICH in treated patients as compared to placebo (6.4% vs. 0.6%). However, overall mortality at 3 months was comparable in the rt-PA and placebo groups. Predictors of ICH include large hemispheric infarcts, National Institutes of Health Stroke Scale (NIHSS) score greater than 23, and the presence of associated severe hypertension [25]. More recently, based on prospective trial (ECASS III) results it may be possible to extend the time window of intravenous rt-PA up to 4.5 hours. The absolute benefits, as expected, were less in this extended time window (ARR of 7%) and the results apply to mild and moderate stroke patients based on the NIHSS (median 8). While the study excluded older patients, those on anticoagulation (irrespective of the INR or PTT), and those with diabetes mellitus and stroke, the validity of these exclusions has not been substantiated and individual management should be decided for individuals based on the physician's judgment [26]. The total dose of 0.9 mg per kg is given as a 60-minute IV infusion, with 10% of the total dose given as an initial bolus. After rt-PA infusion, patients need to be admitted to the ICU. Blood pressure and neurologic status need to be carefully assessed at specified time periods. Systolic blood pressure above 185 mm or mean blood pressure over 130 mm are treated with intravenous labetalol/nicardipine or dose-titrated intravenous sodium nitroprusside. Neurologic worsening should prompt an urgent CT scan to look for possible hemorrhagic conversion of the infarct. Anticoagulants and antiplatelet agents are avoided in the first 24 hours. IV access and invasive procedures should be kept to a minimum in the first 24 hours after rt-PA administration. A recent trial of intra-arterial prourokinase, given within 6 hours of stroke onset, demonstrated improved stroke outcome in middle cerebral artery embolic infarctions [27].

Patients presenting beyond 4.5 hours who are not candidates for intravenous thrombolytic therapy may benefit from intra-arterial thrombolysis or mechanical embolectomy. The results of the Multi Mechanical Embolus Removal in Cerebral Ischemia (Multi MERCI) trial have limited application in the general stroke population because special equipment and trained interventionists are required for such interventions, and the outcomes in the extended time window of up to 8 hours did not demonstrate a result superior to intravenous rt-PA as in the NINDS trial. However, it did demonstrate that results comparable to the rt-PA outcomes were possible with delayed reperfusion [28]. This benefit still remains to be confirmed with the ongoing prospective, randomized trials (IMS 111) and MR and recanalization of stroke clots using embolectomy (MR RESCUE) where IV thrombolysis is followed by intra-arterial interventions if no clinical improvement is demonstrated with the intravenous therapy. The results of a large retrospective analysis of intra-arterial interventions suggested that there was a significant 67% chance of achieving improved outcome (modified Rankin scale [MRS] $\leq$3) in the absence of a combination of older age, blood glucose >150 mg per dL, and NIHSS >18 [29].

Anticoagulation with heparin or low-molecular-weight heparin has been used traditionally without any proof of efficacy. However, heparin has been routinely considered in patients with a clear embolic source, with stroke-in-evolution to prevent progression, and with multiple TIAs to prevent stroke development. However, there is no evidence that supports the use of IV heparin anticoagulation to improve stroke outcome in progressive stroke. Furthermore, the risk of recurrent stroke is low (2% to 3%) in the first few weeks after an acute ischemic stroke (AIS) [30,31]. Cardioembolic stroke patients have a higher risk of recurrence (4.5% to 8.0%) within 2 weeks of the initial event, especially with associated intracardiac thrombi. Heparin therapy may reduce this risk and may be considered within 24 to 48 hours of the initial stroke [30]. Patients with large infarcts should not receive heparin, because they have a higher risk of bleeding into the area of infarction [19,30]. An alternative and safer approach is to begin warfarin as soon as the patient can safely swallow, leading to adequate anticoagulation within 5 to 7 days of stroke onset. The use of heparin therapy in stroke-in-evolution and in multiple TIAs is still under debate. If used, heparin should be initiated as a constant infusion without a bolus (although some stroke neurologists give a small initial bolus of 3,000 to 5,000 U), maintaining the PTT at 1.5 to 2.0 times control. Frequent PTT checks at 6-hour intervals and dose adjustment may reduce the frequency of serious intracranial and systemic hemorrhage [32].

Aspirin may reduce the risk of stroke recurrence after TIA or established stroke and is widely used for this indication [20]. Combined aspirin and extended-release dipyridamole therapy is twice as effective as aspirin alone in reducing stroke recurrence [21]. In aspirin-allergic patients, clopidogrel or ticlopidine can be used. The incidence of serious side effects is greater with ticlopidine, which may cause neutropenia and thrombotic thrombocytopenic purpura. Because thrombotic thrombocytopenic purpura has been reported with both drugs, weekly complete blood count and liver function tests should be done in the first 4 to 6 weeks of initiating therapy [33].

Cerebral edema in ICVD patients is maximal between 48 and 72 hours after onset, and corticosteroids are not effective in ICVD [34]. Osmotic diuretics, such as mannitol, are of uncertain value for cerebral edema associated with ICVD, but we consider using pulse doses (1.00 g per kg, then 0.25 g per kg every 6 hours) if massive edema begins to develop. Intracranial pressure (ICP) monitoring to guide therapy should also be considered. Controlled hyperventilation is perhaps the fastest and most effective temporizing measure to reduce cerebral edema, but its effects are transient and regional cerebral ischemia may worsen due to vasoconstriction. Timely decompressive hemicraniectomy reduces the risk of death by 50% (1 in 2 patients) and improves the outcome by 25% (1 in 4 patients). This has been validated in patients younger than 50 years, although there is no reason not to apply the procedure in older patients. Interestingly enough, the outcomes of this trial were independent of the side of infarction or the presence or absence of aphasia [34].

Recent Advances

Cerebral ischemic insult results in activation of the ischemic cascade. Under these circumstances, reduced reuptake and increased release of glutamate leads to activation of the *N*-methyl-D-aspartate receptors; reduced inhibition of γ-aminobutyric acid and glycine; and increased intracellular calcium influx, lipid peroxidation, and release of free radicals that hasten the process of cell death. Several neuroprotective agents blocking steps of the ischemic cascade have undergone animal studies and human trials. Although almost all reduce the infarct size in animal models of ischemic stroke, so far none have demonstrated any clinical efficacy [35–42]. There were several reasons why neuroprotective therapies have not proven effective in clinical trials. Serious side effects limited the effective doses of medications, the inclusion time to treatment may have been too long, and reperfusion was not established. To overcome these limitations, recent studies have begun to use combination therapies, combining rt-PA with neuroprotective drugs as well as combinations of two neuroprotective drugs with different sites of action [43]. Recently NXY-059, a free radical trapping agent, was reported to improve outcome of AIS, although the phase 3 trial results of the Stroke Acute Ischemic NXY-059 (SAINT) 11 trial conducted in the United States failed to confirm these findings [44]. Induced hypothermia may be useful in limiting damage from large hemispheric infarcts but at present remains an experimental procedure for ischemic stroke. Major problems limiting its use are the lack of availability of appropriate cooling devices, difficulty in obtaining rapid temperature reduction to target values, and complications during subsequent rewarming. Bihemispheric laser therapy of the brain showed promise as a method of improving outcome after ischemic stroke in phase 2 trials but failed to demonstrate efficacy in a subsequent phase 3 randomized trial [45].

Summary

Advances are being made in the treatment of ICVD. It is clear that successful therapy requires early intervention and close assessment for favorable responses and side effects, likely requiring an ICU setting initially. It is recognized that IV thrombolysis may not be effective in large vessel occlusions such as the internal carotid, proximal middle cerebral, and basilar arteries; however, randomized trials are underway to assess this. The current practice of giving full-dose IV rt-PA followed by intervention is widely practiced, but this is neither an FDA-approved therapy nor has it been shown to be beneficial in any case series. Perhaps ECASS 111 and MR RESCUE will provide the answers. Treatment of TIA has undergone a dramatic change since we recognized that the risk of a full-blown ischemic stroke is 10.5% after a cursory ER visit, and the risk can be reduced by 80% with acute in-patient management for 1 to 2 days, as demonstrated by the Oxfordshire study and the 2009 guidelines on management of TIA [46]. The recognition that acute high-dose statins reduce the risk of stroke and improve outcome irrespective of the low-density lipoprotein (LDL) levels is an important addendum to our management strategy within the acute period after an ischemic stroke. In the future, it is probable that a combination of treatments directed at the multiple metabolic and perfusion abnormalities associated with ICVD will be required [47]. Finally, stroke prevention is the most effective means of reducing the first or recurrent stroke. Aggressive use of statins in patients with either hyperlipidemia or elevated C-reactive proteins reduces the risk of progression of atherosclerotic small and large vessel disease and has a cardioprotective role.

INTRACEREBRAL HEMORRHAGE

Nontraumatic ICH occurs less frequently than ICVD but often requires management in the ICU. The majority of cases are due to spontaneous (primary) ICH or rupture of saccular aneurysms and arteriovenous malformations. As the approach to these entities and their management differ considerably, they are discussed separately.

Primary ICH is defined as bleeding within the brain parenchyma without an underlying cause, such as neoplasm, vasculitis, bleeding disorder, prior embolic infarction, aneurysm, vascular malformation, or trauma. One-half of primary ICH cases result from longstanding hypertension. Due to the aggressive control of hypertension, the incidence of ICH has decreased since the mid-1960s. Nonetheless, ICH accounts for 4% to 11% of all stroke cases in the United States and 16% to 26% of all stroke-related deaths [47].

Pathophysiology

ICH is believed to be due to extravasation of arterial blood from ruptured microaneurysms along the walls of small intracerebral arterioles. Microaneurysms known as *Charcot–Bouchard or miliary aneurysms* tend to form on vessels at the usual sites of ICH and develop at sites of vascular branching where mechanical stress is maximal. The aneurysm wall lacks normal vascular histology and is composed mainly of connective tissue layers, which represent a weak point in the arterial system. The formation of these aneurysms is favored by the processes of lipohyalinosis and fibrinoid necrosis, which weaken the walls of arterioles, and are accelerated by chronic hypertension. Although Charcot–Bouchard aneurysms also appear in the normotensive aging brain, their frequency is notably increased in hypertensive patients. They are commonly observed along the lenticulostriate arteries, thalamoperforate arteries, and paramedian branches of the basilar artery. Although this distribution corresponds to the common sites of ICH, it is impossible to prove that these aneurysms are always the cause of bleeding, and the concept of arteriolar microdissection has been raised as an alternative explanation [48].

Continued extravasations of blood result in the formation of a hematoma with secondary accumulation of cerebral edema. The lesion may become massive enough to cause midline shift of cerebral structures followed by transtentorial herniation, which leads to secondary brainstem hemorrhages known as *Duret hemorrhages*. These linear lesions in the midbrain and upper pons are generally multiple and bilateral. Progression of this process results in brainstem dysfunction and death. Depending on the size and location of the ICH, intraventricular extension can occur and lead to the development of acute obstructive hydrocephalus or the later development of a chronic communicating hydrocephalus from impaired cerebrospinal fluid resorption. Some cases of thromboembolic stroke may be misclassified as ICH, because blood may extravasate and accumulate into large hematomas in areas of infarction. This secondary hemorrhage may be mislabeled if an early imaging study is not performed.

Clinical Manifestations

The clinical presentation of ICH is distinctive. In most cases, the onset is during the waking state when the patient is active; it is unusual for ICH to occur during sleep. The onset is abrupt, and the development of neurological deficits occurs progressively over minutes to hours. This contrasts with the fluctuating or stepwise progression of deficits commonly seen in atherothrombotic infarcts, and with the appearance of maximal deficits at onset in cardioembolic strokes. In addition, prior TIA is rare with ICH and relatively common with ischemic stroke. The average age of onset of ICH, 50 to 70 years, is younger than that of other types of stroke. Patients may report lateralized headache; vomiting is common and nuchal rigidity may be present. Seizures are seen more frequently at the onset of ICH (17%) than in ICVD and are more likely to occur if the bleeding involves the cerebral cortex [49]. When first seen by a physician, 44% to 72% of patients are comatose.

The clinical presentation of ICH is monophasic, with active bleeding usually lasting no longer than 2 hours. However, secondary bleeding and subsequent deterioration may occur. Subsequent clinical deterioration is due to the effects of cerebral edema [50]. It was recently suggested that thalamic hemorrhages may bleed further in patients whose hypertension is not adequately controlled [51].

Diagnosis

The diagnosis of ICH can be made by CT scan, which provides accurate information about the size and site of the hematoma as well as the midline shift, and development of cerebral edema. Typically, the hemorrhage is hyperdense on CT scan during the acute phase, although severe anemia or ongoing hemorrhage may make the appearance more iso- or hypodense. The appearance of blood on the MRI scan varies because signal intensity is related to the state of degradation of the hemoglobin. This state changes with time; therefore, MRI is not the study of choice for initial imaging of ICH. In summary, deoxyhemoglobin is found in the first 3 days after ICH and is not well visualized on T1-weighted images but appears as an area of reduced signal intensity on T2-weighted images. Days 3 to 10 after ICH, methemoglobin appears as increased signal intensity of T1-weighted images, but the intracellular portion has reduced signal intensity on T2-weighted images. In the chronic state, the ICH has broken down to hemosiderin, which is poorly visualized on T1-weighted images but appears as reduced signal intensity on T2-weighted images. Magnetic resonance or conventional angiography should be considered in selected cases if an underlying aneurysm or arteriovenous malformation is suspected.

Lumbar puncture is contraindicated in ICH because of the risk of herniation from mass effect. Testing on admission for ICH should include coagulation profile and platelet counts in all patients, as well as bleeding time, if the patient is on aspirin.

Differential Diagnosis

Although the majority of ICH is hypertensive in origin, other etiologies should always be considered. Secondary cerebral hemorrhage may occur after embolic infarction as the lodged embolus fragments and ischemic distal vessels may rupture on reperfusion. This is more common in patients with large embolic infarcts, in patients who are anticoagulated, and in patients with poorly controlled hypertension. ICH secondary to reperfusion may also occur after carotid endarterectomy.

ICH accounts for 0.5% to 1.5% of all bleeding events related to the use of oral anticoagulants. Oral anticoagulation increases the risk of ICH 8- to 11-fold, compared to unanticoagulated patients. Compared with patients with spontaneous ICH, there is a trend toward larger hematomas and a higher mortality rate in patients on anticoagulants [52]. Cerebellar hemorrhage is relatively common in anticoagulated patients, and mortality in these cases may be as high as 65%. Therefore, in anticoagulated patients the onset of focal neurological signs, even if slowly progressive, necessitates CT scan to rule out ICH [53].

The use of fibrinolytic therapy, such as rt-PA, for coronary artery occlusion has also been associated with ICH, especially when concomitant heparin therapy is used. These cases have shown a predilection for the subcortical white matter and lobar areas, generally having a poor prognosis [54]. Surprisingly, the risk for ICH is slightly higher with rt-PA than with streptokinase [55].

ICH associated with the presence of primary or secondary brain tumors is infrequent, accounting for only 2% of all cases of ICH. Higher-grade malignancies, such as glioblastoma multiforme, are more likely to bleed. The presence of thin-walled vessels in areas of neovascularization is thought to be the underlying reason for these hemorrhages. Metastatic lesions with the tendency to bleed include bronchogenic carcinoma, melanoma, renal cell carcinoma, and choriocarcinoma. ICH is frequent in hematologic disorders such as leukemia and reflects both the underlying thrombocytopenia and disseminated intravascular coagulopathy. When disseminated intravascular coagulopathy is due to other organ failures, it can also lead to ICH.

Sympathomimetic drugs, such as methamphetamine, pseudoephedrine, and phenylpropanolamine, have caused ICH in the subcortical white matter. These agents are suspected of inducing a vasculitis. Cocaine, which blocks dopamine and norepinephrine reuptake, has been associated with ICH. Cocaine, especially crack cocaine, appears to incite cerebral vasospasm rather than a vasculitis. The secondary hypertension related to sympathetic stimulation may also cause ICH from any of these agents. This may explain the lack of abnormal angiographic findings in some of these cases [56,57], although recently cerebral vasospasm was demonstrated with magnetic resonance angiography after acute cocaine administration [58]. Acute elevation of blood pressure in otherwise normotensive people, such as that which may follow migraine, is postulated to result at times in ICH.

Specific Syndromes of Intracerebral Hemorrhage

ICH tends to occur in stereotyped locations. In order of descending frequency, these locations are the putamen (30% to 50%), subcortical white matter (15%), thalamus (10%), pons (10%), and cerebellum (10%) [59].

ICH in the putamen is caused by bleeding from a lenticulostriate vessel. Clinically it is manifested by development of flaccid hemiplegia, hemisensory disturbances of all primary modalities, homonymous hemianopia, paralysis of conjugate gaze to the side opposite the lesion, and early alteration in level of consciousness. Subcortical aphasia may occur when a putamen hemorrhage involves the dominant hemisphere, and a hemineglect syndrome when it is on the nondominant side.

Hemorrhages in the subcortical white matter (lobar hemorrhages) are being observed with increasing frequency, particularly in the elderly, and are less commonly related to hypertension than is ICH in other locations. The signs and symptoms depend on the location. Lobar ICH occurs at the gray-white junction and is, therefore, associated with a higher incidence of seizures and headache at onset; it most commonly occurs in the parietal and occipital lobes. Of all ICH locations, lobar hemorrhages have the lowest mortality (approximately 15%) and carry the best prognosis for a good functional recovery. Lobar ICH is frequently caused by cerebral amyloid angiopathy due to the deposition of amyloid in the walls of the small vessels of the cortex and leptomeninges, typically in the frontal and occipital lobes. The process generally spares vessels of the basal ganglia, deep white matter, brainstem, and cerebellum. The abnormal vessel walls take up Congo red stain, thus the alternative term *congophilic angiopathy*. Amyloid angiopathy weakens the walls of many arteries and may be associated with recurrent lobar ICH. Five to ten percent of cases of spontaneous ICH result from amyloid angiopathy, making it second to hypertension as an etiology for ICH [60].

Thalamic ICH is characterized by a unilateral sensorimotor deficit in which sensory findings predominate. A variety of eye signs occur: Parinaud's syndrome, forced disconjugate downgaze deviation medially on the side opposite the lesion, pseudoabducens paresis, up-gaze paralysis, and so forth. The most specific localizing sign is inferomedial disconjugate gaze paresis contralateral to the side of the lesion. A permanent skew deviation, with vertical separation of images, may leave the patient with persistent diplopia. Due to the location, thalamic ICH may rupture into the ventricular system.

Pontine ICH has the highest mortality. Quadriplegia, brainstem dysfunction, and small, unreactive pupils are seen at presentation and many patients rapidly develop coma. Bleeding typically arises from a paramedian branch of the basilar artery and almost always extends into the fourth ventricle. Cases of unilateral pontine ICH have a better outcome [61].

Cerebellar ICH most commonly involves the dentate nucleus (see Fig. 173.5). Alteration of consciousness is unusual at onset, but progressive deterioration with drowsiness typically occurs. The majority of patients initially manifest two of the following: (a) gait, truncal, or limb ataxia; (b) lower motor neuron facial paresis; and (c) an ipsilateral gaze palsy. Other common presenting signs and symptoms are headache, nausea, vomiting, vertigo, nystagmus, and limb ataxia [62]. Early surgical intervention is indicated for lesions larger than 3 cm or in smaller lesions with clinical progression, because cerebellar hemorrhage causes death in up to 60% of cases. Neurologic deterioration due to hemorrhage, causing obstructive hydrocephalus at the level of the fourth ventricle, is not uncommon. Surgical mortality is greatly reduced if the patient is still awake before operation; therefore, early intervention is indicated [62].

Approximately 3% of cases of ICH are primarily intraventricular in location. These events have minimal focal signs, but generally, there is loss of consciousness at onset. Hydrocephalus is a major complication [63].

Treatment

The acute medical management of ICH is aimed at correction of any predisposing systemic factors to prevent further clinical deterioration. Following ICH, there is a hematoma growth of 22% within the first 24 hours and hypertension is a major management problem in these cases. In response to the acute elevation of ICP caused by the hematoma, systemic blood pressure rises to maintain adequate cerebral perfusion pressure. This response, known as *Cushing's reflex*, serves to protect the brain against ischemia, but autoregulation of cerebral blood flow can be impaired after ICH or infarction. In patients with underlying chronic hypertension, the result may be excessively high blood pressure. The best management of this dilemma remains controversial. In chronic hypertension, the lower limit of cerebral autoregulation is shifted toward higher blood pressure; and acute lowering of systolic blood pressure is known to result in unfavorable decreases in cerebral perfusion pressure. Sustained hypertension in the acute phase of ICH, however, can lead to further bleeding or rapid accumulation of cerebral edema [59]. The recommended goal of systolic blood pressure in the acute phase of ICH is between 110 and 160 mm Hg [64]. Blood pressure should be lowered gently, and beta-blockers are the agents of choice. Alternatively, a calcium channel blocker such as intravenous nicardipine may be useful because it does not elevate ICP like other vasodilators [59].

If the hematoma and associated cerebral edema raise ICP, clinical deterioration typically occurs. Acutely, hyperventilation effectively lowers ICP, but only for a matter of hours. Hyperosmolar agents, such as mannitol, sorbitol, and glycerol, provide more sustained reductions in ICP. These drugs reduce the fluid content of the intact brain so that the cranial cavity can accommodate cerebral edema. The osmotic diuresis induced by these agents can lead to dehydration, electrolyte imbalances, and pulmonary edema if the patient is not closely monitored. Treatment of ICH with steroids can be detrimental to overall outcome, so they are not routinely administered [65]. The value of ICP monitoring in these situations remains controversial [65]. Elevation of ICP due to hydrocephalus is treated with ventricular cerebrospinal fluid diversion.

Anticonvulsants are not routinely used in ICH. If seizures are not present at onset, patients are generally at low risk for developing seizures, but hemorrhage into the cortex, regardless of site of origin, predisposes to seizures. Subarachnoid or intraventricular extension of bleeding does not increase the risk of seizures. Seizures have been noted with hemorrhages in the caudate but not with putaminal or thalamic events. Although the incidence of chronic epilepsy from ICH is low (6.5% to 13.0%), any seizures usually begin within the first 2 years after the event [66]. Prophylaxis against peripheral venous thrombosis should be accomplished with pneumatic boots.

After the patient is acutely stabilized, angiography may be performed if there is no history of hypertension or the bleeding is in an atypical location. This is particularly important or pertinent for younger patients, in whom a larger percentage of cases of ICH are due to underlying vascular lesions, such as arteriovenous malformation or aneurysm. At present, surgery may be indicated for lobar ICH in which the patient continues to deteriorate, and for most cerebellar ICH. Emergency ventriculostomy to relieve hydrocephalus should be considered if this condition develops acutely. Surgical intervention for putaminal ICH remains controversial; it is inappropriate for thalamic and pontine hemorrhages.

The prognosis for ICH is worse for larger lesions. By location, pontine ICH has the highest mortality, followed by cerebellar and then basal ganglia lesions. Lobar ICH carries the most favorable outlook for survival and functional recovery [52]. Three factors that have accurately predicted 30-day survival in 92% of ICH patients reviewed are hemorrhage size, Glasgow Coma Scale score, and pulse pressure [46].

Summary and Advances

ICH can be neurologically devastating. Patients with ICH often require an ICU setting because of the severity of disease, particularly when it is complicated by markedly increased ICP. Evacuation of the hematoma was not found to be helpful in randomized trials [67]. However, subgroup analysis suggested a possible role of surgical evacuation in hematoma that are superficial and less than 1 cm from the cortex. A subsequent trial, STICH 2, is underway to address this issue. Recombinant factor VII showed promise in phase 2 trials in reducing hematoma growth and improving outcome but a randomized phase 3 trial did not show any significant improvement in outcome after intracerebral hemorrhage, even though the hematoma growth was reduced [68,69]. Off-label use in reversal of anticoagulation-based ICH is sometimes practiced but with uncertain outcomes.

References

1. Cerebrovascular diseases, in Ropper AH, Brown RH (eds): *Adams and Victor's Principles of Neurology*. 8th ed. New York, McGraw-Hill, 2005, p. 669–748.
2. Sacco S, Marini C, Totaro R, et al: A population-based study of the incidence and prognosis of lacunar stroke. *Neurology* 66:1335, 2006.
3. Bogousslavsky J, Hachinski VC, Boughner DR, et al: Cardiac and arterial lesions in carotid transient ischemic attacks. *Arch Neurol* 43:223, 1988.
4. Asinger RW, Dyken ML, Fisher M, et al: Cardiogenic brain embolism. *Arch Neurol* 46:727, 1989.
5. Messe SR, Silverman IE, Kizer JR, et al: Practice parameter: recurrent stroke with patent foramen ovale and atrial septal aneurysm: report of the Quality Standards Subcommittee of the American Academy of Neurology. *Neurology* 62(7):1042, 2004.
6. Bogousslavsky J, Regli F: Unilateral watershed cerebral infarcts. *Neurology* 36:372, 1988.
7. Chambers BR, Norris JW, Shurvell BL, et al: Prognosis of acute stroke. *Neurology* 27:221, 1987.
8. Bogousslavsky J, Van Melle G, Regli F: The Lausanne stroke registry. *Stroke* 19:1083, 1988.
9. Gilman S: Time course and outcome of recovery from stroke: relevance to stem cell treatment. *Exp Neurol* 199:37–41, 2006.
10. Mohr JP, Caplan LR, Melski JW, et al: The Harvard cooperative stroke registry. *Neurology* 28:754, 1978.
11. Rivers CS, Wardlaw JM, Armitage PA, et al: Do acute diffusion- and perfusion-weighted MRI lesions identify final infarct volume in ischemic stroke? *Stroke* 37:98, 2006.
12. Moonis M, Fisher M: Imaging of acute stroke. *Cerebrovasc Dis* 11(3):143, 2001.
13. Parsons MW, Barber PA, Chalk J: Diffusion- and perfusion-weighted MRI response to thrombolysis in stroke. *Ann Neurol* 57(1):28, 2002.
14. Parsons MW, Barber PA, Chalk J, et al: Diagnostic impact and prognostic relevance of early contrast-enhanced transcranial color-coded duplex sonography in acute stroke. *Stroke* 29:955, 1998.
15. Tegler CH, Burke GL, Dalley GM, et al: Carotid emboli predict poor outcome in stroke. *Stroke* 24:186, 1993.
16. Cerebral Embolism Task Force: Cardiogenic brain embolism. The second report of the Cerebral Embolism Task Force [published erratum appears in *Arch Neurol* 46(10):1079, 1989] [see comments]. *Arch Neurol* 46(7):727, 1989.
17. Dewitt LD, Wechsler LR: Transcranial Doppler. *Stroke* 19:915, 1988.
18. Sacco RL, Adams R, Albers G, et al: Guidelines for prevention of stroke in patients with ischemic stroke or transient ischemic attack: a statement for healthcare professionals from the American Heart Association/American Stroke Association Council on Stroke: co-sponsored by the Council on Cardiovascular Radiology and Intervention: the American Academy of Neurology affirms the value of this guideline. *Circulation* 113:409, 2006.
19. Moonis M, Fisher M: HMG CoA reductase inhibitors (statins): use in stroke prevention and outcome after stroke. *Expert Rev Neurother* 4(2):241, 2004.
20. North American Symptomatic Carotid Endarterectomy Trial Collaborators: Beneficial effects of carotid endarterectomy in symptomatic patients with high grade carotid stenosis. *N Engl J Med* 325:445, 1991.
21. The European Stroke Prevention Study (ESPS): Principal endpoints. The ESPS Group. *Lancet* 2:1351, 1987.
22. Gent M, Blakely JA, Easton JD, et al: The Canadian American Ticlopidine Study (CATS) in thromboembolic stroke. *Lancet* 1:1215, 1989.
23. Sacco RL, Diener HC, Yusuf S, et al; PRoFESS Study Group: Aspirin and extended-release dipyridamole versus clopidogrel for recurrent stroke. *N Engl J Med* 359(12):1238–1251, 2008.
24. Hankey GJ, Klijn CJ, Eikelboom JW: Ximelagatran or warfarin for stroke prevention in patients with atrial fibrillation. *Stroke* 35(2):389, 2004.
25. The National Institute of Neurological Disorders and Stroke rt-PA Stroke Study Group: Tissue plasminogen activator for acute ischemic stroke. *N Engl J Med* 333:1581, 1995.
26. Hacke W, Kaste M, Bluhmki E: Thrombolysis with Alteplase 3 to 4.5 hours after acute ischemic stroke. *N Engl J Med* 359:1317–1329, 2008.
27. Furlan A, Higashida R, Wechsler L, et al: Intra-arterial prourokinase for acute ischemic stroke. The PROACT II study: a randomized controlled trial. Prolyse in Acute Cerebral Thromboembolism [see comments]. *JAMA* 282(21):2003, 1999.
28. Smith WS, Sung G, Saver J, et al: Mechanical thrombectomy for acute ischemic stroke: final results of the Multi MERCI trial. *Stroke* 39(4):1205–1212, 2008.
29. Hallevi H, Barreto AD, Liebeskind D, et al: Identifying patients at high risk for poor outcome after intra-arterial therapy for acute ischemic stroke. *Stroke* 40:1780–1785, 2009.
30. Moonis M, Fisher M: Considering the role of heparin and low-molecular-weight heparins in acute ischemic stroke. *Stroke* 33(7):1927, 2002.
31. Moonis M, Wingard E, Selveraj N, et al: Factors predisposing to secondary hemorrhagic conversion in acute ischemic stroke. *Ann Neurol* 48:497, 2000.
32. Chamorro A, Vila N, Saiz A, et al: Early anticoagulation after large cerebral embolic infarction: a safety study. *Neurology* 45(5):861, 1995.
33. Hankey GJ: Clopidogrel and thrombotic thrombocytopenic purpura. *Lancet* 356(9226):269, 2000.
34. Vahedi K, Hofmeijer J, Juettler C, et al: Early decompressive surgery in malignant infarction of the middle cerebral artery: a pooled analysis of three randomized controlled trials. *Lancet* 6:215–222, 2007.

35. The International Nimodipine Study Group: Meta-analysis of nimodipine trials in acute ischemic stroke. *Stroke* 23:148, 1992.
36. Scatton B, Carter C, Benavides J, et al: *N*-methyl-D-aspartate receptor antagonists. *Cerebrovasc Dis* 1:121, 1991.
37. Smith SE, Meldrum BS: Cerebroprotective effect of a non-*N*-methyl-D-aspartate antagonist, CYKI 52466, after focal ischemia in the rat. *Stroke* 2:861, 1992.
38. Moonis M, Fisher M: Combination therapies, restorative therapies and future directions, in Bogousslavsky J (ed): *Acute Stroke Treatment.* New York, Martin Dunitz, 2003, p 307.
39. The SASS Investigators: Ganglioside GM1 in acute ischemic stroke. *Stroke* 25:1141, 1994.
40. Lenzi GL, Grigoletto F, Gent M, et al: Early treatment of stroke with monosialoganglioside GM1. *Stroke* 25:1552, 1994.
41. Clark WM, Portland OR, Warach SJ; Citicoline Study Group: Randomized dose response trial of citicoline in acute ischemic stroke patients. *Neurology* 46(S1):A425, 1996.
42. Fisher M, Bogousslavsky J: Further evolution toward effective therapy for acute ischemic stroke. *JAMA* 279(16):1298, 1998.
43. Grotta J: Combination therapy stroke trial: rt-PA +/− lubeluzole. *Stroke* 31:278, 2000.
44. Lees KR, Zivin JA, Ashwood T, et al: NXY-059 for acute ischemic stroke. *N Engl J Med* 354(6):354, 2006.
45. Zivin J, Albers G, Bornstein N, et al; NeuroThera Effectiveness and Safety Trial-2 Investigators: Effectiveness and safety of transcranial laser therapy for acute ischemic stroke. *Stroke* 40(4):1359–1364, 2009.
46. Easton D, Saver JL, Albers G, et al: Definition and evaluation of transient ischemic attack: a scientific statement for healthcare professionals from the American Heart Association/American Stroke Association Stroke Council; Council on Cardiovascular Surgery and Anesthesia; Council on Cardiovascular Radiology and Intervention; Council on Cardiovascular Nursing; and the Interdisciplinary Council on Peripheral Vascular Disease: The American Academy of Neurology affirms the value of this statement as an educational tool for neurologists. *Stroke* 40:2273–2296, 2009.
47. Moonis M: Intraarterial thrombolysis within the first three hours after acute ischemic stroke in selected patients. *Stroke* 40:2611–2622, 2009.
48. Mimatsu K, Yamaguchi T: Management of intracerebral hemorrhage, in Fisher M (ed): *Stroke Therapy*. Boston, Butterworth Heinemann, 2001, p 287.
49. Berger AR, Lipton RB, Lesser ML, et al: Early seizures following intracerebral hemorrhage: implications for therapy. *Neurology* 38:1363, 1988.
50. Fisher CM: Clinical syndromes in cerebral hemorrhage, in Fields WS (ed): *Pathogenesis and Treatment of Cerebrovascular Disease.* Springfield, IL, Charles C Thomas, 1961, p 318.
51. Chen ST, Chen SD, Hsu CY, et al: Progression of hypertensive intracerebral hemorrhage. *Neurology* 39:1509, 1989.
52. Radberg JA, Olson JE, Radberg CT: Prognostic parameters in spontaneous hematomas with special reference to anticoagulation treatment. *Stroke* 22:571, 1991.
53. Kase CS, Robinson RK, Stein RW, et al: Anticoagulant-related intracerebral hemorrhage. *Neurology* 35:943, 1983.
54. Kase CS, O'Neil AM, Fisher M, et al: Intracranial hemorrhage after use of tissue plasminogen activator. *Ann Intern Med* 112:17, 1990.
55. ISIS-3 Collaborative Group: A random trial of streptokinase vs tissue plasminogen activator vs anistreplase. *Lancet* 339:753, 1992.
56. Wojak JC, Flamm ED: Intracranial hemorrhage and cocaine use. *Stroke* 18:712, 1987.
57. Toffol GJ, Biller J, Adams HP: Nontraumatic intracerebral hemorrhage in young adults. *Arch Neurol* 44:483, 1987.
58. Kaufman MJ, Levin JM, Ross MH, et al: Cocaine-induced cerebral vasoconstriction detected in humans with magnetic resonance angiography. *JAMA* 279:376, 1998.
59. Duff TA, Ayeni S, Louim AB, et al: Neurosurgical management of spontaneous intracerebral hematomas. *Barrow Neurol Inst Q* 1:29, 1985.
60. Izumihara A, Suzuki M, Ishihara T: Recurrence and extension of lobar hemorrhage related to cerebral amyloid angiopathy: multivariate analysis of clinical risk factors. *Surg Neurol* 64:160, 2005.
61. Chung CS, Park CM: Primary pontine hemorrhage: a new CT classification. *Neurology* 42:830, 1992.
62. Jensen MB, St Louis EK: Management of acute cerebellar stroke. *Arch Neurol* 62:537, 2005.
63. Darby DG, Donnan GA, Saling MA, et al: Primary intraventricular hemorrhage: clinical and neuropsychological findings in a prospective stroke series. *Neurology* 38:68, 1988.
64. Borges LF: Management of nontraumatic brain hemorrhage, in Ropper AM, Kennedy SF (eds): *Neurological and Neurosurgical Intensive Care.* Rockville, MD, Aspen, 1988, p 209.
65. Poungvarin N, Bhoopat W, Viniarejakul A, et al: Effects of dexamethasone in primary supratentorial intracerebral hemorrhage. *N Engl J Med* 316:1229, 1987.
66. Faught E, Peters D, Bartolucci A, et al: Seizures after primary intracerebral hemorrhage. *Neurology* 39:1089, 1989.
67. Mendelow AD, Gregson BA, Fernandes HM, et al: Early surgery versus initial conservative treatment in patients with spontaneous supratentorial intracerebral haematomas in the International Surgical Trial in Intracerebral Haemorrhage (STICH): a randomised trial. *Lancet* 365(9457):387–397, 2005.
68. Mayer S, Brun A, Begtrup NC, et al: Recombinant activated factor VII for acute intracerebral hemorrhage. *N Engl J Med* 352(8):777, 2005.
69. Mayer SA, Bron NC, Begtrup K, et al; FAST Trial investigators: Efficacy and safety of recombinant activated factor VII for acute intracerebral hemorrhage. *N Engl J Med* 358:2127–2137, 2008.

CHAPTER 174 ■ NEURO-ONCOLOGICAL PROBLEMS IN THE INTENSIVE CARE UNIT

N. SCOTT LITOFSKY AND MICHAEL C. MUZINICH

INTRODUCTION

Neuro-oncology encompasses the care of patients with neoplasms affecting the brain, spinal cord, and peripheral nervous system. These tumors may arise either within the nervous system itself or spread from systemic malignancies. Neuro-oncology patients may require care in an intensive care unit (ICU) at a number of different phases of their illnesses. Usually, postoperative patients with brain tumors are admitted to the ICU. Neuro-oncology patients are also admitted to the ICU if they suffer catastrophic or near catastrophic neurologic decline or if they are at high risk to suffer such a change. Lastly, neuro-oncology patients may also suffer from medical processes that require intensive care.

This chapter discusses the intensive care issues that may be encountered in neuro-oncology patients, either following their surgery or as complications of their diseases. These issues include elevated intracranial pressure (ICP), hydrocephalus, seizures, postoperative complications, spinal neoplastic disease, and medical systemic complications.

ELEVATED INTRACRANIAL PRESSURE

Elevated ICP frequently complicates the course of patients with cerebral neoplasms. Both primary and metastatic tumors in the brain can cause elevated ICP. Patients with aggressive brain tumors often succumb as a consequence of uncontrollable elevations in ICP.

Pathophysiology

Normal intracranial pressure ranges between 5 and 15 cm H_2O. This pressure is generated by the volumes of the various components contained in the "closed box" of the skull. These components include brain parenchyma, cerebrospinal fluid (CSF), extracellular water, and blood in vascular spaces. A perturbation of any of these components can increase ICP. Any additional tissue not normally present in the brain, such as a primary or metastatic tumor, or a hemorrhage associated with a tumor, can also increase ICP. While the numerical value of the ICP cannot be ascertained by neurodiagnostic images, some of the perturbations are evident on either computed tomography (CT) scan or magnetic resonance imaging (MRI).

Brain tumors can affect each intracranial component. In addition to the volume of the neoplasm itself, cerebral neoplasms can produce vasogenic edema [1], secondary to increased permeability of blood vessels within or adjacent to the tumor, thereby increasing extracellular water [2,3]. Radiographically, this edema corresponds to hypodensity on CT or hyperintensity on T2-weighted MRI around the enhancing bulk of tumor. Tumor mass, or brain parenchyma displaced by tumor, may obstruct CSF pathways, causing hydrocephalus. Hydrocephalus will be discussed in further detail in the section "Hydrocephalus." Intravascular blood volume also can increase in patients with tumors as a result of hypoventilation. Hypoventilation occurs either related to seizure activity or ICP elevation, both of which can reduce respiratory drive. Hypoventilation increases PCO_2, which causes arterial vasodilation, thereby increasing intravascular volume and ICP. This increase can cause a vicious positive feedback loop by further reducing ventilatory drive.

Signs and Symptoms

Patients can experience a variety of symptoms and signs caused by elevated ICP. These findings do not necessarily correlate with the degree of elevated pressure, though generally the higher the ICP, the more significant the neurologic findings.

As ICP increases, compression of the reticular activating system depresses the patient's level of consciousness. These findings tend to occur sequentially, with the patient progressing from an awake and alert status to progressively more lethargic states and may eventually lead to coma.

Patients may develop a variety of cognitive changes resulting from elevated ICP. Disorientation, short-term memory loss, decreased fund of knowledge, and loss of insight and judgment can occur to varying degrees.

As increasing ICP approaches pressure of the central retinal vein, the patient will usually lose the spontaneous venous pulsations that are seen on routine funduscopic examination. Further elevation of ICP exceeding the central retinal vein pressure causes swelling of the optic disks (papilledema). Papilledema does not usually occur rapidly in the setting of elevated ICP. Usually several days of elevated ICP must ensue before papilledema is evident. A patient with long-standing papilledema may have constriction of his/her visual fields and/or decreased visual acuity.

Brain masses causing elevated ICP can cause brain shifts from one intracranial compartment to another. Usually a brain shift, also known as a "herniation," is away from the mass causing the elevated ICP. Supratentorial masses may cause the brain to herniate inferiorly through the tentorial incisura. With a resulting central diencephalic herniation syndrome, the patient experiences simultaneous bilateral pupillary dilation from compression of the tectum, containing the Edinger–Westphal nucleus of the oculomotor nerve (CN III). A lateral cerebral mass, particularly if in the temporal lobe, forces the uncus of the temporal lobe to herniate through the incisura. This uncal herniation causes compression of CN III between the posterior cerebral artery and the superior cerebellar artery, resulting in unilateral pupillary dilation. In both herniation syndromes, the constrictive phase of the light reflex can also cease to function (unreactive pupils). Usually, though not always, decrease in the patient's level of consciousness precedes pupillary dysfunction.

Patients can also have light-near dissociation. Pressure on the tectum can compress the retinotectal fibers that are part of the afferent limb of the pupillary light reflex; the pupil does not constrict to light appropriately. However, those fibers involved in the afferent limb of pupillary accommodation to near vision, which travel to the tectum through other pathways, are not affected. Patients, therefore, can have pupils that constrict to accommodation but not to light. This is often a very subtle sign of elevated ICP.

Double vision may also be present. The abducens nerve (CN VI), which controls abduction of the eye, has the longest intracranial course of the cranial nerves and is at highest risk of dysfunction when ICP is elevated. Diplopia is usually more pronounced with increasing lateral gaze, either unilaterally or bilaterally.

As the dura and blood vessels are stretched by elevated ICP, the patient may experience headache. Headache is frequently described as "band like" or "pressure like." It tends to occur more commonly in the early morning and may wake the patient from sleep. While the patient is sleeping, the recumbent position decreases venous return to the heart, elevating ICP. In addition, hypoventilation that occurs during sleep will also elevate ICP, increasing the headache.

Not uncommonly, headache is associated with projectile vomiting. Vomiting occurs because of increased pressure on the area postrema.

In addition to the symptoms and signs described earlier, patients with elevated ICP often experience neurologic deficits from the compressive effects of the mass of the tumor on adjacent neural structures. These deficits can include the following: hemiparesis, aphasia, visual field deficits, hearing loss, ataxia (truncal or appendicular), and sensory loss. The presence of these findings is based on the size, location, and rapidity of growth of the mass. Slower growing tumors allow the brain to compensate; focal findings may not be evident until late in the patient's course.

Management

Mechanical and pharmacologic therapies are available to treat elevated ICP, with expectant reduction or elimination of its signs and symptoms. Some require very minimal intervention, while others are much more intensive or invasive.

Head elevation of 30 to 45 degrees is perhaps the easiest treatment available. It increases venous drainage from the brain, thereby reducing blood volume within its intravascular compartment. Head elevation poses minimal risk to the patient. Theoretically, cerebral perfusion could be diminished, but such a reduction is negligible in a patient with normal blood pressure.

Mannitol, an osmotic diuretic, draws fluid out of the brain and into the vascular system by increasing serum osmolarity. From the vascular spaces, the fluid follows the mannitol as the kidney excretes it. Therefore, mannitol reduces intracellular and extracellular water in the brain. Furthermore, mannitol improves blood rheology; ischemic areas of brain adjacent to the tumor mass are better perfused [4]. Mannitol is

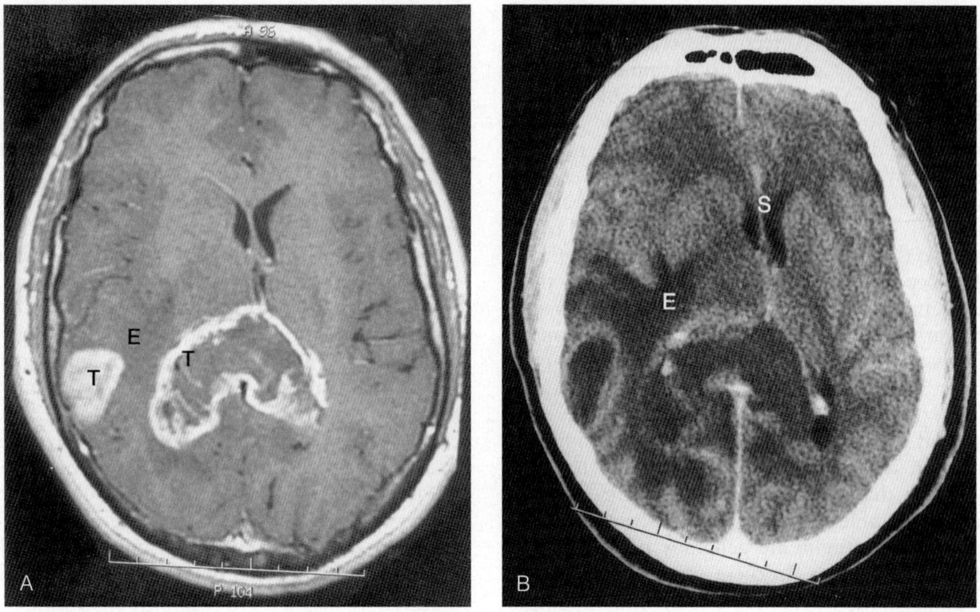

FIGURE 174.1. A: This magnetic resonance imaging, performed on a patient presenting with headache and memory lapses, shows an enhancing mass (T) involving the corpus callosum and right parietal area, with surrounding edema (E). Stereotactic biopsy revealed glioblastoma multiforme. **B:** One week following biopsy, the patient was admitted to the intensive care unit with obtundation and left hemiparesis. His computed tomography shows increased edema (E) and right-to-left midline shift (S)—parafalcine herniation. He required mannitol, increased Decadron, and surgical decompression to improve.

frequently given as an initial resuscitative dose of 1 gm per kg, followed by 0.25 gm per kg every 4 to 6 hours to maintain the diuresis and control ICP. Mannitol is quite effective in lowering ICP and/or reversing early cerebral herniation. It may also be used if patients have significant mass effect identified on neuroimaging studies to stabilize and improve their condition (Fig. 174.1). A number of potential risks are present with long-term mannitol use. Hypotension can occur in already hypovolemic patients. Patients can also become hyperosmolar and hypernatremic. Therefore, mannitol is usually withheld from the patient if serum osmolarity exceeds 320 mOsm per L. Lastly, there is some concern that mannitol may lose effectiveness if used continuously for more than 72 hours.

Furosemide (Lasix), a loop diuretic, rapidly reduces systemic circulating volume. Extracellular and intracellular water in the brain are drawn into the vascular system and are redistributed. Lasix also promotes venous pooling, leading to similar redistribution of fluids. While mannitol is generally used as the first-line agent, Lasix may be used at an initial resuscitative dose of 1 mg per kg in patients with cerebral herniation. Risks are minimal in this setting, as electrolyte abnormalities are unlikely to occur with only a single dose. In a patient who has had frequent vomiting and is already dehydrated, Lasix can cause hypotension from the additional hypovolemia.

Hypertonic saline enhances cerebral blood flow by increasing intravascular osmolarity that creates a gradient to move free water from the interstitial and intracellular compartments to the intravascular space. This is associated with an acute plasma expansion with hemodilution, increase in arterial blood pressure, and reduced vascular resistance [5]. Hypertonic saline has also been found to have some inotropic effects that appear to be derived from improvement in cardiac microcirculation and contractility [6]. However, significant polyuria has been observed in the acute setting which may lead to excessive diuresis and subsequent dehydration. Patients on hypertonic therapy should also have frequent blood draws every 6 hours to monitor serum osmolality and serum sodium. It is generally recommended to have a target serum sodium from 145 to 155 mmol per L and serum osmolality of less than 320 mOsm per L. Serum sodium should not increase more than 15 mmol per L daily and should not be allowed to drop more than 10 mmol per L daily to decrease the risk of central pontine myelinolysis [7].

Glucocorticosteroids can markedly improve symptoms of elevated ICP and/or mass effect in patients with cerebral neoplasms. They work by stabilizing cell membranes and reducing vasogenic edema [8,9]. Dexamethasone (Decadron) is the most commonly used glucocorticosteroid. An initial dose of 10 to 20 mg is followed by 4 to 6 mg every 4 to 6 hours, depending on the severity of the patient's clinical condition. Solu-Medrol (100 mg initially, and then 20 to 40 mg every 4 to 6 hours) is another option. Glucocorticosteroids are the medical mainstay of brain tumor care because their effects are sustained over time. A patient with vasogenic edema from tumor may require steroids for a significant period of time. In the short term, steroids can cause hyperglycemia and exacerbate diabetes mellitus, changing the patient's insulin requirements. Gastrointestinal hemorrhage or ulceration can occur; H_2 blockers, such as Pepcid, Nexium, or Zantac, are frequently given prophylactically. The stimulatory effect of steroids frequently disrupts sleep. Long-term use of steroids may be associated with proximal muscle weakness, avascular necrosis of the femoral head, easy bruising, and other findings of Cushing's syndrome.

In contrast to cerebral vasodilation caused by hypoventilation, hypocarbia from hyperventilation causes cerebral vasoconstriction, which reduces the arterial intravascular blood volume within the brain. Hyperventilation can therefore rapidly reduce ICP and reverse a cerebral herniation syndrome. Although initial hyperventilation can be performed with an AMBU bag valve mask, sustained hyperventilation requires endotracheal intubation and mechanical ventilation of the patient. Moderation of hyperventilation is necessary because at PCO_2 less than 25 mm Hg, cerebral ischemia may result from profound vasoconstriction. A vasodilatory rebound from hyperventilation occurs after approximately 24 hours, thereby negating its positive effects if hyperventilation is used chronically [10].

One of the most effective means of rapidly reducing ICP is to drain CSF. Such a maneuver is effective whether or not the patient has hydrocephalus. In a patient with a brain tumor, the safest method of draining CSF is to place a ventriculostomy, a catheter usually passed into the frontal horn of the lateral ventricle via a small hole drilled through the skull. The procedure can be performed by a neurosurgeon at the bedside. After placement of a ventriculostomy, drainage of CSF into a bag at bedside can reduce ICP. The catheter can also be coupled to a pressure transducer so that ICP can be measured. Usually, CSF is drained if ICP exceeds 15 to 20 mm Hg. The risks of the procedure include hemorrhage and infection. Therefore, coagulation studies are appropriate before the procedure is done, especially in patients who have received recent chemotherapy. The risk of infection increases the longer the catheter remains in place. Sometimes, prophylactic antibiotics are used.

Regardless of what means are necessary to stabilize and/or resuscitate the patient, the best means of controlling ICP in long term is to remove the tumor if possible. Unfortunately, some tumors are unresectable. Gliomas or metastases involving the thalamus or basal ganglia are generally not resected, except in unusual circumstances. In these instances, medical management is necessary to control ICP until adjuvant therapy, such as radiation therapy, can shrink the tumor and reduce its edema-producing capabilities. The same rationale applies to patients with multifocal cerebral masses; patients with more than one metastasis do not usually have multiple operations to resect each tumor, especially if symptoms are controllable with steroids. On the other hand, if the tumor is resectable, its removal can relieve the brain of the extra mass, relieve obstruction to the flow of CSF, and reduce vasogenic edema. In addition to relieving the signs and symptoms of elevated ICP, tumor resection can also relieve the effects of compression on the surrounding brain, improving lateralizing findings. Some tumors can be removed completely. These include meningiomas, vestibular schwannomas, craniopharyngiomas, pituitary adenomas, and metastatic tumors. Microscopic disease may still be present in the tumor bed, particularly in the case of metastases or craniopharyngioma, which may require adjuvant therapy, but ICP can be well controlled. Primary glial neoplasms, however, cannot be completely removed in most cases. The bulk of tumor can be resected, and postoperative neurodiagnostic images may show no residual tumor, but most of these tumors have infiltrating fingers of tumor still present. Even so, removing tumor bulk can alleviate elevated ICP; edema can sometimes be exacerbated with only partial resection, so caution is required.

HYDROCEPHALUS

Brain tumors often can cause hydrocephalus, a situation in which the patient has an increased volume of CSF under increased pressure. Hydrocephalus is typically associated with enlargement of the ventricular system (or a portion thereof) and compression of the normal brain parenchyma. A patient with hydrocephalus may require urgent or emergent intensive care monitoring and treatment. Hydrocephalus is a special case of elevated ICP and warrants separate discussion.

Etiology

Hydrocephalus can occur from a variety of mechanisms in patients with brain tumors. It is as important to identify the etiology of the hydrocephalus as its presence because the definitive treatment of hydrocephalus will be based on its mechanism of formation. Some tumors, as discussed later, are more likely to be associated with certain mechanisms of hydrocephalus than others.

Leptomeningeal infiltration by tumor cells in the subarachnoid space can prevent the absorption of CSF by the arachnoid granulations, either by occluding the granulations or preventing the flow of CSF from the outlet foramen of the fourth ventricle around the dorsolateral convexities to the granulations. Metastatic tumors from the lung, breast, lymphoma, and leukemia are the most frequently involved systemic tumors; primary tumors behaving in this fashion include primitive neuroectodermal tumors (i.e., medulloblastoma), ependymoblastoma, and glioblastoma multiforme. A patient with carcinomatous meningitis will frequently have a stiff neck or cranial neuropathy in addition to symptoms and signs of elevated ICP.

Large extra-axial "benign" tumors, usually in the posterior fossa, can cause hydrocephalus (Fig. 174.2). These tumors include those in the cerebellopontine angle, such as meningioma or vestibular schwannoma. These tumors displace the cerebellar hemisphere and obstruct the fourth ventricle to prevent adequate circulation of CSF. Rarely a choroid plexus papilloma can emerge from the foramen of Luschka and similarly compress the cerebellar hemisphere. Meningiomas of the clivus or tentorium can also displace CSF pathways with resulting hydrocephalus.

Some tumors may originate in a ventricle or protrude into a ventricle and occlude CSF pathways, thus producing hydrocephalus. These tumors include medulloblastoma, ependymoma, choroid plexus papilloma, intraventricular meningioma, colloid cyst, giant cell astrocytoma of tuberous sclerosis, and pineal region tumors.

Parenchymal tumors often can occlude CSF pathways. Primary or metastatic tumors in the thalamus or basal ganglia can displace brain parenchyma and occlude the foramen of Monro or the third ventricle [11]. Tumors in the pineal region may occlude the posterior third ventricle or cerebral aqueduct (Fig. 174.3). Brain stem gliomas or tumors in the cerebellar hemispheres can compress the fourth ventricle [12].

Symptoms and Signs

The clinical picture of a patient with hydrocephalus is frequently the same as that of a patient with elevated ICP. In fact, hydrocephalus must be considered in the differential diagnosis for causes of elevated ICP. Patients with midline masses or carcinomatous meningitis usually do not have lateralizing neurologic deficits such as hemiparesis. Those patients with unilateral brain masses may have lateralizing deficits from compression of the previously normally, but marginally, functioning brain by the progressive hydrocephalus.

Evaluation

If hydrocephalus is suspected, evaluation should proceed promptly. Two questions must be answered—"Does the patient have hydrocephalus?" and "What is the cause of the hydrocephalus?" Either MRI or CT can answer these questions. Because MRI delineates better anatomic definition of the brain, more readily illustrates the relationship of the lesion to CSF pathways, and shows these features in multiple planes, MRI with gadolinium is the preferred study. Sometimes, however, the patient is too ill to obtain an MRI easily, or MRI is not readily available. In these circumstances, a CT scan with IV contrast is sufficient. The purpose of the contrast agent with either study is to characterize the location of the lesion and its relationship to CSF pathways better. The addition of proton magnetic resonance spectroscopy to standard anatomic MRI

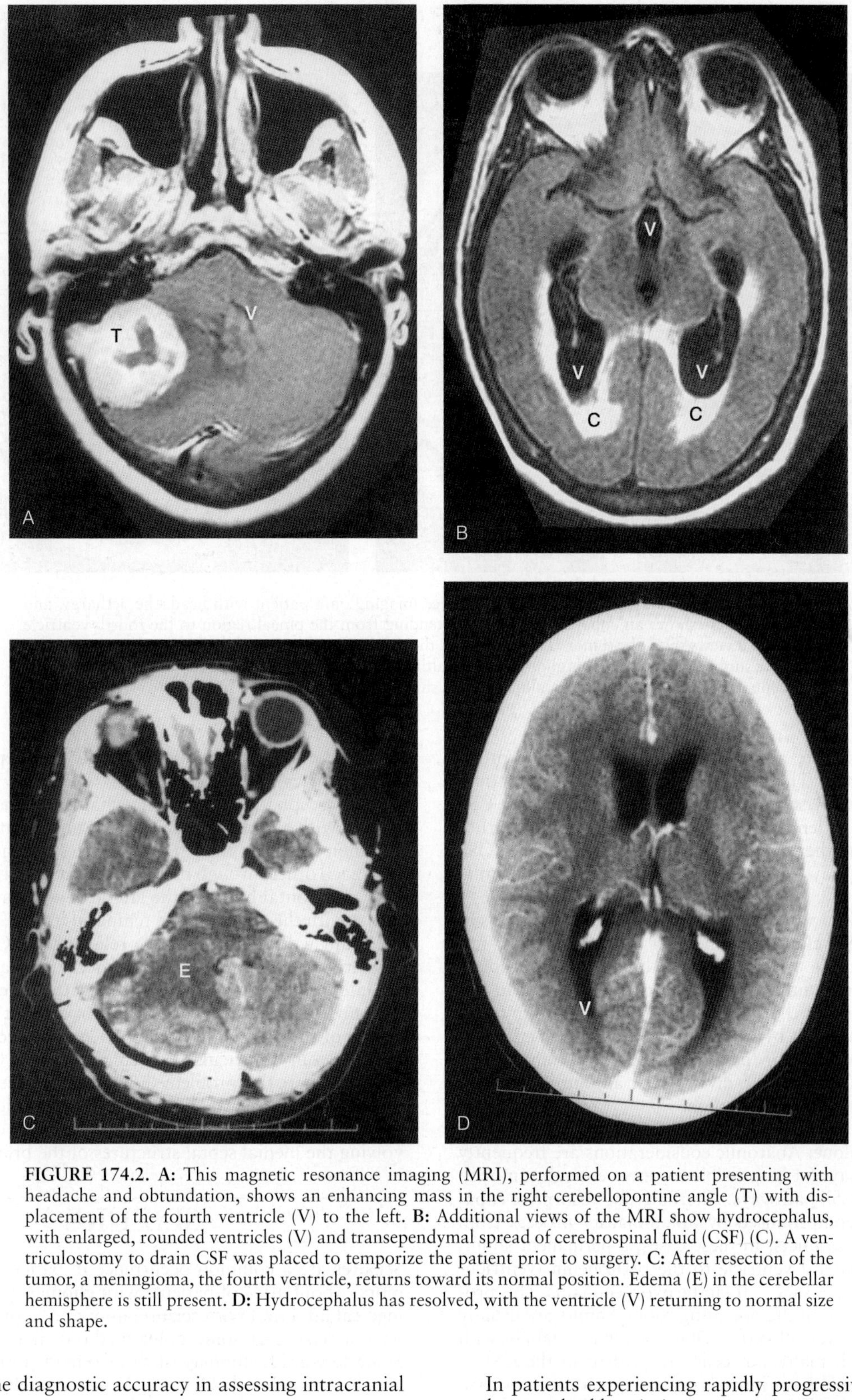

FIGURE 174.2. A: This magnetic resonance imaging (MRI), performed on a patient presenting with headache and obtundation, shows an enhancing mass in the right cerebellopontine angle (T) with displacement of the fourth ventricle (V) to the left. B: Additional views of the MRI show hydrocephalus, with enlarged, rounded ventricles (V) and transependymal spread of cerebrospinal fluid (CSF) (C). A ventriculostomy to drain CSF was placed to temporize the patient prior to surgery. C: After resection of the tumor, a meningioma, the fourth ventricle, returns toward its normal position. Edema (E) in the cerebellar hemisphere is still present. D: Hydrocephalus has resolved, with the ventricle (V) returning to normal size and shape.

may improve the diagnostic accuracy in assessing intracranial mass lesions.

Management

The appropriate intervention for a patient with hydrocephalus depends on several factors. These include the cause of the hydrocephalus, the anatomic location of the obstruction to CSF flow, and the patient's clinical condition.

In patients experiencing rapidly progressive deterioration, such as cerebral herniation, emergent management with a ventriculostomy, as described previously, to divert CSF temporarily can improve the patient's clinical picture. Usually, the drainage chamber is set so that the system can be opened intermittently to drain CSF for ICP greater than 20 mm Hg. Some patients, however, require a lower ICP to achieve neurologic improvement, so the system can be opened for lower pressures. An alternative method of draining CSF in patients with hydrocephalus is to set the system to drain CSF continuously at a particular

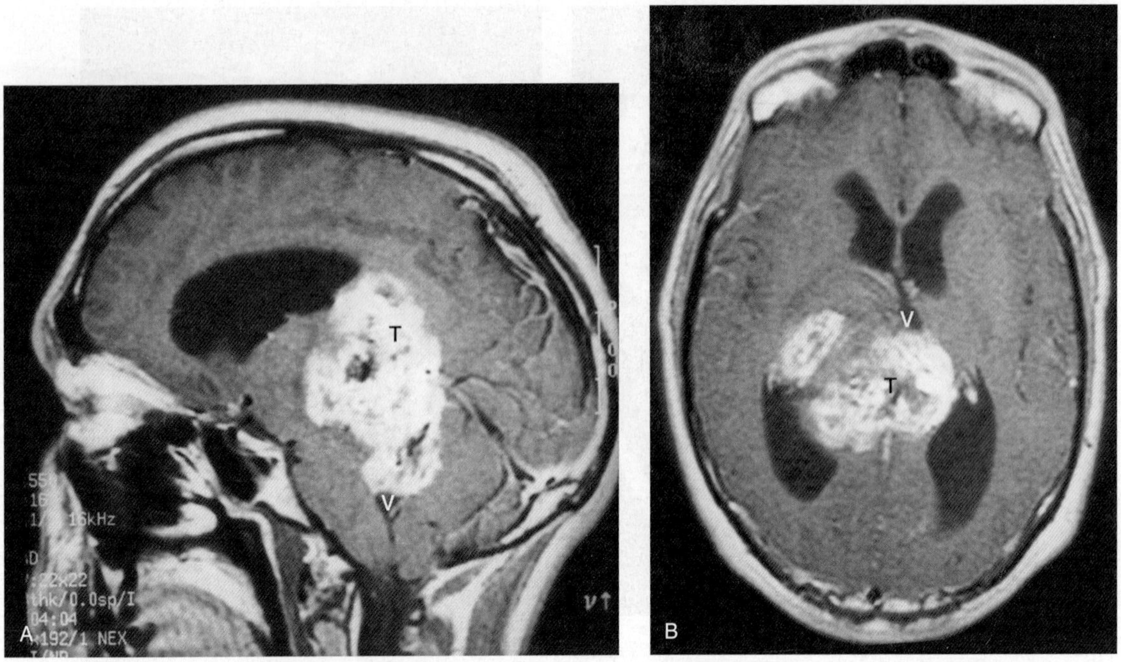

FIGURE 174.3. **A:** This sagittal magnetic resonance imaging on a patient with headache, lethargy, and diffuse weakness shows an enhancing mass (T) extending from the pineal region to the fourth ventricle (V). **B:** Axial views show the tumor (T) compressing the third ventricle (V) with hydrocephalus. Despite an aggressive surgical resection of this glioblastoma multiforme, the patient subsequently developed recurrent hydrocephalus and required a ventriculoperitoneal shunt.

pressure, for instance, at 15 mm Hg. ICP is then recorded on an hourly basis. This technique of CSF drainage should be approached with some caution as large volumes of CSF may drain if the patient strains or coughs, increasing intrathoracic pressure and therefore ICP temporarily. If too much CSF drains, patients may develop subdural or intraparenchymal hemorrhages.

A patient may have only mild hydrocephalus and not be significantly impaired clinically. Emergent intervention may not be necessary, and the patient can be stabilized with Decadron with or without mannitol or other hyperosmolar agent. In this situation, resection of the tumor can provide long-term treatment of hydrocephalus by decompressing the CSF pathways, particularly with posterior fossa or pineal region tumors. The patient may not require CSF diversion at all. Surgery should proceed in a timely fashion, though.

Occasionally, hydrocephalus does not respond to surgical decompression alone. Anatomic considerations are frequently responsible. It may not be possible to resect enough tumor to decompress the CSF pathways. Alternatively, absorptive capabilities may be compromised by inflammatory process from blood or tumor products. In these cases, a permanent shunt, usually from a lateral ventricle to the peritoneum (ventriculoperitoneal), is necessary to treat the hydrocephalus. This procedure is performed in the operating room. Shunts are usually well tolerated and very effective. One concern in a patient with a tumor in which malignant cells are present in the CSF is that the patient will have intraperitoneal spread of tumor via the shunt. This complication occurs uncommonly, though. Persistent symptomatic hydrocephalus dictates that the shunt be placed regardless of this concern.

A more commonly occurring concern in a patient with hydrocephalus who has been shunted is shunt malfunction [13]. Cellular debris, proteinaceous material, or normal choroid plexus can occasionally occlude a shunt. This occurrence is manifested by symptoms and signs of hydrocephalus and elevated ICP. Treatment requires operative revision of the occluded portion of the shunt, usually with replacement of the ventricular catheter or the valve.

Hydrocephalus can be somewhat problematic to treat in a patient with a tumor adjacent to the third ventricle. In this uncommon situation, the lateral ventricles may not communicate with each other through the third ventricle. In the most extreme case, the frontal horns of the lateral ventricles do not communicate with the occipital and temporal horns. Therefore, a single shunt will be ineffective in relieving the CSF obstruction. A ventriculogram, in which intrathecal contrast is placed into the lateral ventricle via a ventricular catheter (either a ventriculostomy or the ventricular portion of a shunt), can define the nature of the obstruction. The patient may require two, three, or even four ventricular catheters to drain CSF adequately. Tumors where this problem should be of concern include craniopharyngioma, central neurocytoma, pilocytic astrocytoma of the hypothalamus, and glioblastoma, among other tumors involving the medial septal structures of the brain.

SEIZURE

Seizures are a common occurrence in patients with brain tumors. About 40% of patients with gliomas initially present to medical attention with seizure; about 55% of glioma patients have a seizure at some point in the course of their disease. Some low-grade gliomas, such as oligodendroglioma, have a very high likelihood of seizure. Approximately 20% of patients with metastatic tumors have a seizure at some time [14,15].

Seizures may be focal or generalized. A patient remains conscious during a focal seizure. The seizure may be a motor seizure in which the patient's mouth twitches or an extremity moves uncontrollably for a period of time. With a dominant hemisphere lesion, aphasia may also occur. During a generalized seizure, the patient loses consciousness. Tonic–clonic movements may occur, and the patient may lose bladder control or bite their tongue. A patient can also experience status epilepticus, a series of seizures occurring in rapid succession with the patient not regaining consciousness between seizures. Status epilepticus is a medical emergency that is addressed in Chapter 172. Occasionally, a patient can have a seizure that is not witnessed or is subclinical in activity. The patient experiences a neurologic deficit, which subsequently improves, leaving healthcare providers puzzled as to the etiology of the transient deficit.

Further evaluation of the known brain tumor patient with seizure is necessary. A seizure can occur in a patient with a known brain tumor for a number of reasons. The most common reason is that the patient's anticonvulsant medication level(s) is (are) subtherapeutic. Drug requirements may change as steroid requirements change; Decadron may interact with Dilantin to lower serum levels [16,17]. Serum drug levels are therefore essential. Other reasons for seizure include a change in the character of the tumor. The tumor may have grown in size [18] or a hemorrhage within the tumor may have occurred. A CT scan of the head without contrast helps to differentiate among these possibilities.

Treatment

While a single generalized seizure usually does not have long-term consequences, such an event may precipitate rapid deterioration in a patient with elevated ICP. The associated hypercarbia from hypoventilation can increase ICP substantially; a stable patient can rapidly deteriorate even to the point of developing a herniation syndrome. Hypoxia can further compromise brain function by causing damage similar to cerebral ischemia, especially in the area already affected by the tumor. Prompt intervention is therefore necessary.

Maintenance of an adequate airway and reestablishment of adequate ventilation is essential. Oxygen should be provided to the patient. Intubation and mechanical ventilation may be required if the patient experiences hypoventilation.

The best medication to stop seizure activity in patients with status epilepticus is Ativan. The initial dose is 2 mg IV, and the dose is repeated acutely every 5 minutes as needed, up to a total of 8 mg until the seizure activity stops. Should 8 mg be required, mechanical ventilation will likely be required. Dilantin (15 mg per kg IV) or phenobarbital (15 mg per kg IV) must be used acutely in conjunction with Ativan, as the Ativan is only for short-term seizure control.

Prophylactic anticonvulsants administered without a seizure having occurred are rarely indicated unless the patient is going to surgery [19]. Following a seizure, the patient should be started on an anticonvulsant, such as Dilantin. The initial loading dose is 15 mg per kg intravenously, with oral or intravenous maintenance dosing of 100 mg three times daily or 200 mg twice a day. Phenobarbital, although more sedating than Dilantin, can also be used. Both Dilantin (or fosphenytoin) and phenobarbital are available in intravenous forms and may be used if the patient is unable to take oral or enteral medications. Tegretol, on the other hand, is only available in an oral form, so it cannot be used in status epilepticus or in patients who cannot tolerate enteral intake. Keppra is available in both oral and intravenous formulas, has fewer interactions with other medications, and tends to have less sedating side effects.

POSTOPERATIVE COMPLICATIONS

One of the most common reasons for a patient with a neuro-oncological illness to be admitted to an ICU is for observation following a neurosurgical procedure. This period of observation may just be overnight or it may be longer, being dictated by the patient's neurologic and/or medical condition. Although perioperative mortality is less than 2%, medical or neurologic complications may occur in up to 30% of cases; older patients and those with increased neurologic deficits are more likely to suffer these morbidities [20]. Therefore, a variety of intraoperative and postoperative complications must be recognized before the patient's neurologic or medical status is irreversibly compromised. Intervention can then proceed promptly.

To anticipate potential complications, vital signs and neurochecks are taken hourly by nurses in the ICU. One of the most important components of the neuro-checks is the patient's level of consciousness, usually denoted by the Glasgow Coma Scale (GCS) score [21,22]. This three-part score consists of patient responses in eye opening, motor, and verbal spheres. Originally developed to document the level of consciousness in patients with head trauma, use of the GCS can readily, reliably, and reproducibly identify changes in the patient's level of consciousness—either deterioration or improvement. Furthermore, its use can help evaluate the effectiveness of interventions by the reported trends. Other components of neuro-checks include pupillary light responses, orientation, and motor function. Any decrement in function warrants prompt evaluation. Such an evaluation should include a CT or MRI scan of the head, serum electrolytes, blood gases, and anticonvulsant level(s). Other tests may be required based on the patient's condition. Recent technological advancements have allowed for production of mobile CT scanners for use in the ICU. While the resolution is significantly less than traditional CT scanning, the mobile CT scanner can be utilized to ascertain gross intracranial pathology in patients who may otherwise be too unstable for transport. Evaluation of the ICU patient for intracerebral hemorrhage or increased ventricular size can be performed at the patient's bedside and allow for rapid diagnosis in patients with acute changes in mental status. Mobile CT scanning has also been utilized intraoperatively during resection of glial tumors, which may allow for more complete resection of intracranial pathology [23].

Intracranial Hemorrhage

One of the most dramatic complications that can occur in the postoperative period is intracranial hemorrhage. Significant hemorrhage usually becomes evident within 6 to 12 hours after the completion of surgery. A patient can bleed into the tumor bed (Fig. 174.4), or into the subdural or epidural spaces. Although steps are taken at surgery to prevent such complications, oozing from small vessels in the tumor bed can occur. Traction by the brain, slackened by tumor removal, mannitol, Lasix, hypertonic saline, hyperventilation, and CSF drainage, can tear or stretch draining veins, leading to blood accumulation in the subdural space. Because the dura is separated from the bone to perform the craniotomy, the epidural space is no longer just a potential space; rather, it is a real space into which blood can ooze from underneath the bone edges and accumulate. Patients who experience significant hypertension or persistent coughing and "bucking" as they emerge from anesthesia are at greater risk for developing postoperative hemorrhage. Hypertension can cause bleeding from arterial-side vessels. The increase in intrathoracic pressure that occurs with coughing or bucking against the endotracheal tube can precipitate venous-side bleeding, as can thrombosis in a draining vein from manipulation.

Postoperative hemorrhage should be suspected in a patient who fails to emerge adequately from anesthesia. Intracranial hemorrhage should also be a concern if the patient deteriorates following emergence from anesthesia and develops progressive decline in level of consciousness, pupillary abnormalities, or

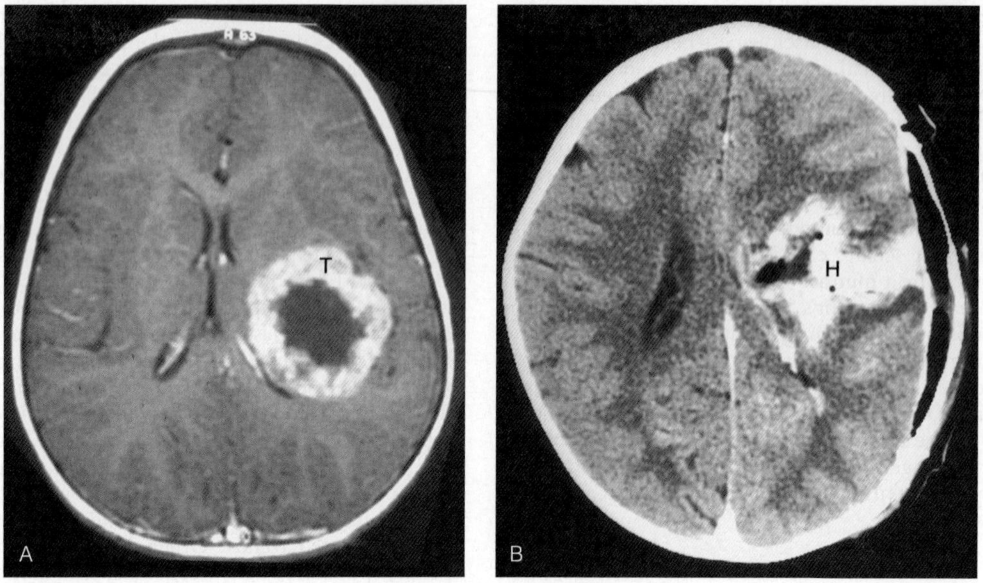

FIGURE 174.4. **A:** This magnetic resonance imaging on a 2-year-old boy shows a large enhancing mass (T) in the left temporoparietal area. **B:** Immediately following surgery to remove the rhabdoid neuroepithelial tumor, the patient had sustained hypertension and awakened slowly from her anesthesia with a mild right hemiparesis. This computed tomography scan shows hemorrhage (H) in the tumor bed. With blood pressure control and observation, the patient recovered to a normal level of consciousness with resolution of her hemiparesis over several days.

new motor deficits. Emergent evaluation with a CT scan is indicated. Coagulation deficits, particularly in patients who have had chemotherapy recently or who have liver disease, should be ruled out with laboratory testing for prothrombin time, partial thromboplastin time, and platelet count.

Should a significant intracranial hemorrhage be identified, the patient may need to return to the operating room to evacuate the hemorrhage. Mannitol and reintubation may be required to stabilize the patient's condition. Occasionally, if the neurologic deterioration is mild, observation or mannitol by itself may be sufficient intervention. As the blood degrades over time and edema subsides, the patient should improve clinically. Frequent follow-up CT scanning is necessary in nonoperative management to evaluate the status of the hemorrhage and surrounding brain.

Cerebral Edema

Manipulation of the tumor and adjacent brain can lead to cerebral edema. Clinical signs can appear quite similar to postoperative hemorrhage, although deficits from edema tend to occur in a more delayed fashion. Prompt treatment with mannitol and Decadron is indicated following a CT scan to confirm the etiology of the patient's neurologic change.

Endocrinopathy

Pituitary tumors may be associated with hypersecretory or hyposecretory states. Other tumors in the sella and parasellar areas may also be associated with endocrinopathy, usually hypopituitarism. Surgery for tumors in these locations can cause endocrine deficits too. Most endocrinopathies encountered in the ICU are related to pituitary hypofunction.

The major neurologically related endocrinopathy evident in the ICU setting is diabetes insipidus, most commonly after craniopharyngioma or pituitary tumor resection. It usually occurs between 18 and 36 hours following surgery. Signs of diabetes insipidus include an increase in urine output greater than 200 mL per hour for 2 consecutive hours, a corresponding drop in urine specific gravity to less than 1.005, and an increase in serum sodium to greater than 147 mEq per L. A patient who is conscious usually experiences increased thirst. Hypotension can occur if the complication is not recognized early. Treatment with DDAVP 0.25 mL (1 mg) subcutaneously or intravenously is indicated when diabetes insipidus is recognized. DDAVP is usually given twice a day. One must be cautious that the patient is actually experiencing diabetes insipidus and is not just mobilizing surgical fluids. In a patient who has had a transsphenoidal resection of a pituitary tumor, increased thirst may be present only because the patient's nasal packs force him/her to mouth-breathe. Diabetes insipidus is usually transient, resolving by about 72 hours postoperatively, so the patient should be permitted to drink freely. For this reason, over the first several days, it is probably better to give the DDAVP only when the patient's findings indicate treatment is appropriate. Occasionally, diabetes insipidus may be permanent. Intranasal DDAVP 0.2 mL at night is an effective dosing regime for these patients in the subacute to chronic phases of diabetes insipidus.

Low serum cortisol is frequently not observed acutely in the ICU as patients are usually on glucocorticosteroids. However, after abrupt cessation of steroid treatment, a patient may experience an Addisonian crisis. Hypotension, weakness, and fatigue are the major findings. Because the steroid depletion is acute, hyponatremia, hyperkalemia, and hyperpigmentation generally are not observed. Treatment should be instituted promptly with hydrocortisone 100 mg IV every 6 hours.

Hypothyroidism usually does not become evident for at least a week following surgical injury to the pituitary gland or hypothalamus. Fatigue, lethargy, and hyporeflexia may be present. Laboratory testing shows low T4 and free thyroxine uptake, as well as low thyroid-stimulating hormone. For a patient with a sellar or parasellar tumor, preoperative recognition and treatment of hypothyroidism help prevent this endocrinopathy from becoming evident postoperatively.

Postoperative Central Nervous System Infections

Infections of the central nervous system are uncommon in neuro-oncology patients. Perioperative antibiotics, such as cefazolin 1 gm IV just prior to the skin incision and then for several doses following surgery, reduce the infection rate [24,25]. The likelihood of a postoperative infection in the absence of CSF leak in a clean operative field (one which does not involve the paranasal or mastoid sinuses) is about 0.8% [26]. Should CSF leak occur or if operative time is extended, the risk of infection increases. Infection can occur in any of the operative spaces.

A patient may develop wound cellulitis. This superficial infection is associated with erythema, induration, and sometimes wound drainage or breakdown. The patient may have a fever and/or elevated white blood cell count. This complication usually occurs within the first week after surgery. It will usually respond to antistaphylococcal antibiotics within several days. A 10-day course of antibiotics is usually sufficient. If drainage from the wound is present, then it should be cultured to tailor antibiotics appropriately.

Bone flap infections are more involved than simple postoperative cellulitis. They tend to occur in a delayed fashion. Drainage from a breakdown in the suture line or from the scalp near the bone flap will usually be present and should be cultured. White blood cell count and erythrocyte sedimentation rate are usually elevated. A CT scan of the head may show an epidural purulent collection or a moth-eaten appearance of the bone. Parenteral antibiotics for several weeks are necessary, though usually insufficient by themselves. Unfortunately, because the bone flap is devascularized, removal of the infected bone flap is usually necessary to eradicate the infection. A cranioplasty can be performed 6 months after the infection has resolved to reconstitute the integrity of the skull.

Postoperative meningitis occurs infrequently, usually in the first week after surgery. Fever without another focus of infection, or "stiff neck" are usually present. Lumbar puncture is essential to rule out meningitis. Usually a CT scan is performed first to rule out a structural cause of the change in level of consciousness that frequently accompanies the infection. The occurrence of meningitis often necessitates the return of the patient from the floor to the ICU. If meningitis is suspected, parenteral antibiotics should be instituted immediately after lumbar puncture. If cultures are positive, or the glucose is low in the presence of a neutrophil pleocytosis in the CSF, then a 14-day course of broad-spectrum antibiotics is appropriate [27]. If the cultures are negative, the antibiotics can be stopped.

A patient with cerebral empyema or abscess after surgery for a brain tumor typically experiences headache and other symptoms and signs of elevated ICP. Lateralizing neurologic deficits are often present. A CT or MRI scan with IV contrast is essential. In subdural or epidural empyema, the dura or arachnoid usually densely enhances with an adjacent low-density fluid collection. An abscess will show ring enhancement at the surgical site, which can look very similar to the original tumor in some cases. Suspicion of empyema or abscess necessitates an urgent return to the operating room to drain the collection of pus and obtain cultures. Six weeks of parenteral antibiotics are then necessary.

Radiation-Related Complications

Most patients with high-grade primary brain tumors or metastatic tumors will receive external beam radiation as an adjuvant therapy to control tumor growth for as long as possible. Although such treatment is usually tolerated without difficulty, a patient may have worsening of his/her neurologic condition during treatment. This "early effect" worsening is usually related to cerebral edema. CT scan and MRI show an increase in low density/intensity signal around the tumor volume. The edema tends to be responsive to high-dose glucocorticosteroids. Once the patient improves, steroids can be slowly tapered to usual maintenance doses.

Much more rarely, a patient may deteriorate in a delayed fashion. "Late effects" occur about 6 to 24 months after completing radiation therapy [28]. Imaging studies show intense enhancement in the area treated. It is often difficult to differentiate radiation necrosis from tumor recurrence solely on the basis of a contrast CT or gadolinium MRI as the two entities, particularly in the case of primary glioma, look similar. Single positron emitting CT, MR spectroscopy, or MR arterial spin labeling studies can often be helpful in establishing the diagnosis; tumor tends to have high metabolic activity and blood flow, while radiation necrosis is metabolically hypoactive. Sometimes, a stereotactic brain biopsy may be required to make a definitive diagnosis. High glucocorticosteroid doses are necessary to treat radiation necrosis. Mannitol may initially be required if the patient has significantly deteriorated in order to stabilize the patient and allow steroids the time to work. Occasionally, a craniotomy to remove the necrotic tissue is required as well.

Single-fraction stereotactic radiosurgery is more likely to be associated with the development of symptomatic radiation necrosis than conventional external beam radiation. In radiosurgery, the patient receives a high dose of radiation to the tumor volume, sparing the surrounding normal brain. Even so, the radiation that the surrounding brain receives may exceed its tolerance if previous radiation therapy was also used. Treatment is as described earlier. Approximately 13% to 50% of gliomas and 10% of metastatic tumors treated with radiosurgery may require subsequent surgical decompression [29,30].

SPINAL TUMORS

Spinal tumors are much less common than intracranial tumors. Most patients with spine tumors do not require ICU treatment. Exceptions include patients with spinal tumors involving the cervical spine or those who have had transthoracic approaches to thoracic spinal neoplasms. These patients will frequently have ICU treatment requirements.

A patient with a cervical spinal cord tumor may have compromise of intracostal musculature or decreased diaphragmatic function with resultant inability to maintain adequate ventilation, depending on the level of the tumor. Vital capacity should be assessed every 6 hours, as its decrement will usually be noted before respiratory insufficiency occurs. A decrease below 10 to 12 cc per kg usually requires semiurgent intubation and mechanical ventilation. Once oxygen desaturation is noted, the patient decompensates rapidly, and emergency resuscitative efforts may be required.

After spinal cord surgery, a patient may experience a temporary ileus. Bowel sounds may stop and the abdomen may become distended. Frequently the patient will need a nasogastric tube. No oral or enteral intake is appropriate until the ileus subsides. Medications will need to be given parenterally.

A spinal cord tumor is not infrequently associated with development of a neurogenic bladder. The patient often requires a Foley catheter to decompress the bladder; although such intervention is necessary, it can mask the findings. Attention to urinary retention following removal of the Foley is in order. Urinary tract infections are also not uncommon, either related to long-term Foley placement or suboptimal bladder emptying.

A long-term intermittent catheterization program to maintain bladder volumes less than 500 cc is necessary if urinary retention persists.

SYSTEMIC COMPLICATIONS

Not infrequently, patients with neuro-oncological primary problems will experience systemic complications necessitating evaluation and treatment in the ICU.

Deep Venous Thrombosis and Pulmonary Embolism

Patients with brain and spinal cord tumors are at risk for development of deep venous thrombosis (DVT) and subsequent pulmonary embolism (PE). Decreased movement of an extremity from a motor deficit predisposes the patient to develop a DVT. Additionally, tumors may be associated with a hypercoagulable state, which can also lead to the development of DVT. Precautions, including TED stockings or sequential leg compression boots, should be taken to prevent DVT from developing. Subcutaneous heparin (5,000 units twice a day) or prophylactic enoxaparin is also an option. Venous duplex scanning can recognize DVT before it becomes symptomatic.

DVT should be suspected if the patient complains of leg pain or has a fever or elevated white count without a clear explanation. PE usually presents with shortness of breath and chest pain. Blood gases show hypocarbia with mild to moderate hypoxia. Administration of oxygen is necessary and prompt evaluation with chest x-ray, V/Q scan, and/or spiral CT of the chest is in order.

Once identified, treatment with anticoagulation may be problematic, especially in the immediate postoperative period [31,32]. In a patient at high risk for PE, some advocate anticoagulation beginning 3 to 5 days after surgery [33], though this time frame is not accepted by all. Most often the patient will have placement of an inferior vena cava (Greenfield) filter to prevent PE until 2 weeks have transpired from surgery. After that time, the use of anticoagulation is much less risky and is the preferred treatment.

Cerebral Infarction

Approximately 15% of cancer patients have significant cerebrovascular pathology noted at autopsy [34]. Patients with primary brain neoplasms are also at risk for cerebral infarction. This complication may be related to the hypercoagulable state present in patients with malignancies. Alternatively, because these patients may be older with premorbid atherosclerosis, they may suffer cerebral infarction. This event should be differentiated from hemorrhage into a tumor or progressive tumor enlargement. CT scan or MRI scanning is essential. The issues regarding anticoagulation must be addressed as with DVT or PE. Daily aspirin is generally safe. Coumadin, if indicated, should be reserved for patients who have not had hemorrhage into the tumor and who are at least 2 weeks postoperative.

Systemic Infections

Systemic infections are not uncommon, and most often include pneumonia, urinary tract infections, or sepsis secondary to line placement. Their management does not differ in the neurooncology patient from any other patient in the ICU.

END OF LIFE IN THE ICU

Unfortunately, despite the variety of available therapies, almost all primary high-grade gliomas will progress, and the patient harboring the tumor will succumb to the disease. A patient with metastatic brain disease may fail tumor treatments as well. Ideally, the patient's physicians will have discussed these possibilities as the patient begins to show signs of decline. The patient and family may decide to limit the intensity of care, and treatment in the ICU is not an issue. However, a patient may deteriorate quickly from the illness and elevated ICP before limits on treatment can be discussed and defined. When these circumstances occur, the physicians in the ICU may need to discuss limiting care with the patient and family. The most intensive interventions—surgery, ventriculostomy, and intubation for hyperventilation—may be most readily decided against. Other interventions, such as mannitol, may be withheld. Sometimes, a decision is made to stop all treatment. Abrupt cessation of Decadron generally leads to a rapid demise of the patient.

On occasion, an aggressively treated patient will continue to deteriorate. Elevated ICP can cause cardiac arrhythmias in the end stage. Prior to the onset of such cardiac difficulties, however, the patient may progress to the point of "brain death." In the United States, the definition of brain death requires that the patient is not hypotensive, hypothermic, or on paralytic or sedative medications. The etiology of the patient's condition should be known. The clinical examination shows the patient to be comatose, without any brainstem reflexes, motor responses, or spontaneous respirations, and on no sedative medications. An apnea test is also necessary. In this test, the patient is provided flow-by oxygen at 100% to maintain adequate oxygenation. The patient is disconnected from the ventilator and observed for the absence of respirations for 10 minutes (until a PCO_2 of 60 mm Hg is reached). Confirmatory tests, such as electrocerebral silence on an electroencephalogram or absence of brain blood flow on a radionucleotide cerebral flow study, can also be helpful [35]. If these criteria are present, the patient should be declared brain dead and removed from life support. Organ donation can be considered and discussed with the family, although systemic malignancy, infection, or specific organ failure would be contraindications to donation.

References

1. Bartkowski H: Peritumoral edema. *Prog Exp Tumor Res* 27:179, 1984.
2. Bruce J, Criscuolo G, Merrill M, et al: Vascular permeability induced by protein product of malignant brain tumors: inhibition by dexamethasone. *J Neurosurg* 67:880, 1987.
3. Black KL, Hoff JT, McGillicuddy JE, et al: Increased leukotriene C4 and vasogenic edema surrounding brain tumors in humans. *Ann Neurol* 19:592, 1986.
4. Muizelaar J, Wei E, Kontos H, et al: Mannitol causes compensatory cerebral vasoconstriction and vasodilation in response to blood viscosity changes. *J Neurosurg* 59:822, 1983.
5. Origitano TC, Wascher TM, Reichman OH, et al: Sustained increase in cerebral blood flow with prophylactic hypertensive hypervolumic hemodilution ("triple-H" therapy) after subarachnoid hemorrhage. *Neurosurg* 27:729–740, 1990.
6. Wildenthal K, Skelton CL, Coleman HN III: Cardiac muscle mechanics in hyperosmotic solutions. *Am J Physiol* 217:302–306, 1969.
7. Peterson B, Khanna S, Fisher B, et al: Prolonged hypernatremia controls elevated intracranial pressure in head-injured pediatric patients. *Crit Care Med* 28:1136–1143, 2000.
8. Shapiro WR, Posner JB: Corticosteroid hormones: effects in an experimental brain tumor. *Arch Neurol* 30:217, 1974.

9. Yamada K, Ushio Y, Hayakawa T, et al: Effects of methylprednisolone on peritumoral brain edema: a quantitative autoradiography study. *J Neurosurg* 59:612, 1983.
10. Muizelaar JP, van der Poel HG, Li ZC, et al: Pial arteriolar vessel diameter and CO_2 reactivity during prolonged hyperventilation in the rabbit. *J Neurosurg* 69:923, 1988.
11. Weaver D, Winn R, Jane J: Differential intracranial pressure in patients with unilateral mass lesions. *J Neurosurg* 55:660, 1982.
12. Raimondi A, Tomita T: Hydrocephalus and infratentorial tumors: incidence, clinical picture and treatment. *J Neurosurg* 55:174, 1981.
13. Sekhar L, Moossy J, Guthkelch N: Malfunctioning ventriculoperitoneal shunts: clinical and pathological features. *J Neurosurg* 56:411, 1982.
14. Ketz E: Brain tumors and epilepsy, in Vinken JPJ, Bruyn GW (eds): *Handbook of Clinical Neurology.* Vol. 16. Amsterdam, Elsevier, 1974, p 254.
15. McKeran R, Thomas D: The clinical study of gliomas, in Thomas DGT, Graham DI (eds): *Brain Tumours: Scientific Basis, Clinical Investigation and Current Therapy.* London, Butterworths, 1980, p 194.
16. Chalk J, Ridgeway K, Brophy T, et al: Phenytoin impairs the bioavailability of dexamethasone in neurological and neurosurgical patients. *J Neurol Neurosurg Psychiatry* 47:1087, 1984.
17. Wong D, Longenecker RG, Liepman M, et al: Phenytoin-dexamethasone: a potential drug interaction. *JAMA* 254:2062, 1985.
18. Glantz M, Recht LD: Epilepsy in the cancer patient, in Vecht CJ (ed): *Handbook of Clinical Neurology. Vol 25(69). Neuro-Oncology, Part III.* New York, Elsevier, 1997, p 9.
19. Cohen N, Stauss G, Lew R, et al: Should prophylactic anticonvulsants be administered to patients with newly-diagnosed cerebral metastases? A retrospective analysis. *J Clin Oncol* 6:1621, 1988.
20. Fadul C, Wood J, Thaler H, et al: Morbidity and mortality of craniotomy for excision of supratentorial gliomas. *Neurology* 38:1374, 1988.
21. Teasdale G, Jennett B: Assessment of coma and impaired consciousness. *Lancet* 2:81–84, 1974.
22. Jennett B, Teasdale G, Galbraith S, et al: Severe head injuries in three countries. *J Neurol Neurosurg Psychiatry* 40:291, 1977.
23. Gumprecht H, Lumenta CB: Intraoperative imaging using a mobile computed tomography scanner. *Minim Invasive Neurosurg* 46(6):317–322, 2003.
24. Haines S: Efficacy of antibiotic prophylaxis in clean neurosurgical operations. *Neurosurgery* 24:401, 1989.
25. Barker FG: Efficacy of prophylactic antibiotics for craniotomy: a meta-analysis. *Neurosurgery* 35:484, 1994.
26. Narotam PK, van Dellen JR, du Trevou MD, et al: Operative sepsis in neurosurgery: a method of classifying surgical cases. *Neurosurgery* 34:409, 1994.
27. Ross D, Rosegay H, Pons V: Differentiations of aseptic and bacterial meningitis in postoperative neurosurgical patients. *J Neurosurg* 69:669, 1988.
28. Leibel SA, Sheline GE: Radiation therapy for neoplasms of the brain. *J Neurosurg* 66:1, 1987.
29. McDermott MW, Chang SM, Keles GE, et al: Gamma knife radiosurgery for primary brain tumors, in Germano IM (ed): *LINAC and Gamma Knife Radiosurgery.* United States, American Association of Neurological Surgeons, 2000, p 189.
30. Alexander EA, Loeffler JS: Radiosurgery using a modified linear accelerator. *Neurosurg Clin N Am* 3:174, 1992.
31. Swann K, Black PM: Management of symptomatic deep venous thrombosis and pulmonary embolism on a neurosurgical service. *J Neurosurg* 64:563, 1986.
32. Choucair A, Silver P, Levin V: Risk of intracranial hemorrhage in glioma patients receiving anticoagulant therapy for venous thromboembolism. *J Neurosurg* 66:357, 1987.
33. Lazio BE, Simard JM: Anticoagulation in neurosurgical patients. *Neurosurgery* 45:838, 1999.
34. Graus F, Rogers L, Posner J: Cerebrovascular complications in patients with cancer. *Medicine* 64:16, 1985.
35. Wijdicks EFM: The diagnosis of brain death. *N Engl J Med* 344:1215, 2001.

CHAPTER 175 ■ GUILLAIN–BARRÉ SYNDROME

ISABELITA R. BELLA AND DAVID A. CHAD

Guillain–Barré syndrome (GBS) was described by Guillain, Barré, and Strohl in 1916 as an acute flaccid paralysis with areflexia and elevated spinal fluid protein without pleocytosis [1]. It is the most common cause of rapidly progressive weakness due to peripheral nerve involvement, with an annual incidence of 0.6 to 2.0 cases per 100,000 population [2]. For decades, GBS has been viewed as an acute inflammatory *demyelinating* polyradiculoneuropathy (AIDP) affecting nerve roots and cranial and peripheral nerves of unknown cause that occurs at all ages. In the past 20 years, the recognition of primary *axonal* forms of GBS has broadened the spectrum of GBS to include both the demyelinating form (AIDP) and axonal forms—acute motor axonal neuropathy (AMAN) and acute motor sensory axonal neuropathy (AMSAN), as well as the Miller–Fisher syndrome. AIDP is the most common subtype in developed countries, while axonal forms are more common in northern China.

Over the years, it has become clear that the condition may be fatal because of respiratory failure and autonomic nervous system abnormalities [3]. It is, therefore, recognized as a potential medical and neurologic emergency that may require the use of intensive care units (ICUs) experienced in handling the complications of the illness [4].

DIAGNOSIS

Clinical Features in Acute Inflammatory Demyelinating Polyradiculoneuropathy

GBS often occurs 2 to 4 weeks after a flulike or diarrheal illness caused by a variety of infectious agents [3], including cytomegalovirus, Epstein–Barr and herpes simplex viruses, mycoplasma, chlamydia, and *Campylobacter jejuni* [5]. It can also be an early manifestation of human immunodeficiency virus (HIV) infection before the development of an immunosuppressed state [6]. Lyme disease may rarely produce a syndrome of polyradiculopathy reminiscent of GBS [7]. Other antecedent events include immunization, general surgery and renal transplantation, Hodgkin's disease, and systemic lupus erythematosus [2,3].

The illness is heralded by the presence of dysesthesias of the feet or hands, or both. The major feature is weakness that evolves rapidly (usually over days) and classically has been described as ascending from legs to arms and, in severe cases, to respiratory and bulbar muscles. Weakness may, however, start in the cranial nerves or arms and descend to the legs or start simultaneously in the arms and legs [2]. Approximately 50% of patients reach the nadir of their clinical course by 2 weeks into the illness, 80% by 3 weeks, and 90% by 1 month [8]. Progression of symptoms beyond 4 weeks but arresting within 8 weeks has been termed *subacute inflammatory demyelinating polyneuropathy* (SIDP) [9], while progression beyond 2 months is designated *chronic inflammatory demyelinating polyradiculoneuropathy* (CIDP), a disorder with a natural history different from GBS [10]. A small percentage of patients (2% to 5%) have recurrent GBS [11].

The extent and distribution of weakness in GBS are variable. Within a few days, a patient may become quadriparetic and respirator dependent, or the illness may take a benign course and after progression for 3 weeks produce only mild weakness of the face and limbs.

Physical Findings

In a typical case of moderate severity, the physical examination discloses symmetric weakness in proximal and distal muscle groups associated with attenuation or loss of deep tendon reflexes (Table 175.1). In the early stage of illness, there is no muscle wasting or fasciculation. If the attack is particularly severe and axons are interrupted, then after a number of months, muscles undergo atrophy and scattered fasciculations may be seen (see later). Sensory loss is usually mild, although a variant of GBS is described in which sensory loss (involving large fiber modalities) is widespread, symmetric, and profound [8]. Respiratory muscles are often involved; between 10% and 25% of patients require ventilator assistance [12] initiated within 18 days (mean of 10 days) after onset [13].

There is often mild to moderate bilateral facial weakness. Mild weakness of tongue muscles and the muscles of deglutition may also develop. Ophthalmoparesis from extraocular motor nerve involvement is unusual in the typical patient with GBS. In the Miller–Fisher variant [14], however, there is ophthalmoplegia in combination with ataxia and areflexia, with little limb weakness per se. Pupillary abnormalities have been noted in GBS [15] and in the Miller–Fisher variant [16]. Papilledema is exceedingly rare [17].

Disturbances of the autonomic nervous system are found in 50% of patients and are potentially lethal [3,4]. Autonomic dysfunction takes the form of excessive or inadequate activity of the sympathetic nervous system or the parasympathetic nervous system, or both [18]. Common findings include cardiac arrhythmias (e.g., persistent sinus tachycardia, bradycardia, ventricular tachycardia, atrial flutter, atrial fibrillation, and asystole), orthostatic hypotension, and transient and persistent hypertension. Other changes include transient bladder paralysis, increased or decreased sweating, and paralytic ileus. These changes are not completely understood but may be due to inflammation of the thinly myelinated and unmyelinated axons of the peripheral autonomic nervous system. A neuropathy predominantly affecting the peripheral autonomic nervous system has been described that may have a pathogenesis similar to that of GBS [19].

TABLE 175.1

FEATURES OF GUILLAIN–BARRÉ SYNDROME

Clinical features	Laboratory features
Rapidly progressive weakness Loss of reflexes Mild dysesthesias (in AIDP) Autonomic dysfunction Respiratory compromise	Elevated cerebrospinal fluid protein Acellular cerebrospinal fluid Electromyogram: In AIDP: slow nerve conduction velocities, conduction block, dispersed responses In axonal GBS: low motor amplitudes, normal conduction velocities, and normal sensory responses in AMAN

AIDP, acute inflammatory demyelinating polyradiculoneuropathy; AMAN, acute motor axonal neuropathy; GBS, Guillain–Barré syndrome.

Clinical Features in Axonal Forms

Axonal forms, like AIDP, present with rapidly progressive weakness, areflexia, and albuminocytological dissociation but differ in the following ways. AMAN patients lack sensory abnormalities and are more commonly found in northern China during summer months among children and young adults. Patients with AMAN also appear to have a more rapid progression to nadir, but recovery times are quicker [20] or similar [21] to AIDP in some patients, while others have a more prolonged course [20].

AMSAN is generally associated with a more severe course and longer time to recovery. In the series by Feasby et al. [22], these patients had a much shorter time to peak severity (1 week), more severe symptoms with more than half requiring mechanical ventilation, inexcitable motor nerves, and most had a poor recovery.

Laboratory Features

The most characteristic laboratory features of GBS are an abnormal cerebrospinal fluid (CSF) profile showing albuminocytologic dissociation (elevated protein without pleocytosis) and abnormal nerve conduction studies.

CSF examination is most helpful in reaching the diagnosis of GBS. Although the CSF profile is usually normal during the first 48 hours after onset [8], by 1 week into the illness, the CSF protein is elevated in most patients, sometimes to levels as high as 1 g per dL. Rarely, even several weeks after onset of GBS, the CSF protein remains normal and the diagnosis must rest on the presence of otherwise typical clinical features [8]. The cell count may be slightly increased but rarely exceeds 10 cells per μL; the cells are mononuclear in nature. When GBS occurs as a manifestation of HIV infection or Lyme disease, the CSF white cell count is generally increased (25 to 50 cells per μL. The CSF glucose is expected to be normal.

Electrodiagnostic studies in AIDP typically disclose slowing (less than 80% of normal) of nerve conduction velocity, most often along proximal nerve segments, with increases in distal motor and sensory latencies [8,23]. The amplitude of the evoked motor responses may be reduced because of axon loss or distal nerve conduction block, and the responses are frequently dispersed because of differential slowing along still-conducting axons [8,23]. Because the pathologic process may be restricted to spinal nerve roots and proximal nerve segments, routine nerve conduction studies may be normal on initial testing. In such cases, however, H-reflexes may be absent and F-responses may be abnormal because of involvement of the most proximal segments of the motor fibers. This, together with a normal sural nerve and abnormal upper extremity sensory action potential, is characteristic of early GBS [24].

Also early in the course of GBS, needle electrode examination electromyography may demonstrate only decreased numbers of motor unit potentials firing on voluntary effort because of nerve conduction block. Several weeks later, active denervation changes, such as fibrillation potentials and positive sharp waves, may be seen if axon loss has occurred.

In patients with the severe axonal form of GBS, AMSAN, motor and sensory nerves may be electrically inexcitable [22]. In AMAN, motor responses are low or absent while conduction velocities and sensory responses are normal [25].

Except for a mild increase in the erythrocyte sedimentation rate, hematologic studies are normal. Serum electrolytes may disclose hyponatremia [3], sometimes to a marked degree, because of inappropriate secretion of antidiuretic hormone caused by a disturbance of peripheral volume receptors. There may be evidence of previous viral or *mycoplasma* infection, such as lymphopenia or atypical lymphocytes. In some cases, evidence of recent viral infection may be sought by measuring antibody (immunoglobulin [Ig] M) titers against specific infectious agents, especially cytomegalovirus, Epstein–Barr virus, and *C. jejuni*. In selected cases, screening for HIV infection should be undertaken.

DIFFERENTIAL DIAGNOSIS

A number of well-defined conditions cause an acute or subacute onset of generalized weakness and must be differentiated from GBS (Table 175.2). These are disorders of the motor unit affecting the neuromuscular junction (e.g., myasthenia gravis and botulism), peripheral nerve (e.g., tick paralysis, shellfish poisoning, toxic neuropathy, acute intermittent porphyria, and diphtheritic neuropathy), motor neuron (e.g., amyotrophic lateral sclerosis, poliomyelitis, and West Nile virus [WNV] neuroinvasive disease), and muscle (e.g., periodic paralysis, metabolic myopathies, and inflammatory myopathies). Other conditions characterized by severe generalized weakness are defined by the setting in which they are encountered—the ICU—and are designated *critical illness polyneuropathy* and the *myopathy of intensive care.*

Intensive Care Unit–Related Weakness

Unlike neuromuscular emergencies such as GBS, myasthenia gravis, or porphyria, in which rapidly progressive weakness develops before admission to the ICU, a number of conditions (polyneuropathy, myopathy, and neuromuscular junction disease) affect patients already in the ICU because of severe systemic illnesses. These conditions are discussed in more detail in Chapter 180. Critical illness polyneuropathy is an axonal sensory-motor polyneuropathy characterized by difficulty weaning from the ventilator, distal greater than proximal muscle weakness, and reduced or absent reflexes that develop in patients with sepsis and multiorgan failure [26]. The development of weakness in the midst of critical illness, as seen in critical illness polyneuropathy, helps differentiate this disorder from axonal GBS, in which weakness develops days to weeks after an infection [27]. A severe necrotizing myopathy can also be seen in critically ill patients [28]. An acute myopathy of intensive care initially described in patients treated with a combination of high-dose corticosteroids (equal to or greater than 1,000 mg methylprednisolone) and neuromuscular blocking agents (NMBAs) for status asthmaticus [29] may also be encountered in the setting of trauma, organ transplantation, burns, and critical illness. Patients have variable degrees of generalized weakness, including respiratory muscles, and this is often recognized when a patient has difficulty weaning from the ventilator. Prolonged neuromuscular blockade after use of the nondepolarizing NMBAs can be seen especially in patients with coexistent renal failure and metabolic acidosis. Presumably, the presence of an active metabolite accounts for the prolonged weakness [30].

TABLE 175.2

CONDITIONS THAT MAY MIMIC GUILLAIN–BARRÉ SYNDROME

Disorder	Major distinguishing features
Myasthenia gravis	Reflexes are spared Ocular weakness predominates Positive response to edrophonium EMG: decremental motor response
Botulism	Predominant bulbar involvement Autonomic abnormalities (pupils) EMG: normal velocities, low amplitudes, incremental response (with high-frequency repetitive nerve stimulation)
Tick paralysis	Rapid progression (1–2 d) Tick present
Shellfish poisoning	Rapid onset (face, finger, toe numbness) Follows consumption of mussels/clams
Toxic neuropathies	EMG: usually axon loss
Organophosphorus	Acute cholinergic reaction toxicity
Porphyric neuropathy	Mental disturbance Abdominal pain
Diphtheritic neuropathy	Prior pharyngitis Slower evolution Palatal/accommodation paralysis Myocarditis
Poliomyelitis	Weakness, pain, and tenderness Preserved sensation Cerebrospinal fluid: protein and cell count elevated
West Nile virus neuroinvasive disease	Associated fever, meningitis, or encephalitis Asymmetric weakness Cerebrospinal fluid: protein and cell count elevated
Periodic paralysis	Reflexes normal Cranial nerves and respiration spared Abnormal serum potassium concentration
Critical illness neuropathy	Sepsis and multiorgan failure >2 wk EMG: axon loss
Acute myopathy of intensive care	Tetraparesis and areflexia Follows prolonged treatment with neuromuscular-blocking agent and corticosteroids Trauma, status asthmaticus, and organ transplantation associated Clinical and EMG features of myopathy

EMG, electromyogram.

Disorders of the Neuromuscular Junction

In patients with myasthenia gravis, limb weakness is predominant proximally and almost always associated with ocular and sometimes pharyngeal muscle weakness (see Table 175.2; see Chapter 176). Muscular fatigability is a hallmark of the disease. Botulism may also cause acute weakness 6 to 36 hours after ingestion of the toxin formed by *Clostridium botulinum*. The condition is characterized by weakness of cranial nerve–innervated muscles, autonomic abnormalities (unreactive pupils and ileus), and occasional respiratory muscle weakness necessitating ventilator assistance.

Disorders of Peripheral Nerve

Tick paralysis is produced by a toxin contained in the head of the tick *Dermacentor andersoni* or *vanabilis* that blocks nerve conduction in the fine terminal portions of motor and sensory nerves. Weakness associated with sensory impairment develops rapidly after the tick has embedded itself into the victim, usually over 1 to 2 days. Shellfish poisoning gives rise to symptoms immediately after contaminated mussels or clams are eaten. Patients complain of face, finger, and toe numbness and then note the development of rapidly progressive descending paralysis, which may involve respiratory muscles.

Toxic neuropathies may be caused by a number of heavy metals, including arsenic, thallium, and lead. These and other potential neurotoxins (e.g., nitrofurantoin) and industrial agents (e.g., the hexacarbons) may produce a rapidly evolving peripheral neuropathy. Most acute toxic neuropathies are axon-loss in character, but in the case of arsenic poisoning, electrodiagnostic features may simulate a demyelinating process identical to some forms of GBS [31]. Organophosphorus insecticide toxicity causes a short-lived acute cholinergic phase marked by miosis, salivation, sweating, and fasciculation followed in 2 to 3 weeks by an acute axon-loss polyneuropathy [32]. An intermediate syndrome occurring 24 to 96 hours after the cholinergic phase and characterized by multiple cranial nerve palsies and respiratory failure has also been described [33]. The latter probably results from a defect at the neuromuscular junction.

Acute intermittent porphyria causes an acute polyneuropathy clinically similar to GBS but differing by its association with mental disturbance and abdominal pain. Attacks of paralysis are precipitated by ingestion of a variety of drugs, including alcohol, barbiturates, estrogens, phenytoin, and sulfonamides. The diagnosis may be established by demonstrating increased levels of porphobilinogen and δ-aminolevulinic acid in the urine.

Diphtheritic neuropathy occurs 2 to 8 weeks after a throat infection. During the height of the infection, there is numbness of the lips and paralysis of pharyngeal and laryngeal muscles. At the time of the neuropathy, diphtheria organisms may be cultured from the throat. Other clues to the diagnosis are clinical and electrocardiographic features of myocarditis.

Disorders of Motor Neurons

Amyotrophic lateral sclerosis is a chronic disorder of the motor system that generally evolves over several years to produce a state of severe generalized muscle weakness, atrophy, and fasciculations. In most instances, respiratory muscle weakness occurs in the latter stages of the illness after the diagnosis has been established. Rarely, however, patients present with acute to subacute respiratory muscle weakness (ventilatory failure) as the first clinical manifestation of this disease. The examination of such patients often discloses some features of lower motor neuron loss (muscle atrophy and fasciculations) in limb and bulbar muscles. The presence of brisk deep tendon reflexes and preserved sensation helps to distinguish this disorder from the neuropathies that might cause acute ventilatory failure. Unlike the situation in GBS where a picture of albuminocytologic dissociation is found, the CSF findings in amyotrophic lateral sclerosis are normal.

Poliomyelitis is rarely seen today, but it has developed in close contacts of newborns immunized with the live attenuated oral vaccine, and individuals whose own immunity to the virus has become inadequate. The disease is characterized by weakness of rapid onset along with severe muscle pain and tenderness. Respiratory muscles are often involved. Deep tendon reflexes are depressed. The illness is distinguished from GBS clinically by the preservation of sensation and the CSF findings. Serum antibody studies may help identify the illness.

A poliomyelitis-like syndrome may also be seen with WNV neuroinvasive disease. Infection of the anterior horn cells by the WNV produces an acute flaccid paralysis, with asymmetric weakness of one or more limbs, particularly the legs, along with hyporeflexia or areflexia. Overt sensory loss is typically absent while loss of bowel and bladder function may occur. Unlike GBS, there may be an associated meningitis, encephalitis, or fever in addition to CSF pleocytosis and elevated CSF protein. Diagnosis depends on detection of WNV-specific antibodies in serum or CSF [34].

Disorders of Muscles

Periodic paralysis (hyperkalemic or hypokalemic) is a disorder of muscle usually inherited in an autosomal-dominant fashion. Patients develop generalized weakness over a period of hours (see Table 175.2). Cranial nerve–supplied muscles are spared, there is generally no respiratory muscle involvement, reflexes are normal, and there is no sensory involvement. Serum potassium measurements aid in the diagnosis.

Rarely, metabolic myopathies may present with the sudden onset of muscle weakness. Patients with abnormalities of glycogen metabolism (e.g., phosphorylase deficiency) or lipid metabolism (e.g., carnitine palmityl transferase deficiency) may develop weakness associated with severe cramps and muscle fiber necrosis; the latter may result in creatine kinase elevations and myoglobinuria.

Dermatomyositis, an inflammatory myopathy, may present with the acute onset of proximal muscle (and, rarely, respiratory muscle) weakness. In contrast to the acute polyneuropathies, deep tendon reflexes are spared, cranial nerves are rarely involved, and serum creatine kinase is elevated.

PATHOGENESIS

AIDP is caused by immunologically mediated demyelination of the peripheral nervous system [3]. It is likely that humoral and cellular components of the immune system participate in macrophage-induced peripheral nerve demyelination [2,35]. Although the histological appearance of AIDP resembles experimental autoimmune neuritis, in which a predominantly T-cell–mediated immune response is directed against peripheral nerve myelin proteins, the role of T-cell–mediated immunity in AIDP remains unclear [35]. The finding of complement activation markers along the outer surface of the Schwann cell [36] have led to the speculation that complement-fixing antibodies directed toward as yet unidentified epitopes on the outer surface of the Schwann cell play a role in AIDP. Axonal degeneration may occur, especially in severe cases, as a "bystander" when there is intense inflammation [37,38].

In axonal subtypes, the immune response is targeted to a different portion of the peripheral nerve, the axon [39]. There is strong evidence that antibodies directed against ganglioside antigens on the axolemma target macrophages to invade the axon at the node of Ranvier [35]. The rapid decline and subsequent quick recovery in many AMAN patients suggests that severe axonal degeneration of the nerve roots is unlikely to be the pathological basis for this disorder; proposed mechanisms include physiological block of conduction or very distal degeneration and subsequent regeneration of the intramuscular motor nerve terminals [21].

The presence of antiganglioside antibodies (GM1 antibodies in both demyelinating and axonal GBS, and GD1 a, GM1b, and GalNAcGD1 a antibodies in axonal GBS) and the finding of ganglioside-like epitopes on some strains of *C. jejuni* have led to the concept of molecular mimicry [40], in which an immune attack occurs on the epitope shared by the nerve fiber and infectious organism [41], as a possible mechanism for GBS, especially *C. jejuni*–associated GBS. There is increasing evidence that anti-GM1 antibodies block sodium ion channels at the nodes of Ranvier, transiently producing conduction failure [42]. In addition, Koga et al. [43] found evidence that the genetic polymorphism of *C. jejuni* determines the production of specific autoantibodies and correlates with the clinical presentation of GBS, possibly through modification of the host-mimicking molecule.

PATHOLOGY

Pathologic studies of nerves in those patients dying with GBS have usually shown infiltration of the endoneurium by mononuclear cells, with a predilection for a perivenular distribution [37]. The inflammatory process occurs throughout the length of the nerve, from its origin at a root level to the distal ramifications of nerve twigs in the substance of muscle fibers. The brunt of the inflammatory process, however, occurs at more proximal levels (e.g., roots, spinal nerves, and major plexuses) and takes the form of discrete foci of inflammation. Macrophages invade intact myelin sheaths and denude the axons [35]. Patients with prominent axon loss are least likely to recover fully and may be left with functionally significant residual motor weakness.

In AMAN and AMSAN, there is evidence of Wallerian-like degeneration of nerve fibers, but only minimal inflammation or demyelination [25]. Macrophages are seen within the periaxonal space especially at the nodes of Ranvier, displacing or surrounding the axon, and leaving the myelin sheath intact [25]. Abnormalities are seen in nerve roots and peripheral nerves; in those with AMSAN, motor and sensory fibers are affected, while only motor fibers are affected in AMAN, with sparing of sensory fibers.

NATURAL HISTORY

The natural history of GBS in the moderately to severely affected patient (i.e., a patient who is unable to walk or who has severe respiratory muscle weakness requiring a ventilator) is usually one of gradual improvement. The ability to walk unassisted returns, on average, in approximately 3 months; in the subset of respirator-dependent patients, the average time to recovery is 6 months [44].

MANAGEMENT

The three major treatment issues in GBS are controlling respiration and deciding when to intubate the patient, recognizing and managing autonomic dysfunction, and determining which patients are candidates for plasmapheresis or intravenous immunoglobulin (IVIG) (Table 175.3).

TABLE 175.3

MANAGEMENT OF GUILLAIN–BARRÉ SYNDROME

General	Monitor respiratory parameters: VC, arterial blood gas Intubate if: VC <12–15 mL/kg Oropharyngeal paresis with aspiration Falling vital capacity over 4–6 h Respiratory fatigue with VC 15 mL/kg Use short-acting medications to control autonomic dysfunction Nursing care: frequent turns to avoid pressure sores Place pads at elbows and fibular head to avoid compression neuropathies Physical therapy Subcutaneous heparin
Treatment:	
Plasmapheresis	Exchange a total of 200 mL plasma/kg body weight over 7–14 d (40–50 mL/kg for 3–5 sessions)[a] Albumin is used as replacement solution, not fresh-frozen plasma During plasmapheresis, monitor blood pressure and pulse every 30 min Obtain complete blood cell count (baseline and before each exchange to calculate plasma volume) Obtain immunoglobulin levels before first exchange and after last exchange; if immunoglobulin G <200 mg/dL after last plasma exchange, infuse 400 mg/kg IVIG
IVIG	2 g/kg divided over 5 consecutive d[b] (0.4 g/kg/d for 5 d)

[a]This is the authors' approach, following the Guillain–Barré Syndrome Study Group guidelines [44]. Other published guidelines recommend two sessions (exchanging 40 mL/kg per session) for ambulatory patients and four sessions (exchanging 40 mL/kg per session) for nonambulatory patients [53].
[b]The authors adhere to the protocol published by the Dutch Guillain–Barré Study Group [54].
IVIG, intravenous immunoglobulin; VC, vital capacity.

Patients with GBS require excellent nursing care, medical management, and emotional support. Respiratory failure is one of the most serious complications of GBS. Need for a ventilator cannot be reliably predicted on the basis of extent of weakness; however, patients who are highly likely to require mechanical ventilation are those with rapid disease progression, bulbar weakness, autonomic dysfunction, and bilateral facial weakness [45]. Patients must be followed carefully with measurements of maximum inspiratory pressure and forced vital capacity (FVC) (Fig. 175.1) until weakness has stopped progressing so the respiratory insufficiency can be anticipated and managed appropriately. A normal FVC is 65 mL per kg; a level of 30 mL per kg is generally associated with a poor forced cough and requires careful observation and management with supplemental oxygen and chest physical therapy. At 25 mL per kg, the sigh mechanism is compromised and atelectasis occurs, leading to hypoxemia. Ropper and Kehne [46] suggest intubation

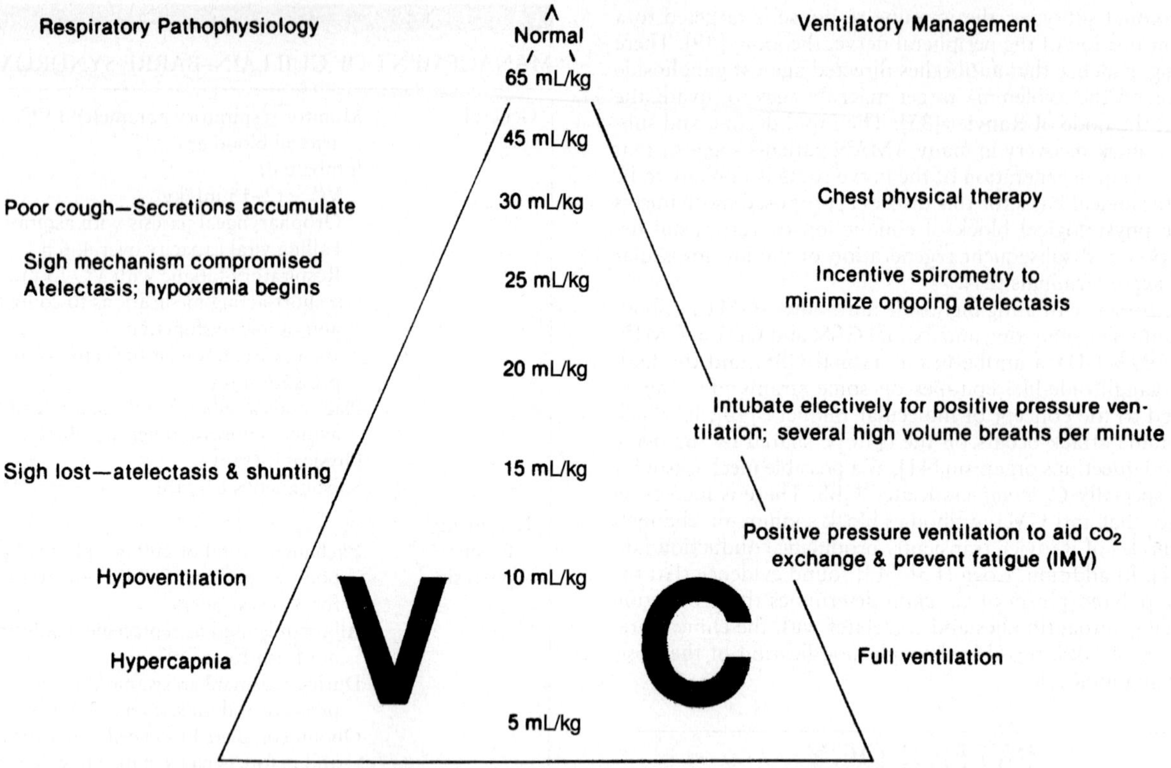

FIGURE 175.1. Relations between vital capacity (VC), pathophysiology of lung function, and suggested therapy in mechanical ventilatory failure. IMV, intermittent mandatory ventilation. [From Ropper AH: Guillain-Barré syndrome, in Ropper AH, Kennedy SK, Zervas NT (eds): *Neurological and Neurosurgical Intensive Care*. Baltimore, University Park Press, 1983, with permission.]

if any one of the following criteria is met: mechanical ventilatory failure with reduced expiratory vital capacity (VC) of 12 to 15 mL per kg, oropharyngeal paresis with aspiration, falling VC over 4 to 6 hours, or clinical signs of respiratory fatigue at a VC of 15 mL per kg. Lawn et al. [45] found the following respiratory factors to be highly associated with progression to respiratory failure: VC less than 20 mL per kg, maximal inspiratory pressure (MIP) less than 30 cm H_2O, maximal expiratory pressure (MEP) less than 40 cm H_2O, or a reduction of more than 30% of VC, MIP, or MEP in 24 hours. Elective intubation may be considered in these patients at particularly high risk for progression to respiratory failure. Intubation should be accomplished with a soft-cuff low-pressure endotracheal tube. A decision to delay tracheostomy for 7 to 10 days is likely to avoid the operation in as many as one-third of patients who improve rapidly and can be extubated after the first few days [46]. Complications of intubation and ventilator assistance are described in Chapters 1 and 58.

The nursing and medical team must also be aware of the many autonomic nervous system disturbances that can occur [18]. Fluctuating blood pressure with transient hypertensive episodes, sometimes associated with extreme degrees of agitation, may be present. Other manifestations of sympathetic nervous system overactivity include sudden diaphoresis, general vasoconstriction, and sinus tachycardia. Evidence of underactivity of the sympathetic nervous system includes presence of marked postural hypotension and heightened sensitivity to dehydration and sedative-hypnotic agents. Excessive parasympathetic nervous system activity is reflected in facial flushing associated with a feeling of generalized warmth and bradycardia. Electrocardiographic changes, consisting of ST- and T-wave changes, also occur. Therefore, careful monitoring of blood pressure, fluid status, and cardiac rhythm is absolutely essential to manage the GBS patient. Hypertension may be managed with short-acting α-adrenergic blocking agents, hypotension with fluids, and bradyarrhythmias with atropine [18]. As noted earlier, hyponatremia may occur and is probably best managed by fluid restriction.

The bedridden patient needs to be turned frequently to avoid the development of pressure sores. Paralyzed limbs require the attention of the physiotherapist so that passive limb movements can be carried out and contractures prevented. The treatment team needs to be aware of the potential for development of compression neuropathies (most commonly of the ulnar and peroneal nerves), and insulating pads should be placed over the usual susceptible sites (the elbow and the head of the fibula). Pain may be treated with standard doses of analgesic agents, but they do not often provide adequate relief. Gabapentin or carbamazepine is particularly helpful in treating the pain in the acute phase [47] and, when disabling, epidural morphine may be necessary [48]. Deep venous thrombosis and pulmonary embolism are ever-present dangers in the bedridden patient with immobilized limbs; for these patients, in addition to physical therapy, subcutaneous heparin (5,000 U twice per day) and support stockings are recommended [47].

A number of multicenter studies [44,49,50] showed that plasmapheresis has a beneficial effect on the course of the illness, even in those patients with several poor prognostic signs [51]. Patients treated with plasmapheresis are able to walk, on average, 1 month earlier than untreated patients; respirator-dependent patients so treated walk 3 months sooner than those who do not receive plasma exchange [44]. The GBS study group guidelines recommend exchanging 200 to 250 mL plasma per kg body weight over 7 to 14 days in three to five treatments [44]. Five percent salt-poor albumin is used as replacement fluid (fresh-frozen plasma should be avoided because of risks of hepatitis, HIV, and occasionally pulmonary edema). It is important to keep in mind, however, that there are also possible risks with albumin, including bleeding, thrombosis, and infection (due to loss of coagulating factors and γ-globulins during plasma exchange, which are not present in the albumin replacement fluid). After each exchange, γ-globulin can be infused to prevent infection.

Plasmapheresis, in general, is recommended for patients who have reached or are approaching the inability to walk unaided, who require intubation or demonstrate a falling VC, and who have weakness of the bulbar musculature leading to dysphagia and aspiration [52]. The French Cooperative Group on Plasma Exchange in Guillain–Barré Syndrome [53] also showed that treatment of patients with mild GBS (i.e., those who are still ambulatory) is beneficial; two plasma exchanges were more beneficial than none in time to onset of motor recovery in patients with mild GBS. Patients with moderate (not ambulatory) or severe (mechanically ventilated) GBS benefited from four exchanges; those with severe GBS did not benefit any further with the addition of two more exchanges. Because of its potential for inducing hypotension, patients who have compromise of their cardiovascular system or autonomic dysfunction may not tolerate this procedure. Plasmapheresis is safe in pregnant women and children [4]. Plasmapheresis is generally not used in patients who are no longer progressing 21 days or more after the onset of GBS.

For many years, plasmapheresis was the gold standard in the treatment of GBS. In 1992, a large randomized trial performed by Dutch investigators demonstrated that treatment with IVIG was at least as effective as plasmapheresis and might be superior [54]. A subsequent large randomized controlled trial (the Plasma Exchange/Sandoglobulin Guillain–Barré Syndrome Trial Group) confirmed the equivalence of IVIG and plasma exchange; in addition, there was no substantial benefit in using a combination of plasma exchange followed by IVIG [55]. In light of these studies, plasma exchange or IVIG may be used to treat GBS. Although both treatments are equally efficacious, IVIG has become the preferred treatment because of its relative ease of administration (plasmapheresis is not available in all centers, and it requires good venous access and a stable cardiovascular system). In 3% to 12% of patients given IVIG, side effects may occur that range from minor reactions such as flulike symptoms, headache, nausea, and malaise to more severe side effects, including anaphylactic reactions in IgA-deficient persons, transmission of hepatitis C, aseptic meningitis, and acute renal failure in those with renal insufficiency. Absolute contraindications to IVIG are unusual, however. For example, patients with IgA deficiency may be given an IgA-poor preparation with precautions (can be pretreated with Benadryl or Tylenol), whereas those with renal insufficiency may be given an IVIG sucrose-poor preparation with close monitoring of their renal status.

A recent American Academy of Neurology practice parameter recommends treatment of GBS patients who are unable to walk with either plasmapheresis or IVIG; treatment is beneficial if given within 4 weeks of onset of neuropathic symptoms for plasmapheresis and within 2 weeks (and possibly 4 weeks) of onset for IVIG [56]. For those patients who are still ambulatory, plasmapheresis may also be considered if given within 2 weeks of onset. Treatment with plasmapheresis followed by IVIG is not recommended.

In a small number of patients (5%), spontaneous relapse occurs within days to weeks after treatment with IVIG or plasmapheresis, oftentimes in those treated early in their illness. Relapse rates are similar in frequency between IVIG and plasmapheresis [57]. Although retreatment with the same therapy is commonly practiced [58], generally with half the initial dose used [59], evidence-based literature is lacking regarding the efficacy of repeat treatment [57].

Although it seems intuitively obvious that treatment of GBS with corticosteroids should be beneficial, corticosteroids are generally ineffective. Hughes and colleagues [60] reviewed six randomized trials of corticosteroid use for GBS; they found no significant difference in disability-related outcome between corticosteroid and placebo groups. Oral corticosteroids delayed recovery while IV methylprednisolone alone was not beneficial or harmful [60]. Although the combination of IVIG and IV methylprednisolone (500 mg per day for 5 days) showed no significant difference over IVIG alone unless adjusted for various factors, there is a trend toward shortened time to independent ambulation with combination treatment [58,61]. Corticosteroids are not recommended in the treatment of GBS.

Finally, it is most important to address the emotional needs of the patient with GBS, who will almost certainly be anxious, fearful, and depressed. The strong likelihood of a good outcome, even in ventilated patients, is noted later in this chapter. Sometimes it is helpful for the patient to speak with a person who has recovered from GBS.

OUTCOME AND PROGNOSTIC FACTORS

In most patients recovery occurs over weeks or months, but in some patients, muscle strength may take 1.5 to 2.0 years to reach its best state with an intensive rehabilitation program [2]. Recovery is not always complete, with only approximately 15% of patients resolving with no residual deficits [4]. Another 50% to 65% of patients are restored to nearly normal function and can resume their work and leisure activities, although some degree of ankle dorsiflexor weakness or numbness of the feet is commonly encountered. Many patients never regain normal stretch reflexes. Severe residual motor weakness or major proprioceptive loss that seriously impairs walking occurs in approximately 10% of patients. Despite close monitoring in the ICU, deaths from GBS do occur, with mortality in the range of 3% to 8% [4]. Causes of fatal outcomes include dysautonomia, sepsis, acute respiratory distress syndrome, and pulmonary emboli [4].

Poor prognostic factors include older age ($\geq$50 years), severe disease at nadir (bedbound or requiring mechanical ventilation), rapid onset of disease, and evidence of axonal loss (reflected on electrodiagnostic studies) [35,42,62]. More recently, elevated CSF neurofilament levels predicted poor outcome, presumably reflecting axonal damage of the proximal motor nerve root [63].

SUMMARY

Careful attention to the patient's history and thorough examination usually point to the diagnosis of GBS, which may be corroborated by the CSF findings (i.e., albuminocytologic dissociation) and results of electrophysiologic testing (i.e., acquired demyelinating or axon-loss polyneuropathy). The mainstay of treatment is excellent nursing and medical care, with close attention to respiratory and autonomic function. Although 10% of patients with GBS are left with substantial residual neurologic deficits, the majority improve and resume their premorbid lifestyles; plasmapheresis and IVIG have been shown to enhance recovery.

Advances in the management of GBS, based on randomized controlled trials or meta-analyses of such trials, are summarized in Table 175.4.

TABLE 175.4

ADVANCES IN MANAGEMENT BASED ON MAJOR CONTROLLED CLINICAL TRIALS OF PLASMAPHERESIS AND INTRAVENOUS IMMUNOGLOBULIN IN GUILLAIN–BARRÉ SYNDROME

References	Purpose	Results
44	Compared PE with supportive care	PE showed beneficial effect in time to improve one clinical grade, time to independent walking, and outcome.
53	Compared various PE treatment schedules in three severity groups	Mild group: 2 PEs more effective than none. Moderate group: 4 PEs more effective than 2 PEs. Severe group: 6 PEs not more beneficial than 4 PEs.
50	(a) To determine effect of PE initiated within 17 d onset and (b) to compare albumin and FFP as replacement fluids	PE beneficial when administered early. No significant difference between albumin and FFP but albumin preferred due to less risks.
54	To determine whether IVIG is as effective as PE	IVIG is as effective as PE and may be superior.
55	Compared IVIG with PE, and combined regimen of PE followed by IVIG	PE and IVIG are equivalent in efficacy when treatment is given within the first 2 weeks of symptoms. The combination of PE followed by IVIG was not more beneficial.

IVIG, intravenous immunoglobulin; FFP, fresh-frozen plasma; PE, plasmapheresis.

References

1. Guillain G, Barré JA, Strohl A: Sur un syndrome de radiculo-nevrite avec hyperalbuminose du liquide cephalo-rachidien sans reaction cellulaire: remarques sur les characteres cliniques et graphiques des reflexes tendineux. *Bull Mem Soc Med Hop Paris* 40:1462, 1916.
2. Ropper AH, Wijdicks EFM, Truax BT: *Guillain-Barré Syndrome*. Philadelphia, FA Davis, 1991.
3. Arnason BGW: Acute inflammatory demyelinating polyradiculoneuropathy, in Dyck PJ, Thomas PK, Griffin JW, et al. (eds): *Peripheral Neuropathy*. Philadelphia, WB Saunders, 1993, p 1437.
4. Ropper AH: The Guillain–Barré syndrome. *N Engl J Med* 326:1130, 1992.
5. Ropper AH: Campylobacter diarrhea and Guillain–Barré syndrome. *Arch Neurol* 45:655, 1988.
6. Cornblath DR, McArthur JC, Kennedy PGE, et al: Inflammatory demyelinating peripheral neuropathies associated with human T-cell lymphotropic virus type III infection. *Ann Neurol* 21:32, 1987.
7. Pachner AR, Steere AC: The triad of neurologic manifestations of Lyme disease: meningitis, cranial neuritis, and radiculoneuritis. *Neurology* 35:47, 1985.
8. Asbury AK, Cornblath DR: Assessment of current diagnostic criteria for Guillain–Barré syndrome. *Ann Neurol* 27[Suppl]:S21, 1990.
9. Oh SJ, Kurokawa K, De Almeida DF, et al: Subacute inflammatory demyelinating polyneuropathy. *Neurology* 61:1507, 2003.
10. Barohn R, Kissel J, Warmolts J, et al: Chronic inflammatory polyradiculoneuropathy. Clinical characteristics, course, and recommendations for diagnostic criteria. *Arch Neurol* 46:878, 1989.
11. Grand Maison F, Feasby TE, Hahn AF, et al: Recurrent Guillain–Barré syndrome: clinical and laboratory features. *Brain* 115:1093, 1992.
12. Hahn A: The challenge of respiratory dysfunction in Guillain–Barré syndrome. *Arch Neurol* 58:871, 2001.
13. Andersonn T, Siden A: A clinical study of the Guillain–Barré syndrome. *Acta Neurol Scand* 66:316, 1982.
14. Fisher CM: Unusual variant of acute idiopathic polyneuritis (syndrome of ophthalmoplegia, ataxia and areflexia). *N Engl J Med* 255:57, 1956.
15. Anzai T, Uematsu D, Takahashi K, et al: Guillain–Barré syndrome with bilateral tonic pupils. *Int Med* 33:248, 1994.
16. Mori M, Kuwabara S, Fukutake T, et al: Clinical features and prognosis of Miller–Fisher syndrome. *Neurology* 56:1104, 2001.
17. Ersahin Y, Mutluer S, Yurtseven T: Hydrocephalus in Guillain–Barré syndrome. *Clin Neurol Neurosurg* 97:253, 1995.
18. Lichtenfeld P: Autonomic dysfunction in the Guillain–Barré syndrome. *Am J Med* 50:772, 1971.
19. Suarez GA, Fealey RD, Camilleri M, et al: Idiopathic autonomic neuropathy: clinical, neurophysiologic, and follow-up studies on 27 patients. *Neurology* 44:1675, 1994.
20. Hiraga A, Mori M, Ogawara K, et al: Recovery patterns and long term prognosis for axonal Guillain–Barré syndrome. *J Neurol Neurosurg Psychiatry* 76:719, 2005.
21. Ho TW, Li CY, Cornblath DR, et al: Patterns of recovery in the Guillain–Barré syndromes. *Neurology* 48:695, 1997.
22. Feasby TE, Gilbert JJ, Brown WF, et al: An acute axonal form of Guillain–Barré polyneuropathy. *Brain* 109:1115, 1986.
23. Albers JW: AAEM Case report #4: Guillain–Barré syndrome. *Muscle Nerve* 12:705, 1989.
24. Gordon PH, Wilbourn AJ: Early electrodiagnostic findings in Guillain–Barré syndrome. *Arch Neurol* 58:913, 2001.
25. Griffin JW, Li CY, Ho TW, et al: Guillain–Barré syndrome in northern China: the spectrum of neuropathological changes in clinically defined cases. *Brain* 118:577, 1995.
26. Zochodne DW, Bolton CF, Wells GA, et al: Critical illness polyneuropathy: a complication of sepsis and multiple organ failure. *Brain* 110:819, 1987.
27. Bolton CF: Critical illness polyneuropathy, in Asbury AK, Thomas PK (eds): *Peripheral Nerve Disorders 2*. Boston, Butterworth–Heinemann, 1995, p 262.
28. Helliwell TR, Coakley JH, Wagenmakers AJM, et al: Necrotizing myopathy in critically-ill patients. *J Pathol* 164:307, 1991.
29. Lacomis D, Giuliani MJ, Cott AV, et al: Acute myopathy of intensive care: clinical, electromyographic, and pathological aspects. *Ann Neurol* 40:645, 1996.
30. Segredo V, Caldwell JE, Matthay MA, et al: Persistent paralysis in critically ill patients after long-term administration of vecuronium. *N Engl J Med* 327:524, 1992.
31. Donofrio PD, Wilbourn AJ, Albers JW, et al: Acute arsenic intoxication presenting as Guillain–Barré syndrome. *Muscle Nerve* 10:114, 1987.
32. Senanayake N, Johnson MK: Acute polyneuropathy after poisoning by a new organophosphate insecticide. *N Engl J Med* 306:155, 1982.
33. Senanayake N, Karalliedde L: Neurotoxic effects of organophosphorus insecticides: an intermediate syndrome. *N Engl J Med* 316:761, 1987.
34. Davis LE, DeBiasi R, Goade DE, et al: West Nile virus neuroinvasive disease. *Ann Neurol* 60:286, 2006.
35. Hughes RA, Cornblath DR: Guillain–Barré syndrome. *Lancet* 366:1653, 2005.
36. Hafer-Macko CE, Sheikh KA, Li CY, et al: Immune attack on the Schwann cell surface in acute inflammatory demyelinating polyneuropathy. *Ann Neurol* 39:625, 1996.
37. Asbury AK, Arnason BG, Adams RD: The inflammatory lesion in idiopathic polyneuritis: its role in pathogenesis. *Medicine* 489:173, 1969.
38. Powell HC, Myers RR: The axon in Guillain–Barré syndrome: immune target or innocent bystander? *Ann Neurol* 39:4, 1996.
39. Hafer-Macko C, Hsieh S, Li CY, et al: Acute motor axonal neuropathy: an antibody-mediated attack on axolemma. *Ann Neurol* 40:635, 1996.
40. Willison HJ: The immunobiology of Guillain–Barré syndromes. *J Peripher Nerv Syst* 10:94, 2005.
41. Sheikh KA, Ho TW, Nachamkin I, et al: Molecular mimicry in Guillain–Barré syndrome. *Ann N Y Acad Sci* 845:307, 1998.
42. Vuvic S, Kiernan MC, Cornblath DR: Guillain–Barré syndrome: an update. *J Clin Neurosci* 16:733, 2009.
43. Koga M, Takahashi M, Masuda M, et al: Campylobacter gene polymorphism as a determinant of clinical features of Guillain–Barré syndrome. *Neurology* 65:1376, 2005.
44. The Guillain–Barré Syndrome Study Group: Plasmapheresis and acute Guillain–Barré syndrome. *Neurology* 35:1096, 1985.
45. Lawn ND, Fletcher DD, Henderson RD, et al: Anticipating mechanical ventilation in Guillain–Barré syndrome. *Arch Neurol* 58:893, 2001.

46. Ropper AH, Kehne SM: Guillain–Barré syndrome: management of respiratory failure. *Neurology* 35:1662, 1985.
47. Hughes RAC, Wijdicks EFM, Benson E, et al: Supportive care for patients with Guillain–Barré syndrome. *Arch Neurol* 62:1194, 2005.
48. Rosenfeld B, Borel C, Henley D: Epidural morphine treatment of pain in the Guillain–Barré syndrome. *Arch Neurol* 43:1194, 1986.
49. Dyck PJ, Kurtzke JF: Plasmapheresis in Guillain–Barré syndrome. *Neurology* 35:1105, 1985.
50. The French Cooperative Group on Plasma Exchange in Guillain–Barré Syndrome: Efficiency of plasma exchange in Guillain–Barré syndrome: role of replacement fluids. *Ann Neurol* 22:753, 1987.
51. McKhann GM, Griffin JW, Cornblath DR, et al: Plasmapheresis and Guillain–Barré syndrome: analysis of prognostic factors and the effect of plasmapheresis. *Ann Neurol* 23:347, 1988.
52. McKhann GM, Griffin JW: Plasmapheresis and the Guillain–Barré syndrome. *Ann Neurol* 22:762, 1987.
53. The French Cooperative Group on Plasma Exchange in Guillain–Barré Syndrome: Appropriate number of plasma exchanges in Guillain–Barré Syndrome. *Ann Neurol* 41:298, 1997.
54. Van der Meche FGA, Schmitz PIM, Dutch Guillain–Barré Study Group: A randomized trial comparing intravenous immune globulin and plasma exchange in Guillain–Barré syndrome. *N Engl J Med* 326:1123, 1992.
55. Plasma Exchange/Sandoglobulin Guillain–Barré Syndrome Trial Group: Randomised trial of plasma exchange, intravenous immunoglobulin, and combined treatments in Guillain–Barré syndrome. *Lancet* 349:225, 1997.
56. Hughes RAC, Widjicks EFM, Barohn R, et al: Practice parameter: immunotherapy for Guillain–Barré syndrome. Report of the Quality Standards Subcommittee of the American Academy of Neurology. *Neurology* 61:736, 2003.
57. Donofrio PD, Berger A, Brannagan TH, et al: Consensus statement: the use of intravenous immunoglobulin in the treatment of neuromuscular conditions. Report of the AANEM ad hoc committee. *Muscle Nerve* 40(5):890–900, 2009.
58. Hughes RAC, Swan AV, Raphaël JC, et al: Immunotherapy for Guillain–Barré syndrome: a systematic review. *Brain* 130:2245, 2007.
59. Asbury AK: New concepts of Guillain–Barré syndrome. *J Child Neurol* 15:183, 2000.
60. Hughes RA, Swan AV, van Koningsveld R, et al: Corticosteroids for treating Guillain–Barré syndrome. *Cochrane Database Syst Rev* (2):CD001446, 2006.
61. Van Koningsveld R, Schmitz PIM, van der Meche FGA, et al: Effect of methylprednisolone when added to standard treatment with intravenous immunoglobulin for Guillain–Barré syndrome: randomized trial. *Lancet* 363:192, 2004.
62. Chiò A, Cocito D, Leone M, et al: Guillain–Barré syndrome: a prospective, population-based incidence and outcome survey. *Neurology* 60:1146, 2003.
63. Petzold A, Brettschenider J, Kin K, et al: CSF protein biomarkers for proximal axonal damage improve prognostic accuracy in the acute phase of Guillain–Barré syndrome. *Muscle Nerve* 40:42, 2009.

CHAPTER 176 ■ MYASTHENIA GRAVIS IN THE INTENSIVE CARE UNIT

ISABELITA R. BELLA AND RANDALL R. LONG

Few physicians have more than a passing acquaintance with myasthenia gravis, although it is by no means rare. The key to handling the emergent problems associated with myasthenia is simply the management of airway and ventilatory support with the same care as in any other instance of respiratory failure (see Chapters 1, 58, and 59). With respiration under control, the treatment of the underlying disease can be unhurried and orderly, and in most patients, it is successful. This chapter reviews briefly the pathogenesis, clinical spectrum, and diagnosis of myasthenia gravis and focuses on the intensive care setting, including management of the patient in crisis and in the perioperative period.

PATHOGENESIS

Myasthenia gravis is an autoimmune disorder of neuromuscular transmission [1]. Circulating antibodies react with components of acetylcholine receptors within postsynaptic muscle membrane and activate complement mediated lysis of the muscle membrane, accelerate receptor degradation, and block receptors (i.e., interfere with normal receptor activation by acetylcholine) [2]. The result is fewer receptors that can be activated at affected neuromuscular junctions, causing weaker muscular contraction. Electrophysiologic study of myasthenic neuromuscular junctions discloses miniature end-plate potentials that are diminished in amplitude [3]. These observations have been clearly linked to the receptor alterations and an altered postsynaptic response to normal quantal transmitter release from the presynaptic nerve terminals. Understanding of this underlying pathophysiology has, in turn, enabled rational approaches to treatment. Various immunosuppressive therapies and acetylcholinesterase inhibitors are primary therapeutic options in managing myasthenia gravis (see later).

EPIDEMIOLOGY

Myasthenia gravis is not rare; its prevalence in Western populations is approximately 1 in 20,000 [4]. The overall female to male ratio is approximately 3:2, although there are two distinct sex-specific incidence peaks, with the incidence among women peaking in the third decade and that among men in the fifth to sixth decades. A mild familial predisposition has been noted, although Mendelian inheritance does not apply.

CLINICAL SPECTRUM

The clinical spectrum of myasthenia gravis is characterized as much by its diversity as it is by its common themes. It may range from a mild and relatively inconsequential disease over a normal lifetime to a fulminant incapacitating disorder. The course of given individuals may also vary widely. The clinical hallmarks of the disease are weakness and exaggerated muscle fatigue. The specific muscles involved and the severity of weakness are highly variable, between individuals and within the same individual over time.

Ocular muscles are most frequently involved; diplopia is common, and various patterns of ophthalmoparesis are seen.

Bulbar muscles are also frequently affected, leading to varying combinations of facial paresis, dysarthria, and dysphagia. Ptosis is common, but the pupils are never affected. Limb muscle involvement may vary from very isolated weakness to generalized (usually proximal) weakness and fatigability. Respiratory muscle weakness is unfortunately not rare, and respiratory insufficiency and the inability to handle oral and upper airway secretions are the critical problems that bring myasthenics to the intensive care setting. Myasthenia should also be considered in any patient who cannot be weaned from ventilator support after an otherwise uncomplicated surgical procedure.

Approximately 15% to 20% of myasthenics have only ocular and eyelid involvement. Longitudinal studies indicate that if an individual manifests only oculomotor weakness for more than 2 years, there is little chance of later limb or respiratory weakness. Although several clinical classification schemes have been devised for categorizing myasthenics according to the distribution and severity of their disease, it is preferable to emphasize the fact that myasthenics often fluctuate over time, with variability rather than constancy being the norm. Some factors contributing to fluctuations of strength are recognizable (see later); many fluctuations appear to be random occurrences.

DIAGNOSTIC STUDIES

The diagnosis of myasthenia gravis is clinically suggested in patients who present with chronic ocular, bulbar, or appendicular weakness, variable over time, with preservation of normal sensation and reflexes. More restricted presentations require a much broader differential diagnosis. Myasthenia gravis should always be considered in the differential diagnosis of isolated ocular or bulbar weakness. Again, prominent muscular fatigability and temporal fluctuation are key features of the disease. Normal pupils, normal sensation, and normal reflexes are to be expected and are helpful in diagnosing myasthenia gravis when coincident with an acute or subacute paralytic illness.

Once the diagnosis of myasthenia gravis is suggested, confirmation rests on the exclusion of other diseases and supporting clinical and laboratory studies. It is important to stress that although abnormal tests may be diagnostic, normal test results do not exclude the diagnosis.

Edrophonium Test

Edrophonium hydrochloride (Enlon; formerly "Tensilon") is a fast, short-acting parenteral cholinesterase inhibitor. It reaches peak effect within 1 minute after intravenous injection and persists to some extent for at least 10 minutes. Myasthenic weakness typically improves transiently after administration of 4 to 10 mg (0.4 to 1.0 mL). The edrophonium test may be blinded, with drug or normal saline being injected. Whether drug or placebo, a 0.2-mL test dose is given to screen for excessive cholinergic side effects, such as cardiac arrhythmia, gastrointestinal hyperactivity, or diaphoresis. A crash cart should always be available, and patients with known cardiac disease and elderly patients warrant electrocardiographic monitoring. The remaining 0.8 mL is given after 1 minute. Interpretation of the test depends on identifying and observing an unequivocal baseline muscular deficit that can be improved following the injection of edrophonium. Ptosis and ophthalmoparesis, if present, are semiquantifiable and well suited; if respiratory compromise is present, monitoring maximum inspiratory pressure (MIP) or vital capacity is useful. As a general rule, positive responses are dramatic; if there is any doubt about the positivity of the test, it should be considered negative. False-positive edrophonium tests are quite rare; false negatives are common. In children, the appropriate test dose is 0.03 mg per kg, one-fifth of which may be given as a test dose.

Neostigmine is a longer-acting parenteral cholinesterase inhibitor that sometimes affects a more obvious clinical response. It is also typically associated with more obvious autonomic side effects. The 1.5-mg test dose (0.04 mg per kg in children) should therefore be preceded by 0.5 mg of atropine; both may be given subcutaneously.

Serological Testing

Recognition of the immune nature of myasthenia gravis has provided a relatively sensitive and highly specific diagnostic study. Approximately 85% of myasthenics have detectable serum antibodies, which bind to acetylcholine receptors (AChR) [5]. The sensitivity drops to 70% in those with purely ocular myasthenia [6]. The antibodies themselves constitute a heterogeneous group, reacting against various receptor subunits. Although the actual antibody titer is of little significance, correlating poorly with the severity of disease or clinical response to therapy, the presence of antibodies is a strong indication of the disease. A normal test does not exclude the diagnosis, especially in the patient presenting with predominantly ocular symptoms and signs. Of note, these antibodies have also been found in a small percentage of patients with Lambert–Eaton myasthenic syndrome, autoimmune liver disorder, and patients with lung cancer without neurologic disease [6].

Among seronegative myasthenic patients, from 30% to 70% may be found to have antibodies directed against muscle-specific tyrosine kinase [MuSK], an enzyme that catalyzes acetylcholine receptor aggregation in the formation of neuromuscular junctions [7]. Animal models have also recently shown that MuSK antibodies may reduce acetylcholine receptor clustering and thus impair neuromuscular transmission [8]. Patients who have antibodies to MuSK are often young women (onset of symptoms before 40 years of age) with prominent bulbar involvement [9] and neck or respiratory muscle weakness [7]. They tend to have more severe disease requiring aggressive immunosuppressive treatment [9] and have a higher frequency of respiratory crisis compared to seronegative or AChR-positive myasthenics [10]. Unlike patients with antibodies to AChR, there appears to be a correlation between MuSK antibody levels and disease severity, with antibody levels often decreasing after various immunosuppressive treatments except thymectomy [11].

Striated muscle antibodies that react with muscle proteins titin and ryanodine receptor have also been found, mainly in patients with thymoma and in those with late onset myasthenia (onset of symptoms >50 years of age) [12]. Thus, they may be helpful in the detection or recurrence of thymoma. In addition, they tend to be associated with more severe disease, and therefore may aid in prognosis [12].

Myasthenics also have an increased incidence of other autoantibodies, including antithyroid antibodies, antiparietal cell antibodies, and antinuclear antibodies, although routine screening for these is not part of the diagnostic evaluation for suspected myasthenia gravis.

Electromyographic Studies

The electromyographic hallmark of myasthenia gravis is a decrement in the amplitude of the muscle potential seen after exercise or slow repetitive nerve stimulation. The decrement should be at least 10% and preferably 15% or more. Routine motor and sensory conduction studies are normal, as is the conventional needle examination. The more severely affected patient is more likely to show a decremental response; responses are most consistently elicited from facial and proximal muscles. If a significant decrement is observed, exercising the muscle briefly for 10 seconds transiently reverses the decrement [13]. Single-fiber electromyography is relatively sensitive, documenting increased jitter [14]—variability in the temporal coupling of single fibers within the same motor unit. Increased jitter, however, is far from specific; most peripheral neurogenic diseases also lead to increased jitter.

MISCELLANEOUS STUDIES

Myasthenia gravis may be associated with either malignant thymoma or thymic hyperplasia. Once a diagnosis is established, chest imaging should be obtained. Because there is also a significant association with thyroid and other autoimmune diseases, appropriate screening studies are indicated in the newly diagnosed myasthenic. Muscle biopsy has no role in the evaluation of myasthenia, unless there is a strong consideration of neurogenic or inflammatory weakness.

CRITICAL CARE OF THE MYASTHENIC PATIENT

Patient in Crisis

Crisis refers to threatened or actual respiratory compromise in a myasthenic patient. It may reflect respiratory muscle insufficiency or inability to handle secretions and oral intake, but it is typically a combination of both. With currently available treatments, myasthenic crisis is not common. An occasional patient presents with fulminating disease; crisis management then coincides with initial evaluation and institution of therapy. Otherwise, crisis may be precipitated by other illnesses, such as influenza or other infections, or by surgery.

General Measures

The respiratory function of any acutely deteriorating or severely weak myasthenic should be monitored compulsively. When the weakening myasthenic reaches a point at which increased respiratory effort is required, fatigue often prevents the effective use of secondary muscles, and respiratory failure rapidly ensues. Arterial blood gas values and even oxygen saturation are poor indicators of incipient failure in the face of respiratory muscle compromise. Forced vital capacity (FVC) and MIP are better indices and should be serially charted. The FVC should be assessed with the patient both sitting and supine, because diaphragmatic paresis may be accentuated in the supine position. MIP measurement requires special care if the patient also has significant facial weakness. An FVC less than 20 mL per kg or an MIP greater than (i.e., not as negative as) −40 cm H_2O suggests impending failure and usually warrants intubation. If a downward trend is noted (greater than 30% decrease) [15], elective intubation should be considered even sooner, unless there is a realistic expectation of rapid reversal.

Acute deterioration in a myasthenic always warrants consideration of contributing circumstances or concurrent illness that may accentuate the underlying defect in neuromuscular transmission. The major considerations are listed in Table 176.1 and discussed later.

TABLE 176.1

CONDITIONS THAT MAY UNDERLIE INTERIM DETERIORATION IN MYASTHENIC PATIENTS

Intercurrent infection; occult infection should be excluded
Electrolyte imbalance (Na, K, Ca, P, Mg)
Cholinergic crisis: if any doubt, discontinue cholinesterase inhibitors
Thyrotoxicosis, hypothyroidism
Medication effects (see Table 176.2)

The possibility of cholinergic crisis in patients receiving anticholinesterase drugs (e.g., pyridostigmine), although no longer common, should not be overlooked. The presence of fasciculations, diaphoresis, or diarrhea should alert the clinician to this possibility. In the past, the importance of differentiating between myasthenic crisis and cholinergic crisis was stressed. Edrophonium testing was used to differentiate between the two; abrupt deterioration after a conventional 10-mg test dose indicated overdosage with cholinesterase inhibitors. One had to be adequately prepared for deterioration and increased respiratory secretions. Because oftentimes it is very difficult to determine the response and because of the potential side effects with overdosage of anticholinesterase drugs of increased pulmonary secretions, many authors now recommend discontinuation of cholinesterase inhibitors at the time of crisis [2,16,17] and reinstituting them when patients are stronger. This assumes that adequate respiratory monitoring and support are in effect. A brief holiday from cholinesterase inhibition also often results in an enhanced response to therapy when reinstituted.

Intercurrent infection is often associated with increased weakness in the myasthenic patient. There should be a comprehensive search for systemic infection in the deteriorating patient, particularly the patient receiving immunosuppressive therapy. Any infections should be treated aggressively. Both hypothyroid and hyperthyroid states are often associated with increased weakness. Again, there is an increased association between thyrotoxicosis and myasthenia gravis. The manifestations of electrolyte imbalance may be enhanced in myasthenics. Otherwise, insignificant electrolyte effects on transmitter release or muscle membrane excitability may be amplified at the myasthenic neuromuscular junction. Potassium, calcium, phosphate, and magnesium alterations should be corrected. Myasthenia gravis may also impart enhanced sensitivity to a number of medications that have only minimal effects on neuromuscular function in normal individuals. Aminoglycoside antibiotics, beta-blockers, and many cardiac antiarrhythmics may have adverse effects. Anticholinergics, respiratory depressants, and sedatives of any kind should be avoided or used only with great caution. *Neuromuscular-blocking agents should never be administered to myasthenics in the intensive care unit (ICU) setting*, because they often have profound and prolonged effects. This increased sensitivity occasionally results in postoperative failure to wean in an undiagnosed mild myasthenic who has undergone surgery for an unrelated problem. Table 176.2 provides a comprehensive listing of medications that may further impair neuromuscular transmission in myasthenic patients.

Some attention should also be given to the general environment in which the myasthenic is managed. The typical noisy, brightly illuminated ICU is not conducive to rest and sleep, which are necessities for the myasthenic patient in whom fatigue may be critical.

Special consideration must be given to respiratory care of the myasthenic. Incentive spirometry should be avoided, because muscular fatigue outweighs any potential benefit, even in the postoperative patient. Careful attention to respiratory toilet is key and can be complicated by cholinesterase inhibitors, which increase respiratory secretions. Atropine may be used to minimize this effect, but its other autonomic side effects, such as ileus, constipation, and delirium, may limit longer-term use.

TABLE 176.2

MEDICATIONS THAT MAY ACCENTUATE WEAKNESS IN MYASTHENIC PATIENTS

Antibiotics	Neuromuscular blockers and muscle relaxants	Antiarrhythmics and antihypertensives	Antirheumatics	Antipsychotics	Others
Amikacin	Anectine (succinylcholine)	Lidocaine	Chloroquine	Lithium	Opiate analgesics
Clindamycin	Norcuron (vecuronium)	Quinidine	D-Penicillamine	Phenothiazines	Oral contraceptives
Colistin	Pavulon (pancuronium)	Procainamide		Antidepressants	Antihistamines
Gentamicin	Tracrium (atracurium)	Beta-blockers			Anticholinergics
Kanamycin	Benzodiazepines	Calcium blockers			
Lincomycin	Curare				
Neomycin	Dantrium (dantrolene)				
Polymyxin	Flexeril (cyclobenzaprine)				
Streptomycin	Lioresal (baclofen)				
Tobramycin	Robaxin (methocarbamol)				
Tetracyclines	Soma (carisoprodol)				
Trimethoprim/sulfamethoxazole	Quinamm (quinine sulfate)				

THERAPY IN MYASTHENIC CRISIS

Therapeutic agents used in the critical care setting parallel those available to the patient with milder myasthenia gravis. Immunosuppressive therapies are the major considerations. Any myasthenic in crisis, if not already receiving immunosuppressive therapy, requires it. Symptomatic therapy with cholinesterase inhibitors is now primarily used on a shorter-term basis, pending response to immunomodulating therapies. Plasmapheresis, intravenous human immune globulin, corticosteroids, and longer-term immunosuppressants and cholinesterase inhibitors are discussed individually.

Plasmapheresis

Recognition of the role of immunoglobulins in the pathogenesis of myasthenia gravis stimulated early, uncontrolled clinical trials of plasmapheresis as soon as efficient pheresis technology became available [18]. The results have been quite favorable, prompting the National Institutes of Health Consensus Conference to support its use despite the lack of controlled trials [19]. Most patients demonstrate a significant clinical response within 48 hours of initiation of plasmapheresis, although the response is short lived unless therapy is continued on an intermittent basis. The rapid response from plasmapheresis can be crucial in the face of crisis, providing a short-term reprieve during which alternative therapy can be initiated or any intercurrent medical problems resolved. Approximately 50 mL per kg should be exchanged per session [20], approximating 60% to 70% of total plasma volume. Plasma removed is replaced by an equal volume of normal saline and 5% albumin, adjusted to maintain physiologic concentrations of potassium, calcium, and magnesium. The usual course of treatment includes three to seven pheresis sessions at 24- to 48-hour intervals. Many patients develop increased sensitivity to cholinesterase inhibitors after plasmapheresis; dosage should be correspondingly reduced. The major potential complications of plasmapheresis include hypotension, arrhythmia, and hypercoagulability due to hemoconcentration. Coincident cardiovascular disease is a relative contraindication to plasmapheresis. Although plasmapheresis is too invasive to be used for long-term therapy in the majority of patients, periodic plasmapheresis has been beneficial in some patients with moderate to severe myasthenia refractory to immunosuppressive agents [21]. Selective removal of acetylcholine receptor antibodies using immunoadsorption columns may also be a promising alternative to plasmapheresis, but further clinical studies are required [22].

Intravenous human immune globulin also frequently leads to rapid yet transient improvement in myasthenics [23]. Intravenous immunoglobulin (IVIG) is a therapeutic option in the event of crisis or in the perioperative period, particularly if the patient's cardiovascular status limits plasmapheresis. Although IVIG and plasmapheresis were found to be equally efficacious in some trials [24], others have reported that plasmapheresis was more efficacious than IVIG; however, complications occurred more often with plasmapheresis [25]. The customary dose is 400 mg per kg per day for 5 consecutive days. More recently, a total dose of 1 gram per kilogram was reported to be equally efficacious to 2 gram per kilogram, although there was a trend toward slight superiority of the higher dose [26]. Maximal improvement occurs by the second week after therapy, and the therapeutic response usually persists for several weeks. Patients should be pretreated with acetaminophen and diphenhydramine to prevent flu-like symptoms that commonly occur during infusion. In addition, adequate hydration will help reduce the potential complication of thrombosis. Renal function should be checked prior to initiation of therapy, as renal failure may occur in those with renal insufficiency. Likewise, an IgA level should be obtained as patients with IgA deficiency may develop anaphylaxis.

Longer-Term Immunosuppression

Corticosteroids have proven to be an effective long-term therapy for almost all myasthenics whose clinical manifestations cannot be well managed with low doses of cholinesterase inhibitors. Despite potential side effects associated with corticosteroid therapy, a response rate of greater than 80% supports its use [27]. Side effects can be minimized with appropriate precautions. Carbohydrate metabolism, electrolytes, blood pressure, and diet should be closely monitored; bisphosphonates (e.g., alendronate sodium, 70 mg weekly), calcium (500 to 1,000 mg per day), and vitamin D supplementation (at least 800 to 1,000 IU per day) as well are prudent to minimize osteopenia. Screening for tuberculosis exposure with skin testing and chest radiographs should be done before initiation of therapy. Occult infection must be excluded in the deteriorating myasthenic.

Recommendations regarding corticosteroid preparation, dose, and regimen vary. Approximately one-third of patients may become transiently weaker before they improve, if given high doses of prednisone initially [3]. Initiation with relatively low doses of prednisone and increasing in a stepwise manner has been advocated by some clinicians to minimize interim deterioration, especially if the patient is not intubated [16]. The authors prefer to begin with 15 to 25 mg of prednisone or its equivalent as a single daily dose, increasing the dose by 5 mg every second or third day until a dose of 1 mg per kg per day is reached. In the critical care setting, concurrent plasmapheresis or IVIG may offset initial steroid-related deterioration; high doses of corticosteroids (1 mg per kg per day) can be initiated in this situation, enabling a more rapid response. Oral corticosteroids are preferable since there is a risk of developing acute steroid-induced myopathy in patients with myasthenia who are given high doses of intravenous corticosteroids [17,28].

Once maximal response is obtained, usually within 1 to 2 months, patients may be gradually shifted to alternate-day therapy by concurrently reducing the off-day dose and increasing the on-day dose, with a 10-mg shift made once each week. Some individuals note a definite off-day adverse effect; this can usually be countered with a 10-mg alternate-day dose. Once stabilized on alternate-day therapy, the on-day dose can be tapered by 5 mg per month. Many patients can be maintained in remission with as little as 20 to 25 mg of prednisone every other day (or alternating with 10 mg). Only rare patients remain in remission if therapy is discontinued, and overenthusiastic tapering of steroids is an all too common precipitant of unnecessary disability or even crisis. Myasthenia sometimes remits spontaneously, and if the patient has undergone thymectomy (see later), the probability of remission increases appreciably, making discontinuation of therapy a more realistic option.

Azathioprine is often used as an alternative agent for longer-term immunosuppression. It is effective in 70% to 90% of patients with myasthenia gravis [2] and is often initiated in patients with an insufficient response to corticosteroids, as a steroid-sparing agent, or in patients in whom corticosteroids are contraindicated [3]. Azathioprine is limited by a relatively long delay before its effects are clinically evident, up to 6 to 12 months, but its side-effect spectrum compares favorably with steroids over a time frame of many years. If a patient tolerates a 50-mg per day test dose, the daily dose can be increased by 50 mg each week up to 2 to 3 mg per kg per day. The dose is reduced if the white blood cell count is less than 3,000 per mm^3; an elevated mean corpuscular volume can also be used to assess adequate response [4,29]. In up to 10% of patients, an influenza-like reaction characterized by fever, malaise, and myalgias occurs within the first few weeks of therapy and resolves after discontinuing the drug [2,29]. Patients should be screened for thiopurine methyltransferase (TPMT) deficiency; those homozygous for TPMT mutations cannot metabolize azathioprine and therefore should not receive the drug. Concurrent treatment with allopurinol should also be avoided as it interferes with the degradation of azathioprine, thereby increasing the risk of bone marrow and liver toxicity [29].

Cyclosporine appears to be as effective as azathioprine in the treatment of myasthenia gravis [30] and is used mainly in patients who are intolerant or refractory to azathioprine. Onset of clinical improvement is quicker than with azathioprine, with most patients noticing improvement after 1 to 3 months, and becoming maximal around 7 months [31]. Its major limitations are renal toxicity and hypertension, which are seen in about one-quarter of patients. To minimize side effects, the starting dose of 5 mg per kg per day can be given in two divided doses 12 hours apart, followed by adjustments to maintain a predose trough level in the range of 100 to 150 ng per L. Subsequent adjustments can be made depending on creatinine levels and clinical improvement, with the aim to reduce the dose as much as possible once maximal improvement is obtained [31]. Renal function (blood urea nitrogen and creatinine) must be continually monitored. Significant hypertension and preexisting renal disease are contraindications to the use of cyclosporine.

Another agent from the realm of transplant medicine, mycophenolate mofetil (CellCept), has also been used effectively for longer-term therapy. Several case series, retrospective analysis, and a small placebo controlled, double-blind trial suggested that mycophenolate mofetil is beneficial in patients with myasthenia gravis [32–34]. Because it is better tolerated than other immunosuppressants, it has become widely used. Recently, however, two large double-blinded randomized controlled trials failed to show any benefit of mycophenolate mofetil over placebo in patients with myasthenia gravis [35,36]. One study showed that mycophenolate mofetil was not superior to placebo during a steroid taper [35], while the other study showed no benefit in taking mycophenolate mofetil with 20 mg prednisone compared to taking prednisone alone [36]. Several factors have been proposed to explain these surprisingly negative results including the short duration of the trials, selection of generally mildly affected patients, and the unexpected significant response to low-dose prednisone [2]. Further studies are warranted to establish the role of mycophenolate mofetil in myasthenia. Despite this, mycophenolate mofetil is still widely used in the treatment of myasthenia gravis. The standard dose is 1,000 mg twice a day, but doses up to 3,000 mg per day may be used. Monthly complete blood counts should be performed to monitor for any evidence of myelosuppression.

In refractory cases in which it has proven difficult to achieve or maintain remission, high-dose cyclophosphamide has proven effective [2]. However, it has significant side effects including bone marrow toxicity, hemorrhagic cystitis, teratogenicity, and increased risk of infections and malignancies. Oral dosage ranges from 1 to 5 mg per kg per day [16]. Recently, Drachman and colleagues reported dramatic clinical improvement by "rebooting the immune system" in patients with refractory myasthenia using high-dose cyclophosphamide 50 mg per kg per day for 4 days, followed by granulocyte colony-stimulating factor; clinical improvement lasted several years in some patients [37].

Several case series have reported a beneficial response of rituximab in patients with refractory myasthenia gravis and in those with MuSK myasthenia gravis [38]. Patients tolerated the treatment without significant side effects, making this a promising drug for the future.

Cholinesterase Inhibitors

Cholinesterase inhibition was the mainstay of pharmacotherapy for myasthenia gravis before the advent of immunosuppressive therapies and thymectomy. Many patients are now maintained in remission on corticosteroids or other immunosuppressive agents, while others, in particular, those with mild nonprogressive or purely ocular disease, require only treatment with an oral anticholinesterase drug, such as pyridostigmine (Mestinon). If an acutely deteriorating patient has been taking a cholinesterase inhibitor, the possibility of cholinergic crisis should be entertained. Overdosage of cholinesterase inhibitors may produce weakness accompanied by muscarinic symptoms such as increased pulmonary and gastric secretions, bradycardia, nausea, vomiting, diarrhea, and nicotinic symptoms such as fasciculations [2,17]. Many authors advocate discontinuing anticholinesterase therapy during myasthenic crisis to minimize secretions, avoid potential exacerbation of weakness due to overdosage of cholinergic medications, and allow easier assessment of response to other therapies [16,17]. It is reasonable to reinstitute anticholinesterase therapy when patients are stronger, starting at a low dosage and gradually increasing the dose until there is clear benefit [16].

The use of intravenous anticholinesterase therapy is controversial. Infusion of intravenous pyridostigmine at 1 to 2 mg per hour during crisis was found in one small retrospective study to be comparable to plasmapheresis [39]. However, intravenous therapy carries the risk of dangerous side effects such as cardiac arrhythmias, myocardial infarction (due to coronary vasospasm), airway obstruction, and increased pulmonary secretions [17,40]. It is therefore more prudent to hold cholinergic drugs until the patient is able to take them orally or through a nasogastric tube [17]. If intravenous anticholinesterase therapy is deemed necessary, neostigmine and pyridostigmine preparations are available in parenteral forms. One milligram of neostigmine given intravenously is roughly equivalent to 120 mg of pyridostigmine taken by mouth. Intravenous pyridostigmine is approximately 1/30th to 1/60th the dose of oral pyridostigmine.

PERIOPERATIVE MANAGEMENT OF THE MYASTHENIC PATIENT

An intercurrent problem requiring surgical intervention was a common source of major morbidity and mortality for myasthenics before the 1960s. Subsequent developments in critical care techniques, especially respiratory care, and in therapy of the underlying disease have dramatically improved this situation. Perioperative management must be compulsive, yet myasthenia gravis should rarely preclude surgical treatment that is otherwise indicated.

Preoperative Considerations

Myasthenia gravis is a major variable in surgical management, whether the surgery is elective or emergent. A neurologist (preferably the neurologist who has been managing the patient) should be considered an integral member of the operative team. If the procedure is elective, the patient's myasthenic status should be optimized before anesthesia and surgery. Pulmonary functions should be reviewed in detail; if respiratory or bulbar muscle function is compromised, therapy adjustments should be undertaken to improve the patient's status. All therapeutic options should be considered, with the possible exception of corticosteroids. If the patient is not receiving steroids, it is prudent to forego or delay this treatment until after surgery, because corticosteroids may increase the risk of infection and retard wound healing. If the patient is already receiving corticosteroids, therapy should be continued, with a short-term increment in dose to compensate for the added stress of anesthesia and surgery. Plasmapheresis or intravenous human immune globulin is often useful in the preoperative setting, providing a transient therapeutic benefit through the preoperative and postoperative periods. Once dose and regimen are optimized, cholinesterase inhibitors may be continued up to the time of surgery. They should then be discontinued because they stimulate respiratory secretions.

It is crucial that all physicians involved in perioperative management of the myasthenic are aware of the particular medications that may accentuate the underlying defect in neuromuscular transmission. It is appropriate to post a warning regarding specific medications on the patient's chart, in a manner analogous to that for medication allergies. Neuromuscular blockade should be avoided during surgery unless absolutely essential; if required, the shortest-acting agents should be used at minimal doses. Accentuated and prolonged effects should be anticipated. Aminoglycoside antibiotics should also be avoided when alternatives are available. There is no clear consensus in favor of any one halogenated anesthetic agent; ether adversely affects neuromuscular transmission. Again, close attention to metabolic homeostasis cannot be overemphasized.

Postoperative Care

Postoperative care of the myasthenic patient should not differ greatly from that of other patients, provided preoperative and intraoperative management has been successful. The patient's status before surgery is often the best indicator of the postoperative course. Intubation and mechanical ventilatory support must be continued until the patient is alert and responsive and demonstrates and maintains adequate pulmonary function. Serial pulmonary functions indicate when the patient can be extubated. An FVC greater than 20 mL per kg and MIP less than (i.e., more negative than) -40 cm H_2O are minimum requirements. If needed, cholinesterase inhibitors may be resumed as a continuous intravenous infusion until bowel function is restored and oral intake allowed. Increased sensitivity to cholinesterase inhibitors is the norm after surgical procedures, especially thymectomy. Resumption at a rate of no more than one-half the preoperative equivalent is often sufficient. Subsequent adjustments should reflect clinical indices. The myasthenic whose neuromuscular function deteriorates during the postoperative period is the exception. In all probability, an intercurrent reversible factor underlies the deterioration. The spectrum of metabolic, infectious, and pharmacologic issues discussed previously should be reviewed.

Thymectomy

After several decades of controversy, there is a consensus that thymectomy favorably alters the natural history of myasthenia gravis, especially in younger patients, independent of the presence or degree of thymic hyperplasia [41]. Thymectomy should be considered early in the course of myasthenia, except in elderly, frail patients. Thymectomy remains an elective procedure, however. The myasthenic with marginal respiratory or bulbar function should be optimally treated before surgery. The perioperative management considerations discussed earlier apply to prethymectomy and postthymectomy management. Some controversy persists regarding the appropriate thymectomy procedure. Most centers favor the transsternal approach. Although more invasive, this approach facilitates recognition and removal of all thymus tissue and avoids postoperative respiratory compromise. There are some proponents of transcervical mediastinoscopic thymectomy; in experienced hands, this remains an alternative. Thymectomy by conventional thoracotomy has no place in the treatment of myasthenia.

CONCLUSION

Respiratory failure is no longer the source of major morbidity and mortality in myasthenia gravis that it once was. When it does occur, appropriate ventilatory support and airway protection provide time for resolution of any intercurrent problems and therapy of the underlying myasthenia. Plasmapheresis and immunosuppression are usually successful; extended intensive care stays should be rare occurrences. Treatment of myasthenia gravis with steroids, immunosuppressive agents, and thymectomy usually enables these patients to lead essentially normal lives.

References

1. Drachman DB, de Silva S, Ramsay D, et al: Humoral pathogenesis of myasthenia gravis, in Drachman DB (ed): *Myasthenia Gravis: Biology and Treatment*. New York, Academy of Sciences, 1987, p 90.
2. Meriggioli MN, Sanders DB: Autoimmune myasthenia gravis: emerging clinical and biological heterogeneity. *Lancet Neurol* 8:475, 2009.
3. Drachman DB: Myasthenia Gravis. *N Engl J Med* 330:1797, 1994.
4. Keesey JC: Clinical evaluation and management of myasthenia gravis. *Muscle Nerve* 29:484, 2004.
5. Hughes BW, Moro De Casillas ML, Kaminski HJ: Pathophysiology of myasthenia gravis. *Semin Neurol* 24:21, 2004.
6. Lennon, VA: Serologic profile of myasthenia gravis and distinction from the Lambert–Eaton myasthenic syndrome. *Neurol* 48[Suppl 5]:S23, 1997.
7. Vincent A, Leite MI: Neuromuscular junction autoimmune disease: muscle specific kinase antibodies and treatments for myasthenia gravis. *Curr Opin Neurol* 18:519, 2005.
8. Shigemoto K, Kubo S, Maruyama N, et al: Induction of myasthenia by immunization against muscle-specific kinase. *J Clin Invest* 116:1016, 2006.
9. Pasnoor M, Wolfe GI, Nations S, et al: Clinical findings in MuSK-antibody positive myasthenia gravis: a U.S. Experience. *Muscle Nerve* 41(3):370–374, 2009.
10. Deymeer F, Bungor-Tuncer O, Yilmaz MS, et al: Clinical comparison of anti-MuSK-vs anti-AchR-positive and seronegative myasthenia gravis. *Neurology* 68:609, 2007.
11. Bartoccioni E, Scuderi F, Minicuci GM, et al: Anti-MuSK antibodies: correlation with myasthenia gravis severity. *Neurology* 67:505, 2006.
12. Romi F, Skeie GO, Gilhus NE, et al: Striational antibodies in myasthenia gravis. *Arch Neurol* 62:442, 2005.
13. Jablecki CK: AAEM Case Report #3: myasthenia gravis. *Muscle Nerve* 14:391, 1991.
14. Sanders DB: Clinical impact of single-fiber electromyography. *Muscle Nerve Suppl* 11:515, 2002.
15. Thieben MJ, Blacker DJ, Liu PY, et al: Pulmonary function tests and blood gases in worsening myasthenia gravis. *Muscle Nerve* 32:664, 2005.
16. Ahmed S, Kirmani J, Janjua N, et al: An update on myasthenic crisis. *Curr Treat Opt Neurol* 7:129, 2005.
17. Lacomis D: Myasthenic crisis. *Neurocrit Care* 3:189, 2005.
18. Pinching AJ, Peters DK, Newson-Davis J: Remission of myasthenia gravis following plasma exchange. *Lancet* 2:1373, 1976.
19. NIH Consensus Conference: The utility of therapeutic plasmapheresis for neurological disorders. *JAMA* 256:1333, 1986.
20. Natarajan N, Weinstein R: Therapeutic apheresis in neurology critical care. *J Intensive Care Med* 20:212, 2005.
21. Triantafyllou NI, Grapsa EI, Kararizou E, et al: Periodic therapeutic plasma exchange in patients with moderate to severe chronic myasthenia gravis non-responders to immunosuppressive agents: an eight year follow-up. *Ther Apher Dial* 13:174, 2009.
22. Zisimopoulou P, Lagoumintzis G, Kostelidou K, et al: Towards antigen-specific apheresis of pathogenic autoantibodies as a further step in the treatment of myasthenia gravis by plasmapheresis. *J Neuroimmunol* 201–202:95, 2008.
23. Donofrio PD, Berger A, Brannagan TH III, et al: Consensus statement: the use of intravenous immunoglobulin in the treatment of neuromuscular conditions. Report of the AANEM Ad Hoc Committee. *Muscle Nerve* 40:890, 2009.
24. Gajdos P, Chevre S, Clair B, et al: Clinical trial of plasma exchange and high-dose intravenous immunoglobulin in myasthenia gravis. *Ann Neurol* 41:789, 1997.
25. Qureshi AI, Choundry MA, Akbar MS, et al: Plasma exchange versus intravenous immunoglobulin treatment in myasthenic crisis. *Neurology* 52:629, 1999.
26. Gajdos P, Tranchant C, Clair B, et al: Treatment of myasthenia gravis exacerbation with intravenous immunoglobulin: a randomized double-blind clinical trial. *Arch Neurol* 62:1689, 2005.
27. Johns TR: Long-term corticosteroid treatment of myasthenia gravis, in Drachman DB (ed): *Myasthenia Gravis: Biology and Treatment*. New York, Academy of Sciences, 1987, p 568.
28. Panegyres PK, Squier M, Mills KR, et al: Acute myopathy associated with large parenteral dose of corticosteroid in myasthenia gravis. *J Neurol Neurosurg Psychiatry* 56:702, 1993.
29. Amato A, Russell J: Disorders of neuromuscular transmission, in Amato A, Russell J (eds): *Neuromuscular Disorders*. New York, McGraw-Hill, 2008, p 457.
30. Schalke BCG, Kappos L, Rohrbach E, et al: Cyclosporine A vs. azathioprine in the treatment of myasthenia gravis: final results of a randomized, controlled double-blind clinical trial. *Neurology* 38[Suppl 1]:135, 1988.
31. Ciafoloni E, Nikhar N, Massey JM, et al: Retrospective analysis of the use of cyclosporine in myasthenia gravis. *Neurology* 55:448, 2000.
32. Chaudhry V, Cornblath DR, Griffin JW, et al: Mycophenolate mofetil: a safe and promising immunosuppressant in neuromuscular diseases. *Neurology* 56:94, 2001.
33. Meriggioli MN, Ciafaloni E, Al-Hayk KA, et al: Mycophenolate mofetil for myasthenia gravis: an analysis of efficacy, safety, and tolerability. *Neurology* 61:1438, 2003.
34. Meriggioli MN, Rowin J, Richman JG, et al: Mycophenolate mofetil for myasthenia gravis: a double-blind, placebo-controlled pilot study. *Ann N Y Acad Sci* 998:494, 2003.
35. Sanders DB, Hart IK, Mantegazza R, et al: An international, phase III, randomized trial of mycophenolate mofetil in myasthenia gravis. *Neurology* 71:400, 2008.
36. The Muscle Study Group: A trial of mycophenolate mofetil with prednisone as initial immunotherapy in myasthenia gravis. *Neurology* 71:394, 2008.
37. Drachman DB, Adams RN, Hu R, et al: Rebooting the immune system with high-dose cyclophosphamide for treatment of refractory myasthenia gravis. *Ann N Y Acad Sci* 1132:305, 2008.
38. Zebardast N, Patwa HS, Novella SP, et al: Rituximab in the management of refractory myasthenia gravis. *Muscle Nerve* 41(3):375–378, 2009.
39. Berrouschot J, Baumann I, Kalischewski P, et al: Therapy of myasthenic crisis. *Crit Care Med* 25:1228, 1997.
40. Chaudhuri A, Behan PO: Myasthenic crisis. *Q J Med* 102:97, 2009.
41. Jaretzki A, Steinglass KM, Sonett JR: Thymectomy in the management of myasthenia gravis. *Semin Neurol* 24:49, 2004.

CHAPTER 177 ■ MISCELLANEOUS NEUROLOGIC PROBLEMS IN THE INTENSIVE CARE UNIT

JING JI, ANN L. MITCHELL AND NANCY M. FONTNEAU

A wide variety of neurologic problems may confront the physician in the intensive care unit (ICU), including several important disorders for which basic information is not readily available. These include

- Suicidal hanging, electrical shock, acute carbon monoxide poisoning, and decompression sickness, which present so blatantly that the diagnosis is rarely in question, yet the range of clinical manifestations and their management may be unanticipated.
- Cerebral fat embolism, which is often not initially suspected if other surgical or medical issues take precedence.
- Singultus (hiccups), which is an all too common secondary problem that may further weaken the severely ill patient.

- Compression neuropathies, which may complicate prolonged bed rest.

SUICIDAL HANGING

Hanging is the second most common means of committing suicide in the United States [1]. Introduced in fifth-century England, hanging proceeded to become the official form of execution. Early on, there was no exact procedure, and most hangings resulted in slow strangulation [2]. Changes in techniques, such that the victim dropped at least his height and the hangman's knot being placed in the submental location, produced a consistently fatal bilateral axis-pedicle fracture, resulting in complete herniation of the disc and severance of the ligaments between C2 and C3 [3]. This injury causes almost immediate death by destroying the cardiac and respiratory centers, lacerating the carotid artery, and injuring the pharynx [2,3].

Suicidal hangings are rarely so expert, and death usually results from strangulation due to interruption of cerebral blood flow [4]. A minimal amount of compression occludes the jugular veins, while an increased force occludes the carotid arteries [5,6]. A much larger force is necessary to arrest blood flow in the vertebral arteries [5]. Pressure on the jugular veins from the noose results in venous obstruction and stagnation of cerebral blood flow, causing hypoxia and loss of consciousness [3]. Cervical muscle tone then decreases, allowing airway obstruction and arterial compression, further worsening hypoxia [3]. In addition, external compression of the carotid bodies or vagal sheath can increase parasympathetic tone, whereas pressure on the pericarotid area stimulates sympathetic tone; either can result in cardiac arrest [4,5]. The altered autonomic tone may also cause a release of catecholamines, resulting in neurogenic pulmonary edema, as well as affect the respiratory smooth muscle tone, causing respiratory acidosis and a further insult to cerebral oxygenation [3].

If blood flow is quickly restored, full recovery can often be expected. If the blood flow is interrupted for more than a few minutes, however, hypoxia causes cell death and cytotoxic and vasogenic edema, with increased intracranial pressure. There is selective vulnerability of the cerebral cortex (particularly the pyramidal cell layer), the globus pallidus, thalamus, hippocampus, and the cerebellar Purkinje cells to anoxia and ischemia.

Diagnosis

Although the diagnosis is rarely in doubt, the patient may show a range of findings, varying from rope burns to coma. In the immediate posthanging period, the patient most commonly shows evidence of an altered level of consciousness, ranging from restlessness, delirium, or violence to lethargy, stupor, or coma. Seizures, and rarely status epilepticus, may occur [4,5]. Hyperthermia may be present because of hypoxic damage to the hypothalamus [6]. Injury to the neck blood vessels occurs in 40% of patients, resulting in carotid dissection, thrombus formation, and distal ischemic infarcts [7]. Venous occlusion may lead to venous congestion, venous ischemia, and hemorrhage [8]. Development of the acute respiratory distress syndrome may result from central nervous system (CNS) catecholamine release, causing constriction of the pulmonary venules [3]. In incomplete hanging, the patient may also show signs of laryngeal and pharyngeal edema, resulting in hoarseness, dysphagia, and stridor [3,8]. Although infrequent in suicidal hangings, fracture of the odontoid and injury to the spinal cord may occur.

Careful neurologic examination should be performed, with particular attention to alterations in the level of consciousness and evidence of spinal cord injury, such as paraparesis, quadriparesis, or urinary retention. There should be frequent monitoring of vital signs for evidence of autonomic instability and stridor. Initial laboratory evaluations should include radiographs of the cervical spine, arterial blood gas determination, electrocardiogram, and cardiac monitoring. CT angiogram should also be considered if suspicious for dissection of the carotid artery [9].

Neuroimaging of the brain may be quite variable, from a normal head computed tomography (CT) scan in many patients, to evidence of edema, hemorrhage, and ischemia. Due to decreased blood flow and the resultant hypoxia, edema may be seen in the white matter tracts [10]. Subcortical and subarachnoid hemorrhages may result from venous occlusion, while ischemic insults may result from venous or arterial occlusion, particularly in the areas of greatest vulnerability: the basal ganglia, cortex, thalamus, and hippocampus [11].

Treatment

The patient may appear dead but might still be resuscitable. Patients quickly lose consciousness with hanging attempts, but may still have cardiac and respiratory function or can quickly regain these with prompt cardiopulmonary resuscitation (CPR). The goals of treatment are to maintain an adequate level of cerebral oxygenation, to decrease the raised intracranial pressure, and to monitor and treat any cardiac arrhythmias or respiratory distress that may develop. In hangings, the mechanical trauma induced by strangulation can also cause hemorrhage and edema in the paratracheal and laryngeal areas and result in a delayed but significant airway obstruction at any time within the first 24 hours. Endotracheal intubation may be required if there is evidence of hypoxia due to acute respiratory distress syndrome, airway obstruction, or increased intracranial pressure [8].

Other concerns in victims of hangings include fractures and thrombi. A fracture of the odontoid requires immediate neurosurgical or orthopedic intervention to stabilize the cervical spine and protect the cord from injury. A carotid thrombus requires prompt vascular intervention to remove the clot and restore patency and blood flow. In addition, assessing the patient for other evidence of self-inflicted injuries and intoxications is also warranted, as is a complete psychiatric evaluation once the patient is able to cooperate.

Course

The prognosis for recovery is not immediately apparent with the first neurologic examination. Many patients have made a full recovery despite an initial Glasgow Coma Scale (GCS) score of 3 [4]. However, the fatality rate for suicidal hangings may range from 60% to 70% [12]. Indicators for a good recovery include a hanging time of less than 5 minutes, a heartbeat present at the scene or in the emergency room, CPR initiated at the scene, a GCS score greater than 3, and an incomplete circumferential ligature [4]. Predictors of a poorer prognosis include evidence of cardiopulmonary arrest, a spontaneous respiratory rate less than 4 per minute, need for intubation, and neurogenic pulmonary edema [5].

Other neurologic sequelae can become manifest either in the immediate posthanging period or after a relatively asymptomatic latent period. The individual may show evidence of a confusional state, a circumscribed retrograde amnesia, Korsakoff's syndrome, or even progressive dementia [8]. Transient hemiparesis, aphasia, abnormal movements, motor restlessness, and myoclonic jerks also can characterize this period [8]. Ear numbness may result from injury to the greater auricular nerve [13]. Three more severe outcomes have also been observed: (a) comatose state with minor neurologic improvement and death; (b) early neurologic recovery, followed by cerebral edema with uncontrollable uncal herniation and severe morbidity or mortality; and (c) complete neurologic recovery, followed by delayed encephalopathy and death [3]. Most patients who survive recover to variable degrees.

ELECTRICAL INJURIES

Approximately 4,000 injuries and 1,000 deaths from electrical shock occur annually in the United States. Most fatalities occur in the workplace, but one third result from contact with household current [14]. Approximately 400 people per year are affected by lightning strikes, with one-third of victims dying due to their exposure [15].

Pathophysiology

Electrical and lightning injuries are exceedingly variable and dependent on a number of factors. Current flowing between two potentials, or amperage, is equal to the voltage divided by the resistance to current flow ($I = V/R$). Current is generated by either an electrical source or a lightning strike. Current may be direct (DC), as with lightning, or alternating (AC), as with most household appliances. Alternating current has a tendency to produce tetanic contractions that prevent voluntary release from the current source, thus prolonging the electrical contact time and increasing the potential for injury. Higher voltages, such as those that occur with lightning or with contact with high-voltage conductors, produce more severe injuries than those due to low voltages. Wet skin and tissues high in water content provide low resistance to current flow and are at a higher risk for injury, while tissues high in fat and air, such as hollow organs, provide high resistance. Nerves and blood vessels have lower than expected resistances, and thus are more sensitive to electrical injury than their water content would suggest [16]. Other variables that affect the severity of damage include the current pathway (i.e., whether it involves the heart, diaphragm, spinal cord, or brain), the area of current contact and exit, and the duration of contact [16].

In addition, lightning injuries are classified according to the type of exposure [17]. "Direct strikes" involve direct contact between the lightning bolt and the highest point of the victim, often the head. "Side flash" involves the spread of electricity from the lightning bolt to a nearby object and then to the patient. Side flash victims are typically exposed to less voltage and current than with a direct strike. Finally, "stride current" involves the spread of electricity from the lightning bolt to the ground and then through contact points in the patient. Stride current patients are more likely to experience spinal cord injuries, as the current crosses through the spinal cord from one limb to another.

Neurologic Complications of Electrical and Lightning Injuries

Neurologic sequelae of electrical injuries affect both the central and peripheral nervous systems, with both immediate and long-term difficulties.

Immediate Effects

Immediate neurologic effects of electrical injuries are noted throughout the neuraxis. Ten percent to 50% of patients experience a brief loss of consciousness, as well as headache, retrograde amnesia, and confusion [18]. Patients with electrical and lightning injuries to the head may also suffer subarachnoid or parenchymal hemorrhages, particularly in the basal ganglia and brainstem [19]. In patients who suffer cardiac or respiratory arrest, posthypoxic encephalopathy may develop in "watershed" areas of the cerebral cortex. Less commonly, patients may present with cerebral infarction or a temporary cerebellar syndrome [19].

Catecholamine release may result in autonomic dysfunction, as evidenced by transitory hypertension, tachycardia, diaphoresis, vasoconstriction of the extremities, and fixed and dilated pupils [20]. Thus, lightning strike victims should receive full resuscitative efforts despite pupillary changes, as these may not indicate brainstem dysfunction. Lightning strike victims may also suffer "keraunoparalysis," a self-limited paralysis more often involving the lower extremities, accompanied by a lack of peripheral pulses, pale and cold extremities, and variable paresthesias [19]. Keraunoparalysis is presumably due to localized vasospasm from catecholamine release.

Acute spinal cord injuries are also seen, particularly with stride current injuries. The spectrum of spinal cord injuries includes paralysis, spasticity, autonomic dysfunction, and, later, chronic pain and pressure ulcers [19]. Acute neuropathies are typically not seen with lightning strikes, but may be seen with electrical injuries in association with compartment syndromes, local burns, or vascular injury [21]. Both electrical and lightning strike victims are vulnerable to the subacute development of cataracts, while lightning strike patients are peculiarly susceptible to tympanic membrane rupture, vertigo, and hearing loss [22,23].

Delayed Effects

Delayed effects of electrical and lightning injuries may also span the neuraxis. Recognized neuropsychiatric effects include depression, posttraumatic stress disorder, fatigue, irritability, and memory and concentration difficulties [24]. Movement disorders have also been described, such as transient dystonias, torticollis, and parkinsonism [19]. Delayed ophthalmologic and otologic consequences include cataracts, conductive and sensorineural hearing loss, and vertigo [22,23]. Delayed autonomic dysfunction may manifest as reflex sympathetic dystrophy, presenting as a limb with burning pain, cutaneous vasoconstriction, swelling, and sweating [20]. Prolonged and permanent spinal cord abnormalities may become manifest in the delayed development of a myelopathy or a motor neuronopathy [14,25]. Peripheral neuropathies may result from compression due to scarring and fibrosis from the original injury or delayed ischemia due to vascular occlusion [26]. Peripheral neuropathies are more likely to occur in areas directly involved by the electrical current, but may also occur in limbs that were not seemingly in the current path [27].

Evaluation

Initial evaluation of the electrical- or lightning-injured patient involves assessment of the scene and evaluation of safety. Disconnect electrical sources before evaluating the patient. Contrary to conventional mythology, lightning-strike victims are not electrically charged and may be examined immediately.

Assessment of cardiopulmonary status is essential, as many victims suffer cardiopulmonary arrest and may recover well if CPR is initiated promptly. Cardiac arrhythmias and asystole commonly accompany these injuries, as does respiratory arrest due to passage of current through the brainstem respiratory centers. Stabilization of the spine is also essential, due to potential spinal cord injuries and fractures from falls.

Neurologic Examination

The neurologic examination should begin with assessment of the level of consciousness. Initially, many patients are comatose, but this is often brief and followed by a period of confusion and amnesia, lasting hours to days [28]. Seizures are uncommon. The cranial nerve examination may reveal fixed and dilated pupils, blindness, papilledema, partial hearing loss, and tinnitus. Rupture of the tympanic membranes may also be present with lightning injuries to the head. Evaluation of the motor system for focal weakness and reflex changes may indicate cerebral injuries, myelopathy, or neuropathy. Cerebral lesions, due to hemorrhage or infarction, may result in contralateral hemiparesis. Spinal cord injuries are more common in the cervical region and produce paraparesis or quadriparesis. Peripheral nerve injuries in the immediate assessment are typically located in areas of extensive burns. Sensory loss is less frequent than motor deficits and is maximal in burned areas.

Laboratory Evaluation

Laboratory evaluations should be focused on the known complications of electrical and lightning injuries. Serial determinations of electrolytes, renal function, and hematocrit are essential for assessing adequate fluid replacement. Serum creatine kinase and urinary myoglobin are useful measures of muscle necrosis. Arterial blood gases may reveal a metabolic acidosis. Electrocardiogram (ECG) and cardiac monitoring are used in patients with cardiopulmonary arrest or with known current pathways through the thorax, as delayed cardiac arrhythmias may develop. Radiologic examinations of the long bones, spine, and skull are indicated when fractures or deep burns are suspected based on the history and physical examination. Magnetic resonance imaging (MRI) or myelography may be used to assess spinal cord damage if signs of myelopathy are present. Cranial imaging is indicated when there is prolonged alteration of consciousness and may reveal intracranial hemorrhages, cerebral edema, or the effect of diffuse cerebral hypoxia. The electroencephalogram (EEG) is also useful to rule out status epilepticus in patients with prolonged unconsciousness. The EEG background may remain slow even when the mental status has returned to baseline. Nerve conduction studies and electromyography may be useful in localizing and following axonal and demyelinating electrical injuries to the peripheral nerves and plexi, although they are not generally used in the acute evaluation.

Management

Evaluation and treatment of medical concerns are essential for good neurologic recovery. Efforts should focus on circulatory volume, hydration status, renal function, acidosis, and electrolyte balance. Because high-voltage electric shock victims usually have myoglobinuria secondary to burns and deep tissue injury, their fluid needs are similar to those of crush injuries. Central venous pressure monitoring is usually needed, and urine output should be maintained at greater than 50 mL per hour. Alkalinization of the urine and osmotic diuresis with mannitol also help to prevent myoglobin nephropathy.

Extensive burns due to direct current or clothing ignition are best treated in specialized burn units. At times, skin grafts are required. Debridement of necrotic muscle and fasciotomy are sometimes necessary to prevent secondary ischemia from a compartment syndrome. Amputation is required if there is significant necrosis. In these patients, arteriography may assist in identifying the level of viability. Tetanus prophylaxis and prevention of superinfection are also needed. Spine and long-bone fractures require stabilization.

Recurrent seizures are treated with phenytoin (18 to 20 mg per kg loading dose followed by 5 to 7 mg per kg per day). Other antiepileptics, such as levetiracetam, could also be considered. Because fluid restriction is contraindicated, patients with signs of increased intracranial pressure require osmotic diuresis with mannitol. Intracranial pressure monitoring may be useful in patients with cerebral edema. Specific treatment for electrical spinal cord injuries is not available, and early institution of physical therapy is recommended. In patients with cardiac arrest, the hypothermia protocol could be considered.

Prognosis

Prognosis is difficult to ascertain for electrical injuries to the nervous system. Patients with deficits at presentation frequently recover fully, whereas those with delayed onset of neurologic deficits may have syndromes that progress over months to years.

CARBON MONOXIDE POISONING

Carbon monoxide is a colorless, tasteless, odorless gas that may give no warning of its presence. It is normally present in the atmosphere in a concentration of less than 0.001%, but a concentration of 0.1% can be lethal [29]. Carbon monoxide is found in automobile exhaust, fires, water heaters, charcoal-burning grills, methylene chloride, volcanic gas, and cigarette smoke. It is also endogenously formed from the degradation of hemoglobin, resulting in baseline carboxyhemoglobin saturation between 1% and 3% [29]. Smoking can raise the endogenous level to 6% to 7% saturation [29]. Carbon monoxide poisoning may occur in the acute and chronic setting. For further information on the pathogenesis, diagnosis, and treatment of carbon monoxide poisoning, see Chapter 64.

Diagnosis

It is important to consider carbon monoxide poisoning in the differential diagnosis of any individual who presents with an altered state of consciousness or headache, particularly in the setting of a long car ride or other exposure to poorly ventilated and incompletely combusted fuel. Of note, the carboxyhemoglobin levels are not indicative of the severity of toxicity and depend on factors such as duration of exposure, comorbid conditions, and ambient carbon monoxide concentration [30]. With mild intoxication, symptoms may include a mild headache, dyspnea on exertion, and fatigability [29]. With increasing levels of toxicity, more severe symptoms may include impaired motor dexterity, blurry vision, irritability, weakness, nausea, vomiting, and confusion [29]. At its most severe, carbon monoxide exposure may cause tachycardia, cardiac irritability, seizures, respiratory insufficiency, coma, and death [29]. In addition, there can be evidence of rhabdomyolysis, flame-shaped superficial retinal hemorrhages, and, occasionally, a cherry-red discoloration best appreciated in the lips, mucous membranes, and skin [29,31].

Furthermore, carboxyhemoglobin levels do not correlate well with the development of delayed neurologic sequelae [32]. In mild carbon monoxide intoxication, in which there is no loss of consciousness and carboxyhemoglobin levels are less than 5% in nonsmokers or less than 10% in smokers, only headache and dizziness at or before presentation were found to correlate with an increased incidence of delayed sequelae, including asthenia, headache, or decreased memory [33].

A head CT scan may be normal early on or show signs of cerebral edema as inferred from narrowed ventricles and effacement of the cerebral sulci. The degree of CT abnormalities does not predict the clinical course [34]. MRI findings may reveal diffuse, confluent diffusion-weighted imaging (DWI), fluid-attenuated inversion recovery, and T_2 (time for

63% of transverse relaxation) hyperintensities bilaterally in the periventricular white matter, centrum semiovale [35,36], basal ganglia, particularly involving the globus pallidus, and the hippocampus [37]. The electroencephalogram usually demonstrates diffuse slowing but is generally of little prognostic value.

Treatment

The criteria for hospital admission include coma, loss of consciousness, or neurologic deficit at any time; any clinical or electrocardiographic signs of cardiac compromise; metabolic acidosis; abnormal chest radiograph; oxygen tension less than 60 mm Hg; and carboxyhemoglobin level greater than 10% in individuals with pregnancy, greater than 15% in those with cardiac disease, or greater than 25% in all other patients [31].

All patients should be treated with 100% oxygen as soon as the diagnosis of carbon monoxide poisoning is even considered. It should be administered through a tight-fitting nonrebreathing mask or after endotracheal intubation in severely sensorium-compromised patients. The administration of 100% oxygen can shorten the half-life of carbon monoxide from 4 to 5 hours to approximately 1 hour [30]. Oxygen should be administered until the carboxyhemoglobin level normalizes [29]. (See Chapters 62 and 64 for a discussion of hyperbaric oxygen therapy.)

Administering 100% oxygen and possibly hyperbaric oxygen therapy are also useful in treating acute cerebral edema, as is mechanical hyperventilation and maintaining fluid and electrolyte homeostasis. Steroids have not been effective in cerebral postanoxic states and may increase the risk of oxygen toxicity seizures if hyperbaric oxygen therapy is being considered [31].

Course

The delayed appearance of neurologic sequelae found in many posthypoxic states occurs with particular frequency and severity after carbon monoxide poisoning. Up to 30% of patients may succumb to the initial exposure and 25% may develop a progressive encephalopathy resulting in a persistent vegetative state, with a 50% mortality rate [34]. Later sequelae may include seizures, cortical blindness, scotomas, Korsakoff's psychosis, irritability, hemiplegia, chorea, and peripheral neuropathy.

Between 10% and 30% of patients develop delayed neurologic sequelae, and there are no guidelines to indicate which patients are at greatest risk [31]. Although there seems to be a rough correlation between duration of initial unconsciousness and increasing age with the development of delayed neurologic sequelae, even patients with mild toxicity can progress to develop the tardive signs [30]. The post–carbon monoxide syndrome begins 7 to 30 days after the initial insult and is characterized by gait disturbances, incontinence, and memory impairment, as well as signs of parkinsonism, mutism, and frontal lobe disinhibition [29,30,38]. The development of isolated cognitive impairment has considerable variability in the literature. Some report memory dysfunction, impaired attention, and affective disorders in moderate to severe carbon monoxide exposure, while other studies suggest that mildly exposed individuals have no cognitive impairments compared to matched controls in neuropsychiatric testing [30,39,40].

On average, 75% of affected individuals largely recover within a year of the insult, although 20% of these individuals continue to show evidence of mild to moderate impairment of memory and extrapyramidal function [41]. Although the specific cause of the delayed syndrome is unknown, it does correlate temporally with the pathologic findings of cerebral white matter demyelination found in the chronic stages of the illness as opposed to the largely gray matter edema, ischemia, and hemorrhagic necrosis found in the acute stage [42]. There is no specific treatment for the delayed neuropsychiatric syndrome, although symptomatic treatment, including cognitive therapies and dopamine agonists, may be of benefit in the short term [41].

DECOMPRESSION SICKNESS

Decompression sickness ("the bends") occurs when gases dissolved in body fluids come out of solution, forming bubbles in tissues and venous blood. Situations in which decompression sickness arises include rapid ascent to the surface by tunnel workers or scuba divers, decompression or rapid ascent in an airplane, and high-altitude flying with inadequate cabin pressurization. In these situations, nitrogen and other inert gases that supersaturate the tissues under high pressure are released as bubbles under conditions of decreased pressure. As the bubbles coalesce, they may cause local tissue ischemia because of compression or venous obstruction. The microcirculation is further compromised by capillary endothelial edema; by activation of platelets, coagulation factors, and complement; and by hemoconcentration due to fluid extravasation [43,44]. Nitrogen, the largest component of inspired air, is lipophilic, and thus gas bubbles are more likely to form in the bone marrow, fat, and spinal cord. Additionally, gas bubbles may result in barotrauma to the pulmonary beds, releasing further air emboli into the venous circulation [43,44].

Symptoms of decompression sickness are variable. In most cases, the onset is within 6 hours of decompression, but may be seen later at 12 to 24 hours [43]. Fulminant cases present earlier. Any organ system can be affected, and symptoms range from a pruritic skin rash ("the creeps"), cough ("the chokes"), and joint pain to paraplegia, vertigo, altered level of consciousness, seizures, shock, and apnea.

Almost 80% of patients with decompression sickness have neurologic symptoms. The most frequent neurologic presentation is with paresthesias, which may be diffuse or focal, and result from gas bubble formation in the skin, joints, peripheral nerves, or spinal cord. Weakness, ranging from monoparesis to quadriplegia secondary to spinal cord involvement, may also occur. Cerebral symptoms are infrequent and range from headache and lethargy to vertigo, visual disturbances, paralysis, and unconsciousness [43,44]. Vertigo, hearing loss, tinnitus, nausea, and vomiting are relatively common complaints, resulting from rupture of the cochlear and semicircular canal membranes.

Air embolism is a more serious decompression illness, and its onset is usually within 5 minutes of decompression. It probably results from tearing of the lung parenchyma secondary to overinflation as the gases in the lungs expand during ascent [43]. The gas escapes into the pulmonary vein and may embolize into large vessels [43]. Venous gas bubbles are effectively filtered by the lungs, but arterial embolism may also result from gas passing through a patent foramen ovale. Based on their buoyancy, the emboli often produce neurologic symptoms by floating into and occluding cerebral arterioles. Unconsciousness and stupor are the most frequent symptoms. Death from cardiopulmonary arrest may also occur. In most patients, improvement in symptoms accompanies the redistribution of the gas emboli to the venous circulation [43].

Recompression is the definitive treatment for decompression diseases. The patient should be transported in a pressurized aircraft to the nearest decompression chamber with minimal delay. (See Chapter 61 for a more detailed discussion of the management and therapy for decompression syndrome.) The Divers Alert Network also maintains a 24-hour phone consultation service to assist with diving accidents, reached at (919) 684-9111.

Remarkable recovery may occur after recompression. Delay in treatment can limit its effectiveness, but recompression should be attempted even up to 2 weeks after the onset of symptoms. Relapses requiring repeated hyperbaric treatment may occur [45]. Patients with long-term sequelae from decompression illnesses should not be re-exposed to conditions that allow their recurrence.

CEREBRAL FAT EMBOLISM SYNDROME

Fat embolism syndrome is characterized by diffuse pulmonary insufficiency with hypoxemia, neurologic dysfunction, and petechiae occurring 12 to 48 hours after trauma [46,47]. At least subclinically, fat embolism is present after all fractures involving the long bones. It is clinically recognized in 0.5% to 2% of patients with long bone fractures and in 5% to 10% of patients who have sustained multiple fractures [48,49]. There are also reports of fat embolism syndrome occurring in the setting of orthopedic procedures, such as hip arthroplasty, intramedullary rods, and leg lengthening procedures [48,50]. There is an increased risk associated with a patent foramen ovale [49].

Pathogenesis

The two main pathogenetic hypotheses of fat embolism syndrome are the mechanical and chemical theories. The mechanical theory posits that physical disruption of bone and blood vessels at the fracture site allows free fat globules to enter venous sinusoids and then to embolize to the lungs [46]. The chemical theory proposes that a trauma-induced catecholamine surge results in lipid mobilization from the fat stores or the coalescence of chylomicrons into fat globules [46,51]. The fat emboli in the circulation may then be broken down by lipases in the lungs or systemic circulation, generating free fatty acids [46,47,52]. The toxic fatty acids stimulate the release of inflammatory mediators, increasing permeability of capillaries, generating acute respiratory distress syndrome (ARDS) and cerebral vasogenic edema [46,47]. Furthermore, the inflammatory mediators may increase platelet adhesion and coagulation [52]. Fat emboli, in conjunction with increased platelet adhesion, may arrest blood flow, resulting in cerebral ischemia and hemorrhage [47,52].

Cerebral fat emboli and ischemia, rather than cerebral anoxia, produce the neurologic damage seen in this condition. The brain is edematous and shows a leptomeningeal inflammatory reaction and cortical surface petechiae. Microscopically, there are fat emboli and ball, ring, and perivascular hemorrhages. The fat emboli are more prevalent in the gray matter, but the hemorrhages are more common in the centrum semiovale, internal capsule, and cerebral and cerebellar white matter [53]. Electron microscopy reveals intravascular fat vacuoles, breakdown of endothelial walls, swollen neurons, and glia [53].

Diagnosis

Characteristically, there is a symptom-free interval of 12 to 48 hours between the inciting trauma and the onset of fat embolism syndrome [46]. Altered consciousness or development of neurological deficits after a lucid interval following trauma should alert the physician to the possibility of fat embolism. The syndrome may present as a spectrum of disability, from subclinical presentations with only a decreased arterial partial pressure of oxygen (PaO_2), decreased platelets or hemoglobin, to a fulminant presentation. Gurd's diagnostic criteria for fat embolism syndrome include one or more major criteria (respiratory insufficiency, neurologic dysfunction, or petechial rash), four or more minor criteria (fever, tachycardia, retinal changes, jaundice, or renal changes), and one or more laboratory criteria (fat macroglobulinemia, decreased hemoglobin or platelets, or increased erythrocyte sedimentation rate) [47]. An alternative diagnostic scheme was proposed by Schonfeld [47], assigning a numerical score to similar criteria with a score of 5 or more suggestive of the diagnosis.

Sudden onset of fever, tachycardia, and tachypnea often herald onset of the syndrome. Respiratory distress and hypoxemia with an oxygen tension less than 60 mm Hg is common and may be the initial or only laboratory abnormality. The chest radiograph may be unremarkable in one-half of the cases, but fine stippling or hazy infiltrates of both lung fields should be sought as they are consistent with fat embolism syndrome [51].

Petechiae are present in 50% to 60% of clinically recognized cases and are most often found on the lower palpebral conjunctivae, neck, anterior axillary folds, and anterior chest wall [47]. There is an associated thrombocytopenia, believed to be caused by the consumption of platelets with their aggregation around the embolic fat droplets, and a progressive anemia with hemoglobin levels commonly less than 9.5 g per 100 mL [51]. Retinal fat emboli and lipuria are each in evidence in more than 50% of patients [51]. The retinal emboli appear as small rosaries of microinfarcts surrounding the macula of both eyes, which over the course of the following 10 to 14 days evolve into yellowish, fatty plaques [51].

The CNS manifestations range from confusion to coma, and although they almost always accompany respiratory insufficiency, they can be the initial and sometimes only symptomatic manifestation of fat embolism syndrome [47]. Impaired consciousness is the earliest recognizable sign. The symptoms can begin with restlessness and confusion and may evolve gradually or abruptly to stupor and coma. Coma, especially if it develops abruptly, portends a poor prognosis [46]. Focal or generalized seizures can occur and may antedate the onset of coma [47]. Decerebrate rigidity is found in up to 15% of cases, and pyramidal signs of hyperreflexia and extensor plantar responses are found in 30% to 70%. Focal neurologic signs, such as aphasia and hemiparesis, are usually restricted to patients with more severe disturbances of consciousness [47].

Neuroimaging of cerebral fat embolism syndrome reveals diffuse vasogenic and cytotoxic edema, as well as areas of hemorrhage and infarct. The most common finding on head CT is evidence of diffuse brain edema, as shown by small ventricles and flattened sulci [54]. Brain MRI performed within 48 hours of a neurologic change may reveal signs of cerebral fat embolism syndrome even earlier than CT. The DWI sequence can exhibit a "starfield" appearance, with dot-like hyperintensities, both patchy and confluent, in border zone areas of territorial gray matter, deep white matter, and basal ganglia [54]. The DWI changes are suggestive of cytotoxic edema. Later, T_2 hyperintensities appear as small subcortical foci in gray and white matter, indicative of vasogenic edema; an increased number of T_2-weighted hyperintensities correlates with a decreased Glasgow Coma Scale [55]. These T_2-weighted hyperintensities disappear with resolution of the neurologic symptoms [56]. The later MRI appearance of brain atrophy and residual multiple infarcts may be present, particularly in patients with a poorer outcome.

Treatment

Rapid immobilization of fractures and their early definitive management decreases the likelihood of fat embolism syndrome [51]. Sequential clinical examinations, chest radiographs, and arterial blood gas determinations in patients believed to be at high risk may help identify early on those needing more aggressive care. These patients should have early and expedient replacement of fluids and blood and administration of 40% oxygen by mask [51].

The support of respiration and maintenance of arterial oxygen levels greater than 70 mm Hg sometimes requires intubation and mechanical ventilation. Placement of a central venous pressure line is useful in monitoring the patient for shock. Steroids have been advocated as treatment to blunt the inflammatory response, to help preserve vascular integrity, and to minimize interstitial edema formation, but there are as yet no controlled trials demonstrating a consistent benefit. A brain CT or MRI is indicated to assess whether there are any direct cerebral traumatic injuries accounting for neurologic symptoms.

Prognosis

Mortality in fat embolism syndrome can reach 10% to 20%, but recent improvements in management have lessened this rate [57]. Twenty-five percent of patients experience permanent neurologic deficits [53]. A favorable prognosis is more likely with normal muscle tone, active deep tendon reflexes, and retention of appropriate pain response [47]. If patients survive the pulmonary insufficiency, neurologic dysfunction is typically reversible [47]. A worse prognosis is portended by coma, severe ARDS, pneumonia, or congestive heart failure [46].

SINGULTUS (HICCUPS)

Hiccups are usually a benign and self-limited condition. Prolonged hiccups can produce fatigue, sleeplessness, weight loss, depression, difficulty in ventilation, and, in postoperative patients, wound dehiscence [58–60]. In intubated patients, persistent hiccups may result in hyperventilation, leading to a respiratory alkalosis [58].

Pathophysiology

Hiccups result from a sudden reflex contraction of the diaphragm, causing forceful inspiration, which is arrested almost immediately by glottic closure, producing the characteristic sound. Afferent pathways include the vagus and phrenic nerves and thoracic sympathetic fibers (T_6 to T_{12}). The efferent pathway includes the phrenic nerve to the diaphragm, the vagus nerve to the larynx, and the spinal nerves to the accessory muscles of inspiration. Although central control of this reflex is not well defined, it probably involves lower brainstem and upper cervical spinal levels, including the respiratory center, phrenic nerve nuclei, medullary reticular formation, and hypothalamus [61].

Etiology

Hiccups may result from a multitude of causes, due to injury or irritation of the afferent or efferent pathways or disease within the central control mechanism. Hiccups most frequently result from irritation of the stomach wall or diaphragm, leading to impulses along the phrenic and vagus nerves. Abdominal disorders causing hiccups include gastric ulceration, gastric distention, gastroesophageal reflux, hiatus hernia, cholecystitis, peritonitis, subdiaphragmatic abscess, ileus, and bowel obstruction. Thoracic disorders that precipitate hiccups include esophagitis, pericarditis, myocardial infarction, pneumonia, and neoplasm. More proximally along the course of the nerves, neck masses, such as neoplasm and goiter, may also result in hiccups. Brainstem neoplasm or ischemia, multiple sclerosis, arteriovenous malformations, and meningoencephalitis are CNS causes. Perioperative causes include neck extension, intubation, visceral traction, and intraoperative manipulation of efferent or afferent nerves [58]. Metabolic disorders, such as uremia, electrolyte abnormalities, alcohol intoxication, diabetes mellitus, and general anesthesia, have also been implicated [58,61]. Medications, most frequently corticosteroids and benzodiazepines, may also induce hiccups [62,63]. Recently, hiccups have been reported in four patients with Parkinson's disease, and dopamine agonists appeared to play a causative role [64,65]. Some patients have idiopathic or psychogenic hiccups.

Evaluation

A history of gastrointestinal, cardiac, pulmonary, or CNS complaints or surgery may assist in determining the etiology of intractable hiccups. The physical examination should rule out inflammation or neoplasm in the thorax, abdomen, CNS, and neck. Chest and abdominal radiographs are obtained routinely, and fluoroscopic evaluation of the diaphragm is sometimes needed. Radiographic or endoscopic evaluation of the gastrointestinal tract is sometimes warranted. If the CNS is implicated, cranial CT or MRI may be useful. Electrocardiography is required. Other investigations include determinations of electrolytes, renal function, glucose, creatine kinase (if myocardial infarction is suspected), and a toxicology screen for alcohol and barbiturates. Lumbar puncture is required if there is a suspicion of CNS infection. Electromyography may be useful if surgical therapy for hiccups is contemplated. Careful review of medications for potential causative agents is indicated.

Management

Initial management includes identification and treatment of disorders that may cause hiccups, such as inflammation, infection, or gastric dilatation. When this is unsuccessful, nonpharmacologic and pharmacologic treatments are available for intractable hiccups.

Nonpharmacologic therapies alter the reflex arc responsible for hiccups. Pharyngeal stimulation may resolve hiccups, either by nasogastric intubation, swallowing dry granulated sugar, or by the introduction of a red rubber catheter through the mouth or nares, followed by a jerky to-and-fro movement [58]. Pharyngeal stimulation tends to be a temporary measure. Counterstimulation of the vagus nerve by pressure on eyeballs, rectal massage, or irritating the tympanic membrane may also alleviate hiccups [61]. Breathing into a paper bag, gasping with fright, Valsalva maneuver, and supramaximal inspiration possibly abolish hiccups by interrupting the stimulus for respiration or increasing the carbon dioxide concentration [66]. Case reports of acupuncture therapy also document effectiveness for refractory hiccups [59].

If nonpharmacologic therapies are ineffective, drug therapy should be initiated. Baclofen 5 mg orally three times a day, increased to 10 mg three times a day, has been effective in decreasing and potentially eliminating hiccups [61]. Alternatively, chlorpromazine taken 25 to 50 mg orally or intramuscularly three or four times a day has also been effective. If this is ineffective in 2 to 3 days, then a slow intravenous infusion of chlorpromazine 25 to 50 mg in 500 to 1,000 mL of normal saline is indicated. Although hypotension may result from intravenous (IV) administration, chlorpromazine may be most effective by this route [67]. If IV chlorpromazine is ineffective, it should be discontinued and 10 mg of metoclopramide given orally four times per day. Other medications used in refractory patients include haloperidol (5 mg three times per day), anticonvulsants (e.g., gabapentin, phenytoin, carbamazepine, and valproic acid), amitriptyline, nifedipine, nimodipine, and amantadine [67].

Most patients respond to mechanical or drug therapy. In refractory cases, transcutaneous stimulation of the phrenic nerve, transesophageal diaphragmatic pacing, vagus nerve stimulation, phrenic nerve block or ablation, or microvascular decompression of the vagus nerve may be useful [60,67–70]. Because there are multiple efferent pathways involved, hiccups may remain even after phrenic nerve ablation.

COMPRESSION NEUROPATHIES

Compression neuropathies are common in the general population. In the ICU population, several nerves are particularly at risk, compression of which may result in delayed morbidity. The ulnar nerve may be compressed in the condylar groove posterior to the medial epicondyle when the arms are positioned in a flexed, pronated, or semipronated fashion, or when the flexed elbows are used by the patient for repositioning. Ulnar nerve palsy causes weakness of the intrinsic muscles of the hand and numbness of the fourth and fifth fingers. The peroneal nerve is also at risk where it courses around the fibular head. The everted immobile position of the leg in severely weak or paralyzed patients contributes to its vulnerability. Other compression neuropathies and brachial plexopathy may result from positions assumed during prolonged coma before hospitalization. Hematomas resulting from clotting disorders, anticoagulation, local injection, arterial puncture, or phlebotomy may also compress the peripheral nerves and plexi. Evaluation of compression neuropathies includes an EMG to localize the lesion. Proper positioning of the limbs to avoid compression of these nerves between the bed and bony prominences is key to prevention.

References

1. Kochanek KD, Murphy SL, Anderson RN, et al: Deaths: final data for 2002. *Natl Vital Stat Rep* 53(5):1–116, 2004.
2. McHugh TP, Stout M: Near-hanging injury. *Ann Emerg Med* 12:774–776, 1983.
3. Kaki A, Crosby ET, Lui ACP: Airway and respiratory management following non-lethal hanging. *Can J Anaesth* 44:445–450, 1997.
4. Matsuyama T, Okuchi K, Seki T, et al: Prognostic factors in hanging injuries. *Am J Emerg Med* 22:207–210, 2004.
5. Gunnell D, Bennewith O, Hawton K, et al: The epidemiology and prevention of suicide by hanging: a systematic review. *Int J Epidemiol* 34(2):433–442, 2005.
6. Calvanese J, Spohr M, Nevada R: Hyperthermia from a near hanging. *Ann Emerg Med* 113:152–155, 1982.
7. Nikolic S, Micic J, Atanasijevic T, et al: Analysis of neck injuries with hanging. *Am J Forensic Med Pathol* 24(2):179–182, 2003.
8. Vander KL, Wolfe R: The emergency department management of near-hanging victims. *J Emerg Med* 12:285–292, 1994.
9. Ikenaga T, Kajikawa M, Kajikawa H, et al: Unilateral dissection of the cervical portion of the internal carotid artery and ipsilateral multiple cerebral infarctions caused by suicidal hanging: a case report. *No Shinkei Geka* 24:853–858, 1996.
10. Ohkawa S, Yamadori A: CT in hanging. *Neuroradiology* 35:591, 1993.
11. Nakajo M, Onohara S, Shinmura K, et al: Computed tomography and magnetic resonance imaging findings of brain damage by hanging. *J Comput Assist Tomogr* 27:896–900, 2003.
12. Spicer RS, Miller TR: Suicide acts in 8 states: incidence and case fatality rates by demographics and method. *Am J Public Health* 90(12):1885–1891, 2000.
13. Arias M, Arias-Rivas S, Perez M, et al: Numb ears in resurrection: great auricular nerve injury in hanging attempt. *Neurology* 64:2153–2154, 2005.
14. Lammertse DP: Neurorehabilitation of spinal cord injuries following lightning and electrical trauma. *NeuroRehabilitation* 20:9–14, 2005.
15. Klein Schmidt-Demasters BK: Neuropathology of lightening-strike injuries. *Semin Neurol* 15(4):323–327, 1995.
16. Cooper MA: Emergent care of lightning and electrical injuries. *Semin Neurol* 15(3):268–278, 1995.
17. Cherington M: Central nervous system complications of lightning and electrical injuries. *Semin Neurol* 15(3):233–240, 1995.
18. Ten Duis HJ: Acute electrical burns. *Semin Neurol* 15(4):381–386, 1995.
19. Cherington M: Spectrum of neurologic complications of lightning injuries. *NeuroRehabilitation* 20:3–8, 2005.
20. Cohen JA: Autonomic nervous system disorders and reflex sympathetic dystrophy in lightning and electrical injuries. *Semin Neurol* 15(4):387–390, 1995.
21. Koumbourlis AC: Electrical injuries. *Crit Care Med* 30[Suppl 11]:S424–430, 2002.
22. Norman ME, Albertson D, Younge BR: Ophthalmic manifestations of lightning strike. *Surv Ophthal* 46(1):19–24, 2001.
23. Ogren FP, Edmunds AL: Neuro-otologic findings in the lightning-injured patient. *Semin Neurol* 15(3):256–262, 1995.
24. Primeau M: Neurorehabilitation of behavioral disorders following lightning and electrical trauma. *NeuroRehabilitation* 20:25–33, 2005.
25. Jafari H, Couratier P, Camu W: Motor neuron disease after electrical injury. *J Neurol Neurosurg Psychiatry* 71:265–267, 2001.
26. Wilbourn AJ: Peripheral nerve disorders in electrical and lightning injuries. *Semin Neurol* 15(3):241–254, 1995.
27. Smith MA, Muehlberger T, Dellon AL: Peripheral nerve compression associated with low-voltage electrical injury without associated significant cutaneous burn. *Plast Reconstr Surg* 109(1):137–144, 2002.
28. Primeau M, Engelstatter GH, Bares KK: Behavioral consequences of lightning and electrical injury. *Semin Neurol* 15(3):279–285, 1995.
29. Ernst A, Zibrak JD: Carbon monoxide poisoning. *N Engl J Med* 339(22): 1603–1608, 1998.
30. Weaver LK: Carbon monoxide poisoning. *Crit Care Clin* 15(2):297–317, 1999.
31. Dinerman N, Huber J: Inhalation injuries, in Rosen P (ed): *Emergency Medicine: Concepts and Clinical Practice*. 2nd ed. St. Louis, Mosby, 1988, p 585.
32. Thom SR, Taber RL, Mendiguren II, et al: Delayed neuropsychiatric sequelae after carbon monoxide poisoning: prevention by treatment with hyperbaric oxygen. *Ann Emerg Med* 25:474–480, 1995.
33. Annane D, Chevret S, Jars-Guincestre C, et al: Prognostic factors in unintentional mild carbon monoxide poisoning. *Intensive Care Med* 27(11):1776–1781, 2001.
34. Lee MS, Marsden CD: Neurological sequelae following carbon monoxide poisoning clinical course and outcome according to the clinical types and brain computed tomography scan findings. *Mov Disord* 9(5):550–558, 1994.
35. Kim JH, Change KH, Song IC, et al: Delayed encephalopathy of acute carbon monoxide intoxication: diffusivity of cerebral white matter lesions. *Am J Neuroradiol* 24(8):1592–1597, 2003.
36. Chu K, Jung KH, Kim H-J, et al: Diffusion-weighted MRI and ^{99m}Tc-HMPAO SPECT in delayed relapsing type of carbon monoxide poisoning: evidence of delayed cytotoxic edema. *Eur Neurol* 51:98–103, 2004.
37. Hopkins RO, Fearing MA, Weaver LK, et al: Basal ganglia lesions following carbon monoxide poisoning. *Brain Inj* 20(3):273–281, 2006.
38. Choi IS: Parkinsonism after carbon monoxide poisoning. *Eur Neurol* 48(1):30–33, 2002.
39. Gale SD, Hopkins RO, Weaver LK, et al: MRI, quantitative MRI, SPECT, and neuropsychological findings following carbon monoxide poisoning. *Brain Inj* 13(4):229–243, 1999.
40. Deschamps D, Geraud C, Julien H, et al: Memory one month after acute carbon monoxide intoxication: a prospective study. *Occup Environ Med* 60:212–216, 2003.
41. Min SK: A brain syndrome associated with delayed neuropsychiatric sequelae following acute carbon monoxide intoxication. *Acta Psychiatr Scand* 73:80–86, 1986.
42. Garland H, Pearce J: Neurological complications of carbon monoxide poisoning. *QJM* 36:445–455, 1967.
43. Neuman TS: Arterial gas embolism and decompression sickness. *News Physiol Sci* 17:77–81, 2002.
44. Tetzlaff K, Shank ES, Muth CM: Evaluation and management of decompression illness—an intensivist's perspective. *Intensive Care Med* 29:2128–2136, 2003.
45. Leach RM, Rees PJ, Wilmshurst P: ABC of oxygen: hyperbaric oxygen therapy. *BMJ* 317:1140–1143, 1998.
46. Levy D: The fat embolism syndrome: a review. *Clin Ortho Relat Res* 261:281–286, 1990.
47. Johnson MJ, Lucas GL: Fat embolism syndrome. *Orthopedics* 19:41–49, 1996.

48. Kamano M, Honda Y, Kitaguchi M, et al: Cerebral fat embolism after a nondisplaced tibial fracture. *Clin Ortho Rel Res* 389:206–209, 2001.
49. Forteza AM, Rabinstein A, Koch S, et al: Endovascular closure of patent foramen ovale in the fat embolism syndrome. *Arch Neurol* 59:455–459, 2002.
50. Dive AM, Dubois PE, Ide C, et al: Paradoxical cerebral fat embolism: an unusual case of persistent unconsciousness after orthopedic surgery. *Anesthesiology* 96(4):1029–1031, 2002.
51. Peltier L: Fat embolism, in Schwartz G (ed): *Principles and Practice of Emergency Medicine*. Philadelphia, WB Saunders, 1986, p 1589.
52. Muller C, Rahn BA, Pfister U, et al: The incidence, pathogenesis, diagnosis and treatment of fat embolism. *Orthop Rev* 23:107–117, 1994.
53. Kamenar E, Burger P: Cerebral fat embolism: a neuropathological study of a microembolic state. *Stroke* 11:477–484, 1980.
54. Ryu CW, Lee DH, Kim TK, et al: Cerebral fat embolism: diffusion-weighted MRI findings. *Acta Radiologica* 46:528–533, 2005.
55. Parizel PM, Demey HE, Veeckmans G, et al: Early diagnosis of cerebral fat embolism syndrome by diffusion-weighted MRI. *Stroke* 32:2942–2944, 2001.
56. Takahashi M, Suzuki R, Osakabe Y, et al: MRI findings in cerebral fat embolism: correlation with clinical manifestations. *J Trauma* 46(2):324–327, 1999.
57. Guenter CA, Braun TE: Fat embolism syndrome. Changing prognosis. *Chest* 79:143–145, 1981.
58. Smith HS, Busracamowongs A: Management of hiccups in the palliative care population. *Am J Hosp Palliat Care* 20(2):149–154, 2003.
59. Liu FC, Chen CA, Yang SS, et al: Acupuncture therapy rapidly terminates intractable hiccups complicating acute myocardial infarction. *South Med J* 98(3):385–387, 2005.
60. Payne BR, Tiel RL, Payne MS, et al: Vagus nerve stimulation for chronic intractable hiccups: case report. *J Neurosurg* 102(5):935–937, 2005.
61. Friedman NL: Hiccups: a treatment review. *Pharmacotherapy* 16:986–995, 1996.
62. Dickerman RD, Jaikumar S: The hiccup reflex arc and persistent hiccups with high-dose anabolic steroids: is the brainstem the steroid-responsive locus? *Clin Neuropharmacol* 24(1):62–64, 2001.
63. Thompson DF, Landry JP: Drug-induced hiccups. *Ann Pharmacother* 31:367–369, 1997.
64. Sharma P, Morgan JC, Sethi KD: Hiccups associated with dopamine agonists in Parkinson disease. *Neurology* 66:774, 2006.
65. Lester J, Beatriz Raina G, Uribe-Roca C, et al: Hiccup secondary to dopamine agonists in Parkinson's disease. *Mov Disord* 15:1667–1668, 2007.
66. Morris LG, Marti JL, Ziff DJ: Termination of idiopathic persistent singultus (hiccup) with supramaximal inspiration. *J Emerg Med* 27(4):416–417, 2004.
67. Kolodzik PW, Eilers MA: Hiccups (singultus): review and approach to management. *Ann Emerg Med* 20:565–573, 1991.
68. Aravot DJ, Wright G, Rees A, et al: Noninvasive phrenic nerve stimulation for intractable hiccups [letter]. *Lancet* 2:1047, 1989.
69. Johnson DL: Intractable hiccups: treatment by microvascular decompression of the vagus nerve. *J Neurosurg* 78:813–816, 1993.
70. Andres DW, Matthews TK: Transesophageal diaphragmatic pacing for treatment of persistent hiccups. *Anesthesiology* 102(2):483, 2005.

CHAPTER 178 ■ SUBARACHNOID HEMORRHAGE

WILEY HALL, MAJAZ MOONIS AND JOHN P. WEAVER

Intracranial hemorrhage after rupture of saccular aneurysms accounts for 6% to 8% of all strokes affecting young adults. Intracranial aneurysms are found in approximately 5% of the population at autopsy and rupture at a rate of 4 to 10 per 100,000 population per year, with a 25% mortality during the first 24 hours [1]. Current mortality rates vary between 35% and 50%. Up to 30% die within the first 2 weeks, and 45% die within 30 days after the initial event. Fifty percent of the survivors are left with significant neurologic impairment [2–4]. As a rule, intensive care medical and surgical interventions are necessary in the management of these cases [5,6].

Subarachnoid hemorrhage (SAH) represents a potentially highly treatable form of stroke. Presently, the usual care of an aneurysmal SAH patient includes early aneurysm repair to limit rebleeding, a calcium channel antagonist to ameliorate cerebral injury secondary to vasospasm, intravascular volume maintenance to address any blood volume deficit, and some form of hemodynamic manipulation. Improvements in functional outcome are due to early intervention, supportive intensive care management, and modern methods of treatment, including cerebral protection, interventional neuroradiology, cerebrospinal fluid (CSF) manipulation, and hemodynamic management [5,6].

PATHOGENESIS

Saccular, or berry, aneurysms must be distinguished from other types of intracerebral aneurysms such as traumatic, dissecting, mycotic, and tumor-related aneurysms. Saccular aneurysms lack the normal muscular media and elastic lamina layers [7]. Eighty-five percent of saccular aneurysms are located in the anterior circulation; 15% are in the posterior circulation [8]. Common sites for aneurysms are at the junction of the anterior cerebral and anterior communicating arteries, the origin of the posterior communicating artery, the middle cerebral artery trifurcation, and at the top of the basilar artery. Less common are those located at the cavernous carotid, the internal carotid bifurcation, the distal anterior cerebral, and the proximal basilar arteries. Twelve percent to 31% of patients have multiple aneurysms. Nine percent to 19% have aneurysms located at identical sites bilaterally (mirror aneurysms), and multiple aneurysms may occur within families [9]. Systemic diseases such as polycystic kidney, Marfan's syndrome, Ehlers–Danlos syndrome, pseudoxanthoma elasticum, fibromuscular dysplasia, and coarctation of the aorta are associated with an increased incidence of intracerebral aneurysms [10,11].

It is unclear at present whether aneurysms have a congenital/hereditary origin or result from subsequent degenerative mechanisms. Supporting a congenital theory for aneurysm occurrence, individuals with a single primary relative with an intracranial aneurysm are at a 1.8 fold increased risk of intracranial aneurysm; those with two primary relatives have a 4.2 fold increased risk. Supporting the degenerative theory, there is an increased incidence of intracranial aneurysms in patients with hypertension, cigarette abuse, and alcohol abuse, and in the majority of cases, a family history of aneurysms is absent [11–14].

Risk of Rupture in Unruptured Intracranial Aneurysms

Ideally, the goal of treatment would be to prevent SAH, which carries a high mortality and morbidity. With increasing use of magnetic resonance angiography (MRA) and high-resolution computed tomography angiography (CTA), incidental or asymptomatic small aneurysms are increasingly recognized before rupture. It is important to estimate the risk of aneurysmal rupture in these cases, which depends on critical size, location, or morphology of the aneurysm itself.

Data from a large, multicenter, prospective study—the International Study of Unruptured Intracranial Aneurysms [15]—suggests that the critical size associated with increased risk of rupture is 10 mm. Patients with unruptured intracranial aneurysms who have not had a prior SAH have a lower risk of aneurysmal rupture than with those in whom another aneurysm has previously ruptured. The annual risk of rupture of unruptured intracranial aneurysms smaller than 10 mm in patients with no previous SAH is 0.05% per year, compared with 0.5% per year in those with a prior SAH. In addition to size, aneurysm location was also predictive of subsequent rupture. Basilar tip aneurysms had the highest risk of rupture [15].

Data from the International Study of Unruptured Intracranial Aneurysms study conflicts with the experience at many centers that the majority of SAHs are attributable to aneurysms less than 10 mm. A smaller study [16] prospectively examining 118 consecutive patients with intracranial aneurysms found that, of 83 ruptured aneurysms, 81.9% and 59% were under 10 and 7 mm, respectively. Mean height and width were 6.7 and 6.1 mm. Seventy-two unruptured aneurysms were found to have similar size distributions, and mean height and width were 5.7 mm. The lack of conclusive evidence regarding prevalence of unruptured intracranial aneurysms in the general population and the absence of a screening tool that is sensitive, cost-effective, and safe enough makes optimal management of unruptured intracranial aneurysms a continuing challenge.

SYMPTOMS

The signs and symptoms of intracranial aneurysms result from their expansion or rupture. Aneurysmal expansion can lead to localized headache, facial pain, pupillary dilatation and ptosis from oculomotor nerve compression, and visual field defects from optic nerve or chiasm compression. Warning leak or "sentinel" hemorrhage occurs in approximately 20% of patients and is characterized by nuchal rigidity or meningismus that usually lasts at least 48 hours. The event is misdiagnosed in 20% to 40% as muscular-tension headache, migraine, sinusitis, viral syndrome, aseptic meningitis, or malingering [17]. Evidence of aneurysmal expansion or warning leak must be regarded with a high index of suspicion because such events precede major hemorrhage. Neurologic and functional outcomes are greatly improved if the patient is treated while neurologically intact before hemorrhage [18].

Aneurysmal rupture typically produces severe headache which is maximal at onset and is associated with neck pain, nausea, vomiting, photophobia, and lethargy. At the time of rupture, patients may lose consciousness and may demonstrate abducens nerve palsy, subhyaloid hemorrhages, or papilledema, reflecting the acute rise in intracranial pressure (ICP) that may transiently equal mean arterial pressure [19]. Other focal symptoms may also develop. Early seizures after SAH (8% to 11%) reflect a rise in ICP and are not indicative of the site or severity of rupture [20,21].

CLINICAL GRADING AND PROGNOSIS

The clinical grading scale developed by Hunt and Hess [22] is useful in estimating the patient's prognosis (Table 178.1). Grades I and II at presentation have a relatively good prognosis, whereas grades IV and V have a poor prognosis, and grade III an intermediate prognosis. The Glasgow Coma Scale is also useful in predicting outcome after early surgical intervention [23].

TABLE 178.1

HUNT AND HESS GRADING SCALE[a]

Grade	Symptoms
I	Asymptomatic or minimal headache and slight nuchal rigidity
II	Moderate-to-severe headache, nuchal rigidity, no neurologic deficit other than cranial nerve palsy
III	Drowsiness, confusion, or mild focal deficit
IV	Stupor, moderate-to-severe hemiparesis, possibly early decerebrate rigidity, and vegetative disturbances
V	Deep coma, decerebrate rigidity, moribund appearance

[a]Serious systemic diseases, such as hypertension, diabetes, severe arteriosclerosis, chronic obstructive pulmonary disease, and severe vasospasm, result in placement of the patient in the next less-favorable category.

DIAGNOSTIC EVALUATION

If SAH is suspected, an urgent noncontrast head CT should be obtained to identify, localize, and quantify the hemorrhage. CT imaging is 98% to 100% sensitive in the first 12 hours after SAH, declining to under 85% sensitive 6 days following a hemorrhage [6]. A lumbar puncture is indicated if the CT is nondiagnostic. CT scan may be negative in up to 35% of patients with sentinel leaks [24]. CT angiography (CTA) is the preferred study in the emergent surgical setting, and is often used when the presence of a large parenchymal clot makes delay for conventional arteriography unacceptable. CTA uses a contrast-enhanced high-speed spiral (helical) CT performed with reconstruction of the axially acquired data into angiographic images. CTA can demonstrate aneurysms of 2- to 3-mm size with sensitivities of 77% to 97% and specificities of 87% to 100% [25,26].

Traumatic lumbar puncture and SAH are distinguished by xanthochromia, demonstrated by spectrophotometric analysis of a centrifuged sample of the CSF [27]. Cell counts remain uniform in all tubes of CSF in a true SAH, and blood clots do not form. The CSF protein is usually elevated and glucose may be very slightly reduced. Opening pressure at the time of lumbar puncture may reflect the elevation of ICP.

Four-vessel cerebral angiography is necessary to localize the aneurysm, define the vascular anatomy, and assess vasospasm and the possible presence of multiple aneurysms. It should be performed within 24 hours after initial hemorrhage. If angiography does not reveal an aneurysm, magnetic resonance imaging and angiography can be performed to reveal aneurysms larger than 3 mm. If these studies are also negative, angiography is repeated in 1 to 3 weeks because acutely, intraluminal thrombus and vasospasm can interfere with angiographic visualization of aneurysms [6,28,29].

GENERAL MEDICAL MANAGEMENT

Complications of SAH are fatal in 25% of cases [15,27]. General preoperative medical management should include provisions for quiet bed rest, head elevation to improve cerebral venous return, good pulmonary toilet to avoid atelectasis and pneumonia, and prophylaxis against thrombophlebitis with pneumatic boots. Patients should receive stool softeners. Nausea and vomiting can be controlled with antiemetics. Pain control is best accomplished with agents such as morphine or fentanyl. Mean arterial pressures higher than 100 mm Hg should be lowered gently until repair of the aneurysm can be achieved, but agents that can depress consciousness such as α-methyldopa should be avoided. Blood pressure is managed with beta-blocking agents; these agents may also reduce the risks of cardiac arrhythmias.

After SAH there may be a salt-wasting diuresis. Suggested mechanisms include an increase in circulating atrial natriuretic peptide. This syndrome is distinguished from the syndrome of inappropriate antidiuretic hormone by urine output and urine chemistry; both may result in hyponatremia. Accordingly, fluid input and output must be followed closely along with serum electrolytes and osmolality.

Seizures have been reported to occur in up to 18% of patients with SAH at onset, and are less common in hospitalized patients, recently reported at 4% [30]. The need for prophylactic anticonvulsants is controversial, and phenytoin remains the most common anticonvulsant used, though recent studies suggest a worse cognitive outcome with its use [31]. Levetiracetam is sometimes substituted if hepatic enzymes rise or suspected drug fever occurs, but data on its efficacy in this setting is as yet unavailable.

Elevation of ICP must be treated promptly with an agent such as mannitol. The use of dexamethasone for cerebral edema is restricted to patients with postoperative edema due to retractor manipulation, and is used to blunt headache caused by meningeal irritation; it has been reported anecdotally to shorten the course of hydrocephalus after SAH as well.

CARDIAC FUNCTION AFTER SUBARACHNOID HEMORRHAGE

Cardiac dysrhythmias may complicate care following SAH; a variety of mechanisms have been proposed. Increased levels of circulating catecholamines influence the α-receptors of the myocardium and can result in prolonged myofibril contraction, eventually causing myofibrillar degeneration and necrosis. An alternative theory of myocardial injury suggests that coronary artery spasm is the mechanism for the myocytolysis. SAH is the most frequent neurologic cause for electrocardiographic changes, which include large upright T waves and prolonged QT intervals (on average, approximately 0.53 seconds). In addition, prominent U waves, inverted T waves, and minor elevation or depression of the ST segment can occur. Despite ST-T changes, the incidence of myocardial ischemia remains low [32,33]. Pathologic Q waves are not common in SAH and suggest the need for further investigations for myocardial infarction. Patients with coronary artery vasospasm have a worse prognosis [34]. Arrhythmias are very common: a prospective study of 120 patients performed by using Holter monitoring indicated a 90% incidence of ventricular and supraventricular arrhythmias in the first 48 hours of hospitalization [35]. These do not appear to account for significant mortality.

NEUROLOGIC COMPLICATIONS

Aneurysmal rebleeding, hydrocephalus, and cerebral vasospasm with ischemia are the three major neurologic complications after SAH.

Rebleeding is a serious and frequent neurologic complication of SAH, carrying a mortality rate from 50% to 70% [5,6,9]. The peak incidence of rebleeding occurs during the first day after SAH, and a secondary peak occurs 1 week later. The rerupture risk for an untreated ruptured aneurysm is 23% at 2 weeks, 35% to 42% at 4 weeks, and 50% within 6 months [29]. Clinically, patients suffer with increasing headache, nausea, vomiting, depressed level of consciousness, and the appearance of new neurologic deficits. Occasionally, seizures occur, but they have not been shown to be a cause of rebleeding. Attempts to prevent rebleeding by drug-induced hypotension and bed rest have not been successful [36]. Antifibrinolytics decrease the rate of rebleeding, but older studies associate their use with increased incidence of ischemic insults from vasospasm [37,38]. Modern approaches including early aneurysm repair and intravascular therapy for vasospasm may ameliorate these issues, but antifibrinolytics are not strongly recommended [6].

Hydrocephalus can develop acutely within the first few hours after SAH because of impaired CSF resorption at the arachnoid granulations or intraventricular blood causing obstruction of CSF outflow. Clinically significant hydrocephalus developing subacutely over a few days or weeks after SAH is manifested by the loss of vertical gaze and progressive lethargy. Patients may appear to be abulic. Ventricular CSF drainage may be indicated if the clinical neurologic examination deteriorates or for any obtunded patient with hydrocephalus. CSF drainage is limited in patients with unprotected aneurysms because there is a danger of rerupture associated with abrupt decreases in ICP. A delayed form of hydrocephalus manifested by cognitive changes and gait disorders may be observed several weeks after the SAH; in these cases, a ventriculoperitoneal shunt may be indicated [5].

Stroke due to vasospasm is a major cause of morbidity and mortality in the postoperative period. Several controlled studies have shown an important role for the calcium antagonist nimodipine in ameliorating neurologic deficits caused by vasospasm. Beneficial effects are probably related to calcium channel–blocking properties, interfering with steps in the ischemic cascade [39–41]. The neurologic outcome and mortality rates of SAH patients prophylactically treated with nimodipine are improved 25% to 50% over control subjects. Fewer infarcts are noted in these patients, although there is no difference in the incidence or extent of arteriographic vasospasm [42–44]. The only adverse effect is mild transient hypotension. Current recommendations are to administer 60 mg of nimodipine orally every 4 hours for a 21-day course beginning at the onset of SAH.

ANEURYSM REPAIR

After acute angiography, patients should undergo aneurysm repair as soon as possible [44–46]. Many centers delay repair in patients who present overnight until the following day to allow approach by a well-rested team. Hemorrhages associated with large parenchymal clots are approached urgently. Delays of longer than 1 to 2 days are no longer common.

Aneurysms may be excluded from the systemic circulation by open surgical or endovascular approach. Open surgery offers definitive repair under direct visualization. The potential benefit of decreased hemorrhage burden in the subarachnoid space following irrigation has been suggested as a means to decrease vasospasm incidence, but this has not been well studied. Endovascular repair offers a less invasive approach, allowing obliteration of aneurysms which may be inaccessiuble to open surgery. Endovascular repair may also be of advantage in higher grade hemorrhages where cerebral edema complicates craniotomy, or in cases where late presentation or diagnosis increases the risk of open surgery. The choice of repair modality is best decided by a team approach combining experts from both interventional neuroradiology and vascular neurosurgery.

SURGICAL MANAGEMENT

Current surgical management necessitates craniotomy for clip occlusion of the aneurysmal neck, using mild systemic intraoperative hypotension, temporary proximal occlusion, and microsurgical techniques [47–49]. Unique problems that dictate the use of specialized techniques include vertebral-basilar system aneurysms, giant aneurysms (greater than 25 mm), and multiple aneurysms. Moreover, some giant aneurysms can be isolated from the intracerebral circulation with an antecedent arterial bypass from the superficial temporal artery, or saphenous vein graft from the cervical or petrous carotid artery. Internal carotid proximal occlusion may still be an effective way to reduce intra-aneurysmal pressure and reduce the occurrence of subsequent hemorrhage in certain aneurysms, but endovascular techniques have mostly replaced surgery to accomplish this treatment.

Postsurgical arteriograms are obtained by most neurosurgeons to assess successful clip placement or to diagnose vasospasm. The availability of portable digital angiography has made the possibility of intraoperative angiography quite practical. Barrow et al. [50] reported a series of 115 procedures with intraoperative arteriography in which 19 studies resulted in an altered surgical plan, presumably saving reoperation. Selection criteria currently rely on the operative difficulty of clip placement, visualization of clip placement, and surgical judgment.

HYPOTHERMIA AND INTRAOPERATIVE CEREBRAL PROTECTION

Hypothermia is a well-known cytoprotective strategy used in cardiac surgery. Animal investigation has demonstrated that a moderate decrease in brain temperature is associated with decreased concentrations of tissue neurotransmitters that might otherwise promote cascades of secondary neuronal and vascular injuries. In addition, the cerebral metabolic rate of oxygen uptake decreases as temperature falls; below 28°C cerebral electrical activity is minimal. While moderate hypothermia (31°C to 34°C) is commonly used as an adjunct to pharmacologic methods for neuroprotection during routine aneurysm surgeries [51,52], larger trials failed to detect an impact on outcome [53].

Deep hypothermia (22°C to 18°C) under barbiturate anesthesia with a short (10- to 15-minute) circulatory arrest is used rarely for reconstruction of giant aneurysms [54]. Previous bleeding disorders, predisposition to hemorrhage, and prior cardiopulmonary disease are all relative contraindications to deep hypothermia; this remains a high-morbidity procedure with fewer than 50% of patients achieving a good outcome. Reported complications include postoperative hemorrhage, deep vein thrombophlebitis, and pulmonary embolism.

INTERVENTIONAL NEURORADIOLOGY

The development of endovascular techniques has allowed increasingly safe and precise access to the cerebral vasculature. Endovascular balloon occlusion, coil technologies, angioplasty, and intraoperative arteriographic definition of vascular reconstruction represent technical advances that have improved outcomes. Endovascular therapy may be used to treat aneurysms by occlusion of the parent artery or by selective occlusion of the aneurysm.

The technique of endovascular balloon occlusion allows the fluoroscopically directed placement of a detachable silicone occlusive balloon within the aneurysmal sac [55]. In recent years, the devices have been abandoned for direct treatment of saccular aneurysms because of complications, including rupture, embolic events, and incomplete aneurysm obliteration. They are used, however, for the treatment of cavernous carotid fistula resulting from a ruptured aneurysm of the intracavernous carotid, and for parent artery occlusion. Temporary occlusion with neurologic monitoring of the patient's condition, electroencephalogram, cerebral blood flow (CBF), and transcranial Doppler (TCD) measurements are used before permanent proximal occlusion.

The most common endovascular approach to aneurysm occlusion is achieved by placing detachable platinum-alloy microcoils into the aneurysm sac. A low positive direct electric current transmitted through the guidewire detaches the coil from the stainless steel microcatheter by electrolysis and promotes intra-aneurysmal electrothrombosis by the attraction of local blood components. Clinical reports demonstrate a relatively high success rate for aneurysm obliteration and lower morbidity and mortality than balloon or free-coil embolization [56–58]. Advanced endovascular techniques, including stent-assisted coiling, balloon remodeling, and multicatheter techniques, allow aneurysms of various morphologies to be treated [59,60].

The International Subarachnoid Aneurysm Trial presented level I evidence supporting endovascular repair of ruptured aneurysms over surgical approach in most patients. The trial reported a 30.9% death or dependency rate in patients undergoing surgical repair, compared with 23.5% in those treated via endovascular approach. Higher rebleed rates at 1 and 4 years in the endovascular group did not offset the improvement in functional outcome [61,62]. The International Subarachnoid Aneurysm Trial was limited by a paucity of posterior circulation aneurysms, possibly because of evolving belief that these aneurysms are better approached via an endovascular approach and thus a perceived lack of clinical equipoise. Aneurysms with ratios of neck size to dome size greater than 0.5 and those with arterial branches arising from their domes or bases may be best treated surgically in most centers due to limitations in endovascular techniques.

POSTOPERATIVE MANAGEMENT

Care following repair of the ruptured aneurysm centers on limiting sequelae of SAH. Patients are monitored in the intensive care unit for evidence of vasospasm and hydrocephalus. Meticulous care to avoid pneumonia, deep venous thrombosis, and skin breakdown are mandatory. Nimodipine is continued for 21 days after hemorrhage [44]. Hypertensive, hypervolemic, hemodilution ("triple-H" or HHT) therapy has not been shown to prevent vasospasm, but is utilized when vasospasm is present to prevent infarction [44,63,64]. Maintenance of hematocrit above 30% is common, but evidence supporting its necessity in patients without evidence of coronary ischemia is lacking.

Cerebral vasospasm is a major cause of morbidity and mortality in patients recovering from SAH. Although noted angiographically in more than 70% of patients, it causes clinically evident symptoms due to cerebral ischemia in only 36% [65]. This difference probably reflects the adequacy of collateral circulation in the individual patient and the degree of vessel narrowing. Unlike rebleeding, the clinical presentation of vasospasm occurs progressively over a period of hours to days. It is rarely seen before the third day after hemorrhage, with a peak between days 4 to 12, and may rarely occur as long as 3 weeks after SAH [5,6]. The neurologic deficits are correlated with the areas of brain supplied by the narrowed arteries. Vasospasm is identified by angiography and noninvasively by TCD techniques.

TCD techniques are now widely used at most cerebrovascular centers. This simple bedside test is sensitive to the onset of cerebral vasospasm as arterial blood flow velocity increases with progressive vessel narrowing. Because the middle cerebral artery has little collateral circulation, diagnosis of vasospasm by TCD measurements is best validated in this vascular territory; TCD has an overall sensitivity of 68% to 94%, specificity of 86% to 100%, positive predictive value of 57% to 95%, and negative predictive value of 80% to 90% [66]. Fewer studies have documented sensitivity of TCD diagnosis for posterior circulation vasospasm [67]. This sensitivity is clinically useful because an elevated blood flow velocity is often detected before the occurrence of ischemic complications of vasospasm. More aggressive treatment aimed to increase cerebral perfusion pressure and improve circulation rheology can be instituted before the onset of neurologic impairment. Use of TCD for large groups of patients has allowed daily charting of the velocity changes that occur with the vasospasm syndrome. The time course of vasospasm onset and duration makes TCD a good tool to stratify patients into risk groups [68].

The amount of blood in the subarachnoid space and its location may predict the degree and location of delayed cerebral ischemic events. In theory, the pathogenesis of spasm is related to products of local erythrocyte breakdown that may be spasmogenic. Potential inducers of spasm include oxyhemoglobin, angiotensin, histamine, serotonin, prostaglandin, and catecholamines [4]. Vasospasm may occur because of endothelial structural changes caused by an inflammatory response, depression of vessel wall respiration, or damage from prolonged active arterial wall contraction. Other theories include impairment of normal vasodilatation, the mechanical effects of arterial compression by clot, and development of a proliferative vasculopathy. Pathologic specimens of affected vessels demonstrate intimal proliferation and medial necrosis. Thus, the pathogenesis of cerebral vasospasm is a complicated multifactorial process. Vasospasm occurs more frequently in patients with a poor clinical grade, thick focal blood clots, or a diffuse layer of blood in the subarachnoid space.

Modern multimodality monitoring of brain tissue oxygen tension and microdialysis of the interstitial space offers the promise of early diagnosis of vasospasm. Early case series suggest that brain tissue chemistry may change up to several days before the onset of vasospasm, best detected by detection of alterations in tissue lactate, lactate/pyruvate ratio, glutamate and other proteins using bedside microdialysis [69–71].

HYPERDYNAMIC THERAPY

Circulatory manipulation is a routine treatment for regional ischemia with predictable benefit [65,72]. Selection criteria for treatment include increasing blood flow velocity signals by TCD measurement, focal deficit, and global impairment of consciousness without hydrocephalus. While there is no proven preventative treatment for cerebral vasospasm, the current mainstay of therapy is hypervolemic hypertensive therapy or HHT. The aim is to augment cerebral perfusion and rheology by raising systolic blood pressure, cardiac output, and intravascular volume. Progress in this area has been predominantly in the area of small cohort studies of intermediate variables, CBF, and systemic blood volume [73–75]. A number of authors have demonstrated that elevation of systemic arterial pressure produces a significant increase in the regional CBF [76–78]. Typically, 20 to 30 mm Hg elevation of the mean arterial pressure increases CBF by 15 to 25 mL per minute per 100 g. In contrast, recent studies have failed to demonstrate a beneficial effect of hemodilution therapy on oxygen delivery in patients with vasospasm [79]. Vasopressors are used to keep systolic blood pressures 20 to 40 points higher than pretreatment levels, and plasma volume is maintained with normal saline and occasionally with albumin, hetastarch, or Plasmanate. This therapy is continued for 48 to 72 hours or until serial imaging studies improve before it is gradually withdrawn under close observation. Risks of therapy include myocardial infarction, congestive heart failure, dysrhythmias, and hemorrhagic infarcts. This treatment can be used most aggressively in the postoperative period because of the risks of aneurysmal rerupture before surgery. Early surgery and careful cardiac monitoring for congestive heart failure are necessary for the prevention of significant complications.

Angioplasty is another proven technique for treatment of cerebral vasospasm [80–82]. Higashida et al. [81] developed a soft silicone balloon that is navigated into the basilar, posterior cerebral (P1), middle cerebral (M1, M2), and anterior cerebral (A1, A2) arteries and provides appropriate pressures to dilate these vessels. Patient selection criteria for treatment include the presence of arteriographic vasospasm without infarction in a patient with a repaired aneurysm. A correlation of symptoms with the anatomy of the vascular narrowing is helpful but not always present because altered mental status is often the presenting symptom of vasospasm. Failure of calcium antagonist prophylaxis or complications of hypertensive hypervolemic therapy are appropriate indications for considering this procedure. Most successful angioplasties are performed in the first 48 hours after onset of major symptoms because the procedure is much less effective as a "salvage" technique after cerebrovascular reserve is depleted and vascular fibrosis occurs. Observations in a rabbit SAH model demonstrated that the initial vessel narrowing is related to vasospasm with subsequent anatomical fibrosis during the next 5 to 7 days, when it accounts for more than 60% of the caliber changes [83]. This identified the timing and extent of alteration of vessel inelastic elements in the production of vasospasm. Thus, angioplasty should be most effective early on before maximal fibrosis occurs. Angioplasty has also been used to treat catheter-induced spasm. Several groups have reported SAH patients who benefited from intra-arterial infusions of papaverine, verapamil, and nicardipine [84–86].

THROMBOLYSIS OF THE SUBARACHNOID SPACE

The degradation of hemoglobin in the cranial subarachnoid space produces a histologic and arteriographic picture consistent with vasospasm, and the severity of spasm/ischemia appears to relate to the amount of blood in the CSF space. Thus, there has been a longstanding interest in removing this spasmogen. A reduced incidence of vasospasm after intrathecal treatment with recombinant tissue-type plasminogen activator within the first 24 hours of onset of SAH, and a drop in the resistance to CSF outflow has been noted after experimental treatment with tissue plasminogen activator [87,88]. The use of intrathecal tissue plasminogen activator has been reported in 109 patients, with one hemorrhagic death due to an epidural hematoma, four nonfatal cases of epidural and intracerebral hematoma, and one extradural hematoma [89]. Arteriographic follow-up demonstrated a decreased incidence of arteriographic vasospasm.

FREE RADICAL SCAVENGERS IN SUBARACHNOID HEMORRHAGE

Free iron from the blood can lead to lipid peroxidation and free radical generation. Free radical scavengers may be useful in preventing further damage [90]. A controlled study in 208 patients using a free radical scavenging agent, nizofenone, demonstrated improvement based on functional recovery, especially in patients with delayed ischemic symptoms, moderate severity of preoperative deficits (Hunt and Hess grades II or III), and diffuse high-density areas in pre- and postoperative CTs [91]. The nonglucocorticoid 21-aminosteroid tirilazad mesylate has been shown to inhibit lipid peroxidation and protect cell membranes by scavenging destructive-free radicals, but positive results of a European trial were not reproduced in a large multicenter North American trial [92–94]. In a post hoc subgroup analysis of the highest dose group, however, mortality was improved from 33% in the vehicle group to 5% in the patient subgroup that included men with admission grades IV and V.

RECOMMENDATIONS

The current literature for unruptured aneurysms has level IV and level V evidence and can support grade C recommendations. Patient factors, biases, and personal preferences influence treatment decisions and should be taken in consideration. Recommendations for ruptured aneurysms are more definite.

1. Management of unruptured intracranial aneurysms.
   a. In general, small incidental aneurysms less than 10 mm require follow-up rather than surgical intervention. Younger patients may require more aggressive management. Small aneurysms in this group may also be treated if there is rapid enlargement, daughter sac formation, or there is a history of familial intracranial aneurysms.
   b. Irrespective of size, coexisting or remaining aneurysms in patients with a previous history of SAH warrant consideration for aneurysm repair.
   c. Patients with basilar tip aneurysms 7 mm or more in diameter have a higher incidence of rupture and treatment should be considered.
   d. Decisions on approach to repair should be made by a team including a vascular neurosurgeon and an interventional neuroradiologist.
2. Management of ruptured aneurysms.

2.1 Aneurysms preferentially treated with surgical clipping include the following:
   a. Patients with poor vascular anatomy for endovascular approach
   b. Acutely ruptured aneurysms with symptomatic intracranial hematoma
   c. Recurrent aneurysms after coil embolization

2.2 Aneurysm preferentially treated by endovascular embolization with detachable coils
   a. Medically unstable patients
   b. Patients with poor neurologic condition (e.g., grade 4 or 5, established vasospasm, or severe brain swelling)
   c. Aneurysms with significant calcification
   d. Residual aneurysms after unsuccessful surgery

2.3 Patients should be monitored for vasospasm postoperatively using clinical examination and TCD if available.
   a. Hyperdynamic therapy is therapeutic but not preventive for vasospasm.
   b. Endovascular therapies for vasospasm should be employed when medical therapies fail.
   c. The calcium channel antagonist nimodipine should be given for the first 21 days following SAH.

3. Giant aneurysms greater than 2.5 cm should be approached on an individual basis. Location, accessibility, and collateral circulation all influence the decision to treat surgically or with endovascular management [15,95,96]. Patients are best approached on an individual basis with direct collaboration between neurosurgeon and interventionalist prior to repair.

References

1. McCormick WF, Nofziger JD: Saccular intracranial aneurysm: an autopsy study. *J Neurosurg* 21:155, 1965.
2. Nieuwkamp DJ, Setz LE, Algra A, et al: Changes in case fatality of aneurysmal subarachnoid haemorrhage over time, according to age, sex, and region: a meta-analysis. *Lancet Neurol* 8:635–642, 2009.
3. Al-Shahi SR, Sudlow CL: Case fatality after subarachnoid haemorrhage: declining, but why? *Lancet Neurol* 8:598, 2009.
4. Ingall TJ, Wiebers DO: Natural history of subarachnoid hemorrhage, in Whisnant JP (ed): *Stroke: Populations, Cohorts, and Clinical Trials*. Boston, Butterworth–Heinemann, 1993.
5. Ropper AH, Gress DR, Diringer MN (eds). Subarachnoid hemorrhage, in *Neurological and Neurosurgical Intensive Care*. Philadelphia. Lippincott Williams & Wilkins, 2004, p 231.
6. Bederson JB, Connolly ES Jr, Batjer HH: Guidelines for the management of aneurysmal subarachnoid hemorrhage. A statement for healthcare professionals from a special writing group of the Stroke Council, American Heart Association. *Stroke* 40:994, 2009.
7. Stebbens WE: Aneurysms, in Stebbens WE, Lie JT (eds): *Vascular Pathology*. London, Chapman Hall, 1995, p 353.
8. Stebbens WE: *Pathology of the Cerebral Blood Vessels*. St. Louis, Mosby, 1972, p 351.
9. Wilkins RM: Subarachnoid hemorrhage and saccular intracranial aneurysm: an update. *Surg Neurol* 15:92, 1981.
10. Schievink WI: Genetics of intracranial aneurysms. *Neurosurgery* 40:651, 1997.
11. Krex D, Shackert HK, Schackert G: Genesis of cerebral aneurysms—an update. *Acta Neurochir* 143:429, 2001.
12. Ruigrok YM, Rinkel GJ, Wijmenga C: Genetics of intracranial aneurysms. *Lancet Neurol* 4:179, 2005.
13. Wang MC, Rubinstein D, Kindt GW, et al: Prevalence of intracranial aneurysms in first degree relatives of patients with aneurysms. *Neurosurg Focus* 13:e2, 2002.
14. Weller RO: Subarachnoid hemorrhage and myths about saccular aneurysms. *J Clin Pathol* 48:1078, 1995.
15. USISA investigators: Unruptured intracranial aneurysms: risk of rupture and risk of surgical intervention. *N Engl J Med* 339:1725, 1998.
16. Beck J, Rohde S, Seifert V, et al: Size and location of ruptured and unruptured intracranial aneurysms measured by 3-dimensional rotational angiography. *Surg Neurol* 65:18, 2006.
17. Juvela S, Hillbom M, Numminen H, et al: Cigarette smoking and alcohol consumption as risk factors for aneurysmal subarachnoid hemorrhage. *Stroke* 24:639, 1993.
18. Jakobsson KE, Säveland H, Hillman J, et al: Warning leak and management outcome in aneurysmal subarachnoid hemorrhage. *J Neurosurg* 85:995, 1996.
19. Fisher CM: Clinical syndromes in cerebral thrombosis, hypertensive hemorrhage and ruptured saccular aneurysms. *Clin Neurosurg* 22:117, 1975.
20. Lin CL, Dumont AS, Lieu AS, et al: Characterization of perioperative seizures and epilepsy following aneurysmal subarachnoid hemorrhage. *J Neurosurg* 99:978, 2003.
21. Byrne JV, Boardman P, Ioannidis I, et al: Seizures after aneurysmal subarachnoid hemorrhage treated with coil embolization. *Neurosurgery* 52:545, 2003.
22. Hunt WE, Hess RM: Surgical risk as related to time of intervention in the repair of intracranial aneurysms. *J Neurosurg* 28:14, 1968.
23. Gotoh O, Tamura A, Yasui N, et al: Glasgow Coma Scale in the prediction of outcome after early aneurysm surgery. *Neurosurgery* 39:19, 1996.
24. Leblanc R: The minor leak preceding subarachnoid hemorrhage. *J Neurosurg* 66:35, 1987.
25. Hsiang JNK, Liang EY, Lam HMK, et al: The role of computed tomographic angiography in the diagnosis of intracranial aneurysms and emergent aneurysm clipping. *Neurosurgery* 38:481, 1996.
26. Hope JKA, Wilson JL, Thomson FJ: Three dimensional CT angiography in the detection and characterization of intracranial berry aneurysms. *AJNR Am J Neuroradiol* 17:439, 1996.
27. Vermeulen M: Subarachnoid haemorrhage: diagnosis and treatment. *J Neurol* 243:496, 1996.
28. Beguelin C, Seiler R: Subarachnoid hemorrhage with normal cerebral panangiography. *Neurosurgery* 13:409, 1983.
29. Kassell NF, Torner JC: The international cooperative study in timing of aneurysm surgery: an update. *Stroke* 15:566, 1984.
30. Rhoney DH, Tipps LB, Murry KR, et al: Anticonvulsant prophylaxis and timing of seizures after aneurysmal subarachnoid hemorrhage. *Neurology* 55:258, 2000.
31. Naidech AM, Kreiter KT, Janjua N, et al: Phenytoin exposure is associated with functional and cognitive disability after subarachnoid hemorrhage. *Stroke* 36:583, 2005.

32. Brouwers PJA, Wijdicks EFM, Hasan D, et al: Serial electrocardiographic recording in aneurysmal subarachnoid hemorrhage. *Stroke* 20:1162, 1989.
33. Hart GK, Humphrey L, Weiss J: Subarachnoid hemorrhage: cardiac complications. *Crit Care Rep* 1:88, 1989.
34. Yuki K, Kodama Y, Onda J, et al: Coronary vasospasm following subarachnoid hemorrhage as a cause of stunned myocardium. *J Neurosurg* 75:308, 1991.
35. Di Pasquale G, Pinelli G, Andreoli A, et al: Holter detection of cardiac arrhythmias in intracranial subarachnoid hemorrhage. *Am J Cardiol* 59:596, 1987.
36. Nibbelink DW, Henderson WG, Torner JC: Intracranial aneurysms and subarachnoid hemorrhage. Report on a randomized treatment study. IV-A. Regulated bedrest. *Stroke* 8:202, 1977.
37. Kassell NF, Torner JC, Adams HP: Antifibrinolytic therapy in the acute period following aneurysmal subarachnoid hemorrhage: preliminary observations from the cooperative aneurysm study. *J Neurosurg* 61:225, 1984.
38. Vermeulen M, Lindsay KW, Murray GD, et al: Antifibrinolytic treatment in subarachnoid hemorrhage. *N Engl J Med* 311:432, 1984.
39. Wong MCW, Haley EC Jr: Calcium antagonists: stroke therapy coming of age. *Curr Concepts Cerebrovasc Dis Stroke* 24:31, 1989.
40. Buchan AM, Sharma M: Experimental study of the pathogenesis and treatment of stroke. *Curr Opin Neurol Neurosurg* 4:38, 1991.
41. Heffez DS, Passonneau JV: Effect of nimodipine on cerebral metabolism during ischemia and recirculation in the mongolian gerbils. *J Cereb Blood Flow Metab* 5:523, 1985.
42. Rinkel GJ, Feigin V, Algra A, et al: Calcium antagonists for aneurysmal subarachnoid hemorrhage. *Cochrane Database Syst Rev* 25:CD000277, 2005.
43. Allen GS, Ahn HS, Preziosi TJ, et al: Cerebral arterial spasm—a controlled trial of nimodipine in patients with subarachnoid hemorrhage. *N Engl J Med* 308:619, 1983.
44. Whitfield PC, Kirkpatrick PJ: Timing of surgery for aneurysmal subarachnoid hemorrhage. *Cochrane Database Syst Rev* 2:CD001697, 2001.
45. Kassel NF, Drake CG: Timing of aneurysm surgery. *Neurosurgery* 10:514, 1982.
46. Kassel NF, Torner JC, Jane JA, et al: The international cooperative study on the timing of aneurysm surgery, part 2: surgical results. *J Neurosurg* 73:37, 1990.
47. Wilson CB, Spetzler RF: Factors responsible for improved results in the surgical management of intracranial aneurysms and vascular malformations. *Am J Surg* 134:33, 1977.
48. Meyer FB, Morita A, Puumala MR, et al: Medical and surgical management of intracranial aneurysms. *Mayo Clin Proc* 70:153, 1995.
49. Barrow DL, Cawley CM: Surgical management of complex intracranial aneurysms. *Neurol India* 52:156, 2004.
50. Barrow DL, Boyer KL, Joseph GJ: Intraoperative angiography in the management of neurovascular disorders. *Neurosurgery* 30:153, 1992.
51. Ogilvy CS, Carter BS, Kaplan S, et al: Temporary vessel occlusion for aneurysm surgery: risk factors for stroke in patients protected by induced hypothermia and hypertension and intravenous mannitol administration. *J Neurosurg* 84:785, 1996.
52. Hindman BJ, Todd MM, Gelb AW, et al: Mild hypothermia as a protective therapy during intracranial aneurysm surgery: a randomized prospective pilot trial. *Neurosurgery* 44:23, 1999.
53. Todd MM, Hindman BJ, Clarke WR, et al: Mild intraoperative hypothermia during surgery for intracranial aneurysm. *N Engl J Med* 352:135, 2005.
54. Spetzler RF, Hadley MN, Rigamonti D, et al: Aneurysms of the basilar artery treated with circulatory arrest, hypothermia, and barbiturate cerebral protection. *J Neurosurg* 68:868, 1988.
55. Weil SM, van Loveren HR, Tomisick TA, et al: Management of inoperable cerebral aneurysms by the navigational balloon technique. *Neurosurgery* 21:296, 1987.
56. Guglielmi G, Vinuela F, Sepetka I, et al: Electrothrombosis of saccular aneurysms via endovascular approach. *J Neurosurg* 75:1, 1991.
57. Guglielmi G, Vinuela F, Dion J, et al: Electrothrombosis of saccular aneurysms via endovascular approach. *J Neurosurg* 75:8, 1991.
58. Picard L, Bracard S, Lehéricy S, et al: Endovascular occlusion of intracranial aneurysms of the posterior circulation: comparison of balloons, free coils and detachable coils in 38 patients. *Neuroradiology* 38:S133, 1996.
59. Pierot L, Spelle L, Vitry F; ATENA Investigators: Immediate clinical outcome of patients harboring unruptured intracranial aneurysms treated by endovascular approach: results of the ATENA study. *Stroke* 39:2497, 2008.
60. Tähtinen OI, Vanninen RL, Manninen HI, et al: Wide-necked intracranial aneurysms: treatment with stent-assisted coil embolization during acute (<72 hours) subarachnoid hemorrhage—experience in 61 consecutive patients. *Radiology* 253:199, 2009.
61. Molyneux A, Kerr R, Stratton I, et al: International Subarachnoid Aneurysm Trial (ISAT) of neurosurgical clipping versus endovascular coiling in 2143 patients with ruptured intracranial aneurysms: a randomized trial. International Subarachnoid Aneurysm Trial (ISAT) Collaborative Group. *Lancet* 360:1267, 2002.
62. Molyneux A, Kerr R, Ly-Mee Y, et al: International Subarachnoid Aneurysm Trial (ISAT) of neurosurgical clipping versus endovascular coiling in 2143 patients with ruptured intracranial aneurysms: a randomized comparison of effects on survival, dependency, seizures, rebleeding, subgroups, and aneurysm occlusion. *Lancet* 366:809, 2005.
63. Treggiari MM, Walder B, Suter PM, et al: Systematic review of the prevention of delayed ischemic neurological deficits with hypertension, hypervolemia, and hemodilution therapy following subarachnoid hemorrhage. *J Neurosurg* 98:978, 2003.
64. Rinkel G, Feigin V, Algra A, et al: Circulatory volume expansion therapy for aneurysmal subarachnoid haemorrhage. *Cochrane Database Syst Rev* 4:CD000483, 2004.
65. Harrod CG, Bendok BR, Batjer HH: Prediction of cerebral vasospasm in patients presenting with aneurysmal subarachnoid hemorrhage: a review. *Neurosurgery* 56:633, 2005.
66. Sloan MA: Detection of vasospasm following subarachnoid hemorrhage, in Babikian VL, Wechsler LR (eds): *Transcranial Doppler Ultrasonography*. St. Louis, Mosby–Year Book, 1993, p 105.
67. Sloan MA, Burch CM, Wozniak MA, et al: Transcranial Doppler detection of vertebrobasilar vasospasm following subarachnoid hemorrhage. *Stroke* 25:2187, 1994.
68. Harders A, Gilsbach J: Hemodynamic effectiveness of nimodipine on spastic brain vessels after subarachnoid hemorrhage evaluated by the TCD method: a review of clinical studies. *Acta Neurochir Suppl* 45:21, 1988.
69. Enblad P, Valtysson J, Andersson J, et al: Simultaneous intracerebral microdialysis and positron emission tomography in the detection of ischemia in patients with subarachnoid hemorrhage. *J Cereb Blood Flow Metab* 16:637, 1996.
70. Cantais E, Boret H, Carre E, et al: Clinical use of bedside microdialysis: a review. *Ann Fr Anesth Reanim* 25:20, 2006.
71. Sarrafzadeh AS, Thomale UW, Haux D, et al: Cerebral metabolism and intracranial hypertension in high grade aneurysmal subarachnoid haemorrhage patients. *Acta Neurochir Suppl* 95:89, 2005.
72. Nibbelink DW: Cooperative aneurysm study: antihypertensive and antifibrinolytic therapy following subarachnoid hemorrhage from ruptured intracranial aneurysm, in Whisnant JP, Sandok BA (eds): *Cerebral Vascular Diseases*. New York, Grune & Stratton, 1975, p 155.
73. Kosnik EJ, Hunt WE: Postoperative hypertension in the management of patients with intracranial arterial aneurysms. *J Neurosurg* 45:148, 1976.
74. Hanley DF, Kirsch JR: Cerebral vasospasm: use of hypervolemic hypertensive therapy. *Crit Care Rep* 1:80, 1989.
75. Ullman JS, Bederson JB: Hypertensive, hypervolemic, hemodilutional therapy for aneurysmal subarachnoid hemorrhage: is it efficacious? Yes. *Crit Care Clin* 12:697, 1996.
76. Muizelaar JP, Becker DP: Induced hypertension for the treatment of cerebral ischemia after subarachnoid hemorrhage: direct effect on CBF. *Surg Neurol* 25:317, 1986.
77. Yonas H, Sekhar L, Johnson DW, et al: Determination of irreversible ischemia by xenon-enhanced computed tomographic monitoring of CBF in patients with symptomatic vasospasm. *Neurosurgery* 24:368, 1989.
78. Volby B: Pathophysiology of subarachnoid hemorrhage: experimental and clinical data. *Acta Neurochir Suppl* 45:1, 1988.
79. Ekelund A, Reinstrup P, Ryding E, et al: Effects of iso- and hypervolemic hemodilution on regional cerebral blood flow and oxygen delivery for patients with vasospasm after aneurysmal subarachnoid hemorrhage. *Acta Neurochir* 144:703, 2002.
80. Nichols DA, Meyer FB, Piegras DG, et al: Endovascular treatment of intracranial aneurysms. *Mayo Clin Proc* 69:272, 1994.
81. Higashida RT, Halbach VV, Cahan LD, et al: Transluminal angioplasty for treatment of intracranial arterial vasospasm. *J Neurosurg* 71:648, 1989.
82. Newell DW, Eskridge JM, Mayberg MR, et al: Angioplasty for the treatment of symptomatic vasospasm following subarachnoid hemorrhage. *J Neurosurg* 71:654, 1989.
83. Vorkapic P, Bevan RD, Bevan JA: Pharmacologic irreversible narrowing in chronic cerebrovasospasm in rabbits is associated with functional damage. *Stroke* 21:1478, 1990.
84. Moragn MK, Jonker B, Finfer S, et al: Aggressive management of aneurysmal subarachnoid haemorrhage based on a papaverine angioplasty protocol. *J Clin Neurosci* 7:305, 2000.
85. Feng L, Fitzsimmons BF, Young WL, et al: Intraarterially administered verapamil as adjunct therapy for cerebral vasospasm: safety and 2 year experience. *Am J Neuroradiol* 23:1284, 2002.
86. Badjatia N, Topcuoglu MA, Pryor JC, et al: Preliminary experience with intra-arterial nicardipine as a treatment for cerebral vasospasm. *Am J Neuroradiol* 25:819, 2004.
87. Findlay JM, Weir BKA, Kassell NF, et al: Intracisternal recombinant tissue plasminogen activator after aneurysmal subarachnoid hemorrhage. *J Neurosurg* 75:181, 1991.
88. Brinker T, Seifert V, Stolke D: Effect of intrathecal fibrinolysis on cerebrospinal fluid absorption after experimental subarachnoid hemorrhage. *J Neurosurg* 74:789, 1991.
89. Mizoi K, Yoshimoto T, Fujiwara S, et al: Prevention of vasospasm by clot removal and intrathecal bolus injection of tissue-type plasminogen activator: preliminary report. *Neurosurgery* 28:807, 1991.
90. Sakaki S, Ohta S, Nakamura H, et al: Free radical reaction and biological defense mechanism in the pathogenesis of prolonged vasospasm in experimental subarachnoid hemorrhage. *J Cereb Blood Flow Metab* 8:1, 1988.
91. Ohta T, Kikuchi H, Hashi K, et al: Nizofenone administration in the acute stage following subarachnoid hemorrhage. *J Neurosurg* 64:420, 1986.
92. Kanamaru K, Weir BKA, Simpson I, et al: Effect of 21-aminosteroid U-74006 F on lipid peroxidation in subarachnoid clot. *J Neurosurg* 74:454, 1991.

93. Kassell NF, Haley EC Jr, Apperson-Hansen C, et al: Randomized, double-blind, vehicle-controlled trial of tirilazad mesylate in patients with aneurysmal subarachnoid hemorrhage: a cooperative study in Europe, Australia, and New Zealand. *J Neurosurg* 84:221, 1996.
94. Haley EC Jr, Kassell NF, Apperson-Hansen C, et al: A randomized, double-blind, vehicle-controlled trial of tirilazad mesylate in patients with aneurysmal subarachnoid hemorrhage: a cooperative study in North America. *J Neurosurg* 86:467, 1997.
95. Bederson JB, Awad IA, Wiebers DO, et al: Recommendations for the management of patients with unruptured intracranial aneurysms. Scientific statement, American Heart Association. *Circulation* 102:2300, 2000.
96. Martin N: Decision making for intracranial aneurysm treatment: when to select surgery and when to select endovascular therapy. *J Stroke Cerebrovasc Dis* 6:253, 1997.

CHAPTER 179 ■ MENTAL STATUS DYSFUNCTION IN THE INTENSIVE CARE UNIT: POSTOPERATIVE COGNITIVE IMPAIRMENT

JOAN M. SWEARER AND SHASHIDHARA NANJUNDASWAMY

Cognitive dysfunction following major surgery is one of the common reasons neurologists are asked to evaluate postoperative patients in the intensive care unit (ICU): patients whose memory and intellectual abilities seem impaired when they otherwise appear to have recovered from the immediate effects of surgery. It is a major concern for the family, patient, and physician when a patient is found not to be intellectually the same on awakening following surgery as he or she was before.

There has been extensive research on cognitive dysfunction following major cardiac surgery and a growing literature from noncardiac surgery. In a literature review of cognitive decline following cardiac surgery published between 1985 and 2005, Newman et al. [1] reported that the incidence of decline noted within the first perioperative week varied from 50% to 70%. The incidence fell to 30% to 50% after 6 weeks, and to 20% to 40% at 6 months and 1 year. Differences in methods between studies (e.g., patient sampling, specific tests used, testing intervals, definitions of cognitive decline) make it difficult to compare the studies in literature reviews and meta-analyses directly. Despite these differences, increased age has been the most consistent factor associated with cognitive dysfunction; prolonged cardiopulmonary bypass has also been noted as a risk factor [1,2].

In a study of major noncardiac surgery [3], 1,064 patients aged 18 years and older completed neuropsychological testing before surgery, at hospital discharge, and 3 months after surgery. At 1 year postsurgery patients were contacted to determine survival status. At hospital discharge 36.6% of the young (18 to 39 years), 30.4% of the middle aged (40 to 59 years), and 41.4% of the elderly (60 years and older) had evidence of postoperative cognitive decline. At 3 months cognitive dysfunction was present in 5.7% young, 5.6% middle aged, and 12.7% elderly patients. Increased age, lower educational level, history of premorbid cerebral vascular accident (with no residual impairment), and cognitive decline at discharge were found to be independent risk factors for postoperative dysfunction at 3 months. Patients with postoperative cognitive decline were at increased risk of death in the first year postsurgery.

Although it is clear from these and other studies that postoperative cognitive decline can occur in elderly patients undergoing both major cardiac and noncardiac surgery, the precise pathophysiologic mechanisms have yet to be elucidated.

MENTAL STATUS EXAMINATION IN THE INTENSIVE CARE UNIT

The primary objectives of a mental status evaluation in the ICU are to screen for the presence of postoperative cognitive decline, to analyze both the nature and extent of the impairment, and to evaluate improvement or worsening over time. Cognitive changes may be obvious when there are gross deficits in learning, memory, attention, or concentration. The decline can also be subtle, with problems in initiative and planning ("executive" functions).

Many mental status screening tests are available [4–7], but none have been specifically developed for, or standardized in, the ICU. A brief screening test may provide a general impression of the patient's mental status, but the clinician must be able to assess areas of relative strength and weakness in greater depth. The following is offered as an outline for a mental status evaluation in the ICU [8–10].

Behavioral Observation and Patient Variables

Determination of the patient's level of wakefulness and arousal is the essential first step in a mental status examination: levels may range from deep coma to stupor, obtundation, normal alertness, hyperalertness, and manic states. Any further interpretation of mental status test results depends on full alertness, and is severely limited if arousal is not normal.

Test performance is also substantially influenced by the patient's ability to sustain attention. A patient who is easily distractible will perform poorly on most cognitive tests. Lack of motivation and effort during testing can have deleterious effects on test performance, and may lead to an overestimation of cognitive impairment. Abnormalities in mood and affect, and behavioral disturbances such as psychosis, disinhibition, hyperactivity, or impulsivity will also negatively impact the patient's test performance.

Other patient variables that can influence test performance include demographic variables (e.g., premorbid cognitive abilities, age, gender, education, cultural background) and medical and psychosocial history (e.g., psychiatric history, social history, present life circumstances). A history from family members is extremely useful in assessing the patient's premorbid abilities.

Finally, test performance is compromised by postoperative pain, use of analgesic and sedating medications, limitations in arm/hand mobility, and possible sensory loss (e.g., hemianopia) or motor impairment (e.g., hemiparesis). Assessment of mental status becomes challenging, and the results uncertain, if the patient is on a ventilator.

Attention

The patient's span of attention can be assessed at the bedside using digit span, which also depends on immediate verbal recall. Repetition of digits both forward and backward should be evaluated. Both tests consist of increasingly longer strings of random number sequences that are presented aloud to the patient. The average score obtained by adults is seven digits forward and five digits backward.

Perseverance or the ability to sustain behavioral output can be measured at the bedside by mental tracking tests. Reciting the alphabet and counting from 1 to 40 by 3s are relatively easy mental tracking tests. Examples of more discriminating tracking tests include serial subtraction of 3s from 100 to 70 and reciting the months of the year backward.

Resistance to interference and response inhibition can be tested with motor sequencing tasks. Examples include the "go-no-go" test (when the examiner taps once, the patient taps twice, but when the examiner taps twice the patient does not tap [11]); and alternating sequences (e.g., copying a sequence of script such as "m n m n m n" [12]). Patients with impaired attention may perseverate on one element of the task rather than alternate between the sequences.

Speech and Language Functions

Speech output should be assessed for fluency (rate and effort of speech), articulation (normal or dysarthric), phrase length, prosody (melody, rhythm, inflection), content (semantics and syntax), and paraphasias (substitutions of rhyming alteration of words). Output can be observed in verbal responses to open-ended questions or by having the patient verbally describe a complex visual scene, such as a photograph ("propositional speech"). Disorders of repetition can be elicited by having the patient repeat phrases that vary in grammatical complexity (e.g., "no ifs, ands, or buts").

Auditory comprehension can be assessed at the bedside in a number of ways. Examples include pointing to named objects, such as body-part identification (e.g., "Point to your left thumb") and following multistage oral commands. Speech comprehension can also be assessed by asking "yes/no" questions such as "Do cows fly?"

Common objects (e.g., watch, pen, eyeglasses) can be used to test naming to confrontation. Component parts (e.g., lens, frame) may detect more subtle naming deficits. Oral reading and comprehension can be tested by having the patient read a brief passage from a newspaper, and then asked "yes-no" questions about its content.

Spontaneous writing and writing to dictation are excellent screening tests for aphasic writing deficits. Comprehension can also be assessed by having the patient follow written directions (e.g., "Point to the ceiling"). Word-list generation by specific category (e.g., animals, items found in supermarket or hardware store) and by specific initial letter is sensitive to both language and attentional sequencing disorders.

Memory Functions

Memory functions include immediate memory span, learning capacity and retention, and retrieval of previously learned information (recent and remote). Immediate memory span is commonly assessed with a digit span forward test (described previously). The ability to learn new information can be investigated in a number of ways. For example, three or four unrelated words are presented and the patient is instructed to remember them. After 5 minutes of other testing, the patient is asked to recall the words. Nonverbal learning can be assessed in a similar fashion using line drawings of simple geometric figures or by pointing to three or four objects in the room and asking the patient to recall them a few minutes later.

Remote memory can be tested by asking questions about political figures (e.g., naming the three previous presidents), dates of major world events (e.g., years of World War II), and personal history (e.g., name of high school attended).

Visuospatial and Visuoconstructive Abilities

Visuoconstructive ability is tested by having the patient copy simple figures (e.g., cube, daisy, interlocking pentagons). Spatial planning can be assessed with clock drawing. The patient is asked to draw the face of a clock and to fill in all the numbers. Left-sided visual inattention or hemispatial neglect is suggested if the patient places all the numerals on one side of the clock, or omits all numerals normally on one side. Capacity to process number/time relationships can be tested by having the patient "set the time to 10 minutes past 11 o'clock."

Executive Functions and Other Cognitive Abilities

Interpretation of proverbs (e.g., "the early bird catches the worm") evaluates concept formation or capacity for abstract thought. Ability to generate abstract thought can be assessed also by asking how word pairs are alike. An example of an easy similarity test pair is "broccoli–cauliflower"; a more difficult pair is "fish–dandelion." Mental arithmetic problems (e.g., "How many quarters are in $1.50?") test reasoning ability as well as immediate memory and concentration. Unfortunately, there are no reliable tests of judgment. Patients may be able to describe an appropriate response to how they would handle a small emergency, but may not behave so in a real emergency.

MENTAL STATUS DYSFUNCTION IN THE INTENSIVE CARE UNIT

Acute Confusional State (Delirium)

Delirium is a very common cause of mental dysfunction in postoperative patients in the ICU. The hallmark features of delirium are inattentiveness, confusion, and psychomotor agitation, although hypoactive delirium is also recognized. An alteration in sleep–wake pattern is evident. Fever, sepsis, metabolic and endocrine disturbances, as well as medication use or withdrawal, or alcohol withdrawal, are among the causes of delirium; this is discussed in more detail in Chapter 197.

Focal Syndromes

Stroke is another adverse neurologic outcome from surgery—especially cardiac surgery [13] or endovascular procedures, such as angioplasty—and is usually recognized by the presence of focal or lateralizing deficits of sudden onset (see Chapter 173). Focal cognitive deficits include aphasia, apraxia, and agnosia; focal motor weakness and/or sensory loss may not be evident if the stroke involves more of the temporal–parietal areas due to low perfusion-border zone ischemia. Wernicke's type of receptive aphasia presents with a speech disturbance when the ischemic zone involves the posterior temporal lobe. In this condition, the patient speaks fluently but unintelligibly, is unable to comprehend speech, and can become agitated.

Postoperative Cognitive Decline/Dysfunction

As previously noted, changes in memory and concentration are often seen in the ICU in the initial postoperative period. These changes can, however, persist well beyond the immediate postoperative period when the effects of anesthesia and analgesia directly affecting cognitive functions have clearly worn off. Most mental status changes improve, but may continue following discharge, even weeks, months, and years later, with associated impaired quality of life and mortality [14,15].

Elderly patients undergoing major cardiac (e.g., coronary artery bypass grafting, thoracic vascular surgery) and major noncardiac (e.g., orthopedic, abdominal) surgery are at the greatest risk for postoperative cognitive decline. Other individual features that increase the risk of mental status dysfunction include previous cerebrovascular disease, previous and undetected cognitive impairment or dementia, and cardiovascular risk factors such as hypertension, diabetes, and peripheral vascular disease [1,2,16–18].

Intraoperative risk factors include surgical technique (e.g., duration of cardiopulmonary bypass, duration of aortic cross-clamping), hypotension, manipulation of diseased aorta, and the effects of general anesthesia and hypothermia. To assess these factors requires close scrutiny of the operative record, and of the anesthesia chart. Atherothromboembolic phenomena (microemboli) and hypoxia with watershed area injury secondary to hypoperfusion are possible causative mechanisms of postoperative cognitive dysfunction due to intraoperative events during surgery [1].

A number of postoperative factors can also affect cognitive status in the ICU, including the use of analgesics, degree of physical discomfort, and depression [16]. These factors may produce short-term but self-limited cognitive change. Nevertheless, they should be taken into account when assessing the mental status of a patient in the ICU.

SUMMARY

Testing for mental status dysfunction of a patient in the ICU can be a complex and difficult task. Interpretation of test results can be confounded by premorbid patient characteristics (e.g., presence of a dementing illness presurgically) and the patient's current status (e.g., drowsiness in the context of high-dose analgesics, sedatives, and other medications). Mental status testing should not be attempted if arousal is abnormal or if the patient is too ill. The approach to testing should be flexible and targeted to the individual patient's complaints and level of functioning. Postoperative cognitive changes range from obvious deficits in concentration and memory to subtle deficits in executive functions. Evidence of abnormality during a screening evaluation warrants a thorough neurologic evaluation.

References

1. Newman MF, Mathew JP, Grocott HP, et al: Central nervous system injury associated with cardiac surgery. *Lancet* 368:695, 2006.
2. Borowicz LM, Goldsborough MA, Selnes OA, et al: Neuropsychological change after cardiac surgery: a critical review. *J Cardiothorac Vasc Anesth* 10:105, 1996.
3. Monk TG, Weldon BC, Garvan CW, et al: Predictors of cognitive dysfunction after major noncardiac surgery. *Anesthesiology* 108:18, 2008.
4. Buschke H, Kuslansky G, Katz M, et al: Screening for dementia with the memory impairment screen. *Neurology* 52:231, 1999.
5. Solomon PR, Hirschoff A, Kelly B, et al: A 7 minute neurocognitive screening battery highly sensitive to Alzheimer's disease. *Arch Neurol* 55:349, 1998.
6. Drachman DA, Swearer JM, Kane K, et al: The Cognitive Assessment Screening Test (CAST) for dementia. *Neurology* 9:200, 1996.
7. Folstein M, Folstein S, McHugh PR: Mini-mental state: a practical method for grading the cognitive state of patients for the clinician. *J Psychiatric Res* 12:189, 1975.
8. Mendez MF, Cummings JL: *Dementia: A Clinical Approach*. 3rd ed. Boston, Butterworth-Heinemann, 2003.
9. Lezak MD, Howienson DB, Loring DW: *Neuropsychological Assessment*. 4th ed. New York, Oxford University Press, 2004.
10. Weintraub S: Neuropsychological assessment of mental state, in Mesulam MM (ed): *Principles of Behavioral and Cognitive Neurology*. 2nd ed. Oxford, Oxford University Press, 2000.
11. Drewe EA: Go-no-go learning after frontal lobe lesions in humans. *Cortex* 11:8, 1975.
12. Luria A: *Human Brain and Psychological Processes*. New York, Harper & Row, 1966.
13. McKhann GM, Grega MA, Borowitz LM, et al: Stroke and encephalopathy after cardiac surgery: an update. *Stroke* 37:562, 2006.
14. Steinmetz J, Christensen KB, Lund T, et al: Long-term consequences of postoperative cognitive dysfunction. *Anesthesiology* 110:548, 2009.
15. Phillips-Bute B, Mathew JP, Blumenthal JA, et al: Association of Neurocognitive function and quality of life 1 year after coronary artery bypass graft (CABG) surgery. *Psychosomatic Med* 68:369, 2006.
16. Newman MF, Croughwell ND, Blumenthal JA, et al: Predictors of cognitive decline after cardiac operation. *Ann Thorac Surg* 59:1326, 1995.
17. Selnes DA, McKhann GM: Neurocognitive complications after coronary artery bypass surgery. *Ann Neurol* 57:615, 2005.
18. Nakamura Y, Kawachi K, Imagawa H, et al: The prevalence and severity of cerebrovascular disease in patients undergoing cardiovascular surgery. *Ann Thorac Cardiovasc Surg* 10:81, 2004.

CHAPTER 180 ■ NEWLY ACQUIRED WEAKNESS IN THE INTENSIVE CARE UNIT: CRITICAL ILLNESS MYOPATHY AND NEUROPATHY

DAVID A. CHAD

Although preexisting neuromuscular disorders (such as myasthenia gravis and the Guillain–Barré syndrome) may cause severe weakness leading to an intensive care unit (ICU) admission, two of the most common causes of *newly acquired weakness arising in the ICU setting* are critical illness myopathy and critical illness polyneuropathy [1,2]. Critical illness myopathy is probably the major contributor to severe ICU-acquired weakness, causing most instances of failure to wean from a respirator in patients with severe systemic diseases in the ICU, while critical illness polyneuropathy affects 70% to 80% of patients with severe sepsis and multiorgan failure [3]. Even experienced clinicians have great difficulty distinguishing between the myopathy and the polyneuropathy of intensive care, especially because the two conditions often coexist in an individual patient [4–6]. In the sections that follow, we discuss each disorder and comment on the differential diagnosis of severe weakness arising in the ICU setting.

CRITICAL ILLNESS MYOPATHY

Diagnosis

The hallmark of critical illness myopathy is weakness that is typically diffuse in distribution, affecting both limb and neck muscles [7]. As is typical of most myopathic disorders, weakness tends to have a proximal predominance in the limbs, but it may also involve distal muscles profoundly. Tendon reflexes tend to be depressed but present, and on occasion, may be absent, possibly due to a generalized reduction in membrane excitability that occurs in sepsis [8]. There may be facial muscle involvement, and rarely, extraocular muscles are affected [9]; other muscles supplied by cranial nerves are usually spared. A serious and common complication of the myopathy is failure to wean from a ventilator due to marked weakness of the diaphragm. Although the majority of affected patients are adults, severe myopathic muscle weakness may occur in children who receive organ transplants [10].

Risk Factors

Critical illness myopathy develops in up to one-third of patients treated for status asthmaticus in the ICU; and in this population, intravenous corticosteroids and neuromuscular blocking agents are considered major risk factors [11]. Occasionally, the myopathy develops in patients who have received high-dose corticosteroids alone, without neuromuscular blocking agents, or in patients who have received neither corticosteroids nor neuromuscular blocking agents, but the latter group typically has severe systemic illness with multiorgan failure and sepsis [8]. Overall, critical illness myopathy accounts for 42% of weakness among patients in the surgical and medical ICU setting [12].

Laboratory Studies

Serum creatine kinase (CK), electromyography (EMG), and muscle biopsy are the most important and revealing studies in the diagnosis of ICU-acquired muscle weakness. An elevated CK level helps to support the diagnosis of a myopathic cause of weakness in an ICU patient, but in the myopathy of intensive care, the CK rise, which is found in about 50% of affected patients, only occurs early in the course of the illness, peaks within a few days of onset, and then declines back into the normal range [7].

EMG Studies

With nerve conduction studies, motor responses are typically low-amplitude or absent, while sensory responses are relatively preserved, with amplitudes that are >80% of normal in two or more nerves (sensory responses may be reduced, however, when ICU polyneuropathy coexists; see following discussion). Sensory responses may also be reduced initially in association with sepsis and increase during clinical recovery [8]. Needle electrode examination shows fibrillation potential activity in resting muscle in some patients. On voluntary muscle activation, motor unit potentials are short in duration and polyphasic in form with early recruitment, but when there is severe weakness or encephalopathy due to sepsis, the patient may be unable to contract muscles sufficiently to permit analysis of motor unit potentials. An interesting observation made of patients with critical illness myopathy, and demonstrated by direct muscle stimulation, is that the condition leads to electrical inexcitability of the muscle membrane [13,14] so that the ratio of nerve-evoked muscle action potential to direct stimulation of muscle is close to 1. In contrast, when weakness stems from severe neuropathy, the ratio of nerve-evoked response to muscle-stimulation–evoked response is less than 1 (and close to 0).

Muscle Biopsy

With a fairly stereotypic clinical presentation, and EMG results typical of a myopathy—often with fibrillation potential activity—the muscle biopsy is usually not necessary to establish the diagnosis of ICU myopathy. When the diagnosis is uncertain, and especially when diseases with specific therapies—such as the Guillain–Barré syndrome—are considered, a muscle biopsy may prove helpful. Biopsy shows muscle fiber atrophy, especially involving the type II fibers; a variable degree of muscle fiber necrosis, the absence of any inflammatory cells; and the hallmark of the disorder: features of a disrupted intramyofibrillar network that manifests as patchy or complete reduction in myosin–adenosine triphosphatase reactivity in nonnecrotic fibers due to a loss of myosin that may be confirmed immunocytochemically or by electron microscopy [8]. There is a spectrum of histopathological severity ranging from a relatively mild myopathy without major structural damage (designated a cachectic myopathy) to a more severe myopathy with selective thick filament loss, and extending to the most severe manifestation of myopathy characterized by pronounced necrotizing features [6].

Pathophysiology

Myosin loss and muscle fiber necrosis probably contribute to persisting weakness. Myosin loss is characteristic of critical illness myopathy, and is essentially pathognomonic of the disorder. Corticosteroids may cause the loss of myosin, but other factors trigger the process, such as an abnormal neuromuscular junction caused by pharmacologic blockade in ICU patients [7]. Consistent with this hypothesis is the observation that a patient with myasthenia developed loss of myosin thick filaments after receiving high-dose corticosteroids [15], and that in an animal model of dexamethasone treatment plus denervation, there was a severe preferential depletion of thick filaments, leading to a reduction in muscle fiber size [16]. Some patients who are not exposed to administered corticosteroids or neuromuscular blocking agents, but who are systemically ill, often with metabolic acidosis, can also develop the myopathy of intensive care. Acidosis may stimulate glucocorticoid production, lead to an increase in muscle protein degradation, and trigger thick filament loss [7]. Finally, as noted earlier, muscle membrane inexcitability is noted in some patients with the disorder. In an animal model of ICU-related myopathy (rats treated with corticosteroids for 7 to 10 days after denervation of muscle in one leg), intracellular recordings in individual muscle fibers demonstrate that many fibers become unable to generate action potentials [17]. Paralysis appears to be due to abnormal inactivation of sodium channels, which suggests that the myopathy of intensive care may be, in part, an acquired disease of ion channel gating.

Treatment

The treatment of critical illness myopathy is essentially symptomatic: treating the underlying systemic illness and to the extent possible, discontinuing or minimizing corticosteroids and neuromuscular blocking agents. There is emerging evidence that intensive insulin therapy might have a role in reducing the incidence of both critical illness myopathy and critical illness polyneuropathy [18], but hypoglycemia remains a major concern. The experience using this modality was based on specific subgroups, which could limit the applicability of the conclusions, and the diagnosis of myopathy was based on EMG criteria alone and did not include information about clinical measures of muscle strength.

Outcome

If patients survive systemic illness, recovery occurs over weeks to months, depending on severity of the myopathy. In patients whose disease severity was pronounced, a recovery period of many months is to be expected along with the need for tracheostomy and long-term ventilatory support; although some motor recovery ultimately occurs in such patients, it is likely that they will be left with residual long-term muscle weakness and atrophy with compromise in daily function and problems with ambulation [19].

CRITICAL ILLNESS POLYNEUROPATHY

Diagnosis

Patients with critical illness polyneuropathy develop a sensorimotor axon-loss polyneuropathy [20]. Although distal muscles may be affected to a greater extent than proximal muscles, more commonly there is generalized flaccid weakness with depressed or absent reflexes. There is usually distal sensory loss, but pain and paresthesias are not typical features. The cranial nerves are generally spared. Many patients with critical illness polyneuropathy have a concomitant encephalopathy stemming from their underlying multiorgan system failure or sepsis, or both [21].

Risk Factors

Approximately 50% of patients admitted to the ICU with sepsis and multiorgan failure for at least 2 weeks will be found to have EMG evidence for an axon-loss polyneuropathy.

Laboratory Studies

EMG Studies

The most important diagnostic test is the EMG. Nerve conduction velocities are normal or only mildly reduced [21], but the amplitudes of sensory and motor responses are reduced, or even absent. This pattern is typical for axon-loss polyneuropathies rather than demyelinating neuropathies and is helpful in distinguishing critical illness polyneuropathy from the Guillain–Barré syndrome, in which, typically, myelin loss leads to slowing of nerve conduction velocities, conduction block and prolonged distal latencies, and delayed late responses (see following discussion). On needle electrode examination, there are typically features of acute denervation—fibrillation potentials and positive sharp wave activity—and reduced recruitment of motor unit potentials; as in many axon-loss polyneuropathies, there may be more pronounced changes seen in distal compared to more proximal muscles.

Pathophysiology

The polyneuropathy appears to be a complication of the systemic inflammatory response syndrome (SIRS) triggered by sepsis, severe trauma, or burns [22]. It may be induced by impaired microcirculation leading to reduced nerve perfusion and endoneurial edema which leads in turn to nerve hypoxia; the neuropathy may also result to a degree from the deleterious effects of cytokines produced by activated leukocytes [23]. There is also evidence that the acute polyneuropathy in critically ill patients stems in part from an abnormality in nerve excitability, caused by increased sodium channel inactivation (similar to what is found in the myopathy of intensive care), without actual nerve damage. This may underlie the reversibility of weakness that occurs in some affected patients [24].

Treatment

Treatment is essentially symptomatic and supportive and comprises attempts to stabilize underlying critical medical and surgical conditions with vigorous treatment of sepsis. A recent study reported a 44% reduction in the incidence of critical illness polyneuropathy in mechanically ventilated critically ill patients who received intensive insulin therapy (IIT) to maintain the blood glucose levels between 4.4 and 6.1 mmol per L [23]. A Cochrane review makes clear, however, that the methodology of this and other studies limits the conclusions regarding the role of IIT in patients with either critical illness myopathy or neuropathy, or both [18].

Outcome

Recovery of sensory and motor function occurs over weeks to months, depending on the severity of the neuropathy. In some of the instances of very slow recovery over months, long-term ventilatory support may be required, even after the underlying critical illness has resolved [19].

DIFFERENTIAL DIAGNOSIS

Certain well-known peripheral neuropathies, neuromuscular junction disorders, and myopathies may present with acutely evolving weakness and simulate critical illness myopathy or polyneuropathy [1,2,25]. Among the acute and severe polyneuropathies, the most common is the Guillain–Barré syndrome, discussed in detail in Chapter 175. In brief, two-thirds of patients have had a preceding viral or bacterial syndrome (especially a *Campylobacter jejuni*-related diarrheal illness), an inoculation, or recent surgery. Most patients present with rapidly progressive areflexic paralysis that typically starts in the legs and spreads proximally, and involves the diaphragm in 25% of cases and the facial muscles in more than 50% of individuals. Most have EMG features of an acquired demyelinating polyneuropathy with slowing of nerve conduction velocity, conduction block, prolonged distal latencies, and prolonged or absent late responses, distinguishing Guillain–Barré syndrome from critical illness polyneuropathy. In most patients with Guillain–Barré syndrome, the cerebrospinal fluid (CSF) examination shows an elevation in protein without increased white cells by the second week of the illness, helping to distinguish Guillain–Barré syndrome from critical illness polyneuropathy, in which the CSF findings are normal. Guillain–Barré syndrome, an immune-mediated disorder, responds to plasma exchange or to intravenous γ-globulin, making early recognition essential in an effort to start treatment early and reduce morbidity.

A rare cause of severe neuropathic weakness is acute intermittent porphyria that may present with attacks of abrupt onset of abdominal pain, psychiatric disturbance, and polyneuropathy. It is generally triggered by drugs that induce the hepatic cytochrome-P450 system (diazepam, theophylline, barbiturates); it is characterized by weakness of the bulbar muscles and the diaphragm, has prominent dysautonomia, and EMG findings reveal features of a severe axon-loss polyneuropathy. Diagnosis is suggested by the presence of urinary porphyrin precursors, notably δ-aminolevulinic acid. The neuropathy responds to oral or parenteral carbohydrate loading and to intravenous hematin.

The most important neuromuscular junction disorder causing acute weakness is myasthenia gravis, described in Chapter 176. In brief, in this immunoglobulin-G immune-mediated postsynaptic condition, in which there is a loss of acetylcholine receptors, most individuals present with ocular muscle weakness (manifested as ptosis and diplopia) and generalized weakness with a fatigable component. More than 90% of patients have antibodies to the acetylcholine receptor, and abnormal EMG findings, with a decremental motor response during repetitive nerve stimulation at 2 to 3 Hz. The acute weakness (defined as myasthenic crisis when respiratory muscles are involved) responds well to plasma exchange or intravenous γ-globulin.

Another neuromuscular junction disorder is prolonged neuromuscular blockade by muscle relaxants. It is virtually always seen in the population of patients with renal or hepatic failure, is often associated with elevated levels of the metabolite of vecuronium (3-desacetylvecuronium), and tends to improve after infusion of acetylcholinesterase inhibitors. Botulism is a presynaptic disorder characterized by rapidly progressive, diffuse, symmetrical weakness with a proximal predominance, dysarthria and dysphagia, respiratory involvement, and a prominent autonomic component including dilated pupils, bradyarrhythmia, orthostatic hypotension, and urinary retention. Management consists of supportive care and administration of trivalent antitoxin.

THE DIAGNOSTIC CHALLENGE: DISTINGUISHING CRITICAL ILLNESS MYOPATHY FROM CRITICAL ILLNESS POLYNEUROPATHY

Favoring the diagnosis of myopathy would be severe generalized weakness, with failure to wean from mechanical ventilation (the latter more likely to be associated with ICU myopathy rather than neuropathy [26]), preservation of reflexes and sensation, a transient rise in CK, and an EMG picture of relatively preserved sensory responses with low or absent motor responses and early recruitment of small, polyphasic motor unit potentials, often with fibrillation potential activity. Favoring a polyneuropathy would be the clinical findings of demonstrable sensory loss and areflexia, and the EMG findings of absent or low motor amplitudes in the company of absent or low sensory responses, along with fibrillation potentials and reduced recruitment of motor unit potentials. Clinically, a polyneuropathy might easily be missed because, in many patients, careful sensory examination is impossible in the ICU setting, especially if there is a coexisting encephalopathy. Further confounding the distinction, reflex loss can occur in either critical illness polyneuropathy or myopathy, fibrillation potentials may be found in both disorders, and voluntary motor unit potentials may not be elicitable either because of inability to activate muscles due to encephalopathy or from severe weakness.

In the final analysis, it may be difficult to distinguish one disorder from another in an individual case: ICU-related myopathy and polyneuropathy arise in a common setting, share the clinical features of severe generalized weakness with areflexia, may have a similar underlying acquired sodium channelopathy (affecting multiple sodium channel isoforms in both nerve and muscle [24]), and cannot always be reliably differentiated by EMG testing. Although a biopsy may be helpful in ambiguous situations, truly distinctive features of either disorder may be difficult to discern. It is likely that in many patients *both* disorders are present in varying degrees [27] and in fact have a combined syndrome of critical illness myopathy and polyneuropathy and may be considered to have critical illness polyneuromyopathy [5] or critical illness myopathy and neuropathy [6]. Personal and collective experience [14,25,28] suggests that in ICU patients with the *most profound weakness and failure to wean,* ICU myopathy probably plays the predominant role.

References

1. Chad DA, Lacomis D: Critically ill patients with newly acquired weakness: the clinicopathological spectrum. *Ann Neurol* 35:257, 1994.
2. Gorson KC: Approach to neuromuscular disorders in the intensive care unit. *Neurocrit Care* 3:195, 2005.
3. Hund E: Critical illness polyneuropathy. A review. *Curr Opin Neurol* 5:649, 2001.
4. De Jonghe B, Sharshar T, LeFaucheur JP, et al: Paresis acquired in the intensive care unit: a prospective multicenter study. *JAMA* 288:2859, 2002.
5. Op de Coul AA, Verheul GA, Leyten AC, et al. Critical illness polyneuromyopathy after artificial respiration. *Clin Neurol Neurosurg* 93:27, 1991.
6. Pati S, Goodfellow JA, Iyadurai S, et al: Approach to critical illness polyneuropathy and myopathy. *Postgrad Med J* 84:354–360, 2008.
7. Lacomis D, Giuliani MJ, Van Cott A, et al: Acute myopathy of intensive care: clinical, electromyographic, and pathological aspects. *Ann Neurol* 40:645, 1996.
8. Lacomis D, Zochodne DW, Bird S: Critical illness myopathy. *Muscle Nerve* 23:1785, 2000.
9. Bella I, Chad DA, Smith TW, et al: Ophthalmoplegia and quadriplegia in the wake of intensive therapy for status asthmaticus. *Muscle Nerve* 17:1122, 1994.
10. Banwell BL, Mildner RJ, Hassall AC, et al: Muscle weakness in critically ill children. *Neurology* 61:1779, 2003.
11. Lacomis D, Smith TW, Chad DA: Acute myopathy and neuropathy in status asthmaticus: case report and literature review. *Muscle Nerve* 16:84, 1993.
12. Lacomis D, Petrella JT, Giuliani MJ: Causes of neuromuscular weakness in the intensive care unit: a study of ninety-two patients. *Muscle Nerve* 21:610, 1998.
13. Rich MM, Bird SJ, Raps EC, et al: Direct muscle stimulation in acute quadriplegic myopathy. *Muscle Nerve* 20:665, 1997.
14. LeFaucheur JP, Nordine T, Rodriguez P, et al: Origin of ICU acquired paresis determined by direct muscle stimulation. *J Neurol Neurosurg Psychiatry* 77:500, 2006.
15. Panegyres PK, Squier M, Mills KR, et al: Acute myopathy associated with large parenteral doses of corticosteroids in myasthenia gravis. *J Neurol Neurosurg Psychiatry* 56:702, 1993.
16. Rouleau G, Karpati G, Carpenter S, et al: Glucocorticoid excess induces preferential depletion of myosin in denervated skeletal muscle fibers. *Muscle Nerve* 10:428, 1987.
17. Rich MM, Pinter MJ: Sodium channel inactivation in an animal model of acute quadriplegic myopathy. *Ann Neurol* 50:26, 2001.
18. Hermans G, De Jonghe B, Bruyninckx F, et al: Interventions for preventing critical illness polyneuropathy and critical illness myopathy. *Cochrane Database Syst Rev* 21 (1):CD006832, 2009.
19. Hemphill JC III, Wade SS: "Chapter 269. Neurologic critical care, including hypoxic-ischemic encephalopathy and subarachnoid hemorrhage." in Fauci AS, Braunwald E, Kasper DL, et al (eds): *Harrison's Principles of Internal Medicine*, 17e: http://www.accessmedicine.com/content.aspx?aID=2888218.
20. Bolton CF, Gilbert JJ, Hahn AF, et al: Polyneuropathy in critically ill patients. *J Neurol Neurosurg Psychiatry* 47:1223, 1984.
21. Zochodne DW, Bolton CF, Wells GA, et al: Critical illness polyneuropathy: a complication of sepsis and multiple organ failure. *Brain* 110:819, 1987.
22. Latronico N, Peli E, Botteri M: Critical illness myopathy and neuropathy. *Curr Opin Crit Care* 11:126, 2005.
23. Sanap MN, Worthley LI: Neurologic complications of critical illness: part II. Polyneuropathies and myopathies. *Crit Care Resusc* 4:133, 2002.
24. Novak KR, Nardelli P, Cope TC, et al: Inactivation of sodium channels underlies reversible neuropathy during critical illness in rats. *J Clin Invest* 119:1150, 2009.
25. Sandrock AW, Louis DN: Case records of the Massachusetts General Hospital. Case 11–1997. *N Engl J Med* 336:1079, 1997.
26. Sander HW, Golden M, Danon MJ: Quadriplegic areflexic ICU illness: selective thick filament loss and normal nerve histology. *Muscle Nerve* 26:499, 2002.
27. Bird SJ, Rich MM: Critical illness myopathy and polyneuropathy. *Curr Neurol Neurosci Rep* 2:527, 2002.
28. Trojaborg W, Weimer LH, Hays AP: Electrophysiologic studies in critical illness associated-weakness: myopathy or neuropathy—a reappraisal. *Clin Neurophys* 112:1586, 2001.

SECTION XIV ■ TRANSPLANTATION

STEPHANIE M. LEVINE

CHAPTER 181 ■ IMMUNOSUPPRESSION IN SOLID-ORGAN TRANSPLANTATION

AMIT BASU, ARTHUR J. MATAS AND ABHINAV HUMAR

Clinically successful solid-organ transplantation required breakthroughs in our understanding of immunology and immunosuppressive therapy. Alexis Carrel, in the early 1900s, described what was to become the modern method of vascular suturing; experimental transplants soon followed [1], but the first successful clinical transplant was not done until five decades later. During that interval, it gradually became apparent that early rapid destruction of allografts was due to an immune process, which came to be known as *rejection*.

Organ transplantation has now become commonplace as the results have improved remarkably with the use of more potent and specific immunosuppressive agents. Progress in nonrenal transplantation has especially accelerated with the use of newer and more potent immunosuppressive agents. Besides the developments in techniques and immunosuppression protocols, progress in tissue typing and cross matching, and in preservation and transportation of harvested organs have played major roles in the rapid development of organ transplantation.

This chapter reviews the clinical use and the adverse reactions associated with commonly used immunosuppressive agents.

PHARMACOLOGIC AGENTS

Calcineurin Inhibitors

Cyclosporine (CSA) and tacrolimus (TAC), although structurally dissimilar, have a similar mechanism of action. Both drugs interfere with the cellular pathway for cytokine production and proliferation. Early events in the T-cell activation process are associated with a rise in the levels of intracellular calcium. The protein calcineurin has been validated as part of the calcium-dependent signal transduction pathway of interleukin-2 (IL-2) production in T cells [2]. CSA and TAC bind to two intracellular receptors, CypA and FKBP12, respectively; these receptors are found in virtually all cell types. The resulting receptor complex binds to calcineurin, blocking its phosphatase ability and thereby stopping the production of IL-2 [2].

The two calcineurin inhibitors (CNIs) currently used are described separately in the following sections.

Cyclosporine

CSA was isolated from a soil sample in Norway and produced by the fungus *Tolypocladium inflatum*. The first formulation of CSA that was approved by the U.S. Food and Drug Administration (FDA) was Sandimmune®; this was modified in the early 1990s by the microemulsion (ME) formulation called Neoral®. In 2000, the first generic versions of CSA were launched. CSA has remained a major component of many transplant regimens.

Pharmacokinetics. CSA is a lipophilic decapeptide, consisting of several amino acids in a ring structure. The original oral formulation (Sandimmune®) is in an olive-oil vehicle, which is necessary to promote absorption [3]. Absorption of Sandimmune® is erratic and it requires the presence of bile in the upper small intestine for absorption. Because many liver transplant recipients require diversion of bile to external drainage, absorption of Sandimmune® is problematic for them [4]. Absorption is also complicated by the presence of food and the length of drug therapy. Neoral® self-emulsifies in water, making absorption much more reliable and much less dependent on the presence of bile.

Studies comparing the two formulations showed these advantages with the ME: a more consistent and linear elimination of CSA; higher area-under-the-curve (AUC) values, leading to reduced dose requirements; reduced effects of diet, and, especially for liver recipients, much better absorption [4]. The side effect profiles were unchanged. The ME has become the primary formulation for CSA. CSA is generally considered a narrow-therapeutic-range drug, so whether generic versions can be used without additional pharmacokinetic study has been controversial.

The oral bioavailability of the ME formulations is approximately 30%. The average half-life of CSA ranges from 6 to 9 hours, with a t_{max} (ME) of approximately 1 hour. CSA is highly bound in plasma to red blood cells. It is extensively metabolized by the liver to multiple metabolites via the cytochrome P450 3A4 enzyme system; however, most of the metabolites are considered essentially inactive. Significant liver impairment can slow the clearance of CSA by the body. Because very little drug is eliminated by the kidney, renal failure does not change CSA elimination [3].

CSA is available as an oral soft gelatin capsule (Neoral®, Sandimmune®), as an oral solution (Sandimmune®, Neoral®), and as an intravenous (IV) preparation (Sandimmune®). To convert to IV use, the IV dose must be calculated as one-third of the daily oral dose. The IV dose can be administered over 6 hours; however, a continuous infusion is usually desired to minimize toxicity.

Adverse Events. The extensive side effect profile of CSA has long been a reason for attempts at minimizing drug exposure. Of most concern is its acute and chronic nephrotoxicity. Acute nephrotoxicity from CSA initially is characterized by vasoconstriction of the intrarenal arterioles, resulting in a reduced glomerular filtration rate. This mechanism of vasoconstriction is not well understood, but may be a result of increase in the vasoactive substance endothelin I [5], the activation of the renin-angiotensin system resulting in increased levels of angiotensin II [6], and possibly a decrease in production of nitric oxide [7]. CSA may also affect prostacyclin levels and induce vasoconstriction by increasing thromboxane A_2 [3].

CSA-induced thrombotic microangiopathy (TMA) was first reported in liver allograft recipients, then in kidney and heart recipients [8]. TMA can present as a full-blown syndrome consisting of hemolytic anemia, thrombocytopenia, neurologic abnormalities, fever, and renal failure. Pathogenic mechanisms include a direct cytotoxic effect on endothelial cells, reduction in prostacyclin synthesis leading to vasoconstriction, platelet aggregation, and thrombus formation. CSA reduces the generation of activated protein C from endothelial cells and increases thromboplastin production from mononuclear and endothelial cells, thus contributing to a prothrombotic effect. Discontinuation of CSA is an important step in management along with plasmapheresis and fresh frozen plasma replacement. TAC or sirolimus (SRL) can be substituted as immunosuppressive agents, although TMA can occur with both these agents.

In heart and lung transplant recipients, the effect of CSA on long-term kidney function has been significant. Kidney biopsies of their native kidneys reveal wrinkling and thickening of the glomerular basement membrane, with some kidneys exhibiting microthrombotic angiopathy and fibrosis. Clinical findings showed that several of these recipients had advanced to end-stage renal disease requiring dialysis; others developed significant proteinuria [9]. However, a study of kidney recipients showed that the incidence of rejection correlated with poorer long-term graft function; higher CSA levels were associated with better, not worse, graft function [10]. Whether or not higher CSA levels are to blame for chronic CSA nephrotoxicity is still a matter of discussion. Transforming growth factor-B type 1 (TGF-B type 1) and platelet-derived growth factor, both fibrogenic cytokines, are produced in increasing amounts by human renal proximal tubular cells by increasing concentrations of CSA [11]. An increase in the activation of the renin-angiotensin system has been linked with the morphological changes that occur in chronic CSA nephrotoxicity by experimental studies [12], and angiotensin II receptor blockers reduce these changes.

Hypertension is another significant adverse event with CSA. Most patients receiving CSA develop hypertension, sometimes requiring multiple drug therapy. The mechanism for CSA-induced hypertension is primarily related to small-vessel vasoconstriction. The renal vasoconstriction may be affected, in part, by increased endothelin production. Patients also develop sodium retention and lower plasma renin levels [13]. Treatment of hypertension has focused on calcium-channel blocker use, because calcium-channel activation induces endothelin vasoconstriction and increases blood pressure. Calcium-channel blockers, such as diltiazem, nifedipine, and amlodipine, have been shown to decrease renal vascular resistance and improve glomerular filtration rate. Given these beneficial renal effects, calcium-channel blockers have been used to try to reduce chronic nephrotoxicity associated with CSA. Clinical evidence of a salutary effect has been conflicting, and further study is needed.

CSA has been associated with several neurologic toxicities, including headaches, tremors, seizures, and encephalopathy. In most instances, but not always, these effects are seen with higher CSA levels. A decrease in dosage may prevent serious tremors and headaches. Reversible posterior leukoencephalopathy can occur after CSA use and affects the posterior white matter and the frontal lobes and gray matter as well [14]. It manifests with confusion, coma, cortical blindness, cerebellar syndrome, hemiplegia, and flaccid paralysis or various combinations of these features. This neurological syndrome and brain imaging abnormalities usually resolve within 2 weeks of stopping CSA, or after dosage reduction if blood levels were high [15]. Hypertrichosis and gingival hyperplasia can reduce patient compliance to CSA. Many patients develop hair growth on their backs and arms; although not life threatening, these cosmetic changes can have emotional and physical repercussions, potentially resulting in graft loss if noncompliance ensues. Electrolyte imbalances may occur with CSA, including hyperkalemia, hyperuricemia, and hypomagnesemia. Patients usually need diet instruction and sometimes electrolyte replacement to control these changes. CSA can increase cholesterol and triglyceride levels, sometimes requiring treatment with lipid-lowering medications [3].

Drug Interactions. CSA is metabolized by the cytochrome P450 3A4 enzyme system that is found not only in the liver but also in the cells lining the intestine; so CSA levels can be increased or decreased by changes in gut absorption or in liver metabolism [16]. Some centers try to manipulate the interaction, intentionally using compounds that inhibit CSA metabolism to decrease the dosage required and, thus, the cost [17]. This practice is controversial, because any change in the interacting drug used affects CSA levels. CSA interactions may also occur with medications that change gut motility and with other nephrotoxic agents [16]. Table 181.1 lists the drugs that affect CSA metabolism, efficacy, and nephrotoxicity.

Clinical Use. CSA was and continues to be extensively used in organ transplantation, especially renal transplant, although now a different CNI, tacrolimus, has become the more commonly used primary immunosuppressive agent [18]. When CSA is used, it is often the ME formulation (Neoral®),

TABLE 181.1

SIGNIFICANT DRUG INTERACTIONS (CYCLOSPORINE, TACROLIMUS, SIROLIMUS)

Inhibitors of metabolism	Inducers of metabolism	Additive nephrotoxicity (cyclosporine and tacrolimus only)
Verapamil	Rifampin	Aminoglycosides
Diltiazem	Phenobarbital	Salicylates
Fluconazole	Phenytoin	Nonsteroidal anti-inflammatory agents
Itraconazole	Carbamazepine	
Ketoconazole	St. John's wort	
Erythromycin		Amphotericin B
Azithromycin		Vancomycin
Clarithromycin		
Grapefruit juice		
Fluvoxamine		
Nefazodone		
Atorvastatin		

although patients with stable allograft function from earlier years may still be using Sandimmune. As Sandimmune® and ME formulations are not considered bioequivalent by the FDA, one cannot be substituted for the other without careful monitoring of doses and serum concentrations. Most centers initiate CSA therapy at 4 to 8 mg per kg per day orally, starting the day after transplant. If the transplanted kidney shows signs of acute tubular necrosis posttransplant, some centers may delay the initiation of CSA. Anti–T-cell preparations may be used during this time to provide T-cell suppression if CSA cannot be started [3]. Because of the better bioavailability of the ME formulation, the need for IV CSA has decreased but still may be necessary if the patient has significant diarrhea or cannot tolerate any oral or nasogastric medications.

Therapeutic Drug Monitoring. Monitoring CSA levels is vital. Maintaining the appropriate levels in the first 6 months posttransplant has a significant effect on graft survival [19]. Monitoring CSA is a challenge because of the differences in bioavailability between patients, the narrow therapeutic range, and the number of compounds available that affect CSA blood concentrations. Several different assays are currently in use to measure CSA. The various methods used today measure whole-blood CSA levels and include radioimmunoassay (RIA), high-performance liquid chromatography (HPLC), and monoclonal antibody assays. HPLC only measures the parent compound of CSA, whereas radioimmunoassay and the monoclonal assays measure CSA plus several metabolites. When deciding whether a blood concentration is appropriate, it is important to know which assay the laboratory is using.

Traditionally, trough concentrations (C0) of CSA have been used to determine the appropriateness of a dosing regimen. Earlier studies were performed with the Sandimmune® formulation, which had quite variable dose-response curves. After the use of the ME preparation became standard, several studies suggested that measuring the AUC would be more predictive of toxicity and rejection (compared with the C0) [20]. AUC monitoring requires more blood samples per measurement, and it is therefore more costly and impractical in clinical practice [20]. A monitoring strategy measuring AUC for the first 4 hours after dosing (AUC 0 to 4 hours) correlates well with clinical outcomes, although it still requires multiple blood samples [21]. A blood sample taken 2 hours after intake of Neoral® (C_2) is the most accurate one-point predictor for AUC 0 to 4 hours and shows less variability than either C0 or C_1. In retrospective analysis, the risk of acute rejection is reduced in patients in whom C_2 were greater than 1,500 μg per L in the 2 weeks following transplantation [22].

In a prospective study, 45% of C_2-monitored patients failed to reach the target levels by day 5 posttransplantation compared with 2.5% of Co-monitored patients [23]; this may explain why the theoretical benefit of C_2 monitoring in the early posttransplant period is not borne out. Due to the lack of prospective evidence showing an advantage for C_2 monitoring in the early posttransplant period, trough levels (C0) remain the standard.

Tacrolimus

With the success of CSA, researchers studied soil samples from around the world, looking for another compound that might turn out to display immunosuppressive properties. TAC, initially known as FK-506, was isolated from a soil sample in Tsukuba, Japan, in May 1984, from the fungus *Streptomyces tsukubaensis* [24]. It has a completely different chemical structure from CSA, yet its effect on the lymphocyte is remarkably similar. A few differences have been found on the cellular level between CSA and TAC. The FKBP12-TAC complex is 10 to 100 times as potent as CSA, possibly due to greater affinity for its binding protein [24,25].

Pharmacokinetics. The pharmacokinetics of TAC are similar to CSA. TAC has an extremely lipophilic, macrocytic lactone structure. Its oral bioavailability ranges anywhere from 4% to 93% (average 25%), with variable dose-response curves between patients. Because of this poor oral bioavailability, the IV dose should be calculated at approximately one-third of the oral daily dose [26]. One significant difference between CSA and TAC is that with TAC the presence or absence of bile in the digestive tract does not significantly alter absorption. This was a problem with Sandimmune® and a reason that TAC was initially studied in the liver transplant population. TAC binds extensively to erythrocytes and exhibits the same temperature-dependent properties as CSA. The metabolism is also similar to CSA, with the cytochrome P450 3A4 system as the primary metabolic pathway. The many metabolites for TAC are still being studied. Less than 1% of active drug is excreted through the urine. The average elimination half-life ranges from 8 to 20 hours, depending on the population studied [26].

TAC is available as a 0.5-mg, 1.0-mg, and 5.0-mg capsule, formulated as a solid dispersion in hydroxymethylcellulose. A suspension can be compounded if necessary for pediatric or nasogastric administration. An IV preparation is solubilized in alcohol and a surfactant. It is available as a 5 mg per mL concentration that must be diluted and administered as a continuous infusion to avoid toxicity [26].

Adverse Events. The adverse event profile of TAC is similar to CSA in many respects. TAC appears to have the same nephrotoxicity seen with CSA, and the mechanism also appears to be the same. However, in one study, mean or median serum creatinine levels in renal transplant recipients were lower in TAC-treated patients, with 5 years follow-up, than in patients treated with cyclosporine ME (or standard formulation) [27]. As with CSA, the nephrotoxicity of TAC is concentration dependent, making drug level monitoring equally important [28].

Hypertension has also been reported with TAC. However, the 5-year follow-up results from the U.S. randomized trial indicate that significantly fewer TAC than CSA recipients were receiving antihypertensive treatment (80.9% vs. 93%, $p < 0.05$) [27]. Immunosuppression with TAC-based regimens is associated with better lipid profiles than is immunosuppression with CSA-based regimens [29]. Neurotoxicity appears to be somewhat worse than with CSA. In randomized trials, liver recipients had more trouble with the neurotoxicity of TAC versus CSA, even when controlling for previous liver failure–induced encephalopathy [30]. Headache, tremor, neuropathy, seizures, blindness, coma, and various other neurologic complaints have been seen with TAC [30]. Patients usually recover when the drug is stopped. The incidence of hyperkalemia appears to be similar to that with CSA, although hypomagnesemia is more likely to occur with TAC-treated patients [31].

TAC-associated TMA has a reported incidence between 1% and 4.7% [32]. All patients have an elevated serum creatinine, but do not always show signs of hemolysis. Renal allograft biopsy provides a conclusive diagnosis. Treatment consists of reduction or discontinuation of TAC, anticoagulation, and/or plasmapheresis with fresh frozen plasma exchange and leads to resolution of TMA in most instances. Rarely, there may be loss of kidney function or patient death.

The incidence of posttransplant diabetes mellitus (PTDM) was significantly higher among TAC-treated patients than CSA-treated patients (9.8% vs. 2.7%) according to a meta-analysis [33]. Many patients with PTDM have reversal of diabetes mellitus, with eventual discontinuation of insulin. In a U.S. trial combining TAC with mycophenolate mofetil (MMF) and corticosteroids, the 10-year incidence was 6.5%, and the 1-year prevalence was 2.2% [34]. TAC does not appear to cause hypertrichosis or gingival hyperplasia, but instead is associated with hair loss. Sometimes these differences become important enough to cause a change in therapy.

Drug Interactions. TAC is metabolized through the same pathway as CSA and has been subject to the same interactions with the cytochrome P450 3A4 system. If the medication is known to alter P450 3A4 activity, it probably alters TAC concentrations. Drugs that cause nephrotoxicity also have the same additive effects with TAC as with CSA (Table 181.1).

Therapeutic Drug Monitoring. As with CSA, careful blood concentration monitoring is required; TAC also has a narrow therapeutic range. TAC is extensively bound to erythrocytes, so whole-blood trough measurements have become the standard for drug monitoring. The primary assay used currently is an automated microparticle enzyme immunoassay, available from Abbott Laboratories (Abbott Park, IL). Several generations of this assay have been used, with the current assay more sensitive at lower drug concentrations. The current suggested therapeutic range for TAC is 5 to 20 ng per mL; however, this range is still controversial and under study [25].

Clinical Use. Because TAC does not require bile to be absorbed, its use has attracted a great deal of interest in liver transplantation. Sandimmune® required bile in the small intestine, and if the bile drainage was being diverted it was almost impossible to obtain adequate CSA blood levels. TAC provided a possible advantage in liver transplantation, so the first major trials were in liver recipients.

The U.S. Multicenter FK-506 Liver Study Group compared the efficacy and safety of a CSA-based regimen (using Sandimmune®) versus a TAC-based regimen in adult and pediatric liver recipients at 12 different centers in the United States [30]. Recipients were randomized to CSA in combination with Azathioprine® (AZA) and steroids, or to TAC in combination with steroids. The investigators looked at patient and graft survival rates as well as the incidence of acute rejection, steroid-resistant rejection, and refractory rejection. At 1 year posttransplant, patient and graft survival rates were similar between the two groups, but TAC was associated with fewer episodes of all categories of rejection. The TAC group did have an increased incidence of adverse events, including nephrotoxicity, neurotoxicity, and hyperglycemia. Follow-up studies using lower doses of TAC have shown a reduction in these adverse events [35,36].

TAC is usually initiated at a dose of 0.05 to 0.10 mg per kg per day. Some centers use a standard starting dose of 2 mg BID, and adjust doses based on the blood concentration. As with CSA, TAC may be delayed after a kidney transplant in the case of graft dysfunction, and started when the kidney is recovering from acute tubular necrosis.

In studies of TAC and CSA in kidney recipients, results have been similar to those with liver recipients (i.e., same graft and patient survival rates, fewer rejection episodes) [37]. This pattern has also been seen in higher-risk patient populations, such as black recipients [38]. Other transplant categories with historically higher rates of rejection, such as pancreas transplant recipients, have seen benefit with TAC-based immunosuppressive regimens [31]. TAC continues to be the primary maintenance immunosuppressive agent in heart, lung, and bowel recipients, and was approved by the FDA for heart transplantation in 2006 [39–42].

Antiproliferative Agents

Antiproliferative agents have been part of transplant protocols since the first transplant was performed in the 1960s. Early antiproliferative agents included radiation, azaserine, and actinomycin D. AZA, developed in the early 1960s, was part of the first successful transplant series reported in 1963. It continues to be used today in maintenance immunosuppressive regimens and for autoimmune diseases. Cyclophosphamide was used when AZA use was not possible, but because of side effects it has never been considered a suitable alternative. A major advance in antiproliferative agents has been the development and use of MMF, released for clinical use in 1995. MMF is now a component of most new transplant regimens, with AZA having been used in transplants performed before 1995.

Azathioprine

Pharmacology. AZA is actually a prodrug of 6-mercaptopurine, an antineoplastic agent used in leukemia regimens. It acts by the inhibition of purine synthesis in the de novo pathway. This purine inhibition leads to the inhibition of the mixed lymphocyte reaction, and to a lesser extent, the antigen–antibody reaction [43].

Pharmacokinetics. AZA is rapidly absorbed after oral administration, with peak levels occurring 1 hour after ingestion. The large first-pass effect after oral administration means that IV doses must be multiplied by a factor of two. AZA is metabolized by xanthine oxidase through several steps to 6-thiouric acid and excreted into the kidneys. Although the half-life of the parent drug is relatively short, the pharmacodynamic effects of the parent drug and metabolites far outlast the time that AZA is present in the bloodstream [43].

Adverse Events. AZA is relatively well tolerated by most patients. The most common side effect is myelosuppression due to suppression of purine synthesis by AZA. The myelosuppression is usually limited to the white blood cells, but occasionally red cell aplasia is observed. Most patients can tolerate this effect by reducing the daily dosage, although some need to discontinue the drug entirely. Liver function tests must be regularly monitored: AZA has been reported to cause hepatic necrosis and liver failure. Pancreatitis or a skin rash may indicate an allergic reaction, in which case AZA may need to be stopped. Hair loss is bothersome to some patients but is reversible. Gastrointestinal (GI) disturbances, including nausea and vomiting, are mild and usually tolerable [43].

Drug Interactions. Severe pancytopenia has been reported when AZA and allopurinol are used together. It is recommended that AZA doses be reduced by 75% if allopurinol is added to the patient's drug regimen. With the development of MMF, the management of this interaction has become easier, as MMF (which is metabolized differently than AZA) can be substituted for AZA when allopurinol is indicated [43].

Clinical Use. AZA is available as a 50-mg tablet that can be split, if necessary. A compounded suspension of 5 mg per mL can be used if tablets are not an option. AZA is also available IV. Most recipients are maintained on a dose of 1.0 to 2.5 mg per kg per day. AZA has an important historical role in transplantation, but its use has declined as newer agents have been introduced. Most likely, recipients currently on AZA were transplanted before 1995 and have done well on that initial regimen. Some centers switched all their recipients when MMF became available, but many are still maintained on AZA due to a significant cost advantage over MMF.

Mycophenolate Mofetil

MMF was approved by the FDA in 1995 to prevent rejection in kidney recipients. Its use has grown to include liver, heart, lung, and pancreas recipients. It has been a major addition to the immunosuppressive arsenal. Many centers have replaced AZA with MMF in their current protocols.

Pharmacology. MMF is also a prodrug, quickly metabolized to the active compound, mycophenolic acid (MPA). MPA acts as a noncompetitive inhibitor of inosine monophosphate dehydrogenase, thereby blocking de novo purine synthesis and proliferation in the T and B lymphocytes [44]. In vitro and in vivo data from rodent models of chronic allograft nephropathy suggest that MMF also decreases vascular smooth muscle cell proliferation, offering theoretical treatment possibilities for the morphology seen in chronic rejection [45].

Pharmacokinetics. Oral MMF is rapidly hydrolyzed in the bloodstream by esterases to MPA, with no measurable parent compound in serum [46]. The oral bioavailability for MPA approaches 100%, so the IV to oral conversion ratio is 1:1. IV administration of MMF provides measurable blood levels of the parent compound during infusion, with levels becoming immeasurable 12 minutes after the end of the infusion. Peak concentrations occur approximately 1 hour after IV or oral administration (but IV has a slightly higher peak than oral) [47]. MPA is subsequently glucuronidated in the liver to inactive metabolic mycophenolic acid glucuronide (MPAG). Enterohepatic cycling recirculates a significant percentage of MPAG secreted in bile back to MPA, displaying a secondary peak in plasma MPA concentration [48]. MPAG is eventually excreted, primarily in the urine; only 6% of MPAG is excreted in the feces [44].

Adverse Events. MMF can cause significant GI problems, including nausea, vomiting, diarrhea, abdominal pain, and gastroesophageal reflux. Persistent diarrhea not accompanied by fever may be associated with an erosive enterocolitis causing malabsorption of nutrients that has been attributed to a toxic action of the acyl MPAG metabolite on absorptive cells [49]. Occurrence of these side effects has more frequently been linked to the MMF dose rather than to the plasma concentration of parent compound or its metabolites. Dividing the total daily dose into four doses instead of two has been effective in reducing GI problems in some recipients. An alternative, enteric-coated form of MPA—mycophenolate sodium (EC-MPS)—has been developed to mitigate the GI toxicities. Patients who had GI intolerance on MMF administration required fewer dose changes of EC-MPS, and showed reduced symptom burden, better functioning, and improved health-related quality of life [50]. Neutropenia and thrombocytopenia can also occur with MMF, requiring a dosage reduction [44]. At 2 g per day, the occurrence rate in the major trials was comparable to AZA. Teratogenic trials of MMF in rabbits showed changes in offspring at doses equivalent to those given to humans. No human teratogenic trials have been performed (but the manufacturer recommends that female patients wait at least 6 weeks after stopping MMF before trying to conceive). Female healthcare workers are also advised by the manufacturer to not open capsules for fear of aerosolization of the drug. It is also recommended that IV MMF be administered using standard chemotherapy precautions [51].

Drug Interactions. MMF is not metabolized by the cytochrome P450 system; therefore, interactions with MMF only affect its absorption, enterohepatic cycling, or renal excretion. As discussed earlier, a significant percentage of the AUC for MMF comes from enterohepatic cycling. Cholestyramine, a bile acid resin, decreases cholesterol by interfering with its enterohepatic cycling. The mixture of cholestyramine and MMF decreases the total AUC by 40%, so the combination of these two drugs is not recommended [51]. Antacids appear to reduce absorption of MMF by 20%, so adjusting dosing times, if possible, is recommended. Ganciclovir and acyclovir compete with MPAG for secretion by the kidney, and animal studies have suggested a possible interaction [51].

Recipients treated with CSA in combination with MMF display lower MPA concentrations than do patients who are not receiving CSA [52]. However, coadministration of MMF with TAC tends to increase MPA levels due to the lack of CSA inhibitory effects, and also possibly due to the inhibition of the uridine diphosphate—glucuronosyl transferase that generates MPAG [53].

Clinical Use. The success of MMF has allowed it to generally replace AZA in many transplant centers. The results of three major trials were instrumental. The U.S., Tricontinental, and European trials compared MMF, in combination with CSA and steroids, with conventional immunosuppression. The U.S. and Tricontinental trials randomized patients to MMF at a low (2 g per day) or high dose (3 g per day) versus AZA, whereas the European study used a placebo instead of AZA [54–56]. All three trials saw significantly reduced rejection in the MMF arm at 6 months posttransplant. The low-dose and high-dose arms demonstrated significantly fewer rejection episodes and clinically significant reductions in the severity and treatment of rejection episodes. Whether long-term MMF changes survival rates is still controversial. The 3-year data from the U.S. trial periods do not yet show a statistically significant difference in patient or graft survival [53].

The high dose (3 g per day) was associated with more side effects in all three trials. Patients on the high dose developed more infections and had a higher rate of GI intolerance and marrow suppression [54–56]. FDA approval of MMF was at a starting dose of 2 g per day, given as a divided dose of 1 g twice daily. In recipients who develop GI or hematologic toxicity, the dosage should be reduced or MMF should be withheld for a few doses. Dividing the daily dose into more than two doses per day can also be beneficial. Recipients may need to discontinue MMF or convert to EC-MPS for GI intolerance.

The major trials used the less effective oil-based form of CSA. A European study using the ME-CSA formulation (Neoral®) showed only modest, insignificant reductions in acute rejection episodes with MMF compared with AZA, questioning the value of using the costlier MMF [57]. These findings which are drawn on low immunologic risk patients ought to be applied cautiously in other situations.

A subgroup analysis of the higher immunological risk African-American patients enrolled in the U.S. pivotal trial showed that the benefit for African-American versus Caucasian recipients was restricted to the MMF 3 g dose versus the MMF 2 g dose or azathioprine cohorts [58]. Thus, African-American recipients should receive 3 g per day unless they are unable to tolerate that dose.

In a multicenter trial, using a combination of TAC with MMF, a MMF dose of 2 g per day reduced the incidence of acute rejection episodes compared with MMF 1 g per day or AZA—the low acute rejection rate of 8.6% using a combination with MMF 2 g per day suggest that a combination with TAC produced superior results to a combination with CSA [59].

Therapeutic Drug Monitoring. Based on initial pharmacokinetics studies, MMF doses have not been calculated on a milligram per kilogram basis [47]. However, there exists a rationale to implement therapeutic drug monitoring for MMF, as pharmacokinetic variability of MMF has been documented due to differences in hepatic/renal function, concurrent drug administration, and the presence of diarrhea, but not to ethnicity [60]. It is the MPA parent compound and not the parent drug MMF that is readily measured in plasma by HPLC, owing to its high predose concentration (C0). Full MPA AUC monitoring with at least seven samples is impractical on a routine basis. Concentration monitoring is most useful early after transplantation when absorption may be slow and incomplete, and clearance more rapid than at 3 months [61].

Sirolimus

The newest immunosuppressive agent to be released by the FDA belongs to a class of compounds known as the mammalian target of rapamycin (mTOR) inhibitors. Sirolimus (SRL), formerly known as rapamycin, was approved in September 1999 to prevent rejection in kidney recipients. It is produced by *Streptomyces hygroscopicus*, a fungus isolated from a soil sample found on Easter Island (Rapa Nui). SRL is the first mTOR inhibitor to be approved in the United States. A derivative of rapamycin, everolimus, was approved by the FDA in August 2004.

Pharmacology. SRL binds to FKBP-12, the same binding protein as TAC. It was initially thought that SRL and TAC could be antagonistic, given that they shared the same binding protein. Further research revealed, however, that the target of SRL is not calcineurin, but rather the target protein mTOR [62]. The inhibition of mTOR prevents cell-cycle progression from G1 to S in T lymphocytes; thus, SRL blocks the rejection pathway at a later stage than CSA or TAC [63].

SRL, because of its inhibition of lymphocyte proliferation at a later stage, may work synergistically with CSA or TAC. Median effect analysis of the pooled data to demonstrate immunosuppression synergy between CSA and SRL shows that administration of SRL allows a twofold reduction in CSA exposure, and conversely CSA allows a fivefold reduction in SRL dose to achieve the same immunosuppressive efficacy [64]. However, SRL reduces the exposure to TAC when the two drugs are coadministered [65].

Pharmacokinetics. SRL is rapidly absorbed, but the systemic bioavailability of the current formulation is approximately 15%. Food can affect systemic absorption, and SRL should be taken consistently with a meal. SRL is extensively distributed among blood components, but unlike CSA or TAC the distribution does not appear to be temperature dependent [66,67]. Only a small fraction of SRL remains unbound. It is extensively metabolized, with seven major metabolites currently identified. The primary pathway for metabolism is the cytochrome P450 3A4 enzyme system. SRL has a much longer half-life than CSA or TAC, with an average terminal half-life of approximately 60 hours. This extended half-life allows it to be dosed on a once-a-day basis. Hepatic impairment can extend the elimination half-life, so patients with mild to moderate liver disease may require dosage adjustment [67].

SRL is currently available as a 2 mg and 1 mg tablet and as a 1 mg per mL suspension. The tablets should not be crushed. For administration, the suspension should be mixed only with water or orange juice; no other liquids have been tested. No IV formulation is commercially available [68].

Adverse Events. SRL has a different profile of adverse events than other immunosuppressive drugs. In one study, SRL used alone in kidney recipients resulted in a lower serum creatinine level and a higher glomerular filtration rate, compared with CSA [68]. SRL use is not entirely bereft of adverse effects on the kidney. TMA has been found to occur with the use of SRL in the absence of CNI use [69]. Proteinuria is a common manifestation of SRL toxicity in patients converted from CNI for renal impairment. Pre-existing renal damage may be necessary before proteinuria manifests [70]. In such cases, proteinuria resolves when patients were converted back to CNI and SRL was stopped [71]. Delayed recovery from ischemia–reperfusion injury has been observed in registry analysis [72] and this occurs due to inhibitors of cell proliferation by SRL affecting tubular repair [73].

Hypertriglyceridemia and hypercholesterolemia are dose-related adverse events of SRL that may be exacerbated by the use of steroids or CNI [74,75]. Their effect appears to peak after 1 month of SRL therapy; in some recipients, lipid levels decreased to near baseline concentrations after 1 year. Fifty-three percent of SRL-treated patients required lipid-lowering agents compared with 24% in the CSA group. The increase in lipids seen with mTOR inhibitors is a long-term concern.

SRL causes dose-dependent thrombocytopenia and leukopenia, particularly during initial therapy; their incidence is variable and usually self-limiting. Significant decreases in platelet or white blood cell counts can be treated by decreasing the dosage. Occurrence of leukopenia and thrombocytopenia correlates with SRL trough concentrations greater than or equal to 16 ng per mL [76]. The incidence of anemia is also increased with the use of mTOR inhibitors. In the global study of primary use of SRL in renal allograft recipients, anemia was observed in 16% of recipients taking 2 mg per day and 27% of recipients taking 5 mg per day of SRL [77].

During clinical trials, other adverse events associated with SRL included hypertension, rash, acne, hypokalemia, diarrhea, aphthous ulcers, and arthralgias [67]. Thirty-one cases of interstitial pneumonitis were reported by the FDA [78], which can occur any time after initiation of SRL treatment and can progress to respiratory failure. A mortality of 12% was noted in this report, although early recognition with immediate discontinuation of SRL should reduce mortality.

Other adverse effects that occur with de novo SRL use in kidney recipients include wound healing problems and lymphoceles [79]. A systemic program based on patient selection with body mass index <32 kg per m^2, the use of closed suction drains, modifications of surgical technique, and avoiding a loading dose of SRL led to a reduction in wound complications and in the incidence of lymphoceles.

Drug Interactions. Most of the drug interactions that have been reported for SRL are related to P450 enzyme inhibition or induction—the same list of drugs that interact with CSA and TAC. Any compound that can affect P450 metabolism may also affect SRL metabolism. As mentioned earlier, significant changes in exposure to TAC or CSA can occur when prescribed along with SRL.

Patients taking SRL have a much higher exposure to MPA, the active constituent of MMF, than do patients taking CSA and MMF [80]; a similar drug interaction is recognized for TAC as well.

Clinical Use. The phase II trials conducted in Europe were among the earliest that used SRL as a principal immunosuppressant. Pooled data from two of these studies showed significantly higher glomerular filtration rates in patients receiving SRL as compared to CSA [81]. A systematic review of randomized trials in which mTOR inhibitors were used in place of CNI as initial therapy after kidney transplantation revealed no difference in the incidence of acute rejection at 1 year, but the serum creatinine was lower in patients receiving mTOR inhibitors [82]. The two large phase III studies of SRL, one conducted in the United States [83] and the second worldwide [77], revealed much about how best to use SRL and its drawbacks. There was a higher incidence of lymphocele formation and wound infection in the SRL arm compared with the control arm. It was also found that the renal function of patients on a combination of SRL and CSA was worse than patients on CSA alone. Regarding the combination of SRL with TAC, registry data suggest poorer graft survival compared to the combination of TAC with MMF [84]. Phase III studies indicated that the combination of either 1.5 mg per day or 3 mg per day of everolimus was better than MMF in the prevention of acute renal allograft rejection when combined with CSA and steroids after kidney transplantation.

The combination of everolimus/CSA was associated with poorer renal function than MMF/CSA combination [85].

Inhibitors of mTOR are potentially attractive agents for use in the maintenance phase of the posttransplant course in patients with CNI toxicity and as a later addition to CNI to enhance immunosuppression in response to acute rejection. A randomized controlled trial suggests that conversion to SRL with impaired graft function results in a rapid improvement in measured glomerular filtration rate at 3 months that was sustained at 2 years; patients remaining on CNI experience deteriorating graft function [86]. Time for conversion in such patients is unclear, but early rather than late conversion is probably best, before the structural changes associated with interstitial fibrosis/tubular atrophy become extensive [87].

Inhibitors of mTOR are known to prevent tumor cell growth. Temsirolimus, an SRL derivative, has been used in phase I/II clinical trials of advanced renal carcinoma, breast cancer, prostate cancer, pancreatic cancer, glioblastoma, and lymphoma. A multivariate analysis of posttransplant malignancies in renal allograft recipients showed a lower incidence of malignancy in patients taking mTOR inhibitors alone or in combination with CNI compared to those taking CNI alone [88]. SRL has been also found to be effective in the treatment of posttransplant lymphoproliferative disorder (PTLD) [89] and Kaposi's sarcoma [90].

Therapeutic Drug Monitoring. Drug level monitoring is extremely important, especially in newer protocols that may not contain CNI or steroids. Making an accurate assay commercially available has been difficult, hindering use of the drug in some instances. Research is ongoing to determine the best assay system. HPLC has been studied and is being used in several centers with good success to date [75]. An immunoassay is also available for SRL therapeutic drug monitoring.

Initial therapeutic drug monitoring of SRL has correlated well with trough concentrations and allograft rejection, such that trough concentrations are generally accepted as a good measure of SRL activity. The therapeutic range is still being debated, but the general agreement is that concentrations between 5 and 15 ng per mL will prevent rejection and toxicity in most patient populations. Higher-risk patients may need to achieve higher trough concentrations [75].

Corticosteroids

Steroids have been a part of transplantation since its inception. It soon became clear, however, that the toxicities of steroids could overshadow their benefits. The role of steroids in transplantation is changing, as experience is gained in the use of newer immunosuppressive medications that are serving to limit corticosteroid use.

Pharmacology

Steroids have many different effects on the immune system. They inhibit T-cell proliferation, T-cell–dependent immunity, and the expression of various cytokines, especially IL-2, IL-6, interferon-γ, and tumor necrosis factor-α (TNF-α) [91]. They also suppress antibody formation and the delayed hypersensitivity response found in allograft rejection [92].

Clinical Use

For years, steroids have been part of any immunosuppressive regimen to prevent and treat rejection. For use in standard immunosuppression, recipients typically begin on a high initial dose [anywhere from 1 mg per kg to 500 mg IV of methylprednisolone (MP)] on the day of the transplant, and then taper over weeks to months to their final maintenance dose. Most centers maintain recipients on 5 to 10 mg daily or every other day. PRED is the oral drug of choice in most programs; however, if IV dosing is required, MP is the drug of choice. The true ratio of MP to PRED potency is 0.8 to 1.0, although for most recipients that difference is small enough to allow a one-to-one conversion [93].

Steroids at high doses have successfully reversed rejection episodes [94]. Most centers use 500 mg to 1 g of IV MP for three doses to reverse a suspected or documented rejection episode. Recipients should be advised that the typical adverse effects for steroids may be magnified at these higher doses. Many centers use three doses of IV MP for mild to moderate rejection episodes. Antibody therapy is used for steroid-resistant rejection or high-grade rejection.

Adverse Effects

Steroid use is associated with a number of problems, acute and long-term. Acute toxicities of corticosteroids include sodium retention, glucose intolerance, mental status changes, and increase in appetite, acne, and gastritis. Most of these problems are magnified with higher doses and are reduced or eliminated once the dosage is reduced. The long-term side effects are costly to treat and reduce quality of life. A cost estimate for the incidence of cataracts, hypertension, osteoporosis, and diabetes in transplant recipients was in the range of $2,500 to $7,500 per patient over 10 years [95]. Graft loss due to rejection is being replaced by death with function, a term referring to recipients who die with a functioning graft. Cardiovascular disease has become one of the leading causes of death with function. Hypertension, hyperlipidemia, and steroid-induced diabetes may be partly responsible for increasing the risk of cardiovascular death. Accordingly, many transplant centers are switching to steroid-withdrawal/steroid-free protocols for many of their recipients.

Steroid Withdrawal Protocols. A meta-analysis of trials where steroid withdrawal had been done in the first year after kidney transplantation showed that although the risk of acute rejection was more than twofold when steroids were withdrawn, there was no significant difference in the incidence of graft failure [96]. Although four of the trials used MMF/CSA and two used MMF/TAC, no attempt was made to differentiate steroid-sparing potential of CSA and TAC. The European TAC/MMF study group randomly assigned immunologically low-risk patients who had undergone transplantation 3 months earlier to continue triple therapy (TAC, MMF, and steroids), withdraw steroid, or withdraw MMF. Incidence of acute rejection was similar in all three groups at 6 months [97] suggesting TAC enables more effective steroid sparing than CSA. Graft and patient survival and the incidence of acute rejection were similar between groups at 3 years, and serum creatinine levels remained stable [98].

A 3-year analysis of a large trial was done of 300 patients receiving basiliximab induction, CNI, and MMF or SRL in which patients were assigned to have steroids withdrawn on day 2 or to continue steroids. No difference was noted in graft function, patient and graft survival, biopsy proven acute rejection, or chronic allograft nephropathy between the two groups [99]. Use of MMF and SRL, with a CNI, may allow safe withdrawal of steroids earlier.

BIOLOGIC IMMUNOSUPPRESSION

Various antibody preparations, both of polyclonal and monoclonal origin, are currently used in clinical immunosuppression. Polyclonal antibodies directed against lymphocytes were developed first and have been used in transplantation since the 1960s. Monoclonal antibody techniques were discovered later, and, in turn, allowed for the development of biologic agents such as OKT3, which target specific subsets of cells. A number of different monoclonal antibodies (mAbs) are currently under development or in various phases of clinical testing; several have been tested and are now in clinical use. Many are directed against functional secreted molecules of the immune system or their receptors, rather than against actual groups of cells.

One disadvantage of early murine-based antibody preparations such as OKT3 is the potential for the development of antimouse antibodies by the recipient—antibodies that may then limit further use of the agent. To address this problem, recent efforts have focused on the development of so-called humanized versions of mAbs. One option is to replace the constant Fc portion of the parental murine antibody with a human Fc component, thus creating a chimeric antibody. These mAbs may be further humanized to preserve only the original complementarity-determining region, the hypervariable region of the antibody that determines antigen specificity. The remainder of the original murine mAb molecule is replaced by human immunoglobulin G. The advantages of these humanized mAbs are a very long half-life, reduced immunogenicity, and the potential for indefinite and repeated use to confer effects over months rather than days [100]. Biologics are used as rescue agents in 20% of all acute rejection episodes, whilst 50% to 70% of patients undergoing kidney transplantation receive biologic induction [18].

Polyclonal Antibodies

Polyclonal antibodies are produced by immunizing animals, such as horses or rabbits, with human lymphoid tissue; allowing for an immune response; removing the resulting immune sera; and purifying the sera in an effort to remove unwanted antibodies. What remain are antibodies that recognize human lymphocytes.

Polyclonal preparations consist of a wide variety of antibodies and detect specificities include many T cell molecules involved in antigen recognition (CD3, CD4, CD8, and TCR), adhesion (CD2, lymphocyte function antigen [LFA]-1, and intracellular adhesion molecule [ICAM]-1), and costimulation (CD28, CD40, CD80, CD86, and CD154), and non-T cell molecules (CD16 and CD20), and class I and class II major histocompatibility complex (MHC) molecules.

After administration of these antibodies, the transplant recipient's total lymphocyte count should fall and hence these are known as depleting antibodies. Lymphocytes, especially T cells, are then lysed, cleared from the circulation, and deposited into the reticular endothelial system. Alternatively, their surface antigen may be masked by the antibody. Polyclonal antibodies have been successfully used to prevent rejection and to treat acute rejection episodes. Two main polyclonal antibody agents are available for clinical use in the United States: ATGAM and Thymoglobulin.

The broad reactivity with adhesion molecules and other receptors upregulated on activated endothelium has led to preferential use of polyclonal antibodies in situations with prolonged ischemia times where endothelial activation and ischemic reperfusion injury is expected [101].

ATGAM®

ATGAM® is obtained by immunizing horses with human thymocytes. It is generally administered at a dose of 10 to 15 mg per kg, in a course lasting 7 to 14 days. ATGAM® must generally be infused into a central vein, because infusion into a peripheral vein is often associated with thrombophlebitis. To avoid the cytokine release syndrome, recipients should be premedicated with MP and diphenhydramine hydrochloride. Side effects include fever, chills, arthralgia, thrombocytopenia, leukopenia, and a serum sickness–like illness. These side effects are more likely related to the release of pyrogenic cytokines such as TNF-α, IL-1, and IL-6 which result from cell lysis due to antibody binding to targeted cellular surface receptors [102]. Increased infection rates are associated with all immunosuppressants, but certain infections, such as cytomegalovirus, are more common after the use of ATGAM® and other antibody preparations [103].

Thymoglobulin (ATG-R)

Thymoglobulin is obtained by immunizing rabbits with human thymocytes. Initial kidney transplant studies show ATG-R® to be statistically superior to ATGAM® in preventing acute rejection episodes and in reversing acute rejection episodes [104,105].

ATG-R® induction and reduced maintenance immunosuppression has been used in closely followed patients and resulting in graft and patient survivals comparable to standard triple immunosuppression [106]. Administration before reperfusion is advocated to maximize antiadhesion molecule effects.

Comparison studies showed that OKT3 reversed a slightly higher number of rejection episodes than ATG-R® in kidney recipients, but both were efficient treatments. First-time use of ATG-R® was associated with fewer side effects than OKT3 [107]. The side effect profiles of ATG-R® and ATGAM® are similar. With ATG-R®, leukopenia and thrombocytopenia may be quite significant. If a significant drop in platelets or white blood cells is noted, the dosage should be halved or the drug temporarily withheld.

Monoclonal Antibodies

The hybridization of murine antibody–secreting B lymphocytes with a nonsecreting myeloma cell line produces mAbs. A number of mAbs are active against different stages of the immune response. OKT3® has been the most commonly used mAb, but the last few years have seen the introduction and wide use of a number of chimeric and humanized mAbs. Chimeric antibodies preserve the specificity of the original antibody better, whereas humanized antibodies are less likely to be neutralized [108]. Both strategies are effective in preventing antibody clearance.

OKT3

On binding to CD3, OKT3® mediates complement-dependent cell lysis and antibody-dependent cell cytotoxicity leading to rapid clearance of T cells from the peripheral circulation [100]. Pan-T cell activation before their elimination results in systemic cytokine release, and a marked cytokine release syndrome which results in most of the adverse effects associated with OKT3®.

Along with T cell depletion, the overall effect of OKT3® is likely to be due to interrupted T cell receptor (TCR) binding and internalization, disrupted trafficking, and cytokine-mediated regulatory changes.

The standard dose of OKT3® is 5 mg per day given IV, although smaller doses may be as effective. Efficacy can be measured by monitoring CD3-positive cells in the circulation. If OKT3® is effective, the percentage of CD3-positive cells should fall to, and stay below, 5%. Failure to reach this level indicates either an inadequate dose or the presence of antibodies directed against OKT3®. Human antimouse antibodies may develop in at least 30% of patients, and render OKT3® ineffective, allowing for the reappearance of CD3-positive cells in the circulation. This scenario is more common with retreatment using OKT3® or with prolonged treatment.

OKT3® is highly effective and versatile. Most commonly, it is used to treat biopsy proven acute rejections in patients who have failed 3 days of therapy with high-dose MP [109]. OKT3® has also been used as induction therapy to prevent acute rejection and as primary treatment for acute rejection associated with vasculitis (Banff 2 or 3) [110]. Use of OKT3® as an induction agent has declined due to its side-effects' profile. Significant, even life-threatening, side effects may be seen with OKT3®. They may occur when cytokines (e.g., TNF, IL-2, and interferon) are released by T cells into the circulation. These side effects usually occur relatively soon after infusion of OKT3®, and they tend to be most severe after the first and second dose, generally abating by the third or fourth dose. Premedication with IV steroids and agents such as diphenhydramine hydrochloride is important to try to minimize these side effects. The most common symptoms are fever and chills, which generally occur within 30 to 60 minutes after the infusion. Generally, only symptomatic treatment is needed. If fever persists beyond the third dose, then an infectious cause should be sought.

The most serious side effect with OKT3® is a rapidly developing, noncardiogenic pulmonary edema that can be life threatening. The risk of this side effect significantly increases if the recipient is fluid overloaded before beginning OKT3®. Pulmonary edema may develop even in euvolemic patients. If patients are fluid overloaded, they should undergo dialysis or ultrafiltration to remove excess volume before they begin OKT3®.

OKT3® is associated with a wide spectrum of neurologic complications. The most common side effect is headache. Aseptic meningitis has also been reported, albeit usually self-limiting. In this situation, a lumbar puncture demonstrates leukocytosis, but the fluid is sterile. Encephalopathy, ranging from mild to severe, has also been described. If severe encephalopathy develops, OKT3® should be discontinued.

Nephrotoxicity occurring with OKT3® therapy is usually self-limiting, and the recipient improves after the first few doses. Allograft thrombosis has also been reported [111]. Late adverse events reported with OKT3® include infections (especially with cytomegalovirus) and lymphomas.

Anti–Interleukin-2 Monoclonal Antibodies

IL-2 is an important cytokine necessary for the proliferation of cytotoxic T cells. Several mAbs have been developed to target the IL-2 receptor, but currently only one agent is available for clinical use: basiliximab (Simulect®). Daclizumab (Zenapax®) was recently withdrawn from clinical use. Binding of these agents to the IL-2 receptor results in blockade of IL-2–mediated responses. Both are humanized antibodies; with basiliximab, the constant region of the antibody is of human origin; the variable region is of murine origin. Therefore, 75% of the antibody is of human origin.

Because major portions of these agents are of human origin, they tend to have much longer half-lives than does OKT3®. Also, unlike OKT3®, they are not associated with a first-dose reaction. The CD25 component of the IL-2 receptor is primarily focused on naive T cell early activation. Based on this effect, clinical trials in kidney recipients have shown these agents to be effective in preventing acute rejection [112]. It is not indicated for the treatment of established acute rejection episodes, however. For basiliximab, two IV doses of 20 mg (one administered preoperatively and the other on postoperative day 4) are recommended.

Comparable outcomes have been seen in studies comparing basiliximab and polyclonal antibodies and maintenance immunosuppression regimens consisting of CSA, MMF, and steroids [113]. Steroid-free maintenance regimens have also been used in kidney transplantation with anti-CD25 induction [114]. CNI monotherapy or avoidance is not facilitated by the use of anti-CD25 preparations [115]. In all clinical trials to date, basiliximab has been shown to be remarkably safe, with minimal side effects ascribed directly to its use.

Alemtuzumab (Campath-1 H®)

The CD52-specific humanized monoclonal antibody alemtuzumab has the advantages of ease of administration, consistency of monoclonal antibodies, and the benefits of humanization. Alemtuzumab rapidly depletes CD-52 expressing lymphocytes centrally and peripherally resulting from bulk T cell depletion with lesser depletion of B cells and monocytes [116].

Although alemtuzumab depletes all T cell subsets, its action is selective for naive cell types [117]. The T cells that are not depleted exhibit a memory phenotype and are most susceptible to CNI. Maintenance regimens using CNI do best following alemtuzumab induction.

Alemtuzumab facilitates reduced maintenance immunosuppression requirements without an increase in infections or malignant complications in kidney, pancreas, lung, and liver transplantations as compared to historical controls [118–123].

With the increasing use of alemtuzumab as an induction agent, there has been increase in its use as an agent for treating steroid-resistant rejection. There have been anecdotal reports of its use in this setting [124]; additional studies are needed to define its role for this indication.

Rituximab (Humanized Anti-CD-20)

This is a chimeric monoclonal antibody specific for CD20, a cell surface glycoprotein involved in B cell activation and maturation. Rituximab rapidly clears CD20+ cells from the circulation. CD20+ cells are precursors to antibody producing plasma cells, but do not produce antibody themselves; neither do they have a direct effector cell role in rejection. Presence of CD20+ infiltrates has been used as a marker for resistant acute rejection [125]. These cells also have a role in intragraft antigen presentation.

Rituximab has been used as an induction agent in lieu of recipient splenectomy in patients undergoing donor desensitization with plasmapheresis and/or intravenous immunoglobulin [126].

Use of rituximab in high-grade rejection remains investigational. Rituximab has a role in the treatment of Banff 2 and 3 rejection and in reducing antibody formations [127].

The most important indication for the area of rituximab in organ transplantation is as a primary treatment of PTLD—somewhere between immunosuppression withdrawal and the aggressive use of chemotherapy.

FUSION PROTEINS

These are made by the fusion of a single receptor targeting a ligand of interest with a secondary molecule, which is typically the Fc portion of an IgG molecule. Fusion proteins can be composed of humanized components limiting their immune clearance and allowing prolonged administration.

Costimulation-Based Agents

Costimulatory molecules alter the threshold for activation of naive T lymphocytes without having a primary activating or inhibitory function. Fusion proteins have been developed that act by blocking costimulation pathways. The two costimulatory receptors on T cells are CD28 and CD152; these serve reciprocal roles—CD28 facilitates a T cell response, whereas CD152 reduces it.

The fusion proteins that act by inhibiting costimulation-based pathways, and have been studied in renal transplantation, inhibit CD28 and CD152 signaling and this leads to immunosuppression.

Belatacept (investigative name LEA29Y) is a second-generation costimulation-blockade agent that has two amino acid substitutions that give slower dissociation rate for binding to the ligands of CD28. It prolongs the onset of acute rejection in nonhuman primates and synergizes with basiliximab and other clinically available agents. The BENEFIT study reported the primary outcomes from a randomized, phase III study of belatacept versus CSA in kidney transplant recipients [128]. At 12 months, belatacept regimes demonstrated superior renal function and similar patient/graft survival versus CSA, despite an increase in acute rejection in the early posttransplant period. Belatacept is a promising, nonnephrotoxic option in kidney transplant recipients and is being developed with the aim of providing CNI avoidance [129]. It is intended for use as an induction agent as well as for maintenance immunosuppression.

OTHER IMMUNOSUPPRESSIVE AGENTS

Leflunomide and Malononitrilamide (MNA)

The potential of overimmunosuppression resulting from the long half-life (15 to 18 days) of leflunomide has been partly overcome by the shorter half-life (6 to 45 hours) of one of its synthetic analogues also known as FK778. Leflunomide and its analogues have strong antiproliferative effects on T lymphocytes and B lymphocytes. Inhibition of pyrimidine synthesis by a direct-leflunomide–mediated inhibition of dihydro-orotate dehydrogenase leads to suppression of DNA and RNA synthesis. This group of medications also acts through inhibition of tyrosine kinase. FK778 and leflunomide possess antiviral effects and have been used successfully to treat cytomegalovirus [130] and BK virus nephropathy [131] in renal transplant patients.

FK778, in combination with TAC and corticosteroids, was used in a phase II multicenter study involving 149 renal transplant patients [132]. Patients receiving FK778 experienced fewer acute rejection episodes, but there was no effect on graft survivals at week 16.

Janus Kinase 3 Inhibitors

Janus kinase 3 (JAK3) is essential for the signal transduction from the cytokine receptors of several cytokines to the nucleus. Being expressed only on immune cell makes it an important target for developing new immunosuppressants. Several JAK3 inhibitors are available, but CP-690559 is the most potent and selective JAK3 inhibitors. In vivo effects of CP-690550 include reduction in natural killer cell and T cell numbers, whilst CD8+ effector memory T cells were unchanged [133]. A randomized, pilot study compared CP690550 (15 mg BID [CP15] and 30 mg BID [CP30], $n = 20$ each) with TAC ($n = 21$) in de novo kidney transplant recipients [134]. Patients received an IL2R antagonist, MMF, and steroids. Coadministration of CP-690550 30 mg BID with MMF was associated with overimmunosuppression. At a dose of 15 mg BID, the efficacy/safety profile was comparable to TAC, although there was higher rate of viral infection. Although, further dose ranging evaluation of CP-690550 is needed, it may become an important component of CNI avoidance regimens.

IMMUNOSUPPRESSIVE STRATEGIES

Immunosuppressive strategies must take into account the risk of an acute rejection episode, the consequences of an acute rejection episode, the side effects of the immunosuppressive agents, and the consequences of graft loss. The relative importance of each factor may vary depending on the organ transplanted. For example, for kidney recipients, an acute rejection episode is a major risk factor for chronic rejection; strategies must minimize the incidence of acute rejection. For liver recipients, an acute rejection episode usually is easily reversed and has little long-term significance; therefore, lower initial doses of immunosuppression can be used and then increased in those patients who suffer a rejection episode. Dialysis provides a backup if a kidney graft fails, whereas there is no recourse (other than a retransplant) for failure of many other solid-organ grafts. Therefore, particularly for heart and lung recipients, early aggressive immunosuppressive strategies are warranted.

Thus, no single approach applies uniformly across all organs to posttransplant immunosuppressive therapy. Immunosuppressive agents can be categorized according to their use:

Induction—those used for a limited interval at the time of transplant;

Maintenance—those used long term for maintenance of immunosuppression; and

Antirejection—those used for a short time or in high doses to reverse an acute rejection episode.

Considerable overlap exists among these categories, however. For example, the monoclonal and polyclonal antibodies can be used for induction or rejection treatment; PRED is used in high doses for induction or antirejection therapy but in low doses for maintenance therapy; and, in some situations, the doses of maintenance therapy drugs (e.g., TAC) are increased to treat rejection.

Finally, many transplant programs individualize immunosuppression depending on the perceived immunologic risk of rejection and graft loss for that recipient. For example, for kidney recipients, immunosuppressive protocols at a single center may vary for human leukocyte antigen–identical living donor recipients, nonidentical living donor recipients, low-risk cadaver donor recipients, and high-risk (e.g., blacks, those with a high panel-reactive antibody or delayed graft function, retransplant) recipients.

Induction

All recipients (except for identical-twin kidney recipients) require immunosuppressive therapy at the time of transplant. Many transplant centers begin with the same immunosuppression that is used for long-term maintenance. Other centers begin using induction therapy with polyclonal (e.g., Thymoglobulin, ATGAM) or monoclonal (e.g., basiliximab, OKT3, alemtuzumab) antibodies. The goal of induction immunosuppression is to provide powerful immunosuppression peritransplant, decrease the overall incidence of rejection, and permit delay in introducing other maintenance agents such as the CNI.

Prospective randomized studies have shown a decreased incidence of acute rejection episodes with early posttransplant induction therapy. The drugs are expensive, however, and a

TABLE 181.2

DRUGS (MONOTHERAPY OR COMBINATION) CURRENTLY USED FOR LONG-TERM MAINTENANCE THERAPY

CSA monotherapy	FK monotherapy
CSA-P	FK-P
CSA-P-MMF	FK-P-MMF
CSA-P-RAPA	FK-P-RAPA
CSA-MMF	FK-MMF
CSA-RAPA	FK-RAPA
CSA-P-AZA	FK-P-AZA
CSA-AZA	FK-AZA
MMF-P	MMF-RAPA
RAPA-P	
RAPA-MMF-P	

AZA, azathioprine; CSA, cyclosporine; FK, tacrolimus; MMF, mycophenolate mofetil; P, prednisone; RAPA, sirolimus.

TABLE 181.3

ADVANCES IN IMMUNOSUPPRESSION OF SOLID-ORGAN TRANSPLANTATION

1. Major emphasis has been in the area of reduction of toxicities of immunosuppressive agents/combinations.
2. With the increasing use of tacrolimus, steroid-free protocols have been used successfully.
3. Use of depletional antibodies like alemtuzumab has allowed the successful use of tacrolimus monotherapy.
4. To circumvent nephrotoxicity of CNIs, several nonnephrotoxic agents like sirolimus, mycophenolate, belatacept, and JAK3 inhibitors have been developed. Use of IL-2 receptor blockers as induction therapy along with combination of nonnephrotoxic agents might one day lead to successful CNI-free immunosuppression.
5. Use of rituximab in the treatment of B-cell (CD20+)–mediated rejection.

CNIs, calcineurin inhibitors.

long-term benefit has not been well documented for low-risk recipients. As a consequence, some centers use induction for all recipients, other centers use it for no recipients, and still others individualize depending on rough calculations of immunologic risk. More recently, the advantages of steroid- or calcineurin-sparing protocols have been touted, so many centers use short-term induction with IV antibodies in an attempt to lower the doses of other immunosuppressive drugs.

One perceived advantage of antibody induction is the ability to use lower doses of CNIs early posttransplant. A frequent concern is perioperative renal function (of the kidney graft for kidney recipients; of the native kidneys for liver, heart, or lung recipients). Because CNIs are nephrotoxic, delaying their introduction until renal function has recovered may be beneficial.

Maintenance Therapy

First Six Months

With the introduction of multiple new agents in the 1990s, immunosuppressive protocols have become more varied. Table 181.2 illustrates the many combinations currently used for long-term posttransplant maintenance therapy. At most centers, CINs (CSA or TAC) form the basis of immunosuppressive protocols. These drugs have been used as monotherapy and/or in combination with PRED or an antimetabolite. Prospective randomized trials have shown a lower incidence of acute rejection when MMF replaces AZA in these combination protocols [54–56]. Similar trials have shown a lower incidence of acute rejection in SRL versus AZA-treated recipients [83]. Additional studies are needed to determine the relative benefits and risks of MMF versus SRL.

Of interest, CNI-free protocols have been devised. The major goal of such protocols is to avoid the nephrotoxicity associated with use of CNIs. The combination of SRL and MMF has been used to achieve these results. Although nephrotoxicity can be avoided, relatively high doses of both drugs need to be used; as discussed previously, they each have their own side effects. In other randomized trials of CNI-free protocols, belatacept [128] and JAK3 inhibitors [133] have been used.

Considerable debate exists as to whether CNI should be used as monotherapy or combined as double or triple therapy for early posttransplant immunosuppression. Preconditioning with alemtuzumab (Campath 1-H) followed by TAC monotherapy has been successfully used in kidney transplantation with low acute rejection rates [121]. It is important to note that for all protocols, monitoring drug levels and maintaining CNI levels within a specified drug range seem critical to prevent acute rejection episodes early posttransplant.

Late Posttransplant

It is unclear whether all agents used for maintenance therapy in the early posttransplant period need to be continued late posttransplant. Meta-analyses have shown no risk to stopping AZA or CNI late posttransplant [135,136]. Meta-analyses of studies of PRED withdrawal in kidney recipients have shown an increased risk of rejection, however, and an increased risk of graft failure in recipients who stopped PRED [136,137]. In addition, single-center studies have shown no impact of stopping MMF in the late posttransplant period.

CONCLUSIONS

Since 1992, following the introduction of a number of new immunosuppressive agents, short-term graft and patient outcomes have improved considerably. However, the side effect of immunosuppressive agents continues to present a major problem. With the increasing use of TAC, steroid-free protocols were used successfully. Development of depleting monoclonal antibodies like alemtuzumab has led to the use of TAC monotherapy as maintenance immunosuppression. In kidney transplantation, long-term outcomes have been affected by the nephrotoxicity of CNI. In nonrenal transplant recipients, CNI toxicity has led to renal insufficiency and failure in a significant number of instances. Development of nonnephrotoxic agents like SRL, MMF, belatacept, and JAK3 inhibitors and their use in combination will some day lead to the successful use of CNI-free immunosuppression. A summary of some of the advances in the field of immunosuppression is shown in Table 181.3.

Another major advantage of the availability of several immunosuppressive agents is that immunosuppression can now be tailored for the individual patient. Those having drug-specific toxicity can be switched to another drug with similar efficacy but differing side effects.

ACKNOWLEDGMENT

We are grateful to Melissa Connell for assistance with the manuscript.

References

1. Hamilton D: Kidney transplantation: a history, in Morris PJ, Knechtle S (ed): *Kidney Transplantation, Principles and Practice*. 6th ed. Philadelphia, WB Saunders, 2008, pp 1–8.
2. Wiederrecht G, Lam E, Hung S, et al: The mechanism of action of FK-506 and cyclosporine A. *Ann N Y Acad Sci* 696:9–19, 1993.
3. Kahan B: Cyclosporine. *N Engl J Med* 321(25):1725–1737, 1989.
4. Friman S, Backman L: A new microemulsion of cyclosporin. *Clin Pharmacokinet* 30(3):181–193, 1996.
5. Perico N, Remuzzi G: Cyclosporine induced renal dysfunction in experimental animals and humans. *Transplant Rev* 5:63, 1991.
6. Lee DB: Cyclosporine and the renin-angiotensin axis. *Kidney Int* 52:248–260, 1997.
7. Morris ST, McMurray JJ, Roger RS, et al: Endothelial dysfunction in renal transplant recipients maintained on cyclosporine. *Kidney Int* 57:1100–1106, 2000.
8. Pham PTT, Peng A, Williamson AH, et al: Cyclosporine and tacrolimus-associated thrombotic microangiopathy. *Am J Kidney Disease* 36(4):844–850, 2000.
9. Griffith M, Crowe A, Papadaki L, et al: Cyclosporin nephrotoxicity in heart and lung transplant patients. *QJM* 89(10):751–763, 1996.
10. Burke J, Pirsch J, Ramos E, et al: Long-term efficacy and safety of cyclosporine in renal-transplant recipients. *N Engl J Med* 331(6):358–363, 1994.
11. Johnson DW, Saunders HJ, Johnson FJ, et al: Cyclosporine exerts a direct fibrogenic effect on human tubulointerstitial cells; roles of insulin like growth factor β_1, and platelet derived growth factor. *J Pharmacol Exp Ther* 289:535–542, 1999.
12. Shihab FS, Bennett WM, Tanner AM, et al: Angiotensin II blockade decreases TGF-β_1 and matrix proteins in cyclosporine nephropathy. *Kidney Int* 52:660–673, 1997.
13. Porter G, Bennett W, Sheldon G, et al: Cyclosporine-associated hypertension. *Arch Intern Med* 150(2):280–283, 1990.
14. Jarosz JM, Howlett DC, Cox TCS, et al: Cyclosporine-related reversible posterior leukoencephalopathy: MRI. *Neuroradiology* 39:711, 1997.
15. Scott VL, Hurrell MA, Anderson TJ: Reversible posterior leukoencephalopathy syndrome: a misnomer reviewed. *Intern Med J* 35:83–90, 2005.
16. Campana C, Regazzi M, Buggia I, et al: Clinically significant drug interactions with cyclosporin. *Clin Pharmacokinet* 30(2):141–179, 1996.
17. Jones T: The use of other drugs to allow a lower dosage of cyclosporin to be used. *Clin Pharmacokinet* 32(5):357–367, 1997.
18. Shapiro R, Young JB, Milford EL, et al: Immunosuppression: evolution in practice and trends, 1993–2003. *Am J Transplant* 5:874, 2005.
19. Johnson E, Canafax D, Gillingham K, et al: Effect of early cyclosporine levels on kidney allograft rejection. *Clin Transplant* 11(6):352–357, 1997.
20. Dumont R, Ensom M: Methods for clinical monitoring of cyclosporine in transplant patients. *Clin Pharmacokinet* 38(5):427–447, 2000.
21. Mahalati K, Belitsky P, West K, et al: Approaching the therapeutic window for cyclosporine in kidney transplantation: a prospective study. *J Am Soc Nephrol* 12(4):828–833, 2001.
22. Keown P (on behalf of the Canadian Neoral Study Group): Absorption profiling of cyclosporine microemulsion (Neoral) during the first two weeks after renal transplantation. *Transplantation* 72:1024–1032, 2001.
23. Kyllonen LE, Salmela KT: Early cyclosporine Co and C_2 monitoring in de novo kidney transplant patients: a prospective randomized single center pilot study. *Transplantation* 81(7):1010–1015, 2006.
24. Goto T, Kino T, Hatanaka H, et al: FK 506: historical perspectives. *Transplant Proc* 23(6):2713–2717, 1991.
25. Scott LJ, McKeage K, Keown SJ, et al: Tacrolimus: a further update of its use in the management of organ transplantation. *Drugs* 63(12):1247–1297, 2003.
26. Venkataramanan R, Swaminathan A, Prasad T, et al: Clinical pharmacokinetics of tacrolimus. *Clin Pharmacokinet* 29(6):404–430, 1995.
27. Vincenti F, Jensik SC, Filo RS, et al: A long term comparison of tacrolimus (FK506) and cyclosporine in kidney transplantation: evidence for improved allograft survival at 5 years. *Transplantation* 73:775, 2002.
28. Shimizu T, Tanabe K, Tokumoto T, et al: Clinical and histological analysis of acute tacrolimus (TAC) nephrotoxicity in renal allografts. *Clin Transplant* 13[Suppl]:48, 1999.
29. Artz MA, Boots JMM, Ligtenberg G, et al: Randomized conversion from cyclosporine to tacrolimus in renal transplant patients: improved lipid profile and unchanged plasma homocysteine levels. *Transplant Proc* 34:1793, 2002.
30. The U.S, Multicenter FK506 Liver Study Group: a comparison of tacrolimus (FK 506) and cyclosporine for immunosuppression in liver transplantation. *N Engl J Med* 331(17):1110–1115, 1994.
31. Webster AC, Woodroffe RC, Taylor RS, et al: Tacrolimus versus ciclosporin as primary immunosuppression for kidney transplant recipients: meta-analysis and meta-regression of randomised trial data. *BMJ* 331:810, 2005.
32. Trimarchi HM, Truong LD, Brennan S, et al: FK 506-associated thrombotic microangiopathy: report of two cases and review of the literature. *Transplantation* 67:539, 1999.
33. Heisel O, Heisel R, Batshaw R, et al: New onset diabetes mellitus in patient receiving calcineurin inhibitors: a systematic review and meta-analysis. *Am J Transplant* 4:583, 2004.
34. Johnson C, Ahsan N, Gonwa T, et al: Randomized trial of tacrolimus (Prograf) in combination with azathioprine or mycophenolate mofetil versus cyclosporine (Neoral) with mycophenolate mofetil after cadaveric kidney transplantation. *Transplantation* 69:834, 2000.
35. Mueller A, Platz KP, Bechstein WO, et al: Neurotoxicity after orthotopic liver transplantation. *Transplantation* 58(2):155–169, 1994.
36. Jindal R, Popescu I, Schwartz M, et al: Diabetogenicity of FK506 versus cyclosporine in liver transplant recipients. *Transplantation* 58(3):370–372, 1994.
37. Pirsch JD, Miller J, Deierhoi MH, et al: For the FK506 kidney transplant study group: a comparison of tacrolimus (FK506) and cyclosporine for immunosuppression after cadaveric kidney transplantation. *Transplantation* 63:977, 1997.
38. Foster CE, Philosophe B, Schweitzer EJ, et al: A decade of experience with renal transplantation in African Americans. *Ann Surg* 236:794, 2002.
39. Sutherland DR, Gruessner RWG, Dunn DL, et al: Lessons learned from more than 1000 pancreas transplants at a single institution. *Ann Surg* 233: 463, 2001.
40. Meiser BM, Pfeiffer M, Schmidt D, et al: Combination therapy with tacrolimus and mycophenolate mofetil following cardiac transplantation: importance of mycophenolic acid therapeutic drug monitoring. *J Heart Lung Transplant* 18:143, 1999.
41. Kur F, Reichenspiner H, Meiser BM, et al: Tacrolimus (FK506) as primary immunosuppressant after lung transplantation. *Thorac Cardiovas Surg* 47:14, 1999.
42. Thompson JS: Intestinal transplantation: experience in the United States. *Eur J Pediatric Surg* 9:271, 1999.
43. Chan G, Canafax D, Johnson C, et al: Therapeutic use of azathioprine in renal transplantation. *Pharmacother* 7(5):165–177, 1987.
44. Fulton B, Markham A: Mycophenolate mofetil. *Drugs* 51(2):278–298, 1996.
45. Moon JI, Kim YS, Kim MS, et al: Effect of cyclosporine, mycophenolic acid, and rapamycin on the proliferation of rat aortic vascular smooth muscle cells: in vitro study. *Transplant Proc* 32:2026, 2000.
46. Bullingham R, Nicholls A, Kamm B: Clinical pharmacokinetics of mycophenolate mofetil. *Clin Pharmacokinet* 34(6):429–455, 1998.
47. Pescovitz M, Conti D, Dunn J, et al: Intravenous mycophenolate mofetil: safety, tolerability and pharmacokinetics. *Clin Transplant* 14(3):179–188, 2000.
48. Bullingham R, Monroe S, Nicholls A, et al: Pharmacokinetics and bioavailability of mycophenolate mofetil in healthy subjects after single-dose oral and intravenous administration. *J Clin Pharmacol* 36(4):315, 1996.
49. Shipkova M, Armstrong VW, Oellerich M, et al: Acyl glucuronide drug metabolites: toxicological and analytical implications. *Ther Drug Monit* 25:1, 2003.
50. Chan L, Mulgaonkar S, Walker R, et al: Patient-reported gastrointestinal symptoms burden and health-related quality of life following conversion from mycophenolate mofetil to enteric-coated mycophenolate sodium. *Transplantation* 81:1290, 2006.
51. Anonymous: Mycophenolate mofetil. Product Monograph. Piscataway, NJ, Roche Pharmaceuticals, 1995.
52. Gregoor PJ, de Sevaux RG, Hene RJ, et al: Effect of cyclosporine on mycophenolate acid trough levels in kidney transplant recipients. *Transplantation* 68:1603, 1999.
53. Zucker K, Tsaroucha A, Olson L, et al: Evidence that tacrolimus augments the bioavailability of mycophenolate mofetil through the inhibition of mycophenolic acid glucuronidation. *Ther Drug Monit* 21(1):35–43, 1999.
54. US Renal Transplant Mycophenolate Mofetil Study Group: Mycophenolate mofetil in cadaveric renal transplantation. *Am J Kidney Dis* 34(2):296–303, 1999.
55. The Tricontinental Mycophenolate Mofetil Renal Transplantation Study Group: A blinded randomized clinical trial of mycophenolate mofetil for the prevention of acute rejection in cadaveric renal transplantation. *Transplantation* 61(7):1029–1037, 1996.
56. European Mycophenolate Mofetil Study Group: Placebo-controlled study of mycophenolate mofetil combined with cyclosporine and corticosteroids for prevention of acute rejection. *Lancet* 345(8961):1321–1325, 1995.
57. Remuzzi G, Lesti M, Gotti E, et al: Mycophenolate mofetil versus azathioprine for prevention of acute rejection in renal transplantation (MYSS): a randomized trial. *Lancet* 364:503, 2004.
58. Neylan J: Immunosuppressive therapy in high-risk transplant patients: dose-dependent efficacy of mycophenolate mofetil in African-American renal allograft recipients. U.S. Renal Transplant Mycophenolate Mofetil Study Group. *Transplantation* 64(9):1277–1282, 1997.
59. Miller J, Mendez R, Pirsch JD, et al: Safety and efficacy of tacrolimus in combination with mycophenolate mofetil (MMF) in cadaveric renal transplant patients. FK506/MMF dose-ranging Kidney Transplant Study Group. *Transplantation* 69:875, 2000.

60. Shaw LM, Korecka M, Aradhye S, et al: Mycophenolic acid area under the curve values in African American and Caucasian renal transplant patients are comparable. *J Clin Pharmacol* 40:624, 2000.
61. Holt DW: Monitoring mycophenolic acid. *Ann Clin Biochem* 39:173, 2002.
62. Heitman J, Movva NR, Hall MN: Targets for cell cycle arrest by the immunosuppressant rapamycin in yeast. *Science* 253:905, 1991.
63. Sehgal S: Rapamune (RAPA, rapamycin, sirolimus): mechanism of action immunosuppressive effect results from blockade of signal transduction and inhibition of cell cycle progression. *Clin Biochem* 31(5):335–340, 1998.
64. Kahan BD, Kramer WG: Median effect analysis of efficacy versus adverse effects of immunosuppressants. *Clin Pharmacol Ther* 70:74, 1991.
65. Balden N, Rigotti P, Furian L, et al: Co-administration of sirolimus alters tacrolimus pharmacokinetics in a dose-dependent manner in adult renal transplant recipients: *Pharmacol Res* 54:181,2006.
66. Yatscoff R, Wang P, Chan K, et al: Rapamycin: distribution, pharmacokinetics, and therapeutic range investigations. *Ther Drug Monitor* 17(6):666–671, 1995.
67. Anonymous: Rapamune oral solution. Product information. Philadelphia, Wyeth-Ayerst Pharmaceuticals, 1999.
68. Groth C, Backman L, Morales JM, et al: Sirolimus (rapamycin)-based therapy in human renal transplantation: similar efficacy and different toxicity compared with cyclosporine. Sirolimus European Renal Transplant Study Group. *Transplantation* 67(7):1036–1042, 1999.
69. Sartelet H, Toupance O, Lorenzato M, et al: Sirolimus-induced thrombotic microangiopathy is associated with decreased expression of vascular endothelial growth factor in kidneys. *Am J Transplant* 5:2441–2447, 2005.
70. Dervaux T, Caillard S, Meyer C, et al: Is sirolimus responsible for proteinuria? *Transplant Proc* 37(6):2828, 2005.
71. Dittrich E, Schmaldienst S, Soleiman A, et al: Rapamycin-associated post-transplantation glomerulonephritis and its remission after reintroduction of calcineurin-inhibitor therapy. *Transpl Int* 17:215–220, 2004.
72. Simon JF, Swanson SJ, Agodoa LYC, et al: Induction sirolimus and delayed graft function after deceased donor kidney transplantation in the United States. *Am J Nephrol* 24:393–401, 2004.
73. Loverre A, Ditonno P, Crovace A, et al: Ischemia-reperfusion induces glomerular and tubular activation of proinflammatory and antiapoptotic pathways: differential modulation by rapamycin. *J Am Soc Nephrol* 15:2675–2686, 2004.
74. Brattstrom C, Wilczek H, Tyden G, et al: Hypertriglyceridemia in renal transplant patients treated with sirolimus. *Transplant Proc* 30(8):3950–3951, 1998.
75. Kahan B, Napoli K, Kelly P, et al: Therapeutic drug monitoring of sirolimus: correlations with efficacy and toxicity. *Clin Transplant* 14(2):97–109, 2000.
76. Hong J, Kahan B: Sirolimus-induced thrombocytopenia and leukopenia in renal transplant recipients: risk factors, incidence, progression, and management. *Transplantation* 69(10):2085–2090, 2000.
77. MacDonald AS, for the Rapamune Global Study Group (RGS): A worldwide, phase III, randomized, controlled, safety and efficacy study of a sirolimus/cyclosporine regimen for prevention of acute rejection in recipients of primary mismatched renal allografts. *Transplantation* 71(2):271–280, 2001.
78. Singer S, Tiernan R, Sullivan E: Interstitial pneumonitis associated with sirolimus therapy in renal-transplant recipients. *N Engl J Med* 343(24): 1815 1816, 2000.
79. Tiong HY, Flechner SM, Zhou L, et al: A systemic approach to minimizing wound problems for de novo sirolimus-treated kidney transplant recipients. *Transplantation* 87:296–302, 2009.
80. Büchler M, Lebranchu Y, Bénéton M, et al: Higher exposure to mycophenolic acid with sirolimus than with cyclosporine cotreatment. *Clin Pharmacol Ther* 78:34–42, 2005.
81. Morales JM, Wramner L, Kreis H, et al: Sirolimus does not exhibit nephrotoxicity compared to cyclosporine in renal transplant recipients. *Am J Transplant* 2(5):436–442, 2002.
82. Webster AC, Lee VW, Chapman JR, et al: Target of rapamycin inhibitors (sirolimus and everolimus) for primary immunosuppression of kidney transplant recipients: a systematic review and meta-analysis of randomized trials. *Transplantation* 81(9):1234–1248, 2006.
83. Kahan BD: Efficacy of sirolimus compared with azathioprine for reduction of acute renal allograft rejection: a randomized multicenter study. *Lancet* 356:194, 2000.
84. Meier-Kriesche HU, Schold JD, Srinivas TR, et al: Sirolimus in combination with tacrolimus is associated with worse renal allograft survival compared to mycophenolate mofetil combined with tacrolimus. *Am J Transplant* 5(9):2273–2280, 2005.
85. Lorber MI, Mulgaonkar S, Butt KMH, et al: Everolimus versus mycophenolate mofetil in the prevention of rejection in de novo renal transplant recipients: a 3-year randomized, multicenter, phase III study. *Transplantation* 80(2):244–252, 2005.
86. Watson CJE, Firth J, Williams PF, et al: A randomized controlled trial of late conversion from CNI-based to sirolimus-based immunosuppression following renal transplantation. *Am J Transplant* 5(10):2496–2503, 2005.
87. Basu A, Falcone JL, Tan HP, et al: Chronic allograft nephropathy score at the time of Sirolimus rescue predicts renal allograft function. *Transplant Proc* 39:94–98, 2007.
88. Kauffman HM, Cherikh WS, Cheng Y, et al: Maintenance immunosuppression with target-of-rapamycin inhibitors is associated with a reduced incidence of de novo malignancies. *Transplantation* 80(7):883–889, 2005.
89. Cullis B, D'Souza R, McCullagh P, et al: Sirolimus-induced remission of posttransplantation lymphoproliferative disorder. *Am J Kidney Dis* 47(5):e67–72, 2006.
90. Stallone G, Schena A, Infante B, et al: Sirolimus for Kaposi's sarcoma in renal-transplant recipients. *N Eng J Med* 352:1317–1323, 2005.
91. Suthanthiran M, Strom T: Renal transplantation. *N Engl J Med* 331(6): 365–376, 1994.
92. Popowniak K, Nakamoto S: Immunosuppressive therapy in renal transplantation. *Surg Clin North Am* 51(5):1191–1204, 1971.
93. Chatterjee S: Immunosuppressive drugs used in clinical renal transplantation. *Urology Suppl* 9(6):52–60, 1977.
94. Alarcon-Zurita A, Ladefoged J: Treatment of acute allograft rejection with high doses of corticosteroids. *Kidney Int* 9(4):351–354, 1976.
95. Veenstra D, Best J, Hornberger J, et al: Incidence and cost of steroid side effects after renal transplantation. *Transplant Proc* 31(1–2):301–302, 1999.
96. Pascual J, Quereda C, Zamora J, et al: Steroid withdrawal in renal transplant patients on triple therapy with a calcineurin inhibitor and mycophenolate mofetil: a meta-analysis of randomized, controlled trials. *Transplantation* 78(10);1548–1556, 2004.
97. Vanrenterghem Y, van Hooff JP, Squifflet JP, et al: Minimization of immunosuppressive therapy after renal transplantation: results of a randomized controlled trial. *Am J Transplant* 5(1):87–95, 2005.
98. Pascual J, van Hooff JP, Salmela K, et al: Three-year observational follow-up of a multicenter, randomized trial on tacrolimus-based therapy with withdrawal of steroids or mycophenolate mofetil after renal transplant. *Transplantation* 82(1):55–61, 2006.
99. Kumar MS, Heifets M, Moritz M, et al: Safety and efficacy of steroid withdrawal two days after kidney transplantation: analysis of results at three years. *Transplantation* 81(6):832–839, 2006.
100. Webster A, Pankhurst T, Rinaldi F, et al: Polyclonal and monoclonal antibodies for treating acute rejection episodes in kidney transplant recipients. *Cochrane Database Syst Rev* 19:CD004756, 2006.
101. Beiras-Fernandez A, Chappell D, Claus Hammer C, et al: Influence of polyclonal anti-thymocyte globulins upon ischemia–reperfusion injury in a non-human primate model. *Transpl Immunol* 15(4):273–279, 2006.
102. Vallhonrat H, Williams WW, Cosimi AB, et al: In vivo generation of 4d, Bb, iC3b, and SC5b-9 after OKT3 administration in kidney and lung transplant recipients. *Transplantation* 67(2):253–259, 1999.
103. Jamil B, Nicholls KM, Becker GJ, et al: Influence of anti-rejection therapy on the timing of cytomegalovirus disease and other infections in renal transplant recipients. *Clin Transplant* 14(1):14–18, 2000.
104. Brennan DC, Flavin K, Lowell JA, et al: A randomized, double-blinded comparison of Thymoglobulin versus Atgam for induction immunosuppressive therapy in adult renal transplant recipients. *Transplantation* 67(7):1011–1018, 1999.
105. Gaber AO, First MR, Tesi RJ, et al: Results of the double-blind, randomized, multicenter, phase III clinical trial of Thymoglobulin versus Atgam in the treatment of acute graft rejection episodes after renal transplantation. *Transplantation* 66(1):29–37, 1998.
106. Starzl TE, Murase N, Abu-Elmagd K, et al: Tolerogenic immunosuppression for organ transplantation. *Lancet* 361(9368):1502–1510, 2003.
107. Regan J, Campbell K, van Smith L, et al: Characterization of anti-Thymoglobulin, anti-Atgam, and anti-OKT3 IgG antibodies in human serum with an 11-min ELISA. *Transpl Immunol* 5(1):49–56, 1997.
108. Delmonico FL, Cosimi AB, Kawai T, et al: Nonhuman primate responses to murine and humanized OKT4 A. *Transplantation* 55(4):722–727, 1993.
109. Tesi RJ, Elkhammas EA, Henry ML, et al: OKT3 for primary therapy of the first rejection episode in kidney transplants. *Transplantation* 55(5):1023–1028, 1993.
110. Kamath S, Dean D, Peddi VR, et al: Efficacy of OKT3 as primary therapy for histologically confirmed acute renal allograft rejection. *Transplantation* 64(10):1428–32, 1997.
111. Abramowicz D, Pradier O, Marchant A, et al: Induction of thromboses within renal allograft by high-dose prophylactic OKT3. *Lancet* 339:777, 1992.
112. Thistlethwaite JR Jr, Nashan B, Hall M, et al: Reduced acute rejection and superior 1-year renal allograft survival with basiliximab in patients with diabetes mellitus. The Global Simulect Study Group. *Transplantation* 70(5):784–790, 2000.
113. Sollinger H, Kaplan B, Pescovitz M, et al: Basiliximab versus antithymocyte globulin for prevention of acute renal allograft rejection. *Transplantation* 72(12):1915–1919, 2001.
114. Rostaing L, Cantarovich D, Mourad G, et al: Corticosteroid-free immunosuppression with tacrolimus, mycophenolate mofetil, and daclizumab induction in renal transplantation. *Transplantation* 79(7):807–814, 2005.
115. Parrott NR, Hammad AQ, Watson CJ, et al: Multicenter, randomized study of the effectiveness of basiliximab in avoiding addition of steroids to cyclosporine a monotherapy in renal transplant recipients. *Transplantation* 79(3):344–348, 2005.
116. Kirk AD, Hale DA, Mannon RB, et al: Results from a human renal allograft tolerance trial evaluating the humanized CD52-specific monoclonal antibody alemtuzumab (CAMPATH-1 H). *Transplantation* 76(1):120–129, 2003.

117. Pearl JP, Parris J, Hale DA, et al: Immunocompetent T-cells with a memory-like phenotype are the dominant cell type following antibody-mediated T-cell depletion. *Am J Transplant* 5:465–474, 2005.
118. Bartosh SM, Knechtle SJ, Sollinger HW: Campath 1-H use in pediatric renal transplantation. *Am J Transplant* 5:1569, 2005.
119. Gruessner RW, Kandaswamy R, Humar A, et al: Calcineurin inhibitor- and steroid-free immunosuppression in pancreas-kidney and solitary pancreas transplantation. *Transplantation* 79:1184–1189, 2005.
120. Kaufman DB, Leventhal JR, Gallon LG, et al: Alemtuzumab induction and prednisone-free maintenance immunotherapy in simultaneous pancreas-kidney transplantation comparison with rabbit antithymocyte globulin induction—long-term results. *Am J Transplant* 6:331–339, 2006.
121. Shapiro R, Basu A, Tan HP, et al: Kidney transplantation under minimal immunosuppression after pretransplant lymphoid depletion with Thymoglobulin or Campath. *J Am Coll Surg* 200:505–515, 2005.
122. McCurry KR, Iacono A, Zeevi A, et al: Early outcomes in human lung transplantation with Thymoglobulin or Campath-1 H for recipient pretreatment followed by posttransplant tacrolimus near-monotherapy. *J Thorac Cardiovasc Surg* 130:528–537, 2005.
123. Tzakis AG, Tryphonopoulos P, Kato T, et al: Preliminary experience with alemtuzumab (Campath-1 H) and low-dose tacrolimus immunosuppression in adult liver transplantation. *Transplantation* 77:1209–1214, 2004.
124. Basu A, Ramkumar M, Tan HP, et al: Reversal of acute cellular rejection (ACR) after renal transplantation with Campath 1 H. *Transplant Proc* 37:923–926, 2005.
125. Sarwal M, Chua MS, Kambham N, et al: Molecular heterogeneity in acute renal allograft rejection identified by DNA microarray profiling. *N Eng J Med* 349:125, 2003.
126. Tydén G, Kumlien G, Genberg H, et al: ABO incompatible kidney transplantations without splenectomy, using antigen-specific immunoadsorption and rituximab. *Am J Transplant* 5:145–148, 2005.
127. Becker YT, Samaniego-Picota M, Sollinger HW, et al: The emerging role of rituximab in organ transplantation. *Transpl Int* 19:621–628, 2006.
128. Vincenti F, Grinyo JM, Charpentier B, et al: Primary outcomes from a randomized, phase III study of belatacept vs cyclosporine in kidney transplant recipients (BENEFIT Study). *Am J Transplant* 9(S2):191, 2009.
129. Vincenti F, Larsen C, Durrbach A, et al: Costimulation blockade with belatacept in renal transplantation. *N Eng J Med* 353:770, 2005.
130. John GT, Manivannan J, Chandy S, et al: Leflunomide therapy for cytomegalovirus disease in renal allograft recipients. *Transplantation* 77:140–1461, 2004.
131. Josephson MA, Gillen D, Javaid B, et al: Treatment of renal allograft polyoma BK virus infection with leflunomide. *Transplantation* 81:704–710, 2006.
132. Vanrenterghem Y, van Hooff JP, Klinger M, et al: The effects of FK778 in combination with tacrolimus and steroids: a phase II multicenter study in renal transplant patients. *Transplantation* 78:9–14, 2004.
133. Paniagua R, Si MS, Flores MG, et al: Effects of JAK3 inhibition with CP-690550 on immune cell populations and their functions in nonhuman primate recipients of kidney allografts. *Transplantation* 80:1283–1292, 2005.
134. Busque S, Leventhal J, Brennan DC, et al: Calcineurin-inhibitor-free immunosuppression based on the JAK inhibitor CP-690550: a pilot study in de novo kidney allograft recipients. *Am J Transplant* 9:1936–1945, 2009.
135. Kunz R, Neumayer HH: Maintenance therapy with triple versus double immunosuppressive regimen in renal transplantation: a meta-analysis. *Transplantation* 63(3):386–392, 1997.
136. Kasiske BL, Chakkera HA, Louis TA, et al: A meta-analysis of immunosuppression withdrawal trials in renal transplantation. *J Am Soc Nephrol* 11(10):1910–1917, 2000.
137. Hricik DE, O'Toole MA, Schulak JA, et al: Steroid-free immunosuppression in cyclosporine-treated renal transplant recipients: a meta-analysis. *J Am Soc Nephrol* 4(6):1300–1305, 1993.

CHAPTER 182 ■ CRITICAL CARE PROBLEMS IN KIDNEY TRANSPLANT RECIPIENTS

MARK L. STURDEVANT AND RAINER W.G. GRUESSNER

INTRODUCTION

A kidney transplant (KTx) remains the most definitive and durable solution for patients reaching end-stage renal disease (ESRD). A successful transplant, as compared with dialysis, can provide a higher quality of life for a longer period at an overall lower cost for the more than 104,000 patients currently awaiting a KTx on the United Network for Organ Sharing waiting list [1,2]. In 2006, in United States KTx centers, the cumulative 1-year graft survival rate was 91.3% for deceased donor recipients and 96.4% for living donor recipients; an analysis of recipients transplanted in 2002 revealed a 5-year graft survival rate of 68.9% for deceased donor recipients and 81.5% for living donor recipients. The half-life graft survival time now projected for deceased donor recipients is approximately 10 years; for living related donor recipients, almost 18 years, depending on the human leukocyte antigen (HLA) match [3–5]. Despite these encouraging results, the waiting list continues to expand, and the living and deceased donor pools have fallen further behind; this divergence results in recipients who can be subjected to the ill effects of uremia and dialysis for more than 5 years pretransplant. Critical care providers therefore face a cohort of patients with a higher acuity of illness than seen even a decade ago. This chapter discusses the salient points of critical care that KTx recipients must receive to optimize their outcomes.

PRETRANSPLANT EVALUATION

Thoughtful patient selection and a thorough pretransplant evaluation of transplant candidates are essential for optimal transplant outcomes; because hypertension, diabetes mellitus, and cardiovascular disease are ubiquitous in this group, risk stratifying is helpful. The pretransplant evaluation should be exhaustive (covering gastrointestinal, pulmonary, neurologic, genitourinary, and infectious disease concerns). The cardiovascular examination is the most important and possibly the most unreliable. Candidates at increased risk for coronary artery disease or cardiac dysfunction, especially those with diabetes, should undergo noninvasive cardiac stress testing. For those with reversible cardiac ischemia, coronary angiography is mandatory to elucidate the need for percutaneous coronary artery balloon dilation or even coronary artery bypass.

The problem lies in the most troublesome deficiency in noninvasive testing—that is, the suboptimal sensitivity for cardiac death and infarction. In a meta-analysis, the sensitivity of the pretransplant cardiac perfusion study for myocardial infarction was only 0.7; for cardiac death, only 0.8 [6,7]. Therefore, the onus remains on transplant physicians to have a high suspicion for life-threatening cardiovascular disease in this patient population; even uremic young adults (<40 years old) should be heavily scrutinized, because more than 90% of them who had renal insufficiency during childhood will have significant cardiac or carotid disease.

Even with an aggressive approach to pretransplant evaluation, cardiac complications occur in 6% of recipients during the first-month posttransplant [6]. Candidates with a history of stroke or transient ischemic attacks (TIAs) require a carotid duplex ultrasound to exclude critical carotid stenoses. Pulmonary function testing should be assessed in candidates with a history of pulmonary disease such as emphysema or asthma. Also, at least one group reported an abnormally high prevalence of pulmonary hypertension (40%) in recipients who were undergoing hemodialysis (HD) via an arteriovenous fistula [8].

Up to 10% of the HD population has antihepatitis C antibodies; therefore, all KTx candidates should be screened, and abnormal liver function test results should stimulate a more thorough evaluation [9]. Cholecystectomy should be considered for candidates with symptomatic cholelithiasis.

Gastrointestinal disease, ranging from gastritis and peptic ulcer disease to colonic diverticulosis, is more common in patients with ESRD. Liberal use of bidirectional endoscopy is justified in this population, and colonoscopy is mandatory in all candidates 50 years and older. Recurrent urinary tract infections or a history of bladder dysfunction mandates a urologic evaluation.

Candidates with a personal or family history of hypercoagulability should undergo a thrombophilia evaluation. If appropriate pretransplant evaluations are readily performed, therapeutic measures can begin in a timely manner to avoid many potential complications (some life threatening).

PERIOPERATIVE CARE

Pretransplant Preparation

Proper pretransplant preparation in the days before the operation is essential for optimal graft and recipient outcome. Ideally, HD-dependent patients can undergo their routine HD session the day before their KTx; appropriate electrolyte panels should be checked within hours of anesthesia induction. Dialysis catheter sites require examination for infection; for recipients on peritoneal dialysis, culture and Gram stains of their peritoneal fluid should be obtained. Each recipient should undergo a repeat history and physical examination, electrocardiogram (ECG), chest x-ray (CXR), and laboratory examination within days before their transplant, to detect any interim health derangements since their last physician visit. A medication list review is mandatory to confirm the cessation of some drugs (e.g., warfarin) and the continuation of others (e.g., beta-blockers), which may affect intraoperative and postoperative outcomes. Bowel preparation occurs at some centers the evening before the operation.

Intraoperative Care

The type of invasive monitoring during the KTx should reflect the nature and degree of the individual recipient's comorbidities. A central venous catheter is often introduced to facilitate monitoring of central venous pressure (CVP), thereby helping to guide intraoperative and postoperative fluid management (particularly in high-risk recipients). Continuous arterial blood pressure monitoring is considered mandatory at most centers, given the high prevalence of hypertension in this population as well as the importance of optimizing the blood pressure at the time of reperfusion. The indications for pulmonary artery pressure monitoring are more controversial, but it may be justifiable for those with significant cardiac dysfunction (e.g., ejection fraction <30%), valvular abnormalities, or known pulmonary artery hypertension. A 20-Fr 3-way Foley catheter is placed in the bladder, which is then filled with saline and antibiotic solution. Compression stockings and sequential compression devices provide deep venous thrombosis prophylaxis.

Communication between the anesthesia and surgical teams is paramount during the KTx. Adequate intravascular volume, especially at the time of reperfusion, is critical to allow the graft to function immediately. The importance of immediate graft function, with avoidance of acute tubular necrosis (ATN) and of delayed graft function (DGF), cannot be overstated: both ATN and DGF have been found to be predictive of increased patient mortality [10]. CVP should be in the range of 10 to 15 mm Hg. Systolic blood pressure, ideally, should be greater than 120 mm Hg at the time of graft reperfusion. Vasopressors (except for low-dose dopamine) should be avoided in lieu of volume expansion. Mannitol at 1 g per kg, when combined with optimal volume expansion, has been shown to decrease the incidence of ATN; it is given concurrently with furosemide at many centers [11]. After the ureteral anastomosis is completed, urine output is measured frequently, which helps guide volume resuscitation in the immediate postoperative period.

Immediate Postoperative Care

Recipients with a higher acuity of illness may require admission to the intensive care unit (ICU) for optimal monitoring; however, the vast majority can receive appropriate care on a solid-organ transplant ward. Serial complete blood counts, coagulation profiles, and chemistries should be obtained; myocardial ischemia should be excluded with serial troponin measurements in the appropriate subgroup of recipients with cardiac risk factors. CXR and ECG are obtained in the immediate postoperative period. Electrolyte abnormalities (hyperkalemia, hypokalemia, hypomagnesemia, and hypocalcemia) are common and should be corrected.

For recipients with initial graft function, fluid management consists of equivalent replacement of urine output, which is measured hourly; if cardiac dysfunction is not present, urine output can initially be replaced milliliter for milliliter. For recipients with high-output diuresis (≥500 mL per hour), 1% dextrose with 0.45% normal saline solution should be administered; potassium replacement may also be necessary, but should not exceed 0.3 mEq per kg per hour intravenously; serum potassium levels should be serially monitored. For recipients with cardiac dysfunction and high-output diuresis (≥500 mL per hour), the volume of fluid replacement should be lower than urine output (i.e., 0.5 mL of replacement for 1 mL of urine). In general, within 24 hours posttransplant, urine output in recipients with initial high-output diuresis is frequently appropriate for the recipient's weight and kidney function; fluid replacement is then converted to a continuous rate of 100 to 150 mL per hour. If initial urine output is less than 500 mL per hour, fluid replacement in nondiabetic recipients should consist of 5% dextrose with 0.45% normal saline solution. In diabetic recipients, 0.45% normal saline solution should be used.

Most KTx recipients are cared for on a surgical ward dedicated to solid-organ transplantation. ICU monitoring may become necessary if complications develop, at any time and at any stage posttransplant. The higher susceptibility of transplant recipients to complications is related to their comorbidities, immunosuppression intensity and duration, and immediacy of graft function. Thus, deceased donor recipients, with their accompanying higher DGF rate and increased immunosuppressant load, are more prone to complications than are living related donor recipients. Deceased donor recipients are also more likely to have felt the effects of prolonged uremia and dialysis, as compared with living donor recipients.

Many risk factors directly correlate with the incidence and severity of posttransplant complications. Between 15% and 30% of high-risk transplant recipients require specific critical care.

CRITICAL EVALUATION OF DYSFUNCTIONAL GRAFTS

Early graft function is affected by numerous factors, such as the quality of the donor (i.e., living vs. deceased), cold and warm ischemia times, and the recipient's volume status and medical stability. Urine output is the most readily apparent parameter to gauge graft function in the initial hours posttransplant, but it may be influenced by a residual effect of diuretics infused during the operation or of urine produced by the recipient's native kidneys. A consistent, downward trend in the serum creatinine level and brisk diuresis (>100 to 200 mL per hour) confirm that the graft is functioning well.

Monitoring the function of an initially delayed or slow functioning graft is more difficult, because urine output is minimal, and the creatinine level may remain at baseline. Doppler ultrasound plays a vital role in surveillance of the newly transplanted kidney and is the most helpful modality in evaluating a dysfunctional graft. Intensivists must be aware of the medical and surgical complications that can occur in the early posttransplant period and that can result in an abrupt change in graft function; graft salvage is only possible with an efficient, expeditious evaluation leading to rapid therapeutic maneuvers.

Medical Complications Leading to Early Graft Dysfunction

Acute Tubular Necrosis

ATN is the most common cause of impaired kidney function immediately posttransplant. Although ATN is rare in living related donor recipients, its incidence averages 35% in deceased donor recipients. It may occur immediately after revascularization or, in grafts with initial diuresis, have a more delayed presentation; dysfunction may last from several days to several weeks. In deceased donor grafts, ATN is usually secondary to prolonged ischemia times, but may also occur in recipients with negative immunologic factors, for example, a high panel-reactive antibody percentage directed against HLAs, a retransplant, and a poor HLA match between donor and recipient. Donor factors such as age, underlying disease (e.g., hypertension), and use of vasopressors (during both procurement and the transplant operation) also contribute to ATN. As stated before, ATN has a detrimental effect not only on later graft function, but also on overall graft survival and postoperative morbidity [12].

Recipients with ATN have a higher incidence of acute rejection, which ultimately lowers graft survival rates by subjecting the kidney to higher rates, and more aggressive progression, of chronic allograft nephropathy [13]. ATN must be differentiated from a vascular catastrophe (renal artery or vein thrombosis) and early acute rejection. Thrombosis should be excluded within 24 hours posttransplant with a Doppler ultrasound to confirm vascular patency. For recipients with ATN, HD frequently must be reinstituted; after a few days to several weeks, kidney function recovers in more than 95% of recipients.

Acute Rejection

A complete discussion of acute kidney graft rejection is beyond the scope of this chapter, however, *acute antibody-mediated rejection* may lead to a rapid decline in early graft function and is therefore relevant. Alloantibodies may form in recipients with a history of blood transfusions, pregnancies, or previous organ transplants; these antibodies can be detected by cross-matching pretransplant, which may, in fact, preclude the transplant. Fortunately, desensitization protocols are in place at many centers that may allow highly sensitized KTx candidates to proceed with a transplant. They do, however, remain at much higher risk for rejection; when these preformed antibodies target capillary endothelium, the complement system may be activated, ultimately resulting in a rapid deterioration of graft function. Only a kidney graft biopsy can confirm the diagnosis; performing the biopsy via an open approach minimizes potential bleeding complications [14,15].

Recurrence of Kidney Disease

Most acute kidney diseases rarely recur, but *focal segmental glomerulosclerosis* (FSGS) and *hemolytic uremic syndrome* (HUS) deserve special mention for their ability to cause profound, early graft dysfunction. Posttransplant nephrotic range proteinuria (i.e., >3.5 g per day) in a recipient with known FSGS should prompt an immediate biopsy, which will likely show diffuse foot process effacement [16]. When graft dysfunction is accompanied by signs of microvascular trauma (i.e., low haptoglobin levels, elevated lactate dehydrogenase levels, and the presence of schistocytes on blood smears), HUS should be suspected. It may be recurrent or de novo: calcineurin inhibitors (CNIs) (i.e., tacrolimus, cyclosporine) have been long implicated as a causative agent [17].

Surgical Complications Leading to Early Graft Dysfunction

Hemorrhage from the venous or arterial anastomosis is rare. Most postoperative bleeding emanates from small vascular tributaries in the renal hilum or from diffuse hemorrhage in the retroperitoneal dissection field. In the confined retroperitoneal space, bleeding usually tamponades, so reexploration is seldom required. Subcapsular bleeding, albeit less common, is considerably more morbid and can lead to significant and irreversible kidney damage if not quickly recognized and controlled. Bleeding should be suspected if recipients are tachycardic, hypotensive, or oliguric, or if they require several units of blood in the early posttransplant period.

Although the incidence of *vascular thrombosis* is low (0.7% to 5%), it almost invariably results in graft loss [18]. Any sudden change in urine output or creatinine levels in the first several weeks posttransplant should prompt urgent Doppler sonography. The best opportunity for graft salvage occurs if the thrombosis is discovered while the patient is in the recovery room; after several hours, salvage is unlikely and nephrectomy is usually necessary.

Causative factors for *renal artery thrombosis* include unidentified intimal flaps, perfusion or preimplantation arterial or graft damage, size discrepancy between donor and recipient vessels, hypotension or hypoperfusion (especially in pediatric recipients with adult donors), and technical difficulties in kidneys with multiple arteries [18]. Other arterial complications include aneurysms and stenosis. Aneurysms may be anastomotic (pseudoaneurysm) or infected (mycotic). Magnetic resonance angiography can usually confirm the diagnosis without exposing the kidney to nephrotoxic contrast; conventional angiography is reserved for equivocal cases. Aneurysms require surgical repair, which can result in graft loss. For recipients with iliac or renal artery stenosis, percutaneous balloon dilation is the treatment of choice; if unsuccessful, surgical repair is necessary.

Renal vein thrombosis, a complication in 0.3% to 4.2% of KTx recipients, may be caused by kinking of the anastomosis, intimal injury during organ procurement, pressure on the vein secondary to a fluid collection (i.e., lymphocele, urinoma, or hematoma), compartment syndrome, and extension of an iliofemoral thrombosis [19]. Renal vein thrombosis usually occurs within the first few posttransplant days and may be characterized by sudden onset of pain and graft swelling, hematuria, and, in the case of iliofemoral thrombosis, an edematous leg. The diagnosis is confirmed by Doppler ultrasound, which will show a pulsatile renal artery (with reversal of blood flow) running into the hilum of an enlarged kidney, possibly surrounded by hematoma. If thrombosis is complete, nephrectomy is necessary, although recovery of function after surgical embolectomy or thrombolytic therapy has been report. If thrombosis is incomplete, immediate thrombectomy is recommended (or, as an alternative, urokinase, and heparin treatment).

Urologic complications are rarely life threatening, but can add significant morbidity and can lead to inferior graft survival rates if not handled in a systematic manner. The incidence of urologic complications ranges from 5% to 14% in most KTx series [20].

Hematuria from the distal ureter or the cystostomy suture line generally ceases within the first 12 to 24 hours posttransplant, but it may result in clot formation in the bladder, especially in grafts with poor initial diuresis. Bladder clots or debris may lead to obstructive uropathy, which presents with a sudden cessation of urine output; obstructive uropathy is the most common cause of new-onset anuria in the immediate postoperative period and should be readily remedied with catheter irrigation. If anuria persists, emergent Doppler ultrasound will (1) confirm renal artery and vein patency and (2) rule out a large retroperitoneal hematoma causing hydronephrosis or a retroperitoneal compartment syndrome. Persistent hematuria due to a bleeding diathesis or technical error in the ureteroneocystostomy may lead to the formation of large bladder clots, which may present with suprapubic pain and "bladder spasms" or with frequent Foley catheter occlusions; if continuous bladder irrigations do not restore diuresis, manual hematoma evacuation is performed via a 20-Fr 6-eye Foley catheter. If hematuria is caused by a posttransplant biopsy, with subsequent clot formation in the renal pelvis, temporary percutaneous placement of a nephrostomy tube may be necessary. Most hematuria-related complications require close urine output monitoring, but rarely ICU admission.

Urine leaks most commonly occur at the ureteroneocystostomy anastomosis and can present in the first few postoperative days (technical error) or during the first several weeks (ureteral necrosis). Symptoms and signs of a urine leak may include graft swelling and tenderness, fever, wound drainage, oliguria, scrotal or labial edema, and ipsilateral thigh swelling. Diagnostic studies that confirm the diagnosis include nephroscintigraphy, retrograde cystography, or pelvic computed tomography (CT) scans. Perirenal fluid collections can be aspirated and sent for fluid creatinine level testing to confirm the diagnosis. Minor urine leaks may spontaneously resolve after several weeks with Foley catheter decompression. Recipients with significant leaks in the early postoperative period are best served by immediate exploration and reimplantation of the ureter. Other investigators advocate for an initial percutaneous maneuvers, namely, a percutaneous nephrostomy and stent placement for 4 to 8 weeks; success rates up to 90% have been reported in some centers with this approach [21,22].

Ureteral stenosis becomes evident months posttransplant and may be secondary to rejection, ischemia, infection, or a tight ureteroneocystostomy. Recipients usually have an elevated creatinine level and hydronephrosis (visualized on ultrasound). A percutaneous nephrostomy elucidates the location and degree of the stenosis and is typically followed by a balloon dilatation with a temporary stent tube. If balloon ureteroplasty and stenting fail, operative repair is required (but fortunately only in the vast minority of recipients). A localized distal ureteral stenosis can be repaired by reimplanting the transplanted ureter, but most stenoses require a ureteroureterostomy (to the native ureter) or an ureteropyelostomy (native ureter to the graft's renal pelvis) because of extensive adhesions and lack of graft mobility [22].

Lymphoceles or hematomas can cause compression of the iliac veins (leading to leg edema or deep venous thrombosis) as well as compression of the ureter (leading to hydronephrosis and impaired graft function). Lymphoceles are a collection of lymph in the retroperitoneal space secondary to disruption of lymphatic vessels along the external iliac artery. The incidence can be decreased with careful ligation of the lymphatic vessels during dissection of the iliac vessels. Symptomatic lymphoceles can be diagnosed by ultrasound and treated with percutaneous drainage. Recurrent lymphoceles are approached laparoscopically [23] or, less commonly, by open laparotomy, to create a peritoneal window for decompression of the lymph leak.

NON-RENAL POST-TRANSPLANT COMPLICATIONS

Cardiovascular Complications

The incidence of *cardiac complications*, the most common cause of death posttransplant [24], depends on the extent of underlying cardiac disease, on the efficacy of the preoperative cardiac evaluation, and on the function of the newly transplanted kidney. Correction of uremia by immediate posttransplant graft function improves the cardiac index, stroke volume, and ejection fraction [25]. In contrast, recipients with ATN experience persistent uremia and oliguria, which may lead to perioperative fluid overload and congestive heart failure if immediate HD is not performed to correct fluid retention and electrolyte derangements. Recipients with diabetes, hypertension, and significant coronary disease are more likely to develop cardiac complications if there is no urine output immediately posttransplant; therefore, such recipients require perioperative ICU monitoring, especially if their left ventricular function is poor (e.g., ejection fraction <30%). Pulmonary artery catheter (PAC) placement to optimize hemodynamics might be prudent, especially in diabetic recipients with coronary artery disease.

Myocardial infarction is uncommon in the perioperative period. It is mostly seen in diabetic recipients with preexisting coronary artery disease who have complicated posttransplant courses with resultant hypotension. ICU admission, serial troponin evaluations, and close monitoring of their hemodynamic parameters are mandatory, especially when complicated by postoperative ATN. Although uncommon in the early posttransplant period, myocardial infarction is one of the major causes of death long-term in transplant recipients. In diabetic recipients, the duration of their diabetes and the presence of preexisting coronary artery disease have an impact on the incidence and severity of posttransplant myocardial infarction, which is the main cause of death in this subgroup. Data suggest that maintaining the hematocrit above 30% is prudent in diabetic recipients: doing so is associated with a 24% decrease in cardiac morbidity in the initial 6 months posttransplant [26].

The incidence of *pericarditis* in the early posttransplant period is 1% to 3% [27]. It has been attributed to infections (e.g., cytomegalovirus [CMV]), fluid overload, and certain medications (e.g., minoxidil). The main factor, however, is uremia. Most episodes of viral or uremic pericarditis occur during the first 8 weeks posttransplant. In contrast, the less frequent bacterial pericarditis develops later, often in recipients with advanced septic complications. Bacterial pericarditis usually requires, besides antibiotic treatment, surgical or ultrasound/CT–guided drainage. Pericardiocentesis is mandatory if cardiac failure, hypotension, or cardiac tamponade develops. Recipients with clinical symptoms of pericarditis require ICU monitoring.

Although *hypertension* is the most common long-term complication posttransplant, with an incidence of up to 50%, it may also require aggressive management immediately posttransplant. Overzealous perioperative hydration may lead to postoperative exacerbation of baseline hypertension. Abrupt cessation of antihypertensive medications should be avoided as well; however, most clinicians do advocate removal of angiotensin-converting enzyme (ACE) inhibitors from the perioperative regimen. CNIs, a part of virtually every immunosuppressive regimen, may also lead to hypertension, especially when they reach toxic levels. The pathophysiology of CNI-induced hypertension has not been fully elucidated, but appears to be multifactorial. CNIs directly lead to systemic vascular constriction by reducing prostacyclin and nitric oxide production while increasing serum levels of endothelin-1; this imbalance favors widespread constriction. Afferent arteriole vasoconstriction in the kidney leads to diminished glomerular filtration, which enhances sodium retention and exacerbates hypertension. Calcium-channel blockers appear to be superior at obviating the renal vasoconstriction induced by CNIs [28–30].

More intensive blood pressure monitoring is warranted in recipients with systolic blood pressure greater than 180 mm Hg or diastolic pressure greater than 100 mm Hg. Treatment often is simply to restart their home regimen, which is typically a combination of calcium-channel blockers, vasodilators, and diuretics. Unless a strong contraindication is noted, perioperative β-blockade is mandatory in this high-risk cohort of surgical patients in order to minimize perioperative cardiac events [31]. Consensus has not been reached on the optimal antihypertensive regimen, given that many drugs interfere with kidney function and CNI metabolism; treatment is based on each individual's response. ICU monitoring and intravenous (IV) antihypertensive infusions (e.g., titration with sodium nitroprusside) may be required, but early posttransplant hypertension can usually be controlled with appropriate oral antihypertensive medications [32].

Hypotension, either intraoperatively or immediately posttransplant, is the single most detrimental nonimmunologic event associated with an increased incidence of graft loss or severe dysfunction. Intraoperative hypotension is usually related to volume depletion or anesthetic agents. Intravascular volume status is assessed most accurately via CVP monitoring, before unclamping, to avoid poor graft perfusion. Posttransplant hypovolemia, especially in recipients with immediate graft function, is often caused by inadequate fluid replacement and should be treated accordingly. Cardiac dysfunction and bleeding must be excluded in recipients with early posttransplant hypotension. Induction immunosuppression (e.g., Thymoglobulin) may lead to hypotension, which is readily reversed by slowing the infusion rate.

As compared with the general population, uremic recipients are more prone to *deep venous thrombosis* (DVT) posttransplant. The incidence of DVT ranges from 1% to 4%. DVT has been linked both to high-dose corticosteroid therapy early posttransplant and to "rebound" hypercoagulability, which is attributed to overcorrection of impaired platelet aggregation and thrombin generation (both associated with uremia). Thrombophilic events of concern within the first few weeks posttransplant include decreased fibrinolytic activity and an increase in plasminogen activation inhibitors. Other risk factors for the development of DVT are postoperative immobilization, increased blood viscosity from posttransplant erythrocytosis, cyclosporine use, and posttransplant hematoma and lymphocele formation (both of which diminish the venous return from the leg and may result in stasis and ultimately thrombosis).

In contrast, neither transient marked elevation nor moderate sustained elevation of hemoglobin levels per se seem to be directly associated with an increased incidence of thromboembolic complications; DVT rarely occurs during periods of peak hemoglobin elevation. Elevated hemoglobin levels (in combination with increased whole blood viscosity, iron deficiency, or hypertension), as well as older recipient age and diabetes, contribute to the occurrence of thrombotic events posttransplant. Aggressive therapeutic phlebotomy to maintain the hematocrit level at less than 55% has been recommended in such recipients. The diagnosis is made clinically and confirmed by Doppler ultrasound to assess the extent of DVT and the potential involvement of the kidney graft in the thrombotic event. Because the kidney is a "high-flow" organ, DVT usually stops at the level of, or distal to, the renal vein anastomosis. About two-thirds of the time, DVT occurs on the graft side.

Once the diagnosis of DVT has been established, standard therapy is systemic heparinization followed by warfarin administration for 3 to 6 months. If DVT occurs in the immediate postoperative period, when heparinization can cause major bleeding, an inferior vena cava filter is an appropriate alternative. Surgical intervention is indicated only if phlegmasia cerulea dolens develops. Venous thrombectomy (with or without creation of a temporary arteriovenous fistula) and, if necessary, fasciotomy are the treatments of choice in that rare situation [33–35].

Pulmonary embolism is rare (<1%) after a KTx, yet more common than in the uremic nontransplant population. In kidney recipients, especially those who were uremic pretransplant, the coagulation system is activated and enhanced during the first-week posttransplant, which may explain the overall higher incidence of pulmonary embolism. In general, quick recovery posttransplant lowers the rate of pulmonary embolism. Pulmonary embolism as a result of DVT occurs in fewer than 1% of kidney recipients, but, if it does occur, the mortality rate is about 40%.

Pulmonary Complications

Most KTx recipients do not require ventilator support postoperatively, but prolonged support may be indicated in case of pulmonary dysfunction secondary to intraoperative fluid overload, cardiac dysfunction, or underlying lung disease.

Pulmonary edema usually is the result of overresuscitation intraoperatively and is more likely to occur in recipients who underwent inadequate pretransplant HD and/or overzealous volume infusion accompanied by a poorly functioning graft. As discussed previously, poor early graft function requires much more precise fluid management to optimize volume status for the graft, without placing the recipient at unacceptable risk for cardiopulmonary complications. Chest radiography in the recovery room to assess pulmonary status should be routine, particularly when anti-CD3 murine monoclonal antibody (OKT3) is given intraoperatively; fluid-overloaded recipients can respond to their first dose of OKT3 with flash pulmonary edema [36,37]. Fortunately, few modern immunosuppressive regimens include OKT3 for induction; its primary role is to combat acute rejection. Recurrent pulmonary edema may be an atypical manifestation of a kidney graft renal artery stenosis.

Pulmonary hypertension (PHT), a known risk factor for death in liver transplant recipients, has now been found to be an independent risk factor for inferior rates of patient survival after a KTx. KTx recipients with known PHT may require ICU care postoperatively, often guided by PAC monitoring [38].

Acute respiratory distress syndrome (ARDS) affects 0.2% of all KTx recipients. It is more likely in recipients with poor initial graft function and in those receiving antithymocyte globulin for induction of immunosuppression. Not surprisingly in this population with a higher acuity of illness, the mortality rate of KTx recipients with ARDS is prohibitive at well over 50% [39].

Metabolic Complications

Hyperkalemia is a frequent perioperative derangement, making serial serum potassium determinations necessary. Surgical trauma and transfusion of banked blood might cause intraoperative hyperkalemia, which can be corrected with intravenous glucose and insulin, thereby driving extracellular potassium into the cells. Posttransplant, hyperkalemia can develop immediately in recipients with ATN and later in those with poor graft function due to severe acute or chronic rejection. Hyperkalemia is frequently secondary to physiologic abnormalities or to medications that decrease potassium excretion in the urine. Such abnormalities include a decrease in the glomerular filtration rate (GFR), injury to distal tubules (which are a major site of potassium secretion in the nephron), and a decrease in plasma aldosterone levels. CNIs cause vasoconstriction of the afferent arterioles and direct damage to distal tubules, leading to hyperkalemia and decreased GFR. Medications that decrease potassium excretion include trimethoprim–sulfamethoxazole (TMP–SMX) (which blocks sodium and potassium exchange in distal tubules), ACE inhibitors, angiotensin-2 receptor-antagonists, and nonsteroidal anti-inflammatory agents (which suppress plasma aldosterone levels leading to higher potassium levels). Hyperkalemia can also be a drug-related side effect (e.g., impeded intracellular potassium entry by a beta-blocker). Therapeutically, a potassium-binding ion exchange resin (e.g., Kayexalate®) can be given or, if a rapid decrease of serum potassium is required, IV glucose, insulin, and bicarbonate infusions. Recipients with hyperkalemia due to poor graft function eventually require HD.

Copious diuresis (>500 mL per hour) immediately posttransplant may result in *hypokalemia,* which requires appropriate potassium replacement. Recipients requiring more than 0.3 mEq per kg per h should be placed on a cardiac monitor.

Less frequently, *hypomagnesemia* and *hypophosphatemia* occur in recipients with high-output diuresis initially. Hypomagnesemia is secondary to drug-related renal wasting (e.g., cyclosporine, tacrolimus, diuretics, aminoglycosides, and amphotericin B), poor dietary intake, and malabsorption from the gastrointestinal tract. Hypophosphatemia is secondary to renal wasting of phosphate, caused by secondary hyperparathyroidism, glucocorticoids (which inhibit the tubular reabsorption of phosphate), and antacids (which bind phosphate in the gastrointestinal tract).

Infectious Complications

A comprehensive review of the role of infectious diseases after a KTx is beyond the scope of this chapter, except for infections known to develop in the immediate posttransplant period (e.g., 1 to 4 weeks). Infections do not occur at random, but rather according to a timetable. Bacterial infections caused by nosocomial pathogens or recipient colonizers tend to occur early posttransplant, affecting the anatomic sites breached during the transplant operation itself, namely, the lungs, blood (indwelling vascular catheters), superficial wounds, and perinephric (deep) space [40].

As compared with all other solid-organ transplant recipients, KTx recipients have the lowest incidence of *pneumonia*; still, it develops in about 16% of KTx recipients and carries with it a mortality rate of 10% to 13%. In the first posttransplant month, 90% of the pneumonic processes are bacterial, particularly staphylococcal and nosocomial Gram-negative species; fungal infections (i.e., *Candida, Aspergillus*) are more frequent when the recipient is on a more intensive immunosuppressive regimen or underwent prolonged antibiotic therapy. Dual fungal and bacterial infections or superinfections have an associated mortality rate as high as 100% [41–43].

Bacterial pneumonias frequently cause fever, along with other expected clinical signs and symptoms making the diagnosis straightforward; however, in the early posttransplant phase it may be difficult to exclude noninfectious thoracic processes (i.e., pulmonary edema, atelectasis, infiltrates). If the CXR reveals abnormal patterns of infiltration, chest CT may be helpful in delineating the cause of the pneumonia. No consensus has been reached on the role of bronchoalveolar lavage (BAL) in the diagnostic evaluation, but it seems prudent for recipients with pneumonia who do not respond to antimicrobial therapy in 48 to 72 hours. No disagreement exists on the degree and rapidity with which to treat a presumed pneumonia; broad-spectrum antibiotics should be initiated immediately to cover the most common culprits mentioned earlier. Antifungals should be considered when appropriate: surveillance cultures should be obtained and reviewed to exclude the presence of multidrug-resistant (MDR) bacteria, for example, methicillin-resistant *Staphylococcus aureus*, vancomycin-resistant enterococci, extended-spectrum beta-lactamase, and MDR *Pseudomonas* or *Klebsiella* [42,43].

The most common posttransplant infectious complication is a *urinary tract infection* (UTI), with an incidence of more than 30% during the initial 90 days posttransplant. UTIs lead to pyelonephritis and bacteremia in more than 10% of immunosuppressed KTx recipients. Gram-negative bacilli are the cause 70% of the time, but *Enterococcus*, *Staphylococcus*, and *Candida* should also be considered as possible etiologic agents. Risk factors for UTI include a history of graft dysfunction, prolonged bladder catheterization, neurogenic bladder, and ureteral surgical complications, including stent placement [44]. Treatment consists of prompt antibacterial therapy even in the cases of asymptomatic bacteruria; for persistent cases, removal of stents and a more thorough evaluation (e.g., voiding cystourethrogram, CT scan) are indicated.

A KTx, a clean-contaminated operation, carries with it a *wound infection* rate of 1% to 6%. This low rate is due to thorough pretransplant skin preparation with chlorhexidine, intravenous administration of a prophylactic antibiotic, irrigation of the urinary bladder with an antibiotic solution, and meticulous attention to hemostasis. If wound infections occur, they are treated according to standard surgical principles of drainage and antimicrobial therapy; exploration and debridement may be necessary for deep-space infections [45].

Most patients undergoing a KTx are HD-dependent and therefore have an indwelling catheter, arteriovenous fistula, or arteriovenous graft, all of which can lead to a *bloodstream infection.* The current national practice guidelines call for goal infection rates of less than 10% at 3 months after catheter placement; unfortunately, most centers fall short of that goal. Catheters should be removed when no longer required. Staphylococcal species and gram-negative bacilli are the most likely pathogens and should be treated aggressively with IV antibiotics and possibly catheter removal [46,47].

Infective endocarditis is rare but may occur in recipients with severe septicemia or longstanding immunosuppression [48]. Cardiac valve vegetations noted on an echocardiogram in recipients with persistent bacteremia confirms the diagnosis; prolonged antibiotic therapy is required.

Viral infections play a prominent role in the intermediate to late posttransplant period, predominantly the herpesvirus genus, for example, CMV, Epstein–Barr virus (EBV), herpes simplex virus (HSV), and varicella-zoster virus (herpes zoster virus [HZV]). Primary HSV infections are rare, but mucocutaneous reactivations of HSV in the early posttransplant period are relatively common, occurring in up to 30% of adult recipients and 8% of pediatric recipients. OKT3 use is associated with an even higher risk of reactivations. HSV is diagnosed by direct immunofluorescent antibody staining, by Tzanck preparation, or by culture of tissue and body fluids. Serodiagnosis is possible if immunoglobin M (IgM) is detected or if a fourfold rise in IgG titers is noted. Symptomatic HSV infections are common with orofacial (virus resides latently in the sensory ganglia) or genital lesions; occasionally, conjunctivitis or corneal ulceration may develop. Topical application of 5% acyclovir ointment accelerates healing and shortens the duration of viral shedding; oral acyclovir (200 mg five times per day) is also effective. If disseminated disease occurs (e.g., hepatitis, meningoencephalitis), IV acyclovir (5.0 mg per kg every 8 hours for 7 to 14 days) is necessary.

CMV infections and disease, while rare during the first posttransplant month, deserve special mention because they affect a large proportion of KTx recipients at some point in their first posttransplant year. In just the initial 100 days posttransplant, up to 60% of recipients develop CMV infections (e.g., viremia), and 25% actually suffer from invasive CMV disease of one or more organ systems. Such infections are associated with chronic graft rejection and decreased graft and patient survival rates. The highest risk of developing CMV infections, up to 60%, is in the donor-seropositive, recipient-seronegative (D+R−) group; the lowest risk, 20% to 40%, is in the D+R+ and D−R+ groups. CMV infections may occur as primary infections (e.g., D+R−) or as a reactivations (e.g., with a seropositive recipient after inception of immunosuppression). CMV superinfections (both primary infections plus reactivations, by separate strains of CMV) in the D+R+ group are associated with the worst graft and patient survival rates among the various groups [49–52].

Success has been achieved in preventing CMV infections with prophylactic 9-[(1,3-dihydroxy-2-propoxy)methyl] guanine (DHPG) in parenteral (ganciclovir) or enteral (valganciclovir) forms. The efficacy of oral DHPG (valganciclovir) was found to be equal to that of oral ganciclovir in preventing CMV disease in high-risk recipients [50]. CMV disease, which is potentially (yet rarely) fatal, has not been eliminated. Symptoms include fever, malaise, headache, myalgia, and arthralgia; leukopenia occurs in more than 70% of infected recipients. CMV infections can present as neuritis, gastritis, or colitis; colitis often causes gastrointestinal tract bleeding. CMV infections can also cause retinitis, hepatitis, pancreatitis, adenopathy, hepatosplenomegaly, and nephritis, frequently during the first 6 months posttransplant.

The gold standard for diagnosis of active CMV disease continues to be growth in tissue culture; however, identification of viremia allows for much earlier diagnosis (<48 hours) and prompt treatment. Two techniques are currently in clinical use: (1) a quantitative polymerase chain reaction assay and (2) an antigenemia assay based on identification of the late structural protein pp65. Both techniques are felt to be equally efficacious in quantifying the viral load of CMV in the serum.

When the diagnosis of CMV disease is established, treatment is initiated with IV DHPG (5 mg per kg every 12 hours if creatinine <1.5 mg per dL, with dose adjusted according to graft function; and 1.2 mg per kg every 48 hours if the recipient is on dialysis). Dose reduction or temporary cessation of DHPG is indicated if leukopenia (white blood cell count <3,000 cells per mm^3) or thrombocytopenia (platelet count <100,000 per mm^3) occurs. DHPG is administered IV for 14 days; the addition of CMV hyperimmune globulin is indicated for recalcitrant and life-threatening cases. Oral DHPG treatment is frequently continued for up to 6 months. For recipients with concurrent CMV and acute rejection, simultaneous treatment is an option: IV ganciclovir should be given at the time of rejection treatment, or if possible, 1 to 2 days before increasing immunosuppression. Since cell-mediated immunity is markedly impaired during CMV infections, superinfections by other opportunistic pathogens are a risk. Graft dysfunction (e.g., glomerulopathy) during or after active CMV infections has been described. Recipients in the D+R− (high-risk) group should receive prophylactic oral DHPG for at least 6 months posttransplant. Currently, oral DHPG is standard for CMV prophylaxis posttransplant and continues for 3 to 6 months.

Varicella-zoster virus, also called HZV, usually presents as dermatomal skin lesions. The diagnosis is frequently made on physical examination alone. HZV can be cultured, and direct immunofluorescent antibody staining or Tzanck preparation can be used. HZV requires systemic therapy with acyclovir, usually over a 7-day period. Varicella-zoster immune globulin is used in seronegative recipients.

EBV infections have been associated with mononucleosis-like symptoms and with fulminant, widespread posttransplant lymphoproliferative disease (PTLD), a form of B-cell lymphoma. Recipients of a kidney from a seropositive donor can seroconvert. Symptoms include EBV-related malaise, fever, headaches, and sore throats. PTLD usually occurs months to years posttransplant in heavily immunosuppressed recipients. Immunosuppression impairs the ability of virus-specific cytotoxic T lymphocytes to control the expression of EBV-infected transformed B cells, leading to polyclonal and monoclonal proliferation of lymphocytes (which constitutes PTLD). Treatment entails cessation of immunosuppression accompanied by anti-CD-20 antibodies (rituximab), and antiviral therapy (e.g., ganciclovir, acyclovir, or anti-CMV immune globulin). Suboptimal responses necessitate conventional lymphoma treatment.

Other viruses causing morbidity after a successful KTx are adenoviruses and influenza viruses (involving the respiratory tract), papovaviruses (progressive multifocal leukoencephalopathy), and hepatitis viruses (in particular hepatitis C). Recipients are also at high risk for developing human papillomavirus infections, which can lead to cancer of the cervix (e.g., invasive squamous cell cancer).

Fungal infections, both local and systemic, are frequent (in up to 14% of KTx recipients), and can occur early posttransplant. Most fungal infections are secondary to *Candida* and *Aspergillus* species. The most common source of *Candida* infections is translocation of organisms from the gastrointestinal tract, followed by infected intravascular catheters. Early posttransplant, *oropharyngeal candidiasis* is the most common fungal infection; it can be prevented and treated with oral nystatin or clotrimazole solutions.

Systemic fungal infections are particularly noted in recipients who are on significant immunosuppression or broad-spectrum antibacterials or who have had multiple rejection episodes and poor graft function; if such infections occur as superinfections, they are associated with a high mortality rate. Patients with cerebral, pulmonary, or visceral involvement, such as meningitis, pneumonia, or endocarditis (most frequently caused by *Candida* or *Aspergillus* species), require reduction or even temporary cessation of immunosuppression [53].

Given their favorable safety profile, the azole antifungals (e.g., fluconazole) are the preferred empiric therapy for fungal infections; however, for life-threatening fungemia, some clinicians favor the echinocandins caspofungin, the newer azole agents or amphotericin B, especially when a *Candida* species other than *Candida albicans* is suspected [54]. Liposomal amphotericin B preparations are now a more palatable option because of their improved safety profile in regards to nephrotoxicity. *Candida* can also cause an uncommon but life-threatening complication: a mycotic pseudoaneurysm. This complication is typically treated with graft nephrectomy, with or without ligation of the external iliac artery, followed by IV amphotericin B. *Cryptococcus* and *Aspergillus* can cause severe pulmonary and cerebral infections requiring systemic amphotericin B. *Pneumocystis jiroveci,* which manifests as interstitial pneumonia, usually late posttransplant [55]. Since the practice of

TMP–SMX prophylaxis was initiated, the incidence of pneumocystic pneumonia (PCP) has decreased significantly. PCP is still seen in heavily immunosuppressed recipients and should be considered in anyone with fever, dyspnea, and nonproductive cough. The CXR will reveal interstitial infiltrate; BAL or lung tissue biopsy (using staining techniques or monoclonal antibodies conjugated with fluorescein) is needed for diagnosis. Therapy consists of IV TMP–SMX (with the dose adjusted according to kidney function) and, in case of sulfa hypersensitivity, pentamidine or dapsone. PCP, like most other severe infections, requires reduction or temporary cessation of immunosuppression.

Mycobacterium tuberculosis infects about 1% of KTx recipients because of prior infections, reactivations, or disseminated disease. Fever, malaise, night sweats, and weight loss usually occur. The diagnosis should be made clinically, because only one-fourth of recipients have a positive tuberculin skin test. Sputum and blood samples should be used to identify acid-fast bacilli and a BAL may be necessary to obtain an appropriate sample. Treatment includes a 2- to 3-drug regimen lasting at least 6 months. Potential agents include isoniazid, rifampin, pyrazinamide, ethambutol, and ciprofloxacin. Despite aggressive treatment, the mortality rate can be high.

Gastrointestinal and Pancreaticobiliary Complications

The incidence of posttransplant gastrointestinal tract complications is 5% to 25%. They are a major cause of morbidity and mortality in the KTx population.

In the *upper gastrointestinal* tract, the most common problem is peptic ulcer disease and its associated complications (bleeding, perforation); evidence suggests a higher prevalence of *Helicobacter* infection in the uremic population. However, the overall incidence of upper gastrointestinal tract complications in KTx recipients has declined considerably over the last two decades, mainly because of the development and ubiquitous use of H_2 blockers and proton-pump inhibitors. Historically, severe upper gastrointestinal tract bleeding episodes occurred in more than 10% of KTx recipients, with a mortality rate of up to 65%; most of these bleeding episodes developed in the early postoperative period, half in the first 3 months [56–58].

Prophylactic gastric operations (various forms of vagotomy) became very popular in the 1970s for patients with chronic kidney failure listed for KTx, in an attempt to decrease the morbidity and mortality rates of peptic ulcer disease posttransplant. With the advent of H_2 blockers (e.g., cimetidine, ranitidine) and inhibitors of the H+–K+ adenosinetriphosphatase (ATPase) enzyme system (e.g., omeprazole, pantoprazole), prophylactic gastric operations are no longer performed [59–62].

If severe upper gastrointestinal tract bleeding occurs despite prophylactic treatment and cannot be controlled by conservative means (including gastroscopy with submucosal injection of epinephrine), the same surgical options (resection, vagotomy) apply as for nontransplant patients. Angiographic embolization for acute hemorrhage has been advocated, and, for anatomic reasons, usually requires embolization of two arteries. The risk of embolization is development of (gastric) necrosis and infection. Patients with severe upper gastrointestinal tract bleeding require ICU monitoring; it is important to stabilize them before they undergo emergency gastric procedures, which have a high mortality rate posttransplant. If extensive gastroduodenal surgery is performed, reduction of immunosuppression is mandatory and postoperative ICU monitoring recommended. An unexpectedly high incidence of CMV infections has been observed in apparent peptic ulcers in KTx recipients. Diagnostic and immunohistochemical improvements have made it easier to detect tissue-invasive CMV infections; for such recipients, DHPG and possibly anti-CMV immune globulin are initiated [63].

The impact of hypercalcemia on the pathogenesis of peptic ulcer disease and on its therapeutic consequences is controversial. Hypercalcemia due to hyperparathyroidism may aggravate peptic ulcer disease. Immediate and permanent cessation of gastric bleeding has been noted after subtotal parathyroidectomy in KTx recipients.

The most common *small bowel* complication is intestinal obstruction. Most kidney grafts are placed retroperitoneally (except in children and in recipients of a simultaneous pancreas-KTx), so obstruction is often related to previous intra-abdominal procedures (e.g., native nephrectomy, splenectomy), infections, or PTLD in the small bowel and mesentery. Obstruction in the early postoperative period may be due to incarceration of small bowel through a peritoneal tear made during retroperitoneal dissection. The same therapeutic principles apply as for nontransplant patients.

The incidence of complications of the *lower gastrointestinal tract* in KTx recipients is 1% to 10%. Colonic perforation and lower gastrointestinal tract hemorrhage are the two most common complications in the immediate posttransplant period and carry considerable morbidity and mortality if not recognized and treated expeditiously.

Colonic perforation, occurring in 1% to 2% of all KTx recipients, is due to (in descending order) diverticulitis, ischemic colitis, and CMV colitis; rarely, stercoral ulceration, fecal impaction, or an undetermined forms of colitis can result in perforation as well. The use of sodium polystyrene sulfonate, given orally or as an enema, has been implicated as a cause of perforation, but only in sporadic case reports, so the practice continues at most centers. About 50% of all colon perforations occur within the first month posttransplant, with a 20% to 38% mortality rate; risk factors for death include age older than 40 years, long-term HD, and exploration more than 24 hours from the time of initial symptoms. Peritoneal signs, the hallmark of hollow organ perforation, are frequently absent in immunosuppressed KTx recipients, mandating a high index of suspicion, liberal use of imaging studies, and a low threshold for exploration; in general, a diverting colostomy has been associated with better outcomes [64–73].

KTx recipients are more susceptible to *colonic diverticulitis* and tend to more readily perforate, as compared with nontransplant patients; KTx recipients with polycystic kidney disease are at even higher risk [74–76]. Steroids are thought to be responsible for the difference in the incidence of diverticulitis between transplant recipients and nontransplant patients; steroids not only mask symptoms but also impair the host's ability to localize and contain the perforation. Furthermore, steroids adversely affect colon wall microcirculation and weaken peritoneal defense mechanisms. Historically, diverticular perforations have been associated with prohibitive (50% to 100%) mortality rates, but a series showed a marked decrease in mortality (12.5%), thanks to increased awareness of the problem and prompt surgical intervention. Recipients with sigmoid diverticulitis require resection of the sigmoid colon, with creation of a colostomy and Hartmann pouch; at least one group of investigators advocates a primary anastomosis and a loop colostomy in appropriate cases. Some transplant surgeons advise a pretransplant partial colectomy for KTx candidates who experience a single episode of documented diverticulitis; however, no consensus has been reached.

Ischemic colitis has been associated with impaired blood flow to the colonic wall, stenosis or occlusion of the inferior mesenteric artery, insufficient vascular collateralization, previous retroperitoneal surgery, immunosuppressive and antibiotic therapy, and diseases such as vasculitis and thrombophilia. Other causative factors are (intermittent or temporary) hypotension and irregular blood volume distribution. Often, however, no explanation is apparent, especially in young KTx recipients with normal mesenteric vessels. Ischemic colitis may be segmental or pancolic; at laparotomy, features suggestive of inflammatory bowel disease may be identified that microscopically lack the typical lesions of Crohn's disease [77,78].

Pseudomembranous colitis caused by the *Clostridium difficile* species is being increasingly recognized, to enhanced surveillance; it can progress to toxic megacolon and perforation. The diagnosis is confirmed via stool toxin assay and culture, or with visualization of the classic pseudomembranes on endoscopy. Such recipients are usually treated conservatively, with metronidazole (250 mg four times daily for 10 days) or oral vancomycin (125 mg every 6 hours for 10 days).

Neutropenic enterocolitis causes mucosal ulceration of the bowel wall. It is associated with profound neutropenia and invasion by clostridial organisms (e.g., *Clostridium septicum*). The course of neutropenic enterocolitis is often progressive, requiring treatment with metronidazole and possibly surgical intervention [79]. *Infectious colitis* is frequently due to CMV infections, which may cause lower gastrointestinal tract hemorrhage; at stated before, CMV rarely is clinically active within the first posttransplant month. Infectious colitis can also be bacterial (e.g., mycobacteria), viral (e.g., herpes), and fungal (e.g., *Candida*) infections. The diagnosis is obtained via endoscopic biopsy and stool cultures, with treatment starting with appropriate and early empiric antimicrobial agents. Surgical intervention is not desirable, given the increased morbidity and mortality rates.

Cecal volvulus is a rare complication but requires prompt surgical intervention [80]. If gangrene is not evident, a cecopexy can be performed; if a perforation has occurred, resection and creation of a colostomy are imperative.

The incidence of posttransplant *acute colonic pseudo-obstruction (Ogilvie's syndrome)* is 1.5% [81]; it causes paralytic colonic ileus resulting in cecal dilation. Usually, it responds to nonoperative therapy consisting of bowel rest and nasogastric decompression, neostigmine, and possibly endoscopic colonic decompression. Like fecal impaction and stercoral ulceration, Ogilvie syndrome can cause colonic perforation, thus necessitating surgical resection. In general, survival rates in recipients with colonic perforation can be improved with early diagnosis and prompt treatment. As with treatment for septicemia, immunosuppression should be markedly reduced. Of interest, rejection in recipients with severe infection is not common. Once the recipient's condition improves, immunosuppression should cautiously be restarted.

Lower gastrointestinal tract *hemorrhage* is most commonly due to opportunistic colitis. Gastrointestinal tract lesions thought to be peptic, particularly when associated with upper gastrointestinal tract bleeding, are frequently the result of CMV infections [82]. Fungal ulceration has also been described as a source of lower gastrointestinal tract hemorrhage, because proton-pump inhibitors, H_2 blockers, and antacids promote fungal overgrowth due to achlorhydria. Another cause of lower gastrointestinal tract bleeding is the ulcerogenic effect of steroids and their tendency to impair the reparative mechanisms of the bowel wall. In addition, conditions such as uremia and diabetes result in colonic distention and impaction, because of autonomic neuropathy; both contribute to the pathogenesis of colonic ulcers. In recipients with lower gastrointestinal tract bleeding, colonoscopy must be undertaken urgently, so that treatment is not delayed. To prevent fungal superinfection dissemination, empiric fluconazole is initiated.

KTx recipients are exposed to numerous risk factors for pancreatitis: (1) immunosuppressants (e.g., corticosteroids, azathioprine, cyclosporine) and diuretics (e.g., furosemide, thiazide diuretics); (2) hypercalcemia with or without hyperparathyroidism [83]; (3) infections (e.g., CMV, HSV) [84]; (4) previous episodes of pancreatitis (uremia); and (5) cholelithiasis (i.e., related to cyclosporine). Therefore, it is hardly surprising that 1% to 6% of recipients suffer a posttransplant episode of pancreatitis. The mortality rate appears to be highest if pancreatitis develops after the first three posttransplant months [85]. Steroids increase the viscosity of pancreatic secretions (theoretically leading to obstruction and dilation of the pancreatic duct) and speed epithelial duct proliferation and peripancreatic fat necrosis. An equally serious side effect of steroids is that they mask abdominal pain during episodes of pancreatitis, thus delaying the diagnosis. Hypercalcemia secondary to tertiary hyperparathyroidism is also considered a major causative factor; excessive serum calcium concentration accelerates the conversion of trypsinogen, promoting pancreatic autodigestion. Infections, especially CMV, are a well-documented cause of posttransplant pancreatitis, but bacterial infections causing pancreatitis have also been reported. The term *rejection pancreatitis* arose from speculation that the host forms antibodies that are reactive not only with the graft (vascular rejection), but also with antigens on the surface of pancreas cells (vascular pancreatitis). Biliary tract disease and alcoholism, the most frequent causes of pancreatitis in nontransplant patients, are of minor importance in KTx recipients [86–89].

The diagnosis of pancreatitis depends mainly on an observed increase in the serum amylase or lipase level. However, hyperamylasemia in uremic recipients is not uncommon (30%), because of reduced amylase clearance in light of insufficient kidney function. The amylase/creatinine clearance ratio appears to be a more sensitive index of pancreatitis in KTx candidates with kidney dysfunction. The degree of hyperamylasemia is not a prognostic factor. A contrast-enhanced CT scan may be helpful in both staging pancreatitis and excluding necrotizing pancreatitis. For the edematous form of pancreatitis, conservative treatment is usually successful. Recipients with hemorrhagic or necrotizing pancreatitis require ICU monitoring, with specific attention to volume replacement and cardiovascular status. In such recipients, reduction of immunosuppression, use of broad-spectrum antibiotics, and ICU monitoring are imperative.

The role of early surgical intervention is still controversial. Recipients with infected pancreatic necrosis are best served with aggressive surgical therapy, including removal of all infected necrotic material, drainage and irrigation of the abdominal cavity, and a low threshold for relaparotomy. Overwhelming sepsis is the most common cause of death, so intensive management of infections is essential. Surgical intervention is also required if pseudocysts develop and do not resolve, although maturation of pseudocysts may take longer in KTx recipients. Pseudocyst complications, such as erosion or obstruction of adjacent vascular and hollow viscus structures, mandate early intervention. The mortality rate from complications of posttransplant pancreatitis appears to be higher than from other forms of pancreatitis. A rapid reduction of immunosuppression is necessary to minimize septic complications.

Pretransplant screening for *cholelithiasis* is variably performed at centers in the United States: the role of prophylactic cholecystectomy for asymptomatic cholelithiasis is controversial. Data generated over the past 15 years failed to strengthen a policy of mandatory pretransplant cholecystectomy for asymptomatic cholelithiasis. *Acute cholecystitis*, especially in uremic diabetic KTx recipients, should be considered if they have sepsis or abdominal pain without a source. *Acalculous cholecystitis* has become more common in recipients with a complicated posttransplant course (e.g., septicemia, multiorgan failure). This diagnosis is established clinically and, especially if recipients are intubated and on the ventilator, by serial ultrasounds and possibly biliary scintigraphy. A cholecystectomy is desirable, but image-guided (ultrasound or CT) cholecystostomy may also be helpful if recipients are too ill to undergo a formal operation [90,91].

Neurologic Complications

Up to 30% of KTx recipients develop neurologic problems posttransplant. The incidence of life-threatening central nervous system (CNS)-related complications in the immediate posttransplant period is 1% to 5% [92–94]. Causative factors are the sequelae not only of the KTx itself, but also of the underlying kidney disease (more common in recipients with diabetes and hypertension) and of pretransplant conditions (e.g., uremia). *Cerebrovascular events* (e.g., infarct, TIA, hemorrhage) are the most frequent complications, usually peaking during the first few months posttransplant. Hypertension, atherosclerosis, diabetes, hyperlipidemia, hypercoagulability, and advanced age—all of which play a major role in the pathogenesis of these complications—are ubiquitous in KTx recipients. For those with strokes or TIAs, conservative treatment (heparinization, aspirin) is best, although carotid endarterectomy can benefit those with ulcerated carotid lesions or with severe but accessible stenoses. The prognosis of intracerebral hemorrhage is poor; posttransplant hypertension is one of the major causative factors and therefore should be aggressively monitored and treated.

All CNS *infections* are considered life threatening, and often result in various degrees of disability. Infections are caused by bacteria (e.g., *Listeria monocytogenes*, *Pseudomonas* species), viruses (e.g., CMV, HSV), fungi (e.g., *Cryptococcus, Aspergillus, Mucor*), and parasites (*Toxoplasma*). *L. monocytogenes* is the most common infectious organism and usually causes meningitis. *Aspergillus* frequently manifests as brain abscesses. Rhinocerebral mucormycosis infection can cause cavernous sinus thrombosis and rapid death. Dissemination of CMV may include the CNS, although the overall incidence is low [95]. Acute polyradiculoneuritis has also been associated with CMV infections [96]. Similarly, dissemination of the VZV can involve the CNS [97] or facial nerve (Ramsay Hunt syndrome). It is crucial to diagnose and treat these infections early and aggressively. Intrathecal administration of antimicrobial drugs or drainage in recipients with brain abscesses may be necessary.

Seizures are associated with excessively high CNI serum levels and affect children at a higher frequency than adults; hypertension and hypomagnesemia may predispose recipients to seizure activity [97–101]. Treatment consists of CNI dose reduction and anticonvulsants; ICU monitoring is mandatory after such events. Other CNI-related complications, such as tremor, dysesthesia, ataxia, and psychologic disorders, usually do not require ICU monitoring. Tacrolimus, more frequently than cyclosporine, causes neurotoxicity in the form of tremor and headaches, both of which can be debilitating; it also can cause paralysis, quadriplegia, coma, and leukoencephalopathy (*posterior reversible encephalopathy syndrome* [PRES]). PRES, occurring in about 0.35% of KTx recipients, is diagnosed by brain magnetic resonance imaging [102]. Another drug-related complication is aseptic meningitis caused by OKT3; treatment consists of discontinuing OKT3 therapy and temporarily administering anticonvulsants.

In contrast to CNS-related problems, peripheral neurologic complications do not require ICU monitoring. Compressive *neuropathy* (involving the femoral nerve or the lateral femoral cutaneous nerve) is due to hematoma, ischemia, or retraction injury at the time of the KTx; all symptoms are confined to the ipsilateral side. This complication has a high degree of reversibility [103]. If a large hematoma is identified, reexploration and evacuation should be performed.

TABLE 182.1

CURRENT CHALLENGES IN KIDNEY TRANSPLANTATION

Clinical dilemma	Management
Higher acuity KTx waiting list	Exhaustive pretransplant evaluation
Age >50: 58%	Intense posttransplant critical care and subspecialty consultation
Diabetic: 28%	
Hypertensive: 22%	Innovative recipient immunomodulation
Waiting list mortality	
Organ scarcity	Desensitization protocols
Sensitized recipients	Complement modulation
	Live donor paired kidney exchange
	National live donor registries

KTx, kidney transplantation.

CURRENT CHALLENGES IN KIDNEY TRANSPLANTATION

Despite the many advances in kidney transplantation, several challenges remain (Table 182.1). During the past decade the proportion of candidates on the active KTx waiting list >50 years of age has increased from 44% to 58% and those with diabetes and hypertension have increased from 24% to 28% and 17 to 22%, respectively. To maintain excellent short-term outcomes, an exhaustive pretransplant cardiovascular evaluation followed by intense posttransplant critical care has become mandatory for this high-acuity cohort of patient [6,7].

Mortality on the waiting list continues to stimulate the adoption of innovative desensitization protocols to allow high-risk recipients an opportunity at transplant. This in turn must be met with equally innovative therapies if antibody-mediated rejection occurs in the early postoperative period. Attempts at modulating the complement system are underway to mitigate early posttransplant injury in the allograft [14].

References

1. Wolfe RA, Ashby VB, Milford EL, et al: Comparison of mortality in all patients on dialysis, patients on dialysis awaiting transplantation, and recipients of a first cadaveric transplant. *N Engl J Med* 341:23, 1999.
2. Organ Procurement and Transplantation Network (OPTN)/Scientific Registry of Transplant Recipients (SRTR) 2008 Annual Report. Available at http://optn.transplant.hrsa.gov/
3. Cecka JM, Terasaki PI: The UNOS scientific renal transplant registry, in Terasaki PI, Cecka JM (eds): *Clinical Transplants.* Los Angeles, UCLA Tissue Typing Laboratory, 2004, p 1.
4. Hariharan S, Johnson CP, Bresnahan BA, et al: Improved graft survival after renal transplantation in the United States, 1988 to 1996. *N Engl J Med* 342:605, 2000.
5. Ishikawa N, Tanabe K, Tokumoto T, et al: Long-term results of living unrelated renal transplantation. *Transplant Proc* 31:2856, 1999.
6. Rabbat CG, Treleaven DJ, Russell JD, et al: Prognostic value of myocardial perfusion studies in patients with end-stage renal disease assessed for kidney or kidney-pancreas transplantation: a meta-analysis. *J Am Soc Nephrol* 14:431, 2003.

7. Humar A, Kerr SR, Ramcharan T, et al: Peri-operative cardiac morbidity in kidney transplant recipients: incidence and risk factors. *Clin Transplant* 15:154, 2001.
8. Yigla M, Nakhoul F, Sabag A, et al: Pulmonary hypertension in patients with end-stage renal disease. *Chest* 123:1577, 2003.
9. Niu MT, Coleman PJ, Alter MJ, et al: Multicenter study of hepatitis C virus infection in chronic hemodialysis patients and hemodialysis center staff members. *Am J Kidney Dis* 22:568, 1993.
10. Dawidson I, Sandor ZF, Coorpender L, et al: Intraoperative albumin administration affects the outcome of cadaver renal transplantation. *Transplantation* 53:774, 1992.
11. van Valenberg PL, Hoitsma AJ, Tiggeler RG, et al: Mannitol as an indispensable constituent of an intraoperative hydration protocol for the prevention of acute renal failure after renal cadaveric transplantation. *Transplantation* 44:784, 1987.
12. Park JH, Yang CW, Kim YS, et al: Clinical impact of slow recovery of renal function in renal transplantation. *Transplant Proc* 31:2841, 1999.
13. Troppmann C, Almond PS, Payne WD, et al: Does acute tubular necrosis affect renal transplant outcome? The impact of rejection episodes. *Transplant Proc* 25:905, 1993.
14. Colvin RB, Smith RN: Antibody-mediated organ-allograft rejection. *Nat Rev Immunol* 5:807, 2005.
15. Racusen LC, Colvin RB, Solez K, et al: Antibody-mediated rejection criteria—an addition to the Banff 97 classification of renal allograft rejection. *Am J Transplant* 3:708, 2003.
16. Artero M, Biava C, Amend W, et al: Recurrent focal glomerulosclerosis: natural history and response to therapy. *Am J Med* 92:375, 1992.
17. Ducloux D, Rebibou JM, Semhoun-Ducloux S, et al: Recurrence of hemolytic uremic syndrome in renal transplant recipients: a meta-analysis. *Transplantation* 65:1405, 1998.
18. Benedetti E, Troppmann C, Gillingham K, et al: Short- and long-term outcome of kidney transplants with multiple renal arteries. *Ann Surg* 221:406, 1995.
19. Englesbe MJ, Punch JD, Armstrong DR, et al: Single-center study of technical graft loss in 714 consecutive renal transplants. *Transplantation* 78:623, 2004.
20. Streeter EH, Little DM, Cranston DW, et al: The urological complications of renal transplantation: a series of 1535 patients. *BJU Int* 90:627, 2002.
21. Bassiri A, Simforoosh N, Gholamrezaie HR: Ureteral complications in 1100 consecutive renal transplants. *Transplant Proc* 32:578, 2000.
22. Waltzer WC, Frischer Z, Shabtai M, et al: Early aggressive management for the prevention of renal allograft loss and patient mortality following major urologic complications. *Clin Transplant* 6:318, 1992.
23. Gruessner RWG, Fasola C, Benedetti E, et al: Laparoscopic drainage of lymphoceles after kidney transplants: Indications and limitations. *Surgery* 117:287, 1995.
24. Matas AJ, Humar A, Gillingham KJ, et al: Five preventable causes of kidney graft loss in the 1990s: a single-center analysis. *Kidney Int* 62:704, 2002.
25. Debska-Slizien A, Dudziak M, Kubasik A, et al: Echocardiographic changes in left ventricular morphology and function after successful renal transplantation. *Transplant Proc* 32:1365, 2000.
26. Djamali A, Becker YT, Simmons WD, et al: Increasing hematocrit reduces early posttransplant cardiovascular risk in diabetic transplant recipients. *Transplantation* 76:816, 2003.
27. Sever MS, Steinmuller DR, Hayes JM, et al: Pericarditis following renal transplantation. *Transplantation* 51:1229, 1991.
28. Laskow DA, Curtis JJ: Posttransplant hypertension. *Am J Hypertens* 3:721, 1990.
29. Textor SC, Taler SJ, Canzanello VJ: Posttransplantation hypertension related to calcineurin inhibitors. *Liver Transplantation* 6:5, 2000.
30. Cauduro RL, Costa C, Lhulier F: Cyclosporine increases endothelin-1 plasma levels in renal transplant recipients. *Transplant Proc* 36:880, 2004.
31. Mangano DT, Layug EL, Wallace E, et al: Effect of atenolol on mortality and cardiovascular morbidity after noncardiac surgery: multicenter study of Perioperative Ischemia Research Group. *N Engl J Med* 335:1713, 1996.
32. Midtvedt K, Neumayer HH: Management strategies for posttransplant hypertension. *Transplantation* 70[Suppl]:SS64, 2000.
33. Murie JA, Allen RD, Michie CA, et al: Deep venous thrombosis after renal transplantation. *Transplant Proc* 19:2219, 1987.
34. Ozsoylu S, Strauss HS, Diamond LK: Effect of corticosteroids on coagulation of the blood. *Nature* 195:1214, 1962.
35. Pasquale MD, Abrams JH, Najarian JS, et al: Use of Greenfield filters in renal transplant patients: Are they safe? *Transplantation* 55:439, 1993.
36. Boyes R, Pur VK, Toledo L, et al: Pulmonary edema in renal transplant patients. *Am Surg* 53:647, 1987.
37. Thislethwaite JR Jr, Stuart JK, Mayes JT, et al: Monitoring and complications of monoclonal therapy: Complications and monitoring of OKT3 therapy. *Am J Kidney Dis* 11:112, 1988.
38. Issa N, Krowka MJ, Griffin MD, et al: Pulmonary hypertension is associated with reduced patient survival after kidney transplantation. *Transplantation* 27:1384, 2008.
39. Shorr AF, Abbott KC, Agadoa LY, et al: Acute respiratory distress syndrome after kidney transplantation: epidemiology, risk factors, and outcomes. *Crit Care Med* 31:1325, 2003.
40. Fishman JA: Infection in solid organ transplant recipients. *N Engl J Med* 357:2601, 2007.
41. Chang GC, Wu CL, Pan SH, et al: The diagnosis of pneumonia in renal transplant recipients using invasive and noninvasive procedures. *Chest* 125:541, 2004.
42. Linden PK: Approach to the immunocompromised host with infection in the intensive care unit. *Infect Dis Clin N Am* 23:535, 2009.
43. Chakinala MM, Trulock EP: Pneumonia in the solid organ transplant patient. *Clin Chest Med* 26:113, 2005.
44. Tolkoff-Rubin NE, Rubin RH: Urinary tract infection in the immunocompromised host. Lessons from kidney transplantation and the AIDS epidemic. *Infect Dis Clin North Am* 11:707, 1997.
45. Patel R, Paya CV: Infections in solid-organ transplant recipients. *Clin Micro Rev* 10:86, 1997.
46. Troidle L, Finkelstein FO: Catheter-related bacteremia in hemodialysis patients: the role of the central venous catheter in prevention and therapy. *Int J Artif Organs* 31:827, 2008.
47. Kidney Disease Outcomes Quality Initiative Clinical Practice Guidelines and Clinical Practice Recommendations: Hemodialysis adequacy, peritoneal dialysis adequacy and vascular access. *Am J Kidney Dis* 48(Suppl 1): S176, 2006.
48. Masutani M, Ikeoka K, Sasaki R, et al: Post transplanted infective endocarditis. *Jpn J Med* 30:458, 1991.
49. Sagedal S, Nordal KP, Hartmann A, et al: A prospective study of the natural course of cytomegalovirus infection and disease in renal allograft recipients. *Transplantation* 70:1166, 2000.
50. Paya C, Humar A, Dominguez E, et al: Efficacy and safety of valganciclovir vs. oral ganciclovir for prevention of cytomegalovirus disease in solid organ transplant recipients. *Am J Transplant* 4:611–620, 2004.
51. Pancholi P, Wu F, Della-Latta P: Rapid detection of cytomegalovirus infection in transplant patients. *Expert Rev Mol Diagn* 4:231–242, 2004.
52. Mengelle C, Pasquier C, Rostaing L: Quantitation of human cytomegalovirus in recipients of solid organ transplants by real-time quantitative PCR and pp65 antigenemia. *J Med Virol* 69:225–231, 2003.
53. Hibberd PL, Rubin RH: Clinical aspects of fungal infection in organ transplant recipients. *Clin Infect Dis* 19[Suppl 1]:S33, 1994.
54. Mora-Duarte J, Betts R, Rotstein C, et al: Comparison of caspofungin and amphotericin B for invasive candidiasis. *N Engl J Med* 347:2020, 2002.
55. Touzet S, Pariset C, Rabodonirina M, et al: Nosocomial transmission of *Pneumocystis carinii* in renal transplantation. *Transplant Proc* 32:445, 2000.
56. Troppmann C, Papalois BE, Chiou A, et al: Incidence, complications, treatment, and outcome of ulcers of the upper gastrointestinal tract after renal transplantation during the cyclosporine era. *J Am Coll Surg* 180:433, 1995.
57. Sarkio S, Halme L, Kyllonen L, et al: Severe gastrointestinal complications after 1,515 adult kidney transplantations. *Transplant Int* 17:505, 2004.
58. Sarosdy MF, Cruz AB, Saylor R, et al: Upper gastrointestinal bleeding following renal transplantation. *Urology* 26:347, 1985.
59. Nardone G, Rocco A, Fiorillo M, et al: Gastroduodenal lesions and *Helicobacter pylori* infection in dyspeptic patients with and without chronic renal failure. *Helicobacter* 10:53, 2005.
60. Bansky G, Huynh Do U, Largiadér F, et al: Gastroduodenal complications after renal transplantation: The role of prophylactic gastric surgery in hyperacid kidney allograft recipients. *Clin Transplant* 1:209, 1987.
61. Uhlschmid G, Largiadér F: Surgical prophylaxis of gastroduodenal complications associated with renal allotransplantation. *World J Surg* 1:397, 1977.
62. Linder MM, Kösters W, Rethel R: Prophylactic gastric operations in uremic patients prior to renal transplantation. *World J Surg* 3:501, 1979.
63. Cohen EB, Komorowski RA, Kauffman HM Jr, et al: Unexpectedly high incidence of cytomegalovirus infection in apparent peptic ulcers in renal transplant recipients. *Surgery* 97:606, 1985.
64. Gautam A: Gastrointestinal complications following transplantation. *Surg Clin N Am* 86:1195, 2006.
65. Scott TR, Graham SM, Schweitzer EJ, et al: Colonic necrosis following sodium polystyrene sulfonate(Kayexalate)-sorbitol enema in a renal transplant patient. Report of a case and review of the literature. *Dis Colon Rectum* 36:607, 1993.
66. Gerstman BB, Kirkman R, Platt R: Intestinal necrosis associated with postoperative orally administered sodium polystyrene sulfonate in sorbitol. *Am J Kidney Dis* 20:159, 1992.
67. Coccolini F, Catena F, Di Saverio L, et al: Colonic perforation after renal transplantation: risk factor analysis. *Transplant Proc* 41:1189, 2009.
68. Konishi T, Watanabe T, Kitayama J, et al: Successfully treated idiopathic rectosigmoid perforation 7 years after renal transplantation. *J Gastroenterol* 39:484, 2004.
69. Flanigan RC, Reckard CR, Lucas BA: Colonic complications of renal transplantation. *J Urol* 139:503, 1988.
70. Lao A, Bach D: Colonic complications in renal transplant recipients. *Dis Colon Rectum* 31:130, 1988.
71. Pirenne J, Lledo-Garcia E, Benedetti E, et al: Colon perforation after renal transplantation: A single-institution review. *Clin Transplant* 11:88, 1997.
72. Church JM, Braun WE, Novick AC, et al: Perforation of the colon in renal homograft recipients. *Ann Surg* 203:69, 1986.
73. Squiers EC, Pfaff WW, Patton PR, et al: Early posttransplant colon perforation: Does it remain a problem in the cyclosporine era? *Transplant Proc* 23:1782, 1991.

74. Scheff RT, Zuckerman A, Harter H, et al: Diverticular disease in patients with chronic renal failure due to polycystic kidney disease. *Ann Int Med* 92:202, 1980.
75. Pirenne J, Lledo-Garcia E, Benedetti E, et al: Colon perforation after renal transplantation: a single-institution review. *Clin Transplant* 11:88, 1997.
76. Dalle Valle R, Capocasale E, Mazzoni MP, et al: Acute diverticulitis with colon perforation in renal transplantation. *Transplant Proc* 37:2507, 2005.
77. Indudhara R, Kochhar R, Mehta SK, et al: Acute colitis in renal transplant recipients. *Am J Gastroenterol* 85:964, 1990.
78. Hellström PM, Rubio C, Odar-Cederlöf I, et al: Ischemic colitis of the cecum after renal transplantation masquerading as malignant disease. *Dig Dis Sci* 36:1644, 1991.
79. Frankel AH, Barker F, Williams G, et al: Neutropenic enterocolitis in a renal transplant patient. *Transplantation* 52:913, 1991.
80. Guerra EE, Nghiem DD: Posttransplant cecal volvulus. *Transplantation* 50:721, 1990.
81. Love R, Sterling JR, Sollinger HW, et al: Colonoscopic decompression for acute colonic pseudo-obstruction (Ogilvie's syndrome) in transplant recipients. *Gastrointest Endosc* 34:426, 1988.
82. Stylianos S, Forde KA, Benvenisty Al, et al: Lower gastrointestinal hemorrhage in renal transplant recipients. *Arch Surg* 123:739, 1988.
83. Frick TW, Fryd DS, Sutherland DER, et al: Hypercalcemia associated with pancreatitis and hyperamylasemia in renal transplant recipients: Data from the minnesota randomized trial of cyclosporine versus antilymphoblast azathioprine. *Am J Surg* 154:487, 1987.
84. Kamalkumar BS, Agarwal SK, Garg P, et al: Acute pancreatitis with CMV papillitis and cholangiopathy in a renal transplant recipient. *Clin Exp Nephrol* 13:389, 2009.
85. Browning NG, Botha JR. Pancreatitis after renal transplantation: A potentially lethal condition. *Clin Transplant* 4:93, 1990.
86. Chapman WC, Nylander WA, Williams LF Sr, et al: Pancreatic pseudocyst formation following renal transplantation: A lethal development. *Clin Transplant* 5:86, 1991.
87. Fernandez JA, Rosenberg JC: Posttransplantation pancreatitis. *Surg Gynecol Obstet* 143:795, 1976.
88. Fernandez-Cruz L, Targarona EM, Alcaraz ECA, et al: Acute pancreatitis after renal transplantation. *Br J Surg* 76:1132, 1989.
89. Johnson WC, Nabseth DC: Pancreatitis in renal transplantation. *Ann Surg* 171:309, 1970.
90. Melvin WS, Meier DJ, et al: Prophylactic cholecystectomy is not indicated following renal transplantation. *Am J Surg* 169:44, 1995.
91. Jackson T, Treleaven D, Arlen D, et al: Management of asymptomatic cholelithiasis for patients awaiting renal transplantation. *Surg Endosc* 19:510, 2005.
92. Adams HP Jr, Dawson D, Coffman TJ, et al: Stroke in renal transplant recipients. *Arch Neurol* 43:113, 1986.
93. Bruno A, Adams H: Neurologic problems in renal transplant recipients. *Neurol Clin* 6:305, 1988.
94. Lee JM, Raps EC: Neurologic complications of transplantation. *Neurologic clinics* 16:21, 1998.
95. Simmons RL, Matas AJ, Rattazzi LC, et al: Clinical characteristics of the lethal cytomegalovirus infection following renal transplantation. *Surgery* 82:537, 1977.
96. Pouteil-Noble C, Vial C, Moreau T, et al: Acute polyradiculoneuritis associated with cytomegalovirus infection in renal transplantation. *Clin Transplant* 7:158, 1993.
97. Peterson LR, Ferguson RM: Fatal central nervous system infection with varicella zoster virus in renal transplant recipients. *Transplantation* 37:366, 1984.
98. McEnery PT, Nathan J, Bates SR, et al: Convulsions in children undergoing renal transplantation. *J Pediatr* 115:532, 1989.
99. Arora P, Kohli A, Kher V, et al: Complex partial seizure: An unusual complication of cyclosporine in renal transplantation. *Clin Transplant* 46:458, 1992.
100. Rubin A: Transient cortical blindness and occipital seizures with cyclosporine toxicity. *Transplantation* 47:572, 1989.
101. Thompson CB, June CH, Sullivan KM, et al: Association between cyclosporine neurotoxicity and hypomagnesaemia. *Lancet* 2:1116, 1984.
102. Bartynski WS, Tan HP, Boardman JF, et al: Posterior reversible encephalopathy syndrome after solid organ transplantation. *Am J Neuroradiol* 29:924, 2008.
103. Kumar A, Dalela D, Bhandari M, et al: Femoral neuropathy: an unusual complication of renal transplantation. *Transplantation* 51:1305, 1991.

CHAPTER 183 ■ SPECIFIC CRITICAL CARE PROBLEMS IN HEART AND HEART–LUNG TRANSPLANT RECIPIENTS

SARA J. SHUMWAY AND EIAS E. JWEIED

The advent of thoracic organ transplantation has brought new hope to patients who were previously doomed by end-stage cardiac, pulmonary, or combined cardiopulmonary disease. The first heart transplant was performed on December 3, 1967. Fourteen years passed before the first successful heart–lung transplant was performed on March 9, 1981. Heart–lung transplantation established the potential for lung transplantation as a viable therapeutic option, and the first successful single-lung transplant was performed in 1983 [1].

HEART TRANSPLANTATION

The United Network for Organ Sharing (UNOS) is a nonprofit organization that maintains the nation's organ transplant waiting list. Patients awaiting cardiac transplants are listed according to severity of illness. Organs are then allocated to those individuals who are severely ill and have waited the longest. Just more than 2,200 heart transplants are performed annually in the United States. There has been a decrease in candidate waiting times, with the average waiting time for a status 1A heart candidate of 50 days and a status 2 candidate of 309 days [2]. A status 1 heart candidate includes those individuals with highest medical urgency. These are patients who have support either via a total artificial heart, ventricular assist device (VAD), intra-aortic balloon pump, or extracorporeal membrane oxygenation. It could also be an individual who has a mechanical assist device in place, either right or left support that is beginning to malfunction. It also includes individuals who are on continuous mechanical ventilation or on high-dose inotropic support and are unable to be weaned. Status 2 candidates are individuals who need a heart transplant but have not been defined as being in the most urgent status. They may be patients who are at home and taking heart-failure medications and are still active and awaiting transplant but are not as critically ill as those individuals in the status 1 category. At any given time, UNOS has approximately 3,000 candidates listed for heart transplant, and most have been waiting for more than a year.

The number of heart transplants performed nationally depends on donor availability. In spite of this, the annual mortality rate on the waiting list has slowly declined during the last 10 years. In the middle to late 1990s, it was not uncommon to have anywhere between 700 and 800 people die from cardiac disease while awaiting a heart transplant. That number has been slowly decreasing to less than 400 each of the last 3 years [2]. This slow decrease is related to the evolution of left ventricular assist devices and their acceptance as a bridge to transplant.

Ninety percent of adult candidates listed for heart transplant have end-stage cardiac disease with some form of cardiomyopathy. Approximately 47% have idiopathic cardiomyopathy, and 35% have ischemic cardiomyopathy. The remaining 15% of heart transplant candidates have end-stage valvular disease, cardiomyopathy associated with congenital heart disease, or graft failure requiring retransplantation. Cardiac retransplantation represents approximately 4% of the adult heart transplant population annually [2,3].

Patient Selection

Many of the specific critical care problems seen in thoracic organ recipients can be reduced by careful patient selection. In well-compensated patients, a weeklong outpatient evaluation is performed. This applies to approximately 80% to 90% of patients seen at a cardiac transplant center. The other 10% to 20% are individuals who are desperately ill and undergo an urgent transplant evaluation.

The recipient assessment consists of a general evaluation, an assessment of the functional and hemodynamic status, and a psychosocial evaluation. All parts are equally crucial. One of the first assessments is an oxygen-consumption treadmill test. For those patients who are capable of performing this test, there are excellent data that demonstrate that a peak oxygen consumption of less than 12 mL per kg per minute is associated with a very poor 1-year survival rate without transplant. Individuals with a peak oxygen consumption of less than 15 mL per kg per minute should be considered for listing [4,5]. The assessment then proceeds with a general evaluation. The patient's medical history is examined to try to determine the cause of the patient's heart disease. General laboratory tests are performed, including a creatinine clearance. Individuals who have a creatinine clearance of less than 50 mL per minute do have a significant increase in the need for postcardiac transplant dialysis and a decrease in survival rate. Individuals with severely abnormal creatinine clearance would be excluded from heart transplant or considered for heart and kidney transplantation. Individuals with diabetes need further end-organ evaluation prior to listing to understand the full scope of their risk.

Nutritional status is also crucial. Those individuals with a body mass index less than 20 kg per m^2 or greater than 35 kg per m^2 would be asked to either gain or lose weight, respectively. Again, individuals at the extremes of the body mass index have an associated increase in postoperative mortality [6,7].

The hemodynamic evaluation consists of an echocardiogram to evaluate function and anatomy, and a cardiac catheterization. The cardiac catheterization includes evaluation of heart function by a right heart catheterization as well as a coronary angiogram. In this assessment, the patient's coronary anatomy is examined for potential intervention, and any abnormalities in the filling pressures, pulmonary capillary occlusion pressure, or pulmonary vascular resistance are identified.

Patients with heart failure and secondary pulmonary hypertension are a group who are of special interest. Pulmonary arterial and capillary wedge pressures are measured to determine the degree to which a patient has secondary pulmonary hypertension and whether or not it is reversible. The patient's hemodynamics should be optimized in the catheterization laboratory in an attempt to decrease the pulmonary arterial pressures to normal levels, and 100% oxygen, nitric oxide, and other pulmonary vasodilators can be used to test for reactivity in the pulmonary bed. The absolute exclusion criteria for heart transplantation are a pulmonary vascular resistance greater than 4 Wood units (WU) and, more importantly, a transpulmonary gradient greater than 15 mm Hg. Individuals with values outside these values would then be listed for heart–lung transplant, or be given a trial of pulmonary vasodilators.

The patient's ABO blood type and panel-reactive antibody (PRA) level is determined to quantitate the patient's preexisting antibodies and sensitization to the general population. If class II (locus D) is greater than 20%, it is recommended that a preoperative cross-match be performed. The patient's HLA typing is also done at that time, and if the PRAs are significantly elevated, the laboratory should be able to identify the particular human leukocyte antigen to which the individual is reacting. Sensitization can occur in many situations. It may occur because of pregnancy, between sexual partners, from prior transplantation, or with transfusions often associated with the placement of a ventricular assist device. Individuals who carry a high PRA level have been treated in the past with plasmapheresis, intravenous immunoglobulin, cyclophosphamide, and mycophenolate mofetil (MMF). There have been inconclusive results with each of these.

The psychosocial evaluation should be centered on evaluating not only the transplant recipient but also the family support for the patient. This needs to be performed by a social worker and, when indicated, other mental health professionals who have a keen understanding of the demands made on a postoperative cardiac transplant patient. Patients need to be medically compliant, have adequate neurocognitive function for the postoperative regimen, and adequate social support.

Once the evaluation has been completed, the patient is evaluated for any relative or absolute contraindication for heart transplant. Those relative contraindications include age greater than 70 years, previous chronic substance abuse, limited social support, limited adaptive ability, mild renal dysfunction, active peptic ulcer disease, cachexia, obesity, and cigarette smoking. It should be noted that to receive a heart transplant, individuals who smoke are required to go through a smoking-cessation program, and many transplant programs require them to sign a contract stating that they will not resume smoking prior to or after the transplant. They also are evaluated for chemical evidence of smoking during their waiting time [8].

Absolute contraindications to cardiac transplantation include ongoing substance abuse, refractory psychiatric conditions, suicidal behavior, severe personality disorder, issues with ongoing medical noncompliance, inadequate neurocognitive ability, irreversible hepatic or renal dysfunction, severe peripheral or cerebral vascular disease, systemic disease that limits rehabilitation, insulin-dependent diabetes with severe end-organ damage, and evidence of severe, fixed, secondary pulmonary hypertension [8–10].

Implantable Cardiac Assist Devices

The proliferation and success of ventricular assist devices probably represent the greatest advance in the treatment of end-stage heart failure and the field of heart transplantation of the past 10 years (Table 183.1). With an assist device implanted, patients who would otherwise not survive long enough to

TABLE 183.1

ADVANCES OF VENTRICULAR ASSIST DEVICES IN HEART FAILURE TREATMENT

Topic	Finding	Reference
Destination therapy trial with pulsatile pumps	Improved survival at one year with mechanical assist device vs. medical management for Class III and IV heart failure	[11]
Bridge to transplant trial with continuous flow pumps	HeartMate II provides effective support to transplant for at least 6 months with 75% survival	[12]
Improved survival with continuous flow pumps	Effective support, improved functional status and quality of life with 72% survival at 18 mo	[48–50]

receive a heart transplant are now living independently at home with reasonably good quality of life until a suitable organ becomes available. Today, at high-volume heart transplant centers, many if not most patients arriving for heart transplantation have an assist device already in place and it can be expected that in the coming years most if not all heart transplant recipients will have had one of these devices implanted by the time they receive an organ.

From their increased use, a corpus of terminology has evolved to categorize and describe the devices themselves, their use, and technical aspects of their function and performance. Most devices are designed to assist the left ventricle and hence are called left ventricular assist devices (LVADs). However, some models are made to be implanted in either ventricle and when implanted on the right side are referred to as a right ventricular assist devices (RVAD). When both ventricles are mechanically assisted, each with its own pump, the whole system together is referred to as a biventricular assist device, or BIVAD.

There are two broad categories of devices in use based on pump mechanism: pulsatile devices that employ some type of pneumatic pump, and continuous, or axial, flow devices that involve a spinning propeller. The cycles of the pulsatile device are measured in beats per minute (bpm) and that of the continuous flow pumps in revolutions per minute (rpm). Each device has an inflow cannula through which the patient's blood is drawn from the heart and into the pump and an outflow cannula that directs the blood back into the patients' circulation.

Further, for both pulsatile pumps and continuous flow pumps, there are two more classifications that can be described on the basis of the location of the pump when implanted: intracorporeal wherein the entire pump is implanted inside the body with the exception of the drive-line that powers the device and passes through an exit site on the abdomen; the other is paracorporeal, or extracorporeal, wherein the pump sits outside the body and the inflow and outflow cannulae enter and exit the skin on the upper abdomen just below the costal margin.

Most LVADs usually involve an inflow cannula placed in the apex of left ventricle and the outflow cannula in the ascending aorta. The only permanent RVAD approved for use in the United States is the Thoratec® Paracorporeal Ventricular Assist Device and its inflow cannula is placed in the right ventricular free wall and the outflow cannula is anastomosed to the pulmonary artery. The Levitronix® CentriMag (now owned by Thoratec®) is approved for temporary right ventricular assistance up to 30 days and its inflow cannula may be placed in either the right atrium or the right ventricle.

Lastly, there is a categorization of devices based upon the intended therapeutic goal for each particular patient. Bridge to transplant (BTT) indicates that the patient is or will become a heart transplant candidate and the device is intended to improve survival and other physiologic parameters until an organ is available. Destination therapy (DT) indicates that the patient is not a transplant candidate but the device is implanted to improve survival and quality of life for the remainder of the patient's life. Bridge to recovery refers to the patient who is expected to recover from heart failure and the device is used to sustain life until the time when it can be weaned off and explanted. Bridge to decision (BTD) refers to those patients for whom survival is not certain and a temporary assist device, such as the AbioMed BVS5000™ or the Levitronix® CentriMag, is used in the critical care setting to prolong life until it can be determined whether the patient ought to be implanted with a long-term device as those used in BTT or DT patients or be disconnected from the BTD device and allowed to expire.

The superior efficacy of VADs over optimal medical management in improving survival in end-stage, New York Heart Association Class 3 or 4 heart failure patients was proven in the REMATCH trial: patients implanted with the Thoratec® HeartMate VE had a 52% survival at one year compared to 25% in the medically managed group [11]. Subsequently the Food and Drug Administration (FDA) approved the HeartMate XVE for destination therapy. The Thoratec® HeartMate II continuous flow pump demonstrated efficacy in bridge to transplantation with 75% survival at 6 months postimplantation and 68% survival at 1 year [12]. It received approval by the FDA in April 2008 for bridge to transplantation and was subsequently approved for destination therapy in January 2010. Smaller devices such as the Jarvik 2000 Flowmaker™ and the HeartWare™ VAD are currently under investigation in the United States with more than two dozens other devices presently in development (Fig. 183.1).

Knowing how these devices work and how these patients are managed will be an important part of the pretransplantation care of the recipient, and indeed any critically ill patient who is admitted with one of these devices. Almost all of these patients will arrive anticoagulated on warfarin. It will be important not to begin administration of plasma and cryoprecipitate until the plan to proceed with the transplant is certain. Administration of blood products without completing the transplant will only sensitize the recipient and increase the PRAs for any subsequent transplant offers [13]. The postoperative course is often complicated by bleeding. Drains for the VAD pocket are necessary and pericardial effusions are more common.

Several studies have examined posttransplant survival and recent studies have shown that recipients of ventricular assist devices have had equal or better posttransplant outcomes [14,15]. One exception is the patient who had VAD-related sepsis prior to transplantation as these patients had a trend to slightly poorer posttransplant survival than those patients who did not have an infection [16].

Donor Criteria

The donor evaluation begins with the pronouncement of brain death. The local organ procurement agency will obtain consent

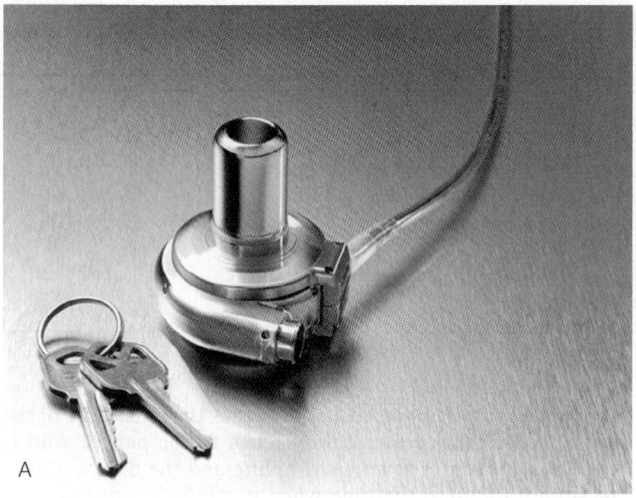

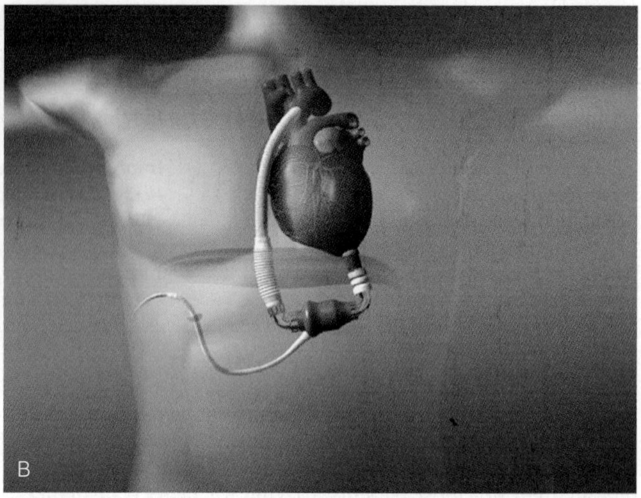

FIGURE 183.1. Continuous flow ventricular assist devices. **A:** HeartWare ventricular assist device. [Reprinted with permission from HeartWare™.] **B:** HeartMate II ventricular assist device. [Reprinted with permission from Thoratec®.]

for donation from the family and proceed with the donor evaluation and support. The donor evaluation consists of taking a general history of any illnesses or risk factors such as heart disease, hypertension, diabetes, or cigarette smoking. Specifics are gathered surrounding the time and mode of death to determine whether there is any potential cardiac injury, down time, cardiopulmonary resuscitation, or cardioversion. The organ-procurement professionals will proceed with a hemodynamic evaluation of the patient. This consists of at least measuring central venous pressures and, potentially, full hemodynamic profiles if pulmonary artery catheter measurement capability exists at the donor hospital. Once the donor is stabilized hemodynamically, further studies are performed. The initial stabilization phase should include endocrine support with the administration of levothyroxine and corticosteroids, reduction of inotropic support if it is appropriate, and, potentially, diuresis or transfusion if needed. A surface echocardiogram is then performed to make sure the heart is structurally normal and that function is normal. A 12-lead electrocardiogram is also obtained. It is not uncommon to find subtle ST changes in individuals who are brain-dead. It is generally accepted that a cardiac catheterization will be necessary in male donors more than 40 years old and female donors more than 45 years old, but catheterization should also be performed in younger donors if the donor has a significant history of hypertension, cigarette smoking, diabetes, or alcohol abuse. Cardiac enzymes need to be carefully evaluated and correlated to any severe hemodynamic instability, the use of cardiopulmonary resuscitation, as well as the time of herniation [17].

A number of studies have demonstrated correlations between elevations of troponin and early graft failure [18,19]. In one study, a cardiac troponin I value greater than 1.6 μg per L was a predictor of early graft failure, with a sensitivity of 73% and a specificity of 94% [18]. These data should be analyzed closely with the patient's hemodynamic function and echocardiographic findings.

A transplant center may request that a second echocardiogram be performed if the first echocardiogram was performed shortly after herniation. Catecholamine-induced left ventricular dysfunction can improve significantly in a short period of time and not preclude excellent short- and long-term outcomes. One must also take into consideration the ischemic time that will be incurred with procurement and travel time. The majority of transplant centers are willing to accept an ischemic time up to 4 hours for adult donors but no more than 6.

Operative Techniques

Donor Operation

Once the donor has been prepared and the abdominal team has started their procedure, the median sternotomy incision is performed. If lungs are being harvested, both pleural spaces are also opened for inspection of both lungs. During this inspection, one should palpate the coronaries to discern any calcifications and also palpate the aortic root for calcifications. External evaluation of the heart is not a reliable evaluation of function unless there is something grossly abnormal, such as severe bruising from a myocardial contusion or a dilated right ventricle. Once it is determined that the heart is appropriate for transplantation and all of the other organ teams are ready, the donor is heparinized and cannulated. The heart is cannulated with a cardioplegia cannula in the ascending aorta. If the lungs are being harvested, a pulmonary artery cannula will be placed in the main pulmonary artery. Once all teams are ready, the aorta is cross-clamped and the flush solution is given. Between 1 and 2 L of cold cardioplegic solution are administered. The heart is vented via the left atrial appendage, excised, and is then submerged in ice slush saline, packaged sterilely, and placed in a cooler for rapid transport to the recipient center.

Recipient Operation

Once the recipient is prepared and draped, the median sternotomy incision is made and the heart is dissected free of any adhesions, and then cardiopulmonary bypass is established.

The recipient is placed on total cardiopulmonary bypass, before the cross-clamp is applied the aorta, and the heart is excised along the atrioventricular groove. The great vessels are divided just above their respective semilunar valves. The anastomoses are performed in the following order: left atrial, right atrial or inferior vena caval, pulmonary arterial, aortic, and, if bicaval anastomoses are being performed, superior vena caval

[20]. Temporary pacing wires are left on the donor right atrium and right ventricle. The organ is reperfused and, once it has recovered, separated from bypass. On separation from bypass, the appropriate inotropic support is administered. Typically, the patient may require dopamine or epinephrine and milrinone for postoperative support. Isoproterenol is used to maintain an appropriate heart rate if bradycardia is a problem or the heart is paced. The pulmonary artery catheter should be floated through the new heart so that pulmonary artery pressures can be monitored closely and any signs of right heart failure can be detected early.

Postoperative Care

The immediate postoperative management of a heart transplant recipient is by and large not unlike that of other cardiac surgery patients. Drips and temporary pacing leads are modified to optimize cardiac index and end-organ perfusion. Typical inotropes used are epinephrine, dopamine, dobutamine, and milrinone. A pulmonary artery catheter is used with continuous mixed venous oximetry and preload is optimized with either volume or diuretic. Usually patients come out of the operating room on Isuprel (isoproterenol) to stimulate the heart rate and/or the temporary pacemaker set to a back-up rate of 90 to 100 bpm or higher. The ideal heart rate for these patients in the first few days postoperatively is 100 to 120 bpm. After the first several days, the heart rate is allowed to drift to its baseline as the cardiac index allows. Occasionally, patients exhibit a distributive shock immediately postoperatively characterized by low systemic vascular resistence and vasopression or neosynephrine are used to treat it.

Ventilatory management varies from patient to patient. The ideal patient who is hemodynamically stable and has no signs of surgical bleeding can be extubated within a few hours. Sometimes patients with right ventricular failure due to pulmonary hypertension need to be treated with inhaled nitric oxide or epoprostenol (Flolan®) and thus mechanical ventilation is continued.

Patients who have had a ventricular assist device placed as a bridge to transplant frequently have had two or more prior sternotomies and arrive to the hospital on Coumadin. These patients have a tendency to bleed more postoperatively and one should keep a low threshold to return to the operating room for exploration if bleeding persists.

Serious ventricular failure after cardiac transplantation is unusual and can be related to poor donor-organ selection, poor graft preservation, a long ischemia time, or rejection due to the presence of preformed antibodies. Early rejection is often heralded by atrial fibrillation and the manifestation of arrhythmias should prompt an immediate work-up and treatment. Plasmapheresis can be very effective in removing preformed antibodies responsible for humoral rejection. Inotropes and pulmonary vasodilators are also often used to manage the right heart failure that frequently accompanies rejection, with the addition of an intra-aortic balloon pump if necessary. In cases of severe graft dysfunction, ventricular assist devices can support the patient until either the donor heart recovers or retransplantation takes place.

Immunosuppression

Balanced triple-drug immunosuppression is still the most commonly used protocol, consisting of calcineurin inhibitors, an antimetabolite, and corticosteroids (Table 183.2). The calcineurin inhibitors include cyclosporine and tacrolimus. Cyclosporine is largely recognized as the agent that moved cardiac transplant from a feasible medical option to an acceptable medical treatment. The physicians at Stanford University performed a randomized control trial in cardiac transplant patients that demonstrated that cyclosporine immunosuppression improved 1-year survival to 80% from the mid-50% range [21]. Patients receiving either cyclosporine or tacrolimus have similar survival rates in heart transplantation, both long and short term [22–24]. However in a controlled clinical trial by Kobashigawa et al. in 2006 studying 343 de novo cardiac transplant patients, tacrolimus in combination with either mycophenolate or sirolimus had fewer occurrences of grade 3 A or greater rejection or hemodynamic compromise rejection at 1 year when compared to cyclosporine and mycophenolate [25]. In addition, median serum creatinine and triglyceride levels were lowest in the tacrolimus and mycophenolate group. Cyclosporine is well known to also cause postoperative hypertension, nephrotoxicity, hepatotoxicity, gingival hyperplasia, hypertrichosis, and tremor. Tacrolimus also causes nephrotoxicity and many of the other side effects of cyclosporine but to a lesser extent, in particular, posttransplant hypertension and gingival hyperplasia.

The antimetabolites include MMF and azathioprine. These inhibit purine synthesis and thus block proliferation of both T and B cells. They are complimentary to the calcineurin inhibitors. Kobashigawa et al. [26] demonstrated considerable benefits to MMF over azathioprine when coupled with cyclosporine in transplants performed in 1998. MMF is current the most widely used antimetabolite in heart transplantation [24].

Corticosteroids remain a cornerstone of therapy. There are multiple regimens for early corticosteroid reduction to avoid the serious side effects of corticosteroids. These include systemic hypertension, obesity, osteoporosis, and glucose intolerance. In spite of the negative side effects, in 2004 approximately 75% of patients were still taking corticosteroids 1 year following their transplants [27]. Monotherapy consisting of tacrolimus is currently being studied in heart transplant recipients. In one study, 75% of recipients were successfully converted to monotherapy [28] and other prospective randomized clinical trials are currently underway to evaluate these findings.

The use of IL-2 receptor blockade has become more prevalent during the last 4 to 5 years. These proliferation signal inhibitors, sirolimus and everolimus, block the activation of the T cell via the engagement of the IL-2 receptor. They have shown promise in significantly reducing the severity of cardiac allograft vasculopathy, the main threat of long-term graft survival. But they remain only a compliment to the calcineurin inhibitors that are still more effective in preventing acute rejection.

Outcomes

The registry of the International Society for Heart and Lung Transplantation (ISHLT) has reported on survival after cardiac transplantation in adult patients transplanted from 2004 to 2008, with survival rates of 85% to 89% at 1 year [29]. The UNOS/OPTN (Organ Procurement and Transplantation Network) database also report survival rates at 1 year of 87.7%. These data were from patients transplanted from 1997 to 2004 [2].

Over the years, the average survival rate for cardiac transplant patients improves. The median survival in patients who were transplanted between 1982 and 1988 was 8.1 years, and that has increased to 9.8 years for individuals transplanted between 1994 and 1998. A significant improvement that has occurred during the current era is the 1-year survival for cardiac retransplantation, which is markedly better than that reported in past eras. The 1-year survival for these patients is 82.4% [2].

TABLE 183.2

BALANCED TRIPLE-DRUG IMMUNOSUPPRESSION PROTOCOL[a]

Drug	Perioperative	Maintenance	Taper	Maintenance	Withdrawal
Corticosteroids					
Methylprednisolone	10 mg/kg intraoperatively or perioperatively; 125 mg IV q8 h three doses postoperatively				
Prednisone	0.5 mg/kg IV/PO qd in two divided doses	0.5 mg/kg IV/PO qd in two divided doses	Decrease dose by 5 mg/d until total daily dose is 0.3 mg/kg/d	1st mo: 0.3 mg/kg/d 2nd mo: 0.2 mg/kg/d 3rd mo: 0.1 mg/kg/d 4th mo: 0.05 mg/kg/d (or 2.5 mg PO qd)	5th mo: total steroid withdrawal (if no rejection for the past 3 mo)
Calcineurin inhibitors					
Tacrolimus	0.05 mg/kg PO preoperatively; 0.1 mg/kg PO qd in two divided doses; dose target levels 0–1 mo, 10–15	Dose target levels 2–6 mo, 10–12 7–12 mo, 10–12 12+ mo, 8–12			
Cyclosporine	2 mg/kg PO preoperatively; 1 mg/kg IV over 24 h., then 3–5 mg/kg PO qd in two divided doses (based on renal function); dose target levels 0–1 mo, 200–250	Dose target levels 2–6 mo, 150–225 7–12 mo, 125–175 12+ mo, 100–125			
Antimetabolite					
Mycophenolate mofetil	1,000 mg PO preoperatively; 2–3 g IV/PO qd in two divided doses; dosage to keep white blood cell count >4.0	2–3 g PO qd in two divided doses			
Azathioprine	34 mg/kg PO preoperatively; 3 mg/kg IV/PO qd postoperatively	1–3 mg/kg PO qd			

[a]Data from Refs. [21–25].
IV, intravenously; PO, orally.

General Complications of Heart Transplantation

Right Heart Failure and Pulmonary Hypertension

Frequently acute right heart failure in the postoperative heart transplant patient is secondary to pulmonary hypertension. As mentioned, patient selection is crucial in identifying those recipients with fixed pulmonary hypertension. Those with a pulmonary vascular resistance ≥4 WU, a systolic pulmonary artery pressure ≥60 mm Hg or a transpulmonary gradient ≥15 mm Hg that does not reverse with vasodilator therapy such as inhaled nitric oxide or a prostacyclin analogue such as epoprostenol should not receive a heart transplant. Despite this, there are still recipients who will have some degree of pulmonary hypertension that will cause right heart strain post-transplantation.

Though right heart failure is frequently accompanied by pulmonary hypertension, other causes include donor selection, poor preservation, or prolonged ischemia time. The main principles of management in all cases of right heart failure are to preserve coronary perfusion, optimize RV preload, and reduce afterload by using high inspired oxygen concentrations, inhaled nitric oxide, and prostacyclin [30]. Intravenous milrinone or dobutamine followed later by oral sildenafil are also mainstays

TABLE 183.3

ISHLT CARDIAC BIOPSY GRADING FOR ACUTE CELLULAR REJECTION

Grade	
0R	No rejection
1R, mild	Interstitial and/or perivascular infiltrate with up to 1 focus of myocyte damage
2R, moderate	Two or more foci of infiltrate with associated myocyte damage
3R	Diffuse infiltrate with multifocal myocyte damage ± edema, ± hemorrhage, ± vasculitis

ISHLT, International Society for Heart and Lung Transplantation.
Data from Stewart S, Winters GL, Fishbein MC, et al: Revision of the 1990 working formulation for the standardization of nomenclature in the diagnosis of heart rejection. *J Heart Lung Transplant* 24:1710, 2005.

of therapy. Finally, in severe cases of right heart failure in the acute postoperative setting, a temporary right ventricular assist device is used to bridge the heart to recovery. The need for mechanical assistance typically lasts only a few days to a week and a low threshold should be kept for implanting a device.

Rejection

Surveillance for rejection in the heart transplant recipient by evaluating endomyocardial biopsies of the right ventricle obtained via the right internal jugular vein is performed frequently during the first year and eventually lessens to two to three times per year. There are four types of rejection: hyperacute, acute cellular, acute humoral, and chronic. The grading scale for rejection was recently revised to simplify it and because there appeared to be little clinical difference between grade 1A and 1B rejection in the old classification and also there was evidence of a benign clinical course for grade 2 rejection in the old classification as well [31]. The new grading system is shown in Table 183.3.

The mainstay of treatment is pulse corticosteroids administered intravenously for 3 days, with or without a subsequent taper. In the case of hemodynamically significant rejection or suspected acute humoral rejection, ultrafiltration, and intravenous immunoglobulin are administered to lower circulating antibodies. The addition of methotrexate or cyclophosphamide also should be considered. Photopheresis has been used to treat patients who have preexistent high levels of PRAs [32]. Late chronic rejection manifests as cardiac allograft vasculopathy, is thought to be due to a combination of humoral and cellular rejection, and is the greatest threat to long-term survival. When a patient has no other options to treat chronic, unrelenting rejection, the last resort is retransplantation.

Infection and Pneumonia

Patients who have undergone thoracic organ transplantation are susceptible to bacterial, fungal, and viral infections. The most morbid viral infection that occurs in thoracic organ transplant recipients is caused by cytomegalovirus (CMV) [33]. Transmission of CMV by a donor organ is very common and hence prophylaxis with ganciclovir is used in CMV-mismatched thoracic transplant recipients. Patients who are seronegative at the time of transplantation and receive a graft from a seropositive donor sustain the highest rate of infection and exhibit the most severe form of CMV disease. Ganciclovir is the treatment of choice.

Pulmonary complications occur in approximately a third of heart transplant recipients [33,34] and is the most common infectious complication in heart transplant recipients. In the first 6 months, hospital acquired bacterial pneumonia is the most common pulmonary complication followed by Aspergillus pneumonia. The overall mortality associated with pneumonia is 35% to 55% and accounts for 40% of all cause mortality. A heightened vigilance for pulmonary infection is critical and the presence of yeast- or mold-positive sputum should be aggressively treated. Risk factors for pulmonary complications are older recipient age, moderate to severe rejection, and development of CMV antigenemia in a previously CMV-seronegative recipient [33].

Coronary Allograft Vasculopathy

The development of coronary allograft vasculopathy can lead to myocardial infarction and sudden death in the cardiac transplant recipient. Routine annual coronary angiography with intravascular ultrasound is performed to permit an accurate assessment of the time of onset and rate of progression of coronary artery disease. Graft atherosclerosis occurs in 30% to 40% of transplant recipients after 3 years and in 40% to 60% of patients by 5 years after transplantation [35]. It remains the major obstacle to long-term survival in cardiac transplant recipients. A correlation between CMV infection and accelerated allograft atherosclerosis has also been identified [36]. Immunologically mediated endothelial damage has been proposed as a stimulus for the development of graft atherosclerosis. Treatment can be temporizing in the form of angioplasty for focal lesions; however, when the disease involves tapering of the distal vessels, only cardiac retransplantation can ultimately treat the problem.

Renal Failure

Renal failure in the perioperative period is often transient, and it may be the direct result of nephrotoxic immunosuppressive drugs. Mild impairment of renal function preoperatively is acceptable as long as the risk of severe renal impairment during the postoperative period is recognized as a possible complication. The lowest acceptable level for creatinine clearance in a potential thoracic organ transplant recipient is 50 mL per minute. For suitable patients, combined heart and kidney transplant can be considered. It is also possible for a patient to be listed for a kidney transplant following thoracic organ transplantation.

Posttransplant Lymphoproliferative Disease

Posttransplant lymphoproliferative disease is a common cause of late death following solid-organ transplantation. It is more commonly seen in the pediatric population and is associated with exposure to the Epstein–Barr virus (EBV). Those at greatest risk for posttransplant lymphoproliferative disease are individuals who are EBV-seronegative before transplant who convert after their transplant. Those individuals who are EBV seropositive before transplant are at a lesser risk but are not risk free. Management includes vigilant monitoring of the patient's EBV status, EBV polymerase chain reaction testing, and regular examinations of lymph node beds for enlargement. Therapy once this problem occurs has not been standardized and runs the gamut of antiviral agents, reduction of immunosuppression, anti-CD20 antibodies (such as rituximab), chemotherapy, and radiation therapy. Many of these have been used in combination.

Gastrointestinal Problems

Approximately 40% of patients experience gastrointestinal complications post-transplant. The majority is related to drug side effects, most notably MMF that can cause nausea, vomiting, and diarrhea [37]. These are most often managed with dose adjustments. Serious complications of the alimentary tract following heart and heart–lung transplantation have been well documented and remain a major source of morbidity and mortality [38]. For that reason, patients with active peptic ulcer disease or diverticular disease are not considered for thoracic organ transplantation, at least until these problems have resolved. Mild liver dysfunction as evidenced by elevation of serum transaminase values and hyperbilirubinemia may occur in patients receiving high doses of cyclosporine. This is a chemical hepatitis that usually responds to a decrease in the dosage. Other immunosuppressants such as azathioprine have been implicated in a similar process. Hepatitis may also be secondary to hepatitis B, CMV, herpes simplex virus, hepatitis A, or hepatitis C.

Biliary tract disease is common in the thoracic organ transplant population. In a series of heart transplant recipients, the incidence of cholelithiasis ranged from 30% to 39%, which is more than twice that expected for age- and gender-matched controls [39]. The primary cause of this problem is thought to be gall bladder stasis and the side effects of specific immunosuppressants [40].

Cardiac Retransplantation

Cardiac retransplantation represents a small fraction of the transplants that are performed annually (the UNOS/OPTN database: 3% to 5% annual retransplant rate) [2]. According to the ISHLT database, approximately 2% of all adult heart transplants internationally are retransplants. In the pediatric heart transplant population, this rate is approximately 6% of all transplants. Current 1-year survival for heart retransplant is 82%, closely approaching the 1-year survival of the original transplant [3]. The primary indications for retransplantation appear to be early graft failure, and in later time periods, chronic rejection or graft atherosclerosis.

HEART–LUNG TRANSPLANTATION

Heart–lung transplants are performed almost exclusively in patients with surgically uncorrectable congenital heart disease and Eisenmenger's physiology [41]. Patients with unrelated severe cardiomyopathy and pulmonary disease may also be candidates for heart–lung transplants. With the difficulty of obtaining a heart–lung block and the outcomes of these procedures, many surgeons repair the congenital heart defect and transplant only the lungs [42]. More and more patients with primary pulmonary hypertension are being treated with bilateral single-lung transplant rather than with heart–lung transplant.

There has been a constant decline in the number of heart–lung transplants performed since the mid-1990s, both nationally and internationally, with fewer than 90 heart–lung transplants being performed annually in the current era [2].

Donor Criteria and Organ Procurement

The donor criteria are similar to the criteria used for heart (as listed previously) and lung transplantation (see Chapter 189). The procurement of the heart–lung block entails simultaneous use of techniques that are otherwise used to procure these same organs separately.

Operative Technique: Heart–Lung Transplant

From the outset, the recipient is placed on cardiopulmonary bypass. The recipient heart is excised first, and then each lung is removed. The phrenic neurovascular bundles are protected bilaterally [39]. The left recurrent laryngeal nerve is also at risk for damage in the region of the ligamentum arteriosum. For that reason, some surgeons leave a portion of the main and left pulmonary artery in situ. The tracheal anastomosis is performed first. Although it can be wrapped with omentum, it does not need to be, because the coronary–bronchial collateral circulation is generally excellent. Performance of the right atrial anastomosis or bicaval anastomoses is followed by the aortic anastomosis. Large aortopulmonary collaterals and bronchial vessels can develop in patients with chronic cyanosis and Eisenmenger's physiology. Extreme care must be taken during the operative procedure in these patients to avoid postoperative bleeding.

Postoperative Care

Postoperative care of patients who have had heart–lung transplantation can be quite complex. Potential complications from the heart or the lungs can arise. The standard postoperative care most closely resembles that of a lung transplant patient, and is discussed in a separate chapter. Postoperative bleeding can be quite profound in this subset of patients, even with careful operative control of collateral vessels.

Outcomes

As of 2009, the current registry reports from ISHLT demonstrate a 1-year survival rate of only 75% for individuals undergoing a heart–lung transplant. The average survival for this group who were transplanted between 1982 and 2003 was 3.2 years. Because of the significant mortality rate that occurred within the first year after the transplant, the conditional half-life was higher at 9 years [27]. Early mortalities were due to technical complications, graft failure, and non-CMV infections accounting for 73% of the deaths. Mortality that occurred beyond the first year was attributed to chronic lung rejection with bronchiolitis obliterans, whereas cardiac rejection or coronary vasculopathy played a minimal role.

In the field of heart–lung transplantation, it was initially thought that endomyocardial biopsy would be the appropriate diagnostic test to detect rejection [43,44]. However, with two organ systems involved, the lungs often reject despite normal findings on endomyocardial biopsy [45]. Transbronchial biopsy reveals what is occurring in the lungs during the perioperative period and, later, complications in the lung grafts may be suggested when there are changes on chest radiograph or in pulmonary function studies, and should be evaluated with transbronchial biopsy [46]. Treatment of recurrent lung rejection consists of pulse corticosteroids with or without a taper. Alternate therapies including lympholytic agents, photopheresis, methotrexate, or cyclophosphamide may be used for refractory cases of rejection [47].

CONCLUSION

The discipline of heart transplantation has recently passed its 40th anniversary, and many major advances have been made.

In spite of the changes that have occurred in recipient criteria, the greater number of potential recipients coming to transplant who are more than 60 years of age, on inotropic support, or using mechanical assist, the outcomes of heart transplantation have improved with each passing year. The field has also enjoyed seeing a decrease in candidate waiting times on the list and the evolution of cardiac assist devices to improve candidates for heart transplant. Clearly, knowledge of cardiac transplant is directly related to the duration of experimental and clinical experience. It is expected that, as understanding continues to expand, long-term survival of transplant recipients will increase.

References

1. Toronto Lung Transplant Group: Unilateral lung transplantation for pulmonary fibrosis. *N Engl J Med* 314:1140, 1986.
2. United Network for Organ Sharing statistics. Available at: http://optn.transplant.hrsa.gov/latestData/step2.asp. Accessed September 19, 2009.
3. Everly M: Cardiac transplantation in the United States: an analysis of the UNOS registry. *Clin Transpl* 35–43, 2008.
4. Mancini DM, Eisen H, Kussmaul W, et al: Value of peak exercise oxygen consumption for optimal timing of cardiac transplantation in ambulatory patients with heart failure. *Circulation* 83:778, 1991.
5. Kao W, Jessup M: Exercise testing and exercise training in patients with congestive heart failure. *J Heart Lung Transplant* 13:S117, 1993.
6. Jimenez J, Edwards L, Jara J, et al: Impact of body mass index on survival following heart transplantation. *J Heart Lung Transplant* 23:S119, 2004.
7. Grady K, White-Williams C, Naftel D, et al: The Cardiac Transplant Research Database (CTRD) Group. Are preoperative obesity and cachexia risk factors for post heart transplant morbidity and mortality: a multi-institutional study of preoperative weight-height indices. *J Heart Lung Transplant* 18:750, 1999.
8. Achuff SC: Clinical evaluation of potential heart transplant recipients, in Baumgartner WA, Reitz BA, Achuff SC (eds): *Heart and Heart-Lung Transplantation*. Philadelphia, PA, WB Saunders, 1990, p 51.
9. Boyle A, Colvin-Adams M: Recipient selection and management. *Semin Thorac Cardiovasc Surg* 16:358, 2004.
10. Miller LW: Listing criteria for cardiac transplantation. *Transplantation* 66:947, 1998.
11. Rose EA, Gelijns AC, Moskowitz AJ, et al: Long-term use of a left ventricular assist device for end-stage heart failure. *N Engl J Med* 345:1435, 2001.
12. Miller LW, Pagani FD, Russell SD, et al: Use of a continuous-flow device in patients awaiting heart transplantation. *N Engl J Med* 357(9):885, 2007.
13. John R, Lietz K, Schuster M, et al: Immunologic sensitization in recipients of left ventricular assist devices. *J Thorac Cardiovasc Surg* 125:578, 2003.
14. Jaski BE, Kim JC, Naftel DC, et al: Cardiac transplant outcomes of patients supported on left ventricular assist device vs. Intravenous inotropic therapy. *J Heart Lung Transplant* 20(4):449, 2001.
15. Radovancevic B, Golino A, Vrtovec B, et al: Is bridging to transplantation with a left ventricular assist device a risk factor for transplant coronary artery disease? *J Heart Lung Transplant* 24(6):703, 2005.
16. Gordon RJ, Quagliarello B, Lowy FD: Ventricular assist device-related infections. *Lancet Infect Dis* 6:426, 2006.
17. John R: Donor management and selection for heart transplantation. *Semin Thorac Cardiovasc Surg* 16:364, 2004.
18. Potapov EV, Ivanitskaia EA, Loebe M, et al: Value of cardiac troponin I and T for selection of heart donors and as predictors of early graft failure. *Transplantation* 71:1394, 2001.
19. Potapov EV, Wagner FD, Loebe M, et al: Elevated donor cardiac troponin T and procalcitonin indicate two independent mechanisms of early graft failure after heart transplantation. *Int J Cardiol* 92:163, 2003.
20. Smith CR: Techniques in cardiac transplantation. *Prog Cardiovasc Dis* 32:383, 1990.
21. Oyer P, Stinson E, Jamieson S, et al: Cyclosporine in cardiac transplantation: a 2 1/2 year follow-up. *Transplant Proc* 15:2546, 1983.
22. Taylor DO, Barr ML, Radovancevic B, et al: A randomized, multicenter comparison of tacrolimus and cyclosporine immunosuppressive regimens in cardiac transplantation: decreased hyperlipidemia and hypertension with tacrolimus. *J Heart Lung Transplant* 18:336, 1999.
23. Reichart B, Meiser B, Vigano M, et al: European multicenter tacrolimus heart pilot study: three year follow-up. *J Heart Lung Transplant* 20:249, 2001.
24. Kobashigawa J, Moriguchi J, Patel J, et al: Five-year results of a randomized single center study of tacrolimus (TAC) vs. microemulsion cyclosporine (CyA) [abstract]. *J Heart Lung Transplant* 23:546, 2004.
25. Kobashigawa JA, Miller LW, Russell SD, et al: Tacrolimus with mycophenolate mofetil (MMF) or sirolimus vs. cyclosporine with MMF in cardiac transplant patients: 1-year report. *Am J Transplant* 6(6):1377, 2006.
26. Kobashigawa J, Miller I, Renlund D, et al: A randomized active-controlled trial of mycophenolate mofetil in heart transplant recipients. Mycophenolate mofetil investigators. *Transplantation* 66:507, 1998.
27. Taylor DO, Edwards LB, Boucek MM, et al: Registry of the International Society for Heart and Lung Transplantation: twenty-second Official Adult Heart Transplant Report—2005. *J Heart Lung Transplant* 24:945, 2005.
28. Baran DA, Zucker MJ, Arrovo LH, et al: Randomized trial of tacrolimus monotherapy: tacrolimus in combination, tacrolimus alone compared (the TICTAC trial). *J Heart Lung Transplant* 26(10):992, 2007.
29. ISHLT Database for North America available at: http://www.ishlt.org/registries/quarterlyDataReportResults.asp?organ=HR&rptType=recip_p_surv&continent=4. Accessed September 22, 2009.
30. Stobierska-Dzierzek B, Awad H, Michler RE: The evolving management of acute right-sided heart failure in cardiac transplant recipients. *J Am Coll Cardiol* 38(4):923, 2001.
31. Stewart S, Winters GL, Fishbein MC, et al: Revision of the 1990 working formulation for the standardization of nomenclature in the diagnosis of heart rejection. *J Heart Lung Transplant* 24:1710, 2005.
32. Sulemanjee NZ, Merla R, Lick SD, et al: The first year post heart transplantation: use of immunosuppressive drugs and early complications. *J Cardiovasc Pharmacol Ther* 13:13, 2008.
33. Atasever A, Bacakoglu F, Uysal FE, et al: Pulmonary complications in heart transplant recipients. *Transplant Proc* 38:1530, 2006.
34. Lenner R, Padilla ML, Teirstein AS, et al: Pulmonary complications in cardiac transplant recipients. *Chest* 120:508, 2001.
35. Hunt SA, Haddad F: The changing face of heart transplantation. *J Am Coll Cardiol* 52:587, 2008.
36. Wang SS: Treatment and prophylaxis of cardiac allograft vasculopathy. *Transplant Proc* 40(8):2609, 2008.
37. Diaz B, Gonzalez Vilchez F, Almenar L, et al: Gastrointestinal complications in heart transplant patients: MITOS study. *Transplant Proc* 39(7):2397, 2007.
38. Kirklin JK, Holm A, Adrete JS, et al: Gastrointestinal complications after cardiac transplantation: potential benefit of early diagnosis and prompt surgical intervention. *Ann Surg* 211:538, 1990.
39. Steck TB, Costanzo-Nordin MR, Keshavarzian A: Prevalence and management of cholelithiasis in heart transplant patients. *J Heart Lung Transplant* 10:1029, 1991.
40. Stief J, Stempfle HU, Gotzberger M, et al: Biliary diseases in heart transplanted patients: a comparison between cyclosporine A versus tacrolimus-based immunosuppression. *Eur J Med Res* 14(5):206, 2009.
41. Spray TL, Huddleston CB: Pediatric lung transplantation, in Patterson GA, Cooper JD (eds): *Lung Transplantation: Chest Surgery Clinics of North America*. Vol 3. Philadelphia, PA, WB Saunders, 1993, p 123.
42. Starnes VA: Heart-lung transplantation: an overview. *Cardiol Clin* 8:159, 1990.
43. Glanville AR, Imoto E, Baldwin JC, et al: The role of right ventricular endomyocardial biopsy in the long-term management of heart-lung transplant recipients. *J Heart Lung Transplant* 6:357, 1987.
44. Griffith BP, Hardesty RL, Trento A, et al: Heart-lung transplantation: lessons learned and future hopes. *Ann Thorac Surg* 43:6, 1987.
45. Starnes VA, Theodore J, Oyer PE, et al: Evaluation of heart-lung transplant recipients with prospective serial transbronchial biopsies and pulmonary function studies. *J Thorac Cardiovasc Surg* 98:683, 1989.
46. Barr M, Meiser B, Eisen H, et al: Photopheresis for the prevention of rejection in cardiac transplantation. Photopheresis Transplantation Study Group. *N Engl J Med* 339:1744, 1998.
47. Glanville A, Baldwin J, Burke C, et al: Obliterative bronchiolitis after heart-lung transplantation: apparent arrest by augmented immunosuppression. *Ann Intern Med* 107:300, 1987.
48. Pagani FD, Miller LW, Russell SD, et al: Extended mechanical circulatory support with a continous-flow rotary left ventricular assist device. *J Am Coll Cardiol* 54(4):312, 2009.
49. John R, Kamdar F, Colvin-Adams M, et al: Improved survival and decreasing incidence of adverse events with the HeartMate II left ventricular assist device as bridge-to-transplant therapy. *Ann Thorac Surg* 86(4):1227, 2008.
50. John R, Kamdar F, Liao K, et al: Low thromboembolic risk for patients with the HeartMate II left ventricular assist device. *J Thorac Cardiovasc Surg* 136(5):1318, 2008.

CHAPTER 184 ■ CARE OF THE PANCREAS TRANSPLANT RECIPIENT

ROBERT M. ESTERL JR, GREGORY A. ABRAHAMIAN, DAVID E.R. SUTHERLAND AND RAJA KANDASWAMY

Type 1 diabetes mellitus has two treatments: (a) exogenous insulin administration or (b) beta cell replacement by pancreas or islet transplantation. The former is burdensome to the patient and gives imperfect glycemic control, predisposing to secondary complications of the eyes, nerves, kidneys, and other systems. The latter, when successful, establishes a constant euglycemic state but requires major surgery—at least for the pancreas transplant—and immunosuppression to prevent rejection, predisposing to complications as well, often compounded by those that are preexisting from diabetes.

The Diabetes Control and Complications Trial [1] showed that intensive insulin therapy (multiple injections per day with doses adjusted by frequent blood sugar determinations) decreased, although rarely normalized, glycosylated hemoglobin levels (HbA1C) and reduced the rate of secondary complications [2]. The threshold for totally eliminating the risks of secondary diabetic complications was perfect glycemic control, an objective that cannot be achieved by even the most sophisticated exogenous insulin-delivery devices available today. Pancreas transplantation induces insulin independence in diabetic recipients without the risk of hypoglycemia and can ameliorate secondary complications. With major advances in the area of management of pancreas transplantation (Table 184.1), the success rate has progressively increased during the past five decades [3]. Today's recipients have a high probability of achieving insulin independence for years, if not indefinitely.

Historically, islet transplants have been less successful than pancreas transplants for a variety of reasons, but the gap is narrowing. In the late 1990s at the University of Alberta, insulin independence was achieved by sequential transplantation of islets from multiple donors and the use of a steroid-free, nondiabetogenic, immunosuppressive regimen [4]. In another series from the University of Minnesota with a similar immunosuppressive regimen, single-donor islet transplants induced insulin independence [5]. In this series, the donors had a high body mass index and the recipients had a low body mass index, so that the net number of islets transplanted per unit weight was similar in the Alberta and Minnesota series. Islet transplants can succeed with strict donor and recipient selection, but are not yet able to supersede pancreas transplants as the mainstay of beta cell replacement. Until islet transplants can consistently succeed from a single donor, regardless of recipient size or insulin requirements, an integrated approach is likely; large donors will be used for islet transplants to recipients with low insulin needs and the remaining donors (the majority) for pancreas transplants to recipients with average- or high-insulin requirements. This strategy will maximize the number of recipients who receive allogeneic beta cells and eliminate surgical complications for at least a subset of patients.

Although short-term islet-graft survival appears promising (even with single donors) [6], long-term graft function after islet transplants (even with multiple donors) continues to be a major impediment to rapid progress. In the University of Alberta series, only 10% of islet transplant recipients were insulin independent at 5 years posttransplant [7].

The main trade-off for recipients of beta cell allografts is the need for immunosuppression. A successful graft makes the recipient euglycemic and normalizes glycosylated hemoglobin levels, but the combined risks of immunosuppression and a major pancreas transplant surgery must be weighed against the long-term risks of imperfect glycemic control with exogenous insulin injection and of development of secondary complications. A randomized prospective trial has not been done to weigh these risks. The burden of daily management of diabetes with the need for multiple sticks to monitor blood sugar levels and to inject insulin tilts the balance in favor of a pancreas or islet transplant for many diabetic patients. Furthermore, antirejection strategies are continually being modified to decrease the complications of immunosuppression. Nevertheless, only a few institutions perform pancreas transplants soon after the onset of diabetic disease [8]; most institutions delay pancreas transplantation until the recipient becomes uremic and needs a kidney transplant.

The main indications for pancreas transplants in patients with normal kidney function are progressive diabetic complications, glycemic lability, and hypoglycemic unawareness, the latter of which may emerge years after the onset of diabetes, particularly in patients with autonomic neuropathy. However, even for nonlabile diabetic patients who attempt tight control by intensive glucose monitoring, the diabetes literature shows a high rate of secondary complications that are just as morbid [9] as complications of chronic immunosuppression in pancreas transplant recipients. Thus, for patients who wish to avoid a lifetime of insulin injections and glucose monitoring and prefer the risks of immunosuppressive complications to the secondary complications of diabetes, a pancreas transplant can be an attractive alternative therapy.

Most pancreas transplant candidates have advanced diabetic nephropathy and require a kidney transplant also. The risks of immunosuppression are already assumed because of the kidney transplant, so a simultaneous or sequential pancreas transplant does not pose significant additional risks other than surgical ones [8]. Although most pancreas transplants are performed in type 1 diabetics with impending or chronic renal failure, some pancreas transplants occur in renal allograft recipients who meet the criteria for type 2 diabetes who want to eliminate the need for exogenous insulin [10].

PANCREAS TRANSPLANT RECIPIENT CATEGORIES

Pancreas transplant candidates are divided into three categories: uremic (need a kidney transplant), posturemic (have a functioning kidney transplant), and nonuremic (do not need a kidney transplant, at least yet). For candidates who are

TABLE 184.1

MAJOR ADVANCES IN THE MANAGEMENT OF PANCREAS TRANSPLANTATION

Topic	Change	References
Organ donation	1) Increased donor pool due to use of organs from donors after cardiac death with comparable graft survival rates to recipients of organs from brain-dead donors 2) Greater application of the expanded donor for pancreas organs	[50,84–90]
Preservation fluids	Improved pancreas preservation fluids/techniques	[92–115]
Pancreas transplant operation	1) Shift from bladder to enteric drainage of pancreatic exocrine secretions 2) Shift from systemic to portal venous drainage 3) Shift toward deceased pancreas transplant after living kidney transplant 4) Increased application of islet cell transplant 5) Increased laparoscopic living donor kidney and segmental pancreas organ procurement	[11,13,14,37,40, 85,124–137]
Immunosuppressive regimens	1) Tacrolimus and mycophenolate mofetil have replaced cyclosporine and azathioprine with improved graft survival 2) Increased use of depleting antibody to encourage innovative immunosuppressive strategies (steroid withdrawal or avoidance, calcineurin withdrawal, monotherapy)	[132–138]

uremic, the options are to receive kidney and pancreas transplants either simultaneously in the same operation or sequentially in separate operations. Which option to take is usually based on the availability and suitability of living and deceased donors for one or both organs at that particular time.

Accordingly, there are three broad categories of pancreas transplants: simultaneous pancreas kidney (SPK) transplant, pancreas after kidney (PAK) transplant, and pancreas transplant alone (PTA).

1. SPK transplants: Most SPK transplants are performed with both organs from the same deceased donor. Because a large number of patients wait on the UNOS list for a kidney organ, unless priority is given to SPK candidates, waiting times tend to be long (years). To avoid two operations and long waiting times, a simultaneous kidney and segmental pancreas transplant from a living donor can be done, but only a few centers offer this option. With successful islet transplantation from a living donor [11], a simultaneous living donor islet-kidney transplant may become a viable option in the future. If a living donor is willing or is medically suitable to give a kidney organ only, another option is a simultaneous living donor kidney and deceased donor pancreas transplant [12]. For this option, the living kidney donor and the recipient must be available at a moment's notice, because the deceased donor pancreas must be transplanted soon after procurement. Alternatively, a recipient of a scheduled living donor kidney transplant could receive a simultaneous deceased donor pancreas organ if it became available fortuitously. If not, and only a living donor kidney is transplanted, the recipient becomes a PAK candidate.
2. PAK transplants: For diabetic patients who have already received a kidney transplant from a living or deceased donor, a PAK transplant can be performed. Most PAK transplants today are performed from a deceased donor in a patient who previously received a living kidney transplant. Although a PAK transplant requires that a uremic diabetic patient undergoes two operations to achieve both a dialysis-free and insulin-independent state, the two transplants done separately are "smaller" procedures than a combined transplant. The time interval between the living donor kidney transplant and the deceased donor pancreas transplant depends on several factors, including recipient recovery from the kidney transplant and donor availability, but the outcomes are similar for all time intervals greater than 1 month duration. Because of the lack of priority of patients who wait for a SPK versus a kidney alone, the PAK is now becoming the most popular pancreas transplant category at many institutions [13,14].
3. PTA: For recipients with adequate kidney function, a solitary pancreas transplant can be performed from either a living or deceased donor. Because the waiting time for a solitary deceased pancreas is relatively short at the present time, living donor solitary pancreas transplants are done infrequently, but are typically indicated if a candidate has a high panel-reactive antibody and a negative cross-match to a living donor. PTA candidates have problems with glycemic control, hypoglycemic unawareness, and frequent insulin reactions but fairly normal renal function. A successful PTA not only obviates these problems, but also probably improves the quality of life, and may ameliorate secondary diabetic complications, thus increasing the applicability of PTA [13–15].

Although the numbers of SPK transplants have remained fairly constant for nearly two decades, the numbers of solitary pancreas transplants (PAK and PTA) have nearly quadrupled [16]. From 2004 to 2008, the most common category of pancreas transplant was the SPK (73%), followed by the PAK (19%) and the PTA (9%); in the PAK category, 76% of the kidney organs came from living donors [3]. Although rare, pancreas transplants can also occur as multiorgan transplants in patients with unique medical problems [17].

HISTORICAL PERSPECTIVES, EVOLUTION, AND IMPROVEMENTS IN PANCREAS TRANSPLANTS

The first clinical pancreas transplant was performed at the University of Minnesota in 1966 [18]. The number of transplants remained low during the 1970s, but progressively increased in the 1980s, due to the introduction of cyclosporine.

By the end of 2008, more than 30,000 pancreas transplants were reported to the International Pancreas Transplant Registry (IPTR) from more than 1,000 centers worldwide, including more that 22,000 in the United States and more than 8,000 outside the United States [3]. In 2010 more than 3,700 patients wait for a pancreas transplant on the UNOS list, and more than 1,200 pancreas transplants have been done annually in the United States [17].

The early history of pancreas transplants involved various surgical techniques, many of which were developed to manage pancreatic exocrine drainage [19]. The first clinical pancreas transplant was performed by Kelly et al. as a duct-ligated, segmental graft at the University of Minnesota in December 1966 [18,20]. In 1973, Lillehei described a series of 13 pancreas transplants at the University of Minnesota where he used enteric drainage (ED) of pancreatic secretions via a cutaneous duodenostomy and a roux-en-y-duodenojejunostomy [20,21]. In the 1970s, Gliedman reported the first segmental pancreas transplant (and then a series of 11 pancreas transplants) with a pancreatic duct–ureter anastomosis for exocrine drainage [20–23]. This technique did not have widespread popularity because of leakage from the pancreatic duct–ureter anastomosis and the cut surface of the pancreas [20].

From the mid-1970s to mid-1980s, segmental pancreas transplants predominated due to a historical belief that the pancreas organ was less antigenic than the duodenal stump [20,21]. With segmental pancreas transplants, two techniques were popularized to manage pancreatic exocrine secretion, including open intraperitoneal drainage by Bewick in 1976 and the University of Minnesota in 1978 [20,24] and synthetic polymer pancreatic duct injection by Dubernard in 1978 [20,25]. In 1983, Sollinger reported the use of direct bladder drainage (BD) to manage pancreatic exocrine secretions in a segmental pancreas graft [26], and the next year he described a series of 10 segmental pancreas transplants with BD that had very few surgical complications, so BD became the predominant technique (Fig. 184.1) [20,27]. In 1982, Groth and Tyden described a segmental pancreas transplant followed by a series of whole-organ pancreas transplants with ED (Fig. 184.2) [28] and this technique ended the predominance of segmental pancreas transplants [20,29].

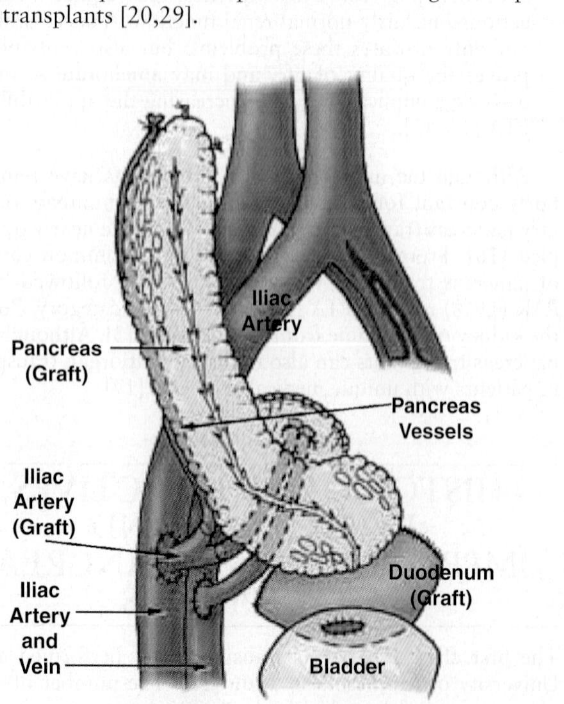

FIGURE 184.1. Bladder-drained pancreaticoduodenal transplant alone from a cadaveric donor.

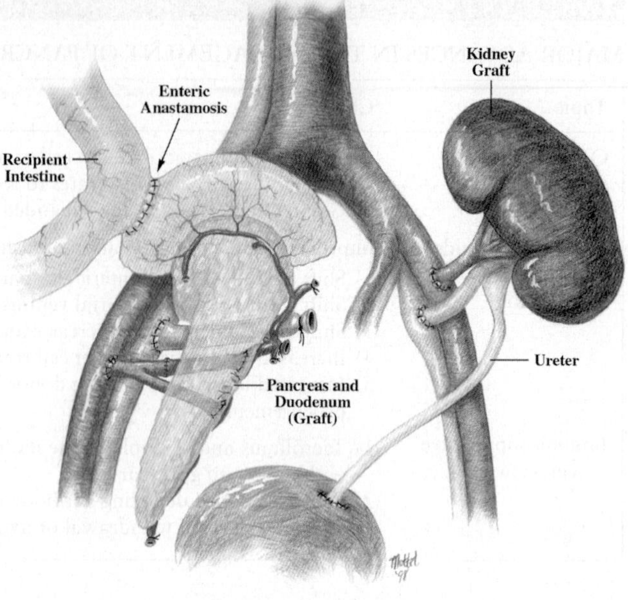

FIGURE 184.2. Enteric-drained simultaneous pancreas and kidney transplant from a cadaveric donor with systemic venous drainage.

In 1987, Nghiem et al. described a whole-organ pancreas transplant with BD via a duodenal stump, a technique that took on widespread acceptance in both Europe and the United States. BD was especially appealing because urinary amylase levels could be tracked to monitor rejection and pancreatitis [20,30]. In mid-1980s, Starzl revived ED of the whole-organ pancreas transplant described by Lellehei 20 years previously [20,31]. In the mid-1980s to the mid-1990s, although BD was popular, urinary complications including cystitis, urethritis, hematuria, metabolic acidosis, and volume depletion led to enteric conversion of whole-organ pancreas transplants in a technique first described by Tom in 1987 [20,32].

Venous drainage of the pancreas has also evolved over the years. Portal drainage was used with segmental grafts in the 1980s [33–36]. In 1989, Mühlbacher described the first case of whole-organ pancreas transplantation with portal venous drainage and exocrine BD [37]. Until 1990s systemic venous drainage had been the norm, until portal drainage gained widespread popularity with ED [38,39] as opposed to BD [37]. By 2004, about 20% of SPK transplants had portal drainage, most commonly to the superior mesenteric vein (Fig. 184.3) and 80% of SPK had ED of pancreatic exocrine secretions [40].

Before standard techniques were developed to procure liver and pancreas grafts with intact blood supplies, segmental pancreas grafts were commonly used. Currently, whole-organ pancreaticoduodenal grafts predominate, although segmental grafts are still used for living donor pancreas transplants. The first living donor pancreas transplant was performed at the University of Minnesota in 1979 [41]. The early series of living donor pancreas transplants consisted of solitary pancreata because the rejection rates for deceased donor pancreata were so high [42]. In the 1990s, living donor pancreas transplants were predominantly performed in combination with a kidney from the same donor (Fig. 184.4) [43–45]. More recently, laparoscopic living donor segmental pancreatectomy has gained popularity [46]. Another approach, as previously mentioned, is to perform a living donor kidney transplant simultaneously with a deceased donor pancreas transplant [12].

Immunosuppressive regimens have made great strides over the years. Most immunosuppressive protocols use antibody

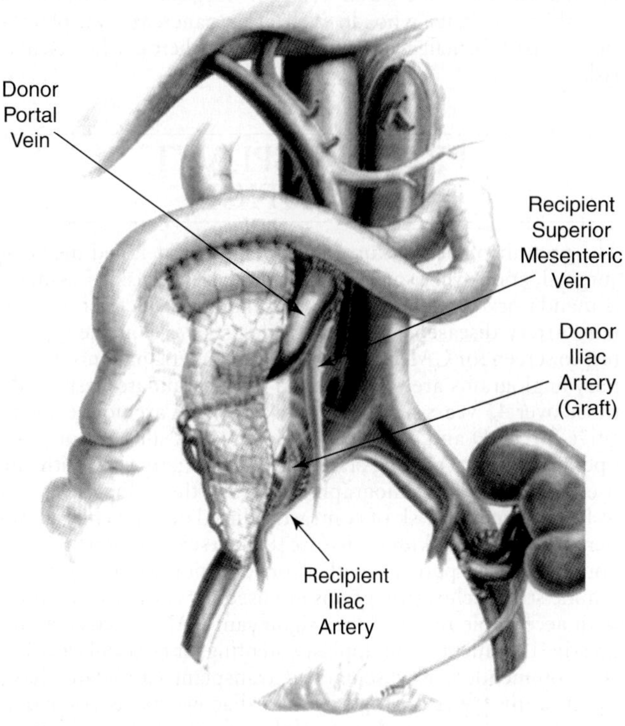

FIGURE 184.3. Enteric-drained simultaneous pancreas and kidney transplants with portal venous drainage of the pancreas graft via the superior mesenteric vein.

induction, followed by maintenance therapy with tacrolimus in combination with mycophenolate mofetil [40]. In the late 1990s and early 2000s some centers such as Northwestern University pushed for steroid-free regimens for pancreas transplants [20]; in fact, of the nearly 25,000 pancreas transplants reported to the IPTR, a third of those in the last 5 years were done with a steroid-free immunosuppressive regimen [20,40]. Today there are more than 140 pancreas transplant centers and 25 islet cell transplant centers in the United States [17]. Some centers have reported extensive experience, including more than 1,000 SPK transplants at the University of

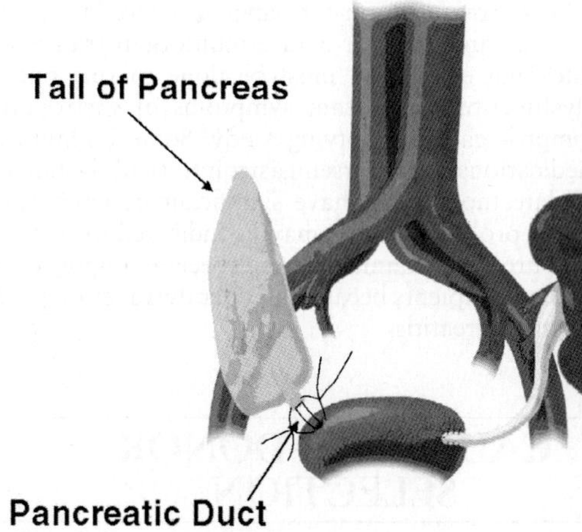

FIGURE 184.4. Simultaneous segmental pancreas and kidney transplant from a living donor. Either bladder- or enteric-drained can be used, but the bladder-drained technique has a lower complication rate and is illustrated.

TABLE 184.2

SUMMARY OF AMERICAN DIABETES ASSOCIATION RECOMMENDATIONS FOR INDICATIONS FOR PANCREAS TRANSPLANTS

Indication for pancreas transplants
1). Imminent or established end-stage renal disease in patients who have had, or plan to have, a kidney transplant
2). History of frequent, acute, and severe metabolic complications (e.g., hypoglycemia, hyperglycemia, ketoacidosis)
3). Incapacitating clinical and emotional problems with exogenous insulin therapy
4). Consistent failure of insulin-based management to prevent acute complications
5). Islet cell transplants hold significant potential advantages over whole-gland transplants but the procedure is experimental and should be performed only within the setting of controlled research studies

Wisconsin [17], and more than 1,900 pancreas transplants of all categories at the University of Minnesota [17]. Since 1980, the IPTR has collected data from all centers in the world [47] and remains an excellent resource for outcome analysis. In addition, the US Transplant Scientific Registry of Transplant Recipients (SRTR), administered through the Arbor Research Collaborative for Health, provides detailed scientific analysis of national, regional, state, and center-specific pancreas graft and patient survival [48].

INDICATIONS AND CONTRAINDICATIONS FOR PANCREAS TRANSPLANTS

The indications for a pancreas transplant have evolved and expanded over the years as the results have improved. The position statement of the American Diabetes Association [49] on indications for a pancreas transplant (Table 184.2) is fairly conservative. A pancreas transplant is also indicated for patients who have developed secondary complications of diabetes including retinopathy, cardiovascular disease, nephropathy, and neuropathy. The progression of many of these complications is halted by a functioning pancreas graft.

With a functioning pancreas transplant improvements with sensory, motor, and autonomic neuropathy and paresthesias have been reported [19,50–55]. Patients with abnormal cardiorespiratory neurologic reflexes have reduced death rates after functioning pancreas transplants [50,56]. There is increased nerve conduction velocity in SPK recipients with functioning pancreas transplants versus those with failed pancreas grafts [51,57,58]. Uremic patients who undergo SPK transplants have improved symptoms of gastroparesis than in patients who have kidney transplants alone [52,59].

Similarly a successful pancreas transplant halts the progression of diabetic changes in the new kidney transplant, and several studies have demonstrated improvement of nephropathy after PTA [50–52]. One study showed that long-term normoglycemia due to a functioning pancreas transplant led to reversal of characteristic diabetic glomerular lesions that occurred in nonuremic PTA recipients who had established nephropathy [52,60]. In addition to improvement in glomerular architecture, this group also showed a reversibility of cortical interstitial expansion and reabsorption of atrophic renal tubules 10 years after PTA [52,61]. These changes in renal architecture may explain the reduction in blood pressure, albuminuria, and nephrotic range proteinuria that some PTA recipients demonstrate [52,62,63], but creatinine clearance can still deteriorate.

Several recent reports have shown stabilization or amelioration of diabetic retinopathy with a functioning pancreas transplant [50–52]. Ramsey et al. reported reduced deterioration in advanced retinopathy with a functioning pancreas transplant at 3 years [52,64]. Wang et al. reported regression of diabetic retinopathy in 43% of SPK recipients versus 23% of kidney transplant alone recipients, although nearly 50% of both groups showed no benefit but follow up was short at 1 year [50,65]. Giannarelli et al. examined 33 type 1 patients who received a pancreas transplant versus 36 type 1 patients who had medical therapy only, and noted that stabilization or amelioration of diabetic retinopathy was 91% versus 43%, respectively [51,66].

Several studies have examined the effects of pancreas transplantation on vasculopathy and cardiovascular risk factors. Severe and advanced vascular disease may be unaffected by a functioning pancreas transplant [50,51]. One series documented improvement in conjunctival microcirculation in 12 SPK patients when compared with five kidney transplant alone recipients [52,67], and other series reported improvement in carotid artery intima-media thickness (which correlates with decreased cardiovascular events) within 2 years of pancreas transplantation [50,52,68,69]. SPK transplants have also shown to improve cardiovascular risk factor profiles, progression of coronary atherosclerotic lesions, left ventricular systolic and diastolic function, and endothelial function [50–52,70–76]. Atherosclerosis regresses in nearly 40% of recipients with a functioning pancreas transplant and this fact may explain improved quality of life and patient survival benefit after pancreas transplantation [50,51,70]. Fiorina et al. demonstrated normalization of left ventricular diastolic function at 4 years after a functioning pancreas graft [50,51,77], which leads to reduction in cardiovascular events [74]. Rates of myocardial infarction and pulmonary edema were lower in SPK recipients than in kidney transplant alone patients, although the kidney alone patients tended to be quite older and the follow up period was short [50,78–80]. Echocardiographic findings 2 years after pancreatic transplantation showed improvement in left ventricular shape and function when compared with kidney transplantation alone. Stabilization [50,56] and even improvement [50,81] in cardiac autonomic dysfunction can occur after pancreas transplantation. A pancreas transplant should really be offered early, before the onset of these complications of diabetes, to interested patients who understand the risks of a significant operation and immunosuppression versus the benefit of insulin independence and freedom from diabetic complications.

Although the most subjective outcome after pancreas transplantation, improved quality of life may be the most important [52]. One study compared the quality of life of diabetic patients who underwent SPK transplants with a kidney transplants alone, and noted that SPK recipients reported improved quality of life in regard to chronic symptoms, effects of kidney disease, cognitive function, pain, physical activity and overall health [82]. Data regarding quality of life in PTA recipients is lacking.

Relative and absolute contraindications include those for any other transplant, such as extremes of age, prohibitive cardiovascular and pulmonary risk, severe hepatic disease, malignancy, active acute and chronic infections, AIDS, severe persistent coagulation disorder, noncompliance, and serious psychosocial problems. Candidates with advanced vascular disease have increased risks of surgical complications, yet, those patients who do well after pancreas transplantation, greatly benefit from stabilization of their cardiovascular risk.

PRETRANSPLANT EVALUATION

The pretransplant workup should include a detailed medical, surgical, and psychosocial evaluation. Cardiac risk assessment is mandatory because diabetes is a major risk factor for coronary artery disease (CAD). Cardiologists vary on the type of test to screen for CAD in pretransplant diabetic patients. Coronary angiograms are performed in most candidates, especially those over 45 years of age. Noninvasive tests are not very sensitive for CAD and are poorly predictive for subsequent postoperative events in long-standing diabetic patients. With the use of iso-osmolar radiographic contrast, there does not seem to be an increased risk of contrast-induced nephropathy in patients with chronic kidney disease [83]. In selected patients (i.e., young, healthy patients with short-duration diabetes) dobutamine stress echocardiograms are used for cardiac evaluation with acceptable results. Once significant CAD is detected, aggressive treatment by angioplasty, stenting, or revascularization is recommended. Revascularized transplant candidates have significantly fewer postoperative cardiac events, as compared with those who received medical therapy alone. The minimum cardiac evaluation should include an ECG, chest radiograph, echocardiogram, and cardiac stress test [50].

A detailed examination must be done to rule out vascular insufficiency in the lower extremities. If such vascular insufficiency is found, it too may need pretransplant correction with angioplasty, endarterectomy, or revascularization, because the transplant operation, often involving an anastomosis to the iliac artery, may further diminish lower extremity blood flow.

Pulmonary function tests are indicated in chronic smokers and patients with a history of chronic pulmonary disease. Postoperative intensive care unit monitoring and perioperative bronchodilator therapy may be indicated in some patients. Liver function tests should be done to rule out hepatic insufficiency and viral hepatitis. The diagnosis of viral hepatitis (especially hepatitis C) is associated with worse long-term outcome after extrahepatic transplantation. Abnormal liver function tests or the diagnosis of viral hepatitis should be followed up with a liver biopsy to rule out cirrhosis. The presence of cirrhosis is a contraindication for pancreas transplant (unless the patient is a candidate for a rare multiorgan transplant). A gastrointestinal evaluation must be done to rule out autonomic dysfunction. Significant symptoms of gastroparesis would prompt a gastric emptying study. Some immunosuppressive medications may worsen gastrointestinal dysfunction (mycophenolate mofetil can have significant gastrointestinal side effects). A prokinetic agent may be indicated to treat gastroparesis. A urologic examination is especially important for bladder-drained recipients because bladder dysfunction predisposes to graft pancreatitis.

CADAVERIC DONOR SELECTION

Pancreas donor selection criteria are not standardized, but instead vary from center to center. Absolute contraindications are the obvious ones applied to most solid organs: active hepatitis

B, hepatitis C (unless the recipient has hepatitis C), human immunodeficiency virus, non-CNS malignancy, surgical or traumatic damage to the pancreas, duodenum or spleen, history of diabetes mellitus, pancreatitis, and extremes of age (less than 10 or more than 60 years). Prolonged intensive care unit stay and duration of brain death have been associated with an increased risk of pancreas graft failure [84]. Other studies have shown that donor age is important. Even middle-aged donors (>45 years old) are associated with pancreas graft failure and increased complications [85–87]. Small donors (<28 kg) have been used for pancreas transplantation with good outcomes [88]. Obesity in the deceased donor is a common cause for refusal of solid-organ pancreas donation, and donors with a BMI >35 kg per m^2 are virtually never used for solid-organ pancreas transplants [50]. Older and obese donors (>50 years old and >30 kg per m^2) are probably more suitable for islet cell than for solid-organ pancreas transplantation [50]. Donors after cardiac death are being used increasingly to expand the donor pool. One survey showed equivalent patient and graft survival at 1, 3, and 5 years in SPK transplant recipients from donors after cardiac death compared with ideal donors after brain death [89]. In general, a pancreas from a so-called marginal donor is associated with good outcome if the pancreas is found to be normal on gross inspection [89,90].

In nearly 3,200 consecutive pancreas donors procured between 2000 and 2005 Vinkers et al. determined the influence of a "preprocurement pancreas suitability" score on the acceptance or refusal of deceased pancreas organs [91]. The investigators assigned a weight for several pre-procurement factors including age, BMI, length of ICU stay, cardiac arrest as cause of death, serum sodium, amylase and lipase levels, and need for vasopressor support to develop a donor score. When the donor score was ≥17, pancreata from these deceased donors were three times more likely to be refused by transplant centers. Donor scoring systems such as this one may provide more objective information about the quality of a deceased pancreas organ to promote wider pancreas donor acceptance.

Pancreas Preservation

University of Wisconsin solution was first used for pancreas preservation in a preclinical model in 1987 [92]. As with most solid organs, in vivo flush followed by simple storage in cold University of Wisconsin solution is still the gold standard for pancreas preservation. In the original canine model, pancreata were preserved for up to 96 hours [93], but in clinical transplantation, pancreas cold preservation exceeding 24 hours has been associated with increased graft dysfunction. Even less than 24 hours, it is evident that the longer the cold ischemia time, the greater the technical complication rate. Therefore, every effort should be made to minimize the cold ischemia time to optimize graft function and to minimize complication rates. The two-layer method (TLM) using University of Wisconsin solution and perfluorochemical [94] has been used in clinical whole pancreas transplantation but more commonly for islet preservation. This method improves pancreas oxygenation, allowing for longer preservation time while providing a mechanism for repair of ischemic damage due to cold storage [95–97]. Some studies show that TLM improves islet yields, islet viability, islet morphology, rates of successful islet isolations and transplants, and islet yields from marginal donors [97–104]. Other studies report that TLM has no effect or is even detrimental for pancreas preservation, and show no difference in islet yields, islet viability or islet transplant outcomes when pancreas organs were preserved with the TLM versus University of Wisconsin solution [97,98,105,106]. More prospective, randomized, controlled trials are needed before the TLM becomes routine procedure.

Three main preservation solutions for pancreas transplantation are available today, including University of Wisconsin solution, Celsior, and histidine–tryptophan–ketoglutarate solution (HTK) [97,98]. HTK has been increasingly used in pancreas transplantation, and its advantages include lower viscosity, less potassium, lower cost and no need for "on-shelf" cold storage, but it requires more solution to flush organs in the multiorgan donor (8 to 12 L of HTK solution vs. 4 to 6 L of Celsior vs. 4 to 6 L of University of Wisconsin solution) [97]. In pancreas transplantation, there have been only one retrospective study [107] and two prospective randomized studies [108,109], which compare University of Wisconsin solution with Celsior and both solutions give similar results. Several reports [110–114] have compared HTK with University of Wisconsin solution and most reports have described equal suitability for perfusion and organ preservation in clinical pancreas transplantation. In an analysis of the UNOS pancreas transplant database from 2004 to 2008, Stewart et al. [115] noted that HTK preservation was associated with a 1.5-fold higher odds of early (<30 days) pancreas graft loss when compared with University of Wisconsin solution, and was independently associated with increased pancreas graft loss in SPK and PTA recipients, especially when cold ischemia times were ≥12 hours. Further prospective, randomized studies will be necessary to determine which perfusion and preservation solution provides the best short-term and long-term pancreas graft survival.

HLA Matching

The impact of HLA matching on outcome varies. HLA matching appears to have little effect on patient, kidney, or pancreas graft survival after SPK transplantation, [116,117], although increased acute rejection rates have been reported with poorer matches [118–120]. For PAK and PTA transplants the data are mixed, ranging from studies showing no impact [121] to registry data showing that higher HLA A and B mismatches are associated with increased immunologic graft loss [117]. Pancreata have been successfully transplanted across rare positive T cell cross-matches, and intravenous immunoglobulin and plasmapheresis have been used to neutralize or eliminate the antibody [50]. A positive T cell cross-match is much more of a risk for immunologic graft loss than is a positive B cell cross-match (especially in a primary pancreas transplant recipient) [50,122].

Anesthetic Considerations in Recipient

A patient with brittle diabetes and secondary complications (e.g., CAD, autonomic neuropathy) can pose special problems for the anesthesiologist. Dysautonomic response to drugs or hypoxia can lead to significant morbidity and even death. It is well documented that long-standing diabetes poses a challenge to the anesthesiologist during intubation. Awareness of these risks and use of an experienced anesthesiology team might help decrease the morbidity and mortality. A major operation such as a pancreas transplant or combined kidney-pancreas transplant is often prolonged and can be associated with significant blood loss. Prompt replacement with blood or colloid solutions should be instituted to avoid hypoperfusion after significant blood loss, because pancreas hypoperfusion can lead to thrombosis. In the intra- and peri-operative period, careful blood glucose monitoring is essential, and continuous intravenous (IV) insulin therapy may be necessary to maintain tight control of blood glucose levels. Blood glucose levels may be high in the immediate postoperative period due to high dose steroids, so continuous IV insulin therapy may be required to control hyperglycemia. Perioperative beta-blockade should be considered for long-standing diabetic patients with a cardiac history.

BACK TABLE PREPARATION OF THE DONOR PANCREAS

Back table preparation of the pancreas organ is necessary before implantation, including these steps:

1. Donor splenectomy (taking care to avoid injury to the pancreatic tail)
2. Shortening the donor duodenum without damage to the main or accessory pancreatic duct (especially important with BD to minimize bicarbonate loss)
3. Ligation of the mesocolic and mesenteric stumps on the anterior aspect of the pancreas
4. Excision of excessive lymphatic and ganglionic tissue in the periportal area
5. Reconstruction of the splenic and superior mesenteric arteries with a donor Y graft including the iliac artery bifurcation (to provide for a single-arterial anastomosis in the recipient)
6. Some mobilization of the portal vein
7. Ligation of the bile duct stump

RECIPIENT OPERATION

Several techniques have been described for the recipient operation [123]. The techniques vary based on whether a solitary pancreas transplant (PTA, PAK) or a combined transplant (SPK) is done. Most SPK transplants are performed through a midline intra-abdominal approach although some are performed through bilateral iliac retroperitoneal incisions.

The major surgical considerations for pancreas transplants include the following:

1. Choice of exocrine secretion of the pancreas, ED versus BD: The 2004 IPTR noted that 81% of SPK, 67% of PAK, and 56% of PTA transplants had ED of pancreatic exocrine secretions [40]. ED is much more physiologic and eliminates the complications of BD (e.g., acidosis, pancreatitis, urinary tract infections, hematuria, urethritis, urinary stricture, urinary disruption). Between 10% and 20% of BD recipients ultimately undergo enteric conversion at 6 to 12 months because of such complications. BD, however, allows for direct measurement of urinary amylase as a marker of exocrine function. A decrease in urinary amylase is sensitive, but not very specific, for acute rejection of the pancreas [40]. Hyperglycemia is a late event in rejection, and a decrease in urinary amylase occurs early in rejection. Thus, rejection episodes may be detected earlier with BD than with ED.

   In clinical practice, the choice of exocrine drainage varies. Some groups always use ED, some always use BD, and others determine the choice of exocrine drainage based on the individual recipient's anatomic constraints and the risk of bowel/urologic complications. Patient and graft survival are similar with both techniques [85,124], but BD is associated with higher rates of urinary tract infections, in addition to urologic and metabolic complications [125,126]. ED is likely to predominate as the major technique in the future, as immunologic strategies to eliminate rejection are further refined. ED usually occurs as an anastomosis between the donor duodenal stump and the recipient proximal jejunum, but graft placement behind the right colon can allow for direct duodenoduodenostomy [125,127].
2. Choice of venous drainage, portal or systemic: The 2004 IPTR reported that in enteric-drained pancreas transplants, 20% of SPK, 23% of PAK, and 35% of PTA cases had venous drainage to the portal vein [40]. Portal drainage is more physiologic than systemic drainage. Theoretically, portal drainage preserves the first-pass metabolism of insulin in the liver. Therefore, pancreas recipients with portal venous drainage will have lower systemic insulin levels than recipients with systemic venous drainage. In one study [128] that compared portal with systemic venous drainage in SPK recipients, there were no significant differences in patient, kidney or pancreas allograft survival rates or early graft loss by pancreatitis or thrombosis. There were no significant differences in early endocrine function, although HbA1C was lower at 6 and 12 months in the portal-drained group.

   Portal venous drainage is difficult to perform with BD unless there is a venous extension graft [37]. However, portal venous drainage is likely to increase in popularity, given some reports that rejection rates are lower in this category [124,129]. Recent modifications include a retroperitoneal portal-enteric drainage technique behind the right colon [130].
3. Choice of graft, whole-organ or segmental: Almost all deceased donor pancreas transplants performed today are whole-organ grafts. Segmental grafts have little role to play in this group, except when a rare anatomic abnormality is noted such that the head of the pancreas cannot be used. A rare instance of a split deceased donor pancreas organ transplanted into two different recipients has been described [131]. All living donor pancreas transplants use segmental grafts (body and tail), which are still capable of maintaining normoglycemia in the recipient.

POSTOPERATIVE CARE

After an uncomplicated pancreas transplant, the recipient is transferred to the postanesthesia care unit or the surgical intensive care unit. Centers that have a specialized monitored transplant unit (with central venous and arterial monitoring capabilities) transition the postoperative recipients through the postanesthesia care unit to the transplant unit. Other centers transfer patients directly to the surgical intensive care unit for the first 24 to 48 hours. Care during the first few hours post transplant is similar to care after any major operative procedure. Careful monitoring of vital signs, central venous pressure, oxygen saturation, urine output, and laboratory parameters is crucial. The following factors are unique to pancreas recipients and should be attended to:

1. Blood glucose levels: Any sudden, unexplained increase in blood glucose levels should raise the suspicion of graft thrombosis. An urgent ultrasound must be done to assess blood flow to the graft. Some centers believe that maintenance of tight glucose control (less than 150 mg per dL) using an IV insulin drip is important to "rest" the pancreas in the early postoperative period.

2. Intravascular volume: Because the pancreas is a "low-flow" organ, intravascular volume must be maintained to provide adequate perfusion to the graft. Central venous pressure monitoring is used to monitor intravascular volume status. In some cases, such as patients with depressed cardiac function, pulmonary artery catheter monitoring may be required during the first 24 to 48 hours. If the hypovolemia is associated with low hemoglobin levels, then packed red cell transfusions should be given; otherwise, crystalloid (and sometimes colloid) replacement should be used to treat hypovolemia.
3. Maintenance IV fluid therapy: The choice of IV fluid therapy can be 5% dextrose in 0.45% normal saline, as long as IV insulin is used to maintain tight blood glucose control, or 0.45% normal saline to maintain acceptable urine output. In SPK recipients, whose IV fluid rate is based on urine output, dextrose should be eliminated if the urine output is high (more than 500 mL per hour), because hyperglycemia may cause an osmotic diuresis leading to worsening hypovolemia. Maintenance IV fluid for BD recipients should also include HCO_3 10 mEq per L to account for the excess HCO_3 loss, or sodium lactate can be used as an alternative.
4. Antibiotic therapy: Broad-spectrum antibiotic therapy (with strong Gram-positive and Gram-negative coverage) and antifungal therapy are instituted in the perioperative period. Antiviral prophylaxis is similar to that for other solid organs and is driven by cytomegalovirus (CMV) status.
5. Anticoagulation: At the University of Texas Health Science Center at San Antonio all pancreas recipients receive enteric-coated aspirin 81 mg started on first postoperative day and continued indefinitely. Recipients of solitary pancreas transplants or "high-risk" SPK transplants also receive an intraoperative dose of heparin (2,500 units), followed by a postoperative regimen of low-dose, continuous IV heparin at 300 units per hour for 24 hours, then 400 units per hour for 24 hours, then 500 units per hour for 5 postoperative days, at which time the IV heparin is discontinued and warfarin begins for 6 months. The partial thromboplastin time for heparin and the international normalized ratio for warfarin are not measured because these drugs are "low dose". Our experience is that therapeutic doses of heparin lead to excessive postoperative hemorrhage that requires reduction in heparin dose, and sometimes red cell transfusion or reoperation.

Immunosuppression

Immunosuppression is essential to thwart rejection in all allotransplant recipients. Before the advent of cyclosporine in the early 1980s, dual therapy with azathioprine and prednisone was the mainstay of immunosuppression for pancreas transplants. From the early 1980s to the mid-1990s, cyclosporine was introduced for maintenance therapy and resulted in significant improvement in immunologic outcomes. Since the mid-1990s, tacrolimus and mycophenolate mofetil have replaced cyclosporine and azathioprine as the primary maintenance immunosuppressive medications. In a prospective, randomized, multicenter study of tacrolimus versus cyclosporine in SPK recipients, Saudek et al. noted that 3-year patient and kidney graft survival were comparable but pancreas graft survival was superior in the tacrolimus-treated cohort (89% tacrolimus vs. 74% cyclosporine) [132]. In addition, with antibody induction steroids have been successfully withdrawn or even avoided in some cases [133,134]. The use of rapamycin in combination with tacrolimus has also allowed for steroid withdrawal or avoidance in some pancreas recipients [135,136]. Specific immunosuppressive regimens vary among different transplant programs. The immunosuppressive protocols for pancreas transplantation for the University of Texas Health Science Center at San Antonio in Table 184.3.

Antibody induction has become mainstay protocol for pancreas recipients. The debate continues as to which antibody preparations are best in pancreas transplant recipients [137]. The administration of depleting agents such as rabbit antithymocyte globulin (rATG) or alemtuzumab has increased dramatically in the last few years, while the use of IL-2 inhibitors has decreased, with the rationale that depleting antibodies provide good immunosuppressive coverage for innovative immunosuppressive strategies including steroid withdrawal or avoidance, minimization of calcineurin inhibitors and even monotherapy in pancreas transplant patients [138]. When combined with steroid withdrawal, minimization of calcineurin inhibitors may require prolonged antibody therapy, which may increase the risk of infection [138].

Results

Outcomes after pancreas transplants have consistently improved over the years. The 2008 SRTR report [48] described pancreas transplant graft and patient survival over the decade from 1997 to 2008. Unadjusted graft survival rates for SPK, PAK, and PTA recipients were 84%, 78%, and 75%, respectively, for year 2006, whereas patient survival rates were similar in all 3 groups (SPK 95%, PAK 97%, PTA 98%) [62]. Those recipients who received SPK transplants experienced the best unadjusted long-term graft survival rates: 73% at 5 years and 53% at 10 years. Graft survival rates for PAK and PTA recipients were statistically lower than SPK recipients, with 5-year rates of 54% and 51%, respectively, and 10-year rates of 35% and 26%, respectively.

The latest report from the IPTR [40] focused on United States pancreas transplants from 2000 to 2004, and included more than 3,800 SPK, more than 600 PAK, and 290 PTA cases. One-year patient survival rates for all three categories were more than 95%. One-year pancreas graft survival rates were higher for SPK (85%) than for PAK (78%) and PTA (76%) recipients. Graft loss from rejection at 1 year was low in all three categories (2% SPK, 8% PAK, 10% PTA). In the majority of all transplants, ED was used for duct management, and of the ED transplants, portal venous drainage was used in 25% of cases. Although overall graft function did not vary with ED or BD, the PTA group had a higher immunologic graft loss rate in ED versus BD cases. BD may result in earlier diagnosis of rejection because of the ability to monitor decreased urinary amylase levels as a marker. Nevertheless, the late rejection rate was higher in the PTA than in other categories.

Donor and Recipient Causes of Pancreas Complications

Donor and recipient factors can influence the postoperative course after pancreas transplantation. In a study of 210 SPK transplants between 1995 and 2007, donor-specific risk factors correlating with postoperative pancreas-related complications included donor age, need for vasopressor support, need for preprocurement blood transfusions, and asystolic events >10 minutes [139]. Increasing donor age and BMI were associated with greater need for postoperative interventions. Graft preservation with HTK solution was associated with significantly higher postoperative complications, as was preexisting cardiac disease in the recipient. The choice of immunosuppression had a significant effect on pancreas-related complications,

TABLE 184.3

UNIVERSITY OF TEXAS HEALTH SCIENCE CENTER AT SAN ANTONIO STANDARD IMMUNOSUPPRESSION-PANCREAS PROGRAM

SPK[a]	PAK[b] and PTA[c]	Rejection
Antithymocyte globulin 1.5 mg/kg: Three doses QOD First dose intraoperatively Give methylprednisolone 250 mg before first dose 100 mg before second dose Give premeds before all doses—diphenhydramine and acetaminophen Monitor ALC[d], platelet count	**Antithymocyte globulin** 1.5 mg/kg: Three doses QOD First dose intraoperatively Give methylprednisolone 250 mg before first dose 100 mg before second dose Give premeds before all doses—diphenhydramine and acetaminophen Monitor ALC, platelet count	***Methylprednisolone*** Day 0–4: 1,000 mg IV[h] Resistant rejection ***Antithymocyte globulin*** 1.5 mg/kg IV up to 7 days Give methylprednisolone 250 mg IV before first dose 100 mg before second dose Give premeds before all doses—diphenhydramine and acetaminophen Monitor ALC, platelet count
Tacrolimus 5 mg po[e] b.i.d.[f] Start when creatinine <4 mg/dL If tacrolimus is delayed continue ATG[g] until tacrolimus levels are therapeutic Levels 8–10 ng/mL for 3 mo Then 5–8 ng/mL	*Tacrolimus* 5 mg po b.i.d. Start postoperatively If tacrolimus is delayed continue ATG until tacrolimus levels are therapeutic Levels 8–10 ng/mL for 3 mo Then 5–8 ng/mL	
Mycophenolate 500 mg po b.i.d. until ATG is removed, then 1 g po b.i.d.	*Mycophenolate* 500 mg po b.i.d. until ATG is removed, then 1 g po b.i.d.	

Round up antithymocyte globulin dose to the nearest 25 mg.
ALC Levels: if zero, hold antithymocyte globulin; if 0.1, give half dose antithymocyte globulin; if 0.2 or above, give full dose.
ATG requires "premeds" with methylprednisolone for first three doses, and diphenhydramine and acetaminophen for all doses.
[a]SPK, simultaneous pancreas kidney.
[b]PAK, pancreas after kidney.
[c]PTA, pancreas transplant alone.
[d]ALC, absolute lymphocyte count.
[e]po, orally.
[f]b.i.d., twice daily.
[g]ATG, antithymocyte globulin.
[h]IV, intravenously.

which were greater after induction therapy with rATG versus daclizumab, and maintenance immunosuppression with tacrolimus/rapamycin or cyclosporine/mycophenolate mofetil versus tacrolimus/mycophenolate mofetil. The duration of the pancreas transplant operation and the presence of elevated C reactive protein were associated with significantly more postoperative complications that required interventions. In another study, donor obesity (BMI >30 kg per m^2) was associated with greater risk of graft thrombosis and deep wound infections [140]. Another trial [141] noted that technical failure of the pancreas graft occurred more commonly when (1) the donor BMI was >30 kg per m^2, (2) the cause of donor death was other than trauma, (3) the preservation time was >24 hours, (4). the duct management was ED versus BD, and (5) recipient BMI was >30 kg per m^2. In other study [142], multivariate analysis showed that technical failure of a pancreas transplant appeared to be the most significant risk factor for kidney graft loss. This evidence underscores that careful donor and recipient selection in addition to improved preservation and surgical techniques play important roles to minimize complications after pancreas transplantation [143].

Surgical Complications

Prevention of surgical complications has critical implications not only on pancreas graft and patient survival, but also on financial impact associated with postoperative care. Early diagnosis and management of surgical complications can limit morbidity; delayed diagnosis, and treatment of pancreas complications can lead not only to pancreas graft loss but also kidney graft loss [143,144]. Common surgical complications in pancreas transplants will now be addressed:

1. Hemorrhage: Postoperative hemorrhage is a frequent reason for early re-laparotomy in pancreas transplant recipients. Hemorrhage can occur from the pancreatic parenchyma, from poorly ligated mesenteric or splenic vascular stumps or from the anastomosis in an enteric-drained or bladder-drained pancreas transplant. The incidence of hemorrhage ranges from 6% to 7% [85], and this risk increases with the use of anticoagulation in the immediate postoperative period. Frequent physical examination and monitoring of hemoglobin help to detect early hemorrhage. Heparin may be temporarily suspended to stabilize the patient. Packed cells should be administered if the recipient has symptomatic anemia. If hemorrhage continues, early operative intervention is indicated. If hemorrhage slows down or ceases, heparin should be resumed at a lower rate and judiciously increased as tolerated.
2. Thrombosis: Thrombosis post transplant ranges from 5% to 6% [85], and remains the most common cause of early pancreas graft failure. The risk increases after segmental

pancreas transplantation because of the small caliber of vessels [145]. Most pancreas transplant thromboses are due to technical causes. Diagnosis is suspected by sudden hyperglycemia and confirmed by sonogram, CT angiogram, formal angiogram, or MRI, which reveals pancreas graft thrombosis. Aggressive anticoagulation will not prevent pancreas transplant thrombosis due to technical reasons. A short portal vein requiring an extension graft or atherosclerotic arteries in the pancreas graft increases the risk for thrombosis. In the recipient, a narrow pelvic inlet with a deeply placed, poorly immobilized iliac vein, atherosclerotic disease of the iliac artery, a technically difficult vascular anastomosis, kinking of the vein by the pancreas graft, significant hematoma formation around the vascular anastomosis, hypovolemia, and a hypercoagulable state are some of the factors that increase the risk for thrombosis. The most common form of hypercoagulable state in the Western population is factor V Leiden mutation. Its incidence ranges from 2% to 5% but may be as high as 50% to 60% in patients with a history (self or family) of vascular thrombosis [146]. Other causes of hypercoagulable state include antithrombin III deficiency, protein C or S deficiency, activated protein C resistance and anticardiolipin antibodies [147]. The transplant surgeon must have a high incidence of suspicion of these hypercoagulable states and treat them aggressively to prevent pancreas graft thrombosis. Thrombosis is diagnosed by sudden hyperglycemia and by imaging studies that show nonpatent pancreatic vessels. Thrombosis usually necessitates transplant pancreatectomy.

3. Duodenal stump leaks: The incidence of duodenal stump leaks ranges from 6% to 7% [85]. A leak from the anastomosis of the duodenum stump to the bowel almost always leads to re-laparotomy. Gross peritoneal contamination due to an enteric leak usually necessitates a graft pancreatectomy. The diagnosis is made by elevated pancreatic enzymes in a patient who has clinical signs of acute abdomen. A plain abdominal radiograph may show free air, and an abdominal CT scan may show free air and extravasation of contrast into the free peritoneal cavity. The differential diagnosis is pancreatitis, abdominal infection, or acute severe rejection. A roux-en-Y anastomosis to the duodenal stump may be a preferred technique, if the risk of leak is thought to be increased during the initial pancreas operation. Other novel techniques such as a venting roux-en-Y-pancreatic duodenojejunostomy have been used in selected recipients [148].

   Small duodenal stump leaks in bladder-drained recipients are usually managed nonoperatively with prolonged catheter decompression of the urinary bladder. The diagnosis of duodenal stump leak is made using plain or CT cystography. Large leaks may require operative intervention, including primary repair, enteric conversion, or even transplant pancreatectomy if there is significant compromise of the duodenal stump.
4. Major intra-abdominal infections: The incidence of significant intra-abdominal infections requiring reoperation ranges from 3% to 4% [85]. Performance of the enteric anastomosis with associated contamination predisposes to this higher rate of intra-abdominal infection, where fungal and Gram-negative organisms predominate. With the advent of percutaneous procedures to drain intra-abdominal abscesses, the incidence of reoperations is fast decreasing. If the infection is uncontrolled or widespread, then graft pancreatectomy followed by frequent washouts may be necessary.
5. Renal pedicle torsion: Torsion of the kidney has been reported after SPK transplants [149,150]. The intraperitoneal location of the kidney (allowing for more mobility) predisposes to this complication. Additional risk factors are a long renal pedicle and a marked discrepancy between the length of artery and vein. Prophylactic nephropexy to the anterior or lateral abdominal wall is recommended with intraperitoneal transplants to avoid this problem. The colon can be mobilized and re-approximated over a kidney transplant in order to prevent torsion also.
6. Others: Other surgical complications that may require re-laparotomy include wound dehiscence, incisional hernia, severe pancreatitis (sometimes hemorrhagic or necrotic), pseudocysts, pseudoaneurysms, arteriovenous (AV) fistula in the graft, severe painful rejection and bowel obstruction [151]. The overall incidence of re-laparotomy for these complications decreased from 32% in the 1980s to 19% in the 1990s, and the mortality rate in recipients requiring re-laparotomy decreased from 9% to 1% over that same period. Improved antibiotic prophylaxis, surgical techniques, immunosuppression, and advances in interventional radiology have all contributed to this decrease [85].

Nonsurgical Complications

1. Pancreatitis: The incidence of posttransplant pancreatitis varies based on the type of exocrine drainage. Bladder-drained recipients with abnormal bladder function are at increased risk of pancreatitis secondary to incomplete bladder emptying and urinary retention causing resistance to flow of pancreatic exocrine secretions. Other causes of pancreatitis include drugs (corticosteroids, azathioprine, cyclosporine), hypercalcemia, viral infections (CMV or hepatitis C), and reperfusion injury after prolonged ischemia. Pancreatitis is usually manifested by an increase in serum amylase and lipase with or without local signs of inflammation. An abdominal ultrasound or CT scan may identify an enlarged, edematous, hypoechoic pancreas transplant. The treatment usually consists of catheter decompression of the bladder for a period of 2 to 6 weeks, depending on the severity of pancreatitis. In addition, octreotide therapy may be used to decrease pancreatic secretions. The underlying urologic problem, if any, should be treated. The patient should be placed on NPO status and total parenteral nutrition should be administered if the pancreatitis is severe. If repeated episodes of pancreatitis occur, enteric conversion of a bladder-drained pancreas transplant may be indicated.
2. Rejection: The incidence of acute rejection ranges from 15% to 30% and immunologic graft loss from 2% to 15% for all types of pancreas transplants at 1 year [3]. The diagnosis is usually based on increased serum amylase and lipase levels in all pancreas transplant patients, and decreased urinary amylase levels in bladder-drained recipients. A sustained drop in urinary amylase levels from baseline should prompt a pancreas biopsy to rule out rejection. In enteric-drained recipients, one has to rely on serum amylase and lipase levels only. A rise in serum lipase levels has shown to correlate well with acute rejection in the pancreas transplant. Other signs and symptoms include tenderness over the graft, unexplained fever, and hyperglycemia (which is usually a late finding). Diagnosis of rejection can be suspected by a hypoechoic, enlarged graft by ultrasound or an enlarged, edematous graft by abdominal CT scan. Diagnosis of rejection can be confirmed by a percutaneous pancreas biopsy [152]. In cases in which percutaneous biopsy is not possible due to technical reasons, empiric therapy for rejection may be started. Rarely, open biopsy is indicated, and transcystoscopic biopsy of a bladder-drained pancreas graft, which was used in the past, has been largely abandoned. Finally, in SPK recipients, isolated pancreas transplant rejection portends a worse renal allograft survival than in patients who experience no rejection [153].

3. Others: Other findings include infectious complications such as CMV, extra-abdominal bacterial or fungal infections, posttransplant malignancy such as posttransplant lymphoproliferative disorder, and other rare complications such as graft-versus-host disease. Many catheter infections are due to Gram-positive organisms, with methicillin resistant coagulase negative isolates quite common [154]. The diagnosis and management of these complications is similar to those of other solid-organ transplants.

Radiologic Studies

1. Ultrasonography: This is the most frequent study used in pancreas recipients. Noninvasive, portable, and relatively inexpensive, it provides prompt information regarding blood flow to the pancreas, the presence of arterial or venous stenosis or occlusion, thrombosis, pseudoaneurysms, AV fistulae, resistance to blood flow within the pancreas (suggestive of either rejection or pancreatitis) and peripancreatic fluid collections.
2. CT scan: A CT scan provides more detail of pancreatic and surrounding anatomy. Use of oral, IV, and bladder contrast (in bladder-drained recipients) is recommended. Thus, a CT cystogram can be combined with an abdominal CT scan. A CT scan is frequently used as a guide in pancreas biopsies or in placement of percutaneous drains for intra-abdominal infection.
3. Fluoroscopy: A contrast cystogram can be performed under fluoroscopy and can be used instead of, or in addition to, a CT cystogram to look for a bladder leak. The combination of the tests increases the sensitivity for detecting bladder leaks.
4. Magnetic resonance angiogram (MRA): An MRA is done if vascular abnormalities are suspected on the ultrasound. MRA provides accurate information about pancreatic vascular patency, but it is inferior to standard angiography in providing fine vascular detail.
5. Angiography: This is the gold standard test for evaluating arterial anatomy in and around the pancreas. However, it is rarely employed, except in cases in which angiographic intervention (such as angioplasty, stenting of a stenotic segment, or coiling of an AV fistula or pseudoaneurysm) is planned. Contrast nephropathy is feared in a solitary pancreas recipient with renal dysfunction, and reasonable alternatives (such as ultrasound) are available.

FUTURE DIRECTIONS

In type 1 diabetic patients with kidney dysfunction, an SPK or PAK transplant is the standard of care. A PTA, however, is less common because the long-term risks of diabetes are weighed against the long-term risks of immunosuppression. A successful pancreas transplant can improve existing neuropathy and nephropathy in diabetic recipients and the survival after a solitary pancreas transplant is better than remaining on the waiting list [155]. As the risks of immunosuppression decrease with novel methods of tolerance and immunomodulation, the balance will tilt in favor of an early transplant. The limiting factor will then be the organ shortage, which could be alleviated if xenotransplantation is able to overcome its current barrier of hyperacute rejection.

The application of islet transplants is rapidly growing. Recent successes suggest that islet transplants can provide all the benefits of pancreas transplants without the risks of major operation. Improvements in islet isolation, islet viability, islet functionality, islet implantation, and immunotherapy will improve islet outcomes, so that only one donor will be necessary to achieve insulin independence [156]. Xenotransplantation of islets may be more readily achievable using encapsulation than with other organs. Prolonged diabetes reversal after intraportal xenotransplant in primates has been documented [157] and may pave the way for human xenotransplant trials. Also, stem cells from numerous sources (e.g., bone marrow, adipose, or cord blood) may be manipulated to differentiate into islets in order to provide a rich supply for transplantation, and islet transplants can be combined with immunomodulation and tolerogenic strategies to minimize or eliminate immunosuppression [156]. This combination would provide for minimally invasive islet cell transplants for all type 1 diabetic patients without the need for long-term immunosuppression. The only scenario that would be better would be the thwarting of autoimmunity before the onset of isletitis, thereby preventing type 1 diabetes mellitus in the first place.

References

1. DCCT Research Group Diabetes control and complications trial (DCCT): The effect of intensive diabetes treatment in long term complications in IDDM. *N Engl J Med* 329:977, 1993.
2. DCCT Research Group Lifetime Benefits and Costs of Intensive Therapy as Practiced in the Diabetes Control and Complications Trial. The Diabetes Control and Complications Trial Research Group. *JAMA* 277:372, 1997.
3. Gruessner AC, Sutherland DER: Pancreas transplant outcomes for United States (US) cases reported to the United Network for Organ Sharing (UNOS) and the International Pancreas Transplant Registry (IPTR). *Clin Transplants* 45–56, 2008.
4. Shapiro AM, Lakey JR, Ryan EA, et al: Islet transplantation in seven patients with type 1 diabetes mellitus using a glucocorticoid-free immunosuppressive regimen. *N Engl J Med* 343:230, 2000.
5. Hering BJ, Kandaswamy R, Harmon JV, et al: Insulin independence after single-donor islet transplantation in type 1 diabetes with hOKT3–1 (ala-ala), sirolimus, and tacrolimus therapy. *Am J Transplant* 1:180, 2001.
6. Hering BJ, Kandaswamy R, Ansite JD, et al: Single-donor, marginal-dose islet transplantation in patients with type 1 diabetes. *JAMA* 293:1594, 2005.
7. Ryan EA, Paty BW, Senior PA, et al: Five-year follow-up alter clinical islet transplantation. *Diabetes* 54:2060, 2005.
8. Sutherland DER, Stratta R, Gruessner A: Pancreas transplant outcome by recipient category: single pancreas versus combined kidney-pancreas. *Curr Opin Organ Transplant* 3:231, 1998.
9. Krolewski AS, Warram JH, Freire MB: Epidemiology of late diabetic complications. A basis for the development and evaluation of preventive programs. *Endocrinol Metab Clin North Am* 25:217, 1996.
10. Light JA, Sasaki TM, Currier CB, et al: Successful long-term kidney-pancreas transplants regardless of C- peptide status or race. *Transplantation* 71:152, 2001.
11. Matsumoto S, Okitsu T, Iwanaga Y, et al: Insulin independence of unstable diabetic patient after single living donor islet transplantation. *Transplant Proc* 37:3427, 2005.
12. Farney AC, Cho E, Schweitzer EJ, et al: Simultaneous cadaver pancreas living-donor kidney transplantation: a new approach for the type 1 diabetic uremic patient. *Ann Surg* 232:696, 2000.
13. Gruessner AC, Sutherland DE, Dunn DL, et al: Pancreas after kidney transplants in posturemic patients with type I diabetes mellitus. *J Am Soc Nephrol* 12:2490, 2001.
14. Humar A, Ramcharan T, Kandaswamy R, et al: Pancreas after kidney transplants. *Am J Surg* 182:155, 2001.
15. Sutherland DER, Gruessner RWG, Humar A, et al: Pretransplant immunosuppression for pancreas transplants alone in nonuremic diabetic recipients. *Transplant Proc* 33:1656, 2001.
16. McCullough KP, Keith DS, Meyer KH, et al: Kidney and pancreas transplantation in the United States, 1998–2007: access for patients with diabetes and end-stage renal disease. *Am J Transplant* 9(part 2):894, 2009.

17. US Department of Health and Human Services, OPTN, HRSA website (2010, April). Retrieved on April 22, 2010, from national data from http://optn.transplant.hrsa.gov.
18. Kelly WD, Lillehei RC, Merkel FK: Allotransplantation of the pancreas and duodenum along with the kidney in diabetic nephropathy. *Surgery* 61:827, 1967.
19. Sutherland DER, Groth CG: The history of pancreas transplantation, in Hakim NS, Papalois VE (eds): *History of Organ and Cell Transplantation*. London, Imperial College Press, 2003, p 120.
20. Squifflet JP, Gruessner RWG, Sutherland DER: The history of pancreas transplant: past, resent and future. *Acta Chir Belg* 108:367, 2008.
21. Lillehei RC, Ruiz JO, Aquino C, et al: Transplantation of the pancreas. *Acta Endocrin* 83[Suppl 205]:303, 1976.
22. Gliedman ML, Gold M, Whittaker J: Clinical segmental pancreatic transplantation with ureter-pancreatic duct anastomosis for exocrine drainage. *Surgery* 74:171, 1973.
23. Gold M, Whittaker JR, Veith FJ, et al: Evaluation of ureteral drainage for pancreatic exocrine secretion. *Surg Forum* 23:375, 1972.
24. Sutherland DER, Goetz FC, Najarian JS: Intraperitoneal transplantation of immediately vascularized segmental grafts without duct ligation: A clinical trial. *Transplantation* 28:485, 1979.
25. Dubernard JM, Traeger J, Neyra P, et al: A new method of preparation of segmental pancreatic grafts for transplantation: trials in dogs and in man. *Surgery* 84:633, 1978.
26. Sollinger HW, Kamps D, Cook K: Segmental pancreatic allotransplantation with pancreatico-cystostomy and high-dose cyclosporine and low-dose prednisone. *Transplant Proc* 15:2997, 1983.
27. Sollinger HW, Cook K, Kamps D, et al: Clinical and experimental experience with pancreaticocystostomy for exocrine pancreatic drainage in pancreas transplantation. *Transplant Proc* 16:749, 1984.
28. Groth CG, Collste H, Lundgren G, et al: Successful outcome of segmental human pancreatic transplantation with enteric exocrine diversion after modifications in technique. *Lancet* 2:522, 1982.
29. Tyden G, Tibell A, Sanberg J, et al: Improved results with a simplified technique for pancreatico-duodenal transplantation with enteric exocrine drainage. *Clin Transplant* 10:306, 1996.
30. Nghiem DD, Corry RJ: Technique of simultaneous renal pancreatoduodenal transplantation with urinary drainage of pancreatic secretion. *Am J Surg* 153:405, 1987.
31. Starzl TE, Iwatsuki S, Shaw BW, et al: Pancreaticoduodenal transplantation in humans. *Surg Gynecol Obstet* 159:265, 1984.
32. Tom WM, Murrda R, First MR, et al: Autodigestion of the penis and urethra by activated pancreatic exocrine enzymes. *Surgery* 102:99, 1987.
33. Calne RY: Paratopic segmental pancreas grafting: a technique with portal venous drainage. *Lancet* 1:595, 1984.
34. Gil-Vernet JM, Fernandez-Cruz L, Caralps A, et al: Whole organ and pancreaticoureterostomy in clinical pancreas transplantation. *Transplant Proc* 17:2019, 1985.
35. Sutherland DE, Goetz FC, Moudry KC, et al: Use of recipient mesenteric vessels for revascularization of segmental pancreas grafts: technical and metabolic considerations. *Transplant Proc* 19:2300, 1987.
36. Tyden G, Lundgren G, Ostman J, et al: Grafted pancreas with portal venous drainage. *Lancet* 1:964, 1984.
37. Mühlbacher F, Gnant MF, Auinger M, et al: Pancreatic venous drainage to the portal vein: a new method in human pancreas transplantation. *Transplant Proc* 22:636, 1990.
38. Rosenlof LK, Earnhardt RC, Pruett TL, et al: Pancreas transplantation. An initial experience with systemic and portal drainage of pancreatic allografts. *Ann Surg* 215:586, 1992.
39. Shokouh-Amiri MH, Gaber AO, Gaber LW, et al: Pancreas transplantation with portal venous drainage and enteric exocrine diversion: a new technique. *Transplant Proc* 24:776, 1992.
40. Gruessner AC, Sutherland DE: Pancreas transplant outcomes for United States (US) cases as reported to the United Network for Organ Sharing (UNOS) and the International Pancreas Transplant Registry (IPTR) as of June 2004. *Clin Transplant* 19;433, 2005.
41. Sutherland DE, Goetz FC, Najarian JS: Living-related donor segmental pancreatectomy for transplantation. *Transplant Proc* 12[4, Suppl 2]:19, 1980.
42. Sutherland DE, Gores PF, Farney AC, et al: Evolution of kidney, pancreas, and islet transplantation for patients with diabetes at the University of Minnesota. *Am J Surg* 166:456, 1993.
43. Gruessner RW, Sutherland DE: Simultaneous kidney and segmental pancreas transplants from living related donors—the first two successful cases. *Transplantation* 61:1265, 1996.
44. Sutherland DE, Najarian JS, Gruessner R: Living versus cadaver donor pancreas transplants. *Transplant Proc* 30:2264, 1998.
45. Gruessner RWG, Sutherland DE, Drangstveit MB, et al: Pancreas transplants from living donors: short-and long-term outcome. *Transplant Proc* 33:819, 2001.
46. Gruessner RWG, Kandaswamy R, Denny R: Laparoscopic simultaneous nephrectomy and distal pancreatectomy from a live donor. *J Am Coll Surg* 193:333, 2001.
47. Sutherland DE: International human pancreas and islet transplant registry. *Transplant Proc* 12[4, Suppl 2]229, 1980.
48. US Transplant Scientific Registry of Transplant Recipients (2010, April). Retrieved on April 22, 2010, from http:/www.ustransplant.org.
49. American Diabetes Association: Pancreas transplantation for patients with type 1 diabetes. *Diabetes Care* 27[Suppl 1]:105, 2004.
50. White SA, Shaw JA, Sutherland DER: Pancreas transplantation. *Lancet* 373:1808, 2009.
51. Gremizzi S, Vergani A, Paloschi V, et al: Impact of pancreas transplantation on type 1 diabetes-related complications. *Curr Opin Organ Transplant* 15:119, 2010.
52. Dean PG, Kudva YC, Stegall MD: Long-term benefits of pancreas transplantation. *Curr Opin Organ Transplant* 13:85, 2008.
53. Kennedy WR, Navarro X, Goetz FC, et al: Effects of pancreatic transplantation on diabetic neuropathy. *N Engl J Med* 322:1031, 1990.
54. Navarro X, Sutherland DE, Kennedy WR: Long-term effects of pancreas transplantation on diabetic neuropathy. *Ann Neurol* 42:727, 1997.
55. Allen RD, Al Harbi IS, Morris JG, et al: Diabetic neuropathy after pancreas transplantation: determinants of recovery. *Transplantation* 63:830, 1997.
56. Navarro X, Kennedy WR, Loewenson RB, et al: Influence of pancreas transplantation on cardiorespiratory reflexes, nerve conduction, and mortality in diabetes mellitus. *Diabetes* 39:802, 1990.
57. Solders G, Tyden G, Persson A, et al: Improvement of nerve conduction in diabetic neuropathy. A follow-up study 4 yr after combined pancreatic and renal transplantation. *Diabetes* 41:946, 1992.
58. Martinenghi S, Comi G, Galardi G, et al: Amelioration of nerve conduction velocity following simultaneous kidney/pancreas transplantation is due to the glycemic control provided by the pancreas. *Diabetologia* 40:1110, 1997.
59. Hathaway DK, Abell T, Cardoso S: Improvement in autonomic neuropathy and gastric function following pancreas-kidney versus kidney-alone transplantation and the correlation with quality of life. *Transplantation* 57:816, 1994.
60. Fioretto P, Steffes MW, Sutherland DE: Reversal of lesions of diabetic nephropathy by pancreas transplantation in man. *N Engl J Med* 339:69, 1998.
61. Fioretto P, Sutherland DER, Najarfian B, et al: Remodeling of renal interstitial and tubular lesions in pancreas transplant recipients. *Kidney Int* 69:907, 2006.
62. Copelli A, Giannarelli R, Vistoli F: The beneficial effects of pancreas transplant alone on diabetic nephropathy. *Diabetes Care* 28:1366, 2005.
63. Coppelli A, Giannarelli R, Boggi U: Disappearance of nephrotic syndrome in type 1 diabetic patients following pancreas transplant alone. *Transplantation* 81:1067, 2006.
64. Ramsay RC, Goetz FC, Sutherland DER, et al: Progression of diabetic retinopathy after pancreas transplantation for insulin-dependent diabetes mellitus. *N Engl J Med* 318:208, 1988.
65. Wang Q, Klein R, Moss SE, et al: The influence of combined kidney-pancreas transplantation on the progression of diabetic retinopathy. *Ophthalmology* 101:1071, 1994.
66. Giannarelli R, Coppelli A, Sartini M, et al: Effects of pancreas-kidney transplantation on diabetic retinopathy. *Transpl Int* 18:619, 2005.
67. Cheung AT, Perez RV, Chen PC: Improvements in diabetic microangiopathy after successful simultaneous pancreas-kidney transplantation; a computer-assisted intravital microscopy study on conjunctival microcirculation. *Transplantation* 68:927, 1999.
68. Larsen J, Ratanasuwan T, Burkman T: Carotid intima media thickness is decreased after pancreas transplantation. *Transplantation* 73:936, 2002.
69. Larsen JL, Colling CW, Ratanasuwan T: Pancreas transplantation improves vascular disease in patients with type 1 diabetes. *Diabetes Care* 27:1706, 2004.
70. Jukema JW, Smets YF, van der Pijl JW, et al: Impact of simultaneous pancreas and kidney transplantation on progression of coronary atherosclerosis in patients with end-stage renal disease due to type 1 diabetes. *Diabetes Care* 25:906, 2002.
71. La Rocca E, Fiorina P, Di CV, et al: Cardiovascular outcomes after kidney-pancreas and kidney-alone transplantation. *Kidney Int* 60:1964–1971, 2001.
72. Coppelli A, Giannarelli R, Mariotti R: Pancreas transplant alone determines early improvement of cardiovascular risks factors and cardiac function in type 1 diabetic patients. *Transplantation* 76:974, 2003.
73. Fiorina P, La Rocca E, Venturini M: Effects of kidney-pancreas transplantation on atherosclerotic risk factors and endothelial function in patients with uremia and type 1 diabetes mellitus. *Diabetes* 50:496, 2001.
74. La Rocca E, Fiorina P, di Carlo V, et al: Cardiovascular outcomes after kidney-pancreas and kidney-alone transplantation. *Kidney Int* 60:1964, 2001.
75. Davenport C, Hamid N, O'Sullivan EP, et al: The impact of pancreas and kidney transplant on cardiovascular risk factors (analyzed by mode of immunosuppression and exocrine drainage). *Clin Transplant* 23:616, 2009.
76. Luan FL, Miles CD, Cibrik DM, et al: Impact of simultaneous pancreas and kidney transplantation on cardiovascular risk factors in patients with type 1 diabetes mellitus. *Transplantation* 84:541, 2007.
77. Fiorina P, LaRocca E, Astorri E, et al: Reversal of left ventricular diastolic dysfunction after kidney-pancreas transplantation in type 1 diabetic uremic patients. *Diabetes Care* 23:1804, 2000.

78. La Rocca E, Fiorina P, Astorri E, et al: Patient survival and cardiovascular events after kidney-pancreas transplantation: comparison with kidney transplantation alone in uremic IDDM patients. *Cell Transplant* 9:929, 2000.
79. Gaber AO, Wicks MN, Hathaway DK, et al: Sustained improvements in cardiac geometry and function following kidney-pancreas transplantation. *Cell Transplant* 9:913, 2000.
80. Biesenbach G, Konigsrainer A, Gross C, et al: Progression of macrovascular events is reduced in type 1 diabetic patients after more than 5 years successful combined pancreas-kidney transplant in comparison to kidney transplantation alone. *Transpl Int* 18:1054, 2005.
81. Cashion AK, Hathaway DK, Milstead EJ, et al: Changes in pattern of 24-hr heart rate variability after kidney and kidney–pancreas transplant. *Transplantation* 68:1846, 1999.
82. Ziaja J, Bozek-Pajak D, Kowalik A, et al: Impact of pancreas transplantation on the quality of life of diabetic renal recipients. *Transplant Proc* 41:3156, 2009.
83. Tadros GM, Malik JA, Manske CL, et al: Iso-osmolar radio contrast iodixanol in patients with chronic kidney disease. *J Invasive Cardiol* 17:211, 2005.
84. Douzdjian V, Gugliuzza KG, Fish JC: Multivariate analysis of donor risk factors for pancreas allograft failure after simultaneous pancreas-kidney transplantation. *Surgery* 118:73, 1995.
85. Humar A, Kandaswamy R, Granger DK, et al: Decreased surgical risks of pancreas transplantation in the modern era. *Ann Surg* 231:269, 2000.
86. Humar A, Harmon JV, Gruessner A, et al: Surgical complications requiring early relaparotomy after pancreas transplantation: comparison of the cyclosporine and FK 506 eras. *Transplant Proc* 31:606, 1999.
87. Kapur S, Bonham CA, Dodson SF, et al: Strategies to expand the donor pool for pancreas transplantation. *Transplantation* 67:284, 1999.
88. Illanes HG, Quarin CM, Maurette R, et al: Use of small donors (<28 kg) for pancreas transplantation. *Transplant Proc* 41:2199, 2009.
89. Salvalaggio PR, Davies DB, Fernandez LA, et al: Outcomes of pancreas transplantation in the United Status using cardiac-death donors. *Am J Transplant* 6:1059, 2006.
90. Bonham CA, Kapur S, Dodson SF, et al: Potential use of marginal donors for pancreas transplantation. *Transplant Proc* 31:612, 1999.
91. Vinkers MT, Rahmel AO, Slot MC, et al: Influence of a donor quality score on pancreas transplantation in the Eurotransplant area. *Transplant Proc* 40:1295, 2008.
92. Wahlberg JA, Love R, Landegaard L, et al: 72-hour preservation of the canine pancreas. *Transplantation* 43:5, 1987.
93. Kin S, Stephanian E, Gores P, et al: Successful 96-hr cold-storage preservation of canine pancreas with UW solution containing the thromboxane A2 synthesis inhibitor OKY046. *J Surg Res* 52:577, 1992.
94. Kuroda Y, Kawamura T, Suzuki Y, et al: A new, simple method for cold storage of the pancreas using perfluorochemical. *Transplantation* 46:457, 1988.
95. Fujita H, Kuroda Y, Saitoh Y: The mechanism of action of the two-layer cold storage method in canine pancreas preservation—protection of pancreatic microvascular endothelium. *Kobe J Med Sci* 41:47, 1995.
96. Tanioka Y, Kuroda Y, Saitoh Y: Amelioration of rewarming ischemic injury of the pancreas graft during vascular anastomosis by increasing tissue ATP contents during preservation by the two-layer cold storage method. *Kobe J Med Sci* 40:175, 1994.
97. Baertschiger RM, Berney T, Morel P: Organ preservation in pancreas and islet transplantation. *Curr Opin Organ Transplant* 13:59, 2008.
98. Iwanaga Y, Sutherland DER, Harmon JV, et al: Pancreas preservation for pancreas and islet transplantation. *Curr Opin Organ Transplant* 13:145, 2008.
99. Matsumoto S, Qualley SA, Goel S, et al: Effect of the two-layer (University of Wisconsin solution-perfluorochemical plus O_2) methods of pancreas preservation on human islet isolation as assessed by the Edmonton Isolation Protocol. *Transplantation* 74:1414, 2002.
100. Fraker CA, Alejandro R, Ricordi C: Use of oxygenated perfluorocarbon toward making every pancreas count. *Transplantation* 74:1811, 2002.
101. Tsujimura T, Kuroa Y, Avila JG, et al: Influence of pancreas preservation on human islet isolation outcomes: impact of the two-layer method. *Transplantation* 78:96, 2004.
102. Salehi P, Mirbolooki M, Kin T, et al: Meliorating injury during preservation and isolation of human islets using the two-layer method with perfluorocarbon and UW solution. *Cell Transplant* 15:187, 2006.
103. Zhang G, Matsumoto S, Newman H, et al: Improve islet yields and quality when clinical grade pancreata are preserved by the two-layer method. *Cell Tissue Bank* 7:195, 2006.
104. Ramachandran S, Desai NM, Goers TA, et al: Improved islet yields from pancreas preserved in perfluorocarbon is via inhibition of apoptosis mediated by mitochondrial pathway. *Am J Transplant* 6:1696, 2006.
105. Kin T, Mirbolooki N, Salehi P, et al: Islet isolation and transplantation outcomes of pancreas preserved with University of Wisconsin solution versus two-layer method using preoxygenated fluorocarbon. *Transplantation* 82:1286, 2006.
106. Collaborative Islet Transplant Registry (CITR) Annual Report, Rockville, MD: The EMMES Corp; August 2007.
107. Manrique A, Jimenez C, Herrero ML, et al: Pancreas preservation with University of Wisconsin versus Celsior solutions. *Transplant Proc* 38:2582, 2006.
108. Boggi U, Vistoli F, del Chiaro M, et al: Pancreas preservation with University of Wisconsin and Celsior solutions: a single-center, prospective, randomized pilot study. *Transplantation* 77:1186, 2004.
109. Nicoluzzi J, Macri M, Fukushima J, et al: Celsior versus Wisconsin solution in pancreas transplantation. *Transplant Proc* 40:3305, 2008.
110. Agarwal A, Murdock P, Pescovitz MD, et al: Follow-up experience using histidine—tryptophan–ketoglutarate solution in clinical pancreas transplantation. *Transplant Proc* 37:3523, 2005.
111. Englesbe MJ, Moyer A, Kim DY, et al: Early pancreas transplant outcomes with histidine–tryptophan ketoglutarate preservation: a multicenter study. *Transplantation* 82:136, 2006.
112. Malek PS, Eghtesad B, Shapiro R, et al: Initial experience using histidine-tryptophan ketoglutarate solution in clinical transplantation. *Clin Transplant* 18:661, 2004.
113. Becker T, Ringe B, Nyibata M, et al: Pancreas transplantation with histidine–tryptophan–ketoglutarate (HTK) solution and University of Wisconsin (UW) solution: is there a difference? *J Pancreas* 8:304, 2007.
114. Schneeberger S, Biebl M, Steurer W, et al: A prospective randomized multicenter trial comparing histidine–tryptophan–ketoglutarate versus University of Wisconsin perfusion solution in clinical pancreas transplantation. *Transplant Int* 22:217, 2009.
115. Stewart ZA, Cameron AM, Singer AL, et al: Histidine–tryptophan ketoglutarate (HTK) is associated with reduced graft survival in pancreas transplantation. *Am J Transplant* 9:217, 2009.
116. Mancini MJ, Connors AF Jr, Wang XQ, et al: HLA matching for simultaneous pancreas-kidney transplantation in the United States: a multivariable analysis of the UNOS data. *Clin Nephrol* 57:27, 2002.
117. Gruessner AC, Sutherland DER, Gruessner RWG: Matching in pancreas transplantation-A registry analysis. *Transplant Proc* 33:1665, 2001.
118. Malaise J, Berney T, Morel P, et al: Effect of HLA matching in simultaneous pancreas-kidney transplantation. *Transplant Proc* 37:2846, 2005.
119. Lo A, Stratta RJ, Alloway RR, et al: A multicenter analysis of the significance of HLA matching on outcomes alter kidney-pancreas transplantation. *Transplant Proc* 37:1289, 2005.
120. Berney T, Malaise J, Morel P, et al: Impact of HLA matching on the outcome of simultaneous pancreas-kidney transplantation. *Nephrol Dial Transplant* 20[Suppl 2]:ii48, 2005.
121. Gruber SA, Katz S, Kaplan B, et al: Initial results of solitary pancreas transplants performed without regard to donor/recipient HLA mismatching. *Transplantation* 70:388, 2000.
122. Khwaja K, Wijkstrom M, Gruessner A, et al: Pancreas transplantation in crossmatch-positive recipients. *Clin Transplant* 17:243, 2003.
123. Krishnamurthi V, Philosophe B, Bartlett ST: Pancreas transplantation: contemporary surgical techniques. *Urol Clin North Am* 28:833, 2001.
124. Stratta RJ, Shokouh-Amiri MH, Egidi MF, et al: A prospective comparison of simultaneous kidney-pancreas transplantation with systemic-enteric versus portal-enteric drainage. *Ann Surg* 233:740, 2001.
125. Boggi U, Amorese G, Marchetti P: Surgical techniques for pancreas transplantation. *Curr Opin Organ Transplant* 15:102, 2010.
126. Jimenez-Romero C, Manrique A, Meneu JC, et al: Comparative study of bladder versus enteric drainage in pancreas transplantation. *Transplant Proc* 41:2466, 2009.
127. De Roover A, Coimbra C, Detry O, et al: Pancreas graft drainage in recipient duodenum: preliminary experience. *Transplantation* 84:795, 2007.
128. Quintela J, Aguirrezabalaga J, Alonso A, et al: Portal and systemic venous drainage in pancreas and kidney-pancreas transplantation: early surgical complications and outcomes. *Transplant Proc* 41:2460, 2009.
129. Philosophe B, Farney AC, Schweitzer EJ, et al: Superiority of portal venous drainage over systemic venous drainage in pancreas transplantation: a retrospective study. *Ann Surg* 234:689, 2001.
130. Boggi U, Vistoli F, Signori S, et al: A technique for retroperitoneal pancreas transplantation with portal-enteric drainage. *Transplantation* 79:1137, 2005.
131. Sutherland DER, Morel P, Gruessner RWG: Transplantation of two diabetic patients with one divided cadaver donor pancreas. *Transplant Proc* 22:585, 1990.
132. Saudek F, Malaise J, Boucek P, et al: Efficiency and safety of tacrolimus compared to ciclosporin microemulsion in primary SPK transplantation: 3-year results of the Euro-SPK 001 trail. *Nephrol Dial Transplant* 20[Suppl 2]:3, 2005.
133. Gruessner RWG, Sutherland DER, Parr E, et al: A prospective, randomized, open-label study of steroid withdrawal in pancreas transplantation-A preliminary report with 6-month follow-up. *Transplant Proc* 33:1663, 2001.
134. Kaufman DB, Leventhal JR, Gallon LG, et al: Pancreas transplantation in the prednisone-free era. *Am J Transplant* 3[Suppl 5]:322, 2003.
135. Salazar A, McAlister VC, Kiberd BA, et al: Sirolimus-tacrolimus combination for combined kidney-pancreas transplantation: effect on renal function. *Transplant Proc* 33:1038, 2001.
136. Kaufman DB, Leventhal JR, Koffron AJ, et al: A prospective study of rapid corticosteroid elimination in simultaneous pancreas-kidney

transplantation: comparison of two maintenance immunosuppression protocols: tacrolimus/mycophenolate mofetil versus tacrolimus/sirolimus. *Transplantation* 73:169, 2002.
137. Singh RP, Stratta RJ: Advances in immunosuppression for pancreas transplantation. *Curr Opin Organ Transplant* 13:79, 2008.
138. Stratta RJ, Alloway RR, Lo A, et al: A multicenter trial of two daclizumab dosing strategies versus no antibody induction in simultaneous kidney-pancreas transplantation: interim analysis. *Transplant Proc* 33:1692, 2001.
139. Fellmer PT, Pascher A, Kahl A: Influence of donor- and recipient-specific factors on the postoperative course after combined pancreas-kidney transplantation. *Langenbeck's Archive of Surgery* 395:19, 2010.
140. Humar A, Ramcharan T, Kandaswamy R, et al: The impact of donor obesity on outcomes after cadaveric pancreas transplants. *Am J Transplant* 4:605, 2004.
141. Humar A, Ramcharan T, Kandaswamy R, et al: Technical failures after pancreas transplants: why graft fail and the risk factors-a multivariate analysis. *Transplantation* 78:1188, 2004.
142. Hill M, Barcia R, Dunn T, et al: What happens to the kidney in an SPK when the pancreas fails due to a technical complication? *Clin Transplantation* 22:456, 2008.
143. Troppmann C: Complications after pancreas transplantation. *Curr Opin Organ Transplant* 15:112, 2010.
144. Goodman J, Becker YT: Pancreas surgical complications. *Curr Opin Organ Transplant* 14:85, 2009.
145. Gruessner RWG, Sutherland DER: Simultaneous kidney and segmental pancreas transplants from living related donors-the first two successful cases. *Transplantation* 61:1265, 1996.
146. Wuthrich RP: Factor V Leiden mutation: potential thrombogenic role in renal vein, dialysis graft and transplant vascular thrombosis. *Curr Opin Nephrol Hypertens* 10:409, 2001.
147. Friedman GS, Meier-Kriesche HU, Kaplan B, et al: Hypercoagulable states in renal transplant candidates: impact of anticoagulation upon incidence of renal allograft thrombosis. *Transplantation* 72:1073, 2001.
148. Zibari GB, Aultman DF, Abreo KD, et al: Roux-en-Y venting jejunostomy in pancreatic transplantation: a novel approach to monitor rejection and prevent anastomotic leak. *Clin Transplant* 14:380, 2000.
149. Roza AM, Johnson CP, Adams M: Acute torsion of the renal transplant after combined kidney-pancreas transplant. *Transplantation* 67:486, 1999.
150. West MS, Stevens RB, Metrakos P, et al: Renal pedicle torsion after simultaneous kidney-pancreas transplantation. *J Am Coll Surg* 187:80, 1998.
151. Troppmann C, Gruessner AC, Dunn DL, et al: Surgical complications requiring early re-laparotomy after pancreas transplantation: a multivariate risk factor and economic impact analysis of the cyclosporine era. *Ann Surg* 227:255, 1998.
152. Malek SK, Potdar S, Martin JA, et al: Percutaneous ultrasound-guided pancreas allograft biopsy: a single-center experience. *Transplant Proc* 37:4436, 2005.
153. Kaplan B, West-Thiekle P, Herren H, et al: Reported isolated pancreas rejection is associated with poor kidney outcomes in recipients of a simultaneous pancreas kidney transplant. *Transplantation* 86:1229, 2008.
154. Kawecki D, Kwiatkowski A, Michalak G, et al: Etiological agents of bacteremia in the early period after simultaneous pancreas-kidney transplantation. *Transplant Proc* 41:3151, 2009.
155. Greussner RW, Sutherland DE, Greussner AC: Mortality assessment for pancreas transplants. *Am J Transplant* 4:2018, 2004.
156. Vardanyan M, Parkin E, Gruessner C, et al: Pancreas vs. islet transplantation: a call on the future. *Curr Opin Organ Transplant* 15:124, 2010.
157. Hering BJ, Wijkstrom M, Graham ML, et al: Prolonged diabetes reversal after intraportal xenotransplantation of wild-type porcine islets in immunosuppressed nonhuman primates. *Nat Med* 12:301, 2006.

CHAPTER 185 ■ MANAGEMENT OF THE ORGAN DONOR

CHRISTOPH TROPPMANN

In 2009, nearly 10,000 patients on the national organ transplant waiting list in the United States died or were de-listed because they had become too ill before a suitable donor organ became available [1]. Almost assuredly, this number underestimates the actual magnitude of the problem. Many patients with end-stage organ failure are currently not even considered for transplantation (and consequently are not listed) because of the strict recipient selection criteria that are being applied—in part as a result of the severe, ongoing organ shortage. The widening gap between available deceased donor organs and the number of patients waiting is a result of the explosive, increased use of organ transplantation therapy over the past 30 years (Tables 185.1 and 185.2), with which the deceased donor pool has not kept pace [1,2] (Fig. 185.1).

The single most important factor that has been identified in this equation is the failure to maximize the conversion of potential deceased donors to actual donors, primarily because of the inability to obtain consent for organ retrieval. The rates of consent granted by families of potential deceased donors range from 0% to 75% and appear to vary widely among geographic regions and ethnic groups [10–12]. The national average is only 54% [12]. Lack of dissemination and poor presentation of information to the public, misperceptions in the general population regarding the beneficial nature of organ transplantation and the necessity of organ retrieval from deceased donors, and inappropriate coordination of the approach to families of potential donors contribute to the stagnation of the organ supply [11–13].

The role of physicians who care for critically ill patients in altering the current situation is crucial. It is their responsibility to seek early referral to an organ procurement organization (OPO) and to ensure that families are adequately approached, thus laying the foundation for obtaining consent (Table 185.3). In the United States alone, approximately 250,000 additional life years could be saved annually if consent for potential deceased donors could be increased to 100% [14]. Intensive care and emergency medicine physicians are obligated ethically and morally to provide the best possible outcome for a very ill

TABLE 185.1

NUMBER OF SOLID ORGAN TRANSPLANTS FROM DECEASED DONORS PER YEAR IN THE UNITED STATES: 1982 VERSUS 2009

Organ	1982	2009
Kidney	3,681	11,296
Liver	62	6,101
Pancreas	38	1,233
Heart	103	2,211
Heart–lung	8	30
Lung	—[a]	1,659
Intestine	—[a]	178

[a]No lung or intestinal transplants were performed in 1982.
Data from references [1–4].

TABLE 185.2

ONE-YEAR GRAFT SURVIVAL RATES (DECEASED DONORS): 1982 VERSUS 2008

Organ	1982[a] (%)	2008 (%)
Kidney	80	91
Liver	35	82
Pancreas	23	86
Heart	65	87
Lung	—[b]	82
Intestine	—[b]	68

[a]Results without cyclosporin A–based immunosuppression.
[b]No lung or intestinal transplants were performed in 1982.
Data from references [4–8] (1982) and [1,2] (2008).

patient. However, after a potential donor has been identified, they are also obligated to seek the best possible outcome for patients with end-stage failure of a vital organ waiting for a transplant by attempting to ensure that organ donation occurs. It is becoming increasingly evident that implementation of critical pathways and standardized donor management protocols play an important role in this context [15–25].

TABLE 185.3

IDENTIFICATION OF POTENTIAL ORGAN DONORS: GUIDELINES FOR REFERRAL TO THE LOCAL ORGAN PROCUREMENT ORGANIZATION

Clinical triggers	All severely neurologically injured patients on a ventilator with any of the following conditions: Head trauma; Cerebral hemorrhage; Primary brain tumor; Hypoxic insult (including prolonged CPR, near drowning, drug overdose, poisoning, cerebral edema, seizures, and asphyxiation injuries)
Referral guidelines	Refer all patients who meet clinical triggers regardless of age and underlying/associated diagnosis Refer all patients who meet clinical triggers *prior* to approaching the family regarding end-of-life decisions Refer patients prior to brain death evaluation Refer patients if the family raises the subject of donation Coroner case status does *not* constitute an exclusion criterion

DONOR CLASSIFICATION

Brain-Dead Deceased Donors

This is by far the most common donor type (currently 90% of all donors belong in this category) [2]. In most Western developed countries, brain death is legally equated with death. The diagnosis of brain death rests on the irreversibility of the neurologic insult and the absence of clinical evidence of cerebral *and* brainstem function. The details of the clinical examination that is required to unequivocally establish brain death are described later in this chapter. Organ procurement proceeds only after brain death has been diagnosed and death has been declared.

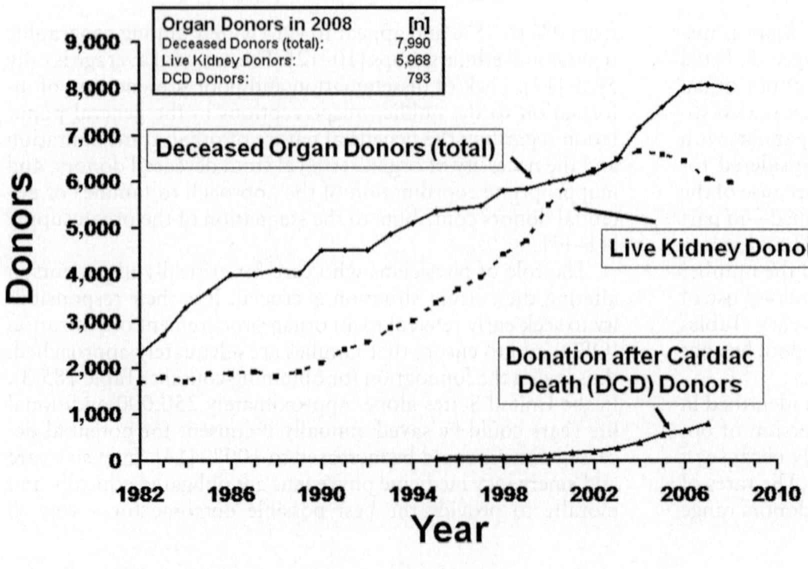

FIGURE 185.1. Evolution of the number of deceased organ donors and living kidney donors between 1982 and 2008 in the United States. (Data from references [1–4,9].)

Donation after Cardiac Death Donors (Formerly Known as Non–Heart-Beating Donors)

Increases in this donor category are to be expected over coming years (Fig. 185.1) [1,2,24,26,27]. Most frequently, families of unconscious patients with severe irreversible traumatic or cerebrovascular brain injury, who do not fulfill the formal criteria of brain death, decide to forgo any further life support treatment and wish to donate the organs of their family member. Time and place of death are therefore controlled. The prospective donor is brought to the operating room and life support treatment is discontinued. Organ procurement is initiated once death has been pronounced by a physician not belonging to the organ recovery and transplant team [26].

An alternative, by far less common scenario—uncontrolled death—involves a patient who expires, for example, in the emergency room following massive trauma or a sudden cardiovascular event. In the interest of minimizing warm ischemia time, flushing cannulas would then have to be inserted and possibly even perfusion of internal organs with cold preservation solution would already have to be started while consent to proceed with organ donation is obtained from the patient's family. Issues that specifically surround this category of donation after cardiac death (DCD) donors have generated considerable debate within the medical community. These issues include ethical concerns centered on when to stop the resuscitation effort and whether it is ethical to perform a procedure (i.e., insertion of flushing cannulas) that presumes consent before actually obtaining it from the family. Other considerations that pertain to both controlled and uncontrolled death DCD donors and that have undergone intense debate, too, include establishing a definition of death after discontinuing life support (there is no commonly accepted definition of, for example, the minimal duration of asystole after the patient expires following withdrawal of support before death can be pronounced; this is currently subject to considerable interinstitutional variation), the possibility of the patient at least temporarily surviving the withdrawal of support systems (backup plans must be clearly defined by each individual institutional DCD donor protocol), and the conflict between providing optimal care for the patient and promoting suitable organ procurement and maintaining donor organ viability [28,29]. Nevertheless, these concerns must be contrasted with the right of self-determination and the final wishes of a competent patient family. Further debate by the medical community and general public is crucial to resolving these complex moral and ethical issues [28,29]. Without such thorough consideration, the deceased donor concept and the donation system that is currently in place might be harmed or discredited.

CURRENT STATUS OF SOLID-ORGAN TRANSPLANTATION

The increased number of solid-organ transplant procedures performed during the last 30 years has been paralleled by a significant improvement in outcome with regard to patient and to allograft survival (Table 185.2). This phenomenon has been attributed to a variety of factors that include (a) the introduction in the early 1980s of the powerful immunosuppressive agent cyclosporin A, followed almost a decade later by tacrolimus, mycophenolate mofetil, and other new immunosuppressants; (b) the availability of antilymphocyte antibody preparations to prevent and treat rejection episodes (e.g., antilymphocyte and antithymocyte globulin); (c) improvements in organ preservation (e.g., use of University of Wisconsin solution); (d) thorough preoperative patient screening for the presence of existing disease processes; and (e) increasing sophistication in the postoperative intensive care of regular as well as high-risk recipients. In addition, the availability of potent, yet nontoxic, antibacterial, antifungal, and antiviral agents has allowed opportunistic infections in immunocompromised transplant patients to be treated more effectively. In combination with refinement of surgical techniques, these factors have led to increasing success of solid-organ replacement therapy.

Thus, transplantation has become the treatment of choice for many patients with end-stage failure of the kidneys, liver, endocrine pancreas, heart, lungs, and small bowel. Successful hand, arm, larynx, and face transplants from deceased donors have also been reported [30–33]. Criteria for potential recipients have been expanded over the past five decades to include infants, children, and individuals previously thought to be at higher risk for complications (e.g., diabetics, elderly patients). Currently, the only patients who are excluded from undergoing transplantation are those with malignancies (metastatic or at high risk for recurrence), uncontrolled infections, those who are unable to withstand major surgery, or those who have a significantly shortened life expectancy due to disease processes unrelated to their organ dysfunction or failure.

Kidney

Currently, patients undergoing kidney transplants from deceased donors exhibit excellent graft survival rates (91% and 68% at 1 and 5 years, respectively) [1,2]. Renal transplantation dramatically improves life expectancy and quality of life, decreases cardiovascular morbidity, and rehabilitates the recipients from a social perspective. Kidney transplants are also less expensive from a socioeconomic standpoint than is chronic hemodialysis. For pediatric patients with chronic renal failure, a functioning renal allograft is the only way to preserve normal growth and ensure adequate central nervous, mental, and motor development.

Liver

Patients with end-stage liver failure die unless they receive a transplant. Liver transplants are an effective treatment for many patients, pediatric and adult, regardless of the cause of liver failure: congenital (i.e., structural or metabolic defects), acquired (i.e., due to infection, trauma, or intoxication), or idiopathic (e.g., cryptogenic cirrhosis, autoimmune hepatitis). A dramatic improvement in graft survival occurred after the introduction of cyclosporin A (Table 185.2). Currently, there are no reliable means to substitute, even temporarily, for a failing liver other than with a transplant. Extracorporeal perfusion, using either animal livers or bioartificial liver devices (e.g., hepatocytes suspended in bioreactors), may someday bridge the gap between complete liver failure and a liver transplant, but these therapeutic modalities are still investigational and are far from becoming standard clinical tools. Use of hepatocyte and stem cell transplants to treat fulminant liver failure and to correct congenital enzyme deficiencies is also in the preliminary stages of study.

Small Bowel

Small bowel transplants are being performed increasingly in patients with congenital or acquired short gut, especially if liver dysfunction occurs because of long-term administration of total parenteral nutrition and if difficulty in establishing or maintaining central venous access occurs. If liver disease is advanced, a combined liver–small bowel or, in highly selected cases, a multivisceral transplant (liver, stomach, small bowel, with or without pancreas) can be performed. Current results are encouraging, and a further increase in the number of small bowel and multivisceral transplants can be expected over the next decade [1,2,34].

Pancreas and Islet

Primary prevention of type 1 insulin-dependent diabetes mellitus is not possible at present, but transplantation of the entire pancreas or isolated pancreatic islets can correct the endocrine insufficiency once it occurs. Glucose sensor systems that *continuously* monitor blood sugar levels coupled with real-time command of an insulin delivery system (implantable pump) are not yet available for routine clinical use. Development of bioartificial and hybrid biomechanical insulin-secreting devices is in the experimental stages. The only effective current option to *consistently* restore continuous near-physiologic normoglycemia, however, is a pancreas transplant [35–37]. Good metabolic glycemic control decreases the incidence and severity of secondary diabetic complications (neuropathy, retinopathy, gastropathy and enteropathy, and nephropathy). Most pancreas transplants are performed simultaneously with a kidney transplant in preuremic patients with significant renal dysfunction or in uremic patients with end-stage diabetic nephropathy. Selected nonuremic patients with brittle type 1 diabetes mellitus (with progression of the autonomic neuropathy to the point of hypoglycemic unawareness, and with repetitive episodes of diabetic ketoacidosis) can benefit from a solitary pancreas transplant (without a concomitant kidney transplant) to improve their quality of life and to prevent the manifestation and progression of secondary diabetic complications. Evidence suggests that a successful pancreas transplant can achieve these goals in uremic and in nonuremic recipients and decrease mortality [35]. Islet transplants are undergoing intensive clinical investigation. Results of transplanting alloislets from deceased donors are encouraging in the short term [36]; however, long-term results have been relatively disappointing [37]. Nonetheless, with further progress to be expected, islet transplants may become a routine form of therapy for patients with complicated diabetes within the next 10 years.

Heart

Heart transplants are the treatment of choice for patients with end-stage congenital and acquired parenchymal and vascular diseases and are recommended generally after all conventional medical or surgical options have been exhausted. After a widely publicized start in 1967, poor results were observed over the ensuing decade. In the 1980s, however, the field of cardiac transplantation experienced dramatic growth (Table 185.1) because of significant improvements in outcome, probably most directly related to immunosuppressive therapy and to refinements in diagnosis and treatment of rejection episodes [38]. Mechanical pumps, such as ventricular assist devices or the bioartificial heart, serve only to bridge the time between end-stage cardiac failure and a transplant and are by no means a permanent substitute for the transplant itself.

Heart–Lung and Lung

Heart–lung and lung transplants are effective treatment for patients with advanced pulmonary parenchymal or vascular disease, with or without primary or secondary cardiac involvement. This field has evolved rapidly since the first single-lung transplant with long-term success was performed in 1983 (Table 185.1). The significant increase in lung transplants is mainly due to technical improvements resulting in fewer surgical complications, as well as to the extremely limited availability of heart–lung donors. Previously, many patients with end-stage pulmonary failure would have waited for an appropriate heart–lung donor. Currently, they undergo a single or a bilateral single-lung transplant instead [39]. Bilateral single-lung transplants are specifically indicated in patients with septic lung diseases (e.g., cystic fibrosis, α_1-antitrypsin deficiency) in which the remaining native contralateral lung could cross-contaminate a single transplanted lung. Double en bloc lung transplants have been abandoned because of technical difficulties related to the bronchial anastomotic blood supply. Mechanical ventilation or extracorporeal membrane oxygenation can be used as a temporary bridge to this type of transplant, but use of these modalities does not obviate the need for organ replacement therapy.

CURRENT STATUS OF ORGAN DONATION

The once steady increases in most types of organ transplant procedures have considerably slowed or reached a plateau over the last several years. This is due to an insufficient augmentation of the donor pool (Tables 185.1 and 185.2; Fig. 185.1). The 55-mile-per-hour speed limit, stricter seat belt and helmet laws, and improved trauma care have all had a significant impact on the number of available brain-dead organ donors [1]. As a consequence, substantial nationwide changes in cause-of-death patterns for brain-dead donors were observed between 1988 and 2008. Head trauma deaths decreased from 34% to 16% of total deaths, whereas cerebrovascular deaths increased from 29% to 41% [1,2]. In 2008, the three leading causes of death among brain-dead donors in the United States were cerebrovascular accidents, blunt head injuries, other cardiovascular events (e.g., myocardial infarctions), followed by gunshot or stab wounds, and other miscellaneous causes [1,2].

To improve organ availability in the face of the donor crisis, the United States Department of Health and Human Services (DHHS) launched at the beginning of the new millennium several national Organ Donation and Organ Transplantation Breakthrough Collaborative initiatives [24,26,40,41]. These were designed to develop and share best practices among donor hospitals, organ procurement organizations, and transplant centers throughout the United States. The initiatives called on the participants to reach a 75% conversion rate (the number of actual donors divided by the number of potential donors) and a 3.75 organs-transplanted-per-donor average yield rate [24,26,40,41]. In large part due to these initiatives and other ongoing national efforts, an encouraging increase of the number of deceased donors in the United States has been observed over the past decade (Fig. 185.1) [1,2,24,26]. Most recently, however, the number of organ donors in the United States has begun to stagnate again (Fig. 185.1) [1,2].

A positive trend that has started to take place is the increasing number of DCD donors (Fig. 185.1) [2,24]. These donors constitute currently 10% of the overall deceased donor pool [2]. Further increases over the coming years are to be expected as the overall organ donor shortage will continue to worsen. In DCD donors, refined surgical techniques allow for fast insertion of cannulas and perfusion of vital organs while these are rapidly excised. Innovative approaches, such as withdrawal of care in the ICU (rather than in the operating room), in the presence of the donor's family, may further increase acceptance of DCD donation among potential donors' families and health care personnel [26,29]. Moreover, refinements of organ perfusion and preservation techniques, including maintenance of the DCD donor on extracorporeal membrane oxygenation (ECMO) until organ recovery can occur, and placement of the recovered organs on pulsatile perfusion pumps during the transport and preservation phase, result in less ischemic organ injury, and allow for better organ preservation and increased use of DCD donor organs, too [24,42–44]. Currently, kidneys and livers are the organs most commonly recovered and transplanted from DCD donors [2].

According to estimates, there are at least 10,500 to 13,800 *potential* brain-dead donors in the United States per year [12]. In 2010, however, there were only 7,944 *actual* deceased organ donors in the United States [1]. In a recent study, the overall consent rate (the number of families agreeing to donate divided by the number of families asked to donate) was 54% in the United States, and the overall conversion rate was 42% [12]. The single most important reason for lack of organ retrieval from 45% to 60% of the potential donor pool is the inability to obtain consent [12,24]. Several studies have shown that family refusal to provide consent and the inability to identify, locate, or contact family members to obtain consent within an appropriate time frame are the leading causes for the nonuse of many potential donors [10–13,24]. A public opinion survey showed that 69% of respondents would be very or somewhat willing to donate their organs, and 93% would honor the expressed wishes of a family member [45]. However, only 52% of these individuals had communicated their wishes to their family. Moreover, 37% of respondents did not comprehend that a brain-dead person should be considered dead and unable to recover, and 59% either believed or were unsure whether or not organs can be bought and sold on the "black market." Also, 42% did not realize that organ donation does not cause any financial cost to the family of the deceased in the United States [45].

Correcting these misperceptions and attempting to increase awareness of the importance of organ transplant must remain the focus of public educational campaigns [24,29]. The family's knowledge of the patient's previous wishes is central to decision making [10,11,13]. Such efforts can be successful, especially among minorities, in whom mistrust and the perception of inequitable access to medical care and organ transplant therapy have led to disappointingly low organ donation and recovery rates [24,46]. It is very important that adequate communication, empathy, and an informative, humane approach to the family of the deceased occur to ensure reasonable consideration of donation. Families are more likely to donate if they are approached by an organ procurement organization coordinator, view the requestor as sensitive to their needs, and experience an optimal request pattern [11,13,21,22]. Educational efforts to enhance organ donation must therefore also be directed at health care professionals and medical students, whose views and knowledge of these issues are often inconsistent and limited [29,47]. Physicians, too, need to be better trained to recognize and refer potential organ donors and to not discuss organ donation until a member of the local organ procurement organization has approached their families [11,13,21,22].

OPTIONS TO INCREASE ORGAN AVAILABILITY

Mechanisms that might serve to increase the number of available organs for transplantation include (a) optimization and maximal use of the current actual donor pool; (b) increasing the number of living donor transplants, including the provision of incentives for live donation; (c) use of other unconventional and controversial donor sources, such as anencephalic donors and executed prisoners; and (d) xenotransplants (e.g., use of animal organs as a potentially unlimited supply for transplantation into humans, particularly after genetic engineering) [48]. The first two mechanisms are of current practical interest, whereas the last two are likely to continue to confront critical care and transplant physicians, nurses, and the lay population over the next years in the form of an ongoing, public debate.

Optimal Use of the Current Donor Pool

As a result of the ongoing organ shortage, transplant surgeons have attempted to refine procurement techniques so that maximal use of the available donor pool occurs [49] (Fig. 185.2). For example, currently more than 85% of all deceased donors are multiple-organ donors. On average, more than three organs are recovered and transplanted from each deceased donor [1,2,24,40,41] (Fig. 185.2). Extension of the organ preservation time by a variety of techniques, including new preservation solutions and pulsatile perfusion preservation, has facilitated allocation of organs to geographically distant transplant centers [44].

Marginal donors—elderly patients, patients with a history of hypertension, poisoning victims, patients with significant organ injury (e.g., liver laceration due to blunt injury), or complications of brain death (e.g., hypotension, oliguria or anuria, disseminated intravascular coagulation)—are now used almost routinely for recovery of kidneys and of extrarenal organs [1,2,24]. Procurement techniques also have been adapted to

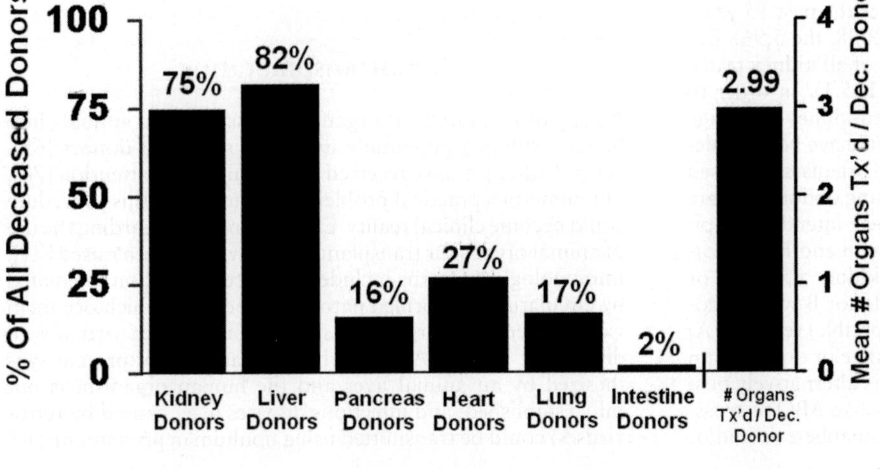

FIGURE 185.2. Organ transplantation rates (by organ) from 8,085 deceased donors (100%) in the United States (2007). The last bar represents the mean number of organs transplanted per deceased donor ("organ yield"). Tx'd, transplanted; Dec., deceased. (Based on data from references [1,2].)

facilitate use of older donors with significant aortic atherosclerosis [50]. Organs with anatomic abnormalities (e.g., multiple renal arteries or ureters, horseshoe kidney, annular pancreas) also are being used routinely. Improvements in operative technique permit the en bloc transplantation of two kidneys from very young donors that would have been too small to be used separately in one recipient [51,52]. Similarly, transplantation of both kidneys from an *adult* donor into one recipient is done to avoid discarding suboptimal kidneys with an insufficient individual nephron mass. To maximize the use of livers, adult donor livers can be split and the two size-reduced grafts transplanted into two recipients (e.g., a pediatric and an adult recipient). A similar principle has also been proposed for the pancreas and has been reported on at least one occasion [53].

Explanted livers from patients undergoing liver transplantation for hepatic metabolic disorders that cause systemic disease without affecting other liver functions (e.g., familial amyloidotic polyneuropathy, hereditary oxalosis) can be used for transplanting other patients ("domino transplant") who are not candidates for deceased livers because of graft shortage (e.g., cirrhotic patients with hepatocellular carcinoma confined to the liver who are not in the group with good expected survival) [54]. The combination of split-liver and domino transplantation can even result in transplantation of three adult patients with one deceased donor graft [55].

The advent of single-lung transplants has made it possible to distribute the heart and lungs of one donor to three recipients. Formerly, transplanting a heart–lung bloc into one recipient was the treatment of choice for end-stage pulmonary disease. If the native heart of a heart–lung recipient is healthy, a domino transplant can be performed: The heart–lung recipient donates his or her heart to another patient in need of a heart transplant. Again, as an attempt to optimize use of scarce donor resources, the reuse of transplanted hearts, kidneys, and livers has been reported [56]. However, all these methods allow only for better use of organs from the existing donor pool. The cornerstone for an effective increase in the number of organ donors remains heightened awareness and education of the public, physicians, and other health care professionals to improve consent and conversion rates [11–13,24,29].

Living Donors

The use of living donors, traditionally limited to kidney transplants, has been expanded to the pancreas, liver, small bowel, and lung [1,2]. In the past, most living donors were genetically related to the recipient—siblings, parents, and adult children. The use of living unrelated kidney donors, who are either emotionally related to the recipient (e.g., spouses, close friends), or emotionally unrelated to the recipient (nondirected, "altruistic" donors) has considerably increased over the past 15 years as a result of the organ shortage [1,2]. In 2008, the 5,968 live donor kidney transplants constituted 34% of all kidney transplants that were done that year [1] (Fig. 185.1). In order to increase that proportion even further, paired-kidney-exchange programs and living donor chain transplants have been implemented [57,58]. In that setting, the supply of organs is increased for instance by exchanging kidneys from living donors who are ABO or cross-match incompatible with their intended recipients, but ABO or cross-match compatible with another donor-recipient pair [donor A would provide a kidney to (ABO or cross-match compatible) recipient B, and donor B would provide a kidney to (ABO or cross-match compatible) recipient A] [57,58]. In cases when paired kidney exchange or donor chain transplants are not available or feasible, it is alternatively possible to precondition the intended recipient of an ABO or cross-match incompatible kidney (by use of plasmapheresis and/or intravenous immunoglobulin and pharmacologic intervention) to still facilitate a successful living donor kidney transplant.

Currently, there is considerable public debate on providing incentives for living kidney donation [59–62]. The debate centers on concerns that reimbursement might lead to the commercialization of organ donation, with the inherent risk of turning potential donors and transplantable organs into a commodity [60–62]. In the United States, those in support of compensating live donors stress that an OPTN-run transparent system of paid living donation would ensure that donors are compensated fairly, eliminate transplant tourism to other countries, greatly diminish the currently existing black market for organs in those countries, and emphasize any potentially interested donor's autonomy—while increasing the organ supply [59,60]. In any case, paid living donation, while a reality in certain regions of the world, remains currently unlawful in the United States and most, if not all, Western Countries.

Even when assuming that (i) public attitudes toward living donation will continue to evolve favorably (Fig. 185.1), (ii) innovative approaches as described above will be increasingly used, and (iii) other alternative means for finding living donors, such as donor solicitation via the internet would ultimately be fully embraced by the transplant community and society, only modest increases of the absolute number of living donors could be expected [60,61,63–66]. Compared with renal transplantation, the proportion of living donor transplants for extrarenal organs is much smaller (less than 5% for liver and less than 0.5% for pancreas, lung, and small bowel) [1]. Thus, living donor transplants will continue to help alleviate the organ shortage for certain organs (kidney, liver) to some extent, but will never be able to completely compensate, even under the best circumstances, for the severe lack of deceased donors.

Other Human Donor Organ Sources

The potential for financial compensation or other rewards for deceased donor families (e.g., compensation for funeral expenses) has been considered as a means to increase donation rates [66].

Certain countries (e.g., China) use organs from executed prisoners. Use of this group would contribute only very small numbers of donors in the United States, and this concept has been rejected by the transplant community here [67]. Likewise, the use of anencephalic babies for solid-organ transplantation would not significantly alleviate the organ shortage because only a few babies fulfill all brain-death criteria. Proposals to use organs from executed prisoners or anencephalic babies would engender a very passionate, emotional debate that could have a negative impact on public opinion and thereby decrease overall organ availability [68]. Therefore, these options are not being actively explored.

Xenotransplantation

Xenotransplantation of organs and tissues from animals into humans offers a potentially unlimited supply of donors [69]. Several attempts have received significant public attention [70], but numerous practical problems remain before this procedure could become clinical reality. Ethical concerns regarding the use of animal organs for transplantation have also been raised [71]. Immunologic concerns include hyperacute rejection (mediated by circulating, preformed natural antibodies), which occurs in vascularized solid-organ transplantation between virtually all discordant species. Also, the biocompatibility of protein synthesized by an animal liver and the human organism is not fully established, and infectious diseases (e.g., caused by retroviruses) could be transmitted using nonhuman primates or pigs as donors. Genetic engineering of animals before their use as donors to overcome the immunologic barriers is an area of intensive investigation. Significant experimental progress in this area could fundamentally change the field of organ transplantation.

Presumed Consent Laws

Presumed consent laws have been implemented in many areas of the world, most notably in several countries in Europe. These laws permit organ procurement unless the potential donor has objected explicitly. A permanently and easily accessible registry of objectors is a prerequisite for such a system. Emphasis is placed on an individual's decision, and family input is limited. In the United States, presumed-consent legislation does not have broad support, and it is uncertain whether the public could reach a consensus on this issue. Moreover, presumed consent would not alleviate the problem of insufficient donor identification and referral [12].

The beneficial impact that such laws can have became evident in Spain. In that country, presumed consent laws coupled with the creation of a decentralized network of mostly hospital-based, specifically trained transplant coordinators (most of them physicians in intensive care units) in the early 1990s led not only to more efficient identification of eligible deceased donors but also to higher consent rates. Accordingly, the annual donation rate in Spain rose from 14.3 donors per million population (pmp) in 1989 to 34.2 pmp in 2008 (United States, 2008: 26.3 pmp) [72–74]. Interestingly, a similar approach (without the presumed consent component) using in-house coordinators at some hospitals the United States did yield greater consent and conversion rates, too, and underscored the advantages that such a system could have, if implemented at a larger scale [75].

REGULATION AND ORGANIZATION OF ORGAN RETRIEVAL AND ALLOCATION

In the early 1980s, the introduction of new immunosuppressive agents engendered a rise in organ transplant activity. Tissue matching (e.g., by use of living-related donor-recipient combinations) became less important, and the use of brain-dead donors increased (Fig. 185.1). In the wake of these developments, consolidation and national regulation of the organ-sharing and allocation organizations, which had previously functioned mainly at a local and regional level, became necessary.

In the United States, the National Organ Transplant Act (NOTA) of 1984 called for a national system to ensure equitable access to transplant therapy for all patients, a major component of which was fair organ allocation. The federal government commissioned a task force on organ transplantation to define such an allocation system. This task force, whose members were appointed by the U.S. Department of Health and Human Services, resolved that human organs are a "national resource to be used for public good" and recommended the creation of a national Organ Procurement and Transplantation Network (OPTN) [3]. In 1986, the U.S. Department of Health and Human Services awarded the OPTN contract to the United Network for Organ Sharing (UNOS). Pursuant to the contract, UNOS was asked to design a network to achieve balance in the goals of equity in organ access and distribution and in optimal medical outcome [76]. In 1986, the Omnibus Budget Reconciliation Act mandated that only hospital members of the OPTN could perform Medicare- and Medicaid-reimbursed transplant procedures. In 1988, the Organ Transplant Amendments reaffirmed the federal interest in equitable organ allocation by locating authority in UNOS as opposed to local transplant organizations.

The national OPTN is currently still operated by the non-profit UNOS and is accountable to the U.S. Department of Health and Human Services. All patients on waiting lists of a transplant program are registered with UNOS, which maintains a centralized computer system linking all OPOs and transplant centers. The United States has been divided into 11 regions for organ procurement, allocation, and sharing purposes (Fig. 185.3). Organs are registered, shared, and allocated through use of the central UNOS computer, which generates a list of recipients for each available organ. Patients awaiting deceased transplantation are ranked according to UNOS policies, based on medical and scientific criteria such as blood type, tissue type, length of time waiting on the list, age (pediatric vs. adult), level of presensitization (percentage of panel reactive antibody), and medical status. National sharing of 0-antigen (A, B, and DR HLA loci) mismatched kidneys is mandated. In

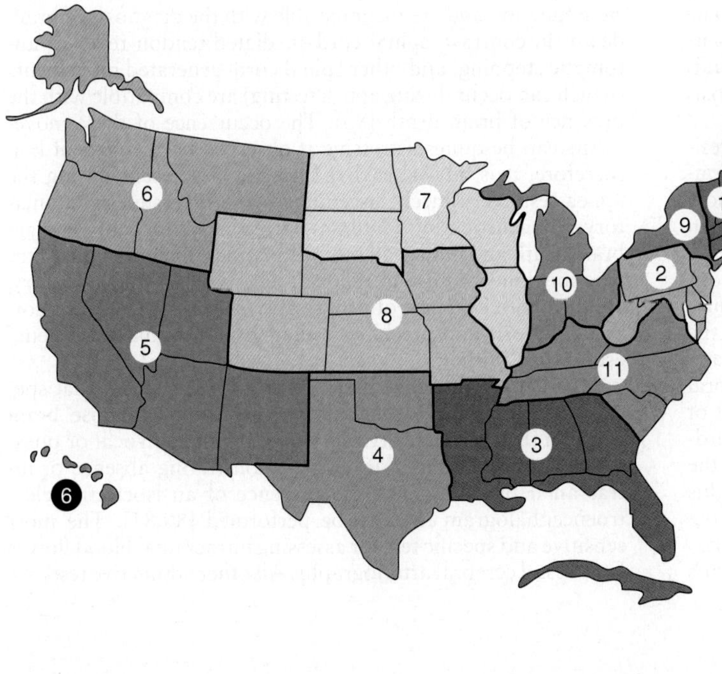

FIGURE 185.3. United Network for Organ Sharing (UNOS) regions in the United States (24-hour access number: 1-800-292-9537). The United States has been divided into 11 regions for organ procurement, allocation, and sharing purposes.

all other cases, and for all other organs, allocation first takes place locally. If no suitable local recipients are available, organs are allocated regionally or nationally [1,76].

LEGAL ASPECTS OF ORGAN DONATION AND BRAIN DEATH

Uniform Anatomical Gift Act

The Uniform Anatomical Gift Act, adopted in 1968 and in force throughout the United States, allows any adult individual (over age 18 years) to donate all or part of the body for transplantation, research, or education. That act provides also the legal basis for procurement of organs from both DCD and brain-dead (vide infra) donors. Explicit consent, which can be revoked at any time, is required. The act also permits legal next of kin to give consent for donation [77]. Donor cards or driver's licenses, on which individuals indicate their consent to postmortem organ donation, are promoted by many states but are legally nonbinding and thus serve ultimately only as a tool to heighten public awareness. In most instances, consent from the next of kin is still sought. Therefore, educational efforts must urge potential donors to make their wishes known to their next of kin [11,13].

Uniform Determination of Death Act

Over the past four decades, brain death has legally become equated with death in most Western developed countries. *Brain death* means that all brain and brainstem function has irreversibly ceased, and circulatory and ventilatory functions are maintained temporarily. The recognition of brain death became possible only after substantial advances in intensive care medicine (e.g., cardiovascular support, prolonged mechanical ventilation). The first classic description of brain death was published in 1959 in France and termed *coma dépassé* (beyond coma). An ad hoc commission of the Harvard Medical School defined brain-death criteria in the United States in 1968 [78]. These criteria were judged by some as being too extensive and too exclusive. In 1981, the President's Commission for the Study of Ethical Problems in Medicine and Biomedical and Behavioral Research formulated the Uniform Determination of Death Act, which established a common ground for statutory and judicial law related to the diagnosis of brain death. The commission stated that "an individual who has sustained... irreversible cessation of all functions of the entire brain, including the brainstem, is dead," and left the criteria for diagnosis to be determined by "accepted medical standards."

Those standards were defined in a related report to the President's Commission on the diagnosis of death by 56 medical consultants in 1981 [79]. The guidelines in that report have now been accepted as the standard for determining brain death in the United States. They are as follows: "Cessation is recognized when (1) all cerebral functions and (2) all brainstem functions are absent. The irreversibility is recognized when (1) the cause of the coma is established and is sufficient to account for the loss of brain functions, (2) the possibility of the recovery of any brain functions is excluded, and (3) the cessation of cerebral and brainstem function persists for an appropriate period of observation and/or trial of therapy" [79]. Confusion regarding this well-founded and accepted medicolegal concept of the equivalence of brain death and death of a human persists to this date among physicians, other health care professionals, and the general public [11,13]. Specifically, in the field of transplantation, it should be unequivocally clear to the potential donor's family and anyone involved in the patient's care that the time of death is the time at which the diagnosis of brain death is established and not the time of cardiac arrest during the organ retrieval. Providing education targeted specifically at these groups and society at large is of paramount importance to optimize consent rates [11,13].

Required Request

Required request laws have now been enacted in all states in the United States. They obligate hospitals to notify an OPO of potential donors and to offer the option of donation to the families of potential donors (brain-dead or DCD donors).

Clinical Diagnosis of Brain Death

The clinical diagnosis of brain death rests on three criteria: (a) irreversibility of the neurologic insult, (b) absence of clinical evidence of cerebral function, and, most important, (c) absence of clinical evidence of brainstem function [79–81] (Table 185.4). Irreversibility is established if structural disease (e.g., trauma, intracranial hemorrhage) or an irreversible metabolic cause is known to have occurred. Hypothermia, medication side effects, drug overdose, or intoxication need to be ruled out when testing for brain death. Plasma concentrations of sedative or analgesic drugs sometimes correlate poorly with cerebral effects. Therefore, residual effects of those drugs can be excluded only by passage of time, if any doubts exist. The observation period (the waiting time between two sequential brain-death examinations) should be at least 6 hours for structural causes and preferably 12 to 24 hours for metabolic causes, drug overdose, or intoxication [80]. Even with potentially reversible metabolic alterations (e.g., hepatic or uremic encephalopathy), recovery has not been described after duration of the brain-death state for more than 12 hours. Clinical testing of cerebral and brainstem function is detailed in Table 185.4 [79–82]. It should be noted that brain-death criteria are more stringent for very young pediatric patients, particularly newborns, in whom criteria for brain death also include demonstration of the absence of blood flow on cerebral flow studies.

After brain death, the pupils become fixed in midposition because sympathetic and parasympathetic input is lost. Decerebrate (abnormal extension) and decorticate (abnormal flexion) responses to painful stimuli imply the presence of some brainstem function and are incompatible with the diagnosis of brain death. In contrast, spinal cord–mediated tendon reflexes, automatic stepping, and other spinal cord–generated movements (which can occur during apnea testing) are compatible with the presence of brain death [83]. The occurrence of these movements can be quite distressing if observed by the next of kin; therefore, it is advisable that they not be present during the apnea test. Very rarely, ascending acute reversible inflammatory polyneuropathy (Guillain–Barré syndrome) can simulate brain death and inhibit all motor functions, including pupillary reactions and brainstem reflexes. The typical clinical history, coupled with evidence of progressive weakness, yields the correct diagnosis and precludes a diagnosis of brain death being established [80].

The American Academy of Neurology has stated that special confirmatory tests are not necessary to diagnose brain death in the vast majority of cases. Only in equivocal or questionable circumstances do tests demonstrating absence of intracranial blood flow or the presence of an isoelectric electroencephalogram need to be performed [80,81]. The most sensitive and specific test for assessing intracranial blood flow is four-vessel cerebral arteriography. All other adjunctive tests are

TABLE 185.4

BRAIN DEATH CRITERIA AND CLINICAL DIAGNOSIS OF BRAIN DEATH

Irreversible, well-defined etiology of unconsciousness
Structural disease or metabolic cause
Exclusion of hypothermia; hypotension; severe electrolyte, endocrine, or acid-base disturbance; and drug or substance intoxication
Sufficient observation period (at least 6 h) between two brain death examinations
No clinical evidence of cerebral function
No spontaneous movement, eye opening, or movement or response after auditory, verbal, or visual commands
No movement elicited by painful stimuli to the face and trunk (e.g., sternal rub, pinching of a nipple, or fingernail bed) other than spinal cord reflex movements
No clinical evidence of brainstem function
No pupillary reflex: pupils are fixed and midposition; no change of pupil size in either eye after shining a strong light source in each eye sequentially in a dark room
No corneal reflex: no eyelid movement after touching the cornea (not the conjunctiva) with a sterile cotton swab or tissue
No gag reflex: no retching or movement of the uvula after touching the back of the pharynx with a tongue depressor or after moving the endotracheal tube
No cough reflex: no coughing with deep tracheal irrigation and suctioning
No oculocephalic reflex (doll's eyes reflex): no eye movement in response to brisk turning of the head from side to side with the head of the supine patient elevated 30 degrees
No oculovestibular reflex (caloric reflex): no eye movements within 3 min after removing earwax and irrigating each tympanic membrane (if intact) sequentially with 50 mL ice water for 30 to 45 seconds while the head of the supine patient is elevated 30 degrees
No integrated motor response to pain: no localizing or withdrawal response, no extensor or flexor posturing
No respiratory efforts on apnea testing ($PaCO_2$ >60 mm Hg or 20 mm Hg higher than the normal baseline value): The patient is preoxygenated with an FIO_2 of 1.0 for 10–15 min, preferably with an arterial line in place for rapid blood gas measurements, while adjusting ventilatory rate and volume such that the $PaCO_2$ reaches ~40–45 mm Hg. After a baseline arterial blood gas value is obtained and the patient is disconnected from the ventilator, O_2 at 6–8 L/min is delivered through a cannula advanced 20–30 cm into the endotracheal tube (cannula tip at the carina). Continuous pulse oximetry is used for early detection of desaturation, which does not usually occur when using this protocol. In most cases, a $PaCO_2$ >60 mm Hg is achieved within 3–5 minutes after withdrawal of ventilatory support; at this point, the patient should be reconnected to the ventilator (or earlier, should hemodynamic instability, desaturation, or spontaneous breathing movements occur). Obtaining an arterial blood gas sample immediately before reinstitution of mechanical ventilation is mandatory. If there is no evidence of spontaneous respirations before reinstitution of mechanical ventilation in the presence of a $PaCO_2$ >60 mm Hg or an increase of >20 mm Hg from the normal baseline value, the criteria for a positive apnea test are met.
Other points
Spinal reflexes, such as deep tendon reflexes and triple flexion responses, can be preserved and do not exclude the diagnosis of brain death
Shivering, goose bumps, arm movements, reaching of the hands toward the neck, forced exhalation, and thoracic respiratory-like movements are possible after brain death and are likely due to neuronal impulse release phenomena of the spinal cord, including the upper cervical cord. All these findings are compatible with the diagnosis of brain death.
Confirmatory tests should be used in cases in which the observation period needs to be shortened (e.g., unstable donors), in equivocal situations in children younger than 1 year old, or if one of the potential pitfalls (Table 185.6) cannot be ruled out (demonstration of absence of intracranial circulation by angiographic contrast or radioisotopic flow studies, transcranial Doppler ultrasonography, or electrocerebral silence documented by an electroencephalogram).

$PaCO_2$, partial arterial carbon dioxide pressure; FIO_2, fraction of inspired oxygen.
From references [79–82].

less sensitive (e.g., digital subtraction angiography, transcranial Doppler ultrasonography), are less specific (e.g., brainstem acoustic evoked potentials), measure only hemispheric flow (e.g., radioisotope angiography), or are indirect (e.g., computed tomography, echoencephalography). If either hemispheric neuronal function (electroencephalogram) or hemispheric flow is assessed, reliable clinical testing of the brainstem must be performed to confirm the diagnosis. The use of a brain-imaging modality, positron emission tomography (using ^{18}F-fluorodeoxyglucose to assess brain metabolism), to diagnose brain death is currently not universally recommended [80]. The decision whether to accept ^{18}F-fluorodeoxyglucose–positron emission tomography as a confirmatory test for determination of brain death is awaiting the results of further studies.

Four-vessel cerebral arteriography is indicated in all conditions that can temporarily cause an isoelectric electroencephalogram (e.g., extreme intoxication). If the indication for cerebral arteriography is unclear, the benefits must be weighed against the potential risks of transporting an unstable patient, hypotension after contrast injection, and the nephrotoxic effects of injection of contrast media that potentially may affect early renal allograft function [82]. Confirmatory tests may serve to shorten the waiting period between the two brain-death examinations, should donor hemodynamic instability occur. Certain potential pitfalls exist in clinical brain-death testing, and the diagnosis should not be considered to have been established until these all have been excluded (Table 185.5). If these cannot be excluded, confirmatory testing is mandatory [80,81].

In summary, the diagnosis of brain death can be established by performance of routine neurologic examinations, including cold caloric and apnea testing on two separate occasions,

TABLE 185.5

PITFALLS IN CLINICAL BRAIN DEATH TESTING AND POTENTIAL REMEDIAL MEASURES[a]

Pitfalls	Remedial measure(s)
Hypotension, shock	Institute fluid resuscitation, use of pressor agents
Hypothermia	Use warmed fluids, ventilatory warmer
Intoxication or drug overdose	If measurable, check drug levels and toxicology screens or increase waiting time between brain death examinations
Neuromuscular and sedative drugs, which can interfere with elicitation of motor responses	Discontinue muscle relaxants and mood- or consciousness-altering medications, increase waiting time between brain death examinations
Pupillary fixation, which may be caused by anticholinergic drugs (e.g., atropine given during a cardiac arrest), neuromuscular blocking agents, or preexisting disease	Discontinue anticholinergic medications and muscle relaxants, increase waiting time between brain death examinations, obtain careful patient history
Corneal reflexes absent due to overlooked contact lenses	Remove contact lenses before brain death examination
Oculovestibular reflexes diminished or abolished after prior use of ototoxic drugs (e.g., aminoglycosides, loop diuretics, vancomycin) or agents with suppressive side effects on the vestibular system (e.g., tricyclic antidepressants, anticonvulsants, and barbiturates) or due to preexisting disease	Obtain careful medication history and patient history

[a]If one of the listed conditions cannot be ruled out, confirmatory testing (cerebral flow studies or electroencephalography) is necessary before brain death is declared.

coupled with prior establishment of the underlying diagnosis and prognosis in most cases. More sophisticated tests are required in cases in which the diagnosis cannot be unequivocally established. However, brain death must be diagnosed in accordance with local regulations and state laws. Details on the locally prevailing regulations are available through the state medical board or the local OPO.

ORGAN DONATION PROCESS

The three key elements leading to successful organ donation are (a) early referral of potential donors, (b) a well-coordinated approach in informing and dealing with the potential donor's family to request and obtain consent, and (c) appropriate critical care therapy of the donor [11,13,15,16]. The optimal course of events for both brain-dead and DCD donors is summarized in Table 185.6.

Early Donor Referral

Early referral of any potential donor to the local OPO minimizes the loss of transplantable organs due to unexpected cardiac arrest and death, hemodynamic instability, serious nosocomial infection, or complications related to intensive care [16,84,85]. For example, an inverse correlation exists between the duration of mechanical ventilation and the suitability of the donor for lung donation.

The evidence is substantial that brain death eventually leads to cardiac arrest, even when cardiorespiratory support is maintained [84,86]. Cardiac arrest occurs in 4% to 28% of potential donors in the maintenance phase. Although approximately 50% of all potential donors die within 24 hours without appropriate support, as many as 25% are not recognized for 48 hours or longer, with identification occurring only at the time of cardiovascular death [86].

The previously outlined clinical guidelines for referral to the local OPO should be applied to any neurologically severely injured patient after admission to the hospital or intensive care unit (Table 185.3). Early contact with the OPO is essential as the latter will provide assistance with further screening and the evaluation of any patient who might potentially become a donor.

Donor Evaluation

General Guidelines

During the initial contact with the OPO, the physician should provide the potential donor's name, age, sex, height, weight, and blood type. Also needed are the date of admission and diagnosis, the nature and extent of any trauma, a concise medical and social history, and the time of brain death (if applicable). Whether local investigative agencies (e.g., medical examiner, coroner) need to be notified also should be specified. The current medical status, including vital signs, urine output, cardiorespiratory status, medications, and culture results, must be communicated. Basic laboratory results should be obtained: arterial blood gas determinations; blood urea nitrogen, creatinine, and electrolyte values; hemoglobin, hematocrit, white blood cell and platelet counts, and tests for serum amylase, total bilirubin, alkaline phosphatase, alanine aminotransferase,

TABLE 185.6

ORGAN DONATION ALGORITHM[a]

1. Early identification of the potential donor by the critical care physician or health care professional (Table 185.3)
2. Early contact with the local or regional OPO for medical, legal, and logistic assistance. If the local OPO's address or phone number is unknown, a 24-h access number to UNOS is available: 1–800-292–9537.
3. Completion of the preliminary screening by the OPO if necessary in consultation with the transplant surgeon for decisions regarding marginal donors

4a. For potential DCD donors: await family decision regarding withdrawal of care. Proceed only if family decides to do so.

4b. For potential brain-dead donors: brain death diagnosis and confirmation (Tables 185.4 and 185.5), certification of death. Family notification and explanation of brain death with its legal and medical implications. Sufficient time for acceptance must be allowed.

5. Request for organ donation. Must be made after, in clear temporal separation, from step 4a or 4b.
6. After consent for organ donation is obtained, the focus switches from treatment of elevated intracranial pressure and cerebral protection to preservation of organ function and optimization of peripheral oxygen delivery (Table 185.8).
7. All remaining laboratory and serologic studies as well as any further studies and tests required in equivocal situations are performed at this point (e.g., coronary angiography for older or marginal heart donors).
8. Final organ allocation by the OPO and UNOS, coordination of the organ recovery operation, notification of the abdominal and thoracic surgical teams. Modification of the final steps may become necessary under special circumstances, for example, in hemodynamically unstable donors.
9. For DCD donors: Support is withdrawn and death is certified (in the ICU or in the operating room).
10. Organ recovery operation (brain-dead and DCD donors).

[a]Steps 4, 5, and 9 should not involve physicians who are part of the transplantation team.
OPO, organ procurement organization; UNOS, United Network for Organ Sharing; DCD, donation after cardiac death.

and aspartate aminotransferase; coagulation profile (including prothrombin time or International Normalized Ratio [INR]); and urinalysis and urine culture should be available, along with electrocardiogram and chest radiograph results. In the case of potential lung donors, chest circumference and radiographic thoracic measurements, as well as the results of an oxygenation challenge [partial arterial oxygen pressure (PaO_2) measurement after ventilation for 10 minutes with a fraction of inspired oxygen (FIO_2) of 1.0], are helpful.

The OPO provides further procedural, administrative, legal, and logistic help. Most importantly, the OPO coordinates how the family is approached. All further testing [including HLA-tissue typing; serologic screening for cytomegalovirus (CMV), for hepatitis A, B, and C viruses, for human immunodeficiency virus (HIV), and for human T-cell lymphotropic virus type I and syphilis; and blood, sputum, and urine cultures] is then coordinated through the OPO if the donor passes the preliminary screening tests. The organ allocation process begins only after the family has decided to withdraw support (DCD donors) or brain death has been declared and consent has been obtained. If prospective tissue typing is to be done, performing a surgical inguinal lymph node biopsy at the donor hospital may be necessary—after consent for organ donation has been obtained but before proceeding with the actual organ recovery several hours later.

The medical status and the life expectancy of the potential recipient without the organ transplant are taken into account when the final decision about transplantation of a specific donor organ is made. The ultimate decision regarding the use of a donor organ is made by the transplant surgeon. At this point, the transplant center may need to obtain further tests to assess the functional status of one or more organ systems. For example, if the heart is to be retrieved, an echocardiogram is usually obtained. In selected donors, coronary angiography is performed. Pulmonary status can be further assessed by bronchoscopy after considering the results of the chest radiograph, oxygenation challenge, and sputum cultures. For potential liver donors who might have fatty liver disease, a percutaneous bedside liver biopsy can be performed. If concern over the suitability of organs arises, direct inspection by the transplant surgeon is necessary at the time of the organ procurement operation. In some cases, an open biopsy (e.g., for kidney or liver) and frozen section pathologic analysis obtained at the time of organ recovery also help in the final decision making. Direct inspection also is important in organ donors who suffered a blunt injury to the head and trunk (e.g., motor vehicle accident). Under these circumstances, intra-abdominal organs have been used successfully despite the presence of parenchymal tears or subcapsular hematomas in either the liver or kidney. Significant injuries to the pancreas preclude its use.

In summary, *each* patient with a severe neurologic injury should be referred to the local OPO as a potential donor, regardless of type of brain injury (e.g., trauma, stroke), history, age, or medical condition (Table 185.3). With few exceptions (vide infra), organ donation should never be excluded a priori because of the clinical situation, the results of imaging studies, or the magnitude of an injury, without first having contacted the local OPO (24-hour access number: 1–800-292–9537).

Organ-Specific Considerations

The use of kidneys from older donors, donors dying of cardiovascular disease, or donors requiring large doses of inotropic drugs for cardiovascular support entails a higher rate of delayed or diminished graft function and is associated with decreased graft survival [87,88]. Nevertheless, organs from these so-called marginal donors are routinely used, given the current prolonged periods (greater than 6 years) that some recipients may wait for available organs, during which their medical condition may deteriorate. Marginal donor kidneys benefit from preservation on a pulsatile perfusion pump, which was shown to improve quality of early graft function and long-term outcomes [44]. In equivocal cases (e.g., donors with elevated baseline serum creatinine levels or a history of hypertension), renal biopsies at the time of organ recovery may quantify the amount of preexisting donor arteriosclerosis or glomerulosclerosis. The critical shortage of organs has led to increasing relaxation of exclusion criteria, with satisfactory long-term results in many recipients. Donor organ function is more important than donor biologic age.

Livers from donors with an abnormal liver enzyme or coagulation profile can frequently still be transplanted. Elevated hepatic enzyme levels may reflect transient hepatic ischemia at the time of resuscitation. The trends observed in the results of serial hepatic enzyme levels are more important than absolute values. Abnormal coagulation test results may be due to disseminated intravascular coagulation (commonly a result of brain injury, not primary hepatic dysfunction). Significant donor hypernatremia (e.g., >155 mg per dL), as commonly observed in under resuscitated brain-dead donors with significant diabetes insipidus, is a risk factor for primary liver graft nonfunction posttransplant. Aggressive intervention prior to procurement is warranted and will ultimately allow for safe transplantation of liver grafts from these hypernatremic donors. The decision to use a liver from a marginal donor has to be made on the basis of relatively crude information. Often, only direct inspection, with or without a biopsy of the liver, at the time of organ recovery provides a final answer and may be the only way to assess a donor with a history of significant ethanol intake. Severe hepatic steatosis is one of the most significant factors predictive of early posttransplant hepatic dysfunction or failure.

In general, donors older than 55 years of age are not considered for pancreas donation. However, donors with hyperglycemia [caused by peripheral insulin resistance, particularly after brain death (see "Endocrine Therapy" section) or hyperamylasemia (which can be a consequence of severe head injury without actual pancreatitis)] [89] are not to be excluded a priori from pancreas donation, because these factors do not necessarily influence posttransplant outcome [90]. A pancreas transplant registry analysis suggested a slightly higher incidence of graft thrombosis for pancreata that had been procured from donors treated with desmopressin (vs. those that did not) [91]. Clearly, further study is necessary to confirm or refute these findings and determine their clinical significance. Currently, the only absolute contraindications to pancreas donation are a history of impaired glucose tolerance or insulin-dependent diabetes mellitus, direct blunt or penetrating trauma to the pancreas, or the finding of acute or chronic pancreatitis at the time of the donor operation.

Regarding heart donation, an important criterion is good donor heart ventricular function immediately before retrieval, as judged by the cardiac surgeon at visual inspection during organ recovery. Ideally, no potential heart donor should be excluded solely on the basis of echocardiographic wall motion abnormalities, a borderline or abnormal ejection fraction, inotropic medication requirements, or heart murmurs, arrhythmias, or other electrocardiographic changes (which often occur in brain-dead individuals in whom no cardiac disease is present) [16].

Risk factors associated with poorer outcome after lung transplantation include a history of smoking, aspiration, purulent secretions observed during bronchoscopy, an abnormal chest radiograph, or an unsatisfactory oxygenation challenge (PaO_2 less than 300 mm Hg after 10 minutes of ventilation with FIO_2 of 1.0 and PEEP of 5 cm H_2O) alone or in combination in lung donors. However, even lungs obtained from such marginal donors have been successfully transplanted [92]. Bronchoscopy often is performed as a final confirmatory test in the operating room by the transplant surgeon immediately before retrieval. Direct intraoperative inspection of the lungs determines whether significant contusions are present, which could preclude use of the organs.

In conclusion, the traditional donor criteria have been considerably expanded over recent years, for both thoracic and abdominal organs, due to the ongoing, severe donor shortage.

Transmission of Infectious Diseases

Transmission of bacterial or fungal infection through organ transplantation can be due to contamination of the organ itself during organ procurement or storage. Published evidence suggests that organs transplanted from bacteremic donors do not transmit bacterial infection or result in poorer recipient outcomes [93]. However, potential donors who exhibit or develop active bacterial or fungal infection that is unresponsive to adequate source control and antibiotic therapy or who have evidence of severe systemic sepsis with positive blood cultures (even without a primary source) should be rejected. Similarly, active tuberculosis is a contraindication to organ donation. Positive urine cultures do not preclude renal donation. Donors with serologic evidence of syphilis have been successfully used.

Absolute contraindications to donation include evidence of significant *acute* viral infections (e.g., viral encephalitis, systemic herpes simplex virus infections, acute viral hepatitis A, B, or C), seropositivity for HIV, and the acquired immunodeficiency syndrome. Individuals known to be at high risk for acquiring such diseases (e.g., intravenous [IV] drug users, prostitutes, or residents of sub-Saharan Africa) are only accepted as donors on a case-by-case basis.

Potential donors that test positive for the hepatitis B virus (HBV) surface antigen (HBsAg) or HBe antigen are usually precluded from donating [16,94]. Serologic positivity for the hepatitis B core antigen antibody (HBcAb) does not constitute an absolute contraindication to proceed with donation [94]. Acceptable organs from donors with any type of serologic evidence of HBV are usually only transplanted into recipients that have demonstrated immunity against HBV (i.e., HBsAb-positivity). Selected recipients may also receive HBV immunoglobulin or lamivudine, or both, beginning at the time of transplant [94]. Ideally, however, all potential organ transplant recipients should receive HBV immunization during the pretransplant evaluation [16].

The use of hepatitis C (HCV)–seropositive donors for selected recipients has become routine [16,95]. For adequate identification of HCV-positive donors, many OPOs now routinely perform nucleic acid testing (by polymerase chain reaction [PCR]) for HCV–RNA. HCV-infected livers and kidneys transplanted into HCV-infected recipients do not convey a worse outcome than HCV-negative grafts [16,95]. In essence, exclusion of all HCV-positive donors would increase the organ shortage while preventing what would appear to be relatively limited disease transmission. As is the case for HBV serology–positive donors, the final decision regarding the use of an HCV serology–positive donor must be made on an individual basis by each transplant surgeon. Factors that are taken into account in such circumstances include the likelihood of disease transmission, the recipient's current medical and serologic status, and whether the organ to be transplanted is life-saving (e.g., liver, heart) [16,95].

CMV also can be transmitted by donor tissue, particularly to CMV-seronegative patients. Effective prophylaxis against and treatment of CMV disease have become a reality with the advent of effective antiviral agents such as ganciclovir and valganciclovir. Positive CMV serologies do not preclude organ donation but have been used to identify high-risk donor-recipient combinations (CMV-seropositive donor–CMV-seronegative recipient) where prophylaxis should be used and careful surveillance for CMV disease is important.

Transmission of Malignancy

Transmission of malignancy via donor organs is very rare [16]. Because donor selection is particularly important in this regard, donors with most types of cancer should not be used. The exceptions are those with low-grade skin malignancies, such as basal cell carcinoma and most squamous cell carcinomas; carcinoma in situ of the uterine cervix; or primary brain tumors, which rarely spread outside the central nervous system (CNS; e.g., grade I astrocytomas, benign meningiomas, and hemangioblastomas, but not medulloblastomas and glioblastomas) [16,96]. It is important to ensure that a CNS tumor does not represent a focus of metastatic disease from the primary site. Metastases from choriocarcinomas, bronchial or renal malignancies, and malignant melanomas may present as what appears to be a primary brain tumor or may bleed and be mistaken for an intracranial hemorrhage because of an arteriovenous malformation or a ruptured aneurysm. Previous treatment of a neoplasm, menstrual irregularities after a pregnancy or a spontaneous abortion in women of childbearing age (suggestive of a choriocarcinoma), or evidence of lesions at other sites in the patient with a purported primary CNS malignancy should preclude organ donation. Donors with primary brain tumors should not be used if they have undergone radiotherapy, chemotherapy, ventriculoperitoneal or ventriculoatrial shunting, or craniotomies, because these treatments either are associated with high-grade malignancies or create potential pathways for the systemic dissemination of tumor cells [16,96].

If a potential donor has had successful cancer treatment in the past, the transplant surgeon must weigh the small potential risk of transmitting micrometastases against discarding a potentially life-saving organ. In general, patients with a history of malignancy with little propensity to recur after therapy (e.g., small, noninvasive lesions treated by complete surgical excision) are considered as organ donors, particularly if they have remained without evidence of recurrence for more than 5 years. Patients who have experienced invasive cancer in which a substantial risk of late recurrence exists (e.g., breast cancer, malignant melanoma), particularly if a large lesion was initially present and chemotherapy or radiation therapy was used, should probably not be considered for donation. Similarly, patients with a history of leukemia or lymphoma should not be considered as donors.

Required Request for Organ Donation and Consent

After the OPO determines the suitability of a potential donor, the next important steps are the brain-death examination (when applicable) and the legally required request for organ donation (Table 185.6). Those steps should *not* involve any of the physicians associated with the transplant team, as this would represent a potential conflict of interest. In 1987, federal required-request legislation became effective and has since been adopted by every state in the United States. Required-request laws mandate that the family of a potential organ donor be offered the option of organ donation. The hospital must notify the local OPO of the presence of a potential organ donor. Several studies have shown that consent rates are highest when an OPO coordinator—rather than a member of the patient's ICU team such as a physician or a nurse—approaches the family about organ donation [11–13,75].

Brain-Dead Donors

For brain-dead donors, it is of the utmost importance to ensure that (a) the family understands and accepts the concept of brain death, including its legal and medical equivalence with death; (b) the request for organ donation is *not* made at the same time that brain death is explained (unless the family voiced the wish to consider donation earlier during the hospitalization); and (c) the approach and request be made by an OPO representative (rather than a member of the potential donor's care team). Sufficient time must be given to the next of kin to begin coping with this information and to accept the loss of the family member. Only then, in clear temporal separation from the explanation of death, should the subject of organ donation be broached and an appropriate request be made [11,13]. As a case in point, within one region of the United States, consent rates were 18% when the discussion of death and the request for donation were combined but rose to 65% when these issues were discussed separately [97]. Also, the family must be informed that after declaration of brain death and consenting to organ donation, all hospital costs relating to donation will be paid by the OPO.

DCD Donors

Families of patients with severe, irreversible brain injuries who do not fulfill the formal criteria of brain death might decide to forgo any further life-sustaining treatment. Only then can the subject of organ donation be broached with the family. As discussed earlier, it is paramount that the approach to the family and the request for organ donation be made by an OPO representative [26,98,99].

Consent

Driver's licenses and signed donor cards are not considered legally binding documents for the purpose of organ donation. Thus, the family's wishes under such circumstances are virtually always honored, even if they are contrary to the donor's wishes expressed on a driver's license or donor card. The Uniform Anatomical Gift Act of 1968 specifies the legal next-of-kin priority for donors over age 18 years in the following order: (a) spouse, (b) adult son or daughter, (c) either parent, (d) adult brother or sister, and (d) legal guardian [79]. Similarly, the order of priority for donors under age 18 years is as follows: (a) both parents, (b) one parent (if both parents are not available and no wishes to the contrary of the absent parent are known), (c) the custodial parent (if the parents are divorced or legally separated), and (d) the legal guardian (if there are no parents). In part in response to the aforementioned dilemma, nearly all states in the United States have now created state donor registries where residents can register their decision to donate (usually on-line) to ensure that they can donate their organs [24]. Such initiatives help to relieve families of making an often difficult decision on the donor's behalf. In contrast to driver's licenses and signed donor cards, an individual's decision to donate that is documented in a state donor registry cannot be overridden by the family [24].

PERIOPERATIVE CRITICAL CARE MANAGEMENT OF THE BRAIN-DEAD ORGAN DONOR

Although some of the critical care issues that pertain to brain-dead organ donors have been met by significant clinical and basic research interest (e.g., hormonal changes and hormonal replacement therapy), there is an overall lack of randomized, controlled studies that could lead to a more evidence-based approach to the care of these patients. The level of evidence provided by these studies is mainly low. It is therefore important to acknowledge that some of the following recommendations may undergo substantial revision as additional, new evidence emerges (Tables 185.7 and 185.8).

Pathophysiology of Brain Death

The majority of our knowledge of the pathophysiologic changes during and after brain death has been derived from experiments performed using animal models. Hemodynamic instability during the phase of impending brain herniation is the result of autonomic dysregulation secondary to the progressive

TABLE 185.7

MAINTENANCE THERAPY ENDPOINTS IN THE BRAIN-DEAD ORGAN DONOR

Variable	Therapeutic endpoint
Systolic blood pressure	100–120 mm Hg or mean arterial pressure ≥60 mm Hg
Central venous pressure	8–10 mm Hg
Urine output	100–300 mL/h
Core temperature	>35°C
Partial arterial oxygen pressure	80–100 mm Hg
Systemic arterial oxygen saturation	95%
pH	7.37–7.45
Hemoglobin	10–12 g/d
Hematocrit	30–35%

loss of central neurohumoral regulatory control of vital functions. The continuous increase in intracranial pressure with worsening brain ischemia leads to severe systemic hypertension (Cushing's response) and frequently is associated with tachyarrhythmias. This process is mediated by an increase in sympathetic activity and an excess of circulating catecholamines ("autonomic storm") [100–102]. A brief period of transient bradycardia associated with the hypertensive response can be seen in the early phase of brain herniation (Cushing's reflex).

During the phase of increased sympathetic activity, there is evidence that coronary blood flow is significantly impaired, resulting in cardiac microinfarcts. Furthermore, decreased hepatic perfusion due to increased intrahepatic shunting has been demonstrated as a result of the excessive sympathetic activity. Neurogenic pulmonary edema is thought to develop during the autonomic storm phase secondary to the temporary elevation of left atrial pressures over the level of pulmonary arterial and alveolar capillary pressures. This causes massive transudation of fluid from the microvasculature into the alveoli and interstitial hemorrhage [100–102]. Within approximately 15 minutes after brain herniation and brain death, catecholamines decrease to below baseline values.

The resting vagal tone is abolished because of destruction of the nucleus ambiguus, eliminating all chronotropic effects of atropine administered after brain death. The total carbon dioxide production after brain death is low, because of the absence of cerebral metabolism and the presence of hypothermia and decreased muscle tone. The subsequent chronic maintenance phase of brain-dead donors is frequently characterized by hypotension, resulting mainly from complete arterial and venous vasomotor collapse with significant peripheral venous pooling.

An increasing body of experimental evidence also shows that brain death leads to activation of proinflammatory and immunoregulatory pathways [102–106]. In small animal brain-death models, messenger ribonucleic acid and protein expression within peripheral solid organs were significantly increased for cytokines (e.g., interleukin-1β, interleukin-6, tumor necrosis factor-α, interferon gamma, tumor growth factor-β), chemokines (e.g., RANTES), adhesion molecules (e.g., P- and E-selectin), and vasoconstrictors (e.g., endothelin) [102–106]. Importantly, brain death has also been associated with enhanced expression of immunoregulatory molecules such as major histocompatibility complex class I and II proteins [103]. Consistent with these findings, increased immunogenicity and accelerated rejection were noted in kidneys and hearts transplanted from brain-dead rodents [102].

Routine Care and Monitoring

Regular nursing care must be continued after brain death. Frequent turning to prevent decubitus ulcers, skin care, dressing changes, urinary and intravascular catheter care, and catheter site care must be meticulous to minimize the risk of infection. Other indwelling devices should be removed, if possible (e.g., ventriculostomies and ventriculoatrial or ventriculoperitoneal shunts, which may have been inserted in certain patients for monitoring or treating of elevated intracranial pressure). Any urinary and intravascular catheters that may have been inserted under suboptimal, emergent conditions without appropriate aseptic technique at the time of original injury should be replaced. A nasogastric tube should always be inserted for gastric decompression and prevention of aspiration.

Arterial lines should be inserted preferentially into peripheral arteries of the upper extremities because femoral arterial line readings can become inaccurate from surgical manipulation of the abdominal aorta during organ procurement. Similarly, central venous catheters should not be inserted through the femoral vein because dissection and manipulation of the inferior vena cava occur during organ procurement. In addition, venous catheters inserted through the femoral vein can cause iliac vein thrombosis. This increases the risk of pulmonary embolization, particularly during surgical venous dissection. Thrombosis can also render the iliac veins unsuitable for use in vascular reconstruction, which may be necessary for some types of abdominal or thoracic organ transplants.

The following parameters must be determined routinely and frequently for all organ donors using various monitoring devices: core temperature (esophageal, rectal, or indwelling bladder catheter temperature probes), heart rate (continuous electrocardiographic monitoring), systemic blood pressure (arterial catheter), central venous blood pressure (subclavian or internal jugular central venous catheter), arterial oxygen saturation (pulse oximetry), and hourly urine output (Foley catheter). Use of a pulmonary artery catheter for measurement of pulmonary arterial and left ventricular wedge pressure and central venous oximetry is not routinely necessary; its use should be reserved for selected unstable donors whose volume status is uncertain or who exhibit persistent acidosis with evidence of tissue hypoperfusion. Laboratory parameters also must be checked regularly, including arterial blood gas, serum electrolytes, blood urea nitrogen, creatinine, lactate, and liver enzyme values; total bilirubin; and hemoglobin, hematocrit, platelet count, and coagulation tests. Testing is adapted to the individual clinical situation—frequent electrolyte determinations if diabetes insipidus has been diagnosed, lactate monitoring in acidotic donors, and repeated coagulation profiles in the presence of disseminated intravascular coagulation.

If infection is suspected, blood, urine, sputum, cerebrospinal fluid, and wound drainage cultures must be obtained. Routine surveillance cultures (usually blood and urine cultures) may be required, depending on the protocol of the local OPO and the organ type. Blood cultures should be obtained using peripheral venipuncture, rather than arterial or central venous catheters, to avoid contamination. Prophylactic antibiotics only should be administered immediately before the retrieval procedure. Any source of infection should be identified, characterized from a microbiologic standpoint, and treated.

General Management Goals

The most important overall goal in the management of brain-dead multiple-organ donors is to optimize organ perfusion and tissue oxygen delivery. Organ viability and function after transplantation are closely correlated with adequacy of resuscitation

TABLE 185.8

MANAGEMENT OF THE DECEASED ORGAN DONOR: SELECTED EVIDENCE PUBLISHED 1993–2009[a]

Study design	Study	Outcome	No. of cases	Level of evidence	Reference
Effect of standardized medical and institutional donor management protocols and pathways					
Individual case control study	Effect of critical donor pathway (including hormonal resuscitation protocol component)	Significant increase of organs procured, organ quality unchanged	270	3b	[15]
Case series	Aggressive hemodynamic monitoring, intervention, and hormonal resuscitation in marginal donors	High organ recovery rates from marginal donors	52	4	[17]
Individual case control study	Impact of hospital-based OPO coordinators on conversion rates	Higher donor conversion rate in hospitals with hospital-based OPO coordinators	NA	4	[75]
Retrospective cohort study	Effect on intensive lung donor management protocol on organ yield	Increased lung yield in the intensive early donor management group	182	4	[23]
Effect of donor pretreatment—Single pharmacologic agents					
Retrospective cohort study	Effect of catecholamine administration to brain-dead donors on graft survival	Catecholamine use associated in dose-dependent manner with significantly better kidney graft survival	3,890	4	[108]
Retrospective cohort study	Effect of dopamine administration on quality of early graft function in the recipients	Lower recipient delayed graft function rates and faster creatinine decrease in the dopamine group	254	4	[107]
RCT	Effect of continuous low-dose dopamine infusion in stable donors with normal renal function on early recipient graft outcomes	Decreased posttransplant need for >1 dialysis session; no effect on rejection and short-term graft survival	265	2b	[109]
Individual case control study	High-dose steroids and aggressive management for marginal lung donors	No graft survival differences for lungs from marginal vs. standard donors	194	3b	[154]
RCT	Effect of high-dose continuous steroid infusion in liver donors on posttransplant outcomes	Improved posttransplant clinical reperfusion parameters (liver enzymes, bilirubin) and less early liver rejection for grafts from the steroid group	100	2b	[153]
RCT	Effect of intensive lung donor management protocol + (steroids or T3 or [steroids + T3] or placebo) on prerecovery lung quality and lung yield	No effect of pharmacologic pre-recovery interventions on lung yield; significantly less extravascular lung water accumulation in steroid groups	60	2b	[23]
Retrospective cohort study	Effect of donor desmopressin use on pancreas graft thrombosis rates (UNOS recipient database)	Higher thrombosis rates in pancreas grafts from donors that had received desmopressin	2,804	4	[91]
Retrospective cohort study	Effect of use of individual drugs on organ yield (UNOS donor database)	Favorable impact of steroids or desmopressin, but not T4, on organ yield	15,601	4	[123]
RCT	Effect of low-dose vasopressin vs. saline on donor hemodynamics and inotrope use	Increase in blood pressure and decrease in inotrope use in vasopressin group	24	2b	[110]
RCT	Effect of T3 infusion (limited to the duration of the organ procurement operation) vs. no T3	No differences for posttransplant liver graft function	25	2b	[124]
RCT	Effect of T3 infusion (within >5 h of organ recovery) vs. none on donor hemodynamics and adenine nucleotide concentration measured in graft biopsy tissue	No differences in hemodynamics and adenine nucleotide levels	52	2b	[145]
Effect of donor pretreatment—Combination hormonal replacement therapy					
Retrospective cohort study	Requirements for adrenergic support of donors receiving thyroxin + steroids + insulin vs. steroids only vs. no hormonal therapy	Less adrenergic support required in donors receiving thyroxin + insulin + steroids	119	4	[127]
Individual case control study	Effect of T3 + steroids + insulin on need for inotropic support and organ yield in unstable donors	Hormonal treatment improved hemodynamics of unstable donors and resulted in similar organ yield as in stable donors	47	4	[127]

(*continued*)

TABLE 185.8

CONTINUED

Study design	Study	Outcome	No. of cases	Level of evidence	Reference
Retrospective cohort study	Impact on organ yield of (T3 or thyroxin) + steroids + vasopressin vs. none	Increased kidney, liver, pancreas, heart, and lung yield rates in donors that received hormonal replacement therapy	10,292	4	[20]
Retrospective cohort study	Impact of (T3 or thyroxin) + steroids + vasopressin vs. all other (>3 hormones) hormonal replacement regimens on heart yield and early heart graft function	Increased number of transplanted hearts and improved early heart graft function	4,543	4	[19]
RCT	Effect of intensive lung donor management protocol and (steroids or T3 or [steroids + T3] or placebo) on lung quality and yield	No effect of steroids + T3 on donor lung quality and yield	60	2b	[23]
Retrospective cohort study	Effect of steroids + T4 on organ yield (UNOS donor database)	No effect of steroids + T4 on organ yield	15,601	4	[123]

[a]Levels of evidence (range: 1A [highest]—5[lowest]) were assigned based on current guidelines published by the Oxford Centre for Evidence Based Medicine (www.cebm.net).
NA, not applicable; OPO, organ procurement organization; RCT, randomized controlled clinical trial; T3, triiodothyronine; T4, thyroxin; UNOS, United Network for Organ Sharing.

and hemodynamic stability during the organ donor maintenance phase.

The events associated with the cause of brain death (e.g., hemorrhagic shock, cardiac arrest) can lead to significant physiologic abnormalities. Head injury preceding brain death is known to induce a hypermetabolic response, equivalent to that observed after a second- or third-degree burn involving approximately 40% of the total body surface area. Significant metabolic stress and impairment of organ perfusion occur during brain herniation, and both events are related to excessive catecholamine release. Any additional circulatory compromise in the time period afterward potentiates the deleterious consequences of these previous adverse events. Posttransplant organ function can be negatively affected by such episodes of cardiovascular dysregulation, particularly in such ischemia-sensitive organs as the heart and liver. For example, even with optimal heart donor management the recipient often needs inotropic support and may exhibit subendocardial myocyte necrosis on biopsy specimens obtained during the early posttransplant period [18,102]. Anticipating these changes associated with brain death and providing optimal management should they occur during the organ donor maintenance phase, as well as optimizing organ function, are of utmost importance [18].

Parameters associated with adequate tissue perfusion in stable donors in the absence of lactic acidosis are listed in Table 185.7. They include systolic blood pressure of 100 to 120 mm Hg, central venous pressure of 8 to 10 mm Hg, oxygen saturation of the arterial blood greater than or equal to 95%, core temperature greater than or equal to 35°C, and hematocrit of 30% to 35% [15,25], the latter balancing the slightly decreased oxygen transport capacity of the red blood cell mass with the beneficial effects of low viscosity on blood flow. Maintaining adequate hemoglobin concentration is also essential in preparation for organ recovery, in which hemodynamic stability throughout the operation is crucial, especially if blood loss occurs.

The use of vasopressors should be minimized if at all possible because of their splanchnic vasoconstrictive effects. Efforts to elevate blood pressure beyond the normal range can adversely affect outcome and should be avoided: High doses of vasopressors can cause arrhythmias and increase myocardial oxygen consumption, and pulmonary edema after excessive fluid administration can render lungs unsuitable for transplantation. After the lung, the pancreas is the organ most prone to tissue edema. Normal central venous pressure and low positive end-expiratory pressure (PEEP) help maintain an adequate perfusion gradient across the hepatic microcirculatory bed (i.e., that between the portal vein and hepatic artery on one side and the inferior vena cava and right atrium on the other).

Selective use of pulmonary artery catheterization must be considered in donors who do not respond to routine management and continue to exhibit hypotension or persistent lactic acidosis after adequate volume loading, particularly in those in whom this occurs despite use of moderate doses of dopamine. Determining pulmonary artery and capillary wedge pressures, cardiac output and index, pulmonary and systemic vascular resistive indices, oxygen availability and consumption, and other parameters helps to differentiate the cause of instability. Appropriate therapy can then be administered (e.g., fluid balance correction or PEEP adjustments, additional inotropic support, preload or afterload reduction). Once the hemodynamic instability has resolved, pulmonary artery catheters should be removed promptly to eliminate the inherent risks of infection, induction of arrhythmias, and mechanical endomyocardial damage.

A potential management conflict exists when the lungs are to be procured in combination with other organs from the same donor. Maintaining a central venous pressure of 8 to 10 mm Hg usually represents an acceptable compromise between the need for sufficient hydration to maintain adequate perfusion and good diuresis versus the dangers of provoking pulmonary edema in potential lung donors. Overall, optimizing hemodynamic parameters is paramount during the donor maintenance phase. Hypotension must be treated aggressively by proper fluid management, while minimizing the use of vasopressors. Hypertensive crises and tachyarrhythmic episodes require prompt intervention. PEEP that exceeds 5 cm H_2O should be used with caution, because hypotension may ensue.

Cardiovascular Support

Hypotension is the most common hemodynamic abnormality seen in brain-dead organ donors. The usual cause is hypovolemia, due to a combination of vasomotor collapse after brain death and the effects of treatment protocols to decrease intracranial pressure, which require minimizing hydration and use of osmotic diuretics (Tables 185.9 and 185.10). After brain death is declared, adequate volume resuscitation of the donor can require several liters of fluid. Until a euvolemic state is achieved, dopamine (greater than 3 μg per kg per minute) can be used temporarily; the dose should be titrated to maintain an adequate systolic blood pressure [15,25]. Infusion rates greater than 10 μg per kg per minute have been associated with increased rates of acute tubular necrosis and decreased renal allograft survival. High infusion rates also lead to decreased perfusion of other organs due to splanchnic vasoconstriction.

Dopamine is also the drug of choice if hemodynamic instability persists after fluid resuscitation and adequate volume loading. Use of isoproterenol and dobutamine should be avoided in this context because of their vasodilatory effects. Drugs with α-adrenergic agonist effects such as phenylephrine (IV infusion 0.15 to 0.75 μg per kg per minute) should be added only if hypotension persists in the face of euvolemia and titration of the dopamine infusion up to 15 μg per kg per minute. α-adrenergic agonists can cause severe peripheral vasoconstriction and reduce renal and hepatic perfusion; for this reason they must be used judiciously. Once these drugs are used, the need for their continued use must be frequently reassessed. Similar considerations apply to the use of epinephrine and norepinephrine (IV infusion up to 0.05 μg per kg per minute) [25]. For the majority (>80%) of donors, adequate hemodynamic goals can be achieved with volume resuscitation and low-to-moderate doses of a single vasopressor agent (dopamine). Interestingly, recent studies have suggested a beneficial impact on early graft function and on graft survival of administration of catecholamines, and in particular of dopamine, to brain-dead patients [107–109]. Several potential mechanisms have been invoked to explain these observations, including a favorable modulatory effect on ischemia-reperfusion and on the upregulation of adhesion molecules that results from the inflammatory state induced by brain death [107–109]. Low-dose arginine vasopressin can serve as an additional or alternative vasopressor. It enhances vascular sensitivity to catecholamines, and may thus allow minimizing their dose and side effects [110–112]. Effective arginine vasopressin doses for improving hemodynamic stability range from 0.01 to 0.1 units per minutes, given as continuous intravenous infusion [111,112].

Measurement of urine output alone as a means of assessing adequacy of fluid resuscitation is notoriously unreliable in brain-dead donors. The presence of a systolic blood pressure between 100 and 120 mm Hg, a central venous pressure between 8 and 10 mm Hg, and the absence of metabolic acidosis (with or without infusion of a small amount of dopamine) with concurrent adequate urine output (at least 1 to 2 mL per kg per hour) are usually better indirect indicators of donor stability and sufficient oxygen delivery to organs and tissues. It is important to remember, however, that the use of vasoconstrictor or inotropic agents does not serve to replace adequate fluid resuscitation. Thus, proper fluid management remains the cornerstone of successful donor management.

When attempting to determine the etiology of hypotension in an organ donor, underlying cardiac disease (e.g., coronary artery disease, valve defects) and factors related to the cause of brain death (e.g., myocardial infarction, cardiac tamponade, or myocardial contusion) must be included in the differential diagnosis. Electrolyte abnormalities such as hypophosphatemia, hypocalcemia, hypokalemia, and hypomagnesemia are common in brain-dead organ donors. The presence of these entities must also be considered when hemodynamic instability is encountered, and frequent testing and correction of these significant electrolyte imbalances are important. Hypophosphatemia and hypocalcemia can decrease myocardial contractility and provoke hypotension [113]; hypokalemia and hypomagnesemia can impair hemodynamics by causing arrhythmias.

As a general rule, medications that possess rapid reversibility and a short half-life should be chosen to treat arrhythmias or hypertension. Hemodynamic instability can be pronounced after brain death, with wide swings between the extremes of hypotension and hypertension, rendering the brain-dead donor more susceptible to cardiovascular drug effects. Hypertension

TABLE 185.9

DIFFERENTIAL DIAGNOSIS OF HYPOTENSION IN THE BRAIN-DEAD ORGAN DONOR

Diagnosis	Common underlying cause(s)
Hypovolemia	See Table 185.10
Hypothermia	Loss of central temperature control, administration of room-temperature intravenous fluids and blood products, heat loss during laparotomies and thoracotomies
Cardiac dysfunction	Arrhythmia (ischemia, catecholamines, hypokalemia, hypomagnesemia) Acidosis Hypo-oxygenation Excessive positive end-expiratory ventilatory pressure Congestive heart failure due to excessive fluid administration Hypophosphatemia Causes related to the injury leading to brain death (cardiac tamponade, myocardial contusion) Myocardial sequelae of autonomic storm Preexisting cardiac disease
Drug side effect or overdose	Long-acting beta-blocker, calcium channel antagonist, antihypertensive agent
Hypocalcemia	Transfusions, hypomagnesemia (e.g., secondary to osmotic diuresis), acute renal failure

TABLE 185.10

DIFFERENTIAL DIAGNOSIS OF HYPOVOLEMIA IN THE BRAIN-DEAD ORGAN DONOR

Arterial and venous vasomotor collapse due to loss of central neurohumoral control
Dehydration (fluid restriction to treat head injury)
Insufficient resuscitation after the injury leading to brain death (e.g., ongoing hemorrhagic shock with coagulopathy after polytrauma)
Polyuria
Osmotic diuresis (mannitol, hyperglycemia)
Diabetes insipidus
Hypothermia
Administration of other diuretics
Massive third spacing in response to the original injury
Decreased intravascular oncotic pressure after excessive resuscitation with crystalloid fluids

can be treated with short-acting vasodilatory agents (e.g., nitroprusside) or a rapidly reversible β-adrenergic antagonist (e.g., esmolol hydrochloride), because hypertension usually is associated with increased circulating catecholamines. Other drugs, such as calcium channel blockers (e.g., verapamil, nifedipine) or longer-acting beta-blockers (e.g., labetalol, propranolol), should be avoided because of their negative inotropic effects and the inability to titrate them precisely. Bradyarrhythmias during the early phase of brain herniation are part of Cushing's reflex and do not usually require any treatment, unless they are associated with hypotension and asystole. Because of the lack of chronotropic effects by atropine after brain death, use of either isoproterenol or epinephrine is required to treat hemodynamically significant bradyarrhythmias.

Tachyarrhythmias are associated with the increased catecholamine release that occurs during and immediately after brain herniation. Administration of short-acting beta-blockers (e.g., esmolol hydrochloride) serves not only to treat arrhythmias but also to mitigate hypertension during the autonomic storm. Use of additional short-acting IV antiarrhythmics (e.g., lidocaine) may become necessary if tachyarrhythmias do not resolve after beta-blocker therapy. Calcium channel blockers (e.g., verapamil) must be avoided under these circumstances because of their negative inotropic effects. Cardiac glycosides (e.g., digoxin) also should not be used because they can induce and potentiate bradyarrhythmias and tachyarrhythmias, and they also have splanchnic vasoconstrictive side effects.

Cardiac arrest occurs in up to 25% of all donors during the maintenance phase after brain death and should be treated by routine measures, with the exception that isoproterenol or epinephrine must be substituted for atropine [84,86]. No intracardiac injections should be given during cardiopulmonary resuscitation because they can render the heart unsuitable for transplantation.

Respiratory and Acid–Base Maintenance

Use of endotracheal suctioning should be minimized during the treatment of cerebral edema to avoid any unnecessary stimulation that would increase intracranial pressure. In contrast, after brain death is declared, vigorous tracheobronchial toilet is important, with frequent suctioning using sterile precautions. Percussion and turning for postural drainage are instituted as well. Even if the lungs are unsuitable for donation, it is important to minimize the risk of atelectasis and infection. Preventing atelectasis facilitates oxygenation and may obviate the need for detrimental high levels of PEEP. Steroids administered to some patients as part of the treatment for increased intracranial pressure predispose to pulmonary infectious complications. The presence of pneumonia can preclude donation of the lungs as well as other organs, depending on its severity and association with systemic sepsis. Routine respiratory care of all donors also includes the use of 5 cm H_2O PEEP to increase alveolar recruitment and prevent microatelectasis [15,25].

In potential lung donors the endotracheal tube should not be advanced more than several centimeters into the trachea, to prevent damage to areas that may become part of an anastomosis. A sample of sputum should be obtained for Gram's stain and cultures to exclude the presence of infection. The samples can be obtained using bronchoscopy, a procedure that is often routinely performed before lung donation. Peak end inspiratory airway pressures should be less than 30 cm H_2O. Traditionally, tidal volumes of 10 to 12 mL per kg have been recommended. However, it is not clear at present to what extent the evidence supporting lung protective strategies for many regular ICU patients—that is, tidal volumes of 6 to 8 mL per kg—also applies to the management of the often injured lungs of brain-dead donors as well [25,114,115]. For now, though, it appears prudent to apply pulmonary management principles that have proven beneficial for general ICU patients also to potential organ donors. For potential lung donors, the lowest FIO_2 that is capable of maintaining a PaO_2 of greater than 100 mm Hg should be selected. If oxygenation is insufficient, PEEP should be increased rather than increasing the FIO_2. High levels of PEEP negatively affect cardiac output, which should be carefully monitored in this setting. If hypotension occurs, PEEP should be reduced. Under these circumstances, use of pulmonary artery catheterization generally should be considered to balance PEEP requirements against those of organ perfusion. In contrast, to correct insufficient arterial oxygenation in non–lung donors, an increase in FIO_2 is preferred over high levels of PEEP [25].

The etiology of pulmonary edema in organ donors can be cardiogenic, neurogenic, aspiration induced, a result of trauma or fluid overload, or a combination of these factors. Neurogenic pulmonary edema usually precludes lung or combined heart–lung donation, but not donation of other organs (e.g., heart, kidney, liver, and pancreas). The treatment for pulmonary edema is supportive and should be directed at maintaining adequate arterial oxygenation without using high levels of PEEP. Fluids must be administered carefully to maintain organ perfusion while avoiding exacerbation of the edema. Excessive use of crystalloid fluids during the initial resuscitation after brain death is declared can render the lungs unsuitable for transplantation. If large amounts of fluid are required, colloids (e.g., albumin solutions) or blood transfusions (if the hemoglobin is less than 8 g per dL) should be considered in addition to the infusion of crystalloid solutions [15].

Respiratory alkalosis can develop in brain-dead organ donors secondary to mechanical hyperventilation as part of the treatment protocol for elevated intracranial pressure. After brain death, the arterial pH should be adjusted to normal values because alkalosis has many undesirable side effects, such as increased cardiac output, systemic vasoconstriction, bronchospasm, and a shift to the left of the oxyhemoglobin dissociation curve [15]. The latter decreases oxygen unloading in the tissues and impairs oxygen delivery, thereby diminishing tissue oxygenation and metabolism. Lactic metabolic acidosis is frequent in brain-dead donors; it should be treated by compensation with a slight respiratory alkalosis until the underlying abnormality has been corrected (e.g., dehydration, tissue ischemia). Administration of sodium bicarbonate should be contemplated only if the increased minute ventilation necessary to induce respiratory alkalosis leads to a decrease in cardiac output. In either situation, the most important aspect of managing metabolic acidosis is to treat the underlying cause. In rare cases, this may require pulmonary artery catheterization to assess the adequacy of hydration, cardiac output, and tissue oxygen delivery.

Renal Function and Fluid and Electrolyte Management

Maintaining adequate systemic perfusion pressure and brisk urine output (greater than 1 to 2 mL per kg per hour), while minimizing the use of vasopressors, contributes to good renal allograft function and reduces the rate of acute tubular necrosis after transplantation. If the urine production is still insufficient (e.g., less than 0.5 mL per kg per hour) after adequate volume loading, loop diuretics (furosemide, ethacrynic acid, bumetanide) or osmotic diuretics (mannitol) can be considered to initiate diuresis. Nephrotoxic drugs (e.g., aminoglycosides) and agents that may exert adverse effects on renal perfusion (e.g., nonsteroidal anti-inflammatory drugs) are contraindicated. Cephalosporins, monobactams, carbapenems, and quinolones are examples of less nephrotoxic but effective antibiotics that can be used if infection occurs.

Polyuria in brain-dead donors is a frequent finding. It can be due to diabetes insipidus, osmotic diuresis (induced by mannitol administered to decrease elevated intracranial pressures or hyperglycemia), physiologic diuresis due to previous massive fluid administration during resuscitation after the original injury with return of third-space fluid into the intravascular space, or hypothermia. Diabetes insipidus often heralds brain death in head-injured patients. It is the most frequent cause of polyuria during the organ donor maintenance phase. Found in up to 80% of all brain-dead bodies [82], it is related to insufficient blood levels of antidiuretic hormone (vasopressin), resulting in the production of large quantities of dilute urine. Diabetes insipidus should be suspected when urine volumes exceed 300 mL per hour (or 7 mL per kg per hour) in conjunction with hypernatremia (serum sodium greater than 150 mEq per dL), elevated serum osmolality (greater than 310 mOsm per L), and a low urinary sodium concentration. In addition to hypernatremia, other electrolyte abnormalities frequently observed during diabetes insipidus include hypokalemia, hypocalcemia, and hypomagnesemia. The appropriate replacement of these electrolyte losses can be guided by urinary electrolyte determinations, which easily allow calculation of the amount of the electrolyte to be replaced. Because diabetes insipidus is so common, mannitol administration should be discontinued after brain death is declared. Other supportive care of patients with diabetes insipidus includes replacing urine output milliliter for milliliter with free water (e.g., 5% solution of dextrose in water IV). Once urine output due to diabetes insipidus exceeds 300 mL per hour, desmopressin (desamino-8-D-arginine vasopressin), a synthetic analog of vasopressin, or arginine vasopressin, should be administered. Desmopressin has a long duration of action (6 to 20 hours) and a high antidiuretic–pressor ratio, avoiding any undesirable splanchnic vasoconstrictive effects that can occur with administration of normal- and high-dose arginine vasopressin [25,110,116]. For example, doses of 1 to 2 μg desmopressin are administered intravenously every 8 to 12 hours to achieve a urine output less than 300 mL per hour [116]. Desmopressin can also be effectively administered subcutaneously, intramuscularly, and intranasally. Vasopressin IV infusion can be started at 0.5 units per hour and titrated up to 6 units per hour, targeting a urine output of 0.5 to 3 mL per kg per hour and a serum sodium of 135 to 145 mEq per L [25,110]. Compared to desmopressin, arginine vasopressin is easier titrated and adds beneficial hemodynamic effects.

During the initial resuscitation phase after brain death is declared, infusion solutions with low sodium content should be used. Subsequently, maintenance fluid should consist of 5% dextrose in 0.45% sodium chloride with 20 mEq potassium added to each liter, administered at a rate of 2 mL per kg per hour during the maintenance phase if urine output is adequate (greater than 1 to 2 mL per kg per hour). If the urine output is greater than 2 mL per kg per hour, IV fluids should be administered at a rate equal to the urine output during the previous hour (IV intake = urine output). If the serum sodium concentration exceeds 150 mEq per dL, the maintenance fluid should consist of 5% dextrose solution with 20 mEq potassium added to each liter. Should the hourly fluid administration rate exceed 500 mL per hour, the dextrose concentration of the maintenance fluid should be decreased to 1% to avoid excessive hyperglycemia. IV maintenance fluids administered to brain-dead organ donors must always contain glucose, which is important to maintain intrahepatic glycogen stores that appear to be associated with normal liver allograft function in the early posttransplant period. The sodium content of certain IV fluids and plasma expanders (e.g., albumin solutions) also must be taken into consideration in hypernatremic patients.

The use of blood transfusions and other blood products should be minimized in organ donors, as in other patients. If transfusion or blood component therapy is necessary, CMV-seronegative blood products or leukocyte filters, or both, should be used whenever possible [15]. All blood must be screened for HIV, HBV, and HCV, and seropositive units should not be used.

Endocrine Therapy

According to previous studies, pituitary hormone blood levels do not uniformly decrease after brain death. Diabetes insipidus develops in approximately 80% of brain-dead donors as a result of low or absent blood levels of vasopressin [82]. These findings are a direct consequence of brain death, which abolishes vasopressin production in the hypothalamic nuclei (supraoptic and paraventricular nuclei) and vasopressin storage and release in the posterior pituitary. In contrast, near normal levels of anterior pituitary hormones, such as thyroid-stimulating hormone, adrenocorticotropic hormone, and growth hormone, have been documented after brain death in some studies [117–120]. Their persistence is probably due to the preservation of small subcapsular areas in the anterior pituitary, the blood supply of which is derived from small branches of the inferior hypophyseal artery. The latter arises from the extradural internal carotid artery, which is relatively protected from increases in intracranial pressure [121]. Recent clinical evidence, however, suggests deficient adrenal cortisol secretion after dynamic stimulation in brain-dead donors, irrespective of the level of pituitary dysfunction [122].

The principle of pharmacologic replacement therapy for deficient posterior pituitary vasopressin after brain death is well established [15,25,110,111,116]. A UNOS database analysis demonstrated a significant association between desmopressin use in donors and organ yield (Table 185.8) [123]. Low-dose vasopressin has been shown to exert beneficial hemodynamic effect in brain-dead donors (Table 185.8) [110,111]. In contrast, controversy still exists regarding the benefits of supplementation with hormones synthesized by organs under anterior pituitary control (i.e., triiodothyronine [T3], thyroxine [T4], and corticosteroids) (Table 185.8) [15,19,20,21,25,123–133]. Initially, the presence of low T3 blood levels was demonstrated after brain death in animal experiments [134]. Administration of exogenous T3 to donor animals improved a variety of metabolic parameters before and after organ preservation [135–137], as well as organ function after transplantation [138]. These findings suggested possibly positive effects of T3 also in human donors. A limited number of uncontrolled clinical trials suggested favorable influences of donor pretreatment with thyroid hormone on hemodynamic and metabolic parameters during the donor maintenance phase [86,139,140] and on outcome after heart transplantation [141–143]. But a number of other investigators failed to observe a significant benefit of thyroid hormone administration on biochemical and hemodynamic donor parameters and on posttransplant outcomes (Table 185.8) [23,123,124,132,144–146].

The latter outcomes could be explained at least in part by the findings of some studies which have suggested that the low T3 levels in human donors do not correlate with the presence of hemodynamic stability [147,148] or outcome after transplantation [149–152] to begin with. The typical thyroidal hormonal pattern after brain death consists of decreased T3, normal or decreased thyroxine, and normal thyroid-stimulating hormone. This pattern is not consistent with acute insufficiency of the hypothalamic–pituitary–thyroid axis or clinically overt hypothyroidism, but is similar to changes observed in other groups of critically ill individuals [130]. Thyroid hormone administration to such patients may not only be ineffective but may theoretically even be detrimental in some cases [130,131]. In summary, there is no conclusive evidence to date that supplementation of organ donors with thyroid hormone *alone* yields a significant clinical benefit.

By contrast, evidence for the potential benefits of routine administration of corticosteroids *alone* is emerging [23,123,153,154]. Normal human serum adrenocorticotropic hormone and cortisol levels have been demonstrated after brain death in some studies [117–120], while others have observed dysfunction of the hypothalamic–pituitary–adrenal axis in patients with traumatic brain injury [119]. Clinically, however, administration of high-dose steroids was noted to stabilize and improve lung function, leading to higher probability of lung recovery from brain-dead patients that had previously not been considered for lung donation, to increase organ yield and to lead to improved outcomes after liver transplantation [15,123,153–156].

Published retrospective evidence suggests that institution of empiric donor management protocols that incorporate *combination* treatment with arginine vasopressin, high-dose corticosteroids, thyroid hormone, and insulin may stabilize and improve cardiac function in brain-dead donors and may result in increased probability of kidney, heart, liver, lung, and pancreas recovery and transplantation and may improve posttransplant outcomes (Table 185.8) [17,19–20,126–129]. These and other findings have served as the basis for recommendations from a national U.S. consensus conference held in 2001 that include: T3: 4 μg bolus, 3 μg per hour continuous infusion; arginine vasopressin: 1 unit bolus, 0.5 to 4.0 units per hour continuous infusion (titrate SVR to 800 to 1,200 using a PA catheter); methylprednisolone 15 mg per kg intravenous bolus, repeat every 24 hours; and insulin continuous intravenous infusion at a minimum rate of 1 unit per hour (titrate blood glucose to 120 to 180 mg per dL) [16,18]. However, given the uncertainty regarding potentially adverse side effects and the absence of high-level evidence, large prospective randomized trials are necessary before routine administration of hormonal combination therapy can be recommended for all donors—particularly because, for example, excellent lung procurement rates from marginal donors and good posttransplant outcomes have also been described in the current era without hormonal supplementation (Table 185.8) [157]. Moreover, the optimal dose and combination, and the contribution of each individual hormone to the observed overall outcome remain yet to be studied and elucidated. The above-mentioned findings have stimulated national prospective multicenter trials that investigate the optimal timing and outcome of combination hormone replacement therapy. Although these trials are ongoing, it appears prudent to reserve routine *combination* hormone replacement therapy for hemodynamically unstable donors that require substantial catecholamine doses (e.g., dopamine >10 μg per kg per min) or have an ejection fraction of less than 45% [16,18,25].

Although brain death is not associated with primary pancreatic endocrine dysfunction, hyperglycemia is frequent in brain-dead donors. Hyperglycemia can be caused by increased catecholamine release, altered carbohydrate metabolism, steroid administration for treatment of cerebral edema, infusion of large amounts of dextrose-containing IV fluids, or peripheral insulin resistance. Treating hyperglycemia in brain-dead donors appears to be important with regard to pancreatic islet cell function. Experimental evidence suggests that high glucose levels may produce transient or irreversible damage to beta cells in the pancreatic islets, in vitro and in vivo [158,159]. This glucose toxicity was attenuated during in vivo experiments by correcting hyperglycemia [160]. Clinical studies in pancreas transplant recipients have demonstrated that donor hyperglycemia is a risk factor for decreased graft survival [90]. It was not established in these studies, however, whether donor hyperglycemia was indicative of marginal or insufficient beta-cell mass or whether impaired pancreatic graft function was related to islet cell dysfunction as a result of hyperglycemia.

Hyperglycemia in and of itself is known to cause insulin resistance [161]. Studies in brain-dead donors have suggested that a state of hyperinsulinemia coupled with peripheral insulin resistance exists, as evidenced by elevated C-peptide–glucose molar ratios [162]. For all the above reasons, it is prudent to maintain blood glucose levels in donors between 120 and 180 mg per dL [163]. Insulin should be administered as needed according to the blood glucose values to mitigate any potential adverse effects of hyperglycemia on pancreatic islets, which could impair glucose homeostasis after transplantation [163]. If hyperglycemia persists despite initial bolus insulin therapy, continuous IV insulin infusion should be instituted to facilitate titration of glucose levels. As in many other critical care patients, good glycemic control is also good standard practice for brain-dead donors, since it acts to prevent ketoacidosis and osmotic diuresis, both of which can be significant problems in the management of brain-dead donors, and since it may contribute to improved overall organ recovery and transplantation rates [164].

Hypothermia

After brain death, the body becomes poikilothermic because of the loss of thalamic and hypothalamic central temperature control mechanisms, and hypothermia usually ensues [165]. Systemic vasodilation causes additional heat loss. Hypothermia can be aggravated by administering room-temperature IV fluids and cold blood products. Adverse effects of hypothermia include decreased myocardial contractility, hypotension, cardiac arrhythmias, cardiac arrest, hepatic and renal dysfunction, and acidosis and coagulopathy [166–168]. Therefore, donor core temperature must be maintained at or above 35°C. It is usually sufficient to use humidified, heated ventilator gases; warmed IV fluids and blood products; and warming blankets to achieve rewarming and to maintain an adequate body temperature. Rewarming with peritoneal dialysis or bladder irrigations generally should not be performed in organ donors.

Coagulation System

Coagulopathy and disseminated intravascular coagulation are common findings in brain-dead donors, particularly after head injuries. Pathologic activation of the coagulation cascade occurs when brain tissue, which is very rich in tissue thromboplastin, comes in contact with blood after trauma. Massive blood transfusions can produce dilutional thrombocytopenia, and subsequent ongoing hemorrhage, hypothermia, and acidosis are all able to trigger or further aggravate coagulopathy. Clinical findings can include pathologic bleeding, abnormal prothrombin time, thrombocytopenia, hypofibrinogenemia, and increased levels of fibrin/fibrinogen degradation products. Treatment of coagulopathy entails use of blood components such as platelets, fresh-frozen plasma, or cryoprecipitate and correction of the underlying pathophysiology (e.g., hypothermia, acidosis, surgical hemorrhage). ε-Aminocaproic acid should not be used because of its potential for inducing microvascular thrombosis, thereby rendering organs potentially unsuitable for transplantation.

Other Aspects

Brain death may also adversely affect the donor's nutritional status. Experimental studies have suggested a hypercatabolic state and decreased hepatic intracellular ATP levels [169].

Moreover, a suboptimal organ energy and redox status along with the inflammatory changes that result from the chemokine and cytokine release associated with brain death may exert a deleterious influence on the magnitude of, and recovery from, ischemia-reperfusion injury and on posttransplant organ function in the recipient. Appropriate nutritional support of the donor may be able to prevent depletion of micro- and macronutrients and may attenuate oxidative stress and ischemia-reperfusion injury. However, currently there is no clinical data available that would directly support routine nutritional supplementation of brain-dead donors [169].

Various pharmacologic donor pretreatment protocols to optimize donor and transplant outcomes have been reported. The clinically beneficial effects of administration of catecholamines, vasopressin (or its analogue desmopressin), and of steroids on both donor and posttransplant outcomes have already been discussed in detail above (Table 185.8) [23,107–109,123,153,154]. In other studies, verapamil mitigated the adverse impact of elevated cytosolic calcium levels on renal allograft function [170] after donor hemodynamic instability. Finally, donor pretreatment with immunosuppressants may have a favorable impact by preventing upregulation of proinflammatory pathways and increased expression of major histocompatibility complex molecules that have been demonstrated to occur after brain death [102,103,104]. The latter pretreatment modalities, however, must be investigated more extensively before they can be routinely applied.

Multiple-Organ Donor Operation

After consent is obtained, the OPO schedules and organizes the organ recovery operation. Often, several surgical teams from different locations participate; their transportation and the preparation of the recipients in the various hospitals must be meticulously coordinated. After certification of death according to the state laws occurs, the brain-dead donor is brought to the operating room. Full cardiovascular and ventilatory support is maintained throughout the operation, until the organs are flushed and cooled. The principles of brain-dead donor management should be reviewed with the anesthesiologist, unless he or she is familiar with the specific clinical aspects of cardiovascular and ventilatory support for brain-dead organ donors. Hemodynamic stability must be maintained during the surgical organ retrieval, which is the equivalent of a combined major abdominal and thoracic operation and can last up to several hours. Transient tachycardia and hypertension may occur while the surgical incision is being made; they most likely reflect spinal reflexes causing vasoconstrictive responses and adrenal stimulation. Subsequently, consideration must be given to the increased heat loss caused by the wide abdominal and thoracic incisions and the duration of the surgery. Vecuronium or pancuronium should be used to inhibit reflex muscular contractions [83]. Tubocurarine should not be used in brain-dead donors because of its association with hypotension as a consequence of histamine release and ganglionic blockade. Maintenance fluid administration throughout the operation must take into account the significant intraoperative fluid losses resulting from extensive dissection with evaporation and blood loss, transsection of lymphatic channels, and massive third-space fluid loss.

All organs to be recovered are completely mobilized, and their vascular pedicles are dissected free. At the end of the operation, systemic heparinization occurs and cannulas are inserted (depending on the organs to be procured) into the abdominal aorta, inferior vena cava, portal vein, aortic arch, and pulmonary artery. Only then is circulatory and respiratory support terminated. The organs are flushed in situ with preservation solution to remove blood and to cool the organs to a temperature of 4°C to 7°C. Simultaneously, topical external cooling is provided by the application of sterile ice slush. The organs are then individually removed, by dividing the remaining attachments and vascular pedicles, and then packaged [49]. Storage in preservation solution at 4°C to 7°C in a cooler surrounded by crushed ice allows maximal preservation times of 4 to 6 hours for heart and lungs, approximately 30 hours for livers and pancreata, and about 40 hours for kidneys. These preservation constraints are taken into consideration as organs are allocated. Critical care of the donor ends when controlled cardiac arrest occurs at the completion of the surgical organ recovery. This finality is ephemeral, however, because it results in the start of new lives for the recipients after a successful organ transplant.

PERIOPERATIVE CRITICAL CARE MANAGEMENT OF THE DONATION AFTER CARDIAC DEATH ORGAN DONOR

Preoperative Care of the Potential DCD Donor (Prior to Obtaining Consent for Organ Donation)

Therapy in those patients must remain primarily aimed at treating the underlying pathology (e.g., head trauma, cerebrovascular accident). Any premature (i.e., prior to the family having made the decision to withdraw care and prior to obtaining consent) change of therapeutic objectives would be unethical and may lead to lower consent rates, thereby further exacerbating the current donor organ shortage [26,28,98].

Preoperative Care of the Actual DCD Donor (After Having Obtained Consent for Organ Donation)

Once consent to proceed with organ donation has been obtained, the focus switches from cerebral protection to preservation of organ function and optimization of peripheral oxygen delivery [26,98]. Maintenance therapy endpoints in DCD donors are identical to those that apply for brain-dead organ donors (Table 185.7). Since DCD donors usually do not exhibit the same pathophysiologic characteristics as brain-dead donors, general management principles for DCD donors are more akin to those that apply to non-brain–dead patients in the ICU that are described elsewhere in this book. Organ-specific considerations (e.g., use of catecholamines) are the same as those described below for brain-dead donors.

Preterminal and Intraoperative Care of DCD Donors

Maintenance therapy as outlined above is continued until support is withdrawn and the patient is extubated (either in the ICU or in the operating room). Any additional premortem interventions (e.g., surgical: insertion of femoral cannulas in preparation of organ recovery; pharmacologic: administration of intravenous heparin, opioids, and phentolamine) must occur in strict accordance with local OPO/hospital DCD protocols and policies [26,98,171–174]. Death is then pronounced by a physician (usually the patient's intensive care physician) not belonging to the organ recovery and transplant team according to criteria that are specified by the local OPO/hospital DCD protocol.

Next, after an additional 2-to-5-minute waiting time, surgical organ recovery begins [26,173,174]. For DCD donors, the use of a rapid procurement technique is mandatory in order to minimize warm ischemia time, particularly when highly ischemia-sensitive organs such as the liver, pancreas, or lungs are to be recovered as well [49].

Disposition of the patient, if death does not occur within a specified waiting time post withdrawal of support, is determined by the local protocol (e.g., return of patient to a nonintensive care hospital floor for comfort care only).

References

1. http://www.optn.org. Accessed April 9, 2011.
2. U.S. Department of Health & Human Services: Deceased Donor Characteristics, Deceased Donors of Any Organ—2008 OPTN/SRTR Annual Report, Transplant Data. http://www.ustransplant.org/annual_reports/current. Accessed May 21, 2010.
3. Report of the Task Force on Organ Transplantation: *Organ Transplantation: Issues and Recommendation.* Washington, DC, US Department of Health and Human Services, 1986, p 36.
4. Heffron TG: Organ procurement and management of the multiorgan donor, in Hall JB, Schmidt GA, Wood LDH (eds): *Principles of Critical Care.* New York, McGraw-Hill, 1992, p 891.
5. Najarian JS, Strand M, Fryd DS, et al: Comparison of cyclosporine versus azathioprine-antilymphocyte globulin in renal transplantation. *Transplant Proc* 15[Suppl 1]:2463, 1983.
6. Starzl TE, Iwatsuki S, Van Thiel DH, et al: Report of Colorado-Pittsburgh liver transplantation studies. *Transplant Proc* 15[Suppl 1]:2582, 1983.
7. Sutherland DER: Pancreas transplantation: overview and current status of cases reported to the registry through 1982. *Transplant Proc* 15[Suppl 1]:2597, 1983.
8. Oyer PE, Stinson EB, Jamieson SW, et al: Cyclosporine in cardiac transplantation: a 2½-year follow-up. *Transplant Proc* 15[Suppl 1]:2546, 1983.
9. Evans RW, Orians CE, Ascher NL: The potential supply of organ donors: an assessment of the efficiency of organ procurement efforts in the United States. *JAMA* 267:239, 1992.
10. Siminoff LA, Arnold RM, Caplan AL, et al: Public policy governing organ and tissue procurement in the United States. *Ann Intern Med* 123:10, 1995.
11. Siminoff LA, Gordon N, Hewlett J, et al: Factors influencing families' consent for donation of solid organs for transplantation. *JAMA* 286:71, 2001.
12. Sheehy E, Conrad SL, Brigham LE, et al: Estimating the number of potential organ donors in the United States. *N Engl J Med* 349:667, 2003.
13. Rodrigue JR, Cornell DL, Howard RJ: Organ donation decision: comparison of donor and nondonor families. *Am J Transplant* 6:190, 2006.
14. Schnitzler MA, Whiting JF, Brennan DC, et al: The life-years saved by a deceased organ donor. *Am J Transplant* 5:2289, 2005.
15. Rosendale JD, Chabalewski FL, McBride MA, et al: Increased transplanted organs from the use of a standardized donor management protocol. *Am J Transplant* 2:761, 2002.
16. Rosengard BR, Feng S, Alfrey EJ, et al: Report of the Crystal City meeting to maximize the use of organs recovered from the cadaver donor. *Am J Transplant* 2:701, 2002.
17. Wheeldon DR: Transforming the "unacceptable" donor: outcomes from the adoption of a standardized donor management technique. *J Heart Lung Transplant* 14:734, 1995.
18. Zaroff JG, Rosengard BR, Armstrong WF, et al: Consensus conference report: maximizing use of organs recovered from the cadaver donor: cardiac recommendations. *Circulation* 106:836, 2002.
19. Rosendale JD, Kauffman HM, McBride MA: Hormonal resuscitation yields more transplanted hearts with improved early function. *Transplantation* 75:1336, 2003.
20. Rosendale JD, Kauffman HM, McBride MA, et al: Aggressive pharmacologic donor management results in more transplanted organs. *Transplantation* 75:482, 2003.
21. Salim A, Velmahos GC, Brown C, et al: Aggressive organ donor management significantly increases the number of organs available for transplantation. *J Trauma* 58:991, 2005.
22. Salim A, Martin M, Brown C, et al: The effect of a protocol of aggressive donor management: implications for the national organ donor shortage. *J Trauma* 61:429–435, 2006.
23. Venkateswaran RV, Patchell VB, Wilson IC, et al: Early donor management increases the retrieval rate of lungs for transplantation. *Ann Thorac Surg* 85:278–286, 2008.
24. Sung RS, Galloway J, Tuttle-Newhall JE, et al: Organ donation and utilization in the United States, 1997–2006. *Am J Transplant* 8 (Part 2): 922–934, 2008.
25. Wood KE, Becker BN, McCartney JG, et al: Care of the potential organ donor. *N Engl J Med* 351:2730, 2004.
26. Reich DJ, Mulligan DC, Abt PL, et al: ASTS recommended practice guidelines for controlled donation after cardiac death organ procurement and transplantation. *Am J Transplant* 9:2004–2011, 2009.
27. Boucek MM, Mashburn C, Dunn SM, et al: Pediatric heart transplantation after declaration of cardiocirculatory death. *N Engl J Med* 349: 709–714, 2008.
28. Doig CJ, Rocker G: Retrieving organs from non-heart-beating organ donors: a review of medical and ethical issues. *Can J Anesth* 50:1069, 2003.
29. D'Alessandro AM, Peltier JW, Phelps JE: Understanding the antecedents of the acceptance of donation after cardiac death by healthcare professionals. *Crit Care Med* 36:1075–1081, 2008.
30. Jones JW, Gruber SA, Barker JH, et al: Successful hand transplantation. One year follow-up. *N Engl J Med* 343:468, 2000.
31. Landin L, Cavadas PC, Nthumba P, et al: Preliminary results of bilateral arm transplantation. *Transplantation* 88: 749–751, 2009.
32. Strome M, Stein J, Esclamado R, et al: Laryngeal transplantation and 40-month follow-up. *N Engl J Med* 344:1676, 2001.
33. Smith CR: Dire wounds, a new face, a glimpse in a mirror. *The New York Times* December 3, 2005:1A.
34. Fishbein TM. Intestinal transplantation. *N Engl J Med* 361:998, 2009.
35. Gruessner RWG, Sutherland DER, Gruessner AC: Mortality assessment for pancreas transplants. *Am J Transplant* 4: 2018–2026, 2004.
36. Shapiro J, Lakey J, Edmond R, et al: Islet transplantation in seven patients with type 1 diabetes mellitus using a glucocorticoid-free immunosuppressive regimen. *N Engl J Med* 343:230, 2000.
37. Ryan EA, Paty BW, Senior PA, et al: Five-year follow-up after clinical islet transplantation. *Diabetes* 54:2060, 2005.
38. Kay MP: The Registry of the International Society for Heart and Lung Transplantation: tenth official report—1993. *J Heart Lung Transplant* 12:541, 1993.
39. Bolman RM III, Shumway SJ, Estrin JA, et al: Lung and heart-lung transplantation: evolution and new applications. *Ann Surg* 214: 456, 1991.
40. Leichtman AB, Cohen D, Keith D, et al: Kidney and pancreas transplantation in the United States, 1997–2006: The HRSA breakthrough collaboratives and the 58 DSA challenge. *Am J Transplant* 8:946–957, 2008.
41. http://www.healthdisparities.net/hdc/html/collaboratives.topics.tgmc.aspx. Accessed November 15, 2009.
42. Gravel MT, Arenas JD, Chenault R II, et al: Kidney transplantation from organ donors following cardiopulmonary death using extracorporeal membrane oxygenation support. *Ann Transplant* 9:57, 2004.
43. Wang C-C, Wang S-H, Lin C-C, et al: Liver transplantation from an uncontrolled non-heart-beating donor maintained on extracorporeal membrane oxygenation. *Transplant Proc* 37:4331, 2005.
44. Moers C, Smits JM, Maathuis M-H J, et al: Machine perfusion or cold storage in deceased-donor kidney transplantation. *N Engl J Med* 360:7–19, 2009.
45. Gallup poll surveys views on organ donation. *Nephrol News Issues* 5:16, 1993.
46. Callender CO, Hall LE, Yeager CL, et al: Organ donation and blacks: a critical frontier. *N Engl J Med* 325:442, 1991.
47. Pollak R: Medical student education and organ donation—a medical school survey. *Clin Transplant* 6:372, 1992.
48. Gridelli B, Remuzzi G: Strategies for making more organs available for transplantation. *N Engl J Med* 343:404, 2000.
49. Brockmann JG, Vaidya A, Reddy S, et al: Retrieval of abdominal organs for transplantation. *Br J Surg* 93:133, 2006.
50. Fukuzawa K, Schwartz ME, Katz E, et al: An alternative technique for in situ arterial flushing in elderly liver donors with atherosclerotic occlusive disease. *Transplantation* 55:445, 1993.
51. Barone GW, Henry ML, Elkhammas EA, et al: Whole organ transplant of an annular pancreas. *Transplantation* 53:492, 1992.
52. Troppmann C, Daily MF, McVicar JP, et al: Hypothermic pulsatile perfusion of small pediatric en bloc kidneys: Technical aspects and outcomes. *Transplantation* 88:289–290, 2009.
53. Sutherland DER, Morel P, Gruessner RWG: Transplantation of two diabetic patients with one divided cadaver donor pancreas. *Transplant Proc* 22:585, 1990.
54. Azoulay D, Didier S, Castaing D, et al: Domino liver transplants for metabolic disorders: experience with familial amyloidotic polyneuropathy. *J Am Coll Surg* 189:584, 1999.
55. Azoulay D, Castaing D, Adam R, et al: Transplantation of three adult patients with one cadaveric graft: wait or innovate. *Liver Transpl* 6:239, 2000.

56. Lowell JA, Smith CR, Brennan DC, et al: The domino transplant: transplant recipients as organ donors. *Transplantation* 69:372, 2000.
57. Ross LF, Rubin DT, Seigler M, et al: Ethics of a paired-kidney-exchange program. *N Engl J Med* 336:1752, 1997.
58. Rees MA, Kopke JE, Pelletier RP, et al: A nonsimultaneous, extended, altruistic-donor chain. *N Engl J Med* 360: 1096–1101, 2009.
59. Starzl T, Teperman L, Sutherland D, et al: Transplant tourism and unregulated black-market trafficking of organs. *Am J Transplant* 9:1484, 2009.
60. Matas AJ, Hippen B, Satel S. In defense of a regulated system of compensation for living donation. *Curr Opin Organ Transplant* 13:379–385, 2008.
61. Radcliffe-Richards J, Daar AS, Guttmann RD et al: The case for allowing kidney sales. *Lancet* 351:1950, 1998.
62. Scheper-Hughes N: The global traffic in human organs. *Curr Anthropol* 41:191, 2000.
63. Jacobs CL, Roman D, Garvey C, et al: Twenty-two nondirected kidney donors: An update on a single center's experience. *Am J Transplant* 4:1110, 2004.
64. Wright L, Campbell M: Soliciting kidneys on Web sites: Is it fair? *Semin Dial* 19:5, 2006.
65. Steinbrook R. Public solicitation of organ donors. *N Engl J Med* 353:441, 2005.
66. Caplan AL, Van Buren CT, Tilney NL: Financial compensation for cadaver organ donation: good idea or anathema. *Transplant Proc* 25:2740, 1993.
67. Guttmann RD: On the use of organs from executed prisoners. *Transplant Rev* 6:189, 1982.
68. Caplan AL: Ethical issues in the use of anencephalic infants as a source of organs and tissues for transplantation. *Transplant Proc* 20:42, 1988.
69. Troppmann C, Gruessner AC, Papalois BE, et al: Discordant xenoislets from a large animal donor undergo accelerated graft failure rather than hyperacute rejection: impact of immunosuppression, islet mass, and transplant site on early outcome. *Surgery* 121:194, 1997.
70. Starzl TE, Fung J, Tzakis A, et al: Baboon-to-human liver transplantation. *Lancet* 341:65, 1993.
71. Caplan AL: Ethical issues raised by research involving xenografts. *JAMA* 254:3339, 1985.
72. Matesanz R, Miranda B, Felipe C, et al: Continuous improvement in organ donation. *Transplantation* 61:1119, 1996.
73. Matesanz R, Marazuela R, Domínguez-Gil B, et al: The 40 donors per million population plan: an action plan for improvement of organ donation and transplantation in Spain. *Transplant Proc* 41:3453–3456, 2009.
74. Council of Europe: International figures on donation and transplantation – 2008. *Newsletter Transplant* 14:14, 2009. http://www.edqm.eu/medias/fichiers/Newsletter_Transplant_Vol_14_No_1_Sept_2009.pdf.
75. Shafer TJ, David KD, Holtzman SM, et al: Location of in-house organ procurement organization staff in level I trauma centers increases conversion of potential donors to actual donors. *Transplantation* 75:1330, 2003.
76. Weimer DL: *Medical Governance: Values Expertise, and Interests in Organ Transplantation.* Washington, D.C.: Georgetown University press, 2010.
77. Sadler AM Jr, Sadler BL, Stason EB: The uniform anatomical gift act: a model for reform. *JAMA* 206:2501, 1968.
78. Beecher HK, Adams RD, Barger AC, et al: A definition of irreversible coma: report of the ad hoc committee of the Harvard Medical School to examine the definition of brain death. *JAMA* 205:337, 1968.
79. Guidelines for the Determination of Death: Report of the medical consultants on the diagnosis of death to the President's Commission for the Study of Ethical Problems in Medicine and Biomedical and Behavioral Research. *JAMA* 246:2184, 1981.
80. Wijdicks EFM: The diagnosis of brain death. *N Engl J Med* 344: 1215, 2001.
81. The Quality Standards Subcommittee of the American Academy of Neurology: Practice parameters for determining brain death in adults. *Neurology* 45:1012, 1995.
82. Darby JM, Stein K, Grenvik A, et al: Approach to management of the heartbeating "brain dead" organ donor. *JAMA* 261:2222, 1989.
83. Saposnik G, Bueri JA, Maurino J, et al: Spontaneous and reflex movements in brain death. *Neurology* 54:221, 2000.
84. Zygun D: Non-neurological organ dysfunction in neurocritical care: impact on outcome and etiological considerations. *Curr Opin Crit Care* 11: 139–143, 2005.
85. Lytle FT, Afessa B, Keegan MT: Progression of organ failure in patients approaching brain stem death. *Am J Transplant* 9: 1446–1450, 2009.
86. Taniguchi S, Kitamura S, Kawachi K, et al: Effects of hormonal supplements on the maintenance of cardiac function in potential donor patients after cerebral death. *Eur J Cardiothorac Surg* 6:96, 1992.
87. Troppmann C, Gillingham KJ, Benedetti E, et al: Delayed graft function, acute rejection, and outcome after cadaver renal transplantation. *Transplantation* 59:962, 1995.
88. Whelchel JD, Diethelm AG, Phillips MG, et al: The effect of high-dose dopamine in cadaver donor management on delayed graft function and graft survival following renal transplantation. *Transplant Proc* 18:523, 1986.
89. Bouwman DL, Altshuler J, Weaver DW. Hyperamylasemia: a result of intracranial bleeding. *Surgery* 94:318, 1983.
90. Gores PF, Gillingham KJ, Dunn DL, et al: Donor hyperglycemia as a minor risk factor and immunologic variables as major risk factors for pancreas allograft loss in a multivariate analysis of a single institution's experience. *Ann Surg* 215:217, 1992.
91. Marques RG, Rogers J, Chavin KD, et al: Does treatment of cadaveric organ donors with desmopressin increase the likelihood of pancreas graft thrombosis? Results of a preliminary study. *Transplant Proc* 36:1048, 2004.
92. Bohrade SM, Vignaswaran W, McCabe MA, et al: Liberalization of donor criteria may expand the donor pool without adverse consequence in lung transplantation. *J Heart Lung Transplant* 19: 1200, 2000.
93. Freeman RB, Giatras I, Falagas ME, et al: Outcome of transplantation of organs procured from bacteremic donors. *Transplantation* 68:1107, 1999.
94. Dodson SF, Bonham CA, Geller DA, et al: Prevention of de novo hepatitis B infection in recipients of hepatic allografts from anti-HBc positive donors. *Transplantation* 68:1058, 1999.
95. Vargas HE, Laskus T, Wang L, et al: Outcome of liver transplantation in hepatitis C virus–infected patients who received hepatitis C virus–infected grafts. *Gastroenterology* 117:149, 1999.
96. Colquhoun SD, Robert ME, Shaked A, et al: Transmission of CNS malignancy by organ transplantation. *Transplantation* 57:970, 1994.
97. Garrison RN, Bentley FR, Raque GH, et al: There is an answer to shortage of organ donors. *Surg Gynecol Obstet* 173:391, 1991.
98. Bernat JL, D'Alessandro AM, Port FK, et al: Report of a national conference on donation after cardiac death. *Am J Transplant* 6:281–291, 2006.
99. Steinbrook R: Organ donation after cardiac death. *N Engl J Med* 357:209–213, 2007.
100. Cooper DKC, Novitzky D, Witcomb WN: The pathophysiological effects of brain death on potential donor organs, with particular reference to the heart. *Ann R Coll Surg Engl* 71:261, 1989.
101. Minnear FL, Barie PS, Malik AB: Effects of transient pulmonary hypertension on pulmonary vascular permeability. *J Appl Physiol Respir Environ Exercise Physiol* 55:983, 1983.
102. Pratschke J, Wilhelm MJ, Kusaka M, et al: Brain death and its influence on donor organ quality and outcome after transplantation. *Transplantation* 67:343, 1999.
103. Takada M, Nadeau KC, Hancock WW, et al: Effects of explosive brain death on cytokine activation of peripheral organs in the rat. *Transplantation* 65:1533, 1998.
104. Bouma HR, Ploeg RJ, Schuurs TA: Signal transduction pathways involved in brain death-induced renal injury. *Am J Transplant* 9: 989–997, 2009.
105. Venkateswaran RV, Dronavalli V, Lambert PA, et al: The proinflammatory environment in potential heart and lung donors: prevalence and impact of donor management and hormonal therapy. *Transplantation* 88: 582–588, 2009.
106. Powner DJ: Effects of gene induction and cytokine production in donor care. *Prog Transplant* 13:9, 2003.
107. Schnuelle P, Yard BA, Braun C, et al: Impact of donor dopamine on immediate graft function after kidney transplantation. *Am J Transplant* 4:419–426, 2004.
108. Schnuelle P, Berger S, De Boer J, et al: Effects of catecholamine application to brain-dead donors on graft survival in solid organ transplantation. *Transplantation* 72:455, 2001.
109. Schnuelle P, Gottmann U, Hoeger S, et al: Effects of donor pretreatment with dopamine on graft function after kidney transplantation. *JAMA* 302: 1067–1075, 2009.
110. Pennefather SH, Bullock RE, Mantle D, et al: Use of low dose arginine vasopressin to support brain-dead organ donors. *Transplantation* 59:58, 1995.
111. Chen JM, Cullinane S, Spanier TB, et al: Vasopressin deficiency and pressor hypersensitivity in hemodynamically unstable organ donors. *Circulation* 100[Suppl II]:II244, 1999.
112. Russell JA, Walley KR, Singer J, et al: Vasopressin versus norepinephrine infusion in patients with septic shock. *N Engl J Med* 358:877–887, 2008.
113. Davis SV, Olichwier KK, Chakko SC: Reversible depression of myocardial performance to hypophosphatemia. *Am J Med Sci* 295:183, 1988.
114. The Acute Respiratory Distress Syndrome Network: Ventilation with lower tidal volumes as compared with traditional tidal volumes for acute lung injury and the acute respiratory distress syndrome. *N Engl J Med* 342:1301, 2000.
115. Avlonitis VS, Fisher AJ, Kirby JA, et al: Pulmonary transplantation: the role of brain death in donor lung injury. *Transplantation* 75:1928, 2003.
116. Richardson DW, Robinson AG: Desmopressin. *Ann Intern Med* 103:228, 1985.
117. Hall GM, Mashiter K, Lumley J, et al: Hypothalamic-pituitary function in the "brain-dead" patient. *Lancet* 2:1259, 1980.
118. Gramm H-J, Meinhold H, Bickel U, et al: Acute endocrine failure after brain death. *Transplantation* 54:851, 1992.
119. Howlett TA, Keogh AM, Perry L, et al: Anterior and posterior pituitary function in brain-stem-dead donors: a possible role for hormonal replacement therapy. *Transplantation* 47:828, 1989.
120. Powner DJ, Hendrich A, Lagler RG, et al: Hormonal changes in brain dead patients. *Crit Care Med* 18:702, 1990.
121. Seeger W (ed): *Atlas of Topographical Anatomy of the Brain and Surrounding Structures.* New York, Springer-Verlag, 1978.
122. Dimopoulou I, Tsagarakis S, Anthi A, et al: High prevalence of decreased cortisol reserve in brain-dead potential organ donors. *Crit Care Med* 31:1113, 2003.

123. Selck FW, Deb P, Grossman EB: Deceased organ donor characteristics and clinical interventions associated with organ yield. *Am J Transplant* 8: 965–974, 2008.
124. Randell TT, Höckerstedt KAV: Triiodothyronine treatment in brain-dead multiorgan donors: a controlled study. *Transplantation* 54:736, 1992.
125. Novitzky D, Cooper DKC, Muchmore JS, et al: Pituitary function in brain-dead patients. *Transplantation* 48:1078, 1989.
126. Van Bakel AB, Pitzer S, Drake P, et al: Early hormonal therapy stabilizes hemodynamics during donor procurement. *Transplant Proc* 36:2573, 2004.
127. Roels L, Pirenne J, Delooz H, et al: Effect of triiodothyronine replacement therapy on maintenance characteristics and organ availability in hemodynamically unstable donors. *Transplant Proc* 32:1564, 2000.
128. Salim A, Vassiliu P, Velmahos GC, et al: The role of thyroid hormone administration in potential organ donors. *Arch Surg* 136:1377, 2001.
129. Reutzel-Selke A, Tullius SG, Zschockelt T, et al: Donor pretreatment of grafts from marginal donors improves long-term graft outcome. *Transplant Proc* 33:970, 2001.
130. Hershman JM: Free thyroxine in nonthyroidal illness. *Ann Intern Med* 98:947, 1983.
131. Hess ML: Letters to the Editor. *J Heart Transplant* 5:486, 1986.
132. Pennefather SH, Bullock RE: Triiodothyronine treatment in brain-dead multiorgan donors: a controlled study. *Transplantation* 55:1443, 1993.
133. Novitzky D, Cooper DKC, Rosendale JD, et al: Hormonal therapy of the brain-dead organ donor: experimental and clinical studies. *Transplantation* 82: 1396–1401, 2006.
134. Novitzky D, Wicomb WN, Cooper DKC, et al: Electrocardiographic, hemodynamic and endocrine changes occurring during experimental brain death in the Chacma baboon. *J Heart Transplant* 4:63, 1984.
135. Novitzky D, Cooper DKC, Morrell D, et al: Change from aerobic to anaerobic metabolism after brain death, and reversal following triiodothyronine therapy. *Transplantation* 45:32, 1988.
136. Novitzky D, Wicomb WN, Cooper DKC, et al: Improved cardiac function following hormonal therapy in brain dead pigs: relevance to organ donation. *Cryobiology* 24:1, 1987.
137. Wicomb WN, Cooper DKC, Novitzky D: Impairment of renal slice function following brain death, with reversibility of injury by hormonal therapy. *Transplantation* 41:29, 1986.
138. Pienaar H, Schwartz I, Roncone A, et al: Function of kidney grafts from brain-dead donor pigs: the influence of dopamine and triiodothyronine. *Transplantation* 50:580, 1990.
139. Washida M, Okamoto R, Manaka D, et al: Beneficial effect of combined 3,5,3-triiodothyronine and vasopressin administration on hepatic energy status and systemic hemodynamics after brain death. *Transplantation* 54:44, 1992.
140. García-Fages LC, Antolín M, Cabrer C, et al: Effects of substitutive triiodothyronine therapy on intracellular nucleotide levels in donor organs. *Transplant Proc* 23:2495, 1991.
141. Orlowski JP, Spees EK: Improved cardiac transplant survival with thyroxine treatment of hemodynamically unstable donors: 95.2% graft survival at 6 and 30 months. *Transplant Proc* 25:1535, 1993.
142. Novitzky D, Cooper DKC, Reichart B: Hemodynamic and metabolic responses to hormonal therapy in brain-dead potential organ donors. *Transplantation* 43:852, 1987.
143. Novitzky D, Cooper DKC, Chaffin JS, et al: Improved cardiac allograft function following triiodothyronine therapy to both donor and recipient. *Transplantation* 49:311, 1990.
144. Goarin J-P, Cohen S, Riou P, et al: The effects of triiodothyronine on hemodynamic status and cardiac function in potential heart donors. *Anesth Analg* 83:41, 1996.
145. Perez-Blanco A, Caturla-Such J, Canovas-Robles J, et al: Efficiency of triiodothyronine treatment on organ donor hemodynamic management and adenine nucleotide concentration. *Intensive Care Med* 31:943, 2005.
146. Schwartz I, Bird S, Lotz Z, et al: The influence of thyroid hormone replacement in a porcine brain death model. *Transplantation* 55:474, 1993.
147. Robertson KM, Hramiak IM, Gelb AW: Endocrine changes and haemodynamic stability after brain death. *Transplant Proc* 21:1197, 1989.
148. Koller J, Wieser C, Gottardis M, et al: Thyroid hormones and their impact on the hemodynamic and metabolic stability of organ donors and on kidney graft function after transplantation. *Transplant Proc* 22:355, 1990.
149. Wahlers T, Fieguth HG, Jurmann M, et al: Does hormone depletion of organ donors impair myocardial function after cardiac transplantation? *Transplant Proc* 20:792, 1988.
150. Macoviak JA, McDougall IR, Bayer MG, et al: Significance of thyroid dysfunction in human cardiac allograft procurement. *Transplantation* 43:824, 1987.
151. Gifford RRM, Weaver AS, Burg JE, et al: Thyroid hormone levels in heart and kidney cadaver donors. *J Heart Transplant* 5:249, 1986.
152. Mariot J, Sadoune L-O, Jacob F, et al: Hormone levels, hemodynamics, and metabolism in brain dead organ donors. *Transplant Proc* 27:793, 1995.
153. Kotsch K, Ulrich F, Reutzel-Selke A, et al: Methylprednisolone therapy in deceased donors reduces inflammation in the donor liver and improves outcome after liver transplantation. *Ann Surg* 248:1042–1050, 2008.
154. Straznicka M, Follette DM, Eisner MD, et al: Aggressive management of lung donors classified as unacceptable: Excellent recipient survival one year after transplantation. *J Thorac Cardiovasc Surg* 124:250, 2002.
155. Follette D, Rudich S, Bonacci R, et al: Importance of an aggressive multidisciplinary management approach to optimize lung donor procurement. *Transplant Proc* 31:169, 1999.
156. Milano CA, Buchan K, Perreas K, et al: Thoracic organ transplantation at Papworth Hospital, in Terasaki PI, Cecka JM (eds): *Clinical Transplants 1999*. Los Angeles, UCLA Tissue Typing Laboratory, 1999.
157. Gabbay E, Williams TJ, Griffiths AP, et al: Maximizing the utilization of donor organs offered for lung transplantation. *Am J Respir Crit Care Med* 160:265, 1999.
158. Dohan FC, Lukens FDW: Lesions of the pancreatic islets produced in cats by administration of glucose. *Science* 105:183, 1947.
159. Collier SA, Mandel TE, Carter WM: Detrimental effect of high medium glucose concentration on subsequent endocrine function of transplanted organ-cultured fetal mouse pancreas. *Aust J Exp Biol Med Sci* 60:437, 1982.
160. Clark A, Bown E, King T, et al: Islet changes induced by hyperglycemia in rats: effects of insulin or chlorpropamide therapy. *Diabetes* 31:319, 1982.
161. Unger RH, Grundy S: Hyperglycemia as an inducer as well as a consequence of impaired islet cell function and insulin resistance: implications for the management of diabetes. *Diabetologia* 28:119, 1985.
162. Massen F, Thicoipe M, Gin H, et al: The endocrine pancreas in brain-dead donors. A prospective study in 25 patients. *Transplantation* 56:363, 1993.
163. Powner DJ: Donor care before pancreatic tissue transplantation. *Prog Transplant* 15:129, 2005.
164. Van den Berghe G, Wouters P, Weekers F, et al: Intensive insulin therapy in critically ill patients. *N Engl J Med* 345:1359, 2001.
165. Powner DJ, Jastremski M, Lagler RG: Continuing care of multiorgan donor patients. *J Intensive Care Med* 4:75, 1989.
166. Swain JA: Hypothermia and blood pH. *Arch Intern Med* 148: 1643, 1988.
167. Koncke GM, Nichols RRD, Mendenhall JT, et al: Ectothermic philosophy of acid-base balance to prevent fibrillation during hypothermia. *Arch Surg* 121:303, 1986.
168. Reuler JB: Hypothermia: pathophysiology, clinical settings, and management. *Ann Intern Med* 89:519, 1978.
169. Singer P, Shapiro H, Cohen J: Brain death and organ damage: the modulating effects of nutrition. *Transplantation* 80:1363, 2005.
170. Korb S, Albornoz G, Brems W, et al: Verapamil pretreatment of hemodynamically unstable donors prevents delayed graft function post-transplant. *Transplant Proc* 21:1236, 1989.
171. Institute of Medicine (IOM): *Report: Non-heart-beating organ transplantation: Practice and protocols*. Washington, DC: National Academy Press, 2000.
172. Institute of Medicine (IOM): Report: Non-heart-beating organ transplantation: medical and ethical issues in procurement. Washington, DC: National Academy Press, 1997.
173. UNOS. Highlights of the June Board Meeting. UNOS Update. 2006. www.unos.org. Accessed November 15, 2009.
174. JCAHOnline. Revised organ procurement and donation standard. http://www.jointcommission.org/Library/JCAHOnline/jo_06.06.htm. Accessed November 15, 2009.

CHAPTER 186 ■ DIAGNOSIS AND MANAGEMENT OF REJECTION, INFECTION, AND MALIGNANCY IN TRANSPLANT RECIPIENTS

TUN JIE, DAVID L. DUNN AND RAINER W.G. GRUESSNER

Allograft rejection in transplant recipients is the side effect of the complex and intricate mammalian immune system, which is intended to defend the host against pathogens. The history of solid-organ transplantation has demonstrated that graft survival depends on manipulating the immune system. However, any modification of the host's defense mechanism can bring unwanted consequences, such as infection and malignancy. Throughout the development of solid-organ transplantation during the 1960s, it became clear that suppressing the immune system of the prospective host would be required for sustained graft function. In the infancy of this field, acute rejection (AR) and graft loss were the rule rather than the exception.

Subsequently, however, successful antirejection treatment and, more important, the ability to markedly reduce the incidence of rejection through preventive strategies allowed solid-organ transplantation to develop beyond its status as a sparingly performed investigational therapy. Specifically, successful allogeneic renal transplantation was achieved using a combination of a high-dose corticosteroid and azathioprine [1]. Contemporaneous observations of those early transplant recipients demonstrated that nonselective immunosuppressive therapy prolonged graft (and patient) survival yet led to an increased susceptibility to infection, often with unusual, opportunistic pathogens [2]. Furthermore, immunosuppressed transplant recipients also had an increased susceptibility to malignancy [3].

In the nearly 50 years since the report of the initial 12 recipients treated for rejection of allogeneic renal grafts, solid-organ transplantation has flourished beyond the expectations of any but the most wildly optimistic pioneers in the field. Kidney, liver, heart, and lung transplants are now standard-of-care therapies for end-stage renal, hepatic, cardiac, and pulmonary disease, respectively. Pancreas and pancreatic islet-cell transplants restore the beta-cell function in patients with diabetes mellitus. Even the small bowel has been successfully transplanted as a treatment for patients with short gut syndrome. Such strides have been made possible by the accumulated advances in organ procurement, preservation, surgical techniques, tissue typing, immunosuppressive therapy, and the use of antibacterial, antifungal, and antiviral agents for both prophylaxis and treatment of posttransplant infection. Table 186.1 lists some of the major advances in the management of rejection, infection, and malignancy in transplant recipients.

Yet even with the expanded immunosuppressive armamentarium of the twenty-first century, it remains difficult to adequately suppress the host immune system (to allow acceptance and even tolerance of the graft) without oversuppressing immune function (and thereby leaving the host vulnerable to opportunistic infection and malignancy). This chapter reviews the complications (namely, graft rejection, infection, and malignancy) of solid-organ transplantation on either side of that delicate balance. Special attention is directed toward opportunistic infections and unusual malignancies that occur in the immunosuppressed patient population.

REJECTION

Unlike the nonspecific innate immune system seen in all living organisms, the adaptive immune system—a unique property of jawed vertebrates—is an evolutionarily more advanced, efficient, "specific," and versatile host defense mechanism against invasion of pathogens. However, a side effect of the ability of the host immune system to recognize and attack "nonself" tissues is rejection of grafted tissues posttransplant. That side effect was observed clinically for centuries before Medawar demonstrated that it was an intrinsic property of the host immune system in response to foreign tissue [4]. The exogenous modulation of the host immune system to allow sustained graft function has proceeded along with—and often preceded—our understanding of the physiologic mechanism of rejection and tolerance.

Integral to our understanding of rejection is its immunologic basis. The immunologic disparity among members of the same species of mammals that leads to lack of recognition of "self" tissue and to rejection of nonself tissue is based on the differences in cell surface molecules that are expressed. In humans, these major histocompatibility antigens were first identified in leukocytes, and hence are termed *human leukocyte antigens* (HLAs). HLAs are subdivided into two classes: class I (HLA-A, -B, and -C), expressed on the surface of all nucleated cells, and class II (HLA-DR, -DQ, and -DP), expressed on the surface of *antigen-presenting cells* (APCs). The recognition of nonself tissue occurs via two distinct immunologic pathways: *direct* and *indirect allorecognition*. Direct allorecognition consists of recipient T-helper cells recognizing donor HLA disparity expressed on the donor cell surface. Indirect allorecognition consists of recipient APCs (generally thought to be activated macrophages, dendritic cells, and B lymphocytes) phagocytosing donor cellular debris, including HLAs, which are then processed and re-presented on the APC surface to be recognized by recipient T- helper cells (CD4+ lymphocytes).

In either pathway, costimulation signals between CD4+ T-helper lymphocytes and CD8+ cytotoxic T lymphocytes trigger a cascade of immunologic events. Interleukin (IL)-2, a crucial and early signal in immune activation, is secreted by activated CD4+ T-helper lymphocytes, engendering increased T-cell responsiveness, clonal expansion of alloreactive T lymphocytes, and acquisition of the cytolytic phenotype by host T lymphocytes. Direct allorecognition leads to a more immediate and vigorous immune response against foreign tissue, but, in both pathways, additional helper T lymphocytes are recruited and secrete a wide array of cytokines (e.g., IL-1, interferon-γ, tumor necrosis factor-α), facilitating the further recruitment of

TABLE 186.1

MAJOR ADVANCES IN MANAGEMENT OF REJECTION, INFECTION, AND MALIGNANCY IN TRANSPLANT RECIPIENTS

Topic	Major advances	Reference
Graft rejection	Desensitization protocols for patients with DSA	[6,32,33]
	Flow cytometry, Luminex-based cross-match	[7,8]
	Induction therapy and biologics reduce rejections	[10–16]
Fungal infection	Caspofungin and voriconazole	[99–102,104]
Viral infection	PCR for CMV and EBV detection	[114,115]
	Preemptive CMV therapy	[120–124,194]
	Liver transplants for patients with HBV or HCV	[137–142]
	Improved outcomes for recipients with HIV	[144–147]
Malignancy	Chemotherapy and rituximab beneficial for PTLD	[170,179,195]
	HHV-8 and posttransplant Kaposi sarcoma	[185–187]
	Liver transplant for patients with HCC	[191–193]

DSA, donor-specific antibody; PCR, polymerase chain reaction; CMV, cytomegalovirus; EBV, Epstein–Barr virus; HBV, hepatitis B virus; HCV, hepatitis C virus; HIV, human immunodeficiency virus; PTLD, posttransplant lymphoproliferative disease; HHV, human herpes virus; HCC, hepatocellular carcinoma.

cytotoxic T lymphocytes, natural killer cells, and B lymphocytes. Then, B lymphocytes begin to secrete antibody directed against the allogeneic tissue in ever-increasing quantities. Infiltration of the graft by such effector cells, the binding of antibody, and the activation of complement lead to rejection in its various forms (vide infra), which, if unchecked, results in graft loss (Fig. 186.1). Donor-recipient mismatches between HLAs may produce an immune response by either the direct or indirect pathways; however, minor non-HLA mismatches typically produce an immune response by the indirect pathway only.

Clinically, rejection is classified according to the temporal relation of graft dysfunction to the transplant operation and the histologic features seen in rejected tissue. The three main types of rejection are *hyperacute (HAR)*, *acute (AR)*, and *chronic (CR)*. Each type is mediated by a different host immune mechanism. Consequently, each type poses different problems for clinicians and researchers.

Hyperacute Rejection

HAR occurs within a few minutes to a few hours after the reperfusion of the graft posttransplant. Preformed antibodies directed against antigens presented by the graft mediate activation of complement, activation of endothelial cells, and formation of microvascular thrombi, leading to graft thrombosis and loss [5]. The process is irreversible; currently, no treatment is available. Because HAR is mediated by circulating preformed antibodies normally directed against ABO system (comprising the four main blood types, i.e., A, B, AB, and O) antigens or against major HLA antigens, thorough screening of potential transplant recipients should prevent nearly all HAR.

The panel-reactive antibody (PRA) assay is a screening test that examines the ability of serum from potential transplant recipients to lyse lymphocytes from a panel of HLA-typed donors. A numerical value, expressed as a percentage, indicates the likelihood of a positive cross-match to the donor population. Therefore, patients lacking preformed antibodies to random donor lymphocytes are defined as having a PRA of 0% and have a very low probability of eliciting a positive lymphocyte cross-match to any donor. The finding of a higher PRA identifies patients at high risk for a positive cross-match and thus for HAR and for subsequent graft loss. Most often, such patients were previously sensitized by childbirth, blood transfusions, or a prior transplant.

Pretransplant, cross-match testing is performed to identify preformed antibodies against class I HLAs (T-lymphocyte cross-match testing) and class II HLAs (B-lymphocyte cross-match testing). A strong positive class I-HLA cross-match immediately pretransplant is ordinarily an absolute contraindication to renal and pancreas transplants. At most centers, heart and liver transplants are performed without a cross-match, unless the recipient is highly sensitized or has previously received a graft possessing major antigens in common with the current donor (i.e., donor-specific antibody [DSA]). A positive B-lymphocyte crossmatch indicates preformed antibodies directed against class II HLAs and is a relative, but not absolute, contraindication to a transplant. Recent studies confirmed the

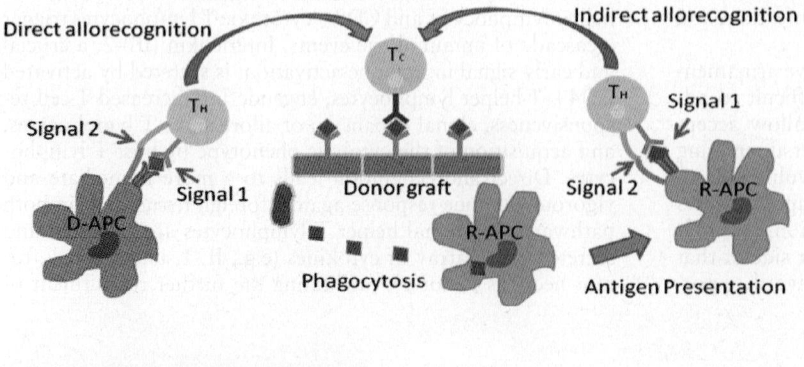

FIGURE 186.1. Direct, indirect pathways of allorecognition. Signal 1 is delivered through the T-cell receptor after engagement by a peptide–HLA complex. Signal 2, also known as costimulatory sign, is delivered by an array of cell-surface molecules on the T helper cell and the antigen-presenting cell (APC). D-APC, donor APC; R-APC, recipient APC; TH, T helper lymphocyte; Tc, cytotoxic T lymphocytes.

efficacy of plasmapheresis followed by administration of immune globulin to reduce PRA levels and to convert strongly positive crossmatch results to weakly positive or negative results, thereby allowing organs to be transplanted across what were previously considered as strong immunologic barriers [6].

Crossmatch testing is a vital tool to identify the presence of antibodies against potential donor antigens and to assess the risks of posttransplant rejection and subsequent graft loss. Ironically, cross-match testing methods are not standardized. Since the mid-1960s, cross-match testing was based on the complement-dependent cytotoxicity (CDC) assay. The CDC assay was further refined by adding a wash step and an antihuman globulin (AHG) step, to increase its sensitivity and specificity. Then, with the introduction of technology based on flow cytometry (FC), the presence of recipient antibody on the surface of donor lymphocytes could be detected independent of complement binding. The FC method further enhances the sensitivity of crossmatch and, since the late 1980s, has been adopted by an increasing number of transplant centers [7].

The latest development in anti-HLA antibody screening was the introduction of Luminex® technology, using HLA-coated fluorescent microbeads and FC. This method in theory pinpoints the DSAs in sera of recipients with high PRA levels. Since all transplant donors are HLA typed nowadays, a negative cross-match for recipients with high PRA levels can be ensured by avoiding the selection of donors carrying unacceptable antigens (virtual cross-match) [8].

The main concerns with these new developments in antibody typing and crossmatch testing are between-center test variability and the thresholds of defining false-negative results (results that could deny recipients with high PRA levels a chance for a potential lifesaving transplant). Currently, it is up to an individual transplant center to implement its own HLA typing and cross-match policy, depending on the center's experience and clinical outcomes.

Although screening has all but eliminated HAR as a clinical problem, active investigation is nonetheless directed at dissecting the underlying pathophysiologic mechanisms of HAR. Another research focus is on the similar rapid rejection of xenoreactive antigens that serve as a barrier to the development of xenotransplantation.

Acute Rejection

AR is the most common form of graft rejection in modern clinical transplantation. It may develop at any time, but is most frequent during the first several months posttransplant. Rarely, it occurs within the first several days posttransplant, a process termed *accelerated acute rejection* (AAR), most likely a combination of amnestic immune response driven by sensitized memory B lymphocytes and activation of the direct allorecognition pathway. Under such circumstances, the donor antigen exposure often occurred in the distant past, so the level of circulating DSAs would have been too low to be detected by conventional crossmatch techniques. Once challenged by the same donor antigens introduced by the organ transplant, dormant memory lymphocytes reactivate, replicate, and differentiate. Within several days, large numbers of antibodies are directed against the donor tissue and result in graft rejection.

Cellular rejection and antibody-mediated rejection (AMR) are not mutually exclusive in AR. Histologically, AR generates an infiltration of activated T lymphocytes into the graft, resulting in gradually progressive endothelial damage, microvascular thrombosis, and parenchymal necrosis. Pathologic grading schemes have been developed regarding the extent to which AR involves vascular damage, cellular infiltration, or a combination of both. Vascular AR is thought to be mediated by the presence of DSAs, albeit not in sufficient numbers to cause HAR. C4 d, a complement split product detected immunohistochemically in the capillaries of biopsied graft specimens, is highly correlated with AMR [9]. Without intervention, AR inevitably progresses to graft loss. The clinical presentation of AR varies markedly, depending on the specific organ, on the level of immunosuppression, and on the attendant reduction of inflammation in the affected tissues.

Unless the host immune system is suppressed pharmacologically, a transplant inevitably leads to AR. A combination of immunosuppressive agents is typically used chronically to prevent AR, including a lymphocyte antagonist (usually a calcineurin inhibitor [CNI] such as cyclosporine or tacrolimus) and an antiproliferative agent (such as azathioprine or mycophenolate mofetil), with or without corticosteroids. Antilymphocyte antibody therapy is often added during induction of immunosuppression or for treatment of "steroid-resistant" AR.

In the last decade, immunosuppression for transplant recipients has been undergoing a paradigm shift. Since the mid-1990s, the use of antibody induction in solid-organ transplant recipients has increased from 25% to more than 60% [10]. In particular, monoclonal antibodies such as basiliximab and daclizumab (both anti-CD25 [IL-2 receptor]) as well as alemtuzumab (Campath-1 H, anti-CD52) were proven to be effective induction agents in preventing AR in renal or pancreas transplantation [11–13]. Furthermore, strategies such as corticosteroid avoidance and CNI-reduced or CNI-free maintenance immunosuppression were shown to be equivalent to traditional triple-drug maintenance [14–16]. Nonetheless, all immunosuppressive agents carry some risk of toxicity and adverse reactions that may complicate therapy (Table 186.2).

Chronic Rejection

CR remains a common yet poorly understood clinical problem, with slightly different manifestations in each type of graft. Over time, the accumulation of microvascular injury in a graft degrades graft function, with eventual graft loss. This process appears to be mediated by multiple mechanisms, likely including both immune and nonimmune factors. Evidence for the contribution to CR of immune factors includes the observation that AR episodes significantly increase the likelihood of CR as well as the correlation, observed in renal transplant recipients, between a poor response to AR treatment and the subsequent development of CR [17]. A similar association between a poor response to AR treatment and the subsequent development of CR has been observed in liver transplant recipients, although reversible AR has little impact. Nonimmune factors likely also contribute to the development and progression of CR, including the toxic effects of immunosuppressive medication and cumulative injury from infection such as that caused by cytomegalovirus (CMV) [18] and polyomavirus [19]. CR nearly always eventuates in graft loss, although the rapidity of the process varies considerably.

Renal Grafts

Current reports indicate that about 10% to 25% of renal transplant recipients experience an episode of AR. Because most episodes are clinically silent, the diagnosis of AR must be considered in recipients whose serum creatinine, blood urea nitrogen, and urinary output values have normalized and whose graft function has been stable in the outpatient setting, but whose serum creatinine and blood urea nitrogen values subsequently rise while their urinary output decreases. The presence of hypovolemia, drug nephrotoxicity (e.g., high calcineurin levels), ureteral obstruction or leak, lymphocele, or vascular anastomotic complications should be excluded, and the diagnosis of

TABLE 186.2

IMMUNOSUPPRESSIVE MEDICATIONS, MECHANISMS OF ACTION, AND COMMON SIDE EFFECTS

Medications	Mechanisms of action	Side effects
Corticosteroids	Upregulate IκB Decrease IL-1, TNF-α, IFN-γ Exert anti-inflammatory effect	Cushing syndrome
Azathioprine	Act as an antimetabolite	Marrow suppression GI, liver toxicity
Mycophenolate mofetil	Specifically affect lymphocytes Act as an antimetabolite	Marrow suppression GI intolerance
Cyclosporine	Act as a calcineurin inhibitor Downregulates IL-2	Nephrotoxicity Neurologic symptoms
Tacrolimus (FK506)	Calcineurin inhibitor Downregulate IL-2, IFN-γ	Nephrotoxicity Neurotoxicity Diabetogenic
Sirolimus (rapamycin)	Block IL-2R, IL-4, IL-6, platelet-derived growth factor signaling	Impaired healing Hypertriglyceridemia
Antilymphocyte globulin	Act as a cytolytic antibody Block and deplete T cells	Leukopenia Thrombocytopenia "Serum sickness"
OKT3	Act as a cytolytic antibody Block T-cell receptor Deplete T cells	Cytokine release Aseptic meningitis
Daclizumab (or basiliximab)	Blocks IL-2R Inhibit T-cell activation	Minimal impact

GI, gastrointestinal; IFN, interferon; IL, interleukin; OKT3, ornithine–ketoacid transaminase-3.

AR should be established via histologic examination of a percutaneous graft biopsy specimen. Rarely, tenderness and swelling in the area of the graft occur, and occasionally fever or other signs of systemic inflammation, although such findings used to be common.

As discussed earlier, most AR episodes occur in the early posttransplant period. Among the subset of recipients who experience delayed graft function, up to 30% exhibit evidence of AR on biopsy [20]; 20% of recipients who require dialysis posttransplant have AR [21]. Intriguingly, up to 30% of recipients with well-functioning grafts also have AR, per early posttransplant protocol biopsies, but whether such findings are clinically important and whether mild episodes should invariably be treated remain controversial [22]. Recent studies have provided data that may allow prediction of individual risk of AR, with the potential for individualizing immunomodulatory therapy. For example, donor IL-6 genetic polymorphism is strongly associated with an increased incidence of AR posttransplant [23], and recipients with elevated levels of serum C-reactive protein (CRP), presumably indicative of systemic inflammation, have a higher rate of AR and a shorter time to AR than those with lower CRP levels [24]. Other biomarkers (such as soluble CD30, gene expression assays on peripheral blood samples, urinary proteomics, and T-lymphocyte subset analysis) were shown to be predictive for rejection or transplant tolerance, and are currently undergoing various clinical investigations [25].

The diagnostic workup for AR includes studies that may identify alternative causes of recipient graft dysfunction (Table 186.3). It is vital to consider alternative diagnoses, particularly in the early postoperative period, including vascular problems with the arterial or venous anastomoses, ureteral obstruction, or urinary leak. Other common causes of apparent graft dysfunction include the acute tubular necrosis associated with delayed graft function, hypovolemia and attendant prerenal azotemia, and the nephrotoxic effects of cyclosporine and tacrolimus. To rule out the vascular and ureteral problems discussed previously, a duplex ultrasound study of the renal graft is commonly obtained. Several ultrasound findings may suggest the diagnosis of AR: increased size of the graft, increased cortical thickness, enlargement of the renal pyramids, and decreased

TABLE 186.3

BASIC WORKUP OF RECIPIENTS WITH GRAFT DYSFUNCTION OR ACUTE REJECTION

History and physical examination	Establish and order differential diagnosis
Doppler ultrasound	Rule out vascular surgical complication Rule out leak (e.g., biliary, ureteral)
Serum chemistry	Evaluate relative blood urea nitrogen and creatinine, amylase, bilirubin Detect and treat electrolyte abnormalities
Drug levels	Evaluate for potential drug toxicity Detect inadequate drug levels
Blood cell count, cultures	Evaluate for potential infection
Graft biopsy	Firmly establish and grade graft rejection

graft renal artery blood flow [26]. The diagnosis of AR is clearly established by percutaneous allograft biopsy and histologic examination. Biopsy is generally safe when performed by experienced practitioners; however, complications include bleeding, hematoma and arteriovenous fistula formation, and ureteral or major vascular injury.

Rejection is graded according to a standardized histologic classification scheme, the modified Banff Criteria, which may be used to guide therapy [27]. Fine-needle aspiration biopsy has been used by some centers to establish the diagnosis of AR; however, some consider the loss of microstructural data, as compared with traditional core biopsy, to be a weakness of the technique. In particular, the diagnoses of acute vascular rejection and CR are difficult to make using fine-needle aspiration biopsy.

The treatment of AR in renal transplant recipients varies between centers. High-dose methylprednisolone (500 to 1,000 mg per day or every other day [2 to 3 doses] is common) is often the initial approach. Corticosteroid-resistant AR, or AR that is histologically graded as severe or vascular, is often treated with potent depleting antilymphocyte antibodies such as murine monoclonal IgG2a antibody (OKT3) or polyclonal antithymocyte globulin (antithymocyte gamma globulin, Thymoglobulin). Alemtuzumab was selectively used to treat AR in some centers [28]. Since some AR episodes occurred while the recipients were on stable immunosuppression, their maintenance therapy was switched from cyclosporine to tacrolimus or from azathioprine to mycophenolate mofetil. Most AR episodes are reversible with current therapies; however, as noted previously, the long-term outlook for preservation of graft function is lessened with each episode, especially when the posttreatment serum creatinine level does not return to the pre-AR baseline.

CR in renal transplant recipients is a persistent clinical problem and appears to be multifactorial, with immunologic and nonimmunologic factors driving the gradual loss of graft function. As described earlier, minimizing the frequency and severity of AR episodes is important in decreasing the likelihood of eventual CR. Nonimmunologic factors thought to contribute to CR include (a) episodes of infection, particularly due to CMV and BK virus (*vide infra*); (b) the nephrotoxicity of CNI therapy; (c) ischemia-reperfusion injury and delayed graft function in the peritransplant period; and (d) innate cell senescence within the graft [29]. Attention is being directed toward identifying inflammatory activity within the graft, in response to both immune and nonimmune insults that may contribute to the development of CR. One of the leading causes of kidney retransplants is CR. It remains a formidable problem that is still poorly understood.

Hepatic Grafts

The hepatic graft is considered to be immunologically "privileged" in that evidence of some degree of immune tolerance occurs in a substantial number of liver transplant recipients over time. Despite that observation, all forms of rejection can occur posttransplant. At one time, it was thought that HAR did not occur in the hepatic graft; this idea is now known to be incorrect, as anti-HLA antibody-mediated HAR has been described in liver transplant recipients [30,31]. Unlike the renal graft, the hepatic graft undergoes HAR over a number of days, not minutes to hours, probably secondary to its ability to absorb a large amount of antibody before the onset of the significant microthrombosis and vascular damage seen in HAR. A more delayed form of antibody-mediated rejection is seen in up to 33% of patients who undergo liver transplants across ABO-incompatible blood groups [32], but even this barrier appears surmountable with the use of plasmapheresis along with aggressive immunosuppression [33].

AR remains an important clinical problem in liver transplantation; even with the use of standard multiagent immunosuppression, the incidence of AR ranges from 30% to 80%. In two large, multicenter trials, double therapy with a CNI and steroids resulted in a 60% to 80% incidence of AR [34,35]. Triple therapy with Neoral® or Sandimmune®, along with azathioprine and prednisone, resulted in a 30% to 45% incidence of AR [36]. Substitution of mycophenolate mofetil for azathioprine further reduced the incidence of AR to 26% [37]. The latest liver transplant regimen, consisting of two doses of a monoclonal anti-IL2 receptor (basiliximab) as induction therapy and dual maintenance therapy with a CNI and mycophenolate mofetil, was shown to lessen the severity of rejection without increase the infection rate [38,39].

The diagnosis of AR in liver transplant recipients is normally suggested by elevated levels of transaminases, bilirubin, or alkaline phosphatase. Among patients with T-tube drainage (which is increasingly uncommon), the biliary drainage may be seen to thicken, darken, and decrease in amount. The suspicion of AR mandates graft biopsy and studies to eliminate other possible causes of early hepatic graft failure. Duplex ultrasonography and, in some cases, cholangiography are increasingly being replaced by magnetic resonance imaging. Biopsy findings are classified, according to a standardized set of criteria, as *mild*, *moderate*, and *severe*, with clear implications for prognosis [40]. AR is normally treated with high-dose corticosteroids, but 5% to 10% of cases are steroid-resistant; such recipients are then treated with an antilymphocyte antibody. Interestingly, in large population studies, the incidence of AR is associated with improved long-term patient survival rates [41], albeit thought to be due to the higher incidence of AR in younger, healthier recipients. Even adjusting for recipient characteristics, AR has not been clearly associated with either decreased graft or patient survival rates; however, frequent AR episodes are a risk factor for subsequent CR, so continued pursuit of immunosuppressive strategies that reduce the risk of AR is imperative.

CR in liver transplant recipients is characterized by vascular obliteration and bile duct loss ("the vanishing duct syndrome"). Seen in 5% to 10% of recipients, it is more common in those with vasculitic findings during AR episodes; if larger vessels are not seen on biopsy, the diagnosis of CR may be misread as AR. The incidence of CR appears to be decreasing, perhaps as a result of changes in immunosuppressive regimens [42]. In addition to multiple AR episodes, other factors associated with an increased risk of CR include CMV infection, chronic hepatitis, increased donor-recipient histocompatibility differences, and increased ischemia time. CR does not always herald graft loss; long-term patient survival and even regeneration of bile ducts have been described. Tacrolimus has been used to salvage grafts in recipients with CR on cyclosporine-based immunosuppression, with a 73% success rate [43].

Pancreas Grafts

At most centers, patients undergoing a pancreas transplant alone or a simultaneous pancreas–kidney transplant receive more potent immunosuppression than do renal transplant recipients, thanks to initial studies demonstrating a higher rate of AR after those two types of pancreas transplant [44]. Overall success rates continue to improve: the risk of AR has been reduced by standardized induction therapy with antilymphocyte antibody preparations, and it may be further reduced with mammalian target of rapamycin (mTOR) inhibitors and/or with IL-2 receptor monoclonal antibodies [45].

Establishing the diagnosis of AR in pancreas transplant recipients may be difficult. Hyperglycemia is a late finding that only occurs with substantial loss of functional islet-cell mass.

By the time hyperglycemia is seen, it may be too late to retain a functional graft. Clinical findings may include fever and graft tenderness; however, pancreas graft rejection is often clinically silent.

For pancreas grafts transplanted along with a renal graft, a rising creatinine level is often used as a surrogate marker of rejection, with antirejection therapy aimed at both the pancreas graft and the renal graft. However, isolated pancreas graft rejection is observed in up to 20% of simultaneous pancreas–kidney transplant recipients who have AR [46].

In pancreas transplant recipients with exocrine bladder drainage, a decreasing urinary amylase level may be used as a marker of graft rejection [47]. Other possible markers of rejection (serum anodal trypsinogen, serum amylase, soluble HLA, and analysis of glucose-disappearance kinetics during a brief glucose tolerance test) have been examined but have failed to gain wide acceptance.

The diagnosis of pancreas graft rejection is confirmed by biopsy, which may be performed percutaneously or, in bladder-drained recipients, through a cystoscopic, transduodenal approach. Complications (bleeding, arteriovenous fistula formation, graft pancreatitis) have been described, but most biopsies do not lead to complications. Pancreas transplant recipients with early evidence of graft dysfunction should undergo Doppler ultrasonography to rule out graft thrombosis, which occurs in up to 10% to 20% of them [48].

Treatment of AR for pancreas transplant recipients is similar to that for renal or liver transplant recipients. High-dose corticosteroids are given initially, but a low threshold is maintained for possibly switching to antibody-based therapy, given the relatively common steroid resistance. Most AR episodes are reversed with treatment.

Cardiac Grafts

Rejection in heart transplant recipients is a major obstacle to long-term success and accounts for up to a third of the deaths. All forms of rejection are seen in heart transplant recipients. Albeit rare, HAR due to preformed antigraft antibodies occurs within minutes to days; it manifests with rapid deterioration of cardiac function, with prolonged need for inotropic support. In recipients whose grafts fail to recover rapidly, an attempt to reverse HAR by plasmapheresis may be made, but success is uncommon, and an immediate retransplant is usually required.

AR in heart transplant recipients is common and usually occurs in the first 3 to 4 months posttransplant. At one time, the diagnosis was made on the basis of the development of congestive heart failure or the elaboration of electrocardiographic abnormalities. However, the present-day use of protocol endomyocardial biopsies has eliminated such late findings of AR, except in noncompliant recipients. Most centers use frequent percutaneous transjugular right ventricular endomyocardial biopsies as part of a standardized surveillance protocol. Biopsies are evaluated histologically, according to an international grading system [49], and therapy is directed accordingly.

Several investigators have developed noninvasive approaches to establishing the diagnosis of AR, including electrocardiographic frequency analysis, nuclear scintigraphic techniques, and echocardiography; however, no approach has attained sufficient sensitivity to eliminate the need for protocol biopsies. The need for continued endomyocardial biopsies later than 1 year posttransplant is controversial, and many centers discontinue performance of biopsies at 1 year unless indicated on clinical grounds.

The treatment of AR is based on histologic findings. Bolus steroid therapy is used in lower-grade rejection without hemodynamic compromise; oral prednisone therapy for mild AR also has been used with success [50]. Salvage therapy with an antilymphocyte antibody agent is most common in recipients with histologic findings of more severe rejection, in recipients with steroid-resistant rejection, and in recipients with signs of hemodynamic compromise. In a series of 100 of such high-risk recipients, AR was reversed in 90% of those treated with 10 to 14 days of OKT3 [51]. However, other investigators have had markedly lower rates of success with OKT3 in the treatment of steroid-resistant rejection [52]. Methotrexate also has been used to reverse AR that fails to respond to steroids or that is refractory to OKT3.

Other approaches include switching from cyclosporine-based to tacrolimus-based immunosuppression as rescue therapy in recipients with refractory AR, a strategy that was proved to be safe and efficacious [50]. Photopheresis has been used in the treatment of recipients with T-cell lymphoma and autoimmune disease. Studies of photopheresis and triple-drug immunosuppression have provided evidence of a decrease in the total number of AR episodes, as compared with triple-drug immunosuppression alone [50]. Of note, photopheresis has reversed refractory high-grade rejection in small numbers of heart transplant recipients [53].

CR manifests in heart transplant recipients as cardiac allograft vasculopathy (CAV), an entity that is the major cause of late-term morbidity and mortality. The pathologic findings of CAV include progressive intimal thickening in a concentric manner, which begins distally within the cardiac vasculature. It is associated with the loss of response to endogenous (and pharmacologic) vasodilators [50]. CAV is thought to be immunologically mediated, because HLA donor-related matching is clearly associated with reduced rates of CAV [54]. Nonimmunologic mechanisms are also thought to be involved; identifiable risk factors for CAV include hyperlipidemia, donor age older than 25 years, recipient weight gain, CMV disease, preexisting donor or recipient coronary artery disease, and increasing time posttransplant [50]. Another nonimmunologic risk factor for CAV is ischemic time during the peritransplant period. As in other solid-organ transplant recipients, the use of mycophenolate mofetil is associated with a reduction in the incidence of CR in heart transplant recipients [55].

Lung Grafts

The lung graft is highly prone to rejection—nearly all lung transplant recipients experience at least 1 AR episode. The clinical difficulty posed by rejection is in distinguishing it from other causes of decreased graft function, most commonly infection.

HAR of the lung graft [56] is mediated by recipient preformed antibodies to the donor graft, in a fashion similar to other organs. The clinical manifestation is similar to the more common ischemia-reperfusion injury, which, unlike HAR, usually resolves. HAR of the lung graft is rare and only described in case reports. To date, we know of no lung transplant recipients who have survived HAR. It must be prevented via initial cross-match testing and exclusion of immunologically unsuitable donor organs.

Most AR episodes occur during the first 3 to 6 months posttransplant. Some recipients experience symptoms, including fever, cough, and dyspnea, but many are asymptomatic. Early diagnosis of AR in lung transplant recipients is essential: untreated AR can lead to respiratory insufficiency or failure, and repeated AR episodes are associated with an increased risk of bronchiolitis obliterans and eventual graft failure [57].

The diagnosis of AR is made by transbronchial biopsy, although less invasive techniques continue to be assessed [58]. Bronchoalveolar lavage (BAL) is also performed to rule out infection before increasing immunosuppression; infection and rejection may occur simultaneously in up to 25% of lung transplant recipients with AR [59]. Early diagnosis of AR may be aided by spirometry; decreases in timed forced expiratory volume, in pulmonary capillary blood volume, and in the diffusing capacity of the lungs for carbon monoxide are associated with AR and should prompt investigation. Radiography is not ordinarily helpful. The histologic findings of AR include lymphocytic infiltrates into the perivascular and interstitial spaces; AR is graded according to histologic findings [60].

The initial treatment of AR in lung transplant recipients typically entails high-dose corticosteroids; if they are not successful, anti–T-cell antibody therapy is tried next. Many recipients initially respond to the steroid pulse therapy, yet it may not completely clear their AR, and secondary episodes are common, so additional therapy may be required. For that reason, surveillance bronchoscopy with transbronchial biopsies and BAL are common after initial treatment [61].

CR in lung transplant recipients is extremely common, affecting up to 40% of recipients at 2 years posttransplant and up to 70% of recipients after 5 years [62]. The mean time to diagnosis of graft dysfunction posttransplant is 16 to 20 months. A definitive histologic diagnosis of early bronchiolitis obliterans may be difficult to obtain, so it must be established largely on clinical grounds. Radiography, again, is not specific. Typical presenting symptoms are cough, progressive dyspnea, and loss of exercise tolerance. The use of home spirometry can point to the diagnosis based on a 20% reduction in timed forced expiratory volume on successive measurements [63]. Factors associated with accelerated bronchiolitis obliterans include multiple episodes of AR, CMV pneumonitis/infection, *Pneumocystis jiroveci* pneumonia (PCP), and episodes of airway ischemia [62,64].

Many different therapies have been tried for recipients with bronchiolitis obliterans, but with little success. Increases in immunosuppression, antilymphocyte antibody therapy, and inhaled cyclosporine have all been tried. Ultimately, the progress of bronchiolitis obliterans is inexorable, with continued loss of graft function and subsequent death. A lung retransplant is the only viable option [65].

INFECTIONS

The suppression of the host immune response is required to establish and maintain a functioning solid-organ graft. The development of immunosuppressive therapies has been impressive, leading to the widespread use of solid-organ transplantation as the primary therapy for a number of organ failure syndromes. This success comes at a price, however, and the successful immunosuppression that allows engraftment leaves the host with an increased susceptibility for a number of serious infectious complications. Up to 80% of solid-organ transplant recipients experience an infectious complication during the first year posttransplant, and infections remain a major cause of morbidity and mortality in the transplant population [66].

The range of potential pathogens that can cause disease in the immunosuppressed host is prodigious. Not only are the common endogenous and nosocomial flora involved, but also "opportunistic" or "atypical" pathogens must be considered in the differential diagnosis of a solid-organ transplant recipient who has evidence of infection. In considering the epidemiology of infectious complications posttransplant, the clinician must assess several factors, including the time posttransplant, the organ transplanted, the type and degree of immunosuppression, the need for antirejection therapy, and the potential occurrence of surgical complications.

The greatest risk of infections corresponds with the period of most intense immunosuppression, which is characteristically during the first 6 to 12 months posttransplant and after antirejection therapy, particularly for repeated AR episodes. Rubin et al. have characterized periods posttransplant during which certain infection patterns may be seen [67]. Infectious complications in the first month posttransplant are typically caused by endogenous or nosocomial flora that would cause disease in an immunocompetent host [68], including (a) bacterial surgical site infections; (b) postoperative or ventilator-associated pneumonia; (c) urinary tract infections (UTIs) associated with prolonged indwelling urinary catheters; (d) intraabdominal infections related to surgical complications; and (e) central venous catheter infections [67,68].

The period between 1 and 6 months posttransplant is typically the time of greatest immunosuppression and, subsequently, the time most opportunistic infections occur. They are frequently caused by fungal or especially viral pathogens that may become activated after lying dormant in the host or may be transferred from the donor with the graft [69,70]. Knowledge of the characteristic patterns of maximal frequency for a number of specific viral pathogens within that 5-month window may be helpful to the clinician in establishing the diagnosis [71].

These infection patterns may be categorized into an *early cluster* of viral agents occurring with peak frequency between 2 and 3 months posttransplant and a *late cluster* more commonly occurring between 4 and 9 months posttransplant. The early cluster includes CMV, adenoviruses, hepatitis B virus (HBV) and hepatitis C virus (HCV), and human herpes virus (HHV)-6 [67–69,71–74]. The late cluster includes varicella zoster and polyoma viruses [19,75]. Epstein–Barr virus (EBV) may cause disease throughout the first year posttransplant [76].

The opportunistic fungi can similarly be observed to cluster with *Candida* and *Aspergillus* species (spp), causing infections in the first 2 to 3 months posttransplant [77,78], whereas *Cryptococcus*, histoplasmosis, coccidioidomycosis, and *P. jiroveci* most often occur later during the first year [79,80].

After the first 6 to 12 months, most transplant recipients exhibit patterns of infectious disease morbidity that are similar to those of the general population, with frequent respiratory infections secondary to pneumococcal infections and influenza, as well as uncomplicated UTIs. However, opportunistic infections can occur anytime. Increased immunosuppression secondary to AR treatment may slightly increase transplant recipients' susceptibility to, and alter the temporal pattern of, various pathogens. When assessing immunosuppressed transplant recipients for infectious diseases, the clinician must maintain a high index of suspicion at all times. The typical localizing signs of infection and inflammation may be blunted, or even absent, because of the anti-inflammatory action of immunosuppressive regimens.

An important component of the solid-organ transplant process is the preoperative assessment of both the recipient and the donor for any underlying infections, or any disease processes that predispose to infections, that could manifest subsequent to administration of exogenous immunosuppression. For the donor, the most important evaluation is the determination of CMV and EBV status, because those two agents are most easily transmitted to a seronegative recipient. Cultures of organ preservation fluid are routinely positive, but appropriate antiviral therapy can ordinarily prevent positive cultures from causing clinically significant disease [81]. For the recipient, a thorough pretransplant history and physical examination are essential to minimize the risk of infectious complications secondary to a latent or indolent infectious process. Routine viral studies should be obtained, vaccinations updated, and prophylaxis administered where indicated (e.g., gut decontamination in liver transplant candidates with end-stage liver disease or prophylactic antibiotics in patients with cystic fibrosis).

Bacterial Infections

In the first 30 days posttransplant, bacterial infections are common. Even in the immunocompetent patient population, bacterial infections are common complications of surgery. The risk of a nosocomial bacterial infection is related to the site of surgery as well as to the continued presence of any catheters, lines, endotracheal tubes, or other breaks in the skin. The most common sites of infection are the urinary tract, the surgical site, the lungs, and the bloodstream. The risk of nosocomial bacterial infections is directly related to host factors (including underlying diseases such as diabetes or cirrhosis, obesity, and chronic pulmonary disease) as well as to technical and management factors (including the length and technique of the operation, the development of a hematoma or seroma, and the need for prolonged urinary catheterization, mechanical ventilation, or central venous catheterization).

Particularly in renal transplant recipients and in bladder-drained pancreas transplant recipients, the urinary tract is a common site of bacterial infections. Bacteriuria may be detected in up to 83% of renal transplant recipients [82], with an attendant increased risk of systemic sepsis and wound infection. The most common pathogens are Gram-negative aerobes, enterococci, and *Candida* spp. The risk factors associated with an increased incidence of UTIs include prolonged catheterization, hemodialysis, and antibiotic prophylaxis in excess of 48 hours [83]. The use of ureteral stents in renal transplant recipients, though it may help reduce ureteral complications, is associated with an increased rate of UTIs [84]. The use of prophylactic trimethoprim-sulfamethoxazole (TMP-SMX) is common in renal transplant recipients, primarily to decrease the risk of UTIs. Long-term prophylaxis helps reduce the incidence of infections due to several opportunistic pathogens, including *P. jiroveci*, *Toxoplasma gondii*, *Listeria monocytogenes*, and *Legionella pneumophila* [85].

Diagnosis of a UTI in transplant recipients is based on clinical suspicion and on urinalysis and culture results. The typical findings of dysuria, hesitance, and frequency may be absent; the only clinical manifestations might be a minimal fever or an elevated white blood cell count. Treatment is often empiric and, because of the risk of bacteremia, should consist of intravenous administration of a third-generation cephalosporin or a quinolone, particularly during the first months posttransplant. Once the causative microbe has been identified and antimicrobial sensitivity data are available, treatment can be refined.

In recipients of solid-organ grafts besides the kidney and bladder-drained pancreas who do not require a long duration of urinary catheterization, an increased risk of bacterial or fungal UTIs is not seen.

Infections of the surgical site are potentially a source of major morbidity and, occasionally, graft loss and mortality in solid-organ transplant recipients. Surgical site or wound infections are classified according to the structures involved. Infections above the fascia are superficial, infections below the fascia are deep, and combined infections involve elements of both the superficial and the deep compartments of the wound [68].

In all solid-organ transplant recipients, immediately before their operation begins, a single dose of an antibiotic should be administered, to decrease the risk of surgical site infections. In pancreas, bowel, lung, and liver transplant recipients, significant degrees of wound contamination may occur, so antibiotics are typically administered for 24 to 72 hours posttransplant, although data to support that practice are lacking. In renal transplant recipients, the surgical site infection rate is very low (1% to 2%) and is comparable to the wound infection rate for other clean-contaminated procedures in immunocompetent patients [86].

However, other transplant procedures are associated with higher rates of infection. The wound infection rate after heart transplants is typically below 8%, which is comparable to the rate for other high-risk cardiac procedures [87]. The rate of wound infections is slightly higher after lung and heart–lung transplants [88]. The rate after liver transplants of superficial wound infections is 6% to 8%; of deep wound infections (most commonly an intra-abdominal abscess secondary to a biliary leak), 15% to 20% [69]. The rate of wound infections after pancreas transplants is high: 10% to 40%, superficial; 15% to 22%, deep; and 8%, combined [89]. Such wound infections confer substantial morbidity, are associated with mortality in some cases, and require a very aggressive approach to diagnosis and therapy.

Pathogenic microbes are predictable, according to the type of operation. In renal transplant recipients, wound infections are caused by the endogenous flora of the skin (Gram-positive aerobes) and the bladder (Gram-negative aerobes), with occasional *Candida* spp and enterococci.

In heart transplant recipients, wound infections are almost invariably due to skin flora such as *Staphylococcus aureus* and *Staphylococcus epidermidis*, although some fungal and atypical pathogens are found.

Lung transplants introduce respiratory flora and the potential for grave infections with *Pseudomonas aeruginosa*.

In liver transplant recipients, wound infections are typically associated with either skin or biliary flora, although any preexisting cirrhosis and end-stage liver disease may result in colonization with drug-resistant nosocomial pathogens.

In pancreas transplant recipients, wound infections are invariably polymicrobial, with gram-positive, fungal, and resistant Gram-negative pathogens frequently present. Treatment generally requires opening of the wound, reexploration, and/or administration of broad-spectrum antimicrobial therapy (with a carbapenem or extended-spectrum penicillin, a β-lactamase inhibitor, and vancomycin) and often antifungal coverage.

Wound infections are often subtle, and findings may be limited to fever, elevated white blood cell count, or wound drainage with a deceptively innocuous appearance. Any wound drainage should be examined by Gram stain and culture; any suspicion or evidence of infections should result in opening of the superficial wound. Additionally, imaging should be undertaken to rule out infections in the deep surgical space; if a fluid collection is identified, percutaneous drainage or prompt exploration is needed. Prolonged, broad-spectrum antimicrobial therapy is used, and immunosuppression is minimized in the face of potentially life-threatening infections.

The development of postoperative pneumonia varies with the type of transplant and is associated with a high mortality rate (20% to 60%) [90]. Renal transplants are associated with the lowest incidence of postoperative pneumonia (1% to 2%); lung transplants, the highest (22%). The most common pathogens are Gram-negative aerobes, staphylococci, and *Legionella* spp. Frequently, *Candida* spp or CMV may be identified along with bacterial pathogens, particularly in the first 2 to 3 months posttransplant. Such findings are clinically significant, and active CMV pneumonitis is a significant risk factor for the development of bacterial pneumonia [90,91].

Several risk factors may predispose solid-organ transplant recipients to the development of pneumonia, including prolonged mechanical ventilation, thoracic surgery, pulmonary edema, and intense immunosuppression or AR treatment. Lung transplant recipients are at increased risk, because of their lungs' preexisting colonization with endogenous flora as well as the loss of the mucociliary clearance function associated with denervation [88]. Those with cystic fibrosis have an additional risk, because their lungs and sinuses are universally colonized with highly drug-resistant flora such as *Pseudomonas aeruginosa* and *Burkholderia cepacia* [92]. The evaluation of suspected pneumonia in lung transplant recipients should be thorough, including bronchoscopy with biopsies and BAL to rule out rejection, as described above. Pleural effusions should be drained and cultured, because the progression of an infected effusion to empyema in lung transplant recipients is associated with a very high mortality rate.

Bacteremia in the transplant population, as in the general hospital population, may occur secondary to seeding along a vascular access device or as a result of hematogenous spread from another source; or, it may be primary (without a source being identified). UTIs, wound infections, and pneumonia are risk factors for the development of bacteremia, as is prolonged vascular catheterization. Additional risk factors include receiving a deceased donor graft, leukopenia, and antirejection therapy. Bacteremia in immunosuppressed patients may present as fever, leukocytosis, leukopenia, or hypotension without other significant manifestations. Consequently, routine blood cultures should be part of any workup for fever in this population. Suspicion of bacteremia should prompt removal and culture of intravascular devices and a search for a source of other sites of infection. The mortality rate of bacterial sepsis and septic shock in transplant recipients exceeds 50%. Consequently, the use of broad-spectrum antimicrobial therapy, an aggressive approach to source control, and the minimization of immunosuppression are indicated.

Several atypical bacterial infections occur in the solid-organ transplant recipients, including mycobacteria such as *Mycobacterium tuberculosis*, *Nocardia* spp, and *Listeria monocytogenes*. Such infections are associated with high rates of morbidity and mortality. Mycobacterial infections are 50 to 100 times more frequent in the transplant population than they are in the general population and are fatal in 30% of cases. Most mycobacterial infections occur within the first 6 to 12 months posttransplant and are associated with intense immunosuppression and antirejection therapy [93]. Infections are typically due to reactivation of latent disease or transmission with the transplanted graft. Their diagnosis is complicated by the typical lack of reaction to skin testing seen with immunosuppression. Consequently, a high index of clinical suspicion is needed. If mycobacterial pulmonary infection is suspected bronchoscopic evaluation with biopsy, acid-fast staining, and culture should be performed. Treatment consists of multidrug therapy with isoniazid, ethambutol, pyrazinamide, and rifampin. Prophylaxis should be considered in patient populations in whom infections are common, in patients with a history of significant exposure without subsequent therapy, and in patients with a history of serious or inadequately treated infections.

Nontuberculous mycobacteria (NTM) such as *Mycobacterium avium complex*, *M. ulcerans*, and *M. xenopi* are environmental mycobacteria that rarely caused disease in humans until the AIDS epidemic two decades ago. NTM infections typically manifest as insidious pulmonary or soft tissue infections in immunosuppressed patients. If NTM infections are suspected, repeat isolations by bronchoscopy or tissue biopsy are required to improve the chance of diagnosis. In addition to acid-fast staining, a special culture for an atypical mycobacterium should be obtained. Besides long-term antimicrobial treatment, wide debridement of the infected site is often required to eradicate such infections [94].

Listeria monocytogenes infection may be associated with pneumonia, bacteremia, or, most ominously, cerebromeningitis in the transplant population. In renal transplant recipients, *Listeria* spp have been associated with a 26% mortality rate. Consequently, if listeriosis (pulmonary or meningitis) is suspected in any immunosuppressed patients, a thorough evaluation must be performed. Empiric therapy for meningitis should include appropriate coverage, such as ampicillin plus an aminoglycoside [95]. The extended-spectrum penicillins also provide adequate coverage.

Nocardial infections most commonly manifest with pulmonary symptoms and signs, but disseminated disease may involve the skin, eyes, and brain, alone or in combination. The clinical manifestations are nonspecific and comprise fever, chills, malaise, occasional cough, dyspnea, headache, or mental status change. Such infections have a mortality rate of 25% to 50% and must be aggressively diagnosed and treated [96]. The diagnosis is made by microscopic examination of sputum or lung (or occasionally brain) biopsy tissue, or by aspiration of a skin nodule using routine, Kinyoun, and Ziehl-Neelsen staining. Treatment consists of high-dose intravenous TMP-SMX, generally in combination with an aminoglycoside, such as amikacin, with continued treatment with oral TMP-SMX, preferably for life. Concurrently, immunosuppression should be curtailed, particularly during treatment of aggressive, disseminated infections.

Fungal Infections

Solid-organ transplants are associated with a significant risk of fungal infections. In the era of broad-spectrum antibacterial prophylaxis and empiric therapy, the incidence of fungi as pathogens is increasing, as is the incidence of azole drug-resistant fungal infections. Fungal infections are most common after liver and pancreas transplants, for which the incidence approaches 40% [97]. But they are less common after renal transplants (only 5%). Nonetheless, all fungal infections are serious infections, with an attendant mortality rate, associated with invasive disease, of 30% to 50%. As described previously, most fungal infections occur during the first 3 to 4 months posttransplant, when immunosuppression is greatest. The source of most fungal pathogens is the oral cavity, the gastrointestinal (GI) tract, or the environment.

The most common fungal pathogens are the *Candida* spp [98]. Candidal overgrowth of the oral and GI tract is common, and prophylaxis consisting of topical nystatin or clotrimazole is often used. Risk factors associated with invasive candidal disease include diabetes, neutropenia, intense immunosuppression, and prolonged administration of antibacterial antibiotics, particularly broad-spectrum agents. Long-term TMP-SMX prophylaxis has not been associated with fungal infections. Despite prophylaxis, invasive candidiasis does occur, most often in transplant recipients with a perforation of the GI tract, an anastomotic breakdown, a deep surgical-site infection, or a concomitant GI infection, such as CMV gastroenteritis or colitis.

Increasing use of triazoles such as fluconazole has led to more frequent isolation of resistant *Candida* species, such as *C. glabrata* and *C. krusei*. Even apart from this observation, most invasive candidal infections should be treated with amphotericin B or the newer agents like echinocandins (see later), because of the attendant morbidity and mortality in the immunosuppressed population [99]. Caspofungin is an echinocandin that acts to block the synthesis of 1,3-β-D-glucan, an essential element of the fungal cell wall. It is well tolerated, with a side effect profile that compares favorably to amphotericin B. Note that caspofungin and amphotericin B appear to act in an additive manner, and cross-resistance has not been identified [100]. Clinical trials of caspofungin versus amphotericin demonstrated equivalent outcomes in the treatment of candidemia [101]. In solid-organ transplant recipients, caspofungin will be an important drug in treating serious fungal infections, particularly because it lacks the nephrotoxicity of amphotericin. Two of the more recently released triazole drugs, itraconazole and voriconazole, also possess activity in vitro against *Aspergillus* spp; the combination of voriconazole and caspofungin has been shown to enhance clinical efficacy [102].

Aspergillosis occurs in 1% to 4% of transplant recipients, most commonly after liver and lung transplants. Half of such patients go on to develop disseminated disease, with a mortality rate in excess of 80% [78,103]. Most patients with aspergillosis present with what appears to be a bacterial pneumonia. In high-risk lung or liver transplant recipients, or in lower risk patients whose supposed pneumonia fails to respond to appropriate antibiotic therapy, an aggressive diagnostic approach is warranted. The diagnosis of aspergillosis is established initially by microscopic examination of samples obtained via bronchoscopy and BAL for the presence of filamentous hyphae. Agents approved by the U.S. Food and Drug Administration (FDA) against invasive aspergillosis include liposomal amphotericin B, itraconazole, voriconazole, posaconazole, and caspofungin. Dissemination to the central nervous system (CNS) may result in brain abscesses, which in the past were nearly uniformly fatal, but more recently have been successfully treated with newer antifungal agents (such as voriconazole) and neurosurgical resection [104].

Infections due to a number of other fungi occur in solid-organ transplant recipients, including *Cryptococcus neoformans, Coccidioides immitis, Blastomyces dermatitidis, Histoplasma capsulatum*, and *Zygomycetes*, *Mucor*, and *Rhizopus* spp. Infections caused by those fungi occur in specific settings and present as specific syndromes that should be considered by the clinician caring for immunosuppressed patients.

Cryptococcus neoformans is the second leading cause of invasive fungal infections in liver transplant recipients. This pathogen may cause pneumonia or meningitis, and patients with pulmonary disease often have CNS involvement as well. It is recommended that immunocompromised patients with cryptococcal infection should undergo lumbar puncture even if asymptomatic neurologically. Skin nodules are occasionally seen. The diagnosis is confirmed by India-ink staining and by testing for cryptococcal antigen in cerebrospinal fluid or sputum. Treatment consists of amphotericin B followed by oral fluconazole [105].

Coccidioides immitis is endemic in the southwestern United States and in Mexico. Between 7% and 9% of solid-organ transplant recipients residing in that area develop coccidioidomycosis, with an associated mortality rate of 25% in pulmonary cases and of up to 70% in disseminated cases [80]. The presentation of disease is variable, as multiple organ systems may be involved. The diagnosis must be made by microscopy, antigen detection, or tissue culture. Lifelong fluconazole prophylaxis for solid-organ transplant recipients who reside in endemic areas is advocated in some centers, though long-term outcome data are lacking. A reduction of calcineurin inhibitor dosage can be an adjunct benefit. The treatment is prolonged amphotericin B administration or azole therapy [106].

Histoplasmosis and blastomycosis infections occur in endemic areas of the American Midwest and in the Mississippi and Ohio River valleys. Invasive disease, either reactivation of latent fungi or a new infection, occurs in up to 2% of solid-organ transplant recipients, with the highest incidence in those areas. Invasive disease spreads from the lungs to the skin and bone marrow. Biopsy and samples for culture analysis may be obtained from skin lesions or from a bone-marrow aspirate. Amphotericin B or itraconazole are appropriate therapeutic agents [79].

Mucor and *Rhizopus* spp in the *Zygomycetes* class are soil fungi that, when inhaled, may cause a highly morbid, invasive rhinocerebral infection in profoundly immunosuppressed patients and in diabetic patients with poor glycemic control [107]. The diagnosis is established by biopsy; treatment is surgical debridement with adjuvant antifungal therapy (amphotericin B with the occasional addition of 5-flucytosine, itraconazole, or rifampin). The mortality rate associated with those types of infections is in excess of 50%.

Pneumocystis jiroveci pneumonia (PCP) is a common cause of pneumonia in immunosuppressed patients. PCP is associated with profound defects in cellular immunity and normally is seen with CD4-positive T-cell counts lower than 200 per μL [108]. Those indices are often seen with OKT3 therapy for AR. Prophylaxis with TMP-SMX or atovaquone (if sulfa allergic) makes PCP a rare entity; however, transplant recipients who have a respiratory illness but did not receive prophylaxis (e.g., because of allergy or noncompliance) should be evaluated promptly for PCP. Untreated PCP has a very high mortality rate. The diagnosis is typically established by bronchoscopy and BAL, with methenamine silver staining of washings, or by transbronchial biopsy. Normal findings should not delay further evaluation and therapy (the characteristic alveolar and interstitial changes seen on a chest radiograph are late findings). Even before the diagnosis of PCP is established, empiric therapy is normally started with intravenous TMP-SMX or inhaled pentamidine. Dapsone is used in patients with a sulfa sensitivity. Concurrent CMV infection is common, so CMV diagnostic studies should be undertaken in patients whose PCP fails to respond promptly to appropriate therapy.

Viral Infections

Viral infections have increasingly been recognized as important causes of morbidity and mortality in solid-organ transplant recipients. Viruses that are endemic and of little clinical concern in the general patient population may produce overwhelming infections in the host with suppressed cellular immunity. The recent appreciation of the immunomodulatory effect of several opportunistic viral pathogens gives even more reason for continued development of effective prophylaxis, diagnosis, and treatment modalities for this class of infectious agents. Immunosuppressed transplant recipients may develop serious viral infections by reactivation of latent virus, by transmission of the virus via the donor graft or via blood transfusion, or by exposure to the virus in the environment.

Pathogens known as the HHVs are important in the solid-organ transplant population (Table 186.4). Those viruses commonly cause disease during periods of intense immunosuppression, particularly early posttransplant and after antirejection therapy. They include many of the most important viral pathogens facing immunosuppressed patients, including CMV, EBV, the herpes simplex viruses (HSVs), and the varicella zoster virus (VZV).

CMV infections affect 30% to 75% of solid-organ transplant recipients, primarily within 2 weeks to 3 months posttransplant. The highest risk for CMV infections is in a CMV-seronegative recipient receiving a graft from a CMV-seropositive donor (the D+/R− graft) [109]. Lung and heart–lung transplant recipients have the highest rate of CMV disease (50% to 80%). Pancreas and pancreas–kidney transplant recipients have a rate of 50%; kidney, heart, or liver transplant recipients, 8% to 35% [110].

The most severe CMV disease is a primary infection in the D+/R− population. A superinfection (due to concurrent reactivation of an endogenous strain and transmission of a serotypically distinct strain of CMV) is typically intermediate in severity, whereas reactivation of latent disease is most often comparatively mild [111]. The range of clinical disease is vast: from asymptomatic infections (detected solely by a change in anti-CMV titer or by shedding of virus or viral DNA in blood, urine, or sputum) to tissue-invasive disease (which may affect the lungs, liver, or intestine). A typical mild infection produces a mononucleosis-like syndrome, including fever, malaise, and

TABLE 186.4

HUMAN HERPES VIRUSES (HHVs)

Virus	Eponym	Clinical syndromes
HHV-1	Herpes simplex virus-1	Mucocutaneous disease Primarily oral–labial symptoms Ocular keratitis Herpes simplex virus encephalitis
HHV-2	Herpes simplex virus-2	Mucocutaneous disease Primarily genital symptoms Ocular keratitis
HHV-3	Varicella zoster virus	Chickenpox, shingles Pneumonitis, encephalitis
HHV-4	Epstein–Barr virus	Infectious mononucleosis Hepatitis, pneumonitis Posttransplant lymphoproliferative disease Burkitt lymphoma
HHV-5	Cytomegalovirus	Mononucleosis, pneumonitis Hepatitis, gastroenteritis, retinitis
HHV-6	Roseola (6B)	Childhood febrile exanthema Mononucleosis, encephalitis Pneumonitis, disseminated disease
HHV-7		No clear clinical entities
HHV-8	Kaposi agent	Cutaneous lymphomas

myalgias, often accompanied by leukopenia. More severe disease clinically manifests with differing signs and symptoms, depending on the site(s) of invasive infection. GI ulceration with occasional hemorrhage is seen in GI disease. CMV pneumonitis may produce respiratory insufficiency and failure. CMV hepatitis may lead to liver failure and to severe pancreatitis can occur. CMV retinitis may produce vision changes, leading to blindness.

Formerly, the presence of CMV was suspected in patients who developed a viral prodrome, with a fourfold increase in anti-CMV titer or by direct observation of CMV inclusion bodies in biopsy specimens. Retrospective confirmation was on the basis of culture analysis that took 2 to 3 weeks. Those inadequate diagnostic techniques have been supplanted by the rapid "shell-vial" culture, in which virus is grown in culture with fibroblasts and examined by immunofluorescence microscopy after incubation with anti-CMV immunofluorescence-linked monoclonal antibodies [112].

A rapid antigenemia assay is also available that measures the levels of the pp65 CMV antigen in sample fluid, but accurate results depend on a normal white blood cell count [113]. Most recently, the polymerase chain reaction has been used to measure viral copy number in peripheral leukocytes and, like the antigenemia assay, may permit very early diagnosis of subclinical CMV infections in at-risk patients [114]. Investigators differ in their preference between those two techniques [115], but both are clearly useful. Overall, the new techniques allow substantiation of CMV infections with greater than 90% to 95% sensitivity and specificity within 24 to 48 hours.

Given the high prevalence and significant morbidity of CMV disease, prophylaxis with ganciclovir, valacyclovir, or valganciclovir for 3 to 6 months posttransplant is common, particularly in high-risk patients. Additional prophylaxis routinely is begun with initiation of antirejection therapy. Several randomized clinical trials have shown ganciclovir prophylaxis to be superior to acyclovir prophylaxis in preventing both reactivation and primary CMV disease in solid-organ transplant recipients [116–119].

A second approach to this problem is the close monitoring of at-risk patients with protocol antigenemia or polymerase chain reaction assays followed by empiric (so-called preemptive) therapy with ganciclovir, if levels rise above a predetermined threshold. This approach, though somewhat more cumbersome, has led to reductions in the burden of CMV disease in liver transplant recipients [120]. Prophylaxis, surveillance with empiric therapy, or a combination of both based on calculated risk is currently practiced in most transplant centers. However, in kidney transplant recipients, surveillance monitoring with preemptive therapy has not been shown to be superior to treatment based on symptomatic disease [121], and, consequently, the main focus in this population is on prophylaxis. Ganciclovir prophylaxis is used for lung, heart–lung, and heart transplant recipients as well [122–124], but data on surveillance, preemptive therapy, and efficacy in such recipients are limited.

Traditionally, treatment of established CMV infections consists of intravenous ganciclovir, followed in most cases by oral ganciclovir. Oral valganciclovir alone can achieve similar clinical outcomes [125]. Anti-CMV immune globulin is available and is commonly added to ganciclovir for the treatment of serious, life-threatening invasive CMV infections, although studies of this agent have been limited to its use in prophylaxis and are equivocal in showing efficacy [126]. Foscarnet (trisodium phosphonoformate) is used in those rare instances where ganciclovir-resistant strains of CMV are isolated. The data that clearly establish the efficacy of foscarnet in treating CMV disease are limited to CMV retinitis; efficacy equivalent to ganciclovir was observed, but foscarnet was associated with a higher rate of adverse effects (e.g., nephrotoxicity) [127].

The HSVs (HSV-1 and HSV-2) commonly cause mucocutaneous disease of the oropharynx (HSV-1) and the genitalia (HSV-2). In profoundly immunosuppressed patients, they may cause disseminated disease, including hepatitis, encephalitis, and pneumonitis. Most such infections are thought to be reactivation of latent virus [128], and the highest risk is in lung and heart transplant recipients. The diagnosis is established by identification of the virus by immunofluorescent monoclonal antibody staining or by Tzanck smear. Culture and rising anti-HSV antibody titers provide evidence as well. Treatment consists of acyclovir; most epidermal lesions respond to oral therapy, but any evidence of disseminated disease requires high-dose intravenous acyclovir and minimization of immunosuppression.

Infections associated with EBV are commonly detectable in solid-organ transplant recipients. The most common manifestations include the typical mononucleosis-type syndrome, pneumonitis, and hepatitis [129]. The diagnosis of EBV infections is made by detection of heterophile immunoglobin M antibodies in serum or by following titers of antibodies to viral capsid antigen or to early antigens. Polymerase chain reaction is also used to monitor viral activity and response to therapy. Treatment consists of acyclovir (or ganciclovir, when a CMV infection is also suspected). Severe invasive disease mandates a reduction in immunosuppressive therapy. The most important aspect of EBV, however, is its association with posttransplant lymphoproliferative disorders (PTLDs) (vide infra).

VZV commonly emerges from latency in immunosuppressed transplant recipients and causes an episode of shingles [75]. More rarely, VZV may cause disseminated infections, such as pneumonitis and encephalitis. The highest risk of disseminated VZV disease is in pediatric transplant recipients who have not been exposed to VZV (e.g., chickenpox); this type of primary infection is associated with a high mortality rate (11%) [130]. Fortunately, the introduction of the varicella vaccine has markedly reduced this type of disease; the vaccine is recommended pretransplant for all pediatric and nonimmunosuppressed transplant candidates [131]. VZV infections are treated with acyclovir; with severe disseminated disease, immunosuppression is reduced [132]. No evidence supports the efficacy of anti-VZV immune globulin for treating severe VZV disease in immunocompromised patients, though it may be considered in nonimmunocompromised individuals.

The role of HHV-6 as a cause of clinical disease is not yet clearly established in solid-organ transplant recipients. Considerable evidence, primarily in bone marrow and stem cell transplant recipients, points to an association between HHV-6 and CNS syndromes, pneumonitis, and a mononucleosis-like immunosuppressive syndrome that may predispose to other opportunistic infections [133]. An association between HHV-6 activation with severe CMV disease has been reported, but understanding causality in this context is difficult. Treatment of neurologic diseases related to HHV-6 includes ganciclovir and foscarnet, either alone or in combination [133]. HHV-7 is not yet clearly associated with clinical syndromes that pose major problems in solid-organ transplant recipients. HHV-8 is linked to the development of Kaposi sarcoma in transplant recipients (vide infra).

Viral hepatitis is a significant problem, particularly in liver transplant recipients, who may have developed end-stage liver disease as a result of HBV or HCV infections. Primary HBV or HCV infections may occur during the transplant operation itself, because of donor graft or blood transfusion transmission.

Would-be donors positive for hepatitis B surface antigen (HBsAg) and/or anti-hepatitis B core antibodies (HBcAbs) are often excluded from donating any organ or tissue [134]. Organs other than the liver have been transplanted from isolated HBcAb-positive donors, without evidence of transmission, but the risk for transmission is unknown [135]. HCV-positive donors are normally excluded from donating any organ [136], except to status-1 patients whose death is imminent or to patients who already have such infections. Liver transplant candidates with HBV or HCV disease are transplanted; currently, their graft and patient survival rates, particularly in the short term, are comparable to those for recipients without HBV or HCV disease. At one time, HBV disease was a contraindication to a liver transplant; however, the use of lamivudine and HBV-immune globulin (HBIG) has significantly reduced the burden of recurrent HBV disease [137,138] and has allowed hundreds of patients with end-stage liver disease secondary to HBV to undergo successful transplants. The optimal duration of HBIG treatment is debatable.

However, the development of recurrent viral disease in patients with HCV is inevitable and may be clinically significant, depending on the severity of the disease [139]. Up to 25% of transplant recipients accelerate to cirrhosis within 5 to 10 years posttransplant, likely related to immunosuppressive therapy and rejection [140]. The care of transplant candidates with HCV includes extending the donor pool, tailoring antiviral treatment pre- and posttransplant, and offering a living donor transplant [141]. The idea of neutralizing human monoclonal antibodies against HCV is currently under clinical investigation [142].

As discussed previously, many of the HSVs are associated with invasive hepatitis, which may progress to fulminant disease. Hepatitis may also be caused by adenovirus infections in solid-organ transplant recipients. Several other viruses cause significant morbidity and mortality in this patient population. Adenoviral infections, though more common in hematopoietic cell transplant patients, do occur in solid-organ transplant recipients. Invasive adenoviral infections most commonly manifest as pneumonitis or hepatitis, both of which carry a poor prognosis [143].

Primary infections with HIV via an organ transplant from an HIV-positive donor have been described; HIV-positive status is ordinarily a contraindication to either donating or undergoing a transplant [144]. However, solid-organ transplant recipients infected with HIV have been identified and have enjoyed long-term survival posttransplant [145], given the success of long-term multidrug therapy for HIV. With the introduction of highly active antiretroviral therapy (HAART), the transplant community has now recognized HIV infections as a chronic condition. In fact, end organ failure develops in HIV-positive individuals as they age and/or from the side effects of their antiviral treatments. Short-term outcomes in HIV-positive transplant recipients have been promising [146]: the HIV load remains suppressed, CD4-positive T-lymphocyte counts are stable, and the risk of opportunistic infection is acceptable. However, major challenges in the care of HIV-positive transplant recipients include high graft rejection rates and multiple drug interactions between HAART and maintenance immunosuppression [147].

The polyomavirus, including BK, JC, and SV40, is a ubiquitous pathogen that has no clinical significance in immunocompetent hosts. BK virus (BKV) is tropic-specific for human transitional and renal tubular epithelial cells. After primary infection, which often occurs in early life, BKV establishes lifelong latency in the host's renal cells. Reactivation takes place when the host's immune system is weakened, such as during pregnancy or posttransplant immunosuppression. The diagnosis is made by detecting free viral particles in the urine, blood, or intranuclear viral inclusion-bearing cells (decoy cells) in urine cytology specimens. BKV nephropathy (BKN) has been increasingly recognized as an important entity in kidney transplant recipients since the mid-1990s; currently, it is seen in 1% to 9% of them within the first year posttransplant [148]. In advanced BKN, the graft failure rate has been reported as high as 60% [149]. Depending on the severity of renal tubule injury, clinical presentations of BKN can include fatigue, fever, mild hydronephrosis, or marked graft dysfunction. In bone marrow transplant recipients, hemorrhagic cystitis has been described. The diagnosis of BKV reactivation is made by urinary cytology, quantitative PCR analysis to measure the viral load in urine or plasma, and kidney biopsy [150]. The mainstays of caring for patients with BKN are to reduce immunosuppression and to closely monitor disease progression. Given the lack of specific antiviral agents against BKV, low-dose cidofovir or leflunomide has been used, with some success, in patients with persistent BKN [151,152].

Human papilloma viruses may cause disease through the development of tissue-specific growth leading to benign or malignant processes, including cervical cancer, cancer of the vulva and perineum, condyloma acuminatum, laryngeal polyposis, and nonmelanotic skin cancer (vide infra). Respiratory syncytial virus may produce a fulminant pneumonia in both adult and pediatric transplant recipients. The diagnosis is made by nasopharyngeal washing. More severe cases should be treated with ribavirin.

Parasitic Infections

Several common parasitic infections are seen in immunosuppressed solid-organ transplant recipients. *Toxoplasma gondii* presents as a brain abscess with neurologic changes [153]. It is seen late posttransplant, whereas a brain abscess in the early posttransplant period is more likely to be fungal [154]. Heart transplant recipients seem to be at greatest risk, possibly due to the presence of *T. gondii* cysts in donor myocardial tissue. If the heart donor was seropositive for *T. gondii*, the recipient normally undergoes prophylactic treatment with pyrimethamine and sulfadiazine for 3 to 6 months posttransplant. Treatment of *T. gondii* infections consists of pyrimethamine and sulfadiazine; the mortality rate is high in transplant recipients who exhibit CNS disease.

MALIGNANCY

Solid-organ transplant recipients have a markedly increased risk of developing malignancy posttransplant. An extensive data collection tracks the epidemiology of tumors in transplant recipients; it was initiated and is maintained by the Israel Penn International Transplant Tumor Registry [155]. The increased incidence of malignancy is multifactorial, probably due to a combination of the activation of latent viruses with oncogenic potential, the direct oncogenic effect of immunosuppressive drugs such as cyclosporine, and, perhaps, environmental factors. Strong but indirect evidence points to the loss of immunologic surveillance as a mechanism of increased oncogenesis. The most common neoplasms in solid-organ transplant recipients are skin cancers, PTLD, lung cancer, Kaposi sarcoma, and carcinoma of the cervix. Of those neoplasms, lung cancer appears to occur at the same frequency as in the general population; the other neoplasms occur at increased frequency in solid-organ transplant recipients. PTLD presents the greatest challenge in terms of attendant high morbidity and mortality rates.

Posttransplant Lymphoproliferative Disorder

The term *PTLD* encompasses a very broad range of pathologies, from simple lymphoid hyperplasia to very aggressive monoclonal B-cell lymphomas. EBV infections play a central causative role. In particular, primary EBV infections posttransplant (EBV D+/R− match) and immunosuppression markedly increase the risk of PTLD [156]. Other risk factors include active CMV disease [157], CMV D+/R− match [158], increasing intensity of immunosuppression [159,160], and, possibly, HCV infections [161] and recipient cytokine gene polymorphisms [162].

PTLD is least common in adult kidney transplant recipients and most common in pediatric small-bowel transplant recipients. It is most common early posttransplant, concurrent with the most intense immunosuppression and with the use of anti–T-cell therapy for AR, particularly repeated courses. However, a subset of PTLD occurs late (several years) posttransplant. These late-occurring neoplasms appear to be related more to patient age, duration, and intensity of immunosuppression, and type of graft than to the more typical risk factors seen in early onset disease.

The clinical presentation of PTLD varies widely, as might be expected from the wide range of pathology encountered with this entity. Many patients experience fever, sweats, and myalgias as the only symptoms. Weight loss, diarrhea, and upper respiratory infection symptoms also are common; some, but not all, patients have lymphadenopathy. CNS involvement, which occurs in up to 20% of patients [163], often manifests as mental status changes. GI disease may be silent or may present as abdominal pain, GI bleeding, perforation with peritonitis, or bowel obstruction. Intrathoracic PTLD has a characteristic radiographic appearance of multiple circumscribed pulmonary nodules, which may or may not be accompanied by mediastinal lymphadenopathy. PTLD in the graft itself can present very similarly to AR; because the therapeutic approach to those two entities is diametrically opposed, a correct diagnosis on biopsy is essential.

Biopsy of suspected lesions is the gold standard in establishing the diagnosis of PTLD. Biopsy specimens are histologically graded (based on cell morphology and nodal architecture) and assessed for clonality (polyclonal or monoclonal) and for the presence of an EBV genome and copy number. Specific cell marker studies are required to establish the cell of origin, but most lesions are EBV positive and of B-cell lineage. Pathologists familiar with PTLD as well as with graft rejection and opportunistic infections should review the biopsy results. Consensus conference standards for the grading and classification of PTLD are used [164]. Histologic classification currently uses the Harris standard formulation [165]. EBV serology does not typically add to the diagnostic workup of PTLD, with many false-negatives in patients with established primary EBV infections [166,167]. Similarly, peripheral cytology is not helpful in making the diagnosis [168]. If PTLD is suspected, patients should undergo imaging of the head, thorax, and abdomen. Fluorodeoxyglucose-positron emission tomography (FDG-PET)/CT scanning has been increasingly used as a diagnostic and/or staging tool and in follow-up studies of PTLD patients [169].

Currently, there is little information to provide direction regarding optimal prophylaxis against PTLD. Clearly, it is important to identify, and closely monitor, high-risk patients (e.g., children; liver and small-bowel transplant recipients; EBV-negative transplant recipients, particularly those with an EBV-positive donor; and transplant recipients on intense antilymphocyte therapy for rejection). Similarly, OKT3 therapy should not be used in high-risk patients without a definitive diagnosis of AR on biopsy. Both antiviral agents and passive immune transfer with anti-EBV immune globulin have been proposed as prophylaxis against PTLD, but data supporting those approaches are lacking. Several trials are ongoing to establish the best prophylactic approach [170]. Intriguingly, the improvements in baseline immunosuppression preventing AR appear to decrease the frequency of PTLD, likely as a byproduct of reducing the frequency of antilymphocyte antibody therapy [171].

Treatment of established PTLD depends on each patient's clinical situation and histologic diagnosis. With few trials to guide therapy, a graded, individualized approach is taken. Ordinarily, immunosuppression is reduced to minimal levels, and specific therapy is directed at the neoplasm. In 25% to 50% of patients, PTLD regresses after their immunosuppression is reduced [172].

Surgical intervention is clearly indicated for patients with GI PTLD that manifests as aggressive disease (e.g., viscus obstruction or perforation). Surgical debulking of the tumor burden has also been used in amenable cases [173], as has radiotherapy [174]. Isolated CNS disease initially should be treated with external beam irradiation.

Medical approaches to treating PTLD include (a) antiviral medications (e.g., acyclovir, ganciclovir) [175]; (b) interferon-α2b [176]; (c) immunoglobulins [75,175]; (d) standard, low-dose, and high-dose chemotherapy protocols [177,178]; and (e) most recently, monoclonal antibodies directed against B-cell surface markers, such as CD19 and CD20 (rituximab) [179]. In unusual cases, immunomodulatory therapy with adoptive transfer of cytotoxic T cells sensitized to EBV has been attempted with some success [180].

Late-onset PTLD, occurring more than 1 to 2 years posttransplant, often does not respond to the reduction in immunosuppression and to the medical therapy typically used in patients with early-onset disease. Often EBV-negative, late-onset PTLD is difficult to treat because of side effects, including infectious complications of the aggressive chemotherapy that is often required. Similarly, CNS involvement may be a marker for PTLD that is potentially refractory to therapy, possibly because of the relatively privileged immune site. Treatment options include intrathecal administration of interferon-α and anti–B-cell antibody therapy along with local radiotherapy, but the prognosis remains guarded [163,181].

Skin Cancer

The most common neoplasms associated with transplants and immunosuppression are nonmelanotic skin cancers. These lesions increase in frequency with sunlight exposure and with increasing time posttransplant. Often-quoted studies show a prevalence of 66% in transplant recipients in Australia after 24 years of surveillance [182] and 40% after 20 years in the Netherlands [183]. Those figures correlate to a 4- to 21-fold increase in prevalence in transplant recipients, as compared with the immunocompetent population, with synergistic increases seen in the areas of highest sunlight exposure.

Most skin cancers in transplant recipients are squamous cell carcinomas. Many recipients develop multiple lesions, and the age at onset is markedly lower than in the general population. The incidence of melanomas is also higher representing 4.8% of skin cancers in kidney transplant recipients, as compared with 2.7% in the general population [155]. Even nonmelanotic squamous cell carcinomas behave more aggressively in transplant recipients, with lymph node metastasis and a 6% mortality rate due to disseminated disease [184]. On identification of skin lesions, prompt surgical extirpation should be undertaken. Solid-organ transplant recipients are instructed to avoid direct exposure to sunlight for any prolonged period and to liberally use sunblock. Clearly, close dermatologic counseling and follow-up are warranted in this patient population.

Kaposi Sarcoma

Kaposi's sarcoma (KS) is a multicentric, vascularized, nodular neoplasm that may affect the skin, visceral tissues (such as the lungs and GI tract), or both. Endemic in the Mediterranean region and Middle East, it is strongly associated with either endogenous or exogenous immunosuppression, as a result both of AIDS and of immunosuppressive therapy. The incidence of this disease in U.S. transplant recipients is 0.4%, which represents a 20-fold increase over the basal rate in the population at large [155]. That figure rises to 1.6% in Italian kidney-transplant recipients and up to 4.0% in Saudi Arabian transplant recipients [185,186]. Recently, human herpes virus (HHV)-8 has been implicated as a causal agent in KS. One small series showed HHV-8 seropositivity pretransplant to be a relative risk factor for development of KS posttransplant [187].

Cutaneous KS is readily identified by clinical appearance and biopsy. But patients with only visceral KS often present with more advanced disease, usually GI bleeding or viscus perforation, sometimes dyspnea related to pulmonary disease. Immunosuppression should be reduced to the extent possible, after which about 30% to 55% of patients will experience remission. Chemotherapy is reserved for patients with visceral KS and for those who do not experience remission after their immunosuppression is reduced. However, of patients with visceral KS, 45% to 50% die of it. Viral studies and antiviral therapy do not yet have any well-established role in fighting this neoplasm, but anecdotal evidence indicates that certain patients may respond to antiviral agents (e.g., ganciclovir).

Cervical Cancer

The rate of development of cervical intraepithelial neoplasia is elevated by 10- to 14-fold in solid-organ transplant recipients and may approach 50% [188,189]. Cervical carcinoma was seen in 10% of all women with posttransplant cancer in the Transplant Tumor Registry [155]. Close surveillance by pelvic examination and Papanicolaou smear is essential in this population, given the increased incidence of disease. In transplant recipients with more advanced cervical cancer, a functioning graft poses complications in selecting and carrying out appropriate therapy. Limited data are available to guide therapy.

Transmitted and Recurrent Malignancy

Case reports have described patients who received grafts that harbored malignant cells, leading to the development of malignancy. Transmission to transplant recipients of renal cell carcinoma, metastatic cancer of the breast or lung, and melanoma has been reported. Currently, cancer or recent history of cancer is a contraindication to organ donation, with the possible exception of some low-grade skin cancers, noninvasive CNS neoplasms, and small, limited, extirpated cancers that are not likely to recur or spread. Nonetheless, some grafts are found to contain foci of neoplasia, which develop into a clinically significant cancer in recipients. This finding emphasizes the need for a thorough examination of donors during organ procurement, particularly considering the present trend toward the use of older donors.

Patients with a history of malignancy clearly are at risk for recurrent disease posttransplant, presumably due to the use of immunosuppression. Data from the Transplant Tumor Registry show a 21% recurrence rate, with the highest rates seen in patients with multiple myeloma (67%), nonmelanotic skin cancer (53%), bladder cancer (29%), soft-tissue sarcoma (29%), renal cell cancer (27%), and breast cancer (23%) [190]. Tumors were least likely to recur if more than 5 years had passed between cancer treatment and the transplant.

Liver transplants to treat patients with primary, well-circumscribed liver tumors represent a special case. In this population, liver tumor size and the number of liver tumors are considered indicative of the likelihood of disease recurrence and patient survival posttransplant [191,192]. Adjuvant techniques, such as cryoablation and radiofrequency ablation, to reduce the tumor burden pretransplant have been used, but currently the data are insufficient to clearly define the ability of adjuvant techniques to reduce posttransplant morbidity and mortality secondary to disease recurrence. Risk factors for recurrence include tumor size >6 cm, number of nodules >5, and vascular invasion per the final pathology report [193]. Clearly, tumor biology dictates the risk of disease recurrence and needs to be further characterized, representing an interesting, perhaps promising experimental arena.

SUMMARY

Over the past several decades, advances in the field of solid-organ transplantation have been significant, such that the primary limitation to further expansion may be considered to be logistic, related to organ availability. Dramatic improvements in medical care and technology have broadened the pool of potential recipients to include those who would have been considered too sick, with too much comorbidity, even a few years ago. Until medical science is able to develop immunosuppression without side effects, the predominant challenges in transplantation will remain the prevention, detection, and treatment of rejection; the prophylaxis, diagnosis, and treatment of infections; and the prevention, detection, and treatment of malignancy. Those clinical problems have only grown in the nearly six decades since the first successful kidney transplant was performed, and they promise to become even more complex throughout the twenty-first century.

References

1. Starzl TE, Marchioro TL, Waddell WR: The Reversal of rejection in human renal homografts with subsequent development of homograft tolerance. *Surg Gynecol Obstet* 117:385–395, 1963.
2. Hill RB Jr, Rowlands DT Jr, Rifkind D: Infectious pulmonary disease in patients receiving immunosuppressive therapy for organ transplantation. *N Engl J Med* 271:1021–1027, 1964.
3. Starzl TE, Penn I, Putnam CW, et al: Iatrogenic alterations of immunologic surveillance in man and their influence on malignancy. *Transplant Rev* 7:112–145, 1971.
4. Medawar PB: The behaviour and fate of skin autografts and skin homografts in rabbits: A report to the war wounds committee of the medical research council. *J Anat* 78(Pt 5):176–199, 1944.
5. Squifflet JP, De Meyer M, Malaise J, et al: Lessons learned from ABO-incompatible living donor kidney transplantation: 20 years later. *Exp Clin Transplant* 2(1):208–213, 2004.
6. Magee CC: Transplantation across previously incompatible immunological barriers. *Transpl Int* 19(2):87–97, 2006.
7. Salvalaggio PR, Graff RJ, Pinsky B, et al: Crossmatch testing in kidney transplantation: patterns of practice and associations with rejection and graft survival. *Saudi J Kidney Dis Transpl* 20(4):577–589, 2009.
8. Taylor CJ, Kosmoliaptsis V, Summers DM, et al: Back to the future: application of contemporary technology to long-standing questions about the clinical relevance of human leukocyte antigen-specific alloantibodies in renal transplantation. *Hum Immunol* 70(8):563–568, 2009.
9. Haas M, Rahman MH, Racusen LC, et al: C4 d and C3 d staining in biopsies of ABO- and HLA-incompatible renal allografts: correlation with histologic findings. *Am J Transplant* 6(8):1829–1840, 2006.
10. Collins AJ, Foley R, Herzog C, et al: Excerpts from the United States Renal Data System 2007 annual data report. *Am J Kidney Dis* 51[1, Suppl 1]:S1–S320, 2008.
11. Kahan BD, Rajagopalan PR, Hall M: Reduction of the occurrence of acute cellular rejection among renal allograft recipients treated with basiliximab, a chimeric anti-interleukin-2-receptor monoclonal antibody. United States Simulect renal study group. *Transplantation* 67(2):276–284, 1999.
12. Vincenti F, Kirkman R, Light S, et al: Interleukin-2-receptor blockade with daclizumab to prevent acute rejection in renal transplantation. Daclizumab triple therapy study group. *N Engl J Med* 338(3):161–165, 1998.
13. Kaufman DB, Leventhal JR, Axelrod D, et al: Alemtuzumab induction and prednisone-free maintenance immunotherapy in kidney transplantation: comparison with basiliximab induction–long-term results. *Am J Transplant* 5(10):2539–2548, 2005.
14. Vincenti F, Schena FP, Paraskevas S, et al: A randomized, multicenter study of steroid avoidance, early steroid withdrawal or standard steroid therapy in kidney transplant recipients. *Am J Transplant* 8(2):307–316, 2008.
15. Vincenti F, Larsen C, Durrbach A, et al: Costimulation blockade with belatacept in renal transplantation. *N Engl J Med* 353(8):770–781, 2005.
16. Ekberg H, Tedesco-Silva H, Demirbas A, et al: Reduced exposure to calcineurin inhibitors in renal transplantation. *N Engl J Med* 357(25):2562–2575, 2007.
17. Matas A: Chronic rejection in renal transplant recipients–risk factors and correlates. *Clin Transplant* 8(3 Pt 2):332–335, 1994.
18. Womer KL, Vella JP, Sayegh MH: Chronic allograft dysfunction: mechanisms and new approaches to therapy. *Semin Nephrol* 20(2):126–147, 2000.
19. Wiseman AC: Polyomavirus nephropathy: a current perspective and clinical considerations. *Am J Kidney Dis* 54(1):131–142, 2009.
20. Gaber LW, Gaber AO, Hathaway DK, et al: Routine early biopsy of allografts with delayed function: correlation of histopathology and transplant outcome. *Clin Transplant* 10(6 Pt 2):629–634, 1996.
21. Jain S, Curwood V, White SA, et al: Weekly protocol renal transplant biopsies allow detection of sub-clinical acute rejection episodes in patients with delayed graft function. *Transplant Proc* 32(1):191, 2000.
22. Veronese FV, Noronha IL, Manfro RC, et al: Protocol biopsies in renal transplant patients: three-years' follow-up. *Transplant Proc* 34(2):500–501, 2002.
23. Marshall SE, McLaren AJ, McKinney EF, et al: Donor cytokine genotype influences the development of acute rejection after renal transplantation. *Transplantation* 71(3):469–476, 2001.
24. Perez RV, Brown DJ, Katznelson SA, et al: Pretransplant systemic inflammation and acute rejection after renal transplantation. *Transplantation* 69(5):869–874, 2000.
25. Sawitzki B, Pascher A, Babel N, et al: Can we use biomarkers and functional assays to implement personalized therapies in transplantation? *Transplantation* 87(11):1595–1601, 2009.
26. Kirkpantur A, Yilmaz R, Baydar DE, et al: Utility of the Doppler ultrasound parameter, resistive index, in renal transplant histopathology. *Transplant Proc* 40(1):104–106, 2008.
27. Solez K, Colvin RB, Racusen LC, et al: Banff 07 classification of renal allograft pathology: updates and future directions. *Am J Transplant* 8(4):753–760, 2008.
28. Clatworthy MR, Friend PJ, Calne RY, et al: Alemtuzumab (CAMPATH-1 H) for the treatment of acute rejection in kidney transplant recipients: long-term follow-up. *Transplantation* 87(7):1092–1095, 2009.
29. Waaga AM, Gasser M, Laskowski I, et al: Mechanisms of chronic rejection. *Curr Opin Immunol* 12(5):517–521, 2000.
30. Bird G, Friend P, Donaldson P, et al: Hyperacute rejection in liver transplantation: a case report. *Transplant Proc* 21(4):3742–3744, 1989.
31. Demetris AJ, Jaffe R, Tzakis A, et al: Antibody-mediated rejection of human orthotopic liver allografts. A study of liver transplantation across ABO blood group barriers. *Am J Pathol* 132(3):489–502, 1988.
32. Gugenheim J, Samuel D, Reynes M, et al: Liver transplantation across ABO blood group barriers. *Lancet* 336(8714):519–523, 1990.
33. Mor E, Skerrett D, Manzarbeitia C, et al: Successful use of an enhanced immunosuppressive protocol with plasmapheresis for ABO-incompatible mismatched grafts in liver transplant recipients. *Transplantation* 59(7):986–990, 1995.
34. European FK506 Multicentre Liver Study Group: Randomised trial comparing tacrolimus (FK506) and cyclosporin in prevention of liver allograft rejection. *Lancet* 344(8920):423–428, 1994.
35. The U. S. Multicenter FK506 Liver Study Group: A comparison of tacrolimus (FK 506) and cyclosporine for immunosuppression in liver transplantation. *N Engl J Med* 331(17):1110–1115, 1994.
36. Otto MG, Mayer AD, Clavien PA, et al: Randomized trial of cyclosporine microemulsion (neoral) versus conventional cyclosporine in liver transplantation: MILTON study. Multicentre International Study in Liver Transplantation of Neoral. *Transplantation* 66(12):1632–1640, 1998.
37. Eckhoff DE, McGuire BM, Frenette LR, et al: Tacrolimus (FK506) and mycophenolate mofetil combination therapy versus tacrolimus in adult liver transplantation. *Transplantation* 65(2):180–187, 1998.
38. Neuhaus P, Clavien PA, Kittur D, et al: Improved treatment response with basiliximab immunoprophylaxis after liver transplantation: results from a double-blind randomized placebo-controlled trial. *Liver Transpl* 8(2):132–142, 2002.
39. Llado L, Fabregat J, Castellote J, et al: Impact of immunosuppression without steroids on rejection and hepatitis C virus evolution after liver transplantation: results of a prospective randomized study. *Liver Transpl* 14(12):1752–1760, 2008.
40. Demetris A, Adams D, Bellamy C, et al: Update of the International Banff Schema for liver allograft rejection: working recommendations for the histopathologic staging and reporting of chronic rejection. An international panel. *Hepatology* 31(3):792–799, 2000.
41. Wiesner RH, Demetris AJ, Belle SH, et al: Acute hepatic allograft rejection: incidence, risk factors, and impact on outcome. *Hepatology* 28(3):638–645, 1998.
42. Pirsch JD, Kalayoglu M, Hafez GR, et al: Evidence that the vanishing bile duct syndrome is vanishing. *Transplantation* 49(5):1015–1018, 1990.
43. Klintmalm GB, Goldstein R, Gonwa T, et al: Use of FK 506 for the prevention of recurrent allograft rejection after successful conversion from cyclosporine for refractory rejection. US Multicenter FK 506 liver study group. *Transplant Proc* 25(1 Pt 1):635–637, 1993.
44. Sollinger HW, Stratta RJ, D'Alessandro AM, et al: Experience with simultaneous pancreas-kidney transplantation. *Ann Surg* 208(4):475–483, 1988.
45. Knight RJ, Kerman RH, Zela S, et al: Pancreas transplantation utilizing thymoglobulin, sirolimus, and cyclosporine. *Transplantation* 81(8):1101–1105, 2006.
46. Sutherland DE, Gruessner R, Moudry-Munns K, et al: Discordant graft loss from rejection of organs from the same donor in simultaneous pancreas-kidney recipients. *Transplant Proc* 27(1):907–908, 1995.
47. Nghiem DD, Gonwa TA, Corry RJ: Metabolic monitoring in renal-pancreatic transplants with urinary pancreatic exocrine diversion. *Transplant Proc* 19(1 Pt 3):2350–2351, 1987.
48. Gruessner AC, Sutherland DE: Pancreas transplant outcomes for United States (US) cases as reported to the United Network for Organ Sharing (UNOS) and the International Pancreas Transplant Registry (IPTR). *Clin Transpl* 45–56, 2008.
49. Billingham ME, Cary NR, Hammond ME, et al: A working formulation for the standardization of nomenclature in the diagnosis of heart and lung rejection: Heart rejection study group. The international society for heart transplantation. *J Heart Transplant* 9(6):587–593, 1990.
50. Hunt SA, Haddad F: The changing face of heart transplantation. *J Am Coll Cardiol* 52(8):587–598, 2008.
51. Haverty TP, Sanders M, Sheahan M: OKT3 treatment of cardiac allograft rejection. *J Heart Lung Transplant* 12(4):591–598, 1993.
52. Wagner FM, Reichenspurner H, Uberfuhr P, et al: How successful is OKT3 rescue therapy for steroid-resistant acute rejection episodes after heart transplantation? *J Heart Lung Transplant* 13(3):438–442, 1994; discussion 442–443.
53. Lehrer MS, Rook AH, Tomaszewski JE, et al: Successful reversal of severe refractory cardiac allograft rejection by photopheresis. *J Heart Lung Transplant* 20(11):1233–1236, 2001.
54. Costanzo-Nordin MR: Cardiac allograft vasculopathy: relationship with acute cellular rejection and histocompatibility. *J Heart Lung Transplant* 11(3 Pt 2):S90–S103, 1992.
55. Kaczmarek I, Ertl B, Schmauss D, et al: Preventing cardiac allograft vasculopathy: long-term beneficial effects of mycophenolate mofetil. *J Heart Lung Transplant* 25(5):550–556, 2006.

56. Choi JK, Kearns J, Palevsky HI, et al: Hyperacute rejection of a pulmonary allograft. Immediate clinical and pathologic findings. *Am J Respir Crit Care Med* 160(3):1015–1018, 1999.
57. Yousem SA, Dauber JA, Keenan R, et al: Does histologic acute rejection in lung allografts predict the development of bronchiolitis obliterans? *Transplantation* 52(2):306–309, 1991.
58. Mamessier E, Milhe F, Badier M, et al: Comparison of induced sputum and bronchoalveolar lavage in lung transplant recipients. *J Heart Lung Transplant* 25(5):523–532, 2006.
59. Higenbottam TW: Lung rejection after transplantation. *Eur Respir J* 2(1): 1–2, 1989.
60. Stewart S, Winters GL, Fishbein MC, et al: Revision of the 1990 working formulation for the standardization of nomenclature in the diagnosis of heart rejection. *J Heart Lung Transplant* 24(11):1710–1720, 2005.
61. Guilinger RA, Paradis IL, Dauber JH, et al: The importance of bronchoscopy with transbronchial biopsy and bronchoalveolar lavage in the management of lung transplant recipients. *Am J Respir Crit Care Med* 152(6 Pt 1):2037–2043, 1995.
62. Coke M, Edwards LB: Current status of thoracic organ transplantation and allocation in the United States. *Clin Transpl* 17–26, 2004.
63. Cooper JD, Billingham M, Egan T, et al: A working formulation for the standardization of nomenclature and for clinical staging of chronic dysfunction in lung allografts. International society for heart and lung transplantation. *J Heart Lung Transplant* 12(5):713–716, 1993.
64. Bando K, Paradis IL, Similo S, et al: Obliterative bronchiolitis after lung and heart-lung transplantation. An analysis of risk factors and management. *J Thorac Cardiovasc Surg* 110(1):4–13, 1995; discussion 13–14.
65. Lama VN: Update in lung transplantation 2008. *Am J Respir Crit Care Med* 179(9):759–764, 2009.
66. Brayman KL, Stephanian E, Matas AJ, et al: Analysis of infectious complications occurring after solid-organ transplantation. *Arch Surg* 127(1):38–47, 1992; discussion 47–48.
67. Rubin RH, Wolfson JS, Cosimi AB, et al: Infection in the renal transplant recipient. *Am J Med* 70(2):405–411, 1981.
68. Dunn DL: Problems related to immunosuppression. Infection and malignancy occurring after solid organ transplantation. *Crit Care Clin* 6(4):955–977, 1990.
69. Kusne S, Dummer JS, Singh N, et al: Infections after liver transplantation. An analysis of 101 consecutive cases. *Medicine (Baltimore)* 67(2):132–143, 1988.
70. Dummer JS, Hardy A, Poorsattar A, et al: Early infections in kidney, heart, and liver transplant recipients on cyclosporine. *Transplantation* 36(3):259–267, 1983.
71. Snydman DR: Epidemiology of infections after solid-organ transplantation. *Clin Infect Dis* 33[Suppl 1]:S5–S8, 2001.
72. Fryd DS, Peterson PK, Ferguson RM, et al: Cytomegalovirus as a risk factor in renal transplantation. *Transplantation* 30(6):436–439, 1980.
73. Singh N, Carrigan DR: Human herpesvirus-6 in transplantation: an emerging pathogen. *Ann Intern Med* 124(12):1065–1071, 1996.
74. McGrath D, Falagas ME, Freeman R, et al: Adenovirus infection in adult orthotopic liver transplant recipients: incidence and clinical significance. *J Infect Dis* 177(2):459–462, 1998.
75. Tan HH, Goh CL: Viral infections affecting the skin in organ transplant recipients: epidemiology and current management strategies. *Am J Clin Dermatol* 7(1):13–29, 2006.
76. Preiksaitis JK, Diaz-Mitoma F, Mirzayans F, et al: Quantitative oropharyngeal Epstein-Barr virus shedding in renal and cardiac transplant recipients: relationship to immunosuppressive therapy, serologic responses, and the risk of posttransplant lymphoproliferative disorder. *J Infect Dis* 166(5):986–994, 1992.
77. Lumbreras C, Cuervas-Mons V, Jara P, et al: Randomized trial of fluconazole versus nystatin for the prophylaxis of Candida infection following liver transplantation. *J Infect Dis* 174(3):583–588, 1996.
78. Kusne S, Torre-Cisneros J, Manez R, et al: Factors associated with invasive lung aspergillosis and the significance of positive Aspergillus culture after liver transplantation. *J Infect Dis* 166(6):1379–1383, 1992.
79. Wheat LJ, Freifeld AG, Kleiman MB, et al: Clinical practice guidelines for the management of patients with histoplasmosis: 2007 update by the Infectious Diseases Society of America. *Clin Infect Dis* 45(7):807–825, 2007.
80. Cohen IM, Galgiani JN, Potter D, et al: Coccidioidomycosis in renal replacement therapy. *Arch Intern Med* 142(3):489–494, 1982.
81. Spees EK, Light JA, Oakes DD, et al: Experiences with cadaver renal allograft contamination before transplantation. *Br J Surg* 69(8):482–485, 1982.
82. Prat V, Horcickova M, Matousovic K, et al: Urinary tract infection in renal transplant patients. *Infection* 13(5):207–210, 1985.
83. Lapchik MS, Castelo Filho A, Pestana JO, et al: Risk factors for nosocomial urinary tract and postoperative wound infections in renal transplant patients: a matched-pair case-control study. *J Urol* 147(4):994–998, 1992.
84. Wilson CH, Bhatti AA, Rix DA, et al: Routine intraoperative ureteric stenting for kidney transplant recipients. *Cochrane Database Syst Rev* (4):CD004925, 2005.
85. Tolkoff-Rubin NE, Cosimi AB, Russell PS, et al: A controlled study of trimethoprim-sulfamethoxazole prophylaxis of urinary tract infection in renal transplant recipients. *Rev Infect Dis* 4(2):614–618, 1982.
86. Judson RT: Wound infection following renal transplantation. *Aust N Z J Surg* 54(3):223–224, 1984.
87. Rabito FJ, Pankey GA: Infections in orthotopic heart transplant patients at the Ochsner Medical Institutions. *Med Clin North Am* 76(5):1125–1134, 1992.
88. Maurer JR, Tullis DE, Grossman RF, et al: Infectious complications following isolated lung transplantation. *Chest* 101(4):1056–1059, 1992.
89. Everett JE, Wahoff DC, Statz C, et al: Characterization and impact of wound infection after pancreas transplantation. *Arch Surg* 129(12):1310–1316, 1994; discussion 1316–1317.
90. Mermel LA, Maki DG: Bacterial pneumonia in solid organ transplantation. *Semin Respir Infect* 5(1):10–29, 1990.
91. Deusch E, End A, Grimm M, et al: Early bacterial infections in lung transplant recipients. *Chest* 104(5):1412–1416, 1993.
92. Snell GI, de Hoyos A, Krajden M, et al: Pseudomonas cepacia in lung transplant recipients with cystic fibrosis. *Chest* 103(2):466–471, 1993.
93. Sinnott JTT, Emmanuel PJ: Mycobacterial infections in the transplant patient. *Semin Respir Infect* 5(1):65–73, 1990.
94. Jie T, Matas AJ, Gillingham KJ, et al: Mycobacterial infections after kidney transplant. *Transplant Proc* 37(2):937–939, 2005.
95. Stamm AM, Dismukes WE, Simmons BP, et al: Listeriosis in renal transplant recipients: report of an outbreak and review of 102 cases. *Rev Infect Dis* 4(3):665–682, 1982.
96. Chapman SW, Wilson JP: Nocardiosis in transplant recipients. *Semin Respir Infect* 5(1):74–79, 1990.
97. Paya CV: Fungal infections in solid-organ transplantation. *Clin Infect Dis* 16(5):677–688, 1993.
98. Nieto-Rodriguez JA, Kusne S, Manez R, et al: Factors associated with the development of candidemia and candidemia-related death among liver transplant recipients. *Ann Surg* 223(1):70–76, 1996.
99. Guery BP, Arendrup MC, Auzinger G, et al: Management of invasive candidiasis and candidemia in adult non-neutropenic intensive care unit patients: Part II. Treatment. *Intensive Care Med* 35(2):206–214, 2009.
100. Groll AH, Walsh TJ: Caspofungin: pharmacology, safety and therapeutic potential in superficial and invasive fungal infections. *Expert Opin Investig Drugs* 10(8):1545–1558, 2001.
101. Wingard JR, Wood CA, Sullivan E, et al: Caspofungin versus amphotericin B for candidemia: a pharmacoeconomic analysis. *Clin Ther* 27(6):960–969, 2005.
102. Singh N, Limaye AP, Forrest G, et al: Combination of voriconazole and caspofungin as primary therapy for invasive aspergillosis in solid organ transplant recipients: a prospective, multicenter, observational study. *Transplantation* 81(3):320–326, 2006.
103. Zeluff BJ: Fungal pneumonia in transplant recipients. *Semin Respir Infect* 5(1):80–89, 1990.
104. Walsh TJ, Anaissie EJ, Denning DW, et al: Treatment of aspergillosis: clinical practice guidelines of the Infectious Diseases Society of America. *Clin Infect Dis* 46(3):327–360, 2008.
105. Saag MS, Graybill RJ, Larsen RA, et al: Practice guidelines for the management of cryptococcal disease. Infectious Diseases Society of America. *Clin Infect Dis* 30(4):710–718, 2000.
106. Galgiani JN, Ampel NM, Blair JE, et al: Coccidioidomycosis. *Clin Infect Dis* 41(9):1217–1223, 2005.
107. Parikh SL, Venkatraman G, DelGaudio JM: Invasive fungal sinusitis: a 15-year review from a single institution. *Am J Rhinol* 18(2):75–81, 2004.
108. Gluck T, Geerdes-Fenge HF, Straub RH, et al: Pneumocystis carinii pneumonia as a complication of immunosuppressive therapy. *Infection* 28(4):227–230, 2000.
109. Dunn DL, Mayoral JL, Gillingham KJ, et al: Treatment of invasive cytomegalovirus disease in solid organ transplant patients with ganciclovir. *Transplantation* 51(1):98–106, 1991.
110. van der Bij W, Speich R: Management of cytomegalovirus infection and disease after solid-organ transplantation. *Clin Infect Dis* 33[Suppl 1]:S32–S37, 2001.
111. Dunn DL, Najarian JS: New approaches to the diagnosis, prevention, and treatment of cytomegalovirus infection after transplantation. *Am J Surg* 161(2):250–255, 1991.
112. Gleaves CA, Smith TF, Shuster EA, et al: Comparison of standard tube and shell vial cell culture techniques for the detection of cytomegalovirus in clinical specimens. *J Clin Microbiol* 21(2):217–221, 1985.
113. Erice A, Holm MA, Gill PC, et al: Cytomegalovirus (CMV) antigenemia assay is more sensitive than shell vial cultures for rapid detection of CMV in polymorphonuclear blood leukocytes. *J Clin Microbiol* 30(11):2822–2825, 1992.
114. Szczepura A, Westmoreland D, Vinogradova Y, et al: Evaluation of molecular techniques in prediction and diagnosis of cytomegalovirus disease in immunocompromised patients. *Health Technol Assess* 10(10):1–176, 2006.
115. Kusne S, Shapiro R, Fung J: Prevention and treatment of cytomegalovirus infection in organ transplant recipients. *Transpl Infect Dis* 1(3):187–203, 1999.
116. Dunn DL, Gillingham KJ, Kramer MA, et al: A prospective randomized study of acyclovir versus ganciclovir plus human immune globulin prophylaxis of cytomegalovirus infection after solid organ transplantation. *Transplantation* 57(6):876–884, 1994.

117. Rubin RH, Kemmerly SA, Conti D, et al: Prevention of primary cytomegalovirus disease in organ transplant recipients with oral ganciclovir or oral acyclovir prophylaxis. *Transpl Infect Dis* 2(3):112–117, 2000.
118. Flechner SM, Avery RK, Fisher R, et al: A randomized prospective controlled trial of oral acyclovir versus oral ganciclovir for cytomegalovirus prophylaxis in high-risk kidney transplant recipients. *Transplantation* 66(12):1682–1688, 1998.
119. Winston DJ, Wirin D, Shaked A, et al: Randomised comparison of ganciclovir and high-dose acyclovir for long-term cytomegalovirus prophylaxis in liver-transplant recipients. *Lancet* 346(8967):69–74, 1995.
120. Singh N, Paterson DL, Gayowski T, et al: Cytomegalovirus antigenemia directed preemptive prophylaxis with oral versus I. V. ganciclovir for the prevention of cytomegalovirus disease in liver transplant recipients: a randomized, controlled trial. *Transplantation* 70(5):717–722, 2000.
121. Brennan DC, Garlock KA, Lippmann BA, et al: Control of cytomegalovirus-associated morbidity in renal transplant patients using intensive monitoring and either preemptive or deferred therapy. *J Am Soc Nephrol* 8(1):118–125, 1997.
122. Duncan SR, Grgurich WF, Iacono AT, et al: A comparison of ganciclovir and acyclovir to prevent cytomegalovirus after lung transplantation. *Am J Respir Crit Care Med* 150(1):146–152, 1994.
123. Merigan TC, Renlund DG, Keay S, et al: A controlled trial of ganciclovir to prevent cytomegalovirus disease after heart transplantation. *N Engl J Med* 326(18):1182–1186, 1992.
124. Hertz MI, Jordan C, Savik SK, et al: Randomized trial of daily versus three-times-weekly prophylactic ganciclovir after lung and heart-lung transplantation. *J Heart Lung Transplant* 17(9):913–920, 1998.
125. Boivin G, Goyette N, Rollag H, et al: Cytomegalovirus resistance in solid organ transplant recipients treated with intravenous ganciclovir or oral valganciclovir. *Antivir Ther* 14(5):697–704, 2009.
126. Ruutu T, Ljungman P, Brinch L, et al: No prevention of cytomegalovirus infection by anti-cytomegalovirus hyperimmune globulin in seronegative bone marrow transplant recipients. The Nordic BMT Group. *Bone Marrow Transplant* 19(3):233–236, 1997.
127. Studies of Ocular Complications of AIDS (SOCA) in collaboration with the AIDS Clinical Trial Group: Cytomegalovirus (CMV) culture results, drug resistance, and clinical outcome in patients with AIDS and CMV retinitis treated with foscarnet or ganciclovir. *J Infect Dis* 176(1):50–58, 1997.
128. Carrier M, Pelletier GB, Cartier R, et al: Prevention of herpes simplex virus infection by oral acyclovir after cardiac transplantation. *Can J Surg* 35(5):513–516, 1992.
129. Langnas AN, Castaldo P, Markin RS, et al: The spectrum of Epstein-Barr virus infection with hepatitis following liver transplantation. *Transplant Proc* 23(1 Pt 2):1513–1514, 1991.
130. Lynfield R, Herrin JT, Rubin RH: Varicella in pediatric renal transplant recipients. *Pediatrics* 90(2 Pt 1):216–220, 1992.
131. Robertson S, Newbigging K, Carman W, et al: Fulminating varicella despite prophylactic immune globulin and intravenous acyclovir in a renal transplant recipient: should renal patients be vaccinated against VZV before transplantation? *Clin Transplant* 20(1):136–138, 2006.
132. Anderson DJ, Jordan MC: Viral pneumonia in recipients of solid organ transplants. *Semin Respir Infect* 5(1):38–49, 1990.
133. Zerr DM: Human herpesvirus 6: a clinical update. *Herpes* 13(1):20–24, 2006.
134. Challine D, Chevaliez S, Pawlotsky JM: Efficacy of serologic marker screening in identifying hepatitis B virus infection in organ, tissue, and cell donors. *Gastroenterology* 135(4):1185–1191, 2008.
135. De Feo TM, Poli F, Mozzi F, et al: Risk of transmission of hepatitis B virus from anti-HBC positive cadaveric organ donors: a collaborative study. *Transplant Proc* 37(2):1238–1239, 2005.
136. Dusheiko G, Song E, Bowyer S, et al: Natural history of hepatitis B virus infection in renal transplant recipients–a fifteen-year follow-up. *Hepatology* 3(3):330–336, 1983.
137. Grellier L, Mutimer D, Ahmed M, et al: Lamivudine prophylaxis against reinfection in liver transplantation for hepatitis B cirrhosis. *Lancet* 348(9036):1212–1215, 1996.
138. Kiyasu PK, Ishitani MB, McGory RW, et al: Prevention of hepatitis B "rerecurrence" after a second liver transplant—the role of maintenance polyclonal HBIG therapy. *Transplantation* 58(8):954–956, 1994.
139. Paik SW, Tan HP, Klein AS, et al: Outcome of orthotopic liver transplantation in patients with hepatitis C. *Dig Dis Sci* 47(2):450–455, 2002.
140. Berenguer M, Prieto M, Rayon JM, et al: Natural history of clinically compensated hepatitis C virus-related graft cirrhosis after liver transplantation. *Hepatology* 32(4 Pt 1):852–858, 2000.
141. Verna EC, Brown RS Jr: Hepatitis C and liver transplantation: enhancing outcomes and should patients be retransplanted. *Clin Liver Dis* 12(3):637–659, 2008, ix–x.
142. Eren R, Landstein D, Terkieltaub D, et al: Preclinical evaluation of two neutralizing human monoclonal antibodies against hepatitis C virus (HCV): a potential treatment to prevent HCV reinfection in liver transplant patients. *J Virol* 80(6):2654–2664, 2006.
143. Carrigan DR: Adenovirus infections in immunocompromised patients. *Am J Med* 102(3A):71–74, 1997.
144. Simonds RJ: HIV transmission by organ and tissue transplantation. *AIDS* 7[Suppl 2]:S35–S38, 1993.
145. Ahuja TS, Zingman B, Glicklich D: Long-term survival in an HIV-infected renal transplant recipient. *Am J Nephrol* 17(5):480–482, 1997.
146. Roland ME, Barin B, Carlson L, et al: HIV-infected liver and kidney transplant recipients: 1- and 3-year outcomes. *Am J Transplant* 8(2):355–365, 2008.
147. Frassetto LA, Tan-Tam C, Stock PG: Renal transplantation in patients with HIV. *Nat Rev Nephrol* 5(10):582–589, 2009.
148. Mengel M, Marwedel M, Radermacher J, et al: Incidence of polyomavirus-nephropathy in renal allografts: influence of modern immunosuppressive drugs. *Nephrol Dial Transplant* 18(6):1190–1196, 2003.
149. Trofe J, Gaber LW, Stratta RJ, et al: Polyomavirus in kidney and kidney-pancreas transplant recipients. *Transpl Infect Dis* 5(1):21–28, 2003.
150. Nickeleit V, Mihatsch MJ: Polyomavirus nephropathy in native kidneys and renal allografts: an update on an escalating threat. *Transpl Int* 19(12):960–973, 2006.
151. Kuypers DR, Bammens B, Claes K, et al: A single-centre study of adjuvant cidofovir therapy for BK virus interstitial nephritis (BKVIN) in renal allograft recipients. *J Antimicrob Chemother* 63(2):417–419, 2009.
152. Leca N: Leflunomide use in renal transplantation. *Curr Opin Organ Transplant* 14(4):370–374, 2009.
153. Luft BJ, Naot Y, Araujo FG, et al: Primary and reactivated toxoplasma infection in patients with cardiac transplants. Clinical spectrum and problems in diagnosis in a defined population. *Ann Intern Med* 99(1):27–31, 1983.
154. Selby R, Ramirez CB, Singh R, et al: Brain abscess in solid organ transplant recipients receiving cyclosporine-based immunosuppression. *Arch Surg* 132(3):304–310, 1997.
155. Penn I: Cancers in renal transplant recipients. *Adv Ren Replace Ther* 7(2):147–156, 2000.
156. Ellis D, Jaffe R, Green M, et al: Epstein-Barr virus-related disorders in children undergoing renal transplantation with tacrolimus-based immunosuppression. *Transplantation* 68(7):997–1003, 1999.
157. Manez R, Breinig MC, Linden P, et al: Posttransplant lymphoproliferative disease in primary Epstein-Barr virus infection after liver transplantation: the role of cytomegalovirus disease. *J Infect Dis* 176(6):1462–1467, 1997.
158. Walker RC: Pretransplant assessment of the risk for posttransplant lymphoproliferative disorder. *Transplant Proc* 27[5 Suppl 1]:41, 1995.
159. Cox KL, Lawrence-Miyasaki LS, Garcia-Kennedy R, et al: An increased incidence of Epstein-Barr virus infection and lymphoproliferative disorder in young children on FK506 after liver transplantation. *Transplantation* 59(4):524–529, 1995.
160. Keay S, Oldach D, Wiland A, et al: Posttransplantation lymphoproliferative disorder associated with OKT3 and decreased antiviral prophylaxis in pancreas transplant recipients. *Clin Infect Dis* 26(3):596–600, 1998.
161. McLaughlin K, Wajstaub S, Marotta P, et al: Increased risk for posttransplant lymphoproliferative disease in recipients of liver transplants with hepatitis C. *Liver Transpl* 6(5):570–574, 2000.
162. Helminen M, Lahdenpohja N, Hurme M: Polymorphism of the interleukin-10 gene is associated with susceptibility to Epstein-Barr virus infection. *J Infect Dis* 180(2):496–499, 1999.
163. Penn I, Porat G: Central nervous system lymphomas in organ allograft recipients. *Transplantation* 59(2):240–244, 1995.
164. Paya CV, Fung JJ, Nalesnik MA, et al: Epstein-Barr virus-induced posttransplant lymphoproliferative disorders. ASTS/ASTP EBV-PTLD Task Force and the Mayo Clinic Organized International Consensus Development Meeting. *Transplantation* 68(10):1517–1525, 1999.
165. Harris NL, Ferry JA, Swerdlow SH: Posttransplant lymphoproliferative disorders: summary of society for hematopathology workshop. *Semin Diagn Pathol* 14(1):8–14, 1997.
166. Cen H, Williams PA, McWilliams HP, et al: Evidence for restricted Epstein-Barr virus latent gene expression and anti-EBNA antibody response in solid organ transplant recipients with posttransplant lymphoproliferative disorders. *Blood* 81(5):1393–1403, 1993.
167. Riddler SA, Breinig MC, McKnight JL: Increased levels of circulating Epstein-Barr virus (EBV)-infected lymphocytes and decreased EBV nuclear antigen antibody responses are associated with the development of posttransplant lymphoproliferative disease in solid-organ transplant recipients. *Blood* 84(3):972–984, 1994.
168. Davey DD, Gulley ML, Walker WP, et al: Cytologic findings in posttransplant lymphoproliferative disease. *Acta Cytol* 34(3):304–310, 1990.
169. Bianchi E, Pascual M, Nicod M, et al: Clinical usefulness of FDG-PET/CT scan imaging in the management of posttransplant lymphoproliferative disease. *Transplantation* 85(5):707–712, 2008.
170. Green M, Reyes J, Webber S, et al: The role of antiviral and immunoglobulin therapy in the prevention of Epstein-Barr virus infection and post-transplant lymphoproliferative disease following solid organ transplantation. *Transpl Infect Dis* 3(2):97–103, 2001.
171. Birkeland SA, Andersen HK, Hamilton-Dutoit SJ: Preventing acute rejection, Epstein-Barr virus infection, and posttransplant lymphoproliferative disorders after kidney transplantation: use of acyclovir and mycophenolate mofetil in a steroid-free immunosuppressive protocol. *Transplantation* 67(9):1209–1214, 1999.
172. Penn I: The role of immunosuppression in lymphoma formation. *Springer Semin Immunopathol* 20(3–4):343–355, 1998.
173. Cacciarelli TV, Green M, Jaffe R, et al: Management of posttransplant lymphoproliferative disease in pediatric liver transplant recipients receiving

primary tacrolimus (FK506) therapy. *Transplantation* 66(8):1047–1052, 1998.
174. Koffman BH, Kennedy AS, Heyman M, et al: Use of radiation therapy in posttransplant lymphoproliferative disorder (PTLD) after liver transplantation. *Int J Cancer* 90(2):104–109, 2000.
175. Pirsch JD, Stratta RJ, Sollinger HW, et al: Treatment of severe Epstein-Barr virus-induced lymphoproliferative syndrome with ganciclovir: two cases after solid organ transplantation. *Am J Med* 86(2):241–244, 1989.
176. Cantarovich M, Barkun JS, Forbes RD, et al: Successful treatment of posttransplant lymphoproliferative disorder with interferon-alpha and intravenous immunoglobulin. *Clin Transplant* 12(2):109–115, 1998.
177. Garrett TJ, Chadburn A, Barr ML, et al: Posttransplantation lymphoproliferative disorders treated with cyclophosphamide-doxorubicin-vincristine-prednisone chemotherapy. *Cancer* 72(9):2782–2785, 1993.
178. Smets F, Vajro P, Cornu G, et al: Indications and results of chemotherapy in children with posttransplant lymphoproliferative disease after liver transplantation. *Transplantation* 69(5):982–984, 2000.
179. Schaar CG, van der Pijl JW, van Hoek B, et al: Successful outcome with a "quintuple approach" of posttransplant lymphoproliferative disorder. *Transplantation* 71(1):47–52, 2001.
180. Rooney CM, Smith CA, Ng CY, et al: Use of gene-modified virus-specific T lymphocytes to control Epstein-Barr-virus-related lymphoproliferation. *Lancet* 345(8941):9–13, 1995.
181. Buell JF, Gross TG, Hanaway MJ, et al: Posttransplant lymphoproliferative disorder: significance of central nervous system involvement. *Transplant Proc* 37(2):954–955, 2005.
182. Sheil AG, Disney AP, Mathew TH, et al: De novo malignancy emerges as a major cause of morbidity and late failure in renal transplantation. *Transplant Proc* 25(1 Pt 2):1383–1384, 1993.
183. Bouwes Bavinck JN, Vermeer BJ, van der Woude FJ, et al: Relation between skin cancer and HLA antigens in renal-transplant recipients. *N Engl J Med* 325(12):843–848, 1991.
184. Penn I: The problem of cancer in organ transplant recipients: an overview. *Transplant Sci* 4(1):23–32, 1994.
185. Montagnino G, Bencini PL, Tarantino A, et al: Clinical features and course of Kaposi's sarcoma in kidney transplant patients: report of 13 cases. *Am J Nephrol* 14(2):121–126, 1994.
186. al-Sulaiman MH, al-Khader AA: Kaposi's sarcoma in renal transplant recipients. *Transplant Sci* 4(1):46–60, 1994.
187. Pica F, Volpi A: Transmission of human herpesvirus 8: an update. *Curr Opin Infect Dis* 20(2):152–156, 2007.
188. Busnach G, Civati G, Brando B, et al: Viral and neoplastic changes of the lower genital tract in women with renal allografts. *Transplant Proc* 25(1 Pt 2):1389–1390, 1993.
189. Ozsaran AA, Ates T, Dikmen Y, et al: Evaluation of the risk of cervical intraepithelial neoplasia and human papilloma virus infection in renal transplant patients receiving immunosuppressive therapy. *Eur J Gynaecol Oncol* 20(2):127–130, 1999.
190. Penn I: Evaluation of transplant candidates with pre-existing malignancies. *Ann Transplant* 2(4):14–17, 1997.
191. Suarez Y, Franca AC, Llovet JM, et al: The current status of liver transplantation for primary hepatic malignancy. *Clin Liver Dis* 4(3):591–605, 2000.
192. Heneghan MA, O'Grady JG: Liver transplantation for malignant disease. *Baillieres Best Pract Res Clin Gastroenterol* 13(4):575–591, 1999.
193. Onaca N, Klintmalm GB: Liver transplantation for hepatocellular carcinoma: the baylor experience. *J Hepatobiliary Pancreat Surg*, 2009.
194. Rayes N, Seehofer D, Schmidt CA, et al: Is preemptive therapy for CMV infection following liver transplantation superior to symptom-triggered treatment? *Transplant Proc* 33(1–2):1804, 2001.
195. Faye A, Quartier P, Reguerre Y, et al: Chimaeric anti-CD20 monoclonal antibody (rituximab) in post-transplant B-lymphoproliferative disorder following stem cell transplantation in children. *Br J Haematol* 115(1):112–118, 2001.

CHAPTER 187 ■ CRITICAL CARE OF THE LIVER AND INTESTINAL TRANSPLANT RECIPIENTS

RUY J. CRUZ JR, WILLIAM D. PAYNE AND ABHINAV HUMAR

INTRODUCTION

The field of liver transplantation has undergone remarkable advances in the last two decades. From an essentially experimental procedure with poor results in the early 1980s, it has progressed to become the accepted treatment of choice for patients with acute and chronic end-stage liver disease. One-year survival rates have increased from 30% in the early 1980s, to more than 85% at present. The major reasons for this dramatic improvement in outcome include improved surgical and preservation techniques, better immunosuppressive regimens, more effective treatment of rejection and infection, and improved care during the critical perioperative period. The field of intestinal transplantation has also made tremendous strides in the last 20 years, though perhaps has not enjoyed the degree of success seen with liver transplantation. Nonetheless, results continue to improve and it is approaching success rates that are not dramatically inferior compared with liver transplantation.

Despite the improved results, both liver and intestinal transplantation remain major undertakings, with potential for complications affecting every major organ system. This chapter focuses on the critical care of these challenging and complicated patients, including preoperative selection and evaluation, intraoperative care, postoperative care, and management of potential complications.

LIVER TRANSPLANTATION

History

The origins of modern clinical liver transplantation date back to the late 1950s, when the surgical techniques were perfected in the dog model [1]. The first human liver transplant was performed by Starzl in 1963 [2], but not until 1967 was the first successful such transplant performed [3]. Little progress was made in the field over the next decade. It remained a dangerous procedure, reserved for terminal patients.

In the early 1980s, liver transplantation proliferated for a variety of reasons, the most important being the introduction of cyclosporine [4]. At that time, it was the most specific immunosuppressive agent and allowed for a dramatic rise in all organ transplants. Patient survival rates for liver recipients on cyclosporine more than doubled. In the late 1980s, the introduction of University of Wisconsin (UW) preservation solution extended the cold preservation time of the cadaver liver from 8 to 24 hours [5].

As the success of liver transplantation grew, so did the indications and the number of people awaiting a transplant. With each passing year, there was an ever increasing disparity between the number of transplants performed and the number of patients awaiting transplant. In 1988, there were approximately 1,500 transplants performed and 3,000 patients awaiting a transplant. In 2008, according to the UNOS Database, 6,319 liver transplants were performed in the United States, while 16,584 patients were listed waiting for an available/suitable organ (UNOS/OPTN, www.optn.transplant.hrsa.gov/, accessed August, 2009) [6].

Given this increasing disparity between the number of actual and potential recipients, recent attempts have been made to expand the donor pool. Some of this increase in donors has been achieved by the use of livers that are considered marginal and would not have been used for transplant a decade ago. Recently, the use of organs from donors after cardiac death (also referred as nonheart beating donors) has emerged as an important source of organs in response to the significant growth of the waiting list. Donation after cardiac death (DCD) involves those donors who present a severe neurological injury and/or irreversible brain damage but still have minimal brain function. In 2000, only 11 centers used DCD livers, increasing to 62 centers in 2007 [7–9].

Innovative surgical procedures have also been used in order to increase the donor pool. These procedures include, but are not limited to, living donor liver transplantation, split-liver transplantation, and dual liver transplantation. Living donor transplants involve transplanting a lobe or part of a lobe from a healthy donor into a potential recipient. Split-liver transplantation involves dividing a cadaver liver into two functional grafts, which can be transplanted into two recipients. Dual liver transplantation involves the use of two lobes (usually two left lobes) from two living donors that are implanted into one adult recipient. These procedures are helping expand the donor pool, but are also associated with unique problems.

Proper allocation of the scarce resource of a deceased donor liver graft has always been an important issue in the development of the field. Recent effects have focused on directing organs to individuals with the greatest need, rather than those with the longest waiting time. In the United States, this lead to the development and adaptation in 2002 of the MELD (Model for End-Stage Liver Disease) and PELD (Pediatric End-Stage Liver Disease) scoring systems [10].

Preoperative Evaluation

A liver transplant is indicated for liver failure, whether acute or chronic. Liver failure is signaled by a number of clinical symptoms (e.g., ascites, variceal bleeding, hepatic encephalopathy, malnutrition) and by biochemical liver test results that suggest impaired hepatic synthetic function (e.g., hypoalbuminemia, hyperbilirubinemia, coagulopathy). The cause of liver failure often influences its presentation. For example, patients with acute liver failure generally have hepatic encephalopathy and coagulopathy, whereas patients with chronic liver disease most commonly have ascites, gastrointestinal (GI) bleeding, and malnutrition.

A host of diseases are potentially treatable by a liver transplant. Broadly, they can be categorized as acute or chronic, and then subdivided by the cause of the liver disease (Table 187.1). Chronic liver diseases account for the majority of liver transplants today. The most common cause in North America is chronic hepatitis, usually due to hepatitis C, less commonly to hepatitis B. Chronic alcohol abuse accelerates the process, especially with hepatitis C. Progression from chronic infection to cirrhosis is generally slow, usually 10 to 20 years. Chronic hepatitis may also result from autoimmune causes, primarily in

TABLE 187.1

DISEASES POTENTIALLY TREATABLE BY A LIVER TRANSPLANT

Cholestatic liver diseases
Primary biliary cirrhosis
Primary sclerosing cholangitis
Biliary atresia
Alagille's syndrome
Chronic hepatitis
Hepatitis B
Hepatitis C
Autoimmune hepatitis
Alcohol liver disease
Metabolic diseases
Hemochromatosis
Wilson's disease
α_1-Antitrypsin deficiency
Tyrosinemia
Cystic fibrosis
Hepatic malignancy
Hepatocellular carcinoma
Neuroendocrine tumor metastatic to liver
Fulminant hepatic failure
Others
Cryptogenic cirrhosis
Polycystic liver disease
Budd–Chiari syndrome
Amyloidosis

women; it can present either acutely over months or insidiously over years [11]. Alcohol often plays a role in end-stage liver disease (ESLD) secondary to hepatitis C, but it may also lead to liver failure in the absence of that viral infection. In fact, alcohol is the most common cause of ESLD in the United States. Such patients are generally suitable candidates for a transplant as long as an adequate period of sobriety can be documented. Most of the centers in the United States require a minimum of 6 months of demonstrated abstinence and an adequate evaluation and treatment period for alcohol addiction. In spite of this strict pretransplant screening the rate of alcohol use after transplant can reach 42% in the first 5 years after transplant [12]

Cholestatic disorders also account for a significant percentage of transplant candidates with chronic liver disease. In adults, the most common causes are primary biliary cirrhosis (PBC) and primary sclerosing cholangitis (PSC). PBC, a destructive disorder of interlobular bile ducts, can progress to cirrhosis and liver failure over several decades. It most commonly affects middle-aged women. PSC, a disease characterized by inflammatory injury of the bile duct, occurs mostly in young men, 70% of whom have inflammatory bowel disease [13]. In children, biliary atresia is the most common cholestatic disorder. It is a destructive, inflammatory condition of the bile ducts; if untreated, it usually results in death within the first 1 to 2 years of life.

A variety of metabolic diseases can result in progressive, chronic liver injury and cirrhosis, including hereditary hemochromatosis (an autosomal recessive disorder characterized by chronic iron accumulation, which may result in cirrhosis, cardiomyopathy, and endocrine disorders including diabetes), α_1-antitrypsin deficiency (which may result in cirrhosis at any age, most commonly in the first or second decade of life), and Wilson's disease (an autosomal recessive disorder of copper excretion, which may present as either fulminant hepatic failure or chronic hepatitis and cirrhosis) [14].

Hepatocellular carcinoma (HCC) may be a complication of cirrhosis from any cause, most commonly with hepatitis B, hepatitis C, hemochromatosis, and tyrosinemia. In 2007, almost 15% of all liver transplants in the United States were performed in patients with a diagnosis of HCC. HCC patients may have stable liver disease, but are not candidates for hepatic resection because of the underlying cirrhosis; they are best treated with a liver transplant. The best transplant candidates are those with a single lesion less than 5 cm in size or with no more than three lesions, the largest no greater than 3 cm in size (known as the Milan criteria). Transplantation outside of these criteria is usually associated with higher recurrence rates, though some centers have shown acceptable 5-year survival in patients that have tumors that slightly exceed the Milan criteria [15,16].

Currently, in the United States, only the patients within Milan criteria are eligible for priority listing for liver transplantation. The amount of waiting list time for patients with HCC remains a critical factor in the success of liver transplantation, as long waiting times may lead to disease progression. Recently downstaging treatment, with transarterial chemoembolization and radiofrequency ablation, has emerged as a possible option for those patients who slightly exceed Milan criteria [17].

A host of other diseases may lead to chronic liver failure and are potentially amenable to treatment with a transplant, including Budd–Chiari (obstruction of the hepatic veins secondary to thrombus, which leads to hepatic congestion, ascites, and eventually liver damage) and polycystic liver disease (in which a large number of cysts, depending on their size, can lead to debilitating symptoms).

Acute liver disease, more commonly termed fulminant hepatic failure (FHF), is defined as the development of hepatic encephalopathy and profound coagulopathy shortly after the onset of symptoms, such as jaundice, in patients without preexisting liver disease. The most common causes in the Western world include acetaminophen overdose, acute viral hepatitis, various drugs and hepatotoxins, and Wilson's disease; often, however, no cause is identified [18]. Treatment consists of appropriate critical care support, giving patients time for spontaneous recovery. The prognosis for spontaneous recovery depends on the patient's age (those younger than 10 and older than 40 years have a poor prognosis), the underlying cause, and the severity of liver injury (as indicated by degree of hepatic encephalopathy, coagulopathy, and kidney dysfunction) (Table 187.2) [19,20]. A subset of patients may have delayed onset of hepatic decompensation that occurs 8 weeks to 6 months after the onset of symptoms. This condition is often referred to as subacute hepatic failure; these patients rarely recover without a transplant.

TABLE 187.2

ADVERSE PROGNOSTIC INDICATORS FOR PATIENTS WITH ACUTE LIVER FAILURE

(I)	Acetaminophen toxicity
	pH <7.30
	Prothrombin time >100 sec (INR >6.5)
	Serum creatinine >300 μmol/L (>3.4 mg/dL)
(II)	No acetaminophen toxicity
	Prothrombin time >100 sec (INR >6.5)
	Age <10 or >40 y
	Non-A, non-B hepatitis
	Duration of jaundice before onset of encephalopathy >7 d
	Serum creatinine >300 μmol/L (>3.4 mg/dL)

TABLE 187.3

INDICATIONS FOR A LIVER TRANSPLANT EVALUATION IN PATIENTS WITH CHRONIC LIVER DISEASE

Clinical indications
Refractory ascites
Spontaneous bacterial peritonitis
Recurrent or severe hepatic encephalopathy
Hepatorenal syndrome
Significant weakness, fatigue, or progressive malnutrition
Recurrent cholangitis or severe pruritus
Progressive bone disease
Biochemical indications
Serum albumin <3.0 g/dL
Serum INR >1.7
Serum bilirubin >2 mg/dL (>4 mg/dL for cholestatic disorders)

Indications for Transplant

Chronic Liver Disease. The simple presence of chronic liver disease with established cirrhosis is not an indication for a transplant (Table 187.3). Some patients have very well-compensated cirrhosis with a low expectant mortality. Patients with decompensated cirrhosis, however, have a poor prognosis without transplant. The signs and symptoms of decompensated cirrhosis include the following:

1. *Hepatic Encephalopathy (HE):* In its early stages, HE may begin with subtle sleep disturbances, depression, and emotional liability. Increasing severity of HE is indicated by increasing somnolence, altered speech, and at the extreme end, coma. Evaluation of the severity of HE is based on the West Haven criteria of altered mental status. A common finding on physical examination is asterixis, an ability to maintain position, which is most commonly tested by having the patients outstretch their arms and hold them in dorsiflexion. However, other simple tests (such as tongue protrusion, dorsiflexion of the foot, or asking the patient to grasp the examiner's fingers) can also trigger the asterixis. Blood tests often reveal an elevated serum ammonia level. HE may occur spontaneously, but is more commonly triggered by a precipitating factor such as infections, GI bleeding, use of sedatives, constipation, diuretics, electrolyte imbalance, or excessive dietary protein intake. The purpose of treatment is to correct the precipitating factor in combination with pharmacological management including nonabsolvable disaccharides (i.e., lactulose), and antibiotics such as neomycin, rifaximin, and metronidazole.
2. *Ascites:* Ascites is generally associated with portal hypertension. The initial approach to the management of ascites is sodium restriction and diuretics. If this approach is not successful, patients may require repeated large-volume (4 to 6 L) paracentesis. A better option to diuretic-resistant ascites requiring frequent paracentesis is transjugular intrahepatic portosystemic shunting (TIPS). A potential complication of TIPS is progression of liver failure or disabling encephalopathy. Patients with signs of far-advanced liver disease such as hyperbilirubinemia, HE, and renal dysfunction are generally not good candidates for TIPS.
3. *Spontaneous Bacterial Peritonitis (SBP):* This complication of chronic liver failure generally signals advanced disease. Anaerobic Gram-negative bacteria (*Escherichia coli, Klebsiella pneumoniae*) account for 60% of the cultured organisms; Gram-positive cocci account for the remainder. Diagnosis is confirmed if a tap of the abdominal fluid shows

a polymorphonuclear neutrophil (PMN) count of >250 per mL. If a traumatic tap is performed (red cells >10,000 per mL), the PMN count should be corrected, subtracting 1 PMN for every 250 red cells. Treatment is generally with a third-generation cephalosporin. The recurrence rate of SBP at 1 year is up to 70%; therefore, prophylaxis with antibiotics (norfloxacin or ciprofloxacin) is highly recommended. The long-term prognosis of patients who develop SBP is extremely poor with mortality rates of 50% to 70% at 1-year follow-up [21].

4. *Portal Hypertensive Bleeding:* The likelihood of patients with cirrhosis developing varices ranges from 35% to 80%. About one-third of those with varices will experience bleeding. The risk of recurrent bleeding approaches 70% by 2 years after the index bleeding episode. Each episode of bleeding is associated with a 30% mortality rate. Thus, urgent treatment of the acute episode and steps to prevent rebleeding are essential. Endoscopy is indicated to diagnose and treat the acute bleed with either band ligation or sclerotherapy. Other therapies include vasoactive drugs such as octreotide or vasopressin, balloon tamponade, TIPS, and emergency surgical procedures (such as a portosystemic shunt or transection of the esophagus). Generally, patients whose endoscopic procedure fails should undergo emergency TIPS, if feasible, to control bleeding. Beta-blockers have been shown to be of value in preventing the first bleeding episode in patients with varices and in preventing rebleeding.
5. *Hepatorenal Syndrome (HRS):* In patients with advanced liver disease and ascites, HRS is characterized by oliguria (<500 mL of urine per day) in association with low urine sodium (<10 mEq per L). It is a functional disorder; the kidneys have no structural abnormalities, and the urine sediment is normal. The differential diagnosis includes acute tubular necrosis, drug nephrotoxicity, and chronic intrinsic renal disease. HRS may be precipitated by volume depletion from diuresis, SBP, or agents such as nonsteroidal anti-inflammatory drugs. Patients may require dialysis support, but the only effective treatment is a liver transplant.
6. *Others:* Other signs and symptoms of decompensated cirrhosis include severe weakness and fatigue, which may sometimes be the primary symptoms. Such weakness can be debilitating, leading to the inability to work or even to carry out day-to-day functions. It may be associated with malnutrition and muscle wasting, which at times may be quite severe. Biochemical abnormalities and loss of synthetic function in advanced ESLD are associated with a low-serum albumin, a high-serum bilirubin, and a rise in the serum international normalized ratio (INR).

The severity of illness and prognosis of patients with chronic liver disease can be estimated by a number of different scoring models including the Childs–Pugh–Turcotte score and the MELD score. The latter is now widely used in the United States for the allocation of organs. It is based on a predicted 3-month mortality for patients awaiting a liver transplant, and uses 3 laboratory values to generate a score which determines priority. The three laboratory values used are serum bilirubin, serum creatinine, and INR. The format is as follows:

$$\begin{aligned}\text{MELD Score} = {} & 0.957 \times \log_e(\text{creatinine mg per dL}) \\ & + 0.378 \times \log_e(\text{bilirubin mg per dL}) \\ & + 1.120 \times \log_e(\text{INR}) \\ & + 0.643\end{aligned}$$

For pediatric patients, the scoring system is somewhat different. The PELD (pediatric end-stage liver disease) score is calculated using the following factors: serum bilirubin, albumin, and INR, the age of the patient (additional points if <1 year old), and if the patient has growth failure [22].

Acute Liver Disease. Patients with FHF should be considered for transplant if they have any one of a number of poor prognostic indicators that predict a low likelihood for spontaneous recovery of liver function (Table 187.2). Generally, FHF patients are more acutely ill than chronic liver failure patients, and thus require more intensive care pretransplant. FHF patients have more severe hepatic parenchymal dysfunction, as manifested by coagulopathy, hypoglycemia, and lactic acidosis. Infectious complications are more common, as is their incidence of kidney failure and neurologic complications, especially cerebral edema.

Coagulopathy is usually secondary to the impaired hepatic synthesis of clotting factors. A component of consumption, as a result of disseminated intravascular coagulation (DIC), may also be associated with FHF. Close attention should be given to the serum glucose level, which is more likely to be decreased in FHF patients. Intravenous (IV) glucose should be administered at a sufficient rate to maintain euglycemia.

The prevalence of bacterial infection in FHF patients is very high, a reflection of the loss of the liver's immunologic functions. The respiratory and urinary systems are the most common sources. In addition, almost one-third of FHF patients develop some form of fungal infection, usually secondary to *Candida* species [23]. Sepsis is generally a contraindication to a transplant; if it is unrecognized pretransplant, the outcome posttransplant is poor.

Multiple organ dysfunction syndrome, characterized by respiratory distress, kidney failure, increased cardiac output, and decreased systemic vascular resistance, is a well-described complication of FHF. It may be due to impaired clearance of vasoactive substances by the liver. Mechanical ventilation and dialysis support may become necessary pretransplant. Hemodynamic abnormalities may manifest as hypotension and worsening tissue oxygenation.

Cerebral edema is substantially more common in FHF patients. As many as 80% of patients dying secondary to FHF have evidence of cerebral edema. The pathogenesis is unclear, but it may be due to potential neurotoxins that are normally cleared by the liver. Diagnosis may be problematic; patients are often sedated and ventilated, making clinical examination difficult. Radiologic imaging is neither sensitive nor specific. Several centers have tried intracranial pressure (ICP) monitoring; therapy (e.g., mannitol, hyperventilation, thiopental) can then be directed to achieve an adequate cerebral perfusion pressure. ICP monitoring also helps predict the likelihood of neurologic recovery posttransplant. Sustained cerebral perfusion pressures of less than 40 mm Hg have been associated with postoperative neurologic death. Disadvantages of ICP monitoring include the risks of performing it in patients with severe coagulopathy; it is also a possible source of infection and may precipitate an intracranial hemorrhage.

Contraindications for Transplant

The indications for a liver transplant are numerous (and are increasing), but the numbers of absolute contraindications are few (and have decreased with time). There are no specific age limits for recipients; their mean age is steadily increasing. Patients must have adequate cardiac and pulmonary function. Other contraindications, as with other types of transplants, include uncontrolled systemic infection and malignancy. HCC patients with metastatic disease, obvious vascular invasion, or significant tumor burden are not good transplant candidates. Patients with other types of extrahepatic malignancy should be deferred for at least 2 years after completing curative therapy before a transplant is attempted.

Currently, the most common contraindication in the United States to a liver transplant is ongoing substance abuse. Before considering patients for a transplant, most centers require a documented period of abstinence, demonstration of compliant behavior, and willingness to pursue a chemical dependency program.

Unique to patients with chronic liver disease, a transplant may be contraindicated in the presence of severe hepatopulmonary syndrome or pulmonary hypertension. Hepatopulmonary syndrome is characterized by impaired gas exchange, resulting from intrapulmonary arteriovenous shunts. These shunts may lead to severe hypoxemia, especially when patients are in the upright position (orthodeoxia). A transplant may be contraindicated if intrapulmonary shunting is severe, as manifested by hypoxemia that is only partially improved with high inspired oxygen concentrations. Pulmonary hypertension (mean pulmonary artery pressure >25 mm Hg in the setting of portal hypertension) is seen in a small proportion of patients with established cirrhosis. Its exact cause is unknown [24]. Diagnosing pulmonary hypertension pretransplant is critical, because major surgical procedures in the presence of nonreversible pulmonary hypertension are associated with a very high risk of mortality. The initial screening is usually performed with transthoracic Doppler echocardiography (TTE) which can estimate pulmonary arterial systolic pressure when tricuspid regurgitation is present. TTE presents a sensitivity of 97% and specificity of 77% in diagnosing pulmonary hypertension in the setting of liver failure. In patients with elevated pulmonary arterial systolic pressure (>50 mm Hg), a more invasive assessment (right heart catheterization) is recommended. It has been shown that perioperative mortality is directly proportional to the mean pulmonary artery pressure (mPAP) and pulmonary vascular resistance. For these reasons, most transplant centers consider a mPAP greater than 35 mm Hg to be an absolute contraindication for transplant. If the mPAP can be lowered below that value using medications (epoprostenol, sildenafil), the patient can still be considered for transplant [24].

Another absolute contraindication for liver transplantation, in case of acute liver failure, is a presence of unresponsive cerebral edema with sustained elevation of intracranial pressure (>50 mm Hg) and a persistent decrease in cerebral perfusion pressure (<40 mm Hg).

Intraoperative Care

A detailed description of the operative procedure and anesthetic management is beyond the scope of this chapter. A basic understanding of the intraoperative course is necessary, however, to aid in postoperative care and monitoring for possible complications.

The operation itself may be divided into three phases: preanhepatic, anhepatic, and postanhepatic. The preanhepatic phase involves mobilizing of the recipient's diseased liver in preparation for its removal. The basic steps include isolating the supra- and infrahepatic vena cava, portal vein, and hepatic artery, and then dividing the bile duct. Given existing coagulopathy and portal hypertension, the recipient hepatectomy may be the most difficult aspect of the procedure. The anesthesia team must be prepared to deal with excessive blood loss during this time.

Once the above-named structures have been isolated, vascular clamps are applied. The recipient's liver is removed, thus beginning the anhepatic phase. This phase is characterized by decreased venous return to the heart because of occlusion of the inferior vena cava and portal vein. Many centers routinely employ a venous bypass system during this time: blood is drawn from the lower body and bowels via a cannula in the common femoral vein and portal vein, and returned through a central venous cannula in the upper body. Potential advantages of bypass include improved hemodynamic stability, reduction of bleeding from an engorged portal system, and avoidance of elevated venous pressures in the renal veins. However, many centers do not routinely use venovenous bypass (VVB). Very few randomized trials have measured specific clinical outcomes with or without VVB. In one randomized trial, postoperative renal function and the need for hemodialysis or hemofiltration were no different between liver recipients with versus without VVB [25]. This, combined with the potential complications of VVB (air embolism, thromboembolism, hypothermia, hemodilution, cannula and incision-related morbidity, trauma to vessels, and incremental costs), have led some centers to adopt a selective use for VVB—reserving it for patients without portal hypertension or for those patients who demonstrate hemodynamic instability with a trial of caval clamping [26].

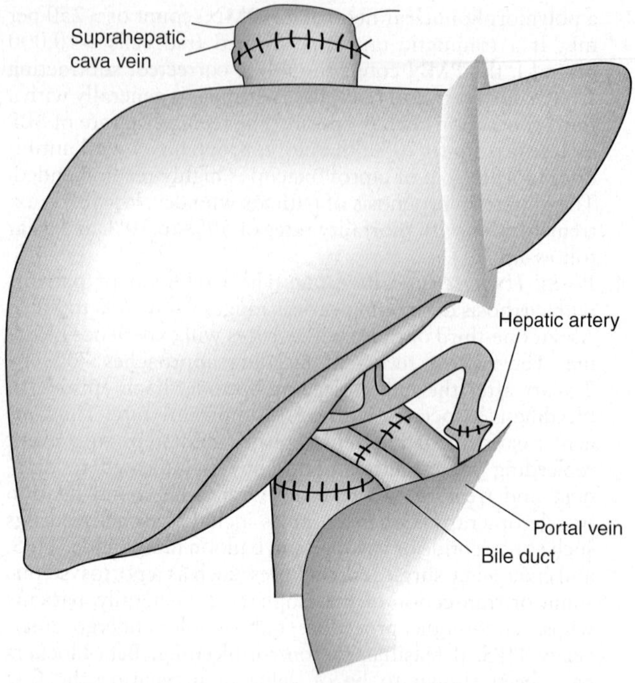

FIGURE 187.1. Illustration of standard liver transplant procedure with replacement of the recipient's inferior vena cava. Typical vascular and biliary anastomoses are shown.

With the recipient liver removed, the donor liver is anastomosed to the appropriate structures to place the new liver in an orthotopic position (Fig. 187.1). The suprahepatic caval anastomosis is performed first, followed by the infrahepatic cava and the portal vein. The portal and caval clamps may be removed at this time, allowing reperfusion of the new liver. Either before or after this step, the hepatic artery may be anastomosed.

With the clamps removed and the new organ reperfused, the postanhepatic phase begins, often characterized by marked changes in the patient's status. The most dramatic changes in hemodynamic parameters usually occur upon reperfusion, with hypotension and the potential for serious arrhythmia. Severe coagulopathy may also develop because of the release of natural anticoagulants from the ischemic liver or active fibrinolysis. Both epsilon aminocaproic acid and aprotinin have been used prophylactically to prevent fibrinolysis and decrease transfusion requirements [27]. Electrolyte abnormalities, most commonly hyperkalemia and hypercalcemia, are often seen after reperfusion; they are usually transient and respond well to treatment with calcium chloride and sodium bicarbonate. After reperfusion of the liver, the final anastomosis is performed, establishing biliary drainage. The recipient's remaining common

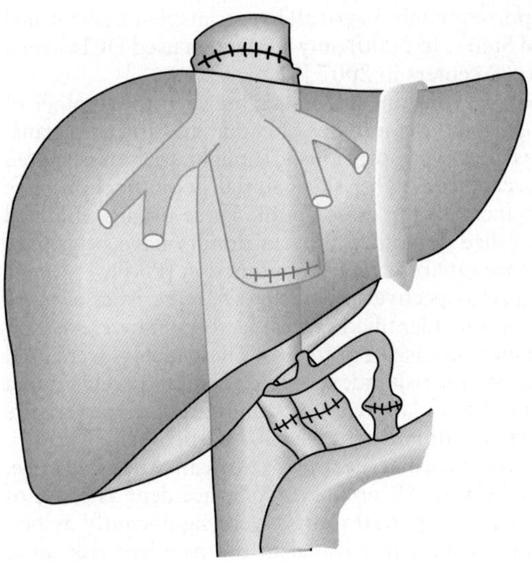

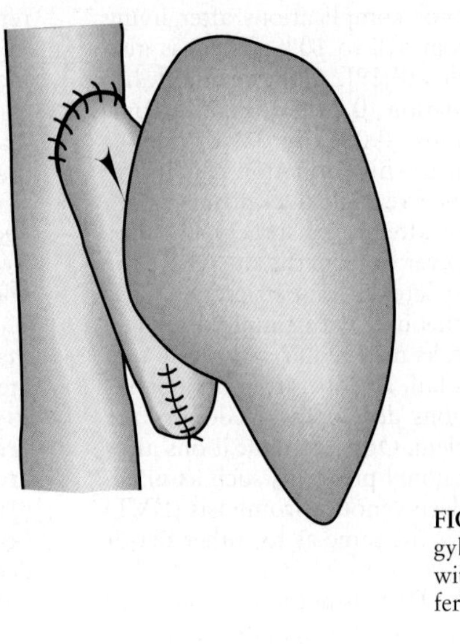

FIGURE 187.2. Illustration of "piggyback" liver transplant procedure with preservation of the recipient's inferior vena cava.

bile duct (choledochoduodenostomy) or a loop of bowel (choledochojejunostomy) may be used.

Several variations of the standard operation have been described, including the "piggyback technique." Here the recipient's inferior vena cava is preserved, the infrahepatic donor cava is oversewn, and the suprahepatic cava is anastomosed to the confluence of the recipient hepatic veins (Fig. 187.2). With this technique, the recipient's cava does not have to be completely crossclamped during anastomosis—thus allowing blood from the lower body to return to the heart uninterrupted, without the need for VVB. In spite of the potential advantages of the "piggyback technique," this procedure is precluded, for obvious reasons, in patients with tumors involving retrohepatic vena cava or main hepatic veins.

The surgical procedure for children does not differ significantly from that for adults. However, the size of the recipient is a significantly more important variable and has an impact on both the donor and the recipient operations.

For pediatric patients (especially infants and small children), the chance of finding a size-matched cadaver graft may be very small: the vast majority of cadaver donors are adults. Accordingly, pretransplant mortality used to be very high in pediatric patients. As a result, three procedures evolved from the principle that a liver is made up of several self-contained segments, each with its own vascular inflow, vascular outflow, and biliary drainage. As a result of these three procedures (namely, reduced-size liver transplants, living related liver transplants, and split-liver transplants), pediatric waiting list mortality rate is now very low.

Reduced-Size Liver Transplants

The earliest efforts involved tailoring a whole-cadaver graft on the back table to fit the recipient. A portion of the liver, such as the right lobe or extended right lobe, was resected and discarded. The remaining left lateral segment was then used for transplant. Reduced-size liver transplant (RSLT) significantly reduced waiting times for children, but negatively affected the adult recipient pool.

Living Donor Liver Transplant

Living donor liver transplant (LDLT) is a natural extension of RSLT. Usually, the left lateral segment from an adult is used (Fig. 187.2), providing sufficient liver tissue for children up to 25 kg. Advantages include the ability to perform the transplant before the recipient deteriorates clinically and the ability to select an ideal donor. The main disadvantage, obviously, is the risk to the donor.

Split-Liver Transplants

With this technique, an adult cadaver liver is divided into two functional grafts: the left lateral segment (which can be transplanted into a child) and the remaining right trisegment (which can be transplanted into an adult). Most split-liver transplants (SLTs) are now performed in vivo: the liver is divided in the cadaver, in a similar fashion to the LDLT procedure. SLT overcomes the disadvantages of both LDLT and RSLT while increasing the donor pool.

Because the severe shortage of organs, partial transplants, either a living donor transplant or a deceased donor split-liver transplant, are being increasingly used for adult recipients also. Usually, in LDLTs for pediatric recipients, the left lateral segment is used; for adult recipients, however, this would be inadequate liver mass and so usually the right lobe is used. Split-liver transplants from deceased donors involve dividing the donor liver into two segments, each of which is subsequently transplanted.

The greatest advantage of a LDLT is that it avoids the waiting time seen with deceased donor organs. In the United States, over 16,500 people are now waiting for liver transplants, but only 6,000 transplants are performed every year (UNOS/OPTN, www.optn.transplant.hrsa.gov/, accessed August, 2009) [6]. Approximately, 15% to 25% of the candidates will die of their liver disease before having the chance to undergo a transplant. For those who do end up receiving a transplant from a deceased donor, the waiting time can be significant, resulting in severe debilitation. With a LDLT, this waiting time can be bypassed, allowing the transplant to be performed before the recipient's health deteriorates further. In 2007, 266 LDLTs were performed in the United States, accounting for 4% of the total liver transplants performed that year.

A partial hepatectomy in an otherwise healthy donor is a significant undertaking, so all potential donors must be very carefully evaluated. Detailed medical screening must ensure that the donor is medically healthy; radiologic evaluation must ensure that the anatomy of the donor's liver is suitable; and a psychosocial evaluation must be done to ensure that the donor is mentally fit and not being coerced. The decision to donate should be made entirely by the potential donor after careful consideration of the risks and of the potential complications, with no coercion from anyone.

The overall incidence of donor complications after living donor liver donation ranges from 5% to 10%. There is also a small risk (<0.5%) of death [28,29]. Of note, mortality is higher for adult-to-adult donation (0.24% to 0.4%) compared with adult-to-child donation (0.09% to 0.2%). This is explained by the fact that adult-to-child donation usually removal of a smaller portion of the liver. Bile duct problems are the most worrisome complication after donor surgery. Bile may leak from the cut surface of the liver or from the site where the bile duct is divided. That site may later become strictured. Generally, bile leaks resolve spontaneously with simple drainage. Strictures and sometimes bile leaks may require an ERCP and stenting. If the above measures fail, a reoperation may be required. Intra-abdominal infections developing in donors are usually related to a biliary problem. Other complications after donor surgery may include incisional problems such as infections and hernias. The risk of deep venous thrombosis (DVT) and pulmonary embolism (PE) is the same as for other major abdominal procedures.

The recipient operation with LDLTs is not greatly different from whole-organ deceased donor liver transplants. The hepatectomy is performed in a similar fashion—the cava should be preserved in all such cases, because the graft will generally only have a single hepatic vein for outflow. This is then anastomosed directly to the recipient's preserved vena cava. Outflow problems tend to be more common with partial versus whole transplants, especially with right lobe transplants (which, again, are usually used for adult recipients). Various methods have been described to improve the outflow of the graft, such as including the middle hepatic vein with the graft, reimplanting accessory hepatic veins, and reimplanting large tributaries that drain the right lobe into the middle hepatic vein [30–32]. Inflow to the graft can be reestablished by anastomosing the donor's hepatic artery and portal vein branch to the corresponding structures in the recipient.

Another method to increase the number of liver transplants is to split the liver from a deceased donor into two grafts, which are then transplanted into two recipients [33]. Thus, a whole adult liver from such a donor can be divided into two functioning grafts. The vast majority of split-liver transplants have been between one adult donor and two pediatric recipients. Splitting one adult liver for two pediatric recipients has no negative impact on the adult donor pool, but it does not increase it either. Adults now account for the majority of patients awaiting a transplant—and the majority of patients dying on the waiting list. Therefore, if split-liver transplants are to have a significant impact on waiting list time and mortality, they must be performed so that the resulting two grafts can also be used in two adult recipients [34]. The worry is that the smaller of the two pieces would not be sufficient to sustain life in a normal-sized adult. However, with appropriate donor and recipient selection criteria, a small percentage of livers from deceased donors could be split and transplanted into two adult recipients.

Recently, the use of organs from donors after cardiac death (also referred as non-heart–beating donors) has emerged as an important source of organs in response to the significant growth of the waiting list. DCD involves those donors who present a severe neurological injury and/or irreversible brain damage but still have minimal brain function. Therefore, DCD offers the patient and the family the opportunity to donate when criteria for brain death will not have been met [7–9]. Two different types of DCD are described. Controlled DCD involves planned withdrawal of ventilatory and organ-perfusion support, most often in the operating room with a surgical team readily available (Maastricht III). In contrast, uncontrolled DCD sustains an unexpected cardiopulmonary arrest and either fails to respond to resuscitation or is declared dead on arrival to the hospital (Maastricht I, II, and IV). The number of DCD liver allografts has gradually increased, and now represents approximately 5% of all liver transplants performed in the United States. In 2000, only 11 centers used DCD livers, increasing to 62 centers in 2007 [8].

Because of the constant imbalance between the number of available organs and the number of candidates for liver transplant, organs that were previously thought to be associated with an unacceptably high risk of initial poor function have been used to increase the donor pool. These organs obtained from the so-called expanded criteria donors have been used with an increase rate of primary nonfunction (PNF).

In 2006, a retrospective study using characteristics of more than 20,000 donors identified several factors that were associated with an increase risk of graft loss. These factors were used to generate a "donor risk index," which is directly related to a predicted rate of graft survival. Six donor/graft characteristics are as follows: (1) donor age over 40 (particularly over 60), (2) donation after cardiac death, (3) African American race, (4) shorter in height, (5) cerebrovascular accident as cause of death and (6) use of partial grafts, were significantly associated with graft failure. In parallel to the recipient risk score (i.e. MELD score) the donor risk index may help to optimize the donor/recipient matching. However, the potential benefit of utilization of this score in organ allocation remains to be determined [35].

Postoperative Care

The postoperative course can range from smooth to extremely complicated, depending mainly on the patient's preoperative status and the development of any complications. The care of all such patients involves (1) stabilization and recovery of the major organ systems (e.g., cardiovascular, pulmonary, renal); (2) evaluation of graft function and achievement of adequate immunosuppression; and (3) monitoring and treatment of complications directly and indirectly related to the transplant.

Initial Stabilization

The initial care immediately posttransplant should be performed in an intensive care unit (ICU) setting. Recipients generally require mechanical ventilatory support for the first 24 to 48 hours. The goal is to maintain adequate oxygen saturation, acid base equilibrium, and stable hemodynamics. Guidelines for extubation are no different from the standard postoperative patient: a level of consciousness sufficient to protect the airway and the ability to maintain adequate oxygenation and ventilation. As well, there should be some indication of function of the new graft prior to attempting extubation. After extubation, it is crucial to continue with aggressive physiotherapy, deep breathing exercises, and ambulation to reduce the typically high incidence of respiratory complications.

Continuous hemodynamic monitoring should be maintained via an arterial line and pulmonary artery catheter. Information obtained should be used to ensure adequate perfusion of the graft and vital organs. The preoperative hyperdynamic circulatory state will often persist into the postoperative period. Later, as hepatic function improves, the cardiac index progressively declines and the SVR increases toward normal values. However, the myocardial dysfunction that is often seen early in the reperfusion phase may persist, with decreased compliance and contractility of the ventricles. The cause of this myocardial depression is unclear, but may be related to the release of vasoactive substances after reperfusion of the ischemic liver and decompression of the portal circulation. The usual treatment is to optimize preload and afterload, and inotropic agents such as dopamine or dobutamine.

To assess for possible bleeding, serial hematocrits should be measured initially every 4 to 6 hours. Coagulation parameters (prothrombin time, partial thromboplastin time, thrombin time) need to be carefully monitored because of frequent coagulopathy, most likely related to intraoperative blood loss and temporary ischemic damage in the revascularized new liver. Other laboratory values to monitor include serum transaminases and serum bilirubin. Normalization of these values, along with improvement in mental status and renal function, are valuable indicators of good graft function.

Fluid management, electrolyte status, and renal function require frequent evaluation after surgery. Most liver recipients have an increased extravascular volume but a reduced intravascular volume. Attention should be given to the potassium, calcium, magnesium, phosphate, and glucose levels. Potassium may be elevated because of poor renal function, residual reperfusion effect, or immunosuppression medications. Diuretics may be required to remove excess fluid acquired intraoperatively, but may result in hypokalemia. Magnesium levels should be kept more than 2 mg per dL to prevent seizures and phosphate levels between 2 and 5 mg per dL for proper support of the respiratory and alimentary tracts. Marked hyperglycemia may be seen secondary to steroids, and should be treated with insulin. Hypoglycemia is often an indication of poor hepatic function.

Nasogastric suction is initially required until normal bowel function resumes (usually 48 hours); patients with a choledochojejunostomy may need more time. Some form of prophylaxis for GI bleeding should be maintained as the physiologic stress after a liver transplant may lead to gastric erosions and ulcerations. The GI tract can be used for nutrition by postoperative day 3 to 5. However, for patients with prolonged ileus or significant intestinal edema—especially if they were malnourished preoperatively—total parenteral nutrition (TPN) should be instituted early.

As soon as the patient enters the ICU, prevention, prophylaxis, and close monitoring of possible infections should begin. Given the magnitude of the operation, the often poor pretransplant medical status, and the need for immunosuppression, it is not surprising that more than 50% of liver recipients develop some infection. Close attention must be given to all invasive monitoring lines, which should be changed every 5 to 7 days. Aggressive pulmonary toilet is needed: the lung is a common source of infection. Perioperative antibiotics with activity against biliary tract pathogens should be employed. All recipients should also receive trimethoprim–sulfamethoxazole to reduce the likelihood of infections secondary to *Pneumocystis* or *Nocardia*. Prophylaxis is also indicated against fungal infections (most commonly *Candida* and *Aspergillus*) and viral infections (most commonly CMV [cytomegalovirus] and herpes virus).

Graft Function and Immunosuppression

A crucial aspect of postoperative care is the repeated evaluation of graft function, which in fact begins intraoperatively, soon after the liver is reperfused. Signs of hepatic function include good texture and color of the graft, evidence of bile production, and restoration of hemodynamic stability. Once the patient arrives in the ICU, evaluation of hepatic function is continued based on clinical signs and laboratory values. The patient who rapidly awakens from anesthesia and whose mental status progressively improves likely has a well-functioning graft. Laboratory values that corroborate good function include normalization of the coagulation profile, resolution of hypoglycemia and hyperbilirubinemia, and clearance of serum lactate. Adequate urine production and good output of bile through the biliary tube (if present) are also indicators of good graft function. Serum transaminase levels will usually rise during the first 48 to 72 hours secondary to preservation injury, and then should fall rapidly over the next 24 to 48 hours.

Induction immunosuppression posttransplant varies from center to center. Many use a triple immunosuppressive regimen based on cyclosporine or tacrolimus, prednisone, and azathioprine or mycophenolate mofetil. Some centers also use antilymphocyte antibody for induction therapy, either for all recipients or only for those with renal dysfunction. The newer humanized monoclonal antibodies (basiliximab or daclizumab) are also being used, usually as part of regimens that involve the withholding of calcineurin inhibitors or steroids [36].

Posttransplant Surgical Complications

Given the magnitude of the operation, surgical complications posttransplant are not uncommon. One important aspect, then, of postoperative care is to be aware of any complications so that they may be quickly recognized and treated. Surgical complications related directly to the operation include postoperative hemorrhage and problems with any of the five anastomoses (five vascular and one biliary).

Postoperative Hemorrhage. Bleeding is common in the postoperative period, and is usually multifactorial. Previously, it has been reported that 15% of patients required a reoperation for bleeding control after transplant. Currently, with the improvement of postoperative treatment of coagulopathy in the ICU, the incidence of reoperation has dropped to 5%. A large raw surface is created during the recipient hepatectomy, often in a patient with significant vascular collaterals secondary to portal hypertension. A number of small persistent bleeding sites may often result. This may be compounded by an underlying coagulopathy resulting from deficits in one or more of the main systems of hemostasis: coagulation, fibrinolysis, and platelet function.

Large volume intraoperative blood transfusions and poor postoperative liver function secondary to ischemic damage of the liver can lead to severe coagulation defects. As liver function improves, coagulation parameters normalize. Fresh frozen plasma (FFP) and cryoprecipitate are used, as needed, until graft function is adequate. Thrombocytopenia is seen in virtually all recipients posttransplant, with lowest levels on postoperative day 3 and 4, then returning to normal by day 7. Platelets are transfused, as needed, for platelet counts less than 50×10^9 per L (depending on the degree of ongoing bleeding), but counts may not increase, because of ongoing deposition of platelets in the spleen. Hyperfibrinolysis, often a problem intraoperatively during the reperfusion phase, may persist into the early postoperative period. Aprotinin, a serine protease inhibitor, may be administered intraoperatively; it decreases hyperfibrinolysis-triggered bleeding in some recipients.

Blood loss should be monitored through the abdominal drains and with serial measurements of hemoglobin and central venous pressures. If bleeding persists despite correction of coagulation deficiencies, an exploratory laparotomy should be performed. Reexploration is especially important if increasing abdominal pressure is evident which may compromise respiratory or renal function. Bleeding complications are generally higher in recipients of reduced-size, split-liver, or living related grafts, because the cut surface of the liver is an additional source of potential blood loss.

Vascular Complications. The incidence of vascular complications after liver transplant is 5% to 10%. Thrombosis is the most common early event; stenosis, dissection, and pseudoaneurysm formation are less common. Any of the four vascular anastomoses may be involved, but the hepatic artery is most common [37].

Hepatic artery thrombosis (HAT) has a reported incidence of 3% to 5% in adults and about 5% to 8% in children. Several risk factors have been reported for early HAT CMV mismatch (seropositive donor liver in seronegative recipient), retransplantation, use of arterial conduits, prolonged operation and cold ischemic times, low recipient weight, severe rejection, variant arterial anatomy, and low-volume transplantation centers. Technical factors that disturb laminar flow of the blood in the arteries (such as intimal dissection, tension on the anastomosis, and kinking of the artery) are also implicated in the development of HAT. Thrombosis rates are higher after split-liver and living related transplants, because of the smaller caliber of vessels and the sometimes complex arterial reconstruction required [38,39].

After HAT, liver recipients may be asymptomatic or they may have severe liver failure secondary to extensive necrosis. Those with thrombosis early postoperatively, especially adults, have the most dramatic signs and symptoms: marked elevation of serum transaminase levels, septic shock, HE, and overall rapid deterioration. Ultrasound with Doppler evaluation is the initial investigation of choice, with more than 90% sensitivity and specificity. Prompt reexploration with thrombectomy and revision of the anastomoses is indicated if the diagnosis is made early. If hepatic necrosis is extensive, a retransplant is indicated. CT or MRI scans may be helpful in determining the extent of necrosis. Some centers have used implantable Doppler probes performing continuous flow monitoring in patients with high risk for development of HAT.

HAT may also present in a less dramatic fashion. The donor bile duct receives its blood supply from the hepatic artery. Thrombosis may therefore render the common bile duct ischemic, resulting in a localized or diffuse bile leak from the anastomosis, or more chronically a diffuse biliary stricture. Late thrombosis may be asymptomatic, especially in children, because of the presence of collaterals (which provide sufficient arterial inflow) along the biliary anastomosis.

Thrombosis of the portal vein is far less frequent (compared with the hepatic artery), occurring in fewer than 2% of recipients. It may be related to a technical factor such as narrowing of the anastomosis or excessive length of the portal vein with kinking. Recipients who require a venous conduit secondary to underlying portal vein thrombosis are also at higher risk for portal vein thrombosis. As with HAT, clinical presentation can vary. Early postoperatively, portal vein thrombosis may result in severe liver dysfunction. Tense ascites and variceal bleeding may be seen secondary to acutely elevated portal and mesenteric venous pressures. If these symptoms develop postoperatively, urgent ultrasound with Doppler evaluation is performed to assess the patency of the portal vein. If the diagnosis is made early, operative thrombectomy and revision of the anastomosis may be successful. If thrombosis occurs late, liver function is usually preserved due to the presence of collaterals. In this case, a retransplant is not necessary, and attention is diverted toward relieving the left-sided portal hypertension.

Complications of the hepatic veins (such as thrombosis and stenosis) are rare, with an incidence of less than 1%. Recurrence of Budd–Chiari syndrome and technical factors such as narrowing of the anastomosis are the most common causes. Presentation is usually with massive ascites and graft dysfunction. Again, ultrasound Doppler will usually demonstrate the problem. The risk of thrombosis is higher in recipients of a left lateral segment, either from a living donor or as part of a split-liver graft. This segment may be quite mobile, and if it is not properly aligned, it may twist on the anastomosis, obstructing flow [40].

Biliary Complications. Complications of the biliary system continue to be common after liver transplantation. The incidence is 10% to 25% with an associated mortality of less than 5% [41]. This incidence may be even higher in partial transplant recipients and recipients of DCD livers. Biliary complications manifest as either a leak or an obstruction. Timing will often determine type and clinical outcome of the complication. Bile leaks tend to occur early postoperatively and often require surgical repair, while obstruction usually occurs later and can often be managed with radiologic or endoscopic techniques.

Most bile leaks occur within the first 30 days posttransplant. Most centers have abandoned the use of external T-tube stents because a leak may occur from the T-tube site when it is removed. In whole liver transplant recipients, biliary leaks occur most commonly at the anastomotic site. The area around the anastomosis has the most tenuous blood supply: both the donor common bile duct (CBD) and the recipient portion of the CBD are supplied by end arteries. Excessive dissection or cauterization around the donor or recipient CBD can further disrupt the blood supply, leading to ischemic complications. Another important cause of biliary tract complications is hepatic artery thrombosis: the donor CBD receives its blood supply from the hepatic artery. With any biliary tract complication, the hepatic artery should be carefully assessed to document patency. Other causes of leaks include poorly placed sutures, excessive number of sutures, and tension on the anastomosis. With partial transplants, the cut surface of the liver represents the most common site for a bile leak.

Clinical symptoms of a bile leak include fever, abdominal pain, and peritoneal irritation. Bile in the abdominal drains is highly suspicious for a leak, but absence of bile in the drains does not preclude the diagnosis. Blood tests may demonstrate an elevation of the white blood cell count, bilirubin, and alkaline phosphatase; unfortunately, no laboratory test is pathognomonic. Ultrasound may demonstrate a fluid collection, but often cholangiography is required for diagnosis. This is simple to perform if an external biliary stent is in place. In the absence of an external stent, options include magnetic resonance cholangiography (MRC), endoscopic retrograde cholangiography (ERC), or percutaneous transhepatic cholangiography (PTC).

Many recommend operative treatment for all early bile leaks. The anastomosis is revised, or for small leaks, additional sutures are placed at the leak site. If there is undue tension in recipients with a CDC, the biliary anastomosis is converted to a CDJ. The increasing popularity of treating nontransplant biliary leaks with endoscopically placed stents has led to their use for transplant-related leaks.

Biliary obstruction is usually secondary to stricture and occurs later in the postoperative period. It is most common at the anastomotic site and is likely related to local ischemia. Nonanastomotic strictures usually have a worse prognosis; they are associated with hepatic artery thrombosis, prolonged cold ischemic times, and ABO-incompatible donors [42]. Patients sustaining biliary obstruction usually present with cholangitis or cholestasis, or both. Ultrasound can be misleading in making the diagnosis, since ductal dilatation may not be seen; however, it is still a crucial test in order to exclude potential hepatic arterial flow complication (which is a potential cause of bile duct stricture). Cholangiography (T-tube cholangiography, ERC, MRC, or PTC, depending on the type of BD reconstruction performed) is always necessary for diagnosis of BD stricture. The treatment is usually not an operation, but rather by percutaneous on internal balloon dilatation and stent placement across the site of stricture. If these initial options fail, surgical revision is required.

Wound Complications. Wound complications, very common in liver transplant recipients, can be a source of significant morbidity. In the general surgical population, risk factors for wound complications have been well described, including a lengthy operative procedure, bowel or biliary contamination, blood transfusions, poor nutritional status, and steroid administration. All of these risk factors are generally present in liver recipients.

The most common problems with the wound are infections and hematomas. Direct bacterial contamination of the wound may occur from bile or bowel contents if a CDJ is performed. Wound hematomas can easily result from large abdominal wall collaterals, compounded by underlying coagulopathy. Wound infections will usually present after postoperative day 5. The infection may be obvious, with fever, chills, erythema, and purulent drainage from the wound. But at times, signs and symptoms may be minimal. Treatment is the same as for nontransplant patients: opening the wound, serial dressing changes, and allowing healing by secondary intention. IV antibiotics should be used with significant cellulitis or systemic symptoms. Necrotizing fasciitis has also been reported, and requires rapid, aggressive debridement plus high-dose IV antibiotics.

Posttransplant Medical Complications

Given the underlying illness and the need for powerful immunosuppression, it is not difficult to see why a significant percentage of liver recipients develop some medical complication before discharge. Medical complications seen early posttransplant may be due to immunosuppression, to residual effects of the liver failure, or to unrelated factors. Almost any organ system may be involved.

Nontechnical Graft Dysfunction. The vascular and biliary complications described earlier can all lead to poor liver function postoperatively. Hepatic dysfunction not related to technical complications may also be seen during this time. Causes may include PNF of the graft, acute rejection, and infection.

PNF is a devastating complication, with a mortality rate of more than 80% without a retransplant. By definition, it is a syndrome that results from poor or no hepatic function from the time of the transplant procedure. Most centers now report the incidence to be less than 5%.

The cause of PNF is unknown, but several retrospective studies have attempted to identify donor risk factors that may predict development of this syndrome. Donor factors that have been associated with PNF include advanced age, increased fat content of the donor liver, longer donor hospital stay before organ procurement, prolonged cold ischemia (>18 hours), and reduced-sized grafts [43].

Early prediction of PNF is valuable in identifying patients that will need a retransplant. It is also important to rule out conditions that may mimic PNF such as hepatic artery thrombosis, accelerated acute rejection, and severe infection. Intraoperative clues may indicate poor graft function. PNF should be considered in recipients who do not stabilize soon after reestablishment of hepatic perfusion, or who have ongoing hemodynamic instability, worsening acidosis and coagulopathy, poor bile production, or poor liver graft color. Upon arrival to the ICU, recipients who do not regain consciousness, or who have increasing renal dysfunction, continued hemodynamic instability, increasing prothrombin time, or persistent hypoglycemia may have PNF. An AST >5,000 IU per L, Factor VIII <60% of normal, PT >20 seconds at 4 to 6 hours postreperfusion, in association with poor bile production, may all suggest PNF.

Unfortunately, no medical treatment is effective for PNF. IV prostaglandin E1 (PGE1) has some useful effect [44], but further evaluation is necessary. Its mechanism of action is presumably a vasodilatory effect on the splanchnic circulation, resulting in enhanced blood flow to the new liver. PGE1 is also immunomodulatory and may lessen the risk of graft rejection. Recipients with suspected PNF should probably be started on a continuous infusion and listed for an urgent retransplant. The starting dose is 0.005 μg per kg per minute, which is increased, as tolerated per blood pressure measurements, to a maximum of 0.03 μg per kg per minute. Ultimately, such recipients do better with a retransplant. However, if a retransplant is to positively influence outcome, it must be done before multiorgan failure develops. In one series of 15 liver recipients with PNF, all those who sustained organ failure in four or more systems died despite a retransplant [45].

Rejection is very common after a liver transplant; 20% to 30% of recipients will have at least one bout at some point posttransplant. Most acute rejection episodes are not seen until at least 1 week posttransplant. Rejection episodes during the first posttransplant week may be seen in recipients of ABO-incompatible grafts, or those with a very strongly positive preoperative cytotoxic cross-match. With current immunosuppressive drugs, signs and symptoms of acute rejection tend to be fairly mild. Most commonly, the serum bilirubin and/or transaminase levels are elevated, which may be completely asymptomatic or may involve mild accompanying symptoms such as fever and malaise. The differential diagnosis must include mechanical complications (such as vascular thrombosis and bile leaks), and underlying sepsis. Ultimately, a histologic assessment of the graft is required to confirm the diagnosis of acute rejection, most commonly via a percutaneous liver biopsy. Mild rejection episodes can usually be treated simply by increasing the level of maintenance immunosuppression. Episodes that are judged to be moderate or severe by histology are usually treated with high-dose IV corticosteroids.

Neurologic Complications. Neurologic complications posttransplant are common, affecting more than 20% of liver recipients. Complications generally manifest as decreased level of consciousness, seizures, or focal neurologic deficits.

Decreased level of consciousness is usually due to oversedation from drugs that have accumulated over days because of impaired hepatic or renal clearance. Benzodiazepines and narcotics are common culprits, but unresponsiveness may also be secondary to calcineurin neurotoxicity. This tends to be more common in patients with previous hepatic encephalopathy.

Multiple metabolic abnormalities are frequent posttransplant, and may diminish alertness. A poorly functioning or nonfunctioning graft with resulting liver failure can lead to hepatic encephalopathy. Other evidence of liver failure is also frequent, such as a marked elevation of liver enzymes, prothrombin time, and ammonia levels. Flumazenil, a benzodiazepine receptor antagonist, improves HE for a short time [46]. It may thus be a useful diagnostic tool when HE is suspected, postoperatively. Renal failure and sepsis may also contribute to a metabolic encephalopathy. After significant periods of perioperative hypotension, a decreased GCS may indicate hypoxic-ischemic encephalopathy. This may be a difficult diagnosis to make, since imaging studies are often normal. Nonspecific abnormalities may be seen on EEG. The clinical scenario is characterized by an initial insult, then a prolonged recovery period, often characterized by decreased alertness.

Central pontine myelinolysis (CPM) is an uncommon cause for failure to awaken posttransplant [47]. Typically, it is seen with marked fluctuations in serum sodium levels and osmolality, or in recovered alcoholics. CT is often normal, but MRI may demonstrate characteristic abnormalities in the pons. Careful attention to shifts in the serum sodium and osmolality may decrease the risk of CPM.

FHF patients, especially those with severe HE and evidence of cerebral edema preoperatively, invariably have a period of diminished level of consciousness posttransplant. Intraoperatively, during the reperfusion phase, their intracranial pressure (ICP) often increases. If untreated and severe, this increase may lead to neurologic death, which is often not diagnosed until in the ICU. Usually, however, the effects of cerebral edema linger over a period of 7 to 10 days postoperatively, with eventual recovery. ICP monitoring pre- and intraoperatively may be of value in detecting cerebral edema and marked elevations of pressure.

Liver recipients, who have an initially normal neurologic course postoperatively, followed by sudden clinical deterioration, should be evaluated for an intracranial hematoma. Predisposing factors include underlying coagulopathy and systolic hypertension.

Postoperative seizures usually occur de novo, tend to be of the generalized tonic clonic variety, and are most common during the first 2 weeks posttransplant. Causes are numerous. Electrolyte abnormalities (such as hyponatremia, hypocalcemia, and hypomagnesemia) and medications, are the most common causes. Structural abnormalities such as intracranial hemorrhage and cerebral infarction may be responsible. Infectious processes (such as meningitis, encephalitis, and a brain abscess) should also be considered.

Immunosuppression medications may sometimes cause significant neurologic changes after transplantation. Several neurotoxic effects have been associated with use of cyclosporine, including tremors, headache, mental status changes, seizures, focal neurological deficits, and/or visual disturbances. Tacrolimus produces neurologic disorders similar to those seen in patients using cyclosporine, but more frequently. Posterior reversible encephalopathy syndrome (PRES) is a rare but serious complication of immunosuppressive therapy after solid organ transplantation (0.5%). In addition to the neurologic symptoms, which range from headaches to mental status changes, this syndrome is associated with a characteristic imaging feature of subcortical white matter lesions on magnetic resonance imaging. The changes in the subcortical white matter are secondary to potentially reversible vasogenic edema. These imaging findings predominate in the territory of the posterior cerebral artery. PRES typically develops in the first 2 months after liver transplantation (90%). A prompt diagnosis of this rare entity with a temporary discontinuation of the calcineurin inhibitor offers the best chance of avoiding long-term sequelae [48].

Cardiovascular Complications. A number of cardiovascular complications (including arrhythmia, ischemia, changes in blood pressure and cardiac arrest) can be seen intra- and postoperatively. They may occur in liver recipients with previously normal cardiac status or in those with underlying comorbid cardiac conditions. The latter group is becoming more important as the increased success of liver transplantation has led to expanded indications and older recipients.

Most intraoperative cardiovascular complications are seen immediately after reperfusion of the liver. About 30% of recipients experience a transient decrease in blood pressure during this phase, which has been termed the postreperfusion syndrome (PRS). This syndrome is defined by a decrease in the mean arterial pressure of at least 30% for 1 minute within the first 5 minutes after reperfusion, accompanied by a decrease in the heart rate and SVR and an increase in the CVP and PCWP. The exact cause of the myocardial depression and decreased contractility seen with PRS is unclear, but is likely multifactorial. Hyperkalemic, cold, acidotic fluid washed out from the graft, combined with existing abnormalities such as hypocalcemia and acidosis, may be the main culprits. Myocardial depressant factors may also be released from the ischemic graft on reperfusion. The effect is generally short-lived; left ventricular function is usually normal within 5 minutes. Some recipients, however, experience extreme bradycardia and hypotension, leading to cardiac arrest; this is rare and small doses of inotropic agents are usually effective. Arrhythmias, such as ventricular tachycardia and ventricular fibrillation, have also been described in the early reperfusion phase.

The incidence of postoperative myocardial ischemia is 5% to 13%. As the age of transplant candidates has increased, so has the likelihood of silent coronary artery disease, leading to perioperative ischemia. Candidates with risk factors and a high probability of coronary artery disease should undergo a pretransplant coronary assessment. Poor exercise tolerance often precludes a formal stress test. Pharmacological stress testing with either dipyridamole thallium imaging or dobutamine echocardiography, may be better. Candidates with positive tests should undergo coronary angiography, with a view toward revascularization procedures (PTCA, CABG) as indicated.

A rare postoperative complication is acute right ventricular failure secondary to severe pulmonary hypertension, but deaths have been reported [49]. The pulmonary hypertension in these recipients was likely present pretransplant. It is an uncommon complication of portal hypertension, affecting less than 1% of patients. The exact cause is unclear, though portal hypertension is the strongest predisposing factor. Histologically, the predominant lesion is a nonspecific plexiform arteriopathy. Pretransplant right heart catheterization may be necessary to establish the diagnosis; severe pulmonary hypertension may contraindicate transplantation.

Pulmonary Complications. The pulmonary system is one of the most common sites of complications posttransplant; infectious and noninfectious pulmonary complications may be seen. Infectious complications predominate after the first posttransplant week, but noninfectious complications (such as pulmonary edema, pleural effusions, atelectasis, and ARDS) predominate prior to that.

Mechanical ventilation, generally short-lived, is required immediately posttransplant in almost all liver recipients. Most patients can be extubated within the first 48 hours. Those with significant preoperative lung disease, malnutrition, or early postoperative pulmonary and hepatic complications tend to require prolonged intubation.

Atelectasis is very common posttransplant, as it is after other major abdominal operations. Significant preoperative ascites and pleural effusions are predisposing factors. Poor nutrition, decreased level of consciousness, and poor lung compliance are other contributing factors. Treatment is generally successful with chest physiotherapy and PEEP, with therapeutic bronchoscopy reserved for recipients with large areas of collapse or persistent atelectasis. Diaphragmatic dysfunction may also be seen posttransplant, with resultant right-sided atelectasis and decreased vital capacity, which may prolong the need for ventilatory support. The cause of this dysfunction is probably a crush injury of the right phrenic nerve, which can occur during surgery when the suprahepatic caval clamp is applied [50]. Usually, the nerve and diaphragmatic function completely recover, but it may take up to 9 months posttransplant.

Pleural effusions are noted in a large number of recipients. The right side is more commonly involved. Usually transudative in origin, pleural effusions may be related to sympathetic fluid accumulation from the operative diaphragmatic dissection or preoperative ascites. Typically, these effusions resolve spontaneously within 1 to 2 weeks. Thoracentesis may be needed to rule out an empyema or hemothorax. If the effusion is large enough to compromise respiratory status, therapeutic thoracentesis or insertion of a small pigtail catheter for drainage should be performed.

All of the above conditions may manifest with arterial hypoxemia postoperatively. A less common cause of hypoxemia is the presence of intrapulmonary vascular dilatations (IPVD). These vascular abnormalities are sometimes seen in patients with chronic liver disease, associated with portal hypertension and spider angiomas of the skin. Common clinical findings are dyspnea, cyanosis, clubbing, exercise desaturation, and orthodeoxia. Two techniques are generally used to confirm intrapulmonary vascular dilatation: transthoracic contrast-enhanced echocardiography, and perfusion body scan with

99mTechnetium-labeled macroaggregated albumin (99mTc-MAA). During transthoracic contrast-enhanced echocardiography, IV injections of microbubbles (diameter <90 μm) are used to visualize intrapulmonary shunts. The timing of the appearance of the microbubbles in the left side of the heart makes the distinction between intracardiac and intrapulmonary shunts. Whole-body scan with 99mTechnetium-labeled macroaggregated albumin allows not only the detection of IPVD, but also its quantification. In normal individuals the macroaggregates (>20 μm in diameter), are normally trapped in the pulmonary circulation. In the presence of cardiac right-to-left shunts or intrapulmonary vascular dilatation, the uptake of 99mTc-MAA in other organs, such as the brain, kidneys, spleen, and liver, can be visualized. The major disadvantage of this technique is the inability to differentiate between intracardiac shunts and IPVD [51,52].

The combination of chronic liver disease, IPVDs, and severe hypoxemia or a markedly increased alveolar arterial oxygen gradient has been termed the hepatopulmonary syndrome (HPS). HPS is reversed in 60% to 90% cases after liver transplantation, and can be documented by a perfusion lung scan [52]. Hypoxemia, requiring supplemental oxygen, can be corrected as early as 6 to 12 months after surgery; however, an increased recovery time is shown in older patients, patients with a preoperative $PaO_2 \leq 52$ mm Hg and/or $AaPO_2 \geq 66$ mm Hg, or if the liver disease is a result of alcohol abuse [51,52].

Patients with significant hypoxemia pretransplant should be investigated for IPVDs. For those with a good response to 100% O_2, the transplant may proceed: the recipient has a good chance for improvement postoperatively. But for those with a poor response, pretransplant pulmonary angiography and embolization might be beneficial. Recipients with documented IPVDs and severe hypoxemia postoperatively may also benefit from embolization, especially if they have large discrete IPVDs.

Renal Complications. Some degree of renal dysfunction is very common after transplant, affecting almost all liver recipients. About 10% have renal failure severe enough to require dialysis. Impairment may already have been present pretransplant, or may develop early or late in the posttransplant period. Early diagnosis, identification of the cause, and appropriate interventions are necessary. Renal failure, whether pre- or posttransplant, increases the mortality rate associated with the procedure.

Postoperative renal problems that may have been present pretransplant are most commonly due to hepatorenal syndrome (HRS) or acute tubular necrosis (ATN). Usually, such problems will improve posttransplant, but recipients with severe pretransplant renal dysfunction are at greater risk for persistent renal impairment posttransplant. Those with prolonged renal impairment pretransplant, or those who are dialysis-dependent and not likely to regain kidney function after a liver transplant, should be considered for a simultaneous liver–kidney transplant. Obtaining a kidney biopsy pretransplant may help determine the reversibility of the underlying renal disease and hence the need for a combined transplant.

Intraoperatively, periods of hypovolemia and hemodynamic instability may contribute to postoperative renal dysfunction secondary to ATN. Such periods can be minimized by invasive cardiac monitoring to maintain adequate blood volumes and cardiac output. A rapid infusion technique is crucial, at times, to allow the anesthesiologist to keep pace with ongoing volume losses. Some surgeons argue that venovenous bypass (VVB) reduces renal vein pressures during the anhepatic phase when the cava is clamped, thus reducing the risk of postoperative renal dysfunction. Several centers routinely use VVB though there is no significant evidence to show a decreased incidence of postoperative renal failure. Several centers have adopted a selective policy, reserving VVB for liver recipients who meet certain criteria, such as hemodynamic instability with caval clamping or preexisting renal dysfunction. Intraoperative administration of verapamil or furosemide has been tried, but there is no good evidence of any significant renal benefit.

Postoperative renal dysfunction is often multifactorial. The cause may be prerenal, renal, or postrenal. Postrenal causes are rare and are usually easy to rule out. Prerenal and renal causes account for the vast majority of dysfunction [53].

Hypoperfusion of the kidneys will lead to a prerenal picture characterized by a low urine output, decreased sodium in the urine (<10 mEq per L), and a fractional excretion of sodium of less than 1%. Hypoperfusion is most common with systemic hypovolemia, often due to ongoing blood loss within the abdomen. Third-space fluid losses into the area of dissection or from bowel wall edema (related to the portal vein clamping) may also lead to intravascular volume depletion and prerenal azotemia. Renal hypoperfusion may also be due to significantly raised intra-abdominal pressure, as with tense ascites or a large volume of intraperitoneal blood and clots.

True HRS will give a picture similar to other prerenal causes, as it is believed to result from renal arterial vasoconstriction. Low sodium and a low fractional excretion of sodium again characterize urinary electrolytes. Generally, HRS is present pretransplant, especially in patients with fulminant hepatic failure or acute deterioration of chronic liver failure. Classically, HRS is considered to be functional, so kidney function should fully recover posttransplant. HRS can be divided into two types (1 and 2) based on prognosis and clinical characteristics. In HRS-1, an abrupt deterioration in the renal function occurs and often develops after a precipitating event (particularly spontaneous bacterial peritonitis). HRS-2 is characterized by a steady or slowly progressive course that occurs mostly in an outpatient setting in patients with refractory ascites. Survival of patients with HRS-1 is shorter than that of patients with HRS-2. The full recovery of kidney function is usually achieved after transplant; however, renal recovery may be delayed, especially in patients with HRS-2 and if some degree of ATN was superimposed. New onset of HRS posttransplant occurs with PNF or severe graft dysfunction, and may indicate the need for an urgent retransplant [54].

Renal causes are most commonly secondary to ischemic ATN, drug nephrotoxicity, or preexisting renal disease. Urinary electrolytes generally reveal a salt-wasting picture, with a high urinary sodium level (>30 mEq per L) and a fractional excretion of sodium >1%. On microscopic urinalysis, granular casts may be identified in the presence of ATN. The cause of ATN in liver recipients is usually ischemia and sustained hypoperfusion of the kidneys. ATN may start preoperatively, especially in acutely ill patients, or may develop secondary to hemodynamic instability intraoperatively. In one study, the predictors of acute renal failure in the immediate postoperative period were poor preoperative clinical conditions (worse Child score), elevated basal creatinine value pretransplant, transfusion of a large volume of blood products, and intraoperative hypotension [53,54]. ATN may also be seen with sepsis and multiple organ dysfunction.

Nephrotoxicity secondary to drugs is also very common. Most liver recipients have some drop in the creatinine clearance posttransplant secondary to cyclosporine or tacrolimus, both of which have significant nephrotoxic properties. Acute renal failure may be more common with high drug levels and with intravenous formulations. These immunosuppressive agents may also worsen existing renal dysfunction. Nephrotoxicity may also be secondary to other drugs, most commonly the aminoglycosides and amphotericin B.

Once renal dysfunction is adequately diagnosed, therapy can be guided appropriately. Invasive monitoring with an arterial line and a pulmonary artery catheter is helpful to optimize hemodynamic parameters and renal perfusion. Hypovolemia should be treated with volume replacement and blood products as necessary. Blood pressure should be kept in the normal range, as determined from preoperative values. For decreased cardiac output secondary to myocardial depression, inotropic agents such as dopamine or dobutamine are indicated. If increased SVR is the main problem, a peripheral vasodilator may be of benefit. Other interventions would depend on the cause of renal dysfunction. Tense ascites can be relieved with paracentesis, while nephrotoxic drugs should be discontinued or their dosage lowered.

Once cardiovascular parameters have been optimized and compounding factors dealt with, efforts should be made to establish diuresis. Prognosis is generally better in recipients with nonoliguric (as opposed to oliguric or anuric) renal failure. The role of diuretic therapy is unclear. Recipients who were on chronic diuretic therapy pretransplant may have "diuretic dependence," and require its continued use posttransplant to maintain urine output. They should be adequately volume-loaded before diuretics are initiated, otherwise renal failure may be exacerbated. A loop diuretic such as furosemide is often the first-line agent. Its delivery to the afferent artery of the kidney depends, in part, on its binding to albumin. Therefore, in recipients with significant hypoalbuminemia, infusion of albumin may be necessary to maximize the effect of the diuretic.

If renal function does not improve, artificial renal support may become necessary. Options include regular hemodialysis or continuous venovenous hemofiltration (CVVH). Intermittent hemodialysis may not be feasible for acutely ill postoperative patients because of the hemodynamic instability it often causes. CVVH imposes a less significant stress on the hemodynamic system. Indications for CVVH or hemodialysis include (1) significant volume overload with evidence of pulmonary edema, (2) persistent or worsening hyperkalemia, and (3) persistent or worsening metabolic acidosis.

In patients with chronic hepatitis C virus (HCV) infection who have undergone a liver transplant, kidney dysfunction can be also associated with type II mixed cryoglobulinemia. Mixed cryoglobulinemia is a systemic vasculitis secondary to circulating immune complex deposition in the small vessels, and is usually triggered by the hepatitis C virus infection. The principal clinical manifestations of glomerular disease (usually membranoproliferative glomerulonephritis, MPGN) are the presence of proteinuria and microscopic hematuria, with impaired kidney function. The diagnosis of HCV-related MPGN is usually made by positive tests for serum HCV antibodies and HCV RNA, high concentrations of cryoglobulins, positive rheumatoid factor assays, and low levels of complement [55].

Infectious Complications. Infections are common after all organ transplants, but the incidence is highest after liver transplantation. More than two-thirds of recipients will experience at least one infective episode. Several factors account for this very high incidence: (1) the length and magnitude of the operation, (2) the high potential for biliary and enteric contamination, and (3) the poor overall medical condition of many recipients.

The incidence of infections has not changed significantly since the early days of liver transplantation. What has changed is the mortality rate. Early series reported mortality rates of 25% to 50% associated with infections. More recent studies, however, suggest that infection-related deaths in most centers are now less than 10%. A better understanding of the immunosuppressed state, identification of risk factors, and more effective means of treatment and prophylaxis have all contributed to an improved prognosis. Nonetheless, infections remain the most common cause of early mortality posttransplant and a significant source of morbidity. Identification of risk factors, preventive measures and effective prophylaxis, rapid diagnosis, and prompt and appropriate treatment are all crucial.

The preoperative workup should include evaluation for any infective diseases. Serologic testing should assess the transplant candidate's CMV, HIV, and hepatitis (B and C) status. Latent infections (such as tuberculosis) that may be reactivated with immunosuppression must be ruled out. Focus should be on active infections that would require treatment pretransplant or even preclude a transplant. Candidates with chronic liver failure are prone to infections such as spontaneous bacterial peritonitis, cholangitis, pneumonia and fungal infections, all of which should be treated appropriately and documented as improved pretransplant. The urgency of the transplant will often determine the length of treatment.

Once the transplant has occurred, efforts should be instituted to prevent infections. Perioperative antibiotics effective against biliary tract pathogens are important. Other prophylactic regimens with proven benefit include trimethoprim–sulfamethoxazole for *Pneumocystis* pneumonia (other options include dapsone, atovaquone, and pentamidine), acyclovir or ganciclovir for CMV and other herpes family viruses, and nystatin or fluconazole/voriconazole for antifungal prophylaxis. Preventive measures that should be followed are no different than for similar, nontransplant patients in a critical care setting: attentive care to indwelling arterial and venous lines, change of central catheters every 7 days, and aggressive pulmonary toilet.

Any postoperative fever should prompt an urgent, thorough evaluation for infection, including culture of blood, urine, sputum, and ascitic fluid, as indicated. A CXR to rule out a pulmonary source should be performed, then bronchoscopy and lavage to evaluate any suspicious infiltrates. A thorough examination with close attention to the wound is important. A wound infection will require opening of the wound and serial dressing changes. If no obvious source of infection is found, a CT scan of the abdomen to look for fluid collections is warranted. A diagnostic aspiration can then be performed to rule out an abscess. If the recipient has a persistent high temperature or toxic appearance, antibiotics should be started, even without identification of the infective source. Generally, a wide-spectrum antibiotic with activity against biliary pathogens is the agent of first choice. Of note, an elevated temperature may also be seen with other conditions, such as acute rejection, graft-versus-host disease, and drug reactions.

Infections posttransplant are broadly categorized into those occurring early (within 1 month) and later. Regardless of the timing, bacterial, viral, or fungal pathogens may be responsible. The relative incidence of these various pathogens differs at different times posttransplant.

Bacterial and fungal organisms account for most infections during the first month. The immunosuppressed state is a risk factor, but these infections are more related to surgical complications, initial graft function, and morbid conditions that existed pretransplant. Risk factors include prolonged surgery, large-volume blood transfusions, PNF requiring a retransplant, and reoperations for bleeding or bile leaks. Common sites for these infections, in decreasing order of frequency, are the abdomen, the respiratory tract, blood, wounds, and the urinary tract.

After the first month, the immunosuppressed state becomes the main risk factor for infection. Immunosuppressive drugs depress cell-mediated immunity, leading to opportunistic infections with viral, fungal, and parasitic pathogens. The risk increases as immunosuppression increases, especially when acute rejection episodes are treated with bolus high-dose steroids or antilymphocyte agents. Bacterial infections generally decline after the first month, except in recipients who have had prolonged ICU stays because of surgical complications or respiratory failure. Other predisposing factors for late bacterial infections are a biliary stricture and hepatic arterial thrombosis.

Bacterial infections usually involve the abdominal cavity, including the wound. Bacterial pathogens often originate from either the biliary tree or from the small bowel. A choledochojejunostomy (CDJ) for biliary drainage is associated with a higher rate of infection than is a duct-to-duct biliary anastomosis. Contamination may occur either at the time of surgery, or later because of biliary complications such as a leak or stenosis. Abdominal infections usually manifest as cholangitis, abscesses (intra- or extrahepatic), peritonitis, or wound infection. Cholangitis often develops with an underlying biliary stricture and may lead to a subsequent ascending infection with development of intrahepatic abscesses. Hepatic artery thrombosis may also lead to ischemia of the allograft and development of intrahepatic abscesses secondary to necrosis of the liver. Peritonitis and an extrahepatic abscess often signal the presence of a bile leak. If an intra-abdominal infection is suspected, a CT scan should be done, with aspiration and culture of any identified fluid collections. If a biliary stent is present, it can be used to evaluate for the presence of a leak or stricture. In the absence of a stent, a nuclear medicine study or cholangiography (percutaneous or endoscopic approach) may be necessary to evaluate the biliary tree. Therapy involves drainage of the abscess, management of any identified biliary complications, and IV antibiotics directed at the most likely pathogens: aerobic Gram-negative bacilli (*E coli, Enterobacter, Pseudomonas*), some aerobic gram-positive cocci (group D *Streptococcus*), and anaerobes.

Fungal infections are a major cause of morbidity and death after all solid-organ transplants. Liver transplants are associated with the highest incidence of fungal infection, with some studies reporting an incidence of about 20%. The cause may be contamination from the biliary tract or small bowel during surgery. Most fungal infections are seen during the first 2 months posttransplant. Risk factors include preoperative renal dysfunction, prolonged duration of surgery, a retransplant, other reoperations, and CMV infection [56]. The vast majority of early fungal infections are secondary to *Candida* or *Aspergillus* species. Less common pathogens include *Cryptococcus* and *Trichosporon*, which are generally seen later in the transplant course because of chronic immunosuppression.

Viral infections generally are not seen until after the first posttransplant month. Common pathogens include CMV, Epstein–Barr virus (EBV), herpes simplex virus (HSV), and the hepatitis viruses (B and C). The mortality rate is generally not as high as with fungal and bacterial infections, yet viral pathogens account for significant morbidity. CMV is the most common pathogen involved. Its presentation ranges from asymptomatic infection to tissue-invasive disease. Asymptomatic infection is characterized by the shedding of virus in urine or saliva plus a change in the recipient's serostatus. CMV disease is suggested by the presence of the virus in the blood and by systemic symptoms such as fever, malaise, arthralgia, and leukopenia, with or without specific end-organ involvement (liver, lungs, bowel, eyes). Tissue-invasive CMV disease (TI-CMV) indicates organ involvement and presents as hepatitis, gastroenteritis, retinitis, or pneumonia.

The introduction and widespread use of IV ganciclovir has significantly altered the prognosis of CMV disease, which now is an uncommon cause of death posttransplant. Treatment with this drug at 10 mg per kg per day for 14 to 21 days posttransplant is effective, with minimal toxicity. Neutropenia may be seen, but usually responds to dose reduction or temporary discontinuation of the drug. If neutropenia remains a problem, then colony-stimulating factor (G-CSF) can be used. IV ganciclovir is also effective prophylaxis against CMV infections. Many different prophylaxis regimens are currently used, including high-dose oral acyclovir for 12 weeks posttransplant and, more recently, newer drugs such as oral ganciclovir, valacyclovir, and valganciclovir.

Viral hepatitis and liver transplantation are closely linked; hepatitis C is a common indication for a transplant. In the vast majority of liver recipients, however, disease eventually recurs in the new graft, representing a persistence or recurrence of preexisting infection. The risk of recurrence is now significantly lower for hepatitis B (versus C), but the former has a significantly worse prognosis. The risk of recurrence for hepatitis B depends in part on pretransplant replicative state. Recipients positive for hepatitis B viral DNA or hepatitis B e antigen have a higher risk of recurrence. Those with fulminant hepatitis B or coexisting hepatitis delta infection have lower recurrence rates. Once infection recurs, the course is characterized by rapid progression and eventual cirrhosis. A retransplant is generally not effective because of the very high recurrence rate in the second graft, especially if disease recurred in the first graft shortly posttransplant. Fortunately, recurrence rates are now very low due to the routine use of infection prophylaxis regimens which include long- and short-term administration of hepatitis B immunoglobulin with or without use of antiviral agents such as lamivudine [57].

Almost all patients transplanted for hepatitis C develop recurrent infection. The prognosis associated with recurrent hepatitis C is not as poor as with recurrent hepatitis B. Many liver recipients will show some histologic evidence of mild hepatic inflammation in the graft by 3 to 6 months posttransplant. However, only about 20% of them progress to cirrhosis requiring a retransplant. Unfortunately, prophylaxis regimens to prevent recurrent hepatitis C are not effective, and so recurrence of hepatitis C liver disease after transplant is becoming an increasingly important problem [58].

Gastrointestinal Complications. GI complications may occur as the direct result of a technical complication from the operation. Bile or enteric leaks from anastomoses can lead to generalized peritonitis or intra-abdominal abscesses. Other GI complications may result from the stress of the operation, an infection, or drug toxicity. Upper GI bleeding is usually secondary to peptic ulcer disease, persistent bleeding from esophageal varices, stress gastritis, or CMV gastroenteritis. Bleeding from gastric and esophageal varices usually settles quickly posttransplant. Persistent bleeding should trigger an assessment of the portal vein to rule out thrombosis or stenosis, which may be the underlying factor. If the recipient recently received sclerotherapy for variceal bleeding, the possibility of postsclerotherapy esophageal ulceration should be considered. Diffuse gastritis secondary to surgical stress is uncommon today, thanks to routine prophylaxis posttransplant with antacids, H2 antagonists, or proton pump inhibitors. Peptic ulcer disease remains a possible cause of upper GI bleeding. High-dose steroids seem to have some causal relationship to its development. Its incidence seems to be highest in the first month posttransplant, perhaps related to the time when steroid doses are generally highest. Ulcerations in the upper GI tract may also be due to infection. Severe esophagitis secondary to *Candida* can progress to frank ulceration with bleeding. Ulcerations may also be of viral origin, most notably CMV. Other unusual causes of GI bleeding are hemobilia after liver biopsy (incidence of 0.03%) and bleeding from the Roux en-Y anastomosis in patients who required choledochojejunostomy.

Lower GI bleeding posttransplant is often secondary to colitis, which is of infectious origin. Usually, opportunistic pathogens such as CMV, *Clostridium difficile*, and fungi (e.g., *Candida*) are responsible. Ulcers of noninfectious origin may also cause colonic bleeding, related to the high-dose steroids used in induction therapy.

Bowel perforation is a devastating complication associated with a high mortality rate. A high index of suspicion is required. The typical signs and symptoms associated with acute peritonitis, such as a high temperature and severe pain, may be masked or hidden by the effects of steroids. Perforation may be of the small or large bowel, with the latter associated with a higher mortality rate. Inadvertent or unrecognized injury to the bowel wall during the operation may later present as a perforation. Perforations may also be spontaneous; these are more common in children, generally occur 7 to 14 days posttransplant, and may be related to the high-dose steroids. As with perforation in nontransplant patients, early diagnosis with prompt reexploration is the best option. The leak can be repaired with irrigation of the abdominal cavity to decrease the degree of contamination.

INTESTINAL TRANSPLANTATION

Intestinal transplants have been performed in the laboratory for years. The first human intestinal transplant was performed in 1966. But it remained essentially an experimental procedure, with dismal results, well into the 1980s. Newer immunosuppressive drugs and advances in the surgical techniques have played a significant role in the successes with the procedure since the mid-1990s. Although intestinal transplants remain the least frequently performed of all transplants, graft survival rates have significantly improved and now approaching those seen with other types of extrarenal transplants. As the early problems with technical graft losses have diminished, immunologic and infectious issues have emerged as the main challenges facing the field today [59].

There are several reasons why the number of intestinal transplants has not increased as dramatically as the other transplants. As with kidney failure patients, a medical alternative exists for patients with intestinal failure, namely, long-term total parenteral nutrition (TPN). Unlike kidney failure patients, however, patients with intestinal failure have no survival advantage with a transplant (vs. medical therapy). Immunologically, the small intestine is the most difficult organ to transplant. It is populated with highly immunocompetent cells, perhaps explaining the reason for the high rejection rates and the need for higher levels of immunosuppression. Moreover, the intestinal lumen is filled with potential infective pathogens, which can gain access to the recipient's circulation if there is any breakdown of the mucosal barrier (which can occur with an acute rejection episode).

Pretransplant Evaluation

Intestinal failure is defined as the inability of the intestine to maintain nutrition or fluid and electrolyte balance without parenteral support. This most commonly results from extensive resection of the small bowel with resultant short bowel syndrome (SBS). Currently intestinal transplant is indicated for patients suffering from irreversible SBS who present with life-threatening complications secondary to the TPN or underlying disease. Traditional criteria for intestinal transplant in patients with SBS on TPN include (i) thrombosis of two major venous access sites, (ii) recurrent line infections and sepsis requiring hospitalization (more than two episodes per year), (iii) imminent liver failure related to TPN, and (iv) severe and frequent electrolyte imbalance and/or dehydration in spite of TPN [60]. At present, patients who are stable on TPN without such complications are generally not considered intestinal transplant candidates, because their estimated annual survival rate may be higher with TPN. However, as results continue to improve with transplant, this may be altered.

Other uncommon indications for intestinal transplant in patients with intestinal failure but without SBS are (i) severe myopathy or neuropathy of the GI tract (hollow visceral myopathy, total intestinal aganglionosis, pseudo-obstruction syndrome), (ii) gut malabsorption syndromes (microvillus inclusion disease, radiation enteritis, selective autoimmune enteropathy), (iii) neoplastic syndromes involving the root of the mesentery (neuroendocrine and desmoid tumors—usually associated with familial adenomatous polyposis or Gardener's syndrome), and (iv) diffuse portomesenteric thrombosis with high risk of GI bleeding [61].

The causes of intestinal failure are different in adult versus pediatric patients. In infants, gastroschisis (21%), volvulus (18%), and necrotizing enterocolitis (12%) account for more than half of the cases. On the other hand, mesenteric vascular thrombosis (22%), Crohn's disease (13%), and trauma (13%) are the most frequent causes of intestinal failure in the adult population [62,63]. Based on data from the International Intestinal Transplant Registry, approximately 60% of the recipients receiving an intestinal transplant had an underlying diagnosis of short bowel syndrome [59]. The development of SBS depends not only on the length of bowel resected, but also on the location of the resection, on the presence or absence of the ileocecal valve, and on the presence or absence of the colon. As a rough guideline, most patients can tolerate resection of 50% of their intestine with subsequent adaptation, avoiding the need for long-term parenteral nutritional support. Loss of greater than 70% of the intestine (considered ultra short gut syndrome), however, usually necessitates some type of parenteral nutritional support. The development of TPN-induced liver failure is much more rapid in children when compared to adults. For these reasons pediatric patients should be considered early for intestinal transplantation before development of irreversible liver injury [64].

The pretransplant evaluation is not too different from that for other transplants. A clear understanding of the anatomy of the patient's GI tract is essential. An upper GI tract series and abdominal CT scan are always necessary in order to plan GI tract reconstruction during the transplant. Hepatic function should be evaluated carefully and a transjugular or percutaneous liver biopsy is often required. If there is evidence of significant liver dysfunction and cirrhosis, a combined liver-intestine or multivisceral transplant may be indicated [65]. Patients with thrombotic disorders need specific hematologic tests to define hypercoagulable states (such as protein C and S deficiency, prothrombin G20210 A and factor V Leiden mutation, and hyperhomocysteinemia). A full abdominal visceral angiography and a comprehensive evaluation of upper and lower central venous system is mandatory in high-risk patients and those with thrombotic disorders. Absolute contraindications such as malignancy, active infection, marked cardiopulmonary insufficiency must be ruled out [62,63,66].

Recently, there has been an increased interest in performing isolated intestine procedures in recipients with early liver failure as there is mounting evidence to suggest that TPN-associated liver disease may be reversed with successful isolated intestine transplant [67,68]. Therefore, early referral of such patients is warranted to see if attempts can be made to salvage the liver.

Surgical Procedure

The indication for transplant and the choice of organs to include in the composite graft are defined by the baseline disease, recipient's anatomy, associated disease (such as diabetes, exocrine pancreatic insufficiency, and renal failure), and functional quality of other abdominal organs. The three most common types of transplants involving the small intestine include isolated intestinal transplantation, combined liver–intestine transplant, and multivisceral transplants [61–63].

The isolated intestine is the graft of choice for patients with irreversible gut failure that is limited to the small bowel. The vascular anastomoses are based on the superior mesenteric vessels. The outflow is usually achieved with the anastomosis of the superior mesenteric vein to the native superior mesenteric vein or splenic vein; however, in some cases a systemic drainage (inferior vena cava) is required. Systemic drainage will lead to certain metabolic abnormalities, but there is no good evidence to suggest that such abnormalities are of any obvious detriment to the recipient. In patients with combined pancreatic dysfunction (i.e., cystic fibrosis, type I diabetes and chronic pancreatitis) the inclusion of the pancreas should be considered. In living donation or in case of severe donor-to-recipient size mismatch (cadaveric adult to pediatric donation), a 200-cm length of the distal small bowel is used; inflow to the graft is via the ileocolic artery, and outflow via the ileocolic vein [61–63,69].

For a combined liver and intestinal transplant, the graft is usually procured intact with an aortic conduit, which contains both the celiac and superior mesenteric arteries. The common bile duct can be maintained intact in the hepatoduodenal ligament along with the first part of the duodenum and whole pancreas. Doing so avoids a biliary reconstruction in the recipient. A partial pancreatectomy, keeping a small rim of the head of the pancreas is also an alternative technique to avoid hilar dissection; however, this procedure has been abandoned by most centers, due to high risk of complications (i.e., pancreatitis and pancreatic fistulas). During the liver–small bowel transplant, the native stomach, duodenum, pancreas, and spleen are left intact and a portocaval shunt is always required for outflow reconstruction of the native organs [61–63].

The third type of transplant including the small bowel is the multivisceral transplant. In general, multivisceral grafts are those which contain a donor stomach, pancreas, and intestine. The common indications for multivisceral transplant include, but are not limited to, hollow visceral myopathy or neuropathy, pseudo-obstruction syndrome, extensive GI polyposis and total symptomatic splanchnic vascular thrombosis. The surgery encompasses the complete splanchnic evisceration and en bloc transplantation of stomach, duodenum, pancreas, liver, and small bowel (full multivisceral transplant). In some occasions, the right and transverse colon can also be included. In patients with preserved liver function, the native liver can be preserved (so called modified multivisceral transplant). In patients with established or impending renal failure, a renal graft (usually right kidney) can also be included in the multivisceral or liver–intestine allografts.

Several factors should be considered in appropriately matching the donor and recipient. Usually ABO-identical grafts are used; ABO nonidentical but compatible grafts are usually avoided because of the higher risk of graft-versus-host disease. Donors should usually be smaller than the recipients, as the latter usually have shrunken peritoneal cavities, and so a smaller graft may be more appropriate because of space constraints. Selective decontamination of the gut (amphotericin B, polymyxin B, and gentamicin) through a nasogastric tube should be attempted in all the donors. CMV enteritis can be a devastating problem in intestinal transplant recipients, and so, if possible, CMV seronegative recipients should receive organs from seronegative donors. Similar viral matching should be performed for EBV, if possible, because of the risk for PTLD [62,69–71].

The recipient operation varies, depending on the graft being implanted. The recipient's surgery is usually a complex procedure due to the presence of abdominal adhesions, stomas, gastrojejunostomies tubes, contracted abdominal cavity, and, in some cases, considerable portal hypertension (patients requiring combined allografts). Generally, arterial inflow to the graft is achieved using the recipient's infrarenal aorta to perform an end-to-side anastomosis (usually an interposition arterial graft is required). This technique is used for all the abovementioned grafts. The venous drainage is achieved either into the portal system or into the inferior vena cava. In full multivisceral or liver–intestine allografts, the venous drainage is established by piggy-back technique or by interpositioning the retrohepatic caval portion.

GI continuity can be achieved by a number of different methods. Commonly the proximal anastomosis of isolated intestine or liver–intestine is a side-to-side jejunojejunostomy. In multivisceral allografts (full or modified), the proximal anastomosis is performed between the stomach to the native esophagus or stomach stump. In multivisceral transplantation a pyloroplasty should be always performed to avoid delayed gastric emptying.

Gastrojejunostomy tubes are usually used permitting gastric decompression and enteral feeding in the early postoperative period. A Bishop–Koop enterostomy (chimney) or loop ileostomy are used to decompress the terminal ileum and to facilitate enteroscopies and biopsies, which is the only reliable method to monitor the allograft and diagnose acute rejection. Finally, the remaining recipient large intestine is anastomosed with the allograft roughly 20 cm proximal to the end ileostomy. Of note, cholecystectomy is performed in all the cases.

Postoperative Care

The early posttransplant care is, in many ways, similar to that of other transplant recipients. Initial care is usually in a critical care setting, so that fluid, electrolytes, and blood product replacement can be carefully monitored. Serial hemoglobin measurements are performed to look for any evidence of bleeding. Serum pH and lactate should also be monitored to look for evidence of intestinal ischemia or injury. In patients who received liver-intestine or multivisceral allografts, pancreatic enzymes and liver function tests should be assessed daily to track the organ functional status. Broad-spectrum antibiotics are routinely administered given the high risk for infectious complications. Routine prophylaxis should also be administered against CMV and EBV infection, especially in the seronegative recipient. Most centers usually use IV ganciclovir with or without the addition of CMV immunoglobulin. The gut decontaminant solution is given enterally, until the enteral feeding is started. Protozoal prophylaxis (i.e., *Pneumocystis* pneumonia) with trimethoprim–sulfamethoxazole should be started in the first week after transplant [62,63].

Immunosuppression should be initiated immediately after surgery. A number of different immunosuppressive protocols have been described. Most centers use lymphoid depleting agents, including Thymoglobulin or alemtuzumab for induction therapy, followed by a tacrolimus-based maintenance regimen [70,71].

Regardless of the protocol, intestinal transplants clearly have a high risk of rejection (incidence of 30% to 50% in the first 90 days after the transplant). It is very important to differentiate enteritis (mostly caused by *Clostridium difficile*, adenovirus, cytomegalovirus and calicivirus) from rejection, since both conditions may be characterized by diarrhea (or increased stoma output), abdominal pain, and low-grade fever. Therefore, careful evaluation of an intestinal biopsy by an experienced pathologist is always necessary. In addition to routine and regular endoscopy and biopsy, other noninvasive markers of intestinal rejection have been described. Recently studies have shown that several molecules, such as calprotectin and citrulline (measured in the stools and blood, respectively), are reliable markers of moderate and severe intestinal rejection [66]. Acute rejection episodes are often associated with infections. Rejection results in damage to the intestinal mucosa, leading to impaired mucosal barrier function and bacterial translocation. Therefore, advanced rejection can be very difficult to treat.

The switch from parenteral to enteral nutrition is gradual and usually occurs in the first 2 weeks after transplant. Antidiarrheic or prokinetic agents are used to modulate the stoma output after transplant, once rejection or enteritis is ruled out.

Short-term results have improved dramatically, mainly due to improvements in surgical technique and in immunosuppression [61,69,71]. Nonetheless, intestinal transplants are still associated with a high complication rate. Potential complications include enteric leaks with generalized peritonitis or localized intra-abdominal abscesses, graft thrombosis, respiratory infections, and life-threatening hemorrhage.

Infectious complications are, unfortunately, very common in intestinal transplant recipients. There are several factors that contribute to this. The intestinal graft itself is a significant source of bacteria, and any process which compromises containment of these bacteria (such as rejection or anastomotic leak) can lead to a systemic infection. Because of the higher risk of rejection, and the consequences associated with rejection, intestinal transplant recipients generally receive higher levels of immunosuppression compared with other organ recipients, usually in a greater immunosuppressed state. Bacteria can translocate from the graft directly into the peritoneal cavity itself, leading to bacterial peritonitis. Bacteria can also spread directly into the portal circulation, and subsequently disseminate to other sites. Besides bacterial infections, viral infections with CMV, EBV, or adenovirus are also more common in intestinal transplant recipients.

Outcomes

According to the UNOS Database, 1,785 intestinal transplants have been performed in the United States since 1990 (UNOS/OPTN, www.optn.transplant.hrsa.gov/, accessed August, 2009). Currently, only eight Medicare-approved centers in the United States perform intestinal/multivisceral transplant. However, 29 centers throughout the country are listed in the International Intestinal Transplant Registry as active small bowel transplant centers [59,60].

Over the past 15 years, there has been a remarkable improvement in short-term patient and graft survival. This is a result of combination of advances in surgical techniques, immunosuppressive strategies, and postoperative management. The 1-year graft and patient survival rates are now about 80%, with no significant difference between the different types of allografts. In spite of the significant improvement of short-term survival, the 5-year survival rate has remained stable at approximately 60%, and the presence of the liver in the composite allograft (liver–intestine and full multivisceral transplants) is associated with a significant improvement in the long-term survival. The most common causes of graft loss and patient death are quite similar and include rejection, technical failure, and infection/sepsis. Other causes of graft loss and death are post-transplant lymphoproliferative disorders (lymphomas), graft-versus-host disease, and pancreatitis (in combined allografts) [61,70,71].

SUMMARY

Care of liver and intestinal transplant recipients, before, during, and after surgery is a significant challenge. The potential is great for an array of complicated medical and surgical problems. Despite dramatic advances in the field, these procedures remain major undertakings with the possibility of complications affecting every major organ system. A systematic approach is necessary to prevent, minimize, and manage these complications. Intensive medical care in an ICU setting may be necessary even pretransplant, especially in patients with fulminant hepatic failure or severely decompensated chronic liver disease. Optimizing the overall medical status of the transplant candidates with chronic liver failure is essential to minimize the likelihood of postoperative problems. Immediately posttransplant, intensive monitoring—with diligent attention to all organ systems—is necessary to ensure a successful outcome. A thorough knowledge of potential complications is required to allow for rapid diagnosis and appropriate treatment.

Improvements in the care of these patients during the critical perioperative period, along with better immunosuppressive regimens, have allowed for remarkable advances (Table 187.4). A liver transplant is the only real treatment of choice for patients with acute and chronic end-stage liver disease. Most centers now report 1-year patient survival rates of about 85% and 5-year survival rates of more than 70%. Intestinal transplants are becoming an increasingly used option for patients with intestinal failure. As results continue to improve, this will become an alternative option to long-term maintenance therapy with TPN. For both liver and intestinal transplants, the future will likely see further improvements in results (with refinements in surgical and preservation techniques and with newer drugs to treat rejection and infections). Care of these patients in the critical perioperative period, however, will remain a crucial aspect of ensuring a successful outcome.

TABLE 187.4

MAJOR ADVANCES OR CHANGES IN THE LIVER TRANSPLANTATION FIELD OVER THE LAST 10 YEARS

Topic	Change	Reference
Allocation system	MELD/PELD utilized widely in the United States with evidence-based analysis showing it to improve patient survival	[10]
Indications for transplant	Extended tumor criteria outside of Milan criteria with equivalent results—for example, UCSF criteria	[16,17]
Surgical technique	Growth in adult-to-adult living donor transplant Donor morbidity for above estimated at 30%–35%	[28,29]
Increasing the donor pool	Increasing use of marginal donors nonheart beating donors, and split livers to expand the donor pool	[7,33,34]
Viral recurrence	Effective prophylaxis regimens to significantly decrease the risk of hepatitis B recurrence after transplant Hepatitis C recurrence becoming an increasing problem	[57,58]

References

1. Moore FD, Wheeler HB, Demissianos HV, et al: Experimental whole organ transplantation of the liver and of the spleen. *Ann Surg* 152:3740, 1960.
2. Starzl TE, Marchioro TL, Von Kaulla KN, et al: Homotransplant of the liver in humans. *Surg Gynecol Obstet* 117:659, 1963.
3. Starzl TE, Iwatsuki S, Von Thiel DH: Evolution of orthotopic liver transplant. *Hepatology* 2:613, 1982.
4. Calne RY, White DJG, Evans DB, et al: Cyclosporin A in cadaveric organ transplantation. *BMJ* 282:934, 1981.
5. Belzer FO, D'Alessandro AM, Hoffman RM, et al: The use of UW solution in clinical transplantation. A 4 year experience. *Ann Surg* 215(6):579–583, 1992.
6. UNOS/OPTN data. http://optn.transplant.hrsa.gov/data. Accessed August 20, 2009.
7. Selck FW, Grossman EB, Ratner LE, et al: Utilization, outcomes, and retransplantation of liver allografts from donation after cardiac death: implications for further expansion of the deceased-donor pool. *Ann Surg* 248(4):599–607, 2008.
8. Reich DJ, Mulligan DC, Abt PL, et al: ASTS recommended practice guidelines for controlled donation after cardiac death organ procurement and transplantation. *Am J Transplant* 9(9):2004–2011, 2009.
9. de Vera ME, Lopez-Solis R, Dvorchik I, et al: Liver transplantation using donation after cardiac death donors: long-term follow-up from a single center. *Am J Transplant* 9(4):773–781, 2009.
10. Weisner R: Evidence-bound evolution of the MELD/PELD liver allocation policy. *Liver Transpl* 11(3):261–263, 2005.
11. Obermayer-Straub P, Strassburg CP, Manns MP: Autoimmune hepatitis. *J Hepatol* 32[1, Suppl]:181–197, 2000.
12. Dawwas MF, Gimson AE: Candidate selection and organ allocation in liver transplantation. *Semin Liver Dis* 29(1):40–52, 2009.
13. Stiehl A, Benz C, Sauer P: Primary sclerosing cholangitis. *Can J Gastroenterol* 14(4):311–315, 2000.
14. Brewer GJ: Recognition, diagnosis, and management of Wilson's disease. *Proc Soc Exp Biol Med* 223(1):39–46, 2000.
15. Mazzaferro V, Regalia E, Doci R, et al: Liver transplantation for the treatment of small hepatocellular carcinomas in patients with cirrhosis. *N Engl J Med* 334(11):693–699, 1996.
16. Yao FY, Ferrell L, Bass NM, et al: Liver transplantation for hepatocellular carcinoma: comparison of the proposed UCSF criteria with the Milan criteria and the Pittsburgh modified TNM criteria. *Liver Transpl* 8(9):765–774, 2002.
17. Yao FY, Kerlan RK Jr, Hirose R, et al: Excellent outcome following downstaging of hepatocellular carcinoma prior to liver transplantation: an intention-to-treat analysis. *Hepatology* 48(3):819–827, 2008.
18. Ostapowicz G, Lee WM: Acute hepatic failure: a Western perspective. *J Gastroenterol Hepatol* 15(5):480–488, 2000.
19. Williams R: Classification, etiology, and considerations of outcome in acute liver failure. *Semin Liver Dis* 16(4):343–348, 1996.
20. O'Grady JG, Alexander GJM, Mayllar KM, et al: Early indicators of prognosis in fulminant hepatic failure. *Gastroenterology* 97:439, 1989.
21. Koulaouzidis A, Bhat S, Saeed AA: Spontaneous bacterial peritonitis. *World J Gastroenterol* 15(9):1042–1049, 2009.
22. McDiarmid SV, Merion RM, Dykstra DM, et al: Selection of pediatric candidates under the PELD system. *Liver Transpl* 10[10 Suppl 2]:S23–S30, 2004.
23. Rolando N, Harvey F, Brahm J, et al: Fungal infection: a common, unrecognized complication of acute liver failure. *J Hepatol* 12:1, 1991.
24. Singh C, Sager JS: Pulmonary complications of cirrhosis. *Med Clin North Am* 93(4):871–883, 2009.
25. Grande L, Rimola A, Cugat E, et al: Effect of venovenous bypass on perioperative renal function in liver transplantation: results of a randomized, controlled trial. *Hepatology* 23(6):1418, 1996.
26. Kuo PC, Alfrey EJ, Garcia G, et al: Orthotopic liver transplantation with selective use of venovenous bypass. *Am J Surg* 170(6):671, 1995.
27. Porte RJ, Molenaar IQ, Begliomini B, et al: Aprotinin and transfusion requirements in orthotopic liver transplantation: a Multicenter randomized double-blind study. EMSALT Study Group. *Lancet.* 355(9212):1303–1309, 2000.
28. Trotter JF, Wachs M, Everson GT, et al: Adult-to-adult transplantation of the right hepatic lobe from a living donor. *N Engl J Med* 346(14):1074—1082, 2002.
29. Brown R Jr, Russo M, Lai M, et al: A survey of liver transplantation from living adult donors in the United States. *N Engl J Med* 348(9):818–825, 2003.
30. Wachs ME, Bak JTE, Karrer FM, et al: Adult living donor liver transplantation using a right hepatic lobe. *Transplantation* 66(10):1313–1316, 1998.
31. Malago M, Molmenti EP, Paul A, et al: Hepatic venous outflow reconstruction in right live donor liver transplantation. *Liver Transpl* 11(3):364–365, 2005.
32. Marcos A, Fisher RA, Ham JM, et al: Right lobe living donor liver transplantation. *Transplantation* 68(6):798–803, 1999.
33. Renz JF, Emond JC, Yersiz H, et al: Split-liver transplantation in the United States: outcomes of a national survey. *Ann Surg* 239(2):172–181, 2004.
34. Humar A, Ramcharan T, Sielaff T, et al: Split liver transplantation for 2 adult recipients: an initial experience. *Am J Transpl* 1(4):366–372, 2001.
35. Feng S, Goodrich NP, Bragg-Gresham JL, et al: Characteristics associated with liver graft failure: the concept of a donor risk index. *Am J Transplant* 6(4):783–790, 2006.
36. Pageaux GP, Calmus Y, Boillot O, et al: Steroid withdrawal at day 14 after liver transplantation: a double-blind, placebo-controlled study. *Liver Transpl* 10(12):1454–1460, 2004.
37. Datsis K, Golling M, Ioannidis P, et al: Vascular complications following 200 liver transplants. *Transplant Proc* 27(5):2607, 1995.
38. Bekker J, Ploem S, de Jong KP: Early hepatic artery thrombosis after liver transplantation: a systematic review of the incidence, outcome and risk factors. *Am J Transplant* 9(4):746–757, 2009.
39. Ozaki CF, Katz SM, Monsour HP Jr, et al: Vascular reconstructions in living-related liver transplantation. *Transplant Proc* 26:167, 1994.
40. Lerut J, Tzakis AG, Bron KM, et al: Complications of venous reconstruction in human orthotopic liver transplantation. *Ann Surg* 205:404, 1987.
41. Tung BY, Kimmey MB: Biliary complications of orthotopic liver transplantation. *Dig Dis* 17(3):133–144, 1999.
42. Colonna JO II, Shaked A, Gomes AS, et al: Biliary strictures complicating liver transplantation: incidence, pathogenesis, management and outcome. *Ann Surg* 216:536, 1992.
43. Maring JK, Klompmaker IJ, Zwaveling JH, et al: Poor initial graft function after orthotopic liver transplantation: can it be predicted and does it affect outcome? An analysis of 125 adult primary transplantations. *Clin Transplant* 11:373–379, 1997.
44. Greig PD, Woolf GM, Sinclair SB, et al: Treatment of primary liver graft nonfunction with prostaglandin E_1. *Transplantation* 48(3):447, 1989.
45. Kamath GS, Plevak DJ, Wiesner RH, et al: Primary non-function of the liver graft: when should we retransplant? *Transplant Proc* 23(3):1954, 1991.
46. Gyr K, Meier R: Flumazenil in the treatment of portal systemic encephalopathy—an overview. *Intensive Care Med* 17:539, 1991.
47. Bronster DJ, Emre S, Boccagni P, et al: Central nervous system complications in liver transplant recipients–incidence, timing, and long-term follow-up. *Clin Transplant* 14(1):1–7, 2000.
48. Bartynski WS, Tan HP, Boardman JF, et al: Posterior reversible encephalopathy syndrome after solid organ transplantation. *AJNR Am J Neuroradiol* 29(5):924–930, 2008.
49. O'Brien JD, Ettinger NA: Pulmonary complications of liver transplantation. *Clin Chest Med* (1):99, 1996.
50. McAlister VC, Grant DR, Roy A, et al: Right phrenic nerve injury in orthotopic liver transplantation. *Transplantation* 55:826, 1993.
51. Herve P, Le Pavec J, Sztrymf B, et al: Pulmonary vascular abnormalities in cirrhosis. *Best Pract Res Clin Gastroenterol* 21(1):141–159, 2007.
52. Krowka MJ, Cortese DA: Hepatopulmonary syndrome. *Chest* 105:1528, 1994.
53. Pascual E, Gomez-Arnau J, Pensado A, et al: Incidence and risk factors of early acute renal failure in liver transplant patients. *Transplant Proc* 25(2):1837, 1993.
54. Garcia-Tsao G, Parikh CR, Viola A: Acute kidney injury in cirrhosis. *Hepatology* 48(6):2064–2077, 2008.
55. D'Amico G: Renal involvement in hepatitis C infection: cryoglobulinemic glomerulonephritis. *Kidney Int* 54:650–671, 1998.
56. Collins LA, Samore MH, Roberts MS, et al: Risk factors for invasive fungal infections complicating orthotopic liver transplantation. *J Infect Dis* 170:644, 1994.
57. Seehofer D, Berg T: Prevention of hepatitis B recurrence after liver transplantation. *Transplantation* 80[1 Suppl]:120–124, 2005.
58. Rodriguez-Luna H, Vargas HE: Management of hepatitis C virus infection in the setting of liver transplantation. *Liver Transpl* 11(5):479–489, 2005.
59. http://www.intestinaltransplant.org. Accessed August 20, 2009.
60. CMS: Medicare national coverage determinations: intestinal and multivisceral transplantation, 2006. Available from www.cms.hhs.gov/transmittals/downloads/R58NCD.pdf. Accessed August 20, 2009.
61. Fishbein TM: Intestinal transplantation. *N Engl J Med* 361(10):998–1008, 2009.
62. Abu-Elmagd K, Bond G: Gut failure and abdominal visceral transplantation. *Proc Nutr Soc.* 62(3):727–737, 2003.
63. Kato T, Ruiz P, Thompson JF, et al: Intestinal and multivisceral transplantation. *World J Surg* 26(2):226–237, 2002.
64. Goulet O, Joly F, Corriol O, et al: Some new insights in intestinal failure-associated liver disease. *Curr Opin Organ Transplant* 14(3):256–261, 2009.
65. Diamanti A, Gambarara M, Knafelz D, et al: Prevalence of liver complications in pediatric patients on home parenteral nutrition: indications for intestinal or combined liver-intestinal transplantation. *Transplant Proc* 35(8):3047–3049, 2003.
66. Selvaggi G, Tzakis AG: Small bowel transplantation: technical advances/updates. *Curr Opin Organ Transplant.* 14(3):262–266, 2009.

67. Fisbein TN, Kaufman SS, Florman SS, et al: Isolated intestinal transplantation: proof of clinical efficacy. *Transplantation* 76(4):636, 2003.
68. Sudan DL, Kafman SS, Shaw BW Jr, et al: Isolated intestinal transplantation for intestine failure. *Am J Gastroenterol* 95(6):1506, 2000.
69. Pascher A, Kohler S, Neuhaus P, et al: Present status and future perspectives of intestinal transplantation. *Transpl Int* 21(5):401–414, 2008.
70. Abu-Elmagd KM, Costa G, Bond GJ, et al: Evolution of the immunosuppressive strategies for the intestinal and multivisceral recipients with special reference to allograft immunity and achievement of partial tolerance. *Transpl Int* 22(1):96–109, 2009.
71. Abu-Elmagd KM, Costa G, Bond GJ, et al: Five hundred intestinal and multivisceral transplantations at a single center: major advances with new challenges. *Ann Surg* 250(4):567–581, 2009.

CHAPTER 188 ■ HEMATOPOIETIC CELL TRANSPLANTATION

PAUL A. CARPENTER, MARCO MIELCAREK AND ANN E. WOOLFREY

GENERAL PRINCIPLES

Hematopoietic cell transplantation (HCT) typically is performed in patients with life-threatening disorders of the hematopoietic system. The procedure has considerable risks of transplant-related morbidity and mortality with a substantial proportion of patients requiring intensive medical care [1,2] (Fig. 188.1). Thus, knowledge of the basic principles of the transplant procedure and an understanding of potential complications including their differential diagnosis are important for improving the outcome of critically ill patients after transplantation.

HCT is potentially curative treatment for diseases including leukemia, lymphoma, myelodysplasia, multiple myeloma, aplastic anemia, hemoglobinopathies, and congenital immune deficiencies. In selected cases, HCT may also have a role in the treatment of solid tumors such as germ cell tumors, renal cell cancer, and breast cancer, and as a type of immunosuppression for patients with life-threatening autoimmune diseases (Table 188.1). In preparation for HCT, high-dose chemotherapy alone, or combined with irradiation therapy, is used to eradicate the underlying disease and to induce transient immunosuppression in the recipient to prevent graft rejection, a possible complication mediated by immunologic host-versus-graft reactions after allogeneic HCT. High-dose chemoradiation is followed by intravenous infusion of the graft, which contains hematopoietic stem cells (HSCs) that home to the bone marrow and reconstitute the hematopoietic system of the patient. In contrast to autologous HCT, allogeneic HCT requires prophylactic immunosuppressive therapy after transplant to prevent or mitigate graft-versus-host disease (GVHD), an inflammatory syndrome that primarily affects the skin, gastrointestinal (GI) tract, and liver.

Classification

HCT can be categorized according to the source of stem cells, the type of donor, or the intensity of the preparative regimen. The type of HCT used in an individual patient is a complex decision based on the patient's age, diagnosis, disease stage, prior treatments, donor availability, and presence of comorbidities.

Stem Cell Source

HSCs capable of reconstituting hematopoiesis in recipients given myeloablative therapy can be obtained from bone marrow, peripheral blood, or umbilical cord blood (UCB). The stem cell products obtained from each of these sources are characterized by distinct kinetics of engraftment and recovery of immune function after transplantation. These features may affect the risks of developing infectious complications and GVHD during the posttransplant period.

Bone Marrow. Bone marrow was historically the most common source of stem cells for HCT but is now used very infrequently for autologous HCT. Bone marrow is harvested from the iliac crest under general anesthesia, from appropriate volunteer donors. Engraftment after bone marrow transplant is evidenced by rising neutrophil and platelet counts and occurs between 3 and 4 weeks after transplant.

"Mobilized" Peripheral Blood. Growth factor–mobilized peripheral blood stem cells (PBSC) are the predominant source of HSC for allogeneic HCT in adults and are almost always used as HSC rescue for autologous HCT [3]. PBSCs are recognized on the basis of their expression of the CD34 surface marker and can be collected from the blood by a semiautomated procedure called leukapheresis. To promote peripheral blood mobilization of PBSC for autologous HCT, patients typically receive chemotherapy followed by administration of G-CSF, which has the benefit of chemotherapy-mediated tumor debulking prior to stem cell collection [4]. For allogeneic HCT, PBSCs are mobilized from healthy donors using growth factor alone.

Engraftment after PBSC transplantation occurs approximately 1 week earlier compared with bone marrow transplantation, which is likely related to the greater proliferative potential of stem and progenitor cells in PBSC. PBSC allografts contain approximately 10 times more T cells than marrow, which influences the development of GVHD, graft rejection, and rate of relapse for malignancies after HCT [5]. Randomized studies of allografts donated from HLA-matched siblings have shown a higher risk for relapse and lower risk for chronic GVHD among recipients of marrow compared with PBSC [3,6].

Umbilical Cord Blood. UCB contains HSC sufficient for reconstitution of hematopoiesis, which can be collected from the placenta and umbilical cord immediately after delivery of a baby. UCB banking has increased the likelihood of donor availability for patients with rare HLA haplotypes. T cells contained in UCB are immunologically naive, which allows for less stringent HLA matching between donor and recipient. The number of HSC contained in a typical UCB unit is several orders of

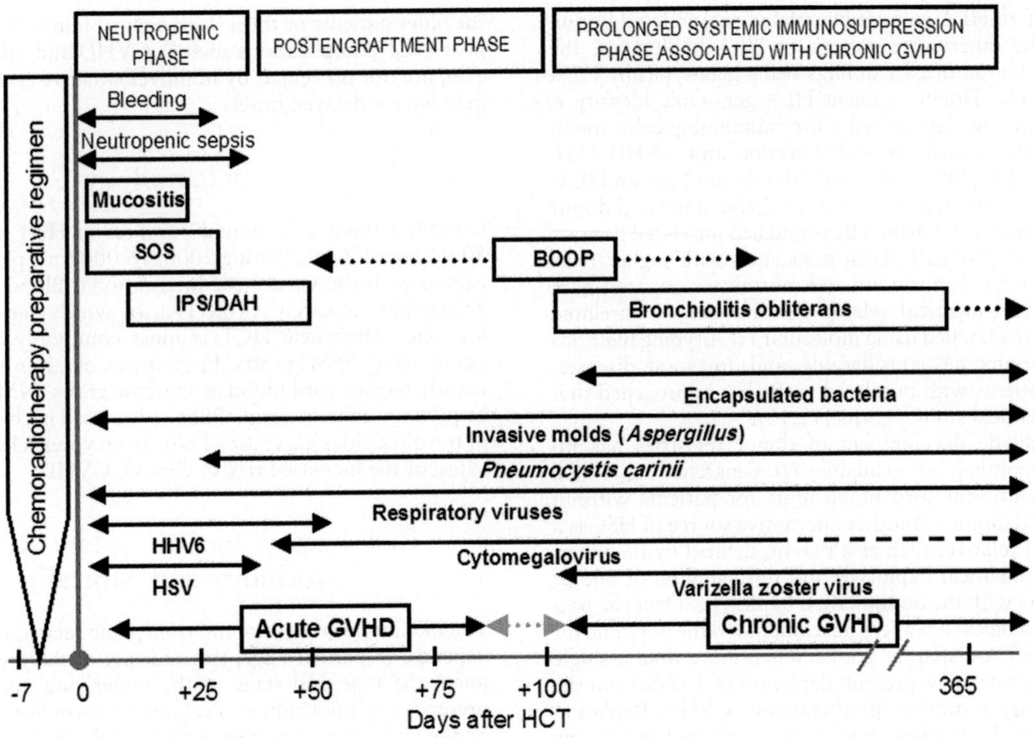

FIGURE 188.1. Complications after myeloablative allogeneic hematopoietic cell transplantation. BOOP, bronchiolitis obliterans with organizing pneumonia; DAH, diffuse alveolar hemorrhage; GVHD, graft-versus-host disease; HHV6, human herpes virus 6; HSV, herpes simplex virus; IPS, idiopathic pneumonia syndrome; SOS, sinusoidal obstruction syndrome.

TABLE 188.1

INDICATIONS FOR ALLOGENEIC OR AUTOLOGOUS TRANSPLANTS

Allogeneic	Autologous
High-risk acute leukemia Acute myeloid leukemia Acute lymphoblastic leukemia	High-risk lymphoma Non-Hodgkin's lymphoma Hodgkin's lymphoma
Chronic leukemia Chronic myeloid leukemia Chronic lymphocytic leukemia	Multiple myeloma
Juvenile myelomonocytic leukemia	Solid tumors Neuroblastoma Poor-risk breast cancer Poor-risk sarcoma
Chronic myelomonocytic leukemia	Investigational Other poor-prognosis tumors Refractory autoimmune disorders
Myelodysplastic syndromes	
Bone marrow failure syndromes Severe aplastic anemia	
Severe immunodeficiency syndromes	
Inborn errors of metabolism	
Hemoglobinopathies Thalassemia major Symptomatic sickle cell disease	

magnitude lower compared with typical bone marrow or PBSC harvests. The smaller number of HSC may result in delayed engraftment, increased risk for graft rejection, and infection [7,8]. Recent studies have shown that infusion of two UCB units increases the total number of HSC, which seems to decrease the risk of graft rejection, thus giving adults as well as children the option of UCB transplantation [9].

Donor Type

Autologous. Transplantation of HSC donated by the patient is termed autologous HCT. Most commonly, autologous PBSC are cryopreserved and then thawed and reinfused once the high-dose preparative therapy has been completed. High-dose chemoradiation is given to kill tumor cells that may not be susceptible to conventional-dose cytotoxic therapy. The success of the autologous transplant procedures relies exclusively on the tumor-eradicating potential of the preparative regimen [10]. The effect the conditioning regimen has on extrahematopoietic tissues determines the dose-limiting toxicity of the procedure. Relapse after autologous HCT may occur from tumor cells that have survived the conditioning therapy or from those that contaminated the graft, although the former mechanism appears to be more important.

Syngeneic. Transplantation of HSCs donated from identical (monozygotic) twins is termed syngeneic HCT. When there is no genetic disparity between donor and recipient, the biology of the transplant is similar to autologous HCT. Compared with allogeneic HCT from HLA-matched related or unrelated donors, relapse rates are higher after syngeneic HCT, which has been attributed to the absence of malignancy-eradicating graft-versus-host reactions.

Allogeneic. Transplantation of HSCs cells donated by another individual is termed allogeneic HCT. Allogeneic HCT requires availability of an HLA-compatible related or unrelated donor. Because of the inheritance pattern of HLA haplotypes, the statistical likelihood of two siblings being genotypically HLA identical is 25%. Donor-recipient HLA genotypic identity is associated with the lowest risks for immunologically mediated complications such as graft rejection and GVHD [11]. For approximately 70% of patients who do not have an HLA-identical sibling donor, a search for a suitable unrelated donor can be considered. HCT from HLA-matched unrelated donors, however, has traditionally been associated with higher risks of transplant-related morbidity and mortality compared with HCT from HLA-identical related donors. Use of unrelated donors who are matched using molecular HLA typing methods can improve outcomes considerably, and, for some diseases, survival of patients with unrelated grafts has approached that with HLA-identical sibling grafts [12,13].

The worldwide development of donor registries has increased the number of available HLA-matched unrelated donors and umbilical cord blood units for patients without suitable related donors. Another alternative source of HSC is a haploidentical relative, such as a parent, defined by the inheritance of one identical haplotype and mismatching of one or more HLA loci with the noninherited haplotype. Over the past decade, technological advances have improved the outcome for recipients of HLA-disparate grafts. When more than a single HLA antigen disparity is present, depletion of T cells from the graft is necessary to prevent life-threatening GVHD. Depletion of T cells from the marrow may be accomplished ex vivo by using immunologic or physical methods to target T cells for removal. Because T cells play an important role in establishment of the graft, early immune reconstitution, and tumor control, T-cell depletion has been associated with higher rates of graft failure, opportunistic infections, and relapse. Strategies to selectively deplete alloreactive T cells remain an active area of research.

Intensity of the Preparative Regimen

Myeloablative

In myeloablative HCT, the preparative regimen ablates the hematopoietic system of the patient and leads to transient but profound myelosuppression with pancytopenia. The transplanted hematopoietic cells reconstitute the ablated hematopoietic system in the recipient. High-dose chemotherapy regimens, with or without doses of total body irradiation (TBI) that exceed 6 Gy, combine different drug combinations that have nonadditive toxicities with radiation. The aim of high-dose therapy is to overcome the genetic heterogeneity of tumors by employing agents with different mechanisms of action. Although the myeloablative regimens used for autologous HCT typically consist of drugs that provide maximum tumor eradication with tolerable toxicity to the patient, regimens used for allogeneic HCT also must provide sufficient recipient immunosuppression to prevent graft rejection. Myeloablative preparative regimens are associated with substantial risks of transplant-related toxicity and mortality, particularly among older or medically ill patients [14].

Nonmyeloablative

Nonmyeloablative preparative regimens for allogeneic HCT are mainly immunosuppressive and aimed at preventing graft rejection. The underlying malignancy is eliminated through the ensuing immunologic graft-versus-tumor effects, provided the tumor expresses antigens that make it a target for immune attack. Compared with myeloablative allogeneic HCT, the extrahematopoietic toxicity from nonmyeloablative preparative regimens is considerably milder, an important consideration for older patients or those with comorbidities [15,16]. Typical post-HCT complications such as GVHD and infections, however, are not prevented by nonmyeloablative conditioning but may have a delayed onset.

Epidemiology

Current estimates of annual numbers of HCT are 45,000 to 50,000 worldwide. During 2006, 16,000 transplants were registered with the Center for International Blood and Marrow Transplant Research (CIBMTR), of which one-half were allogeneic. Allogeneic HCT is most commonly performed in adults using PBSC grafts. In contrast, children now predominantly receive cord blood or marrow grafts (NMDP Web site: http://www.marrow.org/). PBSC is less used in children because of the difficulties harvesting PBSC from young children and because of the increased risk of chronic GVHD.

Risk Factors for Transplant-Related Morbidity and Mortality

The likelihood of developing transplant-related complications depends on patient's age, the intensity of the preparative regimen, the type and stage of the underlying disease, and the presence of comorbidities. Prognosis is most heavily influenced by the underlying disorder. Patients with chronic malignancies and nonmalignant disorders, such as aplastic anemia, have a higher likelihood of survival compared to those with aggressive malignancies, who have a greater tendency to relapse following HCT. Mortality caused by the transplant procedure, and not from disease relapse, termed transplant-related mortality, ranges from 15% to 40% for allogeneic HCT recipients compared to 5% to 10% for autologous HCT recipients. HLA disparity between donor and recipient increases the risk of transplant-related mortality owing to the greater likelihood of developing GVHD and graft rejection. The risk for mortality increases significantly with age, although improvements in supportive care and donor selection and the introduction of nonmyeloablative preparative regimens have increased the proportion of patients older than 60 years who benefit from allogeneic HCT. Recent studies have demonstrated that pretransplant assessment of comorbidities using simple but transplant-specific comorbidity scoring systems has improved the ability to predict subsequent transplant-related mortality and survival [14,17].

TRANSPLANT-RELATED COMPLICATIONS

Transplanted-related complications include infections, regimen-related toxicity (RRT), and complications associated with alloreactivity. More intense conditioning regimens and higher degrees of donor-recipient HLA disparity are associated with greater risk for infection. Regimen-related toxicities include profound cytopenias and organ damage that follow myeloablative conditioning. The complications seen after allogeneic HCT that may occur irrespective of the intensity of the conditioning regimen include rejection, GVHD, and hemolysis.

Regimen-Related Pancytopenia

Reconstitution of hematopoiesis after HCT occurs in an orderly pattern; in general, neutrophil recovery occurs first, followed by recovery of platelets and red blood cells. The tempo of hematopoietic reconstitution varies according to the type of HSC product, being earlier after PBSC grafts and later after UCB grafts, compared with marrow grafts. Transfusions of platelets and red blood cells often are needed until there is marrow recovery. Transfusion of red blood cells should be determined by the clinical condition of the patient, including hemodynamic stability and presence of active hemorrhage. Red blood cell transfusions generally are indicated when the hemoglobin falls below 8 g per dL. Platelet transfusions are indicated when the platelet count falls below 10,000 cells per μL to minimize the risk for spontaneous bleeding [18,19]. Transfusions thresholds should be increased before invasive procedures or in patients with bleeding to a level appropriate for any other intensive care unit (ICU) patient [18]. Platelet consumption may be increased in patients with fever, disseminated intravascular coagulation (DIC), or splenomegaly. Patients who have become alloimmunized to platelet antigens demonstrate poor response to platelet transfusions and may achieve higher platelet counts by limiting the number of donor exposures, controlling fever or DIC, using platelet products that are less than 48 hours old, or use of nonpooled (single-donor) or HLA-matched platelets [20,21].

Precautions should be taken in preparation of blood products for transfusion into HCT patients because passenger lymphocytes pose a risk for generating GVHD and latent viruses may be transferred through leukocytes. Except for the stem cell graft, all other components should be irradiated at a dose of 1,500 to 3,000 cGy to inactivate or eliminate contaminating lymphocytes. Depletion of leukocytes or use of blood components that test seronegative for cytomegalovirus (CMV) is effective for prevention of CMV transmission to CMV-seronegative recipients [21]. Removal of white blood cells from platelet and red blood cell products also decreases the risk for alloimmunization of the patient [22].

Regimen-Related Toxicity

High-dose cytotoxic chemotherapy with or without doses of TBI exceeding 6 Gy may severely disrupt mucosal integrity and has the potential to cause RRT in the skin, GI tract, liver, bladder, lung, heart, kidney, and nervous system. RRT occurs predominantly within the first 3 to 4 weeks after conditioning [23] and is more common after myeloablative than nonmyeloablative conditioning. RRT increases the risk for opportunistic infection, which is already high because of concomitant profound immunosuppression and regimen-related cytopenias. This section will focus on the noninfectious complications of individual organs specifically attributable to conditioning toxicity. Opportunistic infection or, after allografting, GVHD must strongly be considered as etiologies for organ dysfunction in the differential diagnosis of RRT. These alternative diagnoses are covered elsewhere under the appropriate subsection.

Skin

Generalized skin erythema is common after doses of TBI exceeding 12 Gy but is self-limiting and rarely associated with skin breakdown. Regimens that contain cytosine arabinoside (Ara-C), thiotepa, busulfan, etoposide, and carmustine may also cause erythema. Hyperpigmentation typically follows the inflammatory dermatitis, with skin folds often being particularly noticeable. Skin biopsies during the first 3 weeks after transplant often show nonspecific inflammatory changes irrespective of cause, making them frequently unhelpful in distinguishing between RRT, drug allergies, or acute GVHD [24].

Gastrointestinal Tract

Mucositis. Most patients who receive high-dose conditioning regimens develop mucositis. Symptoms include inflammation, desquamation, and edema of the oral and pharyngeal epithelial tissue that typically presents within the first several days after HCT and usually resolves by the third week. Anorexia, nausea, or other intestinal symptoms that persist after day 21 are more likely to be caused by GVHD or infection. Severe mucositis places patients at risk for aspiration and occasionally airway compromise, indicating the need for endotracheal intubation. Damage to the mucosa of the lower GI tract results in secretory diarrhea, cramping abdominal pain, and anorexia, and it facilitates translocation of intestinal bacteria with sepsis [23,25].

Mucositis is treated supportively with total parenteral nutrition, administration of intravenous fluids, and intravenous narcotics for pain control. It is important to recognize an iatrogenic narcotic bowel syndrome, characterized by abdominal pain and bowel dilatation, which occasionally may be a side effect of efforts to control painful symptoms of mucositis or sinusoidal-obstruction syndrome [26].

Acute Upper Esophageal Bleeding. The combination of mucositis, thrombocytopenia, and severe retching may result in a Mallory–Weiss tear, or esophageal hematoma [27]. The latter condition may have associated symptoms of dysphagia and retrosternal pain, and can be diagnosed by computed tomography (CT) scan. These conditions are treated supportively with transfusions to maintain platelet counts of greater than 50,000 per μL and optimal management of nausea and vomiting.

Liver

Sinusoidal Obstruction Syndrome. Sinusoidal obstruction syndrome (SOS; formerly referred to as veno-occlusive disease) develops in 10% to 60% of patients and is a clinical diagnosis based on the triad of tender hepatomegaly, jaundice, and unexplained weight gain usually within 30 days after HCT and in the absence of other explanations for these symptoms and signs [28,29]. It is more likely to be severe in patients with cirrhosis or fibrosis of the liver, or those with a history of hepatitis or liver irradiation (greater than 12 Gy), or chemotherapy-induced SOS [29,30].

Elevations of total serum bilirubin and serum transaminases are sensitive but nonspecific markers for SOS, and urinary sodium levels are typically low. A hepatobiliary ultrasound may show hepatomegaly, ascites, and dilatation of the hepatic vein or biliary system [31]. Doppler ultrasonography may show attenuation, or diagnostic, reversal of hepatic venous flow, but absence of this pattern does not exclude SOS [32]. If the diagnosis remains unclear, a transvenous liver biopsy may be helpful, and simultaneous measurement of hepatic venous pressure showing a gradient of greater than 10 mm Hg is highly specific for SOS [33].

Other causes of jaundice after HCT seldom lead to renal sodium avidity, rapid weight gain, or hepatomegaly. Cyclosporine, methotrexate, and total parenteral nutrition are iatrogenic causes of hyperbilirubinemia, although rarely cause levels greater than 4 mg per dL [34]. Combinations of illnesses that may mimic SOS are cholangitis lenta (cholestatic effects of endotoxin [35], especially when combined with renal insufficiency); cholestatic liver disease with hemolysis and congestive heart failure; GVHD and sepsis syndrome.

Once SOS is established, mathematical models can be used to predict prognosis, based on rates of increase in serum bilirubin and weight according to the elapsed time after transplantation [29,36]. The treatment for the 70% to 85% of patients who are predicted to have a mild or moderate course is largely supportive, with attention to management of sodium and water balance to avoid fluid overload [29]. Diuretics must be used judiciously to avoid depletion of intravascular volume and renal hypoperfusion. Paracentesis is indicated if the degree of ascites threatens respiratory function. There is no universally effective therapy for severe SOS. However, multiple studies, including a recent large international multicenter phase II clinical trial, have demonstrated 30% to 60% complete remission rates with defibrotide, even among patients with severe SOS [37]. There is no support for insertion of peritoneovenous shunts and limited support for use of portosystemic shunts to reduce ascites [38]. Liver transplantation has been successful in a small number of patients [39].

Lung

Pulmonary complications occur in 40% to 60% of patients after HCT [40,41]. Noninfectious pulmonary problems that may occur within 30 days from the transplant include idiopathic pneumonia syndrome (IPS), diffuse alveolar hemorrhage, pulmonary edema [42] due to excessive sodium and fluid administration or associated with SOS, or acute cardiomyopathy induced by cyclophosphamide, and sepsis with adult respiratory distress syndrome (ARDS) [43]. These complications occur more frequently in older patients, those who receive higher-dose conditioning regimens, and those with allogeneic donors, particularly HLA-disparate donors [44]. Although the incidence of life-threatening pulmonary infections has decreased over the past decade due to the introduction of routine antimicrobial prophylaxis, pulmonary complications continue to be a leading cause of death.

Idiopathic Pneumonia Syndrome. IPS is defined as a noninfectious inflammatory lung process that may be triggered by TBI and chemotherapies such as carmustine or busulfan. IPS has been reported in 5% to 10% of patients and occurs with a median onset of 2 to 3 weeks after myeloablative HCT [44,45]. Contributing factors to IPS lung injury may be release of inflammatory cytokines due to alloreactivity or sepsis. The clinical symptoms cannot be distinguished from infection, and may include fever, nonproductive cough, and tachypnea. Hemoptysis is infrequent and more likely related to indicate invasive fungal disease or diffuse alveolar hemorrhage. Radiographic imaging shows diffuse interstitial or multifocal intra-alveolar infiltrates. Arterial blood gases show hypoxemia and the alveolar–arterial oxygen gradient is increased. In the occasional patient who is not too ill to attempt lung function studies, a new restrictive pattern or a reduced diffusing capacity is characteristic. Measurements of pulmonary artery occlusion pressure or echocardiography may be useful to rule out cardiogenic pulmonary edema. Bronchoalveolar lavage or lung biopsy is necessary to exclude bacterial, fungal, or viral infection because *IPS is a diagnosis of exclusion.* Multifocal bronchiolitis obliterans with organizing pneumonia (BOOP) may mimic late-onset IPS and has been more commonly associated with chronic GVHD.

Management of IPS is mainly supportive, including judicious diuresis to decrease pulmonary edema, transfusions of blood components to reverse bleeding diathesis, support of oxygenation, and administration of antibiotics to prevent superinfection with mold and bacteria, particularly in patients receiving high-dose glucocorticoids. Effective therapy for idiopathic pneumonia has not been demonstrated. High-dose glucocorticoids (1 to 2 mg per kg) have been reported to have an adjunctive role in treatment of diffuse alveolar hemorrhage or idiopathic pneumonia, but their efficacy has not been validated in controlled studies [46]. In a recent study of 15 patients who had IPS after allogeneic HCT, combination treatment with soluble tumor necrosis factor receptor (etanercept) and glucocorticoids resulted in an encouraging day-28 survival rate of 73% [47]. More than half of the patients included in this study had required mechanical ventilation at therapy onset. Long-term survival, however, did not appear to be superior compared with historic controls.

The mortality associated with IPS after myeloablative HCT is 50% to 70% [45,48]. Aggressive management, including initiation of mechanical ventilation to identify and treat reversible causes of respiratory failure, is a reasonable approach for most HCT recipients with diffuse or multifocal pulmonary infiltrates. When hemodynamic instability or sustained hepatic and renal failure develop, survival is extremely unlikely. Withdrawal of mechanical ventilation may be appropriate in specific situations.

Acute Respiratory Distress Syndrome. An ARDS-like syndrome also has been described as a presenting feature of acute GVHD, typically early-onset (hyperacute) GVHD. ARDS has an extremely high mortality rate in the transplant population; recovery depends on aggressive treatment of associated infections and support of respiratory and cardiac function [49,50]. The diagnosis of ARDS often is complicated by presence of other illnesses, such as SOS, hemorrhage, or disseminated intravascular hemolysis, which can cause difficulties in fluid management and indicate the need for pulmonary artery catheterization.

Diffuse Alveolar Hemorrhage. Diffuse alveolar hemorrhage may be a manifestation of diffuse alveolar damage. However, the erosion of blood vessels by fungal organisms always needs to be considered [51]. Hemorrhage occurs more frequently in older patients and those with malignancy, severe mucositis, or renal failure [52]. Bloody bronchoalveolar lavage (BAL) fluid with hemosiderin-laden macrophages is characteristic of diffuse alveolar hemorrhage.

Heart

Cardiac complications occur in 5% to 10% of patients after HCT, but death from cardiac failure is uncommon [53,54]. Cardiac injury with hemorrhagic myocardial necrosis is a rare but known adverse effect of high-dose cyclophosphamide, one of the most commonly used chemotherapy agents in conditioning regimens. Acute cardiac failure due to cyclophosphamide has a case mortality rate exceeding 50%. Risk factors for cyclophosphamide cardiotoxicity include use of doses equal to or greater than 120 mg per kg, an underlying diagnosis of lymphoma, prior radiation to the mediastinum or left chest wall, older age, and prior abnormal cardiac ejection fraction [54,55]. Patients who had prior cumulative anthracycline exposures of 550 mg per m^2 doxorubicin equivalents are at an increased risk for developing heart failure. Signs and symptoms of congestive heart failure may occur within a few days of receiving cyclophosphamide, while anthracycline-related cardiomyopathy may have a delayed onset. The electrocardiogram (ECG) may show voltage loss or arrhythmia, and echocardiography may reveal systolic dysfunction, pericardial effusion or tamponade [56]. Older age and a history of abnormal ejection fraction are other factors that predispose to cardiac toxicity [54]. Management includes attention to fluid and sodium balance, afterload reduction, and inotropes.

Kidney and Bladder

Acute Renal Failure. Acute renal failure (ARF), defined by doubling of baseline serum creatinine, occurs in 30% to 50% of all patients during the first 100 days after HCT, and most often during the first 10 to 30 days [57,58]. Occasionally, ARF develops during conditioning or infusion of HSC, as a consequence of tumor or red-cell lysis. ARF occurs most frequently in the setting of SOS and is characterized by low urinary sodium concentration and high blood urea nitrogen to creatinine ratio, similar to the hepatorenal syndrome. Renal hypoperfusion, caused by acute hemorrhage, sepsis, or high-volume diarrhea, may result in ARF. Nephrotoxic drugs like cyclosporine, tacrolimus, all amphotericin products, and aminoglycosides frequently cause renal insufficiency.

Thrombotic microangiopathy (TMA), endothelial damage caused by chemoradiotherapy, cyclosporine, tacrolimus, or sirolimus, occurs in 5% to 20% of patients, more frequently in allograft recipients [59]. The hallmark of thrombotic microangiopathy is red blood cell (RBC) fragmentation (schistocytes) associated with increased RBC turnover (increased reticulocytes; elevations of serum lactate dehydrogenase and indirect bilirubin) without evidence for immune-mediated hemolysis or disseminated intravascular coagulation. The syndrome ranges from subclinical hemolysis to a life-threatening hemolytic syndrome, the latter being seen more frequently when sirolimus therapy is combined with cyclosporine or tacrolimus (calcineurin inhibitors, CNIs) and immediately following conditioning with busulfan and cyclophosphamide. High-therapeutic or supratherapeutic serum levels of CNIs or sirolimus are more prone to be associated with TMA [60]. Management involves careful assessment of volume status and discontinuation or adjustment of the drug levels of the offending agent(s). The use of plasma exchange has been associated with high mortality rates in most series [61] with recent exceptions [62], and may be skewed by selection bias because only the sickest patients are likely to receive the treatment. For this reason, determination of any survival benefit attributable to plasma exchange in the absence of a controlled study is impossible.

Hypertension. Hypertension develops in approximately 60% of patients after HCT, more often in patients given CNIs for GVHD prophylaxis. Glucocorticoid therapy also contributes to the development of hypertension. Uncontrolled hypertension may lead to fatal intracerebral bleeding in thrombocytopenic patients. Therefore, hypertension should be anticipated and controlled medically. Most patients respond to conventional antihypertensive therapy, such as a calcium channel blocker, angiotensin-converting enzyme inhibitor, or beta-blocker. Correction of hypomagnesemia, which often confounds CNI therapy, may improve control of hypertension [63].

Hemorrhagic Cystitis. High-dose cyclophosphamide is commonly used for conditioning, and one of its toxic metabolites, acrolein, accumulates in the urine and may cause a hemorrhagic chemical cystitis during the conditioning regimen or later after HCT [64,65]. Measures to prevent hemorrhagic cystitis include aggressive fluid hydration to increase urine volume that dilutes and minimizes contact of acrolein with the mucosa, and administration of the drug mesna, which provides free thiol groups to detoxify acrolein. Viral infections, particularly adenovirus and BK virus, also have been implicated in the development of hemorrhagic cystitis [66] and the diagnosis is established by viral culture or polymerase chain reaction (PCR) test of a urine sample [66]. Unless there is evidence of disseminated infection, viral cystitis is managed with supportive therapy, including aggressive hydration and platelet transfusions. Intravesicular infusions of ε-aminocaproic acid or prostaglandins have been reported to improve outcome of severe hemorrhagic cystitis [67]. Severe hemorrhagic cystitis caused by BK virus that proves refractory to supportive therapy may respond to therapy with cidofovir [68].

Central Nervous System

Noninfectious complications include cerebrovascular events and encephalopathies due to metabolic, toxic, and immune-mediated causes. Focal symptoms are more indicative of infectious or cerebrovascular mechanisms, while diffuse symptoms such as delirium or coma may have metabolic causes. Fever is not necessarily associated with central nervous system (CNS) infections. Infection should be considered as the cause of any neurologic symptom and should prompt evaluation, including obtaining CT or magnetic resonance imaging (MRI) scans of the head and a sample of cerebrospinal fluid for appropriate cultures, cytochemistry stains, and PCR tests should be undertaken.

Cerebrovascular Events. Thrombocytopenia poses a risk for intracranial hemorrhage, which usually presents as abrupt onset of focal neurologic deficit or mental status changes [69]. Patients with sickle cell disease have a predisposition to CNS hemorrhage after HCT and should be managed carefully by ensuring sufficient platelet and magnesium levels and strict control of hypertension [70]. Ischemic stroke is an unusual complication after HCT but has been reported in patients with *Aspergillus* infections, hypercoagulable states, or TMA [59,71].

Toxic Encephalopathies. Conditioning with high-dose busulfan or carmustine may cause encephalopathy and seizure prophylaxis with phenytoin is usual. High-dose cytarabine may cause cerebellar dysfunction, encephalopathy, and seizures. High-dose cyclophosphamide can be associated with the syndrome of inappropriate antidiuretic hormone (SIADH), rarely causing acute decline in the serum sodium that may prompt seizures. Fludarabine, used frequently in nonmyeloablative conditioning, may cause an encephalopathy.

A rare syndrome of encephalopathy and hyperammonemia without other chemical evidence of liver failure has been reported after HCT [72]. Contributing factors may include hypercatabolism induced by conditioning, glucocorticoids, or sepsis, and high nitrogen loads associated with parenteral nutrition or intestinal hemorrhage. The syndrome is difficult to reverse and has a high mortality rate. Treatment involves hemodialysis and administration of ammonia-trapping agents, such as sodium benzoate or sodium phenylacetate.

Related to a tendency to accumulate in nervous tissues due to their lipophilic characteristics, CNIs can cause a range of neurologic toxicities [73]. Tremor develops in most patients. Seizures have been reported in up to 6% of patients and may present in association with headaches, tremor, or visual disturbances [74]. Seizures should be managed with anticonvulsant therapy and cessation of the drug. When CNIs are essential for management of GVHD, substitution of one agent for the other, or reinstitution of the offending agent at a lower dose, may be feasible [75]. A unique and usually reversible syndrome of cortical blindness has been reported as a complication of cyclosporine treatment; hypertension and hypomagnesemia are thought to be predisposing factors [76]. Toxicity due to calcineurin inhibitor therapy may occur with "therapeutic" drug levels, and clinical suspicion is often confirmed by MRI scans that show multifocal areas of signal hyperintensity on T2 (time for 63% of transverse relaxation) and fluid-attenuated inversion recovery (FLAIR) sequences, most often in the occipital lobe white matter.

Glucocorticoid therapy may be associated with psychosis, mania, or delirium in a dose-dependent fashion. Seizures or altered sensorium may be associated with the use of sedative-hypnotic drugs and have been reported as adverse side effects of many of the commonly used antibiotics and antiviral agents. Metabolic encephalopathy may be associated with Gram-negative sepsis, hypoxic encephalopathy with IPS, and hepatic encephalopathy due to SOS or GVHD.

Treatment of metabolic encephalopathies should be directed at the underlying problem, and offending drugs have to be discontinued. In patients with CNI neurotoxicity, temporary discontinuation of the CNI and the restarting at a lower dose is usually successful. Short-term phenytoin for seizure prophylaxis may be indicated.

Infection

Conditioning regimens and GVHD severely impair host defense mechanisms, and the process of immune reconstitution necessarily requires many months for completion. Together these factors place patients at high risk for acquisition of severe infections. Proper medical care of patients after HCT includes measures to monitor and prevent infection, as it is a leading cause of death.

Prevention of infection is of vital importance to the success of HCT procedures. Hospitalized patients should be housed in single rooms that have positive-pressure airflow and ventilation systems with rapid air exchange and high-efficiency particulate air filtration [77]. Strict visitation, hand washing, and isolation policies should be instituted to prevent introduction or spread of communicable disease. A daily program of skin and oral care should include bathing all skin surfaces with mild soap, brushing teeth with a soft brush, frequent rinsing of the oral cavity with saline, and good perineal hygiene. The diet should exclude foods known to contain bacteria or fungi, and patients should avoid exposure to dried or fresh plants or flowers. Caregivers should be trained in the proper handling of central venous catheters.

Immunologic reconstitution after HCT can broadly be categorized into three phases, which are characterized by a spectrum of opportunistic infections. Advances in management of antimicrobial prevention of opportunistic infections after HCT are outlined in Table 188.2.

Before Engraftment Period

The period before engraftment (less than 30 days posttransplant) is characterized by neutropenia and oral and gastrointestinal mucosal damage. The most common infections are bacterial and fungal. The use of indwelling central venous catheters

TABLE 188.2

ADVANCES IN PREVENTION OF OPPORTUNISTIC INFECTIONS AFTER ALLOGENEIC HEMATOPOIETIC CELL TRANSPLANTATION

Infection	Recommendations for prophylaxis (strength of recommendation)[a]: All patients	Patients with chronic GVHD
Bacteria	Broad-spectrum antibiotic(s) during period of neutropenia (ANC <500/μL). Choices include a single agent, such as levofloxacin or ceftazidime, or a combination of agents, such as piperacillin. [CIII] Patients with hypogammaglobulinemia: Intravenous immunoglobulin administered at 1- to 4-week intervals depending on level. [CIII]	Penicillin VK twice daily for encapsulated organisms. [BIIb] Alternatives: TMP/SMX daily, azithromycin three times per week. [CIII] Patients with hypogammaglobulinemia or repeated sinopulmonary infections: Intravenous immunoglobulin administered at monthly intervals depending on level. [CIII]
Fungi	Fluconazole from start of conditioning to day 75 (allogeneic HCT) or day 30 (autologous HCT). [AIa]	Mold active agents, such as posaconazole when prednisone dose is ≥1 mg/kg. [AI]
PCJ	TMP/SMX is the drug of choice and starts 1–2 wk before transplant until 48 h before HCT, then from engraftment until 6 months after HCT if no chronic GVHD. Alternatives: dapsone, atovaquone, pentamidine. [AIb]	TMP/SMX in a variety schedules. [AIb]
HSV (seropositive patients)	Acyclovir prophylaxis from start of conditioning until day 30. Alternatives: valacyclovir. [AI]	Not indicated
VZV (seropositive)	Acyclovir prophylaxis from start of conditioning until 1 year after HCT for those with a history of natural infection. Alternative: valacyclovir. [AIa]	Acyclovir from start of immune suppression until completion. Alternatives: valacyclovir. [AIa]
CMV (seropositive)	Ganciclovir prophylaxis or preemptive therapy based on plasma CMV DNA detection by PCR between engraftment and day 100. Foscarnet is an equally effective alternative to ganciclovir for preemptive therapy. [AI]	Valganciclovir therapy based on plasma CMV DNA detection by PCR until dose of prednisone is <1 mg/kg. [BIII]
CMV (seronegative)	Preferential use of preemptive therapy with ganciclovir or foscarnet as outlined for seropositive patients. [BII]	Not indicated

[a]Evidence-based grading system adapted from Couriel D, Carpenter PA, Cutler C, et al: Ancillary therapy and supportive care of chronic GVHD: NIH Consensus Development Project on criteria for clinical trials in chronic GVHD: V. Ancillary Therapy and Supportive Care Working Group Report. *Biol Blood Marrow Transplant* 12:375–396, 2006.

Recommendations are "A," should always be offered; "B," should generally be offered; "C," optional; "D," should generally not be offered. Evidence is "level I" if it is derived from ≥1 properly designed randomized, controlled trial; "level II" if it is derived from ≥1 well-designed clinical trial without randomization, from cohort or case-controlled analytical studies, or from multiple time series or dramatic results from uncontrolled experiments; and "level III" if it is derived from opinions of respected authorities based on clinical experience. Qualifiers, "a," indicates that evidence is directly from study(s) in GVHD, or "b" if the evidence was derived indirectly from study(s) in analogous or other pertinent disease.

ANC, absolute neutrophil count; CMV, cytomegalovirus; DS, double strength; GVHD, graft-versus-host disease; HCT, hematopoietic cell transplantation; HSV, herpes simplex virus; IgG, immunoglobulin G; IV, intravenous; max, maximum dose; MTX, methotrexate; PCJ, *Pneumocystis jiroveci* pneumonia; PCR, polymerase chain reaction; SMX, sulfamethoxazole; TMP, trimethoprim; VK, V potassium; VZV, varicella zoster virus.

heightens the risk of blood infections with organisms that colonize the skin, such as coagulase negative *staphylococci* or *Candida spp.*, and gastrointestinal mucosal damage increases the risk of infections with enteric organisms, such as *Escherichia coli. Clostridium difficile* toxic colitis can be a common infection in transplant patients, particularly those patients in intensive care units. Patients with a history of prolonged neutropenia prior to HCT are at risk for developing fungal infections involving the skin, lung, sinuses, which typically are a mold such as *Aspergillus*, or the liver and spleen, typically *Candida* spp. The most likely viral infection in this period is herpes simplex virus. Fever of unknown origin also occurs commonly during the neutropenic period. Prophylactic systemic antibiotics conventionally are administered to reduce the risk of bacteremia during the neutropenic period, although improvement in survival has not been demonstrated [77,78]. Administration of growth factors, such as granulocyte colony-stimulating factor, shortens the duration of neutropenia, but there is little evidence for improvement in outcome [79].

Following Engraftment Period

The period following engraftment (30 to 100 days posttransplant) is characterized by skin and mucosal damage and compromised cellular immunity related to GVHD and its treatment. Viral (CMV) and fungal (*Aspergillus, Pneumocystis jiroveci*) infections predominate during this period. Gram-negative bacteremias related to GVHD-associated mucosal damage and Gram-positive infections due to indwelling catheters remain a risk. Other causes of fever of unknown origin after engraftment include occult sinusitis, hepatosplenic candidiasis, and pulmonary or disseminated *Aspergillus* infection.

Late Phase

The late phase (greater than 100 days posttransplant) is characterized by a persistently impaired cellular immunity in patients with chronic GVHD. Patients with chronic GVHD are highly susceptible to recurrent bacterial infections, especially from encapsulated bacteria, including *Streptococcus pneumonia, Haemophilus influenzae*, and *Neisseria meningitides* (functional asplenia). Bronchopulmonary infections, septicemia, and ear, nose, and throat infections occur. Common nonbacterial infections at this time include varicella zoster, CMV, *P. jiroveci*, and *Aspergillus*.

Evaluation and Treatment

Signs and symptoms of infection may be diminished in patients who are neutropenic or receiving immunosuppressive drugs [80]. Thus, preemptive antibiotic therapy should be instituted promptly for any fever during the neutropenic period, because infections can progress rapidly to a fatal outcome [81]. The febrile patient should be examined thoroughly for source of infection, including the oral cavity, perianal tissue, and skin surrounding the central venous catheter. Cultures should be obtained of blood, urine, and stool if diarrhea is present, and chest radiograph should be performed. Antibiotic therapy should provide empiric coverage for the most common organisms, Gram-positive bacteria that colonize the skin and oral cavity, as well as the less common but more virulent Gram-negative bacteria that arise from the GI tract [78,80,81]. Broad-spectrum antibiotic therapy should be continued through the duration of neutropenia, even if fever resolves. If fever persists, the antibiotic regimen should be broadened after 4 days to provide empiric treatment of fungi. *C. difficile* infection should be considered in patients with diarrhea and can be treated with oral metronidazole.

Evaluation of persistent fevers after granulocyte recovery should consider occult sources of bacterial infection, such as sinuses, perirectal tissue, or central venous lines, as well as viral or fungal etiologies. Removal of the central venous catheter is occasionally required. Viral infections must be considered in patients with GI symptoms and may involve the esophagus, upper and lower intestines, or liver [82]. The diagnosis is established by biopsy or brushings taken from the center of the lesions so as to include infected endothelial cells and submucosal tissue. Host immunosuppression associated with GVHD and its treatment predisposes patients to a variety of opportunistic infections. Patients with active chronic GVHD should receive prophylaxis for *P. jiroveci* pneumonia with trimethoprim–sulfamethoxazole and for encapsulated organisms with daily trimethoprim–sulfamethoxazole, penicillin, or azithromycin. Infectious causes of pulmonary infiltrates must be differentiated from noninfectious causes to ensure prompt institution of appropriate therapy [48,83].

BAL should be performed without delay to establish the etiology of diffuse infiltrates, unless clearly related to pulmonary edema [84]. BAL specimens should be assayed for the presence of common nosocomial bacteria as well as *Legionella, Mycobacteria*, and *Nocardia; P. jiroveci*; fungi other than *P. jiroveci* pneumonia; respiratory viruses; and herpes group viruses by cultures and immunocytochemical stains. Focal pulmonary infiltrates that occur after HCT are most frequently caused by infection, particularly fungal infection [85]. Evaluation of a focal infiltrate should include a CT scan to delineate the number and extent of infiltrates. BAL should be performed as a first step because the procedure is minimally invasive and historically has produced a diagnosis in 50% of patients with fungal lesions using standard diagnostic approaches, although the predictive value of negative results was poor [84]. At some centers, the increasing use of more diagnostic approaches like galactomannan antigen testing [86] or, ongoing development of molecular methods to detect fungi or viral pathogens (e.g., human metapneumovirus [87,88]) continues to improve the yield of BAL. As a result, the number of lung biopsies performed at these centers has declined. Transbronchial biopsy is not recommended because it has not been shown to improve sensitivity in these situations, and often thrombocytopenia precludes the ability to perform the procedure safely. Percutaneous fine-needle aspiration is indicated for diagnosis of peripheral infiltrates that cannot be evaluated by BAL. Fine-needle aspiration has a sensitivity of approximately 67% for diagnosis of fungal infection, but it has a poor negative predictive value. If the diagnosis is not ascertained after BAL or fine-needle aspiration, a biopsy is required [89]. Specimens should be evaluated histologically and undergo testing for bacteria, fungi, and viruses by appropriate cultures and immunocytochemical stains as noted previously. Surgical resection of a solitary fungal lesion may improve the chances for cure [90].

Opportunistic Infections

***Pneumocystis jiroveci* Pneumonia.** Inadequate cell-mediated immunity poses a risk for development of *P. jiroveci* pneumonia infection after HCT [91]. Recommendations for prevention of PJP are found in Table 188.2 [77,92].

Fungal Infections

Factors that predispose to invasive yeast infections include neutropenia, mucosal barrier disruption, and broad-spectrum antibiotics that promote colonization of the GI mucosa [93]. Candidal infections generally occur within the first 3 weeks after HCT, coinciding with the period of neutropenia, although a second period of risk occurs during treatment for chronic GVHD. Invasive candidiasis may involve the liver and spleen, with potential for dissemination to kidneys or rarely, the CNS

[94,95]. The diagnosis of invasive candidiasis is difficult because blood cultures are negative in approximately one half of the cases with organ involvement. Recommendations for prevention of candidiasis are found in Table 188.2. Fluconazole is effective for treatment of the most common *Candida* spp, *C. albicans* and *C. tropicalis* [96,97] (see Table 188.2), but does not prevent or treat infection with *C. glabrata*, *C. krusei*, or *C. parapsilosis*. Removal of the central venous catheter should be considered when *Candida sp*. is isolated from blood cultures. Fungal vegetations on heart valves are possible and echocardiography is often considered. Lipid-complexed amphotericin products, echinocandins, or other azoles may be useful alternatives [98].

Invasive mold infections develop in up to 20% of patients after HCT [99]. The incidence of *Aspergillus* infections is highest within the first month after HCT, and there is a second peak incidence during chronic GVHD. *Aspergillus* infections have been difficult to diagnose by standard methods, and more than 20% of the cases have been diagnosed only at autopsy. Cultures of BAL fluid are negative in 50% of pulmonary disease; therefore, the diagnosis frequently requires a biopsy of affected tissues [85]. The *Aspergillus* Galactomannan Enzyme Immunoassay detects a polysaccharide secreted from *Aspergillus hyphae* and is a useful screening tool, with a sensitivity of 65% and specificity of 95% [100]. High-risk patients, those with severe GVHD treated with high-dose corticosteroids, should be given prophylaxis with agents like voriconazole or posaconazole which is active against aspergillosis and certain other molds. Because invasive aspergillosis is associated with a high mortality rate, documented or suspected infections should be treated aggressively with voriconazole, lipid-complexed amphotericin products, or combination therapy [101,102]. Surgical removal of infected tissue should be restricted to cases of circumscribed disease [103].

Viral Infections

Cytomegalovirus. Protection from exposure by use of seronegative or leukocyte-reduced blood components has reduced the incidence of CMV infection among seronegative patients [21], whereas ganciclovir has been shown to be an effective agent for prevention of CMV disease in seropositive patients [104–106] (see Table 188.2). Ganciclovir should be initiated as prophylaxis after engraftment, with careful monitoring of the patient for marrow suppression, a side effect that can lead to life-threatening infection (Table 188.2) [107]. A reasonable alternative is to monitor for CMV reactivation with serum PCR assays, followed by prompt institution of ganciclovir when the CMV copy number reaches a positive threshold [108–110]. Generally, surveillance CMV PCR testing is performed weekly from transplant day 0 through day 100; however, monitoring generally is continued for CMV positive patients on high-dose corticosteroids.

Although prophylaxis greatly reduces the risk for CMV disease, severe pneumonitis, gastroenteritis, hepatitis, or bone marrow failure continue to occur in a small proportion of patients [111]. The diagnosis of CMV pneumonitis can be established in most patients by PCR assay or rapid shell vial culture of BAL fluid [112]. CMV enteritis is often indistinguishable from GVHD clinically, and the diagnosis relies on endoscopic evaluation [113]. CMV enteritis appears as ulcerations of the esophagus, stomach, or intestines. Viral cultures and histologic stains of the affected tissue are used to establish the diagnosis. Treatment of CMV infection includes ganciclovir (foscarnet or cidofovir are acceptable alternatives) in combination with immune globulin [114,115]. Foscarnet can be used in place of ganciclovir if significant marrow toxicity occurs or drug resistance is identified.

Herpes Simplex Virus. Herpes simplex virus (HSV) is the most common cause of infectious mucositis after HCT and may cause life-threatening encephalitis, hepatitis, or pneumonia in immunocompromised patients [116–118]. HSV pneumonitis or hepatitis is associated with high mortality rates; although less serious, HSV mucositis produces severe local pain and swelling. Acyclovir prophylaxis has been shown to be very effective for prevention of HSV reactivation in seropositive patients and for treatment of established disease [119,120] (see Table 188.2).

Varicella Zoster Virus. Varicella zoster virus (VZV) causes life-threatening disease in immunocompromised patients, as a primary infection or reactivation of endogenous virus [121]. Exposed seronegative patients should receive VZV immune globulin within 96 hours if available, and acyclovir should be administered from days 3 to 22 after exposure [122]. Among seropositive patients, VZV reactivation occurs in approximately 40%, with the highest incidence around 5 months after HCT [121,123]. Prophylaxis with acyclovir is recommended for seropositive patients until 1 year after HCT or until complete discontinuation of immunosuppressive therapy for chronic GVHD immunity [124] (see Table 188.2). VZV infection typically causes local skin involvement, but it can disseminate in immunocompromised patients, resulting in pneumonitis, esophagitis, pancreatitis, hepatitis, or encephalitis [125–128]. VZV hepatitis may present as a syndrome of fever, severe abdominal pain, and elevated aminotransferase levels, and because it is associated with a high mortality rate, should be treated presumptively with high-dose acyclovir [128]. For localized infection, a short course of intravenous acyclovir for 24 to 48 hours can be followed by oral valacyclovir for the duration of therapy.

Respiratory Viruses. Respiratory viruses may spread quickly within HCT patient populations, causing epidemics of life-threatening infection. Respiratory syncytial virus (RSV), influenza, and parainfluenza are the most frequently encountered respiratory viruses in these situations [129]. Symptoms of upper respiratory infection should prompt cultures of nasopharyngeal secretions, careful monitoring for progression of disease, and isolation to prevent spread to other patients. Patients in the period before engraftment are at greatest risk for progression to lower tract disease with RSV. Once lower-tract disease occurs, however, mortality is high regardless of engraftment status [130]. If lower-tract disease is suspected, BAL should be performed to obtain samples for viral fluorescence antibody and PCR tests and viral cultures [131].

Adenovirus. Adenovirus and polyoma BK virus are common causes of hemorrhagic cystitis after HCT [66]. When disseminated, adenovirus can cause hemorrhagic enterocolitis, interstitial pneumonitis, myocarditis, nephritis, meningoencephalitis, or severe hepatitis [132]. Adenoviral infections occur more commonly in children and after allogeneic grafts [133]. Patients with poor T-cell function, such as recipients of T cell–depleted grafts or those receiving intensive immune suppressing therapies, are at greatest risk for disseminated infection. Disseminated infections are often difficult to detect by viral cultures, and PCR assays may be more useful [134]. The most promising treatment results have been reported after administration of cidofovir, although renal insufficiency is a potential side effect [135]. Polyoma BK virus should be considered in the differential diagnosis of renal insufficiency in patients on chronic immune suppression, and can be diagnosed by renal biopsy.

Epstein-Barr Virus. Epstein–Barr virus (EBV) seropositive immunocompromised patients are at risk for development of life-threatening lymphoproliferative disease (LPD) after HCT

[136]. The risk for EBV–LPD is highest among patients who receive T-cell–depleted grafts or who are given intensive immune suppression for treatment of GVHD [137]. The diagnosis is made by biopsy of enlarged nodes or affected tissue. A presumptive diagnosis can be made in high-risk patients who have clinical symptoms and elevated plasma or cellular EBV DNA copy number [138]. The mainstay of therapy is reduction or elimination of immunosuppressive therapy to allow reconstitution of EBV-specific T-cell immunity. However, it may not be feasible to eliminate immunosuppression therapy without risking a flare of life-threatening GVHD. Some studies have shown encouraging results with mAb directed against CD20, which targets EBV-infected B cells [139]. EBV–LPD that develops in recipients of T cell–depleted grafts may be ameliorated by infusion of donor T lymphocytes [140].

Graft Rejection

Graft rejection presents as failure to recover hematopoiesis after transplantation, termed *primary graft failure*, or as the loss of an established donor graft, termed *secondary graft failure*. Persistence of neutropenia (an absolute neutrophil count of more than 100 cells per μL) after day 26 is associated with increased risk of early mortality [141]. Although the molecular and cellular mechanisms are not completely understood, graft rejection appears to be mediated preferentially by recipient T cells [142]. Another described mechanism includes rejection mediated by host natural killer cells which, to some extent, can be overcome by the preparative regimen. Finally, alloimmune antibodies in sensitized recipients may cause rejection in mice but their role in humans is controversial. Donor HLA disparity stimulates strong alloreactive immune responses in the immunocompetent recipient and increases the risk for graft rejection. Donor T cells counteract the rejection responses of host alloreactive cells that have survived the conditioning regimen [143]. Higher stem cell doses facilitate engraftment, particularly when T cell–depleted grafts are used [144,145].

Quantitation of donor engraftment (donor chimerism), using PCR-based techniques to detect donor-specific variable nucleotide tandem repeats (VNTR) sequences, may be helpful in determining whether the graft has been rejected, in which case the peripheral blood T cells will be primarily of host origin, or whether the donor graft is not functioning, in which case the cells will be of donor origin. In the latter case, other causes of graft suppression should be considered, including relapse, medications such as ganciclovir or trimethoprim–sulfamethoxazole, mycophenolate mofetil, or viral infections such as CMV, human herpes virus 6, or parvovirus B19. In either case, graft failure after myeloablative conditioning is a life-threatening complication because autologous reconstitution is uncommon and results in death from hemorrhage or infection. A range of cellular therapies have been used to overcome rejection ranging from donor lymphocyte infusions in the case of declining donor T-cell chimerism, possibly combined with immunosuppressive therapy. In fulminant rejection, retransplantation is necessary, using the same or another donor. Conditioning should preferentially differ from that used at the first transplant to avoid unnecessary toxicity, and a high graft cell dose should be targeted [142].

Graft-Versus-Host Disease

The most significant immunologic barrier to successful HCT is the graft-versus-host reaction, which can result in life-threatening inflammation and tissue destruction. Donor T cells that recognize disparate recipient alloantigens are the central mediators of GVHD. The most important alloantigens are those encoded by the major histocompatibility complex, or HLA system, although non-HLA antigens may certainly be involved. Despite the significance of GVHD as a complication of HCT, patients who develop GVHD have lower relapse rates than patients without GVHD, and this can also be explained by an immunologically mediated graft-versus-tumor (GVT) effect that helps eradicate the underlying malignancy.

Acute Graft-Versus-Host Disease

The incidence and severity of acute GVHD are determined primarily by the degree of HLA disparity and influenced by the nature of GVHD prophylaxis [146–148]. Severe acute GVHD (grades III to IV) develops in 15% of recipients transplanted from HLA-identical sibling donors, and in a greater proportion of those given unrelated or mismatched grafts. Acute GVHD typically begins abruptly at 2 to 4 weeks after myeloablative HCT and generally occurs before day 100, but the onset may be delayed after nonmyeloablative HCT. The clinicopathologic syndrome is consistent with various combinations of inflammatory dermatitis, enteritis, and hepatitis, which reflect the pathophysiology of T-cell activation with generation of cytotoxic lymphocytes and elaboration of inflammatory cytokines that cause tissue damage. The severity of acute GVHD in the three main target organs (skin, liver, and GI tract) is staged 1 through 4 based on accepted criteria that primarily include the extent of rash, magnitude of hyperbilirubinemia, and volume of diarrhea. The various combinations of skin, liver, and GI involvement can then be used to assign an overall grade of GVHD: grade I being mild, and grade IV being life threatening [149,150] (Table 188.3). When cellular injury is severe, GVHD of the skin may manifest with bulla formation and skin ulceration. In the GI tract, symptoms range from mild anorexia, to nausea and vomiting, or to severe bloody diarrhea with cramping periumbilical pain.

Chronic Graft-Versus-Host Disease

Chronic GVHD (CGVHD) occurs in approximately 30% to 60% of transplant recipients, more often when the donor is not an HLA-identical sibling and when there is a history of acute GVHD [151]. There is a higher risk for developing CGVHD with growth factor–mobilized PBSC grafts compared to marrow grafts [152]. CGVHD also is more likely when the recipient or donor is older or CMV seropositive, or in a male patient who receives HSC from a multiparous female donor. Risk factors for mortality at the time of diagnosis of CGVHD include: platelet counts less than 100×10^9 per L, greater than 0.5 mg per kg per day prednisone, serum total bilirubin greater than 34 μmol per L, older recipient, prior acute GVHD, older donor, and graft-versus-host HLA mismatching [153,154].

CGVHD is defined without reference to time after HCT, but by the presence of hallmark CGVHD features, which resemble autoimmune diseases such as systemic sclerosis, Sjogren's syndrome, primary biliary cirrhosis, wasting syndrome, bronchiolitis obliterans, immune cytopenias, and chronic immunodeficiency [155] (Table 188.4). Simply stated, the distinction of chronic from acute GVHD requires the presence of at least one diagnostic clinical sign of CGVHD or presence of at least one distinctive manifestation confirmed by pertinent biopsy or other relevant tests. The overall severity of CGVHD is determined by a 0- to 3-point score (none, mild, moderate, severe) that reflects the clinical effect of CGVHD on the patient's functional status in any number of different organs. CGVHD frequently involves the skin, liver, eyes, mouth, upper respiratory tract, lungs, and esophagus. Less frequently, serosal surfaces, lower GI tract, female genitalia, or fascia are involved. Major causes of morbidity include scleroderma, contractures, ulceration, keratoconjunctivitis, strictures, obstructive pulmonary disease, and weight loss. Uncontrolled chronic GVHD

TABLE 188.3

CLASSIFICATION OF GRAFT-VERSUS-HOST DISEASE

Acute GVHD organ staging			
Organ	**Stage**	**Scores**	**Description**
Skin	1		≤25% body surface area with maculopapular rash
	2		25%–50% body surface area with maculopapular rash
	3		≥50% body surface area with maculopapular rash or erythroderma
	4		Generalized erythroderma with bullae
Liver	1		Bilirubin 2.0–3.0 mg/dL
	2		Bilirubin 3.0–5.9 mg/dL
	3		Bilirubin 6.0–14.9 mg/dL
	4		Bilirubin rise to ≥15 mg/dL
GI tract			Stage is assigned according to a total GI score based on volume of diarrhea, presence of bloody stool, and abdominal pain or cramping
	1		Total GI score of 1
	2		Total GI score of 2
	3		Total GI score of 3–4
	4		Total GI score of 5–7
GI scoring			Diarrhea volume averaged over 3 d
			Adult (mL/d), child[a] (mL/kg/d)
		+1	>500–999, >10–20
		+2	1,000–1,499, >20–30
		+3	>1,500, >30
		+2	Score additional 2 points for presence of abdominal pain or cramping
		+2	Score additional 2 points for presence of bloody stools

Acute GVHD overall grade	Skin stage	Liver stage	GI stage
I	1–2	0	0
II	3 or	1 or	1
III		2–3	2–3
IV	4 or	4 or	4

[a]Children <17 years of age who are <1.73 m^2.
GI, gastrointestinal; GVHD, graft-versus-host disease.
Adapted from Martin PJ, Nelson BJ, Applebaum FR, et al: Evaluation of a CD5-specific immunotoxin for treatment of acute graft-versus-host disease after allogeneic marrow transplantation. *Blood* 88(3):962–969, 1996, with permission.

interferes with immune reconstitution and is strongly associated with increased risks of opportunistic infections and death.

Confirming the Diagnosis of Graft-Versus-Host Disease

Unlike CGVHD, the clinical signs of acute GVHD are not considered sufficiently pathognomonic to establish the diagnosis, especially when there is isolated organ involvement. However, the combination of rash, nausea, and voluminous diarrhea, occurring at the time of, or early after, neutrophil engraftment makes the diagnosis very likely. The differential diagnosis involves ruling out other causes of rash, diarrhea or liver toxicity as listed in Table 188.5. Tissue biopsies of the skin, liver, or stomach are recommended to confirm a histologic diagnosis of GVHD and, most importantly, to exclude opportunistic infection; however, the interpretation of biopsies performed within 3 weeks of myeloablative therapy may be problematic because it is difficult to separate cellular injury induced by chemoradiotherapy from GVHD. The gastric antral mucosa provides the most sensitive site for evaluation of intestinal GVHD and is preferred over duodenal and rectal biopsy because there is less risk for bleeding complications. The histologic hallmark of GVHD-induced cellular injury is apoptosis, observed in epidermal basal keratinocytes, bile duct or intestinal crypt epithelial cells, and often associated with infiltration by lymphocytes [156–158]. Biopsy is unnecessary to confirm the presence of chronic GVHD if at least one diagnostic feature is present, but histologic confirmation or other pertinent testing is necessary when CGVHD features are only distinctive or suggestive (see Table 188.4).

Prevention of Graft-Versus-Host Disease

GVHD prevention strategies are almost always incorporated into the overall treatment plan, and these include optimizing the choice of allogeneic donor and stem cell product based on known risk factors for GVHD, T-cell depletion of the donor HSC graft as discussed earlier, or, most commonly, post-transplant immunosuppression. Adjunctive therapy with ursodeoxycholic acid may improve liver function and a randomized placebo-controlled multicenter study demonstrated that prophylaxis with ursodeoxycholic acid reduced hepatic problems, severe acute GVHD, and improved survival after allogeneic HCT [159].

TABLE 188.4

CLASSIFICATION OF SYMPTOMS AND SIGNS OF CHRONIC GRAFT-VERSUS-HOST DISEASE

Organ or site	Diagnostic	Distinctive[a]	Common[b]
Skin	Poikiloderma Lichen planus-like features Sclerotic features Morphea-like features Lichen-sclerosis–like features	Depigmentation	Erythema Maculopapular rash Pruritus
Nails		Dystrophy Longitudinal ridging, splitting, or brittle features Onycholysis Pterygium unguis Nail loss[c]	
Scalp and body hair		New onset of scalp alopecia Scaling, papulosquamous lesions	
Mouth	Lichen-type features Hyperkeratotic plaques Restriction of mouth opening	Xerostomia Mucocele Mucosal atrophy Pseudomembranes[c] Ulcers[c]	Gingivitis Mucositis Erythema Pain
Eyes		New onset dry, gritty, or painful[d] Cicatricial conjunctivitis Keratoconjunctivitis sicca[d] Confluent punctate keratopathy	
Genitalia	Lichen-planus–like features Vaginal scarring or stenosis	Erosions[c] Fissures[c] Ulcers[c]	
GI tract	Esophageal web Esophageal strictures or stenosis in upper to mid third[c]		Anorexia, nausea vomiting, diarrhea, Failure to thrive
Liver			Bilirubin >2 × ULN Alk Phosp >2 × ULN AST/ALT >2 × ULN
Lung	Bronchiolitis obliterans based on lung biopsy	Bronchiolitis obliterans based on PFTs + radiology[d]	BOOP
Muscles, fascia, joints	Fasciitis Joint stiffness or contractures secondary to sclerosis	Myositis or polymyositis	

Features acknowledged as part of chronic GVHD symptomatology if the diagnosis is already confirmed

Skin	Sweat impairment, ichthyosis, keratosis pilaris, hypopigmentation, hyperpigmentation
Hair	Thinning scalp hair, typically patchy, coarse, dull not explained by endocrine or other causes, premature gray hair
Eyes	Photophobia, periorbital hyperpigmentation, blepharitis
GI tract	Exocrine pancreatic insufficiency
Muscles/Joints	Edema, muscle cramps, arthralgia, or arthritis.
Hematology	Thrombocytopenia, eosinophilia, lymphopenia
Immune	Lymphopenia, hypo- or hypergammaglobulinemia, autoantibodies (AIHA, ITP)
Other	Pericardial/pleural effusions, ascites, peripheral neuropathy, nephrotic syndrome, myasthenia gravis, cardiac conduction abnormality, or cardiomyopathy

[a]Seen in chronic GVHD but are insufficient alone to establish the diagnosis.
[b]Seen in both acute and chronic GVHD alone to establish a diagnosis of chronic GVHD.
[c]In all cases must exclude infection, drug effects, malignancy, or other causes.
[d]Diagnosis of chronic GVHD requires biopsy or radiology confirmation (or Schirmer's test for eyes).
AIHA, autoimmune hemolytic anemia; ALT, alanine aminotransferase; AST aspartate aminotransferase; BOOP, bronchiolitis obliterans with organizing pneumonia; GI, gastrointestinal; ITP, idiopathic (immune) thrombocytopenic purpura; PFTs, pulmonary function tests; ULN, upper limit of normal range for age.
Modified from Filipovich AH, Weisdorf D, Pavletic S, et al: National Institutes of Health consensus development project on criteria for clinical trials in chronic graft-versus-host disease: I. Diagnosis and Staging Working Group report. *Biol Blood Marrow Transplant* 11(12):945–956, 2005, with permission.

TABLE 188.5

DIFFERENTIAL DIAGNOSIS OF ACUTE GRAFT-VERSUS-HOST DISEASE (AGVHD)

AGVHD manifestation	Differential diagnosis
Rash	Drug reaction Allergic reaction Infection Regimen-related toxicity
Diarrhea	Infection (viral, fungal) Narcotic bowel syndrome (opiate withdrawal)
Abdominal pain	Acute pancreatitis Acute cholecystitis (biliary sludge, stones, infection) Narcotic bowel syndrome (opiate withdrawal)
Elevated liver enzymes	Sinusoidal obstruction syndrome Medication toxicities (e.g., cyclosporine) Cholangitis lenta (sepsis) Biliary sludge syndrome Viral infections (CMV, EBV, hepatitis B) Hemolysis

CMV, cytomegalovirus; EBV, Epstein–Barr virus.

Postgrafting Immunosuppression. In the absence of T-cell depletion, posttransplant immune suppression must be administered to control donor alloreactive T cells. Standard prophylaxis regimens deliver a 6-month course of cyclosporine or tacrolimus combined with a short course of methotrexate administered intravenously on the 1st, 3rd, 6th, and 11th days after HCT [147]. After myeloablative conditioning, methotrexate toxicity may exacerbate RRT in high turnover cells such as in oral and intestinal mucosae and hepatocytes. Some patients, particularly those with the C677T polymorphism in the methylene–tetrahydrofolate reductase gene, have more severe mucositis and slower platelet engraftment when given methotrexate [160]. Variations of CNI plus methotrexate include CNI plus mycophenolate mofetil [147,161]. or, tacrolimus and sirolimus, with or without methotrexate [162–164]. Steady-state serum CNI and sirolimus levels require monitoring. Dose reductions should be made when toxicities emerge or when serum trough levels exceed the upper limit of the therapeutic range.

Treatment of Graft-Versus-Host Disease

Despite GVHD prophylaxis regimens, 30% to 80% of allogeneic HCT recipients develop acute GVHD and require additional therapy with glucocorticoids.

Acute Graft-Versus-Host Disease. Glucocorticoids have been the mainstay of primary therapy for acute GVHD. Initial starting doses have been recently calibrated to the severity and extent of organ involvement as demonstrated by one large retrospective study [165]. This approach requires further validation, particularly for grades III and IV acute GVHD. For the one third of patients who develop GVHD without liver involvement, and whose GI symptoms are defined as stage 1 (anorexia, nausea, or vomiting with peak stool volume less than 1,000 mL per day), with or without rash involving less then 50% of the body surface, treatment may reasonably begin at 1 mg per kg per day methylprednisolone (or oral equivalent) combined with topical and minimally absorbed glucocorticoids (beclomethasone or budesonide). When there is liver involvement, or when intestinal and skin GVHD is greater than defined above, methylprednisolone is typically begun at a dose of 2 mg per kg per day for 14 days, by which time rash, diarrhea, abdominal pain, and liver dysfunction usually remit and a glucocorticoid taper is considered appropriate. In patients with GI hemorrhage, surgery very rarely is indicated, and the mainstay of therapy is initiation of immune suppression, along with the infusion of appropriate blood components [166,167]. Several studies, including a randomized trial, have shown no benefit for administration of doses greater than 2 mg per kg per day of methylprednisolone [168,169]. The results of a recent multicenter randomized phase II trial suggested that response and early survival after standard therapy with prednisone might be improved by adding mycophenolate mofetil [170]. A follow-up phase III study to more definitively evaluate this finding is imminent.

Chronic Graft-Versus-Host Disease. In practice, systemic therapy is considered when chronic GVHD is present in more than two organs, or there are moderate to severe abnormalities of a single organ with functional impairment (Table 188.6). In contrast, systemic therapy is generally not warranted for patients with mild abnormalities of one or two organs that do not cause functional impairment. For example, jaundice, or marked elevations of liver enzymes or skin manifestations that are not extensive. However, mild chronic GVHD does warrant systemic therapy when either thrombocytopenia or steroid treatment is present at diagnosis.

Standard primary therapy for clinical extensive CGVHD usually begins with glucocorticoids and extended administration of a CNI. After newly diagnosed CGVHD manifestations have been controlled by daily glucocorticoids, the judicious use of glucocorticoids at the lowest effective dose and alternate-day administration can minimize steroid-related side effects. The median duration of systemic immunosuppression for the treatment of CGVHD approximates 2 to 3 years [153]. Longer therapy tends to be required for recipients of peripheral blood stem cells, male patients with female donors, multiple organ

TABLE 188.6

INDICATION FOR SYSTEMIC IMMUNOSUPPRESSION AT DAY 80

Global severity of chronic GVHD	High-risk features[a]	Systemic therapy
None	Yes	None[b]
Mild (<3 sites[c], no lung)	No	No
Mild	Yes	Yes
Moderate[d] (or mild lung) or severe[e]	Yes or no	Yes

[a]Less than 100,000 platelets/μL, progressive onset (on prednisone).
[b]Need to balance risks and benefits of graft-versus-tumor against risks of developing more severe chronic GVHD based on the coexistence of risk factors, including unrelated or mismatched-related donor, female donor, and peripheral blood stem cell transplant.
[c]No clinically significant functional impairment (score $\leq$1 in each site).
[d]At least one site functionally impaired without major disability (Score 2) or 3 or more sites without clinically significant functional impairment (each with score $\leq$1).
[e]Major disability at any site (score 3, or score $\geq$2 in lung).
GVHD, graft-versus-host disease.

TABLE 188.7

THERAPY OPTIONS FOR STEROID-REFRACTORY ACUTE GRAFT-VERSUS-HOST DISEASE

Therapy	Comments
Systemic	
Polyclonal	
Antithymocyte globulin (ATGAM,[a] Thymoglobulin[b])	Delayed use appears to be very ineffective. Skin responds best.
Monoclonal	
Anti-CD3 (OKT3,[c] visilizumab[d,e])	Currently used infrequently.
Anti-IL2 (daclizumab,[d] basiliximab[f])	Depletes conventional and regulatory T cells.
Anti-TNFα (infliximab[f])	Consider early for refractory lower GI tract.
Anti-CD52 (alemtuzumab[d])	Depletes T & B cells (lower risk EBV PTLD)
Anti-CD2 (alefacept[g])	Depletes memory T cells; needs further study.
Fusion proteins	
Anti-IL2 (denileukin diftitox)	Anti-T cell but also depletes regulatory T cells.
Anti-TNFα (etanercept)	
Macrolides and antimetabolites	
Tacrolimus	Inhibits conventional and regulatory T cells
Sirolimus	Inhibits conventional but not regulatory T cells.
Mycophenolate mofetil	Enteric coated formulation may minimize toxicity but liquid formulation not available
Extracorporeal photopheresis	Mechanism includes facilitation of regulatory T cells Particularly effective in skin, infrequently associated with opportunistic infections.
Mesenchymal stem cells	Mechanism poorly understood but thought to modulate tissue repair.
Topical	
Glucocorticoids	
Budesonide	Useful as steroid-sparing agent in lower GI tract.
Beclomethasone[e]	Useful as steroid-sparing agent in upper GI tract
PUVA	Useful for skin only involvement.

[a]Equine.
[b]Rabbit.
[c]Murine.
[d]Humanized.
[e]Not commercially available.
[f]Chimeric murine–human.
[g]Human IgG1-fusion protein.

involvement at the onset of CGVHD, graft-versus-host HLA mismatching, and hyperbilirubinemia.

Within 3 years of primary therapy, just over one quarter of the patients have resolved CGVHD, 1 out of 10 patients will continue primary therapy beyond 3 years and one-third require secondary treatment with a variety of other immunosuppressive agents [171]. The remaining patients develop recurrent malignancy or die from nonrelapse causes. Infection from a broad array of pathogens is the major cause of nonrelapse mortality, followed by progressive organ failure from CGVHD involvement. Therefore, antibiotic prophylaxis to prevent infection (Table 188.2) and supportive care to minimize morbidity and prevent disability are critically important components of CGVHD management [172].

Steroid-Refractory Graft-Versus-Host Disease. Glucocorticoids often fail to control acute GVHD manifestations such that 40% to 60% of patients have steroid-refractory (SR) acute GVHD. SR-GVHD has been defined operationally as the progression of acute GVHD symptoms beyond 3 days after starting methylprednisolone. Persistence of GVHD beyond 7 to 14 days also should be considered failure of response. The prognosis of acute GVHD can be related to its overall severity (grade) and response to glucocorticoids [173,174]. It is of no surprise that grade III and IV SR acute GVHD, especially with visceral involvement, requires urgent initiation of effective secondary therapy.

Unfortunately, there is no generally accepted therapy for SR acute GVHD. A full review of the various secondary GVHD therapies is beyond the scope of this review but various approaches are listed in Table 188.7 together with a summary of outcomes (Table 188.8). Polyclonal antithymocyte globulins (ATG), and more recently monoclonal antibodies, are generally used to treat life-threatening visceral manifestations where urgent control of GVHD is necessary. Unfortunately, longer term survival has been unusual when visceral manifestations are severe [175–179]. However, early administration of ATG within 14 days of primary therapy was reported in one study to be associated with improved survival [180]. It has remained difficult to improve the survival after SR-refractory acute GVHD because progressive organ dysfunction is often irreversible, and because second-line therapies constitute a "second hit" to an immune system that has already been impaired by cumulative exposure to high-dose prednisone. In this regard, high daily prednisone doses increase the risk for CMV viremia [181]. Similarly, invasive aspergillosis occurs more frequently in patients

TABLE 188.8

ADVANCES IN THERAPY OPTIONS FOR STEROID-REFRACTORY ACUTE GRAFT-VERSUS-HOST DISEASE (AGVHD)

Treatment	Study design/results	Comments	Reference
Antithymocyte globulin (equine ATG)	Single-arm Phase II studies ($N = 29–79$) from 1980 to 1999. CR/PR 30% overall (59%–72% for skin), OS 5%–32%.	Responses considerably better in skin than visceral organs. OS worse in visceral or more severe GVHD. One study found OS better if ATGAM given within 14 d of primary therapy (46% vs. 19%, $p = 0.05$).	[175,180,190,191]
Antithymocyte globulin (rabbit ATG)	Single-arm Phase II ($N = 36$). 89% had mostly three-system Grade III/IV GVHD. CR/PR 59% overall (96% skin, 46% GI, 36% liver. OS 6%.	Very poor survival. Infections, including 25% EBV PTLD rate, were major problems.	[176]
Daclizumab	Single center Phase I/II ($N = 13–57$) from 1990s to 2006. CR/PR 51%–92% overall. OS 25%–46%.	Well tolerated. Responses better in children and in skin GVHD. Significant morbidity and mortality due to infections. Patient selection and aggressive antiviral and fungal prophylaxis advised.	[179,192,193]
Denileukin Diftitox	Single center Phase I/II ($N = 32$). CR/PR 71% overall. OS 30%.	Reversible transaminitis in 22% at MTD. OS 58% (7/12) if achieved CR.	[178]
Infliximab	Single center retrospective ($N = 21–32$) from 1998 to 2004. CR/PR 59%–82% overall. CR 19%–62%. OS 38%–46% at ~1 year.	Well tolerated and active, particularly for GI tract. Better response if age <35 y and longer interval between HCT and infliximab treatment. High rates of opportunistic infection.	[194–196]
Etanercept	Single center retrospective ($N = 13$ with AGVHD) from 1995 to 2005. CR ($N = 4$)/PR ($N = 2$) 46% overall. OS 67% at median 429 d (range: 71–1,007 d); includes 8 other patients with cGVHD.	Well tolerated. Responses most common in GI tract (64%). CMV reactivation (48%), bacterial (14%) and fungal (19%) infections occurred.	[197]
Psoralen and ultraviolet A (PUVA)	Single center retrospective ($N = 103$) from 1994 to 2000. CR 24% by intention to treat. OS 51%.	Generally well tolerated but 8 discontinued because of toxicity. CR 37% if tolerated PUVA for 6 wk. PUVA was steroid sparing; 57% did not require additional therapy for skin GVHD.	[198]
Extracorporeal photopheresis (ECP)	Single-center or multicenter phase II or retrospective ($N = 21–77$) from 1992 to 2006. CR/PR 50%–60%. OS 48%–57%	Best responses in skin (60%–82%) then liver (61%–67%). GI responses variable (0%–75%). Poor Grade IV responses <15%. AEs during ECP: cytopenias. OS 59%–91% among CRs vs. 11%–12% for non-CRs.	[199–203]
Mycophenolate Mofetil	Single-center retrospective ($N = 19–36$). CR/PR 42%–72%. OS 16%*-37%**	Commonest AEs: mild-to-moderate cytopenias. (*at 2 y, **at 5 y including 12 additional patients with cGVHD)	[204,205]
Sirolimus	Single center pilot trial ($N = 21$) from 1996 to 1999. High loading dose and/or high maintenance dosing of sirolimus. CR/PR 28%*. OS 34%	*Frequent expected toxicities (cytopenias, hyperlipidemia, HUS) associated with high-serum concentrations likely limited the efficacy. CR/PR 67% among 18 who received ≥6 doses.	[206]
Pentostatin	Prospective phase I, single center ($N = 23$). CR/PR 76%. OS 26% at a median of 85 d (5–1,258 d).	Universal lymphopenia and late infections were dose-limiting. Best responses in skin. Suggested dose for phase II was 1.5 mg/m^2/d × 3 d.	[207]
Mesenchymal stem cells (hMSCs)	European multicenter phase II ($N = 55$) from 2001 to 2007 of up to 5 doses hMSCs. CR/PR 71%. OS 36% at 2 y. U.S. multicenter phase III hMSC vs. placebo ($N = 260$). Durable CR 35% vs 30% ($p =$ NS)	No infusion toxicities. OS 53% for CRs in the European study. U.S. study found that hMSCs did not improve durable CR rates (primary endpoint) but hMSCs did improve durable liver CRs (29% vs. 5%, $p = 0.046$, $N = 61$) and GI responses (88% vs. 64%, $p = 0.018$, $N = 71$)	[208], written communication, Osiris press release

cGVHD, chronic graft-versus-host disease; CMV, cytomegalovirus; CR, complete response; EBV, Epstein–Barr virus; GI, gastrointestinal; HCT, hematopoietic cell transplantation; HUS, hemolytic uremic syndrome; MTD, maximally tolerated dose; NS, not significant; OS, overall survival; PR, partial response; PTLD, posttransplant lymphoproliferative disorder.

who develop CMV disease and in patients receiving higher doses of prednisone [182]. After nonmyeloablative HCT, high dose prednisone therapy at the time of diagnosis of mold infection has been associated with an increased risk for mold infection-related death [183].

When CGVHD becomes refractory to steroids, in contrast to SR acute GVHD, secondary therapy generally avoids potent antibody therapies unless the manifestations overlap with the disease features typically associated with severe acute GVHD. The time to complete resolution of classical CGVHD manifestations is in the order of weeks to months, and total duration of therapy spans months to years. Therefore, secondary therapies for SR-CGVHD must try to avoid profound T-cell depletion and must generally be more easily delivered chronically in the outpatient setting. Ideally, second-line agents should promote transplantation tolerance so that the morbidity associated with prolonged use of glucocorticoids and other immunosuppressive agents can be minimized.

Promising new agents or strategies that warrant further controlled clinical trials include sirolimus, extracorporeal photophoresis, rituximab, and the platelet-derived growth factor receptor, imatinib, which is of particular interest for the treatment of sclerotic GVHD. A number of ancillary measures that are used with topical intent are often used to target specific organ involvement [172].

Hemolysis

RBC hemolysis may be encountered after HCT and may include more than one etiology. Thrombotic microangiopathy may present as mild hemolysis with RBC fragmentation (schistocytes) or as a more severe form, with thrombocytopenia, renal insufficiency, fever, and altered mental status, similar to hemolytic uremic syndrome (HUS) or thrombotic thrombocytopenic purpura (TTP) [59,184]. Predisposing factors include: endothelial cell injury triggered by chemotherapy, radiation, or immunosuppressive therapy (e.g., CNIs) [59,185]. Drugs such as fludarabine, antithymocyte globulin, or infections with mycoplasma also may produce hemolysis. Unlike the preceding etiologies, hemolysis mediated by major or minor blood group incompatibilities is only seen in recipients of allografts.

Major ABO incompatibility occurs in 30% of allograft recipients and is defined by the presence of isohemagglutinins within recipient plasma that are directed against donor A or B antigens. *Minor* ABO incompatibility also occurs in 30% of recipients and is defined by presence of isohemagglutinins within the donor plasma directed against recipient A or B. *Bidirectional* ABO incompatibility may be present as in the case of a type A recipient and type B donor or vice versa. After successful donor engraftment, the conversion of recipient to donor blood type may take weeks to months because of the relatively long half-life of red blood cells.

Major ABO incompatibility poses a serious risk of severe hemolytic reactions at the time of infusion of the HSC product if preventative steps are not taken. Immediate hemolytic reactions are more likely in the presence of high-level isoagglutinin titers. Therefore, red blood cells are most commonly removed from the graft before infusion to avoid life-threatening hemolysis. Delayed recovery of donor hematopoiesis or hemolysis may occur because recipient plasma cells continue to produce isohemagglutinins for up to several months after HCT [186]. In this case, the diagnosis relies on detection of a positive direct antiglobulin test and the presence of isohemagglutinins directed against donor-type red blood cells. Management of major ABO incompatibility includes the transfusion of group O red blood cells, donor-type platelets, and donor-type plasma until isohemagglutinins against donor-type red blood cells disappear. In the rare cases of ongoing hemolysis due to persistence of donor-directed isohemagglutinins, additional therapy with immunosuppressive agents, erythropoietin, plasma exchange, anti-B-cell antibodies (rituximab), or plasma exchange may be considered [187].

Minor ABO incompatibility poses a risk for mild and self-limited hemolysis at the time of infusion. Delayed hemolysis, seen more commonly after PBSC transplantation, is mediated by clonally expanded donor "passenger lymphocytes" and can present as an abrupt and potentially fatal hemolytic transfusion reaction typically at 1 to 2 weeks after HCT [188,189]. In contrast to major ABO incompatibility, pretransplant donor isohemagglutinin titers do not predict the severity of hemolysis following minor ABO-mismatched HCT. The diagnosis relies again on the detection of a positive direct antiglobulin test and the presence of isohemagglutinins directed against recipient-type red blood cells. To prevent hemolysis, plasma should be removed from the donor HSC product if donor hemagglutinin titers are high. Emergence of donor-derived RBC and isohemagglutinin titers should be monitored after allogeneic HCT. Management of minor ABO incompatibility after HCT includes supportive care with judicious fluid management aimed at preventing acute renal failure, and the transfusion of group O red blood cells and recipient type platelets and plasma. There is no convincing evidence to support the use of plasma exchange.

References

1. Afessa B, Tefferi A, Hoagland HC, et al: Outcome of recipients of bone marrow transplants who require intensive-care unit support. *Mayo Clin Proc* 67:117–122, 1992.
2. Huaringa AJ, Leyva FJ, Giralt SA, et al: Outcome of bone marrow transplantation patients requiring mechanical ventilation. *Crit Care Med* 28:1014–1017, 2000.
3. Bensinger WI, Storb R: Allogeneic peripheral blood stem cell transplantation. *Rev Clin Exp Hematol* 5:67–86, 2001.
4. Reddy RL: Mobilization and collection of peripheral blood progenitor cells for transplantation (Review). *Transfus Apher Sci* 32:63–72, 2005.
5. Korbling M, Anderlini P: Peripheral blood stem cell versus bone marrow allotransplantation: does the source of hematopoietic stem cells matter? *Blood* 98:2900–2908, 2001.
6. Storek J, Gooley T, Siadak M, et al: Allogeneic peripheral blood stem cell transplantation may be associated with a high risk of chronic graft-versus-host disease. *Blood* 90:4705–4709, 1997.
7. Barker JN, Davies SM, DeFor T, et al: Survival after transplantation of unrelated donor umbilical cord blood is comparable to that of human leukocyte antigen-matched unrelated donor bone marrow: results of a matched-pair analysis. *Blood* 97:2957–2961, 2001.
8. Rocha V, Cornish J, Sievers EL, et al: Comparison of outcomes of unrelated bone marrow and umbilical cord blood transplants in children with acute leukemia. *Blood* 97:2962–2971, 2001.
9. Barker JN, Weisdorf DJ, Defor TE, et al: Transplantation of 2 partially HLA-matched umbilical cord blood units to enhance engraftment in adults with hematologic malignancy. *Blood* 105:1343–1347, 2005.
10. Weiden PL, Sullivan KM, Flournoy N, et al: Antileukemic effect of chronic graft-versus-host disease. Contribution to improved survival after allogeneic marrow transplantation. *N Engl J Med* 304:1529–1533, 1981.
11. Anasetti C, Amos D, Beatty PG, et al: Effect of HLA compatibility on engraftment of bone marrow transplants in patients with leukemia or lymphoma. *N Engl J Med* 320:197–204, 1989.
12. Petersdorf EW, Gooley TA, Anasetti C, et al: Optimizing outcome after unrelated marrow transplantation by comprehensive matching of HLA class I and II alleles in the donor and recipient. *Blood* 92:3515–3520, 1998.
13. Woolfrey AE, Anasetti C, Storer B, et al: Factors associated with outcome after unrelated marrow transplantation for treatment of acute lymphoblastic leukemia in children. *Blood* 99:2002–2008, 2002.
14. Sorror ML, Maris MB, Storer B, et al: Comparing morbidity and mortality of HLA-matched unrelated donor hematopoietic cell transplantation after

nonmyeloablative and myeloablative conditioning: influence of pretransplant comorbidities. *Blood* 104:961–968, 2004.
15. Mielcarek M, Leisenring W, Torok-Storb B, et al: Graft-versus-host disease and donor-directed hemagglutinin titers after ABO-mismatched related and unrelated marrow allografts: evidence for a graft-versus-plasma cell effect. *Blood* 96:1150–1156, 2000.
16. McSweeney PA, Niederwieser D, Shizuru JA, et al: Hematopoietic cell transplantation in older patients with hematologic malignancies: replacing high-dose cytotoxic therapy with graft-versus-tumor effects. *Blood* 97:3390–3400, 2001.
17. Sorror ML, Maris MB, Storb R, et al: Hematopoietic cell transplantation (HCT)-specific comorbidity index: a new tool for risk assessment before allogeneic HCT. *Blood* 106:2912–2919, 2005.
18. Anonymous: Consensus conference. Platelet transfusion therapy. *JAMA* 257:1777–1780, 1987.
19. Slichter SJ: Relationship between platelet count and bleeding risk in thrombocytopenic patients (Review). *Transfus Med Rev* 18:153–167, 2004.
20. O'Connell BA, Lee EJ, Rothko K, et al: Selection of histocompatible apheresis platelet donors by cross-matching random donor platelet concentrates. *Blood* 79:527–531, 1992.
21. Bowden RA, Slichter SJ, Sayers M, et al: A comparison of filtered leukocyte-reduced and cytomegalovirus (CMV) seronegative blood products for the prevention of transfusion-associated CMV infection after marrow transplant. *Blood* 86:3598–3603, 1995.
22. Lane TA, Anderson KC, Goodnough LT, et al: Leukocyte reduction in blood component therapy [Review]. *Ann Intern Med* 117:151–162, 1992.
23. McDonald GB, Shulman HM, Sullivan KM, et al: Intestinal and hepatic complications of human bone marrow transplantation. *Gastroenterology* 90:460–477; 770–784, 1986.
24. Sale GE, Shulman HM, Hackman RC: Pathology of hematopoietic cell transplantation, in Blume KG, Forman SJ, Appelbaum FR (eds): *Thomas' Hematopoietic Cell Transplantation.* 3rd ed. Oxford, UK: Blackwell Publishing Ltd., 2004, pp 286–299.
25. Fegan C, Poynton CH, Whittaker JA: The gut mucosal barrier in bone marrow transplantation. *Bone Marrow Transplant* 5:373–377, 1990.
26. Rogers M, Cerda JJ: The narcotic bowel syndrome [Review]. *J Clin Gastroenterol* 11:132–135, 1989.
27. Schwartz JM, Strasser SI, Lopez-Cubero SO, et al: Severe gastrointestinal bleeding after marrow transplantation, 1987–1997: incidence, causes and outcome [Abstract]. *Gastroenterology* 114:A40, 1998.
28. Bearman SI: The syndrome of hepatic veno-occlusive disease after marrow transplantation. *Blood* 85:3005–3020, 1995.
29. McDonald GB, Hinds MS, Fisher LD, et al: Veno-occlusive disease of the liver and multiorgan failure after bone marrow transplantation: a cohort study of 355 patients. *Ann Intern Med* 118:255–267, 1993.
30. Slattery JT, Kalhorn TF, McDonald GB, et al: Conditioning regimen-dependent disposition of cyclophosphamide and hydroxycyclophosphamide in human marrow transplantation patients. *J Clin Oncol* 14:1484–1494, 1996.
31. Hommeyer SC, Teefey SA, Jacobson AF, et al: Sonographic evaluation of patients with venoocclusive disease of the liver: a prospective study. *Radiology* 184:683–686, 1992.
32. Herbetko J, Grigg AP, Buckley AR, et al: Venoocclusive liver disease after bone marrow transplantation: findings at duplex sonography. *Am J Roentgenol* 158:1001–1005, 1992.
33. Shulman HM, Gooley T, Dudley MD, et al: Utility of transvenous liver biopsies and wedged hepatic venous pressure measurements in sixty marrow transplant recipients. *Transplantation* 59:1015–1022, 1995.
34. McDonald GB, Shulman HM, Wolford JL, et al: Liver disease after human marrow transplantation. *Semin Liver Dis* 7:210–220, 1987.
35. Jacobson AF, Teefey SA, Lee SP, et al: Frequent occurrence of new hepatobiliary abnormalities after bone marrow transplantation: results of a prospective study using scintigraphy and sonography. *Am J Gastroenterol* 88:1044–1049, 1993.
36. Bearman SI, Anderson GL, Mori M, et al: Venoocclusive disease of the liver: development of a model for predicting fatal outcome after marrow transplantation. *J Clin Oncol* 11:1729–1736, 1993.
37. Ho VT, Revta C, Richardson PG: Hepatic veno-occlusive disease after hematopoietic stem cell transplantation: update on defibrotide and other current investigational therapies (Review). *Bone Marrow Transplant* 41:229–237, 2008.
38. Fried MW, Connaghan DG, Sharma S, et al: Transjugular intrahepatic portosystemic shunt for the management of severe venoocclusive disease following bone marrow transplantation. *Hepatology* 24:588–591, 1996.
39. Schlitt HJ, Tischler HJ, Ringe B, et al: Allogeneic liver transplantation for hepatic veno-occlusive disease after bone marrow transplantation–clinical and immunological considerations. *Bone Marrow Transplant* 16:473–478, 1995.
40. Soubani AO, Miller KB, Hassoun PM: Pulmonary complications of bone marrow transplantation [Review]. *Chest* 109:1066–1077, 1996.
41. Parimon T, Madtes DK, Au DH, et al: Pretransplant lung function, respiratory failure, and mortality after stem cell transplantation. *Am J Respir Crit Care Med* 172:384–390, 2005.
42. Crawford SW: Noninfectious lung disease in the immunocompromised host [Review]. *Respiration* 66:385–395, 1999.
43. Clark JG, Crawford SW: Diagnostic approaches to pulmonary complications of marrow transplantation. *Chest* 91:477–479, 1987.
44. Meyers JD, Flournoy N, Thomas ED: Nonbacterial pneumonia after allogeneic marrow transplantation: a review of ten years' experience. *Rev Infect Dis* 4:1119–1132, 1982.
45. Kantrow SP, Hackman RC, Boeckh M, et al: Idiopathic pneumonia syndrome: changing spectrum of lung injury after marrow transplantation. *Transplantation* 63:1079–1086, 1997.
46. Metcalf JP, Rennard SI, Reed EC, et al: Corticosteroids as adjunctive therapy for diffuse alveolar hemorrhage associated with bone marrow transplantation. University of Nebraska Medical Center Bone Marrow Transplant Group. *Am J Med* 96:327–334, 1994.
47. Yanik GA, Ho VT, Levine JE, et al: The impact of soluble tumor necrosis factor receptor etanercept on the treatment of idiopathic pneumonia syndrome after allogeneic hematopoietic stem cell transplantation. *Blood* 112:3073–3081, 2008.
48. Crawford SW, Hackman RC: Clinical course of idiopathic pneumonia after bone marrow transplantation. *Am Rev Respir Dis* 147:1393–1400, 1993.
49. Rubenfeld GD, Crawford SW: Withdrawing life support from mechanically ventilated recipients of bone marrow transplants: a case for evidence-based guidelines. *Ann Intern Med* 125:625–633, 1996.
50. Ognibene FP, Martin SE, Parker MM, et al: Adult respiratory distress syndrome in patients with severe neutropenia. *N Engl J Med* 315:547–551, 1986.
51. De Lassence A, Fleury-Feith J, Escudier E, et al: Alveolar hemorrhage. Diagnostic criteria and results in 194 immunocompromised hosts. *Am J Respir Crit Care Med* 151:157–163, 1995.
52. Robbins RA, Linder J, Stahl MG, et al: Diffuse alveolar hemorrhage in autologous bone marrow transplant recipients. *Am J Med* 87:511–518, 1989.
53. Hertenstein B, Stefanic M, Schmeiser T, et al: Cardiac toxicity of bone marrow transplantation: predictive value of cardiologic evaluation before transplant. *J Clin Oncol* 12:998–1004, 1994.
54. Brockstein BE, Smiley C, Al-Sadir J, et al: Cardiac and pulmonary toxicity in patients undergoing high-dose chemotherapy for lymphoma and breast cancer: prognostic factors. *Bone Marrow Transplant* 25:885–894, 2000.
55. Cazin B, Gorin NC, Laporte JP, et al: Cardiac complications after bone marrow transplantation. A report on a series of 63 consecutive transplantations. *Cancer* 57:2061–2069, 1986.
56. Braverman AC, Antin JH, Plappert MT, et al: Cyclophosphamide cardiotoxicity in bone marrow transplantation: a prospective evaluation of new dosing regimens. *J Clin Oncol* 9:1215–1223, 1991.
57. Hingorani SR, Guthrie K, Batchelder A, et al: Acute renal failure after myeloablative hematopoietic cell transplant: incidence and risk factors. *Kidney Int* 67:272–277, 2005.
58. Pulla B, Barri YM, Anaissie E: Acute renal failure following bone marrow transplantation [Review]. *Ren Fail* 20:421–435, 1998.
59. Pettitt AR, Clark RE: Thrombotic microangiopathy following bone marrow transplantation. *Bone Marrow Transplant* 14:495–504, 1994.
60. Cutler C, Henry NL, Magee C, et al: Sirolimus and thrombotic microangiopathy after allogeneic hematopoietic stem cell transplantation. *Biol Blood Marrow Transplant* 11:551–557, 2005.
61. Ho VT, Cutler C, Carter S, et al: Blood and Marrow Transplant Clinical Trials Network Toxicity Committee consensus summary: thrombotic microangiopathy after hematopoietic stem cell transplantation. *Biol Blood Marrow Transplant* 11:571–575, 2005.
62. Worel N, Greinix HT, Leitner G, et al: ABO-incompatible allogeneic hematopoietic stem cell transplantation following reduced-intensity conditioning: close association with transplant-associated microangiopathy. *Transfus Apher Sci* 36:297–304, 2007.
63. June CH, Thompson CB, Kennedy MS, et al: Correlation of hypomagnesemia with the onset of cyclosporine-associated hypertension in marrow transplant patients. *Transplantation* 41:47–51, 1986.
64. Ilhan O, Koc H, Akan H, et al: Hemorrhagic cystitis as a complication of bone marrow transplantation. *J Chemother* 9:56–61, 1997.
65. Seber A, Shu XO, DeFor T, et al: Risk factors for severe hemorrhagic cystitis following BMT. *Bone Marrow Transplant* 23:35–40, 1999.
66. La Rosa AM, Champlin RE, Mirza N, et al: Adenovirus infections in adult recipients of blood and marrow transplants. *Clin Infect Dis* 32:871–876, 2001.
67. Miller LJ, Chandler SW, Ippoliti CM: Treatment of cyclophosphamide-induced hemorrhagic cystitis with prostaglandins [Review]. *Ann Pharmacother* 28:590–594, 1994.
68. Cesaro S, Hirsch HH, Faraci M, et al: Cidofovir for BK virus-associated hemorrhagic cystitis: a retrospective study. *Clin Infect Dis* 49:233–240, 2009.
69. Graus F, Saiz A, Sierra J, et al: Neurologic complications of autologous and allogeneic bone marrow transplantation in patients with leukemia: a comparative study. *Neurology* 46:1004–1009, 1996.
70. Walters MC, Sullivan KM, Bernaudin F, et al: Neurologic complications after allogeneic marrow transplantation for sickle cell anemia (Rapid Communication). *Blood* 85:879–884, 1995.
71. Valilis PN, Zeigler ZR, Shadduck RK, et al: A prospective study of bone marrow transplant-associated thrombotic microangiopathy (BMT-TM) in autologous (AUTO) and allogeneic (ALLO) BMT [Abstract]. *Blood* 86:970a, 1995.

72. Davies SM, Szabo E, Wagner JE, et al: Idiopathic hyperammonemia: a frequently lethal complication of bone marrow transplantation. *Bone Marrow Transplant* 17:1119–1125, 1996.
73. Bechstein WO: Neurotoxicity of calcineurin inhibitors: impact and clinical management [Review]. *Transpl Int* 13:313–326, 2000.
74. Reece DE, Frei-Lahr DA, Shepherd JD, et al: Neurologic complications in allogeneic bone marrow transplant patients receiving cyclosporin. *Bone Marrow Transplant* 8:393–401, 1991.
75. Furlong T, Storb R, Anasetti C, et al: Clinical outcome after conversion to FK 506 (tacrolimus) therapy for acute graft-versus-host disease resistant to cyclosporine or for cyclosporine-associated toxicities. *Bone Marrow Transplant* 26:985–991, 2000.
76. Drachman BM, DeNofrio D, Acker MA, et al: Cortical blindness secondary to cyclosporine after orthotopic heart transplantation: a case report and review of the literature [Review]. *J Heart Lung Transplant* 15:1158–1164, 1996.
77. Centers for Disease Control and Prevention, Infectious Disease Society of America & American Society of Blood and Marrow Transplantation. Guidelines for preventing opportunistic infections among hematopoietic stem cell transplant recipients. *Morb Mortal Wkly Rep* 49:1–125, 2000.
78. Pizzo PA, Hathorn JW, Hiemenz J, et al: A randomized trial comparing ceftazidime alone with combination antibiotic therapy in cancer patients with fever and neutropenia. *N Engl J Med* 315:552–558, 1986.
79. Gisselbrecht C, Prentice HG, Bacigalupo A, et al: Placebo-controlled phase III trial of lenograstim in bone-marrow transplantation [erratum appears in *Lancet* 343(8900):804, 1994]. *Lancet* 343:696–700, 1994.
80. Meyers JD: Infections in marrow recipients, in Mandell GL, Douglas RG, Bennett JE (eds): *Principles and Practice of Infectious Diseases.* 2nd ed. New York: John Wiley and Sons, 1985, pp 1674–1676.
81. Hughes WT, Armstrong D, Bodey GP, et al: 1997 guidelines for the use of antimicrobial agents in neutropenic patients with unexplained fever. Infectious Diseases Society of America [Review]. *Clin Infect Dis* 25:551–573, 1997.
82. Wu D, Hockenbery DM, Brentnall TA, et al: Persistent nausea and anorexia after marrow transplantation: a prospective study of 78 patients. *Transplantation* 66:1319–1324, 1998.
83. Crawford SW, Hackman RC, Clark JG: Open lung biopsy diagnosis of diffuse pulmonary infiltrates after marrow transplantation. *Chest* 94:949–953, 1988.
84. Crawford SW: Fiberoptic bronchoscopy in the critically ill: playing it safe. *Pulmon Perspect* 11:5–8, 1994.
85. Crawford SW, Hackman RC, Clark JG: Biopsy diagnosis and clinical outcome of focal pulmonary lesions after marrow transplantation. *Transplantation* 48:266–271, 1989.
86. Musher B, Fredricks D, Leisenring W, et al: *Aspergillus* galactomannan enzyme immunoassay and quantitative PCR for diagnosis of invasive aspergillosis with bronchoalveolar lavage fluid. *J Clin Microbiol* 42:5517–5522, 2004.
87. Oliveira R, Machado A, Tateno A, et al: Frequency of human metapneumovirus infection in hematopoietic SCT recipients during 3 consecutive years. *Bone Marrow Transplant* 42:265–269, 2008.
88. Englund JA, Boeckh M, Kuypers J, et al: Fatal human metapneumovirus infection in stem cell transplant recipients. Ann Intern Med 144:344 349, 2006.
89. Ellis ME, Spence D, Bouchama A, et al: Open lung biopsy provides a higher and more specific diagnostic yield compared to broncho-alveolar lavage in immunocompromised patients. Fungal Study Group. *Scand J Infect Dis* 27:157–162, 1995.
90. Robinson LA, Reed EC, Galbraith TA, et al: Pulmonary resection for invasive Aspergillus infections in immunocompromised patients. *J Thorac Cardiovasc Surg* 109:1182–1196, 1995.
91. Tuan I-Z, Dennison D, Weisdorf DJ: *Pneumocystis carinii* pneumonitis following bone marrow transplantation. *Bone Marrow Transplant* 10:267–272, 1992.
92. Hughes WT: Use of dapsone in the prevention and treatment of Pneumocystis carinii pneumonia: a review (Review). *Clin Infect Dis* 27:191–204, 1998.
93. Marr KA, Carter RA, Crippa F, et al: Epidemiology and outcome of mould infections in hematopoietic stem cell transplant recipients. *Clin Infect Dis* 34:909–917, 2002.
94. Marr KA, Walsh TJ: Management strategies for infections caused by *candida* species, in Wingard JR, Bowden RA (eds): *Management of Infection in Oncology Patients.* London, UK: Martin Dunitz, 2003, pp 165–177.
95. Goodrich JM, Reed EC, Mori M, et al: Clinical features and analysis of risk factors for invasive candidal infection after marrow transplantation. *J Infect Dis* 164:731–740, 1991.
96. Goodman JL, Winston DJ, Greenfield RA, et al: A controlled trial of fluconazole to prevent fungal infections in patients undergoing bone marrow transplantation. *N Engl J Med* 326:845–851, 1992.
97. Marr KA, Seidel K, White TC, et al: Candidemia in allogeneic blood and marrow transplant recipients: evolution of risk factors after the adoption of prophylactic fluconazole. *J Infect Dis* 181:309–316, 2000.
98. Marr KA: The changing spectrum of candidemia in oncology patients: therapeutic implications. *Curr Opin Inf Dis* 13:615–620, 2000.
99. Wald A, Leisenring W, van Burik JA, et al: Epidemiology of *aspergillus* infections in a large cohort of patients undergoing bone marrow transplantation. *J Infect Dis* 175:1459–1466, 1997.
100. Herbrecht R, Letscher-Bru V, Oprea C, et al: Aspergillus galactomannan detection in the diagnosis of invasive aspergillosis in cancer patients. *J Clin Oncol* 20:1898–1906, 2002.
101. Uchida K, Yokota N, Yamaguchi H: In vitro antifungal activity of posaconazole against various pathogenic fungi. *Int J Antimicrob Agents* 18:167–172, 2001.
102. Manavathu EK, Abraham OC, Chandrasekar PH: Isolation and in vitro susceptibility to amphotericin B, itraconazole and posaconazole of voriconazole-resistant laboratory isolates of Aspergillus fumigatus. *Clin Microbiol Infect* 7:130–137, 2001.
103. Yeghen T, Kibbler CC, Prentice HG, et al: Management of invasive pulmonary aspergillosis in hematology patients: a review of 87 consecutive cases at a single institution. *Clin Infect Dis* 31:859–868, 2000.
104. Goodrich JM, Mori M, Gleaves CA, et al: Early treatment with ganciclovir to prevent cytomegalovirus disease after allogeneic bone marrow transplantation. *N Engl J Med* 325:1601–1607, 1991.
105. Goodrich JM, Bowden RA, Fisher L, et al: Ganciclovir prophylaxis to prevent cytomegalovirus disease after allogeneic marrow transplant. *Ann Intern Med* 118:173–178, 1993.
106. Schmidt GM, Horak DA, Niland JC, et al: A randomized, controlled trial of prophylactic ganciclovir for cytomegalovirus pulmonary infection in recipients of allogeneic bone marrow transplants. *N Engl J Med* 324:1005–1011, 1991.
107. Salzberger B, Bowden RA, Hackman RC, et al: Neutropenia in allogeneic marrow transplant recipients receiving ganciclovir for prevention of cytomegalovirus disease: risk factors and outcome. *Blood* 90:2502–2508, 1997.
108. Boeckh M, Gooley TA, Myerson D, et al: Cytomegalovirus pp65 antigenemia-guided early treatment with ganciclovir versus ganciclovir at engraftment after allogeneic marrow transplantation: a randomized double-blind study. *Blood* 88:4063–4071, 1996.
109. Einsele H, Ehninger G, Steidle M, et al: Polymerase chain reaction to evaluate antiviral therapy for cytomegalovirus disease. *Lancet* 338:1170–1172, 1991.
110. Boeckh M, Gallez-Hawkins GM, Myerson D, et al: Plasma polymerase chain reaction for cytomegalovirus DNA after allogeneic marrow transplantation: comparison with polymerase chain reaction using peripheral blood leukocytes, pp65 antigenemia, and viral culture. *Transplantation* 64:108–113, 1997.
111. Boeckh M, Hoy C, Torok-Storb B: Occult cytomegalovirus infection of marrow stroma. *Clin Infect Dis* 26:209–210, 1998.
112. Springmeyer SC, Hackman RC, Holle R, et al: Use of bronchoalveolar lavage to diagnose acute diffuse pneumonia in the immunocompromised host. *J Infect Dis* 154:604–610, 1986.
113. Cox GJ, Matsui SM, Lo RS, et al: Etiology and outcome of diarrhea after marrow transplantation: a prospective study. *Gastroenterology* 107:1398–1407, 1994.
114. Ljungman P, Engelhard D, Link H, et al: Treatment of interstitial pneumonitis due to cytomegalovirus with ganciclovir and intravenous immune globulin: experience of European bone marrow transplant group. *Clin Infect Dis* 14:831–835, 1992.
115. Reed EC, Bowden RA, Dandliker PS, et al: Treatment of cytomegalovirus pneumonia with ganciclovir and intravenous cytomegalovirus immunoglobulin in patients with bone marrow transplants. *Ann Intern Med* 109:783–788, 1988.
116. Meyers JD, Flournoy N, Thomas ED: Infection with herpes simplex virus and cell-mediated immunity after marrow transplant. *J Infect Dis* 142:338–346, 1980.
117. Johnson JR, Egaas S, Gleaves CA, et al: Hepatitis due to herpes simplex virus in marrow-transplant recipients. *Clin Infect Dis* 14:38–45, 1992.
118. Ramsey PG, Fife KH, Hackman RC, et al: Herpes simplex virus pneumonia: clinical, virological and pathological features in 20 patients. *Ann Intern Med* 97:813–820, 1982.
119. Wade JC, Newton B, McLaren C, et al: Intravenous acyclovir to treat mucocutaneous herpes simplex virus infection after marrow transplantation: a double-blind trial. *Ann Intern Med* 96:265–269, 1982.
120. Gluckman E, Lotsberg J, Devergie A, et al: Prophylaxis of herpes infections after bone marrow transplantation by oral acyclovir. *Lancet* 2:706–708, 1983.
121. Locksley RM, Flournoy N, Sullivan KM, et al: Infection with varicella-zoster virus infection after marrow transplantation. *J Infect Dis* 152:1172–1181, 1985.
122. Zaia JA, Levin MJ, Preblud SR, et al: Evaluation of varicella-zoster immune globulin: protection of immunosuppressed children after household exposure to varicella. *J Infect Dis* 147:737–743, 1983.
123. Han CS, Miller W, Haake R, et al: Varicella zoster infection after bone marrow transplantation: incidence, risk factors and complications. *Bone Marrow Transplant* 13:277–283, 1994.
124. Boeckh M, Kim HW, Flowers MED, et al: Long-term acyclovir for prevention of varicella zoster virus disease after allogeneic hematopoietic cell transplantation—a randomized double-blind placebo-controlled study. *Blood* 107:1800–1805, 2006.

125. Arvin AM: Varicella-zoster virus [Review]. *Clin Microbiol Rev* 9:361–381, 1996.
126. Kleinschmidt-DeMasters BK, Amlie-Lefond C, Gilden DH: The patterns of varicella zoster virus encephalitis. *Hum Pathol* 27:927–938, 1996.
127. Morishita K, Kodo H, Asano S, et al: Fulminant varicella hepatitis following bone marrow transplantation. *JAMA* 253:511, 1985.
128. Verdonck LF, Cornelissen JJ, Dekker AW, et al: Acute abdominal pain as a presenting symptom of varicella-zoster virus infection in recipients of bone marrow transplants. *Clin Infect Dis* 16:190–191, 1993.
129. Bowden RA: Respiratory virus infections after marrow transplant: the Fred Hutchinson Cancer Research Center experience. *Am J Med* 102:27–30, 1997.
130. Harrington RD, Hooton TM, Hackman R, et al: An outbreak of respiratory syncytial virus in a bone marrow transplant center. *J Infect Dis* 165:987–993, 1992.
131. Ghosh S, Champlin RE, Englund J, et al: Respiratory syncytial virus upper respiratory tract illnesses in adult blood and marrow transplant recipients: combination therapy with aerosolized ribavirin and intravenous immunoglobulin. *Bone Marrow Transplant* 25:751–755, 2000.
132. Baldwin A, Kingman H, Darville M, et al: Outcome and clinical course of 100 patients with adenovirus infection following bone marrow transplantation. *Bone Marrow Transplant* 26:1333–1338, 2000.
133. Flomenberg P, Babbitt J, Zuo L, et al: Increasing incidence of adenovirus disease in bone marrow transplant recipients. *J Infect Dis* 169:775–781, 1994.
134. Flomenberg P, Gutierrez E, Piaskowski V, et al: Detection of adenovirus DNA in peripheral blood mononuclear cells by polymerase chain reaction assay. *J Med Virol* 51:182–188, 1997.
135. Legrand F, Berrebi D, Houhou N, et al: Early diagnosis of adenovirus infection and treatment with cidofovir after bone marrow transplantation in children. *Bone Marrow Transplant* 27:621–626, 2001.
136. Orazi A, Hromas RA, Neiman RS, et al: Posttransplantation lymphoproliferative disorders in bone marrow transplant recipients are aggressive diseases with a high incidence of adverse histologic and immunobiologic features. *Am J Clin Pathol* 107:419–429, 1997.
137. Zutter MM, Martin PJ, Sale GE, et al: Epstein-Barr virus lymphoproliferation after bone marrow transplantation. *Blood* 72:520–529, 1988.
138. Hoshino Y, Kimura H, Tanaka N, et al: Prospective monitoring of the Epstein-Barr virus DNA by a real-time quantitative polymerase chain reaction after allogenic stem cell transplantation. *Br J Haematol* 115:105–111, 2001.
139. Kuehnle I, Huls MH, Liu Z, et al: CD20 monoclonal antibody (rituximab) for therapy of Epstein-Barr virus lymphoma after hemopoietic stem-cell transplantation. *Blood* 95:1502–1505, 2000.
140. Papadopoulos EB, Ladanyi M, Emanuel D, et al: Infusions of donor leukocytes to treat Epstein-Barr virus-associated lymphoproliferative disorders after allogeneic bone marrow transplantation. *N Engl J Med* 330:1185–1191, 1994.
141. Offner F, Schoch G, Fisher LD, et al: Mortality hazard functions as related to neutropenia at different times after marrow transplantation. *Blood* 88:4058–4062, 1996.
142. Mattsson J, Ringdén O, Storb R: Graft failure after allogeneic hematopoietic cell transplantation. *Biol Blood Marrow Transplant* 14[Suppl 1]:165–170, 2008.
143. Martin PJ: Prevention of allogeneic marrow graft rejection by donor T cells that do not recognize recipient alloantigens: potential role of a veto mechanism. *Blood* 88:962–969, 1996.
144. Aversa F, Tabilio A, Terenzi A, et al: Successful engraftment of T-cell-depleted haploidentical "three-loci" incompatible transplants in leukemia patients by addition of recombinant human granulocyte colony-stimulating factor-mobilized peripheral blood progenitor cells to bone marrow inoculum. *Blood* 84:3948–3955, 1994.
145. Bachar-Lustig E, Rachamim N, Li HW, et al: Megadose of T cell-depleted bone marrow overcomes MHC barriers in sublethally irradiated mice. *Nat Med* 1:1268–1273, 1995.
146. Beatty PG, Hansen JA, Longton GM, et al: Marrow transplantation from HLA-matched unrelated donors for treatment of hematologic malignancies. *Transplantation* 51:443–447, 1991.
147. Storb R, Deeg HJ, Whitehead J, et al: Methotrexate and cyclosporine compared with cyclosporine alone for prophylaxis of acute graft versus host disease after marrow transplantation for leukemia. *N Engl J Med* 314:729–735, 1986.
148. Beatty PG, Clift RA, Mickelson EM, et al: Marrow transplantation from related donors other than HLA-identical siblings. *N Engl J Med* 313:765–771, 1985.
149. Glucksberg H, Storb R, Fefer A, et al: Clinical manifestations of graft-versus-host disease in human recipients of marrow from HL-A-matched sibling donors. *Transplantation* 18:295–304, 1974.
150. Martin PJ, Nelson BJ, Appelbaum FR, et al: Evaluation of a CD5-specific immunotoxin for treatment of acute graft-versus-host disease after allogeneic marrow transplantation. *Blood* 88:824–830, 1996.
151. Sullivan KM, Shulman HM, Storb R, et al: Chronic graft-versus-host disease in 52 patients: adverse natural course and successful treatment with combination immunosuppression. *Blood* 57:267–276, 1981.
152. Cutler C, Giri S, Jeyapalan S, et al: Acute and chronic graft-versus-host disease after allogeneic peripheral-blood stem-cell and bone marrow transplantation: a meta-analysis. *J Clin Oncol* 19:3685–3691, 2001.
153. Stewart BL, Storer B, Storek J, et al: Duration of immunosuppressive treatment for chronic graft-versus-host disease. *Blood* 104:3501–3506, 2004.
154. Akpek G, Zahurak ML, Piantadosi S, et al: Development of a prognostic model for grading chronic graft-versus-host disease. *Blood* 97:1219–1226, 2001.
155. Filipovich AH, Weisdorf D, Pavletic S, et al: National Institutes of Health consensus development project on criteria for clinical trials in chronic graft-versus-host disease: I. Diagnosis and Staging Working Group report. *Biol Blood Marrow Transplant* 11:945–956, 2005.
156. Sale GE, Shulman HM, McDonald GB, et al: Gastrointestinal graft-versus-host disease in man. A clinicopathologic study of the rectal biopsy. *Am J Surg Pathol* 3:291–299, 1979.
157. Sale GE: Pathology and recent pathogenetic studies in human graft-versus-host disease. *Surv Synth Path Res* 3:235–253, 1984.
158. Sale GE, Shulman HM, Gallucci BB, et al: Young rete ridge keratinocytes are preferred targets in cutaneous graft-versus-host disease. *Am J Pathol* 118:278–287, 1985.
159. Ruutu T, Eriksson B, Remes K, et al: Ursodeoxycholic acid for the prevention of hepatic complications in allogeneic stem cell transplantation. *Blood* 100:1977–1983, 2002.
160. Ulrich CM, Yasui Y, Storb R, et al: Pharmacogenetics of methotrexate: toxicity among marrow transplantation patients varies with the methylenetetrahydrofolate reductase C677T polymorphism. *Blood* 98:231–234, 2001.
161. Yu C, Seidel K, Nash RA, et al: Synergism between mycophenolate mofetil and cyclosporine in preventing graft-versus-host disease among lethally irradiated dogs given DLA-nonidentical unrelated marrow grafts. *Blood* 91:2581–2587, 1998.
162. Alyea EP, Li S, Kim H, et al: Sirolimus, tacrolimus and reduced-dose methotrexate as graft versus host disease (GVHD) prophylaxis after non-myeloablative stem cell transplantation: low incidence of acute GVHD compared with tacrolimus/methotrexate or cyclosporine/prednisone [Abstract]. *Blood* 104(Part 1): 209a, #730, 2004.
163. Antin JH, Lee SJ, Neuberg D, et al: Sirolimus (RAP), tacrolimus (FK), and low dose methotrexate (MTX) for GVHD prophylaxis in mismatched related donor or unrelated donor transplantation. *Blood* 98[Suppl 1]:857a, #3559, 2001.
164. Antin JH, Kim HT, Cutler C, et al: Sirolimus, tacrolimus, and low-dose methotrexate for graft-versus-host disease prophylaxis in mismatched related donor or unrelated donor transplantation. *Blood* 102:1601–1605, 2003.
165. Mielcarek M, Storer BE, Boeckh M, et al: Initial therapy of acute graft-versus-host disease with low-dose prednisone does not compromise patient outcomes. *Blood* 113:2888–2894, 2009.
166. McDonald GB, Bouvier M, Hockenbery DM, et al: Oral beclomethasone dipropionate for treatment of intestinal graft-versus-host disease: a randomized, controlled trial. *Gastroenterology* 115:28–35, 1998.
167. Fried RH, Murakami CS, Fisher LD, et al: Ursodeoxycholic acid treatment of refractory chronic graft-versus-host of the liver. *Ann Intern Med* 116:624–629, 1992.
168. Vogelsang GB, Hess AD, Santos GW: Acute graft-versus-host disease: clinical characteristics in the cyclosporine era. *Medicine* 67:163–174, 1988.
169. van Lint MT, Uderzo C, Locasciulli A, et al: Early treatment of acute graft-versus-host disease with high- or low-dose 6-methylprednisolone: a multicenter randomized trial from the Italian Group for Bone Marrow Transplantation. *Blood* 92:2288–2293, 1998.
170. Alousi AM, Weisdorf DJ, Logan BR, et al: Etanercept, mycophenolate, denileukin, or pentostatin plus corticosteroids for acute graft-versus-host disease: a randomized phase 2 trial from the Blood and Marrow Transplant Clinical Trials Network. *Blood* 114:511–517, 2009.
171. Carpenter PA, Sanders JE: Steroid-refractory graft-vs.-host disease: past, present and future. *Pediatr Transplant* 7[Suppl 3]:19–31, 2003.
172. Couriel D, Carpenter PA, Cutler C, et al: Ancillary therapy and supportive care of chronic graft-versus-host disease: national institutes of health consensus development project on criteria for clinical trials in chronic graft-versus-host disease: V. Ancillary Therapy and Supportive Care Working Group report. *Biol Blood Marrow Transplant* 12:375–396, 2006.
173. Martin PJ, Schoch G, Fisher L, et al: A retrospective analysis of therapy for acute graft-versus-host disease: initial treatment. *Blood* 76:1464–1472, 1990.
174. Hings IM, Severson R, Filipovich AH, et al: Treatment of moderate and severe acute GVHD after allogeneic bone marrow transplantation. *Transplantation* 58:437–442, 1994.
175. Khoury H, Kashyap A, Adkins DR, et al: Treatment of steroid-resistant acute graft-versus-host disease with anti-thymocyte globulin. *Bone Marrow Transplant* 27:1059–1064, 2001.
176. McCaul KG, Nevill TJ, Barnett MJ, et al: Treatment of steroid-resistant acute graft-versus-host disease with rabbit antithymocyte globulin. *J Hematother Stem Cell Res* 9:367–374, 2000.
177. Couriel DR, Saliba RM, Giralt S, et al: Acute and chronic graft-versus-host disease after ablative and nonmyeloablative conditioning for allogeneic hematopoietic transplantation. *Biol Blood Marrow Transplant* 10:178–185, 2004.

178. Ho VT, Zahrieh D, Hochberg E, et al: Safety and efficacy of denileukin diftitox in patients with steroid-refractory acute graft-versus-host disease after allogeneic hematopoietic stem cell transplantation. *Blood* 104:1224–1226, 2004.
179. Przepiorka D, Kernan NA, Ippoliti C, et al: Daclizumab, a humanized anti-interleukin-2 receptor alpha chain antibody, for treatment of acute graft-versus-host disease. *Blood* 95:83–89, 2000.
180. MacMillan ML, Weisdorf DJ, Davies SM, et al: Early antithymocyte globulin therapy improves survival in patients with steroid-resistant acute graft-versus-host disease. *Biol Blood Marrow Transplant* 8:40–46, 2002.
181. Nichols WG, Corey L, Gooley T, et al: Rising pp65 antigenemia during preemptive anticytomegalovirus therapy after allogeneic hematopoietic stem cell transplantation: risk factors, correlation with DNA load, and outcomes. *Blood* 97:867–874, 2001.
182. Marr KA, Carter RA, Boeckh M, et al: Invasive aspergillosis in allogeneic stem cell transplant recipients: changes in epidemiology and risk factors. *Blood* 100:4358–4366, 2002.
183. Fukuda T, Boeckh M, Carter RA, et al: Risks and outcomes of invasive fungal infections in recipients of allogeneic hematopoietic stem cell transplants after nonmyeloablative conditioning. *Blood* 102:827–833, 2003.
184. Qu L, Kiss JE: Thrombotic microangiopathy in transplantation and malignancy. *Semin Thromb Hemost* 31:691–699, 2005.
185. Rabinowe SN, Soiffer RJ, Tarbell NJ, et al: Hemolytic-uremic syndrome following bone marrow transplantation in adults for hematologic malignancies. *Blood* 77:1837–1844, 1991.
186. Rowley SD, Donaldson G, Lilleby K, et al: Experiences of donors enrolled in a randomized study of allogeneic bone marrow or peripheral blood stem cell transplantation. *Blood* 97:2541–2548, 2001.
187. Bolan CD, Leitman SF, Griffith LM, et al: Delayed donor red cell chimerism and pure red cell aplasia following major ABO-incompatible nonmyeloablative hematopoietic stem cell transplantation. *Blood* 98:1687–1694, 2001.
188. Bolan CD, Childs RW, Procter JL, et al: Massive immune haemolysis after allogeneic peripheral blood stem cell transplantation with minor ABO incompatibility. *Br J Haematol* 112:787–795, 2001.
189. Oziel-Taieb S, Faucher-Barbey C, Chabannon C, et al: Early and fatal immune haemolysis after so-called 'minor' ABO-incompatible peripheral blood stem cell allotransplantation. *Bone Marrow Transplant* 19:1155–1156, 1997.
190. Remberger M, Aschan J, Barkholt L, et al: Treatment of severe acute graft-versus-host disease with anti-thymocyte globulin (Review). *Clin Transplant* 15:147–153, 2001.
191. Arai SM: Poor outcome in steroid-refractory graft-versus-host disease with antithymocyte globulin treatment. *Biol Blood Marrow Transplant* 8:155–160, 2002.
192. Perales MA, Ishill N, Lomazow WA, et al: Long-term follow-up of patients treated with daclizumab for steroid-refractory acute graft-vs-host disease. *Bone Marrow Transplant* 40:481–486, 2007.
193. Miano M, Cuzzubbo D, Terranova P, et al: Daclizumab as useful treatment in refractory acute GVHD: a paediatric experience. *Bone Marrow Transplant* 43:423–427, 2009.
194. Couriel D, Saliba R, Hicks K, et al: Tumor necrosis factor-alpha blockade for the treatment of acute GVHD. *Blood* 104:649–654, 2004.
195. Patriarca F, Sperotto A, Damiani D, et al: Infliximab treatment for steroid-refractory acute graft-versus-host disease. *Haematologica* 89:1352–1359, 2004.
196. Sleight BS, Chan KW, Braun TM, et al: Infliximab for GVHD therapy in children. *Bone Marrow Transplant* 40:473–480, 2007.
197. Busca A, Locatelli F, Marmont F, et al: Recombinant human soluble tumor necrosis factor receptor fusion protein as treatment for steroid refractory graft-versus-host disease following allogeneic hematopoietic stem cell transplantation. *Am J Hematol* 82:45–52, 2007.
198. Furlong T, Leisenring W, Storb R, et al: Psoralen and ultraviolet A irradiation (PUVA) as therapy for steroid-resistant cutaneous acute graft-versus-host disease. *Biol Blood Marrow Transplant* 8:206–212, 2002.
199. Greinix HT, Volc-Platzer B, Kalhs P, et al: Extracorporeal photochemotherapy in the treatment of severe steroid-refractory acute graft-versus-host disease: a pilot study. *Blood* 96:2426–2431, 2000.
200. Greinix HT, Knobler RM, Worel N, et al: The effect of intensified extracorporeal photochemotherapy on long-term survival in patients with severe acute graft-versus-host disease. *Haematologica* 91:405–408, 2006.
201. Messina C, Locatelli F, Lanino E, et al: Extracorporeal photochemotherapy for paediatric patients with graft-versus-host disease after haematopoietic stem cell transplantation. *Br J Haematol* 122:118–127, 2003.
202. Calore E, Calo A, Tridello G, et al: Extracorporeal photochemotherapy may improve outcome in children with acute GVHD. *Bone Marrow Transplant* 42:421–425, 2008.
203. Perfetti P, Carlier P, Strada P, et al: Extracorporeal photopheresis for the treatment of steroid refractory acute GVHD. *Bone Marrow Transplant* 42:609–617, 2008.
204. Basara N, Kiehl MG, Blau W, et al: Mycophenolate Mofetil in the treatment of acute and chronic GVHD in hematopoietic stem cell transplant patients: four years of experience. *Transplant Proc* 33:2121–2123, 2001.
205. Nash RA, Furlong T, Storb R, et al: Mycophenolate mofetil (MMF) as salvage treatment for graft-versus-host-disease (GVHD) after allogeneic hematopoietic stem cell transplantation (HSCT): safety analysis [Abstract]. *Blood* 90[Suppl 1]:105a, #459.
206. Benito AI, Furlong T, Martin PJ, et al: Sirolimus (Rapamycin) for the treatment of steroid-refractory acute graft-versus-host disease. *Transplantation* 72:1924–1929, 2001.
207. Bolanos-Meade J, Jacobsohn DA, Margolis J, et al: Pentostatin in steroid-refractory acute graft-versus-host disease. *J Clin Oncol* 23:2661–2668, 2005.
208. Le Blanc K, Frassoni F, Ball L, et al: Mesenchymal stem cells for treatment of steroid-resistant, severe, acute graft-versus-host disease: a phase II study. *Lancet* 371:1579–1586, 2008.

CHAPTER 189 ■ CRITICAL CARE OF THE LUNG TRANSPLANT RECIPIENT

LUIS F. ANGEL AND STEPHANIE M. LEVINE

Over the past three decades, lung transplantation (LT) has become a successful therapeutic option for patients with end-stage pulmonary parenchymal or vascular disease. In the early era of LT, the primary complications associated with the procedure were dehiscence and impaired healing of the bronchial anastomosis and early graft failure; these complications occurred in most patients who survived for more than 1 week. Improvements in donor and recipient selection and surgical techniques, the development of new immunosuppressive drugs, and better management of complications, such as primary graft dysfunction (PGD), rejection, and infections have all contributed to advancing the field (Table 189.1). Despite these advances, LT is still associated with numerous complications, often requiring intensive care management.

According to the 2009 report of the International Society for Heart and Lung Transplantation (ISHLT), more than 2,700 lung transplants were performed in 2007 alone. The ISHLT Registry reports that the 1-year survival rate for lung transplant recipients is 79%, the 3-year rate is 64%, and the 5-year rate is 52% [1]. There has been an improvement in median survival in the recent years to 5.7 years over the 4.7 years found in previous years. The most common cause of mortality is PGD in the

TABLE 189.1

MAJOR ADVANCES OR CHANGES IN LUNG TRANSPLANTATION OVER THE PAST FIVE YEARS

Topic	Change	Reference
Transplant procedures by indication	More BLT procedures performed for COPD	[1]
Allocation system	Organs allocated by necessity, not time on waiting list	[7]
Increasing the donor pool	Increasing the use of marginal/extended donors	[15–18]
Primary graft dysfunction	No proven benefit of inhaled nitric oxide administered prophylactically for the prevention of PGD	[31]
	New staging system for PGD	[26]
Immunosuppression	Possible benefit from inhaled cyclosporine	[59]
Rejection	Revision of the staging system for bronchiolitis obliterans syndrome	[62]
Infection prophylaxis	PCR used to monitor for CMV infection following transplant	[74]
	Effective antifungal prophylactic regimens available	[81]
	Twelve months of oral valganciclovir is effective for CMV prophylaxis	[76]
Revision of staging of pathologic rejection	Restaging of lymphocytic bronchiolitis	[58]

BLT, bilateral lung transplantation; CMV, cytomegalovirus; COPD, chronic obstructive pulmonary disease; PCR, polymerase chain reaction; PGD, primary graft dysfunction.

first 30 days following transplantation, non-cytomegalovirus (CMV) infection in the first year following transplantation, and chronic rejection at all subsequent time intervals.

INDICATIONS

Single-lung transplantation (SLT) is performed for obstructive nonsuppurative lung disease, such as emphysema resulting from tobacco use or α_1-antitrypsin deficiency. It is also indicated for fibrotic lung diseases such as idiopathic pulmonary fibrosis (29%), familial pulmonary fibrosis, drug- or toxin-induced lung disease, occupational lung disease, sarcoidosis, limited scleroderma, lymphangioleiomyomatosis, eosinophilic granuloma, and other disorders resulting in end-stage fibrotic lung disease [1].

The most frequent indications for bilateral lung transplantation (BLT) are suppurative pulmonary lung disease, cystic fibrosis and bronchiectasis (31%) and severe chronic obstructive pulmonary disease (COPD) resulting from tobacco use (26%), or α_1-antitrypsin deficiency (8%). In addition, more than 90% of transplant centers prefer to perform BLT when patients have idiopathic pulmonary hypertension (5%) [1].

Heart–lung transplantation (HLT) is performed at only a few transplantation centers and should be reserved for patients who cannot be treated by LT alone. The most frequent indications for HLT are Eisenmenger syndrome with a cardiac anomaly that cannot be corrected surgically and severe end-stage lung disease with concurrent severe heart disease. HLT is discussed in more detail in Chapter 183.

GUIDELINES FOR RECIPIENT SELECTION

There has been a revision of the original consensus-based guidelines for the selection of lung transplant candidates [2]. Any patient with end-stage pulmonary or cardiopulmonary disease with the capacity for rehabilitation can be considered for transplantation. The patient should have untreatable end-stage pulmonary disease, no other significant medical illness, have a limited life expectancy, and be psychologically stable and compliant.

Age

The 2006 international guidelines for the selection of transplant candidates [2] now suggest an age limit of 65 years regardless of procedure type. Although this is somewhat arbitrary, numerous patients with end-stage pulmonary disease are young to middle-aged, and there is a relative lack of available donors.

Relative Contraindications

Transplantation is not contraindicated in patients with systemic diseases that are limited to the lungs such as scleroderma, systemic lupus erythematosus, polymyositis, and rheumatoid arthritis. These cases should be considered on an individual basis. Osteoporosis has become a significant problem in the post-transplant period, and preexisting symptomatic osteoporosis has also been identified as a relative contraindication to transplantation.

Patients with active sites of infection are not considered to be good transplant candidates. Treated tuberculosis and fungal disease pose a particular problem but are not contraindications for LT. Many centers will not consider performing a transplant in a patient who is chronically colonized with a resistant organism (e.g., *Burkholderia species*, methicillin-resistant Staphylococcus, atypical mycobacterium, or Aspergillus) and it is recommended to try to eradicate these organisms in the pre-transplant period and to consider each patient on an individual basis. However, if considered, these patients should be candidates only for BLT procedures since the remaining colonized lung could pose a serious threat to the new graft in the case of an SLT. This issue is of particular concern in cystic fibrosis patients who are often infected with drug resistant organisms. Both *Burkholderia cenocepacia* (specific strains) and *Burkholderia gladioli* are of concern due to poor posttransplant outcomes [3].

A requirement for invasive mechanical ventilation is a strong relative contraindication to transplantation, although LT has been performed successfully in small numbers of mechanically ventilated patients with CF, and other end-stage lung disease [4,5]. In one small series there was a longer time on postoperative mechanical ventilation and a longer ICU stay following LT. Rates of PGD, survival, and total hospital stay were similar to those in patients undergoing LT not on mechanical ventilation [4]. Recently venoarterial extracorporeal membrane oxygenation (ECMO) has been used in end-stage lung disease patients during transplantation with good short-term function and survival rates [5]. In a large review of the United Network Organ sharing (UNOS) database of patients undergoing LT on mechanical respiratory support 586 on mechanical ventilation and 51 on ECMO as a bridge to LT, the authors found that patients on mechanical ventilation or ECMO have lower survival rates following LT compared to those not requiring support [6]. Noninvasive ventilatory support is not considered a relative contraindication to transplantation

To be considered for transplantation, patients should have an ideal body weight of >70% or ≤130% predicted (BMI 18 to 30 kg per m^2). Those patients with poor nutritional status may be too weak to withstand the surgical procedure; those patients who are obese make more difficult surgical candidates and may have higher mortality rates than nonobese patients.

Pretransplant low-dose therapy with corticosteroids has been proven to be acceptable for patients who cannot have therapy with corticosteroids completely discontinued. Initial data implicated corticosteroids as a cause of tracheal bronchial dehiscence. Currently, transplant programs will consider patients who can be maintained in the long term on a regimen of prednisone of ≤20 mg per day and may consider patients who are receiving higher doses.

Prior thoracotomy or pleurodesis was once considered to be a relative contraindication to transplantation due to increased technical difficulties and increased bleeding. Despite this, transplantation can be successfully performed in these patients.

Absolute Contraindications

The 2006 international guidelines [2] identified several absolute contraindications to LT including major organ dysfunction (i.e., renal creatinine clearance of ≤50 mg per mL per minute), HIV infection, hepatitis B antigen positivity, and hepatitis C with biopsy-documented liver disease. Active malignancy within the prior 2 years is also a contraindication to transplantation. For patients with a history of breast cancer greater than stage 2, colon cancer greater than Duke A stage, renal carcinoma, or melanoma greater than or equal to level 2, the waiting period should be at least 5 years. Restaging is suggested prior to transplant listing.

Severe nonosteoporotic skeletal disease, such as kyphoscoliosis, is often an absolute contraindication to transplantation, primarily because of the technical difficulties encountered during surgery.

Drug abuse and alcoholism are considered to be contraindications to transplantation because patients with these conditions are at high risk for noncompliance. Patients who continue to smoke despite having end-stage pulmonary disease are not candidates for LT. Transplant centers require patients to abstain from cigarette smoking, alcohol use, or narcotics use for 6 months to 2 years before being considered for lung transplant evaluation.

The patient must be well motivated and emotionally stable to withstand the extreme stress of the pretransplant and perioperative period. A history of noncompliance or significant psychiatric illness is an absolute contraindication

DONOR ALLOCATION AND SELECTION

Until the spring of 2005, as established by the United Network of Organ Sharing, lungs were allocated primarily by time on the waiting list, and not by necessity. In the spring of 2005, the system for donor allocation for lungs was revised, and assigned priority for lung offers became based on a benefit or need-based Lung Allocation Score [7]. The LAS is calculated using the following measures: (1) waitlist urgency measure (i.e., the expected number of days lived without a transplant during an additional year on the waitlist); (2) posttransplant survival measure (i.e., the expected number of days lived during the first year posttransplant); and (3) the transplant benefit measure (i.e., the posttransplant survival measure minus waitlist urgency measure) [8]. Although it is still too early to determine the long-term effects that this new allocation system will have on LT, it appears that many of the goals of the system (decreased waiting list deaths, and times, prioritizing patients by urgency rather than time on the list) are being accomplished, with comparable survival rates except in those with the very high LAS scores (>46 in one study) [9,10]. There appears to be a stepwise decline in posttransplant survival as the LAS score increases. In patients with high LAS scores there was also higher morbidity including requirements for dialysis, infections, and longer lengths of stay [11]. Since the implementation of the LAS, the distribution of patient diagnoses on the list, and those transplanted, has also shifted from a majority of COPD patients to an increasing number of patients with pulmonary fibrosis. In addition, sicker patients are being transplanted.

Donor lungs are first distributed locally, then regionally, and finally nationally. Currently, the average time spent on the waiting list is approximately 18 to 24 months, and therefore close management of the listed transplant patient is required. Despite this close attention, a small percentage of patients die while awaiting transplantation.

A shortage of donor organs remains the primary factor limiting the number of LTs performed. Contributing to this shortage is the estimate that lungs for transplantation are procured from only 19% of multiorgan donors [12]. The vast majority of transplanted lungs are from brain-dead donors. A small number of LT procedures involving living related donors and non–heart-beating lung donors (also called donation after cardiac death [DCD]) have been performed at institutions specializing in these procedures [13]. In a small group of DCD donors lung transplant recipients, rates of PGD, acute rejection, bronchiolitis obliterans, and 2-year survival rates were comparable to those of lung transplant recipients from cadaveric donors during the same period. Graft function was better preserved in the DCD recipients [14].

The usual donor selection criteria are age younger than 60 to 65 years, no history of clinically significant lung disease, normal results from a sputum Gram stain, and a limited history of smoking (less than 20 pack-years). In addition, the lung fields should be clear as demonstrated by chest radiograph, and gas exchange should be adequate as demonstrated by a partial pressure of arterial oxygen (PaO_2) more than 300 mm Hg, while receiving fractional inspired oxygen (FIO_2) equal to 1, or a PaO_2/FIO_2 ratio of more than 300 with a positive end expiratory pressure (PEEP) of 5 cm H_2O. Bronchoscopy is also part of the evaluation of the donor. The main goal of the endobronchial evaluation is to rule out gross aspiration or purulent secretions in the distal airways.

Lungs from extended donors (i.e., those who do not meet all of the criteria listed earlier) are now more frequently being transplanted in an attempt to expand the donor pool [15–18], and some centers are actively engaged in developing protocols for optimizing marginal donor lungs, thereby rendering them transplantable. By instituting a protocol including educational and donor management interventions, and changing donor classification and selection criteria, a single-organ procurement organization was able to increase the percentage of lungs procured from 11.5% to 22.5% with an increase in the number of procedures performed, without adverse recipient outcomes [15].

Donors are excluded from potential lung donation if there is evidence of active infection, human immunodeficiency virus, hepatitis, or malignancy. Donor and recipient compatibility is assessed by matching A, B, and O blood types and chest wall size. Human leukocyte antigen (HLA) matching is not routinely performed in LT except in patients with history of preformed donor-specific antibodies.

SURGICAL TECHNIQUES

Initially, double-lung transplantation was the procedure of choice; the anastomosis was placed at the level of the trachea. However, the rate of ischemic airway complications was prohibitive. Now, SLT or BLT (essentially sequential SLT) with anastomoses at the level of the mainstem bronchi is the preferred surgical technique. At the time of cardiac harvest, the donor lung is usually removed through a median sternotomy. The pulmonary veins are detached from the heart with a residual 5-mm cuff of left atrium. The pulmonary artery is transected from the main pulmonary trunk, and the mainstem bronchus is transected between two staple lines. During transportation to the recipient site, the partially inflated donor lung graft is placed into preservation solution, usually a low-potassium dextran solution with extracellular electrolyte composition or a modified Euro-Collins solution with an intracellular electrolyte composition at 4°C.

For SLT, the recipient surgery is performed through a posterolateral thoracotomy or sternotomy, or vertical axillary muscle-sparing minithoracotomy. Most centers start with the bronchial anastomosis, without a vascular anastomosis of the bronchial circulation of the recipient and donor lungs. Initially, most transplant procedures involved an end-to-end anastomosis, which was wrapped with a piece of omentum or pericardial fat with an intact vascular pedicle for assistance in bronchial revascularization. Subsequently, a telescoping technique was recommended, with the recipient and donor bronchi overlapping by approximately one cartilaginous ring. This procedure allowed the recipient's intact bronchial circulation to supply the donor bronchus. More recently, most anastomoses are performed with an end-to-end single suture in the membranous portion and a single or continuous suture in the cartilaginous portion, without omental wrap, and telescoping is performed when the donor and recipient bronchi differ in size and there is a natural, unforced telescoping of both bronchi [19,20].

After the bronchial anastomosis has been performed, the donor pulmonary veins are anastomosed end-to-end to the recipient's left atrium, and the pulmonary arteries are attached with an end-to-end anastomosis.

BLT is usually performed through a transverse thoracosternotomy (clamshell incision) or a median sternotomy followed by sequential single-lung procedures. Cardiopulmonary bypass may be required for patients with pulmonary hypertension or those who cannot tolerate single-lung ventilation or perfusion and who experience marked hypoxemia or hemodynamic instability. Although center specific, an increasing number of cases (nearly 50% of LT procedures at some institutions) are performed with the use of cardiopulmonary bypass.

GENERAL POSTOPERATIVE MANAGEMENT

After LT, patients usually remain intubated, require mechanical ventilation, and are transferred to the ICU. Most patients are ventilated in a volume-control mode, although in recent years some transplant centers have changed to pressure-control ventilation, or airway pressure release ventilation. In general, low tidal volume ventilation strategies are used. Airway pressures are kept as low as possible so that barotrauma and anastomotic dehiscence can be avoided. Many institutions use routine pharmacologic sedation. Patients are generally maintained with tidal volumes of 6 to 8 mL per kg postoperatively. At most institutions, a low level of PEEP (5.0 to 7.5 cm H_2O) is applied immediately after lung expansion in the operating room and is continued after transplantation. Early extubation is one of the main goals after LT, and lung transplant recipients who do not experience complications are extubated within the first 12 to 24 hours postoperatively if they meet the commonly accepted weaning criteria. Some centers may attempt to extubate immediately postoperatively [21]. Both postural drainage and chest physiotherapy can be routinely employed without concern for mechanical complications at the anastomosis, and patients should perform incentive spirometry soon after extubation.

Certain patient populations require special ventilator management. Most patients with idiopathic pulmonary hypertension undergo BLT; however, at a few centers some patients undergo SLT for pulmonary hypertension with an increased risk of reperfusion pulmonary edema because nearly all of the perfusion is going to the newly implanted lung.

Patients with obstructive lung disease can encounter problems if the delivered tidal volume or the required levels of PEEP are high. Occasionally, clinically significant acute native lung hyperinflation can occur and can compromise the newly transplanted lung and lead to hypotension and hemodynamic instability. To reduce this problem, some transplant centers avoid PEEP for patients undergoing SLT for obstructive disease. However, the problem is magnified when patients experience reperfusion injury or pneumonia after transplantation; in such cases the compliance of the transplanted lung is decreased and higher PEEP is required for maintaining oxygenation. As a consequence, the more compliant emphysematous lung becomes overexpanded and can herniate toward the contralateral hemithorax [22]. Attempts to prevent this possible complication by using selective independent ventilation with a double-lumen endotracheal tube have been tried. Lung hyperinflation is associated with a significantly longer stay in the intensive care unit (ICU), a longer duration of mechanical ventilation, and a trend toward higher mortality [23].

Pain control is usually provided by opiates, usually fentanyl, administered intravenously or morphine sulfate via an epidural catheter with a patient-regulated pain-control system.

Because many patients are nutritionally depleted before transplantation as a result of their underlying disease, postoperative nutrition is important. Ideally, enteral nutrition should be provided as soon as tolerated.

Antibiotics are routinely administered for the first 48 to 72 hours after transplantation. Antibiotic regimens include broad-spectrum antibiotic coverage for both Gram-negative and Gram-positive bacteria. Most centers advocate empiric anaerobic coverage. Gram stains and cultures of sputum from the donor and the recipient may be used when available to guide the choice of appropriate antibiotics. Many centers routinely use antifungal agents such as inhaled amphotericin B, voriconazole, or itraconazole postoperatively. Most transplantation programs administer ganciclovir and, more recently, valganciclovir for CMV prophylaxis if either the patient or the donor is CMV-positive before surgery.

Immunosuppression is begun preoperatively with tacrolimus or cyclosporine and corticosteroids. Corticosteroids are administered in the operating room as intravenous methylprednisolone 0.5 to 1 g (usually administered at the time of reperfusion) and then at doses of 1 to 3 mg per kg daily for the next 3 days, followed by 0.8 mg per kg daily and then conversion to an equivalent oral dose. In the past, lympholytic medications, such as intravenous antithymocyte globulin (ATG) at 1.5 mg per kg daily for 3 to 5 days or muromonab-CD3 (Orthoclone OKT3) at 5 mg per day for the first 5 to 10 days, were used as induction therapy after transplantation; however, more recently the use of these medications has been limited. Some centers currently use interleukin (IL)-2 receptor blockers (e.g., basiliximab) for induction. A retrospective registry analysis of the impact of induction therapy on survival following LT showed a survival advantage with the use of interleukin-2- receptor antagonists in both SLT and BLT recipients and in BLT recipients treated with ATG [24]. After the transplantation procedure, most patients begin a triple immunosuppression protocol with a combination of prednisone, a calcineurin agent, tacrolimus or cyclosporine, and a cell cycle inhibiting agent, mycophenolate mofetil or azathioprine [25].

POSTOPERATIVE PROBLEMS

Primary Graft Dysfunction

Perhaps the most serious problem in the postoperative period after LT is PGD [26]. It is estimated that as many as 80% of patients will experience some degree of PGD and as many as 15% of cases can be severe [27]. A 2005 consensus conference attempted to standardize the grading of PGD on the basis of gas exchange and the presence of radiographic infiltrates (Table 189.2). When the acute lung injury definition of acute respiratory distress syndrome (ARDS)—a PaO_2/FIO_2 ratio of less than 200 is used to define the most severe form of PGD (grade 3), the reported incidence is 10% to 25%. PGD is a diagnosis of exclusion; the condition usually occurs hours to 3 days after LT, whereas rejection and infection are more common after the first 24 hours. A stenosis at the venous anastomosis presents with similar signs and symptoms, but this diagnosis can be excluded by transesophageal echocardiography. However, because the timing of these disorders may vary, differentiation may be difficult [26].

TABLE 189.2

GRADING OF THE SEVERITY OF PRIMARY GRAFT DYSFUNCTION

Grade	PaO_2/FIO_2	Radiographic infiltrates consistent with pulmonary edema
0	>300	No
1	>300	Yes
2	200–300	Yes
3	<200	Yes

Adapted from Christie JD, Carby M, Bag R, et al: Report of the ISHLT Working Group on Primary Lung Graft Dysfunction part II: definition. A consensus statement of the International Society for Heart and Lung Transplantation. *J Heart Lung Transplant* 24(10):1454–1459, 2005, with permission.

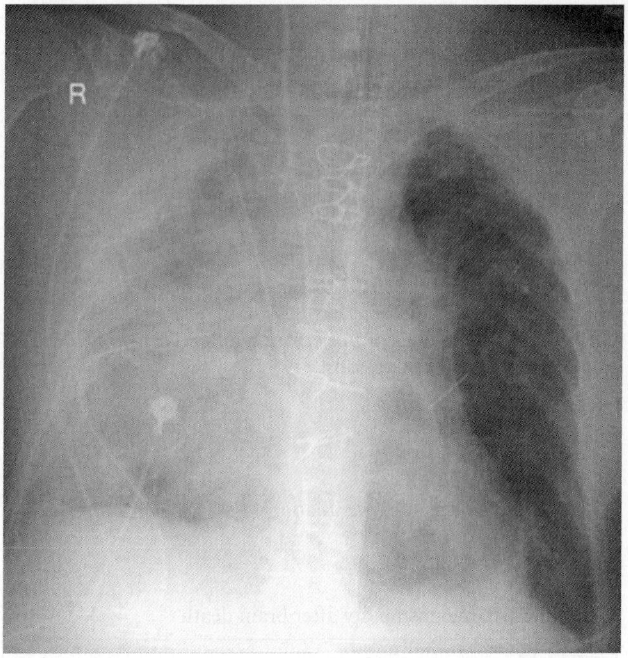

FIGURE 189.1. Severe primary graft dysfunction in the transplanted lung following a right single-lung transplant for idiopathic pulmonary fibrosis.

PGD can persist to various degrees for hours to days after LT. Clinically, PGD is characterized by the appearance of new alveolar or interstitial infiltrates on radiographs, a decrease in pulmonary compliance, an increase in pulmonary vascular resistance, and a disruption in gas exchange. Radiographic findings in these patients include a perihilar haze, patchy alveolar consolidations, and, in the most severe form, dense perihilar and basilar alveolar consolidations on air bronchograms (Fig. 189.1). Pathology reports from biopsy specimens, autopsies, or lung explants removed during retransplantation indicate diffuse alveolar damage. PGD usually stabilizes over the next 2 to 4 days and then begins to resolve, or worsens with all cause mortality rates at 30 days exceeding 40% in some studies.

PGD is managed supportively with diuretics and mechanical ventilation, often with protective ventilatory strategies [28]. Because endogenous nitric oxide (NO) activity decreases after LT, there are several reports of the successful use of inhaled NO for hypoxemia and for pulmonary hypertension as a consequence of graft dysfunction after transplantation [29–32]. However, in one randomized, placebo-controlled trial (84 patients), the prophylactic inhalation of NO 10 minutes after reperfusion and for a minimum of 6 hours, was not shown to be beneficial for hemodynamic variables, reperfusion injury, oxygenation, time to extubation, length of intensive care or hospital stay, or 30-day mortality [31]. A similar study beginning NO at the onset of ventilation supported these findings [30]. The use of artificial surfactant replacement has also been examined [33–35]. An open randomized prospective trial studying the use of instilled bovine surfactant immediately after establishment of the bronchial anastomosis, showed improved oxygenation and decreased PGD, shortened intubation time, and enhanced

TABLE 189.3

POSSIBLE RISK FACTORS FOR PRIMARY GRAFT DYSFUNCTION AFTER LUNG TRANSPLANTATION

Recipient characteristics
Pulmonary hypertension
Diffuse parenchymal lung disease diagnosis
Body mass index >25 kg/m^2
Operative factors
Cardiopulmonary bypass during surgery
Prolonged ischemic time for the organ
Methods/techniques of preservation and reperfusion
Blood product transfusions
Donor characteristics
Female gender
African American race
Age <21 y or >45 y
Prolonged mechanical ventilation
Aspiration pneumonia
History of tobacco use
Trauma
Hemodynamic instability after brain death

Adapted from references [27,43–48].

early post-LT recovery in the treatment group, although an unusually high incidence of PGD was found in the control group [34]. The use of ECMO for severe early graft dysfunction [36] has also been described, with a hospital survival rate of 42% in an analysis of the Extracorporeal Life Support Organization registry study [37]. High-frequency oscillatory ventilation and independent lung ventilation have been used in some cases. Retransplantation has also been performed, but the outcome for patients undergoing retransplantation for PGD has been very poor.

Severe PGD usually leads to compromised short-term outcomes, including increase in the duration of mechanical ventilation and lengths of stay, poor 1-year survival rates (40% for patients with PGD in one single-center study), and compromised function among survivors [38,39]. Long-term outcomes, such as pulmonary function and the incidence of bronchiolitis obliterans, are also impacted, and more severe PGD and longer duration of PGD significantly increases the development of bronchiolitis obliterans syndrome (BOS) [40,41].

Although the mechanisms of PGD have not been completely delineated, several contributing factors have been postulated, including the disruption of lymphatics, bronchial vasculature, or nerves, and lung injury occurring either during preservation of the graft or after reperfusion [42]. Multiple risk factors (Table 189.3) may be associated with the development of PGD [27,43–48]. Some have borne out in multivariate analysis. Donor variables include: female gender, African American race, donor age less than 21 years and more than 45 years, prolonged mechanical ventilation, aspiration pneumonia, history of tobacco use, trauma, and hemodynamic instability following brain death. The technique used for graft preservation and the perfusion solution (e.g., Eurocollins), the use of cardiopulmonary bypass, prolonged ischemic times, and blood product transfusions may also be risk factors for PGD. Recipient factors contributing to PGD include: a diagnosis of pulmonary hypertension, elevated pulmonary artery pressures at the time of transplant, body mass index (BMI) >25 kg per m^2, and diffuse parenchymal lung disease. Humoral rejection has recently been postulated to be a risk factor for PGD [48]. Since the institution of the LAS, some studies have shown an increase in the incidence of PGD [49] but others have not supported this finding [50].

Intensive Care Unit Outcomes

Few data are available for predicting outcomes and length of ICU stay after LT. It is known that the duration of mechanical ventilation is prolonged and the ICU mortality increased for patients who experience PGD [38]. One study found that an immediate postoperative PaO_2/FIO_2 ratio of less than 200 predicted an ICU stay of 5 days or more [51]. In another study, poor nutritional status (BMI below the 25th percentile) in patients remaining in the ICU for more than 5 days was associated with a higher ICU mortality rate [52]. In this same study, a preoperative diagnosis of pulmonary hypertension or restrictive lung disease and BLT rather than SLT were associated with longer ICU stays. Another study examined the value of intravascular volume status and central venous pressure (CVP) in predicting ICU outcomes; the results indicated that a CVP higher than 7 mm Hg after transplantation was associated with a longer duration of mechanical ventilation, longer ICU and hospital stays, and higher 2-month mortality rates [53].

Among patients requiring prolonged ICU stays, those who underwent tracheostomy were more likely to have undergone BLT, to have required cardiopulmonary bypass during the procedure, to have experienced postoperative pneumonia, to have had more significant reperfusion injury at 48 hours, to have had longer initial periods of mechanical ventilation, and to have required reintubation more often [54].

Late Complications Requiring Admission to the Intensive Care Unit

The number of lung transplant recipients who are admitted to the ICU is expected to increase as the number of long-term survivors increases. The postoperative mortality rate has decreased because of improved surgical techniques and perioperative care, and approximately 90% to 95% of patients are discharged alive after transplantation. However, after this immediate posttransplantation period, lung transplant recipients are more likely than some other solid-organ transplant recipients to experience infection or rejection that often requires readmission to the ICU.

Nearly 25% of lung transplant recipients require an ICU admission after the initial hospital discharge. The most common admission diagnoses are respiratory failure and sepsis. These patients frequently require mechanical ventilation (53%), and the mortality rate is generally close to 40%. Prognostic factors for mortality include higher acute physiology and chronic health evaluation (APACHE) scores, a forced expiratory volume in one second (FEV_1) lower than the patient's best posttransplantation FEV_1, nonpulmonary organ dysfunction, low-serum albumin level, and longer duration of mechanical ventilation [55]. Patients admitted with a diagnosis of BOS who require mechanical ventilation are at the highest risk of mortality. The long-term survival of patients who recover from the ICU stay is also compromised; however, a high percentage of patients (50%) can still enjoy long-term survival after an ICU admission.

Airway Complications

Because of the lack of revascularization of the bronchial circulation, anastomotic complications, such as bronchial dehiscence, bronchial stenosis, and bronchial infection, are the main airway complications reported in the first few weeks to months after LT. The incidence of anastomotic complications has decreased as surgical techniques have improved and surgeons have gained experience with the procedure. The reported incidence of this complication ranges widely: some studies report it to be as high as 33%; others, as low as 1.6%. However, in reality, most recent series suggest a range of 7% to 18% [56], with a related mortality rate of 2% to 4%. Risk factors for airway complications include ischemia of the donor bronchus during the posttransplant period, due to loss of bronchial blood flow (only the pulmonary vessels are revascularized during LT surgery), surgical techniques for the anastomosis, length of the donor bronchi, acute rejection, and bronchial infections.

Airway complications can be classified as early or late. Early airway complications usually occur during the first 4 to 12 weeks after transplantation and manifest themselves as a partial or complete anastomotic dehiscence or a fungal (usually *Aspergillus* or *Candida* species) or bacterial (usually *Staphylococcus* or *Pseudomonas* species) anastomotic infection. These conditions can subsequently result in anastomotic strictures or bronchomalacia. Clinically, bronchial dehiscence may cause prolonged air leaks in the early posttransplantation period. In some cases, the dehiscence may also lead to infection or the formation of peribronchial abscesses or fistulas. The results of chest radiographs and computed tomography (CT) scans are usually nonspecific; however, the appearance of extraluminal air on chest CT scans is very sensitive and specific for the diagnosis of anastomotic dehiscence. Bronchoscopy is the preferred diagnostic method for evaluating the bronchial anastomosis. This procedure may be performed routinely (surveillance bronchoscopy) or because of pulmonary symptoms, usually during the first 6 months after transplantation. During this period, the anastomosis should be evaluated carefully, the integrity of the mucosa should be assessed, and specimens from a bronchial wash or brush should be sent for cultures and cytologic examination. If there is any evidence of infection, antibiotics and antifungals (usually inhaled amphotericin with or without itraconazole or voriconazole) should be administered based on culture results.

Late bronchial anastomotic complications, including stenosis (most common), bronchomalacia, and development of exophytic granulation tissue are often the result of infection or dehiscence during the early weeks after transplantation. These complications manifest themselves as cough, shortness of breath, wheezing, dyspnea on exertion, and worsening obstruction as documented by pulmonary function testing. The characteristic flow volume loop demonstrates a concave appearance in both the inspiratory loop and the expiratory loop. Bronchial strictures or stenoses may also be seen on chest radiographs or CT scans, or by bronchoscopy. Therapeutic options for anastomotic complications include balloon dilation of a stricture, stent placement, cryotherapy, argon beam coagulation, laser procedures, and, rarely, surgery.

Rejection

Graft rejection is categorized clinically according to the time of onset after transplantation and the histopathologic pattern. The three types of rejection are hyperacute, acute, and chronic. Hyperacute rejection is mediated by preexisting alloantibodies that immediately bind to the donor vascular epithelium and lead to vessel thrombosis because of complement activation. This was thought to be a rare complication after LT. However, humoral or antibody mediated rejection is currently an area of active research in the field of LT [57]. Humoral rejection is characterized by local complement activation or the presence of antibody to donor HLAs and may be a risk factor for BOS. Treatment of humoral rejection includes plasmapheresis, intravenous immunoglobulin and/or rituximab, a monoclonal antibody against the CD-20 antigen.

Acute Rejection

As many as 50% to 55% of patients experience acute rejection during the first postoperative month, and as many as 90% will experience at least one episode of acute rejection within the first year [57]. Acute rejection usually occurs between 10 and 90 days after LT. It is not uncommon (20% of lung transplant recipients) for a single patient to experience either recurrent (more than two episodes) and/or persistent (failure to resolve with standard therapy) rejection. Acute rejection usually does not occur as frequently after the first postoperative year. Risk factors for acute rejection are poorly defined, but HLA mismatches may be correlated with its occurrence.

Clinically, acute rejection manifests itself as cough, shortness of breath, malaise, and fever. Occasionally, the presentation is asymptomatic; 68% of transplantation centers advocate surveillance bronchoscopy for the detection of this condition, although outcome data are not available [25]. Physical examination may detect rales or wheezing. The usefulness of chest radiography depends on the time since transplantation. Typically, during the first month the results of chest radiography can be abnormal in as many as 75% of rejection episodes; however, the results of radiography are abnormal in only 25% of rejection episodes that occur more than 1 month after transplantation. The most common radiographic patterns associated with acute rejection are a perihilar flare, and alveolar or interstitial localized or diffuse infiltrates with or without associated pleural effusion. In addition, CT may show ground glass opacities, septal thickening, and volume loss. New pleural fluid or increases in the amount of pleural fluid produced during the second to sixth week after LT is common among patients with acute lung rejection. The characteristics of the fluid are consistent with those of an exudate: the total lymphocyte count is often more than 80% of the total number of white blood cells.

Physiologic findings during periods of acute rejection include hypoxemia and deterioration in pulmonary function. Pulmonary function abnormalities are characterized by at least a 10% to 15% decline in FEV_1 from baseline and/or at least a 20% decline in forced expiratory flow (FEF) over 25% to 75% of expired vital capacity. Once again, these changes are nonspecific and can also be seen with infectious processes and graft complications.

Because clinical criteria alone cannot differentiate acute rejection from infection and less common graft complications, transbronchial biopsy (TBBx) with BAL has become the primary diagnostic procedure. The sensitivity of diagnosing acute rejection by TBBx ranges from 61% to 94%, and the specificity ranges from 90% to 100%. A histologic grading system for acute pulmonary rejection was proposed in 1990 and revised in 1996 and 2007 [58]. Pathologically, acute rejection is characterized by perivascular, mononuclear lymphocytic infiltrates with or without airway inflammation; histologically, it is graded from A_0 to A_4 on the basis of the degree of perivascular inflammation. In addition, the airway can be involved by lymphocytic bronchitis or bronchiolitis, which is graded from B_0 to B_x [58]. As rejection progresses, the perivascular lymphocytic infiltrates surrounding the venules and arterioles become dense and extend into the perivascular and peribronchiolar alveolar septa. Severe rejection may involve the alveolar space; parenchymal necrosis, hyaline membranes, and necrotizing vasculitis have been described [58]; and respiratory failure requiring mechanical ventilation can occur.

Once acute rejection has been diagnosed, treatment consists of augmenting the level of immunosuppression. Intravenous methylprednisolone (10 to 15 mg per kg daily for 3 days) followed by an increase in the maintenance regimen of prednisone regimen to 0.5 to 1 mg per kg daily, with tapering over the next several weeks, is a standard treatment regimen. Maintenance immunosuppression should also be augmented. Typically, symptoms resolve in days, and histologic follow-up 3 to 4 weeks later should demonstrate resolution. Recurrent or persistent acute rejection may require conversion in the baseline immunosuppressive regimen. Lympholytic therapy, methotrexate, photophoresis, total lymphoid irradiation, and aerosolized cyclosporine have been used with varied success [59].

Obliterative Bronchiolitis

Chronic rejection has been equated with the histologic finding of obliterative bronchiolitis (OB); it is a primary cause of morbidity and mortality after LT and the leading single cause of death more than 1 year after transplantation [1]. The incidence of OB ranges from 35% to 50% at various centers. OB has been defined clinically by an obstructive functional defect and histologically by obliteration of terminal bronchioles. OB generally occurs in a mean of 16 to 20 months after LT, but it has been reported as early as 3 months after transplantation. More than 50% of recipients will experience some degree of OB by 5 years after transplantation [1].

The causes of and risk factors for OB remain unclear. Several possible causes have been proposed, including uncontrolled acute rejection, lymphocytic bronchiolitis, CMV pneumonitis, CMV infection without pneumonitis, community acquired respiratory viruses, gastroesophageal reflux disease, PGD, antibody-mediated rejection, HLA-A mismatches, total HLA mismatches, absence of donor antigen-specific hyporeactivity, non-CMV infection, older donor age, and bronchiolitis obliterans with organizing pneumonia [40,41,60–63]. The most consistently identified risk factor is acute rejection, particularly in those patients who experience recurrent, high-grade episodes of acute rejection.

Clinically, OB can manifest itself as an upper respiratory tract infection and can be mistakenly treated as such. Other patients exhibit no clinical symptoms, but pulmonary function testing demonstrates gradual obstructive dysfunction. FEV_1 has been the standard spirometric parameter used for diagnosis, but midexpiratory flow rates may be a more sensitive parameter for early detection.

Typically, chest radiographs are not helpful in the diagnosis of OB because their results are unchanged from the results of baseline posttransplantation radiographs. High-resolution CT scans may show peripheral bronchiectasis, patchy consolidation, decreased peripheral vascular markings, air trapping, mosaicism, tree-in-bud changes, and bronchial dilation; these findings may aid in the diagnosis of OB [64]. Air trapping on end-expiratory high-resolution CT scans has been shown to be a sensitive (91%) and accurate (86%) radiologic indicator of OB, but it may not be able to provide an early diagnosis of this disorder. As with acute rejection, TBBx is used to diagnose OB, but primarily to exclude other diagnoses. The classic pathologic finding is constrictive bronchiolitis. Unfortunately, the sensitivity of TBBx for diagnosing OB is low (range: 15% to 87%), and the diagnosis of OB is often made by exclusion. OB is graded physiologically on the basis of the degree of change in pulmonary function (FEV_1) from baseline [61,62]. Because of the variability in obtaining bronchioles by TBBx, the ISHLT has established a staging system for BOS [62]. This staging is based on a reduction in FEV_1 of more than 20% from baseline after transplantation and is associated with a decrease in the FEF 25% to 75%, with or without the pathologic documentation of OB.

Once OB has been diagnosed histologically or clinically by excluding alternative diagnoses, treatment involves administering high-dose methylprednisolone followed by a tapering course of oral corticosteroids. Lympholytic depleting agents such as ATG, OKT_3, alemtuzumab, and basiliximab can be considered if there is no clinical response to corticosteroid treatment. Therapy may stabilize pulmonary function, but it only rarely results in substantial improvement. Alternative immunosuppressants such as sirolimus have also been associated with stabilization of pulmonary function when used as rescue treatment for BOS. Methotrexate, total lymphoid radiation, aerosolized cyclosporine, photophoresis, and newer immunosuppressants have been used to treat refractory cases of OB. Inhaled cyclosporine may be added for cases of lymphocytic bronchiolitis. Several studies have shown stabilization and/or improvement in BOS when a macrolide agent, such as azithromycin or clarithromycin is added to the regimen, likely due to the immunomodulating effects [65–67].

Infection, including bronchiectasis, frequently complicates intensive immunosuppression for OB and may result in death. Pseudomonas is a common offender, and aerosolized aminoglycoside antibiotics or suppressive quinolone treatment may be considered. Because most cases of OB can only be stabilized, strategies directed at prevention, early diagnosis, and treatment are necessary for the preservation of lung function. Retransplantation has been performed with varied results. Survival rates are somewhat lower than those after the initial transplantation and are superior when performed for the indication of BOS (1 year 62% and 5 year 45%), than for PGD [68,69].

Infectious Complications

Infections are an important cause of early and late morbidity and mortality after transplantation and are the leading single specific cause of death during the first year after transplantation [1]. The incidence of infection is significantly higher among recipients of lung transplants than among recipients of most other solid organ transplants; this higher incidence may be related to the continuous exposure of the allograft to the environment. Other predisposing factors include a diminished cough reflex because of denervation, poor lymphatic drainage, decreased mucociliary clearance, recipient-harbored infection, and, occasionally, transfer of infection from the donor organ. Nosocomial infections, such as urinary tract infections, ventilator-assisted pneumonia, and infections at the site of the surgical wound or the vascular access, also occur during the early postoperative period. However, in most circumstances the allograft is the primary site of infection.

Bacterial Infections

Bacterial pneumonia is the most common life-threatening infection that develops during the early postoperative period. Its incidence during the first two postoperative weeks is reported to be as high as 35% [70–72]. Common organisms include *Pseudomonas aeruginosa* and *Staphylococcus species*. The incidence of perioperative bacterial pneumonia has been reduced to as low as 10% by prophylaxis with broad-spectrum antibiotics, usually an antipseudomonal cephalosporin and clindamycin, and by routine culture of the trachea of both the donor and the recipient at the time of transplantation. Prophylactic antibiotics are usually discontinued after 3 days if the results of cultures are negative; the antibiotics are tailored to the cultured organisms if the results are positive. For transplant recipients with bronchiectasis, postoperative bacterial prophylaxis is usually continued for 14 days. The incidence of bacterial pneumonia is high during the first 6 months after transplantation but decreases thereafter, although a second late peak in incidence often occurs when immunosuppression is augmented for the treatment of chronic rejection. During the early posttransplantation period, bacterial infection due to Staphylococcus or, less commonly, Pseudomonas can develop at or distal to the site of the anastomosis.

It is often difficult to distinguish pneumonia from other early graft complications, such as reperfusion injury, pulmonary edema, rejection, and other causes of infection. In addition, differentiating between colonization and invasion may be difficult and often requires invasive procedures such as bronchoscopy with BAL, quantitative sterile brush sampling, or TBBx.

Other Infections

Atypical pneumonias, including those due to Legionella, mycobacteria, and Nocardia, are uncommon during the first month after transplantation but occur among 2% to 9% of recipients of lung or heart–lung transplants. At transplantation centers that routinely administer prophylaxis with trimethoprim–sulfamethoxazole during the first year after transplantation and reinitiate it when immunosuppression is augmented, the incidence of Pneumocystis pneumonia is less than 1%.

Most opportunistic infections occur within 6 months after transplantation. Sustained immunosuppression leading to a decrease in cell-mediated immunity predisposes the patient to infection with opportunistic organisms such as Aspergillus, Mycobacterium, Nocardia, and geographically endemic fungi.

Viral Infections

Viral infections are a primary cause of morbidity and mortality among long transplant recipients. During the first 6 months after transplantation, CMV accounts for most of the viral infections among these patients [72,73]. The typical time period for the development of CMV infection is 30 to 150 days postoperatively; the incidence of illness (i.e., infection and disease) is approximately 50%. Risk factors for CMV disease depend on the serology of the donor and the recipient and on the use of high-intensity immunosuppressive therapy, including cytolytic therapy. Approximately 15% to 35% of CMV-positive patients who receive grafts from either CMV-positive or CMV-negative donors experience CMV disease, whereas approximately 55% of CMV-negative patients who receive a graft from a CMV-positive donor may experience CMV disease. Most studies indicate that CMV pneumonitis contributes to the development of chronic rejection [62].

CMV can cause a wide spectrum of disease, ranging from asymptomatic infection, such as shedding of the virus in the urine or BAL, to widespread dissemination. The most common presentation of CMV among lung transplant recipients is pneumonitis, but the infection may also present as gastroenteritis, hepatitis, or colitis. CMV pneumonitis can often be confused with acute rejection. Clinical findings of CMV pneumonitis include fever, cough, flu-like illness, hypoxemia, an interstitial or alveolar infiltrate, and leukopenia. A definitive diagnosis of invasive disease requires cytologic or histologic changes in cell preparation or tissue. Therefore, diagnosis often requires flexible bronchoscopy with TBBx and BAL; this combination can detect 60% to 90% of CMV pneumonias. Currently, plasma-based polymerase chain reaction (PCR) assays are used to screen patients and to detect CMV infection [74]. The risk of CMV pneumonitis after LT is usually related to the serum concentration of CMV DNA, and this measure is used in many programs for the preemptive management of CMV [75].

The pathologic hallmark of CMV infection is a cytomegalic 250-nm cell containing a large central basophilic intranuclear inclusion. This inclusion is referred to as an "owl's eye" because it is separated from the nuclear membrane by a halo. Identifying CMV cytologically is very specific (98%) but lacks sensitivity (21%) for detecting the presence of infection. Other pathologic findings in the lung parenchyma of patients with CMV pneumonia include a lymphocytic and mononuclear-cell interstitial pneumonitis.

Ganciclovir (oral or intravenous) and oral valganciclovir are currently the mainstays of therapy for invasive CMV disease [73]. Bone marrow toxicity is one of the primary limiting side effects of ganciclovir therapy and may necessitate conversion to an alternative agent such as foscarnet. Most centers also use CMV-specific hyperimmunoglobulin to treat CMV disease.

Prophylaxis against CMV infections has become an important strategy at most transplantation centers. Initially, some centers attempted to match CMV-negative recipients with CMV-negative donors; however, the limited donor supply did not allow the continuation of this practice. The use of CMV-negative blood products is advocated. Prophylaxis with ganciclovir or valganciclovir seems to be effective in delaying the onset of CMV infection. Most centers give prophylaxis to all patients except CMV-negative recipients who receive grafts from CMV-negative donors. Prophylaxis is usually recommended for at least 90 days, particularly for CMV-negative recipients of grafts from CMV-positive donors. A recent randomized, controlled, multicenter study examined the efficacy of extending valganciclovir prophylaxis from the standard 3 months to 12 months in at risk (either donor or recipient CMV positive) patients. The investigators found a significant reduction in CMV infection, disease, and disease severity without increased ganciclovir resistance or toxicity in those patients receiving the longer course of therapy [76]. For patients at highest risk of infection, CMV hyperimmunoglobulin may be added to the regimen. Preemptive strategies, such as initiating treatment when a high level of CMV DNA is detected by PCR, may also delay and decrease the severity of CMV infection and may become the standard of care.

Other viruses that affect lung transplant recipients include herpes simplex virus (early after transplantation), community acquired respiratory viruses, such as respiratory syncytial virus, other paramyxoviruses (such as parainfluenza), influenza virus, metapneumovirus, and adenovirus [77]. Some transplantation programs initiate prophylaxis with acyclovir for herpes infection after the discontinuation of ganciclovir.

Fungal Infections

Fungal infections are more common among recipients of lung transplants than among recipients of other solid-organ transplants [78,79]. The overall incidence of invasive fungal infection after LT ranges from 15% to 35%. Such infections usually develop during the first few months after transplantation. Fungal infections carry the highest morbidity and mortality rates of all infections after transplantation; mortality rates can range from 40% to 70%.

Aspergillus species such as *A. fumigatus, A. flavus, A. terreus,* and *A. niger* can be colonizing organisms, can cause an infection that suggests an indolent, progressive pneumonia, or can cause an acute fulminant infection that disseminates rapidly. Aspergillus can invade blood vessels and may appear as an infarct on chest imaging or present with hemoptysis. The radiographic findings of pulmonary aspergillosis include focal lower-lobe infiltrates, patchy bronchopneumonic infiltrates, single or multiple nodules with or without cavitation, thin wall cavities, and opacification of the entire lung graft. High-resolution CT scans may reveal a halo sign that is believed to be pathognomonic for angioinvasive fungal infections such as aspergillosis [80]. Other manifestations of Aspergillus infection include pseudomembranous tracheobronchitis, often at and distal to the site of the anastomosis. Diagnosing invasive aspergillosis requires identifying organisms within tissues. These organisms can appear as septate hyphae that branch at acute angles and can be detected on hematoxylin-eosin and methenamine silver stains.

Survival rates for patients with Aspergillus infection have been improved by the early initiation of broad-spectrum azoles (such as voriconazole or itraconazole), high-dose amphotericin, or both, sometimes with the addition of an echinocandin, and a reduction in immunosuppressive therapy. Surgical resection may rarely be required to maximize cure rates in patients with aspergillosis. A lipid formulation of amphotericin B should also be considered for the management of invasive fungal infections among patients who cannot tolerate conventional amphotericin B or who experience nephrotoxicity with conventional amphotericin B, and among patients with progressive fungal infection despite therapy with conventional amphotericin. Prophylaxis with the azoles (voriconazole or itraconazole) for 3 to 6 months, and/or with amphotericin or aerosolized amphotericin, has shown promise in decreasing the incidence of Aspergillus infection after transplantation [81].

Candidal infections may occur during the early postoperative period but usually do not cause invasive disease. *Candida* species can cause a variety of syndromes among lung transplant recipients; these syndromes include mucocutaneous disease, line sepsis, wound infection, and, rarely, pulmonary involvement. Fluconazole and caspofungin have emerged as effective alternatives for treating infections caused by *Candida albicans*, but amphotericin B may still be considered for widespread disease. Fluconazole appears to be less active against other *Candida* species such as *C. glabrata* and *C. krusei.*

Less common causes of fungal infections among lung transplant recipients include *Cryptococcus neoformans* and the dimorphic fungi (*Coccidioides, Histoplasma*, and *Blastomyces*). Amphotericin B or the newer broad-spectrum azole agents are the initial therapeutic choices for treating serious infections with the invasive mycoses. The dose, duration of therapy, and alternative therapies differ depending on the organism.

Immunosuppression

After LT, a typical regimen for the maintenance of immunosuppression consists of tacrolimus at a dose of approximately 0.1 mg per kg orally every day in two divided doses (adjusted to maintain a serum concentration of 8 to 15 ng per mL), or cyclosporine 5 mg per kg orally every day in two divided doses (with dose adjusted to maintain serum concentrations of 250 to 350 ng per mL), and mycophenolate mofetil at a dose of 1 to 3 g daily, or azathioprine 1 to 2 mg per kg daily (adjusted to maintain a leukocyte count higher than 4,000 to 4,500 per mm^3), and prednisone approximately 0.5 mg per kg daily for the first month and then tapered by 5 mg per week over the next few months to a final maintenance dose of 5 mg per day. A minority of transplantation programs completely discontinue the administration of prednisone approximately 1 year after transplantation. The role of sirolimus after LT remains to be established. It is recommended that sirolimus not be used in the early perioperative period due to impaired wound healing.

Physicians caring for transplant recipients must be aware of the numerous drugs that can interact with tacrolimus and cyclosporine. For example, the azoles cause a significant increase in the serum concentrations of cyclosporine and tacrolimus. Likewise, discontinuing azole agents without increasing the dose of cyclosporine or tacrolimus can cause an acute and life-threatening decrease in the therapeutic concentrations of these drugs. Interactions with macrolide antibiotics, calcium channel blockers, and gastric motility drugs have also been reported. The concentrations of cyclosporine and tacrolimus are decreased by rifampin and anticonvulsants.

All immunosuppressants are associated with toxicity and drug interactions [82]. The details of these complications are discussed in a separate chapter.

Miscellaneous Complications

Another possible complication of LT is postoperative hemorrhage requiring reexploration. One of the early clues to this diagnosis is radiographic evidence of a hemothorax or what appears to be a retained clot, or a large volume of blood draining from the thoracostomy tubes. This complication may occur more frequently among patients who require cardiopulmonary bypass with its attendant requirement for anticoagulation or among patients with pleural adhesions from previous procedures such as pleurodesis or diagnostic or therapeutic lung surgery. Persistent air leaks can occasionally occur but are unlikely unless the bronchial anastomosis loses its integrity, because the lung parenchyma is normally not entered during a routine LT procedure [83].

In addition to the bronchial anastomotic complications discussed earlier, vascular anastomotic complications can occur. A stenosis at the venous anastomosis is indicated by radiographic evidence of pulmonary edema and infiltrates; this condition can be confused with PGD and is usually diagnosed by transesophageal echocardiography. A stenosis at the arterial anastomosis is suggested by unexplained gas exchange abnormalities and pulmonary hypertension.

Phrenic nerve dysfunction and diaphragmatic paralysis, which occur in conjunction with other types of cardiothoracic surgery, occur after LT with an incidence of 3% to 9.3% and are associated with a prolongation in the number of days for which mechanical ventilation is required, an increase in the length of stay in the ICU, an increase in the use of ICU resources, and an increase in the need for tracheostomy [84]. An inability to wean the patient from mechanical ventilation may indicate phrenic nerve dysfunction; the diagnosis can be confirmed by phrenic nerve conduction studies. For patients who do not require ventilation, the diagnosis of phrenic nerve dysfunction can be made with a fluoroscopic "sniff test." If the injury is the result of stretching of the phrenic nerve or trauma to the nerve during the surgical procedure but the nerve is not completely transected, a slow recovery can be anticipated. Complete transection is rare, but the damage is permanent. Diaphragmatic plication or pacing can be performed in some cases.

Pleural effusions can develop and/or persist following LT. The characteristics of these effusions are usually lymphocyte predominant exudates and can be associated early on with severing of the lymphatics (i.e., chylous effusion) or with rejection. A single-center study of a large number of lung transplant patients found that 27% of pleural effusions in these patients required drainage. 96% of the effusions were exudates, 27% of patient had infected pleural effusions with organisms such as fungal pathogens (specifically Candida most commonly), followed by bacterial etiologies. These infected effusions were characterized by high lactate dehydrogenase levels and neutrophilia [85]. Other causes of pleural effusions include heart failure, pulmonary embolism, and trapped lung. Rarely pleurodesis or decortication may be required.

Lung transplant recipients also experience gastroparesis, severe gastroesophageal reflux resulting in aspiration pneumonia, and an increased incidence of gastrointestinal emergencies [86]. These conditions include colonic perforation, small-bowel obstruction, diverticulitis, CMV colitis, megacolon, prolonged ileus, ischemic bowel, and pancreatitis [87]. Gastroesophageal reflux may be more severe among transplant recipients with cystic fibrosis.

Renal insufficiency is also a frequent complication among lung transplant recipients. This complication results from a combination of infections leading to sepsis and acute tubular necrosis, or from medication-related renal toxicity.

Cardiac arrhythmias, especially supraventricular arrhythmias such as atrial fibrillation, commonly develop in the perioperative period [88].

In one series of lung transplant recipients, the incidence of deep venous thrombosis and pulmonary embolism was reported to be 8.6%. This complication was believed to be related to alterations in coagulability leading to a hypercoagulable state or hypercoagulability due to their underlying disease [89,90].

Posttransplant lymphoproliferative disease (PTLD) and other malignancies can occur among lung transplant recipients. The incidence of PTLD after LT reportedly ranges from 1.8% to 9.4% [91]. PTLD comprises a heterogenous group of lymphoid proliferations, usually of the B-cell form, that are strongly associated with the Epstein–Barr virus (EBV). Patients for whom the results of pretransplantation serological studies are negative for EBV but who receive an organ from an EBV-positive donor and experience seroconversion are at a higher risk of PTLD. Clinically, PTLD usually occurs during the first year after transplantation; it involves the allograft and manifests itself as radiographic findings of solitary or multiple pulmonary nodules. Treatment includes reducing the level of immunosuppression, institution of antiviral therapy, and administering the anti-CD20 monoclonal antibody rituximab. In some cases, chemotherapy or surgery may be indicated.

Significant advances have been made in the field of LT since its inception more than 30 years ago, allowing this procedure to be a successful therapeutic option for patients with end-stage parenchymal or vascular lung disease. However, despite these improvements, numerous complications, many of which are managed by critical care professionals, can arise in this group of patients, and the unique aspects of their care are important.

References

1. Christie JD, Edwards LB, Aurora P, et al: The Registry of the International Society for Heart and Lung Transplantation: Twenty-sixth Official Adult Lung and Heart-Lung Transplantation Report-2009. *J Heart Lung Transplant* 28:1031–1049, 2009.
2. Orens JB, Estenne M, Arcasoy S, et al: International guidelines for the selection of lung transplant candidates: 2006 update—a consensus report from the Pulmonary Scientific Council of the International Society for Heart and Lung Transplantation. *J Heart Lung Transplant* 25:745–755, 2006.
3. Murray S, Charbeneau J, Marshall BC, et al: Impact of Burkholderia infection on lung transplantation in cystic fibrosis. *Am J Respir Crit Care Med* 178:363–371, 2008.
4. Vermeijden JW, Zijlstra JG, Erasmus ME, et al: Lung transplantation for ventilator-dependent respiratory failure. *J Heart Lung Transplant* 28:347–351, 2009.
5. Hsu HH, Chen JS, Ko WJ, et al: Short-term outcomes of cadaveric lung transplantation in ventilator-dependent patients. *Crit Care* 13:R129, 2009.
6. Mason DP, Thuita L, Nowicki ER, et al: Should lung transplantation be performed for patients on mechanical respiratory support? The US experience. *J Thorac Cardiovasc Surg* 139:765–773, e761, 2010.
7. United Network for Organ Sharing [Internet] Richmond: [cited June 16, 2010]. Available at: http://www.unos.org/resources/frm_LAS_Calculator.asp
8. Davis SQ, Garrity ER Jr: Organ allocation in lung transplant. *Chest* 132:1646–1651, 2007.
9. Merlo CA, Weiss ES, Orens JB, et al: Impact of U.S. Lung Allocation Score on survival after lung transplantation. *J Heart Lung Transplant* 28:769–775, 2009.
10. Takahashi SM, Garrity ER: The impact of the lung allocation score. *Semin Respir Crit Care Med* 31:108–114, 2010.
11. Russo MJ, Iribarne A, Hong KN, et al: High lung allocation score is associated with increased morbidity and mortality following transplantation. *Chest* 137:651–657, 2010.
12. United Network for Organ Sharing [Internet] Richmond: [cited June 16, 2010]. Available at: http://optn.transplant.hrsa.gov/latestData/rptData.asp
13. De Oliveira NC, Osaki S, Maloney JD, et al: Lung transplantation with donation after cardiac death donors: long-term follow-up in a single center. *J Thorac Cardiovasc Surg* 139:1306–1315, 2010.
14. Erasmus ME, Verschuuren EA, Nijkamp DM, et al: Lung transplantation from nonheparinized category III non-heart-beating donors. A single-centre report. *Transplantation* 89:452–457, 2010.
15. Angel LF, Levine DJ, Restrepo MI, et al: Impact of a lung transplantation donor-management protocol on lung donation and recipient outcomes. *Am J Respir Crit Care Med* 174:710–716, 2006.
16. Bhorade SM, Vigneswaran W, McCabe MA, et al: Liberalization of donor criteria may expand the donor pool without adverse consequence in lung transplantation. *J Heart Lung Transplant* 19:1199–1204, 2000.
17. Gabbay E, Williams TJ, Griffiths AP, et al: Maximizing the utilization of donor organs offered for lung transplantation. *Am J Respir Crit Care Med* 160:265–271, 1999.
18. Venkateswaran RV, Patchell VB, Wilson IC, et al: Early donor management increases the retrieval rate of lungs for transplantation. *Ann Thorac Surg* 85:278–286, 2008; discussion 286.
19. Boasquevisque CH, Yildirim E, Waddel TK, et al: Surgical techniques: lung transplant and lung volume reduction. *Proc Am Thorac Soc* 6:66–78, 2009.
20. Schmid RA, Boehler A, Speich R, et al: Bronchial anastomotic complications following lung transplantation: still a major cause of morbidity? *Eur Respir J* 10:2872–2875, 1997.
21. Augoustides JG, Watcha SM, Pochettino A, et al: Early tracheal extubation in adults undergoing single-lung transplantation for chronic obstructive pulmonary disease: pilot evaluation of perioperative outcome. *Interact Cardiovasc Thorac Surg* 7:755–758, 2008.
22. Ahya VN, Kawut SM: Noninfectious pulmonary complications after lung transplantation. *Clin Chest Med* 26:613–622; vi, 2005.
23. Angles R, Tenorio L, Roman A, et al: Lung transplantation for emphysema. Lung hyperinflation: incidence and outcome. *Transpl Int* 17:810–814, 2005.
24. Hachem RR, Edwards LB, Yusen RD, et al: The impact of induction on survival after lung transplantation: an analysis of the International Society for Heart and Lung Transplantation Registry. *Clin Transplant* 22:603–608, 2008.
25. Levine SM: A survey of clinical practice of lung transplantation in North America. *Chest* 125:1224–1238, 2004.
26. Christie JD, Carby M, Bag R, et al: Report of the ISHLT Working Group on Primary Lung Graft Dysfunction part II: definition. A consensus statement of the International Society for Heart and Lung Transplantation. *J Heart Lung Transplant* 24:1454–1459, 2005.
27. Lee JC, Christie JD, Keshavjee S: Primary graft dysfunction: definition, risk factors, short- and long-term outcomes. *Semin Respir Crit Care Med* 31:161–171, 2010.
28. Shargall Y, Guenther G, Ahya VN, et al: Report of the ISHLT Working Group on Primary Lung Graft Dysfunction part VI: treatment. *J Heart Lung Transplant* 24:1489–1500, 2005.
29. Ardehali A, Laks H, Levine M, et al: A prospective trial of inhaled nitric oxide in clinical lung transplantation. *Transplantation* 72:112–115, 2001.
30. Botha P, Jeyakanthan M, Rao JN, et al: Inhaled nitric oxide for modulation of ischemia-reperfusion injury in lung transplantation. *J Heart Lung Transplant* 26:1199–1205, 2007.
31. Meade MO, Granton JT, Matte-Martyn A, et al: A randomized trial of inhaled nitric oxide to prevent ischemia-reperfusion injury after lung transplantation. *Am J Respir Crit Care Med* 167:1483–1489, 2003.
32. Perrin G, Roch A, Michelet P, et al: Inhaled nitric oxide does not prevent pulmonary edema after lung transplantation measured by lung water content: a randomized clinical study. *Chest* 129:1024–1030, 2006.
33. Amital A, Shitrit D, Raviv Y, et al: Surfactant as salvage therapy in life threatening primary graft dysfunction in lung transplantation. *Eur J Cardiothorac Surg* 35:299–303, 2009.
34. Amital A, Shitrit D, Raviv Y, et al: The use of surfactant in lung transplantation. *Transplantation* 86:1554–1559, 2008.
35. Struber M, Fischer S, Niedermeyer J, et al: Effects of exogenous surfactant instillation in clinical lung transplantation: a prospective, randomized trial. *J Thorac Cardiovasc Surg* 133:1620–1625, 2007.
36. Oto T, Rosenfeldt F, Rowland M, et al: Extracorporeal membrane oxygenation after lung transplantation: evolving technique improves outcomes. *Ann Thorac Surg* 78:1230–1235, 2004.
37. Fischer S, Bohn D, Rycus P, et al: Extracorporeal membrane oxygenation for primary graft dysfunction after lung transplantation: analysis of the Extracorporeal Life Support Organization (ELSO) registry. *J Heart Lung Transplant* 26:472–477, 2007.
38. Thabut G, Vinatier I, Stern JB, et al: Primary graft failure following lung transplantation: predictive factors of mortality. *Chest* 121:1876–1882, 2002.
39. Arcasoy SM, Fisher A, Hachem RR, et al: Report of the ISHLT Working Group on Primary Lung Graft Dysfunction part V: predictors and outcomes. *J Heart Lung Transplant* 24:1483–1488, 2005.
40. Daud SA, Yusen RD, Meyers BF, et al: Impact of immediate primary lung allograft dysfunction on bronchiolitis obliterans syndrome. *Am J Respir Crit Care Med* 175:507–513, 2007.
41. Huang HJ, Yusen RD, Meyers BF, et al: Late primary graft dysfunction after lung transplantation and bronchiolitis obliterans syndrome. *Am J Transplant* 8:2454–2462, 2008.
42. Schnickel GT, Ross DJ, Beygui R, et al: Modified reperfusion in clinical lung transplantation: the results of 100 consecutive cases. *J Thorac Cardiovasc Surg* 131:218–223, 2006.

43. Barr ML, Kawut SM, Whelan TP, et al: Report of the ISHLT Working Group on Primary Lung Graft Dysfunction part IV: recipient-related risk factors and markers. *J Heart Lung Transplant* 24:1468–1482, 2005.
44. Bobadilla JL, Love RB, Jankowska-Gan E, et al: Th-17, monokines, collagen type V, and primary graft dysfunction in lung transplantation. *Am J Respir Crit Care Med* 177:660–668, 2008.
45. Christie JD, Kotloff RM, Pochettino A, et al: Clinical risk factors for primary graft failure following lung transplantation. *Chest* 124:1232–1241, 2003.
46. de Perrot M, Bonser RS, Dark J, et al: Report of the ISHLT Working Group on Primary Lung Graft Dysfunction part III: donor-related risk factors and markers. *J Heart Lung Transplant* 24:1460–1467, 2005.
47. Kuntz CL, Hadjiliadis D, Ahya VN, et al: Risk factors for early primary graft dysfunction after lung transplantation: a registry study. *Clin Transplant* 23:819–830, 2009.
48. Westall GP, Snell GI, McLean C, et al: C3d and C4d deposition early after lung transplantation. *J Heart Lung Transplant* 27:722–728, 2008.
49. Kozower BD, Meyers BF, Smith MA, et al: The impact of the lung allocation score on short-term transplantation outcomes: a multicenter study. *J Thorac Cardiovasc Surg* 135:166–171, 2008.
50. McCue JD, Mooney J, Quail J, et al: Ninety-day mortality and major complications are not affected by use of lung allocation score. *J Heart Lung Transplant* 27:192–196, 2008.
51. Guillen RV, Briones FR, Marin PM, et al: Lung graft dysfunction in the early postoperative period after lung and heart lung transplantation. *Transplant Proc* 37:3994–3995, 2005.
52. Plochl W, Pezawas L, Artemiou O, et al: Nutritional status, ICU duration and ICU mortality in lung transplant recipients. *Intensive Care Med* 22:1179–1185, 1996.
53. Pilcher DV, Scheinkestel CD, Snell GI, et al: High central venous pressure is associated with prolonged mechanical ventilation and increased mortality after lung transplantation. *J Thorac Cardiovasc Surg* 129:912–918, 2005.
54. Padia SA, Borja MC, Orens JB, et al: Tracheostomy following lung transplantation predictors and outcomes. *Am J Transplant* 3:891–895, 2003.
55. Hadjiliadis D, Steele MP, Govert JA, et al: Outcome of lung transplant patients admitted to the medical ICU. *Chest* 125:1040–1045, 2004.
56. Santacruz JF, Mehta AC: Airway complications and management after lung transplantation: ischemia, dehiscence, and stenosis. *Proc Am Thorac Soc* 6:79–93, 2009.
57. Martinu T, Howell DN, Palmer SM: Acute cellular rejection and humoral sensitization in lung transplant recipients. *Semin Respir Crit Care Med* 31:179–188, 2010.
58. Stewart S, Fishbein MC, Snell GI, et al: Revision of the 1996 working formulation for the standardization of nomenclature in the diagnosis of lung rejection. *J Heart Lung Transplant* 26:1229–1242, 2007.
59. Iacono AT, Johnson BA, Grgurich WF, et al: A randomized trial of inhaled cyclosporine in lung-transplant recipients. *N Engl J Med* 354:141–150, 2006.
60. Glanville AR, Aboyoun CL, Havryk A, et al: Severity of lymphocytic bronchiolitis predicts long-term outcome after lung transplantation. *Am J Respir Crit Care Med* 177:1033–1040, 2008.
61. Weigt SS, Wallace WD, Derhovanessian A, et al: Chronic allograft rejection: epidemiology, diagnosis, pathogenesis, and treatment. *Semin Respir Crit Care Med* 31:189–207, 2010.
62. Estenne M, Maurer JR, Boehler A, et al: Bronchiolitis obliterans syndrome 2001: an update of the diagnostic criteria. *J Heart Lung Transplant* 21:297–310, 2002.
63. Sharples LD, McNeil K, Stewart S, et al: Risk factors for bronchiolitis obliterans: a systematic review of recent publications. *J Heart Lung Transplant* 21:271–281, 2002.
64. de Jong PA, Dodd JD, Coxson HO, et al: Bronchiolitis obliterans following lung transplantation: early detection using computed tomographic scanning. *Thorax* 61:799–804, 2006.
65. Gerhardt SG, McDyer JF, Girgis RE, et al: Maintenance azithromycin therapy for bronchiolitis obliterans syndrome: results of a pilot study. *Am J Respir Crit Care Med* 168:121–125, 2003.
66. Gottlieb J, Szangolies J, Koehnlein T, et al: Long-term azithromycin for bronchiolitis obliterans syndrome after lung transplantation. *Transplantation* 85:36–41, 2008.
67. Shitrit D, Bendayan D, Gidon S, et al: Long-term azithromycin use for treatment of bronchiolitis obliterans syndrome in lung transplant recipients. *J Heart Lung Transplant* 24:1440–1443, 2005.
68. Aigner C, Jaksch P, Taghavi S, et al: Pulmonary retransplantation: is it worth the effort? A long-term analysis of 46 cases. *J Heart Lung Transplant* 27:60–65, 2008.
69. Kawut SM, Lederer DJ, Keshavjee S, et al: Outcomes after lung retransplantation in the modern era. *Am J Respir Crit Care Med* 177:114–120, 2008.
70. Lease ED, Zaas DW: Complex bacterial infections pre- and posttransplant. *Semin Respir Crit Care Med* 31:234–242, 2010.
71. Fishman JA: Infection in solid-organ transplant recipients. *N Engl J Med* 357:2601–2614, 2007.
72. Remund KF, Best M, Egan JJ: Infections relevant to lung transplantation. *Proc Am Thorac Soc* 6:94–100, 2009.
73. Zamora MR, Davis RD, Leonard C: Management of cytomegalovirus infection in lung transplant recipients: evidence-based recommendations. *Transplantation* 80:157–163, 2005.
74. Hadaya K, Wunderli W, Deffernez C, et al: Monitoring of cytomegalovirus infection in solid-organ transplant recipients by an ultrasensitive plasma PCR assay. *J Clin Microbiol* 41:3757–3764, 2003.
75. Sanchez JL, Kruger RM, Paranjothi S, et al: Relationship of cytomegalovirus viral load in blood to pneumonitis in lung transplant recipients. *Transplantation* 72:733–735, 2001.
76. Palmer SM, Limaye AP, Banks M, et al: Extended valganciclovir prophylaxis to prevent cytomegalovirus after lung transplantation: a randomized, controlled trial. *Ann Intern Med* 152:761–769, 2010.
77. Kumar D, Erdman D, Keshavjee S, et al: Clinical impact of community-acquired respiratory viruses on bronchiolitis obliterans after lung transplant. *Am J Transplant* 5:2031–2036, 2005.
78. Hosseini-Moghaddam SM, Husain S: Fungi and molds following lung transplantation. *Semin Respir Crit Care Med* 31:222–233, 2010.
79. Sole A, Salavert M: Fungal infections after lung transplantation. *Curr Opin Pulm Med* 15:243–253, 2009.
80. Pinto PS: The CT Halo Sign. *Radiology* 230:109–110, 2004.
81. Minari A, Husni R, Avery RK, et al: The incidence of invasive aspergillosis among solid organ transplant recipients and implications for prophylaxis in lung transplants. *Transpl Infect Dis* 4:195–200, 2002.
82. Taylor JL, Palmer SM: Critical care perspective on immunotherapy in lung transplantation. *J Intensive Care Med* 21:327–344, 2006.
83. Ferrer J, Roldan J, Roman A, et al: Acute and chronic pleural complications in lung transplantation. *J Heart Lung Transplant* 22:1217–1225, 2003.
84. Ferdinande P, Bruyninckx F, Van Raemdonck D, et al: Phrenic nerve dysfunction after heart-lung and lung transplantation. *J Heart Lung Transplant* 23:105–109, 2004.
85. Wahidi MM, Willner DA, Snyder LD, et al: Diagnosis and outcome of early pleural space infection following lung transplantation. *Chest* 135:484–491, 2009.
86. Sodhi SS, Guo JP, Maurer AH, et al: Gastroparesis after combined heart and lung transplantation. *J Clin Gastroenterol* 34:34–39, 2002.
87. Lyu DM, Zamora MR: Medical complications of lung transplantation. *Proc Am Thorac Soc* 6:101–107, 2009.
88. Mason DP, Marsh DH, Alster JM, et al: Atrial tibrillation after lung transplantation: timing, risk factors, and treatment. *Ann Thorac Surg* 84(6):1878–1884, 2007.
89. Izbicki G, Bairey O, Shitrit D, et al: Increased thromboembolic events after lung transplantation. *Chest* 129:412–416, 2006.
90. Yegen HA, Lederer DJ, Barr RG, et al: Risk factors for venous thromboembolism after lung transplantation. *Chest* 132:547–553, 2007.
91. Reams BD, McAdams HP, Howell DN, et al: Posttransplant lymphoproliferative disorder: incidence, presentation, and response to treatment in lung transplant recipients. *Chest* 124:1242–1249, 2003.

SECTION XV ■ METABOLISM/NUTRITION

DOMINIC J. NOMPLEGGI

CHAPTER 190 ■ NUTRITIONAL THERAPY IN THE CRITICALLY ILL PATIENT

DOMINIC J. NOMPLEGGI

The nutritional management of critically ill patients has changed dramatically over the past 10 years. Changes in the areas of nutritional assessment, guidelines for total energy provided, disease-specific feeding, and immune-enhancing enteral nutrition have been the most prominent. The rationale for nutrition support comes from the knowledge that critically ill patients are prone to develop malnutrition, which is known to be associated with serious complications such as sepsis and pneumonia, leading to a poor outcome and even death [1].

Although guidelines continue to be in evolution, there are sufficient data on clinically proven principles and methods of nutrition support to permit practical and useful recommendations for the specific problems and questions confronted by the intensivist.

The Society of Critical Medicine and the American Society for Parenteral and Enteral Nutrition convened an expert panel to review all available data in the literature to establish guidelines for the provision and assessment of nutrition support therapy in the adult critically ill patient [2]. These recommendations concluded that now after more then 30 years of investigation, nutrition *support* in critically ill patients, once regarded as adjunctive care designed to preserve lean body mass, maintain immune function, and avoid metabolic complications should now be considered nutrition *therapy* specifically aimed at attenuating the metabolic response to stress, prevent oxidative injury and improve the immune response [2]. Table 190.1 does not list all of the recommendations of the panel but summarizes all the recommendations supported by randomized trials.

WHAT IS MALNUTRITION AND HOW DO WE RECOGNIZE IT?

Malnutrition in ICU patients is common and can be present on admission or develop as a result of the metabolic response to injury. This response to injury can lead to changes in substrate metabolism, causing alterations in body composition and nutrient deficiencies that become clinically evident [3]. During starvation, the body uses fat and muscle protein as a source of energy in order to preserve visceral protein [4]. Mobilization of fat for fuel is an important adaptive response for survival because glucose stores, in the form of glycogen, provide only 1,200 kcal in the first 24 hours of starvation. The body attempts to use muscle protein rather than visceral protein because visceral protein is essential for vital functions of the body. Skeletal muscle mass decreases steadily, and its rate of loss exceeds that of weight loss [5]. Because these changes are difficult to assess, intensivists have had to resort to a variety of tools such as clinical, anthropometric, chemical, and immunological parameters that reflect altered body composition [6].

Nutritional Assessment

It is not known how long a critically ill patient can tolerate lack of nutrient intake without adverse consequences, but because critical depletion of lean tissue can occur after 14 days of starvation in severely catabolic patients, it is recommended that nutrition support be instituted in patients who are not expected to resume oral feeding for 7 to 10 days [7]. A recent study conducted by the European Society of Intensive Care Medicine (ESICM) surveyed intensivists from 35 countries using a 49-item questionnaire to determine how they cope with these issues and to assess the current practice of nutritional management in intensive care units (ICUs) [8].

In the ESICM study, 45% of the patients were fed within 24 hours and 47% between 24 and 48 hours of admission to the ICU [8]. The need for nutritional support is determined by the balance between endogenous energy reserves of the body and the severity of stress. The best clinical markers of stress are fever, leukocytosis, hypoalbuminemia, and a negative nitrogen balance.

The purpose of nutritional assessment is to identify the type and degree of malnutrition to devise a rational approach to treatment. Percentage weight loss in the patient's past 6 months, serum albumin level, and total lymphocyte count are readily available, commonly used measures to assess nutritional status. A 10% or 10-lb weight loss over the previous 12 months is an indicator of protein calorie malnutrition. This results from inadequate caloric intake. Hypoalbuminemic malnutrition or kwashiorkor is due to severe stress or profound malnutrition. Albumin is not a very sensitive indicator of malnutrition in ICU patients because its synthesis is influenced by numerous factors other than nutritional status such as protein losing states, hepatic function, and acute infection or inflammation [9]. Normal concentrations of albumin are unattainable in many critically ill patients because of large fluid shifts and inadequate synthesis to meet demands. Hypoalbuminemia should be viewed as a marker of injury and not as an indicator of impaired nutrition. Most critically ill patents have a combination of the two. The protein calorie malnutrition can be easily treated by supplying adequate caloric intake. The hypoalbuminemic malnutrition is most effectively treated by nutrition support and treatment of the stresses that led to this severe catabolic condition.

Traditionally, weight loss of 10 lb or 10% of usual weight is clinically important, weight loss of 20% to 30% suggests moderate protein calorie malnutrition, and greater than 30%, severe protein calorie malnutrition. Unfortunately, in many critically ill patients, total body weight is often an insensitive parameter because of progressive total body salt and water retention. Anthropometrics (i.e., measurement of triceps skinfold thickness and midarm muscle circumference) are reasonably accurate even in the presence of excess body water because edema accumulates to a lesser extent in the upper extremities

TABLE 190.1

SUMMARY OF EVIDENCE-BASED GUIDELINES FOR NUTRITION SUPPORT

- Enteral Nutrition (EN) is preferred over parenteral nutrition (PN) for critically ill patients who require nutrition support.
- Bowel sounds are not required for the initiation of enteral feeding.
- Immune modulating enteral formulations should be used for critically ill patients on mechanical ventilation but with caution in patients with severe sepsis.
- Patients with ARDS and severe acute lung injury require enteral feeding containing anti-inflammatory lipids (i.e., omega-3 fish oil, borage oil) and antioxidants.
- Antioxidant vitamins and trace minerals, specifically containing selenium, should be given to all critically ill patients receiving nutrition therapy
- EN regimens not containing glutamine should be supplemented with glutamine in burn, trauma and mixed critically ill patients.
- Protocols to promote moderately strict control of serum glucose levels (110–150 mg/dL) when providing nutrition support are recommended.

Adapted from McClave SA, Martindale RG, Vanek VW, et al: Guidelines for the provision and assessment of nutrition support therapy in the adult critically ill patient: Society of Critical Care Medicine (SCCM) and American Society for Parenteral and Enteral Nutrition (A.S.P.E.N.) *J Parent Enteral Nutr* 33:277–318, 2009.

[10]. However, they are difficult to perform in critically ill patients, time consuming, and not routinely performed. The general appearance of the patient, with emphasis on evidence of temporal, upper body, and upper extremity wasting of skeletal muscle mass, provides a quick, inexpensive, and clinically useful measure of nutritional status. For the reasons above, clinicians have found that body mass index may be a more practical way to assess nutritional status. As presented in Chapter 191, Driscoll suggests that a patient weight less than 85% of the ideal body weight (IBW) or BMI less than 18.5 indicates moderate malnutrition. Severe malnutrition would be considered likely if weight is less than 75% of IBW or BMI is less than 16 kg per m^2. Thus, a greater sense of urgency to intervene with nutrition support is present under these conditions and should be undertaken within several days of the acute injury.

Malnutrition is closely correlated with alterations in immune response as measured by skin test reactivity and total lymphocyte count. A total lymphocyte count less than 1,000 per mm^3 is indicative of altered immune function and is associated with decreased skin test reactivity. Loss of delayed cutaneous hypersensitivity to common antigens is a measure of impaired cellular immunity, which has consistently been found to be associated with malnutrition [9].

Subjective global assessment (SGA) is a method for evaluating nutritional status that uses clinical parameters like history, physical findings, and symptoms [11,12]. The SGA determines whether (a) nutritional assimilation has been restricted because of decreased food intake, maldigestion, or malabsorption, (b) any effects of malnutrition on organ function and body composition have occurred, and (c) the patient's disease process has influenced nutrient requirements [7].

As stated by the advisory committee convened by the National Institutes of Health, the American Society for Parenteral and Enteral Nutrition, and the American Society for Clinical Nutrition, "there is no 'gold standard' for determining nutritional status because (a) there is no universally accepted clinical definition of malnutrition, (b) all current assessment parameters are affected by illness and injury, (c) it is difficult to isolate the effects of malnutrition from the influence of the disease on clinical outcome, and (d) it is not clear which of the commonly used nutrition assessments techniques is the most reliable because of the paucity of comparative data" [7].

According to the ESICM questionnaire, the critical care community appears to most commonly assess nutritional status using the SGA and laboratory parameters [8]. Although there are no data to attest to the reliability of this approach in critically ill patients, serum albumin, stress level, weight loss in excess of 10% of ideal body weight, and SGA have been shown to be reasonable markers of nutritional status in noncritically ill hospitalized patients. Until future studies show otherwise, weight loss, serum albumin, and SGA are likely to be reliable parameters to follow in patients who are not volume overloaded. They are simple to measure, generally accepted, and commonly used.

HOW MUCH SHOULD YOU FEED?

Macronutrients

Body cell mass is the major determinant of the total caloric requirement. Energy needs can be estimated or measured directly using indirect calorimetry. Because estimated energy requirements have been shown to be adequate in most patients, direct measurement is usually reserved for patients in whom estimating energy needs are difficult or when patients do not appear to respond to therapy (e.g., worsening respiratory function, continued weight loss, or a decrease in prealbumin levels, a more sensitive marker of protein synthesis than albumin).

The general principle of macronutrient support is to provide enough energy to promote anabolic functions and avoid caloric overload. Caloric requirements of 25 to 30 kcal per kg should be based on the usual body weight and are adequate for most patients [2,9]. If patients are not responding to therapy as indicated by the parameters listed above, or if they are in a severe catabolic state as occurs in multiple trauma or burns patients, they may need 30 or even 40 kcal per kg.

Protein

The usual protein requirement has been estimated to be 1.2 to 1.5 g per kg per day for actual body weight. Nitrogen retention can be monitored and protein adjusted to support protein synthetic functions. Protein should be reduced when the blood urea nitrogen rises to 100 mg per dL or an elevated ammonia level is associated with clinical encephalopathy to limit the impact of the uremia and to avoid worsening encephalopathy associated with elevated ammonia levels [9].

Carbohydrates

Generally patients will need about 25 to 30 kcal per kg per day to meet there energy requirements. Approximately 20 kcal per kg per day of the actual body weight can be provided as carbohydrate. Levels of carbohydrate above 30 kcal per kg per day increase the risk of hyperglycemia. Hyperglycemia should be avoided because it is associated with abnormalities in granulocyte adhesion, chemotaxis, phagocytosis and intracellular killing, and poor clinical outcomes.

Hyperglycemia is a major contributing factor to postoperative infection. Blood sugars greater than 220 mg per dL on postoperative day 1 have been associated with a fivefold increased risk of serious infection [13]. A recent study in patients requiring total parenteral nutrition (TPN) to determine whether the frequency of hyperglycemia and infectious complications can be reduced by an underfeeding strategy (1,000 kcal with 70 g per kg as protein) provision of 1.5 g per kg of protein in conjunction with 25 kcal per kg was not associated with more hyperglycemia or infections than deliberate underfeeding. However, a regimen of 25 kcal per kg in conjunction with 1.5 g per kg of protein did provide significant nutritional benefit in terms of nitrogen balance as compared with hypocaloric TPN [14]. This suggests that it is not a hypocaloric low carbohydrate formula that protects against infection but rather the avoidance of hyperglycemia. Alternatively, TPN can be adjusted and regular insulin given, as needed, to maintain a blood glucose level from 110 to 150 mg per dL [2].

Fat

Usually no more than 15% to 20% of total calories per day should be provided as fat. This will avoid infectious complications that may be due to dysfunction of the reticuloendothelial system, which has been associated with the administration of excess lipids [15]. Omega-6 polyunsaturated fatty acids should be provided in doses adequate to prevent essential fatty acid deficiency (at least 7% of total calories). Medium-chain triglycerides (MCT) can be administered with long-chain triglycerides (LCT). MCTs are more water soluble and require less lipase activity and bile salts for absorption. Patients with malabsorption, pancreatic insufficiency, and chronic liver disease can absorb them more easily. The ratio of MCT to LCT depends on the route of administration and product availability [9].

Electrolytes, Micronutrients, and Fluid

Potassium, magnesium, phosphate, and zinc should be provided in amounts necessary to maintain normal serum levels. The absolute requirements for vitamins, minerals, and trace elements have not yet been determined. Normal serum and blood levels of vitamins have been established but may vary with the laboratory in which the measurement is obtained [9]. In general, patients should receive 25 mL of fluid per kg actual dry body weight to avoid dehydration. Three milliliters of trace elements injection 5 (Multitrace-5®) and 10 mL of multiple vitamin infusion (Infuvite Adult®) will provide adequate vitamins, trace elements, and minerals and should be added to TPN daily. The required daily allowance (RDA) for all vitamins and minerals are usually provided in 1,000 to 1,500 mL of most enteral formulas. If the patient is receiving less than a liter of enteral feeding, vitamin supplementation may be necessary. Spot electrolyte measurements (aliquots of urine, ostomy, nasogastric, or fistulous output) may be very helpful in determining proper replacement. If the total daily volume of the lost fluid is measured, the daily loss of any electrolyte in that fluid can be estimated using the following equation: mmol per L $\times$ volume output per 24 hours (in liters) = mmol per 24 hours (e.g., 20 mL of urine contains 100 mmol per L, the daily urine output is 2 L; therefore, the 24 hour urine sodium output is 200 mmol).

WHICH ROUTE OF ADMINISTRATION?

Enteral Feeding

Enteral feeding has been shown in clinical studies to reduce infection and preserve gut integrity, barrier, and immune function. It is the preferred route of nutrient administration because it is more physiologic, safer, and less expensive than parenteral feeding. Current recommendations support initiation of enteral nutrition as soon as the patient is hemodynamically stable [2]. The only contraindication is a nonfunctioning gut. For example, intragastric feeding requires adequate gastric motility. Gastric residuals should be checked hourly and a volume greater than 200 mL necessitates modification of the infusion rate to minimize reflux and aspiration. Supplemental parenteral nutrition to meet caloric requirements or small bowel feeding to potentially decrease the risk of aspiration will be necessary until normal gastric function returns. Gastric atony and colonic ileus do not preclude enteral feeding but may require gastric decompression and small bowel feeding.

Initiation of enteral feeding does not require active bowel sounds or the passage of flatus or stool. Small bowel feedings can be given in the presence of mild or resolving pancreatitis and low output enterocutaneous fistulas (less than 500 mL per day) [2,8]. Recently, even patients with severe acute pancreatitis (acute physiology and chronic health evaluation [APACHE] II score 12 to 13) receiving enteral nutrition were found to have significantly fewer total complications and septic complications than patients receiving parenteral nutrition [16]. Worsening abdominal distention or diarrhea in excess of 1,000 mL per day requires a medical evaluation. If distention is present, enteral feedings should be discontinued. If no infectious cause for the diarrhea is found, antidiarrheals can be administered and feedings continued [9]. Nasogastric feeding is appropriate for most patients except those with a history of aspiration pneumonia associated with reflux. Those patients should be fed postpylorically or via a G-tube to minimize nasogastric tube-associated reflux of gastric contents and aspiration. Although there are some recent data suggesting it is just as safe to feed patients with severe pancreatitis intragastrically, the bulk of existing evidence favors feeding intrajejunally to minimize pancreatic stimulation [17].

Standard isotonic polymeric formulations can meet most patients' nutritional needs. The use of elemental formulas should be reserved for patients with severe small bowel absorptive dysfunction. The "American Gastroenterological Association Medical Position Statement: Guidelines for the use of enteral nutrition" has concluded that disease or organ-specific specialty formulations generally are more expensive and have a limited clinical role, and they will require more data to justify their practicality and effectiveness [18].

There are numerous issues that arise when providing enteral nutrition to critically ill patients. We provide guidelines to help the readers of this review overcome the problems that often arise when administering enteral tube feeding.

In general, most complications associated with the use of feeding tubes relate to placement, displacement, or malfunction of the tubes. It is important to remember that these tubes require frequent maintenance to avoid complications. The position of nasogastric or nasoenteric feeding tubes placed at the bedside should be confirmed endoscopically or radiographically before use because clinical assessment is unreliable. The use of promotility drugs has not been shown to be consistently beneficial and although they can increase the volume of feeding the overall impact is small [2,9]. Excessive force during insertion, which can result in malposition, should be avoided. Tubes need to be flushed regularly to avoid clogging with medications or tube feeding. Cycled tube feeding is recommended, if possible, to facilitate this. Little is known about compatibility of most medications with tube feeding and, therefore, medications should not be mixed with tube feedings since this can lead to precipitation of the medication with blockage of the tube and decreased absorption of the medication.

Placement of tubes across the gastroesophageal junction or pylorus can lead to incompetence of the sphincter, reflux, and aspiration. In patients at risk for or with a history of aspiration associated with reflux we recommend percutaneously placed gastric or jejunal feeding tubes. Gastric tubes are preferred because the smaller caliber of the jejunal tubes makes them likely to clog with administration of anything except liquid medications. Percutaneously placed tubes that fall or are pulled out should be replaced cautiously. Unlike noncritically ill patients who usually have had their feeding tubes in place long term, critically ill patients are likely to have had their tube placed recently or may have impaired healing and, therefore, may not have a fully developed cutaneous fistula. For these reasons we recommend confirming placement with a contrast-enhanced radiograph before use when replacing these tubes at the bedside.

Elevating the head of the bed 30 degrees and checking for gastric residuals to avoid increases in the volume of the gastric contents, which can lead to hypersecretion and reflux of gastric contents, is also recommended.

Stress gastritis, also known as stress-related erosive syndrome (SRES), is a term used to describe gastrointestinal mucosal injury associated with serious systemic disease. Most patients at risk cannot have oral feedings. Histamine H_2 receptor antagonists (H2RAs) have been shown to protect against significant gastrointestinal hemorrhage. There are less data on the efficacy of proton pump inhibitors (PPIs). A reasonable suggestion has been to wait 6 to 12 hours between stopping parenteral H2RAs before starting to feed and initiating therapy with a PPI [19].

Parenteral Feeding

Parenteral nutrient administration is recommended when the gastrointestinal tract is nonfunctional or inaccessible or enteral feeding is insufficient. Although parenteral nutrient admixtures are not as nutritionally complete as enteral formulations, nutritional goals are achieved more often with the former than the latter. This is usually attributable to a variety of barriers. A recent study of four university-based ICUs at two hospitals found that physicians ordered a daily volume of enteral feeding that was 66% of the requirement, but because only 78% of the ordered volume was infused, patients received only 52% of target calories. Sixty-six percent of the time the reasons given for stopping the infusion were determined to be avoidable. Half the patients whose tube feedings were checked every 4 hours had their feedings held for residual volumes less than 200 mL, when the guideline for stopping the tube feeding was a residual of greater than 200 mL [20]. Protocols for delivery of enteral feeding can avoid this.

Parenteral nutrition is associated with an increased risk of infectious complications, especially line infection, and increased cost. Strict adherence to protocols emphasizing aseptic techniques and limiting central line interruption can decrease complications. Peripheral indwelling central catheters or central subclavian or internal jugular lines should be considered and implanted permanent lines should be avoided [9]. Management of infected temporary lines is easier and has fewer complications.

HOW DO YOU PREVENT COMPLICATIONS AND MAXIMIZE BENEFITS?

Anticipating potential complications leads to early recognition, minimizes the impact of the complications, and improves outcome. Adherence to general guidelines for energy requirements, mentioned above, should help avoid overfeeding. Overfeeding can lead to a number of problems, such as cholestatic liver disease, hyperglycemia, increased infections, and worsening hypercapnic respiratory failure. When there is doubt, expired gas analysis can be used to assess caloric requirements. A respiratory quotient (R/Q) greater than 1 generally indicates overfeeding. R/Q is the quotient of mL CO_2 produced per mL O_2 consumed. Increased CO_2 production will cause a rise in the R/Q from 0.80, a normal, average steady state. Reducing total calories (glucose and fat) may benefit patients with chronic lung disease fed parenterally who develop worsening hypercapnia. Assessment of nitrogen balance (the difference between nitrogen produced and nitrogen eliminated in urine and stool) every 5 to 7 days may be useful for adjusting the protein dose. Prerenal azotemia from excessive protein administration is an indication to decrease nitrogen intake. Patient outcome following acute renal failure (creatinine greater than twice normal) does not improve with the administration of specialized formulations.

Monitoring triglycerides and adjusting continuous fat infusion to keep triglycerides less than 500 mg per dL will avoid hypertriglyceridemia. Monitoring of prealbumin because of its short half-life (i.e., 2 days) can be used to assess response to feeding in the ICU setting. Monitoring of fluid and electrolytes is essential particularly in patients receiving TPN to avoid volume overload. Deficiencies in potassium or calcium can lead to cardiac arrhythmias. Hypophosphatemia can precipitate rhabdomyolysis, severe muscle weakness, and respiratory failure. Hypomagnesemia can cause muscle weakness and even seizures. Zinc deficiency can lead to impaired wound healing, diarrhea, and cutaneous anergy. Routine monitoring of vitamins and minerals in patients on short-term parenteral nutrition support is not useful because deficiencies are usually only associated with long-term therapy. Monitoring on a selected case basis when there are clinical signs or symptoms of a vitamin deficiency (e.g., hyperkeratosis [vitamin A], megaloblastic anemia [folate/vitamin B_{12}]) is more practical. Although liver enzymes should be monitored weekly to determine if biliary or liver disease has developed, specialized formulations are not indicated unless there are signs of encephalopathy [9].

WHAT IS THE IMPORTANCE OF PROVIDING SPECIAL KEY NUTRIENTS?

Effects of special nutrients on regulation of the processes of inflammation and repair and immune function have been the object of many recent studies. Although specialized nutrients added to parenteral or enteral formulas have been shown to modulate a variety of cellular responses, their precise clinical utility is still unresolved. For example, arginine is an amino acid that participates in a variety of metabolic processes, including synthesis of nitrous and nitric oxide, compounds known to protect the liver from damage in a murine model of endotoxin-induced hepatic necrosis [21], urea synthesis, lymphocyte proliferation, and wound healing. Other studies have shown that diets rich in fish oils increased survival in guinea pigs challenged with endotoxin [22,23].

The branched chain amino acids leucine, isoleucine, and valine are essential amino acids required for protein synthesis. Although improvement in nitrogen balance can be observed when these are given in combination with other essential amino acids in doses of 0.5 to 1.2 g per kg per day, their efficacy in improving patient outcomes remains to be defined [9,24].

The importance of glutamine to normal cellular function and its unique function in amino acid metabolism, in both health and disease, has recently been elucidated [25]. The skeletal muscle-free amino acid pool is 61% glutamine, and accelerated mobilization of glutamine occurs during catabolic states. In such states, glutamine depletion occurs despite administration of standard parenteral amino acids, which do not contain glutamine because of their instability in aqueous solution. In rats, decline of the intracellular pool of glutamine in skeletal muscle has been shown to correlate with skeletal muscle protein degradation. The majority of glutamine released from skeletal muscle is taken up by intestinal cells. Rat studies have shown that glutamine-supplemented parenteral nutrition improves gut mucosal metabolism and nitrogen balance in sepsis and also increases villus height and mucosal thickness in starved rats, suggesting that mucosal barrier defense is improved [26,27]. However, in humans, a randomized trial of glutamine supplementation in parenteral nutrition detected no difference in infectious complications or median length of hospital stay between groups [28].

Addition of specialized key nutrients to enteral formulas to enhance immune function has been suggested for the reasons outlined earlier. A meta-analysis of 12 studies that used either of the two most common commercially available enteral feeding preparations enriched with the "immunonutrients" arginine and omega-3 fatty acids concluded that they had no effect on mortality [29]. However, significant reductions in infection rates, ventilator days, and hospital length of stay in patients fed these formulas are sufficient to justify their use. These benefits were most pronounced in surgical patients, although they were present in all groups of patients [29]. Although the relative efficacy of any single immune-enhancing component versus its combination with another is impossible to state on the basis of the presently available evidence [30], commercially available formulas fortified with "immunonutrients" are clearly beneficial and we recommend their use [2].

Although the administration of growth hormone can attenuate the severe catabolic state induced by the metabolic response to injury, surgery, and sepsis, two randomized placebo-controlled clinical trials found that in-hospital mortality, length of stay in the ICU, and duration of mechanical ventilation were greater in patients receiving growth hormone [31].

In summary, nutrition support should be considered essential to the treatment of any critical illness. We have provided some useful guidelines for the nutritional assessment, estimation of energy requirement, route of nutrient delivery, estimations of the effectiveness of nutrition provided in critically ill patients, and also suggested some practical points to simplify delivery and avoid associated complications related to parenteral and enteral feeding.

References

1. Giner M, Laviano A, Meguid MM, et al: In 1995 a correlation between malnutrition and poor outcome in critically ill still exists. *Nutrition* 12:23–29, 1996.
2. McClave SA, Martindale RG, Vanek VW, et al: Guidelines for the provision and assessment of nutrition support therapy in the adult critically ill patient: Society of Critical Care Medicine (SCCM) and American Society for Parenteral and Enteral Nutrition (A.S.P.E.N.) *J Parent Enteral Nutr* 33:277–318, 2009.
3. Wolfe RR, Durkot MJ, Allsop JR, et al: Glucose metabolism in severely burned patients. *Metabolism* 28:1031–1039, 1979.
4. McMahon M, Bistrian BR: The physiology of nutritional assessment and therapy in protein-calorie malnutrition. *Dis Mon* 36:378–417, 1990.
5. Heymsfield SB, McManus C, Stevens C, et al: Muscle mass: reliable indicator of protein-energy malnutrition severity and outcome. *Am J Clin Nutr* 35:1192–1199, 1982.
6. Jahoor F, Shangraw RE, Miyoshi H, et al: Role of insulin and glucose oxidation in mediating the protein catabolism of burns and sepsis. *Am J Physiol* 257:E323–E331, 1989.
7. Klein S, Kinney J, Jeejeebhoy K, et al: Nutrition support in clinical practice: review of published data and recommendations for future research direction. *J Parenter Enteral Nutr* 21:133–156, 1997.
8. Preiser JC, Berre J, Carpentier Y, et al: Management of nutrition in European intensive care units: results of a questionnaire. *Intensive Care Med* 25:95–101, 1999.
9. Cerra FB, Benitez MR, Blackburn GL, et al: Applied nutrition in ICU patients: a consensus statement of the American College of Chest Physicians. *Chest* 111:769–778, 1997.
10. Hehir DJ, Jenkins RL, Bistrian BR, et al: Nutrition in patients undergoing orthotopic liver transplantation. *J Parenter Enteral Nutr* 9:695–700, 1985.
11. Baker JP, Detsky AS, Wesson DE, et al: Nutritional assessment: a comparison of clinical judgment and objective measures. *N Engl J Med* 306:969–972, 1982.
12. Detsky AS, McLaughlin JR, Baker JP, et al: What is subjective global assessment of nutritional status? *J Parenter Enteral Nutr* 11:8–13, 1987.
13. Pomposelli JJ, Baxter JK III, Babineau TJ: Early postoperative glucose control predicts nosocomial infection rate in diabetic patients. *J Parenter Enteral Nutr* 22:77–81, 1998.
14. McCowen KC, Friel C, Sternberg J, et al: Hypocaloric total parenteral nutrition: effectiveness in prevention of hypoglycemia and infectious complications—a randomized clinical trial. *Crit Care Med* 28:3606–3611, 2000.
15. Seidner DL, Mascioli EA, Istfan NW, et al: Effects of long-chain triglyceride emulsions on reticuloendothelial system function in humans. *J Parenter Enteral Nutr* 13:614–619, 1989.
16. Kalfarentzos F, Kehagias J, Mead N, et al: Enteral nutrition is superior to parenteral nutrition in severe acute pancreatitis: results of a randomized prospective trial. *Br J Surg* 84:1665–1669, 1997.
17. Eatock FC, Chong P, Menezes N, et al: A randomized study of early nasogastric versus nasojejunal feeding in severe acute pancreatitis. *Am J Gastroenterol* 100:432–439, 2005.
18. Kirby DF, Delegge MH, Fleming CR: American Gastroenterological Association Medical Position Statement: Guidelines for the use of enteral nutrition. *Gastroenterology* 108:1280–1301, 1995.
19. Wolfe MM, Sachs G: Acid suppression: optimizing therapy for gastroduodenal ulcer healing, gastroesophageal reflux disease, and stress-related erosive syndrome. *Gastroenterology* 118:S9–S31, 2000.
20. McClave SA, Sexton LK, Spain DA, et al: Enteral tube feeding in the intensive care unit: factors impeding adequate delivery. *Crit Care Med* 27:1252–1256, 1999.
21. Billiar TR, Curren RD, Stueh DJ, et al: Inducible cytosolic enzyme activity for the production of nitric oxides from L-arginine. *Biochem Biophys Res Commun* 168:1034–1040, 1990.
22. Mascioli EA, Leader L, Flores E, et al: Enhanced survival to endotoxin in guinea pigs fed IV fish oil. *Lipids* 23:623–625, 1988.
23. Mascioli EA, Iwasa Y, Trimbo S, et al: Endotoxin challenge after menhaden oil to diet: effects on survival of guinea pigs. *Am J Clin Nutr* 49:277–282, 1989.
24. Nompleggi DJ, Bonkovsky HL: Nutritional supplementation in chronic liver disease: an analytical review. *Hepatology* 19:518–533, 1994.
25. Lacey JM, Wilmore DW: Is glutamine a conditionally essential amino acid? *Nutr Rev* 48:297–309, 1990.
26. Chen K, Okuma T, Okuma K, et al: Glutamine-supplemented parenteral nutrition improves gut mucosal metabolism and nitrogen balance in septic rats. *J Parenter Enteral Nutr* 18:167–171, 1994.
27. Inoue Y, Grant JP, Synder PJ: Effect of glutamine-supplemented total parenteral nutrition on recovery of small intestine after starvation atrophy. *J Parenter Enteral Nutr* 17:165–170, 1993.
28. Powell-Tuck J, Jamieson CP, Bettany EA, et al: A double blind randomized controlled trial of glutamine supplementation in parenteral nutrition. *Gut* 45:82–88, 1999.
29. Beale RJ, Bryg DJ, Bihari DJ: Immunonutrition in the critically ill: a systematic review of clinical outcome. *Crit Care Med* 27:2799–2805, 1999.
30. Bistrian BR: Enteral nutrition: just a fuel or an immunity enhancer? *Minerva Anestesiol* 65:471–474, 1999.
31. Takala J, Ruokonen E, Webster N, et al: Increased mortality associated with growth hormone treatment in critically ill adults. *N Engl J Med* 341:785–792, 1999.

CHAPTER 191 ■ PARENTERAL AND ENTERAL NUTRITION IN THE INTENSIVE CARE UNIT

DAVID F. DRISCOLL AND BRUCE R. BISTRIAN

Nutritional and metabolic support during acute illness is an integral part of the clinical care of critically ill patients. The significance of such interventions is predicated on three main factors: (a) degree of metabolic stress; (b) dysfunction of major organ systems; and/or (c) presence of protein-calorie malnutrition (PCM). In the first case, metabolic stress can arise from a variety of sources including, for example, severe injuries sustained by major trauma such as closed head injury, multiple long-bone fractures, third-degree burns of greater than 25% body surface area, and severe sepsis and stress of lesser intensity such as thoracoabdominal surgery, pulmonary infection, systemic infection, or any source of active systemic inflammation. Often, more than one form of metabolic stress may be present that can accentuate and/or dysregulate the injury response. Concerning the second factor, metabolically stressed patients may develop acute failure of vital organs during the critical care period or have underlying chronic end-organ dysfunction. Acute or chronic disease, particularly of the cardiopulmonary, renal, or hepatic system, often further complicates the clinical course and requires modification of nutritional support during critical illness, especially in the elderly [1]. Finally, the presence of preexisting or the likely early development of PCM is key to identifying those patients who will derive the greatest clinical benefits from nutritional and metabolic support therapy.

Approximately 35 years ago, the prevalence of PCM in hospitalized general medical and surgical patients was reported to be as high as 50% of all adult admissions to a large teaching hospital [2,3]. More recent reports continue to document high rates of malnutrition in hospitalized patients [4–9]. When moderate to severe PCM accompanies severe metabolic stress, an increase in nutrition-related complications can be expected to occur, including wound dehiscence, nosocomial infections, and severe fluid, electrolyte, and acid–base disturbances. During stress, substantial catabolism of both endogenous and exogenous protein and energy occurs coincident with the injury response. In support of the metabolic response to injury, the breakdown of body protein, principally from muscle and connective tissue stores, supports amino acid and energy needs to mount various beneficial components of the systemic inflammatory response by the release of amino acids for accelerated synthesis of such proteins as leukocytes, hepatic acute phase and cellular proteins, and wound tissue, and gluconeogenesis for the optimization of energy requirements for such tissues as cardiac, leukocytes, and fibroblasts. An assessment of the degree of this response can be estimated by application of the catabolic index [10]. However, if protein calorie malnutrition complicates injury or infection, the systemic inflammatory response is less intense than that found in normally nourished individuals with a similar degree of injury. Consequently, the degree and duration of the metabolic response, with respect to nitrogen breakdown, is greatly diminished. In terms of the degree of catabolism, for example, a malnourished elderly patient with significant catabolic injury could manifest nitrogen losses that may be as a much as 50% less than normally nourished younger counterparts with the same injury [1]. Although this might imply a less severe catabolic response sparing lean tissue, the pathologic consequences are more severe as a result of the muting of the beneficial aspects of the systemic inflammatory response, and these adverse effects tend to occur sooner. Moreover, the time course to intervene with nutritional and metabolic support to limit the likelihood of nutrition-related complications is also shortened by as a much as 50% (i.e., 5 to 7 days) in the moderate to severely malnourished versus normally nourished individuals (i.e., 7 to 10 days) with the same metabolic stress. Ultimately, the consequences of ongoing depletion of the metabolically active body cell mass in the malnourished reduce the ability to recover from acute illness, can be associated with severe deficiencies in minerals that are typically found in muscle (potassium, magnesium, and phosphorus), and often lead to severe impairments in immunocompetence, wound healing, and organ repair.

Once the decision to provide nutrition support is made, parenteral or enteral nutritional therapies are available options. In every case, if the gastrointestinal tract is functional and the patient is hemodynamically stable, enteral nutrition (EN) should be instituted. However, if significant malnutrition also exists and a prolonged recovery is anticipated, it should be recognized that the time frame to achieve eucaloric intakes for EN often takes much longer due to associated gastrointestinal intolerance, compared with parenteral nutrition (PN). As central venous access is generally necessary during critical illness, EN support can often be supplemented with PN [11] so as to avoid the prolongation of caloric deficits during acute illness, which are particularly of concern in initially malnourished patients or the most critically ill with closed head injury, multiple trauma, major burns, and severe sepsis. In such patients it appears that early feeding within the first 72 hours, whether by enteral, parenteral, or the combination, has the greatest impact on outcome in terms of mortality. Although mild decrements in energy balance in the critical care setting may well be tolerated and in certain circumstances appropriate, at least 1 g of protein per kg and 15 kcal per kg advancing to 1.5 g protein per kg and 20 to 25 kcal per kg as soon as possible should be the goal to avoid adverse, nutrition-related outcomes. Moreover, intensive metabolic support (i.e., the provision of electrolytes and acid–base therapy) can also be accomplished efficiently through the PN admixture. The amount of parenteral nutrients can be gradually reduced as the patient is transitioned to EN coincident with remission of the stress response and return of full gastrointestinal tolerance to tube feeding. Thus, in the intensive care unit (ICU), nutrition support is often provided to patients using both enteral and parenteral means, especially during the acute care period. The purpose of supplying both EN and PN where appropriate should not be motivated by attempts to meet protein and energy needs as soon as possible, but rather as a means of providing trophic stimulation to enterocytes and hopefully a quicker transition to full enteral feedings, while PN is used to treat severe metabolic disorders such as hypokalemia, hypophosphatemia, and metabolic alkalosis, that can only be safely and effectively addressed by the intravenous route of administration. The greatest challenge facing the critical care clinician is to appropriately identify those patients who are in greatest need of nutrition support therapy and to provide it in a manner that is both effective and does not produce iatrogenic complications.

CLINICAL CONSEQUENCES OF DELAYING NUTRITION SUPPORT

Although at times it is difficult to pinpoint the cause and effect of nutrition-related complications during critical illness, it should be intuitively obvious that withholding nutrition will ultimately lead to death from starvation. This message was poignantly illustrated in the deaths of Maze prisoners in Belfast, Ireland, as detailed in a report from Leiter and Marliss [12] in 1982. Ten Irish Republican Army prisoners went on a hunger strike that led to their deaths over a period of 45 to 73 days of fasting. All were young lean males and the critical weight loss that resulted in death was approximately 35% calculated from the first day of the fast. It is also generally acknowledged that patients who approach 35% to 40% losses from their ideal or usual body weight through inadequate nutritional intake are at greatest risk of malnutrition-related death. Presumably, at these extreme levels of body mass depletion, both the size and function of vital organs of the viscera are considerably diminished. At some critical point, presumed to be when fat stores become limited, protein catabolism now coming from both skeletal and visceral organs accelerates. If one discontinues providing life-sustaining needs for energy, the loss of a critical mass of body protein is ultimately reached and death from organ failure is imminent.

The effects on the vital organs can be catastrophic, since oxygen consumption of the visceral organs is much higher than that of resting skeletal muscle. The imbalance between loss of skeletal muscle and visceral organ mass initially favoring visceral organs has also been suggested to explain the higher energy expenditures per body weight seen in severely depleted hospitalized patients (average of approximately 70% of ideal body weight) as a result of an approximate 10-fold difference in resting oxygen consumption between skeletal muscle compared to visceral tissues such as the liver [13]. During starvation (with adequate water intake), and in the absence of metabolic stress, a normally nourished, thin individual can survive for periods of approximately 6 to 10 weeks. In terms of total body nitrogen, it is estimated that the loss of 350 to 500 g of nitrogen is potentially lethal. In terms of body mass index (BMI), which is weight in kg per height in meters squared, it is generally considered that a BMI less than 13 kg per m^2 in males and less than 11 kg per m^2 in females is incompatible with life [14]. However, the rapidity of weight loss is also a factor, since lesser degrees of semistarvation (i.e., smaller energy deficits) are better tolerated. Table 191.1 depicts the relationship of BMI with nutritional status.

By way of comparison, the metabolically stressed patient experiences greater catabolism coincident with acute illness and can lose as much as 30 g of nitrogen per day, representing about 1 kg of lean tissue from the breakdown of lean body mass. Generally, the majority of these losses can be measured in a 24-hour urine collection as urea nitrogen and used for nitrogen balance estimation. Nitrogen balance studies assess the difference between dietary protein (nitrogen) intake and nitrogen excretion. Healthy individuals consuming an adequate diet in terms of essential nutrients including protein (0.8 g protein per kg per day) and sufficient energy to provide energy balance will be in zero nitrogen balance. That is the nitrogen in is equaled by the nitrogen out in urine (mostly) and feces, reflecting no net change in lean body mass. Net nitrogen losses in patients receiving parenteral or enteral feeding can vary from 0 to 30 g per day, depending on the extent of the injury response and the level of feeding. With the systemic inflammatory response, the utilization of protein to maintain lean body mass is impaired, making the daily requirement increase to about 1.5 g protein per kg per day. Similarly, energy requirements increase, which are offset to some degree by the reduction in physical activity characteristic of the hospitalized patient. With the development of renal dysfunction, the proportionate amounts of nitrogen found in the urine become substantially less, with a concomitant rise in blood urea nitrogen (BUN). In general, in a 70-kg male every 5 mg% change in BUN represents 2 g of nitrogen catabolized and not excreted, and 1.5 g of nitrogen for a 60-kg female, based on average total body water of 60% and 50% for males and females, respectively. Protein intakes must be adjusted to limit the rise in BUN, but nutrition efficacy should not be sacrificed to renal function beyond a reduction to the 1 g protein per kg for other than very brief periods. Renal replacement therapy such as dialysis or hemofiltration should be considered in those circumstances. Once the BUN becomes stable, even if elevated by impaired renal function, a 24-hour urine urea nitrogen excretion represents the amount catabolized over that period. The catabolic index (CI) (CI = 24-hour urine urea nitrogen − [0.5 × dietary nitrogen + 3]), adjusts for the effects of dietary intake and obligatory nitrogen loss on urinary urea nitrogen excretion. The catabolic index is the difference between measured and predicted urine urea nitrogen excretion. For example, the major catabolic stresses that produce the highest nitrogen losses and catabolic indices include burns, head injury, severe sepsis, and multiple trauma. The clinical application of nitrogen balance and CI assessments are illustrated in Table 191.2.

There are potential clinical scenarios that may affect the accuracy of nitrogen balance studies. This is especially true in patients with renal dysfunction that may reduce nitrogen output and could erroneously suggest an improvement in nitrogen balance. A correction of the nitrogen balance study can be applied to account for the nitrogen losses that do not appear in the urine, but result in an increase in the BUN concentration. Assuming nitrogen intake remains constant, two important pieces of data are required to correct for the nitrogen losses not appearing in the urine and include the patient's BUN and body weight at the beginning and end of the 24-hour collection period. These are important because most of the urea is distributed in total body water. A clinical example that applies to this method of correction appears in Table 191.3.

In terms of lean body mass, each gram of nitrogen lost represents approximately 30 g of (hydrated) lean tissue (hydration ratio: approximately 4 or 5 to 1). For patients with daily

TABLE 191.1

BODY MASS INDEX AND NUTRITIONAL STATUS

Body mass index	= weight in kg ÷ (height in m)^2
Assumptions:	weight: 75 kg; height: 1.84 m
BMI	= 75/(1.84)^2
	= 22.2
Body mass index	Nutritional status
≥30	Obese
≥25–<30	Overweight
20–<25	Normal
<18.5	Moderate malnutrition
<16	Severe malnutrition
<13	Lethal in males
<11	Lethal in females

TABLE 191.2

CLINICAL APPLICATION OF THE NITROGEN BALANCE AND CATABOLIC INDEX ASSESSMENTS[a]

Nitrogen balance	$= \frac{\text{protein intake (g)}}{6.25} - (24\text{ h UUN} + 4)$
	$= \frac{105\text{ g}}{6.25} - (20 + 4)$
	$= -7.2$ g
Catabolic index	$=$ UUN (g) $-$ ($\frac{1}{2} \times$ dietary nitrogen $+ 3$)
	$= 20$ g $- (0.5 \times 16.8$ g $+ 3)$
	$= 8.6$ (severe stress)
<0 no significant stress	
0–5 significant stress	
>5 severe stress	

[a]Assumptions: 70 kg male; 105 g protein intake; 20 g UUN over 24 hours.
UUN, urine urea nitrogen.

nitrogen losses of 30 g, which represents the highest catabolic nitrogen loss in the absence of dietary protein intake, approximately 1 kg of lean tissue would be lost each day. Such losses cannot be sustained for protracted periods, and under these circumstances, nutrition support is clearly indicated within the first 24 to 36 hours even in the previously well-nourished patient to address this extraordinary rate of loss. Using cumulative nitrogen deficits of 350 to 500 g, a sustained loss of this magnitude could theoretically result in death in approximately 2 to 3 weeks, although catabolic rates usually diminish in the later weeks of injury. For the severely malnourished patient of 75% ideal body weight, one can estimate the critical survival period to be in the range of 1.5 to 2 weeks under the same circumstances. Finally, a cumulative caloric deficit of 10,000 kcal or more during acute illness has been associated with significant morbidity and mortality in the surgical ICU [15]. However, it is likely that the associated protein deficit played the larger role, since normal individuals have more than 150,000 stored calories as fat, which always makes up the greater proportion of the caloric deficit. A study in the medical ICU has shown that intakes of less than 25% of requirements were associated with a higher rate of bloodstream infections [16].

Of course, projections of survival or complications are estimates and may be highly variable depending on other factors (i.e., nutritional status, metabolic stress[es], end-organ function, and so forth). Moreover, in the clinical setting, such high outputs of nitrogen over long periods will not likely be sustained, as medical and surgical therapies will usually be successful in reducing the stress response. Furthermore, both the rate of reduction in lean body mass and the intensity of the systemic inflammatory response diminish as PCM develops. Such patients will invariably receive calories (dextrose) and electrolytes from various parenteral infusions, so that some form of supplementation is given, which also slows the loss of lean tissue. Consequently, the outcome of death from the total lack of nutrition support is rare. However, nutrition-related complications, such as impaired wound healing and immunocompetence leading to nosocomial infection, are the common proximate causes of increased morbidity and mortality under such circumstances.

IDENTIFYING PATIENTS IN NEED OF NUTRITION SUPPORT

In the ICU setting, it is often difficult to identify those patients who are at greatest risk of developing nutrition-related

TABLE 191.3

NITROGEN BALANCE CORRECTION IN RENAL DYSFUNCTION[a]

Prenitrogen balance data	
BUN = 31 mg/dL; weight = 70 kg; 105 g protein intake	
Prestudy	
Total body water @ 70 kg	= 42 L
Total BUN @ 31 mg/dL	= 42 L × 310 mg/L (or 310 mg/L)
	= **13,020 mg or 13 g**
Postnitrogen balance data	
BUN = 51 mg/dL; weight = 74 kg; 105 g protein intake; 24 h UUN = 20 g	
Poststudy	
Total body water @ 74 kg	= 42 L + 4 L
	= 46 L
Total BUN @ 51 mg/dL (or 510 mg/L)	= 46 L × 510 mg/L
	= **23,460 mg or 23.5 g**
Nitrogen balance	$= \frac{\text{protein intake (g)}}{6.25} - (24\text{ h UUN} + 4)$
	$= \frac{105\text{ g}}{6.25} - (20 + 4)$
	= −7.2 g
Corrected N-balance	= 13.02 g −23.5 g urea nitrogen (blood)
	= −10.5 g not excreted in urine
	= −10.5 g (BUN) + (−7.2 g UUN)
	= **−17.7 g**

[a]Assumptions: Total body water = 60% (for males).
BUN, blood urea nitrogen; UUN, urine urea nitrogen.

complications due to preexisting malnutrition. Such patients are often volume overloaded due to massive administration of parenteral fluids from multiple drug therapies and often acute volume resuscitation, as well as maintenance intravenous therapy to support intravascular volume. This fluid retention and weight gain is often compounded by the hormonal consequences of the systemic inflammatory response such as enhanced insulin, aldosterone, and antidiuretic hormone secretion, which favor salt and water retention. Consequently, the weight of the patient is artificially high, and major efforts of the ICU team are often directed at reducing volume intake in order to mobilize third-space fluids. A weight history may be difficult to obtain or overlooked entirely because of more acute clinical issues. Moreover, an accurate patient weight is also important to optimize drug therapy. Under these circumstances, a moderately to severely malnourished patient may escape detection by the primary care team, and only be recognized as malnourished after fluid homeostasis is achieved, or worse, a potentially preventable nutrition-related complication, such as wound breakdown, occurs. Clearly, at this point, the opportunity to minimize such complications from expert nutrition support has passed, and the course toward rehabilitation may be long and costly.

To avoid this scenario, a more substantial effort must be undertaken to identify the patients at greatest risk. Nutrition screening programs on admission, especially by dieticians, can greatly assist in identifying these patients, but many patients, especially acute admissions for emergent care, may escape this surveillance process. In these cases, the premorbid weight is very important and should be obtained if at all possible. It will at least provide a baseline prior to the numerous medical and surgical maneuvers that may take place over the ensuing 24 to 48 hours that could dramatically change the patient's weight in the critical care setting.

If the admission weight is not obtained, then the clinician may need to estimate the patient's body weight from available hospital data. Estimations may be made based on the most recent weight recorded, and then backtracked through the medical chart using the intake and output records to reconstruct the original weight history. For critically ill patients, such records are usually reliable, and a reasonable estimate may be made. This estimate may be confirmed by subsequent discussions with the patient or family. When confirmed, the body weight can then be compared to standard measures for population-based body weight for height tables such as the ideal body weight or the BMI. A patient weight less than 85% of the ideal body weight (IBW) or BMI less than 18.5 indicates moderate malnutrition. Severe malnutrition would be considered likely if weight is less than 75% of IBW or BMI is less than 16 kg per m^2. Thus, a greater sense of urgency to intervene with nutrition support is present under these conditions and should be undertaken within several days of the acute injury. If the patient is deemed well nourished, then intervention may be delayed unless the systemic inflammatory response is severe (i.e., major third-degree burns, closed head injury with a Glasgow Coma Score less than 8, multiple trauma with very high acute physiology and chronic health evaluation [APACHE] or injury severity scores, severe pancreatitis with a positive CT scan and more than three Ranson criteria, and so forth). Then, because the systemic inflammatory response is likely to endure beyond 1 week, very early nutritional support is indicated. The serum albumin level, which reflects the presence of a recent systemic inflammatory response, is not often helpful in this setting because the invariable systemic inflammatory response and common disturbances in volume status make hypoalbuminemia universal. However, severe hypoalbuminemia (less than 2.4 g per dL) usually reflecting a greater degree and/or longer duration of systemic inflammation identifies a population at much greater nutritional risk. Finally, if the weight-based data are not reliable, a formal nutrition support consult or indirect calorimetry may be indicated.

NUTRITIONAL REQUIREMENTS

Protein

The amount and type of protein administered to the critically ill depend on the clinical circumstances of each patient. Nevertheless, there is an upper limit to the quantity of protein that can be given based on net protein utilization during metabolic stress. In general, providing protein in amounts above 1.75 g per kg per day exceeds the capacity of the body to use the administered protein to increase synthesis [17,18]. Amounts above this level of intake are essentially completely converted to urea and serve no nutritional purpose. At intakes ranging between 0.6 to 1.75 g per kg per day, each increment of intake increases net protein synthesis at a cost of increasing the proportion going to ureagenesis. In patients with nitrogen accumulation disorders (of either renal or hepatic origin), a compromise must often be made between greatest rates of net protein synthesis and lowest rates of urea or ammoniagenesis. For example, as the BUN increases, especially above 100 mg%, the risk of uremic complications increases, including bleeding, or, increasing the production of ammonia in encephalopathic patients. Generally, the optimal protein intake in critically ill patients is given at twice the recommended daily amount (approximately 0.8 g per kg per day) of normal adults, at approximately 1.5 g per kg per day. With renal impairment, at least 1 g per kg should be provided and greater amounts given if tolerated or dialysis is initiated. In patients with liver failure at least 1 g per kg of standard protein should be provided and up to 1.5 g per kg if tolerated. This is done recognizing the overall impairments in protein utilization that accompanies metabolic stress, as well as the heightened needs during catabolism.

The type of protein administered varies with the patient's condition and the route of administration. For PN support, standard protein mixtures are given in their monomeric form as individual crystalline amino acids and levorotatory isomers, which comprise the essential amino acids (histidine, isoleucine, leucine, lysine, methionine, phenylalanine, threonine, tryptophan, and valine) and the nonessential amino acids (alanine, aminoacetic acid, arginine, cysteine, proline, serine, and tyrosine). In standard amino acid formulations, the branched-chain amino acids (leucine, isoleucine, and valine) comprise approximately 18% to 25% of the amino acid profile. Collectively, they are available in commercial intravenous solutions in concentrations ranging from 3% to 15%. On average, for every 6.25 g of the amino acids in the mixture, 1 g of nitrogen is available, although this number is lower with a number of the specialized amino acid formulas. The caloric value of protein is 4.1 kcal per g, and such calories should be counted in critically ill patients when tracking energy intakes.

Specialized amino acid mixtures have evolved that include selected profiles. For example, renal formulations have been devised that principally provide the essential amino acids (histidine, isoleucine, leucine, lysine, methionine, phenylalanine, threonine, tryptophan, and valine), while hepatic formulations have eliminated or reduced aromatic amino acids (phenylalanine, tryptophan, and tyrosine) and the sulphur-containing amino acid methionine and increased the proportion of branched-chain amino acids (BCAAs) (isoleucine, leucine, and valine). However, the routine use of these expensive formulations in these conditions over conventional or standard amino acid mixtures has not been convincingly demonstrated, and in certain cases when used to meet full protein needs, may be harmful [19]. For patients with nitrogen accumulation disorders, the use of branched-chain enriched amino acid formulas in the range of 45% to 50% of the total amino acid profile have been shown to improve protein utilization when total amino acid intakes are given in the 40- to 70-g range and may reduce the risk of encephalopathy when compared to a standard formula. Finally, other attempts at modifying the profiles of amino acid mixtures, such as the extemporaneous preparation by the hospital pharmacy of sterile glutamine in total parenteral nutrition (TPN), have shown some benefits in selected settings but they require a considerable level of parenteral compounding expertise. In addition, in order to safely provide this compounded sterile preparation, ongoing quality assurance measures as outlined by the *United States Pharmacopeia* must be performed and therefore such practices are subject to Federal Drug Administration oversight [20]. A glutamine-containing dipeptide formulation, which is commercially available in Europe, has been the subject of some positive trials, but its ultimate place in the care of the critically ill is not yet established.

For EN support, protein is typically provided in either an oligomeric form as protein hydrolysates containing various peptides ranging from di- and tripeptides to polymers of eight or more, or as whole protein usually provided as casein or in its polymeric form as, for example, casein hydrolysates. Less commonly, they can even be provided as the individual amino acids. Most formulations contain a fixed amount of protein in the range of 30 to 40 g per L and thus for fluid-restricted patients in the ICU cannot meet the protein needs of most patients. Alternatively, more concentrated enteral formulae exist that may be used, or the clinician may opt to add protein modules to conventional products to increase protein density. However, in either case, both approaches result in higher osmolarities that may affect gastrointestinal tolerance.

Carbohydrate

The amount and type of energy provided to improve the utilization of the prescribed protein intake also varies with the individual patient. As well, there are physiologic limits to the amounts given, beyond which significant complications are more likely. For most patients, providing 25 kcal per kg per day is sufficient to support the protein synthetic response to metabolic stress. This is the total energy expenditure of most critically ill, postoperative patients. Amounts above 30 kcal per kg per day exceed the energy expenditure of most hospitalized patients except those with severe burns, closed head injury, and multiple trauma where measured caloric expenditures are usually 30 to 40 kcal per kg. However, providing nutritional support in amounts greater than 30 kcal per kg leads to higher rates of hyperglycemia in both types of patients; in the postoperative setting, due to overfeeding, and in the trauma unit, due to the severity of systemic inflammatory response. Although better glycemic control through the use of insulin would be one way to reduce the infectious risk in the latter instance, it is interesting to note that in several trials of immune-enhancing diets that improved outcomes and reduced infection rates have been seen at energy intakes at 30 kcal per kg or less, in diets that are likely to have been hypocaloric [21]. For carbohydrates, the physiologic limits are linked to the normal endogenous hepatic production rates for glucose, which approximate 2 mg per kg per minute or about 200 g per day for a 70-kg healthy adult [22]. This is the amount of glucose needed by the body to meet the obligate needs of tissues dependent on glucose (i.e., brain, renal medulla, red blood cells, and so forth), and it is derived from body stores of glycogen (glycogenolysis) or made from noncarbohydrate sources such as from protein breakdown to gluconeogenic amino acid precursors (gluconeogenesis). Glycogen stores are limited and therefore can be rapidly depleted during acute metabolic stress (i.e., within 24 hours) [23]. Thus, the major source of glucose in the hypocaloric state following stress comes from gluconeogenesis, and higher amounts than usual are produced to support the metabolic response to injury, accelerated by the hormonal milieu produced by the increased secretion of catecholamines, glucagon, cortisol, and growth hormone [24]. The judicious provision of nutrition support is designed to attenuate the extent of protein breakdown without exacerbating significant changes in nutritional and metabolic homeostasis. Similar to the case with protein, as carbohydrate intake increases net oxidation occurs, but with an increasing proportion going to nonoxidative pathways (glycogen synthesis and particularly de novo lipogenesis). However, glycogen synthesis is limited by available storage capacity of about 500 g in normal adults and perhaps 1,000 g in a critically ill patient receiving TPN, with its resultant very high insulin levels. There is effectively no limit for fat storage. The optimal balance is at intakes at about 400 g per day, with maximal glucose oxidized of 700 g per day. Thus, in a 70-kg adult, glucose to amino acid of 2:1 TPN formula providing glucose at 400 g per day and 1.5 g of protein per kg per day represents about 25 kcal per kg per day.

For PN, glucose is the only reasonable carbohydrate fuel or energy source that is widely available for intravenous administration. Generally, it is provided as a monohydrate and its caloric equivalent is therefore 3.4 kcal per g rather than 4 kcal per g for its anhydrous form. It is commercially available in a variety of concentrations ranging from 2.5% to 70% in sterile water for injection. Glucose is the primary energy source of any PN admixture prescribed for central venous alimentation and typically is given in final admixture concentrations from 10% to 25%. Higher concentrations can be given, but are associated with an increase in the number of dextrose-associated complications if the amounts given are too large.

For EN, carbohydrates may be given in a number of chemical forms. For example, they can be given as the monosaccharide, glucose, frequently found in monomeric or elemental formulas. Alternatively, in less refined formulas, carbohydrates may be provided as oligosaccharides, such as hydrolyzed cornstarch, or more complex polysaccharides, such as corn syrup, are frequently used. The selection of a particular enteral formula is largely based on a number of clinical factors such as gastrointestinal function, fluid status, and end-organ function.

Fat

Lipids serve as an alternative energy source that is used to substitute for a portion of the carbohydrate calories. PN support prescribed in this fashion, it is referred to as a total nutrient admixture, all-in-one or 3-in-1 mixed-fuel system [25]. As with protein and carbohydrates, the amount and type of lipids used will vary depending on the clinical condition of the patient. For the most part, long-chain triglycerides (LCTs) derived from vegetable oils have been the principal source of lipid calories used in the clinical setting. Specifically, soybean oil, which is rich in polyunsaturated omega-6 fatty acids, has been extensively used, especially for intravenous nutrition. It is a major source of the essential fatty acids, linoleic, and alpha linolenic acids. However, ill-considered prescribing habits, where either excessive quantities or infusion rates have been used, have led to clinically significant adverse effects such as immune dysfunction and pulmonary gas diffusion abnormalities in critically ill patients. The excessive administration of intravenous lipid emulsions (IVLE) can accumulate in the liver and impair Kupffer cell function, thus interfering with a major component of the reticuloendothelial system [26,27]. In addition, lipid injectable emulsions are composed of various oils that serve as prostaglandin precursors that are immunosuppressive, especially those of the n6 series such as PGE_2, which suppresses lymphocyte proliferation and natural killer cell activity [28], and can reverse hypoxic vasoconstriction in patients with adult respiratory distress syndrome [29]. In contrast, the oxidation and subsequent plasma clearance of lipids is significantly improved when IVLEs are given over 24 hours versus briefer intervals [30]. Impaired plasma clearance of lipids can result in fat overload syndrome and is a particularly significant clinical issue in children [31–42]. Fat overload syndrome can result from the administration of a stable fat emulsion over brief intervals [29,30,43–47] or from more modest doses of lipid that might be physicochemically unstable [48]. In fact, a review of the literature regarding *stable* fat emulsions has concluded that virtually all of the adverse effects associated with LCTs have occurred when the infusion rate exceeds 0.11 g per kg per hour [49]. For a 70-kg adult this limit would be approximately 13 hours for 500 mL of 20%, which makes 3-in-1 admixture infusions safer and easier to administer as a continuous infusion over 24 hours rather than as a separate "IV piggyback" over a brief period, which would require an infusion rate almost twice as fast. In addition, piggyback infusion of lipids is not recommended beyond 12 hours [50].

Recent reports regarding the clinical significance of unstable fat emulsions have emerged. On December 1, 2007, the United States Pharmacopeia (USP), which is recognized by the Food and Drug Administration (FDA) as the official compendium for drug standards, was the first pharmacopeia worldwide to establish globule size limits for intravenous lipid emulsions [51]. This is notable because intravenous lipid emulsions had been used clinically in the United States for more than 30 years (and Europe for more than 45 years), when most drugs have official USP specifications within 5 years of FDA approval [52]. The USP limits specified two size limits: (i) mean droplet size (MDS $<0.5\ \mu$m) and (ii) large diameter tail, expressed as the percent of fat globules $>5\ \mu$m ($PFAT_5 <0.05\%$). The primary motivation for these limits was to avoid the development of microvascular pulmonary embolism from an excessive population of large-diameter fat globules indicating instability of the emulsion.

Around the time the USP announced its intentions to adopt these limits in 2004 [53], a major lipid emulsion product also changed its conventional packaging from glass to plastic containers. With this change in packaging, the lipid emulsion product now failed the large-diameter globule limits of the USP [54]. Lipid emulsions failing USP limits were also shown to produce less stable emulsions when packaged in syringes for neonates [55], when mixed in TPN admixtures [56] and when used in a multichamber bag premixed for TPN therapy [57]. Moreover, lipid emulsions not meeting pharmacopeial limits were also shown to be associated with significant hypertriglyceridemia in premature neonates when compared to lipid emulsions meeting USP limits [58], although this has not been confirmed in a randomized clinical trial. Finally, in animal studies lipid emulsions failing USP limits were shown to be hepatotoxic [59]. A recent study intended to explore the extent of physiologic damage from the infusion of unstable lipid emulsions produced evidence of hepatic accumulation of fat associated with oxidative stress, liver injury and a low-level systemic inflammatory response [60].

Triglyceride clearance is maximal at serum triglyceride levels of up to about 400 mg per dL, and patients who initially have serum triglycerides at this level will tolerate even lesser amounts of fat without adverse consequences. In patients who have normal serum triglyceride levels at initiation of TPN, serum triglyceride levels are usually not monitored. For those with levels greater than 200 mg per dL it is reasonable to check the triglyceride again after a stable regimen has been attained with lipids below 0.11 g per kg per hour. Stable levels below 400 mg per dL are acceptable while receiving lipid emulsions.

For PN therapy, soybean oil emulsions continue to dominate the United States market. However, there are a number of different lipid compositions presently available in Europe and under investigation in the United States [61]. They include various mixtures of soybean oil with medium-chain triglycerides (MCTs), olive oil, and fish oil. In nearly every case, soybean oil is included in sufficient proportions to provide adequate amounts of the essential fatty acids [62].

For EN therapy, a number of the lipid types available for parenteral use in Europe are widely available in the United States for enteral administration in complete nutritional diets. Typically, they contain 30% to 40% of the total calories as fat and often contain blends of corn and soy oil. However, in the more specialized enteral formulas, MCTs, fish oil, and even structured lipids are available. Moreover, in some of these products the fat content is either severely restricted (i.e., 3% to 10% of total calories for the fat-intolerant patient) or may be as high as 55% for the patient with pulmonary compromise.

Volume

The maintenance of fluid homeostasis is an important goal in critical care. At times, many patients in the ICU become severely volume-overloaded as a consequence of parenteral fluid administration and the fluid-retentive state characteristic of critical illness [63–65]. For this reason, when assessing fluid status, it is important to bear in mind the usual contribution of water to body weight or total body water (TBW) of the patient under normal, unstressed conditions. In normal adults, TBW comprises approximately 50% to 60% of body weight. As lean body mass is hydrated in a ratio of approximately 4 parts water to 1 part protein, lean tissue is a significant component of TBW. In the clinical setting, acute changes in weight over short intervals primarily reflect net changes in TBW which almost never reflect lean tissue gains in the hospital setting. For example, a 10% increase in weight over 24 to 48 hours represents a proportional increase in TBW and may be associated with adverse clinical consequences, such as greater ventilator dependence, impaired cardiovascular function, and disturbances in electrolyte homeostasis. Even when the patient is considered euvolemic, the contributions to volume from nutrition support are generally limited to approximately 25 mL per kg per day, as other reasons for fluid administration are usually indicated.

Depending on the volume assessments by the primary care team, the amount of nutrition support that may be provided by either PN or EN may be affected. The most significant effect occurs when volume restrictions are imposed. When this happens, hypocaloric nutrition is usually provided due to the limitations associated with caloric density. Caloric or macronutrient density is the sum total of calories from protein, carbohydrates, and fat, expressed in kilocalories per milliliter (kcal per mL). Generally, the caloric density of typical formulations routinely prescribed for either PN or EN support is approximately 1 kcal per mL, but special forms of each therapy are available that reasonably allow up to 1.5 kcal per mL to be formulated. However, most enteral formulations are commercially available in fixed concentrations and therefore are less easily manipulated to the specific needs of the critically ill patient than with the PN admixture. For example, with a 1,000 mL fluid restriction allotted for PN support, the increased macronutrient density could be achieved to attain eucaloric nutrition for adult patients weighing up to 60 kg (25 kcal per kg). Of course, these special dosage forms are generally more expensive than conventional products, and the cost-to-benefit ratio has not been fully demonstrated. The usual parenteral formula provided when fluid restriction is necessary is a more standard PN admixture [66], providing 70 g of amino acids and 210 g of glucose (A7D21) approximating 1,000 kcal in a 1 L final volume when

TABLE 191.4

HYPOCALORIC 1,000 mL TOTAL PARENTERAL NUTRITION REGIMENS AS A SINGLE- VERSUS MIXED-FUEL SYSTEM IN INTENSIVE CARE UNIT PATIENTS

Weight (kg)	Total kcal/d[a]	Single-fuel		Mixed-fuel		
		Amino acids[b] (%)	Glucose[c] (%)	Amino acids (%)	Glucose (%)	Lipids[d] (%)
40	600	40 g or 266 mL (4)[e]	128 g or 183 mL (12.8)[e]	40 g or 266 mL (4)[e]	75 g or 107 mL (7.5)[e]	20 g or 100 mL (2)[e]
50	750	50 g or 333 mL (5)[e]	160 g or 228 mL (16)[e]	50 g or 333 mL (5)[e]	96 g or 137 mL (9.6)[e]	24 g or 120 mL (2.4)[e]
60	900	60 g or 400 mL (6)[e]	192 g or 275 mL (19.2)[e]	60 g or 400 mL (6)[e]	115 g or 164 mL (11.5)[e]	29 g or 145 mL (2.9)[e]
70	1,050	70 g or 466 mL (7)[e]	224 g or 320 mL (22.4)[e]	70 g or 466 mL (7)[e]	135 g or 192 mL (13.5)[e]	34 g or 170 mL (3.4)[e]
80	1,200	80 g or 533 mL (8)[e]	256 g or 366 mL (25.6)[e]	80 g or 533 mL (8)[e]	154 g or 220 mL (15.4)[e]	39 g or 195 mL (3.9)[e]

[a]Calories from the hypocaloric regimen consists of 1 g/kg/day of protein and 15 kcal/kg/day total or approximately 50% to 60% of needs. Hypocaloric regimens that are intended as permissive underfeeding are often intended for patients whose present weight is within 10% of ideal body weight.
[b]Assumes a stock bottle of 15% amino acids at 4.1 kcal/g.
[c]Assumes a stock bottle of 70% hydrated dextrose at 3.4 kcal/g.
[d]Assumes a stock bottle of 20% lipid emulsion at 9 kcal/g and providing approximately 20% of total calories.
[e]Final concentration of nutrient in 1,000 mL of total parenteral nutrition fluid.
From Driscoll DF: Formulation of enteral and parenteral mixtures, in Pichard C, Kudsk KA (eds): *Update in Intensive Care Medicine*. Brussels, Springer-Verlag, 2000, pp 138–150, with permission.

compounded from the standard 10% amino acid (700 mL) and 70% dextrose (300 mL) stock solutions, and is usually given for short periods of up to 10 days. Such a formula offers a compromise of the usual desired protein and caloric goals and may provide for a clinical outcome not distinguishable from higher protein, eucaloric regimens [67]. Tables 191.4 and 191.5 provide examples of PN formulations that may be used in the acute critical care setting in adult patients who are fluid restricted (i.e., 1,000 mL for TPN), whose regimens are often hypocaloric for clinical and practical reasons (see Table 191.4), as well as for goal amounts of nutrients in TPN in the absence of fluid restrictions [68]. A recent analysis of highly concentrated TPN admixtures, using a 16% crystalline amino acid solution containing lipid injectable emulsions in eucaloric amounts, showed them to be stable for up to 30 hours with a net fluid savings of approximately 20% compared with conventional 10% amino acids [69]. Patient-specific PN therapy for pediatric patients (premature, neonate, infant, and adolescent) may be devised using specific practice guidelines [70].

Electrolytes

There are seven key electrolytes that must be monitored and provided as necessary in nutritional admixtures. In some cases, certain electrolytes must be given in *standard* quantities as part of the recommend dietary allowance, while others are given in *variable* amounts and replaced according to the clinical needs of the patient. However, in both cases, the daily requirements can be highly variable especially during acute illness for a variety of reasons, including drug therapy [71,72]. As well, in all cases certain electrolytes may be deliberately omitted because of retention disorders associated with certain disease states. This, of course is more difficult to accomplish with enteral formulas that contain fixed amounts of nutrients and electrolytes. Nevertheless, avoiding the consequences of wide fluctuations in serum electrolyte concentrations that may assume clinical significance in the critical care setting is an important and necessary goal.

TABLE 191.5

EUCALORIC, EUVOLEMIC TOTAL PARENTERAL NUTRITION REGIMENS AS A SINGLE- VERSUS MIXED-FUEL SYSTEM IN INTENSIVE CARE UNIT PATIENTS

Weight (kg)	Total kcal/d[a]	Single-fuel		Mixed-fuel		
		Amino acids[b]	Glucose[c]	Amino acids	Glucose	Lipids[d]
40	1,000	60 g or 400 mL	222 g or 317 mL	60 g or 400 mL	166 g or 237 mL	21 g or 105 mL
50	1,250	75 g or 500 mL	277 g or 396 mL	75 g or 500 mL	208 g or 297 mL	26 g or 130 mL
60	1,500	90 g or 600 mL	333 g or 476 mL	90 g or 600 mL	250 g or 357 mL	31 g or 155 mL
70	1,750	105 g or 700 mL	388 g or 554 mL	105 g or 700 mL	290 g or 414 mL	37 g or 185 mL
80	2,000	120 g or 800 mL	444 g or 634 mL	120 g or 800 mL	333 g or 476 mL	42 g or 210 mL

[a]Calories from the eucaloric and euvolemic regimen consists of 1.5 g/kg/day of protein and 25 mL/kg/day respectively. Eucaloric and euvolemic regimens are in conformance with the ASPEN Guidelines for safe total parenteral nutrition formulations and intended for patients whose present weight is within 10% of ideal body weight.
[b]Assumes a stock bottle of 15% amino acids at 4.1 kcal/g.
[c]Assumes a stock bottle of 70% hydrated dextrose at 3.4 kcal/g.
[d]Assumes a stock bottle of 20% lipid emulsion at 9 kcal/g and providing approximately 25% of total calories.
From Driscoll DF: Formulation of enteral and parenteral mixtures, in Pichard C, Kudsk KA (eds): *Update in Intensive Care Medicine*. Brussels, Springer-Verlag, 2000, pp 138–150, with permission.

Standard Additives

Calcium. Approximately 98% of total body calcium is present in the skeleton. Thus, the extracellular concentration in plasma is but a fraction of total calcium stores and is tightly regulated by parathyroid hormone. As absorption of calcium from the gastrointestinal tract diminishes because of impaired absorption or decreased or absent intake, and serum levels begin to fall, the parathyroid glands sense these changes and secrete parathormone that promotes calcium mobilization from bone to restore normal serum concentrations. However, critical illness disturbs normal calcium homeostasis and mild depressions of total and free calcium concentrations are common [73]. The parenteral equivalent of the recommended dietary allowance (pRDA) for adults is about 25% of the oral recommended dietary allowance (RDA) or 200 mg (10 mEq or 5 mmol) of elemental calcium daily. Higher amounts may be used if needed when seeking to maintain calcium at the lower limit of normal, but this does increase the risk of incompatibility with phosphate salts that could produce fatal pulmonary emboli [74–76]. Therefore, if higher amounts are needed, it may be necessary to use fat emulsion-free formulas that allow greater amounts of calcium and phosphate to be infused safely. The other alternative, separate infusions of calcium should be done with great care especially if given by the peripheral veins, as extravasation injury can be severe [77–79]. In addition, the separate administration of parenteral calcium may be incompatible as a coinfusion with other common infusions applied in the critical care setting such as sodium bicarbonate. Moreover, if parenteral calcium is given intermittently and the same intravenous line is to be used for other medications, it should be flushed with saline or other suitable parenteral fluid (i.e., D_5 W) immediately following termination of the calcium infusion. Parenteral forms of calcium are commercially available in three forms, including the gluconate, acetate, and chloride salts. Of these, the gluconate form is preferred in PN admixtures, as it is least capable of forming insoluble products. However, for immediate delivery of calcium in emergency situations such as severe hypocalcemia, the chloride form is the best form for bioavailability reasons, although it is the most reactive salts with respect to compatibility with nutrient formulas and therefore should not be employed when compounding TPN formulas.

Magnesium. Another predominant intracellular cation, magnesium, plays a pivotal role in calcium metabolism. For parathyroid hormone to be secreted in response to hypocalcemia, magnesium is required [80]. In certain instances, corrections of serum magnesium concentrations have been sufficient to normalize hypocalcemia [81]. Such responses have been viewed as an indication of the extent of magnesium deficiency [82]. Furthermore, similar to calcium, hypomagnesemia is commonly seen in critical illness, and the goal is similar (i.e., to maintain levels at about the lower limit of normal). The pRDA is about 33% of the oral RDA or 120 mg (10 mEq or 5 mmol) for elemental magnesium per day. The only parenteral form of magnesium available is as the sulfate salt.

Phosphorus. Phosphorus is an essential element involved in numerous life-sustaining metabolic processes. For example, if omitted from a PN admixture, a life-threatening hypophosphatemia may ensue within days of initiating therapy. Like magnesium and calcium, it is too predominantly found in the intracellular compartment. However, because its gastrointestinal absorption is highly efficient, the pRDA for phosphorus is the same as its oral RDA at 1,000 mg (30 mmol) daily. The use of milliequivalent units to describe phosphorus concentrations in a solution is often mistakenly applied. At this time, the only parenteral form of phosphorus commercially available in the United States is a mixture of inorganic salts of monobasic ($H_2PO_4^-$) and dibasic (HPO_4^-) phosphate ions. Milliequivalents are defined as the molecular weight (in mg) divided by the valence of a single ion, which is determined by the pH of the final solution. As the pharmaceutical dosage form is a mixture of two ions and has a finite yet variable pH range, the dosage form cannot be accurately described in mEq units. However, because sodium and potassium are the accompanying anions, it has become traditional to order them in terms of mEq units where, for example, 30 mmol of phosphorus is found in about 40 mEq of the commonly available formulations.

Variable Additives

Sodium. Sodium is often prescribed in daily amounts ranging from 60 to 100 mEq each day. However, certain clinical conditions preclude the use of sodium beyond minute quantities (i.e., 0 to 20 mEq per day) such as found with florid congestive heart failure, end-stage liver disease, and during attempts to reduce massive volume overload characterized by extensive third-spacing of fluids by volume restriction and active diuresis. In contrast, patients with severe sodium deficits can require daily amounts that may be as much as three to four times higher than typical quantities given to those without sodium restrictions. There is limited to no impact of sodium amounts on nutritional efficacy. Parenteral forms of sodium are available as chloride, acetate, and phosphate salts.

Potassium. Potassium is often prescribed in daily amounts ranging from 40 to 80 mEq each day. As described earlier, there are extreme clinical conditions that may require either severe restriction or expansion of the daily dose so that ranges of potassium intake may be from 0 to 400 or more mEq per day. For instance, a severe amphotericin-induced renal loss of potassium of 100 mEq per L with a 4 L urine output can be managed by placing an equivalent amount in the parenteral formula so long as close monitoring of potassium in the serum and urine output is provided. In all cases, serum potassium concentrations should be closely monitored, as the safe clinical range is narrow and levels outside may produce severe and even life-threatening cardiovascular complications. Like sodium, parenteral forms of potassium are available as chloride, acetate, and phosphate salts.

Chloride. Chloride salts are widely used in nutrition support. Most often they are provided as sodium and potassium salts and quantitatively constitute the majority of anions present in nutritional formulations. In the past, an emphasis on chloride salts with parenteral crystalline amino acid formulations had tended to produce an iatrogenic metabolic acidosis. However, these formulations have since been revised and balanced with an appropriate amount of acetate ions. Thus, it is not necessary to include the inherent concentrations of chloride and acetate present in amino acid products in the additive calculation for the final PN admixture.

Acetate. Acetate salts are primarily used when clinically indicated for the treatment of metabolic acidemia. They are the only suitable alkalinizing salt for use in nutritional formulations. With respect to alkalinizing power, acetate is equivalent to bicarbonate, but this requires cellular metabolism to be effective. Bicarbonate salts should never be used in PN admixtures as they can form insoluble carbonates with calcium ions that are present in most nutritional admixtures and as such could result in the formation of fatal pulmonary emboli [83].

Trace Minerals

To provide a balanced nutritional formulation, trace minerals are generally included in most nutritional formulations. These include chromium, copper, manganese, selenium, and zinc. In addition, iodine, and molybdenum may also be present in certain formulations. However, for most acute situations, the absence of trace minerals for brief periods (days to weeks) will not produce clinically significant adverse effects. In contrast, the absence of trace minerals in the patient receiving long-term PN support may lead to significant deficiency [84]. However, since manganese is excreted in bile, there is some concern about manganese overload when chronically provided to patients receiving long-term home TPN. Iron is a special case, since hypoferremia is an invariable consequence of the systemic inflammatory response. Furthermore, large amounts of parenteral iron supplementation may worsen septic states. For this reason, iron is not usually provided in TPN formulas during critical illness and when provided to nonseptic patients in home, PN should only be provided when clinically necessary, since iron overload can result in patients with short gut syndromes who have substantial enteral intake. Iron is incompatible in fat emulsion-containing formulas.

Vitamins

Multivitamins are an essential component of all nutritional formulations. This is particularly true for PN formulations. During the national vitamin shortage that occurred in the summer of 1988, three patients died as a result of receiving vitamin-free PN in a matter of 3 to 5 weeks [85]. Ultimately, the cause of death was related to acute thiamine deficiency producing a refractory lactic acidosis. As a water-soluble vitamin, thiamine is an important cofactor in the entry of pyruvate into the Krebs cycle as well as facilitating the processing of glucose within the Krebs cycle. In the absence of thiamine, pyruvate cannot enter the Krebs cycle and is therefore converted to lactic acid. The administration of hypertonic dextrose, the major energy component of PN therapy, accelerates the consumption of thiamine and thus accentuates the clinical course of the condition. Therefore, multivitamins are an essential part of any nutrition support regimen.

The Food and Drug Administration has mandated a change in the composition of adult parenteral multivitamins after nearly 30 years of clinical use [86]. The concentrations of four vitamins (thiamine, pyridoxine, ascorbic acid, and folate) were increased by 50% to 100% of previous amounts and for the first time, vitamin K has been added at 150 mcg per vial. This latter addition may well have some impact on therapeutic doses of warfarin for full anticoagulation as well as for low-dose warfarin therapy for home TPN patients. Lastly, with respect to enteral feeding formulas, the RDA for vitamins is generally met when caloric intakes are between 1,500 to 2,000 kcal per day.

Immunonutrients

There have been a number of nutritional additives that have been alternatively given in supraphysiologic amounts in an effort to improve outcome. The main ones would include lipids composed of high concentrations of the unsaturated long-chain fatty acids (LCFA) containing n3 or n9 fatty acids, medium-chain saturated fatty acids (MCFA), and certain "conditionally essential" amino acids. Historically, soybean oil, containing polyunsaturated fatty acids (PUFAs), rich in the 18-carbon essential (cannot be synthesized endogenously) n6 fatty acid linoleic acid and n3 fatty acid alpha linolenic acid, has been the main source of fat used in lipid injectable emulsions. These fatty acids are the precursors to the true "necessary" fatty acids, arachidonic and eicosapentaenoic acids from the n6 and n3 families, respectively, whereas the n9 fatty acid, oleic acid is nonessential (i.e., can be synthesized endogenously) [87].

Unfortunately, however, the n6 fatty acids from soybean oil can be proinflammatory and potentially detrimental when provided in large amounts to the critically ill, especially in patients with adult respiratory distress syndrome [29,44–45,88–92]. Therefore, substitution of a portion of the conventional n6 fatty acids with alternative lipid fuels such as the n3 fatty acids (20- and 22-carbon PUFAs) from fish oil, or 18-carbon monounsaturated n9 fatty acids from olive oil, or saturated MCFAs from coconut oil (mostly comprises 8- to 10-carbons), may modulate the proinflammatory response. Thus, one benefit of these alternative lipid sources is a reduction in the intake of the highly vasoactive n6 PUFA precursors to ones with less pronounced effects on eicosanoid metabolism by changing the fatty acid composition of cell membranes. The n6 PUFAs produce proinflammatory eicosanoids (i.e., prostaglandins, prostacyclins, thromboxanes, leukotrienes) and increase the responsiveness of cytokines (i.e., interleukin [IL]-1, IL-6, and TNF) which subsequently lead to an increased systemic inflammatory response. Meanwhile, the n3 and n9 lipids lead to eicosanoids that are less proinflammatory and even anti-inflammatory. Another benefit is related to a unique metabolic action of the substituted lipid(s) that may have favorable clinical implications. In the case of MCFAs, their metabolism is independent of carnitine transport into the mitochondria with rapid oxidation and less interference with the reticuloendothelial system (RES), while olive oil may be better tolerated with respect to liver function in certain patients receiving conventional soybean oil–based formulations [93].

Of the amino acids used in clinical nutrition, arginine and glutamine have been shown to exert favorable immune effects in patients receiving nutrition support. Arginine has been shown to stimulate T-cell function and wound healing, but may be harmful in certain patients under certain conditions depending on dose [94,95]. Thus, its role in immune enhancement has not been clearly defined, and it is most often given as part of a complex nutritional formula containing other potential immunonutrients. Nonetheless, there appears to be a correlation of demonstrable benefits at doses exceeding 4% of the total energy intake [95]. Glutamine is the most abundant amino acid in the human body, and it is an important nutrient for rapidly dividing immune cells such as lymphocytes and macrophages. Despite its abundance, serum and tissue glutamine concentrations fall during critical illness, which largely reflects its diverse needs during acute metabolic stress. Its role in clinical nutrition is also not well defined, and in a large clinical trial in ICU patients, no differences in outcomes were noted between groups receiving 20 g per L versus a conventional enteral formula that was isonitrogenous and isocaloric [96]. Data with parenteral glutamine tend to be more positive in the critically ill, which may reflect the prominent first pass clearance of enteral glutamine limiting systemic appearance of the amino acid.

DIFFERENCES BETWEEN ENTERAL AND PARENTERAL NUTRITION

Nutrition support may be provided in a variety of ways ranging from noninvasive approaches such as dietary counseling for food and oral supplements to invasive forms of therapy. Of the interventional approaches to nutrition support, these can be accomplished by aseptic placement of intravascular catheters (i.e., PN), or by extravascular devices placed into the gastrointestinal tract (i.e., EN). Each invasive form of nutrition support has its advantages and disadvantages, and the selection of either approach must be individualized.

Routes of Administration

Enteral Nutrition Options

Like PN therapy, EN can be delivered in a variety of ways with some distinct advantages of one access route over the other. The options include gastric, duodenal, and jejunal placement of various enteral feeding catheters. The simplest technique is the nasogastric placement of a feeding tube into the stomach. However, this approach is often associated with the greatest degree of gastrointestinal intolerance. A higher degree of successful feeding is likely with fluoroscopic, endoscopic, or surgical placement of the feeding catheter beyond the ligament of Treitz. Furthermore, enteral feeding catheters placed in the upper jejunum may even allow feeding in patients with severe pancreatitis [97]. However, placement of feeding tubes in the jejunum postinjury rarely occurs spontaneously and generally requires fluoroscopic or endoscopic assistance, which is expensive and delays feeding.

Parenteral Nutrition Options

PN may be provided by either peripheral or central venous access. Peripheral venous access is clearly less invasive and has minimal complications. The most significant complications are related to maintenance of the patency of the venous catheter and thrombophlebitis and the limited use of each venipuncture site for a relatively short duration. Most peripheral vein catheters will last between 48 to 72 hours from the time of the initial insertion, and therefore a systematic rotation of other infusion sites must be performed. Ultimately, however, the number of viable peripheral venipuncture sites is limited and generally of little practical value in the ICU setting. Moreover, due to the osmolarity limits of these low-flow blood vessels, very large fluid volumes are required to approach protein and energy requirements for most patients, which is not practical in the ICU setting. Peripherally inserted central (venous) catheters (PICCs) generally last longer and can even be used to provide hypertonic PN admixtures. However, the inability to change catheters over guidewires for PICCs for suspected infections, and a greater likelihood of mechanical complications makes this a less desirable alternative to a central venous catheter.

By far, central venous catheterization is most commonly used to deliver PN therapy. Invariably, central venous access is necessary for virtually all patients requiring ICU care, so the delivery of PN therapy does not introduce unique clinical risks associated with catheter placement (i.e., pneumothorax, catheter malposition, catheter infections, and so forth). In addition to supplying nutrition support, the PN admixture can also be used as a vehicle to provide intensive metabolic support such as replacement of large amounts of electrolytes and correction of acid–base balance, which otherwise could not be accomplished by peripheral vein or EN therapy, largely due to osmolarity limitations. Moreover, it has also been used as a vehicle for selected pharmacotherapies, which can also assist in reducing excess fluid intakes associated with multiple diluents (i.e., D_5W, saline, and so forth) used to deliver drugs [98].

Parenteral Versus Enteral Nutrition and Complications

Approximately 15 years ago, there was a significant push toward the use of EN over PN as being a safer mode of nutrient supplementation. The principal benefit purportedly associated with the use of EN is reduced infectious complications compared with PN support in the critically ill. Three key investigations conducted in trauma patients were largely responsible for promoting enteral over PN, showing that patients receiving the latter mode of nutrition support had significantly higher rates of infectious complications [99–101]. In addition, this association appeared to be subsequently confirmed by meta-analysis [102]. However, as eloquently pointed out by Jeejeebhoy [103] in 2001, studies such as these are significantly flawed in that the groups receiving PN have significantly higher energy intakes that are associated with significantly higher blood glucose levels, which predisposes them to nosocomial infections. Higher energy intakes are easily obtainable via PN, whereas they are more difficult to achieve with EN during acute illness due to gastrointestinal intolerance [104].

Subsequently, Simpson and Doig [105] conducted a more sensitive approach to meta-analysis comparing studies of parenteral versus EN only in the critically ill. Previous systematic reviews of the risks and benefits of nutrition support have relied on a composite scales technique that combines certain dimensions of the quality of the selected trial used in the metaanalysis into a combined summary score. Consequently, important differences in methodologic quality (i.e., concealment of allocation, appropriate blinding, and analysis according to the intention-to-treat principle) may be overlooked, making well-conducted studies appear poorly conducted [106]. In contrast, the approach by Simpson and Doig in assessing parenteral versus EN, using the intent-to-treat principle, applied a component scale technique and demonstrated increased infectious complications with PN, but more importantly, reduced mortality by 50% compared with enteral feeding. This impressive benefit was also shown to be largely the effect of early feeding, since a post hoc analysis of TPN versus early enteral feeding showed no difference in mortality [105]. The latter finding was in contradistinction to previous analyses applying the composite scales approach in assessing the benefits and risks of PN [102,107]. Finally, the seminal publication by Van den Berghe et al. [108] in 2001 showed a significant morbidity and mortality benefit in surgical ICU patients receiving adequate nutrition either enterally, parenterally, or by combination when blood glucose levels were aggressively managed with the intravenous infusion of insulin, and the clinical significance of hyperglycemia in nutritional support was clearly established. Two groups of patients were studied ($n = 1{,}548$) to receive either "intensive" or "conventional" insulin therapy concurrent with PN. Blood glucose management assigned to the "intensive" insulin therapy group was treated with an insulin infusion if levels were above 110 mg%, whereas in the "conventional" insulin therapy group, insulin was initiated at levels above 215 mg%. The standard infusion consisted of 50 units of insulin in 50 mL of 0.9% sodium chloride solution (1 U per mL), and the maximum insulin dose was arbitrarily set at 50 U per hour for all groups. Hypoglycemia was defined as a blood glucose determination of 40 mg% or less. Within 24 hours, on average, all patients received approximately 1 g of protein and 19 kcal per kg per 24 hours, respectively. Significant reductions in in-hospital morbidity (e.g., renal and hepatic function, bloodstream infections, polyneuropathy) and mortality were observed in the "intensive" versus "conventional" insulin therapy group, where, for example, control of the morning blood glucose levels for all patients were significantly different between groups (103 ± 33 mg% vs. 153 ± 19 mg%, respectively). Additional significant clinical benefits (e.g., days on ventilator, lower TISS-28 scores) were also noted for those patients with ICU stays exceeding 5 days.

A follow-up study by Van den Berghe et al. [109] in 2006 was conducted, but this time it was performed in medical ICU patients receiving EN. Unfortunately, the nutrition support data were not as clearly presented as in the 2001 study, but inferences are made as to how it was supplied. The nutritional goals stated from the outset was 22 to 30 kcal per kg per 24 hours (with approximately 20% to 40% of energy as fat calories) and protein at between 0.5 to 1.5 g per kg per 24 hours, with EN beginning as early as possible, once the patient was hemodynamically stable. Subsequently, in the results, two figures are shown that give more details about the success of achieving the stated nutritional goals during this study. One depicts the "total intake of nonprotein calories (kcal per 24 hours)" versus "day" showing that by days 3 and 4 of the study a steady amount of calories (between approximately 1,500 to 1,600 calories per day) were achieved over the 14-day profile. The other depicts the "fraction of kilocalories administered by enteral route" versus "day" showing achievement of 50% of total calories via EN at day 7 and roughly 70% by day 12 of the 14-day profile. The slow progression of enteral nutritional support is expected in critically ill patients, as contrasted from their previous PN study showing rapid advancement of protein and calories [108]. No significant improvements in mortality were noted, but morbidity (e.g., acute renal failure, days on ventilator) was reduced for patients receiving "intensive" insulin therapy. Of note, for the patients staying in the ICU for less than 3 days (n = 433) ("and for whom data were censored after randomization") [109], 56 deaths occurred in the "intensive" versus 42 deaths in the "conventional" insulin infusion group. Moreover, although the severity of hypoglycemia was similar between groups, hypoglycemia was more common in the "intensive" insulin treatment group. A subsequent logistic regression analysis revealed hypoglycemia to be an independent risk factor for death, prompting the investigators to speculate "that the benefit from intensive insulin therapy requires time to be realized" [109]. For patients staying 3 days or more, the mortality benefits seen in the previous study [108] were similarly observed and may support their theory of a time-dependent benefit of aggressive blood glucose management. From a nutritional perspective, the slow progression of protein and calories via the enteral route suggests significant caution in applying aggressive insulin therapy in medical ICU patients receiving EN support only, since parenteral glucose may make hypoglycemia less likely.

A closer evaluation of the manuscript and the table provided in a supplemental appendix reveals that rather marginal amounts of protein and adequate calories were given to the "intention-to-treat group (n = 1,200)" at approximately 40 g of protein and 1,200 kcal daily, whereas in the "long-stayers (in ICU 3 days or more)," approximately 50 g of protein and 1,500 kcal daily were given. It is also obvious from this table that the parenteral infusions were glucose only and not TPN, and that the protein intake in the first 72 hours was about 10 g protein per day. Thus, these critically ill patients did not receive early, adequate feeding, which should be the goal in the critically ill. Furthermore, this less than optimal nutritional therapy was provided at a rather high cost in terms of hypoglycemia with an incidence of 25.1% versus 3.9% in the intensive versus conventional treatment in the long stayers in the ICU.

In conclusion, much of the increase in morbidity related to PN and EN is due to hyperglycemia, which can be significantly reduced by intensive insulin therapy. The level of glycemia necessary to accomplish this goal, whether <110 mg per dL or only <150 mg per dL, is not yet defined. Surgical patients being adequately fed may benefit from the lower range, but a recent large study of intensive insulin therapy alone without full feeding in mixed populations of medical and surgical patients have significantly lower mortality with looser control of <180 mg per dL versus tighter control (81–108 mg per dL) [110]. A possible interpretation is that to accomplish early, adequate feeding requires some parenteral feeding in many critically ill patients who also may serve to minimize the risks of hypoglycemia when employing tighter glucose control.

Tolerance

Enteral Nutrition

Tolerance to nutrition support interventions is highly variable and principally depends on the clinical condition of the patient and the mode of administration. In general, critically ill patients are least able to tolerate all forms of nutrition support. This is particularly true with EN and often limits the amount of protein and calories that can be provided, as gastrointestinal intolerance to feeding is common. As well, a number of other factors associated with ICU care can also interfere with its efficacious delivery [111]. The use of specialized formulations that provide elemental forms of the macronutrients, or are of reduced osmolarity, or of low fat content, may reduce the degree of gastrointestinal intolerance. Moreover, the use of antimotility agents will benefit some patients as well. Nevertheless, despite these preventive measures, gastrointestinal intolerance cannot be successfully managed in all patients. Other maneuvers, such as diluting the enteral feeding formula rarely alleviate the problem and generally should not be undertaken. Rather, providing monomeric or oligomeric formulations with reduced fat content at full strength, given at low rates (i.e., 20 mL per hour) and slowly advanced (i.e., 10 mL per hour every 6 to 12 hours as tolerated) will define those patients who will likely succeed with EN. As a general rule, patients who suffer multiple trauma excluding head injury are usually more tolerant of enteral feeding and allow quicker advancement than those critically ill patients who have closed head injury, sepsis, or are postoperative. Consequently, the time course to achieve eucaloric nutrition is usually longer than with PN.

Parenteral Nutrition

In contrast, patients receiving PN will physically tolerate large amounts of nutrients when given by intravenous administration. The "physiologic brake" that obviously limits EN is not readily apparent. Metabolic abnormalities, such as hyperglycemia and electrolyte and acid–base disturbances, can be easily ascribed to the consequences of the metabolic response to injury, rather than recognizing the contribution of overly aggressive PN support. Furthermore, these iatrogenic metabolic abnormalities are often addressed independently from the PN admixture, such as by separate infusions of insulin, fluid, electrolytes, and so forth, without modifying the PN regimen. The net effect of parenteral overfeeding can unnecessarily complicate the critical care of such patients and lead to significant increases in morbidity and even mortality. However, once metabolic homeostasis is achieved, the time course to reach eucaloric nutrition support is usually brief compared with EN therapy.

Fixed Versus Variable Amounts of Nutrients

Enteral Nutrition

There is limited opportunity to manipulate the contents of EN formulations as these products are premade as "complete" commercial products. Of course, they may be modified by the addition of various nutrient modules, but cannot easily be specifically tailored to the patient, especially during acute illness. For example, a number of electrolyte additives may precipitate the complex feeding formulas and cause clogging of the feeding tube. The addition of other components to the enteral formulation increases the osmolarity, which is an important consideration for enteral feeding, as well as increasing the risk of incompatibilities [68]. Thus, the flexibility of enteral therapy is limited, which may make it difficult to achieve the proper balance of nutrients during severe metabolic stress. Once the stress response remits and major organ function improves, this becomes a less pressing concern.

Parenteral Nutrition

Major stability issues associated with PN admixtures preclude the manufacture of ready-to-use commercial products. Of these, the interaction between certain amino acids with dextrose forming oxidized end products, known as the Maillard reaction is generally acknowledged [70]. The use of multicompartment bags offer a possible alternative to these reactions, but as with enteral products, they too become clinically limiting in the unstable patient in the acute care setting. Thus, PN admixtures are most often made extemporaneously from individual commercial ingredients (i.e., amino acids, dextrose, lipids, electrolytes, and so forth) by qualified pharmacy personnel. The introduction of automated compounding devices and their subsequent widespread use has made the practice of patient-specific admixtures a relatively easy task [112]. Thus, even the sickest of ICU patients can receive some form of nutrition support by the prescribing of unique and specifically designed formulations to support the protein synthetic response to injury.

Costs

Enteral Nutrition

Historically, EN formulations have been a fraction of the cost of PN admixtures as they are ready-to-use and largely comprised of polymeric forms of macronutrients. However, with refinements in these products to construct oligomeric or monomeric forms of protein and carbohydrates, the so-called elemental formulas, the costs have increased substantially. Moreover, the addition of novel nutrients, such as omega-3 fatty acids, glutamine, arginine, and others to produce nutritional supplements that may have pharmacologic effects, particularly with respect to immune function, has increased costs that now exceed most PN formulations per kcal. Although the data are promising for these innovative formulations in terms of their potential to reduce length of stay and possibly infectious complications, the full extent of these claims have not been fully substantiated.

Parenteral Nutrition

By historical comparison, PN was always more expensive than EN therapy. There were many good reasons for this [113], considering the product had to be specially compounded under aseptic conditions to be suitable and safe for intravenous administration. As the methods of commercial production improved and became more efficient and competition increased, the costs of PN therapy have significantly declined. Compared with specialized formulas that contain immunonutrients or certain concentrated enteral products, the present costs of PN therapy are equal or in many cases less expensive. In contrast, for conventional, polymeric EN supplements, the cost of the formulations is still substantially less than PN formula costs. However, the placement of an enteral feeding tube and components (pumps, sets, and so forth) are dedicated to the provision of nutrition support, whereas central venous lines are already being used for the provision of intravenous fluids, medications, and blood tests. Therefore, additional costs of even conventional EN therapy must be considered.

Complications

The complications or adverse patient events associated with parenteral and EN include mechanical, septic, and metabolic misadventures [114]. For example, mechanical complications of invasive nutrition support are often associated with the misplacement of various types of feeding access devices (i.e., vascular injury or pneumothorax). With experienced clinicians, the incidence of such complications is substantially reduced and clinically acceptable at about 1% to 2%.

Metabolic and associated septic complications are more common and can have a significant impact on patient outcome. Severe disturbances in fluid, electrolyte, and acid–base homeostasis are commonly associated with high rates of morbidity and mortality in the ICU. This is especially true in patients with significant heart disease [115]. As well, septic complications in association with hyperglycemia and infections in critically ill patients receiving parenteral or EN are at least equally significant, if not even more so [116]. Therefore, a more modest provision of energy intake (i.e., approximately 25 total kcal per kg per day) should be the overall goal of therapy by whatever route of delivery and is most likely to succeed, and with this, fewer nutrition-related complications are likely. However in the first 3 to 7 days of enteral and PN providing at least 50% of the estimated energy requirement along with protein intake of at least 1 g per kg may be a reasonable compromise meeting the definition or early, adequate feeding while lowering the risk of metabolic and infectious complications.

Appropriate Application of Nutrition Support

Nutrition support does not improve outcome in operative patients who are well nourished, no matter what route of administration it is given. A number of examples appear in the medical literature supporting this contention. For example, a randomized clinical trial of perioperative nutrition support only found significant improvement in the malnourished group irrespective of feeding mode [117]. Heslin et al. [118] reported no benefit with enteral tube feeding in patients with gastrointestinal cancer without significant weight loss. In fact, the routine provision of EN in well-nourished patients may cause significant impairments in ventilatory function and mobility [119]. Finally, an extensive review of the literature has corroborated the lack of benefits in the standard prescription of nutrition support in patients who initially are well nourished and undergoing moderate stress as following major thoracoabdominal surgery [120]. There is reasonable support for early and adequate feeding in the most critically stressed even when initially well-nourished such as those with closed head injury, severe multiple trauma, major third degree burns, and severe sepsis, not to prevent the development of malnutrition but presumably to limit the severity of the systemic inflammatory response.

In contrast, invasive feeding in the malnourished patient is likely to be effective in a variety of clinical scenarios. This is particularly true during acute metabolic stress, where ongoing catabolism results in significant daily losses of body protein. Patients with weight loss classified as moderate (i.e., 10% or more) or severe (i.e., 20% or more) from usual or IBW are most susceptible to nutrition-related complications such as infection or wound dehiscence. The absence of nutritional intervention in this vulnerable population for protracted periods of time (i.e., greater than 7 to 10 days) may have a significant impact on outcome. Moreover, even the initially well-nourished patient cannot sustain the protein synthetic response to injury for long periods. For example, in a randomized study of the effects on outcome of postoperative feeding with TPN, those who were inadequately fed for 14 days had a significant increase in morbidity and mortality [121]. Patients who suffer multiple traumas, major burns, or closed head injury are a unique group. Although generally well nourished at the outset, the severity of catabolic response and the likely duration of substantially longer than 7 days make early nutritional intervention within the first few days beneficial.

MONITORING PARAMETERS FOR NUTRITION SUPPORT

Electrolytes

During critical illness, severe electrolyte disorders are common and are primarily the result of various concomitant etiologies, including changes in (a) the function of major organ systems, especially the kidneys; (b) fluid balance affecting intravascular volume and the hormonal milieu produced as a result of the metabolic response to severe stress(es); (c) intra- or extracellular shifts of ions associated with acid–base disturbances; and (d) multiple drug therapies. Renal dysfunction has profound effects on electrolyte balance by influencing the absorption and excretion of most notably, sodium, potassium, magnesium, phosphorus, and titratable acids. As renal function declines, the excretion of these electrolytes decreases and the PN admixture must be adjusted accordingly. For example, in some cases, electrolytes are significantly reduced, while in other circumstances they are entirely omitted from the daily admixture. As well, chloride ions are often substituted with alkalinizing anions such as acetate to combat the metabolic acidosis associated with renal failure.

Fluid overload is a common finding in critically ill patients related to intraoperative support of renal blood flow and function, acute volume resuscitation with crystalloids in the ICU, and the administration of multiple intravenous medications that may produce its own set of complications. For example, acute increases of 10% or greater above usual body weight over short intervals clearly reflect a significant expansion of total body water that may impede the weaning of the patient from mechanical ventilation. Thus, clinical efforts to return to the patient's premorbid weight, such as by aggressive diuretic therapy and concentrating intravenous medications in the least diluent volume possible, are often used. In certain severe circumstances, the use of colloids for acute volume expansion, followed by aggressive diuretic therapy as a "push–pull" method of fostering diuresis is undertaken to achieve a net negative fluid balance. More recently, the use of hemofiltration procedures to accomplish this goal has proven quite effective. Despite "third-spacing" of fluids, the consequences of the antidiuretic and antinatriuretic responses of stress often present as a hyponatremia and can be mistakenly treated by the parenteral administration of sodium salts in an effort to correct the serum sodium concentration. However, given that sodium essentially distributes in total body water, one can easily calculate that, in fact, the patient is both fluid and total body sodium overloaded. Hence, clinical maneuvers to address the problem should be directed at increasing both sodium and free water losses, with gradual restoration of serum sodium concentrations. A clinical example of this estimation appears in Table 191.6.

The acute intra- or extracellular shifting of electrolytes is primarily the result of the effects of changes in acid–base homeostasis and serum insulin concentrations. In the former case, serum potassium concentrations are most affected by changes in acid–base status. Potassium is predominantly an intracellular ion whose concentration in the intracellular compartment is much higher than its extracellular concentration. When arterial pH falls below normal, potassium shifts to the extracellular compartment and hyperkalemia occurs, and conversely, metabolic alkalosis produces hypokalemia.

Insulin also has a profound effect on the shifting of potassium, magnesium, and phosphorus between the intra- and extracellular environments. In fact, the life-threatening refeeding syndrome that occurs in severely malnourished patients is associated with the shifting of these electrolytes from the extracellular to the intracellular compartments [122]. In the atrophic heart muscle characteristic of severe malnutrition (i.e., greater than 30% below ideal body weight), severe reductions of serum potassium (i.e., less than 3 mEq per L) and serum phosphorus (i.e., less than 0.2 mg per L) related to feeding may have life-threatening electrophysiologic consequences [123].

Finally, critically ill patients commonly receive multiple drug therapies intravenously for a variety of clinical reasons and include, for example, cardiovascular agents, vasopressors, diuretics, anesthesia/sedation therapy, crystalloids, colloids, antibiotics, anticoagulants, and so forth. These can cause clinically significant effects by altering intended drug actions (i.e., toxic synergism, reduced drug effects) or by addition of substantial diluent volumes (i.e., greater than 500 mL), worsening a fluid-overloaded state. The clinical care of acutely ill patients with severe fluid and electrolyte disorders can be optimally managed through intensive metabolic monitoring and selective manipulations of PN admixture components [71,72,123].

TABLE 191.6

ESTIMATING TOTAL BODY SODIUM IN THE ACUTE CARE SETTING[a]

Premorbid total body sodium	
Total body water @ 70 kg	= 42 L
Total body sodium	= 42 L × 140 mEq/L
	= **5,880 mEq**
Present total body sodium	
Total body water @ 91 kg	= 42 L + (91 kg − 70 kg)
	= 63 L
Total body sodium	= 63 L × 130 mEq/L
	= **8,190 mEq**
Excess total body sodium	
8,190 − 5,880	= **2,310 mEq**

[a] Assumptions: Premorbid weight = 70 kg male; presently = 91 kg; serum sodium = 140 mEq/L (normal); presently = 130 mEq/L; total body water = 60% (for males).

Insulin and Glucose Homeostasis

Notwithstanding its regulatory role in glucose homeostasis in terms of glucose production and breakdown in the liver, as well as its facilitated transport of glucose into muscle and other obligatory tissues, insulin is a complex hormone that exhibits numerous metabolic effects that may be of significant clinical consequences in critically ill. The mechanisms by which abnormally elevated blood glucose concentrations in critically ill patients produce metabolic dysfunction have been described [124]. With respect to infectious risk, the ability of mononuclear (macrophages and monocytes) and polymorphonuclear neutrophils to exert phagocytic, oxidative bursts, and killing functions is significantly impaired. Thus, infections of the bloodstream, lungs, and superficial wounds (i.e., any surgical incision site, intra-, and extravascular catheter sites, or other topical sites of injury) are significantly increased following periods of hyperglycemia.

Glucose homeostasis is best achieved when parenteral insulin is given in an effective manner. A review of the methods of administration employed emphasize that the route of insulin delivery should be commensurate with the means of administration of carbohydrate calories [125]. In the acute phases of critical illness, patients receiving PN should receive intensive insulin therapy [108]. Once, stabilized (i.e., patients receiving the largest source of glucose as parenteral calories), insulin should be given in the TPN admixture in amounts sufficient to cover the caloric intake from this source over 24 hours. When exclusive PN therapy is given, 24-hour glucose intake may account for as much as 150 to 300 g per L daily (510 to 1,020 kcal), requiring substantial amounts of insulin in the admixture, and can be effectively accomplished [125]. As well, in some cases supplemental "low-volume, full-strength" EN may provide 50 to 150 g per 24 hours (170 to 510 kcal), which should be managed with subcutaneous insulin provided based on blood glucose determinations taken on a regular basis and algorithm-based insulin doses.It should be emphasized that, the insulin should be administered subcutaneously as an intravenous dose has a serum half-life of approximately 5 to 7 minutes. The same principles may be applied to patients receiving substantial amounts of glucose in the peritoneal dialytic regimens, where insulin is often best provided in the dialysis solution. Thus, in some cases, such as a patient undergoing both peritoneal dialysis and PN or EN, insulin is given via multiple routes to cover the administration of glucose from various sources to link the insulin administration to the source of exogenous glucose. When hyperglycemia is severe due to severity of the stress response or severity of insulin deficiency (type 1) or insulin resistance (type 2), it is reasonable to employ continuous intravenous insulin and close blood glucose monitoring to quickly establish glucose homeostasis, whatever the source of exogenous glucose.

Goals of Nitrogen Balance

Achieving positive nitrogen balance is an unrealistic goal in the critically ill early in the clinical course. Rather, the principal aim of nutritional intervention is to support the protein synthetic response to injury and, therefore, narrow the negative nitrogen gap (where output exceeds input) that occurs during severe metabolic stress. Even when the metabolic stress has subsided, it should be recognized that nutritional rehabilitation of the moderate to severe malnourished patient occurs at a limited rate equivalent to approximately 1 kg of body weight per week and generally much of this repletion will occur outside the hospital after discharge. This estimation is based on a maximum rate of repletion of a positive nitrogen balance (i.e., approximately +5 g per day) that represents 150 g of lean tissue (hydrated protein) and a calorically equivalent amount of fat (13 g) per day. Weight increases above this rate of repletion can only reflect increases in total body water.

Finally, it should be mentioned that when expending the effort to obtain a 24-hour urine collection, additional laboratory measurements should be performed on this specimen such as for the determination of creatinine excretion and certain electrolytes (sodium, potassium, chloride). In this way, important additional clinical information may be provided including creatinine clearance, urea clearance, fractional excretion of sodium, and quantification of electrolyte losses, among other possible data that may be used in the clinical and nutritional/metabolic care of critically ill patients.

EVIDENCE-BASED GUIDELINES FOR NUTRITION SUPPORT THERAPY

In 2009, the Society of Critical Care Medicine (SCCM) and the American Society for Parenteral and Enteral Nutrition (ASPEN) developed and copublished "Guidelines for the Provision and Assessment of Nutrition Support Therapy in the Adult Critically Ill Patient" [126,127]. The last statement of the introduction of this document is noteworthy: "*Delivering early nutrition support therapy, primarily using the enteral route, is seen as a proactive therapeutic strategy that may reduce disease severity, diminish complications, decrease length of stay in the ICU, and favorably impact patient outcome.*" Of the 12 categories or conditions (sections A through L), nine sections related to EN, two sections on PN, and one section (L) relating to end-of-life situations. It is the authors' opinion that this document is unfortunately biased against the potential utility of PN in many circumstances. The assessment system applied in the guidelines consisted of "Levels of Evidence" and "Grades of Recommendation." "Levels of Evidence" were from I to V, with "Level I" being the strongest evidence and "Level V" being the weakest evidence. The "Grades of Recommendation" were from A to E, with "A" being the highest and "E" being the lowest. If, for example, one scores the grades according to a quality point average (QPA) as applied in education with $A = 4.0, B = 3.0 \ldots E = 0.0$, the evidence is poor for both EN and PN. For example, in the SCCM/ASPEN 2009 guidelines, the QPA for all EN sections was 1.21 and the QPA for all PN sections was 1.25. We selected three controversial statements in the guideline:

A3. "EN is the preferred route of feeding over parenteral nutrition (PN) for the critically ill patient who requires nutrition support therapy. Grade B"

The statement is correct, and fits Dr. Dudrick's original thesis "if the guts works, use it," but the principal rationale for its preference, that is, reduced infectious morbidity is misidentified. Although previous studies have shown this association to be true, the premise overlooks the importance of blood glucose control and caloric intake in these studies. Invariably, the PN group in many of the supporting studies received significantly more calories than the EN group and consequently, had higher blood glucose values that clearly increase infectious complications. This is not surprising since EN is often not well tolerated in eucaloric amounts as PN, and is frequently interrupted for various clinical maneuvers or diagnostic tests in the critical care setting. As well, the insulin required to maintain glucose homeostasis is greater for parenteral compared to enteral glucose. Furthermore, the data supporting this statement was essentially derived before the subsequent eras of reduced energy provision and tight glucose control in the critically ill.

G1. "If the patient is deemed to be a candidate for PN, steps to maximize efficacy (regarding dose, content, monitoring, and choice of additives) should be used. Grade C"

In accordance with the thesis of "do no harm," it would seem intuitively obvious that the safety and efficacy of PN would be accomplished by optimizing the formulation. A "Grade C" recommendation diminishes the importance of dosing nutrients, which unfortunately, is associated with a long history of overfeeding and its attendant complications. In the same section (G6), the use of extemporaneously prepared parenteral glutamine is given the same "Grade C," despite the fact that such an additive is classified as a "HIGH RISK" compounded sterile preparation by the United States Pharmacopeia [20].

H3. "Serum phosphate levels should be monitored closely and replaced appropriately when needed. Grade E"

The literature is replete with data on the importance of serum phosphate levels is the critically ill, especially with respect to the risks associated with hypophosphatemia on myocardial performance and respiratory function [128]. Moreover, the provision of hypertonic glucose in a PN admixture produces a supraphysiologic increase in serum insulin levels that will cause significant intracellular shifts that may produce life-threatening hypophosphatemia in susceptible patients. A "Grade E" recommendation is inappropriate in this circumstance. Also in 2009, the European Society of Parenteral and Enteral Nutrition (ESPEN) produced "Guidelines on Parenteral Nutrition: Intensive Care" [129]. Seventeen statements (categories or conditions) are included and there are three Grades of Recommendation (A, B, C) with the strongest evidence being "Grade A" versus the weakest evidence with a "Grade C." Only two statements received "Grade A." We selected three controversial statements in this guideline.

Under "Requirements"

> "During acute illness, the aim should be to provide energy as close as possible to the measured energy expenditure in order to decrease negative energy balance. Grade B"

In the ICU setting, particularly during the early phases of critical illness, hypocaloric regimens often seem to be most prudent. Maintenance of normal blood glucose values should take precedence over energy balance in most critical care settings, and then once achieved, judicious increases in calories can commence.

> "In the absence of indirect calorimetry, ICU patients should receive 25 kcal/kg/day increasing to target over the next 2–3 days. Grade C"

As already stated, caloric intakes in the ICU should be advanced slowly after the initial provision of 50% of energy and 1.0 to 1.2 g protein per kg to avoid hyperglycemia and infectious morbidity. As stated earlier, for most patients, providing 25 kcal per kg per day is sufficient to support the protein synthetic response to metabolic stress. The guideline, as stated, implies that 25 kcal per kg per day is the starting point, when in fact, for most adult patients, it is the target range [130], and is gradually reached after initiating lesser amounts of calories from the outset.

Under "Amino Acids"

> "When PN is indicated in ICU patients the amino acid solution should contain 0.2–0.4 g/kg/day of L-glutamine (e.g., 0.3–0.6 g/kg/day alanyl-glutamine dipeptide). Grade A"

Although there is a commercial product in Europe that is available to provide glutamine supplementation, a recommendation of Grade A seems to be overly optimistic. This is especially true given the recent assessment of L-glutamine in the ICU of an "area of uncertainty" from one of the leading investigators in the field [130]. Thus, such a recommendation seems premature at this time.

At this time, the data is unclear for several reasons. First, the guidelines and methods of assessment must be standardized between organizations. Second, "mining of data" from past studies, many of which are significantly flawed with respect to design and endpoints, cannot yield meaningful guidelines, despite the use of statistical tools, such as meta-analyses. Third, critically ill patients are not homogenous. As recently pointed out, EN is contraindicated in 10% to 15% of ICU patients; there are very few well-designed, randomized controlled studies of PN efficacy, and preexisting malnutrition, combined with numerous pathophysiologic factors in ICU patients which greatly complicate the role of nutrition support [130].

Thus, it seems that to definitively address the evidence for nutrition support therapy in the ICU setting will require designing better studies in the future rather than the current methods to rehash old data from a previous era using statistical tools. A major emphasis should clearly be on the design (randomized controlled trial, sufficient power, APACHE score, etc.) and specific endpoints for future studies to answer the question of the impact of nutritional therapy in the critically ill on morbidity and mortality and clinical outcome. For example, multicenter studies should focus on the potential role of early (within 72 hours of ICU admission) and adequate energy (>50%, but <110% of energy requirements) and protein (at least 1.2 g per kg per day) by whatever means necessary (enteral, parenteral, or both). Only then can we have a true understanding of the role of nutrition support therapy in the critically ill.

CONCLUSIONS

Nutritional and metabolic support is an essential component of the clinical care of critically ill patients. However, if applied in an overly aggressive manner without thought to the nutritional status, amounts of nutrients, route of administration, and the clinical condition of the patient, significant iatrogenic complications may occur and little clinical benefit can be expected. Thus, nutritional support of the critically ill must be carefully integrated into the overall clinical care of the patient, with specific and measurable outcome measures in order to obtain the maximum benefits of this important therapy.

References

1. Driscoll DF, Bistrian BR: Special considerations required for the formulation and administration of total parenteral nutrition in the older patient. *Drugs Aging* 2:395–405, 1992.
2. Bistrian BR, Blackburn GL, Hallowell E, et al: Protein nutritional status of general surgical patients. *JAMA* 230:858–860, 1974.
3. Bistrian BR, Blackburn GL, Vitale J, et al: Prevalence of malnutrition in general medical patients. *JAMA* 235:1567–1570, 1976.
4. Reilly JJ, Hull SF, Albert N, et al: Economic impact of malnutrition: a model system for hospitalized patients. *J Parenter Enteral Nutr* 12:371–376, 1988.
5. McWhirter JP, Pennington CR: Incidence and recognition of malnutrition in hospital. *BMJ* 308:945–948, 1994.
6. Shahar A, Feiglin L, Sharar DR, et al: High prevalence and impact of subnormal serum vitamin B_{12} levels in Israeli elders admitted to a geriatric hospital. *J Nutr Health Aging* 5:124–127, 2001.
7. Kyle UG, Genton L, Pichard C: Hospital length of stay and nutritional status. *Curr Opin Clin Nutr Metab Care* 8:397–402, 2005.
8. Singh H, Watt K, Veitch R, et al: Malnutrition is prevalent in hospitalized medical patients: are housestaff identifying the malnourished patient? *Nutrition* 22:350–354, 2006.
9. Kuzu MA, Terzioglu H, Genc V, et al: Preoperative nutritional risk assessment in predicting postoperative outcome in patients undergoing major surgery. *World J Surg* 30:378–390, 2006.
10. Bistrian BR: A simple technique to estimate severity of stress. *Surg Gynecol Obstet* 148:675–678, 1979.
11. Driscoll DF, Blackburn GL: Total parenteral nutrition 1990: a review of its current status in hospitalized patients. The need for patient-specific feeding. *Drugs* 40:346–363, 1990.
12. Leiter LA, Marliss EB: Survival during fasting may depend on fat as well as protein stores. *JAMA* 248:2306–2307, 1982.
13. Ahmad A, Duerksen DR, Munroe S, et al: An evaluation of resting energy expenditure in hospitalized, severely underweight patients. *Nutrition* 15:384–388, 1999.
14. Henry CJ: Body mass index and the limits of human survival. *Eur J Clin Nutr* 44:329–335, 1990.
15. Bartlett RH, Dechert RE, Mault JR, et al: Measurement of metabolism in multiple organ failure. *Surgery* 92:771–779, 1982.
16. Rubinson L, Diette GB, Song X, et al: Low caloric intake is associated with nosocomial blood stream infections in patients in the medical intensive care unit. *Crit Care Med* 32:350–357, 2004.
17. Shaw JHF, Widmore M, Wolfe RR: Whole body protein kinetics in severely septic patients: the response to glucose infusion in total parenteral nutrition. *Ann Surg* 205:66–72, 1987.
18. Shaw JHF, Wolfe RR: Whole body protein kinetics in patients with early and advanced gastrointestinal cancer: the response to glucose infusion and total parenteral nutrition. *Surgery* 103:148–155, 1988.

19. Lamiell JJ, Ducey JP, Freese-Kepczyk BJ, et al: Essential amino acid-induced hyperammonemic encephalopathy and hypophosphatemia. *Crit Care Med* 18:451–452, 1990.
20. *Pharmaceutical Compounding—Sterile Preparations. Physical Tests.* United States Pharmacopeia 34/National Formulary 29. Rockville, MD, United States Pharmacopeia Convention, Inc, 2011, pp. 336–373.
21. Bistrian BR: Hyperglycemia and infection: which is the chicken and which is the egg? [Editorial]. *J Parenter Enteral Nutr* 25:180–181, 2001.
22. Cahill GF: Starvation in man. *N Engl J Med* 282:668–675, 1970.
23. Wolfe RR: Carbohydrate metabolism in critically ill patients. *Crit Care Clin* 3:11–24, 1987.
24. Douglas RG, Shaw JHF: Metabolic response to trauma and sepsis. *Br J Surg* 76:115–122, 1989.
25. Driscoll DF: Clinical issues regarding the use of total nutrient admixtures. *Ann Pharmacother* 24:296–303, 1990.
26. Seidner DL, Mascioli EA, Istfan NW, et al: Effects of long-chain triglyceride emulsions on reticuloendothelial system function in humans. *J Parenter Enteral Nutr* 13:614–619, 1989.
27. Jensen GL, Mascioli EA, Seidner DL, et al: Parenteral infusion of long and medium-chain triglycerides and reticuloendothelial system function in man. *J Parenter Enteral Nutr* 14:467–471, 1990.
28. Hwang D: Essential fatty acids and the immune response. *FASEB J* 3:2052–2061, 1989.
29. Mathru M, Dries DJ, Zecca A, et al: Effect of fast vs. slow intralipid infusion on gas exchange, pulmonary hemodynamics, and prostaglandins metabolism. *Chest* 99:426–429, 1991.
30. Abbott WC, Grakauskas AM, Bistrian BR, et al: Metabolic and respiratory effects of continuous and discontinuous lipid infusions. *Arch Surg* 119:1367–1371, 1984.
31. Belin RP, Bivins BA, Jona JZ, et al: Fat overload with a 10% soybean oil emulsion. *Arch Surg* 111:1391–1393, 1976.
32. Periera GR, Fox WW, Stanley CA, et al: Decreased oxygenation and hyperlipemia during intravenous fat infusions in premature infants. *Pediatrics* 66:26–30, 1980.
33. Heyman MB, Storch S, Ament ME: The fat overload syndrome. Report of a case and literature. *Am J Dis Child* 135:628–630, 1981.
34. Haber LM, Hawkin EP, Seilheimer DK, et al: Fat overload syndrome. An autopsy study with evaluation of the coagulopathy. *Am J Clin Pathol* 90:223–227, 1988.
35. Puntis JW, Rushton DI: Pulmonary intravascular lipid in neonatal necropsy specimens. *Arch Dis Child* 66:26–28, 1991.
36. Schulz PE, Weiner SP, Haber LM, et al: Neurological complications from fat emulsion therapy. *Ann Neurol* 35:628–630, 1994.
37. Toce SS, Keenan WJ: Lipid intolerance in newborns is associated with hepatic dysfunction but not infection. *Arch Pediatr Adolesc Med* 149:1249–1253, 1995.
38. Jasnosz KM, Pickeral JJ, Graner S: Fat deposits in the placenta following maternal total parenteral nutrition with intravenous lipid emulsion. *Arch Pathol Lab Med* 119:555–557, 1995.
39. Gohlke BC, Fahnenstich H, Kowalewski S: Serum lipids during parenteral nutrition with a 10% lipid emulsion with reduced phospholipid emulsifier content in premature infants. *J Pediatr Endocrinol Metab* 10:505–509, 1997.
40. Colomb V, Jobert-Giraud A, Lacaille F, et al: Role of lipid emulsions in cholestasis associated with long-term parenteral nutrition in children. *J Parenter Enteral Nutr* 24:345–350, 2000.
41. Kadowitz PJ, Spannhake EW, Levin JL, et al: Differential effects of prostaglandins on the pulmonary vascular bed. *Prostaglandin Thromboxane Res* 7:731–744, 1980.
42. Driscoll DF, Bistrian BR, Demmelmair H, et al: Pharmaceutical and clinical aspects of lipid emulsions in neonatology. *Clin Nutr* 27:495–503, 2008.
43. Hwang TL, Huang SL, Chen MF: Effects of intravenous fat emulsion on respiratory failure. *Chest* 97:934–938, 1990.
44. Smyrniotis VE, Kostopanagiotou GG, Arkadopoulos NF, et al: Long-chain versus medium-chain lipids in acute pancreatitis complicated by acute respiratory distress syndrome: effects on pulmonary hemodynamics and gas exchange. *Clin Nutr* 20:139–143, 2001.
45. Suchner U, Katz DP, Furst P, et al: Effects of intravenous fat emulsions on lung function in patients with acute respiratory distress syndrome or sepsis. *Crit Care Med* 29:1569–1574, 2001.
46. Venus B, Prager R, Patel CB, et al: Hemodynamic and gas exchange alterations during Intralipid infusion in patients with adult respiratory distress syndrome. *Chest* 95:1278–1281, 1989.
47. Skeie B, Askanazi J, Rothkopf MM, et al: Intravenous fat emulsions and lung function: a review. *Crit Care Med* 16:183–194, 1988.
48. Hulman G: The pathogenesis of fat embolism. *J Pathol* 176:3–9, 1995.
49. Klein S, Miles JM: Metabolic effects of long-chain and medium-chain triglycerides in humans. *J Parenter Enteral Nutr* 18:396–397, 1994.
50. Sacks GS, Driscoll DF: Does lipid hang time make a difference? Time is of the essence. *Nutr Clin Pract* 2002;17:284–290.
51. *Globule Size Distribution in Lipid Injectable Emulsions. Physical Tests.* United States Pharmacopeia 32/National Formulary 27. Rockville, MD, United States Pharmacopeia Convention, Inc, 2009, pp 283–285.
52. Driscoll DF: Lipid injectable emulsions: Pharmacopeial and safety issues. *Pharm Res* 23:1959–1969, 2006.
53. *Globule Size Distribution in Lipid Injectable Emulsions. Pharm Forum* 30:2235–2240, 2004.
54. Driscoll DF: The pharmacopeial evolution of Intralipid injectable emulsions in plastic containers: From a coarse to a fine dispersion. *Int J Pharm* 368:193–198, 2009.
55. Driscoll DF, Ling PR, Bistrian BR: Physical stability of 20% lipid injectable emulsions via simulated syringe infusion: Effects of glass vs. plastic product packaging. *J Parenter Enteral Nutr* 31:148–153, 2007.
56. Driscoll DF, Silvestri AP, Mikrut BA, et al: Stability of adult-based Total nutrient admixtures with soybean oil-based lipid injectable emulsions: The effect of glass versus plastic packaging. *Am J Health-Syst Pharm* 64:396–403, 2007.
57. Driscoll DF, Thoma A, Franke R, et al: Fine vs. Coarse All-In-One (AIOs) as 3-chamber plastic (3-C-P) bags over 48 hours. *Am J Health-Syst Pharm* 66:649–656, 2009.
58. Martin CR, Dumas GJ, Zheng Z, et al: Incidence of hypertriglyceridemia in critically ill neonates receiving lipid injectable emulsions in glass vs. plastic containers: A retrospective analysis. *J Pediatr* 152:232–236, 2008.
59. Driscoll DF, Ling PR, Silvestri AP, et al: Fine vs. coarse total nutrient admixture infusions over 96 hours in rats: Fat globule size and hepatic function. *Clin Nutr* 27:889–894, 2008.
60. Driscoll DF, Ling PR, Andersson C, et al: Hepatic indicators of oxidative stress and tissue damage accompanied by systemic inflammation in rats following a 24-hour infusion of an unstable lipid emulsion admixture. *J Parenter Enteral Nutr* 33:327–335, 2009.
61. Driscoll DF, Adolph M, Bistrian BR: Lipid emulsions in parenteral nutrition, in Rombeau JL, Rolandelli R (eds): *Parenteral Nutrition*. Philadelphia, PA, WB Saunders, 2001, pp 35–59.
62. Driscoll DF: Lipid injectable emulsions: 2006. *Nutr Clin Pract* 21:381–386, 2006.
63. Simmons RS, Berdine GG, Seidenfeld JJ, et al: Fluid balance and adult respiratory distress syndrome. *Am Rev Respir Dis* 135:924–929, 1987.
64. Lowell JA, Schifferdecker C, Driscoll DF, et al: Postoperative fluid overload: not a benign problem. *Crit Care Med* 18:728–733, 1990.
65. Nahtomi-Shick O, Kostuik JP, Winters BD, et al: Does intraoperative fluid management in spine surgery predict intensive care unit length of stay? *J Clin Anesth* 13:208–212, 2001.
66. Echenique MM, Bistrian BR, Blackburn GL: Theory and techniques of nutritional support in the ICU. *Crit Care Med* 10:546–559, 1982.
67. McCowen KC, Friel C, Sternberg J, et al: Hypocaloric total parenteral nutrition: effectiveness in prevention of hyperglycemia and infectious complications. *Crit Care Med* 28:3606–3611, 2000.
68. Driscoll DF: Formulation of enteral and parenteral mixtures, in Pichard C, Kudsk KA (eds): *Update in Intensive Care Medicine*. Brussels, Springer-Verlag, 2000, pp 138–150.
69. Driscoll DF, Silvestri AP, Nehne J, et al: The physicochemical stability of highly concentrated total nutrient admixtures (TNAs) intended for fluid-restricted patients. *Am J Health Syst Pharm* 63:79–85, 2006.
70. National Advisory Group on Standards and Practice Guidelines for Parenteral Nutrition: Safe practices for parenteral nutrition formulations. *J Parenter Enteral Nutr* 22:49–66, 1998.
71. Driscoll DF: Drug-induced metabolic disorders and parenteral nutrition in the intensive care unit: a pharmaceutical and metabolic perspective. *Ann Pharmacother* 23:363–371, 1989.
72. Driscoll DF: Drug-induced electrolyte disorders in a patient receiving parenteral nutrition [Editorial]. *J Parenter Enteral Nutr* 24:174–175, 2000.
73. Zivin JR, Gooley T, Zager RA, et al: Hypocalcemia: a pervasive metabolic abnormality in the critically ill. *Am J Kidney Dis* 37:689–698, 2001.
74. Flurkey H: A case presentation: precipitate in the central venous line: what went wrong? *Neonatal Netw* 13:51–55, 1994.
75. Hill SE, Heldman LS, Goo EDH, et al: Fatal microvascular pulmonary emboli from precipitation of a total nutrient admixture solution. *J Parenter Enteral Nutr* 20:81–87, 1996.
76. Shay DK, Fann LM, Jarvis WR: Respiratory distress and sudden death associated with receipt of a peripheral parenteral nutrition admixture. *Infect Control Hosp Epidemiol* 18:814–817, 1997.
77. Yoscowitz P, Ekland DA, Shaw RC, et al: Peripheral intravenous infiltration necrosis. *Ann Surg* 182:553–556, 1975.
78. Goldminz D, Barnhill R, McGuire J, et al: Calcinosis cutis following extravasation of calcium chloride. *Arch Dermatol* 124:922–925, 1988.
79. Kagen MH, Bansal MG, Grossman M: Calcinosis cutis following the administration of intravenous calcium therapy. *Cutis* 65:193–194, 2006.
80. Anast CS, Mohs JM, Kaplan SL, et al: Evidence for parathyroid failure in magnesium deficiency. *Science* 177:606–607, 1972.
81. Hermans C, Lefebvre C, Devogelaer JP, et al: Hypocalcemia and chronic alcohol intoxication: transient hypoparathyroidism secondary to magnesium deficiency. *Clin Rheumatol* 15:193–196, 1996.
82. Rude RK, Oldham SB, Sharp CF Jr, et al: Parathyroid hormone secretion in magnesium deficiency. *J Clin Endocrin Metab* 47:800–806, 1978.
83. Food and Drug Administration: Safety alert: hazards of precipitation associated with parenteral nutrition. *Am J Hosp Pharmacol* 51:1427–1428, 1994.
84. Baptista RJ, Bistrian BR, Blackburn GL, et al: Utilizing selenious acid to reverse selenium deficiency in total parenteral nutrition patients. *Am J Clin Nutr* 39:816–820, 1984.

85. Anonymous: Deaths associated with thiamine-deficient total parenteral nutrition. *Morb Mortal Wkly Rep* 38:43–46, 1989.
86. Food and Drug Administration: Parenteral multivitamin products; drugs for human use; drug efficacy implementation; amendment. *Fed Regist* 65:21200–21201, 2000.
87. Bistrian BR: Clinical aspects of essential fatty acid metabolism: Jonathan Rhoads lecture. *J Parenter Enteral Nutr* 27:168–175, 2003.
88. Masclans JR, Iglesia R, Bermejo B, et al: Gas exchange and pulmonary haemodynamic responses to fat emulsions in acute respiratory distress syndrome. *Intensive Care Med* 24:918–923, 1998.
89. Moore FA: Caution: use fat emulsions judiciously in intensive care patients. *Crit Care Med* 29:1569–1574, 2001.
90. Suchner U, Katz DP, Furst P, et al: Impact of sepsis, lung injury, and the role of lipid infusion on circulating prostacyclin and thromboxane A(2). *Intensive Care Med* 28:122–129, 2002.
91. Faucher M, Bregeon F, Gainnier M, et al: Cardiopulmonary effects of lipid emulsions in patients with ARDS. *Chest* 124:285–291, 2003.
92. Lekka ME, Liokatis S, Nathanail C, et al: The impact of intravenous fat emulsion administration in acute lung injury. *Am J Respir Crit Care Med* 169:638–644, 2004.
93. Reimund JM, Arondel Y, Joly F, et al: Potential usefulness of olive oil-based lipid emulsions in selected situations of home parenteral nutrition-associated liver disease. *Clin Nutr* 23:1418–1425, 2004.
94. Grimble RF: Immunonutrition. *Curr Opin Gastroenterol* 21:216–222, 2005.
95. Bistrian BR, McCowen KC: Nutritional and metabolic support in the adult intensive care unit: key controversies. *Crit Care Med* 34:1525–1531, 2006.
96. Hall JC, Dobb G, Hall J, et al: A prospective randomized trial of enteral glutamine in critical illness. *Intensive Care Med* 29:1710–1716, 2003.
97. Fushiki T, Iwai K: Two hypotheses on the feedback regulation of pancreatic enzyme stimulation. *FASEB J* 3:121-128, 1989.
98. Driscoll DF, Baptista RJ, Mitrano FP, et al: Parenteral nutrient admixtures as drug vehicles: theory and practice in the critical care setting. *Ann Pharmacother* 25:276–283, 1991.
99. Moore FA, Moore EE, Jones TN, et al: TEN versus TPN following major abdominal trauma-reduced septic morbidity. *J Trauma* 29:916–923, 1989.
100. Kudsk KA, Croce MA, Fabian TC, et al: Enteral versus parenteral feeding. *Ann Surg* 215:503–513, 1992.
101. Moore F, Feliciano D, Andrassy R, et al: Early enteral feeding compared with parenteral, reduces postoperative septic complications. *Ann Surg* 216:172–183, 1992.
102. Heyland D: Parenteral nutrition in the critically-ill patient: more harm than good? *Proc Nutr Soc* 59:457–466, 2000.
103. Jeejeebhoy KN: Total parenteral nutrition: potion or poison? *Am J Clin Nutr* 74:160–163, 2001.
104. Bistrian BR: Update on total parenteral nutrition [Editorial]. *Am J Clin Nutr* 74:153–154, 2001.
105. Simpson F, Doig GS: Parenteral versus enteral nutrition in the critically ill: a meta-analysis of trials using the intent to treat principle. *Intensive Care Med* 31:12–23, 2005.
106. Huwiler-Muntener K, Juni P, Junker C, et al: Quality of reporting of randomized trials as a measure of methodologic quality. *JAMA* 287:2801–2804, 2002.
107. Heyland DK, MacDonald S, Keefe L, et al: Total parenteral nutrition in the critically ill patient: a meta-analysis. *JAMA* 280:2013–2019, 1998.
108. Van den Berghe G, Wouters P, Weekers F, et al: Intensive insulin therapy in critically ill patients. *N Engl J Med* 345:139–167, 2001.
109. Van den Berghe G, Wilmer A, Hermans G, et al: Intensive insulin therapy in medical ICU. *N Engl J Med* 354:449–461, 2006.
110. The NICE-SUGAR Study Investigators: Intensive versus conventional glucose control in critically ill patients. *N Engl J Med* 360:1283–1297, 2009.
111. McClave SA, Sexton LA, Spain DA, et al: Enteral tube feeding in the intensive care unit: factors impeding adequate delivery. *Crit Care Med* 27:1252–1256, 1999.
112. Driscoll DF, Sanborn MD, Giampietro K: ASHP guidelines on the safe use of automated compounding devices for the preparation of parenteral nutrition admixtures. *Am J Health Syst Pharm* 57:1343–1348, 2000.
113. Anonymous: Follow-up on septicemias associated with contaminated Abbott intravenous fluids. *Morb Mortal Wkly Rep* 20:91–92, 1971.
114. Nehme AE: Nutrition support of the hospitalized patient: the team concept. *JAMA* 243:1906–1908, 1980.
115. Cohen MC, Driscoll DF, Bistrian BR: Parenteral nutrition in patients with cardiac diseases, in Rombeau JL, Caldwell MD (eds): *Parenteral Nutrition*. Philadelphia, PA, WB Saunders, 1993, pp 617–630.
116. Khaodhiar L, McCowen K, Bistrian BR: Perioperative hyperglycemia, infection or risk? *Curr Opin Clin Nutr Metab Care* 7:79–82, 1999.
117. Von Meyenfeldt M, Meijerink W, Rouflart M, et al: Perioperative nutritional support: a randomized clinical trial. *Clin Nutr* 11:180–186, 1992.
118. Heslin M, Lattany L, Leung D, et al: A prospective randomized trial of early enteral feeding after resection of upper gastrointestinal malignancies. *Ann Surg* 226:567–577, 1997.
119. Watters J, Krikpatrick S, Norris S, et al: Immediate postoperative enteral feeding results in impaired respiratory mechanics and decreased mobility. *Ann Surg* 226:369–377, 1997.
120. Klein S, Kinney J, Jeejeebhoy KN, et al: Nutrition support in clinical practice: review of published data and recommendations for future research directions. *Am J Clin Nutr* 66:683–706, 1997.
121. Sandstrom R, Drott C, Hyltander A, et al: The effect of postoperative intravenous feeding (TPN) on outcome following major surgery evaluated in a randomized study. *Ann Surg* 217:185–195, 1993.
122. Apovian C, McMahon MM, Bistrian BR: Guidelines for refeeding the marasmic patient. *Crit Care Med* 18:1030–1033, 1990.
123. Matarese LE, Speerhas R, Seidner DL, et al: Foscarnet-induced electrolyte abnormalities in a bone marrow transplant patient receiving parenteral nutrition. *J Parenter Enteral Nutr* 24:170–173, 2000.
124. Van den Berghe G, Wouters PJ, Bouillon R, et al: Outcome benefit of intensive insulin therapy in the critically ill: insulin dose versus glycemic control. *Crit Care Med* 31:359–366, 2003.
125. McMahon MM, Manji N, Driscoll DF, et al: Parenteral nutrition in patients with diabetes mellitus. Theoretical and practical considerations. *J Parenter Enteral Nutr* 13:545–553, 1989.
126. Martindale RG, McClave SA, Vanek VW, et al: Guidelines for the provision and assessment of nutrition support therapy in the adult critically ill patient. *Crit Care Med* 37:2679–2709, 2009.
127. McClave SA, Martindale RG, Vanek VW, et al: Guidelines for the provision and assessment of nutrition support therapy in the adult critically ill patient. *J Parenter Enteral Nutr* 33:277–316, 2009.
128. Knochel JP: The clinical status of hypophosphatemia. *N Engl J Med* 313:447–449, 1985.
129. Singer P, Berger MM, Van den Burghe G, et al: ESPEN Guidelines on parenteral nutrition: Intensive care. *Clin Nutr* 28:387–400, 2009.
130. Ziegler TR: Parenteral nutrition in the critically ill patient. *N Engl J Med* 361:1088–1097, 2009.

CHAPTER 192 ■ DISEASE-SPECIFIC NUTRITION

MICKEY M. OTT, BRYAN R. COLLIER AND DOUGLAS SEIDNER

INTRODUCTION

In the critically ill patient, the constant barrage of multiple physiologic derangements quickly leads to malnutrition. The hypermetabolic response to stress changes the nutritional requirements of these individuals, but failure of the various organ systems complicates the issue. Renal, hepatic, and pulmonary function must be considered when prescribing nutritional therapy in the intensive care unit (ICU). This chapter will discuss the metabolic abnormalities associated with these disease processes, the nutritional assessment of the patient in organ failure, and propose evidence-based guidelines for nutritional support in these disease-specific populations.

RENAL FAILURE

Despite many recent advances in medical therapy, management of the critically ill patient with renal failure remains a challenging endeavor. Acute renal failure (ARF) is associated with an overall mortality rate of 50% to 90%, depending on its derivations and comorbid conditions [1]. Hypotension and hypovolemia, secondary to excessive fluid losses, inadequate fluid replacement, or decreased cardiac output are the leading causes of renal failure in the ICU. Factors such as shock or sepsis and exposure to nephrotoxic drugs or blood transfusions can also predispose patients to renal dysfunction. Early diagnosis and restoration of circulating blood volume to the kidneys may decrease the risk of permanent damage; however, the course to renal recovery is often a complicated one. The patient in chronic renal failure (CRF) is also at increased risk for morbidity, as these patients will likely present with protein-calorie malnutrition at baseline. Moreover, the nutritional support of the patient on dialysis will offer a unique challenge to the critical care physician.

Malnutrition and Hypermetabolism

In general, renal failure is characterized by altered nutrient metabolism, defective metabolic waste excretion, inadequate nutrient intake, and excessive nutrient losses. Approximately 10% to 70% of patients with CRF undergoing maintenance dialysis are severely malnourished [2,3]. In these patients, malnutrition is most often the result of poor dietary intake secondary to uremia-induced gastroparesis, poor-tasting highly restrictive diet prescriptions, and medications with gastrointestinal side effects. Diminishing creatinine clearance levels have been linked to a spontaneous decline in the dietary protein intake of CRF patients as well [3,4]. In addition, patients with acute renal failure and critical illness represent by far the largest group receiving supplemental nutrition [5].

The dialysis dose also plays a significant role in the development of malnutrition. The protein catabolic rate of patients undergoing dialysis can be calculated to estimate daily protein intakes of these individuals [6]. In a 1983 investigation by Acchiardo et al., daily protein intakes of less than 0.8 g per kg, as measured by protein catabolic rate, correlated with an increased morbidity and mortality rate compared to patients with greater protein intakes [7]. A subsequent study by Lindsey and Spanner demonstrated a strong linear relationship between dialyzer urea clearance, duration of dialysis, and volume dialyzed (collectively expressed as *Kt/V*) and protein catabolic rate [8]. It is suggested by this correlation that an adequate dose of dialysis is influential on sufficient nutrient intake and the prevention of malnutrition in chronic dialysis patients [9].

Critical illness imposes an even greater metabolic stress and nutritional demand on the patient with renal dysfunction. Protein-calorie malnutrition (PCM) is reportedly present in 25% to 60% of individuals undergoing continuous renal replacement therapy (CRRT) within the intensive care unit [10]. It is important to note that the increased energy expenditure seen in these patients is a direct result of the hypermetabolic response to infection and injury and not of the renal failure itself. Indirect calorimetry has been used to show that the intensity of renal dysfunction has no direct bearing on energy expenditure [11]. Renal failure is, however, the root of several metabolic alterations that often interfere with nutritional status and overall stability of the critically ill patient.

Metabolic Abnormalities

Common metabolic abnormalities associated with ARF include glucose intolerance, impaired lipolysis, increased protein catabolism, decreased protein synthesis, fluid and electrolyte imbalance, and metabolic acidosis (Table 192.1). Although renal excretion of insulin is diminished, insulin resistance coupled with the stress of sepsis or injury can lead to significant hyperglycemia in this patient population. Decreased activity of lipolytic enzymes, such as hepatic triglyceride lipase and lipoprotein lipase, may reduce clearance of parenterally infused triglycerides by as much as 60% in ARF patients versus controls with intact renal function [12]. Adequate energy provision may thus be hindered by altered carbohydrate and fat metabolism. Nonprotein calorie requirements in ARF patients are best met with formulas providing mixed substrates in the ratio of 50% to 70% as carbohydrate and 30% to 50% as fat [13].

TABLE 192.1

METABOLIC RESPONSES TO ACUTE RENAL FAILURE

Nutrient	Metabolic abnormalities
Glycemic	Diminished metabolism of insulin and glucagon Glucose intolerance (hyperglycemia) Peripheral insulin resistance Increased glycogenolysis and gluconeogenesis
Lipid	Increased lipolysis with reduced clearance of serum lipids Hypercholesterolemia Hypertriglyceridemia
Protein and amino acid	Increased catabolism of skeletal muscle and visceral proteins Diminished amino acid uptake Reduced insulin-mediated protein and amino acid synthesis Azotemia
Fluid and electrolyte	Anuria Anasarca Ascites Altered serum concentrations of sodium, phosphorus, or potassium Hypocalcemia Metabolic acidosis

Data compiled from references [8,12,17,19,26].

Several factors contribute to increased protein catabolism and overall negative nitrogen balance in ARF patients. In accordance with the metabolic response to injury, patients with renal failure experience an increase in gluconeogenesis, leading to the breakdown of skeletal muscle proteins for use as energy and for synthesis of acute-phase proteins. Metabolic acidosis, frequently seen in renal failure, can trigger skeletal muscle protein breakdown as well. Reduction in muscle protein synthesis in this population has been linked to diminished cellular uptake of glucose and amino acids secondary to insulin resistance, altered cellular ion transport mechanisms, and defective intracellular synthesis [14,15].

Varying protein and energy provisions also influence protein catabolism and nitrogen balance in ARF patients. A 1996 investigation of 40 ICU patients with ARF receiving continuous venovenous hemofiltration revealed that at levels of protein administration above 1.5 g per kg per day, increasing energy provisions are associated with an increase in protein catabolism [16] (Fig. 192.1). Increasing energy provisions had a protein-sparing effect at lower levels of protein administration. Net nitrogen balance was also examined in this population (Fig. 192.2). Protein administration rates of 1.5 to 2.0 g per kg per day were associated with a positive net nitrogen balance,

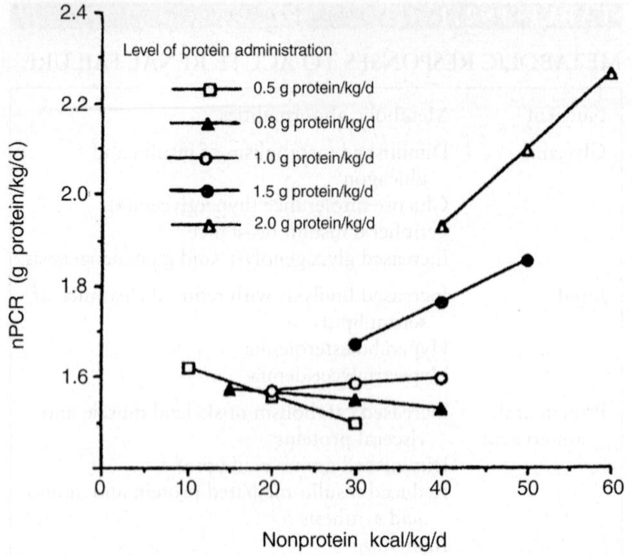

FIGURE 192.1. Effect of varying energy and protein provisions on protein catabolism. At higher levels of protein administration (>1.5 g/kg/d), increasing energy provisions are associated with increased net protein catabolic rate (nPCR). At lower levels of protein administration (<0.5 g/kg/d), increasing energy provisions promote protein sparing. [Adapted from the American Society for Parenteral and Enteral Nutrition (ASPEN) and Macias WL, Alaka KJ, Murphy MH, et al: Impact of nutritional regimen on protein catabolism and nitrogen balance in patients with acute renal failure. *JPEN J Parenter Enteral Nutr* 20(1):56–62, 1996, with permission. ASPEN does not endorse the use of this material in any form other than its entirety.]

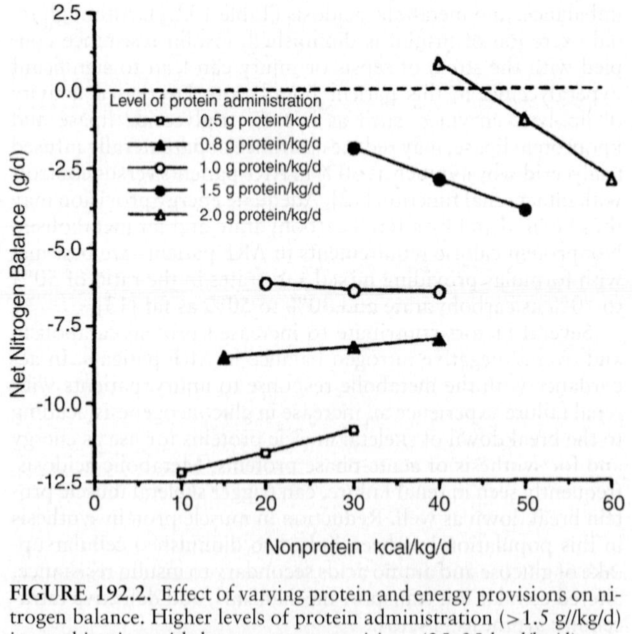

FIGURE 192.2. Effect of varying protein and energy provisions on nitrogen balance. Higher levels of protein administration (>1.5 g//kg/d) in combination with lower energy provisions (25–35 kcal/kg/d) promote a more favorable net nitrogen balance. [Adapted from the American Society for Parenteral and Enteral Nutrition (ASPEN) and Macias WL, Alaka KJ, Murphy MH, et al: Impact of nutritional regimen on protein catabolism and nitrogen balance in patients with acute renal failure. *JPEN J Parenter Enteral Nutr* 20(1):56–62, 1996, with permission. ASPEN does not endorse the use of this material in any form other than its entirety.]

although at these elevated levels of protein provision, lower-energy administration rates were necessary to prevent protein catabolism and promote more favorable nitrogen balance. Final nutrient recommendations were for 1.5 to 1.8 g protein per kg per day with energy levels between 25 to 35 kcal per kg per day in critically ill ARF patients on continuous venovenous hemodialysis (CVVHD) [5,16].

Close monitoring of fluid status is crucial to the maintenance of adequate intravascular volume and renal perfusion. Fluid is typically restricted to 1.0 to 1.5 L per day in nondialysis anuric or oliguric patients. Concentrated enteral or parenteral formulas are often required to meet daily nutrient needs under these circumstances. Dialysis, with special emphasis on CRRT, allows for a liberalization of fluid provisions to thereby permit an adequate supply of protein and energy to the renal patient. In the ICU setting, ARF patients tend to be severely volume overloaded with fluid shifting to the extravascular space secondary to hypoalbuminemia. Even while on some form of CRRT, maintenance of fluid balance is challenging in these patients and importance should be given to adequate protein provision for repletion and reversal of the effects of low serum albumin levels. In CRRT, there is a loss of at least 0.2 g amino acids per liter of ultra filtrate (up to 10 to 15 g amino acids per day), and of 5 to 10 g per day of proteins. Vitamins are also lost in significant amounts; however, there does not appear to be lipid losses across the filter [5].

Serum electrolyte levels fall within a wide range of highs to lows depending on renal excretion, extent of catabolism, and type and duration of dialysis [17]. Increased catabolism of skeletal muscle protein releases phosphorus, potassium, and magnesium into the bloodstream, leaving elevated serum electrolyte values. Because of this, parenteral nutrition (PN) formulations for renal patients are often made with low levels of these cations. A 1998 case report demonstrated the dangers of undershooting electrolyte needs in a frequently malnourished CRF population [18]. Introducing a carbohydrate load parenterally or even enterally to a malnourished patient stimulates insulin release and cellular anabolism, thereby enhancing intracellular ion transport [19]. The subsequent decline in serum electrolyte levels with resulting clinical complications is referred to as the *refeeding syndrome*. This case study reported four CRF patients who developed significant hypophosphatemia after starting PN due to inadequate electrolyte provisions in combination with intracellular shifts [18]. It is thus recommended that dextrose infusions be started gradually and serum electrolytes be monitored closely to correct for potential abnormalities in this population. Depressed serum ionized calcium levels are a common result of hyperphosphatemia and uremia. Supplementation is most often necessary to prevent release of calcium from the bone. Multivitamin preparations standard to enteral and parenteral formulas are adequate for most ARF and CRF patients. Support exists in the literature that vitamin C should not exceed 30 to 50 mg per day, because inappropriate supplementation may result in secondary oxalosis. If signs of vitamin A or other toxicities are observed, daily provision may need to be withheld. The kidney normally excretes trace elements; however, excess accumulation in renal failure is unlikely as gastrointestinal tract losses also occur. The micronutrient milieu may also be affected by the mode and dose of renal replacement therapy. Recent data show that prolonged CRRT results in selenium and thiamine depletions despite supplementation at recommended amount [5].

Standard daily doses of trace elements may be safely given to most patients in renal failure. Iron deficiency anemia is a commonly documented finding among end-stage renal disease patients. Recent research has focused on anemia and carnitine, an amino acid with a central role in long-chain fatty acid oxidation. Deficiency of carnitine has been associated with dialysis, and supplementation of L-carnitine has led to the improvement of hematocrit levels in HD patients [20]. Metabolic acidosis in this population is a result of diminished acid excretion, increased protein catabolism, and daily protein intake [21]. Bicarbonate should be given enterally or intravenously to maintain pH more than 7.2 or serum bicarbonate more than 17 mEq per L. When supplementing by PN, sodium or potassium acetate is given because bicarbonate forms an insoluble precipitate with calcium in PN solutions.

Nutrition Assessment

The identification of malnutrition and timely initiation of nutrition support in critically ill patients with renal failure may not only reduce their degree of protein depletion but also increase their chances for survival [1]. Unfortunately, common measures of nutritional status, such as serum albumin, serum transferrin, weight changes, and anthropometrics tend to fluctuate with the alterations in fluid balance inherent to this patient population. Despite this, serum albumin is considered the strongest laboratory predictor of mortality for hospitalized patients with renal failure [22]. Daily monitoring of weight and intake and output records can help to assess fluid balance in these individuals. It is essential to use a dry weight (i.e., free of edema or ascites) when examining alterations in weight status. The dry or adjusted body weight of a renal patient may then be used to more closely estimate daily nutrient needs.

Continuous Renal Replacement Therapy (CRRT) Versus Intermittent Hemodialysis (HD)

It is commonly thought that dialysis therapy can be relied on to correct many of the metabolic derangements associated with acute and chronic renal failure. This may be true under most circumstances; however, research and patient care experience have shown that patients receiving intravenous (IV) nutrition are at greater risk for fluctuating serum chemistries despite regular dialysis treatments [1,18]. HD can also increase the risk of hypotension and may add to the hemodynamic instability of the ICU patient by limiting the removal of adequate fluid. CRRT is useful for 24-hour-per-day clearance of nitrogenous wastes, metabolic by-products, and excess fluids. CRRT is often preferable to HD in the critical care setting because it reduces the risks for fluid and electrolyte disorders and hypotension while allowing for more liberal fluid and nutrient provisions. In patients with severe fluid intolerance, slow continuous ultrafiltration may be necessary. Protein losses can be as high as 10 to 13 g per HD session versus 5 to 10 g per day in CRRT [23,24]. Amino acids can be added to the hemodialysate solution to promote retention of nitrogen balance [25]. Consideration should be given to typical glucose content of the dialysate, as this may make a significant contribution to the caloric load of patients already exhibiting some form of glucose intolerance. Dialysate of CRRT is approximately 1.5% glucose, thereby contributing up to 600 glucose calories during a 10-L per day dialysis infusion [26].

Enteral and Parenteral Formulations

A wide array of enteral nutrition products has been designed for patients in varying stages of renal disease (Table 192.2). Formula selection depends largely on the individual's fluid allowance [27]. For predialysis ARF patients in need of short-term enteral nutrition, a formula containing only essential amino acids and histidine with little or no vitamins, minerals, and electrolytes may be appropriate. Products with reduced levels of protein, phosphorus, potassium, magnesium, and vitamin A are useful for patients with chronic renal insufficiency, yet not on dialysis. Moderate protein formulas with low electrolyte content are often indicated for patients receiving intermittent dialysis treatments. All enteral products designed for use in renal dysfunction are concentrated in volume (2 kcal per mL) to aid in fluid management. It is best to initiate tube feedings at a slow rate in this population and advance the feeding rate gradually to prevent osmotic diarrhea. Because patients on CRRT demonstrate improved clearance of nitrogenous wastes, fluid, and electrolytes, standard enteral formulas may be used. In this case, selection likely depends more on accompanying clinical conditions than on renal status. For example, a low-carbohydrate formula may be more appropriate for the CRRT patient with glucose intolerance than the typical calorically dense renal formulas.

Delayed gastric emptying related to dialysis treatment, diabetes, high blood urea nitrogen levels, hyperglycemia, or postoperative gastrointestinal complications can lead to enteral feeding intolerance in patients with renal failure. PN is indicated when the enteral route cannot safely be used to fully meet daily nutritional requirements. In general, standard amino acid solutions can be used. When fluid volume restriction is necessary, concentrated 15% amino acids solutions are helpful. A parenteral amino acid solution of equal amounts of essential amino acids and standard amino acids at a dose of 1 g per kg

TABLE 192.2

SPECIALTY ENTERAL PRODUCTS FOR USE IN RENAL FAILURE

Manufacturer	Product	Caloric density (kcal/mL)	NPC:N	Protein (g/L)	Carbohydrate of total kcal (%)	Fat of total kcal (%)	PO_4 (mg/L)	K (mg/L)	Na (mg/L)
Nestle[a]	Renalcal	2.0	338:1	34.4	58	35	—	—	—
Nestle[a]	NutriRenal	2.0	143:1	70	40	46	700	1,256	740
Abbott[b]	Nepro	2.0	154:1	70	43	43	685	1,060	845
Abbott[b]	Suplena	2.0	393:1	30	51	43	730	1,120	790
Nestle[a]	Novasource Renal	2.0	140:1	74	40	45	650	810 or 1,100[c]	1,000 or 1,600[c]

[a]Nestle Healthcare Nutrition (Minnetonka, MN).
[b]Abbott Nutrition (Columbus, OH).
K, potassium; Na, sodium; NPC:N, nonprotein calorie to nitrogen ratio; PO_4, phosphorus; —, negligible amounts.

per day may be given in cases of severe intolerance to standard mixtures despite intensive dialysis. Patients receiving enteral or parenteral preparations using essential amino acids as the sole source of nitrogen have demonstrated conflicting results concerning improvement in nitrogen balance and overall recovery of renal function [14,28,29]. Also, nonessential amino acids may become conditionally essential for protein synthesis and ammonia detoxification when the patient is under the stress of certain disease states. Thus, the use of formulations containing only essential amino acids should be reserved for less than 2 weeks of treatment in quantities less than 0.5 g per kg per day for patients with worsening renal function who are unable to begin dialysis.

Intradialytic parenteral nutrition (IDPN) is another means of nutritional support designed for use in malnourished HD patients unable to meet full protein and energy requirements by the oral or enteral route. IDPN may offer some advantages over PN in that dedicated vascular access is not needed and administration is done during dialysis therapy to avoid fluid overload. On the other hand, IDPN alone cannot provide adequate daily nutrition; it places the patient at high risk for hyperglycemia with insulin resistance, and expenses of the treatment are comparable to PN [30]. Several trials have attempted to demonstrate the efficacy of IDPN with favorable results; however, limitations in study design have left health care professionals wary of supporting its use in clinical practice [31]. A recent prospective study of 16 malnourished HD patients receiving IDPN revealed a significant weight gain after 6 months of IDPN treatment [32]. No control group was used in this study and no other outcome variables (i.e., morbidity, mortality) were adequately evaluated. At present IDPN should not be used as a substitute for total PN, especially in the critical care setting.

Summary of Nutritional Recommendations

Primary efforts of the caregiver should be directed toward management of the various nutritional and metabolic disorders commonly associated with renal failure. Adequate nutrient provision may optimize renal function, improve nutritional status, and raise the chances of survival in ARF patients [33]. Protein and energy requirements are largely dependent on the underlying causes of renal failure in the critically ill patient. ARF secondary to sepsis or severe injuries places a far greater nutrient demand on patients than that of nephrotoxic drug-induced ARF. The Harris–Benedict equation is used to calculate basal energy requirements, which is then multiplied by an activity and stress factor to determine total energy expenditure. Estimates of total energy expenditure in a critically ill population are typically between 30 and 45 kcal per kg per day. Increasing energy above this does not improve nitrogen balance [34]. Patients with a prolonged stay in the ICU may benefit from the more accurate predictions of energy expenditure afforded by indirect calorimetry [35]. Nondialyzed patients with ARF require a protein restriction of less than 0.5 g per kg of essential amino acids or 0.6 to 1.0 g per kg per day of mixed protein sources. However, such severe restrictions should not be imposed for longer than 2 weeks, and importance should be given to adequate energy provision for protein sparing. Patients receiving intermittent HD require 1.2–1.5 g per kg per day of mixed protein sources, whereas those undergoing CRRT can tolerate protein levels of up to 2.5 g per kg per day. Serum electrolytes should be monitored daily with additives adjusted on an individual basis. Standard vitamins and trace minerals can safely be provided to renal failure patients in the ICU. Fluid allowances for nondialyzed or HD patients are based on 24-hour urine output with an additional 500 mL for insensible losses. Those undergoing CRRT should be permitted additional fluid for provision of full nutritional support. A summary of recommendations supported by randomized controlled trials is included in Table 192.3.

TABLE 192.3

NUTRITION SUPPORT IN ACUTE KIDNEY INJURY

Increasing energy intake from 30 to 40 kcal/kg/d does not improve nitrogen balance and results in elevated levels of triglycerides and blood sugars [34].
Protein intake of 2.5 g/kg/d is recommended to achieve positive nitrogen balance in patients on CRRT.
Indirect calorimetry can improve the accuracy of energy provision in patients on CRRT.

LIVER FAILURE

As the central regulatory organ of the body, the liver is responsible for the metabolism, storage, activation, transport, and synthesis of many vital nutrients. Biochemical reactions fundamental to carbohydrate metabolism such as glycogenesis and gluconeogenesis are carried out in the liver. Albumin, transferrin, prealbumin, and prothrombin are a few of the major serum proteins generated in the liver. Fatty acid oxidation as well as the production of bile salts, triglycerides, and cholesterol for lipid absorption and transport is part of the normal hepatic function. The liver is also responsible for the catabolism of various potentially toxic substances including ammonia, alcohol, and acetaminophen. Liver damage can lead to the disruption of many of these processes; however, due to the large capacity for hepatic reserve, dysfunction is not usually seen until 80% to 90% of the liver cells have been injured [36].

A number of insults can initiate the cellular degeneration of acute or chronic liver disease. Viral infection, alcohol use, medications or other hepatotoxic agents, cardiac shock, chronic cholestasis, metabolic disorders, and autoimmune diseases are all potential instigators of liver injury. The damage can be so sudden and severe that it results in fulminant hepatic failure (FHF), a rare disease involving extensive liver necrosis and often culminating in death. Complications of FHF include metabolic abnormalities such as hypoglycemia or acidosis, hemodynamic instability, cerebral edema, sepsis or immunosuppression, and the hepatorenal syndrome. The presence of hepatic encephalopathy (HE), manifested by several neurologic, behavioral, and neuromuscular changes, may be able to predict the prognosis of FHF depending on the severity of the impairment [37]. Treatment of FHF often involves nutritional intervention; however, no controlled studies have been done to assess the benefits of nutrition therapy in this population.

Patients with acute hepatitis tend to be highly catabolic in the setting of severe gastrointestinal distress. Nausea, vomiting, and anorexia with occasionally concurrent acute pancreatitis may preclude the ability for oral intake. Short-term nutrition support is often necessary until causes of the acute injury to the liver have been identified and treated.

The end stage of most chronic liver diseases is the development of cirrhosis. Cirrhosis is characterized by repeated episodes of necrosis, followed by regrowth and formation of connective scar tissue. The resulting disruption of normal hepatic structure increases resistance of blood flow to the liver. Portal hypertension, esophageal varices with gastrointestinal bleeding, and ascites often stem from altered hepatic circulation in cirrhotic patients. Clinical evidence of cirrhosis can progress from elevated serum transaminases and jaundice to hypoalbuminemia and HE. Malnutrition has been documented in up to 100% of hospitalized patients with alcoholic liver cirrhosis [38]. It is important to note that the presence of esophageal varices or ascites does not preclude the use of small bowel nasoenteric tube feeding in malnourished cirrhotic patients [39]. Several controlled trials using enteral nutrition in this population have demonstrated improvements in liver function tests, nutritional status, nitrogen balance, length of hospitalization, and overall prognosis [40–42]. The achievement of positive nitrogen balance did not have a negative impact on encephalopathy, azotemia, edema, or ascites among the study groups.

Malnutrition and Metabolic Alterations

Malnutrition in acute and chronic liver disease is the result of a combination of factors. A decrease in oral intake is common in the patient with prolonged gastrointestinal distress, early satiety secondary to ascites, or excessive alcohol consumption. Maldigestion and malabsorption leading to steatorrhea is often seen with cholestasis or chronic pancreatitis. Malnutrition in liver failure is also closely linked to the presence of severe metabolic derangements characteristic of hypercatabolic states of organ injury. Impaired glycogen synthesis and storage as well as decreased hepatic degradation of stress hormones lead to the preferential use of lipid and protein reserves for gluconeogenesis [43]. Insulin resistance and glucose intolerance are usual complications of early liver failure. Hypoglycemia can occur in decompensated cirrhosis or FHF as a result of hepatic glycogen depletion and impaired gluconeogenesis.

Hepatic steatosis with concurrent depletion of adipose tissue stores is a frequent consequence of the imbalance between lipid uptake, fatty acid oxidation, and the release of lipoproteins by the damaged liver. It is important to note that hepatic steatosis is often preventable by avoiding overfeeding. Lipids are the primary source of energy in enteral nutrition supplements designed for use in liver failure patients. IV lipids are also metabolized well by critically ill patients with hepatic failure when given in amounts not to exceed the energy needs of the individual patient. A recent study by Druml et al. found no significant difference in uptake, hydrolysis, or oxidation of a 20% IV lipid emulsion in septic patients with hepatic failure versus in healthy controls [44].

Altered protein metabolism is by far the most challenging aspect of providing nutrition therapy to the critically ill patient with liver disease. Cirrhosis has long been established as a catabolic disease, with unremitting protein degradation and inadequate resynthesis leading to depletion of visceral protein stores and muscle wasting [45]. Under ordinary circumstances, the skeletal muscle collects circulating branched-chain amino acids (BCAAs) for the synthesis of glutamine and alanine, amino acids that are released into the bloodstream and taken up by the liver for use in hepatic gluconeogenesis. Glutamine is also a carrier for ammonia, a potentially toxic by-product of protein metabolism. Ammonia is normally converted into urea by the liver and excreted by the kidneys. As liver function declines, uptake of serum glutamine is diminished and the degradation of ammonia into urea is impaired. In this case, excess serum glutamine and ammonia is diverted to renal pathways for direct excretion by the kidneys.

Adequate protein intake is therefore essential in the liver patient not only for the provision of energy by gluconeogenesis but also for the preservation of skeletal muscle mass and the prevention of HE. The clinical practice of protein restriction in patients with liver damage is common, for fear of precipitating or worsening central nervous system changes associated with HE. Several protein-related theories have been proposed regarding the development of HE, although it is of significance that the occurrence of encephalopathy has not been observed to directly correlate with protein intake in cirrhotic patients [46]. IV protein solutions with higher concentrations of BCAAs have been developed for use in liver disease based on the following hypothesis. As the use of BCAAs by skeletal muscle increases, serum levels decrease, thereby leaving an imbalance of BCAAs and aromatic amino acids at the blood–brain barrier. With less opposition from BCAA, aromatic amino acids readily cross into the central nervous system to form "false neurotransmitters." The false neurotransmitters compete with actual neurotransmitters for binding sites and disrupt normal central nervous system function to cause symptoms of HE [47].

Elevated serum ammonia concentrations have also been implicated in the pathogenesis of HE. Ammonia metabolites such as glutamine in cerebrospinal fluid have been correlated with the severity of encephalopathy [48]. Plauth et al. evaluated differences in serum ammonia levels between enterally and parenterally fed cirrhotic patients' status post–transjugular intrahepatic portosystemic shunt placement [49]. The small intestinal metabolism of enterally fed glutamine was found to produce significantly greater serum ammonia levels than the direct systemic infusion of parenterally fed glutamine. This suggests that PN may allow for a safer way to provide protein to encephalopathic patients. Enteral or parenteral administration of glutamine, however, is not recommended in patients with moderate to severe liver disease [50].

Zinc plays an important role in the regulation of nitrogen metabolism and zinc deficiency has been implicated in the pathogenesis of hepatic encephalopathy. Zinc supplementation therefore would seem to be a potential target for therapy and many studies have tried to address this question with conflicting results. To date there is no clear evidence of a beneficial effect for zinc supplementation for patients with hepatic encephalopathy [51].

Enteral and Parenteral Formulations

As mentioned previously, enteral and parenteral formulas for use in liver failure are designed to normalize plasma amino acid concentrations and improve encephalopathic symptoms. Hepatic enteral nutrition products are generally calorically dense, enriched with BCAAs, and of low-to-moderate fat content (Table 192.4). IV solutions for use in hepatic failure consist of 8% amino acids with 36% of total amino acids provided as BCAA (e.g., valine, isoleucine, and leucine) and only 2% as aromatic amino acids (e.g., tryptophan, phenylalanine, and tyrosine). These include Aminosyn-HF (Hospira, Inc., Lake Forest, IL), Hepatasol (Clintec Nutrition, Deerfield, IL), and HepatAmine (B. Braun Medical, Inc., Irvine, CA). Several leaders of nutrition-related research have published studies, reviews, and meta-analyses on the topic of oral or enteral BCAAs and HE, although consensus is still lacking among them [52–54]. Differences in the degree of encephalopathy, duration of treatment, type of control therapy, and amount of BCAAs supplied have limited the ability to draw distinct conclusions. Numerous research trials have also been conducted in an attempt to demonstrate clinical benefits of BCAA-enriched PN. A meta-analysis of seven such trials concluded that encephalopathy and survival rates were significantly improved among patients treated with BCAAs versus the control groups treated mainly with large doses of dextrose and lactulose or neomycin [55]. It should be noted, however, that improvement in encephalopathy did not always correlate with changes in serum amino acid levels. Other factors may have influenced mental status and mortality in these patients. A Cochrane Review from 2003 looked at 11 randomized trials (556 patients) regarding the effect of BCAA on hepatic encephalopathy [56]. Compared to the control regimens, the BCAA arms showed improvement

TABLE 192.4

SPECIALTY ENTERAL PRODUCTS FOR USE IN HEPATIC FAILURE

Manufacturer	Product	Caloric density (kcal/mL)	NPC:N	Protein (g/L)	BCAA of total protein (%)	Carbohydrate of total kcal (%)	Fat of total kcal (%)	MCT of total fat (%)	PO_4 (mg/L)	Na (mg/L)
Nestle[a]	NutriHep	1.5	209:1	40	50	77	12	66	1,000	320
Hormel[b]	Hepatic-Aid II	1.2	148:1	44.1	46	57	28	0	0	<585

[a]Nestle Healthcare Nutrition (Minnetonka, MN).
[b]Hormel Health Labs, Inc. (Savannah, GA).
BCAA, branched-chain amino acids; MCT, medium-chain triglyceride; Na, sodium; NPC:N, nonprotein calorie to nitrogen ratio; PO_4, phosphorus.

in encephalopathy at the end of the treatment. There was no effect on survival. Given the lack of follow-up, poor quality, and the small sample size of these studies, however, the reviewers concluded that there is no convincing evidence that BCAA have a beneficial effect on patients with hepatic encephalopathy [57]. In one large, randomized trial by Muto et al, oral BCAA given to patients with cirrhosis improved the combined rate of death and progression to liver failure [56]. Iwasa et al. showed improvement in regional cerebral blood flow in patients with cirrhosis treated with BCAA [58]. In regards to PN, few published studies exist to date comparing BCAA-enriched TPN to parenteral solutions containing standard amino acids [59–61]. No differences in outcome were noted in each of these studies.

Nevertheless, recommendations for clinical practice may be made from the evidence at hand. A primary focus in the management of HE should be on treatment of the underlying causes [9]. Dehydration, infection, electrolyte abnormalities, gastrointestinal bleeding, acid–base imbalances, and medications have been implicated in the occurrence of encephalopathy among critical care patients. In most acute cases, mental status improves with correction of precipitating abnormalities. Use of lactulose or neomycin, or both, for bowel cleansing and sterilization is the first line of treatment for hyperammonemia. The practice of restricting dietary protein in cirrhotic patients, especially those with HE, may seem prudent given the clear relationship between serum ammonia levels and poor outcomes. However, Cordoba et al. showed in a randomized controlled trial that restricting protein intake during encephalopathy had no beneficial effect [62]. When nutrition support is needed, a standard protein formula can be initiated at doses of 0.6 to 0.8 g per kg per day [63]. Restriction of protein is only necessary until the causes of encephalopathy have been identified and treated. To maintain nitrogen balance, nutrition support should be advanced as tolerated to goals of 1.0 to 1.5 g per kg per day in critical care situations [64]. BCAA-enriched formulas are solely reserved for use in severe encephalopathy refractory to standard treatment, but evidence for their role as a first choice is mounting.

Nutrition Assessment

Traditional parameters of nutritional status such as weight loss and depletion of visceral protein stores are frequently masked among liver failure patients by the presence of ascites or edema. Serum albumin, prealbumin, and transferrin levels are more reflective of disease-related intravascular volume expansion and increased protein catabolic rate than the severity of nutritional deficit. Despite this, albumin remains an important marker of PCM among liver patients. Because the upper extremities tend to escape the fluid retention often seen in liver patients, mid-arm muscle circumference and triceps skinfold measurements are considered to be the most accurate tools for nutrition assessment in this population. Recent investigations have centered on the detection of those nutritional parameters most predictive of survival, indicative of PCM, and responsive to treatment in liver failure patients. A prospective study of 271 mildly to severely malnourished patients with chronic alcoholic hepatitis revealed significant improvements in visceral proteins and mid-arm muscle mass in response to intensive nutrition therapy along with oral administration of oxandrolone, an androgenic anabolic steroid [46]. Severe reduction in mid-arm muscle circumference and triceps skinfold measurement, suggestive of muscle mass and body fat depletion were found to be independent predictors of survival in a study of 212 hospitalized cirrhotic patients. In this study, Alberino et al. also advised the inclusion of upper-arm anthropometry to improve prognostic accuracy of the Child-Pugh score, a commonly used classification of the severity of liver disease [65]. A comprehensive analysis of all available data, including physical examination, anthropometric measurements, and laboratory values, may therefore be the best determinant of nutritional status in liver disease.

Summary of Nutritional Recommendations

In devising a plan for nutritional management of the critically ill patient with liver disease, one must consider the etiology of the disease, associated complications and metabolic abnormalities, and concurrent disease processes (Table 192.5). Despite the inherent difficulties in obtaining an accurate dry weight, the Harris-Benedict equation with stress factors may be used in most liver patients to estimate basal energy expenditure. Requirements for most patients are met with 25 to 35 kcal per kg per day or basal energy expenditure times 1.2 to 1.4, and standard protein doses of 1.0 to 1.5 g per kg per day [66]. Nonprotein calories are generally supplied in proportions of 50% to 70% carbohydrate and 30% to 50% fat in the setting of glucose intolerance. Patients demonstrating symptoms of persistent encephalopathy despite aggressive medical management require a temporary protein restriction of 0.6 to 0.8 g per kg per day pending treatment of underlying causes. If the patient does not respond to protein restriction, a BCAA-enriched formula should be used to promote nitrogen balance. Sodium and fluid restriction are indicated with ascites or edema. Recommended daily allowances of vitamins, minerals, and trace elements are usually sufficient in this population, although additional supplementation of thiamine and folate is customary in alcoholic cirrhosis. Pescovitz et al. document an elevated rate of profound zinc deficiency among patients with end-stage liver disease [67]. Supplementation of zinc in these cases may improve HE; however, efficacy of zinc as a routine therapy for encephalopathy is still controversial [68].

In the case of severe liver disease such as FHF, indirect calorimetry is a more accurate method of determining energy

TABLE 192.5

NUTRIENT REQUIREMENTS IN VARIOUS STAGES OF LIVER DISEASE

Degree of liver injury	Total energy (kcal/kg/d)	Protein or amino acids (g/kg/d)
Compensated cirrhosis	25–35	1.0–1.2 for maintenance, 1.2–1.5 for repletion
Decompensated cirrhosis	25–35	Begin with 0.6–0.8 of standard protein If improvement, advance to 1.2–1.5 as tolerated If refractory, supplement with BCAA until positive nitrogen balance is achieved
Fulminant hepatic failure	35–40	0.6–0.8, if improvement advance
Post–liver transplant	25–35	1.2–1.5

BCAA, branched-chain amino acids.
Data compiled from references [8,34,48,56,59,62].

requirements. Because patients in FHF have limited gluconeogenesis capacity, nutrition support should be initiated peripherally with 10% dextrose to limit the possibility of hypoglycemia and limit catabolism. To provide more substantial dextrose concentrations parenterally, central access is required. Fluid restriction is often necessary to prevent exacerbation of cerebral edema. However, with the use of peripheral 10% dextrose solution, large volumes are required to achieve nutritional goals. Protein administration should begin with 0.6 to 0.8 g per kg per day of a standard amino acid solution. Standard protein provisions should be advanced as tolerated to 1.2 to 1.5 g per kg per day if the encephalopathy improves. If the patient remains in negative nitrogen balance with severe encephalopathy, BCAA formulas should be used and advanced as tolerated to achieve positive nitrogen balance. Protein requirements in FHF are 1.5 to 1.75 grams per kg per day, and basal energy requirements in FHF are 35 to 40 kcal per kg per day provided as a mixture of carbohydrate and lipid substrates. A summary of recommendations supported by randomized controlled trials is included in Table 192.6.

TABLE 192.6

NUTRITION SUPPORT IN LIVER DISEASE: SUMMARY OF CONTROLLED TRIALS

Cirrhosis and severe malnutrition:

Total enteral tube feeding, compared to a regular diet, improves liver function and reduces mortality in hospitalized patients [40].

Alcoholic liver disease:

Protein calorie malnutrition correlates significantly with mortality, clinical severity of the liver disease, and biochemical liver dysfunction [42].

Supplemental enteral tube feeding, in addition to an oral diet, results in more rapid improvement of liver function in hospitalized patients [102].

Hepatic encephalopathy (acute):

Branched-chain amino acid enriched nutrition support leads to a more rapid resolution of hepatic encephalopathy, but has no affect on mortality [56].

Normal protein intake is well tolerated and results in less protein breakdown when compared to low protein intakes [62].

Note: Studies did not specifically focus on patients in the critical care setting and most were small in size.

Liver Transplantation

Currently, the best therapy for unsalvageable liver failure is liver transplantation [50]. It is important to note that not only must the nutritional status of the liver transplant recipient be considered, but also that of the donor. There is evidence to suggest that infusion of large quantities of dextrose can restore glycogen stores, that feeding the donor patient improves protein synthesis, that fish oils may increase hepatic energy content, and that glutamine offers some graft protection in ischemia-and-reperfusion injury [69,70].

Liver transplant candidates should undergo a comprehensive nutritional assessment to uncover signs of poor nutritional status. Once moderate-to-severe PCM has been established, nutrition support should be initiated to promote improved postoperative outcomes [50,71]. Nutrition support is also of value in the immediate posttransplant period. Hasse et al. randomized 50 posttransplant patients to receive standard enteral nutrition or parenteral electrolyte solutions until oral diets were tolerated [72]. A decreased incidence of infection and faster recovery of nitrogen balance was found in the enterally fed group during the first 21 days after undergoing orthotopic liver transplantation. Posttransplant patients are often faced with impaired glucose tolerance and hyperlipidemia, although standard lipid infusion is generally well tolerated and necessary to maintain glycemic control in this population. Tight blood glucose control with special emphasis on the increased risk for hypoglycemia may help reduce the chances for postoperative septic complications. Energy requirements are estimated using the Harris-Benedict equation multiplied by stress factors of 1.2 to 1.3, with protein needs estimated at 1.2 g per kg per day. No specific advantages have been found with regard to the use of BCAA-enriched amino acids solutions or fat emulsions containing medium- and long-chain triglycerides in this population [72].

PULMONARY FAILURE

Optimal functioning of the pulmonary system is essential to the maintenance of adequate nutritional status. Through the process of gas exchange, the lungs and supporting respiratory structures provide oxygen to vital tissues for nutrient metabolism. The respiratory system also plays a major role in regulation of acid–base balance. Pulmonary injury or insufficiency can lead to malnutrition and dependence on mechanical ventilation in the critically ill patient. Acute respiratory distress syndrome (ARDS), characterized by severe progressive hypoxemia and mechanical ventilation, is a frequent result of trauma, sepsis, or surgery in the critical care setting. The patient with chronic obstructive pulmonary disease (COPD) may also undergo periods of acute exacerbation requiring intensive care. Malnutrition has been documented in up to 60% of this population, with the highest incidence occurring in the mechanically ventilated. In a 1996 study by Vitacca et al., nutritional prognostic indicators such as weight loss and percentage of ideal body weight were able to significantly predict the need for mechanical ventilation among hospitalized COPD patients. Decreased survival rates have been observed in malnourished, critically ill COPD patients as well [73,74].

Malnutrition may result from a variety of factors inherent to the pulmonary disease process. Hyperinflation of the lung with an associated decrease in abdominal volume often leads to anorexia, early satiety, and tube feed intolerance. Oral intake may also be hindered by dyspnea and fatigue during meal times. Significant weight loss is found in 20% to 40% of patients with forced expiratory volume in 1 second (FEV_1) of less than 50% [75]. Energy expenditure is reported to be up to 20% above normal in COPD due to the increased work of breathing [76]. Patients with significant COPD spend 430 to 720 kcal per day in the task of breathing, whereas normal subjects use only 36 to 72 kcal per day toward the same goal [9]. Impaired gas exchange with inadequate delivery of oxygen to body tissues has been implicated as a cause of malnutrition in COPD [77]. Increased levels of tumor necrosis factor, an inflammatory mediator, may additionally lead to alterations in energy expenditure and the development of anorexia in this population [78].

Effects of Malnutrition on Pulmonary Function

Just as pulmonary disease influences the onset of malnutrition, poor nutritional status may significantly impair several structural and functional components of the respiratory system [79]. Respiratory muscles display reduced efficiency and endurance during nutrition deprivation due to loss of muscle mass and depletion of energy reserves. Impaired respiratory muscle function eventually results in decreased ventilatory drive and inefficient gas exchange or hypercapnia and hypoxemia. Severe hypophosphatemia, often seen during rapid refeeding of malnourished patients, also adversely affects respiratory muscle function resulting in decreased delivery of oxygen to the tissues [80]. Hypoalbuminemia, associated with critical illness and malnutrition, decreases osmotic pressure, leading to the expansion of extracellular fluid and increased interstitial lung fluid or pulmonary edema. A reduction in pulmonary functional reserve capacity accompanies fluid retention in the lungs [81]. Immunity from respiratory tract infection relies heavily on the preserved integrity of the pulmonary system. Nosocomial pneumonia is the most common fatal infection among hospitalized individuals. Malnutrition in the setting of critical illness not only impairs immune response but also damages specific pulmonary defense mechanisms. Decreased secretion of immunoglobulin A, reduced alveolar macrophage recruitment, increased bacterial adherence to respiratory epithelium, and a weakened lung matrix are all potential outcomes of malnutrition leading to increased risk of pneumonia and mortality in the critically ill patient [9].

Nutritional Assessment

As previously mentioned, common indicators of nutritional status have correlated with the duration of mechanical ventilation and mortality in hospitalized COPD patients. Several recent studies have focused on uncovering specific parameters most predictive of nutritional status and outcome in this population. A large-scale, prospective study conducted by Landbo et al. observed strong associations between low body mass index (BMI) and increased mortality in subjects with severe COPD [82]. In a similar study, Hallin et al. demonstrated that patients who were under weight (BMI < 20) had a lower FEV_1 and a higher risk of dying within the next 2 years following their hospital admission [83]. It is unclear, however, if nutritional support in the chronic COPD patient can improve these outcomes.

In regard to defining nutritional status, Faisy et al. compared changes in bioelectrical impedance analysis with various anthropometric and biologic parameters among ICU patients with COPD and acute respiratory failure [84]. Bioelectrical impedance analysis more accurately detected severe alterations in nutritional status in those patients requiring mechanical ventilation, whereas anthropometric data were inconclusive. Low serum albumin levels were also significantly associated with increased mortality among patients in this study. Weight changes, serum albumin levels, and bioelectrical impedance analysis, if available, are thus used as valuable tools in assessment of nutritional status and prediction of outcome in patients with severe respiratory insufficiency.

An accurate measure of energy expenditure is of utmost importance in the nutritional care of the patient with pulmonary disease. Underfeeding, with the consequence of malnutrition, may increase risk of infection, prolong ventilator dependence, delay wound healing, and increase overall hospital morbidity and mortality. An overestimation of energy needs is associated with several metabolic, hepatic, and respiratory complications, including increased carbon dioxide production with inability to wean from mechanical ventilation (Table 192.7). McClave et al. demonstrated an inverse correlation between the degree of feeding in mechanically ventilated adults and the amount of air inspired and expired over the period of 1 minute [85]. Patients receiving greater than 100% up to 300% of nutritional needs as estimated by indirect calorimetry showed significant decreases

TABLE 192.7

POTENTIAL COMPLICATIONS OF OVERFEEDING

System	Complications
Metabolic	Hypermetabolism
	Hyperglycemia
	Increased lipogenesis
	Fluid overload
	Hypophosphatemia
	Hypokalemia
	Hypomagnesemia
Hepatic	Hepatic steatosis
	Cholestatic liver disease
	Elevated serum transaminases
Respiratory	Increased carbon dioxide production
	Hypercapnia
	Increased minute ventilation
	Increased ventilatory drive
	Decreased oxygen saturation
	Increased respiratory quotient
	Weakened respiratory muscles
	Difficulty weaning from mechanical ventilation

Data compiled from references [8,56,70,77,79,83,94,95].

in minute ventilation, whereas those receiving less than 100% of their caloric requirements had significant increases in minute ventilation. Ventilatory settings may be adjusted to account for minor discrepancies in provision of nutrient requirements without much setback; however, this study also revealed that only approximately 25% of hospitalized patients actually receive calories within 10% of energy requirements [86,87].

Indirect calorimetry is a clinical tool by which measurements of respiratory gas exchange are used to determine energy requirements and substrate utilization for a given subject. It continues to be the gold standard for establishing nutritional goals. Several researchers have examined the benefits of using indirect calorimetry over predictive equations to assess energy expenditure in critically ill patients with acute respiratory failure [85,87,88]. Flancbaum et al. found poor correlation between various predictive formulas and indirect calorimetry measurements. A 1997 review by Brandi et al. concluded that although several sources of error exist, indirect calorimetry remains the most appropriate measure of energy expenditure in mechanically ventilated patients. Recommendations were also made to obtain several measurements throughout the course of a patient's illness to more closely approximate nutritional requirements under fluctuating metabolic states. In cases in which indirect calorimetry is not available or not feasible, the Harris-Benedict equation may be used to estimate resting energy expenditure (REE), which is then multiplied by a stress factor of 1.3 to 1.5 to approximate energy requirements in this population.

Nutrient Requirements and Nutrient Impact on Pulmonary Function

Substrate utilization as assessed by indirect calorimetry is the ratio of oxygen consumed to carbon dioxide produced on metabolism of various macronutrients. This ratio is referred to as the respiratory quotient (R/Q). The oxidation of fat, protein, and carbohydrate produces an R/Q of 0.7, 0.8, and 1.0, respectively. Ideally, the R/Q of a given patient should approximate 0.85 to reflect metabolism of mixed substrates. When carbohydrate or total calorie provisions exceed energy requirements, R/Q levels rise above 1.0 to suggest fat synthesis. An R/Q of less than 0.7 is indicative of inadequate nutrition support with breakdown of bodily fat and protein stores. This information is useful for the adjustment of fuel mixtures within the nutrient prescription to avoid potentially harmful effects of over or underfeeding the ventilator-dependent patient.

The provision of carbohydrate in excess of 5 mg per kg per minute in severely stressed patients increases carbon dioxide production ($\dot{V}CO_2$) and may delay weaning from mechanical ventilation. Jih et al. reported the case of a septic ARDS patient who developed increased respiratory distress and hypercapnic acidosis in response to hypercaloric carbohydrate infusion [89]. Hypercapnia resolved as carbohydrate and total calories were decreased to levels consistent with indirect calorimetry measurements of REE. Talpers et al. maintain that total caloric intake has more of an impact on respiratory function in mechanically ventilated patients than excessive carbohydrate calories [90]. No difference in ($\dot{V}CO_2$) was observed upon variation in carbohydrate provisions with consistent total caloric intake (1.3 × REE). In contrast, increasing total caloric provisions (1.5 to 2.0 × REE) with fixed carbohydrate content led to a significant progressive increase in ($\dot{V}CO_2$). Administration of PN at a calorie level equal to indirect calorimetry measurements did not increase ($\dot{V}CO_2$) or ventilatory demand in a 1994 analysis of mechanically ventilated patients by Kiiski and Takala [91]. In many cases, sustained hyperglycemia in the critically ill mechanically ventilated patient signifies a need for decrease in carbohydrate or total calorie provisions rather than an incremental increase in insulin dosage.

The substitution of fat for carbohydrate calories may lower R/Q and decrease ($\dot{V}CO_2$) to ease weaning from the ventilator [92]. The use of IV fat emulsions (IVFE) is not without its drawbacks, however. Rapid infusion of IVFE may adversely affect gas exchange by decreased rate of clearance, deposition of lipid particles within the reticuloendothelial system, and subsequent reduction in pulmonary diffusion capacity. This effect is most often seen in patients with existing pulmonary dysfunction and with rates of lipid administration more than 1 kcal per kg per hour [93]. Immune function is also compromised by rapid infusion of IVFE in patients with pulmonary insufficiency. Specific omega-6 polyunsaturated fatty acids, including linoleic acid, serve as precursors for synthesis of vasoconstrictive prostaglandins and proinflammatory eicosanoids. The resulting activation of pulmonary neutrophils limits bacterial clearance from systemic circulation and increases uptake of bacteria into the lungs [94]. Inflammatory cells, possibly activated by lipids, release phospholipase A[2] and platelet-activating factor, enhancing edema formation, inflammation, and surfactant alterations [95]. Specialized enteral formulas designed to decrease production of proinflammatory agents and enhance immune function in pulmonary patients are discussed in the following section.

Battistella et al. examined the effects of withholding IVFE for 10 days in 57 polytrauma patients requiring total PN [96]. Results indicated a significantly greater length of ICU and hospital stay, longer duration of mechanical ventilation, and higher incidence of infection in patients receiving IVFE. It is, however, impossible to fully assign the differences to the withholding of lipids, as this group did not receive extra calories to account for the absence of lipid. The group with IVFE received 25% more total calories, which could have contributed to the increase in adverse outcomes in this group of patients. Clinical experience has shown that IVFE may be given safely in the range of 20% to 40% of nonprotein calories infused over a period of 12 to 24 hours in the critically ill patient [9].

Protein requirements in critically ill patients with pulmonary failure are elevated in accordance with the hypercatabolism of stressed states. Consequences of protein malnutrition, including loss of diaphragmatic muscle mass, are significant enough to warrant 1.5 to 2.0 g per kg per day of protein depending on the need for repletion [97]. Unfortunately, an increase in ventilatory drive and minute ventilation may be seen with protein infusion. BCAA formulas, in particular, may result in severe respiratory distress [98]. It is therefore recommended that protein provisions be advanced slowly with close attention to respiratory function in mechanically ventilated patients.

Enteral and Parenteral Nutrition

The use of enteral nutrition or PN is necessary in nearly every patient that requires prolonged ventilator support. However, the use of PN in the patient with pulmonary failure has become increasingly scrutinized. Plurad et al. showed that the administration of PN was independently associated with late onset ARDS [99]. In general, parenteral nutrition should be avoided in this patient population. In those patients in whom PN must be used secondary to inability to use the gastrointestinal tract, there is new evidence to suggest that omega-3 fatty acids-supplemented parenteral nutrition may be better than standard formulas [100]. Currently, these formulas are not available in the United States.

Although the intubated and sedated patient is at increased risk of aspiration, enteral nutrition is clearly the preferred route of feeding due to improved outcomes, lower costs, decreased

TABLE 192.8

SPECIALTY ENTERAL PRODUCTS FOR USE IN PULMONARY FAILURE

Manufacturer	Product	Caloric density (kcal/mL)	NPC:N	Protein (g/L)	Carbohydrate of total kcal (%)	Fat of total kcal (%)	MCT of total fat (%)	PO_4 (mg/L)	Na (mg/L)
Nestle[a]	Nutrivent	1.5	114:1	67.5	27	55	40	1,200	1,170
Abbott[b]	Pulmocare	1.5	125:1	62.6	28	55	20	1,060	1,310
Abbott[b]	Oxepa	1.5	125:1	62.5	28	55	N/A	1,060	1,310
Nestle[a]	Novasource Pulmonary	1.5	102:1	75	40	40	N/A	1,070	1,290
Nestle[a]	Respalor	1.5	102:1	75	40	40	N/A	1,000	1,270

[a]Nestle Healthcare Nutrition (Minnetonka, MN).
[b]Abbott Nutrition (Columbus, OH).
MCT, medium-chain triglycerides; N/A, data not available; Na, sodium; NPC:N, nonprotein calorie to nitrogen ratio; PO_4, phosphorus.

risk of sepsis, and improved preservation of gut mucosal barrier. Proposed mechanisms by which risks for aspiration may be reduced include timely weaning of the patient off pressor support, maintenance of the patient in a semirecumbent body position, and the use of transpylorically placed feeding tubes [80,101]. Gastric feedings may work equally as well if gut motility is intact. Kearns et al. [102] found no clear difference between the use of small bowel and gastric feeding tubes in the prevention of ventilator-associated pneumonia [102]. Despite this, small bowel tube placement remains the preferred method of feeding for improved nutrient intake in a population frequently hindered by gastric ileus.

Standard enteral formulas may be used in most patients with pulmonary dysfunction, however, current recommendations advise that specialized nutritional support is indicated in the critically ill who are unable to consume an oral diet within 5 to 10 days [103]. Fluid and sodium-restricted tube feedings are often necessary until the risk for pulmonary edema resolves. Enteral products designed specifically for use in pulmonary disease should be reserved for patients with existing COPD and increasing difficulty weaning off the ventilator (Table 192.8). These formulas are typically nutrient dense with moderate to high levels of fat (40% to 60%). Akrabawi et al. examined the effects of a moderate fat (Respalor; 41% fat) (Novartis Nutrition, Minneapolis, MN) versus high fat (Pulmocare; 55% fat) (Abbott Nutrition, Columbus, OH) enteral formula on gastric emptying times and pulmonary function in 36 patients with COPD [104]. Although no differences were found in pulmonary function between the two feedings, gastric emptying times were significantly enhanced with the moderate-fat meal. This implies possible benefits, including improved tolerance and overall increased nutrient intake and absorption with the use of a moderate-fat enteral nutrition product providing 30% of total fat as medium-chain triglycerides.

A specialty enteral feeding was designed to counteract the inflammatory cascade and improve oxygenation in the patient with ARDS. This product (Oxepa, Abbott Nutrition, Columbus, OH) is supplemented with eicosapentaenoic acid and gamma-linolenic acid, two fatty acids with anti-inflammatory properties. Gadek et al. compared the effects of this specialized enteral formula (Oxepa) with a control feeding (Pulmocare) in 98 critically ill patients with ARDS [105]. The two formulas differed only in terms of lipid composition and increasing levels of antioxidants in the experimental product. Significant beneficial effects on oxygenation (partial arterial pressure of oxygen/fraction of inspired oxygen: 203 vs. 168), minute ventilation, duration of mechanical ventilation (11 vs. 16.3 days; $p = 0.011$), and length of ICU stay (12.8 vs. 17.5 days; $p = 0.016$) were demonstrated in patients fed the specialized diet compared with controls. Further studies are necessary to clearly identify the benefits of these specialized formulas, but based on the recommendations by several nutritional organizations, these formulas should be chosen in patients with ARDS [106,107].

Immunonutrition has also received substantial recent attention. Possible advantages include reduced duration of mechanical ventilation and decreased incidence of pulmonary infection among the critically ill. Atkinson et al. conducted a prospective, double-blind, controlled trial on the use of IMN Impact (Nestle, Minnetonka, MN), an enteral formula supplemented with arginine, purine nucleotides, and omega-3 fatty acids [108]. Three hundred and sixty-nine ICU patients were randomized to receive IMN Impact or an isocaloric, isonitrogenous enteral feed. There was no difference in hospital mortality rate between the two groups. Those patients receiving more than 2.5 L of IMN Impact within 72 hours of ICU admission ($n = 50$ IMN Impact vs. $n = 51$ control formula) had a significant reduction in median duration of mechanical ventilation (6.0 vs. 10.5 days; $p = 0.007$) and median length of hospital stay (15.5 vs. 20.0 days; $p = 0.03$). Mendez et al. found opposite effects when comparing an immune-enhancing formula (Perative, Abbott Nutrition, Columbus, OH) with an essentially isonitrogenous, isocaloric standard feeding [109]. Overall mortality was again identical between the two groups; however, those receiving immunonutrition remained longer on the ventilator (16.4 vs. 9.7 days) and in the hospital (32.9 vs. 22 days) than the control group. It is important to note that Perative does not contain purine nucleotides and delivers omega-3 fatty acids in the form of canola oil rather than fish oils. A recent review of 23 clinical trials involving immune-enhancing formulas concluded that immunonutrition has established a reduced need for ventilation and a decreased risk of infectious complications in malnourished postsurgical ICU patients with known COPD [110]. According to the most recently published guidelines, the use of specialized enteral formulas with anti-inflammatory profiles is now recommended in patients with ARDS with the potential to improve outcomes [107].

Summary of Nutritional Recommendations

Sustained nutrition therapy in mechanically ventilated patients has demonstrated several benefits including increased serum albumin, reduced anasarca, improved respiratory function, and facilitated weaning from the ventilator. Overfeeding can be highly detrimental to the ventilator-dependent critically ill patient. However, it appears that more often than not, nutritional requirements for these patients are underestimated. Daily energy needs are best determined by indirect calorimetry; although, approximations may be made with predictive equations and stress factors of 1.3 to 1.5 × REE or 25 to 30 kcal per kg. Careful monitoring of intake and output, weight changes, and respiratory status is required when indirect calorimetry is not available. Protein needs generally range between 1.5 to 2.0 g per kg per day, with cautious advancement to goal levels. Carbohydrate dosages should not exceed 5 mg per kg per minute provided as 60% to 80% of nonprotein calories. A conservative dose of fat emulsion is recommended in the range of 20% to 40% of nonprotein calories infused over 12 to 24 hours. Enteral feedings with roughly 30% fat, 50% carbohydrate, and 20% protein are generally well tolerated, provided nutrient requirements are not exceeded. Modified and immune enhanced formulas are gaining favor, but should be reserved for those with ARDS and obvious difficulties weaning off the respirator. Maintenance of fluid balance is also of primary importance in the critically ill patient with pulmonary insufficiency. Concentrated parenteral solutions and enteral formulas should be used as necessary. Sodium restriction is indicated in patients with pulmonary edema or congestive heart failure. Hypophosphatemia may be avoided by gradual advancement of nutrition support in severely malnourished patients. Serum phosphorus, potassium, and magnesium levels should be monitored routinely and deficiencies should be corrected aggressively in the critically ill patient. A summary of recommendations supported by randomized controlled trials is included in Table 192–9.

TABLE 192.9

NUTRITION SUPPORT IN PULMONARY DISEASE

Early enteral nutrition (within 24–48 h admission) decreases infectious complications, including pneumonia.
Enteral formulas with anti-inflammatory lipid profiles and antioxidants improve oxygenation, decrease duration of mechanical ventilation, and shorter intensive care unit length of stay in acute respiratory distress syndrome or acute lung injury [105].
Enteral formulas that provide immunonutrition (arginine, glutamine, nucleic acids, omega-3 fatty acids, antioxidants) decrease duration of mechanical ventilation, organ failure, hospital and intensive care length of stay, and mortality [108, 111].

Note: Early enteral nutrition is not a part of this chapter but a general concept that has been indirectly related to decrease pneumonia.

References

1. Kopple JD: The nutrition management of the patient with acute renal failure. *JPEN J Parenter Enteral Nutr* 20:3–12, 1996.
2. Kopple JD: Effect of nutrition on morbidity and mortality in maintenance dialysis patients. *Am J Kidney Dis* 24:1002–1009, 1994.
3. Toigo G, Aparicio M, Attman PO, et al: Expert Working Group report on nutrition in adult patients with renal insufficiency (part 1 of 2). *Clin Nutr* 19:197–207, 2000.
4. Ikizler TA, Greene JH, Wingard RL, et al: Spontaneous dietary protein intake during progression of chronic renal failure. *J Am Soc Nephrol* 6:1386–1391, 1995.
5. Cano NJ, Aparicio M, Brunori G, et al: ESPEN Guidelines on Parenteral Nutrition: adult renal failure. *Clin Nutr* 28:401–414, 2009.
6. Gotch FA, Sargent JA: A mechanistic analysis of the National Cooperative Dialysis Study (NCDS). *Kidney Int* 28:526–534, 1985.
7. Acchiardo SR, Moore LW, Latour PA: Malnutrition as the main factor in morbidity and mortality of hemodialysis patients. *Kidney Int Suppl* 16:S199–S203, 1983.
8. Lindsay RM, Spanner E: A hypothesis: the protein catabolic rate is dependent upon the type and amount of treatment in dialyzed uremic patients. *Am J Kidney Dis* 13:382–389, 1989.
9. Seidner D: Nutrition support in liver, pulmonary and renal disease, in Shikora S, Blackburn G (eds): *Nutrition Support, Theory and Therapeutics.* New York: Chapman and Hall, 1997, pp 556–557.
10. Moore LW, Acchiardo SR, Smith SO, et al: Nutrition in the critical care settings of renal diseases. *Adv Ren Replace Ther* 3:250–260, 1996.
11. Schneeweiss B, Graninger W, Stockenhuber F, et al: Energy metabolism in acute and chronic renal failure. *Am J Clin Nutr* 52:596–601, 1990.
12. Druml W, Fischer M, Sertl S, et al: Fat elimination in acute renal failure: long-chain vs medium-chain triglycerides. *Am J Clin Nutr* 55:468–472, 1992.
13. Wolk R: Nutrition in renal failure, in Gottschlich MM (ed): *The Science and Practice of Nutrition Support. A Case-Based Core Curriculum.* Dubuque, IA: American Society for Parental and Enteral Nutrition, 2001, pp 575–599.
14. Feinstein EI, Blumenkrantz MJ, Healy M, et al: Clinical and metabolic responses to parenteral nutrition in acute renal failure. A controlled double-blind study. *Medicine (Baltimore)* 60:124–137, 1981.
15. Mitch WE: Mechanisms causing loss of lean body mass in kidney disease. *Am J Clin Nutr* 67:359–366, 1998.
16. Macias WL, Alaka KJ, Murphy MH, et al: Impact of the nutritional regimen on protein catabolism and nitrogen balance in patients with acute renal failure. *JPEN J Parenter Enteral Nutr* 20:56–62, 1996.
17. Rodriguez D, Lewis SL: Nutritional management of patients with acute renal failure. *ANNA J* 24:232–241, 1997.
18. Duerksen DR, Papineau N: Electrolyte abnormalities in patients with chronic renal failure receiving parenteral nutrition. *JPEN J Parenter Enteral Nutr* 22:102–104, 1998.
19. Solomon SM, Kirby DF: The refeeding syndrome: a review. *JPEN J Parenter Enteral Nutr* 14:90–97, 1990.
20. Matsumoto Y, Amano I, Hirose S, et al: Effects of L-carnitine supplementation on renal anemia in poor responders to erythropoietin. *Blood Purif* 19:24–32, 2001.
21. Caravaca F, Arrobas M, Pizarro JL, et al: Metabolic acidosis in advanced renal failure: differences between diabetic and nondiabetic patients. *Am J Kidney Dis* 33:892–898, 1999.
22. Lowrie EG, Lew NL: Death risk in hemodialysis patients: the predictive value of commonly measured variables and an evaluation of death rate differences between facilities. *Am J Kidney Dis* 15:458–482, 1990.
23. Davenport A, Roberts NB: Amino acid losses during continuous high-flux hemofiltration in the critically ill patient. *Crit Care Med* 17:1010–1014, 1989.
24. Seidner DL, Matarese LE, Steiger E: Nutritional care of the critically ill patient with renal failure. *Semin Nephrol* 14:53–63, 1994.
25. Chazot C, Shahmir E, Matias B, et al: Dialytic nutrition: provision of amino acids in dialysate during hemodialysis. *Kidney Int* 52:1663–1670, 1997.
26. Mehta RL: Therapeutic alternatives to renal replacement for critically ill patients in acute renal failure. *Semin Nephrol* 14:64–82, 1994.
27. Jordi Goldstein-Fuchs DMB: Renal failure, in *Contemporary Nutrition Support Practice: A Clinical Guide.* St. Louis: Saunders, 2003.
28. Freund H, Atamian S, Fischer JE: Comparative study of parenteral nutrition in renal failure using essential and nonessential amino acid containing solutions. *Surg Gynecol Obstet* 151:652–656, 1980.
29. Naylor CD, Detsky AS, O'Rourke K, et al: Does treatment with essential amino acids and hypertonic glucose improve survival in acute renal failure?: a meta-analysis. *Ren Fail* 10:141–152, 1987.
30. Chertow GM: Modality-specific nutrition support in ESRD: weighing the evidence. *Am J Kidney Dis* 33:193–197, 1999.
31. Wolfson M, Foulks CJ: Intradialytic parenteral nutrition: a useful therapy? *Nutr Clin Pract* 11:5–11, 1996.
32. Mortelmans AK, Duym P, Vandenbroucke J, et al: Intradialytic parenteral nutrition in malnourished hemodialysis patients: a prospective long-term study. *JPEN J Parenter Enteral Nutr* 23:90–95, 1999.
33. Cerra FB: Hypermetabolism, organ failure, and metabolic support. *Surgery* 101:1–14, 1987.
34. Fiaccadori E, Maggiore U, Rotelli C, et al: Effects of different energy intakes on nitrogen balance in patients with acute renal failure: a pilot study. *Nephrol Dial Transplant* 20:1976–1980, 2005.
35. Scheinkestel CD, Kar L, Marshall K, et al: Prospective randomized trial to assess caloric and protein needs of critically Ill, anuric, ventilated patients requiring continuous renal replacement therapy. *Nutrition* 19(11–12):909–916, 2003.
36. Delich PC, Siepler JK, Parker P: Liver disease, in Gottschlich MM (ed): *The ASPEN Nutrition Support Core Curriculum: A Case-Based Approach – The Adult Patient.* Silver Spring, MD: American Society for Parenteral and Enteral Nutrition, 2007, pp 540–557.

37. Raup SM KP: Hepatic failure, in *Contemporary Nutrition Support Practice. A Clinical Guide.* Philadelphia: WB Saunders, 1998.
38. Marsano L, McClain CJ: Nutrition and alcoholic liver disease. *JPEN J Parenter Enteral Nutr* 15:337–344, 1991.
39. de Lédinghen V, Beau P, Mannant PR, et al: Early feeding or enteral nutrition in patients with cirrhosis after bleeding from esophageal varices? A randomized controlled study. *Dig Dis Sci* 42:536–541, 1997.
40. Cabre E, Gonzalez-Huix F, bad-Lacruz A, et al: Effect of total enteral nutrition on the short-term outcome of severely malnourished cirrhotics. A randomized controlled trial. *Gastroenterology* 98:715–720, 1990.
41. Kearns PJ, Young H, Garcia G, et al: Accelerated improvement of alcoholic liver disease with enteral nutrition. *Gastroenterology* 102:200–2005, 1992.
42. Mendenhall CL, Tosch T, Weesner RE, et al: VA cooperative study on alcoholic hepatitis. II: Prognostic significance of protein-calorie malnutrition. *Am J Clin Nutr* 43:213–218, 1986.
43. Bugianesi E, Kalhan S, Burkett E, et al: Quantification of gluconeogenesis in cirrhosis: response to glucagon. *Gastroenterology* 115:1530–1540, 1998.
44. Druml W, Fischer M, Ratheiser K: Use of intravenous lipids in critically ill patients with sepsis without and with hepatic failure. *JPEN J Parenter Enteral Nutr* 22:217–223, 1998.
45. McCullough AJ, Tavill AS: Disordered energy and protein metabolism in liver disease. *Semin Liver Dis* 11:265–277, 1991.
46. Mendenhall CL, Moritz TE, Roselle GA, et al: Protein energy malnutrition in severe alcoholic hepatitis: diagnosis and response to treatment. The VA Cooperative Study Group #275. *JPEN J Parenter Enteral Nutr* 19:258–265, 1995.
47. Fischer JE, Funovics JM, Aguirre A, et al: The role of plasma amino acids in hepatic encephalopathy. *Surgery* 78:276–290, 1975.
48. Latifi R, Killam RW, Dudrick SJ: Nutritional support in liver failure. *Surg Clin North Am* 71:567–578, 1991.
49. Plauth M, Roske AE, Romaniuk P, et al: Post-feeding hyperammonaemia in patients with transjugular intrahepatic portosystemic shunt and liver cirrhosis: role of small intestinal ammonia release and route of nutrient administration. *Gut* 46:849–855, 2000.
50. Li SD, Lue W, Mobarhan S, et al: Nutrition support for individuals with liver failure. *Nutr Rev* 58:242–247, 2000.
51. Sundaram V, Shaikh OS: Hepatic encephalopathy: pathophysiology and emerging therapies. *Med Clin North Am* 93:819–836, vii, 2009.
52. Fabbri A, Magrini N, Bianchi G, et al: Overview of randomized clinical trials of oral branched-chain amino acid treatment in chronic hepatic encephalopathy. *JPEN J Parenter Enteral Nutr* 20:159–164, 1996.
53. Marchesini G, Bianchi G, Rossi B, et al: Nutritional treatment with branched-chain amino acids in advanced liver cirrhosis. *J Gastroenterol* 35[Suppl 12]:7–12, 2000.
54. Mizock BA: Nutritional support in hepatic encephalopathy. *Nutrition* 15:220–228, 1999.
55. Naylor CD, O'Rourke K, Detsky AS, et al: Parenteral nutrition with branched-chain amino acids in hepatic encephalopathy. A meta-analysis. *Gastroenterology* 97:1033–1042, 1989.
56. Als-Nielsen B, Koretz RL, Kjaergard LL, et al: Branched-chain amino acids for hepatic encephalopathy. *Cochrane Database Syst Rev* CD001939, 2003.
57. Muto Y, Sato S, Watanabe A, et al: Effects of oral branched-chain amino acid granules on event-free survival in patients with liver cirrhosis. *Clin Gastroenterol Hepatol* 3:705–713, 2005.
58. Iwasa M, Matsumura K, Watanabe Y, et al: Improvement of regional cerebral blood flow after treatment with branched-chain amino acid solutions in patients with cirrhosis. *Eur J Gastroenterol Hepatol* 15:733–737, 2003.
59. Kanematsu T, Koyanagi N, Matsumata T, et al: Lack of preventive effect of branched-chain amino acid solution on postoperative hepatic encephalopathy in patients with cirrhosis: a randomized, prospective trial. *Surgery* 104:482–488, 1988.
60. Michel H, Bories P, Aubin JP, et al: Treatment of acute hepatic encephalopathy in cirrhotics with a branched-chain amino acids enriched versus a conventional amino acids mixture. A controlled study of 70 patients. *Liver* 5:282–289, 1985.
61. Rocchi E, Cassanelli M, Gibertini P, et al: Standard or branched-chain amino acid infusions as short-term nutritional support in liver cirrhosis? *JPEN J Parenter Enteral Nutr* 9:447–451, 1985.
62. Cordoba J, Lopez-Hellin J, Planas M, et al: Normal protein diet for episodic hepatic encephalopathy: results of a randomized study. *J Hepatol* 41:38–43, 2004.
63. Teran JC: Nutrition and liver diseases. *Curr Gastroenterol Rep* 1:335–340, 1999.
64. Fischer JE: Branched-chain-enriched amino acid solutions in patients with liver failure: an early example of nutritional pharmacology. *JPEN J Parenter Enteral Nutr* 14:249S–56S, 1990.
65. Alberino F, Gatta A, Amodio P, et al: Nutrition and survival in patients with liver cirrhosis. *Nutrition* 17:445–450, 2001.
66. Lochs H, Plauth M: Liver cirrhosis: rationale and modalities for nutritional support–the European Society of Parenteral and Enteral Nutrition consensus and beyond. *Curr Opin Clin Nutr Metab Care* 2:345–349, 1999.
67. Pescovitz MD, Mehta PL, Jindal RM, et al: Zinc deficiency and its repletion following liver transplantation in humans. *Clin Transplant* 10:256–260, 1996.
68. Marchesini G, Fabbri A, Bianchi G, et al: Zinc supplementation and amino acid-nitrogen metabolism in patients with advanced cirrhosis. *Hepatology* 23:1084–1092, 1996.
69. Driscoll DF, Palombo JD, Bistrian BR: Nutritional and metabolic considerations of the adult liver transplant candidate and organ donor. *Nutrition* 11:255–263, 1995.
70. Singer P, Cohen J, Cynober L: Effect of nutritional state of brain-dead organ donor on transplantation. *Nutrition* 17:948–952, 2001.
71. Weimann A, Plauth M, Bischoff SC, et al: Nutrition of liver transplant patients. *Can J Gastroenterol* 14[Suppl D]:85D–88D, 2000.
72. Hasse JM, Blue LS, Liepa GU, et al: Early enteral nutrition support in patients undergoing liver transplantation. *JPEN J Parenter Enteral Nutr* 19:437–443, 1995.
73. Gray-Donald K, Gibbons L, Shapiro SH, et al: Nutritional status and mortality in chronic obstructive pulmonary disease. *Am J Respir Crit Care Med* 153:961–966, 1996.
74. Vitacca M, Clini E, Porta R, et al: Acute exacerbations in patients with COPD: predictors of need for mechanical ventilation. *Eur Respir J* 9:1487–1493, 1996.
75. Schols AM, Soeters PB, Dingemans AM, et al: Prevalence and characteristics of nutritional depletion in patients with stable COPD eligible for pulmonary rehabilitation. *Am Rev Respir Dis* 147:1151–1156, 1993.
76. Donahoe M, Rogers RM, Wilson DO, et al: Oxygen consumption of the respiratory muscles in normal and in malnourished patients with chronic obstructive pulmonary disease. *Am Rev Respir Dis* 140:385–391, 1989.
77. Sridhar MK, Carter R, Lean ME, et al: Resting energy expenditure and nutritional state of patients with increased oxygen cost of breathing due to emphysema, scoliosis and thoracoplasty. *Thorax* 49:781–785, 1994.
78. de Godoy I, Donahoe M, Calhoun WJ, et al: Elevated TNF-alpha production by peripheral blood monocytes of weight-losing COPD patients. *Am J Respir Crit Care Med* 153:633–637, 1996.
79. Schwartz DB: Pulmonary and cardiac failure, in *The ASPEN Nutrition Support Core Curriculum: A Case-Based Approach—The Adult Patient.* Silver Spring, MD: American Society of parenteral and Enteral Nutrition, 2007.
80. Schwartz DB: Pulmonary failure, in *Contemporary Nutrition Support Practice: A Clinical Guide.* St. Louis: Saunders, 2003.
81. Benotti PN, Bistrian B: Metabolic and nutritional aspects of weaning from mechanical ventilation. *Crit Care Med* 17:181–185, 1989.
82. Landbo C, Prescott E, Lange P, et al: Prognostic value of nutritional status in chronic obstructive pulmonary disease. *Am J Respir Crit Care Med* 160:1856–1861, 1999.
83. Hallin R, Gudmundsson G, Suppli UC, et al: Nutritional status and long-term mortality in hospitalised patients with chronic obstructive pulmonary disease (COPD). *Respir Med* 101:1954–1960, 2007.
84. Faisy C, Rabbat A, Kouchakji B, et al: Bioelectrical impedance analysis in estimating nutritional status and outcome of patients with chronic obstructive pulmonary disease and acute respiratory failure. *Intensive Care Med* 26:518–525, 2000.
85. McClave SA, Lowen CC, Kleber MJ, et al: Are patients fed appropriately according to their caloric requirements? *JPEN J Parenter Enteral Nutr* 22:375–381, 1998.
86. Heyland DK, Drover JW, Dhaliwal R, et al: Optimizing the benefits and minimizing the risks of enteral nutrition in the critically ill: role of small bowel feeding. *JPEN J Parenter Enteral Nutr* 26:S51–S55, 2002.
87. Brandi LS, Bertolini R, Calafa M: Indirect calorimetry in critically ill patients: clinical applications and practical advice. *Nutrition* 13:349–358, 1997.
88. Flancbaum L, Choban PS, Sambucco S, et al: Comparison of indirect calorimetry, the Fick method, and prediction equations in estimating the energy requirements of critically ill patients. *Am J Clin Nutr* 69:461–466, 1999.
89. Jih KS, Wang MF, Chow JH, et al: Hypercapnic respiratory acidosis precipitated by hypercaloric carbohydrate infusion in resolving septic acute respiratory distress syndrome: a case report. *Zhonghua Yi Xue Za Zhi (Taipei)* 58:359–365, 1996.
90. Talpers SS, Romberger DJ, Bunce SB, et al: Nutritionally associated increased carbon dioxide production. Excess total calories vs high proportion of carbohydrate calories. *Chest* 102:551–555, 1992.
91. Kiiski R, Takala J: Hypermetabolism and efficiency of CO_2 removal in acute respiratory failure. *Chest* 105:1198–1203, 1994.
92. Kuo CD, Shiao GM, Lee JD: The effects of high-fat and high-carbohydrate diet loads on gas exchange and ventilation in COPD patients and normal subjects. *Chest* 104:189–196, 1993.
93. Klein S, Miles JM: Metabolic effects of long-chain and medium-chain triglyceride emulsions in humans. *JPEN J Parenter Enteral Nutr* 18:396–397, 1994.
94. Grant JP: Nutrition care of patients with acute and chronic respiratory failure. *Nutr Clin Pract* 9:11–17, 1994.
95. Lekka ME, Liokatis S, Nathanail C, et al: The impact of intravenous fat emulsion administration in acute lung injury. *Am J Respir Crit Care Med* 169:638–644, 2004.
96. Battistella FD, Widergren JT, Anderson JT, et al: A prospective, randomized trial of intravenous fat emulsion administration in trauma victims requiring total parenteral nutrition. *J Trauma* 43:52–58, 1997.

97. Malone AM: Acute respirator distress syndrome: pathophysiology, treatment, and nutrition intervention. *Support Line* 2:8–14, 1998.
98. Laaban JP, Kouchakji B, Dore MF, et al: Nutritional status of patients with chronic obstructive pulmonary disease and acute respiratory failure. *Chest* 103:1362–1368, 1993.
99. Plurad D, Green D, Inaba K, et al: A 6-year review of total parenteral nutrition use and association with late-onset acute respiratory distress syndrome among ventilated trauma victims. *Injury* 40:511–515, 2009.
100. Wang X, Li W, Li N, et al: Omega-3 fatty acids-supplemented parenteral nutrition decreases hyperinflammatory response and attenuates systemic disease sequelae in severe acute pancreatitis: a randomized and controlled study. *JPEN J Parenter Enteral Nutr* 32:236–241, 2008.
101. Drakulovic MB, Torres A, Bauer TT, et al: Supine body position as a risk factor for nosocomial pneumonia in mechanically ventilated patients: a randomised trial. *Lancet* 354:1851–1858, 1999.
102. Kearns PJ, Chin D, Mueller L, et al: The incidence of ventilator-associated pneumonia and success in nutrient delivery with gastric versus small intestinal feeding: a randomized clinical trial. *Crit Care Med* 28:1742–1746, 2000.
103. Malone AM: The use of specialized enteral formulas in pulmonary disease. *Nutr Clin Pract* 19:557–562, 2004.
104. Akrabawi SS, Mobarhan S, Stoltz RR, et al: Gastric emptying, pulmonary function, gas exchange, and respiratory quotient after feeding a moderate versus high fat enteral formula meal in chronic obstructive pulmonary disease patients. *Nutrition* 12:260–265, 1996.
105. Gadek JE, DeMichele SJ, Karlstad MD, et al: Effect of enteral feeding with eicosapentaenoic acid, gamma-linolenic acid, and antioxidants in patients with acute respiratory distress syndrome. Enteral Nutrition in ARDS Study Group. *Crit Care Med* 27:1409–1420, 1999.
106. Martindale RG, McClave SA, Vanek VW, et al: Guidelines for the provision and assessment of nutrition support therapy in the adult critically ill patient: Society of Critical Care Medicine and American Society for Parenteral and Enteral Nutrition: Executive Summary. *Crit Care Med* 37:1757–1761, 2009.
107. McClave SA, Martindale RG, Vanek VW, et al: Guidelines for the Provision and Assessment of Nutrition Support Therapy in the Adult Critically Ill Patient: Society of Critical Care Medicine (SCCM) and American Society for Parenteral and Enteral Nutrition (A.S.P.E.N.). *JPEN J Parenter Enteral Nutr* 33:277–316, 2009.
108. Atkinson S, Sieffert E, Bihari D: A prospective, randomized, double-blind, controlled clinical trial of enteral immunonutrition in the critically ill. Guy's Hospital Intensive Care Group. *Crit Care Med* 26:1164–1172, 1998.
109. Mendez C, Jurkovich GJ, Garcia I, et al: Effects of an immune-enhancing diet in critically injured patients. *J Trauma* 42:933–940, 1997.
110. Hillhouse J: Immune-enhancing enteral formulas: effect on patient outcome. *Support Line* 23:16–22, 2001.
111. Pontes-Arruda A, Aragao AM, Albuquerque JD: Effects of enteral feeding and eicosapentaenoic acid, gamma-linolenic acid, and antioxidants in mechanically ventilated patients with severe sepsis and septic shock. *Crit Care Med* 34:2325–2333, 2006.

SECTION XVI ■ RHEUMATOLOGIC, IMMUNOLOGIC, AND DERMATOLOGIC PROBLEMS IN THE INTENSIVE CARE UNIT

NANCY Y.N. LIU

CHAPTER 193 ■ RHEUMATOLOGIC DISEASES IN THE INTENSIVE CARE UNIT

NANCY Y.N. LIU AND JUDITH A. STEBULIS

Patients with established rheumatologic diseases are rarely admitted to the intensive care unit (ICU) because of their inflammatory joint disease. However, since many of these diseases include systemic involvement, organ system failure and complications of therapy are common reasons for ICU admission. Other musculoskeletal problems frequently encountered in the intensive care setting include (a) patients whose underlying rheumatic diseases may pose certain problems in the planning and execution of certain critical care procedures, such as endotracheal intubation or (b) patients in whom acute rheumatic syndromes develop during their hospitalization.

ACUTE RHEUMATIC DISEASES IN THE INTENSIVE CARE SETTING

Several acute musculoskeletal disorders occur with increasing frequency in selected populations of hospitalized patients, including those in the ICU. The most common is crystal-induced arthritis due to monosodium urate, calcium pyrophosphate dihydrate, basic calcium phosphate (BCP)-hydroxyapatite, or calcium oxalate crystals. Two other acute arthritides include septic arthritis from bacteremia and spontaneous hemarthrosis due to complications from anticoagulation therapy or bleeding diathesis.

Gout

Pathogenesis

Gout is characterized by initial intermittent attacks of mono- or polyarticular arthritis in the setting of prolonged hyperuricemia. Over many years, attacks become more frequent and chronic arthropathy may develop. Acute gout is triggered by precipitation or shedding of monosodium urate crystals in the joint space or nearby soft tissues, provoking an intense inflammatory reaction. Regardless of a primary or secondary etiology of hyperuricemia, marked fluctuations in serum urate levels increase the risk of acute gout.

Although the specific triggering event that initiates an isolated attack may be difficult to define, many factors produce serum urate fluctuations and result in an increased incidence of secondary gout in ICU patients. A reduction in glomerular filtration rate from either intrinsic renal disease or decreased effective arteriolar blood volume will result in reduced filtered load of urate, hyperuricemia, and an increased risk of gout. In addition, a reduction in effective arteriolar blood volume results in enhanced tubular reabsorption of urate. Since organic acids such as lactic acid, β-hydroxybutyric acid, and acetoacetic acid may competitively inhibit the renal tubular secretion of uric acid, conditions in which these acids accumulate will also lead to hyperuricemia. Mechanisms of hyperlacticacidemia in the critically ill patient are multiple.

Drug-induced hyperuricemia is a common cause of gout in both hospitalized and nonhospitalized patients. Diuretic therapy decreases effective arteriolar blood volume and also may directly inhibit renal tubular secretion of uric acid. Although thiazide diuretics are the most commonly implicated cause of hyperuricemia and gout, other diuretics including furosemide, acetazolamide, ethacrynic acid, and diazoxide are also potential culprits. Furosemide and diazoxide may also induce hyperlacticacidemia.

In addition to diuretics, other drugs associated with hyperuricemia include low-dose salicylates (less than 2.0 g per day), pyrazinamide, levodopa, α-methyldopa, and cyclosporine. Because of the uricosuric effect of radiocontrast media, a contrast study might precipitate an attack of acute gout. Finally, a hyperuricemic patient who undergoes any surgical procedure is at risk for postoperative gout.

Clinical Features

Gout is easily identifiable and treatable. Classically, the patient with acute gout complains of sudden onset of an exquisitely painful joint that involves one or more sites in an asymmetric pattern. The attack is sometimes accompanied by low-grade fever, particularly in a polyarticular presentation. The great toe is involved in more than 50% of the initial acute attacks and in 90% of acute attacks at some time in the course of the disease. Other common sites of involvement in order of observed frequency include insteps, ankles, knees, wrists, fingers, and elbows. Periarticular sites of urate deposition in bursae, tendons, and soft tissues may be similarly inflamed during an acute attack. On examination, the involved area is erythematous, swollen, warm, and exquisitely painful on palpation, and sometimes with joint motion. The overlying erythema and edema often extends beyond the joint capsule and can mimic cellulitis or bursitis. The presence of lymphangitis or lymphadenopathy and the absence of pain on joint motion are more consistent with cellulitis. Bursitis can be distinguished from true arthritis since full joint extension is preserved in bursitis, and the region of erythema is not within the borders of the joint compartment. If clinical suspicion of joint infection is low then diagnostic arthrocentesis should be avoided until a therapeutic trial of appropriate antibiotics for cellulitis has been completed. Otherwise, there may be a risk of introducing organisms into a sterile joint. However, if motion is restricted or if radiography suggests an effusion, a diagnostic arthrocentesis should be performed before the institution of any therapy.

The diagnosis of gout is confirmed when aspirated synovial fluid or soft tissue site reveals negatively birefringent monosodium urate crystals within polymorphonuclear neutrophils (PMNs) under polarizing light microscopy. Gouty synovial fluid is inflammatory, with more than 2,000 leukocytes per μL, occasionally as high as 100,000 per μL, and PMNs predominate in the cell differential. Since gout and septic arthritis have similar clinical features and rarely coexist, aspirated synovial fluid should always be Gram stained for microorganisms and cultured. Elevations in erythrocyte sedimentation rate (ESR), C-reactive protein (CRP), and peripheral leukocytosis cannot distinguish gout from other inflammatory states. Serum urate may be normal during an acute attack, while an elevated level does not confirm the diagnosis without crystal identification.

Therapy

Once the diagnosis of acute gout is established, the immediate aim of therapy is to terminate the attack by interruption of the inflammatory response. Long-term management (e.g., prevention of recurrent attacks, sequelae of tophaceous disease or renal stones) need not be considered in the ICU setting. In fact, the initiation or discontinuation of any drugs that alter urate levels (i.e., allopurinol, febuxostat, probenecid, or salicylates) may prolong the acute attack. Asymptomatic hyperuricemia should not be treated.

Corticosteroids. Systemic and intra-articular steroids are effective for the treatment of gout. Intravenous (IV) methylprednisolone (100 to 150 mg IV daily for 1 to 3 days) or intramuscular triamcinolone acetonide (60 to 80 mg daily for 1 to 3 days) is the preferred agent in critically ill patients [1]. Oral prednisone may also be effective in doses of 20 to 30 mg twice per day initially and tapered over 7 to 14 days with decrements of 10 mg every two days [1]. Potential complications of steroid treatment include hyperglycemia, fluid retention secondary to mineralocorticoid effects, and hypothalamic-pituitary-adrenal suppression. Intra-articular corticosteroid injections are an excellent choice for acute gouty arthritis if few joints are involved since systemic side effects are avoided. Steroid injections provide rapid resolution of symptoms, usually within 12 to 24 hours, but if infection is suspected, corticosteroid injection should be delayed until culture results are available. Intra-articular corticosteroids are quite effective in small joints if performed by physicians skilled in these injections. Dosing ranges from 10 to 60 mg methylprednisolone or equivalent triamcinolone, depending on the size of the joint involved.

Adrenocorticotropic Hormone. Adrenocorticotropic hormone (ACTH) has been used for more than 40 years for the treatment of gout. Dosing regimens vary, starting at 40 to 80 IU intramuscularly, subcutaneously, or intravenously 1 to 3 times a day until symptoms abate. Adverse effects include mild hyperglycemia and fluid overload. Although the overall safety profile and efficacy of ACTH are excellent, its use is limited by its lack of availability and prohibitive cost. Its anti-inflammatory effects are result of interruptions of microtubule function in multiple cell types but particularly PMNs' function in chemotaxis, adhesion, phagocytosis, and production of cytokines.

Colchicine. Colchicine is one of the established treatments for gout. Its main mechanism of action involves formation of a reversible complex with the tubulin subunit of microtubules leading to reduced activation and migration of PMNs. Oral colchicine is absorbed in the small intestine and excreted in the bile and urine, reaching a peak serum level in 2 hours. Gastrointestinal side effects, most notably diarrhea, occur in up to 80% of patients, resulting in electrolyte imbalances and fluid losses. In the critically ill patient, oral colchicine may not be feasible and is potentially toxic. Renal and hepatic insufficiencies are risk factors for colchicine related neuromyopathy and bone marrow suppression. In addition, potential drug–drug interactions, including macrolide antibiotics, HMG-CoA reductase inhibitors, fibric acid derivatives, verapamil and diltiazem, and cyclosporine may potentiate colchicine toxicities.

A recent study reports equal efficacy in reducing pain of acute gout with low dose colchicine (1.2 mg orally followed in 1 hour by another 0.6 mg orally) to traditional oral loading of colchicine (1.2 mg orally followed by 0.6 mg every hour for 6 hours) [2]. In addition, the gastrointestinal side effects are significantly reduced with the low dose regimen. Thus, if an ICU patient with an acute onset of gout has normal renal and hepatic function and is able to take oral colchicine, the low dose regimen is a reasonable choice. However, if there is renal insufficiency, dose adjustment is necessary and colchicine is probably best avoided if creatinine clearance is less than 10 mL per minute. A more appropriate use of oral colchicine is the prevention of subsequent attacks once the acute attack is treated. Dosages of 0.6 mg orally once or twice a day have been effective (again dose adjustment is necessary based on GFR) [3]. The most common side effects include nausea, diarrhea, and proximal myopathy with elevated creatinine kinase levels. The risk of myotoxicity correlates with a creatinine clearance of less than 50 mL per minute.

Intravenous colchicine has been used in the past for acute gout. However, due to numerous deaths and inappropriate use of the intravenous route, the United States Food and Drug Administration has recommended the discontinuation of production of intravenous colchicine since 2008 and it is unavailable at this time.

Nonsteroidal Anti-inflammatory Drugs. Nonsteroidal anti-inflammatory drugs (NSAIDs) are effective in the treatment of acute gout. However, the mechanism of action involves prostaglandin inhibition, which can interfere with gastric mucosal integrity and worsen renal function by reducing renal perfusion in the setting of volume contraction. NSAIDs may also cause other side effects, including decreased coronary flow and mental status changes. Although the cyclooxygenase-2 inhibitor agents offer the possibility of fewer adverse events, their safety profile is based on outpatient experience. Serious adverse effects with these newer agents have been reported. Given the fact that many patients in the ICU have some degree of renal disease and are at risk for gastrointestinal bleeding, NSAIDs are rarely a first-line agent in the treatment of gout in the ICU.

Other Microcrystalline Arthropathies

Although gout is the best-defined and most common crystalline arthropathy, several other crystalline-induced syndromes may mimic gout and cause potential diagnostic confusion. These include calcium pyrophosphate dihydrate (CPPD), BCP-hydroxyapatite, or calcium oxalate crystals.

Pathogenesis

The pathophysiology of these entities appears to be similar to that of gouty arthritis, involving a complex series of biochemical reactions that lead to an inflammatory response within the involved joint or periarticular region. Similar to gout, each of these disorders may be more common in a specific subset of ICU patients.

The acute, self-limited form of CPPD deposition (also known as *pseudogout*) may be precipitated by surgery of any type and is related to downward fluxes in serum calcium levels that lead to crystal shedding into intra-articular spaces. Attacks commonly occur several days postoperatively and often involve the knee or wrist. Severe medical illnesses, such as ischemic heart disease, cerebral infarction, and thrombophlebitis, may also provoke attacks of CPPD arthritis.

Patients on chronic intermittent peritoneal dialysis have a high incidence of acute arthritis that is secondary to CPPD or

BCP-hydroxyapatite deposition in articular cartilage. In contrast, chronic hemodialysis patients are at risk for acute arthritis from calcium oxalate crystals.

Clinical Features

Clinically, each of the above crystalline arthropathies is indistinguishable from acute gout. The presence of radiographic calcification in hyaline or articular cartilage of the involved joint (i.e., chondrocalcinosis) suggests the diagnosis of pseudogout, but the diagnosis is confirmed by visualizing weakly positively birefringent, rhomboid-shaped CPPD crystals within synovial fluid PMN under polarizing microscopy. Calcium oxalate crystals, likewise, are positively birefringent, but they are pleomorphic, bipyramidal, or rod-like in shape. Smaller BCP-hydroxyapatite crystals, however, are not visible under polarizing microscopy, and a presumptive diagnosis is made given the clinical setting, the exclusion of other diagnoses, and the occasional presence of periarticular, amorphous calcifications on radiographs.

Therapy

Therapeutic options are limited in the ICU patient if NSAIDs are contraindicated. Isolated joints can be aspirated and injected with corticosteroids once infection is excluded. Alternatively, a regimen of tapering corticosteroids similar to acute gout is effective. Pseudogout may also respond dramatically to colchicine in dosing similar to gout. Low dose colchicine is also used to prevent recurrent attacks in patients who have frequent events.

Septic Arthritis

Joint infection is the most critical diagnosis to establish and treat in any ICU patient who develops acute mono- or oligoarthritis. A delay in the diagnosis and treatment of septic arthritis may lead to destruction of articular cartilage and loss of joint function. Furthermore, a diagnosis of septic arthritis may help identify and initiate early treatment of the source of septicemia, such as endocarditis (see Chapter 80).

Pathogenesis

Risk factors for development of septic arthritis include diabetes mellitus, age over 80, skin infections, rheumatoid arthritis (RA), intravenous drug abuse, alcoholism, recent joint surgery, low socioeconomic status, and presence of prosthetic joints [4]. In addition, patients in the ICU often have multiple invasive procedures, indwelling lines, or catheters that are potential portals of infection. Whether or not these predisposing factors exist, acute septic arthritis usually develops from hematogenous seeding from another site of infection. Direct inoculation or local extension from adjacent soft tissue infection or osteomyelitis is less common. Prosthetic joints or damaged joints from rheumatoid or osteoarthritis are particularly susceptible to hematogenous seeding. Once an infection is established within a joint, a complex cascade of physiologic responses occurs that leads to a severe inflammatory reaction with subsequent cartilage degradation and bone destruction. The rapidity and severity of this process depends on the virulence of the organism and the length of time delay before appropriate antibiotics are started.

Clinical Features

Clinically, septic arthritis may be indistinguishable from crystalline arthritis or other inflammatory joint diseases. The presentation is often acute and monoarticular with physical findings of warmth, swelling, tenderness, and erythema within the confines of the joint margins, and markedly limited joint motion. The knee, hip, shoulder, elbow, and ankle are the most common joints involved. Atypical joints such as the sternoclavicular, symphysis pubis, or sacroiliac joints are common sites of infection in younger patients, or those with a history of intravenous drug use. Polyarticular infections may occur in 20% of the cases in reported studies [4], particularly in patients with rheumatoid arthritis. Fever is a variable finding and when present, it may be low grade.

High clinical suspicion remains essential to the diagnosis of septic arthritis. Unless physical examination indicates extra-articular features (e.g., cellulitis), any ICU patient with an acutely swollen, painful joint needs a diagnostic arthrocentesis to exclude infection. In the case of suspected cellulitis, appropriate antibiotics should be administered and arthrocentesis performed only if symptoms or findings do not improve within 48 hours. The diagnosis of septic arthritis is supported by an elevated white blood cell count (WBC), ESR, and CRP, but these studies cannot reliably differentiate infection from other inflammatory processes. Conversely, the absence of fever or normal ESR or CRP cannot exclude septic arthritis. Thus, synovial fluid analysis can confirm septic arthritis and identify organisms on Gram's stain or in culture. The fluid should be transferred immediately to the laboratory, both anaerobic and aerobic cultures should be ordered routinely, and special requests for fungus or other organisms that require a special growth medium (e.g., *Neisseria gonorrhoeae*) are ordered if clinically indicated. In addition, synovial fluid analysis for WBC with differential and crystal search may support a diagnosis of infection before microbiology results are available. Although leukocyte counts under 20,000 per μL have been associated with septic arthritis, the WBC generally exceeds 50,000 per μL and on occasion may be as high as 200,000 per μL with a marked PMN predominance. A meta-analysis of various laboratory studies in septic arthritis suggests that the likelihood ratio of septic arthritis increases incrementally with higher synovial leukocyte counts [5]. However, since septic arthritis has been associated with WBC as low as 2,000 per μL to 50,000 per μL, the absolute number cannot differentiate septic arthritis from other inflammatory states such as rheumatoid, psoriatic, or crystalline arthritis.

Although initial radiographs of the infected joint are often normal, baseline x-rays are useful to identify preexisting joint abnormalities and for comparison to identify subsequent changes of septic damage. MRI imaging may be helpful to evaluate joints that are difficult to assess clinically (i.e. spine, sacroiliac, or hip), bone for underlying osteomyelitis, and soft tissue for sinus tracts. Classic late radiographic findings include juxta-articular osteopenia, joint-space narrowing, or subchondral bone loss.

Therapy

Once the diagnosis of septic arthritis is either strongly suspected on clinical grounds or documented by positive Gram's stain or culture, treatment requires adequate drainage in addition to appropriate antibiotics. *N. gonorrhoeae* is the most common cause of septic arthritis in patients under the age of 30, but overall, *Staphylococcus aureus (S. aureus)*, including methicillin resistant *S. aureus* (MRSA), is the most common organism in the immunocompetent patient, followed in frequency by *Streptococcal* species. Together, these Gram-positive organisms made up 91% of septic arthritis in a prospective study [6]. Gram negative and anaerobic organisms occur less frequently but must be suspected in patients at risk (elderly, immunocompromised, recent hospitalization or surgery, prior antibiotics, and possible urogenital or abdominal infections) [4]. In the critically ill patient with multiple risk factors, broad-spectrum antibiotic coverage against staphylococcus and streptococcus, Gram-negative bacteria, and pseudomonas should be initiated until culture results are available. Fungal or mycobacterial septic arthritis is often subacute or chronic and thus unlikely to be initially considered but remains the possible cause if symptoms persist. *Candida* organisms have caused acute arthritis and the Gram stain may be positive before cultures are available. The duration of antibiotic therapy varies according to the clinical situation, but antibiotics should be continued intravenously for at least 2 weeks. Further route and duration of therapy depend on the specific type and sensitivity of identified organism and the patient's clinical response. However, the length of treatment is usually at least 4 weeks for nongonococcal septic arthritis. Please refer to Chapter 77 for appropriate antibiotic treatment and dosing for presumptive or identified infectious organisms.

Drainage of the infected joint either with serial percutaneous needle aspirations or surgical intervention is also crucial. Since there are no prospective studies comparing these options, controversy exists regarding the optimal approach. The physical removal of inflammatory cells, cellular debris, lysosomal enzymes, and bacterial byproducts reduce the potential damage to the joint. Prosthetic joints and other native joints such as hip, shoulder, wrist, finger, sacroiliac or sternoclavicular joints require immediate surgical intervention, while native septic knees may respond to serial percutaneous needle aspiration. Arthroscopy or arthrotomy has the advantage of more complete debridement of fibrin, infected synovium, and loculations. However, percutaneous drainage may be the only option in a critically ill patient who is unstable for surgery. Indications for surgical intervention include initial delay in diagnosis, established joint damage from RA or osteoarthritis, failure to sterilize the joint fluid after 3 to 5 days of antibiotics, difficult percutaneous aspirations due to loculations, or infection with Gram-negative bacterium. Thus, the ideal approach is to consult both the orthopedist and rheumatologist at the time of diagnosis to decide on optimal management.

The affected joint should be immobilized in functional position in the first few days. Once antibiotics are given and drainage has been performed, early physical therapy with passive range of motion and graduation to active range of motion will improve outcome [7].

Finally, since septic arthritis usually occurs as a consequence of bacteremia from a distant primary source of infection, investigation for these sites must be pursued. Unless an obvious site of local inoculation is present, cultures from blood, urine, sputum, indwelling lines, and catheters should be obtained before the institution of antibiotics. In addition, imaging studies such as echocardiography, tomography (CT), or gallium scanning might locate the source of infection.

Septic Arthritis in the Prosthetic Joint

Although rates of prosthetic joint infections (PJI) are generally quite low, 0.8% to 1.9% and 0.3% to 1.7% for knees and hips, respectively [8], RA patients have an increased risk of developing infected prosthetic joints. Risk factors are similar for native septic arthritis discussed previously as well as a history of prior infection of prosthetic joint at the same site or revision arthroplasty. Early infection, usually within 3 months of surgery, is usually due to *S. aureus* or more virulent organisms from direct inoculation at the time of surgery; chronic infections with less aggressive bacterium including coagulase-negative staphylococci occur often months to years after the replacement. Bacteremia with seeding of a prosthetic joint can occur anytime. Causative organisms for PJI are predominantly Gram-positive cocci (65%); aerobic Gram-negative bacilli and anaerobes contribute 10%, while 20% are polymicrobial infections [8].

Clinical features of acute PJI include localized pain, fever (occurring in $<50\%$), and elevation of ESR, while more chronic infections may present with only pain and loosening of hardware on radiograph. CRP elevation of more than 5 mg per L has a sensitivity of 95% and specificity of 62% in the diagnosis of PJI [9]. Plain radiographs cannot distinguish aseptic periprosthetic loosening from infection. Computed tomography and magnetic imaging may be distorted by ferromagnetic prostheses. The imaging of choice for the diagnosis of PJI is indium-111 labeled WBC in combination with technetium-99m-labeled sulfur colloid bone scan [10]. Synovial fluid studies are as useful in prosthetic joint infections as native joint infections. However, a synovial fluid WBC more than 1,700 cells per μL from the prosthetic knee joint or more than 4,200 cell per μL from the prosthetic hip joint with predominantly PMNs on the differential is enough to suggest infection [8]. If aspiration is not done before surgery, then intraoperative sampling of multiple periprosthetic tissue sites will increase the yield of an organism. Culture of the removed prosthesis may also provide additional microbial information.

Treatment of suspected PJI should initially cover both Gram-negative and Gram-positive organisms with a regimen such as vancomycin and an aminoglycoside until microbiology results and antibiotic sensitivities are available (see Chapter 77). Initial infectious disease consultation will help guide therapy.

Antibiotics alone without surgical intervention, however, are rarely successful. If the patient is a surgical candidate, options include: (1) resection arthroplasty, (2) one or two stage surgery with prosthesis removal and reimplantation, or (3) surgical debridement with retention of prosthesis with or without long-term oral antibiotic suppression. The first option is rarely performed unless the patient has failed previous surgical attempts at eradicating the infection or is likely to have minimal functional improvement after replacement. Chronic PJI requires resection arthroplasty with one or two stage exchanges. The latter usually entails removal of the infected prosthesis, treatment with antibiotics with or without an antibiotic loaded spacer for a period of 6 to 12 weeks, and then subsequent reimplantation. Debridement with retention of the infected prosthesis is an option only if (i) age of the prosthesis is less than 3 months; (ii) symptoms have been present for less than 3 weeks; (iii) absence of sinus tract communicating with joint space; (iv) no radiographic evidence of prosthetic loosening; (v) infection not involving *S. aureus, Pseudomonas aeruginosa*, enterococcus, fungal or multidrug resistant organisms; and (vi) absence of comorbidities such as diabetes and rheumatoid arthritis [11]. Prolonged oral antibiotics (3 months for hips and 6 months for knees) are recommended in patients treated with debridement with implant retention [8].

Hemarthrosis

In the absence of an underlying inherited disorder of coagulation, hemarthrosis in the intensive care setting is most likely a complication of anticoagulation therapy, most frequently described in patients receiving an oral anticoagulant (sodium warfarin). Since hemarthrosis may occur spontaneously in an anticoagulated patient, a history of trauma is often absent. Clinically, a patient develops a monoarticular, painful, swollen, warm, and tense effusion. A prolongation of coagulation parameters suggests the diagnosis, but diagnostic arthrocentesis is essential to confirm the diagnosis of hemarthrosis and exclude septic arthritis, crystalline disease, or other causes. When performed aseptically and carefully, arthrocentesis is safe and free of significant long-term morbidity. It is unnecessary to reverse the anticoagulant state prior to arthrocentesis.

A precise definition of hemarthrosis has not been established, but the diagnosis is suggested by a synovial fluid hematocrit exceeding 3%. Causes of hemarthrosis other than anticoagulation include trauma (especially with intra-articular fracture), blood dyscrasias, Charcot joint, synovial tumors such as pigmented villonodular synovitis or other primary or metastatic neoplasms, myeloproliferative disease, CPPD arthropathy, septic arthritis, sickle cell trait or disease, and scurvy.

Despite the fact that hemophiliac patients with repeated hemarthrosis have significant joint abnormalities, an isolated episode of spontaneous hemarthrosis has a benign prognosis. Treatment of hemarthrosis from hemophilia or other bleeding diathesis is discussed elsewhere (see Chapters 108,109, and 114). Management of spontaneous hemarthrosis from anticoagulation consists of immobilization, analgesia, and if possible, temporarily reducing or correcting clotting parameters with fresh frozen plasma if the patient is not at high risk of thromboembolism. If the patient is at high risk (i.e., prosthetic valve), allowing the INR to drift toward the lower therapeutic range is one option. Arthrocentesis may reduce the pressure of joint distension. Once the hemarthrosis improves, close monitoring of coagulation parameters to values within the therapeutic range minimizes the chance of recurrence.

ASPECTS OF RHEUMATIC DISEASES COMPLICATING INTENSIVE CARE PROCEDURES

Difficult endotracheal intubations may be encountered in patients with RA, juvenile idiopathic arthritis (JIA), ankylosing spondylitis (AS), or systemic sclerosis (SSc). Involvement of the cervical spine, temporal mandibular joints, or oral aperture may limit adequate positioning, visualization, or successful endotracheal intubation with conventional techniques. The use of fiberoptic intubation, laryngoscopy, or blind nasotracheal intubation may suffice in some instances (see Chapter 1), although a tracheostomy may be required for satisfactory tracheal cannulation (see Chapter 15), particularly in emergent situations. Potentially more serious neurological sequelae are anterior atlantoaxial subluxation or a staircase cervical subluxation that involves many cervical vertebrae.

The prevalence of atlantoaxial instability in RA patients is estimated to be anywhere from 23% to 60% depending on the subpopulation studied and is associated with duration and severity of disease [12]. This instability also occurs in certain subgroups of patients with JIA and ankylosing spondylitis. Although the majority of patients with cervical spine involvement are asymptomatic, forced manipulation of the neck (e.g., during intubation, endotracheal suctioning, nasogastric tube placement, bronchoscopy, or endoscopy) may precipitate symptoms and signs of spinal cord compression.

Cervical instability and dislocations most commonly occur at the atlantoaxial (first and second cervical vertebrae) junction due to laxity or erosion of the transverse ligament caused by synovitis. Subsequently, the odontoid (superior peg of the second cervical vertebra) moves more freely and can protrude posteriorly, particularly during neck flexion, and compress the spinal cord, lower medulla, or vertebrobasilar arteries. Fracture or erosive destruction of the odontoid may allow the atlas (first cervical vertebra) to slide posteriorly on the second cervical vertebrae, a process termed posterior atlantoaxial subluxation. Destruction of the lateral atlantoaxial joints and of the bones of the foramen magnum may allow the axis to sublux cephalad, so-called vertical subluxation. Symptoms suggestive of cervical myelopathy include Lhermitte's sign, neck pain radiating up to the occiput, paresthesias in the hands or feet, loss of arm or leg strength, and urinary incontinence or retention.

Patients at risk are identified with lateral cervical spine radiographs in flexed and extended views. The normal distance between the odontoid process and the arch of the atlantis is less than 4 mm. If this distance is exceeded, care should be taken to avoid sudden or forced neck flexion during any intensive care procedure. A soft cervical collar to maintain the neck in slight extension helps prevent sudden forced flexion and is a reminder to all caregivers that any neck manipulation should proceed with caution. Open-mouth posterior-to-anterior views will exclude odontoid fracture and severe subluxation, but MRI scanning is the best imaging procedure to exclude cord compression.

In patients with ankylosing spondylitis where multilevel cervical fusion exists, large anterior cervical osteophytes can prevent adequate visualization of the larynx or successful endotracheal intubation. Fixed cervical flexion deformities can hinder appropriate neck positioning for intubation. The ankylosed spine is often osteoporotic and brittle. Minor forces in flexing or extending the neck can result in inadvertent fracture. Thus, plain radiograph imaging with lateral views before any procedure can help establish potential barriers to endotracheal intubation and the need for fiberoptic nasotracheal intubation [13].

Patients with JIA (and RA more rarely) may have established micrognathia due to temporomandibular joint disease that restricts lower jaw motion and limits access to the oropharynx. Micrognathia may also cause upper respiratory tract obstruction and sleep apnea, both of which occur more commonly in patients with JIA. In contrast, patients with systemic sclerosis (SSc) may have facial tissue fibrosis and atrophy that reduce the oral aperture and make orotracheal intubation impossible. In these situations, early awareness of the need for nasotracheal intubation will prevent potential complications in routine or emergency endotracheal intubation.

Nearly 50% to 75% of patients with longstanding RA have involvement of the cricoarytenoid joints on CT scans, but only half have symptoms [14]. These synovial joints allow adduction and abduction of the vocal cords. Symptoms of cricoarytenoid involvement include throat pain, sensation of a foreign object in the throat, odynophagia, dysphagia, hoarseness, shortness of breath, and stridor. As a result of acute or chronic inflammation, the vocal cords may become fixed in a position of adduction, resulting in upper airway obstruction and respiratory failure. The diagnosis may be made and distinguished from recurrent laryngeal nerve paralysis, tumor, and thyroiditis by visualizing the vocal cords either by indirect laryngoscopy or fiberoptic nasopharyngoscopy. In the patient with chronically restricted motion of the cricoarytenoid joints, a superimposed insult, like an upper respiratory tract infection or trauma from intubation, may cause sufficient soft tissue swelling to cause laryngospasm or airway obstruction. Treatment of life-threatening airway obstruction includes establishing an airway by cricothyroidotomy or tracheostomy, high-dose systemic corticosteroids, systemic antirheumatic therapy, and topical aerosolized corticosteroids.

RHEUMATOID ARTHRITIS

Rheumatoid arthritis (RA) is a chronic, autoimmune, inflammatory disorder that affects synovial joints and extra-articular organ systems. The patient with RA may require admission to the ICU because of airway obstruction due to cricoarytenoid arthritis or atlantoaxial subluxation (discussed previously); septic arthritis; respiratory distress from large pleural effusions or parenchymal lung disease; cardiac dysfunction due to pericardial, myocardial, or endocardial involvement; necrotizing vasculitis; or mononeuritis. The approach to the RA patient in the ICU includes knowledge of the diverse complications of rheumatoid disease and the potential toxicities of RA medications including NSAIDs, corticosteroids, traditional disease modifying agents, and the newer biologic agents.

Pathogenesis

Rheumatoid arthritis is characterized by chronic synovial inflammation with subsequent articular cartilage and bone destruction in a genetically susceptible host. The initial triggering antigen, whether exogenous or self, has not been identified, but the subsequent CD4 T-cell activation initiates the process of recruitment of other cells to the joint space, including macrophages, neutrophils, and B cells. Fibroblast-like and macrophage-like synovial cells perpetuate synovial inflammation through elaboration of cytokines that have paracrine and autocrine activity. In addition to cytokines, the products of several cell types also induce adhesion molecules and stimulate angiogenesis. Activated synovial cells also release metalloproteinases responsible for degradation of articular cartilage and erosion of bone.

Joint Infections Complicating Rheumatoid Arthritis

One indication for admission of the RA patient to an ICU is sepsis, particularly involving joints. RA patients are more susceptible to developing septic arthritis, often polyarticular and more severe than in patients without RA. A variety of factors, including immunosuppressive drugs, general debility, immobility, and cutaneous ulcers predispose the rheumatoid patient to developing bacterial infections in other sites, which hematogenously seed inflamed rheumatoid joints. Normal protective mechanisms, PMN leukocyte bacterial killing, PMN chemotaxis, and complement and serum bactericidal activity are all decreased in the rheumatoid joint. Although joint sepsis after arthrocentesis or intra-articular steroid injection is a rare complication, infection has been reported in this context and may be more resistant to treatment.

A delay in diagnosing joint sepsis in RA patients may also contribute to their increased morbidity and mortality. Other factors include: 1) masking of joint pain and inflammation by NSAIDs, corticosteroids, and immunosuppressive agents; 2) generalized debility and malnutrition; and 3) attributing the joint inflammation to RA rather than infection by the patient or physician. Failure to recognize septic arthritis complicating RA may have disastrous effects. When a single or few joints are more inflamed than others in a rheumatoid patient, joint sepsis should be excluded by arthrocentesis, Gram's stain, and cultures of synovial fluid, blood, and other appropriate sites guided by the patient's signs and symptoms. Inspection of the skin for a possible portal of bacterial entry and a thorough general examination are of the utmost importance.

The microbiology of septic arthritis complicating RA includes a wide range of organisms, but in approximately 80% of cases, the organism is *S. aureus*. Streptococcal species are also common pathogens. Gram-negative organisms (*Pseudomonas aeruginosa*, *Escherichia coli*, *Proteus mirabilis*, and others), anaerobes, fungi, mycobacterium, and polymicrobial infection, have all been reported as causes of septic arthritis in the rheumatoid joint.

Management of septic arthritis in a rheumatoid patient is identical to patients without RA. However, the septic rheumatoid joint more frequently fails percutaneous needle aspiration. Early surgical drainage with synovectomy may be the preferred treatment since there is more proliferative synovitis and an increased tendency for loculations to develop in this population.

Pulmonary Involvement in Rheumatoid Arthritis

The respiratory system in the patient with RA can be involved in numerous ways, including upper airway, bronchi, pleura, parenchyma, vasculature, and diaphragmatic muscles. Pulmonary infections are common, particularly in the patient with poor mucociliary clearance, ineffective cough, on immunosuppressive therapy, or with associated Sjögren's syndrome. Table 193.1 summarizes respiratory tract involvement in RA and other connective tissue disorders. In addition, certain antirheumatic drugs are associated with potential pulmonary toxicities. Angioedema and bronchospasm induced or aggravated by aspirin or other NSAIDs is most common followed by hypersensitivity pneumonitis from methotrexate or sulfasalazine, or interstitial fibrosis from methotrexate.

Pleural Disease

Pleuritis and interstitial disease are the most common pulmonary manifestations of RA, and the former is most common in a subset of male patients who are seropositive and have nodules. Although involvement may be asymptomatic, acute febrile pleurisy or large pleural effusions impairing respiratory function may occur and result in ICU admission. The differential diagnoses of the pleural effusions include malignancy, pulmonary infarction, viral or bacterial infection, tuberculosis, and empyema. Infectious empyema occurs with increased frequency in patients with preexisting rheumatoid pleural effusions and should be suspected in debilitated, anemic, or hypoproteinemic patients who have been treated with corticosteroids and have persistent fever and pleural effusions. In patients on anti–tumor necrosis factor alpha (anti-TNF-α therapies), reactivation of (or new infection with) tuberculosis is of major concern and needs to be excluded with pleural biopsy.

Pleural effusions and sterile empyemas associated with RA are exudative and have characteristic features: elevated lactic dehydrogenase (often >700 IU per L), total protein (>4 g per dL), low glucose (<40 mg per dL), and pH <7.2. Other characteristics include clear yellow to green-yellow appearance, white blood cell count of 100 to 7,000 cells per μL (predominantly lymphocytes), reduced complement levels, cholesterol crystals, and immune complexes [15]. Chylous effusions may occur if necrotic subpleural nodules rupture into the pleural space.

Once infections including tuberculosis and malignancy are excluded, symptomatic pleural effusions are managed with NSAIDs and thoracentesis. In recurrent pleuritis or sterile empyema, intrapleural corticosteroids, systemic corticosteroids in moderate doses, and additional disease modifying agents are recommended. Rarely, surgical pleurodesis or decortication is required if chronic adhesive fibrothorax develops. There are no prospective trials to evaluate the efficacy of many of these recommendations [15]. High-dose corticosteroid therapy may not be effective and carries an increased risk of an empyema.

Lung Disease

ILD occurs in up to 40% to 60% of patients with RA depending on the subpopulations studied and screening tests used to make the diagnosis. In a prospective European study of newly diagnosed RA patients, the annual incidence was 4 in 1,000 patients but over 20 years, mortality was over 75% in those patients with interstitial lung disease, with the majority of deaths due to ILD [16]. Thus after infection, pulmonary disease is the second most common cause of mortality in RA patients. Pathologically, usual interstitial pneumonia(UIP) is more common than nonspecific interstitial pneumonitis (NSIP). Lymphocytic interstitial pneumonitis (LIP), organizing pneumonia (OP), and acute interstitial pneumonia are less common.

Symptoms include dyspnea on exertion, cough, and chest discomfort. Physical and laboratory findings include dry crackles, diminished diffusion capacity, and restrictive physiology, as well as desaturation with exercise. Chest radiographs may show an interstitial pattern, but high-resolution CT scanning (HRCT) is a more sensitive test in assessing pneumonitis and fibrosis. Bronchoalveolar lavage (BAL) is not particularly helpful except to rule out infection, while thoracoscopy guided lung biopsy provides the best pathologic details. Treatment of ILD due to RA is extremely challenging. Some patients may respond

TABLE 193.1

RESPIRATORY INVOLVEMENT IN CONNECTIVE TISSUE DISEASES

	Common	Rare (<10%)
Upper airway involvement		
Cricoarytenoid arthritis	RA	SLE
Laryngeal nodules	RA	
Bronchial tree		
Obliterative bronchiolitis		RA
Bronchiectasis	SSc	RA, SS, SLE
Follicular or constrictive bronchiolitis		RA, SS
Bronchiolitis obliterans with organizing pneumonia	RA	SLE, PM/DM
Parenchyma		
Interstitial lung disease	RA, SSc, SS, PM/DM	SLE
Acute pneumonitis		SLE, PM/DM
Bronchiolitis obliterans with organizing pneumonia	RA	PM/DM
Cryptogenic organizing pneumonia		RA, SLE, PM/DM, SSc
Rheumatoid nodules ± cavitation	RA	
Aspiration	SSc, PM/DM	RA
Drugs: methotrexate, sulfasalazine, minocycline		
Infections	All	
Pleura		
Pleuritis	RA, SLE	
Pleural effusions	RA, SLE	
Pleural thickening	RA	SLE
Respiratory muscle disease		
Myositis	PM/DM	RA
Diaphragm dysfunction	PM/DM	SLE
Vascular		
Pulmonary hypertension	SSc	SLE, RA, PM/DM, APS
Vasculitis	SLE	PM/DM, RA
Diffuse alveolar hemorrhage		SLE, RA, PM/DM, APS
Pulmonary Embolism	APS, SLE	

RA, rheumatoid arthritis; SLE, systemic lupus erythematosus; SSc, systemic sclerosis; SS, Sjogren syndrome; PM/DM, polymyositis/dermatomyositis; APS, antiphospholipid syndrome.

to corticosteroids alone but the progressive nature of the disease may require treatment with cytotoxic agents although it is unclear which immunosuppressant is most effective [17]. In those patients with ground glass opacities on HRCT scanning, IV cyclophosphamide is being used increasingly, although no large controlled trial exists to support this approach. Case reports on the use of biologic agents are conflicting.

Other less common manifestations of rheumatoid lung disease may require treatment in the ICU when patients develop respiratory distress. These include bronchiolitis obliterans with organizing pneumonia (BOOP), obliterative bronchiolitis (OB), cryptogenic organizing pneumonia, pulmonary vasculitis, spontaneous pneumothorax, and lung toxicity secondary to antirheumatic therapy. It is particularly important to distinguish BOOP from ILD and OB, and only lung biopsy will provide histological distinction.

Obliterative alveolitis is often characterized by the abrupt onset of dyspnea and a dry cough with inspiratory crackles, sometimes with a mid-inspiratory squeak, a clear chest radiograph or finding of hyperinflation, irreversible airflow obstruction at low volumes on pulmonary function testing, mild-to-moderate arterial hypoxemia with a respiratory alkalosis, and progressive obliteration of small airways (1 to 6 mm in diameter) with constrictive bronchiolitis [18]. The prognosis is generally poor with a fairly rapid rate of progressive airflow obstruction. Despite the lack of adequate therapeutic trials, when patients present with rapidly progressive deterioration, recommendations based on expert opinion include bronchodilators and inhaled and oral corticosteroids (1 to 1.5 mg per kg per day). Macrolides, pulse intravenous cyclophosphamide, or etanercept (with methotrexate) may be considered as second-line therapy [18]. Progression to respiratory failure is common. In contrast, BOOP is more responsive to corticosteroid therapy.

Rarely, chronic vasculitis may involve pulmonary as well as bronchial arterioles and result in pulmonary hypertension and cor pulmonale. Therapy consists of corticosteroids in combination with cytotoxic agents (see Chapter 196).

Although pulmonary manifestations of RA are frequent, they are rarely the primary reason for admission to the ICU. Infectious pneumonia is particularly frequent and the major cause of mortality in rheumatoid patients. Since the advent of TNF-α agents, atypical infections and reactivation of tuberculosis have been of great concern.

Rheumatoid Cardiac Involvement

RA may involve all structures of the heart as a result of granulomatous proliferation or vasculitis. Pericarditis, myocarditis, endocarditis (valvulitis), coronary arteritis, aortitis, and cardiac conduction abnormalities have all been reported. Cardiac involvement may be the principal reason for intensive care hospitalization, or may complicate the course of the rheumatoid patient hospitalized in the ICU for other medical or surgical problems.

Pericarditis, the most common of the rheumatoid cardiac manifestations (approximately 50% by autopsy studies) rarely causes impairment of left ventricular function. However, constrictive pericarditis or a large pericardial effusion may rarely cause cardiac tamponade. The pericardial fluid has the same characteristics as pleural fluid (see the section Pulmonary Involvement in Rheumatoid Arthritis). Pericarditis generally responds to the administration of 30 to 40 mg prednisone per day over a several-week period. Corticosteroids alone are less likely to be effective in the setting of cardiac tamponade. Pericardiocentesis should be performed early if tamponade is suspected (see Chapters 7 and 35) or if there is a question of septic or suppurative pericarditis. Aspiration of pericardial fluid may temporarily improve cardiac function, but often the viscosity of the fluid, loculations, and thickness of the pericardium necessitate pericardiectomy. In cases of constrictive pericarditis, pericardiectomy is the only effective therapy.

The myocardium may be affected by granulomatous inflammation and by vasculitis. Cardiac conduction abnormalities, including complete heart block, may develop because of subcutaneous nodules. Arteritis may affect the coronary arteries and the aorta. In patients with active systemic vasculitis, coronary arteritis may be the cause of myocardial infarction. Involvement of the aorta, either by rheumatoid granulomas or inflammation of the aortic vasa vasorum, may result in dilatation of the aortic root and aortic valvular insufficiency.

Rheumatoid arthritis patients die prematurely from cardiovascular events that include (i) ischemic heart disease, often silent; (ii) congestive failure, often in the setting of preserved ejection fraction; and (iii) sudden death. When compared to non-RA patients, these increased cardiovascular complications are not explained by traditional risk factors alone. Other factors, including poor primary or secondary preventive care and comorbid conditions along with the chronic inflammatory or immunologic state contribute to premature cardiac deaths [19]. Thus, in the ICU setting, silent cardiovascular disease with atypical presentations must be considered in the rheumatoid patient.

Rheumatoid Vasculitis

The vasculitis that complicates RA is a panarteritis with mononuclear cell infiltrates in all layers of the involved blood vessels, fibrinoid necrosis in active lesions, and thrombosis associated with intimal proliferation. Rheumatoid vasculitis tends to occur in patients with severe deforming RA, subcutaneous nodules, and high-titer rheumatoid factor, and in patients with Felty's syndrome. The clinical features of rheumatoid vasculitis are variable and include palpable purpura, cutaneous ulceration including pyoderma gangrenosum, distal arteritis ranging from fingernail-fold infarcts and splinter hemorrhages to digital gangrene, and arteritis of major organs including the bowel, kidneys, heart, lungs, liver, spleen, pancreas, and components of the nervous system in a manner similar to polyarteritis nodosa. Severe necrotizing forms of rheumatoid vasculitis, manifested as digital gangrene, intestinal bleeding or perforation, myocardial or renal infarction, and mononeuritis multiplex, are associated with a poor prognosis and are treated aggressively in a manner similar to that of polyarteritis and Wegener's granulomatosis (see Chapter 196) with high-dose corticosteroids, cytotoxic agents, and occasionally plasmapheresis.

Neurologic Complications of Rheumatoid Arthritis

All components of the nervous system can be affected by RA. The brain and meninges, spinal cord, peripheral nerves, and muscles may be involved with granulomatous inflammation in the form of rheumatoid nodules or vasculitis; the spinal cord and cranial and peripheral nerves may also be compressed by skeletal and soft tissue structures, and the nervous system may be affected by hyperviscosity syndrome and medications.

Spinal cord compression is one of the most common neurologic complications in patients with RA is discussed in previous section. Manifestations that require immediate intervention include the sensation of anterior instability of the head during neck flexion, drop attacks, loss of urinary bladder and anal sphincter control, dysphagia, vertigo, hemiplegia, dysarthria, nystagmus, changes in level of consciousness, and peripheral paresthesias without evidence of a peripheral cause. Although RA patients may have radiographic evidence of cervical subluxation without symptoms, once signs of cord compression become apparent, myelopathy may progress rapidly. For patients with manifestations of spinal cord and brainstem compression, surgical reconstruction of normal alignment and stabilization are treatments of choice. For the nonsurgical candidate, a firm collar can be used in an effort to immobilize the neck and prevent further subluxation.

SYSTEMIC LUPUS ERYTHEMATOSUS

Systemic lupus erythematosus (SLE) is an autoimmune disease characterized by excessive autoantibody production and immune complex deposition in multiple organ systems. The clinical result of these varied immune abnormalities is a disease with tremendous variation in signs and symptoms that range from arthralgias, rash, and fatigue to life-threatening renal, central nervous system (CNS), cardiac, pulmonary, or hematological manifestations. Diagnosis of SLE is based on the clinical criteria set forth by the American College of Rheumatology [20]. Mortality of SLE patients admitted to the ICU is much higher than the general ICU population (47% vs. 27%) [21]. In the ICU patient with established SLE, it is essential to differentiate problems caused directly by SLE activity from those with secondary causes such as infections, drug-induced lupus, NSAID-induced renal dysfunction, aseptic meningitis, and corticosteroid-induced psychosis. Diseases associated with SLE include avascular necrosis, hypertensive encephalopathy, pseudotumor cerebri, amyloidosis, myasthenia gravis, and thrombotic thrombocytopenic purpura. In ICU patients without a prior history of autoimmune disease, SLE should be considered in the differential diagnosis of patients presenting with acute renal failure, seizures, myocarditis, acute pulmonary deterioration, hemolytic anemia, or thrombocytopenia.

Renal Disease

Renal involvement is the major cause of disease-related mortality in SLE patients. The frequency of renal involvement ranges from 38% to nearly 80% depending on definition, but clinical lupus nephritis (LN) occurs in approximately 50% of the patients. Advances in diagnostic and therapeutic modalities have dramatically improved the survival of lupus patients with renal disease. Glomerulonephritis and progressive renal failure, however, remain major sources of morbidity and mortality. LN constitutes approximately 3% of all end-stage renal failure in patients on dialysis or requiring transplantation. Recent data from one transplant group with predominantly white patients found no difference in overall 15-year patient survival (80%) and graft survival (69%) in SLE patients compared with controls [22]. Early graft thrombosis occurred more frequently in patients with antiphospholipid antibodies (APAs) and recurrence of LN was around 8% [23].

Classification of lupus-associated glomerulonephritis (GN) is based on histopathologic, immunofluorescent, and electron microscopic changes according to the 2003 revised classification by the International Society of Nephrology and the Renal Pathology Society (ISN/RPS) classification [24]. The classification includes: Class I: mesangial GN; Class II: mesangial proliferative GN; Class III: focal proliferative GN; Class IV: diffuse proliferative GN with two subclasses, segmental and global; Class V: membranous GN; and Class VI: advanced sclerosing GN. Renal lesions are commonly pleomorphic, vary from one glomerulus to another, and temporally transition from one class to another over time. The tubulointerstitium and vasculature are often involved. Semiquantitative scoring to define activity and chronicity may provide information on prognosis and guidelines for therapeutic options. In particular, the presence of proliferative lesions and chronic lesions are associated with greater mortality.

The clinical manifestations of renal involvement vary from rapidly progressive renal failure with attendant fluid overload, to congestive heart failure or accelerated hypertension, and are common events precipitating an ICU admission. A sudden deterioration in an SLE patient's renal function warrants careful consideration of other causes of acute renal insufficiency (see Chapter 73) before attributing the deterioration to active SLE. In particular, hypovolemia, drug-induced interstitial nephritis or renal insufficiency, renal vein thrombosis, and contrast-induced acute tubular necrosis must be excluded. Physical examination may reveal evidence of SLE activity in other organ systems. Laboratory studies should include routine tests to assess renal status and fluid balance, and immunologic studies, including double-stranded DNA (dsDNA) antibody, total hemolytic complement, third (C3) and fourth (C4) complement components, and ESR. Active serologies suggest SLE flare, but normal values do not exclude active disease.

Management of LN depends on the patient's renal histopathology and functional parameters. Thus, a patient with mesangial glomerulonephritis with normal creatinine clearance requires no specific therapy, whereas a patient with increasing azotemia, active urinary sediment, and impaired clearance requires aggressive therapy. It is now established that in patients with severe glomerulonephritis (ISN/RPS class III or IV), the combination of high dose prednisone with monthly intravenous pulse cyclophosphamide (IVCY) for 6 months followed by quarterly infusions for additional 6 months stabilizes renal function and improves survival. This regimen is the standard for comparison in all other LN drug trials [25,26]. In the past few years, several trials in different populations have documented the equivalency of mycophenolate mofetil (MMF) up to 3 g per day to monthly IVCY as induction therapy for class III, IV, or V LN [27]. More recently, a large international trial conducted by the ALMS group (Aspreva Lupus Management Study) confirmed this equivalence of both induction regimens at the end of 24 weeks with a response rate of 56% in each group [28]. However, only 8% from either treatment group reached complete remission. This study also supported the racial and ethnic differences in LN and the response to therapy reported in other studies. Patients of Hispanic and African descent had a much better response to MMF than IVCY (60% vs. 38%), while whites and Asian patients responded equally to either regimen. The risk for gonadal failure was less with MMF but other toxicities such as infections were similar. Given the currently available evidence, it appears that MMF and IVCY are equivalent induction therapies for severe LN. Durability of remission is being assessed in a continuation of the ALMS trial in which responders were randomized to either MMF or azathioprine (AZA) for maintenance therapy [28]. Another recent study demonstrated better efficacy and fewer long-term toxicities in maintenance therapy with AZA or MMF rather than the traditional quarterly IVCY after initial monthly IVCY induction [29].

In an acutely ill ICU patient with LN and/or other organ system involvement, IVCY along with pulse IV methylprednisolone at 500 to 1,000 mg daily for 3 days may be the regimen of choice since many of the studies have not stratified for disease severity. The protocol for administration of IVCY therapy is outlined in Table 193.2. Dose adjustments for renal insufficiency are outlined and subsequent monthly dosing is based on nadir white blood cell counts. Another option for IVCY induction is the low dose regimen from the Euro-Lupus Nephritis Trial, which demonstrated equal efficacy and less gonadal toxicity between low dose IVCY (500 mg every 2 weeks for six doses) and high dose IVCY (500 to 750 mg per M^2 with maximum of 1,500 mg, monthly for 6 months, followed by every 3 month infusion until a year) [30]. Both groups then received AZA at 2 mg per kg per day for maintenance. The long-term outcomes measured by death, end-stage renal disease, and doubling of serum creatinine were similar in both groups after 10 years [31].

TABLE 193.2

INTRAVENOUS CYCLOPHOSPHAMIDE THERAPY (IVCY)

1. Initiate IV hydration at 200–500 mL/h
   Normal or ½ NS for 1 L over 1–2 h if CrCl >50 mL/min and depending on cardiac status. (If medical status prevents adequate hydration, MESNA can be substituted—see below.)
2. Antiemetic treatment:
   a. Ondansetron, 8 mg IV <30 min (or PO <60 min), prior to CY and then 8 mg every 8 h for 24 h
   b. Granisetron, 1–2 mg IV <30 min (or <60 min PO) prior to CY and then every 12 h PO for 24 h
3. MESNA (for CrCl <50 mL/min or inadequate prehydration due to cardiopulmonary status)
   Give 60% of total CY dose in divided doses: Infuse over 15 min 20% of CY dose (mixed in 50 mL of D_5 W) 30 min prior to CY and repeat same doses 4 and 8 h following CY.
4. Cyclophosphamide: Initial dose is 500–750 mg/M^2 in 250 mL NS over 60 min. Subsequent dose is based on nadir WBC obtained at days 7, 10, 14 after infusion.
   Dose adjustments
   a. CrCl 10–50 mL/min: 75% of CY dose
   b. CrCl <10 mL/min: 50% of CY dose
   c. Hemodialysis patients: 50% of CY dose after dialysis
   d. Subsequent month dose: increase or decrease by 10%–20% of previous dose
5. Posthydration fluid is identical to prehydration. Monitor adequate urine output and encourage frequent voiding for 24 h after IVCY. In patients without indwelling Foley catheter, avoid CY infusion after 4 PM to reduce prolonged bladder contact with CY metabolites over night.

CY, cyclophosphamide; D_5 W, dextrose 5% in water; IV, intravenous; MESNA, sodium 2-mercaptoethane sulfonate, NS, normal saline; PO, by mouth; WBC, white blood cells.

Membranous GN (Class V), which constitutes 20% of LN, is less aggressive than Class IV GN. While renal survival rate is at 80% at 10 years, it is still associated with significant comorbidities of hyperlipidemia, cardiovascular and thromboembolic diseases [32]. Angiotensin-converting enzyme (ACE) inhibitors have been used successfully to reduce proteinuria. Treatment with corticosteroids, AZA, and cyclosporine has been studied in small series. More recently, the pooled subset of Class V patients from two prospective randomized studies on treatment of GN demonstrated equivalent efficacy and safety profile of MMF and IVCY [33]. Adjunctive renoprotective therapies that include aspirin, statins, ACE inhibitors, or angiotensin receptor blockers should also be instituted.

Advances in biologic therapies for RA and psoriatic arthritis have also stimulated investigations for SLE. Initial open label studies and case reports suggest promising results with the use of rituximab (RTX), an anti-CD20 B-cell depleting monoclonal antibody, for reducing SLE activity. Surprisingly, a randomized trial comparing RTX to placebo with a background of MMF for active proliferative LN revealed no additional benefit, and another study on active nonrenal SLE was also negative [34,35]. Trials of other potential therapies are underway, including a human monoclonal against B-lymphocyte stimulator (BLyS).

Neuropsychiatric Disease

Neuropsychiatric systemic lupus erythematosus (NPSLE), which encompasses involvement of the central, peripheral, and autonomic nervous systems along with psychiatric syndromes, occurs in 25% to 80% of SLE patients depending on the criteria applied or methods used for diagnosis. Although NPSLE was considered a poor prognostic indicator in the older literature, it does not seem to have significant impact on survival rates. Active CNS disease contributed primarily or secondarily to death in only small percentage of patients.

Neuropsychiatric manifestations of SLE can be classified into central versus peripheral nervous system involvement. Due to the limitations of the ACR classification criteria of CNS involvement, an ad hoc neuropsychiatric lupus nomenclature committee of the American College of Rheumatology defined 19 manifestations that included 12 in the CNS and 7 in the peripheral nervous system [36] (Table 193.3). The wide range of prevalence for the more diffuse CNS syndromes (cognitive dysfunction, anxiety, acute confusional states, and psychosis) and headache is due to the definition, criteria, or diagnostic parameters used in reported studies. This proposed nomenclature attempts to define the spectrum of NPSLE but is not a substitute for clinical diagnosis. An individual SLE patient may have multiple neuropsychiatric manifestations and these can develop prior to the formal diagnosis of SLE or during an inactive disease state. Frank psychosis is relatively rare, estimated at 5%. Often, it is difficult to separate active lupus psychosis from other causes such as functional disorders, uremia, illicit drugs, metabolic disturbances, medications, or infections.

Focal central nervous system disease, including seizures that occur in 15% to 35% of SLE patients, can antedate the diagnosis of SLE or develop any time during the disease course. Grand mal seizures are the most common, but essentially all types have been reported. Secondary causes of seizures must be sought since in several prospective studies of SLE patients with neurologic events, a majority of seizures were due to associated infection, uremia, hypertension, and metabolic abnormalities.

Cerebrovascular accidents (5% to 18%) include infarctions secondary to intracranial hemorrhage or arteritis, thrombosis from lupus anticoagulant (LAC) or APA-associated hypercoagulable states, or embolism from Libman-Sacks endocarditis. Movement disorders including chorea, ataxia, and hemiballismus are rare (<1%) [37]. Transverse myelitis is an unusual but devastating complication of SLE characterized by acute or subacute paraplegia or quadriplegia associated with sensory level deficit and loss of sphincter control. Cerebrospinal fluid (CSF) analysis reveals pleocytosis, low CSF glucose, and high CSF protein. T2-weighted magnetic resonance imaging (MRI) usually demonstrates increased signal intensity and cord edema. Meningitis, usually infectious, may develop in SLE patients. However, aseptic meningitis can be idiopathic or secondary to administration of ibuprofen or AZA.

Peripheral nervous system syndromes include cranial neuropathies (4% to 49%) such as facial palsies and ocular muscle dysfunction. Pure sensory or motor abnormalities based on electromyography/nerve conduction studies (EMG/NCS) occur in up to 47% but plexopathy, Guillain-Barré syndrome, and autonomic neuropathy are rare.

The differentiation of NPSLE from other CNS disorders is difficult and remains a process of elimination. CSF pleocytosis and low glucose require exclusion of infections. Electroencephalography generally reveals diffuse brain wave slowing, but focal activity suggests seizures. Serum antiribosomal P antibodies are associated with lupus psychosis. The gold standard for imaging the central nervous system in SLE is conventional MRI with gadolinium. CT scans are less sensitive and should be reserved for patients in whom MRI is contraindicated or for emergent situations to document bleed, infarct, cerebral edema, or masses. Focal lesions in the subcortical white matter

TABLE 193.3

NEUROPSYCHIATRIC MANIFESTATIONS OF SYSTEMIC LUPUS ERYTHEMATOSUS

Central nervous system
Diffuse neuropsychiatric syndromes
Cognitive dysfunction (50%–80%)
Anxiety disorders (7%–70%)
Mood disorders (14%–57%)
Psychosis as defined by *DSM-IV* related to medical condition (5%–8%)
Acute confusional state (4%–7%)
Focal neurological syndromes
Headache (24%–72%): range from migraine, tension, or benign intracranial hypertension
Seizures (15%–35%): grand mal, petit mal, temporal lobe, focal
Cerebrovascular disorders (5%–18%): infarcts, transient ischemic attacks
Movement disorders (<1%): chorea
Transverse myelitis (<1%)
Demyelinating syndrome (<1%)
Aseptic meningitis (<1%)
Peripheral nervous system
Peripheral neuropathy
Polyneuropathy (3%–28%)
Mononeuropathy, single or multiplex
Plexopathy (<1%)
Cranial neuropathies (4%–49%)
Acute inflammatory demyelinating polyradiculoneuropathy (Guillain-Barré syndrome) <1%
Autonomic neuropathy (<1%)
Myasthenia gravis (<1%)

Adapted from The ACR nomenclature and case definitions for neuropsychiatric lupus syndromes. *Arthritis Rheum* 42:599–608, 1999; Hanly JG. Neuropsychiatric lupus. *Rheum Dis Clin N Am* 31:273, 2005.

are the most common MRI findings and correlate with ischemic changes. Changes in the gray matter that brighten on T2-weighted imaging suggest more acute events and may improve with therapy. However, it is often difficult to distinguish acute from chronic MRI lesions, and subcortical lesions are found in up to 50% of patients without any neuropsychiatric symptoms. Angiography is invasive and rarely results in an accurate diagnosis of active CNS lupus. Since the sensitivity of MRI in patients with cognitive or affective symptoms is low, additional imaging with single-photon emission computerized tomography (SPECT), which measures functional cerebral blood flow, is attractive. Although sensitivity is high (positive in 86% to 100% of patients with major NPSLE manifestations), specificity is low since nearly half of SLE patients without neuropsychiatric involvement have positive SPECT scans [38]. Magnetic resonance angiography is not sensitive enough to delineate the smaller vessels involved in NPSLE. Newer imaging techniques such as magnetic resonance spectroscopy, magnetic transfer imaging, and perfusion and diffusion weighted imaging are still viewed only as research tools and their roles in assessment of NPSLE remain to be determined.

Management of SLE patients with neuropsychiatric manifestations should focus on specific neurologic symptoms. Non-SLE causes of CNS disease, including infections, uremia, hypertension, metabolic disturbances, hypoxia, or drug toxicities, must be identified and treated appropriately. If steroid psychosis is suspected, a brief doubling of the steroid dose for 3 days may exclude the possibility of a diffuse CNS syndrome. If no improvement or evidence of active lupus is noted, the steroid dose should be tapered. Seizures are treated with appropriate anticonvulsant medications. Status epilepticus is treated with anticonvulsants and high-dose steroids. Psychotic patients should receive antipsychotic agents. High-dose steroids have been recommended for neuropsychiatric lupus; dosages range from 1.0 to 1.5 mg per kg per day, or its equivalent. In severe cases, pulse IV methylprednisolone in a dose of 1,000 mg per day for 3 days is preferred. As for immunosuppressive agents, few prospective studies of treatment of NPSLE have been performed. A recent Cochrane database review of therapy for neuropsychiatric lupus found only one controlled clinical trial that suggested better outcomes with monthly IVCY than steroids alone [39,40]. Limited case reports of rituximab therapy in NPSLE suggest efficacy but no randomized studies are available. Transverse myelitis has been treated successfully with pulse methylprednisolone, IVCY, and plasmapheresis.

Pulmonary Disease

The pleuropulmonary manifestations of SLE are common and can involve the pleura, parenchyma, vasculature, diaphragm, or airways (see Table 193.1). Acute pulmonary symptoms can be the initial presentation of SLE that results in an ICU admission, while the prevalence of long-term lung damage (11.6% by 10 years of disease duration) can contribute to the SLE morbidity and mortality [41].

Pleuritis with or without effusions has been reported in 30% to 50% of patients with SLE, depending on the method of study (i.e., clinical history, radiograph findings, or autopsy findings) [42]. Pleural effusions are usually small and bilateral, but massive collections can occur. Thoracentesis is indicated when the etiology of the fluid is uncertain or if respiratory compromise is present. Pleural fluid is characteristically exudative with high protein, pH more than 7.35, and glucose normal or slightly decreased in contrast to the uniformly low glucose and pH seen in rheumatoid pleural effusions. White blood cell counts are elevated and consist predominantly of PMNs. The presence of lupus erythematosus cells on Wright stain is infrequent but highly specific for SLE. Antinuclear antibodies (ANAs) are frequently present in pleural fluids. Mild pleuritis usually responds to NSAIDs or low-dose corticosteroids (0.5 mg per kg per day prednisone or its equivalent). The latter is used only after infection has been excluded.

Acute lupus pneumonitis (ALP), although uncommon (0% to 14%), can be life threatening [42] and may be the initial presentation of SLE. It cannot be differentiated from other forms of bronchopneumonia, and thus infectious etiologies should be excluded by appropriate studies. Clinically, patients present with fever, severe dyspnea, tachypnea, and hypoxemia. Chest radiographs reveal patchy alveolar infiltrates, usually basilar in location. Mortality is as high as 50%. Transbronchial brushings with biopsies and bronchoalveolar lavage may help distinguish infections from acute immunologically mediated pneumonitis. High frequency of anti-SSA/SSB antibodies has been associated with ALP. Given the poor prognosis, therapy requires high-dose corticosteroids (1 to 2 mg per kg per day) or pulse IV methylprednisolone (1,000 mg IV daily for 3 days) along with broad-spectrum antibiotics until final cultures return. Case reports suggest the use of IVCY, plasmapheresis, or immunoglobulins in patients who respond poorly to steroids.

Pulmonary hemorrhage is a rare but potentially fatal complication. Patients characteristically present with acute dyspnea, tachycardia, severe hypoxemia, rales, sudden drop in hematocrit, and hemoptysis. Rarely, diagnosis is delayed due to the absence of hemoptysis. BAL provides the most reliable confirmation with the presence of bloody fluid, hemosiderin-laden macrophages, purulent sputum, and absence of pathogenic organisms on culture and Gram stain. Pathologic findings include intra-alveolar hemorrhage sometimes associated with interstitial pneumonitis or capillaritis. Immunopathologic studies may reveal granular deposition of immunoglobulin G (IgG) in alveolar septal walls and pulmonary vessels, thus suggesting a possible immune complex–mediated process. Therapy is generally aggressive with IV methylprednisolone at 1,000 mg daily for 3 days followed by tapering high-dose oral (1 mg per kg per day) corticosteroids. The addition of IVCY should be considered in patients who are critically ill or fail pulse corticosteroids. Plasmapheresis has been added in case reports, but whether it offers any additional benefit is unclear. Mortality remains high at 80% despite such treatment. (See Chapter 53 for an in-depth discussion of intrapulmonary hemorrhage and pulmonary-renal syndromes.)

The prevalence of ILD is less than 3% in several studies and may occur before or after ALP. Patients usually present with dyspnea on exertion, productive cough, pleuritis, and rales. Pulmonary function tests reveal a restrictive pattern and marked reduction in diffusing capacity. High-resolution thin-section CT may differentiate earlier-stage alveolitis from end-stage fibrosis. The presence of dense alveolar opacities or "ground-glass" appearance suggests active inflammation and may guide therapy. Treatment for ILD is challenging, and there are no prospective randomized trials. Therapy for symptomatic disease begins with high-dose corticosteroid therapy and again, IVCY or AZA has been used in clinically progressive ILD.

Pulmonary arterial hypertension (PAH) in SLE is less common in SLE than other connective tissue diseases and is estimated at 0.9% [43]. Pathologically, changes of intimal thickening and fibrosis, medial hypertrophy, altered elastic laminae, and periadventitial fibrosis have been similar to changes seen in idiopathic pulmonary hypertension. Necrotizing arteritis has been reported. Patients usually present with severe dyspnea on exertion and fatigue. Patients with PAH have a greater frequency of Raynaud's phenomenon than SLE patients without PAH (75% vs. 25%) [44]. In addition, the prevalence of APAs is higher in SLE-associated PAH than in other connective tissue diseases with PAH (47% vs. 19%) [45]. Because symptoms often develop late in the clinical course, assessment with Doppler echocardiography is useful to monitor for progressive disease requiring therapy.

Therapy for primary pulmonary hypertension is evolving rapidly with the use of IV prostacyclin (epoprostenol), a prostacyclin analog (iloprost), and endothelin-receptor antagonist (bosentan). IV prostacyclin has provided significant benefit in idiopathic PAH, and these therapies have been applied to PAH secondary to systemic sclerosis and less so SLE (also see the section Systemic Sclerosis). Sildenafil (a phosphodiesterase isoenzyme 5 inhibitor that enhances endothelial nitric oxide and cyclic GMP, resulting in selective pulmonary, bronchial, and coronary artery vasodilation) is effective for lupus-related PAH [46]. Calcium channel blockers are ineffective. A retrospective, open-labeled study compared the use of IVCY alone versus IVCY with vasodilator therapy in patients with SLE-related PAH. The patients given IVCY alone had less severe PAH (New York Heart Association, Class II/III) and 50% responded [47]. It is postulated that there may be a role of immune or inflammatory mechanisms in PAH associated with connective tissue disorders. This is an intriguing but yet not proven pathogenesis.

Pulmonary embolism and peripheral vasoocclusive disease are well-known risks in SLE. One prospective study documented the risk of deep vein thrombophlebitis at approximately 12%, with a 9% risk for pulmonary embolism. The risk of thromboembolic events is increased in patients with LAC and APAs (see "Antiphospholipid Syndrome" section).

Other rare pulmonary syndromes occur in SLE. Dyspnea from shrinking lung syndrome can be either acute or chronic and has a prevalence of 0.9% [42]. Postulated mechanisms include myopathy of respiratory skeletal muscles or diaphragm, phrenic neuropathy, or pleural inflammation. Pulmonary function tests reveal reduced total lung volumes with a restrictive pattern while chest radiographs reveal low lung volumes. Acute reversible hypoxemia, possibly secondary to pulmonary leukocyte aggregation, has been described in acutely ill SLE patients. Patients present with severe hypoxemia, hypocapnia, and increased alveolar-arterial PO_2 gradient without obvious parenchymal lung disease. Treatment with high dose glucocorticoids improves oxygenation. Cricoarytenoid or laryngeal involvement causing upper airway obstruction varies from 0.3% to 30% [42]. Bronchiectasis is common but usually clinically asymptomatic.

Cardiac Disease

Cardiovascular involvement in SLE ranges from 29% to 66%. This tremendous range reflects whether data is based on clinical parameters or pathologic findings at autopsy. Often, the latter studies document significant findings in the heart without clinical correlation. However, a multisite international SLE cohort study confirmed that circulatory disease (including cardiac, arterial, and cerebral vascular disease) is the major cause of mortality [48].

Pericardial disease is by far the most common cardiac manifestation of SLE (see Chapter 35) but less common than lupus pleuritis. Subclinical pericarditis is often documented only at autopsy. Pericarditis usually presents in association with other organ system activity, rather than as an initial manifestation of SLE. Classic symptoms include an anterior or substernal pleuritic chest pain that is characteristically relieved by leaning forward. A pericardial rub may be heard. Although objective radiographic, electrocardiogram (ECG), and echocardiographic findings of pericarditis are similar to idiopathic pericarditis, some patients may have relatively normal findings.

Life-threatening complications of pericarditis include cardiac tamponade and constriction. Both entities are rare; the incidence of tamponade is reported at 1% to 2.5% while constriction is described in case reports [49]. Since hemodynamically significant pericarditis is rare, pericardiocentesis fluid data are limited. Typically, pericardial fluid is exudative with high protein and normal-to-low glucose, compared with serum. The total WBC counts from various reports have ranged from 544 to 199,600 cells per μL, with predominantly PMN cells. Thus, suppurative pericarditis becomes a significant and important differential in SLE patients with pericarditis. Other reported pericardial fluid features include low or absent complement levels, lupus erythematosus (LE) cells on Wright stains, and positive ANA titers, but none of these findings can differentiate infectious from lupus pericarditis. Constrictive pericarditis may develop after successful treatment of pericarditis with or without corticosteroids.

Once other causes of pericarditis, including uremia, drugs, or viral infections, have been eliminated, hemodynamically stable but symptomatic pericarditis can be successfully treated with NSAIDs or, occasionally, moderate dose (15 to 30 mg per day) oral corticosteroids. If fever is present and the etiology of the pericardial effusion is not clear, a diagnostic pericardiocentesis may be necessary to rule out bacterial or opportunistic infections. Hemodynamically compromising effusions require pericardiocentesis and high-dose IV corticosteroids (e.g., equivalent of 1 mg per kg per day of prednisone). IVIg has been used for the treatment of life-threatening pericarditis. If effusions recur despite the use of high-dose steroids, repeat drainage, pericardial window, or even pericardial stripping may be required.

Another common cardiac manifestation of SLE is valvular heart disease involving the mitral, aortic, or tricuspid valves, often asymptomatic and picked up on echocardiography. Thickened leaflets are common findings but nonbacterial, verrucous lesions (Libman-Sacks endocarditis) may result in embolic events, secondary infectious endocarditis, or valvular insufficiency or stenosis. At autopsy, 15% to 60% of SLE patients have lesions composed of immune complexes, fibrin, platelets, and fibrotic changes on the ventricular surface of the mitral valve (and less commonly, aortic valve), ventricular endocardium, chordae tendineae, and papillary muscle. Clinically, the presence of these lesions does not correlate with murmurs. Prevalence varies from 11% by transthoracic echocardiogram to 43% by transesophageal approach [50]. If significant valvular dysfunction occurs, valve repair or replacement may be required, but complications include rapid calcification of the repaired valve or bioprosthesis. Ongoing anticoagulation is recommended in some cases.

Since the mid-1980s, the presence of Libman-Sacks endocarditis has been associated with the presence of APAs in SLE and primary antiphospholipid syndrome (APS). However, other studies have not confirmed this association in all patients. Whether valvular lesions associated with APA are different in morphology and location remains unclear. Lifelong anticoagulation is indicated if thromboembolic events occur.

Myocardial involvement in SLE is the least frequent manifestation of cardiac disease and should be categorized as primary or secondary. Primary myocarditis is rare, clinically occurring in 2.1% to 14.0% of SLE patients [51]. *Myocarditis* has been defined as unexplained tachycardia, congestive heart failure, ventricular arrhythmias, conduction defects, ST- or T-wave changes, or cardiomegaly without evidence of valvular or pericardial disease. Congestive heart failure from myocarditis is rare and is estimated to occur in 4% of cases. In most studies cardiac function was evaluated by echocardiography, thallium stress tests, and, rarely, invasive hemodynamic studies. Secondary myocardial dysfunction in SLE includes systemic hypertension, valvular disease, pulmonary disease, coronary artery ischemia (see following discussion), drug toxicity, and amyloidosis. These secondary causes are often more important than true lupus myocarditis. Management of patients with evidence of carditis rests on distinguishing primary from secondary disorders. In the rare patient who does have myocarditis from SLE, high-dose corticosteroids are indicated. Data regarding the use of immunosuppressive agents is scarce.

Primary coronary artery involvement in SLE includes embolic events, thromboses, or a true vasculitis of the vessels as opposed to secondary changes of premature atherosclerosis. Coronary arteritis is rare and difficult to distinguish from atherosclerosis on arteriographic studies unless repetitive studies are performed. In a prospective study of 100 SLE patients, 5% of those with clinical ischemic symptoms responded to increases in steroid dosage, suggesting active arteritis [51]. This can occur in the absence of extracardiac SLE activity. Thrombosis associated with APAs may contribute to myocardial ischemia.

Myocardial infarction from accelerated atherosclerosis, however, occurs more frequently in SLE patients and especially in the age group between 35 to 44 years. Circulatory diseases including heart disease, arterial disease, and cerebral vascular events is the major cause of death in a large multinational SLE cohort, with a standardized mortality ratio (ratio of deaths observed to deaths expected) of 1.7 [48]. SLE patients in the Nurses' Health Study had a more than twofold age adjusted relative risk for cardiovascular disease [52]. Another large lupus cohort reports 9% to 10% incidence of atherosclerotic disease [53]. The mean age of these patients was 48 years, and lupus was quiescent at the time of angina or myocardial infarction. Subclinical atherosclerotic disease is estimated at 37% to 43% of SLE patients based on arterial calcifications by ultrasound or electronic beam CT. Traditional risk factors are more prevalent in the SLE population but SLE is also an additional major risk. Other identified factors include hyperlipidemia, older age at SLE onset, duration of SLE, hypertension, and duration of corticosteroid use.

The management of SLE patients with acute myocardial ischemia initially should be similar to any patient with atherosclerotic coronary artery disease. However, the etiology of the ischemia must be determined since management of coronary arteritis differs from management of atherosclerotic disease. Evidence of extracardiac SLE activity may be helpful. Laboratory tests, including ANA, anti-dsDNA, complement levels, complete blood count with differential and platelet counts may provide some indicators of SLE activity. LAC and APAs should be checked. ECG, echocardiogram, and thallium stress tests do not distinguish arteritis from atherosclerosis. Coronary arteriogram may be helpful in separating thrombosis and vasculitis from atherosclerosis. However, arteriographic distinction of the latter two may be difficult. If arteriography reveals thrombosis without evident atherosclerosis and the presence of APAs is documented, therapy should consist of anticoagulation and antiplatelet medications.

Conduction abnormalities and arrhythmias due to SLE are usually clinically insignificant. The incidence of atrioventricular nodal block is estimated at 5%. Sinus tachycardia without underlying pathology (fever, dehydration, congestive heart failure, thyroid disease, drug abuse) may be a subtle manifestation of lupus activity. If acute conduction disease is suspected clinically to be secondary to myocarditis or arteritis, a short trial of corticosteroids could be initiated in the hemodynamically compromised patient.

Hematologic Disease

Hematological abnormalities constitute one of the major criteria for SLE. These include hemolytic anemia, thrombocytopenia, leukopenia, and lymphopenia. Anemia is present in 50% of SLE patients, with anemia of chronic disease being the most common etiology [54]. Other causes of anemia include iron deficiency (from menses, gastrointestinal bleeding, or poor iron absorption), autoimmune hemolytic anemia (AIHA), drug induced (cyclophosphamide or AZA), pure red cell aplasia, and chronic renal insufficiency. Rarely, other syndromes including thrombotic thrombocytopenia purpura and macrophage activation syndrome have been reported in SLE patients who have more than two cell lines affected [55].

Only 8% to 28% of lupus patients develop AIHA sometime during the course of their disease. While 18% to 65% of SLE patients have a positive direct Coombs assay, significant hemolytic anemia develops in only 10% [54]. The presence of warm IgG autoantibodies and complement on the red cell surface is characteristic of SLE AIHA. Clinically, AIHA is accompanied by an elevated reticulocyte count and indirect bilirubin and decreased haptoglobin levels. Severe hemolytic anemia, defined as hemoglobin less than 8 g per dL, is often associated with concomitant seizures, nephritis, serositis, and other cytopenias [56]. In addition, 74% of patients with AIHA will have APAs. Over 75% to 96% of patients with AIHA respond rapidly to high-dose corticosteroids (60 to 100 mg per day prednisone orally or with intravenous methylprednisolone at 1.5 mg per kg per day) [57,58]. Prednisone is tapered slowly after 3 weeks, based on laboratory results. If active hemolysis persists after 3 weeks, other therapeutic modalities include danazol, dapsone, immunosuppressive agents, and splenectomy; however, splenectomy induces permanent remission in fewer than 50% of patients. Combination of high-dose steroids and danazol, 800 to 1,200 mg per day, is an alternative treatment for severe AIHA, with subsequent gradual steroid tapering. One retrospective study of SLE patients treated for AIHA suggests that danazol was most effective in long-term treatment [58,59]. The efficacy of IVIg is short term and not sustained. Uncontrolled trials or case reports with AZA, cyclophosphamide, plasmapheresis, or rituximab have shown therapeutic response.

Leukopenia, defined as a total white blood cell count of less than 4,000 per μL, occurs in 50% to 60% of SLE patients, but associated infectious complications are rare unless CD4 counts are below 200. In the febrile, severely neutropenic patient, granulocyte-stimulating factor has been used. *Lymphopenia*, defined as counts lower than 1,500 per μL, is seen in 84% of SLE patients during active disease.

Thrombocytopenia, or platelet counts lower than 100,000 per μL, is observed in 20% to 40% of SLE patients and is severe (less than 50,000 per μL) in 10% of patients. Idiopathic thrombocytopenic purpura (ITP) may be the initial presentation of SLE. In evaluating any patient with thrombocytopenia, underlying causes including drug toxicities, ineffective thrombopoiesis, congestive splenomegaly, dilutional effects, and abnormal platelet destruction by disseminated intravascular coagulation (DIC), thrombotic thrombocytopenic purpura (TTP), hemolytic-uremic syndrome (HUS), vasculitis, drug-induced infection, or hematological excluded. The pathologic mechanism is usually antiplatelet antibodies, with resultant splenic sequestration and decreased platelet life span, although there is association with elevated APA as well. A bone marrow biopsy is helpful in distinguishing various forms of thrombocytopenia. SLE-associated ITP is characterized by an increased number of megakaryocytes.

Once TTP, HUS, DIC, and drug toxicities are excluded, therapy of severe SLE-associated ITP (less than 50,000 per μL) is similar to that of idiopathic autoimmune thrombocytopenia. Corticosteroid therapy at 1 mg per kg per day is the recommended initial therapy. Subsequent tapering is guided by platelet counts. Administration of IVIg may result in a rapid increase in platelet counts. Recommended doses range from 0.4 to 1.0 g per day or 6 to 15 mg per kg per day for 4 to 7 days, but success at maintaining platelet counts is variable. Splenectomy is an option for patients who fail medical therapy, although sustained remission is seen in only 64% of patients after splenectomy [60]; thus, the long-term benefit of splenectomy is still questioned. For refractory disease, danazol, 800 to 1,200 mg per day alone or in conjunction with corticosteroids, has been effective in several studies [58]. Immunosuppressive agents include various combinations of vincristine or vinca-loaded platelets, cyclophosphamide, and AZA. Anecdotal evidence and open case reports suggest that rituximab (RTX) is effective for intractable disease [61].

Lupus anticoagulant (LAC) interferes with the activation of prothrombin activator complex (factors Xa and V, Ca^{2+}, and phospholipid) of the intrinsic and extrinsic pathways. The laboratory findings are markedly prolonged partial thromboplastin time and normal or mildly prolonged prothrombin time that cannot be corrected by mixing with normal plasma. In addition, patients may also have false-positive reactions in the test for syphilis (VDRL). (Please see the section Antiphospholipid Syndrome for clinical details.) Although many SLE patients have both LAC and APA, subsets of patients have only one or the other laboratory abnormality.

Gastrointestinal Disease

The gastrointestinal involvement in SLE is not frequently considered because many gastrointestinal symptoms can be attributed to complications of drug therapy, particularly salicylates, NSAIDs, corticosteroids, hydroxychloroquine, and AZA. SLE-related gastrointestinal disease varies from of 8% to 22% and includes serositis, mesenteric vasculitis or thrombosis, pancreatitis, cholecystitis, inflammatory bowel disease, protein losing enteropathy, intestinal pseudo-obstruction, and pneumatosis intestinalis [62,63].

The most serious but rare (<1%) gastrointestinal complication of SLE is mesenteric vasculitis or thrombosis with subsequent large or small intestinal ischemia. The severity and extent of involvement vary and symptoms may be chronic or acute in presentation. Intestinal involvement ranges from segmental edema or ulcerations to perforations. Evaluation should include plain films, paracentesis (to rule out perforation or bacterial peritonitis), CT scans, or angiography. Although features of dilated bowel, bowel wall edema or enhancement, or edema of the mesentery or its vessels are nonspecific, multiple vessel involvement, often in the areas of ileum and jejunum, is found in SLE mesenteric vasculitis [64]. However, angiographic results may be normal due to small vessel disease. Direct visualization with endoscopy or colonoscopy may also provide useful information.

Lupus peritonitis is less devastating but often quite dramatic in presentation. Peritoneal fluid may be present, and is usually transudative and sterile with a low cell count. Other causes of ascites must be ruled out, including constrictive pericarditis, nephrotic syndrome, and spontaneous bacterial peritonitis. Pancreatitis attributed to active SLE is rare and more often related to usual causes of pancreatitis in non-SLE patients (e.g., drugs, hepatobiliary infection, alcohol, etc.) [63]. In a recent report, protein losing enteropathy and intestinal pseudo-obstruction were the most common gastrointestinal manifestations in hospitalized SLE patients [62].

Management of the SLE patient with abdominal pain does not differ significantly from that for non-SLE patients. In patients with mild to moderate pain with a chronic course, medications and intercurrent disease should be considered first as the cause of pain and surgical consult obtained. If no etiology is found, peritonitis should be considered and treated with a moderate increase in steroids. In patients who present acutely, supportive care should be started and appropriate laboratory and imaging studies performed. Paracentesis should be done to exclude perforated viscus or infection. A therapeutic trial of high-dose steroids can then be instituted if mesenteric vasculitis is suspected. Rapid (12 to 48 hours) response usually is consistent with vasculitis or peritonitis, although complete response is often delayed; if a patient deteriorates clinically, exploratory laparotomy is necessary. If studies suggest mesenteric vasculitis, IVCY may be necessary along with the corticosteroids.

Drug-Induced Lupus

The syndrome of drug-induced lupus (DIL) should be considered in ICU patients if systemic symptoms of fever, arthralgias, arthritis, pleuropericarditis, or, less commonly, rash develop. Because many ICU patients receive medications that potentially induce SLE (Table 193.4), the diagnosis must be excluded. Although some medications, particularly procainamide, hydralazine, and TNF-α inhibitors, produce positive ANA tests, this does not necessarily imply that drug-induced lupus is present. Symptoms typically develop several months after the institution of the offending medication. Although CNS and renal manifestations are rare, case reports of more atypical drug-induced lupus have been reported. Males and females are equally susceptible. DIL is more common in older patients, except for minocycline related DIL. Laboratory values reveal an elevated ESR, mild leukopenia or thrombocytopenia, and positive ANA; antihistone antibodies are present in 90% of patients; and specific antibodies to dsDNA and Smith (Sm) antigen are uncommon. However, TNF-α inhibitors such as etanercept or infliximab have been associated with anti-dsDNA, anti-Ro, anti-Sm, and antineutrophil cytoplasmic antibodies (ANCA) [65]. Discontinuation of the offending medication results in gradual diminution of symptoms that may last as long as a year. NSAIDs or low-dose steroids may control the symptoms, and in patients with severe organ system involvement, treatment is similar to idiopathic lupus.

Most rheumatologists believe that patients with idiopathic SLE who require hydralazine, procainamide, isoniazid, phenytoin, beta-blockers, or other medication that can potentially induce lupus can take these medications. TNF-α inhibitors, however, are relatively contraindicated in SLE. It is advisable to document the clinical and serologic status of the patient before starting the medication.

ANTIPHOSPHOLIPID SYNDROME

Antiphospholipid syndrome (APS) is defined by vascular thrombosis or pregnancy complications in the presence of moderate-to-high titer IgG or IgM anticardiolipin antibodies (APAs), lupus anticoagulant (LAC), or high titer anti-β_2 glycoprotein-I antibody, documented at least twice 12 or more weeks apart (Table 193.5). Other features often associated with APS, but not included in the classification criteria, include livedo reticularis, skin ulcers, endocardial disease, thrombocytopenia, Coombs-positive hemolytic anemia, and false-positive tests for syphilis [66]. Primary APS occurs in the absence of other connective tissue disease. When APS is associated with SLE or other connective tissue disorders, it is referred to as *secondary APS*. Patients with *catastrophic APS* (CAPS) present with acute multiorgan failure from occlusive vasculopathy of small vessels in the kidney, lungs, brain, heart, adrenal glands, and liver. Large vessel occlusions have also been reported.

The LAC, APAs, and anti-β_2 glycoprotein-I antibody all bind to negatively charged phospholipids. How these antibodies induce thrombosis remains unknown, but interaction with endothelial cells, coagulation factors, and platelets, and complement activation, all play a role. Thromboses and emboli occur in all vessel sizes and organ systems. Nonthrombotic associations include valvular lesions similar to Libman-Sacks, hemolytic anemia, thrombocytopenia, and livedo reticularis.

TABLE 193.4

MEDICATIONS ASSOCIATED WITH DRUG-RELATED LUPUS

Type	Definite	Possible	Rare[a]
Cardiovascular	Methyldopa Hydralazine Procainamide Quinidine Practolol Diltiazem	Captopril Beta-blockers Hydrochlorothiazide Amiodarone Ticlopidine	Reserpine Minoxidil Chlorthalidone Clonidine HMG CoA inhibitors Spironolactone Disopyramide Prazosin
Anticonvulsants or neurologic medications		Phenytoin Mephenytoin Primidone Carbamazepine Trimethadione	Levodopa Ethosuximide Valproate
Psychiatric	Chlorpromazine	Lithium carbonate	Lamotrigine
Antibiotics	Isoniazid Minocycline	Sulfonamides Nitrofurantoin Rifampin	Streptomycin Tetracycline Penicillin Nalidixic acid Griseofulvin, terbinafine
Endocrine		Methimazole Propylthiouracil, Methylthiouracil Glyburide	Tolazamide
Rheumatic	Penicillamine TNF-α inhibitors	Sulfasalazine	Gold salts Allopurinol *p*-Aminosalicylic acid NSAIDs: tolmetin, ibuprofen, sulindac, diclofenac, tolmetin
Others	Interferon gamma	Danazol, dapsone	Psoralen Quinine Leuprolide acetate Promethazine Timolol eye drops Olsalazine, mesalamine Zafirlukast Interleukin 2 Docetaxel

[a]Rare: usually case reports.

The APS manifestations that most likely require ICU admission are cerebrovascular disease, pulmonary embolism, major abdominal or extremity arterial or venous thrombosis, myocardial infarctions, severe valvular disease (insufficiency or thrombotic valvular vegetations), and intracardiac thrombosis. Renal manifestations of APS include hypertension, proteinuria, acute or subacute renal insufficiency, and end-stage renal failure [67]. The classic renal lesion is thrombotic microangiopathy, but the entire renal vasculature can be affected: renal artery lesions can cause renal artery stenosis, cortical ischemia, and infarct, while thrombosis of the renal vein and inferior vena cava result in nephrotic range proteinuria. Hemodialysis patients with APS are at increased risk of vascular access thrombosis. CAPS, which occurs in less than 1% of APS, is the most serious and devastating subset with multisystem small vessel thromboses occurring within a short time period, usually less than 1 week [68]. Differentiation from TTP and DIC is imperative but sometimes difficult since microangiopathic hemolytic anemia or elevated fibrin split products are sometimes present in CAPS. Precipitating factors include infection, surgery, malignancy, subtherapeutic anticoagulation, and SLE flares. Mortality is high, nearly 48%, with death most often associated with renal, pulmonary, splenic, or adrenal involvement, or underlying SLE [69].

APS patients with *venous* thrombosis are treated with heparin anticoagulation followed by conversion to warfarin with an international normalized ratio (INR) target of 2.0 to 3.0. Lifelong anticoagulation is supported by a high incidence of recurrent thrombosis when warfarin is discontinued. A prospective trial comparing two intensities of warfarin for prophylaxis suggests that moderate dose (INR 2.0 to 3.0) is comparable to high dose (INR 3.1 to 4.0) in preventing further thrombosis and equal in bleeding complications [70]. However, in this study, only 24% of patients had arterial thrombosis and thus controversy still exists as to whether high intensity warfarin (INR 3.1 to 4.0) is necessary for patients with arterial clots. In APS patients with recurrent thrombosis despite therapeutic anticoagulation, treatment options include standard dose warfarin plus an antiplatelet agent, high intensity warfarin, unfractionated heparin, or low-molecular-weight heparin. For CAPS, combination therapy with high-dose corticosteroids, high intensity anticoagulation, and IVIg or plasmapheresis has the

TABLE 193.5

MODIFIED SAPPORO CLASSIFICATION CRITERIA FOR ANTIPHOSPHOLIPID SYNDROME

Clinical criteria
1. Vascular thrombosis involving any size vessel (arterial, venous, or capillary)
2. Pregnancy complications
a. Three or more sequential spontaneous miscarriages before 10 weeks gestation (without obvious causes)
b. One or more unexplained death of normal fetus beyond 10 weeks gestation
c. Preterm delivery of normal fetus <34 weeks due to preeclampsia, eclampsia, or placental insufficiency
Laboratory criteria (measured at least on two occasions, 12 weeks apart)
1. Moderate-to-high titer IgM or IgG anticardiolipin antibodies by ELISA
2. Lupus anticoagulant defined by guidelines from International Society on Thrombosis and Hemostasis
3. High titer (>99 percentile) IgM or IgG anti-β_2 glycoprotein-I antibody by ELISA
Diagnosis is based on the presence of one clinical and one laboratory criteria. The laboratory finding should not be less than 12 weeks or more than 5 years apart from the clinical event.

Adapted from Miyakis S, Lockshin MD, Atsumi T, et al: International consensus statement on an update of the classification criteria for definite antiphospholipid syndrome. *J Thromb Haemost* 4(2):295–306, 2006.

best survival data [68]. There is no evidence to support anticoagulation as primary prevention in individuals who have antiphospholipid antibodies or LAC without thrombotic manifestations [71].

Other causes of hypercoagulability associated with venous thrombosis include deficiencies of protein C, protein S, plasminogen, and antithrombin III; factor V Leiden; prothrombin mutation and homocystinemia; nephrotic syndrome; and paraneoplastic syndrome. In patients with arterial thromboses, homocystinemia, and other nongenetic causes including cocaine use, valvular heart disease, atrial myxoma, and arterial stenosis should be excluded.

SYSTEMIC SCLEROSIS

SSc, or scleroderma, is an immune-mediated disease characterized by progressive fibrosis of the vasculature and viscera resulting in end-organ damage in the skin, heart, lungs, kidneys, and gastrointestinal tract. There are two subsets of scleroderma: (a) limited cutaneous disease, often associated with the anticentromere antibody and (b) systemic/diffuse disease, associated with the presence of antitopoisomerase 1 (SCL-70) or anti-RNA polymerase. Both subsets have potential end-organ complications that result in ICU admission, including severe digital ischemia from Raynaud's phenomenon, respiratory failure, cardiac dysfunction, or renal insufficiency. The following discussion is limited to these areas.

Severe Raynaud's Phenomenon

Although primary Raynaud's phenomenon (RP) is common in the general population (up to 5%), severe secondary RP associated with connective tissue disease often is more difficult to treat and digital ulceration or gangrene may occur in 25% of SSc patients. Dihydropyridine-type calcium channel blockers, usually nifedipine, reduce the frequency and severity of RP attacks, and are considered first-line therapy [72]. Bosentan, a dual endothelin receptor antagonist, is effective in reducing the number of new digital ulcers [73,74]. Limited evidence suggests that sildenafil, a phosphodiesterase inhibitor, reduces the frequency and severity of attacks and promotes healing of digital ulcers [75,76]. Topical nitrates, ACE inhibitors, and α-adrenergic receptor blockade are additional therapies with modest benefit. Intravenous prostacyclin (epoprostenol) or iloprost (a prostacyclin analog) are effective in patients with severe digital ischemia refractory to other therapies (Table 193.6) [77]. Oral prostanoids are less effective. Use of intravenous prostaglandins should be avoided in patients with pulmonary hypertension unless closely monitored. Chemical sympathectomy with lidocaine provides short-term pain relief, but surgical digital sympathectomy is a last alternative when medical therapies fail.

Pulmonary Disease

Pulmonary involvement in SSc is now the major cause of death (more than 50%). The prevalence of lung disease ranges from 25% to 90% [78]. Clinically significant disease from interstitial fibrosis or pulmonary arterial hypertension (PAH) is estimated at 40% (see Table 193.1).

Exertional dyspnea, cough, and basilar crackles are the predominant clinical features of ILD. Radiographs may reveal pulmonary fibrosis in 33% to 40%, with a characteristic basilar reticulonodular or honeycombing pattern [78]. High-resolution CT scans (HCRT) are more sensitive in documenting the reticular and ground glass opacities of ILD when plain radiographs are relatively normal. Pulmonary function tests may reveal abnormalities even before radiographic or clinical findings. The classic pattern is restrictive, with decreased total lung capacity and forced vital capacity. These findings correlate with fibrosis of the chest wall, diaphragm, and pleura. A decrease in diffusing capacity (D_LCO) may occur in either ILD or pulmonary hypertension and has been reported in isolation without other pulmonary function test abnormalities. Patients with ILD may develop secondary PAH, but the degree of PAH is disproportionate to the degree of ILD.

Prevention of progressive fibrotic disease is the goal of treatment for SSc-associated ILD. In one study, the extent of disease on CT was predictive of mortality and FVC decline, suggesting that patients with more advanced CT abnormalities should be treated [79]. Patients with less extensive disease should be monitored closely and treated if there is evidence of radiographic progression or decline in pulmonary function. BAL cellularity does not predict disease progression or response to treatment, and currently has a limited role in the evaluation of ILD, but is useful to rule out infection [80]. A randomized, placebo controlled study of oral cyclophosphamide (1 mg per kg per day titrated to maximum of 2 mg per kg per day) found small but statistically significant improvement in forced vital capacity (FVC), skin score, and subjective symptoms [81]. Another randomized, placebo controlled study of IVCY (0.5 to 0.7 g per M^2 monthly) demonstrated improvement in FVC [82]. Although there are no controlled trials to compare efficacy of oral versus intravenous CY, the IV route is most practical initially in the critically ill ICU patient. Debate exists as to whether concomitant high-dose prednisone or prednisolone provides additional benefit. Case reports and small open studies of mycophenolate mofetil are encouraging, but larger studies are needed.

Isolated PAH is more common in limited scleroderma, but also occurs in patients with diffuse disease, with a prevalence of 12% to 15% [83]. Pulmonary vasospasm and

TABLE 193.6

DRUG THERAPY FOR SEVERE RAYNAUD'S AND PULMONARY HYPERTENSION IN SSC

Drug	Route of administration	Pulmonary arterial hypertension[a]	Severe digital ischemia[a]	Side effects
Epoprostenol	Continuous, intravenous	2 ng/kg/min titrated to 11 ng/kg/min [90]	2 ng/kg/min titrated up to 4–8 ng/kg/min over 5 d [77]	Catheter related; flushing, nausea, jaw pain, diarrhea, depression
Iloprost	Inhalant	5 μg 6–9 times/d [116]	Ineffective	Flushing, jaw pain, ? syncope
Iloprost[b]	Intravenous		0.5–2 ng/kg/d for 6 h for over 3–5 d [117]	Infusion site pain, headache, nausea, diarrhea, vomiting, jaw pain
Treprostinil	Continuous infusion, or subcutaneous	2 ng/kg/min titrated up to 40 ng/kg/min [118]	2 ng/kg/min titrated up to 40 ng/kg/min (case reports)	Jaw pain, headache, diarrhea, nausea, infusion site pain
Treprostinil	Inhalant	6–18 μg 4 times/d		
Bosentan	Oral	125 mg b.i.d. [84,85]	62.5 mg b.i.d. then increased to 125 mg b.i.d. [73,74]	Hepatotoxicity, anemia, edema, male infertility, teratogenicity
Ambrisentan	Oral	5–10 mg/d [86]		Hepatotoxicity, anemia, edema, male infertility, teratogenicity
Sitaxsentan[b]	Oral	100 mg/d [87,88]		Hepatotoxicity, anemia, edema, male infertility, teratogenicity
Sildenafil	Oral	20 mg t.i.d. to 80 mg t.i.d. [89]	50 mg b.i.d. [75,76]	Headache, diarrhea, dyspepsia, flushing

[a]Numbers in brackets are reference numbers.
[b]Not currently available in the United States.

endothelial cell activation with subsequent arterial wall proliferative changes contribute to the development of PAH. Symptoms include exertional dyspnea, fatigue, reduced exercise tolerance, chest pain, syncope, and lower extremity edema, but patients may be asymptomatic until the disease is advanced. The most sensitive tests are decreased diffusing capacity, often with preserved lung volumes, and Doppler echocardiography showing increased pulmonary pressures and right atrial and ventricular hypertrophy. Right heart catheterization is the gold standard for confirmation of suspected PAH and allows vasodilator trials to assess the degree of pulmonary vascular responsiveness to iloprost or epoprostenol, inhaled nitric oxide, or adenosine. General measures include the use of supplemental oxygen for hypoxic patients, diuretics for management of volume overload, and digoxin for atrial arrhythmias. Anticoagulation is recommended for advanced PAH, but controlled studies have not been done.

Treatment for PAH has recently advanced with oral agents in addition to intravenous or subcutaneous prostacyclin (epoprostenol, iloprost, and treprostinil). Bosentan, a dual endothelin receptor A and B antagonist, maintains vasodilation in the pulmonary arterial bed and clearance of endothelin, improves exercise tolerance, reduces symptoms, and stabilizes hemodynamics [84,85]. Bosentan is currently approved by the FDA for treatment of New York Heart Association (NYHA) class II, III, and IV PAH. Ambrisentan, a selective endothelin-A receptor antagonist, recently has been approved for treatment of NYHA Class II and III PAH [86]. Sitaxsentan is another selective endothelin-A antagonist only approved in Europe [87,88]. Sildenafil, a phosphodiesterase-5 inhibitor, increases vascular smooth muscle cyclic guanosine monophosphate (cGMP) with subsequent vasodilation, improves hemodynamic measures, and improves exercise capacity at doses of 20 mg to 80 mg three times a day [89]. Since these oral agents cause fewer side effects and eliminate the need for intravenous or subcutaneous delivery, they now are the preferred initial drugs of choice for treatment of PAH. Intravenous prostacyclin, epoprostenol, and a subcutaneous prostacyclin analog, treprostinil, are approved for treatment of NYHA class III and IV PAH, and epoprostenol has approval for use in SSc PAH [90]. Given the problems associated with the need for continuous delivery and the associated adverse effects, both agents are reserved for patients who have failed oral therapy. Inhaled prostacyclin, iloprost, 2.5 to 5.0 μg dosed six to nine times per day, also has been approved for the treatment of NYHA class III and IV PAH. Combination therapy with inhaled iloprost, intravenous or subcutaneous prostacyclin, and oral agents may provide even greater benefit, but controlled studies are not available. Table 193.6 summarizes the current therapies available for treatment of PAH.

Surgical interventions include atrial septostomy or transplantation. The former is viewed as a bridge to transplantation since it creates a right-to-left shunt to reduce right heart pressures. However, with recent advances in medical therapy, time to transplantation has been prolonged in the PAH population.

Cardiac Disease

Cardiac involvement in SSc may be a primary process within the heart or secondary to other major organ involvement (i.e., pulmonary, renal, vascular, thyroid). Primary cardiac disease in SSc includes pericardial disease, myocardial disease, conduction abnormalities, and arrhythmias. Because the most common symptoms are dyspnea, orthopnea, atypical chest pain, palpitations, fatigue, and dizziness, the clinical manifestations of cardiac disease can be confused with those of other organ systemic involvement. Recent studies have also shown an increased burden of atherosclerotic coronary disease in SSc [91].

Pericardial disease is the most common cardiac manifestation, and as in SLE, asymptomatic pericardial disease based on autopsy series or echocardiographic data has a much higher prevalence than symptomatic disease (33% to 71% vs. 7% to 20%). Pericardial effusions are usually small and do not influence prognosis. Larger effusions (>200 mL), however, are associated with poor prognosis. Pericardial tamponade with hemodynamic compromise is rare. Pericardiocentesis is rarely required unless the patient is hemodynamically compromised or febrile and an infectious etiology must be excluded. Pericardial fluid tends to be serous with a wide range of leukocyte counts and with normal complement levels. Corticosteroids are rarely required for treatment.

Myocardial involvement is the most common cardiac finding in patients with SSc at autopsy, ranging from 12% to 89%; however, symptomatic disease occurs less frequently than pericarditis. Pathologically, the most common findings are patchy, focal myocardial fibrosis equally distributed in both ventricles and all three layers of the heart [92]. Autonomic cardiac neuropathy may also contribute to cardiac morbidity in SSc patients.

Clinically, myocardial disease may result in cardiomyopathy, left ventricular diastolic dysfunction, congestive heart failure, angina, conduction abnormalities, or malignant arrhythmias. A high percentage of SSc patients without cardiac symptoms have an abnormal resting ECG, chest radiograph, Holter monitor, or echocardiogram. Electrophysiological studies reveal a high incidence of reentrant supraventricular tachyarrhythmias and atrioventricular conduction delays. Ventricular tachycardia occurs in 10% to 13% of patients and may be the cause of sudden death. Advanced myocardial fibrosis, rather than selective fibrosis of the conduction system, appears to be responsible for conduction abnormalities and arrhythmias.

Evaluation of acutely ill SSc patients for suspected heart disease should include a routine ECG and chest radiograph. Doppler echocardiography provides information regarding the pericardium, valvular function, systolic and diastolic ventricular function, chamber size, wall thickness, and the presence of pulmonary hypertension. Nuclear scanning may reveal subclinical myocardial disease; cardiac catheterization is useful for accurate assessment of pulmonary arterial pressures but is otherwise unremarkable unless the patient has arteriosclerosis. Negative endoyocardial biopsies cannot exclude myocardial fibrosis since the pathologic process tends to be patchy.

Treatment of SSc cardiac disease is tailored to the specific syndrome. Pericarditis can be treated with NSAIDs or low-dose corticosteroids. Diuresis should be pursued with caution in patients with large pericardial effusions. Renal failure has been reported in patients after vigorous diuresis, presumably secondary to hypovolemia superimposed on low cardiac output resulting in decreased renal cortical blood flow. Congestive heart failure is treated as outlined in Chapter 33. However, if echocardiography reveals evidence of diastolic dysfunction, ACE inhibitors or calcium channel blockers may be more appropriate than inotropic agents. A high index of suspicion for coronary artery disease and aggressive management of modifiable risk factors are important aspects of therapy for all patients.

Renal Disease

In addition to cardiac and pulmonary involvement in diffuse scleroderma, significant morbidity and mortality result from renal disease. The onset of accelerated to malignant hypertension accompanied by signs of microangiopathic hemolytic anemia, hyperreninemia, and rapidly progressive renal failure describes a syndrome referred to as *scleroderma renal crisis* (SRC). SRC may develop in up to 15% to 20% of patients with diffuse scleroderma [93]. SRC typically occurs early in the course of disease in patients with diffuse disease, often in the setting of other organ system involvement. Predictors for development of SRC include high skin score, large joint contractures (wrists, elbows, knees), enlarged cardiac silhouette, and prednisone use [93].

Although the pathophysiology of SRC is unknown, several factors contribute to its evolution. The primary event is endothelial cell injury, leading to intimal proliferation and luminal narrowing. Combined with other contributing factors such as vasospasm, decreased renal blood flow leads to increased renin release and clinical development of malignant hypertension and SRC. Moderate-to-high dose corticosteroid use is associated with the development of SRC, possibly because of the inhibition of prostacyclin production. Microangiopathic hemolytic anemia and thrombocytopenia develop with associated elevation of fibrin degradation products, decreased haptoglobin, elevated reticulocyte count, and the presence of urinary hemosiderin. The urinary sediment contains small amounts of protein (<2.5 g per 24 hours) but typically no red blood cell casts.

The diagnosis of SRC should be strongly considered in the SSc patient with accelerated hypertension. Symptoms of malignant hypertension include headache, confusion, altered vision, and seizures. However, SRC may occur rarely in normotensive patients. Examination of peripheral blood smears for microangiopathy rapidly confirms the syndrome of SRC in a hypertensive patient. Virtually all patients with SRC have elevated plasma renin activity, although serial tests of renin levels in patients with scleroderma are not predictive of the onset of this syndrome.

Since the advent of aggressive management with ACE inhibitors, conservation or improvement in renal function is possible. It is now clear that this class of drugs is the standard of care in SRC. Short-acting ACE inhibitors should be started and titrated upward every 6 to 12 hours. Blood pressure should be controlled within 48 hours. Additional antihypertensives, including calcium channel blockers, can be added. In many patients treated with ACE inhibitors, there may be a transient reduction in glomerular filtration rate and a rise in serum creatinine. In a large prospective observational study of patients with SRC who were treated with ACE inhibitors, 61% had good outcomes (defined as no or temporary dialysis) and only 4% progressed to renal failure or dialysis [94]. In patients with good outcomes after the initial renal crisis, continuing ACE inhibitors indefinitely may provide further benefit to maintain renal function. Survival data of patients with good outcomes after SRC are similar to those of SSc patients without renal crisis. SRC accounts for only 8% of deaths in SSc, but in a retrospective review of SSc patients, those patients with SRC had a long-term survival of only 50% [93]. There is no evidence to support the use of ACE inhibitors for primary prevention of SRC.

Gastrointestinal Disease

Gastrointestinal tract involvement is common in SSc, affecting 50% to 80% of patients. The most common physiologic abnormalities, esophageal dysmotility and decreased lower esophageal sphincter (LES) pressure, are manifested by symptoms of dysphagia and heartburn, respectively. Pathologically, impaired microvascular perfusion initially alters myoelectrical function of the smooth muscle layer and later, hypoperfusion results in fibrotic changes in muscularis, submucosa, and lamina propria [95]. Although dysphagia and heartburn can be treated symptomatically, serious complications include strictures and Barrett's esophagus.

Gastric involvement is less common but can include gastroparesis with symptoms of early satiety, bloating, and vomiting. Telangiectasias are a common source of gastrointestinal blood loss, and gastric antral vascular ectasia (GAVE) may present with acute bleeding and antedate the diagnosis of SSc.

However, other causes of gastrointestinal bleeding also must be excluded.

Small and large intestinal involvement usually occurs concomitantly and results in malabsorption with symptoms of bloating, cramping, and intermittent or severe diarrhea. Hypomotility due to progressive smooth muscle atrophy and fibrosis results in bacterial overgrowth. In addition, adynamic ileus or pseudo-obstruction may occur. Although barium studies reveal wide-mouth sacculations or diverticula on the antimesenteric border, most patients have relatively few symptoms. Fecal incontinence and constipation are common but underreported. Rare complications include obstruction due to fecal impaction, megacolon, and volvulus. Pneumatosis cystoides intestinalis (PCI), or intramural air-filled cysts in the small or large intestines, may be found incidentally or cause abdominal pain, diarrhea, or bloody rectal discharge. Rupture of these cysts results in pneumoperitoneum without peritonitis.

Primary biliary cirrhosis is the most common liver disease associated with SSc. Up to 18% of patients with primary biliary cirrhosis have SSc, usually the limited cutaneous form, whereas 8% of all SSc patients have antimitochondrial antibodies. The liver disease most often follows the diagnosis of SSc but can precede it.

Treatment of gastroesophageal dysmotility and reflux includes modifications in eating and high-dose proton pump inhibitors. Treatment for GAVE includes various therapeutic endoscopic procedures such as cautery, sclerotherapy, and laser ablation. Prokinetic agents, including metoclopramide and macrolide antibiotics, have been reported to be useful in treatment of esophageal, gastric, and intestinal disease. Intestinal malabsorption has been treated with antibiotics, low-residue diets, medium-chain triglycerides, fat-soluble vitamins, and total parenteral nutrition. Octreotide improves intestinal peristalsis in pseudo-obstruction, and in combination with erythromycin may have additive benefits [96]. An investigational 5-HT4 receptor agonist, prucalopride, improves symptoms and gut transport in SSc [97]. Prucalopride recently was approved for use in Europe, but is not yet available in the United States. Cisapride, another 5-HT4 receptor agonist, is severely restricted in the US because of concerns regarding severe cardiac arrhythmias. PCI is usually managed conservatively without surgery, but both malabsorption and PCI are poor prognostic indicators [98].

IDIOPATHIC INFLAMMATORY MYOPATHIES

Polymyositis (PM), *dermatomyositis* (DM), and *inclusion body myositis* (IBM), the most common acquired inflammatory myopathies, are characterized by progressive symmetric proximal muscle weakness and elevated muscle enzymes. Each subtype also has unique clinical and histologic features. In both PM and DM, other organ system involvement is common. DM has classic skin findings including a heliotrope rash on the upper eyelids, scaly erythematous patches called Gottron's papules overlying the MCP and PIP joints and the extensor surfaces of the knees and elbows, and erythema typically in a V shape and mantle distribution on the neck and chest. PM and IBM have no skin manifestations. Both PM and DM may have pulmonary, cardiac, or gastrointestinal involvement. IBM differs from PM/DM in many ways including older age at onset, more indolent course with poor response to treatment, more frequent asymmetric and distal muscle involvement, and often only mild creatinine kinase elevation. The diagnosis of PM/DM is based on criteria established by Bohan and Peter [99]: symmetric proximal muscle weakness, typical rash of DM, elevated serum muscle enzymes, myopathic changes on electromyography, and characteristic muscle biopsy abnormalities. Muscle biopsy is usually required to establish the diagnosis and exclude other causes of muscle weakness. The biopsy should be taken from a muscle that is weak on exam, usually the quadriceps or deltoid. Obtaining the biopsy from a muscle contralateral to one with myopathic changes on EMG may improve the diagnostic yield. T2-weighted MRI with fat suppression can also be useful for identifying an actively inflamed muscle for biopsy [100]. A number of myositis-specific antibodies (MSAs) and myositis-associated antibodies (MAAs) have been identified that correlate with specific clinical presentations and may contribute diagnostic and prognostic information [101,102]. Anti–Mi-2, found in up to 10% of patients with myositis, is associated with classic DM, and is a marker for a more favorable prognosis. Antibodies against a signal recognition particle (SRP) occur in only 5% of myositis patients but are associated with acute, severe myositis with an overall poor prognosis. Table 193.7 summarizes the various clinical and laboratory features of these three idiopathic inflammatory myopathies.

Inflammatory myositis is also associated with other connective tissue diseases (SSc, SLE, mixed connective tissue disease), malignancy, inborn errors of metabolism, lipid storage disease, and mitochondrial myopathies, but these will not be discussed here. Numerous drugs can cause myopathy or myositis that is sometimes difficult to distinguish from inflammatory myositis. These drugs include lipid lowering agents, glucocorticoids, antipsychotics, antimalarials, colchicine, nucleoside reverse transcriptase inhibitors (NRTIs), alcohol, and cocaine. Bacterial infections (*S. aureus, Streptococcus pyogenes, Clostridium perfringens, Borrelia burgdorferi*) and viruses (coxsackievirus A and B, echovirus, influenza A and B, adenovirus 2 and 21, hepatitis B and C, and HIV) can cause a myopathy that may be confused with PM or DM. Parasites including trichinosis, toxoplasmosis, cysticercosis, toxocariasis, and amebiasis may all cause myositis. Muscular dystrophies, neuropathic disease, and metabolic/endocrine diseases also need to be excluded in patients with muscle weakness.

PM and DM are primarily disorders of skeletal muscle, but involvement of the pulmonary, cardiac, articular, gastrointestinal, or vascular systems sometimes lead to catastrophic illness requiring support in an ICU. Moreover, organ dysfunction may occur in patients with overlap syndromes. Respiratory failure, cardiac abnormalities, or comorbidities related to immunosuppression are the most common reasons for ICU admission. A complete discussion of the presentation, diagnosis, management, and differential diagnosis is beyond the scope of this chapter but excellent reviews exist [103–105].

Pulmonary Involvement

Lung disease in PM/DM patients is common (20% to 30% of patients; see Table 193.1) and includes (a) respiratory insufficiency due to weakness of intercostal or diaphragmatic muscles; (b) aspiration pneumonia; (c) pneumonia from neither aspiration nor opportunistic infection; and (d) ILD. Pulmonary vasculitis, pleuritis, pulmonary edema, alveolar hemorrhage, secondary pulmonary hypertension, and bronchiolitis obliterans with organizing pneumonia have also been reported but are uncommon. Dyspnea, cough, and chest pain, are the usual symptoms.

Respiratory failure from intercostal muscle weakness or diaphragmatic dysfunction occurs in 7% of PM/DM patients. Thus, pulmonary mechanics (spirometry, inspiratory force) should be evaluated when respiratory symptoms develop. Serial measurements often predict impending respiratory failure that might necessitate intubation and mechanical ventilation. Management of respiratory failure resulting from muscle weakness is supportive (oxygen, mechanical ventilation) and

TABLE 193.7

FEATURES OF IDIOPATHIC INFLAMMATORY MYOPATHIES

	Polymyositis	Dermatomyositis	Inclusion body myositis
Mean age at onset	45	Childhood or 40	65
Sex (M:F)	1:2	1:2	2:1
Mode of onset	Insidious over months	Insidious over months	Insidious over years
Distribution of muscle involvement	Proximal >> distal symmetric	Proximal >> distal symmetric	Variable, may be primarily distal, asymmetric
Dermatologic findings (see text)	No	Yes	No
Raynaud's	Yes	Yes	No
Pulmonary disease	Yes	Yes	No
Cardiac disease	Yes, rare	Yes, rare	No
Arthritis	Yes	Yes	No
Gastrointestinal tract	Yes	Yes	Cricopharyngeal dysfunction
Creatine kinase	Highly elevated	Highly elevated-classic DM Normal-amyopathic DM	Normal or minimally elevated
Electromyogram/nerve conduction studies	Myopathic features	Myopathic features	Myopathic features but also some neurogenic changes
Histopathology	Endomysial CD8 cells, without vascular inflammation	Perivascular infiltrate of B and CD4 cells and late complements (C_{5-9}, membrane attack complex); perifascicular atrophy	Similar to PM but also presence of intracellular lined vacuoles and inclusions; EM with microtubular filaments
Autoantibodies	Jo-1 (20%), U1-RNP (10%), PM-Scl (10%), SRP (<5%)	Jo-1 (5%); Mi-2 (10%); U1-RNP (5%); PM-Scl (0.5%)	Rare
Malignancy association	Yes (twofold increase)	Yes (sixfold increase)	No
Response to therapy	Good	Good	Poor

DM, dermatomyositis; EM, electron microscopy; PM, polymyositis; RNP, ribonuclear protein; Scl, scleroderma.

accompanied by therapy directed at the underlying myositis (see Chapter 49).

Bronchopneumonia occurs in up to 24% of PM/DM patients. Contributing factors include pharyngeal incompetence and poor airway protection with subsequent aspiration, iatrogenic immunosuppression, and often a weakened cough. Infectious agents include virulent bacteria and opportunistic organisms. Myositis occurring in the setting of acquired immunodeficiency further expands the possible spectrum of infectious agents. Hence, respiratory symptoms should be evaluated aggressively with chest radiographs and routine and specialized microbiologic techniques (culture for bacteria, mycobacteria, fungi, and smears for *Pneumocystis jiroveci*).

The most common type of parenchymal lung disease in PM/DM is ILD with a prevalence of 20% to 60%. Patients develop progressive dyspnea with or without a nonproductive cough and bibasilar rales. Ground glass opacities and reticulonodular infiltrates may be present on HRCT scans. Pulmonary function tests reveal decreased lung volumes and reduced diffusing capacity. Histopathology usually reveals nonspecific interstitial pneumonia (NSIP) or usual interstitial pneumonia (UIP). Patients with Jo-1 and other antiaminoacyl-tRNA synthetase antibodies have a high incidence of ILD, along with prominent arthritis, fever, Raynaud's phenomenon, and dry, cracking skin lesions referred to as *mechanic's hands*. Fulminant ILD has occurred in amyopathic DM without anti-Jo antibodies.

Myocardial Involvement

Cardiac and pulmonary diseases are the main prognostic factors for PM/DM mortality [106]. Up to 70% of patients have cardiac abnormalities on noninvasive testing, but clinically, few are symptomatic. Myocarditis may manifest as heart failure, arrhythmias, cardiac arrest, or myocardial infarction. It is difficult to diagnose since levels of creatine kinase and muscle brain fractions are elevated as a result of skeletal muscle inflammation. Cardiac troponin I is the most specific marker for myocardial involvement. Cardiac imaging techniques (echocardiogram, gallium citrate or indium-labeled antimyosin antibody detection, and scintigraphic studies) are insensitive and nonspecific for detecting myositis. Contrast enhanced cardiac MRI may provide more information, but large-scale evaluation of its sensitivity and specificity is lacking in PM/DM patients. The gold standard of diagnosis requires endomyocardial biopsy but is invasive. Although previous literature suggested an association of anti-SRP antibodies with myocarditis, recent studies contradict this.

The extent to which any cardiac abnormality is iatrogenic or arises as a complication of the disease is unclear. For example, steroid therapy accelerates atherosclerosis and may exacerbate hypertension, diabetes mellitus, and electrolyte disturbances. Similarly, hypoxia from pulmonary involvement contributes to arrhythmias, axis shifts, and strain patterns on ECG.

Other Organ System Involvement

The major gastrointestinal manifestation of inflammatory myopathies is weakness of the upper pharyngeal striated muscles, resulting in dysphonia, dysphagia, and regurgitation of fluids. Smooth muscle involvement of the distal esophagus is rare, and intestinal vasculitis, commonly seen in childhood dermatomyositis, is also uncommon.

Renal failure and its attendant metabolic abnormalities are the result of rhabdomyolysis, myoglobinemia, and subsequent myoglobinuria. Myoglobinuric renal failure is rare but tends to occur in patients with acute or hyperacute presentations as a result of widespread muscle necrosis and release of sarcoplasmic materials, including myoglobin. Therapy is directed toward the underlying muscle disease while maintaining an adequate urinary output.

Malignancy

The relationship of PM/DM to malignancy has been established by several epidemiologic studies [107]. DM is associated with the highest risk (sixfold increase compared to age and gender-matched population), while PM has a twofold increase. The risk decreases with time but even at 5 years, the risk is still measurable. Identified risk factors include female sex, later age at diagnosis, cutaneous necrosis and leukocytoclastic vasculitis, and capillary damage. Malignancies commonly associated with DM/PM include breast, ovarian, lung, colon, gastric, pancreatic, nasopharyngeal, and non-Hodgkin's lymphoma [103].

Treatment

High-dose corticosteroids are the first-line therapy for PM/DM, although there are no clinical trials to support this approach. Treatment is usually begun with prednisone 1 to 1.5 mg per kg per day for 6 to 8 weeks, then tapered based on clinical response. In more severe cases (dysphagia, alveolitis, myocarditis, or impending respiratory failure from muscle weakness), IV methylprednisolone may be given at a dose of 1,000 mg daily for 3 days followed by the usual high-dose oral corticosteroid regimen. In steroid responsive patients, a steroid-sparing agent (methotrexate, AZA, mycophenolate mofetil, tacrolimus, cyclophosphamide, or cyclosporine) may be added to facilitate steroid tapering, but efficacy is based on small case series or clinical experience as no randomized clinical trials have been done. IVIg is recommended for patients with severe weakness refractory to steroids based on proven efficacy in a randomized, placebo-controlled trial in patients with DM [108]. Therapy for progressive or severe ILD usually requires the use of corticosteroids and cyclophosphamide. Cyclosporine and tacrolimus can be used in refractory cases. A number of case reports suggest that rituximab can be effective for PM/DM resistant to other therapies, and a placebo-controlled trial is underway. There is conflicting data regarding the use of TNF inhibitors; anecdotal reports suggest benefit for some patients with PM/DM, but lack of efficacy and a high frequency of disease flares were reported in one open-label pilot study [109].

Therapy for IBM is more difficult since it responds to steroids poorly and slowly. IVIg and methotrexate have not been effective in double-blind, placebo-controlled trials. Current recommendations include a trial of steroids if muscle biopsies reveal significant inflammation and physical therapy to help maintain strength and function.

DRUGS USED IN RHEUMATIC DISEASE

Nonsteroidal Anti-inflammatory Drugs

NSAIDs are the cornerstone of therapy in patients with rheumatic diseases. Numerous NSAIDs with variable dosing regimens are currently available. In the intensive care setting, however, comorbidities are often present in the acutely ill patient, and thus limit their use. Potential NSAID toxicities (gastrointestinal bleeding, exacerbation of cardiac and renal dysfunction) may far outweigh their benefits. NSAIDs are contraindicated in patients who are anticoagulated, further restricting their use in critically ill patients.

Corticosteroid Therapy

Although NSAIDs are the drugs of choice in the initial treatment of nonseptic inflammatory joint disease, corticosteroids are more effective for the vasculitides and inflammatory, multisystem autoimmune diseases such as SLE. The physiology and mechanism of action of corticosteroids are beyond the scope of this chapter.

Exogenous corticosteroids at a dose equivalent to prednisone 5.0 to 7.5 mg per day inhibit the hypothalamic-pituitary-adrenal axis. Thus, patients who are on corticosteroids chronically require increased stress doses when situations such as surgery, sepsis, trauma, or other serious medical complications occur. Several corticosteroid preparations are available, which differ in potency, half-life, and mineralocorticoid activity. In the ICU, the most commonly used corticosteroids are hydrocortisone, methylprednisolone, and prednisone. There are few indications to use the long-acting corticosteroids, such as dexamethasone, in patients with rheumatic diseases. At physiologic concentrations, corticosteroids are primarily bound by transcortin, but at higher levels, plasma concentrations of albumin-bound and free corticosteroid are increased. In hypoalbuminemic patients, a greater percentage of corticosteroid is free, thus increasing the anti-inflammatory effects and the toxicities. Since corticosteroids are metabolized in the liver, the concomitant administration of drugs that increase hepatic microsomal enzyme activity (phenytoin, barbiturates) also accelerates corticosteroid metabolism.

The dosage and mode of administration of corticosteroids depend on the clinical situation. In rheumatoid arthritis patients without evidence of vasculitis, joint symptoms usually can be controlled with less than 10 mg per day of prednisone. In contrast, a patient with newly diagnosed DM requires high-dose prednisone (1 to 1.5 mg per kg per day) to achieve disease control. The more usual situation in the ICU is the patient with multisystem involvement from SLE or vasculitis. In these patients, high-dose parenteral methylprednisolone can be initiated at 50 to 100 mg per day.

For acutely ill patients who fail conventional high-dose steroids (i.e., 1.0 to 1.5 mg per kg per day), pulse IV methylprednisolone at 1,000 mg per day infused over 60 minutes and repeated daily for 3 consecutive days may be more effective. Pulse IV methylprednisolone may produce minor side effects, such as metallic taste, facial flushing, transient hypertension, and hyperglycemia. More significant (but rare) toxicities include seizures, anaphylaxis, intractable hiccups, arrhythmias, hemiplegia, psychosis, and sudden death. In four reported deaths, patients were receiving furosemide concurrently. Theories on the mechanism of death include an electrolyte imbalance resulting in cardiac arrhythmias, cardiovascular collapse due to hypovolemia and vasodilation, and anaphylaxis. Data are limited on the actual mechanism of action by pulse methylprednisolone in suppressing SLE or vasculitis activity. In addition, the long-term toxicities are unknown. Thus, these factors must be weighed against the patient's clinical status.

High-dose daily corticosteroids are usually continued for 4 to 6 weeks. If disease activity remains controlled, further tapering should be attempted. Switching to alternate-day steroids reduces hypothalamic-pituitary-adrenal axis suppression and reduces or prevents Cushing's syndrome. This regimen, however, does not prevent steroid-induced osteopenia. If the patient does not improve with high-dose or pulse corticosteroids, the addition of other immunosuppressive agents must be considered.

Immunosuppressive Therapy

Immunosuppressive agents were initially used in rheumatic diseases as steroid-sparing agents. However, convincing evidence exists that these agents can produce dramatic improvement or induce remission in many different rheumatic diseases. The most commonly used drugs include methotrexate, AZA, cyclophosphamide, leflunomide, and mycophenolate mofetil. Cytotoxic drugs should be initiated in patients with life-threatening or organ-threatening diseases that have failed to respond to conventional therapy. In addition, the patient should have reversible lesions rather than end-stage disease. Many of the drugs are teratogens contraindicated during pregnancy. Thus, in any patient starting cytotoxic therapy, pregnancy needs to be excluded. Active infection cannot be present at the start of cytotoxic therapy. Patients with a positive PPD require further evaluation and treatment for active versus latent tuberculosis. Once therapy is initiated, laboratory studies need to be monitored carefully.

The dosing of immunosuppressive agents for the different rheumatic diseases has been discussed in previous sections. In the ICU setting, adjustment to conventional dosing may be necessary based on renal or hepatic function since many of these agents are metabolized or excreted through the kidney or liver. Drug interactions such as allopurinol with AZA or trimethoprim with methotrexate are also important considerations.

Mechanism of Action and Metabolism

All immunosuppressive agents interfere with the cell cycle, and the cytotoxic effects occur through inhibition of cell division.

Azathioprine (AZA), a purine analog, prevents biosynthesis of the purine bases, adenine, and guanine. AZA is a prodrug that is metabolized in the liver to 6-mercaptopurine and then, through the enzyme thiopurine S-methyltransferase (TMPT), to its active metabolites. A genetic polymorphism of TMPT results in variable enzyme activity and predicts greater risk of myelosuppression in patients with low or absent levels. TMPT genotype testing is recommended before initiating AZA therapy [110]. Since 45% of the prodrug is renally excreted, the dose should be reduced in patients with renal insufficiency, but specific recommendations are not available. AZA should be avoided, or the dose markedly reduced, in patients taking allopurinol, which interferes with its metabolism by inhibiting xanthine oxidase.

Mycophenolate mofetil (MMF) is a reversible inhibitor of inosine monophosphate dehydrogenase, whose effects also result in reduced purine synthesis and consequent inhibition of T- and B-cell proliferation. The antiproliferative effects of MMF are relatively specific for lymphocytes. Other potential mechanisms of MMF-induced immunosuppression include induction of T lymphocyte apoptosis and inhibition of adhesion molecule expression. Most of the MMF dose (90%) is excreted renally and the remainder by enterohepatic elimination. Dose adjustment is necessary in patients with renal insufficiency.

Methotrexate (MTX) inhibits dihydrofolate reductase, thus reducing intracellular tetrahydrofolate levels and interfering with tetrahydrofolate dependent metabolic pathways, which include purine and pyrimidine metabolism. Potential mechanisms whereby MTX exerts an anti-inflammatory effect include increased extracellular adenosine concentrations, reduction of inflammatory cytokines (IL-1B and IL-6), inhibition of cyclooxygenase and lipoxygenase activity, and induction of apoptosis. MTX and its metabolites are excreted by the kidney. Methotrexate should not be used in patients whose estimated glomerular filtration rate is less than 30 mL per minute.

Leflunomide (LEF) selectively inhibits dihydroorotate dehydrogenase, an enzyme critical in the de novo synthesis of pyrimidine ribonucleosides. By reducing the pyrimidine pool and thus inhibiting DNA synthesis, LEF is postulated to modulate pathogenic T-cell proliferation and the subsequent inflammatory cascade. LEF has a very long half-life, is highly protein bound, undergoes enterohepatic recirculation, and is eliminated by the gastrointestinal tract and kidneys. It should not be used in patients with hepatic or severe renal impairment.

Cyclophosphamide (CY) is an alkylating agent that binds to DNA and prevents cell replication. CY is cytotoxic to both resting and dividing lymphocytes. It globally reduces T-cell function, and reduces B-cell numbers and antibody production. CY is metabolized by the liver to several active and inactive compounds that are also excreted in the urine. Dose adjustment is recommended for patients with renal insufficiency (Table 193.2.) Hepatic impairment does not appear to alter CY clearance. Hepatic and renal function should be monitored.

Toxicities

Toxicities common to all immunosuppressive agents include bone marrow suppression, infections, and gastrointestinal irritation. Bone marrow toxicity may occur anytime, as early as 1 or 2 weeks after institution of therapy. Leukopenia, especially granulocytopenia, is common. Anemia and thrombocytopenia may occur in conjunction with leukopenia but rarely alone. Infections secondary to immunosuppression occur with any drug but do not necessarily correlate with the degree of leukopenia, duration of drug therapy, or concomitant corticosteroid therapy. MTX and LEF are rated as pregnancy class X (contraindicated, risk outweighs benefits), and should not be used during pregnancy. AZA, rated as class D (positive evidence of risk), is considered safer than many other immunosuppressive agents during pregnancy based on literature in the transplant population. When the benefit of immunosuppression appears to outweigh the risks (e.g., in renal transplant recipients, active lupus, or inflammatory bowel disease), AZA is preferred over other immunosuppressive medications. We strongly recommend avoidance of CY and MMF (both pregnancy class D) during pregnancy except in life-threatening medical conditions in which no alternative therapy is available.

Specific toxicities of AZA include hypersensitivity hepatitis characterized by elevated transaminases and cholestasis that usually resolve after drug discontinuation, but irreversible damage has been reported. Pancreatitis has also been associated with AZA. Azoospermia, anovulation, and teratogenesis are unusual. TPMT levels do not predict these toxicities, in contrast to the known association of low enzyme level with risk of myelosuppression. It is uncertain whether neoplasia occurs at a greater incidence in rheumatic patients treated with AZA as compared to transplant patients. However, relative risk of lymphoproliferative disorders in RA patients receiving AZA is estimated at 2.2% to 8.7%.

The toxicity profile of MMF is similar to AZA and includes hepatitic abnormalities and myelosuppression. Gastrointestinal intolerance with nausea, vomiting, and diarrhea may improve over time and seldom requires drug discontinuation. A delayed release formulation is available that may improve GI tolerance. There is some evidence that MMF provides protection against fungal infections. As with other immunosuppressive medications, there may be an increased risk of malignancies, including lymphoma.

MTX's minor toxicities include nausea, vomiting, anorexia, diarrhea, and weight loss. Stomatitis occurs with variable severity. Alopecia, photosensitivity to ultraviolet light, urticaria, and cutaneous vasculitis may occur. Major hematological toxicities include megaloblastic anemia and, rarely, pancytopenia. Elevations in hepatitic enzymes also occur and require careful monitoring. Hepatic fibrosis is an infrequent but concerning complication. Acute interstitial pneumonitis is the most common pulmonary toxicity associated with MTX. Other pulmonary toxicities include interstitial fibrosis, pleuritis, noncardiogenic pulmonary edema, and increased pulmonary nodulosis. Opportunistic infections, including *P. jiroveci* pneumonia, cryptococcosis, and disseminated herpes zoster, have occurred with low-dose weekly MTX therapy for RA. Small series have reported development of lymphoproliferative disorders in MTX-treated patients, and it is well established that RA patients are at greater risk for lymphoma. However, a study reviewing a national data bank for rheumatic disease in over 18,000 patients did not identify a significantly higher risk of lymphoma in patients treated with MTX [111]. Risk factors for MTX toxicity include renal insufficiency, viral infections, folic acid deficiency, and concurrent use of trimethoprim-sulfamethoxazole and probenecid. For a MTX overdose, folinic acid (leucovorin), in a dose equal to the MTX dose, should be given every 4 to 6 hours until the serum MTX level is no longer detectable.

Toxicities associated with LEF include diarrhea, alopecia, rash, hypertension, and peripheral neuropathy. Liver enzymes may be elevated but usually return to normal with dose reduction or drug discontinuation. In patients who experience severe side effects or who wish to become pregnant, elimination of LEF and its metabolites can be accelerated by the administration of cholestyramine, 8 g three times a day for 11 days.

The major side effects of CY are infertility, bladder toxicity, carcinogenicity, and bone marrow suppression. Oral and IV regimens induce gonadal dysfunction in men and women because of injury to germinal epithelium. Azoospermia in males and amenorrhea in premenopausal women is dose related and is usually permanent. The risk may be reduced by the induction of gonadal quiescence during CY treatment. Leuprolide was shown to preserve ovarian function in women treated with CY for LN [112]. Leuprolide was ineffective in men, but a small study has shown a reduced risk of azoospermia in men treated with testosterone [113]. Sperm banking is also recommended for men undergoing CY therapy. Cryopreservation of ova or embryos is usually not practical as it entails hormonal manipulation and significant delay in treatment. Hemorrhagic cystitis due to acrolein, a metabolite of CY, occurs in 20% to 30% of patients receiving oral CY. Bladder carcinoma occurs in 10% of patients who receive long-term CY therapy, even 20 years after exposure. IVCY may have fewer bladder complications than the oral regimen. Adequate hydration for all patients and concomitant use of sodium 2-mercaptoethane sulfonate (MESNA) during IVCY infusion in patients with renal insufficiency reduce the risk of hemorrhagic cystitis. The regimen is outlined in Table 193.2. Skin and hematologic malignancies and premalignant and malignant changes of the cervix are also associated with CY. Hepatotoxicity is rare, but nausea or vomiting with IVCY is common. Other toxicities include infections, cardiomyopathy, and pulmonary fibrosis. *P. jiroveci* pneumonia has also occurred in patients with autoimmune diseases treated with CY and steroids. PCP prophylaxis is recommended for all patients treated with CY.

Biological Modifiers

In addition to the above traditional immunosuppressive agents, this past decade has witnessed the development of multiple biologic modifiers for the treatment of rheumatic diseases including anticytokine therapies, T-cell costimulation blockade, and B-cell depletion (see Table 193.8). Biologic agents are increasingly used to treat rheumatoid arthritis (RA), psoriatic arthritis (PsA), and ankylosing spondylitis (AS). Use of biologic agents in other rheumatologic diseases is still in investigational stages. It is unlikely that the ICU physician will initiate any of these agents for therapeutic indications. However, if a patient is receiving one of these agents chronically, it is important for the

TABLE 193.8

BIOLOGIC AGENTS FOR THE TREATMENT OF RHEUMATIC DISEASES

Drug	Mechanism of action	Half-life	Side effects
Etanercept	Soluble p75 TNF-α receptor fusion protein	72–132 h	Injection site/infusion reaction, Tb reactivation, opportunistic infections, fungal and mycobacterial infections, demyelinating syndromes, drug-induced lupus, pancytopenia, aplastic anemia, hepatotoxicity, CHF, possible increased risk of lymphoma and nonmelanoma skin cancer
Infliximab	Chimeric anti-TNF-α monoclonal antibody	7–12 d	
Adalimumab	Human anti-TNF-α monoclonal antibody	10–20 d	
Golimumab	Human anti-TNF-α monoclonal antibody	14 d	
Certolizumab pegol	Human anti-TNF-α antibody Fab' fragment coupled to polyethylene glycol	14 d	
Abatacept	CTLA4-Ig soluble fusion protein, inhibits T-cell activation by blocking costimulatory signal	8–25 d	Infusion reactions, infections, COPD exacerbation, possible increased risk of lung cancer and lymphoma
Tocilizumab	Humanized IgG1 IL-6 receptor antibody	6–13 d	Infusion reactions, infections similar to TNF-α inhibitors, hypertension, hypercholesterolemia, elevated hepatotoxicity gastrointestinal perforation
Anakinra	Human recombinant IL-1 receptor antagonist	4–6 h	Injection site reactions, serious infections
Rituximab	B-cell depleting chimeric monoclonal CD20 antibody	19 d	Infusion reactions, PML, new or reactivated viral infections, including fulminant hepatitis B

TNF, tumor necrosis factor; Tb, tuberculosis; Fab, fragment antigen binding; CTLA4, cytotoxic T lymphocyte-associated antigen; CHF, congestive heart failure; COPD, chronic obstructive pulmonary disease; IL, interleukin; PML, progressive multifocal leukoencephalopathy.

ICU team to understand the mechanism of action and the potential complications or toxicities of these therapies [114].

Five biologic agents that inhibit TNF-α, one IL-6 inhibitor, and one IL-1 receptor antagonist are currently available to treat rheumatoid arthritis (RA). The TNF-α inhibitors are also used to treat psoriatic arthritis (PsA) and ankylosing spondylitis (AS). Because antigen-activated T cells initiate the cell-mediated immune response and the cytokines TNF-α, IL-1, and IL-6 promote the inflammatory processes in inflammatory joint diseases, these anticytokine therapies control signs and symptoms of inflammatory arthritis, and in RA and PsA, have been shown to retard the progression of joint damage.

Four TNF-α inhibitors (etanercept, infliximab, adalimumab, and golimumab) are currently approved in the treatment of moderate-to-severe RA, psoriatic arthritis, and ankylosing spondylitis. Certolizumab pegol, the newest of the TNF-α inhibitors, is currently approved for RA and is being studied for use in other types of inflammatory arthritis. Although TNF-α has many diverse cellular effects in RA and other inflammatory arthropathies, it acts as a potent inflammatory cytokine by binding to one of its receptors, p55 or p75, on chondrocytes, fibroblasts, and osteoclasts in the rheumatoid synovium and stimulates the production of metalloproteinases and other effector molecules that damage the joint. In addition, TNF-α–activated endothelial cells express adhesion molecules, which promote the ingress of PMN cells into the joint. Naturally occurring soluble TNF-α receptors, which theoretically should neutralize TNF-α, exist in high concentrations in rheumatoid synovial fluid but may be inadequate in concentration to neutralize TNF-α in this disease.

Etanercept, a fusion protein comprised of two recombinant p75-soluble TNF-α receptors combined with the Fc portion of human IgG, is administered in subcutaneous injections (25 mg twice a week or 50 mg weekly) alone or in combination with methotrexate. Adalimumab and golimumab are recombinant human IgG_1 monoclonal antibodies against TNF-α. Adalimumab is administered as a 40 mg subcutaneous injection every other week, and golimumab is given in a single monthly 50 mg subcutaneous injection. Infliximab, a chimeric (human and mouse) monoclonal antibody against TNF-α, is administered intravenously at starting doses of 3 mg per kg at weeks 0, 2, and 6, followed by maintenance infusion every 8 weeks. The dose can be titrated to response with maximal dosage of 10 mg per kg. Certolizumab is a human anti-TNF-α antibody Fab' fragment that is chemically linked to polyethylene glycol. Certolizumab is administered by subcutaneous injection at 2- or 4-week intervals. Methotrexate is recommended in combination with infliximab and adalimumab to reduce the frequency of neutralizing human/antichimeric antibodies or human/antihuman antibodies respectively. All five TNF-α inhibitors have been demonstrated in controlled studies to provide clinical benefit and, more importantly, halt the progression of joint damage in RA and PsA.

Short-term toxicities of etanercept, adalimumab, golimumab, and certolizumab include injection site reactions with local urticarial lesions that often resolve with subsequent repeated dosing. Mild hypersensitivity reactions with infliximab infusion occur in 20% of patients, but 2% will experience severe infusion reactions. There is an increased risk of serious infections in patients taking TNF-α inhibitors, including opportunistic, fungal, and mycobacterial infections. All patients should be tested for latent TB prior to initiating therapy with a TNF-α inhibitor and patients with known hepatitis B infection should not receive these drugs.

Demyelinating syndromes have been reported in patients treated with TNF-α inhibitors. Immunogenicity, low-titer anti-dsDNA antibody, and drug-induced lupus syndromes have been documented in patients treated with TNF-α inhibitors. Pancytopenia, aplastic anemia, elevated liver function tests, and exacerbation of preexisting or new onset congestive heart failure have all been reported. Long-term toxicities, including increased risk for malignancy, are an ongoing concern, although the data is inconclusive. Initial surveillance suggested a higher incidence of lymphoma and nonmelanoma skin cancers. Recent meta-analysis of published articles on TNF-α inhibitors suggests a higher rate of malignancy than patients in placebo or methotrexate groups [115]. However, other studies from large patient data bank registries from the United States and Europe have not shown increased malignancy rates associated with TNF-α inhibitors [111].

IL-1, produced by rheumatoid synovial macrophages, acts synergistically with TNF-α on synovial fibroblasts, chondrocytes, endothelial cells, and osteoclasts to promote influx of PMNs into the joint, release of metalloproteinases and collagenases from chondrocytes, and activation of osteoclastic bone resorption. IL-1 binds to two types of cell-surface receptors, but only type I is capable of intracellular activation. Anakinra, a human recombinant IL-1–receptor antagonist, competitively inhibits IL-1 binding to type 1 receptors and is approved for treatment of moderate-to-severe RA. Because of its short half-life, anakinra must be administered daily as a 100 mg subcutaneous injection. Toxicities include injection site reactions and an increase in serious infections. Due to the need for daily injections, modest benefit in RA, and the availability of other biologic agents, anakinra is seldom used for RA, although it remains an effective therapy for some cryopyrin-associated periodic syndromes.

IL-6, a proinflammatory cytokine expressed in RA synovial tissues, promotes the activation of B-cells, T-cells, and macrophages, and upregulation of endothelial adhesion molecule expression. IL-6 also stimulates osteoclast maturation and promotes bone erosion. Tocilizumab, a humanized IgG1 anti-IL-6 receptor antibody, is approved for treatment of RA in patients who fail to respond to DMARDs and TNF-α inhibitors. Tocilizumab is administered as a monthly IV infusion either alone or in combination with weekly methotrexate. The risk of serious infection is similar to the TNF-α inhibitors. TB has been reported, but there is insufficient data to quantify the risk. To date, there is no evidence of an increased incidence of malignancies in RA patients treated with tocilizumab, but long-term data is not available. In clinical trials, tocilizumab has also been associated with hypertension, hypercholesterolemia, elevated liver transaminases, and lower gastrointestinal perforation.

Rituximab (RTX), a chimeric monoclonal antibody to CD20 that results in depletion of mature B cells and disruption of T-cell activation, has been used for treatment of non-Hodgkin lymphoma (NHL). Rituximab is approved for treatment of RA in combination with methotrexate in patients who failed other disease modifying antirheumatic drugs (DMARDs) including anti-TNF-α therapies. Toxicities include infusion reactions with hypotension, fever, and nausea. Serious and potentially fatal viral infections, either new or reactivated, including reactivation of hepatitis B with fulminant hepatitis and hepatic failure, have been reported. There does not appear to be an increased risk of serious bacterial infections in RA patients treated with rituximab, but of the infections reported, respiratory tract infections are the most common. No opportunistic infections or tuberculosis, and no increased risk of malignancy have been reported in the limited follow up of treated RA patients. Data from the NHL database on rituximab has been reassuring in that serious adverse events were infrequent. However, there are case reports of progressive multifocal leukoencephalopathy (PML) in patients with RA and SLE.

Abatacept, a selective modulator of T-cell activation, is approved for the treatment of moderate-to-severe RA in patients who have an inadequate response to methotrexate, other DMARDs, or TNF-α inhibitors. In addition to cognate binding of the T-cell receptor to MHC/antigen on the antigen presenting cell (APC), T-cell activation requires a second costimulatory

TABLE 193.9

MANAGEMENT OF RHEUMATIC DISEASES: AVAILABLE TRIALS AND STRENGTH OF EVIDENCE

	Treatment recommendations	Strength of evidence[a]
Systemic lupus erythematosus (SLE): Lupus nephritis (LN)	Improved long-term preservation of renal function in proliferative glomerulonephritis with CY, AZA, or combination therapy when compared with high doses steroid alone [25]	A
	Combination therapy of IVCY with high-dose methylprednisolone improves renal outcome without significant toxicities [26]	A
	MMF is as effective as IVCY in induction of remission of class III and IV LN without differences in toxicity; MMF more effective than IVCY in patients of Hispanic or African origin [27,28]	A
	Low dose IVCY is equivalent to high dose IVCY efficacy for induction, sustained stabilization, toxicity profile over 10 years in LN (Class III, IV, V) [31]	A
	Short-term induction with IVCY followed by MMF or AZA for maintenance, if better at maintaining remission of lupus glomerulonephritis than long-term IVCY [29]	A
	MMF is equivalent to IVCY in induction of remission of Class V LN [33]	A
SLE: Neuropsychiatric (NSPLE)	IVCY is more effective than pulse methylprednisolone alone for severe NPSLE [39]	A
Antiphospholipid syndrome (APS)	High intensity warfarin therapy is not superior to moderate intensity warfarin therapy in patients with APS [70]	B
	Asymptomatic, persistently APA-positive individuals do not benefit from low-dose aspirin for primary thrombosis prophylaxis [71]	B
Systemic sclerosis (SSc): Raynaud's phenomena (RP)	Intravenous prostanoids are effective in healing digital ulcers in patients with SSc RP [77,117]	A
	Bosentan is effective in preventing new digital ulcers in patients with SSc RP [73,74]	A
	Sildenafil reduces the frequency and severity of attacks and promotes healing of digital ulcers in SSc RP [75,76]	B
SSc: Interstitial lung disease	Both IVCY and oral CY provide modest improvement in SSc lung function, dyspnea, and skin scores compared to placebo [81,82]	A
SSc: Pulmonary hypertension (PAH)	Continuous infusion of epoprostenol for SSc related PAH improves exercise capacity and hemodynamics compared to conventional therapy [90]	B
	Oral bosentan improves exercise capacity, dyspnea index, and functional class when compared with placebo in patients with PAH [84,85]	A
	Sildenafil improves exercise tolerance, functional class, and hemodynamics compared to placebo in patients with PAH [89]	B
	Ambrisentan improves exercise capacity, functional class, and hemodynamics in patients with PAH [86]	B
	Sitaxsentan improves exercise capacity, functional class, and hemodynamics in patients with PAH [87,88]	A

[a]*Strength of Evidence* (based on Ebell MH, Siwek J, Weiss BD, et al: Strength of Recommendation Taxonomy (SORT): A patient-centered approach to grading evidence in the medical literature. *Am Fam Physician* 69:548–556, 2004).
Level A recommendation is based on consistent and good-quality patient-oriented evidence; *Level B* recommendation is based on inconsistent or limited-quality patient oriented evidence.
APA, antiphospholipid antibody; AZA, azathioprine; IVCY, intravenous cyclophosphamide; MMF, mycophenolate mofetil.

signal delivered by binding of the T-cell CD28 receptor to an APC-bound B7 molecule. Abatacept (CTLA4-Ig) is a soluble fusion protein comprised of the extracellular domain of CTLA4 and the Fc portion of IgG1 that interferes with T-cell activation by binding to CD80 (B7-1) or CD86 (B7-2), thereby inhibiting the required costimulatory signal. Toxicities include hypersensitivity infusion reactions, infections, exacerbation of COPD, and potential concerns about malignancies including lymphoma and lung cancer.

An admitted ICU patient who has recently received one of these biologic agents should be approached as an immunocompromised host. Atypical or opportunistic infections are high on the differential if the patient is febrile. In addition, other toxicities of these drugs (although rare), including cytopenias, liver function abnormalities, atypical neurological symptoms, and congestive heart failure, may contribute to the patient's overall medical status. Given the critical nature of the illness that requires ICU care, it is prudent to postpone patients' scheduled doses of these biologic agents until their medical status is more stable. The biologic agents should not be used in patients with active infections. There are no well-controlled studies of the use of these agents in pregnant women. The TNF-α inhibitors and anakinra are rated pregnancy class B (no evidence of risk). Abatacept, rituximab, and tocilizumab are all class C (risk cannot be ruled out). Use of these biologic agents should be avoided during pregnancy unless no alternative therapies are available. Given the limited data on long-term toxicities of biologic therapies, vigilance in surveillance of toxicities is imperative and ongoing.

Advances in management of rheumatologic diseases, based on randomized controlled trials or meta-analyses of such trials, are summarized in Table 193.9.

References

1. Terkeltaub RA: Clinical practice. *Gout. N Engl J Med* 349(17):1647–1655, 2003.
2. Terkeltaub RA, Furst DE, Bennett K, et al: High versus low dosing of oral colchicine for early acute gout flare: twenty-four-hour outcome of the first multicenter, randomized, double-blind, placebo-controlled, parallel-group, dose-comparison colchicine study. *Arthritis Rheum* 62(4):1060–1068, 2010.
3. Terkeltaub R: Colchicine Update: 2008. *Semin Arthritis Rheum* 38:411–419, 2008.
4. Mathews C, Weston V, Jones A, et al: Bacterial septic arthritis in adults. *Lancet* 375:846–855, 2010.
5. Martgaretten M, Kohlwes J, Moore D, et al: Does this adult have septic arthritis. *JAMA* 297:1478–1488, 2007.
6. Gupta MN SR, Field M: Prospective 2-year study of 75 patients with adult-onset septic arthritis. *Rheumatology (Oxford)* 40:24–30, 2001.
7. Donatto K: Orthopedic management of septic arthritis. *Rheum Dis Clin North Am* 24(2):275–286, 1998.
8. Del Pozo J, Patel R: Infection associated with prosthetic joints. *N Engl J Med* 361:787–794, 2009.
9. Muller M, Morawietz L, Hasart O, et al: Diagnosis of periprosthetic infections following total hip arthroplasty: evaluation of the diagnostic values of pre- and intraoperative parameters and the associated strategy to preoperatively select patients with high probability of joint infections. *J Orthop Surg* 8:31, 2008.
10. Love C, Marwin S, Palestro C: Nuclear medicine and the infected joint replacement. *Semin Nucl Med* 39:66–78, 2009.
11. Marculescu CE, Berbari EF, Hanssen AD, et al: Outcome of prosthetic joint infections treated with debridement and retention of components. *Clin Infect Dis* 42(4):471–478, 2006.
12. Neva M, Hakkinen A, Makien H: High prevalence of asymptomatic cervical spine subluxation in patients with rheumatoid arthritis waiting for orthopedic surgery. *Ann Rheum Dis* 65:884–888, 2006.
13. Sciubba D, Nelson C, Hsieh P: Perioperative challenges in the surgical management of ankylosing spondylitis. *Neurosurg Focus* 24:E1–E10, 2008.
14. Geterud A, Ejnele H, Mansson I: Severe airway obstruction caused by laryngeal rheumatoid arthritis. *J Rheumatol* 13(5):948–951, 1986.
15. Balbir-Gurman A, Yigla M, Nahir AM, et al: Rheumatoid pleural effusion. *Semin Arthritis Rheum* 35(6):368–378, 2006.
16. Koduri G, Norton S, Young A, et al: Interstitial lung disease has a poor prognosis in rheumatoid arthritis: results from an inception cohort. *Rheumatology (Oxford)* 49(8):1483–1489, 2010.
17. Brown KK: Rheumatoid lung disease. *Proc Am Thorac Soc* 4(5):443–448, 2007.
18. Devouassoux G, Cottin V, Liote H: Characterisation of severe obliterative bronchiolitis in rheumatoid arthritis. *Eur Respir J* 33(5):1053–1061, 2009.
19. Gabriel SE: Why do people with rheumatoid arthritis still die prematurely? *Ann Rheum Dis* 67[Suppl 3]:iii30–iii34, 2008.
20. Hochberg M: Updating the American College of Rheumatology revised criteria for the classification of systemic lupus erythematosus. *Arthritis Rheum.* 40:1725, 1997.
21. Hsu CL, Chen KY, Yeh PS, et al: Outcome and prognostic factors in critically ill patients with systemic lupus erythematosus: a retrospective study. *Crit Care* 9(3):177–183, 2005.
22. Moroni G, Tantardini F, Gallelli B, et al: The long-term prognosis of renal transplantation in patients with lupus nephritis. *Am J Kidney Dis* 45(5):903–911, 2005.
23. Ponticelli C, Moroni G: Renal transplantation in lupus nephritis. *Lupus* 14(1):95–98, 2005.
24. Weening JJ, D'Agati VD, Schwartz MM, et al: The classification of glomerulonephritis in systemic lupus erythematosus revisited. *Kidney Int* 65(2):521–530, 2004.
25. Steinberg AD, Steinberg SC: Long-term preservation of renal function in patients with lupus nephritis receiving treatment that includes cyclophosphamide versus those treated with prednisone only. *Arthritis Rheum* 34(8):945–950, 1991.
26. Illei GG, Austin HA, Crane M, et al: Combination therapy with pulse cyclophosphamide plus pulse methylprednisolone improves long-term renal outcome without adding toxicity in patients with lupus nephritis. *Ann Intern Med* 135(4):248–257, 2001.
27. Ginzler EM, Dooley MA, Aranow C, et al: Mycophenolate mofetil or intravenous cyclophosphamide for lupus nephritis. *N Engl J Med* 353(21):2219–2228, 2005.
28. Appel GB, Contreras G, Dooley MA, et al: Mycophenolate mofetil versus cyclophosphamide for induction treatment of lupus nephritis. *J Am Soc Nephrol* 20(5):1103–1112, 2009.
29. Contreras G, Tozman E, Nahar N, et al: Maintenance therapies for proliferative lupus nephritis: mycophenolate mofetil, azathioprine and intravenous cyclophosphamide. *Lupus.* 14[Suppl 1]:s33–s38, 2005.
30. Houssiau FA, Vasconcelos C, D'Cruz D, et al: Immunosuppressive therapy in lupus nephritis: the Euro-Lupus Nephritis Trial, a randomized trial of low-dose versus high-dose intravenous cyclophosphamide. *Arthritis Rheum* 46(8):2121–2131, 2002.
31. Houssiau FA, Vasconcelos C, D'Cruz D, et al: The 10-year follow-up data of the Euro-Lupus Nephritis Trial comparing low-dose and high-dose intravenous cyclophosphamide. *Ann Rheum Dis* 69(1):61–64, 2010.
32. Austin HA, Illei GG: Membranous lupus nephritis. *Lupus* 14(1):65–71, 2005.
33. Radhakrishnan J, Moutzouris DA, Ginzler EM, et al: Mycophenolate mofetil and intravenous cyclophosphamide are similar as induction therapy for class V lupus nephritis. *Kidney Int* 77(2):152–160, 2010.
34. Furie R, Looney RJ, Rovin B, et al: Efficacy and safety of rituximab in subjects with active proliferative lupus nephritis (LN): results from the randomized double-blind phase III Lunar study. *Arthritis Rheum* 60[Suppl]:S429, 2009.
35. Merrill JT, Neuwelt CM, Wallace DJ, et al: Efficacy and safety of rituximab in moderately-to-severely active systemic lupus erythematosus: the randomized, double-blind, phase II/III systemic lupus erythematosus evaluation of rituximab trial. *Arthritis Rheum* 62(1):222–233, 2010.
36. American College of Rheumatology nomenclature and case definitions for neuropsychiatric lupus syndromes. *Arthritis Rheum* 42(4):599–608, 1999.
37. Hanly J: Neuropsychiatric Lupus. *Rheum Dis Clin N Am* 31:273–298, 2005.
38. Govoni M, Castellino G, Padovan M, et al: Recent advances and future perspective in neuroimaging in neuropsychiatric systemic lupus erythematosus. *Lupus* 13(3):149–158, 2004.
39. Barile-Fabris L, Ariza-Andraca R, Olguin-Ortega L, et al:. Controlled clinical trial of IV cyclophosphamide versus IV methylprednisolone in severe neurological manifestations in systemic lupus erythematosus. *Ann Rheum Dis* 64(4):620–625, 2005.
40. Trevisani VF, Castro AA, Neves Neto JF, et al: Cyclophosphamide versus methylprednisolone for treating neuropsychiatric involvement in systemic lupus erythematosus. *Cochrane Database Syst Rev* 2006(2):CD002265.
41. Bertoli AM, Vila LM, Apte M, et al: Systemic lupus erythematosus in a multiethnic US Cohort LUMINA XLVIII: factors predictive of pulmonary damage. *Lupus* 16(6):410–417, 2007.
42. Pego-Reigosa JM, Medeiros DA, Isenberg DA: Respiratory manifestations of systemic lupus erythematosus: old and new concepts. *Best Pract Res Clin Rheumatol* 23(4):469–480, 2009.
43. Coghlan JG, Handler C: Connective tissue associated pulmonary arterial hypertension. *Lupus* 15(3):138, 2006.
44. McMillan E, Martin WL, Waugh J, et al: Management of pregnancy in women with pulmonary hypertension secondary to SLE and anti-phospholipid syndrome. *Lupus* 11(6):392–398, 2002.
45. Assous N, Allanore Y, Batteux F, et al: Prevalence of antiphospholipid antibodies in systemic sclerosis and association with primitive pulmonary arterial hypertension and endothelial injury. *Clin Exp Rheumatol* 23(2): 199–204, 2005.
46. Badesch DB, Hill NS, Burgess G, et al: Sildenafil for pulmonary arterial hypertension associated with connective tissue disease. *J Rheumatol* 34(12):2417–2422, 2007.
47. Jais X, Launay D, Yaici A, et al: Immunosuppressive therapy in lupus- and mixed connective tissue disease-associated pulmonary arterial hypertension: a retrospective analysis of twenty-three cases. *Arthritis Rheum* 58(2):521–531, 2008.
48. Bernatsky S, Boivin JF, Joseph L, et al: Mortality in systemic lupus erythematosus. *Arthritis Rheum* 54(8):2550–2557, 2006.
49. Rosenbaum E, Krebs E, Cohen M, et al: The spectrum of clinical manifestations, outcome and treatment of pericardial tamponade in patients with systemic lupus erythematosus: a retrospective study and literature review. *Lupus* 18(7):608–612, 2009.
50. Roldan CA, Qualls CR, Sopko KS, et al: Transthoracic versus transesophageal echocardiography for detection of Libman-Sacks endocarditis: a randomized controlled study. *J Rheumatol* 35(2):224–229, 2008.
51. Mandell B: Cardiovascular involvement in systemic lupus erythematosus. *Semin Arthritis Rheum* 17:126, 1987.
52. Hak AE, Karlson EW, Feskanich D, et al: Systemic lupus erythematosus and the risk of cardiovascular disease: results from the nurses' health study. *Arthritis Rheum* 61(10):1396–402, 2009.
53. Bruce IN, Gladman DD, Urowitz MB: Premature atherosclerosis in systemic lupus erythematosus. *Rheum Dis Clin North Am* 26(2):257–278, 2000.
54. Giannouli S, Voulgarelis M, Ziakas PD, et al: Anaemia in systemic lupus erythematosus: from pathophysiology to clinical assessment. *Ann Rheum Dis* 65(2):144–148, 2006.
55. Lambotte O, Khellaf M, Harmouche H, et al: Characteristics and long-term outcome of 15 episodes of systemic lupus erythematosus-associated hemophagocytic syndrome. *Medicine (Baltimore).* 85(3):169–182, 2006.
56. Jeffries M, Hamadeh F, Aberle T, et al: Haemolytic anaemia in a multi-ethnic cohort of lupus patients: a clinical and serological perspective. *Lupus* 17(8):739–743, 2008.
57. Gomard-Mennesson E, Ruivard M, Koenig M, et al: Treatment of isolated severe immune hemolytic anaemia associated with systemic lupus erythematosus: 26 cases. *Lupus* 15(4):223–231, 2006.
58. Avina-Zubieta JA, Galindo-Rodriguez G, Robledo I, et al: Long-term effectiveness of danazol corticosteroids and cytotoxic drugs in the treatment of hematologic manifestations of systemic lupus erythematosus. *Lupus* 12(1):52–57, 2003.

59. Letchumanan P, Thumboo J: Danazol in the treatment of systemic lupus erythematosus: a qualitative systematic review. *Semin Arthritis Rheum* 40(4):298–306, 2011.
60. You YN, Tefferi A, Nagorney DM: Outcome of splenectomy for thrombocytopenia associated with systemic lupus erythematosus. *Ann Surg* 240(2):286–292, 2004.
61. Eisenberg R, Albert D: B-cell targeted therapies in rheumatoid arthritis and systemic lupus erythematosus. *Nat Clin Pract Rheumatol* 2(1):20–27, 2006.
62. Xu D, Yang H, Lai CC, et al: Clinical analysis of systemic lupus erythematosus with gastrointestinal manifestations. *Lupus* 19(7):866–869, 2010.
63. Sultan SM, Ioannou Y, Isenberg DA: A review of gastrointestinal manifestations of systemic lupus erythematosus. *Rheumatology (Oxford)* 38(10): 917–932, 1999.
64. Lee CK, Ahn MS, Lee EY, et al: Acute abdominal pain in systemic lupus erythematosus: focus on lupus enteritis (gastrointestinal vasculitis). *Ann Rheum Dis* 61(6):547–550, 2002.
65. Olsen NJ: Drug-induced autoimmunity. *Best Pract Res Clin Rheumatol* 18(5):677–688, 2004.
66. Levine JS, Branch DW, Rauch J: The antiphospholipid syndrome. *N Engl J Med* 346(10):752–763, 2002.
67. D'Cruz D: Renal manifestations of the antiphospholipid syndrome. *Curr Rheumatol Rep* 11(1):52–60, 2009.
68. Cervera R, Font J, Gomez-Puerta JA, et al: Validation of the preliminary criteria for the classification of catastrophic antiphospholipid syndrome. *Ann Rheum Dis* 64(8):1205–1209, 2005.
69. Bucciarelli S, Espinosa G, Cervera R, et al: Mortality in the catastrophic antiphospholipid syndrome: causes of death and prognostic factors in a series of 250 patients. *Arthritis Rheum* 54(8):2568–2576, 2006.
70. Crowther MA, Ginsberg JS, Julian J, et al: A comparison of two intensities of warfarin for the prevention of recurrent thrombosis in patients with the antiphospholipid antibody syndrome. *N Engl J Med* 349(12):1133–1138, 2003.
71. Erkan D, Harrison MJ, Levy R, et al: Aspirin for primary thrombosis prevention in the antiphospholipid syndrome: a randomized, double-blind, placebo-controlled trial in asymptomatic antiphospholipid antibody-positive individuals. *Arthritis Rheum* 56(7):2382–2391, 2007.
72. Kowal-Bielecka O, Landewe R, Avouac J, et al: EULAR recommendations for the treatment of systemic sclerosis: a report from the EULAR Scleroderma Trials and Research group (EUSTAR). *Ann Rheum Dis* 68(5):620–628, 2009.
73. Korn JH, Mayes M, Cerinic MM: Digital ulcers in systemic sclerosis: prevention by treatment with bosentan, an oral endothelin receptor antagonist. *Arthritis Rheum* 50(12):3985–3993, 2005.
74. Seibold J, Matucci-Cerinic M, Denton CP, et al: Bosentan reduces the number of new digital ulcers in patients with systemic sclerosis. *Ann Rheum Dis* 65[Suppl]:90, 2006.
75. Fries R, Shariat K, von Wilmowsky H, et al: Sildenafil in the treatment of Raynaud's phenomenon resistant to vasodilatory therapy. *Circulation* 112:2980–2985, 2005.
76. Brueckner C, Becker MO, Kroencke T, et al: Effect of sildenafil on digital ulcers in systemic sclerosis: analysis from a single centre pilot study. *Ann Rheum Dis* 69(8):1475–1478, 2010.
77. Simms RW, Farber H, Kissin E, et al: Intravenous epoprostenol for severe digital ischemia in scleroderma. *Arthritis Rheum* 50[Suppl 9]:1702, 2004.
78. White B: Interstitial lung disease in scleroderma. *Rheum Dis Clin North Am* 29(2):371–390, 2003.
79. Goh NS, Desai SR, Veeraraghavan S, et al: Interstitial lung disease in systemic sclerosis: a simple staging system. *Am J Respir Crit Care Med* 177(11):1248–1254, 2008.
80. Goh NS, Veeraraghavan S, Desai SR, et al: Bronchoalveolar lavage cellular profiles in patients with systemic sclerosis-associated interstitial lung disease are not predictive of disease progression. *Arthritis Rheum* 56(6):2005–2012, 2007.
81. Tashkin DP, Elashoff R, Clements PJ, et al: Cyclophosphamide versus placebo in scleroderma lung disease. *N Engl J Med* 22;354(25):2655–2666, 2006.
82. Hoyles RK, Ellis RW, Wellsbury J, et al: A multicenter, prospective, randomized, double-blind, placebo-controlled trial of corticosteroids and intravenous cyclophosphamide followed by oral azathioprine for the treatment of pulmonary fibrosis in scleroderma. *Arthritis Rheum* 54(12):3962–3970, 2006.
83. Denton C, Black C: Pulmonary hypertension in systemic sclerosis. *Rheum Dis Clin North Am* 29(2):335–349, 2003.
84. Rubin LJ, Badesch DB, Barst RJ, et al: Bosentan therapy for pulmonary arterial hypertension. *N Engl J Med* 346(12):896–903, 2002.
85. Channick RN, Simonneau G, Sitbon O, et al: Effects of the dual endothelin-receptor antagonist bosentan in patients with pulmonary hypertension: a randomised placebo-controlled study. *Lancet* 358(9288):1119–1123, 2001.
86. Galie N, Olschewski H, Oudiz RJ, et al: Ambrisentan for the treatment of pulmonary arterial hypertension: results of the ambrisentan in pulmonary arterial hypertension, randomized, double-blind, placebo-controlled, multicenter, efficacy (ARIES) study 1 and 2. *Circulation* 117(23):3010–3019, 2008.
87. Barst RJ, Langleben D, Frost A, et al: Sitaxsentan therapy for pulmonary arterial hypertension. *Am J Respir Crit Care Med* 169(4):441–447, 2004.
88. Barst RJ, Langleben D, Badesch D, et al: Treatment of pulmonary arterial hypertension with the selective endothelin-A receptor antagonist sitaxsentan. *J Am Coll Cardiol* 47(10):2049–2056, 2006.
89. Galie N, Ghofrani HA, Torbicki A, et al: Sildenafil citrate therapy for pulmonary arterial hypertension. *N Engl J Med* 353(20):2148–2157, 2005.
90. Badesch DB, Tapson VF, McGoon MD, et al: Continuous intravenous epoprostenol for pulmonary hypertension due to the scleroderma spectrum of disease. A randomized, controlled trial. *Ann Intern Med* 132(6):425–434, 2000.
91. Khurma V, Meyer C, Park GS, et al: A pilot study of subclinical coronary atherosclerosis in systemic sclerosis: coronary artery calcification in cases and controls. *Arthritis Rheum* 59(4):591–597, 2008.
92. Ferri C, Giuggioli D, Sebastiani M, et al: Heart involvement and systemic sclerosis. *Lupus* 14(9):702–707, 2005.
93. Demarco P, Weisman M, Seibold J, et al: Predictors and outcomes of scleroderma renal crisis: the high-dose versus low-dose D-penicillamine in early diffuse systemic sclerosis trial. *Arthritis Rheum* 46(11):2983–2989, 2002.
94. Steen VD, Medsger TA: Long-Term outcome of scleroderma renal crisis. *Ann Intern Med* 133:600–603, 2000.
95. Ebert EC: Gastric and enteric involvement in progressive systemic sclerosis. *J Clin Gastroenterol* 42(1):5–12, 2008.
96. Perlemuter G, Cacoub P, Chaussade S, et al: Octreotide treatment of chronic intestinal pseudoobstruction secondary to connective tissue diseases. *Arthritis Rheum* 42(7):1545–1549, 1999.
97. Boeckxstaens GE, Bartelsman JF, Lauwers L, et al: Treatment of GI dysmotility in scleroderma with the new enterokinetic agent prucalopride. *Am J Gastroenterol* 97(1):194–197, 2002.
98. Jaovisidha K, Csuka ME, Almagro UA: Severe gastrointestinal involvement in systemic sclerosis: report of five cases and review of the literature. *Semin Arthritis Rheum* 34:689–702, 2004.
99. Bohan A, Peter JB: Polymyositis and dermatomyositis I. *N Engl J Med* 292:344–347, 1975.
100. Walker UA: Imaging tools for the clinical assessment of idiopathic inflammatory myositis. *Curr Opin Rheumatol* 20(6):656–661, 2008.
101. Targoff IN: Myositis specific autoantibodies. *Curr Rheumatol Rep* 8(3): 196–203, 2006.
102. Gunawardena H, Betteridge ZE, McHugh NJ: Newly identified autoantibodies: relationship to idiopathic inflammatory myopathy subsets and pathogenesis. *Curr Opin Rheumatol* 20(6):675–680, 2008.
103. Christopher-Stine L, Plotz PH: Adult inflammatory myopathies. *Best Pract Res Clin Rheumatol* 18(3):331–344, 2004.
104. Oddis C, Medsger T: *Clinical Features, Classification, and Epidemiology of Inflammatory Muscle Disease.* 4th ed. Edinburgh, Mosby, 2008.
105. Iorizzo LJ III, Jorizzo JL: The treatment and prognosis of dermatomyositis: an updated review. *J Am Acad Dermatol* 59(1):99–112, 2008.
106. Dankó K, Ponyi A, Constantin T, et al: Long-term survival of patients with idiopathic inflammatory myopathies according to clinical features: a longitudinal study of 162 Cases. *Medicine (Baltimore)* 83:35–42, 2004.
107. Buchbinder R, Forbes A, Hall S, et al: Incidence of malignant disease in biopsy-proven inflammatory myopathy. A population-based cohort study. *Ann Intern Med* 134(12):1087–1095, 2001.
108. Dalakas MC, Illa I, Dambrosia JM, et al: A controlled trial of high-dose intravenous immune globulin infusions as treatment for dermatomyositis. *N Engl J Med* 329(27):1993–2000, 1993.
109. Dastmalchi M, Grundtman C, Alexanderson H, et al: A high incidence of disease flares in an open pilot study of infliximab in patients with refractory inflammatory myopathies. *Ann Rheum Dis* 67(12):1670–1677, 2008.
110. Clunie G, Leonard L: Relevance of thiopurine methyltransferase status in rheumatology patients receiving azathioprine. *Rheumatology (Oxford)* 43:13–18, 2004.
111. Wolfe F, Michaud K: Lymphoma in rheumatoid arthritis: the effect of methotrexate and anti-tumor necrosis factor therapy in 18,572 patients. *Arthritis Rheum* 50(6):1740–1751, 2004.
112. Dooley M, Patterson CC, Hogan SL, et al: Preservation of ovarian function using depot leuprolide acetate during cyclophosphamide therapy for severe lupus nephritis. *Arthritis Rheum* 43[Suppl]:2858, 2000.
113. Masala A, Faedda R, Alagna S, et al: Use of testosterone to prevent cyclophosphamide-induced azoospermia. *Ann Intern Med* 15;126(4):292–295, 1997.
114. Furst DE, Keystone EC, Fleischmann R, et al: Updated consensus statement on biological agents for the treatment of rheumatic diseases. *Ann Rheum Dis* 69[Suppl 1]:i2–i29, 2009.
115. Bongartz T, Sutton AJ, Sweeting MJ, et al: Anti-TNF antibody therapy in rheumatoid arthritis and the risk of serious infections and malignancies: systematic review and meta-analysis of rare harmful effects in randomized controlled trials. *JAMA* 295(19):2275–2285, 2006.
116. Olschewski H, Simonneau G, Galie N, et al: Inhaled iloprost for severe pulmonary hypertension. *N Engl J Med* 347(5):322–329, 2002.
117. Wigley FM, Wise RA, Seibold JR, et al: Intravenous iloprost infusion in patients with Raynaud phenomenon secondary to systemic sclerosis: a Multicenter, placebo-controlled, double-blind study. *Ann Intern Med* 120(3):199–206, 1994.
118. Tapson VF, Gomberg-Maitland M, McLaughlin VV, et al: Safety and efficacy of IV treprostinil for pulmonary arterial hypertension: a prospective, multicenter, open-label, 12-week trial. *Chest* 129(3):683–6838, 2006.

CHAPTER 194 ■ ANAPHYLAXIS

FREDERIC F. LITTLE AND HELEN M. HOLLINGSWORTH

Anaphylaxis is the most severe and potentially fatal form of the immediate hypersensitivity reactions. The term *anaphylaxis* (antiphylaxis) is derived from the Greek and means "against protection" [1]. It describes the shock-like state that is caused by contact with a substance and contrasts with the term *prophylaxis*, which denotes a beneficial or protective state resulting from contact with a substance.

The clinical features of anaphylactic reactions are the physiologic sequelae of release of chemical mediators from tissue-based mast cells and circulating basophils and include a potential for life-threatening vascular collapse and respiratory obstruction [2,3]. A clinically and physiologically indistinguishable hypersensitivity reaction, which is called an anaphylactoid reaction, differs from anaphylactic reactions only because the chemical mediators are released by nonimmunologic mechanisms. Since the clinical features are indistinguishable, both will be referred to collectively as anaphylactic reactions [4].

Estimation of the annual incidence of anaphylactic reactions is hampered by complex coding and incomplete reporting. A recent European study estimated annual incidences of severe and fatal anaphylaxis at 1 to 3 per 10,000 and 1 to 3 per million, respectively [5]. Extrapolations from a comprehensive study of emergency department visits in a geographically defined U.S. population predict about 245,000 outpatient episodes of severe anaphylaxis annually. The additional cases consequent to medicines and radiocontrast media in hospitalized patients would at least equal the emergency room number. An estimated 1,500 people die of anaphylaxis per year, stressing the importance of prevention, as well as prompt diagnosis and treatment [6,7].

PATHOPHYSIOLOGY OF ANAPHYLACTIC REACTIONS

Mechanisms of Release of Chemical Mediators

In humans, anaphylaxis involves a series of steps that result in the release of chemical mediators from tissue-based mast cells and circulating basophils. First, contact with an antigen stimulates the generation of antibodies of the immunoglobulin E (IgE) class. Next, the IgE molecules bind by way of their Fc receptor to a glycoprotein receptor on the cell-surface membrane of tissue mast cells and blood-borne basophils, the so-called target cells. As many as 4,000 to 100,000 IgE molecules normally bind to a single target cell, and up to 100,000 to 500,000 in atopic individuals [8,9]. This binding may remain for weeks to months. When two IgE molecules with the same Fab binding (antigen recognition) specificity are in close proximity on the surface of mast cells and basophils, the cells are termed *sensitized*.

For subsequent antigenic exposure to stimulate the release of mediators from mast cells and basophils, the specific antigen must bind to the Fab portion of two IgE molecules fixed to the surface of the target cell. This bridging of two IgE molecules initiates a series of biochemical modifications called the activation–secretion response (Fig. 194.1). This sequence causes secretion of preformed primary mediators of anaphylaxis from cytoplasmic granules in target cells, including histamine, serotonin, eosinophil chemotactic factor of anaphylaxis (ECF-A), heparin, neutrophil chemotactic factor, and proteolytic enzymes that include tryptase [10].

The activation–secretion response also stimulates synthesis of kallikrein [11,12] and newly generated, secondary lipid mediators, which include platelet-activating factor (PAF) [1]; prostaglandin D_2 (PGD_2), a product of the cyclooxygenase pathway of arachidonic acid metabolism [12]; and leukotrienes C_4, D_4, and E_4 (LTC_4, LTD_4, and LTE_4), products of the lipoxygenase pathway of arachidonic acid metabolism. Several cytokines are also released after activation, including interleukins (IL-1, IL-2, IL-3, IL-4, IL-5, and IL-6), tumor necrosis factor, endothelin-1, and granulocyte-macrophage colony stimulating factor [13].

A variety of substances may induce IgE antibody formation and, on subsequent challenge, provoke anaphylactic reactions [14]. The most common substances are drugs, insect venoms, foods, and allergen extracts used in specific immunotherapy (SIT) [15,16]. These and other less common causes of IgE-mediated anaphylaxis are outlined in Table 194.1.

Non–IgE-mediated anaphylaxis occurs when certain ingested or infused substances cause direct mast cell and basophil activation. Clinically significant examples of non–IgE-mediated anaphylaxis are noted in Table 194.2. The administration of blood, serum, or immunoglobulins to patients who are IgA deficient can result in immune complex formation between donor IgA and recipient IgG anti-IgA antibodies [4,17]. These immune complexes fix complement causing activation of the complement cascade with release of the C3a and C5a complement fragments. C3a and C5a are anaphylatoxins and can directly activate mast cells and basophils.

Physiologic Properties of the Chemical Mediators of Anaphylaxis

The most important chemical mediators of anaphylaxis are histamine, cysteinyl leukotrienes (LTC_4, LTD_4, and LTE_4), PAF, and bradykinin. Physiologically, these substances increase arteriolar vasodilatation, enhance capillary permeability, recruit other inflammatory cells, and precipitate bronchoconstriction (reviewed in [18]). The contribution of multiple mediators other than histamine explains the limited benefit of antihistamines *alone* in treating anaphylaxis.

Histamine (reviewed in [19]) acts to (a) increase capillary permeability by stimulating terminal arteriolar dilatation and contraction of endothelial cells in postcapillary venules, which opens intercellular gaps, and, as a result, causes the development of urticaria and angioedema; (b) increase secretion from nasal and bronchial mucous glands; (c) stimulate

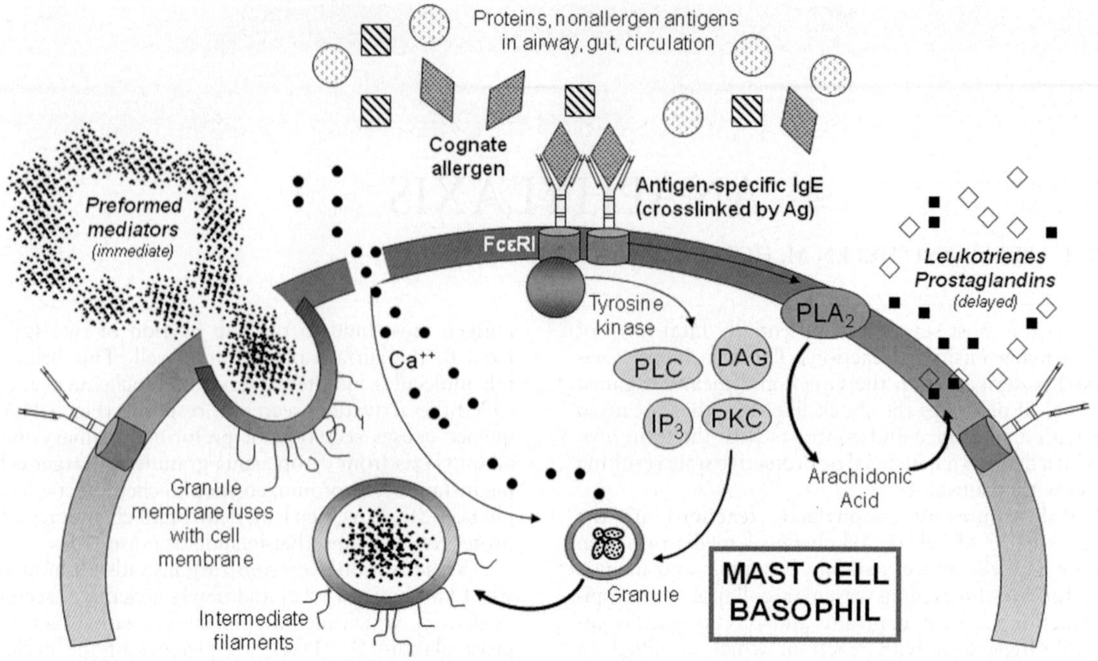

FIGURE 194.1. Chemical mediator release. When two IgE molecules are bridged by an antigen that is specifically recognized by those IgE molecules, a cascade of transmembrane and intracellular events is triggered. The end result is the extrusion of granule contents (mediators) into the extracellular space and elaboration of other, newly formed mediators. Tyrosine kinase appears to be an important intramembrane messenger that initiates the intracellular cascades. At least one cascade involves PLC, which mediates calcium influx into the cell and catalyzes hydrolysis of phosphatidylinositol into the secondary messengers 1,4,5-IP_3 and 1,2-DAG. IP_3 plays a role in calcium mobilization; DAG mediates production of arachidonic acid metabolites and activates PKC. PKC, in turn, participates in the fusion of granules within the cell membrane. PLA_2 mediates the conversion of membrane phospholipid into arachidonic acid, resulting in elaboration of prostaglandins and leukotrienes. Ag, antigen; DAG, diacylglycerol; IgE, immunoglobulin E; IP_3, inositol triphosphate; PKC, protein kinase C; PLA_2, phospholipase A_2; PLC, phospholipase C.

TABLE 194.1

CAUSES OF IMMUNOGLOBULIN E–MEDIATED ANAPHYLAXIS[a]

Type	Agent	Example
Proteins	Allergen extracts	Pollen, dust mite, mold
	Vaccines	Influenza
	Venoms	Hymenoptera
	Heterologous serum	Tetanus antitoxin [16], antithymocyte globulin, snake antivenom
	Others	Heparin, latex [113], thiobarbiturates, seminal fluid
Hormones		Insulin [140], ACTH, TSH [16] progesterone, salmon calcitonin
Haptens	Antibiotics	Beta-lactams [73], ethambutol, nitrofurantoin, sulfonamides [74], streptomycin, vancomycin [143]
Disinfectants		Ethylene oxide
Local anesthetics[b] [144]		Benzocaine, tetracaine, Xylocaine, mepivacaine
Others		Aminopyrine, sulfobromophthalein

[a]Numbers in brackets are reference citations.
[b]Precise mechanism not established.
ACTH, adrenocorticotropic hormone; TSH, thyroid-stimulating hormone.

TABLE 194.2

CAUSES OF NON–IMMUNOGLOBULIN E-MEDIATED ANAPHYLAXIS[a]

Complement activation
Blood product transfusion in IgA-deficient patient [17]
Hemodialysis with cuprophane membrane [145]
Direct release of chemical mediators of anaphylaxis
Protamine [146][b]
Radiographic contrast media [147]
Dextran [148][b]
Hydroxyethyl starch [149]
Muscle relaxants [150]
Ketamine [151]
Local anesthetics [144][b]
Codeine and other opiate narcotics [150,152]
Highly charged antibiotics, including amphotericin B [143]
Generation of leukotrienes
Nonsteroidal anti-inflammatory drugs [132]
Indomethacin [133]
Acetylsalicylic acid (aspirin) [153]
Sulindac [134]
Zomepirac sodium [135]
Tolmetin sodium [136]
Other
Antineoplastic agents (e.g., platinum-based [154,155])
Sulfiting agents
Exercise [120]
Idiopathic recurrent anaphylaxis [124,126]

[a]Numbers in brackets are reference citations.
[b]Precise mechanism not established.

contraction of smooth muscle; (d) enhance prostaglandin synthesis; (e) chemotactically modulate eosinophil migration; and (f) regulate parasympathetic afferent nerve stimulation (a process blocked by atropine), which increases airway resistance and decreases lung compliance. Studies of histamine infusion in normal human volunteers suggest that vasodilatation is mediated by both H_1 and H_2 receptors, whereas bronchoconstriction and tachycardia are mediated by H_1 receptors alone [20].

In anaphylaxis, LTC_4, LTD_4, and LTE_4 (a) induce a prolonged constrictive effect, on bronchial smooth muscle, which affects the peripheral more than the central airways, (b) increase vascular permeability, and (c) act as chemotactic agents for other inflammatory cells [21,22]. In fact, leukotrienes are far more potent bronchoconstrictors than histamine.

Two additional modulators of anaphylaxis are bradykinin, which appears to be activated by mast cell kallikrein and PAF. Bradykinin stimulates a slow, sustained contraction of bronchial and vascular smooth muscles while increasing vascular permeability and secretion from mucous glands [15]. PAF contributes to the pulmonary and cardiovascular manifestations of anaphylaxis by inducing platelet aggregation with release of serotonin, adenosine triphosphate, and lysosomal enzymes from preformed granules [23,24]. In addition, PAF is a potent chemotactic factor for eosinophils and can directly increase vascular permeability [25].

Thus, the physiologic consequences of chemical–mediator release in anaphylaxis are (a) an increased vascular permeability; (b) an increased secretion from nasal and bronchiolar mucous glands; (c) smooth muscle contraction in the blood vessels, the bronchioles, the gastrointestinal tract, and the uterus; (d) migration–attraction of eosinophils and neutrophils; (e) bradykinin generation stimulated by kallikrein substances; and (f) induction of platelet aggregation and degranulation. These events coordinate to increase the vascular permeability that in turn permits the access of a variety of plasma proteins (antibodies, complement, kinins, and coagulation proteins) to tissue sites, which further contributes to the observed inflammation. Substances such as PAF and Hageman factor potentially contribute to local coagulation abnormalities, which may also be seen in anaphylactic reactions [20].

CLINICAL AND LABORATORY FEATURES

Mast cells are concentrated in the skin, in the mucous membranes of the respiratory and gastrointestinal tracts, and in the perivenular tissue, while basophils are located in the bloodstream, all of which are potential sites of exposure to offending antigens (e.g., food, drugs, insect venom, and diagnostic agents) [26]. These sites are also most commonly involved in the manifestations of anaphylaxis. Urticaria, angioedema, respiratory obstruction, and vascular collapse are the most important clinical features of anaphylaxis, and these signs and symptoms are due to the direct effects of mast cell and basophil-derived mediators on affected organ systems. Other clinical manifestations may include (a) a sense of fright or impending doom, (b) weakness or dizziness, (c) sweating, (d) sneezing, (e) rhinorrhea, (f) conjunctivitis, (g) generalized pruritus and swelling, (h) cough, (i) wheezing, stridor, or breathlessness, (j) choking, (k) dysphagia, (l) vomiting or diarrhea, (m) abdominal pain, (n) incontinence, (o) uterine cramps, and (p) loss of consciousness.

Profound hypotension and shock may develop as a result of significant arteriolar vasodilatation, increased vascular permeability, cardiac arrhythmias [27,28], or irreversible cardiac failure [29], even in the absence of respiratory or other symptoms [3,30]. Furthermore, transient or sustained hypotension may result in local tissue ischemia, stroke, myocardial infarction, or death [30,31]. Intravascular coagulation, evidenced by a fall in the levels of factors V, VIII, fibrinogen, kininogen, and complement components, has also been described [32].

Anaphylaxis-induced fatalities most often result from involvement of the respiratory tract [31,33,34]. Structures throughout the respiratory tract may be affected, but respiratory failure is generally the result of upper respiratory tract obstruction due to laryngeal edema or obstruction of small airways due to bronchoconstriction, mucosal edema, and hypersecretion of mucus [35,36]. Intra-alveolar hemorrhage and acute respiratory distress syndrome have been reported [36,37].

The physical examination of a patient with anaphylactic shock often reveals a rapid, weak, irregular, or unobtainable pulse; tachypnea, respiratory distress, cyanosis, hoarseness, stridor, or dysphagia secondary to laryngeal edema; diminished breath sounds, crackles, cough, wheezes, and hyperinflated lungs due to severe bronchoconstriction; urticaria; angioedema or conjunctival edema (Table 194.3) [38]. Any patient may manifest only a subset of these findings, sometimes only cardiovascular collapse or only stridor and breathlessness.

Laboratory findings in anaphylaxis are varied. Biochemical abnormalities in anaphylaxis include elevation of serum histamine and tryptase levels, depression of serum complement components, and decreased levels of high-molecular-weight kininogen. Although these biochemical abnormalities codify our understanding of the pathophysiology of anaphylaxis, they are rarely evaluated in the management of clinically established anaphylaxis. As discussed in the next section, serum tryptase may be helpful retrospectively when the diagnosis is uncertain [39].

Although there have been no systematic reviews of electrocardiographic findings, reports describe disturbances in rate,

TABLE 194.3

CLINICAL MANIFESTATIONS OF ANAPHYLACTIC REACTIONS

System	Reaction	Symptoms	Signs
Respiratory tract	Rhinitis	Nasal congestion and itching	Mucosal edema
	Laryngeal edema	Dyspnea	Laryngeal stridor, edema of vocal cords
	Bronchoconstriction	Cough, wheezing, and sensation of chest tightness	Crackles, respiratory distress, tachypnea, and wheezes
Cardiovascular	Hypotension	Syncope, feeling of faintness	Hypotension, tachycardia
	Arrhythmias	Palpitations	ECG changes: nonspecific ST segment and T-wave changes, nodal rhythm, and atrial fibrillation
Skin	Urticaria	Pruritus, hives	Urticarial lesions
	Angioedema	Nonpruritic swelling of extremity or perioral, or periorbital region	Nonpruritic, frequently asymmetric swelling of extremity, perioral, or periorbital region
Gastrointestinal tract	Smooth muscle contraction, Mucosal edema	Nausea, vomiting, abdominal pain, and diarrhea	Abdominal tenderness, distention
Eye	Conjunctivitis	Ocular itching, lacrimation	Conjunctival inflammation

ECG, electrocardiogram.
Summarized from references [38] and [1].

rhythm, repolarization, and ectopy [40–42], as well as myocardial infarction [28,43]. Chest radiography may reveal hyperinflation caused by severe bronchoconstriction.

DIAGNOSIS AND DIFFERENTIAL DIAGNOSIS OF ANAPHYLAXIS

Development of the characteristic clinical features of anaphylaxis shortly after exposure to an antigen or other inciting agent usually establishes the diagnosis of an anaphylactic reaction [2]. The setting is often suggestive as well: a patient who has just received an antibiotic injection or radiographic contrast media infusion or one who presents to the emergency room after a yellow jacket sting.

The clinical disorders that may be confused with anaphylaxis are sudden, acute bronchoconstriction in an asthmatic, vasovagal syncope, tension pneumothorax, mechanical airway obstruction, pulmonary edema, cardiac arrhythmias, myocardial infarction with cardiogenic shock, aspiration of a food bolus, pulmonary embolism, seizures, acute drug toxicity, hereditary angioedema, cold or idiopathic urticaria, septic shock, and toxic shock syndrome [15].

Initial laboratory testing often is not helpful. However, serum obtained during the acute episode can be assayed subsequently for tryptase and histamine. Total serum tryptase levels include both α- and β-tryptase. The former is increased in systemic mastocytosis and the latter can be elevated for up to 6 hours after suspected anaphylaxis onset [44]. However, the sensitivity of serum β-tryptase is suboptimal as levels can be normal after documented anaphylaxis, especially if caused by foods [45]. There may be a role for serial measurements in documenting the course of systemic mast cell and basophil degranulation [38]. Serum histamine is rarely assessed clinically because it must be obtained within the first hour after a reaction and requires special handling.

Retrospectively, measurement of antigen (allergen)-specific IgE antibodies by an ImmunoCAP (or similar assay, which have replaced radioallergosorbent tests [RAST]) may be helpful. Specific skin tests may also define allergic sensitivity. Skin testing must be done in a carefully controlled setting due to the risk of provoking another severe reaction. Cutaneous assessment for the presence of antigen-specific IgE may be negative for several days after a reaction, because mast cell and basophil degranulation at the time of the initial reaction may lead to a refractory period. This can be avoided by delaying testing for 4 to 6 weeks [46].

CLINICAL COURSE OF ANAPHYLACTIC REACTIONS

Clinical criteria that make the diagnosis of anaphylaxis "highly likely" have been codified [2]. The characteristic features of anaphylactic reactions are (a) the rapid onset of clinical manifestations that follow contact with or the administration of antigen and (b) the rapid progression of symptoms to a severe and potentially fatal outcome. Recognition of the early signs and symptoms of anaphylaxis and prompt treatment are imperative in preventing progression to irreversible shock and death [38].

The constellation of clinical symptoms as well as their severity and duration is variable but will depend to some extent on the mode of antigen exposure. Anaphylaxis may occur within seconds following parenteral introduction of antigen [32] and usually occurs within 30 minutes. In contrast, anaphylaxis that follows oral administration of an antigen may develop within minutes to several hours [47]. Generally, the more rapid the onset of symptoms, the more severe will be the reaction [1]. Mild systemic reactions often last for several hours, rarely more than 24 hours. Severe manifestations, such as laryngeal edema, bronchoconstriction, and hypotension, if not fatal, may persist or recur for several days. However, even severe manifestations may resolve within minutes of treatment. About 5% to 20% of patients will experience biphasic or protracted anaphylaxis, with signs and symptoms recurring up to 24 hours or persisting beyond 24 hours after initial presentation [38]. This highlights the need for close observation after initial response to treatment.

TREATMENT OF ANAPHYLAXIS

The key to successful treatment of anaphylaxis is prompt intervention to support cardiopulmonary function and prevent further exposure to the inciting stimulus when possible. The prompt administration of epinephrine is critical, and should be supplemented with aggressive use of vasopressors, fluid replacement, and medications as indicated to counteract the effects of released chemical mediators [38]. Injectable epinephrine, tourniquets, intravenous infusion materials and fluids, antihistamines, intubation equipment, a tracheostomy set, and individuals trained to use these materials should be available. Since symptoms of a systemic anaphylactic reaction may be followed by potentially fatal manifestations, patients must be serially examined and continuously monitored [38]. Many therapeutic and diagnostic agents frequently employed in intensive care settings (e.g., antibiotics, radiographic contrast) may induce anaphylactic reactions. Thus, the anticipation and the preparedness to deal with these potential reactions are very important.

Emergency Measures

The evaluation of individuals who are suspected of having anaphylaxis must be performed rapidly. The cause and mechanism of antigen exposure should be ascertained to assess how long the inciting antigen has been present and, when possible, to limit further absorption. A history of previous allergic reactions and former treatment may help to guide immediate therapy, obviating the need to try previously failed regimens in a life-threatening situation [48].

Supportive Cardiopulmonary Measures

Particular attention to the respiratory and cardiovascular systems is paramount and must include assessment for laryngeal edema and bronchoconstriction, as well as monitoring oxygenation, blood pressure, and cardiac rhythm [48].

Ensuring adequate ventilation and oxygenation is essential. Supplemental oxygen should be administered and pulse oximetry monitored. Intubation and assisted ventilation may be necessary in cases of severe bronchoconstriction, and ventilator management strategies such as those used for treatment of status asthmaticus may be necessary. These techniques are discussed in Chapters 48 and 58.

Although intubation is usually feasible, edema of the tongue, larynx, or vocal cords may obstruct the upper airway and preclude oropharyngeal or nasopharyngeal intubation. To ensure a patent airway in such instances, cricothyroidotomy or tracheotomy may be necessary (see Chapter 12) [49]. Cricothyroidotomy is preferred to tracheotomy when performed in an emergent situation, as the former is easier to perform and is usually safer [49]. Contraindications to cricothyroidotomy include a suspected neck fracture or a serious injury to the larynx or cricoid cartilage.

Close electrocardiographic monitoring is indicated because the sequelae of anaphylaxis and its therapy are both potentially arrhythmogenic [41]. Hypotension, acidosis, hypoxia, vasopressors, and bronchodilators are well-described predisposing factors for cardiac arrhythmias (see Chapter 42). Adequate intravenous access should be established as soon as possible, initially with two 18-gauge or larger peripheral catheters.

Pharmacologic Therapy

The mainstay of therapy is parenteral epinephrine (adrenaline), which acts on bronchial and cardiac β-receptors, causing bronchial dilatation and both chronotropic and inotropic cardiac stimulation. An equally important effect of epinephrine is stimulation of α-adrenergic receptors on blood vessels, which causes vasoconstriction. This is important in reversing anaphylaxis-induced hypotension and in delaying antigen absorption when infiltrated locally into an injection or sting site [48]. In addition, epinephrine increases the intracellular levels of cyclic adenosine monophosphate (AMP) and thereby inhibits the activation of tissue-based mast cells and circulating basophils [20,50,51]. Inhaled β_2-adrenergic agents, such as albuterol sulfate or salbutamol, complement the actions of epinephrine by reversing bronchoconstriction and reducing bronchial mucus secretion [52].

Antihistamines, particularly the H_1-receptor blocker diphenhydramine, are useful for treating cutaneous manifestations of anaphylaxis, but are slower in onset than epinephrine and not helpful for hemodynamic compromise. Thus, they are considered adjunctive therapy to epinephrine. Given their beneficial safety profile, they may be administered empirically unless there is a specific contraindication (e.g., known prior hypersensitivity). Glucocorticoids, although not immediately active in anaphylactic shock, are effective pharmacologic agents that are capable of increasing tissue response to β-adrenergic agonists as well as inhibiting basophil activation and phospholipase-mediated generation of LTC_4, LTD_4, and LTE_4 [53,54].

The guidelines for pharmacologic therapy of anaphylaxis are listed in Table 194.4.

Specific Therapy

Epinephrine. Epinephrine should be administered first to treat all initial manifestations of anaphylaxis [38,55]. When administered alone, it may reverse rhinitis, urticaria, bronchoconstriction, and hypotension. The failure to administer epinephrine or a delay in its administration may be fatal. There is compelling evidence, both from animal and human studies, that epinephrine is more rapidly absorbed when given intramuscularly (IM) rather than subcutaneously (SC) [56,57]. The IM route is definitely preferred for patients who are hypotensive (see below) or when adequate SC absorption is in doubt [58]. The dose is 0.2 to 0.5 mL of a 1:1,000 dilution (0.2 to 0.5 mg) and should be repeated in 5 to 15 minutes if improvement is equivocal, usually not more than three times [38,48]. Absorption of parenterally introduced antigens (e.g., stinging insect venom, vaccines) may be retarded by infiltrating the site with approximately half the dose of epinephrine. Tourniquet application proximal to the site of antigen exposure that is sufficient to occlude venous and lymphatic returns without interfering with arterial blood flow may also retard absorption of the antigen [1]. The tourniquet should be loosened for approximately 15 to 30 seconds every 10 to 15 minutes.

If shock develops, IM or SC epinephrine is unlikely to be absorbed. In this setting, epinephrine should be given intravenously: 1 mg (1 mL of a 1:1,000 solution or 10 mL of a 1:10,000 solution) diluted in 500 mL of D_5W and infused at a rate of 0.5 to 2.0 mL per minute (1 to 4 μg per minute) with continuous electrocardiographic monitoring. If intravenous access is not easily obtained, epinephrine should be given by endotracheal tube (10 mL of a 1:10,000 solution). If hypotension persists, continuous infusion of a pressor, such as norepinephrine, dopamine, or phenylephrine, is typically initiated (see Chapters 32, 148, and 157).

Volume resuscitation is also important, as described below. If no response to pressors and initial volume resuscitation occurs, the central venous pressure (CVP) may provide guidance regarding further fluid resuscitation. A CVP between 0 and 12 cm H_2O suggests that more intravenous fluids should be given, whereas a CVP more than 12 cm H_2O suggests that the hypotension may be based on myocardial failure. For refractory hypotension, pulmonary artery catheterization (see Chapter 4) can help guide further fluid, inotropic, and vasopressor therapy, as outlined in Chapters 32,148, and 157.

Preexisting β-adrenergic blockade with noncardioselective or cardioselective agents is another potential cause of refractory anaphylactic shock [14,59]. In the presence of beta-blockade, anaphylaxis is characterized by bradycardia with or without atrioventricular nodal delay (in contrast to the usual tachycardia), profound and refractory hypotension, urticaria, and angioedema [59]. Whether beta-blockade truly increases the chance of developing anaphylaxis or just the severity is not known. Beta-blockade appears to increase anaphylactic mediator synthesis and release, as well as altering end-organ responsiveness. Although α-adrenergic agents may increase in vitro release of mast cell mediators in the presence of beta-blockade [60], the drug of first choice for treating anaphylaxis in the presence of beta-blockade remains epinephrine [59]. Dopamine, which has combined α, β, and dopaminergic activities, may be useful for shock refractory to epinephrine. The dose of β agonists will likely have to be more than usual to overcome the beta-blockade. Several case reports note the success with glucagon, often used in the treatment of beta-blocker overdose, in treating refractory shock. Glucagon appears to increase cardiac cyclic AMP independent of β-receptors and to increase heart rate despite beta-blockade [59,61].

Bronchodilators. Bronchoconstriction is treated with a nebulized short-acting β-agonist (typically albuterol 0.5 mL of 0.5% solution diluted in 3 mL of normal saline), often in addition to parenteral epinephrine, as described above. Nebulizer treatments should be repeated every 15 to 20 minutes until bronchoconstriction abates. In addition, a methylxanthine may be given: 250 to 500 mg of aminophylline may be infused over 20 minutes (see Chapter 48), although scientific data supporting this are limited. Methylxanthines are not recommended in hypotensive patients, as they may worsen hypotension and cause unpredictable cardiovascular toxicity [1]. Their exact mechanism of action is not well defined and they are not first-line agents in the treatment of bronchoconstriction.

Volume Resuscitation. Given the distributive nature of shock in anaphylaxis, aggressive volume resuscitation should accompany epinephrine (and other vasoactive medications) if hypotension develops. Prompt initiation of intravenous fluids is more important than whether the fluid is colloid or crystalloid. As noted earlier, refractory hypotension may warrant invasive hemodynamic monitoring to guide therapy.

Antihistamines. Parenteral administration of histamine receptor antagonists is preferred over oral administration. The H_1-receptor-blocker diphenhydramine (1 to 2 mg per kg up to 50 mg for an adult) can be given intravenously as a bolus [1]. The H_2-receptor-blockers cimetidine (300 mg for adult) or ranitidine (150 mg for adult) can be infused over 3 to 5 minutes [62]. Antihistamines are more effective in prevention than in treatment of full-blown anaphylaxis and should never be used as the primary therapy for anaphylactic shock. H_2-receptor-blocking antihistamines prevent the fall in diastolic blood pressure induced by experimental histamine infusion [54], and the H_2-blocker cimetidine has been reported to reverse refractory systemic anaphylaxis [62]. However, the evidence that H_2-receptor-blocking antihistamines are effective in the treatment of anaphylaxis is anecdotal.

Glucocorticoids. Although glucocorticoids are not of immediate clinical benefit, they help to reduce bronchoconstriction and laryngeal edema and provide blood pressure support when used in high doses and for prolonged attacks (see Table 194.4 for recommended doses). The generally recommended initial dose of aqueous hydrocortisone is 5 mg per kg to a maximum of 200 mg given intravenously, followed by 2.5 mg per kg to 200 mg given intravenously every 4 to 6 hours [1,4], for 24 to 48 hours.

Despite the theoretical basis for glucocorticoids preventing late recurrences of anaphylaxis, biphasic anaphylaxis has been reported to occur in 20% of anaphylactic reactions in spite of glucocorticoid therapy [63,64]. In this report, after an initial response to therapy, life-threatening symptoms recurred up to 8 hours later. Whether glucocorticoid therapy helped prevent recurrences after 8 hours, is not known. Because of the possibility of a late recurrence, patients should be monitored in the intensive care setting for 8 to 12 hours after resolution of symptoms. Roughly 30% of anaphylaxis cases may have protracted symptoms for 5 to 32 hours despite vigorous therapy including glucocorticoids [64]. One characteristic of patients with biphasic or protracted anaphylaxis is oral ingestion of the offending antigen. On this basis, it would be reasonable to include enteral activated charcoal and sorbitol in the therapy of such patients to reduce the absorption and duration of exposure to the antigen (see Chapter 117 on drug overdose).

TABLE 194.4

TREATMENT OF ANAPHYLAXIS IN ADULTS [2,38,156]

Mandatory and immediate
General measures
Aqueous epinephrine (1:1,000), 0.2 to 0.5 mL IM; up to 3 doses at 1- to 5-min intervals
Tourniquet proximal to antigen injection or sting site
Aqueous epinephrine (1:1,000), 0.1 to 0.3 mL infiltrated into antigen injection or sting site (unless anatomic region with terminal circulation, e.g., fingertip)
For laryngeal obstruction or respiratory arrest
Establish airway: endotracheal intubation, cricothyroidotomy or tracheotomy
Supplemental oxygen
Mechanical ventilation
After clinical appraisal
General measures
Diphenhydramine, 1.25 mg/kg to maximum of 50 mg, IV or IM
Aqueous hydrocortisone, 200 mg, or methylprednisolone, 50 mg, IV every 6 h for 24–48 h
Ranitidine, 150 mg, IV over 3–5 min
For hypotension
Aqueous epinephrine (1:1,000), 1 mL in 500 mL of saline at 0.5–2.0 mL/min, or 1–4 μg/min, preferably by a central venous line
Normal saline, lactated Ringer's, or colloid volume expansion
Glucagon, if patient is receiving beta-blocker therapy and hypotension is refractory, 1 mg/mL IV bolus or infusion of 1 mg/L of D_5W at a rate of 5–15 mL/min
For bronchoconstriction
Supplemental oxygen
Albuterol (0.5%), 0.5 mL in 2.5 mL of saline, by nebulizer
Aminophylline, only if patient *not* in shock and unresponsive to albuterol and epinephrine, 5 mg/kg to maximum or 500 mg IV over 20 min, then 0.3–0.8 mg/kg/h IV

D_5W, dextrose in 5% water; IM, intramuscular; IV, intravenous.

PREVENTION OF ANAPHYLACTIC REACTIONS

In view of the potential morbidity and mortality from anaphylactic reactions, prevention is of primary importance. Prevention includes obtaining a careful history to identify possible precipitants of anaphylaxis. Both physicians and patients should be aware of potential cross-reacting agents. For example, individuals with anaphylaxis secondary to aspirin are frequently sensitive to nonsteroidal anti-inflammatory drugs, such as ibuprofen, naproxen, ketorolac, and sulindac. Other preservatives, such as metabisulfite, ethylenediamine, and methylparaben, have been associated with anaphylactic reactions. It is therefore helpful to review the inactive ingredients contained in medications temporally associated with anaphylaxis [65].

Prevention of reactions to specific agents (e.g., antibiotics) is discussed below. In general, patients with a history of anaphylaxis should wear a Medic-Alert bracelet or necklace, which detail offending precipitants and potential cross-reacting agents. In addition, patients should be provided with and instructed in the use of anaphylaxis kits (e.g., EpiPen, Dey, Napa, CA) for prompt treatment in future reactions. Finally, consultation with an allergist can clarify the offending trigger (if unknown) and guide appropriate further evaluation and treatment plans. These three actions are the most relevant elements of post-anaphylaxis care from the intensive care perspective.

MANAGEMENT OF ANAPHYLAXIS TO SPECIFIC AGENTS AND PRECIPITANTS

Beta-Lactam Antibiotic Anaphylaxis

One of the most common causes of anaphylaxis in the United States is penicillin. Systemic reactions complicate approximately 1% to 2% of penicillin courses. Approximately 10% of the population will have positive skin tests to penicillin. Thus, a substantial portion of the population is at risk for developing anaphylactic reactions to the drug. About 10% of these reactions are life-threatening and 2% to 10% are fatal [16]. Seventy-five percent of the patients who die of penicillin anaphylaxis have experienced previous allergic reactions to the drug. As with other medications, the risk of a severe reaction is greater with parenteral administration than with oral administration [16]. On the other hand, about 80% of individuals who report penicillin allergy are found to be nonallergic on subsequent evaluation [66].

Skin testing for penicillin hypersensitivity with the major determinant benzylpenicilloyl-poly-L-lysine (BPO, PRE-PEN®, and ALK-Abello) and minor determinants benzylpenicillin (Pen-G), benzylpenicilloate, and benzylpenilloate is effective at detecting IgE-mediated sensitivity and thereby identifying individuals at risk for developing acute allergic reactions to penicillin [16]. The negative predictive value of skin testing when both major and minor determinants of penicillin are used is excellent for immediate hypersensitivity reactions to penicillin [66,67]. This testing does not evaluate other types of sensitivity, such as serum sickness reactions, morbilliform rashes, hemolytic anemia, and interstitial nephritis. In addition, it does not evaluate patients who may have specific allergy to a beta-lactam side chain of a penicillin derivative, for example, cephalosporins or carbapenems [68]. Cross-reactivity between beta-lactams and monobactams, for example, aztreonam, is rare. For critically ill patients, who need a beta-lactam drug and who have a history of beta-lactam antibiotic allergy, the best strategy is to use an alternate, non cross-reacting antibiotic or to proceed with a rapid desensitization protocol [69] (Table 194.5). A retrospective review of antibiotic desensitization for IgE-mediated allergy found that it was successful in 75% of patients [70].

TABLE 194.5

DESENSITIZATION SCHEDULE FOR BETA-LACTAM ANTIBIOTICS

Dose no.	Concentration of stock solution (mg/mL)[a]	Concentration of infused solution (mg/mL)[b]
1	0.0005	0.00001
2	0.005	0.0001
3	0.05	0.001
4	0.5	0.01
5	5	0.1
6	50	1
7	500	10

[a] Stock solution is prepared by solubilizing the antibiotic with nonbacteriostatic saline to a final concentration of 500 mg/mL. Dilutions of 1 mL of each preceding antibiotic dilution to 9 mL of diluent.
[b] One milliliter of stock solution is further diluted into 50 mL of saline and infused during 20 minutes.
From Borish L, Tamir R, Rosenwasser LJ: Intravenous desensitization to beta-lactam antibiotics. *J Allergy Clin Immunol* 80:314–319, 1987, with permission.

The incidence of anaphylactic reactions to cephalosporins is infrequent, but increasing [16,71]. Patients with a history of penicillin allergy have been reported to have allergic reactions to cephalosporins at a rate of 5.4% to 16.5%, compared with patients with a negative history, whose reaction rate was 1% to 2% [72,73]. The rate of cross-reactivity is lower with second- and third-generation than with first-generation cephalosporins. However, not all of these reactions reflect true cross-reactivity, as only 15% to 40% of patients with a positive history react to penicillin on subsequent testing [72,74]. In a study of 30 patients with immediate-type hypersensitivity reactions to second- and third-generation cephalosporins, 25 of 36 reactions were anaphylactic shock [75]. Only 13% of individuals had either a positive skin test or *in vitro* evidence of antigen-specific IgE to penicillin determinants, while all but three reactions were correlated with a positive skin test to culprit cephalosporins. Unfortunately, skin testing with cephalosporin derivatives is not reliable; severe allergic reactions have occurred in patients with negative cephalosporin skin tests and cephalosporin antigenic determinants for skin testing have not been standardized. On the other hand, patients with negative penicillin skin tests have no greater risk of allergic reaction to cephalosporins than the general population [73]. Several protocols for desensitization to cephalosporins have been outlined in a review [76]. Cross-reactivity between cephalosporins appears related to the degree of similarity of the R1 side chains, and 90% of patients allergic to second- and third-generation cephalosporins do not react to penicillin derivatives [71].

As noted earlier, monobactams (e.g., aztreonam) do not show cross-reactivity with penicillin, but do show some cross-reactivity with the cephalosporins (i.e., ceftazidime) [71]. Carbapenems (e.g., imipenem, meropenem), in comparison, have historically shown significant *in vivo* cross-reactivity with penicillin, and desensitization in penicillin-allergic patients was recommended when there was no reasonable alternative [77]. More recent reports in PCN skin test–positive patients have suggested that carbapenems can be given safely to young

[78,79] and adult [80] patients, who have negative skin tests to the proposed carbapenem. In urgent settings and/or where skin testing and graded challenge are not feasible, a desensitization protocol should be employed with the same precautions as if giving the patient penicillin [73].

Food Anaphylaxis

Food allergy occurs in approximately 6% of children and 3.7% of adults [47]; however, fatal anaphylactic reactions are much less common. Due to variable patterns of absorption, biphasic and/or prolonged anaphylaxis occurs in about 20% of cases. However, the delayed phase is rarely associated with a mild acute phase, where hypotension and bronchoconstriction are readily apparent [81]. A review of fatal and severe nonfatal anaphylactic reactions to foods revealed several important features of the fatal anaphylactic reactions: all occurred in patients with asthma, all were in a public setting rather than in the home, and all were associated with delayed administration of epinephrine [82]. The foods that caused these severe reactions were peanuts, cashews, milk, filberts, walnuts, and eggs. In another review of the causes of anaphylaxis, the five most common foods were pine nuts, peanuts, soy, shellfish, and other nuts [83]. A survey of food-related anaphylactic fatalities reported to an association registry confirmed the association between asthma and severe anaphylaxis; 90% of fatalities in this group were due to peanuts and tree nuts [34]. A methodical approach to the diagnosis and treatment of food hypersensitivity has been outlined by Sicherer and Sampson [47].

Processed foods may contain significant amounts of milk products, despite a lack of mention of this on the label ingredient lists [84]. This is important to remember in patients with milk allergy who appear to experience a cryptogenic anaphylactic episode. Standards for food labeling instituted in 2006 by the U.S. Food and Drug Administration have assisted patients with food allergy and their providers by requiring identification of possible trace allergen contaminants in processed foods. Other food additives, such as preservatives, have been implicated as causes of anaphylaxis [85].

Anesthetic Anaphylaxis

Immediate hypersensitivity reactions to local anesthetics are rare, despite them being one of the most commonly used groups of drugs in medicine [86,87]. Cell-mediated reactions that manifest as contact dermatitis are more common. Local anesthetics are divided into two classes: group I (para-aminobenzoic acid ester) consists of benzocaine, tetracaine, and procaine; group II (non–ester-containing) consists of Xylocaine, mepivacaine, dibucaine, and cyclomethycaine. Cross-reactivity between the two groups is very rare and cross-reactivity between the amides is also rare [88,89]. Skin testing, using a progressive challenge protocol, can help determine whether sensitivity exists and which drugs are likely to be safe in the future [87,89].

General anesthetics, such as neuromuscular blocking agents and thiobarbiturates, also cause anaphylaxis [90]. A skin test protocol has been described for evaluating patients with possible allergy to general anesthetics [91]. Other etiologies of perioperative anaphylaxis include allergy to antibiotics, latex, glutaraldehyde, and opioids.

Since neuromuscular blocking agents are used in intensive care units, anaphylaxis to these agents should be considered in the differential diagnosis of unexplained hypotension in the intensive care unit.

Radiocontrast Media Anaphylaxis

Radiocontrast dye studies are frequently necessary in critically ill patients, so it is important to know when a reaction is likely to occur and how to prevent it. Unfortunately, the likelihood of an anaphylactic reaction to radiocontrast dye cannot be predicted by pretesting with oral, conjunctival, or intradermal skin tests [92]. Although the overall adverse reaction rate ranges from 1% to 12% [93], patients with a history of a previous anaphylactic reaction to radiocontrast dye have a repeat reaction rate of 35% to 60% [94]. Patients with a general history of allergies, whether to inhalant allergens, foods, or medications, also have an increased reaction rate of serious reactions compared with nonallergic individuals [95]. The majority of contrast dye reactions are non-IgE mediated, although evidence is accumulating to suggest that an IgE-mediated mechanism may be contributory in some cases [96,97]. Although exceedingly rare, there have been several confirmed reports of anaphylactic reactions to iodinated oral contrast: Gastrografin (sodium and meglumine diatrizoate), Hypaque (sodium diatrizoate), barium sulfate, and gadolinium [98–102].

Nonionic, low-osmolal radiocontrast agents have largely replaced high ionic contrast media due to a decreased incidence of overall adverse reactions [103,104], although not all studies have found a reduction in life-threatening reactions or death [105,106]. Currently, for patients who have had a prior anaphylactic reaction to contrast media and who require a contrast study, the use of nonionic, low-osmolal contrast is recommended in addition to pretreatment with glucocorticoids, diphenhydramine with or without ephedrine [107], as outlined below. Iso-osmolal and noniodinated contrast are also being explored as alternatives to low-osmolal agents [107,108].

Pretreatment protocols have been developed for patients with a history of a prior anaphylactic reaction who require additional intravascular dye studies [92,94,109]. In one study of 192 procedures in patients with previous anaphylactic reactions to contrast media, pretreatment with prednisone, 50 mg orally at 13 hours, 7 hours, and 1 hour before the procedure, diphenhydramine, 50 mg orally or intramuscularly at 1 hour before the procedure, and ephedrine, 25 mg orally at 1 hour before the procedure resulted in a reaction rate of 3.1% [94]. A multicenter study of nonselected patients receiving intravenous contrast media reported a reaction rate of 5.4% in 2,513 patients given oral methylprednisolone, 32 mg at 12 hours and again at 2 hours before the procedure [109]. In this same study, a single dose of methylprednisolone, 32 mg 2 hours before the procedure, was no better than placebo, with a reaction rate of 9.4% in 1,759 patients. This finding raises the question of how to manage patients with a prior history of anaphylaxis requiring an urgent radiocontrast study. In a small study, nine such patients were treated with hydrocortisone, 200 mg intravenously immediately and every 4 hours until the procedure was completed, and diphenhydramine, 50 mg intravenously 1 hour before the procedure [110]. Roughly half of the patients received one dose of hydrocortisone, and the other half received two doses. No reactions occurred in these patients. Given that this study evaluated only nine patients, it remains unknown whether additional therapy with ephedrine or an H_2-receptor blocking agent, or both, would provide better protection.

Latex-Induced Anaphylaxis

Latex allergy, caused by sensitivity to *Hevea brasiliensis* proteins, can take several forms: contact dermatitis, asthma, urticaria, and anaphylaxis. Perioperative anaphylaxis caused by latex exposure has been described in several children with *spina bifida* and in patients with a history of multiple surgical procedures [111]. In addition, latex allergy has become an occupational hazard in the health profession since the institution of universal precautions [112]. Sensitivity seems to be increased in atopic individuals with frequent exposure to latex. Unexplained perioperative or nosocomial urticaria, bronchoconstriction, or hypotension should raise concern for latex anaphylaxis. Mucosal and parenteral exposures have the highest risk of anaphylaxis.

Patients with latex allergy often have cross sensitivity with certain fruits and vegetables, including banana, kiwi, avocado, chestnut, papaya, potato, and tomato. Latex is found in a wide spectrum of health care products, including elastic thread, rubber bands, condom catheters, Foley catheters, surgical/examination gloves, enema bags, tubing on blood pressure cuffs, rubber stoppers on medication vials and intravenous line tubing, as well as some surgical drapes, drains, and gowns [113–116].

Establishing a diagnosis of latex allergy in a patient who is at high risk based on prior exposures or who may have had latex-induced anaphylaxis is important to guide future prevention efforts. However, skin test extracts are not yet commercially available in the United States and noncommercial latex extracts have been associated with systemic reactions. In addition, the specificity and sensitivity of noncommercial extracts may vary. A preferred alternative is serological testing by Phadia ImmunoCAP or the Siemens Immulite autoanalyzer; these tests have about 80% sensitivity [114,115].

The most important steps in prevention of future anaphylactic reactions to latex are careful patient education and in-hospital latex avoidance through the use of alert bracelets and latex-free kits [90]. Verbal and written information should be provided regarding potential sources of latex exposure and sources of latex-free gloves for patients to take to dentist and doctor visits. In addition, patients should understand the importance of alerting health care professionals who may care for them in the future and the need to carry an EpiPen kit in case of inadvertent exposure.

Stinging Insect Venom Anaphylaxis

Venom extracts for yellow jacket, white-faced hornet, yellow-faced hornet, wasp, honeybee, and fire ant are available for skin testing to confirm specific IgE mediation and for desensitization. Results with venom desensitization suggest more than 95% protection against anaphylaxis on subsequent stings [85]. The duration of desensitization therapy necessary for long-term protection is probably 5 years [117,118]. The geographic distribution of fire ants is expanding, making systemic allergic reactions to these insects a growing concern [119].

Exercise-Induced Anaphylaxis

Exercise-induced anaphylaxis syndrome is distinct from cold and cholinergic urticaria and exercise-induced asthma and usually occurs in individuals who engage in vigorous exercise [120,121]. A subgroup of these patients is allergic to a specific food, such as shrimp or celery, which acts as a cofactor; manifestations of anaphylaxis only occur if ingestion of the specific food is accompanied by exercise. Other potential cofactors include nonsteroidal anti-inflammatory drugs (NSAIDs), alcoholic beverages, and exposure to high pollen counts [122,123]. Typically, these patients can either ingest the food/NSAID or perform the exercise without adverse effect.

Anaphylaxis can be prevented by delaying exercise by at least 2 and preferably 4 hours after eating (48 hours after ingesting a food cofactor) and stopping exercise at the onset of pruritus. When NSAIDs are a cofactor, they should not be taken for at least 24 hours prior to exercise. Exercising with someone who is capable of administering epinephrine is also recommended. Antihistamines are occasionally of benefit in prevention.

Idiopathic Anaphylaxis

A group of patients has been described who experience recurrent anaphylaxis without an identifiable precipitant, the so-called *idiopathic anaphylaxis* [124]. In these patients, a careful review of all foods, preservatives, and drugs ingested prior to the episodes, as well as physical factors such as exercise, fails to reveal a cause for recurrent life-threatening anaphylaxis. These patients should be evaluated for possible systemic mastocytosis [125]. Maintenance therapy with antihistamines,

TABLE 194.6

MANAGEMENT OF ANAPHYLAXIS—QUALITY OF THE EVIDENCE

History of exposures and timing is the most important information to determine whether a set of symptoms was due to anaphylaxis and what tripper precipitated the event. (C)

The appropriate dose of epinephrine should be administered promptly at the onset of anaphylaxis. (A/D)

Intravenous infusion of crystalloid or colloid is essential for patients who are unstable or refractory to initial therapy with epinephrine. (B)

Specific situations

The extent of allergic cross-reactivity between penicillin and cephalosporins is low. (C)

Aztreonam cross-reacts with ceftazidime by shared R-group side chain. (B)

The three groups at increased risk for latex anaphylaxis are health care workers, children with *spina bifida* and genitourinary problems, and workers with occupational exposure to latex. (B)

Precautions for latex-allergic patients undergoing anesthesia include avoiding latex gloves, latex blood pressure cuffs, latex tourniquets, latex intravenous tubing ports, and rubber stoppers on vials. (B)

The greatest number of anaphylactic reactions in children has involved peanuts, tree nuts, fish, shellfish, milk, and eggs. (C)

Anaphylactic reactions to foods almost always occur immediately, but may recur hours later. (A)

Strength of recommendation

A. Directly based on meta-analysis of randomized controlled trials or from at least one randomized controlled trial or systematic review of randomized controlled trials/body of evidence.
B. Directly based on at least one controlled trial without randomization or at least one other type of quasi-experimental study or extrapolated recommendation from A.
C. Directly based on at least one other type of quasi-experimental or descriptive/comparative study or extrapolated recommendation from A or B.
D. Directly based on evidence from expert committee report or opinions or clinical experience of respected authorities or both.

Summarized from reference [38] and others.

oral glucocorticoids, and sympathomimetics has been shown to reduce the frequency and severity of episodes of this disorder [126,127].

Angiotensin-Converting Enzyme Inhibitor Angioedema

Severe, potentially life-threatening facial and oropharyngeal angioedema may occur in individuals with hypersensitivity to angiotensin-converting enzyme (ACE) inhibitors [128–130]. Onset of angioedema usually starts within the first several hours or up to a week after beginning therapy, but angioedema can develop after months to years of asymptomatic usage [128]. Subsequent episodes may occur after days to weeks of continued usage. A late onset of symptoms, 12 to 24 hours after the last dose, has been reported with the long-acting ACE inhibitors lisinopril and enalapril [130]. As with ACE-induced cough, cross-reactivity is the rule among different ACE inhibitors. The mechanism is unknown but is suspected to be related to an alteration in bradykinin metabolism or, possibly, an interaction with components of the complement cascade (e.g., complement 1-esterase inhibitor) [131].

Aspirin and NSAIDs

Acetylsalicylic acid (aspirin) and nonsteroidal anti-inflammatory agents cause urticaria, flares of urticaria in patients with chronic idiopathic urticaria, anaphylaxis, and aspirin-exacerbated respiratory disease (AERD) [132–136]. Most patients have either the urticaria/anaphylaxis pattern or the respiratory disease pattern, but a few patients have both. Some patients with the urticaria/anaphylaxis pattern appear to have sensitivity to a particular NSAID, but most have cross-sensitivity that is related to an abnormality of prostaglandin/leukotriene metabolism [137]. Desensitization protocols for patients with coronary artery disease, who need the antiplatelet effects of aspirin, have been published [138,139].

Miscellaneous Causes of Anaphylaxis

Insulin therapy has been associated with an increased risk of anaphylaxis, particularly when a patient on insulin therapy has a history of local wheal-and-flare reactions at the site of insulin injections and interrupts insulin therapy for more than 48 hours and then resumes it [16,140]. Anaphylaxis has also been described with recombinant DNA insulin [141] and to protamine in neutral protamine Hagedorn (NPH) insulin [142].

The injection of heterologous serum carries a significant risk of anaphylaxis. Human serum (homologous) should be used whenever available. If heterologous serum must be used (antitoxin for snake bites, passive rabies immunization in developing countries, and antilymphocytic serum for organ transplantation), patients are usually evaluated for cutaneous sensitivity by first performing a scratch test with antitoxin or normal horse serum. If there is no reaction, 0.02 mL of a 1:10 serum dilution can be injected intradermally. As with all skin testing, the physician must be prepared to treat any systemic reactions that arise [1].

Patients with mastocytosis appear to be at greater risk for developing anaphylaxis from Hymenoptera stings (even in the absence of IgE mediation) and from mast cell degranulating agents (see Table 194.2). These patients should carry an epinephrine kit during Hymenoptera season. Administration of diagnostic and therapeutic agents that might cause mast cell activation should be avoided in these patients.

The quality of evidence and recommendations for diagnosis and management of anaphylaxis are summarized in Table 194.6.

References

1. McGrath K. Anaphylaxis. In: Patterson R, Grammer LC, Greenberger PA (eds). *Allergic Diseases – Diagnosis and Management*. Philadelphia: Lippincott-Raven, 1997, pp 439–458.
2. Sampson HA, Munoz-Furlong A, Campbell RL, et al: Second symposium on the definition and management of anaphylaxis: summary report–Second National Institute of Allergy and Infectious Disease/Food Allergy and Anaphylaxis Network symposium. *J Allergy Clin Immunol* 117(2):391–397, 2006.
3. Austen KF: Systemic anaphylaxis in the human being. *N Engl J Med* 291(13):661–664, 1974.
4. Sheffer AL: Anaphylaxis. *J Allergy Clin Immunol* 75(2):227–233, 1985.
5. Moneret-Vautrin DA, Morisset M, Beaudouin E, et al: Epidemiology of life-threatening and lethal anaphylaxis: a review. *Allergy* 60(4):443–451, 2005.
6. Neugut AI, Ghatak AT, Miller RL: Anaphylaxis in the United States: an investigation into its epidemiology. *Arch Intern Med* 161(1):15–21, 2001.
7. Yocum MW, Butterfield JH, Klein JS, et al: Epidemiology of anaphylaxis in Olmsted County: A population-based study. *J Allergy Clin Immunol* 1999; 104(2 Pt 1):452–456.
8. Conroy MC, Adkinson NF Jr, Lichtenstein LM: Measurement of IgE on human basophils: relation to serum IgE and anti-IgE-induced histamine release. *J Immunol* 118(4):1317–1321, 1977.
9. Oettgen HC, Geha RS: IgE regulation and roles in asthma pathogenesis. *J Allergy Clin Immunol* 107(3):429–440, 2001.
10. Kemp SF, Lockey RF: Anaphylaxis: a review of causes and mechanisms. *J Allergy Clin Immunol* 110(3):341–348, 2002.
11. Newball HH, Talamo RC, Lichtenstein LM: Anaphylactic release of a basophil kallikrein-like activity. II. A mediator of immediate hypersensitivity reactions. *J Clin Invest* 64(2):466–475, 1979.
12. Hamberg M, Svensson J, Hedqvist P, et al: Involvement of endoperoxides and thromboxanes in anaphylactic reactions. *Adv Prostaglandin Thromboxane Res* 1:495–1501, 1976.
13. Kaliner M, Lemanske R: Rhinitis and asthma. *JAMA* 268(20):2807–2829, 1992.
14. Austen KF: Systemic anaphylaxis in man. *JAMA* 192:108–110, 1965.
15. Frick OL: Immediate hypersensitivity. In: Fudenberg H, Stites DP, Caldwell JL, et al (eds). *Basic and Clinical Immunology*. Philadelphia, Saunders, 1980 pp 274–303.
16. Anderson JA: Allergic reactions to drugs and biological agents. *JAMA* 268(20):2844–2857, 1992.
17. Vyas GN, Perkins HA, Fudenberg HH: Anaphylactoid transfusion reactions associated with anti-IgA. *Lancet* 2(7563):312–315, 1968.
18. Busse WW, Lemanske RF Jr: Asthma. *N Engl J Med* 344(5):350–362, 2001.
19. Simons FE: Advances in H1-antihistamines. *N Engl J Med* 351(21):2203–2217, 2004.
20. Kaliner M, Austen KF: Cyclic AMP, ATP, and reversed anaphylactic histamine release from rat mast cells. *J Immunol* 112(2):664–674, 1974.
21. Kanaoka Y, Boyce JA: Cysteinyl leukotrienes and their receptors: cellular distribution and function in immune and inflammatory responses. *J Immunol* 173(3):1503–1510, 2004.
22. Drazen JM: Leukotrienes as mediators of airway obstruction. *Am J Respir Crit Care Med* 1998; 158(5 Pt 3):S193–S200.
23. Pinckard RN, Halonen M, Palmer JD, et al: Intravascular aggregation and pulmonary sequestration of platelets during IgE-induced systemic anaphylaxis in the rabbit: abrogation of lethal anaphylactic shock by platelet depletion. *J Immunol* 119(6):2185–2193, 1977.
24. Henson PM, Gould D, Becker EL: Activation of stimulus-specific serine esterases (proteases) in the initiation of platelet secretion. I. Demonstration with organophosphorus inhibitors. *J Exp Med* 144(6):1657–1673, 1976.
25. Townley RG, Hopp RJ, Agrawal DK, et al: Platelet-activating factor and airway reactivity. *J Allergy Clin Immunol* 83(6):997–1010, 1989.
26. Roberts LJ, Lewis RA, Lawson JA, et al: Arachidonic acid metabolism by rat mast cells: Departments of Medicine and Pharmacology, Vanderbilt University, Nashville, Tennessee, and Department of Medicine, Harvard University, Boston, Massachusetts. *Prostaglandins* 15(4):717, 1978.
27. Bernreiter M: Electrocardiogram of patient in anaphylactic shock. *J Am Med Assoc* 170(14):1628–1630, 1959.
28. Levine HD: Acute myocardial infarction following wasp sting. Report of two cases and critical survey of the literature. *Am Heart J* 91(3):365–374, 1976.

29. Delage C, Mullick FG, Irey NS: Myocardial lesions in anaphylaxis. A histochemical study. *Arch Pathol* 95(3):185–189, 1973.
30. Hanashiro PK, Weil MH: Anaphylactic shock in man. Report of two cases with detailed hemodynamic and metabolic studies. *Arch Intern Med* 119(2):129–140, 1967.
31. James LP, Austen KF: Fatal systemic anaphylaxis in man. *N Engl J Med* 270:597–603, 1964.
32. Smith PL, Kagey-Sobotka A, Bleecker ER, et al: Physiologic manifestations of human anaphylaxis. *J Clin Invest* 66(5):1072–1080, 1980.
33. Pumphrey R: Anaphylaxis: can we tell who is at risk of a fatal reaction? *Curr Opin Allergy Clin Immunol* 4(4):285–290, 2004.
34. Bock SA, Munoz-Furlong A, Sampson HA: Fatalities due to anaphylactic reactions to foods. *J Allergy Clin Immunol* 107(1):191–193, 2001.
35. Barnard JH: Allergic and pathologic findings in fifty insect-sting fatalities. *J Allergy* 40(2):107–114, 1967.
36. Delage C, Irey NS: Anaphylactic deaths: a clinicopathologic study of 43 cases. *J Forensic Sci* 17(4):525–540, 1972.
37. Edde RR, Burtis BB: Lung injury in anaphylactoid shock. *Chest* 63(4):637–638, 1973.
38. Joint Task Force on Practice Parameters; American Academy of Allergy, Asthma and Immunology; American College of Allergy, Asthma and Immunology; Joint Council of Allergy, Asthma and Immunology: The diagnosis and management of anaphylaxis: an updated practice parameter. *J Allergy Clin Immunol* 115[3, Suppl 2]:S483–S523, 2005.
39. Schwartz LB, Metcalfe DD, Miller JS, et al: Tryptase levels as an indicator of mast-cell activation in systemic anaphylaxis and mastocytosis. *N Engl J Med* 316(26):1622–1626, 1987.
40. Patel SC, Detjen PF: Atrial fibrillation associated with anaphylaxis during venom and pollen immunotherapy. *Ann Allergy Asthma Immunol* 89(2):209–211, 2002.
41. Booth BH, Patterson R: Electrocardiographic changes during human anaphylaxis. *JAMA* 211(4):627–631, 1970.
42. Petsas AA, Kotler MN: Electrocardiographic changes associated with penicillin anaphylaxis. *Chest* 64(1):66–69, 1973.
43. Yildiz A, Biceroglu S, Yakut N, et al: Acute myocardial infarction in a young man caused by centipede sting. *Emerg Med J* 23(4):e30, 2004.
44. Kanthawatana S, Carias K, Arnaout R, et al: The potential clinical utility of serum alpha-protryptase levels. *J Allergy Clin Immunol* 103(6):1092–1099, 1999.
45. Brown SG, Blackman KE, Heddle RJ: Can serum mast cell tryptase help diagnose anaphylaxis? *Emerg Med Australas* 16(2):120–124, 2004.
46. Goldberg A, Confino-Cohen R: Timing of venom skin tests and IgE determinations after insect sting anaphylaxis. *J Allergy Clin Immunol* 100(2):182–184, 1997.
47. Sicherer SH, Sampson HA: 9. Food allergy. *J Allergy Clin Immunol* 117 [2, Suppl Mini-Primer]:S470–S475, 2006.
48. Valentine MD: Anaphylaxis and stinging insect hypersensitivity. *JAMA* 268(20):2830–283, 1992.
49. Boyd AD, Romita MC, Conlan AA, et al: A clinical evaluation of cricothyroidotomy. *Surg Gynecol Obstet* 149(3):365–368, 1979.
50. Orange RP, Austen WG, Austen KF: Immunological release of histamine and slow-reacting substance of anaphylaxis from human lung. I. Modulation by agents influencing cellular levels of cyclic 3',5'-adenosine monophosphate. *J Exp Med* 134(3 Pt 2):136s–48s, 1971.
51. Sutherland EW, Robison GA. The role of cyclic-3',5'-AMP in responses to catecholamines and other hormones. *Pharmacol Rev* 18(1):145–161, 1966.
52. Lichtenstein LM, Margolis S: Histamine release in vitro: inhibition by catecholamines and methylxanthines. *Science* 161(844):902–903, 1968.
53. Austen KF: Tissue mast cells in immediate hypersensitivity. *Hosp Pract (Off Ed)* 17(11):98–108, 1982.
54. Sullivan JJ, Kulczycki A: Immediate hypersensitivity responses. In: Parker CW (ed). *Clinical Immunology*. Philadelphia, Saunders, 1980 pp 130–148.
55. Simons FE: Anaphylaxis. *J Allergy Clin Immunol* 121[2, Suppl]:S402–S407, 2008.
56. Gu X, Simons FE, Simons KJ: Epinephrine absorption after different routes of administration in an animal model. *Biopharm Drug Dispos* 20(8):401–405, 1999.
57. Simons FE, Roberts JR, Gu X, Simons KJ: Epinephrine absorption in children with a history of anaphylaxis. *J Allergy Clin Immunol* 101(1 Pt 1): 33–37, 1998.
58. Hughes G, Fitzharris P: Managing acute anaphylaxis. New guidelines emphasise importance of intramuscular adrenaline. *BMJ* 319(7201):1–2, 1999.
59. Toogood JH: Risk of anaphylaxis in patients receiving beta-blocker drugs. *J Allergy Clin Immunol* 81(1):1–5, 1988.
60. Jacobs RL, Rake GW Jr, Fournier DC, et al: Potentiated anaphylaxis in patients with drug-induced beta-adrenergic blockade. *J Allergy Clin Immunol* 68(2):125–127, 1981.
61. Zaloga GP, DeLacey W, Holmboe E, et al: Glucagon reversal of hypotension in a case of anaphylactoid shock. *Ann Intern Med* 105(1):65–66, 1986.
62. Yarbrough JA, Moffitt JE, Brown DA, et al: Cimetidine in the treatment of refractory anaphylaxis. *Ann Allergy* 63(3):235–238, 1989.
63. Lee JM, Greenes DS: Biphasic anaphylactic reactions in pediatrics. *Pediatrics* 106(4):762–766, 2000.
64. Lieberman P: Biphasic anaphylactic reactions. *Ann Allergy Asthma Immunol* 95(3):217–226, 2005.
65. Twarog FJ, Leung DY: Anaphylaxis to a component of isoetharine (sodium bisulfite). *JAMA* 248(16):2030–2031, 1982.
66. Salkind AR, Cuddy PG, Foxworth JW: The rational clinical examination. Is this patient allergic to penicillin? An evidence-based analysis of the likelihood of penicillin allergy. *JAMA* 285(19):2498–2505, 2001.
67. Sogn DD, Evans R III, Shepherd GM, et al: Results of the National Institute of Allergy and Infectious Diseases Collaborative Clinical Trial to test the predictive value of skin testing with major and minor penicillin derivatives in hospitalized adults. *Arch Intern Med* 152(5):1025–1032, 1992.
68. Torres MJ, Romano A, Mayorga C, et al: Diagnostic evaluation of a large group of patients with immediate allergy to penicillins: the role of skin testing. *Allergy* 56(9):850–856, 2001.
69. Borish L, Tamir R, Rosenwasser LJ: Intravenous desensitization to beta-lactam antibiotics. *J Allergy Clin Immunol* 1987; 80(3 Pt 1):314–319.
70. Turvey SE, Cronin B, Arnold AD, et al: Antibiotic desensitization for the allergic patient: 5 years of experience and practice. *Ann Allergy Asthma Immunol* 92(4):426–432, 2004.
71. Antunez C, Blanca-Lopez N, Torres MJ, et al: Immediate allergic reactions to cephalosporins: evaluation of cross-reactivity with a panel of penicillins and cephalosporins. *J Allergy Clin Immunol* 117(2):404–410, 2006.
72. Anderson JA: Cross-sensitivity to cephalosporins in patients allergic to penicillin. *Pediatr Infect Dis* 5(5):557–561, 1986.
73. Saxon A, Beall GN, Rohr AS, et al: Immediate hypersensitivity reactions to beta-lactam antibiotics. *Ann Intern Med* 107(2):204–215, 1987.
74. DeSwarte RD, Patterson R: Drug allergy. In: Patterson R, Grammer LC, Greenberger PA (eds). *Allergic Diseases – Diagnosis and Management.* Philadelphia, Lippincott-Raven, 1997 pp 317–401.
75. Romano A, Mayorga C, Torres MJ, et al: Immediate allergic reactions to cephalosporins: cross-reactivity and selective responses. *J Allergy Clin Immunol* 106(6):1177–1183, 2000.
76. Kelkar PS, Li JT: Cephalosporin allergy. *N Engl J Med* 345(11):804–809, 2001.
77. Saxon A, Adelman DC, Patel A, et al: Imipenem cross-reactivity with penicillin in humans. *J Allergy Clin Immunol* 82(2):213–217, 1988.
78. Atanaskovic-Markovic M, Gaeta F, Medjo B, et al: Tolerability of meropenem in children with IgE-mediated hypersensitivity to penicillins. *Allergy* 63(2):237–240, 2008.
79. Atanaskovic-Markovic M, Gaeta F, Gavrovic-Jankulovic M, et al: Tolerability of imipenem in children with IgE-mediated hypersensitivity to penicillins. *J Allergy Clin Immunol* 124(1):167–169, 2009.
80. Romano A, Viola M, Gueant-Rodriguez RM, et al: Imipenem in patients with immediate hypersensitivity to penicillins. *N Engl J Med* 354(26):2835–2837, 2006.
81. Golden DB: Patterns of anaphylaxis: acute and late phase features of allergic reactions. *Novartis Found Symp* 257:101–110, 2004.
82. Sampson HA, Mendelson L, Rosen JP: Fatal and near-fatal anaphylactic reactions to food in children and adolescents. *N Engl J Med* 327(6):380–384, 1992.
83. Wiggins C: A. Characteristics and etiology of 30 patients with anaphylaxis. *Immunol Allergy Practice* 13:313, 1991.
84. Gern JE, Yang E, Evrard HM, et al: Allergic reactions to milk-contaminated "nondairy" products. *N Engl J Med* 324(14):976–979, 1991.
85. Moffitt JE, Golden DB, Reisman RE, et al: Stinging insect hypersensitivity: a practice parameter update. *J Allergy Clin Immunol* 114(4):869–886, 2004.
86. Haugen RN, Brown CW: Case reports: type I hypersensitivity to lidocaine. *J Drugs Dermatol* 6(12):1222–1223, 2007.
87. Gall H, Kaufmann R, Kalveram CM: Adverse reactions to local anesthetics: analysis of 197 cases. *J Allergy Clin Immunol* 97(4):933–937, 1996.
88. Schatz M: Skin testing and incremental challenge in the evaluation of adverse reactions to local anesthetics. *J Allergy Clin Immunol* 74(4, Pt 2):606—616, 1984.
89. Chandler MJ, Grammer LC, Patterson R: Provocative challenge with local anesthetics in patients with a prior history of reaction. *J Allergy Clin Immunol* 79(6):883–886, 1987.
90. Lieberman P: Anaphylactic reactions during surgical and medical procedures. *J Allergy Clin Immunol* 110[2, Suppl]:S64–S69, 2002.
91. Moscicki RA, Sockin SM, Corsello BF, et al: Anaphylaxis during induction of general anesthesia: subsequent evaluation and management. *J Allergy Clin Immunol* 86(3 Pt 1):325–332, 1990.
92. Shehadi WH: Adverse reactions to intravascularly administered contrast media. A comprehensive study based on a prospective survey. *Am J Roentgenol Radium Ther Nucl Med* 124(1):145–152, 1975.
93. Canter LM: Anaphylactoid reactions to radiocontrast media. *Allergy Asthma Proc* 26(3):199–203, 2005.
94. Greenberger PA: Contrast media reactions. *J Allergy Clin Immunol* 74 (4, Pt 2):600—605, 1984.
95. Morcos SK: Review article: Acute serious and fatal reactions to contrast media: our current understanding. *Br J Radiol* 78(932):686–693, 2005.
96. Dewachter P, Mouton-Faivre C, Felden F: Allergy and contrast media. *Allergy* 56(3):250–251, 2001.
97. Laroche D, imone-Gastin I, Dubois F, et al: Mechanisms of severe, immediate reactions to iodinated contrast material. *Radiology* 209(1):183–190, 1998.

98. Miller SH: Anaphylactoid reaction after oral administration of diatrizoate meglumine and diatrizoate sodium solution. *AJR Am J Roentgenol* 168(4):959–961, 1997.
99. Marik PE, Patel SY: Anaphylactoid reaction to oral contrast agent. *AJR Am J Roentgenol* 168(6):1623–1624, 1997.
100. Seymour PC, Kesack CD: Anaphylactic shock during a routine upper gastrointestinal series. *AJR Am J Roentgenol* 168(4):957–958, 1997.
101. Skucas J: Anaphylactoid reactions with gastrointestinal contrast media. *AJR Am J Roentgenol* 168(4):962–964, 1997.
102. Li A, Wong CS, Wong MK, et al: Acute adverse reactions to magnetic resonance contrast media–gadolinium chelates. *Br J Radiol* 79(941):368–371, 2006.
103. Barrett BJ, Parfrey PS, McDonald JR, et al: Nonionic low-osmolality versus ionic high-osmolality contrast material for intravenous use in patients perceived to be at high risk: randomized trial. *Radiology* 183(1):105–110, 1992.
104. Cochran ST: Anaphylactoid reactions to radiocontrast media. *Curr Allergy Asthma Rep* 5(1):28–31, 2005.
105. Cochran ST, Bomyea K, Sayre JW: Trends in adverse events after IV administration of contrast media. *AJR Am J Roentgenol* 176(6):1385–1388, 2001.
106. Wolf GL, Arenson RL, Cross AP: A prospective trial of ionic vs nonionic contrast agents in routine clinical practice: comparison of adverse effects. *AJR Am J Roentgenol* 152(5):939–944, 1989.
107. Greenberger PA, Patterson R: The prevention of immediate generalized reactions to radiocontrast media in high-risk patients. *J Allergy Clin Immunol* 87(4):867–872, 1991.
108. Coche EE, Hammer FD, Goffette PP: Demonstration of pulmonary embolism with gadolinium-enhanced spiral CT. *Eur Radiol* 11(11):2306–2309, 2001.
109. Lasser EC, Berry CC, Talner LB, et al: Pretreatment with corticosteroids to alleviate reactions to intravenous contrast material. *N Engl J Med* 317(14):845–849, 1987.
110. Greenberger PA, Halwig JM, Patterson R, et al: Emergency administration of radiocontrast media in high-risk patients. *J Allergy Clin Immunol* 77(4):630–634, 1986.
111. Landwehr LP, Boguniewicz M: Current perspectives on latex allergy. *J Pediatr* 128(3):305–312, 1996.
112. Liss GM, Sussman GL, Deal K, et al: Latex allergy: epidemiological study of 1351 hospital workers. *Occup Environ Med* 54(5):335–342, 1997.
113. Jaeger D, Kleinhans D, Czuppon AB, et al: Latex-specific proteins causing immediate-type cutaneous, nasal, bronchial, and systemic reactions. *J Allergy Clin Immunol* 89(3):759–768, 1992.
114. Biagini RE, Krieg EF, Pinkerton LE, et al: Receiver operating characteristics analyses of Food and Drug Administration-cleared serological assays for natural rubber latex-specific immunoglobulin E antibody. *Clin Diagn Lab Immunol* 8(6):1145–1149, 2001.
115. Biagini RE, MacKenzie BA, Sammons DL, et al: Latex specific IgE: performance characteristics of the IMMULITE 2000 3gAllergy assay compared with skin testing. *Ann Allergy Asthma Immunol* 97(2):196–202, 2006.
116. Kelly KJ, Sussman G, Fink JN: Rostrum. Stop the sensitization. *J Allergy Clin Immunol* 98(5, Pt 1):857–858, 1996.
117. Reisman RE, Lantner R: Further observations of stopping venom immunotherapy: comparison of patients stopped because of a fall in serum venom-specific IgE to insignificant levels with patients stopped prematurely by self-choice. *J Allergy Clin Immunol* 83(6):1049–1054, 1989.
118. Golden DB, Kwiterovich KA, Kagey-Sobotka A, et al: Discontinuing venom immunotherapy: outcome after five years. *J Allergy Clin Immunol* 97(2):579–587, 1996.
119. deShazo RD, Butcher BT, Banks WA: Reactions to the stings of the imported fire ant. *N Engl J Med* 323(7):462–466, 1990.
120. Sheffer AL, Austen KF: Exercise-induced anaphylaxis. *J Allergy Clin Immunol* 66(2):106–111, 1980.
121. Volcheck GW, Li JT: Exercise-induced urticaria and anaphylaxis. *Mayo Clin Proc* 72(2):140–147, 1997.
122. van Wijk RG, de GH, Bogaard JM: Drug-dependent exercise-induced anaphylaxis. *Allergy* 50(12):992–994, 1995.
123. Shadick NA, Liang MH, Partridge AJ, et al: The natural history of exercise-induced anaphylaxis: survey results from a 10-year follow-up study. *J Allergy Clin Immunol* 104(1):123–127, 1999.
124. Wong S, Dykewicz MS, Patterson R: Idiopathic anaphylaxis. A clinical summary of 175 patients. *Arch Intern Med* 150(6):1323–1328, 1990.
125. Webb LM, Lieberman P: Anaphylaxis: a review of 601 cases. *Ann Allergy Asthma Immunol* 97(1):39–43, 2006.
126. Wong S, Yarnold PR, Yango C, et al: Outcome of prophylactic therapy for idiopathic anaphylaxis. *Ann Intern Med* 114(2):133–136, 1991.
127. Lenchner KI, Ditto AM: Idiopathic anaphylaxis. *Allergy Asthma Proc* 25[4, Suppl 1]:S54–S56, 2004.
128. Roberts JR, Wuerz RC: Clinical characteristics of angiotensin-converting enzyme inhibitor-induced angioedema. *Ann Emerg Med* 20(5):555–558, 1991.
129. Israili ZH, Hall WD: Cough and angioneurotic edema associated with angiotensin-converting enzyme inhibitor therapy. A review of the literature and pathophysiology. *Ann Intern Med* 117(3):234–242, 1992.
130. Bielory L, Lee SS, Holland CL, et al: Long-acting ACE inhibitor-induced angioedema. *Allergy Proc* 13(2):85–87, 1992.
131. Dykewicz MS: Cough and angioedema from angiotensin-converting enzyme inhibitors: new insights into mechanisms and management. *Curr Opin Allergy Clin Immunol* 4(4):267–270, 2004.
132. Friedlaender S: Adverse reactions to aspirin and non-steroidal antiinflammatory drugs. *Immunol Allergy Practice* 2:73, 1980.
133. Vane JR: Inhibition of prostaglandin synthesis as a mechanism of action for aspirin-like drugs. *Nat New Biol* 231(25):232–235, 1971.
134. Burrish GF, Kaatz BL: Sulindac-induced anaphylaxis. *Ann Emerg Med* 10(3):154–155, 1981.
135. Corre KA, Rothstein RJ: Anaphylactic reaction to zomepirac. *Ann Allergy* 48(5):299–301, 1982.
136. Moore ME, Goldsmith DP: Nonsteroidal anti-inflammatory intolerance. An anaphylactic reaction to tolmetin. *Arch Intern Med* 140(8):1105–1106, 1980.
137. Mastalerz L, Setkowicz M, Sanak M, et al: Hypersensitivity to aspirin: common eicosanoid alterations in urticaria and asthma. *J Allergy Clin Immunol* 113(4):771–775, 2004.
138. Gollapudi RR, Teirstein PS, Stevenson DD, et al: Aspirin sensitivity: implications for patients with coronary artery disease. *JAMA* 292(24):3017–3023, 2004.
139. Silberman S, Neukirch-Stoop C, Steg PG: Rapid desensitization procedure for patients with aspirin hypersensitivity undergoing coronary stenting. *Am J Cardiol* 95(4):509–510, 2005.
140. Lieberman P, Patterson R, Metz R, et al: Allergic reactions to insulin. *JAMA* 215(7):1106–1112, 1971.
141. Grammer LC, Roberts M, Buchanan TA, et al: Specificity of immunoglobulin E and immunoglobulin G against human (recombinant DNA) insulin in human insulin allergy and resistance. *J Lab Clin Med* 109(2):141–146, 1987.
142. Gruchalla RS: 10. Drug allergy. *J Allergy Clin Immunol* 111[2, Suppl]: S548–S559, 2003.
143. Wong JT, Ripple RE, MacLean JA, et al: Vancomycin hypersensitivity: synergism with narcotics and "desensitization" by a rapid continuous intravenous protocol. *J Allergy Clin Immunol* 94(2, Pt 1):189–194, 1994.
144. Thomas AD, Caunt JA: Anaphylactoid reaction following local anaesthesia for epidural block. *Anaesthesia* 48(1):50–52, 1993.
145. Craddock PR, Fehr J, Brigham KL, et al: Complement and leukocyte-mediated pulmonary dysfunction in hemodialysis. *N Engl J Med* 296(14): 769–774, 1977.
146. Olinger GN, Becker RM, Bonchek LI: Noncardiogenic pulmonary edema and peripheral vascular collapse following cardiopulmonary bypass: rare protamine reaction? *Ann Thorac Surg* 29(1):20–25, 1980.
147. Lieberman P, Siegle RL, Taylor WW: Anaphylactoid reactions to iodinated contrast material. *J Allergy Clin Immunol* 62(3):174–180, 1978.
148. Fanous LH, Gray A, Felmingham J: Severe anaphylactoid reactions to dextran 70. *Br Med J* 2(6096):1189–1190, 1977.
149. Ring J, Messmer K: Incidence and severity of anaphylactoid reactions to colloid volume substitutes. *Lancet* 1(8009):466–469, 1977.
150. Fisher MM: Severe histamine mediated reactions to intravenous drugs used in anaesthesia. *Anaesth Intensive Care* 3(3):180–197, 1975.
151. Mathieu A, Goudsouzian N, Snider MT: Reaction to ketamine: anaphylactoid or anaphylactic? *Br J Anaesth* 47(5):624–627, 1975.
152. Schoenfeld MR: Acute allergic reactions to morphine, codeine, meperidine hydrochloride, and opium alkaloids. *N Y State J Med* 60:2591–2593, 1960.
153. Berkes EA: Anaphylactic and anaphylactoid reactions to aspirin and other NSAIDs. *Clin Rev Allergy Immunol* 24(2):137–148, 2003.
154. Basu R, Rajkumar A, Datta NR: Anaphylaxis to cisplatin following nine previous uncomplicated cycles. *Int J Clin Oncol* 7(6):365–367, 2002.
155. Sliesoraitis S, Chikhale PJ: Carboplatin hypersensitivity. *Int J Gynecol Cancer* 15(1):13–18, 2005.
156. Simons FE: Anaphylaxis: Recent advances in assessment and treatment. *J Allergy Clin Immunol* 124(4):625–636, 2009.

CHAPTER 195 ■ DERMATOLOGY IN THE INTENSIVE CARE UNIT

NIKKI A. LEVIN, DORI GOLDBERG, LAUREN ALBERTA-WSZOLEK, MEGAN BERNSTEIN AND ALEXIS C. PERKINS

INTRODUCTION

Patients in the intensive care unit (ICU) often present with cutaneous findings. Their reason for admission to the ICU may be primarily dermatologic, as in the case of toxic epidermal necrolysis (TEN) or pemphigus vulgaris, two diseases in which large areas of the epidermis are shed. Or they may have skin findings that provide diagnostic clues to their internal disease, as when a patient with systemic lupus erythematosus presents with a classic malar rash. Patients with life threatening infections, such as Rocky Mountain spotted fever and Meningococcemia, may present with characteristic skin lesions that suggest the correct diagnosis and allow prompt institution of lifesaving treatment.

Skin conditions in ICU patients are often iatrogenic, being caused by drugs (e.g., TEN, drug reaction with eosinophilia and systemic symptoms (DRESS), acute generalized exanthematous pustulosis (AGEP)), procedures (e.g., cholesterol emboli), dressings (e.g., contact dermatitis), or inattentive care (e.g., pressure ulcers). At other times, patients may have skin conditions which, although relatively minor, may complicate their ICU stay, put other patients and health care workers at risk (e.g., scabies), or make patients uncomfortable (e.g., miliaria, Grover's disease).

In this chapter, we give an overview of serious illnesses with prominent cutaneous findings, including drug reactions, exfoliative erythrodermas, infections, blistering disorders, vascular disorders, connective tissue disorders, and graft-versus-host disease (GVHD). In addition, we provide a brief description of more common but less serious dermatoses that may coexist in ICU patients, with suggestions for their management. We emphasize the importance of lesion morphology, that is, the shape, color, size, arrangement, and distribution of skin lesion in making a correct diagnosis. Table 195.1 provides a list of skin diseases arranged by morphology to assist in formulating a differential diagnosis.

Dermatologic consultation is often helpful for diagnosis and management of skin diseases in ICU patients. The dermatologic consultant may be able to help sort out multiple potential differential diagnoses by inspection of morphology, skin biopsy, or use of other diagnostic tests (skin scrapings for scabies, potassium hydroxide preparations for fungus, viral and bacterial cultures, direct fluorescent antibody tests for viral infections, etc.) Since morphology evolves with the natural course of disease and with attempted therapeutic measures, it is helpful to request consultation early in the course of cutaneous disease.

DRUG ERUPTIONS

Cutaneous drug reactions are frequently encountered in ICU patients. Certain drug reactions such as toxic epidermal necrolysis (TEN), Stevens–Johnson syndrome (SJS), DRESS, and acute generalized exanthematous pustulosis (AGEP) may be the primary cause for admission to the ICU. These reactions will be discussed in depth following a brief overview of more commonly occurring drug reactions. The exanthematous or morbilliform drug eruption is the most common (Fig. 195.1). It typically appears 7 to 14 days after introduction of the offending agent. Clinically it appears as symmetric macules that may become slightly papular on the trunk and upper extremities, and may become confluent with time. Low-grade fever and pruritus are sometimes present. The differential diagnosis includes viral exanthem, Kawasaki's disease, GVHD, and the more serious drug reactions discussed below (TEN, SJS, DRESS, and AGEP). Facial edema, mucosal lesions, blisters or sloughing of the skin, and laboratory abnormalities such as neutrophilia, eosinophilia, and elevated liver function tests may indicate the presence of a more serious drug reaction. Withdrawal of the causative drug is the most important treatment, although topical corticosteroids and oral antihistamines may be used for symptomatic relief. Exanthematous drug eruptions resolve without sequelae 1 to 2 weeks after the offending drug has been discontinued.

Toxic Epidermal Necrolysis/ Stevens–Johnson Syndrome

Toxic epidermal necrolysis (TEN) and Stevens–Johnson syndrome (SJS) are entities on a spectrum of severe cutaneous reactions that are most commonly caused by medications. They exhibit severe blistering and sloughing of the skin (Fig. 195.2) with mucosal involvement (Fig. 195.3), and may have high morbidity and mortality. The distinction between TEN and SJS is based on the percentage of skin involved with SJS being <10%, TEN being >30%, and SJS/TEN overlap being 10% to 30% of the body surface area affected. The cumulative annual incidence of these entities has been estimated at 1.89 per million people. SJS is more common in children, whereas TEN is more common in adults. TEN is more common in women, and the incidence increases with age and immunosuppression [1]. HIV infection increases the risk of SJS/TEN with the incidence of TEN in HIV patients receiving trimethoprim-sulfamethoxazole, 8.4 per 100,000 exposures as opposed to 2.6 per 100,000 exposures in non-HIV infected individuals [2]. There appears to be a genetic component to SJS/TEN, as multiple studies have demonstrated HLA alleles related to hypersensitivity to specific medications, however, at this time human leukocyte antigen (HLA) testing is not clinically useful due to its expense [2].

Ninety five percent of patients with TEN have a history of drug exposure and there is a clear relationship to a drug in 80% of cases. Only half of SJS cases are related to medications with the remainder being attributed to infections, including mycoplasma, which may present as mucositis without typical skin manifestations. The most common causative medications along with relative risks listed in parentheses include: trimethoprim-sulfamethoxazole (172), carbamazepine

TABLE 195.1

DIFFERENTIAL DIAGNOSIS OF SKIN ERUPTIONS BY MORPHOLOGY

Fever and rash
- Infectious disease (bacterial, fungal, viral)
- Rheumatologic disease (SLE, rheumatoid arthritis, juvenile rheumatoid arthritis, Still's disease, mixed connective tissue disease)
- Pustular psoriasis
- Drug eruption
- Leukemia/lymphoma
- Lofgren's syndrome (acute sarcoidosis with erythema nodosum, hilar adenopathy, fever, and arthritis)
- Sweet's syndrome
- Polyarteritis nodosa

Morbilliform (maculopapular)
- Drug eruption
- Viral exanthem
- Graft-versus-host disease
- Rickettsial infections

Generalized erythema
- Staphylococcal scalded skin syndrome
- Exfoliative erythroderma

Localized erythematous papules and plaques
- Psoriasis
- Seborrheic dermatitis
- Contact dermatitis
- Pityriasis rosea
- Tinea
- Scabies
- Dermatomyositis
- Lupus erythematosus
- Secondary syphilis
- Urticaria
- Still's disease
- Disseminated candidiasis
- Erythema nodosum
- Grover's disease

Annular (ring-shaped) erythematous lesions
- Tinea
- Erythema multiforme
- Urticaria
- Granuloma annulare
- Sarcoid
- Subacute cutaneous lupus
- Sweet's syndrome
- Erythema chronicum migrans (Lyme disease)
- Leprosy

Pustules
- Pustular psoriasis
- Steroid acne
- Folliculitis
- Acute generalized exanthematous pustulosis (AGEP)

Vesicles/Bullae
- Herpes simplex
- Varicella zoster
- Miliaria
- Bullous infections (impetigo, tinea, cellulitis)
- Erythema multiforme/Stevens–Johnson syndrome/TEN
- Pemphigus
- Paraneoplastic pemphigus
- Bullous pemphigoid
- Linear IgA dermatosis
- Epidermolysis bullosa acquisita
- Porphyria cutanea tarda
- Dermatitis herpetiformis

Purpura
- Vasculitis
- Purpura fulminans
- Calciphylaxis
- Heparin or Coumadin necrosis
- Cryoglobulinemia
- Cholesterol emboli
- Myeloproliferative disease
- Antiphospholipid syndrome

Ulcers
- Vasculopathy
- Infectious
- Neoplastic
- Bullous disorders
- Panniculitis
- Neuropathy
- Bites
- Aphthae
- Trauma

(90), NSAIDS (72), corticosteroids (54), phenytoin (53), allopurinol (52), phenobarbital (45), valproic acid (25), cephalosporins (14), quinolones (10), and aminopenicillins (6.7), with more recent reports implicating lamotrigine, rituximab, imatinib, lenalidomide [3]. The time from drug ingestion to clinical symptoms is generally 1 to 3 weeks, except for the aromatic anticonvulsants that can take up to 2 months to cause disease [4].

The cutaneous eruption may be heralded by a 1 to 3 day prodrome of fever and flu-like symptoms. The initial cutaneous finding is irregularly shaped erythematous to purpuric macules with irregular size and shape distributed on the face and trunk. This may evolve into flaccid blisters that may be easily enlarged with lateral pressure. The skin can become gray, which usually heralds full thickness epidermal sloughing. Mucosal involvement is present in 90% of patients with SJS and TEN, with the most common affected areas being the conjunctiva, oral cavity, and genitalia. Symptoms include severe skin pain and difficulty swallowing and urinating. Respiratory epithelium may also be involved with resultant dyspnea, pulmonary edema, and hypoxia.

The differential diagnosis includes staphylococcal scalded skin syndrome (SSSS), acute generalized exanthematous pustulosis (AGEP), severe acute GVHD, drug-induce linear IgA bullous dermatosis, and paraneoplastic pemphigus. The appropriate clinical setting and skin biopsy easily differentiate SJS/TEN from these entities. Two skin biopsies are recommended, one for frozen section and the other for routine H&E. Early lesions demonstrate necrotic keratinocytes, while advanced lesions reveal full-thickness epidermal necrosis, and a recent study indicates that the density of the dermal mononuclear cell infiltrate correlates with the severity of disease and mortality rate [5].

Prompt diagnosis and rapid cessation of the causative medication along with supportive therapy is the cornerstone of

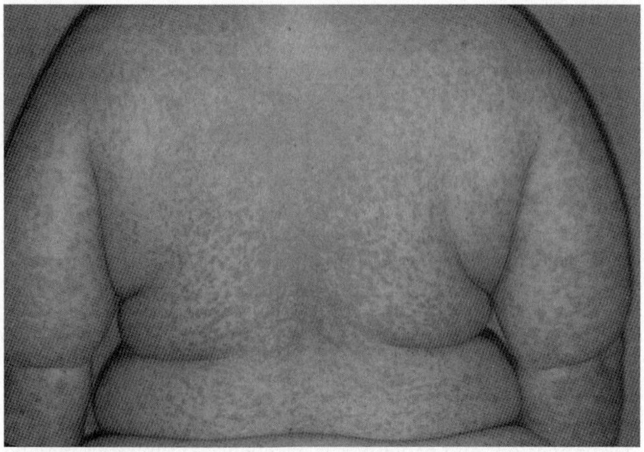

FIGURE 195.1. Morbilliform (maculopapular) drug eruption. Note the pink blanchable papules and plaques with areas of confluence over the trunk and extremities.

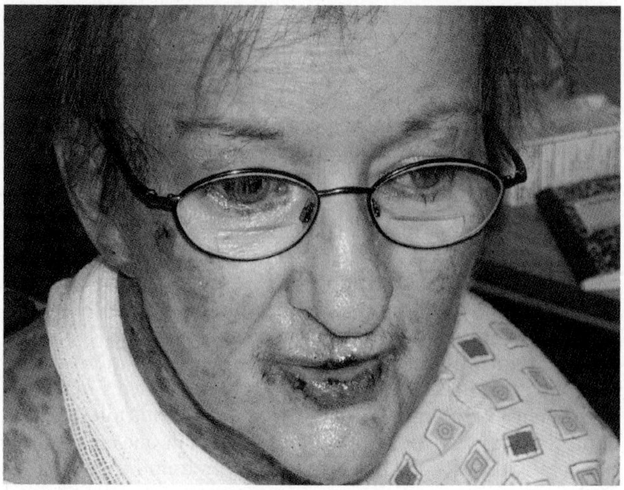

FIGURE 195.3. Stevens–Johnson syndrome. Bullae over the left top eyelid and erythematous and edematous plaques on the neck and shoulders. Note the erosions over the lips.

therapy. Careful monitoring of fluid volume, electrolytes, renal function, nutritional status, and evaluation for signs of sepsis should be performed. For extensive body surface involvement, care should be provided in an ICU with staff accustomed to caring for patients with fragile and denuded skin, usually a burn unit. Uninvolved skin should not be manipulated, while involved skin should be covered with Vaseline impregnated gauze and a topical antibiotic ointment. Debridement of necrotic skin may be followed by placement of artificial membranes or biologic dressings such as xenografts or allografts. Daily bacterial cultures should be performed of involved skin and mucosa as well as blood, urine, and any intravenous catheters, as sepsis is the most common cause of mortality in patients with SJS/TEN. Systemic antibiotics should not be started unless signs of sepsis are present because of the risk of selecting for antibiotic resistant organisms, and prophylactic use of antibiotics has not been shown to improve outcome [2]. Patients should be followed by an ophthalmologist to avoid conjunctival scarring. Currently, there is no gold standard systemic therapy for TEN/SJS. Intravenous immunoglobulin (IVIG) has been used, based on its ability to bind Fas receptors, thought to be a major mediator of apoptosis in TEN/SJS. Unfortunately, there are no randomized double-blind trials to support its use, and while some studies have shown mortality benefit with doses more than 1 g per kg per day, others have shown no benefit or even increased mortality associated with its use [6]. Systemic corticosteroid pulse therapy early in the disease course has been shown to have benefit in preventing ocular complications, and topical high potency corticosteroids appear to prevent corneal epithelial stem cell loss and scarring [7]. There is some emerging evidence that high dose (1.5 mg/kg/day) pulse corticosteroids decreased TEN-associated mortality [2]. Other systemic treatments have been tried, but none are recommended at this time [8].

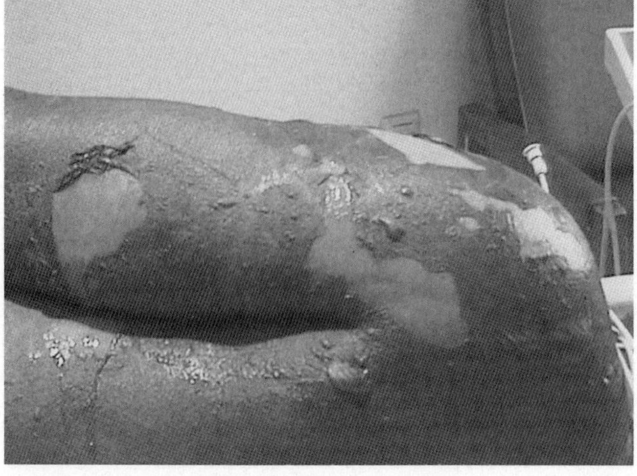

FIGURE 195.2. Toxic epidermal necrolysis. Bullae and sheets of epidermal sloughing leaving behind red denuded areas are seen.

The mortality rate for SJS and TEN is 5% and 30%, respectively, and is directly related to the percentage of skin involved. Risk of mortality can be predicted using the SCORTEN algorithm. One point each is assigned for the presence of the following seven criteria: age >40 years, presence of malignancy, heart rate >120, initial epidermal detachment >10%, serum urea nitrogen >10 mmol per L, serum glucose >14 mmol per L, and serum bicarbonate <20 mmol per L. The points are added and the predicted mortality based upon this total is 0 to 1 (3.2%), 2 (12.1%), 3 (35.8%), 4 (58.3%), and 5 or more (90%) [9]. Healing of sloughed epidermis usually takes 3 weeks and survivors may experience ocular scarring and visual loss. If the causative medication is reintroduced, the disease may recur in less than 48 hours. Notably, a patient who experiences TEN to one class of medication is not predisposed to TEN in response to other medication classes; however, cross-reactivity may be seen between related drug classes such as penicillins and cephalosporins.

Drug Rash with Eosinophilia and Systemic Symptoms

Drug rash with eosinophilia and systemic symptoms (DRESS) is a potentially fatal hypersensitivity reaction to medication, most commonly anticonvulsants [10]. The incidence is between 1/1,000 to 1/10,000 exposures and it is thought to occur with higher frequencies in patients of African ancestry [11].

Although the etiology of DRESS is not understood completely, alteration in drug detoxification pathways and a causative role for human herpesvirus 6 have been proposed [12,13]. DRESS is most commonly caused by the aromatic anticonvulsants, including phenobarbital, phenytoin, and carbamazepine. Of note, these drugs may cross-react. Other common causes include allopurinol, sulfonamides, minocycline, and dapsone.

In contrast to other drug reactions, DRESS may develop as late as 4 to 6 weeks after the offending medication has been introduced. DRESS has even been reported to occur more than 1 year after initiating allopurinol. The rash is usually morbilliform, though erythroderma, pustules, vesicles, and purpuric areas may also be present. High fever and edema of the face are hallmarks of this entity. Systemic involvement may include pharyngitis, lymphadenopathy, hepatosplenomegaly, peripheral eosinophilia, abnormal liver function tests, arthralgias, pulmonary infiltrates, and interstitial nephritis. Allopurinol and minocycline are associated with severe DRESS, the former frequently causing renal failure, and the latter causing pneumonitis [14]. Circulating atypical lymphocytes may also be present [11]. High eosinophil count and multiple medical comorbidities were poor prognostic factors in one series of 30 patients with DRESS [15]. Another study found that vitamin D deficiency was common among patients with DRESS, and that myocarditis is an underdiagnosed systemic manifestation, which may be detected by cardioselective biomarkers, echo, or cardiac MRI [16].

The differential diagnosis includes AGEP, SJS, TEN, Kawasaki's disease, and the hypereosinophilic syndrome. Histopathology of skin biopsies taken from patients with DRESS is variable and therefore not diagnostic [15]. The history of recent initiation of a suspect drug, the presence of atypical lymphocytes, peripheral eosinophilia, increased liver function tests, abnormal serum creatinine or urinalyses, and cutaneous eruption as described above, especially with facial edema, suggest the diagnosis of DRESS.

The most effective treatment is prompt diagnosis and cessation of the offending drug. Antipyretics may be used to treat the fever but they have no impact on disease outcome. Multiple independent case reports have suggested that systemic corticosteroid therapy may halt internal disease progression. Additionally, the disease has been reported to recur upon stopping corticosteroid treatment too soon. This has led many authorities to suggest treatment with systemic corticosteroids when there is internal involvement. However, no case control or randomized controlled trial data are available [17]. Thus, primary and secondary prevention of DRESS is of utmost importance. One must have knowledge of the most common causative drugs and an understanding of the cross-reactivity among the aromatic hydrocarbons. Mortality rates up to 10% have been reported and are primarily due to fulminant hepatitis.

Acute Generalized Exanthematous Pustulosis

Acute generalized exanthematous pustulosis (AGEP), also known as toxic pustuloderma [18] or pustular drug rash [19] is a very rare drug reaction that presents with fever, leukocytosis, and multiple pustules on a background of generalized erythema. There appears to be no sexual predilection and AGEP may occur at any age. Incidence rates have been estimated at 1 to 5 cases per million per year [20].

Drugs are responsible for at least 90% of AGEP cases. In a report of 97 cases from Europe, aminopenicillins (odds ratio [OR] = 23), macrolides (OR = 11), quinolones (OR = 33), hydroxychloroquine (OR = 39), calcium channel blockers (OR = 15), anticonvulsants (OR = 8), and corticosteroids (OR = 12) were the most common causative agents [21]. More recently, spider bites have been reported as triggers [22]. Patch testing with the offending agent is frequently positive reflecting the dominant role of T cells in the disorder.

The eruption is frequently sudden in onset and the majority of cases appear within 24 hours to several days of exposure to the offending agent. A fever of more than 38°C is followed by the appearance of tiny nonfollicular pustules on a background of generalized erythema and edema. Petechiae, purpura, vesicles, or target lesions may be present, and oral lesions may be observed in 20% of patients. The face and intertriginous areas are the most common presenting locations. Neutrophilia occurs in 90% and eosinophilia in 30% of patients. Liver function tests are usually normal and there is typically no systemic involvement, but lymphadenopathy is sometimes seen. The differential diagnosis includes pustular psoriasis, subcorneal pustular dermatosis, DRESS, and in severe cases, TEN. An acute onset and clinical history of a new drug favors AGEP over pustular psoriasis, whereas DRESS and TEN exhibit systemic involvement.

Discontinuation of the causative drug is the definitive treatment. Once the diagnosis is made and the causative drug is stopped, the pustules will resolve in less than 15 days with desquamation, and prognosis is excellent. Antipyretics may be used for symptomatic treatment of the fever and topical steroids may be used for symptomatic treatment of the rash, although neither will hasten the resolution of the eruption.

EXFOLIATIVE ERYTHRODERMA

Erythroderma (Fig. 195.4) is a rare, life-threatening skin condition characterized by erythema involving at least 90% of the body surface area with variable degrees of scaling [23–25]. While age at presentation varies with the underlying cause, patients are typically over 40 or 45 years. Male to female ratio and reported incidence are also variable, and there is no racial predilection [25–27].

The causes of erythroderma may be categorized into preexisting skin conditions (psoriasis, atopic dermatitis, contact dermatitis, and seborrheic dermatitis), drug reactions, malignancy, skin infections and infestations, and idiopathic etiology [23,25,27]. Over 60 topical and systemic medications have been implicated in erythroderma, including ACE inhibitors, anticonvulsants, penicillin, vancomycin, antifungals, and barbiturates [26,27]. Leukemias and lymphomas constitute up to 40% of malignancy-related erythrodermas. Cutaneous T cell lymphoma (CTCL) and Sezary syndrome represent most of these cases. Primary blood vessel malignancy and solid organ cancers are also reported in association with erythroderma [27]. SSSS, HIV seroconversion, superficial dermatophyte and candidal infections, scabies infestation, lupus erythematosus, sarcoidosis,

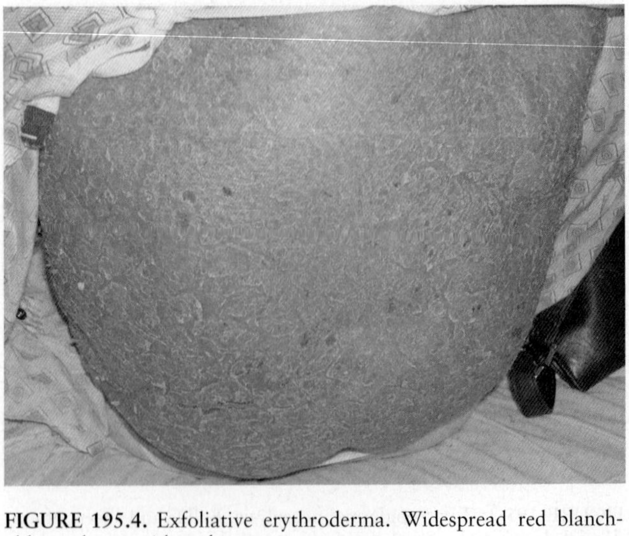

FIGURE 195.4. Exfoliative erythroderma. Widespread red blanchable erythema with scale.

and mastocytosis may rarely cause erythroderma as well. Up to 46% of cases have no identifiable trigger [23,26].

Varying degrees of scaling, which often begin at flexural surfaces, follow intense widespread erythema within 2 to 6 days. Erythroderma associated with psoriasis and atopic dermatitis has a more indolent course than the more rapidly progressive form linked to malignancy, drugs, and SSSS [26]. Along with intense erythema, patients may have fever, hyperkeratosis of the palms and soles, nail dystrophy, cheilitis, alopecia, edema of the face and legs, dermatopathic lymphadenopathy, hepatomegaly, and splenomegaly [25,26].

Erythrodermic patients have dramatic disturbances in the body's regulatory mechanisms. Increased cutaneous blood flow results in exaggerated heat and fluid losses with a compensatory increase in the body's basal metabolic rate. This, in conjunction with the shedding of 20 to 30 g per day of proteinaceous scale, can result in a hypoalbuminemia that exacerbates edema and nutritional deficits [26,27]. Complications include electrolyte imbalance, dehydration, high output cardiac failure, and secondary infections.

Identification of the underlying trigger is important in the evaluation and management of erythrodermic patients. Early examination of the skin with corroborating evidence from skin biopsy may be helpful in establishing the etiology, but in the majority of adult cases, the underlying dermatosis is obscured by widespread erythema and scaling. Skin biopsy has recently been shown to be more useful in detecting some underlying triggers for infantile and neonatal cases of erythroderma [28].

Erythroderma should be managed as a dermatologic emergency in the inpatient setting. Initial treatment, regardless of the underlying cause, consists of temperature regulation, hemodynamic support and monitoring, and skin care. Topical therapies include low-to-mid potency corticosteroids such as triamcinolone 0.025% to 0.1% cream under wet dressings. Tap water soaked gauze dressings may be changed every 2 to 3 hours, and tepid baths may provide additional relief. As the skin condition improves, emollients can be substituted for corticosteroids. Systemic corticosteroids can be helpful, but must be used with caution in atopic dermatitis and are contraindicated in infection and psoriasis. Additional therapy is targeted at the triggering disease and may include systemic retinoids, cyclosporine, or methotrexate in the case of psoriasis, and psoralen with UVA phototherapy in the case of CTCL [26,27]. Regardless of the underlying cause, relapses of erythroderma are common. Mortality rates range from 4.6% to 64% and are influenced by advanced age and comorbidities [25].

INFECTIONS

Toxic Shock Syndrome

Toxic shock syndrome (TSS) is an acute febrile illness caused by toxin-producing strains of *Staphylococcus aureus*, presenting with fever, rash, and hypotension and often progressing to multiorgan failure [29]. A similar syndrome caused by *Streptococcus pyogenes* has also been described, known as streptococcal toxic shock syndrome (STSS) [30]. TSS is rare and more often seen in young women (yearly incidence of 1/100,000 women of reproductive age) than men, most likely due to its association with tampon use. Predisposing factors for TSS include menstruation, recent childbirth or surgery, burn wounds, intravenous drug use, pneumonia, and influenza. STSS has an estimated yearly incidence of 10 cases/100,000 population and shows no gender predilection [29]. Pathophysiology of both entities involves massive release of cytokines due to bacterial toxins acting as superantigens.

Both TSS and STSS present with high fever, headache, nausea and vomiting, and myalgias and arthralgias. Hypotension, metabolic acidosis, acute renal failure, elevated transaminases, thrombocytopenia, leukocytosis, disseminated intravascular coagulation, cardiomyopathy, and acute respiratory distress syndrome (ARDS) are often seen. Most patients with TSS do not have an obvious localized *S. aureus* infection. In contrast, 80% of patients with STSS have a clinically evident painful streptococcal soft tissue infection, often necrotizing fasciitis, usually of an extremity [29].

Skin findings are especially prominent in TSS, which classically presents with generalized macular (sunburn-like) erythema, but a scarlatiniform rash with accentuation of the flexures can also be seen. Erythema of the palms and soles, conjunctivae, and mucous membranes is also observed. The patient may develop a bright red "strawberry" tongue. The eruption is followed 1 to 2 weeks later by desquamation, especially of the palms and soles.

The differential diagnosis includes Rocky Mountain spotted fever, meningococcemia, Kawasaki's disease, SSSS, scarlet fever, or a medication hypersensitivity reaction. Blood cultures are positive in 60% of cases of STSS, less often (<15%) in TSS [29]. Diagnosis is on clinical grounds and requires four major criteria (fever >38.9°C, diffuse macular erythroderma, desquamation 1 to 2 weeks later, hypotension, and poor peripheral perfusion) and at least three minor criteria (vomiting or diarrhea; severe myalgia or CPK twice normal; hyperemic mucous membranes; elevated urea or creatinine; elevated bilirubin, ALT, or AST; platelets $<100 \times 10^9$/L; and disorientation or altered consciousness). TSS also has a specific T cell signature with early depletion of the V beta 2 subset followed by massive expansion, which can aid in early diagnosis [31]. Skin biopsy showing a neutrophilic and eosinophilic perivascular and interstitial infiltrate with scattered necrotic keratinocytes can be helpful.

Treatment is with supportive care (intravenous fluids and vasopressors), penicillinase-resistant antibiotics, and intravenous immunoglobulin (IVIG) or fresh frozen plasma (FFP). Nafcillin 1 to 2 g intravenously every 4 hours is the first line antibiotic for TSS and clindamycin 600 to 900 mg intravenously every 8 hours for STSS. As cases of TSS due to methicillin-resistant *S. aureus* (MRSA) are increasing in frequency, treatment with vancomycin (1 to 2 g IV every 24 hours) may sometimes be necessary [32]. In addition, prompt surgical exploration and drainage of suspected deep tissue infections is critical in cases of STSS in which necrotizing fasciitis may be present.

In one study of IVIG in STSS, 30 day survival improved from 34% to 67% and in the only randomized placebo controlled study of treatments for STSS, IVIG decreased mortality by 3.6-fold [33]. TSS has a case fatality rate of less than 5%, whereas mortality in STSS ranges from 30% to 70%, and significant morbidity, including renal failure, amputation, or hysterectomy may also occur [29,30].

Cellulitis and Erysipelas

Cellulitis is an acute bacterial infection of the skin and subcutaneous tissues. Erysipelas is a superficial form of cellulitis that is more indurated and well demarcated than other forms of cellulitis, in which the border between involved and uninvolved skin is indistinct. Cellulitis is common and more frequently affects men than women. The lower extremities are most often involved (73% of cases), followed by the upper extremities (19%), and head and neck (7%) [34].

Cellulitis is usually caused by group A beta-hemolytic streptococci or *S. aureus*, including MRSA [35], although it may also be caused by Group B streptococci, *Haemophilus influenzae*, *Pseudomonas aeruginosa*, and other bacteria, in certain settings. Erysipelas is almost always caused by Group A streptococci. Predisposing factors for cellulitis include venous stasis disease, lymphedema, lower extremity ulceration, tinea pedis, and obesity. Bacteria on the skin surface enter through breaks in the skin and proliferate in the dermis and subcutaneous tissues, causing inflammation.

Patients with cellulitis present with erythema, swelling, warmth, and tenderness of a poorly demarcated area, usually on the leg, often in the setting of lower extremity swelling or dermatitis. If a line is drawn around the involved area, the area of redness is often seen to spread outward over hours to days. Patients frequently have tender local lymphadenopathy and/or lymphangitis. Fever or myalgias are sometimes present. In erysipelas, the skin is bright red and the borders are elevated and sharply demarcated from the uninvolved skin.

Cellulitis has a broad differential diagnosis, including contact dermatitis, superficial thrombophlebitis, deep venous thrombosis, necrotizing fasciitis, lipodermatosclerosis, and insect bites or stings [36,37]. One of the most commonly confused entities is simple stasis dermatitis, which is usually bilateral with scaling and hyperpigmentation of the distal lower extremities in addition to erythema and swelling. It is usually not tender unless ulceration is present.

Diagnosis of cellulitis and erysipelas is generally on clinical grounds. Blood cultures are of low yield (4% positive) unless the patient has signs of sepsis, and tissue cultures from needle aspirates are positive in only 10% to 20% of cases [38]. However, if the patient has an active ulcer, this may be cultured. Radiographic studies are usually unnecessary, although plain films or computed tomography (CT) may be of value to evaluate underlying osteomyelitis, and magnetic resonance imaging (MRI) may be used to differentiate cellulitis from necrotizing fasciitis [36]. If necrotizing fasciitis is strongly suspected, surgical debridement and intravenous antibiotics should be initiated immediately without waiting for radiologic or microbiologic studies.

Treatment of cellulitis is directed at the most likely bacterial causes, which are Streptococci and *S. aureus*. Initial treatment of the hospitalized patient is with beta-lactamase-resistant penicillins or cephalosporins such as cefazolin 1 g IV every 6 hours, nafcillin 1 to 1.5 g IV every 4 to 6 hours, or ceftriaxone 1 g IV every 24 hours. If MRSA is suspected, treatment is with vancomycin 1 to 2 g IV every 24 hours. As the cellulitis begins to resolve and the patient becomes afebrile, the patient may be converted to oral dicloxacillin or cephalexin 500 mg every 6 hours, for a total course of 7 to 14 days of antibiotics [36].

Local treatment of a cellulitic limb with elevation to reduce swelling and saline dressings to any open wounds may be helpful. Prognosis of patients with uncomplicated cellulitis is excellent but recurrences are common. Treatment of underlying tinea pedis with topical azole antifungals and of venous stasis or lymphedema with compression hosiery can help prevent recurrences [36].

Necrotizing Fasciitis

Necrotizing fasciitis (NF) is a rapidly progressive infection involving the subcutis and fascia that typically occurs in the elderly, diabetics, alcohol abusers, and those with chronic cardiac disease or peripheral vascular disease. It is increasing in frequency among young, previously healthy individuals. NF may occur *de novo*, after surgery, or after penetration or even blunt trauma. Injection drug use is not an infrequent cause of NF [39]. The extremity is the usual site of involvement. When NF originates in the scrotum, it is known as Fournier's gangrene. Most cases result from a polymicrobial infection. Pathogens may include Streptococci, *S. aureus*, enterococci, *Escherichia coli, Pseudomonas, Bacteroides, and* Clostridium *spp*. Community acquired MRSA has been reported more recently [40]. Invasive Group A *Streptococcus* is implicated in previously healthy patients. Other less frequent pathogens include *Pseudomonas aeruginosa*, *Aeromonas hydrophila*, and *Vibrio vulnificus, Haemophilus influenzae* type b.

The skin is initially shiny, erythematous, hot, tender, swollen, and tense. Pain is out of proportion to physical findings. Within 24 to 36 hours, skin color changes from red to dusky gray-blue, and bullae may develop. Deeper soft tissue may feel firm. With the destruction of cutaneous nerves, skin becomes anesthetic. The area becomes gangrenous by the fourth or fifth day, and patients appear toxic with fever, chills, tachycardia, shock, and leukocytosis.

NF may be difficult to differentiate from cellulitis, especially early in the course of disease. Features that suggest NF include: severe pain which may be out of proportion to physical findings, anesthesia of involved skin, rapid spread, edema and bulla formation, associated varicella infection, signs of shock, elevated creatine phosphokinase level, or NSAID use. NSAID use is implicated in disease progression through attenuation of signs and symptoms of inflammation that leads to a delay of diagnosis and treatment. MRI may help to discern extent of involvement. A newer tool called the laboratory risk indicator for necrotizing fasciitis uses a scoring system based on C-reactive protein, total white cell count, hemoglobin, sodium, creatinine, and glucose levels to help distinguish between necrotizing soft tissue infections and non-necrotizing infections, and in one retrospective study, was noted to predict mortality and amputation rate [41].

Early fasciotomy and immediate intravenous antimicrobial therapy based on initial Gram stain are crucial. Initial therapy usually involves a beta-lactam/beta-lactamase inhibitor. Hyperbaric oxygen therapy for anaerobic gram negative infection is controversial. Supportive care and attention to nutrition are important in optimizing postoperative wound healing. Even with early treatment, mortality may be between 20% and 40%. Poor prognostic factors include age over 50, diabetes, arteriosclerosis, delay of more than 7 days in diagnosis and surgical intervention, and infection involving the trunk rather than the extremity [42]. Other factors associated with mortality include STSS and immunocompromised state [39,43].

Staphylococcal Scalded Skin Syndrome

Staphylococcal scalded skin syndrome (SSSS) is a blistering, desquamative skin condition caused by the exfoliative toxins of *S. aureus*. Infants and young children are the most commonly affected, likely due to their immature immune and renal function, resulting in a lack of antitoxin antibodies and accumulation of exfoliative toxin. A few cases have been reported in adults who generally have underlying renal impairment or immunosuppression [44,45].

Two toxins, ETA and ETB, have been detected in human disease, with the majority caused by ETA. These toxins bind to and cleave desmoglein 1, a desmosomal protein in the superficial epidermis critical for binding between keratinocytes. Cleavage of this protein causes separation between keratinocytes in the upper layers of the epidermis and also of the superficial epidermis from deeper layers, with resulting fragile blisters and denuded skin [44,45].

In the localized form of SSSS, bullous impetigo, *S. aureus* enters the skin through a break or tear and elaborates exfoliative toxin that results in the development of blisters. Further spread is prevented by antibodies to the toxin. In generalized SSSS, the focus of infection is at a distant site, such as an abscess, pneumonia, osteomyelitis, or endocarditis. Frequently, however, a focus of infection is not found. A lack of protective antibodies allows the toxin to reach the epidermis by hematogenous spread and cause widespread skin disease [44–46].

Whereas bullous impetigo has no associated systemic symptoms, generalized SSSS is associated with a prodrome of fever, malaise, and generalized erythema. This is followed by the formation of large blisters with clear or purulent fluid that easily rupture, leaving extensive areas of denuded skin. The degree of skin involvement may vary from focal blistering to entire body exfoliation. Significant pain and tenderness, hypothermia, fluid losses, secondary infection with *Pseudomonas* and other species, bacteremia, and sepsis may complicate the disease course [44,45].

SSSS should be considered for any presentation of fever and diffuse skin erythema. While the main differential diagnosis is toxic epidermal necrolysis, other conditions to consider include pemphigus foliaceus, scalding or chemical burns, GVHD, and epidermolysis bullosa. A thorough evaluation should include determination of the degree of denudation, identification of the source of infection, determination of fluid status, and a search for signs of secondary infection. Culture and Gram stain of the skin and focus of infection may identify *S. aureus*, but alone do not confirm the diagnosis of SSSS. Enzyme-linked immunosorbent assay (ELISA) can detect production of exotoxin from isolated *S. aureus* species, but should be used as confirmation of SSSS only, as false negatives can easily result if the pathogenic strain of bacteria is not detected on culture. Blood cultures are frequently positive in adults with SSSS [44,45].

Skin biopsy is the most useful diagnostic test, since it further distinguishes between SSSS and TEN. SSSS shows cleavage in the mid-epidermis with minimal associated inflammation. In TEN, cleavage occurs at the dermo-epidermal junction and there is cellular necrosis of the epidermis. TEN can also be distinguished clinically by the presence of mucosal involvement, a finding that is not seen in SSSS. Pemphigus foliaceus, an autoimmune blistering disorder caused by autoantibodies against desmoglein-1, can be difficult to distinguish both clinically and by routine histology [44,45]. Direct immunofluorescence will demonstrate anti-desmoglein antibodies in the epidermis of pemphigus foliaceus patients [47].

Treatment of generalized SSSS is with intravenous antibiotics targeting penicillin-resistant *S. aureus*. Aminoglycosides may be added if there are signs of secondary infection. Analgesia, fluid resuscitation, and wound care are other key elements of treatment. Use of steroids is contraindicated [44,45].

Exfoliation continues for 24 to 48 hours after institution of appropriate antibiotics. MRSA must be considered in any patient not responding to therapy after this time. Although the disease is rarely fatal in children, mortality in adults, even with treatment, is upward of 50% to 60%, when there are serious underlying medical conditions [44,45].

Meningococcemia

Neisseria meningitidis is a major cause of meningitis and sepsis in the United States, with an annual incidence of approximately 1 in 100,000. Meningococcal disease is often rapidly fatal due to shock and multiorgan failure. The majority of cases occur in winter and early spring. Infants and teenagers have the highest rates of infection. Meningococcal disease often occurs in localized outbreaks such as in schools or military barracks [48]. Most affected patients are previously healthy, but those with HIV, immunoglobulin deficiencies, asplenia, or inherited and acquired deficiencies of terminal complement components C5–C9 are at increased risk [48,49].

N. meningitidis is an aerobic gram positive diplococcus that only infects humans. Thirteen serotypes have been identified, of which groups A, B, C, Y, and W-135 are the major pathogens. A vaccine against types A, C, Y, and W-135 is in use for high-risk individuals. The bacteria inhabit the respiratory mucosa and are spread person to person through respiratory secretions. They possess virulence factors that allow invasion through the respiratory epithelium and into the bloodstream. There, they damage endothelium directly and release lipopolysaccharide endotoxin, which provokes massive release of tumor necrosis factor alpha, interleukins-1 and –6, and interferon-gamma. These cytokines promote vascular permeability, hypotension, and eventually multiorgan failure and disseminated intravascular coagulation [48,49].

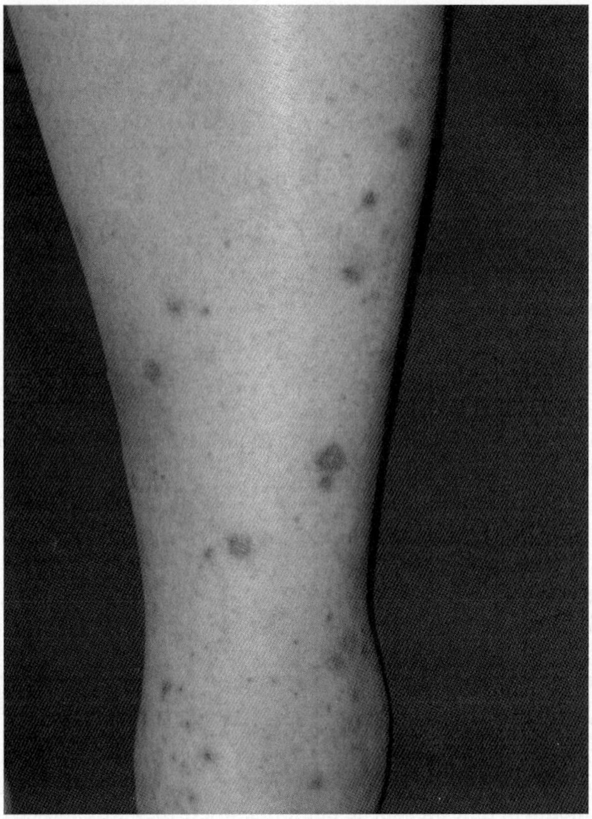

FIGURE 195.5. Meningococcemia. Purpuric papules and plaques, some of which have a dusky or gunmetal gray center.

Meningococcal disease may present in mild cases as a viral syndrome with fever, headache, nausea, vomiting, and arthralgias, but in fulminant cases, patients are severely ill with high fever, hypotension, and a hemorrhagic rash. Half of the cases will have meningitis with headache, stiff neck, and photophobia. Cutaneous findings are prominent in as many as 60% of patients with meningococcemia, with petechiae or purpura beginning at points of pressure on the trunk and extremities, but spreading to involve any body area. Urticarial and maculopapular lesions may also be observed early in the clinical course. As meningococcemia progresses, large areas of irregular gunmetal gray hemorrhage and necrosis may develop (Fig. 195.5) due to disseminated intravascular coagulation. In 10% to 20% of children with meningococcemia, purpura fulminans in combination with multiorgan failure and adrenal hemorrhage, the Waterhouse–Friderichsen syndrome, may occur [50].

The differential diagnosis of meningococcemia includes Rocky Mountain spotted fever, leukocytoclastic vasculitis, toxic shock syndrome, erythema multiforme, and other forms of bacterial sepsis. Diagnosis is usually based on blood or cerebrospinal fluid cultures, and in cases of meningococcal meningitis, gram staining of CSF is up to 90% sensitive. Newer polymerase chain reaction (PCR) tests for meningococcus are available, including the IS-1106, nspA, and ctrA TaqMan tests

[50,51]. Because meningococcal sepsis progresses rapidly and has a case fatality rate of up to 40%, treatment should never be delayed pending diagnosis.

Prompt treatment with an appropriate antibiotic is critical in treating meningococcal disease. First line treatment in adults 18 to 50 years of age is a broad-spectrum cephalosporin, such as ceftriaxone (2 g IV q12 hours). In adults over 50 years of age, ampicillin is given concomitantly. Once the diagnosis of meningococcemia is confirmed, patients in the United States may be switched to penicillin G (4 million units IV Q 4 hours), as penicillin-resistant strains have not been identified there [50]. Intensive supportive care with intravenous fluids, pressors, and ventilatory support is usually needed. Prognosis for untreated cases is very poor, with 70% dying before antibiotics were available. Overall case fatality of meningococcal disease is now around 10%, though it remains 40% for those with sepsis. Up to 19% of survivors have severe sequelae such as deafness or loss of a limb [48].

Rocky Mountain Spotted Fever

Rocky Mountain spotted fever (RMSF) is a life-threatening tick-borne febrile illness caused by the intracellular pathogen, *Rickettsia rickettsi*. Despite its name, RMSF is most commonly reported in the Southeast to Midwest states. Cases occur most often in the summer months, when humans are most likely to be exposed to ticks. RMSF is a rare disease, with an annual incidence of 2.2 cases per million [52]. The disease is most common in children, due to the relatively large amount of time they spend outdoors, where they are exposed to ticks.

RMSF is caused by *R. rickettsi*, a pleomorphic coccobacillary obligate intracellular parasite, which is transmitted to humans by the American dog tick (*Dermacentor variabilis*) in the Eastern United States and the wood tick (*Dermacentor andersoni*) in the mountain West.

R. rickettsi infects vascular endothelium and smooth muscle cells where it can replicate and spread to other cells, causing vascular and tissue injury. Vasculitis may occur in the gastrointestinal tract, lungs, kidneys, liver, heart, brain, and skin, leading to multiorgan failure. In addition, *R. rickettsi* promotes the coagulation cascade, leading to hypercoagulability and thrombocytopenia.

Most patients with RMSF present within 14 days of a tick bite with fever and severe headache. Rash usually occurs 2 to 5 days later. Roughly half of all patients will present with the classic triad of fever, rash, and headache. The rash of RMSF is initially blanching pink to red macules on the wrists and ankles, spreading to the palms and soles and then to the arms, legs, and trunk. The face is usually spared. Over several days, the rash becomes purpuric with areas of hemorrhage and necrosis [53]. In addition to fever and headache, patients frequently present with abdominal pain, nausea and vomiting, myalgias, and shortness of breath. Respiratory failure, myocardial edema, renal failure, liver dysfunction, and altered mental status may occur [54].

The differential diagnosis of RMSF includes other febrile illnesses with rash, such as ehrlichiosis, meningococcemia, toxic shock syndrome, measles, drug fever, idiopathic thrombocytopenic purpura, and various viral syndromes. In cases where no rash occurs, the differential diagnosis would include appendicitis, gastroenteritis, and other causes of acute abdomen. Several diagnostic tests are helpful, but in no case should treatment be delayed pending results once RMSF is suspected. The indirect fluorescent antibody test for *R. rickettsi* is 94% sensitive and specific but requires 7 to 14 days to become positive. Skin biopsy shows a lymphohistiocytic vasculitis with extravasation of red blood cells and occasional fibrin thrombi. *R. rickettsi* may be identified intracellularly by Giemsa staining. Nonspecific laboratory findings include thrombocytopenia and elevated transaminases.

Treatment of RMSF is with doxycycline 100 mg twice daily (or 3 mg/kg of body weight, whichever is higher) for at least 7 days, given orally for outpatients and intravenously for hospitalized patients. Doxycycline should be used even in children (at a dose of 4.4 mg/kg per day divided into BID doses), as the risk of tooth staining has been shown to be quite low for short-term therapy. This regimen will cover other tick-borne illnesses such as Lyme disease and ehrlichiosis, as well as RMSF. Chloramphenicol (at a dose of 50 to 75 mg per kg per day divided into four doses) is an alternative choice for pregnant women and patients with documented allergy to doxycycline, but is reportedly less effective [55]. Treatment should be continued until the patient has been afebrile for 2 to 3 days.

Case fatality rates range from 0.6% to 9%, with worse prognosis in older patients. Untreated RMSF has a mortality of 25%, whereas patients receiving appropriate treatment within 5 days of symptom onset have a mortality of 5% [52].

Disseminated Herpes Simplex Virus Infection

Herpes simplex virus (HSV), a member of the human herpes virus family, is a common cause of dermatologic disease. HSV-1 and HSV-2 have seroprevalence rates as high as 80% and 25% of U.S. adults respectively [56].

Infection is spread by close physical contact of mucous membranes or open skin with infected fluids or skin that is actively shedding virus. After initial infection, the virus remains latent in the dorsal root ganglion. Reactivation may be triggered by stress, illness, trauma (such as from intubation), intense UV exposure, and pregnancy. Grouped vesicles on an erythematous base, often with associated pain or pruritus, appear with reactivation. Rupture of vesicles leaves characteristic punched-out ulcers with scalloped edges [56,57].

Infection in immunocompetent patients is self-limited [58]. Immunocompromised patients (HIV, malignancy, medications, or pregnancy) have more frequent, more severe reactivations and there is an increased risk of disseminated cutaneous and visceral disease [56,58]. Reactivation of genital HSV in immunocompromised and pregnant individuals is associated with an increased risk of visceral dissemination and high mortality. Patients with disrupted skin secondary to eczema, TEN, burns or other conditions, are at risk for disseminated cutaneous disease known as Kaposi's varicelliform eruption or eczema herpeticum [56].

Patients with vesicular eruptions should be examined carefully for clustered lesions or erosions suspicious of HSV. A high index of suspicion is essential. The differential diagnosis includes herpes zoster, varicella, contact dermatitis, bullous impetigo, and other causes of vesiculation of the skin. Confirmatory tests include Tzanck smear, direct fluorescent antibody (DFA), viral culture, PCR, and ELISA. All studies are most sensitive when performed on vesicles less than 48 hours old. DFA and culture should be performed together to increase sensitivity from approximately 50% for each alone, to almost 80% [59]. PCR is the most sensitive test, but it is not always available.

Although there are no controlled studies for treatment of disseminated disease and no evidence that treatment decreases mortality, intravenous acyclovir at 8 to 10 mg per kg every 8 hours for 7 to 10 days is generally employed [57]. The dose is adjusted for patients with renal insufficiency. Alternatives for acyclovir-resistant cases include foscarnet, vidarabine, and cidofovir [58]. Secondary bacterial infection may complicate the course of HSV infection and should be treated with appropriate antibiotic therapy.

Disseminated Herpes Zoster

Varicella zoster virus (VZV) causes both chicken pox (varicella), representing a primary infection, and shingles (zoster), a manifestation of reactivated latent infection. After initial exposure, the virus remains dormant in the dorsal root ganglion [60] or in cranial nerve root ganglia [61]. Medications, aging, malignancy, bone marrow transplant, HIV, and poor nutrition can affect immune status and thereby increase the risk of reactivation. Incidence is approximately 5 per 1,000 per year, with no sex predilection, but there is significantly higher occurrence in at-risk populations and the elderly. A vaccine that is 50% to 64% effective against zoster is now in clinical use, but is not universally administered [60].

Upon reactivation, VZV tracks along sensory nerves to affect a particular dermatome, most commonly the thoracic dermatome. A prodrome of pain, pruritus, and paresthesia in the affected dermatome is noted by up to half of the patients. This is followed by an eruption of erythematous macules and/or papules. Over 24 hours, the lesions begin to vesiculate, and over the next 48 to 72 hours, crust over. Pain is the most common symptom, present in 90% to 95% of patients. Prior to onset of skin lesions, involvement of the thoracic dermatome may be mistaken for acute coronary syndrome.

Immunocompromised hosts may have atypical presentations with unusual lesion morphology, distribution, greater ulceration, and dissemination. Disseminated disease, defined as more than 20 lesions outside the primary dermatome, may present with multiple contiguous or non-contiguous dermatomes. Visceral dissemination can involve the lung, liver, and brain [61], but even in immunocompromised hosts, visceral disease is a low likelihood [60]. Cases of VZV reactivation and visceral dissemination without cutaneous lesions have been rarely reported [60,62].

Uveitis, keratitis, corneal ulcers, and blindness may result from reactivation along the ophthalmic division of the trigeminal nerve. Myelitis or encephalitis may result in weakness and altered mental status. Rarely, motor nerves may be involved with resulting weakness [60].

Differential diagnosis includes HSV infections, bullous drug eruption, contact dermatitis, and erythema multiforme. Tzanck smear, direct fluorescent antibody, or viral culture should be performed if the diagnosis is in question. However, treatment should not be delayed pending results. Patients should be treated if they present within 1 week of onset of their lesions or if they still have any lesions that have not crusted over [61].

Oral acyclovir or valacyclovir is appropriate for healthy individuals who can take oral treatment and for uncomplicated cases in immunocompromised patients. The dosing regimen is 1 g of valacyclovir or 500 mg of famciclovir every 8 hours, or acyclovir 800 mg 5 times a day, with dose adjustment for renal insufficiency. The duration of treatment is 7 to 10 days. IV acyclovir is the treatment of choice in immunocompromised patients with ophthalmic, disseminated, or HIV-associated disease or those with significant comorbidities [60,61]. Acyclovir resistance is more prevalent in immunocompromised populations and should be suspected if new lesions are forming on acyclovir or a related drug (famciclovir, valacyclovir). Viral sensitivities should be checked in this setting. Resistant strains are treated with foscarnet, 180 mg per kg per day divided into two or three doses and renally adjusted [61]. CNS, ophthalmologic, or atypical cutaneous presentations should trigger neurology, ophthalmology, and dermatology consultation [60,61].

Disseminated Candidiasis

Systemic candidiasis may occur as candidemia or as an infection involving a single or multiple organs. It is the fourth most common cause of bloodstream infection in hospitalized patients, with *C. albicans* and *C. glabrata* comprising 70% to 80% of these cases [63]. Immunosuppression and granulocytopenia are important risk factors for candidemia. Patients at high risk include those with hematologic malignancies, those undergoing chemotherapy, and organ and stem cell transplant recipients. Other risk factors for systemic candidiasis include ICU stay, presence of a central venous catheter, parenteral nutrition, broad-spectrum antibiotics, severe trauma, burns, hemodialysis, abdominal surgery, and GI perforation.

Skin lesions are present in up to 35% of patients with systemic candidiasis [63,64]. The eruption appears as pink or violaceous, firm papules or nodules most commonly on the trunk and extremities, but can also involve the face [64]. The lesions are often purpuric, which may be due to concurrent thrombocytopenia or vascular damage from the candida [64]. Other presentations include hemorrhagic or necrotic lesions, pustules, and abscesses. The eyes, kidney, liver, heart, and meninges may also be affected by hematogenous spread of the organism.

Blood cultures are positive in only 50% to 60% of patients with disseminated candidiasis; therefore, biopsy of a skin lesion is a more sensitive approach in early diagnosis and should be submitted for both pathology and tissue culture. Histopathology demonstrates aggregates of hyphae and spores in the dermis. The 1–3 D-glucan detection assay, which was approved by the FDA in 2004, measures the level of glucan in the fungal cell wall and therefore detects fungi, including candida, with a high degree of sensitivity and specificity.

Treatment requires extended courses of a systemic antifungal, usually fluconazole, caspofungin, or less commonly amphotericin B. Intravenous micafungin is a newer agent for invasive candidiases, which was well tolerated in clinical trials [65]. Intravenous catheters should also be removed and replaced, as should other potential sources of infection. With a mortality rate of 30% to 40%, systemic candidiasis causes more fatalities than any other systemic mycosis [63].

BLISTERING DISEASES

Pemphigus vulgaris, paraneoplastic pemphigus, and bullous pemphigoid are autoimmune blistering disorders characterized by autoantibodies directed at cell–cell adhesion molecules or components of the basement membrane zone.

Pemphigus Vulgaris

Pemphigus vulgaris is a rare but potentially fatal bullous disorder that affects the skin and mucous membranes. The worldwide incidence is 0.76 to 5 per million population. However, the incidence is much higher in those of Jewish ancestry [66]. Pemphigus typically affects middle-aged or older individuals. Pemphigus is caused by autoantibodies against the desmosomal proteins, desmoglein 1 and 3, which are required to maintain cellular adhesion between keratinocytes in the epidermis.

Virtually all patients with pemphigus develop painful oral erosions, which are usually the presenting signs. Hoarseness and dysphagia may be a sign of pharyngeal and esophageal involvement, respectively. Cutaneous lesions develop in more than half of the patients, usually after the onset of oral erosions. Vesicles or bullae in pemphigus are fragile and rupture easily since blistering occurs within the epidermis. Consequently, it is more likely to encounter erosions rather than intact blisters on the skin. Blistering may be induced by rubbing intact, normal appearing skin near areas of blistering, a phenomenon known as the Nikolsky sign. Extensive loss of epidermal barrier function in pemphigus may be complicated further by secondary systemic bacterial infection and fluid loss.

TABLE 195.2

SUMMARY OF RECOMMENDATIONS BASED UPON RANDOMIZED CONTROLLED CLINICAL TRIALS FOR PEMPHIGUS VULGARIS

Intervention	Year	Study	No. of Patients	Findings	Reference
Oral prednisolone, high dose (120 mg/d) versus low dose (60 mg/d) regimens	1990	Prospective, randomized trial over 5 y	22	High dose regimen had no long-term benefit over low dose regimen in terms of frequency of relapse or incidence of complications	Ratnam et al. [67]
Adjuvant oral dexamethasone pulse therapy (300 mg pulses 3 d/mo) versus placebo in conjunction with conventional oral prednisolone (80 mg/d) and azathioprine sodium (3 mg/d)	2006	Multicenter, randomized, placebo-controlled trial	20	No benefit of oral dexamethasone pulse therapy given in addition to conventional treatment	Mentink et al. [68]
Comparison of four treatment regimens for pemphigus vulgaris: prednisolone alone, prednisolone plus azathioprine, prednisolone plus mycophenolate mofetil, and prednisolone plus intravenous cyclophosphamide pulse therapy	2007	Randomized, controlled open-label trial over 1 y	120 (30 pts/ arm)	Efficacy of prednisolone is enhanced when combined with cytotoxic agent. Azathioprine was found to be the most efficacious cytotoxic drug to reduce steroid, followed by cyclophosphamide and mycophenolate mofetil.	Chams-Davatchi et al. [69]
Comparison of oral methylprednisolone plus azathioprine or mycophenolate mofetil	2006	Prospective, multicenter, randomized, non-blinded trial	33	Azathioprine and mycophenolate mofetil have similar efficacy, corticosteroid-sparing effects and safety profiles as adjuvant treatments.	Beissert S et al. [70]
High dose intravenous immunoglobulin (IVIG) over 5 consecutive days in patients relatively resistant to systemic steroids	2009	Multicenter, randomized, placebo-controlled, double-blind trial	61 (includes pemphigus foliaceus)	IVIG (400 mg/kg/day for 5 days) is safe and effective for relatively steroid resistant patients.	Amagai M et al. [71]
Dapsone versus placebo in patients already on conventional systemic steroids	2008	Multicenter, randomized, placebo-controlled, double-blind trial	19	"Trend to efficacy" of dapsone but not statistically significant.	Werth et al. [72]
Cyclosporine as adjuvant to systemic corticosteroids	2000	Concurrently randomized trial	29	Cyclosporine ineffective as adjuvant to corticosteroids.	Ioannides D et al. [73]

For patients with only oral disease, the differential diagnosis includes oral HSV, aphthous ulcers, oral lichen planus, and systemic lupus erythematosus. With cutaneous disease, further consideration should be given to bullous impetigo, bullous drug eruptions, and other autoimmune blistering disorders. Drug-induced pemphigus has been associated with the use of various medications, in particular penicillamine and captopril [66].

Diagnosis of pemphigus is made by routine histology, which demonstrates loss of cell–cell adhesion of keratinocytes (acantholysis) and retained attachment of basal cells to the basement membrane along the dermal-epidermal junction. Immunofluorescence of perilesional tissue shows intercellular deposits of IgG. Serum sent for indirect immunofluorescence or ELISA assays will demonstrate circulating antibodies, and titers in pemphigus usually correlate with disease activity [66].

Standard treatment of pemphigus is oral prednisone at 1 mg per kg per day. Studies of corticosteroid-sparing agents for pemphigus, including azathioprine, mycophenolate mofetil, cyclosporine, cyclophosphamide, and IVIG, are reviewed in Table 195.2 [67–73]. Plasmapheresis and rituximab have also been reported to be effective in case series. However, based on a Cochrane review [74], the optimal therapeutic strategy has not been established. Most patients require maintenance treatment for sustained remission. Prior to treatment with oral corticosteroids, most patients died within 5 years of disease onset. Current mortality rate is about 5% to 15%, mostly due to complications from immunosuppressive therapy such as sepsis [66].

Paraneoplastic Pemphigus

Paraneoplastic pemphigus is a variant of pemphigus associated with benign or malignant neoplasms. Most commonly associated conditions include non-Hodgkin's lymphoma, chronic lymphocytic leukemia, Castleman's disease, thymoma, sarcoma, and Waldenstrom's macroglobulinemia. Autoantibodies in paraneoplastic pemphigus are directed against a variety of proteins including desmogleins 1 and 3, Bullous Pemphigoid Antigen 230, as well as the plakin family of proteins [75].

The disease usually presents with a recalcitrant stomatitis involving the mouth and characteristically, the lips. Other mucous membranes, including the eyes, genitalia, nasopharynx, and esophagus, may be involved. Cutaneous lesions are polymorphic and may resemble pemphigus vulgaris, bullous pemphigoid, erythema multiforme, or lichen planus. Some patients develop bronchiolitis obliterans, which may be fatal as a result of respiratory failure [75].

Two thirds of patients diagnosed with paraneoplastic pemphigus have a known underlying neoplasm. In the other third, mucocutaneous disease precedes the diagnosis of an associated neoplasm, and these patients must be carefully followed. Severe, intractable stomatitis is a clue in differentiating paraneoplastic pemphigus from other bullous disorders.

Disease associated with benign neoplasms such as thymoma or Castleman's disease may improve or clear completely with treatment of the underlying condition. The course of disease and prognosis in malignancy-associated paraneoplastic pemphigus is poor. The stomatitis is often refractory to treatment with corticosteroids and immunosuppressants [75].

Bullous Pemphigoid

Bullous pemphigoid (BP) is a chronic subepidermal blistering disorder that usually affects the elderly. It has an incidence of 6 to 7 cases per million. It is usually not life-threatening but often requires long-term use of immunosuppressive agents, which can lead to morbidity and mortality.

Subepidermal blisters in BP result from autoantibodies directed against the hemidesmosomal proteins BP180 and BP230, which are located at the epidermal-dermal junction. BP may be induced by medications, the most common of which are penicillamine and furosemide. Other reported associations include captopril, bumetanide, phenacetin, amoxicillin, ciprofloxacin, potassium iodide, and gold [76].

BP has a variety of clinical manifestations, including a nonbullous prodromal phase characterized by severe pruritus, either alone or associated with excoriated eczematous or urticarial lesions. The bullous phase is characterized by tense vesicles and bullae on normal or erythematous skin. Unlike pemphigus, numerous blisters in bullous pemphigoid are found intact. The lesions are frequently symmetric and are most commonly found in flexural areas on the limbs, the lower trunk, and abdomen. The oral mucosa is involved in 10% to 30% of patients [76].

The differential diagnosis includes pemphigus, bullous lupus erythematosus, dermatitis herpetiformis, bullous erythema multiforme, cicatricial pemphigoid, linear IgA dermatosis, and epidermolysis bullosa acquisita. Diagnosis is made by skin biopsy from the edge of a blister, which shows a subepidermal blister with an eosinophil-rich dermal inflammatory infiltrate. Direct immunofluorescence of perilesional skin shows linear deposits of IgG and/or C3 along the basement membrane zone. Indirect immunofluorescence will detect circulating autoantibodies in 60% to 80% of patients [76].

Bullous pemphigoid has a tendency toward remission and can be controlled more easily than pemphigus. Treatment with high-potency topical corticosteroids may be effective with fewer side effects than the usually employed therapy with oral corticosteroids. Other immunosuppressive agents such as azathioprine, mycophenolate mofetil, cyclophosphamide, and methotrexate may be added for recalcitrant cases or for steroid sparing. The combination of nicotinamide and minocycline or tetracycline has been successful in small case series. Dapsone, IVIG, plasmapheresis, and extracorporeal photopheresis have all been reported to be effective as well.

VASCULAR DISORDERS

Cutaneous Vasculitis

Vasculitis is defined by inflammation of the blood vessel wall and may involve any sized vessel. Since this subject is covered in more depth in Chapter 196, the present discussion will focus on cutaneous findings. Vasculitis may be limited to the skin, or there may be multiorgan involvement involving most commonly the kidneys, the gastrointestinal tract, and/or the joints. It is important to recognize that skin involvement may be a sign of more serious internal organ involvement. The pathogenesis involves immune complex deposition in the affected vessel walls leading subsequent activation of complement. Vasculitis may primary, or secondary to infections (15% to 20%), medications (10% to 15%), malignancy (2% to 5%), or inflammatory disorders including connective tissue disease, inflammatory bowel disease, and others (15% to 20%) [77]. Commonly associated infections include *Streptococcal* and other bacterial acute respiratory infections, bacterial endocarditis, gonococcemia, chronic meningococcemia, hepatitis B and C, HIV, CMV, and mycobacteria. Implicated medications include antibiotics, allopurinol, thiazide diuretics, hydantoins, propylthiouracil, NSAIDs, and anti-TNF agents. Malignancies associated with vasculitis include lymphoproliferative, hematologic, and solid organ cancers. Among connective tissue diseases, systemic lupus erythematosus and rheumatoid arthritis are most likely to be complicated by cutaneous and systemic vasculitis. The underlying etiology may remain unidentified in up to 50% of patients [77].

Vasculitis affecting the skin may be a clue to involvement of other organs. Recognition of cutaneous morphologies associated with vasculitis allows for early recognition and classification of disease, timely workup and diagnosis, and prompt treatment. Cutaneous findings in vasculitis correlate with the size of vessels involved.

Cutaneous small vessel vasculitis includes Henoch-Schonlein purpura, urticarial vasculitis, septic vasculitis, and essential mixed cryoglobulinemia in which HCV may precipitate an immune response. The morphologic hallmark of small vessel vasculitis in the skin is palpable purpura. Red to purple, nonblanching macules and papules are concentrated over dependent areas of the skin such as the ankles and lower legs (Fig. 195.6), or over pressure areas such as the buttocks. There may be significant associated edema. Other morphologies include urticarial lesions, which are less evanescent than typical hives. The patient may have associated constitutional symptoms and arthralgias. Although most cases of cutaneous small vessel leukocytoclastic vasculitis affect only the skin, further consideration should be given to involvement of the renal, gastrointestinal, and central nervous system vasculature. The eruption typically resolves over weeks with hyperpigmentation. It is important to monitor for systemic disease, even after the cutaneous signs have resolved.

Polyarteritis nodosa, Wegener's granulomatosis, and Churg-Strauss syndrome are conditions in which there is inflammation of small and medium sized arteries. Mucocutaneous findings may be found in Churg-Strauss syndrome (55%) and Wegener's granulomatosis (40%). These conditions may present with painful subcutaneous nodules that often ulcerate, typically on the dependant areas such as the lower legs. Other mucocutaneous findings may include a necrotizing livedo reticularis, digital ischemia with gangrene, and oral ulcers. Palpable purpura, splinter hemorrhages, and pustules may also be

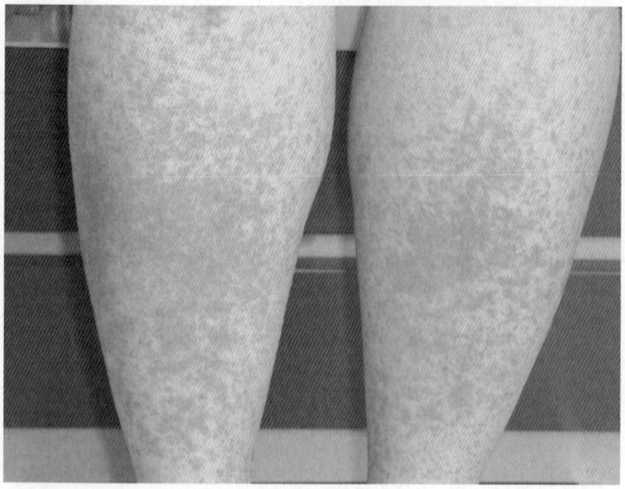

FIGURE 195.6. Vasculitis. Nonblanching, red to purple papules and plaques over the legs associated with edema.

present when there is concomitant small vessel disease. There may be associated constitutional symptoms, myalgias, and arthralgias. Peripheral sensorimotor neuropathy, cardiomyopathy or myocardial infarction, gastrointestinal symptoms and intestinal infarction, seizures, hemiplegia, and necrosis of major organs may also result from inflammation of larger vessels.

Disorders with large vessel vasculitis are usually diagnosed when bruits, asymmetric pulses, claudication, or neurologic deficits are present. Some patients also have cutaneous findings that serve as clues to underlying pathology. In giant cell arteritis (GCA), the temporal artery is tender, swollen, indurated, or pulseless. The tongue may be tender, atrophic, swollen, or cyanotic. Rarely, patients with GCA may have tender nodules overlying other superficial arteries. In less than 20% of cases of Takayasu's arteritis, erythema nodosum-like nodules or pyoderma gangrenosum like ulcers may be present. Cutaneous findings, although present in 80% of patients, are nonspecific in Kawasaki's disease, a syndrome associated with coronary artery aneurysms in 12% of affected children. The eruption of Kawasaki's disease is polymorphous, and patients may present with macules, papules, wheals, targetoid plaques, papulovesicles, pustules, or a scarlatiniform eruption most commonly on the abdomen, groin, perineum, and buttocks. There is often desquamation of the fingertips and mucous membrane involvement may include conjunctival injection, dryness of the lips, erythema of the mouth, and prominent tongue papillae (strawberry tongue). Most patients have enlarged cervical lymph nodes and high fever.

Histopathologic evaluation is important for diagnosis and early lesions are most revealing on biopsy. Thus, timely consultation of the dermatology service is important. Along with determining size of vessel disease, microscopic evaluation of tissue vessels distinguishes inflammatory from noninflammatory vessel disease. Furthermore, immunofluorescence studies of sampled tissue may help confirm a diagnosis of IgA vasculitis associated with Henoch-Schonlein purpura.

It is important to consider coagulopathies and other occlusive vascular diseases in the differential diagnosis of vasculitis since the management of noninflammatory vessel disease differs from that of vasculitis. Purpura, livedo reticularis, ulcers, and necrosis are manifestations of coagulopathies such as immune thrombocytopenic purpura (ITP), thrombotic thrombocytopenic purpura (TTP), drug-induced thrombocytopenia, inherited platelet dysfunction, warfarin and heparin necrosis, disseminated intravascular coagulation (DIC), gammopathies, protein C and S deficiencies, and the antiphospholipid syndrome. In bland occlusive disorders in which vessels may be occluded by fibrin, cryoglobulins, or emboli, the purpura may be palpable as in leukocytoclastic vasculitis, so the clinical distinction is not always apparent.

Treatment is directed at the underlying etiology and preventing the progression of inflammation. It is always important to evaluate and treat any underlying cause, whether it is infection, malignancy, or drug. With early intervention, morbidity and mortality from vasculitis may be reduced. For disease limited to the skin, supportive care with rest, leg elevation, and analgesics is usually sufficient. NSAIDs, colchicine, dapsone, or prednisone are helpful for patients with recalcitrant or progressive skin disease. Severe intractable skin disease or involvement of organs other than the skin requires immunosuppressive therapy with high dose prednisone 1 to 2 mg per kg per day, sometimes with steroid sparing support from methotrexate, cyclosporine, azathioprine, or cyclophosphamide [77].

Purpura Fulminans

Purpura fulminans (PF) is characterized by extensive purpura and necrosis of the skin associated with fever, DIC, sepsis, and hypotension. PF is seen mostly in three clinical settings: acute infections, inherited or acquired coagulopathies, and idiopathic. Meningococcemia, in which 3% of cases develop PF, is the most commonly associated infection. Varicella and pneumococcal sepsis are less frequently associated and rare or isolated reports include *H. influenza* [78] and other organisms. Asplenism is a risk factor for infection associated with PF. PF in the newborn period is usually due to an inherited coagulopathy and results in high mortality. PF has also been reported in association with acquired coagulopathies seen in inflammatory bowel disease [79,80]. Idiopathic disease is the mildest variant [81–83].

The pathophysiology of PF depends on the underlying trigger. The common endpoint is that of extensive microvascular thrombosis that affects cutaneous and visceral blood supply. In meningococcemia, endotoxin results in release of cytokines and activation of coagulation pathways, and infection is associated with substantially decreased levels of protein C [81].

Initially in PF, there is pain and erythema in affected areas. Irregular areas of blue–black discoloration develop within the center of erythematous patches, and lesional skin becomes indurated. There is progression to hemorrhagic vesicles and bullae, and finally to tissue necrosis. Lesions associated with infection tend to involve distal parts first and spread proximally, while idiopathic and coagulopathy-associated disease may remain localized to the lower extremities. Idiopathic PF usually affects only the skin; however, other forms may result in widespread necrosis with multiorgan failure. Disease complications include scarring, secondary infection, digital or limb necrosis, and autoamputation [81–83].

Differential diagnosis of PF includes Henoch-Schonlein purpura and post-infectious thrombocytopenic purpura, although these are both associated with milder disease than seen in PF. The presence of DIC helps distinguish PF from other causes of cutaneous necrosis [82].

Early recognition of disease and underlying trigger is essential in this rapidly progressive condition. Appropriate antimicrobials are instituted for infection. Supportive care includes aggressive fluid resuscitation, electrolyte monitoring, and replacement of blood products. If deficient, protein C and antithrombin III may be replaced. Other treatment options include fresh frozen plasma, heparin, plasmapheresis, topical nitroglycerin (for local vasodilation), and recombinant tissue plasminogen activator [82]. Surgical consultation may be necessary for debridement and grafting.

Antiphospholipid Antibody Syndrome

Antiphospholipid antibody syndrome (APS) is characterized by a hypercoagulable state with venous or arterial thrombosis, recurrent fetal loss, thrombocytopenia, and elevated titers of the antiphospholipid antibodies (anticardiolipin antibodies, lupus anticoagulant, anti-β-2 glycoprotein I antibodies). Up to 2% of the normal population exhibits detectable titers of these antibodies and 0.2% have elevated titers. APS may be primary, or it may be seen in conjunction with systemic lupus erythematosus, malignancy, drugs, infection, or hematologic disease [84–86].

Cutaneous manifestations in APS, although highly variable, are common and often the presenting sign of disease. Therefore, recognition of these findings is essential for early diagnosis and prompt evaluation for more extensive disease. Skin lesions are thought to be a direct result of arterial or venous occlusion and subsequent ischemia. The most common finding is livedo reticularis or livedo racemosa, seen in up to 40% of patients, and up to 70% of patients who have systemic lupus. These present as a netlike pattern of dusky erythema often found on the upper or lower extremities; they are thought to be more common in cases with underlying arterial disease and are less often seen in veno-occlusive disease [87]. Other associated findings include cyanotic macules, ecchymoses and purpura, ulcerations of the ears, face, and legs, porcelain-white scars (atrophie blanche) at the ankles, thrombophlebitis, Raynaud's phenomenon, digital ischemia, and gangrene. Any major organ systems can be affected by thrombosis [84–86].

The differential diagnosis of APS includes other disorders with associated livedo reticularis and cutaneous necrosis including vasculitis, warfarin-induced skin necrosis (WISN), cholesterol emboli, and cryoglobulinemia. Similar to other vaso-occlusive disorders, APS shows bland thrombosis of small dermal vessels. APS is distinguished from other noninflammatory vaso-occlusive disorders by the presence of elevated antiphospholipid antibody titers [84,86]. Although cutaneous findings are common, they are not among the diagnostic criteria for APS, which require positive antibodies on two occasions at least 6 weeks apart in addition to a history of vascular thrombosis or pregnancy complications [88].

Both treatment and prophylaxis consist of anticoagulation. Some advocate the use of aspirin in those without a history of thrombosis or with superficial venous thrombosis only. Otherwise, long-term warfarin anticoagulation with an INR goal of 3 to 4 is recommended. Immunosuppressive agents and immunotherapy (plasmapheresis, intravenous immunoglobulin, cyclophosphamide) may help reduce antibody levels, but is likely to rebound once treatment is discontinued [84,86].

Warfarin-Induced Skin Necrosis

Warfarin-induced skin necrosis (WISN) is seen in 0.01% to 0.1% of individuals on warfarin, 3 to 10 days after starting therapy. Women are affected four times more frequently than men, and are most often middle-aged and obese. Three quarters of patients with WISN are being treated for deep venous thrombosis or pulmonary embolism. Atrial fibrillation, valve replacement, and arterial occlusion are disorders in which anticoagulation with warfarin less commonly results in WISN [89].

Although the pathophysiology of WISN is not understood completely, the generally accepted mechanism involves the imbalance between intrinsic procoagulant and anticoagulant factors created early on during warfarin therapy. Due to their short half-lives, anticoagulant protein C and factor VII are depleted before procoagulant factors II, IX, and X, and this results in an initial hypercoagulability that is thought to trigger onset of WISN [89]. Most individuals on warfarin do not experience this complication, and therefore additional risk factors are likely required to induce necrosis. Protein C and S deficiency, activated protein C resistance, Factor V Leiden, antithrombin III deficiency, or prothrombin gene mutations, and heparin-induced thrombocytopenia may be contributory. Protein C deficiency, either inherited or acquired, is a significant risk factor [89], and has been implicated in more than 50% of cases of WISN. High loading doses of warfarin and inadequate overlap with heparin therapy are also thought to increase risk of early WISN. There are rare reports of cases occurring up to years after the onset of warfarin therapy, and delayed-onset WISN may be related to poor compliance with warfarin, broken up courses of interacting medications, or changing liver synthetic function [89].

WISN generally occurs 3 to 10 days after initiation of therapy. Patients experience pressure or pain in the involved area of skin. Poorly demarcated, indurated erythema develops asymmetrically over fatty areas such as the breast, buttock, thighs, and lower abdomen. Induration progresses over 24 to 72 hours to edema with a *peau d'orange* surface, blue–black discoloration, and hemorrhagic bullae. Localized or widespread full thickness skin necrosis ensues. Histology of involved skin shows noninflammatory thrombosis and fibrin deposition in small dermal vessels with necrosis of the dermis and subcutaneous fat [89].

Differential diagnosis of WISN includes necrotizing fasciitis, APS, DIC or purpura fulminans, calciphylaxis, gangrene, embolic disease, cellulitis, and pyoderma gangrenosum. Recent initiation of warfarin should raise suspicion of WISN.

Screening for hypercoagulable states before anticoagulation is neither predictive of WISN risk nor cost-effective. Low initial loading doses and gradual increases in warfarin levels may decrease risk of WISN. WISN is treated by discontinuation of warfarin, administration of FFP and vitamin K to reverse its effects, and anticoagulation with heparin. Small lesions may be treated conservatively. Extensive involvement may necessitate debridement, grafting, and in extreme cases, amputation. Deep tissue necrosis, secondary infection, and multiorgan failure are more likely with more widespread disease. Even with treatment, the mortality rate is 15% within 3 months of onset. Prior episodes of WISN are not predictive of future occurrences. In most patients with WISN, future warfarin therapy may be reinstituted with caution, avoiding loading doses and overlapping with heparin initially [89].

Cryoglobulinemia

Cryoglobulinemia (CG) is characterized by precipitation of immunoglobulins from serum in cold temperatures. It is classified into three subtypes. Type I CG constitutes 5% to 25% of cases and presents with monoclonal immunoglobulinemia. It is associated with underlying hematologic disease such as multiple myeloma or Waldenstrom's macroglobulinemia. Types II and III CG are the mixed cryoglobulinemias. Type II constitutes 40% to 60% of cases and is associated with a mixture of polyclonal and monoclonal immunoglobulins. It generally occurs in patients with persistent viral infections such as hepatitis C and HIV. Type III CG represents 40% to 50% of cases. It is associated with a polyclonal immunoglobulinemia and with connective tissue disorders.

Two distinct syndromes are seen with CG depending on the subtype. In type I disease, monoclonal cryoglobulins result in hyperviscosity of blood, which may manifest on the skin as livedo reticularis or Raynaud's phenomenon. Cryoglobulins precipitate in cold and result in vascular occlusion or immune complex-mediated vasculitis which may cause digital ischemia and purpura, respectively.

The mixed cryoglobulinemias are seen in association with infectious and inflammatory diseases. These underlying conditions are thought to trigger B cell hyperactivation, which promotes production of cryoglobulins. Meltzer's triad of palpable purpura, arthralgia, and myalgia may be apparent in 25% to 30% of patients. Other findings include fatigue, neuropathy (70% to 80%), and cutaneous vasculitis. The course in these patients fluctuates. Organ systems other than the skin may be involved as well. The kidneys may be affected in any of the three forms. Bone marrow may be involved in Type I disease, while the peripheral nervous system may be affected in Types II and III.

Diagnosis is based on clinical signs and symptoms and elevated serum cryoglobulin levels. Blood samples should be collected into prewarmed vials and maintained at 37 °C to prevent precipitation of cryoglobulins. While involved skin characteristically shows noninflammatory occlusion of dermal vessels by immunoglobulin precipitates, leukocytoclastic vasculitis may be apparent in up to 50% of cases.

Treatment of mild disease is supportive in nature and otherwise focused on any underlying disease process. For more severe disease, options include immunosuppressive agents, plasmapheresis, rituximab, and radiation or chemotherapy to treat associated hematologic malignancy.

Cryoglobulinemia itself does not typically worsen clinical outcomes of associated disease. Morbidity and mortality are attributed to associated diseases, and death is often due to cardiac disease or infection [90].

Embolic Diseases

Embolization of cholesterol or atheromatous material, fat, or tumor may result in striking systemic and cutaneous findings. Cholesterol embolization is typically a result of interventional vascular procedures such as left heart catheterization or angiograms, and can also be associated with cardiac surgery, thrombolysis, and aortic dissection. Less frequently, patients with severe and extensive atherosclerotic disease may experience spontaneous embolization, or emboli triggered by coughing or straining. Showers of cholesterol and atherosclerotic material travel distally and lodge in small arteries of the CNS, lungs, GI tract, kidneys, and skin. Presenting signs and symptoms of embolic disease include mental status changes, pulmonary edema, heme positive stools, and acute renal failure. Cutaneous findings are striking when apparent and include livedo reticularis, a coarse netlike pattern of violaceous erythema evident on the lower extremities and abdomen (Fig. 195.7). The erythema may be more prominent when the patient is standing compared to the supine position. Tender blue discoloration, petechiae, ecchymoses, ulceration, and gangrene of the feet and toes may eventuate. Pedal pulses are generally intact but bruits may be audible over the femoral artery and abdominal aorta. Calf tenderness is variable. Similar findings on the arm and hands may result from aortic embolization to the upper extremities [91–93].

Fat embolization, seen most commonly after fractures of the long bones or following surgical procedures, is a less common source of embolic disease that presents with the classic triad of pulmonary, neurologic, and cutaneous symptoms. It has rarely been reported following liposuction. Petechiae distributed on the upper body (head, neck, chest, and subconjunctiva) are thought to be pathognomonic and are seen about 50% of the time [94]. Emboli from atrial myxoma, a benign cardiac hamartoma, may result in cyanosis, ecchymoses, splinter hemorrhages, and tender violaceous lesions of the digits [95].

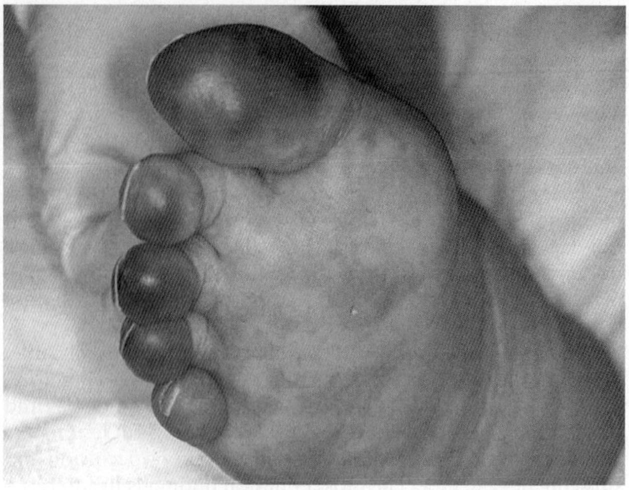

FIGURE 195.7. Cholesterol emboli. Purpuric plaques involving the toes represent areas of necrosis. Note the livedoid (reticulated) pattern on the sole of the foot, an earlier sign of vascular occlusion.

The diagnosis of emboli should be highly suspected in any patient with characteristic skin findings, acute onset end-organ failure, and a recent invasive vascular procedure. Biopsy of the affected organ will show occlusion of vessels with needle-shaped clefts representing cholesterol crystals. Skin is the most accessible and easiest tissue to sample. Atrial myxoma is evident on echocardiogram, and sampling of affected skin will demonstrate the embolized myxomatous material. Laboratory parameters such as BUN, creatinine, CBC and ESR, presence of hematuria, and heme positive stools will be reflective of the organs involved. Treatments include surgical removal or bypass of emboli, amputation of gangrenous digits, and anticoagulation if disease is not thrombolytic-induced [92,95].

Calciphylaxis

Calciphylaxis, or calcific uremic arteriolopathy, is a rare but serious disorder involving calcification of cutaneous arteries and resultant tissue necrosis, usually in the setting of end-stage renal disease (ESRD) and dialysis. Other risk factors include hyperparathyroidism, obesity, white race, female sex, liver disease, malignancy, hypercoagulability, and use of corticosteroids or vitamin D [96]. An elevated calcium phosphate product is not a prerequisite for calciphylaxis, nor is there a correlation between the degree of elevation of calcium, phosphate, or parathyroid hormone levels and the likelihood of developing calciphylaxis. Among patients with ESRD, 1% to 4% develop this disorder.

Calciphylaxis presents with the acute onset of intensely painful indurated purpuric to necrotic skin lesions on a background of livedo reticularis, erythematous papules, plaques, and subcutaneous nodules. Lesions are most common on the thighs, buttocks, and lower abdomen, but may even occur on the digits.

The differential diagnosis of calciphylaxis includes vasculitis, warfarin necrosis, atheroemboli, cryoglobulinemia, APS, protein C or S deficiency, polyarteritis nodosa, and disseminated intravascular coagulation. A deep incisional skin biopsy is usually diagnostic. Calcification is seen in the subcutaneous fat, especially in the medial layer of arterioles, associated with endovascular fibrosis, thrombosis, and necrosis of the subcutaneous fat and overlying skin. Vasculitis is not seen. Laboratory studies addressing causes of hypercoagulability can be helpful as can plain radiographs or technetium 99 bone scans showing vascular calcification.

Treatment of calciphylaxis is controversial and no controlled studies have been performed. Most sources recommend normalization of calcium and phosphorus levels using diet, binding agents, low-calcium dialysis, and sometimes parathyroidectomy [97]. Good wound care and pain control are important. Precipitating factors such as intravenous infusions, oral calcium supplements, or corticosteroids should be avoided or discontinued. Recent studies suggest that use of cinacalcet (30 to 60 mg daily) or sodium thiosulfate (25 gm IV given three times weekly after hemodialysis) may be useful [98]. Overall mortality in calciphylaxis is 80% [97].

CONNECTIVE TISSUE DISORDERS

Systemic Lupus Erythematosus (SLE)

Lupus erythematosus may involve the skin in many forms. Patients with the acute form of cutaneous lupus erythematosus are most likely to have systemic disease, which may be encountered in an ICU setting.

Approximately 80% of patients with SLE have cutaneous manifestations that, although they appear in a multitude of ways, are helpful in identifying affected patients. In fact, 4 of the 11 American Rheumatism Association criteria for diagnosing SLE are cutaneous findings (malar rash, photosensitivity, discoid rash, and oral ulceration). The most characteristic eruption is a transient facial erythema involving the malar area and the bridge of the nose that follows sun exposure (Fig. 195.8). The redness, which may be accompanied by edema, lasts between hours and several weeks before resolving without scarring. This "butterfly" rash may be an indicator of internal disease as it may be associated with anti-dsDNA antibody and lupus nephritis [99].

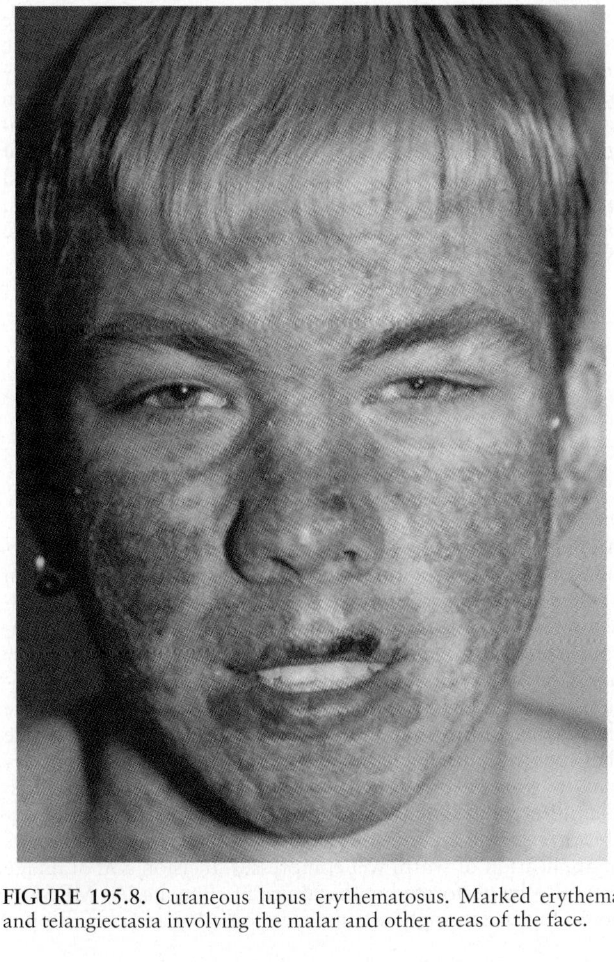

FIGURE 195.8. Cutaneous lupus erythematosus. Marked erythema and telangiectasia involving the malar and other areas of the face.

Erythema and poikiloderma (hyperpigmentation, hypopigmentation, telangiectasia, and atrophy) also occurs over other sun-exposed surfaces such as the V neck area of the chest as well as the back. On the hands, this erythema characteristically spares the knuckles. Tense bullae, also triggered or worsened by sun exposure, may appear in a similar distribution. Mucous membrane lesions occur in about 20% to 30% of patients with SLE. Petechiae or shallow ulcerations may be noted on the hard palate and may accompany malar erythema. Gingival, nasal, and vaginal ulcerations may also be seen.

Scalp hair shedding occurs diffusely and is not associated with scarring. Fragile hairs on the periphery of the scalp break and appear short. Hair shedding may also result from telogen effluvium associated with a chronic illness. Patients with SLE are also more likely to have alopecia areata [99], which typically manifests as oval patches of scalp alopecia.

Vascular lesions, although not specific for SLE, occur in 50% of patients and are highly suggestive of connective tissue disease. The presence of Raynaud's phenomenon, persistent palmar erythema, periungual telangiectasias, purplish plaques over the tips of fingers and toes with cold exposure, and persistent erythema over the palms, soles, elbows, knees, or buttocks should prompt a search for systemic disease.

Vasculitis involving postcapillary venules in the skin manifests as palpable purpura or hemorrhagic wheals. Nodules that ulcerate along the course of arteries reflect deeper, larger vessel involvement. Vascular thrombosis as a consequence of an associated APS causes punched out ulcers that typically appear over malleolar and pretibial surfaces. The presence of livedo reticularis, thrombosis, and cutaneous infarction also warrants consideration of a prothrombotic state.

Less common cutaneous findings in SLE include a symmetric eruption of erythematous papules on the extremities, which demonstrate palisaded granulomatous inflammation with or without vasculitis on light microscopy. Calcinosis cutis, rarely present in SLE, presents as reddish or violaceous firm plaques or nodules on the head, trunk, or extremities.

Other connective tissue diseases should be considered in the differential diagnosis of the acute lupus syndrome. Eruptions of lupus localized to the head and neck may be difficult to differentiate from rosacea, dermatomyositis, drug induced photosensitivity, and sunburn. Drug eruptions or exanthems appear similar when lupus manifests diffusely on the skin.

Treatment of cutaneous lupus is difficult. Strict sun protection along with topical corticosteroids and calcineurin inhibitors are a mainstay of treatment. Antimalarial drugs with or without corticosteroids or steroid-sparing immunosuppressives may be required for systemic or severe skin disease.

Dermatomyositis

Dermatomyositis is a rare disease characterized by a proximal muscle myositis with skin changes. It has a bimodal age distribution and is more common in female and black patients. Initial cutaneous manifestations include swelling of the face and eyelids with a characteristic violaceous erythema. These changes become more widespread with erythema and telangiectasia spreading to the neck and sun-exposed area of the chest, to the back in a shawl distribution, as well as to the scalp, elbows, and knees. These eruptions are usually photosensitive, and pruritus or burning is a common complaint. Gottron's sign, which consists of scaly reddish papules over the knuckle, is considered pathognomonic of dermatomyositis. Hands may take on the appearance of mechanics' hands with hyperpigmentation, scaling, fissuring of the fingertips, ragged cuticles, and enlarged proximal nail fold capillaries. Intermittent malaise, anorexia, weight loss, and arthralgias are often apparent at this stage. Cutaneous disease usually precedes myositis by months. Juvenile dermatomyositis is relatively rare, and has a better prognosis, but requires aggressive treatment to prevent calcinosis of affected skin. Dermatomyositis may be drug-induced, with hydroxyurea being the most common culprit [100].

Aggressive treatment at this early stage allows for better disease control with lower immunosuppression. Early treatment also reduces the development of disfiguring calcium deposition in the skin and muscle. Initial treatment of skin disease is sunscreen with topical corticosteroids or calcineurin inhibitors, but resistant skin disease may require methotrexate or antimalarials. With evident myositis, therapy requires the use of prednisone (0.5 to 1.5 mg/kg/d tapered slowly over 1 to 2 years) and the addition of a steroid-sparing immunosuppressive such as azathioprine or methotrexate. It is important to also consider the coexistence of other connective tissue diseases such as scleroderma, systemic lupus erythematosus, and rheumatoid arthritis in a patient with dermatomyositis. With appropriate and timely therapy, patients may become disease-free and off therapy within 2 to 4 years. Patients should be surveyed for an occult visceral malignancy which is associated with dermatomyositis in up to 25% of adult cases. Poor prognostic factors include malignancy, older age, initiating therapy after 24 months of muscle weakness, extensive cutaneous lesions, dysphagia, and cardiac or pulmonary issues [101]. A discussion of myositis and systemic disease associated with dermatomyositis is detailed in Chapter 193.

DERMATOLOGIC ISSUES RELATED TO BONE MARROW TRANSPLANTATION

Graft-Versus-Host Disease

Graft-versus-host disease (GVHD) occurs in 30% to 80% of hematopoietic cell transplant recipients and is regarded as the primary cause of morbidity and mortality in these patients [102]. Although it is typically a complication of bone marrow and hematopoietic stem cell transplantations, GVHD may also occur in the setting of unirradiated blood product infusion, solid organ transplantation, and maternal–fetal transfusions [103]. Risk factors for GVHD include unrelated donor, HLA mismatch, older age of recipient, female donor with a male recipient, and suboptimal dosing of immunosuppressive drugs. Patients who develop GVHD appear to be at a reduced risk of recurrence of their malignancy, probably due to graft-versus-leukemia or graft-versus-malignancy reactions.

GVHD can occur when immunologically competent donor T cells are transferred to a host that is incapable of rejecting them. The pathogenesis is incompletely understood, but the mediators include donor CD4+ and CD8+ T cells, NK cells, host dendritic cells, macrophages, major and minor histocompatibility antigens on immune and epithelial cells, and cytokines including TNF-α, and IFN-γ [102].

GVHD can be divided into acute and chronic forms, with the acute form developing within the first 100 days after transplantation and the chronic form developing after about day 100.

Acute GVHD

Acute GVHD occurs in 25% to 40% of patients receiving transplants from HLA matched siblings, and it increases to 60% to 80% with 1 HLA mismatch [103]. There is decreased survival from acute GVHD after allogeneic bone marrow transplant. Acute GVHD is classified into four grades based on the extent of skin involvement, serum bilirubin level, and the amount of diarrhea per 24 hours. Skin findings begin with painful or pruritic erythematous macules on the palms, soles, and ears and evolve into a diffuse morbilliform eruption which is often folliculocentric. In severe cases, there may be progression with bullae formation, erythroderma, and skin necrosis. There have been rare reports of acquired ichthyosis as a manifestation of acute GVHD [104]. The differential diagnosis of acute GVHD includes drug eruptions, viral exanthems, and the eruption of lymphocyte recovery. Mucous membrane lesions may be difficult to distinguish from mucositis caused by chemotherapy.

Histopathology of involved skin classically shows an interface dermatitis and apoptotic keratinocytes. However, the utility of a skin biopsy in diagnosing GVHD is controversial. In a small case series, the presence of eosinophils in biopsy specimens was not a reliable marker favoring drug hypersensitivity reaction over GVHD [105]. In three bone marrow transplant recipients with acute skin eruptions, biopsy led to an initial diagnosis of drug eruption, and immunosuppressive therapy was delayed until additional features of GVHD appeared, resulting in considerable morbidity and two deaths.

Chronic GVHD

Chronic GVHD occurs in 30% to 60% of patients and is more common in hematopoietic stem cell transplants compared to bone marrow transplants [102]. A patient's risk of developing chronic GVHD is 11 times higher with a prior history of acute GVHD, but 20% to 30% of patients can develop chronic GVHD without prior acute GVHD [103].

There are two forms of chronic cutaneous GVHD, lichenoid and sclerodermoid. The lichenoid variant is characterized by erythematous and violaceous papules and plaques, often distributed on flexural surfaces that resemble lichen planus. The sclerodermoid form presents with sclerotic, indurated white to yellow plaques that involve the dermis. The process may extend to fascia and result in significant tightening of skin and joint contractures. Lichen sclerosis and eosinophilic fasciitis can also be presentations of the sclerodermoid variant of chronic GVHD [106]. The oral mucosa is often involved and may demonstrate redness and atrophy of mucosal surfaces, lacy white reticulations of buccal mucosa, and ulcerations. Xerostomia is frequently present as well.

COMMON DERMATOLOGIC CONDITIONS COEXISTING IN ICU PATIENTS

Abscess

A cutaneous abscess is a painful, fluctuant, walled-off collection of pus found within the skin. A furuncle represents an abscess associated with a hair follicle and a carbuncle is a collection of multiple furuncles. Abscesses and furuncles are typically caused by *S. aureus*. Patients may carry *S. aureus* in their nares or have Staphylococcal folliculitis as preceding conditions. The clinical presentation consists of a small red papule that evolves into a tender, erythematous deep-seated nodule that may become fluctuant with time. The surrounding area may be warm to the touch if there is an associated cellulitis. The differential diagnosis includes an inflamed epidermal inclusion cyst and an insect bite. Conservative treatment consists of application of warm wet compresses. Incision and drainage may also be performed with culture of contents. As MRSA is becoming increasingly common, lesions that recur or do not respond to conservative treatment may necessitate appropriate antibiotic treatment based on culture results.

Folliculitis

Folliculitis is a very common disorder characterized by inflammation or irritation of hair follicles. Although cultures are usually negative, Staphylococci, Pseudomonas, or Malassezia furfur are commonly causative. Herpes virus and dermatophytes are less commonly implicated. Folliculitis presents as papules or pustules on an erythematous base with a centrally extruding hair. The lesions may be pruritic and are most often found on the face, scalp, thighs, axillae, and inguinal area. Pseudomonal folliculitis may be more inflammatory and localized to a distribution that would be covered by a bathing suit. Pityrosporum folliculitis may be localized to the upper back and chest and be extremely pruritic. A follicular papulopustular eruption on the face, chest, and upper back has been associated with EGF-R inhibitors and correlates with a positive response to chemotherapy [107]. Diagnostic tools include a potassium hydroxide preparation, Gram stain, and bacterial, fungal, and viral cultures. Treatment is directed at the underlying etiology. Most cases will respond to appropriate topical and/or oral antibiotics (most commonly anti-staphylococcal). Pityrosporum folliculitis requires topical or oral antifungals and Pseudomonal folliculitis may require fluoroquinolones. The prognosis is generally good, but some patients experience recurrent disease [107].

Steroid Acne

Administration of either topical or systemic corticosteroids can lead to the abrupt appearance of an acneiform eruption. In a prospective study of 51 patients receiving intravenous corticosteroids in the setting of acute spinal cord injury, one subject (2%) developed steroid acne [108]. Lesions of steroid acne are usually monomorphic inflammatory papules and pustules that appear on the chest and back. The eruption resolves within weeks of discontinuing the corticosteroids.

Peripheral Edema

Peripheral edema, which is commonly seen in the elderly and hospitalized patients, occurs when capillary hydrostatic pressure and filtration exceeds the lymphatic drainage rate. Common causes of edema include heart failure, renal failure, nephrotic syndrome, cirrhosis, venous thrombosis, or medications, particularly calcium channel blockers. Acute exacerbations of chronic edema may cause edema blisters which present as asymptomatic, noninflammatory tense vesicles and bullae with clear fluid, usually on the distal lower extremities. Edema blisters can be distinguished from other blistering disorders by clinical history and physical examination. If needed, a biopsy for routine histopathology and immunofluorescence may help exclude other blistering disorders. Acute peripheral edema may also produce local dermal edema, leading to induration of the skin and dimpling, known as *peau d'orange*.

Stasis Dermatitis

Stasis dermatitis occurs in the setting of venous hypertension due to valvular incompetence. Risk factors include conditions that exacerbate lower extremity edema such as obesity, congestive heart failure, cirrhotic liver disease, and chronic renal insufficiency. Typically, there is reddish mottling and a yellowish or brown discoloration of the medial lower legs, corresponding to the location of major communicating veins. There may be an eczematous component as well that often results from contact sensitization to topical medicaments applied to the legs. There are often other signs of venous hypertension, including edema, varicose veins, and venous leg ulcers. Over years, the legs may develop lipodermatosclerosis, which occurs when adipose tissue becomes indurated and adherent to fascia, and lower legs take on the appearance of an inverted wine bottle.

The diagnosis is evident in the right clinical context. However, asteatotic eczema, contact dermatitis, and cellulitis may also be considered in the differential. Relief of itching is attained through the regular application of emollients and the use of class IV or V topical steroids. Long-term management involves improving venous return through various measures such as leg elevation above the level of the heart, elastic compression, and exercises to strengthen calf muscles. Care should be taken to avoid trauma to the leg that would facilitate ulcer formation. In severe cases, ligation of incompetent communicating veins may be necessary.

Pressure Ulcers

Pressure ulcers are areas of ischemic soft tissue necrosis resulting from prolonged pressure, shearing force, or friction anywhere on the body. Sites that are most frequently involved include skin overlying bony prominences of the sacrum, ischial tuberosities, heels, greater trochanters, and lateral malleoli. Nonblanching erythema of skin overlying a bony prominence may signify impending ulceration. Other early indicators include warmth, edema, or induration of skin. Initial ulcers appear punched out. Ulceration may occur as partial thickness skin loss, full thickness skin loss involving subcutaneous tissue, or full thickness skin loss extending to muscle, tendon, or bone. Associated pain may be severe and should be managed aggressively. Treatment involves relief of pressure, which may be accomplished through frequent position changes and supportive surfaces such as air, liquid, or foam cushions. Local wound care includes cleansing with normal saline, debridement, and occlusive hydrocolloid dressings to optimize healing. Operative repair is necessary in some cases. Wounds should be monitored for local infection and treated accordingly. Sepsis and osteomyelitis may further complicate ulceration.

Psoriasis

In its most common form (chronic plaque psoriasis), psoriasis presents as chronic well-demarcated erythematous plaques with adherent silvery scale, most commonly over the elbows, knees, and scalp. In guttate psoriasis, there are smaller psoriatic papules and plaques diffusely over the body, and this is often triggered by streptococcal infections. Sudden onset of pustules that coalesce to form "lakes of pus" at the edges of psoriatic plaques associated with fever typifies the more generalized form of pustular psoriasis (Fig. 195.9). Hypocalcemia and pregnancy may be triggering factors in pustular psoriasis. In erythrodermic psoriasis, there is bright red erythema involving $\geq 90\%$ of the skin. These patients are itchy and also complain of chills from the extensive heat loss due to dilatation of cutaneous vessels. In both pustular and erythrodermic forms, patients are generally toxic and may have associated acute respiratory distress syndrome, congestive heart failure, pneumonia, or viral hepatitis (see "Exfoliative Erythroderma" section).

There is a newly recognized association of psoriasis, particularly severe disease, with increased risk of cardiovascular, cerebrovascular, and peripheral vascular disease [109,110].

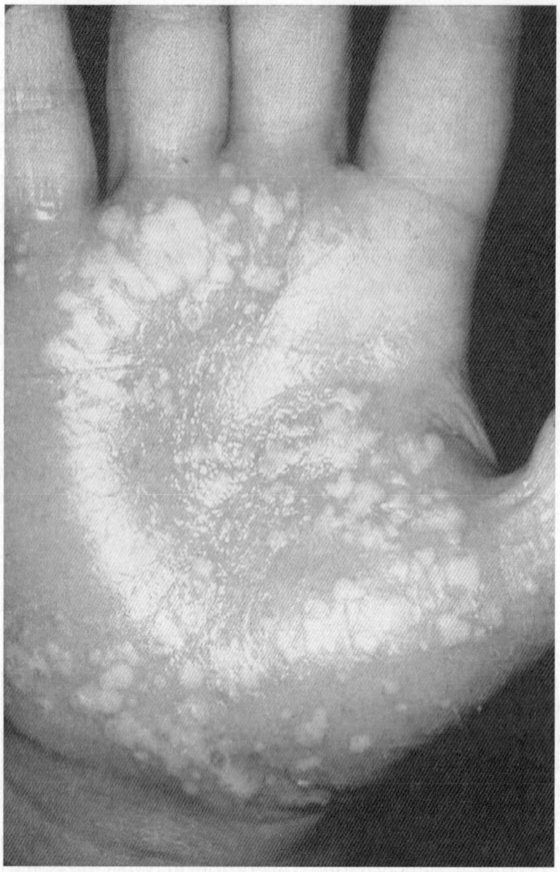

FIGURE 195.9. Pustular psoriasis. Large pustules coalescing to form "lakes of pus" over an area of well-demarcated erythema of the palm.

Treatment of routine cases is with topical corticosteroids and the vitamin D derivative, calcipotriene (Dovonex), whereas more severe cases require ultraviolet phototherapy, methotrexate, systemic retinoids, or TNF-α blocking agents.

Atopic Dermatitis

Atopic dermatitis is characterized by eczematous skin changes and typically involves flexor surfaces in adults, although any body area may be involved. Atopic dermatitis, asthma, and hayfever constitute the atopic triad. The disease is most common in young children in whom the tendency for atopic dermatitis is to gradually improve with age; however, in a minority of patients, disease persists into or manifests in adulthood. In the most severe cases, eczematous dermatitis may evolve into erythroderma (see "Exfoliative Erythroderma" section). Other complications of this disease include secondary bacterial infection (impetigo) or herpetic infection, a condition known as eczema herpeticum. Treatment of atopic dermatitis includes topical corticosteroids, emollients, oral antihistamines, antibiotics as needed, and management of coexisting asthma and allergies.

Contact Dermatitis

Contact dermatitis occurs when direct contact with a substance triggers an inflammatory response in the skin. Irritant contact dermatitis, which accounts for 80% of contact cases, occurs when a chemical directly induces damage to the skin. Common irritants include soap, water, and solvents. The remaining cases represent an immunologically mediated, delayed (Type IV) hypersensitivity reaction. Causes of allergic contact dermatitis in hospitalized patients include adhesives, topical medications, frequently topical antibiotics, preservatives, fragrances, metals, and rubber components.

Acute contact dermatitis, whether irritant or allergic in nature, presents with pruritic papules and weepy vesicles on an erythematous base, initially localized to the area of contact. Chronic lesions are erythematous plaques of thickened skin with accentuated skin markings, scale, and occasionally fissuring. The differential diagnosis may vary depending on the location of the eruption, but generally includes atopic dermatitis, seborrheic dermatitis, stasis dermatitis, and tinea.

History and physical examination are usually sufficient to make the diagnosis. Patch testing may be useful in identifying potentially relevant contact allergens. Treatment involves avoidance of the offending agents. For mild to moderate cases, topical steroids and bland emollients are used. For extensive and severe cases, a 2- to 3-week tapering course of oral prednisone, along with an oral antihistamine to relieve pruritus, is appropriate. For lesions that are oozing and crusting, wet-to-dry or aluminum acetate compresses may be helpful.

Seborrheic Dermatitis

Seborrheic dermatitis is a very common, usually asymptomatic, scaly eruption of the oil-gland bearing skin of the scalp, face, and trunk. It may present in mild cases as common dandruff and in severe cases as a florid erythematous scaling eruption involving the scalp, eyebrows, eyelids, paranasal folds, chest, and axillae. Seborrheic dermatitis typically occurs in perfectly healthy individuals, but is usually most severe in immunocompromised patients, such as those infected with HIV, and in patients with neuropsychiatric disorders. An acute severe presentation should prompt testing for HIV. *Malassezia* yeasts are frequently seen at high levels on the skin of patients with seborrheic dermatitis, but their pathogenic role is unclear. Nonetheless, treatment with antifungals is quite effective.

Diagnosis of seborrheic dermatitis is clinical. The differential diagnosis includes psoriasis, tinea capitis, rosacea, and atopic or contact dermatitis.

Treatment is with antidandruff shampoos containing selenium sulfide, zinc pyrithione or ketoconazole, and topical antifungals (ketoconazole cream, etc.) or mild corticosteroids (hydrocortisone cream). If the patient is not bothered by this rash, it need not be treated.

Transient Acantholytic Dermatosis (Grover's Disease)

Transient acantholytic dermatosis (TAD) is a common eruption consisting of discrete variably pruritic red to brown nonfollicular scaly keratotic papules of the upper trunk seen typically in middle-aged white men, more often in the wintertime. TAD is often seen in bedbound patients and is associated with malignancies. Like miliaria, TAD is often associated with heat and excessive sweating; however, its histopathology, clinical appearance, and treatment are different. Lesions of TAD are more keratotic and scaly than those of miliaria, and histopathology reveals epidermal acantholysis rather than spongiosis. TAD may also be confused with folliculitis, which consists of follicular nonscaly papules and pustules. Treatment of TAD consists of mitigation of heat and sweating, application of midstrength topical corticosteroids (such as triamcinolone cream

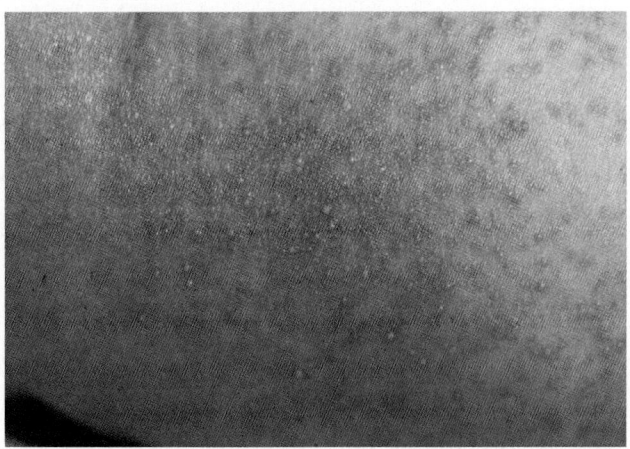

FIGURE 195.10. Miliaria rubra. Tiny nonfollicular inflammatory papules and pustules.

0.1%) twice daily for up to 2 weeks, topical lotions containing pramoxine or menthol, and oral antihistamines (such as hydroxyzine 10 to 25 mg every 6 hours as needed). In severe cases, oral retinoids such as isotretinoin (0.5 to 1 mg per kg daily) may be used. The condition usually remits slowly over weeks to months but can recur.

Miliaria

Miliaria is a common skin eruption in hospitalized patients, caused by blockage of eccrine sweat ducts that occurs with fever and excessive sweating. It occurs in three main forms: miliaria crystallina, which presents as tiny clear asymptomatic superficial vesicles on the trunk, head, and neck; miliaria rubra, which presents as uniform, small pruritic erythematous papules on the trunk, neck, and flexural extremities (Fig. 195.10); and miliaria profunda, which presents as firm, flesh-colored asymptomatic nonfollicular papules or pustules on the trunk and extremities of patients who have had repeated episodes of miliaria rubra. It is important to be able to recognize miliaria to distinguish it from more medically significant entities such as disseminated herpes simplex, varicella, or candidiasis. The distribution of miliaria in areas where the skin is occluded and where excessive sweating occurs is helpful for the diagnosis. Miliaria crystallina does not need to be treated, as it is self-limited and asymptomatic. Miliaria rubra may be treated by decreasing the heat and humidity of the patient's environment. Some reports state that oral ascorbic acid and topical lanolin can be helpful, but no controlled trials have been done [111].

Tinea Corporis

Tinea corporis is a common, superficial fungal infection found on the skin excluding the palms, soles, scalp, and groin. *Trichophyton rubrum* is the most common causative organism, although any dermatophyte may be responsible. Tinea corporis presents as one or multiple annular lesions with erythematous scaly borders that exhibit centrifugal spread and leave a central clearing. Other clinical presentations include Tinea profunda, which exhibits a granulomatous or verrucous appearance due to an excessive host inflammatory response, and Majocchi's granuloma, which presents as follicular-based pustules or papules. The differential diagnosis includes nummular eczema, subacute cutaneous lupus erythematosus, and granuloma annulare. The diagnosis is easily confirmed by potassium hydroxide examination of scale or fungal cultures. Limited disease may be treated with topical agents such as naftifine 1% cream, terbinafine 1% cream, or clotrimazole 1% cream applied twice daily for 2 to 4 weeks. More extensive or recalcitrant disease may require systemic treatment such as itraconazole 100 mg daily or terbinafine 250 mg daily for 2 weeks. Prognosis is excellent with 70% to 100% cure after treatment, but recurrence is common [112].

Scabies

Scabies is a common, extremely pruritic dermatosis caused by infestation with the mite, *Sarcoptes scabiei*. It spreads from person-to-person through direct skin contact, although it can rarely spread through fomites such as bedding or towels. Scabies should be considered in the differential diagnosis of any patient with severe generalized itching, especially if they have had contact with residential institutions such as nursing homes, where it may be epidemic.

Patients with scabies present with severe generalized pruritus, sparing the head and neck, which is worst at night. The pathognomonic lesions are linear burrows (Fig. 195.11), most often found on the hands and feet, especially in the web spaces. Papules, pustules, vesicles, and nodules may also occur, the last being especially common in children. Scabies has a predilection for the hands, feet, wrists, axillae, abdomen, buttocks, and genitalia. Immunocompromised and neurologically impaired patients may present with the crusted or "Norwegian" variant of scabies, in which the skin is markedly thickened and crusted. These crusts are filled with thousands of mites and the patients are highly infectious.

Definitive diagnosis of scabies is made by observing skin scrapings microscopically for mites, eggs, or mite feces. First line treatment of scabies is with topical 5% permethrin cream applied from neck down and left on overnight, with special attention to the genitalia, web spaces, and under the fingernails. All household members or suspected contacts should be treated simultaneously. All bedding, clothing, and towels are then laundered. The application is repeated after 1 week. When topical treatment is impractical, oral ivermectin may be given as a single dose of 200 μg/kg of body weight, repeated in 1 week. Itching usually resolves within 6 weeks of adequate treatment [113].

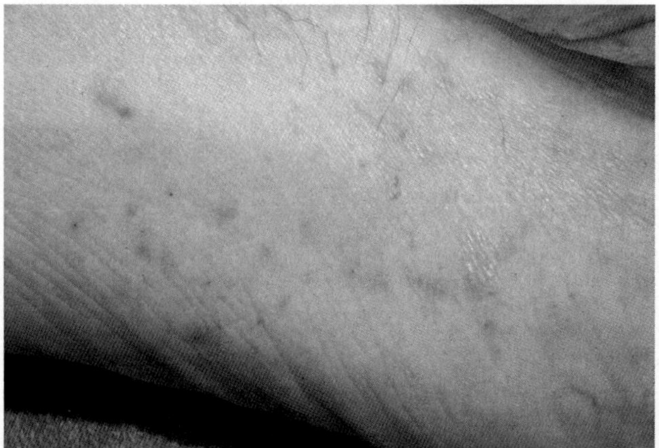

FIGURE 195.11. Scabies. Pink excoriated papules and linear burrows on the foot.

References

1. Klein PA: Stevens-Johnson syndrome and toxic epidermal necrolysis. Emedicine, 2009. Available at: http://emedicine.medscape.com/article/1124127-overview. Accessed August 24, 2009.
2. Pereira FA, Mudgil AV, Rosmarin DM: Toxic epidermal necrolysis. *J Am Acad Dermatol* 56:181–200, 2007.
3. Mockenhaupt M, Viboud C, Dunant A, et al: Stevens–Johnson syndrome and toxic epidermal necrolysis: Assessment of medication risks with emphasis on recently marketed drugs. The EuroSCAR-Study. *J Invest Derm* 128(1):35–44, 2008.
4. Roujeau JC, Kelly JP, Naldi L, et al: Medication use and the risk of Stevens–Johnson syndrome or toxic epidermal necrolysis. *N Engl J Med* 333(24):1600, 1995.
5. Quinn AM, Brown K, Bonish BK, et al: Uncovering histologic criteria with prognostic significance in toxic epidermal necrolysis. *Arch Dermatol* 141:683–687, 2005.
6. Faye O, Roujeau JC: Treatment of epidermal necrolysis with high-dose intravenous immunoglobulins (IVIG): Clinical experience to date. *Drugs* 65(15):2085, 2005.
7. Araki Y, Sotozono C, Inatomi T, et al: Successful treatment of Stevens–Johnson syndrome with steroid pulse therapy at disease onset. *Am J Opthalmol* 147:1004–1011, 2009.
8. Chave TA, Mortimer NJ, Sladden MJ, et al: Toxic epidermal necrolysis: Current evidence, practical management and future directions. *Br J Dermatol* 153(2):241, 2005.
9. Bastuji-Garin S, Fouchard N, Bertocchi M, et al: SCORTEN: a severity-of-illness score for toxic epidermal necrolysis. *J Invest Dermatol* 115(2):149, 2000.
10. Bocquet H, Bagot M, Roujeau JC: Drug-induced pseudolymphoma and drug hypersensitivity syndrome (drug rash with eosinophilia and systemic symptoms: Dress). *Semin Cutan Med Surg* 15(4):250, 1996.
11. Roujeau JC: Clinical heterogeneity of drug hypersensitivity. *Toxicology* 209(2):123, 2005.
12. Sullivan JR, Shear NH: The drug hypersensitivity syndrome: What is the pathogenesis? *Arch Dermatol* 137(3):357, 2001.
13. Descamps V, Valance A, Edlinger C, et al: Association of human herpesvirus 6 infection with drug reaction with eosinophilia and systemic symptoms. *Arch Dermatol* 137(3):301, 2001.
14. Eshki M, Allanoire L, Musette P, et al: Twelve-year analysis of severe cases of DRESS. A cause of unpredictable multiorgan failure. *Arch Dermatol* 145:67–72, 2009.
15. Chiou CC, Yang LC, Hung SI, et al: Clinicopathological features and prognosis of DRESS: a study of 30 cases in Taiwan. *J Eur Acad Dermatol Venereol* 22:1044–1049, 2008.
16. Ben m'rad M, Leclerc-Mercier S, Blanch P, et al: Drug-induced hypersensitivity syndrome. Clinical and biologic disease patterns in 24 patients. *Medicine* 88:131–140, 2009.
17. Tas S, Simonart T: Management of drug rash with eosinophilia and systemic symptoms (DRESS syndrome): an update. *Dermatology* 206(4):353, 2003.
18. Staughton RC, Payne CM, Harper JI, et al: Toxic pustuloderma—a new entity? *J R Soc Med* 77[Suppl 4]:6, 1984.
19. Macmillan AL: Generalised pustular drug rash. *Dermatologica* 146(5):285, 1973.
20. Sidoroff A, Halevy S, Bavinck JN, et al: Acute generalized exanthematous pustulosis (AGEP)–a clinical reaction pattern. *J Cutan Pathol* 28(3):113, 2001.
21. Sidoroff A, Dunant A, Viboud C, et al: Risk factors for acute generalized exanthematous pustulosis – results of a multi-national case-control study (EuroSCAR). *Br J Dermatol* 157:989–996, 2007.
22. Davidovici BB, Pavel D, Cagnano E, et al: Acute generalized exanthematous pustulosis following a spider bite: report of 3 cases. *J Am Acad Dermatol* 55(3):525–529, 2006.
23. Sigurdsson V, Toonstra J, Hezemans-Boer M, et al: Erythroderma. A clinical and follow-up study of 102 patients, with special emphasis on survival. *J Am Acad Dermatol* 35(1):53, 1996.
24. Sigurdsson V, Toonstra J, van Vloten WA: Idiopathic erythroderma: a follow-up study of 28 patients. *Dermatology* 194(2):98, 1997.
25. Rym BM, Mourad M, Bechir Z, et al: Erythroderma in adults: a report of 80 cases. *Int J Dermatol* 44(9):731, 2005.
26. Umar SH, Kelly AP: Erythroderma (generalized exfoliative dermatitis). Emedicine, 2009. Available at: http://emedicine.medscape.com/article/1106906-overview. Accessed August 25, 2009.
27. Sehgal VN, Srivastava G, Sardana K: Erythroderma/exfoliative dermatitis: A synopsis. *Int J Dermatol* 43(1):39, 2004.
28. Leclerc-Mercier S, Bodemer C, Bourdon-Lanoy E, et al: Early skin biopsy is helpful for the diagnosis and management of neonatal and infantile erythrodermas. *J Cutan Pathol*, 37(2): 249–255, 2010.
29. Stevens DL: The toxic shock syndromes. *Infect Dis Clin North Am* 10: 727, 1996.
30. Wolf JE, Rabinowitz LG: Streptococcal toxic shock-like syndrome. *Arch Dermatol* 131:73, 1995.
31. Ferry T, Thomas D, Bouchut JC, et al: Early diagnosis of Staphylococcal toxic shock syndrome by detection of the TSST-1 Vbeta signature in peripheral blood of a 12-year-old boy. *Pediatr Infect Dis J* 27(3):274–277, 2008.
32. Andrews JI, Shamshirsaz AA, Diekema DJ: Nonmenstrual toxic shock syndrome due to methicillin-resistant staphylococcus aureus. *Obstet Gyn* 112(4):933–938, 2008.
33. Young AE, Thornton KL: Toxic shock syndrome in burns: diagnosis and management. *Arch Dis Child Educ Pract Ed* 92:97–100, 2007.
34. Baddour LM, Eason JH, Lunde PA, et al: Case report: acute cellulitis and lymphadenitis caused by mucoid streptococcus pyogenes. *Am J Med Sci* 312(1):40, 1996.
35. McKinnon PS, Paladino JA, Grayson ML, et al: Cost-effectiveness of ampicillin/sulbactam versus imipenem/cilastatin in the treatment of limb-threatening foot infections in diabetic patients. *Clin Infect Dis* 24(1):57, 1997.
36. Swartz MN: Clinical practice. Cellulitis. *N Engl J Med* 350(9):904, 2004.
37. Falagas ME, Vergidis PI: Narrative review: diseases that masquerade as infectious cellulitis. *Ann Intern Med* 142(1):47, 2005.
38. Cox NH: Management of lower leg cellulitis. *Clin Med* 2(1):23–27, 2002.
39. Rieger U, Gugger CY, Farhadi J, et al: Prognostic factors in necrotizing fasciitis and myositis: analysis of 16 consecutive cases at a single institution in Switzerland. *Annals of Plastic Surgery* 58(5):523, 2007.
40. Miller LG, Perdreau-Remington F, Reig G, et al: Necrotizing fasciitis caused by community-acquired methicillin-resistant staphylococcus aureus in Los Angeles. *N Engl J Med* 352(14):1445, 2005.
41. Su Y, Chen H, Hong U, et al: Laboratory risk indicator for necrotizing fasciitis score and the outcomes. *ANZ J Surg* 78(11):968, 2008.
42. Hasham S, Matteucci P, Stanley PR, et al: Necrotising fasciitis. *BMJ* 330(7495):830, 2005.
43. Golger A, Ching S, Goldsmith C, et al: Mortality in patients with necrotizing fasciitis. *Plastic & Reconstructive Surg* 119(6):1803–1807, 2007.
44. Ladhani S: Recent developments in staphylococcal scalded skin syndrome. *Clin Microbiol Infect* 7(6):301, 2001.
45. Ladhani S: Understanding the mechanism of action of the exfoliative toxins of staphylococcus aureus. *FEMS Immunol Med Microbiol* 39(2):181, 2003.
46. King RW, Victor PDS: Staphylococcal scalded skin syndrome. Emedicine, 2009. Available at: http://emedicine.medscape.com/article/788199-overview. Accessed July 20, 2009.
47. Patel GK, Varma S, Finlay AY: Staphylococcal scalded skin syndrome in healthy adults. *Br J Dermatol* 142(6):1253, 2000.
48. Rosenstein NE, Perkins BA, Stephens DS, et al: Meningococcal disease. *N Engl J Med* 344(18):1378, 2001.
49. Tanzi E, Silverberg N: Meningococcemia. Emedicine, 2007. Available at: http://emedicine.medscape.com/article/1052846-overview. Accessed July 20, 2009.
50. Gondim FDAA, Singh MK, Croul SE: Meningococcal meningitis. Emedicine, 2009. Available at: http://emedicine.medscape.com/article/1165557-overview. Accessed July 20, 2009.
51. Cummings KC, Louie J, Probert WS, et al: Increased detection of meningococcal infections in California using a polymerase chain reaction assay. *Clin Infect Dis* 46(7):1124–1126, 2008.
52. Lacz N, Schwarz R: Rocky Mountain spotted fever. Emedicine, 2009. Available at: http://emedicine.medscape.com/article/1054826-overview. Accessed July 20, 2009.
53. McGinley-Smith DE, Tsao SS: Dermatoses from ticks. *J Am Acad Dermatol* 49(3):363, 2003.
54. Singh-Behl D, La Rosa SP, Tomecki KJ: Tick-borne infections. *Dermatol Clin* 21(2):237, 2003.
55. Masters EJ, Olson GS, Weiner SJ, et al: Rocky Mountain spotted fever: a clinician's dilemma. *Arch Intern Med* 163(7):769, 2003.
56. Torres G: Herpes simplex. Emedicine, 2007. Available at: http://emedicine.medscape.com/article/1132351-overview. Accessed August 25, 2009.
57. Corey L: Herpes simplex virus, in Mandell GL, Bennett JE, Dolin R (eds): *Principles and practice of infectious diseases*. 6th ed. New York, Churchill Livingstone, 2005, p. 1762.
58. Chilukuri S, Rosen T: Management of acyclovir-resistant herpes simplex virus. *Dermatol Clin* 21(2):311, 2003.
59. Lafferty WE, Krofft S, Remington M, et al: Diagnosis of herpes simplex virus by direct immunofluorescence and viral isolation from samples of external genital lesions in a high-prevalence population. *J Clin Microbiol* 25(2):323, 1987.
60. Anderson WE: Varicella-zoster virus. Emedicine, 2009. Available at: http://emedicine.medscape.com/article/231927-overview. Accessed August 25, 2009.
61. Ahmed AM, Brantley JS, Madkan V, et al: Managing herpes zoster in immunocompromised patients. *Herpes* 14(2):32, 2007.
62. Grant RM, Weitzman SS, Sherman CG, et al: Fulminant disseminated varicella zoster virus infection without skin involvement. *J Clin Virol* 24(1–2):7, 2002.

63. Hidalgo JA, Vazquez JA: Candidiasis. Emedicine, 2008. Available at: http://emedicine.medscape.com/article/213853-overview. Accessed August 24, 2009.
64. Bae GY, Lee HW, Chang SE, et al: Clinicopathologic review of 19 patients with systemic candidiasis with skin lesions. *Int J Dermatol* 44(7):550, 2005.
65. Cross SA, Scott LJ: Micafungin: a review of its use in adults for the treatment of invasive and oesophageal candidiasis, and as prophylaxis against candida infections. *Drugs* 68(15):2225, 2008.
66. Zeina B, Mansour S: Pemphigus vulgaris. Emedicine, 2009. Available at: http://emedicine.medscape.com/article/1064187-overview. Accessed August 24, 2009.
67. Ratnam KV, Phay KL, Tan CK: Pemphigus therapy with oral prednisolone regimens. A 5-year study. *In J Dermatol* 29:363–367, 1990.
68. Mentink LF, Mackenzie MW, Tóth GG, et al: Randomized controlled trial of adjuvant oral dexamethasone pulse therapy in pemphigus vulgaris: PEMPULS trial. *Arch Dermatol* 142:570–576, 2006.
69. Chams-Davatchi C, Esmaili N, Daneshpahooh M, et al: Randomized controlled open-label trial of four treatment regimens for pemphigus vulgaris. *J Am Acad Dermatol* 57:622–628, 2007.
70. Beissert S, Werfel T, Frieling U, et al: A comparison of oral methylprednisolone plus azathioprine or mycophenolate mofetil for the treatment of pemphigus. *Arch Dermatol* 142:1447–1454, 2006.
71. Amagai M, Ikeda S, Shimizu H, et al: A randomized double-blind trial of intravenous immunoglobulin for pemphigus. *J Am Acad Dermatol* 60:595–603, 2009.
72. Werth VP, Fivenson D, Pandya AG, et al: Multicenter randomized, double-blind, placebo-controlled, clinical trial of dapsone as a glucocorticoid-sparing agent in maintenance-phase pemphigus vulgaris. *Arch Dermatol* 144:25–32, 2008.
73. Ioannides D, Chrysomallis F, Bystryn JC: Ineffectiveness of cyclosporine as an adjuvant to corticosteroids in the treatment of pemphigus. *Arch Dermatol* 136:868–872, 2000.
74. Martin LK, Werth V, Villanueva E, et al: Interventions for pemphigus vulgaris and pemphigus foliaceus. *Cochrane Database Syst Rev* 1:CD006263, 2009.
75. Goldberg LJ, Nisar N: Paraneoplastic pemphigus. Emedicine, 2008. Available at: http://emedicine.medscape.com/article/1064452-overview. Accessed August 24, 2009.
76. Chan L: Bullous pemphigoid. Emedicine, 2008. Available at: http://emedicine.medscape.com/article/1062391-overview. Accessed August 24, 2009.
77. Callen JP: Hypersensitivity vasculitis (Leukocytoclastic vasculitis). Emedicine, 2009. Available at: http://emedicine.medscape.com/article/1083719-overview. Accessed August 24, 2009.
78. Gast T, Kowal-Vern A, An G, et al: Purpura fulminans in an adult patient with Haemophilus influenzae sepsis: case report and review of the literature. *J Burn Care Res* 27(1):102, 2006.
79. Kennedy KJ, Walker S, Pavli P, et al: What may underlie recurrent purpura fulminans? *Med J Aust* 186(7):373, 2007.
80. Kempton CL, Bagby G, Collins JF: Ulcerative colitis presenting as purpura fulminans. *Inflamm Bowel Dis* 7(4):319, 2001.
81. Smith OP, White B: Infectious purpura fulminans: diagnosis and treatment. *Br J Haematol* 104(2):198, 1999.
82. Nolan J, Sinclair R: Review of management of purpura fulminans and two case reports. *Br J Anaesth* 86(4):581, 2001.
83. Grill F, Munoz P, Jofre R, et al: Clinical microbiological case: a necrotic skin lesion in a patient with renal failure. *Clin Microbiol Infect* 9(6):538, 2003.
84. Gibson GE, Su WP, Pittelkow MR: Antiphospholipid syndrome and the skin. *J Am Acad Dermatol* 36(6):970–982, 1997.
85. Nahass GT: Antiphospholipid antibodies and the antiphospholipid antibody syndrome. *J Am Acad Dermatol* 36(2):149–171, 1997.
86. Sharkey MP, Daryanani II, Gillett MB, et al: Localized cutaneous necrosis associated with the antiphospholipid syndrome. *Australas J Dermatol* 43(3):218–220, 2002.
87. Weinstein S, Piette W: Cutaneous manifestations of antiphospholipid antibody syndrome. *Hematol Oncol Clin North Am* 22(1):67–77, 2008.
88. Kriseman YL, Nash JW, Hsu S: Criteria for the diagnosis of antiphospholipid syndrome in patients presenting with dermatologic symptoms. *J Am Acad Dermatol* 57(1):112–115, 2007.
89. Nazarian RM, Van Cott EM, Zembowicz A, et al: Warfarin-induced skin necrosis. *J Am Acad Dermatol* 61(2):325, 2009.
90. Ainsworth C, Edgerton CC: Cryoglobulinemia. Emedicine, 2009. Available at: http://emedicine.medscape.com/article/329255-overview. Accessed August 25, 2009.
91. McGevna LF, Hogan MT, Raugi J: Cutaneous manifestations of cholesterol embolism. Emedicine, 2009. Available at: http://emedicine.medscape.com/article/1096593-overview. Accessed August 24, 2009.
92. Donohue KG, Saap L, Falanga V: Cholesterol crystal embolization: an atherosclerotic disease with frequent and varied cutaneous manifestations. *J Eur Acad Dermatol Venereol* 17(5):504, 2003.
93. Hitti WA, Wali RK, Weinman EJ, et al: Cholesterol embolization syndrome induced by thrombolytic therapy. *Am J Cardiovasc Drugs* 8(1):27, 2008.
94. Wang H, Zheng J, Deng C, et al: Fat embolism syndromes following liposuction. *Aesth Plast Surg* 32(5):731, 2008.
95. Garcia FVMJ, Sanz-Sanchez T, Aragues M, et al: Cutaneous embolization of cardiac myxoma. *Br J Dermatol* 147(2):379, 2002.
96. Kalajian AH, Malhotra PS, Callen JP, et al: Calciphylaxis with normal renal and parathyroid function: Not as rare as previously believed. *Arch Dermatol* 145(4):451–458, 2009.
97. Hafner J, Keusch G, Wahl C, et al: Uremic small-artery disease with medial calcification and intimal hyperplasia (so-called calciphylaxis): A complication of chronic renal failure and benefit from parathyroidectomy. *J Am Acad Dermatol* 33(6):954, 1995.
98. Raymond CB, Wazny LD: Sodium thiosulfate, bisphosphonates, and cinacalcet for treatment of calciphylaxis. *Am J Health-Syst Pharm* 65:1419–1429, 2008.
99. Bartels CM, Muller D: Systemic lupus erythematosus. Emedicine, 2009. Available at: http://emedicine.medscape.com/article/332244-overview. Accessed August 24, 2009.
100. Seidler AM, Gottleib AB: Dermatomyositis induced by drug therapy: a review of case reports. *J Am Acad Dermatol* 59:872–880, 2008.
101. Jorizzo LJ, Jorizzo JL: The treatment and prognosis of dermatomyositis: an updated review. *J Am Acad Dermatol* 59:99–112, 2008.
102. Gilliam AC: Update on graft versus host disease. *J Invest Dermatol* 123(2):251–257, 2004.
103. Scheinfeld NS, Kuechle MK: Graft versus host disease. Emedicine, 2008. Available at: http://emedicine.medscape.com/article/1050580-overview. Accessed August 24, 2009.
104. Huang J, Pol-Rodriguez M, Silvers D, et al: Acquired ichthyosis as a manifestation of acute cutaneous graft-versus-host disease. *Pediatr Dermatol* 24(1):49–52, 2007.
105. Marra DE, McKee PH, Nghiem P: Tissue eosinophils and the perils of using skin biopsy specimens to distinguish between drug hypersensitivity and cutaneous graft-versus-host disease. *J Am Acad Dermatol* 51(4):543, 2004.
106. Schaffer JV, McNiff JM, Seropian S, et al: Lichen sclerosus and eosinophilic fasciitis as manifestations of chronic graft-versus-host disease: expanding the sclerodermoid spectrum. *J Am Acad Dermatol* 53(4):591–601, 2005.
107. Satter EK: Folliculitis. Emedicine, 2008. Available at: http://emedicine.medscape.com/article/1070456-overview. Accessed August 24, 2009.
108. Fung MA, Berger TG: A prospective study of acute-onset steroid acne associated with administration of intravenous corticosteroids. *Dermatology* 200:43–44, 2000.
109. Gelfand JM, Neimann AL, Shin DB, et al: Risk of myocardial infarction in patients with psoriasis. *JAMA* 296(14):1735–1741, 2006.
110. Prodanovich S, Kirsner RS, Kravetz JD, et al: Association of psoriasis with coronary artery, cerebrovascular, and peripheral vascular diseases and mortality. *Arch Dermatol* 145(6):700–703, 2009.
111. Levin NA: Miliaria. Emedicine, 2009. Available at: http://emedicine.medscape.com/article/1070840-overview. Accessed August 10, 2009.
112. Lott MER, Zember G: Tinea corporis. Emedicine, 2008. Available at: http://emedicine.medscape.com/article/1091473-overview. Accessed August 10, 2009.
113. Cordoro KM, Wilson BB, Kauffman CL: Scabies. Emedicine, 2008. Available at: http://emedicine.medscape.com/article/1109204-overview. Accessed August 10, 2009.

CHAPTER 196 ■ VASCULITIS IN THE INTENSIVE CARE UNIT

PAUL F. DELLARIPA AND DONOUGH HOWARD

The vasculitides are a group of disorders characterized by the presence of destructive inflammation in vessel walls [1–4]. The possibility of systemic vasculitis should be considered in a patient with systemic complaints and dysfunction of multiple organ systems, frequently in the context of constitutional symptoms such as fever, malaise, and weight loss (Table 196.1). Patients hospitalized in the intensive care unit (ICU) may present with symptoms related to the clinical features associated with a specific vasculitis but may also present with a known diagnosis of vasculitis and complications of treatment, most notably infection.

Vasculitic syndromes typically are classified by the size of vessel involved. Though there may be overlap in the vessel size, diseases may affect predominately large vessels (Takayasu's arteritis), medium-size arteries (such as polyarteritis nodosa and central nervous system [CNS] vasculitis), and small vessels (Wegener's granulomatosis, microscopic polyangiitis, Churg-Strauss syndrome, cryoglobulinemia, and drug-induced vasculitis). These particular vasculitides will be the focus of this chapter. For a more general discussion of vasculitis, other references are noted [1–4].

Disorders not discussed but that may simulate presentation of vasculitis include embolism due to endocarditis, cardiac myxoma, hypercoagulable states including the antiphospholipid antibody syndrome, hyperviscosity syndromes, chronic ergotism, radiation arteriopathy, and, less commonly, Ehlers–Danlos syndrome, neurofibromatosis, Sweet's syndrome, pseudoxanthoma elasticum, and Köhlmeier–Danlos diseases [5,6].

POLYARTERITIS NODOSA

Polyarteritis nodosa (PAN) is a systemic necrotizing arteritis involving predominately medium-size vessels, although sometimes affecting smaller vessels. Vasculitic lesions characteristically occur at the bifurcations or branches of vessels and are often segmental. Almost any organ can be involved, but frequently the skin, peripheral nerves, kidneys, gastrointestinal (GI) tract, and joints are the principal organs affected [7].

Clinical manifestations vary from mild localized disease to multisystem organ failure. Patients generally complain of malaise, weight loss, fevers, abdominal or lower-extremity pain, myalgias, or arthralgias. Clinical parameters include hypertension and azotemia with proteinuria but rarely glomerulonephritis. Peripheral neuropathy occurs in up to 60% of cases, usually involving a mixed sensorimotor and mononeuritis multiplex [8]. Sudden-onset paresthesias associated with motor deficits are common manifestations. CNS involvement, including seizures, focal events, and altered mental status, are less common [9]. Musculoskeletal symptoms including arthralgias (50%), and less frequently, arthritis can occur [7]. Vasculitis of skeletal muscles may cause severe myalgias, and muscle biopsy can be useful diagnostically [10]. Abdominal pain may have a variety of causes, including intestinal angina, mesenteric thrombosis, and localized gallbladder or liver disease. Acute GI bleeding, perforation, and infarction are rare but are associated with a high mortality if the diagnosis is not established promptly [11]. Cardiac involvement, observed in nearly 60% of autopsy series, is often clinically silent and includes congestive heart failure, pericarditis, myocardial infarctions, and conduction abnormalities [12,13]. Cutaneous lesions include nonspecific palpable purpura, livedo reticularis, tender nodular lesions, digital infarcts, and ulcers [14]. Arteritis of the eye, testes, pancreas, ovaries, breasts, and involvement of the temporal arteries may develop rarely.

The pathogenesis of polyarteritis is unknown. Hepatitis B surface antigen has been found in a minority of patients with PAN. The presence of circulating immune complexes of hepatitis B surface antigen and deposition of surface antigen and immunoglobulin in vessel walls has suggested that immune mechanisms may play a role in some forms of polyarteritis [15,16]. Hepatitis C has rarely been associated with PAN [17]. Pathologically, fibrinoid necrosis and pleomorphic cellular infiltration, predominantly with lymphocytes, macrophages, and varying degrees of polymorphonuclear leukocytes involve the entire wall of small and medium muscular arteries. Thromboses and aneurysms can be found in lesions [18].

The diagnosis of PAN focuses on the most frequent areas of involvement, namely, nerve, skin, and GI systems. Laboratory parameters usually include elevated sedimentation rate, elevated C-reactive protein (CRP), and thrombocytosis. Antineutrophil cytoplasmic antibody (ANCA), antinuclear antibody (ANA), and rheumatoid factor are not typically present in PAN. Mesenteric angiography often shows evidence of aneurysms including the renal, hepatic, and mesenteric arteries, and areas of arterial stenosis alternating with normal or dilated vessels [18]. Sural nerve biopsies are easily accessible sources of nerve tissue when a mononeuritis is present, although the location of biopsy may be guided by electromyography.

Although there is no consensus for treatment of PAN, administration of corticosteroids at 1 mg per kg per day orally is indicated in nearly all cases. In fulminant disease, daily intravenous (IV) methylprednisolone, 1 g per day for 3 days, is reasonable followed by daily oral or intravenous corticosteroids. In the presence of GI involvement, intravenous dosing may need to be continued especially in life-threatening cases. The use of a second drug is guided by the severity of presentation and if there is failure to respond to steroids alone. A severity of illness scoring system (the Five Factor Score) has been developed based on five different parameters, namely, proteinuria more than 1 g per day, azotemia, GI involvement, cardiomyopathy, and CNS involvement. The presence of two or more of these factors portends a mortality of nearly 50% [7]. A review of long-term follow-up of these patients suggests that those with more severe illness as defined with one of the above factors have a higher survival rate when treated with cyclophosphamide [19]. Cyclophosphamide may be given orally, usually 2 mg per kg per day, though adjustment should be made for renal failure (Table 196.2). If the oral route is not feasible, then intravenous dosing of 500 to 1,000 mg per m^2 monthly is

TABLE 196.1

NOTABLE PHYSICAL SIGNS, SYMPTOMS, AND LABORATORY FEATURES OF DIFFERENT VASCULITIC SYNDROMES

Constitutional Symptoms (WG, MPA, CSS, BS, TA, PAN, GCA)	Pulmonary infiltrates/nodules (WG, MPA, CSS)
Sinusitis/epistaxis (WG, MPA, CSS)	Pulmonary hemorrhage (WG, MPA, rarely CSS, BS, Cryo)
Cough, hemoptysis (WG, MPA, CSS, rarely Cryo)	Subglottic stenosis (WG)
Otitis/hearing loss (WG)	Cardiac involvement (CSS, PAN, WG, TA)
Ocular involvement (WG, BS, GCA, TA)	Mononeuritis (WG, PAN, MPA, Cryo)
Cutaneous lesions (WG, PAN, MPA, Cryo, CSS, BS)	Glomerulonephritis (WG, MPA, rarely Cryo)
Claudication (TA, GCA)	Hypertension (PAN, TA)
Arthritis/arthralgia (WG, CSS, MPA, Cryo, PAN)	ANCA positivity (WG, MPA, CSS)
Abdominal pain/GI bleeding (PAN, CSS, BS, MPA)	Angiographic abnormalities (PAN, TA)

ANCA, antineutrophil cytoplasmic antibody; BS, Behcet's syndrome; Cryo, cryoglobulinemia; CSS, Churg-Strauss syndrome; GCA, giant cell arteritis; MPA, microscopic polyangiitis; PAN, polyarteritis nodosa; TA, Takayasu's arteritis; WG, Wegener's granulomatosis.

appropriate (see Table 196.3). Plasmapheresis (PE) in combination with antiviral therapy is indicated in hepatitis B-associated PAN, though PE does not improve outcome in non–hepatitis B virus PAN [29,30].

A variety of drugs, viral infections, connective tissue diseases such as rheumatoid arthritis, and underlying malignancies may cause a necrotizing angiitis that may be indistinguishable from polyarteritis [31–36].

MICROSCOPIC POLYANGIITIS

Microscopic polyangiitis is a necrotizing vasculitis that involves small vessels, including arterioles, capillaries, and venules. As noted previously, cases of microscopic polyangiitis previously classified as part of the PAN classification were distinguished mainly by the presence of segmental necrotizing glomerulonephritis. Clinical presentations may involve concomitant capillaritis with or without alveolar hemorrhage and rapidly progressive glomerulonephritis, the so-called pulmonary renal syndrome, although more indolent and slower presentations have been described. Glomerulonephritis occurs in nearly all cases, and pulmonary involvement ranging from cough and dyspnea to frank hemoptysis occurs in up to 30% of cases. Neuropathy and cutaneous vasculitis occur in up to 50% of cases [14,35,36].

Pathologically, renal lesions show segmental necrosis, minimal immune or pauci-immune deposition, and crescent formation. In the lung, there is edema of the alveolar wall, neutrophilic invasion, type II epithelial cell hyperplasia, and a paucity of immune deposits. These findings may not be histologically different from those found in patients with Wegener's granulomatosis, and clinically the two entities may be difficult to distinguish. ANCA is found in about 75% of cases, mostly specific for myeloperoxidase (MPO), though occasionally ANCA proteinase 3 (PR3) has been described [36].

Diagnosis is typically made with a biopsy of lung, kidney, skin, or nerve in conjunction with a positive ANCA result. Treatment is similar as described for Wegener's granulomatosis, with corticosteroids at 1 mg per kg per day oral or intravenous methylprednisolone, and cyclophosphamide orally or intravenously [36]. Recent studies comparing rituximab with cyclophosphamide therapy for initial remission induction suggest similar efficacy and toxicities, while rituximab maybe more effective for relapsing disease [27,28]. PE may have a role in the treatment of severe renal disease with evidence suggesting a lower reduced frequency of dialysis, but no mortality benefit [21]. There are no prospective data available regarding the efficacy of PE in diffuse alveolar hemorrhage (DAH), although retrospective data suggest a benefit [37]. In the face of DAH and severe respiratory failure in the setting of a systemic vasculitis, PE in addition to corticosteroids and cyclophosphamide is reasonable as long as every effort has been made to exclude infection. In relapsing disease, intravenous immunoglobulin may be of benefit [20].

TABLE 196.2

DOSAGE ADJUSTMENTS OF ORAL CYCLOPHOSPHAMIDE WITH RENAL IMPAIRMENT

Creatinine clearance (mL/min)	Oral cyclophosphamide dose (mg/kg/d)
>100	2.0
50–99	1.5
25–49	1.2
15–24	1.0
<15 or on dialysis	0.8

From WGET Research Group: Design of the Wegener's Granulomatosis Etanercept Trial (WGET). *Control Clin Trials* 23(4):450–468, 2002, with permission.

CHURG-STRAUSS SYNDROME

Churg-Strauss syndrome (CSS) is characterized by the presence of eosinophilic infiltrates and granulomas in the respiratory tract and necrotizing vasculitis in the setting of asthma and peripheral eosinophilia. Typically, patients have a preceding history of asthma and allergic rhinitis and then develop constitutional symptoms of fatigue and weight loss followed by systemic symptoms such as mononeuritis, cardiomyopathy, pulmonary infiltrates, or abdominal pain [14]. Pulmonary disease includes fleeting or diffuse infiltrates and nodular lesions,

TABLE 196.3

RANDOMIZED TRIALS IN THE TREATMENT OF VASCULITIS

Study	Types of vasculitis	Study design	Results	Comment
Gayraud et al. [19]	PAN, MPA, CSS	Meta-analysis of randomized trials	Survival benefits of CYC in addition to CS with FFS $\geq$2	Meta-analysis of four different prospective trials; mixed patient population
Jayne et al. [20]	WG, MPA	Prospective double-blinded placebo controlled, using IVIG in patients with persistent disease activity	Reduced disease activity in IVIG treated group	Short-term follow-up (3 mo)
Gaskin and Jayne [21]	WG, MPA all with renal failure	Randomized controlled trial using either plasmapheresis or pulse CS in addition to standard CS/CYC	Lower rate of dialysis dependence in plasmapheresis treated group	1 year follow-up data only
De Groot et al. [22]	WG, MPA	Prospective, randomized, unblinded comparing MTX to CYC in both induction and maintenance of remission in nonrenal AAV	No difference in the number of patients achieving remission, but higher rates of relapse noted in the MTX treated group	MTX may still maintain remission if initial induction is with CYC
Jayne et al. [23]	WG, MPA	Prospective, randomized, unblinded comparing CYC and AZA in remission maintenance	Relapse rate was not significantly different between the two groups; no difference in AEs	Supports standard of care of changing to AZA once remission induced with CYC
WGET [24]	WG	Prospective, randomized, double-blinded, placebo-controlled trial looking at maintenance of remission with the addition of etanercept or placebo to standard treatment	No increase in remission–maintenance noted in the etanercept group; possible increased malignancy rate in the etanercept group	Shows no role for TNF inhibitors in the maintenance of remission
deGroot K et al. [25]	ANCA associated vasculitis	Prospective randomized controlled trial using oral or IV CYC for induction of remission	No difference in time to remission or proportion of patients who achieved remission	Total dose of CYC less in IV group. Study not powered to detect differences in relapse rates amongst the two groups.
Pagnoux C et al. [26]	WG, MP	Prospective, open label, multicenter trial using either methotrexate or azathioprine as maintenance therapy after remission achieved with CYC and CS.	Relapse rates similar in both groups and AE were similar in both groups.	
Jones RB, et al. [27]	WG, MP: nephritis only	Prospective, open label, multicenter, parallel trial comparing RTX to standard intravenous CYC for induction therapy	Sustained remission rates were similar in both groups and adverse events in both groups were similar	12 month follow-up; small number (44 pts) Patients in RTX group also received IV CYC 15 mg/kg with first and third infusions
Stone, et al. [28]	WG, MP	Randomized, double-blinded, double-dummy multicenter trial comparing RTX to oral CYC for induction therapy	RTX is equivalent to oral CTX in remission induction; no difference in adverse events; RTX may be superior to CYC in relapsing disease	6 months follow-up only and data on maintenance of remission with AZA not available yet 197 patients total

AAV, ANCA-associated vasculitis; AEs, adverse events; AZA, azathioprine; CS, corticosteroid; CSS, Churg-Strauss syndrome; CYC, cyclophosphamide; IVIG, intravenous immunoglobulin; MPA, microscopic polyangiitis; MTX, methotrexate; PAN, polyarteritis; RTX, rituximab; TNF, tumor necrosis factor; WG, Wegener's granulomatosis; WGET, Wegener's granulomatosis etanercept trial.

and peripheral infiltrates occur in up to 75% of patients [38]. The diagnosis of eosinophilic pneumonia may be suggested in the context of peripheral infiltrates and peripheral eosinophilia. Rarely alveolar hemorrhage may occur. Peripheral neuropathy occurs in up to 75% of patients with CSS, whereas renal involvement is much less common than in microscopic polyangiitis and Wegener's granulomatosis. Other sources of morbidity and mortality include GI involvement with bleeding and bowel perforation, cardiac involvement causing arrhythmias, myocarditis, pericarditis, and congestive heart failure [38,39]. The etiology of CSS is unknown. ANCA is positive in approximately 38% to 60% of cases, mostly myeloperoxidase [40–42]. As mentioned earlier, the presence of more than one of the five prognostic factors (i.e., proteinuria ≥1 g, azotemia, GI involvement, cardiomyopathy, and CNS involvement) has been associated with a higher mortality and should guide the choice of treatment, suggesting corticosteroids as mentioned above for limited disease and addition of cyclophosphamide in the setting of severe disease [19].

CRYOGLOBULINEMIC VASCULITIS

Cryoglobulins are immunoglobulins that precipitate below 37°C. There are three types: Type I, seen in myeloproliferative disorders; type II, or mixed essential cryoglobulins; and type III, mixed polyclonal. Types II and III are most closely associated with hepatitis C infection. Typical involvement includes cutaneous vasculitis, arthritis, and peripheral neuropathy. Abnormal liver enzymes suggest hepatitis C infection; complement levels, especially C4, are decreased [43,44]. Infrequently, cryoglobulinemic vasculitis may be life threatening with severe renal, GI, and pulmonary involvement including alveolar hemorrhage [45,46]. Therapy in severe cases consists of corticosteroids and cyclophosphamide with careful attention to the potential risk of increased hepatitis C replication. In severe cases involving progressive glomerulonephritis, PE or cryofiltration may be of additional benefit [47–49]. The use of rituximab combined with pegylated interferon and ribavirin may be useful in refractory cases [50].

WEGENER'S GRANULOMATOSIS

Wegener's granulomatosis is a disease of unknown etiology characterized by granulomatous vasculitis of the upper and lower respiratory tract, segmental necrotizing glomerulonephritis, and systemic vasculitis of small blood vessels [51]. A subset of patients may have disease isolated to the upper respiratory tract or have less severe organ involvement and are referred to as having "limited" Wegener's granulomatosis. Although the disease may affect individuals of a wide range of ages, the disease most commonly affects persons in their fourth or fifth decades of life with a slight predominance for men over women [52,53]. Patients most frequently require intensive care treatment for severe pneumonitis, glomerulonephritis, stroke, myocardial infarction, multiorgan system dysfunction secondary to necrotizing vasculitis, and infection due to immunosuppression and anatomic abnormalities secondary to the granulomatous inflammation.

The etiology of Wegener's granulomatosis is unknown. Possible infectious etiologic associations with *Staphylococcus aureus* have been proposed but are as yet unproven [54]. ANCA is present in more than 90% of patients with systemic Wegener's granulomatosis, and in 70% to 80% with active limited disease. In Wegener's granulomatosis, the pattern noted on immunofluorescence is C-ANCA or cytoplasmic staining, and the specific antigen in most cases is the PR3 antigen, although in 10% of cases or more, there may be a P-ANCA or perinuclear staining with MPO (myeloperoxidase) as the specific antigen [55]. Correlation of ANCA titers with clinical remission is controversial, with the most recent data suggesting that relapse is unlikely in treated patients with negative titers, whereas those with rising or recurrently positive titers have a higher risk of relapse, although the timing of relapse is not predictable [56,57]. There is also increasing evidence of the pathogenicity of ANCA in the vasculitic component of Wegener's granulomatosis [58].

Pathologically, the vessels involved in Wegener's granulomatosis include small arteries and veins; these vessels are often adjacent to granuloma. The pathology of vasculitis includes fibrinoid necrosis with inflammatory mononuclear cell infiltrates of vessel walls, focal destruction of the elastic lamina, and narrowing or obliteration of vessel lumens. Granulomatous lesions are characterized by areas of central necrosis surrounded by epithelial fibroblasts and scattered multinucleated giant cells [59]. Granulomatous vasculitis may involve the lung, skin, CNS, peripheral nerves, heart, and other organs.

Most patients (approximately 85% to 90%) present with symptoms referable to the upper respiratory tract, including sinusitis, nasal obstruction, rhinitis, otitis, hearing loss, ear pain, gingival inflammation, epistaxis, sore throat, laryngitis, and nasal septal deformity. Fever, in addition to being caused by the underlying disease, may be due to suppurative otitis or *S. aureus* sinusitis [60]. Granulomatous vasculitis of the upper respiratory tract may lead to damage of nasal cartilage, resulting in the "saddle-nose" deformity, sore throat, and oral and nasal mucosal ulcers [61]. In addition, chondritis of the nose or ear may develop [62]. Laryngeal involvement may result in severe narrowing of the upper respiratory tract [63,64]. Approximately 10% of patients present with only nonspecific constitutional symptoms such as arthralgias, myalgias, fever, and weight loss. Unusual manifestations of Wegener's granulomatosis include distinctive punched-out ulcerative skin lesions appearing as pyoderma gangrenosum [65] and painless subcutaneous nodules occurring in approximately 2% to 5%.

Although only one third of patients present with symptomatic lung involvement (including cough, sputum production, dyspnea, chest pain, hemoptysis, and even life-threatening pulmonary hemorrhage), lower respiratory tract disease is found in almost all patients after evaluation. The characteristic chest radiographic findings are multiple, nodular, bilateral cavitary infiltrates, but infiltrates without sharp margins occur more frequently than distinct nodules. Cavitation may occur in distinct nodules and in infiltrates with less-defined borders. Nodules may have thick or thin walls. Infiltrates may involve the lower or upper lobes. In approximately 50% of patients, the infiltrates are bilateral. Infiltrates may be transient [64,66]. Less common chest radiographic abnormalities include paratracheal masses, large cavitary lesions, a miliary pattern, massive pleural effusion, calcified nodule, and masses between the trachea and esophagus [67]. Computed tomography (CT) of the chest may reveal pulmonary lesions not well demonstrated on plain radiographs.

Wegener's granulomatosis may also be associated with inflammation and subsequent scarring/stenosis of the subglottic region, in about 25% of patients [68]. This complication is distinctly more common in younger adult and pediatric populations and may sometimes be difficult to differentiate from relapsing polychondritis where tracheal and subglottic inflammation is the major presenting feature.

Although renal manifestations are often asymptomatic, urinalysis reveals renal involvement in approximately 80% of patients at presentation. The typical renal lesion is segmental necrotizing glomerulonephritis. Functional renal impairment may progress rapidly if appropriate therapy is not instituted promptly [69,70].

The vasculitis of Wegener's granulomatosis may cause a variety of other clinical manifestations, including arthralgias and less commonly arthritis, most frequently affecting the knees [71,72]; perinephric hematoma; renal artery aneurysms;

ureteral obstruction [73]; a variety of cutaneous lesions, including ulcers, papules, vesicles, and subcutaneous nodules [66]; episcleritis; conjunctivitis; scleritis; uveitis; optic nerve vasculitis [74]; mononeuritis multiplex or polyneuritis; cranial nerve dysfunction; meningitis [75]; cerebral infarction [76]; subarachnoid hemorrhage; abdominal pain; intestinal perforation; and diarrhea [77].

Typically, diagnosis is based on the clinical findings of upper and lower respiratory tract noninfectious inflammation [78] with glomerulonephritis and positive anti-PR3 antibodies and rarely MPO antibodies. In cases with more limited involvement or where ANCA titers are negative or show the less typical MPO specificity, tissue diagnosis may be necessary.

Recent advances in the treatment of Wegener's granulomatosis have led to the development of a biphasic approach with an initial remission–induction phase using a combination of cyclophosphamide and corticosteroids for 3 to 6 months followed by a remission–maintenance phase using a less toxic immunosuppressive agent, usually methotrexate or azathioprine, for a further 12 to 24 months [79].

Initial treatment with corticosteroid is generally given as prednisone 1 mg per kg per day orally. In the critically ill ICU patient with severe systemic involvement, pulse corticosteroid with IV methylprednisolone 1 g per day for 3 days is advocated, transitioning to prednisone 1 mg per kg per day orally or its IV equivalent. Prednisone therapy is maintained at 60 mg for 1 month and then weaned to 20 mg over 2 to 3 months and then to zero over 6 months.

Cyclophosphamide can be administered as monthly intravenous boluses or as a daily oral dose. Both approaches have shown similar rates of remission–induction at 6 months, 78% with daily oral treatment versus 89% with monthly IV boluses [25]. However, relapse rates were much higher in the monthly IV group, 52% compared with 18% in the daily oral group. In the clinically ill patient, initial treatment with an IV bolus of cyclophosphamide 500 to 1,000 mg per m^2 body surface area is recommended followed by transitioning to daily oral cyclophosphamide 2 mg per kg 4 weeks later. Oral or intravenous doses need to be adjusted for renal impairment. Table 196.2 outlines renal adjustments in oral cyclophosphamide doses. Table 196.3 outlines a standard protocol for the use of IV cyclophosphamide.

Cyclophosphamide therapy is associated with significant morbidity and with patients or their proxy needs to be counseled prior to consent for treatment. There is overall a 2.4-fold increase in malignancy with 11-fold increase in the risk of leukemia or lymphoma and a significant increased risk of bladder cancer occurring in 1% to 3% of Wegener's granulomatosis patients treated with cyclophosphamide [80]. Hemorrhage cystitis has been reported in 12% to 43% of patients treated for Wegener's granulomatosis. In one NIH study, 57% of women of childbearing years became infertile [80]. Opportunistic infection, particularly with *Pneumocystis jiroveci*, was reported in 6% of patients in initial trials with combination cyclophosphamide and corticosteroids and it is now the standard of care for patients to be prophylactically treated with double strength trimethoprim/sulfamethoxazole, 3 times weekly.

Due to these significant morbidities with cyclophosphamide, two recent randomized trials explore the efficacy and safety of rituximab versus cyclophosphamide (one study with intravenous dosing and the second with oral dosing) as induction therapy for ANCA-associated vasculitis. The results in both studies suggest equivalency in inducing remission but also similar adverse event profile [27,28]. Thus, rituximab represents an alternative in induction therapy for patients with ANCA associated vasculitis. The precise role of rituximab in rapidly progressive vasculitis in the critically ill patient is unknown as this was not the focus of the two prospective trials utilizing this agent.

Once remission has been achieved over the first 3 to 6 months, the aim of ongoing therapy is to maintain remission using a less toxic immunosuppressive agent and monitoring the patient closely for signs of relapse. Typical remission–maintenance agents are methotrexate 15 to 25 mg per week orally or subcutaneously or azathioprine 1.5 mg per kg per day orally. Both drugs have been shown to have similar efficacy and side effect profiles in this setting [26]. Mycophenolate mofetil has also shown promise both in remission induction and maintenance [81].

A prospective placebo controlled trial in the use of the tumor necrosis factor inhibitor etanercept as a remission–maintenance agent showed no added efficacy over standard therapy [24]. Treatment of relapsing disease with rituximab may be more effective than repeat cyclophosphamide [28]. Other treatment considerations include management of concomitant upper and lower respiratory tract infections, which are common and difficult to diagnose when superimposed on inflammatory disease.

As mentioned earlier, Wegener's granulomatosis is specifically associated with subglottic stenosis. Optimal treatment of this is best achieved with localized treatment, with bronchoscopic mechanical dilatation, and transbronchial corticosteroid injection of the involved area [82].

DRUG-INDUCED VASCULITIS

Cases of vasculitis associated with the use of certain drugs, vaccines, and toxins have long been recognized. Previously these were described as hypersensitivity reactions causing small vessel vasculitis [83]. More recent work in drug-induced vasculitis has broadened the group to include a large variety of small- and medium-vessel syndromes. There are no specific pathological or clinical features that distinguish this group from other forms of vasculitis. Cases ranging from self-limiting cutaneous involvement to severe multiorgan failure have been reported. Diagnosis is based simply on the development of vasculitis where a causal drug/agent can be identified, which in most cases leads to resolution of the vasculitis after drug discontinuation. There is great variation in the length of drug exposure before symptoms develop, with many reports of years of exposure before the apparent sudden onset of vasculitis.

The most commonly reported medications causing drug-induced vasculitis include, propylthiouracil, allopurinol, hydralazine, cefaclor, minocycline, D-penicillamine, phenytoin, isotretinoin, and methotrexate with colony stimulating factors [84], quinolone antibiotics, and leukotriene inhibitors more recently added to the list [85]. Other cases have been reported following vaccination, particularly hepatitis B [86] and influenza [87].

The pathophysiology of drug-induced vasculitis appears to be varied. Recently, cases of drug-induced vasculitis have been shown to be associated with temporary production of ANCA antibodies, typically against the MPO antigen and most notable with propylthiouracil and allopurinol [88]. Antibody titers also decrease in these cases following the discontinuation of medication, supporting its causal role [89].

Drug-induced vasculitis can involve medium or small vessels and therefore can present with a variety of clinical features depending on the site and size of vessel involved. Drug-induced vasculitis can present with clinical manifestations similar to any other systemic vasculitis, and there are no clinical findings specific to the syndrome. Skin involvement is common, most commonly in the form of palpable purpura. Although 33% of patients have no symptoms associated with the lesions, 40% complain of burning or pain. Bowel and nervous system involvement is also well recognized along with arthralgias and myalgias. Renal involvement is present in 40% of cases.

Treatment involves the withdrawal of potential causative medications. With mild skin involvement alone, no specific treatment is advocated. Where skin breakdown occurs, skin lesions are very symptomatic, or if internal organ involvement is identified, treatment with corticosteroids is beneficial. In rare cases, particularly those associated with ANCA production, other immunosuppressive agents may be necessary but usually only for short periods of time.

CENTRAL NERVOUS SYSTEM VASCULITIS

CNS vasculitis is a rare condition that can present as a primary form confined to the CNS, known as primary angiitis of the CNS (PACNS) or as a secondary form associated with a systemic vasculitis or other systemic illness. Although many of the systemic vasculitides and rheumatologic diseases can result in CNS involvement and are discussed briefly in other sections, this section focuses on the CNS manifestations of PACNS. Other secondary causes of CNS vasculitis and syndromes mimicking CNS vasculitis include sarcoidosis, antiphospholipid antibody syndrome, lymphoma, atrial myxoma, atheroemboli, reversible vasoconstrictive syndrome, Lyme disease, HIV infection, herpes zoster, tuberculosis, and drugs including cocaine, methamphetamines, ergotamine, pseudoephedrine, and heroin [90].

The clinical presentation associated with PACNS is broad and includes subacute memory loss, acute encephalopathy, and other cognitive and behavioral changes. Seizures, cranial nerve abnormalities, focal deficits involving the cerebrum, cerebellum, and brainstem, spinal cord lesions, meningismus, headache, auditory and vestibular disturbances, intracranial or subarachnoid hemorrhage, and reduced visual acuity or blindness due to retinal and optic nerve vasculitis have been described [91,92]. Frequently, patients have hypertension that aggravates their underlying disease or raises questions about their primary diagnosis. Disease manifestations may develop precipitously but often can present with a long prodrome over months involving subtle mental status changes and cognitive dysfunction [91,92]. The disease has a predilection for the small and medium vessels, especially of the leptomeninges and appears more common in men.

The diagnostic approach to CNS vasculitis includes a careful, frequently repeated neurologic examination, laboratory studies including cultures, viral and bacterial serologies, ANCA, cryoglobulins, antinuclear antibodies, antiphospholipid antibodies, and complement levels, which may help to establish secondary causes of CNS vasculitis related to infections, connective tissue disorders, and systemic vasculitides. CSF abnormalities seen in PACNS, including elevated protein levels and elevated cell counts, mostly lymphocytes, occurs in 80% of patients [92]. Angiographic changes showing alternating areas of stenosis and ectasia are suggestive of the disease but can be seen with other diagnoses including vasospasm and infection. In biopsy proven cases of PACNS, angiography is normal in 40% of cases [92,93]. Magnetic resonance imaging (MRI) can additionally be suggestive of ischemic lesions due to vasculitis if lesions are seen in different vascular distributions, although this finding is not specific for PACNS. A negative MRI and normal CSF make CNS vasculitis less likely, although cases of PACNS have been described with a negative MRI [94,95]. In most cases, unless angiography is highly suggestive in the correct clinical context, pathologic confirmation is necessary. Biopsy of the leptomeninges and other areas guided by previous imaging is necessary to rule out other diagnoses including infection, malignancy, and sarcoidosis, among other diagnoses. In PACNS, the inflammatory infiltrate is predominately mononuclear cells, but neutrophils, plasma cells, and histiocytes are also noted [96].

Treatment of PACNS involves corticosteroids (CS) as the initial treatment of choice, ranging from doses of 1 mg per kg per day orally to 1 g intravenously daily for 3 days followed by oral CS. Cyclophosphamide is used in most cases although absolute recommendations are limited by a lack of prospective trials [97].

There are other vasculitic syndromes that can cause similar presentations, as discussed above, although they typically will present with CNS manifestations in the context of other systemic features such as fever, weight loss, peripheral neuropathy, glomerulonephritis, arthritis, or other organ involvement. PAN, Wegener's granulomatosis, and Churg-Strauss syndrome can all present with CNS involvement including seizure, cranial nerve deficit, cerebral vascular events, and subarachnoid hemorrhage [98–101].

OTHER VASCULITIDES

Takayasu's arteritis is a large vessel vasculitis that affects the aortic arch and branches, affecting mainly women up to the age of 50. Patients typically present with constitutional symptoms of fatigue, weight loss, elevated erythrocyte sedimentation rate, and evidence of limb claudication and bruits. Patients can present with stroke due to inflammation and subsequent stenosis of the extracranial vessels [102]. Behcet's disease is characterized by aphthous stomatitis, genital ulcers, and can sometimes present with vasculitis that can affect various-sized blood vessels. Meningoencephalitis, seizure, intracranial hemorrhage, and cerebral vascular events have been reported [103]. Connective tissue disease such as systemic lupus erythematosus (SLE), rheumatoid arthritis, and Sjögren syndrome can all be associated with a variety of CNS manifestations including stroke, seizure, encephalopathy, and aseptic meningitis [104–106].

CHOLESTEROL EMBOLISM

Cholesterol crystal embolization can produce a clinical picture very similar to that of a systemic vasculitis [107,108] with the gradual onset of peripheral skin lesions, typically blue toe or livedo reticularis [109], with worsening renal function [110]. Bowel ischemia, acute confusional states [111], and retinal embolization may also be present.

The syndrome occurs due to the release of cholesterol crystals from eroded atherosclerotic plaques. It occurs most frequently following percutaneous endovascular interventions [112,113], but spontaneous episodes or those following anticoagulant [114] or thrombolytic therapy [115] have also been reported.

The chronology of impaired renal function after angiography may help distinguish radiocontrast dye-induced renal failure from renal failure due to atheromatous microemboli. Renal failure caused by radiocontrast dye tends to appear soon after the study, reaches maximal severity within 7 to 10 days, and then improves, with renal function returning to baseline over several weeks. In contrast, renal failure due to atheromatous microemboli to the kidney generally develops over 1 to 4 weeks or even over several months after the angiographic procedure and may not be reversible.

To establish the diagnosis of atheromatous emboli, one must have a high degree of suspicion based on the clinical presentation, history, physical findings, and laboratory results. The diagnosis is confirmed by the demonstration on histologic samples of biopsied skin, muscle, and kidney or amputated tissue of the characteristic biconvex needle-shaped clefts representing the "ghosts" of the cholesterol crystals within arteries and arterioles that are dissolved during routine histologic preparation [116]. With special histologic preparation, the cholesterol crystals display birefringence when viewed with a polarized light microscope.

Treatment of atheromatous emboli consists of controlling pain and blood pressure, and measures to increase local blood flow with topical glyceryl trinitrate (2% Nitrol) ointment, sympathetic blockade, calcium channel blockers to reduce vasospasm, and perhaps pentoxifylline to improve the rheostatic properties of red blood cells. Newer vasodilator agents such as iloprost and phosphodiesterase inhibitors are also being tried [117,118]. There are also case reports of improvements in cholesterol emboli-associated renal disease with statins [119]. Corticosteroid therapy has also been reported to be helpful in several case reports [120]. There are, however, no controlled trials in the use of any of these agents.

A number of modalities are ineffective for the treatment of atheromatous emboli, including the use of antiplatelet drugs and low-molecular-weight dextran. The use of heparin and warfarin is controversial. The general consensus, however, is that these drugs are contraindicated, because by preventing the formation of an organized thrombus over ulcerated atheromatous plaques, anticoagulants may allow continued breakdown and embolization of material [121]. In cases of chronic distal embolization from abdominal aortic aneurysm, surgical repair or endovascular stent-graft repair usually leads to definitive resolution [122].

TREATMENT STRATEGIES IN UNDIFFERENTIATED RHEUMATIC DISEASES PRESENTING WITH CRITICAL ILLNESS AND RELAPSE OR WORSENING KNOWN RHEUMATIC DISEASE

In certain circumstances, patients present to the hospital or ICU with overwhelming respiratory failure or hemodynamic instability without a previously defined rheumatic disorder. For example, patients with undiagnosed SLE or vasculitis may present with respiratory failure, alveolar hemorrhage, and rapidly progressive renal failure but no specific historical clues or previous serologic data supporting any particular diagnosis, and the results of laboratory and tissue evaluation biopsy may not yet be available. In this situation, one cannot be certain whether the underlying process is an immune complex–mediated disease, such as SLE, Goodpasture's syndrome, or cryoglobulinemia, or a pauci-immune process such as Wegener's granulomatosis or microscopic polyangiitis. The appropriate laboratory evaluation would include an ANCA, ANA, anti-glomerular basement membrane antibody, and cryoglobulins prior to initiating therapy. Initial therapy might include PE, which may transiently remove autoantibodies, cytokines, and complement associated with the inflammatory process, in addition to high-dose methylprednisolone, 1 g intravenously per day for 3 days, and then initiation of intravenous or oral cyclophosphamide [123,124]. The benefit of intravenous immunoglobulin in relapsing or life-threatening vasculitis is not well understood due to a paucity of controlled trials [125,126].

In the face of known rheumatic disease treatment failure, caution must be exercised to exclude infectious sources that may mimic worsening of the underlying disease process. Especially in patients on chronic or high-dose corticosteroids and or cyclophosphamide, particular attention must be paid to exclude opportunistic infections such as *P. jiroveci* and fungal infections such as *Aspergillus* while deciding whether disease activity is escalating and becoming unresponsive to therapy. Once infection has been thoroughly excluded, one can consider either higher doses of a standard or novel immunosuppressive agent or addition of other therapies such as immunoglobulin or PE.

Due to the rarity of systemic vasculitis, there have previously been few prospective clinical trials evaluating accepted treatments. In recent years due to establishment of several investigator consortiums, multicenter prospective studies are now beginning to be performed. The more important of these studies are summarized in Table 196.3.

References

1. Frankel SK, Sullivan EJ, Brown KK: Vasculitis: Wegener's granulomatosis, Churg-Strauss syndrome, microscopic polyangiitis, polyarteritis nodosa and Takayasu's arteritis. *Crit Care Clin* 18:855–879, 2002.
2. Saleh A, Stone JH: Classification and diagnostic criteria in systemic vasculitis. *Best Pract Res Clin Rheumatol* 19(2):209–221, 2005.
3. Pallan L, Savage CO, Harper L: ANCA associated vasculitis: from bench research to novel treatments. *Nat Rev Nephrol* 5(5):278–286, 2009.
4. Jayne D: The diagnosis of vasculitis. *Best Pract Res Clin Rheumatol* 23(3): 445–453, 2009.
5. Lie JT: Vasculitis simulators and vasculitis look-alikes. *Curr Opin Rheumatol* 4:47–55, 1992.
6. O'Keefe ST, Woods BO, Breslin DJ, et al: Blue toe syndrome. Causes and management. *Arch Intern Med* 152:2197–2202, 1992.
7. Guillevin L, Lhote F, Gayraud M, et al: Prognostic factors in polyarteritis nodosa and Churg-Strauss syndrome: a prospective study of 342 patients. *Medicine* 75:17–28, 1996.
8. Griffin J: Vasculitis neuropathies. *Rheum Dis Clin North Am* 27:751–760, 2001.
9. Moore PM, Fauci AS: Neurologic manifestations of systemic vasculitis: a retrospective and prospective study of clinicopathologic features and responses to therapy in 25 patients. *Am J Med* 71:517–524, 1981.
10. Said G, Lacroi-Ciaudo C, Fujimura H, et al: The peripheral neuropathy of necrotizing arteritis: a clinical pathologic study. *Ann Neurol* 23:461–465, 1988.
11. Levine SM, Hellman DB, Stone JH: Gastrointestinal involvement in polyarteritis nodosa (1986–2000); presentation and outcomes in 24 patients. *Am J Med* 112:386–391, 2002.
12. Holsinger DR, Osmundson PJ, Edwards JE: The heart in periarteritis nodosa. *Circulation* 25:610–618, 1962.
13. Schrader ML, Hochman JS, Bulkley BH: The heart in polyarteritis nodosa: a clinicopathologic study. *Am Heart J* 109:1353–1359, 1985.
14. Lhote F, Guilliven L: Polyarteritis nodosa, microscopic polyangiitis, Churg-Strauss syndrome: clinical aspects and treatment. *Rheum Dis Clin North Am* 21:911–947, 1995.
15. Fye KH, Becker MJ, Theofilopoulos AN, et al: Immune complexes in hepatitis B antigen-associated periarteritis nodosa: detection by antibody independent cell–mediated cytotoxicity and the Raji cell assay. *Am J Med* 62:783–791, 1977.
16. Tsukada N, Koh C, Owa M, et al: Chronic neuropathy associated with immune complexes of hepatitis B virus. *J Neurol Sci* 61:193–211, 1983.
17. Carson CW, Conn AJ, Czaja AJ, et al: Frequency and significance of antibodies to hepatitis C virus in polyarteritis nodosa. *J Rheumatol* 20:304–309, 1993.
18. Cid MC, Grau JM, Casademont J, et al: Immunohistochemical characterization of inflammatory cells and immunologic activation markers in muscle and nerve biopsy specimens from patients with polyarteritis nodosa. *Arthritis Rheum* 37:1055–1061, 1994.
19. Gayraud M, Guillevin L, Toumelin P, et al: Long-term follow-up of polyarteritis nodosa, microscopic polyangiitis, and Churg-Strauss syndrome. *Arthritis Rheum* 44(3):666–675, 2001.
20. Jayne DRW, Chapel H, Adu D, et al: Intravenous immunoglobulin for ANCA-associated systemic vasculitis with persistent disease activity. *Q J Med* 93:433–439, 2000.
21. Gaskin G, Jayne D: Adjunctive plasma exchange is superior to methylprednisolone in acute renal failure due to ANCA-associated glomerulonephritis. *J Am Soc Nephrol* 13[Suppl S]:2A–3A, 2002.
22. De Groot K, Rasmussen N, Bacon PA, et al: Randomized trial of cyclophosphamide versus methotrexate for induction of remission in early systemic antineutrophil cytoplasmic antibody-associated vasculitis. *Arthritis Rheum* 52(8):2461–2469, 2005.
23. Jayne D, Rasmussen N, Andrassy K, et al: A randomized trial of maintenance therapy for vasculitis associated with antineutrophil cytoplasmic autoantibodies. *N Engl J Med* 349(1):36–44, 2003.

24. WGET Research Group: Etanercept plus standard therapy for Wegener's granulomatosis. *N Engl J Med* 352:351–356, 2005.
25. deGroot K, Harper L, Jayne DR, et al: Pulse versus daily oral cyclophosphamide for induction of remission in antineutrophil cytoplasmic antibody-associated vasculitis. *Ann Int Med* 150(10):670–680, 2009.
26. Pagnoux C, Mahr A, Hamidou MA, et al: Azathioprine or methotrexate maintenance for ANCA-associated vasculitis. *N Engl J Med* 359(26):2790–2803, 2008.
27. Jones RB, Tervaert JW, Hauser T, et al: Rituximab versus cyclophosphamide in ANCA-Associated Renal Vasculitis. *N Engl J Med* 363:211–220, 2010.
28. Stone JH, Merkel PA, Spiera R, et al: Rituximab versus cyclophosphamide for ANCA-Associated Vasculitis. *N Engl J Med* 363:221–232, 2010.
29. Guillevin L, Mahr A, Cohen P, et al: Short-term corticosteroids then lamivudine and plasma exchanges to treat hepatitis B virus related polyarteritis nodosa. *Arthritis Rheum* 51(3):482–487, 2004.
30. Guillevin L, Fain O, Lhote F, et al: Lack of superiority of steroids plus plasma exchange to steroids alone in the treatment of polyarteritis nodosa and Churg-Strauss syndrome. A prospective randomized trial in 78 patients. *Arthritis Rheum* 35:208–215, 1992.
31. Citron BP, Halpern M, McCarron M, et al: Necrotizing angiitis associated with drug abuse. *N Engl J Med* 283(19):1003–1111, 1970.
32. Luqmani R, Watts RA, Scott DGI, et al: Treatment of vasculitis in rheumatoid arthritis. *Ann Intern Med* 145:566–576, 1994.
33. Mertz LE, Conn DL: Vasculitis associated with malignancy. *Curr Opin Rheumatol* 4:39–46, 1992.
34. Somer T, Finegold SM: Vasculitides associated with infections, immunizations, and antimicrobial drugs. *Clin Infect Dis* 20:1010–1036, 1995.
35. Falk RJ, Nachman PH, Hogan SL, et al: ANCA glomerulonephritis and vasculitis: a Chapel Hill perspective. *Semin Nephrol* 20(3):233–243, 2000.
36. Jayne D: Challenges in the management of microscopic polyangiitis: past, present and future. *Curr Opin Rheumatol* 20(1):3–9, 2008.
37. Klemmer PJ: Plasmapheresis for diffuse alveolar hemorrhage in patients with systemic vasculitis. *Am J Kidney Dis* 42(6):1149–1153, 2003.
38. Guillevin L, Cohen P, Gayraud M, et al: Churg-Strauss syndrome: clinical study and long-term follow-up in 96 patients. *Medicine (Baltimore)* 78:26–37, 1999.
39. Neuman T, Manger B, Schmid M, et al: Cardiac involvement in Churg Strauss syndrome: impact of endomyocarditis. *Medicine (Baltimore)* 88(4):236–243,2009.
40. Guillevin L, Visser H, Noel LH, et al: Antineutrophilic cytoplasm antibodies in systemic polyarteritis nodosa with and without hepatitis B virus infection and Churg-Strauss syndrome—62 patients. *J Rheumatol* 20:1345–1349, 1993.
41. Solans R, Bosch JA, Perez-Bocanegra C, et al: Churg-Strauss syndrome: outcome and long-term follow-up of 32 patients. *Rheumatology* 40:763–771, 2001.
42. Sable-Fourtassou R, Cohen P, Mahr A, et al: Antineutrophil cytoplasmic antibodies and Churg-Strauss syndrome. *Ann Intern Med* 143:632–638, 2005.
43. Agnello V, Ghung RT, Kaplan LM: A role for hepatitis C virus in type II cryoglobulinemia. *N Engl J Med* 327:1490–1495, 1992.
44. Lamprecht P, Moosig F, Gause A, et al: Immunologic and clinical follow-up of hepatitis C virus associated cryoglobulinemic vasculitis. *Ann Rheum Dis* 60:385–390, 2001.
45. Tarantino A, Campise M, Banfi G, et al: Long-term predictors of survival in essential mixed cryoglobulinemic glomerulonephritis. *Kidney Int* 47:618–623, 1995.
46. Bombardieri S, Paoletta P, Ferri C, et al: Lung involvement in essential mixed cryoglobulinemia. *Am J Med* 66:748–756, 1979.
47. Gomez-Tello V, Onoro-Canaveral JJ, de la Casa Monje RM, et al: Diffuse recidivant alveolar hemorrhage in a patient with hepatitis C virus related mixed cryoglobulinemia. *Intensive Care Med* 25(3):319–322, 1999.
48. Rieu V, Cohen P, Andre MH, et al: Characteristics and outcome of 49 patients with symptomatic cryoglobulinemia. *Rheumatology (Oxford)* 41:290–300, 2002.
49. Guillevin L, Pagnoux C: Indications of plasma exchanges for systemic vasculitides. *Ther Apher Dial* 7(2):155–160, 2003.
50. Saadoun D, Resche-Rigon M, Sene D, et al: Rituximab combined with Peg-interferon -ribavirin in refractory hepatitis C virus-associated cryoglobulinaemia. *Ann Rheum Dis* 67(10):1431–1436, 2008.
51. Cupps TR, Fauci AS: *Wegener's Granulomatosis: The Vasculitides*. Philadelphia, WB Saunders, 1981.
52. Fauci AS, Wolff SM: Wegener's granulomatosis: studies in eighteen patients and a review of the literature. *Medicine* 52(6):535–561, 1973.
53. Wolff SM, Fauci AS, Horn RG, et al: Wegener's granulomatosis. *Ann Intern Med* 81(4):513–525, 1974.
54. Popa ER, Tervaert JW: The relationship between *Staphylococcus aureus* and Wegener's granulomatosis: current knowledge and future directions. *Intern Med* 42(9):771–780, 2003.
55. Franssen C, Stegeman CA, Kallenberg CG, et al: Antiproteinase 3 and antimyeloperoxidase-associated vasculitis. *Kidney Int* 57(6):2195–2206, 2000.
56. Finkielman JD, Merkel PA, Schroeder D, et al: Antiproteinase 3 antineutrophil cytoplasmic antibodies and disease activity in Wegener's granulomatosis. *Ann Intern Med* 147(9):611–619, 2007.
57. Sanders JS, Huitma MG, Kallenberg CG, et al: Prediction of relapse in PR3-ANCA-associated vasculitis by assessing responses of ANCA titres to treatment. *Rheumatology (Oxford)* 45(6):724–729, 2006.
58. Falk RJ, Jennette JC: ANCA are pathogenic—oh yes they are! *J Am Soc Nephrol* 13(7):1977–1979, 2002.
59. Godman GC, Churg J: Wegener's granulomatosis: pathology and review of literature. *Arch Pathol* 58:533–553, 1954.
60. Fauci AS, Haynes BF, Katz P, et al: Wegener's granulomatosis: prospective clinical and therapeutic experience with 85 patients for 21 years. *Ann Intern Med* 98(1):76–85, 1983.
61. Schramm VL Jr, Myers EN, Rogerson DR: The masquerade of vasculitis: head and neck diagnosis and management. *Laryngoscope* 88(12):1922–1934, 1978.
62. Goldenberg DL, Goodman ML: Case 26-1985. Case records of the Massachusetts General Hospital: weekly clinicopathological exercises. *N Engl J Med* 312:1695–1697, 1985.
63. Harrington JT, McCluskey RT: Case 24-1979. Case records of the Massachusetts General Hospital: weekly clinicopathological exercises. *N Engl J Med* 300:1378–1380, 1979.
64. McDonald TJ, DeRemee RA: Wegener's granulomatosis. *Laryngoscope* 93(2):220–231, 1983.
65. Bernhard JD, Mark EJ: Case 17–1986. Case records of the Massachusetts General Hospital: weekly clinicopathological exercises. *N Engl J Med* 314:1170–1173, 1986.
66. McGregor MG, Sandler G: Wegener's granulomatosis. A clinical and radiological survey. *Br J Radiol* 37:430–439, 1964.
67. Maguire R, Fauci AS, Doppmann JL, et al: Unusual radiographic features of Wegener's granulomatosis. *Am J Roentgenology* 130(2):233–238, 1978.
68. Langford CA, Sneller MC, Hallahan CW, et al: Clinical features and therapeutic management of subglottic stenosis in patients with Wegener's granulomatosis. *Arthritis Rheum* 39(10):1754–1760, 1996.
69. Weiss MA, Crissman JD: Renal biopsy findings in Wegener's granulomatosis: segmental necrotizing glomerulonephritis with glomerular thrombosis. *Hum Pathol* 15(10):943–956, 1984.
70. Horn RG, Fauci AS, Rosenthal AS, et al: Renal biopsy pathology in Wegener's granulomatosis. *Am J Pathol* 74(3):423–440, 1974.
71. Pritchard MH: Wegener's granulomatosis presenting as rheumatoid arthritis (two cases). *Proc R Soc Med* 69(7):501–504, 1976.
72. Noritake DT, Weiner SR, Bassett LW, et al: Rheumatic manifestations of Wegener's granulomatosis. *J Rheumatol* 14(5):949–951, 1987.
73. Baker SB, Robinson DR: Unusual renal manifestations of Wegener's granulomatosis. Report of two cases. *Am J Med* 64(5):883–889, 1978.
74. Haynes BF, Fishman ML, Fauci AS, et al: The ocular manifestations of Wegener's granulomatosis. Fifteen years' experience and review of the literature. *Am J Med* 63(1):131–141, 1977.
75. Parker SW, Sobel RA: Case 12–1988. Case records of the Massachusetts General Hospital: weekly clinicopathological exercises. *N Engl J Med* 318:760, 1988.
76. Satoh J, Miyasaka N, Yamada T, et al: Extensive cerebral infarction due to involvement of both anterior cerebral arteries by Wegener's granulomatosis. *Ann Rheum Dis* 47(7):606–611, 1988.
77. Camilleri M, Pusey CD, Chadwick VS, et al: Gastrointestinal manifestations of systemic vasculitis. *Q J Med* 52(206):141–149, 1983.
78. Lynch JP, Matteson E, McCune WJ: Wegener's granulomatosis: evolving concepts. *Med Rounds* 2:67, 1989.
79. Regan M, Hellmann D, Stone J: Treatment of Wegener's granulomatosis. *Rheum Dis Clin North Am* 27(4):863–886, 2001.
80. Hoffman G, Kerr G, Leavitt R: Wegener's granulomatosis: an analysis of 158 patients. *Ann Intern Med* 116:488–498, 1992.
81. Stassen PM, Cohen Tervaert JW, Stegeman CA: Induction of remission in active antineutrophil cytoplasmic antibody-associated vasculitis with mycophenolate mofetil in patients who cannot be treated with cyclophosphamide. *Ann Rheum Dis* 66(6):798–802, 2007.
82. Langford CA, Sneller MC, Hallahan CW, et al: Clinical features and therapeutic management of subglottic stenosis in patients with Wegener's granulomatosis. *Arthritis Rheum* 39:1754–1760, 1996.
83. Calabrese LH, Michel BA, Bloch DA, et al: The American College of Rheumatology 1990 criteria for the classification of hypersensitivity vasculitis. *Arthritis Rheum* 33(8):1108–1113, 1990.
84. Bonilla MA, Dale D, Zeidler C, et al: Long-term safety of treatment with recombinant human granulocyte colony-stimulating factor in patients with severe congenital neutropenias. *Br J Haematol* 88(4):723–730, 1994.
85. Merkel P: Drug-induced vasculitis. *Rheum Dis Clin North Am* 27(4):849–862, 2001.
86. Ascherio A, Zhang SM, Hernan MA, et al: Hepatitis B vaccination and the risk of multiple sclerosis. *N Engl J Med* 344(5):327–332, 2001.
87. Blumberg S, Bienfang D, Kantrowitz FG, et al: A possible association between influenza vaccination and small vessel vasculitis. *Arch Intern Med* 140(6):847–848, 1980.
88. Choi HK, Merkel P, Walker AM, et al: Drug-induced ANCA-positive vasculitis: prevalence amongst patients with high titers of anti-myeloperoxidase antibodies. *Arthritis Rheum* 43(2):405–413, 2000.
89. Dedeoglu F: Drug-induced autoimmunity. *Curr Opin Rheumatol* 21(5): 547–551, 2009.
90. Siva A: Vasculitis of the nervous system. *J Neurol* 248:451–468, 2001.

91. Younger DS, Calabrese LH, Hays AP: Granulomatous angiitis of the nervous system. *Neurol Clin* 15:821–834, 1997.
92. Calabrese LH, Furlan AJ, Gragg LA, et al: Primary angiitis of the central nervous system (PACNS): a reappraisal of diagnostic criteria and revised clinical approach. *Cleve Clin J Med* 59:293–306, 1992.
93. Duna GF, Calabrese LH: Limitations of invasive modalities in the diagnosis of primary angiitis of the central nervous system. *J Rheumatol* 222:662–667, 1995.
94. Harris K, Tram D, Skekels W, et al: Diagnosing intracranial vasculitis: the roles of MRI and angiography. *Am J Neuroradiol* 15:317–330, 1994.
95. Stone JH, Pomper MG, Roubenoff R, et al: Sensitivities of noninvasive tests for central nervous system vasculitis: a comparison of lumbar puncture, computed tomography, and magnetic resonance imaging. *J Rheumatol* 21(7):1277–1282, 1994.
96. Lie JT: Primary (granulomatous) angiitis of the central nervous system: a clinical pathologic analysis of 15 new cases and a review of the literature. *Hum Pathol* 23:164–171, 1992.
97. Hajj-Ali RA, Ghamande S, Calabrese LH, et al: Central nervous system vasculitis in the intensive care unit. *Crit Care Clin* 18:897–914, 2002.
98. Moore PM, Cupps T: Neurologic complications of vasculitis. *Ann Neurol* 14:155–157, 1983.
99. Moore PM, Fauci AS: Neurologic manifestations of systemic vasculitis: a retrospective and prospective study of clinicopathologic features and responses to therapy in 25 cases. *Am J Med* 71:517–524, 1981.
100. Sigal LH: The neurologic presentation of vasculitic and rheumatologic syndromes. A review. *Medicine (Baltimore)* 66:157–180, 1987.
101. Nishino H, Rubino F, DeRemee R, et al: Neurological involvement in Wegener's granulomatosis: an analysis of 324 consecutive cases at the Mayo Clinic. *Ann Neurol* 33:4–9, 1993.
102. Takano K, Sadoshima S, Ibayashi S, et al: Altered cerebral hemodynamics and metabolism in Takayasu's arteritis with neurological deficits. *Stroke* 24(10):1501–1506, 1993.
103. Siva A, Altintas A, Saip S: Behcet's syndrome and the nervous system. *Curr Opin Neurol* 17(3):347–357, 2004.
104. Alexander EL: Neurologic disease in Sjögren's syndrome: mononuclear inflammatory vasculopathy affecting the central/peripheral nervous system and muscle. *Rheum Dis Clin North Am* 19:869–908, 1993.
105. Neamtu L, Belmont M, Miller DC, et al: Rheumatoid disease of the central nervous system with meningeal vasculitis presenting with seizure. *Neurology* 56(6):814–815, 2001.
106. Ellis SG, Verity MA: Central nervous system involvement in systemic lupus erythematosus: a review of neuropathologic findings in 57 cases. *Semin Arthritis Rheum* 8:212–221, 1979.
107. Cappiello RA, Espinoza LR, Adelman H, et al: Cholesterol embolism: a pseudovasculitic syndrome. *Semin Arthritis Rheum* 18(4):240–246, 1989.
108. Anderson RW: Necrotizing angiitis associated with embolization of cholesterol. *Am J Clin Pathol* 43:65, 1965.
109. Applebaum RM, Kronzon I: Evaluation and management of cholesterol embolization and the blue toe syndrome. *Curr Opin Cardiol* 11(5):533–542, 1996.
110. Hara S, Asada Y: Atheroembolic renal disease: clinical findings of 11 cases. *J Atheroscler Thromb* 9(6):288–291, 2002.
111. Thadhani RI, Camargo CA, Xavier RJ, et al: Atheroembolic renal failure after invasive procedures. Natural history based on 52 histologically proven cases. *Medicine* 74:350–358, 1995.
112. Paraskevas KI, Koutsias S, Mikhailidis DP, et al: Cholesterol crystal embolization: a possible complication of peripheral endovascular interventions. *J Endovasc Ther* 15(5):614–625, 2008.
113. Fukumoto Y, Tsutsui H, Tsuchihashi M, et al: The incidence and risk factors of cholesterol embolization syndrome, a complication of cardiac catheterization: a prospective study. *J Am Coll Cardiol* 42(2):211–216, 2003.
114. Moll S, Huffman J: Cholesterol emboli associated with warfarin treatment. *Am J Hematol* 77(2):194–195, 2004.
115. Hitti WA, Wali RK, Weinman EJ, et al: Cholesterol embolization syndrome induced by thrombolytic therapy. *Am J Cardiovasc Drugs* 8(1):27–34, 2008.
116. Manganoni AM, Venturini M, Scolari F, et al: The importance of skin biopsy in the diverse clinical manifestations of cholesterol embolism. *Br J Dermatol* 150(6):1230–1231, 2004.
117. Grenader T, Lifschitz M, Shavit L: Iloprost in embolic renal failure. *Mt Sinai J Med* 72(5):339–341, 2005.
118. Elinav E, Chajek-Shaul T, Stern M, et al: Improvement in cholesterol emboli syndrome after iloprost therapy. *BMJ* 324(7332):268–269, 2002.
119. Yonemura K, Ikegaya N: Potential therapeutic effect of simvastatin on progressive renal failure and nephrotic-range proteinuria caused by renal cholesterol embolism. *Am J Med Sci* 322(1):50–52, 2001.
120. Graziani G, Santostasi S, Angelini C, et al: Corticosteroids in cholesterol emboli syndrome. *Nephron* 87(4):371–373, 2001.
121. Belenfant X, d'Auzac C, Bariety J, et al: Cholesterol crystal embolism during treatment with low-molecular-weight heparin. *Presse Med* 26(26):1236–1237, 1997.
122. Carroccio A, Olin JW, Ellozy SH, et al: The role of aortic stent grafting in the treatment of atheromatous embolization syndrome: results after a mean of 15 months follow-up. *J Vasc Surg* 40(3):424–429, 2004.
123. Soding PF, Lockwood CM, Park GR: The intensive care of patients with fulminant vasculitis. *Anaesth Intensive Care* 22:81–89, 1994.
124. Schmitt WH, Gross WL: Vasculitis in the seriously ill patient: diagnostic approaches and therapeutic options in ANCA-associated vasculitis. *Kidney Int* 53(64):S39–S44, 1998.
125. Martinez V, Cohen P, Pagnoux C, et al: Intravenous immunoglobulins for relapses of systemic vasculitides associated with antineutrophil cytoplasmic autoantibodies: results of a multicenter, prospective, open label study of twenty two patients. *Arthritis Rheum* 58(1):308–317, 2008.
126. Fortin PM, Tejani AM, Bassett K, et al: Intravenous immunoglobulins as adjuvant therapy for Wegener's granulomatosis. *Cochrane Database Syst Rev* 8(3):CD007057, 2009.

SECTION XVII ■ PSYCHIATRIC ISSUES IN INTENSIVE CARE

JOHN QUERQUES

CHAPTER 197 ■ DIAGNOSIS AND TREATMENT OF AGITATION AND DELIRIUM IN THE INTENSIVE CARE UNIT PATIENT

JASON P. CAPLAN

> ...patients are attacked with insomnolency, so that the disease is not concocted; they become sorrowful, peevish, and delirious; there are flashes of light in their eyes, and noises in their ears; their extremities are cold, their urine unconcocted; the sputa thin, saltish, tinged with an intense color and smell; sweats about the neck, and anxiety; respiration, interrupted in the expulsion of the air, frequent and very large; expression of the eyelids dreadful; dangerous deliquia [syncope]; tossing of the bed-clothes from the breast; the hands trembling, and sometimes the lower lip agitated. These symptoms, appearing at the commencement, are indicative of strong delirium, and patients so affected generally die, or if they escape, it is with a deposit, hemorrhage from the nose, or the expectoration of thick matter, and not otherwise. Neither do I perceive that physicians are skilled in such things as these; how they ought to know such diseases as are connected with debility, and which are further weakened by abstinence from food, and those aggravated by some other irritation; those by pain, and from the acute nature of the disease, and what affections and various forms thereof our constitution and habit engender, although the knowledge or ignorance of such things brings safety or death to the patient.
>
> *Hippocrates, 400 B.C.*

In *On Regimen in Acute Diseases*, Hippocrates identified agitation as a harbinger of severe illness and poor outcome [1]. His admonition that physicians understand the causes and treatments of agitation remains vital today, for the safety not only of patients but also of hospital staff attending to them. Nowhere is this more pertinent than in the intensive care unit (ICU) and its finely balanced environment of invasive and often delicate treatment modalities, interference with which is rarely as easily corrected as is "tossing of the bed-clothes." The sudden pulling of precisely placed central lines, intra-aortic balloon pumps, or endotracheal tubes can carry profound consequences for patients and those responsible for their care.

The term "ICU psychosis" has unfortunately entered common medical parlance in reference to agitation and confusion in the ICU patient [2]. This misnomer is inaccurate for several reasons. Classifying agitation as psychosis is usually diagnostically incorrect; moreover, drawing an etiologic connection between the patient's geography and the development of agitation is nonsensical. Historically, sensory deprivation and interruption of normal sleep patterns alone were thought to result in behavioral disturbances in the ICU, but modern research has not confirmed this relationship [2]. The causal attribution of mental status changes to the environment of the ICU is dangerous because it obviates the need for further diagnostic inquiry that could reveal a previously unidentified pathologic process. As with all new symptoms, careful diagnosis is the first step toward effective treatment.

This chapter reviews the causes, presentations, and treatments of common causes of agitation in the ICU patient, focusing on delirium.

DELIRIUM

Perhaps the most common cause of agitation in the general hospital as a whole, and the ICU in particular, delirium is a neuropsychiatric manifestation of a systemic disturbance (Table 197.1) [3]. As such, the paramount task in its treatment is the identification of its underlying cause(s).

Epidemiology

Prospective studies of all patients admitted to the ICU regardless of pathology have found incidence rates of delirium of 31% on admission [4] and 82% when limited to the population requiring intubation and mechanical ventilation [5].

A diagnosis of delirium exacts a profound toll on both the immediate and long-term well-being of patients and the economic resources required for their care. One study of mechanically ventilated patients in the ICU demonstrated significant increases in length of hospital stay and 6-month mortality, even after adjustment for age, severity of illness, comorbidities, coma, and medication exposure [5]. Another study of patients—limited to those who did not require mechanical ventilation—found that a diagnosis of delirium independently predicted longer hospital stay, even after correction for relevant covariates [6]. When framed in fiscal terms, delirium has been associated with 39% higher ICU costs and 31% higher hospital costs overall [7]. Delirium predicts greater hospital costs across multiple domains, including professional, technical, consultative, and nursing [8].

Disruptive behavior poses a grave risk of acute injury to the delirious ICU patient because of the extensive use of invasive technology in the ICU. This hazard has been specifically studied in patients who extubate themselves. Restlessness and agitation—two of the most frequent concomitants of delirium—independently predict self-extubation, which results in laryngeal and vocal cord trauma, emesis, aspiration, cardiac arrhythmia, respiratory arrest, and death [9].

Etiology

An exhaustive review of conditions that may precipitate delirium would likely cover the breadth of medical and surgical practice. Given the near limitless number of possible etiologies,

TABLE 197.1

DIAGNOSTIC CRITERIA FOR DELIRIUM

Alteration of consciousness and attention
Change in cognition (e.g., memory deficit, disorientation, language or perceptual disturbance) that is not due to dementia
Development over hours to days
Fluctuation during the course of the day
Precipitation by a medical condition or its treatment

Adapted from American Psychiatric Association: *Diagnostic and Statistical Manual of Mental Disorders*. 4th ed. Text Revision. Washington, DC, American Psychiatric Association, 2000.

when searching for a possible cause of delirium, it often proves useful to scan the clinical data searching for broad categories of pathology. The mnemonic "I WATCH DEATH" (Table 197.2) lists the processes most commonly related to delirium; the mnemonic "WWHHHHIMPS" (Table 197.3) aids recall of immediately life-threatening causes.

With complicated conditions requiring interventions on multiple fronts, patients in the ICU are often subjected to polypharmacy. A review of the patient's medication list with an eye toward certain categories of medications frequently causative of, or contributory to, delirium is warranted (Table 197.4). Particular offenders include anticholinergics, antihistamines, corticosteroids, opioids, and benzodiazepines [10,11].

Pathology

Alertness is subserved by the ascending reticular activating system (RAS) and its bilateral thalamic projections; attention is mediated by neocortical and limbic inputs to this system [12]. Structural or neurochemical interference with these pathways could theoretically result in the deficits in alertness and attention that are the hallmarks of delirium. Because the primary neurotransmitter of the RAS is acetylcholine, the relative deficit of cholinergic reserve in the elderly (e.g., due to microvascular disease or due to atrophy) may be the neural basis of the heightened risk of delirium in the geriatric population. Medications with anticholinergic activity are likely to disrupt this system's functioning even further.

In the setting of impaired oxidative metabolism, dopaminergic neurons have been found to release excess amounts of dopamine; its subsequent reuptake and extracellular metabolism are also disrupted. Because, at high levels, dopamine is theorized to facilitate the excitatory effects of glutamate [13], this dopaminergic hypothesis constitutes a proposed mechanism for the agitation seen in delirium. In fact, oxidative dysfunction predicts increased risk of delirium [14].

TABLE 197.2

I WATCH DEATH: A MNEMONIC FOR COMMON CAUSES OF DELIRIUM

*I*nfections	Pneumonia, urinary tract infection, encephalitis, meningitis, syphilis
*W*ithdrawal	Alcohol, sedative–hypnotics
*A*cute metabolic	Acidosis, alkalosis, electrolyte disturbances, hepatic or renal failure
*T*rauma	Heat stroke, burns, postoperative state
*C*entral nervous system pathology	Abscess, tumor, hemorrhage, seizure, stroke, vasculitis, normal pressure hydrocephalus
*H*ypoxia	Hypotension, pulmonary embolus, pulmonary or cardiac failure, anemia, carbon monoxide poisoning
*D*eficiencies	Vitamin B_{12}, niacin, thiamine
*E*ndocrinopathies	Hyper- or hypoglycemia, hyper- or hypoadrenalism, hyper- or hypothyroidism, hyper- or hypoparathyroidism
*A*cute vascular	Hypertensive encephalopathy, shock
*T*oxins or drugs	Medications, drugs of abuse, pesticides, solvents
*H*eavy metals	Lead, manganese, mercury

Adapted from Wise MG, Trzepacz PT: Delirium (confusional states), in Rundell JR, Wise MD (eds): *The American Psychiatric Press Textbook of Consultation-Liaison Psychiatry*. Washington, DC, American Psychiatric Press, 1996, pp 258–274.

TABLE 197.3

WWHHHHIMPS: A MNEMONIC FOR LIFE-THREATENING CAUSES OF DELIRIUM

*W*ithdrawal
*W*ernicke's encephalopathy
*H*ypoxia or hypoperfusion of the brain
*H*ypertensive crisis
*H*ypoglycemia
*H*yper- or hypothermia
*I*ntracranial hemorrhage or mass
*M*eningitis or encephalitis
*P*oisons (including medications)
*S*tatus epilepticus

Adapted from Wise MG, Trzepacz PT: Delirium (confusional states), in Rundell JR, Wise MD (eds): *The American Psychiatric Press Textbook of Consultation-Liaison Psychiatry*. Washington, DC, American Psychiatric Press, 1996, pp 258–274.

Risk Factors and Detection

Risk factors for delirium can be divided into three broad categories: properties of the illness (acute physiologic), preexisting properties of the patient (chronic physiologic), and properties of the environment (iatrogenic) (Table 197.5) [15].

The majority of patients suffering from delirium present with the hypoactive subtype. Withdrawn and psychomotorically retarded, the patient with hypoactive delirium is frequently thought by caretakers and family to be depressed. Although these patients cause little disruption to the ICU environment and provoke less acute distress in their treaters, they are no less subject to the adverse outcomes of an altered sensorium. Although the immediate threat to safety may be less apparent in these cases, hypoactive delirium can rapidly and unpredictably evolve into acute agitation as a result of unchecked, upsetting delusions. Moreover, the subjective experience of hypoactive delirium is as intense and distressing as the agitated variety [16].

Two delirium screening scales have been validated for use by nonpsychiatric personnel in the ICU. The Confusion Assessment Method for the ICU (CAM-ICU) features a four-domain assessment that can be administered in less than 1 minute [17]. Both sensitivity and specificity are >90%, and it has been translated into several languages. The Intensive Care Delirium Screening Checklist (ICDSC) features eight items, each scored present or absent. Sensitivity and specificity of the ICDSC are

TABLE 197.4

COMMON ICU DRUGS ASSOCIATED WITH DELIRIUM

Antiarrhythmics	Beta-blockers
Disopyramide	Calcium channel blockers
Lidocaine	Digitalis preparations
Mexiletine	Diuretics
Procainamide	Acetazolamide
Quinidine	Dopamine agonists
Tocainide	Amantadine
Antibiotics	Bromocriptine
Aminoglycosides	Carbidopa
Amodiaquine	Levodopa
Amphotericin	Selegiline
Cephalosporins	H_2-Blockers
Fluoroquinolones	Immunosuppressants
Gentamicin	Azacitidine
Isoniazid	Chlorambucil
Metronidazole	Cyclosporine
Rifampin	Cytosine arabinoside
Sulfonamides	Dacarbazine
Tetracyclines	FK-506
Ticarcillin	5-Fluorouracil
Vancomycin	Hexamethylmelamine
Anticholinergics	Ifosfamide
Atropine	Interleukin-2
Benztropine	L-Asparaginase
Chlorpheniramine	Methotrexate
Diphenhydramine	Procarbazine
Eye and nose drops	Tamoxifen
Scopolamine	Vinblastine
Anticonvulsants	Vincristine
Phenytoin	Ketamine
Sodium valproate	Nonsteroidal anti-inflammatory drugs
Antidepressants	Ibuprofen
Antiemetics	Indomethacin
Promethazine	Naproxen
Metoclopramide	Opioids
Antiviral agents	Propylthiouracil
Acyclovir	Salicylates
Efavirenz	Steroids
Interferon	Sympathomimetics
Ganciclovir	Aminophylline
Nevirapine	Theophylline
Baclofen	Phenylpropanolamine
Barbiturates	Phenylephrine
Benzodiazepines	

Adapted from Cassem NH, Murray GB, Lafayette JM, et al: Delirious patients, in Stern TA, Fricchione GL, Cassem NH, et al (eds): *Massachusetts General Hospital Handbook of General Hospital Psychiatry*. 5th ed. Philadelphia, PA, Mosby, 2004, pp 119–134.

99% and 64%, respectively [18]. The minimal time required to complete either of these scales allows for scoring several times daily, which is an important feature, given the waxing and waning nature of delirium. Both scales are available at www.icudelirium.org. Careful screening and early detection can limit the sequelae of delirium and forestall the additional consequences attendant to the evolution of hypoactive delirium into agitation.

Diagnostic Evaluation

In ambiguous cases of delirium, an electroencephalogram (EEG) may provide objective data to aid diagnosis. Although the association of delirium and EEG changes was first described in the 1940s, no objective test since has demonstrated better performance in accurately detecting delirium. In their classic studies, Engel and Romano described three landmark electrographic findings in delirious patients: generalized slowing, consistency of this slowing despite wide-ranging underlying conditions, and resumption of a normal rhythm with treatment [19]. For all presentations of delirium, generalized slowing in the delta-theta range (delta: 0 to 4 Hz, theta: 4 to 8 Hz), poor organization of the background rhythm, and loss of reactive changes to eye opening and closing are considered diagnostic [20]. Recent studies have estimated the sensitivity of EEG in the diagnosis of delirium to be approximately 75%, with false–negative results likely a result of slowing not sizable enough to drop the patient's baseline rhythm from one range to the next.

EEG may also prove helpful in discerning the etiology of a delirium, since delirium tremens (DTs) as a result of alcohol or sedative–hypnotic withdrawal is associated with low-voltage fast activity superimposed on slow waves, while sedative–hypnotic toxicity is associated with fast beta activity (>12 Hz) [20]. EEG may also detect previously undiagnosed deliriogenic conditions, including nonconvulsive status epilepticus, complex partial seizures, or cerebral lesions that may act as seizure foci.

Once delirium is confirmed, the search for an underlying medical cause should commence. A careful step-by-step approach can help prune a near-endless list of possible etiologies. Although no evidence-based protocol of diagnostic studies most likely to identify a culprit exists, broad-based, relatively inexpensive, and noninvasive laboratory testing can often be informative (Table 197.6).

In most circumstances, psychiatric consultation is beneficial to the patient and the consultee. A consultation psychiatrist's familiarity with delirium and its causes and treatments usually speeds diagnosis and intervention. Delay in psychiatric consultation predicts lengthier hospitalization [21].

Pharmacologic Management

The definitive treatment of delirium is the identification and treatment of the underlying cause(s). In addition, numerous interventions may reduce its potentially harmful sequelae.

Cholinergic Agents

Given the hypocholinergic/hyperdopaminergic neurophysiological model of delirium, the intuitive goals of pharmacologic treatment are to increase cholinergic and decrease dopaminergic activities. By reversibly inhibiting metabolism of acetylcholine, the cholinesterase inhibitor physostigmine has been shown to reverse delirium resulting from multiple etiologies, but its clinical utility is limited by a brief duration of efficacy and a narrow therapeutic window. Therefore, physostigmine is usually used only when delirium is known (or highly suspected) to be caused by anticholinergic toxicity, for which it is considered the agent of choice [22].

Some small studies and case series of dementia-treating cholinesterase inhibitors have demonstrated possible delirioprotective effects [23,24], but these agents' utility in the acute setting is hampered by their long half-lives and subsequent extended interval before therapeutic serum levels are reached. Two randomized, double-blind, placebo-controlled trials failed to demonstrate any benefit of donepezil in either preventing or treating postoperative delirium [25,26]. An additional randomized, placebo-controlled trial of rivastigmine for delirium prevention also failed to demonstrate any such benefit [27].

TABLE 197.5

RISK FACTORS FOR DELIRIUM

Properties of illness (acute physiologic)	Properties of patient (chronic physiologic)	Properties of environment/treatment (iatrogenic)
Hyper- or hyponatremia	Age >70 y	Administration of psychoactive medication
Hyper- or hypoglycemia	Transfer from a nursing home	Tube feeding
Hyper- or hypothyroidism	History of depression	Bladder catheter
Hyper- or hypothermia	History of dementia	Rectal catheter
BUN/creatinine ratio ≥18	History of stroke	Central venous catheter
Renal failure (creatinine >2 mg/dL)	History of seizure	Physical restraints
Liver disease (bilirubin >20 mg/dL)	Alcohol abuse within 1 mo	
Cardiogenic shock	Drug overdose or illicit use within 1 wk	
Septic shock	History of congestive heart failure	
Hypoxia	Human immunodeficiency virus infection	
	Malnutrition	

Adapted from Ely EW, Siegel MD, Inouye SK: Delirium in the intensive care unit: an under-recognized syndrome of organ dysfunction. *Semin Respir Crit Care Med* 22:115–126, 2001.

TABLE 197.6

ASSESSMENT OF THE PATIENT WITH DELIRIUM

Basic laboratory tests—consider for all patients with delirium	Electrolytes Glucose Albumin Blood urea nitrogen Creatinine Aspartate aminotransferase Alanine aminotransferase Alkaline phosphatase Albumin Complete blood count Electrocardiogram Chest radiograph Arterial blood gases Urinalysis Thyroid stimulating hormone Vitamin B_{12} Folate Rapid plasma reagin
Additional laboratory tests—consider as clinically indicated	Heavy metal screen Lupus erythematosus preparation Antinuclear antibody Urine porphyrins Urine culture Urine drug screen Ammonia Human immunodeficiency virus antibody Venereal Disease Research Laboratory test Blood culture Serum medication levels (e.g., digoxin, theophylline, cyclosporine, phenobarbital, carbamazepine, FK-506) Lyme titer Cerebrospinal fluid analysis Brain computed tomography or magnetic resonance imaging Electroencephalogram

Adapted from American Psychiatric Association: Practice guideline for the treatment of patients with delirium. *Am J Psychiatry* 156[5, Suppl]: 1–20, 1999.

Haloperidol

As dopamine receptor antagonists, neuroleptics are theoretically suited to the task of dampening dopaminergic activity. Through decades of clinical experience and published data, haloperidol, a butyrophenone neuroleptic, has shown itself to be the agent of choice in the treatment of acute delirium [28,29]. It is ideal for use in the ICU since it can be administered by the oral, intramuscular (IM), or intravenous (IV) route. Although the U.S. Food and Drug Administration (FDA) has not approved the IV administration of haloperidol, FDA regulations permit the use of any approved drug for a non-approved indication or by an unsanctioned route in the context of innovative therapy. IV administration is preferable to the oral and IM routes for multiple reasons, including improved absorption; limitation of pain as a consequence of injection; minimization of apprehension on the part of the patient; and reduction in extrapyramidal side effects (EPS), including acute dystonia, parkinsonism, and akathisia [30]. Although there is no standard dosing regimen for the use of IV haloperidol, treatment is usually initiated with a bolus dose ranging from 0.5 mg (in the elderly) to 10 mg (for severe agitation). A 30-minute interval should be observed between doses to gauge the effect of the previously administered dose. If the initial dose does not achieve the desired effect, then the next dose can be effectively doubled until appropriate sedation is achieved (i.e., 1 mg, 2 mg, 5 mg, 10 mg, and so on). Although a randomized, double-blind comparison trial did not support the use of benzodiazepines alone for the management of delirium (except when due to alcohol or sedative–hypnotic withdrawal), IV lorazepam in doses of 1 or 2 mg can be coadministered with haloperidol to achieve more rapid sedation [31]. The combination of haloperidol and lorazepam has been shown to allow for lower total doses of each drug [32] and to minimize EPS further [33].

Complete absence of agitation should be targeted, and the regimen should be adjusted to achieve this goal. Once agitation is effectively quelled, haloperidol can be given 2 or 3 times daily, with additional doses provided as needed for breakthrough agitation. The total dose can be gradually decreased; it is usually wise to wean the evening dose last to provide some prophylaxis of "sundowning."

Side Effects of Haloperidol. As with all pharmacologic interventions, the use of haloperidol is not without risk. Neurologic sequelae—EPS, seizures, neuroleptic malignant syndrome, and tardive dyskinesia—have all been associated with the chronic use of haloperidol. In practice, however, these are rare and are minimized by IV administration [30]. Of these neurologic symptoms, akathisia is often most problematic in the setting of delirium since the sense of having to be in motion at all times is noxious, tiring, and likely to exacerbate agitation. Treatment with β-blockade is often effective. In clinical practice, haloperidol's reported lowering of the seizure threshold appears negligible [34].

Hypotension, a rare complication, is easily detected by routine monitoring in the ICU. Haloperidol has been shown in some cases to prolong the QT interval, resulting in increased risk for torsade de pointes and possible death [35,36]. An electrocardiogram should be ordered to measure the baseline corrected QT (QTc) interval, and serum potassium, magnesium, and calcium levels should be checked and monitored [28]. Once treatment begins, a QTc >500 milliseconds or an increase >25% from baseline may warrant telemetry, cardiologic consultation, and reduction or discontinuation of haloperidol. In these cases, it is advisable to calculate the QTc manually, since the automated reading may overestimate the value and result in the needless interruption of necessary treatment. The minimization of other drugs with the potential to prolong the QTc should also be considered to allow the ongoing effective treatment of delirium. Other antipsychotics, including the newer agents, have also been associated with QT prolongation [37].

Other Dopamine Receptor Antagonists

Droperidol, the other member of the butyrophenone family of neuroleptics, had been used extensively for the treatment of delirium, but its use was constrained by the 2001 FDA-mandated black-box warning regarding QT prolongation, torsade de pointes, and death [38].

Phenothiazines, the other major class of so-called conventional or first-generation neuroleptic medications (e.g., chlorpromazine, fluphenazine, thioridazine, mesoridazine, perphenazine, and trifluoperazine), are poorly suited to the treatment of delirium due to sedation, anticholinergic effects, and α-adrenergic blockade.

With the exception of clozapine, all of the so-called atypical or second-generation neuroleptic agents (i.e., risperidone, olanzapine, quetiapine, ziprasidone, and aripiprazole) have been studied in the treatment of delirium [39–42]. Single case reports, case series, retrospective analyses, and open-label studies have found these medications to be safe, well tolerated, and effective.

Quetiapine may have a niche role in the treatment of delirium in patients with Parkinson's disease or Lewy body dementia, since its action at various subtypes of dopamine receptors is less likely to exacerbate these disorders [43]. The strict regulation of clozapine due to the risk of agranulocytosis effectively precludes its use in delirium.

In 2005, the FDA required that a black-box warning be placed on all atypical neuroleptics indicating an increased risk of death when used to treat behavioral problems in elderly patients with dementia and, in 2008, broadened this warning to encompass conventional neuroleptics. In addition, risperidone, olanzapine, and aripiprazole carry warnings regarding a potential increased risk of cerebrovascular events in elderly patients with dementia-related psychosis. The benefits of neuroleptics in treating delirium often outweigh their risks.

Randomized, Controlled Trials of Dopamine Receptor Antagonists in Delirium

To date, there have been five randomized, controlled trials investigating neuroleptics in the management of acute delirium, and two randomized, double-blind, placebo-controlled trials of a neuroleptic for the prophylaxis of delirium (Table 197.7) [31,44–49]. Of the five treatment studies, four demonstrated clinical improvement in delirium with the use of neuroleptics (specifically haloperidol, chlorpromazine, risperidone, olanzapine, and quetiapine). The remaining study by Girard and colleagues used only presence or absence of delirium as a measure

TABLE 197.7

RANDOMIZED, CONTROLLED TRIALS OF NEUROLEPTIC AGENTS IN DELIRIUM

Study	Response examined	Oral agents compared	Total number of patients	Results
Breitbart et al. [31]	Treatment	Haloperidol Chlorpromazine Lorazepam	30	Both neuroleptics significantly improved delirium. No improvement was seen with lorazepam. The lorazepam arm was terminated early due to adverse effects.
Han et al. [44]	Treatment	Haloperidol Risperidone	24	No significant difference was found in efficacy or response rate between haloperidol and risperidone.
Skrobik et al. [45]	Treatment	Haloperidol Olanzapine	73	Clinical improvement was similar for both agents. Haloperidol was associated with extrapyramidal side effects not seen with olanzapine.
Devlin et al. [46]	Treatment	Quetiapine Placebo	36	Scheduled quetiapine resulted in more rapid resolution of delirium, reduced agitation, and improved rates of transfer to home or a rehabilitation facility. Both groups received as-needed intravenous haloperidol.
Girard et al. [47]	Treatment	Haloperidol Ziprasidone Placebo	101	All patients were mechanically ventilated. Neither neuroleptic significantly decreased duration of delirium.
Kalisvaart et al. [48]	Prophylaxis	Haloperidol Placebo	430	Low-dose haloperidol did not reduce the incidence of postoperative delirium. It decreased severity and duration of delirium and length of stay.
Prakanrattana et al. [49]	Prophylaxis	Risperidone Placebo	126	Single-dose risperidone following cardiac surgery significantly reduced the incidence of postoperative delirium.

of clinical status [47]. Since the definitive treatment of delirium requires identification and treatment of the underlying cause, it may not be reasonable to expect that a neuroleptic will completely eradicate all symptoms of a delirium to the point that it is undetectable. Rather, neuroleptics are intended to manage the symptoms of delirium and to reduce the likelihood of further harm to the patient or ICU staff.

Dexmedetomidine

Dexmedetomidine is a selective α_2-adrenergic receptor agonist used as a sedative and analgesic in the ICU. A number of randomized, controlled trials have demonstrated a significantly lower incidence of delirium when ICU patients were sedated with dexmedetomidine compared with midazolam, lorazepam, or propofol [50–52]. An additional study comparing dexmedetomidine with morphine found a comparable incidence but a shorter duration of delirium with dexmedetomidine [53]. A randomized, open-label trial comparing dexmedetomidine infusion with IV haloperidol for the management of delirious intubated patients demonstrated significantly shortened time to extubation and length of ICU stay with dexmedetomidine [54]. Despite the relatively high cost of the drug, two studies have demonstrated it to be cost-effective due to the offset of time spent ventilated, time in the ICU, and the sparing of other expensive sedating agents [52,55].

Prevention

When possible, patient education limits distress from the experience of delirium. If a patient is to undergo a procedure that carries a high risk of delirium, or has multiple risk factors for delirium, preemptively informing the patient of the risk of delirium, describing its clinical course, and emphasizing it may be experientially distressing but that it is not uncommon or permanent have proven helpful in limiting the emotional dysregulation that may lead to behavioral problems later in the course. Similarly, education of the patient's family and reduction of their distress can result in an environment that is more reassuring to the patient and less likely to foment paranoia.

Environmental cues in the ICU can prove invaluable in helping the patient maintain a sense of temporal continuity, thus reducing disorientation. Maintenance of a regular sleep–wake cycle is vital, with lighting cues adjusted to simulate night and day as closely as possible. Noise should be limited at night, although in a busy ICU this may not always be tenable. Televisions should be turned off, and noises from monitors, pumps, and pagers adjusted to a reasonable minimum.

Efforts should be made to orient the patient with a clock, a calendar, and a clearly visible sign indicating the name of the hospital. Measures to increase the familiarity of the milieu with photographs, items from home, and visits from family members can also limit disorientation and distress. Because some patients may be unwilling to report the presence of perceptual disturbances because of fear or shame, frequent reassurance that such phenomena are not a sign of going "crazy" can prevent a frightened patient from acting injudiciously.

One randomized, double-blind, placebo-controlled study examined the use of haloperidol started preoperatively in elderly patients undergoing hip surgery as prophylaxis against postoperative delirium [48]. Results indicated that, while there was no statistically significant decrease in the incidence of delirium, there were significant decreases in severity and duration of delirium and in the length of hospital stay. Another study examined the administration of a single dose of risperidone after cardiac surgery and demonstrated a significant decrease in the incidence of delirium [49].

OTHER CAUSES OF AGITATION

Dementia is a predisposing risk factor for the development of delirium. The demented patient, however, is also at risk of becoming agitated in the ICU as a result of unfamiliar surroundings and possible delusional beliefs. Behavioral measures should be employed to help the patient orient to the milieu. In cases of acute agitation, haloperidol is the treatment of choice; however, in cases of Lewy body dementia, quetiapine is less likely to exacerbate parkinsonian symptoms.

Similarly, the patient with preexisting schizophrenia may have difficulty in understanding and adapting to an ICU stay. Preemptive behavioral measures should be taken to make the ICU as familiar and comfortable as possible.

TABLE 197.8

DIFFERENTIAL DIAGNOSIS OF AGITATION

	Delirium	Dementia	Depression	Schizophrenia
Onset	Acute	Insidious[a]	Variable	Variable
Course	Fluctuating	Progressive[b]	Variable	Variable
Reversibility	Usually	Not usually	Usually	Not usually
Level of consciousness	Impaired	Unimpaired until late stages	Unimpaired	Unimpaired[c]
Attention and memory	Both poor	Poor memory without marked inattention	Attention usually intact, memory intact	Poor attention, memory intact
Hallucinations	Usually visual but can occur in any sensory modality	Visual or auditory	Usually auditory	Usually auditory
Delusions	Fleeting, fragmented, usually persecutory	Paranoid, often fixed	Complex and mood-congruent	Frequent, complex, systematized, and often paranoid

[a] Except when due to strokes, when the onset is acute.
[b] Lewy body dementia often presents with a waxing and waning course imposed on an overall progressive decline. Vascular dementia follows a stepwise pattern, worsening with each successive stroke.
[c] Except when complicated by catatonia.
Adapted from Trzepacz PT, Meagher DJ: Delirium, in Levenson JL (ed): *The American Psychiatric Publishing Textbook of Psychosomatic Medicine.* Washington, DC, American Psychiatric Publishing, 2005, pp 91–130.

Inadequately controlled pain, panic-like anxiety, and a sense of hopelessness resulting from depression can also present with agitation. Anxiety and depression are discussed in Chapters 198 and 199, respectively. Once the trigger for agitation is understood, the appropriate course of treatment is often relatively straightforward. Table 197.8 compares and contrasts several diagnostic traits characteristic of different causes of agitation.

Various substance-withdrawal syndromes may present with agitation and delirium. These often require specific treatment (usually featuring replacement of the dependence-inducing agent and gradual taper) and are covered in Chapter 145.

NONPHARMACOLOGIC TREATMENT OF AGITATION

Despite all efforts to curtail agitated or disruptive behavior, some patients may ultimately require physical intervention to prevent injury to themselves or hospital staff. Interventions range from relatively unobtrusive (e.g., use of mitts to prevent interference with equipment or constant observation to minimize wandering) to more restrictive (e.g., soft limb restraints, Posey vests, four-point locked leather restraints) [28]. Most states and individual institutions have protocols governing the application and documentation of such procedures. Since the application of physical restraints can, in itself, be disquieting to the patient, such intervention should be accompanied by the administration of sedating medication.

LONG-TERM SEQUELAE

Patients diagnosed with delirium are at greater risk for a multitude of neuropsychiatric sequelae long after their discharge from the hospital. Multiple studies have demonstrated increased risk of longstanding cognitive impairment in delirious patients when compared to matched controls [56–58]; one study reported that a diagnosis of delirium resulted in an almost doubled risk of cognitive impairment at 2 years [59]. A review of the available literature by Jackson and colleagues concluded that the presence of delirium (regardless of severity or duration) predicts a greater risk of long-term cognitive impairment, including the development of dementia [60]. Post-traumatic stress disorder (PTSD) has been reported in up to 44% of patients admitted to the ICU [61]. While PTSD may result from the experience of actual physical experiences in the ICU, it has also been reported to occur as the sole result of frightening, hallucinatory, or delusional symptoms experienced in the context of delirium [62]. PTSD is fully discussed in Chapter 198.

CONCLUSION

Agitation in the ICU patient jeopardizes the immediate safety of the patient and may signify a potentially unidentified pathologic process. Delirium is the most frequent cause of agitation and is associated with poorer outcomes across multiple facets of patient care. Careful evaluation of possible causes of delirium is vital, since its only definitive cure is identification and treatment of the responsible underlying condition. Management may involve both pharmacologic and environmental measures, with manipulation of the dopaminergic and cholinergic axes, the primary targets of pharmacologic intervention.

Agitation may also be a symptom of other psychiatric disorders. Preexisting diagnoses of dementia, depression, or psychosis do not rule out the presence of delirium; however, active delirium does rule out the possibility of being able to diagnose a new dementia, depression, or psychosis. Given this level of diagnostic primacy and its manifold associated deleterious sequelae, delirium should be at the cornerstone of any investigation of agitation in the ICU.

References

1. Hippocrates: *On Regimen in Acute Diseases* (Part 11), in Adams F (trans): *The Internet Classics Archive*. Available at: http://classics.mit.edu/Hippocrates/acutedis.html. Accessed February 3, 2010.
2. McGuire BE, Basten CJ, Ryan CJ, et al: Intensive care unit syndrome: a dangerous misnomer. *Arch Intern Med* 160:906–909, 2000.
3. American Psychiatric Association: *Diagnostic and Statistical Manual of Mental Disorders*. 4th ed. Text Revision. Washington, DC, American Psychiatric Association, 2000.
4. McNicoll L, Pisani MA, Zhang Y, et al: Delirium in the intensive care unit: occurrence and clinical course in older patients. *J Am Geriatr* Soc 51:591–598, 2003.
5. Ely EW, Shintani A, Truman B, et al: Delirium as a predictor of mortality in mechanically ventilated patients in the intensive care unit. *JAMA* 291:1753–1762, 2004.
6. Thomason JW, Shintani A, Peterson JF, et al: Intensive care unit delirium is an independent predictor of longer hospital stay: a prospective analysis of 261 non-ventilated patients. *Crit Care* 9:R375–R381, 2005.
7. Milbrandt EB, Deppen S, Harrison PL, et al: Costs associated with delirium in mechanically ventilated patients. *Crit Care Med* 32:955–962, 2004.
8. Franco K, Litaker D, Locala J, et al: The cost of delirium in the surgical patient. *Psychosomatics* 42:68–73, 2001.
9. Atkins PM, Mion LC, Mendelson W, et al: Characteristics and outcomes of patients who self-extubate from ventilatory support: a case-control study. *Chest* 112:1317–1323, 1997.
10. Tuma R, DeAngelis LM: Altered mental status in patients with cancer. *Arch Neurol* 57:1727–1731, 2000.
11. Gaudreau JD, Gagnon P, Harel F, et al: Psychoactive medications and risk of delirium in hospitalized cancer patients. *J Clin Oncol* 23:6712–6718, 2005.
12. Querques J: An approach to acute changes in mental status, in Stern TA (ed): *The Ten-Minute Guide to Psychiatric Diagnosis and Treatment*. New York, Professional Publishing Group, 2005, pp 97–107.
13. Brown TM: Basic mechanisms in the pathogenesis of delirium, in Stoudemire A, Fogel BS, Greenberg D (eds): *Psychiatric Care of the Medical Patient*. 2nd ed. New York, Oxford University Press, 2000, pp 571–580.
14. Seaman JS, Schillerstrom J, Carroll D, et al: Impaired oxidative metabolism precipitates delirium: a study of 101 ICU patients. *Psychosomatics* 47:56–61, 2006.
15. Ely EW, Siegel MD, Inouye SK: Delirium in the intensive care unit: an under-recognized syndrome of organ dysfunction. *Semin Respir Crit Care Med* 22:115–126, 2001.
16. Breitbart W, Gibson C, Tremblay A: The delirium experience: delirium recall and delirium-related distress in hospitalized patients with cancer, their spouses/caregivers, and their nurses. *Psychosomatics* 43:183–194, 2002.
17. Ely EW, Inouye SK, Bernard GR, et al: Delirium in mechanically ventilated patients: validity and reliability of the confusion assessment method for the intensive care unit (CAM-ICU). *JAMA* 286:2703–2710, 2001.
18. Bergeron N, Dubois MJ, Dumont M, et al: Intensive care delirium screening checklist: evaluation of a new screening tool. *Intensive Care Med* 27:859–864, 2001.
19. Engel G, Romano J: Delirium, a syndrome of cerebral insufficiency. *J Chronic Dis* 9:260–277, 1959.
20. Jacobson S, Jerrier H: EEG in delirium. *Semin Clin Neuropsychiatry* 5:86–92, 2000.
21. Bourgeois JA, Wegelin JA: Lagtime in psychosomatic medicine consultations for cognitive-disorder patients: association with length of stay. *Psychosomatics* 50:622–625, 2009.
22. Burns MJ, Linden CH, Graudins A, et al: A comparison of physostigmine and benzodiazepines for the treatment of anticholinergic poisoning. *Ann Emerg Med* 35:374–381, 2000.
23. Dautzenberg PL, Wouters CJ, Oudejans I, et al: Rivastigmine in prevention of delirium in a 65 year old man with Parkinson's disease. *Int J Geriatr Psychiatry* 18:555–556, 2003.
24. Dautzenberg PL, Mulder LJ, Olde Rikkert MG, et al: Delirium in elderly hospitalized patients: protective effects of chronic rivastigmine usage. *Int J Geriatr Psychiatry* 19:641–644, 2004.
25. Liptzin B, Laki A, Garb JL, et al: Donepezil in the prevention and treatment of post-surgical delirium. *Am J Geriatr Psychiatry* 13:1100–1106, 2005.

26. Sampson EL, Raven PR, Ndhlovu PN, et al: A randomized, double-blind, placebo-controlled trial of donepezil hydrochloride (Aricept) for reducing the incidence of postoperative delirium after elective total hip replacement. *Int J Geriatr Psychiatry* 22:343–349, 2007.
27. Gamberini M, Bolliger D, Lurati Buse GA, et al: Rivastigmine for the prevention of postoperative delirium in elderly patients undergoing elective cardiac surgery—a randomized controlled trial. *Crit Care Med* 37:1762–1768, 2009.
28. American Psychiatric Association: Practice guideline for the treatment of patients with delirium. *Am J Psychiatry* 156[5, Suppl]:1–20, 1999.
29. Cassem NH, Murray GB, Lafayette JM, et al: Delirious patients, in Stern TA, Fricchione GL, Cassem NH, et al (eds): *Massachusetts General Hospital Handbook of General Hospital Psychiatry*. 5th ed. Philadelphia, PA, Mosby, 2004, pp 119–134.
30. Menza MA, Murray GB, Holmes VF, et al: Decreased extrapyramidal symptoms with intravenous haloperidol. *J Clin Psychiatry* 48:278–280, 1987.
31. Breitbart W, Marotta R, Platt MM, et al: A double-blind trial of haloperidol, chlorpromazine, and lorazepam in the treatment of delirium in hospitalized AIDS patients. *Am J Psychiatry* 153(2):231–237, 1996.
32. Adams F, Fernandez F, Andersson BS: Emergency pharmacotherapy of delirium in the critically ill cancer patient. *Psychosomatics* 27[1, Suppl]:33–38, 1986.
33. Menza MA, Murray GB, Holmes VF, et al: Controlled study of extrapyramidal reactions in the management of delirious, medically ill patients: haloperidol versus intravenous haloperidol plus benzodiazepines. *Heart Lung* 17:238–241, 1988.
34. Pisani F, Oteri G, Costa C, et al: Effects of psychotropic drugs on seizure threshold. *Drug Saf* 25:91–110, 2002.
35. Metzger E, Friedman R: Prolongation of the corrected QT and torsades de pointes cardiac arrhythmia associated with intravenous haloperidol in the medically ill. *J Clin Psychopharmacol* 13:128–132, 1993.
36. Hunt N, Stern TA: The association between intravenous haloperidol and torsades de pointes: three cases and a literature review. *Psychosomatics* 36:541–549, 1995.
37. Stöllberger C, Huber JO, Finsterer J: Antipsychotic drugs and QT prolongation. *Int Clin Psychopharmacol* 20:243–251, 2005.
38. Kao LW, Kirk MA, Evers SJ, et al: Droperidol, QT prolongation, and sudden death: what is the evidence? *Ann Emerg Med* 41:546–558, 2003.
39. Alao AO, Soderberg M, Pohl EL, et al: Aripiprazole in the treatment of delirium. *Int J Psychiatry Med* 35:429–433, 2005.
40. Boettger S, Breitbart W: Atypical antipsychotics in the management of delirium: a review of the empirical literature. *Palliat Support Care* 3:227–238, 2005.
41. Lacasse H, Perreault MM, Williamson DR: Systematic review of antipsychotics for the treatment of hospital-associated delirium in medically or surgically ill patients. *Ann Pharmacother* 40:1966–1973, 2006.
42. Straker DA, Shapiro PA, Muskin PR: Aripiprazole in the treatment of delirium. *Psychosomatics* 47:385–391, 2006.
43. Lauterbach EC: The neuropsychiatry of Parkinson's disease and related disorders. *Psychiatr Clin North Am* 27:801–825, 2004.
44. Han CS, Kim YK: A double-blind trial of risperidone and haloperidol for the treatment of delirium. *Psychosomatics* 45:297–301, 2004.
45. Skrobik YK, Bergeron N, Dumont M, et al: Olanzapine vs haloperidol: treatment of delirium in the critical care setting. *Intensive Care Med* 30:444–449, 2004.
46. Devlin JW, Roberts RJ, Fong JJ, et al: Efficacy and safety of quetiapine in critically ill patients with delirium: a prospective, multicenter, randomized, double-blind, placebo-controlled pilot study. *Crit Care Med* 38:419–427, 2010.
47. Girard TD, Pandharipande PP, Carson SS, et al: Feasibility, efficacy, and safety of antipsychotics for intensive care unit delirium: the MIND randomized, placebo-controlled trial. *Crit Care Med* 38:428–437, 2010.
48. Kalisvaart KJ, de Jonghe JF, Bogaards MJ, et al: Haloperidol prophylaxis for elderly hip-surgery patients at risk for delirium: a randomized placebo-controlled study. *J Am Geriatr Soc* 53:1658–1666, 2005.
49. Prakanrattana U, Prapaitrakool S: Efficacy of risperidone for prevention of postoperative delirium in cardiac surgery. *Anaesth Intensive Care* 35:714–719, 2007.
50. Pandharipande PP, Pun BT, Herr DL, et al: Effect of sedation with dexmedetomidine vs lorazepam on acute brain dysfunction in mechanically ventilated patients: the MENDS randomized controlled trial. *JAMA* 298:2644–2653, 2007.
51. Riker RR, Shehabi Y, Bokesch PM, et al: Dexmedetomidine vs midazolam for sedation of critically ill patients: a randomized trial. *JAMA* 301:489–499, 2009.
52. Maldonado JR, Wysong A, van der Starre PJ, et al: Dexmedetomidine and the reduction of postoperative delirium after cardiac surgery. *Psychosomatics* 50:206–217, 2009.
53. Shehabi Y, Grant P, Wolfenden H, et al: Prevalence of delirium with dexmedetomidine compared with morphine based therapy after cardiac surgery: a randomized controlled trial (DEXmedetomidine COmpared to Morphine-DEXCOM Study). *Anesthesiology* 111:1075–1084, 2009.
54. Reade MC, O'Sullivan K, Bates S, et al: Dexmedetomidine vs. haloperidol in delirious, agitated, intubated patients: a randomised open-label trial. *Crit Care* 13:R75, 2009.
55. Dasta JF, Kane-Gill SL, Pencina M, et al: A cost-minimization analysis of dexmedetomidine compared with midazolam for long-term sedation in the intensive care unit. *Crit Care Med* 38:497–503, 2010.
56. Francis J, Kapoor WN: Prognosis after hospital discharge of older medical patients with delirium. *J Am Geriatr Soc* 40:601–606, 1992.
57. McCusker J, Cole M, Dendukuri N, et al: Delirium in older medical inpatients and subsequent cognitive and functional status: a prospective study. *CMAJ* 165:575–583, 2001.
58. Katz IR, Curyto KJ, TenHave T, et al: Validating the diagnosis of delirium and evaluating its association with deterioration over a one-year period. *Am J Geriatr Psychiatry* 9:148–159, 2001.
59. Dolan MM, Hawkes WG, Zimmerman SI, et al: Delirium on hospital admission in aged hip fracture patients: prediction of mortality and 2-year functional outcomes. *J Gerontol A Biol Sci Med Sci* 55:M527–M534, 2000.
60. Jackson JC, Gordon SM, Hart RP, et al: The association between delirium and cognitive decline: a review of the empirical literature. *Neuropsychol Rev* 14:87–98, 2004.
61. Kapfhammer HP, Rothenhausler HB, Krauseneck T, et al: Posttraumatic stress disorder and health-related quality of life in long-term survivors of acute respiratory distress syndrome. *Am J Psychiatry* 161:45–52, 2004.
62. DiMartini A, Dew MA, Kormos R, et al: Posttraumatic stress disorder caused by hallucinations and delusions experienced in delirium. *Psychosomatics* 48:436–439, 2007.

CHAPTER 198 ■ DIAGNOSIS AND TREATMENT OF ANXIETY IN THE INTENSIVE CARE UNIT PATIENT

SHELLEY A. HOLMER AND ROBERT M. TIGHE

Anxiety is a normal, adaptive biological response to threat. It occurs when a person feels helpless and apprehensive about an uncertain future due to a perceived inability to predict or control a desired outcome. In contrast, *pathologic anxiety* is normal anxiety run amok. It occurs spontaneously or amid usually benign circumstances, is excessive in intensity or duration, and impairs functioning and behavior. Anxiety manifests in a variety of ways, resulting in physical, affective, behavioral, and cognitive symptoms and signs (Table 198.1).

Patients admitted to the intensive care unit (ICU) commonly experience anxiety in response to pain, invasive procedures, an unfamiliar setting, and the fear of death. In moderation, anxiety

TABLE 198.1

SYMPTOMS AND SIGNS OF ANXIETY

Physical	Behavioral
Tachycardia	Restlessness
Tachypnea	Agitation
Hypertension	Compulsiveness
Diaphoresis	Avoidance
Light-headedness	Noncompliance with diagnostic or therapeutic interventions
Tremulousness	Fidgetiness
Affective	Cognitive
Uneasiness	Apprehension
Edginess	Worry
Nervousness	Fear of emotional or bodily damage
Fright	Denial
Panic	Obsessiveness
Terror	Preoccupation with harm
	Thoughts about death

can promote healthful behaviors, just as pain can lead to protection from future injury. In excess, however, anxiety can complicate diagnosis, interfere with treatment, and contribute to poor outcomes by increasing both morbidity and mortality. Anxiety can complicate the clinical picture, as symptoms and signs of many medical problems overlap with those of anxiety (e.g., chest pain, palpitations, tachycardia, diaphoresis, tremulousness). Overwrought patients may refuse tests or procedures they fear will cause pain or will lead to bad news. Patients with phobias of blood, needles, and confined spaces (e.g., as in computed tomography and magnetic resonance imaging machines) may forego necessary interventions. Pathologic anxiety may contribute to the need for ICU admission in the first place.

This chapter reviews the physiologic concomitants of anxiety, medical causes of anxiety, critical medical conditions particularly affected by anxiety, anxiety disorders specific to the ICU setting, and the treatment of anxiety.

PHYSIOLOGIC EXPRESSIONS OF ANXIETY

The physiologic expressions of anxiety are myriad. By activating the *fight or flight response*, anxiety recruits the entire autonomic nervous system to respond to an unknown enemy. Multiple organ systems—endocrine, gastrointestinal, musculoskeletal, immune, cardiovascular, and respiratory—are involved [1]. Anxiety increases blood levels of cortisol, prolactin, and growth hormone [2]. A disquieted patient has enhanced gastric motility and gastric secretions, vasoconstriction of the splanchnic and cutaneous circulations, and vasodilation of striated muscle groups [3]. Anxiety also has direct effects on the immune system: a reduction in the chemotaxis of lymphocytes and neutrophils, a decrease in the phagocytic ability of neutrophils, and an increase in plasma levels of tumor necrosis factor α and superoxide anion [4]. This suggests a complex physiologic effect of anxiety in the critically ill population.

The organ systems adversely affected by anxiety of most concern to the intensivist are the cardiovascular and respiratory systems. Anxiety affects the cardiovascular system by altering normal autonomic tone, manifested as increases in heart rate, blood pressure, cardiac output, and cardiac irritability [1]. The stress of simply being hospitalized augments urinary excretion of catecholamines, which represents activation of the sympathetic nervous system and contributes to cardiac arrhythmias [5]. In the fight or flight response, augmentation of cardiac output prevents cardiovascular collapse, but, in heart failure and myocardial infarction (MI), excessive cardiac output can be detrimental. Anxiety increases respiratory rate, tidal volume, and airway resistance [6] and can induce hyperventilation and syncope. These data suggest that anxiety, while exacting a psychological toll, also significantly alters cardiorespiratory physiology, especially in the critical care setting.

MEDICAL CAUSES OF ANXIETY

Because failure to identify and treat *organic* (i.e., *medical* or *secondary*) causes of anxiety can result in increased morbidity and mortality, the distinction between organic and *functional* (i.e., *psychiatric* or *primary*) causes is vitally important. The presence of an organic cause is suggested when anxiety occurs autonomously in the absence of an apparent psychologically charged situation or of a discrete physical event (e.g., acute pain or tachyarrhythmia). However, in any given patient, determination of what constitutes an appropriate or sufficient psychological precipitant for anxiety is difficult. Life history, cultural background, and prior behavioral conditioning are often unknown to clinicians in the fast-paced ICU setting. Therefore, when anxiety is present and no clear psychological or medical cause is obvious, a thorough search for an organic cause is indicated.

Anxiety is a symptom of hundreds of medical conditions; Table 198.2 provides a list of conditions common in the ICU. Two syndromes that are particularly difficult to distinguish from primary anxiety are delirium and substance withdrawal.

Delirium

Treating delirious patients solely with anxiolytics (e.g., benzodiazepines) can exacerbate their confusion, so it is important to distinguish delirium from anxiety by doing a brief cognitive examination. In delirium, performance of tasks of attention, orientation, memory, and language is often impaired; rarely does an anxious patient have these deficits. By definition, delirium always has a medical cause; therefore, determination of its cause, rather than simply treating its symptoms, is vital. Recognition and management of delirium are discussed in Chapter 197.

TABLE 198.2

COMMON MEDICAL CAUSES OF ANXIETY

Neurologic	Respiratory
Delirium	Respiratory failure
Substance withdrawal syndromes	Asthma
Complex partial seizures	Hypoxia
Traumatic brain injury	Hyperventilation
Pain	Pneumothorax
Cardiac	Pulmonary edema
Acute myocardial infarction	Pulmonary embolism
Shock	Toxic
Paroxysmal tachycardia	Illicit drug intoxication
Metabolic	Anticholinergic intoxication
Hypoglycemia	Prednisone
Hyperthyroidism	Isoniazid
Pheochromocytoma	Caffeine
Cushing's syndrome	
Addison's disease	

Substance Withdrawal Syndromes

Because withdrawal from central nervous system depressants (e.g., opioids, benzodiazepines, alcohol) can be life-threatening, it should always be high on the differential diagnosis of anxiety. This diagnosis can be missed because patients either under-report their substance use or are unable to communicate. Patients can also withdraw from sedatives and opioids prescribed during a lengthy period of mechanical ventilation. Recognition and treatment of withdrawal syndromes are discussed in Chapter 145.

SCENARIOS IN WHICH ANXIETY SIGNIFICANTLY AFFECTS OUTCOMES OF MEDICAL ILLNESS

Acute Myocardial Infarction

As heart disease remains the leading cause of mortality in the United States, *acute coronary syndrome* is a common reason for admission to the coronary care unit (CCU). Prevention and treatment have focused on awareness and alteration of traditional risk factors (e.g., hyperlipidemia, hypertension, family history). A developing literature supports consideration of psychosocial factors as well, most frequently, anxiety, depression, and personality traits [7–11].

Anxiety is a frequent occurrence in the CCU, both related to MI itself and as a premorbid condition contributing to the development of MI [12]. In the general hospital, anxiety has been noted to occur in 24% to 31% of patients after MI [13]. The stress of being cared for in an ICU, particularly the relinquishing of control and privacy, in addition to dealing with a potentially life-threatening disease, contribute to anxiety in this setting [9]. Anxiety in the CCU after MI rapidly rises and peaks within the first 12 hours; declines, though persists, during the next 36 hours; and then increases again as patients face transfer out of the CCU and ultimately discharge from the hospital [14]. Physicians and nurses often under-recognize anxiety and underestimate its severity after MI [15]. Anxiolysis should be an early consideration in post-MI patients.

Physiologically, anxiety-disordered patients have decreased heart rate variability, which may result in an alteration in cardiac autonomic tone [16,17], either by heightened sympathetic stimulation or diminished vagal control [7]. Enhanced sympathetic stimulation is associated with arrhythmias [18], and reduced vagal control is linked with impairment in the baroreflex control of the heart; both perturbations are associated with sudden death [19]. These physiologic changes may explain why anxiety—especially phobic anxiety—enhances risk for sudden death [20,21]. In addition, elevated anxiety is associated with poor implementation of important risk-reducing recommendations after MI, particularly stress reduction, greater socialization, smoking cessation, and adherence to carrying supplies [22].

Two groups demonstrated that anxiety, independent of depressive symptoms, was associated with in-hospital complications after acute MI, including recurrent ischemia, reinfarction, congestive heart failure, and ventricular arrhythmias [9,10]. Further trials are required to determine the nature of this relationship; whether the effect of anxiety is "dose"-dependent; and whether effective anxiety treatment improves cardiac outcomes acutely.

Several studies have looked at the correlation between anxiety and post-MI outcomes in the long term. Some [12,23,24], but not all [25–28], prospective trials demonstrated that high levels of anxiety predicted cardiac events (unstable angina, reinfarction) and/or mortality. Meyer et al. [11] showed that anxiety predicted greater mortality in post-MI patients only if left ventricular function was reduced. These reports suggest that the data for hard cardiac endpoints over the long term remain unclear.

Weaning from Mechanical Ventilation

Respiratory failure and consequent need for mechanical ventilation are common causes of admission to the ICU. Nearly three fourths of patients resume spontaneous, unassisted breathing with little difficulty [29]. However, patients who require prolonged mechanical ventilation have longer hospital stays, face higher morbidity and mortality, and require lengthier rehabilitation. Therefore, the goal is to wean patients as soon as possible.

The experience of shortness of breath has been well associated with anxiety and is one of the most commonly reported symptoms in panic disorder. In fact, anxiety and panic have been shown to lead to hyperventilation, which, when performed voluntarily, induces panic attacks and mediates a wide variety of psychosomatic symptoms [6]. Chronic hyperventilation due to anxiety and panic leads to hypocapnia and slowed recovery from changes in respiratory status. The integral connection between anxiety and respiratory physiology suggests anxiety may contribute to respiratory failure.

Given the limitations of communication and easy fatigability in patients with critical illness, the evaluation of anxiety in this setting remains difficult. Nearly 60% of patients on a ventilator may experience moderate levels of anxiety. The highest levels occur in patients intubated for primary respiratory disorders (e.g., chronic obstructive pulmonary disease [COPD]) and in those on prolonged (>22 days) artificial ventilation, the very groups who are most at risk for difficulty weaning from mechanical ventilation [30].

Although the physiologic measures used to determine readiness to wean from the ventilator are well known and several of them have been studied closely in clinical trials, information about the effect of the patient's psychological state, specifically anxiety, on weaning from the ventilator is scant. Anxiety may cause shortness of breath and a fear of death or abandonment, especially as ventilatory support is withdrawn. This can stimulate the sympathetic nervous system; cause bronchoconstriction; and increase airway resistance, work of breathing, and oxygen demand. This cascade can become a perpetuating cycle of anxiety, muscle fatigue, and thus weaning failure [31].

Anxiety should be considered in all patients during the weaning process, especially those who are intubated for primary respiratory causes and for a prolonged period. Given the paucity of data regarding the effect of anxiety on ventilator weaning, no clear treatment guidelines exist; however, it is well appreciated that weaning should be approached from a multidisciplinary standpoint. Treatment includes pharmacologic, environmental, and educational approaches, and is enhanced when both patient and nursing staff are involved in the decision to wean and in the process of weaning.

Because anxiety and respiratory distress due to fatiguing respiratory muscles can produce similar cardiorespiratory manifestations, it is important to try to distinguish between these two syndromes. Only if one is convinced that anxiety is the cause should one consider pharmacotherapy for anxiety because pharmacotherapy with benzodiazepines can potentially prolong weaning due to central pump fatigue from respiratory depression (see Chapter 60 on Mechanical Ventilation Part III: Discontinuation). Although this class of medications is associated with respiratory depression and altered level of consciousness, benzodiazepines can be quite effective when used judiciously in the correct setting. Neuroleptics are less associated with respiratory depression and may be more beneficial than benzodiazepines, especially for patients whose weaning failure is due to fear or to delirious agitation.

More recent evidence suggests a role for dexmedetomidine, an α_2-adrenergic receptor agonist, which causes a rapid onset of sedation and analgesia but not respiratory depression [32–34]. The lack of respiratory-depressant effects allows patients to be extubated while remaining on dexmedetomidine, whereas benzodiazepines require discontinuation or reduction prior to extubation. Though not specifically studied in anxious patients, dexmedetomidine demonstrates adequate sedation and decreased time on the ventilator, suggesting that it may be a useful agent in the anxious patient attempting to wean from the ventilator.

Nursing support is critical in successful weaning. Staffing should remain as consistent as possible with an individual patient, and during active weaning, a 1:1 nurse-to-patient ratio should be maintained. Weaning is more successful when patients are aware of their environment and engaged in discussions of the plan and process of weaning. Patients should be told and reminded that weaning without extubation does not represent a failure but is part of the process. Music therapy has been associated with decreased anxiety levels in ICU patients and may facilitate weaning [35].

Asthma

Up to 8.9% of adults in the United States have been diagnosed with asthma; of those, 3.4% have experienced an episode in the preceding 12 months [34]. In a multicenter study in 2000, 10% of 29,430 admissions for asthma were to the ICU and 2.1% of these patients were intubated [36]. Despite the advent of inhaled corticosteroids in 1972, there continues to be a population of patients with brittle or near-fatal asthma that follows a poor clinical course even with aggressive use of anti-inflammatory agents. This has re-heightened attention to psychological factors (e.g., anxiety, depression, and denial) as a possible focus of intervention in these patients.

Anxiety has a strong association with asthma, particularly in severe cases admitted to the hospital. Anxiety-spectrum disorders have been identified among individuals suffering near-fatal asthma attacks, and patients who deny the disease process are more likely to develop near-fatal asthma attacks [37,38]. A prospective study of children with asthma identified a relationship between stressful life events and new asthma attacks both immediately and 5 to 7 weeks after a stressful event [39]. Despite this, there appears to be no difference in anxiety or other psychological parameters in adults with severe, life-threatening asthma compared to asthma patients requiring hospital admission [40]. Due to the retrospective reporting in many of these studies, however, a causal relationship between anxiety and asthma cannot be confirmed; moreover, whether the association is due to a direct physiologic impact on airway resistance or reflects a comorbid disease process is not known [41]. Despite the lack of answers, it is clear that asthmatic patients suffer from higher rates of anxiety. For this reason, anxiolysis in ICU patients admitted for asthma exacerbations may need to be considered.

ANXIETY DISORDERS SPECIFIC TO THE INTENSIVE CARE UNIT

Patients with a variety of anxiety disorders present to the ICU. Symptoms associated with these conditions can be exacerbated by the acute medical or surgical problem that led to the ICU admission. In addition, medications used to treat a preexisting anxiety disorder may be discontinued on admission, or their bioavailability may be altered by interactions with newly prescribed medications. Both discontinuation and pharmacokinetic changes may significantly worsen preexisting primary anxiety disorders. In addition to exacerbating established psychiatric illnesses, the experience of the ICU can lead to new, longstanding anxiety disorders [42]. Anxiety disorders particularly relevant in the ICU include acute stress disorder (ASD), posttraumatic stress disorder (PTSD), and panic disorder.

Acute and Posttraumatic Stress Disorders

The experience of treatment in the ICU—which includes frightening confusion, painful invasive procedures, and fear of death—can be traumatic for many patients. Often, especially in the surgical ICU, patients are admitted due to a traumatic event (e.g., motor vehicle accident, severe burn, and assault). These circumstances predispose patients to the development of ASD and PTSD.

Diagnosis of both ASD and PTSD requires clinically significant distress following an experience of threatened death or serious injury, which engenders intense fear, helplessness, or horror in the traumatized person. That event is then re-experienced through dreams, intrusive memories, flashbacks, or intense distress when exposed to reminders of the event. Other characteristic symptoms include emotional numbing, anhedonia, amnesia, restricted affect, and symptoms of autonomic arousal (e.g., irritability, hypervigilance, and exaggerated startle response). For a diagnosis of ASD, these symptoms must occur within the first month after the trauma; if symptoms persist beyond 1 month, a diagnosis of PTSD should be considered.

Some patients develop syndromes consistent with both ASD and PTSD consequent to events that occur in the ICU. The prevalence of PTSD in ICU patients has been widely studied. A systematic review of the literature found the median point prevalence of clinically significant PTSD symptoms to be 22% (range 8% to 51%), significantly higher than the 3.5% prevalence of PTSD in the general population [43,44]. The risk of developing ASD and PTSD is presumed to be even higher in patients who are admitted to the ICU after a trauma.

There is a burgeoning literature about the prevention of PTSD related to critical care. Several studies have attempted to identify risk factors for developing ICU-related PTSD; the most robust risks are: preexisting anxiety and depression, greater ICU benzodiazepine administration, and memories of in-ICU frightening experiences, nightmares, and delusions [43]. The positive correlation between benzodiazepines and PTSD symptoms may be due to the need for higher doses of these medications in patients with preexisting psychiatric conditions. However, benzodiazepines are likely an independent risk factor for PTSD because they often result in delirium and prolonged sedation, both of which may spawn frightening agitation and delusions and necessitate physical restraint. When patients with ICU-associated PTSD report the content of their intrusive memories and nightmares, they are commonly false memories laid down during periods of delirium or sedation. These false memories fill in memory gaps such that true memories of the ICU stay become interwoven with fragments of dreams, delusions, and hallucinations [45]. Isoflurane may have an advantage over midazolam for sedation in reducing memories of delusions and hallucinations [46]. Studies indicate that false memories of the ICU stay are correlated with higher rates of PTSD and worse health-related quality of life [47–49]. Therefore, interventions that target delirium, disorientation, and faulty reality testing may prevent the development of PTSD. Though the provision of a self-help rehabilitation manual did not reduce anxiety or PTSD symptoms compared to usual care, patients who read a daily-event log recorded for them during their critical care

TABLE 198.3

SYMPTOMS OF A PANIC ATTACK

Neurologic	Respiratory
Feeling dizzy, unsteady, light-headed, or faint	Dyspnea
Feeling unreal or detached from oneself	Sensation of smothering
Fear of losing control, going crazy, or dying	Feeling of choking
Paresthesias	Gastrointestinal
Cardiovascular	Nausea
Palpitations	Abdominal distress
Pounding heart	Miscellaneous
Tachycardia	Diaphoresis
Chest pain or discomfort	Trembling
	Shaking
	Chills
	Hot flashes

Adapted from reference 65.

admission had less anxiety compared to patients who did not read such a diary [50,51].

Even in the absence of delirium, prolonged sedation may contribute to the development of PTSD. Studies comparing daily sedation withdrawal to continuous sedation and light versus deep sedation showed fewer PTSD symptoms with sedation withdrawal and light sedation [52,53].

Studies of psychopharmacologic intervention for the prevention of PTSD have yielded mixed results. Several studies have demonstrated a decrease in the prevalence of PTSD in critically ill patients treated with stress doses of corticosteroids, which are thought to have an effect on traumatic-memory retrieval [54–57]. There is also evidence that treatment with β-receptor antagonists may protect against the development of PTSD, perhaps by blocking catecholamines, which enhance memory of emotionally arousing experiences [58–61]. However, this benefit was not seen in a randomized, controlled trial of critically ill patients [62]. Further research is necessary before prophylactic treatment with either corticosteroids or β-blockers becomes a standard intervention.

In the ICU, acute trauma should be treated with supportive reassurance and symptom-targeted medications. Clinicians should identify and treat delirium, make efforts to reduce unnecessary sedation, and help orient patients to what is happening around them. A recent study identified other modifiable predictors of PTSD: memories about pain, lack of control, and inability to express needs [63]. These can be addressed with appropriate pain assessment and management, allowing patients more choices in their care, and helping patients to communicate (e.g., using Passy-Muir valves in tracheostomized patients). Psychiatric consultation can be useful for both acute management and recommendations for outpatient treatment, especially in patients with preexisting psychiatric illnesses.

Panic Disorder

Panic disorder is one of the most common psychiatric disorders in patients who are high users of medical services. The risk for development of panic disorder is higher in patients with mitral valve prolapse, asthma, COPD, and migraine [64]. As defined

TABLE 198.4

SOME INTRAVENOUS MEDICATIONS FOR THE TREATMENT OF ANXIETY

Drug	Typical dose	Onset (min)	Drug interactions	Side effects
Lorazepam	0.04 mg/kg	5–15	Fewer drug interactions than other benzodiazepines	Respiratory depression, mixed in propylene glycol solution, venous irritation
Diazepam	0.1–0.2 mg/kg	1–3	Effects increased by cimetidine, erythromycin, isoniazid, ketoconazole, metoprolol, propranolol, valproate Effects decreased by rifampin and theophylline	Respiratory depression, mixed in propylene glycol solution, venous irritation
Midazolam	0.025–0.35 mg/kg	1–3	Same as diazepam	Respiratory depression, accumulates with prolonged (>48 h) use, excessive sedation
Propofol	0.25–1 mg/kg (loading dose) then 1–6 mg/kg (continuous infusion)	<1	Minimal	Respiratory depression, vasodilation particularly with bolus dosing and in hemodynamically unstable patients
Haloperidol	1–5 mg	20–30	Effects decreased by rifampin Medications that widen QT interval	QT interval prolongation, neuroleptic malignant syndrome, EPS (less with IV than with oral use)
Dexmedetomidine	Initial recommended dose: 0.8 μg/kg/h titrated to a dose between 0.2 and 1.4 μg/kg/h	6	Minimal but has the potential to augment bradycardia induced by vagal stimuli or negative chronotropic drugs and may increase the effects of vasodilators	Hypotension, bradycardia

EPS, extrapyramidal symptoms; IV, intravenous.
Adapted from Marino PL (ed): *The ICU Book*. 2nd ed. Baltimore, Lippincott Williams & Wilkins, 1998; and Eisendrath SJ, Shim JJ: Management of psychiatric problems in critically ill patients. *Am J Med* 119:22, 2006.

by the *Diagnostic and Statistical Manual of Mental Disorders* [65], a panic attack is a discrete period of fear or discomfort that develops suddenly, reaches a peak within 10 minutes, and is associated with the symptoms listed in Table 198.3. Panic disorder consists of recurrent panic attacks accompanied by persistent fear of having additional attacks, worry about the implications and consequences of the episodes, and a significant change in behavior related to the attacks. Many panic-disordered patients are hypervigilant to internal bodily stimuli, and some fear that their attacks indicate the presence of an undiagnosed, life-threatening illness. These concerns are assuaged only when the panic disorder is accurately diagnosed and effectively treated.

Risks for developing panic attacks include separation, disruption of important relationships, and medical illness—all endemic in the ICU. Timely diagnosis and treatment of panic disorder can circumvent unnecessary medical procedures and decrease morbidity and mortality. Additionally, the physiologic consequences of panic may exacerbate symptoms of preexisting medical conditions and lead to more frequent medical hospitalizations. However, because its presentation is similar to that of several medical conditions (e.g., MI, stroke, gastrointestinal conditions, respiratory compromise), especially in the ICU, panic disorder must be considered a diagnosis of exclusion. Treatment for panic disorder includes psychotherapy and medication. Cognitive-behavioral techniques (e.g., psychoeducation, anxiety management skills, cognitive reframing, and exposure to somatic cues) have been well studied. Benzodiazepines and antidepressants—specifically the selective serotonin reuptake inhibitors (SSRIs)—are the standard of care for the psychopharmacological management of panic disorder.

TREATMENT OF ANXIETY IN THE INTENSIVE CARE UNIT

Treatments for anxiety in the ICU include both nonpharmacologic and pharmacologic options. Additionally, the stress placed on medical and nursing staff attending to anxious patients in an emotionally charged treatment setting must be acknowledged and addressed to improve the overall care of anxious patients in the ICU. This topic is reviewed in Chapter 202.

Nonpharmacologic methods that have been explored include education, environmental manipulation, muscle relaxation, and music therapy. The data supporting these practices are limited and equivocal. Nonetheless, these therapeutic modalities have been useful in clinical practice.

TABLE 198.5

RANDOMIZED TRIALS OF ANXIETY TREATMENTS IN CRITICALLY ILL PATIENTS

Study	Enrollment	Intervention	Results
Sackey et al. [46]	40 mechanically ventilated ICU patients	Isoflurane vs. midazolam	Trend toward fewer memories of delusions/hallucinations in the isoflurane group. No differences between groups in memories of feelings or factual events or in anxiety, depression, and well-being scores.
Jones et al. [50]	126 ICU patients	Self-help rehabilitation manual vs. routine follow-up	Trend toward a lower rate of depression in intervention group. No differences in anxiety and PTSD symptoms between groups.
Knowles et al. [51]	36 ICU patients	Prospective diary reviewed postdischarge vs. standard of care	Improvement in both depression and anxiety symptoms in experimental group.
Kress et al. [52]	32 mechanically ventilated ICU patients	Daily sedation withdrawal vs. continuous sedation	Fewer PTSD symptoms in daily sedation withdrawal group.
Treggiari et al. [53]	137 mechanically ventilated ICU patients	Light vs. deep sedation	Fewer symptoms in the light sedation group at 4 weeks. No differences in anxiety and depression between groups.
Schelling et al. [55]	91 patients undergoing cardiac surgery, 48 followed up in 6 months	High-dose corticosteroids perioperatively vs. standard care	Reduced PTSD symptoms in the steroid group. No difference in traumatic memories between groups.
Weis et al. [56]	36 patients undergoing cardiac surgery	Stress-dose hydrocortisone vs. placebo	Reduced incidence of chronic stress symptoms and better health-related QoL in steroid group. No difference in traumatic memories between groups.
Schelling et al. [57]	20 patients with septic shock	Stress-dose hydrocortisone vs. placebo	Lower incidence of PTSD in intervention group. No difference in traumatic memories between groups.
Stein et al. [62]	48 patients admitted to a surgical trauma center	Propranolol vs. gabapentin vs. placebo	No differences in PTSD symptoms, depression, or ASD at 1, 4, and 8 months after injury.
Ziemann et al. [66]	41 CAD patients admitted to a CCU	Individualized contact with nurse vs. usual care	Significantly less anxiety, depression, and hostility in the experimental group.
Corbett et al. [67]	89 mechanically ventilated patients after nonemergent CABG	Propofol vs. dexmedetomidine	No differences in pain, anxiety, and sleep/rest between groups.

ASD, acute stress disorder; CABG, coronary artery bypass grafting; CAD, coronary artery disease; CCU, coronary care unit; ICU, intensive care unit; PTSD, posttraumatic stress disorder; QoL, quality of life.

Patients should be made aware of their clinical situation and oriented to their environment. Provision of ambient light, a clock, and a calendar promotes accurate orientation and a normal sleep–wake cycle. In addition, to foster a sense of control and mastery of their situation, patients should be made an integral part of decision-making. In a randomized, controlled trial of 41 CCU patients, those who were given choices about family visits, daily hygiene schedule, physical activity, and their room environment enjoyed significant improvement in anxiety and depression measures after 48 hours [66]. Muscle relaxation has been used with some success in weaning patients from ventilators. In limited studies, relaxed, nonpercussion music decreased anxious symptoms and associated physiologic measures. These methods should be considered adjunctive to pharmacotherapy and may help reduce the need for medications.

Benzodiazepines represent the standard for anxiolysis in the ICU; of these, lorazepam is the most widely used. Available in an intravenous formulation, it undergoes little hepatic metabolism, has no active metabolites, and is more appropriate for use in patients with liver disease or with poor liver function. Lorazepam is also useful for long-term sedation in ventilated patients as it is not associated with heart block (as is propofol) or with wide body storage (as is midazolam). However, lorazepam is mixed with propylene glycol, and prolonged use of high doses can precipitate an osmolar-gap acidosis.

Another agent of recent interest and increasingly used in the ICU is dexmedetomidine, which inhibits the central and peripheral effects of norepinephrine and epinephrine, resulting in sedation and analgesia. While dexmedetomidine may cause bradycardia and hypotension, trial data suggest that clinically significant adverse hemodynamic changes are rare [33,34]. Dexmedetomidine and propofol performed equally in pain and anxiety reduction and sleep/rest promotion [67].

Other agents that may prove useful in the anxious patient are SSRIs, neuroleptic agents, and propofol. SSRIs have been shown to decrease the sense of dyspnea in anxious patients with COPD [68]. Neuroleptics are beneficial in patients who are fearful, delirious, or so anxious that they are nearly psychotic [69]. Use of neuroleptic agents is discussed in Chapter 197. Propofol continues to be the most commonly used medication for sedation in the ICU but is impractical for routine anxiolysis given its significant respiratory-depressant effects [70]. Table 198.4 contrasts various agents commonly used to quell anxiety in critically ill patients. Table 198.5 presents a summary of randomized trials of anxiety treatments in critically ill patients.

CONCLUSION

Ubiquitous in the ICU, anxiety has a broad range of physiologic and psychological consequences. Although it can be difficult to diagnose in the acutely ill, current evidence suggests that identification and treatment of anxiety enhance patient comfort and compliance and improve morbidity and mortality. Therefore, anxiety should be routinely assessed in critically ill patients. Psychiatric consultation should be considered whenever anxiety complicates the clinical course.

References

1. Hoehn-Saric R, McLeod DR: The peripheral sympathetic nervous system: its role in normal and pathologic anxiety. *Psychiatr Clin North Am* 11:375, 1988.
2. Gerra G, Zaimovic A, Mascetti GG, et al: Neuroendocrine responses to experimentally-induced psychological stress in healthy humans. *Psychoneuroendocrinology* 26:91, 2001.
3. Lader MH: Behavior and anxiety: physiologic mechanisms. *J Clin Psychiatry* 44:5, 1983.
4. Arranz L, Guayerbas N, De la Fuente M: Impairment of several immune functions in anxious women. *J Psychosom Res* 62:1, 2007.
5. Lown B, Verrier RL, Corbalan R: Psychologic stress and threshold for repetitive ventricular response. *Science* 182:834, 1973.
6. Wilhelm FH, Gevirtz R, Walton RT: Respiratory dysregulation in anxiety, functional cardiac, and pain disorders: assessment, phenomenology, and treatment. *Behav Modif* 25:513, 2001.
7. Rozanski A, Blumenthal JA, Kaplan J: Impact of psychological factors on the pathogenesis of cardiovascular disease and implications for therapy. *Circulation* 99:2192, 1999.
8. Strik JJ, Denollet J, Lousberg R, et al: Comparing symptoms of depression and anxiety as predictors of cardiac events and increased health care consumption after myocardial infarction. *J Am Coll Cardiol* 42:1801, 2003.
9. Moser DK, Riegel B, McKinley S, et al: Impact of anxiety and perceived control on in-hospital complications after acute myocardial infarction. *Psychosom Med* 69:10, 2007.
10. Huffman JC, Smith FA, Blais MA, et al: Anxiety, independent of depressive symptoms, is associated with in-hospital cardiac complications after acute myocardial infarction. *J Psychosom Res* 65:557, 2008.
11. Meyer T, Buss U, Herrmann-Lingen C: Role of cardiac disease severity in the predictive value of anxiety for all-cause mortality. *Psychosom Med* 72:9, 2009.
12. Moser DK, Dracup K: Is anxiety early after myocardial infarction associated with subsequent ischemic and arrhythmic events? *Psychosom Med* 58:395, 1996.
13. Lane D, Carroll D, Lip GY: Anxiety, depression, and prognosis after myocardial infarction: is there a causal association? *J Am Coll Cardiol* 42:1808, 2003.
14. An K, De Jong MJ, Riegel BJ, et al: A cross-sectional examination of changes in anxiety early after acute myocardial infarction. *Heart Lung* 33:75, 2004.
15. Huffman JC, Smith FA, Blais MA, et al: Recognition and treatment of depression and anxiety in patients with acute myocardial infarction. *Am J Cardiol* 98:319, 2006.
16. Francis JL, Weinstein AA, Krantz DS, et al: Association between symptoms of depression and anxiety with heart rate variability in patients with implantable cardioverter defibrillators. *Psychosom Med* 71:821, 2009.
17. Yeragani VK, Tancer M, Seema KP, et al: Increased pulse-wave velocity in patients with anxiety: implications for autonomic dysfunction. *J Psychosom Res* 61:25, 2006.
18. Anderson KP: Sympathetic nervous system activity and ventricular tachyarrhythmias: recent advances. *Ann Noninvasive Electrocardiol* 8:75, 2003.
19. La Rovere MT, Bigger JT Jr, Marcus FI, et al: Baroreflex sensitivity and heart-rate variability in prediction of total cardiac mortality after myocardial infarction. *Lancet* 351:478, 1998.
20. Albert CM, Chae CU, Rexrode KM, et al: Phobic anxiety and risk of coronary heart disease and sudden cardiac death among women. *Circulation* 111:480, 2005.
21. Watkins LL, Blumenthal JA, Davidson JR, et al: Phobic anxiety, depression, and risk of ventricular arrhythmias in patients with coronary heart disease. *Psychosom Med* 68:651, 2006.
22. Kuhl EA, Fauerbach JA, Bush DE, et al: Relation of anxiety and adherence to risk-reducing recommendations following myocardial infarction. *Am J Cardiol* 103:1629, 2009.
23. Frasure-Smith N, Lesperance F, Talajic M: The impact of negative emotions on prognosis following myocardial infarction: is it more than depression? *Health Psychol* 14:388, 1995.
24. Denollet J, Brutsaert DL: Personality, disease severity, and the risk of long-term cardiac events in patients with a decreased ejection fraction after myocardial infarction. *Circulation* 97:167, 1998.
25. Mayou RA, Gill D, Thompson DR, et al: Depression and anxiety as predictors of outcome after myocardial infarction. *Psychosom Med* 62:212, 2000.
26. Lane D, Carroll D, Ring C, et al: Effects of depression and anxiety on mortality and quality-of-life 4 months after myocardial infarction. *J Psychosom Res* 49:229, 2000.
27. Lane D, Carroll D, Ring C, et al: Do depression and anxiety predict recurrent coronary events 12 months after myocardial infarction? *QJM* 93:739, 2000.
28. Welin C, Lappas G, Wilhelmsen L: Independent importance of psychosocial factors for prognosis after myocardial infarction. *J Intern Med* 247:629, 2000.
29. Brochard L, Rauss A, Benito S, et al: Comparison of three methods of gradual withdrawal from ventilatory support during weaning from mechanical ventilation. *Am J Respir Crit Care Med* 150:896, 1994.
30. Chlan LL: Description of anxiety levels by individual differences and clinical factors in patients receiving mechanical ventilatory support. *Heart Lung* 32:275, 2003.
31. Blackwood B: The art and science of predicting patient readiness for weaning from mechanical ventilation. *Int J Nurs Stud* 37:145, 2000.
32. Reade MC, O'Sullivan K, Bates S, et al: Dexmedetomidine vs. haloperidol in delirious, agitated, intubated patients: a randomized open-label trial. *Crit Care* 13:R75, 2009.

33. Riker RR, Shehabi Y, Bokesch PM, et al: Dexmedetomidine vs midazolam for sedation of critically ill patients: a randomized trial. *JAMA* 301:489, 2009.
34. Gerlach AT, Murphy CV, Dasta JF: An updated focused review of dexmedetomidine in adults. *Ann Pharmacother* 43:2064, 2009.
35. Lee OK, Chung YF, Chang ME, et al: Music and its effect on the physiological responses and anxiety levels of patients receiving mechanical ventilation: a pilot study. *J Clin Nurs* 14:609, 2005.
36. Rose D, Mannino DM, Leaderer BP: Asthma prevalence among US adults, 1998–2000: role of Puerto Rican ethnicity and behavioral and geographic factors. *Am J Public Health* 96:880, 2006.
37. Vazquez I, Romero-Frais E, Blanco-Aparicio M, et al: Psychological and self-management factors in near-fatal asthma. *J Psychosom Res* 68:175, 2010.
38. Barton C, Clarke D, Sulaiman N, et al: Coping as a mediator of psychosocial impediments to optimal management and control of asthma. *Respir Med* 97:747, 2003.
39. Sandberg S, Jarvenpaa S, Penttinen A, et al: Asthma exacerbations in children immediately following stressful life events: a Cox's hierarchical regression. *Thorax* 59:1046, 2004.
40. Kolbe J, Fergusson W, Vamos M, et al: Case-control study of severe life threatening asthma (SLTA) in adults: psychological factors. *Thorax* 57:317, 2002.
41. Rietveld S, Everaerd W, Creer TL: Stress-induced asthma: a review of research and potential mechanisms. *Clin Exp Allergy* 30:1058, 2000.
42. Sukantarat K, Greer S, Brett S, et al: Physical and psychological sequelae of critical illness. *Br J Health Psychol* 12:65, 2007.
43. Davydow DS, Gifford JM, Desai SV, et al: Posttraumatic stress disorder in general intensive care unit survivors: a systematic review. *Gen Hosp Psychiatry* 30:421, 2008.
44. Kessler RC, Chiu WT, Demler O, et al: Prevalence, severity and comorbidity of 12-month DSM-IV disorders in the National Comorbidity Survey Replication. *Arch Gen Psychiatry* 62:617, 2005.
45. Nelson BJ, Weinert CR, Bury CL, et al: Intensive care unit drug use and subsequent quality of life in acute lung injury patients. *Crit Care Med* 28:3626, 2000.
46. Sackey PV, Martling CR, Carlsward C, et al: Short- and long-term follow-up of intensive care unit patients after sedation with isoflurane and midazolam—a pilot study. *Crit Care Med* 36:801, 2008.
47. Jones C, Griffiths RD, Humphris G, et al: Memory, delusions, and the development of acute posttraumatic stress disorder-related symptoms after intensive care. *Crit Care Med* 29:573, 2001.
48. Ringdal M, Plos K, Lundberg D, et al: Outcome after injury: memories, health-related quality of life, anxiety, and symptoms of depression after intensive care. *J Trauma* 66:1226, 2009.
49. Ringdal M, Plos K, Lundberg D, et al: Memories and health-related quality of life after intensive care: a follow-up study. *Crit Care Med* 38:38, 2010.
50. Jones C, Skirrow P, Griffiths RD, et al: Rehabilitation after critical illness: a randomized, controlled trial. *Crit Care Med* 31:2456, 2003.
51. Knowles RE, Tarrier N: Evaluation of the effect of prospective patient diaries on emotional well-being in intensive care unit survivors: a randomized controlled trial. *Crit Care Med* 37:184, 2009.
52. Kress JP, Gehlbach B, Lacy M, et al: The long-term psychological effects of daily sedative interruption on critically ill patients. *Am J Respir Crit Care Med* 168:1457, 2003.
53. Treggiari MM, Romand JA, Yanez ND, et al: Randomized trial of light versus deep sedation on mental health after critical illness. *Crit Care Med* 37:2527, 2009.
54. Schelling G, Roozendaal B, De Quervain DJ: Can posttraumatic stress disorder be prevented with glucocorticoids? *Ann N Y Acad Sci* 1032:158, 2004.
55. Schelling G, Kilger E, Roozendaal B, et al: Stress doses of hydrocortisone, traumatic memories, and symptoms of posttraumatic stress disorder in patients after cardiac surgery: a randomized study. *Biol Psychiatry* 55:627, 2004.
56. Weis F, Kilger E, Roozendaal B, et al: Stress doses of hydrocortisone reduce chronic stress symptoms and improve health-related quality of life in high-risk patients after cardiac surgery: a randomized study. *Thorac Cardiovasc Surg* 131:277, 2006.
57. Schelling G, Briegel J, Roozendaal B, et al: The effect of stress doses of hydrocortisone during septic shock on posttraumatic stress disorder in survivors. *Biol Psychiatry* 50:978, 2001.
58. Pitman RK, Sanders KM, Zusman RM, et al: Pilot study of secondary prevention of posttraumatic stress disorder with propranolol. *Biol Psychiatry* 51:189, 2002.
59. Vaiva G, Ducrocq F, Jezequel K, et al: Immediate treatment with propranolol decreases posttraumatic stress disorder two months after trauma. *Biol Psychiatry* 54:947, 2003.
60. Krauseneck T, Padberg F, Roozendaal B, et al: A beta-adrenergic antagonist reduces traumatic memories and PTSD symptoms in female but not male patients after cardiac surgery. *Psychol Med* 20:1, 2009.
61. Schelling G, Richter M, Roozendaal B, et al: Exposure to high stress in the intensive care unit may have negative effects on health-related quality-of-life outcomes after cardiac surgery. *Crit Care Med* 31:1971, 2003.
62. Stein MB, Kerridge C, Dimsdale JE, et al: Pharmacotherapy to present PTSD: results from a randomized controlled proof-of-concept trial in physically injured patients. *J Trauma Stress* 20:923, 2007.
63. Myhren H, Toien K, Ekeberg O, et al: Patients' memory and psychological distress after ICU stay compared with expectations of the relatives. *Intensive Care Med* 35:2078, 2009.
64. Muller JE, Koen L, Stein DJ: Anxiety and medical disorders. *Curr Psychiatry Rep* 7:245, 2005.
65. American Psychiatric Association: *Diagnostic and Statistical Manual of Mental Disorders*. 4th ed. Washington, DC, American Psychiatric Association, 1994.
66. Ziemann KM, Dracup K: Patient-nurse contracts in critical care: a controlled trial. *Prog Cardiovasc Nurs* 5:98, 1990.
67. Corbett SM, Rebuck JA, Greene CM, et al: Dexmedetomidine does not improve patient satisfaction when compared with propofol during mechanical ventilation. *Crit Care Med* 33:940, 2005.
68. Smoller JW, Pollack MH, Systrom D, et al: Sertraline effects on dyspnea in patients with obstructive airway disease. *Psychosomatics* 39:24, 1998.
69. McDougle CJ, Epperson CN, Pelton GH, et al: A double-blind, placebo-controlled study of risperidone addition in serotonin reuptake inhibitor-refractory obsessive-compulsive disorder. *Arch Gen Psychiatry* 57:794, 2000.
70. Wunsch H, Kahn JM, Kramer AA, et al: Use of intravenous infusion sedation among mechanically ventilated patients in the United States. *Crit Care Med* 37:3031, 2009.

CHAPTER 199 ■ DIAGNOSIS AND TREATMENT OF DEPRESSION IN THE INTENSIVE CARE UNIT PATIENT

EDITH S. GERINGER, JOHN QUERQUES, MEGHAN S. KOLODZIEJ, TUESDAY E. BURNS AND THEODORE A. STERN

Intense emotions are evoked routinely in intensive care units (ICUs), where life-and-death decisions occur daily. In the ICU, depression can be a psychological reaction to an acute medical illness, a manifestation of a primary affective disorder, a mood disorder associated with a specific organic disease or its treatment, or a result of the confusing overlap of somatic symptoms of depression and symptoms of medical illnesses.

In this chapter, the term depression refers not to being transiently sad, discouraged, disappointed, despondent, or grief-stricken but refers to major depressive disorder (MDD), defined in the 4th edition of the *Diagnostic and Statistical Manual of Mental Disorders* (DSM-IV) [1] as a syndrome of distinct and persistent dysphoria associated with neurovegetative changes and functional impairment. Varied in presentation, course, and response to treatment, depressive disorders remain a pathophysiological enigma, despite centuries of recognition and more recent investigation of their possible genetic, neurochemical, neuroanatomic, endocrine, and immune underpinnings [2,3].

Many physicians believe that depression is appropriate in the ICU because severe illness devastates a person's life. However, we believe that while being dispirited may be an understandable response to critical illness, having a depressive disorder is not; therefore, it is always important to treat the latter. In fact, compelling evidence shows that untreated depression increases morbidity and mortality from cardiac and neurologic conditions and has detrimental effects on other—perhaps all—organ systems.

In this chapter, we focus on the links between depressive and medical conditions and the diagnosis, evaluation, and treatment of depression in critically ill patients.

LINKS BETWEEN DEPRESSION AND MEDICAL CONDITIONS

Cardiovascular Disease

That depression is associated with the development and the progression of coronary heart disease (CHD), and with worse prognosis in CHD patients, is well established [4]. Not proven thus far is that treatment of depression can improve or prevent these outcomes. After two trials—the Enhancing Recovery in Coronary Heart Disease Patients (ENRICHD) study [5] and the Myocardial Infarction and Depression–Intervention Trial (MIND–IT) [6]—failed to show this, attention turned to isolating those attributes of a depressive episode that portend greater risk. Secondary analyses of these and other trials have examined symptom type, episode onset before or after an index event [7,8], recurrence [9,10], treatment responsiveness [11], and persistence of the cardiotoxic effects of depression [12]. For example, some studies suggested that worse cardiac outcomes are associated with somatic/affective symptoms (e.g., insomnia, fatigability, and diminished libido) more than with cognitive/affective symptoms (e.g., pessimism, self-dislike, and suicidal ideas) [13–15].

Possible explanations for the greater rates of cardiac death among patients diagnosed with depression include hypothalamic–pituitary–adrenal axis hyperactivity, elevation in inflammatory markers (e.g., interleukin 6, tumor necrosis factor α), diminished heart rate variability, decreased parasympathetic tone, increased sympathetic tone, and enhanced platelet activation causing more avid platelet aggregation and plaque formation [16]. Interestingly, sertraline decreases platelet and endothelial activation in depressed patients after an acute coronary syndrome (ACS) [17,18]. The Heart and Soul Study, a prospective cohort study of 1,017 patients with stable CHD, found that behavioral factors, especially physical inactivity, were most responsible for the greater rate of adverse cardiac events in patients with depressive symptoms [19].

Cerebrovascular Disease

As with cardiovascular disease, there appear to be bidirectional links between cerebrovascular disease and depressive illness. The Caerphilly Study of 2,201 men found that psychological distress predicted fatal stroke but not nonfatal stroke or transient ischemic attack (TIA) [20]. The Framingham Heart Study of 4,120 men and women found that depressive symptoms were a risk factor for stroke or TIA before, but not after, age 65 [21].

Poststroke depression (PSD) has been extensively studied during the past 3 decades. Robinson [22] pooled the available data and found the mean prevalence of poststroke affective illness to be 19.3% for major depression and 18.5% for minor depression. Risk factors for the development of PSD include stroke severity, extent of physical disability, presence of cognitive impairment, and poor social support [23].

In the early 1980s, Robinson et al. [24,25] reported that the severity of PSD correlated with the proximity of the lesion to the frontal pole in the left, but not the right, hemisphere. This finding has been replicated by some [26,27], but not all [28], researchers; this localization may hold only during the first few months after stroke [29].

DIAGNOSIS OF DEPRESSION

Important questions for the intensivist are "What is depression?" and "What does a patient experiencing depression look like in the ICU?" To qualify for a diagnosis of MDD according to the DSM-IV, a patient must have five of the nine symptoms listed in Table 199.1, one of which must be either depressed mood or anhedonia, most of the day, nearly every day, for at least 2 weeks. The mnemonic—SIG: E CAPS (where SIG [abbreviation for the Latin, *signa*] refers to the instructions on a prescription, E refers to energy, and CAPS refers to capsules)—is a helpful guide to remember the eight neurovegetative symptoms associated with depressed mood. The mnemonic—ABCs of depression—portrays more richly the myriad affective, behavioral, and cognitive aspects of the condition (Table 199.2). Each symptom should be asked about, and questions about suicide should be raised directly. If a patient has thoughts of suicide, he or she should be asked whether there is a specific plan; the physician should then make a judgment about the likelihood of the patient's acting on the plan. If an active plan for suicide exists, psychiatric consultation is imperative (see Chapter 200).

Four of the nine diagnostic criteria (i.e., insomnia, fatigue or loss of energy, diminished ability to think or concentrate, and anorexia or weight loss) are difficult to attribute exclusively to depression in the medically ill patient. However, in terminally ill cancer patients, Chochinov et al. [30] found that inclusion of these somatic symptoms in the diagnostic criteria did not artifactually increase rates of diagnosis, as long as the cardinal symptoms of depressed mood and anhedonia were held to the strict requirement of presence most of the day, nearly every day, for at least 2 weeks.

TABLE 199.1

SIG: E CAPS—A MNEMONIC FOR DIAGNOSTIC CRITERIA FOR MAJOR DEPRESSIVE DISORDER

Depressed mood
*S*leep, increased or decreased
*I*nterest or pleasure in activities, markedly decreased (anhedonia)
*G*uilt or feelings of worthlessness
*E*nergy, decreased
*C*oncentration, decreased
*A*ppetite or weight, increased or decreased
*P*sychomotor agitation or retardation
*S*uicidal thinking

Adapted from American Psychiatric Association: *Diagnostic and Statistical Manual of Mental Disorders*. 4th ed. Washington, DC, American Psychiatric Association, 1994.

TABLE 199.2

ABCs OF DEPRESSION—AFFECTIVE, BEHAVIORAL, AND COGNITIVE FEATURES

Affective	Behavioral	Cognitive
Depressed mood	Crying	Suicidal thinking
"Blue" mood	Increased or decreased sleep	Thoughts of death
Sadness	Increased or decreased appetite	Somatic preoccupation
Blunted affect	Decreased energy	Guilty rumination
Hopelessness	Psychomotor agitation or retardation	Confusion
Emptiness	Increased or intractable pain	Decreased concentration
Irritability	Deliberate self-injury	
Anger	Impulsivity	
Decreased interest	Poor eye contact	
	Noncompliance	

Patients Who are Unable to Speak

It may be particularly difficult to diagnose depression in a patient who is being mechanically ventilated or who has aphasia. However, much can be learned about a patient even when he or she is mute. It is important to watch facial expressions, observe hand gestures and other body language, and read lips. An individual who averts his or her eyes from the examiner's gaze may be demoralized, discouraged, or depressed. Slow, sighing respirations may indicate depression rather than respiratory insufficiency. The astute clinician can also watch vital-sign monitor screens, looking for changes that can signify intense affect.

Does the patient respond to the mention of a favorite hobby or a grandchild with a smile or with tears? Is the patient's affect labile or consistent with the content of the discussion? Emotional lability is not usually an indicator of MDD; instead, it suggests frontal lobe dysfunction. One can probe for affect by joking and observing the patient's reaction.

A patient who can move his or her arms can be asked to write, draw, or point to a letter or a picture board. One simple screening test that can be used is human figure drawing (i.e., having the patient draw a picture of a person and another of what the patient thinks is wrong with the person). Typically, drawings by depressed patients convey their sense of dejection or a disordered understanding of their dilemma.

TABLE 199.3

METHODS OF ASSESSING DEPRESSION IN SENSORIALLY COMPROMISED PATIENTS

- Watch facial expressions and gestures
- Write questions
- Have patients write answers
- Use letter or picture board
- Observe whether facial expressions are consistent with content of discussion
- Observe rate of change of affect
- Ask about and observe neurovegetative features of depression
- Ask about known sources of the patient's enjoyment (e.g., favorite hobby, grandchildren, sports) and observe whether the patient takes pleasure in these things
- Joke with the patient or tell a funny story and observe the patient's reaction
- Ask the patient to draw a picture of himself or herself and what is wrong, then assess the pictures for a sense of demoralization or hopelessness
- Make a fist and ask the patient, "What would you do if you had one of these?", and assess emotions in response to this maneuver

Some tracheostomized patients may have the oxygenation status, control of respiratory muscles, and ability to manage secretions sufficient to use a Passy-Muir valve, which permits exhaled air to pass the larynx and thus allows the patient to speak. Alternatively, electronic voice-output communication aids may be used. These devices pair prerecorded messages or synthesized speech with labeled icons; patients communicate messages by touching buttons on display screens or on touch-sensitive keyboards. Speech pathologists have knowledge of and access to such technology. Methods of assessing depression in sensorially compromised patients are summarized in Table 199.3.

DIFFERENTIAL DIAGNOSIS OF DEPRESSION

Causes Related to Medical Conditions

A variety of medical illnesses can cause affective disorders, contribute to their occurrence, and worsen their severity (Table 199.4). Clues that depression is due to a medical illness include

TABLE 199.4

MEDICAL CONDITIONS ASSOCIATED WITH DEPRESSIVE SYMPTOMS

Cardiovascular	Metabolic
Cardiac tumors	Acid–base problems
Congestive heart failure	Hypokalemia
Hypertensive encephalopathy	Hyper- or hyponatremia
	Renal failure
Collagen-vascular	Neoplastic
Polyarteritis nodosa	Carcinoid
Systemic lupus erythematosus	Pancreatic carcinoma
Endocrine	Neurologic
Diabetes mellitus	Brain tumor
Hyper- or hypoadrenalism	Multiple sclerosis
Hyper- or hypoparathyroidism	Parkinson's disease (especially with on/off phenomenon)
Hyper- or hypothyroidism	Temporal lobe epilepsy
	Stroke
	Subcortical dementia
Infectious	Nutritional
Hepatitis	Vitamin B_{12} deficiency
Human immunodeficiency virus	Wernicke's encephalopathy
Mononucleosis	
Influenza	

older age at onset of symptoms, lower incidence of a family history of depression, and changes in personality and cognition. A thorough history (including a review of systems), physical (including neurologic) examination, and laboratory testing can distinguish between primary (i.e., due to a psychiatric condition) and secondary (i.e., due to a medical condition) causes of depression. For secondary causes, treatment of the underlying illness is usually more effective than is the use of psychotropic medications.

Perhaps the most important differential diagnosis to consider in a patient who appears to have MDD is hypoactive delirium. The key feature that distinguishes it from depression is inattention (i.e., an inability to focus and sustain alertness on a given stimulus and to resist distraction by other stimuli). Delirium is discussed in Chapter 197.

Causes Related to Medical Treatments

The pharmacologic agents most often responsible for depression in the ICU are antihypertensives, beta-blockers, antiarrhythmics, and steroids (Table 199.5). Some medications may cause depression only after several weeks or even months of continuous use. If a drug regimen or a dosage increase appears to be temporally related to the patient's depression, the dose should be lowered or the medication eliminated entirely. If the medication cannot be stopped without serious risk to the patient, the depression should be treated.

Steroids

Depression, mania, psychosis, and delirium are frequent side effects of corticosteroid therapy. Mood symptoms are dose-dependent and usually occur within the first 2 weeks of therapy, although they can arise on the first day. A practical rule of thumb holds that neuropsychiatric adverse effects are common with prednisone $\geq$80 mg per day (or equivalent), uncommon $\leq$30 mg per day, and not uncommon in between. Although it has been suggested that women are more likely to develop steroid-induced adverse effects, the apparent increased frequency may be due to the higher prevalence of rheumatologic diseases in women. Corticosteroid-induced mood disorders are generally reversible with dosage reduction or discontinuation of the medication.

TABLE 199.5

DRUGS ASSOCIATED WITH DEPRESSIVE SYMPTOMS

Acyclovir (especially at high doses)
Alcohol
Amphetamine-like drugs (withdrawal): fenfluramine, phenmetrazine, phenylpropanolamine
Anabolic steroids: methandrostenolone, methyltestosterone
Anticonvulsants (at high doses or plasma levels): carbamazepine, phenytoin, primidone
Antihypertensives: clonidine, hydralazine, methyldopa, reserpine, thiazides
Asparaginase
Baclofen
Barbiturates
Benzodiazepines: alprazolam, clonazepam, clorazepate, diazepam, lorazepam, triazolam
Beta-blockers: atenolol, betaxolol, propranolol, timolol
Bromides
Bromocriptine
Cimetidine
Cocaine (withdrawal)
Oral contraceptives
Corticosteroids
Cycloserine
Dapsone
Digitalis (at high doses or in elderly patients)
Diltiazem
Disopyramide
Ethionamide
Halothane (postoperatively)
Heavy metals
Histamine-2 receptor antagonists: cimetidine, ranitidine
Interferon α
Isoniazid
Isotretinoin
Levodopa (especially in the elderly)
Mefloquine
Metoclopramide
Metrizamide
Metronidazole
Nalidixic acid
Narcotics: meperidine, methadone, morphine, pentazocine, propoxyphene
Nifedipine
Nonsteroidal anti-inflammatory drugs
Norfloxacin
Phenylephrine
Prazosin
Procaine derivatives: lidocaine, penicillin G procaine, procainamide
Thyroid hormones
Trimethoprim-sulfamethoxazole

LABORATORY EVALUATION OF DEPRESSION

Although the clinical interview and mental status examination are the most important components of psychiatric diagnosis, the use of laboratory tests is essential to exclude organic causes of depression. Although there is no consensus on the laboratory tests necessary in a patient with new-onset mood disorder, Table 199.6 lists those tests that should be considered. Thyroid-stimulating hormone is not on this list because many critically ill patients have abnormal thyroid biochemical profiles but do not have intrinsic thyroid disease. Syphilis and hypovitaminosis are rarely the sole causes of depression; tests for these conditions should be ordered only when there is a specific indication for them. Neuroimaging, electroencephalography, and cerebrospinal fluid analysis are relatively indicated in patients with new-onset psychiatric symptoms, altered cognition, new neurologic symptoms, seizures, and fever. The more of these features a patient has, the more important these additional tests become.

TREATMENT OF DEPRESSION

Patients who meet the criteria for MDD are usually treated with a somatic therapy (including pharmacotherapy and electroconvulsive therapy [ECT]), alone or in combination with psychotherapy (Table 199.7). In critical care units, somatic therapies are the most widely used treatments for depression. Pharmacotherapy may be used in critical care units also for patients who have an adjustment disorder with depressed mood, particularly when these patients have several neurovegetative symptoms. A patient who is neither eating nor sleeping and who lacks the energy to participate in his or her rehabilitation may be helped considerably by antidepressants, especially psychostimulants.

Each type of pharmacotherapy has its own indications and contraindications, but general rules are available when

TABLE 199.6

LABORATORY EVALUATION OF DEPRESSION

Complete blood count with differential
Complete blood chemistries
Serum and urine toxicology
Urinalysis
Vitamin B_{12}
Folate
Rapid plasma reagin
Neuroimaging
Electroencephalogram
Cerebrospinal fluid analysis

selecting an antidepressant [31,32]. The most common rule is to choose a medication with a side-effect profile that best fits a patient's needs. For instance, a patient who is having trouble sleeping will benefit from a sedating antidepressant. Conversely, a patient who has severe psychomotor retardation may benefit from a more stimulating antidepressant. With the exception of the psychostimulants, all antidepressants require approximately 4 to 6 weeks until full antidepressant effects are noted, although some response can occur in 1 to 2 weeks. Obviously, in critical care units, quicker effects are generally needed. Stimulants and ECT work more quickly, usually within several days. Patients with depression may also manifest considerable anxiety and may be helped by the use of an anxiolytic while awaiting response to an antidepressant. Psychotically depressed patients (with delusions or hallucinations) may need antipsychotics for control of symptoms.

Psychostimulants

Psychostimulants have been used to treat depressive symptoms since their development in the 1930s, but they fell into disrepute when they became known as drugs of abuse in the 1950s and 1960s. Since then, there have been numerous reports on the use of stimulants in the treatment of depressed patients, particularly apathetic and geriatric patients; recently, there has been a renewed interest in the use of psychostimulants in depressed, medically ill patients who are intolerant of other medications

TABLE 199.7

COMPARATIVE PROPERTIES OF SOME ANTIDEPRESSANTS

Drug	Metabolism	ACh	Sedation	OH	Cardiac arrhythmia	Seizure risk	Target dose range (mg/d)	Drug interactions
Stimulants	Renal	0	0	0	Rare	Rare	5–20	
SSRIs								Risk of serotonin syndrome
Citalopram	Hepatic	+	+	+	Rare	Rare	20–60	Relatively few
Escitalopram	Hepatic	0–+	0–+	0–+	Rare	Rare	10–30	Relatively few
Fluoxetine	Hepatic	+	+	+	Rare	Rare	≥20	Increased levels of TCAs
Fluvoxamine	Hepatic	+	+	+	Rare	Rare	50–250	
Paroxetine	Hepatic	+	+	0	Rare	Rare	≥20	
Sertraline	Hepatic	0	0	0	Rare	Rare	50–200	
SNRIs								Risk of serotonin syndrome
Duloxetine	Hepatic	+	+	0–+	Rare	Rare	30–90	
Venlafaxine	Hepatic	0	0	0	Rare	Rare	150–300	
TCAs								
Amitriptyline	Hepatic	+++	+++	+++	Yes	Increased	≥150	
Amoxapine	Hepatic	+	++	+	Yes	Increased	≥200	
Desipramine	Hepatic	+	+	+++	Yes	Increased	≥150	
Doxepin	Hepatic	++	+++	++	Yes	Increased	≥200	
Imipramine	Hepatic	++	++	+++	Yes	Increased	≥200	
Maprotiline	Hepatic	+	+++	+	Yes	Increased	≥150	
Nortriptyline	Hepatic	++	++	+	Yes	Increased	≥100	
Protriptyline	Hepatic	+++	+	++	Yes	Increased	≥30	
MAOIs	Hepatic	0	+	+++	Rare	Rare	45–90	Hypertensive crisis with tyramine or sympathomimetics; avoid narcotics
Others								
Bupropion	Hepatic	+	0	0	Rare	Increased	IR, 200–300; SR/XL, 150–300	
Mirtazapine	Hepatic	+	+++	+	Rare	Rare	30–45	
Trazodone	Hepatic	0	+++	++	Yes	Increased	≥150	Digitalis toxicity

+, low; ++, moderate; +++, high; ACh, anticholinergic effects; IR, immediate release; MAOIs, monoamine oxidase inhibitors; OH, orthostatic hypotension; SNRIs, serotonin–norepinephrine reuptake inhibitors; SR, sustained release; SSRIs, selective serotonin reuptake inhibitors; TCAs, tricyclic antidepressants; XL, extended release.
Adapted, in part, from Mann JJ: The medical management of depression. *N Engl J Med* 353:1819, 2005.

[33]. Thought to be particularly effective in patients with cancer and stroke, their rapid onset is of great use in any setting, including the ICU, where speed of recovery is crucial. For example, they are valuable in patients who are difficult to wean from mechanical ventilation [34].

The psychostimulants most commonly used are dextroamphetamine (Dexedrine) and methylphenidate (Ritalin). Both appear to work through the direct neuronal release of dopamine and norepinephrine; dextroamphetamine blocks catecholamine reuptake and weakly inhibits monoamine oxidase. Both of these psychostimulants are predominantly excreted by the kidneys, although dextroamphetamine also undergoes a complex biotransformation.

The usual effects of stimulants are to increase motor behavior, increase arousal, and decrease appetite; however, in patients who are anorexic on the basis of depression, appetite is paradoxically increased, likely through dopaminergic stimulation of the nucleus accumbens. Their antidepressant effect is usually evident in the first 2 days of treatment, if not earlier. In a review of 66 patients hospitalized on medical-surgical wards at Massachusetts General Hospital, 93% achieved maximum benefit within 2 days of use [35,36]. Stimulants do not show anticholinergic effects or cause orthostatic hypotension. They can increase heart rate and blood pressure and can cause coronary spasm and cardiac arrhythmias; however, these effects are rare (even with preexisting cardiac abnormalities) at the low doses (5 to 20 mg/day) usually used for the treatment of depression [35]. In fact, stimulants have been used safely and effectively in a broad spectrum of patients, including those with critical illness, and have shown little potential for abuse or dependence. Contraindications to stimulant use include the concurrent use of α-methyldopa (which becomes a sympathoamine when metabolized), monoamine oxidase inhibitors (MAOIs), and bronchodilators; and pregnancy, seizures, delirium, psychosis, significant hypertension, and active angina [37].

Psychostimulants should be the first consideration in treating depression in critically ill patients. Patients are started on 5 mg of methylphenidate or 2.5 to 5 mg of dextroamphetamine in the morning. The dose is increased by 5 mg per day (for methylphenidate) or 2.5 to 5 mg per day (for dextroamphetamine) until a therapeutic effect is detected or until a maximum dose of 20 mg has been reached. Heart rate and blood pressure should be monitored as closely as necessary. Stimulants are usually given for at least 1 to 2 weeks after depressive symptoms have fully remitted. In most cases, after stimulants are stopped, depression does not recur.

Stimulants taken in overdose may cause seizures, coma, hallucinations, paranoia, hyperthermia, hypertension, cardiac arrhythmias, angina, and circulatory collapse. The major treatment for overdose is to acidify the urine (which enhances renal excretion) and to use supportive measures for all other abnormalities.

Modafinil (Provigil)—a wakefulness-promoting medication approved for narcolepsy, shift work sleep disorder, and obstructive sleep apnea/hypopnea syndrome—may be a beneficial alternative to the psychostimulants.

Selective Serotonin Reuptake Inhibitors

The SSRIs are a class of antidepressants that causes a potent and selective blockade of serotonin reuptake. Since the introduction of fluoxetine (Prozac) in 1987, SSRIs have become the most widely prescribed class of antidepressants. Other SSRIs include sertraline (Zoloft), paroxetine (Paxil), fluvoxamine (Luvox), citalopram (Celexa), and escitalopram (Lexapro). They are far less anticholinergic, antihistaminergic, and anti-α_1-adrenergic than the older tricyclic antidepressants (TCAs) and, therefore, are associated with far fewer side effects. They also have fewer cardiovascular effects and do not commonly cause orthostatic hypotension.

Pharmacokinetics

SSRIs are well absorbed from the gastrointestinal tract, and absorption is generally unaffected by food and antacids. They have a large volume of distribution and are highly protein-bound. They are extensively metabolized in the liver, where they are oxidized, methylated, and conjugated. The elimination half-lives of sertraline, paroxetine, fluvoxamine, and citalopram are approximately 1 day (although sertraline has a mildly active metabolite with a half-life of 66 hours); this allows once-a-day dosing. Fluoxetine has a half-life of 2 to 3 days and a highly active metabolite (norfluoxetine) with a mean half-life of 6.1 days. Fluoxetine takes a much longer time to reach steady state and, more importantly for drug overdoses, can take weeks to months to be fully cleared. Elimination half-lives are dose-dependent (i.e., higher doses and lengthier usage are associated with higher plasma levels and longer half-lives). SSRIs show wide interindividual variation in pharmacokinetics and do not yet have a clearly established dose-response curve.

Metabolic Impairment

Fluoxetine, sertraline, fluvoxamine, and citalopram are unaffected by renal dysfunction [38,39]. Paroxetine, although minimally excreted in the urine (like other SSRIs), shows increased plasma concentrations in the setting of renal disease [38]. Fluoxetine, sertraline, paroxetine, and citalopram doses should be reduced by at least half in patients with liver disease [38]. Fluvoxamine has been used in patients with cirrhosis and hepatic encephalopathy without adverse effects [40]. The hepatic clearance, not the plasma concentration, of fluvoxamine is affected by cirrhosis. Therefore, the dosage frequency, rather than the total dosage, should be altered [40]. In elderly individuals, fluoxetine does not have altered pharmacokinetics; in contrast, sertraline and paroxetine have increased plasma levels and slower clearance. Although citalopram has a 30% longer half-life in the elderly, the frequency and severity of side effects are not higher in this group [41].

Side Effects

SSRIs can cause tremulousness, agitation, irritability, insomnia, anorexia, nausea, vomiting, diarrhea, excess sweating, and sexual dysfunction (i.e., decreased libido, erectile and orgasmic dysfunction). The syndrome of inappropriate antidiuretic hormone is an uncommon adverse effect reported with all of the SSRIs; especially in critically ill patients, other causes of hyponatremia should be sought before attributing the metabolic derangement to the SSRI. The SSRIs do not typically cause clinically significant changes in heart rate, blood pressure, or the electrocardiogram (ECG). Overdoses of SSRIs are discussed in Chapter 124.

Theoretically, SSRIs can cause angina or myocardial infarction (MI) due to the direct vasoconstrictive effects of serotonin on damaged myocardium. When fluoxetine therapy is initiated, serum serotonin levels rise for the first 2 weeks and then return to baseline. This mechanism has been implicated in 3 cardiac deaths that occurred 10 days after initiation of fluoxetine [42]. This theoretical concern should extend to other SSRIs as well.

Drug–Drug Interactions

The SSRIs are extensively metabolized by the cytochrome P450 system. All of them also inhibit various isoenzymes in this system and consequently raise the plasma levels of other drugs metabolized by those isoenzymes; sertraline, citalopram, and escitalopram do this the least. The interactions most likely to

TABLE 199.8

SELECTED SUBSTRATES AND INHIBITORS OF CYTOCHROME P450 ISOENZYMES

1A2	2C	2D6	3A3/4
		Substrates	
Acetaminophen	Barbiturates	Codeine	Amiodarone
Aminophylline	Diazepam	Encainide	Astemizole
Haloperidol	Mephenytoin	Flecainide	Calcium-channel blockers
TCAs	Omeprazole	Haloperidol	Cisapride
Theophylline	Phenytoin	Hydrocodone	Diazepam
	Propranolol	Metoprolol	Disopyramide
	TCAs	Propafenone	Lidocaine
		Propranolol	Loratadine
		TCAs	Macrolide antibiotics
		Timolol	Omeprazole
			Propafenone
			Quinidine
			Steroids
			Terfenadine
			TCAs
		Inhibitors	
Fluoxetine	Fluoxetine[a]	Fluoxetine[a]	Fluoxetine
Fluvoxamine[a]	Fluvoxamine[a]	Paroxetine[a]	Fluvoxamine[a]
Paroxetine	Sertraline	Sertraline	Nefazodone[a]
			Sertraline

[a]Strong inhibitor.
TCAs, tricyclic antidepressants.

occur in an ICU are listed in Table 199.8. Attention to drug dosage can mitigate the harmful effects of these interactions.

Drug Discontinuation

The usually mild symptoms of the SSRI discontinuation syndrome (e.g., headache, dizziness, myalgias, and nausea) are generally eclipsed by more pressing issues in critically ill patients.

Atypical Antidepressants

Bupropion

A monocyclic ketone antidepressant, bupropion (Wellbutrin) blocks norepinephrine and dopamine reuptake. As such, it can be activating and used in place of psychostimulants for patients who cannot tolerate these agents or in whom they are contraindicated. Its major side effects are agitation, insomnia, tremulousness, nausea, vomiting, and diarrhea. The immediate-release formulation is associated with an increased risk of seizures, but this risk in the sustained-release (SR) and extended-release (XL) preparations is comparable to that associated with other antidepressants. It carries a low risk of cardiac toxicity, though, in overdose, sinus tachycardia and intraventricular conduction delays have been reported [43]. Bupropion has gained widespread use as an aid to smoking cessation.

Mirtazapine

Mirtazapine (Remeron) is an analog of the tetracyclic antidepressant, mianserin. As an antagonist at presynaptic and postsynaptic α_2-adrenergic receptors and at postsynaptic 5-HT_2 and 5-HT_3 receptors, it enhances both norepinephrine and serotonin transmission. It has few anticholinergic and anti-α_1-adrenergic effects. Mirtazapine is a potent histamine blocker and can cause significant sedation, an increase in appetite, and weight gain—a side-effect profile that is often exploited to advantage in medically ill patients. Mirtazapine is devoid of significant effects on the cytochrome P450 system, making it less apt to cause drug–drug interactions.

Venlafaxine

Venlafaxine (Effexor) is a selective serotonin and norepinephrine reuptake inhibitor (SNRI). It is very similar to the SSRIs in most clinical and pharmacologic aspects. It has few anti-α_1-adrenergic, anticholinergic, and antihistaminergic side effects. Venlafaxine has a 6- to 8-hour half-life and must be given 2 to 3 times daily, but an extended-release preparation (Effexor XR) allows once-daily dosing. It causes a dose-dependent increase in systolic and diastolic blood pressure (up to 7.5 mm Hg), occurring in approximately 7% of patients taking daily doses between 200 and 300 mg and in up to 13% of patients taking >300 mg [44]. The major active metabolite of venlafaxine, desvenlafaxine, is now available as a primary compound (Pristiq); its advantages over its parent compound are uncertain.

Duloxetine

Another SNRI, duloxetine (Cymbalta) is indicated for MDD, generalized anxiety disorder, diabetic neuropathy, and fibromyalgia. Its half-life is 12 hours, and it can be given once or twice daily. Like venlafaxine, it has little effect on α_1-adrenergic, cholinergic, and histaminergic receptors. Any therapeutic advantage over venlafaxine, particularly in critically ill patients, has yet to be demonstrated.

Trazodone

A triazolopyridine derivative, trazodone (Desyrel) is an atypical antidepressant usually used as a sleep aid. It has a more benign cardiac profile than the TCAs and rarely causes cardiac dysrhythmias. The most common cardiovascular effect of trazodone is orthostatic hypotension. Priapism is a rare adverse event.

Tricyclic Antidepressants

TCAs work by blocking reuptake of norepinephrine and serotonin at presynaptic sites. The most common side effects of TCAs are sedation, orthostatic hypotension, and anticholinergic effects (including confusion, blurred vision, dry mouth, constipation, and urinary hesitancy or retention). The tertiary-amine parent compounds, amitriptyline (Elavil) and imipramine (Tofranil), are more apt to produce these adverse effects than are their respective secondary-amine metabolites, nortriptyline (Pamelor) and desipramine (Norpramin).

Because of this extensive side-effect profile, including adverse effects on cardiac conduction and cardiac rhythm, the TCAs have largely been eclipsed in recent times by the SSRIs and other newer agents, which are safer and better tolerated. For example, in a head-to-head comparison of nortriptyline and fluoxetine in patients with cardiac disease, patients taking nortriptyline had 5 times the incidence of adverse cardiac effects compared to those in the fluoxetine group (20% vs. 4%) [45]. TCAs are relatively contraindicated in patients with cardiac disease and are not recommended in the acute post-MI period. In fact, some data even suggest that TCAs may precipitate arrhythmias and sudden death in cohorts other than just the post-MI population [46].

As a result, it is relatively unusual to see a patient on a TCA at an antidepressant dose in the ICU and highly unusual to start a TCA in an ICU patient. TCAs are still used with some regularity for neuropathic pain syndromes; when used in this situation, doses are much lower than those used in depression treatment. Overdoses with TCAs may be treated in the ICU and are discussed in Chapter 123.

Monoamine Oxidase Inhibitors

The MAOIs (isocarboxazid [Marplan], phenelzine [Nardil], tranylcypromine [Parnate]) work by blocking the oxidative deamination of biogenic amines (e.g., norepinephrine, serotonin) and have been used for the treatment of depression since the 1950s. MAOIs may cause a profound hypertensive crisis when a patient taking MAOIs also takes a sympathomimetic medication (e.g., reserpine, guanethidine, pseudoephedrine, and ephedrine) or ingests tyramine-containing foods (e.g., aged cheeses, pickled foods, and yeast extracts). Coadministration with opioids, particularly meperidine, also may lead to hypertensive crises and to elevated blood levels of meperidine and its neurotoxic metabolite, normeperidine. The use of beta-blockers with MAOIs may lead to unopposed α-adrenergic activity and also cause severe hypertension. For these reasons, similar to TCAs, MAOIs are infrequently used in recent times, even by psychiatrists, and it would be highly unusual to begin an MAOI in an ICU patient. Overdoses with MAOIs may be treated in the ICU and are discussed in Chapter 123.

Pharmacologic Treatment of Depression in Heart Disease

Several studies have examined the effect of antidepressant treatment on psychiatric or cardiovascular outcome or both in patients with CHD. These include the Sertraline Antidepressant Heart Attack Randomized Trial (SADHART), ENRICHD, MIND–IT, and the Canadian Cardiac Randomized Evaluation of Antidepressant and Psychotherapy Efficacy (CREATE) trial. The basic details and findings of these landmark studies, as well as two other randomized trials [47,48], are summarized in Table 199.9.

In SADHART, response to sertraline was independently predicted by each of the following factors: (a) onset of the current depressive episode before the ACS, (b) a history of MDD, and (c) greater severity of depression [49]. Moreover, in the cohort with recurrent MDD, quality of life and several functional status scores were significantly improved in the sertraline group [50]. SADHART was designed to evaluate only the safety and efficacy of sertraline, not its effect on cardiac outcomes. Nevertheless, the number of severe cardiac events (e.g., death, MI, congestive heart failure [CHF], recurrent angina, stroke) was lower in patients treated with sertraline (14.5%) compared with those receiving placebo (22.4%) [51]. After a median follow-up of almost 7 years, baseline MDD severity and persistence of depression despite active or placebo treatment in the 6 months immediately after ACS independently predicted more than a doubling of mortality risk [7].

ENRICHD was the first trial of the effect of depression treatment on mortality and reinfarction in post-MI patients [5]. The differential improvement in depression between the intervention and the usual-care groups was only modest and was short-lived. Most notably, the intervention yielded no cardiac benefit. This negative result may have occurred because many of the patients in the usual-care arm received antidepressant medication, thus potentially obscuring any between-group differences. In fact, a secondary analysis found that patients exposed to SSRIs had a lower risk of death or recurrent MI and of all-cause mortality compared to patients who did not take SSRIs [52]. In addition, patients with mild, transient depressions likely to have improved on their own were included in the study, and the treatment duration of 6 months may have been too short to discern a salutary effect.

Thus Carney et al. [53] undertook a subgroup analysis of patients with full (rather than modified) criteria for MDD or minor depression, a baseline Beck Depression Inventory (BDI) score ≥ 10, and a history of at least one episode of MDD and completed the follow-up evaluation 6 months after enrollment (i.e., those patients who completed the intervention). While the difference in the mean change in BDI score from baseline to 6 months between groups was higher in this narrowed sample than in the entire cohort, this enhanced improvement did not translate into a survival benefit. While patients who responded to the intervention experienced a reduction in mortality, the authors recommended caution in evaluating this finding as it was based on small numbers.

MIND–IT examined the effects of antidepressant treatment on cardiac prognosis and on the long-term course of depression [6]. The active treatment arm included three possibilities: randomization to mirtazapine or placebo, open treatment with citalopram, or treatment at the discretion of the treating psychiatrist. Those randomized to mirtazapine or placebo were given the option to switch to unblinded citalopram if there was no response after 8 weeks. Similar to ENRICHD, no significant differences between active treatment and usual care were found in depressive or cardiac outcome. In a separate analysis of just the patients who received mirtazapine, this agent yielded a therapeutic advantage over placebo [54]. In a three-way comparison of responders and nonresponders to either antidepressant (mirtazapine or citalopram) and patients who received no treatment, responders had the least cardiac events, followed by the untreated patients and then the nonresponders, leading the authors to suggest that persistence of depression may be the crucial "cardiotoxic" attribute of depressive illness, for which treatment resistance may be a marker [55].

TABLE 199.9

RANDOMIZED, CONTROLLED TRIALS OF DEPRESSION PHARMACOTHERAPY IN PATIENTS WITH CARDIOVASCULAR DISEASE

Study	Enrollment	Intervention	Results
Berkman et al. [5]	2,481 patients with modified[a] DSM-IV major or minor depression and/or low perceived social support within 28 d after MI	Intervention (CBT ± sertraline 50–200 mg/d or other medication) vs. usual care for 6 mo	The intervention yielded a significant, though modest, improvement in depression and in social support after 6 mo. This effect was insignificant for depression after 30 mo and for social support after 42 mo. There was no significant difference between groups in death or nonfatal MI, all-cause mortality, cardiac mortality, or recurrent nonfatal MI after an average follow-up of 29 mo.
van Melle et al. [6]	331 patients with ICD-10 depression 3–12 mo after MI	Intervention (mirtazapine, citalopram, or nonpharmacological treatment) vs. usual care for 6 mo	There was no difference between groups in mean BDI scores, presence of depression, and incidence of cardiac events at 18 mo.
Roose et al. [47]	81 patients with MDD and stable ischemic heart disease	Paroxetine 20–30 mg/d vs. nortriptyline for 6 wk	61% of the patients on paroxetine improved compared to 55% of those on nortriptyline. Those on SSRI had fewer adverse cardiac events.
Strik et al. [48]	54 patients with MDD 3–12 mo after a first MI	Fluoxetine vs. placebo	The response rate in the fluoxetine group was significantly greater at week 25, especially in patients with mild depression. There was no decrease in cardiac function in the fluoxetine group.
Glassman et al. [51]	369 patients with MDD and ACS (either MI or unstable angina)	Sertraline 50–200 mg/d vs. placebo for 24 wk	Sertraline had no significant effect on mean LVEF, increase in PVCs, QTc prolongation, and other cardiac measures. In cohorts with recurrent or severe MDD, depression scores were significantly lower in the sertraline group.
Honig et al. [54]	91 patients with DSM-IV depression 3–12 mo after MI	Mirtazapine vs. placebo for 24 wk	Mirtazapine was superior to placebo on two of three depression scales at 8 and 24 wk. There was no assessment of effect on cardiac outcomes.
Lespérance et al. [56]	284 patients with DSM-IV MDD and CAD	Twelve weekly sessions of IPT with CM vs. CM alone, and citalopram 20–40 mg/d vs. placebo for 12 wk	The addition of IPT to clinical management conferred no therapeutic advantage. Citalopram was significantly more effective than placebo in reducing depression.

[a]Symptoms of ≥7 days' duration if there was ≥1 prior depressive episode, 14 days if not.
ACS, acute coronary syndrome; BDI, Beck Depression Inventory; CBT, cognitive-behavioral therapy; CM, clinical management; DSM-IV, *Diagnostic and Statistical Manual of Mental Disorders*, 4th edition; ICD-10, *International Classification of Diseases*, 10th edition; IPT, interpersonal therapy; LVEF, left ventricular ejection fraction; MDD, major depressive disorder; MI, myocardial infarction; PVCs, premature ventricular contractions; QTc, QT interval corrected for heart rate; SSRI, selective serotonin reuptake inhibitor.

CREATE, the first and only study designed to evaluate paired psychological and pharmacological interventions for depression treatment in CHD patients, failed to show a therapeutic advantage for interpersonal therapy, a manualized, short-term therapy focused on loss, grief, life transitions, interpersonal conflicts, and social isolation [56]. It demonstrated, however, that citalopram is an effective antidepressant in this population.

Several additional studies in this area are currently underway. The Safety and Efficacy of Sertraline for Depression in Patients with CHF (SADHART–CHF) study will evaluate the effects of 12 weeks of sertraline compared to placebo on depression and cardiac prognosis in approximately 500 patients with MDD and chronic systolic heart failure [57]. The Bypassing the Blues (BtB) study will randomize 450 patients after coronary artery bypass grafting (CABG) to either an 8-month nurse-delivered telephone-based collaborative care intervention or usual care and evaluate the effect on mood, cardiac morbidity, health-related quality of life, and other outcomes [58]. The first study of the prevention of depression in CHD patients, the Depression in Coronary Artery Disease (DECARD) trial will randomize 240 patients with ACS, but without depression, to 1 year of escitalopram or placebo [59].

Pharmacologic Treatment of Depression in Stroke

Table 199.10 summarizes findings from the randomized, controlled trials of depression treatment and prophylaxis in patients with cerebrovascular disease [60–79]. In a randomized, double-blind, placebo-controlled study of poststroke patients, nortriptyline was more effective than fluoxetine or placebo

TABLE 199.10

RANDOMIZED, CONTROLLED TRIALS OF DEPRESSION PHARMACOTHERAPY IN PATIENTS WITH CEREBROVASCULAR DISEASE

Study	Enrollment	Intervention	Results
Lauritzen et al. [60]	20 poststroke patients with depression	Imipramine and mianserin[a] vs. desipramine and mianserin for 6 wk	The imipramine arm was superior to the desipramine arm.
Rampello et al. [61]	31 patients with "retarded" depression within 12 mo after CVA	Reboxetine[b] 4 mg twice daily vs. placebo for 16 wk	Reboxetine showed good efficacy, safety, and tolerability. There was a significant difference in change in HDRS and BDI scores between groups.
Robinson et al. [62]	159 patients with MDD 10 d to 3 mo after CVA	Nefiracetam[c] 600 or 900 mg/d vs. placebo	Both arms showed response rates >70% and remission rates >40%. Patients in the top quintile of HDRS scores showed a significant effect with 900 mg compared to 600 mg or placebo.
Robinson et al. [63]	104 poststroke patients with and without depression	Nortriptyline 25–100 mg/d, fluoxetine 10–40 mg/d, or placebo for 12 wk	Nortriptyline resulted in a significantly higher response than fluoxetine or placebo in reversing depression, reducing anxiety, and improving functional status. Neither active treatment improved cognitive or social functioning in depressed or nondepressed patients.
Wiart et al. [64]	31 poststroke patients with MDD	Fluoxetine 20 mg/d vs. placebo for 6 wk	Fluoxetine produced a significant improvement in depression but not in motor, cognitive, or functional scores.
Fruehwald et al. [65]	50 poststroke patients with depression	Fluoxetine 20 mg/d vs. placebo for 3 mo	Both groups showed significant improvement, with no between-group difference, after 1 mo. At 18 mo, the fluoxetine group had significantly less depression.
Choi-Kwon et al. [66]	152 patients 3–28 mo after CVA with depression, emotional incontinence, or anger proneness	Fluoxetine 20 mg/d vs. placebo for 3 mo	Fluoxetine produced significantly higher scores in the mental health, general health, and social functioning domains of QOL after 12 mo.
Li et al. [67]	150 poststroke patients with moderate to severe depression	FEWP[d] vs. fluoxetine vs. placebo for 8 wk	The active arms showed a higher clinical response than placebo, but no difference between FEWP and fluoxetine was discernible at the end of the study.
Choi-Kwon et al. [68]	152 poststroke patients with depression, emotional incontinence, or anger proneness	Fluoxetine 20 mg/d vs. placebo for 3 mo	Fluoxetine significantly improved emotional incontinence and anger proneness but not depression.
Andersen et al. [69]	66 patients with depression 2–52 wk after CVA	Citalopram 10–40 mg/d vs. placebo for 3 and 6 wk	Citalopram yielded greater improvement than placebo.
Rampello et al. [70]	74 poststroke patients with depression	Citalopram 20 mg/d vs. reboxetine 4 mg/d for 16 wk	Both agents showed good safety and tolerability. Citalopram showed a greater effect on anxious depression, reboxetine on retarded depression.
Cravello et al. [71]	50 poststroke patients with depression	Venlafaxine SR 75–150 mg/d vs. fluoxetine 20–40 mg/d for 8 wk	Both agents yielded similar improvement in depressive symptoms. Venlafaxine showed more improvement on an alexithymia scale.
Grade et al. [72]	21 poststroke patients admitted to a rehabilitation facility	Methylphenidate 5–30 mg/d vs. placebo for 3 wk	Methylphenidate yielded lower HDRS and Zung[e] scores.
Murray et al. [73]	123 poststroke patients with MDD or minor depression	Sertraline 50–100 mg/d vs. placebo for 26 wk	Both groups improved substantially. There was no difference in depression between groups and significantly less emotional distress and better QOL in the treatment group.
Narushima et al. [74]	48 poststroke patients who were not depressed at baseline	Nortriptyline 25–100 mg/d, fluoxetine 10–40 mg/d, or placebo for 12 wk for prophylaxis	Significantly fewer depressive episodes occurred in the treatment groups. However, more nortriptyline-treated patients developed depression in the 6 months after treatment was stopped compared to the other two groups.
Robinson et al. [75]	176 patients without depression within 3 mo after CVA	Escitalopram vs. placebo vs. problem-solving therapy for 1 y for prophylaxis	Patients who received either escitalopram or therapy were significantly less likely to develop depression. In an intention-to-treat analysis, escitalopram, but not therapy, was significantly superior to placebo in depression prevention.

(continued)

TABLE 199.10

CONTINUED

Study	Enrollment	Intervention	Results
Niedermaier et al. [76]	70 poststroke patients who were not depressed	Mirtazapine 30 mg/d vs. placebo for 1 y for prophylaxis and treatment	Significantly fewer patients in the treatment group developed depression. Fifteen out of 16 patients who developed depression were treated effectively with mirtazapine.
Rasmussen et al. [77]	137 poststroke patients who were not depressed at baseline	Sertraline 50–150 mg/d vs. placebo for 1 y for prophylaxis	Significantly fewer patients in the sertraline group developed depression compared to the placebo group.
Almeida et al. [78]	111 patients without depression <2 wk after CVA	Sertraline 50 mg/d vs. placebo for 24 wk for prophylaxis	There was no significant difference in development of depressive symptoms.
Palomäki et al. [79]	100 patients with acute ischemic CVA	Mianserin 60 mg/d vs. placebo for 1 y as prophylaxis	Prevalence of depression did not differ between groups. No difference in stroke outcome or functional outcome was found.

[a] An antagonist at α_2-adrenergic pre- and postsynaptic receptors and 5-HT_2 receptors, similar to mirtazapine, available in Europe.
[b] A norepinephrine reuptake inhibitor available in Europe.
[c] A so-called cognitive enhancer used in patients with Alzheimer's disease.
[d] A Chinese herbal antidepressant.
[e] A depression rating scale.
CVA, cerebrovascular accident; FEWP, Free and Easy Wanderer Plus; HDRS, Hamilton Depression Rating Scale; MDD, major depressive disorder; PSD, poststroke depression; QOL, quality of life; SR, sustained release.

in reversing depression, reducing anxiety, and improving performance of daily activities [63]. Treatment with either antidepressant significantly increased the survival of depressed patients and, interestingly, nondepressed patients as well [80]. Other studies [64–67], although not all [68], found that fluoxetine was more effective than placebo for PSD. Citalopram [69,70], venlafaxine [71], and methylphenidate [72] also have been beneficial. Recently, Jorge et al. [81] found that poststroke patients who received escitalopram showed more improvement in global cognitive functioning than did patients who received placebo or problem-solving therapy. Moreover, this effect was independent of the antidepressant effect of the SSRI. Fluoxetine and sertraline may be more effective for emotional incontinence and anger proneness after stroke than for depression [68,73]. Nortriptyline [74], fluoxetine [74], escitalopram [75], and mirtazapine [76] were effective in preventing PSD; sertraline had mixed results [77,78], and mianserin was ineffective [79].

Electroconvulsive Therapy

ECT is a safe and effective treatment that may be used in cases of severe or delusional depression or when more conventional therapies cannot be used or are ineffective or intolerable to patients. Found to be particularly helpful in the depressive states accompanying stroke, Parkinson's disease, and dementia, ECT has become part of the standard of care for treatment of severe depression in the medically ill [82]. ECT is also used to treat catatonia.

There are no absolute contraindications to ECT, but patients with unstable cerebro- or cardiovascular disease or increased intracranial pressure warrant closer scrutiny [83–85]. The decision to proceed with ECT or not is made after a careful weighing of the risks of the treatment itself on any underlying physical morbidity against the risks of ongoing untreated depressive illness. This calculation is best done by a psychiatrist experienced in ECT in consultation with an anesthesiologist and other specialists. The latest research in this area has examined the memory impairment associated with ECT and the relationship of lead placement (e.g., bifrontal, bitemporal, and unilateral) to cognitive function [86–89].

Psychological Management

Although pharmacologic treatments are the mainstay of treatment for depression in the ICU, psychological remedies are also important. Patients often benefit from information, clarification, reassurance, and support. Psychological therapies are most useful in cases of adjustment disorder with depressed mood, often as an adjunct to pharmacologic interventions. Evidence has shown that brief psychotherapy at the bedside can give way to increased resilience and hope [90].

When patients come to the ICU, they are often terrified about the outcome of the illness that brings them there. They frequently believe that the illness, no matter how well controlled in the ICU, will continue to be life-threatening after discharge. Some patients believe that their illness will necessitate a radical change in lifestyle. For example, many cardiac patients secretly believe that having had an MI means they will never be able to have sex again. One way to help patients with such concerns is to ask specific questions about how they believe their illness will affect daily life in the future. In this way, one will hear the patient's specific fears and be able to educate the patient about the real effects of the illness. Another example is the patient who is physically weak after an MI and thinks he or she is a cardiac cripple. The patient does not understand that the physical debility is the result of muscle wasting from prolonged bed rest. Education often reassures patients.

Another way to help patients cope with depression in the ICU involves learning about a patient's premorbid activities. Because patients in the ICU feel stripped of their identities and are demoralized, showing interest in who they are and what is important to them can remind them that they are respected and have lives outside the hospital. Families also can be helped to have realistic expectations. Strategies to help patients and families cope effectively in the ICU are discussed in Chapter 201.

CONCLUSION

Treatment of depression in ICUs is multifaceted. Many difficulties are involved in treating depression. Nevertheless, aggressive treatment of depression in the ICU can drastically improve a patient's sense of well-being and transform a demoralized, hopeless patient into an active participant in treatment. In this chapter, we have outlined the recognition, differential diagnosis, and treatment of depression in ICUs. We strongly advocate that depression be treated as a serious illness; although a depressed mood is sometimes understandable, a depressive disorder is never appropriate.

References

1. American Psychiatric Association: *Diagnostic and Statistical Manual of Mental Disorders*. 4th ed. Washington, DC, American Psychiatric Association, 1994.
2. Belmaker RH, Agam G: Major depressive disorder. *N Engl J Med* 358:55, 2008.
3. Dowlati Y, Herrmann N, Swardfager W, et al: A meta-analysis of cytokines in major depression. *Biol Psychiatry* 67:446, 2010.
4. Frasure-Smith N, Lespérance F: Depression and cardiac risk: present status and future directions. *Heart* 96:173, 2010.
5. Berkman LF, Blumenthal J, Burg M, et al: Effects of treating depression and low perceived social support on clinical events after myocardial infarction: the Enhancing Recovery in Coronary Heart Disease Patients (ENRICHD) Randomized Trial. *JAMA* 289:3106, 2003.
6. van Melle JP, de Jonge P, Honig A, et al: Effects of antidepressant treatment following myocardial infarction. *Br J Psychiatry* 190:460, 2007.
7. Glassman AH, Bigger JT, Gaffney M: Psychiatric characteristics associated with long-term mortality among 361 patients having an acute coronary syndrome and major depression: seven-year follow-up of SADHART participants. *Arch Gen Psychiatry* 66:1022, 2009.
8. Rafanelli C, Milaneschi Y, Roncuzzi R, et al: Dysthymia before myocardial infarction as a cardiac risk factor at 2.5-year follow-up. *Psychosomatics* 51:8, 2010.
9. de Jonge P, van den Brink RHS, Spijkerman TA, et al: Only incident depressive episodes after myocardial infarction are associated with new cardiovascular events. *J Am Coll Cardiol* 48:2204, 2006.
10. Carney RM, Freedland KE, Steinmeyer B, et al: History of depression and survival after acute myocardial infarction. *Psychosom Med* 71:253, 2009.
11. Carney RM, Freedland KE: Treatment-resistant depression and mortality after acute coronary syndrome. *Am J Psychiatry* 166:410, 2009.
12. Carney RM, Freedland KE, Steinmeyer B, et al: Depression and five year survival following acute myocardial infarction: a prospective study. *J Affect Disord* 109:133, 2008.
13. de Jonge P, Ormel J, van den Brink RHS, et al: Symptom dimensions of depression following myocardial infarction and their relationship with somatic health status and cardiovascular prognosis. *Am J Psychiatry* 163:138, 2006.
14. Linke SE, Rutledge T, Johnson BD, et al: Depressive symptom dimensions and cardiovascular prognosis among women with suspected myocardial ischemia: a report from the National Heart, Lung, and Blood Institute–sponsored Women's Ischemia Syndrome Evaluation. *Arch Gen Psychiatry* 66:499, 2009.
15. Schiffer AA, Pelle AJ, Smith ORF, et al: Somatic versus cognitive symptoms of depression as predictors of all-cause mortality and health status in chronic heart failure. *J Clin Psychiatry* 70:1667, 2009.
16. Goldston K, Baillie AJ: Depression and coronary heart disease: a review of the epidemiological evidence, explanatory mechanisms and management approaches. *Clin Psychol Rev* 28:288, 2008.
17. Serebruany VL, Gurbel PA, O'Connor CM: Platelet inhibition by sertraline and N-desmethylsertraline: a possible missing link between depression, coronary events and mortality benefits of SSRIs. *Pharmacol Res* 43:453, 2001.
18. Serebruany VL, Glassman AH, Malinin AI, et al: Platelet/endothelial biomarkers in depressed patients treated with the selective serotonin reuptake inhibitor sertraline after acute coronary events: the Sertraline Antidepressant Heart Attack Randomized Trial (SADHART) platelet substudy. *Circulation* 108:939, 2003.
19. Whooley MA, de Jonge P, Vittinghoff E, et al: Depressive symptoms, health behaviors, and risk of cardiovascular events in patients with coronary heart disease. *JAMA* 300:2379, 2008.
20. May M, McCarron P, Stansfeld S, et al: Does psychological distress predict the risk of ischemic stroke and transient ischemic attack? the Caerphilly Study. *Stroke* 33:7, 2002.
21. Salaycik KJ, Kelly-Hayes M, Beiser A, et al: Depressive symptoms and risk of stroke: the Framingham Study. *Stroke* 38:16, 2007.
22. Robinson RG: Poststroke depression: prevalence, diagnosis, treatment and disease progression. *Biol Psychiatry* 44:376, 2003.
23. Hackett ML, Anderson CS: Predictors of depression after stroke. *Stroke* 36: 2296, 2005.
24. Robinson RG, Szetela B: Mood changes following left hemispheric brain injury. *Ann Neurol* 9:447, 1981.
25. Robinson RG, Kubos KL, Starr LB, et al: Mood disorders in stroke patients: importance of location of lesion. *Brain* 107:81, 1984.
26. Morris PLP, Robinson RG, Beverley R, et al: Lesion location and poststroke depression. *J Neuropsychiatry Clin Neurosci* 8:399, 1996.
27. Vataja R, Pohjasvaara T, Leppävuori A, et al: Magnetic resonance imaging correlates of depression after ischemic stroke. *Arch Gen Psychiatry* 58:925, 2001.
28. Carson AJ, MacHale S, Allen K, et al: Depression after stroke and lesion location: a systematic review. *Lancet* 356:122, 2000.
29. Shimoda K, Robinson RG: The relationship between post-stroke depression and lesion location in long-term follow-up. *Biol Psychiatry* 45:187, 1999.
30. Chochinov HM, Wilson KG, Enns M, et al: Prevalence of depression in the terminally ill: effects of diagnostic criteria and symptoms threshold judgments. *Am J Psychiatry* 151: 537, 1994.
31. Mann JJ: The medical management of depression. *N Engl J Med* 353:1819, 2005.
32. Unützer J: Late-life depression. *N Engl J Med* 357:2269, 2007.
33. Orr K, Taylor D: Psychostimulants in the treatment of depression: a review of the evidence. *CNS Drugs* 21:239, 2007.
34. Rothenhäusler H-B, Ehrentraut S, von Degenfeld G, et al: Treatment of depression with methylphenidate in patients difficult to wean from mechanical ventilation in the intensive care unit. *J Clin Psychiatry* 61:750, 2000.
35. Kaufmann M, Murray G, Cassem N: Use of psychostimulants in medically ill depressed patients. *Psychosomatics* 23:817, 1982.
36. Woods SW, Tesar GE, Murray GB, et al: Psychostimulant treatment of depressive disorders secondary to medical illness. *J Clin Psychiatry* 47:12, 1986.
37. Baldessarini RJ: Drugs and the treatment of psychiatric disorders, in Goodman GA, Goodman LS, Gilman A (eds): *The Pharmacological Basis of Therapeutics*. 6th ed. New York, Macmillan, 1980.
38. Hale AS: New antidepressants: use in high-risk patients. *J Clin Psychiatry* 54[Suppl]:61, 1993.
39. Spigset O, Hagg S, Stegmayr B, et al: Citalopram pharmacokinetics in patients with chronic renal failure and the effect of haemodialysis. *Eur J Clin Pharmacol* 56:9, 2000.
40. DeVane CL, Gill HS: Clinical pharmacokinetics of fluvoxamine: applications to dosage regimen design. *J Clin Psychiatry* 58[Suppl]:3, 1997.
41. Gutierrez M, Abramowitz W: Steady-state pharmacokinetics of citalopram in young and elderly subjects. *Pharmacotherapy* 20:1441, 2000.
42. Fricchione GL, Woznicki RM, Klesmer J, et al: Vasoconstrictive effects and SSRIs [letter]. *J Clin Psychiatry* 54:71, 1993.
43. Shrier M, Diaz J, Tsarouhas N: Cardiotoxicity associated with bupropion overdose [letter]. *Ann Emerg Med* 35:100, 2000.
44. Thase ME: Effects of venlafaxine on blood pressure: a meta-analysis of original data from 3744 depressed patients. *J Clin Psychiatry* 59:502, 1998.
45. Roose SP, Glassman AH, Attia E, et al: Cardiovascular effects of fluoxetine in depressed patients with heart disease. *Am J Psychiatry* 155:660, 1998.
46. Witchel HJ, Hancox JC, Nutt DJ: Psychotropic drugs, cardiac arrhythmias and sudden death. *J Clin Psychopharmacol* 23:58, 2003.
47. Roose SP, Laghrissi-Thode F, Kennedy JS, et al: Comparison of paroxetine and nortriptyline in depressed patients with ischemic heart disease. *JAMA* 279:287, 1998.
48. Strik JJMH, Honig A, Lousberg R, et al: Efficacy and safety of fluoxetine in the treatment of patients with major depression after first myocardial infarction: findings from a double-blind, placebo-controlled trial. *Psychosom Med* 62:783, 2000.
49. Glassman AH, Bigger JT, Gaffney M, et al: Onset of major depression associated with acute coronary syndromes: relationship of onset, major depressive disorder history, and episode severity to sertraline benefit. *Arch Gen Psychiatry* 63:283, 2006.
50. Swenson JR, O'Connor CM, Barton D, et al: Influence of depression and effect of treatment with sertraline on quality of life after hospitalization for acute coronary syndrome. *Am J Cardiol* 92:1271, 2003.
51. Glassman AH, O'Connor CM, Califf RM, et al: Sertraline treatment of major depression in patients with acute MI or unstable angina. *JAMA* 288:701, 2002.
52. Taylor CB, Youngblood ME, Catellier D, et al: Effects of antidepressant medication on morbidity and mortality in depressed patients after myocardial infarction. *Arch Gen Psychiatry* 62:792, 2005.
53. Carney RM, Blumenthal JA, Freedland KE, et al: Depression and late mortality after myocardial infarction in the Enhancing Recovery in Coronary Heart Disease (ENRICHD) study. *Psychosom Med* 66:466, 2004.

54. Honig A, Kuyper AMG, Schene AH, et al: Treatment of post-myocardial infarction depressive disorder: a randomized, placebo-controlled trial with mirtazapine. *Psychosom Med* 69:606, 2007.
55. de Jonge P, Honig A, van Melle JP, et al: Nonresponse to treatment for depression following myocardial infarction: association with subsequent cardiac events. *Am J Psychiatry* 164:1371, 2007.
56. Lespérance F, Frasure-Smith N, Koszycki D, et al: Effects of citalopram and interpersonal psychotherapy on depression in patients with coronary artery disease: the Canadian Cardiac Randomized Evaluation of Antidepressant and Psychotherapy Efficacy (CREATE) trial. *JAMA* 297:367, 2007.
57. Jiang W, O'Connor C, Silva SG, et al: Safety and efficacy of sertraline for depression in patients with CHF (SADHART–CHF): a randomized, double-blind, placebo-controlled trial of sertraline for major depression with congestive heart failure. *Am Heart J* 156:437, 2008.
58. Rollman BL, Belnap BH, LeMenager MS, et al: The Bypassing the Blues treatment protocol: stepped collaborative care for treating post-CABG depression. *Psychosom Med* 71:217, 2009.
59. Hansen BH, Hanash JA, Rasmussen A, et al: Rationale, design and methodology of a double-blind, randomized, placebo-controlled study of escitalopram in prevention of Depression in Acute Coronary Syndrome (DECARD). *Trials* 10:20, 2009.
60. Lauritzen L, Bendsen BB, Vilmar T, et al: Post-stroke depression: combined treatment with imipramine or desipramine and mianserin: a controlled clinical study. *Psychopharmacology* 114:119, 1994.
61. Rampello L, Alvano A, Chiechio S, et al: An evaluation of efficacy and safety of reboxetine in elderly patients affected by "retarded" post-stroke depression: a random, placebo-controlled study. *Arch Gerontol Geriatr* 40:275, 2005.
62. Robinson RG, Jorge RE, Clarence-Smith K: Double-blind randomized treatment of poststroke depression using nefiracetam. *J Neuropsychiatry Clin Neurosci* 20:178, 2008.
63. Robinson RG, Schultz SK, Castillo C, et al: Nortriptyline versus fluoxetine in the treatment of depression and in short-term recovery after stroke: a placebo-controlled, double-blind study. *Am J Psychiatry* 157:351, 2000.
64. Wiart L, Petit H, Joseph PA, et al: Fluoxetine in early poststroke depression: a double-blind placebo-controlled study. *Stroke* 31:1829, 2000.
65. Fruehwald S, Gatterbauer E, Rehak P, et al: Early fluoxetine treatment of post-stroke depression: a three-month double-blind placebo-controlled study with an open-label long-term follow-up. *J Neurol* 250:347, 2003.
66. Choi-Kwon S, Choi J, Kwon SU, et al: Fluoxetine improves the quality of life in patients with poststroke emotional disturbances. *Cerebrovasc Dis* 26:266, 2008.
67. Li L-T, Wang S-H, Ge H-Y, et al: The beneficial effects of the herbal medicine Free and Easy Wanderer Plus (FEWP) and fluoxetine on post-stroke depression. *J Altern Complement Med* 14:841, 2008.
68. Choi-Kwon S, Han SW, Kwon SU, et al: Fluoxetine treatment in poststroke depression, emotional incontinence, and anger proneness: a double-blind, placebo-controlled study. *Stroke* 37:156, 2006.
69. Andersen G, Vestergaard K, Lauritzen L: Effective treatment of poststroke depression with the selective serotonin reuptake inhibitor citalopram. *Stroke* 25:1099, 1994.
70. Rampello L, Chiechio S, Nicoletti G, et al: Prediction of the response to citalopram and reboxetine in post-stroke depressed patients. *Psychopharmacology* 173:73, 2004.
71. Cravello L, Caltagirone C, Spalletta G: The SNRI venlafaxine improves emotional unawareness in patients with post-stroke depression. *Hum Psychopharmacol* 24:331, 2009.
72. Grade C, Redford B, Chrostowski J, et al: Methylphenidate in early post-stroke recovery: a double-blind, placebo-controlled study. *Arch Phys Med Rehabil* 79:1047, 1998.
73. Murray V, von Arbin M, Bartfai A, et al: Double-blind comparison of sertraline and placebo in stroke patients with minor depression and less severe major depression. *J Clin Psychiatry* 66:708, 2005.
74. Narushima K, Kosier JT, Robinson RG: Preventing poststroke depression: a 12-week double-blind randomized treatment trial and 21-month follow-up. *J Nerv Ment Dis* 190:296, 2002.
75. Robinson RG, Jorge RE, Moser DJ, et al: Escitalopram and problem-solving therapy for prevention of poststroke depression: a randomized controlled trial. *JAMA* 299:2391, 2008.
76. Niedermaier N, Bohrer E, Schulte K, et al: Prevention and treatment of poststroke depression with mirtazapine in patients with acute stroke. *J Clin Psychiatry* 65:1619, 2004.
77. Rasmussen A, Lunde M, Poulsen DL, et al: A double-blind, placebo-controlled study of sertraline in the prevention of depression in stroke patients. *Psychosomatics* 44:216, 2003.
78. Almeida OP, Waterreus A, Hankey GJ: Preventing depression after stroke: results from a randomized placebo-controlled trial. *J Clin Psychiatry* 67:1104, 2006.
79. Palomäki H, Kaste M, Berg A, et al: Prevention of poststroke depression: 1 year randomized placebo controlled double blind trial of mianserin with 6 month follow up after therapy. *J Neurol Neurosurg Psychiatry* 66:490, 1999.
80. Jorge RE, Robinson RG, Arndt S, et al: Mortality and poststroke depression: a placebo-controlled trial of antidepressants. *Am J Psychiatry* 160:1823, 2003.
81. Jorge RE, Acion L, Moser D, et al: Escitalopram and enhancement of cognitive recovery following stroke. *Arch Gen Psychiatry* 67:187, 2010.
82. Christopher EJ: Electroconvulsive therapy in the medically ill. *Curr Psychiatry Rep* 5:225, 2003.
83. American Psychiatric Association: *The Practice of Electroconvulsive Therapy: Recommendations for Treatment, Training, and Privileging*. 2nd ed. Washington, DC, American Psychiatric Association, 2001.
84. Lisanby SH: Electroconvulsive therapy for depression. *N Engl J Med* 357:1939, 2007.
85. Tess AV, Smetana GW: Medical evaluation of patients undergoing electroconvulsive therapy. *N Engl J Med* 360:1437, 2009.
86. UK ECT Review Group: Efficacy and safety of electroconvulsive therapy in depressive disorders: a systematic review and meta-analysis. *Lancet* 361:799, 2003.
87. Kellner CH, Knapp R, Husain MM, et al: Bifrontal, bitemporal and right unilateral electrode placement in ECT: randomised trial. *Br J Psychiatry* 196:226, 2010.
88. Sienaert P, Vansteelandt K, Demyttenaere K, et al: Randomized comparison of ultra-brief bifrontal and unilateral electroconvulsive therapy for major depression: cognitive side-effects. *J Affect Disord* 122:60, 2010.
89. Smith GE, Rasmussen KG, Cullum CM, et al: A randomized controlled trial comparing the memory effects of continuation electroconvulsive therapy versus continuation pharmacotherapy: results from the Consortium for Research in ECT (CORE) study. *J Clin Psychiatry* 71:185, 2010.
90. Griffith JL, Gaby L: Brief psychotherapy at the bedside: countering demoralization from medical illness. *Psychosomatics* 46:109, 2005.

CHAPTER 200 ■ MANAGING THE SUICIDAL PATIENT IN THE INTENSIVE CARE UNIT

SAORI A. MURAKAMI AND HOA THI LAM

The assessment of the suicidal patient is a significant challenge for any intensive care team. Even when a psychiatrist is consulted to conduct an expert assessment of risk and to assist with the formulation of a treatment plan, the intensivist's ability to evaluate, manage, and safeguard the patient's safety is essential. The evaluation and management of a patient—whether contemplating suicide or recovering from a suicide attempt—require an understanding of risk factors, protective factors, the interplay among these various elements, and the relationship between staff and patient. In addition, the primary medical team should be aware of the necessity for ongoing psychiatric care during and after the stabilization of acute medical issues.

This chapter reviews the epidemiology of suicide, risk and protective factors, parasuicide, and intervention and management strategies for suicidal patients in the intensive care unit (ICU).

EPIDEMIOLOGY OF SUICIDE

Suicide is the 11th leading cause of death in the United States (8th in men, 16th in women) [1]. In 2006, suicide was responsible for 33,300 deaths, with higher rates among whites, youths, and individuals more than 65 years of age [2]. Although no recent national estimates of the number of admissions to ICUs due to suicide attempts are available, in 2008, 376,306 people presented to an emergency department for treatment of self-harm, and 163,489 people were hospitalized due to self-inflicted injuries [1].

RISK AND PROTECTIVE FACTORS

Although appraisals of suicide risk are incapable of absolute predictions of suicidal behavior, careful history-taking, detailed examination, and astute clinical judgment allow a comprehensive understanding and evaluation of risk factors, protective factors, and the interplay among them (Table 200.1).

The first set of factors is sociodemographic, including age, gender, race, marital status, and religion. In general, men are more likely to complete suicide, whereas women are more likely to make attempts [1,3,4]. White men are more likely to attempt suicide than nonwhites; among nonwhite populations, rates vary [1,3]. Suicide rates increase in two particular age distributions: late adolescence to young adulthood and older than age 65 [1,2,5]. In general, the suicide rate is greatest among divorced and widowed people, followed by single individuals, and married people [5]. The combination of age, gender, and marital status also plays a role; young widowed men have a particularly high rate of suicide [5].

Some evidence suggests that religious beliefs and the strength of one's religious convictions protect against suicide; however, for some, religion may increase suicide risk. For example, an individual who believes he will be reunited with his lost loved ones when he himself dies may be comforted by the idea of dying. Thus, the various meanings religion can have in different people's lives mandate careful exploration with the patient of the role of religion in death and suicide [5,6].

Psychiatric illness contributes significantly to the risk for suicide. Retrospective studies have identified one or more psychiatric disorders in individuals who have completed suicide or presented following a suicide attempt [7,8]. In addition, conditions often comorbid with psychiatric illnesses (e.g., substance use disorders) increase the risk for suicide. The presence of a past history of suicide attempts, suicidal thinking, self-injurious behavior, impulsivity, assaultiveness, and trauma (physical or emotional) is an important component of risk assessment. Whether a patient is in active outpatient psychiatric treatment—and compliant with it—is also critical. Psychological factors—coping skills, tolerance of emotions, personality traits, insight, and judgment—figure prominently in the estimation of how a patient handles stress.

The presence of a physical illness contributes to the risk for suicide, with the number of physical illnesses increasing the risk for suicide in a linear fashion [9]. Suicide risk is greater in patients with neurologic disorders (e.g., Huntington's chorea, organic brain syndromes, multiple sclerosis, spinal cord injuries), and suicide attempts are more common in patients with epilepsy [5,10,11]. In addition, head trauma is associated with an enhanced risk for suicide, particularly when behavioral or cognitive sequelae result. Executive function deficits due to delirium, dementia, or mental retardation also contribute to the risk for suicide. Other illnesses of significance are listed in Table 200.1 [5,12].

TABLE 200.1

RISK AND PROTECTIVE FACTORS FOR SUICIDE

Sociodemographic factors
Age
Gender
Race
Marital status
Religion
Psychiatric history and present psychiatric conditions
Psychiatric disorders
Substance abuse/dependence
History of suicide attempts
History of self-injurious behavior
History of homicidal or assaultive behavior
Impulsivity
History of physical or emotional trauma
Psychiatric treatment, both outpatient and inpatient
History of treatment adherence
Psychological factors
Medical history and present medical conditions
Neurologic disorders
Head trauma, with or without cognitive and behavioral sequelae
Executive function deficits
Malignancies
Human immunodeficiency virus infection
Acquired immune deficiency syndrome
Peptic ulcer disease
Chronic inflammatory diseases
Hemodialysis-treated chronic renal failure
Heart disease
Chronic pulmonary disease
Family history
Psychiatric illness
Substance abuse/dependence
History of completed suicide
Psychosocial stressors
Family life
Work life
Relationships
Finances
Recent real or perceived loss

Adapted from American Psychiatric Association: Practice Guideline for the Assessment and Treatment of Patients with Suicidal Behaviors. Arlington, VA, American Psychiatric Association, 2003. Available at: www.psych.org/psych_pract/treatg/pg/Practice%20Guidelines8904/SuicidalBehaviors.pdf. Accessed January 2, 2010.

Psychosocial stressors—including states of family life, work life, relationships, finances, and losses—are important considerations when assessing risk. A family history of psychiatric disturbances, substance use, or completed suicide may indicate potential genetic vulnerabilities in management of these stressors and response to interventions.

Protective factors include the presence of supports (e.g., family, friends, faith) and the absence of risk factors.

Risk and protective factors must be understood on a case-by-case basis [13–15]. Despite the significance of each factor, the weight to attribute to each element must be individualized, as the interaction among these features defines each patient's unique risk. For example, a 70-year-old unmarried white man with an incurable malignancy may be protected from suicide by his religion's prohibition against it and by his three grandchildren's frequent visits.

PARASUICIDE

Some physicians may differentiate "genuine" suicide attempts (in which the person's aim was to kill himself) from parasuicide, a term introduced by Kreitman meaning "a non-fatal act in which the individual deliberately causes self-injury or ingests a substance in excess of any prescribed or generally recognized therapeutic dosage" [16]. Often, parasuicide is not a failed attempt to kill oneself per se, but could be either a maladaptive way to cope with emotions or an effort to elicit a specific reaction from someone else, whether an emotional response (e.g., feeling hurt or sorry) or a behavioral one (e.g., forestalling abandonment or providing nurturance). As such, a physician may be tempted to construe parasuicide as less concerning than an authentic attempt to end one's life. However, these individuals require equal attention and caution because parasuicide often recurs; when repeated often enough, such behavior may prove lethal, even if death is unintended. Furthermore, parasuicide may leave the person subsequently suicidal [17,18]. For example, a man who commits parasuicide in an attempt to keep his wife from divorcing him may feel genuinely suicidal if his wife ends up leaving him.

TREATMENT OF THE SUICIDAL PATIENT

Nonpharmacologic Interventions

A patient's verbalization of intent to harm himself or herself poses a unique challenge for the ICU physician. Although such utterances can be variously motivated and belie different intentions, any such statement should be taken seriously and viewed as the patient's request for help and support. Suicidal statements may take the form of explicit declaration or implicit action (e.g., refusal to eat or to cooperate with care). The suicidal act can be impulsive or deliberate. Because accurate prediction of which statements will result in action is impossible, the ICU team must institute effective precautions whenever a patient avows suicide.

The ICU team should implement close monitoring, in the form of constant observation by a one-to-one sitter or more frequent checks of the patient. Physical restraint of a patient at ongoing risk may be necessary when constant observation is not possible [12]. Staff should be aware of potential means by which patients may harm themselves. Any opportunity of jumping from windows or of hanging should be minimized, if not eliminated. All material that a person may use to harm himself or herself (e.g., razors, scissors, needles, glass, medications, and eating utensils) must be removed and any personal belongings searched for these items. Staff should also be aware of items brought in by visitors. The team should review medications and consider decreasing or discontinuing medications that may heighten impulsivity or disinhibition. Estimations of safety should be made at least daily.

The primary team must also identify and address among themselves any negative feelings they have about the patient. Emotional reactions to dealing with psychological problems in the ICU can include helplessness, insecurity, fear, anxiety, guilt, and sympathy. People who repeatedly attempt suicide or whose motives have been deemed "manipulative" can engender frustration, anger, and exhaustion with demands for constant attention, thereby creating distance between the patient and the treatment team. It is important to understand these feelings and to prevent them from hampering patient care and clouding recognition of a potentially unsafe patient. For example, patients with borderline personality disorder can "split" the staff (i.e., behave well for one subset of the staff and badly for another) [19]. Regular communication among staff members and between the staff and the patient can minimize splitting and prevent team members from feeling defensive or apologetic in the face of a critical and demanding patient.

An empathic approach that seeks to understand what the patient feels can prevent these emotions from instigating countertherapeutic responses. Even if a "suicide attempt" is an effort to elicit a particular response from others (rather than a genuine attempt to end one's life), the desperation required to put one's life at risk is nonetheless sobering. For people whose intent was to die, waking up from an unsuccessful suicide attempt can be accompanied by despair, shame, guilt, fear, anger, a sense of inferiority, and ambivalence about having survived [20]. The physical discomfort of the life-sustaining measures employed in the ICU only compounds such patients' pain.

Medications

The question of whether and when to restart psychiatric medications following a suicide attempt can be a difficult one, particularly if the person attempted to kill himself or herself by overdose on these agents. The decision to resume outpatient medicines must be guided first and foremost by accurate psychiatric diagnosis. They should not be restarted reflexively just because they had been prescribed previously; they should be ordered only if the patient has a bona fide psychiatric condition. Psychiatric consultation can be beneficial when the diagnosis is uncertain.

The next consideration is the patient's physical condition and the medications' effects on organs that the suicidal act may have compromised. Medications that are potentially toxic to impaired organs should not be restarted. Attention should also be paid to the patient's level of arousal and the risks for seizures and arrhythmias because psychiatric medications may enhance these risks.

Anxiety is a potent risk factor for suicide and should be treated to prevent recurrence of suicidal behavior and intensification of suicidal thinking. Benzodiazepines can be particularly helpful in quelling anxiety, whereas neuroleptic medications—both conventional and atypical—are preferred when anxiety escalates into outright fear. For full discussions of the use of neuroleptic agents and benzodiazepines in the ICU, see Chapters 197 and 198, respectively.

Psychiatric Consultation

Psychiatric consultation is strongly recommended whenever a patient's safety is questionable. The consultant will address psychiatric diagnosis, suicide risk, medications, and disposition. Consultation can also be helpful in understanding the psychological dynamics between patient and staff. The patient who may be thinking about, or at risk of, self-harm but has not articulated a specific thought may also benefit from expert consultation; elderly patients often do not report suicidal thoughts to caretakers [21,22].

When requesting a consultation, it is helpful to provide the consultant with as many details of the suicide attempt as possible (e.g., method, number of pills in cases of ingestion, likelihood of rescue). The exact words used by a patient who makes a suicidal comment, as well as the context in which the statement was made, are critically important and should be included in the consultation request. Basic elements of the patient's mental status (e.g., level of wakefulness, affect, presence of psychosis, and ongoing suicidal thinking) should be determined and relayed to the psychiatrist.

Clear documentation from the nursing staff and physicians will help the consultant follow the patient's course and identify points of intervention. The existence of a suicide note can be of particular help in the assessment of suicide and in intervention planning [23]. However, whether to keep the suicide note in the permanent medical record is not clear. The suicide note can be of help to subsequent treaters; yet, in deference to the patient's privacy, a brief and general discussion of the note's existence and content may be all that is necessary for the medical record. The resolution of this matter should be made in consultation with the psychiatrist.

Disposition

When medically and surgically stable, patients face two options for discharge—home or psychiatric facility. Patients who may benefit from or require continued treatment in a psychiatric facility are those whose risk factors outweigh their protective factors. This decision is usually made with the psychiatric consultant, who will also assist with placement, prior authorization (which is required by some insurance plans), and the handling of any legal matters (e.g., if the patient is unwilling to be hospitalized psychiatrically and thus requires involuntary commitment).

CONCLUSION

Suicide is a tragic consequence of mental and physical illness that represents a relatively small number of ICU admissions. Nonetheless, the care of a patient who is suicidal or has just attempted suicide requires attention to a number of details not usually considered in the management of a typical ICU patient. The ICU team must be cognizant of their emotional reactions to the patient and of patient–staff dynamics, vigilant for potentially dangerous objects in the physical environment, and knowledgeable about specific interventions, including constant observation of the potentially self-harming patient. Psychiatric consultation can be helpful in managing important aspects of care for this patient population, from diagnosis and safety assessment to medication management and disposition.

References

1. Centers for Disease Control and Prevention, National Center for Injury Prevention and Control: Web-based Injury Statistics Query and Reporting System (WISQARS). Available at: http://www.cdc.gov/ncipc/wisqars. Accessed January 2, 2010.
2. Heron M, Hoyert D, Murphy, SL, et al: Deaths: final data for 2006. *Natl Vital Stat Rep* 57:14, 2009.
3. Institute of Medicine: Reducing Suicide: A National Imperative. Washington, DC, National Academies Press, 2002. Available at: http://books.nap.edu/books/0309083214/html/index.html. Accessed January 2, 2010.
4. Moscicki E: Epidemiology of suicide, in Goldsmith S (ed): *Risk Factors for Suicide*. Washington, DC, National Academy Press, 2001, p 1.
5. American Psychiatric Association: Practice Guideline for the Assessment and Treatment of Patients with Suicidal Behaviors. Arlington, VA, American Psychiatric Association, 2003. Available at: www.psych.org/psych_pract/treatg/pg/Practice%20Guidelines8904/SuicidalBehaviors.pdf. Accessed January 2, 2010.
6. Gearing RE, Lizardi D: Religion and suicide. *J Relig Health* 48:332, 2009.
7. Henriksson MM, Aro HM, Marttunen MJ, et al: Mental disorders and comorbidity in suicide. *Am J Psychiatry* 150:935, 1993.
8. Moscicki EK. Epidemiology of completed and attempted suicide: toward a framework for prevention. *Clin Neurosci Res* 1:310, 2001.
9. Goodwine RD, Marusic A, Hoven CW: Suicide attempts in the United States: the role of physical illness. *Soc Sci Med* 56:1783, 2003.
10. Bell GS, Sander JW: Suicide and epilepsy. *Curr Opin Neurol* 22:174, 2009.
11. Jones JE, Hermann BP, Barry JJ, et al: Rates and risk factors for suicide, suicidal ideation, and suicide attempts in chronic epilepsy. *Epilepsy Behav* 4:S31, 2003.
12. Stern TA, Perlis RH, Lagomasino IT: Suicidal patients, in Stern TA, Fricchione GL, Cassem NH, et al. (eds): *Massachusetts General Hospital Handbook of General Hospital Psychiatry*. 5th ed. St. Louis, Mosby, 2004, p 93.
13. Dumais A, Lesage AD, Alda M, et al: Risk factors for suicide completion in major depression: a case-control study of impulsive and aggressive behaviors in men. *Am J Psychiatry* 162:2116, 2005.
14. Cassells C, Paterson B, Dowding D, et al: Long- and short-term risk factors in the prediction of inpatient suicide: review of the literature. *Crisis* 26:53, 2005.
15. Bryan CJ, Rudd DM: Advances in the assessment of suicide risk. *J Clin Psychol* 62:185, 2006.
16. Ojehagen A, Regnell G, Traskman-Bendz L: Deliberate self-poisoning: repeaters and nonrepeaters admitted to an intensive care unit. *Acta Psychiatr Scand* 84:226, 1991.
17. Brown GK, Steer RA, Henriques GR, et al: The internal struggle between the wish to die and the wish to live: a risk factor for suicide. *Am J Psychiatry* 162:1977, 2005.
18. Comtois KA: A review of interventions to reduce the prevalence of parasuicide. *Psychiatr Serv* 53:1138, 2002.
19. American Psychiatric Association: *Diagnostic and Statistical Manual of Mental Disorders*. 4th ed. Washington, DC, American Psychiatric Association, 1994.
20. Wolk-Wasserman D: The intensive care unit and the suicide attempt patient. *Acta Psychiatr Scand* 71:581, 1985.
21. Duberstein PR, Conwell Y, Seidlitz L, et al: Age and suicidal ideation in older depressed inpatients. *Am J Geriatr Psychiatry* 7:289, 1999.
22. Conwell Y, Thompson C: Suicidal behaviors in elders. *Psychiatr Clin North Am* 31:333, 2008.
23. Foster T: Suicide note themes and suicide prevention. *Int J Psychiatry Med* 33:323, 2003.

CHAPTER 201 ■ PROBLEMATIC BEHAVIORS OF PATIENTS, FAMILY, AND STAFF IN THE INTENSIVE CARE UNIT

CRAIGAN T. USHER

> The ear says more
> Than any tongue.
>
> *W.S. Graham, "The Hill of Intrusion"*

Whether a patient being treated in the intensive care unit (ICU), a supportive family member, or a physician or other healthcare professional working there, it is clear that the ICU is a stressful environment [1–5]. Problematic communication among patients, their families, and the hospital staff can hinder the restoration and maintenance of basic life functions that are the hallmark of intensive care. Occasionally, such difficult patient–staff or family–staff interactions stem from problems with care providers themselves. Depression, anxiety, overwork, sleep deprivation, longstanding interpersonal rigidity, and the cumulative effects of stress may cause some physicians and nurses to fail to address adequately the emotional needs of their patients and patients' families [6–8]. In other instances, patients and families become overwhelmingly stressed, their judgment and interpersonal skills rent asunder by longing, shame, rage, and despair. Such patients and family members may then act in ways that are irritating or even dangerous.

This chapter presents approaches to problematic patient conduct in the ICU, details common patterns of exasperating behavior in critically ill patients, provides practical ways of dealing with them empathically, and outlines some effective modes of communication with families of patients in the ICU. Above all, this chapter emphasizes that listening to patients and family members, paying special attention to the psychological needs underlying problematic behavior, and attempting to meet those needs make better patient–doctor/family–doctor relationships possible.

APPROACH TO PROBLEMATIC BEHAVIORS

Critically ill patients can behave in disruptive ways that jeopardize ICU activity and treatments. Some patients become childlike, cry or whimper, turn away from care providers, and refuse examinations or procedures. A number of patients grow demanding of nurses' and physicians' attention; they hurl insults when providers are not as attentive as they would like. Others may be violent, threatening staff, even punching and kicking caretakers.

Before deciding how to approach the disruptive patient, one must first answer the questions "Do I feel safe?" and "Is the patient safe?" ICU personnel learn to override their fears as they perform procedures that demand brisk, decisive action. Unfortunately, such denial occasionally leads to failure to heed an internal alarm regarding patient behavior, resulting in injury to patients and staff. Hence, it is key to "tune-in" to this sense of peril when acute danger to a patient or others exists and then to administer calming medications, summon security personnel, and apply physical restraints if necessary [9]. Physical confrontation with a non-delirious patient can sometimes be avoided by calling security personnel expeditiously, as merely seeing several officers, patients recognize the seriousness with which staff is approaching their threats or actions—and then relax.

For example, emerging from delirium after a near-lethal toxic ingestion, an impetuous adolescent threatened to "beat up" staff if not permitted to leave the ICU immediately. When hospital security arrived and the physician informed the young patient he would have to wait, the teenager quickly sat back in bed. Asked by the psychiatric consultant why he had calmed, the young man explained: "When it was just the nurses and doctor, I thought I could take them. But I knew I wasn't going anywhere when the police arrived. So I chilled."

Once the safety of the patient, other patients, and staff is ensured, examination of underlying causes of a patient's taxing behavior follows. As irritability and emotional lability are the final common pathway of myriad medical and psychiatric conditions and of normal emotional responses, precise determination of the cause of a patient's disruptive behavior is often vexing. Asking and answering the questions listed in Table 201.1 can be helpful in narrowing the vast differential diagnosis.

Delirium is a common source of troublesome patient behavior in the ICU. Patients who are hallucinating or harboring persecutory delusions that ICU staff is torturing them can be immensely problematic. Due to its potentially lethal nature [10], delirium should be ruled out first as the driving force behind a patient's disruptiveness. A full discussion of delirium is provided in Chapter 197.

After delirium has been excluded, it is important to look for major psychiatric illnesses, which are frequently exacerbated by the chaos, vulnerability, and prolonged inner tension associated with being treated in the ICU [11]. The intensivist should discern if the patient has a history of psychotic disorder, affective illness, or anxiety disorder and, in the absence of contraindications, should order any medications that have been effective in treating these conditions in the past. As part of this psychiatric workup, a substance-use history is also imperative; data from collateral sources may be necessary to confirm the patient's report. At any step in the process of assessing the roots of patients' problematic behaviors, psychiatric consultation may be useful in establishing and confirming diagnoses and in guiding treatment.

While gathering data about psychiatric conditions and substance use, common sources of patient stress in the ICU (e.g., pain, sleeplessness, and isolation) should be eliminated, as much as possible. Biancofiore et al. showed that liver transplant recipients and patients who underwent major abdominal surgery identified "being unable to sleep, being in pain, having tubes in nose/mouth, missing husband/wife, and

TABLE 201.1

KEY QUESTIONS ABOUT BEHAVIORAL PROBLEMS IN THE INTENSIVE CARE UNIT

Safety
- Is the patient's behavior dangerous? If so, how can I keep the patient and others safe?

Delirium
- Is the patient delirious? If so, am I effectively treating the underlying causes of delirium?

Psychiatric illness
- Does the patient have an anxiety, mood, or psychotic disorder or other psychiatric illness? If so, am I providing adequate treatment for these conditions?

Intoxication and withdrawal
- Is the patient intoxicated with or withdrawing from alcohol or other substance? Am I addressing the untoward effects of withdrawal?

Psychosocial stressors
- Can I reduce pain, sleeplessness, isolation, and other stressors related to being in the ICU?

Personality problems
- What is the patient's predominant mode of coping? How can I best manage this patient's uniquely taxing coping strategies?

seeing family and friends only a few minutes a day as the major stressors" [12]. Provision of adequate analgesia, effective sleep aids, anxiolytic agents, and uninterrupted interaction with significant others often substantially curtails problematic behaviors.

COMMON PATTERNS OF PROBLEMATIC BEHAVIOR

Critical illness leads many patients to feel lonely, dependent, or anxious about the prospect of death; traumatic memories may be reawakened as well. To keep these unpleasurable feelings and recollections at bay, ICU patients deploy a broad array of psychological defenses. Some patients' patterns of defense—that is, their personalities—are quite adaptive, even at times of stress. Other patients are devoid of the healthy emotional protoplasm, reliable social supports, and ample psychological armamentarium required to deal well with adversity. Such patients may be said to suffer from *psychosocial insufficiency*. Through denial, devaluation, passive-aggressiveness, and other primitive defenses [13], these patients are prone to wreak havoc in the ICU.

Psychosocially insufficient patients fall into two categories: (a) those with personality disorders who were difficult to deal with even before becoming critically ill and (b) those who have simply regressed and use primitive coping mechanisms that, outside the ICU, would be less apparent. Because the focus in the ICU is on the "here and now," distinguishing between these two categories is unnecessary. More important is recognition of pathologic personality styles [14] that frequently engender loathing in ICU personnel and require limit-setting, validation, and a commitment on the part of the physician to have a different, less unpleasant type of relationship with the patient (Table 201.2).

The Dependent Patient

Dependent patients demand assistance in nearly every aspect of their ICU experience. Through urgent requests for

TABLE 201.2

COMMON PROBLEMATIC COPING STYLES OF PATIENTS AND FAMILY MEMBERS IN THE INTENSIVE CARE UNIT

Personality type	Core deficit	Characteristic behavior	Suggested response
Dependent	Hypersensitive to abandonment, inadequacy, and aloneness	Craves attention Demands special care Childlike Cries easily and complains of abandonment and inadequate care	Schedule examination and rounding times Anticipate nursing staff changes, physician care shifts, transfer to floor Validate patient's plight and offer to help within reason
Narcissistic	Hypersensitive to loss of control and stature Defended against looking weak	Denies severity of illness Shows bravado Critical of ICU staff and care	Acknowledge patient's stature Enlist patient as active partner in care and decision-making
Obsessive	Hyperaware of loss of control Defended against looking weak	Excessive focus on medical facts and minutiae Restricted affect Not apt to "show emotional cards"	Schedule patient and family meetings Have a set amount of information to share with patient and family Provide factual explanations of data Avoid emotional commentary or inquiry
Dramatic	Difficulty feeling cared for or thought of except within emotionally extreme exchanges	Engaging and charming to some staff, denigrating and caustic to others May have multiple allergies and phobias May "fire" some staff and take exception to rules	Acknowledge patient's positive attributes Validate patient's plight and offer to help within reason Set limits as a team

Adapted from Kahana RJ, Bibring GL: Personality types in medical management, in Zinberg NE (ed): *Psychiatry and Medical Practice in a General Hospital*. New York, International Universities Press, 1965, p 108.

spoon-feeding, bedpan assistance, pillow adjustment, analgesia, and better food, among sundry other entreaties, dependent patients drive nurses and house officers to distraction. Yet, when examined through a sympathetic lens, one finds that dependent patients are incredibly fearful and leverage demands for care to keep their nurses and doctors in sight, thus reducing their anxiety. In this way, demanding patients are like the infant who, unable to hold onto the mental image of his mother, wails when she leaves the room. These patients are hypersensitive to aloneness. To mitigate these fears, nurses and doctors should keep such patients informed (e.g., when they plan to return, when rounds will take place, and when family will visit).

Still, for many dependent patients, basic information of this sort is insufficient to quiet their incessant demands for instant anxiety reduction. In these situations, validation of these patients' feelings, communication that their requests are understood, and explanation that the staff is unable to provide everything these patients want are key. These tasks are often accomplished through "I wish" statements. For example, a particularly dependent and anxious patient in a busy ICU pled for her ICU team to stay in the room. Respecting that the patient felt she needed more security than she was experiencing, the team leader responded: "While I wish we could stay here longer to explore your questions and provide further reassurance, unfortunately we need to complete rounds. However, I will return at noon to check on you." By validating the patient's needs, acknowledging her personal limitations, and providing reassurance about the time of return, this physician better met the patient's dependency needs.

The Narcissistic Patient

Being critically ill in the ICU can lead the most psychologically healthy person to feel infantilized; hence, for most patients, regaining a sense of control is extremely important. For some patients, however, this need to regain control takes the form of entitled demands and scathing critique. These patients often admonish nurses ("You're not doing that the right way!"), belittle their doctors (e.g., calling young house staff "Doogie Howser"), and name-drop ("Dr. Smith is an expert cardiologist I play golf with, and he would never allow that").

With such patients, it is best to appeal to, rather than to confront, their narcissism. When the narcissistic patient looks around the ICU, all he sees are his inadequacy, inability, and incapacity. The intravenous pump reminds him he cannot feed himself, the ventilator brings to mind that he cannot breathe unaided, and the bedside commode or bedpan becomes a glaring reminder of his inability to move about nimbly. By using words that remind the patient that, despite his infirmities, he is still a valuable person, one then "joins" the patient and incurs less wrath and invective. Such "joining" can be done by respectfully calling patients "Mr.," "Ms.," and "Dr.," as appropriate. It is also helpful to ask them about their lives outside the hospital, promoting the notion that they are not frail and infantile but able-bodied adults endowed with personal agency despite their current debility.

The narcissistic patient, with his sense of specialness and need for excessive admiration, appreciates any control he can be afforded. Even if this means controlling the light switch, choosing the hour the physical therapist will arrive, or using patient-controlled analgesia, the narcissistic patient revels in being a partner in his care. Finally, avoidance of power struggles and sharing of dilemmas are key to working with these patients effectively. For example, an astute medical intern said to a "very important person" (VIP) in the ICU: "While I realize the catheter is completely uncomfortable, if I were to remove it right now, it is likely I would have to replace it tomorrow. I can do this if you'd like—it is your decision—but I am concerned that this would cause you even greater pain." Knowing he had a choice, the VIP felt greater self-agency and was thus able to defer to the doctor's educated opinion, electing to leave the catheter in for the time being.

The Obsessive Patient

The obsessive patient is rules-based and acts much like an early school-age child clinging to the rules of a board game. Following the obsessive mantra "a place for everything and everything in its place" [15], the obsessive patient wants to know what his radiograph shows before it is even taken. His day can rise and fall on laboratory minutiae. Like the narcissistic patient, the obsessive individual feels his control slipping away at times of illness. However, rather than acting in a haughty manner to deny that illness is stripping him of his control, the obsessive patient attempts to attain mastery over his condition through excessive focus on detail. A master of "losing the forest for the trees," the obsessive patient gets mired in the fine points. He asks questions incessantly and wants to manage his own treatment. For example, one obsessive patient with myasthenia gravis espied an "L" next to her hematocrit and demanded to know why she was not being transfused when her hematocrit was 32.3%. When her nurse sat down at her bedside and provided a synopsis of her laboratory results and the team's rationale for management, the patient was soothed. For all patients, but particularly for obsessive ones, it is helpful to: (a) have in mind a set amount of information that the team wants to share with the patient, thus allowing the patient the mastery over illness he or she craves but without overwhelming him or her; (b) announce a regular time when nurses and physicians will share a progress report; and (c) use scientific/deductive reasoning to explain each step in treatment.

The Dramatic Patient

With intense difficulty identifying their own affective state and the thoughts and feelings of others [16], extremely dramatic patients or family members, many of whom may suffer from borderline personality disorder, make erroneous assumptions about their caregivers' intentions. Based on little data, such patients sense that they are loved and appreciated by some, while loathed and apt to be mistreated or abandoned by others. The dramatic patient or family member thus idealizes and praises some staff members while alienating others with toxic devaluation and belligerence. Even the most mindful, well-meaning, intelligent physician or nurse can find himself or herself suddenly on the wrong side of this idealization/devaluation "split." Validating patients' feelings but not necessarily their beliefs can be helpful. For example, one family member berated a physician: "You must hate our family!" The physician responded: "I am surprised to hear you say that, because I am not aware of having bad feelings toward you or your family. I wonder what gives you that impression." The family member then explained that the doctor seemed to turn away from the family when he passed by the visitors' lounge and "did not do nearly enough family meetings." Now understanding that this person required more information and dialogue than he customarily provided, the physician agreed to have more frequent meetings and made a concerted effort to acknowledge the family's presence when passing them, and thus enjoyed a more positive working relationship with this family member.

When clinicians who have had completely different experiences with a dramatic patient or family member confer, they are at odds over how to handle the dramatic individual's demands. This discord creates tremendous tension among treatment team members and can be relieved when clinicians acknowledge they

TABLE 201.3

PRINCIPLES OF ESTABLISHING LIMITS AND NEGOTIATING CONFLICTS IN THE INTENSIVE CARE UNIT

Acknowledge the patient's real struggles.
Explain limits in a clear and concise manner. Avoid jargon such as, "You are demonstrating unsafe behavior, sir. This is a nonsmoking environment," and simply offer, "You can't smoke while you're in the unit."
Before speaking with the patient, know what areas, if any, are flexible and make concessions to the patient in those areas.
Determine consequences for transgressing limits in advance.
Avoid long, drawn-out arguments as they are rarely, if ever, useful. Leaving the patient's bedside to cool down, thinking of a new strategy, or consulting a colleague is better than acting impulsively.

Adapted from Winnick JA, Wool CA, Geringer ES, et al: Problematic behavior of patients, family, and staff in the intensive care unit, in Irwin RS, Rippe JM (eds): *Irwin and Rippe's Intensive Care Medicine*. 5th ed. Philadelphia, Lippincott Williams & Wilkins, 2003, p 2192.

have had divergent emotional experiences with a patient. Once this "split" is named, the team can then strategize how best to set limits (Table 201.3).

COMMUNICATION WITH FAMILIES

Almost always for better, but occasionally for worse, family members are not mere visitors to the ICU [17]. Families play an integral role in encouraging and comforting critically ill patients and informing distant loved ones of patients' progress or problems. With the exception of those patients who, prior to hospitalization, expressed their preferences for medical care, relatives are also responsible for learning about a patient's diagnosis and prognosis and making decisions for critically ill patients who lack the capacity to make medical choices for themselves.

It can be difficult to function in these roles, as the experience of having a family member in the ICU takes a psychological toll. One study revealed that 69% of family members of intensive care patients suffered depressive symptoms and 35% had anxious symptoms [2]. Azoulay and colleagues reported that up to one third of family members suffered posttraumatic stress symptoms 3 months after their family member was discharged from the ICU [3].

Adequate communication between ICU staff and patients' family members is central to reducing family stress and dissatisfaction [18,19], decreasing conflict around end-of-life decisions [20], limiting futile interventions [21], and reducing strife between families and ICU staff [22]. Some general principles of communication with families in the ICU include providing clear and concise medical information, scheduling and keeping appointment times to meet with families, respecting the uniqueness of the family and the patient, attending to special aspects of the patient's and family's life story, and providing early diagnostic and prognostic information, even if this means saying, "I'm not sure" [23,24] (Table 201.4).

Even with good communication, problems arise. Occasionally, before the physician can provide information regarding prognosis, family members will foreclose discussion and disagree with the doctor or other family members about how

TABLE 201.4

***CORE* PRINCIPLES OF COMMUNICATION WITH FAMILIES IN THE INTENSIVE CARE UNIT**

*C*lear Provide family members with clear, concise descriptions of the patient's condition. Avoid jargon. Ask if you have adequately addressed the family's questions and concerns.
*O*n time Schedule appointments for family conferences or treatment updates and try, as best as possible, to be on time. Send a representative if you must.
*R*espect the patient's uniqueness These appointments are as much about what you say as how well you listen. Pay close attention to people's names and what makes the patient special.
*E*arly diagnosis and prognosis Even if it means saying, "I'm not sure," try to inform the family early in the ICU stay.

much workup or end-of-life treatment to pursue. Some special situations related to the emotional life of family members bear examination in further detail. These include the guilty family member, the family member compelled to preserve the dignity or "fighter status" of the patient, and the vindictive family member. Physician interventions or "conversational reframes" in these situations are aimed not at coercion but at enhancement of doctor–family and family–family conversation about how best to proceed with a critically ill family member's care.

Occasionally, a sibling, parent, or child of an ICU patient who has played little role in the ailing family member's life attempts to rectify this estrangement by coming to the rescue at the 11th hour. To assuage their guilt, these family members demand that "everything" be done for their relative, to the point of pushing for futile assessments and treatments. Reframing the dilemma for these family members, giving them a sense of authority, and explaining how they can be helpful can shift the family–staff dialogue. For example, one intensivist told a particularly guilt-ridden son whose mother had suffered a severe stroke: "I know you've had to be away for several years and not been able to play a day-to-day role in your mother's care. However, this is a really big opportunity to help support your dying mother and your struggling sister. You can help your sister and the rest of your family come to a well thought-out decision about your mother's care." By suggesting how this young man could help in the here and now and indirectly addressing his guilt, the physician altered this concerned son's attitude.

When dealing with end-of-life care, some family members will demand that everything be done because they do not want their loved one to seem weak. "But he's a fighter," some relatives protest. In these situations, one should listen closely to why it is important that the patient's status as a "fighter" be maintained. Once this information is obtained, the ICU staff member might illustrate how the patient remains a fighter even as heroic measures are scaled back. For example, a 78-year-old World War II naval veteran was admitted to the ICU with a massive myocardial infarction from which a meaningful recovery was extremely unlikely. The patient's daughter touted the fact that her father had made it through polio, the Pacific campaign, and a kidney transplant, and refused even to discuss withdrawing ventilator support. Wed to the picture of her father as a warrior, this loving daughter asserted, "He's made it this far and he'll keep fighting." When the intensivist told the daughter he understood her father had made it through these trying illnesses and battles, detailed the extent of her father's myocardial damage, and emphasized that it took a "remarkably massive" heart attack to bring him down, the daughter's vision of her father as a "fighter till the end" was affirmed. She was then more amenable to discussing end-of-life care and relaxed her terse "do everything" commands.

Some family members may be angry with the patient. Wasserman studied responses provided by relatives of patients who had attempted suicide and found that a family's request for "do not resuscitate" orders sometimes reflected anger toward the patient [25]. Eliciting these feelings during a family meeting may help family members to acknowledge the hostile origins of their decisions and to feel they have acted less impulsively and more thoughtfully about how to proceed with a loved one's care.

Communication between ICU staff and a patient's family may be disrupted when a family member does not want to make decisions on behalf of a loved one or suffers symptoms of anxiety, depression, or other psychiatric illness [26]. Such family members may derive great benefit from consultation with the ICU's social worker or an outpatient psychiatrist. When discussions over care reach a standstill and interventions spur little movement, referral to an ethics consultant or committee (particularly with regard to end-of-life care) or patient-rights advocate (regarding a family member's grievance) may help resolve the conflict.

CONCLUSION

Physicians, nurses, and other members of the critical care team are often confronted with patients and families whom they find taxing or even dangerous. Establishment of safety, exclusion of causes of disruptive behavior amenable to medical intervention, examination of the patient's and family member's predominant defense mechanisms, and attempts to address the patient's or family member's psychological needs better can improve such difficult interactions. Patients with personality problems often respond to validation of their distress and to limit-setting, entailing a description of how they are expected to act and what they can expect from their caregivers. Family members and loved ones play a crucial role in critical care; ensuring that they are part of the ICU team involves providing clear diagnostic information early on, conveying respect for the uniqueness of patients and their families, and providing regular, scheduled updates.

References

1. Rattray JE, Johnston M, Wildsmith JA: Predictors of emotional outcomes of intensive care. *Anaesthesia* 60:1085, 2005.
2. Pochard F, Azoulay E, Chevret S, et al: Symptoms of anxiety and depression in family members of intensive care unit patients: ethical hypothesis regarding decision-making capacity. *Crit Care Med* 29:1893, 2001.
3. Azoulay E, Pochard F, Kentish-Barnes N, et al: Risk of post-traumatic stress symptoms in family members of intensive care unit patients. *Am J Respir Crit Care Med* 171:987, 2005.
4. Coomber S, Todd C, Park G, et al: Stress in UK intensive care unit doctors. *Br J Anaesth* 89:873, 2002.
5. Fischer JE, Calame A, Dettling AC, et al: Experience and endocrine response in neonatal and pediatric critical nurses and physicians. *Crit Care Med* 28:3281, 2000.
6. Krebs EE, Garrett JM, Konrad TR. The difficult doctor? Characteristics of physicians who report frustration with patients: an analysis of survey data. *BMC Health Serv Res* 6:128, 2006.
7. Rincon HG, Granados M, Unutzer J, et al: Prevalence, detection, and treatment of anxiety, depression, and delirium in the adult critical care unit. *Psychosomatics* 42:391, 2001.
8. Curtis JR, Engleberg RA, Wenrich MD, et al: Missed opportunities during family conferences about end-of-life care in the intensive care unit. *Am J Respir Crit Care Med* 171:844, 2005.
9. Trenoweth S: Perceiving risk in dangerous situations: risk of violence among mental health inpatients. *J Adv Nurs* 42:278, 2003.
10. Ely EW, Shintani A, Truman B, et al: Delirium as a predictor of mortality in mechanically ventilated patients in the intensive care unit. *JAMA* 291:1753, 2004.
11. Granberg A, Bergbom Enberg I, Lundber D: Patients' experience of being critically ill or severely injured and cared for in an intensive care unit in relation to the ICU syndrome. Part I. *Intensive Crit Care Nurs* 14:294, 1998.
12. Biancofiore G, Bindi ML, Romanelli AM, et al: Stress-inducing factors in ICUs: what liver transplant recipients experience and what caregivers perceive. *Liver Transpl* 11:967, 2005.
13. Vaillant GE: *Adaptation to Life*. Boston, Little, Brown, 1977.
14. Bibring GL, Kahana RJ. *Lectures in Medical Psychology: An Introduction to the Care of Patients*. New York, International Universities Press, 1968.
15. Dor J. *The Clinical Lacan*. New York, Other Press, 1999.
16. Fonagy P: Attachment and borderline personality disorder. *J Am Psychoanal Assoc* 48:1129, 2000.
17. Molter NC: Families are not visitors in the critical care unit. *Dimens Crit Care Nurs* 13:2, 1994.
18. Malacrida R, Bettelini R, Molo C, et al: Reasons for dissatisfaction: a survey of relatives of intensive care patients who died. *Crit Care Med* 26:1187, 1998.
19. Curtis JR, Patrick DL, Shannon SE, et al: The family conference as a focus to improve communication about end-of-life care in the intensive care unit: opportunities for improvement. *Crit Care Med* 29[2, Suppl]:N26, 2001.
20. Lilly CM, De Meo DL, Sonna LA, et al: An intensive communication intervention for the critically ill. *Am J Med* 109:469, 2000.
21. Rivera S, Kim D, Garone S, et al: Motivating factors in futile clinical interventions. *Chest* 119:1944, 2001.
22. Fins JJ, Solomon MZ: Communication in intensive care settings: the challenge of futility disputes. *Crit Care Med* 29[2, Suppl]:N10, 2001.
23. McDonagh JR, Elliot TB, Engleberg RA, et al: Family satisfaction with family conferences about end-of-life care in the intensive care unit. *Crit Care Med* 32:1484, 2004.
24. Leclaire MM, Oakes JM, Weinert CR: Communication of prognostic information for critically ill patients. *Chest* 128:1728, 2005.
25. Wasserman D: Passive euthanasia to attempted suicide: one form of aggressiveness of relatives. *Acta Psychiatr Scand* 79:460, 1989.
26. Azoulay E, Pochard F, Chevret S, et al: Half the family members of intensive care unit patients do not want to share in the decision-making process: a study in 78 French intensive care units. *Crit Care Med* 32:1832, 2004.

CHAPTER 202 ■ RECOGNITION AND MANAGEMENT OF STAFF STRESS IN THE INTENSIVE CARE UNIT

GUY MAYTAL

Intensive-care settings reveal humanity at its best and at its worst. This is as true for the staff as it is for the patients. We who serve in intensive care settings in a true sense risk our own lives in these settings—our feelings, our self-esteem, our self-respect. By risking these daily we grow; by avoiding the risk we must face the dehumanization of ourselves or of our patients.

Cassem and Hackett [1]

The intensive care unit (ICU) is a structurally, functionally, and socially complex entity with its own culture, personnel, protocols, and problems [2,3]. Today, such units are routinely filled to capacity with complicated patients suffering from multiple life-threatening illnesses. As technology has advanced, patients with once-terminal illnesses are surviving longer, raising ever more complicated ethical issues [4].

For patients and their families, time spent in an ICU can lead to physical and psychological trauma [5–7]. The overall "hostile" environment of the ICU—with its multiple, complicated devices, lack of patient comforts, lack of privacy, and elevated ambient noise—contributes to negative psychological outcomes for patients [8].

This same environment also affects ICU staff. The psychological pressures on ICU personnel are myriad: increasingly sophisticated technological advances, overwhelming amounts of data, burdensome demands on caretakers, long hours, nursing shortages, and trying ethical issues. Staff may not be prepared to handle their emotional reactions to these challenges while simultaneously tending to the technical and clinical aspects of intensive care.

This chapter reviews the general concepts of stress and burnout, the tensions associated with training and working as a physician or a nurse in an intensive care setting, and strategies for managing staff stress in the ICU.

STRESS

The physiologic, cognitive, and affective facets of stress are based on the seminal early work of Selye [9] on the *general adaptation syndrome*. Selye defined stress as the nonspecific result of any demand on the body, and observed that different organisms and biological systems respond to stress in a stereotyped and predictable three-part pattern. The initial alarm reaction (characterized by activation of the sympathetic nervous system and various hormonal, immunologic, and psychological responses) is followed by the stage of resistance, during which the organism establishes a temporary homeostasis by marshalling various reserves to adapt to the new situation. However, the body's ability to adapt is finite, and, with continued exposure to the stressor, its reserves become depleted and the organism enters a stage of exhaustion.

Researchers in biology and sociology have expanded this work to encompass processes ranging from individual cellular responses to stress, to the reactions of individuals and social systems to external and internal stressors. The study of occupational stress (i.e., stress due to one's work situation) has grown substantially since the 1960s, expanding to professions ranging from factory work to nursing. Research during the past four decades has consistently demonstrated the significant adverse impact of excessive occupational stress on physical health, mental health, and decision-making. Regardless of the field, low job satisfaction is often predicted by a small number of factors: little participation in decision-making, ambiguity about job security, poor use of skills, and lack of clarity about role. These stressors are consistent with the *demand–control model* of the effects of job demands on worker's well-being. This model predicts that the fewer demands and more control a worker has on the job, the less stress he will experience [10,11]. For example, an analysis from the Swedish National Registry of 958,000 people found that hospitalization rates for myocardial infarction (MI) were higher among men and women with high-demand, low-control jobs [11].

Other well-recognized occupational stressors include noise-related stress, dangerousness of the work environment, nonstandard work hours, and excessive fatigue [10]. Of these stressors, work overload and a poor social environment at work are the most significant determinants of work-related health problems. Cross-sectional associations between work overload and health complaints are consistently reported [12,13]. Furthermore, work overload and overall low job satisfaction are strongly associated with the development of psychiatric (particularly affective) problems. A meta-analysis of job satisfaction and health outcomes examined 485 studies (267,995 individuals) and concluded that poor job satisfaction was strongly associated with the development of depressive and other affective illnesses [14].

In addition to physical and mental health, decision making also can be adversely affected by high levels of stress. Awareness of one's limited knowledge and problem-solving capabilities, fear that bad outcomes will occur regardless of which choice is made, worry about making a fool of oneself, and fear of loss of self-esteem if the decision is wrong can force decision-makers to come to "premature closure." Fearing a negative assessment of their sense of helplessness, otherwise rational decision-makers foreclose the decisional dilemma before a search for, and an unbiased assimilation of, all relevant information and generation and careful appraisal of all alternatives can be completed [15].

Such premature closure can lead to incorrect or even harmful decisions [15]. For example, in their classic study of patients with acute MI, Hackett and Cassem [16] noted that the majority of patients experiencing what they thought might be an MI delayed calling for help for 4 to 5 hours. In an effort to avoid

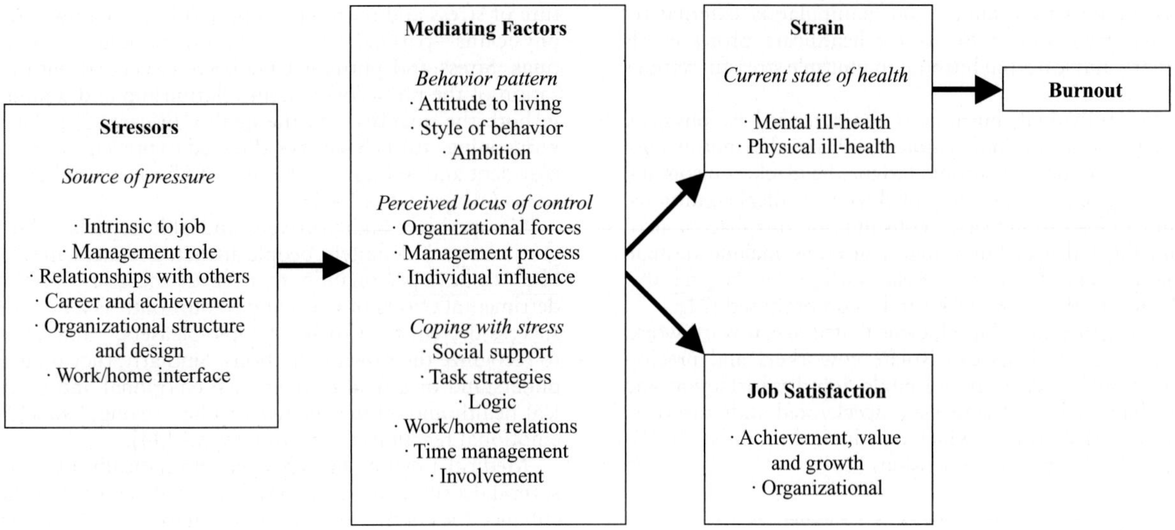

FIGURE 202.1. Stress–strain model of occupational stress. [Adapted from Cooper CL, Sloan SJ, Williams S: *Occupational Stress Indicator: Management Guide*. Windsor, UK, NFER-Nelson, 1988.]

the anxiety of a potentially devastating diagnosis and its implications, these patients came to premature closure and made potentially deleterious decisions about when to seek medical attention [17].

In a work environment, including the ICU, stressors (both work- and nonwork-related, both internal and external) affect each individual in a unique manner as mediated by a variety of factors. The interaction between stressors and mediating factors leads the individual to experience either strain or job satisfaction (Fig. 202.1) [18]. When this interaction leads to strain that is chronic or particularly intense (or both), burnout occurs.

BURNOUT SYNDROME

Coined by the clinical psychologist Herbert Freudenberger [19] in 1974, *burnout syndrome* has been viewed as a behavioral or a psychological condition as well as a process or a syndrome [20]. Research during the past 2 decades (especially by Maslach and colleagues) has narrowed the current definition to encompass the spheres of emotional exhaustion, depersonalization (i.e., negative or cynical attitudes regarding work), and the absence of personal accomplishment—particularly among individuals who do "people work" (Table 202.1) [21]. While emotional exhaustion is the key component of the syndrome, people with all three symptoms experience the greatest degree of burnout [22]. Ultimately, this definition describes a process whereby highly motivated and committed individuals lose their spirit, their motivation for creativity, and, in the ICU, their belief in their ability to help people [23,24].

Burnout varies in intensity and duration, although it often has an insidious onset [25]. Even if an individual's experience of burnout does not reach consciousness initially, it may affect others, burdening the system with another source of stress.

Many have argued that the cause of burnout lies in our need to believe that our lives are meaningful and that what we do is useful and important [23]. Work takes on a central role in providing some people with this sense of meaning in their lives. When individuals who derive such meaning from work think they have failed in their jobs, they may experience burnout. Burnout tends to afflict people who enter their professions with high motivation and idealism; it is particularly common in occupations often seen as "callings" [26]. In a supportive environment, highly motivated individuals reach their goals and achieve success, which leads to a sense of meaningfulness that itself increases the original motivation. However, in an unsupportive environment, these individuals cannot accomplish what they set out to do and consequently fail. For people who expect a sense of meaningfulness from work, such failure often leads to burnout.

Everyone experiences stress, but only those who start their careers with high levels of idealism, motivation, and commitment are at risk for burning out: "You cannot burn out unless you were 'on fire' initially" [23]. Burnout occurs almost exclusively in individuals who work with people, arising from the emotional stress that such interactions engender. ICU staff tend to be idealistic, committed, and driven—the very attributes which render them susceptible to burnout. In assessing and managing burnout, attention should be paid to the impact of job-related stressors and their ramifications, as well as the individual's personality style. The character trait of hardiness (i.e., initiative, willingness to take risks, ability to face uncertainty,

TABLE 202.1

THREE COMPONENTS OF BURNOUT

Emotional exhaustion	Reduced energy and job enthusiasm Emotional and cognitive distancing from the job
Depersonalization	Cynicism Lack of engagement and distancing from patients Treatment of patients as inanimate, unfeeling objects
Absence of personal accomplishment	A significantly diminished sense of efficacy, effectiveness, involvement, commitment, engagement, and capacity to innovate, change, and improve

Adapted from McManus IC, Keeling A, Paice E: Stress, burnout and doctors' attitudes to work are determined by personality and learning style: a twelve year longitudinal study of UK medical graduates. *BMC Med* 2:29, 2004.

and assertiveness in attaining and manipulating external rewards) has been shown to protect healthcare professionals (particularly nurses) from burnout in multiple stressful settings [27].

For the individual, burnout is characterized by physical, emotional, and attitudinal symptoms. Physical symptoms are nonspecific and include chronic fatigue, headaches, insomnia, weight changes, and worsening of chronic medical conditions. Burnout can lead to increased consumption of tobacco, alcohol, and illicit drugs. Emotional symptoms include despair, hopelessness, and depression. Relationships can become disrupted and the ability to work can be compromised [21].

On an organizational level, cynical attitudes toward work, colleagues, and patients can isolate coworkers and precipitate staff conflicts. At some hospitals, job dissatisfaction and burnout have led to absenteeism, accelerated staff turnover, and severe staff shortages, which may limit the number of ICU beds available for patient admissions [28].

STRESS AND BURNOUT IN HEALTHCARE PROFESSIONALS

Stress is a common aspect of medical practice for physicians, nurses, and trainees. Not surprisingly, studies over the past several decades have reported a high prevalence rate of burnout in healthcare professionals. Rates of burnout among physicians range from 25% to 60%, depending on working conditions and medical specialty [29–34]; burnout can develop at any stage of a physician's career. Nurses also experience high levels of burnout. Studies in nurses indicate rates of 35% to 50%, depending on working conditions, clinical setting, and level of autonomy experienced [22]. Multiple factors have been associated with burnout in healthcare professionals, but the best characterized include: heavy workload, stressful work environments (e.g., ICUs), severity of patients' illnesses, and conflicts with coworkers or patients [35,36].

Physicians who experience burnout suffer physical (e.g., anorexia, insomnia, tachycardia, and hypertension) and psychological (e.g., irritability, frustration, apathy, indecision, and depression) symptoms. Burnout leads to increased nurse distress, decreased patient satisfaction, increased mortality in the ICU, and substance abuse [37,38]. Furthermore, approximately 10% of physicians develop a substance-related disorder in their lifetimes; the risk of narcotic abuse in physicians is ten times that of the general population. Substance abuse often leads to sanctions and to loss of license and livelihood [39]. The primary risk factors for addiction in physicians include high stress levels, access to drugs, and chronic fatigue, all pronounced in ICU settings. Often shielded by a "code of silence" among fellow practitioners, impaired physicians often come to clinical attention in an advanced stage of addiction.

Just as concerning are the statistics on physician suicide. Male physicians are two times more likely to commit suicide than average Americans; female physicians are three times as likely [40]. Furthermore, physicians' personal relationships with spouses and children are damaged by burnout: "Being a physician is one of the few socially acceptable reasons for abandoning a family" [41].

STRESS AND ITS CONSEQUENCES IN PHYSICIAN TRAINING

During the past 20 years, the medical and sociological literatures have documented the impact that work-related stress has on physicians and on their ability to care for patients. Consequently, efforts have been made to understand the nature of stress and burnout in house officers, fellows, and staff physicians—particularly those who work in intensive care settings. Stress and burnout have been associated with deterioration of the physician–patient relationship and a diminution in both the quantity and the quality of care [37]. Therefore, burgeoning efforts have been directed to prevent stress and impairment and to improve the care of physicians suffering from stress or burnout [42–44].

Competitive, highly driven, and able to delay short-term gratification indefinitely, people attracted to medicine are more likely to have personalities that render them susceptible to the detrimental effects of stress and to burnout. As a rule, they are success-driven, tend to be "people-pleasers," and are unable to recognize their own limitations. Similarly, they do not often understand or attend to their own emotional and psychological health and, citing the need to be "strong," squelch their emotional reactions to stressful events [44].

Medical practice has changed dramatically over the past several decades, and many physicians who entered medicine to enhance their sense of control and mastery find themselves in a medical system that is increasingly out of their control [44]. Physicians have experienced a decline in status and autonomy alongside increased work pressures. Under closer scrutiny by regulatory agencies and insurance companies, physicians have had to contend with ever growing amounts of paperwork. Due to increased pressure to discharge patients, the acuity of patients in hospital settings has increased, "turnover" is more rapid, and interventions are more aggressive.

House officers, in particular, face a unique constellation of stressors. According to a review of the stresses of residency by Colford and McPhee [42], the stressors faced by house officers are varied, including those related to the nature and educational structure of residency, being a female resident, and perceptions about work. Among the most potent stressors are sleep deprivation, information overload, long work hours, and confrontation with chronic and fatal diseases. Others include financial debt (including from educational loans), personal relationships, and anxiety about malpractice. These researchers also found that alcohol and drug abuse was a significant problem in 7% to 10% of physicians. They cited studies verifying high levels of stress due to physicians' relationships, psychological problems (e.g., anxiety and depression), and professional dissatisfaction.

In recent years, more quantitative evaluations of the effects of stress and burnout on house officers have implicated residency-related stressors in contributing to psychiatric and physical impairment. Such stressors include overnight call, responsibility for four or five times as many patients at night as during daytime hours, lack of supervision while on call, the inability to complete a task without interruptions, and lack of substantive patient interactions [45–47].

In a longitudinal study that examined the impact of job stress on house officers, Tyssen and colleagues [45] followed 371 medical students from their last semester through the end of their internship. They found that 11% of these interns had mental health problems. Predictors of mental health problems included prior mental health problems, a high level of neuroticism, and experience of a serious negative life event during internship. Most important among these factors was perceived job stress. Furthermore, perceiving oneself as deficient in clinical skills or knowledge at the end of medical school was related to a mental health problem during internship. Importantly, gender, number of hours worked weekly, and lack of sleep were not linked to mental health problems.

In a similar study, Newbury-Birch and Kamali [46] examined the relationship among work-related stress, job satisfaction, and personality factors in 109 medical house officers. They found that 24% of the men and 38% of the women suffered from psychological stress. Levels of depression and anxiety were significant among these house officers. The personality characteristic of neuroticism was a predisposing factor for stress and anxiety.

Shanafelt and colleagues [47] examined the relationship between burnout and self-reported patient care practices in a university-based internal medicine residency program. They found that 87 (76%) of the residents surveyed met criteria for burnout. Those residents who were burned out were much more likely to be depressed, have low career satisfaction, and report significantly more "suboptimal patient practices."

Stress and burnout are associated not only with work hours but with a variety of internal and external factors; quality of teamwork, personality characteristics, and trouble with the work/home interface all contribute to the development of stress and burnout in house officers. A 12-year longitudinal study of medical school graduates found that specific personality traits (e.g., high neuroticism, low extraversion, and low conscientiousness) measured while in medical school strongly predicted the development of stress, burnout, and job satisfaction as a staff physician [48].

Despite work-hour restrictions, house officers and fellows continue to shoulder stressful workloads that have a significant impact on their physiology and psychology [46]. Gopal and coworkers [48] studied a single cohort of residents before (2003) and after (2004) restrictions on work hours were implemented. Residents in 2004 had less burnout, emotional exhaustion, sleep deprivation, and depression. However, the residents did not perceive any significant changes in their quality of life, and their learner satisfaction was significantly reduced.

Parshuram and colleagues [49] prospectively studied 11 critical care fellows in Toronto, Canada, working within the Ontario guidelines limiting work hours and overnight call shifts. The researchers thoroughly examined the amount of work performed by the fellows (e.g., number of hours, admissions, procedures, pages). They also used Holter monitors to screen for arrhythmias, pedometers to measure distance walked, and urinalysis to evaluate hydration. The results showed that, despite work-hour restrictions, the fellows continued to work long shifts, with little sleep (average, 1.9 hours per night), frequent pages (average, 41 per shift), many admissions, and many procedures. Furthermore, they walked an average of 6.3 km per shift. More alarming was that abnormalities in heart rate and rhythm occurred in all participants. Ketonuria was found in 21% of the shifts during which it was measured, indicating dehydration and suggesting self-neglect.

STRESS AND BURNOUT AMONG INTENSIVISTS

Stress and burnout are not limited to house officers and fellows. Staff physicians—in particular those who work in ICUs—have a high prevalence of burnout syndrome. The protracted stress of working as a physician can lead to lower-quality patient care, disruptions in personal relationships, and even impairment of physical health [50]. Intensivists labor in an atmosphere of perpetual stress and often limited rewards. In addition, society often has unrealistic expectations of the physician not only as a professional but also as a spouse, parent, employer, and community member. Failure to live up to any of these can lead to a sense of failure [50]. A 2001 survey by the Canadian Medical Association found a significant decline in physician morale, due to volume of work, sleep deprivation, teaching and research demands, potential for litigation, and greater demands from the public [44].

In recent years, researchers have attempted to better quantify the way in which these stressors affect physicians who work in intensive care settings. Coomber and coworkers [38] surveyed all members of the Intensive Care Society in the United Kingdom (85% response rate, 758 respondents) to identify "distressed" doctors and to relate this state to "repeated and long-term exposure to job stressors." They found that nearly 30% of the physicians surveyed were distressed, 12% were depressed, and 3% had suicidal thoughts. These physicians reported that the most stressful aspects of their work were the feeling of being overstretched, the effect of work hours and stress on personal/family life, and the pressure to compromise standards when resources were limited. Other important stressors included perceiving a lack of peer recognition, feeling alone in making important decisions, and occasionally having too much responsibility.

In a recent survey of 978 French intensivists, Embriaco and colleagues [35] found that 46.5% had a high level of burnout syndrome. Risk factors included female sex, increased workload, and conflicts with coworkers. Similarly, in a survey of 6000 American physicians, female physicians were 60% more likely to report burnout than their male counterparts [51]. Furthermore, in the Embriaco study, workload (as measured by number of shifts per month and length of time from the last day off) was associated with higher rates of burnout. Lastly, conflicts with coworkers are associated with higher levels of burnout, while good relationships with nurses are a protective factor [35,36,52].

Given the high frequency of burnout in physician populations, the Academy of Professors of Medicine analyzed survey data from more than 4,000 physicians in the United States and the Netherlands and formulated a model to predict burnout. Their model (Fig. 202.2) lists factors specific to physicians that place them at risk for developing burnout, and suggests areas of intervention to help prevent the development of this burdensome and costly syndrome [37].

STRESS AND BURNOUT AMONG INTENSIVE CARE UNIT NURSES

Although nurses and physicians work in the same physical environment, nurses have unique working conditions, emphasize

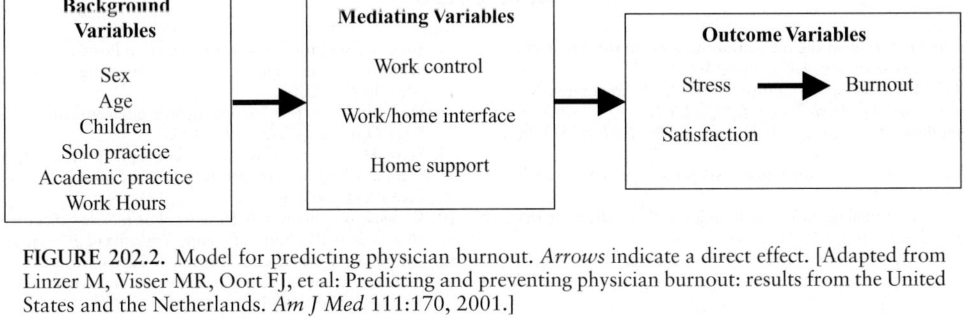

FIGURE 202.2. Model for predicting physician burnout. *Arrows* indicate a direct effect. [Adapted from Linzer M, Visser MR, Oort FJ, et al: Predicting and preventing physician burnout: results from the United States and the Netherlands. *Am J Med* 111:170, 2001.]

different aspects of clinical care, and experience different stresses. As one nurse stated in a study on burnout: "There is a mutual goal in your work as a nurse, no matter where you work, and that is to take care of the patient. Nursing is a job in which you are always under pressure. You are dealing with life and death issues on a daily basis. You can't come to work and say: I slept only five hours tonight and I'm tired. You have to be on full alert at all times. You work under incredible pressure with little rewards" [53].

Nurses usually work in the ICU indefinitely, compared to residents, and even critical care fellows and attendings, who rotate through different units in the hospital. Despite their relative permanence in the ICU, nurses do not generally accrue as much autonomy and stature as do physicians, which may lead to stress over career and organizational structure [54]. Poncet and colleagues [36] surveyed 2,392 French nurses working in 165 ICUs (mean time from graduation was 40 months and mean time working in the ICU was 36 months). Severe burnout was identified in 33% of the nurses surveyed. Four characteristics were independently associated with this outcome: younger age, organizational factors (e.g., less autonomy in scheduling days off), poor quality of working relationships, and factors related to end-of-life decisions. Other studies also have demonstrated that concerns surrounding ethical decisions are consistently the most important issues of ICU nurses [55]. In situations in which nurses attempt to reconcile their ideals regarding ethical dilemmas with the reality of their limited autonomy, stress can develop. Nurses with fewer workplace restrictions and thus greater autonomy have less anxiety and are more likely to advocate for their patients [56].

The personality trait of hardiness also can protect against stress and burnout among ICU nurses [57–59]. Aiming not merely at survival in the face of difficult circumstances but at the enrichment of life, hardiness consists of the triad of commitment (a sense of purpose expressed by becoming an active rather than a passive participant in life), control (the tendency to behave in a way that influences life events rather than to feel impotent in the face of adversity), and challenge (the belief that change, instead of stability, is normal and a stimulus to enhance maturity rather than a threat to security) [60]. Wright and colleagues [61] found a strong inverse relationship between hardiness and burnout in 31 intensive care nurses. Any interventions to reduce stress and burnout among nurses should include efforts to augment hardiness [62].

MANAGEMENT OF STAFF STRESS AND BURNOUT IN THE INTENSIVE CARE UNIT

Stress and burnout are common and deleterious to the ICU team. Therefore, preventing and ameliorating burnout syndrome in the ICU should be a priority. Ample descriptive reports of interventions to address stress and burnout in the ICU exist, but there are few outcome studies. Their general aim is to reduce stressors for staff, employing individual, interpersonal, and organizational strategies. The use of humor, support groups, and a system for outside referral are important in preventing and managing stress [45].

Individual strategies proposed to prevent burnout include relaxation training, time management, assertiveness training, team building, and meditation [21]. The aim of all such strategies is to enhance individuals' capacity to cope with the demands of their jobs [49,63]. For example, Isaksson Rø and colleagues studied the effectiveness of a 1-day individual session or a 1-week group intervention aimed to prevent burnout in 227 Norwegian physicians. They found that participants in either intervention had a significantly reduced level of emotional exhaustion as compared to physicians who did not participate [64].

Given that interpersonal conflict is a risk factor for severe burnout, improving the quality of relationships among doctors and nurses protects against burnout [35,36]. Groups and workshops have been reported as useful in managing stress [1,62,65,66]. Cassem and Hackett [1] described weekly and impromptu group meetings to explore ICU staff reactions to crises, to resolve conflict, and to discuss feelings, experiences, and knowledge. McCue and Sachs [62] described the effectiveness of a stress management workshop for medical and pediatric residents; it cost little, was positively received, and demonstrated significant short-term improvement in stress and burnout scores.

On the organizational level, reducing work hours and improving work organization is a first step toward burnout prevention [49]. Furthermore, ensuring adequate staffing, shared decision-making, active review of unit policies and procedures, freeing up time for patient care or research, bolstering administrative support, and allowing flexibility to curtail work/home conflict may help reduce stress and increase job satisfaction [37,67].

CONCLUSION

Recognizing and attending to staff stress in the ICU are necessary to ensure the continued effectiveness and well-being of each individual and of the unit as a whole. Left unaddressed, staff stress and burnout can exact a heavy price. As Civetta [68] wrote:

> We must accentuate the positive qualities of human capabilities that are beyond technological advancement. . . . A smile, a touch, confidence and security are still beyond our programming capabilities. . . . We must focus on our distinct human qualities of insight and caring. In this way, the popular view that intensive care is a depersonalizing environment can be replaced by the recognition that human beings are caring for human beings.

References

1. Cassem NH, Hackett TP: Stress on the nurse and therapist in the intensive-care unit and the coronary-care unit. *Heart Lung* 4:252, 1975.
2. Conway J, McMillan M: Exploring the culture of an ICU: the imperative for facilitative leadership. *Nurs Leadersh Forum* 6:117, 2002.
3. Sharp S: Understanding stress in the ICU setting. *Br J Nurs* 5:369, 1996.
4. Winkenwerder W: Ethical dilemmas for house staff physicians. *JAMA* 254: 3454, 1984.
5. Daley L: The perceived immediate needs of families with relatives in the intensive care setting. *Heart Lung* 13:231, 1984.
6. Cuthbertson BH, Hull A, Strachan M, et al: Post-traumatic stress disorder after critical illness requiring general intensive care. *Intensive Care Med* 30:450, 2004.
7. Jones C, Skirrow P, Griffiths RD, et al: Posttraumatic stress disorder-related symptoms in relatives of patients following intensive care. *Intensive Care Med* 30:456, 2004.
8. Donchin Y, Seagull FJ: The hostile environment of the intensive care unit. *Curr Opin Crit Care* 8:316, 2002.
9. Selye H: History of the stress concept, in Goldberger L, Breznitz S (eds): *Handbook of Stress: Theoretical and Clinical Aspects*. 2nd ed. New York, Free Press, 1993, p 7.
10. Karasek R, Theorell T: *Healthy Work: Stress, Productivity and the Reconstruction of Working Life*. New York, Basic Books, 1990.
11. Alfredsson L, Spetz CL, Theorell T: Type of occupation and near-future hospitalization for myocardial infarction and some other diagnoses. *Int J Epidemiol* 14:378, 1985.

12. Landsbergis PA: Occupational stress among health care workers: a test of the job demand-control mode. *J Organ Behav* 9:217, 1988.
13. Karasek R, Gardell B, Lindell J: Work and non-work correlates of illness and behavior in male and female Swedish white collar workers. *J Occup Behav* 8:187, 1987.
14. Faragher EB, Cass M, Cooper CL: The relationship between job satisfaction and health: a meta-analysis. *Occup Environ Med* 62:105, 2005.
15. Janis IL: Decision making under stress, in Goldberger L, Breznitz S (eds): *Handbook of Stress: Theoretical and Clinical Aspects*. 2nd ed. New York, Free Press, 1993, p 56.
16. Hackett TP, Cassem NH: Psychological management of the myocardial infarction patient. *J Human Stress* 1:25, 1975.
17. Kasl SV, Cobb S: Health behavior, illness behavior, and sick role behavior. *Arch Environ Health* 12:246, 1966.
18. Cooper CL, Sloan SJ, Williams S: *Occupational Stress Indicator: Management Guide*. Windsor, UK, NFER-Nelson, 1988.
19. Freudenberger HJ: Staff burnout. *J Soc Issues* 30:159, 1974.
20. Paine WS (ed): *Job Stress and Burnout*. Beverly Hills, CA, Sage Publications, 1982.
21. Maslach C, Schaufeli WB, Leiter MP: Job burnout. *Annu Rev Psychol* 52:397, 2001.
22. Embriaco N, Papazian L, Kentish-Barnes N, et al: Burnout syndrome among critical care healthcare workers. *Curr Opin Crit Care* 13:482, 2007.
23. Pines AM: Burnout, in Goldberger L, Breznitz S (eds): *Handbook of Stress, Theoretical and Clinical Aspects*. 2nd ed. New York, Free Press, 1993, p 386.
24. Marshall RE, Kasman C: Burnout in the neonatal intensive care unit. *Pediatrics* 65:1161, 1980.
25. Carroll JFX, White WL: Theory building: integrating individual and environmental factors within an ecological framework, in Paine WS (ed): *Job Stress and Burnout*. Beverly Hills, CA, Sage Publications, 1982, p 41.
26. Freudenberger HJ: *Burn-out: The High Cost of High Achievement*. Garden City, NY, Doubleday, 1980.
27. Ouellette SC: Inquiries into hardiness, in Goldberger L, Breznitz S (eds): *Handbook of Stress: Theoretical and Clinical Aspects*. 2nd ed. New York, Free Press, 1993, p 386.
28. Maslach C, Pines A: Burnout, the loss of human caring, in Pines A, Maslach C (eds): *Experiencing Social Psychology*. New York, Random House, 1979.
29. Ramirez AJ, Graham J, Richards MA, et al: Burnout and psychiatric disorder among cancer clinicians. *Br J Cancer* 71:1263, 1995.
30. Grassi L, Magnani K: Psychiatric morbidity and burnout in the medical profession: an Italian study of general practitioners and hospital physicians. *Psychother Psychosom* 69:329, 2000.
31. Lemkau J, Rafferty J, Gordon R: Burnout and career-choice regret among family practice physicians in early practice. *Fam Pract Res J* 14:213, 1994.
32. Keller KL, Koenig WJ: Management of stress and prevention of burnout in emergency physicians. *Ann Emerg Med* 18:42, 1989.
33. Deckard GJ, Hicks LL, Hamory BH: The occurrence and distribution of burnout among infectious diseases physicians. *J Infect Dis* 165:224, 1992.
34. Gallery ME, Whitley TW, Klonis LK, et al: A study of occupational stress and depression among emergency physicians. *Ann Emerg Med* 21:58, 1992.
35. Embriaco N, Azoulay E, Barrau K, et al: High level of burnout in intensivists: prevalence and associated factors. *Am J Respir Crit Care Med* 175:686, 2007.
36. Poncet MC, Toullic P, Papazian L, et al: Burnout syndrome in critical care nursing staff. *Am J Respir Crit Care Med* 175:698, 2007.
37. Linzer M, Visser MR, Oort FJ, et al: Predicting and preventing physician burnout: results from the United States and the Netherlands. *Am J Med* 111:170, 2001.
38. McCall SV: Chemically dependent health professionals. *West J Med* 174:50, 2001.
39. Roy A: Suicide in doctors. *Psychiatr Clin North Am* 8:377, 1985.
40. Clever LH: Who is sicker: patients—or residents? Residents' distress and the care of patients. *Ann Intern Med* 136:391, 2002.
41. Colford JM, McPhee SJ: The raveled sleeve of care: managing the stresses of residency training. *JAMA* 261:889, 1989.
42. Butterfield PS: The stress of residency: a review of the literature. *Arch Intern Med* 148:1428, 1988.
43. Gundersen L: Physician burnout. *Ann Intern Med* 125:125, 2001.
44. Tyssen R, Vaglum P, Gronvold NT, et al: The impact of job stress and working conditions on mental health problems among junior house officers: a nationwide Norwegian prospective cohort study. *Med Educ* 34:374, 2000.
45. Newbury-Birch D, Kamali F: Psychological stress, anxiety, depression, job satisfaction, and personality characteristics in preregistration house officers. *Postgrad Med J* 77:109, 2000.
46. Shanafelt TD, Bradley KA, Wipf JE, et al: Burnout and self-reported patient care in an internal medicine residency program. *Ann Intern Med* 136:358, 2002.
47. McManus IC, Keeling A, Paice E: Stress, burnout and doctors' attitudes to work are determined by personality and learning style: a twelve year longitudinal study of UK medical graduates. *BMC Med* 2:29, 2004.
48. Gopal R, Glasheen JJ, Miyoshi TJ, et al: Burnout and internal medicine resident work-hour restrictions. *Arch Intern Med* 165:2595, 2005.
49. Parshuram CS, Dhanani S, Kirsh JA, et al: Fellowship training, workload, fatigue and physical stress: a prospective observational study. *CMAJ* 170:965, 2004.
50. Coomber S, Todd C, Park G, et al: Stress in UK intensive care unit doctors. *Br J Anaesth* 89:873, 2002.
51. McMurray JE, Linzer M, Konrad TR, et al: The work lives of women physicians results from the physician work life study. *J Gen Intern Med* 15:372, 2000.
52. Stehle JL: Critical care nursing stress: the findings revisited. *Nurs Res* 30:182, 1981.
53. Pines AM, Kanner AD: Nurses' burnout: lack of positive conditions and presence of negative conditions as two independent sources of stress. *J Psychosoc Nurs Ment Health Serv* 20(8):30, 1982.
54. Goodfellow A, Varnam R, Rees D, et al: Staff stress on the intensive care unit: a comparison of doctors and nurses. *Anaesthesia* 52:1037, 1997.
55. Spoth R, Konewko P: Intensive care staff stressors and life event changes across multiple settings and work units. *Heart Lung* 16:278, 1987.
56. Erlen JA, Sereika SM: Critical care nurses, ethical decision-making and stress. *J Adv Nurs* 26:953, 1997.
57. Daines PA: Personality hardiness: an essential attribute for the ICU nurse? *Dynamics* 11:18, 2000.
58. Larrabee JH, Janney MA, Ostrow CL, et al: Predicting registered nurse job satisfaction and intent to leave. *J Nurs Adm* 33:271, 2003.
59. Judkins SK, Ingram M: Decreasing stress among nurse managers: a long-term solution. *J Contin Educ Nurs* 33:259, 2002.
60. Kobasa S, Maddi S, Courington S: Personality and constitution as mediators in the stress-illness relationship. *J Health Soc Behav* 22:368, 1981.
61. Wright TF, Blache CF, Ralph J, et al: Hardiness, stress, and burnout among intensive care nurses. *J Burn Care Rehabil* 14:376, 1993.
62. Fein SL: Burnout in nursing: prevention and management, in Fein IA, Strosberg MA (eds): *Managing the Critical Care Unit*. Rockville, MD, Aspen, 1987, p 96.
63. Rø KE, Gude T, Tyssen R, et al: Counselling for burnout in Norwegian doctors: one year cohort study. *BMJ* 337:a2004, 2008.
64. Simon NM, Whitely S: Psychiatric consultation with MICU nurses: the consultation conference as working group. *Heart Lung* 6:497, 1977.
65. McCue JD, Sachs CL: A stress management workshop improves residents' coping skills. *Arch Intern Med* 151:2273, 1991.
66. Stern TA, Prager LM, Cremens MC: Autognosis rounds for medical housestaff. *Psychosomatics* 34:1, 1993.
67. Firth-Cozens J, Moss F: Hours, sleep, teamwork, and stress: sleep and teamwork matter as much as hours in reducing doctors' stress. *BMJ* 317:1335, 1988.
68. Civetta JM: Beyond technology: intensive care in the 1980s. *Crit Care Med* 9:763, 1981.

DORRIE K. FONTAINE • SHAWN CODY

CHAPTER 203 ■ USE OF NURSING-SENSITIVE QUALITY INDICATORS

MARGARET LACCETTI AND CHERYL H. DUNNINGTON

INTRODUCTION

Nursing care does make a difference to the patient, to the families, to the healthcare team and in determining patient outcomes. Functions of nursing in the critical care environment include: ongoing assessment of the patient, therapeutic interaction with the family, facilitation of communication across multiple healthcare disciplines, and engaging in activities directly impacting the patient clinical outcome. A critical care nurse is a registered nurse who has been specially oriented and educated concerning the needs and acute physiology of a critically ill patient. Through the application of scientific knowledge, the critical care nurse reacts to the full range of human experiences, within the context of a caring relationship. One focus of nursing care in the ICU is the concept of quality. Quality includes the promotion of safe, efficient, and effective care based on scientific principles demonstrated through evidence that culminates in satisfaction for the patient, family, and the nurse.

The scope of practice for a nurse is determined by the level of formal education or preparation, area of clinical practice, competency validation, hospital or facility policy, and education or training as part of or required for a particular job. Scope of practice may also be mandated by the individual State Board of Nursing or through legislation. Critical care nurses receive more intensive orientation in preparation for patient care, and may be required to hold certifications in areas such as advanced life support. The American Association of Critical Care Nurses has developed a set of standards of care (Table 203.1) and defines the scope of practice for the critical care nurse, using the principles developed by the American Nurses Association (ANA) [1]. Utilization of these standards provides a framework for the delivery of comprehensive, high quality care.

CRITICAL CARE NURSES: PAST TO PRESENT

In 1854, Florence Nightingale was the first to identify the need to segregate the sickest patients needing the most intensive care in an area she referred to as her Monitoring Unit. Here, patients wounded in battle were able to receive nursing care with greater regularity, from women she had trained specifically. Through delivery of more consistent care from better trained nurses, she was able to demonstrate significantly decreased battlefield mortality, from 40% to 2% [2].

Caring for the most critically ill patients separate from other patients allows nurses to meet the complex needs of patients and families. This is accomplished through application of specific training and education with regard to disease process, treatment modalities, and the psychology of devastating injury or illness. Additionally, sequestering critically ill patients for care facilitates changes in nurse-to-patient ratio. A critical care nurse is commonly responsible for the nursing care of one or two patients.

Critical care nursing, as we know it today, emerged after World War II. The increase in medical specialization and improvement of technology influenced the development of this specialty [3]. The first intensive care or critical care units were established in the 1960s. Preparation to care for these patients resulted in development of curricula addressing nurses as well as intensivists, physicians specifically trained in critical care.

Nurses are the largest group of healthcare providers caring for patients daily in the critical care unit. As members of the healthcare team, nurses are responsible to provide nursing and medical interventions, as ordered, and evaluate the effect of those interventions on patients. An enormous part of the demand of patient care is the work of nurses, based on standards of care supported by appropriate resource allocation, enhanced nursing knowledge, accountability, and institutional policies and procedures. Clinical decision making is grounded in evidence-based practice that grows from the nurse's commitment to lifelong learning. Developing and implementing a plan of care allows interventions to be provided in a safe, systematic way, tailored to the condition of each individual patient. As a result of a holistic approach and long periods of time at the bedside in critical care, it is the nurse who gives voice to the patient and family, including them in planning for care. Communication and collaboration among healthcare professionals are essential in planning and delivering care, as well as in maintaining a healthy work environment, one that promotes safe, efficient, effective care for patients. Interdisciplinary communication and collaboration are critical to prevent errors and omissions in the plan of care. The American Association of Critical Care Nurses, in a 2005 study [4], described the consequences of poor communication behaviors among healthcare professionals. These consequences include medication errors, infections, falls, increasing complications of both disease and treatment, and death. Seven areas were specified to be contributing to poor outcome: broken rules, mistakes, lack of support, incompetence, poor teamwork, disrespect, and micromanagement. Participants in this study described a resistance to communicating with others regarding these areas. Only through promotion of enhanced communication can patient safety and improved outcomes be expected. The Joint Commission on Accreditation of Healthcare Organizations identifies poor communication as a primary factor in sentinel events [5]. The Institute of Medicine described communication as a contributor to the harm patients experience in the course of their care [6].

The result of poor nursing care in relation to poor patient outcomes has been evaluated. These poor outcomes result in higher overall cost, low rates of nursing job satisfaction,

TABLE 203.1

CRITICAL CARE NURSING: STANDARDS OF CARE

Assessment	The nurse caring for the critically ill patient collects all data that is pertinent to the patient. This data is collected from the patient, family, and other members of the healthcare team to develop a holistic view of the patient and their issues. Data collection is driven by the priorities of the patient's immediate condition and anticipated concerns for care. The critical care nurse uses analytical models and problem solving tools when collecting assessment data. All relevant data is documented and communicated to other healthcare providers.
Diagnosis	The critical care nurse uses the assessment data to develop diagnosis and care issues directly related to this individual patient. These diagnoses are prioritized according to the immediate needs of the patient.
Planning	The critical care nurse is sometimes seen as the coordinator of the plan of care for the individual patient. They take into account the patients' individualized needs and situation. This care plan is developed in conjunction with the patient, family, and other members of the healthcare team. The plan establishes priorities, provides continuity of care, and considers resources available.
Implementation	Once the plan of care has been developed, it is the responsibility of the critical care nurse to implement the care. The interventions are developed to promote comfort and reduce or prevent suffering.
Evaluation	The critical care nurse must evaluate all plans of care once they have been implemented. They must evaluate the effectiveness of interventions and check if the desired outcome was achieved.

decreased patient and family satisfaction, accreditation issues, and lower rates of reimbursement [7]. For example, cost per case will increase in medical patients with urinary tract infection and pressure ulcers and in surgical patients with urinary tract infection and pneumonia. Provision of safe, high quality patient care is motivated by both professional accountability and growing financial pressure. By evaluating the quality of patient care, opportunities for poor patient outcomes can be eliminated or prevented. Use of Nursing-Sensitive Quality Indicators (NSQI) provides an opportunity to evaluate and improve care in the critical care unit. Quality and Nurse sensitive indicators are defined as measures and indicators that reflect the impact of nursing actions on outcomes. Although the entire scope of nursing-sensitive indicators includes structure, process, and outcome of nursing, nursing-sensitive indicators in critical care are primarily outcome driven.

Nursing-sensitive quality indicators identify and allow measurement of structures of nurse-specific patient care, the processes by which this care is accomplished, and the outcomes of that care. They are performance measures that quantify the work of nursing and the outcomes of that work. These indicators are particularly useful in the critical care setting, where intensive nursing care directly influences patient safety and outcome. In addition to measurement, the use of NSQI promotes identification of best practice and accountability for practice, and points out gaps in research, education, and practice within the discipline of nursing and in interdisciplinary patient care. NSQI, as they measure nursing's impact on the quality of patient care, are instrumental in helping hospitals to reduce misdirection of nursing time to nonproductive or non-patient care tasks or activities. By allowing nurses to engage in the work of nursing, patient outcomes are improved, appropriate staffing decisions are made, and nurse job-satisfaction is enhanced [8].

The American Nurses Association (ANA) Nursing Safety and Quality Initiative began in 1994, aimed at the development of hospital quality indicators. Data from this initiative was stored in the National Database of Nursing Quality Indicators (NDNQI), at the Midwest Research Institute and University of Kansas School of Nursing in 1998. The initial outcome measures included nosocomial infection rate (bacteremia), rate of patient falls with injury, patient satisfaction with nursing care, patient satisfaction with pain management, patient satisfaction with educational information, and patient satisfaction with care. Process measures included maintenance of skin integrity. The NDNQI has developed nationally accepted measures to assess quality of nursing care, identifying and promoting best practice around specific indicators. The database provides members the transparency of quality outcomes, motivating nursing leaders to implement practice that can maintain or improve those outcomes. Current NDNQI indicators can be found in Table 203.2.

NSQI IN CRITICAL CARE NURSING PRACTICE

Infection is one complication critical care patients are particularly at risk for, as the result of invasive procedures, disease process, and exposure to multiple infective organisms. Specific NSQI address behaviors aimed at avoiding this risk. The most common potential infections in the ICU are catheter-associated urinary tract infection, central line related blood stream infection (BSI), and ventilator-associated pneumonia.

Urinary Tract Infections

Catheter-associated urinary tract infections (CAUTI) contribute to almost half of all nosocomial infections, resulting in increased hospital stays and cost of treatment. Placement of urinary catheters in the critically ill patient facilitates determination of urinary output. They are also essential in managing incontinence in the unresponsive or immobile patient, preventing moisture-related skin breakdown. However, an indwelling urinary catheter enhances the risk of UTI.

Urinary catheter care is a direct responsibility of nursing, including proper placement, assessment, maintenance of a closed system, use of aseptic technique when obtaining a urine sample, management of the collecting bag system, and appropriate delegation of tasks. The critical care nurse is well prepared to provide care as necessary for UTI prevention, as well as to delegate care tasks such as catheter hygiene, appropriately and safely to ancillary staff. It has been proposed that one important aspect of CAUTI prevention may include increases in the number of registered nurses (RN) at the bedside to provide patient care. In one study, a large and significant inverse relationship was found between full-time-equivalent RNs per adjusted inpatient day and urinary tract infections after major surgery [9].

Proper placement of a urinary catheter mandates that strict asepsis be maintained throughout insertion. Choice of an appropriately sized catheter is critical in proper placement. The

TABLE 203.2

NDNQI NURSING INDICATORS

Nursing hours per patient day	■ Registered nurse (RN) hours per patient day ■ Licensed practical/vocational nurses (LPN/LVN) hours per patient day ■ Unlicensed assistive (UAP) hours per patient day
Nursing turnover	
Nosocomial infections	
Patient falls	
Patient falls with injury	■ Injury level
Pressure ulcer rate	■ Community acquired ■ Hospital acquired ■ Unit acquired
Pediatric pain assessment, intervention, reassessment cycle	
Pediatric peripheral intravenous infiltration	
Psychiatric physical/sexual assault	
RN/education/certification	
RN survey	■ Job satisfaction scales ■ Practice environment scale
Restraints	
Staff mix	■ RN ■ LPN/LVN ■ UAP ■ Percent agency staff

NDNQI, National Database of Nursing Quality Indicator.

smallest possible catheter to promote bladder drainage reduces opportunities for infection by reducing damage to urethral mucosa during insertion.

Assessment of the patient with a urinary catheter should, at least, address the presence of adequate urinary production, as well as placement of the collecting bag at an appropriate place below the level of the patient's body. The catheter should be secured to the patient's thigh (or abdomen, in male patients only) with a catheter strap or anchoring system to prevent pulling and tugging. Pulling on the catheter can cause damage to the tissue in the urethra. Damage to this area can lead to a bladder infection. Use of skin prep under the anchoring system may help to prevent skin irritation and breakdown [10]. Care of the patient with a urinary catheter includes cleaning the catheter with soap and water or peri spray as part of daily hygiene and following a bowel movement, and avoiding powders and creams on or around the catheter or insertion area. CAUTI prevention is enhanced when the collection bag is emptied consistently prior to moving or ambulating the patient, and maintaining the drainage bag and tubing below the bladder level to facilitate urine flow and prevent backward flow into the bladder. It is important to never place the collecting bag on top of the patient when transferring him to or from a stretcher, as this allows backflow of urine to the patient.

Three main sites of potential infection in patients with a urinary catheter are: along the urethral wall (avoided by providing catheter care), at the junction between catheter and drainage bag if the system is opened (avoided by maintaining a closed system and not disconnecting the catheter from drainage bag), and at the drainage outlet (avoided with appropriate aseptic technique).

Through conscientious and evidence-based nursing care for the patient with an indwelling urinary catheter, it is possible to prevent CAUTI, thereby reducing the patient's risk of increased length of stay in the hospital, infection-related complications, and increased cost of patient care.

Blood Stream Infection

As the result of multiple invasive procedures that will occur in the care of a patient in the critical care unit, as well as conditions or treatments that may compromise the patient's ability to resist infection, the critically ill patient is at greater risk for nosocomial infection. Catheter-related BSIs are one example of an infectious complication that occurs in patients cared for in critical care units. These catheter-related BSIs are responsible for increased healthcare costs, longer critical care unit stays, longer hospital stays, and death.

A central venous line is a catheter that delivers fluids directly into the central circulation. Three primary functions of this catheter in critically ill patients are large volume fluid resuscitation, hemodynamic monitoring, and administration of hyperosmolar intravenous fluids, such as total parenteral nutrition. They may be an alternative when the patient has poor peripheral access, and specifically with multi-lumen catheters that allow for administration of complex medication regimens and solutions simultaneously. In critically ill patients, the advantages of central vascular access over peripheral access are many. Central access allows medications and solutions administered directly into central circulation, promoting rapid systemic distribution. Blood flow at the right atrium or superior vena cava is rapid, large volume, quickly diluting hyperosmolar solutions. The patient's peripheral vasculature is preserved intact for later access, when the patient is no longer a resident of the critical care unit.

Catheter-related BSIs are identified by positive blood culture with the catheter suspected as the infective site clinically or in light of the microbiology. Through excellent nursing care, the critical care nurse is instrumental in preventing these infections from the process of insertion, attending to aseptic technique during dressing changes and catheter use, and by comprehensive assessment of the site and patient status, as long as the catheter remains in place.

Preventive measures essential for the nurse to facilitate at insertion of a central catheter include appropriate hand hygiene for aseptic procedures, full barrier precautions, and skin preparation with 2% chlorhexidine or the institutional policy driven choice. Use of gloves does not eliminate the need for hand washing.

Regular assessment of the insertion site for drainage, redness, oozing or swelling, and assessment of the dressing for integrity are part of comprehensive nursing care of the critically ill patient. Hub or injection cap contamination is another source of potential infection. Thorough cleansing with an antimicrobial is required prior to every access. Cleansing is mechanical, as well as chemical, and it is important to allow antimicrobial solutions to dry before accessing the port. All connectors should be regularly inspected for integrity, and antimicrobial disinfection should be used at connection sites whenever the closed system is broken. The nurse can also determine when it may be appropriate to remove a central catheter. If a central line is not being used, or the patient's condition or treatments support vascular access peripherally, removing the central catheter may be a good choice to reduce the patient's risk of catheter-related BSI [11].

Given the need for multiple opportunities to utilize vascular access in critically ill patients, multi-lumen catheters are the norm in critical care units. There is evidence that multi-lumen central venous catheters put patients at slightly higher risk of infection compared with single-lumen catheters. However, this increased risk is justified for the critically ill patient by the convenience and improved vascular access afforded by multi-lumen vascular catheters [12].

Finally, documentation is a nursing function vital to prevention, prompt identification, and treatment of catheter-related BSIs. Documentation is a primary form of communication between members of the healthcare team. It provides history and context to clinical findings. Nursing documentation of process and procedure during insertion or use of a central line, and routine assessment findings provide the basis for prevention and early intervention.

Ventilator-Associated Pneumonia

Ventilator-associated pneumonia (VAP) is the most common type of hospital-acquired infection, impacting approximately 9% to 27% of all mechanically ventilated patients [13]. VAP can increase the average length of stay for an ICU patient by 7 to 9 days. It may also increase mortality by up to 43% when the patient has an antibiotic resistant microbe [14]. This translates to an additional cost of $40,000 to each hospital stay and can be estimated to cost hospitals $1.2 billion per year. Approximately 50% of all antibiotic use in the hospital setting is for the treatment of VAP [15].

VAP is defined as a pneumonia that occurs 48 hours after mechanical intubation. The endotracheal tube provides a direct link for the bacteria to the lungs. Upper airway and oral secretions pool above the cuff on the endotracheal tube, forming a biofilm that can be dislodged into the lungs during routine nursing tasks such as suctioning, turning the patient, or repositioning the endotracheal tube. The body is unable to prevent entry of these bacteria into the lungs, enhancing the risk of pneumonia. Diagnosis of VAP is based upon radiographic findings, clinical, laboratory, and microbiology results. Symptoms to be considered in diagnosis include fever, elevated white count, and purulent sputum [16].

Nursing plays an integral role in the prevention of VAP. The CDC recommends that all patients receive a pneumococcal vaccine every 5 years, except those who received the vaccination over the age of 65 [17]. Critical care nurses are the front line against the prevention of VAP. It is the care that the bedside nurse provides that has the greatest impact. Things as basic as hand washing prior to patient contact will contribute to prevention.

Mouth care, a basic nursing intervention, is thought to decrease VAP by reducing the amount of bacteria in a patient's mouth. Mouth care is described as not only rinsing the mouth but also brushing the teeth, gums, and tongue to remove plaque. The use of pharmacological agents (such as chlorhexidine) has shown to decrease VAP in the cardiac surgery population, but these protocols remain untested in other patient populations [18].

The old habit of using saline lavages down the endotracheal tube prior to suctioning is related to an increase in the VAP rate. Rather than liquefying secretions, the saline lavage actually dislodges bacteria from the endotracheal tube and pushes the bacteria into the lungs [19].

Turning patients who are intubated on a routine basis not only improves pulmonary status, it also helps prevent pressure ulcers. The position of the patient is critical in VAP prevention; studies have shown that having the bed elevated to between 30 and 45 degrees prevents reflux and aspiration of stomach contents into the lungs [19]. It is imperative to not only have the patient at more than 30 degrees while in bed, but also during transport, or during CT scan or MRI, if it is possible to maintain the elevation of the head of the bed.

The use of standardized orders and clinical pathway guidelines are an important part of the prevention of VAP. All disciplines must be aware of the standards of care and practice to those standards.

Lastly, even in the busiest of ICU's, it is important that the patient's pneumococcal vaccine status be assessed and addressed.

Pressure Ulcers

Pressure ulcers are the direct result of decreased capillary perfusion to the skin and subcutaneous tissues as the result of compression. They range from areas of redness and irritation to frank tissue necrosis. Mortality is related to pressure ulcer development, particularly in elderly patients, with some studies describing rates of mortality as high as 60% in older persons within 1 year of hospital discharge [20]. More often, pressure ulcers occur with changes in health status, particularly as mobility, perfusion, and nutritional status are negatively affected. Pressure ulcers result in increased length of stay and increased hospital costs related to treatment. The Healthcare Cost and Utilization Project, in 2006, determined the average charge for pressure ulcer treatment per hospital stay to be $37,800 [21].

Multiple risk factors are associated with the development of pressure ulcers, including host-specific factors such as nutritional status and disease process and systemic factors such as preventive resources and workload of direct caregivers. Risk factor identification, preventive measures, and treatment of existing pressure ulcers to decrease exacerbation and progression and promote healing are all within the purview of the critical care nurse. Disease states putting the patient at risk to develop pressure ulcers include diabetes mellitus, cardiovascular and peripheral vascular disease, stroke, renal failure, sepsis, febrile illnesses, cancer, and hypotension. Patients who are hypovolemic are at risk because of decreased perfusion, as are those who are malnourished. Illness states directly affect nutritional status by increasing metabolic need. Any physiologic process that impedes the microcirculation, whether locally or systematically increases the risk for pressure ulcer development. (Smoking is an important contributor to impairment of the microcirculation, so a current smoking history is a significant risk factor to add to the patient's risk profile.)

Previous history of pressure ulcer is a clinical risk indication. Any condition or treatment that impairs patient mobility directly enhances the patient risk, including use of physical restraints. Pressure ulcer development has been associated with low body mass index, where the boney prominences do not have the protective benefit of adipose tissue, and with obesity, where increased weight directly impedes capillary flow and perfusion. Both localized and generalized edema can also contribute to the risk of ulcer development. Incontinence, both urinary and fecal, and diuresis put the patient at risk of moisture-related ulcer development, as will poor hygiene. In the critical care area, the presence of multiple tubes, lines, and catheters also put the patient at risk by adding new areas of perfusion compression. Pressure ulcers form below the nostrils or behind the ears as a result of pressure from a nasal oxygen cannula or elsewhere, when IV tubing or urinary catheters lay under body parts. This short list of risk factors just begins to describe patients in critical care.

The work of the critical care nurse is in both prevention and treatment; the essential starting point is assessment. Preventive assessment includes identification of those patients at high risk to develop pressure ulcers by defining the risk factors present, so that preventive measures can be instituted to address as many of these factors as possible. A variety of tools have been developed for this purpose, with the Norton and Braden scales most popular in hospitals in the United States. Regardless of the tool chosen, the importance is to use it consistently for comprehensive risk assessment and to document and communicate both the findings from the scale or tool and the plans in place for prevention. Additionally, patients at risk must be assessed regularly for areas of redness, poor capillary refill or skin tears, all of which indicate the beginnings of pressure ulcer formation.

Prevention can be especially challenging for the nurse caring for the critically ill patient. Many of the risk factors identified may be directly related to either disease or treatment and may be difficult to modify. Therefore, the consequences of disease or treatment must be considered in the prevention plan. For example, the patient with low body mass index and protuberant boney prominences will be managed through frequent turning, positioning, and use of assistive devices to promote mobility or maintain positioning. Longer term interventions to address nutritional needs may or may not be possible for a particular patient at a particular time.

Considerations for preventive interventions include skin care, hygiene, support surfaces to reduce pressure distribution, nutrition and hydration, and mobility and mechanical loading. Although there is no current agreement on what preventive skin care exactly entails, bathing to promote good basic hygiene, particularly in cases of incontinence, and use of protective or barrier products in areas prone to moisture, friction, irritation, or compression are essential. Barrier skin products are essential to managing pressure ulcer prevention in the incontinent patient, as urine or stool can chemically promote skin breakdown in certain conditions, or complicate pressure ulcers through the potential for infection. The bathing process also promotes mobility, even if only passive mobility, repositioning during bathing and application of skin protection products, and an opportunity to assess for developing ulcers or areas of potential hazard, such as wrinkles or rolls in bedding or tubes and catheters in place underneath the patient's body. It is important to address dry skin as a risk but avoid traditional lotions or creams. They may promote moisture-associated ulcers, and may even promote bacterial growth.

Assessing for and addressing hydration issues are important in the critically ill patient. Hypovolemia or hypotension directly affects capillary perfusion, decreasing oxygen delivery to areas of compression, enhancing the risk for pressure ulcers at those points. Hypervolemia may result in edema, also increasing the risk of compression.

In critical care units, nurses are particularly apt to utilize 'special beds' to prevent skin breakdown. There are a variety of choices currently available, with much variation depending on the facility. However, the goals of any of these special surfaces are redistribution of weight or pressure, reducing incidence of compression and promoting capillary perfusion. As risk factors mount in preventive assessment, the more beneficial a specialized support surface becomes. Little research currently supports which is the best surface to use, and patients with different clinical conditions may have widely different needs. Drawbacks to use of special support surface beds, whether dynamic air or particle beds, or static surfaces such as foam, are expense, availability, and sometimes, ease of use for the nurse.

Enhanced mobility as prevention may include using assistive devices to promote patient-assisted mobility or the traditional nursing approach of frequent turning and positioning. Providing an over bed trapeze for the bedbound patient may give a patient who is strong enough the leverage assistance to be able to move about in bed more frequently. Even maintaining both upper side rails in a raised position when not directly caring for the patient may give him the opportunity to use those side rails as assistive devices in being able to move, sit up, or turn side to side.

For the patient unable to move himself in the bed, turning and positioning at least every 2 hours to reduce compression over potential areas of breakdown over time is essential. A sentinel study evaluating time between repositioning has added to the science of nursing in identifying the 2-hour window as being the most beneficial for most patients [22], but even Florence Nightingale described turning and repositioning her patients in the quest for optimal return to health. Turning and repositioning in a timely fashion can be a challenge in the critical care setting. The patient's clinical condition, as well as equipment used for treatment may impede options for positioning. Patients who are unconscious, paralyzed, or immobile for other reasons may be unable to remain in position once turned or moved. So, it becomes vital for the nurse to use mobility aids and positioning devices to effectively move the patient. Mobility devices may be as simple as using the draw sheet or more sophisticated, such as air driven hover devices or lifts. Although mobility aids protect the patient, just as importantly, they are designed to protect the nurse from injury while repositioning the patient. Once moved, wedges, pillows, splints, or other devices may be used to retain that position. Please be certain that those devices do not contribute to new areas of compression on their own.

With critically ill patients, the most carefully implemented prevention regimen may fail, or the patient who arrives in the critical care unit in a state of progressively declining health may already have one or several pressure ulcers. At that point, using agency procedures or clinical guidelines, cleaning, staging, consistent assessment and restaging as required. A variety of treatment measures including those interventions useful for prevention, are used to prevent exacerbation, stage advancement, and promote healing.

Specialized interventions may include debridement, whether surgically or mechanically, such as the use of a wet to dry dressing. Large ulcers may be treated using wound vacuum dressings to promote closure but retard abscess formation. As pressure ulcers are often particularly painful, assessment and pain management is another essential part in managing pressure ulcers in the critical care unit.

Falls

More than one third of persons over the age of 65 fall every year, and half of these falls are recurrent. By 2020, the estimated cost related to falls and subsequent injuries is $34 billion dollars [23]. The Joint Commission has identified falls as high risk and requires all facilities to develop a fall prevention program. This initiative was instituted because of the increase of patient deaths due to falls (sentinel events): in 2008, the Joint Commission reported 60 sentinel events related to falls and this trend has been rising since 1996 [24].

While the ICU frequently treats patients post fall, it is important to monitor and prevent falls during their ICU stay. Every patient must be assessed for fall risk upon admission, at least daily and when there is a change in status. Multiple tools are available for assessing risk, such as Heinrich II and Morse scales. All tools consider age, comorbidities, fall history, physical limitations, cognitive impairment, and current medications [25,26]. The majority of all ICU patients classify as high risk.

It is the responsibility of the critical care nurse to identify those patients at risk for falling and institute measures to prevent falls. Based upon assessed needs of the patient, the bedside team needs to initiate measures to prevent falls that may include physical and psychosocial needs as well as environmental concerns.

Addressing physical needs includes provision of adequate pain management, intervention with sensory deficiencies such as sight or hearing, interventions preventing or alerting changes in position of rising from the bed or chair such as wedge cushions, lap belts, or tab (bed exit) alarms. Other interventions to meet physical needs may include repositioning for both safety and comfort, and adequately meeting toileting needs. Toileting includes instituting a schedule based on patient need, frequent offering of assistance, commode or bedpan, and teaching regarding urinary catheterization.

Providing for psychosocial needs includes management of anxiety, frequent reminders to request help before moving about, enlisting the aid of family members or sitters to alert staff-to-patient movement, or using distraction techniques to minimize the effects of the critical care environment.

Environmental issues that may add to the risk of falls in the critical care unit include noise and lightning as well as inconsistent patient observation. Initiatives to control noise, normalize lighting, promote quiet time or rest, or simply moving the patient closer to the nurses' station for more consistent observation may be useful interventions to reduce the risk of falling.

THE CHALLENGE OF FOCUSING ON ONE NSQI AS IT IMPACTS ON OTHERS

Use of NSQI in clinical practice is not just an exercise in measurement, but a true clinical tool in improving patient outcomes. Nurses do, indeed, influence patient care and patient outcomes. Even focus on a single NSQI promotes preventive or health promoting action in other areas of the patient's health, even on other measurable NSQI [27]. Focused nursing measures on prevention of catheter-related urinary tract infections may address issues such as incontinence, directly affecting risk for pressure ulcers. Helping the patient to increase or enhance mobility, finding ways to eliminate catheter need and enhance bladder emptying may also address mobility-associated risks for pressure ulcer formation. Conversely, interventions aimed at preventing VAP may confound or prohibit efforts intended to address another NSQI. For example, maintaining the head of the bed at a 45 degree angle as a preventive measure for ventilator-associated pneumonia may prevent efforts at early removal of indwelling urinary catheter, as the patient is unable to move and position effectively to promote use of a bed pan or urinal, thus putting the patient at greater risk for UTI. The critical care nurse's holistic approach to caring for the patient allows for consideration and balance in prevention and intervention to facilitate optimal patient outcomes through enhancing preventive measures to consider other interventions necessary.

References

1. Bell L: *AACN Scope and Standards for Acute and Critical Care Nursing Practice.* Aliso Veijo, CA, American Association of Critical-Care Nurses, 2008.
2. Mundinger O'Neil, Nightingale F, et al: *Florence Nightingale: Measuring Hospital Care Outcomes.* Joint Commission on Accreditation of Health Care Outcomes, Oakbrook Terrace: IL, Joint commision, 1999.
3. Zalumas J: *Caring in Crisis: An oral History of Critical Care Nursing.* Philadelphia, University of Pennsylvania Press, 1995.
4. Maxfield D, Grenny J, McMillan R, et al: Silence kills: the seven crucial conversations for healthcare. Available at: http://www.silencekills.com. Accessed September 3, 2009.
5. The Joint Commission: *Improving Handoff Communication.* Oakbrook Terrace, IL: Joint Commission Resources, 2007.
6. Institute of Medicine: *Keeping Patients Safe: Transforming the Work Environment of Nurses.* Washington, DC, National Academy Press, 2004.
7. Pappas SH: The cost of nurse-sensitive adverse events. *J Nurs Adm* 38(5): 230–236, 2008
8. Kovner C, Gergen PJ: Nurse staffing levels and adverse events following surgery in U.S. hospitals. *Image J Nurs Sch* 30(1):315, 1998.
9. Gray ML: Securing the indwelling catheter. *Am J Nurs* 108(12):44–50, 2008.
10. Mercer-Smith J: Indwelling catheter management: From habit-based to evidence-based practice. *Ostomy Wound Manage* 49(12):34–45, 2003.
11. Byrnes MC, Coopersmith CM: Prevention of catheter-related blood stream infection. *Curr Opin Crit Care* 13(4):411–415, 2007.
12. Dezfulian C, Lavelle J, Nallamothu BK, et al: Rates of infection for single-lumen versus multilumen central venous catheters: a meta-analysis. *Crit Care Med* 31(9):2385–2390, 2003.
13. Seneff MG, Zimmerman JE, Knaus WA, et al: Predicting the duration of mechanical ventilation. The importance of disease and patient characteristics. *Chest* 110(2):496–479, 1996.
14. Craven DE: Epidemiology of ventilator-associated pneumonia. *Chest* 117(4, Suppl 2):186S–187S, 2000.
15. Wood CG, Swanson JM: Managing ventilator-associated pneumonia. *AACN Adv Crit Care* 20(4):309–316, 2009.
16. Kollef MH: The prevention of ventilator-associated pneumonia. *N Engl J Med* 340(8):627–634, 1999.
17. Tablan OC, Anderson LJ, Besser R, et al: Guidelines for preventing health-care associated pneumonia, 2003: recommendations of CDC and Healthcare Infection Control Practices Advisory Committee. *MMWR Recomm Rep* 53(RR 3):1 36, 2004.
18. Munro CL, Grap MJ: Oral health and care in the intensive care unit: state of the science. *Am J Crit Care* 13:25–33, 2004.
19. Moore T: Suctioning techniques for the removal of respiratory secretions. *Nurs Stand* 18(9):47–55, 2003.
20. Allman RM, Goode PS, Patrick MM, et al: Pressure ulcer risk factors among hospitalized patients with activity limitations. *JAMA* 273:865–870, 1995.
21. Russo CA, Elixhauser A: Hospitalizations related to pressure sores, 2003 Healthcare Cost and Utilization Project. Rockville, MD: Agency for Healthcare Research and Quality. Available at: http://hcup-as.arhrq.gov/reports/statbriefs/sb3.pdf. Accessed October 27, 2009.
22. Norton D, McLaren R, Exton-Smith A: *An Investigation of Geriatric Nurse Problems in Hospitals.* Edinburgh UK, Churchill Livingston, 1975.

23. The Costs of Fall Injuries Among Older Adults Fact Sheet; Centers for Disease Control and Prevention, National Center for Injury Prevention and Control, 2009.
24. Joint Commission for the Accreditation of Hospitals website: Sentinel Event Statistics. Available at: http://www.jointcommission.org/SentinelEvents/Statistics/. Accessed 2010.
25. Hendrich A, Nyhuis A, Kippenbrock T, et al: Hospital falls: Development of a predictive model for clinical practice. *Appl Nurs Res* 8(3):129–139, 1995.
26. Morse J: *Preventing Patient Falls*. Thousand Oaks, CA, Sage, 1997.
27. Needleman J, Kurtzman ET, Kizer KW: Performance measurement of nursing care. *Med Care Res Rev* 64(2):10S–43S, 2007.

CHAPTER 204 ■ ROLE OF THE ADVANCED PRACTICE NURSE IN CRITICAL CARE

THERESA R. MACFARLAN

INTRODUCTION

Advanced practice nurses (APNs) are registered nurses prepared at the master's or doctoral level. They function in a multitude of inpatient and outpatient settings across the health care continuum. APN roles include Clinical Nurse Specialist (CNS), Nurse Practitioner (NP), Certified Nurse–Anesthetist, and Nurse Midwife. Though their practice environments, patient populations, specialty knowledge-base and skill sets vary greatly, all APNs share core competencies of direct clinical practice, expert coaching and guidance, consultation, research, clinical and professional leadership, collaboration, and ethical decision-making [1]. CNSs and Acute Care Nurse Practitioners (ACNPs) possess education and expertise in areas that uniquely equip them to practice in the critical care environment. All APN roles require advanced nursing knowledge and skills; the roles are not the same as those held by physicians, although APN practice may be similar to physicians in many medical therapeutic realms [1]. When APNs begin to transfer new skills or interventions into their practice, they become nursing skills, informed by the clinical practice values of the nursing model: "*the advanced practice of nursing is not the junior practice of medicine* [1]."

This chapter describes the Acute Care CNS and ACNP roles, scope of practice, certification, credentialing, and reporting mechanisms. In addition, the science related to outcomes of APN practice and co-practice with other providers is discussed.

ROLE AND SCOPE OF PRACTICE

CNS—A CNS is an expert clinician in a specialized area of nursing practice. The specialty may be defined by a population (women), a setting (critical care unit), a disease or medical subspecialty (cardiovascular disease), a type of care (rehabilitation), or a type of problem (wounds) [1,2]. The CNS approaches the APN role through three spheres of influence: at the patient level in direct care, at the nurse level with staff development, and at the institution level providing oversight of care [1]. Staff education and system change responsibilities represent a large percentage of the CNS's role [1]. In each of the spheres of influence, the primary goal of the CNS is continuous improvement of patient outcomes and nursing care. Key elements of CNS practice are to create environments through mentoring and system changes that empower nurses to develop caring, evidence-based practices. The CNS is responsible and accountable for diagnosis and treatment of health-illness states, disease management, health promotion, and prevention of illness and risk behaviors among individuals, families, groups, and communities [3].

ACNP—Of the APN categories, nurse practitioners (NPs) have undergone the broadest expansion in practice arenas. Emerging from the primary care setting, NPs began to expand their role into specialty and subspecialty areas in response to population changes in health care. Preparing NPs for acute care practice began in the early 1990s as a response to the need for advanced level practitioners in the inpatient, acute and critical care settings. Only ACNPs have been educated and trained to manage critically ill patients in ICU settings, but NPs with other educational preparation (such as family, adult, or gerontology) may practice in other hospital areas. However, this use of other NPs in the acute care setting has been questioned, as their scope of practice (academic preparation and experience) does not always include acute care patient management [4].

Though both CNS and ACNP are targeted to a patient-centered approach to care for patient populations, the continuous on-unit presence of the ACNP at the bedside of patients often differentiates the role of the ACNP from the CNS role [1]. In a 2006 American Association of Critical Care Nurses (AACN) study of APN practice, ACNPs reported spending 74% of their practice time directed toward individual patient management, while CNSs divided their time between nursing personnel (36%), populations of patients (21%), and other disciplines, organizations, or systems (17%) [4]. The primary responsibilities of ACNPs involve activities related to direct management of patient care, accounting for 85% to 88% of time spent in the role [5]. Key elements of the ACNP role include conducting physical examinations and comprehensive health assessments, gathering patients' medical histories, ordering and interpreting the full spectrum of diagnostic tests and procedures, use of differential diagnoses to reach a medical diagnosis, prescribing medications, providing and evaluating the outcomes of interventions, conducting rounds, initiating transfers and consultations, and preparing patients for discharge [6,7]. ACNP care includes health promotion, disease prevention, health education, and counseling as well as the diagnosis and management of acute and chronic diseases [3].

CREDENTIALING

Credentialing is furnishing the documentation necessary to be authorized by a regulatory body or institution to engage in certain activities and to use a certain title [1]. In all states, APN regulation for practice is based on basic nursing licensure, but many states have additional rules and regulations that delineate requirements and define and limit who can use a specific advanced practice nursing title [1,7]. Nurse practice acts are administered under the authority of state governments to assure public safety [7]. In 23 states, the board of nursing has sole authority over advanced practice nursing; in others, there is joint authority with the board of medicine, the board of pharmacy, or both [8]. Advanced practice nursing certification is national in scope, and it is a mandatory requirement for APNs to obtain and maintain credentialing in most states [9]. APNs must fulfill continuing education (CE) and practice requirements to successfully maintain their national certification, although requirements differ from specialty to specialty. Each advanced practice nursing certification entity clearly lays out the requirements and time frame for recertification. National certifications for most specialties last from 5 to 8 years, and require that the candidate retest unless established parameters are met [1].

Credentialing and licensure for prescriptive authority also occur at the state level. Pharmacology requirements vary from state to state, with most states requiring a core advanced pharmacotherapeutics course during the graduate APN educational program, and yearly continuing education credits to maintain prescriptive privileges [1].

The requirement for APN hospital privileges varies according to the nurse's practice. Many hospitals have different levels of hospital privileges, ranging from "full" privileges to modified privileges for specific functions [1]. A collaborative practice agreement exists between an APN and physician to define parameters of practice for the APN. Many states require this as part of APN licensure [8]. This agreement may take many forms, from a one-page written agreement defining consultation and referral patterns to a more specific prescribed protocol for specific functions based on state statues for APNs. These agreements should be written as broadly as possible to allow for practice variations and new innovations [1].

CERTIFICATION

CNS—Upon completion of an accredited graduate CNS program, certification by examination is available through the American Nurses Credentialing Center (ANCC), or through the certification boards of specialty organizations. The American Association of Critical Care Nurses (AACN) offers a Critical Care Nurse Specialist exam [2]. However, certification exams are not available for many CNS specialties. This is a major regulatory barrier for many CNS specialties in those states that require CNS certification for second licensure [1]. Creating a universal CNS certification examination is in the forefront of current efforts to address this problem. Some states allow prescriptive authority for CNSs.

ACNP—Upon completion of an accredited graduate ACNP program, a national certification exam is available through ANCC or AACN. National certification for acute care nurse practitioner practice began in 1995 [1]. For licensure, many states do not differentiate between NP specialties (such as family and acute care) [1]. ACNPs are granted full prescriptive authority, regulated by state statutory and regulatory bodies [1].

REPORTING MECHANISM

Reporting structures for APNs vary widely within health care organizations [1]. In organizations with many APNs, an APN may report to another APN. In the critical care setting, APNs may report to a nursing administrator responsible for critical care, to a physician, or both. This type of dual reporting may maximize support for the role and clarify role expectations [9]. As licensed independent providers, ACNPs in many institutions must obtain privileges through the credentialing committee. This process may require a designated physician supervisor/collaborator [1]. The degree of supervision needed may change as the APN becomes more experienced in the role.

FACTORS AFFECTING THE GROWTH OF THE ACNP IN CRITICAL CARE

Major factors that contributed to integrating ACNPs into the critical care arena occurred in the late 1990s as a result of a decrease in the number of medical residents and an increase in the acuity of the patient population. Strict guidelines have been placed on resident work hours by the Accreditation Council of Graduate Medical Education (ACGME) and the Residency Review Committee [10]. Instituted in 2003 [5], the 80-hour workweek restriction has especially challenged surgical residents who must balance operative and nonoperative care time in managing critically ill patients [10]. This has contributed to the almost impossible task of providing appropriate level 24-hour intensive care unit coverage by surgical house staff. In a national survey, Gordon et al. [10] found that the use of Physician Assistants (PAs) or NPs may be one effective strategy in allowing surgical residents to care more efficiently for critically ill patients under the new ACGME guidelines. Critical care units that employ ACNPs report being able to meet the ACGME standard for the 80-hour workweek for residency training programs [11]. ACNPs are uniquely equipped to bridge the gap between the nursing and medical models of care, providing seamless continuity of care to patients and their families.

EVIDENCE-BASED OUTCOMES DRIVEN CARE

Evidence-based practice for ACNPs can be described as using the best scientific evidence and clinical expertise to influence patient outcomes [12]. APNs should be adept in the search and critical review of published material, including familiarity with grading systems that indicate the strength of the evidence. Multiple clinical studies have demonstrated cost-containment, decreased days on mechanical ventilation, and decreased length of stay (LOS) as a result of direct APN involvement in managing patients in critical care units [13–20]. Cardiovascular (CV) surgeon and ACNP collaborative practice decreased the LOS for specific diagnosis-related group (DRGs) and decreased total cost for the episode of care when compared to CV surgeon alone. Cowan et al. (2005) [21] demonstrated that physician/NP collaboration focused on enhancing continuity, multidisciplinary team planning, discharge coordination and assessment after discharge, and reduced LOS and hospital costs without negatively affecting readmissions or mortality. In a study that compared outcomes in chronically critically ill patients admitted to a subacute Medical Intensive Care Unit (MICU) who were collaboratively managed by an ACNP/attending physician team or a team composed of fellows and an attending physician, no significant differences were reported in LOS, duration of mechanical ventilation, number of patients who had been weaned at discharge, and disposition [22]. After adding two ACNPs to their trauma service, one teaching hospital was able to obtain compliance with residency work hour limitations by decreasing the average number of hours worked per trauma resident per week from 86 to 79 hours, as well as decreasing overall hospital LOS [23]. In the area of patient/family satisfaction, NPs have been shown to score higher than resident or attending physicians [24–31]. It has been shown that MD/NP collaboration can enhance continuity of care, multidisciplinary team planning, discharge coordination and assessment after discharge, reducing LOS and hospital costs without affecting readmissions or mortality [21].

COLLABORATIVE PROVIDERS

ACNPs and CNSs sometimes practice collaboratively with other providers in critical care, especially in teaching hospitals and university settings. Brief descriptions of physician assistants and intensivists are included to differentiate clinical roles.

Physician Assistant (PA)

The first formalized physician assistant program was implemented at Duke University in 1965 [32]. PA programs were first developed to augment the practice of primary care physicians, fill service gaps in underserved areas, and help control health care costs [33]. PAs emerged from a medical model of care, as compared to APNs whose identity and practice is shaped by the nursing model of care [34]. The PA role is rapidly expanding beyond primary care to specialty and inpatient practice, including critical care [4].

Intensivists

The Leapfrog Group (founded in November, 2000) recommendations emerged from the growing evidence supporting dedicated intensivist staffing in ICUs. A review of studies revealed that ICUs in which an intensivist manages or co-manages all patients, there were improved patient outcomes, including a reduction in hospitality mortality [35]. Leapfrog recommends at least 8 hour per day intensivist on-unit presence as one of four hospital safety standards supported by evidence-based research. ACNPs provide expert, collaborative care with the intensivists. The AACN has described the importance of effective communication in critical care practice as a core element for patient safety, seamless care, and healthy work environments [36].

CONCLUSION

The complexity of multilayered chronic diseases upon acute illness states, additional regulatory burden for documentation and outcome measurements, the explosion of information and medical technologies, and the astronomical cost of health care poses challenges unforeseen by our nursing predecessors. The enormous workforce and economic burden associated with long-stay ICU patients mandates innovative approaches for their care provision. Nursing practice continues to evolve, striving to keep pace with the needs of an increasingly complex and aging population. Nursing has always been a dynamic profession, evolving with the needs of the population and the capacities of health care systems' resources. Creative visioning and the passion to deliver skilled and compassionate care continue to drive nursing's capacity to meet health care needs. With the current health care crisis of unsustainable cost escalation, it is imperative that healthcare organizations deliver high quality care that is highly efficient and cost effective. Provision of intensive care is one of the largest and most costly aspects of health care in the United States [22]. We are entering a period of unprecedented growth in the number of individuals likely to need ICU services. With current levels of growth, the U.S. health care system will fall far short in the ability even to provide the current level of care, let alone increase the access for the critically ill to intensivists by the year 2020 [35,37]. APN-friendly cultures do not occur by chance, but are created when committed organizations and APNs share common vision and values. An APN friendly culture is one in which all professionals are valued and recognized as possessing unique contributing knowledge and skill-sets necessary to provide excellent, collaborative patient and family-centered care [38]. As we move forward into the uncertain health care climate of the future, ACNPs and CNSs can deliver cost-effective, competent, collaborative, and compassionate care to the growing critical care population.

References

1. Hamric AB, Spross JA, Hanson CM: *Advanced Practice Nursing: An Integrative Approach*. St Louis, Elsevier Saunders, 2009.
2. National Association of Clinical Nurse Specialists Web site. www.nacns.org/AboutNACNS/FAQS/tabid/109/Default.aspx. Accessed December 12, 2009.
3. Consensus Model for APRN Regulation: Licensure, Accreditation, Certification and Education. Available at: www.tnaonlince.org/Media/pdf/aprn-consensus model-08.pdf. Updated 2008. Accessed December 12, 2009.
4. Kleinpell RM, Ely EW, Grabenkort R: Nurse practitioners and physician assistants in the intensive care unit: an evidence-based review. *Crit Care Med* 36(10):2888–2897, 2008.
5. Howie-Esquivel J, Fontaine DK: The evolving role of the acute care nurse practitioner in critical care. *Curr Opin Crit Care* 12(6):609–613, 2006.
6. Kleinpell RM: Acute care nurse practitioner practice: results of a 5-year longitudinal study. *Am J Crit Care* 14(3):211–219; quiz 220–221, 2005.
7. Advanced Practice Work Group: *Scope and Standards of Practice for the Acute Care Nurse Practitioner.* 2006, p 50.
8. Lugo NR, O'Grady E, Hodnicki D, et al: Ranking state NP regulation: practice environment and consumer health care choice. *Am J Nurse Pract* 11(4):8–24, 2007.
9. Bryant-Lukosius D, Dicenso A: A framework for the introduction and evaluation of advanced practice nursing roles. *J Adv Nurs* 48(5):530–540, 2004.
10. Gordon CR, Axelrad A, Alexander JB, et al: Care of critically ill surgical patients using the 80-hour Accreditation Council of Graduate Medical Education work-week guidelines: a survey of current strategies. *Am Surg* 72(6):497–499, 2006.
11. Caserta FM, Depew M, Moran J: Acute care nurse practitioners: the role in neuroscience critical care. *J Neurol Sci* 261(1–2):167–171, 2007.
12. Kleinpell RM, Gawlinski A, Burns SM: Searching and critiquing literature essential for acute care NPs. *Nurse Pract* 31(8):12–13, 2006.
13. Burns SM, Earven S: Improving outcomes for mechanically ventilated medical intensive care unit patients using advanced practice nurses: a 6-year experience. *Crit Care Nurs Clin North Am* 14:231–243, 2002.
14. Burns SM, Earven S, Fisher C, et al: Implementation of an institutional program to improve clinical and financial outcomes of mechanically ventilated patients: one-year outcomes and lessons learned. *Crit Care Med* 31(12):2752–2763, 2003.
15. Cusson RM, Buus-Frank ME, Flanagan VA, et al: A survey of the current neonatal nurse practitioner workforce. *J Perinatol* 28(12):830–836, 2008.
16. Heward Y: Advanced practice in paediatric intensive care: a review. *Paediatr Nurs* 21(1):18–21, 2009.
17. Hicks GL Jr: Cardiac surgery and the acute care nurse practitioner—"the perfect link". *Heart Lung* 27(5):283–284, 1998.
18. Jensen L, Scherr K: Impact of the nurse practitioner role in cardiothoracic surgery. *Dynamics* 15(3):14–19, 2004.
19. Kleinpell RM: APNs: invisible champions? *Nurs Manage* 38(5):18–22, 2007.
20. Russell D, VorderBruegge M, Burns SM: Effect of an outcomes-managed approach to care of neuroscience patients by acute care nurse practitioners. *Am J Crit Care* 11:353–364, 2002.
21. Cowan MJ, Shapiro M, Hays RD, et al: The effect of a multidisciplinary hospitalist/physician and advanced practice nurse collaboration on hospital costs. *J Nurs Adm* 36(2):79–85, 2006.
22. Hoffman LA, Tasota FJ, Zullo TG, et al: Outcomes of care managed by an acute care nurse practitioner/attending physician team in a subacute medical intensive care unit. *Am J Crit Care* 14(2):121–130; quiz 131–132, 2005.

23. Christmas AB, Reynolds J, Hodges S, et al: Physician extenders impact trauma systems. *J Trauma* 58(5):917–920, 2005.
24. Bryant R, Graham MC: Advanced practice nurses: a study of client satisfaction. *J Am Acad Nurse Pract* 14:88–92, 2002.
25. Chang E, Daly J, Hawkins A, et al: An evaluation of the nurse practitioner role in a major rural emergency department. *J Adv Nurs* 30:260–268, 1999.
26. Green A, Davis S: Toward a predictive model of patient satisfaction with nurse practitioner care. *J Am Acad Nurse Pract* 17(4):139–148, 2005.
27. Lenz ER, Mundinger MO, Kane RL, et al: Primary care outcomes in patients treated by nurse practitioners or physicians. Two year follow up. *Med Care Res Rev* 61:332–351, 2004.
28. Litaker D, Mion LC, Planarsky L, et al: Physician-nurse practitioner teams in chronic disease management: the impact on costs, clinical effectiveness and patients' perception of care. *J Interprof Care* 17:223–237, 2003.
29. Moore S, Corner J, Haviland J, et al: Nurse led followup and conventional medical followup in management of patients with lung cancer: a randomized trial. *Br Med J* 325:1145–1147, 2002.
30. Sidani S, Doran D, Porter H, et al: Outcomes of nurse practitioners in acute care. *Internet J Adv Nurs Pract* 8, 2006.
31. Sidani S, Doran D, Porter H, et al: Processes of care: comparison between nurse practitioners and physician residents in acute care. *Nurs Leadersh* 19:69–85, 2006.
32. Thourani VH, Miller JI Jr: Physicians assistants in cardiothoracic surgery: a 30-year experience in a university center. *Ann Thorac Surg* 81(1):195–199; discussion 199–200, 2006.
33. Physician Assistant History Center. Available at: http://www.pahx.org/index.htm. Updated 2004. Accessed August 20, 2009.
34. Cooper RA: New directions for nurse practitioners and physician assistants in the era of physician shortages. *Acad Med* 82(9):827–828, 2007.
35. Angus DC, Shorr AF, White A, et al: Critical care delivery in the United States: distribution of services and compliance with Leapfrog recommendations. *Crit Care Med* 34(4):1016–1024, 2006.
36. Becker D, Kaplow R, Muenzen PM, et al: Activities performed by acute and critical care advanced practice nurses: American Association of Critical-Care Nurses Study of Practice. *Am J Crit Care* 15(2):130–148, 2006.
37. Shorr AF, Angus DC: Do intensive care unit patients have intensive care unit physicians? Unfortunately not. *Crit Care Med* 34(6):1834–1835, 2006.
38. Richmond TS, Becker D: Creating an advanced practice nurse-friendly culture: a marathon, not a sprint. *AACN Clin Issues* 16(1):58–66, 2005.

CHAPTER 205 ■ INTERPROFESSIONAL COLLABORATION AMONG CRITICAL CARE TEAM MEMBERS

DEBRA GERARDI AND DORRIE K. FONTAINE

"In the ICU, nurses and physicians stand at a patient's bedside initially as strangers, thrown together by a combination of choice and circumstance. With each interaction, they assess one another's knowledge, openness to suggestion, and commitment to patient care. They learn each other's strengths and weaknesses and, over time, forge relationships that become the bedrock of effective collaboration. They communicate, negotiate, and compromise [1]."

INTERPROFESSIONAL COLLABORATION IN CRITICAL CARE

Collaboration among critical care professionals is essential to the provision of safe and effective care in the Intensive Care Unit (ICU). Outcomes associated with effective collaboration include patient safety, improved quality indicators, retention of healthcare providers, and patient and family satisfaction with care. In 1994, a joint position statement was issued by the Society of Critical Care Medicine (SCCM) and the American Association of Critical Care Nurses (AACN) promoting a multidisciplinary approach for managing and providing intensive care services as the preferred model of care [2]. Since that time, an increasing number of mandates and standards issued from national organizations reinforce interprofessional collaboration as a necessary component of care delivery in complex clinical environments.

This chapter describes the principles and importance of interprofessional collaboration, the integration of teamwork as a means of achieving collaborative outcomes, and strategies for cultivating environments in which collaborative delivery of safe patient care can flourish.

DEFINING COLLABORATION

Collaboration is the process of working together toward common goals through joint communication and joint decision-making [3]. Collaboration is both a process and a style that blends high levels of assertiveness and cooperation. Interprofessional collaboration is defined as the process in which different professional groups work together to positively impact health care and relies on negotiated agreements to bring the valued and unique contributions of experts to patient care. Interprofessional collaboration involves understanding what enables effective collaboration as well as understanding barriers to collaboration including: unhealthy power dynamics, poor communication patterns, lack of understanding of one's own and others' roles and responsibilities, and conflicts due to varied approaches to patient care that are inherent within diverse clinical teams [4]. Collaboration is vital, difficult, and learnable [5]. True collaboration is relational and requires skilled communication, trust, knowledge, shared responsibility, mutual respect, optimism, and coordination [6].

COLLABORATION AS A CORE COMPETENCY FOR HEALTH PROFESSIONALS

Health professionals are required to possess core competencies (knowledge, skills, and attitudes) associated with interprofessional collaboration including communication, negotiation, and conflict resolution as a component of academic training and professional practice [7–9]. The Accreditation Council for Graduate Medical Education and the Association for American Medical Colleges include aspects of communication, coordination, and collaboration among the required physician competencies [10]. Explicit guidelines for collaboration are embedded in professional codes of ethics for nurses and physicians [11,12]. Understanding of and respect for the professional contributions of colleagues across the professions is a necessary precursor to effective collaboration. Slow progress is being made to incorporate these competencies into curricula across the health professions to better teach the concepts of collaboration that support patient safety and improved care coordination [9,13].

MANDATES FOR INTERPROFESSIONAL COLLABORATION

The need for improved interprofessional collaboration has been discussed for decades among professional associations—particularly among critical care associations. The past decade has seen a shift from discussion to concerted action, as multiple calls for improvement in care delivery from the Institute of Medicine (IOM) have emerged, resulting from data linking poor clinical outcomes to ineffective teamwork and inadequate care coordination [14–16]. There is substantial evidence that the leading contributors to medical errors and unsafe care are breakdowns in teamwork, communication, and the overriding culture of health care itself [17,18]. Hundreds of billions of dollars are wasted on medical errors and ineffective care coordination each year [19]. In addition to poor patient outcomes, ineffective collaboration has been linked to perceptions of hostile work environments [20], low morale, and job stress among health professionals [21], increased turnover of clinical staff [22], and moral distress [23]. As such, new mandates are emerging to focus attention within healthcare organizations on strategies for developing interprofessional collaboration as a component of safe patient care.

The National Quality Forum (NQF) added teamwork training and interventions to their 2006 consensus report, Safe Practices for Better Healthcare, which are now represented in the 2009 Report as Safe Practice #3—Teamwork Training and Skill Building [24]. The Joint Commission, through their Patient Safety Goals [25], their sentinel event alerts [17], and their accreditation standards, requires improved teamwork, collaboration, and conflict management across the healthcare organization. Calls for conversation and dialogue to begin to address the challenges to working together are growing [26–28]. With this increased interest comes a growing database of empirical evidence associated with teamwork, collaboration, and improved conflict management in the clinical setting. This culture shift creates a golden opportunity for researchers interested in elucidating the impact of professional subcultures, human factors, team training, and conflict dynamics on the effectiveness of interprofessional collaboration and its impact on clinical outcomes, quality of work environments, and the resilience of health professionals.

INTERPROFESSIONAL COLLABORATION—EMERGING RESEARCH

The complexity of delivering critical care services requires ongoing integration of skills and knowledge from multiple professions. Emerging research highlights several areas including: perceptions of health professionals; the impact of collaboration and teamwork on clinical outcomes, quality indicators, retention of health professionals, patient satisfaction, and the quality of the work environment; characteristics of effective teams; and the influence of conflict on team effectiveness. Much of the research is based on self-reports combined with only a few observational or controlled trials. Several key studies will be reported here that serve as the foundation for future strategies.

Perceptions of Health Professionals

Physicians and nurses often state the importance of collaboration, communication, and cooperation in delivery of clinical care. Until recently, however, there has been little evidence as to how each of the professions defines these key components of the practice environment. In a 2009 study, health professionals indicated understanding and appreciation of professional roles and responsibilities, and communicating effectively to be two core competencies necessary for patient-centered collaborative practice [29]. Studies where both physicians and nurses were queried about collaboration and communication in their specific units suggest that their perspectives are often far apart. Using the Safety Attitude Questionnaire, Sexton and colleagues found that nurses' and anesthesiologists' perceptions of teamwork in the operating room were significantly lower than that reported by surgeons in the same area [30]. One study measuring communication in four ICUs in the United Kingdom noted that, while a majority of senior physicians reported a highly positive open communication style between nurses and physicians, only one third of nurses reported the same [31]. Thomas et al. investigated critical care nurses and physicians' attitudes about teamwork in eight ICUs in six hospitals. Findings of the 320 subjects suggested that while over 70% of physicians viewed collaboration as very high, only one third of the nurses felt the same [32]. These studies indicate that the two professions experience the organizational climate very differently. This begs the question, what underlies these varying perceptions, given that those surveyed were working together in the same units?

A review of the various codes of ethics for the professions of nursing, pharmacy, medicine, occupational therapy, social work, physical therapy, respiratory care, and chaplaincy indicate that the levels of ethical responsibility associated with interprofessional practice fall into five categories: professional conduct (citizenship), acknowledgement of others, cooperation, collaboration, and conflict engagement. The categories reflect a progression in depth of professional engagement and they provide a glimpse into the perceptions each profession acquires regarding interprofessional practice [33]. The discrepancy highlighted in the studies above suggests that differing approaches found in the professional codes of ethics may impact the way in which each profession is defining and perceiving collaboration. This idea proves likely based on the results of a 2006 survey measuring teamwork among nurses and physicians in the OR (operating room) setting. Discussions with survey respondents indicated that, "nurses often described good collaboration as 'having their input respected,' whereas physicians often described good collaboration as having nurses, 'who anticipate their needs and follow instructions' [30]." Research into effective teamwork indicates that having shared mental models and a common language are key for working well together. A good starting point for enhancing collaboration is the joint development of shared models for collaboration that provide a common language for working together.

Impact on Quality, Safety, and Retention

Research that examines the impact of interprofessional teams on patient safety is limited. Most reports either are anecdotal or include a limited description of the methods used to measure team effects [16]. A 2009 Cochrane review of clinical trials measuring the impact of interprofessional collaboration practice-based interventions designed to improve the work interactions or processes among various types of health professionals yielded five studies that fit the review criteria [4]. The five studies evaluated the effects of interprofessional rounds, interprofessional meetings, and an externally facilitated interprofessional audit. Three of the studies found that the interventions led to improvements in patient care, such as drug use, length of hospital stay and total hospital charges, while one study showed no impact, and one study showed mixed outcomes. The results of other studies suggest a positive correlation between interprofessional practice and clinical outcomes. Recent studies looking at the impact of teams in critical care and primary care have linked teamwork to increased survival to discharge, decreased readmission to the intensive care unit (ICU), fewer adverse events, shorter lengths of stay, and decreased mortality rates following surgical interventions [34]. Research assessing system failures in ORs and ICUs found that positive perceptions of team coordination among ICU staff were associated with lower error rates, that is, when the staff perceived timely transfer of information, role clarity, and awareness of team member activities [35]. Thomas et al. assessed the relationship between teamwork and noncompliance with neonatal resuscitation standards in 132 videotaped resuscitations and found a weak correlation between team behaviors (information sharing, inquiry, treatment planning, and leadership) and compliance [36]. There is also evidence that good team behaviors are linked to decreased turnover among nursing staff in the OR [30] and survey research has shown a link between high levels of cooperation between ICU nurses and physicians and reports of staff burnout [37]. Greater perceived relational coordination has been associated with patient perceptions of higher quality of care, less postoperative pain, greater postoperative functioning, and shorter length of stay [16].

The 2004 Institute of Medicine report, *Keeping Patients Safe*, addresses the work environment of nurses and its impact on patient safety. The report provides an extensive review of the literature on interprofessional collaboration in its *Appendix B: Interdisciplinary Collaboration, Team Functioning, and Patient Safety* [16]. Additional research is needed to differentiate the impact of team behaviors, organizational context, team composition, and team stability on clinical outcomes. In addition, the next phase of research should further elaborate strategies for cultivating team effectiveness [34].

Interprofessional Collaboration and End-of-Life Care

End-of-life care in the ICU is a complex and oftentimes an emotion-filled, process. Much work has been done to examine how to improve end-of-life care. In a 2005 special report from the Hastings Center, three areas were identified as needing greater attention to improve end-of-life care. The authors suggested a rethinking of assumptions related to (i) the end-of-life care delivery system, (ii) the approach to advance directives and surrogate decision making, and (iii) how to manage conflict and disagreement [38]. Each of these has implications for collaborative practice among ICU team members. Difficulties for clinicians in providing end-of-life care include: variability in practice, poor communication among providers, lack of consensus regarding plan of care, incomplete documentation, and differences of opinion regarding the definition of futility [39]. According to a statement released from the Consensus Conference in Critical Care, "The principles of shared end-of-life decision making between patients, family members, and clinicians can be achieved only through full participation of all ICU healthcare professionals in the communication and decision-making process [40]."

Critical care nurses have consistently described one of the greatest stressors in their work to be related to decision-making regarding futile treatment [41]. The most important factor enabling nurses to move from cure to comfort-oriented care is developing a consensus about the treatment plan. A survey of 864 critical care nurses revealed barriers to good end-of-life care as being disagreement about the direction of the dying patient's care, actions that prolonged a patient's suffering, and physicians who were evasive and avoided talking with patient's families [42]. When nurses believe that they are powerless to impact decisions related to a course of treatment they perceive to be unethical or harmful to the patient, it leads to moral distress [43]. According to the American Association of Critical Care Nurses, moral distress has a significant impact on the clinical work environment. Studies indicate that one in three nurses experiences moral distress and in one study, nearly half of the nurses surveyed left their unit, and for some their profession, as a result of moral distress [44]. Incorporation of shared goal setting, protocols for managing end of life care, collaborative decision-making processes, and interprofessional dialogue related to complex cases can alleviate some of the stress experienced by all clinicians in the critical care environment and improve care for patients and their families at a very difficult time in their lives.

STRATEGIES FOR ADVANCING INTERPROFESSIONAL COLLABORATION

There can be no assurance of safe, effective, quality care without collaboration that begins with a trusting, respectful relationship. Addressing what some consider these "soft" issues may in reality be the solution to many of the hardest challenges in critical care settings. In the complex environment of the ICU, the challenge to focus full attention on the patient experience and create systems of care where clear communication from respectful collaboration is the norm is crucial [45]. The history of critical care in the United States is replete with the concept of teams and reliance on expertise from many professionals—the hallmark of the ICU [46]. Relationship-centered care, where the primacy of relationship of patient and healthcare provider exists, cannot occur without skilled partnerships of all members of the healthcare team, especially physicians and nurses [47].

Given the broad impact of interprofessional collaboration and the growing application of teamwork to provision of critical care, it is important to better understand the current strategies for advancing collaborative practices and team effectiveness. Bronstein describes a model for interprofessional collaboration that includes: interdependence, professional activities (work structures and acts), flexibility in traditional roles, collective ownership of goals, and reflection on process (how well the team is working together) [48]. Reader et al. in a review of the literature linking teamwork to outcomes in intensive care generated a performance framework categorizing the various team behaviors that had an impact on clinical care. These behaviors can be categorized as: team communication, team leadership, team coordination, and team decision making [49]. Clarifying models for observing and evaluating collaborative practices provides a baseline for improving performance and elucidating what works. An overview of some of the emerging areas of interest associated with interprofessional collaboration is described below.

Attitudes and Attributes Indicative of Effective Interprofessional Practice

A blend of relational qualities, personal characteristics, skills, and activities constitute collaborative practice. The give and take between team members is in constant flux and resides within the context of the organizational environment. Team factors are divided into task, process, and relationship components. Processes include methods for communicating and sharing information, managing conflict, goal setting, and decision-making. Relationship factors include trust, respect, shared mental maps, status differentials, and attitudes toward teamwork [33]. Increasing emphasis on relational aspects of teamwork is emerging as principles from complexity science further define the necessary elements for high quality care in complex systems. In a study assessing factors that contribute to higher quality outcomes in complex primary care practices, Lanham et al. found trust, mindfulness, heedfulness, respectful interaction, diversity, social/task relatedness, and rich/lean communication to be important factors for the emergence of high-quality care. In addition, they determined that effective reflection, learning, and sense making were requisite behaviors among members of the clinical team [50].

Research indicates that attitudes toward teamwork impact the presence of collaborative practice [51]. Favorable attitudes toward team performance and collaborative patient management approaches maximized team outcomes [16]. There is a significant amount of literature addressing the relational aspects of trust and respect as components of collaborative practice [52]. The Society for Critical Care Medicine describes the attributes of interprofessional teams to be: trust and transparency, collaboration and communication, appreciation of complimentary roles for a shared purpose, leadership, action, and accountability [53].

Team Effectiveness

Collaborative patient-centered care is associated primarily with work in interprofessional teams [54]. In addition to the attitudes and attributes necessary for teamwork, there are specific skills and processes that enable a diverse collection of professionals to work in concert to provide care to critically ill patients. High functioning teams are characterized as having good communication, low levels of interpersonal conflict, high levels of collaboration, coordination, cooperation, and participation [34]. Team coordination is the concerted and synchronous performance of patient care tasks by team members. Coordination requires each team member to maintain an awareness of the work accomplished by the others on the team [49].

Collaboration, as an ongoing process, occurs across a continuum requiring a range of skills for engaging at various levels of depth and nuance. These skills include the capacity for self-reflection, the ability to communicate effectively across professional groups, the ability to give and receive feedback and engage in shared decision-making, consensus building, and the ability to engage in and resolve conflicts [33]. Work processes that support engagement across this continuum are essential as is effective team leadership.

A great deal of research has been conducted on teamwork and team behaviors. One model that has emerged as a foundation for addressing team performance is the Salas framework. This model specifies five core aspects of teamwork which include (i) team leadership (formal and informal), (ii) collective orientation (cohesiveness, common goals, and team success), (iii) mutual performance monitoring (awareness of others and understanding and appreciation of various roles), (iv) backup behavior (helping one another), and (v) adaptability (ability to adjust strategies and resources on the basis of situational assessment) [55]. These areas of teamwork are supplemented by three coordinating activities that include (i) establishing shared mental models, (ii) closed loop communication, and (iii) mutual trust. This model serves as the foundation for the evidence-based TeamSTEPPS training curriculum developed by the Department of Defense and the Agency for Healthcare Research and Quality (AHRQ) [56].

The construct of "team" has multiple definitions. In a recent literature review assessing the impact of teams on clinical and organizational effectiveness, team was defined as, "a collection of individuals who are interdependent in their tasks, who share responsibility for outcomes, who see themselves and who are seen by others as an intact social entity embedded in one or more larger social systems (for example, business unit or corporation), and who manage their relationships across organizational boundaries [34]." Impacting team effectiveness is the continuous morphing of team membership. The idea of team in a traditional work setting is much different in the clinical setting where shift changes, floating, locum tenens, trainee rotations, cross-covering, consultation, procedural specialists, and interdepartmental support staff all impact team configuration at any point in time. This dynamic creates challenges for communication and development of trust among team members. The forming and re-forming of the team requires establishment of relationships on an ongoing, quick-time basis [57]. Team dynamics and organizational complexity require clear communication among team members and effective methods for collaborative decision-making.

Team Communication and Decision Making

Physicians and nurses speak different languages, approach patient care from different frames of reference, and carry out their work very differently from each other (shift work vs. case-based work). The holistic model of nursing, with its emphasis on relational practice and sensitivity to patients' needs as primary, is a different framework from the scientific and objective model of medicine and its emphasis on disease process and diagnosis. As such communication difficulties are predictable. Schmitt identifies the key interprofessional communication patterns that contribute to errors in diagnosis and treatment as (i) counterproductive hierarchical communication; (ii) disjunctions in distribution of authority, responsibility, and accountability across disciplines; and (iii) issues of lack of respect and lack of clarity with regard to legal and ethical obligations across disciplines [58]. Additionally, nurses and physicians evaluate each other's competence in different ways. In a study reported by Schmalenberg et al., physicians tended to judge the competence of the nurses by the quality of the information given, particularly in emergency situations when the patient's condition had changed. Nurses tended to judge the competence of the physician by patient outcomes and the absence of complications, consultation with the nurse prior to writing orders, and the extent to which the physician listened and collaborated in determining the patient's plan of care [59,60]. The need for bridging these world views to ensure effective communication and decision-making is obvious. A look at communication patterns during patient care rounds demonstrates both the status differential between physicians and nurses and the differing perceptions of information sharing. In a 9-month study in which researchers observed 2,391 intensive care interactions, it was noted that nurses made only 12% of comments during rounds and only 10% of the team discussion was directed toward the nurses [61]. The observed nurses were asked their opinion by the medical staff only four times in the nine-month period, and when interviewed, the nurses portrayed themselves as assertive during rounds. Physicians rely on the surveillance function of nurses who are present with the patient a larger portion of the time and they rely on timely reporting of information by the nurse to make critical treatment decisions.

Team communication is the ongoing sharing of information, ideas, and opinions among members of the team. Reader reviewed 35 studies on teamwork in the ICU and found that errors in patient care occurred most often when team communication failed, particularly after shift change and handoffs, with 37% of the observed errors associated with nurse/physician communication [49]. In a 2008 survey of over 5,000 critical care nurses, 40% of those responding rated communication with physicians as only fair or poor with close to 60% noting verbal abuse [62]. Pronovost and colleagues analyzed ICU adverse event and critical incident data and found that critical incidents were associated with reluctance among nursing staff to report observed errors and patient care issues, a lack of communication between physicians and nurses regarding changes in treatment, inaccurate transfer of information between ICU teams, and inadequate information transfer when new patients were admitted to the unit [63].

Such results have led to initiatives that help the various professions communicate more effectively with each other. These include the use of electronic medical records, practice protocols, procedural checklists designed together by the team, and the use of SBAR for reports from one clinician to another. SBAR, which stands for Situation-Background-Assessment-Recommendation is a script developed by the military as a means of communicating necessary information in a concise and uniform manner so that the receiver of the information can make prompt decisions in response [64]. These efforts help to reinforce the aspects of effective teamwork identified previously including shared mental models, collective orientation, and closed loop communication.

Team decision-making occurs as information and perceptions from the various team members are integrated. Decisions can be made together as the members confer or may be made by the team leader on behalf of the team [49]. Complex decision-making requires the integration of divergent viewpoints within the team that represent a rich array of perspectives, experience, and information. Negotiating through the differences to come to agreement regarding the plan of care is an essential skill for critical care teams. Doing so is dependent upon the relational factors previously described including trust and respect. Teams that adopt competitive, rather than collaborative approaches are not only less effective, but they also create environments in which there are lower levels of team member satisfaction [65]. When negotiations are cooperative, team members are better able to remain flexible and open to the ideas of others leading to more creative problem solving. When conflict levels are high and negotiations are competitive, cognitive flexibility decreases and defensive postures prevent effective collaboration. Team member support for team decisions is predicated on the perceived level of procedural fairness experienced during the decision-making process [16]. Those teams where senior members seek out and incorporate the perspectives and opinions of junior members are more likely to have members who remain engaged with the group, follow through on team decisions, and who continue to be cooperative in future negotiations.

Self-Reflection and Self-Correction

Effective critical care teams are capable of giving and receiving feedback among the various team members and they are able to self-correct, that is, adapt their actions to changes in the patient's condition or to changes in team performance [55]. Reflective practice enables clinicians to evaluate their own responses to situations and to identify areas that need attention. Reflective practice techniques have increasingly been integrated into the teaching of communication skills in medical schools to improve clinician–patient interactions [66]. Developing team practices that allow for self-reflection, observation, and evaluation of group process, and incorporation of what is learned into performance improvement activities, greatly enhances team effectiveness and develops improved trust as the team discovers what qualities and activities enable them to function effectively. Mechanisms for reflecting on performance include: use of team debriefs, case reviews, facilitated reflection with mentors or coaches, and informal conversations among team members.

Professional practice entails continuous learning and adaptation as feedback is received to improve performance and provide increasingly sophisticated care. Improving clinical abilities is just one aspect of self-corrective behavior. A more difficult component of professional practice is the giving and receiving of feedback among colleagues, particularly feedback related to professional conduct and team behaviors [45]. In the seminal 2005 study, *Silence Kills*, researchers sampled critical care staff and physicians in 13 ICUs nationwide. The researchers discovered that the majority of critical care staff and physicians surveyed had concerns about competence of some of their colleagues, had witnessed shortcuts and mistakes, and had experienced disrespect and insufficient team support with very few speaking up to address these concerns [67]. The reasons given by those surveyed for not speaking up include: fear of retaliation, lack of conflict skills, deference to authority, and the belief that nothing will come from speaking up. Avoidance of these difficult conversations led to elaborate workarounds, by physicians and nursing staff, which compromised patient care. In most cases, team members were aware of a colleague's poor performance, often for over a year, and they allowed it to continue rather than provide the necessary feedback needed for improving performance.

Failing to address clinical performance is not the only area of difficulty for health professionals. In July 2008, the Joint Commission released Sentinel Event Alert #40, *Behaviors that Undermine a Culture of Safety* [17]. The alert cites evidence of the correlation between intimidating and disruptive behaviors and the incidence of medical errors and preventable adverse events, patient satisfaction, costs of care, and retention of qualified personnel. The alert goes on to indicate that there is a history of tolerance and indifference to such behaviors and that failure to address these behaviors at both the individual and system levels contributes to unsafe care.

Increasingly, research indicates a large prevalence of unprofessional conduct that could contribute to patient harm. Such behavior also impacts the quality of the work environment. The results from Rosenstein's studies indicate that more than 90% of clinicians surveyed felt that disruptive behaviors invoked feelings of stress and frustration, with more than 80% feeling that disruptive behaviors caused a loss of concentration, reduced team collaboration, and impaired information transfer. In addition, more than 90% felt that disruptive behaviors contributed to poor communication and impaired nurse–physician relationships [68]. A 2009 study among experienced labor and delivery nurses indicates that despite their knowledge of proper clinical actions based on evidence and national practice standards in five high-risk scenarios, the nurses chose to delay or work around the physician when the physician was difficult to deal with. This was particularly true when the nurses believed that their manager or hospital administration would not back them up [69].

The findings of these studies add to the growing literature base that calls for a reexamination of what it means for nurses and physicians to authentically collaborate for patients to receive expert coordinated care. Improving the capacity of clinicians across the professions to engage in conflict situations and give difficult feedback to colleagues is an essential step in improving the safety of patient care and the quality of clinical work environments [26]. Since January 2009, the Joint Commission has required accredited healthcare organizations to (i) develop a universal code of conduct, (ii) implement a process for dealing with lapses in professional conduct, and (iii) to develop and implement a conflict management process for addressing conflicts among the three top leadership groups (executives and senior management, medical staff, and the governing body) [70]. This increased focus on improving conflict management in the clinical setting is a powerful step in helping to cultivate conflict competent organizations.

Conflict Competence Among Team Members

In addition to managing day-to-day team processes, critical care teams must also manage the competing agendas that inherently exist in interprofessional teams [71]. Just as with perceptions of collaboration and communication, there are differing perspectives among physicians and nurses regarding the presence of conflict. "Studies indicate that physicians do not always recognize nurses' perspectives on conflict. In a study of conflict in intensive care units, nurses identified nearly twice as many conflicts as were identified by both the physician and the nurse [72]." Again, developing a shared mental model of conflict and developing the skills of team members to constructively engage with each other is crucial.

Health professionals identify high levels of conflict in the workplace and much of that conflict is with each other. In a 2009 survey sent to 13,000 physicians and nurses, nearly 98% of the survey respondents reported witnessing behavior problems between doctors and nurses in the past year, with 30% indicating they saw such behaviors weekly and 10% indicating daily occurrences [73]. Among ICU intensivists responding to a survey published in 2009, 70% reported conflict in the past week, with half of the incidents perceived as "severe" and those reporting indicated that the conflict was associated with increased job strain [21].

Physicians and nurses identify a desire for increased opportunities for training and open dialogue that focuses on teamwork and conflict engagement [74,75]. Expertise in conflict management ranges from novice to expert and incorporates capacity for addressing personal conflict, as well as skill in facilitating and mediating conflicts among others. Foundational to skill acquisition is the development of non-adversarial (dialogic) mindsets, cognitive roadmaps for approaching conflict, and expanded capacity for self-reflection and self-correction of ineffective behaviors [76]. Maine Medical Center in Portland, ME and the UMass Memorial Medical Center in Worcester, MA are examples of institutions that have invested in systematic communications training for healthcare providers, leading to sustained improvements in safety and quality [77].

Difficulties that can contribute to conflict within the team include role boundary issues, perceptions of unfair decision-making processes, autonomy versus team needs, feeling that one's contribution is not valued, miscommunication of information, and inappropriate use of hierarchy [78]. Not all conflict is bad and in fact conflict is often necessary for obtaining the best decisions in complex cases. Evidence of the impact of variable types of conflict indicates that some types of conflict (task-related) can improve social capital (trust) within the team and thereby improve coordination of patient care [79].

Conflict within the critical care team may be associated with serious medical errors. An analysis of a national survey of over 6,000 residents (multispecialty sample) indicated that just over 20% reported "serious conflict" with another staff member with nearly 10% of those conflicts being between the resident and nursing staff, and 10% being with another resident. Among those residents who reported no conflict with professional colleagues, 23.8% reported having made a serious medical error, and among those who reported conflict with two or more colleagues, the serious medical error rate was 51%. Further research is needed to determine the empirical association but the significant difference in error rates is enough to prompt further attention [80].

Developing conflict competence across the clinical team to better manage interpersonal conflict is a key aspect of effective team performance. Training and coaching can help to develop conflict engagement skills that enable productive conversations around difficult issues [76]. In addition, ensuring that team leaders and senior professionals model constructive conflict behaviors is even more powerful as a means of embedding conflict competence among team members. Assisting team members and team leaders by incorporating system-wide policies that address conflict and unprofessional conduct provides a starting place for difficult conversations to occur. In addition, embedding conflict experts within the organization whose job is to help facilitate or mediate disputes is another means of supporting safe patient care.

Team Training and Simulation

The growing emphasis on teamwork and interprofessional practice within academic training will have a positive impact on future generations of clinicians. However, there is a lack of team orientation and skills among practicing clinicians. To respond to this need, many organizations are implementing team training and simulation to help promote safe care and more effective clinical coordination, particularly in complex or high risk areas such as the OR, ICU, ED, and Labor and Delivery [81]. In 2007, the AHRQ launched a national effort to support team training to improve communication and teamwork skills among health professionals [56]. Known as TeamSTEPPS™, the program curriculum reflects more than 20 years of research and applied knowledge from other industries including aviation, nuclear power, and the military. Another approach for improving team skills is the use of high fidelity simulation in which clinical teams are given scenarios to enact within a highly sophisticated simulation environment, much as astronauts or pilots would do. The simulations are videotaped and the clinical scenario is adjusted during the training session to assess not only clinical knowledge but also team skills, leadership, and crisis management. Debriefs following the simulations provide for a discussion among team members as to what worked and what could be done to improve performance. Designing training programs that provide for interprofessional learning promotes collaboration and understanding of roles, concentrates the group's efforts toward the needs of patients, and promotes development of trust and respect within the team [82].

Organizational Supports for Interprofessional Collaboration

Even teams that have excellent skills in communication, decision-making, and clinical expertise need support from the organization in which they reside. Design of work processes, policies, and the broader culture of the organization all play a role in supporting effective collaborative practice. Intentionally developing team leaders and supporting them with mentors and coaches is one means of organizational support [83]. Additionally, creating dyadic leadership models, or "productive pairs," in which there is co-leadership of the ICU by both a medical director and a nursing director, can provide direct support to the clinical teams and also provides a means for modeling interprofessional collaboration and setting a culture of collaboration within the unit. A joint task force from the American Association of Critical-Care Nurses (AACN) and the Society of Critical Care Medicine (SCCM) developed a collaborative practice leadership model in 1983 that resulted in 10 principles outlining the interdependent nature of the two professions in the critical care environment and also outlined the complimentary roles of the two leaders [84]. Such partnerships enable the leaders to more fully address the complex integration of competing demands that range from clinical operations to financial management, risk management, and professional development of new clinicians.

Broader efforts to embed effective interprofessional collaboration across the entire healthcare organization are also underway. The ANCC Magnet certification process specifically emphasizes effective collaboration practices and communication among the professions and those organizations seeking this coveted designation must demonstrate what they have done to ensure adequate mechanisms are in place [85]. Research evaluating nurse–physician relationships within Magnet hospitals has demonstrated better relationships and more collegial work climates than non-Magnet designated hospitals [28]. Hospitals celebrating their Magnet credential now number over 300 with many more seeking certifications.

An innovative model developed to support interprofessional collaboration across the medical center has been implemented by the University of Virginia and makes use of the social technology Appreciative Inquiry [86]. Initiated in 2005, the Center for Appreciative Practice has developed collaborative efforts by the Schools of Medicine, Nursing, and the Health System as a method of supporting ongoing efforts to identify what works best using an appreciative focus. This enables professionals to develop solutions together while enhancing their appreciation of the accomplishments and contributions of colleagues from other professional groups. Such innovative approaches are highly indicative of organizational cultures that fully support interprofessional collaboration and the impact it can have on improving patient care and the quality of work environments.

PERSONAL WELL-BEING AND RESILIENCE

Collaborative environments are not only good for patients, but they also support the well-being of the health professionals who provide care to the seriously ill. A growing area of research related to resilience and personal well-being emphasizes the importance of self-care and collegial support as a means of providing safe care and enabling health professionals to continue in their work for the duration of their career. In a study published in 2008, residents from nine separate residency programs indicated that personal well-being not only impacted the quality of their work, but that high levels of personal well-being resulted in greater patience and collegiality with other health professionals and that low levels of personal well-being contributed to increased interpersonal conflict with colleagues [87]. The residents cited the ability to talk with colleagues as one means of maintaining their sense of personal well-being. Surveys of ICU and OR physicians and nurses indicate that the majority of them seriously underestimate the effect of stress on their professional performance and the likelihood of making an error [16]. Increasingly, emphasis on interprofessional collaboration as a means of improving resilience will emerge as health professionals look for ways to decrease stress, better manage conflict, and effectively navigate the growing complexity of healthcare organizations.

CONCLUSION

There is a growing emphasis on interprofessional collaboration in critical care environments as a means of improving the safety and quality of patient care, to support the development of healthy work environments, and to further the resilience and well-being of health professionals. A great deal more research is needed to further these efforts. Training and academic preparation that reinforces team skills and an appreciation of the contributions of the various professions provides a first step in the promotion of effective collaboration. The development of new models for implementing clinical teamwork, joint leadership, and organization-wide supports will continue to shift the culture of health care toward one in which the various professions are working together, and not just side-by-side.

References

1. Dracup K: Changing partners. *Am J Crit Care* 16:104–105, 2007.
2. Brilli RJ, Spevetz A, Branson RD, et al: Critical care delivery in the intensive care unit: defining roles and the best practice model. *Crit Care Med* 29(10):2007–2019, 2001.
3. Wakefield MK: Putting patients first: improving patient safety through collaborative education. Collaborative education to ensure patient safety—Joint meeting of the Council on Graduate Medical Education and the National Advisory Council on Nurse Education and Practice. Report to the Secretary of U.S. Department of Health and Human Services and U.S. Congress. 2000.
4. Zwarenstein M, Goldman J, Reeves S: Interprofessional collaboration: effects of practice-based interventions on professional practice and healthcare outcomes. *Cochrane Database Syst Rev* 8(3):CD000072, 2009.
5. Linden RM: *Leading Across Boundaries: Creating Collaborative Agencies in a Networked World.* San Francisco, CA, John Wiley & Sons, 2010.
6. American Association of Critical Care Nurses. AACN standards for establishing and sustaining healthy work environments: a journey to excellence. Available at: http://www.aacn.org/WD/HWE/Docs/HWEStandards.pdf. Updated 2005. Accessed June 12, 2010.
7. American Association of Colleges of Nursing. Essentials of Baccalaureate Education for Professional Practice. Available at: http://www.aacn.nche.edu/Education/pdf/BaccEssentials08.pdf. Published 2008. Updated 2008. Accessed May 31, 2010.
8. Institute of Medicine. Health Professions Education: A Bridge to Quality. Available at: http://www.nap.edu/openbook.php?isbn=0309087236. Updated 2003. Accessed May, 31, 2010.
9. Cronenwett L, Sherwood G, Barnsteiner J: Quality and safety education for nurses. *Nurs Outlook* 55:122–131, 2007.
10. Accreditation Council for Graduate Medical Education. ACGME Outcome Project-General Competencies. Available at: http://www.acgme.org/outcome/comp/GeneralCompetenciesStandards21307.pdf. Updated 2007. Accessed May 31, 2010.
11. America Nurses Association: *Nursing Code of Ethics with Interpretive Statements.* Washington, DC, American Nurses Association, 2001.
12. American Medical Association Committee on Ethics and Judicial Affairs. Opinions on inter-professional relations—nurses, 2004. Available at: http://www.ama-assn.org/ama1/pub/upload/mm/code-medical-ethics/ceja-3i09.pdf. Updated 2004. Accessed May 31, 2010.
13. Blue A, Zoller J, Stratton T, et al: Interprofessional education in US medical schools. *J Interprof Care* 24:204–206, 2010.
14. Institute of Medicine. To Err is Human—Building a Safe Healthcare System. Available at: http://www.nap.edu/openbook.php?record_id=9728. Updated 2000. Accessed 5/31, 2010.
15. Institute of Medicine. *Crossing the Quality Chasm—A New Health System for the 21st Century.* Available at: http://www.nap.edu/openbook.php?isbn=0309072808. Published 2001. Updated 2001. Accessed May 31, 2010.
16. Institute of Medicine. *Keeping patients safe: Transforming the work environment of nurses.* Available at: http://www.nap.edu/openbook.php?isbn=0309090679. Updated 2004. Accessed May 31, 2010.
17. Joint Commission. Joint Commission Sentinel Event Alert # 40, Behaviors that undermine safe patient care. Available at: http://www.jointcommission.

org/sentinelevents/sentineleventalert/sea_40.htm. Updated 2008. Accessed June 12, 2010.
18. Joint Commission. Joint Commission Sentinel event #30, Preventing infant death and injury during delivery. Available at: http://www.jointcommission.org/SentinelEvents/SentinelEventAlert/sea_30.htm. Updated 2004. Accessed June 12, 2010.
19. Thomson Reuters. Waste in the U.S. Healthcare System Pegged at $700 Billion. Available at: http://thomsonreuters.com/content/press_room/tsh/waste_US_healthcare_system. Updated 2009. Accessed June 12, 2010.
20. Donchin Y, Seagull FJ: The hostile environment of the intensive care unit. *Curr Opin Crit Care* 8:316–320, 2002.
21. Azouley E, Timsit JF, Sprung CL, et al: Prevalence and factors in intensive care unit conflicts-The Conflicus Study. *Am J Respir Crit Care Med* 180:853–860, 2009.
22. Rosenstein AH: Disruptive physician behavior contributes to nursing shortage: study links bad behavior by doctors to nurses leaving the profession. *Physician Exec* 28(6):8–11, 2002.
23. Hamric AB, Blackwell LJ: Nurse-physician perspectives on the care of dying patients in intensive care units: collaboration, moral distress, and ethical climate. *Crit Care Med* 35:422–429, 2007.
24. National Quality Forum: *Safe Practices for Better Healthcare-2009 Update: A Consensus Report*. Washington, D.C., NQF, 2009.
25. Joint Commission Resources. National Patient Safety Goals. Available at: http://www.jcrinc.com/National-Patient-Safety-Goals/. Accessed May 2009.
26. Fontaine DK, Gerardi D: Healthier hospitals? *Nurs Manage* 36(10):34–44, 2005.
27. Reeves S, Zwarenstein M: The doctor-nurse game in the age of interprofessional care: a view from Canada. *Nurs Inq* 15(1):1–2, 2008.
28. Schmalenberg C, Kramer M: Nurse-Physician relationships in hospitals: 20,000 nurses tell their story. *Crit Care Nurse* 29:74–83, 2009.
29. Suter E, Arndt J, Arthur N, et al: Role understanding and effective communication as core competencies for collaborative practice. *J Interprof Care* 23:41–51, 2009.
30. Sexton JB, Makary MA, Tersigni AR, et al: Teamwork in the operating room: frontline perspectives among hospitals and operating room personnel. *Anesthesiology* 105:877–884, 2006.
31. Reader TW, Flin R, Mearns K, et al: Interdisciplinary communication in the intensive care unit. *Br J Anaesth* 98:347–352, 2007.
32. Thomas EJ, Sexton JB, Helmreich RL: Discrepant attitudes about teamwork among critical care nurses and physicians. *Crit Care Med* 31:956–959, 2003.
33. Gerardi D: The emerging culture of health care: improving end-of-life care through collaboration and conflict engagement among health care professionals. *Ohio St J Disp Resol* 23:105, 2007.
34. Lemieux-Charles L, McGuire WL: What do we know about health care team effectiveness? A review of the literature. *Med Care Res Rev* 63:263–300, 2006.
35. van Beuzekom M, Akerboom SP, Boer F: Assessing system failures in the operating rooms and intensive care units. *Qual Saf Health Care* 16:45–50, 2007.
36. Thomas EJ, Sexton JB, Lasky R, et al: Team-work and quality during neonatal care in the delivery room. *J Perinatol* 26:163–169, 2006.
37. Poncet M, Toullic P, Papazian L, et al: Burnout syndrome in critical care nursing staff. *Am J Respir Crit Care Med* 175:698–704, 2007.
38. Murray TH, Jennings B: The quest to reform end of life care: rethinking assumptions and setting new directions. *Hastings Cent Rep* 35(Suppl 6):s52–s57, 2005.
39. Carlet J, Thijs LG, Antonelli M, et al: Challenges in end-of-life care in the ICU-Statement of the 5th International Consensus Conference in Critical Care: Brussels, Belgium April 2003. *Intensive Care Med* 30:770–784, 2004.
40. Boyle DK, Miller PA, Forbes-Thompson SA: Communication and end-of-life care in the intensive care unit: patient, family, and clinician outcomes. *Crit Care Nurs Q* 28:302–316, 2005.
41. Badger JM: Factors that enable or complicate end of life care. *Am J Crit Care* 14:513–521, 2005.
42. Ferrell BR: Understanding the moral distress of nurses witnessing medically futile care. *Oncol Nurs Forum* 33:922–930, 2006.
43. Meltzer LS, Huckaby L: Critical care nurses' perceptions of futile care and its effect on burnout. *Am J Crit Care* 13:202–208, 2004.
44. American Association of Critical Care Nurses. AACN Position Statement on moral distress. Available at: http://www.aacn.org/WD/Practice/Docs/Moral_Distress.pdf. Updated 2008. Accessed June 12, 2010.
45. Gerardi D, Fontaine DK: True collaboration: envisioning new ways of working together. *AACN Adv Crit Care* 18(1):10–14, 2007.
46. Fairman J, Lynaugh JE: *Critical Care Nursing: A History*. Philadelphia, PA, University of Pennsylvania Press, 1998.
47. Suchman AL: A new theoretical foundation for relationship-centered care: complex responsive processes of relating. *J Gen Intern Med* 21:S40–S44, 2006.
48. Bronstein LR: A model for interdisciplinary collaboration. *Soc Work* 48:297–306, 2003.
49. Reader TW, Flin R, Mearns K, et al: Developing a team performance framework for the intensive care unit. *Crit Care Med* 37:1787–1793, 2009.
50. Lanham HJ, McDaniel RR, Crabtree BF, et al: How improving practice relationships among clinicians and nonclinicians can improve quality in primary care. *Jt Comm J Qual Patient Saf* 35:457–466, 2009.
51. Kaissi A, Johnson T, Kirschbaum M: Measuring teamwork and patient safety attitudes of high risk areas. *Nurs Econ* 21:211–218, 2003.
52. Pullon S: Competence, respect, and trust: key features of successful interprofessional nurse-doctor relationships. *J Interprof Care* 22:133–147, 2008.
53. Society of Critical Care Medicine. Available at: http://www.sccm.org/Professional_Development/Quality_Initiatives/Pages/Paragon.aspx. Accessed June 12, 2010.
54. D'Amour D, Ferrada-Videla M, San Martin Rodriguez L, et al: The conceptual basis for interprofessional collaboration: core concepts and theoretical frameworks. *J Interprof Care* 19[Suppl 1]:116–131, 2005.
55. Baker DP, Day R, Salas E: Teamwork as an essential component of high-reliability organizations. *Health Serv Res* 4:1576–1598, 2006.
56. U.S. Department of Health and Human Services. AHRQ TeamSTEPPS Program. Available at: http://teamstepps.ahrq.gov/. Accessed June 12, 2010.
57. Hawryluck LA, Espin SL, Garwood KC, et al: Pulling together and pushing apart: tides of tension in the ICU Team. *Acad Med* 77[Suppl]:S73–S76, 2002.
58. Yeager S: Interdisciplinary collaboration: the heart and soul of health care. *Crit Care Nurs Clin North Am* 17:143–148, 2005.
59. Schmalenberg C, Kramer M, King CR, et al: Excellence through evidence, securing collegial/collaborative nurse-physician relationships. Part 1. *J Nurs Adm* 35:450–458, 2005.
60. Schmalenberg C, Kramer M, King CR, et al: Excellence through evidence: securing collegial/collaborative nurse-physician relationships, part 2. *J Nurs Adm* 35:507–514, 2005.
61. Coombs M, Ersser S: Medical hegemony in decision-making: a barrier to interdisciplinary working in intensive care? *J Adv Nurs* 46:245–252, 2004.
62. Ulrich BT, Lavandero R, Hart KA, et al: Critical care nurses' work environments 2008: a follow-up report. *Crit Care Nurse* 29:93–101, 2009.
63. Pronovost PJ, Thompson D, Holzmueller CR, et al: Toward learning from patient safety reporting systems. *J Crit Care* 21:305–315, 2006.
64. Leonard M, Graham S, Bonacum D: The human factor: the critical importance of effective teamwork and communication in providing safe care. *Qual Saf Health Care* 13[Suppl 1]:85–90, 2004.
65. De Dreu CK, Weingart LR: Task versus relationship conflict, team performance, and team member satisfaction: a meta-analysis. *J Appl Psychol* 88:741–749, 2003.
66. Fryer-Edwards K, Arnold RM, Baile W, et al: Reflective teaching practices: an approach to teaching communication skills in a small-group setting. *Acad Med* 81:638–644, 2006.
67. Maxfield D, Grenny J, McMillan R, et al: Silence Kills: The seven crucial conversations for healthcare. Available at: http://www.aacn.org/WD/Practice/Docs/PublicPolicy/SilenceKillsExecSum.pdf. Updated 2005. Accessed June 10, 2010.
68. Rosenstein AH, O'Daniel M: Survey of the impact of disruptive behaviors and communication defects on patient safety. *Jt Comm J Qual Patient Saf* 34(8):464–471, 2008.
69. Simpson KR, Lyndon A: Clinical disagreements during labor and birth: how does real life compare to best practice? *MCN Am J Matern Child Nurs* 34(1):31–39, 2009.
70. Joint Commission. Joint Commission Leadership Standards. Available at: http://www.jcrinc.com/Books-and-E-books/The-Joint-Commissions-Leadership-Standards/1734/. Updated 2009. Accessed June 12, 2010.
71. Lingard LA, Espin SL, Evans C, et al: The rules of the game: Interprofessional collaboration in the intensive care unit team. *Crit Care* 8:R403–R408, 2004.
72. Back A, Arnold RM: Dealing with conflict in caring for the seriously ill, "It was just out of the question." *JAMA* 293:1374–1383, 2005.
73. Johnson C: Bad blood: doctor-nurse behavior problems impact patient care. Special report: 2009 Doctor-Nurse Behavior Survey. Available at: http://net.acpe.org/Services/2009_Doctor_Nurse_Behavior_Survey/index.html. Accessed June 12, 2010.
74. Dewitty V, Osborne JW, Friesen MA, et al: Workforce conflict—what's the problem? *Nurs Manage* 40(5):31–37, 2009.
75. Zweibel R, Goldstein J, Manwaring J, et al: What sticks: how medical residents and academic health care faculty transfer conflict resolution training from the workshop to the workplace. *Conflict Resolution Quarterly* 25(3):321–350, 2008.
76. Gerardi D: Conflict training for health professionals—strategies for cultivating conflict competent organizations. Available at: http://ehcco.com/news.php. Accessed June 12, 2010.
77. Fontaine DK: Danger in Disruption. *AHRQ WebM&M [serial online]*. October 2009.
78. Kvarnstrom S: Difficulties in collaboration: a critical incident study of interprofessional healthcare teamwork. *J Interprof Care* 22:191–203, 2008.
79. Lipsky D, Avgar A: Toward a strategic theory of workplace conflict management. *Ohio St J Disp Resol* 24:143, 2008.
80. Baldwin D, Daugherty S: Interprofessional conflict and medical errors: results of a national multi-specialty survey of hospital residents in the U.S. *J Interprof Care* 22:573–586, 2008.
81. Baker DP, Salas E, King H, et al: The role of teamwork in the professional education of physicians: current status and assessment recommendations. *Jt Comm J Qual Patient Saf* 31(4):185–202, 2005.

82. Baker DP, Gustafson S, Beaubien JM, et al: Medical team training programs in health care. *Advances in patient safety*. Volume 4-Programs, tools, and products. Available at: http://www.ncbi.nlm.nih.gov/bookshelf/br.fcgi?book=aps4&part=A7246. Accessed June 12, 2010.
83. Boyle DK, Kochinda C: Enhancing collaborative communication of nurse and physician leadership in two intensive care units. *J Nurs Adm* 34(2):60–70, 2004.
84. Disch J, Beilman G, Ingbar D: Medical directors as partners in creating healthy work environments. *AACN Clin Issues* 12:366–377, 2001.
85. American Nurses Credentialing Center. Magnet Recognition Program. Available at: http://www.nursecredentialing.org/. Accessed June 12, 2010.
86. University of Virginia. Appreciative practice at the University of Virginia. Available at: http://appreciativeinquiry.virginia.edu/. Accessed June 10, 2010.
87. Ratanawongsa N, Wright SM, Carrese JA: Well-being in residency: effects on relationships with patients, interactions with colleagues, performance, and motivation. *Patient Educ Couns* 72:194–200, 2008.

CHAPTER 206 ■ HEALTHY WORK ENVIRONMENTS: NECESSARY FOR PROVIDERS AND PATIENTS

KATHLEEN M. McCAULEY

Envision the following scenario: you are a recent graduate of your basic educational program or fellowship, have successfully passed your boards and certification examinations, are armed with superb references from your mentors and faculty, and have identified two job openings in which you can work with the leaders in your specialty. The locations are perfect, close enough to family and friends, and the salary is competitive. You have scheduled interviews at each site and are excited about the opportunities to launch your career and are ready to convince the interviewers that you are the perfect new addition to their team. Your mentors have coached you in competitive strategies to stand out from the other applicants. Given that both interviewers are eager to hire you, how will you choose?

In launching a new career or accepting a new position to further an established career, clinicians would be wise to consider the health of the work environment as important in their final decision. The responsibilities of succeeding in a complex healthcare provider role coupled with demands of personal lives, particularly when complicated by caring for children and/or aging parents, contribute to stress. An analysis of sources of stress for women physicians revealed that expectations at both work and home were key factors, but also that the quality of the work environment was important as well [1].

Results of an expanding body of research and anecdotal reports from a wide range of stakeholders argue that the health of the work environment is critical to both professional satisfaction and patient outcomes. In this chapter, the consequences of toxic work places and knowledge about characteristics of healthy work environments will be reviewed. Differing communication norms between physicians and nurses, inaccurate perceptions about the reality of the ways that team members contribute to critical patient care decisions, significant deficits in conflict management skills, and tolerance for disrespectful treatment of colleagues all contribute to unnecessary and dangerous tension in the workplace that can harm patients. This chapter presents strategies for creating healthy work places, including widespread adoption of national standards.

A sense of what constitutes a toxic versus healthy work environment was clarified by Heath and colleagues [2]. They conducted a series of focus groups with nurses, who were asked to consult with multiple colleagues prior to their discussion. Consensus emerged that toxic environments lack effective communication as well as trust. Hazing behaviors were reported in toxic environments that included withholding critical information, setting each other up to fail, and sometimes actual physical violence. When there is a lack of vision and leadership, arguments over conflicting values are common. In toxic environments, poor behavior is exhibited by all healthcare providers and these problematic behaviors extend to patients and families both as perpetrators and victims.

In times of documented shortages of key healthcare providers, work environments that drive talented clinicians from direct care roles require serious attention. In a study examining job satisfaction rates of nurses in the United States (U.S.), Canada, England, Scotland, and Germany, Aiken and colleagues found that with the exception of German nurses, job dissatisfaction was high, ranging from 33% to 41%. These dissatisfaction rates are much higher than those reported by other professional (10%) and general workers (15%). Of particular concern is the effect of the work environment on younger nurses since one out of three U.S. nurses in this study planned to leave the hospital job within the next year [3]. Factors contributing to job dissatisfaction included insufficient staff to deliver high quality care or simply to get the work done, inadequate support services, failure of administrators to listen to nurses' concerns, minimal opportunity to participate in policy decisions, lack of recognition of contributions, and poor opportunities for advancement [4]. Dr. Julie Sochalski, an expert in health policy who has conducted research on the shortage of nurses and consulted for the federal government about healthcare reform, argues that the current shortage cannot be remedied by enhanced recruitment alone. We must retain our best and brightest clinicians and it means that our work environments must be healed (J. Sochalski, personal communication, 2010).

Positive nurse–physician relationships coupled with adequate staffing and strong support from hospital administrators are associated with significantly lower rates of nurse burnout and with patients who were twice as likely to report higher levels of satisfaction with their care [5]. Conversely, in a study conducted in Switzerland, nurses caring for an average of eight patients daily felt that they needed to ration nursing care. Rationing was related to adverse patient outcomes such as medication errors, falls, avoidable critical incidents, and pressure ulcers. Rationing included nurses' perceptions that they were unable to deliver needed nursing interventions such as feeding and hygiene, patient education and rehabilitation, monitoring, support and advocacy, and documentation of care and preventive functions such as appropriate hand washing. The Swiss investigators found that even low levels of rationing were associated with poor outcomes and yet they acknowledged that some rationing is inevitable. Further research is needed to identify a threshold in which truly unacceptable rationing occurs. It is likely that rationing of care, since it directly affects the patient, may be an important variable in understanding the influence of staffing and work environments on patient outcomes [6]. Burnout and dissatisfaction with rationing of care are clearly negative influences on a healthy work environment.

HEALTHY WORK ENVIRONMENT STANDARDS

In 2003, the Board of Directors of the American Association of Critical-Care Nurses (AACN) embarked on a strategic planning initiative to identify the three most pressing issues in which AACN's influence and voice could have the greatest impact on members. Consensus emerged that nurse staffing, healthy work environments, and end-of-life care were pivotal issues. Staffing and healthy work environments were seen as critical issues for nursing's largest specialty organization because of evidence that strong and supportive environments contribute to lower patient mortality rates [7]. Healthy work environments are those in which professionals work as team members, respect each other, and display caring for patients and families as well as each other. In these environments, effective collaboration provides opportunities for shared problem solving and emergence of shared mental models that support new solutions [2]. Professionals are empowered to practice according to the standards of their professions, including making decisions about their practice. They are led by leaders with the skills and power to design and implement a vision for superb practice. This was the vision that motivated the AACN Board of Directors to charge a work group, led by past president Connie Barden to develop healthy work environment standards [8]. These standards, listed in Table 206.1, were designed to give a strong message that immediate change in current practice settings was needed. Research identifying factors foundational to healthy work environments support AACN's decision to select these standards as the framework to drive widespread change.

TABLE 206.1

AACN STANDARDS FOR ESTABLISHING AND SUSTAINING HEALTHY WORK ENVIRONMENTS: A JOURNEY TO EXCELLENCE

Skilled Communication: Nurses must be as proficient in communication skills as they are in clinical skills
True Collaboration: Nurses must be relentless in pursuing and fostering true collaboration
Effective Decision Making: Nurses must be valued and committed partners in making policies, directing and evaluating clinical care, and leading organizational operations
Appropriate Staffing: Staffing must ensure effective match between patient needs and nurse competencies
Meaningful Recognition: Nurses must be recognized and should also recognize others for the value each brings to the work of the organization
Authentic Leadership: Nurse leaders must fully embrace the imperative of a healthy work environment, authentically live it, and engage others in its achievement

Adapted from American Association of Critical-Care Nurses: AACN Standards for establishing and sustaining healthy work environments: a journey to excellence. *Am J Crit Care* 14(3):187–197, 2005.

ENHANCING COMMUNICATION AND COLLABORATION: EFFECTIVE DECISION MAKING

There is evidence that nurses and physicians who work together differ significantly in their perceptions of collaborative decision making. In a large French study involving over 3,000 nurses and over 500 physicians, over 90% of the total sample agreed that decisions involving patients' end-of-life care should be made collaboratively. In practice, however, physicians were nearly twice as likely as nurses to report that nurses were involved in decision making (50% vs. 27%) and were significantly more satisfied with decision processes (73% vs. 33%, $p < 0.001$). These uneven perceptions were paralleled by strong differences in reports of physician consultation with nurses in the decision making process (79% vs. 31%, $p < 0.001$). Nurses were much more likely to feel that their presence in the meeting with the family was important. They valued being there more than the physicians valued their presence (56% vs. 36%, $p < 0.05$). The importance of these findings to clinical practice was evident in that significant linkages were found between satisfaction with decision making, perception of the unit's commitment to high ethical standards, and nurses' involvement in achieving these standards ($p < 0.0001$) [9]. Understanding that providers have disparate views of successful collaboration provides insight into potential root causes of communication problems both in day-to-day practice and when providers and patients face tough decisions. Efforts to achieve an ethical solution to practice dilemmas using processes that respect and value the input of the entire healthcare team are needed to achieve truly healthy work environments.

Effective communication has been shown to affect prevention of adverse outcomes. In particular, timeliness of nurse–physician communication was related to decreased incidence of pressure ulcers in a critical-care patient population, and conversely, when nurses perceived variability in communication with physicians, ventilator associated pneumonia (VAP) rates were higher [10]. Given the importance of preventing adverse events, it is reasonable to consider changes in care processes to foster clear and effective communication. System changes such as use of multidisciplinary rounds, appointment of a hospitalist medical director, and addition of a nurse practitioner (NP) to support the care interface between staff nurses and physicians are becoming more common, particularly in tertiary care hospitals. In a setting with these values in place, when care in that environment was compared with standard practice on a similar acute medical care unit, it was found that attending physicians and house staff perceived nurse collaboration to be significantly better but both the physicians and nurses rated collaboration with the NPs to be significantly better than with each other. No differences were found between nurses' perceived communication and collaboration with physicians on the model unit versus the standard practice unit. However, physicians on the model unit reported improved communication with each other. Improved patient outcomes included reduction in patient length of stay and care costs without reductions in quality of care or increased readmissions [11]. A possible explanation for the positive outcomes of physician/NP collaboration may lie in an appreciation of skills gained through NP versus MD education. It has been argued that NPs may be more adept at managing patients through chronic care protocols in primary care. This is supported by their nursing background with its focus on patient education and use of communication skills [12]. Hence, the NP lives in both worlds and can easily translate and fill in gaps.

Why would physicians and nurses perceive care processes so differently? As was evident in Vazirani and colleagues' study [11], staff nurses may have difficulty being freed from direct care responsibilities to be able to participate in patient rounds or may be uncomfortable presenting their data and recommendations and thus avoid participation. Clear expectation for each provider's role in rounds, support for their participation through patient coverage, and providing adequate mentoring of young professionals in effective participation strategies are needed. Dialogue to ensure clarity about the characteristics of good collaboration and to develop respect and recognition of the value of each others' contributions are important steps in achieving benefits for patients and providers. Without this preparation, physicians may view improved collaboration to mean simply receiving accurate patient information and nurses following through on physician orders versus actual sharing in the decision making process. Addition of an NP to the team may serve as a bridge between nurses and physicians, improving the flow of information but may have the unintended effect of predisposing the nurses to communicate with the NP at times when they otherwise may call a physician [11].

Nurse–physician communication difficulty may have its roots in disparate educational systems. In their basic education, nurses are expected to present a broad, comprehensive picture of the patient's situation, in contrast to the targeted, specific problem focus that drives physician communication [13]. Nursing case summaries are graded highly if they thoroughly addressed the patient's physical health problems, including supporting pathophysiology, emotional and coping reactions, family and community support systems, and the interrelationships between all of these, resulting in a comprehensive nursing care plan that also integrates the nurse's support of the medical plan. Parsimonious, concise descriptions tend to be graded as missing key information and insights. Those training exercises, while designed to educate the nurses to view the patient holistically as a being with vast nursing needs beyond the medical illness, do not prepare them for a concise, problem-specific and action-driven health system, particularly as exists in critical-care settings. Thus, vastly different and ingrained way of thinking about patients' problems coupled with hierarchical power differentials can lead to pervasive dysfunctional norms of communication. Fear of reprisal or ridicule blocks interjection of critical information into the dialogue. Reliance on vague, imprecise communication styles may exclude critical information or urgency in message delivery. Leonard and colleagues [13] refer to this as the "hint and hope" model—one that holds a strong potential to harm patients.

Similarly, if a culture of perfection, personal failure, and blame exists rather than one of analysis of human and systems factors that contribute to errors, the tendency to bury errors and near misses rather than discuss them openly and correct root causes, further impede effective communication and harm patients [13]. Effective communication skills are needed. Given the authentic team leadership and implementation of skill building strategies, nurses can learn to participate effectively in interdisciplinary rounds, to summarize concisely changes in patients' conditions and to advocate for their needs, and to diffuse the inevitable conflicts that emerge among the healthcare team and with patients and families [14].

A widely used communication tool, SBAR (situation, background, assessment, recommendation) supports concise and organized communication between providers. It is a structure that guides a nurse's explanation of the situation, focusing on relevant background information, an assessment of what is happening and recommendations for corrective action. This technique has been criticized, however, for its failure to ensure that each provider fully understands the patient's problem and recommended action. Consequently, another tool gaining acceptance, STICC, adds a requirement for feedback and clarification of misunderstanding. With this tool, S describes the situation (Here's what I think we face), T is the task (This is what I think we should do), I refers to intent (This is why we should do it), C describes concern (What we should keep our eyes on), and C provides an opportunity to calibrate (Now let's talk; tell me what you don't understand, can't do, or if you see something I don't) [15]. Outcomes improve in settings in which nurses are empowered to state clearly that the patient requires immediate attention and can expect that this message will receive an immediate response, no matter the time of day or day of the week. While techniques such as SBAR and STICC improve the clarity of the message, the sense that "something isn't right" should be recognized as a call to action. Borrowing techniques in critical language from the airline industry such as the CUS system (I'm concerned, I'm uncomfortable, this is unsafe or I'm scared) provides a shorthand way of alerting colleagues that the problem is serious and demands attention. It is inevitable that false alarms will occur but a culture of effective communication and collaboration further supports strengthening nurses' assessment and communication skills [13].

STAFFING

An emerging body of research demonstrates strong connections between nurse staffing, particularly RN staffing, and patient outcomes. For surgical patients in acute care hospitals, increasing Registered Nurse (RN) care hours by 1 hour per day resulted in an 8.9% reduction in the patients' odds of developing pneumonia. The importance of the RN's role in care, as compared to less skilled nursing personnel, was further validated by a reduction in the risk of pneumonia by 9.5% when the proportion of RNs to overall nursing personnel increased by 10% [16]. Turnover of nursing staff has been shown to affect how a healthcare team learns from experiences with each other so that their abilities develop and they grow in behavioral skills and that, in turn, affects patient outcomes. Higher levels of workgroup learning were associated with higher patient satisfaction and fewer severe medication errors. Conversely, workgroup learning was found to be lower when turnover levels were moderate (3.31% to 4.5%) [17].

Evidence is also emerging that the educational level, skill set of the nurse, and quality of nurse–physician relationships make a difference. A 10% increase in the number of nurses prepared with a baccalaureate or higher degree resulted in a 5% decrease in both the likelihood that a surgical patient would die within 30 days of admission or that a failure to rescue event would occur [18]. These results occurred even after adjusting for patient characteristics such as comorbid conditions, hospital characteristics such as size, teaching status, and technology level, nurse staffing and experience, and the board certification status of the surgeon. Similarly, substituting unlicensed aids for RNs has been shown to reduce quality outcomes in a large study (18,142 patients) of patients with common cardiovascular and pulmonary diagnoses. The largest part of the variance in 30-day mortality rate was attributed to patient age and illnesses (44.2%). However, hospital and nursing factors accounted for an additional 36.9% of the variance. Lower 30-day patient mortality rate was found in settings with a higher proportion of baccalaureate nurses (OR, 0.81; 95% CI [0.68, 0.96]), presence of more RNs versus less skilled nursing personnel (OR, 0.83; 95% CI [0.73, 0.96]), and healthy nurse–physician relationships (OR, 0.74; 95% CI [0.60, 0.91]).

The use of temporary nurses was associated with a higher 30-day mortality rate (OR, 1.26; 95% CI [1.09, 1.47]) [19].

Nurses, however, perceive that staffing to deliver quality care involves more than simple nurse-to-patient ratios. In a study based on interviews conducted with 279 nurses from 14 Magnet Hospitals, nurses perceived staffing to be adequate when all providers worked as members of a team, collaboration was strong, and nurses possessed the knowledge, experience, and skills to meet patient needs. Empowerment to make autonomous clinical decision and control of their practice environment were crucial factors as were support strategies such as computerized documentation, order entry systems, and well trained, motivated, assistive personnel and support services. Patient acuity influenced staffing perceptions but these nurses perceived that high patient acuity was best handled when other positive work environment characteristics were present. Nurses valued administrators' recognition of the need to factor patient acuity into staffing allocations [20]. In a study of nearly 8,600 Canadian nurses, an analysis of nurses' perceptions about their work environment found a direct causal relationship between poor staffing and nurses' emotional burnout, and a direct positive relationship between the presence of a nursing model of care, one that values nurses' personal and professional ideals, and personal accomplishments [21].

The notion that perceived staffing adequacy is not as simple as nurse–patient ratios was addressed in a significant way by AACN and the AACN Certification Corporation when they charged a workgroup with developing and refining a new paradigm for clinical practice. Initially designed as a framework to guide development of a conceptually redefined certification examination, the model became a driving force to articulate nurses' contribution in achieving AACN's vision—*a healthcare system driven by the needs of patients and families where acute and critical-care nurses make their optimal contribution* [22]. The Synergy Model for Clinical Excellence identifies patient characteristics and nurse competencies that, when matched appropriately, enable patient outcomes to be optimized [23]. Table 206.2 describes the patient characteristics and Table 206.3 identifies the competencies of the nurses caring for these patients.

TABLE 206.2

AACN'S SYNERGY MODEL FOR CLINICAL EXCELLENCE: PATIENT CHARACTERISTICS

Resiliency: The patient's capacity to rebound or return to function using compensatory physiological and other coping mechanisms; a history of adapting to significant stressors; reserve capacity
Vulnerability: Degree of susceptibility to real or potential stressors; affected by physiological capacity, coping ability, pre-illness health status; the person's ability to protect themselves from threats
Stability: Capacity to maintain a steady state, maintain equilibrium; influenced by responsiveness to therapies
Complexity: Interconnectedness of two or more systems; can be physiological, psychological, family interactions or environmental impact; with greater numbers of systems affected, complexity increases
Resource Availability: Supports available to the patient by the family, community, and the patient himself/herself; resources are broadly defined: physical, emotional, fiscal, social, personal; in general, more resources are linked to better outcomes
Participation in Care: Engagement by the patient and family in care processes; influenced by educational levels/health literacy, cultural background and resources
Participation in Decision Making: Ability to comprehend and act on information and to contribute to decisions; influenced by cultural background, degree of physiologic function, beliefs and values
Predictability: Accuracy in anticipating responses and course of illness; facilitates use of diagnostic indices and evidence-based pathways to plan care

Adapted from Hardin S, Kaplow R: *Synergy for Clinical Excellence. The AACN Synergy Model for Patient Care.* Sudbury, MA, Jones and Bartlett Publishers, 2005, pp 3–54.

TABLE 206.3

AACN'S SYNERGY MODEL FOR CLINICAL EXCELLENCE: NURSE COMPETENCIES

Clinical Judgment: Nursing skill, clinical reasoning, and critical thinking abilities developed over time through education, practice, and attention to evidence-based care; ability to integrate patient-specific knowledge into care planning and delivery
Advocacy: Serve as a moral agent, one who intervenes to support another who cannot voice her/his own rights and needs; helps to resolve ethical conflicts and clinical problems for patients and families
Caring Practices: A large collection of nursing practices that provide a therapeutic, supportive, and compassionate environment that promotes healing and prevents unnecessary suffering; applies to patients, families, and staff
Collaboration: Cooperative engagement among all members of healthcare team, along with patients and families to achieve optimal and realistic patient goals
Systems Thinking: Ability to see the real causes of problems; knowledge and skills to manage the environment and resources for the betterment of the patient, family, and health care team, within and across health and non-healthcare systems
Response to Diversity: Recognition, appreciation, and incorporation of differences among racial, ethnic, marginal, and vulnerable populations to support individuality, cultural attributes, spirituality, family, and lifestyle preferences into the provision of care.
Clinical Inquiry: Persistent process of questioning and evaluating practice to ensure that practice is informed by current research and experiential learning
Facilitator of Learning: Recognition of patient and family needs for knowledge and skill development and use of standardized and patient appropriate materials and creative strategies to ensure that patients and families are prepared to handle their healthcare needs; valuing and promoting life-long learning among all members of the team.

Adapted from Hardin S, Kaplow R: *Synergy for Clinical Excellence. The AACN Synergy Model for Patient Care*. Sudbury, MA, Jones and Bartlett Publishers, 2005, pp 57–107.

RECOGNIZED POSITIVE WORK ENVIRONMENTS: MAGNET HOSPITALS AND BEACON UNITS

During the 1980s, nursing administrators noted that some hospitals continued to maintain adequate staffing even during nursing shortages. Subsequent research identified the positive practice environment characteristics of these hospitals and the term "Magnet" was applied to them since they served as a magnet for nurses. The knowledge gained from this research was used by the American Nurses Association and its accrediting arm, the American Nurses Credentialing Center (ANCC), to develop a Magnet Recognition program to identify those hospitals with the quality indicators and standards of care that result in excellence in patient care and an exemplary practice environment for nurses. Of the prestigious *U.S. News & World Report* Honor Roll of top hospitals, 71% of medical centers and 90% of the Children's Hospitals achieving that designation are Magnet organizations [24].

In 2003, AACN launched the Beacon Award for Critical-Care Excellence. This highly competitive award recognizes individual critical care and progressive care units whose staff has achieved high levels of quality patient and family care and excellent care outcomes within a healthy work environment. The award recognizes outstanding outcomes in recruiting and retaining a staff that values ongoing education and training to sustain competent practice, research and evidence-based practice, strong leadership and commitment to organizational ethics, and a sustained healing environment [25]. While nurses tend to lead the movement to attain Beacon status, this honor cannot be achieved or sustained without significant interdisciplinary collaboration and authentic leadership to transform the practice environment.

The benefits of a healthy work environment and factors associated with sustaining it can be understood by examining work environment research conducted in Magnet institutions. For example, when work environment characteristics of 23 Magnet institutions were compared with 156 non-Magnet hospitals, Magnet designation was associated with significantly more decentralized decision making involving nurses, collegial nurse/physician relationships, adequate staffing, presence of nurse managers with good leadership skills, and a preceptor program for newly hired RNs. Without Magnet designation, only 17.3% of the hospitals scored well on practice environment measures and all scored lower on all characteristics than the ANCC Magnet hospitals [26]. Similarly, a survey of over 2300 nurses from 110 ICUs in 68 hospitals revealed that nurses in Magnet hospitals perceived their work environment to be significantly better than those in non-Magnet facilities [27].

In a study of over 4,000 nurses, Ulrich and colleagues [25] examined perceptions of work environments within agencies that had Magnet or Beacon status, were actively pursuing either status, or had neither status. Nurses in Magnet or Beacon agencies had significantly more positive appraisals of the work environment, greater current job satisfaction, a higher rated skill set of the nursing leadership team, and improved quality of care compared with non–Magnet/ Beacon agencies. They also rated quality of interdisciplinary team communication and collaboration more positively, as well as respect for RNs, organizational support for education and certification, and nursing career satisfaction. Shared governance structures were significantly more likely to be in place in Magnet or Beacon organizations. In many of the parameters measured, units and organizations on the journey to Magnet or Beacon fared significantly better than those groups not pursuing that designation [25].

Insight into factors that staff nurses, physicians, and nurse managers perceive to be most important in the work place may help colleagues understand differences in expectations and emphasis in effort. In a survey of all three groups working together in Magnet institutions, Schmalenberg and colleagues [20] found that physicians overwhelmingly viewed a competent nurse as a colleague who was able to make timely, correct, and independent decisions to support patients. These physicians reported that they rely on nurses who can quickly discern what patients need and implement the required care, particularly when physicians were unable to be physically present.

TABLE 206.4

SPECIFIC STRATEGIES TO IMPLEMENT HEALTHY WORK ENVIRONMENTS

1. Empower nurses to control practice through strong physician and team collaborative decision making and active participation in interdisciplinary rounds; teamwork becomes a core value.
2. Shared governance models included members from multiple departments and disciplines resulting in an "integrated" model that is far more efficient and empowering than single discipline "silo" governance models (p. 82).
3. Staffing structures that allow nurses the time to attend rounds and governance meetings. Governance structures that support nurses' input into decisions by administrators, physicians, and others.
4. Groups own the outcomes of decisions and care improvement efforts; a culture exists that appreciates individual and group contributions
5. Quality patient care is based on the best scientific evidence and is morally and ethically congruent with the patient's wishes and professional standards.
6. Safe care is the minimum but goals demanded excellent, high quality patient/family centered care.
7. Competence, ongoing education, personal accountability for evidence-based practice, and certification were valued and expected.
8. Camaraderie and a family orientation among team members resulted in a nurturing work environment where expression of concerns and feelings was the norm. Team members supported and filled in for each other without grumbling.
9. Respect, trust, and treating each other as equals and with dignity were valued. The same principles applied to interactions with patients and families.
10. Honesty and integrity as core values were reflected in communication; team members are reluctant to place blame, seeking instead root causes of problems. Willingness to acknowledge mistakes and short comings is valued.
11. Patient advocacy and clinical autonomy are supported by appropriate surveillance to prevent complications or rescue patients and a passion to get patients what they need.
12. Stewardship means that the team values the patient's and each other's time and energy; appropriately uses and conserves resources and delivers quality outcomes.
13. Active transmission of core values and unit norms to new members of the team happens because managers and team members develop and implement a conscious plan to ensure that the values and norms become entrenched in the culture of the team.

Adapted from Kramer M, Schmalenberg C, Maguire P, et al: Walk the talk: promoting control of nursing practice and a patient-centered culture. *Critical Care Nurse* 29(3):77–93, 2009.

These comments clearly demonstrated that competent nurses earned the trust and respect of physicians [14].

Nurse manager expectations were similar in that they valued the vigilance, advocacy, and persistence of competent nurses. While correctly interpreting what is happening and acting on it was critical in their view, they also valued nurses who demonstrated commitment to ongoing competence through education. The managers expected that nurses request increasingly challenging assignments, incorporate the latest evidence-based practice standards into care, and manage both complexity and volume of care responsibilities. Organizational skills of priority setting and multitasking are needed to manage the demands of busy units, but competent care demands complex thought processes and decision making skills while retaining empathy and concern for the individual patient [14]. Thus, managers' view of competence is much broader than that reported by physicians in this study. While physicians and staff nurses agreed on the importance of clinical knowledge and decision making and physicians welcomed and expected the input of competent nurses, they may have failed to comprehend the full range of nursing duties, particularly with a full caseload of acute and critically ill patients. Hence, the importance that nurses and nurse managers place on multitasking is understandable [14]. These findings support the notion that healthcare today is characterized by "complexity compression," a term that describes the challenges inherent in taking on additional responsibilities while simultaneously providing highly complex care in a condensed time frame [28]. For today's work environments to become healthy, recognizing that complexity compression affects all providers is a critical step. As our reliance on each others' expertise grows, our appreciation for the demands on each other and our support for each other must grow as well. Specific characteristics demonstrating achievement of a healthy work environment are described in Table 206.4.

TRANSFORMING WORK PLACES: AUTHENTIC LEADERSHIP

Achieving and sustaining the change described in these studies requires leaders with the skills to build teams and motivate staff to develop a broad set of competencies in communication, collaboration, decision making, as well as evidence-based practice. Individual as well as team competencies are needed to transform work places and sustain positive change. One strategy that was found to increase significantly collaborative communication, problem solving, and conflict management skills was a 24-hour program using a modular format that offered leadership and communication training to physician and nurse leaders in an organization. Strong engagement was reflected in attendance rates of over 90% of the sessions and positive evaluations about the usefulness of the learning. While this study involved a small sample, it demonstrates that investing in joint physician–nurse leadership competency development is effective [29].

Efforts to create healthy work environments through systems improvements and enhanced skills in communication, collaboration, and leadership are likely to have additional payoff in terms of patient outcomes and satisfaction. To turn our current silo-driven, fragmented health systems into centers of patient-focused care, we must ensure that sustained commitment to collaborative care is based on effective communication and is led by authentic leaders [30].

CONCLUSIONS AND NEXT STEPS

Let's return to where we began—the job interview scenario. Thriving in today's difficult practice world demands that we acquire a strong base in the evidence supporting clinical care. Colleagues who share that commitment will contribute to our growth in knowledge and clinical decision-making skills. Evidence is also growing that patient outcomes are not controlled only by the clinical decisions we make but by the environment where those decisions are implemented. Healthy workplaces promote collaborative decision making, leading to better informed decisions and avoidance of incomplete or inaccurate information that contributes to adverse events and poor outcomes. Therefore, gather as much information as you can about the practice climate, interprofessional relationships, and skills of the leadership team. Ask to speak with members of the disciplines you will be practicing with to understand the real level of collaboration that exists. Interview the managers and leaders you will be working with to ascertain their commitment to achieving a work environment where you will make your optimum contribution and thrive. Finally, be a force for a positive environment that supports each other as well as patients and families. The factors listed in Table 206.4 provide a start. We all have a stake in the process and the outcomes.

References

1. Stewart DE, Ahmad F, Cheung AM, et al: Women physicians and stress. *J Wom Health Gend Base Med* 9(2):185–190, 2000.
2. Heath J, Johanson W, Blake N: Healthy work environments: A validation of the literature. *Journal of Nursing Administration* 34(11):524–530, 2004.
3. Aiken LH, Clarke SP, Sloane DM, et al: An international perspective on hospital nurses' work environments: the case for reform. *Policy Polit Nurs Pract* 2(4):255–263, 2001.
4. Aiken LH, Clarke SP, Sloane DM, et al: Nurses' reports on hospital care in five countries. *Health Aff* 20(3):43–53, 2001.
5. Vahey DC, Aiken LH, Sloane DM, et al: Nurse burnout and patient satisfaction. *Med Care* 42[2, Suppl]:II-57–II-64, 2004.
6. Schubert M, Glass T, Clarke S, et al: Rationing of nursing care and its relationship to patient outcomes: the Swiss extension of the International Hospital Outcomes Study. *Int J Qual Health Care* 20(4):227–237, 2008.
7. Aiken L, Smith H, Lake E, et al: Lower Medicare mortality among a set of hospitals known for good nursing care. *Medical Care* 32:771–787, 1994.
8. American Association of Critical Care Nurses: AACN Standards for establishing and sustaining healthy work environments: a journey to excellence. *Am J Crit Care* 14(3):187–197, 2005.
9. Ferrand E, Lemaire F, Regnier B, et al: Discrepancies between perceptions by physicians and nursing staff of intensive care unit *end-of-life decisions. Am J Respir Crit Care Med* 167:1310–1315, 2003.
10. Manojlovich M, Antonakos CL, Ronis DL, et al: Intensive care units, communication between nurses and physicians, and patients' outcomes. *Am J Crit Care* 18(1):21–30, 2009.
11. Vazirani S, Hays R, Shapiro M, et al: Effect of a multidisciplinary intervention on communication and collaboration among physicians and nurses. *Am J Crit Care* 14(1):71–76, 2005.
12. Grumbach K, Bodenheimer T: Can health care teams improve primary care practice? *JAMA* 291(10):1246–1251, 2004.
13. Leonard M, Graham S, Bonacum D: The human factor: the critical importance of effective teamwork and communication in providing safe care. *Qual Saf Health Care* 13:i85–i90, 2004.
14. Schmalenberg C, Kramer M, Brewer B, et al: Clinically competent peers and support for education: structures and practices that work. *Critical Care Nurse* 28(4):54–65, 2008.
15. Sutcliffe KM, Lewton E, Rosenthal MM: Communication failures: an insidious contributor to medical mishaps. *Acad Med* 79(2):186–194, 2004.
16. Cho S-H, Ketefian S, Barkauskas V, et al: The effects of nurse staffing on adverse events, morbidity, mortality and medical costs. *Nursing Research* 52(2):71–79, 2003.
17. Bae S-H, Mark B, Fried B: Impact of nursing unit turnover on patient outcomes in hospitals. *J Nurs Sch* 42(1):40–49, 2010.
18. Aiken LH, Clarke SP, Cheung RB, et al: Educational level of hospital nurses and surgical patient mortality. *JAMA* 290(12):1617–1623, 2003.

19. Estabrooks C, Midodzi W, Cummings G, et al: The impact of hospital nursing characteristics on 30-day mortality. *Nursing Research* 54(2):74–84, 2005.
20. Schmalenberg C, Kramer M: Perception of adequacy of staffing. *Critical Care Nurse* 29(5):65–71, 2009.
21. Leiter MP, Spence Laschinger HK: Relationships of work and practice environment to professional burnout. *Nursing Research* 55(2):137–146, 2006.
22. American Association of Critical-Care Nurses (2010) *Vision*. Available at: http://www.aacn.org/wd/memberships/content/mission_vision_values_ethics.pcms?menu=membership#vision. Accessed April 9, 2010.
23. Hardin S, Kaplow R: *Synergy for Clinical Excellence. The AACN Synergy Model for Patient Care*. Sudbury, MA: Jones and Bartlett Publishers, 2005, pp 3–54.
24. American Nurses Credentialing Center (2010). Magnet Recognition Program in the News. Available at: http://www.nursecredentialing.org/Headlines/MagnetRecognitionPrograminthеNews.aspx. Accessed April 9, 2010.
25. Ulrich BT, Woods D, Hart KA, et al: Critical care nurses' work environments value of excellence in Beacon and Magnet organizations. *Critical Care Nurse* 27(3):68–77, 2007.
26. Lake E, Friese C: Variations in nursing practice environments: relation to staffing and hospital characteristics. *Nursing Research* 55(1):1–9, 2006.
27. Choi J, Bakken S, Larson E, et al: Perceived nursing work environment of critical care nurses. *Nursing Research* 53(6):370–378, 2004.
28. Krichbaum K, Diemert C, Jacox L, et al: Complexity compression: nurses under fire. *Nurs Forum* 42(2):86–94, 2007.
29. Boyle DK, Kochinda C: Enhancing collaborative communication of nurse and physician leadership in two intensive care units. *J Nurs Adm* 34(2):60–70, 2004.
30. McCauley K, Irwin RS: Changing the work environment in ICUs to achieve patient focused care: the time has come. *Chest* 130(5):1–8, 2006.

CHAPTER 207 ■ ICU NURSING IN THE TELEMEDICINE AGE

REBECCA J. ZAPATOCHNY RUFO, TERESA A. RINCON AND SHAWN CODY

INTRODUCTION

In the 1999 publication by the Institute of Medicine, *To Err Is Human*, the authors painted a grim picture of medical errors in hospitalized patients [1]. The report stated tens of thousands of patients each year suffer a preventable medical error. Errors can lead to death, physical impairment, increased length of stay, and cost increases amounting to billions of dollars. The Institute of Medicine (IOM) estimated that almost 100,000 American patients die yearly from medical errors making it the eighth leading cause of death in the United States.

Historically, Intensive Care Units (ICUs) are major sites for medical errors and complications. Patient safety experts cite outmoded systems of work as the reason for many of healthcare's errors and quality problems [2]. It is believed that redesigned systems will yield safer, better care. According to the Leapfrog Group, a healthcare advisory board for Fortune 500 companies [3], more than four million patients are admitted to the ICUs and approximately 500,000 die annually. They estimated that providing a dedicated, intensivist-based care model could save between 50,000 and 100,000 lives annually [4] and that mortality could be reduced by 15% to 20%.

Modern ICUs are complex and prone to errors [5]. In 1999, Doering described what she termed as threats to effective collaboration in the critical care setting [6]. These threats included the complexity of the environment and the increasing workloads of staff at the bedside. She suggested that the process of effective collaboration required a commitment of administrators and staff alike when both are facing competition for scarce resources. Effective communication and collaboration required time and nurturing from all involved. It should be built on a concept of trust and could not be rushed and is often the first thing to be omitted when outside forces pull caregivers in different directions.

AGING WORKFORCE

Long lengths of stay, higher rates of infection, and failure to rescue are patient care outcomes that have been linked with nurse staffing levels [7]. Concerns related to the implications of a projected nursing shortage has influenced interest in how staffing mix as well as sheer loss of numbers of critical care nurses could lead to an increase in errors in patient care. This led to the passing of the Nurse Reinvestment Act (NRA), Public Law 107–205 in 2002 by Congress. This legislation was aimed at stimulating the growth of the nursing profession [8].

The composition of the registered nurses (RNs) workforce was predicted to shift to the largest group of RNs being in the 50- to 60-year-old age group by 2010 and according to a recent study by Auerbach et al., RNs in their 50s will outnumber all other age groups in this profession by 2012 [9]. The demand for RNs is predicted to accelerate at the same time as the nation's eighty million baby boomers begin to reach the age of 65. By 2020, the gap between supply and demand of RNs is estimated at over 400,000 [10].

Although some progress has been made in recruitment and retention of nurses, the future projections still fall short of the goal of maintaining a supply and demand balance for this vital workforce. Discovering more innovative solutions to leverage nursing expertise and practice is needed. The Sixth report by the National Advisory Council on Nurse Education and Practice (NACNEP) recommended the use of simulation-based education as well as utilization of interactive Internet-based learning programs to enhance effectiveness of nursing education and critical thinking skills. Strategic use of technology to not replace the nursing workforce but to enhance skill mix and staffing as well as to prepare and support the novice nurse was also recommended [11]. Leveraging nursing practice and expertise through the use of technology is the essence of telenursing.

A task force was commissioned by the Robert Wood Johnson Foundation to publish a white paper in 2006 to identify strategies and opportunities for retaining the experienced nursing workforce. This paper examined the effects of loss of knowledge that occurs when older experienced nurses leave the profession [12]. Leading experts are convinced that organizations suffer detrimental effects on productivity and performance with loss of older employees. Shifting the ratio of experienced nurses to less experienced nurses will have serious implications on quality and safety of patient care according to national experts [12]. If the emerging role development of the telemedicine team is fostered by internal driving forces of clinical competence, independent decision making, and strong interpersonal skills, then can telemedicine enable a new care delivery model that embraces empowerment through leveraging of critical resources?

What happens to nursing knowledge, if as projected, large numbers of experienced nurses leave the field all at once? Bleich et al. warns that the implications of loss of knowledge will be devastating to not only performance and productivity but the shift from "experienced to less experienced nurses will have serious implications for quality and safety of patient care" [13]. The authors go on to explain that more than just "rudimentary skills and routine know-how about common processes" are required, these nurses also have "deep-smarts," a "tacit knowledge" that is difficult but not impossible to articulate into formal language. It is a knowledge that is gained through the maturation process of being a nurse; a synthesis of learned knowledge, deep insight, and intuition that allows the experienced nurse to incorporate multiple assessment variables rapidly into an assessment and a plan of care. It is the "state of knowing" that could be lost as nurses leave the profession if we do not find innovative and creative solutions to maintain and leverage it.

IS TELEMEDICINE THE ANSWER?

According to leading experts, telemedicine may be leveraged to support a multidisciplinary intensivist-led team and incorporates re-engineering of workflow processes, outcome measurement, collaboration and professional role development to facilitate efforts to change behavior for improved patient quality [14]. Telemedicine is defined as the transmission of electronic data from one location to another to allow for remote evaluation of the data by a medical professional [15–17]. Data may include pictures, EKGs, radiology studies, or audio–video feeds. The remote medical professional then communicates back to the sending facility with an opinion using one of several means, including fax, audio, video, or other electronic means.

The concept of telemedicine has been around for several decades. Telemedicine in its current form can be found in the literature as far back as the 1950s [15]. The National Aeronautics and Space Administration monitored astronauts' heart rate and respirations while in space from a remote location or during test runs on the earth. NASA continued to monitor astronauts and to develop computer software over the ensuing years [15]. Several projects were funded by government agencies in the 1960s, 1970s, and 1980s to bring medical care to remote or hard to reach locations both nationally and internationally, often using microwave audio and video communication. Most of these early projects could not be sustained due primarily to the prohibitive cost of the microwave communication technology [16].

During the 1990s, the availability and transmission of digital radiological studies allowed the efficient reading of images remotely, allowing a single radiologist from a different location to interpret studies when an on-site radiologist was not available. Another use that gained favor around the same time was the use of psychiatric staff doing remote evaluations. Telemedicine has also allowed neurologists to remotely review studies and allow for real-time decision making in the treatment of acute stroke care [17]. This along with changes to the laws required for consults to allow for neurologists to bill for their remote services has greatly enhanced the care of these patients.

Today telemedicine is a significant component of the Department of Veterans Affairs strategic plan to care for veterans [18]. According to the American Psychiatric Association, "Telepsychiatry is currently one of the most effective ways to increase access to psychiatric care for individuals living in underserved areas" [19]. The Department of Health and Human Services, Health Resources and Services Administration (HRSA), supports the use of telehealth to meet the needs of underserved people [20].

Over the past 10 years the advancement of computer systems of relatively low cost and of faster transmission has greatly enhanced what data can be viewed from a remote location. The advent of clinical documentation systems at the bedside have further made the data readily available using electronic means. Over the past 35 years, research scientists have worked to develop computer systems to assist clinicians in making decisions related to patient care [21]. This coupled with high-resolution audio–video technologies have led to the emergence of telemedicine in the intensive care unit or tele-ICU care.

TELE-ICU STAFFING PATTERNS

A modern tele-ICU center is typically staffed by both clinical and nonclinical members. The fundamental component to the remote clinical team includes experienced critical care nurses and physicians specializing in Critical Care Medicine. Other board certified specialty physicians such as cardiothoracic, pulmonary medicine, cardiology, and trauma/surgery may serve as the tele-ICU physician. Affiliate practitioners such as Nurse Practitioners and Pharmacists are adjunctive team members in some tele-ICUs to leverage resources in patient monitoring, management, and performance improvement. Operational processes are supported by nonclinical staff in the tele-ICU center through timely, current data entry and by facilitation of communication between remote and onsite teams.

The number of clinical and nonclinical staff required for each program is dependent upon the volume of monitored beds and the off-site team's level of involvement with the bedside. At least one physician along with several nurses and nonclinical support consist of the core team members each shift. An additional physician or mid-level practitioner such as an advanced practice nurse may be needed to meet the demands of monitoring larger patient volumes. The tele-ICU care team composition is dependent on the type of service provided. There are specialty physicians providing consultative care models using telemedicine technology to support the care of critically ill patients. Some of these care modalities use telenursing support in their programs.

Tele-ICU staffing is impacted by several factors including the ratio of patients monitored per tele-ICU nurse. Typically, one tele-ICU nurse monitors approximately 35 to 50 patients. The ratio affects the number of nurses required each shift to staff the tele-ICU.

One consideration of staffing is the degree of integration and effort needed by the tele-ICU nurse to maintain timely data for monitoring and interventional purposes. Another consideration in managing this many patients is the degree of electronic documentation performed at the bedside versus the remote site. Fragmentation of documentation (paper, electronic, combination) impacts monitoring abilities of the tele-ICU nurse and demands greater oversight to maintain accuracy of data.

TELE-ICU NURSING

The ICU nurse is a key leader to clinical transformation and the re-engineering of care processes. Therefore, it would follow that the tele-ICU nurse would and should be an integral part of the tele-ICU team. What makes the tele-ICU nurse think differently than the bedside ICU nurse? How does the tele-ICU nurse use or draw upon innate cognitive abilities when processing information? Drawing from previous experience, training and knowledge the expert critical care nurse uses tacit knowledge to synthesize complex physiological information and care modalities into nursing diagnoses and recommendations for optimizing patient care. Information technologies (ITs) allow nurses to not only view information remotely but to observe pertinent data in an organized, real-time manner enhance the efficiency in which clinicians can amalgamate information.

TRANSITION FROM THE BEDSIDE

The tele-ICU nurse requires a transitioning process to fulfill role development. The transitioning period or role development may last several months past orientation. A fundamental aspect of this period is learning new responsibilities as a tele-ICU nurse versus an ICU nurse. Role development encompasses expanded functions as mentor, preceptor, educator, leader, and program advocacy. Unlike bedside care, the tele-ICU nurse must learn to transition from hands-on care to technology-driven care.

Conceptual development is important to understanding role transition of the tele-ICU nurse. Discussion of conceptual development of the tele-ICU nurse is limited to absent in the literature. Understanding what makes the tele-ICU nurse transition into an emerging new breed of caregiver is important to the future of nursing practice. A paradigm shift occurs in care delivery once the bedside ICU nurse transitions into a tele-ICU nurse. The shift in traditional care delivery of one to three ICU patients is now dozens of patients per shift. How does the tele-ICU nurse begin to conceptualize and synthesize from managing individual patients to whole populations of patients occur? Benner [22] identifies five stages of nursing development and the teaching/learning needs at each stage. These stages are congruent with the professional role development and transition period of the tele-ICU nurse. Unlike a new graduate nurse at the novice stage of professional bedside practice, the tele-ICU nurse possesses clinical experience but is new to the emerging role of the remote environment as well as to using IT to drive decision making and assessment practices. All nurses transition to some degree through these five stages of development regardless of their specialty area. The time spent in each developmental stage will vary with each nurse and the ability to adapt to the complexity of the new role.

The case could be made that these expert nurses should be physically present at the bedside caring for complex patients and providing face to face mentorship of novice nurses. How could taking more nursing expertise away from the bedside actually serve to enhance staff mix? Because of nurse supply and demand trends and predictions, finding alternative ways to leverage nursing expertise across the over 6,000 ICU in the nation will take a creative and innovative approach [23].

Expertise and knowledge working in isolation from caring can hinder execution of high level nurse practice. Therefore, it is imperative to include a balance of knowledge and caring in the development of the emerging discipline of virtual or tele-ICU nursing. Dr. Jean Watson's Theory of Human Caring contain 10 factors that are described by her as "those aspects of nursing that actually potentiate therapeutic healing processes and relationships; they affect the one caring and the one-being-cared-for" [24]. She describes the soul or spirit within human beings as "greater than the physical, mental, and emotional existence of a person at any given point in time." According to Watson, this inner spirit allows each individual to achieve a "higher degree of consciousness, an inner strength, and a power that can expand human capacities." The virtual nurse should possess a deep-rooted attribute of caring that extends to not only patients but also to the care providers at the bedside.

TELE-ICU COLLABORATION

The tele-ICU nurse needs to balance caring with power to meet the needs of the patient–family unit through negotiation and advocacy. The concept of power is frequently associated with negative connotations such as restricting freedom, authoritative leadership, and hierarchical status [25]. Power also is referenced to coercion and domination of others. Leaders may display various forms of power or a lack of power depending on the situation and degree of empowerment. Legitimate power is when one person relinquishing power to another individual. This power is associated with action and expertise. Power can be connected with knowledge, coercion or conditioned.

The empowered tele-ICU nurse exhibits effectual use of clinical knowledge and innovative technology. Virtual rounding is an example of empowerment and is a principle mechanism to immediately serve as a clinical resource for assessment, intervention, or mentoring. Nurses should conduct virtual patient and environmental rounds proactively to assess for potential sources of complications, errors and interventional effectiveness. Understanding the concepts of social presence can effectuate acceptance from caregivers at the bedside and mitigate interaction issues related to critical missing communication cues.

Empowerment inherent in organizations where individuals are encouraged to assume responsibility and act in line with organizational goals is an approach that allows staff to retain control over their work, where responsibility is delegated within the hierarchy and resources are readily available [26,27]. Hence, organizational development for a tele-ICU service should begin with a vision and strategy that empowers the remote team to work toward the best care practices within an integrated team model. If this is not present then virtual teams will struggle against entrenched loyalties and hierarchical power structures that are prohibitive to safe and collaborative patient care. Some examples of integrated team approaches with a tele-ICU team are the following:

- Decreased ventilator days [28])
- Implementation of evidence-based best practice strategies at system levels [29,30]
- Ability to provide real-time feedback or reports to guide clinician practice
- Improved compliance to best practice standards [31,32]
- Increased cost effectiveness of critical care
- Prevention of cardiac arrest and complication prevention/management [33–36]

The virtual presence of the tele-ICU nurse may further complicates effective communication due to the lack of direct person to person contact and inability to read the body language. For decades, the healthcare industry has known that ineffective communication has been a significant factor in adverse events in hospitals and in critical care. Inadequate communication was cited as one of the main findings of the 1999 IOM *To Err Is Human* publication [1]. A 2003 study examined the attitudes of critical care nurses and physicians regarding collaboration and teamwork [37]. The results described that physicians predominantly found collaboration to be satisfactory yet the nursing staff interviewed found collaboration lacking. It is thought that communication and collaboration throughout critical care among caregivers is not what it should be [38]. This is important to keep in mind from a tele-ICU perspective as the camera and microphone may be viewed as intrusive. We are reminded of this in George Orwell's 1949 novel "1984" [39]. Written at the end of World War II, it described a fictional society run by The Party, and it's affect on the main character, Winston Smith. In the novel, all thoughts and actions are controlled by the party, through the use of spies, cameras, and microphones. The controlling Party, and its leader, Big Brother, are attempting to control everything in the people's lives, from where they work to how they think. This "1984" mentality of technology connecting everyone in the world could contribute to a reluctance of care providers and consumers in embracing telemedicine as sound method of care delivery. Understanding this mind-set is important as telemedicine care providers address the communication and collaboration barriers that can surface when using technology-enhanced care modalities.

The tele-ICU nurse is in a unique position to view variation or gaps in care across and within health systems. As the tele-ICU nurse finds these opportunities for improvement this along with Appreciative Intelligence (AI) creates "survival anxiety" which can influence or prompt change to occur [40]. This leads to unfreezing of prior perceptions of care delivery and with AI, tele-ICU nurses can then reframe situations for better negotiating or problem solving in more creative ways. They can use concepts of AI to enhance critical thinking and drive interventions in order to achieve patient safety goals. For example, the tele-ICU nurse has the potential to view continuous vital sign trending. The bedside vital sign data is processed through decision support software that identifies early trends in deterioration. When a vital sign alert is triggered the tele-ICU nurse evaluates the alert for potential patient deterioration, using an audio–video assessment, review of laboratory values, and other pertinent clinical data to assist in the critical thinking and assessment processes. The tele-ICU nurse rapidly processes these data using tacit knowledge which leads to decision making related to evidence-based practice.

COMPUTER-ENHANCED CARE

Social presence (SP) using computer-mediated communication (CMC) has been studied in education disciplines [41–43] and its learnings can be applied to the telemedicine arena. Communication mediums can determine how well people communicate but that individual perceptions often have a powerful influence on acceptance of these mediums. SP has been described as the state of being "real" in mediated communication and is based in telecommunication literature. Social presence relates to how a person is perceived as being real and being there or present in communication [42].

The aspects of SP influence how well communication occurs. Although the degree of saliency and the quality of the social medium can assist in influencing satisfaction of users in using technology as a vehicle of communication, individual perspectives have been shown to be a powerful dynamic [43]. Factors that influence the degree of social presence are: verbal or nonverbal cues, physical proximity, formality of dress, facial expressions, eye contact, humor, and personal topics of conversation. CMC is considered low in the order of social presence [44]. Given previous statistics that highlight the role of communication in errors that harm patients, understanding the impact of modes of communication is important to this discussion. Tele-ICU nurses should receive advanced training in communication techniques and nursing leadership should design communication algorithms that enhance collaboration and mitigate negative perceptions. Further research is needed in the area of telenursing and social presence.

Since the tele-ICU nurse can manage 35 to 50 patients per shift, thoughtful strategies must be employed to accomplish efficient, comprehensive rounding. Studer, a nationally recognized healthcare management thought leader identified nine steps to standardize rounding [45]. These nine steps are applicable in various settings where rounding is present.

1. Give staff a heads-up. The tele-ICU nurse should inform the bedside caregivers of their presence and purpose for rounding.
2. Prepare a scouting report. Understand specific issues or situations within each unit that may impact rounding such as staffing constraints, new nurses.
3. Make a personal connection. Identify a common connection with bedside caregivers to facilitate compassion and genuine personal concern.
4. Identify an issue or concern raised on a previous rounding episode. Demonstrates your follow through to resolve an issue or problem.
5. Remember five questions framed in a positive manner. Script five basic questions that are communicated in a positive and inviting approach for rounding purposes.
6. When an individual identifies a problem, assure him or her that you will do the best to resolve their concern(s). Develops the foundation for open and trusted relationships.
7. Record issues that arise in a rounding log. This will allow for accurate accountability of issues and needs of the bedside caregivers or patients.
8. Recognize and reward those who are identified a high performers. Extending words of thanks for superior work and positive interactions develops strong relationships.
9. Repeat process. The tele-ICU nurse gains repeated experience with rounding since this is an essential function of their role.

TELEMEDICINE AND EVIDENCED-BASED PRACTICE

An expert committee formed by the IOM found that "current care is insufficiently reliable in its use of the best science and best-known practices because it lacks IT systems that put that knowledge at the point of use and because it honors and protects unscientific variations in care based on local habits, unquestioned forms of autonomy, and insufficient curiosity" [46]. According to leading nursing experts the acquisition and implementation of evidence-based practice is lacking in nursing practice [47]. Data also suggests that social interaction and experience are the two most utilized sources of practice knowledge for nurses [48]. Nurses in the virtual environment should maintain a high level of competency through attainment of advance certifications in critical care. Given this, the tele-ICU nurse has a unique opportunity to maintain and disseminate a high level of evidence-based practice knowledge.

CONCLUSION

As discussed previously, the expert nurse can rapidly put together the whole patient picture integrating the patient's needs into timely and appropriate nursing interventions while others may be focused on the next task or a technical skill [49]. This ability to synthesize knowledge into appropriate decision-making skills can then facilitate effective support to the bedside nurse practice. Nurses make hundreds of decisions a day when caring for patients [50]. The tele-ICU nurse can serve as not only a sounding board for bedside nurses as they make these decisions they can use influence and negotiating skills to facilitate evidence-based care practices. Within this context the virtual clinicians function autonomously yet collaboratively with bedside caregivers in clinical decision-making. The autonomy and independence of the virtual team is cultivated from years of professional experiences, personal attributes, hardiness, and exceptional tacit knowledge synthesis skills. In this virtual environment, nurses and physicians are challenged differently than at the bedside. Monitoring patient data and intervening without physical presence demand skillful communication and expertise in critical care.

Leveraging scarce critical care nursing expertise is just one of the benefits of tele-ICU care models. An expert nursing team can coach and mentor novice ICU nurses remotely, reinforcing care practices, assisting in establishing patient goals, and enhancing critical thinking and assessment skills. Experience is a prerequisite for becoming an expert, according to research that focused on critical care nurses and the learning process [51]. Experts have the ability to go beyond the tasks to read and respond to the global needs of the patient. This allows for the ability to avert potential catastrophe or "failure to rescue" [49,51]. Most sites report that nurses working in a tele-ICU have on average 10 to 15 years of experience in various fields of critical care nursing.

Multidisciplinary integration of the tele-ICU technology and care delivery method through empowerment contributes to organizational acceptance and utilization [52]. Widespread integration with nurses, physicians, respiratory therapists, dieticians, physical medicine, and other care givers will leverage clinical and technical expertise. Data transparency can be enhanced across disciplines with immediate availability of electronic clinical documentation tools within software applications.

Using standardized reporting metrics to evaluate severity adjusted mortality and length of stay as well as compliance with best practice standards is a benefit to centralized data collection. Quality assurance/improvement oversight can be enhanced and efficiency improved with technological tools and tele-ICU processes [53]. This can lead to development of system wide clinical risk reduction strategies that can in turn improve patient safety and quality. Tele-ICU systems allow providers to extract reports from the software application in real-time to evaluate and intervene on patients at multiple intervals each day.

Robust health IT systems employ clinical decision support tools to prompt the clinician to institute evidence-based best practices at the point of care. These systems can provide real-time feedback and reports to alert the physician/nurse to any gaps in care that need to be filled. These "smart" systems coupled with collaboration between on-site and tele-ICU teams empower clinicians to implement best care processes effectively and consistently [54,55].

References

1. Kohn LT, Corrigan J, Donald MS, eds: *To Err is Human: Building a Safer Health System*. Washington, DC, National Academy Press, 2000.
2. Kozar R, Shackford S, Cocanour C: Challenges to the care of the critically ill: novel staffing paradigms. *J Trauma* 64:366–373, 2008.
3. The Leapfrog Group About Us: Available at: http://www.leapfroggroup.org/about_us. Accessed December 30, 9009.
4. Birkmeyer JD, Birkmeyer CM, et al: *Leapfrog Safety Standards: the Potential Benefits of Universal Adoption*. Washington, DC: The Leapfrog Group, 2000.
5. Yeager S: Interdisciplinary collaboration: the heart and soul of health care. *Crit Care Nurs Clin North Am* 17:143–148, 2005.
6. Doering LV: Nurse-physician collaboration: at the crossroads of danger and opportunity. *Crit Care Med* 27(9):2066–2067, 1999.
7. Needleman J, Buerhaus P, Mattke S, et al: Nurse staffing levels and the quality of care in hospitals. *N Engl J Med* 346(22):1715–1722, 2002.
8. U.S. Department of Health and Human Services: *NACNEP: Third Report to the Secretary of Health and Human Services and the Congress*. 2000. Healthy People 2010. 2nd ed. Washington, DC, U.S. Government Printing Office. Available at: http://bhpr.hrsa.gov/nursing/nac/nacreport.htm. Accessed January 25, 2010.
9. Auerbach DI, Buerhaus PI, Straiger DO: Better late than never: workforce supply implications of later entry into nursing. *Health Aff* 26:178–185, 2007.
10. Buerhaus PI, Needleman J, Mattke S, et al: Strengthening hospital nursing. *Health Aff* 21(5):123–132, 2002.
11. U.S. Department of Health and Human Services: *NACNEP: Sixth Report to the Secretary of Health and Human Services and the Congress*. Washington, DC, U.S. Government Printing Office. Available at: http://ftp.hrsa.gov/bhpr/nursing/sixth.pdf. Accessed January 25, 2010.
12. Hatcher BJ, Bleich MR, Connolly C, et al: Wisdom at work: the importance of the older and experienced nurse in the workforce. Robert Wood Johnson Foundation, 2006.
13. Bleich MR, Cleary BL, Davis K, et al: Mitigating knowledge loss, a strategic imperative for nurse leaders. *J Nurs Adm* 39(4):160–164, 2009.
14. The Leap Frog Group: ICU Physician Staffing (IPS) Factsheet. Available at: http://www.leapfroggroup.org/media/file/FactSheet_IPS.pdf. Accessed July 4, 2010.
15. Brown N: A brief history of telemedicine. Telemedicine Information Exchange. 1995. Available at: http://tie.telemed.org/articles/article.asp?path=articles&article=tmhistory_nb_tie95.xml. Accessed July 27, 2009.
16. Perednia P, Allen A: Telemedicine, technology and clinical applications. *JAMA* 273(6):483–488, 1995.
17. Schwamm L, Audebert H, Amarenco P, et al: Recommendations for the implementation of telemedicine within stroke systems of care. *Stroke* 40:2635–2660, 2009.
18. Department of Veterans Affairs: Approaches to make health information systems available and affordable to rural and medically underserved communities, in Principi AJ (ed.). 2004.
19. American Psychiatric Association: (2010). Topic 4: Telepsychiatry. Available at: http://www.psych.org/Departments/HSF/UnderservedClearinghouse/Linkeddocuments/telepsychiatry.aspx. Accessed July 4, 2010.
20. Health Resources and Services Administration: Telehealth. Available at: http://www.hrsa.gov/telehealth/. Accessed June 18, 2010.
21. Mark DB: Decision making in clinical medicine, Chapter 3, in Fauci AS, Kasper DL, Hauser SL, et al. (eds): *Harrison's Principles of Internal Medicine*. 17th ed. 2008. Available at: http://www.accessmedicine.com.proxy.kumc.edu:2048/content.aspx?aid=2858216. Accessed June 22, 2010.
22. Benner P: *From Novice to Expert*. New Jersey, Prentice Hall Health, 2001.
23. Critical Care Workforce Partnership position statement: The aging of the U.S. population and increased need for critical care services. AACN/ACCP/ATS/SCCM. Available at: http://www.sccm.org/sccm/Public+Health+and+Policy/AgingUSPopulation2001.pdf. Published November 2001. Accessed July 22, 2010.
24. Watson J: The theory of human caring: retrospective and prospective. *Nurs Sci Q* 10(1):49–52, 1997.
25. Kuokkanen L, Leino-Kilpi H: Power and empowerment in nursing: three theoretical approaches. *J Adv Nurs* 31(1):235–241, 2000.
26. Vogt J, Murrell K: *Empowerment in Organizations. How to Spark Exceptional Performance*. San Diego, CA, Pfeiffer & Company, 1990.
27. Clutterbuck D: *The Power of Empowerment. Release the Hidden Talents of Your Employees*. London: Kogan Page, 1994.
28. Raitz-Cowboy E, Rajamani S, Jamil MG, et al: Impact of remote ICU management on ventilator days. *Crit Care Med* 33(12):A1, 2005.
29. Ikeda D, Hayatdavoudi S, Winchell J, et al: Implementation of a standard protocol for the surviving sepsis 6 and 24 hour bundles in patients with an APACHE III admission diagnosis of sepsis decreases mortality in an open adult ICU. *Crit Care Med* 34(12):A2, 2006.
30. Rincon T, Bourke G, Ikeda D, et al: Screening for severe sepsis: an incidence analysis. *Crit Care Med* 34(12):A257, 2007.
31. Aaronson ML, Zawada ET, Herr P: Role of a telemedicine intensive care unit program (TISP) on glycemic control (GC) in seriously ill patients in a rural health system. *Chest* 130:(4) 226s, 2006.
32. Youn B: ICU process improvement: using telemedicine to enhance compliance and documentation for the ventilator bundle. *Chest* 130:(4):226S, 2006.
33. Shaffer J, Johnson JW, Kaszuba F, et al: Remote ICU management improves outcomes in patients with cardiopulmonary arrest. *Crit Care Med* 33:A5, 2005.
34. Hayatdavoudi S, Ikeda D, Seiver A, et al: Impact of a protocol treating severe sepsis on renal function and survival of septic shock patients in an open ICU. *Crit Care Med* 34(12):A18, 2006.
35. Breslow MJ: Remote ICU care programs: current status. *J Crit Care* 22:66–76, 2007.
36. Reis M: Tele-ICU: a new paradigm in critical care. *Int Anesthesiol Clin* 47(1):153–170, 2009.
37. Thomas EJ, Sexton JB, Helmreich RL: Discrepant attitudes about teamwork among critical care nurses and physicians. *Crit Care Med* 31(3):956–959, 2003.
38. Surgenor SD, Blike GT, Corwin HL: Teamwork and collaboration in critical care: lessons from the cockpit. *Crit Care Med* 31(3):992–993, 2003.
39. Orwell G: *Nineteen Eighty-Four*. London, Martin Secker & Warburg Ltd, 1949.

40. American Library Association: The Information Literacy Competency Standards for Higher Education (2000). Available at: http://www.ala.org/acrl/ilcomstan.
41. Thatchenkery T, Metzker C: *Appreciative Intelligence*. San Francisco, CA, Berrett-Koehler Publishers, 2006.
42. Lowenthal PR: Social presence, in Rogers P, Berg G, Boettcher J, et al. (eds): *Encyclopedia of Distance and Online Learning*.
43. Virginia Commonwealth University Center for Teaching Excellence: Online Teaching and Learning Resource Guide: Social Presence/Cognitive Presence/Teaching Presence (2009). Available at: https://elearning.kumc.edu/section/default.asp?id=410603081025. Accessed May 25, 2010.
44. Cobb SC: Social presence and online learning: a current view from a research perspective. *J Interact Online Learn* 8(3):241–254, 2009.
45. Studor Q: *Hardwiring Excellence*. Florida, Fire Starter Publishing, 2003.
46. Berwick DM: A user's manual for the IOM's 'quality chasm' report; patients' experiences should be the fundamental source of the definition of "quality". *Health Affairs* 21(3):80–90.
47. Achterberg T, Schoonhoven L, Grol R: Nursing implementation science: how evidence-based nursing requires evidence-based implementation. *J Nurs Scholarsh* 40(4):302–310, 2008.
48. Estabrooks CA, Rutakumwa W, O'Leary KA, et al: Source of practice knowledge among nurses. *Qual Health Res* 15(4):460–476, 2005.
49. Dracup K, Bryan-Brown CW: From novice to expert to mentor: shaping the future. *Am J Crit Care* 13:448–450, 2004.
50. Benner P: *From Novice to Expert: Excellence and Power in Clinical Nursing Practice*. Menlo Park, CA, Addison-Wesley, 1984.
51. Dracup K, Morris PE: How will they learn? *Am J Crit Care* 17:306–309, 2008.
52. Zapatochmy-Rufo RJ: Virtual ICUs foundations for healthier environments. *Nurs Manag* 38(2):32–39, 2007.
53. Rincon T, Welcher B, Srikanth D, et al: Economic implications of data collection from a remote center utilizing technological tools. *Crit Care Med* 34(12):Abstract Supplement A161, 2007.
54. Rincon T, Bourke G, Ikeda D: Centralized, remote care improves sepsis identification, bundle compliance, and outcomes. *Chest* 132(4):Abstract Supplement 557S, 2007.
55. Zawada ET, Aaronson ML, Herr P, et al: Relationship between levels of consultative management and outcomes in a telemedicine intensivist staffing program in a rural health system. *Chest* 130(4):226S, 2006.

SECTION XIX ■ CONTEMPORARY CHALLENGES IN THE INTENSIVE CARE UNIT

CRAIG M. LILLY

CHAPTER 208 ■ ICU ORGANIZATION AND MANAGEMENT

THOMAS L. HIGGINS AND JAY S. STEINGRUB

INTRODUCTION

Organization is the act of assembling elements into an orderly, functional whole. Management is the ongoing revision and renovation of that careful assembly to cope with change. The concept of "bedside management" is familiar to clinicians who titrate vasopressors or adjust ventilator settings; intensive care unit (ICU) management is itself a form of titration and continuous adjustment. ICU management extends beyond simply implementing policies and procedures, organizing service and teaching rounds, preparing budgets, and complying with regulations. The successful ICU manager must also innovate and facilitate change. Creativity is important, but perseverance may be more essential because of the ways a typical organization will resist change. Knowing how to navigate the obvious and subtle impediments to change is a key skill for the ICU manager.

The already staggering cost of health care continues to escalate, and now represents 16% of the gross domestic product (GDP) in the United States, with estimates that unchecked, it could double again to 31% of GDP in the next 25 years [1]. Hospital costs are roughly a third of total health care costs, and intensive care alone consumes between 4% and 10% of total healthcare costs, or 0.56% to 1.5% of GDP [2–4]. One-third of Medicare patients spend part of their hospital stay in the ICU or coronary care unit, at an average unit cost per day of $2,616 (in 2004 US dollars) [5]. Discrepancies exist between the Medicare Provider Analysis and Review File (MedPAR) and the Hospital Cost Report Information System (HCRIS), two federal databases used to assess inpatient and critical care costs in the Medicare population [6]. In fact, critical care days may have decreased by 4.5% between 1995 and 2000 based on HCRIS data, while an increase of 7.2% was seen using MedPAR data, which includes "post/intermediate" billing codes [6]. Nonetheless, the Center for Medicare and Medicaid Services continues to forecast a substantial increase in the rate of growth in volume and intensity of medical services as the leading edge of the "baby boom" generation enters retirement [7]. Physician and nursing shortages [8] and increasing costs will constrain growth of intensive care services, while consumer demand (fueled in part by easy internet access to information) and an aging population with chronic disease will exacerbate existing capacity issues. New, unpredictable risks (e.g., novel bacterial and viral threats, terrorism) require preparedness and the ability to ramp up critical care capacity in a crisis. Meanwhile, attention continues to be focused on preventable medical errors. This confluence of events implies that attention must be paid to the health and well-being of the ICU in addition to addressing the needs of individual patients [9].

The conceptual frameworks [10] and business skills for successful ICU leadership must somehow be acquired, whether in business school or on-the-job. Important characteristics of leaders include self-awareness, self-regulation, motivation, empathy, and social skill [11]. The American College of Physician Executives is one organization that provides information on how to prepare for and succeed in medical management [12]. A formal Masters of Business Administration (MBA) program will typically include courses on accounting, data analysis, ethics, financial analysis, human resource management, information systems, marketing, production/operations management, organizational behavior, organizational planning and strategy, quality improvement, team building, and leadership. Given the difficulty in compressing a multiyear MBA curriculum into a book chapter, we will focus on typical ICU organization patterns, human resource issues, the roles of the ICU director, methods for monitoring clinical ICU care, and ancillary management issues.

ICU ORGANIZATION

In broad terms, there are three common models for ICU organization:

- **Open Unit:** Any physician with privileges to admit patients to the hospital may admit and care for patients in the ICU. Patient care decisions are made by the admitting physician, often with the input of consultants. Admission and discharge (triage) decisions fall to the unit director only in event of a bed or staffing shortage. Intensivists may be available for consultation at the request of the attending physician. The major perceived benefit of this model is continuity of care, and it remains prevalent in the United States, particularly in smaller hospitals.
- **Closed Unit:** All patients entering the ICU are transferred to the care of an intensivist (critical care specialist) for the duration of the ICU stay. Depending on local custom, the admitting physician may remain closely involved or collaborate from a distance. Benefits of this model include documented reductions in mortality, rates of complications, and ICU and hospital length of stay. This model is more common in Europe and Australia, but is gaining acceptance in the United States, based on research findings and response to external pressure from the Leapfrog Group [13] and payers.
- **Transitional (Semiclosed) Unit:** Patients are referred for ICU admission to an intensivist, who reviews all admissions for appropriateness (gate-keeping). Final decisions regarding admission, discharge and triage rest with the physician unit director or his or her designee. Either automatically, or by specific consultation, the intensivist may participate in some or all of the patient's care in conjunction with the patient's attending physician of record. The intensivist's role may be limited to triage functions and emergency response, but more often encompasses hemodynamic, respiratory, fluid,

nutritional, and safety management. This model is seen in the transition phase between open and closed structures, and remains common in surgical practices where the attending surgeon addresses the specific operative aspects of a patient's care (e.g., wound care, transplant immunosuppressive regimens) while delegating resuscitation, physiologic monitoring, organ system support and ICU safety issues to the intensivist.

Pronovost et al. [14] conducted a systematic review of articles examining physician staffing patterns and clinical outcomes published through 2001. The model of care in each of 17 studies was classified as low intensity (no intensivist or elective consultation) or high intensity (mandatory critical care consultation or closed ICU). The high-intensity model was associated with lower ICU mortality (pooled mortality risk estimate 0.61) and lower hospital mortality (pooled mortality risk estimate 0.71). Although the literature overwhelmingly favors intensivist staffing models, a recent retrospective analysis of the Project IMPACT database by Levy et al. [15] demonstrated *higher* odds for hospital mortality in patients managed by critical care physicians. These counterintuitive findings have been challenged as being caused by unmeasured confounders including case mix differences [16] and the role of trainees and part-time academic faculty [17]. The higher risk-adjusted mortality in *teaching* hospitals where more invasive interventions are performed [18] may also counteract beneficial effects of full-time intensivists.

Case-control studies, where outcomes have been examined before and after implementing a closed model, offer additional insight into the value of intensivists. Patients admitted to closed units tend to be sicker [19,20], as might be expected with tighter triage criteria, although average severity scores are not necessarily higher in closed units [21]. Nursing confidence in physician clinical judgment improves [18], as a closed system allows the nurse to contact one managing physician rather than having to call the pulmonologist for ventilator changes, the nephrologist for fluid and electrolyte issues, and the cardiologist for arrhythmias. (Although, as Marik et al. [17] have pointed out, detrimental "parceling out" of care may occur in an academic setting even when full-time intensivists are present). These efficiencies are generally reflected in shorter ICU and hospital LOS [19]. The effect of dedicated intensivist staffing on ICU LOS remains significant after case-mix is adjusted for risk factors such as patient age, admission severity of illness, pre-ICU length of stay and percentage of patients requiring mechanical ventilation [22].

Staffing patterns, in terms of in-house, overnight coverage, also vary widely [23]. The benefits of around-the-clock (versus business hours) in-house intensivist coverage is uncertain, despite outcome differences documented as a function of ICU admission time and day of week [24–28]. At the hospital level, there is no statistically significant mortality difference based on time of admission for most (77%) diagnoses [29], including acute myocardial infarction, congestive heart failure, pneumonia, stroke, gastrointestinal bleeding, and many surgical conditions. Mortality was higher, though, in patients with ruptured abdominal aortic aneurysms, acute epiglottitis, and pulmonary embolus, when these patients presented on the weekend. This suggests that for at least some conditions, adverse effects occur because of decreased weekend staffing, lack of patient familiarity with cross-coverage, and perhaps less supervision. Around-the-clock intensivist coverage may reduce severity-adjusted mortality [30] but there is debate if the on-site physicians need to be intensivists, especially given the current shortage of specialists [31]. Introduction of continuous on-site intensivists improves processes of care and staff satisfaction, and decreases ICU complications and hospital length of stay [32].

Remote intensive care, using a telemedicine approach, has been proposed as a partial solution to the shortage of intensivists. Using intensivists and physician extenders to provide supplemental monitoring and management of ICU patients between noon and 7 AM, Breslow et al. were able to demonstrate reductions in hospital mortality (RR 0.73), ICU length of stay (3.63 vs. 4.35 days) and lower variable costs per case [33]. Given the critical care shortage of intensivists, tele–ICU systems can potentially permit these specialists to monitor more patients, and those patients who might not otherwise have access to an intensivist. Despite the shortage of data, Leapfrog Group and the University Health System Consortium have encouraged the application of tele-ICU [34]. Results from the first federally funded multicenter evaluation of tele-ICU of approximately 4,000 patients from before and after activation of a tele-ICU did not demonstrate any differences in adjusted hospital and ICU mortality, length of stay or ICU complications with telemedicine intervention [35]. Of interest, improved survival rates were observed in the sicker population while mortality for less severely ill patients was increased. A major limitation of this multicenter trial include limited authority delegated to the tele-ICU by the majority of attending physicians; that is choosing to limit the remote specialists to monitoring rather than direct intervention authority. In addition, the inability to share the ICU electronic medical records with the central facility could have potentially delayed implementation of tele-ICU orders. The mixed outcome benefit of telemedicine for the ICU noted in recent trials [36] may indicate that the actual mechanisms of implementing telemedicine in ICU may play a significant role as to its effectiveness. Understanding and identifying local hospital wide operations including ICU staffing levels, evaluation of standardized care processes if any and availability of computerized order entry capability may help identify which ICUs benefit from tele-ICU.

A hospital's approach to ICU organization will depend on its patient population, existing professional talent, physical facilities, and economies of scale. Reimbursement for critical care and evaluation/management services typically cannot cover the cost of a dedicated intensivist in smaller units. Triage functions and general management of the unit (as opposed to management of individual patients) cannot be billed to patients, and thus does not generate professional revenue. However, there is ample evidence that hospital investment in physician intensivist services is recouped with better patient flow (reducing the need for additional ICU beds) and lower utilization of pharmacy, laboratory, and radiology services. Simply having an intensive care physician round daily on postoperative patients shortens LOS, reduces complications and lowers total hospital cost in patients undergoing esophageal resection [37] or abdominal aortic surgery [38]. Organizational restructuring of a cardiothoracic unit with an attending physician dedicated to ICU care resulted in reduced pharmacy, radiology, and laboratory utilization, and a per-patient decrease in hospital costs of $2,285 [39]. Pronovost et al. developed a financial model for 6-, 12-, and 18-bed intensive care units for hospitals transitioning over a 1-year period to the Leapfrog Group ICU physician staffing standard. Cost savings ranged from $510,000 to $3.3 million, depending on bed size [40]. Their best-case scenario results could generate up to $13 million in annual savings, while a worst-case scenario imposed net costs of $1.3 million.

PHYSICIAN HUMAN RESOURCE ISSUES

Hiring full-time critical care specialists is already a challenge with the growing shortage of intensivists. Critical care work force needs have not been adequately addressed by public policy [41]. Medicare payments often do not cover the costs of providing critical care [42,43]. Angus et al. predicted in 2000 that supply and demand of intensivists would remain in equilibrium until 2007, but that demand would subsequently grow, producing serious shortfalls by 2020 [44]. The Society of Critical Care Medicine conducted a survey of 731 critical care physicians in 2004. These respondents planned to retire at an average age of 62 years, and to change focus or reduce patient load beginning in their fifties [45]. Nearly 40% of the respondents were already over the age of 45. Their average workweek was 66 hours, with a typical shift of 10 to 12 hours, providing clinical care an average of 48 weeks per year. It is unclear that the next generation of intensivists will continue to work at this level of intensity, or that critical care will be a viable career choice when remuneration is better for specialties with shorter working hours and less stress.

Current Leapfrog Group standards call for *in-house* intensivist staffing for a minimum of 8 hours, 7 days per week [13,46] or ≥2,920 hours per year to cover one ICU, with requirements for off-hours coverage met by an intensivist on beeper call, with an FCCS-certified physician or physician extender immediately available in-house. Hospitalists with FCCS certification can also potentially provide off-hours ICU coverage. In a retrospective study of care provided during after-hours coverage of a pediatric intensive care unit, Tenner et al. found improved survival with hospitalists compared with housestaff [47].

It is helpful to consider the concept of a clinical full-time equivalent (FTE) to represent the amount of work done by one individual working only on direct patient-care tasks in the intensive unit. In reality, some ICU clinicians will also allocate professional time to research, administration, or education; choose to work part time, or spend part of their clinical time on the trauma team, in the pulmonary clinic, or administering anesthesia. A full-time physician working only in the ICU might have grant funding for 0.25 FTE, and another 0.25 stipend for administrative and educational activity, leaving 0.5 FTE for ICU clinical activity.

How many hours will one FTE work in a year? The SCCM respondents' reports annual work hours from less than 1,000 to more than 4,000, but most commonly 2,000 to 2,500 hours [44]. Since attractive jobs currently offer at least 4 weeks vacation, about 10 paid holidays and at least 5 days of meeting time, we'll consider annual work to be 45 weeks with 10-hour days, yielding 2,250 hours, in accord with the range reported in the SCCM survey. If in-house coverage for the ICU is around-the-clock, 365 days per year, with 30 minutes overlap at the beginning and end of 12-hour shifts, then annual hours to be covered are 9,490. Thus, 4.2 FTEs would be needed to cover the clinical workload. This workload might be met by five physicians, assuming each worked full time and 0.8 FTE was sufficient to attend to administrative and quality assurance activities. If coverage is only during the daytime (3,650 hours per year) fewer FTEs would be required; although on-call hours must still be staffed.

Staffing calculations must consider intensivist-to-patient staffing ratios, which are not well-defined. In England and Wales, where intensivists staff 80% of ICU's, the average six-bed general ICU has three consultants committed to the unit, and another three consultants participating in the on-call rotation [48]. A retrospective study from the Mayo Clinic [49] did not find differences in the severity-adjusted mortality rate at daytime intensivist-to-bed ratios between 1:7.5 and 1:15 although ICU length of stay increased at the higher extreme. Larger hospitals with closed units may take advantage of cross-coverage between units, providing daytime care at intensivist to patient ratios of 1:8 to 1:12; and increasing the ratio during off-hours when there are fewer acute interventions or procedures to be accomplished.

MULTIDISCIPLINARY MODELS: PHYSICIAN EXTENDERS

The enormous work force requirements and economic burdens of providing round-the-clock critical care staffing has led physician leaders, hospital administrators, and insurance companies to re-examine models of health care delivery. Some medical centers now employ physician extenders on the critical care team as a response to physician shortage at both the attending and house-staff level. Physician extender is a broad term covering mid-level health care providers such as nurse practitioners (NPs) and physician assistants (PAs). Physician assistants must complete an accredited education program, usually 2 years in duration, but often requiring prior college and health care experience. PAs must pass a national examination to obtain a license, and always work under a physician's supervision. A nurse practitioner is a registered nurse who has completed advanced training and must be licensed in the state where practicing. Following state licensure, NPs may seek national certification from professional nursing boards and/or pursue specialty certification. NPs have more latitude to practice independently.

Driving forces that have accelerated employment of the physician extenders include cutbacks in federal funding for residency training, identifiable patient care needs, and ACGME standards placing strict limits to the number of hours that medical trainees can participate in providing care. Physician extenders can provide safe and cost-effective care as part of a collaborative medical management team in acute care settings and they are well received by patients, nurses, physicians, and administrators. A limited number of studies suggest that introduction of NP/intensivist team-based care is beneficial to patient outcomes, financial outcomes, length of stay, and patient satisfaction [50]. An attending physician/NP team can safely manage former ICU patients admitted to a subacute unit therefore allowing the intensivist/fellow team time to care for higher acuity ICU patients [51]. Decreased overall length of stay and ICU length of stay, lower rates of UTI and skin breakdown, and a shorter time to mobilization have been documented after introduction of an NP team to neuroscience ICUs [52]. NP participation in weaning protocols for mechanical ventilation has been associated with greater reductions in mechanical ventilation days, ICU length of stay, and hospital length of stay when compared to pre-NP participation [53]. NPs and physicians in training had equivalent efficacies in performing required tasks but residents spend more time in nonunit activities (lectures, rounds) and NPs spend more time monitoring patients, talking to families, and collaborating with other health team members [54].

A team-oriented culture characterized by timely communication is associated with a shorter length of ICU stay, greater ability to accommodate the needs of patient families, and a higher quality of technical care [55]. Including PAs on housestaff-directed ICU teams does not appear to affect rates of occupancy, mortality, or complications [56].

Intensive care services are among the most urgent and costly aspects of healthcare in the United States, and national surveys indicate the need to accommodate about 50,000 patients a day [43]. Professional societies are projecting an inability to meet this demand with intensivists, so the role of physician extenders will need to be further examined as a major component of the healthcare delivery model for critically ill patients.

ROLE OF THE ICU DIRECTOR

The Joint Commission on Accreditation of Health Care Organizations (JCAHO) requires that an individual be designated as the ICU Director, but actual job descriptions vary. At one extreme, the medical director may simply approve critical care policies and serve as a resource for questions that cannot be solved by nursing administration. He or she may triage only in times of high census, and may have very little role in the delivery of critical care, other than to his or her own patients. At the other extreme, the medical director may lead the team of intensivists that assumes total responsibility for all patients occupying ICU beds. Nonclinical duties may consume more work effort than clinical responsibilities when committee membership, administrative tasks, budget preparation, educational activities, and the business of running the ICU physician practice are included. When the medical director is heavily involved in day-to-day operations, ICU occupancy rates and number of patients misallocated to ICU beds decline [57]. ICU admission decisions are only part of the triage function. One in six patients experience ICU discharge issues (unexpected medical deterioration, level of care issues, administrative problems [58]) that demand executive resolution.

Larger hospitals typically have multiple intensive care units, each with its own director. The directors or designees may participate in a hospital-wide Critical Care Committee that sets overall policies and procedures. In some units, the medical director may delegate administrative tasks, quality improvement, education, and research to associate medical directors. Typically, the ICU director(s) will have a close working relationship with the nursing unit manager in each unit. Multidisciplinary units will involve interaction with other professionals (pharmacists, dieticians, social workers, clergy, utilization management specialists) and the medical director may have an overall coordinating role. Essential character traits of the successful ICU director include willingness to collaborate, ability to delegate, trust in colleagues, and excellent communication skills.

Tasks performed by the ICU Director can best be divided into strategic versus tactical (Table 208.1). Strategic tasks involve the "big picture": recognition of patterns and trends, setting priorities, considering alternatives, and implementing change. The ICU Director is often the champion for process improvement projects. Areas deserving of strategic consideration include cost containment, the overall culture of the ICU, quality improvement efforts, education of physicians, nurses and other health professionals, and coping with change driven by ICU, hospital and external factors [59]. Developing a strategic vision and communicating it well are essential roles. Yet, it is equally important to lead by example, particularly when it comes time to drive change, such as implementing electronic medical records or computerized physician order entry.

TABLE 208.1

STRATEGIC VERSUS TACTICAL DUTIES OF THE ICU DIRECTOR

Strategic	Tactical
Creating ICU vision and mission statement	Conflict resolution, communicating vision
Evaluating and improving quality of care	Implementing care "bundles" and protocols
Right-sizing physician workload	Hiring new staff; creating call schedule
Fostering interdisciplinary relationships	Interdisciplinary rounds. Joint conferences
Planning for the future	Budgeting; space and equipment needs
Delivering value	Specific cost-containment initiatives
Economic self-sufficiency of practice	Monthly review of financial statements
Professional development	Physician and nursing education
Efficient resource management	Bed triage: written policies
Exploiting advanced technology	Implementing electronic medical records

Tactical chores consist of the day-to-day, "hands-on" running of the unit. Leaving aside patient care, which in itself can fill the day, there are issues of personnel coordination, patient triage, bed allocation, and conflict resolution [60]. The ICU director is often granted by hospital policy the authority to intervene in any patient's care, and may be charged with evaluating issues and complaints that originate from family members, nursing staff, other physicians, or hospital administration. Tools to assist with the tactical aspects of patient care include checklists [61] and computerized systems. The danger is that tactical chores multiply to occupy all available time, leaving little time for strategic direction. Implementation of computerized order sets, therapist-directed protocols, and other "bundles" of care help to minimize the individual, routine tactical decisions, and leave more time for strategic thinking.

The difference between strategy and tactics reflects the difference between leading and managing. Applied to academic teaching rounds as an example, the residents or physician assistants should be patient managers responding to the information flow of physical exam findings, laboratory tests, and radiology reports. They collect and analyze this data, and develop a daily or even hourly plan. In contrast, the attending physician or fellow should not get lost in the details, but rather should be planning at a higher level exactly what broad changes and interventions will be required to get the patient recovered and discharged from the unit. It is difficult to concentrate on both tactics and strategy at the same time, which argues for dividing the effort with a team approach. The strategic leader should not be isolated from patient contact, however, for it is the experienced interpretation of clues and subtleties that define the expert [62].

The job responsibilities of the ICU Director (and by delegation, the triage physician of the day) create an inherent conflict of interest. A treating physician's fiduciary responsibility is to advocate for an individual patient's best interest. As the ICU manager, however, there is a responsibility to do the most good for the greatest number of patients. The essence of triage is to maximize benefits for the group, even at the expense of an individual. In times of bed shortages, the ethical principle of beneficence ("do good") conflicts with the ethical principle of social justice. For example, a 92-year-old patient has a cardiac arrest at home, and arrives intubated and ventilated in the emergency room with fixed pupils but slight respiratory effort. Although the outcome is uncertain, it certainly does not look promising. Should the last remaining ICU bed go to this patient who is unlikely to survive, if it means refusing a complex hospital transfer, canceling an operating room procedure, or denying ICU admission to a septic patient on a regular nursing floor? These ethical issues are discussed elsewhere in this text, but it is essential for the ICU director to recognize these conflicts and preemptively construct ICU and hospital policy to address how such conflicts are to be handled.

BUDGET AND PROFESSIONAL REIMBURSEMENT ISSUES

The ICU director may be responsible for managing the budget of the entire critical care unit, including the nursing and respiratory therapy components, but if so, will usually have administrative assistance. More typically, the division chief in an academic ICU or the director of a practice group will be particularly concerned with revenue from physician professional activity. Particular attention must be paid to actual revenue received since the net collected will always be less than gross professional billing, a problem that is increasingly worse with the current system for physician payment based on the Medicare sustainable growth rate [63].

In the United States, critical care revenue is generated by billing critical care codes (CPT code 99291 and 99292) when the patient qualifies for time-based bedside critical care, or otherwise for Evaluation and Management Codes (typically CPT code 99232–33 for subsequent hospital care, and 99251–53 inpatient consultation) [64,65]. Various procedures have specific codes, and each code is associated with relative value units (RVU) that form the basis for eventual payment. Further information on CPT coding is available on the AMA Web site [66] and through the American College of Chest Physicians [67], among other sources. The relationship between total RVU and CPT codes change over time. For example, insertion of a pulmonary artery catheter generated 3.79 total facility RVU in 2006, but only 3.08 RVU in 2009. On the other hand, CPT 99291 (Critical Care, first hour) was worth 5.99 RVU in 2009, up from 5.48 in 2006. Despite the 9% increase in RVU for this code, however, reimbursement only increased a little over 1%. Critical care physicians must constantly monitor the coding and reimbursement landscape. As of January 1, 2010, the Center for Medicare and Medicaid services (CMS) eliminated all inpatient and outpatient consultation codes. It is anticipated that other insurance carriers may adopt these changes going forward, but as of this writing, consultation codes are still valid for most non-CMS claims. In the interim, providers (or their billing offices) have to pay careful attention to how claims are submitted, depending on a patient's insurance status. Demonstration projects are already underway to move away from RVU piece-work to a global, or bundled, payment system [68].

The connection between RVU generation and effort in the ICU setting in any case is tenuous at best, in part due to the difficulty in documenting and billing the multitude of small tasks accomplished over the course of the day. The bulk of billable services may occur during the normal business day. Thirty-one to seventy-four minutes of bedside attention to one patient will justify a single CPT 99291 code. Additional services rendered to that patient throughout a 24-hour period would have to exceed 74 total minutes to additionally bill CPT 99292. As a result, off-hours interventions may generate less income than what it costs to staff those hours, although revenue will depend on the number of patients seen, their severity of illness, and the reimbursement rate for a particular locale. In many institutions, revenue received may be 50% or less of what was actually billed, owing to indigent patients and contractual agreements with insurers. Thus, under systems of reimbursement used in the United States, it may not be possible for a critical care physician group to be self-funding on patient care revenue alone especially when providing extended hours of in-house coverage.

The ICU director plays an increasingly important role in managing the business aspects of the critical care practice. It is helpful to have a tracking system to ensure that each physician is submitting his or her patient care charges in a timely manner, and that the billing service is properly submitting and capturing these charges. On a monthly basis, patient care volume, charges submitted and relative value units (RVU) should be reviewed and compared with budgeted amounts. Individual physician performance by billing code should be tracked, not only for productivity, but also to ensure that codes are being used appropriately and in line with the practice's usual profile. It would be unusual for all patients to qualify for critical care codes; some percentage of patients may only qualify for E&M billing, with or without additional procedures. Periodic internal audits help confirm physician compliance with Medicare and insurer billing rules; it is easier and less costly to identify and rectify any issues internally. The alternative may be an external audit, where any errors detected in a small sample of charts will be applied proportionately over a multiyear period to demand a large retrospective repayment for billing errors. A provision in the 2009 American Recovery and Reinvestment Act of 2009 mandates annual fraud and abuse training for health care providers.

The Centers for Medicare and Medicaid Services (CMS) have recently implemented a Recovery Audit Contractor (RAC) program to review billing and identify over- and underpayment [69]. Four regional auditing firms will be paid on a contingency basis to review medical record documentation, especially the diagnostic specificity of admitting and discharge diagnoses, listings of comorbidities, and evidence of medical necessity as patients transition from care environments (operating room, recovery room, emergency department, inpatient vs. observation status). Service level is likely to drive reimbursement more than patient location. The coding of diagnosis-related groups (DRGs) will come under particular scrutiny. DRGs likely to trigger review include many common ICU conditions including sepsis (versus infection alone); acute respiratory failure (versus acute systolic or diastolic heart failure), pneumonia, chest pain, and stroke (versus transient ischemic attack).

ICU directors are frequently asked to represent the ICU on multiple hospital committees, particularly pharmacy and therapeutics, informatics oversight, quality improvement, peer-review, and technology assessment. Depending on the hospital's structure, the ICU director may report to the chair of Medicine, Surgery, or Anesthesia (or all three!) and frequently interact with Emergency Medicine, Obstetrics, Radiology, Laboratory Medicine, Clinical Engineering, Information Systems, Risk Management, and Nursing. A "virtual" critical care department can monitor and manage all critical care activities, while retaining a traditional academic reporting structure [70]. Responsibilities of the ICU director include developing a team performance framework for the unit [71], and addressing the physical, emotional and professional elements that create an attractive and rewarding ICU work environment [9]. These communication and collaboration activities take time, and, not surprisingly, administrative and other non-patient care activities may consume 50% or more of the ICU Director's work hours. Since this time is not revenue generating, these activities must be supported by other means such as a hospital stipend.

MONITORING CLINICAL CARE

Good structure (attributes of the setting in which care occurs) facilitates good process (what is actually done), which promotes good outcome (or results) [72]. Although the JCAHO historically focused on structural elements such as medical staff organization, available equipment, and human resources, emphasis has now shifted to analysis of process and outcome. Performance variables (appropriateness and effectiveness of care) may offer advantages over outcome variables for ICU evaluation, but are less well developed [73]. Most benchmarking currently takes place by outcome assessment, commonly using mortality and resource utilization as endpoints. Because patients present with different levels of disease and physiologic reserve, raw outcome measures such as mortality must be adjusted for severity of illness [74]. For the ICU, tools include the Acute Physiology and Chronic Health Evaluation (APACHE) system [75–77], and the Mortality Probability Models (MPM) [78,79]; the Simplified Acute Physiology Score (SAPS) [80,81], and the Intensive Care National Audit and Research Centre (ICNARC) model [82]. These systems are based on large databases, report acceptable discrimination and calibration, and have been extensively examined in the peer-reviewed literature. However, only a minority of hospitals (about 10% of acute care hospitals in the United States) consistently collect this type of data. Although APACHE and MPM are generally used in North America, SAPS in Europe, and ICNARC in Great Britain, models can be employed in any location as long as the model is recalibrated for the local environment [83].

ICU severity models facilitate comparisons between intensive care units, and are most useful for retrospective analysis of performance, with limited but improving utility for real-time management. (APACHE, for example, offers a "bed-board" that displays both current severity of illness and daily predictions for mortality, discharge, and next-day resource utilization but unless this is interfaced to the electronic medical record, updates depend on coordinators entering updated information.) Project IMPACT (which uses the MPM prediction model) and the APACHE system each carefully define data elements and outcomes to be collected, and thus facilitate comparison of local outcomes with national data. APACHE provides the ability to run local comparison reports on an ad hoc basis; comparison reports from Project IMPACT are centrally generated on a quarterly schedule. APACHE, SAPS, and MPM have all recently transitioned from models based on 1990's data to updated versions that reflect changes and improvement in medical practice over the past 15 years [76,78,80].

An APACHE IV score comprises the Acute Physiology Score ("APS," see later), age, and chronic health items. The APS is generated by summing point values based on physiologic derangement in 17 variables and then adding points for age and chronic health status [76]. The APS is interpreted in light of the main patient diagnosis, patient location, and duration of hospital stay prior to admission to the ICU. Mechanical ventilation during the first ICU day and emergency surgical status also influence an individual's predicted mortality. Although the error bars around the mortality estimate are modestly large for any individual patient, the APACHE system has been shown to be quite reliable at assessing outcome for groups of patients [76]. APACHE IV is also useful for assessing ICU length of stay in groups of patients even though utility is limited for individuals [84].

Project IMPACT, developed by the Society of Critical Care Medicine, began collecting data in 1996 and providing benchmarking with the MPM-II model, SAPS-II, and APACHE II. Beginning in 2007, Project IMPACT transitioned to the updated MPM-III model [85]. Project IMPACT data collectors must pass a certification examination to access the data entry module. The MPM-III model has been prospectively validated using recent Project IMPACT data from 55,459 patients at 103 participating ICU's in North America [86]. As of this writing, plans are underway to consolidate the APACHE system and Project IMPACT into a single critical care information system that will take advantage of the ease and immediacy of the MPM score (generated on admission) with the more detailed, disease-specific predictions of the APACHE system at 24 hours and beyond.

Specialized scoring systems are more appropriate for pediatric [87], trauma [88,89], or cardiac surgical units [90]. Pediatric scoring (e.g., PRISM) differs from adult scoring due to expected differences in normal physiologic ranges. Cardiac surgical systems downplay acute physiology, which is deliberately controlled by the operating room team, and emphasize variables such as left ventricular function, IABP use, and cardiopulmonary bypass (CPB) time that might not be available or clinically relevant in other patient groups. Performance of the general severity models deteriorates when case-mix in an ICU becomes skewed [91]. APACHE-IV accommodates case-mix differences by including disease-specific coefficients. MPM-III provides sub-group models for use when an individual ICU's case-mix is skewed from average [92], although the general model is essentially as good as specialized models for identifying outliers.

The primary clinical limitation of all outcome-adjustment models is that they apply to analysis of outcome in groups of patients, but not when making individual therapeutic decisions. At best, the prognostic estimates for an individual patient may be used in a probabilistic manner to predict bed or other resource utilization, but could be inaccurate if applied as a prediction for application or denial of individual medical therapy, because of the uncertainty of individual estimates. A patient's risk will change over time, making it problematic, for example, to use the admission severity score to determine eligibility for later therapy [42]. In fact, ICU physicians discriminate between survivors and non-survivors more accurately than scoring systems, at least in the initial 24 hours of care [93].

Groups of patients can be compared by generating predicted mortality rates with APACHE, ICNARC, MPM, or SAPS as a tool, and comparing the prediction with actual results. The ratio of observed mortality to predicted mortality is called standardized mortality ratio (SMR), and an ICU with a SMR close to 1.0 would be exhibiting expected performance based on their case-mix of patients. SMRs significantly greater than 1 indicate a higher than expected mortality whereas SMRs less than 1 suggest outcomes better than expected. The sample size and distribution of patient acuities will determine exactly how far from 1.0 (in either direction) the SMR becomes significant.

Events and therapy prior to ICU admission that alter physiology at admission creates a "lead time" bias which has a measurable effect on outcome [75,94]. Because the SMR will be affected by differing use of postacute facilities and the percentage of patients with DNR orders, it may not always be valid in interhospital comparisons, unless applied to similar types of hospitals with similar policies [95].

Both clinical performance and cost-effectiveness should be considered when defining high-quality ICU care [96]. Rapoport and Teres initially described a method, since updated [97] that graphically displays both severity-adjusted clinical outcome and cost-effectiveness, using weighted hospital days as a proxy for cost. With this method, normalized severity-adjusted mortality is displayed on the x axis, and normalized weighted hospital days on the y axis (Fig. 208.1). Standard deviations of the normalized scale are displayed relative to the group mean at the origin (0,0). Units performing significantly better than predicted for both dimensions of care will chart in the right upper quadrant of the graph.

CRITICAL CARE OUTREACH SERVICE AND EARLY WARNING SYSTEMS

Illness is commonly heralded by a constellation of quantifiable changes in physiologic and biochemical measurements. Abnormal values of selected physiologic measurements are useful as an objective indication of a patient's risk level (as with severity scores) but may also be used "real-time" to predict subsequent clinical deterioration on hospital wards. In theory, if hospital staff were to identify and provide intervention to these patients at an earlier stage, outcomes could improve, in terms of reduced intensive care admissions and length of stay. Critical Care outreach services include the employment of a Rapid Response Team (RRT) and/or an Early Warning System (EWS) to identify and provide intervention to potentially deteriorating hospitalized patients. The fundamental concept behind the evolution of Critical Care Outreach Programs is that significant vital sign abnormalities occur in many patients in the hours prior to acute cardiorespiratory events [98,99]

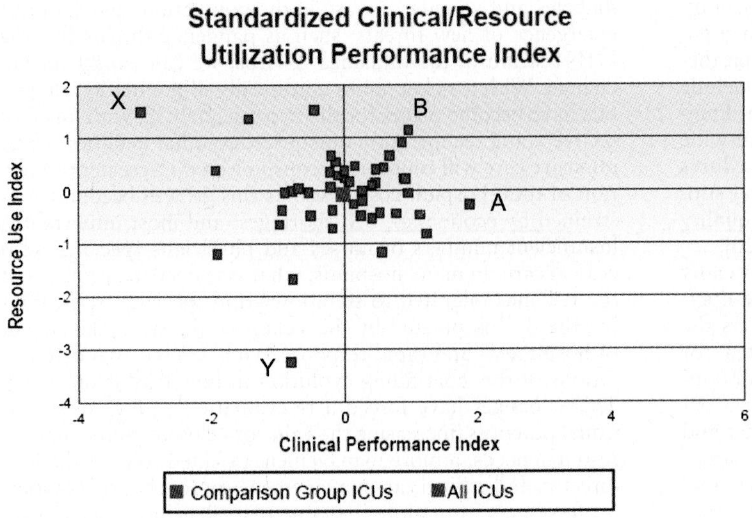

FIGURE 208.1. Standardized Clinical/Resource Utilization Performance Index. Hospital A has superior risk-adjusted mortality, while hospital B has superior risk-adjusted length-of-stay. Both hospitals are in the desirable right upper quadrant. Hospital X has a short length of stay, but coupled with risk-adjusted mortality that is worse than predicted. Hospital Y has length-of-stay issues while remaining within the expected severity-adjusted mortality range.

Analysis postimplementation of a RRT model of care (also called Medical Emergency Team or MET) on hospital wards demonstrates 17% to 50% fewer cardiorespiratory arrests [97,98,100]. The composition of a RRT/MET varies by hospital but frequently includes an ICU nurse and/or physician, a hospitalist, and a respiratory therapist. The Institute for Healthcare Improvement has recommended that hospitals establish RRTs as one of the six strategies of the 100,000 Lives Campaign [101]. Though the purpose of the RRT is to reduce preventable deaths [102], evidence supporting their effectiveness remains controversial [103–105]. Clinical trial results have suffered from methodologic limitations, varying staffing models, and limited number of randomized control trials. A recent trial could not document reductions in hospital-wide code rates or mortality but did demonstrate fewer cardiorespiratory arrests outside the ICU [106]. It is possible that the RRT involvement may propel end-of-life discussions in patients on the wards that might otherwise not have taken place. Further comprehensive investigations of the expanding RRT model will require better data on hospital characteristics, assessment of patient–family satisfaction, assessment of end-of-life issues, and nursing and physician satisfaction on the wards.

EWS incorporate technology to provide earlier identification of patients at risk of clinical deterioration on general hospital wards [107,108]. Although clinicians generally excel at detecting acute change, incremental changes in vital signs may not be clinically apparent, but become obvious using tracking software. A "track and trigger" EWS is designed to secure the timely presence of skilled clinical assistance by the bedside of patients exhibiting physiologic signs compatible with impending critical illness [109]. Although RRT responses might be triggered by a single dramatic physiologic vital sign change, EWS responds to simultaneous multiple parameters using patterns of subtle alterations in vital signs to identify patients at risk [110]. An automated EWS score is calculated from a handful of traditional physiologic parameters (mental status, heart rate, blood pressure, respiratory rate, temperature, urine output) recorded with traditional bedside or electronic charting [111]. Several readings over time may be more informative than isolated recordings. Newer bedside physiologic monitors (for example, Philips MP Series with ProtocolWatch) [112] can automate this process without requiring a full electronic medical record. Although recent data indicates that EWS integrating information from multiple physiologic variables is better at detecting physiologic instability [113], the diversity and methodologic limitations of most studies to date limit the ability to interpret the effectiveness of EWS application in hospitals.

Failure to identify clinical emergencies may be becoming more frequent as sick patients cannot always be accommodated in critical care units. High-quality multicenter research will be needed to determine the most appropriate triggers for activation of the EWS and/or RRTs and the effect of these interventions on patient outcomes. Because EWS and RRT deployment will affect ICU resource utilization, ICU leaders need to be involved in planning, implementing, and maintaining these systems.

OPERATIONAL ISSUES

Nursing staffing levels are now subject to public scrutiny, and literature supports a link between staffing levels and patient outcome. Excessive nursing workload has been shown to correlate with increased mortality [114], longer hospital length of stay and increased complications [60], and the spread of resistant bacterial organisms in the ICU [115]. Adverse events have been reported to occur in about 20% of critically ill patients, with roughly half reportedly being preventable [116]. The most common cause of an adverse event is failure to carry out intended treatment correctly, often because of miscommunication or poor coordination of care [117]. Some hospitals have explored crew resource management training, adapted from the aviation industry, to improve team collaboration and coordination, and ultimately improve patient safety. The medical director, in conjunction with the nurse manager and other professionals, will play a major role in defining and maintaining the organizational culture of the ICU. Disruptive physician behavior adversely affects nursing retention [118] and occasionally will require the intervention of the medical director, perhaps with the assistance of the hospital's Physician Health or Medical Staff Health committee. Effective teamwork is essential, and team leadership is vital in promoting team interaction and coordination [70].

Interdisciplinary communication is fostered by a number of formal and informal efforts. At a basic level, the format for daily ICU rounds should encourage all members of the team to contribute information, ask questions, and make suggestions for the direction of care. Formal multidisciplinary rounds, often held weekly, are useful when discussing the needs of long-term patients in the ICU, and offer an opportunity to step back from acute physiologic concerns to collect additional insight from allied health professional, social service and clergy. Conferences, journal club, lectures, and research projects offer opportunities for beneficial interdisciplinary interaction. Some hospitals have established a Critical Care Practice Committee (CCPC), composed of physician and nursing representatives from each intensive care unit, the emergency department, and the postanesthesia recovery unit. Members of this committee may also include representatives from Pharmacy, Central Supply, Clinical Engineering, Respiratory Therapy, and Purchasing. A hospital-wide CCPC facilitates standardization of policies and procedures [69,119], implementation of care bundles, decisions on supplies to be stocked, maintenance of "Code" carts, and quality improvement initiatives relevant to the membership [120].

Patient families deserve special consideration; especially since the family is likely to notice and appreciate the operational efficiencies and communication style that reflects the ICUs culture. A multicenter evaluation of a scoring system for family satisfaction [121] identifies the key components for family satisfaction as assurance (the need to feel hope for a desired outcome), proximity (the need for personal contact and to be physically and emotionally near the patient), information (which should be consistent, realistic and timely), personal comfort, and support (resources, support systems and ventilation). Written materials (booklets, information sheets) can help meet family informational needs, especially with older, better educated relatives [122].

SUMMARY

Economic considerations continue to drive the agenda in hospitals and intensive care units, and with the wave of "baby boomers" reaching retirement, increasing incidence of obesity, diabetes and vascular disease in the population, and sporadic emergence of new threats, such as pandemic threats like the H1N1 strain of the Influenza A virus, we can expect further change. With a sicker, more chronically ill population, hospitals have become places for the hyper-acutely ill, with much of recovery and recuperation outsourced to other facilities. Thus, intensive care will continue to consume an ever-greater proportion of total hospital costs, even as this growth becomes constrained by economics, bed shortages, and most importantly, insufficient numbers of nurses and physicians specializing in critical care. In many hospitals, what was once the province of the ICU has migrated to step-down and specialty units, leaving the ICU populated by the sickest of the sick. The advent of hospitalists and rapid response teams are but two manifestations of this continuing evolution in how care is delivered. These changes have forced a re-evaluation of ICU organizational practices (increasing the value of "closed" units), human resource needs, a more management oriented role for the ICU director, and critical care management approaches that involve professionals from more than one ICU. Benchmarking critical care outcome becomes essential in managing the increasingly complex world of the ICU, and we are on the threshold of having computerized real-time systems to automate some of the tactical decisions that occupy too much professional time. Telemedicine, increased automation, use of physician extenders and protocol supported care are all potential solutions to the impending crisis in critical care delivery. Continued change emphasizes the need for clinically and managerially competent physicians to organize and manage the increasingly complex world of critical care.

References

1. Bartlett B: Health Care: Costs and reform. Available at: www.forbes.com/2009/07/02/health-care-costs-opinions-columnists-reform_print.html. Accessed September 4, 2009.
2. Angood PB: Right care, right now—you can make a difference. *Crit Care Med* 33:2729–2780, 2005.
3. Halpern NA, Pastores SM, Greenstein RJ: Critical care medicine in the United States 1985–2000: An analysis of bed numbers, use, and costs. *Crit Care Med* 32:1254–1259, 2004.
4. Bloomfield EL: The impact of economics on changing medical technology with reference to critical care medicine in the United State. *Anesth Analg* 96:418–425, 2003.
5. Milbrandt EB, Kersten A, Rahim M, et al: Growth of intensive care unit resource use and its estimated cost in Medicare. *Crit Care Med* 36:2505–2510, 2008.
6. Halpern NA, Pastores SM, Thaler HT, et al: Critical care medicine use and cost among Medicare beneficiaries 1995–2000: major discrepancies between two United States federal Medicare databases. *Crit Care Med* 35:692–699, 2007.
7. Social Security and Medicare Boards of Trustees: Status of the Social Security and Medicare Programs: A summary of the 2009 Annual Reports. Social Security Online. Available at: http://www.ssa.gov/OACT/TRSUM/index.html. Accessed September 4, 2009.
8. Kelley MA, Angus D, Chalfin DB, et al: The critical care crisis in the United States: a report from the profession. *Chest* 125:1514–1517, 2004.
9. Alameddine M, Dainty KN, Deber R, et al: The intensive care unit work environment: current challenges and recommendations for the future. *J Crit Care* 24:243–248, 2009.
10. Bekes CE, Dellinger RP, Brooks D, et al: Critical care medicine as a distinct product line with substantial financial profitability: The role of business planning. *Crit Care Med* 32:1207–1214, 2004.
11. Goleman D: What makes a leader? Harvard Business Review, November–December 1998.
12. American College of Physician Executives: Available at: http://www.acpe.org/ACPEHome/index.aspx. Accessed September 5, 2009.
13. Leapfrog Group Web site: Available at: http://www.leapfroggroup.org. Accessed February 17, 2006.
14. Pronovost PJ, Angus DC, Dorman TD, et al: Physician staffing patterns and clinical outcomes in critically ill patients: a systematic review. *JAMA* 288:2151–2162, 2002.
15. Levy MM, Rapoport J, Lemeshow S, et al: Association between critical care physician management and patient mortality in the intensive care unit. *Ann Intern Med* 148:801–809, 2008.
16. Higgins TL, Nathanson B, Teres D: What conclusions should be drawn between critical care physician management and patient mortality in the ICU? *Ann Intern Med* 149:767, 2008.
17. Marik P, Myburgh J, Annane D, et al: What conclusions should be drawn between critical care physician management and patient mortality in the ICU? *Ann Intern Med* 149:770–771, 2008.
18. Metnitz PG, Reiter A, Jordan B, et al: More interventions do not necessarily improve outcome in critically ill patients. *Intensive Care Med* 30:1586–1593, 2004.
19. Topeli A, Laghi F, Tobin MJ: Effect of closed unit policy and appointing an intensivist in a developing country. *Crit Care Med* 33:299–306, 2005.
20. Carson SS, Stocking C, Podsadecki T, et al: Effect of organizational change in the medical intensive care unit of a teaching hospital: a comparison of "open" and "closed" formats. *JAMA* 276:322–328, 1996.
21. Multz AS, Chalfin DB, Samson IM, et al: A "closed" medical intensive care unit (MICU) improves resource utilization when compared with an "open" MICU. *Am J Respir Crit Care Med* 157:1468–1473, 1998.
22. Higgins TL, McGee WT, Steingrub JS, et al: Early indicators of prolonged intensive care unit stay: impact of illness severity, physician staffing, and pre-intensive care unit length of stay. *Crit Care Med* 31:45–51, 2003.
23. Parshuram CS, Kirpalani H, Mehta S, et al: In-house, overnight physician staffing: a cross-sectional survey of Canadian adult and pediatric intensive care units. *Crit Care Med* 34:1674–1678, 2006.
24. Barnett MJ, Kaboli PJ, Sirio CA, et al: Day of the week of intensive care admission and patient outcomes: a multisite regional evaluation. *Med Care* 40:530–539, 2002.
25. Uusaro A, Kari A, Ruokonen E: The effects of ICU admission and discharge times on mortality in Finland. *Intensive Care Med* 29:2144–2148, 2003.
26. Wunsch H, Mapstone J, Brady T, et al: Hospital mortality associated with day and time of admission to intensive care units. *Intensive Care Med* 30:895–901, 2004.
27. Morales IJ, Peters SG, Afessa B: Hospital mortality rate and length of stay in patients admitted at night to the intensive care unit. *Crit Care Med* 31:858–863, 2003.
28. Ensminger SA, Morales IJ, Peters SG, et al: The hospital mortality of patients admitted to the ICU on weekends. *Chest* 126:1292–1298, 2004.
29. Bell CM, Redelmeier DA: Mortality among patients admitted to hospitals on weekends as compared with weekdays. *N Engl J Med* 345:663–668, 2001.
30. Blunt MC, Burchett KR: Out-of-hours consultant cover and case-mix-adjusted mortality in intensive care. *Lancet* 356:735–736, 2000.

31. Burchardi H, Moerer O: Twenty-four hour presence of physicians in the ICU. *Crit Care* 5:131–137, 2001.
32. Gajic O, Afessa B, Hanson AC, et al: Effect of 24-hour mandatory versus on-demand critical care specialist presence on quality of care and family and provider satisfaction in the intensive care unit of a teaching hospital. *Crit Care Med* 36:36–44, 2008.
33. Breslow MJU, Rosenfeld BA, Doerfler M, et al: Effect of a multiple site intensive care unit telemedicine program on clinical and economic outcomes: an alternative paradigm for intensivist staffing. *Crit Care Med* 32:31–38, 2004.
34. FACTSHEET: ICU Physician Staffing (IPS): The Leapfrog Group. Available at: www.leapfroggroup.org. Accessed July 1, 2009.
35. Thomas EJ, Lucke JF, Wueste L, et al: Association of Telemedicine for remote monitoring of intensive care patients with mortality, complications and length of stay. *JAMA* 302(24):2671–2678, 2009.
36. Morrison JL, Cai Q, Davis N, et al: Clinical and economic outcomes of the electronic intensive care unit: Results from two community hospitals. *Crit Care Med* 38:2–8, 2010.
37. Dimick JB, Pronovost PJ, Heitmiller RF, et al: Intensive care unit physician staffing is associated with decreased length of stay, hospital cost, and complications after esophageal resection. *Crit Care Med* 29:753–758, 2001.
38. Pronovost PK, Jenckes MW, Dorman T, et al: Organizational characteristics of intensive care units related to outcomes of abdominal aortic surgery. *JAMA* 281:1310–1317, 1999.
39. Cannon MA, Beattie C, Spreoff T, et al: The economic benefit of organizational restructuring of the cardiothoracic intensive care unit. *J Cardiothorac Vasc Anesth* 17:565–570, 2003.
40. Pronovost PJ, Needham DM, Waters H, et al: Intensive care unit physician staffing: financial modeling of the Leapfrog standard. *Crit Care Med* 32:1247–1253, 2004.
41. Grover A: Critical care workforce: a policy perspective. *Crit Care Med* 34:S7–S11, 2006.
42. Gerber DR, Bekes CE, Parrillo JE: Economics of critical care: Medicare part A versus part B payments. *Crit Care Med* 34:S82–S87, 2006.
43. Higgins TL, Steingrub JS, Tereso G, et al: Drotrecogin Alfa (activated) in sepsis: initial experience with patient selection, cost and clinical outcomes. *J Intensive Care Med* 20:291–297, 2005.
44. Angus DC, Kelley MA, Schmitz RJ, et al: Current and projected workforce requirements for car of the critically ill and patients with pulmonary disease: can we meet the requirements of an aging population. *JAMA* 284:2762–2770, 2000.
45. Society of Critical Care Medicine: *Compensation of Critical Care Professionals*. Des Plains, IL, 2005, p 9.
46. Manthous CA: Leapfrog and critical care: evidence and reality based intensive care for the 21st century. *Am J Med* 115:188–193, 2004.
47. Tenner P, Dibrell H, Taylor RP: Improved survival with hospitalists in a pediatric intensive care unit. *Crit Care Med* 31:847–852, 2003.
48. Audit Commission: *Critical to Success: the Place of Efficient and Effective Critical Care Services Within the Acute Hospital*. London, England, Audit Commission, 1999.
49. Dara SI, Afesso B: Intensivist-to-bed ratio. Association with outcomes in the medical ICU. *Chest* 128:567–572, 2005.
50. Rudy EB, Davidson LJ, Daly B, et al: Care activities and outcomes of patients cared for by acute nurse practitioners, physician assistants, and resident physicians: a comparison. *Am J Crit Care* 7:267–281, 1998.
51. Hoffman LA, Tasota FJ, Zullo TG, et al: Outcomes of care managed by an acute care nurse practitioner/attending physician team in a subacute medical intensive care unit. *Am J Crit Care* 14:121–132, 2005.
52. Russell D, VorderBruegge M, Burns SM: Effect of an outcomes-managed approach to care of neuroscience patients by acute care nurse practitioners. *Am J Crit Care* 11:353–362, 2002.
53. Burns SM, Earven S: Improving outcomes for mechanically ventilated medical intensive care unit patients using advanced practice nurses: a 6-year experience. *Crit Care Nurs Clin North Am* 14:231–243, 2002.
54. Hoffman LA, Tasota FJ, Scharfenberg C, et al: Management of patients in the intensive care unit: comparison via work sampling analysis of an acute care nurse practitioner and physicians in training. *Am J Crit Care* 12:436–443, 2003.
55. Hoffman LA, Happ MB, Scharfenberg C, et al: Perceptions of physicians, nurses and respiratory therapists about the role of acute care nurse practitioners. *Am J Crit Care* 13:480–488, 2004.
56. Dubayo B, Samson M, Carlson R: The role of physician assistants in critical care units. *Chest* 99:89–91, 1991.
57. Mallick R, Strosberg M, Lambrinos J, et al: The intensive care unit medical director as manager: impact on performance. *Med Care* 33:611–624, 1995.
58. Levin PD, Worner TM, Sviri S, et al: Intensive care outflow limitation—frequency, etiology and impact. *J Crit Care* 18:206–211, 2003.
59. Higgins TL, Teres D: External forces shaping critical care, in Irwin RS, Rippe JM (eds): *Intensive Care Medicine*. 5th ed. Philadelphia, PA, Lippincott Williams and Wilkins, 2003, pp 2224–2231.
60. Leape LL, Fromson JA: Problem doctors: is there a system-level solution? *Ann Intern Med* 144:107–115, 2006.
61. Pronovost P, Berenholt S, Dorman T, et al: Improving communication in the ICU using daily goals. *J Crit Care* 18:71–75, 2003.
62. Klein G: Power to see the invisible, in: *Sources of Power. How People Make Decisions*. Cambridge, MA, The MIT Press, 1999, pp 147–175.
63. Dorman T: Unsustainable growth rate: physician perspective. *Crit Care Med* 34:S78–S81, 2006.
64. McLain T: Tackling four common myths about critical care service codes. *Today's Hospitalist* 4–5; August 2004.
65. Dorman T, Loeb L, Sample G: Evaluation and management codes: from current procedural terminology through relative update commission to Center for Medicare and Medicaid Services. *Crit Care Med* 34:S71–S77, 2006.
66. AMA CPT Code: Available at: https://catalog.ama-assn.org/Catalog/cpt/cpt_search.jsp. Accessed January 11, 2010.
67. American College of Chest Physicians Web site: Coding for Chest Medicine. Available at: https://accp.chestnet.org/storeWA/StoreAction.do?method=view&pcrNum=23. Accessed January 11, 2010.
68. Hackbarth G, Reischauer R, Mutti A: Collective accountability for medical care—toward bundled medicare payments. *N Engl J Med* 359:3–5, 2008.
69. Centers for Medicare and Medicaid Services, RAC Web site. Available at: http://www.cms.hhs.gov/RAC/. Accessed September 10, 2009.
70. McCauley K, Irwin RS: Changing the work environment in ICUs to achieve patient-focused care. *Chest* 130:1571–1578, 2006.
71. Reader TW, Flin R, Mearns K, et al: Developing a team performance framework for the intensive care unit. *Crit Care Med* 37:1787–1793, 2009.
72. Donabedian A: The quality of care. How can it be assessed? *JAMA* 260:1743–1748, 1988.
73. Rotondi AJ, Sirio CA, Angus DC, et al: A new conceptual framework for ICU performance appraisal and improvement. *J Crit Care* 17:16–28, 2002.
74. Nathanson BH, Higgins TL: An introduction to statistical methods used in binary outcome modeling. *Semin Cardiothorac Vasc Anesth* 12:153–166, 2008.
75. Knaus WA, Draper EA, Wagner DP, et al: APACHE II: a severity of disease classification system. *Crit Care Med* 13:818–829, 1985.
76. Knaus WA, Wagner DP, Draper EA, et al: The APACHE III prognostic system. Risk prediction of hospital mortality for critically ill hospitalized adults. *Chest* 100:1619–1636, 2005.
77. Zimmerman JE, Kramer AA, McNair DS, et al: Acute physiology and chronic health evaluation (APACHE) IV: hospital mortality assessment for today's critically ill patients. *Crit Care Med* 34:2674–2676, 2006.
78. Lemeshow S, Teres D, Klar J, et al: Mortality probability models (MPM II) based on an international cohort of intensive care unit patients. *JAMA* 270:2478–2486, 1993.
79. Higgins TL, Teres D, Copes W, et al: Assessing contemporary intensive care unit outcome: an updated Mortality Probability Model (MPM0-III). *Crit Care Med* 35:827–835, 2007.
80. Le Gall J-R, Lemeshow S, Saulnier F: A new simplified acute physiology score (SAPS II) based on a European/North American multicenter study. *JAMA* 270:2957–2963, 1993.
81. Moreno RP, Metnitz PGH, Almeida E, et al: SAPS 3—from evaluation of the patient to evaluation of the intensive care unit. Part 2: Development of a prognostic model for hospital mortality at ICU admission. *Intensive Care Med* 31:1345–1355, 2005.
82. Harrison DA, Parry GJ, Carpenter JR, et al: A new risk prediction model for critical care: The Intensive Care National Audit & Research Centre (ICNARC) model. *Crit Care Med* 35:1091–1098, 2007.
83. Harrison DA, Brady AR, Parry GJ, et al: Recalibration of risk prediction models in a large multicenter cohort of admissions to adult, general critical care units in the United Kingdom. *Crit Care Med* 34:1378–1388, 2006.
84. Zimmerman JE, Kramer AA, McNair DS, et al: Intensive care unit length of stay: benchmarking based on acute physiology and chronic health evaluation (APACHE) IV. *Crit Care Med* 34:2517–2529, 2006.
85. Cerner Critical Care Outcomes: Available at: www.cerner.com/public/Cerner_3.asp?id=27087. Accessed September 4, 2009..
86. Higgins TL, Kramer AA, Nathanson BH, et al: Prospective validation of the intensive care unit admission Mortality Probability Model (MPM_0-III). *Crit Care Med* 37:1619–1623, 2009.
87. Pollack MM, Ruttimann UE, Getson PR: Pediatric risk of mortality (PRISM) score. *Crit Care Med* 16:1110–1116, 1988.
88. Baker SP, O'Neil B, Haddon W, et al: The injury severity score: a method for describing patients with multiple injuries and evaluating emergency care. *J Trauma* 14:187–196, 1974.
89. Champion HR, Sacco WJ, Copes WS, et al: A revision of the trauma score. *J Trauma* 33:417–423, 1992.
90. Higgins TL, Estafanous FG, Loop FD, et al: Stratification of morbidity and mortality outcome of preoperative risk factors in coronary artery bypass patients. *JAMA* 267:2344–2348, 1992.
91. Murphy-Filkins RL, Teres D, Lemeshow S, et al: Effect of changing patient mix on the performance of an intensive care unit severity-of-illness model: how to distinguish a general from a specialty intensive care unit. *Crit Care Med* 24:1968–1973, 1996.
92. Nathanson B, Higgins TL, Kramer AA, et al: Subgroup mortality probability models: are they necessary for specialized intensive care units? *Crit Care Med* 37:2375–2386, 2009.
93. Sinuff T, Adhikari NK, Cook DJ, et al: Mortality predictions in the intensive care unit: comparing physicians with scoring systems. *Crit Care Med* 34:878–885, 2006.
94. McQuillan P, Pilkington S, Allan A, et al: Confidential inquiry into quality of care before admission to intensive care. *BMJ* 316:1853–1858, 1998.

95. Teres D, Higgins TL, Steingrub JS, et al: Defining a high-performance ICU system for the 21st century: a position paper. *J Intensive Care Med* 13:195–205, 1998.
96. Rapoport J, Teres D, Lemeshow S, et al: A method for assessing the clinical performance and cost effectiveness of intensive care units: a multi-center inception cohort study. *Crit Care Med* 22:1385, 1994.
97. Nathanson BH, Higgins TL, Teres D, et al: A revised method to assess intensive care unit clinical performance and resource utilization. *Crit Care Med* 35:1853–1862, 2007.
98. Franklin C, Mathew J: Developing strategies to prevent in-hospital cardiac arrest: analyzing responses of physicians and nurses in the hours before the event. *Crit Care Med* 22:244–247, 1994.
99. Schein RM, Hazday N, Pena M, et al: Clinical antecedents to in-hospital cardiopulmonary arrest. *Chest* 98:1388–1392, 1990.
100. Buist MD, Moore GE, Bernard SA, et al: Effects of a medical emergency team on reduction of incidence of and mortality from unexpected cardiac arrests in hospital: preliminary study. *BMJ* 324:387–390, 2002.
101. Berwick DM, Calkins DR, McCannon CJ, et al: The 100,000 Lives Campaign: setting a goal and a deadline for improving health care quality. *JAMA* 295:324–327, 2006.
102. Bellomo R, Goldsmith D, Uchino S, et al: Prospective controlled trial of effect of medical emergency team on postoperative morbidity and mortality rates. *Crit Care Med* 32:916–921, 2004.
103. Hillman K, Chen J, Cretikos M, et al: Introduction of the medical emergency team (MET) system: a cluster-randomised controlled trial. *Lancet* 365:2091–2097, 2005.
104. Wachter RM, Pronovost PJ: The 100,000 Lives Campaign: a scientific and policy review. *Jt Comm J Qual Patient Saf* 32:621–627, 2006.
105. Winters BD, Cuong J, Hunt EA, et al: Rapid response systems: a systemic review. *Crit Care Med* 35:1238–1243, 2007.
106. Chan PS, Khalid A, Longmore LS, et al: Hospital-wide code rates and mortality before and after implementation of a rapid response team. *JAMA* 300:2506–2513, 2008.
107. Morgan RJM, Williams F, Wright MM: An early warning system for detecting developing critical care illness. *Clin Intensive Care* 8:100, 1997.
108. Stenhouse C, Coates S, Tivey M, et al: Prospective evaluation of a modified early warning score to aid earlier detection of patients developing critical illness on a general surgical ward. *Br J Anaesth* 84:663, 2000.
109. Subbe CP, Gao H, Harrison DA: Reproducibility of physiological track-and-trigger warning systems for identifying at-risk patients on the ward. *Intensive Care Med* 33:619–624, 2007.
110. Tarassenko L, Hann A, Young D: Integrated monitoring and analysis for early warning of patient deterioration. *Br J Anaesth* 97:64–68, 2006.
111. Whittington J, White R, Haig KM, et al: Using an automated risk assessment report to identify patients at risk for clinical deterioration. *Jt Comm J Qual Patient Saf* 33:569–574, 2007.
112. Philips ProtocolWatch Web site. Accessed September 10, 2009.
113. Hravnak M, Edwards L, Clontz A, et al: Defining the incidence of cardiorespiratory instability in patients in step-down units using an electronic integrated monitoring system. *Arch Intern Med* 168:1300–1308, 2008.
114. Tarnow-Mordi WO, Hau C, Warden A, et al: Hospital mortality in relation to staff workload: a 4-year study in an adult intensive care unit. *Lancet* 356:185–189, 2000.
115. Vicca AF: Nursing staff workload as a determinant of methicillin-resistant Staphylococcus aureus spread in an adult intensive therapy unit. *J Hosp Infect* 43:109–113, 1999.
116. Rothschild JM, Landrigan CP, Cronin JW, et al: The critical care safety study: the incidence and nature of adverse events and serious medical errors in intensive care. *Crit Care Med* 33:1694–1700, 2005.
117. Baggs JG, Schmitt MH, Mushlin AI, et al: Association between nurse-physician collaboration and patient outcomes in three intensive care units. *Crit Care Med* 27:1991–1996, 1999.
118. Rosenstein A: Nurse-physician relationships: impact on nurse satisfaction and retention. *Am J Nurs* 102:26–34, 2002.
119. Niemi K, Geary S, Larrabee M, et al: Standardized vasoactive medications: a unified system for every patient, everywhere. *Hosp Pharm* 40:984–993, 2005.
120. Curtis JR, Cook DJ, Wall RJ, et al: Intensive care unit quality improvement: a "how-to" guide for the interdisciplinary team. *Crit Care Med* 34:211–218, 2006.
121. Wasser T, Matchett S, Ray D, et al: Validation of a total score for the critical care family satisfaction survey. *J Clin Outcomes Manage* 11:502–507, 2004.
122. Soltner C, Lassalle V, Galienne-Bouygues S, et al: Written information that relatives of adult intensive care unit patients would like to received—a comparison to published recommendations and opinion of staff members. *Crit Care Med* 37:2197–2202, 2009.

CHAPTER 209 ■ CRITICAL CARE INFORMATION SYSTEMS: STRUCTURE, FUNCTION, AND FUTURE

WILLIAM F. BRIA, JOSEPH J. FRASSICA, RICHARD KREMSDORF, M. MICHAEL SHABOT AND VIOLET L. SHAFFER

INTRODUCTION

In over five decades since the first implementation of the electronic health record (EHR) in the United States, there have been both the rise, definition, and establishment of critical care medicine as a specialty and important force in health care both in research and practice.

Although technology has played an essential role in the very creation of the specialty (e.g., ventilators, cardiovascular monitoring), the implementation of the EHR in U.S. hospitals, and, as per available data sources, in intensive care units (ICUs), remains at a meager 1.5% [1].

With the American Recovery and Reinvestment Act (ARRA), the HITECH section promises to stimulate "meaningful use" of information technology (IT) in U.S. hospitals. This is the greatest single transformation ever undertaken of the information infrastructure of U.S. health care.

This chapter reviews a number of key components of IT in the modern U.S. ICU. The reader is introduced to some of the most important innovative technologies that have been brought to bear on the safe, effective, and efficient delivery of critical care medicine.

General information on the electronic medical record, departmental information systems, and coding and billing information systems has been extensively documented elsewhere and we assume a working knowledge of these basic components of the modern healthcare information infrastructure. Instead, we concern ourselves with the ICU-specific IT of greatest interest to the practicing critical care physician.

In this chapter, we address (i) telemedicine in the ICU, (ii) clinical decision support systems, and (iii) outcomes' prediction information systems.

TELEMEDICINE AND THE INTENSIVE CARE UNIT

According to the Military Health System Web site, telemedicine may be defined as "an umbrella term that encompasses various technologies as part of a coherent health service information resource management program [2]. Telemedicine is the capture, display, storage and retrieval of medical images and data towards the creation of a computerized patient record and managed care. Advantages include: move information, not patients or providers; enter data ONCE in a health care network; network quality specialty health care to isolated locations; and build from hands-on experience."

Critical care information systems (CCIS) have largely overcome the technical barriers to their implementation. While there are enormous amounts of data available and opportunities to enhance the delivery of critical care, it remains challenging to marshal those resources in ways that meet the needs of both hands-on caregivers and overall delivery system efficiency and quality.

There are two large categories in which clinical information systems technology can be deployed and each is enhanced by the use of the other approaches. These are (i) single-patient–focused tools and (ii) multiple-patient–focused tools.

Single-Patient–Focused Tools

The most mature implementation of critical care clinical information systems consists of tools which meet the needs of the hands-on caregivers. Historically, massive amounts of data documenting an ICU patient's clinical status and treatment have been recorded on large double-sided paper flow sheets, which are plagued with problems of legibility, inaccurate calculations, and use restricted to a single person at a time. By replacing this document with computer screens, each customized to a specific purpose, these problems have been essentially solved.

Going beyond simple replacement of paper documents provides an opportunity to present information such that patterns are more easily recognized. For example, correlation of measures of physiologic status, clinical status (such as urinary output and body weight), and administration of medications can facilitate clinical analysis by juxtaposing interdependent variables. Less obviously, trends over longer periods of time can be easily displayed while these could only be laboriously drawn by hand.

Optimal use of clinical information systems should also guide the hands-on caregivers to provide care using evidence-based protocols. Simply creating a place to document the position of head of the bed underscores that this is important issue to be managed in prevention of ventilator-associated pneumonia (VAP). Explanatory information can also be provided on a just-in-time basis to encourage protocol compliance. Computer provider order entry prompts and order sets can also facilitate standardization of care.

Simply collecting and displaying information electronically, while an advance over a paper record, vastly underutilizes the capability of the computer system. The data are being gathered in a computable form and consequently are subject to continuous analysis, enabling detection of patterns that could signify clinical decompensation. Vastly larger datasets than can be retained and analyzed in the human brain can be evaluated and, furthermore, it can be done continuously on all monitored patients, simultaneously. Such an early warning system could trigger evaluation that might otherwise be delayed.

Finally, computable information that describes in detail both the patient's status and treatment can be used to analyze compliance with protocols for optimal care, resource utilization, and outcomes. Monitoring on a near real-time basis provides timely feedback and is an opportunity to intervene to improve ongoing care.

Once all of these capabilities are available and used by the hands-on caregiving team, their individual capabilities can be optimized. Nonetheless, the realities of the critical care environment are such that patients may be critically ill and yet not be in a setting where their care needs can be expeditiously met. For example, a patient might be in a distant hospital where intensivist coverage is not available. Or, even in a sophisticated medical center, patients may decompensate outside the ICU and, indeed, even in the ICU after hours, an intensivist might not be physically available to respond.

Two technological approaches to dealing with this problem have developed, each dependent on a suitably trained intensivist sitting at a remotely located computer that is equipped with a microphone and speaker and a high-bandwidth Internet connection. Each approach also has one or more high-resolution cameras which can be controlled by a remote physician and means to communicate with caregivers and patients and family who are in the patient's room. Medical devices such as stethoscopes can sometimes be connected as well.

Connectivity to additional clinical information systems varies according to institutional capabilities. For example, some systems have as many as eight monitors arrayed such that the remote physician can see the real-time electrocardiogram tracing, access the institution's image archiving and communication systems, and review all elements of a comprehensive clinical information system, simultaneous with viewing and talking with the patient. Without question, availability of this full suite of technological capabilities allows a comprehensive evaluation of the patient that far surpasses the limited verbal interaction between the bedside caregiver and a physician connecting by telephone. It is now well documented that such interactions can provide for more timely and therapeutically appropriate interventions [3]. Nonetheless, such evaluations are still limited in that hands-on physician diagnostic and therapeutic maneuvers are not available when the physician is remote. It has been documented that remote proctoring of a procedure being performed by a house officer who is in the hospital is a practical alternative when immediate interventions are required. Furthermore, even in the case where the physician or patient will need to travel to the point of care, useful temporizing measures may be deployed.

A form of technology that is particularly well suited for the interaction with an individual patient is a mobile robot, offering what is referred to as "robotic telepresence." One form of this device can actually be driven remotely by the physician from its storage location to the patient's location in the appropriately equipped facility. Using wireless connectivity, the robot establishes a similar connection to that which exists in rooms that have been specifically hardwired for these capabilities. Because of the costs of connectivity, institutions frequently limit fixed installations to ICUs. Nonetheless, it is clear that patients in other patient care locations can decompensate and care may be needed elsewhere. Such robots provide a lower cost means to provide similar capabilities and could be used to augment the expertise of rapid response teams.

Interactions may be initiated by the caregiving staff from any care location. In such circumstances acceptance has been generally very favorable. Nurses feel that there are trained physicians who are awake and available in the middle of the night and can be provided with all of the information needed to provide care. As a consequence, nurses may be more confident that the patients are receiving quality care. A limitation is that the remote physician may have less of an appreciation for the patient's clinical course than a physician who has seen the patient daily. However, in some ICUs, the physician on call at night at home and using the robot may be the same person who rounded on the patient that day. Interaction between remote and primary treating physicians remains an essential element of care.

Multiple-Patient–Focused Tools

In institutions where multiple ICUs have been equipped with cameras in each room and connectivity to clinical information systems and other clinical data sources has been established, a team is established at a central monitoring location which may be distant from the ICUs and hospital(s), frequently off campus in less-expensive commercial office space. Analysis of signals from bedside monitors and other devices as well as the results of laboratory tests alert off-site providers to perform patient assessments. Alternatively, bedside providers can request evaluation and off-site management. Interventions, including the ordering of diagnostic tests, medications or consultations, or the manipulation of life support devices can be done by off-site providers or by on-site providers. Thus, a single patient interaction may be initiated by the remote physician as well as by hands-on caregivers. Like any team endeavor, effectiveness is determined in part by communication timeliness and dynamics of trust and responsibility among the bedside and off-site team members.

The primary responsibilities of the remote monitoring team are identification of unfavorable trends and to intervene to enhance best practice adherence, perform care plan reviews for patients admitted after day time hours and provide ICU pharmacist [4] review of after hours provider medications orders which provides an additional safety net for patients in the ICU [3,4]. Bedside caregivers have the potential to be overwhelmed by the need to care for multiple patients, and the requirement to deal with the mechanics of providing care may interfere with always maintaining perspective on the patient's course.

Information systems that power the central monitoring station have been equipped with series of rules that evaluate clinical information as it is being gathered at the bedside and returned from the laboratory. By correlating this data, alerts can be fired to draw the attention of the remote monitoring team. The team then has the clinical information available to judge whether this is a new or serious development which then prompts interactions with the bedside caregiving team. Such tools may also be available to the bedside caregiving team; however, their many clinical duties can often result in a delayed response. Furthermore, many bedside clinical information systems are much less sophisticated in this area than are the systems designed for use in monitoring a population of patients.

An important capability is the opportunity to perform virtual rounds on the sickest patients. The acuity status is used to identify which patients might most benefit from closer observation. In this way, the remote physician can perform virtual rounds at intervals to judge the effect of medications which may have been administered to determine if physiologic responses are improving or deteriorating. This surveillance can be an important complement to bedside care.

An essential element for the success of remote monitoring of critically ill patients is the effective collaboration between the hands-on caregivers in the central monitoring team. The bedside critical care multidisciplinary team that is responsible for the patient and sees the patient and family on an ongoing basis is best positioned to establish the daily plan of care for each patient. The role of the off-site team members is to keep the patient on the intended trajectory and to communicate with the bedside providers when the patent's course has deviated from that path. In ICUs where full-time 24-hour day coverage is not available, which is the vast majority of ICUs, physician interaction that may be necessary to ensure that the goals of care are achieved may be sporadic and untimely. The remote team serves as a surrogate for the bedside team at times when they are not able to attend to the patient. In recent years, evidence has accumulated that ongoing availability of intensivist is associated with improved outcomes. If there are an insufficient number of trained intensivists to cover the ICUs that exist, such remote monitoring is being used to increase the availability of trained staff.

It has also been established that implementing certain protocols for care of critically ill patients is associated with better outcomes in the management of sepsis and the avoidance of VAP. Nonetheless, it has proven challenging not only to achieve initial compliance with such protocols, but even more difficult to maintain compliance at a high level. An additional role played by a central monitoring team is to identify when patients who are eligible for a protocol are not receiving such care.

To the extent that the remote monitoring team functions completely independently from the on-site caregivers, there is opportunity for miscommunication and compromise of trust. Indeed, bedside caregivers have been reported to feel threatened by the sense of someone looking over their shoulders all the time and the primary treating physicians could resent intrusions that alter the plan of care set out by them [5]. A substantial investment in relationship building and acceptance by all members of the on-site and remote teams of the importance of minimizing medical errors is thought to be associated with larger improvements in outcomes.

In the fall of 2009, a new technological sea change is that the Blackberry and Apple iPhone are beginning to not only take over the previous place of the medical pager, but, due to their ubiquitous access to high-speed Internet, provide the means to deliver high-resolution bedside monitoring device (BMDI) data, as well as complete access to the electronic medical record from any location at any time. Although telemedicine has enabled new healthcare structures, as mentioned earlier, these new technologies delivered to the individual practitioner are likely to transform medicine just as has happened in the business world [6].

ANALYSIS OF DELIVERY SYSTEM PERFORMANCE WITH REAL-TIME FEEDBACK

Clinical Decision Support

Clinical decision support (CDS) has been defined as a system that uses two or more items of patient data to generate case-specific advice [7]. In practical terms, CDS includes a wide range of functions, including predefined rules, alerts, reminders, workflow, and collaboration tools—and associated content—for improved medical decision making. CDS is often intended to facilitate the introduction of and conformance to evolving evidence-based medical protocols and standards of care while enabling appropriate individual physician discretion (such as during order entry). Rules are, at their core, built on IF/THEN logic statements that allow a tremendous amount of flexibility and power to be added to systems within critical care and across the hospital or integrated health system.

Over the past decade, the business end (e.g., the user experience) of CDS has been the alert box. A growing number of studies are beginning to reveal the critical limitation of alerts that, by design, interrupt the clinician's workflow, in particular, during order entry [8,9]. The primary reason for this limitation lies in CDS systems designed mainly to alert post hoc after the clinician has requested a particular item (e.g., drug dosage, test).

CDS has the potential to provide special value in settings like the ICU due to the density of data assailing the busy critical care physician and the ability of computers to combine, synthesize, and correlate these data and then create more complex rules and information interpretation displays [10]. Studies have demonstrated that critical care rounds may challenge the physician with 20 times more data elements than the human brain can simultaneously process [11]. In the past, we have relied on the team approach to cope with this onslaught. In the current practice reality of competing priorities of intensivist time, numerous handoffs among providers, the need for IT to take more of a facilitation role for the ICU physician and nurse is substantial. The next emerging developments in CCIS are likely to be in both the areas of visual design and complex rules and algorithms to predict and inform clinicians about patient circumstances by multiple means. This is discussed, along with emerging techniques for ICU performance management and related metrics, in a later section of this chapter.

Stepwise Plan of Implementation of a Critical Care Information System

The following steps enable the physician, in combination with other stakeholders such as nurses and pharmacists, to evaluate, select, and obtain maximal benefits from CCIS systems, with the assistance of a professionally certified and experienced project manager (typically from the IT department). It is the project manager who coordinates overall project planning, ensures that the required technical resources will be available on time, and monitors tasks and milestones among the project team. Technical needs such as interfaces to other IT systems and to medical devices, hardware, power, physical space, network access, and system security are necessary parts of this coordinated planning in addition to software delivery and configuration.

1. Goal setting: Considerations for valued, realistic goals. Experience has shown that the most important goal for achieving successful CCIS implementation is improvement in the quality of patient care. An ICU team is well versed in the concept of change, usually in the context of changes in patient condition. However, deploying and leveraging a CCIS implementation is a different kind of change. It should enable and will require reengineering of certain processes and a reduction in productivity during transition should be anticipated. An ICU team is not expected to tolerate delays in patient care, and needs to plan carefully and set realistic expectations around workflow issues that typically occur in the context of the learning curve necessary to use a new CCIS. With the goal of improved quality of patient care as the guiding light, the sequence of introduction of CCIS and the speed of implementation can be considered. An improved structure of order sets that have the support of virtually all clinicians and that interface with other department's systems (e.g., laboratory, pharmacy, radiology) is key [12].
2. CCIS users must have understanding and input into CCIS design before implementation. The history of CCIS implementation has shown that physicians are the most likely group to be surprised by CCIS structure and function. Reasons include lack of physician attendance at planning meetings, and therefore little direct input in CCIS planning and configuration, due to physician perception of systems as being solely clerical. The importance of involving clinically influential physician leaders in a successful CCIS process has been shown in the literature [21]. The chief medical informatics officer (CMIO), serving as a bridge between physicians and IT through design, training, support, and enhancement, improves clinical IT deployments. Note that about 7% of CMIOs come from the ranks of intensive care medicine, according to recent survey data [13].
3. Preemptive workflow and practice reengineering. The knowledge base necessary for a successful CCIS implementation is not limited to learning about the system itself. More important is the timely recognition that the workflow changes engendered by implementation can be both tolerated and supportive of the central goal of improved patient care.
4. Minimize changes to base system before implementation. This step is really a caveat of step 2. Yes, users should have some time to learn the out-of-the-box system and suggest changes before implementation, but that has to be balanced with the actual experience of the "shake-down cruise" period with the new system during the daily operations of the ICU. Veteran computer analysts of many CCIS implementations will attest to the frequency of changes of some components of a system back to factory specs after a few weeks or months of use. Nothing can replace time and experience in using a system in the actual ICU environment to truly recognize what would or would not be a helpful modification.
5. Establish implementation milestones. Implementation of a complex system should be phased in gradually, with each step building on the foundation of the previous component. Starting with results reporting, to computerized physician order entry (CPOE), then to decision support, workflow is increasingly affected and the changes take time to be absorbed effectively. This process is necessary to avoid any adverse impact on the all-important central goal of improved patient care.
6. Establish a backup/back-out plan for each milestone. It needs to be recognized that a successful implementation may require some temporary delays for extra training or system reconfiguration. Daily clinical operations of the ICU must always be paramount.
7. CCIS should be viewed as a system of patient-centered reminders, not an attempt to control providers. CCIS systems should be a helpful aid in optimizing patient care; for example, memory aids and consistent care reminders can be helpful. Components that may be perceived as attempting to control user behavior are not well accepted, and systems have been rejected on these grounds [14].

Critical Care Specific Technologies

Concurrent Process Monitoring

On the most basic level, CCIS put an end to juggling the awkwardly large flow sheet. Like CPOE, they eliminate the confusion and potential errors that can result from illegible handwriting and from fluid contamination, including the familiar coffee spill. The truly significant contributions CCIS makes to patient safety are in the areas of care processes and medical decision making. First among these is the ease of access to data. Access to a paper record can be problematic in the ICU, where multiple clinicians need to assess the patient's clinical condition and response to treatment. Electronic records allow multiple caregivers to view the data at the same time, without waiting to access the one-and-only paper chart. Clinicians not in the ICU can check on a patient's status without physically having to be in the unit, allowing them to be consulted at the very moment their expertise is needed. When timeliness is critical, access is a critical enabler.

The impact of access on patient safety is enhanced when clinicians have confidence that the data provided are accurate and timely. By automating calculations, CCIS ensures that measures such as input/output are computed correctly, and provides multiple measures, including those too time-consuming to compute routinely on paper such as hemodynamic calculations incorporating many variables. In addition, CCIS can automatically acquire data directly from monitoring equipment and ventilators, eliminating delays and errors in data gathering.

Unlike the paper flow sheet, with its fixed format, CCIS offer multiple displays of data. Each display provides a problem-oriented view suitable for analysis of the issue at hand. Constrained to one view of the data, physicians using paper-based systems on occasion resort to duplicate data entry, a practice nurses are trained to disallow. By contrast, CCIS allows the clinician to select from multiple displays, each providing a problem-oriented view suitable for analysis of the issue at hand.

CCIS further supports the clinician by easing trend recognition. Specific displays establish the correlation of events in time, offsetting the possibility that it might be less apparent on the computer screen than on the paper flow sheet. Other displays provide multi-day views, which are critical for measures like fluid balance and fever curves, surpassing the paper flow sheet's view of only one day at a time. The displays on CCIS integrate multiple data elements that stand in isolation on the existing flow sheet. By combining vital signs, laboratory results, ventilator settings, medication drips, and medication administration, CCIS enables clinicians to address the complicated clinical scenarios characteristic of critically ill patients in ICUs. This integrated record also assures attention to details that can be lost in a frenetic setting; for example, by issuing a warning that a medication is overdue or being dosed earlier than appropriate per orders.

In the ICU and throughout the hospital, specialized tools can address "failure to rescue," which has been identified by the Agency for Healthcare Research and Quality (AHRQ) as accounting for the majority of patient-safety Medicare deaths. These tools provide proactive clinical surveillance; they interpret patient data (which are collected by the CCIS) and act as early warning systems.

In failure to rescue, the patient experiences clinical decompensation over a period of hours, without intervention by caregivers. This error of omission occurs for any of several reasons. The changes in the patient's condition may be subtle; for example, a physiologic value may be decreased, but not alarmingly so unless viewed as part of a trend. In other cases, changes may not be appreciated for what they signify. Clinicians may lack the necessary expertise to discern such changes or may be overwhelmed with other tasks. Indeed, according to the AHRQ, there is strong evidence that level of staffing and the nursing skill-mix are both factors in this failure.

Delays in detecting changes are of grave concern for a simple reason: the earlier the intervention, the greater the likelihood for a better clinical outcome. Intervening at the first signs of decompensation may make it possible to avert cardiorespiratory renal failure or address a more treatable complication. For example, stabilizing a patient whose heart rate is reaching dangerous levels (less than 40, more than 130 beats per minute) is more likely to succeed and less likely to involve additional complications than resuscitating a patient in a state of cardiac arrest.

There are warnings, if caregivers are able to recognize critical data among the numerous data elements on every patient. Studies of clinical instability suggest that patients experience symptoms in advance of critical events like cardiac arrest. In one study, 70% showed evidence of respiratory deterioration within 8 hours of arrest; in another, 66% of patients showed abnormal signs and symptoms within 6 hours [15].

Proactive clinical surveillance systems highlight trends and out-of-bounds values and conditions for further scrutiny. They provide displays—"dashboards"—that integrate different data elements to optimize evaluation of clinical problems. An additional feature offers severity scoring for the purpose of early detection of decompensation, issuing modified early warning scores to alert clinicians to problems as they develop.

These dashboards function both inside and outside the ICU to identify patients whose conditions are worsening, putting them in critical condition. Depending on their resources, hospitals may respond in several different ways.

In many hospitals, ICUs are staffed with nurse specialists and have high nurse-to-patient ratios. Yet most hospitals in the United States do not have a full-time intensivist on staff, ready to step in when a patient decompensates in the ICU or in another unit elsewhere in the hospital. In some instances, physicians in other specialties who practice in the ICU choose not to have an intensivist on staff, even if their hospital has the financial resources to recruit one. Nationally, there are more ICUs than intensivists. In 2001, staffing every ICU sufficiently would have required 35,000 to 40,000 intensivists, and there were less than 10,000 of these specialists.

Outside critical care areas, nurse-to-patient ratios are typically lower. Moreover, general medical/surgical areas are staffed by nurses who are not trained in the care of the critically ill. When a patient decompensates, the nurse is less likely to recognize this has happened, and the patient is less likely to receive appropriate interventions. Failure to recognize and respond quickly to patients with deteriorating conditions not only results in cardiac arrests and death, but is also associated with serious complications and prolongation of hospital length of stay. For patients and professionals in these units, the dashboards provided by hospital-wide proactive clinical surveillance systems improve safety, if in fact there is a mechanism for responding.

One approach is to create what the Institute for Healthcare Improvement [16] calls a rapid response team (RRT), also known as medical emergency team. The RRT consists of clinicians and nurses with critical care expertise that can be called anywhere in the hospital if a patient experiences acute change(s) in physiologic conditions; for example, in respiratory rate (more than 8 or less than 28 per minute), systolic blood pressure (less than 90), oxygenation, and neurologic status. As structured by the Institute for Healthcare Improvement, the program is contingent on a nurse to request help.

Whether or not a hospital has RRTs, a computerized surveillance system could function to alert clinicians that a patient is decompensating. Studies show a 50% reduction in non-ICU cardiac arrests, reduced postoperative emergency ICU transfers (58%) and deaths (37%), and reduction in arrest prior to ICU transfer (4% vs. 30%). With RRTs, one 750-bed community hospital reported a 23% decrease in their overall code rate per 1,000 discharges, a 44% decrease in codes occurring outside their ICU, and a 48% increase in the percentage of coded patients surviving at discharge.

Whether or not a hospital has RRTs, surveillance systems function to alert clinicians that a patient is decompensating. In either situation, the decision may be made to move the patient to critical care. Survival in the ICU is enhanced if patients are brought to the ICU in less critical condition and are less likely to experience severe complications. Moving patients into the ICU reduces the incidence of codes in areas outside the ICU that are less skilled at responding to them. Effective patient triage, management of potentially seriously ill patients prior to development of progressive physiologic deterioration, and reduction of unanticipated ICU admissions may also result in savings that can neutralize the cost of maintaining an RRT.

Another capability provided by CCIS that has the potential to improve patient safety includes concurrent process monitoring. This relies on details of care that define how a process is being implemented. When data are captured electronically and stored as discrete data elements, they can become available for analysis. When analyses are concurrent (e.g., done as care is delivered), they allow managers and caregivers to have visibility into global processes of care. In the ICU, concurrent process monitoring allows evaluation of whether a particular practice is actually being implemented and whether it is affecting outcomes, such as elevation of the head of the bed to reduce the likelihood of VAP.

Historically, organizations are good at creating policies and procedures, but much less effective in deploying them. Although it is easy to sit in a conference room and discuss them, it is harder to get people to follow them. If data are extracted and tabulated manually, it is laborious to figure out whether a particular practice is being implemented and the reporting is done long after the events being studied have occurred. In such cases, caregivers may believe "It used to be that bad, but now we're better." With more retrospective analysis, the same pattern repeats.

In contrast, concurrent process analyses allow the implementation of evidence-based practices by identifying and reinforcing practice patterns as they occur. Moreover, concurrent monitoring takes advantage of data already being gathered in the course of care, eliminating the need for duplicate data entry or chart abstraction.

Critical Care Decision Support Systems

The ICU is routinely acknowledged by hospital executives as a high-cost, high-risk hospital center. Intensive care and the role of intensive care-trained professional have been far less well appreciated as the service that often is the difference between effective and profitable hospital care for seriously ill patients. Ironically, despite great challenges of data collection and a general lack of payer and care-delivery organization support, ICU researchers have been among the real pioneers in trying to understand how to impact the effectiveness and efficiency of ICU and overall hospital care. As clinical automation and the resulting routine and standardized data collection are becoming more common, it is likely that these important methods for measuring, comparing, and improving care will find their way into mainstream medical practice.

ICU PERFORMANCE MANAGEMENT

Since the Institute of Medicine published its 1999 "expose" on patient safety [17], the ICU has received increased national attention as an important target for medical error reduction and improved quality. Both the Leapfrog Group collaborative of large employers and the Joint Commission accreditation organization have focused on developing national ICU performance measurement metrics [18]. IT can be used to more easily gather patient, process, and outcomes data and facilitate improvement. Performance measures are typically categorized as structural (how care is organized), process (what is done), or outcomes (including medical/functional, such as death or the ability to perform specific functions of daily life); experiential, which covers both patients/families and providers; and financial, which includes both cost/resource use and profitability perspectives.

Structure and process measures are used on the presumption that their variance causes a specific significant variance in one or more outcomes. Examples of popular structural ICU measurable processes are intensivist coverage [19] and appropriate levels of nurse staffing. Head-of-bed elevation in mechanically ventilated patients to prevent nosocomial pneumonia and associated increased mortality is an example of a contemporary measurable process [12].

One of the most significant challenges in quality improvement efforts is the lack of trust or alignment that can exist among clinicians, hospital administrators, insurance companies, and government over the motivation behind measurement. Clinicians believe that the purpose of measurement should be to understand and improve—while they too often, and too often rightly, assume payers' and overseers' plan to use metrics only to judge and to penalize—not to reward superior performance or improve patient care but only to drive down cost.

Given this environment, without standardized measures of meaningful medical outcomes that are defined, understood, and accepted by the relevant clinical community, making significant progress is difficult. Business intelligence systems, including performance dashboard techniques, that combine clinical data from computer-based patient records with financial data for analysis and reporting are predicted to be an area of increased interest. As this evolution occurs, critical care leaders will want to assure that their unique information needs are met in these systems and that appropriate attention is given to elements like risk adjustment and critical care-specific process analysis. Niche ICU analytic systems such as the Virtual Pediatric Intensive Care Unit (PICU) Performance System/National Association of Children's Hospitals and Related Institutions, the Vermont-Oxford Network for neonatal intensive care, and Cerner Corporation's Acute Physiology, Age, Chronic Health Evaluation (APACHE) prognostic, concurrent, and retrospective decision support system focused on adult ICU units are also available [20].

RISK-ADJUSTMENT MODELS FOR COMPARING INTENSIVE CARE OUTCOMES

Risk adjustment, severity adjustment, or case-mix adjustment are terms used to describe mathematical models derived from large datasets of a particular population whose purpose is to represent the relative risks individual patients bring at the entry point to care process. Patient risk factors of course impact what care processes and resources are required to produce similar outcomes and what the best realistically achievable outcomes are. Modeling research needs to define three elements: (a) the binary or continuous outcome variable(s) to be modeled (e.g., lived/died, length of stay), (b) the beginning and end points in time (e.g., at admission to the ICU, at discharge from the hospital, at 100 days), and (c) the specific risk factors to be included (e.g., age/gestational age, weight/birth weight, diagnosis, physiology). Because most hospital patient records are still paper-based, the most viable data source developing risk adjustment has been those using administrative (claims) data, examples being APR-DRGs (all patient refined diagnosis-related groups) and disease staging. Model developers juggle the collection cost versus the desirability of capturing specific data, but unequivocally more detailed patient data than that included in claims is required to adequately represent patient-risk variance in the ICU population. Model developers also struggle with defining reasonable end points for capturing outcomes. They also need to consider and factor in relationships among institutions and settings, potentially "gaming of the system." A report card that inadequately adjusts for patient risk might harm hospitals and physicians who take on the highest risk patients, or encourage entities to transfer dying patients to reduce their mortality [20]. As an example, a recent analysis of several Pennsylvania hospitals pointed out a facility with higher reported stroke mortality rates, in part because it kept more terminal stroke patients in the hospital rather than discharging them to home or hospice [22]. As Iezonni [23] notes, "developing risk adjusters de novo is complicated and often frustrating." Risk models for adult, pediatric, and neonatal ICU populations have been sufficiently vetted and have sufficiently evolved to serve as the foundation for nationally standardized outcomes measurement in an increasingly automated hospital environment. Risk models need to be reevaluated periodically to assure that they remain consistent with current patient factor, care process improvements, and outcomes' experience. They should also be evaluated for their appropriateness in geographies not included in their modeling datasets.

There are multiple risk-adjustment models in current use. Representative examples of ICU risk-adjustment models based primarily on U.S. patient data include

1. APACHE IV (Acute Physiology, Age, Chronic Health Evaluation, 4th version) [24,25]
2. PRISM (Pediatric Risk of Mortality) [26]
3. SNAP/SNAPPE (Score for Neonatal Acute Physiology) [27]
4. Neonatal Risk Models of the Vermont-Oxford Network

EVALUATING RISK-ADJUSTED OUTCOMES INFORMATION

Because risk-adjusted assessments are based on mathematical models, taking an objective approach to understanding the causes of variance data is logical. For example, there are four main causes of variance, and sequentially evaluating them helps clinicians gain familiarity with the models and acceptance of variance between actual and predicted results. These models include (i) data randomness (small sample), (ii) existence of patient risk factors not incorporated or (iii) adequately weighted in the particular model, and (iv) variance likely attributable to differences in care.

Emerging Trends: Predictive Modeling and Data Visualization

Predictive analytics enable an organization to estimate or anticipate the risk of future events, and are used increasingly in other industries, such as for predicting consumer behavior. In health care, these techniques are often applied for planning demand for healthcare services and facilities, for identification of at-risk populations, and for actuarial projection of healthcare utilization or life span.

Clinical decision support systems in the future will take more advantage of larger databases of increasingly granular patient data to drive pattern recognition engines that will help clinicians predict physiologic deterioration progressively earlier in its course. Examples of predictive models in use today include the individual patient predictions components of the APACHE IV ICU models referenced previously [25], and the Northern New England Cardiovascular Disease Study Group's preoperative mortality risk and cerebrovascular accident and risk of vascular complication models [28]. Not intended to replace but to support physician judgment, such predictive models have to date focused on evaluating the appropriateness of ICU admission and readiness for discharge, assessing patient progress and effectiveness of current therapies, building care team consensus around prognosis and care strategies, identifying patients for palliative care assessments, and improving

Unit Abbreviation	[redacted]-CV
Unit Name	CV Surgery
Medical Director	[redacted], MD
Nursing Director	[redacted], RN

	December	November	October	6 Month Avg	12 Month Avg	Current vs. 12-mo Trend	Notes
Operating Beds	8.0	8.0	8.0	8.0	8.0	No Change (<1%)	
Discharges	47.0	54.0	50.0	47.0	47.4	No Change (<1%)	
Occupancy	62.6%	65.9%	62.6%	58.2%	62.4%	No Change (<1%)	
Average ICU Length of Stay (days)	3.30	2.93	3.11	3.04	3.20	Increase of 3.1%	
Average Hospital Length of Stay (days)	5.30	5.19	5.58	5.01	5.44	Decrease of 2.5%	
% IMU/Routine Room Charges	24.2%	18.9%	19.0%	17.2%	16.0%	Increase of 51%	
ICU Glucose Monitoring							
Bedside glucose measurements per day	5.79	6.84	3.54	4.20	3.54	Increase of 63.7%	All measurements
Euglycemia (80-150 mg/dL)	78.0%	73.6%	69.0%	68.3%	56.5%	Increase of 38%	Only post-24-hour samples
Hypoglycemia <60 mg/dL	0.9%	1.4%	0.5%	1.1%	0.9%	Decrease of 2.1%	Excludes first 24 hrs
60-79 mg/dL	6.1%	5.0%	3.7%	4.4%	3.1%	Increase of 98.4%	Excludes first 24 hrs
Euglycemia 80-150 mg/dL	78.0%	73.6%	69.0%	68.3%	56.5%	Increase of 38%	Excludes first 24 hrs
Hyperglycemia >150 mg/dL	15.1%	59.1%	68.3%	63.1%	74.2%	Decrease of 79.7%	Excludes first 24 hrs
ICU HAI Bundle Compliance							
VAP Bundle Compliance - MD	NA	100.0%	100.0%	100.0%	100.0%	-	
VAP Bundle Compliance - Nursing	NA	100.0%	0.0%	50.0%	33.3%	-	
CR-BSI Insertion Bundle Compliance	100.0%	90.0%	92.3%	97.1%	97.3%	Increase of 2.8%	
CR-BSI Line Maintenance Compliance	100.0%	44.4%	25.0%	47.7%	51.4%	Increase of 94.6%	
ICU Utilization							
Epotin cost per ICU day	$0.00	$2.17	$2.95	$1.74	$1.60	Decrease of 100%	Procrit & Aranesp for non-ESRD
Nicardipine cost per ICU day	$5.93	$3.39	$6.91	$5.29	$9.25	Decrease of 35.9%	Cardene only
Propofol cost per ventilator day	$4.92	$9.69	$13.15	$9.49	$8.42	Decrease of 41.6%	
Antibiotics cost per day	$20.97	$44.71	$37.38	$35.31	$30.39	Decrease of 31%	
Average # Ventilator Days	1.62	2.67	2.89	2.27	2.10	Decrease of 22.9%	For ventilated patients only
Vent-to-Trach Days	0.00	0.00	0.00	0.00	10.00	Decrease of 100%	Excludes same-day trachs
% Avoidable ICU Days	0.0%	0.0%	0.0%	0.0%	0.0%	-	*Subject to reporting revision*
ICU Costs & Margin							
Total Indirect cost per patient day	$[redacted]	$[redacted]	$[redacted]	$[redacted]	$[redacted]	Increase of 53.7%	
Total Direct cost per Patient day	$[redacted]	$[redacted]	$[redacted]	$[redacted]	$[redacted]	Decrease of 7.5%	
Laboratory	$306	$325	$340	$361	$350	Decrease of 12.7%	
Chargeable Supplies	$1,621	$1,804	$1,667	$1,790	$1,774	Decrease of 8.6%	
Pharmacy	$305	$383	$334	$357	$315	Decrease of 3.4%	
Radiology	$30	$28	$32	$30	$29	Increase of 5.4%	
Respiratory	$30	$44	$42	$37	$37	Decrease of 19.4%	
Room & Other	$1,370	$1,474	$1,340	$1,438	$1,454	Decrease of 5.8%	
Contribution Margin per ICU Case[1]	$[redacted]	$[redacted]	$[redacted]	$[redacted]	$[redacted]	Increase of 42.8%	
ICU Outcomes							
% Readmissions	0.0%	4.0%	2.0%	2.1%	2.6%	Decrease of 100%	
Within 48 hrs leaving ICU	0.0%	4.0%	0.0%	0.7%	1.8%	Decrease of 100%	
After 48 hrs leaving ICU	0.0%	0.0%	2.0%	1.4%	0.9%	Decrease of 100%	
% Mortality	0.0%	1.9%	0.0%	2.1%	1.9%	Decrease of 100%	
High Risk[a] (APR-DRG)	NA	1.9%	0.0%	2.1%	1.8%	-	APR-DRG ROM = 3 or 4
Low Risk[a] (APR-DRG)	NA	0.0%	0.0%	0.0%	0.2%		APR-DRG ROM = 1 or 2

FIGURE 209.1. ICU metrics dashboard. Courtesy of Memorial Hermann Healthcare System, Houston, Texas.

communications and setting realistic expectations with patients and families. Additional efforts now underway include a database being developed at the Mayo Clinic that incorporates clinical patient data along with genomic data. The expectation is that powerful prediction models will result from analysis of this large-scale aggregated patient history, outcomes, and genomic dataset [29].

Another large-scale database is currently being collected and analyzed by a collaborative of industrial, medical, and academic partners (MIT, Philips Medical Systems, and the Beth Israel Deaconess Medical Center) [30]. To date analysis of this dataset (MIMIC II) has resulted in several prediction models that provide a rudimentary "early warning system" for several specific types of physiologic deterioration. One such model consists of a rule set that, when applied to near real-time patient physiologic data, is capable of predicting hemodynamic deterioration hours before its occurrence [31]. Early warning alerts from advanced clinical decision support systems hold the promise of improving response times to patient events. Although it seems to logically follow that such early identification of physiologic deterioration would allow earlier intervention and prevention of patient crises, the effects of these interventions on patient outcomes are yet to be studied.

It is important to note that the use of individual patient risk prediction for concurrent or prospective decision support has been challenging to incorporate into physicians' workflow, and has struggled to obtain widespread physician acceptance.

ADVANCES IN DATA VISUALIZATION TECHNIQUES

Although many organizations have successfully applied performance metrics, severity scores, and predictive risk models for improved quality and decision making, data collection/calculation and integrated display is likely to expand more in the next decade than in all previous ones. Designers have much work to do to accomplish meaningful display of the most important patient, process, alerting, and predictive information without overloading the clinician's ability to absorb and respond. Two examples of the application of modern data visualization techniques are represented in Figures 209.1 and 209.2. Figure 209.1 illustrates a comprehensive ICU performance management dashboard, as used by the Memorial Hermann Healthcare System in Houston, Texas. Note the integration of different categories of metrics, such as census, occupancy, glycemic control, infection prevention bundle compliance, medication and ventilator utilization, financial data, and patient outcomes. This is a fully automated monthly report that is electronically distributed to ICU and executive management across the health system. Figure 209.2 displays a comprehensive real-time ICU hospital-acquired infection (HAI) dashboard, including HAI rates and detailed bundle compliance results for prevention of catheter-related blood stream infection and VAP. This is a live intranet web display that is

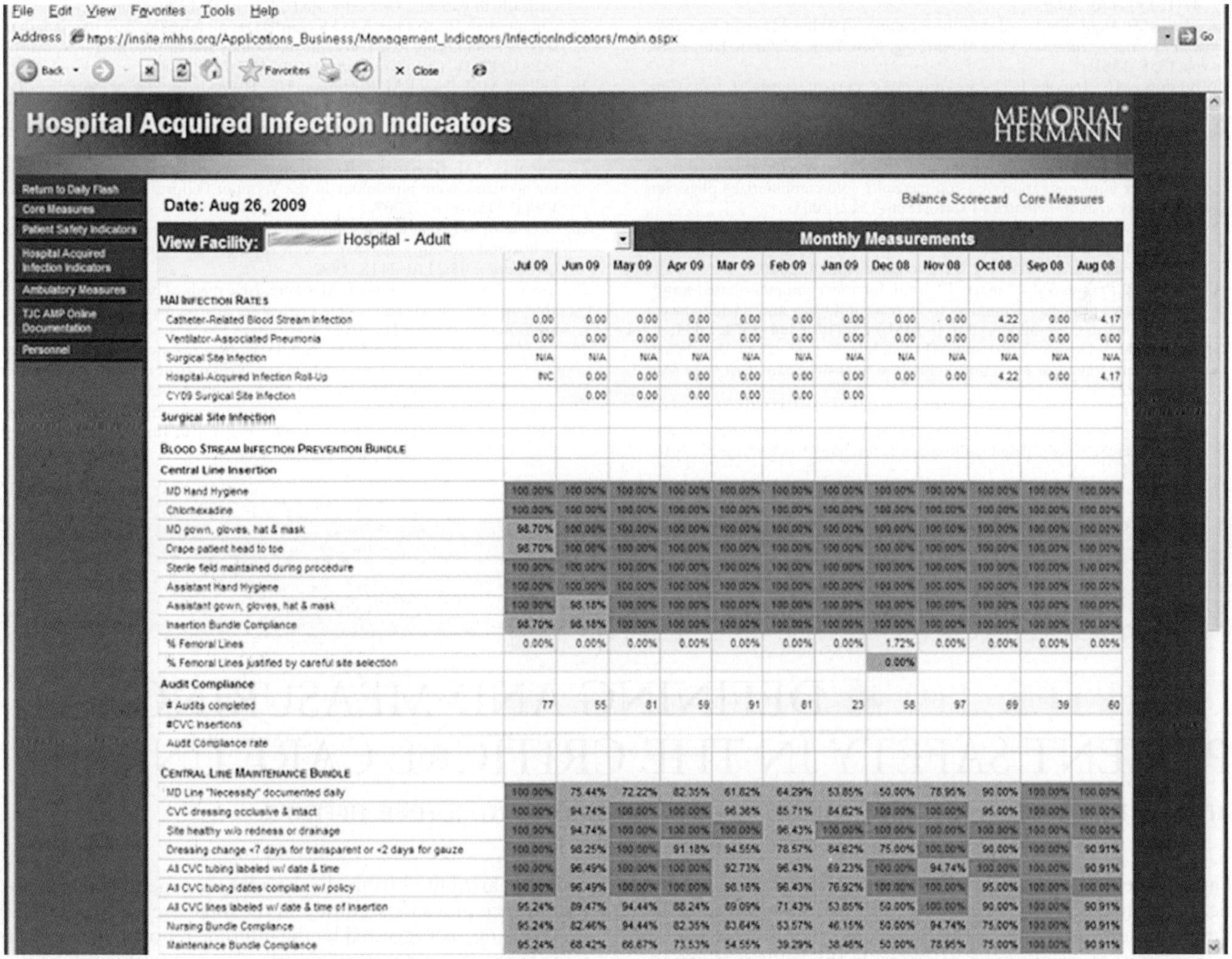

	Jul 09	Jun 09	May 09	Apr 09	Mar 09	Feb 09	Jan 09	Dec 08	Nov 08	Oct 08	Sep 08	Aug 08
HAI INFECTION RATES												
Catheter-Related Blood Stream Infection	0.00	0.00	0.00	0.00	0.00	0.00	0.00	0.00	0.00	4.22	0.00	4.17
Ventilator-Associated Pneumonia	0.00	0.00	0.00	0.00	0.00	0.00	0.00	0.00	0.00	0.00	0.00	0.00
Surgical Site Infection	N/A	N/A	N/A	N/A	N/A	N/A	N/A	N/A	N/A	N/A	N/A	N/A
Hospital-Acquired Infection Roll-Up	INC	0.00	0.00	0.00	0.00	0.00	0.00	0.00	0.00	4.22	0.00	4.17
CY09 Surgical Site Infection		0.00	0.00	0.00	0.00	0.00	0.00					
Surgical Site Infection												
BLOOD STREAM INFECTION PREVENTION BUNDLE												
Central Line Insertion												
MD Hand Hygiene	100.00%	100.00%	100.00%	100.00%	100.00%	100.00%	100.00%	100.00%	100.00%	100.00%	100.00%	100.00%
Chlorhexadine	100.00%	100.00%	100.00%	100.00%	100.00%	100.00%	100.00%	100.00%	100.00%	100.00%	100.00%	100.00%
MD gown, gloves, hat & mask	98.70%	100.00%	100.00%	100.00%	100.00%	100.00%	100.00%	100.00%	100.00%	100.00%	100.00%	100.00%
Drape patient head to toe	98.70%	100.00%	100.00%	100.00%	100.00%	100.00%	100.00%	100.00%	100.00%	100.00%	100.00%	100.00%
Sterile field maintained during procedure	100.00%	100.00%	100.00%	100.00%	100.00%	100.00%	100.00%	100.00%	100.00%	100.00%	100.00%	100.00%
Assistant Hand Hygiene	100.00%	100.00%	100.00%	100.00%	100.00%	100.00%	100.00%	100.00%	100.00%	100.00%	100.00%	100.00%
Assistant gown, gloves, hat & mask	100.00%	98.18%	100.00%	100.00%	100.00%	100.00%	100.00%	100.00%	100.00%	100.00%	100.00%	100.00%
Insertion Bundle Compliance	98.70%	98.18%	100.00%	100.00%	100.00%	100.00%	100.00%	100.00%	100.00%	100.00%	100.00%	100.00%
% Femoral Lines	0.00%	0.00%	0.00%	0.00%	0.00%	0.00%	0.00%	1.72%	0.00%	0.00%	0.00%	0.00%
% Femoral Lines justified by careful site selection								0.00%				
Audit Compliance												
# Audits completed	77	55	81	59	91	81	23	58	97	69	39	60
#CVC Insertions												
Audit Compliance rate												
CENTRAL LINE MAINTENANCE BUNDLE												
MD Line "Necessity" documented daily	100.00%	75.44%	72.22%	82.35%	61.82%	64.29%	53.85%	50.00%	78.95%	90.00%	100.00%	100.00%
CVC dressing occlusive & intact	100.00%	94.74%	100.00%	100.00%	96.36%	85.71%	84.62%	100.00%	100.00%	95.00%	100.00%	100.00%
Site healthy w/o redness or drainage	100.00%	94.74%	100.00%	100.00%	100.00%	96.43%	100.00%	100.00%	100.00%	100.00%	100.00%	100.00%
Dressing change <7 days for transparent or <2 days for gauze	100.00%	98.25%	100.00%	91.18%	94.55%	78.57%	84.62%	75.00%	100.00%	90.00%	100.00%	90.91%
All CVC tubing labeled w/ date & time	100.00%	96.49%	100.00%	100.00%	92.73%	96.43%	69.23%	100.00%	94.74%	100.00%	100.00%	90.91%
All CVC tubing dates compliant w/ policy	100.00%	96.49%	100.00%	100.00%	98.18%	96.43%	76.92%	100.00%	100.00%	95.00%	100.00%	100.00%
All CVC lines labeled w/ date & time of insertion	95.24%	89.47%	94.44%	88.24%	89.09%	71.43%	53.85%	50.00%	100.00%	90.00%	100.00%	90.91%
Nursing Bundle Compliance	95.24%	82.46%	94.44%	82.35%	83.64%	53.57%	46.15%	50.00%	94.74%	75.00%	100.00%	90.91%
Maintenance Bundle Compliance	95.24%	68.42%	66.67%	73.53%	54.55%	39.29%	38.46%	50.00%	78.95%	75.00%	100.00%	90.91%

FIGURE 209.2. Hospital-acquired infection indicators dashboard. Courtesy of Memorial Hermann Healthcare System, Houston, Texas.

updated constantly. Both reports are widely available within the Memorial Hermann system and have helped drive performance excellence.

Most importantly, to taking advantage of these new possibilities, though, is that senior medical executives, ICU directors, and clinicians must "own" responsibility for localizing and embracing performance metrics and the advancing base of evidence-based decision support being made available.

In conclusion, the modern CCIS is a dynamic information instrument, extending the capabilities of the intensive care physician and staff in ways that would be considered science fiction only a generation ago. The rapid adoption of these new information tools is now anticipated, as the complexity of medical care, particularly in the ICU setting, becomes increasingly demanding and evidence-based decision making moves from a goal to an expectation of acute medical care.

References

1. Jha AK, Des Roches CM, Campbell EG, et al: Use of electronic health records in U.S. hospitals. *N Engl J Med* 360(16):1628–1638, 2009.
2. MHS Optimization and Population Health Support Center: Glossary Terms and Abbreviations/Acronyms. Available at: http://www.tricare.mil/mhsophsc/mhs_supportcenter/glossary/Tg.htm. Accessed April 1, 2010.
3. Lilly CM, Cody S, Zhao H, et al: Hospital mortality, length of stay, and preventable complications among critically ill patients before and after tele-ICU reengineering of critical care processes. *JAMA* 305(21), 2011.
4. Forni A, Skehan N, Hartman CA, et al: Evaluation of the impact of a tele-ICU pharmacist on the management of sedation in critically ill mechanically ventilated patients. *Ann Pharmacother* 44(3): 432-438, 2010.
5. Groves RHJ, Holcomb BWJ, Smith ML: Intensive care telemedicine: evaluating a model for proactive remote monitoring and intervention in the critical care setting. *Stud Health Technol Inform* 131:131–146, 2008.
6. Thomas E, Lucke JF, Wueste L, et al: Association of telemedicine for remote monitoring of intensive care patients with mortality, complications, and length of stay. *JAMA* 302(24):2671–2678, 2009.
7. Berenson RA, Grossman JM, November EA: Does telemonitoring of patients—the eICU—improve intensive care? *Health Aff (Millwood)* 28(5): w937–w947, 2009.
8. Ries M: Tele-ICU: a new paradigm in critical care. *Int Anesthesiol Clin* 47(1):153–170, 2009.
9. Morris A: Algorithm-based decision- making, in Tobin MJ (ed): *Principles and Practice of Intensive Care Monitoring*. New York, McGraw-Hill, 1998, pp 1355–1381.
10. Breslow MJ: Remote ICU care programs: current status. *J Crit Care* 22(1):66–76, 2007.
11. Miller GA: The magical number seven plus or minus two: some limits on our capacity for processing information. *Psychol Rev* 63(2):81–97, 1956.
12. Han YY, Carcillo JA, Venkataraman ST, et al: Unexpected increased mortality after implementation of a commercially sold computerized physician order entry system. *Pediatrics* 116(6):1506–1512, 2005.
13. Shaffer V, Lovelock J: Results of the Gartner-AMDIS survey of chief medical informatics officers. Available at: http://www.gartner.com/DisplayDocument?id=1121012. Last accessed April 1, 2010.
14. Dexter PR, Perkins SM, Maharry KS, et al: Inpatient computer-based standing orders vs physician reminders to increase influenza and pneumococcal vaccination rates: a randomized trial. *JAMA* 292(19):2366–2371, 2004.
15. Rosenfeld BA, Dorman T, Breslow MJ, et al: Intensive care unit telemedicine: alternate paradigm for providing continuous intensivist care. *Crit Care Med* 28(12):3925–3931, 2000.
16. Institute for Healthcare Improvement: Building rapid response teams. Available at: http://www.ihi.org/IHI/Topics/CriticalCare/IntensiveCare/ImprovementStories/BuildingRapidResponseTeams.htm. Accessed April 1, 2010.
17. Homsted L: Institute of medicine report: to err is human: building a safer health care system. *Fla Nurse* 48(1):6, 2000.
18. The Joint Commission: National hospital quality measures—ICU, March 2009. Available at: http://www.jointcommission.org/PerformanceMeasurement/MeasureReserveLibrary/Spec+Manual+-+ICU.htm. Accessed April 1, 2010.
19. Leapfrog Group: The Leapfrog Group for patient safety. Available at: http://www.leapfroggroup.org/home. Accessed April 1, 2010.
20. Knaus WA, Wagner DP, Draper EA, et al: The APACHE III prognostic system. Risk prediction of hospital mortality for critically ill hospitalized adults. *Chest* 100(6):1619–1636, 1991.
21. Baker DW, Einstadter D, Thomas CL, et al: Mortality trends during a program that publicly reported hospital performance. *Med Care* 40(10):879–890, 2002.
22. Heard B: Customized data helps the Reading Hospital face clinical issues and improve outcomes. Available at: https://www.readinghospital.org/wtn/Page.asp?PageID=WTN001750.PDF. Accessed April 1, 2010.
23. Iezzoni L: *Risk Adjustment for Measuring Healthcare Outcomes*. 3rd ed. Chicago, IL, Health Administration Press, 2003.
24. Zimmerman JE, Kramer AA, McNair DS, et al: Acute physiology and chronic health evaluation (APACHE) IV: hospital mortality assessment for today's critically ill patients. *Crit Care Med* 34(5):1297–1310, 2006.
25. Zimmerman JE, Kramer AA, McNair DS, et al: Intensive care unit length of stay: benchmarking based on acute physiology and chronic health evaluation (APACHE) IV. *Crit Care Med* 34(10):2517–2529, 2006.
26. Pollack MM, Patel KM, Ruttimann UE: The pediatric risk of mortality III—acute physiology score (PRISM III-APS): a method of assessing physiologic instability for pediatric intensive care unit patients. *J Pediatr* 131(4):575–581, 1997.
27. Zupancic JAF, Richardson DK, Horbar JD, et al: Revalidation of the score for neonatal acute physiology in the Vermont Oxford Network. *Pediatrics* 119(1):e156–e163, 2007.
28. O'Connor GT, Plume SK, Olmstead EM, et al: Multivariate Prediction of in hospital mortality associated with coronary artery bypass graft surgery. *Circulation* 85:2110–2118, 1992.
29. Mayo Clinic: Mayo Clinic, IBM aim to drive medical breakthroughs. Available at: http://www.mayoclinic.org/feature-articles/mayoibmcollaboration.html. Accessed April 12, 2010.
30. Saeed M, Lieu C, Raber G, et al: MIMIC II: a massive temporal ICU patient database to support research in intelligent patient monitoring. *Comput Cardiol* 29:641–644, 2002. NASA: Grant numbers: NASA NCC9–58.
31. Eshelman LJ, Lee KP, Frassica JJ, et al: Development and evaluation of predictive alerts for hemodynamic instability in ICU patients. *AMIA Annu Symp Proc* 6:379–383, 2008.

CHAPTER 210 ■ DEFINING AND MEASURING PATIENT SAFETY IN THE CRITICAL CARE UNIT

ALAN M. FEIN, STEVEN Y. CHANG, SARA L. MERWIN, DAVID OST AND JOHN E. HEFFNER

Patient safety has become a major concern of the general public, policy makers, and local, state, and national government. Frequent news coverage has been devoted to individuals who were victims of serious medical errors. In the 1999 publication of the Institute of Medicine, *To Err Is Human: Building a Safer Health Care System* [1], the risks of medical care were highlighted, particularly the nearly 100,000 deaths per year that could be attributed to medical errors. A general sense of the importance of a safety culture in the intensive care unit (ICU) is increasing, as suggested by the multiple reports and publications in the lay and scientific media devoted to this topic [2].

The high-risk environment of the ICU benefits from integrated and coordinated systems that identify patient safety problems and report them to providers so they can improve their performance. To maintain high-quality care, critical care teams need to know not only what to do but also how they are doing and what they need to do to improve their structure, processes, and outcomes of care. Donabedian [3] first described these three domains—structure, process, and outcome—as necessary elements for measuring the quality of health care. They also serve as a conceptual framework for measuring patient safety in the ICU.

On a broad scale, ICU patient safety-reporting systems identify trends and patterns allowing health care organizations, governmental agencies, and private accreditation organizations to monitor the quality and safety of health care delivery, which facilitates public reporting of data and increases transparency [4]. Patient safety-reporting systems also have the potential to create large data repositories that inform the development of strategies that reduce the risk of preventable medical incidents [5,6].

Effective reporting systems require definitions and methods that are standardized throughout the community of providers, so that information can be shared and meaningful comparisons can be made. In the 2003 report, *Patient Safety: Achieving a New Standard of Care,* the Institute of Medicine (IOM) emphasized the importance of standardizing and better managing information on patient safety to improve outcomes of care [5]. A critical element of this standardization is the development of a common taxonomy of patient safety terms. In the absence of standardized terminology, health care providers have no way to know what events to capture and how to describe those events in consolidated reports [7]. Also, fragmented approaches for defining and classifying near misses, adverse events, and other patient safety concepts prevent aggregation of data in formats that allow analysis and summary reporting [1,8]. To date, governmental and private sector accrediting bodies have not coordinated their efforts to develop actionable, integrated, validated, and reliable systems to measure and report medical errors and patient safety [9].

SAFETY LESSONS FROM OTHER INDUSTRIES

Safety and error prevention in the health care setting compares unfavorably with that in aviation, banking, chemical manufacturing, and military services in peacetime. Lessons from these industries are now being applied to the health care industry. Approaches to safety in these industries are characterized by well-defined strategies to protect workers and customers. Technology-based approaches are part of this strategy, but organizational and psychologic aspects are contributing factors as well. For example, developing a culture of safety has been identified as one important method of improving safety. The aviation industry has focused on the importance of teamwork in reinforcing a safety culture.

Although technical, organizational, and psychologic interventions are effective, it is also worth noting the limits of the existing method. Persistence of fatalities in aviation and auto transportation suggest that safety efforts may be counterbalanced by other competing risk factors such as high volumes, greater complexity of the product, cost-pressure, and rapidly changing designs. This is particularly relevant to health care because the population is changing (higher number of increasingly older and higher-risk patients) and the technology is changing at a very rapid rate [10].

Thus, there is probably an upper limit in terms of cost-effective health care safety that can be reached, but has not been attained. Health services are being encouraged by the IOM report to aim for an error rate of less than 3.4 per million, that is, "six-sigma quality." The discipline of anesthesiology in particular has made substantial contributions through its development of a safety culture and equipment-manufacturing standardization that resulted in a reduction in anesthesia-related deaths to 4.4 per million, that is, "five-sigma standard."

To achieve this standard in the ICU, there must be a precise definition of the terms needed to study patient safety, their methods of measurement, how these can be applied to the special problems of ICU organization, physician training, and development of a culture of safety, and finally how these concepts apply to governmental regulations.

DEFINITIONS

The basic terms in common use to define concepts of patient safety are listed in Table 210.1 and show the working definitions that have entered into the lexicon of the patient safety industry [11]. Health care quality is defined by the IOM as "the degree to which health services for individuals and populations increase the likelihood of desired health outcomes and are consistent with current professional knowledge" [12]. This definition conforms to two (process and outcome) of the three constructs (structure, process, and outcome) proposed by Donabedian [3] to be necessary for measuring the quality of health care. The IOM has also listed several attributes of quality care that define quality care as being safe, patient-centered, timely, effective, efficient, and equitable [13]. Thus, patient safety is one domain within the broader concept of quality.

Patient safety has been variously defined by the Agency for Health Care Research and Quality (AHRQ) as "the absence of the potential for, or the occurrence of, healthcare associated injury to patients created by avoiding medical errors as well as taking action to prevent errors from causing injury" [14] and "freedom from accidental or preventable injuries produced by medical care" [15].

Within this context of safety, medical errors are defined as "mistakes made in the process of care that result in or have the potential to result in harm to patients. Mistakes include the failure of a planned action to be completed as intended or the use of a wrong plan to achieve an aim. These can be the result of an action that is taken (error of commission) or an action that is not taken (error of omission)" [14]. Errors of commission (e.g., ordering an incorrect drug dose) as compared with errors of omission (e.g., failure to order heparin for venous thromboembolism prophylaxis) are more readily noted. Errors are further classified as *active* or *latent* [16,17]. Active errors occur at the interface between a human provider and a care-delivery system (e.g., mechanical ventilator, intravenous pump) and typically involve readily apparent actions (e.g., adjusting a dial incorrectly). Latent errors define a less obvious failure of a health care organization or structure that contributed to errors or allowed the errors to harm patients. An example of a latent error would be understaffing of nurses in an ICU. Other typologies include domains that ascribe characteristics of preventability, seriousness and whether the error was intercepted before affecting a patient [18] (Table 210.1).

Errors have also been classified as *slips* or *mistakes*. Slips are failures of automatic behaviors, or lapses in concentration (e.g., forgetting to perform a routine task due to a lapse in memory) and often occur from fatigue or distractions in the workplace. Mistakes represent incorrect choices, such as choosing the wrong drug for a clinical condition, and typically result from inexperience or lack of knowledge or training. The remedies for these two types of errors differ, with slips being more responsive to removing distractions from the workplace or automating monotonous tasks and mistakes respond to increased training or supervision.

Incidents are defined as unexpected or unanticipated events or circumstances not consistent with the routine care of a particular patient, which could have or did lead to an unintended

TABLE 210.1

GENERAL TERMS USED IN PATIENT SAFETY

Quality: The degree to which health services for individuals and populations increase the likelihood of desired health outcomes and are consistent with current professional knowledge

Patient safety: The absence of the potential for, or the occurrence of, health care-associated injury to patients created by avoiding medical errors as well as taking action to prevent errors from causing injury. Freedom from accidental or preventable injuries produced by medical care

Medical errors: Mistakes made in the process of care that result in or have the potential to result in harm to patients. Mistakes include the failure of a planned action to be completed as intended or the use of a wrong plan to achieve an aim. These can be the result of an action that is taken (error of commission) or an action that is not taken (error of omission)

Active errors: Errors that occur at the interface between a human provider and a care-delivery system (e.g., mechanical ventilator, intravenous pump) and typically involve readily apparent actions (e.g., adjusting a dial incorrectly).

Latent errors: Less obvious failures of a health care organization or structure that contributed to errors or allowed the errors to harm patients. An example of a latent error would be understaffing of nurses in an intensive care unit.

Serious medical errors: A medical error that causes harm (or injury) or has the potential to cause harm. Includes preventable adverse events, intercepted serious errors, and nonintercepted serious errors. Does not include trivial errors with little or no potential for harm or nonpreventable adverse events.

Intercepted serious error: A serious medical error that is caught before reaching the patient

Nonintercepted serious error: A serious medical error that is not caught and therefore reaches the patient but because of good fortune or because the patient had sufficient reserves to buffer the error, it did not cause clinically detectable harm

Nonpreventable adverse event: Unavoidable injury due to appropriate medical care

Preventable adverse event: Injury due to a nonintercepted serious error in medical care.

Slips: Failures of automatic behaviors, or lapses in concentration (e.g., forgetting to perform a routine task due to a lapse in memory) and often occur from fatigue or distractions in the workplace.

Mistakes: Incorrect choices, such as choosing the wrong drug, a clinical condition and typically result from inexperience or lack of knowledge or training.

Incident: An event or circumstance that could have, or did lead to, unintended and/or unnecessary harm to a person.

Harm: Death, injury, suffering, dissatisfaction, or disability experienced by a person.

Near miss: Any incident that could potentially lead to patient harm.

Adverse event: Any injury due to medical management, rather than the underlying disease.

Adapted from references [11,12,14–18].

or unnecessary harm to a person, or a complaint, loss, or damage. Adverse events are different, and are defined as an "untoward and usually unanticipated outcome that occurs in association with health care" [14] or more broadly stated by the IOM as "an injury resulting from a medical intervention" [1]. The Critical Care Safety Study defines adverse events as "Any injury due to medical management, rather than the underlying disease [18]. Describing an event as an adverse event does not imply poor-quality care or that an error occurred. An adverse event only indicates that an undesirable outcome resulted from a medical intervention rather than an underlying disease process [19]. As an example, if proper procedures are followed for central line placement but the patient develops a pneumothorax, this would constitute an adverse event even though all the elements of quality care were met.

Most existing typologies of definition related to patient safety pertain to medical interventions. Errors of diagnosis are emerging as relatively uninvestigated but equally important causes of unsafe patient management in the ICU [20].

MEASUREMENT OF SAFETY IN THE INTENSIVE CARE UNIT

The science of measuring and reporting patient safety remains immature and can be viewed from the perspective of whether the measure identifies a structure, process, or outcome related to safety. Different methods of measurement focus on one or more of these elements and may be more or less efficient at identifying safety risks in one or more of these domains. The primary methods of measurement include incident reporting, targeted monitoring, use of discharge data sets, process of care measurement, trigger tools, ICU audits, and direct observation [18].

Incident Reporting

In terms of collecting safety measurement data, traditional methods based on incident reporting of specific adverse events have been largely ineffective for several reasons [21]. First, reports have been generated in a punitive environment that focuses on the provider who committed an error rather than systems of care and discourages self-reporting of errors [5]. Second, each report of an error represents a "numerator" value that does not give insight into the denominator pool of patients at risk for similar errors. In the absence of these values, the incidence of errors and the overall safety of an ICU cannot be assessed. Third, definitions of errors used in incident-reporting systems vary, which impedes data synthesis, analysis, collaborative work, and evaluation of the impact of changes in health care delivery [22]. And fourth, appropriate functional data spanning the domains of structure, process, and outcome are not collected, which impedes the ability to "deconstruct" an error to understand its root causes and patient impact.

Recent advances to incident reporting have enhanced the detection and analysis of errors. Internet-based systems allow anonymous reporting of errors to encourage providers who have either committed an error or have knowledge of an error to enter related information into a central data repository. Institutional commitment to a "culture of safety" has a motivational effect on error reporting because health care providers note the impact that a reported error can generate in terms of improved quality of care. This culture requires several essential process elements to enhance error reporting: A team (a) convenes to develop preventative solutions to a reported error, (b) generates plans to improve the care, and (c) has a method for implementing and measuring the impact of their plan [23]. The Intensive Care Unit Safety Reporting System (ICUSRS) is an anonymous reporting system that focuses on "systems factors" rather than "person factors" and provides expert analysis with feedback and guidance to improve processes of care and prevent error recurrences [11,24]. The University Health Systems Consortium's Safety Net reporting system can generate consolidated reports with application to the ICU [24].

However, problems remain with incident reporting in terms of the taxonomy used to describe errors and adverse events. The Joint Commission (JC) published a patient safety event taxonomy and classification schema for near misses, errors, and adverse events [11]. The taxonomy was designed to conform to an analytical framework and common word usages to promote its use and the understanding of its output. Data entered allows classification of a patient safety event within five complementary primary groups: *impact*—the outcome or effects of medical error and systems failure, commonly referred to as harm to the patient; *type*—the implied or visible processes that were faulty or failed; *domain*—the characteristics of the setting in which an incident occurred and the type of individuals involved; *cause*—the factors and agents that led to an incident; and *prevention and mitigation*—the measures taken or proposed to reduce incidence and effects of adverse occurrences.

The ICUSRS reporting platform similarly uses a framework for evaluating factors that contribute to an incident [11]. Both the JC and ICUSRS systems recognize that errors are multifactorial and therefore include multiple variables along the three domains of structure, process, and outcomes, such as caregiver performance, systems of care, resource availability, functioning of teams, and the environment of care. These systems describe events with a multidimensional taxonomy to allow the comprehensive description and full deconstruction of errors to determine their root causes [9]. However, even if taxonomy issues of incidence reporting are improved, the problem of determining the true incidence rate remains. A comprehensively described and deconstructed incident only gives insight into the numerator; it does not provide information on the number of patients at risk and does not allow determination of true incidence rates.

Targeted Monitoring

A complementary approach to incident reporting is targeted monitoring. ICUs can measure their patient safety outcomes by monitoring a specific indicator, such as the incidence of *Clostridium difficile* infection in the ICU or ventilator-associated pneumonia. In so doing, ICUs are challenged to define their denominators and select indicators that can be readily detected and counted to provide an accurate numerator. The denominator is especially difficult to determine because the measurement has major impact on interpretation [11]; for instance, *C. difficile* infection rates can be described per ICU patient, patient ICU days, or at-risk patient ICU days. The numerator data are equally challenging because of the time and expense of chart extraction needed for their collection. If the characteristics of the patient population change over time, then these factors must be accounted for as well. For example, if the patient population changes or new services such as transplant are offered by a given hospital, then the patient mix will change and adjusted hazard rates will be needed. Thus, for this approach to work, a multidisciplinary team that includes people with ICU training, organizational skills, database management, and epidemiology are needed.

Discharge Data

Discharge data represents a potential source of information to allow the retrospective collection of quality and safety indicators to profile ICU performance [25–27]. Recently, AHRQ has developed empiric measures of quality and safety from multistate discharge data in a redesign of the original Healthcare Cost and Utilization Project Quality Indicators [28]. The Patient Safety Indicators are relevant to ICU safety of care. Although most of these indicators relate to surgical patients, newer indicators are being designed to measure the safety of care for medical patients with critical illnesses, such as myocardial infarction, stroke, and congestive heart failure.

Although this method is powerful and can be quite useful, it is important to also recognize its limitations. Discharge data analysis gives insight into outcomes, but little information on structure or process. Large datasets such as these also have limited data quality for clinically relevant covariates, so controlling for confounders is difficult. Because all of the clinically relevant covariates are not included, the problem of residual confounding is always a problem and caution should be exercised when interpreting results. Making interinstitutional comparisons is therefore difficult, and even when trending data over time, results must be analyzed with caution. When patient populations and their problems are relatively homogenous and stable over time, this is a good system (e.g., surgical patients). When there is marked heterogeneity in terms of clinical problems and rapid changes in process of care over time, this approach will have difficulty. Having said this, discharge datasets can be an important tool for hypothesis generation so that ICU leaders can then launch more systematic studies into particular problems.

Process of Care Measurement

Safety can also be measured through determination of the proportion of patients who receive certain processes of care that have a strong evidentiary base for improving clinical outcomes. However, it may be difficult to isolate and to ascertain the contributory effect of influential factors, that is, adherence to best practice by the caregiving team, the role of complications, or level of care. Physicians and other clinicians often have a stronger sense of accountability toward a process measure than an outcome measure because the process measure can be more strongly linked to a particular care provider or team [29]. Also, physicians may believe that outcomes can be overly influenced by severity of disease and prove resistant to quality improvement efforts. To serve as an accurate measure of safety and to influence quality improvement, process measures must have a causal relationship with the outcome they are intended to represent.

Examples of process measures include approaches for ordering therapy in the ICU. Medication errors and adverse drug events occur commonly in the ICU [30] and can be limited by the use of formatted drug-ordering forms [31]. Computerized physician order entry for drugs has the potential to decrease the rate of serious medication errors [32] and to improve clinical outcomes when applied to antibiotic prescribing [33]. Additional care processes that should be in place to support patient safety can be constructed by reviewing evidence-based clinical practice guidelines [34], such as standardizing orders for ventilator management in the ICU [35].

Process of care measurement is often very effective for certain types of problems, like computerized order entry, but it is important to recognize some of the limitations and difficulties inherent in the system when applied to more complex problems. When strong evidence-based clinical practice guidelines are available, this is a feasible strategy, but often this is not the case. In addition, properly identifying those patients eligible for a particular protocol in the appropriate time period is critical. Examples include the use of thrombolytics for myocardial infarction and stroke, as well as recombinant activated protein C for sepsis. Determining the numerator for such process of care measures is fairly easy (who actually received the drug), but determining the denominator can be more difficult and can be costly because of the time and expense needed for data collection (e.g., reviewing every chart in the emergency department of a patient presenting with angina or suspected myocardial infarction). In addition, chart abstraction in such cases usually requires a high level of expert judgment, which makes it even more difficult. Thus, process of care measurement, because of cost and time considerations, may be a suitable approach to improving safety for those problems in which there is a strong-evidence base and in which the costs of identifying the patient population (both numerator and denominator) are sustainable and warranted by the value of information obtained.

Intensive Care Unit Audits

An audit of the existing structure of an ICU can also measure patient safety. Evidence supports improved outcomes in ICUs staffed by sufficient numbers of board-certified intensivists [36,37]. Additional structure measures of safety include the presence of resources to establish ongoing competency of medical staff and residents [38], adequate nurse staffing and skill sets [39,40], and appropriate technology resources, such as smart pumps and bar coding [41]. And, most importantly, the presence of a culture of safety represents a central structure within an ICU for promoting safety. Such a culture emerges from the presence of leaders who are committed to safety and staff who understand that errors are inevitable, acknowledge that errors are to be reported, dedicate time to learn about new risks and hazards, support teamwork and open communication, and upgrade procedures and implement safeguards on a continuing basis [16]. Organizational characteristics of safe programs with low accident rates include successful safety programs with strong management commitment, safety training as part of new employee's training, frequent open contacts between workers and management, general environmental control and good housekeeping, a stable workforce, and positive reinforcement for good safety practices. Surveys exist that allow ICU directors to assess the status of their units' culture of safety [42–45]. Pronovost and Sexton [44] recommend measuring the entire hospital annually with the full Safety Attitudes Questionnaire, which has construct validity and sufficient reliability for measuring the single construct of safety culture. Once measured, the culture of safety can be improved with focused interventions for any low-scoring hospital areas, such as an ICU.

Trigger Tools

Trigger tools refer to techniques used to detect organizational signals for adverse events. For instance, orders for flumazenil may identify patients who were given an overdose of a benzodiazepine drug. The flumazenil order therefore would serve as a trigger to perform a chart review. A trigger or set of triggers can be used to identify medical records for retrospective review to assess organizational safety or used in "real time" as a tool to identify a specific patient at risk for an adverse outcome. Trigger tools for the ICU have been shown to be practical approaches to enhance detection of adverse events in critically ill patients [46].

INTENSIVE CARE UNIT ORGANIZATION

Because patient safety and quality of care are intricately related, it is vital that intensive care medicine be effective and efficient at delivering safe, high-quality care at a low cost, especially as between 0.66% and 1% of the gross domestic product in the United States is spent on critical care services [47–49]. As with any critical activity, the organization and structure of services affect its delivery [50].

The Committee on Manpower for Pulmonary and Critical Care Societies was sponsored by the American Thoracic Society, the American College of Chest Physicians, and the Society of Critical Care Medicine to make supply–demand projections about pulmonary and critical care services and physicians [51]. It was estimated that by 2020 there would be a deficit of pulmonologists equal to 35% of demand and that by 2030 the deficit would be equal to 46% of demand. The calculated shortfalls for intensivists were 22% and 35% for 2020 and 2030, respectively.

Given these shortages in physician personnel resources, it is imperative that ICUs optimize their organization and utilization of personnel. Thus, several issues regarding organization and staffing of the ICU are relevant (see Chapter 208). Current controversies in this area include whether around-the-clock intensivist staffing are required for quality care, whether closed or open ICU formats are better, and whether regional intensive care centers are necessary.

Intensivist Staffing

Twenty-four hours a day, 7 days a week (24/7) attending intensivist coverage was available in only 6% of American ICUs in a 1991 survey, and such coverage was available in 72% of European ICUs in the European Prevalence of Infection in Intensive Care survey [52,53]. Given the discordance in around-the-clock coverage across the Atlantic Ocean, there is surprisingly little evidence to support the benefit of 24/7 coverage of ICUs by senior intensivists. In fact, many academic institutions in the United States offer 24/7 coverage by dedicated house staff and other physician extenders with critical care attending backup, either by pager or mobile phone, without any temporal changes in mortality or utilization of resources [54].

There has been much speculation regarding the benefits of continuous, on-site attending physician coverage in the ICU [55–58]. Hypothesized benefits might include decreased mortality, decreased length of stay, decreased global costs (although ICU costs might be higher), decreased complications, improved nutritional management, efficient admission and discharge policies, improved reimbursement, and improved ICU team functioning. Within the context of patient safety, improved staffing ratios would presumably tend to reduce latent errors and mistakes. A single, retrospective pre- and postintervention study examining 24/7 intensivist coverage in the United Kingdom did show a decline in mortality with institution of continuous, on-site attending coverage [59]. Others studies have continued to support the benefits of intensivist involvement in critical care, even in ICUs where control was maintained by primary care physicians. Intensivist involvement also has been demonstrated to improve outcome in settings involving surgery of the abdominal aortic and esophagus, pediatric critical care and combat injuries. On balance, however, there are little data supporting the hypothesis that attending intensivists need to be on-site on a continuous basis to provide cost-effective quality care. In fact, a multicenter retrospective analysis suggested that there was a higher mortality rate when critically ill patients were managed by intensivists [60]. Although issues of confounding and controlling for these factors are always at issue in retrospective analysis, this study (Project Impact) has only reinforced the need to further study optimal staffing and training for critical care personnel.

Higher staffing ratios, whether nursing or physician, should theoretically eventually improve quality of care; for example, 1:1 patient-to-nurse ratios and continuously available on-site physicians from all specialties. The real issue centers around the incremental costs and benefits of improved staffing ratios compared with the current ratios (generally, 2:1 patients-to-nurse and variable attending coverage). We can restate the question as, given the finite and constrained resources we have, what is the optimal physician staffing ratio and organization for ICUs from a societal cost-effectiveness perspective? Currently, there are insufficient data to answer this question and indeed the "correct" answer is probably contingent on many other factors, including societal values, economic resources, physician manpower considerations, nursing costs and availability, nurse training, availability of house staff, house staff training, organizational culture, technology costs, and legal considerations.

As an example, if resident and fellow house staff are available, ICU nurses have advanced training and good organization, the number of patients in the ICU is small, and the clinical population has relatively straightforward problems, then in-house, 24/7 intensivist coverage is less likely to be cost-effective compared to intensivist backup (on-call). However, if ICU size goes up, complexity of patient problems increase, house staff training for ICU-related problems goes down, and there is a high amount of nursing staff turnover, which limits their expertise, then 24/7 intensivist coverage may have more benefits. The interaction of many of these variables makes study of this field complex because multiple variables have an impact on each other as well as an impact on safety and outcomes, but the issues of patient safety and the potentially high costs of instituting 24/7 coverage warrant further prospective studies.

ICU Models

The 24/7 intensivist staffing variable is a critical element of several variables determining ICU safety as it impacts errors of omission and recognition and can reduce critical mistakes. However, in addition to the actual number and availability of intensivists, how they are organized is equally and possibly even more important if cost-effective quality care is to be delivered.

One aspect of organization that can impact care is whether an ICU uses an open or closed model. Much evidence suggests that in an open ICU, intensivist consultation should be required for critically ill patients [61]. More ideally, however, critical care services should be delivered in closed units with dedicated intensivist staffing with administrative structures that allow for rapid implementation of protocols that have been proven to be beneficial to patients [54,62,63]. It might even be possible that a closed ICU functions efficiently without implementation of protocols as suggested by a nonblinded study [64,65]. Closed units also allow for strong leadership coupled with a multidisciplinary team approach to patient care, which might allow for effective and efficient delivery of services in the manner envisioned by the Society for Critical Care Medicine [50,66,67].

From a patient safety perspective, strong evidence-based protocols offer many potential advantages. They can help to minimize both slips and mistakes. For instance, daily assessment of patients to determine if they should undergo weaning from mechanical ventilation is important, but in the busy ICU environment, this can easily be overlooked. The liberation of patients from mechanical ventilation via protocols has been studied by Ely et al. (1996 and 1999) [63,68]. In a randomized, controlled trial of 300 intubated adult patients, Ely et al. [68] showed that early identification of patients capable of spontaneous breathing via daily screening by other physicians, respiratory therapists, and nurses could decrease the duration of mechanical ventilation by 1.5 days when compared to patients in whom their attending physicians made decisions about extubation on an individual basis, despite the fact that the intervention (e.g., daily screening) group was more ill. In a subsequent study, Ely et al. [63] showed a respiratory therapist-directed weaning protocol *without direct physician supervision* could be instituted in the ICUs of their university medical center with modest degrees of success. This would constitute one example in which protocols, disseminated through a closed ICU organization, can improve safety by limiting slips.

Other management strategies, such as sedation and ventilator management of ARDS/ALI are well suited for development of protocols and may further limit mistakes, such as over- or undersedation in the ICU [69,70] and enhance use of lower tidal volume ventilation. Nurse-driven protocols with specific sedation targets and daily lightening of sedation have been shown to impact duration of mechanical ventilation.

Intuitively, it seems that protocols would be easier to institute using a closed ICU organizational structure rather than an open structure. Protocol development, dissemination, and implementation are all facilitated by having a stable, smaller number of physician providers rather than having many providers with varying practice patterns. In addition, development and implementation of protocols allows for process of care measures to be built into the system, so that the measurement of safety in the ICU can be achieved in a more cost-effective manner.

Regional Intensive Care Unit Centers and Telemedicine

The Leapfrog group (http://www.leapfroggroup.org) is a consortium "made up of more than 170 companies and organizations that buy health care." The consortium's overarching objectives are to improve the quality, safety, and affordability of health care, including the way critical care medicine is practiced. What distinguishes Leapfrog from other quality-improvement organizations is its tremendous economic clout. Their current recommendations for ICU organization are that (a) ICUs should be managed or co-managed by intensivists who are dedicated to the unit and who are physically present during daytime hours, and that at other times, (b) the intensivists can return pages within 5 minutes, and (c) that the intensivists can either reach the ICU or can arrange for physician extenders to be on-site within 5 minutes. Whether or not one agrees with these recommendations (often misinterpreted as requiring on-site 24/7 intensivist coverage), many hospitals are attempting to adhere to the standards set forth by the Leapfrog group. Their recommendations for ICU staffing and practice are primarily based on "common sense and rational extrapolation of the data"[71]. Because *there are not* and will not be enough pulmonologists and intensivists to staff all hospitals in the fashion suggested by the Leapfrog group [51], there will need to be alternative acceptable schemes for the delivery of critical care services.

One potential solution is the regionalization of intensive care services in a hub-and-spoke pattern similar to airports [67,72]. In 1994, the American College of Critical Care Medicine challenged the medical community to study the regionalization of ICUs [36]. Since then, however, only a few studies have directly examined the issue of transferring adult critically ill patients from community hospitals to larger tertiary care centers [73,74]. In a retrospective, case-controlled study, Rogers et al. [73] showed that trauma patients could be safely stabilized at smaller, outlying community hospitals prior to transfer to a level I trauma center. Similarly, Surgenor et al. [74] showed in a prospective fashion that interhospital transfers of patients requiring high-level critical care were as safe as intrahospital transfers. Both of these studies hint at the feasibility of safely regionalizing critical care services as one method for partially dealing with the likely shortage of physicians trained and dedicated to critical care medicine [51]. In addition, higher volume centers have been demonstrated to have improved outcomes in patients with sepsis and respiratory failure requiring mechanical ventilation, thereby reinforcing the case for transfer to regional centers of critical care excellence.

However, even if transfers can be accomplished safely, it is not clear that regionalization can deal with the significant shortages projected. Regionalization of high-level services may allow some economies of scale to be recognized, but it is unlikely that these benefits could fully offset the shortages projected.

Another increasingly used model involves telemedicine [75]. In this paradigm, one or several ICUs are electronically linked to a central and remote site where intensivists monitor critically ill patients. For instance, ICUs (patient rooms and nursing stations) can be linked to the remote site via cameras, speakers, and microphones. The hospital computer and data system, order-entry system, ICU and telemetry monitors, digital radiography, and any other required information systems can be linked remotely to intensivists. This allows for oversight of ICU activities without actually requiring that critical care physicians be physically on-site. Procedures can then be performed by on-site physician extenders while the ICU nurses can carry out orders. The patients' primary physicians or daytime intensivists can then choose to be involved to varying degrees during off-hours.

Two studies have been published examining the feasibility of ICU telemedicine and the associated patient outcomes [76,77]. Rosenfeld et al. [77], compared a single prospective intervention arm to two retrospective baseline arms (one arm to exclude seasonal variations and the second to account for temporal changes in outcome) of surgical ICU patients, and found that severity-adjusted ICU mortality, severity-adjusted hospital mortality, ICU length of stay, and complication rates all decreased by a statistically significant amount while concurrently lowering costs. Breslow et al. [76] demonstrated similar benefits when linking multiple ICUs to a remote monitoring site using commercially available equipment. Nonetheless, another study of the effectiveness of telemedicine failed to conclusively demonstrate improved outcomes or length of stay [78].

In a previously well staffed critical care system, the addition of an supplementary layer of telemedicine monitoring improved hospital and ICU mortality and length of stay. Adherence to critical care "best practices" was also improved [79].

PHYSICIAN TRAINING AND DEVELOPMENT OF A CULTURE OF SAFETY

It is during residency training that physicians acquire not only their clinical knowledge, but also their familiarity with system-based practice attitudes toward patient safety. Because development of a culture of safety is one of the key elements to solving patient safety issues, the training of residents is central to developing long-term solutions to patient-safety problems. However, the ICU experience can be one in which residents themselves become a safety issue. Residents need to acquire the body of knowledge, skills, and experience necessary to function as attending physicians, and as part of this training they need to develop a culture of safety. Yet, lack of supervision, experience, and resident fatigue can adversely affect patient safety, especially in the ICU setting. It is thus useful to separate the issues of safety into those related to proper resident training, which affects the culture of safety in the long term, and those related to resident performance, which impacts patient safety in the short term.

Teaching a Culture of Safety

Poor outcomes related to resident errors have been documented by up to 45% of house officers queried, with nearly one third of the incidents associated with patients' death [80]. Resident cross-coverage and hand-offs also increases the risk of medical errors. The harried work environment and heavy workloads add to the risk of medical mishaps. It is within this context that residents are also acquiring their attitudes and the habits that determine their culture of patient safety. There is typically limited integration of safety practice into work routines [81]. To address these issues, governmental, local, and educational organizations have focused on how patient safety can be integrated into the continuum of medical education. Only a small proportion of clerkships and directors of clerkships, in the medical student setting, have patients' safety content as part of course curricula. Limited exposure of medical students to quality management, quality improvement, and organizational problem solving, has prompted curriculum guidelines that require residents to develop competency in six areas, including; patient care, medical knowledge, patient-based learning, personal and group communication skills, professionalism, and system-based practice [81,82]. Patient-based learning and system-based practice are the areas most relevant to patient safety and the development of a culture of safety.

The traditional morbidity and mortality conference in medical school-teaching hospitals has been an important training forum, for discussion of adverse events and errors as well as inculcating a safety culture. Data show that Internal medicine conferences were longer than surgery conferences and allowed more time for listening to invited speakers but had less time in audience discussion. Problematic cases in medicine were less often attributed to root causes. There was less frequent acknowledgement of specific errors in the medical cases compared with those in surgery [83].

Resident and Trainee Performance

Optimal resident and trainee performance requires adequate rest, supervision, and sufficient training to perform increasingly complex problem-solving tasks. Each of these areas can contribute to safety as they represent potentially latent medical errors (errors due to the design of the educational system as well as the health care delivery system).

Preparing for work by getting sufficient sleep and enhancing alertness is a recognized responsibility of the clinician. Despite this seemingly obvious axiom, extended work hours and extreme fatigue among trainees are long-standing traditions in medical education and have often been the hallmarks of "excellence" in educational programs. Prolonged work hours and being on call was exceedingly common, with workweeks of 120 hours and on-call shifts of 48 hours not unusual. However, resulting fatigue has been associated with altered moods, depression, anxiety, confusion, and anger, and, most recently, impairment in clinical performance [84,85]. Among documented impairments were decreased technical dexterity, impaired clinical reasoning, and inability to learn and accommodate new information. In a recent study of medical house staff in which work was limited to 16 and fewer consecutive hours, trainees slept more and had less than half the rate of attention failures compared to traditional "long" schedules. Interns working extended shifts of 24 to 30 hours had greater attention failures and performance associated with significantly more medical errors compared to those scheduled to work only 16 consecutive hours [86,87]. These findings have been observed across medical specialties with prolonged shifts associated with decreased attention, vigilance, and simulated driving performance similar to blood alcohol level of up to 0.05%. In addition, the odds of having a motor vehicle crash were significantly increased after prolonged work shifts. Extended shifts increased the amount of risk of any motor vehicle crash and falling asleep at the wheel [88]. Although preliminary studies have demonstrated significant improvement in mortality in common hospital diagnoses (acute myocardial infarction, congestive heart failure and gastrointestinal bleeding) in the first 2 years following these reform measures, cost estimates for these reforms have been estimated at $1.7 billion [89,90].

An assumption that improved work schedules will lead to improved patient outcomes has led to significant regulatory intervention to limit trainee work schedules. Following the 1984 Libby Zion case, New York State, adopted regulations that limit resident work hours to 80 hours per week, and with increased supervision [91]. The Accreditation Council for Graduate Medical Education (ACGME) has set standards for work hours and time off, although these vary among the specialties. The Association of American Medical Colleges issued duty hour regulations in July 2003. The purpose of these rules was to limit the number of weekly work hours, continuous hours, call frequency and set a minimum time between on call and insuring days off in between [92]. Direct federal regulation of work hours and duty periods for house staff has been introduced to the United States Congress [88], but federal policy also requires ACGME certification. In addition to regulating trainees, other proposed JC standards for 2008 may include recommendations to set limits on physician and nurse work schedules to reduce fatigue and thereby the frequency of medical errors.

Even when trainees have sufficient rest, they still require adequate training and supervision. The question becomes how to acquire sufficient experience while minimizing patient risks. Previous paradigms of critical care education have emphasized knowledge acquisition over performance. The critical care unit poses unique educational obstacles. Limitations of current training practices include difficulty in procuring cadavers, and tissues. There are ethical and financial barriers to utilization of animals. "Real" patients are increasingly reluctant to be used as a training tool. Critical care procedures are often dangerous and extremely difficult to learn and teach. Because of the learning curve, patients may be harmed, and the phrase "see one, do one, teach one" may no longer be relevant to modern practice.

One option that is being increasingly used in the ICU is simulation. Simulation is the imitation or representation of a potential situation in an experimental setting. It can be used to train physicians in the cognitive, procedural, and problem-solving aspects of critical care. Simulation has been increasingly used as an effective tool for training in medical settings [85]. First pioneered by Edward Leap, who designed a flight simulator for pilots in the 1920s, simulators are used today by all commercial airlines, by astronauts, the military, and the nuclear power industry. Medical simulators today frequently incorporate computers and virtual reality, but it is important to recognize that simulation training does not necessarily imply use of a computer. Simulators have traditionally focused on cardiopulmonary resuscitation models and normal/abnormal heart sounds, but many forms of simulation training are becoming available. Other simulators relevant to the ICU include mechanical models of the airway to teach basic bronchoscopy as well as newer bronchoscopy simulators with virtual reality augmentation [93]. The type of simulator (computer driven, mechanical, or a combination) depends upon the task being learned. For critical care, tasks can be broadly grouped into cognitive tasks (e.g., knowledge of physiologic responses to ventilator changes, analysis of cardiac rhythms in ACLS), mechanical-procedural tasks (e.g., bag-valve mask ventilation [94], intubation [95,96], bronchoscopy [93], central line placement [97]), and team performance tasks (e.g., respiratory failure using the Anesthesia Crisis Resource Management (ACRM) course [98], ACLS [99]). Simulation has been applied to all three areas. The incremental benefit of simulation training as compared with standard teaching methods on real-life performance has been demonstrated in only a few studies [93,97,100]. However, there is a much larger body of evidence in which surrogate outcomes (not real-life performance per se) have been used to demonstrate the positive effects of simulation training. Surrogate outcomes in these cases have included measures of student confidence [97] or performance on a model [94–96,99]. On balance, while the current evidence base is still incomplete with only a few randomized trials documenting superior real-life performance after simulation training, it reasonable to conclude that simulation training will play an increasingly important role in critical care education. The advantages hypothesized for simulation include safety, efficiency, and availability. Intricate elements of difficult procedures and potential complications as well as the response to equipment malfunction can be selectively and repeatedly rehearsed. The ability to provide immediate feedback and train teams is also enhanced. Employing simulation models may positively impact direct and indirect costs associated with training and educating personnel through reduced use of operating rooms and may potentially reduce malpractice claims. It is anticipated that as the expense of such equipment diminishes, simulators will be increasingly adopted in medical school curriculums and residency training.

The Agency for Health Care Quality and Research has made development of simulation devices and protocols an important priority. At the present time, there is only limited clinical evidence supporting the efficacy of simulators on improving patient-based outcomes such as length of stay and mortality.

REGULATION AND GOVERNMENT IMPACT ON PATIENT SAFETY

The role of government and nongovernmental regulation has increased during the past decade and taken on an international scope. As the public has become more aware of the need for patient safety and quality improvement within health care, there have been many new regulatory and reimbursement initiatives originating from the public sector (federal and state governments and agencies [e.g., www.ahrq.com]), state and county health departments, purchasers, and nongovernmental organizations (e.g., JC, ACGME), and international organizations (e.g., World Health Organization [WHO]). The hypothesis that significant mortality can be attributed to medical error has facilitated the implementation of rules and guidelines. Regulatory efforts encompass rules and regulations but also accreditation of organizations, certification of providers, and reimbursement programs based on patient safety processes and outcomes. Purchasers, led by the Centers for Medicare and Medicaid Services have adopted pay-for-performance reimbursement models [101] and nonreimbursement strategies for complications of care-related to specific "never events" [102]. A new area of interest pertains to appropriate levels of regulatory oversight for patient safety research that ensures patient protection yet fosters the acquisition of new knowledge necessary to improve patient care in the ICU [103].

Many regulatory initiatives are likely to improve outcomes, but others overlap thereby presenting a risk for causing confusion and malaise in health care providers as they attempt to comply with conflicting rules, mandates, and guidelines, and may actually become impediments to patient safety. Two trends include greater collaboration in developing safety efforts between relevant organizations and emergence of international partnerships of regulatory organizations. These efforts may result in improved harmonization of standards and regulations.

In regard to physician-related accreditation and certification, the ACGME has included patient safety concerns in its resident program accreditation process both in mandating duty hour limitations and requiring the inclusion of patient safety in educational curricula. The American Board of Medical

Specialties requires evidence of practice improvement efforts for maintenance of certification. Some of the required modules include patient safety domains. Regarding organizational-level regulations, the JC publishes annually an update of its national patient safety goals in support of their standards for accreditation, which include ICU-related processes of care [104]. In 2005, the JC and Joint Commission International were designated by the World Health Organization (WHO) as the first members of the WHO Collaborating Centre for Patient Safety Solutions. The Collaborating Centre has organized an international network to identify, evaluate, adapt, and disseminate patient safety solutions (http://www.ccforpatientsafety.org/WHO-Collaborating-Centre-for-Patient-Safety-Solutions-continued/). This effort demonstrates the international intent to create linkages with key organizations and individuals with expertise in patient safety, which include accrediting bodies, national patient safety agencies, professional societies, and others.

Independent, not-for-profit organizations, such as the Institute for Healthcare Improvement (IHI), develop programs to accelerate improvement by promoting cultures for change, stimulating promising concepts for improving quality and safety, and assisting health care organizations to implement these new concepts. The IHI has had considerable influence on regulatory organizations with respect to adoption of IHI initiatives, such as ventilator bundles, central line bundles, sepsis bundles, intensivist staffing models, and rapid response teams (http://www.ihi.org/IHI/Topics/CriticalCare/IntensiveCare/Changes/IntensiveCareChangesIndex.htm). Because of the emphasis on rapid promotion of promising new interventions, such organizations have occasionally endorsed interventions prematurely, such as tight glycemic control, ahead of supporting evidence.

Other proposed areas of regulation include minimum nursing staffing ratios to meet workload demands [105] for Medicare-participating hospitals and limitations of excessive work hours for nurses and residents. Hospitals have also been required to implement specific improvements and to develop a program for quality assessment. The IHI has also suggested that a patient safety officer needs to be an important component of all large health care organizations [106].

Safety has become a major concern in the high-risk environment of the ICU. Integrated and coordinated systems that identify patient safety problems and report them back to providers so they can improve their performance and so that they can improve "their structure, processes and outcomes of care" are being implemented. ICU reporting systems identify trends and patterns that facilitate health care improvement and reduction of preventable medical incidents. Because safety and error prevention in the health care setting compares unfavorably with those of other industries, a major thrust has been to adopt strategies and technologies that have proved successful in other settings and to apply them to the ICU. Common definitions of health care-related safety concepts and systems for safety monitoring and reporting will improve individual and group capability to improve patient safety. Approaches that have been implemented to some extent in the ICU community include incident reporting, targeted monitoring of process of care and discharges, trigger tools and ICU audits. Integration of electronic ICU patient data, such as hospital admissions information, laboratory results, progress notes, imaging and authentication data, with non-ICU patient data across a hospital computerized medical record is a prerequisite for promoting patient safety. ICU organization and staffing models also impact safety in the ICU and continue to be studied [107] along with team-training efforts [108] and programs in critical care telemedicine. Hospital design with placement of the ICU adjacent to emergency departments and surgical suites to facilitate rapid transfer of unstable patients will come under increased review. Although regulation by public sector agencies will impact the safety of the critical care environment, developing a culture of safety through graduate and postgraduate medical education will also be a major part of an ongoing program of quality improvement.

References

1. Kohn L, Corrigan J, Donaldson MS (eds): *To Err is Human: Building a Safer Health System*. Washington, DC, National Academies Press, 2000.
2. Berwick DM: Health for life 6 keys to safer hospitals. *Newsweek*, December 12, 2005, p 76.
3. Donabedian G: A evaluating the quality of medical care. *Milbank Mem Fund Q* 44[Suppl]:166, 1966.
4. Centers for Medicare and Medicaid Services: Hospital Quality Information Initiative. Available at: http://cms.hhs.gov/quality/hospital/hqii.asp. Accessed December 29, 2005.
5. Institute of Medicine: *Patient Safety: Achieving a New Standard of Care*. Washington, DC, National Academies Press, 2003.
6. Needham DM, Sinopoli DJ, Thompson DA, et al: A system factors analysis of "line, tube, and drain" incidents in the intensive care unit. *Crit Care Med* 33:1701, 2005.
7. Hofer TP, Kerr EA, Hayward RA: What is an error? *Eff Clin Pract* 3:261, 2000.
8. Runciman WB, Webb RK, Helps SC, et al: A comparison of iatrogenic injury studies in Australia and the USA. II: reviewer behavior and quality of care. *Int J Qual Health Care* 12:379, 2000.
9. Chang A, Schyve PM, Croteau RJ, et al: The JCAHO patient safety event taxonomy: a standardized terminology and classification schema for near misses and adverse events. *Int J Qual Health Care* 17:95, 2005.
10. Guarnieri M: Landmarks in the history of safety. *J Safety Res* 23:151, 1992.
11. Pronovost PJ, Thompson DA, Holzmueller CG, et al: Defining and measuring patient safety. *Crit Care Clin* 21:1, 2005.
12. Lohr KN, Schroeder SA: A strategy for quality assurance in medicare. *N Engl J Med* 322:707, 1990.
13. Institute of Medicine: *Crossing the Quality Chasm: A New Health System for the 21st Century*. Washington, DC, National Academies Press, 2001.
14. AHRQ: AHRQ's Patient safety initiative: building foundations, reducing risks. Interim Report to the Senate Committee on Appropriations. *AHRQ Publications* 04-RG005, 2003.
15. PSNet Patient Safety Net: Glossary. Available at: http://psnet.ahrq.gov/glossary.aspx. Accessed June 19, 2009.
16. Reason J: *Human Error*. New York: Cambridge University Press, 1990.
17. Reason J: Human error: models and management. *BMJ* 320:768, 2000.
18. Rothschild JM, Landrigan CP, Cronin JW, et al: The Critical Care Safety Study: The incidence and nature of adverse events and serious medical errors in intensive care. *Crit Care Med* 33:1694–1700, 2005.
19. Sax HC, Browne P, Mayewski RJ: Can aviation-based team training elicit sustainable behavioral change? *JAMA* 303(2):159–161, 2010.
20. Newman-Toker DE, Pronovost PJ: Diagnostic errors—the next frontier for patient safety. *JAMA* 301:1060–1062, 2009.
21. Garland A: Improving the ICU: part 2. *Chest* 127:2165–2179, 2005.
22. Kaplan HS, Battles JB, Van der Schaaf TW, et al: Identification and classification of the causes of events in transfusion medicine. *Transfusion* 38:1071, 1998.
23. Nolan T: A primer on leading improvement in health care. Presented at the Fifth European Forum on Quality Improvement in Health Care; November 2000; Berlin.
24. Needham DM, Thompson DA, Holzmueller CG, et al: A system factors analysis of airway events from the Intensive Care Unit Safety Reporting System (ICUSRS). *Crit Care Med* 32:2227, 2004.
25. Poniatowski L, Stanley S, Youngberg B: Using information to empower nurse managers to become champions for patient safety. *Nurs Admin Q* 29:72, 2005.
26. Romano PS, Geppert JJ, Davies S, et al: A national profile of patient safety in U.S. hospitals. *Health Aff (Millwood)* 22:154, 2003.
27. Zhan C, Miller MR: Excess length of stay, charges, and mortality attributable to medical injuries during hospitalization. *JAMA* 290:1868, 2003.
28. Agency for Healthcare Research and Quality: AHRQ Quality Indicators. Available at: http://www.qualityindicatorsahrq.gov/. Accessed June 19, 2009.
29. Rubin HR, Pronovost P, Diette GB: The advantages and disadvantages of process-based measures of health care quality. *Int J Qual Health Care* 13:469, 2001.

30. Leape LL, Cullen DJ, Clapp MD, et al: Pharmacist participation on physician rounds and adverse drug events in the intensive care unit. *JAMA* 282:267, 1999.
31. Wasserfallen JB, Butschi AJ, Muff P, et al: Format of medical order sheet improves security of antibiotics prescription: the experience of an intensive care unit. *Crit Care Med* 32:655, 2004.
32. Bates DW, Leape LL, Cullen DJ, et al: Effect of computerized physician order entry and a team intervention on prevention of serious medication errors. *JAMA* 280:1311, 1998.
33. Pestotnik SL, Classen DC, Evans RS, et al: Implementing antibiotic practice guidelines through computer-assisted decision support: clinical and financial outcomes. *Ann Intern Med* 124:884, 1996.
34. Pronovost PJ, Berenholtz SM, Ngo K, et al: Developing and pilot testing quality indicators in the intensive care unit. *J Crit Care* 18:145, 2003.
35. Krimsky WS, Mroz IB, McIlwaine JK, et al: A model for increasing patient safety in the intensive care unit: increasing the implementation rates of proven safety measures. *Qual Saf Health Care* 18:74–80, 2009.
36. Carson SS, Stocking C, Podsadecki T, et al: Effects of organizational change in the medical intensive care unit of a teaching hospital: a comparison of "open" and "closed" formats. *JAMA* 276:322, 1996.
37. Dara SI, Afessa B: Intensivist-to-bed ratio: association with outcomes in the medical ICU. *Chest* 128:567, 2005.
38. Sherertz RJ, Ely EW, Westbrook DM, et al: Education of physicians-in-training can decrease the risk for vascular catheter infection. *Ann Intern Med* 132:641, 2000.
39. Carayon P, Gurses AP: A human factors engineering conceptual framework of nursing workload and patient safety in intensive care units. *Intensive Crit Care Nurs* 21:284, 2005.
40. Tibby SM, Correa-West J, Durward A, et al: Adverse events in a paediatric intensive care unit: relationship to workload, skill mix and staff supervision. *Intensive Care Med* 30:1160, 2004.
41. Husch M, Sullivan C, Rooney D, et al: Insights from the sharp end of intravenous medication errors: implications for infusion pump technology. *Qual Saf Health Care* 14:80, 2005.
42. Zohar D: Safety climate in industrial organizations: theoretical and applied implications. *J Appl Psychol* 65:96, 1980.
43. Pronovost PJ, Weast B, Holzmueller CG, et al: Evaluation of the culture of safety: survey of clinicians and managers in an academic medical center. *Qual Saf Health Care* 12:405, 2003.
44. Pronovost P, Sexton B: Assessing safety culture: guidelines and recommendations. *Qual Saf Health Care* 14:231, 2005.
45. Kho ME, Carbone JM, Lucas J, et al: Safety climate survey: reliability of results from a multicenter ICU survey. *Qual Saf Health Care* 14:273, 2005.
46. Resar RK, Rozich JD, Simmonds T, et al: A trigger tool to identify adverse events in the intensive care unit. *Jt Comm J Qual Patient Saf* 32:585–590, 2006.
47. Berenson RA: Intensive care units (ICUs): clinical outcomes, costs, and decision-making. *Health Technology Case Study 28, prepared for the Office of Technology Assessment, US Congress*. Washington, DC, US Government Printing Office, 1984. Publication No. OTA-HCS-28.
48. Chalfin DB, Cohen IL, Lambrinos J: The economics and cost-effectiveness of critical care medicine. *Intensive Care Med* 21:952, 1995.
49. Halpern NA, Pastores SM: Critical care medicine in the United States 2000–2005: an analysis of bed numbers, occupancy rates, payer mix, and costs. *Crit Care Med* 38:65, 2010.
50. Zimmerman JE, Shortell SM, Rousseau DM, et al: Improving intensive care: observations based on organizational case studies in nine intensive care units: a prospective, multicenter study. *Crit Care Med* 21:1443, 1993.
51. Angus DC, Kelley MA, Schmitz RJ, et al: Caring for the critically ill patient. Current and projected workforce requirements for care of the critically ill and patients with pulmonary disease: can we meet the requirements of an aging population? *JAMA* 284:2762, 2000.
52. Groeger JS, Strosberg MA, Halpern NA, et al: Descriptive analysis of critical care units in the United States. *Crit Care Med* 20:846, 1992.
53. Vincent JL, Suter P, Bihari D, et al: Organization of intensive care units in Europe: lessons from the EPIC study. *Intensive Care Med* 23:1181, 1997.
54. Morales IJ, Peters SG, Afessa B: Hospital mortality rate and length of stay in patients admitted at night to the intensive care unit. *Crit Care Med* 31:858, 2003.
55. Burchardi H, Moerer O: Twenty-four hour presence of physicians in the ICU. *Crit Care* 5:131, 2001.
56. Carlson RW, Weiland DE, Srivathsan K: Does a full-time, 24-hour intensivist improve care and efficiency? *Crit Care Clin* 12:525, 1996.
57. Crippen D: The dilemma of full-time ICU physician coverage. *Cost Qual Q J* 3:38, 1997.
58. Lustbader D, Fein A: Emerging trends in ICU management and staffing. *Crit Care Clin* 16:735, 2000.
59. Blunt MC, Burchett KR: Out-of-hours consultant cover and case-mix-adjusted mortality in intensive care. *Lancet* 356:735, 2000.
60. Levy MM, Rapoport J, Lemeshow S: Association between critical care physician management and patient mortality in the intensive care unit. *Ann Intern Med* 148:801, 2008.
61. Manthous CA, Amoateng-Adjepong Y, al-Kharrat T, et al: Effects of a medical intensivist on patient care in a community teaching hospital. *Mayo Clin Proc* 72:391, 1997.
62. Carson SS, Stocking C, Podsadecki T, et al: Effects of organizational change in the medical intensive care unit of a teaching hospital: a comparison of 'open' and 'closed' formats. *JAMA* 276:322, 1996.
63. Ely EW, Bennett PA, Bowton DL, et al: Large scale implementation of a respiratory therapist-driven protocol for ventilator weaning. *Am J Respir Crit Care Med* 159:439, 1999.
64. Krishnan JA, Moore D, Robeson C, et al: A prospective, controlled trial of a protocol-based strategy to discontinue mechanical ventilation. *Am J Respir Crit Care Med* 169:673, 2004.
65. Tobin MJ: Of principles and protocols and weaning. *Am J Respir Crit Care Med* 169:661, 2004.
66. Azocar RJ, Lisbon A: Captaining the ship during a storm: who should care for the critically ill? *Chest* 120:694, 2001.
67. Parrillo JE: A silver anniversary for the society of critical care medicine—visions of the past and future: the presidential address from the 24th educational and scientific symposium of the society of critical care medicine. *Crit Care Med* 23:607, 1995.
68. Ely EW, Baker AM, Dunagan DP, et al: Effect on the duration of mechanical ventilation of identifying patients capable of breathing spontaneously. *N Engl J Med* 335:1864, 1996.
69. The Acute Respiratory Distress Syndrome Network: Ventilation with lower tidal volumes as compared with traditional tidal volumes for acute lung injury and the acute respiratory distress syndrome. *N Engl J Med* 342:1301, 2000.
70. Kress JP, Pohlman AS, O'Connor MF, et al: Daily interruption of sedative infusions in critically ill patients undergoing mechanical ventilation. *N Engl J Med* 342:1471, 2000.
71. Manthous CA: Leapfrog and critical care: evidence- and reality-based intensive care for the 21st century. *Am J Med* 116:188, 2004.
72. Thompson DR, Clemmer TP, Applefeld JJ, et al: Regionalization of critical care medicine: task force report of the American College of Critical Care Medicine. *Crit Care Med* 22:1306, 1994.
73. Rogers FB, Osler TM, Shackford SR, et al: Study of the outcome of patients transferred to a level I hospital after stabilization at an outlying hospital in a rural setting. *J Trauma* 46:328, 1999.
74. Surgenor SD, Corwin HL, Clerico T: Survival of patients transferred to tertiary intensive care from rural community hospitals. *Crit Care* 5:100, 2001.
75. Breslow MJ: ICU telemedicine. Organization and communication. *Crit Care Clin* 16:707, 2000.
76. Breslow MJ, Rosenfeld BA, Doerfler M, et al: Effect of a multiple-site intensive care unit telemedicine program on clinical and economic outcomes: an alternative paradigm for intensivist staffing. *Crit Care Med* 32:31, 2004.
77. Thomas EJ, Lucke JF, Wueste L, et al: Association of telemedicine for remote monitoring of intensive care patients with monitoring, complications, and length of stay. *JAMA* 302:2671–2678, 2009.
78. Rosenfeld BA, Dorman T, Breslow MJ, et al: Intensive care unit telemedicine: alternate paradigm for providing continuous intensivist care. *Crit Care Med* 28:3925, 2000.
79. Lilly CM, Cody S, Zhao H, et al: Hospital mortality, length of stay, and preventable complications among critically ill patients before and after tele-ICU reengineering of critical care processes. *JAMA* 305(21):2175–2183, 2011.
80. Shaughnessy AF, Nickel RO: Prescription-writing patterns and errors in a family medicine residency program. *J Fam Pract* 29:290, 1989.
81. Heffner JE, Ellis R, Zeno B: Safety in training and learning in the intensive care unit. *Crit Care Clin* 21:129, 2005.
82. Batalden P, Leach D, Swing S, et al: General competencies and accreditation in graduate medical education. *Health Aff (Millwood)* 21:103, 2002.
83. Pierluissi E, Fischer M, Campbell A, et al: Discussion of medical errors in morbidity and mortality conferences. *JAMA* 290:2838, 2003.
84. Buysse DJ, Barzansky B, Dinges D, et al: Sleep, fatigue and medical training: setting an agenda for optimal learning and patient care. *Sleep* 26:218, 2003.
85. Grenvik A, Schaefer JJ, DeVita MA, et al: New aspects on critical care medicine training. *Curr Opin Crit Care* 10:233, 2004.
86. Lockley SW, Cronin JW, Eans EE, et al: Effect of reducing interns' weekly work hours on sleep and attentional failures. *N Engl J Med* 351:1829, 2004.
87. Drazen J: Awake and informed. *N Engl J Med* 351:1829, 2004.
88. Gaba DM, Howard SK: Fatigue among clinicians and the safety of patients. *N Engl J Med* 347:1249, 2002.
89. Volpp KG, Rosen AK, Rosenbaum PR, et al: Mortality among patients in VA hospitals in the first 2 years following ACGME resident duty hour reform. *JAMA* 298(9):984–992, 2007.
90. Nuckols TK, Bhattacharya J, Wolman DM, et al: Cost implications of reduced work hours and workloads for resident physicians. *N Engl J Med* 360:2202–2215, 2009.
91. Robins NS: *The Girl Who Died Twice: Every Patient's Nightmare. the Libby Zion Case and the Hidden Hazards of Hospitals*. New York, Delacorte Press, 1995.
92. Resident duty hours language: final requirements Accreditation Council for Graduate Medical Education: Available at: http://www.acgme.org. Accessed July 27, 2003.
93. Ost D, DeRosiers A, Britt EJ, et al: Assessment of a bronchoscopy simulator. *Am J Respir Crit Care Med* 164:2248–2255, 2001.

94. Kory PD, Eisen LA, Adachi M, et al: Initial airway management skills of senior residents: simulation training compared with traditional training. *Chest* 132:1927–1931, 2007.
95. Lim TJ, Lim Y, Liu EH: Evaluation of ease of intubation with the GlideScope or macintosh laryngoscope by anaesthetists in simulated easy and difficult laryngoscopy. *Anaesthesia* 60:180–183, 2007.
96. Kovacs G, Bullock G, Ackroyd-Stolarz S, et al: A randomized controlled trial on the effect of educational interventions in promoting airway management skill maintenance. *Ann Emerg Med* 36:301–309, 2000.
97. Britt RC, Novosel TJ, Britt LD, et al: The impact of central line simulation before the ICU experience. *Am J Surg* 197:533–536, 2009.
98. Lighthall GK, Barr J, Howard SK, et al: Use of a fully simulated intensive care unit environment for critical event management training for internal medicine residents. *Crit Care Med* 31:2437–2443, 2003.
99. Wayne DB, Butter J, Siddall VJ, et al: Simulation-based training of internal medicine residents in advanced cardiac life support protocols: A randomized trial. *Teach Learn Med* 17:202–208, 2005.
100. Crabtree NA, Chandra DB, Weiss ID, et al: Fibreoptic airway training: correlation of simulator performance and clinical skill. *Can J Anaesth* 55:100–104, 2008.
101. Rosenthal MB: Beyond pay for performance—emerging models of provider-payment reform. *N Engl J Med* 359:1197–1200, 2008.
102. Milstein A: Ending extra payment for "never events"—stronger incentives for patients' safety. *N Engl J Med* 360:2388–2390, 2009.
103. Kass N, Pronovost PJ, Sugarman J, et al: Controversy and quality improvement: lingering questions about ethics, oversight, and patient safety research. *Jt Comm J Qual Patient Saf* 34:349–353, 2008.
104. Commission J: National Patient Safety Goals. [Internet]. Oak Brook, IL: JC, 2009. Available at: http://www.JointCommission.org/PatientSafety/NationalPatientSafetyGoals/. Accessed June 18, 2009.
105. Carayon P, Alvarado CJ: Workload and patient safety among critical care nurses. *Crit Care Nurs Clin North Am* 19:121–129, 2007.
106. Patient Safety Officer Executive Development Program. Available at: http://www.ihi.org/IHI/Programs/ProfessionalDevelopment/PatientSafetyOfficerTraining. Accessed June 19, 2009.
107. Gajic O, Afessa B: Physician staffing models and patient safety in the ICU. *Chest* 135:1038–1044, 2009.
108. Dunn EJ, Mills PD, Neily J, et al: Medical team training: applying crew resource management in the veterans health administration. *Jt Comm J Qual Patient Saf* 33:317–325, 2007.

CHAPTER 211 ■ MEDICAL ETHICS, END OF LIFE CARE, AND CLINICAL RESEARCH IN THE INTENSIVE CARE UNIT

MARK TIDSWELL, PAUL G. JODKA AND JAY S. STEINGRUB

Scientific knowledge and technology dominate the intensive care unit (ICU) environment and the practice of critical care medicine. Caring for the critically ill person challenges our ability to apply knowledge in the best interest of the individual. The critical care physician is confronted by complex medical decisions, life-and-death circumstances, and a person who is frequently unable to communicate. This makes it difficult to intimately understand their moral values and wishes at the time when these values are most meaningful. Moral issues are inescapable in the course of critical care and occur so frequently that resolving some issues becomes a matter of routine. Deciding what we should do for the welfare of our patients is guided not only by scientific knowledge, but also by understanding numerous other complex and evolving attributes of the physician–patient relationship including: moral responsibilities to patients, legal obligations, and the role of the patient in decision making. This chapter provides an overview of current practice of guiding patients or families in making decisions about critical care, withdrawing life-sustaining treatments, and participating in clinical research.

Moral obligations of physicians to their patients have been recognized for millennia, and are described in the Hippocratic Oath (400 BC), the Oath and Prayer of Maimonides (1783), Nuremberg code (1947), The Belmont Report for protection of human subjects in research (1979), and contemporary guidelines and codes for physicians [1–3]. Whereas ancient and traditional descriptions of physician responsibilities emphasized trust, compassion, fairness, caring, and acting in the best interest of patients, contemporary conceptions of the patient-physician relationship emphasize the patient's individualism, or autonomy in decision making. This change in emphasis appears to have evolved along with social, political, and judicial prominence of respect for individuals along with a growing social mistrust of commercialized medical care and clinical research during the past 40 years. Humane care based on a foundation of trust remains the responsibility of the physician, particularly in the ICU where patients may have lost their ability to advocate and to be self-governing due to their illness, fear of dying, and limited understanding the scientific basis of their treatment.

Ethics is a branch of philosophy that concerns the analysis of moral obligations, values, and choices. Ethics involves deliberation and reasoning about the best course of action and results in a clearly delineated path to a decision. Critical care physicians apply ethical reasoning to make moral decisions with patients in the ICU. The ethical questions that confront physicians are practical, not theoretical, and the answers lead to decisions about the best choices in the care of patients.

PRINCIPLES OF BIOETHICS

Medical ethics is a one branch of bioethics. The ethical framework generally used for medical decision making is reasoning from ethical principles [4–6] (Table 211.1). The oldest principles are *beneficence* and *nonmaleficence*, and other principles have been described in recent decades. *Justice*, or fairness, implies that patients will be given the treatment that is indicated for their condition without regard to social, economic, ethnic, or other attributes. Unfortunately, there may be times when resources such as ICU beds or mechanical ventilators are limited and ICU physicians may need to work with hospital administration and the community to clarify how care may be rationed [7]. At the time this chapter was written, a global influenza pandemic was predicted [8,9]. *Patient autonomy* has, in recent years, become foremost among ethical principles. This emphasis on the importance of individual choice has been

TABLE 211.1

PRINCIPLES OF BIOETHICS

Beneficence: physicians act in the best interests of the patient
Nonmaleficence: physicians exercise caution when providing treatment
Justice: physicians allocate resources fairly
Autonomy: physician and patient deliberate about patient goals when deciding on medical therapy or research participation

influenced by numerous social changes and increasing distrust of the corporations and medical centers. Several highly publicized instances of inappropriate medical research in the United States during 1960 to 1980 led to legislation and policies defining the place of informed consent in research and in medical care. Autonomy is the foundation for the practice of informed consent for medical research and clinical care. Autonomy is exercised by patients but must be enabled by physicians and is based on an assumption that the competent informed person can weigh risks and benefits and make a decision that balances their medical needs and personal values. Autonomy requires that the patient or surrogate is able to deliberate about personal goals and act under their own direction (self-governance). The joint participation of physician and patient in "shared decision making" is recommended [10,11]. Unfortunately, it is usually not possible for ICU patients to share decision making due to the nature of their illness and life support devices. The physician plays a role by acknowledging the importance of autonomy and ensuring that a surrogate is identified as a decision maker.

Acknowledging the importance of autonomy emphasizes the role of the individual patient in decision making. To make decisions, the patient or surrogate must have information about the possible risks and benefits of an intervention. The ICU physician must provide information about the diagnosis and prognosis of the critical illness that will be used in a decision of consent or refusal. The competent and informed patient has the ability to consent to, or refuse, medical interventions or research. Because autonomy means that a person has ability to make decisions on all aspects of their life, the autonomous person may choose to not only oppose the advice of physicians, family, and friends, but may also choose to act contrary to their own previously expressed wishes and can change their mind. If a person lacks autonomy then their ability to speak for themselves can be protected by referring to a substitute such as previously expressed wishes or a surrogate decision maker.

Patient autonomy alone is not sufficient to describe the patient–physician relationship and the physician remains obligated to their own moral responsibilities and to acknowledging the values of the patient. In practice, the principles already described represent different values that must be considered and balanced against each other when reasoning toward a treatment decision by asking the question: how much potential benefit at how much risk is acceptable to this critically ill person? Beyond these generally accepted principles there are many other perspectives that may influence decision making, such as religious authority, the importance of relationships, the rights of the patient, or the value of patient care to society. It is possible that patients, families, or ICU staff will appeal to other ethical perspectives when reasoning toward a treatment decision, and while the patient is free to reason from their own ethical value system to guide their choices, the four principles are the standard guiding principles for the ICU physician.

DETERMINING DECISION-MAKING CAPACITY

To exercise autonomy, a patient must have the capacity to make a choice. Determining whether a patient has capacity occurs daily in the ICU and the critical care physician should be adept at this assessment. Physicians use criteria listed in Table 211.2 [12,13] and also must comply with local hospital policy and state law when determining decision-making capacity. Decision making capacity is decision specific; that is, patients may have the capacity to make some decisions but not other decisions. Capacity is determined one decision at a time by a physician (in contrast to competency that is determined by the courts).

All of the criteria listed in Table 211.2 must be present, or the patient lacks capacity. When the critically ill person is unable to make decisions, the physician must document lack of capacity and plans for making decisions. Historically, physicians and/or a capable family member made decisions. Currently, patients are likely to use advance directives or assign surrogate decision makers to make medical decisions should they become incapacitated. Patients with terminal disease can address situations where death is imminent and there is no hope of recovery by preparing advanced directives, or living wills. Advance directives are also useful for patients who indicate that they would refuse life support under any circumstance. However, in many cases, the circumstances of a patient's critical illness may be unanticipated, prognosis may be unknown, and written directives may be ambiguous. In the absence of a clear advanced directive, surrogate decision makers provide a "substituted judgment" for the incapacitated patient based on their knowledge of the patient's values and previous statements made by the patient. Surrogates are most often relatives of the patient either through legal authorization by the patient prior to their illness, or as permitted by state laws. To fulfill the role, a surrogate must disregard their own values and represent the values of the patient. An incapacitated patient can accept or refuse therapy through a surrogate. Refusal of therapy has been legally guaranteed to patients for decades, and the results of landmark cases of permanently incapacitated patients in persistent vegetative states refusing therapy through surrogates can be extended to ICU patients. Cases such as *Quinlan* (1976), *Cruzan* v. *Missouri* (1990), and *Schiavo* (2003–2005) led to laws that permit refusal of therapy through a surrogate. In many states, surrogates are required to now bring forward "clear and convincing evidence" in verbal statements from the patient prior to incapacitation to justify refusal of therapy [14–17].

PHYSICIAN RESPONSIBILITY FOR THE INCAPACITATED PATIENT

Physicians identify lack of capacity and confirm the need for a surrogate decision maker. Physicians may have discussed with the patient their understanding of, and wishes for, life support prior to critical illness. But, although obligated to act in the best

TABLE 211.2

CRITERIA FOR DECISION-MAKING CAPACITY

1. The patient communicates a choice
2. The patient understands the relevant information
3. The patient understands the situation and consequences
4. The patient manipulates the information rationally

interest of patients, there is a limit to the authority of physicians and they cannot make value decisions without taking into account the wishes of the patient. Physicians may have limited information about the values of a patient, they may have a very different set of personal values, or may have financial conflicts of interest with patient wishes [4]. Physicians cannot function as a patient surrogate to make decisions, but, in the capacity as treating physician, can refuse to perform procedures or provide care that they believe are unnecessary or non-beneficial [18–21]. Usually patients or surrogates can be dissuaded from unnecessary care by engaging in a thorough discussion of the appropriate care, reasons for refusing care, and offering a second opinion. Physicians are not compelled to perform services that violate their own moral values and can arrange for another physician to care for the patient. When patient wishes are known or communicated through a surrogate, the physician should attempt to carry these out, and obtain consent for procedures. Although some procedures can be justified without consent in the absence of previously expressed wishes on an emergency and life-saving basis, unless there is a justification physicians risk the charges of battery or negligence if procedures or other interventions are provided without consent or after refusal of consent [5,22,23].

Remarkably, surveys of ICU physicians have found that decision making practice varies greatly and often does not involve the patient. Some physicians report that they continue life support even when there is little hope of benefit from intensive care. The results of the SUPPORT study indicated that physicians did not consistently document or write a DNR order for patients that did not wish to have cardiopulmonary resuscitation (CPR) [24]. A survey in 1999 of ICU physicians from 16 European countries indicated that 73% of ICU's frequently admitted patients with no hope of survival. DNR orders were followed only 58% of the time. Yet, on the other hand, many physicians withheld therapy for patients who had no prospect of meaningful life, or deliberately administered large doses of drugs until death ensued. Only 41% of physicians surveyed felt ethical issues should involve patient and/or family [25].

Many patients with terminal illnesses will come to the ICU for resuscitation or monitoring prior to their deaths. CPR has little likelihood of improving survival of patients with terminal illnesses, and is usually regarded as nonbeneficial. Such a procedure with a low likelihood of success can be regarded as not in the best interest of the patient. This differs from medical futility, since futile care is defined as having no physiological rationale or care to which the patient has already failed to respond [4,18]. The term "futile" carries an important meaning and should be used carefully and accurately. When death is imminent and treatment has failed, then withholding futile care is supported by legal precedent. However, when death is not imminent, physicians may not be able to predict outcome. In one study, daily surveys of ICU staff found that physicians and nurses were unable to predict survival and quality of life 6 months after ICU. Nurses were incorrect in 58% of 45 patients and physicians were incorrect in 27% of 26 patients. Only one of the survivors about whom physicians believed care was futile reported poor quality of life 6 months after ICU [26]. A larger study that investigated determinants of withdrawal of mechanical ventilation found that physician's prediction of low likelihood of survival (<10%) was a factor associated with withdrawal of mechanical ventilation and/or death [27]. In this study 3.6% of patients survived to hospital discharge after withdrawal of mechanical ventilation. A decision to withdraw support in this study was associated significantly with physician's perception of the patient's preferences about the use of life support. The ICU physician needs to know the precise hospital and legal definitions for "futility" and avoid invoking the term in cases where care is perceived as carrying a low likelihood of success or sustaining an unacceptable quality of life that is better termed nonbeneficial. If there is a plan to withhold support or procedures, for example, CPR, and the procedure is not strictly futile, then information should be provided about the procedure and rationale should be explained to the patient/surrogate [20,21,28].

ETHICS COMMITTEES

Ethics committees or ethics consultants provide an additional resource for resolving ethical conflicts. The committee is an objective "third party" not previously involved in disputes of the case. Committees review the medical and ethical and psychosocial aspects of the case and provide an ethical analysis. Committees can also provide social and emotional support to families and may be able to discuss and explain the ethical issues for longer periods of time than physicians and nurses. Since most ethics consultants are employed by the hospital, families may perceive a bias in favor of physicians or an attempt to protect the interests of the hospital. However, ethics consultants are usually well received by both physicians and patients/surrogates [28,29]. In addition to resolving conflicts, ethics consultations are associated with decrease in the duration of ICU length of stay and use of life-prolonging treatments for patients who ultimately do not survive [29].

COMMUNICATION WITH PATIENTS AND SURROGATES

Numerous studies and ICU practice guidelines over the past decade emphasize the importance of effective communication with, and support of, families of critically ill patients. Communication about plans for patient care most often takes place between physicians and family members, rather than between physicians and patients [30]. Discussions with families frequently occur when physicians have decided that continuation of care will be ineffective, but interviews with families indicate that more than half of family and patient representatives do not fully understand the prognosis and treatment plan [31]. To facilitate shared decision making, in which physician and family jointly reach a decision, communication must be more effective and needs to begin early during the ICU stay [10,11].

Physicians are more likely to achieve effective communication when meetings begin earlier in the course of care. In one study, proactive, formal, multidisciplinary meetings were held within 72 hours of ICU admission for patients with clinical features including a predicted ICU stay longer than 5 days, or predicted mortality greater than 25%. In these meetings the medical facts, the patient's perspectives on death dying and critical care, the care plan and the criteria for determining success of the care plan, were discussed. Intensive communication decreased ICU length of stay and allowed earlier access to palliative care [32]. Consistent proactive communication with families for updates on progress and encouragement to use advanced support when appropriate is recommended [10,11]. Improved communication can also be facilitated by using a private place for discussion, listening, empathic statements, acknowledging family emotions, focus on patient values and treatment wishes, clear explanation of the principle of surrogate decision making, assurance that the patient will not suffer, and support for the decisions made by the family [32–37]. A simplified mnemonic for important elements of effective physician–family communication is VALUE (Value and appreciate what is said by family members, Acknowledge the family members' emotions, Listen, Understand who the patient is as a person, Elicit questions from the family members) [39].

Families of ICU patients suffer and may develop long-term mental health issues related to the trauma of witnessing the ICU treatment or end-of-life care of a loved one. Symptoms can include posttraumatic stress disorder (PTSD), anxiety, and depression [33,40]. It is now clear that physicians have an opportunity to lessen the suffering of the family members through effective communication with families about prognosis and care of ICU patients. In one multicenter trial [38], proactive end-of-life conferences with relatives of patients dying in French ICUs resulted in better long-term psychological outcomes in the family members when compared with customary end-of-life conferences. The proactive communication intervention followed detailed guidelines [41], physicians focused on achieving the elements of effective communication summarized by the mnemonic VALUE, and family members received a brochure on bereavement. Physician–family conferences were longer (median 30 minutes vs. 20 minutes) and relatives spent more time talking (median 14 minutes vs. 5 minutes) in the intervention group. Relatives that participated in the proactive intervention had lower prevalence of PTSD symptoms, depression, and anxiety when interviewed 90 days later [38].

Ethical reasoning is part of shared decision making about ICU care for individual patients usually conducted together with a patient surrogate. Family conferences are important for facilitating care of the incapacitated ICU patient and are a forum for providing accurate prognostic information; whether the prognosis is that the patient is expected to survive or, at the other extreme, unlikely to benefit from critical care [32,42]. When a decision is made to forgo life-sustaining treatments and change to end-of-life care, effective communication serves the best interests of the patient and can improve the psychological well being of the surviving relatives.

Discussions that prepare families for the death of a patient or to discuss withdrawal of life support are an increasingly important part of a critical care physician's practice [30,43–45]. Interviews with surrogate decision makers suggest that accurate and timely prognostic information is preferred [46]. There was, however, no clear preference among surrogates (with surrogates divided for and against) about whether it was appropriate for physicians to make a recommendation about withdrawing life support [47]. Surrogate perceptions of communication and end-of-life care can be improved [48,49] and quality improvement can be assessed by means of several survey tools or outcome measures [50–52].

Among the ethical principles described in the preceding section, autonomy is emphasized in the United States. In contrast, this may not always be the case in European countries, where regional and national practices regarding the role of families in decision making, and legal and medical opinions about withholding or withdrawing life support, vary widely [25,53–57].

END-OF-LIFE CARE IN THE INTENSIVE CARE UNIT

Death remains a common occurrence in ICUs, with an estimate suggesting that as many as one in five Americans die during an episode of care that included an ICU admission [58]. Data from North America as well as Europe suggest that the percentage of patients dying following a decision to withdraw or withhold life-sustaining treatments is substantial, and increasing. Thus, critical care clinicians are effectively "managing" the process of death and dying in ICUs with increasing frequency [43,53,59–61]. A number of problems and challenges have been described in ICU end-of-life care, including the inability to predict outcomes for individual patients early in their ICU course, the difficulty in assessing patient preferences with the attendant challenges of surrogate decision making, communication problems between families and ICU staff, as well as concerns regarding the adequacy of symptom management for dying patients [24,43,59,62,63]. Wide variability in physician preferences and practices regarding withdrawal of life-sustaining therapies has been described [27,64,65].

A number of recommendations and guidelines to enhance care-delivery for dying ICU patients [45,66–73] are currently being incorporated into instruction in end-of-life skill to a broad range of trainees in and residency and fellowship training programs [74]. Quality indicators for end-of-life care in ICUs include domains of care focusing on patient and family-centered decision making, communication, continuity of care, emotional, practical, and spiritual support for patients and families, symptom management, as well as the creation of support systems for ICU clinicians. Ideally, the future of end-of-life care in the ICU will incorporate a range of validated palliative care-derived principles and allow for the development of a more robust evidence-based structure for the provision of such care.

End-of-Life Decision Making

General principles regarding the ethical framework surrounding decision making in the ICU setting are outlined in prior sections of this chapter. In the United States, there is substantive consensus, as well as legal support, for several ethical principles of particular relevance to ICU practice. These are (i) a distinction can be drawn between acts of killing, and allowing patients to die; (ii) withholding and withdrawing life-sustaining treatments can be considered equivalent; and (iii) the "doctrine of double effect" permits assertive symptom treatment with medications at the end-of-life even if death might be inadvertently hastened (an unintended, albeit foreseen potential consequence of such medication use) [43,75–79].

Patient- and family-centered care is increasingly being viewed as an ideal model for patient care in ICUs, and this naturally extends into the arena of end-of-life decision making as well [43,80,81]. Involving patients' families and surrogates in this process is of obvious importance, given the high percentage of ICU patients lacking decisional capacity [82,83]. A number of factors may influence physicians' attitudes and recommendations regarding end-of-life questions, but most importantly, clinicians must integrate their patients' views and values into a given care plan to establish goals of treatment that meet the needs of patients and families, in addition to being clinically realistic. Communication between all parties involved in a given case is the means to achieve this goal. Effective communication with clinicians is of great importance to family members, and in fact, families may rate a given caregiver's communication skills as equally or more important than their clinical skills [84,85]. Yet, despite the importance assigned by families of critically ill patients to communication issues, data suggest that ICU caregivers frequently fall short of family expectations in this regard [31,74,84–86].

A variety of strategies for improving end-of-life communication have been evaluated, and there is an evolving set of recommendations for the conduct of clinician-family conferences in the ICU [34,36,38,43]. In general, clinicians should focus on spending more time listening to families during conferences, acknowledge and address families' emotions, as well as encourage questions from family members. The use of the mnemonic VALUE during family meetings has been examined as a tool for the conduct of these meetings, and there is data suggesting that such structured approaches to communication not only facilitate real-time communication, but also reduce psychological morbidity of ICU patients' families [38].

The largest issue for all parties involved is ultimately the *content* and *focus* of these discussions, namely, how best to meet the needs of a given patient. For families, the acute onset of life-threatening critical illness may be a singular, unprecedented event, whereas ICU staffs encounter death and dying on an almost routine basis. Therefore, it is of particular importance to consider communication an ongoing, dynamic process with a timeline that will vary from case to case, as families grapple with the need to fathom the patient's wishes (if not explicitly known) in addition to dealing with their own responses to a given situation. Clearly, there is no universal "blueprint" to delineate how to best guide patients, families, or surrogates through the process of decision making in the ICU, as every individual case has unique aspects. Conflict may arise at any point in a patient's care, and it may occur among members of the care team, among family members, or between the clinicians and family members. Timely, open, and honest communication may be the best strategy to avoid or ameliorate such conflicts, although on occasion outside agents may need to be engaged for mediation (e.g., ethics committees).

Changing Treatment Goals at the End of Life

The perspective that intensive care and palliative care are incompatible with each other is being replaced by the opinion that the need for restorative and palliative care coexists along the illness trajectory, with varying emphasis being placed on one versus the other as treatment goals are re-defined [80,87,88]. Once a decision has been made to forgo further curative treatment endeavors, any treatment or intervention ought to be scrutinized regarding its potential to advance the goal of maximizing comfort [89,90]. In general terms, the needs for pain relief, freedom from anxiety and agitation, relief of dyspnea, and the provision of spiritual support, if desired, become the predominant focus of care [90,91]. Ideally, clinicians should explore individual circumstances and adjust their approach on a case-by-case basis as needed.

Withdrawal of Life-Sustaining Treatments: Practical Considerations

Prior to the withdrawal of life-sustaining treatments, clinicians must inform the patient (if interactive) and the patient's family/surrogates about what to expect during this process. They need to be reassured that the patient's comfort will determine medication administration and the tempo with which the withdrawal process occurs. Family members and friends must have as much access to the patient as needed, and can be encouraged to participate in caregiving to an extent commensurate with their abilities and desires. The ICU staff should attempt to modify the patient's immediate environment to create as peaceful a setting as possible. Any unnecessary equipment, monitors, tubes, drains, and lines should be removed. The withdrawal of mechanical ventilation is unique in that its abrupt cessation can potentially cause suffering. Interventions such as pacemakers, defibrillators, vasopressors, intravenous fluids and nutrition, renal replacement therapy, as well as any medications that do not further the goal of maximizing comfort should therefore be discontinued prior to ventilator withdrawal. The cessation of artificial nutrition and hydration at times raises concerns for clinicians and families alike, potentially for a multitude of reasons [92]. Thirst, for example, may be a concern that can be managed without enteral or parenteral hydration by ice chips or other methods moistening the mouth [93]. Despite such concerns, there is little evidence to suggest that the maintenance of artificial nutrition and hydration contributes to a dying patient's comfort, and it may in fact be associated with complications (e.g., feeding tube malfunction, unintentional dislodgement, nausea) [93–95].

As these initial steps are taken, the patient must be closely observed for any signs of distress, such as grimacing, tachycardia, hypertension, accessory muscle use, sweating, and restlessness. Such symptoms can be treated with opioids (for relief of pain and dyspnea) and sedatives (e.g., benzodiazepines), often in combination. Clinical practice guidelines for the use of sedatives and analgesics in critically ill patients have been devised, applying to patients who are expected to recover, as well as those who are dying [91,96]. Clearly, the situation of the dying patient differs from that of the patient for whom curative therapies continue, but some common themes remain. Systematic symptom assessment with documentation and individualized medication administration is of utmost importance. Once the patient is comfortable, ventilator support can be withdrawn. This can occur either by immediate extubation of the patient, or through a process of gradual reduction in ventilator settings. Either approach is acceptable, assuming that clinicians use anticipatory medication dosing appropriate to the change in level of patient comfort that is predicted in response to a given intervention. In actual practice, a range of physician preferences has been reported [97]. Whether or not to ultimately extubate the patient (if the weaning approach is employed) depends on a variety of factors, including the patient's and/or family/surrogates preferences and airway considerations (e.g., edema, volume of secretions), among others.

Systematic investigation of clinical practice and patient preferences has improved the care of ICU patients. The studies cited above have our enhanced ethical reasoning and decision making for patients during all phases of their ICU care.

AN ETHICAL GUIDE TO RESEARCH

Clinical research involving critically ill persons is necessary and poses important ethical challenges. Significant research efforts in critical care medicine have enabled clinicians to improve outcomes and quality of life of those lives saved. Although the ICU remains the ideal environment to evaluate the effects of novel therapeutic agents and cutting-edge technologies, clinical research in this setting raises considerable ethical challenges. We continue to apply ethical principles to support the risks, benefits, and possible burdens of research protocols, yet many legal and ethical aspects of critical care research remain ambiguous. Ethical issues elicited by research require an acceptable balance of benefit and risk, the requirement for clinical equipoise, and the requisite for a valid informed consent process [98]. Nonetheless, concerns about the clarification of the boundary edge between research and clinical care continue to exist, with ethicists debating approaches that may help subjects better recognize the distinction between research and treatment [99]. This failure to understand which parts of ICU activity is research constitutes the *therapeutic misconception* [100] and may result in an overestimate of research benefits and an underestimate of risks. The next section discusses contemporary issues challenges encompassing research and medical ethics in the ICU.

ETHICAL PRINCIPLES APPLIED TO RESEARCH

Research involving critically ill persons is governed by ethical principles. In response to flagrant exploitation during human experimentation in the course of the World War II, The Nuremburg Code set standards for medical experimentation on humans, establishing that voluntary consent of the human subject is absolutely essential. Subsequently, the Declaration of Helsinki asserted a voluntary consent requirement, and further affirmed that participants in research must possess the right to self-determination (choose to participate) and the right to make informed decisions regarding participation in research, both initially and during the course of the research [101]. The Belmont Report in 1979 articulated the boundaries between research and clinical practice, and identified the principles of autonomy, beneficence, and justice as the ethical underpinnings of ethical research [1]. Defining the boundaries between research and practice, the Belmont Report stated that *practice* refers to interventions intended to better the well-being of a patient and that these interventions have a likely expectation of success, whereas the term *research* was defined as activity designed to test a hypothesis, allow conclusions to be made, and therefore contributes to generalized knowledge. Three basic principles were described, including respect for persons (autonomy), beneficence, and justice. Applying these principles into practice and at the same time adhering to federal regulations, researchers must execute these concepts in an unbiased fashion and with proper clinical judgment to protect the interests of the research subject and assure the integrity of a study.

Autonomy

The informed consent process is an application of the principles of autonomy, with features highlighting disclosure, comprehension, voluntariness, and competence in making a decision to participate in research. The first principle, autonomy, or the right to render independent decisions, requires that the researcher discuss the trial fully in terms that the subject or their designee will understand the process of informed consent and will protect those persons unable to make an informed decision [82]. During these discussions, study risks, procedures, benefits, alternative treatment options, and study-related questions are reviewed. The informed consent process should document understanding and agreement to study participation by a subject who is competent and independent. Ongoing communication with the subject or their designee during the trial is necessary to maintain informed consent and avoid potential conflicts.

Beneficence

Beneficence in research differs from beneficence in clinical care since the actual benefits of research procedures are frequently unknown. Many participants in research trials remain unaware of study design implications, including the possibility of random assignment to a placebo control or comparison group. Although some subjects may participate in research to promote societal benefits, most enroll to achieve direct benefits [102]. Potential study participants may believe they will receive the treatment that is best for them rather than what is best for science. This perception of benefit could inadvertently induce subjects to enroll in research. Consequently, the investigator must attempt to challenge the "therapeutic misconception," the mistaken belief that the research will directly benefit the subject, which draws subjects to research trials. To do so, the investigator must clearly define benefits (if any) and risks, and the study must be monitored for occurrence of anticipated and unexpected risks.

One commonly accepted ethical requirement of randomized controlled trials is uncertainty or equipoise about the interventions being compared. Clinical equipoise [103] ensures a genuine parity in terms of benefit, harm, and uncertainty between therapeutic interventions that subjects would receive as part of clinical practice and the associated potential risks of nontherapeutic interventions (research) of a clinical trial [104]. Investigators should always inform subjects or their surrogates of the difference between an established therapeutic intervention and a nontherapeutic research intervention.

Justice

The principle of justice in research deals with who should receive the benefits of research and who bears the burden. These risks and benefits should be shared equally among all eligible patients in our society. Recruitment of both underserved and underrepresented groups assure each participant's ethical participation in research trials as well as securing the practical objectives of recruiting and retaining a wide range of study participants so as to ensure that the results from clinical trials are generalizable to larger populations. It is the investigator's responsibility to ensure that each subject fully comprehends the study, inclusive of any man, woman, or minority that speaks or reads a language other than English.

Informed Consent for Intensive Care Unit Research

Informed consent is an essential prerequisite for most human trials and is a process for patients and the research staff to come to a common understanding about the uncertainties of the research trial. The five elements of informed consent [82] require the following:

1. The person consenting must be competent in making medical decisions.
2. The information relevant to the person and his or her situation must be disclosed.
3. The person consenting must be able to understand the information.
4. Consent must be voluntary and free from undue influence or coercion.
5. The person must authorize treatment in a clinical investigation.

Because patients are frequently unable to give their own consent, and ICU research is often complex and unfamiliar, it is more difficult to fulfill the five elements of consent for research on ICU patients than for most other groups of patients. Legal experts and ethicists have continually emphasized the importance of transmitting information to potentially participating subjects during the entire process of consent. This process also requires several evaluations including the assessment of the decision-making capacity and competence of the prospective research volunteer. The ability of individuals to incorporate the information needed for providing effective informed consent must be established by assessment for decision-making capacity [105]. The decision making capacity doctrine refers to determination that the potential participating subject has the following abilities:

1. Possesses a comprehensive understanding of the study objectives relevant to the decision to volunteer;
2. Has the ability to weigh the possible risks and benefits of the study and alternative options to participating in a study;
3. Reasoning ability to incorporate the information with personal priorities, values, and consequences;
4. Awareness of their (subject's) right to withdraw from a trial at any time.

Decision-making capacity is generally interpreted to be task specific. That is, a prospective subject may make an informed decision about participating in a trial involving a simple procedure, but not a more complex process. As an illustration, though a potential subject for a trial may be judged legally incompetent to manage their financial affairs, they may maintain sufficient decision-making capacity to make meaningful decisions about participating in a clinical study or choice of medical treatment. A variety of assessment scales (i.e., mini mental state exam) may be employed to determine decisional capacity; formal and less formal assessments are allowable and the relevancy of the exam will depend on the specific research protocol to be done [106]. When prospective participants are temporarily incompetent or lack decision-making capacity due to serious illnesses, either the subject cannot be enrolled or a designated surrogate can provide consent.

A barrier to enrolling ICU patients in research studies is the information that must be provided to obtain consent. Studies of the consent process show that patients and surrogates frequently fail to understand consent documents, and many cannot distinguish between research and routine care [107]. At the center of the issue is a fundamental conflict between two components of informed consent: full disclosure of relevant information, and understanding of the information by the prospective participant of the study. With the scientific language and complexity of clinical trial methodology, it is highly likely that most participants with insufficient skills will have difficulty totally understanding the study's objective(s) and the consent form. Moreover, when developing an informed consent document that enhances readability, simplification of the document may unintentionally render it ambiguous or perhaps too appealing. Though informed consent documentation is essential to obtain, time spent in conversation with prospective study subjects to assist the subject in better understanding the research project is vital. Informed consent is not only a brief discussion to obtain a signed document, but is a process that continues throughout the clinical trial. Consequently, improving the consent process is an important challenge to the immediate future of critical care research.

SURROGATE CONSENT

Federal regulations for the protection of human subjects defined under the "common rule" state that "no institution may involve a human being as a subject in research unless the investigator has obtained the legally effective informed consent from the subject or the subject's legally authorized representative" [108]. The term *legally authorized representative* (LAR) may be interpreted specifically to mean a court-appointed guardian, or more broadly to mean individuals who are authorized under state law or rules of the institution to serve as a proxy decision maker for clinical decisions. Consequently, all research trials must require that surrogate consent be obtained from the subject's legally authorized representative/surrogate decision maker in conditions of critical illnesses in which potentially effective therapies or research interventions need to be initiated within a specific time frame and that documentation of the presence of cognitive impairment, lack of capacity, or serious life-threatening diseases and/or conditions of the prospective subject exists. Currently, most institutional review boards (IRBs) in the United States with laws that sanction surrogate consent for overall medical treatment permit family members to serve as LAR for research. Surrogate consent for participation in a research study should be employed to the extent that it is consistent with the intent of the Common Rule 45 CFR 46, (Subpart A) and all other federal and state laws pertaining to the protection of human subjects participating in research [109].

One approach to recruit patients in studies, while simultaneously preserving sound ethical research and patient autonomy, is to include employing a consent option [110], whereby surrogate consent is initially obtained to enroll a patient in a trial, and the consent process is repeated (continuing consent) when the subject regains competence. This consent option allows a patient to refuse continuing participation but can preserve important collected data.

Some acute care research can proceed under a waiver of informed consent for interventions that may be medically necessary or require emergency treatment. In 1996, federal regulations established a policy for a waiver of informed consent for a limited class of research in human subjects who require emergency therapy and due to the subject's medical condition and the unavailability of a LAR, no legally effective informed consent can be obtained. This amendment (21 CFR 50.24) [111] permits a waiver of informed consent so that the patient may become a subject in a random assignment emergency research project that may include a placebo arm. Under the terms of the waiver, consent would be waived in certain life-threatening circumstances, including: the person requiring emergent action to save his or her life; the person is not capable to provide informed consent as a result of the condition; a surrogate is not readily available to obtain consent within the clinical trial window; the available therapies are unproven for this life-threatening condition; or the collection of scientific evidence is appropriate and necessary to evaluate safety and effectiveness of a particular intervention. A recent survey indicated that a majority of those surveyed concur with the potential benefit of allowing subjects to participate in an emergency research study without prior consent. Yet approximately 30% of persons would not be willing to choose to participate in emergency research or provide consent for their family members despite knowledge about the process [112].

INSTITUTIONAL REVIEW BOARD

Local review boards (IRB) at each institution in the United States represent one essential component of the multiple protections for research subjects. IRBs are overseen by the Office for Human Research Protections (OHRP), the agency responsible for evaluating local IRB compliance with federal regulations for protection of human research subjects, and by the Food and Drug Administration [113]. IRBs assure that research protocols are conducted ethically, that the research question is potentially beneficial and scientifically sound, and that risks to the subjects are minimized. In practice, much of the focus of an IRB review is the adequacy and accuracy of the information provided in the informed consent document to permit potential subjects to understand risks and procedures in a research study.

Individual IRBs have latitude to interpret and apply the federal regulations. The process of approving research protocols differs among institutions and may be attributable to state and local practice (laws, institutional polices, professional, and community standards). Variability in approving IRB research proposals can also be due to differences in the interpretation of the federal regulations [114]. It may be necessary for the OHRP to clarify regulations if IRB decisions deviate from the original intent of federal regulations. Review of multicenter clinical trials by a central IRB is another method to reduce unwarranted variations among IRBs and to also address ambiguities of the federal regulations.

QUALITY IMPROVEMENT INITIATIVE OR RESEARCH?

In recent years, quality improvement (QI) initiatives have become more interventional and are often tied to cost-containment efforts. Review of the federal definitions of research related to typical QI activity suggest that much QI activity should be categorized as research because it may not benefit the patient and may represent a potential burden or risk. Without informed consent, much QI activity could be considered a violation of the principles of the Belmont Report. The purpose of QI activity is generalizable knowledge, but defining when this is research is difficult. Casarett et al. [115] suggest that a QI intervention is appropriately called research if the research subjects need protection as the patients involved in the project are not expected to benefit from the knowledge gained and are subjected to additional risks beyond usual clinical practice. Bellin and Dubler [116] concluded that studies using a control group are considered research; projects that carry minimal risk (data collection) are more readily characterized as not research, whereas riskier projects require independent review. Generally speaking, quality improvement initiatives are not anticipated to have any application beyond the specific organization in which they are conducted. If the goal of the project is to evaluate the accomplishments of an established program and information acquired from the evaluation improves a local program, the activity should not be deemed as research activity. On the contrary, when a quality improvement project involving human participants is testing a newly modified or untested intervention or program to establish its effectiveness and is applicable elsewhere, whether in published form or not, this activity would be considered human participant research and subject to IRB review. QI research has recently been addressed by the OHRP in response to a quality improvement research project seeking at reducing catheter-related infections in 103 ICUs at 67 Michigan hospitals [117]. The initial OHRP conclusion that the initiative constituted human subjects research requiring IRB review was based on the doctrine that informed consent was necessary for quality improvement research involving multiple centers. Given that informed consent for this study evaluating a protocol designed to routinely implement five evidence-based procedures could not have been obtained, does the absence of consent violate any important infringement of patient autonomy? A further review by the OHRP concluded that the initiative was being used solely for "clinical purposes and was not considered medical research or experimentation" [118]. In this specific case, the quality improvement interventions were not experimental but rather safe and demonstrated compliance with evidence-based procedures. Accordingly, patients were not rendered to be at greater risk than that provided by routine clinical care. Further discussions are warranted to reach consensus on the ethical and regulatory viewpoint to waive informed consent for low-risk research where the logistical situation may not allow for consent to be obtained, and consent would not necessarily offer significant protection for subjects.

HEALTH INSURANCE PORTABILITY AND ACCOUNTABILITY ACT

The Health Insurance Portability and Accountability Act (HIPAA) regulations established a federal minimum on the protection of patient privacy [119]. HIPAA regulations mandate appropriate confidentiality safeguards for medical records research without subject authorization. Recent proliferation of electronic health records and computerized research of these records have raised concerns about privacy of health information. Some argue that informed consent should not be required for research of databases because of the potential benefits to society, the minimal risks to the patients involved, and the impracticability of obtaining consent from all patients. One approach is to acquire a limited dataset, omitting information that might permit patient identification. An IRB may authorize a waiver of consent under specific regulations including when a study intervention is minimal risk (e.g., collection of routine data) and does not alter routine care. The rationale for study without consent is that the research involves minimal risk to the subject and these patients would consent if they could be informed, the waiver will not adversely affect the subject's rights and welfare, the research could not be performed without a waiver, or the subjects will eventually be provided with additional relevant information after participation. In our publicly funded health system, patients have a social obligation to allow their de-identified health care data to be used without their consent so that the health care system can be monitored and benefit all. For certain data registry subcomponents such as collection and storage of biological samples and direct patient interviews, consent should be obtained. Some critics suggest that the HIPAA regulations or restrictive interpretation of these regulations will lead to further barriers to clinical research, diminish the volume of research, and discourage institutions from making medical records available for research. In one national survey, HIPAA, researchers reported that privacy rules have added significant costs and delays to the conduct of research in the United States and negatively influenced the conduct of clinical research [120].

SUMMARY

Decision making about goals of critical care, end-of-life care, and participating in clinical research is influenced by a long history of ethical reasoning, legal judgments, and clinical considerations. The evolving practice of shared decision making for critically ill persons is being shaped by our understanding societal values and the impact of ICU care on patients and their families.

References

1. National Commission for the Protection of Human Subjects of Biomedical and Behavioral Research: Belmont Report: Ethical Principles and Guidelines for the Protection of Human Subjects of Research. Washington, DC: US Government Printing Office, 1979.
2. Code of medical ethics current opinions with annotations. American Medical Association, Council on Ethical and Judicial Affairs; annotations prepared by the Southern Illinois University Schools of Medicine and Law, 2004.
3. Beauchamp TL, Childress JF: Principles of Biomedical Ethics. 5th ed. Oxford University Press, 2001.
4. Lo B: Resolving Ethical Dilemmas: A Guide for Clinicians. 3rd ed. Lippincott Williams & Wilkins, 2005.
5. Annas GL: The Rights of Patients. 3rd ed. New York University Press, 2003.
6. Steinbock B, Arras JD, London AJ: Ethical issues in modern medicine. Belmont Report, 2003.
7. Truog RD, Brock DW, Cook DJ, et al: Rationing in the intensive care unit. *Crit Care Med* 34:958–963, 2006.
8. The ANZIC Influenza Investigators: Critical care services and 2009 H1N1 influenza in Australia and New Zealand. *N Engl J Med* 361:1925–1934, 2009.
9. Christian MD, Hawryluck L, Wax RS, et al: Development of a triage protocol for critical care during an influenza pandemic. *CMAJ* 175(11):1377–1381, 2006.
10. Carlet J, Thijs LG, Antonelli M, et al: Challenges in end-of-life care in the ICU: statement of the 5th International Consensus Conference in Critical Care. Brussels, Belgium, April 2003. *Intensive Care Med* 30:770–784, 2004.
11. Davidson JE, Powers K, Hedayat KM, et al: Clinical practice guidelines for support of the family in the patient centered intensive care unit: American College of Critical Care Medicine Task force 2004–2005. *Crit Care Med* 35(2):605–622, 2007.

12. Applebaum PS, Grisso T: Assessing patients' capacities to consent to treatment. *N Engl J Med* 319:1635–1638, 1988.
13. Lo B: Assessing decision-making capacity. *Law, Med Health Care* 18:193–201, 1990.
14. *In the matter of Karen Quinlan*. 70 NJ 10, 335 A. 2D 647 (1976).
15. *Cruzan v Director, Missouri Department of Health*, 497 US 261 (1990).
16. *Schindlers v. Michael Schiavo*, US District Court case no. 8:05-CV-530-T-27TBM (22 March 2005), and other cases available at: www.miami.edu/ethics2/ (accessed May 1, 2006).
17. Hook CC, Mueller PS: The Terri Schiavo saga: the making of a tragedy and lessons learned. *Mayo Clin Proc* 80(11):1449–1460, 2005.
18. Helft PR, Siegler M, Lantos J: The rise and fall of the futility movement. *New Eng J Med* 348(4):293–296, 2000.
19. Consensus statement of the Society of Critical Care Medicine's Ethics Committee regarding futile and other possibly inadvisable treatments. *Crit Care Med* 25:887–891, 1997.
20. Luce JM: Physicians do not have a responsibility to provide futile or unreasonable care if a patient or family insists. *Crit Care Med* 23:760–766, 1995.
21. Medical futility in end-of-life care: report of the Council on Ethical and Judicial Affairs. *JAMA* 281:937–941, 1999.
22. Davis N, Pohlman A, Gehlbach B, et al: Improving the process of informed consent in the critically ill. *JAMA* 289:1963–1968, 2003.
23. *Perry v. Shaw* (2001) 88 Cal. App. 4th 658, 106 Cal. Rptr. 2d 70.
24. The SUPPORT Principal Investigators: A controlled trial to improve care for seriously ill hospitalized patients: the study to understand prognoses and preferences for outcomes and risks of treatments (SUPPORT). *JAMA* 274:1591–1598, 1995.
25. Vincent JL: Forgoing life support in western European intensive care units: the results of an ethical questionnaire. *Crit Care Med* 27(8):1626–1633, 1999.
26. Frick S, Uehlinger DE, Zuercher Zenklusen RM: Medical futility: predicting outcome of intensive care unit patients by nurses and doctors—a prospective comparative study. *Crit Care Med* 31:456–461, 2003.
27. Cook D, Rocker G, Marshall J, et al: Withdrawal of mechanical ventilation in anticipation of death in the intensive care unit. *N Engl J Med* 349:1123–1132, 2003.
28. Schneiderman LJ, Gilmer T, Teetzel HD, et al: Effect of ethics consultations on nonbeneficial life-sustaining treatments in the intensive care setting: a randomized controlled trial. *JAMA* 290:1166–1172, 2003.
29. Schneiderman LJ, Gilmer T, Teetzel HD: Impact of ethics consultations in the intensive care setting: a randomized, controlled trial. *Crit Care Med* 28:3920–3924, 2000.
30. Prendergast TJ, Luce JM: Increasing incidence of withholding and withdrawal of life support from the critically ill. *Am J Respir Crit Care Med* 155: 15–20, 1997.
31. Azoulay E, Chevret S, Leleu G, et al: Half the families of intensive care unit patients experience inadequate communication with physicians. *Crit Care Med* 28:3044–3049, 2000.
32. Lilly CM, De Meo DL, Sonna LA, et al: An intensive communication intervention for the critically ill. *Am J Med* 109:469–475, 2000.
33. Pochard F, Azoulay E, Chevret S, et al: Symptoms of anxiety and depression in family members of intensive care unit patients: ethical hypothesis regarding decision-making capacity. *Crit Care Med* 29:1893–1897, 2001.
34. McDonagh JR, Elliott TB, Engelberg RA, et al: Family satisfaction with family conferences about end-of-life care in the intensive care unit: increased proportion of family speech is associated with increased satisfaction. *Crit Care Med* 32:1484–1488, 2004.
35. Curtis JR, Engelberg RA, Wenrich MD, et al: Missed opportunities during family conferences about end-of-life care in the intensive care unit. *Am J Respir Crit Care Med* 171:844–849, 2005.
36. Stapleton RD, Engelberg RA, Wenrich MD, et al: Clinician statements and family satisfaction with family conferences in the intensive care unit. *Crit Care Med* 34:1679–1685, 2006.
37. Glavan BJ, Engelberg RA, Downey L, et al: Using the medical record to evaluate the quality of end-of-life care in the intensive care unit. *Crit Care Med* 36:1138–1146, 2008.
38. Lautrette A, Darmon M, Megarbane B, et al: A communication strategy and brochure for relatives of patients dying in the ICU. *N Engl J Med* 356: 469–478, 2007.
39. Curtis JR, White DB: Practical guidance for evidence-based ICU family conferences. *Chest* 134(4):835–843, 2008.
40. Azoulay E, Pochard F, Kentish-Barnes N, et al: Risk of post-traumatic stress symptoms in family members of intensive care unit patients. *Am J Respir Crit Care Med* 171:987–994, 2005.
41. Curtis JR, Patrick DL, Shannon SE, et al: The family conference as a focus to improve communication about end-of-life care in the intensive care unit: opportunities for improvement. *Crit Care Med* 29(Suppl 2):N26–N33, 2001.
42. White DB, Engelberg RA, Wenrich MD, et al: Prognostication during physician-family discussions about limiting life support in intensive care units. *Crit Care Med* 35:442–448, 2007.
43. Truog RD, Campbell ML, Curtis JR, et al: Recommendations for end-of-life care in the intensive care unit: a consensus statement by the American Academy of Critical Care Medicine. *Crit Care med* 36:953–963, 2008.
44. Way J, Back AL, Curtis JR: Withdrawing life support and resolution of conflict with families. *BMJ* 325:1342–1345, 2002.
45. Clarke EB, Curtis JR, Luce JM, et al: Quality indicators for end-of-life care in the intensive care unit. *Crit Care Med* 31(9):2255–2262, 2003.
46. Apatira L, Boyd EA, Malvar G, et al: Hope, truth, and preparing for death: perspectives of surrogate decision makers. *Ann Intern Med* 149:861–868, 2008.
47. White DB, Evans LR, Bautista A, et al: Are physicians' recommendations to limit life support beneficial or burdensome? Bringing empirical data to the debate. *Am J Respir Crit Care Med* 180:320–325, 2009.
48. Abbott KH, Sago JG, Breen CM, et al: Families looking back: one year after discussion of withdrawal or withholding of life sustaining support. *Crit Care Med* 29:197–201, 2001.
49. Studdert DM, Mello MM, Burns JP, et al: Conflict in the care of patients with prolonged stay in the ICU: types, sources, and predictors. *Intensive Care Med* 29:1489–1497, 2003.
50. Curtis JR, Engelberg RA: Measuring success of interventions to improve the quality of end-of-life care in the intensive care unit. *Crit Care Med* 34(11, Suppl):S341–S347, 2006.
51. Heyland DK, Rocker GM, Dodek PM, et al: Family satisfaction with care in the intensive care unit: results of a multiple center study. *Crit Care Med* 30:1413–1418, 2002.
52. Wasser T, Matchett S: Final version of the Critical Care Family Satisfaction Survey questionnaire. *Crit Care Med* 29:1654–1655, 2001.
53. Sprung CL, Cohen SL, Sjokvist P, et al: End of life practices in European intensive care units: the Ethicus Study. *JAMA* 290:790, 2003.
54. Bell D: The legal framework for end of life care: a United Kingdom perspective. *Intensive Care Med* 33:158–162, 2007.
55. Michalsen A: Care for dying patients—German legislation. *Intensive Care Med* 33:1823–1826, 2007.
56. Zamperetti N, Proietti R: End of life in the ICU: laws, rules and practices: the situation in Italy. *Intensive Care Med* 32:1620–1622, 2006.
57. Vincent JL: End-of-life practice in Belgium and the new euthanasia law. *Intensive Care Med* 32:1908–1911, 2006.
58. Angus DC, Barnato AE, Linde-Zwirble WT, et al: Use of intensive care at the end of life in the United States: an epidemiologic study. *Crit Care Med* 32:638, 2004.
59. Prendergast TJ, Claessens MT, Luce JM: A national survey of end of life care for critically ill patients. *Am J Respir Crit Care Med* 158:1163, 1998.
60. Smedira NG, Evans BH, Grais LS, et al: Withholding and withdrawal of life support from the critically ill. *N Engl J Med* 322:309, 1990.
61. Prendergast TJ, Luce JM: Increasing incidences of withholding and withdrawal of life support from the critically ill. *Am J Respir Crit Care Med* 155: 15, 1997.
62. Nelson JE, Danis M: End of life in the intensive care unit: where are we now? *Crit Care Med* 29:N2, 2001.
63. Nelson JE, Meier DE, Oei EJ, et al: Self-reported symptom experience of critically ill cancer patients receiving intensive care. *Crit Care Med* 29:449, 2001.
64. Bach PB, Carson SS, Leff A: Outcomes and resources utilization for patients with prolonged critical illness managed by university-based or community-based subspecialists. *Am J Respir Crit Care Med* 158:1410, 1998.
65. Kollef MH: Private attending physician status and the withdrawal of life-sustaining interventions in a medical intensive care unit population. *Crit Care Med* 24:968, 1996.
66. Curtis RJ, Rubenfeld GD (eds): *Managing Death in the Intensive Care Unit: The Transition from Cure to Comfort*. New York, Oxford University Press, 2001.
67. Campbell ML, Curtis JR (Eds): *End-of-Life Care. Critical Care Clinics*. Philadelphia, Elsevier Saunders, 2004.
68. Hawryluck LA, Harvey WRC, Lemieux-Charles L, et al: Consensus guidelines on analgesia and sedation in dying intensive care unit patients. *BMC Med Ethics* 3:1, 2002.
69. Rubenfeld GD, Curtis JR: Beyond ethical dilemmas: improving the quality of end-of-life care in the intensive care unit. *Crit Care* 7:11, 2003.
70. Robert Wood Johnson Foundation: Promoting excellence, in EOLC via University of Montana. Available at: http://www.promotingexcellence.org. Accessed April 28, 2006.
71. EPERC: End-of-life/Palliative Education Resource Center. Available at: http://www.mew.edu. Accessed April 28, 2006.
72. Center to Advance Palliative Care: *Palliative care in the ICU*. Available at: www.capc.org/palliative-care-across-the-continuum. Accessed April 28, 2006.
73. Brody H, Campbell ML, Faber-Langendoen K, et al: Withdrawing intensive life-sustaining treatment—recommendations for compassionate clinical management. *N Engl J Med* 336:652, 1997.
74. Levy MM: End-of-life care in the intensive care unit: Can we do better? *Crit Care Med* 29:N56, 2001.
75. Brock DW: Death and dying, in Veatch RM (ed), *Medical Ethics*. Boston, Jones and Bartlett, 1989, pp 329–356.
76. Quill TE, Dresser R, Brock DW: The rule of double effect—a critique of its role in end-of-life decision making. *N Engl J Med* 337:1768, 1997.
77. Lo B, Rubenfeld G: Palliative sedation in dying patients: "we turn to it when everything else hasn't worked". *JAMA* 294:1810, 2005.
78. Quill TE: The ambiguity of clinical intensions. *N Engl J Med* 329:10390, 1993.

79. Sulmasy DP: Commentary: double effect—intension is the solution, not the problem. *J Law med Ethics* 28:26, 2000.
80. Institute of Medicine: Committee on Care at the End of Life: Approaching Death. Washington, DC, National Academy Press, 1997.
81. National Consensus Project for Quality Palliative Care: Clinical Practice Guidelines for Quality Palliative Care, Pittsburgh, National Consensus Project, 2004.
82. Luce JM: Is the concept of informed consent applicable to clinical research involving critically ill patients? *Crit Care Med* 31:S153, 2003.
83. White DB, Curtis JR, Lo B, et al: Decisions to limit life-sustaining treatment for critically ill patients who lack both decision-making capacity and surrogate decision-makers. *Crit Care Med* 34:2053, 2006.
84. Curtis RJ, Rubenfeld GD (eds): *Managing Death in the Intensive Care Unit: The Transition from Cure to Comfort*. New York, Oxford University Press, 2001, p 85.
85. Hickey M: What are the needs of families of critically ill patients? A review of the literature since 1976. *Heart Lung* 19(4):401, 1990.
86. Heyland DK, Rocker GM, Dodek PM, et al: Family satisfaction with care in the intensive care unit: results of a multiple center study. *Crit Care Med* 30(7):1413, 2002.
87. Danis M: Improving end-of-life care in the intensive care unit: what's to be learned from outcomes research? *New Horizons* 6:110, 1998.
88. Danis M, Federman D, Fins JJ, et al: Incorporating palliative care into critical care education: principles, challenges and opportunities. *Crit Care Med* 27:2005, 1999.
89. Mancini I, Body JJ: Assessment of dyspnea in advanced cancer patients. *Support Care Cancer* 7:229, 1999.
90. McCann RM, Hall WJ, Groth-Juncker A: Comfort care for terminally ill patients: the appropriate use of nutrition and hydration. *JAMA* 272:1263, 1994.
91. Troug RD, Berde CB, Mitchell C, et al: Barbiturates in the care of the terminally ill. *N Engl J Med* 327:1678, 1992.
92. Gillick MR: Rethinking the role of tube feeding in patients with advanced dementia. *N Engl J Med* 342:206, 2000.
93. Viola RA, Wells GA, Peterson J: The effects of fluid status and fluid therapy on the dying: a systematic review. *J Palliat Care* 13:41, 1997.
94. Steinbrook R, Lo B: Artificial feeding—solid ground, not a slippery slope. *N Engl J Med* 318:286, 1998.
95. Cook DJ, Guyatt GH, Jaeschke R, et al: Determinants in Canadian health care workers of the decision to withdraw life support from the critically ill. Canadian Critical Care Trials Group. *JAMA* 273:703, 1995.
96. Christakis NA, Asch DA: Biases in how physicians choose to withdraw life support. *Lancet* 342:642, 1993.
97. Asch DA, Christakis NA: Why do physicians prefer to withdraw some forms of life support over others? Intrinsic attributes of life-sustaining treatments are associated with physicians' preferences. *Med Care* 34:103, 1996.
98. American Thoracic Society documents: The ethical conduct of clinical research involving critically ill patients in the United States and Canada. *Am J Respir Crit Care Med* 170:1375–1384, 2004.
99. Levine RJ: Boundaries between research involving human subjects and accepted and routine professionals practices, in Bogomolny RL (ed), *Human Experimentation*. Dallas, TX, Southern Methodist University Press, 1976, pp 3–20.
100. Appelbaum PS, Lidz CW, Grisso T: Therapeutic misconception in clinical research: frequency and risk factors. *IRB* 26:1–8, 2004.
101. World Medical Association: Declaration of Helsinki: recommendations guiding physicians in biomedical research involving human subjects. *JAMA* 277:925–926, 1997.
102. Appelbaum PS, Roth LH, Lidz CW, et al: False hopes and best data: consent to research and the therapeutic misconception. *Hastings Cent Rep* 17:20–24, 1987.
103. Miller FG, Brody H: A critique of clinical equipoise. Therapeutic misconception in the ethics of clinical trials. *Hastings Cent Rep* 33:19–28, 2005.
104. Lidz CW, Appelbaum PS, Grisso T, et al: Therapeutic misconception and the appreciation of risks in clinical trials. *Soc Sci Med* 58:1689–1697, 2004.
105. Etchells E, Darzins P, Silberfeld M, et al: Assessment of patient capacity to consent to treatment. *J Gen Intern Med* 14:27–34, 1999.
106. Dunn LB, Nowrangi MA, Palmer BW, et al: Assessing decisional capacity for clinical research or treatment: a review of instruments. *Am J Psychiatry* 163:1323–1334, 2006.
107. Howard JM, DeMets D: How informed is informed consent: the BHAT experience. *Control Clin Trials* 2:287–303, 1981.
108. Silverman HJ, Luce JM, Schwartz J: Protecting subjects with decisional impairment in research: the need for a multifaceted approach. *Am J Respir Crit Care Med* 169:10–14, 2004.
109. Department of Health and Human Services: Common rule, 45 CF 46. Federal policy for the protection of human subjects: notices and roles. *Fed Regist* 50:28003–29032.
110. Wendler D, Rackoff J: Consent for continuing research participation. What is it and when should it be obtained? *IRB* 24:1–6, 2002.
111. Department of Health and Human Services, Food and Drug Administration: Protection of human subjects: informed consent and waiver of informed consent requirements in certain emergency research. Final Rules. Title 21, Code of Federal Regulations. Part 50:24. *Fed Regist* 61:51528–51533, 1996.
112. Longfield JN, Morris MJ, Moran KA, et al: Community meetings for emergency research community consultation. *Crit Care Med* 36:731–736, 2008.
113. Koski G: Ethics, science, and oversight of critical care research: the Office for Human Research Protections. *Am J Respir Crit Care Med* 169:982–986, 2004.
114. Silverman H, Hull SC, Sugarman J: Variability among institutional review boards' decisions within the context of a multicenter trial. *Crit Care Med* 29:235–241, 2001.
115. Casarett D, Karlawish JHT, Sugarman J: Determining when quality improvement initiatives should be considered research: proposed criteria and potential implications. *JAMA* 283:2275–2280, 2000.
116. Belin E, Dubler NN: The quality improvement-research divide and the need for external oversight. *Am J Public Health* 19:1512–1517, 2001.
117. Pronovost P, Needham D, Berenholtz S, et al: An intervention to decrease catheter related bloodstream infections in the ICU. *N Engl J Med* 355:2725–2732, 2006.
118. Miller FG, Emanuel EJ: Quality-improvement research and informed consent. *N Engl J Med* 358:765–767, 2008.
119. US Department of Health and Human Services: OCR Privacy Brief: Summary of the HIPAA Privacy Rule. Washington, DC, Office for Civil Rights, HIPAA Compliance Assistance, 2003.
120. Ness RB, for the Joint Policy Committee, Societies of Epidemiology: Influence of the HIPAA Privacy Rule on Health Research. *JAMA* 298: 2164–2170, 2007.

CHAPTER 212 ■ ASSESSING THE VALUE AND IMPACT OF CRITICAL CARE IN AN ERA OF LIMITED RESOURCES: OUTCOMES RESEARCH IN THE INTENSIVE CARE UNIT

ANDREW F. SHORR, WILLIAM L. JACKSON JR AND DEREK C. ANGUS

During the last three decades, critical care has matured to a distinct medical specialty. Sepsis, respiratory failure, and the care of the complicated postoperative patient are now perceived as the purview of the intensivist. Concomitant with this evolution in critical care medicine has been a growing focus on health care outcomes. This emphasis on the end points and effects of medical care generally and critical care specifically reflects the realization that critically ill subjects face a high risk of death and that many interventions applied in the intensive care unit (ICU) are expensive. Some older studies estimate that nearly 1% of the gross national product of the United States is consumed in the ICU and, relative to days spent on hospital wards, others suggest that ICU costs are nearly three times greater [1,2]. Whether it is mechanical ventilation (MV), extensive nursing care, or acute dialysis, many of the technologies and medications used in the ICU are associated with substantial economic costs. In addition, many often perceive that ICU interventions only delay mortality rather than prevent mortality, or that mortality reduction in the ICU comes only at the price of significant morbidity. Thus, there is increasing pressure to carefully evaluate and to understand the results of ICU care. This pressure becomes even more evident when one considers that ICU outcomes must be evaluated from both patient and societal perspectives. In other words, the emphasis on outcomes in the ICU reflects an underlying question about value.

Outcomes research reflects a systematic effort to address these issues and concerns. According to a recent position statement on outcomes research in critical care, "Outcomes research is employed to formulate clinical practice guidelines, to evaluate the quality of care, and to inform health policy decisions" [3]. Like clinical critical care, outcomes research draws on many different tools and expertise in multiple disciplines. More than only an issue of economics, outcomes research requires expertise in psychology and anthropology (to understand patient and physician behavior), epidemiology (to identify disease patterns and burdens), and health services research (to appreciate process) [3]. Use of a term like *outcomes*, though, presupposes a question: Outcomes for whom? At the bedside, the clinician or the investigator focuses on pathophysiology of a sole patient. Outcomes research addresses broader issues. Rather than being either centered on a particular disease or a physiologic measure, outcomes research deals with the overall results of care for the patient, for the family, and for society. Also in distinction to traditional clinical research, outcomes research has clear policy aspects as well; it attempts to facilitate debates about competing plans for resource allocation, research priorities, and national health policy. As an example, a randomized clinical trial deals with issues of efficacy (Does intervention "*x*" in a controlled environment have an independent impact?) and outcomes research is more concerned with effectiveness (What are the implications of intervention "*x*" applied outside a controlled setting and in the "real world" for the patient and society?). Traditional clinical research, moreover, often employs experimental approaches, and observational methods are routinely used in outcomes research. In short, outcomes research attempts to use methods from the social sciences to augment the understanding of health care as opposed to using only methods from conventional "hard" sciences. As a recent summary regarding outcomes research in sepsis indicated, the outcomes researcher seeks to answer a question separate from traditional research [4]. The clinical investigator essentially asks, "Does this work?" and outcomes researchers deal with the concern, "Does it help?" [4].

Readers should note that outcomes research is now a key component of the biomedical enterprise. It is no longer seen as an option or an add-on. It fits with mechanistic and clinical work in building the triumvirate of information needed to translate research findings into clinical practice. The absence of outcomes studies can lead to the failure to adopt what otherwise might be useful interventions.

METHODS IN OUTCOMES RESEARCH

Outcomes research relies on multiple methods for exploring patient-centered concerns. Generally, researchers employ both qualitative and quantitative methods [3]. Qualitative approaches are only occasionally used but can offer insight into complex processes that do not easily lend themselves to standard hypothesis testing. As such, qualitative work often results in the generation of important hypotheses for more formal testing. Quantitative methods are more standard in outcomes research in critical care and have two general aspects. First, they use some tool to measure a particular outcome (e.g., mortality, quality of life, functional status, cost). Second, quantitative techniques then seek to compare the outcome of interest between at least two alternatives. Unlike the controlled environment of the bench laboratory or even the randomized controlled trial (RCT), outcomes research is necessarily exposed to multiple potential confounders that can and do affect the primary measure of interest. Because critical care outcomes research remains patient-centered, it is important to acknowledge that these subjects bring with them complexities that may alter their mortality, quality of life, and function. Moreover, the impact of these preceding factors may affect a researcher's end point of interest in ways that have little to do with the intervention under study. Similarly, after any intervention in the ICU, many post-ICU variables come into play that might affect the results of an outcomes study.

To address these complexities requires adoption of various techniques, all of which must be rigorous and reproducible. Therefore, outcomes research relies on more than simply RCTs. RCTs are well suited for deciding if specific interventions or agents can alter an easily ascertainable end point such as mortality. For example, use of large sample sizes combined with both block randomization techniques and protocols for patient care help to ensure that the potential confounders previously noted are minimized and, in turn, allows one to explore questions such as how low tidal volume MV affects mortality at day 28. But if the policy or research query deals with the functional status or total cost of care for survivors of acute respiratory distress syndrome (ARDS) more than a year after their hospital discharge, one may require additional approaches other than an RCT. In any event, critical care outcomes research begins by defining a particular question. The investigator can subsequently determine which approach is most appropriate.

In fact, sometimes outcomes research requires entirely separate study designs and major modifications to traditional models of clinical research. In other cases, more traditional models of investigation can be expanded to incorporate outcomes measures. This generally requires building these measures into the trial during the study inception phase. Therefore, outcomes research can be seen as an extension and complement to standard research practices. In other areas of medicine, such as rheumatology, patient-centered measures such as quality of life have come to serve as the primary end point in clinical studies.

Observational Studies

Of the various types of observational studies (e.g., case series, case-control, cross-sectional, and cohort), two are particularly important in critical care outcomes. A cross-sectional design has the advantage of looking at one precise time or over a short period of time at a specific disease or practice. This snapshot-in-time approach can provide important insight into both epidemiology and health services research. For example, a recent 1-day international survey of respiratory failure in the ICU demonstrated the burden of this disease relative to other diseases treated in the ICU and also documented the wide range in practice style with respect to the use of MV [5]. The Sepsis Occurrence in Acutely Ill Patients (SOAP) study, a European sepsis registry using an essentially cross-sectional design (it covered a set 2-week period) confirmed the burden of sepsis in the ICU and underscored the variability in the use of various medical therapies in the care of these patients [6]. Hence, these cross-sectional analyses generated important information about the current state of affairs and therefore provided a potential benchmark for use in future comparisons.

In addition, cohort studies are valuable components in outcomes research. With this strategy, subjects are selected based on some common characteristic (e.g., a diagnosis, a risk factor) and then observed [7]. Thus, cohort analyses have the advantage of being prospective. Cohort studies also specify a set starting time for the observation (e.g., time zero) from which observations proceed forward. Researchers can then look at the interplay of certain predefined risk factors or interventions and the characteristics that defined the cohorts to see how these affect the outcome. Often a cohort design is used to either describe the natural history of a disease or to assess quality of life. Although theoretically straightforward, cohort studies pose important challenges to the researcher. Selection bias and the inherent heterogeneity of critically ill patients can confound efforts to create a homogeneous cohort. Similarly, one needs to ensure means for capturing multiple potential exposure variables and acknowledge that the interaction between risk factors, exposures, and time is complex.

As Needham et al. [7] and Dowdy et al. [8] indicate in a recent review of methodologic issues associated with cohort studies, this study design has three key components: subjects, outcomes and exposures, and time. Subjects must be carefully identified, but the cohort study gives the researcher flexibility to define the population as sharing particular characteristics, such as common diagnoses, or risk factors. Alternatively, cohorts can be developed such that two groups emerge: individuals exposed to a particular event or variable and those not exposed. As a result, one can, using this technique, begin to draw conclusions about causal relationships. Generally, because the cohort shares some common time of designation (e.g., time zero) by observing the population one can evaluate the strength of the relationship between the given exposure and the outcome. Unlike the rigidity of an RCT, in which randomization works to ensure study groups are similar except for the intervention in question, a cohort design provides the researcher the chance to explore multiple exposures simultaneously, and how they interact with each other. To the point, in an RCT of a novel treatment for sepsis, any differences seen in outcomes should be a function of the particular intervention experimentally introduced. The ICU organization, pre-ICU care, and posthospital events should not affect the outcome because randomization should ensure that the impact of these variables is equalized between the active and comparator groups.

The purpose of a cohort study is to enhance the RCT by providing information that cannot, by definition, be gleaned from the RCT. Expanded adoption of cohort studies can also facilitate better understanding of natural history by shifting the focus back to a time prior to ICU admission. Without some initial work with adopting a cohort approach, we cannot hope to address significant questions relating to what determines which patients get admitted to the ICU, who most likely benefits from ICU care, and the outcomes for those never admitted to the ICU.

INTERVENTIONS AND END POINTS IN CRITICAL CARE OUTCOMES RESEARCH

Unlike traditional biomedical research, which looks at either novel technologic interventions (new drugs, new devices) or perhaps management strategies, the interventions studied in outcomes research are more diverse. Certain clinical measures have significant outcomes implications for the patient and society. However, managerial and organizational changes may be equally important. The issue of management and organization of critical care services is particularly acute at present, given current (and conflicting) data suggesting that the model of ICU administration affects both mortality and cost [9,10]. The question of organization and management is broader than simply whether one uses a closed, full-time intensivist model or a more traditional open ICU model. Under the rubric of organization and management are questions of nurse-to-patient ratios, the role for respiratory therapy, and the value of a dedicated critical care pharmacy group. Measuring how these types of potential features of the ICU work and whether they help patients and society is perhaps as important a question as if a new molecule for sepsis alters mortality. Issues of management and organization can provide feedback to affect the conduct of traditional research. Whether it is studies of resuscitation strategies or rapid response teams, these types of interventions include service, delivery, and organizational aspects. If any one of these components of the trial collapses, the entire venture may be jeopardized.

Mortality

With respect to end points, mortality remains the center of investigative efforts because it has tangible meaning to the patient, to health care institutions, and to society. When outcomes research addresses mortality, it tries to do it in an appropriate context. In other words, the question of mortality begs the question of when? Is the appropriate timeframe survival to ICU discharge or to hospital discharge? Are these time points too myopic? Altering long-term mortality (e.g., 2 years after ICU admission) would be an admirable goal. Historically, 28-day all-cause mortality has served as the primary end point for trials in critical care. However, after some period of time it seems reasonable to postulate that occurrences and interventions in the ICU diminish in their impact while the patient's age [11] and health state prior to his or her ICU admission [3] become the main drivers of outcomes. Thus, the issue revolves around the timeframe chosen for measurement and its likely mechanistic link to the intervention under evaluation [12].

It is important to be cautious, though, since one can artificially alter ICU mortality by early use of certain interventions (e.g., tracheotomy in order to facilitate transfer to a chronic ventilator care facility). Likewise, decisions about when to suggest withdrawal of care can alter the apparent timing of death in the ICU. The central limitation is that with all time-dependent end points, there can be confounding by multiple factors. As the recent American Thoracic Society position statement on outcomes research appropriately observes, "The 'correct' mortality endpoint depends on the specific research question, the mechanisms and timing of the disease and/or treatment under study, and the study design" [3]. In addition, if a disease state is not associated with significant mortality, use of this measure may simply fail to capture the value of a particular intervention. Finally, mortality as the sole end point of any research ignores the entire concern about morbidity and the tradeoff between mortality and morbidity. Similarly, it fails to address the quality of life of the survivor.

Mortality, moreover, has limitations as a tool for comparing outcomes across different ICUs. Although recorded and tracked nearly uniformly in ICUs throughout the world, ICU mortality is a relatively uninformative measure of ICU performance. Extensive variability exists in not only the types of patients admitted to different ICUs but also in admission and discharge policies [12]. Some ICUs serve as major referral centers for and receive multiple transfers from other hospitals. These patients tend to be sicker or in need of specialized care. Hence, the mortality rates of the ICUs that send these persons elsewhere may be artificially low compared to the ICUs that accept such high-risk cases. Similarly, ICUs with intermediate-care facilities can transition individuals out of the ICU at different rates than ICUs lacking access to these resources. This fact can alter apparent ICU mortality rates because one might essentially be able to transition patients receiving comfort care only out of the ICU so that when they die the death is not captured as an ICU-related event.

One could correct for these possible variables by employing a definition of ICU mortality (for benchmarking performance) that removed transfers from both the numerator and denominator of the crude mortality rate. Adjusting for differences for availability of "stepdown" wards can be made by limiting comparisons to like-sized hospitals. However, even these efforts would be insufficient for purposes of performance and quality assessments because issues of case-mix remain unaddressed. Case-mix as a concept tries to capture that different ICUs admit different types of patients with differing severity of illnesses. It is important to note that case-mix as a concept describes more than differences in disease severity [13]. Case-mix adjusting tries to balance issues with underlying diagnosis, comorbidity, age, and severity of illness [13]. To illustrate the breadth of the aspects related to case-mix one need only consider an ICU that cared for only postoperative cardiothoracic patients should report low mortality rates and an ICU that admitted mainly immunocompromised persons would certainly describe different outcomes, even after one adjusted for severity of illness. As a corollary, comparing mortality between similar types of ICUs that admit similar types of patients, after controlling for disease severity, can prove helpful [13].

Severity of Illness Tools

To address disease severity, multiple tools exist. They differ with respect to the variables they measure, when they measure these variables, and if they try to describe ICU mortality or hospital mortality. The Acute Physiology and Chronic Health Evaluation (APACHE) score is commonly used in the United States and the Simplified Acute Physiology Score (SAPS) system is more regularly employed in Europe [14–16]. Severity of illness scores have been developed for application in specific types of patients (e.g., pediatrics, trauma) and others try to deal with a broader range of subjects. Other modeling systems include the Sequential Organ Failure Assessment (SOFA) score and the Multiple Organ Dysfunction Score [17,18]. A major limitation of all scoring systems is that they are developed and validated on large patient populations. Therefore, predicted mortality estimates for individual patients cannot and should not be translated into decisions at the bedside as to whether, based solely on predicted mortality, one should withhold or offer aggressive care.

Another concern with severity of illness tools as they relate to mortality is that some were initially created many years ago. Over time, new interventions and technologies have altered patient care and morality. Hence, older iterations of certain models may not longer apply and no longer have adequate calibration to be informative. Like many scales, they require recalibration. As an example, the APACHE system is now on its fourth revision, and with APACHE II versus APACHE IV, there are significant differences in terms of the explanatory power [19]. Nonetheless, in critical care research many have adopted the APACHE II and III approach as its equations are published. Researchers and administrators need therefore be cautious when assuming that similar scores computed by an older rubric necessarily translate into similar predicted mortalities among populations or across ICUs. APACHE generally functions by exploring historical cohorts of patients and creating prediction scores based on this "control" population. Alternatively one can also use the acuity measures used in these instruments to derive from predictions that are specific for the population of interest or under study.

Calculations of the actual scores for patients can also be prone to error. Several studies document significant interobserver variability among even trained researchers as to the calculation of severity of illness scores [20]. With APACHE II, one project revealed that the interrater agreement was strikingly poor ($\kappa = 0.20$) [21]. The main sources of variability appeared to be in assessment of the Glasgow Coma Score but variability was evident even in the determination of the blood pressure. Changes in practice can also have unpredicted effects on severity of illness scores. Nearly all scoring systems rest on measurement of physiologic parameters such as blood pressure, platelet count, and hemoglobin. The more extreme the actual value from the "normal" range, the greater the negative impact of this factor on the individual's composite severity of illness score. As an example, a low hemoglobin is associated with more APACHE II points than a normal hemoglobin. Clinicians, though, may now be more tolerant of lower hemoglobins than they were when APACHE II was created. In fact, a restrictive transfusion strategy that necessarily allows the hemoglobin to drift lower may improve outcomes [22]. Consequently, APACHE II scores may be rising in ICU patients over time, reflecting this change in practice because physicians are not transfusing as frequently. This increase in APACHE II-predicted mortality when actual mortality might improve because of a change in clinical practice based on a large randomized trial underscores a significant assumption and limitation of severity of illness scoring classifications.

Severity of Illness and Performance Assessment

Mortality prediction equations can also result in calculation of a standardized mortality ratio (SMR) [13]. This ratio compares observed mortality to predicted mortality. Conceptually, the SMR can be calculated irrespective of the severity of illness system used to determine the predicted mortality. Ratios greater than 1 suggest excess mortality and those less than 1 imply enhanced survivorship. Implicitly, an SMR greater than 1 indicates an ICU with inferior outcomes after adjusting for severity of illness case mix. Alternatively, though, differences in SMR can reflect more than quality. First, scoring systems may be generally imprecise (see previous discussion) and may not capture some aspects of disease severity or other case-mix issues. Second, the SMR can be affected by the quality of data collection and by the sample size. There is also discordance in the published literature exploring if and how well the SMR correlates with other markers of ICU quality. Some investigators suggest the SMR sufficiently captures aspects of quality and others conclude that the relationship between other markers of quality and the SMR is less clear [13]. It is likely that no one SMR calculation method accurately reflects quality. Therefore, as policy makers, third-party payers, and patients demand simple report cards that allegedly capture quality, it is important that the intensivist resist the urge to simply publish SMRs without references to case-mix. Some more recent scoring systems address this (i.e., APACHE IV) but still may be imprecise as they derive from historical cohorts. We need to encourage the use of multiple measures beyond the SMR to describe qualitative differences in ICUs.

Nevertheless, the SMR can be used over time to assess interventions within an ICU or group of relatively homogenous ICUs [13]. Although one may not be able to conclude that SMR differences across institutions reflect true differences in quality and performance, when used as a benchmarking tool the SMR can be insightful. If one ICU has historical data about its case-mix and performance, it can then track over time how the SMR varies in response to interventions. Conversely, an increasing SMR can suggest the presence of some change in practice or structure that is adversely affecting mortality. By identifying these trends and investigating them, ICU staff can elucidate potentially harmful changes that have transpired and attempt to address them.

Organ Failures

One effort to move beyond mortality as the primary outcome measure in critical care has been the evolution of the concept of organ failure-free days [3]. The free-day paradigm recognizes that reducing mortality in the ICU may not always reduce morbidity. In fact, reductions in mortality may only increase morbidity by keeping alive for several additional days patients who otherwise would have died but then, nonetheless, succumb to the acute illness. From a different vantage, some interventions may appear attractive on a superficial level because they decrease the duration of either MV or vasopressor support. However, a shorter duration of MV in one population may only reflect a higher death rate in that cohort. In other words, there is a competing impact of mortality in the assessment of such time-to-event (e.g., liberation from MV) phenomena.

These two facts promoted the development of the failure-free day paradigm. As a consensus conference on sepsis stated, this concept evolved out of a need to evaluate "the net effects of therapy" and to try to "integrate mortality with morbidity" [3]. Failure-free days are computed so that each day alive free of the organ failure in question is counted during the specified observation period. If a patient dies before the study termination or requires support beyond this time point, he or she is assigned 0 failure-free days. Historically, failure-free days are measured up to day 28 following the start of an investigation. The 28-day cutpoint, however, is arbitrary and reflects that most trials in critical care use the 28-day mark as the final date for ascertaining vital status. One could follow subjects out further if there were a biologically plausible reason to believe that the intervention under analysis could have an impact to that time point. As an example, if one were interested in MV-free days accrued during the 28 days following a patient's enrollment in a study and the patient died on day 7, he or she would be credited with no ventilation-free days. If the individual required 7 days of ventilation and was alive at day 28, he or she would have earned 21 MV-free days. If remaining on the ventilator for all 28 days, no ventilator-free days would accrue.

The failure-free day approach has the potential advantage of capturing morbidity that transpires outside the ICU, such as the need for continued dialysis, as it is organ system-specific rather than defined purely based on the subject's location of care. It can further account for shifts in a patient's clinical status that might not be measured accurately if a researcher only recorded mortality. A patient with chronic obstructive pulmonary disease, for instance, might require 2 days of ventilatory support initially, be liberated from MV, but then several days later deteriorate and need to be placed back on ventilatory support. This waxing and waning in clinical status can potentially be accurately described from an outcomes perspective with the use of ventilator-free days.

Is it appropriate to pool death with requiring 28 days of MV but still surviving? The fundamental struggle in this question illustrates why organ failure-free days can only be used as an adjunct to other measures of outcomes in critical care. It is certainly not clear that organ failures correlate with meaningful clinical outcomes or if surviving 28 days on a ventilator with a respiratory organ failure is comparable with death. On the other hand, the concept of organ failure-free days allows one to examine if and how a novel approach or therapy might accelerate recovery. In turn, it lays the foundation for the use of pooled end points in clinical trials in critical care. If mortality remains the only primary end point for studies in critical care, then investigators may fail to pursue options that may prove valuable in other ways. The organ failure-free day concept also allows one to capture the effect of interventions on markers of resource utilization and cost. Differences in the use of ventilation, dialysis, and vasopressors have important implications for patients. Simultaneously, because of the costs associated with these interventions, decreasing organ failures and morbidity has ramifications for health care institutions, third-party payers, and policy makers. Future work in this area may in fact move beyond organ failure and try to develop metrics that incorporate this with mortality into a form of quality-adjusted survival measure.

Health Status

From the patient's perspective, surviving the ICU raises many issues. Most patients will require some additional time for further recovery along with the potential need for rehabilitation. Moreover, some physical impairment persists after ICU care, and this impairment can affect functional status, mental health, and quality of life. Globally, each of these concepts (functional state, mental health, quality of life) all attempt to capture the concept of health status. The need for adequate assessments of health status is made more acute given the limitations evident if one has only a sole focus on mortality.

Readers should note that, although the concepts are intertwined, functional status (either physical or mental) is distinct from quality of life [23]. Functional status depicts the subject's capacities and quality of life attempts to gauge an individual's satisfaction and state of well-being. As a result of this subtle distinction, someone who has a major functional limitation may rate his or her quality of life as high while another patient with relatively minor limitations might describe his or her quality of life as poor. Moreover, quality of life essentially relies on using the individual as his or her own control. Persons necessarily rate their quality of life relative to what they perceive it was prior to needing ICU therapy. Functional status, on the other hand, generally measures capabilities relative to a fixed scale of performance that is set irrespective of what the person's prior functional status might have been. As such, functional status tends to be more objective. Quality of life, alternatively, is influenced by a person's values, perceptions, and preferences [24]. Quality of life also is measured in a social context. Assessing an ARDS survivor's lung function provides no insight into how having physical limitations after surviving ARDS alters one's interactions with their family and friends.

Functional status captures physiologic assessments of impairment along with global and mental/neuropsychologic performance. Early outcomes studies in critical care and functional status explored the long-term pulmonary complications of ARDS [25]. Researchers examined how gas exchange and radiographs varied over time in ARDS survivors. Other investigators have used general measures of functional status to describe survivors of ICU care [25]. Often-used tools for this include the 6-minute walk test and the activities of daily living (ADL) system. ADL assessments as a tool have the advantage of being widely familiar to clinicians and easy to implement. Some, though, question their applicability to critical care outcomes [23]. ADLs may be of limited value because they were developed specifically for the elderly. Young survivors of critical illness may recover to a state of function beyond what the ADLs can possibly capture. The information that does exist indicates that severe functional impairment results following ICU care and that it may resolve slowly. For example, Herridge et al. [26], in a prospective observational analysis of ARDS survivors, noted that only 50% had returned to work by 1 year and many reported persistent limitations in their ADLs.

Evaluation of cognitive impairment complements appraisals of functional status. Again, because of the difficulty in assembling cohorts of critical care survivors, the heterogeneity of these patients, and the lack of validated tests appropriate for ICU survivors, limited information exists regarding this as an outcome parameter. In a comprehensive review of this issue, Hopkins and Brett [27] reported that at 1 year nearly a third of ARDS patients had cognitive limitations. A more recent study of a cohort of 51 ICU subjects suggested that 35% of these subjects scored at or below a level similar to the lowest fifth percentile of a normal population [28]. However, over time, 95% had experienced significant improvements in cognitive function [28].

The implications of persistent cognitive impairment are significant because they may portend difficulties with future employment and return to work. Hence, improved evaluations of cognitive recovery after critical illness in clinical trials, and the time course of that recovery, may help identify interventions that can have major implications for our patients. Again, if not incorporated into outcomes research, one cannot determine if and how what we do affects this variable. Likewise, it seems that different approaches to care in the ICU can alter neuropsychologic recovery from critical illness. Specifically, posttraumatic stress disorder (PTSD) is an emerging concern in outcomes research. The incidence of PTSD following an ICU course is unknown, but some survivors report disturbing memories and meet the clinical criteria for PTSD. Outcomes researchers have linked the development of PTSD to previous delusional memories while hospitalized, suggesting that our approach to sedation during the acute phase of a subject's illness can affect the rates of PTSD [29]. Confirming this, Kress et al. [30] observed that the incidence of PTSD approached 33% in persons randomized to standard sedation practices in the ICU and there was no PTSD in those allocated to a strategy relying on a daily interruption of sedation.

Quality of Life

In distinction to functional parameters such as the 6-minute walk distance or even cognitive function, estimating quality of life posses several unique challenges. Determining both the validity and reliability of quality-of-life measures, for example, is difficult. In addition, quality-of-life evaluations represent an intersection of clinical science with social science because many of the tools for rating quality of life rely on psychometrics for their theoretical foundations. Furthermore, the results of quality-of-life determinations can be affected by who is asking the questions and how they are asked. Research documents clearly that a patient and his spouse may score the patient's quality of life differently.

In general, quality-of-life tests attempt to score this on some form of a scale, which may be either continuous or categorical. The survey tool itself is often composed of select items that ask about certain aspects of life, functionality, quality, and so forth [24]. Items that inquire about certain, specific categories or aspects of quality of life are considered to fall within the same domain. Examples of domains routinely used to classify quality of life include pain and impairment, functional status, social role, satisfaction, and death. In reporting the results of quality-of-life testing, both aggregate scores and scores within a certain domain may be reported. The aggregate score often gives a sense of the overall health-related quality of life. Breaking out scores across the various dimensions can presents a profile of how an illness impacts quality of life. In addition, two distinct types of quality-of-life data are regularly collected: health profiles and utility measures [31]. The former generates information regarding the impact of disease and therapies for it on a unique patient. Utility measures, on the other hand, represent the preferences of groups of individuals who share certain common characteristics, such as exposure to like treatments or similar underlying disease states.

Quality-of-life scales may be either generic or disease-specific. Generic scales, such as the Sickness Impact Profile (SIP) or the Short-Form 36 (SF-36), have been developed in large diverse populations so that normal values exist [31]. Using these types of instruments allows comparisons across multiple disease states and various populations. Disease-specific instruments, such as the St. George's Respiratory Disease Questionnaire, may be better calibrated to detect changes over time as they focus on only one disease state or organ system [31]. These disease-specific measures are also focused on aspects of

TABLE 212.1

EXAMPLES OF QUALITY-OF-LIFE MEASURES

Name	Goal	Description	Concepts assessed
Sickness Impact Profile (SIP)	To asses health-related dysfunction	136 items in 12 domains	Physical, psychosocial, other (e.g., sleep, rest)
Short-Form 36 (SF-36)	Survey of general health status	36 items in 8 domains and a summary score	Physical, mental
Nottingham Health Profile	To determine perceived physical, social, and emotional health	Initial part of 38 items and second section of 7 items	Physical mobility, energy, pain, social isolation, emotional
EuroQuol	To measure health state and to determine preferences for 14 hypothetical health states	5 items measured at 3 levels	Physical and mental functioning

Adapted from Chaboyer W, Elliot D: Health-related quality of life in ICU survivors: review of the literature. *Intensive Crit Care Nurs* 16:88, 2000.

quality of life that may be of most concern to that specific group of patients. In other words, there is a tradeoff among rubrics between generalizability and resolution. Therefore, understanding critical care outcomes and ICU care's impact on quality of life necessitates studies using both approaches. Examples of various quality-of-life measures are shown in Table 212.1.

Despite using differing tools, examination of different types of patient cohorts, and issues with follow up evaluation, most quality-of-life research indicates that this is substantially impaired initially in ICU survivors. For example, Tian and Miranda [32] evaluated more than 3,500 ICU patients 1 year after initial admission. Employing the SIP, they observed that scores were substantially reduced among survivors. The main source of the impairment in quality-of-life assessment arose in the area of physical functioning. Interestingly, there was no correlation between the extent of the limitation in quality of life and either severity of illness at ICU admission or the duration of stay in the ICU. Others have confirmed this observation that severity of illness does not explain the limited quality of life reported by some persons. In a cohort of elderly survivors of prolonged MV, Chelluri et al. [33] observed that initial severity of illness as measured by the APACHE III score failed to explain both subsequent functional limitations and lower quality-of-life scores during the year following ICU discharge. Using the SF-36 rather than the SIP, Heyland et al. [34] concentrated on sepsis survivors. Compared to the general U.S. population, scores were significantly lower in nearly all domains. Both physical functioning and social functioning were rated at approximately two-thirds the level noted in a general U.S. sample. However, when analyzed against a cohort of subjects with chronic disease such as either chronic obstructive pulmonary disease or congestive heart failure, the self-reported quality of life of sepsis survivors was similar.

More recent studies have explored how quality of life changes over time after ICU discharge. Most surveys of quality of life represent cross-sectional efforts measuring this at only one time point and therefore provide little information about rates of change in quality of life or how pre-ICU quality of life affects quality of life after discharge. Addressing these limitations, Cuthbertson and coworkers [35] prospectively followed 300 consecutive patients admitted to their ICU. They measured quality of life using two different tools at 3, 6, and 12 months after ICU discharge. At 3 months, quality of life was substantially reduced compared to the subjects' premorbid states. During the ensuing year, quality of life improved and approached the pre-ICU level. Unfortunately, at 1 year, the quality of life of survivors still remained lower than that reported for a general population. Among 109 persons with ARDS, Herridge et al. [26] reported similar patterns in the recovery of quality of life. During 12 months, scores on the SF-36 for physical functioning doubled and those for social functioning rose by 75%.

Several general themes appear in the quality-of-life literature relating to ICU care. First, quality of life is substantially impaired in ICU survivors, but this improves with time after ICU discharge. Second, despite changes in quality of life, this may not return to preadmission levels and the time course of any recovery may be slow. Third, it is unclear what factors contribute to the quality of life of ICU survivors and how interventions in the ICU can affect subsequent quality of life.

Hence, many issues remain unresolved in this area of critical care outcomes research. Plaguing efforts to better comprehend this important patient-centered measure are multiple methodologic issues. As one systematic review of quality-of-life studies concluded: "There is no agreement as to the optimal instrument and [that] differences between studies preclude meaningful comparisons or pooling of results" [36]. These concerns explain why there has been a paucity of work in this area and why one group of investigators observed that fewer than 2% of all articles dealing with general critical care published from 1992 to 1995 dealt with this topic [37]. Despite all these concerns, an expert panel on surviving sepsis endorsed the SF-36 as best suited for outcomes research in critical care [4].

ECONOMIC OUTCOMES

A final aspect of critical care outcomes deals with economic and financial issues. The ICU remains a major focus for concerns relating to cost. Part of this arises from the fact that many expensive technologies are applied in the ICU. Simultaneously, ICU bed days are disproportionately expensive compared with costs related to general ward bed days. Adding to increased cost, sensitivity is a growing demand for ICU care. With the aging of the population, the need for critical care resources will escalate. For example, during the next three decades, the incidence of severe sepsis and septic shock has been projected to rise by 30% [38].

Relative to the entire U.S. economy, it was estimated that, approximately two decades ago, ICU costs accounted for nearly 1% of the nation's gross national product [1]. In a similar analysis, total critical care costs by the year 2000 had nearly tripled from 1984 and now exceeded $55.5 billion annually [39]. As a function of the national economy, however, the proportion of the gross domestic product devoted to the ICU had decreased to 0.56% [39]. Despite this relative fall in the resources consumed by critical care, which essentially reflects the growth of the U.S. economy, the ICU now accounts for one in seven dollars spent on hospital care in the United States [39]. On a per-day basis, the most recent analyses indicate that costs for the initial day of MV in the ICU exceed $10,000 and fall to $4,000 per day by ICU day 3 when most subjects are clinically stable [2]. In short, from any perspective, whether societal or local, critical care remains exceedingly expensive.

As a result of this economic pressure, patients, physicians, third-party payers, and policy makers are all demanding improved efficiency and optimization of resource allocation. In the United Kingdom, formal cost analyses have become the purview of regulatory agencies, and recommendations from these authorities influence the adoption of new therapies. In the United States, legislation to require formal economic analyses for the approval of new pharmaceuticals is under consideration. Critical care practitioners, therefore, require an appreciation of economics and finance in order to advocate for their patients and the resources they need to care for the critically ill.

A Primer on Economic Analysis

Economic analysis represents a means for understanding and appreciating value in order to facilitate the efficient allocation of scare resources in light of competing claims for those resources. In many scenarios, the criteria employed to determine how to spend limited dollars may not be evident or may be filled with assumptions and bias. The essential goal of economic analysis is to make explicit both the means and criteria used for decision-making. Reflecting the growing significance of economic issues, multiple formal position statements now exist describing both the means to conduct and the implications of financial studies in health care [40,41].

There are several basic varieties of economic analysis in health care: cost-minimization, cost–benefit, cost-effectiveness, and cost-utility. Cost-minimization presupposes that the outcome of interest is fixed and competing approaches are equally efficacious. The main issue, therefore, is which alternative costs less. In critical care, though, few interventions achieve similar results, so a more complex means for comparing options is required. When both costs and outcomes differ, it is necessary to assign the distinct options a value in some common schema (such as dollars). After converting potential results of interventions into dollars, one can proceed with cost–benefit analysis. Cost–benefit analysis is rarely used in health care because many end points are not easily converted into dollar values (e.g., the dollar value of a life) and because cost–benefit approaches may inadvertently assign more value to those who have higher earning potential. Cost-effectiveness acknowledges the limitations of cost–benefit and thus leaves the outcome (or denominator) in clinical terms such that one is now comparing costs per common measure of effectiveness. Often-used examples of this in critical care explore costs per year of life saved or per ICU days avoided. Cost-utility analysis builds on cost-effectiveness analysis by adjusting the clinical outcome for the quality that results from the intervention.

The standard denominator for these types of studies is the quality-adjusted life-year (QALY). The QALY concept acknowledges that a year of life spent in a long-term ventilator facility is not viewed by the patient as being of the same quality as a year lived being fully functional. Although arbitrary, most consider cost-effective interventions that yield a price per QALY saved of between $50,000 and $100,000.

One source of confusion and controversy in economic analysis is estimation of costs. Given the market structure of health care, charges rarely reflect cost. In fact, formal means exist to convert charges to cost based on published cost-to-charge ratios. Analytically, costs can be computed through microcosting, in which the unique costs for each component of care are determined and then summed. Costs can also be estimated based on average bed-day costs. Both approaches have limitations: Microcosting may underestimate the fixed costs associated with care delivery and a bed-day approach assumes that costs remain similar despite the intensity of care the patient requires.

Any conversation about cost, though, has an underlying central question: Cost to whom? This issue of perspective is key in all economic analyses. Some intervention may appear cost-effective to an institution because it shifts costs to a third-party payer. For the payer, though, the intervention will be seen as less than optimal. To address this fact, formal recommendations for the conduct of cost-effectiveness analyses encourage adoption of a societal perspective [40,41]. Utilization of a common societal perspective can also facilitate comparisons across alternatives. However, in critical care, a societal perspective poses specific challenges. As one review notes: "The societal perspective forces consideration of outcomes and costs not usually considered in critical care studies and a time horizon longer than most critical care studies" [13,41].

Uncertainty represents a final aspect of cost-effectiveness and outcomes that merits mention. All estimates for any study's inputs are bracketed by assumptions and uncertainty. The issue then becomes how one's conclusions are affected by this inherent uncertainty. If the costs of an ICU day are half what one assumes, does it alter the outcome of an analysis? Determining the impact of this uncertainty is best done through sensitivity analysis. Sensitivity analysis is a tool for varying a model's inputs across a range of assumptions and seeing if and how the results vary in response to this. If introducing such variability fails to affect the conclusions, one can be more confident as to the strength of the outcomes.

Disease-Specific Costs

Multiple studies in the last several years have attempted to gauge the costs of various diseases commonly encountered in the ICU. These reports help provide estimates of disease-state costs, which can be then used for cost-effectiveness analyses of preventive interventions or be relied on for budget planning.

With respect to nosocomial infection, Warren et al. [42] calculated the attributable cost of a catheter-related blood stream infection (CRBSI) to be nearly $12,000 per event. Their study prospectively followed a cohort of critically ill subjects and compared those developing CRBSIs to those not suffering this complication. In addition, they controlled for multiple potential confounders such as severity of illness, use of MV, and need for dialysis. Blot et al. [43], in a retrospective case-controlled study in Europe, reached similar conclusions. They reported that a CRBSI significantly prolonged the duration of MV and ICU length of stay and resulted in net excess costs totaling €14,000 [43]. Reflecting these high costs, multiple preventive strategies have been shown to be cost-effective. In an analysis of a multifaceted educational intervention emphasizing the pathogenesis, implications, and prevention of CRBSI, researchers from Washington University demonstrated that their efforts saved approximately $500,000 during the course of a year [44]. Likewise, use of chlorhexidine rather than povidone, adherence to the need for full barrier drapes, and adoption of antibiotic-impregnated catheters have been shown to yield net savings despite their initially high acquisition costs.

Ventilator-associated pneumonia also represents a common and costly ICU-acquired infection. Rello and coworkers [45] observed that the costs of this disease exceeded $40,000 per case. This analysis, though, was limited because it was a retrospective assessment of a large administrative database such that the definition of pneumonia employed might have led to selection bias. Alternatively, Warren et al. [46], in a prospective study of a community ICU, suggested that the costs of ventilator-associated pneumonia were similar to those reported by Rello et al. Hence, two distinct studies using different approaches reached similar conclusions.

For non-ICU acquired processes, community-acquired pneumonia (CAP) represents a major driver of national health care expenditures by the U.S. government. Describing outcomes in a cohort of patients with severe CAP, Angus et al. [47] suggested that persons with CAP needing ICU care generated total hospital costs in excess of $21,000. Strikingly, this amount was more than 3 times greater than the costs for inpatient CAP not needing ICU admission. From a societal perspective, Kaplan et al. [48] reviewed data from Medicare and calculated that national ICU costs for CAP surpassed $2.1 billion. The financial implications of sepsis are also staggering. Multiple reports document hospital costs per case at approximately $30,000 to $40,000 [49,50]. Costs in Europe seen somewhat lower than those noted in the United States. For example, Adrie et al. [51] prospectively recorded costs for sepsis in six French ICUs. The mean cost of severe sepsis equaled €22,800. They further described that sepsis costs varied based on whether the infection was community-acquired or evolved while the subject was hospitalized. In attempting to determine cost drivers in sepsis, Burchardi and Schneider [52] reviewed multiple costing reports and concluded that direct costs account for only 20% to 30% of overall costs in sepsis.

Cost-Effectiveness Studies in Critical Care

Coincident with the growing interest in cost-containment in critical care has been a rise in the number of formal cost-effectiveness analyses published in this field. Examples of such analyses have explored multiple resource-intense processes such as the use of MV in ARDS, reliance on renal replacement therapies (RRT) for acute renal failure in the ICU, and drotrecogin alfa (activated) (APC) for severe sepsis.

In ARDS, Hamel et al. [53] used information from the Study to Understand the Prognoses and Preferences for Outcomes and Risks of Treatments (SUPPORT) to investigate the value of MV. They estimated that ventilatory support was a cost-effective strategy overall, but that the cost-effectiveness ratio varied from $29,000 per QALY saved to $110,000 per QALY based on the subject's initial risk of death. Their analysis was insensitive to patient age as the cost-effectiveness ratio in subjects younger than 65 years was $32,000 versus $46,000 per QALY in those older than 75 years. One strength of this analysis was its close follow-up of patients, and thus the ability to more precisely account for postdischarge health care utilization.

Also using similar techniques, Korkeila et al. [54] investigated RRT. They tracked patients needing RRT and calculated that the costs per 6-month survivor were $80,000. In a comparable study to the one by Hamel et al., the SUPPORT investigators reported that the cost per QALY saved by initiating dialysis and continuing aggressive care was $128,000 [55]. Again, underlying prognosis, not surprisingly, affected the cost-effectiveness ratio. In the best prognosis group, cost per QALY approached $68,000. In the worse prognosis group, it measured $274,000 per QALY saved. The authors concluded that, except in those with exceedingly good prognoses, this approach was not cost-effective. Readers should note that these cost estimates are from nearly a decade ago, and if updated to reflect health care inflation would only reinforce the impression that acute RRT has substantial financial implications for society.

Finally, much emphasis has been placed on estimating the cost-effectiveness of APC because of its acquisition costs. Different groups of researchers have approached this issue from differing national perspectives (e.g., Canada vs. Europe vs. United States) [56–58]. Using data from their own ICU and results from the pivotal clinical trial for APC, Manns et al. [56] concluded that the cost per year of life gained with APC in severe sepsis was $28,000. APC was more cost-effective in persons at higher risk of death as determined by the APACHE II score ($25,000 per year of life gained). Even in older patients with more severe sepsis, APC was cost-effective. Looking at QALYs as a more traditional end point, Angus et al. [57] reached similar results. They computed that APC therapy yielded a cost of $49,000 per QALY gained. This ratio improved further if therapy was restricted to those at higher risk of death ($27,000 per QALY) [57]. Their analysis was most sensitive to the likely duration of survival with the cost-effectiveness of APC deteriorating to more than $100,000 QALY if survivors lived less than 4.6 years. Cost-effectiveness studies conducted from both UK and German perspectives have confirmed the findings of these two analyses [58,59].

Although not a definitive review of the many cost-effectiveness analyses performed in critical care outcomes research, these three examples illustrate that this approach can be used successfully to inform both professional and policy dialogue. They also help to demonstrate the value of ICU care despite its seemingly expensive implications for third-party payers and national governments. Uniformly, these reports illustrate that it is possible to measure proxies for cost rather easily and hence should become routine in the conduct of clinical research. Cost researchers, alternatively, need to be cautious as the time period they choose to study (e.g., short term, intermediate term, and long term) can affect their results and conclusions. Short-term costs may be saved with a novel intervention. Over the longer term, though, what might have appeared attractive economically could result in major costs to society.

CONCLUSION

Outcomes research remains an emerging field in critical care. As appreciation of patient-centered issues expands along with improved understanding of the diseases treated in the ICU, the need for more extensive and refined outcomes research will grow. Outcomes research, fortunately, encompasses a wide area of interest, and patient-centered outcomes can now be better folded into end points of clinical trials. Although methodologic issues continue to exist and further refinement in analytic techniques is required, the practicing intensivist needs to grasp the issues central to outcomes research.

References

1. Berenson RA: Intensive care units: clinical outcome, costs, and decision making (Health Technology Case Study 28). Prepared for the Office of Technology Assessment, US Congress, OTA_HCS_28. Washington, DC, 1984.
2. Dasta JF, McLaughlin TP, Mody SH, et al: Daily cost of an intensive care unit day: the contribution of mechanical ventilation. *Crit Care Med* 33:1266, 2005.
3. Rubenfeld GD, Angus DC, Pinsky MR, et al: Outcomes research in critical care: results of the American Thoracic Society Critical Care Assembly workshop on outcomes research. The Members of the Outcomes Research Workshop. *Am J Respir Crit Care Med* 160:358, 1999.
4. Marshall JC, Vincent JL, Guyatt G, et al: Outcome measures for clinical research in sepsis: a report of the 2nd Cambridge Colloquium of the International Sepsis Forum. *Crit Care Med* 33:1708, 2005.
5. Esteban A, Anzueto A, Frutos F, et al: Characteristics and outcomes in adult patients receiving mechanical ventilation: a 28-day international study. *JAMA* 287:345, 2002.
6. Vincent JL, Sakr Y, Reinhart K, et al: Is albumin administration in the acutely ill associated with increased mortality? Results of the SOAP study. *Crit Care* 9:R745, 2005.
7. Needham DM, Dowdy DW, Mendez-Tellez PA, et al: Studying outcomes of

intensive care unit survivors: measuring exposures and outcomes. *Intensive Care Med* 31:1153, 2005.
8. Dowdy DW, Needham DM, Mendez-Tellez PA, et al: Studying outcomes of intensive care unit survivors: the role of the cohort study. *Intensive Care Med* 31:914, 2005.
9. Pronovost PJ, Angus DC, Dorman T, et al: Physician staffing patterns and clinical outcomes in critically ill patients: a systematic review. *JAMA* 288:2151, 2002.
10. Levy MM, Rapoport J, Lemeshow S, et al: Association between critical care physician management and patient mortality in the intensive care unit. *Ann Intern Med* 148:801, 2008.
11. Feng Y, Amoateng-Adjepong Y, Kaufman D, et al: Age, duration of mechanical ventilation, and outcomes of patients who are critically ill. *Chest* 136:759, 2009.
12. Beck D: Mortality probabilities and case-mix adjustment by prognostic models, in Ridley S (ed): *Outcomes in Critical Care*. Oxford, Reed Elsevier, 1992.
13. Boyd O: Case-mix adjustment and prediction of mortality—the problems with interpretation, in Ridley S (ed): *Outcomes in Critical Care*. Oxford, Reed Elsevier, 1992.
14. Knaus WA, Draper EA, Wagner DP, et al: APACHE II: a severity of disease classification system. *Crit Care Med* 13:818, 1985.
15. Zimmerman JE, Kramer AA: Outcome prediction in critical care: the Acute Physiology and Chronic Health Evaluation models. *Curr Opin Crit Care* 14:491, 2008.
16. Le Gall JR, Loirat P, Alperovitch A, et al: A simplified acute physiology score for ICU patients. *Crit Care Med* 12:975, 1984.
17. Vincent JL, Moreno R, Takala J, et al: The SOFA (Sepsis-related Organ Failure Assessment) score to describe organ dysfunction/failure. On behalf of the Working Group on Sepsis-Related Problems of the European Society of Intensive Care Medicine. *Intensive Care Med* 22:707, 1996.
18. Marshall JC, Cook DJ, Christou NV, et al: Multiple organ dysfunction score: a reliable descriptor of a complex clinical outcome. *Crit Care Med* 23:1638, 1995.
19. Zimmerman JE, Kramer AA, Douglas S, et al: Acute Physiology and Chronic Health Evaluation (APACHE) IV ICU length of stay benchmarks for today's critically ill patients. *Chest* 128[Suppl 1]:297S, 2005.
20. Ledoux D, Finfer S, McKinley S: Impact of operator expertise on collection of the APACHE II score and on the derived risk of death and standardized mortality ratio. *Anaesth Intensive Care* 33:585, 2005.
21. Booth FV, Short M, Shorr AF, et al: Application of a population-based severity scoring system to individual patients results in frequent misclassification. *Crit Care* 9(5):R522, 2005.
22. Hebert PC, Wells G, Blajchman MA, et al: A multicenter, randomized, controlled clinical trial of transfusion requirements in critical care. transfusion requirements in critical care investigators, Canadian Critical Care Trials Group. *N Engl J Med* 340:409, 1999.
23. Ridley S: Non-mortality outcomes measures, in Ridley S (ed): *Outcomes in Critical Care*. Oxford, Reed Elsevier, 1992.
24. Koutsogiannis DJ, Noseworthy T: Quality of life after critical care, in Ridley S (ed): *Outcomes in Critical Care*. Oxford, Reed Elsevier, 1992.
25. Herridge MS: Long-term outcomes after critical illness. *Curr Opin Crit Care* 8:331, 2002.
26. Herridge MS, Cheung AM, Tansey CM, et al: One-year outcomes in survivors of the acute respiratory distress syndrome. *N Engl J Med* 348:683, 2003.
27. Hopkins RO, Brett S: Chronic neurocognitive effects of critical illness. *Curr Opin Crit Care* 11:369, 2005.
28. Jackson JC, Gordon SM, Ely EW, et al: Research issues in the evaluation of cognitive impairment in intensive care unit survivors. *Intensive Care Med* 30:209, 2004.
29. Nickel M, Leiberich P, Nickel C, et al: The occurrence of posttraumatic stress disorder in patients following intensive care treatment: a cross-sectional study in a random sample. *J Intensive Care Med* 19:285, 2004.
30. Kress JP, Gehlbach B, Lacy M, et al: The long-term psychological effects of daily sedative interruption on critically ill patients. *Am J Respir Crit Care Med* 168:1457, 2003.
31. Chaboyer W, Elliott D: Health-related quality of life of ICU survivors: review of the literature. *Intensive Crit Care Nurs* 16:88, 2000.
32. Tian ZM, Miranda DR: Quality of life after intensive care with the sickness impact profile. *Intensive Care Med* 21:422, 1995.
33. Chelluri L, Pinsky MR, Donahoe MP, et al: Long-term outcome of critically ill elderly patients requiring intensive care. *JAMA* 269:3119, 1993.
34. Heyland DK, Hopman W, Coo H, et al: Long-term health-related quality of life in survivors of sepsis. Short Form 36: a valid and reliable measure of health-related quality of life. *Crit Care Med* 28:3599, 2000.
35. Cuthbertson BH, Scott J, Strachan M, et al: Quality of life before and after intensive care. *Anaesthesia* 60:332, 2005.
36. Hennessy D, Juzwishin K, Yergens D, et al: Outcomes of elderly survivors of intensive care: a review of the literature. *Chest* 127:1764, 2005.
37. Heyland DK, Guyatt G, Cook DJ, et al: Frequency and methodologic rigor of quality-of-life assessments in the critical care literature. *Crit Care Med* 26:591, 1998.
38. Angus DC, Linde-Zwirble WT, Lidicker J, et al: Epidemiology of severe sepsis in the United States: analysis of incidence, outcome, and associated costs of care. *Crit Care Med* 29:1303, 2001.
39. Halpern NA, Pastores SM, Greenstein RJ: Critical care medicine in the United States 1985–2000: an analysis of bed numbers, use, and costs. *Crit Care Med* 32:1254, 2004.
40. Siegel JE, Weinstein MC, Russell LB, et al: Recommendations for reporting cost-effectiveness analyses. Panel on cost-effectiveness in health and medicine. *JAMA* 276:1339, 1996.
41. Understanding costs and cost-effectiveness in critical care: report from the Second American Thoracic Society Workshop on Outcomes Research. *Am J Respir Crit Care Med* 165:540, 2002.
42. Warren DK, Zack JE, Elward AM, et al: Nosocomial primary bloodstream infections in intensive care unit patients in a nonteaching community medical center: a 21-month prospective study. *Clin Infect Dis* 33:1329, 2001.
43. Blot SI, Depuydt P, Annemans L, et al: Clinical and economic outcomes in critically ill patients with nosocomial catheter-related bloodstream infections. *Clin Infect Dis* 41:1591, 2005.
44. Warren DK, Zack JE, Mayfield JL, et al: The effect of an education program on the incidence of central venous catheter-associated bloodstream infection in a medical ICU. *Chest* 126:1612, 2004.
45. Rello J, Ollendorf DA, Oster G, et al: Epidemiology and outcomes of ventilator-associated pneumonia in a large US database. *Chest* 122:2115, 2002.
46. Warren DK, Shukla SJ, Olsen MA, et al: Outcome and attributable cost of ventilator-associated pneumonia among intensive care unit patients in a suburban medical center. *Crit Care Med* 31(5):1312, 2003.
47. Angus DC, Marrie TJ, Obrosky DS, et al: Severe community-acquired pneumonia: use of intensive care services and evaluation of American and British Thoracic Society diagnostic criteria. *Am J Respir Crit Care Med* 166:717, 2002.
48. Kaplan V, Angus DC, Griffin MF, et al: Hospitalized community-acquired pneumonia in the elderly: age- and sex-related patterns of care and outcome in the United States. *Am J Respir Crit Care Med* 165:766, 2002.
49. Wood KA, Angus DC: Pharmacoeconomic implications of new therapies in sepsis. *Pharmacoeconomics* 22:895, 2004.
50. Piacevoli Q, Palazzo F, Azzeri F: Cost evaluation of patients with severe sepsis in intensive care units. *Minerva Anestesiol* 70:453, 2004.
51. Adrie C, Alberti C, Chaix-Couturier C, et al: Epidemiology and economic evaluation of severe sepsis in France: age, severity, infection site, and place of acquisition (community, hospital, or intensive care unit). *J Crit Care* 20:46, 2005.
52. Burchardi H, Schneider H: Economic aspects of severe sepsis: a review of intensive care unit costs, cost of illness and cost effectiveness of therapy. *Pharmacoeconomics* 22:793, 2004.
53. Hamel MB, Phillips RS, Davis RB, et al: Outcomes and cost-effectiveness of ventilator support and aggressive care for patients with acute respiratory failure due to pneumonia or acute respiratory distress syndrome. *Am J Med* 109(8):614, 2000.
54. Korkeila M, Ruokonen E, Takala J: Costs of care, long-term prognosis and quality of life in patients requiring renal replacement therapy during intensive care. *Intensive Care Med* 26(12):1824, 2000.
55. Hamel MB, Phillips RS, Davis RB, et al: Outcomes and cost-effectiveness of initiating dialysis and continuing aggressive care in seriously ill hospitalized adults. SUPPORT Investigators. Study to understand prognoses and preferences for outcomes and risks of treatments. *Ann Intern Med* 127:195, 1997.
56. Manns BJ, Lee H, Doig CJ, et al: An economic evaluation of activated protein C treatment for severe sepsis. *N Engl J Med* 347:993, 2002.
57. Angus DC, Linde-Zwirble WT, Clermont G, et al: Cost-effectiveness of Drotrecogin alfa (activated) in the treatment of severe sepsis. *Crit Care Med* 31:1, 2003.
58. Davies A, Ridley S, Hutton J, et al: Cost effectiveness of Drotrecogin alfa (activated) for the treatment of severe sepsis in the United Kingdom. *Anaesthesia* 60:155, 2005.
59. Neilson AR, Burchardi H, Chinn C, et al: Cost-effectiveness of Drotrecogin alfa (activated) for the treatment of severe sepsis in Germany. *J Crit Care* 18:217, 2003.

SECTION XX ■ CRITICAL CARE CONSEQUENCES OF WEAPONS (OR AGENTS) OF MASS DESTRUCTION

LAWRENCE C. MOHR JR

CHAPTER 213 ■ BIOLOGICAL AGENTS OF MASS DESTRUCTION

ANGELINE A. LAZARUS, ASHA DEVEREAUX AND LAWRENCE C. MOHR JR

OVERVIEW

The use of biological agents in warfare has been recorded throughout history. The first reported biological attack occurred in 1346 when the Tartar army used catapults to throw plague-infected corpses into the city of Kaffa. During the French and Indian War, British forces supplied blankets laden with smallpox to Native Americans supportive of the French. This caused a widespread epidemic of smallpox, leading to the surrender of Fort Carillon by Native American defenders and subsequent outbreaks of smallpox among tribes in the Ohio region [1]. In World War II, a Japanese plane reportedly dispersed rice and fleas infected with the plague organism over the city of Chu Hsien, China. An epidemic of bubonic plague developed in the Chu Hsien region shortly after this event [1].

In 1972, the United States and 161 other nations signed the Convention on the Prohibition of the Development and Stockpiling of Biological and Toxin Weapons. This international treaty prohibits the production of biological weapons and mandates the destruction of existing stockpiles. However, in 1979, there was an accidental release of aerosolized anthrax from the Institute of Microbiology and Virology at Sverdlovsk in the former Soviet Union. This resulted in an outbreak of inhalational anthrax and at least 66 deaths among the local civilian population [1].

In 1999, the Centers for Disease Control and Prevention (CDC) was designated as the lead agency in the United States for planning the public health response to a bioterrorism attack. Several reports published about that same time indicated that the risk of biological terrorism was increasing and that the use of biological agents, as both large-scale and small-scale weapons, was being actively explored by many nations and terrorist groups [2–6]. The concern expressed in these reports was realized after the attack on the World Trade Center in the fall of 2001, and when 22 cases of anthrax occurred in the United States as a result of anthrax spores being sent through the U.S. mail. There were 5 deaths among the 22 patients with anthrax [7,8]. These attacks demonstrated significant vulnerabilities of the United States to bioterrorism and the need for healthcare providers to be prepared to deal with bioterrorism attacks in their respective communities.

In 2002, the CDC published the *Public Health Assessment of Potential Biological Terrorism Agents* [9]. In this publication, potential bioterrorism agents were placed in one of three categories for the planning of public health preparedness. The agents in each category are summarized in Table 213.1. *Category A* agents have the greatest potential for the production of mass casualties and a major adverse public health impact. *Category B* agents have some potential for large-scale dissemination and mass casualties, but would be expected to cause less illness and death than Category A agents. *Category C* agents are those that do not pose a high bioterrorism threat at the present time, but could emerge as a future threat. This chapter focuses on Category A agents that have the greatest ability to cause mass casualties and significant loss of life. The Category B agent, ricin, is also discussed because of its unique potential to be used as a clandestine agent of terrorism.

SMALLPOX

The last case of endemic smallpox occurred in Somalia in 1977. In 1980, the World Health Organization (WHO) declared that the disease was eradicated. However, in recent years there has been renewed concern about the variola virus, the causative agent of smallpox, primarily due to the potential of the variola virus to be used as a biological weapon of mass destruction and the possibility for such a weapon to cause a major smallpox epidemic among infected populations. As a result of this concern, the WHO has restricted the number of laboratories officially authorized to serve as repositories for the variola virus to two: the CDC in Atlanta, Georgia, and the Vektor Institute in Novosibirsk, Russia [10].

Although smallpox has been officially declared to be eradicated, there is a possibility for its reemergence. In the nineteenth century, a major epidemic of smallpox appeared in the icy Sakha Republic in Russia, resulting in significant mortality. In the event of unusual thawing or flooding in that region, there is concern that infected corpses might be a potential source for the reemergence of smallpox. Although no live variola viruses have been isolated in the Sakha region, there is historical evidence of smallpox virus survival in interred and exhumed individuals from the eighteenth century [11].

With the increasing concern of bioterrorism and the possibility for the variola virus to be weaponized, the U.S. Military began smallpox vaccination of its troops on December 13, 2002 [12]. Much has been learned regarding the indications, contraindications, and efficacy of the vaccine since this mass immunization process began. Considerable thought has also been given to the dire consequences of a smallpox attack and the preparations necessary to manage a large-scale epidemic resulting from such an attack [13]. This section focuses on those aspects of smallpox infection that are most relevant to the critical care physician.

Virology

The causative agent of smallpox, the variola virus, is a member of the *Poxviridae* family, subfamily *Chordopoxvirinae*, and genus *Orthopoxvirus*. This genus also includes vaccinia (used in the smallpox vaccine), monkeypox virus, camelpox, and cowpox. The variola virus, like other members of the *Poxviridae* family, is a large, enveloped, DNA virus. *Poxviridae* viruses

TABLE 213.1

BIOTERRORISM AGENTS AND THREAT CATEGORIES

Category A	Category B	Category C
Bacillus anthracis (anthrax)	*Coxiella burnetii* (Q fever)	Nipah virus
Yersinia pestis (plague)	*Brucella* species (brucellosis)	Hantavirus
Variola major (smallpox)	*Burkholderia mallei* (Glanders)	Tickborne hemorrhagic fever viruses
Clostridium botulinum (botulism)	Ricin	Tickborne encephalitis viruses
Francisella tularensis (tularemia)	*Clostridium perfringens*	Yellow fever
Viral hemorrhagic fevers	Epsilon toxin	Multidrug-resistant tuberculosis
	Staphylococcal enterotoxin B	

Adapted from Rotz LD, Khan AS, Lillibridge SR, et al: Public health assessment of potential biological terrorism agents. *Emerg Infect Dis* 8:225, 2002.

are the only viruses that can replicate in the cytoplasm of cells without involvement of the cell nucleus. The variola virus has a brick-shaped morphology, measures 260 by 150 nm, and has one of the largest viral genomes known. Its large genome makes it difficult to genetically engineer or synthesize the virus in the laboratory. Humans are the only known reservoir for the variola virus, although monkeys are susceptible to infection [14]. The variola virus is very stable and maintains infectivity for long periods of time outside the human host [15]. There are two strains of variola, variola major and variola minor. Variola major is more virulent with a mortality rate between 20% and 50% in infected individuals. Variola minor causes a similar illness, but the mortality is less than 1% [16].

Transmission and Pathogenesis

Transmission of variola occurs from person to person by respiratory droplet nuclei dispersion. Transmission is enhanced by infected individuals who have a cough. Although infrequent, infection has also been known to occur following contact with infected clothing, bedding, or other contaminated fomites [17,18].

Following inhalation, the variola virus seeds the mucus membranes of the upper and lower respiratory tract and then migrates to regional lymph nodes, where viral replication occurs. Viral replication in regional lymph nodes leads to viremia, which results in systemic dissemination of the virus to other organs including the liver, spleen, skin, lung, brain, and bone marrow, where it continues to replicate. Clinical symptoms typically develop after an incubation period of 7 to 17 days.

Clinical Manifestations

Following the initial infection period of 1 to 4 days in which viremia occurs, the clinical manifestations of smallpox appear in a series of distinct phases [18]. These phases that are uniquely characteristic of smallpox are summarized here.

Incubation Phase

The incubation phase of smallpox lasts for 7 to 17 days after infection. During this phase, the virus replicates in regional lymph nodes of the upper and lower respiratory tract. During the incubation phase, infected individuals will most likely be asymptomatic but may have minimal symptoms, such as low-grade temperature elevation or a mild, erythematous rash. Smallpox is not contagious during the incubation phase.

Prodrome Phase

Approximately 7 to 17 days after exposure and initial infection, viremia develops and the variola virus spreads systematically to mucous membranes of the oropharynx, lungs, liver, spleen, bone marrow, and dermal layer of skin. The prodrome phase is characterized by the abrupt onset of high fever (greater than 40°C), headache, nausea, vomiting, and backache. These symptoms are sometimes accompanied by abdominal pain and delirium [19]. These prodromal symptoms typically last for 2 to 4 days. Smallpox may be contagious during the prodrome phase.

Eruption Phase

The eruption phase occurs 2 to 4 days after the onset of prodromal symptoms. Enanthema of the tongue, mouth, and oropharynx precedes the eruption phase by about 1 day. The eruption phase usually begins as small, red maculopapular lesions approximately 2 to 3 mm in diameter. The lesions first appear on the face, hands, and forearms. Lower extremity lesions appear shortly thereafter. The fever usually fades as the skin lesions appear. Symptoms of the prodrome phase may continue and patients can appear very ill. During the next 2 days, the skin lesions become distinctly papular and spread centrally to the trunk. Lesions also appear on the mucous membranes of the oropharynx, and oropharyngeal sections become highly infectious. Smallpox is most contagious during the eruption phase. Healthcare workers, family members, and other close contacts are at greatest risk of contracting smallpox from an infected individual during this phase.

Vesicular Phase

In 2 to 3 days after the eruption of skin lesions, the papular lesions begin to appear vesicular. The vesicles are filled with a thick, opaque fluid and typically range from 2 to 5 mm in diameter. The vesicles are most abundant on the face and extremities. The vesicular phase usually lasts for 2 to 3 days. Humoral antibodies become detectable during this period. Smallpox is contagious during the vesicular phase.

Pustular Phase

The vesicular lesions become pustules approximately 4 to 7 days after the onset of rash. The pustules are sharply raised, firm to the touch, and may have a depressed center and become umbilicated after several days. The pustular phase lasts for 5 to 8 days. Smallpox is contagious during the pustular phase.

Crust Phase

The umbilicated pustules eventually desiccate and become crusted scabs. During this time, there may be a fever spike that may indicate the presence of a superimposed bacterial infection. The crust phase lasts for 5 to 7 days. The crusts contain virus particles and smallpox remains contagious during this phase.

Desquamation Phase

Approximately 2 weeks after the eruption of the rash, desquamation begins. During this phase, the crusts separate from the skin and begin to fall off. Crusts on the palms and soles persist the longest and typically desquamate last. Virus particles are found in the fallen-off crusts and patients are infectious until all crusts separate and fall off. The desquamation phase typically lasts for several weeks. After the crusts fall off the skin, lesions heal and form depressed, depigmented scars.

There are several important characteristics of the smallpox skin lesions that can help to distinguish smallpox from varicella infections (chickenpox). The sequential appearance of the various types of skin lesions described previously is one important characteristic. The distribution of the skin lesions is also characteristic. Smallpox lesions appear first on the face and hands, then on the upper and lower extremities and, over the course of approximately 1 week, eventually spread to the trunk. In all phases of smallpox, there is a predominance of skin lesions on the face and extremities. Another important characteristic of smallpox is that skin lesions are mostly of the same type and same stage of development throughout each clinical phase. The synchronous and centrifugal nature of the smallpox skin lesions is the hallmark of this disease. In contrast, the skin lesions associated with varicella infections are greatest on the trunk, spare the hands and soles, and are at multiple stages at any given time, with papules, vesicles, and crusts all present simultaneously [18].

The mortality rate from the usual variety of smallpox is 3% in vaccinated individuals and 30% in those who are unvaccinated [20]. Death from smallpox is presumed to be secondary to a systemic inflammatory response syndrome caused by overwhelming quantities of immune complexes and soluble variola antigen. Smallpox-associated systemic inflammatory response syndrome results in severe hypotension that usually occurs in the second week of illness. Respiratory complications, including pneumonia and bronchitis, are common [18]. Due to fever and fluid shifts during the vesicular stage of the rash, severe intravascular volume and electrolyte imbalance may occur, which can lead to the development of renal failure. Encephalitis (less than 1% affected) and bacteremia may arise, with the risk of each increasing with the severity of the disease and contributing to mortality. Osteomyelitis, arthritis, and orchitis are other rare manifestations.

There are two atypical manifestations of smallpox that have very high mortality rates [17]. Hemorrhagic smallpox occurs in less than 3% of infected individuals. The hemorrhagic form is characterized by a short incubation period and an erythematous skin eruption that later becomes petechial and hemorrhagic, similar to the lesions seen in meningococcemia. Most individuals with the hemorrhagic form of smallpox die in 5 to 6 days after onset of the rash. The malignant form, or "flat smallpox," is characterized by a fine-grained, reddish, nonpustular, and confluent rash, occasionally with hemorrhage. The malignant form occurs in 2% to 5% of infected individuals. Patients with the malignant form have severe systemic illness and most die within several days. Pulmonary edema occurs frequently in both hemorrhagic and malignant smallpox and contributes to the high mortality rates [20].

The primary long-term sequela of smallpox is the "pockmarks" that affect the skin. These are pitted lesions that permanently scar the face due to infection of sebaceous glands. Panophthalmitis, viral keratitis, and corneal ulcers can cause permanent blindness in 1% of infected individuals. Infection with smallpox results in lifelong immunity [20].

Diagnosis

The differential diagnosis of papulovesicular lesions that can be confused with smallpox includes chickenpox (varicella), shingles (varicella-zoster), disseminated herpes simplex, monkeypox, drug eruptions, generalized vaccinia, eczema vaccinatum, impetigo, bullous pemphigoid, erythema multiforme, molluscum contagiosum, and secondary syphilis. Severe chickenpox (varicella) is the most common eruption that can be confused with smallpox. Table 213.2 delineates clinical features that can help to distinguish chickenpox from smallpox.

Confirmation of smallpox can be performed by the analysis of skin scrapings, vesicular fluid, and oropharyngeal swabs. Specimens should be collected using respiratory and contact isolation procedures, ideally by previously vaccinated personnel. Specimen collection techniques and guidelines are available from public health departments, the CDC, and the WHO [18]. If smallpox is suspected, the local public health department should be notified immediately. Public health departments can provide valuable assistance in collecting specimens and getting them to an appropriate laboratory for analysis. The brick-shaped variola virus is distinguished from varicella-zoster by electron microscopy. However, polymerase chain reaction (PCR) assays are the mainstay of diagnosis at the present time. Serologic testing is not useful in differentiating the variola virus from other orthopoxviruses. Laboratory specimens

TABLE 213.2

DISTINGUISHING CLINICAL FEATURES IN SMALLPOX AND CHICKENPOX

Feature	Smallpox	Chickenpox
Prodrome	2–4 days of high fever, headache backache, vomiting, abdominal pain	Absent-to-mild, 1 day
Rash	Starts in oral mucosa, spreads to face, and expands centripetally	Starts on trunk and expands centrifugally
Palms/soles	Common	Rare
Timing	Lesions appear and progress at same time	Lesions occur in crops; lesions at varied stages of maturation
Pain	May be painful	Often pruritic
Depth	Pitting and deep scars	Superficial; does not scar

should only be manipulated and processed at laboratories with Biosafety Level 4 facilities [17]. Again, local public health departments can assist in getting specimens to an appropriate laboratory.

Infection Control

Although the primary transmission of smallpox is via respiratory droplet nuclei, infected clothing and bedding can also transmit disease [11]. Individuals with smallpox are most infectious within the first 7 to 10 days of the rash, but the disease is contagious until all crusted lesions have fallen off [17]. Secondary cases occur in family members or healthcare workers who are exposed to an infectious individual. If a new outbreak were to occur, it is anticipated that the rate of transmission may be as high as 10 new cases for every infected person. All individuals who have direct contact with the index case should be quarantined for 17 days in respiratory isolation. Home quarantine will be necessary in mass casualty situations. Healthcare workers caring for infected individuals should be vaccinated and use strict airborne and contact isolation procedures. Infected patients should be placed in respiratory isolation and managed in a negative-pressure isolation room, if possible. Patients should remain isolated until all crusted lesions have fallen off. Patients should also be vaccinated if the disease is in the early stage. If performed early, vaccination may significantly decrease the severity of smallpox symptoms [18].

Treatment

There is no U.S. Food and Drug Administration (FDA)-approved drug for the treatment of smallpox. At the present time, treatment is primarily supportive. Supportive care includes maintaining general hygiene, appropriate antibacterial therapy for secondary skin infections, daily eye irrigation for severe cases, and ensuring that the patient receives adequate nutrition and hydration. Topical treatment with idoxuridine can be considered for the treatment of corneal lesions.

Animal studies have suggested that cidofovir has activity against orthopoxviruses, including variola. Cidofovir given at the time of, or immediately following, exposure has the potential to prevent cowpox, vaccinia, and monkeypox. Aerosolized cidofovir has been shown to protect mice against intranasal challenge with the cowpox virus [21]. Additional animal studies are being conducted with other antiviral agents. A new class of potent antipoxviral drugs (ST-246 and lipid-soluble cidofovir CMX001) has been developed and stockpiled [22]. It has been demonstrated that vaccinia immune globulin decreases pulmonary viral loads and pneumonitis in animals with vaccinia or cowpox. However, there is no evidence that the use of vaccinia immune globulin offers any survival or therapeutic benefit in patients infected with smallpox.

Immunization

Smallpox eradication was possible due to a successful worldwide vaccination program with live vaccine viruses. Vaccination continues to be the mainstay of smallpox prevention. First-generation live virus vaccines (Dryvax, APSV, Lancy-Vaxina, L-IVP) were administered by puncturing the skin of the upper arm with a bifurcated needle to induce a robust humoral immunity. Many side effects, reactions, and contraindications resulted from the use of these vaccines. Second-generation vaccines produced in the last 5 to 10 years still contain replication-competent viruses produced in tissue culture and elicit an immunity level similar to first-generation vaccines. A lyophilized preparation of live vaccinia virus (Dryvax, Wyeth Laboratories, Lancaster, PA) that contains polymyxin B, streptomycin, tetracycline, and neomycin was used in the 2004–2005 U.S. vaccination program. Third-generation vaccine formulations have utilized attenuated vaccinia strains (LC16m8, MVA, NYVAC, DVVL) with the hope of an improved safety profile [23]. There has been considerable discussion regarding the efficacy of pre-exposure mass vaccination to protect the public against smallpox in the event of a bioterrorism attack. At the present time, the CDC recommends voluntary vaccination for those likely to be exposed to smallpox and "ring vaccination" in the event of a smallpox outbreak [24,25].

Within 1 week of primary vaccination, the Jennerian pustule develops a gray-white loculated pustule with central umbilication. This marks a "major reaction" and implies successful vaccination. The Jennerian pustule will then crust and darken and remain for approximately 3 weeks following immunization. Successful revaccination is marked by mild induration at the inoculation site. A repeat vaccination attempt is suggested for any equivocal responses. Due to the shortage of vaccine supply in early 2002, dilution studies showed that the vaccinia virus diluted to a titer as low as $10^{7.0}$ plaque-forming units (pfu) per mL (approximately 10,000 pfu per dose) will result in vesicle formation in 97% of inoculated individuals [26]. Dilutions to a titer of $10^{6.5}$ pfu per millimeter were only effective in 70% of those immunized. Lower doses decrease success to as low as 15% [27]. A successful primary vaccination offers full immunity for 5 to 10 years in 95% of those immunized. Successful revaccination is likely to be effective for 10 to 20 years.

The WHO and CDC instructions for the administration of smallpox vaccine are as follows [17,18,28]:

- *Site of vaccination*: Outer aspect of upper arm over the insertion of the deltoid muscle.
- *Preparation of skin*: None, unless the site is obviously dirty. Use water to cleanse the site because the use of a disinfectant can kill the virus.
- *Withdrawal of vaccine from the ampule*: A cool, sterile bifurcated needle is inserted into the reconstituted vaccine ampule. A droplet is sufficient for vaccination and is contained within the fork of the needle. Never dip the same needle back into the ampule to avoid contamination.
- *Application*: The needle is held at 90 degrees perpendicular to the skin; the needle then touches the skin to release the droplet. For primary vaccination, three strokes are made in a 5-mm area. For revaccination, 15 up/down, perpendicular strokes of the needle are rapidly made in the area of 5 mm diameter (through the drop of vaccine deposited on the skin). The strokes should be sufficiently vigorous so that a trace of blood appears at the site. If blood does not appear, the procedure (three strokes) should be repeated with the same needle.
- *Dressing*: Although the WHO does not recommend a dressing, the CDC recommends a loose sterile gauze dressing covered by a semipermeable dressing to prevent transmission of the virus. Absorb the excess blood and vaccine with gauze, and dispose the gauze in a biohazard receptacle.
- *Unused Vaccine*: Unused vaccine is good for 90 days after reconstitution and should be refrigerated without any special light precautions.

The most common adverse reactions following smallpox vaccination are tenderness and erythema at the injection site and secondary bacterial infections. Fever, malaise, local lymphadenopathy, erythema multiforme, Stevens–Johnson syndrome, urticaria, exanthems, contact dermatitis, and erythematous papules have been reported [29]. Inadvertent autoinoculation of another body site, generalized vaccinia (vesicles or pustules appearing on normal skin distant from the vaccination site), eczema vaccinatum, vaccinia keratitis, and progressive vaccinia have been reported in primary vaccinations. Postvaccinia encephalitis is a very rare complication. Myopericarditis was reported in 200 cases from the recent military vaccination program, at a rate of 117 cases per million vaccinees [12,30]. The cause of postvaccination myopericarditis is not well understood but is probably immunologically mediated and not from direct viral infection of the myocardium. As a result, the CDC has recommended that routine vaccination should not be given to anyone with known previous cardiac disease or three or more risk factors for coronary artery disease [18,31]. The reported rate of cardiac mortality is 1.1 deaths per million primary vaccines. A review of approximately 39,000 people vaccinated against smallpox (36% primary vaccinations and 64% revaccinations) reported the following adverse reactions: encephalitis in 1 individual, myopericarditis in 21 individuals, generalized vaccinia in 2 individuals, inadvertent inoculation in 7 individuals, and ocular vaccinia in 3 individuals [32].

Contraindications to smallpox vaccination are infants less than 1 year of age, immune suppression, eczema, exfoliative skin conditions, pemphigus, cardiac disease as previously described, allergy to any component of the vaccine, and pregnant or breastfeeding women. Individuals who are taking, or have taken, high-dose corticosteroids should not be vaccinated within 1 month of completing corticosteroid therapy. Although testing for human immunodeficiency virus (HIV) is not mandatory prior to smallpox vaccination, the Advisory Committee on Immunization Practices has recommended that HIV testing be readily available to all individuals considering smallpox vaccination [25]. Individuals with a contraindication to vaccination should avoid people who have been recently vaccinated, due to possible transmission of vaccinia from viral shedding at the vaccination site. A small number of deaths (12/68) in the 1960s were attributed to unvaccinated persons exposed to recently vaccinated friends or family members [33].

Healthcare workers must be aware of the possibility for the nosocomial transmission of vaccinia during the hospitalization of a recently vaccinated patient. Nosocomial infection can result in mortality up to 11%. Direct carriage of the virus on the hands, nasal mucosa, fomites, contaminated equipment, and laundry has been implicated in the transmission of vaccinia [34]. Risk of the nosocomial transmission can be mitigated by several simple precautions. Semipermeable dressings should be applied to the site of a recent vaccination and changed frequently if there is evidence of the accumulation of purulent material. Gloves should be worn during dressing changes and meticulous handwashing with antimicrobial soap should be performed by all healthcare providers, both before and after contact with a recently vaccinated patient. Contaminated dressings should be disposed of in a biohazard container. Care should be taken to avoid contact of the vaccination site with material or equipment that could transmit the virus to other individuals. Clothing, towels, and other cloth materials that have contact with the site can be decontaminated by routine laundering with hot water. If at all possible, healthcare workers who are responsible for dressing changes should be vaccinated against smallpox, but nonvaccinated individuals are acceptable as long as appropriate precautions are observed [25]. Sexual transmission of vaccinia virus from a recently immunized active duty military member to a civilian has been recently reported following immunization [34].

Treatment of adverse effects following smallpox vaccination include supportive therapy; administration of vaccinia immune globulin; cidofovir; and an antiviral ophthalmic ointment, such as trifluridine or vidarabine, for eye involvement. Vaccinia immune globulin is available from the CDC, although the supply is limited. Cidofovir is available at no cost from the CDC under investigational use if a patient fails to respond to vaccinia immune globulin, the patient is near death, or all inventories of vaccinia immune globulin are depleted. The dose of cidofovir is 5 mg per kg, given intravenously, during 60 minutes as a single dose [18].

Due to the adverse effects of vaccinia, the federal government contracted with Acambis (Cambridge, England) and Baxter Healthcare (Cambridge, MA) to purchase a cell culture-derived smallpox vaccine that has demonstrated 94% efficacy in phase II clinical trials. Further research on the development of safer smallpox vaccines is currently in progress. In August 2007, the ACAM2000 vaccine was licensed by the FDA for administration to people at high risk of smallpox or other orthopoxvirus diseases. Over 200 million doses of the vaccine have been purchased by the U.S. Strategic National Stockpile (covers approximately 62% of the population), but it is not available for commercial use. Clinical trials show similar efficacy and side effects profile to the Dryvax vaccination, but ACAM200 cannot be diluted [18,22].

In the event of an international release of variola virus, the priority of vaccination is as follows [24,25,35]:

- *Group 1*: Individuals directly exposed to the release.
- *Group 2*: Individuals with face-to-face household contact with a directly exposed individual.
- *Group 3*: Personnel directly involved in the evaluation, care, or transport of infected patients.
- *Group 4*: Laboratory personnel responsible for handling and processing specimens, and others who may be exposed to infectious materials.

ANTHRAX

In the fall of 2001, 22 cases of anthrax with 5 deaths occurred in the United States as a result of anthrax spores in envelopes sent through the U.S. mail. Early recognition and treatment of anthrax by astute clinicians was responsible for preventing additional deaths [7,8]. Anthrax is thought to be the most likely biological agent to be used in a bioterrorism attack. Identification of a single case should prompt notification of local, state, and national public health authorities [36]. The CDC has rapid response teams with specialized expertise, training, and equipment that can be deployed immediately to assist local authorities in the event of a bioterrorism attack [8]. Cases of anthrax in animals have been reported to occur sporadically in North America. In 2006, an outbreak was reported in Canada that affected over 900 animals. Two cases of cutaneous anthrax and one case of inhalational anthrax in humans were reported in the United States from occupational exposure associated with drum making using animal hides from West Africa [37].

Microbiology

Bacillus anthracis (from the Greek word for coal, *anthrakis*) is a large, Gram-positive, aerobic, spore-forming, nonmotile bacillus. *B. anthracis* is found in the soil of many regions of the world, where it exists in the endospore form. Its virulence is determined by two plasmids. One plasmid involves the synthesis of a poly D glutamic acid capsule that inhibits phagocytosis of vegetative bacilli and the other contains genes for the synthesis of exotoxins. The exotoxins are known as *protective antigen*, *edema factor*, and *lethal factor*. The *protective antigen* is a binding protein that is necessary for entry into the host cell and combines with both edema factor and lethal factor to produce "edema toxin" and "lethal toxin" [38]. Edema toxin converts adenosine triphosphate to cyclic adenosine monophosphate (cAMP), resulting in high intracellular cAMP levels that impair water homeostasis and thereby cause cellular edema. Lethal toxin stimulates the overproduction of cytokines, primarily tumor necrosis factor-α and interleukin-1-β that cause macrophage lysis. The sudden release of inflammatory mediators appears to be responsible for the marked clinical toxicity of the bacteremic form of anthrax.

Clinical Manifestations

There are three forms of anthrax infection. The clinical characteristics of each form are determined by the route of entry of the anthrax spores. *Cutaneous anthrax* is the most common naturally occurring form, comprising approximately 95% of cases reported. Spores enter the body through breaks in the skin and begin low-level germination within days, resulting in soft tissue or mucosal edema and localized necrosis. Initially, a painless, pruritic macule appears, followed by vesiculation, ulceration, and a black, "coal-like" painless eschar, from which anthrax gets its name. The eschar sloughs within 2 to 3 weeks of onset [39]. Abscess formation occurs only with superinfection. Endospores phagocytosed by macrophages are often transported to regional lymph nodes causing painful lymphadenopathy and lymphangitis. Infrequently, cutaneous anthrax may spread hematogenously with significant morbidity and death in a small number of individuals. Cutaneous anthrax has been reported to cause microangiopathic hemolytic anemia, renal dysfunction, and coagulopathy [40].

Gastrointestinal and *oropharyngeal anthrax* usually occur following the ingestion of contaminated meat. This is a rare manifestation of anthrax, with most cases occurring in Africa. Mucosal ulcers, edema, and regional lymphadenopathy are initial manifestations. In the oropharyngeal form, pseudomembranes are seen in the oropharynx and upper airway obstruction can develop. In the gastrointestinal form, a necrotizing infection progresses from the esophagus to the cecum. Fever, nausea, vomiting, abdominal pain, gastrointestinal bleeding, and bloody diarrhea are typical symptoms. Anemia, electrolyte abnormalities, and hypovolemic shock may follow. Massive ascites that is occasionally purulent has been reported. Death results from intestinal perforation or septicemia [20].

The third form of anthrax infection is *inhalational anthrax*. Anthrax spores are 1 to 1.5 μm in size and easily deposit in the alveoli following inhalation. There, the endospores are phagocytosed by the pulmonary macrophages and transported via lymphatics to the mediastinal lymph nodes, where they may remain dormant as "vegetative cells" for approximately 10 to 60 days or longer. Once germination in the lymph nodes is complete, bacterial replication occurs. The replicating bacteria release edema and lethal toxins that produce a hemorrhagic mediastinitis.

In some patients, the initial symptoms are relatively mild and nonspecific, resembling an upper respiratory tract infection. Fever, chills, fatigue, nonproductive cough, nausea, dyspnea, chest pain, and myalgias are common presenting complaints (Table 213.3) [36,37]. These symptoms typically last for 2 to 3 days and then progress to a more severe, fulminant illness. However, some patients present with fulminant illness without any prodromal symptoms. Dyspnea and shock characterize the fulminant phase of inhalational anthrax. The number of spores inhaled, age of the patient, and the underlying immune status most likely affect the clinical course of the disease [41]. Chest radiographs show mediastinal widening and pleural effusions that may be massive (Fig. 213.1). *B. anthracis* bacilli, bacillary fragments, and anthrax antigens can be identified by immunohistochemistry testing of the pleural fluid [42]. Although parenchymal infiltrates are not prominent, a focal hemorrhagic necrotizing pneumonitis, resembling the Ghon complex of tuberculosis, was noted in 11 of 42 autopsy patients from the accidental release of anthrax in Sverdlovsk, USSR, in 1979. Almost 50% of patients with inhalational anthrax develop hemorrhagic meningitis as a result of the hematogenous spread of *B. anthracis*. Massive bacteremia, with up to 10^7 to 10^8 bacteria per mL of blood, causes overwhelming septic shock and death within hours after the onset of symptoms. According to the Defense Intelligence Agency, the lethal dose to kill 50% of persons exposed (LD_{50}) to weapons-grade anthrax is 2,500 to 55,000 spores [43]. However, as few as one to three spores may be sufficient to cause infection [36].

TABLE 213.3

CLINICAL FEATURES OF INHALATIONAL ANTHRAX (U.S. OUTBREAK 2001, $n = 10$)

Feature	Incidence (%)
Fever and chills	100
Fatigue, malaise, lethargy	100
Cough	90
Nausea/vomiting	90
Dyspnea	80
Sweats-drenching	70
Chest discomfort	70
Myalgias	50
Headache	50
Confusion	40
Abdominal pain	30
Sore throat	20
Rhinorrhea	10

Adapted from Inglesby TV, O'Toole T, Henderson DA, et al: Anthrax as a biological weapon. *JAMA* 287:2236, 2002.

Diagnosis

A high index of suspicion is necessary to make the diagnosis of anthrax when patients present with a severe flulike illnesses. Laboratory findings from the U.S. outbreak in 2001 showed that patients had a mild neutrophil-predominant leukocytosis,

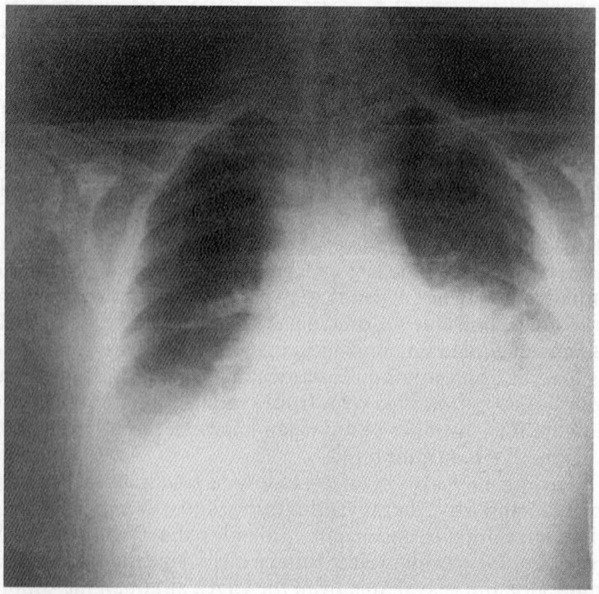

FIGURE 213.1. Chest radiograph from a patient with anthrax showing mediastinal widening and a pleural effusion. [From the CDC Web site: http://www.bt.cdc.gov/agent/anthrax/anthrax-images/inhalational.asp.]

in the range of 7,500 to 13,300 per μL. Peak white blood cell count during illness ranged from 11,900 to 49,600 per mm^3. Elevated transaminases, hyponatremia, and hypoxemia were also noted [7,37,41,43]. One hundred percent of these patients had an abnormal chest radiograph with mediastinal widening, pleural effusions, consolidation, and infiltrates predominating. The presence of mediastinal widening that may require computed tomography scanning to elucidate should be considered diagnostic of anthrax until proven otherwise [44–46]. Hemorrhagic necrotizing lymphadenitis and mediastinitis are pathognomonic of anthrax, but these are autopsy findings of these conditions [19]. *B. anthracis* is easily cultured from blood, cerebral spinal fluid, ascites, and vesicular fluid with standard microbiology techniques. The laboratory should be notified when the diagnosis of anthrax is being considered, as many hospital laboratories will not further characterize *Bacillus* species unless requested. Biosafety Level 2 conditions apply for workers handling specimens because most clinical specimens have spores in the vegetative state that are not easily transmitted [36]. The presence of large Gram-positive rods in short chains that are positive on India ink staining is considered presumptive of *B. anthracis*, until the results of cultures and other confirmatory tests are obtained. Confirmatory testing can be performed by the CDC Laboratory Response Network. Rapid detection tests based on immunohistochemistry, and PCR techniques are available via the Laboratory Response Network [37]. Nasal swabs are not recommended because they are not reliable for making the diagnosis of anthrax. Following the 2001 anthrax attack, there were negative nasal swab results in patients with fatal inhalational anthrax [43]. In June 2004, the FDA approved the Anthrax Quick ELISA test (Immunetics, Inc., Boston, MA) that detects antibodies to the protective antigen of *B. anthracis* exotoxin. The test can be completed in less than 1 hour and is available to hospital and commercial laboratories by the manufacturer [37].

Treatment

Due to the fulminant course of inhalational anthrax, prompt initiation of therapy is essential for survival. Ciprofloxacin (400 mg) or doxycycline (100 mg) given intravenously every 12 hours with one to two other antibiotics that have predicted efficacy against anthrax is currently recommended. Additional antibiotics that are effective against anthrax include rifampin, vancomycin, imipenem, chloramphenicol, penicillin, ampicillin, clindamycin, and clarithromycin. Two survivors of anthrax during the U.S. outbreak received parenteral ciprofloxacin, clindamycin, and rifampin. The addition of clindamycin may attenuate toxin production [44]. There are limited data regarding treatment of pregnant women for anthrax. However, the limited information that is available suggests that the use of ciprofloxacin during pregnancy is unlikely to be associated with a high risk for structural birth defects [47]. Therefore, ciprofloxacin should be given to pregnant women for the treatment of inhalational anthrax unless otherwise contraindicated. Doxycycline is relatively contraindicated in pregnancy and should only be considered if ciprofloxacin is unavailable or absolutely contraindicated. Therapy with ciprofloxacin or doxycycline should continue for 60 days. Patients can be switched to oral therapy with ciprofloxacin (500 mg twice daily) or doxycycline (100 mg twice daily) after fulminant symptoms have resolved and they are stable. The use of systemic corticosteroids has been suggested for meningitis, severe edema, and airway compromise. Parenteral ciprofloxacin and another antibiotic with good central nervous system penetration, such as rifampin, should be part of the initial treatment regimen for anthrax meningitis. Cutaneous anthrax with systemic involvement, significant edema, and lesions of the head and neck should be treated similarly. Uncomplicated cutaneous anthrax can be treated with oral ciprofloxacin or doxycycline for 7 to 10 days, but, due to the possibility of concomitant inhalational exposure, a 60-day course is recommended [36,37].

A review of anthrax cases in adults from 1900 to 2004 noted that fulminant inhalational anthrax is often fatal despite advances in medical care. Early diagnosis and initiation of therapy during the prodromal phase improved survival and are pivotal for decreasing mortality in inhalational anthrax [48]. Similarly, a review of anthrax cases in children from 1900 to 2005 shows that early diagnosis and treatment of all forms of anthrax are critical for improved survival in children [49].

Prophylaxis

All patients exposed to anthrax should receive prophylaxis with oral ciprofloxacin (500 mg twice daily), levofloxacin (500 mg daily), or doxycycline (100 mg twice daily) for 60 days, regardless of laboratory test results. Nasal swabs can confirm exposure to anthrax, but cannot exclude it. High-dose penicillin or ampicillin may be an acceptable alternative for 60 days in patients who are allergic or intolerant to the recommended antibiotics [36,37]. More than 5,000 people received postexposure prophylaxis following the 2001 U.S. outbreak, but only about half completed the 60-day course. The main reasons for discontinuing therapy were gastrointestinal or neurologic side effects (75%) or a low perceived risk (25%).

The anthrax vaccine (AVA-Biothrax) manufactured by BioPort Corporation in Lansing, Michigan, is the only licensed human anthrax vaccine in the United States. The vaccine consists of supernatant material from cultures of a toxigenic, nonencapsulated strain of *B. anthracis*. A six-dose series has been used by the U.S. Military. The anthrax vaccine is not available to the general public at the present time. Although efficacy data are limited to goat hair mill workers from the 1950s to 1974, fully vaccinated individuals did not contract anthrax as compared to those who did not participate in the vaccine program [50]. Approximately 95% of vaccinated individuals seroconvert after the third dose of vaccine. Data regarding vaccine safety from more than 1 million doses administered to members of the U.S. Military reveal that the adverse events were without any significant pattern or association. The vaccine is generally considered to be safe by the FDA [50]. A review by the U.S. Army Medical Research Institute of Infectious Diseases reported a 1% (101/10,722) incidence of systemic symptoms, most commonly headache. Local or injection site reactions occurred in 3.6% [36]. A study comparing four subcutaneous injections of anthrax vaccine adsorbed (AVA) with three and four intramuscular injections of AVA showed similar immunoprotection at 7 months with less adverse effects at the injection site. Following an aerosolized *B. anthracis* attack, postexposure prophylactic vaccination and antibiotic therapy remain the most effective and least expensive strategies [51].

TULAREMIA

Tularemia is a zoonosis found in a wide range of animals, primarily small mammals such as rodents and rabbits. In 1922, tularemia was reported to cause fatal illness in humans [52]. In the late 1920s, tularemia was recognized as a threat to laboratory workers. Tularemia is caused by *Francisella tularensis*, an intracellular, nonspore-forming, aerobic Gram-negative coccobacillus. In the mid-twentieth century, both the United States and the former Soviet Union developed biological weapons that could disperse *F. tularensis* [53]. Biological weapons have now been banned and are no longer in production. However, there is concern that *F. tularensis* could be used as an agent of bioterrorism. In a 1970 report, the WHO estimated that 50 kg of aerosolized *F. tularensis* dispersed over a metropolitan area of 5 million people could cause 19,000 deaths and 250,000 incapacitating illnesses [19,54]. The impact of such an attack would probably linger for several weeks to months due to disease relapses [54].

Microbiology

F. tularensis is a nonsporulating, nonmotile, Gram-negative coccobacillus. It is a hardy organism, which makes it well suited for use as an agent of bioterrorism. It can survive in moist soil, water, and animal carcasses for many weeks. However, chlorination of water prevents its spread through water contamination. *F. tularensis* can be aerosolized and inhalation of aerosolized organisms poses a threat to those exposed. The most common isolate, and the most virulent form, is *F. tularensis* biovar *tularensis* (Group A). Inoculation or inhalation of as few as 10 organisms may cause clinical disease [55–57]. *F. tularensis* biovar *palaearctica* is found mostly outside of the United States, most notably in Europe. Transmission of *F. tularensis* to humans occurs predominantly through tick and fleabites, handling of infected animals, ingestion of contaminated food and water, and inhalation of the aerosolized organism. There is no human-to-human transmission of *F. tularensis*. As a biological weapon, the organism would most likely be dispersed as an aerosol and cause mass casualties from an acute febrile illness that may progress to severe pneumonia [19].

Epidemiology

Tularemia occurs worldwide but is rare in Africa, Central, South America, and the United Kingdom, with highest incidence in Russia and Scandinavian countries [57–59]. In the United States, tularemia cases are reported most often from the south central and western states (Arkansas, Illinois, Missouri, Oklahoma, Tennessee, Texas, Utah, Virginia, and Wyoming). The predominant mode of transmission to humans in the United States is by tick bites, and most cases are reported in spring and summer. Hunters and trappers exposed to animal reservoirs are at high risk for exposure [57–59]. In Europe and Japan, mosquito bites and the handling of infected animals appear to cause the disease. A large outbreak of tularemia in 2003 along with small summer outbreaks between 1995 and 2005 in Sweden suggests environmental sources clustering around recreational areas [60]. Tularemia epidemics may have a seasonal presentation. *F. tularensis* var *tularensis*, often seen in summer, is tick-borne, while *F. palaearctica*, seen in fall and winter, is commonly transmitted from contaminated water, rodents, or aquatic animals. An outbreak of tularemia in Martha's Vineyard, Massachusetts, during the summer of 2000 was associated with lawn mowing and brush cutting [61,62]. A waterborne outbreak resulting in 21 cases of oropharyngeal and 5 cases of glandular tularemia was reported in Georgia [63].

Pathogenesis

F. tularensis enters the human host via the eye, respiratory tract, gastrointestinal tract, or a break in the skin. The virulence of the organism depends on its ability to replicate within the macrophage. On entering the macrophage, the organism proliferates. This is followed by apoptosis of the macrophage and the release of a larger number of organisms, leading to involvement of the local lymph nodes and bacteremia. Once bacteremia develops, *F. tularensis* infects the lungs, pleura, spleen, liver, and kidney. The host defense against *F. tularensis* is reported to be T-cell independent in the first 3 days and T-cell dependent after 3 days of infection. Initially, a focal suppurative necrosis with polymorphonuclear cells, macrophages, epithelioid cells, and lymphocytes are noted. The predominant protective mechanism in containing the disease comes from cell-mediated immunity. On histopathology, granulomas with necrosis may be seen in infected organs. Following inhalational exposure, hemorrhagic airway inflammation progressing to bronchopneumonia, pleuritis, and pleural effusion have been reported [55–57]. The mucosal immunopathogenesis of *F. tularensis* in animal models has shown that the antibodies may provide both prophylactic and therapeutic protection against pulmonary infection when there is active cell-mediated immunity [64].

Clinical Features

The clinical manifestations of tularemia depend on the site of entry, exposure dose, virulence of the organism, and host immune factors. Hematogenous spread may occur from any of the initial clinical presentations. Tularemia can have various clinical presentations that have been classified as primary pneumonic, typhoidal, ulceroglandular, oculoglandular, oropharyngeal, and septic. The *ulceroglandular form* is the most common naturally occurring form of tularemia. After an incubation period of 3 to 6 days (range, 1 to 25 days) following a vector bite or animal contact, patients present with symptoms of high fevers (85%), chills (52%), headache (45%), cough (38%), and myalgias (31%). They may also have malaise, chest pain, abdominal pain, nausea, vomiting, and diarrhea. A pulse-temperature dissociation is often seen. At the site of inoculation, a tender papule develops that later becomes a pustule and ulcerates. Lymph nodes draining the inoculation site become enlarged and painful (85%). Infected lymph nodes may become suppurative, ulcerate, and remain enlarged for a long period of time. Exudative pharyngitis and tonsillitis may develop following ingestion of contaminated food or inhalation of the aerosolized organism. Pharyngeal ulceration and regional lymphadenopathy may be present. A systemic disease caused by *F. tularensis* without lymph node enlargement and presenting with fever, diarrhea, dehydration, hypotension, and meningismus is referred to as the *typhoidal form*. The *pneumonic form* of tularemia may occur as a primary pleuropneumonia following the inhalation of aerosolized organisms. The pneumonic form may also occur as a result of hematogenous spread from other sites of infection or following oropharyngeal tularemia. After an inhalational exposure, constitutional symptoms, such as fever and chills, typically precede the onset of respiratory symptoms. The respiratory symptoms include a dry or minimally productive cough, pleuritic chest pain, shortness of breath, and hemoptysis. Pleural effusions, either unilateral or bilateral, can occur. Pneumonic tularemia can rapidly progress to respiratory failure with acute respiratory distress syndrome, multiorgan failure, disseminated intravascular coagulation, rhabdomyolysis, renal failure, and hepatitis [55–57,65]. Rarely, peritonitis, pericarditis, appendicitis, osteomyelitis, erythema nodosum, and meningitis have been reported to occur in tularemia. It has been reported that delays in diagnosis and failure to institute prompt aminoglycoside therapy results in higher morbidity [66]. The mortality rate of untreated tularemic pneumonia is 60%, but with proper antibiotic therapy the mortality rate is significantly reduced to 1% to 2.5% [55,56].

Laboratory and Radiographic Findings

A high index of suspicion is needed in order to make an early diagnosis of tularemia. Lack of response to conventional treatment for skin ulcers or community-acquired pneumonia, along

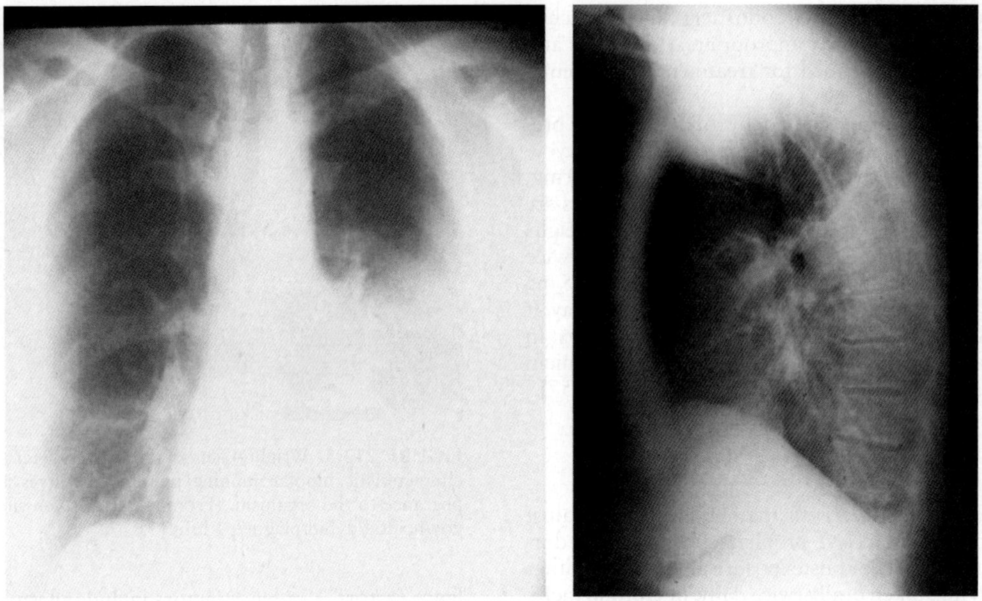

FIGURE 213.2. Chest radiograph from a 27-year-old man who contracted tularemic pneumonia after skinning a rabbit that he had hunted. [Courtesy of Angeline A. Lazarus, MD.]

with a history of exposure to animals, may alert the clinician to think of tularemia. Routine laboratory tests, such as a complete blood count and serum chemistry panels, are generally nondiagnostic. A complete blood count may show a leukocytosis with a normal differential or mild lymphocytosis. Mild elevations of lactic dehydrogenase, transaminases, and alkaline phosphatase may be seen on a serum chemistry panel. If rhabdomyolysis is present, an elevated serum creatine kinase concentration and urine myoglobin may be seen. Sterile pyuria has been reported. Mild abnormalities in cerebrospinal fluid cell counts, protein, and glucose have also been reported [54,56,65].

Tularemia can present with multiple abnormalities on a chest radiograph (Fig. 213.2). A report of the chest radiographic findings in 50 patients who had a confirmed diagnosis of tularemia showed the following abnormalities: patchy airspace opacities (74%, unilateral in 54%); hilar adenopathy (32%, unilateral in 22%); pleural effusion (30%, unilateral in 20%); unilateral lobar or segmental opacities (18%); cavitation (16%); oval opacities (8%); and cardiomegaly with a pulmonary edema pattern (6%). Rare findings such as apical infiltrates, empyema with bronchopleural fistula, miliary pattern, residual cyst, and residual calcification occurring in less than 5% of patients were also reported [67].

Diagnosis

It is possible to isolate *F. tularensis* from sputum, blood, and other body fluids, but the organism can be difficult to culture. Culture media must contain cysteine or sulfhydryl compounds for *F. tularensis* to grow. Notification of laboratory personnel that tularemia is suspected can be helpful in enhancing the yield of culture. Notification of laboratory personnel will also help to ensure that they observe appropriate biosafety procedures when manipulating specimens. Routine diagnostic procedures can be performed in Biosafety Level 2 conditions. Examination of cultures in which *F. tularensis* is suspected should be done in a biological safety cabinet. Manipulation of cultures and other procedures that might produce aerosols or droplets should be conducted under Biosafety Level 3 conditions [56].

Examination of secretions and biopsy specimens with direct fluorescent antibody or immunochemical stains may help to identify the organism. The diagnosis is often made through serologic testing using enzyme-linked immunosorbent assay (ELISA). Serologic titers may not be elevated early in the course of disease. A fourfold rise is typically seen during the course of illness. A single tularemia antibody titer of 1:160 or greater is supportive of the diagnosis [55,56,65]. The combined use of ELISA and confirmatory Western blot analysis was found to be the most suitable approach to the serological diagnosis of tularemia [67,68]. Other diagnostic methods include antigen detection assays and PCR [68–70]. A multitarget real-time TaqMan PCR assay (Applied Biosystems, Foster City, CA) has been reported to have high sensitivity and specificity for the diagnosis of tularemia and may be a valuable tool for the analysis of clinical specimens and field samples following a bioterrorism attack [71].

Treatment

The antibiotic of choice for the treatment of tularemia is streptomycin, 1 g, given intramuscularly (IM) twice daily. Gentamicin, 5 mg per kg, given IM or intravenously (IV) once daily, can be used instead of streptomycin. For children, the preferred antibiotics are streptomycin, 15 mg per kg, given IM twice daily (not to exceed 2 g per day) or gentamicin, 2.5 mg per kg, given IM or IV thrice daily. Alternate choices for adults are doxycycline, 100 mg, given IV twice daily; chloramphenicol, 15 mg per kg, given IV four times daily; or ciprofloxacin, 400 mg, given IV twice daily. For children, alternate choices are doxycycline, 100 mg, given IV twice daily if the child weighs 45 kg or more, and doxycycline, 2.2 mg per kg, given IV twice daily for children weighing less than 45 kg. Chloramphenicol and ciprofloxacin can also be used as alternate antibiotics in children. The ciprofloxacin dose in children should not exceed 1 g per day. Gentamicin is preferred over streptomycin for treatment during pregnancy. Chloramphenicol should not be given to pregnant patients. Treatment with streptomycin, gentamicin, or ciprofloxacin should be continued for 10 days. Treatment with doxycycline or chloramphenicol should be continued for 14 to 21 days. Patients beginning treatment with doxycycline, chloramphenicol, or ciprofloxacin can be switched to oral antibiotics when clinically appropriate. β-Lactams and macrolides are not recommended for treatment of tularemia [56,72].

In a mass casualty setting caused by tularemia, the preferred antibiotic for adults and pregnant women is doxycycline, 100 mg, taken orally twice daily, or ciprofloxacin 500 mg, taken orally twice daily. For children, the preferred choices are doxycycline, 100 mg, taken orally twice daily if the child weighs 45 kg or more; doxycycline, 2.2 mg per kg, taken orally twice daily if the child weighs less than 45 kg; or ciprofloxacin, 15 mg per kg, taken orally twice daily and not to exceed 1 g per day. It is recommended that therapy be continued for 3 to 14 days. In immunosuppressed patients, either streptomycin or gentamicin is the preferred antibiotic in mass casualty situations [56,57].

Prophylaxis

Individuals exposed to *F. tularensis* may be protected against systemic infection if they receive prophylactic antibiotics during the incubation period. For postexposure prophylaxis, either doxycycline, 100 mg, taken orally twice daily, or ciprofloxacin, 500 mg, taken orally twice daily for 14 days, is recommended. Both doxycycline and ciprofloxacin can be taken by pregnant women for postexposure prophylaxis, but ciprofloxacin is preferred. Postexposure prophylaxis for children is the same as treatment during mass casualty situations [56,57].

Immunization

In Russia, a live attenuated vaccine has been used to offer protection to those living in tularemia-endemic areas. In the United States, a live attenuated vaccine has been given to laboratory personnel working with *F. tularensis*. The currently available vaccine does not offer total protection against inhalational exposure to *F. tularensis*. Therefore, vaccination is not recommended for postexposure prophylaxis. The intranasal administration of an attenuated live vaccine has been shown to provide protection against intranasal infection with *F. tularensis* biovar A in mice. The use of such a vaccine in humans requires further investigation [55,56,73,74].

PLAGUE

Plague is a zoonotic infection, primarily seen in rodents and rabbits. Humans are infected as an accidental host. Historically, three pandemics with bubonic plague occurred in the sixth, fourteenth, and nineteenth centuries, killing millions of people in Europe, Africa, and Central and Southern Asia. The fourteenth century pandemic became known as the "Black Death." This pandemic reportedly took the lives of more than 40 million people [75]. In recent years, the highly contagious nature of plague has raised concern about its possible use as an agent of bioterrorism.

Microbiology

Plague is caused by *Yersinia pestis*, a Gram-negative, nonmotile coccobacillus of the family *Enterobacteriaceae*. *Yersinia pestis* has a bipolar staining pattern with Wright–Giemsa or Wayson stain that gives a "safety pin" appearance to the stained organism (Fig. 213.3). From recent genetic studies of *Yersinia pestis*, it appears that there are three biovars and that the original organism has undergone chromosomal rearrangements over the years, leading to new ribotypes of the biovars. Three plasmids of *Yersinia pestis* have been identified as the source of virulence factors. Virulence factors include plasminogen activator, lipopolysaccharide endotoxin, V antigen, F1 antigen, and W antigen. These virulence factors confer antiphagocytic activity, cytotoxicity, and facilitate use of host nutrients to escape other host defense mechanisms [76–81]. The lipopolysaccharide endotoxin is responsible for the systemic inflammatory response, acute respiratory distress syndrome, and multiorgan failure [77,82].

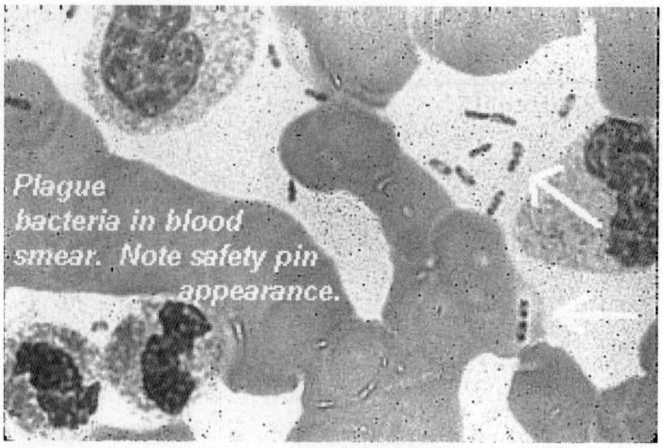

FIGURE 213.3. Wright–Giemsa stain of *Yersinia pestis* showing the characteristic bipolar staining pattern that gives a "safety pin" appearance to the organism. [From the CDC Web site: http://www.cdc.gov/ncidod/dvbid/plague/p1.htm.]

Plague is naturally transmitted by the bite of a plague-infected flea. Rodents, particularly rats and squirrels, are the natural reservoirs that transmit *Yersinia pestis* to fleas. After ingestion of blood from an infected animal, bacteria multiply in the digestive tract of the flea. Hundreds of bacteria are then regurgitated into the next animal or human victim of the plague-infected flea. Plague can be transmitted by all species of fleas; protection against fleabites is an important preventive measure in endemic areas and during epidemics. In the United States, the most common vector for the transmission of plague to humans is the *Diamanus montanus* flea. The most important reservoirs in the United States include ground squirrels, rock squirrels, and the prairie dog. Transmission to humans also occurs by direct contact with infected live or dead animals, inhalation of respiratory droplets from patients with pneumonic plague, or from direct contact with infected body fluids or tissue [76–78,82,83].

Plague as a Bioweapon

The use of plague as an intentional agent of warfare first occurred in 1346 with the Tartars catapulting the plague-infected corpses of their troops to the Christian Genoese troops during the siege of Kaffa. Since that time, plague has been used by the military forces of Russia against Sweden, and Japan against China. The biowarfare program of United States had plague in its arsenal before destroying biological weapons in the early 1970s. The CDC has classified plague as a Category A threat agent. Aerosolized droplets of *Yersinia pestis* could be used as a biowarfare agent, resulting in the highly fatal pneumonic form of plague [76,77,84]. Plague is contagious from person to person and can result in a greater number of casualties than those initially exposed and infected. The WHO estimates that 50 kg of *Yersinia pestis* aerosolized over a population of 5 million people may result in 150,000 infections and 36,000 deaths [53]. Intentional dispersion of *Yersinia pestis* as an aerosol will lead to pneumonic plague, while the release of infected fleas will usually result in bubonic or septicemic plague [53,76,77,84].

Epidemiology

Plague has been reported worldwide, with most human cases occurring in the developing countries of Africa and Asia. The WHO reports global occurrence of 1,000 to 3,000 cases per year. More than 90% of plague cases reported in the United States come from the states of Arizona, New Mexico, California, and Colorado, with rare cases from Texas. The majority of cases occur in spring and summer, when people come in contact with rodents and fleas while outdoors. In endemic areas of the United States, there is a higher incidence of plague among Native Americans compared to non-Native Americans [76,77,85–88]. In Uganda, 127 clinical cases of plague (88% bubonic, 12% pneumonic) were identified in 2006. Of these, 28 patients (22%) died and 11 of these had pneumonic plague. In one family, four members died of pneumonic plague [89]. Two small outbreaks of oropharyngeal plague were reported from the Middle East from the eating of raw camel liver and meat [90,91]. The WHO reported an outbreak of plague in the Democratic Republic of the Congo, consisting of 130 cases of pneumonic plague, 61 of which were fatal [92]. Smaller outbreaks of plague continue to occur throughout the world [93]. Recent studies have suggested that the Black Death pandemic probably led to mutations in the chemokine receptor CCR5. These mutations may confer immunity to certain individuals against plague and other infections, such as HIV-1 [94].

Pathogenesis

The common forms of naturally acquired human plague are *bubonic, septicemic*, and *primary pneumonic* forms. The bubonic and septicemic forms are the most common presentations. After entering the body through a fleabite, bacteria migrate via cutaneous lymphatics to the regional lymph nodes and are subjected to phagocytosis. If not killed by host defense systems, the bacteria proliferate within the macrophages with the aid of fraction I, an envelope antigen of *Yersinia pestis*. Other virulence factors secreted by the bacteria facilitate extracellular spread and resistance to destruction. The initial infection in lymph nodes causes lymphadenitis and local swelling that is referred to as the "bubo"; hence, the name "bubonic plague." Most buboes develop in the groin, axilla, or neck. Virulence factors perpetuate the progression of disease, leading to septicemia and the infection of other organs. Endotoxins released by *Yersinia pestis* result in the septic state and increased resistance to host defenses [76–82].

Inhalation of infected droplets of *Yersinia pestis* results in primary pneumonic plague. The primary pneumonic form is rapid in onset with an incubation period of 1 to 6 days (mean, 2 to 4 days). Presenting features are fevers, chills, cough, and blood-tinged sputum. Following inhalation into the lungs, *Yersinia pestis* organisms are engulfed by macrophages and transported to the lymphatic system and regional lymph nodes. This is followed by transient bacteremia that results in the seeding of other organs such as the spleen, liver, skin, and mucous membranes. Secondary pneumonic plague occurs as sequelae of bubonic or primary septicemic plague. Primary septicemic plague occurs when there is direct entry of *Yersinia pestis* bacilli into the bloodstream. The early recognition of primary septicemic plague is difficult because it resembles other febrile illnesses with septicemia. Other rare forms of plague are *plague meningitis* and *plague pharyngitis*. Plague meningitis occurs following the hematogenous spread of *Yersinia pestis* bacilli to the meninges. Plague pharyngitis may occur following the ingestion or inhalation of *Yersinia pestis* bacilli. Both plague meningitis and plague pharyngitis cause cervical lymphadenitis [76,78].

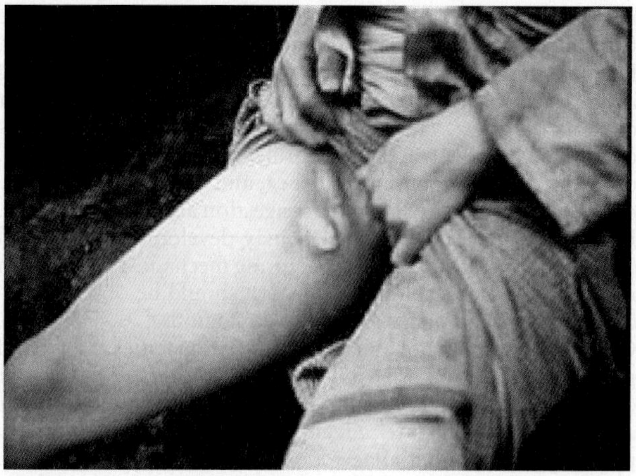

FIGURE 213.4. Bubonic plague with the characteristic bubo. [From CDC Web site: http://www.cdc.gov/ncidod/dvbid/plague/diagnosis.]

Clinical Presentation

The incubation period and clinical manifestations of plague vary according to mode of transmission. Of the plague cases seen in the United States, 85% are bubonic plague, 10% to 15% are primary septicemic plague, and less than 1% are primary pneumonic plague. Bubonic plague may progress to septicemic or pneumonic plague in 23% and 9% of cases, respectively. The clinical presentation of plague in children is similar to that of adults. There are little data regarding unique manifestations of plague in pregnant women [76,77,82,89,95,96].

Bubonic Plague

Following the bite of an infected flea, fever, chills, and headache will develop in 1 to 8 days. Nausea, vomiting, malaise, altered mentation, cough, abdominal pain, and chest pain may also be present. Patients then develop lymphadenitis, buboes (Fig. 213.4), and severe pain. Based on site of inoculation, palpable, regional buboes appear in the groin, axillae, or cervical regions, with erythema of the overlying skin. These enlarged lymph nodes are necrotic and contain dense concentrations of *Yersinia pestis* bacilli [76,77,95].

Septicemic Plague

A minority of patients exposed to *Yersinia pestis* develop septicemic plague, either as a primary form (without buboes) or secondary to the hematogenous spread of bubonic or primary pneumonic plague. The clinical features are similar to those of Gram-negative sepsis, with fever, chills, nausea, vomiting, and hypotension. Abdominal pain from hepatosplenomegaly, acral cyanosis, disseminated intravascular coagulation, and purpura has been reported. Severe anxiety and confusion may occur. Endotoxin released from *Yersinia pestis* may produce severe hypotension, oliguria, anuria, and acute respiratory distress syndrome. Gangrenous changes of the fingers, toes, and nose may occur. As a result of these manifestations, septicemic plague has been called the Black Death. Without treatment, the mortality rate of septicemic plague is 100% [75–77,87–89].

Pneumonic Plague

Primary pneumonic plague occurs by inhaling respiratory droplets from infected humans or animals and is characterized by a severe, rapidly progressive pneumonia with septicemic features that is rapidly fatal if not treated within 24 hours. Plague is highly contagious by the airborne route. Following an incubation period of 1 to 6 days, there is a rapid onset of fever, dyspnea, chest pain, and cough that may be productive of bloody, watery, or purulent sputum. Tachycardia, cyanosis, nausea, vomiting, diarrhea, and abdominal pain may occur. Intra-alveolar edema and congestion are commonly seen. Buboes are generally absent, but may develop in the cervical area. Acute respiratory failure requiring mechanical ventilation may occur. Strict respiratory isolation should be observed because pneumonic plague is highly contagious [76,77,97–99]. Chest radiographs show bilateral alveolar opacities (89%) and pleural effusions (55%). Cavitations may occur [98]. Alveolar opacities in secondary pneumonic plague may have a nodular appearance. Mediastinal adenopathy is very rare in primary pneumonic plague but hilar node enlargement is often present. This can help to distinguish primary pneumonic plague from anthrax if bioterrorism is suspected and a causative agent has not been identified [100,101]. Without prompt treatment, the mortality rate of primary pneumonic plague is 100% [75].

Secondary pneumonic plague occurs in approximately 12% of individuals with bubonic plague or primary septicemic plague. It develops as a result of the hematogenous spread of *Yersinia pestis* bacilli to the lungs. It typically presents as a severe bronchopneumonia. Common symptoms include cough, dyspnea, chest pain, and hemoptysis. Chest radiographs typically show bilateral, patchy alveolar infiltrates that may progress to consolidation. In contrast to primary pneumonic plague, mediastinal, cervical, and hilar adenopathy may occur [76,100,101]. A chest radiograph from a patient with secondary pneumonic plague is shown in Figure 213.5.

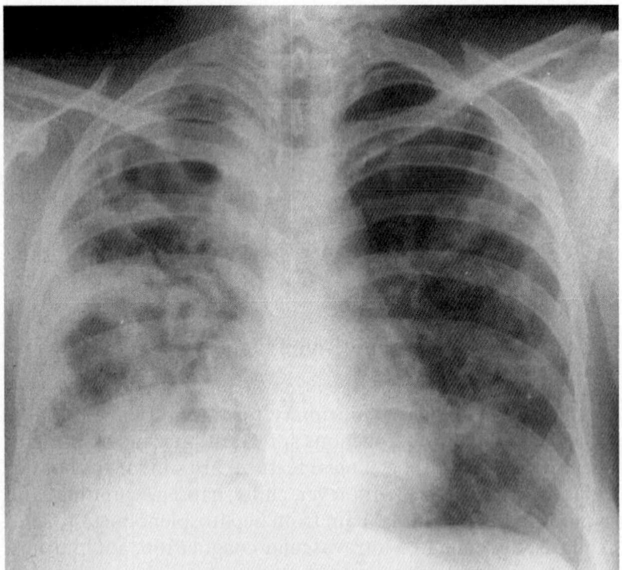

FIGURE 213.5. A 38-year-old man from Himachal Pradesh was admitted with complaints of fever, cough, hemoptysis, and dyspnea. There is endemicity of pneumonic plague where the patient came from due to the prevalent custom of hunting wild rats and rodents. Sputum examination was positive for *Yersinia pestis*. The patient was successfully treated with antibiotics. [Chest radiograph courtesy of Sanjay Jain, MD, Department of Internal Medicine, and Surinder K. Jindal, MD, Professor of Medicine, Postgraduate Institute of Medical Education and Research, Chandigarh, India.]

Diagnosis

The diagnosis of septicemic and pneumonic plague is challenging when buboes are not present. A high index of suspicion is critical in making an early diagnosis so that appropriate therapy can be started as soon as possible. The presence of Gram-negative rods in bloody sputum of an immunocompetent host should suggest pneumonic plague. In the event of multiple, simultaneous cases of rapidly progressive pneumonia, pneumonic plague should be considered in the differential diagnosis. For suspected bubonic plague, the differential diagnosis includes tularemia, cat scratch disease, suppurative adenitis, scrub typhus, tuberculosis, chancroid, and lymphogranuloma venereum [76,77].

Laboratory Diagnosis

A mild-to-moderate leukocytosis with neutrophil predominance and toxic granulations are seen in all forms of plague. In severe cases, elevated transaminases, azotemia, and coagulopathy with disseminated intravascular coagulation are often seen. The sputum is usually purulent, often blood-tinged, and contains *Yersinia pestis* bacilli. A Gram's stain of sputum, blood, or lymph node aspirate may show Gram-negative coccobacilli. Identification of the organism may be difficult by Gram's stain alone because an improperly decolorized specimen can cause *Yersinia pestis* to resemble a Gram-positive diplococcus as a result of its bipolarity. Microscopic examination of a sputum specimen prepared with Wright–Giemsa stain will show the characteristic bipolar staining pattern more clearly (Fig. 213.3). Cultures may be positive for *Yersinia pestis* within 24 to 48 hours. Misidentification of *Yersinia pestis* may occur with automated bacterial identification devices [76,77]. Rapid diagnostic tests such as immunoglobulin-M immunoassay, direct fluorescent antibody testing, and PCR are available in certain laboratories. Direct fluorescent antibody staining for *Yersinia pestis* (Fig. 213.6) and dipstick antigen detection tests are highly specific and are available at some centers [76,77,102–105]. A rapid diagnostic test using monoclonal antibodies to the F1 antigen has recently been field-tested in Madagascar and was shown to be comparable in specificity and sensitivity to detection by ELISA in both bubonic and pneumonic plague. This rapid diagnostic test shows promise for the early on-site diagnosis of

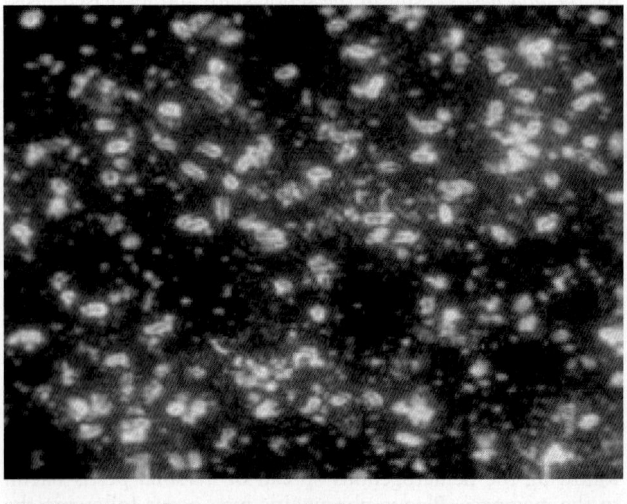

FIGURE 213.6. Fluorescence antibody positivity for *Yersinia pestis* is seen as bright, intense green staining around the bacterial cell. [From CDC Web site: http://www.cdc.gov/ncidod/dvbid/plague/bacterium.htm.]

plague [103]. Additional tests for detection and confirmation that are available through the Laboratory Response Network include PCR assays, molecular-based subtyping, and immunohistochemistry on formalin-fixed tissues [77].

The CDC recommends that plague should be suspected in persons with symptoms of fever and lymphadenopathy if they reside in, or have recently traveled to, a plague-endemic area and if Gram-negative and/or bipolar-staining coccobacilli are seen on a smear taken from affected tissues or other specimens. The diagnosis of plague should be presumed if immunofluorescence staining of smear or material is positive for the presence of *Yersinia pestis* F1 antigen and/or a single serum specimen shows the anti-F1 antigen in a titer of greater than 1:10 by agglutination. In order to confirm the diagnosis of plague, the CDC recommends that one or more of the following criteria be met: isolation of *Yersinia pestis* from a clinical specimen, a single *Yersinia pestis* antibody titer of more than 1:128 dilution, or a fourfold rise in paired sera antibody titer to *Yersinia pestis* F1 antigen. Antibody susceptibility testing should be done at a reference laboratory because there are no standardized procedures for such testing [76,77,105]. Plague as a bioterrorism agent should be suspected when multiple cases of severe and rapidly progressive pneumonic plague cases are seen with fulminant systemic symptoms and hemoptysis.

Treatment

Traditionally, streptomycin or gentamicin has been the mainstay of therapy for *Yersinia pestis*. Other acceptable antibiotics are ciprofloxacin, tetracycline, doxycycline, and chloramphenicol [75–77,82,83,106–109]. The recommendations of the Working Group on Civilian Biodefense for treatment of adult patients with plague in a small, contained casualty setting is streptomycin 1 g IM, given twice daily; gentamicin, 5 mg per kg IM or IV, once daily; or a 2 mg per kg loading dose of gentamicin followed by 1.7 mg per kg IM or IV thrice daily. The dosing of aminoglycosides must include adjustment for renal function. Alternate choices include doxycycline, 100 mg IV, given twice daily or 200 mg IV given once daily; ciprofloxacin, 400 mg IV, given twice daily; or chloramphenicol, 25 mg per kg IV, given four times daily. For pregnant women with plague, the treatment of choice is adult dosing with gentamicin, as described previously. Alternative choices for pregnant women include ciprofloxacin or doxycycline with dosing similar to that of other adults. It should be noted that doxycycline is relatively contraindicated in pregnancy and should only be given to pregnant women if other antibiotics are unavailable or contraindicate. For children, the preferred antibiotics are streptomycin, 15 mg per kg IM, given twice daily (maximum dose of 2 g per day), or gentamicin, 2.5 mg per kg IM or IV, given thrice daily. Alternate antibiotics for children include doxycycline at the adult dose if the child weighs more than 45 kg; doxycycline, 2.2 mg per kg IV, given twice daily if the child weighs under 45 kg; ciprofloxacin, 15 mg per kg IV, given twice daily; or chloramphenicol, 25 mg per kg IV, given four times daily. The duration of treatment is 10 days. For breastfeeding mothers and infants, treatment with gentamicin is recommended. Alternate therapy with fluoroquinolones can be used in either setting. The treatment of immunosuppressed individuals is similar to that of immunocompetent individuals [76,77].

Mass Casualty Treatment and Prophylaxis

In a mass casualty situation from the intentional release of plague, the urgency to initiate prompt treatment of infected individuals, as well as prophylaxis for those exposed but uninfected, may cause a significant stress on healthcare capabilities. The ability to administer parenteral streptomycin or gentamicin will be limited. The Working Group on Civilian Biodefense recommends the use of ciprofloxacin, 500 mg, taken orally twice daily or doxycycline, 100 mg, taken orally twice daily for adults and pregnant women, both for treatment and postexposure prophylaxis. The alternate choice is chloramphenicol, 25 mg per kg, taken orally four times daily. For children, the preferred choices are the adult dose of doxycycline if the child weighs more than 45 kg and 2.2 mg per kg orally twice daily for child weighing less than 45 kg. Children may also be given ciprofloxacin, 20 mg per kg, orally twice daily, or chloramphenicol, 25 mg per kg, orally four times daily. For breastfeeding mothers and infants, treatment with doxycycline is recommended. The duration of treatment is 7 days. All individuals who come within 2 m of a patient with pneumonic plague should receive postexposure prophylaxis. These recommendations are consensus-based for treating plague following an intentional release or bioterrorism attack and may not reflect the FDA-approved use or indications [76,77].

Immunization

Vaccination with a killed, whole-cell vaccine against plague was available in the United States until 1999 for those at high risk for exposure, such as military personnel, those working in endemic areas, and laboratory personnel working with *Yersinia pestis*. The vaccine was not effective against pneumonic plague, and adequate protection in a biowarfare setting is doubtful. Several studies of newer vaccines against plague are ongoing. Vaccines using F1 capsular antigen of doxycycline, 100 mg, taken orally twice daily *pestis* and monoclonal antibodies specific to the F1 and V antigens have shown promising results against pneumonic plague in animal models. Phase I studies with recombinant F1 and V antigens are underway. However, there is no approved vaccine for use against plague available in the United States at the present time [77,110–112].

Infection Control

Patients suspected of plague should be isolated and antibiotic therapy should be instituted promptly. Universal exposure precautions, respiratory isolation using CDC droplet precautions, and special handling of blood and discharge from buboes must be followed. In cases of pneumonic plague, strictly enforced respiratory isolation in addition to the use of masks, gloves, gowns, and eye protection must be continued for the first few days of antibiotic therapy. Following 2 to 4 days of therapy with appropriate antibiotics, patients with both nonpneumonic plague and pneumonic plague may be removed from isolation [113–115]. Laboratory workers should be warned of potential plague infection because cases of laboratory-acquired plague have been reported [98].

Preventive Measures

For naturally occurring cases, the primary preventive measure for plague is rodent and flea control. In endemic areas, the use of insect repellant, the wearing of gloves while handling wild animals, and avoiding rodent burrows will reduce exposure to *Yersinia pestis* [113,114].

BOTULINUM TOXIN

Botulinum is an extremely potent toxin produced by *Clostridium botulinum*, an anaerobic, spore-forming bacterium that is present in the soil. Unlike botulinum toxin that is inactivated by temperatures above 85°C for 5 minutes, *Clostridium* spores can survive temperatures of 105°C for up to 4 hours, but are readily destroyed by chlorine. Spores may remain viable for over 30 years in a dry state and are resistant to ultraviolet light exposure [116,117]. The botulinum toxin produced by *Clostridium botulinum* is the most poisonous substance known. It can cause a serious, life-threatening paralytic illness in exposed individuals, is easily produced in a laboratory, and can be easily transported. In view of these properties, botulinum toxin has been identified as a major bioterrorism threat [116,118]. It has been designated as a Category A bioterrorism threat by the CDC [10]. There are reports that several countries may have stockpiled or are developing botulinum toxin for use as a bioweapon [116,118]. The general features and management of botulism are presented in Chapters 88 and 175, but the implications of botulism as a bioterrorist weapon are discussed here.

Botulinum Toxin as an Agent of Bioterrorism

There are three forms of naturally occurring botulism: *Foodborne botulism, wound botulism*, and *intestinal (infant and adult) botulism*. All forms of botulism can produce a serious paralytic illness that can lead to respiratory failure and death.

Botulinum toxin solution is a colorless, odorless, tasteless liquid that is easily inactivated by heating at a temperature greater than 85°C for 5 minutes. There are seven different antigenic types that are named botulinum A, B, C, D, E, F, and G. Given its extreme potency, botulinum toxin can produce devastating effects and mass casualties if intentionally dispersed by aerosol or used to contaminate the water supply. One gram of botulinum toxin has the capacity to kill more than 1 million persons if aerosolized [117,118]. Botulinum toxin types A, B, E, and F have been associated with naturally occurring foodborne botulism. Types C and D botulinum toxin cause natural disease in birds and cattle. Type G botulinum toxin is found in South America, but it has not been associated with foodborne botulism. Inhalational challenge studies with aerosolized botulinum toxin in monkeys have demonstrated the development of illness following exposure to types C, D, and G. Researchers suspect that humans are also susceptible to these types [118–120].

The intentional use of botulinum toxin can be either inhalational or foodborne. In the 1930s, the Japanese reportedly executed a number of Manchurian prisoners by feeding them cultures of *Clostridium botulinum*. During World War II, there was concern that Germany had weaponized botulinum toxin for use as a biowarfare agent. This led to the production of more than 1 million doses of botulinum toxoid vaccine for allied forces in Europe, but the vaccine was never given. Botulinum toxin was produced by the United States for use as a bioweapon from World War II to the early 1970s when the bioweapon program was terminated. Following the 1972 Convention on the Prohibition of the Development and Stockpiling of Biological and Toxin Weapons, both the former Soviet Union and Iraq continued to develop botulinum toxin as a biowarfare agent. After the 1991 Persian Gulf War, Iraq admitted to U.N. weapons inspectors that it had produced and stockpiled biological weapons containing botulinum toxin. It has been reported that several countries may continue to produce or stockpile botulinum toxin for use as a bioweapon [118].

At the present time, there is considerable concern about the potential use of botulinum toxin as an agent of bioterrorism. Contamination of either a food or a beverage source that can retain the potency of botulinum toxin can result in mass casualties, serious illness among affected individuals, the overwhelming of hospitals, enormous stress on intensive care units, and significant anxiety among the general population [117,118]. It has been estimated that 1 g of botulinum toxin added to milk that is commercially distributed and consumed by 568,000 individuals can result in 100,000 cases of botulism [121]. It has also been estimated that 1 g of aerosolized botulinum toxin could potentially kill more than 1 million people [118]. The dispersion of aerosolized botulinum toxin in the unsuccessful terrorist attacks in Japan during the early 1990s suggests that botulinum toxin could be used in future bioterrorism attacks.

Pathogenesis

Following exposure by inhalation or ingestion, the toxin is activated, enters the circulation, and the heavy chain of the toxin gets bound to the neuronal membrane on the presynaptic side of the neuromuscular junction. The toxin then enters the neuronal cell, after which the light chain of the toxin cleaves the synaptic proteins that form the synaptic fusion complex. Disruption of the synaptic fusion complex prevents release of acetylcholine release into the synaptic cleft. Without acetylcholine, the affected muscle becomes paralyzed. Muscle paralysis can last for several months. Death from botulism is caused by failure of the respiratory muscles to contract. The central nervous system is unaffected as botulism toxin does not cross the blood–brain barrier. A prospective, observational cohort study of 91 botulism patients in Thailand showed that those individuals presenting with dyspnea, moderate-to-severe ptosis, and papillary changes were likely to progress to respiratory failure, while a long incubation period before symptoms appeared was associated with a more favorable prognosis [122].

Treatment

The treatment of botulism includes supportive care, mechanical ventilation if necessary, and the administration of botulinum antitoxin. In an outbreak following an intentional release, the healthcare demands may overwhelm current capabilities, especially with regard to the availability of mechanical ventilators and critical care providers. At present, there is an ongoing U.S. government effort to stockpile mechanical ventilators that can be deployed in the event of a mass casualty.

Rega et al. suggest an algorithm to assess the severity of botulism cases that may be helpful in mass casualty situations [123]. Specific therapy for botulism involves the administration of botulinum antitoxin. Early suspicion of botulism and the prompt administration of botulinum antitoxin can reduce nerve damage and disease severity. However, any muscle paralysis existing prior to antitoxin administration will not be reversed. The goal of antitoxin therapy is to prevent further paralysis by neutralizing unbound botulinum toxin in the circulation. If the type of botulinum toxin is known, a type-specific antitoxin can be given. If the toxin type is not known, the trivalent antitoxin containing neutralizing antibodies against botulinum toxin types A, B, and E should be given. Botulinum antitoxin is available from the CDC through state and local health departments. If another type of toxin is intentionally dispersed during a bioterrorism attack, consideration may be given for the use of an investigational heptavalent antitoxin (ABCDEFG) that is in the possession of the U.S. Army. Physicians should review the package insert prior to administering the antitoxin to familiarize themselves with the dose, dilution, and mode of administration. A new heptavalent botulinum antitoxin (HBAT) approved by the FDA replaced the former botulinum antitoxin in 2010. This heptavalent antitoxin contains equine-derived antibody to all the seven botulinum toxins from A to G. If a case of botulism is suspected, prompt diagnosis is essential. If botulism is confirmed, the CDC will provide the new heptavalent antitoxin and detailed instructions for its intravenous administration [124]. Additional doses of botulinum antitoxin will be needed if multiple cases of botulism occur after an intentional release. Following the initial administration of botulinum antitoxin, patients should be carefully assessed for refractory problems, such as rapidly progressing paralysis, severe airway obstruction, or overwhelming respiratory tract secretions, which may indicate the need for an additional dose. Hypersensitivity reactions to botulinum antitoxin may occur. These include anaphylaxis, serum sickness, chills, fever, dyspnea, cutaneous erythema, and edema of the tongue. The incidence of hypersensitivity with the recommended one-vial dose is about 1%. A small dose can be given initially to screen for hypersensitivity, but this would be impractical in a mass casualty situation [116–118,125–127].

Prophylaxis

In the United States, a pentavalent botulinum toxoid is available from the CDC for the immunization of laboratory workers who may be exposed to botulinum toxin and for the protection of military personnel in the event of a biowarfare attack. It may be obtained on an investigational basis for others at high risk for botulinum toxin exposure. Botulinum toxoid, 0.5 mL, is given subcutaneously at 0, 2, and 12 weeks, followed by a booster dose at 1 year. Adequate immunity against botulinum toxin is assessed by measuring antitoxin titers. In one study, an adequate response was noted in 91% of those immunized against toxin A and 78% of those immunized against toxin B. In an animal study, the intranasal administration of botulinum toxin in mice, with and without prechallenge immunization with pentavalent toxoid, showed intra-alveolar hemorrhage and interstitial edema in both groups, but the immunized mice were protected from lethality and nervous system changes in comparison to nonimmunized mice [128].

Mass immunization of the public with botulinum toxoid is not recommended and is not currently available. It takes several months to attain acquired immunity following the administration of botulinum toxoid and, therefore, it is not effective for postexposure prophylaxis. Recent evidence suggests that a recombinant oligoclonal antibody may have efficacy in preventing and treating botulism. Animal studies have shown promise for using the heavy chain of the botulinum toxin molecule as an inhalational agent for the treatment of botulism [116–118,125,128].

RICIN

Ricin is a potent toxin that belongs to the broad family of ribosome-inhibiting proteins and is easily extracted from seeds contained in the bean of the castor plant, *Ricinis communis*. "Ricinus" is the Latin word for tick and the plant was given this name for the resemblance of castor bean seeds to engorged ticks [129]. The castor plant, a native plant of Africa, is a common outdoor plant in warm climates and is also used for ornamental purposes. Castor bean seeds, castor oil, and the castor plant itself have been used for many centuries for their medicinal (laxative and purgative), lubricant, and decorative properties. Castor bean seeds contain high concentrations of ricin. Ingestion of as few as three seeds can be fatal. Ricin is an immunotoxin, allergen, and toxic enzyme that inhibits protein synthesis. As a result of its biochemical properties, ricin has antitumor effects and has undergone phase I and phase II clinical trials as a chemotherapeutic agent. Ricin can be inactivated by heating to 175°F for 10 minutes. It can be produced in liquid, crystalline, or dry powder forms. Both the liquid and powder forms have the potential to be aerosolized [130,131].

Toxicology

Ricin is an enzyme consisting of two sulfide-linked polypeptide chains, A and B. The A-chain enters the cytosol of a cell, inactivates the 28S ribosomal subunits, inhibits protein synthesis, and causes cell death. The B-chain binds to the cell surface at galactose-containing sites and facilitates entry of the A-chain into the cell [132,133]. Most of the data regarding the toxicity of ricin come from animal experiments. Both the toxicity and the lethality of ricin depend on the exposure dose and the route of administration. In experiments using mice, the LD_{50} and time of death are 3 to 5 μg per kg and 60 hours by inhalation, 5 μg per kg and 90 hours by intravenous injection, and 20 mg per kg and 85 hours by intragastric administration. The lethal doses of ricin in humans have been calculated to be approximately 5 to 10 μg per kg by inhalation and 1 to 10 μg per kg by injection [134–137]. On exposure to lethal doses of ricin by inhalation, rats develop a necrotizing tracheobronchitis and pneumonia with parenchymal inflammation and pulmonary edema. These pathologic changes lead to alveolar flooding and hypoxemia. Immunohistochemical stains show that ricin binds to bronchiolar cells, macrophages, and alveolar lining cells. In nonhuman primates, inhalation of ricin leads to death within 48 hours of exposure, and autopsy shows diffuse necrosis of airways, severe pulmonary edema, severe fibrinopurulent pneumonia, and mediastinal lymphadenitis [135]. Animal data show that the Kupffer cells are the primary targets of ricin-induced injury to the liver [134]. Ricin toxicity is not contagious to other individuals.

Ricin as an Agent of Bioterrorism

The high toxicity, relative ease of production, ease of dissemination, and stability of ricin in ambient conditions make it a potential agent of bioterrorism. Ricin can be dispersed as an aerosol or as a contaminant of food and beverages for the purpose of causing multiple casualties. Most experts agree that it would be logistically difficult to use ricin for the production of large-scale mass casualties because it would take a very large amount to do so [138]. However, ricin may be an ideal agent for small-scale bioterrorism attacks against high-value targets. Dozens of people could be killed in such attacks and the psychological impact on a community could be enormous.

There have been several reports of the use or intended use of ricin in terrorist activities. In 1978, a Bulgarian diplomat, Georgi Markov, was killed in London by a ricin-containing pellet fired from an umbrella-based weapon [139,140]. In January 2003, British authorities arrested 10 individuals from North Africa who were residing in a London apartment where ricin was found [140]. In October 2003, ricin was identified in an envelope at a Greenville, South Carolina, post office [140–142]. In November 2003, an envelope addressed to the White House was reportedly intercepted by the Secret Service and was found to contain ricin [140]. In February 2004, ricin was reportedly detected in the Dirksen Senate Office Building [140]. These events highlight the need for critical care providers to be familiar with the recognition and management of ricin poisoning.

Ricin Toxicity in Humans

The pathologic changes and clinical symptoms caused by ricin exposure depend on the exposure dose and the route of exposure. The clinical effects of ricin in humans have been described following cases of castor seed ingestion and parenteral use in chemotherapeutic clinical trials. There are limited clinical data regarding ricin toxicity via inhalational route in humans. The clinical findings observed in animal models after the oral or parenteral administration of ricin appear to correlate with the clinical findings of humans exposed to oral or parenteral ricin. Therefore, the findings from animals following inhalational exposure are presumed to be similar to those that would be experienced by humans following ricin inhalation. Leukocytosis appears to be a constant finding, regardless of the route of exposure. Ricin toxicity by any route of exposure can produce hallucinations and seizures.

Gastrointestinal Route

The ingestion of castor seeds can cause human illness that ranges from mild to severe, based on the amount of ricin ingested. Compared to other routes of ricin exposure, the gastrointestinal route is the least toxic. A review of 751 cases of castor seed ingestion reported symptoms consisting of nausea, vomiting, and abdominal cramping within a few hours after ingestion, followed by diarrhea that may become bloody and lead to both dehydration and volume depletion. Patients developed hypotension, severe fluid and electrolyte loss, tachypnea, tachycardia, and sweating. There were case fatality rates of 8.1% for untreated individuals and 0.4% for treated individuals. Death occurred approximately 72 hours after exposure. In addition, sore throat, dilation of the pupils, altered mental status, hallucinations, and seizures were noted in some patients. On autopsy, hepatic necrosis, renal necrosis, necrosis of the gastrointestinal mucosa with local hemorrhage, and mesenteric lymph node necrosis were found. The hepatic and renal damage may be secondary to vascular collapse rather than the result of direct toxin injury [131,143–146].

Parenteral Route

In cases of ricin toxicity produced by parenteral administration, pain at the site of injection, fatigue, malaise, headache, rigors, and fever were noted in the first 24 hours. Patients also showed local necrotic lymphadenopathy. Ricin, when used as a chemotherapeutic agent at a dose of 18 to 20 μg per kg, caused nausea, vomiting, myalgia, and fatigue [131]. More serious adverse effects may include pulmonary edema, hypoalbuminemia, cardiac failure, hypotension, hypovolemic shock, acute hepatorenal failure, gastrointestinal bleeding, thrombocytopenia, and bleeding diathesis [131–133,143,147–149].

Inhalational Route

Patients with inhalational exposure of ricin may develop symptoms within 3 to 24 hours. The only information regarding human exposure to the inhalational form comes from exposure to castor seed dust. Reported symptoms from dust inhalation include itchy eyes, nasal and bronchial congestion, urticaria, chest tightness, and wheezing. Severe bronchospasm has been reported [131]. In an accidental exposure, ricin caused fever, chest tightness, dyspnea, cough, nausea, and arthralgias in 4 to 8 hours. These symptoms are suggestive of an allergic syndrome. Based on animal data following high-dose inhalational exposures, one may expect humans to develop cough, dyspnea, chest pain, cardiac dysfunction, cyanosis, arthralgias, airway necrosis, alveolitis, high permeability pulmonary edema, adult respiratory distress syndrome, and acute respiratory failure. The mortality rate in animals is high following ricin inhalation and usually occurs within 36 to 72 hours. It appears that ricin causes endothelial cell damage with fluid and protein leak with edema [131–133,143].

Ricin as an Allergen

Allergic responses of types I and IV have been reported following dermal exposure to castor seeds and castor seed dust. A case report describes an anaphylactic-type reaction in a woman when one of the seeds from her castor-bean necklace disintegrated in her fingers. The woman experienced rhinitis, sneezing, periorbital edema, and facial urticaria requiring a subcutaneous injection of epinephrine [150–152]. Urticaria has been reported following the inhalation of castor seed dust [150]. Although the incidence of ricin-associated allergic reactions is unknown, they may be relatively frequent among exposed individuals because of the immunogenic properties of the ricin molecule.

Diagnosis

The diagnosis of ricin toxicity is challenging. The differential diagnosis includes exposure to staphylococcal enterotoxin, phosgene, oxides of nitrogen, and organohalides. If a bioterrorism attack is suspected, anthrax, plague, and tularemia should also be considered. Ricin intoxication by the inhalational route can be confirmed by ELISA analysis of nasal mucosal swabs taken within 24 hours of exposure. Specific ricin antigen testing or immunochemical staining of serum and respiratory secretions can also be performed. Because ricin is an immunogenic toxin, a significant increase in the antiricin antibody titer 2 weeks after exposure may also be helpful in confirming the diagnosis. It is recommended that acute and convalescent antibody titers be obtained in all individuals suspected of ricin intoxication. However, antiricin antibodies are rapidly metabolized and excreted, so the absence of a significant increase in titer does not exclude the diagnosis [131,153,154].

Neutrophilic leukocytosis is usually present in peripheral blood. Pleural effusions and bilateral alveolar infiltrates, indicative of pulmonary edema, may be seen on chest radiographs. Arterial blood gases should be monitored to assess oxygenation, the adequacy of ventilation, and acid–base status. Myocardial ischemia, cardiac dysrhythmias, and cardiac conduction abnormalities may occur. Therefore, an electrocardiogram and cardiac biomarkers should be obtained. An echocardiogram may be helpful in assessing myocardial contractility if heart failure is suspected [131,155].

Treatment

The management of ricin intoxication is largely supportive, regardless of the route of exposure [130,132,133]. All patients suspected of ricin intoxication should be decontaminated by removing all clothing and washing the skin with soap and water. Careful attention to fluid and electrolyte balance is essential, especially in patients with pulmonary edema. Vasopressors may be needed for the management of severe hypotension. If ricin ingestion has occurred, gastric lavage may be helpful in removing ricin from the gastrointestinal tract. If the patient is alert, activated charcoal can be given. Blood transfusion with packed red blood cells may be needed if severe anemia is caused by bloody diarrhea. If inhalation is the route of exposure, careful airway management is essential. Bronchospasm should be treated with a nebulized bronchodilator. Patients with severe pulmonary edema will require intubation and mechanical ventilation. Oxygen should be administered at a concentration sufficient to keep the arterial oxygen tension (PaO_2) greater than 60 mm Hg. Myocardial infarction, myocardial ischemia, cardiac dysrhythmias, and cardiac conduction abnormalities should be treated as appropriate. A temporary pacemaker may be required for severe conduction abnormalities, such as complete heart block. Mild allergic reactions can be treated with an antihistamine. Epinephrine should be given for anaphylaxis. A nonsteroidal anti-inflammatory drug can be given for arthralgias and myalgias [131].

There is no specific antitoxin for ricin. Animal studies have shown that active immunization or passive prophylaxis can be effective against the parenteral or intraperitoneal administration of ricin if administered within a few hours following exposure. One animal study showed that the administration of aerosolized antiricin antibody can offer protection against the effects of ricin inhalation. The intratracheal administration of ricin toxoid led to reduction in lung inflammation in another animal study. There are no clinical trials or reports regarding the use of these agents in humans; therefore, their therapeutic efficacy in the clinical setting is unknown [130–133,146].

Most patients with ricin intoxication should survive the acute effects if appropriate supportive care is given promptly after exposure. However, because the clinical effects of ricin intoxication are dose-related, individuals exposed to high concentrations may die from cardiopulmonary arrest in spite of the best supportive care.

Immunization

Animal studies have shown that rats immunized against ricin with formalin-treated toxoids administered subcutaneously survived acute inhalation challenges with lethal doses of ricin [137,156,157]. Another animal study showed that the immunization of mice with an oral ricin-toxoid vaccine encapsulated in polymeric microspheres offered protection against inhalational exposure to ricin [158]. Several studies using a rat model have shown that antibody-mediated immunity to ricin following ricin-toxoid vaccination offered protection against lethal doses of ricin. There are also animal data that indicate that secretory antibodies are important in preventing injury to the lung after an aerosol challenge with ricin. Although ricin-toxoid vaccines have been shown to be protective in animal models, they may not be clinically useful in humans due to safety concerns. Researchers are working on the development of a vaccine against ricin that can be given to humans prior to exposure. The future use of such a vaccine in humans will depend on its safety profile and its efficacy in stimulating protective antibodies against ricin, especially in the mucosal layers of the respiratory and intestinal tracts [131,159–162].

References

1. Eitzen EM, Takafuji ET: Historical overview of biological warfare, in Sidell FR, Takafuji ET, Franz DR (eds): *Medical Aspects of Chemical and Biological Warfare*, in Zajtchuk R, Bellamy RF (eds). *Textbook of Military Medicine, Part I. Warfare, Weaponry and the Casualty*. Washington, DC, United States Department of the Army, Office of the Surgeon General and Borden Institute, 1997, p 415.
2. Report of the Center for Strategic and International Studies Homeland Defense Project: Combating chemical, biological, radiological, and nuclear terrorism: a comprehensive strategy. Center for Strategic and International Studies. December 2000. Available at: http://www.csis.org./homeland/reports/combat-chembiorad.pdf. Accessed December 29, 2005.
3. United States Commission on National Security/21st Century: Phase I report on the emerging security environment for the first quarter of the 21st century: New world coming; American security in the 21st century. September 15, 1999, pp 1–11. Available at: http://www.nssg.gov/Reports/nwc.pdf. Accessed December 29, 2005.
4. United States Commission on National Security/21st Century: Phase II report on a U.S. National Security Policy for the 21st Century: seeking a national strategy; a concept for preserving security and promoting freedom. April 15, 2000, p 1. Available at: http://www.nssg.gov/PhaseII.pdf. Accessed December 29, 2005.
5. United States Commission on National Security/21st Century: Phase III report of the U.S. Commission on National Security/21st Century: roadmap for a national security/21st century; imperative for change. February 15, 2001, p 1. Available at: http://www.nssg.gov/PhaseIIIFR.pdf. Accessed December 29, 2005.
6. Davis CJ: Nuclear blindness: an overview of the biological weapons programs of the former Soviet Union and Iraq. *Emerg Infect Dis* 5:509, 1999.
7. Bush LM, Abrams BH, Beall A, et al: Index case of fatal inhalational anthrax due to bioterrorism in the United States. *N Engl J Med* 345:1607, 2001.
8. Hughes J, Gerberding JL: Anthrax bioterrorism: lessons learned and future directions. *Emerg Infect Dis* 8:1013, 2002.
9. Rotz LD, Khan AS, Lillibridge SR, et al: Public health assessment of potential biological terrorism agents. *Emerg Infect Dis* 8:225, 2002.
10. MCFadden G: Killing a killer. *PLoS Pathog* 29:6, 2010.
11. Ambrose C: Osler and the infected letter. *Emerg Infect Dis* 11:689, 2005.
12. Grabenstein JD, Winkenwerder W: U.S. military smallpox vaccination program experience. *JAMA* 289:3278, 2003.
13. Henderson DA, Inglesby TV, Bartlett JG, et al: Smallpox as a biological weapon: medical and public health management. *JAMA* 281:2127, 1999.
14. Horgan ES, Ali HM: Cross immunity experiments in monkey between variola, alastrim and vaccinia. *J Hygiene* 39:615, 1939.
15. Noble J, Rich JA: Transmission of smallpox by contact and by aerosol routes in Macaca irus. *Bull World Health Organ* 40:279, 1969.
16. Breman JG, Henderson DA: Diagnosis and management of smallpox. *N Engl J Med* 346:1300, 2002.
17. Smallpox. Geneva, Switzerland: World Health Organization; 2006. Available at: http://www.who.int/mediacentre/factsheets/smallpox/en/print.html. Accessed January 31, 2006.
18. Center for Infectious Disease Research and Policy: Smallpox: current, comprehensive information on pathogenesis, microbiology, epidemiology, diagnosis, treatment, and prophylaxis. Minneapolis, MN, University of Minnesota; Updated February 6, 2009. Available at: http:// www.cidrap.umn.edu/cidrap/content/bt/smallpox/biofacts/smllpx-summary.html. Accessed August 31, 2009.
19. Marik PE, Bowles SA: Medical aspects of biologic and chemical agents of mass destruction, in Irwin RS, Rippe JM (eds): *Intensive Care Medicine*. 5th ed. Philadelphia, *Lippincott Williams & Wilkins*, 2003, p 823.
20. McClain DJ: Smallpox, in Sidell FR, Takafuji ET, Franz DR (eds): *Medical Aspects of Chemical and Biological Warfare*, in Zajtchuk R, Bellamy RF (eds). *Textbook of Military Medicine, Part I: Warfare, Weaponry and the Casualty*. Washington, DC, United States Department of the Army, Office of the Surgeon General and Borden Institute, 1997, p 539.
21. Bray M, Martinez M, Smee DF, et al: Cidofovir protects mice against lethal aerosol or intranasal cowpox viral challenge. *J Infect Dis* 181:10, 2000.
22. Handley L, Buller RM, Frey SE, et al: The new ACAM2000^{TM}vaccine and other therapies to control orthopoxvirus outbreaks and bioterror attacks. *Expert Rev Vaccines* 8:841, 2009.
23. Kennedy RB, Ovsyannikova IG, Jacobson RM, et al: The immunology of smallpox vaccines. *Curr Opin Immunol* 21:314, 2009.
24. Fauci A: Smallpox vaccination policy—the need for dialogue. *N Engl J Med* 346:1319, 2002.
25. Centers for Disease Control and Prevention: Recommendations for using smallpox vaccine in a pre-event vaccination program: supplemental recommendations of the Advisory Committee on Immunization Practices (ACIP) and the Healthcare Infection Control Practices Advisory Committee (HICPAC). *MMWR Morb Mortal Wkly Rep* 52(RR07):1, 2003. Available at: http://www.cdc.gov.mmwr/preview/mmwrhtml/rr5207al.htm. Accessed January 29, 2006.
26. Frey SE, Newman FK, Cruz J, et al: Dose-related effects of smallpox vaccine. *N Engl J Med* 346:1275, 2002.
27. Frey SE, Couch RB, Tacket CO, et al: Clinical responses to undiluted and diluted smallpox vaccine. *N Engl J Med* 346:1265, 2002.
28. Fulginiti VA, Papier A, Lane JM, et al: Smallpox vaccination: a review, part I. Background, vaccination technique, normal vaccination and revaccination, and expected normal reactions. *Clin Infect Dis* 37:241, 2003.
29. Greenberg RN, Schosser RH, Plummer EA, et al: Urticaria, exanthems, and other benign dermatologic reactions to smallpox vaccination in adults. *Clin Infect Dis* 38:958, 2004.
30. Mientka M: DoD Smallpox Policy Revised After Deaths. Lambertville, NJ: U.S. Medicine, 2003, p 8.
31. Butler M: CDC Advises States not to Vaccinate Heart Patients Against Smallpox. Lambertville, NJ: U.S. Medicine, 2003, p 9.
32. Casey CG, Iskander JK, Roper MH, et al: Adverse effects associated with smallpox vaccination in the United States, January–October 2003. *JAMA* 294:2734, 2005.
33. Sepkowitz KA: How contagious is vaccinia? *N Engl J Med* 348:439, 2003.
34. Washington 2010 Weekly, July 2, 2010, 59(25): p 773.
35. Bozette SA, Boer R, Bhatnagar V, et al: A model smallpox-vaccination policy. *N Engl J Med* 348:416, 2003.
36. Inglesby TV, O'Toole T, Henderson DA, et al: Anthrax as a biological weapon. *JAMA* 287:2236, 2002.
37. Center for Infectious Disease Research and Policy: Anthrax: current, comprehensive information on pathogenesis, microbiology, epidemiology, diagnosis, treatment, and prophylaxis. Minneapolis, MN, University of

Minnesota, Last updated on July 28, 2010. Available at: http://www.cidrap.umn.edu/cidrap/content/bt/anthrax/biofacts/anthraxfactsheet.html. Accessed August 20, 2010.

38. Friedlander AM: Anthrax, in Sidell FR, Takafuji ET, Franz DR (eds): *Medical Aspects of Chemical and Biological Warfare*, in Zajtchuk R, Bellamy RF (eds): *Textbook of Military Medicine, Part I: Warfare, Weaponry and the Casualty*. Washington, DC, United States Department of the Army, Office of the Surgeon General and Borden Institute, 1997, p 467.
39. Shafazand S, Doyle R, Ruoss S, et al: Inhalational anthrax: epidemiology, diagnosis and management. *Chest* 116:1369, 1999.
40. Freedman A, Afonja O, Chang MW, et al: Cutaneous anthrax associated with microangiopathic hemolytic anemia and coagulopathy in a 7-month-old infant. *JAMA* 287:869, 2002.
41. Barakat LA, Quentzel HL, Jernigan JA, et al: Fatal inhalational anthrax in a 94-year-old Connecticut woman. *JAMA* 287:863, 2002.
42. Guarner J, Jernigan JA, Shieh WJ, et al: Pathology and pathogenesis of bioterrorism-related inhalational anthrax. *Am J Pathol* 163:701, 2003.
43. Borio L, Frank D, Mani V, et al: Death due to bioterrorism-related inhalational anthrax. *JAMA* 286:2554, 2001.
44. Mayer T, Bersoff-Matcha S, Murphy C, et al: Clinical presentation of inhalational anthrax following bioterrorism exposure-report of 2 surviving patients. *JAMA* 286:2549, 2001.
45. Krol CM, Uszynski M, Dillon EH, et al: Dynamic CT features of inhalational anthrax infection. *Am J Roentgenol* 178:1063, 2002.
46. Earls JP, Cerva D, Berman E, et al: Inhalational anthrax after bioterrorism exposure: spectrum of imaging findings in two surviving patients. *Radiology* 222:305, 2002.
47. Cono J, Cragun JD, Jamieson DJ, et al: Prophylaxis and treatment of pregnant women for emerging infections and bioterrorism emergencies. *Emerg Infect Dis* 12(11):1631, 2006.
48. Holty JE, Kim RY, Bravata DM: Anthrax: a systematic review of atypical presentations. *Ann Emerg Med* 48:200, 2006.
49. Bravata, Holty JE, Wang E, Lewis R, et al: Inhalational, gastrointestinal, and cutaneous anthrax in children. A systematic review of cases: 1900–2005. *Arch Pediatr Adolesc Med* 161(9):896, 2007.
50. Friedlander AM, Pittman PR, Parker GW: Anthrax vaccine: evidence for safety and efficacy against inhalational anthrax. *JAMA* 282:2104, 1999.
51. Marano N, Plikaytis BD, Martin SW, et al: Effects of a reduced dose schedule and intramuscular administration of anthrax vaccine adsorbed on immunogenicity at 7 months. A randomized trial. *JAMA* 300(13):1532, 2008.
52. Francis E: Tularemia: a new disease of man. *JAMA* 78:1015, 1922.
53. Christopher GW, Cieslak TW, Pavlin JA, et al: Biological warfare: a historical perspective. *JAMA* 278:412, 1997.
54. World Health Organization: Health aspects of chemical and biological weapons. Geneva, Switzerland, World Health Organization, 1970. Available at: http://www.who.int/csr/delibepidemics/biochem1stenglish/en. Accessed November 22, 2005.
55. Evans ME, Friedlander AM: Tularemia, in Sidell FR, Takafuji ET, Franz DR (eds): *Medical Aspects of Chemical and Biological Warfare*, in Zajtchuk R, Bellamy RF (eds). *Textbook of Military Medicine, Part I. Warfare, Weaponry and the Casualty*. Washington, DC, United States Department of the Army, Office of the Surgeon General and Borden Institute, 1997, p 503.
56. Dennis DT, Inglesby TV, Henderson DA, et al: Tularemia as a biological weapon: medical and public health management. *JAMA* 285:2763, 2001.
57. Center for Infectious Disease Research and Policy: Tularemia: current, comprehensive information on pathogenesis, microbiology, epidemiology, diagnosis, treatment, and prophylaxis. Last updated March 16, 2010. Available at: http://www.cidrap.umn.edu/cidrap/content/bt/tularemia/biofacts/tularemiafactsheet.html. Accessed May 1, 2010.
58. Farlow J, Wagner DM, Dukerich M, et al: *Francisella tularensis* in the United States. *Emerg Infect Dis* 11:1835, 2005.
59. Sjostedt A: Tularemia: History, epidemiology, pathogen physiology, and clinical manifestations. *Ann New York Acad Sci* 1105:1, 2007.
60. Svensson K, Back E, Eliasson H, et al: Landscape epidemiology of tularemia outbreaks in Sweden. *Emerg Infect Dis* 15:1937, 2009.
61. Feldman KA, Enscore RE, Lathrop SL, et al: An outbreak of primary pneumonic tularemia on Martha's Vineyard. *N Engl J Med* 345:1601, 2001.
62. Matyas BT, Nieder HS, Telford SR: Pneumonic tularemia on Martha's Vineyard. Clinical, epidemiologic, and ecological characteristics. *Ann New York Acad Sci* 1105:351, 2007.
63. Chitadze N, Kuchuloria T, Clark DV et al: Water-borne outbreak of oropharyngeal and glandular tularemia in Georgia: investigation and follow-ups. *Infection* 37:514, 2009.
64. Metzger DW, Bakshi CS, Kirimanjeswara G: Mucosal immunopathogenesis of *Francisella tularensis*. *Ann New York Acad Sci* 1105:266, 2007.
65. Evans ME, Gregory GW, Schaffner W, et al: Tularemia: a 30-year experience with 88 cases. *Medicine* 64:251, 1985.
66. Penn RL, Kinasewitz GT: Factors associated with a poor outcome in tularemia. *Arch Intern Med* 147:265, 1987.
67. Rubin SA: Radiographic spectrum of pleuropulmonary tularemia. *AJR Am J Roentgenol* 131:277, 1978.
68. Porsch-Ozcurumez M, Kischel N, Priebe H, et al: Comparison of enzyme-linked immunosorbent assay, western blotting, microagglutination, indirect immunofluorescence assay, and flow cytometry for serological diagnosis of tularemia. *Clin Diagn Lab Immunol* 11:1008, 2004.
69. Lamps LW, Havens JM, Sjostedt A, et al: Histologic and molecular diagnosis of tularemia: a potential bioterrorism agent endemic to North America. *Mod Pathol* 17:489, 2004.
70. Johansson A, Forsman M, Sjostedt A: The development of tools for diagnosis of tularemia and typing of *Francisella tularensis*. *APIMS* 112:898, 2004.
71. Versage JL, Severin DD, Chu MC, et al: Development of a multitarget real-time TaqMan PCR assay for enhanced detection of *Francisella tularensis* in complex specimens. *J Clin Microbiol* 41:5492, 2003.
72. Enderlin G, Morales L, Jacobs RF, et al: Streptomycin and alternative agents for the treatment of tularemia: review of the literature. *Clin Infect Dis* 19:42, 1994.
73. Oyston PC, Griffiths R: Francisella virulence: significant advances, ongoing challenges and unmet needs. *Expert Rev Vaccines* 8(11):1575–1585, 2009.
74. Conlan JW, Oyston PCF: Vaccines against *Francisella tularensis*. *Ann New York Acad Sci* 1105:325, 2007.
75. McGovern TW, Friedlander AM: Plague, in Sidell FR, Takafuji ET, Franz DR (eds): *Medical Aspects of Chemical and Biological Warfare*, in Zajtchuk R, Bellamy RF (eds). *Textbook of Military Medicine, Part I. Warfare, Weaponry and the Casualty*. Washington, DC, United States Department of the Army, Office of the Surgeon General and Borden Institute, 1997, p 479.
76. Inglesby TV, David T, Dennis DT, et al: Plague as a biological weapon: medical and public health management. *JAMA* 283:2281, 2000.
77. Center for Infectious Disease Research and Policy: Plague: current, comprehensive information on pathogenesis, microbiology, epidemiology, diagnosis, and treatment. Last updated April 29, 2010. Available at: http://www.cidrap.umn.edu/cidrap/content/bt/plague/biofacts/plaguefactsheet.html. Accessed June 1, 2010.
78. Smego RA, Frean J, Koornhof HJ: Yersiniosis I: microbiological and clinicoepidemiological aspects of plague and non-plague *Yersinia* infections. *Eur J Clin Microbiol Infect Dis* 18:1, 1999.
79. Straley SC, Skrzypek E, Plano GV, et al: Yops of *Yersinia* spp. pathogenic for humans. *Infect Immunol* 61:3105, 1993.
80. Sodeinde O, Subrahmanyam Y, Stark K, et al: A surface protease and the invasive character of plague. *Science* 258:1004, 1992.
81. Straley SC: The plasmid-encoded outer-membrane proteins of *Yersinia pestis*. *Rev Infect Dis* 10[Suppl 2]:S323, 1988.
82. Poland JD, Dennis DT: Plague, in Evans AS, Brachman PS (eds): *Bacterial Infections of Humans: Epidemiology and Control*. New York, *Plenum Medical Book Company*, 1998, p 545.
83. Galimand M, Guiyoule A, Gerbaud G, et al: Multidrug resistance in *Yersinia pestis* mediated by a transferable plasmid. *N Engl J Med* 337:667, 1997.
84. Centers for Disease Control and Prevention: Recognition of illness associated with the intentional release of a biologic agent. *MMWR Morbid Mortal Wkly Rep* 50:893, 2001.
85. Centers for Disease Control and Prevention: Human plague—United States, 1993–1994. *MMWR Morbid Mortal Wkly Rep* 43:242, 1994.
86. Centers for Disease Control and Prevention: Pneumonic plague—Arizona, 1992. *MMWR Morbid Mortal Wkly Rep* 41:737, 1992.
87. Hull HF, Montes JM, Mann JM: Septicemic plague in New Mexico. *J Infect Dis* 155:113, 1987.
88. World Health Organization: Plague, in *WHO Report on Global Surveillance of Epidemic-prone Infectious Diseases*. Geneva, Switzerland, World Health Organization, 2000, p 25. Available at: http://www.who.int/csr/resources/publications/surveillance/en/plague.pdf. Accessed November 24, 2005.
89. Centers for Disease Control and Prevention: Bubonic and pneumonic plague—Uganda 2006. *MMWR Morbid Mortal Wkly Rep* 58:778–781, 2009.
90. Bin Saeed AA, Al-Hamdan NA, Fontaine RE: Plague from eating raw camel liver. *Emerg Infect Dis* 11:1456, 2005.
91. Arbaji A, Kharabsheh S, Al-Azab S, et al: A 12-case outbreak of pharyngeal plague following the consumption of camel meat, in north-eastern Jordan. *Ann Trop Med Parasitol* 99:789, 2005.
92. World Health Organization: Plague, Democratic Republic of the Congo. *Wkly Epidemiol Rec* 80:65, 2005.
93. World Health Organization: Human plague in 2002 and 2003. *Wkly Epidemiol Rec* 79:301, 2004.
94. Stephens JC, Reich DE, Goldstein DB, et al: Dating the origin of the CCR5-Delta 32 AIDS-resistance allele by the coalescence of haplotypes. *Am J Hum Genet* 62:1507, 1998.
95. Crook LD, Tempest B: Plague: a clinical review of 27 cases. *Arch Intern Med* 152:1253, 1992.
96. Wong TW: Plague in a pregnant patient. *Tropical Doctor* 16:187, 1986.
97. Ratsitorahina M, Chanteau S, Rahalison L, et al: Epidemiological and diagnostic aspects of the outbreak of pneumonic plague in Madagascar. *Lancet* 355:111, 2000.
98. Burmeister RW, Tigertt WD, Overholt EL: Laboratory-acquired pneumonic plague. *Ann Intern Med* 56:789, 1962.
99. Davis KJ, Fritz DL, Pitt ML, et al: Pathology of experimental pneumonic plague produced by fraction 1-positive and fraction 1-negative *Yersinia pestis* in African green monkeys (*Cercopithecus aethiops*). *Arch Pathol Lab Med* 120:156, 1996.
100. Alsofrom DJ, Mettler FA, Mann JM: Radiographic manifestations of plague in New Mexico, 1975–1980. A review of 42 proved cases. *Radiology* 139:561, 1981.

101. Ketai L, Alrahji AA, Hart B, et al: Radiologic manifestations of potential bioterrorist agents of infection. *Am J Roentgenol* 180:565, 2003.
102. Rahalison L, Vololonirina E, Ratsitorahina M, et al: Diagnosis of bubonic plague by PCR in Madagascar under field conditions. *J Clin Microbiol* 38:260, 2000.
103. Williams JE, Gentry MK, Braden CA, et al: Use of an enzyme-linked immunosorbent assay to measure antigenemia during acute plague. *Bull World Health Organ* 62:463, 1984.
104. Chanteau S, Rahalison L, Ralafiarisoa L, et al: Development and testing of a rapid diagnostic test for bubonic and pneumonic plague. *Lancet* 361:211, 2003.
105. Centers for Disease Control and Prevention: *Plague: diagnosis*. Atlanta, GA, Centers for Disease Control and Prevention, 2006. Available at: http://www.cdc.gov/NCIDOD/DVBID/plague/diagnosis.htm. Accessed January 29, 2006.
106. Russell P, Eley SM, Green M: Efficacy of doxycycline and ciprofloxacin against experimental *Yersinia pestis* infection. *J Antimicrob Chemother* 41:301, 1998.
107. Rasoamanana B, Coulanges P, Michel P, et al: Sensibilité de *Yersinia pestis* aux antibiotiques: 277 souches isolées à Madagascar entre 1926 et 1989. *Arch Inst Pasteur Madagascar* 56:37, 1989.
108. Smith MD, Vinh DX, Nguyen TT, et al: In vitro antimicrobial susceptibilities of strains of *Yersinia pestis*. *Antimicrob Agents Chemother* 39:2153, 1995.
109. Wong JD, Barash JR, Sandfort RF, et al: Susceptibilities of *Yersinia pestis* strains to 12 antimicrobial agents. *Antimicrob Agents Chemother* 44:1995, 2000.
110. Garner JS: Hospital Infection Control Practices Advisory Committee: guideline for isolation precautions in hospitals. *Infect Control Hosp Epidemiol* 17:53, 1996.
111. Titball RW, Williamson ED: *Yersinia pestis* (plague) vaccines. *Expert Opin Biol Ther* 4:965, 2004.
112. Williamson ED, Flick-Smith HC, LeButt C, et al: Human immune response to a plague vaccine comprising recombinant F1 and V antigens. *Infect Immunol* 73:3598, 2005.
113. Dennis DT, Gage KL, Gratz N, et al: *Plague Manual: Epidemiology, Distribution, Surveillance and Control*. Geneva, Switzerland, *World Health Organization*, 1999.
114. Centers for Disease Control and Prevention: *Plague: Prevention and Control*. Atlanta, GA, Centers for Disease Control and Prevention, 2006. Available at: http://www.cdc.gov/NCIDOD/DVBID/plague/prevent.htm. Accessed January 29, 2006.
115. Kool JL: Risk of person-to-person transmission of pneumonic plague. *Clin Infect Dis* 40:1166, 2005.
116. Middlebrook JL, Franz DR: Botulinum toxins, in Sidell FR, Takafuji ET, Franz DR (eds): *Medical Aspects of Chemical and Biological Warfare*, in Zajtchuk R, Bellamy RF (eds). *Textbook of Military Medicine, Part I. Warfare, Weaponry and the Casualty*. Washington, DC, United States Department of the Army, Office of the Surgeon General and Borden Institute, 1997, p 643.
117. Center for Infectious Disease Research and Policy: Botulism: current, comprehensive information on pathogenesis, microbiology, epidemiology, diagnosis, treatment, and prophylaxis. February 5, 2009. Available at: http://www.cidrap.umn.edu/cidrap/content/bt/botulism/biofacts/botulismfactsheet.html. Accessed June 14, 2010.
118. Arnon SS, Schechter R, Inglesby TV, et al: Botulinum toxin as a biological weapon: medical and public health management. *JAMA* 285:1059, 2001.
119. Centers for Disease Control and Prevention: Botulism in the United States, 1899–1996. *Handbook for epidemiologists, clinicians, and laboratory workers*. Atlanta, GA, Centers for Disease Control and Prevention, 1998.
120. Hatheway CL, Johnson EA: Clostridium: the spore-bearing anaerobes, in Collier L, Ballows A, Sussman M (eds): *Topley & Wilson's Microbiology and Microbial Infections*. 9th ed. New York, Oxford University Press, 1998, p 731.
121. Wein LM, Liu Y: Analyzing a bioterror attack on the food supply: the case of botulinum toxin in milk. *Proc Natl Acad Sci USA* 102:9984, 2005.
122. Witoonpanich R, Vichayanrat E, Tantisiriwit K, et al: Survival analysis for respiratory failure in patients with food-borne botulism. *Clin Toxicol* 48:177, 2010.
123. Rega P, Burkholder-Allen K, Bork C: An algorithm for the evaluation and management of red, yellow, and green patients during a botulism mass casualty incident. *Am J Disaster Med* 4:192, 2009.
124. CDC: Investigational heptavalent botulinum antitoxin (HBAT) to replace licensed botulinum antitoxin AB and investigational botulinum antitoxin E. *MMWR Morb Mortal Wkly Rep* 19: 299, 2010.
125. Sobel J: Botulism: *Clin Infect Dis* 41:1167, 2005.
126. Black RE, Gunn RA: Hypersensitivity reactions associated with botulinal antitoxin. *Am J Med* 69:567, 1980.
127. Dembeck ZF, Smith LA, Rusnak JM: Botulism: cause, effects, diagnosis, clinical and laboratory identification, and treatment modalities. *Dis Med Public Health Prepared* 2007 1:122, 2007.
128. Taysse L, Daulon S, Calvet J, et al: Induction of acute lung injury after intranasal administration of toxin botulinum a complex. *Toxicol Pathol* 33:336, 2005.
129. Armstrong WP: The castor bean: a plant named after a tick, in Armstrong WP (ed): *Wayne's World: An On-Line Textbook of Natural History*. Noteworthy Plants, March, 1999. Available at: http://waynesword.palomar.edu/plmar99.htm. Accessed December 2, 2005.
130. Centers for Disease Control and Prevention: *Facts About Ricin*. Atlanta, GA: Centers for Disease Control and Prevention, February 5, 2004.
131. Franz DR, Jaxx NK: Ricin toxin, in Sidell FR, Takafuji ET, Franz DR (eds): *Medical Aspects of Chemical and Biological Warfare*, in Zajtchuk R, Bellamy RF (eds). *Textbook of Military Medicine, Part I. Warfare, Weaponry and the Casualty*. Washington, DC, United States Department of the Army, Office of the Surgeon General and Borden Institute, 1997, p 631.
132. Audi J, Belson M, Patel M, et al: Ricin poisoning: a comprehensive review. *JAMA* 294:2342, 2005.
133. Spivak L, Hendrickson RG: Ricin. *Crit Care Clin* 21:815, 2005.
134. Derenzini M, Bonetti E, Marionozzi V, et al: Toxic effects of ricin: studies on the pathogenesis of liver lesions. *Virchows Arch B Cell Pathol* 20:15, 1976.
135. Balint GA: Ricin: the toxic protein of castor oil seeds. *Toxicology* 2:77, 1974.
136. Wilhelmsen CL, Pitt ML: Lesions of acute inhaled lethal ricin intoxication in rhesus monkeys. *Vet Pathol* 33:296, 1996.
137. Griffiths GD, Rice P, Allenby AC, et al: Inhalation toxicology and histopathology of ricin and abrin toxins. *Inhal Toxicol* 7:269, 1995.
138. Kortepeter MG, Parker GW: Potential biological weapons threats. *Emerg Infect Dis* 5:523, 1999.
139. Crompton R, Gall D: Georgi Markov—death in a pellet. *Med Leg J* 48:51, 1980.
140. Shea D, Gottron F: Ricin: technical background and potential role in terrorism. CRS Report for Congress. Washington, DC, Congressional Research Service, February 4, 2004.
141. Ricin found at South Carolina postal facility. Atlanta, GA: CNN.com; October 30, 2003. Available at: http://www.cnn.com/2003/US/10/22/ricin.letter/index.html. Accessed December 6, 2005.
142. Schier JG, Patel MM, Belson MG, et al: Public health investigation after the discovery of ricin in a south Carolina Postal facility. *Am J Pub Health* 97:S152, 2007.
143. Centers for Disease Control and Prevention: *Toxic syndrome description: ricin or abrin poisoning*. Atlanta, GA: *Centers for Disease Control and Prevention*; March 26, 2005. Available at: http://www.bt.cdc.gov/agent/ricin/pdf/ricinabrintoxidrome.pdf. Accessed December 6, 2005.
144. Bradbury SM, Dickers KJ, Rice P: Ricin poisoning. *Toxicol Rev* 22:65, 2003.
145. Ingle NV, Kale VG, Talwalkar YB: Accidental poisoning in children with particular reference to castor beans. *Indian J Pediatr* 33:237, 1966.
146. Alpin PJ, Eliseo T: Ingestion of castor oil plant seeds. *Med J Aust* 168:423, 1997.
147. Fine DR, Shepherd HA, Griffiths GD, Green M: Sub-lethal poisoning by self-injection with ricin. *Med Sci Law* 32:70, 1992.
148. Schnell R, Borchmann P, Staak JO, et al: Clinical evaluation of ricin A-chain immunotoxins in patients with Hodgkin's lymphoma. *Ann Oncol* 14:729, 2003.
149. Frankel AE, Kreitman RJ, Sausville EA: Targeted toxins. *Clinical Cancer Rev* 6:326, 2000.
150. Topping MD, Henderson RT, Luczynska CM, et al: Castor bean allergy among workers in the felt industry. *Allergy* 37:603, 1982.
151. Kanerva L, Estlander T, Jolanki R: Long-lasting contact urticaria. Type I and type IV allergy from castor bean and a hypothesis of systemic IgE-mediated allergic dermatitis. *Dermatol Clin* 8:181, 1990.
152. Lockey SD, Dunkelberger L: Anaphylaxis from an Indian necklace. *JAMA* 206:2900, 1968.
153. *Fact Sheet: Laboratory Testing for Ricin*. Atlanta, GA, Centers for Disease Control and Prevention; February 23, 2006. Available at: http://www.bt.cdc.gov/agent/ricin/pdf/ricinlabtesting.pdf. Accessed February 23, 2006.
154. United States Army Medical Research Institute of Infectious Diseases: Ricin, in Kortepeter M, Christopher G, Cieslak T, et al (eds): *Medical Management of Biological Casualties Handbook*, 4th ed. Fort Detrick, MD, United States Army Medical Research Institute of Infectious Diseases, February 2001, p 70. Available at: http://www.nbc-med.org/SiteContent/HomePage/WhatsNew/MedManual/Feb01/handbook.htm. Accessed December 3, 2005.
155. Ma L, Hsu CH, Patterson E, et al: Ricin depresses cardiac function in the rabbit heart. *Toxicol Appl Pharmacol* 138:72, 1996.
156. Hewetson J, Rivera V, Lemley P, et al: A formalinized toxoid for protection of mice from inhaled ricin. *Vaccine Research* 4:179, 1996.
157. Cieslak TJ, Christopher GW, Kortepeter MG, et al: Immunization against potential biological warfare agents. *Clin Infect Dis* 30:843, 2000.
158. Kende M, Yan C, Hewetson J, et al: Oral immunization of mice with ricin toxoid vaccine encapsulated in polymeric microspheres against aerosol challenge. *Vaccine* 20:1681, 2002.
159. Mantis NJ: Vaccines against the category B toxins: Staphylococcal enterotoxin B, epsilon toxin and ricin. *Adv Drug Deliv Rev* 57:1424, 2005.
160. Lord JM, Roberts LM, Robertus JD: Ricin: structure, mode of action, and some current applications. *FASEB J* 8:201, 1994.
161. *Summary of the NIAID Ricin Expert Panel Workshop*. Bethesda, MD: National Institute of Allergy and Infectious Diseases, April 1–2, 2004. Available at: http://www.niaid.nih.gov/Biodefense/ricin_meeting.pdf. Accessed December 3, 2005.
162. Vitetta ES, Smallshaw JE, Coleman E, et al: A pilot clinical trial of a recombinant ricin vaccine in normal humans. *Proc Natl Acad Sci USA* 103:2268, 2006.

CHAPTER 214 ■ CHEMICAL AGENTS OF MASS DESTRUCTION

JAMES GEILING AND LAWRENCE C. MOHR JR

If supposedly civilized nations confined their warfare to attacks on the enemy's troops, the matter of defense against warfare chemicals would be purely a military problem, and therefore beyond the scope of this study. But such is far from the case. In these days of total warfare, the civilians, including women and children, are subject to attack at all times.

Colonel Edgar Erskine Hume, Medical Corps, U.S. Army, 1943 [1]

Chemical agents of terror have moved to the forefront of concern for healthcare providers as weapons of mass destruction (WMD) have become readily available to both domestic and international terrorists. Critical care physicians must be familiar with these agents, their impact on patients, and the potential dangers these compounds can cause to healthcare workers.

Although terrorists have traditionally focused their efforts on the use of conventional explosives, chemical agents have emerged as attractive weapons of terrorism for a variety of reasons:

- Raw materials for their production are readily available throughout the world.
- Raw materials are inexpensive.
- A chemical weapon of mass destruction can be produced with relatively small amounts of raw materials.
- They may be odorless, colorless, and tasteless.
- They are poorly detected.
- They do not destroy infrastructure.
- They possess a latency period between the time of exposure and the development of clinical symptoms.
- Their use produces a mass media response [2].

Hospital-based physicians normally, at some time in their medical career, study the skills and procedures needed to treat mass casualties. The focus, however, has traditionally centered on large numbers of casualties presenting to the emergency department as a result of multisystem trauma, such as that sustained in an explosion, airplane crash, or natural disaster. The event of September 11, 2001, and subsequent terrorist threats have changed the nature of physician training and preparation requirements. The scope of preparation now requires knowledge of the mass care of victims following a WMD event. This chapter focuses on the recognition and management of patients exposed to common chemical agents of mass destruction.

HISTORY

Chemical agents of mass destruction are gaseous, liquid, or solid substances that are employed against a population because of their direct toxic effects. Virtually any toxic substance can be used as an agent of mass destruction. However, those that have been successfully weaponized are characterized by ease of production, ease of handling during weapon assembly, dispersion properties, and ability to cause injury and death in relatively low concentrations [3].

Although the first reported use of chemical agents dates back to 1000 BC, when Chinese forces used arsenical smokes, the use of chemical agents in warfare began in earnest during World War I when German forces seeking a breakout from the stalemate of trench warfare released 150 tons of chlorine gas from 6,000 cylinders on the afternoon of April 15, 1915, near Ypres, Belgium. The chlorine gas resulted in 800 deaths and caused the retreat of 15,000 Allied troops, largely because of the psychological terror produced by the gas attack.

The next major use of chemical weapons took place more than 2 years later, on July 12, 1917, again near Ypres. On that date, German forces attacked Allied troops with artillery shells containing sulfur mustard. This attack resulted in 20,000 casualties. Although many casualties had debilitating injuries, less than 5% of the troops died as a result of the chemical attack. Persistent and nonvolatile, sulfur mustard caused a host of new problems for Allied forces, including a latency period before the effects appeared and the need for men, and their horses, to wear protective overgarments [4].

The Geneva Convention of 1925 banned the use of chemical warfare agents because of the physical and psychological trauma they imposed on their victims.

Nerve agents appeared in the 1930s when the German industrial chemist, Dr. Gerhard Schrader, began research into the development of stronger insecticides, the first two of which were tabun and sarin. German forces stockpiled these for use in World War II, but never used them.

Chemical agents were used sporadically in the second half of the twentieth century. The United States used defoliants and riot-controlled agents in Vietnam. Iraq used mustard, tabun, and eventually sarin against Iran in the Iran–Iraq war of the 1980s. Later in the 1980s, reports implicated Iraq in the use of cyanide against the Kurdish population in northern Iraq [5].

The most recent publicized use of chemical agents took place in Japan when the Aum Shinrikyo religious cult released sarin gas on two occasions. The first took place on June 27, 1994, in Matsumoto and resulted in 600 persons exposed, 58 admitted to the hospital, and 7 deaths [6]. The more famous and larger event took place the following year, on March 20, 1995, when the cult released sarin gas in the Tokyo subway system during rush hour. The subway system attack resulted in the deaths of 11 commuters and the medical evaluation of approximately 5,000 individuals [7].

In 1997 the Chemical Weapons Convention (CWC) went into effect as an international treaty that bans the use, development, production, acquisition, transfer, stockpiling, and retention of chemical weapons by signatory nations. At the time of this writing, the CWC was ratified by 175 nations, including the United States. The CWC is administered by the Organization for the Prohibition of Chemical Weapons, which conducts regular inspections and monitors compliance with provisions of the treaty [8].

DETECTION AND DECONTAMINATION

Initial steps in the management of chemical agent casualties include detection of the chemical agent used in the attack and the decontamination of casualties. Detailed discussions on detection and decontamination are beyond the scope of this chapter. However, hospital-based critical care physicians should understand basic concepts of these topics to better care for their patients and protect themselves and their facilities from potential harm.

The most important tool in detecting the use of these agents is accurate and timely intelligence from military or law enforcement agencies. Unfortunately, hospitals are not usually in the information-sharing and decision-making circles with these groups. As a result, initial awareness of a chemical agent attack typically occurs with the first patient presenting to the emergency department. Hospitals and physicians can improve their preparedness for the management of chemical agent casualties by actively participating in disaster-planning activities in their respective communities.

Various types of sensing devices can be used for the detection of chemical agents in the environment. At the present time, all commercially available detection equipment uses point source technology; that is, proximity to the substance is required. The handheld Chemical Agent Monitor uses ion mobility spectrometry to detect mustard and nerve agents. Chemical agent detection papers, such as the M8 and M9 papers (Anachemia, Lachine, Quebec, Canada), can be used to detect mustard and nerve agents. The M256 Detection Kit (Anachemia, Lachine, Quebec, Canada) can detect mustard, nerve agents, phosgene, and cyanide. Standoff capability, that is, detecting agents from as far away as 5 km, has been developed to detect contaminated areas without being exposed [9]. Newer chemical agent detection technologies will continue to evolve in response to the terrorism threat. These can only help ensure hospitals and providers have quicker, more accurate information to meet the needs of victims.

Ideally, the decontamination of chemical agent casualties should be accomplished by first responders or hazardous material personnel prior to evacuation or transport to a medical facility. Unfortunately, most disaster victims bypass emergency medical system transport and arrive unannounced at the closest hospital. As a result, hospitals must be prepared to decontaminate chemical agent casualties prior to admission. Facilities and protocols to decontaminate such casualties should be developed by all hospitals. Such processes are needed to protect the victims from further exposure and to prevent the spread of chemical agents within the hospital and among healthcare providers. Critical care physicians, nurses, and support personnel may be called on to help develop decontamination protocols and assist in the decontamination process. It is imperative that all individuals designated to serve on decontamination teams be thoroughly trained in the procedures, precautions, and protective clothing required in the decontamination process. Attempting to provide help in a contaminated environment without prior training puts the healthcare provider at risk of being exposed to a chemical agent and could impede the delivery of effective medical care for the victims of a chemical attack.

The sarin gas release in Tokyo provides a clear example of the need for preparation and training prior to a chemical attack. Of the 1,364 emergency personnel who responded to the attack, 135 (9.9%) became symptomatic and required medical support themselves. None of the first responders wore protective clothing or face masks and off-gassing of the chemical agent from clothing of victims played a significant role in their complaints. These effects were evident among hospital staff as well first responders. It was reported that 23% of the staff at the hospital that received the patients also experienced symptoms [10].

The Occupational Safety and Health Administration (OSHA) mandates that all healthcare providers be trained to perform their duties without jeopardizing the health and safety of themselves or coworkers. It provides guidance for the use of personal protective equipment and requires that written plans be developed for hospitals to train teams in the use of personal protective equipment to receive contaminated victims [11]. Most medical facilities prepare their decontamination teams to operate in OSHA personal protective equipment Level C; that is, full-face mask with an air-purifying canister respirator and chemical-resistant clothing.

In most situations, effective chemical decontamination can be performed by carefully removing the victim's clothing and thoroughly washing the victim with soap and water. It has been reported that removing contaminated clothing alone can eliminate 85% to 90% of chemical contaminants [12]. Recently developed for the military and soon to be used by first responders is Reactive Skin Decontamination Lotion (RSDL) (O'Dell Engineering Ltd/E-Z-EM Canada Inc., Canada). It is not used for prophylactic protection or total body decontamination, but, if applied early following exposure, is effective in neutralizing chemical warfare agents and T2 mycotoxins [13]. However, in exposures associated with trauma, RSDL may interfere with normal wound healing [14]. EasyDECON (Envirofoam Technologies, Huntsville, Alabama) can be used to decontaminate exposed environmental surfaces. Normally employed as a foam, it effectively neutralizes a variety of chemical agents including nerve gases and mustard [15]. Finally, medical facilities must consider environmental variables such as wind direction, wind velocity, temperature, and water runoff when setting up decontamination areas. These environmental considerations are important in protecting patients and employees from exposure to chemical agents, as well as minimizing the risk of contaminating buildings and equipment during the patient decontamination process.

CLASSIFICATION OF CHEMICAL AGENTS

Chemical agents are normally classified into broad categories based on their mechanism of action and physiologic effects. The most common classification scheme divides them into the following categories:

- Nerve agents
- Vesicants
- Cyanide agents or "blood" agents
- Pulmonary agents or "choking" agents
- Nonlethal incapacitating agents

Nerve Agents

Because they are the most toxic, nerve agents are the most feared of chemical agents. All nerve agents are organophosphorus compounds, which inhibit butyrylcholinesterase in the plasma, acetylcholinesterase in the red blood cell (RBC), and acetylcholinesterase at cholinergic receptor sites in the central and peripheral nervous systems. The chemical bond between nerve agent molecules and acetylcholinesterase is irreversible; thus, acetylcholinesterase activity returns only with new acetylcholinesterase synthesis or RBC turnover (1% per day) [16]. The decrease in acetylcholinesterase activity results in the accumulation of acetylcholine at both muscarinic and nicotinic receptors in the central nervous system and neuromuscular junctions of the peripheral nervous system. Cholinergic overstimulation resulting from the accumulation of excess acetylcholine in the central and peripheral nervous systems is responsible for the clinical manifestations of nerve agent toxicity [17].

After an acute exposure to nerve agents, RBC acetylcholinesterase reflects nervous system acetylcholinesterase activity better than the activity of butyrylcholinesterase in the plasma. The measurement of RBC acetylcholinesterase activity is principally a research tool at the present time, and it is not useful in the management of mass casualties from nerve agent exposure. However, its measurement in blood samples collected from victims of a chemical attack may be useful in forensic investigations.

Several different nerve agents currently exist, each characterized by a unique molecular structure that irreversibly inhibits acetylcholinesterase. Compounds that were originally developed in Germany have been designated as the "G" series of nerves agents. The "V" series of agents are better absorbed through the skin than the "G" agents and are so designated because they are more "venomous." The most common nerve agents include:

- GA (tabun): ethyl N,N-dimethylphosphoramidocyanidate
- GB (sarin): isopropyl methyl phosphonofluoridate
- GD (soman): pinacolyl methyl phosphonofluoridate
- GF: O-cyclohexyl-methylphosphonofluoridate
- VX: O-ethyl S-(2-(diisopropylaminoethyl) methyl phosphonothiolate

The "G" agents are volatile, whereas VX is a persistent, oily substance with better percutaneous absorption. Each of these agents can be dispersed through a variety of weapons and munitions.

Inhalation of nerve gas is the most effective means of producing clinical effects, although it can also be ingested. High doses of persistent nerve agents, such as VX, can be absorbed through the skin. The clinical effects of nerve agent toxicity occur as a result of acetylcholine accumulating at both nicotinic sites (autonomic ganglia and skeletal muscle) as well as muscarinic sites (including postganglionic parasympathetic fibers, glands, and pulmonary and gastrointestinal smooth muscles). Nicotinic receptors appear to be most sensitive to the effects of nerve agents, with inactivation of acetylcholinesterase in autonomic ganglia and the neuromuscular junction of skeletal muscle responsible for many symptoms and signs of nerve agent exposure. The typical clinical manifestations of nerve agent toxicity are similar to those produced by organophosphate insecticides, although nerve agents are up to 1,000 times more toxic [17].

The basic clinical syndrome produced by nerve agents can be remembered by the acronym "SLUDGE": salivation, lacrimation, urination, defecation, gastric distress, and emesis. Alternatively, "DUMBELS" (diarrhea, urination, miosis, bradycardia/bronchorrhea/bronchospasm, emesis, lacrimation, salivation/secretion/sweating) provides a more detailed tool to remember the muscarinic signs and symptoms [18]. Specific signs and symptoms in various organ systems depend on the dose of nerve agent received. Inhalation of a nerve agent usually produces immediate effects that occur within seconds to minutes after exposure. Dermal absorption usually produces delayed effects that can develop at any time between 10 minutes and 18 hours after skin exposure, depending on the dose. Common signs and symptoms in each organ system are summarized here.

Inhalation of a nerve agent typically results in the development of rhinorrhea, bronchorrhea, and bronchoconstriction soon after exposure. Dyspnea and chest tightness are common early symptoms. Coughing and wheezing may occur. The volume of airway secretions, the magnitude of bronchoconstriction, and the severity of airway symptoms all increase with higher exposure doses. High-dose or prolonged exposure may result in diaphragmatic weakness and centrally mediated apnea, which can result in ventilatory failure [16,17].

Although vagally mediated bradycardia is the expected heart rate response from cholinergic overstimulation of muscarinic receptors, this is commonly overridden by tachycardia resulting from nicotinic-mediated adrenergic stimulation and hypoxia. First-, second-, and third-degree heart block may occur [16,17]. Prolongation of the QTc interval can precipitate Torsade de pointes that has a poor prognosis [19]. Although hypertension may occur as a result of nicotinic-mediated adrenergic stimulation, blood pressure usually remains normal. A decline in blood pressure is typically a sign of impending death [4].

Muscarinic and nicotinic stimulation of the peripheral nervous system typically results in muscle fasciculations and profuse sweating, respectively. Muscle weakness and muscle paralysis may occur following high-dose exposures. Seizures can develop suddenly. The seizures may resolve spontaneously, but can be prolonged with status epilepticus [16,17]. Smaller-exposure doses typically result in nonspecific neurologic findings including an inability to concentrate, insomnia, irritability, and depression. A variety of psychological and behavioral changes, ranging from mild confusion to severe anxiety, can also occur [15]. Hallucinations or complete disorientation do not appear. Mild exposure also may result in a slight decline in memory function, as observed in first responders in the Tokyo sarin gas release of 1995 [20]. In the decade since that event, those exposed continue to have mild cerebellar effects and principally posttraumatic stress disorder [21].

Direct contact of the eyes with nerve agent vapor causes miosis that is usually associated with intense ocular pain. Patients also complain of blurred or dim vision and typically have injected conjunctivae with significant lacrimation.

Nausea and vomiting may be among the first signs of nerve agent toxicity. Abdominal cramping and diarrhea may also occur [16,17].

Unfortunately, few of the clinical signs or symptoms listed here may appear following exposure to a high dose of nerve agent. This is due to the fact that the range of exposure of doses, which produce clinical symptoms, is only slightly less than those which cause death. Therefore, central nervous system collapse with seizures, loss of consciousness, and central apnea may be the first signs of nerve agent toxicity following a high-dose exposure [16].

Management of all nerve agent casualties begins with the traditional "ABCs" of resuscitation: airway, breathing, and circulation support. Contaminated patients should be managed in the following order:

- Airway management
- Breathing support
- Circulation and hemorrhage control
- Antidote administration
- Decontamination
- Wound dressing
- Evacuation to a noncontaminated treatment location [22]

Ventilatory failure is the primary cause of death following nerve agent exposure [23]. As a result, airway management and breathing support are extremely important in the management of nerve agent casualties. The nausea and vomiting that these patients typically experience must be considered in their airway management. In this regard, all patients should be considered to have a full stomach. Endotracheal intubation and assisted ventilation are required for the management of ventilatory failure. High airway resistance necessitating the need of pressures up to 50 to 70 cm of water may complicate ventilatory support [17]. Because of high airway pressures, if a cuffed endotracheal tube cannot be placed, a double-lumen Combitube (Tyco

Healthcare, Pleasanton, CA) is preferable to a laryngeal mask airway [24]. Once an effective airway has been established, ventilatory assistance can be provided by manual ventilation using a bag-valve device or by mechanical ventilation. Nebulized ipratropium can be used for the treatment of bronchospasm that may, in turn, result in decreased airway resistance [16]. Frequent suctioning is necessary to remove the copious airway secretions associated with nerve agent exposure. The use of depolarizing neuromuscular blocking agents during ventilatory assistance should be avoided [25].

The principal antidote for nerve agents is atropine. Atropine is an anticholinergic drug that blocks acetylcholine receptor sites. As a result, atropine blocks the pathophysiologic effects of the excess acetylcholine that accumulates as a result of nerve gas exposure; it is most effective at muscarinic sites. Atropine is primarily used for the purpose of drying up the copious airway secretions that patients develop following nerve agent exposure. The standard adult dosing regimen is 2 mg, administered intramuscularly, every 5 to 10 minutes, titrated to the patient's secretions. The recommended pediatric dose is 0.05 mg per kg, with a minimum dose of 0.1 mg, administered intravenously every 2 to 5 minutes, titrated to effect [17,23]. In severe cases, adult patients may require 10 to 20 mg of atropine in the first hour to control secretions. The administration of atropine to a hypoxemic patient could precipitate the development of ventricular fibrillation. Therefore, oxygen should be administered and hypoxemia corrected before atropine is given [22,26]. Miosis will not respond to parenteral atropine. Topical tropicamide is effective for the treatment of miosis and the relief of ocular pain [23]. Atropine alone may not be an effective treatment for terminating seizures or reversing ventilatory failure [17,26]. Bulk atropine is available for reconstitution and may be required in the setting of mass nerve agent casualties.

Pralidoxime chloride is the other major antidote for nerve agents. It functions by "prying off" the nerve agent molecule from acetylcholinesterase, thereby rendering the enzyme active again. Unfortunately, it must be given early, before the agent–enzyme bond matures or "ages," that occurs in as little as 2 minutes for soman but takes 3 to 4 hours for sarin. Once the agent–enzyme bond completely ages, the bond is irreversible and pralidoxime chloride has no therapeutic effect. Pralidoxime chloride is only effective at nicotinic sites and, therefore, helps to increase muscle strength. The standard adult dose is 15 to 25 mg per kg or 1 g, given intravenously (in 100 to 250 mL of 0.9% saline) during 20 to 30 minutes. The initial dose may be followed by an infusion of 200 to 500 mg per hour, if necessary. Higher dosing with a 2 g load followed by 1 g per hour for 48 hours has been shown to significantly decrease atropine requirements and the duration of mechanical ventilation in patients poisoned by organophosphate pesticides [27]. Severe hypertension is a potential side effect of pralidoxime chloride, and this can be rapidly reversed by a 5-mg intravenous infusion of phentolamine. The recommended pediatric dose is 15 to 25 mg per kg administered intravenously during 30 to 40 minutes [23].

Atropine and pralidoxime chloride come packaged as two autoinjectors in commercially available kits, called MARK-I Nerve Agent Antidote Kits (Meridian Medical Technologies, Columbia, MD). Each kit contains one AtroPen Auto-Injector containing 2 mg of atropine and one pralidoxime chloride Auto-Injector containing 600 mg of pralidoxime chloride. The same company also now produces DuoDote™, a single autoinjector 2.1 mg of atropine and 600 mg of pralidoxime chloride [28].

Historically, diazepam has been the anticonvulsant recommended for the management of seizures associated with nerve agent exposure. In the hospital setting, diazepam may be given intravenously. The adult intravenous dose is 5 to 10 mg every 10 to 20 minutes until seizures resolve, but not to exceed 30 mg in an 8-hour period. The pediatric dose is 15 to 25 mg per kg [23]. Autoinjectors that contain 10 mg of diazepam are available for use in the field (Meridian Medical Technologies). In both hospital and prehospital settings, healthcare providers must carefully monitor patients for signs of ventilatory failure following the administration of diazepam. Lorazepam and midazolam that are typically used in a critical care environment are also effective in controlling seizures following nerve agent exposure [29,30].

Decontamination is a key step in the treatment of nerve agent casualties because minimizing exposure to the agent decreases the severity of toxic effects. Removal of all clothing, rinsing the eyes with water or normal saline for 10 minutes, and washing the entire body once with soap and water should suffice. Decontamination should be conducted as soon as possible after ventilatory and circulatory support has been initiated and antidotes have been administered. Rapid decontamination is especially important for nerve agents that can be absorbed through the skin. It is important for healthcare providers to wear protective clothing and face masks prior to and during contamination of nerve agent casualties [10,16].

Vesicants

The two principal vesicants or "blister agents" are sulfur mustard and lewisite. This section focuses on the more notable sulfur mustard (bis-[2-chloroethyl] sulfide) that is commonly referred to as *mustard*. Lewisite has similar health effects except for the immediacy of its action in comparison to mustard, which has a latency period. It normally takes several hours between contact with mustard and the onset of signs and symptoms, with the specific latency period depending on the exposure dose. In general, the higher the exposure dose, the shorter the latency period. Mustard is an oily liquid that ranges from clear to pale yellow to dark brown in color. It classically smells like onion, garlic, or mustard, which is allegedly how it got its name. At temperate conditions, it is a persistent liquid that volatilizes slowly. At temperatures greater than 100°F, however, mustard evaporates and mustard vapor becomes a major hazard. As a weapon, mustard will most likely be employed as a contact agent [31].

On entering living cells, mustard alkylates and cross-links DNA that causes DNA strand breaks and eventually leads to cell death. Mustard damages any skin that it contacts, resulting in vesicle or bullae formation within 4 to 24 hours after exposure. Vesicle formation typically peaks within several days after contact with the skin; of note, the bullae fluid is not toxic and therefore not a threat to providers. As the most sensitive organ to low dosage exposures, contact with the eyes may result in painful irritation, conjunctivitis, blepharospasm, and corneal opacity related to edema and pannus formation. Blindness can occur if the corneal pannus is severe and covers the visual axis. Eyelid burns may be first or second degree. Mild-to-severe airway damage can occur following mustard inhalation. The extent and severity of airway damage is dose-dependent, with lower doses primarily affecting the upper airways and higher doses affecting both upper and lower airways. At all doses, the proximal and upper airways are affected more than lower airways. High inhalational doses can cause severe inflammation, inflammatory exudate, necrosis of mucous membranes, mucosal sloughing, and pseudomembrane formation. Sloughed mucosal tissue and pseudomembranes can cause obstruction of the lower airways and serve as a nidus for respiratory tract infections, principally *Pseudomonas*. Other pulmonary problems include asthma, laryngospasm, acute bronchitis, chronic bronchitis, bronchiectasis, tracheobronchial stenosis, pulmonary fibrosis, and bronchiolitis obliterans [32,33]. Hypoxia and hypercarbia may occur as a result of ventilation-perfusion mismatching caused by airway mucosal sloughing and hyperreactive or bronchitic airways. Severe gastrointestinal side effects and bone marrow suppression can occur following ingestion of high doses of mustard. Leukopenia with a cell count less than 200 cells per mm^3 portends a poor prognosis. Sepsis may occur as a result of leukopenia and the breakdown of skin, respiratory epithelium, and gastrointestinal mucosa [34].

Decontamination is a critical component in the management of mustard casualties. Indeed, decontamination within 1 to 2 minutes after exposure is the most effective means of reducing serious skin and tissue damage from mustard. Because of its persistence, removal of mustard from casualties must occur before admission to a medical treatment facility so healthcare workers do not become contaminated. In general, the medical care of mustard casualties is supportive. Areas of denuded skin should be treated like burns and liberally covered with silver sulfadiazine ointment [12]. Calamine lotion may soothe mild burning and itching in erythematous areas of skin. Nonsteroidal anti-inflammatory drugs may help to mitigate pain associated with cutaneous inflammation. Cooling the skin to 15°C and applying deferoxamine or zinc oxide may also be beneficial [35]. Skin healing following mustard exposure takes longer than skin healing following thermal burns. Some patients may require skin grafts and reconstructive surgery.

Respiratory care is mostly supportive. Bronchodilators may be helpful for the treatment of asthma-like symptoms related to hyperreactive airways. Corticosteroids may also be helpful, but should be used with caution because of the risk of superinfection. Intubation and ventilatory support may be necessary for the management of severe laryngospasm or respiratory failure following high doses of inhaled mustard. Bronchoscopy may be necessary to remove pseudomembrane fragments from the airway. Chronic, progressive tracheobronchial stenosis has been reported following mustard inhalation, and may require periodic bronchoscopy with bougienage and laser photoresection to maintain airway patency [36].

For systemic toxicity, early treatment with nonsteroidal anti-inflammatory agents may be useful. Thiosulfate decreases toxicity in animals; also in animal models, granulocyte colony stimulating factor has been shown to reduce the duration of neutropenia by approximately half [37].

In summary, acute mortality is relatively low, but morbidity is high following exposure to mustard. The severity and duration of illness and injuries following mustard exposure are directly related to the exposure dose and routes of exposure. Because of the persistence of mustard, decontamination is critically important in the management of mustard casualties and for protecting healthcare workers from being exposed. Victims of mustard exposure will consume significant healthcare resources in the management of their acute care needs and some will require prolonged periods of treatment and rehabilitation for chronic sequelae.

Cyanide

Cyanide can exist either as gas or as a colorless, volatile liquid that easily vaporizes. In both physical states, it typically has the smell of bitter almonds, although 40% to 60% of the population is unable to detect this odor. It is a chemical asphyxiant of the type that is historically classified as a "blood" agent. Cyanide can be used as an agent of mass destruction in two chemical forms: hydrogen cyanide and cyanogen chloride. Although very lethal in high doses, the volatility of cyanide makes it difficult to weaponize and it ranks among the least lethal of the common chemical agents of mass destruction. Cyanide produces its pathologic effects by binding to iron-containing sites on cytochrome a_3 in the mitochondria that inhibits the enzyme's activity. The binding of cyanide to cytochrome a_3 can occur very rapidly. Cytochrome a_3 is a key enzyme in the cytochrome oxidase system involved in aerobic metabolism within the mitochondria of cells. Inhibition of cytochrome a_3 by cyanide effectively stops cellular respiration and forces affected cells into anaerobic metabolism. Cyanide also has an increased affinity for the ferric ion in methemoglobin that is a property exploited for treatment of cyanide poisoning [38].

The clinical manifestations of cyanide poisoning result from the inability of cells to extract and use oxygen. The onset of signs and symptoms occurs rapidly following inhalation (within 15 seconds), whereas a delayed response of up to 30 minutes follows ingestion. Metabolic acidosis develops as a consequence of increased lactate production from anaerobic metabolism. Compensatory mechanisms to increase oxygen delivery to tissues include tachycardia and increased minute ventilation, which are the earliest clinical signs. Dyspnea may occur as a result of the hyperpnea. Other signs include agitation, anxiety, vertigo, headache, muscle weakness, and trembling. Diaphoresis and flushing sometimes occur. Seizures have been reported. Dilated, unresponsive pupils and coma are late signs of cyanide poisoning and portend a poor prognosis. Without treatment, cyanide victims eventually develop apnea and cardiac dysrhythmias, followed by death from cardiac arrest [38].

Both the administration of specific antidotes and supportive care should be given as soon as possible after exposure to cyanide. Sodium nitrite and sodium thiosulfate are the traditional antidotes used to treat cyanide poisoning. This treatment's objectives focus on detoxifying and excreting the cyanide, as well as on preventing its reentry into the cell. One ampule containing 300 mg of sodium nitrite in 10 mL of diluent (30 mg per mL) is administered intravenously for 2 to 4 minutes to form methemoglobin. The pediatric dose of sodium nitrite is 0.33 mL per kg of a 3% solution given intravenously for 2 to 4 minutes, not to exceed 10 mL. Cyanide binds more effectively and preferentially to the ferric ion site on methemoglobin in comparison to cytochrome a_3. Therefore, the methemoglobin generated by sodium nitrite removes cyanide from cytochrome a_3-binding sites and frees the enzyme to once again participate in the processes of cellular respiration and aerobic metabolism. Following sodium nitrite administration, 12.5 g of sodium thiosulfate in 50 mL of diluent is administered intravenously at a rate of 3 to 5 mL per minute. The pediatric dose of sodium thiosulfate is 412.5 mg per kg (1.65 mL per kg), given intravenously at a rate of 3 to 5 mL per minute. Sodium thiosulfate acts as substrate for rhodanese, converting the cyanide to thiocyanate that is then excreted in the urine. Sodium nitrite and sodium thiosulfate are very effective antidotes for the treatment of cyanide poisoning if they are given before the cessation of cardiac activity [38,39].

A specific challenge in managing these patients is in the prehospital environment, specifically in hypoxia environments such as fires or smoke, inhalation where decreased oxygen-carrying capacity can be exacerbated by the induction of methemoglobinemia. Hydroxocobalamin, a precursor of vitamin B_{12}, provides an alternative treatment option for both pre- and in-hospital management. Cyanokit® (Dey L.P., Napa CA., www.cyanokit.com) contains two vials of 2.5 g of lyophilized hydroxocobalamin that is reconstituted in 100 cc saline for administration. The standard initial adult dose is 5 g infused over 15 minutes with an additional 5 g given depending on the patient's condition. Hydroxocobalamin binds with cyanide to form cyanocobalamin that is then excreted in the urine. It is well tolerated with no known major toxicities. Of note, the red molecule results in red mucous membranes, skin, and urine [40]. A major impediment to widespread use of this modality is its cost which is over twice as expensive as the sodium nitrite/sodium thiosulfate kit [41].

Supportive care for cyanide poisoning includes the administration of oxygen that has been shown to be effective in managing hypoxia, even though the poor cellular uptake and utilization of oxygen found in cyanide toxicity would suggest supplemental oxygen to be of little efficacy. Hyperbaric oxygen may also be beneficial in select severely ill patients, though this therapy would be difficult to institute in a mass casualty setting [12]. Ventilatory support should be provided as needed. Consideration should be given to the administration of sodium bicarbonate for the treatment of severe lactic acidosis in patients who are unconscious or hemodynamically unstable. The recommended dose of sodium bicarbonate intravenously is 1 to 2 mg per kg intravenously, for both adults and children. Arterial blood gas analysis is used to guide the need for repeat doses of sodium bicarbonate to ensure that a metabolic alkalosis does not develop. In most cases of cyanide poisoning, appropriate supportive care in conjunction with the administration of sodium nitrite and sodium thiosulfate or hydroxocobalamin before cardiac arrest occurs can result in a complete recovery over a period of several days [38,40,42].

Pulmonary or "Choking" Agents

Pulmonary or "choking" agents cause acute lung injury after inhalation. The acute lung injury produced by these agents typically results in the development of pulmonary edema. Phosgene and chlorine are the two most common chemical agents in this category. Both were used as chemical warfare agents in World War I. Their effects relate, in part, to their water solubility. Highly water-soluble gases like ammonia, hydrogen chloride, and sulfur dioxide affect primarily the eyes and upper airway mucous membranes. Chlorine, a moderately water-soluble gas, affects the upper airway less but also damages the lower airway. Finally, slightly water-soluble gases like phosgene affect primarily the lower airways.

Phosgene is a colorless gas at room temperature, but becomes a volatile liquid on cooling or compression. The gaseous form has an odor of green corn or freshly mown hay. The gas is denser than air and accumulates in low-lying areas. On exposure to water, phosgene hydrolyzes to form carbon dioxide and hydrochloric acid. These hydrolyzation products may cause phosgene gas to appear as a white cloud when it comes into contact with water vapor in the air [43].

Initial symptoms of phosgene poisoning are primarily related to inflammatory irritation of the eyes and mucous membranes of the oronasopharynx. The irritation is caused by the hydrochloric acid that is formed when phosgene reacts with tissue water. Initial symptoms occur shortly after exposure and include burning sensation in eyes, conjunctival erythema, increased lacrimation, soreness of the throat and nasal membranes, rhinorrhea, coughing, choking, and tightness in the chest. Nausea, occasional vomiting, and headache have also been reported to occur shortly after phosgene exposure. These may be the only symptoms that occur following a low-concentration exposure. However, a life-threatening illness, characterized by noncardiogenic pulmonary edema and respiratory failure, can develop after exposure to higher concentrations.

Inhaled phosgene causes the formation of hydrochloric acid in the airways and alveoli that causes direct inflammatory injury to epithelial cells and endothelial cells of pulmonary capillaries. In addition, phosgene causes an acylation reaction with amino, hydroxyl, and sulfhydryl groups on cellular macromolecules, resulting in oxidative injury to lung tissues. It also stimulates the synthesis of lipoxygenase-derived leukotrienes that results in the chemotactic attraction of neutrophils and their accumulation in the lung. In the lung, the damaged alveolar-capillary membrane leads to pulmonary edema. This effect only occurs through direct inhalation.

As noted earlier, inhaled phosgene affects primarily the lower respiratory tract, causing diffuse bronchoalveolar injury, bronchospasm, and noncardiogenic pulmonary edema. Exertion tends to decrease the latency period between phosgene inhalation and the development of pulmonary symptoms, as well as exacerbate pulmonary symptoms once they occur. Phosgene-produced pulmonary edema may begin as early as 2 to 6 hours after inhalation. Although the pulmonary edema may appear to be mild at first, it can become extensive and life threatening. Normal pulmonary lymphatic drainage may be overwhelmed by increasing pulmonary edema that leads to the development of the acute respiratory distress syndrome (ARDS) in some individuals. The onset of ARDS may be delayed for up to 48 hours after phosgene inhalation [44].

Chlorine is a greenish-yellow, noncombustible gas at room temperature and normal atmospheric pressure. It is heavier than air and gravitates to low-lying areas if released in the environment. Chlorine has a strong, pungent odor similar to bleach that is usually detectable by smell, even in low concentrations. It is a highly reactive element and, like phosgene, forms hydrochloric acid on contact with water [43].

Initial symptoms of chlorine exposure are similar to the initial symptoms following exposure to phosgene. Again, these symptoms are caused by irritation produced by the hydrochloric acid that is formed when chlorine comes into contact with tissue water. Initial symptoms occur within minutes after exposure and include burning of the eyes, redness of the conjunctivae, increased lacrimation, soreness of the throat and nasal membranes, rhinorrhea, coughing, choking, and tightness in the chest. Burning and blistering of the skin can occur shortly after contact of chlorine with exposed areas [45].

Inhalation of chlorine, even in low concentrations, causes immediate coughing and choking that can be severe. The coughing and choking tend to prevent some of the inhaled chlorine from reaching the peripheral airways and lung tissue. Thus, inhaled chlorine typically affects the upper airway primarily, causing laryngeal edema, laryngospasm, and bronchospasm. Hoarseness and aphonia may occur. Dyspnea is the first sign of upper airway involvement, followed by copious secretions, productive cough, and chest tightness. Wheezing typically occurs with bronchospasm. Individuals with a history of asthma or airway hyperactivity may have particularly severe bronchospasm. Severe bronchospasm may cause mediastinal and subcutaneous emphysema secondary to air trapping. Inhalation of high concentrations of chlorine may produce laryngospasm that is severe enough to cause sudden death [43].

Noncardiogenic pulmonary edema can occur within 2 to 4 hours following the inhalation of chlorine, especially in high concentrations [46]. Frothy sputum and rales may be the first clinical signs of pulmonary edema. Radiographic signs of pulmonary edema typically lag behind the development of clinical symptoms [47]. The development of ARDS with hypoxemic respiratory failure may eventually occur. The fluid losses associated with severe pulmonary edema and ARDS can be so profound that hypovolemic shock develops.

Management of individuals exposed to inhaled phosgene and chlorine is essentially the same. There is no specific antidote for either agent and treatment is supportive. In all cases, the patient must be removed from the contaminated environment and contaminated clothing as soon as possible. Decontamination should be performed by washing the patient with soap and copious amounts of water for 3 to 5 minutes. The eyes should be flushed with normal saline. Exertion should be minimized during transport and hospitalization.

Aggressive bronchodilator therapy with a nebulized β_2 agonist is the mainstay of therapy for bronchospasm. Nebulized ipratropium may be added if the β_2 agonist alone is ineffective. Systemic corticosteroids may be useful in the treatment of severe bronchospasm, particularly in individuals who have a history of asthma or airway hyperreactivity. Animal studies have shown that inhaled corticosteroids improve oxygenation and attenuate the development of acute lung injury, especially when given in conjunction with an inhaled bronchodilator [48]; this has not, however, been validated in humans. Thus, although systemic corticosteroids are recommended for life-threatening situations, there is no definitive clinical evidence for their efficacy in reducing the severity of acute lung injury or pulmonary edema.

Bacterial superinfection of the airways can lead to the development of severe tracheobronchitis and pneumonia 3 to 5 days after toxic irritant exposure. The presence of persistent fever, elevated white blood, or the production of thick, purulent sputum should prompt the physician to obtain cultures of sputum, blood, and any pleural fluid that is evident on chest radiograph. Empiric antibiotics should be given in accordance with the guidelines for intensive care unit patients with community-acquired pneumonia. The antibiotic regimen should be adjusted on the basis of the culture and antibiotic sensitivity results [43].

Intubation and mechanical ventilation may be required for severe bronchospasm, laryngospasm, and pulmonary edema. They are usually required for the management of ARDS and respiratory failure. Given the rapidity with which these problems can develop, preparations for intubation and mechanical ventilation should take place during the latency period, before serious respiratory problems develop. Nasotracheal intubation should not be performed because of nasal inflammation. Orotracheal intubation under direct visualization of the airways is the recommended technique. During mechanical ventilation, an appropriate amount of positive end-expiratory pressure, typically in the range of 5 to 10 cm H_2O, and inverse ratio ventilation may be helpful in improving oxygenation in patients with pulmonary edema or ARDS (see Chapters 47 and 58). In animal models, protective ventilation strategies with 6 mL per kg tidal volumes improve oxygenation, decrease shunt fraction, and improve mortality [49].

Careful attention must be given to fluid balance and the administration of intravenous fluids in patients with pulmonary edema and ARDS. Vasopressors may be required for the treatment of hypovolemic shock. Both ibuprofen and acetylcysteine aerosol have demonstrated some efficacy in preventing phosgene-induced lung injury in animal models, although there are no human clinical trials regarding their use [50,51].

Pulmonary edema that appears within 4 hours after phosgene or chlorine exposure is a poor prognostic sign. Some individuals may develop the reactive airways dysfunction syndrome (RADS) following phosgene or chlorine inhalation [52,53]. This disorder is characterized by chronic, nonspecific airway hyperreactivity that persists after the patient has recovered from the effects of an acute exposure. Patients who develop RADS should receive prompt treatment with oral prednisone (40 to 80 mg daily for 10 to 15 days) followed by treatment with a high dose of an inhaled corticosteroid, such as beclomethasone (2,000 μg per day). RADS patients should be followed closely with serial methacholine bronchial challenge testing, and the dose of oral corticosteroid should be tapered in accordance with improvements in airway hyperresponsiveness. It may take years for some individuals with RADS to show significant improvement in airway hyperresponsiveness [54]. However, most individuals who survive phosgene or chlorine exposure will recover completely with no long-term effects [43].

Nonlethal Incapacitating Agents

Chemical agents that cause temporary incapacitation are commonly classified as nonlethal agents. These chemical agents, although potentially lethal in high concentrations, are typically employed in doses that cause temporary injury or confusion to individuals or groups of individuals. They are commonly used to incapacitate unruly groups in military or riot control situations. However, they could be used in a terrorist attack. In this regard, they could be used alone, they could be used prior to an attack with conventional weapons, or they could be used in conjunction with other chemical, biological, or radiological agents of mass destruction.

The most common incapacitating agent is BZ (QNB; 3-quinuclidinyl benzilate), a competitive inhibitor of acetylcholine at postsynaptic and postjunctional muscarinic receptors. BZ is a stable, odorless, persistent crystalline solid. It is usually dispersed as a fine solid powder, although it can be dissolved in a liquid substrate and dispersed as a liquid aerosol. Both the powder and aerosolized forms can be readily ingested or inhaled. Ingestion and inhalation of BZ particles that are 1 μm in size result in bioavailabilities that are approximately 80% and 50% of a parental dose, respectively [55].

The clinical effects of BZ are similar to those of atropine, although BZ is approximately 25 times more potent and has a much longer duration of action. Symptoms of BZ exposure include mydriasis, blurred vision, dry mouth, indistinct speech, dry skin, increased deep tendon reflexes, poor coordination, decreased level of concentration, illusions, and short-term memory deficits. The most prominent central nervous system effects of BZ are related to so-called "anticholinergic delirium." The delirium typically occurs after high-dose BZ exposure and has been described as a "walking dream." This syndrome is characterized by periods of staring, unintelligible muttering, occasional shouting, and bizarre hallucinations. The degree of delirium can fluctuate frequently from minute to minute, with periods of lucidity and appropriate responses interspersed among periods of severely altered mental status [4,55].

The intensity and duration of anticholinergic symptoms associated with BZ exposure are dose-dependent, with higher doses causing more severe symptoms and a longer duration of effect. Incapacitating symptoms typically appear within 1 hour after exposure, peak at approximately 8 hours after exposure, and subside gradually during the next 48 to 72 hours. All individuals exposed to BZ should be decontaminated by washing the entire body with soap and water. Medical therapy is mostly supportive, to include control of the patient for the prevention of accidents, removal of dangerous objects from the patient's environment to prevent self-inflicted harm during delirium, moist swabs or hard candy for dryness of the mouth, keeping the room temperature at 75°F or below to prevent the development of hyperthermia, and the use of topical antibiotics and sterile dressings for abrasions of dry, parched skin. Severe signs and symptoms of BZ exposure can be treated with physostigmine. Physostigmine temporarily raises acetylcholine concentrations by binding reversibly to anticholinesterase on postsynaptic or postjunctional membranes. Physostigmine can be administered either intravenously or intramuscularly. The recommended intravenous dose is 30 μg per kg by slow infusion at a rate of 1 mg per minute. The recommended intramuscular dose is 45 μg per kg in adults and 20 μg per kg in children. The patient should be evaluated every hour for improvement in signs and symptoms, with physostigmine readministered periodically at a dose and time interval that is titrated to the severity of clinical signs. Physostigmine can cause a precipitous decrease in heart rate and patients should be carefully monitored during its administration. It should not be administered to any patient with cardiopulmonary instability, hypoxemia, electrolyte imbalance, or acid–base disturbances that predispose to cardiac dysrhythmias and seizures. It is recommended that an intravenous test dose of 1 mg be administered to adults if the diagnosis of BZ exposure is in doubt. If slight improvement is noted and there are no adverse effects within 1 hour, the full dose can be given [4,55].

Riot control agents are intended to produce unpleasant but nonpersistent medical effects. They are sometimes referred to as *irritants*. The two riot control agents most commonly used are 2-chloro-1-phenylethanone (CN or MACE; MACE Security International, Bennington, VT) and 2-chlorobenzalmalononitrile (CS or tear gas). Another product used for riot control or security is oleoresin capsaicin (OC or pepper spray). All riot control agents cause significant irritation to the eyes, upper airways, and skin. In addition to burning of the eyes and increased lacrimation, exposed individuals may experience temporary blepharospasm with transient blindness. Upper airway symptoms include rhinorrhea, sneezing, salivation, and tightness of the chest. Exposed individuals with preexisting reactive airway disease may develop bronchospasm, which can progress to respiratory failure [56]. Because riot control agents are dispersed as a solid powder, decontamination consists of getting the victims into fresh air, removing their clothing, and irrigating their eyes and mucous membranes with normal saline. Treatment is nonspecific and supportive. Most symptoms resolve in 15 to 30 minutes. Episodes of acute bronchospasm in susceptible individuals should be treated with a short-acting β_2 agonist administered by nebulizer [57].

Finally, a variety of other readily available compounds can be aerosolized and need to be considered as potential incapacitating agents. Nausea-producing agents such as diphenylaminearsine (DM or "adamsite") can produce incapacitating gastrointestinal symptoms. Psychedelic drugs, such as 3,4-methylenedioxymethamphetamine and phencyclidine, are easily obtained and could be used as aerosolized incapacitating agents. In October 2002, carfentanil, a potent aerosolized derivative of fentanyl, was probably employed in combination with halothane in an attempt by Russian authorities to release more than 800 hostages held by terrorists in Moscow's Dubrovka Theater. Unfortunately, 127 hostages in the theater died and more than 650 were hospitalized after being exposed to the chemicals that were used in the rescue attempt [58]. This is a good example of how readily available pharmaceutical agents can be used to incapacitate, or even kill, a large number of individuals.

SUMMARY

Chemical agents pose a significant threat to populations throughout the world, whether accidentally released from an industrial or transportation accident, or released intentionally as part of a crime or terrorist event. Regardless of the cause of release, they have the potential to produce a large number of casualties in a short period of time. However, the terminology *weapons of mass destruction* does not entirely reflect the impact that a terrorist attack with such agents could have on the general population. Even a relatively small number of casualties from a terrorist attack would be likely to cause significant psychological trauma, resulting in anxiety and behavioral changes among large numbers of "worried well." Such psychological trauma could significantly disrupt normal business and community activities for a long period of time. Instilling widespread fear and anxiety in the general population is a primary goal of terrorism and, unfortunately, the use of chemical agents is an efficient method of achieving that goal.

Critical care providers must be prepared to deal with the recognition, decontamination, transport, medical treatment, and psychological trauma of casualties resulting from chemical agents. They must also be prepared to protect themselves and colleagues from contamination with chemical agents during the course of patient care. Training in the medical management of chemical agent casualties and planning for mass casualty situations are essential to ensure that the best possible care is provided to the victims of a chemical exposure or chemical attack.

DECLARATION

The opinions and assertions contained herein are those of the authors and do not necessarily reflect the views or position of the Department of Veterans Affairs, Dartmouth Medical School, or the Medical University of South Carolina.

References

1. Hume EE: *Victories of Army Medicine*. Philadelphia, JB Lippincott, 1943, p 10.
2. Cieslak TJ: *Biological Warfare and Terrorism*. USA, Fort Detrick, Frederick, MD, U.S. Army Medical Research Institute of Infectious Diseases, 2000.
3. White SM: Chemical and biological weapons. Implications for anaesthesia and intensive care. *Br J Anaesth* 89:306, 2002.
4. U.S. Army Medical Research Institute of Chemical Defense: *Medical Management of Chemical Casualties Handbook*. 3rd ed. Aberdeen Proving Ground, MD, U.S. Army Medical Research Institute of Chemical Defense, 2000.
5. Smart JK: History of chemical and biological warfare: an American perspective, in Sidell FR, Takafuji ET, Franz DR (eds): *Medical Aspects of Chemical and Biological Warfare*, in Zajtchuk R, Bellamy RF (eds): *Textbook of Military Medicine, Part I: Warfare, Weaponry and the Casualty*. Washington, DC, United States Department of the Army, Office of the Surgeon General and Borden Institute, 1997, p 9.
6. Okudera H, Morita H, Iwashita T, et al: Unexpected nerve gas exposure in the city of Matsumoto; report of rescue activity in the first sarin gas terrorism. *Am J Emerg Med* 15:527, 1997.
7. Okumura T, Takasu N, Ishmatsu S, et al: Report on 640 victims of the Tokyo subway sarin attack. *Ann Emerg Med* 28:129, 1996.
8. Convention on the Prohibition of the Development, Production, Stockpiling and Use of Chemical Weapons and on their Destruction (Chemical Weapons Convention). Available at: http://www.opcw.org/chemical-weapons-convention/. Accessed September 9, 2009.
9. Mobile Chemical Agent Detector. Available at: http://www.es.northropgrumman.com/solutions/mcad/. Accessed September 9, 2009.
10. Okamura T, Suzuki K, Fukuda A, et al: The Tokyo subway sarin attack: disaster management, Part 2: hospital response. *Acad Emerg Med* 5:618, 1998.
11. Horton D, Berkowitz Z, Kaye WE: Secondary contamination of ED personnel from hazardous materials events, 1995–2001. *Am J Emerg Med* 21:199, 2003.
12. Kales SN, Christiani DC: Acute chemical emergencies. *N Engl J Med* 350:800, 2004.
13. RSDL Skin Decontamination Product. Available at: http://www.rsdecon. [illegible] Accessed September 9, 2009.
14. Walters T, Kauvar D, Reeder J, et al: Effect of reactive skin decontamination lotion on skin wound healing in laboratory rats. *Mil Med* 172:318, 2007.
15. Lindsey J: Amazing terrorism tool: new foam could revolutionize decon. *JEMS* 28:84, 2003.
16. Leikin JB, Thomas RG, Walter FG, et al: A review of nerve agent exposure for the critical care physician. *Crit Care Med* 30:2346, 2002.
17. Sidell FR: Nerve agents, in Sidell FR, Takafuji ET, Franz DR (eds): *Medical Aspects of Chemical and Biological Warfare*, in Zajtchuk R, Bellamy RF (eds): *Textbook of Military Medicine, Part I: Warfare, Weaponry and the Casualty*. Washington, DC, United States Department of the Army, Office of the Surgeon General and Borden Institute, 1997, p 129.
18. Thomas RG: Chemoterrorism: nerve agents, in Walter FB, Klein R, Thomas RG (eds): *Advanced Hazmat Life Support Provider Manual*. 3rd ed. Tucson, AZ, University of Arizona Board of Regents, 2003, p 302.
19. Chuang FR, Jang SW, Lin JL, et al: QTc prolongation indicates a poor prognosis in patients with organophosphate poisoning. *Am J Emerg Med* 14:451, 1996.
20. Nishiwaki Y, Maekawa K, Ogawa Y, et al: Effects of sarin on the nervous system in rescue team staff members and police officers 3 years after the Tokyo sarin attack. *Environ Health Perspect* 109:1169, 2001.
21. Hoffman A, Eisenkraft A, Finkelstein A, et al: A decade after Tokyo sarin attack: a review of neurological follow-up of the victims. *Mil Med* 172:607, 2007.
22. Berkenstadt H, Marganitt B, Atsmon J: Combined chemical and conventional injuries—pathophysiological, diagnostic, and therapeutic aspects. *Isr J Med Sci* 27:623, 1991.
23. Lee EC: Clinical manifestations of sarin nerve gas exposure. *JAMA* 290:659, 2003.

24. De Jong RH: Nerve gas terrorism: a grim challenge to anesthesiologists. *Anesth Analg* 96:819, 2003.
25. Cosar A, Kenar L: An anesthesiological approach to nerve agent victims. *Mil Med* 171:7, 2006.
26. Marik P, Bowles S: Management of patients exposed to biological and chemical warfare agents. *J Int Care Med* 17:147, 2002.
27. Pawar K, Bhoite R, Pillay C, et al: Continuous pralidoxime infusion versus repeated bolus injection to treat organophosphorus pesticide poisoning: a randomized controlled trial. *Lancet* 368:2136, 2006.
28. DuoDote Auto-Injector. Available at: www.duodote.com. Accessed September 12, 2009.
29. Wiener SW, Hoffman RS: Nerve agents: a comprehensive review. *J Intensive Care Med* 19:22, 2004.
30. McDonough J, McMonagle J, Copeland T, et al: Comparative evaluation of benzodiazepines for control of soman-induced seizures. *Arch Toxicol* 73:473, 1999.
31. Sidell FR, Urbanetti JS, Smith WJ, et al: Vesicants, in Sidell FR, Takafuji ET, Franz DR (eds): *Medical Aspects of Chemical and Biological Warfare*, in Zajtchuk R, Bellamy RF (eds): *Textbook of Military Medicine, Part I: Warfare, Weaponry and the Casualty*. Washington, DC, United States Department of the Army, Office of the Surgeon General and Borden Institute, 1997, p 197.
32. Emad A, Rezaian GR: The diversity of the effects of sulfur mustard gas inhalation on respiratory system 10 years after a single, heavy exposure: analysis of 197 cases. *Chest* 112:734, 1997.
33. Thomason JW, Rice TW, Milstone AP: Bronchiolitis obliterans in a survivor of a chemical weapons attack. *JAMA* 290:598, 2003.
34. Wattana M, Bey T: Mustard gas or sulfur mustard: an old chemical agent as a new terrorist threat. *Prehosp Disaster Med* 24:19, 2009.
35. Karayilanoglu T, Gunhan O, Kenar L, et al: The protective and therapeutic effects of zinc chloride and desferrioxamine on skin exposed to nitrogen mustard. *Mil Med* 168:614, 2003.
36. Freitag L, Firusian N, Stamatis G, et al: The role of bronchoscopy in pulmonary complications due to mustard gas inhalation. *Chest* 100:1436, 1991.
37. Anderson D, Holmes W, Lee R, et al: Sulfur mustard-induced neutropenia: treatment with granulocyte colony-stimulating factor. *Mil Med* 171:448, 2006.
38. Baskin SI, Brewer TG: Cyanide poisoning, in Sidell FR, Takafuji ET, Franz DR (eds): *Medical Aspects of Chemical and Biological Warfare*, in Zajtchuk R, Bellamy RF (eds): *Textbook of Military Medicine, Part I: Warfare, Weaponry and the Casualty*. Washington, DC, United States Department of the Army, Office of the Surgeon General and Borden Institute, 1997, p 271.
39. Berlin CM: The treatment of cyanide poisoning in children. *Pediatrics* 6:793, 1970.
40. Guidotti T: Acute cyanide poisoning in prehospital care: new challenges, new tools for intervention. *Prehosp Disaster Med* 21:s40, 2005.
41. BoundTree Medical. Available at: www.boundtree.com. Accessed September 15, 2009.
42. Brivet F, Delfraissy JF, Bertrand P, et al: Acute cyanide poisoning: recovery with non-specific supportive therapy. *Intensive Care Med* 9:33, 1983.
43. Urbanetti JS: Toxic inhalational injury, in Sidell FR, Takafuji ET, Franz DR (eds): *Medical Aspects of Chemical and Biological Warfare,* in Zajtchuk R, Bellamy RF (eds): *Textbook of Military Medicine, Part I: Warfare, Weaponry and the Casualty*. Washington, DC, United States Department of the Army, Office of the Surgeon General and Borden Institute, 1997, p 247.
44. Prevention and treatment of injury from chemical warfare agents. *Med Lett Drugs Ther* 44:1, 2002.
45. Kaufman J, Burkons D: Clinical, roentgenological and physiological effects of acute chlorine exposure. *Arch Environ Health* 23:29, 1971.
46. Das R, Blanc PD: Chlorine gas exposure and the lung. *Toxicol Ind Health* 9:439, 1993.
47. Bunting H: The pathology of chlorine gas poisoning, in *Fasciculus on Chemical Warfare Medicine*. Washington, DC, Committee on Treatment of Gas Casualties, National Research Council, 1945, p 24 (vol 2).
48. Wang J, Winskog E, Walther SM: Inhaled and intravenous corticosteroids both attenuate chlorine gas-induced lung injury in pigs. *Acta Anaesthesiol Scand* 49:183, 2005.
49. Parkhouse D, Brown R, Jugg B, et al: Protective ventilation strategies in the management of phosgene-induced acute lung injury. *Mil Med* 172:295, 2007.
50. Sciuto AM, Strickland PT, Kennedy TP, et al: Protective effects of N-acetylcysteine treatment after phosgene exposure in rabbits. *Am J Respir Crit Care Med* 151:768, 1995.
51. Sciuto AM, Hurt HH: Therapeutic treatments of phosgene-induced lung injury. *Inhal Toxicol* 16:565, 2004.
52. Currie GP, Ayres JG: Assessment of bronchial responsiveness following exposure to inhaled occupational and environmental agents. *Toxicol Rev* 23:75, 2004.
53. Evans RB: Chlorine: state of the art. *Lung* 183:151, 2004.
54. Malo JL, Chan-Yeung M, Lemiere C, et al: Reactive airways dysfunction syndrome and irritant induced asthma. *Up To Date* September 8, 2005, update. Available at: www.uptodate.com. Accessed February 9, 2007.
55. Ketchum JS, Sidell FR: Incapacitating agents, in Sidell FR, Takafuji ET, Franz DR (eds): *Medical Aspects of Chemical and Biological Warfare,* in Zajtchuk R, Bellamy RF (eds): *Textbook of Military Medicine, Part I: Warfare, Weaponry and the Casualty*. Washington, DC, United States Department of the Army, Office of the Surgeon General and Borden Institute, 1997, p 287.
56. Thomas R, Smith P: Riot control agents, in Roy MJ (ed): *Physician's Guide to a Terrorist Attack*. Totowa, NJ, Human Press, 2004, p 325.
57. Sidell FR: Riot control agents, in Sidell FR, Takafuji ET, Franz DR (eds): *Medical Aspects of Chemical and Biological Warfare,* in Zajtchuk R, Bellamy RF (eds): *Textbook of Military Medicine, Part I: Warfare, Weaponry and the Casualty*. Washington, DC, United States Department of the Army, Office of the Surgeon General and Borden Institute, 1997, p 307.
58. Wax PM, Becker CE, Curry SC: Unexpected "gas" casualties in Moscow: a medical toxicology perspective. *Ann Emerg Med* 41:700, 2003.

CHAPTER 215 ■ THE MANAGEMENT OF ACUTE RADIATION CASUALTIES

LAWRENCE C. MOHR JR

INTRODUCTION

It has been stated by the nation's political and military leadership that it is not a matter of "if" but "when" another terrorist attack will occur within the continental United States. Such future attacks could include the use of a radiological dispersion device, commonly called a "dirty bomb," an attack on a nuclear power plant or the detonation of a nuclear weapon. Indeed, a nuclear attack by a group of rogue terrorists is the single greatest risk to our homeland security. The objective of this chapter is to become familiar with the medical consequences of a radiological or nuclear attack and the management of casualties that could result from such an attack. It is to help you to think about the "unthinkable."

RADIOLOGICAL WEAPONS OF TERRORISM

Radiological dispersion devices, or "dirty bombs," consist of radioactive materials that are placed around a high explosive charge. The radioactive material is released and dispersed by detonation of the high explosive charge. Dirty bombs are easy to make and raw materials are readily available throughout the world. It is important to note that dirty bombs are not nuclear weapons and are not weapons of mass destruction. Their adverse health effects depend on the type and amount of explosive used, the type and amount of radioactive material used, and atmospheric conditions at the time of detonation. Most injuries from a dirty bomb will come from the blast effects of the conventional explosion [1,2]. Acute radiation health effects are very unlikely. Delayed health effects, such as the development of cancer, are also unlikely. The risk of developing cancer following a dirty bomb attack is related to the radiation exposure dose and to the amount of internal radiation that results from the inhalation, ingestion, and absorption of radioactive material through the skin or open wounds. Long-term psychological trauma is likely to occur among some members of a population who have been exposed to radioactive material from a dirty bomb [2,3].

A nuclear explosion results from nuclear fission or from thermonuclear fusion, in which a tremendous amount of energy is suddenly released in the form of heat, blast, and radiation. Human injury is caused by exposure to a combination of these three forms of energy following a nuclear detonation. The radiation exposure from a nuclear explosion can be very intense and lead to a life-threatening acute radiation syndrome, radiation burns, thermal burns, and blast injuries. Such radiation exposure can also result in the development of various types of cancer and leukemia over a period of many years if an individual survives the short-term initial effects of a nuclear explosion [4–6].

The life-threatening acute radiation syndrome may develop in some radiation-exposed individuals following a nuclear explosion. The acute radiation syndrome consists of a continuum of complex and unique medical sub-syndromes that involve the hematopoietic, gastrointestinal, and central nervous systems in a dose-related fashion. Patients who develop any of the acute radiation sub-syndromes require prompt assessment and critical care management in order to minimize loss of life. It is essential that any physician who may be called upon to treat patients following a nuclear explosion be familiar with the diagnosis and management of these unique sub-syndromes [7]. The acute radiation syndrome and its associated sub-syndromes are discussed in detail later in the chapter.

BASIC RADIATION PHYSICS

In order to understand the medical aspects of radiation exposure, it is important to review some basic principles of radiation physics. *Radiation* is defined, simply, as energy that is transmitted through space. The transmitted energy may be in the form of high-speed particles or electromagnetic waves. There are two general types of radiation: ionizing radiation and nonionizing radiation. Ionizing radiation has enough energy, so that when it interacts with an atom, it can remove tightly bound electrons from their orbits and cause the atom to become charged. Nonionizing radiation, on the other hand, does not have enough energy to remove electrons from their orbits. Ionizing radiation is more harmful to humans than nonionizing radiation and is the type of radiation that would be expected to be released in a radiological or nuclear attack.

Ionizing radiation can take four forms: alpha, beta, gamma, and neutron radiation. Alpha radiation consists of the emission of a helium nucleus from a parent nucleus, such as ^{235}Uranium; it is a particle that has an atomic mass of four and a charge of plus one. Beta radiation is the emission of a small negatively charged particle from a parent nucleus, such as ^{40}Potassium. Beta particles have a mass that is almost undetectable and a charge of minus one, similar to that of an electron. Gamma radiation is the emission of high-energy electromagnetic waves from a parent nucleus, such as ^{60}Cobalt. Gamma rays have no mass, no charge, and frequently accompany the emission of alpha or beta particles. Neutrons are very high-energy particles that are emitted from parent nuclei, such as ^{235}Uranium and ^{239}Plutonium during a nuclear chain reaction. Nuclear chain reactions can be controlled, such as the kind found in a nuclear reactor, or they can be uncontrolled, such as the type that causes a nuclear explosion. Neutrons are very damaging to human cells and tissues [8,9].

Each specific type of ionizing radiation has a different penetrating distance with respect to inert material and human tissues. Alpha particles will not penetrate paper or human skin. Indeed, you can safely hold an alpha-emitter, such as ^{240}Plutonium, in your hand as long as you do not have any breaks in the skin. However, if alpha particles are ingested, inhaled, or internalized through a break in the skin, they can do a tremendous amount of internal damage to human cells and tissues [8,9].

Beta radiation will penetrate paper, thin layers of skin, and the conjunctiva of the eye, but will not penetrate thin layers of plastic or aluminum foil. Beta particles travel relatively short distances and will be stopped by most clothing. As with alpha particles, beta radiation is more damaging to human tissues if inhaled or ingested [8,9].

Gamma rays can travel significant distances and are a highly penetrating type of ionizing radiation. They readily penetrate skin and clothing. Gamma radiation can cause considerable damage to human cells and tissues after penetration. Several inches of lead or several feet of concrete are required to stop gamma rays [8,9].

Neutrons are high-energy nuclear particles that have no charge. Neutron radiation easily penetrates skin and clothing and can cause significant damage to internal tissues and organs. Neutrons primarily cause biological damage by colliding with other particles. They transfer the most energy when they collide with particles that are about the same size, especially protons. These high-energy, subatomic collisions result in the dislodgement of both protons and tightly bound electrons from atoms that are bombarded by neutrons, with ionization of atoms in surrounding cells and tissues. Neutron radiation is extremely harmful to humans. It is not stopped by plastic, glass, or lead; it can only be stopped by several feet of concrete [8,9].

Ionizing radiation causes damage to human cells and tissues through two biological mechanisms: (i) direct high-energy damage to DNA molecules and (ii) the generation of free radicals, which secondarily damage DNA molecules by superoxide radicals generated from ionized water. The fate of irradiated human cells is dependent on the dose of radiation exposure. Low-dose exposures are characterized by DNA and cellular repair. Moderate-dose exposures are characterized by permanently damaged DNA and significantly altered cells, which may be eliminated by apoptosis, or reproduce abnormally and eventually lead to the development of cancer. High-dose radiation exposures typically result in cell death, which causes several serious, acute radiation syndromes that can result in death of the organism [10,11].

Human radiation exposure can be categorized as either external or internal. External exposure, which involves exposure to the skin, may be either whole body or partial body depending on the surface area exposed to radiation. Internal exposure may occur from the inhalation, ingestion, or transdermal penetration of radioactive material. Combined radiation injuries may also occur in cases where radiation exposure and trauma occur concurrently. In combined radiation injuries, radioactive material is introduced through open wounds [8].

RADIATION DOSES

There are two units of radiation dose that physicians must be familiar with: the Rad and the Gray. It is not essential for physicians to understand the physics that underlie the determination of these doses, but it is important for them to know that these are the units which are used to express the amount of radiation that is absorbed by human tissues. The Rad is the traditional unit of radiation absorbed dose. One Rad is defined as 100 ergs per g. The Gray (abbreviated Gy) is the newer Standard International unit of radiation exposure. One Gy is equal to 100 Rads, which is defined as 1 J per kg. One hundred centi-Gray (100 cGy) are equal to 1 Gray [12].

Radiation doses can be measured by several techniques. A radiac meter is an instrument that directly measures radiation dose using a Geiger–Müller tube or similar device. There are many different types of radiac meters, each of which may be more sensitive to specific types of radiation, such as alpha, gamma, or neutrons, than to other types of radiation. It is important, therefore, to know both the capabilities and limitations of any radiac meter that one uses to determine radiation doses. Most radiac meters in use today are highly portable and will accurately measure alpha, beta, gamma, and neutron radiation. The measurement of the lymphocyte count between 24 and 48 hours after exposure can provide a useful biological estimate of radiation dose, especially in the clinical setting [13]. The dose range in Gy and the estimated lethality associated with each dose range is illustrated in Table 215.1.

TABLE 215.1

LYMPHOCYTE COUNT BETWEEN 24 AND 48 HOURS AFTER RADIATION EXPOSURE, ESTIMATED DOSE RANGE (Gy), AND ESTIMATED LETHALITY (%)

Lymphocyte count ($\times$1,000/mm^2)	Dose range (Gy)	Lethality (%)
3.0	0–0.25	—
1.2–2.0	1–2	<5
0.4–1.2	2.0–3.5	<50
0.1–0.4	3.5–5.5	50–99
0–0.1	>5.5	99–100

From Walden TL, Farzaneh MS. Biological assessment of radiation damage, in Walker RI,, Cerveny TJ (eds): *Medical Consequences of Nuclear Warfare,* in Zajtchuk R Bellamy RF (eds): *Textbook of Military Medicine, Part I: Warfare, Weaponry and the Casualty.* Washington, DC, *United States Department of the Army, Office of the Surgeon General and Borden Institute,* 1996, p 87. Available at: http://www.usuhs.mil/afrri/outreach/pdf/tmm/chapter6/chapter6.pdf.

Chromosomal aberrations and translocations in lymphocytes can provide a useful estimate of both the type of radiation that one has been exposed to as well as the radiation dose [14]. This method requires considerable expertise in fluorescent in situ hybridization techniques as well as expertise in the interpretation of the chromosomal abnormalities. As a result, the analysis of chromosomal aberrations is primarily used as a research tool at the present time.

OVERVIEW OF RADIATION CASUALTIES

Radiation casualties consist of two general types: an acute radiation syndrome and delayed illnesses that may occur many years after radiation exposure. Acute radiation syndrome is a life-threatening condition consisting of a continuum of dose-related sub-syndromes that occur shortly after a high-dose radiation exposure, such as may occur following the detonation of a nuclear weapon. Delayed illnesses include leukemia, lymphoma, and various solid tumors, which may occur later in life following radiation exposure doses that are lower than those needed to produce acute radiation illness. In general, the higher the radiation dose, the more severe the acute effects of radiation exposure, the greater the probability of delayed illnesses, and the higher the mortality rate [4,7,15].

In considering the human dose-response to radiation exposure, a measurement known as the $LD_{50/60}$ is commonly used. The $LD_{50/60}$ is the radiation dose that causes a 50% mortality rate in an exposed population within 60 days following exposure. For whole-body radiation exposure, the $LD_{50/60}$, with no treatment, is 3 to 4 Gy. Therefore, 50% of a population that receives a radiation dose of 3 to 4 Gy will die within 60 days unless they receive treatment. With appropriate treatment and supportive care following radiation exposure, the $LD_{50/60}$ is 4 to 5 Gy [7,12].

ACUTE RADIATION SYNDROME AND SUB-SYNDROMES

Acute radiation syndrome is a continuum of dose-related organ system sub-syndromes that develop after an acute radiation exposure of greater than 1 Gy. There are three main sub-syndromes that occur: the hematopoietic sub-syndrome, the gastrointestinal sub-syndrome, and the central nervous system sub-syndrome. Each of these sub-syndromes occurs in a dose-related fashion. The hematopoietic sub-syndrome occurs with radiation exposures greater than 1 Gy. The gastrointestinal sub-syndrome occurs in addition to the hematopoietic sub-syndrome at radiation exposures greater than 6 Gy. The central nervous system sub-syndrome occurs in addition to the hematopoietic and gastrointestinal sub-syndromes at radiation exposures greater than or equal to 20 Gy.

All acute radiation sub-syndromes begin with a *prodromal phase* that lasts for 2 to 6 days. This phase is characterized by nausea, vomiting diarrhea, and fatigue. The higher the radiation dose, the more rapid the onset, and the more severe the symptoms of the prodromal phase. After 2 to 6 days of the prodromal phase, the patient enters a *latent phase*, in which he or she appears to recover and is totally asymptomatic. The latent phase lasts for several days to 1 month, with the time period inversely proportional to the radiation exposure dose, that is, the higher the dose, the shorter the latent period. After the asymptomatic latent period, the patient enters the *manifest illness phase*. This phase of acute radiation illness lasts from several days to several weeks and is characterized by the manifestation of the hematopoietic, gastrointestinal, and central nervous system sub-syndromes, according to the exposure dose that the patient received [16].

Some individuals may develop a radiation-associated multiple organ dysfunction syndrome in association with the organ-specific clinical syndromes mentioned in the previous paragraph. Multiple organ system dysfunction typically occurs in the manifest illness phase, but may also occur early after a sublethal radiation exposure. Patients with hematopoietic, gastrointestinal, central nervous system, and multiple organ dysfunction syndromes will require management in an intensive care unit [17,18].

The Hematopoietic Sub-Syndrome

The hematopoietic sub-syndrome typically occurs with a radiation dose of greater than 1 Gy. It is characterized by bone marrow suppression resulting from the radiation-induced destruction of hematopoietic stems cells within the bone marrow. Hematopoietic stem cell destruction results in pancytopenia, which is characterized by a progressive decrease in lymphocytes, neutrophils, and platelets in the peripheral blood. Both the magnitude and the time course of the pancytopenia are related to the radiation dose. In general, the higher the radiation dose, the more profound and the quicker the pancytopenia occurs [7,16].

Lymphocytic stem cells are exquisitely sensitive to radiation and circulating lymphocytes decrease rapidly following radiation exposure and remain low for a long period of time. Erythrocytic stem cells, on the other hand, seem to be more resistant to radiation than lymphocytic, neutrophilic, and thrombocytic stem cells. Therefore, the red blood cell count and hemoglobin concentration typically do not decrease to the same extent as lymphocytes, neutrophils, and platelets following radiation exposure. Hematological effects that occur in the manifest illness phase of the hematopoietic sub-syndrome following radiation exposures of 1 Gy and 3 Gy are depicted in Figure 215.1.

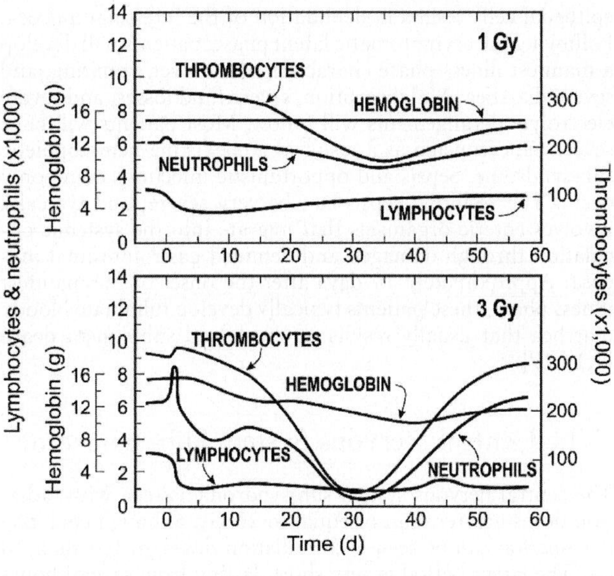

FIGURE 215.1. Hematological effects in the manifest illness phase of the hematopoietic sub-syndrome following radiation exposures of 1 and 3 Gy, respectively. [From Cerveny TJ, McVitte TJ, Young RW: Acute radiation syndrome in humans, in Walker RI, Cerveny TJ (eds): *Medical Consequences of Nuclear Warfare*, in Zajtchuk R, Bellamy RF (eds): *Textbook of Military Medicine, Part I: Warfare, Weaponry and the Casualty*. Washington, DC, United States Department of the Army, Office of the Surgeon General and Borden Institute, 1996, p 19. Available at: http://www.usuhs.mil/afrri/outreach/pdf/tmm/chapter2/chapter2.pdf. Accessed April 14, 2010.

As seen in Figure 215.1, the hematological effects of acute radiation exposure are dependent on the radiation dose. A radiation exposure of 3 Gy or more results in significant hematological effects than a radiation exposure of 1 Gy. Lymphocytes will decrease very rapidly following a radiation exposure of 3 Gy, and they will stay low for a relatively long period of time. Typically, it takes about 90 days before lymphocytes begin to recover from a 3 Gy radiation exposure. Neutrophils, after an initial period of intravascular demargination, will also begin to decline fairly rapidly following a 3 Gy exposure. Neutrophils do not fall as rapidly as lymphocytes, but between 3 and 5 days following exposure, such patients will be significantly neutropenic. Platelets also decrease steadily following a 3 Gy exposure and patients will become significantly thrombocytopenic at 2 to 3 weeks. Both platelets and neutrophils will reach a nadir, with values close to zero, at about 30 days following a 3 Gy exposure. Platelets and neutrophils then recover gradually during the next 30 days. Lymphocytes remain low for a long period of time, however, and typically do not begin to recover for at least 90 days following a 3 Gy exposure. Thus, there is a period of about a month following a 3 Gy exposure when patients will be significantly lymphopenic, neutropenic, and thrombocytopenic. Such patients are susceptible to developing serious infections and serious bleeding problems during that time [7].

The Gastrointestinal Sub-Syndrome

The gastrointestinal sub-syndrome typically occurs following a radiation dose of greater than 6 Gy. It develops as a result of radiation damage to intestinal epithelial cells. The loss of epithelial cells results in denudation of the intestinal mucosa. Following the asymptomatic latent phase, patients will develop a manifest illness phase characterized by fever, vomiting, and severe diarrhea. Malabsorption, severe fluid losses, and severe electrolyte derangements will follow. Most patients will have severe pancytopenia as a result of a coexisting hematopoietic sub-syndrome. Sepsis and opportunistic infections commonly occur. The resulting sepsis can be very severe, and typically involves enteric organisms that migrate into the systemic circulation through damaged and denuded gastrointestinal mucosa. Approximately 10 days after the onset of the manifest illness phase, these patients typically develop fulminate bloody diarrhea that usually results in shock and subsequent death [7,16,19].

The Central Nervous System Sub-Syndrome

The central nervous system sub-syndrome is seen with radiation doses greater than or equal to 20 Gy, although cognitive dysfunction can be seen with radiation doses greater than 10 Gy. The latent period is very short, lasting from several hours to 3 days. Following the asymptomatic latent period, patients typically develop nausea, vomiting, diarrhea, and confusion. Microvascular leaks in the cerebral circulation result in cerebral edema. Elevated intracranial pressure and cerebral anoxia may develop rapidly. Mental status changes develop early in the manifest illness phase and the patient eventually becomes comatose. Seizures and burning dysesthesia may occur. Patients typically die within hours after onset of the manifest illness phase of the central nervous system sub-syndrome [1,7,20,21].

Multiple Organ Dysfunction Syndrome

As mentioned previously, some patients may develop multiple organ system dysfunction following exposure to ionizing radiation. This was first reported following a 1999 nuclear accident in Japan [22–24]. Idiopathic pneumonia syndrome, acute respiratory distress syndrome, diffuse alveolar hemorrhage, fluid and electrolyte abnormalities, bacteremia, and acute renal insufficiency may occur [17]. The specific causes of radiation-associated multiple organ system dysfunction are unknown. Similarly, there is no well-defined dose–effect relationship that has been associated with its development. However, there are several clues to possible pathogenic mechanisms. It is known that whole body radiation exposure causes severe inflammation, which is probably mediated by the generation of reactive oxygen species and cytokines [25–27]. Increased permeability of blood vessels has also been observed shortly after radiation exposure [22,25]. Furthermore, hemorrhagic shock, the inability to increase oxygen consumption with adequate oxygen delivery, and sepsis, all of which may occur following radiation exposure, have been associated with multiple organ system dysfunction [25,28,29]. From a clinical perspective, it is important to understand that all of these phenomena may contribute to the unpredictable and rapid development of multiple organ system dysfunction in some patients following acute radiation exposure. Such patients will require prompt supportive care and treatment in an intensive care unit in order to maximize the potential for survival [17].

Prognosis

The prognosis of patients who develop acute radiation sub-syndromes depends on the radiation dose to which they were acutely exposed. Patients who are exposed to 1 to 2 Gy will probably survive. Survival is possible in patients who are exposed to doses of 2 to 5.5 Gy, but many of these patients will require prompt treatment and intensive care in order to survive. Survival is possible, but improbable, in patients who are exposed to doses of 5.5 to 10 Gy. Even with the most aggressive treatment, survival is extremely rare following exposure doses above 10 Gy and impossible following doses greater than 20 Gy [30].

Management

All patients should receive basic supportive care following acute radiation exposure. This consists of fluid and electrolyte balance, antiemetic agents to manage vomiting, antidiarrheal agents to manage diarrhea, proton pump inhibitors for gastrointestinal ulcer prophylaxis, pain management, psychological support, and pastoral care if death is likely. In patients with any of the acute radiation sub-syndromes, it is important not to instrument the gastrointestinal tract, since this could result in perforations that precipitate fulminate bleeding or sepsis [31,32].

Cytokine therapy with a colony-stimulating factor should be given to certain patients in order to stimulate neutrophil production in the bone marrow [30]. If there are less than 100 casualties, cytokines should be given to patients with no other injuries who have had a radiation exposure of 3 to 10 Gy. If patients in this category have multiple injuries or burns, they should receive cytokine therapy if they received a radiation dose of 2 to 6 Gy. If, on the other hand, the number of casualties is greater than 100, cytokines should be given to patients with no other injuries who have had a radiation exposure dose of 3 to 7 Gy and to patients with multiple injuries or burns who have had an exposure dose of 2 to 6 Gy [30–32].

Various types of granulocyte colony-stimulating factor (G-CSF) can be given: G-CSF (Filgrastim), pegylated G-CSF (Pegfilgrastim), or GM-CSF (Sargramostim). These are all commercially available preparations and they are all effective. The recommended doses of the various cytokines for the treatment of acute radiation sub-syndromes in adults are summarized in Table 215.2.

There are also guidelines for the use of antibiotics following acute radiation exposure [26–28]. If the total number of casualties is 100 or less, patients with no other injuries should be given antibiotics if they have been exposed to a radiation dose of 2 to 10 Gy. Patients in this category with multiple injuries or burns should be given antibiotics if they have received a radiation exposure dose of 2 to 6 Gy. In a mass casualty situation, in which there are more than 100 casualties, patients with no other injuries should be given antibiotics if they received a radiation exposure of 2 to 7 Gy. Patients in a mass casualty situation who have multiple injuries or burns should be given antibiotics if they received a radiation exposure dose of 2 to 6 Gy [30–32].

The specific antibiotic regimen used in the management of an acute radiation sub-syndrome should depend on the antibiotic susceptibilities of any specific organisms that are able to be isolated from blood or tissue cultures. It is generally recommended that a fluoroquinolone with streptococcal coverage be used, along with acyclovir or one of its congeners for viral coverage, and fluconazole for the coverage of fungi and candida. Once culture results are obtained, specific antibiotic treatment should be given according to the sensitivities of any organisms that are isolated. Antibiotics should be continued until the absolute neutrophil count is greater than 0.5×10^9 cells per L, until they are no longer effective, or for the duration indicated for specific organisms that have been isolated [30–32].

Blood transfusions are indicated for patients with an acute radiation sub-syndrome who have severe bone marrow damage or who require concurrent trauma resuscitation. The purpose

TABLE 215.2

RECOMMENDED DOSES OF CYTOKINES

Cytokine	Adults	Children	Pregnant women[a]	Precautions
G-CSF or filgrastim	Subcutaneous administration of 5 μg/kg of body weight per day, continued until ANC >1.0 × 10^2 cells/L	Subcutaneous administration of 5 μg/kg/d, continued until ANC >1.0 × 10^2 cells/L	Class C (same as adults)	Sickle-cell hemoglobinopathies, significant coronary artery disease, ARDS; consider discontinuation if pulmonary infiltrates develop at neutrophil recovery
Pegylated G-CSF or pegfilgrastim	1 subcutaneous dose, 6 mg	For adolesoents >45 kg, 1 subcutaneous dose, 6 mg	Class C (same as adults)	Sickle-cell hemoglobinopathies, significant coronary artery disease, ARDS
GM-CSF or sargramostim	Subcutaneous administration of 250 μg/m²/d, continued until ANC >1.0 × 10^2 cells/L	Subcutaneous administration of 250 μg/m²/d, continued until ANC >1.0 × 10^2 cells/L	Class C (same as adults)	Sickle-cell hemoglobinopathies, significant coronary artery disease, ARDS; consider discontinuation if pulmonary infiltrates develop at neutrophil recovery

[a]Express in biodosimetry must be consulted. Any pregnant patient with exposure to radiation should be evaluated by a health physicist and maternal-fetal specialist for an assessment of risk to the fetus. Class C refers to U.S. Food and Drug Administration Pregnancy Category C which indicates that studies have shown animal, teraragenic, or embryocidal effects, but there are no adeqate controlled studies in women; or no studies are available in animals or pregnant women.

ANC, absolute neutrophil count; ARDS, acute respiratory distress syndrome; G-CSF, granulocyte colony-stimulating factor; GM-CSF, granulocyte-macrophage colony-stimulating factor.

of blood transfusions in such patients is to provide erythrocytes for the improvement of oxygen-carrying capacity, blood volume to improve hemodynamic parameters, and platelets to help prevent bleeding. Cytokines, not blood transfusions, are used to increase absolute neutrophil counts, according to the criteria and doses previously discussed. All cellular products in the blood to be transfused should be leukoreduced and irradiated to 25 Gy in order to prevent a graft versus host reaction. Leukoreduction also helps to protect against platelet alloimmunization and the development of cytomegalovirus infections [17,30].

Stem cell bone marrow transplantation should be considered for certain patients with acute radiation illness. Allogenic stem cell transplantation is indicated for individuals who have a radiation exposure dose of 7 to 10 Gy. If a patient is fortunate enough to [illegible] or a syngenetic donor, preferably an identical twin, stem cell transplantation should be considered if they have had radiation exposure doses of 4 to 10 Gy [30,31].

ACUTE RADIATION ILLNESS AND TRAUMA

The blast from a nuclear detonation can produce powerful, high-pressure winds that have greater velocities than the most powerful hurricane winds. These winds can extend miles from the point of detonation. They can cause large numbers of seriously injured casualties from missiles caused by flying debris or from individuals being blown against objects in the environment.

The combination of an acute radiation syndrome and trauma presents some special challenges to the physician. There is a significant increase in mortality among patients who have this combination of illness and injury and such patients require prompt medical and surgical care in order to survive. They should receive the standard treatment for acute radiation syndromes, as described earlier. They are also very susceptible to operative and postoperative infections as a result of decreased neutrophil and lymphocyte counts and require 2 to 3 months for the bone marrow to recover after acute radiation exposure. This greatly complicates the management of such patients, especially those with multiple, serious injuries. Most importantly, if a patient with a combination of an acute radiation syndrome and trauma requires surgery, the operation should be performed within 48 hours after the initial radiation exposure. If surgery is not performed in this "window of opportunity" following acute radiation exposure, it may have to be postponed for up to 2 to 3 months [31,33]. Therefore, all radiation-exposed patients with life-threatening traumatic injuries should be transported to a surgical care facility and receive emergency surgery as soon as possible within the 48-hour "window."

ACUTE RADIATION DERMATITIS

An acute radiation dermatitis may occur in conjunction with acute radiation illness. The symptoms and signs of acute radiation dermatitis typically appear several days *after* an acute radiation exposure. Although acute radiation dermatitis is essentially a radiation burn, it is different from the thermal burns that may occur *immediately* after exposure of the skin to a nuclear explosion. In this regard, radiation burns and thermal burns are different. Exposure of the skin to radiation causes loss of the epidermal layer at radiation doses greater than 2 Gy. This leads to erythema and blisters. Loss of the dermis occurs at radiation exposure doses of greater than 10 Gy, and this results in the development of skin ulcers. Skin ulcerations that result from radiation doses greater than 10 Gy heal very slowly over a period of many months, if they heal at all. Chronic skin ulcers in patients with acute radiation illness predispose these patients to the development of serious infections. Such ulcers should be debrided early in their development to help prevent infection. Topical antibiotics, such as mafenide acetate or silver sulfadiazine, should be applied prophylactically. However, since these topical antibiotics can cause neutropenia, they should be used judiciously with careful monitoring of the absolute neutrophil count in severely neutropenic patients. Although no studies have been conducted on the efficacy of skin grafting in radiation burn patients, it is recommended that an attempt should be made to graft full-thickness burns and ulcers [33,34].

INTERNAL CONTAMINATION

In the assessment of patients with acute radiation exposure, it is important to ascertain whether or not they have experienced any internal contamination. Internal radiation contamination can occur by the inhalation, ingestion, or the transdermal penetration of radioactive material. It can occur via a variety of portals, such as the nose, the mouth, a wound, or, with a large enough dose, by the penetration of gamma rays or neutrons directly through intact skin. Internal organs commonly affected by internal radiation contamination are the thyroid, the lung, the liver, adipose tissue, and bone. These are the areas where radioactive isotopes tend to accumulate within the human body. Leukemia and various types of cancers can develop in these organs many years after an acute radiation exposure with internal contamination.

Assessment of Potential Internal Radiation Contamination

The patient history is crucial to determining whether or not they may have experienced internal contamination. Any history which suggests that a patient may have inhaled, ingested, or internalized radioactive material through open wounds should prompt further evaluation for internal contamination. This assessment should attempt to identify both the radiation dose received and, if possible, the specific isotopes that cause the internal contamination. An initial survey of the patient should be performed with a radiac meter, especially around the mouth, nose, and wounds, to give some idea of the extent of any possible internal exposure. The diction of radioactive isotopes on nasal swabs can be very helpful to determine whether or not a patient has been exposed internally. If it is suspected that a person has inhaled a significant amount of radioactive material, bronchoalveolar lavage can be considered for the purposes of identifying inhaled radioactive isotopes as well as for removing residual radioisotopes from the lungs. Bronchoalveolar lavage has been shown to be effective in removing inhaled radioactive isotopes from the lungs of animals. The collection of stool and urine samples can be very helpful in determining both the type and the amount of internal radiation that an individual might have received. Chest and whole-body radiation counts can also be helpful in determining the extent of any internal radiation contamination. Unfortunately, however, most medical institutions do not have the capability to do either chest or whole-body radiation counts. The analysis of nasal swabs, stool samples, and urine samples are the most practical methods of determining the type and extent of internal radiation contamination by hospital-based physicians [35,36].

Treatment of Internal Radiation Contamination

Patients who have experienced internal radiation contamination should be promptly treated in order to reduce the absorbed radiation dose and prevent the development of future health problems. The goals of treatment are to reduce absorption and enhance elimination of the internal radionuclide contaminant. There are three main categories of agents that are used to treat internal radiation contamination: purgative agents, blocking agents, and chelation agents. Specific agents are used to treat internal contamination by specific radioactive isotopes. Such treatment is most effective when given as soon as possible after the radiation exposure. Gastric lavage can be used to empty the stomach completely after the potential ingestion of radionuclides. If promptly performed, it could decrease the concentration of radionuclides in the gastrointestinal tract. This could result in a decrease of the absorbed radiation dose. In deciding whether or not to treat a patient for internal radiation contamination, the physician may need to act on preliminary information and may have to treat potentially exposed individuals empirically, based on the information that is available [35,36].

Purgative Agents

Purgative agents help to remove radionuclides from the gastrointestinal tract. The most common purgatives are laxatives and enemas, which are helpful in reducing the residence time of radionuclides in the colon. Prussian blue (ferric ferrocyanide) is an ion exchange resin that binds ^{137}cesium in the gastrointestinal tract and facilitates its secretion. Patients who have experienced internal ^{137}cesium contaminate should be treated with oral Prussian blue (3 g, three times daily) for at least 3 weeks. Aluminum phosphate binds ^{90}strontium in the gastrointestinal tract. A single, 100 mL oral dose of aluminum phosphate gel will reduce the gastrointestinal absorption of ^{90}strontium by 85%. Oral aluminum phosphate should be used if internal contamination with ^{90}strontium is expected [35,36].

Blocking Agents

Blocking agents block both the uptake and bioavailability of internal radionuclide contaminants. The most important blocking agent is potassium iodide, which is used for the treatment of internal contamination with $^{125/131}$iodine. Potassium iodide blocks the uptake of radioactive iodine by increasing the uptake of nonradioactive isotope. Since the thyroid gland is very sensitive to the effects of internal contamination with $^{125/131}$iodine, potassium iodine should be given as soon as possible after radioactive iodine exposure. It is recommended that patients take 300 mg of potassium iodide per day for 7 to 14 days following a potential $^{125/131}$iodine exposure. Potassium iodide can also be taken prophylactically if there is sufficient warning of a potential $^{125/131}$iodine exposure. The standard prophylactic regimen is a single 130 mg dose of potassium iodide [35,36].

Chelation Agents

Chelation agents are the mainstay of treatment for internal radiation contamination. Chelation agents are substances that bind strongly with certain metals to form a stable, soluble complex that can be excreted by the kidneys. Diethylenetriaminepentaacetic acid (DTPA) is the most effective and commonly recommended chelation agent for the treatment of internal radiation contamination. DTPA complexes are very stable and water soluble and are unlikely to release bound radionuclides prior to renal excretion. DTPA chelation therapy is especially effective for the treatment of internal radiation contamination with ^{241}americium, ^{60}cobalt, and ^{239}plutonium. DTPA is administered as an intravenous solution of 1 g dissolved in 250 mL of saline or 5% glucose, infused over 1 hour per day for up to 5 days. DTPA can be used for the treatment of all internal radiation contaminants except $^{238-235}$uranium. The use of DTPA is contraindicated for treatment of $^{238-235}$uranium contamination because of an increased risk of renal damage. It is

TABLE 215.3

AGENTS USED TO TREAT COMMON INTERNAL RADIATION CONTAMINANTS

Radionuclide	Primary toxicity	Treatment	Agent category	Route
^{241}Americium	Bone, liver	DTPA	Chelation	IV infusion
^{137}Cesium	Total body	Prussian blue	Purgative	Oral
^{60}Cobalt	Total body	DTPA	Chelation	IV infusion
$^{125/131}$Iodine	Thyroid	Potassium iodide blocking	Oral	
^{239}Plutonium	Bone, lung	DTPA	Chelation	IV infusion
^{210}Polonium	Lung, kidney	Dimercaprol	Chelation	IM injection
^{90}Strontium	Bone	Aluminum phosphate	Purgative	Oral
$^{238-235}$Uranium	Kidney	$NaHCO_3$ and diuretic	Chelation	Oral

recommended that internal contamination with $^{238-235}$uranium be treated with oral sodium bicarbonate, with the dose regulated to maintain an alkaline urine pH. Excretion of $^{238-235}$uranium can be enhanced with the addition of a diuretic, such as furosemide [35,36].

Dimercaprol is a chelation agent that is particularly useful for the treatment of internal contamination with ^{210}polonium. Dimercaprol has been used for many years as an effective chelation agent for mercury poisoning. For ^{210}polonium contamination, 5 mg per kg of dimercaprol should be given initially, followed by 2.5 mg per kg two times daily for 10 days. Dimercaprol should be given by deep intramuscular injection only; it should not be given intravenously. Dimercaprol is very nephrotoxic and should always be used with caution. It is recommended that oral sodium bicarbonate be given to maintain an alkaline urine pH, which decreases the risk of nephrotoxicity by preventing the dissociation of the dimercaprol-^{210}polonium complex in the urine. Serum creatinine and urine pH should be carefully monitored during treatment with dimercaprol [35,36].

Need for Rapid Treatment

In order to be most effective, treatment for internal contamination should begin within hours after the radiation exposure. Early information on the history of a radiation exposure incident may or may not identify the major isotopes involved. Patients will likely present with no clinical symptoms other than conventional trauma. Therefore, critical decisions regarding the initial, empirical treatment of potential internal radiation contamination may have to be based on the historical information that is provided. It is imperative that physicians who could be involved in the management of radiation casualties be familiar with the agents used for treatment of the most likely internal radiation contaminants. These agents are summarized in Table 215.3.

DECONTAMINATION

In order to prevent contamination of other patients and medical staff, radiation casualties must be decontaminated prior to admission to a hospital. However, life-saving emergency medical care should be performed as soon as possible and before decontamination takes place. Therefore, a special emergency treatment area, where potentially contaminated patients can be treated and stabilized, will have to be set up outside the hospital. Once a patient has been stabilized, decontamination can occur in another specially designated area that is also outside the hospital. It is recommended that the designated decontamination area be at least 50 yards downwind from the hospital or other treatment area.

All healthcare workers should protect themselves with scrubs, gowns, masks, double gloves, and shoe covers during the treatment and decontamination of radiation casualties. These measures provide sufficient protection from any radioactive isotopes that could be contaminating a patient. It is recommended that healthcare workers continue to observe these measures after decontamination of a radiation casualty, since it is possible that the decontamination could be incomplete and residual radioactive material could remain on the patient. Similarly, it is best to assume that every patient in close proximity to a radiation-exposure event is contaminated, even if no radiation is detected by a radiac meter. Such patients should be decontaminated as usual and members of the decontamination team and medical treatment staff should wear protective clothing.

The decontamination process is quite simple. All of the patient's clothing must be removed and discarded into a clearly labeled and secure container, so that it does not further contaminate people and surroundings after removal. If the clothing needs to be cut off the patient, the scissors should be washed with soap and water between each cut to avoid spreading contamination on subsequent cuts. After all clothing has been removed, the patient is thoroughly washed with soap and water. This simple soap-and-water process has been shown to be effective in removing more than 95% of residual radioactive material from radiation-exposed patients [37].

Once a radiation-exposed patient has been stabilized and decontaminated, he or she should be admitted to the hospital or other treatment facility for definitive care. Again, it is best to assume that hospitalized radiation-exposed patients may still be contaminated, even after the decontamination process has been completed. Thus, it is recommended that all radiation casualties be admitted to specially designated areas of the hospital and that the staff in these areas wear appropriate protective clothing, as described earlier.

Patients exposed to potentially life-threatening doses of radiation will require critical care management during the manifest illness phase of an acute radiation sub-syndrome. In order to reduce the potential of radioactive contamination, it is recommended that such patients be cared for in specially designated areas of intensive care units or in a designated hospital area that has been converted to an intensive care unit for the management of radiation casualties.

References

1. McCann DGC: Radiation poisoning: Current concepts in the acute radiation syndrome. *Am J Clin Med* 3:13, 2006.
2. Radiation dispersion device and industrial contamination situations, in *Medical Management of Radiological Casualties*. 2nd ed. Bethesda, MD, Armed Forces Radiobiology Research Institute, 2003, p 41. Available at: http://www.afrri.usuhs.mil/outreach/pdf/2edmmrchandbook.pdf. Accessed April 14, 2010.
3. Mickley AG: Psychological factors in nuclear warfare, in Walker RI, Cerveny TJ (eds): *Medical Consequences of Nuclear Warfare,* in Zajtchuk R, Bellamy RF (eds): *Textbook of Military Medicine, Part I: Warfare, Weaponry and the Casualty*. Washington, DC, United States Department of the Army, Office of the Surgeon General and Borden Institute, 1996, p 165. Available at: http://www.usuhs.mil/afrri/outreach/pdf/tmm/chapter8/chapter8.pdf. Accessed April 14, 2010.
4. Walden TL: Long-term and low-level effects of ionizing radiation, in Walker RI, Cerveny TJ (eds): *Medical Consequences of Nuclear Warfare*, in Zajtchuk R, Bellamy RF (eds): *Textbook of Military Medicine, Part I: Warfare, Weaponry and the Casualty*. Washington, DC, United States Department of the Army, Office of the Surgeon General and Borden Institute, 1996, p 19. Available at: http://www.usuhs.mil/afrri/outreach/pdf/tmm/chapter9/chapter9.pdf. Accessed April 14, 2010.
5. Carcinogenesis, in *Medical Management of Radiological Casualties*. 2nd ed. Bethesda, MD, Armed Forces Radiobiology Research Institute, 2003, p 4. Available at: http://www.afrri.usuhs.mil/outreach/pdf/2edmmrchandbook/pdf. Accessed April 14, 2010.
6. Hoel DG, Li P: Threshold models in radiation carcinogenesis. *Health Phys* 75:107, 1998.
7. Cerveny TJ, McVitte TJ, Young RW: Acute radiation syndrome in humans, in Walker RI, Cerveny TJ (eds): *Medical Consequences of Nuclear Warfare*, in Zajtchuk R, Bellamy RF (eds): *Textbook of Military Medicine, Part I: Warfare, Weaponry and the Casualty*. Washington, DC, United States Department of the Army, Office of the Surgeon General and Borden Institute, 1996, p 19. Available at: http://www.usuhs.mil/afrri/outreach/pdf/tmm/chapter2/chapter2.pdf. Accessed April 14, 2010.
8. Types of ionizing radiation, in *Medical Management of Radiological Casualties*. 2nd ed. Bethesda, MD, Armed Forces Radiobiology Research Institute, 2003, p 4. Available at: http://www.afrri.usuhs.mil/outreach/pdf/2edmmrchandbook.pdf. Accessed April 14, 2010.
9. Radiation, in *Principles of Nuclear Physics*. Sandia Base, Albuquerque, New Mexico, Atomic Weapons Training Group, 1960, p 86.
10. Begg AC: Radiobiology: State of the present art. A conference report. *Int J Radiat Biol* 86:71, 2010.
11. Sedelnikova OA, Redon CE, Dickey JS, et al: Role of oxidatively induced DNA lesions in human pathogenesis. *Mutat Res* 704:152, 2010.
12. Units of radiation, in *Medical Management of Radiological Casualties*. 2nd ed. Bethesda, MD, Armed Forces Radiobiology Research Institute, 2003, p 6. Available at: http://www.afrri.usuhs.mil/outreach/pdf/2edmmrchandbook.pdf. Accessed April 14, 2010.
13. Walden TL, Farzaneh MS: Biological assessment of radiation damage, in Walker RI, Cerveny TJ (eds): *Medical Consequences of Nuclear Warfare,* in Zajtchuk R, Bellamy RF (eds): *Textbook of Military Medicine, Part I: Warfare, Weaponry and the Casualty*. Washington, DC, United States Department of the Army, Office of the Surgeon General and Borden Institute, 1996, p 87. Available at: http://www.usuhs.mil/afrri/outreach/pdf/tmm/chapter6/chapter6.pdf. Accessed April 14, 2010.
14. Agrawala PK, Adhikari JS, Chaudhury NK: Lymphocyte chromosomal aberration assay in radiation biodosimetry. *J Pharm Bioall Sci* 2:197, 2010.
15. Anno GH, Young RW, Bloom RM, et al: Dose response relationships for acute ionizing-radiation lethality. *Health Phys* 84:565, 2003.
16. Berger ME, Christensen DM, Lowry PC, et al: Medical management of radiation injuries: current approach. *Occup Med* 56:162, 2006.
17. Jackson WL, Gallhager G, Myhand RC, et al: Medical management of patients with multiple organ dysfunction arising from acute radiation syndrome. *BJR Suppl* 27:161, 2005.
18. Meineke V, Fliedner TM: Radiation-induced multi-organ involvement and failure: challenges for radiation accident medical management and future research. *BJR Suppl* 27:196, 2005.
19. Gastrointestinal kinetics, in *Medical Management of Radiological Casualties*. 2nd ed. Bethesda, MD, Armed Forces Radiobiology Research Institute, 2003, p 11. Available at: http://www.afrri.usuhs.mil/outreach/pdf/2edmmrchandbook.pdf. Accessed April 14, 2010.
20. Clinical acute radiation syndrome, in *Medical Management of Radiological Casualties*. 2nd ed. Bethesda, MD, Armed Forces Radiobiology Research Institute, 2003, p 15. Available at: http://www.afrri.usuhs.mil/outreach/pdf/2edmmrchandbook.pdf. Accessed April 14, 2010.
21. Centers for Disease Control and Prevention. Acute Radiation Syndrome: A Fact Sheet for Physicians. March 18, 2005. Available at: http://www.bt.cdc.gov/radiation. Accessed April 18, 2010.
22. Akashi M, Hirama T, Tanosaki S, et al: Initial symptoms of acute radiation syndrome in the JCO criticality accident in Tokai-mura. *J Radiat Res* 42[Suppl]:S1, 57, 2001.
23. Ishii T, Futami S, Nishida M, et al: Brief note and evaluation of acute-radiation syndrome and treatment of a Tokai-mura criticality accident patient. *J Radiat Res* (Supplement) 42:S1, 67, 2001.
24. Hirama T, Tanosaki S, Kandatsu S, et al: Initial medical management of patients severely irradiated in the Tokai-mura criticality accident. *Br J Radiol* 76:246, 2003.
25. Akashi M: Role of infection and bleeding in multiple organ involvement and failure. *BJR Suppl* 27:17, 2005.
26. Akashi M, Hachiya M, Osawa Y, et al: Irradiation induces WAF1 expression through a p53-independent pathway in KG-1 cells. *J Biol Chem* 270:19181, 1995.
27. Akashi M, Hachiya M, Paquette RL, et al: Irradiation increases manganese superoxide dismutase mRNA levels in human fibroblasts. Possible mechanisms for its accumulation. *J Biol Chem* 270:15864, 1995.
28. Rhee P, Waxman K, Clark L, et al: Tumor necrosis factor and monocytes are released during hemorrhagic shock. *Resuscitation* 25:249, 1993.
29. Moore FA, Sauaia A, Moore EE: Postinjury multiple organ failure: a bimodal phenomenon. *J Trauma* 40:501, 1996.
30. Waselenko JK, MacVittie TJ, Blakely WF, et al: Medical management of acute radiation syndrome: Recommendations of the Strategic National Stockpile Radiation Working Group. *Ann Intern Med* 140:1037, 2004.
31. Dons RF, Cerveny TJ: Triage and treatment of radiation-injured casualties, in Walker RI, Cerveny TJ (eds): *Medical Consequences of Nuclear Warfare,* in Zajtchuk R, Bellamy RF (eds): *Textbook of Military Medicine, Part I: Warfare, Weaponry and the Casualty*. Washington, DC, United States Department of the Army, Office of the Surgeon General and Borden Institute, 1996, p 19. Available at: http://www.usuhs.mil/afrri/outreach/pdf/tmm/chapter3/chapter3.pdf. Accessed April 14, 2010.
32. Management protocol for acute radiation syndrome, in *Medical Management of Radiological Casualties*. 2nd ed. Bethesda, MD, Armed Forces Radiobiology Research Institute, 2003, p 27. Available at: http://www.afrri.usuhs.mil/outreach/pdf/2edmmrchandbook.pdf. Accessed April 14, 2010.
33. Blast and thermal biological effects, in *Medical Management of Radiological Casualties*. 2nd ed. Bethesda, MD, Armed Forces Radiobiology Research Institute, 2003, p 33. Available at: http://www.afrri.usuhs.mil/outreach/pdf/2edmmrchandbook.pdf. Accessed April 14, 2010.
34. Walker RI: Infectious complications of radiation injury, in Walker RI, Cerveny TJ (eds): *Medical Consequences of Nuclear Warfare,* in Zajtchuk R, Bellamy RF (eds): *Textbook of Military Medicine, Part I: Warfare, Weaponry and the Casualty*. Washington, DC, United States Department of the Army, Office of the Surgeon General and Borden Institute, 1996, p 19. Available at: http://www.usuhs.mil/afrri/outreach/pdf/tmm/chapter5/chapter5.pdf. Accessed April 14, 2010.
35. Cerveny TJ: Treatment of internal radionuclide contamination, in Walker RI, Cerveny TJ (eds): *Medical Consequences of Nuclear Warfare,* in Zajtchuk R, Bellamy RF (eds): *Textbook of Military Medicine, Part I: Warfare, Weaponry and the Casualty*. Washington, DC, United States Department of the Army, Office of the Surgeon General and Borden Institute, 1996, p 19. Available at: http://www.usuhs.mil/afrri/outreach/pdf/tmm/chapter4/chapter4.pdf. Accessed April 14, 2010.
36. Internal contamination, in *Medical Management of Radiological Casualties*. 2nd ed. Bethesda, MD, Armed Forces Radiobiology Research Institute, 2003, p 54. Available at: http://www.afrri.usuhs.mil/outreach/pdf/2edmmrchandbook.pdf. Accessed April 14, 2010.
37. General aspects of decontamination, in *Medical Management of Radiological Casualties*. 2nd ed. Bethesda, MD, Armed Forces Radiobiology Research Institute, 2003, p 68. Available at: http://www.afrri.usuhs.mil/outreach/pdf/2edmmrchandbook.pdf. Accessed April 14, 2010.

CHAPTER 216 ■ PLANNING AND ORGANIZATION FOR EMERGENCY MASS CRITICAL CARE

JAMES GEILING, ROBERT M. GOUGELET AND LAWRENCE C. MOHR JR

HOSPITAL AND COMMUNITY DISASTER RESPONSE

The Importance of Hospitals in Disaster Response

Hospitals and their critical care units play important roles in a community's response to a disaster, whether the disaster is sudden in nature, such as an explosion, or a more prolonged event, such as pandemic influenza. First of all, hospitals are the major source of a community's medical care and provide rapid access to health care. Most likely, the first response of an individual with a disaster-related medical problem will be to go to the closest hospital. Similarly, emergency medical system ambulances will routinely transport critically ill or injured patients to the nearest hospital. Second, hospitals are capable of managing critically ill or injured patients in a timely manner if adequate staff and resources are available. Third, it is especially difficult to provide critical care outside of the hospital setting during a disaster. For example, it may be possible to provide medical care in a building of opportunity, such as a school gymnasium, for low-acuity patients. However, providing critical care in such a setting would require significant amounts of medical equipment, supplies, and specially trained staff. It would be logistically difficult, costly, and time consuming to move critical care resources to a nonhospital facility during a disaster. Finally, hospitals which are accredited by the Joint Commission or other accrediting agencies must meet specific requirements for disaster preparedness. These requirements include continuity-of-operations plans, an internal operations center with an incident command structure, and the planning and conduct of disaster response exercises in coordination with the neighboring community.

In summary, the hospital is the major healthcare asset in disaster response and is likely to be the only facility where critical care is provided. In order to maintain its capability to respond to the most critical patients during a disaster, the hospital must be part of a community-based healthcare response system that can be efficiently mobilized during a catastrophic event.

The large numbers of patients requiring care immediately after a disaster, the continued flow of patients during a prolonged disaster, or the loss of hospital infrastructure as a result of a disaster, all have the potential to overwhelm available resources at any hospital. Thus, it is possible that there will be limits to the number of patients that can be cared for and the level of care that can be provided by a hospital during a catastrophic event.

Surge capacity generally refers to the ability to manage a sudden or prolonged increase in numbers of patients that would otherwise severely challenge or exceed the present capacity of the facility. Medical surge capacity may be defined, more technically, as "the quantifiable amount of community or regional resources and services available for providing medical care in emergencies that overwhelm the normal medical infrastructure" [1]. To provide adequate surge capacity and maintain medical system resiliency during disasters, hospitals and communities must have medical preparedness plans, as well as carefully planned command and control systems that will efficiently manage the medical response.

Local Community Medical Response

Incident Command Systems

In the United States, both hospitals and community governments are required to adhere to the requirements of the National Incident Management System, which is managed by the Federal Emergency Management Agency [2]. This includes the requirement that both hospitals and communities have an Incident Command System (ICS) [3]. The currently used ICS model for disaster response is a modular system that follows the basic principles of organizational leadership, with one person in charge of a command section that supervises the activities of 3 to 7 subsections. Most ICS structures have five principal components:

1. *Leadership*—This is the command section, chaired by the leader of the response effort (the incident commander). The incident commander is supported by special staff, such as public affairs, public safety, legal counsel, etc.
2. *Operations*—This section oversees and coordinates the immediate response and ongoing operational activities. This tends to be the most active section during a disaster.
3. *Planning*—This section assesses the potential for future events, develops contingency plans for future events, and plans timelines for the deployment of critical resources. These planning activities permit the operations branch to focus on managing the response to active events.
4. *Logistics*—This section focuses on the logistical support that every event requires, including equipment, personnel, supplies, and infrastructure support.
5. *Finance*—This section accounts for and manages all money that is spent during responding to a disaster. While immediate costs and purchases during a disaster tend to be supported by affected communities and hospitals, accurate purchasing records, inventory records, personnel costs, and transportation costs must be carefully managed in order to recoup costs after the event.

The Hospital Incident Command System (HICS) manages the response within the hospital and coordinates the hospital's efforts with the overall community response. The HICS is led by an incident commander within the hospital. The hospital's incident commander and the community incident commander communicate with each other directly through telephone, radio, computer, or via liaison personnel. The organization and leadership of the HICS is usually different than organizational structure and leadership of day-to-day hospital operations [4]. What works for managing the daily business of a hospital oftentimes does not work well for managing the response to a crisis. Therefore, hospitals, and their intensive care units (ICUs), must assign personnel to specific HICS positions as part of their disaster preparedness planning. Each individual assigned to an HICS position has specific duties that must be performed prior to, during, and following the disaster response. It is imperative that all HICS personnel be fully trained for the duties they are required to perform.

Modular Emergency Medical Systems

The Modular Emergency Medical System, or MEMS, is a community emergency medical care system consisting of temporary facilities that can be quickly set up to supplement hospital care during a disaster. This system provides a conceptual framework for managing a surge in patients who require screening, triage, antibiotic treatment, immunizations, prophylaxis, or noncritical inpatient care. The MEMS helps hospitals to maximize their critical care capacity during a disaster by providing temporary, alternate facilities that can care for noncritical patients in their respective communities.

The major MEMS components are Neighborhood Emergency Help Centers (NEHC) and Acute Care Centers (ACC). Both types of centers can provide screening and triage. The NEHC provides routine, nonurgent outpatient care. The ACC can provide inpatient care to acutely ill noncritical patients. The ACC can receive patients directly from the incident, or be a facility to which hospitals can offload stable inpatients in order to free up hospital critical care bed space during overwhelming events. Local or regional authorities can open an NEHC or an ACC under two scenarios: (i) when a federal public health incident or a federal disaster is declared or (ii) when the state governor has issued a state of emergency. Both types of temporary facilities will operate under the command and control of the local community ICS with support from a Regional Multiagency Command [5].

How Does Critical Care Fit into the MEMS Plan?

The hospital is only place where critical care can be provided immediately after a disaster. Therefore, the community's medical surge plan must address how to protect the hospital from being overwhelmed with patients during a disaster. A carefully executed MEMS plan allows hospitals to offload stable patients to an ACC. This will help to prevent the hospital from being overwhelmed during a disaster and allow the hospital to expand its critical care capabilities by utilizing non-ICU hospital beds for critical care, if necessary.

Refining Surge Capacity

Hick and colleagues suggest a classification for surge capacity that may aid hospitals and communities in their planning for a major disaster [6]. They categorize surge capacity into three levels:

- *Conventional capacity*—This level would be implemented in major mass-casualty incidents that trigger activation of the hospital emergency operations plan. The resources used (spaces, staff, and supplies) would be consistent with the hospital's usual care levels.
- *Contingency capacity*—This level would be used temporarily during a major mass casualty incident, or on a longer-term basis during a disaster whose medical demands exceeded community resources. The resources would require adaptations to medical care spaces, staffing constraints, and supply shortages, but without significant impact on the medical care that is delivered.
- *Crisis capacity*—This level would be implemented in catastrophic situations that result in a significant impact on standard of medical care that can be provided. Severe limitations of space, staff, and supplies would not allow hospitals to provide the usual standard of medical care. If surge capacity reaches the crisis level, resources would be allocated in a way that facilitates the best possible medical care with the limited resources that are available.

It is recommended that hospitals and their critical care units develop disaster preparedness plans that contain specific criteria for each level of surge capacity. It is important to note that the same disaster event might have very different effects on different hospitals, depending on the institution's size. For example, an eight-victim automobile crash may require a conventional level of surge capacity for a large hospital that has a level 1 trauma center, but could require a contingency or crisis level of surge capacity for a small community hospital.

CRITICAL CARE IN DISASTERS

Current Status

From 2002 to 2007, the Hospital Preparedness Program of the U.S. Department of Health and Human Services spent $2.2 billion to support medical preparedness goals, which included improvement of hospital surge capabilities [7]. However, in 2008 the U.S. General Accounting Office reported that many states are still not adequately prepared to respond effectively to a catastrophic event, such as pandemic influenza, in which medical resources could become overwhelmed and there would be a need to change the way medical care is provided by altering or adjusting the care pathways [8]. During a major disaster, nothing will challenge hospitals more than attempting to provide high-quality critical care with limited resources.

Traditionally, most hospitals have focused their disaster planning on trauma care capabilities. However, the advent of severe acute respiratory syndrome (SARS) and the risk of an H1N1 influenza pandemic have caused hospitals to consider their overall critical care capability, to include medical critical care, as an important component of disaster response plans. For example, it is estimated that without adequate critical care resources during the 2003 SARS outbreak in Toronto, the case fatality rate would have been approximately 20%, compared to the 6.5% case fatality rate that actually occurred [9]. These data highlight the importance of including the overall critical care capabilities of hospitals in disaster planning efforts, not just the capabilities for trauma care.

At present, it is estimated that the average daily occupancy rate of critical care beds in the United States is 65%. This suggests that some hospitals may have the capability to expand critical care services during a disaster, assuming that staff and supplies are available [10]. However, even with normal excess capacity, there does not appear to be a sufficient number of critical care beds to meet the demands of a pandemic that might affect the entire nation at the same time. It is estimated that critically ill patients who are not cared for in an ICU have a threefold mortality rate compared with those who are cared for in an ICU [11]. Thus, if critical care capabilities become overwhelmed by large numbers of critically ill or injured patients during a disaster, high mortality rates are likely to occur.

Surging Assets to Optimize Critical Care Capability

In planning for surge capacity during disasters, hospitals need to prepare for events that have a sudden impact and are of relatively short duration, such as transportation accidents,

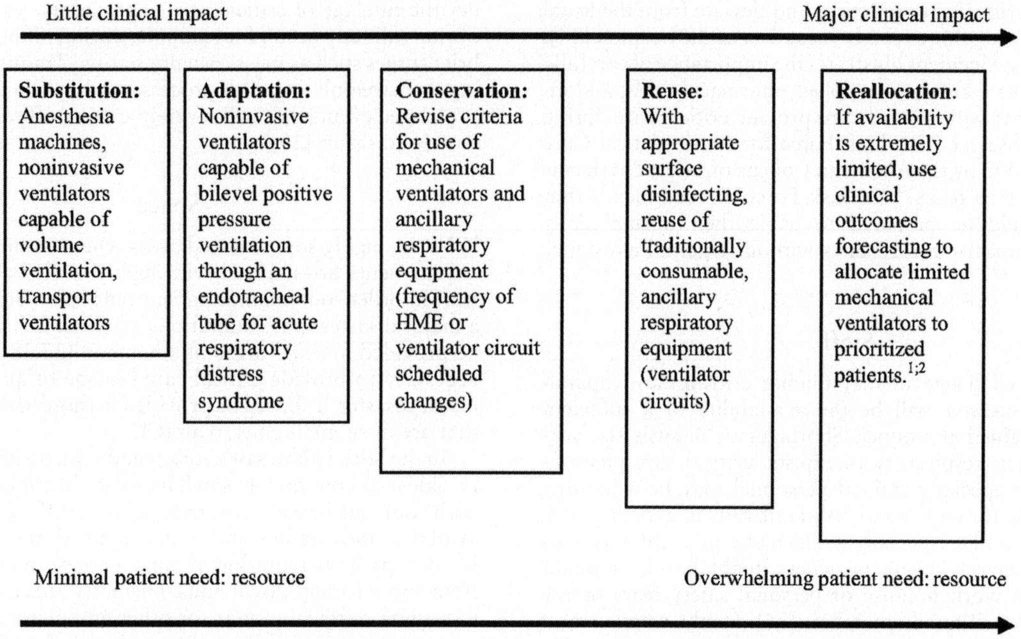

Little clinical impact
Major clinical impact
Substitution: Anesthesia machines, noninvasive ventilators capable of volume ventilation, transport ventilators
Adaptation: Noninvasive ventilators capable of bilevel positive pressure ventilation through an endotracheal tube for acute respiratory distress syndrome
Conservation: Revise criteria for use of mechanical ventilators and ancillary respiratory equipment (frequency of HME or ventilator circuit scheduled changes)
Reuse: With appropriate surface disinfecting, reuse of traditionally consumable, ancillary respiratory equipment (ventilator circuits)
Reallocation: If availability is extremely limited, use clinical outcomes forecasting to allocate limited mechanical ventilators to prioritized patients.1;2
Minimal patient need: resource
Overwhelming patient need: resource

FIGURE 216.1. Stepwise modifications in resource use to maintain positive-pressure ventilation. HME, heat and moisture exchanger. [From Rubinson L, Hick JL, Hanfling DG, et al: Definitive care for the critically ill during a disaster: a framework for optimizing critical care surge capacity. *Chest* 133:18S–31S, 2008.]

explosions, bombings, as well as more prolonged events, such as earthquakes, hurricanes, and influenza pandemics [12,13].

A common rubric for the planning of critical care surge capacity places critical care resources into three categories: "*stuff*"—the medical supplies and equipment necessary for providing critical care; "*staff*"—the availability of trained critical care providers and support personnel; and "*space*"—the physical space within the hospital that can be used to provide critical care to a large number of critically ill or injured patients [14]. In all disaster situations, the effective utilization of critical care surge capacity will ultimately depend on the training and effectiveness of the hospital and community incident command systems which must execute surge capacity plans [15].

Stuff

Patients requiring care beyond the levels available on medical-surgical wards are generally admitted to ICUs because of monitoring needs, the need for intensive-care nursing, or the need for treatment with special equipment. The provision of mechanical ventilation is the most common requirement needed to manage critically ill patients with respiratory compromise. The main challenge in providing this important therapeutic modality during a disaster is the availability of mechanical ventilators.

The United States has approximately 62,000 full-feature ventilators or 20 of these per 100,000 residents (52 pediatric full-feature ventilators per 100,000 children under age 14). Approximately 100,000 ventilators that are less than full-feature are also available [16]. In any disaster with a large number of critically ill patients, it is likely that the availability of mechanical ventilators will rapidly decrease. Thus, in preparing to provide mechanical ventilation to a large number of critically ill disaster casualties, planners need to consider other options, such as anesthesia machines or noninvasive positive-pressure ventilation. Although these alternatives are not ideal for infection control, and their use may be limited by a lack of skilled respiratory therapists, they may be the best available options in a major disaster [17,18,19]. A systematic stepwise approach for providing positive-pressure ventilator support as resources become progressively scarce during a disaster is illustrated in Figure 216.1.

In considering the use of mechanical ventilators during a disaster, it is recommended that emergency response personnel should not rely on ventilators that operate on high-pressure medical gas. This is because such devices typically require a large amount of oxygen, which is likely to be in short supply during a prolonged event, especially if there are large numbers of casualties with respiratory problems. The most common form of hospital oxygen is liquid oxygen. The technical difficulties involved in supplying, storing, generating, and concentrating this kind of oxygen make it virtually impossible to increase supplies to a level that will meet the high demand caused by a large number of critically ill patients [20]. Finally, both mechanical ventilator and oxygen vendors may have multiple contracts with different hospitals within a region; such contract duplication could result in major shortages if all hospitals in a region require increased support simultaneously.

In order to support the need for additional mechanical ventilators during a disaster, both the United States and Canada have prepositioned stockpiles of sophisticated transport ventilators throughout their respective countries. The United States has at least 4,600 prepositioned ventilators at the present time [21]. Three types of transport ventilators are currently available in the United States stockpiles: Impact 754, Pulmonetic Systems LTV-1200, and Puritan Bennett LP-10 [22]. Access to these ventilators during a disaster would be provided by the federal government through a formal request from an affected state [23]. In addition, many states and regions are developing their own mechanical ventilator stockpiles along with plans for distributing the stockpiled ventilators to affected areas during a disaster.

The provision of critical care during a disaster will also require that a large quantity of supplies and pharmaceuticals be on hand and readily available to critical care providers. In 2005, during the Hurricane Katrina disaster in New Orleans, the lack of available supplies, pharmaceuticals, and operational equipment forced the dedicated providers at Charity Hospital to improvise critical care practices and deviate from the usual standards of care prior to final evacuation of the hospital [24]. This unfortunate incident illustrates the importance of carefully planning for the increase in supplies, pharmaceuticals, and infrastructure that will be needed to provide critical care during a prolonged disaster. The Task Force for Mass Critical Care convened in 2007 by the American College of Chest Physicians (hereafter referred to as "the Task Force") recommends that hospitals should be prepared to triple their normal daily critical care capacity for 10 days without external assistance [25].

Staff

A significant challenge in maintaining critical care capability during a disaster will be the availability of a sufficient number of trained personnel. Shortages of intensivists, critical care nurses, respiratory therapists, critical care pharmacists, or other specially trained personnel may be a limiting factor in caring for large numbers of critically ill patients. Such limitations could be especially problematic in settings such as pandemic influenza, where providers might be ill, or might choose not to work because of personal safety fears or the need to care for ill family members [26]. Lastly, many critical care providers also play important emergency response roles in their communities; this is especially prevalent in nonurban settings. Such "dual-hat" responsibilities could impact the availability of critical care providers in hospitals during a major disaster.

In reviewing critical care staffing requirements during a disaster, the Task Force endorsed previously published recommendations on the surging of staff [14]. In short, the most experienced providers should perform direct patient care, if feasible. Those providers not normally operating in critical care settings should be cross-trained, or retrained, on essential bedside skills in the ICU as part of a hospital's disaster preparedness program. Finally, systematic procedures (such as protocols) should be instituted and understood by all critical care providers, in order to standardize processes, maximize good outcomes, and maximize safety to patients and staff during a disaster.

While intensivists are the most highly trained critical care physicians and should provide direct patient care to the extent feasible, in surge conditions they will need to focus part of their effort on supervising cross-trained physicians from other specialties. In such a situation, intensivists should only provide direct care for patients who require complex treatment or procedures. Nonintensivist physicians who are skilled in proving hands-on care, such as hospitalists, inpatient pediatricians, general surgeons, or anesthesiologists, could be assigned six patients each. Intensivists could supervise 4 to 8 such providers, thereby extending their critical care expertise to almost 50 patients. Similarly, critical care nurses understand the need for matching nursing staff with patient acuity. ICU charge nurses could, therefore, match several non-ICU nurses to appropriate patients within a "pod" of patients that are overseen by an ICU nurse, leaving only the most complex patients under the sole care of other ICU nurses. Another approach could be to assign specific bedside care procedures to non-ICU nurses (bathing, vital signs, catheter management, medication delivery, etc.), thereby permitting ICU nurses to oversee the provision of specific critical nursing care to several patients. Respiratory therapists usually provide care to four to six ICU patients, in accordance with the American Association for Respiratory Care Uniform Reporting Manual. Surge requirements may mandate a higher ratio of patients per therapist, ICU therapists supervising outpatient or non-ICU therapists, or even ICU therapists directing non-therapists in basic respiratory care. Finally, oncology, outpatient, radiation, or other non-ICU pharmacists may similarly be asked to support critical care operations under the tutelage of critical care pharmacists. Variants of these options already occur, for example, during off hours, or during brief surges such as mass casualty setting. Training for, rehearsing and streamlining such processes will become necessary for prolonged events that will severely strain staff resources during a major disaster [20].

Space

ICUs are highly sophisticated areas where complex equipment requirements are married with highly skilled and specialized staff in order to maximize patient outcomes. However, during a major disaster space limitations may require that critical care be provided in other areas of a hospital [27,28]. If it becomes necessary to provide critical care outside of an ICU during a major disaster, it should be provided in those areas of a hospital that are most analogous to an ICU.

In the initial phases of a surge requirement, hospitals should be able to accommodate small increases in critically ill patients with minimal impact, assuming that "stuff" and "staff" are available and the hospital is not at maximum capacity. Stable ICU patients requiring minimal care or monitoring can be transferred to step-down units, telemetry areas, postanesthesia care units, surgical centers, or other ambulatory care settings, as appropriate. In this event, the hospital bed space should be decompressed by transferring stable ward patients to home care, to skilled nursing facilities, or to alternate community facilities such as an ACC. As an emergency mass critical care event progresses, formal critical care space will need to expand into other areas of the hospital, with the hospital continuing to make room for critically ill patients by transferring the most stable inpatients elsewhere.

An alternative to expanding internal ICU capability is for communities to develop and deploy "field" ICUs. Critical care has been provided in such settings before, and can be especially relevant and appropriate when hospitals have been physically destroyed or incapacitated [29–31]. However, because of the logistical requirements for specialized equipment, infection control support, and the relocation of trained personnel, critical care should only be provided in "field" settings as a last resort. In most major disaster situations, such facilities can be best used for the management of noncritically ill patients who are transferred from hospitals in order to free up space for the management of the critically ill. The Task Force recommends using alternate sites, or buildings of convenience, for critical care only if a region's medical facilities are physically destroyed or rendered unsafe to occupy [20].

RESOURCE ALLOCATION AND TRIAGE DURING TIMES OF OVERWHELMING DEMAND

The Greatest Good for the Greatest Number of Victims

The goal of surging critical care resources during a disaster is to provide the greatest good for the greatest number of event victims. Critical care providers and institutions should strive to manage resources within their own facility and region with the goal of providing usual critical care practices to the extent possible. However, in a major disaster, as resources become increasingly limited, healthcare providers and leaders must have a plan in place to change the focus of critical care from the needs of the individual to the needs of the population as a whole. This requires a defined triage plan to be developed, communicated, and implemented fairly.

Ethical and Legal Principles

Utilitarian principles guide the theory of the "greatest good for the greatest number." In times of overwhelming resource constraints, limited capabilities should be targeted to those with the greatest likelihood of benefitting from the care. Those who are unlikely to recover or improve with the available care are not abandoned, but are provided with appropriate palliative care. This fundamental principle guides the implementation of a mass-casualty triage system during major disasters [32].

The Task Force supports the concept that if surge measures do not meet demand, then individual autonomy will be limited. It mandates a fair and just rationing of resources, based on objective information and decision-making, in order to benefit the population as a whole, rather than individual patients. Such a shift in healthcare priorities requires active community involvement and an open, transparent decision-making processes. Ideally, plans for the fair and just rationing of critical care resources during periods of overwhelming demand should be developed prior to the disaster. "Procedural justice" requires absolute conformity to the agreed-upon process, which itself must be repeatedly reevaluated and validated through ongoing, real-time epidemiological investigation [33].

Importantly, in order to implement such processes, providers must feel secure in their legal protection. Hence, providers must be legally protected from local and state law if there is a need to deviate from the usual standards of care during periods of scarce resources. The need for such legal protection was poignantly highlighted in New Orleans during the Hurricane Katrina disaster, as palliative care was provided to some patients as evacuation attempts were repeatedly delayed and hospital capabilities were overwhelmed [34]. Several states have begun efforts to address this important issue [35,36]. The Task Force recommends that uniformly accepted, predetermined algorithms be developed for triaging critically ill patients during a disaster, with adherence to these algorithms being sufficient to provide necessary legal protection to providers and other decision makers [33].

Critical Care Triage

Triage processes have been well described for the prehospital and emergency department mass-casualty events, such as the use of START (Simple Triage and Rapid Treatment) cards [37]. However, ICU triage processes and procedures have not been well studied or validated in overwhelming critical care disasters. The Task Force recommends that planning for the triage of critically ill patients during a major disaster should include well-defined "triggers" that promptly alert hospital and community leadership to the fact that critical care resources are being overwhelmed and there is a need to direct the use of a triage process. Such triggers would include a lack of critical equipment or medical supplies, inadequate critical care spaces, inadequate staff, and inadequate capability to transfer noncritically ill patients to other facilities.

Once the requirement to triage care has been directed, critical care providers must determine which patients should receive critical care and which patients should not. This process needs to be carefully planned and evaluated with community

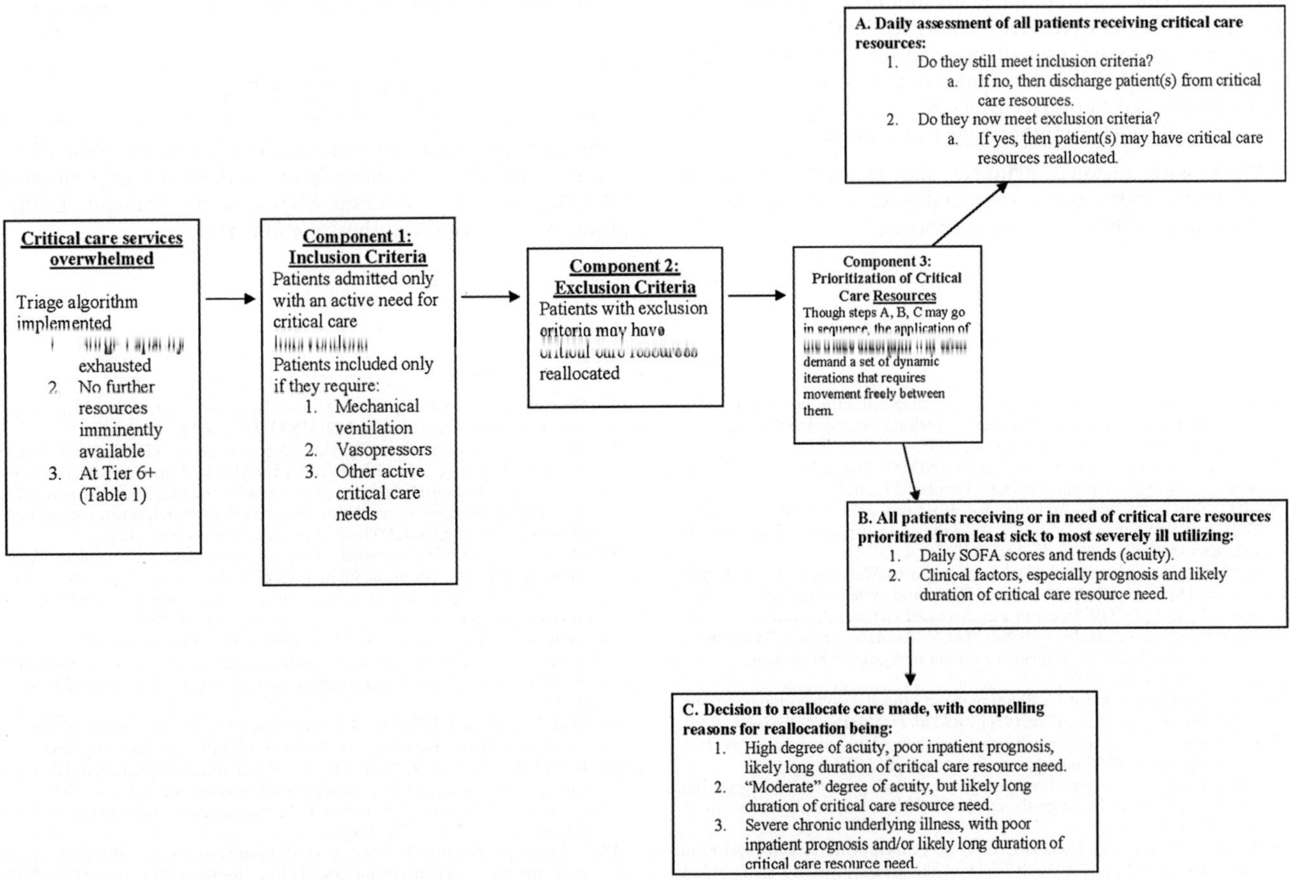

FIGURE 216.2. Critical care triage algorithm. [From Devereaux AV, Dichter JR, Christian MD, et al: Definitive care for the critically ill during a disaster: a framework for allocation of scarce resources in mass critical care. *Chest* 133:51S–66S, 2008.]

involvement prior to a catastrophic event. If, for example, a healthcare system or region proposes to exclude critical care to the very elderly during a major disaster, then community representatives from the elderly population would need to be included in such decisions. That is, the elderly would participate in advance planning with providers on how to triage the elderly in future mass-casualty emergencies.

Several severity-of-illness models have been developed for the ICU setting that may be applied to the triage process. However, all have similar limitations in that they have not been rigorously evaluated in emergency mass critical-care scenarios. The Task Force and other groups have advocated the use of the Sequential Organ Failure Assessment (SOFA) score because of its demonstrated effectiveness in the ongoing assessment of critically ill patients and the ease with which it can be calculated with minimal laboratory requirements [33,38].

The Task Force recommends that hospitals establish a critical care triage team for the effective and ethical triage of critically ill patients. It recommends that the triage team consist of a small group of experienced providers to include an intensivist, a critical care nurse, a respiratory therapist or pharmacist, and a hospital administrator. This group, operating independently from the bedside clinicians, would gather periodic SOFA scores to determine the severity of illness and document improvement, stability, or deterioration of critically ill patients over time. The Task Force recommends that patients with high SOFA scores (>11) not be offered critical care. Similarly, patients who deteriorate or fail to improve over time would have their critical care resources reallocated to other patients (Fig. 216.2). The availability of an experienced critical care triage team has the advantage of removing the burden of triage decisions from busy clinicians who are providing critical care at the bedside. In the HICS, the critical care triage team should operate under the command of the Hospital Operations Section Chief.

In order to assure compliance and integrity of the triage process, the Task Force recommends that a review committee be established to oversee triage plans and operations. This committee, distinct from the triage team, would:

- Work with regional planners and maintain situational awareness in the community and state, regarding the ongoing use and need of triage protocols;
- Review the implementation of the local triage protocol, to ensure compliance and integrity of triage operations;
- Serve as a forum for appeals by patients, families, and staff regarding the accurate and ethical implementation of the triage tool; and
- Participate in the real-time epidemiological evaluation of the catastrophic event, to help public health and other officials determine the ongoing validity of the SOFA score as a triage tool for critically ill patients.

SUMMARY

Preparing ICUs for disasters requires a methodical approach within a defined organizational structure in order to optimize care for large numbers of critically ill patients. Ideally, hospitals are the optimal setting to provide critical care for severely ill and injured patients. During major disasters, hospitals should coordinate with community medical response systems to offload patients with minor injuries or illnesses so that hospital resources can be focused on the care of critically ill patients.

Predisaster planning and training are essential for mitigating the adverse effects of an overwhelming disaster on hospitals and their communities. Carefully developed plans for surging critical care "stuff, staff, and space" will facilitate continuation of usual critical care processes for as long as possible. However, if surge procedures fail to meet the critical care demands of an overwhelming patient influx, processes to triage and alter the usual standards of critical care must be implemented. The planning concepts and guidelines outlined in this chapter can help guide critical care practitioners to care for their patients under the challenging conditions of a catastrophic disaster.

DECLARATION

The opinions and assertions contained herein are those of the authors and do not necessarily reflect the views or position of the Department of Veterans Affairs, or the academic institutions with which the authors are affiliated.

References

1. NH Medical Surge Capacity Guidelines. Available at: http://www.dhhs.state.nh.us/DHHS/CDCS/LIBRARY/Policy-Guideline/ppcc-NHMedicalSurgeGuidelines.htm. Accessed October 30, 2009.
2. National Incident Management System (NIMS). Available at: http://www.fema.gov/emergency/nims/. Accessed October 29, 2009.
3. NIMS Implementation Activities for Hospitals and Healthcare Systems. Released September 12, 2006. Available at: http://www.fema.gov/pdf/emergency/nims/imp_hos.pdf. Accessed May 2, 2011.
4. California Emergency Medical Services Authority Web site, Disaster Medical Services Division—Hospital Incident Command System: Available at: http://www.emsa.ca.gov/HICS/default.asp. Accessed October 30, 2009.
5. Multiagency coordination systems (MACS): Available at: http://www.fema.gov/emergency/nims/MultiagencyCoordinationSystems.shtm#item1. Accessed October 31, 2009.
6. Hick J, Barbera J, Kelen G: Refining surge capacity; conventional, contingency, and crisis capacity. *Disast Med and Pub Health Prepar* 3:S1–S9, 2009.
7. GAO Report on Emergency Preparedness: Available at: http://www.gao.gov/new.items/d08668.pdf. Accessed October 30, 2009.
8. GAO: Emergency preparedness: states are planning for medical surge, but could benefit from shared guidance for allocating scarce medical resources. GAO-08-668, 2008.
9. Booth C, Matukas L, Tomlinson G, et al: Clinical features and short-term outcomes of 144 patients with SARS in the greater Toronto area. *JAMA* 289:644–654, 2003.
10. Halpern N, Pastores S, Greenstein R: Critical care medicine in the United States 1985–2000; an analysis of bed numbers, use, and costs. *Crit Care Med* 32:1254–1259, 2004.
11. Sinuff T, Kahnamoui K, Cook D, et al: Rationing critical care beds: a systematic review. *Crit Care Med* 32:1588–1597, 2004.
12. Homeland Security Council, U.S. Department of Homeland Security: National Planning Scenarios: Created for Use in National, Federal, State and Local Homeland Security Preparedness. Available at: http://media.washingtonpost.com/wpsrv/nation/nationalsecurity/earlywarning/NationalPlanningScenariosApril2005.pdf. Accessed October 29, 2009.
13. Overview of MSCC, Emergency Management and the Incident Command System. In: *Medical Surge Capacity Handbook*; September 2007, pp 1–32. Available at: http://www.hhs.gov/disasters/discussion/planners/mscc/chapter1/1.1.html#1.1.2. Accessed October 29, 2009.
14. Rubinson L, Nuzzo J, Talmor D: Augmentation of hospital critical care capacity after bioterrorist attacks or epidemics: recommendations of the working group on emergency mass critical care. *Crit Care Med* 33:2393–2403, 2005.
15. Hick J, Barbera J, Kelen G: Refining surge capacity: conventional, contingency, and crisis capacity. *Disast Med Pub Health Prep* 3:S1–S9, 2009.
16. Rubinson L, Vaughn F, Nelson S, et al. Mechanical ventilators in US acute care hospitals. *Disaster Med Public Health Preparedness*. 4:1–8, 2010.
17. Daugherty E, Branson R, Rubinson L: Mass casualty respiratory failure. *Curr Opin Crit Care* 13:51–56, 2007.
18. Rubinson L, Branson R, Pesik N, et al: Positive-pressure ventilation equipment for mass casualty respiratory failure. *Biosecur Bioterror* 4:183–194, 2006.
19. Cheung T, Yam L, So L, et al: Effectiveness of non-invasive positive pressure ventilation in the treatment of acute respiratory failure in severe acute respiratory syndrome. *Chest* 126:845–850, 2004.

20. Rubinson L, Hick J, Curtis R, et al: Definitive care for the critically ill during a disaster: medical resources for surge capacity. *Chest* 133:32S–50S, 2008.
21. Christian M, Devereaux A, Dichter J, et al: Definitive care for the critically ill during a disaster: current capabilities and limitations. *Chest* 133:8S–17S, 2008.
22. Train the Trainer—Ventilators of the National Stockpile: Summary of a Workshop presented at the 55th International Respiratory Congress; San Antonio Texas: December 4, 2009. Available at: http://www.aarc.org/education/meetings/congress_09/advance_program/workshops.cfm. Accessed December 14, 2009.
23. Office of Public Health Preparedness and Response: Strategic National Stockpile. Available at: http://www.bt.cdc.gov/stockpile/. Accessed October 30, 2009.
24. deBoisblanc B: Black hawk, please come down: reflections on a hospital's struggle in the wake of Hurricane Katrina. *Am J Respir Crit Care Med* 172:1239–1240, 2005.
25. Rubinson L, Hick JL, Hanfling DG, et al: Definitive care for the critically ill during a disaster: a framework for optimizing critical care surge capacity. *Chest* 133:18S–31S, 2008.
26. Qureshi K, Gershon R, Sherman M, et al: Healthcare worker's ability and willingness to report to duty during catastrophic disaster. *J Urban Health* 82:378–388, 2005.
27. Simchen E, Sprung C, Galai N, et al: Survival of critically ill patients hospitalized in and out of intensive care units. *Crit Care Med* 35:449–457, 2007.
28. Gomersall C, Tai D, Loo S, et al: Expanding ICU facilities in an epidemic: recommendations based on experience from the SARS epidemic in Hong Kong and Singapore. *Int Care Med* 32:1004–1013, 2006.
29. Grissom T, Farmer J: The provision of sophisticated critical care beyond the hospital: lessons from physiology and military experiences that apply to civil disaster medical response. *Crit Care Med* 33:S13–S21, 2005.
30. Halpern P, Rosen B, Carasso S, et al: Intensive care in a field hospital in an urban disaster area: lessons from the August 1999 earthquake in Turkey. *Crit Care Med* 31:1410–1414, 2003.
31. Eastman A, Rinnert K, Nemeth I, et al: Alternate site surge capacity in times of public health disaster maintains trauma center and emergency department integrity: hurricane Katrina. *J Trauma* 63:253–257, 2007.
32. Lin J, Anderson-Shaw L: Rationing of resources: ethical issues in disasters and epidemic situations. *Prehosp Disas Med* 24:215–221, 2009.
33. Devereaux AV, Dichter JR, Christian MD, et al: Definitive care for the critically ill during a disaster: a framework for allocation of scarce resources in mass critical care. *CHEST* 133:51S–66S, 2008.
34. Strained by Katrina, a Hospital Faced Deadly Choices. New York Times Magazine, August 30, 2009. Available at: http://www.nytimes.com/2009/08/30/magazine/30doctors.html. Accessed October 30, 2009.
35. The Louisiana State Legislature. Regular Session, 2008. Senate Bill Number 301. Available at: http://legis.state.la.us./billdata/byinst.asp?sessionid=08rs&billtype=SB&billno=301. Accessed October 30, 2009.
36. Utah Pandemic Influenza Hospital and ICU Triage Guidelines for Adults; Prepared by Utah Hospitals and Health Systems Association for the Utah Department of Health Hospitals and Health Systems Association, Version 3, September 29, 2009; http://www.pandemicflu.utah.gov/.
37. START Triage: The Race Against Time. Available at: http://www.start-triage.com/index.htm. Accessed October 30, 2009.
38. Christian MD: Critical care during a pandemic; final report of the Ontario Health Plan for Influenza Pandemic (OHPIP) working group on adult critical care admission, discharge and triage criteria, April 2006.

APPENDIX

JOSEPH J. FRASSICA

CALCULATIONS COMMONLY USED IN CRITICAL CARE

JOSEPH J. FRASSICA

TABLE OF CONTENTS

ABBREVIATIONS USED IN THE APPENDIX

A	Alveolar	atm	Atmosphere
D	Dead	BSA	Body surface area
E	Expiration	cap	Capillary
I	Inspiration	cr	Creatinine
P	Pressure	dyn	Dynamic
$\dot{Q}$	Net liquid flow	is	Interstitium
R	Respiratory quotient	st	Static
T	Tidal	ICP	Intracranial pressure
V	Volume	a	Arterial
Δ	Change	d	Distribution
H	Viscosity	l	Length
Π	Oncotic pressure	r	Radius
Σ	Permeability	t	Time
		$\bar{v}$	Mixed venous

FAHRENHEIT AND CELSIUS TEMPERATURE CONVERSIONS

°C	°F	°C	°F
45	113.0	32	89.6
44	111.2	31	87.8
43	109.4	30	86.0
42	107.6	29	84.2
41	105.8	28	82.4
40	104.0	27	80.6
39	102.2	26	78.8
38	100.4	25	77.0
37	98.6	24	75.2
36	96.8	23	73.4
35	95.0	22	71.6
34	93.2	21	69.8
33	91.4	20	68.0

DOSAGE AND ACTION OF COMMON INTRAVENOUS VASOACTIVE DRUGS

	Dosage	α	β_1	β_2
Dopamine	1–2 μg/kg/min	+	+	0
	2–10 μg/kg/min	++	+++	0
	10–30 μg/kg/min	+++	++	0
Dobutamine	2–30 μg/kg/min	+	+++	++
Norepinephrine	0.05–1 mg/kg/min titrate to effect	+++	++	+
Epinephrine	0.1–1.0 mg/kg/min	++	+++	+++
Isoproterenol	2–10 μg/min	0	+++	+++
Phenylephrine	0.1–0.5 mg/kg/min	+++	0	0
Milrinone	(Loading dose 50 mg/kg over 10–15 min)			
	0.375–0.75 mg/kg/min	—	—	—
Labetolol	2 mg/min; max dose 300 mg	—	—	—
Esmolol	50–300 mg/kg/min	—	—	—

HEMODYNAMIC CALCULATIONS

MEAN BLOOD PRESSURE (mm Hg)

$= \overline{BP}$

$= \dfrac{\text{Systolic BP} + (2 \times \text{Diastolic BP})}{3}$

$= \text{Diastolic BP} + \dfrac{1}{3}(\text{Systolic BP} - \text{Diastolic BP})$

Normal values: 85–95 mm Hg

THE FICK EQUATION FOR CARDIAC INDEX ($L/min/m^2$)

$= \text{CI}$

$= \dfrac{\text{CO}}{\text{BSA}}$

$= \dfrac{\text{Oxygen consumption}}{\text{Arterial } O_2 \text{ contemt} - \text{Venous } O_2 \text{ content}}$

$= \dfrac{10 \times \dot{V}O_2\,(mL/min/m^2)}{\text{Hgb}\,(g/dl) \times 1.39}$

$\times(\text{Arterial \% saturation} - \text{Venous \% saturation})$

Normal values: 2.5–4.2 $L/min/m^2$

STROKE INDEX ($mL/beat/m^2$)

$= \dfrac{\text{CI}\,(L/min/m^2) \times 1{,}000}{\text{Heart rate (beats/ min)}}$

Normal values: 33–47 $mL/beat/m^2$

SYSTEMIC VASCULAR RESISTANCE ($dyne/sec/cm^5$)

$= \text{SVR}$

$= \dfrac{80 \times (\text{Arterial } \overline{BP} - \text{Right atrial } \overline{BP})}{\text{CO (L/min)}}$

Normal values: 770–1,500 $dyne/sec/cm^5$

PULMONARY VASCULAR RESISTANCE ($dyne/sec/cm^5$)

$= \text{PVR}$

$= \dfrac{80 \times (\text{Pulmonary artery } \overline{BP} - \text{Pulmonary capillary wedge pressure})}{\text{CO (L/min)}}$

Normal values: 20–120 $dyne/sec/cm^5$

TOTAL PULMONARY RESISTANCE ($dyne/sec/cm^5$)

$= \text{TPR}$

$= \dfrac{80 \times \text{Pulmonary artery } \overline{BP}}{\text{CO (L/min)}}$

CAPILLARY FLUID FILTRATION

$= \dot{Q}_f$

$= k(P_{cap} - P_{is}) - k\sigma(\pi_{cap} - \pi_{is})$

NUTRITIONAL CALCULATIONS

BODY MASS INDEX

$= \text{BMI}$

$= \dfrac{\text{Weight (kg)}}{(\text{Height [cm]})^2}$

CALORIC CONTENT OF FOODS

Food type	kcal/g	Range
Carbohydrate	3.4	3.4–4.1
Protein	4.0	3.3–4.7
Fat	9.1	9.1–9.5

RESPIRATORY QUOTIENT

$= \dfrac{CO_2 \text{ production (mL/ min)}}{O_2 \text{ consumption (mL/ min)}}$

$= \dfrac{\dot{V}_{CO_2}}{\dot{V}_{O_2}}$

RELATIONSHIP OF FUEL BURNED TO RESPIRATORY QUOTIENT

Fuel	*R*
Ketones	<0.6
Fat	0.7
Carbohydrate	1.0
Lipogenesis	>1.0

NITROGEN BALANCE

$= \text{Nitrogen consumed} - \text{Nitrogen excreted}$

$= \dfrac{\text{Protein calories (kcal/day)}}{25}$

$- \text{Urine nitrogen (g/day)} - 5\,(g/day)$

HARRIS–BENEDICT EQUATION OF RESTING ENERGY EXPENDITURE (kcal/day)

$\text{Males} = 66 + (13.7 \times \text{Weight [kg]}) + (5 \times \text{Height [cm]}) - (6.8 \times \text{Age})$

$\text{Females} = 655 + (9.6 \times \text{Weight [kg]}) + (1.8 \times \text{Height [cm]}) - (4.7 \times \text{Age})$

WEIR EQUATION (MODIFIED) OF ENERGY EXPENDITURE (kcal/day)

$= (3.94 \times \dot{V}_{O_2}\,[mL/min]) + (1.11 \times \dot{V}_{CO_2}\,[mL/min])$

TYPICAL DRUG DOSAGES FOR RAPID SEQUENCE INTUBATION

Muscle relaxants	
Rocuronium	0.6–1.2 mg/kg
Succinylcholine	1 mg/kg
Vecuronium	0.1–0.20 mg/kg
Sedatives	
Etomidate	0.3–0.4 mg/kg
Ketamine	1–2 mg/kg
Propofol	1–2 mg/kg
Thiopental	3–4 mg/kg

PULMONARY CALCULATIONS

TIDAL VOLUME

$$= V_T$$
$$= \text{Dead space} + \text{Alveolar space}$$
$$= V_D + V_A$$

ALVEOLAR GAS EQUATION

$$PAO_2 = PIO_2 - \frac{PaCO_2}{R}$$
$$= FIO_2(P_{atm} - P_{H_2O}) - \frac{PaCO_2}{R}$$
$$= 150 - \frac{PaCO_2}{R}\text{(room air, sea level)}$$

ALVEOLAR ARTERIOLAR GRADIENT

$$= A - a \text{ gradient}$$
$$= PAO_2 - PaO_2$$

Normal values (upright): $2.5 + (0.21 \times \text{age})$

ALVEOLAR VENTILATION (L/min)

$$= \dot{V}_E$$
$$= k\frac{\dot{V}CO_2}{PaCO_2}$$
$$= \frac{0.863 \times \dot{V}_{CO_2}(\text{mL/ min})}{Pa_{CO_2}(1 - V_D/V_T)}$$

Normal values: 4–6 L/min

BOHR EQUATION OF DEAD SPACE

$$V_D/V_T = \frac{PACO_2 - PECO_2}{PACO_2}$$

Normal values: 0.2–0.3

PHYSIOLOGIC DEAD SPACE

$$V_D/V_T = \frac{PaCO_2 - PECO_2}{PaCO_2}$$

Normal values: 0.2–0.3

OXYGEN DISSOLVED IN BLOOD (mL/dL)

$$= DO_2$$
$$= 0.003\,(\text{mL } O_2/\text{dL}) \times PaO_2\,(\text{mm Hg})$$

OXYGEN CAPACITY OF HEMOGLOBIN (mL O_2/dL)

$$= 1.39\,(\text{mL } O_2) \times \text{Hgb}\,(\text{g/dL})$$

Normal values: 17–24 mL/dL

OXYGEN CONTENT OF THE BLOOD (mL/dL)

$$= C_{O_2}$$
$$= D_{O_2} + (1.39 \times \text{Hgb [g/dL]} \times [\% \text{ Hgb saturated with } O_2])$$
$$= D_{O_2} + (1.39 \times \text{Hgb [g/dL]} \times S_{O_2})$$

Normal values: 17.5–23.5 mL/dL

PERCENTAGE OF SATURATION OF HEMOGLOBIN WITH OXYGEN

$$= SO_2$$
$$= 100 \times \frac{CO_2 - DO_2}{1.39 \times \text{Hgb (g/dL)}}$$

Normal values: >95%

PHYSIOLOGIC SHUNT

$$= \dot{Q}_S/\dot{Q}_T$$
$$= \frac{C_{capO_2} - C_{O_2}}{C_{capO_2} - C_{\bar{v}O_2}}$$
$$= \frac{1.39 \times \text{Hgb (g/dL)} + 0.003 \times PaO_2 - CaO_2}{1.39 \times \text{Hgb (g/dL)} + 0.003 \times PaO_2 - C\bar{v}O_2}$$

Normal values: <5%

COMPLIANCE

$$= \Delta V/\Delta P\ (\text{mL/cm } H_2O)$$

On Mechanical Ventilation

$$\text{Static compliance} = C_{st} = \frac{V_T}{P_{plateau} - P_{end\ exp}}$$
$$\text{Dynamic effective complicance} = C_{dyn} = \frac{V_T}{P_{peak} - P_{end\ exp}}$$

During Spontaneous Breathing

$$\text{Compliance of the lung} = C_L = \frac{V_T}{P_{alveolus} - P_{pleura}}$$
$$\text{Compliance of the chest wall} = CW_{cw} = \frac{V_T}{P_{pleura} - P_{atm}}$$
$$\text{Compliance of the respiratory system} = C_{rs} = \frac{V_T}{P_{alveolus} - P_{atm}}$$

Normal values: $C_{st} > 60$ mL/cm H_2O; $C_{dyn} > 60$ mL/cm H_2O
$C_L > 200$ mL/cm H_2O; $C_{rs} > 100$ mL/cm H_2O

RESISTANCE—OHM'S LAW

$$= \Delta P/\text{flow} = \Delta P/\dot{Q}$$

Normal values: airway resistance of the lung at functional residual capacity (FRC) = 2 cm H_2O/L/sec

WORK-OF-BREATHING

$$W_{\text{Thorax}} = \int_{t_1}^{t_2} (P_{\text{aw}} - P_{\text{atm}})\dot{V}\text{dt}$$

$$W_{\text{Lung}} = \int_{t_1}^{t_2} (P_{\text{aw}} - P_{\text{es}})\dot{V}\text{dt}$$

$$W_{\text{Chest wall}} = \int_{t_1}^{t_2} (P_{\text{es}} - P_{\text{atm}})\dot{V}\text{dt}$$

Normal values: $W_{\text{thorax}} = 0.5$ kg-M/min

LAPLACE'S LAW OF SURFACE TENSION OF A SPHERE

$$P = 2T/r$$

POISEUILLE'S LAW OF LAMINAR FLOW

$$\dot{V} = \frac{P\pi r^4}{8\eta l}$$

COMPOSITION AND PROPERTIES OF COMMON INTRAVENOUS SOLUTIONS

Solution	Na^+	Cl^-	K^+	Ca^+	Lactate	Kcal/L	mOsm/L
D5W	0	0	0	0	0	170	252
D10W	0	0	0	0	0	240	505
D50W	0	0	0	0	0	1,700	2,530
½ NS	77	77	0	0	0	0	154
NS	154	154	0	0	0	0	308
3% NaCl	513	513	0	0	0	0	1,026
Ringer's lactate	130	109	4	3	28	0	308
10% mannitol	0	0	0	0	0	0	1,098

ELECTROLYTE AND RENAL CALCULATIONS

ANION GAP

$$= [Na^+] - [Cl^-] - [HCO_3^-]$$

Normal values: 9–13 mEq/L

EXPECTED ANION GAP IN HYPOALBUMINEMIA

$$= 3 \times (\text{albumin [g/dL]})$$

CALCULATED SERUM OSMOLALITY

$$= 2[Na^+] + \frac{[\text{Glucose}]}{18} + \frac{[\text{BUN}]}{2.8}$$

Normal values: 275–290 mOsm/kg

OSMOLAR GAP

= Serum osmolality measured – Serum osmolality calculated

Normal values: 0–5 mOsm/kg

Na^+ AND GLUCOSE

$[Na^+]$ decreases 1.6 mEq/L for each 100 mg/dL increase in [glucose]

TOTAL CALCIUM AND ALBUMIN

Corrected calcium (mg/dL) = Measured total calcium (mg/dL) + 0.8(4.0 – serum albumin)

GLOMERULAR FILTRATION RATE = GFR

$$\text{Measured} = \text{Creatinine clearance} = \frac{U_{\text{Creat}}V}{P_{\text{Creat}}}$$

$$= \frac{[\text{Creatinine}]_{\text{urine}}\ (\text{g/dL}) \times \dfrac{\text{Urine volume (mL/day)}}{1{,}440\ \text{(minute/day)}}}{[\text{Creatinine}]_{\text{plasma}}\ (\text{mg/dL})}$$

$$\text{Estimated for males} = \frac{(140 - \text{Age}) \times (\text{Lean body weight [kg]})}{P_{\text{Creat}} \times 72}$$

Estimated for females = 0.85 × Male estimate

Normal values: 74–160 mL/min

WATER DEFICIT IN HYPERNATREMIA (L)

$$= 0.6 \times (\text{Body weight [kg]}) \times \left(\frac{[Na^+]}{140} - 1\right)$$

WATER EXCESS IN HYPONATREMIA (L)

$$= 0.6 \times (\text{Body weight [kg]}) \times \left(1 - \frac{[Na^+]}{140}\right)$$

FRACTIONAL EXCRETION OF SODIUM

$$= F_E\ \text{Na}$$

$$= \frac{\text{Excreted Na}^+}{\text{Filtered Na}^+} \times 100$$

$$= \frac{U_{Na^+} \times V}{\text{GFR}} \times [Na^+] \times 100$$

$$= \frac{U_{Na^+}/[Na^+]}{U_{\text{Creat}}/[\text{Creat}]}$$

ACID–BASE FORMULAS

HENDERSON–HASSELBALCH EQUATION

$$\text{pH} = \text{p}K + \log \frac{[HCO_3^-]}{0.03 \times PaCO_2}$$

HENDERSON'S EQUATION FOR CONCENTRATION OF H^+

$$[H^+](\text{nM/L}) = 24 \times \frac{PaCO_2}{[HCO_3^-]}$$

METABOLIC ACIDOSIS

Bicarbonate deficit (mEq/L) = 0.5 × (Body weight [kg]) ×(24 – [HCO_3^-])

Expected $PCO_2 = 1.5 \times [HCO_3^-] + 8 \pm 2$

METABOLIC ALKALOSIS

Bicarbonate excess = 0.4 × (Body weight [kg]) × ([HCO_3^-] – 24)

RESPIRATORY ACIDOSIS

$$\text{Acute: } \frac{\Delta H^+}{\Delta PaCO_2} = 0.8$$

$$\text{Chronic: } \frac{\Delta H^+}{\Delta PaCO_2} = 0.3$$

NEUROLOGIC CALCULATIONS

GLASGOW COMA SCALE (3–15)

= Eyes (1 – 4) + Motor (1 – 6) + Verbal (1 – 5)

Normal value: 15

TABLE A.1

SPECIFIC COMPONENTS OF THE GLASGOW COMA SCALE

Eye opening	
Spontaneous	4
To speech	3
To pain	2
Nil	1
Motor response	
Obeys commands	6
Localizes	5
Withdraws	4
Exhibits abnormal flexion	3
Exhibits abnormal extension	2
Nil	1
Verbal response	
Oriented	5
Confused, conversant	4
Uses inappropriate words	3
Uses incomprehensible sounds	2
Nil	1

CEREBRAL PERFUSION PRESSURE (mm Hg)

$= \overline{BP} - ICP$

BODY SURFACE AREA FORMULA AND NOMOGRAM

BODY SURFACE AREA (BSA)

$= (\text{Height [cm]})^{0.718} \times (\text{Weight [kg]})^{0.427} \times 74.49$

See Figure A.1 for the nomogram for calculating BSA.

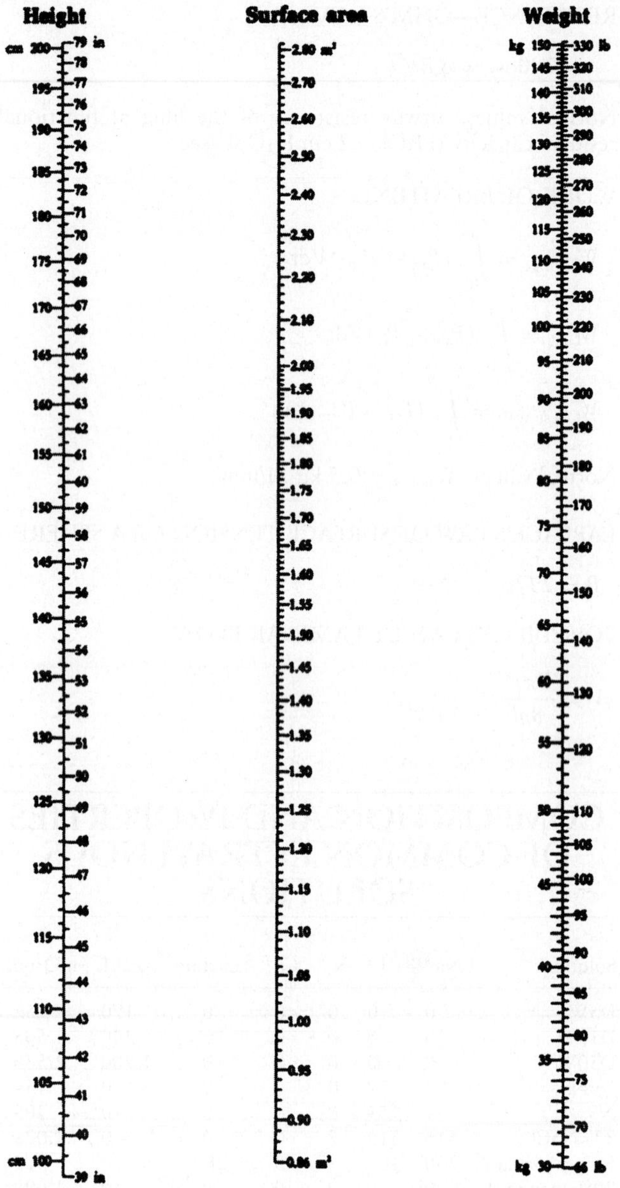

FIGURE A.1. Nomogram for calculation of body surface area (BSA) in square meters by height and weight.

PHARMACOLOGIC CALCULATIONS

DRUG CLEARANCE

$= V_d \times K_{el}$

DRUG HALF-LIFE

$= t_{1/2}$

$$= \frac{0.693}{K_{el}}$$

DRUG ELIMINATION CONSTANT

$= K_{el}$

$$= \frac{\ln\left(\frac{[\text{Peak}]}{[\text{Trough}]}\right)}{t_{peak} - t_{trough}}$$

DRUG LOADING DOSE

$= V_d \times$ [Target peak]

DRUG DOSING INTERVAL

$$= \frac{-1}{K_{el}} \times \ln\left(\frac{\text{Desired trough}}{\text{Desired peak}}\right) + \text{Infusion time (hours)}$$

See ICU Acuity Scoring for the calculation of APACHE scores.

ICU ACUITY SCORING

SAPS II Score [1,2]

Type of admission		Points
	Scheduled surgery	0
	Unscheduled surgery	8
	Medical	6
Chronic diseases	None	0
	Metastatic carcinoma	9
	Hematologic malignancy	10
	AIDS	17
Age	<40	0
	40–59	7
	60–69	12
	70–74	15
	75–79	16
	≥80	18
Temperature	<39°C	0
	>39°C	3
Heart rate	<40	11
	40–69	2
	70–119	0
	120–159	4
	≥160	7
Systolic blood pressure	<70 mm Hg	13
	70–99	5
	100–199	0
	≥200	2
Urine output	<500 cc/24 h	11
	500–999 cc/24 h	4
	>1,000 cc/24 h	0
Glasgow Coma Score	<6	26
	6–8	13
	9–10	7
	11–13	5
	14–15	0
Serum urea or BUN	<10	0
	10–29.9	6
	≥30	10
Serum sodium	>146 mEq/L	1
	125–144 mEq/L	0
	<125 mEq/L	5
Serum potassium	<3 mEq/L	3
	3–4.9 mEq/L	0
	>5 mEq/L	3
WBC	<1,000/mm^3	12
	1,000–19,000/mm^3	0
	>20,000/mm^3	3
HCO_3^-	<15 mEq/L	6
	15–19 mEq/L	3
	≥20	0
Bilirubin	<4 mg/dL	0
	4–5.9 mg/dL	4
	≥6	9
PaO_2/FIO_2 (if ventilated or CPAP)	<100	11
	100–199	9
	≥200	6

(continued)

CONTINUED

SAPS II, Simplified Acute Physiology Score II.

APACHE IV VARIABLES (NON-CABG PATIENTS) [3]

Age **Chronic Health Issues on Admission** *Use the one with the highest point value that is present* *Nonoperative and emergency surgery patients only otherwise = 0*	**Points**
AIDS	23
Hepatic failure	16
Lymphoma	13
Metastatic cancer	11
Leukemia/multiple myeloma	10
Immunosuppression	10
Cirrhosis	4
None/not available	0

Acute Physiology Score
P_aO_2/FIO_2 ratio (or $P(A–a)O_2$ for intubated patients with $FIO_2 > = 0.5$
Ventilated anytime during day 1 Y/N
ICU admission information
Admit to ICU from floor
Transfer to ICU from other hospital
Admit to ICU from OR/PACU

Emergency surgery Y/N
Pre-ICU length of stay (# of days between ICU and hospital admission)
Admitting diagnosis (see Diagnosis Tables)
If DX is acute MI is the patient on thrombolytic therapy? Y/N
Unable to obtain GCS (due to meds, anesthesia or sedation) Y/N
GCS

Acute Physiology Score (APS Score)

Pulse (beats/min)
Select heart rate furthest from 75

≤39	8
40–49	5
50–99	0
100–109	1
110–119	5
120–139	7
140–154	13
≥155	17

Mean blood pressure (MAP)
Select MAP furthest from 90

≤39	23
40–59	15
60–69	7
70–79	6
80–99	0
100–119	4
120–129	7
130–139	9
≥140	10

Temperature (degrees centigrade)
Select core temperature furthest from 38
Add 1 degree centigrade to axillary temps prior to selecting worst value

≤32.9	20
33–33.4	16
33.5–33.9	13
34–34.9	8
35–35.9	2
36–39.9	0
≥40	4

Respiratory rate (breaths/min)
Select respiratory rate furthest from 19
For patients on mechanical ventilation no points are given for respiratory rates of 6–12

≤5	17
6–11	8
12–13	7
14–24	0
25–34	6
35–39	9
40–49	11
≥50	18

PaO_2 (mm Hg)
Use only for nonintubated patients or intubated patients with FIO_2 <0.5 (50%)

≤49	15
50–69	5
70–79	2
≥80	0

OR

A-aDO_2
Only use A-aDO_2 for intubated patients with FIO_2 ≥0.5 (50%)
Do not use PaO_2 weights for these patients

<100	0
100–249	7
250–349	9
350–499	11
≤500	14

Hematocrit (%)
Select hematocrit furthest from 45.5

≤40.9	3
41–49	0
≥50	3

WBC (cu/mm)
Select WBC furthest from 11.5

<1.0	19
1.0–2.9	5
3.0–19.9	0
20–24.9	1
≥25	5

Creatinine without ARF (mg/dL)
Select creatinine furthest from 1

≤0.4	3
0.5–1.4	0
1.5–1.94	4
≥1.95	7

OR

Creatinine with ARF (mg/dL)
Acute renal failure (ARF) is defined as creatinine ≥1.5 mg/dL as creatinine ≥1.5 mg/dL and urine output <410 cc/d and no chronic dialysis

0–1.4	0
≥1.5	10

Urine Output (cc/day)
Total for day

≤399	15
400–599	8
600–899	7
900–1,499	5
1,500–1,999	4
2,000–3,999	0
≥4,000	1

BUN (mg/dL)
Select highest BUN

≤16.9	0
17–19	2
20–39	7
40–79	11
≥80	12

Sodium (mEq/L)
Select sodium furthest from 145.5

≤119	3
120–134	2
135–154	0
≥155	4

Albumin (g/dL)
Select albumin furthest from 3.5

≤1.9	11
2–2.4	6
2.5–4.4	0
≥4.5	4

Bilirubin (mg/dL)
Select highest bilirubin furthest from 0

≤1.9	0
2–2.9	5
3–4.9	6
5–7.9	8
≥8	16

Glucose (mg/dL)
Select glucose furthest from 130
Glucose ≤39 mg/dL is lower weight than 40–59

≤39	8
40–59	9
60–199	0
200–349	3
≥350	5

Neurological Abnormalities Score (see matrix)
Acid–Base Abnormalities Score (see matrix)

Adapted from Cerner Apache. *Apache IV Calculations.xls* with permission.
APACHE IV Score Calculator available at: http://www.cerner.com/public/filedownload.asp?LibraryID=40394. Accessed July 26, 2010.
Note: Mortality prediction calculations based on the APACHE IV are different for the day of ICU admission and subsequent days.

MPM0 III VARIABLES [4]

Category	Variable
Physiology	
	Coma or deep stupor at admission not due to drug overdose
	Heart rate >150 beats/min
	Systolic blood pressure ≤90 mm Hg
Chronic diagnoses	
	Chronic renal compromise or insufficiency
	Cirrhosis
	Metastatic malignant neoplasm
Acute diagnoses	
	Acute renal failure
	Cardiac dysrhythmia
	Cerebrovascular accident
	Gastrointestinal bleeding
	Intracranial mass effect
Other variables	
	CPR within 24 hours prior to admission
	Mechanical ventilation within one hour of admission
	Medical or unscheduled surgery admission
	Full code status
	Age (years)

MPM_0-III variables are collected at the time of ICU admission or within 1 hour of admission.
Calculator available at: http://www.cerner.com/public/filedownload.asp?LibraryID=25783. Last accessed July 26, 2010.
Adapted from White Paper Report. Available at: http://www.cerner.com/public/filedownload.asp?LibraryID=34399. Accessed July 26, 2010.

TABLE A.2

APACHE IV NONOPERATIVE DIAGNOSES [3]

Diagnostic group

Cardiovascular diagnoses
- AMI
- Anterior
- Inferior/lateral
- Non-Q
- Other
- Cardiac arrest
- Cardiogenic shock
- Cardiomyopathy
- Congestive heart failure
- Chest pain, rule out AMI
- Hypertension
- Hypovolemia/dehydration (not shock)
- Hemorrhage (not related to GI bleeding)
- Aortic aneurysm
- Peripheral vascular disease
- Rhythm disturbance
- Sepsis (by infection site)
- Cutaneous
- Gastrointestinal
- Pulmonary

(*continued*)

TABLE A.2

CONTINUED

- Urinary tract
- Other location
- Unknown location
- Cardiac drug toxicity
- Unstable angina
- Cardiovascular, other

Respiratory diagnoses
- Airway obstruction
- Asthma
- Aspiration pneumonia
- Bacterial pneumonia
- Viral pneumonia
- Parasitic/fungal pneumonia
- COPD (emphysema/bronchitis)
- Pleural effusion
- Pulmonary edema (noncardiac)
- Pulmonary embolism
- Respiratory arrest
- Respiratory cancer (oral, larynx, lung, trachea)
- Restrictive lung disease (fibrosis, sarcoidosis)
- Respiratory disease, other

GI diagnoses
- GI bleeding, upper
- GI bleeding lower/diverticulitis
- GI bleeding, varices
- GI inflammatory disease
- Neoplasm
- Obstruction
- Perforation
- Vascular insufficiency
- Hepatic failure
- Intra/retroperitoneal hemorrhage
- Pancreatitis
- Gastrointestinal, other

Neurologic diagnoses
- Intracerebral hemorrhage
- Neurologic neoplasm
- Neurologic infection
- Neuromuscular disease
- Drug overdose
- Subdural/epidural hematoma
- Subarachnoid hemorrhage, intracranial aneurysm
- Seizures (no structural disease)
- Stroke
- Neurologic, other

Trauma diagnoses
- Trauma involving the head
- Head trauma with either chest, abdomen, pelvis, or spine injury
- Head trauma with extremity or facial trauma
- Head trauma only
- Head trauma with multiple other injuries
- Trauma, chest and spine trauma
- Trauma, spine only
- Multiple trauma (excluding head trauma)

Metabolic/endocrine diagnoses
- Acid–base, electrolyte disorder
- Diabetic ketoacidosis
- Hyperglycemic hyperosmolar nonketotic coma
- Metabolic/endocrine, other

Hematologic diagnoses
- Coagulopathy, neutropenia, thrombocytopenia, pancytopenia
- Hematologic, other

Genitourinary diagnoses
- Renal, other

Miscellaneous diagnoses
- General, other

TABLE A.3

APACHE IV SURGICAL DIAGNOSES [3]

Diagnostic group

Cardiovascular surgery
- Valvular heart surgery
- CABG with double or redo valve surgery
- CABG with single valve surgery
- Aortic aneurysm, elective repair
- Aortic aneurysm, rupture
- Aortic aneurysm, dissection
- Femoral–popliteal bypass graft
- Aortoiliac, aortofemoral bypass graft
- Peripheral ischemia (embolectomy, thrombectomy, dilation)
- Carotid endarterectomy
- Cardiovascular surgery, other

Respiratory surgery
- Thoracotomy, malignancy
- Neoplasm, mouth, larynx
- Thoracotomy, lung biopsy, pleural disease
- Thoracotomy, respiratory infection
- Respiratory surgery, other

GI surgery
- GI malignancy
- GI bleeding
- Fistula, abscess
- Cholecystitis, cholangitis
- GI inflammation
- GI obstruction
- GI perforation
- GI, vascular ischemia
- Liver transplant
- GI surgery, other

Neurologic surgery
- Craniotomy or transsphenoidal procedure for neoplasm
- Intracranial hemorrhage
- Subarachnoid hemorrhage (aneurysm, arteriovenous malformation)
- Subdural/epidural hematoma
- Laminectomy, fusion, spinal cord surgery
- Neurologic surgery, other

Trauma surgery
- Head trauma only
- Multiple trauma sites including the head
- Surgery for extremity trauma
- Multiple trauma (excluding the head)

Genitourinary surgery
- Renal/bladder/prostate neoplasm
- Renal transplant
- Hysterectomy
- Genitourinary surgery, other

Miscellaneous surgery
- Amputation (nontraumatic)

NORMAL VALUES OF EXPIRATORY PEAK FLOW [5]

There is a wide variability in peak expiratory flows due to individual differences. Values also vary slightly depending on the peak flow meter used.

TABLE A.4

NORMAL VALUES OF EXPIRATORY PEAK FLOW FOR MEN

	Height				
Age (y)	60 Inches	65 Inches	70 Inches	75 Inches	80 Inches
20	554	602	649	693	740
25	543	590	636	679	725
30	532	577	622	664	710
35	521	565	609	651	695
40	509	552	596	636	680
45	498	540	583	622	665
50	486	527	569	607	649
55	475	515	556	593	634
60	463	502	542	578	618
65	452	490	529	564	603
70	440	477	515	550	587

TABLE A.5

NORMAL VALUES OF EXPIRATORY PEAK FLOW FOR WOMEN

	Height				
Age (y)	55 Inches	60 Inches	65 Inches	70 Inches	75 Inches
20	390	423	460	496	529
25	385	418	454	490	523
30	380	413	448	483	516
35	375	408	442	476	509
40	370	402	436	470	502
45	365	397	430	464	495
50	360	391	424	457	488
55	355	386	418	451	482
60	350	380	412	445	475
65	345	375	406	439	468
70	340	369	400	432	461

From Higgins TL, Teres D, Copes WS, et al: Assessing contemporary intensive care unit outcome: An updated Mortality Probability Admission Model (MPM0-III). *Crit Care Med* 35(3):827–835, 2007, with permission.

References

1. Le Gall J, Lemeshow S, Saulnier F: A new simplified acute physiology score (SAPS II) based on a European/North American multicenter study. *JAMA* 270:24, 1993.
2. French Society of Anesthesia and Intensive Care: SAPS II calculator. Available at: http://www.sfar.org/scores2/saps2.html. Accessed August 2, 2006.
3. Zimmerman JE, Kramer AA, McNair DS, et al: Acute Physiology and Chronic Health Evaluation (APACHE) IV: hospital mortality assessment for today's critically ill patients. *Crit Care Med* 34(5):1297–1310, 2006.
4. Higgins TL, Teres D, Copes WS, et al: Assessing contemporary intensive care unit outcome: An updated Mortality Probability Admission Model (MPM0-III). *Crit Care Med* 35(3):827–835, 2007.
5. Leiner GC, Abramowitz S, Small MJ, et al: Expiratory peak flow. Standards for normal subjects. Use as a clinical test of ventilatory function. *Am Rev Respir Dis* 86:644, 1963.

TABLE OF THERAPEUTIC AGENTS USED AS ANTIDOTES IN MEDICAL TOXICOLOGY

Luke Yip, MD*, Jeremy S. Helphenstine, DO, Jerry D. Thomas, MD, FACMT, FACEP, Ian M. Ball, MD, FRCPC, DABEM

*The views expressed do not necessarily represent those of the agency or the United States.

This is a list of therapeutic agents that are used in medical toxicology and has been organized into a table format to facilitate rapid access to concise information guiding indication and dosing of a therapeutic agent. This table is divided into four columns. The first column is alphabetically organized in terms of a specific agent; individual agents appear alphabetically in the Index. The second column focuses on indications and uses in medical toxicology. The third column provides guidelines for adult dosing of the therapeutic agent. The fourth column highlights caveats and potential complications. The content of this table is not intended to be a comprehensive list of therapeutic agents and is not a substitute for reference textbooks in medical toxicology (e.g., Goldfrank's Toxicologic Emergencies and Medical Toxicology) and does not address envenomations by exotic venomous creatures or envenomations outside the United States. Some of the listed therapeutic agents may not be available to every clinician, and it may be prudent to be familiar with the therapeutic agents that are available in the respective clinician's practice.

This table that appears on the next 11 pages, comprehensively covers the topic.

Therapeutic agent	Uses	Dosing	Caveat/Complications
Activated charcoal	GI decontamination ■ Multiple dose consideration: Carbamazepine, dapsone, phenobarbital, quinine, or theophylline.	Oral/nasogastric single dose: 1–2 g/kg Oral/nasogastric multiple dose: Hourly, every 2 h, or every 4 h at a dose equivalent to 12.5 g/h for 12–24 h.	GI decontamination considerations (after patient stabilized and precautionary measures to minimize aspiration). Should not be administered in patients with decreased bowel sounds/ileus.
	Theophylline poisoning	Activated charcoal 1–2 g/kg followed by hourly, every 2 h, or every 4 h at a dose equivalent to 12.5 g/h until serum theophylline <15 μg/mL; alternatively, 0.25–0.5 g/kg/h via continuous nasogastric infusion; not in patients with decreased bowel sounds/ileus.	Co-administration of cathartics with multiple dosing may produce hypernatremia, hypokalemia, hypermagnesemia, and metabolic acidosis. Aspiration Constipation; bowel obstruction
Antivenom	Known or suspected coral snake envenomation	Coral snake ■ IV coral snake antivenom 4–6 vials with each vial diluted in 50 to 100 mL of normal saline and administered over 1 h; if signs/symptoms appear or progress, administer 4–6 more vials of antivenom.	Precaution: Be prepared to manage acute anaphylactic (shock) and anaphylactoid reactions. Antivenom: Equine origin; may be effective in late presenters. Serum sickness: May occur 7–21 days following antivenom therapy.
	Crotalidae (Subfamily Crotalinae: pit vipers, e.g., rattle snake)	Crotalidae ■ IV CroFab® (Protherics, Inc., London): Administer 4–6 vials; carefully monitor for further progression of local effects and systemic symptoms, and laboratory studies (i.e., CBC, PT/INR, fibrin, fibrin degradation products) are repeated one hour after completing antivenom infusion; administer additional rounds of antivenom (4–6 vials) if initial control (i.e., reversal or marked attenuation of all venom effects) has not been achieved; continue this pattern until control is evident then administer 2 vials of CroFab every 6 h for 3 additional doses; most cases 8–12 vials to establish initial control. ■ Reconstituted each CroFab vial with normal saline 10 mL and roll vials between hands; dilute total dose to be administered in normal saline 250 mL and infused over 1 h.	Precaution: See **Coral snake.** Antivenom: Ovine origin; most effective within first 24 h following envenomation, may be beneficial in late presenters with severe findings (e.g., coagulopathy); limited efficacy in preventing wound necrosis or reversing cellular damage; thrombocytopenia may be resistant to antivenom therapy. Serum sickness: See **Coral snake.**

	Widow spider (*Latrodectus* sp., e.g., black widow)	*Lactrodectus* IV antivenom (preferable) 1 reconstituted vial further diluted in 50–100 mL of normal saline over 30 min or IM one reconstituted vial in the anterolateral thigh; a second vial can be administered if necessary. The physician should be in immediate attendance to observe for any sign of adverse drug events; signs/symptoms should completely resolve within a few hours.	Precaution: See **Elapidae.** Antivenom: Equine origin; most effective in the acute setting, may be beneficial in late presenters (e.g., 96 h) with prolonged symptoms. Serum sickness: See **Elapidae.**
Atropine	Cholinesterase inhibitors (e.g., organic phosphorus agents, nerve agents)	IV atropine 1–4 mg, double the dose every 5–10 min as needed until pulmonary secretions are controlled (tachycardia is *not* a contraindication to atropine); once stabilized start atropine infusion (10–20% of total dose for stabilization per hour); restart atropine at the first signs of cholinergic excess. [See **Pralidoxime**]	To be administered with pralidoxime following organophosphate or nerve agent poisoning. Carbamates and other reversible cholinesterase inhibitors: Atropine *and* pralidoxime are used to treat acutely ill patients unless carbaryl (Sevin) is known to be involved, then just atropine and supportive care. Atropine requirement following nerve agent poisoning may be significantly less than for organophosphate poisoning. Atropine has no effect on muscle weakness or paralysis and will not affect acetylcholinesterase regeneration rate.
Botulinum antitoxin	Botulism	Botulinum antitoxin for treatment of naturally occurring noninfant botulism is available only from Centers for Disease Control (CDC). Heptavalent botulinum antitoxin (HBAT) contains equine-derived antibody to the seven known botulinum toxin types (A-G) and replaces a licensed bivalent botulinum antitoxin AB and an investigational monovalent botulinum antitoxin E (BAT-AB and BAT-E). The HBAT FDA IND treatment protocol includes specific, detailed instructions for intravenous administration of antitoxin and return of required paperwork to CDC. Health-care providers should report suspected botulism cases immediately to their state health department; all states maintain 24-hour telephone services for reporting of botulism and other public health emergencies. Additional emergency consultation is available from the CDC botulism duty officer via the CDC Emergency Operations Center, telephone, 770–488-7100. Additional information regarding CDC's botulism treatment program is available at http://www.bt.cdc.gov/agent/botulism.	The lethality of botulinum toxin outweighs the risk of adverse events from antitoxin treatment, and treatment is considered acceptable for anyone with presumed illness or potentially exposed to the toxin. Available from local health department or CDC Precaution: Be prepared to manage acute anaphylactic (shock) and anaphylactoid reactions. Antivenom: Equine origin; antitoxin administration within 24 h after exposure have resulted in shorter clinical course of botulism without regression of symptoms, but a comparable mortality rate to later antitoxin administration. Serum sickness: May occur 7–21 days following antivenom therapy.
Calcium	Calcium channel antagonist poisoning	IV calcium gluconate (10%) 0.6 mL/kg bolus (0.2 mL/kg 10% calcium chloride) over 5–10 min followed by continuous calcium gluconate infusion at 0.6–1.5 mL/kg/h (0.2–0.5 mL/kg/h 10% calcium chloride), titrate infusion to affect improved blood pressure/contractility, follow ionized calcium levels every 30 min initially and then every 2 h maintaining ionized calcium twice normal.	Mixed clinical response (disappointing at times), primarily inotropic effect.

(*continued*)

CONTINUED

Therapeutic agent	Uses	Dosing	Caveat/Complications
	Hydrofluoric acid		
	■ Digital exposure and pain	Apply a 2.3–2.5% calcium gluconate preparation in a water-soluble gel to exposed area(s) $\geq$30 min or until symptoms resolve. Pain unrelieved by gel therapy ■ Regional intra-arterial: Place catheter in direction of blood flow by Seldinger technique, continuously monitor arterial waveform (arteriography if any concern as to adequate placement), infuse 50 mL of 2.5% calcium gluconate in normal saline over 4 h; repeated doses may be required over 12–24 h. Or ■ Administer 40 mL of a 2.5% calcium gluconate solution by Bier block technique (i.e., catheterize a distal vein and exsanguinate extremity by elevation and compression with an Esmarch bandage, inflate blood pressure cuff to 100 mm Hg above systolic pressure and maintain for 15–20 min following calcium administration, gradually deflate cuff over 5 min).	
	■ Symptomatic inhalation exposure	Nebulized 25% calcium gluconate may improve symptoms following mild exposure.	
	■ History suggestive of a substantive dermal or oral exposure that may lead to systemic toxicity	Oral calcium or magnesium containing antacids 30–60 mL. IV calcium chloride 1 g over 30 min; patients with normal vital signs and remain stable should be monitored with serum calcium levels every 30 min for the first 2–3 h; IV calcium chloride 1 g boluses to maintain serum calcium concentration in the high normal laboratory reference range, repeat as needed; a fall in serum calcium concentration below the normal range, dysrhythmias or a fall in blood pressure is treated with IV calcium chloride 2–3 g boluses every 15 min *or* IV magnesium sulphate [See **Magnesium**]	
Carnitine	Valproic acid overdose		
	■ Coma, symptomatic hyperammonemia, symptomatic hepatotoxicity, or rising serum ammonia levels	IV L-carnitine 100 mg/kg (max 6 g) over 30 min followed by 15 mg/kg every 4 h over 10–30 min until clinical improvement; consider treatment for patients with serum VPA >450 μg/mL.	
	■ Acute overdose without hepatic enzyme abnormalities or hyperammonemia	Consider oral L-carnitine 100 mg/kg/d (max 3 g) divided every 6 h.	

Chelators ■ Dimercaprol (BAL, British Anti-Lewisite) ■ Edetate calcium disodium (Calcium disodium versenate, $CaNa_2$ EDTA) ■ Deferoxamine (DFO) ■ Diethylenetriamine-pentaacetate (DTPA) ■ Prussian blue (ferric hexacyanoferrate) ■ Succimer (2,3-dimercaptosuccinic acid, DMSA)	Arsenic (As): Suspected acute symptomatic As poisoning	IM BAL 3–5 mg/kg every 4 h, gradually tapering to every 12 h over several days; switched to DMSA 10 mg/kg every 8 h for 5 d, reduced to every 12 h for another 2 wk; additional course of treatment may be considered based on posttreatment results: 24-h urinary As excretion is followed before, during, and after chelation with continued chelation therapy until the urinary As excretion <25 μg/24 h or during the recovery period when urinary inorganic As concentration <100 μg/24 h or total blood As <200 μg/L.
	Lead (Pb) ■ Symptomatic Pb encephalopathy	IM BAL is 75 mg/m^2 (3 to 5 mg/kg) every 4 h. After 4 h have elapsed since the priming dose of BAL start IV $CaNa_2$ EDTA 1,500 mg/m^2/d (30 mg/kg/d). In cases of cerebral edema and or increased intracranial pressure associated with encephalopathy, administer $CaNa_2$ EDTA (same dosage) by deep IM injection (extremely painful) along with procaine 0.5% in two to three divided doses every 8–12 h. Continue BAL and $CaNa_2$ EDTA 5 days. Cessation of chelation is often followed by a rebound in blood Pb concentration, a second chelation course may be considered based on whole blood Pb concentration after 2 days' interruption of BAL and $CaNa_2$ EDTA treatment, and the persistence or recurrence of symptoms. A third course may be required if the whole blood concentration rebounds ≥ 50 μg/dL within 48 h after second chelation treatment. If chelation is required for the third time, it should begin a week after the last dose of BAL and $CaNa_2$ EDTA.
	■ Symptomatic patients who are not overtly encephalopathic	IM BAL is 50 mg/m^2 (2 to 3 mg/kg) every 4 h. After 4 hours have elapsed since the priming dose of BAL, start IV $CaNa_2$ EDTA 1,000 mg/m^2/d (20 to 30 mg/kg/d) or in two to three divided doses every 8–12 h. BAL and $CaNa_2$ EDTA should be continued for 5 days with daily monitoring of whole blood Pb concentrations. BAL may be discontinued any time during these 5 days if the whole blood Pb level <50 μg/dL but $CaNa_2$ EDTA treatment should continue for 5 days. A second or third course of chelation may be considered based on the same guidelines as in the previous paragraph.
	■ Asymptomatic patients with whole blood Pb levels ≥ 70 μg/dL	BAL and $CaNa_2$ EDTA in the same doses and with the same guidelines as for treatment of symptomatic Pb poisoning without encephalopathy. A second course of $CaNa_2$ EDTA chelation alone may be necessary if whole blood Pb concentration rebounds ≥ 50 μg/dL within 5–7 days after chelation has ceased. Alternative: Oral DMSA 10 mg/kg (350 mg/m^2) every 8 h for 5 d then every 12 h for 2 wks. Additional course of treatment may be considered based on posttreatment whole blood Pb concentrations, and the persistence or recurrence of symptoms. An interval ≥ 2 wks may be indicated to assess the extent of posttreatment rebound in whole blood Pb concentration.

(continued)

CONTINUED

Therapeutic agent	Uses	Dosing	Caveat/Complications
	Mercury (Hg) ■ Elemental Hg poisoning	Oral DMSA (10 mg/kg every 8 h, tapering to every 12 h over the next several days and continued until urinary Hg concentration approaches background) may enhance urinary Hg excretion and reduce nephrotoxicity after GI absorption of elemental Hg.	No proven chelation effect on improving clinical outcome. BAL may redistribute Hg to the brain. Confirming elemental Hg exposure: 24-hour urinary Hg excretion <50 μg/24 h most useful tool in diagnosing acute exposure (normal whole blood mercury concentration <2 μg/dL and "spot" urine mercury Hg concentration <10 μg/L).
	■ Suspected acute inorganic Hg poisoning	BAL and DMSA; See **Arsenic.**	BAL is most effective within 4 hours of ingestion. Confirming Hg exposure: See **Elemental Hg**; whole blood Hg concentrations >50 μg/dL in acute poisoning associated with gastroenteritis and acute renal tubular necrosis.
	■ Organic Hg poisoning	No proven effect on improving clinical outcome. DMSA appears promising in animal studies; [See **Elemental Hg**].	Confirmatory Hg exposure: Whole blood Hg concentrations >20 μg/dL associated with symptoms; urinary Hg concentration not useful.
	Iron (Fe) poisoning: Symptomatic patient (e.g., recurrent vomiting or diarrhea, acidosis, shock and decreased level of consciousness or coma) regardless of serum Fe concentration or asymptomatic patient with serum Fe concentration ≥ 500 μg/dL (90 μmol/L)	IV DFO initiated slowly and gradually increased to 15 mg/kg/h over 20–30 min and continued for 24 h; continuous IV DFO therapy >24 h (rarely needed) is interrupted for 12 of every 24 h; treatment endpoints include resolution of systemic signs/symptoms, correction of acidosis, and return of urine color to normal (if patient developed vin rosé colored urine during therapy).	Rapid infusion associated with tachycardia, hypotension, shock, generalized beet red flushing of the skin, blotchy erythema, and urticaria. Acute renal failure can result when deferoxamine is administered to hypovolemic patients. Pulmonary toxicity associated with continuous infusion therapy over days. Deferoxamine therapy may increase risk for *Yersinia* infections.
	Known or suspected internal contamination with radioactive cesium (Cs) or radioactive/nonradioactive thallium (Tl).	Adults/adolescents: Oral Prussian blue 3 g t.i.d.; treatment should continue for 30 d minimum and patient reassessed for residual whole body radioactivity and duration of treatment should be guided by the level of contamination and clinical judgment.	Treatment with Prussian blue should be initiated as soon as possible after suspected contamination; contamination should be verified as soon as possible. Prussian blue does not treat the complications of radiation exposure. Obtain quantitative baseline of the internalized radioactive contamination by whole-body counting and/or bioassay (e.g., Biodosimetry) or feces/urine sample. Obtain weekly radioactivity counts in urine and fecal samples to monitor radioactive elimination rate. Prussian blue capsules can be opened and mixed with food or drinks. Complications of Prussian blue treatment include constipation, hypokalemia, blue-colored stools, and blue discoloration of mouth/teeth.

	Known or suspected internal contamination with plutonium, americium, or curium.	Day 1: IV calcium-DTPA (CaDTPA) 1 g in 5 mL over 3–4 min *or* in 100–250 mL D5W, normal saline, or LR over 30 min. Day 2: IV zinc-DTPA (ZnDTPA) 1 g in 5 mL over 3–4 min *or* in 100–250 mL D5W, normal saline, or LR over 30 min every day (continue with daily CaDTPA dosing if ZnDTPA not available); treatment duration based on individual response and weekly radioactivity in blood, urine, and fecal samples.	Treatment with DTPA should be initiated as soon as possible after suspected contamination; contamination should be verified as soon as possible. ZnDTPA should be used for any further chelation after the first dose of CaDTPA; monitor CBC with differential, BUN, serum chemistries and electrolytes, and urinalysis regularly; if using more than one CaDTPA dose, monitor these laboratory tests carefully and consider mineral supplementation containing zinc as appropriate. Obtain quantitative baseline of the internalized radioactive contamination by whole-body counting and/or bioassay (e.g., Biodosimetry) or feces/urine sample. Obtain weekly radioactivity counts in blood, urine, and fecal samples to monitor radioactive contaminant elimination rate. Nebulized therapy may exacerbate asthma or precipitate respiratory adverse events
	Internal plutonium, americium, or curium contamination is only by inhalation.	Day 1: Nebulize diluted CaDTPA 1 g at a 1:1 ratio with sterile water or saline. Day 2: Nebulize diluted ZnDTPA 1 g at a 1:1 ratio with sterile water or saline; after nebulization, encourage individuals not to swallow any expectorant; treatment duration based on individual response and weekly radioactivity in blood, urine, and fecal samples.	
Cyanide "antidote" ■ Dicobalt edetate ■ Hydroxocobalamin ■ Cyanide antidote kit ■ 4-dimethylaminophenol (4-DMAP)	Known or suspected CN toxicity (e.g., occupation, fire in an enclosed space), severe and unexplainable anion gap metabolic acidosis	IV dicobalt edetate 300 mg over 1–5 min if certain of the diagnosis particularly when patient is unconscious with deteriorating vital signs; repeat one to two dose base on clinical response; adverse events include hypotension, cardiac dysrhythmias, angioedema, OR IV hydroxocobalamin 5 g over 15–30 min, repeat one to two doses base on clinical response; transient pink discoloration of mucous membranes, skin, urine; may interfere with colorimetric determinations of serum iron, bilirubin, creatinine concentration, OR Cyanide antidote kit: Amyl nitrite (broken in gauze and held close to the nose and mouth of spontaneously breathing patients, or can be placed into the face mask lip or inside the resuscitation bag) should be inhaled for 30 seconds of each min with a fresh pearl used every 3–4 min and IV sodium nitrite 300 mg (10 mL of a 3% solution) over 5–20 min and IV sodium thiosulfate 12.5 g (50 mL of a 25% solution) over 10 min; repeat one to two doses of sodium nitrite and thiosulfate base on clinical response, OR IV 4-DMAP 3–5 mg/kg; precise extent of induced methemoglobinemia may not be predictable.	Initial resuscitation: Ventilate and oxygenate patient with 100% oxygen. When diagnosis is uncertain, administer IV sodium thiosulfate. Nitrates should be cautiously used in cases of suspected concomitant carbon monoxide exposure (e.g., house fires). Nitrate dosing based on Hgb concentration: Hgb (g/dL) — Sodium nitrite (3%) (cc/kg) 7.0 — 0.19 8.0 — 0.22 9.0 — 0.25 10.0 — 0.27 11.0 — 0.30 12.0 — 0.33 13.0 — 0.36 14.0 — 0.39
Dextrose	Hypoglycemia	Bolus: IV dextrose 0.5–1.0 g/kg (D50W 1.0–2.0 mL/kg).	Repeat bolus(es) may be indicated depending on clinical response.

(continued)

CONTINUED

Therapeutic agent	Uses	Dosing	Caveat/Complications
Digoxin-specific antibody fragments	Digoxin overdose: Symptomatic patients, cardiac dysrhythmias that threaten or result in hemodynamic compromise, serum potassium >5.0 mmol/L, serum digoxin concentration >10.0 ng/mL (12.8 nmol/L) 6 h after overdose or >15 ng/mL (19.2 nmol/L) at any time.	DigFab dosing: ■ From dose ingested: One vial of DigFab (40 mg) binds 0.6 mg of digoxin; Example: Ingestion of 3 mg of digoxin [bioavailability 80% (0.8)] requires four vials. ■ From serum digoxin concentration: See Box I at the end of this Table on page 2254 ■ By titration: Administer four to six vials of DigFab and repeat depending on clinical effect.	May be effective treatment following naturally occurring cardioactive steroid (e.g., plants or animals origin) poisoning. DigFab (1,200 mg) are safe and effective treatment for yellow oleander induced cardiac dysrhythmias (e.g., bradycardia (<40 per min), sinus arrest or block, atrial Tachydysrhythmias, second- or third-degree atrioventricular block.
Ethanol	Toxic alcohol (e.g., methanol, ethylene glycol) poisoning	IV ethanol (10% solution in D5W) 10 mL/kg over 1 h followed by 1.5 mL/kg/h, target serum ethanol 100 mg/dL until toxic alcohol is undetectable and clear clinical-biochemical recovery. Hemodialysis consideration: Increase ethanol infusion to 3.0 mL/kg/h at the time of hemodialysis and decrease to 1.5 mL/kg/h after hemodialysis; closely monitor serum ethanol and glucose level; adverse events include hypoglycemia, fluid overload, inebriation. Continue ethanol treatment until undetectable serum toxic alcohol level (significant toxic alcohol may rebound following hemodialysis).	Ethanol only *inhibits* metabolism of toxic alcohols.
	Known, suspected, or symptomatic monofluoroacetate exposure	Oral ethanol (96%) 40–60 mL, followed by IV ethanol (10% solution in D5W) 10 mL/kg over 1 h and 1.5 mL/kg/h for the next 6–8 h.	
Euglycemic clamp (hyperinsulinemia euglycemia therapy)	Calcium channel and beta-adrenergic antagonist poisoning with hypodynamic myocardium.	IV regular insulin 1 IU/kg bolus followed by infusion 0.5 IU/kg/h titrated every 30 min to desired effect on contractility or blood pressure (echocardiography for measuring myocardial response); euglycemia = serum glucose 100–250 mg/dL (5.5–14 mmol/L) is maintained by IV dextrose 25 g bolus with initial insulin bolus [unless serum glucose >400 mg/dL (22 mmol/L)] followed by dextrose infusion 0.5 g/kg/h titrated based on bedside glucose monitoring every 20–30 min until serum glucose is stable and then every 1–2 h; replace potassium if <2.5 mmol/L *and* a source of potassium loss.	Clinical response not immediate and increase chance of benefit with early detection of hypodynamic myocardium and early initiation of therapy; numerical hypoglycemia, hypokalemia, hypophosphatemia, hypomagnesemia.
Flumazenil	Diagnostic aid in assessing benzodiazepine (BZD) poisoning	IV flumazenil 0.1–0.2 mg followed by 0.1 to 0.2 mg every minute (max 2 mg) until awake, failure to respond makes BZD unlikely cause.	Flumazenil: Half-life 1–2 h; reverses sedative/anxiolytic effects, inconsistent in reversing BZD-induced respiratory depression; precipitate abrupt BZD withdrawal syndrome in patients on chronic BZD therapy or BZD dependent patients; unmask epileptogenic effects of polypharmacy overdoses.

Folinic acid (leucovorin)	Methotrexate (MTX) overdose		Leucovorin infusion rate should be <160 mg/min. Most beneficial when administered within 1 h of exposure. Monitor serum MTX concentrations at 12, 24, and 48 h postexposure so folinic acid therapy can be adjusted accordingly.
	■ Known amount of MTX ingested or administered	Initial IV leucovorin dose in milligram doses is equal to or greater than the estimated ingested MTX dose, repeat the folinic acid dose 3–6 h until serum MTX concentration $<10^{-8}$ molar.	
	■ Unknown MTX dose	IV leucovorin 10 mg/m^2.	
	■ Leucovorin dosing based on serum MTX drug concentration.	MTX 5×10^{-5} M: IV leucovorin 1,000 mg/m^2 MTX $5 \times 10^{-5} - 5 \times 10^{-6}$ M: IV leucovorin 100 mg/m^2 every 3 h MTX $5 \times 10^{-6} - 5 \times 10^{-7}$ M: IV leucovorin 30 mg/m^2 every 6 h or 10 mg/m^2 every 3 h MTX $<5 \times 10^{-7}$ M: Oral leucovorin 10 mg/m^2 every 6 h until MTX $<5 \times 10^{-8}$ M. Folinic acid is continued until serum MTX concentration <0.1 μmol/L in patients undergoing chemotherapy and <0.01 μmol/L in patients without cancer; therapy is continued until marrow recovery in severe cases even when serum MTX becomes undetectable.	
	Methanol and ethylene glycol poisoning	IV leucovorin 2 mg/kg every 4 to 6 h until toxic alcohol is undetectable, clear clinical–biochemical recovery; if leucovorin not available IV folic acid 50–70 mg every 4 h; leucovorin preferred over folic acid Hemodialysis consideration: Administer additional leucovorin dose at end of hemodialysis.	
Fomepizole	Toxic alcohol (e.g., methanol, ethylene glycol)	IV fomepizole 15 mg/kg followed by 10 mg/kg every 12 h × 4 doses, then 15 mg/kg every 12 h thereafter until toxic alcohol is undetectable and clear clinical-biochemical recovery; all infusions over 30 min. Hemodialysis consideration: Administer next scheduled fomepizole dose if ≥6 h since last dose; during hemodialysis dosing is every 4 h; end of dialysis and time of last dose 1 to 3 h administer half of next scheduled dose, >3 h administer next scheduled dose. Continue fomepizole treatment until undetectable serum toxic alcohol level (significant toxic alcohol may rebound following hemodialysis).	Fomepizole only *inhibits* metabolism of toxic alcohols.
Glucagon	Calcium channel and beta-adrenergic antagonist poisoning with associated bradycardia.	IV glucagon 5 mg bolus, titrate to heart rate by doubling the bolus dose every 5–10 min and if an effective dose is achieved start an infusion to deliver the effective bolus dose each hour (e.g., heart rate increased after two successive 5 mg boluses, then administer 10 mg/h).	More of a chronotropic than ionotropic effect.

(*continued*)

CONTINUED

Therapeutic agent	Uses	Dosing	Caveat/Complications
Lipid emulsion therapy	Local anesthetic (e.g., bupivacaine) toxicity	IV lipid emulsion (e.g., Intralipid, Liposyn III 20%, 500 mL bottle) ■ 1–2 mL/kg over 1 min and infusion 0.25 mL/kg/min ■ Repeat bolus at 3–5 min intervals 2–3 × if circulation not been restored ■ After another 5 min increase infusion rate to 0.5 mL/kg/min if circulation not been restored ■ Continue infusion until hemodynamic recovery (>8 mL/kg unlikely to be effective?)	Laboratory data and accumulating clinical experience with lipid emulsion therapy in bupivacaine, levobupivacaine, mepivacaine, prilocaine, and ropivacaine toxicity suggests early lipid therapy to attenuate progression of local anesthetic toxic syndrome. Consider lipid emulsion therapy in patients with severe lipophilic drug toxicity.
Magnesium	Hydrofluoric acid: Oral exposure	Oral calcium or magnesium containing antacids 30–60 mL. History suggestive of a substantive exposure that may lead to systemic toxicity: IV magnesium sulfate 2–6 g over 30 min follow by an infusion 1–4 g/h; additional magnesium boluses as indicated by careful clinical assessments and laboratory investigations *or* IV calcium chloride [see **Calcium**]	
Methylene blue (1% solution)	Symptomatic methemoglobinemia or methemoglobin >20%	IV methylene blue 1–2 mg/kg over 5 min, repeat doses may be needed; onset of action ≤30 min.	Repetitive or continuous methylene blue dosing and GI decontamination may be needed when there is continued absorption or slow elimination of an agent producing methemoglobinemia: IV methylene blue 0.05% (in normal saline) 0.1 mg/kg/h *or* 3–7 mg/h has been suggested. Potential to cause hemolyic anemia in patients with glucose-6-phosphate dehydrogenase deficiency. Chlorate inactivates glucose-6-phosphate dehydrogenase
***N*-acetylcysteine** (NAC)	Acetaminophen (APAP) Other causes of liver failure	Oral: 140 mg/kg followed by 70 mg/kg every 4 h (dilute 3:1 with carbonated/fruit beverage for palatability); repeat the same oral dose if vomiting occurs within 1 h. OR IV: 150 mg/kg in 200 mL D5W over 1 h followed by 50 mg/kg in 500 mL D5W over 4 h followed by 100 mg/kg in 1 L D5W over 16 h (6.25 mg/kg/h).	Oral NAC: IV antiemetic (e.g., ondansetron 8 mg for associated nausea/vomiting. Anaphylactoid reaction
Naloxone	Opioid overdose with respiratory, CNS, or cardiovascular compromise	IV naloxone 0.04–0.1 mg if opioid dependent otherwise 2 mg; 10–20 mg may be required for high potency opioids (e.g., methadone, pentazocine, propoxyphene, diphenoxylate); repeat IV naloxone boluses may be required every 20–60 min Therapeutic IV naloxone infusion: Multiply the effective naloxone bolus dose by 6.6, adding that quantity to 1,000 mL normal saline, infuse solution at 100 mL/h, titrated to maintain adequate spontaneous ventilation without precipitating opioid withdrawal, empirically continued for 12–24 h; carefully observed for 2–4 h for recurrent respiratory depression after discontinuing naloxone infusion; allow naloxone to abate in acute iatrogenic opioid withdrawal.	Goal is to re-establish adequate spontaneous ventilation; intralingual/endotracheal/ intraosseous administration acceptable if no immediate IV access; IM/SC less desirable in urgent situation. May be effective following clonidine overdose.

Octreotide	Oral hypoglycemic agent-induced hypoglycemia	IV octreotide 50 μg/h *or* IM octreotide 100 μg every 6 h.	Acute hypoglycemia should be treated with IV dextrose. [See **Dextrose**]
Physostigmine	Physostigmine diagnostic aid: Selective use in anticholinergic agitation and delirium resulting from unknown ingestion; a positive response (e.g., patient awakens, provides history consistent with anticholinergic toxicity) obviates additional testing (e.g., cranial computed tomography and lumbar puncture)	IV physostigmine 0.5 to 2 mg at ≤0.5 mg/min, if no reversal of anticholinergic effect within 10–20 min administer an additional 1–2 mg.	Contraindications include bronchospasm, mechanical intestinal or urogenital tract obstruction, early (<6 h) cyclic antidepressant overdose, overdose with cardiac conduction delay, cyclic antidepressant poisoning with high-dose/drug-level phenomena (e.g., hypotension, coma, seizures, cardiac conduction delays, and dysrhythmias).
Polyethylene glycol electrolyte (PEG) solution	Whole bowel irrigation (WBI) for gastrointestinal decontamination following oral ingestion/overdose (e.g., modified-release drug formulation, heavy metal)	See Box II at the end of this Table on page 2254	WBI: After patient stabilization, patient is able to tolerate charcoal/WBI, and precautionary measures to minimize aspiration.
Pralidoxime	Cholinesterase inhibitors (e.g., organic phosphorus agents, nerve agents, physostigmine poisoning.	IV pralidoxime 30 mg/kg over 30 min followed by a continuous infusion 8–10 mg/kg/h with empiric dose adjustment based on clinical response, continue until atropine has not been required for 24–48 h and patient extubated; restart pralidoxime if recurrent signs/symptoms. [See **Atropine**]	To be administered with atropine following organophosphate or nerve agent poisoning. Carbamates and other reversible cholinesterase inhibitors: Atropine *and* pralidoxime are used to treat acutely ill patients unless carbaryl (Sevin) is known to be involved, then just atropine and supportive care.
Protamine	Known amount of heparin administered	IV protamine dose is calculated from the dose of heparin administered and heparin's approximate half-life (i.e., 60–90 min), such that the amount of protamine does not exceed the expected intravascular amount of heparin at the time of infusion. Slowly administer protamine over 15 min.	Precaution: Be prepared to manage acute anaphylactic (shock) and anaphylactoid reactions. Protamine administered in the absence of heparin or in an amount exceeding that necessary for heparin neutralization can act as an anticoagulant and may inhibit platelet function with a resultant weaker clot. 1 mg of protamine sulfate neutralizes 100 U (1 mg) of heparin. Incomplete neutralization of low-molecular-weight heparins.
	When faced with a patient believed to have received an overdose of an unknown quantity of heparin, the decision to use protamine should be made when the setting is correct and a prolonged partial thromboplastin time (PTT) and persistent bleeding are present. Empiric protamine dosing based on activated coagulation time (ACT)	ACT 200–300 sec: IV protamine 0.6 mg/kg ACT 300–400 sec: IV protamine 1.2 mg/kg Repeat ACT 5–15 min following protamine dose and in 2–8 h to evaluate heparin rebound, further dosing based on these values.	

(continued)

CONTINUED

Therapeutic agent	Uses	Dosing	Caveat/Complications
	■ ACT is not available	IV protamine 25–50 mg (adult) and adjusted accordingly. Repeat dosing in several hours may be necessary if heparin rebound occurs.	
Pyridoxine	Ethylene glycol poisoning	IV Pyridoxine 3–5 mg/kg/d *or* 50 mg every 6 h until toxic alcohol is undetectable and acidemia resolved.	
	Isoniazid (INH) overdoses ■ First sign of neurotoxicity	IV diazepam or equivalent *and* pyridoxine in milligram doses equal to the amount of INH ingested or 5 g in cases of unknown amount of ingestion administered over 30–60 min.	
	■ Seizures or status epilepticus	IV diazepam or equivalent *and* pyridoxine in milligram doses equal to the amount of INH ingested or 5 g in cases of unknown amount of ingestion at 500 mg/min until seizures terminate and remainder of dose infused over next few hours; repeat pyridoxine dose if seizures persist or recur.	
Silibinin	Amanita mushroom poisoning	An open-label clinical trial using an *investigational new drug*, IV silibinin, in the treatment of suspected amatoxin-mushroom poisoning is available in the United States, call the Legalon® SIL hotline: 866–520-4412; http://sites.google.com/site/legalonsil/home	
Sodium bicarbonate	Ethylene glycol and methanol poisoning	IV sodium bicarbonate 1–2 mmol/kg boluses, target blood pH 7.40, and urine pH 7.0–8.0.	Large doses may be needed to treat metabolic acidosis and may produce hypocalcemia. Potassium replacement/supplement.
	Type I antidysrhythmic drug toxicity (sodium channel antagonist effect, e.g., tricyclic antidepressants, quinidine)	ECG (maximal limb-lead) QRS $\geq$120 msec or RaVR $\geq$3 mm or R/SaVR $\geq$0.7: IV sodium bicarbonate 1–2 mmol/kg bolus $\times$ 2; repeat ECG every 3–5 min; IV sodium bicarbonate 1–2 mmol/kg bolus until QRS duration stabilized.	
	Salicylate poisoning	Urine alkalinization: IV sodium bicarbonate 1–2 mmol/kg bolus followed by continuous infusion of sodium bicarbonate 150 mmol mixed in 1,000 mL D5W starting at 1.5 to 2.0 times maintenance rate, adjusted to maintain urinary pH 8.0 and arterial pH <7.55; assess clinical status/laboratory parameters (e.g., electrolytes, acid-base, urine pH) hourly; terminate when clear clinical-biochemical recovery and serial decline in serum ASA concentration towards therapeutic range.	
	Methotrexate and chlorpropamide overdoses, symptomatic chlorophenoxy herbicide poisoning, known or symptomatic pentachlorophenol poisoning	Urine alkalinization: IV sodium bicarbonate 1–2 mmol/kg bolus followed by continuous infusion of sodium bicarbonate 150 mmol mixed in 1,000 mL D5W starting at 1.5 to 2.0 times maintenance rate, adjusted to maintain urinary pH 8.0 and arterial pH <7.55; reassess clinical status/laboratory parameters (e.g., electrolytes, acid-base, urine pH) hourly; terminate when clear clinical-biochemical recovery.	

Thiamine	Ethylene glycol poisoning	IV thiamine 100 mg/d *or* every 6 h until toxic alcohol is undetectable and acidemia resolved.	
Vitamin K_1	Patients with or suspected major anticoagulant-related hemorrhage or INR >20	IV vitamin K_1 10 mg (diluted with 5% dextrose, 0.9% sodium chloride, or 5% dextrose in 0.9% sodium chloride; administered at ≤1 mg/min; be prepare to treat anaphylaxis) *or* oral/nasogastric vitamin K_1 7 mg/kg/d divided every 6 h. Endpoint of vitamin K_1 therapy: Discontinue therapy at an arbitrary time and obtain serial INR/PT, restart vitamin K_1 when INR/PT is elevated *or* monitor serum factor VII concentration when vitamin K_1 therapy is withheld, restart vitamin K_1 when a progressive decrease in factor VII levels to 30% of normal *or* serum brodifacoum concentration <10 ng/mL, *or* when serum vitamin K 2,3-epoxide concentration begins to fall.	IV prothrombin complex concentrate (PCC) 50 U/kg *or* IV fresh frozen plasma (FFP) 10–20 mL/kg *or* IV recombinant activated factor VII (rFVIIa) 15–90 μg/kg is concurrently administered with vitamin K_1. IV vitamin K is associated with anaphylaxis.

D50W = dextrose 50% water; D25W = dextrose 25% water; D10W = dextrose 10% water; h = hours; IM = intramuscular; IV = intravenous; LR = Lactated Ringer's; max = maximum; NS = normal saline; RaVR = terminal R wave in lead aVR; R/SaVR = R-wave/S-wave ratio in lead aVR; wks = weeks.

Box I. Digoxin antibody dosing calculator.

$$\text{Number of vials} = \frac{\text{Digoxin body burden to be neutralized in ng/mL (nmol/L} \times 1.28) \times \text{weight (kg)} \times \text{volume of distribution (Vd)}}{1{,}000 \times 0.6\ \text{mg/vial}}$$

V_d: Adults 8 L/kg

Box II. Polyethylene glycol solution (PEG) whole bowel irrigation.
Insert nasogastric/oral tube and administer PEG solution at 2 L/h for 5 h and clear rectal effluent is evident; doubtful patients would be cooperative or tolerate oral PEG.

INDEX

Note: Page numbers followed by *f* and *t* indicates figure and table respectively.